To

Dr. Mike & Dr. Paul Saxton

With Appreciation

For your Kindness & Care

of my late Husband & myself

I Thank you

Marta Haynes

17th edition

CECIL TEXTBOOK OF MEDICINE

Edited by

JAMES B. WYNGAARDEN, M.D.

Director, National Institutes of Health,
Bethesda, Maryland

LLOYD H. SMITH, Jr., M.D.

Chairman, Department of Medicine,
University of California, San Francisco, School of Medicine,
San Francisco, California

1985

W. B. SAUNDERS COMPANY Philadelphia/London/Toronto/Mexico City/Rio de Janeiro/Sydney/Tokyo

W. B. Saunders Company: West Washington Square
Philadelphia, PA 19105

1 St. Anne's Road
Eastbourne, East Sussex BN21 3UN, England

1 Goldthorne Avenue
Toronto, Ontario M8Z 5T9, Canada

Apartado 26370—Cedro 512
Mexico 4, D.F., Mexico

Rua Coronel Cabrita, 8
Sao Cristovao Caixa Postal 21176
Rio de Janeiro, Brazil

9 Waltham Street
Artarmon, N.S.W. 2064, Australia

Ichibancho, Central Bldg., 22-1 Ichibancho
Chiyoda-Ku, Tokyo 102, Japan

Listed here is the latest translated edition of this book together with the language of the translation and the publisher.

Chinese (7th Edition)—Chinese Medical Association, Shanghai, China
Italian (9th Edition)—Societa Editrice Universo, Rome, Italy
(15th Edition, in preparation)—Piccin Editore, Padova, Italy
Japanese (14th Edition)—Igaku Shoin Ltd., Tokyo, Japan
Polish (9th Edition)—Panstwowy Zaklad Wydawnictw Lekarskich, Warsaw, Poland
Portuguese (14th Edition)—DISCOS CBS Industria e Comercio Ltda., Rio de Janeiro, Brazil
Serbo-Croat (11th Edition)—Medicinska Knjiga, Belgrade, Yugoslavia
Spanish (14th Edition)—Nueva Editorial Interamericana Ltda., Mexico City
(15th Edition, in preparation)—Nueva Editorial Interamericana Ltda., Mexico City

Library of Congress Cataloging in Publication Data
Main entry under title:

Textbook of Medicine.

Simultaneously published in 1 v.
Includes bibliographies and index.
1. Internal medicine. I. Cecil, Russell L. (Russell La Fayette), 1881–1965. II. Wyngaarden, James B., 1924– . III. Smith, Lloyd H. (Lloyd Holly), 1924– . IV. Title: Cecil Textbook of Medicine.
[DNLM: 1. Medicine. WB 100 T354]
RC46.T35 1985 616 84-20225
ISBN 0-7216-9629-5 (set)
ISBN 0-7216-6927-9 (v. 1)
ISBN 0-7216-9628-7 (v. 2)

Library of Congress Cataloging in Publication Data
Main entry under title:

Textbook of Medicine.

Simultaneously published in 2 v.
Includes bibliographies and index.
1. Internal medicine. I. Cecil, Russell L. (Russell La Fayette), 1881–1965. II. Wyngaarden, James B., 1924– . III. Smith, Lloyd H. (Lloyd Holly), 1924– . IV. Title: Cecil Textbook of Medicine.
[DNLM: 1. Medicine. WB 100 T354]
RC46.T35 1985b 616 84-20226
ISBN 0-7216-9626-0

ISBN 0-7216-9626-0 Single Volume
ISBN 0-7216-9627-9 Volume 1
ISBN 0-7216-9628-7 Volume 2
ISBN 0-7216-9629-5 Set

Textbook of Medicine

Last digit is the print number: 9 8 7 6 5 4 3 2

DOSAGE NOTICE

Extraordinary efforts have been made by the authors, the editors, and the publisher of this book to ensure that dosage recommendations are precise and in agreement with the highest standards of practice.

However, dosage schedules are changed from time to time in the light of accumulating clinical experience and continuing laboratory studies. This is most likely to occur in the case of recently introduced products.

We urge, therefore, that you check the package information data for the manufacturer's recommended dosage. In addition, there are some quite serious situations, each encountered only rarely, in which drug therapy must be individualized and expert judgment advises the use of a higher dosage or administration by a different route than is included in the manufacturer's recommendations. Throughout the text many such instances are indicated by a footnote.

THE EDITORS

Preface

Both the science and the practice of medicine change rapidly. This has been true throughout the twentieth century; it has been particularly true during these last decades of the century. Since it first appeared in 1927, the *Cecil Textbook of Medicine* has reflected that change in its successive editions appearing every three to four years. This seventeenth edition represents a continuation of that long tradition.

The theme of the book has always been to provide an "authoritative clinical guidance and a reasoned, scientific basis for the pursuit of medicine." This can be accomplished only by a rigorous periodic reexamination of the content, organization, and balance of the book, which, despite its large scope, cannot be truly comprehensive. Judgments must be made as to what to exclude, as well as what to include and what is likely to be of greatest interest and importance in the early future. As an editorial responsibility, a plan must then be developed to best translate these ideas into improvements in the book. In arriving at these judgments for the seventeenth edition, we have been greatly assisted by a talented group of eight Consulting Editors and by Fred Plum, Editor for *Neurologic and Behavioral Diseases.*

In this edition we are privileged to have four new Consulting Editors: Thomas E. Andreoli (Renal Disease), Charles C. J. Carpenter (Infectious Diseases), Robert J. Lefkowitz (Principles of Therapeutics), and William E. Paul (Diseases of the Immune System). They join four editorial colleagues from previous editions who have continued in this important role: John F. Murray (Respiratory Diseases), David G. Nathan (Hematologic Diseases), Marvin H. Sleisenger (Gastrointestinal Diseases), and Andrew G. Wallace (Cardiovascular Diseases). The Consulting Editors have carried out extensive reviews of their respective sections for content, presentation, and organization. In concert with them we have selected the individual authors who have contributed the specific chapters: the concise, scholarly reviews that, after all, collectively compose the substance of such a book.

In keeping with past tradition there has been a significant turnover of participants in the book in order to ensure fresh approaches to specific topics. In this edition, for example, there are 109 new contributors or previous contributors with newly assigned areas of responsibility. As such, approximately 40 per cent of the individual chapters have been completely rewritten under new authorship, in addition to the extensive editorial changes to be found in chapters that have remained under previous authorship. This type of "programmed regeneration" requires that, in addition to the usual editorial scrutiny of all parts of the book, each individual chapter be completely recast every two to three editions. In addition to advising on the selection of the new participants, the Consulting Editors have been particularly concerned with reviewing these new chapters and sections of the book. The contributors who collectively compose the authorship of this seventeenth edition of *Cecil* represent a remarkably broad source of collaborators from more than 100 institutions. It is to them that we are particularly indebted for the substance of this large compendium of the science and practice of medicine.

What changes have been introduced in this newest edition of a venerable book? The most important changes are dispersed throughout the book as the painstaking updating of all of the chapters. Particular attention has been directed to the selection of recent references in readily available journals and books to supplement the necessarily compressed summaries offered in the chapters. As before, the references have been annotated to make them more useful for the reader. Beyond these general improvements throughout the book, some more specific changes have been introduced, a few of which will be noted here. Part II, *Human Growth, Development, and Aging,* has important new chapters on "Management of Common Problems in the Elderly" (T. Franklin Williams) and on "Care of Dying Patients and Their Families" (Sylvia A. Lack). These thoughtful chapters, and that on "Ethics in the Practice of Medicine" (Albert R. Jonsen), concern themselves with issues of increasing importance to medicine and to society at large. A new Part III has been introduced on the topic *Personal Health Care and Preventive Medicine.* It has become increasingly clear that maintenance of health is greatly influenced by factors under the control of the individual. At the extremes this is a topic that shades into the faddism and cultism of certain "life styles" and that is tinged with shamanism, commercialism, and unfounded claims. Nevertheless, there is a large body of scientific information to buttress our intuitive sense that the individual can have a considerable influence on his or her health through daily decisions concerning diet, exercise, the use of tobacco, alcohol or other drugs, the use of automobile seat belts, and many other factors. Therefore, seven brief chapters have been devoted to these topics with which all physicians must be concerned.

A new Part IV on *Principles of Diagnosis* has also been introduced, composed of three essays: "Clinical Approach to the Patient" (William L. Morgan, Jr.), "The Use and Interpretation of Laboratory-Derived Data" (James B. Wyngaarden), and "Overview of Imaging Techniques and Projection for the Future" (Alexander R. Margulis). Of course the specifics of diagnosis are discussed in the chapters concerning individual diseases and further outlined in the introductory chapters for each organ system. Nevertheless, this Part offers a valuable overview of how clinical and laboratory medicine can be integrated by the clinician in pursuing a diagnosis. Part XXVI on *Occupational and Environmental Medicine* comprises a series of chapters that relate to the increasingly important role of the environment, whether ambient or in the workplace, in the health of the individual or of the public. These physical, chemical, and even psychological factors may be overt or they may be extraordinarily elusive unless they are specifically looked for by history or laboratory investigation.

In addition to the above newly organized Parts of this seventeenth edition of *Cecil,* novel chapters have been introduced within other Parts to reflect the changing importance of areas of biological science and medical practice. For example, Part VI on *Principles of Human Genetics* contains new chapters on "Expectations from Recombinant DNA Research" (W. French Anderson) and "Contributions of Recombinant DNA Research to Diagnosis of Heritable Disease" (C. Thomas Caskey). Together these chapters offer a broad overview of this remarkable area of molecular biology and its relevance to clinical medicine. Similarly, Part XXI, entitled *Diseases of the Immune System,* now contains a new chapter on "Acquired Immunodeficiency Syndrome" (Anthony S. Fauci) to reflect current progress in our understanding of the etiology, pathogenesis, and clinical manifestations of AIDS, perhaps the most alarming and baffling epidemic related to an infectious agent in the United States in the past generation.

Cecil is a very large book, but still it cannot hope to cover all of medicine or medical science. Three current books are linked to *Cecil* by design, format, and joint editorial responsibility and serve to extend its breadth. All three will appear in new editions in 1985. *Pathophysiology: The Biological Principles of Disease* (Volume I of the *International Textbook of Medicine*), edited by Lloyd H. Smith, Jr. and Samuel O. Thier, summarizes the most pertinent aspects of basic science relevant to medical practice. Similarly, *Medical Microbiology and Infectious Diseases* (Volume II of the *International Textbook of Medicine*), edited by Abraham I. Braude, contains a more comprehensive summary of the world experience with the infectious and parasitic diseases. *Review of General Internal Medicine*, edited by the editors of *Cecil*, will appear in a third edition linked to the seventeenth edition of *Cecil*. As before, its *1200* questions and answers are designed to be of intrinsic educational benefit as well as to reinforce the value of *Cecil* as a reference text. *Cecil* can stand alone, but it is further enhanced by members of its extended family.

"Language is the armoury of the human mind; and at once contains the trophies of its past, and the weapons of its future conquests." As all editors know, the weaponry of language, in Coleridge's image above, does not always come fully burnished in submitted manuscripts. We have been privileged to work with skilled editorial assistants at all stages of planning and preparation of this book. Margaret Quinlan in Bethesda and Judith Serrell in San Francisco have been invaluable collaborators working directly with the editors on a daily basis. Lorraine Kilmer, Donna Walker, Edna Dick, and Frank Polizzano at the W. B. Saunders Company have brought long experience and admirable professionalism to this large and complex enterprise. In the course of this project the overall editorial responsibility for *Cecil* at the W. B. Saunders Company was shifted from John J. Hanley to J. Dereck Jeffers. Both of these seasoned editors have been of immense help to us in planning and in bringing this seventeenth edition to completion. We express our deepest appreciation to all of our collaborators above, with whom it has been a pleasure to work in maintaining the traditions of a book that has itself become an institution in medicine.

JAMES B. WYNGAARDEN

LLOYD H. SMITH, JR.

Contributors

FRANÇOIS M. ABBOUD, M.D.
Professor of Internal Medicine, Professor of Physiology and Biophysics, University of Iowa College of Medicine. Head, Department of Internal Medicine, University of Iowa Hospitals and Clinics, Iowa City, Iowa.
Shock

DAVID H. ALPERS, M.D.
Professor of Medicine, Washington University of School of Medicine. Physician, Barnes Hospital, St. Louis, Missouri.
Enteral Nutritional Therapy

DAVID F. ALTMAN, M.D.
Associate Clinical Professor of Medicine and Associate Dean of Student Affairs, University of California, San Francisco School of Medicine. Director of Gastroenterology Clinic, University of California, San Francisco, Hospitals and Clinics, San Francisco, California.
Food Poisoning; Diseases of the Rectum and Anus

WILLIAM J. C. AMEND, Jr., M.D.
Clinical Professor of Medicine and Surgery, University of California, San Francisco, School of Medicine. Attending Physician, Moffitt-Long Hospitals, San Francisco, California.
Renal Transplantation

W. FRENCH ANDERSON, M.D.
Adjunct Professor of Genetics, George Washington University, Washington, D.C. Chief, Laboratory of Molecular Hematology, National Heart, Lung and Blood Institute, National Institutes of Health, and Attending and Admitting Physician, Clinical Center, National Institutes of Health, Bethesda, Maryland.
Expectations from Recombinant DNA Research

THOMAS E. ANDREOLI, M.D.
Professor and Chairman, Department of Internal Medicine, University of Texas Medical School at Houston. Chief of Medicine, The Hermann Hospital, and Medical Director, Texas Kidney Institute, Hermann Hospital, Houston, Texas.
Approach to the Patient with Renal Disease; Disorders of Fluid Volume, Electrolyte, and Acid-Base Balance; Posterior Pituitary

VINCENT T. ANDRIOLE, M.D.
Professor of Medicine, Yale University School of Medicine. Attending Physician, Yale–New Haven Hospital, New Haven, Connecticut.
Urinary Tract Infections and Pyelonephritis

CLAUDE D. ARNAUD, M.D.
Professor of Medicine and Physiology, University of California, San Francisco, School of Medicine. Chief, Endocrine Section, San Francisco Veterans Administration Medical Center, San Francisco, California.
Mineral and Bone Homeostasis; The Parathyroid Glands, Hypercalcemia, and Hypocalcemia; The Ultimobranchial Cells and Calcitonin

K. FRANK AUSTEN, M.D.
Theodore B. Bayles Professor of Medicine, Harvard Medical School. Chairman, Department of Rheumatology and Immunology, Brigham and Women's Hospital, Boston, Massachusetts.
Polyarteritis Nodosa Group

BERNARD M. BABIOR, M.D., Ph.D.
Professor of Medicine, Tufts University School of Medicine. Physician, New England Medical Center Hospital, Boston, Massachusetts.
Function of Neutrophils and Mononuclear Phagocytes; Disorders of Neutrophil Function

H. J. M. BARNETT, M.D., LL.D.
Professor and Chairman, Faculty of Medicine, Department of Clinical Neurological Sciences, University of Western Ontario. Chief, Department of Clinical Neurological Sciences, University Hospital, London, Ontario, Canada.
Cerebrovascular Diseases: Introduction, Cerebral Ischemia and Infarction, Intracranial Hemorrhage

D. W. BARRY, M.D.
Adjunct Associate Professor of Medicine, Duke University School of Medicine, Durham, North Carolina. Head, Departments of Clinical Investigation and Virology, Wellcome Research Laboratories, Burroughs Wellcome Company.
Antiviral Therapy

JOHN G. BARTLETT, M.D.
Professor of Medicine, Johns Hopkins University School of Medicine. Chief, Division of Infectious Diseases, Johns Hopkins Hospital, Baltimore, Maryland.
Lung Abscess; Bronchiectasis and Cystic Fibrosis; Clostridial Myonecrosis and Other Clostridial Diseases; Pseudomembranous Colitis; Botulism

MICHAEL BARZA, M.D.
Professor of Medicine, Tufts University School of Medicine. Attending Physician, Infectious Disease Division, New England Medical Center Hospital, Boston, Massachusetts.
Diseases Caused by Pseudomonads; Listeriosis; Erysipeloid

DAVID A. BASS, M.D., D.Phil.
Professor of Medicine, Bowman Gray School of Medicine of Wake Forest University. Attending Physician, Infectious Diseases, North Carolina Baptist Hospitals, Inc., Winston-Salem, North Carolina.
Eosinophilic Syndromes

STEPHEN G. BAUM, M.D.
Professor of Medicine, Cell Biology, Microbiology and Immunology, Albert Einstein College of Medicine of Yeshiva University. Attending Physician, Bronx Municipal Hospital Center and Hospital of The Albert Einstein College of Medicine, Bronx, New York.
Mycoplasmal Infections; Adenovirus Diseases

JOHN D. BAXTER, M.D.
Professor of Medicine and Biochemistry and Biophysics, University of California, San Francisco, School of Medicine. Chief, Division of Endocrinology, Director, Metabolic Research Unit, University of California, San Francisco, Moffit-Long Hospitals, San Francisco, California.
Principles of Endocrinology; Disorders of the Adrenal Cortex

WILLIAM S. BECK, M.D.
Professor of Medicine, Harvard Medical School. Physician and Director, Hematology Research Laboratory, Massachusetts General Hospital, Boston, Massachusetts.
Megaloblastic Anemias

CHARLES E. BECKER, M.D.
Professor of Medicine, University of California, San Francisco, School of Medicine. Chief, Occupational Medicine and Clinical Pharmacology and Toxicology, San Francisco General Hospital Medical Center, San Francisco, California.
Principles of Occupational Medicine

DONALD P. BECKER, M.D.
Professor and Chairman, Division of Neurological Surgery, Virginia Commonwealth University Medical College of Virginia. Chief of Neurosurgery, Medical College of Virginia Hospitals; Consultant Neurosurgeon, McGuire Veterans Administration Medical Center, Richmond, Virginia.
Head Injuries; Injuries to the Spine

VICTOR S. BEHAR, M.D.
Professor of Medicine, Duke University School of Medicine. Director, Cardiovascular Laboratory, Duke University Hospital, Durham, North Carolina.
Diseases of the Myocardium

MICHAEL D. BENDER, M.D.
Associate Clinical Professor of Medicine, University of California, San Francisco, School of Medicine, San Francisco. Attending Physician, Director of Medical Education, Peninsula Hospital and Medical Center, Burlingame, California.
Diseases of the Peritoneum; Diseases of the Mesentery and Omentum

J. CLAUDE BENNETT, M.D.
Professor and Chairman, Department of Medicine, University of Alabama School of Medicine. Physician-in-Chief, University of Alabama Hospitals, Birmingham, Alabama.
Rheumatoid Arthritis

JOHN E. BENNETT, M.D.
Head, Clinical Mycology Section, Laboratory of Clinical Investigation, National Institute of Allergy and Infectious Diseases, National Institutes of Health, Bethesda, Maryland.
Brucellosis

PAUL D. BERK, M.D.
Albert A. and Vera G. List Professor of Medicine (Hematology), Mt. Sinai School of Medicine of the City University of New York. Attending Physician, The Mount Sinai Hospital, New York; Consultant, Veterans Administration Hospital, Bronx, New York, and National Institutes of Health, Bethesda, Maryland.
Erythrocytosis and Polycythemia; Myeloproliferative Disorders

ROBERT N. BERK, M.D.
Professor and Chairman, Department of Radiology, University of California, San Diego, School of Medicine. Director, Department of Radiology, University of California, San Diego, University Hospital, La Jolla, California.
Diagnostic Imaging Procedures in Gastroenterology

ERNEST BEUTLER, M.D.
Clinical Professor of Medicine, University of California, San Diego, School of Medicine. Chairman, Department of Basic and Clinical Research, and Head, Division of Hematology/Oncology, Scripps Clinic and Research Foundation, La Jolla, California.
Galactosemia

EDWIN L. BIERMAN, M.D.
Professor of Medicine and Head, Division of Metabolism, Endocrinology and Nutrition, University of Washington School of Medicine. Attending Physician, University of Washington Affiliated Hospitals, Seattle, Washington.
Obesity

DANIEL D. BIKLE, M.D., Ph.D.
Assistant Professor of Medicine, University of California, San Francisco, School of Medicine. Codirector, Special Diagnostic and Treatment Unit, San Francisco Veterans Administration Medical Center, San Francisco, California.
Vitamin D; Osteomalacia and Rickets

J. MICHAEL BISHOP, M.D.
Professor of Microbiology and Immunology, University of California, San Francisco, School of Medicine. Director, The George Williams Hooper Research Foundation, University of California, San Francisco, California.
Oncogenes

ALAN L. BISNO, M.D.
Professor of Medicine, Department of Medicine, Division of Infectious Diseases, University of Tennessee College of Medicine. Attending Physician, Memphis Regional Medical Center and The University of Tennessee Medical Center; Consulting Physician, Baptist Memorial Hospital, Memphis, Tennessee.
Rheumatic Fever

D. MONTGOMERY BISSELL, M.D.
Associate Professor of Medicine, University of California, San Francisco, School of Medicine. Attending Physician, University of California, San Francisco Hospitals and Clinics and San Francisco General Hospital Medical Center, San Francisco, California.
Porphyria

LEO F. BLACK, M.D.
Professor of Internal Medicine, Mayo Medical School. Consultant in Internal Medicine and Thoracic Diseases, Mayo Clinic, Rochester, Minnesota.
Neoplasms of the Lung

DANIEL S. BLUMENTHAL, M.D.
Associate Professor of Community Medicine and Family Practice, Morehouse School of Medicine. Attending Physician, Southwest Community Hospital and Hughes Spalding Pavilion, Grady Memorial Hospital, Atlanta, Georgia.
Nematodes: Introduction; Strongyloidiasis; Capillariasis; Hookworm Diseases; Cutaneous Larva Migrans; Trichostrongyliasis; Gnathostomiasis; Primate Nematodiases; Ascariasis; Toxacariasis; Anisakiasis; Trichuriasis; Enterobiasis; Angiostrongyliasis

DANE R. BOGGS, M.D.
Professor of Medicine, University of Pittsburgh School of Medicine. Staff Physician, Presbyterian University Hospital, Pittsburgh, Pennsylvania.
The Leukopenic State; Leukemoid Reactions

GILES G. BOLE, M.D.
Professor of Internal Medicine and Physician-in-Charge, Rheumatology Division and Rackham Arthritis Research Unit, University of Michigan Medical School. Chief, Rheumatology Division, Department of Medicine, University of Michigan Medical Center, Ann Arbor, Michigan.
Diseases With Which Arthritis is Frequently Associated; Miscellaneous Forms of Arthritis; Nonarticular Rheumatism; Synovial Tumors

THOMAS D. BOYER, M.D.
Associate Professor of Medicine, University of California, San Francisco, School of Medicine. Chief of Gastroenterology, San Francisco Veterans Administration Medical Center, San Francisco, California.
Cirrhosis of the Liver; Major Sequelae of Cirrhosis

PHILIP S. BRACHMAN, M.D.
Clinical Professor of Community Health and Clinical Instructor in Medicine, Emory University School of Medicine, Atlanta, Georgia.
Anthrax

JEROME S. BRODY, M.D.
Professor of Medicine, Boston University School of Medicine. Chief, Pulmonary Section, University Hospital and Boston City Hospital, Boston, Massachusetts.
Diseases of the Pleura, Mediastinum, Diaphragm, and Chest Wall

JOHN D. BRUNZELL, M.D.
Professor of Medicine, Division of Metabolism, University of Washington School of Medicine, Seattle, Washington.
The Hyperlipoproteinemias

ANTHONY D. M. BRYCESON, M.D., D.T.M. & H.
Senior Lecturer, London School of Hygiene and Tropical Medicine. Consultant Physician, Hospital for Tropical Diseases, London, England.
Tropical Phagedenic Ulcer

REBECCA H. BUCKLEY, M.D.
James B. Sidbury Professor of Pediatrics and Professor of Immunology, Duke University School of Medicine. Chief, Division of Allergy and Immunology, Department of Pediatrics, Duke University Medical Center, Durham, North Carolina.
Primary Immunodeficiency Diseases

WARD E. BULLOCK, M.D.
Arthur Russell Morgan Professor of Medicine and Director, Division of Infectious Diseases, University of Cincinnati College of Medicine, Cincinnati, Ohio.
Leprosy (Hansen's Disease)

DAVID M. BURNS, M.D.
Assistant Professor of Medicine, University of California, San Diego, School of Medicine. Division of Pulmonary and Critical Care Medicine, University of California, San Diego, Medical Center, La Jolla, California.
Tobacco and Health

BENJAMIN BURROWS, M.D.
Professor of Internal Medicine, University of Arizona College of Medicine. Attending Pulmonologist, Arizona Health Sciences Center, Tucson, Arizona.
Chronic Airways Diseases; Abnormalities of Lung Aeration

THOMAS BUTLER, M.D.
Associate Professor of Medicine, Case Western Reserve University School of Medicine, Cleveland, Ohio. Consultant, International Centre for Diarrheal Diseases Research, Dhaka, Bangladesh.
Yersinia Infections; Nonsyphilitic Treponematoses; Relapsing Fever

JOEL N. BUXBAUM, M.D.
Professor of Medicine, New York University School of Medicine. Chief, Rheumatology Section, Veterans Administration Hospital; Associate Attending Physician, Bellevue Hospital Center, New York, New York.
The Amyloid Diseases

ANDREI CALIN, M.D.
Consultant Rheumatologist, Royal National Hospital for Rheumatic Diseases, Bath, Ireland.
The Spondyloarthropathies

GEORGE P. CANELLOS, M.D.
Professor of Medicine, Harvard Medical School. Chief of Medical Oncology, Dana-Farber Cancer Institute, Brigham and Women's Hospital, Boston, Massachusetts.
Carcinoma of the Breast

CHARLES C. J. CARPENTER, M.D.
Professor and Chairman, Department of Medicine, Case Western Reserve University School of Medicine. Physician-in-Chief, University Hospitals, Cleveland, Ohio.
Introduction to Microbial Diseases; Extraintestinal Infections Caused by Enteric Bacteria; Shigellosis

C. THOMAS CASKEY, M.D.
Professor of Medicine, Cell Biology, and Biochemistry, Baylor College of Medicine. Attending Physician, St. Luke's Episcopal Hospital and The Methodist Hospital, Houston, Texas.
Contributions of Recombinant DNA Research to Diagnosis of Heritable Disease

JOHN P. CELLO, M.D.
Associate Professor of Medicine, University of California, San Francisco, School of Medicine. Chief, Gastroenterology, San Francisco General Hospital Medical Center, San Francisco, California.
Carcinoma of the Pancreas

BRUCE A. CHABNER, M.D.
Director, Division of Cancer Treatment, National Cancer Institute, National Institutes of Health, Bethesda, Maryland.
Principles of Cancer Therapy

ROBERT M. CHANOCK, M.D.
Chief, Laboratory of Infectious Diseases, National Institute of Allergy and Infectious Diseases, National Institutes of Health, Bethesda, Maryland.
Respiratory Syncytial Virus; Parainfluenza Viral Diseases

BAYARD CLARKSON, M.D.
Professor of Medicine, Cornell University Medical College. Chief, Hematology/Lymphoma Service, Memorial Sloan-Kettering Cancer Center, New York, New York.
The Chronic Leukemias

RAY E. CLOUSE, M.D.
Assistant Professor of Medicine, Washington University School of Medicine. Assistant Physician, Barnes Hospital, St. Louis, Missouri.
Parenteral Nutrition

CHARLES G. COCHRANE, M.D.
Member, Department of Immunopathology, Scripps Clinic and Research Foundation; Adjunct Professor, Department of Pathology, University of California, San Diego, School of Medicine, La Jolla, California.
Immune Complex Diseases

MARTIN G. COGAN, M.D.
Assistant Professor of Medicine, University of California, San Francisco, School of Medicine. Attending Physician and Medical Director, Acute Hemodialysis Unit, Moffitt-Long Hospitals, San Francisco, California.
Specific Renal Tubular Disorders: Introduction; Renal Tubular Acidosis

ALAN S. COHEN, M.D.
Conrad Wesselhoeft Professor of Medicine, Boston University School of Medicine. Chief of Medicine and Director, Thorndike Memorial Laboratory, Boston City Hospital, Boston, Massachusetts.
Specialized Diagnostic Procedures in the Rheumatic Diseases

WILLIAM G. COUSER, M.D.
Professor of Medicine and Head, Division of Nephrology, University of Washington School of Medicine, Seattle, Washington.
Glomerular Disorders

JAMES D. CRAPO, M.D.
Associate Professor of Medicine, Duke University School of Medicine. Chief, Division of Allergy, Critical Care, and Respiratory Medicine, Duke University Medical Center, Durham, North Carolina.
Physical, Chemical, and Aspiration Injuries of the Lung

PHILIP E. CRYER, M.D.
Professor of Medicine, Washington University School of Medicine. Physician, Barnes Hospital, St. Louis, Missouri.
The Adrenal Medullae and the Sympathetic Nervous System; The Carcinoid Syndrome

RONALD G. CRYSTAL, M.D.
Chief, Pulmonary Branch, National Heart, Lung and Blood Institute, National Institutes of Health, Bethesda, Maryland.
Interstitial Lung Disease

RONALD P. DANIELE, M.D.
Professor of Medicine and Pathology, University of Pennsylvania School of Medicine. Attending Physician and Director of the Interstitial Lung Disease Program, Hospital of the University of Pennsylvania, Philadelphia, Pennsylvania.
Asthma

THOMAS E. DAVIS, M.D.
Associate Professor of Human Oncology and Medicine, University of Wisconsin Medical School. Associate Director for Clinical Programs, Wisconsin Clinical Cancer Center, Madison, Wisconsin.
Non-Hodgkin's Lymphomas

VINCENT W. DENNIS, M.D.
Associate Professor of Medicine, Duke University School of Medicine, Durham, North Carolina.
Investigations of Renal Function

IVAN DIAMOND, M.D., Ph.D.
Director, Ernest Gallo Clinic and Research Center; Professor and Vice-Chairman, Department of Neurology; Professor of Pediatrics and Pharmacology, University of California, San Francisco, School of Medicine, San Francisco, California.
Alcohol-Related and Nutritional Disorders of the Nervous System

CHARLES A. DINARELLO, M.D.
Associate Professor of Medicine and Pediatrics, Tufts University School of Medicine. Physician, New England Medical Center Hospital, Boston, Massachusetts.
Pathogenesis of Fever

RAPHAEL DOLIN, M.D.
Professor of Medicine, University of Rochester School of Medicine and Dentistry. Physician with Admitting Privileges, The Strong Memorial Hospital, Rochester, New York.
Enteroviral Diseases: Introduction; Paralysis and Other Neurologic Complications of Nonpolio Enteroviruses; Epidemic Pleurodynia; Myocarditis and Pericarditis Caused by Enteroviruses; Mucocutaneous Infections Caused by Enteroviruses; Acute Hemorrhagic Conjunctivitis; Respiratory Tract Illness Associated with Enteroviruses; Viral Gastroenteritis

C. T. DOLLERY, M.B.
Professor of Clinical Pharmacology, Royal Postgraduate Medical School, University of London. Consultant Physician, Hammersmith and Ealing Hospitals, London, England.
Arterial Hypertension

R. GORDON DOUGLAS, Jr., M.D.
Professor and Chairman, Department of Medicine, Cornell University Medical College. Physician-in-Chief, The New York Hospital, New York, New York.
Immunization; Influenza; Herpes Simplex Virus Infections

BRIAN O. L. DUKE, M.D., S.D., D.T.M. & H.
Chief, Unit for Filarial Infections, World Health Organization, Geneva, Switzerland.
Onchocerciasis; Streptocerciasis

DAVID T. DURACK, M.B., D.Phil.
Professor of Medicine and Professor of Microbiology and Immunology, Duke University School of Medicine. Chief, Division of Infectious Diseases, Duke University Medical Center, Durham, North Carolina.
Pneumococcal Pneumonia; Infective Endocarditis

DAVID J. DRUTZ, M.D.
Professor of Medicine and Microbiology and Chief, Division of Infectious Diseases, University of Texas Medical School at San Antonio. Chief, Infectious Diseases Section, and Attending Physician, Audie L. Murphy Memorial Veterans Hospital; Attending Physician, Medical Center Hospital and St. Luke's Lutheran Hospital, San Antonio, Texas.
Actinomycosis; Nocardiosis; The Mycoses: Introduction: Histoplasmosis; Coccidioidomycosis; Blastomycosis; Paracoccidioidomycosis; Cryptococcosis; Sporotrichosis; Candidiasis; Aspergillosis; Mucormycosis; Mycetoma; Chromomycosis

THEODORE C. EICKHOFF, M.D.
Professor of Medicine, University of Colorado School of Medicine. Director of Internal Medicine, Presbyterian Medical Center, Denver, Colorado.
Bartonellosis; Trench Fever; Q Fever; Colorado Tick Fever

BRYAN T. EMMERSON, M.D., Ph.D.
Professor of Medicine, University of Queensland Medical School. Department of Medicine, Princess Alexandra Hospital, Brisbane, Queensland, Australia.
Toxic Nephropathy

EDWARD A. EMMETT, M.B., B.S., M.S.
Professor and Director, Division of Occupational Medicine, Department of Environmental Health Sciences, Johns Hopkins University School of Hygiene and Public Health. Active Part-time Staff, Johns Hopkins Hospital and Wyman Park Health System, Baltimore, Maryland.
Occupational Diseases of the Skin

JEROME ENGEL, Jr., M.D., Ph.D.
Professor of Neurology and Anatomy, Department of Neurology, University of California, Los Angeles, School of Medicine. Neurologist, UCLA Hospital, Los Angeles, California.
The Epilepsies

STANLEY FAHN, M.D.
H. Houston Merritt Professor of Neurology, Columbia University College of Physicians and Surgeons. Attending Neurologist, Neurological Institute and Presbyterian Hospital, New York, New York.
The Extrapyramidal Disorders: Parkinsonism; Essential Tremor; The Choreas; Other Extrapyramidal Disorders; The Dystonias

ANTHONY S. FAUCI, M.D.
Chief, Laboratory of Immunoregulation, National Institute of Allergy and Infectious Diseases, National Institutes of Health, Bethesda, Maryland.
Glucocorticosteroid Therapy; Familial Mediterranean Fever; Acquired Immunodeficiency Syndrome; The Vasculitic Syndromes; Wegener's Granulomatosis and Midline Granuloma

DOUGLAS T. FEARON, M.D.
Associate Professor, Harvard Medical School. Rheumatologist and Immunologist, Brigham and Women's Hospital, Boston, Massachusetts.
Complement

HARVEY FEIGENBAUM, M.D.
Distinguished Professor of Medicine, Indiana University School of Medicine. Director of Hemodynamic Laboratories; Senior Research Associate, Krannert Institute of Cardiology, Indianapolis, Indiana.
Echocardiography

MARK FELDMAN, M.D.
Associate Professor of Internal Medicine, University of Texas Southwestern Medical School at Dallas. Associate Chief of Staff for Research and Development, Dallas Veterans Administration Medical Center, Dallas, Texas.
Peptic Ulcer: Complications

PHILIP J. FIALKOW, M.D.
Professor and Chairman, Department of Medicine, University of Washington School of Medicine. Physician-in-Chief, University Hospital, and Attending Physician, Harborview Medical Center, Seattle, Washington.
Clonal Development and Stem Cell Origin of Proliferative Disorders

ALFRED P. FISHMAN, M.D.
William Maul Measey Professor of Medicine, University of Pennsylvania School of Medicine. Director, Cardiovascular-Pulmonary Division, Department of Medicine, Hospital of the University of Pennsylvania, Philadelphia, Pennsylvania.
Heart Failure; Pulmonary Hypertension

JOHN S. FORDTRAN, M.D.
Chief, Department of Internal Medicine, Baylor University Medical Center, Dallas, Texas.
Diarrhea

BERNARD G. FORGET, M.D.
Professor of Medicine and Human Genetics, Chief of Hematology Section, Department of Medicine, Yale University School of Medicine. Attending Physician, Yale–New Haven Hospital, New Haven, Connecticut.
Sickle Cell Anemia and Associated Hemoglobinopathies

NOBLE O. FOWLER, M.D.
Professor of Medicine and Director, Division of Cardiology, University of Cincinnati College of Medicine. Attending Physician, Christian R. Holmes and Cincinnati General Hospitals, University of Cincinnati Medical Center, Cincinnati, Ohio.
Diseases of the Aorta

DAVID W. FRASER, M.D.
President, Swarthmore College, Swarthmore, Pennsylvania; Adjunct Professor of Medicine, University of Pennsylvania School of Medicine, Philadelphia, Pennsylvania.
Legionellosis

F. CLARKE FRASER, Ph.D., M.D., D.Sc. (Acadia)
Professor of Clinical Genetics, Memorial University of Newfoundland Faculty of Medicine. Attending Physician, Department of Medicine, General Hospital, and Department of Medicine and Therapeutics, Janeway Child Health Centre, St. John's, Newfoundland, Canada.
Genetic Counseling

JOSEPH F. FRAUMENI, Jr., M.D.
Associate Director for Epidemiology and Biostatistics, National Cancer Institute, National Institutes of Health. Adjunct Professor of Epidemiology, Department of Preventive Medicine and Biometrics, School of Medicine, Uniformed Services University of the Health Sciences, Bethesda, Maryland.
Epidemiology of Cancer

GARY D. FRIEDMAN, M.D.
Assistant Director for Epidemiology and Biostatistics, Department of Medical Methods Research, Kaiser-Permanente Medical Care Program, Oakland, California. Associate Clinical Professor of Medicine and of Family and Community Medicine, University of California, San Francisco, School of Medicine, San Francisco; Lecturer in Epidemiology, School of Public Health, University of California, Berkeley, California.
The Preventive Health Examination

JAMES F. FRIES, M.D.
Associate Professor of Medicine, Stanford University School of Medicine. Attending Physician, Stanford University Hospital, Stanford, Palo Alto Veterans Administration Medical Center, Palo Alto, and Santa Clara Valley Medical Center, San Jose, California.
Approach to the Patient with Musculoskeletal Disease

LAWRENCE A. FROHMAN, M.D.
Professor of Medicine and Director, Division of Endocrinology and Metabolism, University of Cincinnati College of Medicine. Attending Physician, University Hospital; Consultant Endocrinologist, Veterans Administration Hospital and Jewish Hospital, Cincinnati, Ohio.
Neuroendocrine Regulation and Its Disorders; The Anterior Pituitary

JOHN J. GALLAGHER, M.D.
Physician, Charlotte Memorial Hospital; Research Associate, Heineman Medical Research Center and Sanger Clinic, Charlotte, North Carolina.
Cardiac Arrhythmias

JOHN I. GALLIN, M.D.
Chief, Bacterial Diseases Section, Laboratory of Clinical Investigation, National Institute of Allergy and Infectious Diseases, National Institutes of Health, Bethesda, Maryland.
The Compromised Host

KENNETH D. GARDNER, Jr., M.D.
Professor of Medicine, University of New Mexico School of Medicine. Chief, Division of Renal Diseases, University of New Mexico Teaching Hospital/Bernalillo County Medical Center, Albuquerque, New Mexico.
Cystic Diseases of the Kidney

JEFFREY A. GELFAND, M.D.
Associate Professor of Medicine, Tufts University School of Medicine. Physician, Infectious Diseases Service, New England Medical Center Hospital, Boston, Massachusetts.
Advice to Travelers

JOHN W. GITTINGER, Jr., M.D.
Associate Professor of Surgery and Neurology and Chairman, Division of Ophthalmology, University of Massachusetts Medical School. Chief of Ophthalmology, University of Massachusetts Medical Center, Worcester, Massachusetts.
Eye Diseases: Introduction; Cataract; Glaucoma; Disc Swelling and Optic Atrophy; Ocular Inflammation; Ocular Infections; Orbital Disease and Tumors; Intraocular Tumors; Rheumatoid and Connective Tissue Diseases; Ocular Vascular Disease; The Eye and Medications

RICHARD J. GLASSOCK, M.D.
Professor of Medicine, University of California, Los Angeles, School of Medicine, Los Angeles. Chairman, Department of Medicine, Harbor-UCLA Medical Center, Torrance, California.
Mechanisms of Renal Injury

JOHN H. GLICK, M.D.
Professor of Medicine, University of Pennsylvania School of Medicine, and Associate Director for Clinical Research, University of Pennsylvania Cancer Center. Attending Physician, Hospital of the University of Pennsylvania, Philadelphia, Pennsylvania.
Hodgkin's Disease

ROBERT M. GLICKMAN, M.D.
Samuel Bard Professor of Medicine and Chairman, Department of Medicine, Columbia University College of Physicians and Surgeons. Director, Medical Service, Presbyterian Hospital, New York, New York.
Malabsorption: Pathophysiology and Diagnosis

MARTIN GOLDBERG, M.D.
Gordon and Helen Hughes Taylor Professor of Medicine, University of Cincinnati College of Medicine, and Director, Department of Internal Medicine, University of Cincinnati Medical Center. Physician-in-Chief, University Hospital, Cincinnati, Ohio.
Tubulo-interstitial Disease: Introduction to Interstitial Nephritis and Interstitial Nephropathy; Analgesic-Associated Nephropathy

DAVID W. GOLDE, M.D.
Professor of Medicine, University of California, Los Angeles, School of Medicine. Chief, Division of Hematology-Oncology, UCLA Center for the Health Sciences, Los Angeles, California.
Development and Morphology of Granulocytes and Macrophages

RALPH GOLDMAN, M.D.
Professor of Medicine in Residence, University of California, Los Angeles, School of Medicine. Associate Chief of Staff for Education, Wadsworth Veterans Administration Medical Center, West Los Angeles, California.
Aging and Geriatric Medicine

SHERWOOD L. GORBACH, M.D.
Professor of Medicine and Microbiology, Tufts University School of Medicine. Chief, Infectious Diseases Division, New England Medical Center Hospital, Boston, Massachusetts.
Diseases Caused by Non–Spore-Forming Anaerobic Bacteria; Typhoid Fever

JARED J. GRANTHAM, M.D.
Professor of Medicine and Director, Division of Nephrology, University of Kansas College of Health Sciences and Hospital, Kansas City, Kansas. Attending Physician, Veterans Administration Hospital, Kansas City, Missouri.
Acute Renal Failure

JOSEPH C. GREENFIELD, Jr., M.D.
James B. Duke Professor of Medicine, Duke University School of Medicine. Chairman, Department of Medicine, and Chief, Division of Cardiology, Duke University Medical Center and Veterans Administration Hospital, Durham, North Carolina.
Electrocardiography

B. M. GREENWOOD, M.D.
Director, Medical Research Council Laboratories, Fajara, Banjul, Gambia.
African Trypanosomiasis

JAMES H. GRENDELL, M.D.
Assistant Professor of Medicine and Physiology, University of California, San Francisco, School of Medicine. Attending Physician, San Francisco General Hospital Medical Center, San Francisco, California.
Vascular Diseases of the Intestine

JEROME E. GROOPMAN, M.D.
Assistant Professor of Medicine, Harvard Medical School. Attending Hematologist-Oncologist, New England Deaconess Hospital, Boston, Massachusetts.
Langerhans Cell (Eosinophilic) Granulomatosis

CARL GRUNFELD, M.D., Ph.D.
Assistant Professor of Medicine, University of California, San Francisco, School of Medicine. Co-Director, Special Diagnostic and Treatment Unit, San Francisco Veterans Administration Medical Center, San Francisco, California.
Pancreatic Islet Cell Tumors

ROGER GUILLEMIN, M.D., Ph.D.
Professor and Chairman, Laboratories for Neuroendocrinology, The Salk Institute; Adjunct Professor of Medicine, University of California, San Diego, School of Medicine, La Jolla, California.
Endorphins, Enkephalins and Other Opioid Peptides: Their Significance in Physiology and Medicine

J. CAULIE GUNNELLS, Jr., M.D.
Professor of Medicine, Division of Nephrology, Duke University School of Medicine, Durham, North Carolina.
Vascular Disorders of the Kidney

JOHN L. HAMERTON, D.Sc.
Professor of Pediatrics and Human Genetics, University of Manitoba Faculty of Medicine. Scientific Staff, Health Sciences Centre and St. Boniface Hospital, Winnipeg, Manitoba, Canada.
Chromosomes and Their Disorders

EDWARD D. HARRIS, Jr., M.D.
Professor and Chairman, Department of Medicine, University of Medicine and Dentistry of New Jersey, Rutgers Medical School, Piscataway. Chief, Medical Services, Middlesex General-University Hospital, New Brunswick, New Jersey.
Systemic Sclerosis (Scleroderma)

DONALD C. HARRISON, M.D.
Professor of Medicine and William G. Irwin Professor of Cardiology, Stanford University School of Medicine. Chief of Cardiology, Stanford University Medical Center, Stanford, California.
Cardiac Catheterization and Cineangiography

DONALD H. HARTER, M.D.
Charles L. Mix Professor of Neurology and Chairman, Department of Neurology, Northwestern University Medical School. Chairman, Department of Neurology, and Attending Neurologist, Northwestern Memorial Hospital, Chicago, Illinois.
Parameningeal Infections

WILLIAM L. HASKELL, Ph.D.
Associate Professor of Medicine, Stanford University School of Medicine, Stanford, California.
Exercise and Health

MICHAEL A. W. HATTWICK, M.D.
Clinical Assistant Professor, Department of Community and Family Medicine, Georgetown University School of Medicine, Washington, D.C. Attending Physician, The Fairfax Hospital, Falls Church, and Arlington Hospital and Northern Virginia Doctors Hospital, Arlington, Virginia.
Rabies

JOHN P. HAYSLETT, M.D.
Professor of Medicine, and Chief, Section of Nephrology, Yale University School of Medicine, New Haven. Attending Physician, Yale–New Haven Hospital, New Haven, and Veterans Administration Hospital, West Haven, Connecticut.
Renal Disease in Pregnancy

LOUIS A. HEALEY, M.D.
Clinical Professor of Medicine, University of Washington School of Medicine. Rheumatologist, Virginia Mason Hospital, Seattle, Washington.
Polymyalgia Rheumatica and Giant Cell Arteritis

DONALD A. HENDERSON, M.D., M.P.H.
Dean and Professor of Health Policy and Management, The Johns Hopkins University School of Hygiene and Public Health, Baltimore, Maryland.
Variola and Vaccinia

J. ALLAN HOBSON, M.D.
Professor of Psychiatry, Harvard Medical School. Director, Laboratory of Neurophysiology, Massachusetts Mental Health Center, Boston, Massachusetts.
Sleep and Its Disorders

EDWARD W. HOLMES, M.D.
Professor of Medicine, Assistant Professor of Biochemistry, Duke University School of Medicine. Chief of the Division of Metabolism, Endocrinology, and Genetics, Duke University Medical Center, Durham, North Carolina.
Other Disorders of Purine Metabolism

LEWIS B. HOLMES, M.D.
Associate Professor of Pediatrics, Harvard Medical School. Associate Pediatrician and Chief, Embryology-Teratology Unit, Massachusetts General Hospital; Consultant in Pediatrics (Genetics), Brigham and Women's Hospital, Boston, Massachusetts.
Congenital Malformations

PHILIP C. HOPEWELL, M.D.
Associate Professor of Medicine, Scientific Staff of Cardiovascular Research Institute, University of California, San Francisco, School of Medicine. Staff Physician, San Francisco General Hospital Medical Center, San Francisco, California.
Critical Care Medicine

DONALD R. HOPKINS, M.D., M.P.H.
Assistant Director for International Health, Centers for Disease Control, Atlanta, Georgia.
Dracunculiasis

RICHARD B. HORNICK, M.D.
Chairman, Department of Medicine, University of Rochester School of Medicine and Dentistry. Physician in Chief, The Strong Memorial Hospital, Rochester, New York.
Salmonella Infections Other Than Typhoid Fever; Tularemia

DONALD W. HOSKINS, M.D.
Clinical Associate Professor of Medicine, Cornell University Medical College. Associate Attending Physician (Medicine), The New York Hospital; Attending Physician and Chief of Medicine, Doctors Hospital, New York, New York.
Trichinellosis (Trichinosis)

DAVID S. HOWELL, M.D.
Professor of Medicine, Director of Arthritis Division, Department of Medicine, University of Miami School of Medicine. Medical Investigator, Veterans Administration Medical Center; Attending Physician, James M. Jackson Memorial Hospital, Miami, Florida.
Osteoarthritis (Degenerative Joint Disease); The Painful Shoulder; The Painful Back

R. RODNEY HOWELL, M.D.
David R. Park Professor and Chairman, Department of Pediatrics, University of Texas Medical School at Houston. Pediatrician-in-Chief, The Herman Hospital and University of Texas Health Science Center at Houston; Consultant in Pediatrics, M. D. Anderson Hospital and Tumor Institute and Shriners Hospital for Crippled Children, Houston, Texas.
The Glycogen Storage Diseases; Pentosuria; Essential Fructosuria and Hereditary Fructose Intolerance

STEPHEN B. HULLEY, M.D., M.P.H.
Professor of Epidemiology, University of California, San Francisco, School of Medicine, San Francisco, California.
Principles of Personal Medicine

JULIANNE IMPERATO-McGINLEY, M.D.
Associate Professor of Medicine, Division of Endocrinology, Cornell University Medical College. Associate Attending Physician, The New York Hospital, New York, New York.
Disorders of Sexual Differentiation

HARRY S. JACOB, M.D.
Professor and Chief, Division of Hematology, University of Minnesota Medical School—Minneapolis. Attending Physician, University of Minnesota Hospitals and Clinics of the University of Minnesota Health Sciences Center and Veterans Administration Medical Center, Minneapolis, Minnesota.
Hemolysis Due to Intracorpuscular Abnormalities

D. GERAINT JAMES, M.D., LL.D. (Hon.)
Senior Physician and Dean, Royal Northern Hospital, London. Consultant Physician, Medical Ophthalmology Unit, St. Thomas' Hospital, London; Consulting Physician, Royal Navy.
Sarcoidosis

KARL M. JOHNSON, M.D.
U.S. Army Medical Research Institute for Infectious Diseases, Ft. Detrick, Frederick, Maryland.
Arthropod-Borne Viral Fevers: Introduction; Viral Hemorrhagic Fevers: Introduction; Hemorrhagic Fever Caused by Dengue Viruses; Tick-Borne Flavivirus Diseases; Crimean Hemorrhagic Fever; Hemorrhagic Diseases Caused by Arenaviruses; African Hemorrhagic Fever; Hemorrhagic Fever with Renal Syndrome

KENNETH P. JOHNSON, M.D.
Professor and Chairman, Department of Neurology, University of Maryland School of Medicine. Attending Physician, University of Maryland Hospital, Baltimore, Maryland.
Syphilitic Infections of the Central Nervous System

MARIE-LOUISE JOHNSON, M.D., Ph.D.
Clinical Professor of Dermatology, Yale University School of Medicine. Attending Physician, Yale–New Haven Hospital, New Haven, Connecticut; Director of Medical Education, Benedictine Hospital, Kingston, New York.
Cutaneous Manifestations of Internal Malignancy; Skin Diseases: Introduction; Pathophysiology; Examination of the Skin; Principles of Therapy; Differential Diagnosis; Significant Dermatologic Signs of Disease; Selected Significant Dermatologic Diagnoses

RICHARD T. JOHNSON, M.D.
Dwight D. Eisenhower Professor of Neurology and Professor of Microbiology and Neuroscience, Johns Hopkins University School of Medicine. Neurologist, Johns Hopkins Hospital, and Consulting Neurologist, Baltimore City Hospitals, Baltimore, Maryland.
Viral Infections of the Nervous System: Introduction; Viral Meningitis and Encephalitis; Herpes Simplex Encephalitis; Herpes Zoster; Acute Anterior Poliomyelitis; Slow Viral Infections of the Nervous System

ALBERT R. JONSEN, Ph.D.
Professor of Ethics in Medicine, Department of Medicine, University of California, San Francisco, School of Medicine, San Francisco, California.
Ethics in the Practice of Medicine

JOHN P. KANE, M.D., Ph.D.
Professor of Medicine, Cardiovascular Research Institute and Department of Medicine, University of California, San Francisco, School

of Medicine. Attending Physician, Moffitt-Long Hospitals, San Francisco, California.
The Judicious Diet

ALBERT Z. KAPIKIAN, M.D.
Head, Epidemiology Section, Laboratory of Infectious Diseases, National Institute of Allergy and Infectious Diseases, National Institutes of Health, Bethesda, Maryland.
The Common Cold

JERRY G. KAPLAN, M.D.
Assistant Professor of Neurology, Albert Einstein College of Medicine of Yeshiva University, Bronx, New York.
Nerve Biopsy in Peripheral Nerve Disease

MANUEL E. KAPLAN, M.D.
Professor of Medicine, University of Minnesota Medical School—Minneapolis. Chief, Hematology/Oncology Section, Veterans Administration Medical Center, Minneapolis, Minnesota.
Hemolytic Disorders: Introduction; Acquired Hemolytic Disorders

SAMUEL KAPLAN, M.D.
Professor of Pediatrics and Medicine, University of Cincinnati College of Medicine. Director, Division of Cardiology, Children's Hospital Medical Center, Cincinnati, Ohio.
Congenital Heart Disease

HERANT A. KATCHADOURIAN, M.D.
Professor of Psychiatry and Behavioral Sciences, Vice Provost for Undergraduate Education, Stanford University, Stanford, California.
The Life-Cycle Perspective in Medicine; Development to Adulthood; Adulthood

SAMUEL L. KATZ, M.D.
Wilburt C. Davison Professor and Chairman, Department of Pediatrics, Duke University School of Medicine. Chief of Pediatrics, Children's Medical and Surgical Center, Duke University Medical Center, Durham, North Carolina.
Whooping Cough; Measles; Rubella

ALAN S. KEITT, M.D.
Associate Professor of Pathology and Medicine, University of Florida College of Medicine. Director, Hematology Laboratories, Shands Teaching Hospital and Clinics; Attending Hematologist, Veterans Administration Medical Center, Gainesville, Florida.
Introduction to the Anemias; Anemia Due to Failure of Progenitor Cells

JOHN H. KERR, D.M.
Clinical Lecturer in Anaesthetics and Fellow of Green College, University of Oxford. Consultant in Anaesthetics and Intensive Care, Nuffield Department of Anaesthetics, Oxfordshire Health Authority, John Radcliffe Hospital, Oxford, England.
Tetanus

SIDNEY KIBRICK, M.D., Ph.D.
Professor Emeritus of Pediatrics and Microbiology and Associate Professor Emeritus of Medicine, Boston University School of Medicine. Visiting Physician for Pediatrics, Boston City Hospital, Boston, Massachusetts.
Varicella and Herpes Zoster

EDWIN D. KILBOURNE, M.D.
Professor and Chairman, Department of Microbiology, Mount Sinai School of Medicine of the City University of New York, New York.
Introduction to Viral Diseases

BENJAMIN KISSIN, M.D.
Professor in Psychiatry, Downstate Medical Center College of Medicine, State University of New York. Attending Physician, University Hospital, New York University Medical Center, and Kings County Hospital Center, Brooklyn, New York.
Alcohol Abuse and Alcohol-Related Illness

SAULO KLAHR, M.D.
Professor of Medicine and Director, Renal Division, Washington University School of Medicine. Physician, Barnes Hospital; Staff Physician and Consultant in Nephrology, The Jewish Hospital, St. Louis, Missouri.
Structure and Function of the Kidneys

JAMES P. KNOCHEL, M.D.
Vice Chairman and Professor of Internal Medicine, University of Texas Southwestern Medical School at Dallas. Chief, Medical Service, Dallas Veterans Administration Medical Center; Senior Attending Physician, Parkland Memorial Hospital, Dallas, Texas.
Disorders Due to Heat and Cold

JUHA KOKKO, M.D., Ph.D.
Professor of Internal Medicine, Chief of Nephrology Division, University of Texas Southwestern Medical School at Dallas. Chief of Nephrology, Parkland Memorial Hospital, Dallas, Texas.
Chronic Renal Failure

EDWIN H. KOLODNY, M.D.
Associate Professor, Department of Neurology, Harvard Medical School, Boston. Associate Neurologist, Massachusetts General Hospital, Boston; Acting Director, Eunice Kennedy Shriver Center for Mental Retardation, Waltham, Massachusetts.
Gaucher's Disease; Niemann-Pick Disease

HERMES A. KONTOS, M.D., Ph.D.
Professor of Medicine, Health Science Division, Virginia Commonwealth University Medical College of Virginia. Attending Physician, Medical College of Virginia Hospitals, and Consultant, McGuire Veterans Administration Medical Center, Richmond, Virginia.
Vascular Diseases of the Limbs

STEPHEN M. KRANE, M.D.
Professor of Medicine, Harvard Medical School. Physician and Chief, Arthritis Unit, Massachusetts General Hospital, Boston, Massachusetts.
Connective Tissue Structure and Function

RICHARD M. KRAUSE, M.D.
Director, National Institute of Allergy and Infectious Diseases, National Institutes of Health, Bethesda, Maryland.
Streptococcal Diseases

WILLIAM L. KRINSKY, M.D., Ph.D.
Associate Professor of Epidemiology, Section of Medical Entomology, Yale University School of Medicine, New Haven, Connecticut.
Arthropods and Leeches

DONALD J. KROGSTAD, M.D.
Associate Professor of Medicine and Pathology, Washington University School of Medicine. Co-Director, Microbiology and Serology Laboratories, Barnes Hospital, St. Louis, Missouri.
Amebiasis and Amebic Meningoencephalitis

JAMES P. KUSHNER, M.D.
Professor of Medicine, University of Utah School of Medicine. Attending Physician, University Hospital and Veterans Administration Hospital, Salt Lake City, Utah.
Normochromic Normocytic Anemias; Hypochromic Anemias

SYLVIA A. LACK, M.D.
Consultant in Hospice Care, St. Mary's Hospital, Waterbury, Connecticut.
Care of Dying Patients and Their Families

DAVID J. LANG, M.D.
Chairman of Pediatrics, City of Hope Medical Center, Duarte, California.
Cytomegalovirus Infection

P. REED LARSEN, M.D.
Professor of Medicine, Harvard Medical School. Investigator, Howard Hughes Medical Institute; Senior Physician, Brigham and Women's Hospital, Boston, Massachusetts.
The Thyroid

JOHN LASZLO, M.D.
Professor of Medicine, Duke University School of Medicine, Durham, North Carolina. Attending Physician, Hematology-Oncology, Duke University Hospital, Durham, and Veterans Administration Hospital, Oteen, North Carolina.
Oncology: Introduction

GERALD S. LAZARUS, M.D.
Milton B. Hartzell Professor and Chairman, Department of Dermatology, University of Pennsylvania School of Medicine, Philadelphia, Pennsylvania.
Panniculitis and Disorders of the Subcutaneous Fat

ROBERT J. LEFKOWITZ, M.D.
James B. Duke Professor of Medicine, Duke University School of Medicine, Durham, North Carolina.
Pharmacologic Principles Related to the Autonomic Nervous System

BERNARD LEVIN, M.D.
Associate Professor of Medicine, University of Chicago Pritzker School of Medicine. Attending Physician, University of Chicago Hospitals and Clinics, Chicago, Illinois.
Ulerative Colitis

MICHAEL D. LEVITT, M.D.
Professor of Medicine, University of Minnesota Medical School—Minneapolis. Associate Chief of Staff for Research, Veterans Administration Medical Center, Minneapolis, Minnesota.
Pancreatitis

ROBERT I. LEVY, M.D.
Professor of Medicine, Columbia University College of Physicians and Surgeons. Attending Physician, Presbyterian Hospital, New York, New York.
Prevalence and Epidemiology of Cardiovascular Disease

ROBERT A. LEWIS, M.D.
Associate Professor of Medicine, Harvard Medical School. Immunologist and Rheumatologist and Associate Physician, Brigham and Women's Hospital, Boston, Massachusetts.
Mastocytosis

LAWRENCE M. LICHTENSTEIN, M.D.
Professor of Medicine, Johns Hopkins University School of Medicine, Baltimore, Maryland.
Anaphylaxis; Insect Sting Allergy

MORTIMER B. LIPSETT, M.D.
Director, National Institute of Child Health and Human Development, National Institutes of Health. Clinical Professor of Medicine, Uniformed Services University of the Health Sciences, Bethesda, Maryland.
The Testis

JOHN N. LOEB, M.D.
Professor of Medicine, Columbia University College of Physicians and Surgeons. Attending Physician, Presbyterian Hospital, New York, New York.
Polyglandular Disorders

D. LYNN LORIAUX, M.D., Ph.D.
Clinical Director, National Institute of Child Health and Human Development, National Institutes of Health, Bethesda, Maryland.
Hirsutism

DONALD B. LOURIA, M.D.
Chairman, Department of Preventive Medicine and Community Health, New Jersey Medical School. Attending Physician, UMD-University Hospital, Newark, New Jersey.
Trace Metal Poisoning

ROBERT G. LUKE, M.D.
Professor of Medicine, Director, Division of Nephrology, and Director, Nephrology Research and Training Center, University of Alabama School of Medicine. Attending Nephrologist, University of Alabama Hospitals and Children's Hospital, Birmingham, Alabama.
Dialysis

VANIZE MACÊDO, M.D.
Professor of Tropical Medicine, University of Brasilia. Physician, University Hospital, Brasilia, Brazil.
Chagas' Disease (American Trypanosomiasis)

ADEL A. F. MAHMOUD, M.D., Ph.D.
Professor of Medicine and Molecular Biology and Microbiology, Department of Medicine; Chief, Division of Geographical Medicine, Case Western Reserve University School of Medicine. Physician, University Hospitals, Cleveland, Ohio.
Introduction to Protozoan Diseases and Helminthic Diseases; Schistosomiasis

STEPHEN E. MALAWISTA, M.D.
Professor of Medicine and Chief, Section of Rheumatology, Department of Medicine, Yale University School of Medicine. Attending Physician, Yale–New Haven Hospital, New Haven, and Veterans Administration Hospital, West Haven, Connecticut.
Infectious Arthritis

PETER F. MALET, M.D.
Assistant Professor of Medicine, University of Pennsylvania School of Medicine. Attending Physician, Hospital of the University of Pennsylvania and Veterans Administration Hospital, Philadelphia, Pennsylvania.
Normal Physiology of Bile Formation; Pathophysiology of Gallstone Disease; Roentgenologic and Other Imaging Tests; Chronic Cholecystitis; Biliary Stricture; Other Causes of Bile Duct Obstruction; Benign Tumors and Pseudotumors of the Gallbladder

HENRY J. MANKIN, M.D.
Edith M. Ashley Professor of Orthopaedic Surgery, Harvard Medical School. Orthopaedist in Chief, Massachusetts General Hospital, Boston, Massachusetts.
Bone Tumors

AARON J. MARCUS, M.D.
Professor of Medicine, Cornell University Medical College. Chief, Hematology-Oncology, and Attending Physician, Veterans Administration Medical Center; Attending Physician, New York Hospital, New York, New York.
Hemorrhagic Disorders: Abnormalities of Platelet and Vascular Function

ANDREW M. MARGILETH, M.D.
Professor and Vice Chairman, Department of Pediatrics, Uniformed Services University of the Health Sciences, Bethesda, Maryland. Senior Attending Physician, Naval Hospital, Bethesda, Maryland, and Walter Reed Army Medical Center and Children's Hospital National Medical Center, Washington, D.C.
Cat Scratch Disease

ALEXANDER R. MARGULIS, M.D.
Professor and Chairman, Department of Radiology, University of California, San Francisco, School of Medicine. Radiologist in Chief, University of California, San Francisco Hospitals and Clinics, San Francisco, California.
Overview of Imaging Techniques and Projection for the Future

ERROL B. MARLISS, M.D.
Garfield Weston Professor of Nutrition and Professor of Medicine, McGill University Faculty of Medicine, Montreal. Senior Physician, Royal Victoria Hospital, Montreal, Quebec, Canada.
Protein-Calorie Undernutrition

ROBERT J. MASON, M.D.
Professor of Medicine, University of Colorado School of Medicine. Head, Pulmonary Division, National Jewish Hospital and Research Center/National Asthma Center; Co-Head, Pulmonary Division, University of Colorado Health Sciences Center, Denver, Colorado.
Occupational Lung Disease

HENRY MASUR, M.D.
Deputy Chief, Critical Care Medicine Department, Clinical Center, National Institutes of Health, Bethesda, Maryland.
Toxoplasmosis; Pneumocystosis

J. BRUCE McCLAIN, M.D.
Assistant Professor of Medicine, Uniformed Services University of the Health Sciences, School of Medicine, Bethesda, Maryland. Chief, Infectious Disease Service, Walter Reed Army Medical Center, Washington, D.C.
Rat Bite Fevers; Leptospirosis

RICHARD V. McCLOSKEY, M.S., M.D.
Professor of Medicine, Jefferson Medical College of Thomas Jefferson University, Philadelphia. Former Chairman, Department of Medicine, Daroff Division, Albert Einstein Medical Center, Philadelphia, Pennsylvania.
Diphtheria

HUGH O. McDEVITT, M.D., Ph.D.
Professor of Medical Microbiology and Medicine, Stanford University School of Medicine. Physician, Stanford University Hospital, Stanford, California.
The Major Histocompatibility Complex and Disease Susceptibility

PAUL R. McHUGH, M.D.
Henry Phipps Professor of Psychiatry, Johns Hopkins School of Medicine. Psychiatrist-in-Chief and Director, Department of Psychiatry, Johns Hopkins Hospital, Baltimore, Maryland.
Psychologic Illness in Medical Practice

PATRICK A. McKEE, M.D.
Investigator, Howard Hughes Medical Institute; Professor of Medicine and Assistant Professor of Biochemistry, Duke University School of Medicine. Chief, Division of General Internal Medicine, Duke University Medical Center, Durham, North Carolina.
Disorders of Blood Coagulation

RONALD P. MESSNER, M.D.
Professor of Internal Medicine and Director, Section of Rheumatology-Clinical Immunology, University of Minnesota Medical School—Minneapolis. Consulting Rheumatologist, Veterans Administration Medical Center and Hennepin County Medical Center, Minneapolis, Minnesota.
Dermatomyositis and Polymyositis

LOUIS H. MILLER, M.D.
Head, Malaria Section, Laboratory of Parasitic Diseases, National Institute of Allergy and Infectious Disease, National Institutes of Health, Bethesda, Maryland.
Malaria

ROBERT B. MILLMAN, M.D.
Clinical Professor of Public Health and Associate Professor of Clinical Psychiatry, Cornell University Medical College. Director, Alcohol and Drug Abuse Programs, The New York Hospital-Cornell Medical Center, New York, New York.
Drug Abuse and Dependence

THOMAS P. MONATH, M.D.
Director, Division of Vector-Borne Viral Diseases, Center for Infectious Diseases, Centers for Disease Control, Public Health Service, Fort Collins, Colorado.
Arthropod-Borne Viral Encephalitides; Yellow Fever

WILLIAM L. MORGAN, Jr., M.D.
Professor of Medicine, University of Rochester School of Medicine and Dentistry. Associate Chairman, Department of Medicine, The Strong Memorial Hospital, Rochester, New York.
Clinical Approach to the Patient

ARNO G. MOTULSKY, M.D., D.Sc. (Hon.)
Professor of Medicine and Genetics, University of Washington School of Medicine. Attending Physician, University and Providence Hospitals; Consulting Physician, Children's Orthopedic Hospital, Seattle, Washington.
Hemochromatosis (Iron Storage Disease); Hereditary Syndromes Involving Multiple Organ Systems

S. HARVEY MUDD, M.D.
Laboratory of General and Comparative Biochemistry, Department of Health and Human Services, National Institutes of Health, Bethesda, Maryland.
Homocystinuria

MAURICE A. MUFSON, M.D.
Professor and Chairman, Department of Medicine, Marshall University School of Medicine, Huntington, West Virginia. Associate Chief of Staff for Research, Veterans Administration Medical Center; Active Staff, Cabell-Huntington and St. Mary's Hospitals, Huntington, West Virginia.
Viral Pharyngitis, Laryngitis, Croup, and Bronchitis

JOHN F. MURRAY, M.D.
Professor of Medicine of the Senior Staff, Cardiovascular Research Institute, University of California, San Francisco, School of Medicine. Chief of Chest Service, San Francisco General Hospital Medical Center, San Francisco, California.
Respiratory Diseases: Introduction; Respiratory Structure and Function; Respiratory Failure

BRYAN D. MYERS, M.D.
Associate Professor of Medicine, Stanford University School of Medicine. Director of Clinical Nephrology, Stanford University Medical Center, Stanford, California.
Diabetes and the Kidney

DAVID G. NATHAN, M.D.
Robert A. Stranahan Professor of Pediatrics, Harvard Medical School. Pediatrician-in-Chief, Dana Farber Cancer Institute; Chief, Division of Hematology and Oncology, The Children's Hospital, Boston, Massachusetts.
Hematologic Diseases: Introduction

FRANKLIN A. NEVA, M.D.
Chief, Laboratory of Parasitic Diseases, and Member, Laboratory of Clinical Investigation, National Institute of Allergy and Infectious Diseases, National Institutes of Health. Attending Physician, Clinical Center, National Institutes of Health, Bethesda, Maryland.
Leishmaniasis

ARTHUR W. NIENHUIS, M.D.
Chief, Clinical Hematology Branch, National Heart, Lung, and Blood Institute, National Institutes of Health, Bethesda, Maryland.
Hemoglobin Synthesis; The Thalassemias

ALAN S. NIES, M.D.
Professor of Medicine and Pharmacology, University of Colorado School of Medicine. Attending Physician, University Hospitals, The University of Colorado Health Sciences Center, Denver, Colorado.
Principles of Drug Therapy; Interactions Between Drugs; Adverse Reactions to Drugs

JOHN A. OATES, M.D.
Chairman, Department of Medicine, and Professor, Medicine and Pharmacology, Vanderbilt University School of Medicine. Physician-in-Chief, Vanderbilt University Hospital, Nashville, Tennessee.
Prostaglandins, Thromboxane A_2, and Leukotrienes

ROBERT K. OCKNER, M.D.
Professor of Medicine, Director of Liver Center, University of California, San Francisco, School of Medicine. Chief of Gastroenterology, Moffitt-Long Hospitals, San Francisco, California.
Clinical Approach to Liver Disease; Hepatic Metabolism in Liver Disease; Laboratory Tests in Liver Disease; Approaches to the Diagnosis of Jaundice; Acute Viral Hepatitis; Toxic and Drug-Induced Liver Disease; Chronic Hepatitis

WILLIAM D. ODELL, M.D., Ph.D.
Professor of Medicine and Physiology and Chairman, Department of Medicine, University of Utah School of Medicine and Affiliated Hospitals, Salt Lake City, Utah.
Endocrine Manifestations of Tumors: "Ectopic" Hormone Production

JERROLD M. OLEFSKY, M.D.
Professor of Medicine, University of California, San Diego, School of Medicine, La Jolla, California.
Diabetes Mellitus

ERIC A. OTTESEN, M.D.
Head, Clinical Parasitology Section, Laboratory of Clinical Investigation, and Senior Investigator, Laboratory of Parasitic Diseases, National Institute of Allergy and Infectious Diseases, National Institutes of Health, Bethesda, Maryland.
Filariasis: Introduction; Lymphatic Filariasis; Tropical Eosinophilia; Loiasis; Mansonella ozzardi *Infection; Perstans Filariasis; Dirofilariasis; Possible Human Meningonemiasis*

CHARLES Y. C. PAK, M.D.
Professor of Internal Medicine, University of Texas Southwestern Medical School at Dallas, Dallas, Texas.
Renal Calculi

WILLIAM W. PARMLEY, M.D.
Professor of Medicine, University of California, San Francisco, School of Medicine. Chief of Cardiology, Moffitt-Long Hospitals, San Francisco, California.
Circulatory Function and Control

WILLIAM E. PAUL, M.D.
Chief, Laboratory of Immunology, National Institute of Allergy and Infectious Diseases, National Institutes of Health, Bethesda, Maryland.
Introduction: The Immune System

HERBERT A. PERKINS, M.D.
Clinical Professor of Medicine, University of California, San Francisco, School of Medicine. Scientific Director, Irwin Memorial Blood Bank of the San Francisco Medical Society, San Francisco, California.
Blood Transfusion

WALTER L. PETERSON, M.D.
Associate Professor of Internal Medicine, University of Texas Southwestern Medical School at Dallas. Assistant Chief, Medical Service, Dallas Veterans Administration Medical Center, Dallas, Texas.
Peptic Ulcer: Medical Therapy; Gastrointestinal Hemorrhage

SIDNEY PHILLIPS, M.D.
Professor of Medicine, Mayo Medical School. Director, Gastroenterology Unit, Mayo Clinic, Rochester, Minnesota.
Disorders of Gastrointestinal Motility

THEODORE L. PHILLIPS, M.D.
Professor and Chairman, Department of Radiation Oncology, University of California, San Francisco, School of Medicine. Attending Physician, Moffit-Long Hospitals and Veterans Administration and Mt. Zion Medical Centers, San Francisco, California.
Radiation Injury

NATHANIEL F. PIERCE, M.D.
Professor of Medicine, Johns Hopkins University School of Medicine. Chief, Infectious Diseases, Baltimore City Hospitals, Baltimore, Maryland.
Cholera

SHELDON R. PINNELL, M.D.
Professor of Medicine and Chief, Division of Dermatology, Duke University School of Medicine, Durham, North Carolina.
Marfan's Syndrome; Ehlers-Danlos Syndrome

FRED PLUM, M.D.
Titzell Professor and Chairman, Department of Neurology, Cornell University Medical College. Neurologist-in-Chief, The New York Hospital, New York, New York.
Approach to the Patient Including General Management; Principles of Diagnosis; The Neurologic Examination; Acute Central Nervous System Poisoning; Prognosis in Severe Brain Damage and Diagnosis of Brain Death; Brief Loss of Consciousness; Regional Diagnosis of Cerebral Disorders; Focal Disturbances of Higher Function; Amentia and Dementia; Autonomic Disorders and Their Management; Smell and Taste; Neuro-ophthalmology; Asthenia, Fatigue, and Weakness; Ataxia and Related Gait Disorders.

CHARLES E. POPE II, M.D.
Professor of Medicine, University of Washington School of Medicine. Chief, Gastroenterology, Seattle Veterans Administration Medical Center, Seattle, Washington.
Diseases of the Esophagus

CAROL S. PORTLOCK, M.D.
Associate Professor of Medicine, Yale University School of Medicine. Staff Physician, Yale–New Haven Hospital, New Haven, Connecticut.
Introduction to Neoplasms of the Immune System; Burkitt's Lymphoma

JEROME B. POSNER, M.D.
Professor of Neurology, Cornell University Medical College. Chairman, Department of Neurology, Memorial Sloan-Kettering Cancer Center, New York, New York.
Nonmetastatic Effects of Cancer on the Nervous System; The Neurologic History; Sustained Impairment of Consciousness; Hearing and Equilibrium; Episodic Loss of Motor Function; Disorders of Sensation; Differential Diagnosis of Muscle, Nerve Root, and Spinal Disorders; Intervertebral Disc Disease; Neoplasms of the Spinal Canal; Inflammatory Diseases of the Spinal Canal; Vascular Disorders of the Spinal Canal; Congenital Anomalies of the Craniovertebral Junction, Spine, and Spinal Cord

BASIL A. PRUITT, Jr., M.D.
Commander and Director, U.S. Army Institute of Surgical Research, Brooke Army Medical Center, Fort Sam Houston, Texas.
Electric Injury

CHARLES PUTMAN, M.D.
Chairman and Professor, Department of Radiology, and James B. Duke Professor of Radiology and Professor of Medicine, Duke University School of Medicine. Chief of Staff, Duke University Hospital, Durham, North Carolina.
Radiography of the Heart

CHARLES E. RACKLEY, M.D.
Anton and Margaret Fuisz Professor and Chairman, Department of Medicine, Georgetown University School of Medicine. Physician-in-Chief, Georgetown University Medical Center, Washington, D.C.
Valvular Heart Disease

SAMUEL RAPOPORT, M.D., Ph.D.
Assistant Professor of Neurology and Chief, Division of Clinical Neurophysiology, Cornell University Medical College. Assistant Attending Neurologist, The New York Hospital, New York, New York.
Neurologic Diagnostic Procedures

FLOYD C. RECTOR, Jr., M.D.
Professor of Medicine and Physiology and Senior Scientist, Cardiovascular Research Institute, University of California, San Francisco, School of Medicine, San Francisco, California.
Obstructive Nephropathy

CHARLES E. REED, M.D.
Professor of Internal Medicine, Mayo Medical School. Attending Physician, Saint Mary's Hospital and Rochester Methodist Hospital, Rochester, Minnesota.
Drug Allergy

SEYMOUR REICHLIN, M.D., Ph.D.
Professor of Medicine, Tufts University School of Medicine. Chief, Endocrine Division, and Senior Physician, New England Medical Center Hospital, Boston, Massachusetts.
The Pineal

HERBERT Y. REYNOLDS, M.D.
Professor of Medicine and Head, Pulmonary Section, Yale University School of Medicine. Attending Physician, Yale–New Haven Hospital, New Haven, and Veterans Administration Hospital, West Haven, Connecticut.
Introduction to Pneumonia; Pneumonia Due to Klebsiella (Friedländer's Pneumonia); Pneumonia Caused by Other Aerobic Gram-Negative Bacilli; Aspiration Pneumonia

CHARLES T. RICHARDSON, M.D.
Professor of Medicine, University of Texas Southwestern Medical School at Dallas. Chief, Gastroenterology, Dallas Veterans Administration Medical Center, Dallas, Texas.
Gastritis; Pathogenesis of Peptic Ulcer; Zollinger-Ellison Syndrome

RONALD F. RIEDER, M.D.
Professor of Medicine and Director of Hematology, State University of New York, Downstate Medical Center College of Medicine. Attending Physician, Kings County Hospital Center and State University Hospital, Brooklyn, New York.
Unstable Hemoglobins; Abnormal Hemoglobins with Altered Oxygen Affinity; Methemoglobinemia and Sulfhemoglobinemia

RICHARD A. RIFKIND, M.D.
Chairman, Sloan-Kettering Institute for Cancer Research, Memorial Sloan-Kettering Cancer Center. Attending Physician, Memorial Hospital for Cancer and Allied Diseases, Memorial Sloan-Kettering Cancer Center, New York, New York.
Diseases of the Spleen

B. LAWRENCE RIGGS, M.D.
Professor of Medicine, Mayo Medical School. Chairman, Division of Endocrinology and Metabolism, Mayo Clinic, Rochester, Minnesota.
Osteoporosis

RICHARD S. RIVLIN, M.D.
Professor of Medicine, Cornell University Medical College. Chief, Nutrition Service, Memorial Sloan-Kettering Cancer Center, and Chief, Nutrition Division, New York Hospital–Cornell University Medical Center, New York, New York.
Disorders of Vitamin Metabolism: Deficiencies, Metabolic Abnormalities, and Excesses

WILLIAM O. ROBERTSON, M.D.
Professor of Pediatrics, Department of Pediatrics, University of Washington School of Medicine. Medical Director, Seattle Poison Center, Washington Poison Network, and Children's Orthopedic Hospital and Medical Center, Seattle, Washington.
Common Poisonings

IRWIN H. ROSENBERG, M.D.
Professor of Medicine and Co-Director, Section of Gastroenterology, University of Chicago Pritzker School of Medicine, Chicago, Illinois.
Inflammatory Bowel Disease: Introduction; Crohn's Disease

ROGER N. ROSENBERG, M.D.
Professor and Chairman, Department of Neurology, and Professor of Physiology, University of Texas Southwestern Medical School at Dallas. Chief, Neurological Services, Parkland Memorial Hospital and Children's Medical Center, Dallas, Texas.
Striatonigral Degeneration; Motor Neuron Diseases; Spinocerebellar Degenerations; Syringomyelia; The Phakomatoses or Neurocutaneous Syndromes

GRIFF T. ROSS, M.D., Ph.D.
Director, Division of Reproductive Sciences, Department of Obstetrics, Gynecology and Reproductive Sciences, University of Texas Medical School at Houston, Houston, Texas.
The Ovaries

DAVID A. ROTTENBERG, M.D.
Associate Professor of Neurology, Cornell University Medical Center. Associate Attending Neurologist, The New York Hospital and Memorial Hospital for Cancer and Allied Diseases, Memorial Sloan-Kettering Cancer Center, New York, New York.
Intracranial Hypotension; Intracranial Hypertension; Pseudotumor Cerebri; Hydrocephalus

DAVID W. ROWE, M.D.
Associate Professor of Pediatrics, University of Connecticut School of Medicine, and Head, Director of Pediatric Endocrinology/Diabetes, University of Connecticut Health Center; Attending Physician, John Dempsey Hospital, University of Connecticut Health Center, Department of Pediatrics, Farmington, Connecticut.
Osteogenesis Imperfecta

LEWIS P. ROWLAND, M.D.
Henry and Lucy Moses Professor and Chairman, Department of Neurology, Columbia University College of Physicians and Surgeons. Director, Neurology Service, Presbyterian Hospital, New York, New York.
Diseases of Muscle and Neuromuscular Junction: Introduction; Inherited Diseases; Sporadic Disorders

GERALD F. M. RUSSELL, M.D., D.P.M.
Professor of Psychiatry, Institute of Psychiatry, University of London. Honorary Consultant Psychiatrist, Bethlem Royal and Maudsley Hospitals, London, England.
Anorexia Nervosa

ROBERT M. RUSSELL, M.D.
Associate Professor of Medicine, Tufts University School of Medicine. Director of Human Studies, U.S.D.A. Human Nutrition Research Center on Aging, Tufts University, and Staff Physician, New England Medical Center Hospital, Boston, Massachusetts.
Nutrient Requirements; Nutritional Assessment

DAVID C. SABISTON, Jr., M.D.
James B. Duke Professor of Surgery and Chairman of the Department, Duke University School of Medicine, Durham, North Carolina.
Surgical Treatment of Coronary Artery Disease

SYDNEY E. SALMON, M.D.
Professor of Internal Medicine, and Director, Cancer Center, University of Arizona College of Medicine, Tucson, Arizona. Attending Physician in Hematology and Oncology, University Hospital, Arizona Health Sciences Center, Tucson, Arizona.
Plasma Cell Disorders

JOHN E. SALVAGGIO, M.D.
Henderson Professor and Chairman, Department of Medicine, Tulane University School of Medicine. Senior Physician, Charity Hospital at New Orleans; Chief of Medicine, Tulane University Hospital; Active Staff, Touro Infirmary and Veterans Administration Medical Center, New Orleans, Louisiana.
Allergic Rhinitis

JAY P. SANFORD, M.D.
Professor of Medicine and Dean, Hibert School of Medicine, Uniformed Services University of the Health Sciences, Bethesda, Maryland. Attending Physician, Walter Reed Army Medical Center, Naval Hospital (Bethesda), and Consultant, Clinical Center, National Institutes of Health, Bethesda, Maryland.
Snake Bites

WILLIAM SCHAFFNER, M.D.
Professor and Chairman, Department of Preventive Medicine, and Professor and Chief, Division of Infectious Diseases, Department of Medicine, Vanderbilt University School of Medicine, Nashville, Tennessee.
Psittacosis

BRUCE F. SCHARSCHMIDT, M.D.
Associate Professor of Medicine, University of California, San Francisco, School of Medicine. Attending Physician, University of California, San Francisco Hospitals and Clinics, San Francisco, California.
Bilirubin Metabolism and Hyperbilirubinemia; Parasitic, Bacterial, Fungal, and Granulomatous Liver Disease; Inherited, Infiltrative, and Metabolic Disorders Involving the Liver; Acute and Chronic Hepatic Failure with Encephalopathy; Hepatic Tumors

HERBERT H. SCHAUMBURG, M.D.
Professor and Acting Chairman of Neurology, Albert Einstein College of Medicine of Yeshiva University. Attending Neurologist, Bronx Municipal Hospital Center and Hospital of the Albert Einstein College of Medicine, Bronx, New York.
Diseases of the Peripheral Nervous System: Introduction and Basic Terminology; Anatomic Classification of Neuropathy; Inflammatory Polyneuropathy; The Diabetic Neuropathies; Neuropathy Associated with Uremia; Neuropathy Associated with Endocrine Diseases; Hereditary Neuropathies; Toxic Neuropathy: Pharmaceutical Agents; Toxic Neuropathy: Occupational Biological and Environmental Agents; Miscellaneous Disease-Specific Neuropathies; Acute Physical Injury and Chronic Compression-Entrapment Neuropathies; Bell's Palsy, Brachial Neuritis, and Trigeminal Neuropathy

ALAN N. SCHECHTER, M.D.
Professorial Lecturer in Biochemistry, George Washington University School of Medicine and Health Sciences, Washington, D.C.; Professor, Department of Biology, Johns Hopkins University, Baltimore, Maryland. Chief, Laboratory of Chemical Biology, National Institute of Arthritis, Diabetes, and Digestive and Kidney Diseases, National Institutes of Health, Bethesda, Maryland.
Hemoglobin Structure and Function

PHILIP S. SCHEIN, M.D.
Professor of Medicine and Pharmacology, Georgetown University School of Medicine, Washington, D.C. Vice President, Clinical Research and Development, Smith Kline and French Laboratories, Philadelphia, Pennsylvania.
Biologic Effects of Tumors; Tumor Markers

LAWRENCE R. SCHILLER, M.D.
Assistant Professor of Internal Medicine, University of Texas Southwestern Medical School of Dallas. Staff Physician, Dallas Veterans Administration Medical Center, and Attending Physician, Parkland Memorial Hospital, Dallas, Texas.
Peptic Ulcer: Epidemiology, Clinical Manifestations, and Diagnosis

ROBERT W. SCHRIER, M.D.
Professor and Chairman, Department of Medicine, University of Colorado School of Medicine. Attending Physician, University Hospitals, The University of Colorado Health Sciences Center, Denver, Colorado.
Other Renal Tubular Disorders

H. RALPH SCHUMACHER, Jr., M.D.
Professor of Medicine, University of Pennsylvania School of Medicine. Director, Rheumatology-Immunology Center, Veterans Administration Medical Center, and Staff Rheumatologist, Hospital of the University of Pennsylvania, Philadelphia, Pennsylvania.
Calcium Crystal Deposition Arthropathies; Relapsing Polychondritis; Multifocal Fibrosclerosis

CHARLES R. SCRIVER, M.D.C.M.
Professor, Departments of Pediatrics and Biology and Center for Human Genetics, McGill University Faculty of Medicine. Senior Physician and Director, Division of Medical Genetics, Montreal Children's Hospital, Montreal, Quebec, Canada.
Hyperaminoaciduria

S. K. K. SEAH, M.D., Ph.D.
Associate Professor of Medicine, McGill University Faculty of Medicine. Attending Physician, The Montreal General Hospital, Montreal, Quebec, Canada.
Hermaphroditic Flukes

F. JOHN SERVICE, M.D., Ph.D.
Professor of Medicine, Mayo Medical School. Consultant in Internal Medicine and Endocrinology and Metabolism, Mayo Clinic, Rochester, Minnesota.
Hypoglycemic Disorders

WILLIAM R. SHAPIRO, M.D.
Professor of Neurology, Cornell University Medical College; Attending Neurologist, Memorial Sloan-Kettering Center and The New York Hospital, New York, New York.
Intracranial Tumors

JOHN N. SHEAGREN, M.D.
Associate Dean and Professor of Internal Medicine, University of Michigan Medical School. Attending Physician, University of Michigan Hospitals, Ann Arbor, Michigan.
Shock Syndromes Related to Sepsis; Staphylococcal Infections

PAUL SHERLOCK, M.D.
Professor and Vice Chairman, Department of Medicine, Cornell University Medical College, New York, New York. Chairman, Department of Medicine, Memorial Sloan-Kettering Cancer Center; Attending Physician, The New York Hospital; Visiting Physician, The Rockefeller University Hospital, New York, New York; and Consulting Staff, North Shore University Hospital, Manhasset, New York.
Gastrointestinal Endoscopy; Neoplasms of the Stomach

DONALD H. SILBERBERG, M.D.
Professor and Chairman, Department of Neurology, University of Pennsylvania School of Medicine. Chairman, Department of Neurology, Hospital of the University of Pennsylvania; Consultant, Children's Hospital of Philadelphia and Pennsylvania Hospital, Philadelphia, Pennsylvania.
The Demyelinating Diseases

SOL SILVERMAN, Jr., M.A., D.D.S.
Professor and Chairman, Department of Oral Medicine, University of California, San Francisco, School of Dentistry. Attending Dentist, Moffitt-Long Hospitals, San Francisco, California.
Oral Medicine

FREDERICK R. SINGER, M.D.
Professor of Medicine and Orthopaedic Surgery, University of Southern California School of Medicine. Associate Program Director, U.S.P.H.S. General Clinical Research Center, Los Angeles County (LAC)—USC Medical Center, and Director, Endocrine Laboratory, Orthopaedic Hospital—USC Bone and Connective Tissue Laboratories, Los Angeles, California.
Paget's Disease of Bone (Osteitis Deformans)

EDUARDO SLATOPOLSKY, M.D.
Professor of Medicine, Washington University School of Medicine. Director, Chromalloy American Kidney Center; Physician, Barnes Hospital; Consulting Physician, Jewish Hospital of St. Louis, St. Louis, Missouri.
Renal Osteodystrophy

MARVIN H. SLEISENGER, M.D.
Professor and Vice Chairman, Department of Medicine, University of California, San Francisco, School of Medicine. Chief, Medical Service, San Francisco Veterans Administration Medical Center; Attending Physician, Moffitt-Long Hospitals, San Francisco, California.
Gastrointestinal Diseases: Introduction; Malabsorption: Management; Miscellaneous Inflammatory Diseases of the Intestine

WILLIAM S. SLY, M.D.
Chairman, E. A. Doisy Department of Biochemistry, St. Louis University School of Medicine. Pediatrician, Cardinal Glennon Memorial Hospital for Children, St. Louis, Missouri.
The Mucopolysaccharidoses

LLOYD H. SMITH, Jr., M.D.
Chairman, Department of Medicine, University of California, San Francisco, School of Medicine, San Francisco, California.
Medicine as an Art; Renal Hyperaminoacidurias; Primary Hyperoxaluria; The Hyperphenylalaninemias; Histidinemia; The Hyperprolinemias and Hydroxyprolinemia; Diseases of the Urea Cycle; Branched-Chain Aminoaciduria; Disorders of Pyrimidine Metabolism; Phosphorus Deficiency and Hypophosphatemia; Disorders of Magnesium Metabolism

GORDON L. SNIDER, M.D.
Professor of Medicine and Director, Pulmonary Center, Boston University School of Medicine; Lecturer in Medicine, Tufts University School of Medicine. Chief, Pulmonary Medicine Section, Boston Veterans Administration Medical Center; Member, Evans Department of Clinical Research, University Hospital; Attending Physician, Boston City Hospital, Boston, Massachusetts.
Special Diagnostic Procedures in Pulmonary Disease

RALPH SNYDERMAN, M.D.
Frederic M. Hanes Professor of Medicine, Professor of Immunology, and Chief, Division of Rheumatic and Genetic Diseases, Department of Medicine, Duke University School of Medicine. Investigator, Howard Hughes Medical Institute; Attending Physician, Duke University Hospital and Veterans Administration Hospital, Durham, North Carolina.
Mechanisms of Inflammation and Tissue Destruction in the Rheumatic Diseases; Behçet's Disease

ROGER D. SOLOWAY, M.D.
Professor of Medicine, University of Pennsylvania School of Medicine. Associate Chief, Gastrointestinal Section, Hospital of the University of Pennsylvania, Philadelphia, Pennsylvania.
Asymptomatic Gallstones; Acute Cholecystitis; Gallstone Ileus; Choledocholithiasis and Cholangitis; Carcinoma of the Gallbladder; Tumors of the Bile Duct; Postcholecystectomy Syndrome

NICHOLAS A. SOTER, M.D.
Professor of Dermatology, New York University School of Medicine. Medical Director, Skin and Cancer Unit, Department of Dermatology, New York University Medical Center, New York, New York.
Urticaria and Angioedema

P. FREDERICK SPARLING, M.D.
Chairman, Department of Microbiology and Immunology, and Professor of Microbiology and Medicine, University of North Carolina at Chapel Hill School of Medicine. Attending Physician, The North Carolina Memorial Hospital, Chapel Hill, North Carolina.
Sexually Transmitted Diseases: Introduction and Common Syndromes; Gonococcal Infections; Lymphogranuloma Venereum; Granuloma Inguinale; Chancroid; Syphilis

WALTER E. STAMM, M.D.
Associate Professor of Medicine, University of Washington School of Medicine. Head, Infectious Disease Division, Harborview Medical Center, Seattle, Washington.
Diseases Caused by Chlamidiae: Introduction; Trachoma; Neonatal Chlamydial Infections

ALFRED D. STEINBERG, M.D.
Chief, Section on Cellular Immunology, Arthritis and Rheumatism Branch, National Institute of Arthritis, Diabetes, and Digestive and Kidney Diseases, National Institute of Health. Medical Director, United States Public Health Service, National Institutes of Health, Bethesda, Maryland.
Systemic Lupus Erythematosus

DAVID P. STEVENS, M.D.
Associate Clinical Professor of Medicine, Case Western Reserve University School of Medicine. Assistant Physician, University Hospitals of Cleveland, Ohio.
Other Protozoan Diseases

DANIEL P. STITES, M.D.
Professor of Laboratory Medicine and Medicine; Director, Immunology Laboratory, and Vice Chairman, Department of Laboratory Medicine, University of California, San Francisco, School of Medicine. Attending Physician, University of California, San Francisco Hospitals and Clinics, San Francisco, California.
Diseases of the Thymus

RAINER STORB, M.D.
Professor of Medicine, Department of Medicine, Division of Oncology, University of Washington School of Medicine. Program Head, Transplantation Biology Department, Fred Hutchinson Cancer Research Center, Seattle, Washington.
Bone Marrow Transplantation

GORDON J. STREWLER, M.D.
Assistant Professor of Medicine, University of California, San Francisco, School of Medicine. Clinical Investigator, San Francisco Veterans Administration Medical Center; Attending Physician, University of California, San Francisco Hospitals and Clinics, San Francisco, California.
Osteonecrosis, Osteosclerosis, and Other Disorders of Bone

WADI N. SUKI, M.D.
Professor of Medicine and Physiology and Chief, Renal Section, Department of Medicine, Baylor College of Medicine. Senior Attending Physician and Chief, Renal Service, The Methodist Hospital, Houston, Texas.
Hereditary Chronic Nephropathies

MORTON N. SWARTZ, M.D.
Professor of Medicine, Harvard Medical School. Chief, Infectious Disease Unit, Massachusetts General Hospital, Boston, Massachusetts.
Bacterial Meningitis; Meningococcal Disease; Infections Caused by Hemophilus Species; Babesiosis

NORMAN TALAL, M.D.
Professor of Medicine and Microbiology, University of Texas Health Science Center at San Antonio. Chief, Clinical Immunology Section, Audie L. Murphy Memorial Veterans Hospital, San Antonio, Texas.
Sjögren's Syndrome

CLIFFORD TASMAN-JONES, B.Sc., M.B., Ch.B.
Associate Professor in Medicine, Medical School, University of Auckland. Consultant Physician and Gastroenterologist, Auckland Public Hospital, Auckland, New Zealand.
Disturbances of Trace Mineral Metabolism

ROBERT B. TESH, M.D.
Associate Professor of Epidemiology, Yale University School of Medicine, New Haven, Connecticut.
Dengue; West Nile Fever; Phlebotomus Fever; Rift Valley Fever; Fevers Caused by Alphaviruses

SAMUEL O. THIER, M.D.
Sterling Professor and Chairman, Department of Internal Medicine, Yale University School of Medicine. Chief of Medicine, Yale–New Haven Hospital, New Haven, Connecticut.
Cystinuria

RICHARD C. THIRLBY, M.D.
Assistant Professor of Surgery, University of Texas Health Science Center at Dallas. Staff Surgeon, Dallas Veterans Administration Medical Center and Parkland Memorial Hospital, Dallas, Texas.
Peptic Ulcer: Surgical Therapy

LEWIS THOMAS, M.D.
Professor, State University of New York at Stony Brook, New York. President Emeritus, Memorial Sloan-Kettering Cancer Center, New York, New York.
Medicine as a Very Old Profession

NORBERT W. TIETZ, Ph.D.
Professor of Pathology, University of Kentucky College of Medicine. Director of Clinical Chemistry, University of Kentucky Medical Center, Lexington, Kentucky.
Reference Ranges and Laboratory Values of Clinical Importance

GEORGE TOLIS, M.D., M.Sc.
Associate Professor of Medicine, Obstetrics and Gynecology, McGill University Faculty of Medicine, Montreal, Quebec, Canada. Director, Division on Endocrinology, Hippokrateion Hospital, Athens, Greece.
Nonmalignant Diseases of the Breast

ARA TOURIAN, M.D.
Associate Professor of Neurology, Duke University School of Medicine. Attending Neurologist, Duke University Medical Center, Durham, North Carolina.
Wilson's Disease

H. RICHARD TYLER, M.D.
Professor of Neurology, Harvard Medical School. Director of Neurological Services, Brigham and Women's Hospital, Boston, Massachusetts.
Acute Transverse Myelitis

J. BLAKE TYRRELL, M.D.
Associate Clinical Professor of Medicine, University of California, San Francisco School of Medicine, San Francisco, California.
Disorders of the Adrenal Cortex: Laboratory Evaluation of Adrenocortical Function; Cushing's Syndrome

JOUNI UITTO, M.D., Ph.D.
Professor of Medicine, University of California, Los Angeles, UCLA School of Medicine, Los Angeles. Associate Chief and Director of Research, Division of Dermatology, Department of Medicine, Harbor-UCLA Medical Center, Torrance, California.
Pseudoxanthoma Elasticum

FRANCIS A. WALDVOGEL, M.D.
Professor of Medicine, University of Geneva. Chief, Infectious Disease Division, and Physician-in-Chief, Clinique Médicale Thérapeutique, University Hospital, Geneva, Switzerland.
Osteomyelitis

ANDREW G. WALLACE, M.D.
Professor of Medicine, Duke University School of Medicine. Chief Executive Officer, Duke University Hospital, Durham, North Carolina.
Approach to the Patient with Cardiovascular Disease

PATRICK C. WALSH, M.D.
Professor and Director, Department of Urology, The Johns Hopkins University School of Medicine. Urologist-in-Chief, The James Buchanan Brady Urological Institute, Johns Hopkins Hospital, Baltimore, Maryland.
Diseases of the Prostate

HOWARD J. WEINSTEIN, M.D.
Associate Professor of Pediatrics, Harvard Medical School. Associate in Medicine, The Children's Hospital; Assistant Physician, Dana Farber Cancer Institute, Boston, Massachusetts.
The Acute Leukemias

RICHARD P. WENZEL, M.D.
Professor of Medicine, University of Virginia School of Medicine, and Chairman and Professor, Department of Epidemiology, University of Virginia Graduate School of Arts and Sciences. Hospital Epidemiologist, University of Virginia Hospital, Charlottesville, Virginia.
Prevention and Treatment of Hospital-Acquired Infections

ROBERT E. WHALEN, M.D.
Professor of Medicine and Director, Cardiovascular Disease Service, Duke University School of Medicine, Durham, North Carolina.
Disorders of the Pericardium; Tumors of the Heart

CATHERINE M. WILFERT, M.D.
Professor of Pediatrics and Microbiology, Duke University School of Medicine. Pediatrician, Duke University Hospital; Consultant, Cabarrus County Hospital and Durham County General Hospital, Durham, North Carolina.
Foot and Mouth Diseases; Mumps

JAMES T. WILLERSON, M.D.
Professor of Medicine and Director, Cardiology Division, University of Texas Southwestern Medical School at Dallas. Staff Physician, Parkland Memorial Hospital, Dallas, Texas.
Angina Pectoris; Acute Myocardial Infarction; Sudden Cardiac Death

RICHARD D. WILLIAMS, M.D.
Professor and Head, Department of Urology, University of Iowa School of Medicine, Iowa City, Iowa.
Urinary Tract Anomalies; Tumors of the Kidney, Ureter, and Bladder

T. FRANKLIN WILLIAMS, M.D.
Director, National Institute on Aging, National Institutes of Health, Bethesda, Maryland. Professor of Medicine, University of Rochester,

Rochester, New York; Lecturer in Medicine, Johns Hopkins University School of Medicine, Baltimore, Maryland.
Management of Common Problems in the Elderly

JOHN WILLIAMSON, B.Sc. (Biochem.), M.B., B.S. (Qd.), D.A. (Melb.)
Honorary Clinical Teacher, Faculty of Medicine, University of Queensland, and Lecturer in Resuscitation, James Cook University of North Queensland. Visiting Anaesthetist, Townsville General and Mater Hospitals, Townsville, North Queensland, Australia.
Venemous and Poisonous Marine Animals

JAMES E. WILSON III, M.D.
Late Professor of Medicine, Jefferson Medical College of Thomas Jefferson University. Late Director of the Pulmonary Division, Department of Medicine, Thomas Jefferson University Hospital, Philadelphia, Pennsylvania.
Pulmonary Embolism; Fat Embolism Syndrome

SIDNEY J. WINAWER, M.D.
Professor of Clinical Medicine, Cornell University Medical College. Chief and Attending Physician, Memorial Sloan-Kettering Cancer Center, New York, New York.
Neoplasms of the Large and Small Intestine

CHARLES L. WISSEMAN, Jr., M.D.
Professor and Chairman, Department of Microbiology, University of Maryland School of Medicine, Baltimore, Maryland.
Rickettsial Diseases: Introduction; The Typhus Group; Rocky Mountain Spotted Fever; Tick-Borne Rickettsioses of the Eastern Hemisphere; Rickettsialpox; Scrub Typhus

MARTIN S. WOLFE, M.D.
Clinical Professor of Medicine, George Washington University School of Medicine and Health Sciences, and Clinical Associate Professor of Medicine, Georgetown University School of Medicine. Attending Physician, George Washington University Medical Center and Georgetown University Hospital, Washington, D.C.
The Cestodes: Introduction; Diphyllobothrium latum *(Fish Tapeworm);* Taenia saginata *(Beef Tapeworm);* Taenia solium *(Pork Tapeworm; Human Cysticercosis);* Hymenolepis nana *(Dwarf Tapeworm); Echinococcosis (Hydatid Disease); Other Rarer Tapeworms; Treatment of Tapeworm Infections*

SHELDON M. WOLFF, M.D.
Endicott Professor and Chairman, Department of Medicine, Tufts University School of Medicine. Physician-in-Chief, New England Medical Center Hospital, Boston, Massachusetts.
The Febrile Patient

EMANUEL WOLINSKY, M.D.
Professor of Medicine and Pathology, Case Western Reserve University School of Medicine. Acting Director, Department of Pathology, Cleveland Metropolitan General Hospital, Cleveland, Ohio.
Tuberculosis; Other Mycobacterioses

HARVEY WOLINSKY, M.D., Ph.D.
Clinical Professor of Medicine, Mount Sinai School of Medicine of the City University of New York. Attending Physician, The Mount Sinai Hospital, New York, New York.
Atherosclerosis

JERRY S. WOLINSKY, M.D.
Professor of Neurology, University of Texas Medical School at Houston. Attending Neurologist, Hermann Hospital, Houston, Texas.
Central Nervous System Complications of Viral Infections and Vaccines; Reye's Syndrome; Neurologic Complications in the Immunologically Compromised Host

JAMES B. WYNGAARDEN, M.D.
Director, National Institutes of Health, Bethesda, Maryland.
Medicine as a Science; Medicine as a Public Service; The Use and Interpretation of Laboratory-Derived Data; Human Heredity; Biochemical Genetics; Inborn Errors of Metabolism; Metabolic Diseases: Introduction; Fabry's Disease; Alcaptonuria; Gout; Acatalasia

LOWELL S. YOUNG, M.D.
Professor of Medicine, Division of Infectious Diseases, University of California, Los Angeles, School of Medicine. Attending Physician, UCLA Center for the Health Sciences, Los Angeles, California.
Antimicrobial Therapy

JOHN A. ZAIA, M.D.
Associate Clinical Professor of Pediatrics, University of Southern California School of Medicine, Los Angeles, California. Director, Virology and Infectious Diseases, Division of Pediatrics, City of Hope Medical Center, Duarte, California.
Infectious Mononucleosis

BARRY L. ZARET, M.D.
Professor of Internal Medicine and Diagnostic Radiology and Chief, Section of Cardiology, Yale University School of Medicine. Professor of Internal Medicine and Diagnostic Radiology, Yale–New Haven Hospital, New Haven, Connecticut.
Nuclear Cardiology

CONTENTS

	COLOR PLATES	xxxii
PART I	MEDICINE AS A LEARNED AND HUMANE PROFESSION	1
PART II	HUMAN GROWTH, DEVELOPMENT, AND AGING	15
PART III	PERSONAL HEALTH CARE AND PREVENTIVE MEDICINE	35
PART IV	PRINCIPLES OF DIAGNOSIS	57
PART V	PRINCIPLES OF THERAPEUTICS	69
PART VI	PRINCIPLES OF HUMAN GENETICS	117
PART VII	CARDIOVASCULAR DISEASES	150
PART VIII	RESPIRATORY DISEASES	368
PART IX	CRITICAL CARE MEDICINE	463
PART X	RENAL DISEASES	483
PART XI	GASTROINTESTINAL DISEASES	645
PART XII	DISEASES OF THE LIVER, GALLBLADDER, AND BILE DUCTS	803
PART XIII	HEMATOLOGIC DISEASES	866
PART XIV	ONCOLOGY	1059
PART XV	METABOLIC DISEASES	1103
PART XVI	NUTRITIONAL DISEASES	1174
PART XVII	ENDOCRINE AND REPRODUCTIVE DISEASES	1219
PART XVIII	DISEASES OF BONE AND BONE MINERAL METABOLISM	1415
PART XIX	INFECTIOUS DISEASES	1469
PART XX	DISEASES CAUSED BY PROTOZOA AND METAZOA	1775
PART XXI	DISEASES OF THE IMMUNE SYSTEM	1846
PART XXII	MUSCULOSKELETAL AND CONNECTIVE TISSUE DISEASES	1891
PART XXIII	NEUROLOGIC AND BEHAVIORAL DISEASES	1965
PART XXIV	EYE DISEASES	2217
PART XXV	SKIN DISEASES	2227
PART XXVI	OCCUPATIONAL AND ENVIRONMENTAL MEDICINE	2277
PART XXVII	LABORATORY REFERENCE RANGE VALUES OF CLINICAL IMPORTANCE	2315

(Detailed Table of Contents begins on the following page)

Contents

PART I MEDICINE AS A LEARNED AND HUMANE PROFESSION

1 Medicine as an Art, *Lloyd H. Smith, Jr.* 1
2 Medicine as a Science, *James B. Wyngaarden* 4
3 Medicine as a Public Service, *James B. Wyngaarden* 7
4 Medicine as a Very Old Profession, *Lewis Thomas* 9
5 Ethics in the Practice of Medicine, *Albert R. Jonsen* 11

PART II HUMAN GROWTH, DEVELOPMENT, AND AGING

6 The Life-Cycle Perspective in Medicine, *Herant A. Katchadourian* 15
7 Development to Adulthood, *Herant A. Katchadourian* 16
8 Adulthood, *Herant A. Katchadourian* 20
9 Aging and Geriatric Medicine, *Ralph Goldman* 22
10 Management of Common Problems in the Elderly, *T. Franklin Williams* 26
11 Care of Dying Patients and Their Families, *Sylvia A. Lack* 30

PART III PERSONAL HEALTH CARE AND PREVENTIVE MEDICINE

12 Principles of Personal Medicine, *Stephen B. Hulley* 35
13 The Judicious Diet, *John P. Kane* 37
14 Exercise and Health, *William L. Haskell* 40
15 Immunization, *R. Gordon Douglas, Jr.* 42
16 Tobacco and Health, *David M. Burns* 46
17 Alcohol Abuse and Alcohol-Related Illnesses, *Benjamin Kissin* 50
18 The Preventive Health Examination, *Gary D. Friedman* 55

PART IV PRINCIPLES OF DIAGNOSIS

19 Clinical Approach to the Patient, *William L. Morgan, Jr.* 57
20 The Use and Interpretation of Laboratory-Derived Data, *James B. Wyngaarden* 61
21 Overview of Imaging Techniques and Projection for the Future, *Alexander R. Margulis* 64

PART V PRINCIPLES OF THERAPEUTICS

22 Principles of Drug Therapy, *Alan S. Nies* 69
23 Interactions Between Drugs, *Alan S. Nies* 79
24 Adverse Reactions to Drugs, *Alan S. Nies* 82
25 Common Poisonings, *William O. Robertson* 84
26 Pharmacologic Principles Related to the Autonomic Nervous System, *Robert J. Lefkowitz* 90
27 Antimicrobial Therapy, *Lowell S. Young* 96
28 Antiviral Therapy, *D. W. Barry* 108
29 Glucocorticosteroid Therapy, *Anthony S. Fauci* 111

PART VI PRINCIPLES OF HUMAN GENETICS

30 Human Heredity, *James B. Wyngaarden* 117
31 Biochemical Genetics, *James B. Wyngaarden* 122
32 Inborn Errors of Metabolism, *James B. Wyngaarden* 127
33 Expectations from Recombinant DNA Research, *W. French Anderson* 132
34 Contributions of Recombinant DNA Research to Diagnosis of Heritable Disease, *C. Thomas Caskey* 135
35 Chromosomes and Their Disorders, *John L. Hamerton* 138
36 Congenital Malformations, *Lewis B. Holmes* 144
37 Genetic Counseling, *F. Clarke Fraser* 147

PART VII CARDIOVASCULAR DISEASES

38 Approach to the Patient with Cardiovascular Disease, *Andrew G. Wallace* 150
39 Prevalence and Epidemiology of Cardiovascular Disease, *Robert I. Levy* 155
40 Circulatory Function and Control, *William W. Parmley* 158
41 Specialized Diagnostic Procedures 164
41.1 Radiography of the Heart, *Charles E. Putman* 164
41.2 Electrocardiography, *Joseph C. Greenfield, Jr.* 169
41.3 Echocardiography, *Harvey Feigenbaum* 175
41.4 Nuclear Cardiology, *Barry L. Zaret* 179
41.5 Cardiac Catheterization and Cineangiography, *Donald C. Harrison* 183
42 Heart Failure, *Alfred P. Fishman* 189
43 Shock, *François M. Abboud* 211
44 Congenital Heart Disease, *Samuel Kaplan* 225
45 Valvular Heart Disease, *Charles E. Rackley* 242
46 Pulmonary Hypertension, *Alfred P. Fishman* 256
47 Arterial Hypertension, *C. T. Dollery* 266
48 Atherosclerosis, *Harvey Wolinsky* 281
49 Disorders of Coronary Arteries 284
49.1 Angina Pectoris, *James T. Willerson* 284
49.2 Acute Myocardial Infarction, *James T. Willerson* 288
49.3 Sudden Cardiac Death, *James T. Willerson* 296
49.4 Surgical Treatment of Coronary Artery Disease, *David C. Sabiston, Jr.* 297
50 Cardiac Arrhythmias, *John J. Gallagher* 300
51 Diseases of the Myocardium, *Victor S. Behar* 329
52 Disorders of the Pericardium, *Robert E. Whalen* 339
53 Diseases of the Aorta, *Noble O. Fowler* 345
54 Vascular Diseases of the Limbs, *Hermes A. Kontos* 353
55 Tumors of the Heart, *Robert E. Whalen* 366

PART VIII RESPIRATORY DISEASES

56 Introduction, *John F. Murray* 368
57 Respiratory Structure and Function, *John F. Murray* 372
58 Special Diagnostic Procedures in Pulmonary Disease, *Gordon L. Snider* 381
59 Asthma, *Ronald P. Daniele* 390
60 Chronic Airways Diseases, *Benjamin Burrows* 396
61 Abnormalities of Lung Aeration, *Benjamin Burrows* 404
62 Interstitial Lung Disease, *Ronald G. Crystal* 406
63 Lung Abscess, *John G. Bartlett* 419
64 Bronchiectasis and Cystic Fibrosis, *John G. Bartlett* 422
65 Pulmonary Embolism, *James E. Wilson III* 426
66 Fat Embolism Syndrome, *James E. Wilson III* 431
67 Sarcoidosis, *D. Geraint James* 432
68 Neoplasms of the Lung, *Leo F. Black* 439
69 Diseases of the Pleura, Mediastinum, Diaphragm, and Chest Wall, *Jerome S. Brody* 447
70 Respiratory Failure, *John F. Murray* 454

PART IX CRITICAL CARE MEDICINE

71 Critical Care Medicine, *Philip C. Hopewell* 463

PART X RENAL DISEASES

72 Approach to the Patient with Renal Disease, *Thomas E. Andreoli* 483
73 Structure and Function of the Kidneys, *Saulo Klahr* 490

74 Mechanisms of Renal Injury, *Richard J. Glassock* 501
75 Investigations of Renal Function, *Vincent W. Dennis* 507
76 Disorders of Fluid Volume, Electrolyte, and Acid-Base Balance, *Thomas E. Andreoli* 515
77 Acute Renal Failure, *Jared J. Grantham* 544
78 Chronic Renal Failure, *Juha Kokko* 549
79 Treatment of Irreversible Renal Failure 559
79.1 Dialysis, *Robert G. Luke* 559
79.2 Renal Transplantation, *William J. C. Amend, Jr.* 563
80 Glomerular Disorders, *William G. Couser* 568
81 Tubulointerstitial Diseases 589
81.1 Introduction to Interstitial Nephritis and Interstitial Nephropathy, *Martin Goldberg* 589
81.2 Analgesic-Associated Nephropathy, *Martin Goldberg* 592
81.3 Toxic Nephropathy, *Bryan T. Emmerson* 594
82 Obstructive Nephropathy, *Floyd C. Rector, Jr.* 604
83 Specific Renal Tubular Disorders 608
83.1 Introduction, *Martin G. Cogan* 608
83.2 Renal Tubular Acidosis (RTA), *Martin G. Cogan* 608
83.3 Renal Hyperaminoacidurias, *Lloyd H. Smith, Jr.* 610
83.4 Cystinuria, *Samuel O. Thier* 611
83.5 Other Renal Tubular Disorders, *Robert W. Schrier* 613
84 Diabetes and the Kidney, *Bryan D. Myers* 616
85 Urinary Tract Infections and Pyelonephritis, *Vincent T. Andriole* 619
86 Vascular Disorders of the Kidney, *J. Caulie Gunnells, Jr.* 623
87 Renal Disease in Pregnancy, *John P. Hayslett* 624
88 Hereditary Chronic Nephropathies, *Wadi N. Suki* 627
89 Renal Calculi, *Charles Y. C. Pak* 628
90 Cystic Diseases of the Kidney, *Kenneth D. Gardner, Jr.* 633
91 Anomalies of the Urinary Tract, *Richard D. Williams* 638
92 Tumors of the Kidney, Ureter, and Bladder, *Richard D. Williams* 639

PART XI GASTROINTESTINAL DISEASES

93 Introduction, *Marvin H. Sleisenger* 645
94 Diagnostic Imaging Procedures in Gastroenterology, *Robert N. Berk* 650
95 Gastrointestinal Endoscopy, *Paul Sherlock* 658
96 Oral Medicine, *Sol Silverman, Jr.* 662
97 Diseases of the Esophagus, *Charles E. Pope II* 667
98 Gastritis, *Charles T. Richardson* 677
99 Peptic Ulcer 681
99.1 Pathogenesis, *Charles T. Richardson* 681
99.2 Epidemiology, Clinical Manifestations, and Diagnosis, *Lawrence R. Schiller* 684
99.3 Medical Therapy, *Walter L. Peterson* 688
99.4 Surgical Therapy, *Richard C. Thirlby* 691
99.5 Complications, *Mark Feldman* 693
99.6 Zollinger-Ellison Syndrome, *Charles T. Richardson* 696
100 Neoplasms of the Stomach, *Paul Sherlock* 697
101 Disorders of Gastrointestinal Motility, *Sidney Phillips* 702
102 Diarrhea, *John S. Fordtran* 712
103 Malabsorption 719
103.1 Pathophysiology and Diagnosis, *Robert M. Glickman* 719
103.2 Management, *Marvin H. Sleisenger* 729
104 Inflammatory Bowel Disease 740
104.1 Introduction, *Irwin H. Rosenberg* 740
104.2 Crohn's Disease, *Irwin H. Rosenberg* 740
104.3 Ulcerative Colitis, *Bernard Levin* 748
105 Vascular Diseases of the Intestine, *James H. Grendell* 756
106 Neoplasms of the Large and Small Intestine, *Sidney J. Winawer* 761
107 Pancreatitis, *Michael D. Levitt* 771
108 Carcinoma of the Pancreas, *John P. Cello* 777
109 Food Poisoning, *David F. Altman* 780
110 Diseases of the Rectum and Anus, *David F. Altman* 783
111 Diseases of the Peritoneum, *Michael D. Bender* 786
112 Diseases of the Mesentery and Omentum, *Michael D. Bender* 790
113 Gastrointestinal Hemorrhage, *Walter L. Peterson* 791
114 Miscellaneous Inflammatory Diseases of the Intestine, *Marvin H. Sleisenger* 796

PART XII DISEASES OF THE LIVER, GALLBLADDER, AND BILE DUCTS

115 Clinical Approach to Liver Disease, *Robert K. Ockner* 803
116 Hepatic Metabolism in Liver Disease, *Robert K. Ockner* 804
117 Bilirubin Metabolism and Hyperbilirubinemia, *Bruce F. Scharschmidt* 806
118 Laboratory Tests in Liver Disease, *Robert K. Ockner* 809
119 Approaches to the Diagnosis of Jaundice, *Robert K. Ockner* 812
120 Acute Viral Hepatitis, *Robert K. Ockner* 813
121 Toxic and Drug-Induced Liver Disease, *Robert K. Ockner* 820
122 Chronic Hepatitis, *Robert K. Ockner* 824
123 Parasitic, Bacterial, Fungal, and Granulomatous Liver Disease, *Bruce F. Scharschmidt* 827
124 Inherited, Infiltrative, and Metabolic Disorders Involving the Liver, *Bruce F. Scharschmidt* 832
125 Cirrhosis of the Liver, *Thomas D. Boyer* 835
126 Major Sequelae of Cirrhosis, *Thomas D. Boyer* 840
127 Acute and Chronic Hepatic Failure with Encephalopathy, *Bruce F. Scharschmidt* 845
128 Hepatic Tumors, *Bruce F. Scharschmidt* 848
129 Diseases of the Gallbladder and Bile Ducts 851
129.1 Normal Physiology of Bile Formation, *Peter F. Malet* 851
129.2 Pathophysiology of Gallstone Disease, *Peter F. Malet* 852
129.3 Roentgenologic and Other Imaging Tests, *Peter F. Malet* 853
129.4 Clinical Categories of Gallbladder and Biliary Tract Disease 855
Asymptomatic Gallstones, *Roger D. Soloway* 855
Chronic Cholecystitis, *Peter F. Malet* 855
Acute Cholecystitis, *Roger D. Soloway* 857
Gallstone Ileus, *Roger D. Soloway* 859
Choledocholithiasis and Cholangitis, *Roger D. Soloway* 859
Biliary Stricture, *Peter F. Malet* 861
Other Causes of Bile Duct Obstruction, *Peter F. Malet* 862
Carcinoma of the Gallbladder, *Roger D. Soloway* 863
Benign Tumors and Pseudotumors of the Gallbladder, *Peter F. Malet* 863
Tumors of the Bile Duct, *Roger D. Soloway* 863
Postcholecystectomy Syndrome, *Roger D. Soloway* 864

PART XIII HEMATOLOGIC DISEASES

130 Introduction, *David G. Nathan* 866
131 Introduction to the Anemias, *Alan S. Keitt* 870
132 Anemia Due to Failure of Progenitor Cells, *Alan S. Keitt* 876
133 Normochromic Normocytic Anemias, *James P. Kushner* 882
134 Hypochromic Anemias, *James P. Kushner* 885
135 Megaloblastic Anemias, *William S. Beck* 893
136 Hemolytic Disorders: Introduction, *Manuel E. Kaplan* 900
137 Hemolysis Due to Intracorpuscular Abnormalities, *Harry S. Jacob* 902
138 Acquired Hemolytic Disorders, *Manuel E. Kaplan* 907
139 Hemoglobin Structure and Function, *Alan N. Schechter* 915
140 Hemoglobin Synthesis, *Arthur W. Nienhuis* 918
141 The Thalassemias, *Arthur W. Nienhuis* 920
142 Sickle Cell Anemia and Associated Hemoglobinopathies, *Bernard G. Forget* 927
143 Unstable Hemoglobins, *Ronald F. Rieder* 932
144 Abnormal Hemoglobins with Altered Oxygen Affinity, *Ronald F. Rieder* 933

145 Methemoglobinemia and Sulfhemoglobinemia, *Ronald F. Rieder* 934
146 Blood Transfusion, *Herbert A. Perkins* 936
147 Development and Morphology of Granulocytes and Macrophages, *David W. Golde* 940
148 Function of Neutrophils and Mononuclear Phagocytes, *Bernard M. Babior* 942
149 Disorders of Neutrophil Function, *Bernard M. Babior* 949
150 The Leukopenic State, *Dane R. Boggs* 953
151 Leukemoid Reactions, *Dane R. Boggs* 958
152 Clonal Development and Stem Cell Origin of Proliferative Disorders, *Philip J. Fialkow* 961
153 Erythrocytosis and Polycythemia, *Paul D. Berk* 963
154 Myeloproliferative Disorders, *Paul D. Berk* 972
155 The Chronic Leukemias, *Bayard Clarkson* 975
156 The Acute Leukemias, *Howard J. Weinstein* 986
157 Introduction to Neoplasms of the Immune System, *Carol S. Portlock* 992
158 Non-Hodgkin's Lymphomas, *Thomas E. Davis* 994
159 Burkitt's Lymphoma, *Carol S. Portlock* 999
160 Hodgkin's Disease, *John H. Glick* 1000
161 Langerhans Cell (Eosinophilic) Granulomatosis, *Jerome E. Groopman* 1009
162 Eosinophilic Syndromes, *David A. Bass* 1011
163 Plasma Cell Disorders, *Sydney E. Salmon* 1013
164 Diseases of the Spleen, *Richard A. Rifkind* 1023
165 Bone Marrow Transplantation, *Rainer Storb* 1025
166 Hemorrhagic Disorders: Abnormalities of Platelet and Vascular Function, *Aaron J. Marcus* 1028
167 Disorders of Blood Coagulation, *Patrick A. McKee* 1040

PART XIV ONCOLOGY

168 Introduction, *John Laszlo* 1059
169 Oncogenes, *J. Michael Bishop* 1066
170 Epidemiology of Cancer, *Joseph F. Fraumeni, Jr.* 1069
171 Biologic Effects of Tumors, *Philip S. Schein* 1073
172 Tumor Markers, *Philip S. Schein* 1075
173 Endocrine Manifestations of Tumors: "Ectopic" Hormone Production, *William D. Odell* 1077
174 Nonmetastatic Effects of Cancer on the Nervous System, *Jerome B. Posner* 1081
175 Cutaneous Manifestations of Internal Malignancy, *Marie-Louise Johnson* 1084
176 Principles of Cancer Therapy, *Bruce A. Chabner* 1086

PART XV METABOLIC DISEASES

177 Introduction, *James B. Wyngaarden* 1103

Disorders of Carbohydrate Metabolism

178 Galactosemia, *Ernest Beutler* 1104
179 The Glycogen Storage Diseases, *R. Rodney Howell* 1105
180 Pentosuria (Essential Pentosuria), *R. Rodney Howell* 1107
181 Essential Fructosuria and Hereditary Fructose Intolerance, *R. Rodney Howell* 1108
182 Primary Hyperoxaluria, *Lloyd H. Smith, Jr.* 1108

Disorders of Lipoprotein Metabolism

183 The Hyperlipoproteinemias, *John D. Brunzell* 1109
184 Fabry's Disease (Glycosphingolipidosis), *James B. Wyngaarden* 1116
185 Gaucher's Disease (Glucosyl Ceramide Lipidosis), *Edwin H. Kolodny* 1117
186 Niemann-Pick Disease (Sphingomyelin Lipidosis), *Edwin H. Kolodny* 1119

Inborn Errors of Amino Acid Metabolism

187 Hyperaminoaciduria (With a Classification of the Inborn and Developmental Errors of Amino Acid Metabolism), *Charles R. Scriver* 1120
188 The Hyperphenylalaninemias, *Lloyd H. Smith, Jr.* 1126
189 Alcaptonuria, *James B. Wyngaarden* 1128
190 Histidinemia, *Lloyd H. Smith, Jr.* 1129
191 The Hyperprolinemias and Hydroxyprolinemia, *Lloyd H. Smith, Jr.* 1129
192 Diseases of the Urea Cycle, *Lloyd H. Smith, Jr.* 1129
193 Branched-Chain Aminoaciduria, *Lloyd H. Smith, Jr.* 1130
194 Homocystinuria, *S. Harvey Mudd* 1131

Disorders of Purine and Pyrimidine Metabolism

195 Gout, *James B. Wyngaarden* 1132
196 Other Disorders of Purine Metabolism, *Edward W. Holmes* 1142
197 Disorders of Pyrimidine Metabolism, *Lloyd H. Smith, Jr.* 1145

Inherited Disorders of Connective Tissue

198 The Mucopolysaccharidoses, *William S. Sly* 1146
199 Marfan's Syndrome, *Sheldon R. Pinnell* 1149
200 Ehlers-Danlos Syndrome, *Sheldon R. Pinnell* 1150
201 Osteogenesis Imperfecta, *David W. Rowe* 1151
202 Pseudoxanthoma Elasticum, *Jouni Uitto* 1152

Disorders of Porphyrins or Metals

203 Porphyria, *D. Montgomery Bissell* 1153
204 Acatalasia, *James B. Wyngaarden* 1158
205 Wilson's Disease (Hepatolenticular Degeneration), *Ara Tourian* 1158
206 Hemochromatosis (Iron Storage Disease), *Arno G. Motulsky* 1160
207 Phosphorus Deficiency and Hypophosphatemia, *Lloyd H. Smith, Jr.* 1163
208 Disorders of Magnesium Metabolism, *Lloyd H. Smith, Jr.* 1165

Other Hereditary Disorders

209 Familial Mediterranean Fever, *Anthony S. Fauci* 1167
210 The Amyloid Diseases, *Joel N. Buxbaum* 1168
211 Hereditary Syndromes Involving Multiple Organ Systems, *Arno G. Motulsky* 1172

PART XVI NUTRITIONAL DISEASES

212 Nutrient Requirements, *Robert M. Russell* 1174
213 Nutritional Assessment, *Robert M. Russell* 1179
214 Protein-Calorie Undernutrition, *Errol B. Marliss* 1183
215 Anorexia Nervosa, *Gerald F. M. Russell* 1188
216 Obesity, *Edwin L. Bierman* 1191
217 Disorders of Vitamin Metabolism: Deficiencies, Metabolic Abnormalities, and Excesses, *Richard S. Rivlin* 1197
218 Disturbances of Trace Mineral Metabolism, *Clifford Tasman-Jones* 1209
219 Enteral Nutritional Therapy, *David H. Alpers* 1211
220 Parenteral Nutrition, *Ray E. Clouse* 1215

PART XVII ENDOCRINE AND REPRODUCTIVE DISEASES

221 Principles of Endocrinology, *John D. Baxter* 1219
222 Endorphins, Enkephalins, and Other Opioid Peptides: Their Significance in Physiology and Medicine, *Roger Guillemin* 1234
223 Prostaglandins, Thromboxane A_2, and Leukotrienes, *John A. Oates* 1237
224 Neuroendocrine Regulation and Its Disorders, *Lawrence A. Frohman* 1241
225 The Anterior Pituitary, *Lawrence A. Frohman* 1251
226 The Posterior Pituitary, *Thomas E. Andreoli* 1266
227 The Pineal, *Seymour Reichlin* 1273
228 The Thyroid, *P. Reed Larsen* 1275
229 Disorders of the Adrenal Cortex, *J. Blake Tyrrell* and *John D. Baxter* 1300
  Structure and Development of the Adrenal Cortex, *John D. Baxter* 1300
  Synthesis, Circulation, and Metabolism of Adrenal Steroids, *John D. Baxter* 1300
  Regulation of Adrenal Steroid Production, *John D. Baxter* 1303
  Actions of Adrenal Steroids, *John D. Baxter* 1305

Laboratory Evaluation of Adrenocortical Function, *J. Blake Tyrrell* 1307
Adrenocortical Hypofunction, *John D. Baxter* 1310
Cushing's Syndrome, *J. Blake Tyrrell* 1313
Mineralocorticoid Excess States, *John D. Baxter* 1317
230 Diabetes Mellitus, *Jerrold M. Olefsky* 1320
231 Hypoglycemic Disorders, *F. John Service* 1341
232 Pancreatic Islet Cell Tumors, *Carl Grunfeld* 1348
233 Disorders of Sexual Differentiation, *Julianne Imperato-McGinley* 1351
234 The Testis, *Mortimer B. Lipsett* 1365
235 Diseases of the Prostate, *Patrick C. Walsh* 1375
236 The Ovaries, *Griff T. Ross* 1379
237 Hirsutism, *D. Lynn Loriaux* 1395
238 Nonmalignant Diseases of the Breast, *George Tolis* 1398
239 Carcinoma of the Breast, *George P. Canellos* 1402
240 Polyglandular Disorders, *John N. Loeb* 1405
241 The Adrenal Medulla and the Sympathetic Nervous System, *Philip E. Cryer* 1408
242 The Carcinoid Syndrome, *Philip E. Cryer* 1413

PART XVIII DISEASES OF BONE AND BONE MINERAL METABOLISM

243 Mineral and Bone Homeostasis, *Claude D. Arnaud* 1415
244 Vitamin D, *Daniel D. Bikle* 1423
245 Osteomalacia and Rickets, *Daniel D. Bikle* 1425
246 The Parathyroid Glands, Hypercalcemia, and Hypocalcemia, *Claude D. Arnaud* 1431
247 The Ultimobranchial Cells and Calcitonin, *Claude D. Arnaud* 1451
248 Renal Osteodystrophy, *Eduardo Slatopolsky* 1453
249 Osteoporosis, *B. Lawrence Riggs* 1456
250 Paget's Disease of Bone (Osteitis Deformans), *Frederick R. Singer* 1461
251 Osteonecrosis, Osteosclerosis, and Other Disorders of Bone, *Gordon J. Strewler* 1463
252 Bone Tumors, *Henry J. Mankin* 1466

PART XIX INFECTIOUS DISEASES

Section 1 Introduction

253 Introduction to Microbial Diseases, *Charles C. J. Carpenter* 1469
254 The Febrile Patient, *Sheldon M. Wolff* 1470
255 Pathogenesis of Fever, *Charles A. Dinarello* 1471
256 Shock Syndromes Related to Sepsis, *John N. Sheagren* 1473
257 The Compromised Host, *John I. Gallin* 1477
258 Prevention and Treatment of Hospital-Acquired Infections, *Richard P. Wenzel* 1485
259 Advice to Travelers, *Jeffrey A. Gelfand* 1492

Section 2 Bacterial Diseases

Pneumonia

260 Introduction to Pneumonia, *Herbert Y. Reynolds* 1494
261 Pneumococcal Pneumonia, *David T. Durack* 1498
262 Mycoplasmal Infections, *Stephen G. Baum* 1505
263 Pneumonia Due to Klebsiella (Friedländer's Pneumonia), *Herbert Y. Reynolds* 1509
264 Pneumonia Caused by Other Aerobic Gram-Negative Bacilli (Pseudomonas, Escherichia coli, and Serratia), *Herbert Y. Reynolds* 1510
265 Aspiration Pneumonia, *Herbert Y. Reynolds* 1513
266 Legionellosis, *David W. Fraser* 1516

Streptococcal Diseases

267 Streptococcal Diseases, *Richard M. Krause* 1519
268 Rheumatic Fever, *Alan L. Bisno* 1527

Endocarditis

269 Infective Endocarditis, *David T. Durack* 1533

Staphylococcal Infections

270 Staphylococcal Infections, *John N. Sheagren* 1543

Bacterial Meningitis, Morton N. Swartz

271 Bacterial Meningitis 1551
272 Meningococcal Disease 1557
273 Infections Caused by Hemophilus Species 1563

Osteomyelitis

274 Osteomyelitis, *Francis A. Waldvogel* 1566

Whooping Cough

275 Whooping Cough (Pertussis), *Samuel L. Katz* 1568

Diphtheria

276 Diphtheria, *Richard V. McCloskey* 1571

Clostridial Diseases

277 Clostridial Myonecrosis and Other Clostridial Diseases, *John G. Bartlett* 1573
278 Pseudomembranous Colitis, *John G. Bartlett* 1576
279 Botulism, *John G. Bartlett* 1577
280 Tetanus, *John H. Kerr* 1579

Anaerobic Bacteria

281 Diseases Caused by Non–Spore-Forming Anaerobic Bacteria, *Sherwood L. Gorbach* 1583

Typhoid Fever and Salmonellosis

282 Typhoid Fever, *Sherwood L. Gorbach* 1587
283 Salmonella Infections Other Than Typhoid Fever, *Richard B. Hornick* 1589

Other Bacterial Infections

284 Extraintestinal Infections Caused by Enteric Bacteria, *Charles C. J. Carpenter* 1592
285 Shigellosis, *Charles C. J. Carpenter* 1596
286 Cholera (Asiatic Cholera), *Nathaniel F. Pierce* 1598
287 Yersinia Infections, *Thomas Butler* 1600
288 Tularemia, *Richard B. Hornick* 1603
289 Anthrax, *Philip S. Brachman* 1606
290 Diseases Caused by Pseudomonads, *Michael Barza* 1608
291 Listeriosis, *Michael Barza* 1609
292 Erysipeloid, *Michael Barza* 1611
293 Actinomycosis, *David J. Drutz* 1612
294 Nocardiosis, *David J. Drutz* 1613
295 Brucellosis, *John E. Bennett* 1614
296 Bartonellosis, *Theodore C. Eickhoff* 1617

Presumptive Bacterial Disease

297 Cat Scratch Disease, *Andrew M. Margileth* 1618

Diseases Due to Mycobacteria

298 Tuberculosis, *Emanuel Wolinsky* 1620
299 Other Mycobacterioses, *Emanuel Wolinsky* 1631
300 Leprosy (Hansen's Disease), *Ward E. Bullock* 1634

Sexually Transmitted Diseases, P. Frederick Sparling

301 Introduction and Common Syndromes 1639
302 Gonococcal Infections 1644
303 Lymphogranuloma Venereum 1648
304 Granuloma Inguinale (Donovanosis) 1649
305 Chancroid 1650
306 Syphilis 1650

Spirochetal Diseases Other Than Syphilis

307 Nonsyphilitic Treponematoses, *Thomas Butler* 1661
308 Relapsing Fever, *Thomas Butler* 1662
309 Tropical Phagedenic Ulcer, *Anthony D. M. Bryceson* 1664
310 Rat Bite Fevers, *J. Bruce McClain* 1665
311 Leptospirosis, *J. Bruce McClain* 1666

Diseases Caused by Chlamydiae

312 Introduction, *Walter E. Stamm* 1668
313 Trachoma, *Walter E. Stamm* 1669
314 Neonatal Chlamydial Infections, *Walter E. Stamm* 1670
315 Psittacosis (Ornithosis, Parrot Fever), *William Schaffner* 1671

Rickettsial Diseases

316 Introduction, *Charles L. Wisseman, Jr.* 1672
317 The Typhus Group, *Charles L. Wisseman, Jr.* 1678
318 Rocky Mountain Spotted Fever, *Charles L. Wisseman, Jr.* 1680
319 Tick-Borne Rickettsioses of the Eastern Hemisphere, *Charles L. Wisseman, Jr.* 1682
320 Rickettsialpox, *Charles L. Wisseman, Jr.* 1683
321 Scrub Typhus, *Charles L. Wisseman, Jr.* 1684
322 Trench Fever, *Theodore C. Eickhoff* 1685
323 Q Fever, *Theodore C. Eickhoff* 1686

Section 3 Viral Diseases

324 Introduction to Viral Diseases, *Edwin D. Kilbourne* 1687

Viral Infections of the Respiratory Tract

325/326 The Common Cold, *Albert Z. Kapikian* 1691
327 Viral Pharyngitis, Laryngitis, Croup, and Bronchitis, *Maurice A. Mufson* 1695
328 Respiratory Syncytial Virus, *Robert M. Chanock* 1696
329 Parainfluenza Viral Diseases, *Robert M. Chanock* 1698
330 Influenza, *R. Gordon Douglas, Jr.* 1700
331 Adenovirus Diseases, *Stephen G. Baum* 1705

RNA Viral Infections Characterized by Cutaneous Lesions

332 Measles (Morbilli, Rubeola), *Samuel L. Katz* 1706
333 Rubella (German Measles), *Samuel L. Katz* 1709
334 Foot and Mouth Disease (Aphthous Fever, Epizootic Stomatitis), *Catherine M. Wilfert* 1711
335 Mumps (Epidemic Parotitis), *Catherine M. Wilfert* 1712

Diseases Caused by Herpes-Type Viruses

336 Herpes Simplex Virus Infections, *R. Gordon Douglas, Jr.* 1714
337 Cytomegalovirus Infection, *David J. Lang* 1717
338 Infectious Mononucleosis, *John A. Zaia* 1719
339 Varicella and Herpes Zoster, *Sidney Kibrick* 1721
340 Variola and Vaccinia, *Donald A. Henderson* 1724

Enteroviral Diseases, Raphael Dolin

341 Introduction 1728
342 Paralysis and Other Neurologic Complications of Nonpolio Enteroviruses 1730
343 Epidemic Pleurodynia (Bornholm Disease, Epidemic Myalgia, Devil's Grip, Sylvest's Disease) 1730
344 Myocarditis and Pericarditis Caused by Enteroviruses 1731
345 Mucocutaneous Infections Caused by Enteroviruses 1732
346 Acute Hemorrhagic Conjunctivitis 1733
347 Respiratory Tract Illness Associated with Enteroviruses 1734

Viral Disease of the Gastrointestinal Tract

348 Viral Gastroenteritis (Acute Infectious Nonbacterial Gastroenteritis, Epidemic Diarrhea, Winter Vomiting Disease), *Raphael Dolin* 1734

Arthropod-Borne Viral Fevers

349 Introduction, *Karl M. Johnson* 1736

Undifferentiated Fevers

350 Dengue, *Robert B. Tesh* 1737
351 West Nile Fever, *Robert B. Tesh* 1738
352 Phlebotomus Fever, *Robert B. Tesh* 1738
353 Rift Valley Fever, *Robert B. Tesh* 1739
354 Fevers Caused by Alphaviruses: Chikungunya, O'Nyong-Nyong, Mayaro, Ross River, and Ockelbo, *Robert B. Tesh* 1740
355 Colorado Tick Fever, *Theodore C. Eickhoff* 1740
356 Arthropod-Borne Viral Encephalitides, *Thomas P. Monath* 1742

Viral Hemorrhagic Fevers

357 Introduction, *Karl M. Johnson* 1750
358 Yellow Fever, *Thomas P. Monath* 1750
359 Hemorrhagic Fever Caused by Dengue Viruses (DHF), *Karl M. Johnson* 1754
360 Tick-Borne Flavivirus Diseases: Kyasanur Forest Disease and Omsk Hemorrhagic Fever, *Karl M. Johnson* 1755
361 Crimean Hemorrhagic Fever, *Karl M. Johnson* 1755
362 Hemorrhagic Diseases Caused by Arenaviruses: Argentine and Bolivian Hemorrhagic Fevers and Lassa Fever, *Karl M. Johnson* 1756
363 African Hemorrhagic Fever (Marburg-Ebola Disease), *Karl M. Johnson* 1757
364 Hemorrhagic Fever with Renal Syndrome (HFRS), *Karl M. Johnson* 1757

Section 4 The Mycoses, *David J. Drutz*

365 Introduction 1758
366 Histoplasmosis 1759
367 Coccidioidomycosis 1761
368 Blastomycosis (North American Blastomycosis, Gilchrist's Disease) 1762
369 Paracoccidioidomycosis 1764
370 Cryptococcosis 1765
371 Sporotrichosis 1767
372 Candidiasis (Candidosis) 1768
373 Aspergillosis 1770
374 Mucormycosis (Phycomycosis, Zygomycosis) 1771
375 Mycetoma (Maduromycosis) 1773
376 Chromomycosis 1773

PART XX DISEASES CAUSED BY PROTOZOA AND METAZOA

377 Introduction to Protozoan and Helminthic Diseases, *Adel A. F. Mahmoud* 1775

Section 1 Protozoan Diseases

378 Malaria, *Louis H. Miller* 1776
379 African Trypanosomiasis (Sleeping Sickness), *B. M. Greenwood* 1780
380 Chagas' Disease (American Trypanosomiasis), *Vanize Macedo* 1783
381 Leishmaniasis, *Franklin A. Neva* 1786
382 Toxoplasmosis, *Henry Masur* 1792
383 Pneumocystosis, *Henry Masur* 1796
384 Babesiosis (Piroplasmosis), *Morton N. Swartz* 1798
385 Amebiasis and Amebic Meningoencephalitis, *Donald J. Krogstad* 1799
386 Other Protozoan Diseases, *David P. Stevens* 1802

Section 2 Helminthic Diseases

387 Introduction, *Adel A. F. Mahmoud* 1804

The Cestodes, Martin S. Wolfe

388 Introduction 1804
389 Diphyllobothrium Latum (The Fish Tapeworm) 1805
390 Taenia Saginata (The Beef Tapeworm) 1806
391 Taenia Solium (The Pork Tapeworm; Human Cysticercosis) 1806
392 Hymenolepis Nana (The Dwarf Tapeworm) 1807
393 Echinococcosis (Hydatid Disease) 1807
394 Other, Rarer Tapeworms 1808
395 Treatment of Tapeworm Infections 1809

The Trematodes

396 Schistosomiasis (Bilharziasis), *Adel A. F. Mahmoud* 1809
397 Hermaphroditic Flukes, *S. K. K. Seah* 1815

The Nematodes

398 Introduction, *Daniel S. Blumenthal* 1819
399 Strongyloidiasis, *Daniel S. Blumenthal* 1819
400 Capillariasis, *Daniel S. Blumenthal* 1820
401 Hookworm Disease, *Daniel S. Blumenthal* 1820
402 Cutaneous Larva Migrans, *Daniel S. Blumenthal* 1821
403 Trichostrongyliasis, *Daniel S. Blumenthal* 1822
404 Gnathostomiasis, *Daniel S. Blumenthal* 1822
405 Primate Nematodiases, *Daniel S. Blumenthal* 1822
406 Ascariasis, *Daniel S. Blumenthal* 1822
407 Toxocariasis, *Daniel S. Blumenthal* 1823
408 Anisakiasis, *Daniel S. Blumenthal* 1824
409 Trichuriasis, *Daniel S. Blumenthal* 1824
410 Enterobiasis, *Daniel S. Blumenthal* 1824
411 Trichinellosis (Trichinosis), *Donald W. Hoskins* 1825
412 Angiostrongyliasis, *Daniel S. Blumenthal* 1826

Filariasis

413 Introduction, *Eric A. Ottesen* 1827
414 Dracunculiasis, *Donald R. Hopkins* 1828
415 Lymphatic Filariasis (Wuchereria bancrofti, Brugia malayi, and Brugia timori), *Eric A. Ottesen* 1828
416 Tropical Eosinophilia, *Eric A. Ottesen* 1830
417 Loiasis, *Eric A. Ottesen* 1830
418 *Mansonella ozzardi* Infection, *Eric A. Ottesen* 1831
419 Perstans Filariasis, *Eric A. Ottesen* 1831
420 Dirofilariasis, *Eric A. Ottesen* 1831
421 Possible Human Meningonemiasis, *Eric A. Ottesen* 1832
422 Onchocerciasis (River Blindness), *Brian O. L. Duke* 1832
423 Streptocerciasis, *Brian O. L. Duke* 1833

Section 3 Arthropods and Animal Poisons

424 Arthropods and Leeches, *William L. Krinsky* 1833
425 Snake Bites, *Jay P. Sanford* 1841
426 Venomous and Poisonous Marine Animals, *John Williamson* 1843

PART XXI DISEASES OF THE IMMUNE SYSTEM

427 Introduction: The Immune System, *William E. Paul* 1846
428 Complement, *Douglas T. Fearon* 1852
429 Primary Immunodeficiency Diseases, *Rebecca H. Buckley* 1855
430 Acquired Immunodeficiency Syndrome (AIDS), *Anthony S. Fauci* 1861
431 Urticaria and Angioedema, *Nicholas A. Soter* 1863
432 Allergic Rhinitis, *John E. Salvaggio* 1867
433 Anaphylaxis, *Lawrence M. Lichtenstein* 1870
434 Insect Sting Allergy, *Lawrence M. Lichtenstein* 1872
435 Immune Complex Diseases, *Charles G. Cochrane* 1874
436 The Major Histocompatibility Complex and Disease Susceptibility, *Hugh O. McDevitt* 1877
437 Drug Allergy, *Charles E. Reed* 1883
438 Mastocytosis, *Robert A. Lewis* 1887
439 Diseases of the Thymus, *Daniel P. Stites* 1889

PART XXII MUSCULOSKELETAL AND CONNECTIVE TISSUE DISEASES

440 Approach to the Patient with Musculoskeletal Diseases, *James F. Fries* 1891
441 Connective Tissue Structure and Function, *Stephen M. Krane* 1894
442 Mechanisms of Inflammation and Tissue Destruction in the Rheumatic Diseases, *Ralph Snyderman* 1898
443 Specialized Diagnostic Procedures in the Rheumatic Diseases, *Alan S. Cohen* 1906
444 Rheumatoid Arthritis, *J. Claude Bennett* 1911
445 The Spondylarthropathies, *Andrei Calin* 1917
446 Infectious Arthritis, *Stephen E. Malawista* 1922
447 Systemic Lupus Erythematosus, *Alfred D. Steinberg* 1924
448 Systemic Sclerosis (Scleroderma), *Edward D. Harris, Jr.* 1932
449 Sjögren's Syndrome, *Norman Talal* 1936
450 The Vasculitic Syndromes, *Anthony S. Fauci* 1937
451 Polyarteritis Nodosa Group, *K. Frank Austen* 1941
452 Wegener's Granulomatosis and Midline Granuloma, *Anthony S. Fauci* 1943
453 Polymyalgia Rheumatica and Giant Cell Arteritis, *Louis A. Healey* 1946
454 Dermatomyositis and Polymyositis, *Ronald P. Messner* 1947
455 Calcium Crystal Deposition Arthropathies, *H. Ralph Schumacher, Jr* 1950
456 Relapsing Polychondritis, *H. Ralph Schumacher, Jr* 1951
457 Osteoarthritis (Degenerative Joint Disease), *David S. Howell* 1951
458 The Painful Shoulder, *David S. Howell* 1954
459 The Painful Back, *David S. Howell* 1955
460 Diseases with which Arthritis is Frequently Associated, *Giles G. Bole* 1957
461 Miscellaneous Forms of Arthritis, *Giles G. Bole* 1958
462 Nonarticular Rheumatism, *Giles G. Bole* 1959
463 Synovial Tumors, *Giles G. Bole* 1960
464 Behçet's Disease, *Ralph Snyderman* 1960
465 Panniculitis and Disorders of the Subcutaneous Fat, *Gerald S. Lazarus* 1962
466 Multifocal Fibrosclerosis (Multicentric Fibrosclerosis, Fibrosing Syndromes), *H. Ralph Schumacher, Jr.* 1963

PART XXIII NEUROLOGIC AND BEHAVIORAL DISEASES

Section 1 Clinical Study of the Patient with Neurologic Symptoms

467 Approach to the Patient, Including General Management, *Fred Plum* 1965
468 Principles of Diagnosis, *Fred Plum* 1965
469 The Neurologic History, *Jerome B. Posner* 1966
470 The Neurologic Examination, *Fred Plum* 1967
471 Neurologic Diagnostic Procedures, *Samuel Rapoport* 1968

Section 2 Disorders of Cerebral Function

472 Disturbances of Consciousness and Arousal 1971
- 472.1 Sustained Impairment of Consciousness, *Jerome B. Posner* 1971
- 472.2 Acute Central Nervous System Poisoning, *Fred Plum* 1979
- 472.3 Prognosis in Severe Brain Damage and Diagnosis of Brain Death, *Fred Plum* 1981
- 472.4 Brief Loss of Consciousness, *Fred Plum* 1983
- 472.5 Sleep and Its Disorders, *J. Allan Hobson* 1986

473 Regional Diagnosis of Cerebral Disorders, *Fred Plum* 1991
474 Focal Disturbances of Higher Function, *Fred Plum* 1993
475 Amentia and Dementia, *Fred Plum* 1998
476 Psychologic Illness in Medical Practice, *Paul R. McHugh* 2001
477 Drug Abuse and Dependence, *Robert B. Millman* 2015

Section 3 Pathophysiology and Management of Major Neurologic Symptoms

478 Autonomic Disorders and Their Management, *Fred Plum* 2025
479 The Special Senses and Related Functions 2031
- 479.1 Smell and Taste, *Fred Plum* 2031
- 479.2 Neuro-ophthalmology, *Fred Plum* 2032
- 479.3 Hearing and Equilibrium, *Jerome B. Posner* 2037

480 Disorders of Motor Function 2044
- 480.1 Asthenia, Fatigue, and Weakness, *Fred Plum* 2044
- 480.2 Ataxia and Related Gait Disorders, *Fred Plum* 2044
- 480.3 Episodic Loss of Motor Function, *Jerome B. Posner* 2046

481 Disorders of Sensation, *Jerome B. Posner* 2047

Section 4 Alcohol-Related and Nutritional Disorders of the Nervous System

482 Alcohol-Related and Nutritional Disorders of the Nervous System, *Ivan Diamond* 2064

Section 5 The Extrapyramidal Disorders, *Stanley Fahn*

483 Parkinsonism 2070
484 Essential Tremor (Familial or Senile Tremor) 2073
485 The Choreas 2074
486 Other Extrapyramidal Disorders 2076
487 The Dystonias 2077

Section 6 Inherited, Congenital, and Idiopathic Degenerative Diseases of the Nervous System, *Roger N. Rosenberg*

488 Striatonigral Degeneration 2079
489 Motor Neuron Diseases 2079
490 Spinocerebellar Degenerations 2080
491 Syringomyelia 2084
492 The Phakomatoses or Neurocutaneous Syndromes 2084

Section 7 Cerebrovascular Diseases, *H. J. M. Barnett*

493 Introduction 2086
494 Cerebral Ischemia and Infarction 2090
495 Intracranial Hemorrhage 2103

Section 8 Infectious and Inflammatory Disorders of the Nervous System

496 Parameningeal Infections, *Donald H. Harter* 2111
497 Syphilitic Infections of the Central Nervous System, *Kenneth P. Johnson* 2118

Viral Infections of the Nervous System

498 Introduction, *Richard T. Johnson* 2121
499 Viral Meningitis and Encephalitis, *Richard T. Johnson* 2122
500 Herpes Simplex Encephalitis, *Richard T. Johnson* 2126
501 Herpes Zoster, *Richard T. Johnson* 2128
502 Acute Anterior Poliomyelitis, *Richard T. Johnson* 2130
503 Rabies, *Michael A. W. Hattwick* 2132
504 Slow Viral Infections of the Nervous System, *Richard T. Johnson* 2135

Section 9 Neurologic Disorders Associated with Altered Immunity or Unexplained Host-Parasite Alterations

505 Acute Transverse Myelitis, *H. Richard Tyler* 2138
506 Central Nervous System Complications of Viral Infections and Vaccines, *Jerry S. Wolinsky* 2139
507 Reye's Syndrome, *Jerry S. Wolinsky* 2141
508 Neurologic Complications in the Immunologically Compromised Host, *Jerry S. Wolinsky* 2141

Section 10 The Demyelinating Diseases

509 The Demyelinating Diseases, *Donald H. Silberberg* 2143

Section 11 The Epilepsies

510 The Epilepsies, *Jerome Engel, Jr.* 2149

Section 12 Intracranial Tumors and States of Altered Intracranial Pressure

511 Intracranial Tumors, *William R. Shapiro* 2161
512 Intracranial Hypotension, *David A. Rottenberg* 2166
513 Intracranial Hypertension, *David A. Rottenberg* 2167
514 Pseudotumor Cerebri, *David A. Rottenberg* 2168
515 Hydrocephalus, *David A. Rottenberg* 2169

Section 13 Injury to the Head and Spine, *Donald P. Becker*

516 Head Injuries 2170
517 Injuries to the Spine 2175

Section 14 Mechanical Lesions of Nerve Roots and Spinal Cord, *Jerome B. Posner*

518 Differential Diagnosis of Muscle, Nerve Root, and Spinal Disorders 2178
519 Intervertebral Disc Disease 2182
520 Neoplasms of the Spinal Canal 2184
521 Inflammatory Diseases of the Spinal Canal 2186
522 Vascular Disorders of the Spinal Canal 2187
523 Congenital Anomalies of the Craniovertebral Junction, Spine, and Spinal Cord 2187

Section 15 Diseases of the Peripheral Nervous System

524 Introduction and Basic Terminology, *Herbert H. Schaumburg* 2188
525 Anatomic Classification of Neuropathy, *Herbert H. Schaumburg* 2189
526 Inflammatory Polyneuropathy (Guillain-Barré Syndrome and Related Disorders), *Herbert H. Schaumburg* 2190
527 The Diabetic Neuropathies, *Herbert H. Schaumburg* 2192
528 Neuropathy Associated with Uremia, *Herbert H. Schaumburg* 2193
529 Neuropathy Associated with Endocrine Diseases (Other Than Diabetes), *Herbert H. Schaumburg* 2194
530 Hereditary Neuropathies, *Herbert H. Schaumburg* 2194
531 Toxic Neuropathy: Pharmaceutical Agents, *Herbert H. Schaumburg* 2195
532 Toxic Neuropathy: Occupational, Biological, and Environmental Agents, *Herbert H. Schaumburg* 2195
533 Miscellaneous Disease-Specific Neuropathies, *Herbert H. Schaumburg* 2195
534 Acute Physical Injury and Chronic Compression-Entrapment Neuropathies, *Herbert H. Schaumburg* 2196
535 Bell's Palsy, Brachial Neuritis, and Trigeminal Neuropathy, *Herbert H. Schaumburg* 2197
536 Nerve Biopsy in Peripheral Nerve Disease, *Jerry G. Kaplan* 2198

Section 16 Diseases of Muscle and Neuromuscular Junction, *Lewis P. Rowland*

537 Introduction 2198
538 Inherited Diseases 2201
539 Sporadic Disorders 2209

PART XXIV EYE DISEASES, *John W. Gittinger, Jr.*

540 Introduction 2217
541 Cataract 2217
542 Glaucoma 2217
543 Disc Swelling and Optic Atrophy 2219
544 Ocular Inflammation 2219
545 Ocular Infections 2220
546 Orbital Disease and Tumors 2221
547 Intraocular Tumors 2222
548 Rheumatoid and Connective Tissue Diseases 2222
549 Ocular Vascular Disease 2223
550 The Eye and Medications 2225

PART XXV SKIN DISEASES, *Marie-Louise Johnson*

551 Introduction 2227
552 Pathophysiology 2227
553 The Examination of the Skin 2232
554 Principles of Therapy 2239
555 The Differential Diagnosis 2241
556 Significant Dermatologic Signs of Disease 2250
557 Selected Significant Dermatologic Diagnoses 2267

PART XXVI OCCUPATIONAL AND ENVIRONMENTAL MEDICINE

558 Principles of Occupational Medicine, *Charles E. Becker* 2277
559 Occupational Lung Disease, *Robert J. Mason* 2279

560 Physical, Chemical, and Aspiration Injuries of the Lung, *James D. Crapo* 2287
561 Occupational Diseases of the Skin, *Edward A. Emmett* 2295
562 Radiation Injury, *Theodore L. Phillips* 2297
563 Electric Injury, *Basil A. Pruitt, Jr.* 2303
564 Disorders Due to Heat and Cold, *James P. Knochel* 2304
565 Trace Metal Poisoning, *Donald B. Louria* 2307

PART XXVII LABORATORY REFERENCE RANGE VALUES OF CLINICAL IMPORTANCE

566 Reference Ranges and Laboratory Values of Clinical Importance, *Norbert W. Tietz* 2316
Index i

COLOR PLATES

PLATE 1 DIABETES MELLITUS (Part XVII, pages 1320–1341)

PLATE 2 HEMATOLOGIC DISEASES (Part XIII, pages 866–1058)

PLATE 3 HEMATOLOGIC DISEASES (Part XIII, pages 866–1058)

PLATE 4 MEASLES (Part XIX, pages 1706–1711)

PLATE 5 PROTOZOAN DISEASES (Part XX, pages 1776–1803)

PLATE 6 SKIN DISEASES (Part XXV, pages 2227–2276)

PLATE 7 SKIN DISEASES (Part XXV, pages 2227–2276)

PLATE 8 MENINGOCOCCAL DISEASE (Part XIX, pages 1557–1563)

PLATE 9 RHEUMATIC FEVER (Part XIX, pages 1527–1532)

PLATE 1 DIABETES MELLITUS

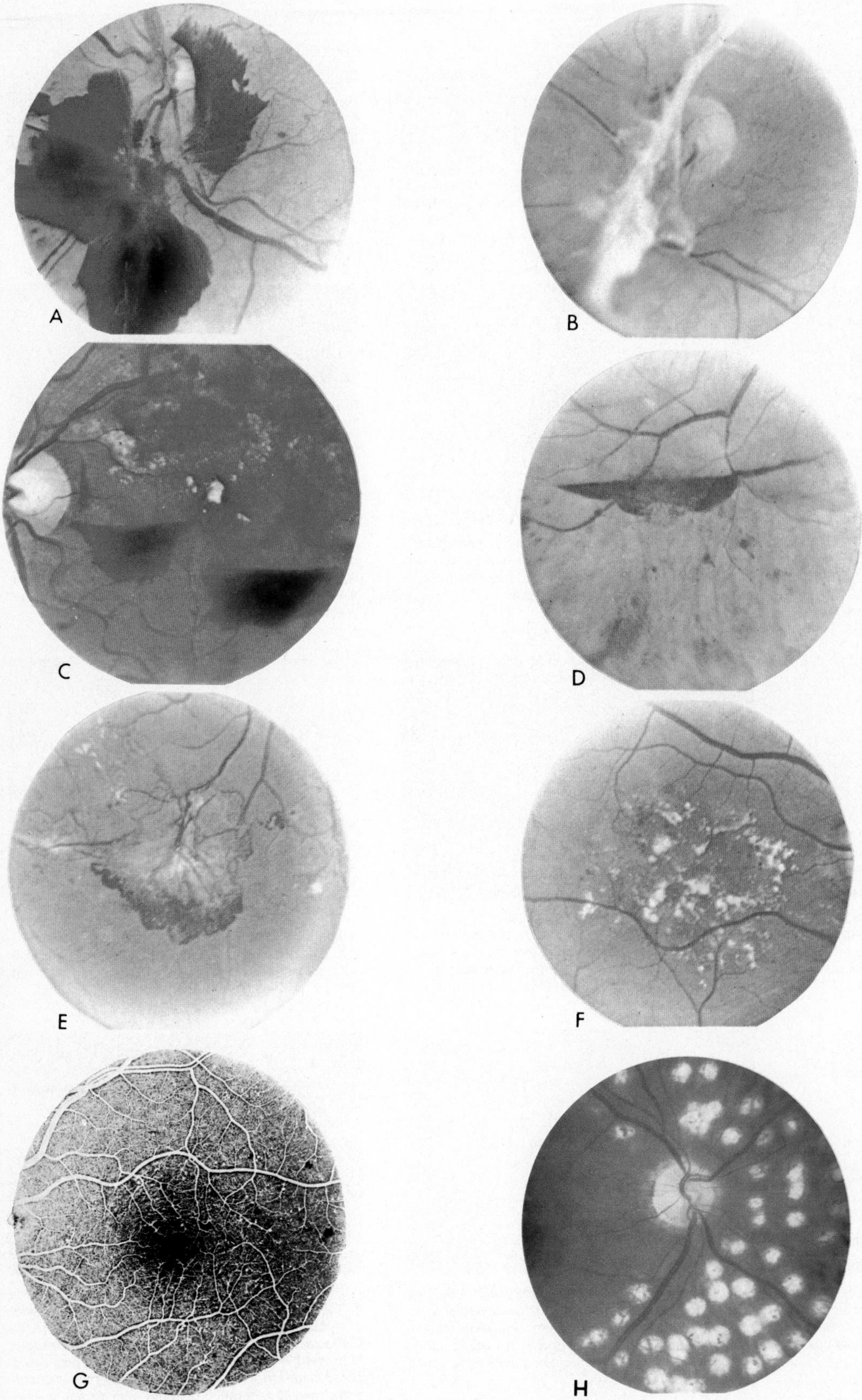

A, Vitreous and preretinal hemorrhage from the disc area secondary to disc neovascularization.

B, Fibrous band resulting from going into a quiescent stage of retinopathy one year after slide *A* was taken. Patient maintained quiescent stage for eight years until he died a cardiac death.

C, Preretinal hemorrhages in region of macula which also has exudates and superficial hemorrhages. Note boat-shaped dependency type of hemorrhage.

D, Preretinal hemorrhage at site of frond of neovascularization. Note the new vessel fan underneath the boat-shaped preretinal hemorrhage. It is these new vessels which rupture spontaneously or with minimal stress.

E, Extensive fan of new vessels with fibrous network elevated forward into vitreous. Feeding vessels come from multiple arteries and veins at the retinal level, the entire process being analogous to an angioma.

F, Characteristic waxy exudates in macular zone accounting for decrease in vision, apparently due to incompetent capillaries and leaking from central areas of rings of waxy exudates where the red blotches are noted.

G, Fluorescein angiography in a diabetic, showing some very fine microaneurysms and some tiny areas of capillary closure but with good parafoveal network of vessels and 20/20 vision. These are early changes of diabetic retinopathy probably not seen on ophthalmoscopy. (Courtesy of Dr. L. Aiello.)

H, Photograph of retina following laser therapy, showing circumscribed areas of destruction and fibrous replacement. (Courtesy of Dr. M. B. Landers, III.)

PLATE 2 HEMATOLOGIC DISEASES

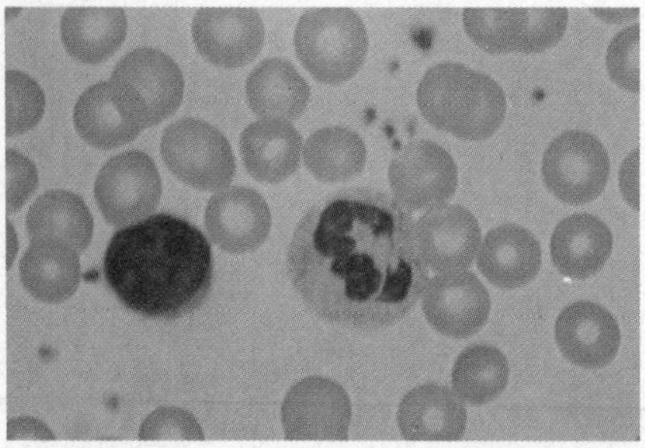

A, Normal peripheral blood smear showing an adult lymphocyte at the left, a mature segmented poly in the center, scattered platelets in the background, and normal appearing red blood cells. Note the normal central one-third pallor of the red cells (× 1200).

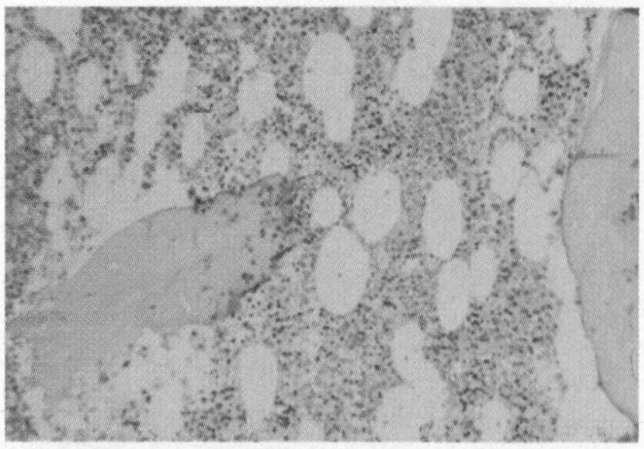

B, Normal bone marrow biopsy, low power. Note the normal fat content, about 50 per cent of the marrow. Normal hematopoietic cells are seen, including scattered megakaryocytes (× 100).

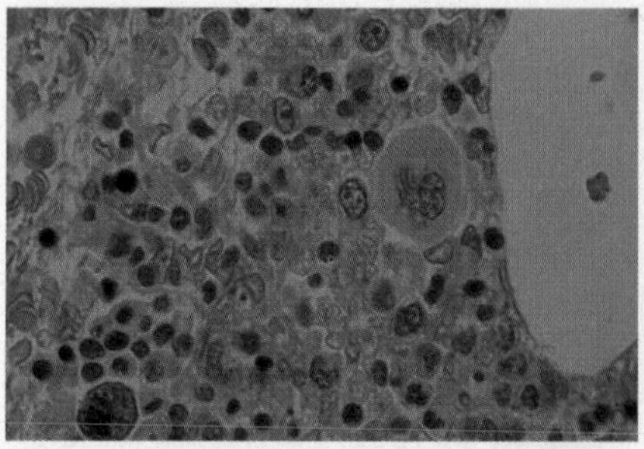

C, Normal bone marrow biopsy, high power. Note the detail of the background megakaryocytes, as well as scattered myeloid and erythroid cells in a ratio of approximately 3:1 (× 1000).

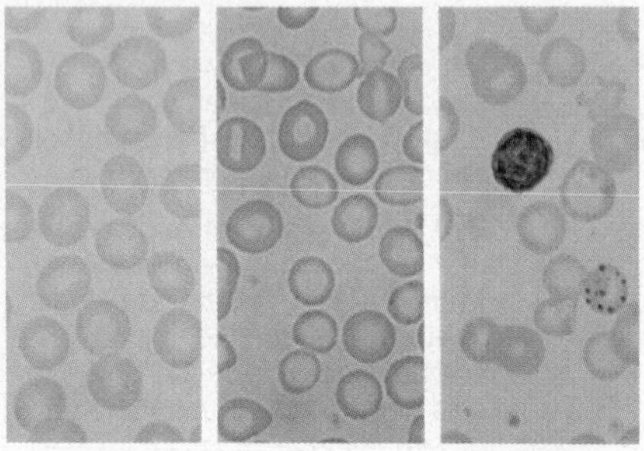

D, Peripheral blood smear showing normal red blood cells (left panel) compared with hypochromic cells of iron deficiency (central panel) or chronic lead poisoning (right panel). In the right panel note the prominent basophilic stippling. The cells are hypochromic as well as macrocytic (× 1200).

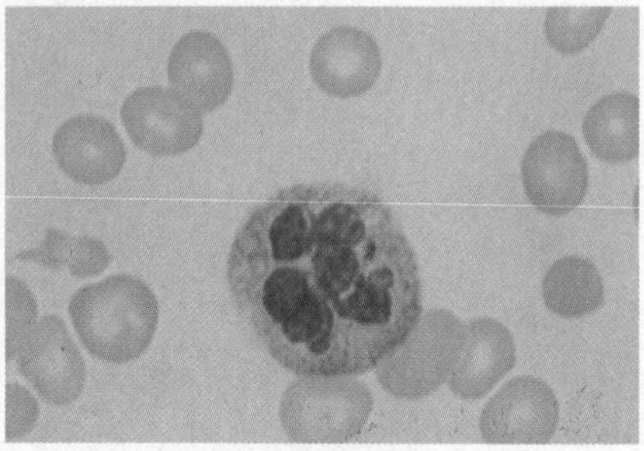

E, Peripheral blood smear showing a gigantic poly (macrocytic hypersegmented poly) in a patient with pernicious anemia. A few macrocytic red cells are noted, along with mild poikilocytes (× 1200).

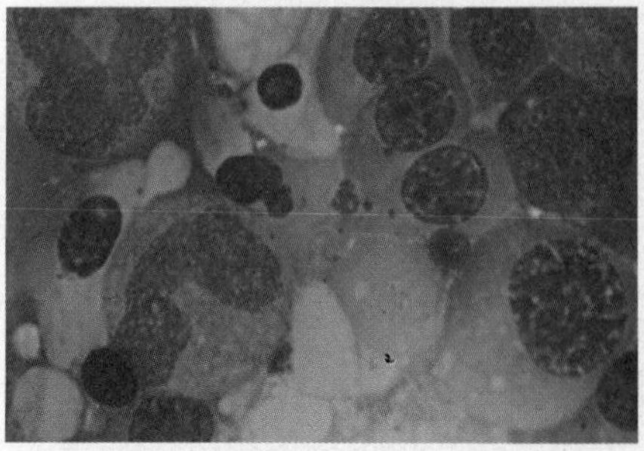

F, Marrow showing megaloblastic findings. Note the megaloblastic erythroid cells, characterized by maturation arrest. Nuclei have open chromatin while the cytoplasm shows early normal hemoglobinization. Several giant metamyelocytes are noted as well.

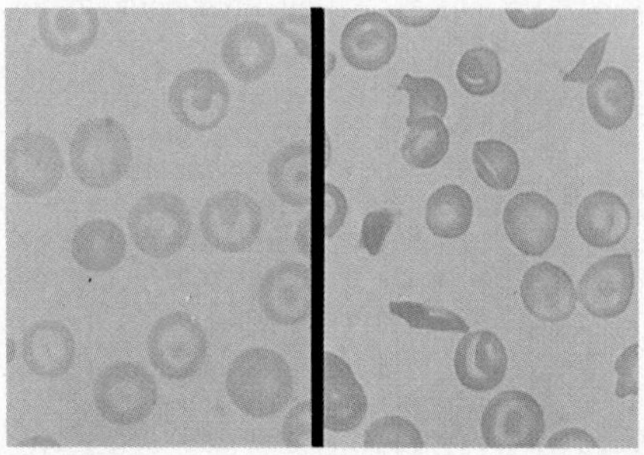

G, Thalassemia major showing marked anisocytosis, poikilocytosis, hypochromia, and target cell formation in the peripheral blood (left panel) and striking erythroid hyperplasia in the right panel, from the bone marrow (× 1200).

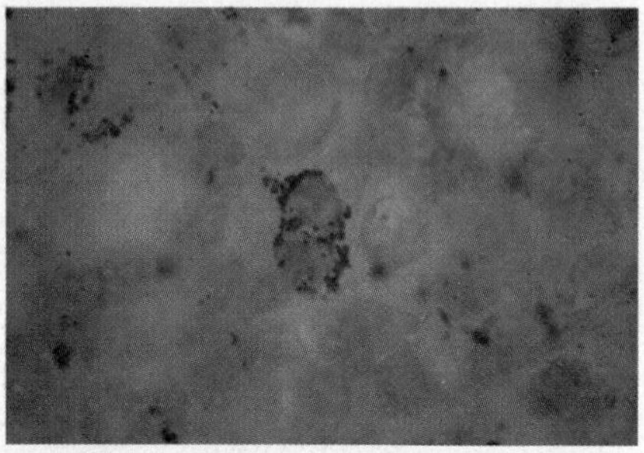

H, Bone marrow smear showing classic ringed sideroblasts. The normoblasts show clumps of iron (hemosiderin) surrounding the nucleus, resulting in a "ring." Physiologically, no more than two or three dots of iron are normally present. Prussian blue stain (× 1200).

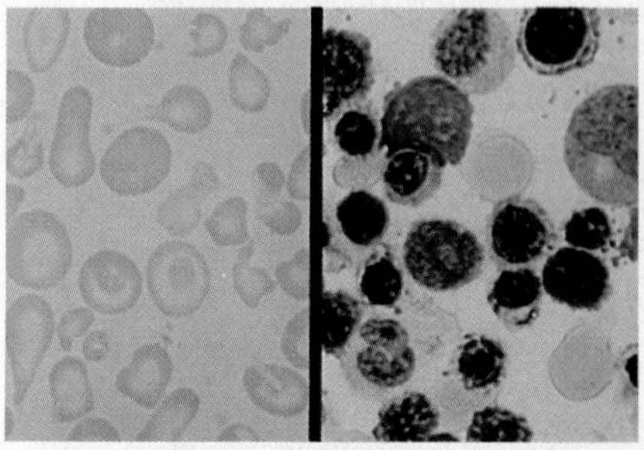

I, Peripheral blood smears from hemoglobin C, A trait (left panel) showing target cells and a few spherocytes, and hemoglobin S-C disease (right panel) showing sickled cells as well as target cells and other deformed red cells (× 1200).

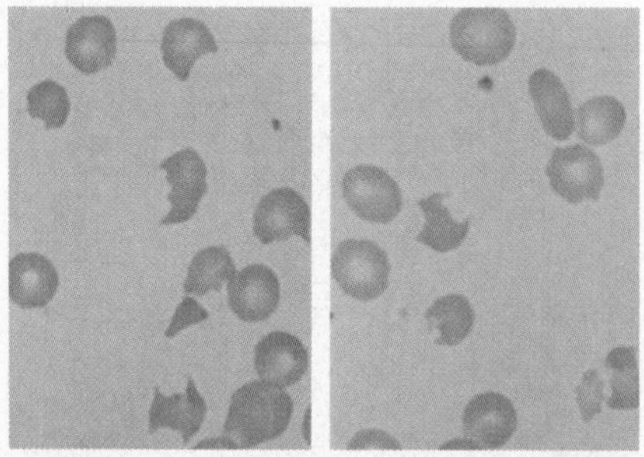

J, Peripheral blood smear from a patient with the hemolytic-uremic syndrome, showing striking schistocytes, also called helmet cells. Note the ragged and deformed red cells caused by rapid intravascular hemolysis due to physical factors (× 1200).

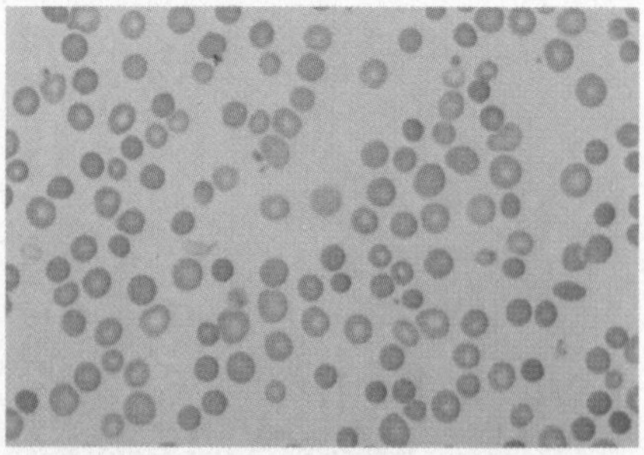

K, Peripheral blood smear from a patient with hereditary spherocytosis showing numerous spherocytes characterized by small size and dense hemoglobin stain. Scattered normal size red cells are also noted, along with occasional larger erythrocytes representing young cells (reticulocytes) (× 400).

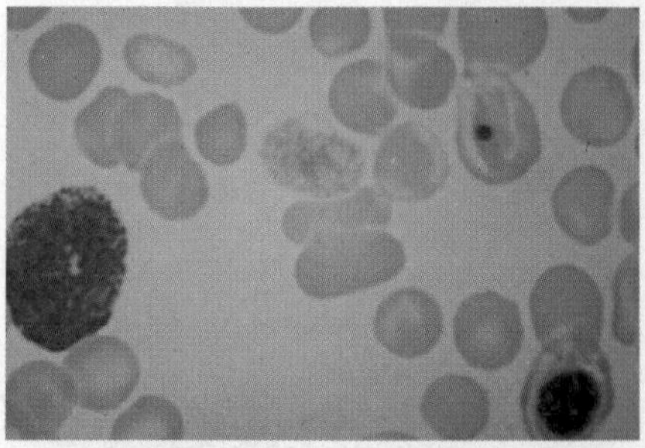

L, Peripheral blood smear showing a Howell-Jolly body in the erythrocyte in the right upper area of the slide. The round, dense granule represents nuclear DNA. At the lower right is a nucleated red cell. A giant platelet is present in the middle of the slide and a basophil is noted in the lower left corner. The patient had an underlying myeloproliferative disorder with a recent splenectomy (× 1200).

PLATE 3 HEMATOLOGIC DISEASES

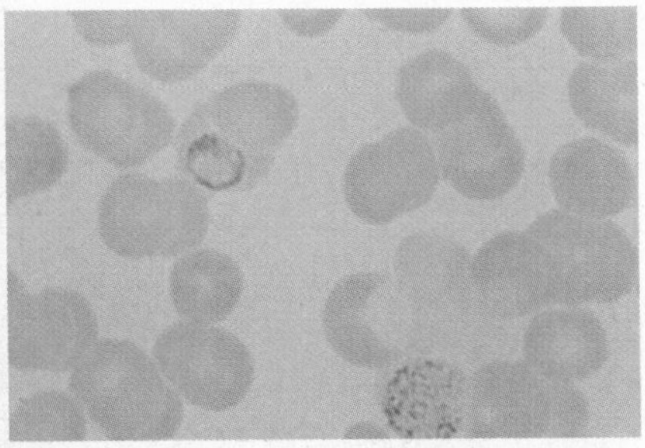

A, Peripheral blood showing malaria parasites within two red blood cells. Note the ringed form in the upper red cell and the numerous parasites in the lower red cell (× 1200).

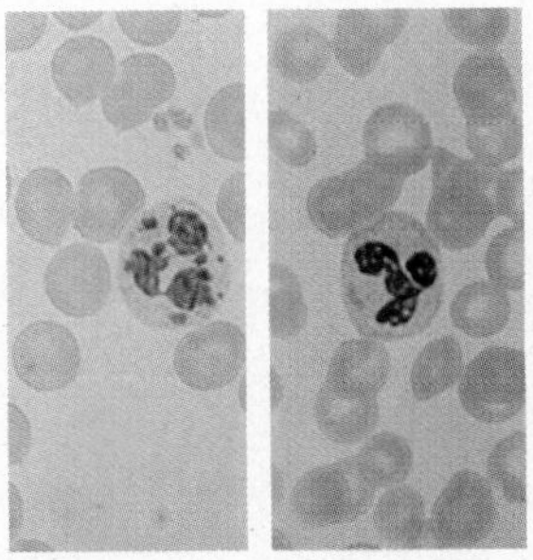

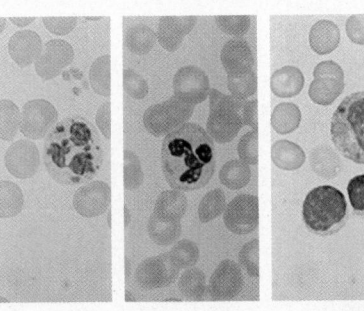

B, Leukocyte inclusions. *Left,* Giant basophilic granules in the Chediak-Higashi anomaly. *Center,* Basophilic inclusions (Döhle's bodies) within immature granulocytes. *Right,* Myelocyte with basophilic granules in Chediak-Higashi syndrome (× 1200).

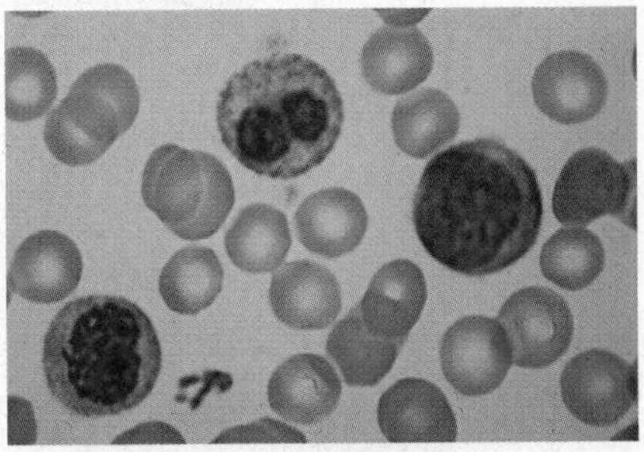

C, Pelger-Huët cells in the peripheral blood of a patient with chronic myeloid leukemia. Note the mature neutrophil in the center with an unsegmented adult poly in the lower left corner. A myeloblast is seen in the right of the slide (× 1200).

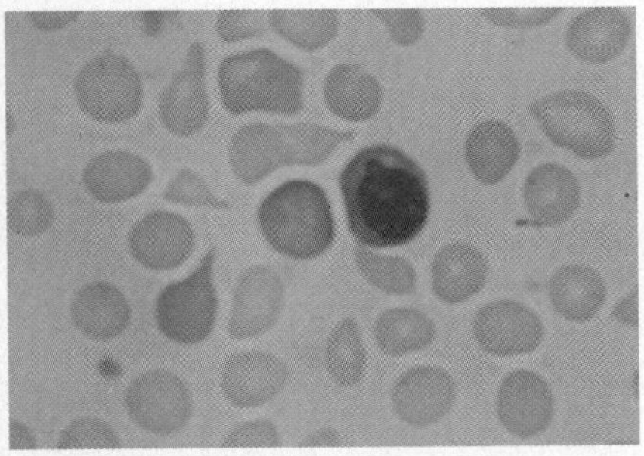

D, Peripheral blood smear showing leukoerythoblastic features, from a patient with myeloid metaplasia. Note the large nucleated red cell along with numerous tear drop–shaped red cells. Polychromatophilia is also present. Not seen in this slide are immature myeloid cells (× 1200).

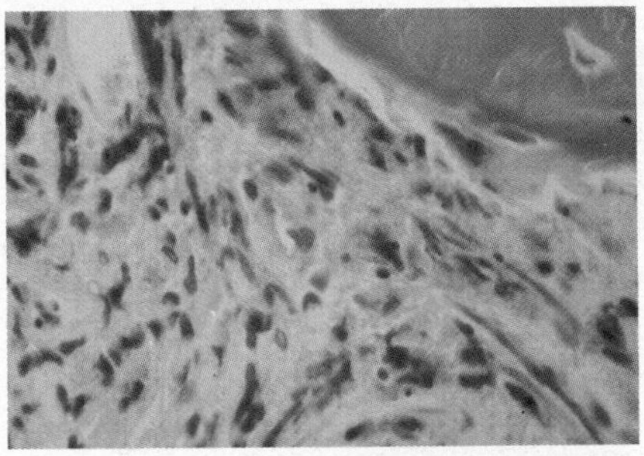

E, Myelofibrosis. Bone marrow biopsy showing intense fibrous tissue and primitive marrow reticulum cells replacing normal bone marrow elements (× 1000).

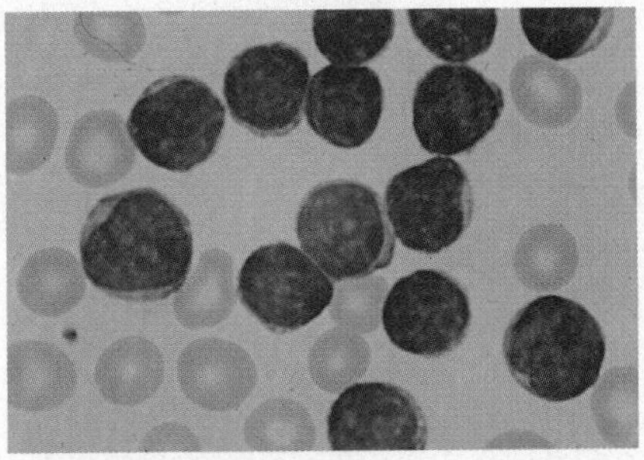

F, Chronic lymphocytic leukemia. Peripheral blood smear showing a majority of small mature-appearing lymphocytes, characterized by clumped nuclear chromatin and a rim of cytoplasm (× 1200).

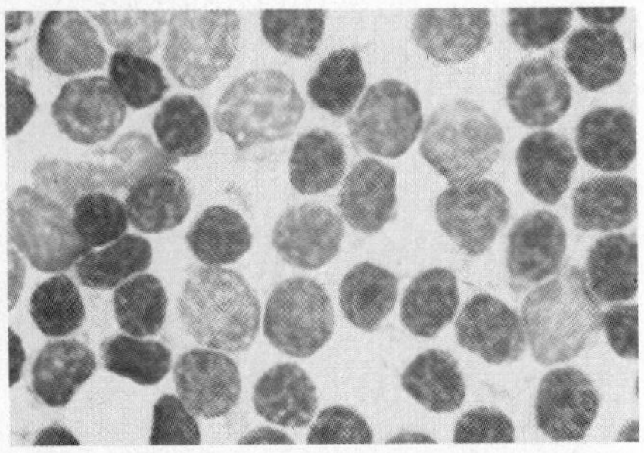

G, Bone marrow. Chronic lymphocytic leukemia showing dense infiltration by small mature-appearing lymphocytes with clumped chromatin and scanty cytoplasm (× 1200).

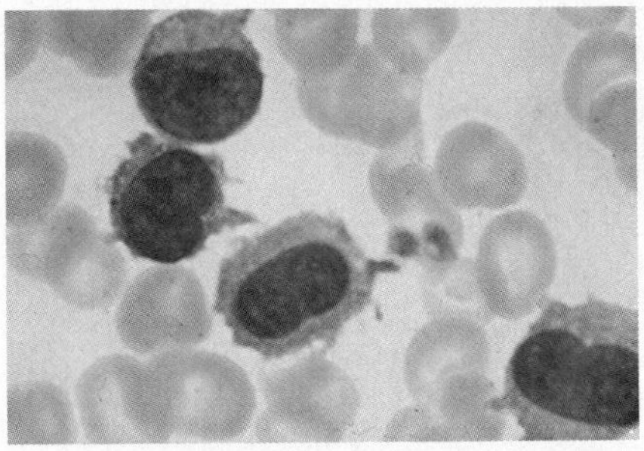

H, Hairy cell leukemia. Peripheral blood showing medium sized lymphoid cells with cytoplasmic strands or "hairs." Nuclei are somewhat immature (light staining) and indented in some of the cells. Indistinct nuclei are evident (× 1200).

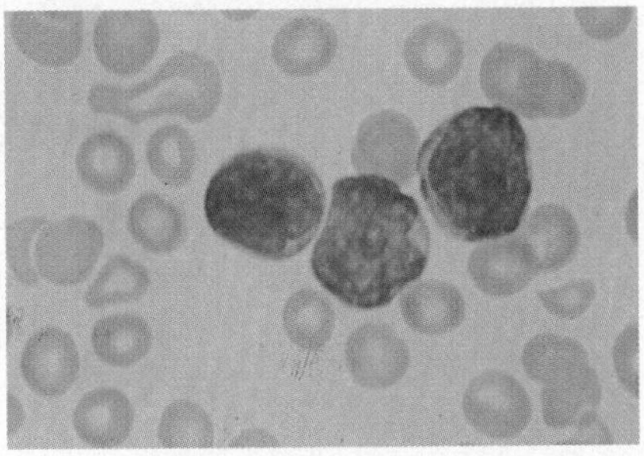

I, Acute lymphocytic leukemia. Peripheral blood showing three lymphoblasts, characterized by small size, immature light staining chromatin pattern, indistinct nuclei, and scanty cytoplasm (× 1200).

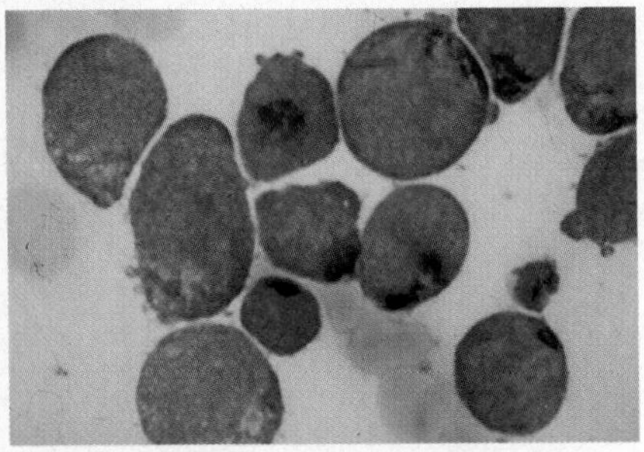

J, Acute myelogenous leukemia. Peroxidase stain showing marked positive activity in the majority of blasts, including the presence of Auer rods (× 1200).

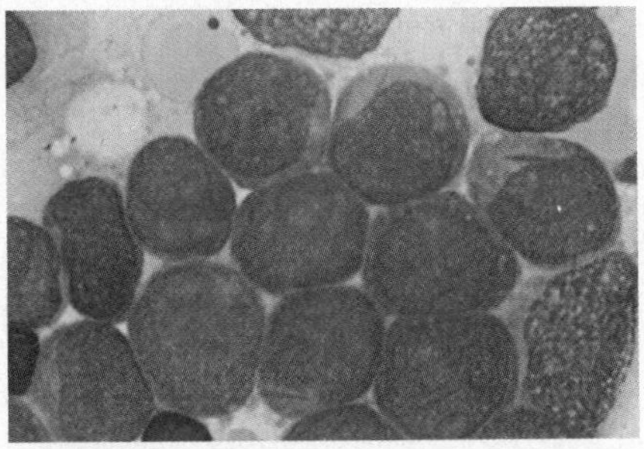

K, Acute myelogenous leukemia. Bone marrow, Giemsa stained, showing myeloblasts, some with prominent Auer rods (× 1200).

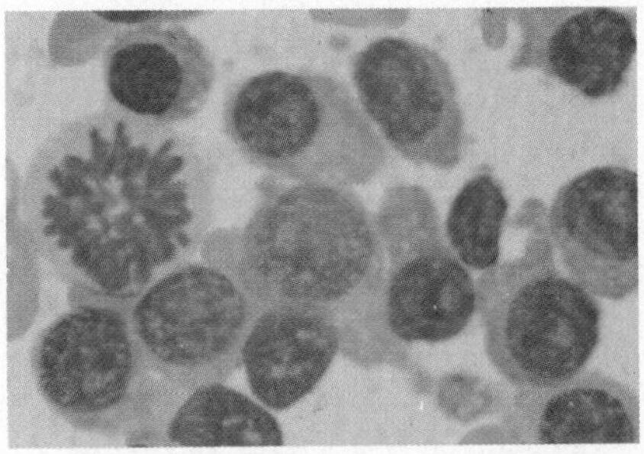

L, Multiple myeloma. Marrow shows a clump of immature plasma cells with eccentric nucleus, prominent nucleoli, and deep blue cytoplasm. A mitosis is present (× 1200).

PLATE 4 MEASLES

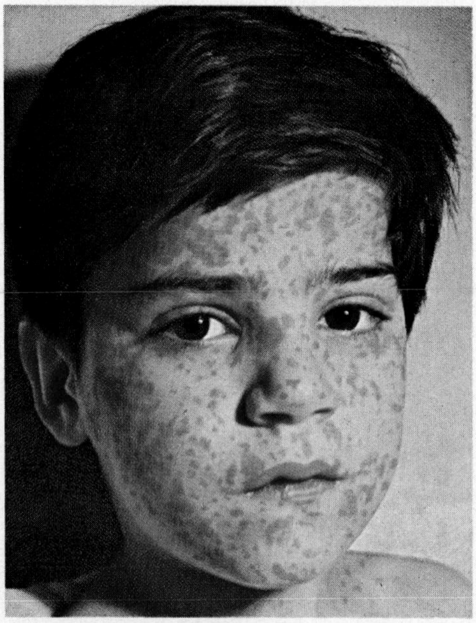

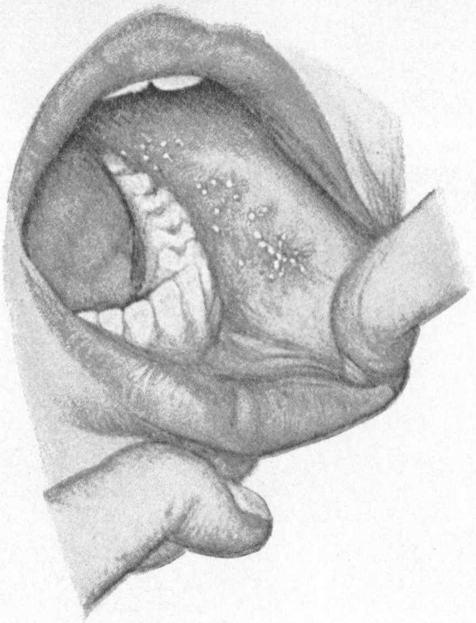

Upper, Early measles eruption. (Reproduction from Therapeutic Notes, by Courtesy of Parke, Davis & Company.)

Lower, Koplik's spots in measles (Hecker, Trumpp, and Abt).

PLATE 4. *See figure on the opposite page.*

A to *D* show various erythrocyte forms of falciparum or vivax malaria (× 1500).

A, "Ring forms" of *Plasmodium falciparum.* Note the delicate rings and an erythrocyte containing two organisms.

B, Trophozoite of *Plasmodium vivax.* The red cell is enlarged, Schüffner's dots are seen, and the parasite is large and ameboid.

C, Schizont of *Plasmodium vivax* with at least 18 merozoite nuclei.

D, Gametocyte of *Plasmodium falciparum.* The crescent or banana shape is characteristic.

E, Trypanosoma rhodesiense in the peripheral blood. It has a nucleus, posterior kinetoplast, undulating membrane, and flagellum (× 1500).

F, Spleen smear showing a cell filled with *Leishmania donovani.* The rod-shaped kinetoplast and large round nucleus appear as two adjacent red dots.

G, Methenamine silver nitrate stain of clump of *Pneumocystis* cysts. They appear as black circles against the blue background (× 800).

H, Stool sample observed by light microscopy, showing a motile *Entamoeba histolytica* moving in a straight line across the field. The ameba contains lucent vacuoles and shows a pseudopod directed to the upper right (× 500).

(*A, C, D,* and *F* are photographs taken by T. C. Jones from the Cornell Parasitology teaching slides; *B* is from the collection of H. Zaiman, originally photographed by M. Wittner; *E* and *G* were provided by R. B. Roberts; *H* is a photograph of fresh material provided by T. C. Jones.)

PLATE 5 PROTOZOAN DISEASES

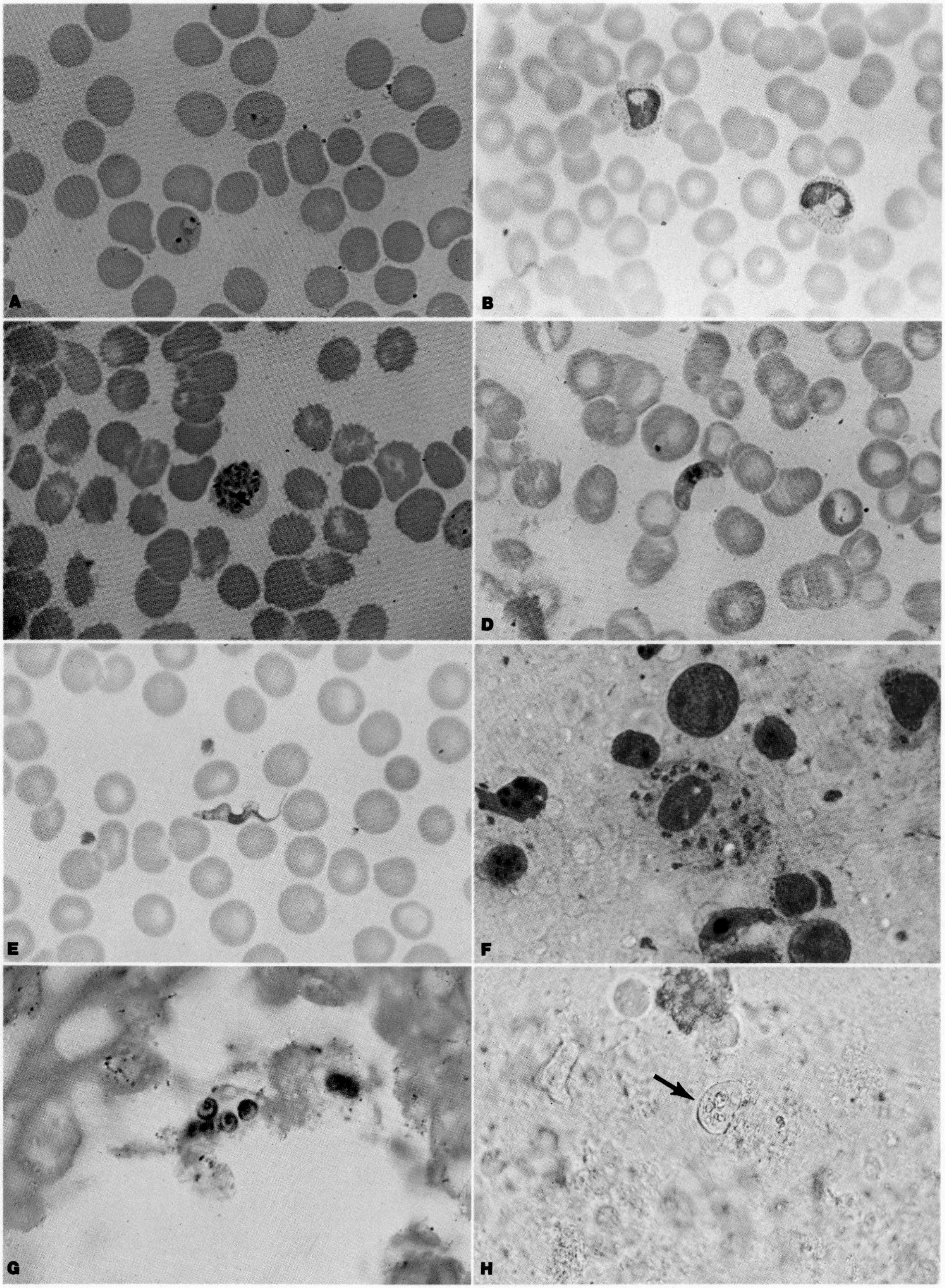

See legend on the opposite page.

PLATE 6 SKIN DISEASES

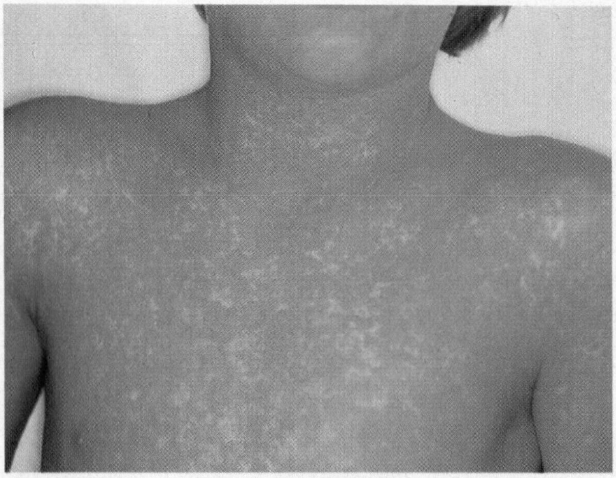

A, Drug eruption.

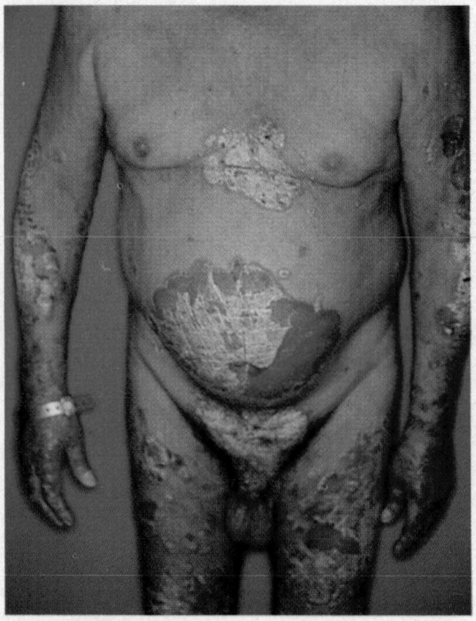

B, Psoriasis.

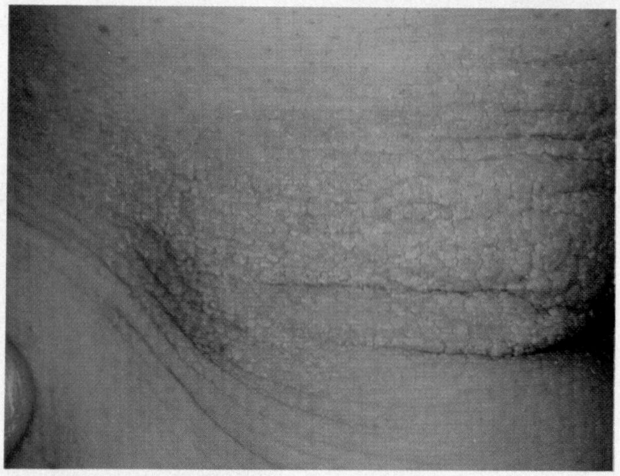

C, Acanthosis nigricans.

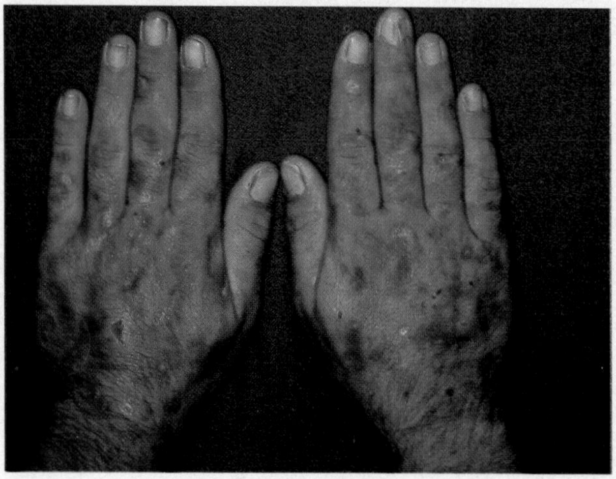

D, Porphyria cutanea tarda.

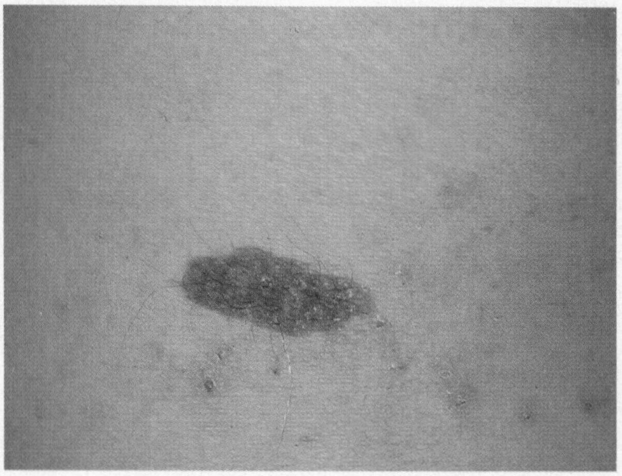

E, Junctional nevus.

PLATE 7 SKIN DISEASES

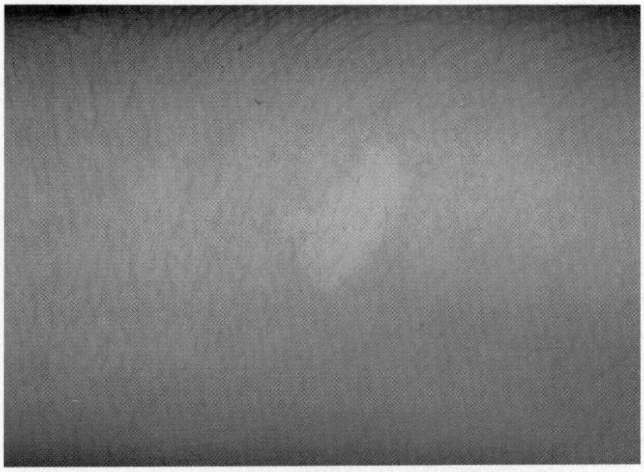

F, Tuberous sclerosis ash leaf.

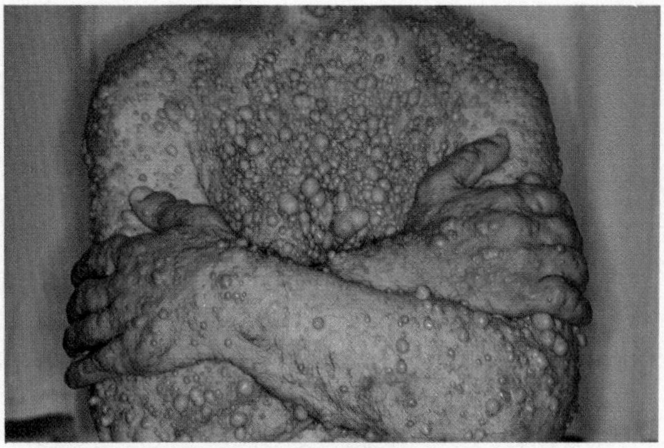

G, Neurofibromatosis—von Recklinghausen's disease.

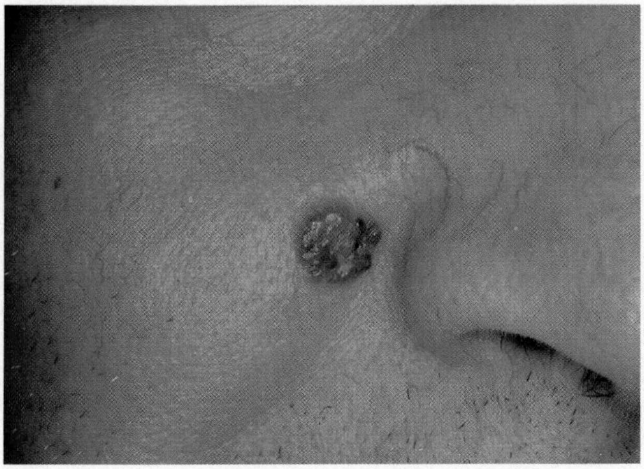

H, Basal cell carcinoma.

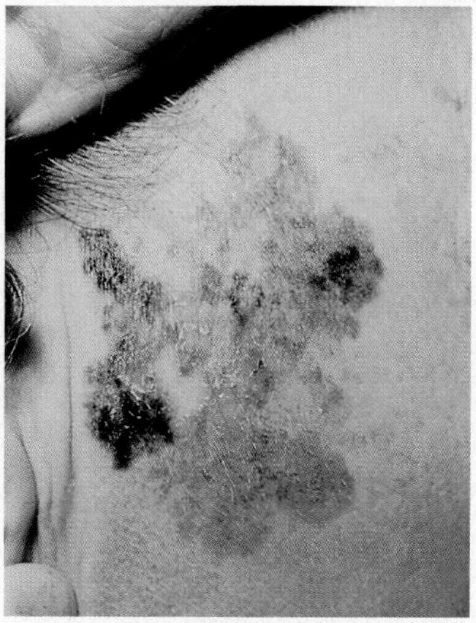

I, Lentigo maligna.

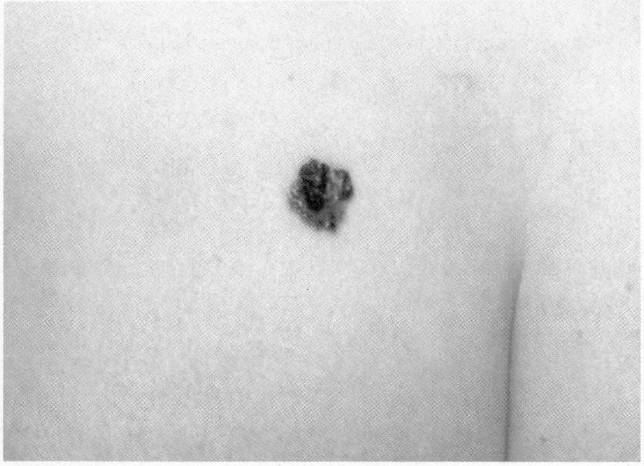

J, Nodular melanoma.

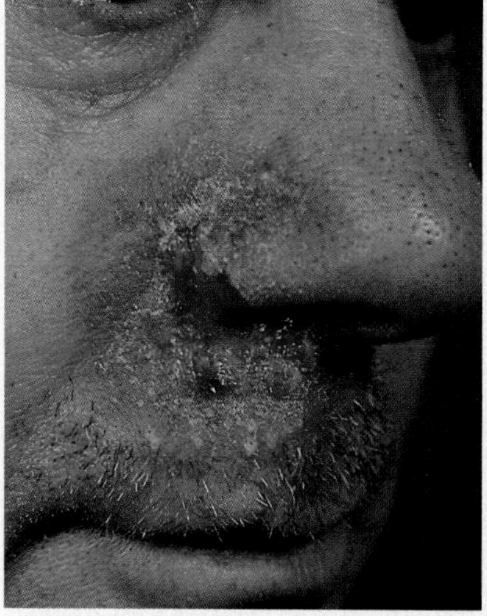

K, Squamous cell carcinoma.

PLATE 8 MENINGOCOCCAL DISEASE

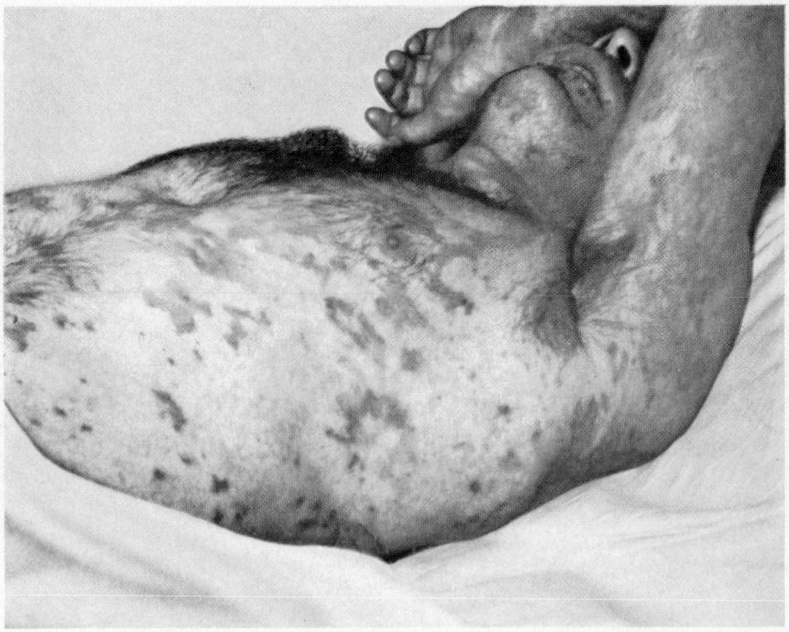

Skin lesions in fulminating meningococcemia (Courtesy of Dr. Worth B. Daniels).

PLATE 9 RHEUMATIC FEVER

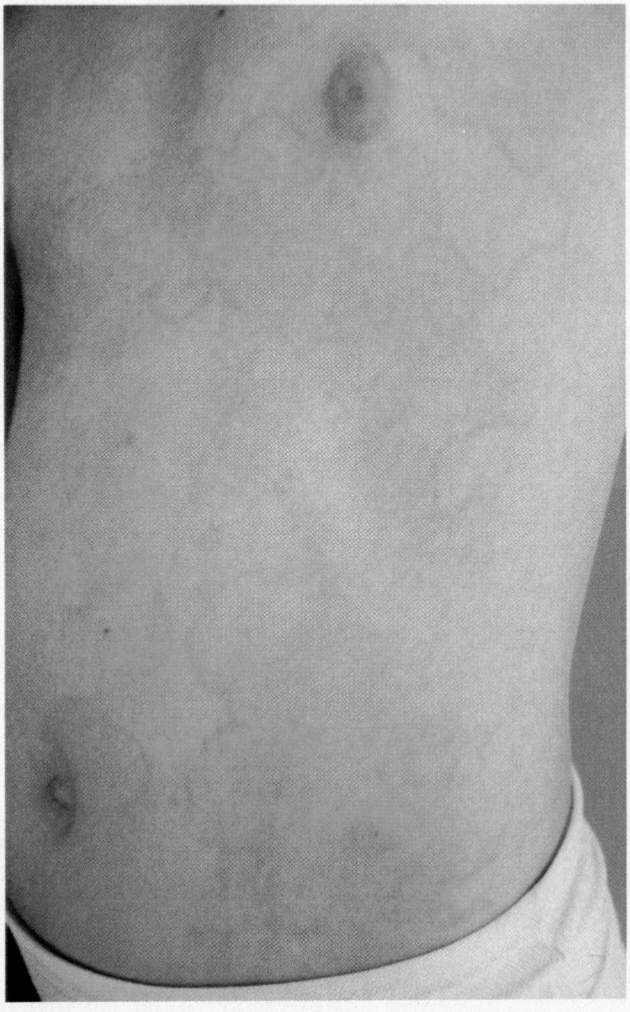

Erythema marginatum (Courtesy of Solomon E. Levin, M.D.).

CECIL
TEXTBOOK OF MEDICINE

Part I
MEDICINE AS A LEARNED AND HUMANE PROFESSION

The *Cecil Textbook of Medicine* is addressed to medical students, residents, fellows, and practitioners of all ages. It deals with the body of knowledge of human disease. In contrast, these introductory essays are presented mainly for those now entering the profession, for students deserve a broader perspective of medicine than is offered by its subject matter alone.

1. MEDICINE AS AN ART

Lloyd H. Smith, Jr.

What is medicine? "Medicine is not a science but a learned profession, deeply rooted in a number of sciences and charged with the obligation to apply them for man's benefit." In this eloquent statement from an earlier edition of this book, Walsh McDermott defined medicine as a human activity undertaken for the benefit of others whether in the area of public health, "statistical compassion," or in the care of the individual patient.

Medicine can also be defined in other terms. It is a mutable body of knowledge, skills, and traditions applicable to the preservation of health, the cure of disease, and the amelioration of suffering. The boundaries of medicine blend into psychology, sociology, economics, and even into cultural heritage. Disease may be encoded in the genome; disease may also be encoded by the deprivations of poverty and ignorance. Medicine must therefore be concerned not only with an abnormal molecule but also with an abnormal childhood. As such it is open ended in a way that is both humbling and exhilarating to those who pursue it as a career.

Medicine is continually changing. The honored verities of one generation become the shopworn shibboleths of the next. Much of what we now so confidently espouse, including that compressed within this edition, will amuse our successors as being remarkably bizarre in its naiveté. Medical competence is based on the continuing pursuit of ever changing concepts. It must be renewed as the substance of medicine itself is transformed.

The practice of medicine is far more than the application of scientific principles to a particular biologic aberration. Its focus is on the patient whose welfare is its continuing purpose. That purpose of medicine is self evident in theory, but more difficult to sustain under the pressures of medical practice. For example, it is tragically easy for the patient to become merely the repository in which a disease or a syndrome has chosen to manifest its particular silhouette. During the training years every physician has subconsiously participated in what might be termed the personification of disease. A case of meningitis is admitted through the emergency room; a pheochromocytoma will be discussed at Grand Rounds. It is perhaps inevitable that a disease becomes symbolically an entity to the physician who must become familiar with all of its manifestations and guises. In the art of medicine the physician must be the advocate of the patient as well as the adversary of disease. It is the patient who is personified rather than the disease.

THE PATIENT. The description of a patient is simply that of a fellow human being in need of help. The patient comes seeking help because of a problem relating to his or her health. This subjective judgment carries with it disquieting concerns, although these may be unexpressed. Anxiety is present even in the most stoical of patients; this fact must never be forgotten or disregarded by the physician. The patient's anxiety may be specific—for example, in a fear of cancer with all that implies in the public mind concerning pain, degradation, and inexorable death. More often the anxiety is amorphous: fear of loss of independence or employment; fear of failure to meet obligations to one's family or to retain the regard of a loved one; or fear of an inability to maintain a life of dignity and significance. In the rush to crystallize a chief complaint and present illness the physician too often brushes aside these considerations.

The patient presents to the physician on alien and unfamiliar ground—in the structured and artificial setting of an office, a clinic, or a hospital bed. This form of health care of the individual, as opposed to health care in the aggregate, is often described by the unfelicitous phrase "the personal encounter system." Unfortunately it often seems distressingly like confrontation to the patient, who comes after all for comfort, not for encounter. Each human being is unique within a life that is enormously complex—in heredity, early experiences, cultural and psychologic environment, education, opportunities, successes, failures, fantasies, emotional commitments, motivations, and in the adjustments and compromises that serve to cripple or to mature. Living, therefore, is the ultimate personal encounter system. With an extensive and diverse experience the patient comes to the physician with "a problem." A chief complaint is requested. Defenses must be lowered and the emotions that spill out may be distressing. The patient's response must be selective and brief; as a result it is not infrequently distorted, perhaps even misleading.

What does the patient want when coming to see a physician? There are certain common hopes and expectations. Patients want to be listened to, so that their fears and concerns can be fully expressed and the burden shared. They want physicians to be interested in them as fellow human beings in a compassionate but nonjudgmental fashion. They expect professional competence incorporating the best in medical science and technology. They want to be reasonably informed as to the probable cause of their concerns and what the future is likely to hold. They want not to be abandoned. To each patient these desires and expectations vary in relative importance. It is notable that not all patients expect to be cured. These expectations will be further discussed in the light of how the physician should endeavor to meet them.

TRADITIONAL EXPECTATIONS OF PATIENTS. *Patients want to be listened to and understood.* This has been well expressed by Wilfred Trotter, a great English neurosurgeon:

". . . As long as medicine is an art, its chief and characteristic instrument must be human faculty. We come therefore to the very practical question of what aspects of human faculty it is necessary for the good doctor to cultivate. . . . The first to be named must always be the power of attention, of giving one's whole mind to the patient without the interposition of oneself. It sounds simple but only the very greatest doctors ever fully attain it. It is an active process and not either mere resigned listening or even politely waiting until you can interrupt. Disease often tells its secrets in a casual parenthesis. . . ."

Eventually the medical record must be organized in a logical and consistent fashion. But a history rarely unfolds that way. Patients do not divulge their fears in neat paragraphs or in direct responses to a cascade of queries. It is important to let patients tell their own stories. The manner of formulation and expression of symptoms and anxieties may be as informative as the medical data transmitted. The good physician is an attentive listener, with an ear for Trotter's "casual parenthesis."

Patients want physicians to be interested in them as fellow human beings. This interest cannot be that of the unusual "case" of the carcinoid syndrome or of hairy cell leukemia; the center of interest must be the patient as a person. It is difficult for the physician to feign such an interest, for patients are very perceptive, especially during the vulnerability that illness induces. In the practice of medicine the physician will encounter all of the virtues and vices to which mankind is heir. The physician need not be morally neutral in personal judgments, but these must be stringently excluded from professional activities. The response of the physician to human frailty and fallibility should be that of compassion rather than cynicism, of interest in the infinite variety of human experience rather than of repulsion from its aberrations.

Patients expect professional competence in medical science and technology. The physician must be a scholar both to attain professional competence and to sustain it during times of revolutionary changes in science and technology. All of the other attributes of the good physician will be of little avail in the absence of sound scholarship. Compassion is no substitute for knowing what should be done. The education of the physician and the role of the physician as a scientist will be discussed more fully below.

Patients want to be kept reasonably informed. The physician must listen to and communicate with the patient. Time must be set aside for this. Failure to do so is a serious error, for silence is a form of communication that is usually adverse. The physician should voluntarily answer questions of concern to the patient. The physician must also inform the patient concerning the illness and what it implies. A number of books have been developed to assist in patient education and are often quite effective in translating medical terminology into lay terms. Furthermore, clubs for mutual support and education have been formed by patients who share their common experiences with such chronic disabilities as ileostomies or amputations. Admirable and important as these are, they do not obviate the need for patients to learn from their own physicians about their particular illnesses and what they may mean in and for their future lives. This need extends beyond the legal confines of informed consent, which is now an important issue in medical practice.

Patients want not to be abandoned. Death comes to everyone. There are finite limits to what can be accomplished by medical science and technology in the alleviation of suffering and the prolongation of life. This fact is well known to both patients and physicians. When that limit is reached, the physician often feels powerless and even guilty that no more can be done. As a consequence there is a tendency to withdraw attention and direct it elsewhere. Nothing could be a greater mistake. It is at the margins of medical science that the role of the physician is enhanced. It is here that the art of medicine comes to the forefront in the care of the patient, whether it be by emotional support, relief of pain, small adjustments in medicines or diet, daily conversation and examination, or other methods to show that the patient is still someone of dignity and worth in whom interest has not been lost and for whom hope has not been abandoned. And when no more can be done for the patient it is time to care for the family. It is this caring role rather than the curing role of the physician that is so well described in Ch. 4 by Lewis Thomas. At this stage, as Walsh McDermott has written, "it is up to each of us to follow to the fullest measure the charge laid down long ago for the physician to become himself the treatment."

THE PHYSICIAN. The physician has both chosen and been chosen to enter an arduous and demanding profession, the origins of which stretch back to antiquity. Part priest, part shaman, part mystic, part alchemist, the physician of the past reflected the beliefs and expectations of the time and met a perceived need of fellow men. The history of medicine is part of the heritage of every physician and reflects the cultural history of each society.

The physician enters a profession with established values and traditions of ethical conduct and responsibilities. But each physician, as each patient, is unique. The physician is not a disembodied instrument that can be passively shaped by the profession, but rather a human being with innate strengths and weaknesses that must be recognized in order to meet the expectations of patients and of the profession, not least of which are those standards established for oneself. The qualities of the ideal physician are easy to state but difficult to attain: compassion, sincere interest in one's fellow man, knowledge of human nature, tact, equanimity, sustained scholarship, curiosity, and high ethical standards. Physical and mental vigor might be added to those traits, for the life of the physician is not for the languid or the disengaged. No one has been endowed with or ever fully achieves excellence in all of these qualities. One must first know oneself and judge how one can most closely approach those ideals in one's professional life.

THE EDUCATION OF THE PHYSICIAN. Barriers are encountered at the very beginning in the initial selection for medical school as many seek entry for few positions. Undergraduate education is sometimes distorted and breadth of personal experience curtailed in a grim and often distasteful race for competitive acceptance. This inadvertent feedback inhibition not infrequently results from erroneous conceptions of what may or may not impress admission committees of medical schools. Nevertheless, the phenomenon remains as a concern to all who are interested in the future of our profession. Admission committees of medical schools too often exercise allosteric control over the higher education of those destined to enter our profession.

The Basic Science Years. In the standard curriculum of medical school in the United States two years are largely devoted to the sciences basic to medicine and two years to clinical training. Fortunately there are a number of interesting variations on this thematic progression which diminish its rigidity and permit the student to re-explore basic science after an introductory clinical experience.

In the United States students usually arrive at medical school after an intensive four-year experience at a college or a university. They anticipate a scholarly atmosphere of a graduate school which will prepare them to enter the practice of a profession for which they hold idealistic expectations. Instead they are immediately assailed with a formidable array of "basic sciences" linked to the structure and function of the human organ systems. New facts constitute not so much an intellectual feast as an engorgement. Each discipline is attended by devotees who are passionately persuaded of the seminal role of their segment of science in the future of the profession. This commitment is translated into the basic academic commodity, curricular time, in which these cluttered wares are exhibited. Awed by the dimensionless task, students struggle with uneven success to assimilate and survive, conscious always that their receptor mechanisms are overloaded and of a continuing sense of high output failure. They look forward in hope that subsequent years will reward their endurance in the more congenial atmosphere of the clinic.

This is patently a caricature, as all will recognize. It can be said, as Mark Twain said of Wagner's music, " it is not as bad as it sounds." The quality of basic science in medical schools is often superb; the substance of modern science has a certain grandeur; many faculty members are gifted in imparting a sense of intellectual adventure to their students; finally, many students now arrive at medical school with a mature understanding of one or more of the fundamental disciplines of biology. Nevertheless this caricature contains elements of truth as seen from the perspective of medical students. The central question is not whether basic science is necessary for medical research, since few would deny its importance there, but whether it is relevant in the education of every physician to the degree to which it is currently emphasized. In the real world of patient care, public health, and medical economics, should the student have to struggle with the intricacies of post-transcriptional modifications of messenger RNA, or is this merely a rite of passage prescribed by a science-obsessed faculty? This is a reasonable question and calls for a response other than a simple reference to flexnerian orthodoxy.

A knowledge of the scientific underpinnings of medicine is clearly necessary in order to marshal the basic information required to understand a patient's illness and to be able to reason logically about the problems of diagnosis and therapy. If there were any doubt on that point, it would be quickly dispelled by random perusal of this book. Much of the basic science which seems abstruse and irrelevant today will find its way into clinical practice in the not too distant future. Medical research is only one step removed from patient care.

Beyond the assimilation of scientific information, there is an even more important consideration. Many of you will have most of your professional experience in the twenty-first century. The changes in medical science and technology will be enormous and largely unpredictable. Only the scientific method will remain unaltered as an invaluable instrument with which fallible man can acquire new knowledge and, equally important, debride that which proves fallacious. It is imperative that students learn the scientific method as part of their education if they are to participate critically and effectively in a changing profession. How can this be done? Perhaps the best method is to participate personally, even for a relatively brief period of time, in a research project so that learning comes from first hand experience. If that does not prove practical, one can pursue some scientific topic in depth and write a critical analysis of it. It is important to learn one area of inquiry in great detail, even though it may have to be a limited area, in order to penetrate to its frontier. It is only there that science can be understood as a process rather than as a repository.

The Clinical Years. In his perceptive essay "On Becoming a Clinician," in an earlier edition of this textbook, Paul B. Beeson described many of the disquieting stresses to which the student is subjected on entry into the clinical years. Every medical student will benefit from reading those thoughts from one of America's most distinguished physicians. Most students enter the clinical years with a sense of relief, but it is relief linked with anxieties. Some of these anxieties cluster around the following questions:

How can I cope with the uncertainties of clinical medicine?

What are the boundaries of clinical medicine? How much and what am I supposed to learn?

How will I function in my interactions with patients?

How will I measure up to the expectations of my colleagues?

How will I be able to maintain my own identity as an individual in a profession that so obsessively dominates my time and energy?

Other questions could be formulated. Each student possesses a unique idiotype of anxieties that cannot be purged by platitudes. Each will arrive at personal answers, or more likely at personal accommodations, through experience.

THE UNCERTAINTY PRINCIPLE OF CLINICAL MEDICINE. There is an "uncertainty principle" in medicine as there is in physics. The practice of medicine is inexact and will remain so. If it were not, it would be a science or a technology rather than an art. The measuring instrument is personal and unique. Subjective mensuration defies precision. Who can quantify nausea or the severity of pain? Symptoms may be forgotten, suppressed, or amplified when filtered through the grid of personality. Available data are often indirect, incomplete, or even contradictory. Patients respond in varying fashions to treatment across the range from simple reassurance (which is rarely simple) to surgical or pharmaceutical interventions. Clinical medicine is often based on experience and judgment—which are largely euphemisms for a knowledge of probabilities.

The process of formulating a diagnosis or selecting a therapy is not as arbitrary as it first seems. There are rational means for narrowing the range of diagnostic possibilities: a precise description of symptoms; an accurate and thorough characterization of physical findings; selective laboratory studies to evaluate the functions of organ systems; a synthesis of information to define syndromic patterns; a marshaling of information on etiology and pathogenesis. All of this requires attention to detail, consistency of work habits, and good intellect.

Hypotheses are formed and algorithms branch away from various entry points as new data are obtained which support or fail to support a working diagnosis. This process of clinical reasoning is often best displayed in the Clinicopathologic Conference (CPC). In the absence of certainty, best guesses must be utilized and in making informed guesses, generally dignified as judgments, the clinician actually relies upon subliminal statistics.

Medical decisions based on probabilities are necessary but also perilous. Even the most astute physician will occasionally be wrong. The wise physician will often recognize that a decision is erroneous and discard or modify the hypothesis on which it is based. The best decision may be approached only by successive approximations. Action may have to be taken despite lack of confirmation of a hypothesis (working diagnosis). Chester M. Jones, a noted clinical teacher, used to say: "If you cannot make a diagnosis, make a decision." Despite the remarkable contributions of science and technology, clinical medicine is frequently inexactitude in action. The student entering the clinical years will quickly realize the dangers to the welfare of the patient of dogmatism in clinical practice. The ambiguities and errors that you will encounter in your own experience and observe in the work of others should be an antidote to arrogance. Some errors are inevitable and should not humiliate you, but they should teach humility.

CLINICAL MEDICINE AS A DISCIPLINE WITHOUT BOUNDARIES. The basic sciences are demanding but, as taught in medical schools, they have reasonably defined margins. It is true that these margins are somewhat artificial, since the disciplines of modern biology merge almost imperceptibly into one another. Nevertheless, the educational responsibilities of the medical student can often be designated within the subject material of a lecture course, syllabus, and textbook. Not so in clinical medicine. The student emerges into an open-ended system of bewildering complexity in which science is blurred by sociology, psychology interacts with economics, traditions and ethical concepts are buffeted by new imperatives. Within this complicated system, the practice of clinical medicine goes forward. The student does not encounter a theoretical discipline to be observed and analyzed in tranquility, but is abruptly thrown into the structured workings of the second largest industry in the United States where the health and even the survival of many people are at stake on a daily basis.

Based on previous educational experiences, students often ask, "How much am I expected to learn in this course?" No one can supply a satisfactory answer. The student stands on the threshold of a learning experience in clinical medicine that will extend over the remainder of an active career as a physician. Learning must have that stretch if the student is to meet the responsibilities of a physician. The course is merely a contrived entry point into that longitudinal experience. More advanced faculty members, medical residents, or even senior students in other rotations in medicine seem remarkably well informed. Yet no single individual has a balanced knowledge in all aspects of medicine. The specialist will often be adept only within a defined subset of medicine, and even the generalist will be uneven in many areas of information. Within this confusing and sometimes overwhelming setting the student must become an independent scholar in medicine—independent in the sense that never again will others outline or circumscribe the subject material.

Most students adapt themselves remarkably quickly to the changed environment of clinical medicine. The new language of the hospital, including its acronymic barbarisms (SOB, PERLA, COPD, etc.), no longer jar the ear, and the concepts of pathophysiology being applied at the bedside awaken latent memories. The student learns that there are habits of thought and clusters of associations so that the physician does not laboriously go back to first principles to meet each new clinical problem. These thought patterns are efficient and useful if they do not gel into medicine by reflex and aphorism. The student learns by listening, participating, observing, arguing, reading, and reflecting. As earlier generations of students have discovered, the intensity of the experience and the special chemistry of confronting the clinical problem of a specific patient serve to fix the information received in one's memory with a vividness far beyond that obtained from even the most brilliant lecture.

Beyond the required participation in clinical rotations, how should the student approach the study of medicine? It would be presumptuous to give a doctrinaire answer. Medical students have usually been seasoned by five or six years of higher education before they begin the study of clinical medicine and during those years have developed their own best methods of learning. In approaching internal medicine, in contrast perhaps to some more circumscribed specialties, it will usually prove most valuable to study in depth the specific problems presented by one's own patients rather than beginning with a systematic approach to cover all of the discipline. In this way one can exploit the intense immediacy of those experiences which, supplemented by conferences, rounds, seminars, conversations, and all of the other ways of learning on the fly, will usually converge to give a broad familiarity with the subject. A share in the responsibility of caring for a patient is a powerful stimulus to learning.

What is the role of the *Cecil Textbook of Medicine* in the learning process? This book attempts to provide the student or the physician with succinct but authoritative summaries about diseases or groups of diseases. Essays written by more than 250 acknowledged experts in their respective fields represent collectively a systematic approach to internal medicine. The chapters are designed to give a basic, lucid, and up-to-date consensus concerning the state of the art in our understanding of specific diseases, but they cannot be all inclusive. Many of the topics discussed within a few pages have received more extended treatment elsewhere as separate monographs. Each of the subspecialty areas (cardiology, gastroenterology, endocrinology, etc.) is the subject of textbooks similar in size to this one. The student should therefore cultivate the habit of consulting at least some of the carefully selected references that extend the information supplied in this basic text.

In general it is also wise for students to begin reading medical journals early in their study of clinical medicine. In this way a start can be made toward the regular study of current medical literature and also the foundations of one's own medical library can be laid. Each student may have a personal preference. The most frequently read medical journal by students and practitioners is the *New England Journal of Medicine.* It is particularly useful for the student with its CPC, surveys of medical progress, editorial comments on current topics, original articles, and lively correspondence. In this manner the student establishes an early acquaintance with the frontiers of medicine and with its issues, uncertainties, and controversies.

THE STUDENT AND THE PATIENT. One of the student's earliest concerns on entering clinical medicine is how to interact with patients and how to assume the traditional role of a physician. The student is concerned that personal insecurities will impair effective communication with patients in whose care he or she is now called upon to participate. Rarely does this turn out in practice to be a serious problem. The expectations of most patients in the physician-patient interaction, discussed above, are realistic ones. Patients are usually aware of the progression of assigned responsibilities in the student-house staff-faculty team and do not expect omniscience or authoritarianism from the student. Not infrequently the patient forms a special attachment to the student, especially if the student has been perceptive enough to listen in the sense described above by Wilfred Trotter. If the student respects the personal dignity of the patient as a fellow human being, and listens in a sensitive manner, the patient responds with gratitude and returns that respect. Even when patients are initially perceived as hostile or belligerent, the student must maintain equanimity and try to understand the sources of these reactions. Do not allow yourself to be drawn into the flippant cynicism that sometimes passes for sophistication in the subculture of student and house staff training. Francis Peabody's sentient summary is still most apt, "for the secret of the care of the patient is in caring for the patient."

STUDENTS AND THEIR COLLEAGUES. Beginning in the clinical years the relationships of students with their colleagues in medicine undergo a subtle change. No longer are they merely the passive recipients of data and concepts supplied by the faculty through lectures, conferences, syllabi, or laboratories. They are participating with graduated responsibilities in the practice of medicine. A point in the medical history or a question asked by the student may prove decisive in arriving at the solution of a clinical problem. Frequently the most effective teachers of students are the house staff or more advanced students. Students will find many residents to be splendid teachers who not only make them feel at home on the service but also take the extra time to include them in all of the discussions. On most teaching services there is a certain amount of badinage or gamesmanship which enlivens interactions. If this is recognized as such, and not taken too seriously, it can serve to enhance rather than demean the learning experience. As a student you must not hesitate to ask questions or bring up new points of view and must not be intimidated by your current position in this shifting hierarchy. Even the chief medical resident faced similar qualms only a few years ago. But above all, remember that it is the patient's welfare, and not your own ego, that is paramount.

THE PHYSICIAN AS A NONPHYSICIAN. Beginning in the basic science years but exacerbated in the clinical years, students often become concerned about the level of commitment demanded of them. How much of a life that is finite in time and energy must be devoted to medicine? What is the boundary between dedication and obsession? After all one does not really become a physician; one remains a human being who has acquired certain knowledge and skills that allow one to function as a physician during specific periods of time. What should those times be? How and when does one shift roles from being a physician to being a "nonphysician"? This is, of course, a generic question that is as applicable to science, art, business, or any other human activity as it is to medicine.

The student will not readily find an all-embracing answer to this question. Each student will most likely evolve a personal answer and it will be an operational one representing the integral of microcompromises and adjustments made throughout one's subsequent career. The "complete physician," narrowly construed, would be a very poor physician if he were merely an observer rather than a participant in the pageantry of his time. Physicians owe it to themselves, to their families, to society, and to their patients not to become simply skilled but detached automatons. On the other hand, the practice of medicine is not a job but a profession that cannot be sealed off into convenient hours for earning one's living. To attempt to do so smacks of dilettantism. Between these extremes one must decide for oneself where the compromises will be made along the varying border between personal and professional life. Tensions will remain, but properly channeled they can be creative and rewarding.

2. MEDICINE AS A SCIENCE

James B. Wyngaarden

The practice of medicine rests firmly upon a foundation of biologic and behavioral sciences, which in turn trace their evolution to chemistry, physics, mathematics, psychology, anthropology, and epidemiology. The physician must acquire both an extensive knowledge base in science, and a comfortable familiarity with the ways of science. Preservation of professional competence requires a continuing growth of knowledge, an analytical approach to problem solving, and a critical assessment of new hypotheses and scientific advances.

The substance of biologic science underlies most of the medical progress of the past half century which has so remarkably advanced the ability of the physician to intervene in illness. Much of this progress has been in fundamental or "basic" science, conducted in the pursuit of truth for its own sake. Significant progress has also resulted from research conducted by physician-scientists with a specified clinical goal in mind—for example, the elucidation of a disease mechanism. Advances in medicine also continue to occur through serendipity or by astute clinical observations concerning patients or groups of patients and their illnesses, but these are now the exceptions. The only rational approach to finding new methods for prevention or treatment is based on scientific explanations of the causes and mechanisms of disease.

Some years ago, Comroe and Dripps* traced the origins of ten major clinical innovations in cardiovascular and pulmonary medicine to document the actual antecedents of medical progress. Over 60 per cent of the enabling discoveries were in the category of basic science; over 40 per cent were the result of research carried out without any particular clinical application in mind.

The major health care problem of our time lies in the continued existence of diseases for which we can do little. At least in the more economically advanced countries of the world, it does not lie in the cost of health care or in its distribution, inequitable and serious as these problems may be. Even if the best of contemporary medicine were universally available without financial barriers, cancer would continue to kill, rheumatoid arthritis would continue to cripple, and schizophrenia would continue to render insane. We have no definitive answers for these diseases and for many more the descriptions of which constitute the substance of this book—or else we have what Lewis Thomas has called a "halfway technology," capable of modification but not of prevention or cure. Medicine as a science is incomplete. It will remain so, for science itself is by its nature incomplete.

The present bioscientific character of medical practice is a relatively recent development. Throughout most of recorded history medicine was anything but scientific, being dominated by empiricism and shackled by dogma. Diagnoses were inexact, causes of diseases poorly understood, and therapies frivolous and haphazard. Interventions by physicians consisted of bleeding, purging, cupping, administration of infusions of every known plant and of solutions of every known metal, and prescription of every possible diet—with no scientific foundation for these practices. Nor could there be such a foundation in the absence of a body of scientific biomedical knowledge.

Harbingers of change emerged slowly in the early nineteenth century, as new principles of physics and chemistry were applied to medicine. Physiologists stressed functions of organs and tissues. Its exemplars, especially Claude Bernard (1813–1878), emphasized the experimental method in establishing biologic knowledge and the necessity of basing medical practice in such knowledge. Pathologists, led by Virchow (1821–1902), stressed the critical study of normal and abnormal tissues and the correlation of features of disease with precise anatomic observations. Bacteriologists, with Pasteur (1822–1895) and Koch (1843–1910) in the vanguard, began to identify the microorganisms and to implicate specific organisms in specific diseases—the anthrax bacillus in anthrax, the tubercle bacillus in consumption, the pneumococcus in lobar pneumonia, the streptococcus in puerperal fever. The groundwork for future therapies was being laid by these great Western European scientists, but there was relatively little that physicians could do about most illnesses at the time. Their major contributions were diagnostic, prognostic, and supportive. By correct diagnosis they could advise concerning outcome. By common-sense supportive measures they could provide comfort and maximize opportunities for recovery. But interventions were as likely as not to make things worse. The first edition of Osler's *Textbook of Medicine* in 1892 was revolutionary for its skepticism and its therapeutic nihilism, as this remarkable physician condemned the majority of nostrums and remedies as useless, even harmful.

*Comroe JH, Dripps RD: The top ten clinical advances in cardiovascular-pulmonary medicine and surgery between 1945 and 1975: How they came about. Bethesda, Md., Public Inquiries and Reports Branch, National Heart, Lung, and Blood Institute, National Institutes of Health, 1977.

Slowly, specific therapies—insulin for diabetes, liver extract for pernicious anemia—or specific immunizations—diphtheria antitoxin, pneumococcic antisera—appeared. But it was not until the decade 1935–1945 that the entry of sulfonamides and penicillin into clinical medicine made curable a large number of previously lethal and untreatable diseases. It is customary to date the beginnings of modern medicine from these relatively recent events.

The language of contemporary biologic science has become increasingly biochemical. The compositions of organs, tissues, cells, organelles, and membranes have been defined. The biosynthesis and catabolism of hundreds of compounds have been elucidated. The regulation of body processes has been described at progressively finer levels, and in chemical language. Many pharmacologic agents are now understood in terms of specific loci and mechanisms of action. The expansion of new knowledge continues at a pace that is bewildering to all but experts in a given field. Current advances are particularly rapid in immunology, molecular biology, and peptide research. A beginning has been made in explaining human behavior in mechanistic terms, as more and more chemical mediators and pharmacologic modifiers are discovered.

We have entered a molecular age of basic biologic science, and molecular biology is now a well-recognized discipline. The molecular influence pervades all the traditional disciplines underlying clinical medicine. Approximately 200 inborn errors are now understood in terms of specific missing or abnormal enzymes or other proteins. There are more than 240 known abnormal human hemoglobins, and for each of these the precise structural defect in the DNA of the mutant gene can be defined. Membrane, cytoplasmic, and nuclear receptors for hormones and drugs are exploding upon us, and old as well as new diseases are being defined in terms of receptor abnormalities—for example, type II hypercholesterolemia and nephrogenic diabetes insipidus. Recognition of opiate receptors has led to the discovery of endogenous peptides (endorphins) with analgesic activity. Their localization gives promise of further understanding of the limbic system, affective states, and addictions. The number and function of neurotransmitters has greatly increased, and these and other advances in neuroscience portend exciting developments in understanding how the brain works. DNA sequencing techniques and restriction endonucleases now permit precise identification of the exact structural alteration of the gene in an increasing number of hereditary diseases. Gene therapy—both pharmacologic modification of specific gene action and physical replacement of damaged genetic segments—is now possible in experimental systems.

Much of the recent fundamental information in science has been obtained by the process of reductionism—the exploring of details, and the details of details, until all the smallest bits of the structure, or the smallest parts of the mechanism, are exposed to scrutiny. The scientists responsible for our evolving understanding of biologic systems know that the reductionist approach must often precede reconstitutive endeavors. Scientific progress rests on myriads of small observations, tedious measurements, and the findings of investigators asking humble, answerable questions. Instead of reaching for the whole truth, the scientist examines small, defined, and clearly separable phenomena. The pattern of science is a stepwise extension of what came before, with an occasional quantum leap forward through great discovery.

The examples of advances in medical science mentioned above have been largely drawn from the areas of ultrastructure, biochemistry, and molecular biology. In biology these disciplines have arbitrary and porous boundaries: physiology, pharmacology, neurosciences, cell biology, molecular biology, biochemistry, immunology, biophysics—all are in a phase of confluence, and the common language is chemistry. Medicine is not only a branch of applied biology, however. It also subsumes many aspects of psychology, sociology, anthropology, and economics. These disciplines, too long neglected or denigrated as "soft science," are now increasingly recognized as germane to medicine as a discipline and the practice of medicine as a profession.

Critics of the bioscientific strategy of medicine have claimed that the great advances that have dramatically reduced mortality rates consist in the improvement of the environment, the correction of malnutrition, and the control of infectious diseases through immunizations and antimicrobial agents, and that the relevant medical breakthroughs largely occurred before the prodigious expansion of federal support of biomedical science began in the early 1950's. They contend that the enormous expenditures that have made the United States preeminent in biomedical research have produced too little in the way of medical advance to justify their continuation, and have instead fostered the development of an extremely costly technology which has had only a minimal effect upon mortality statistics. They propose that the bioscientific strategy of medicine should be replaced by an ecologic strategy for health.

These critics ignore several important realities: (1) A bioscientific strategy for medicine and an ecologic strategy for health are not mutually exclusive, and both may be valid. (2) Major advances have occurred since 1950 that have revolutionized the outlook in individual diseases or disease groups—for example, in Hodgkin's disease, acute lymphocytic leukemia of children, Parkinson's disease, and Wilson's disease. (3) Such advances have rested in most instances on a deeper and clearer understanding of underlying disease mechanisms. (4) The elucidation of a disease mechanism and the devising of rational therapy usually depend upon the application of basic scientific knowledge to a clinical problem in the laboratory or clinic—for instance, the definition of pathways and rates of purine synthesis led to the development of a xanthine oxidase inhibitor (allopurinol) for the control of hyperuricemia and hyperuricaciduria. (5) The expansion of the knowledge bank of the past quarter century justifies great optimism for the eventual control and cure of major diseases and the possible elimination of premature death from illness.

The list of human diseases for which there are as yet no definitive measures for prevention or cure is still formidable. Fresh insights into the nature of these diseases are needed. These insights can come only from continued basic research. Those who believe that there is an abundance of scientific information locked in the laboratory merely awaiting a new emphasis on human application are mistaken. Those who believe that a series of crash programs will lead to ready cures of cancer and heart, vascular, arthritic, emotional, and mental disease are misled. The essential pieces of background information are not merely awaiting assembly; most have yet to be discovered.

The practice of medicine is both a science and an art. A skilled physician must have extensive medical knowledge, which is the bedrock of technical competence. In addition, he or she must have judgment, tact, decisiveness, restraint, compassion, interest, time, and other personal qualities of caring and dedication. The science and the art of medicine must always be intimately linked. The student studies the science of medicine first, masters it early, and returns to it frequently. The student acquires the art of medicine—the skillful application of medical knowledge and judgment in the optimal care of the patient—more gradually and with experience.

THE PHYSICIAN AS A SCIENTIST. Since medicine is derived from a number of sciences relevant to the health of individuals or of groups, physicians must be trained as scientists to utilize these complex disciplines effectively.

To be a scientist the physician must have more than rote scientific knowledge, or even fluency in its particular jargon. Physicians must be conversant with the processes of scientific inquiry—how data are obtained and evaluated; how hypotheses are framed, modified, or discarded; the uses and limitations of inductive reasoning. In short they must understand science as an intellectual instrument which has been slowly perfected over centuries. Only in this way can they remain attentive to medical progress as a critical and independent participant. Otherwise they will be in danger of being the passive purveyor of medical fashions. Both the spirit and rigor of science are necessary for the physician to become and remain a scholar in medicine. Medical practice itself contains many of the elements of scientific inquiry in the pursuit and evaluation of data (history, physical examination, laboratory studies) and in framing a hypothesis (tentative clinical diagnosis).

As a scientist the physician is the beneficiary of both the fruits of scientific research and of the mental discipline of the scientific method. To a greater or lesser degree the physician also has the opportunity to contribute personally to medical progress. Most medical research is now carried out by teams of participating investigators in elaborately equipped laboratories which utilize the advanced instrumentation and technology of modern science. There is still scope, however, for scientific contributions made by inquiring physicians based on their own experiences in patient care. Much of medical progress has derived from this kind of curiosity in the past. In addition this form of clinical research, on whatever modest scale it may be engaged in, adds excitement and zest to professional life. As Thomas Hobbes has written: "Desire to know why, and how, curiosity, which is a lust of the mind, that by a perseverance of delight in the continued and indefatigable generation of knowledge, exceedeth the short vehemence of any carnal pleasure."

THE PHYSICIAN AS A HUMANIST. Since the physician deals with fellow human beings in need of help, the patient and the public logically assume that the physician is a humane and caring person as well as a competent practitioner. Yet a crisis of confidence appears to have beset modern medicine.* As the technology and complexity of medicine have increased, medical care has become more institutionalized and its delivery depersonalized. A widely held view, particularly among nonphysicians, is that the science and technology of medicine are responsible for the perceived decline of compassion in medicine. They seem to suggest that there is something inherently contradictory between science and humanity, between technology and compassion. There is, of course, no reason that scientific knowledge and compassion should be in conflict. Science and technology underlie most of the advances of medicine that enable contemporary physicians to render more effective medical care than their professional forebears were able to offer. Glick even views computed tomography as a technologic advance of extraordinary compassion. Its use has spared patients many more difficult, painful, and dangerous procedures, and has permitted definitive diagnoses to be made earlier. Physicians cannot be made more compassionate by downgrading science any more than students can be made more humanistic by study of the humanities, desirable though such studies may be in their own right. Nor can one validly claim a dehumanizing effect for long and arduous hours of training, for the arduousness of training has declined during the period of alleged loss of compassion in medicine. Glick suggests that "the fundamental problems lie for the most part outside the medical establishment, within society as a whole. The physician is largely a reflection of society. . . .Basic human character traits are well developed by the time a student enters medical school." He suggests that the prime examples of humane medicine are to be found in persons in whom service to humanity ranks as a higher priority than personal gratification. That characteristic is a reaffirmation of Hippocrates and of Osler, and of every other truly great physician. Its expression is enhanced, not hindered, by good science and complex technology, applied for the benefit of the patient.

*Glick SM: Humanistic medicine in a modern age. N Engl J Med 304:1036, 1981.

3. MEDICINE AS A PUBLIC SERVICE

James B. Wyngaarden

Medicine is a serving profession, one that exists not for its own sake but for the benefit of others. "The responsibilities of medicine are threefold: to generate scientific knowledge and to teach it to others; to use the knowledge for the health of an individual or a whole community; and to judge the moral and ethical propriety of each medical act that directly affects another human being" (McDermott).

We have already discussed the generation of scientific knowledge and the way in which scientific advances continually modify and extend the practice of medicine. It is in the application of an increasingly scientific medicine in a rapidly changing society that new and sometimes discomfiting issues arise. This chapter will briefly introduce selected issues faced by the physician in the practice of medicine as a member of modern society.

PATTERNS OF MEDICAL PRACTICE. Practitioners who apply medical knowledge for the benefit of patients are of two sorts: those who deal personally with individual patients, and those who deal with people as groups. We call the latter activity *community medicine*, which is a component of public health. In community medicine, group membership is usually determined by geographical location, or census tract. The members of such a community are not self-selected on the basis of perception of disease; rather, they are identified as members of the community on the basis of other common characteristics, usually location. At any one time a community will comprise many more people who are healthy than who are ill. Important functions of community medicine are the provision of appropriate health services for its members, the continuous surveillance of the population for discovery of individuals in need of care, and the creation of entry points for those so identified. These are large social challenges, as yet imperfectly attained. Marked unevenness in access to and in utilization of physician services remains a problem in most countries. In the United States these problems have been ameliorated but by no means solved by Medicare and Medicaid programs for financing of hospital and physician services. Important though these topics are, they are beyond the scope of this book, which is principally oriented toward the care of the individual patient. By and large the constituency described in this book consists of self-selected patients who consult a physician because of *dis-ease*, i.e., concern about their personal health.

Physicians who render personal medical care do so in a variety of practice patterns, ranging from solo practices to partnerships, to multispecialty groups, to full-time situations in an organized clinic or a medical school faculty, to Health Maintenance Organizations (HMO's) or Independent Practice Associations (IPA's). The traditional doctor-patient relationship, in which the patient identifies a specific physician as his or her own personal doctor, may exist within any of these practice patterns. Many patients want a personal physician who knows them, who is available for first contact and continuing care, and who offers a portal of entry to specialists for those conditions warranting referral. This type of practice, termed "primary care," characterizes activities of general practitioners, family physicians, and general internists, as well as of many pediatricians and obstetricians. Often their services are complemented by nurse-clinicians or physician associates. Physicians who see patients in referral for common conditions that do not require high technology, and who characteristically see them in an office or community hospital setting, are said to be offering "secondary care." Those who manage patients with complex illnesses requiring high technology, or the use of powerful, high-risk drugs or procedures, or highly specialized knowledge of limited availability, are said to be rendering "tertiary care." University hospitals and many large urban referral hospitals frequently function as "tertiary care centers." But categories of activities are not always clearly separable. Family practitioners and generalist internists and pediatricians normally concentrate on primary care. Community hospitals and subspecialists often practice a mixture of primary and secondary care medicine. Large teaching hospitals generally offer a full spectrum of services—primary care in their clinics, secondary care as a community referral center, tertiary care for patients who have complex medical problems or who are critically ill.

The provision of continuing comprehensive care has traditionally required a high order of accessibility on the part of the primary care physician. In the following essay, Dr. Thomas eloquently describes the repetitive interruptions of sleep that characterized the nights of his general practitioner father. In recent decades physicians have sought relief from the overwhelming physical and emotional drain of continuous availability with its potentially excessive cost to personal and family life. Solo practitioners arrange to cross-cover each other, partners arrange on-call schedules, and metropolitan physicians often refer nocturnal and weekend patients to emergency rooms. In some group practices, individual doctor-patient relationships have been supplanted by a team approach. These changes in professional mores reflect evolving attitudes on the extent to which compassionate behavior in the practice of medicine should be allowed to dominate a physician's time and personal life. The availability of the individual physician has diminished as the scientific competence of the profession has increased. Perhaps there is a relationship here. When no one in the profession had many answers to illness, and treatment consisted largely of evaluation and prognosis, the reassuring presence of the physician constituted in itself the fulfillment of the Hippocratic Oath. As the science and technology of medicine expand, no one doctor can any longer be expert in all areas and the care of the patient, when something is seriously wrong, necessarily becomes a collective effort. The personal interest of each physician continues to be essential, however, so that there may be a series of satisfying doctor-patient relationships. The patient usually wants one doctor as his or her personal advocate, regardless of the extent of sharing of medical responsibility.

THE PATIENT AS A CONSUMER. Some of the traditional and universal expectations of patients have been discussed in the initial essay, Medicine as an Art. The general trend toward greater consumer awareness has created many new patient expectations. For example, patients now understand a great deal more about the human body and its disorders than they did a generation ago. As a consequence they expect more detailed information from the physician. Science teaching has improved; even the principles of molecular biology are now taught in the grade schools. Newspapers, magazines, and television regularly inform the public of advances in medicine. Many communities offer health seminars to the general public. Home medical encyclopedias are widely available. The individual has been admonished to take personal responsibility for his or her own health through weight control, dietary discretion, limitation of intakes of saturated fats and of salt, regular exercise, moderation in or abstinence from smoking and drinking, attention to the purity of water and of air, and appropriate diversions from work. These measures are widely accepted as contributing to physical and mental health. For those with chronic illnesses there are primers prepared by voluntary health agencies or the U.S. Public Health Service. In many instances there are clubs to join, organized about a diagnosis (e.g, lupus erythematosus clubs) or a procedure (e.g., laryngectomy clubs). One can send a coupon and urine sample to test for diabetes, or have one's blood pressure checked at the supermarket. Ethnic groups at increased risk for certain diseases can avail themselves of screening programs for sickle cell disease or Tay-Sachs carrier status. Such measures and others have publicized medical progress and have kindled high expectations for imminent "breakthroughs." Such anticipations are often fanned by an overly exuberant press. All of these factors combine to place increased demands upon the physician to inform in greater detail, and to anticipate increasingly sophisticated inquiries from patients and relatives.

The public is also well aware that substantial tax dollars have been spent on medical research and on the production of more physicians since World War II. They have come to view excellent medical care and access to it as a birthright. For the majority of Americans these birthrights have been achieved, but important segments of our society and of many societies throughout the world are still excluded from optimal medical care by poverty, location, or both. For many of those with access to care the costs have become a preoccupation. The percentage of the American gross national product spent on medical care has risen substantially for two decades and is now about 10 per cent. In part this reflects the extension of medical care to many individuals for whom it was only marginally available in the past. In larger part this reflects the costs of progress in medicine. Drugs are now available to treat conditions that in times past could only be observed. New technologies in medicine permit diagnostic and therapeutic procedures scarcely dreamed of a decade or two ago. The rising costs of medical care are particularly pronounced in circumstances in which partial solutions are much more expensive than the ultimate cure is likely to be. The classic example is poliomyelitis. Current examples include the expensive technology of renal dialysis and transplantation for chronic kidney failure and of coronary bypass surgery and heart transplantation for coronary artery disease. Doctors control many of the expenditures in medical care and therefore must share in the serious concerns about its escalating costs. They decide on hospitalization, order diagnostic studies, prescribe the drugs patients take, or recommend surgery. Control of costs of medical care is a lively topic in the public arena.

The advancing technology of medicine has enabled more and more interventions in the natural course of disease. An increasing number of parts of the body can be replaced by transplanted organs or mechanical substitutes. The term "invasive procedure" has become commonplace in our lexicon. The potential of such procedures for diagnostic information or therapeutic achievement is awesome. Benefits of scientific medicine can now be proffered to patients thought beyond help only several years ago. When all goes well one is exhilarated by the wonder of the success. But high risk procedures in high risk patients cannot always go well. There are unanticipated complexities of disease, adverse biologic responses, genetic differences, flaws of judgment, variations in physicians' skills, mechanical failures. Often the doctor, or the hospital, or the pharmaceutical company is held responsible, sometimes for events beyond anyone's control. An example is the Guillain-Barré syndrome that followed influenza vaccination a few years ago.

DEFENSIVE MEDICINE. High technology medicine has carried with it a lowering of the threshold for litigation on the part of patients when something does go wrong. Some physicians respond by the practice of "defensive medicine." This has at least three components, each of which earns mixed reviews. The first is informed consent. In concept this is unassailable. The patient clearly has the right to have anything that is proposed fully explained in advance, and the right to give or withhold consent. Three or four decades ago informed consent was largely limited to anesthesia and operating permits. Today, in dual response to the consumer's rights movement and defensive medical postures, informed consent often involves written descriptions of procedures that include explicit accounts of every conceivable misfortune that has ever followed a given diagnostic test, drug therapy, or surgical procedure. Many alert, intelligent persons appreciate such candor, but some recoil in apprehension and forego needed therapy. A patient may acknowledge understanding the form and its attendant discussion, sign, and minutes later be completely unable to explain what was "understood" and approved. In such instances the practice clearly is not achieving its intended goals.

Defensive medicine also may extend the medical workup that a prudent physician will perform in a given circumstance. When clinical concern results in a thorough history, a careful and complete physical examination, and appropriate laboratory studies, roentgenograms, or special diagnostic procedures, the patient is clearly the beneficiary. But when studies of marginal validity are ordered or excessive consultations are requested, solely because of fear of potential litigation, the costs of medical care are driven upward to no good end. Yet physicians are often on the horns of a dilemma, often forced by the perception of their own best interests to exceed what is in the patient's best interest. Experienced physicians who are secure in their knowledge and competence will rely less on extensive studies and wide-ranging consultations than will more apprehensive or tentative doctors.

Defensive medicine also mandates the keeping of more thorough records. In case of challenge to adequacy or competence of care, the written record is the physician's defense. The record should contain all relevant data pertaining to the patient. It should also contain all important data pertaining to the doctor's opinions or conclusions, decisions, prescriptions, actions, and communications. The evolution of thoughts and responses should be clearly discernible from the record. If such entries are recorded at appropriately frequent intervals, an effective reconstruction of events is possible, should the need arise. These are, of course, all benchmarks of good medical practice. But the growing necessity for increasingly detailed documentation has its cost in time. When added to other items of escalating paper work in medical practice, this translates into reduced professional productivity. If defensive medicine benefits the patient the additional costs may be justified, but in terms of the aforementioned responses the cost-benefit ratio is at present unknown.

PUBLIC ACCOUNTABILITY. The privilege of practicing medicine is increasingly being coupled with accountability in the exercise of this stewardship. Private accountability has always been implied in the doctor-patient relationship. The entry of substantial public money into the field of medical care has also brought with it new forms of public accountability and regulation of medical practice. Facilities and equipment to be used for care that is subject to federal reimbursement require "Certificates of Need" and approval from the Health Systems Agency. Professional Standards Review Organizations now establish admission criteria, minimal and maximal limits of medical workup, and rules for documentation of medical practice activities. Federally sponsored patients admitted to hospital require "certification," and continuing stays in hospital require frequent additional justifications. If the validity of a more extended stay is challenged, the patient risks "decertification" and personal liability for subsequent expenses. These measures were enacted to assure quality of care according to consistent standards; the hidden agenda was cost control. Membership on hospital staffs involves clear delineation of departmental assignments, and of clinical privileges, also in the interest of "quality assurance." But in the final analysis quality assurance depends upon the ability of the physician; the quality of professional education and training; personal standards of performance, integrity, and dedication; and a lonely and resolute self-discipline. This is not to say that medical practices should not be exposed to public view and public accountability. They should and they will continue to be. Perhaps in time mechanisms will be found that are less onerous and distracting than those currently in use. The Federal role in medical care and practice will remain, although it may change. But the ultimate contract is between the patient and the doctor, and this relationship must be based on mutual trust and mutual respect. No amount of third party surveillance must be allowed to supplant that venerable tradition.

4. MEDICINE AS A VERY OLD PROFESSION

Lewis Thomas

I first heard the term "medical ethics" in my childhood, a long time ago. Then, it referred to a small set of unambiguous, nonphilosophical matters worried over only by doctors and their families and related exclusively to money. Doctors who advertised, overcharged their patients, surreptitiously took over the care of patients already being looked after by another doctor, or split fees with other doctors were unethical and that was what the word meant. Doctors who performed abortions were not unethical, they were immoral or criminal, or both. Human experimentation was not unethical because there was no such activity, or perhaps it is better to say that it was not realized, even by practicing doctors, that experiments were performed on patients in the normal course of medical practice.

This was a time ago and medicine has changed a great deal, more than is remembered by most people, changed so much that even those old enough to have lived though the whole period have difficulty in recognizing the connections between the old enterprise and the new one. For, in a certain sense, it is like that: it is as though we gave up altogether one kind of profession called medicine and then took up another one. A long look backward is needed to see the change.

I am just old enough to take that sort of view, first-hand, having been born into a doctor's family during the last decades of the profession's former existence as an applied art, then growing up in a household sustained by that endeavor, then being trained as a doctor at the very turning point when it began to change into something like a science, and finally pursuing a career in the profession which was the result of that evolution. In those years it was easier to shift from one field to another, perhaps because the requirements for deep expertise were less demanding in the absence of so many detailed facts to comprehend. Thus, I had a close professional look at several disciplines along the way: pediatrics, internal medicine, pathology, infectious disease, immunology, and administration. All of these have changed so much in recent years that I cannot imagine people climbing over departmental walls and specialty boards so easily. On the other hand, I do envision a time ahead when the clinical sciences will come to share the same ground in their base of knowledge. Before long, a post-M.D. period of training in internal medicine and molecular genetics might serve to prepare a young graduate for almost any discipline, in the kind of medicine that lies somewhere ahead.

My father began the practice of medicine in 1905. He was a busy and successful general practitioner for most of his life, switching to become a self-trained and self-certified surgeon in his latter years, as was the custom at that time. During all his years in general practice he possessed only small bits of science, used solely for the purpose of diagnosis, and almost no science at all for therapy. What he did, for treating disease, was to "look after" people. This was all he, or anyone else, knew how to do, and it had little to do with technology. Indeed, if it became known in the small town I grew up in that a doctor had become locally famous for his technical capacity to treat this or that disease, the question of medical ethics was automatically raised by the local establishment. Claims for being able to treat disease were almost, not quite but almost, grounds for being charged with quackery, and usually the charge was warranted. In those days quackery abounded.

Not to say that treatments for illness were not used by doctors, but these were more like gestures of reassurance, sometimes like incantations or amulets. Prescriptions were written in Latin of great complexity for numberless compounds, most of them green and bitter-tasting but without any known biologic properties, issued for all kinds of complaints, but neither my father nor other doctors of this time had any real faith in them. The best that could be said for the treatments was that they did no harm, which, by the way, was considerably more than could be said for the medicine of his father's time, or his grandfather's. I don't recall ever hearing about a suit for malpractice during my father's professional lifetime. The question simply didn't arise. Nobody could possibly have been damaged by the therapy available, even less by omitting it.

The doctors of his generation were mostly passive, and the things they did in their practices were mostly watching and waiting. They had been educated at the end of the first great revolution in medicine, and a large part of their education emerged out of the destruction and abandonment of masses of misinformation which preceding generations of physicians had taken for granted.

For a great many centuries, the technology of therapeutic medicine had been based on something rather like pure guesswork, and anybody's theory stood a good chance of being incorporated into dogma for the generations to follow. It was taken for granted that medicine, to be effective, had to be a strenuous, perilous sort of enterprise, and if things like these were not done the most ordinary kinds of illness would surely end fatally. There was no disease for which a treatment was not recommended. It is sometimes complained by today's medical students that the mountains of reductionist facts to be learned and set in memory are more than the mind can cope with, but the students just before my father's generation had a lot more to complain about. Looking through any textbook of medicine or pediatrics in the last years of the nineteenth century must have caused the learner's heart to sink. Every other page is filled with bizarre, esoteric pieces of therapy, each one to be performed exactly as laid out and learned (since none of them made any intrinsic sense) by rote. Poliomyelitis had to be treated by injections of strychnine, the application of leeches over the spine, the administration by mouth of extracts of belladonna and ergot, potassium iodide, huge doses of mercurial purgatives, faradic stimulation of the muscles, bleeding, and cupping. Meningitis required all these things, plus the spreading of cantharides ointment over the head and spine, strong enough to produce large blisters. Since all patients were treated more or less alike, there were almost no controlled investigations, and chance observations were quickly turned from anecdotes to tradition. Even so esteemed and skilled a pediatrician as Abraham Jacobi wrote in his famous 1896 textbook, concerning erysipelas, "The recovery of a young man observed with such symptoms lately I attribute solely to the large quantities of brandy administered."

Bleeding had been the sovereign therapy throughout the century before my father's entry into practice. The conventional treatment for tuberculosis and rheumatic fever was the removal each day of about a pint of blood, or enough to cause blanching, weakness, faintness, and a palpable weakening of the pulse: early *shock,* in short, facilitated even more by calomel and antimony in doses arranged to produce violent diarrhea and vomiting. George Washington, by the way, is reported to have been treated for a peritonsillar abscess by the removal of 82 ounces of blood in his last, fatal illness. The point of all this was the doctrine, passed down through the centuries from Galen, that disease—any disease—was caused by the congestion of blood in one organ or another.

Protests against this kind of medicine had been raised as early as the 1830's, and a few observant physicians, here and abroad, took a careful look at what doctors were doing in the treatment of typhoid fever and delirium tremens and realized that they were doing a lot more harm than good. It very slowly dawned on the profession that a great many patients with various illnesses were capable of getting well all by themselves, without any treatment, and that many of the treatments then popular were probably making matters worse, but it took long decades before this kind of medicine was given up. At the same time, a genuine scientific activity, equivalent to the natural history of that day, got underway. Reliable classifications of human disease were constructed, based on careful clinical observations and correlated with the discoveries being made in the emerging field of pathology. Slowly but surely, during the latter part of the nineteenth century, the natural history of disease came to dominate medical education, and the art of making an accurate diagnosis and forecasting the likely outcome of every illness became the highest skill and the indispensable craft of the practicing physician.

This is what the doctors of my father's generation were trained to do. At the same time, largely under the influence of Sir William Osler, they were trained to be skeptical about treating disease. There were a few things they could do, but only a few. Malaria could be treated with quinine, digitalis was used with skill for heart failure, and morphine was the great standby—the most respected of all the drugs in the pharmacopoeia—for pain.

By the time I arrived in medical school in the mid-1930's there had been a few genuine advances, but still only a few: liver extract for pernicious anemia, insulin for diabetes, the early vitamins, immunization against diphtheria and tetanus, antiserum for pneumococcal pneumonia, not much else. I was taught at Harvard Medical School, as my father had been taught at Columbia, that treating disease would be the least of my future responsibilities. The doctor's job was to recognize the nature of disease with precision, so that he could explain to the patient, and to the patient's family, what was happening to him and how it was most likely to turn out.

This task, the explaining of illness, was the most important part of what was then called the art of medicine. It still is. Indeed, it has been a central duty of medicine, justifying all those millennia of the profession's existence, dating all the way back to our origins in shamanism. When you think about it, the first thing a sick person wants to know—and the sicker he is the more urgently he wants to know it—is "What's gone wrong?" And, in the same breath, "What happens next?" "Am I going to live?"

The quality of medicine's answers to these questions, and therefore the very usefulness of the doctor, were always matters of doubt until the great medical reform of the late nineteenth century. By the time of Osler, and in the decades that followed, science became the basis for explanation, and the answers became correspondingly more reliable.

It is easy to see why the mere act of explaining was so important, once you realize what being ill was like in the era before the discovery of antibiotics and the nearly successful conquest of infectious disease. Living was a considerably more chancy enterprise then. If you developed typhoid fever, which was still a common illness in the early years of my father's practice, you knew you were in for two months of constant high fever, deep malaise and debilitation, and the risk at any time of hemorrhage or perforation of the intestine. You had about one chance in four of dying. If it was lobar pneumonia, which was the most common serious infection when I was a medical student, you had the prospect of dying or recovering spectacularly on your own within a shorter period—two weeks or so. The greatest danger of all, feared by everyone, was tuberculosis. People worried then about TB as they worry now about cancer, but for better reasons; people of all ages died from tuberculosis, and there was nothing at all to be done about it. Rheumatic fever, the cause of rheumatic heart disease, was the first thing to worry about whenever a young child developed a sore throat, and if you didn't worry about this you had to worry about poliomyelitis. The chief cause of insanity, filling the state hospitals of that time, was syphilis of the brain.

It was an enormous relief to be told that you or your family had none of these things the matter, and this was the function of a good doctor. But there was, of course, a lot more to the practice of medicine than simply explaining things.

When I was starting out as an intern, swept off my feet by the new demands for science in treating infectious disease, I used to wonder what my father did to keep so busy in his practice back in the days when there were no sulfonamides, no penicillin, no way of treating anything. Throughout my childhood, the telephone rang all day and all night in our house, and I remember waking up most nights at the sound of my father heaving out of bed and off in the family car on house calls, carrying along his black doctor's bag which contained almost nothing of any real value. There was nothing exceptional about his practice; this is what life was like for all the doctors in town when I was growing up. And yet, there was very little that he could do. He was, by the way, fully aware of this himself, as were his colleagues; he used to complain sometimes that most of the time he felt helpless; he was never really convinced that anything he did made a real difference to the outcome of an illness, in any of his patients, in all his life in medicine.

There is a mystery here, and it is an aspect of medicine that has been forgotten by too many people, doctors and patients alike. Once the nature of the illness had been identified for what it was, and the news conveyed to the patient, several other things happened. First of all, the doctor took on the responsibility for the outcome, for better or worse. And, perhaps most important of all, he stood by. Standing by was, getting down to brass tacks, what the doctor did: he might not have anything much in that black bag, and no magical potions to serve up, and certainly nothing that he could put into or get out of a computer, but he did have his presence, and that made a difference. Sir William Osler used to teach that it could make all the difference in the world: if the doctor understood what was occurring in his patient, and made that understanding available, and made himself available at the same time as a source of hope and strength, these acts of professional skill could turn the tide. I believe these things, even though I do not understand them.

I have one other piece of reminiscence about the medicine of 50 years ago, which has some bearing on the general problem of the future of medicine and medical science. It is this: 50 years ago, just before the profession underwent its transformation and the art began to incorporate science and technology, no one had the ghost of an idea that anything was about to happen. It was taken for granted by my generation that the medicine we were being taught in the year 1935 was precisely the medicine that would be with us for the rest of our lives. We expected nothing to change. If anyone had tried to tell us that the power to control bacterial infections was just around the corner, or that open-heart surgery or kidney transplants would be possible within two decades, or that some kinds of cancer would be cured by chemotherapy, or that there would soon be within reach a comprehensive biochemical explanation, in the most reductionist detail, for genetics and genetically determined diseases, we would have reacted in blank disbelief. We had no reason to believe that medicine would ever change. We knew that subacute bacterial endocarditis and tuberculous meningitis were always fatal; we regarded schizophrenia as a totally unapproachable and insoluble problem; we believed that mental retardation was an act of nature for which we would never have an explanation, much less a treatment. All this has, of course, changed. Tuberculosis has vanished as a threat to the life of young children. There are so many new clues to the underlying mechanism of neoplasia that it is now a problem to make the right choice of a research line to pursue; senile dementia is out in the open, recognized now as one of the great challenges to medical science in our time.

And so forth. What this recollection tells me is that we should keep our minds wide open to the future. It is going to be different, whatever we think today. And, since change is inevitable, we should be spending more of our thought and energy making sure that the air is right for changes that seem to be in the right direction. This means, from my point of view, which I acknowledge as being self-interested and wholly prejudiced, more science.

We cannot go back to the old days in medicine. We should never allow ourselves to forget the healing property of a physician's presence and we should hang on to this mysterious gift even though we cannot explain it, but we cannot return to the era when that was all there was in medicine. We are nowhere near yet to where we should be; we are beset all around by the imperfections in our profession; we do a lot of things the wrong way and neglect doing essential things we could be doing better; even so, there is no prospect for changing medicine for the better in the years ahead except through science, more and profounder science.

But when people in my position say things like this we are well advised to add a cautionary footnote or two. We are always at risk of sounding like making too many promises, and speaking out of hubris, and we are not as candid as we ought to be about the extent of our ignorance. We are not about to change the world, nor are we in possession of a level of scientific understanding so powerful as to frighten people with what we might do next. We are, I'd say, *pretty* good at using science in medicine, but, thus far, only pretty good.

I wish there were some formal courses in medical school on Medical Ignorance; textbooks as well, although they would have to be very heavy volumes. We have a long way to go.

It is easy, these days, to look ahead. Medicine is being transformed before our eyes, and the power of our technologies for diagnosis and treatment is increasing with every month's new journal.

But I do not foresee any real change in the fundamental responsibility of doctors. Whatever they may gain in the way of technology in the decades ahead, I hope that they will be bound by the same deeply personal obligation to serve their patients. I hope my profession will never lose the memory of this obligation, for it is all we have in the way of historical continuity, the only real link to our professional ancestors.

I remember a short story from real life which illustrates an aspect of the responsibility of doctoring which does not find emphasis in many textbooks of medicine. Some years back I was invited to give a lecture on antibiotics at the annual meeting of a county medical society in a remote part of Mississippi. The audience was almost entirely made up of general practitioners, real country doctors. For the president of the society, a man in his 40's, this meeting was the major event of the year and one of the major occasions in his professional life; he was to be inducted formally into the office of president and had his speech prepared and ready. Just as the meeting began he was handed a note and left the auditorium to take a telephone call. That was the last I saw of him until three hours later, when he came back looking tired and worn out. I knew that he was deeply disappointed to have missed what should have been his own professional triumph, and I asked him what had happened. It was a call from a family of an elderly patient of his who had just died, he said. He felt that he ought to be there, to help the family, and to be useful. He simply had to be there, he said.

This was about 30 years ago, but I've never been able to forget that doctor and his example of good doctoring that evening. It's not quite the same thing as open-heart surgery or curing meningitis, but if I were looking around for a role model for today's medical students to look at very closely, I'd pick that country doctor in the backwoods countryside of Mississippi, if I could find him.

5. ETHICS IN THE PRACTICE OF MEDICINE

Albert R. Jonsen

"The responsibilities of medicine are threefold: to generate scientific knowledge and to teach it to others; to use the knowledge for the health of an individual or a whole community; and to judge the moral and ethical propriety of each medical act that directly affects another human being." With these words, Dr. Walsh McDermott opened his chapter, Medicine in Modern Society, in earlier editions of this textbook. Textbooks of medicine communicate the knowledge that con-

stitutes the science of medicine and explain its application in the art of medicine. The third responsibility, "to judge the moral and ethical propriety of each medical act," is not expounded in the textbooks. Yet no one enters the profession of medicine without becoming vividly aware of its ethical tradition. The science and the art are imparted to students along with implicit ethical imperatives: to seek the patient's benefit, to avoid harm, to be respectful and compassionate, to preserve confidences, and to maintain competence. Medical students see these values embodied in their best professors, although as Louis Lasagna has said, students "may quickly absorb the moral atmosphere around them without questioning it." Physicians praise these values in their best colleagues, past and present. Some physicians fail to honor this ethical tradition; social and financial influences exert counterforces against it. Still, the ideals are clear and their vitality in the behavior of many individual physicians is remarkable.

The current revivial of interest in medical ethics was not stimulated by a plague of immorality among physicians. It has not arisen because there is general disdain of, or disagreement about, the general principles of medical ethics. Rather, it has been fostered by a growing awareness on the part of physicians and the public that these general principles often seem inadequate to new situations. In some instances, widely publicized events have dramatized this inadequacy: the "God Committee," which selected patients "of social worth" in the early days of chronic hemodialysis; the Karen Ann Quinlan case; the Willowbrook hepatitis studies. In addition, interested scholars from medicine, philosophy, theology, sociology, and the law have attempted to analyze critically the general principles and to discern how they apply to the contemporary science and practice of medicine. In this way, a new discipline has arisen, sometimes called "bioethics."

Although the issues discussed in this new discipline are compelling, the discussions are necessarily general and abstract. The physician, however, must make decisions about the care of patients; often, those decisions will have ethical implications. The general and abstract must become particular and concrete. It is not enough to have a sincere attitude about, for example, discontinuing life-support systems. It is not sufficient to read a moving essay on allowing the dying "to die in dignity." Attitudes and information must be transformed into choices and practice. When the occasion arises, the ethical problems in the care of a patient must be assessed as skillfully as the patient's medical problem.

Every physician is familiar with the method of organizing clinical information: presenting symptoms and signs, history, physical exam, laboratory data. The competent physician evaluates these elements in seeking a diagnosis and selecting a treatment. A parallel method for reaching an ethical decision can be formulated. In almost any sort of clinical-ethical problem—be it withdrawing treatment, obtaining informed consent, preserving a confidence, or allocating a scarce resource—the facts and values necessary for a careful assessment can be displayed and evaluated under four headings: (1) indications for medical intervention, (2) patient's preferences, (3) patient's quality of life, and (4) external factors. This chapter will briefly explain how these four topics can be helpful in reaching an ethical decision. Thoughtful review of the relevant facts and values can put order into what is often a very confused consideration. Orderly consideration may not, of course, always reach the most suitable conclusion, but it should help avoid the two extremes that often distort clinical-ethical decisions: rash and precipitate action or paralyzing indecision. Both extremes can lead to tragedy for the physician, the patient, the family, and the institution.

INDICATIONS FOR MEDICAL INTERVENTION. Patients approach physicians with the hope of receiving the benefit of improved health or care in illness. The habitual activity of a physician is to gather information from and about the patient and to evaluate it with a view to determining whether or not medical intervention can benefit the patient. Clinical judgment, in which informed and careful estimates are made of the probable benefits and risks of each step in diagnosis and therapy, reflects the primary ethical responsibility of the physician. The most ancient rule of medical ethics is the Hippocratic dictum, "As to diseases, make a habit of two things—to help, or at least to do no harm." This duty manifests the "principle of beneficence," which ethicists designate as one of the fundamental ethical principles. They define it as "the duty to help others further their important and legitimate interests. . . ."

In most encounters between physician and patient, fulfillment of this duty is ethically unproblematic (although it may be medically difficult). Patients can inform the physician of the legitimate interests they wish furthered: they wish their health restored, their pain and symptoms relieved, their disabilities alleviated, their fears allayed. Physicians often respond with actions which have as their goal some specific benefit corresponding to those interests: elimination of meningococci by administration of penicillin G, control of blood pressure of 180/115 by an antihypertensive agent, prevention of the symptoms of celiac sprue by a gluten-restricted diet, and so forth. The interests of the patient and the response of physician center on benefits which reflect the goals of medical intervention: (1) restoration of health, (2) relief of symptoms, (3) restoration of function or maintenance of impaired function, (4) saving endangered life, and (5) supporting the patient by counseling and education. While all of these goals are seldom fully attained, they are the objectives which define the benefits of medicine.

At times, however, it might be asked whether one or another of these benefits is, in truth, a "benefit" for a particular patient. This question may occur to physician or to family in circumstances in which the patient is no longer able to declare his or her own interests. Typical clinical situations in which this sort of problem appears are as follows:

Case 1. A 46-year-old man, with Hodgkin's disease, Stage IV, has been unresponsive to chemotherapy and is now profoundly immunodeficient. He goes into bacteremic shock and renal failure. Should antibiotics and vasopressors be used? Should the patient be dialyzed?

Case 2. A 69-year-old woman has multiple sclerosis, diagnosed 30 years ago. She is now paraplegic and has begun to experience mood disturbance and to show signs of intellectual deterioration. She is brought to the hospital for treatment of pneumonia. Should she be treated?

In these cases, the first important ethical consideration is also the important clinical consideration: what objectives can be achieved by medical intervention? The answer must not be sought in the expected immediate results of some specific clinical intervention, but in those fundamental goals of medicine noted above.

The first formulation of the ethical question must be a realistic assessment of what might be accomplished by intervention (both in terms of the nature of the accomplishment and the probability of its occurrence). In Case 1, the only goal likely to be accomplished is the prolonging of organic life. It can be argued that this, in and of itself, is not a proper goal of medicine. It is highly questionable that the physician has a duty to sustain and prolong human life when no prospect for any other human function is in view. The duty to prolong life in this sense has no roots in the history of medical ethics; it is an "artifact" of modern intensive care techniques. The physician's ethical obligation to initiate or continue treatment arises from the real probability that treatment will produce genuine benefit to the patient.

In Case 2, several of the goals of medicine can be achieved. Despite the woman's ultimate prognosis, she can be restored to her previous condition and be helped in a number of ways. In terms of medical indications, she should be treated. However, her own preferences and the future quality of her life are added considerations. These are treated under the next two headings.

THE PREFERENCES OF THE PATIENT. If benefiting the patient means furthering that person's best interests, the patient's preferences, in general, should determine what constitutes benefit and harm. Individuals are usually the best advocates for their own interests. Recent critics of medicine accuse physicians of "paternalism," of assuming, because of their dominance over patients, the right to judge what is in that person's interest. Certainly, the history of medicine reveals an ethic colored by paternalism. The Hippocratic Oath states, "I will use treatment to help the sick, according to my ability and judgment." The patient's "ability and judgment" are not mentioned. In the past, "compassionate deception" was recommended "for the patient's good." Informed consent is a modern notion. Contemporary medical ethics, in the opinion of some of its proponents, consists almost entirely of the debate over paternalism and autonomy.

Autonomy, the personal liberty to make one's own choices and plan one's own life, is one of the central concepts of ethics. All of us value it highly in our own lives. An ethicist has written, "To respect autonomous agents is to recognize with due appreciation their own considered value judgments and outlooks even when it is believed that their judgments are mistaken."

In the practice of modern physicians, paternalism and autonomy are seldom in stark contrast. Physicians may be deficient in communicating information; often patient's preferences are not elicited or are disregarded. However, most modern physicians consider themselves advisors and, when important questions arise about diagnosis, prognosis, and therapy, they will inform patients of their options and respect their preferences. The practice of informed consent is growing and the practice of deception waning. Still, there are situations in which serious ethical questions about autonomy must be asked. Two, in particular, occur from time to time in clinical practice: the refusal of recommended treatment for disorders felt by the physician to be critical for the patients, and the decision to treat or not to treat incompetent patients.

The problem of refusal may appear in two ways:

Case 3. A 46-year-old woman has all of the indications for coronary angiography. She is known to the physician as timid and fearful. In the office, she is extremely nervous. Her physician fears she may refuse angiography if told the risks. Should she be told?

Case 4. A 54-year-old man, brought to the emergency room, has signs and symptoms strongly indicative of myocardial infarction. He is alert and oriented. He refuses hospitalization and insists on returning home. Should he be restrained?

The physician's anticipation that the patient may refuse recommendations (Case 3) does not justify deception, even though disclosure should be careful and sympathetic. Grounds for this anticipation may be weak. Should the patient suffer adverse experience about which she was not informed, trust in the physician would be shaken. Deception fails to respect the patient. It undermines confidence in the profession. Should the informed patient actually refuse an intervention, efforts can be made to ascertain the motive and, if it is fear or misunderstanding, to deal with these. Actual refusal by an alert and competent person (Case 4) should be respected once the physician has made serious efforts to assure understanding and to ascertain competence. Similarly, if the woman with multiple sclerosis (Case 2) had no mental deficit, her refusal of treatment for acute disease should be respected.

Autonomy implies competence. Competence consists in the ability to deliberate about information and to draw conclusions: the conclusions need not be "true" or "sensible" or "correct." Clinical evidence of disorientation, confusion, psychosis, or even "peculiar judgments" when metabolic disturbance is suspected can cast doubt on competence. In the absence of clinical evidence of incompetence, it should not be presumed.

Case 5. A 32-year-old man known to his physician as a Jehovah's Witness has been treated for four years for peptic ulcer. He arrives at the hospital bleeding severely and refuses blood. He is lethargic and somewhat disoriented.

Case 6. A 19-year-old college student comes to the infirmary complaining of severe headache, malaise, and stiff neck. She has a fever of 39.4, and her pupils are contracted. Spinal fluid shows gram-positive diplococci. She refuses antibiotics but offers no reason.

In Case 4, the refusal of the patient with myocardial infarction to be hospitalized, no solid evidence of incompetence exists. The refusal of hospitalization possibly arises from denial, a common human psychologic mechanism rather than a mark of incompetence. The decision may be foolish and its consequences tragic. But the physician, after attempts at explanation and persuasion, does not bear responsibility for that patient's autonomous choice. Case 5 reveals a patient who is not, at that moment, competent. However, his history verifies long commitment to a doctrine of which, it can be presumed, he accepts the consequences. His refusal should be respected. The "reasonableness" of that doctrine, in the eyes of others, is irrelevant. Case 6 shows a person who, while appearing oriented, might be presumed incompetent. She has a high fever; she offers no reason for refusal, and the consequences of refusal are certain and serious.

Most ethicists acknowledge that if a person truly is incapable of deciding rationally and freely, a form of limited paternalism is ethical. It involves making judgments in a person's best interest *temporarily*—until such persons are again capable of doing so for themselves. Thus, restraining a person in the hospital whose insistence on leaving appears to arise from a metabolically altered mental state could be justified, but only until the condition clears. However, such paternalism is justified only when there is solid evidence to suspect lack of competence. Vague affirmations, such as "It's his sickness talking," or "She is too emotional to make the right decision," hardly meet this standard. In general, the ethical principle of respect for autonomy requires a physician to formulate a judgment about the best interest of the patient, to offer that judgment to the patient for consideration, and to abide by the patient's considered decision. When the patient has no ability to express such a decision, the physician should formulate a judgment based upon the best available evidence of that person's preferences: from past experience with the patient, from family and friends, from written directives, and so forth.

QUALITY OF LIFE. The phrase "quality of life" is used when people make judgments about the goodness or satisfaction of the life they are living, or about some part of it. It is a very subjective judgment: one arthritic patient might say, "My life is pretty poor quality. I've a lot of pain and not much mobility."; another might say, "I've got a lot of pain and not much mobility, but I have good quality life, since I can still read and listen to my music." At times it may be quite vague, as when one reads in a chemotherapy research consent form, "This treatment is intended to improve your quality of life; however, any treatment may decrease your quality of life." Doctors and patients alike are interested in life of high quality. In their dealings with each other, that interest dictates efforts to alleviate pain and symptoms, to stop the ravages of disease, and to allay fear and anxiety. Individuals are the best judges of the quality of their own lives. In recent years, however, the phrase has taken on a rather special meaning in medical discussions.

Those discussions often take place about a patient who is severely ill and whose only prospects are a life of pain or extreme limitation. At times, the patient's limitations may not be the result of a current acute illness, but of some other disorder, such as congenital retardation. Again, the patient's life might be one of deprivation or degradation. Still again, the patient may exist in a persistent vegetative state. In such cases, when acute medical intervention is needed, the question may be asked, "Is a life of such quality worth saving?"

The problems raised by this question are extremely complex. In general, three points should be made about the use of "quality of life" as a factor in clinical decisions. First, reports by the person who is living the life should be distinguished from the observations of other parties: the former have a higher claim to validity than the latter.

Second, physicians may be inclined to view only those features of life that are most prominent in their contact with patients, namely, the physical and the psychological. Yet persons with severe physical limitations may have vital intellectual lives. Persons with intellectual limitations may enjoy supportive social relationships. Persons suffering great pain may live profound spiritual lives.

Third, all quality of life judgments are value judgments. Some of these value judgments can be amply supported by reference to certain manifest facts, such as the perception that someone is in great pain or is depressed. Other value judgments are less dependent on facts and more on personal or social predilections or prejudices, such as disdain for persons of low intelligence, the unproductive, and the unsuccessful.

In clinical decisions, the former sort of value judgments legitimately carry considerable weight; the latter, in general, should not be influential (often such "moralistic" attitudes are implicit and have to be uncovered). There are two reasons for this: medicine has long attempted to eliminate moralistic judgments from clinical decisions and to care for suffering persons simply because they are suffering. Reliance on any such criteria starts one down the slippery slope: the terminally ill are judged worthless, then the mentally ill, then the chronically ill, and so forth. The tragic consequences of this reasoning have marred medicine's history in this century. The less dramatic, but still tragic consequences for patients of certain social and economic status or of certain "unacceptable" life styles have been frequently documented. Quality of life is, then, an extraordinarily subtle notion. Its meaning in clinical decisions must be carefully scrutinized and cautiously applied.

EXTERNAL FACTORS. The three previous themes bear on the well-being, the preferences, and the qualities of the patient as an individual. In addition to these, it is sometimes necessary to consider the factors external to the patient. These are the effects created in others' lives or in society by decisions made about the patient. Some of these are burdens: costs incurred by families, institutions, or society; hardships imposed upon relatives; dangers posed to other parties. Some are benefits: relief from hardships, protection of others, teaching and research potential associated with treatment. How are these external factors to be weighed in clinical decisions?

Certain external factors have long been branded as unethical: a physician prolonging useless treatment for profit alone; a family allowing a relative to die for the sake of inheritance. Others have been closely scrutinized and their role in ethical decisions carefully delineated: the use of patients for research purposes, the revealing of confidences for the benefit of others. The general rules are clear in these instances (although their application is often unclear). Except in very special circumstances, patients can be used for research only with their express consent, and, should the research procedure increase their risks, there should be some expectation of compensatory benefit to the patient. Confidences obtained in the course of care must be maintained unless there is well-founded anticipation that, because of lack of that information, notable harm is very likely to come to another party.

The influence of cost of care on clinical decisions is currently being debated. The import of this external factor on clinical decisions must be viewed even more cautiously than quality of life considerations. In principle, it is safe to say that only when patient preferences are unclear or unknown, when likelihood of benefit is low, and when the quality of the expected outcome is poor, the costs of continued care, for the family and for society, may become a legitimate consideration in deciding to forego life-sustaining treatment.

At the level of policy rather than of clinical decision, there may be determinations whether certain classes of patients should receive certain treatments, e.g., persons over or under a given age will not receive chronic hemodialysis; whether certain modalities of treatment will be developed and made available, e.g., a totally implantable artificial heart; whether a preventive modality should be developed in preference to a high-technology therapy. These policies should be designed not only in view of efficiency but also in view of the imperatives of distributive justice, the fair distribution of burdens and benefits throughout a society. At present, "the just allocation of health care" is being studied intensely by those concerned about medical ethics.

In general, policy determinations should not be decisive in clinical decisions about particular patients. Policy determinations should be made at that level where authority is properly situated, where public scrutiny can take place, and where information is available. External factors, while important, deserve the lowest priority in ethical decisions about patient care. Only when the objectives of honoring the patient's wishes and providing a benefit to the patient cannot be reasonably met should these factors be considered as important and decisive. Obviously, in any particular case, there will be discussion about the nature of these objectives and the probability of their attainment.

CONCLUSIONS. Ethical positions are neither entirely a matter of private preference nor a matter of general principles. They are a mixture of preferences, principles, and facts. The mixture is often confused. If it is the responsibility of the competent practitioner "to judge the moral and ethical propriety of medical acts," the confusion should be dispelled as much as possible. In each difficult case, the ethical perplexity should be clearly stated, the facts carefully discerned, personal prejudices exposed, and the relevant principles thoughtfully examined. This chapter has suggested a method for organizing these elements in view of a clinical decision. However, a method alone will not resolve the problems. Content, in the form of appreciation of ethical values and understanding of ethical principles, must be inserted into the method. Some reading should be done in the now voluminous and valuable literature in medical ethics. Consultation with persons familiar with these issues should be sought. Frank conversation with all involved, the patient, the family, house officers, and nurses, should be promoted. In this way, the practitioner will deserve to be called not only competent but also responsible.

Beauchamp TL, Childress JF: Principles of Biomedical Ethics. New York, Oxford University Press, 1979. *An excellent systematic treatment, more philosophical than practical, of the basic principles which should underlie medical practice and health care.*

Jonsen AR, Cassel C, Lo B, Perkins H: The ethics of medicine: An annotated biography of recent literature. Ann Intern Med 92:136, 1980. *A selection of articles from medical literature on the major ethical problems encountered by the practitioner of internal medicine.*

Jonsen AR, Siegler M, Winslade W: Clinical Ethics: A Practical Approach to Ethical Decisions in Clinical Medicine. New York, Macmillan, 1981. *A practical guide to frequent ethical problems posed to the practitioner; explains the four considerations of medical indications, patient preferences, quality of life, and external factors.*

Reich W (ed.): Encyclopedia of Bioethics. New York, The Free Press-Macmillan, 1978. *An invaluable reference work of comprehensive, concise entries on most of the issues of biomedical ethics.*

Reiser SJ, Dyck AJ, Curran WF (eds.): Ethics in Medicine: Historical Perspectives and Contemporary Concerns. Cambridge, Mass., The MIT Press, 1977. *The most complete anthology of historical and current literature about the leading issues of medical ethics.*

Walters L (ed.): Bibliography of Bioethics. Book Tower, Detroit, Gale Research Company, six volumes, 1975-. *A comprehensive compilation of citations of English language literature in medical ethics. Issued annually and available as Bioethicsline, a computerized information system of the National Library of Medicine.*

SUMMARY

These introductory essays have been both discursive and eclectic. Medicine is almost boundless in scope as we move well into the last two decades of the twentieth century. Although much has changed, there is much that has remained the same in its traditions and common purposes. Eight centuries ago Moses ben Maimon (Maimonides) prayed:

"Grant me an opportunity to improve and extend my training, since there is no limit to knowledge. Help me to correct and supplement my educational defects as the scope of science and its horizon widen day by day. Give me the courage to realize my daily mistakes so that tomorrow I shall be able to see and understand in a better light what I could not comprehend in the dim light of yesterday."

The *Cecil Textbook of Medicine* has been dedicated to furnishing "a better light" for more than one half a century. It is a privilege to be associated with this 17th edition of a book that has become an institution in medical education.

JAMES B. WYNGAARDEN AND LLOYD H. SMITH, JR.

Part II
HUMAN GROWTH, DEVELOPMENT, AND AGING

6. THE LIFE-CYCLE PERSPECTIVE IN MEDICINE

Herant A. Katchadourian

The perception of the individual in the context of the life cycle is essential for understanding patients and for dealing efficiently with their ailments and infirmities. In the seventeenth century Sir Thomas Browne wrote:

"Confound not the distinctions of thy Life which Nature hath divided, that is, Youth, Adolescence, Manhood, and old Age; nor in these divided Periods, wherein thou art in a manner Four, conceive thyself but One. Let every division be happy in its proper Virtues, nor one Vice run through all. Let each distinction have its salutary transition, and critically deliver thee from the imperfections of the former; so ordering the whole, that Prudence and Virtue may have the largest Section."

It is not merely convention that requires case histories to begin with a statement of the patient's age. Considerations related to chronologic age enter into the interpretation of the history of illness and the findings of physical examinations and laboratory tests. Since the prevalence and manifestations of illness are often age related, the fact that one is dealing with a child or an adult, an adolescent or an elderly person, significantly influences probabilistic judgments in differential diagnosis. At an even more fundamental level, the developmental phase itself determines the fact and nature of illness. Bedwetting or the presence of immature blood cells in the circulation does not carry the pathologic connotations in an infant that it would in an adult. Treatment, too, is age dependent, because the choice of procedure and dosage and even the expected outcome are significantly linked to age.

Even though a person's age is a chronologic fact, to declare that someone is a child or an adult implies that the life span is divisible into phases and that childhood and adulthood are definable periods within it. But despite their pervasive use, terms like *child, adolescent,* or *adult* have no precise medical definition. Even more ambiguous are terms that refer to various subphases of these periods, such as *late adolescence* or *middle age.*

Until the seventeenth century, there was no special emphasis on childhood as a separate phase of life in Western societies. In the Middle Ages, as soon as children could look after themselves, they simply joined the world of adults, dressed like adults, and shared adult work and play. Although some went to school, there was no age grading in classrooms, and the ten- and twenty-year-olds could be taught together.

The shift away from viewing children as miniature adults began with the Reformation and the Counter Reformation in the seventeenth century. The philosophies of John Locke (1632–1704) and Jean Jacques Rousseau (1712–1778) were important early influences in shaping modern views of childhood. It was only after children had been recognized by society as a class of individuals different from adults that physicians began to make the same distinction systematically. Thus, although references to diseases of children can be found even in the most ancient of medical texts (such as the Ebers Papyrus of 1550 B.C.), medical specialization based on the age of the patient dates back only to the middle of the nineteenth century, when pediatrics began to emerge as a distinct field.

Since the turn of the century, both social and medical perspectives of the life span have tended toward further differentiation. Our modern concept of adolescence was greatly influenced by Granville Stanley Hall (1844–1924), a leading figure in American psychology and education. During the last several decades, adolescent medicine and geriatrics have become fairly well established subspecialties, and there is growing interest in the specific processes and problems of adulthood itself.

There are several advantages to a life-cycle or life-span view. First is the extension of the developmental focus beyond childhood and adolescence, so that adulthood and old age also can be seen as dynamic and changing phases of life. This approach allows not only a more coherent longitudinal view of life but also a better understanding of its components over time and in a broader context. For example, sexual physiology and behavior make better sense if understood in terms of their varied manifestations at different phases of life and in relation to other significant biologic and psychosocial events occurring concurrently.

The second advantage of a life-cycle perspective is that it facilitates a multidisciplinary, integrative approach to human development and behavior. It furnishes a conceptual umbrella broad enough to incorporate a variety of views and approaches toward making cumulative sense out of the diversity of human life.

Finally, when the field of life-span developmental psychology has reached sufficient maturity, it may provide useful indices of the normative tasks and critical events that characterize the various nodal points and transitional periods of the life cycle. Such indices will help the physician assess the patient in a set of normative contexts and will facilitate more intelligent judgments in pathology. Furthermore, to the extent that such normative crises are predictable, there is allowance for anticipation and preparation to cope with them. The physician stands to gain from such knowledge not only in dealing with patients but also in the conduct of his or her own life. Although we share our patients' experiences only infrequently, in living out our own lives we are basically no different from those we set out to help.

On the other hand, the concept of the life cycle, like any other model or theory, is not a panacea. When theory becomes dogma, it entraps us into expectations that become self-fulfilling prophecies. By accepting the notion of "growing pains," we may be inclined to take lightly serious pain in a growing person. If adolescence is considered a turbulent period, then adolescents will oblige us by becoming turbulent. If middle age is expected to be a time for finding new directions, then middle-aged people may be inclined to throw away the worthwhile with the worthless in their vocational and personal lives.

Concepts like the cycle are useful at best as modest aids to our understanding the awesome complexity of human beings. Such concepts are not meant to be devices with which to wrap up life and put it in our pockets.

Brim OG, Kagan J (eds.): Constancy and Change in Human Development. Cambridge, Mass., Harvard University Press, 1980. *Contributions on topics in personality developments and socialization from a life-span perspective.*

Browne T: Part III, Sect. 8 of Christian Morals. *In* Religio Medici, Letter to a Friend, Urn-burial and Other Papers. Boston, 1878. *A classic in medical philosophy.*

Engel GL: Psychological Development in Health and Disease. Philadelphia, W. B. Saunders Company, 1962. *Psychological development in health and disease through the life span. Highly readable, psychoanalytically based synthesis by a distinguished psychoanalyst and specialist in psychosomatic medicine. Written primarily for medical students.*

Lidz T: The Person: His and Her Development Throughout the Life Cycle. New York, Basic Books, 1983. *A well-written, integrated account of human development through the life cycle by a well-known psychoanalyst and specialist in family therapy.*

Simons RC, Pardes H: Understanding Human Behavior in Health and Illness. Baltimore, Williams & Wilkins Company, 1977. *A multi-authored book by psychiatrists on human behavior through the life span with specific focus on each major phase. Readable and illustrated. Aimed primarily at medical students.*

Steinberg LD (ed.): The Life Cycle. New York, Columbia University Press, 1981. *An anthology organized around five life cycle periods for each of which the developmental issues of mastery and competence, identity and the self, and relations with others are examined.*

Sze WC: Human Life Cycle. New York, Jason Aronson, Inc., 1977. *An extensive collection of articles on psychosocial approaches to the human life cycle. Primarily written for social workers. Authors include well known past and current figures from psychiatry and the social sciences.*

7. DEVELOPMENT TO ADULTHOOD

Herant A. Katchadourian

The terms "adolescent" and "adult" are both derived from the Latin "to grow" *(adolescere)*: an adolescent is someone who is growing up, and an adult is someone who has grown up. Although this designation is overly simple to encompass the complex changes entailed in attaining adulthood, bodily growth and reproductive maturation are in fact among the cardinal events in this process. The period of life during which these biologic changes occur is properly referred to as "puberty," to differentiate it from the psychosocial developmental phase of "adolescence" with which it overlaps but does not coincide.

BIOLOGIC PROCESSES IN PUBERTY

The changes that constitute puberty have been classified by Marshall and Tanner as follows: (1) Acceleration and then deceleration of skeletal growth (the adolescent growth spurt). (2) Altered body composition as a result of skeletal and muscular growth, together with changes of the quantity and distribution of fat. (3) Development of the circulatory and respiratory systems, leading, particularly in boys, to increased strength and endurance. (4) The development of the gonads, reproductive organs, and secondary sex characteristics. (5) A combination of factors, not yet fully understood, which modulates the activity of those nervous and endocrine elements that initiate and coordinate all these changes.

These changes result in two major biologic outcomes that have profound psychosocial repercussions. First, the child attains the physique and physiologic characteristics of the adult, including reproductive capacity. Second, most of the major adult physical sex differences become established through this process, greatly enhancing sexual dimorphism in adulthood.

These changes are virtually universal but with important differences between normal individuals in the onset, order, and rate of growth at puberty. We shall be mainly concerned here with the general patterns.

SOMATIC CHANGES. One usually becomes aware of the onset of puberty through its somatic manifestations. But these are preceded by hormonal changes, which in turn are triggered by activities in hypothalamic and other brain centers. The precise mechanisms that determine the onset of puberty are as yet unknown.

Among contemporary Western youth, the first signs of puberty become apparent at about age 10 to 11 among girls and 11 to 12 among boys (see Fig. 7–1). There is, however, a wide range of normal variability extending from 8½ to 13 years for girls and 9½ to 15 for boys. Most children do enter puberty within these ages (95 per cent of girls show at least one sign of puberty by age 13½), yet perfectly normal exceptions are possible at both extremes.

Puberty entails a whole host of changes, some of which are shown in Figure 7–1. Each of these events has its own schedule and range of variability. The general sequence of these events is more predictable than the ages at which they are likely to unfold. Girls enter puberty consistently earlier than boys by about two years, but here again the magnitude of discrepancy depends on what is being compared; girls grow pubic hair a year and a half earlier, but breast budding antedates testicular enlargement by six months.

It is essential to appreciate the normality of this wide range of variability during puberty. The physician must be prepared to encounter adolescents of the same chronologic age with dramatic differences in physical appearance, depending on

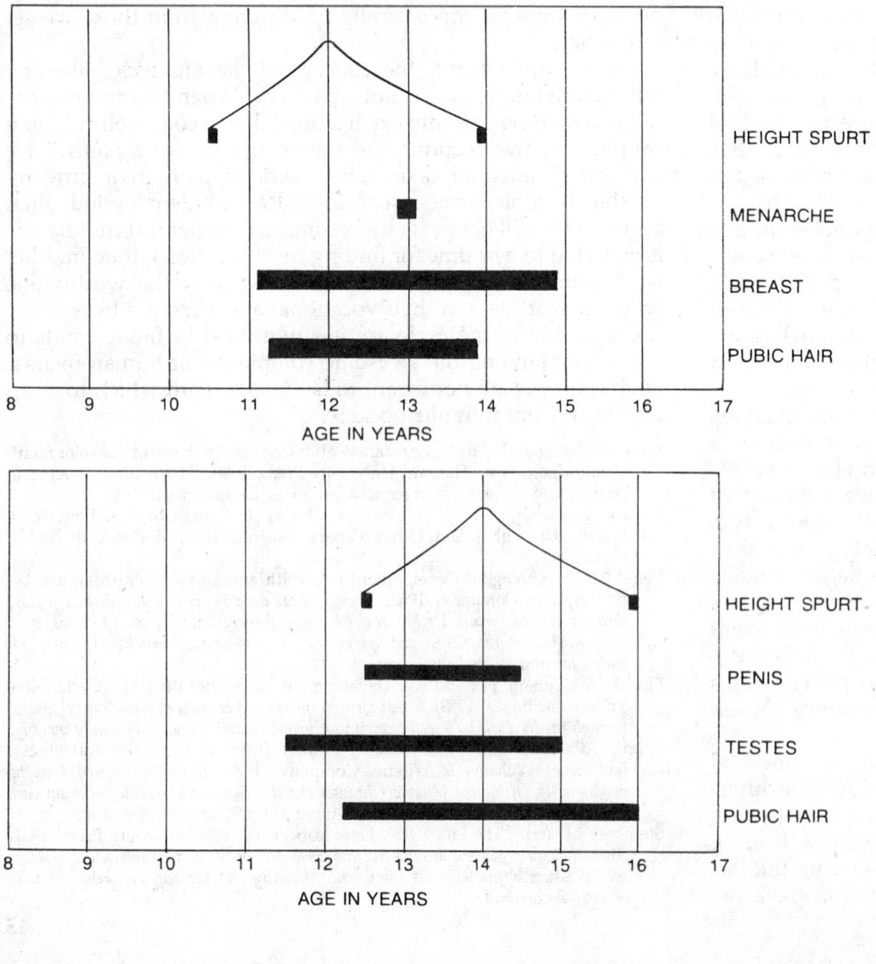

Figure 7–1. Sequence of events of puberty in girls (above) and boys (below). (From Tanner JM: Sci Am 229:40, 1973. Copyright © 1973 by Scientific American, Inc. All rights reserved.)

whether they have entered puberty, are part way through it, or have completed the process.

Height and Weight. The pubescent growth spurt is among the more dramatic events encountered during development. Growth in stature is in progress throughout childhood. Actually, by age 10, boys have already attained 78 per cent and girls 84 per cent of their adult height. What makes the growth spurt at puberty noteworthy is mainly its rate rather than its magnitude. The height spurt typically starts at about 10½ years among girls, reaches peak velocity at 12, and ends by 14. But it may start as early as 9½ or end as late as 15 years. Among boys, the onset is usually at about 12 to 13 (or as early as 10½ and as late as 16), the peak at 14, and the end at 16 (or between 13½ and 17½). During the year of peak height velocity, a boy grows on an average of 3 to 5 inches and a girl somewhat less. This means an actual doubling in velocity of growth and approximates the rapid growth rate of the two-year-old child. Following the growth spurt, the rate of growth decelerates rapidly. Most girls at 14 years and most boys at 16 years reach 98 per cent of their ultimate adult height. Further noticeable growth in stature ceases at about 18 years in women and at 20 years in men.

Stature is determined by a host of genetic and environmental factors. It varies among children as it does among adults. During puberty further differences emerge which are transient artifacts of discrepant rates of growth. Thus early maturing adolescents may move ahead of their peers but eventually end up no taller. How tall a youngster will be as an adult is generally of considerable consequence to the individual and the family. Boys are usually worried about not being tall enough and girls about growing to be too tall.

The gain in weight during puberty follows a similar pattern to height, but it is a more labile index of development than height. The nonskeletal growth increments are more marked than those for skeletal growth; by age 10, boys have gained only 55 per cent and girls 59 per cent of their adult weight. The factors that contribute to gain in weight are the increased size of the skeleton, muscles, and internal organs, and the amount of fat.

There is a marked sex difference between the amount and distribution of subcutaneous fat which contributes to shaping bodily contours. Infants accumulate subcutaneous fat (more in the case of females), but children gradually lose their chubbiness until shortly before puberty when they regain some of it. With the growth spurt a negative fat balance is established among boys, but not among girls, who usually enter adulthood with more body fat than males, particularly in the region of the pelvis and breasts.

Musculature and Strength. There is a marked increase in the size and strength of the musculature at puberty in both sexes but more so for males. This is the result of muscle cells becoming more numerous and larger. Among boys, the increase in number of cells is fourteen-fold; among girls, tenfold. In females, maximum muscle cell size is reached by age 10½, whereas in males muscle cells continue to enlarge until the end of the third decade.

Body Proportions. The difference between the physique of the child and the adult is determined by variation in body proportions as well as size. During puberty body proportions undergo marked changes, and when these are in progress they may become sources of concern and distress to adolescents who feel that they look neither like their former childhood selves nor quite like adults. For example, legs accelerate in growth a year before the trunk, contributing to the stereotype of the gangling adolescent. Leg growth itself is not uniform; the foot accelerates first (though it stops growing soon), followed by the calf and the thigh. Similarly, hand and forearm grow ahead of the upper arm.

The adult face becomes distinctive through changes undergone during puberty. The neural pattern of growth, which also characterizes the growth of the cranium, places it ahead of other systems in the developmental schedule. Thus, throughout the growth period the size of the head becomes progressively smaller relative to the rest of the body. With the growth spurt at puberty, which affects the size of the cranium much less than the other parts of the skeleton, this trend is further exaggerated.

Other changes affect the head itself. The bones of the face grow faster than those of the cranial vault, so that at puberty the face is said to "emerge from under the skull." The profile of the adult becomes straighter, the nose and the jaw more prominent, and the lips fuller. Facial appearance is further altered by the recession of the hairline and in males by the growth of facial hair. All these changes are more marked among males.

Some sex differences in physical features are present at birth and become further exaggerated at puberty. For example, the male forearm is longer relative to height and contributes to his stronger hand grip. Other differences that emerge at puberty include the male's broader shoulders, narrower hips, and longer legs relative to trunk length.

Internal Changes. Numerous internal changes accompany the more evident manifestations of puberty. The heart, like other muscles of the body, participates in the growth spurt and its weight nearly doubles. The steady rise of systolic blood pressure throughout childhood accelerates and soon attains adult values. The concurrent decline in pulse rate is checked, and there may even be a slight increase in the resting heart rate. Blood volume, hemoglobin, and the number of red blood cells are all increased. Lung size and respiratory capacity increase during puberty, whereas respiratory rate continues to decrease. These changes are more marked in the male, including a greater efficiency in oxygen exchange.

The net effect of these and related physiologic alterations in puberty greatly increases the capacity for physical exertion and allows quicker recovery from its effects. Greater exercise tolerance combined with superior strength permits individuals of both sexes to vastly outperform their prepubescent selves in physical effort.

Not all changes at puberty are in the direction of growth and better performance. The lymphoid system regresses markedly. Myopic children become more so, and many new cases of myopia appear during this time.

Reproductive Maturation. The maturation of the reproductive system is the quintessential mark of puberty. It involves the accelerated growth of the internal sex organs and the external genitalia, accompanied by the development of secondary sexual characteristics, which include the development of the female breast, the sprouting of pubic and axillary hair, the lowering pitch of the voice, and the appearance of facial hair in the male. In physiologic terms, the key events are the activation of ovulation and the menstrual cycle in females and the production of sperm and the ability to ejaculate in males. At least some prepubescent children have orgasmic capability but do not ejaculate semen prior to the development at puberty of the prostate gland, which produces most of the seminal fluid.

FEMALE REPRODUCTIVE MATURATION. Breast development is usually the first visible sign of female puberty; it starts between the ages of 8 and 13 and is completed between 13 and 18. Transient asymmetry is not unusual. Pubic hair ordinarily appears next, starting at age 11 to 12 and developing into the adult pattern by about 14; it precedes the growth of axillary hair by about a year. Breast and pubic hair growth follow predictable patterns that have been standardized and are used as indices of pubertal development.

The external genitalia become enlarged and their erotic sensitivity heightened. The internal sex organs rapidly increase in weight. Uterine musculature develops more fully, and the endometrium undergoes its elaborate cyclical changes following menarche. The vagina enlarges, with thickening of its epithelium.

Menarche does not commonly herald puberty as is sometimes erroneously assumed, but it is one of the late events. In the

United States, the average age at menarche currently ranges from about 9 to 18 years (mean, 12.83). Contrary to earlier assumptions that a secular trend of decreasing ages at menarche was in progress, current data show that the age at menarche has not changed for the past three decades at least among American middle class girls.

MALE REPRODUCTIVE MATURATION. The onset of puberty in males is signaled by enlargement of the testes, which usually starts between 10 and 13½ and remains in progress until ages 14½ to 18. Pubic hair growth occurs between 12 and 16. The growth of the facial and axillary hair lags behind by two years. The first ejaculation usually occurs at 11 or 12, but mature sperm take a few more years to appear. This relative pubescent sterility in girls and boys who have otherwise matured sexually does not amount to reliable contraceptive security.

The penis begins to grow markedly about a year after testicular and pubic hair development. Deepening of the voice results from enlargement of the larynx. It is a late event in puberty and much less marked among females. Some breast enlargement may be observed in males, which eventually regresses as a rule.

NEUROENDOCRINE CONTROL OF PUBERTY. A complex set of neuroendocrine mechanisms underlies the initiation and control of puberty. They involve the interaction of hypothalamic hormones, anterior pituitary hormones (somatotropin, gonadotropins—FSH, LH), and steroid hormones from the gonads and adrenal cortex (estrogens, progestins, androgens). Other substances such as thyroid hormones and insulin also take part in these regulating mechanisms.

The nature and actions of these hormones are discussed elsewhere (see Ch. 234 and 236). The precise mechanism that initiates puberty is not known. The hypothalamus, pituitary, gonads, and body tissues have the capacity to be stimulated into adult function long before the normal ages of puberty. This means that puberty is due to the further activation of an already functional system.

The current postulate is that as the child matures, the hypothalamic receptor sites become less sensitive to inhibition by circulating low levels of steroid hormones. Consequently, under hypothalamic prompting, larger amounts of gonadotropins are produced by the pituitary, which in turn increases gonadal hormonal output. Through continuing readjustment of the equilibrium between pituitary and gonadal activities, gonadal steroids required to suppress the hypothalamus reach a level that exceeds the threshold of sensitivity of peripheral tissues to these hormones, and the physical changes of puberty are set into motion.

FACTORS AFFECTING PUBERTY. A wide range of genetic and environmental factors influence the onset and course of events in puberty. The human pattern of puberty is the culmination of an evolutionary process starting with primates. The current pattern of puberty in humans probably evolved early and has basically not changed except for relatively minor aspects such as its time of onset.

The presence of racial differences in pubertal patterns remains unsettled. The force of genetic factors is discernible in familial tendencies. Randomly chosen girls reach menarche differing on the average by 19 months; for sisters who are not twins, the difference is 13 months; for nonidentical twins, it is 10 months; for identical twins, 2.8 months.

The influence of climate is dubious; that of seasons more certain: height increases twice as fast in the spring, and growth in weight is four or five times as fast in the autumn; during spring there is a significant reduction in the incidence of menarche.

Malnutrition stunts growth and will interfere with the pubertal process. The effects are selective, as growth of sexual organs is relatively less retarded than that of other tissues. Boys are more vulnerable than girls. Differences in menarchal age in various countries and between social classes are due at least in part to nutritional factors. The effects of illness are highly variable. Most acute conditions have no lasting effect; disorders specific to the endocrine systems in question will have profound influence (see Ch. 234 and 236). Finally, emotional factors have considerable bearing on the developmental process, but in ways that are as yet poorly understood.

PSYCHOSOCIAL DEVELOPMENT

A comprehensive account of psychosocial aspects of normal adolescence would include psychologic reactions to the changes of puberty; emotional maturation; sexual behavior; cognitive and ideologic development; identity formation; restructuring of parental, sibling, and peer relationships; school experiences and vocational choice; participation in the youth subculture; and socialization into the adult world. These events include so many complex variables and uncertainties that no concise and generally acceptable account of adolescent development is currently feasible.

A central question in adolescent psychology is whether normal adolescence is characterized by psychological turmoil. The concept that adolescence constitutes a stormy stage of life was dominant in psychiatric thinking (referred to as *Sturm und Drang*, or storm and stress); the view that "coming of age" need not necessarily entail turmoil has recently gained more credence through research involving adolescent populations at large rather than relying on extrapolations from clinical experience. A sensible compromise is to view adolescence as a labile period when emotional turmoil may occur, without either expecting that it necessarily do so or viewing youngsters who show no such distress as problematic.

Adolescent development is often assessed in terms of "tasks" the person must accomplish in order to successfully emerge from this stage. Beyond obvious requirements, such as the need to move toward economic self-sufficiency, the tasks that are set forth usually reflect a particular theoretical view or social value system. Some of these schemes are nevertheless quite useful for the clinician, because they provide a convenient framework in which to assess the young individual.

STAGES OF ADOLESCENT DEVELOPMENT. Tasks of adolescence are often subdivided as characterizing one of three subphases of adolescence. Thus, in *early adolescence* there is the task of psychologically integrating the ongoing somatic changes of puberty. Changes in body proportions and body image, menstruation, and enhancement of the sexual drive are among the developments that require psychologic adaptation and adjustment.

There is some reshuffling of peer relationships, but these remain largely nonsexual. Intense outside relationships begin to form as exemplified by strong attachments and "crushes." But the home still remains the center of the youngster's life.

The adolescent makes important strides in cognitive development at this time, constituting Piaget's stage of "formal operations." Starting with age 11 to 12 and going on to 14 or 15, this process endows the adolescent with the capacity to use propositional and deductive logic. The person can now reason abstractly, formulate hypotheses, and manipulate ideas in sophisticated adult fashion.

Similarly, Kohlberg has categorized stages of moral development that begin with "premoral" concern with avoiding punishment which is a carryover from childhood. The teenager then moves on to conventional role conformity to remain in the good graces of the family and to win approval. Only by about 16 or 17 are right and wrong understood as self-accepted moral principles.

Mid-adolescence raises the issues of dealing with family attachments and controls, revolt and conformity, participation in youth subcultures, further differentiation of gender identity, sexual experiences, and falling in love. *Late adolescence* is preoccupied by the task of self-definition and the identity crisis which, according to Erikson, is the phase-specific task of adolescence. The capacity for intimacy and more mature forms of love and sexual relationships characterizes adolescents approaching the threshold of adulthood.

RESTRUCTURING RELATIONSHIPS. Common social expectations require that the adolescent increasingly relate to others as an adult. This implies being less dependent and more dependable, along with a host of other expectations that are by no means consistently fulfilled by the majority of adults themselves. The most crucial set of relationships to be redefined involves parents or other adults on whom the adolescent is economically and psychologically dependent.

Anna Freud has proposed that this detachment or emancipation from childhood ties is managed through a number of psychologic mechanisms. One such mechanism is for adolescents to detach themselves from the parents by displacing their intense feelings of attachment for them onto other people and interests. If this occurs slowly, the youngsters experience periods of moodiness and other reactions akin to those seen in mourning over a serious loss. The need to become separate may make them act seclusive or be "like strangers" in the home. These feelings need not entirely dominate their lives and may well be hidden under the continuing cordiality they maintain with their parents as well as the new and rewarding experiences they begin to develop in relating to them more like adults.

A more abrupt expression of detachment is to run away from home. Some homes are so intolerable that this move is no less than an act of self-preservation. There are also many socially approved forms of leaving home, such as going away to boarding school or college, joining the armed forces, marrying prematurely, and so on, which may be at least in part motivated by the need to break away.

The attachment to others may take the form of friendships with peers, teachers, employers, or more distant figures such as rock stars or sports or movie figures to whom adolescents become uncritically and helplessly attached as they were earlier to parents.

A second mechanism is to reverse the feelings held toward the parents whereby love, dependence, and respect turn into various intensities of hate, revolt, and contempt. More often, positive feelings simply become tinged with ambivalence. This process is in part the result of seeing parents as they really are and in part a means of facilitating giving them up by dwelling on their shortcomings. Since it is safer and less painful for the conflict to be shifted from the private to the public arena, the fault finding may become focused on parental substitutes, public institutions, society, and the world at large. But youth can also be critical of society on justifiable grounds quite apart from personal considerations.

Another mechanism involves adolescents turning inward as it were and investing their own selves with the intense feelings formerly reserved for parents. This would account for the narcissism and selfishness of young people, their preoccupation with their bodies, and their inflated ideas of beauty, strength, and competence.

DEALING WITH DRIVES. Sexual behavior antedates adolescence, yet there is a distinct upsurge of sexual interest and behavior at this time. The forms that adolescent sexuality takes are influenced by culturally determined norms that vary widely in their level of permissiveness.

Masturbation is the most frequent means to orgasm among adolescents. Although this practice has lost most of its earlier condemnation, it remains a source of some embarrassment. Homosexual experimentation is not uncommon, but in only a minority of cases does homosexuality become the dominant sexual orientation. Currently, petting and coitus are an important part of the sexual life of many adolescents. Below the age of 15, fewer than one in ten has had sexual intercourse, but by age 17 one out of three high school students reports such experience. A national probability sample of 15- to 19-year-old never-married women (studied in 1976) showed 27 per cent to have had premarital sex (63 per cent for blacks, 31 per cent for whites). An estimated two out of five women and three out of five men attending college have engaged in coitus. A million teenage pregnancies a year and high rates of sexually transmitted diseases among youth confront physicians with serious challenges in dealing with the unfolding of sexuality in adolescence.

The expression of aggression in adolescence is a very serious social and medical problem. Violent deaths such as those resulting from accidents represent by far the leading cause of death in the second decade of life, accounting for over half of all deaths from all causes between the ages of 10 and 19. Homicide is the fifth most common cause of death among 10- to 14-year-olds. In 15- to 19-year-olds, homicide ranks second and suicide fourth. Young men aged 15 to 19 have the highest rates of committing rape; women in the same age group are the most frequent victims of rape.

IDENTITY FORMATION. Mainly as a result of Erikson's work, the concept of identity as the central task of adolescence has gained wide currency. The psychosocial transition to adulthood is accomplished during adolescence through the achievement of a sense of ego identity. In everyday terms, identity refers to a person's individuality, the response to the question of "Who am I?" The issue of identity is not settled once and for all during adolescence. What occurs at best is a clarification and reworking of earlier solutions and enough of a consolidation to provide the person with a self-sameness, even though many aspects of the personality continue to be reworked and refined in successive phases of the life cycle.

Two important components of identity are gender identity and gender or sex roles. Whereas biologic sex defines one as male or female, gender identity extends this definition to the realm of masculinity and femininity. Gender roles in turn express the public expectations of how one ought to behave based on these definitions. These culturally elaborated components of identity are closely interrelated. Thus, gender identity is said to be the private experience of gender role, and gender role the public expression of gender identity. All these facets of being a man or woman have profound effects on personality development and on behavior in health and in disease.

In more global terms, the criterion of attaining adulthood may be phrased in terms of achieving competence in a variety of spheres. Biologically, this means completing growth and becoming endowed with reproductive capacity. Psychologically, it requires a sufficient differentiation of the self whereby one can perceive the uniqueness of oneself in the context of other relationships. It implies the ability to recognize people as they are and to relate to them effectively. As a minimum, it entails being able to look after oneself as well as being able to look after others in one or another context of one's choosing. It involves the capacity to help run society and be run by it.

In the final analysis, the task of becoming adult and what it means to be adult resolve into philosophical quests about the meaning and purpose of life. These are not primarily medical issues; but to the extent that the physician at some level must deal with the patient as a person within a given social context, these considerations become relevant to medical practice.

Adelson J (ed.): Handbook of Adolescent Psychology. New York, John Wiley & Sons, 1980. *Comprehensive and in-depth coverage of all aspects of adolescent development.*

Erikson EH: Identity, Youth and Crisis. New York, W. W. Norton, 1968. *Chapter 3 provides a comprehensive account of the identity formation through the life cycle.*

Freud A: Adolescence. *In* The Psychoanalytic Study of the Child. New York, International Universities Press, 13:255, 1958. *A classic psychoanalytic contribution to the psychology of adolescent development.*

Grumbach MM, Grave GD, Mayer FE: Control of the Onset of Puberty. New York, John Wiley & Sons, 1974. *A detailed exposition of the physiologic mechanisms that trigger and control the process of puberty.*

Katchadourian HA: The Biology of Adolescence. San Francisco, W. H. Freeman, 1977. *A college level text on the somatic changes and hormonal regulation of puberty and the common ailments and health hazards during adolescence.*

Katchadourian HA (ed.): Human Sexuality: A Comparative and Developmental Perspective. Berkeley, University of California Press, 1979. *Sexuality, with special focus on gender identity and sex roles viewed from evolutionary, biologic, psychologic, sociologic, and anthropologic perspectives.*

Litt IF (ed.): Adolescent Medicine. Pediat Clin North Am Vol 27, No 1. Philadelphia, W. B. Saunders Company, 1980. *A symposium with numerous contributions on various facets of adolescent medicine.*

Money J, Ehrhardt AA: Man and Woman, Boy and Girl. Baltimore, The Johns Hopkins Press, 1972. *A comprehensive account of differentiation and dimorphism of gender identity from conception to maturity.*

Tanner JM: Fetus into Man. Cambridge, Mass., Harvard University Press, 1978. *A comprehensive account of physical growth and development from conception to maturity by an internationally recognized British authority.*

8. ADULTHOOD

Herant A. Katchadourian

INTRODUCTION

Unlike the pediatrician, who can turn to a vast literature on child development, physicians who deal with adults can find no comparable source of information on normative adult development. Until recently the prevailing view was that after childhood and adolescence, nothing of major consequence happened in developmental terms until toward the latter part of the normal life span, when the individual began to age. Currently gaining credence is an alternative viewpoint, whereby adulthood is seen not as a simple plateau interposed between the ascending steps of childhood and the descending steps of old age, but rather as a phase of life with its own discernible normative tasks and predictable transitions and stages. Although there is as yet no generally accepted developmental sequence for the adult years, and considerable disagreement over whether a stage theory for adulthood has any validity, knowledge accumulated in this field is of potential usefulness to the physician in understanding and treating adults.

ISSUES, CHANGES, AND STAGES

In attempting to understand the unfolding of adult life, the simplest approach is to identify those issues pertinent to adult life that are readily observable among a wide sector of the adult population. More ambitious is the attempt to delineate stages of adult development through which most individuals pass and which therefore constitute significant nodal points and predictable landmarks of adult life.

Factors within the first category are easier to identify, but because of their ubiquity and high variability they are also more difficult to systematize. Similarly, innumerable variables can be identified in the social realm in terms of the various adult roles individuals take on, maintain, change, or abandon. For example, a large segment of the adult population goes through the sequence of courtship, marriage, parenthood, and separation from grown-up children. Similar sequences exist in vocations and other social realms. Yet the voluminous social science literature that elucidates these issues does not always help us understand how these events fit into a life-cycle perspective.

Investigators have identified certain trends that are characteristic of some phases of adult life. Neugarten, for example, has described an increased tendency during middle age toward "interiority," which consists of increased emphasis upon introspection and stock-taking and conscious reappraisal of the self. Another characteristic of middle age is a change in one's perception of time. Whereas in earlier years the individual reckons time in terms of "time lived," with middle age the focus shifts to "time left to live." Although younger individuals are quite aware of their mortality, it is experienced in more personal terms during middle age and later, when a shift occurs from more abstract concern about death to a more personalized perception of its certainty and significance to one's everyday life. Additional discriminations between age groups center on attitudes toward the self and others. For instance, age-related responses have been obtained to questions such as whether marriage has been a good thing, whether parents are a cause of problems, and the possibility of changing careers (Gould).

Of various stage theories, the most widely known is Erikson's eight phases of the life cycle. In Erikson's view, the psychosocial transition to adulthood is accomplished during adolescence (Stage V) through the achievement of a sense of Identity, which in turn makes possible the establishment of a sense of Intimacy, the first phase-specific task of adulthood proper (Stage VI). Erikson defines these phase-specific tasks in terms of polar opposites of successful outcome or failure. Thus the counterpart to Intimacy is Isolation. Stage VII revolves around the issue of Generativity versus Stagnation. Using a heterosexual paradigm, Erikson sees as the central task at this phase the establishment of the next generation through the production and care of offspring, or, alternatively, through other altruistic and creative acts. The final phase of adult life confronts the task of Integrity versus Despair and Disgust. Integrity is the outcome of having taken care of things and people, originated others and generated things and ideas, and adapted to triumphs and disappointments. Because adulthood has received less attention in Erikson's work than adolescence, a great deal of Erikson's thinking about the derivatives and precursors of these adult stages of development has yet to be enunciated.

A more recent attempt to delineate stages in development comes from the work of Levinson and his associates. So far, this investigation has reported on male subjects between the ages of 18 and 45 only. Developmental phases in the lives of these men have been discerned to consist of the following: First is a transitional phase ("leaving the family") that usually stretches from the end of high school into the early twenties. During this period the young man may go through a phase of institutional living outside the home, such as in college or the military. Or, should he join the labor force, he may continue living at home but substantially outside parental control. Next is the phase of "getting into the adult world," which extends from the early twenties to the end of the twenties. During this period an initial definition of oneself as an adult is attained, and the individual fashions an initial life structure providing a link between the self and the adult world. This is a time of exploration and choice, when provisional commitments are made to an occupation. Those who resist making even tentative choices tend to develop a desperate need to settle down later on, or forfeit the chances of ever forming a reasonably satisfying life structure. Next is the "age 30 transition," a phase one passes through between the ages of 28 and 32. Like all transitional periods, this phase may be characterized by considerable turmoil, confusion, and struggle within oneself and with others, or it may simply entail a quiet reassessment of one's state and moving on.

The next period, "settling down," extends to the end of the thirties. The person now makes deeper commitments, investing more of himself in work, family, and other interests. There is a strong tendency toward maintaining order, stability, and security, while simultaneously striving to move ahead in order to "make it." In conflict with both these tendencies is the residual need to be free and unfettered. An important component of the settling-down period is "becoming one's own man," which typically is accomplished between the ages of 35 and 39 and represents the high point of early adulthood. During this phase a man has a profound need to be affirmed by society in the roles that he values most. In most instances this need involves some key event in the person's vocational career.

The "mid-life transition" ushers in another turning point, in which, irrespective of past accomplishments, the person confronts the issue of disparity between what has been gained and what one wants for himself. Major issues include the sense of bodily decline and recognition of one's mortality. There is a more acute sense of aging and further reorganization of the person's sense of gender identity. The crucial issue at mid-life is the changing relationship to the self. The mid-life transition occurs around the age of 40 and usually encompasses several years. By the mid-forties there is a period of restabilization that ushers the individual into middle adulthood.

CRISES OF ADULT LIFE

Traditionally the menopause has served as an example of mid-life crisis. It represents a fairly discrete biologic event, and its psychologic repercussions have been taken to constitute a coherent entity. Physicians who treat middle-aged women could testify to having seen countless such cases (see Ch. 236). Yet when examined within a broader population base of women at large, the menopause emerges as a very different entity. For instance, in one nonmedical sample studied by Neugarten, only a few of the women viewed the menopause as a major source of worry. (The women were much more concerned about getting older, developing cancer, or losing their husbands.) Although many women presumably experience the symptoms of vasomotor instability ("hot flashes") and other physiologic signs of hormonal withdrawal, the majority seem to take these events in stride without major loss of feminine identity or sexual function. Furthermore, women who have difficulty during the menopause turn out to be the same women who had difficulty with menarche, menstrual periods, and pregnancy, which would indicate that the problem is idiosyncratic, rather than related to a normative developmental crisis.

Another crisis commonly assumed to affect women predominantly is related to the "empty nest" created when grown-up children leave home. But investigation reveals that the postparental stage of life is associated with a higher, rather than lower, level of life satisfaction for women. Some studies show that marital adjustment improves for both sexes during middle age, possibly because of increased companionship after the children have left home (Burr; Rollins and Feldman).

The question has been raised repeatedly whether men undergo a counterpart of the female menopause. In a literal sense, of course, they do not; but the question is more difficult to answer in the broader sense of a climacterium encompassing bodily and psychic involutional changes during the transition from middle age to old age. Unlike ovarian function, which generally ceases between the ages of 48 and 50, testicular function declines gradually if at all in adulthood, so that the production of sperm and testosterone declines gradually over decades. Yet many of the psychologic symptoms associated with the female menopause, such as irritability and depression, seem to characterize significant numbers of middle-aged males also.

Sexual function in middle life is another common source of concern. It has long been observed that potency generally suffers with age, but age is only one factor that has a bearing on this issue, and it is by no means clear that declining potency is predominantly due to aging as such rather than illness. Without denying the possibility that a fundamental biologic process related to aging affects sexual function, one can also assume that in a large number of cases failing potency with increasing age is an artifact of psychologic factors and social expectations. It is also important to recognize the changing nature of sexual response without equating such altered responses with sexual failure. The middle-aged or older male generally requires more physical stimulation to attain erection, for example, although in his younger years psychologic arousal would often have been sufficient. But once having attained an erection, an older man is likely to maintain it longer or delay ejaculation at will, thus enhancing his lasting capacity during sexual intercourse. Other changes of sexual function at the physiologic level for aging men and women have been described (Masters and Johnson). None of these alterations in sexual function can yet be linked to a particular stage or phase of adult life.

Numerous other issues critical to mid-life have been proposed in the realms of economic life, social roles, and intrapsychic processes (Butler). On reviewing the more current literature, Brim derives the following six statements that sum up theories of the male mid-life crisis and may possibly be extrapolated to women crossing the threshold of middle life:

First, the mid-life male is likely to be undergoing profound personality changes.

Second, these changes will have more than one cause.

Third, a "male mid-life crisis" will occur for some men if there are multiple, simultaneous demands for personality change; if, for instance, during the same month or year the man throws off his last illusions about great success; accepts his children for what they are; buries his father and his mother and yields to the truth of his mortality; recognizes that his sexual vigor and, indeed, interest, are declining, and even finds relief in the fact.

Fourth, these challenges may be stretched out over ten or twenty years. Some men are obsessed about their achievements, but not yet confronting the fact of death; other men are sharply disappointed in their children's personalities but not yet concerned about sexual potency. The events come sooner for some men, much later for others. There is no evidence that they are related to chronologic age in any but the most general sense—e.g., "sometime during the forties."

Fifth, there is as yet no evidence for either developmental periods or "stages" in the mid-life period, in which one event must come after another or one personality change brings another in its wake. The existence of "stages," if proved true, would be a powerful concept in studying mid-life; meanwhile, there is a danger of our using this facile scheme as a cover for loose thinking about human development, without carrying forward the necessary hard-headed analyses of the evidence.

Sixth, the "growing pains" of mid-life, like those of youth and of old age, are transitions from one comparatively steady state to another, and these changes, even when they occur in crisis dimensions, bring for many men more happiness than they found in younger days.

Block J: Lives Through Time. Berkeley, Bancroft Books, 1971. *A longitudinal study of 171 men and women, focused on character formation and change. Serious research monograph.*

Brim OG Jr: Theories of the male mid-life crisis. Counseling Psychologist 6:2, 1976. *A thoughtful critique of current concepts of mid-life crisis by a distinguished social psychologist.*

Burr WR: Satisfaction with various aspects of marriage over the life cycle: A random middle class sample. J Marriage Family 32:29, 1970.

Butler RN: Psychiatry and psychology of the middle-aged. *In* Freedman AM, Kaplan HK, Sadock BJ (eds.): Comprehensive Textbook of Psychiatry. Vol 2. 2nd ed. Baltimore, Williams & Wilkins Company, 1975, pp 2390–2404. *A good review of middle-age related crises from a psychiatric perspective.*

Erikson EH (ed.): Adulthood. New York, W. W. Norton, 1978 (originally published as an issue of Daedalus in 1976). *Essays on adulthood by a wide range of authors, many of whom approach the subject from philosophical and literary perspectives. Contributors include two psychiatrists: Coles (Work and Self Respect) and H. Katchadourian (Medical Perspectives in Adulthood).*

Gould RL: Transformations. New York, Simon & Schuster, 1978. *An investigation of adulthood based on a sample of psychiatric outpatients and other subjects not in therapy.*

Kimmel DC: Adulthood and Aging. New York, John Wiley & Sons, 1974. *An introductory level textbook on adulthood.*

Levinson DJ, Darrow CN, Klein EB, Levinson MD, McKee B: The Seasons of a Man's Life. New York, Alfred A. Knopf, 1978. *One of the major studies of adulthood based on a sample of 40 males from four vocational backgrounds.*

Lowenthal MF, Thurnher M, Chiriboga D: Four Stages of Life. San Francisco, Jossey-Bass, 1975. *A study of adults of both sexes in four transitional phases of life: high school seniors, young newlyweds, middle-aged parents, and an older group about to retire.*

Maas HS, Kuypers JA: From Thirty to Seventy. San Francisco, Jossey-Bass, 1975. *Based on interviews with a sample of elderly men and women, focusing on their personality, life style, and health, and comparisons with data on the same persons from a project started in 1929.*

Masters WH, Johnson VE: Human Sexual Response. Boston, Little, Brown & Company, 1966. *The first major investigation of the physiology of human sexual response. Includes changes that occur with aging in normal sexual functions.*

Neugarten BL (ed.): Middle Age and Aging. Chicago, University of Chicago Press, 1968. *A rich selection of contributions by well-known authors, including the editor, who is among the foremost investigators of adulthood.*

Rollins BC, Feldman R: Marital satisfaction over the life cycle. J Marriage Family 32:20, 1970.

Valiant GE: Adaptation to Life. Boston, Little, Brown & Company, 1977. *A longitudinal study of a group of Harvard freshmen into middle age. Presented through fascinating biographies.*

White RW: Lives in Progress. New York, Holt, Rinehart and Winston, 1966. *A study of adult personality, focusing on three case histories (one of whom is a physician).*

9. AGING AND GERIATRIC MEDICINE

Ralph Goldman

Few individuals live to maturity in a world of great environmental danger. The persistence of a species requires that enough members survive and reproduce so that a balance can be established. Once this is assured, individual survival is no longer essential. In humans the control of infections and malnutrition, improved management of trauma, and the reduction in death associated with reproduction have produced a profound social as well as scientific revolution. Figure 9–1 shows changes in survival over a prolonged historical period. During the sixteenth century, in the city of York, England, only 45 per cent of girls survived their first year, 18 per cent reached age 20, 11 per cent reached age 40, and 3 per cent reached age 65. These data are worse than what must have been the norm for that period, but similar statistics in other cities existed into the current century. In the United States and most developed countries, 97 per cent of white women will now reach age 40, 84 per cent will reach age 65, and 38 per cent will reach age 85. The outlook for men is less favorable, yet 94 per cent will reach age 40 and 72 per cent will reach age 65.

The very existence of a large older population means that deaths from serious injury and disease at younger ages have decreased. Thus, although medical researchers and practitioners have been chiefly concerned with acute injuries and illnesses of younger patients, the focus of their activities must now be shifted to chronic conditions, including their acute episodes, and to a consideration of the nature and implications of the aging process itself.

The word *gerontology* derives from the Greek *gerontos,* old man, and *logos,* discourse upon, and refers to the study of the aging process. The word *geriatrics* is derived from *gerontos,* and *iatros,* physician, or *iatreia,* cure, literally physician or treatment of old men. The age at which a patient becomes eligible for geriatric care is artificial and arbitrary and usually relates to a statutory criterion, such as eligibility for Social Security or the age of mandatory retirement. Geriatrics uses the knowledge of gerontology, but the latter must study the aging process, which starts much earlier in life. Aging can be said to start at conception, but for practical purposes growth and development are associated with incremental processes, whereas during maturity and senescence decremental processes predominate.

Life span refers to the longest survival for a member of a species and serves as an index of maximum potential under ideal natural conditions. *Life expectation* refers to the average length of survival from a specific age, most commonly from birth, for a given cohort. Scientific and social improvements have increased life expectancy, but have not altered life span.

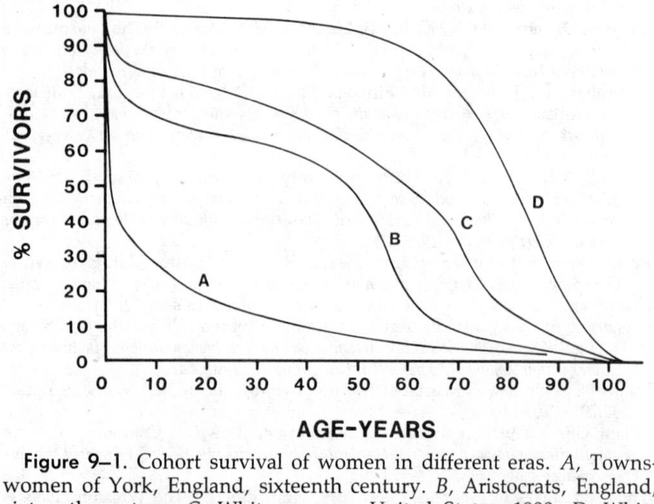

Figure 9–1. Cohort survival of women in different eras. *A,* Townswomen of York, England, sixteenth century. *B,* Aristocrats, England, sixteenth century. *C,* White women, United States, 1900. *D,* White women, United States, 1978. (*A* and *B* from Cowgill UM: Sci Am 222:104, 1970. *C* and *D* from Statistical Abstract, US, 1982-83).

Geriatrics is not limited to management of deterioration, dementia, and death. A large portion of the practice of medicine must, by the very fact of general survival to advanced age, be with older patients not usually thought of as a geriatric clientele. It is necessary for the concept of geriatric care to include both ambulatory and acute, as well as chronic, disease. The role of geriatrics is to integrate the information developed by gerontology with traditional medical knowledge to increase the well-being of aging patients.

STRUCTURAL AND FUNCTIONAL CHANGES WITH AGE

A primary problem of gerontology is to identify changes that are due to age alone and to differentiate these changes, if they exist, from pathologic processes. Growth and development are universal and proceed according to an intrinsically determined pattern that can be modified by the environment within limits compatible with survival. Changes caused by aging must also be universal. They should be unidirectional, and experience indicates that they are decremental. Although there is no a priori reason that age change should be either extrinsic or intrinsic in origin, the evidence now supports an intrinsic mechanism. The following are some of the major structural and functional changes with age which have been observed in humans and most mammals.

CELLS. Postmitotic cells, primarily muscle and nerve cells, are incapable of multiplication; they are not replaced when lost, and their number decreases with age. Mitotic cells have a limited capacity for replacement and are not immortal, as was once thought. Some cells, particularly the postmitotic cells, accumulate pigment within storage granules, and all cells show degeneration of intracellular organelles.

TISSUES. The regularity of tissue structure is lost, the individual cells enlarge, but the total number of cells decreases approximately 30 per cent. Fat deposition increases and conceals much of the loss of active cell mass. Intercellular collagen and elastin increase. The proportion of soluble collagen decreases, and there may be increased cross-linking between the long-chain collagen macromolecules. Elastin loses its discrete structure and elasticity and has an increased calcium content.

HEART. There is myocardial hypertrophy and fibrosis, and the valves become stiffer with age. The maximum cardiac rate and stroke volume, and thus the cardiac output, are well maintained in the absence of coronary heart disease. The isometric contraction and relaxation times are prolonged. Although there is a statistically valid increase in ECG intervals, there is no visually discernible abnormality in the normal pattern.

BLOOD VESSELS. The increased collagen, altered elastin, and increased calcium result in arterial rigidity with elevation of the systolic pressure, accelerated pulse wave velocity, and a loss of 10 per cent in cardiac systolic efficiency. The peripheral resistance is increased, whether because of arteriolar atrophy or spasm is not established, and the diastolic pressure is slightly elevated. The capillary basement membrane thickness increases from 700 to 1100 Angstroms between youth and old age.

EXCRETORY SYSTEM. The number of nephrons decreases 30 to 40 per cent between 25 and 85 years. The filtration rate, renal blood flow, and tubular functions are proportionately reduced, although the serum creatinine level is maintained because of reduced release from the decreasing muscle mass. The capacity for compensatory hypertrophy diminishes with age and increasingly depends upon cellular hypertrophy rather than hyperplasia.

RESPIRATORY SYSTEM. Upper respiratory infections become less frequent because of immunologic experience. The compliance of the chest wall is decreased. The total lung capacity is unchanged, but the residual volume is doubled and the vital capacity is reduced. The maximum breathing capacity decreases about 50 per cent between the third and ninth decades. The reduced cough efficiency, decreased ciliary activity of the bronchial epithelium, and increased dead space enhance the potential for mechanical and infectious respiratory complications of surgery and enforced bed rest in the aged individual.

GASTROINTESTINAL SYSTEM. Hiatus hernia, atrophic gastritis, appendiceal involution, and colonic diverticulosis are increasingly common. Motility may be disorganized, and fecal incontinence is frequent in the mentally impaired. Salivary, gastric, and fasting pancreatic secretion are decreased, but after stimulation pancreatic secretion is normal. Digestion and absorption are generally adequate, although iron and calcium may be less well absorbed. The liver shows characteristic change and atrophy. Bromsulphalein storage in hepatic cells is linearly decreased, but the secretory transport maximum is unchanged. The frequency of cholelithiasis approaches 40 per cent by the eighth decade.

ENDOCRINE SYSTEM. Blood levels of GH may be decreased and those of TSH, ACTH, and ADH are maintained. Blood levels of FSH are increased fifteen-fold and LH three-fold in postmenopausal women, whereas in men these changes are marginal. Large doses of estrogen fail to suppress FSH, and the feedback control mechanism in women is probably impaired. The serum T_4 remains normal, although the rate of turnover is decreased; T_3 is reduced 25 to 40 per cent. Responses to stress and to TSH are normal. The status of PTH is not certain, but the postmenopausal decrease in estrogen may allow an unopposed PTH effect and predispose to osteoporosis. The glucose tolerance decreases with age, and if the usual standards are used, 50 per cent of all individuals aged 70 or older would have diabetes. An adjustment in diagnostic criteria is obviously necessary. This reduced tolerance may be due to a delay in insulin release by the beta cells. Glucagon levels are unchanged. The plasma cortisol level and the circadian cycle persist, but a decreased secretion rate is matched by reduced disposal and excretion rates. The response of cortisol secretion to stress still needs clarification. The blood level and urinary excretion of aldosterone decrease 50 per cent between youth and old age, and the response to sodium depletion is reduced two thirds. The secretion of renin has a similar age-related decrease. Adrenal androgen also decreases progressively to less than one half of young adult values. There is a decrease in norepinephrine and an increase in monamine oxidase and serotonin in the brain with age. Stimulation results in a delayed but quantitatively normal increase in the excretion of epinephrine. After the menopause all female estrogen is adrenal in origin and thus decreases markedly; in males there is little age-related change. Since progesterone is a precursor of cortisol, adrenal production is probably sustained in both sexes. The production and clearance of testosterone decline, but there is no agreement that blood levels are reduced.

BLOOD. There is no decrease in the blood volume before age 80, red cell survival time is normal, and anemia is usually secondary to chronic disease or iron depletion. The number and distribution of leukocytes is unchanged, except for T lymphocytes, which are probably decreased. The leukocytosis of inflammation and immunoglobulin production after antigenic challenge are both decreased. Immune surveillance is markedly decreased despite an increase in total gamma globulin. Platelets may have increased adhesiveness and fibrinogen may be increased, but there is no conclusive evidence of hypercoagulability. The erythrocyte sedimentation rate may be markedly accelerated without evidence of disease.

MUSCULOSKELETAL SYSTEM. Muscle cell loss and disorganization cause a progressive reduction in muscle strength. The poor reparative characteristics of cartilage lead to deterioration as early as the third decade, with progressive loss of joint surfaces and resultant degenerative arthritis. Throughout life there is a continuous remodeling of bone by reabsorption of interior surfaces and formation on exterior surfaces. By age 40 the reabsorption exceeds bone formation. Both the protein matrix and the bone mineral are involved, and clinical osteoporosis may result. In women 25 per cent of the bone is lost. Fractures of the vertebral body and femoral neck may result. The cumulative risk of hip fracture by age 90 approaches 25 per cent for women and 10 per cent for men.

THE INTEGUMENT. Wrinkling and sagging of the skin and graying of the hair are hallmarks of aging. The epidermis thins and contains less melanin, and cell replacement slows, resulting in delayed healing. The epidermal glands are reduced in number and function, and the skin is dry. A significant reduction in subcutaneous fat, increased collagen, and fragmented, inelastic elastin cause the observed wrinkling. The blood supply is reduced, and capillary fragility results in the common subcutaneous senile purpura. The loss of subcutaneous fat, reduction of vascularity, and slowed cell replacement contribute to the frequency and severity of decubitus ulceration. Hair distribution is subject to genetic and racial variation, but in each individual is determined by the number of active and resting hair follicles in local areas more than by follicular atrophy. Luxuriant scalp hair in youth decreases with age; facial hair appears at puberty and may persist in males, but it may appear after the menopause in Caucasian women; axillary and pubic hair appears at puberty and, in women, decreases after the menopause. Graying is due to decreased melanin production by the hair follicle. The rate of nail growth decreases 40 per cent.

NERVOUS SYSTEM. Nerve cells are postmitotic and are not replaced when lost.The weight of the brain is essentially constant, but careful studies have shown not only a significant loss of cells, as many as 45 per cent in some cortical areas, but, more important, a loss of cellular integrity and of cellular interconnections. A consensus of several studies shows that from age 17 to age 80 years the cerebral blood flow declines from 79 to 46 ml per minute per 100 grams of brain tissue and the cerebral oxygen consumption rate decreases from 3.6 to 2.7 ml per minute per 100 grams of brain. The mean arterial pressure is constant at 90 to 100 mm Hg, but the derived cerebrovascular resistance increases from 1.3 to 2.1 mm Hg per ml blood per minute per 100 grams of brain. Patients with senile dementia cluster at the lowest levels of blood flow and oxygen utilization, but there is overlap with subjects lacking overt intellectual deterioration. Motor nerve conduction velocity decreases about 15 per cent, and sensory nerve conduction velocity may decrease 30 per cent between 20 and 95 years. Sleep levels 3 and 4 become less prominent and brief arousals more frequent with age, but total sleep time may be little affected. A reciprocal increase of monamine oxidase and decrease of norepinephrine in brain tissue may be causal to the depression and apathy so often associated with aging.

SENSORY ORGANS. Visual acuity decreases with age, primarily because of reduction in transparency of the optical portions of the system. There is also loss in the extent of the visual fields, decrease in the speed of dark adaptation, elevation in the minimal threshold of light perception, and reduction in the critical speed of flicker fusion. There is a continuous, but decelerating, formation of cells on the lens surface, which gradually lose their nuclei and become transparent. Thus the lens thickens with age and there is progressive loss of the elasticity needed to deform the lens adaptively. Between ages 42 and 45 years, previously normal individuals will need corrective glasses for near vision. Hearing decreases, particularly for high tones after age 60, especially in men. There is a decrease in the senses of taste, smell, and touch. Pain fibers appear to be intact, but pain threshold may be reduced.

THE GOMPERTZ CONCEPT

In 1825, Benjamin Gompertz, a British actuary, proposed a concept that at advanced ages the age-specific risk of death increased geometrically, and could be computed by the formula:

$$q_x = q_o e^{ax}$$

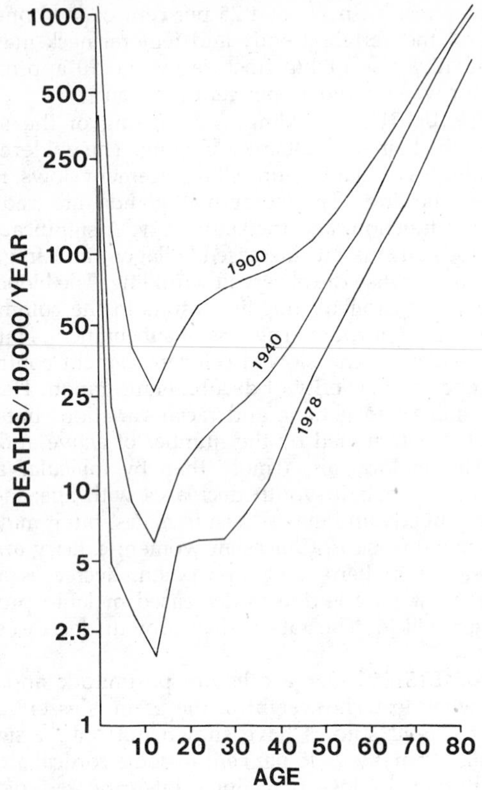

Figure 9–2. Mortality rates for white women, United States, 1900, 1940, and 1978.

where q_x is the death rate at age x, q_o is the death rate at age o, and a is a constant. When age is plotted against the log of the age-specific death rate, the portion of the curve that corresponds to Gompertz's formula is essentially a straight line (Fig. 9–2). Thus at these ages the risk of death is determined by age. The Gompertz concept has been found to be valid for all mammals.

Figure 9–2 shows the changes in age-specific mortality during the present century for American white women and demonstrates features that would be magnified by a longer time frame. The biggest gains have resulted from the reduction of infections and infant and maternal mortality and from the better management of trauma. Since the slope accelerates as the risk is reduced at lower ages, the benefits at advanced age are less prominent, and there may be a limit to the amount of reduction that can be achieved without modification of the aging process itself.

THEORIES OF AGING

The search for perpetual youth and immortality has given rise to many theories of aging, most now only of historical interest. Genetic factors are undoubtedly important, because each species has a characteristic life span, and within species there are strain differences in survival distribution. Genetic theories raise the possibilities of programmed senescence or of program exhaustion. Recent knowledge of genetic mechanisms has resulted in the development of a number of error theories based on the concept that defects in protein synthesis can accumulate over time. Postmitotic cells, because of their long life, should be vulnerable particularly at the levels of transcription and translation, whereas mitotic cells should be vulnerable to somatic mutation during replication. Chromosome studies show an increase in gross abnormalities visible by light microscopy.

Another group of theories has arisen from developments in immunology. Both humoral and cellular immunocompetence decline, but autoimmune manifestations increase with age and amyloid deposits become common, particularly in the walls of blood vessels. The constant occurrence of somatic mutations could result in an ongoing immunologic response, possibly to a cell product from within a cell otherwise not distinguishable on its surface as alien, and thus free to continue producing its aberrant product. Mutation of immunocompetent cells that no longer recognize "self" would produce a graft-versus-host reaction.

Several other theories, not necessarily mutually exclusive, have attained some support. The finite limit of the reproductive capacity of mitotic cells, now very conclusively established by Hayflick, indicates that some limits to mortality exist on a cellular level. The accumulation of storage granules within the cellular cytoplasm, particularly lipofuscin, may interfere with cellular functions. Quantitative increases in the amount and cross-linkage of collagen and related macromolecules have been shown for the connective tissue matrices. A similar cross-linkage of intracellular macromolecules, particularly DNA and RNA, could impair cell function. The existence of free radicals and exposure to natural radiation could produce irreversible changes in genetic and protein structures.

The accumulating evidence makes it unlikely that aging is a unitary phenomenon for which a specific therapy may be found. For the present it may be more practical to reconcile the observations of aging with certain clinical phenomena. Since aging is conceived as universal, any process that affects only a segment of the population has been considered to be a disease. However, if every individual has a potential for cancer which is held in check by immunosurveillance, the development of cancer would depend upon the level of the defense and the strength of the carcinogenetic mechanisms. Since immune competence decreases with age, cancer should occur when the defense is no longer adequate to cope with the stress. The rate of development of atherosclerosis has been linked to risk factors, particularly blood pressure, glucose tolerance, and blood lipid levels. Each increment in arterial pressure is linked with a statistical increase in mortality. Whether an individual dies of a vascular complication, cancer, or some other cause depends upon the individual vulnerability of a particular system. The risk for each potential cause of aging death and the likelihood that more than one will be present increases geometrically with age, as does the risk of death. The phenomenon of the one-horse shay, in which all parts wore out at the same moment, is just as improbable in biology as in mechanics.

PSYCHOSOCIAL PROBLEMS OF THE AGED

Very few members of migratory, hunting societies lived to old age, and those few must have had unique qualities. Despite the obvious value of their wisdom, they probably were not spared if their incapacity endangered the group. The development of fixed, agricultural communities increased the security of the aged, especially after the development of property rights and rules of inheritance. Science and technology further increased the number of survivors to old age. However, the industrial revolution also broke up the family as a social and economic unit, increased social and geographic mobility, and so altered the social position of the aged that new social models have become necessary.

The popular image of the aged is negative. They are thought of as reduced in intelligence, limited in memory, rigid in concept, and uncongenial in personality. In fact, intellectual competence usually persists until quite late in life, and established knowledge and experience compensate for slowness of learning. Even flexibility of thought is greater than was once believed. The increasing level of general education is improving the ability of the aged to adapt and to maintain interests.

Nevertheless, aging is associated with losses. There is the loss of occupation, as a source both of income and of meaningful activity. The loss of income may be more important because of reduced social leverage than lowered standard of living. Yet, with adequate income noneconomic activities can often become significant and satisfying. The loss of friends and family and separation from children become increasingly painful. The loss of vigor and attractiveness and, ultimately, the loss of health are the final reminders that the cycle is closing. Women now live eight years longer than men and are several years younger at the time of marriage. Geriatrics as a specialty must deal largely with older women who will be widowed for an average of ten years with reduced economic resources and social contacts.

Under these conditions it is not surprising that depression is common and is often manifest as dementia or insomnia. The apparent intellectual decline is really a loss of attention created by the depression, and effective therapy can be gratifying.

In caring for aging patients, the physician must be aware of a range of problems which are less important in other age groups. First, the life experience of the patient encompasses a time period which the younger physician knows only indirectly, and the patient may be conditioned by lifetime social and ethnic considerations which also may be quite alien to him. Second, the patient may not have the economic or social resources to adhere to a prescribed regimen. Third, the patient has an increased probability of multiple problems which may be self-treated or lie in the area of another specialist. Multiple medications may be utilized with potential incompatibilities. Fourth, the patient may be incompetent, and both the history and the therapy may suffer as a result. Fifth, the longer the survival, the more likely the loss or absence of a spouse or companion. Sixth, the need for social welfare, visiting nurse, homemaker, and related services is extensive, and when properly used can often help maintain an older patient at home as the preferred medical, social, and economic solution.

Despite the enumerated decrements associated with aging, most older individuals live remarkably active and satisfying lives. Social Security, pensions, Medicare and health insurance, and a long period of relative economic prosperity have greatly improved the economic aspects. If the individual survives, the general enfeeblement of aging is infrequently incapacitating before age 75 or 80. It is becoming usual to speak of early and late old age, since the two periods may be quite different.

It is during advanced old age that the stereotypes may be more typical. Significant senile dementia may be present in 20 per cent. Losses of hearing and vision reduce sensory input and with reduced physical mobility may aggravate the other problems of social isolation. These patients are often best managed in a home for the aged or in a skilled nursing facility if they are unable to perform the activities of daily living. The residents in these homes now average more than 80 years.

SPECIAL PROBLEMS OF MANAGEMENT

See also Ch. 11.

DIET. There is little evidence that age alters the need for specific nutrients, but the total calories should be reduced to compensate for decreased metabolic activity and cell mass. Because a reduced total diet may result in an inadequate intake of vitamins, calcium, and iron, appropriate supplements may be prescribed. No specific diet to promote longevity has yet been confirmed. The older patient will have an increased probability of need for a specific therapeutic diet, and the ability to conform to the dietary prescription must be determined.

MEDICATION. The age-related concerns of clinical pharmacology are those of drug level, receptor and effector competence, and drug toxicity. Drug levels are determined by absorption, volume of distribution, biodegradation, and excretion. Quantitatively, the 40 to 50 per cent decrease in renal function is the most important age-related factor for substances which are excreted in active form in the urine. The decrease in renal function may produce a significant increase in blood levels if dose is not adjusted. An important factor in dose level is patient compliance. Reliable information requires frequent review of all drugs taken, including over-the-counter medications. Each patient should be instructed periodically to bring in all actively used drugs in their containers to determine the exact drugs taken and their amounts. This is a most instructive exercise for both patient and physician.

Recent studies have shown quantitative and qualitative changes in the receptor sites, particularly of the nervous system, heart, and muscle. The reduced number and integrity of effectors are the natural result of the changes previously described. Further information should do much to rationalize geriatric pharmacology.

Drug misadventures increase in frequency with age. The patient has had more opportunity for prior sensitization. In addition, the multiple medical problems increase the number of drugs to be administered. The frequency of pharmacologic incompatibilities and of drug-drug interactions increases geometrically with the number taken (see Ch. 24). Safe and effective drug therapy requires knowledge of the drugs used, their probable pharmacologic changes with age, tests for blood level, and close titration for effect. In addition, drug prescription should be selective and minimal and the patients closely observed for untoward responses.

INSTITUTIONALIZATION. Approximately 1.25 million of those over 65 years, about 5 per cent, now reside in nursing homes, and many others live in sheltered settings. The major determinants of need are inadequate social supports coupled with intellectual impairment, physical disability, or both. Over 90 per cent of women and almost 80 per cent of men in nursing homes have no spouse, and more than half have significant dementia. Need increases rapidly with age, especially after age 80. Ideally, home maintenance should be continued as long as possible. Homemaker and visiting nurse or other home health services may be helpful. Day care centers, day hospitals, and access to brief placement may provide "respite care" to alleviate caretaker stress.

Placement usually becomes necessary when the individual is alone and cannot provide self-care. Individuals with families are usually placed only when there is serious stress, as when the caretaker becomes incapacitated or the patient's dementia seriously disrupts the household. The exact costs of home care are not well documented, but recent data suggest that in many cases with severe disability the costs may exceed those of a nursing home.

The majority of nursing homes have been constructed within the past 20 years, and standards of construction have been greatly improved. Two levels of care are now recognized. The skilled nursing facility (SNF) provides for patients requiring specific nursing procedures or total care, and the intermediate care facility (ICF) cares for patients requiring a lesser level of care. Nursing homes must be licensed, and they must be inspected by Medicare and Medicaid to be eligible for these programs. Checklists are available to guide the patient and the family in appropriate selection. Many communities also have residential care programs, including homes for the aged, board and care facilities, and home placement for individuals capable of this level of independence yet unable to manage totally alone. Placement must be carefully individualized, with full regard for all physical, psychiatric, social, and economic factors.

THE PHYSICIAN'S RESPONSIBILITY

The inevitability of death and the presence of incurable disease should not lull the physician into nihilism or neglect. Most individuals are socially competent and lead active and enjoyable lives until their terminal illnesses. Many conditions, as with younger patients, are either self-limited or curable. Chronic disease is often subject to control, and symptoms can usually be reduced if not eliminated. Much can be done to assist the patient in maintaining independence and dignity as long as possible and to meet death with the least discomfort.

Humans are mortal. Not all diseases will be cured or deaths prevented. It is only within this century that the physician's intervention has been decisive in more than occasional situations. We must not allow our new-found technical competence to separate us from our larger role as physicians. Now that our patients live out their life spans, the more frequently we will be unable to cure and to prevent death. Yet, as with physicians in millenia past, we are not freed of our responsibilities to comfort, to console, to reassure, to be available. This is a responsibility which cannot be delegated; it is the essence of medical practice.

Binstock RH, Shanas E (eds.): Handbook of Aging and the Social Sciences. New York, Van Nostrand Reinhold Company, 1976. *Current opinion of leaders in the social sciences, with comprehensive coverage and good relevant bibliographies. Basically a reference source.*

Birren JE, Schaie KW (eds.): Handbook of the Psychology of Aging. New York, Van Nostrand Reinhold Company, 1977. *A wide-ranging handbook that includes good discussions of age changes in the nervous system and the sense organs.*

Brocklehurst JC (ed.): Textbook of Geriatric Medicine and Gerontology. 2nd ed. Edinburgh and London, Churchill Livingstone, 1978. *British experience and point of view. Scholarly coverage with extensive bibliographies.*

Finch CE, Hayflick L (eds.): Handbook of the Biology of Aging. New York, Van Nostrand Reinhold Company, 1977. *A reference text with excellent presentations. Most of the organ systems are covered in detail.*

Fries JF, Crapo LM: Vitality and Aging. San Francisco, W. H. Freeman and Company, 1981. *A modern statement of the limits of life.*

Reichel W (ed.): Clinical Aspects of Aging. Baltimore, Williams & Wilkins Company, 1978. *A comprehensive, readable text. Well-recognized contributors.*

Rossman I (ed.): Clinical Geriatrics. 2nd ed. Philadelphia, J. B. Lippincott Company, 1979. *Broad and authoritative coverage. Strong bibliographies.*

Strehler BL: Time, Cells and Aging. 2nd ed. New York, Academic Press, 1977. *An extensively revised edition of a classic monograph on aging theory.*

10. MANAGEMENT OF COMMON PROBLEMS IN THE ELDERLY

T. Franklin Williams

A physician must approach the care of elderly persons with an informed, comprehensive, balanced perspective about aging itself and about the diseases and disabilities that commonly occur in older people. The previous section has described the physiologic changes that normally occur with aging. From the clinical perspective it is important to keep in mind that most older people are in reasonably good health and, despite some decline in maximum functional ability, can still function well at all ordinary activities. There are many persons in their eighties and nineties who can and do carry on all usual living activities, take long walks, are intellectually sharp with good memories, continue to be sexually active, and most of the time are symptom-free. Thus when someone, no matter how old, comes to a physician with a complaint of discomfort or dysfunction, the complaint should not be dismissed as being simply "old age," but should be investigated and treated appropriately. Sir Ferguson Anderson of Glasgow, the "dean" of geriatricians, tells the story of the old man who came to his doctor complaining of pain in his right knee. "Why, John," the doctor said, "what do you expect at your age? This pain is just due to old age." To which John replied, "But doc, my left knee is just as old and it isn't hurting."

At the same time, a physician must understand that with increasing age people do accumulate chronic diseases and disabilities. Over the age of 65, 80 per cent have one or more chronic conditions; among the most common are some form of arthritis (present in 40 per cent in national surveys), hearing impairment (30 per cent), and chronic cardiac conditions (20 per cent). One in five persons over the age of 75 may be expected to have diabetes. In those 75 or older, four or more identifiable chronic problems are commonly present.

In addition to recognizing and treating the acute and chronic *diseases* that occur, the physician must give attention to the functional losses, the *disabilities* that are present, and attempt to reverse or minimize them no matter what can or cannot be done about underlying chronic diseases. The ultimate goal of care for elderly persons should be to restore or maintain as much function as possible—to help the patient to maintain as much independence of living, as much of a preferred life style, as possible. Such a rehabilitative approach is an essential part of the therapy.

In those elderly patients who have some irreversible functional losses and thus need regular assistance in functioning, an additional part of the plan for care must be identification of who will provide the needed help and where. The extent and quality of family support and the potentials for community or institutional support services must be determined and worked into the overall, ongoing therapeutic program.

SPECIAL FEATURES OF THE WORKUP OF ELDERLY PATIENTS

HISTORY-TAKING. Special attention should be given to the history of other (chronic) conditions that are likely to be present in addition to the immediate chief complaint, and to obtaining additional historical information from close relatives and previous records. An older person, like any patient consulting a physician, is most interested in having the immediate problem addressed and may tend to downplay past history and other chronic but less obviously troubling conditions. It is the interaction of multiple diseases, the necessity to deal simultaneously with these multiple problems, that is one of the distinguishing characteristics of geriatric medicine. A closely related necessity is to obtain complete information on all drugs the patient is taking, both prescribed and over-the-counter medications. The numbers and variety are often astounding, and unfavorable drug interactions commonly contribute to the patient's discomfort and dysfunctions. A good technique is to have the patient (or responsible family member) bring in all the medications the patient is taking, for review, on each office visit.

Certain common functional problems should be explicitly inquired about: any history of falling, any episodes of urinary incontinence, any disturbances in sleep.

It is a good practice whenever possible to talk with one or more close family members to obtain their observations on the patient's functional status, mood, and daily routines, including intake of food and medicines. Such additional information is absolutely essential if there is evidence of dementia or depression in the patient—in such circumstances the patient may give quite a misleading story. If the patient is living alone (as a third or more of older women are), then it will be desirable or even necessary to have the benefit of observations from a home visit by the physician or by a visiting nurse or social worker. The help that a home visit can provide toward obtaining an accurate, complete picture of an older person's status and circumstances—whether living alone or with family—is considered to be so important by geriatricians in the United Kingdom that such a visit is an almost invariable first step in the workup of a referred patient; in the United States we should include such visits in our evaluations more often than we do.

Any person who has lived 70 years or more will almost always have had previous medical or surgical care, in or out of the hospital, and may well have seen several specialists. It should be routine practice, when taking on the care of such a patient (as primary physician or consultant) to obtain summaries or copies of all previous records, including results of all diagnostic tests. Such information is important in understanding current problems and reducing the extent of further diagnostic tests that are needed. In particularly complex or unclear situations, there should be direct discussion with physicians who have previously seen the patient.

PHYSICAL EXAMINATION. As part of a regular complete physical examination of an older patient, certain features should receive special attention, depending in part on clues from the history. These include evaluation of mobility, of mental status, and of mood. The ability of the patient to move around adequately and the degree of stability in balance and gait can be appraised to a degree from simple observation of the patient as he or she arrives. But because of the commonness of gait and balance disturbances in old people, and in particular if there is any history of falls or near-falls, these characteristics should be explicitly evaluated through observing the patient taking a prescribed walk down the corridor, turning and returning. Does each foot carry through a full swing with each step? Is there any limp? Is there any tendency to lean or fall to one side? Is the pace at a usual speed? One should perform the Romberg test and test the patient's ability to maintain balance when purposely given a moderate shove. If there is any history of falls and near-falls, special attention should also be given to checking for orthostatic hypotension and for any evidence of arrhythmia.

In assessing mental status, it is a good practice to use a standard short mental status examination as a screening test for any degree of mental impairment. A number of such tests have been developed; the commonly used ones are described and critically appraised by Kane and Kane (1981). Such a short mental status questionnaire should be used only for screening purposes in the course of a regular physical examination: the identification of any degree of mental inadequacy on such a test should be followed by a thorough investigation of the extent and possible causes of the dementia (see below).

A similar approach is to be recommended in assessing the mood of an older patient, in particular if there is any clue in the history to possible depression. Several short, standardized tests for depression are available. Again, any suggestion of depression on such a screening test should lead to a thorough evaluation of the extent and possible causes.

In light of the frequency of poor eating practices by older persons, particularly those living alone, special attention should be given to any indications of poor nutrition—weight loss, anemia, vitamin deficiency. Also in light of the frequency of functionally limiting problems, hearing and vision should be adequately tested; joint mobility and muscular strength should be thoroughly evaluated; and any evidence of peripheral neuropathy should be sought.

ASSESSMENT OF FUNCTIONAL STATUS. All aspects of daily functioning should be evaluated by history and physical examinations. Loss of ability to carry out such functions makes the older person dependent on others, at home or in institutional care. These functional characteristics include the usual activities of daily living (ADL): feeding oneself, bathing, dressing, toileting, ambulation, and continence. In addition the person, particularly if living alone, may need to be able to carry out the "instrumental" activities of daily living (IADL), i.e., those activities necessary for maintenance of the immediate environment: obtaining food, cooking, laundering, housecleaning, transportation, use of telephone, managing medications.

ADDITIONAL DIAGNOSTIC TESTS. The same general principles for choosing diagnostic tests for younger patients should apply in the workup of older patients as well: the aim is to obtain any information that will help in clarifying the cause of disease or the functional loss, *if* this information will likely lead to effective therapy. The special circumstances that arise more often in older than in younger patients are those in which, because of the other chronic complicating problems that are present, the best judgment may be not to proceed with any form of treatment that may be risky or unpleasant and offers only minimal chance for improvement. Such judgments should be weighed in consultation with the patient and close family before embarking on diagnostic procedures: if the treatment plans will not be changed by the outcome of the procedure then it should not be done.

However, because of the tendency, referred to earlier, to dismiss treatable problems of elderly patients as being simply the concomitants of old age, it is important to try to identify any potentially reversible condition and to use relevant diagnostic aids. An adequate use of diagnostic tests is especially indicated in the common, functionally disabling conditions faced by older people. These are discussed below.

ASSESSMENT OF FAMILY AND COMMUNITY SUPPORTS. A final essential element in the workup of a frail, elderly person, i.e., a patient who may face the necessity of ongoing help with daily activities, is the collection of information about the home environment, the family relationships, the degree of supporting services potentially available, the degree of "burn-out" or exhaustion that may have already occurred, and the availability of home care services and institutional services in the community. A visiting nurse or social worker can be very helpful in obtaining some of these services and in helping to integrate them into an overall plan.

DIAGNOSIS AND MANAGEMENT OF MAJOR COMMON PROBLEMS OF ELDERLY PATIENTS

EPISODES OF ACUTE ILLNESS. Older people with diminished reserves and chronic diseases are more prone to injuries, acute infections (especially respiratory), and other acute illnesses than are younger people, and are also more likely to decompensate at such times. It is a common observation that an old person, previously mentally competent at home, may become quite confused on admission to the strange environment of a hospital under the stresses of an acute illness. Careful attention must be given to every aspect of the patient's status, looking for the appearance of heart failure, overt diabetes, delirium, or increased risk of falling. Drug regimens should be kept simple and the possibility of deleterious effects of overdosage or drug interactions should be continuously reviewed (Steel, 1981).

Recovery from an acute illness will also take longer than in a younger person, and there is real risk that the previous functional level may not be regained. As early as possible in an episode of acute illness the older patient should be helped to be up and about, to keep joints supple and muscular strength as intact as possible, to retain or regain urinary continence through use of regular toilet facilities, to dress and feed oneself and engage in social exchanges in usual ways, i.e., out of bed and dressed. The patient should remain in familiar home surroundings or return there as quickly as possible. Convalescent and rehabilitative efforts should be continued as long as any progress is being made.

DEMENTIA. The loss of mental competence is one of the most common and most distressing of functional disabilities in older persons, affecting about 5 per cent of those over age 65 and 20 per cent of those over age 80. We now know that dementia is *not* a feature of normal aging but instead is due to one or another of several disease processes. The most common form of dementia in old people is that of the Alzheimer's type, accounting for 50 per cent or more of cases. This is a (usually) progressive dementia associated with considerable cerebral atrophy and characteristic pathologic changes in selected regions of the brain, with neurofibrillary tangles within neurons and degenerating plaques at end-plates. As a result of much recent research, it now seems clear that these damaged neurons are producing far less of the neurotransmitter acetylcholine (and possibly other neurotransmitters also) than normal. With the accumulating evidence that the deficiency in this neurotransmitter is the cause of the failure in mental function, various research efforts are in progress to find ways to achieve more production of acetylcholine (for example, through providing substrate) or to delay its destruction or prolong its effectiveness. Thus far, results, while promising, are inconclusive.

Other causes of dementia in the elderly include damage from multiple small infarcts or one or more larger infarcts secondary to cerebrovascular disease, metabolic or endocrine disorders such as hypothyroidism and vitamin B_{12} deficiency, brain tumors, brain injury (such as the late dementia that may appear in professional boxers, which has the same pathologic changes as Alzheimer's disease), the Korsakoff's dementia of chronic alcoholism, and the condition known as normal pressure hydrocephalus. Most importantly, severe depression can present as dementia, reversible with successful treatment of the depression. Indeed, a number of the possible causes are potentially reversible or treatable. Thus it is essential, when confronted by an older person with any signs of dementia, to conduct a thorough differential diagnostic evaluation. This should include comprehensive mental testing to define the extent of the dementia, specific tests for all of the treatable causes, and in most instances, a CT scan that can usually identify or exclude infarcts and tumors and can help diagnose normal pressure hydrocephalus. The finding of cerebral atrophy alone on the CT scan would be consistent with but not diagnostic of dementia of Alzheimer's type, inasmuch as a significant degree of atrophy occurs in the normal aging process without loss of mental function.

The physician should be aware of and sensitive to the alarm older patients and family members may have at the least sign of any aberration in mentation and should be able to recognize "benign forgetfulness" as a common trait at all ages and reassure patient and family that this is not the first stage of progressive dementia. Benign forgetfulness characteristically is the inability to recall a name or some specific element of a prior experience, when one thinks one should be able to do so. The person can recall many related features of the person or episode and knows precisely what element or name is not being recalled. Usually recall of that element will occur later, unexpectedly. In contrast, a person with progressive dementia will have no recollection of the entire episode, as if it never happened, or can make only feeble, ineffective efforts to reconstruct the identity of the forgotten person.

If the final diagnosis is dementia of the Alzheimer's type or one of the other irreversible dementias, the physician, nurses, and social workers must treat the family as well as the patient and help them to make the best of a distressing situation (Steele, 1982). The long-established daily activities of the patient in familiar surroundings should be maintained as much as possible, with avoidance of surprises or new and different decisions to be made. Family members should be helped to understand the disease and the fact that the patient will probably not understand it or the burden they carry in responsibility for whatever the patient can no longer do for himself or herself. They should be helped to accept the services of home support personnel to assist in the care of the patient—housekeeper, personal care aide, home health aide, or nurse—as needed to help prevent "burn-out" on their part; to accept respite care for the patient (temporary full-time care given in the home or a temporary nursing home admission) so that the family members may get away for a vacation or a special occasion; and to accept permanent nursing home care for the patient if this becomes best for everyone. They should be informed of support groups like the Alzheimer's Disease and Related Dementias Association (ADRDA), chapters of which now exist in most larger communities, and should be put in touch with social agencies and legal resources if necessary to help in making various legal and financial arrangements. The physician's involvement in all of these aspects may seem to some to be peripheral to the practice of medicine but in fact is central to the physician's primary goals of maintaining the health and functioning of the patient and the patient's family to the maximum extent possible. In working with problems like these the physician needs the close participation of well-informed nurses and social workers who can take the lead in management of many aspects.

DEPRESSION. Depressive reactions of varying degrees of severity are much more common in elderly persons than has been recognized and warrant more attention in diagnosis and treatment. As a person lives into later years losses are inevitable—death of family members and friends, usually "loss" of job through retirement, usually less income, often loss of some degree of health, less vigor, possibly loss of familiar home environment through moving. Some degree of grief and reactive depression is to be expected in response to such losses, but emotionally healthy older persons will work through such grief and return to their usual level of mood, outlook, and activity. Persistence of depressive symptoms may represent activation of a longer-standing depressed state or appearance of a new disorder.

If depression is suspected, it should be thoroughly evaluated with psychiatric consultation, and perhaps treated by therapeutic trials of antidepressant drugs. In severe instances not responsive to drugs, electroshock therapy has been found to be successful in many elderly patients.

FALLS. Falling is a very common event as people become older, occurring as often as once a year or more in half of those over age 75. In addition to the accompanying risk of injury—with up to 5 per cent of falls there may be fracture of the hip or arm—one or more falls may lead to such a fear of further falling that an older person will severely limit mobility and activities. Falls are often also a harbinger of other diseases or disabilities; one study in the United Kingdom has reported twice the overall mortality from various causes in the year following a first fall in older people, compared to age- and sex-matched persons who did not fall.

A number of risk factors contribute to the likelihood of falling, and it is typically the multiplicity of such risk factors in the same person that makes falling highly likely, rather than any one of them. These include diminished distant vision, disturbances in balance, abnormal gait, weakness in the lower extremities, decreased mental status, orthostatic hypotension, depression, and effects of drugs on alertness. All such factors should be searched for and as many as possible corrected as a part of regular preventive care and especially at the time of any fall.

Environmental hazards also contribute to the risk. As already noted, a home visit by at least one of the professionals helping to care for frail older persons can be invaluable and should include observation and recommendations for correcting such environmental hazards as poor lighting, rugs that can slide, objects blocking usual walkways, lack of nonslipping strips and hand grips in bath tubs, and lack of handrails on stairs.

A person who has fallen should be thoroughly examined for even subtle signs of injury or fracture and for any underlying or associated disease condition, including a new febrile illness, painless myocardial infarction, and stroke. If any of the risk factors listed above is present and not fully correctable, the patient should be helped to use an appropriate walking aid such as a cane or walker.

URINARY INCONTINENCE. Lack of control of urination is far more common than generally recognized by health professionals; some studies suggest that up to 50 per cent of older women have this problem. It has been referred to as the "closet disease" of old age because of the high frequency of denial of its presence—out of embarrassment or the mistaken view that nothing can be done about it. Older persons living alone may become oblivious to its presence, unaware of the odors around their house and on their clothes which are obvious to visitors. Frequent urinary incontinence, particularly night-time incontinence, by a person living with family is a major cause of caregiver exhaustion and the precipitating reason for their seeking institutional care. Within long-term care institutions, the presence of urinary incontinence in a resident means that such a person must be cared for at a skilled nursing or high-intensity intermediate level of care, even if otherwise the person might manage well in a minimal care setting.

For all of these reasons it is important for the physician, in evaluating any older patient, to determine (from patient and family or other sources such as visiting nurse) whether the patient has any problem with urinary incontinence, and if so to conduct a thorough diagnostic workup and, based on the findings, to undertake appropriate treatment (Williams and Pannill, 1982). In most instances the problem can be eliminated or controlled.

A good first step in evaluating reported or suspected urinary incontinence is to arrange tc have an "incontinence diary" kept by the patient or caregiver—a daily record for several days of just when episodes of incontinence occur, roughly how much urine is spilled, the circumstances—while up and about or in bed or while on the way to the bathroom but "didn't quite make it"—and whether the patient is aware of the episode. In some instances simply keeping such a diary leads a previously careless person to achieve satisfactory control. The diary provides information on the magnitude of the problem and clues to possible causes.

Further workup of the incontinence should proceed from simple to more complex tests, as needed. Urinalysis and culture may indicate a urinary tract infection that, if eliminated, will result in restoration of continence. Observing whether there is any urinary spillage with coughing or straining in the upright position (after preparing the patient with sufficient fluid intake to be sure there is urine to spill) may point to stress incontinence. Catherization after the patient has attempted to void completely can provide evidence for an obstructed or atonic bladder and overflow incontinence.

The most common cause of urinary incontinence in older people is instability of the detrusor system of the bladder—the loss of normal neurologic inhibiting influences as the bladder fills. The detrusor muscle, if uninhibited, will begin to contract spontaneously when filling has reached relatively small volumes, 150 ml or less, and the patient will find it difficult or impossible to suppress the tendency to void. Unequivocal diagnosis of this condition requires cystometric studies and such should be done when needed; some physicians who are thoroughly familiar with the differential diagnosis of incontinence may choose to use first a trial of therapy for the presumptive diagnosis of instability, once other causes such as those referred to above have been eliminated.

In persons with stress incontinence or detrusor instability, the use of biofeedback and other training exercises has been found to help a number of patients to control this problem. Assuring quick access to a toilet, such as use of a bedside toilet at night, can help a person with detrusor instability reach the toilet in time. If the stress incontinence in women is associated with major anatomical changes, e.g., severe uterine prolapse, or when prostatic obstruction in men is the apparent cause, then surgical intervention may be indicated.

Drugs with anticholinergic effects are successful in decreasing detrusor instability in some patients; their use is often limited by undesirable anticholinergic effects in other organ systems, such as dry mouth and disturbances in gastrointestinal function. At least theoretically, anticholingeric drugs could worsen dementia of the Alzheimer's type (see above). Efforts have been made to identify drugs of this type whose effects are mainly on the bladder.

The use of imipramine for detrusor instability warrants special note because this antidepressant has both anticholinergic and sympathomimetic actions and may be helpful both through relaxing the bladder (anticholinergic effect) and through contracting or tightening the urethral sphincter (sympathomimetic effect). Whether it is actually more effective than other anticholinergic drugs has not been established.

When overflow incontinence secondary to a distended, atonic bladder is present (as occurs with diabetic neuropathy), cholinergic drugs may be helpful.

Even if none of the above approaches is effective, acceptable management of the incontinence may be achieved through use of special waterproof pants with absorbent liners, the use of special absorbent pads on the bed, specially fitted collecting devices in women, and in selected patients the use of intermittent straight catheterization. The use of chronic indwelling catheters is rarely indicated.

PRESSURE ULCERS AND CONTRACTURES. These are unfortunate and for the most part preventable common complications of chronic illness in frail older people. Even a few hours of total immobility, as after a stroke or in the recovery period following surgery, will likely result in pressure damage to the skin and subcutaneous tissues; as little as a day or two of immobility in a joint may lead to contracture formation. Once these problems develop, correcting them is a long, tedious, and expensive process.

Preventive measures for any patient at risk of developing pressure (decubitus) ulcers or contractures should include regular, frequent passive or active movement of joints and turning, assiduous skin care, careful attention to avoiding potential damage from wrinkled bed clothes, and care in lifting, not pulling, a patient while changing his or her position. A patient should be sitting in a chair and also walking as much as possible; while sitting he or she should shift weight at least every 15 to 20 minutes.

Once pressure ulcers have developed, even greater attention should be paid to the preventive practices just described. The ulcer should be kept clean, with scrubbing and soaking three to four times a day; mild antiseptic cleansing solutions such as half-strength povidone are better than stronger agents, which may cause further tissue damage. A good practice is to leave wet-to-dry gauze dressings on the wound. Surgical debridement of any necrotic tissue should be done.

As important as local care of the wound is attention to adequate general nutrition and to the treatment of any systemic disease that may cause a general catabolic response. With good wound care in a patient who is adequately nourished and otherwise well or recovering, ulcers will heal rapidly; the presence of chronic infection elsewhere, or poor nutrition, can thwart the effectiveness of even the best wound care. With large ulcers, once the wound surface is thoroughly healthy, skin grafting may be indicated.

Minor degrees of contractures can often be corrected with regular, frequent, careful stretching exercises, following a regimen established for the patient by a physical therapist. More severe and unresponsive contractures may require surgical correction. Such a step can be valuable and justified if it helps to restore mobility and independence or significantly eases the nursing care burdens of family or professionals.

DECISIONS ABOUT LONG-TERM CARE. Elderly persons who acquire chronic, irreversible functional losses must have appropriate ongoing supportive services: the goal should be to substitute help by others only to the extent necessary, thus preserving the maximum possible degree of independence for the patient. Arriving at sound decisions about such long-term care requires a complete evaluation of the patient, as described above.

Often the need for decisions arises at a time of crisis: already borderline functional capabilities of the older person may have further deteriorated owing to a new condition, e.g., injury, stroke, etc., or the caregiving spouse or child may become ill or unable to continue the previous extent of care. The physician, in collaboration with other professionals (e.g., visiting nurse, social worker) and the patient and family, must weigh the relative merits and feasibility of maintaining the patient at home with support services, or arranging care in a long-term care institution, i.e., nursing home or intermediate care facility. Most older people strongly prefer to continue living in their familiar home settings, and most families desire to help the patient to stay there. Through thoughtful use of various supportive services—meals on wheels, housekeeper, personal care or home health aides, day programs—it is possible to maintain many such patients at home whose care needs would have equally well justified nursing home admission. The cost of the external supporting services in such instances may be only 50 to 60 per cent as much as the nursing home alternative would cost; the family clearly makes up the difference through their own provision of personal care, meals, etc. These features are discussed here because with the continually growing numbers of very elderly persons in our society there will be major increases in the pressures on our long-term care systems, and physicians will continue to be involved at the critical points of decision-making where careful efforts to help stabilize and maintain many patients at home will be most important.

CARE OF TERMINALLY ILL ELDERLY PERSONS. "Aging" and "dying" are so often throught of as almost synonymous that the problems of how to approach terminal care and how far to go in heroic or extraordinarily expensive diagnosis and treatment are considered by many to be issues that primarily appear in the care of the aged. The actual picture is somewhat different. Almost all of the circumstances in which inevitable death can be predicted in a fairly short time occur in patients with advanced cancer, at any age. For elderly patients with terminal cancer the same principles of care apply as for younger patients: when patient, family, and the responsible physician have agreed that no further efforts at curative therapy are warranted, the primary goal should be comfort care, avoiding heroics.

Similar decisions can be made in instances in which an older person has had such irreversible loss of mental function that he or she has little if any remaining apparent contact with surroundings and communication with others, especially family or nursing personnel. If those who are closest to the patient agree on the hopelessness of further curative or extraordinary treatment, including their view that this is also what the patient would say for himself or herself (or perhaps did say earlier, verbally or in writing such as a "living will"), then comfort care should be the practice. In fact, despite frequently expressed views that physicians order too much heroic, expensive care in elderly patients in hopeless situations, one study has found evidence for this in only 10 per cent of instances in two hospitals (and in most of those it was the family that insisted on such efforts); in 90 per cent of the cases everyone involved agreed that putting primary emphasis on comfort care had been appropriately accomplished (Loomis and Williams, 1983).

What is comfort care? The precise details will vary with the condition of each individual patient. Overall, the physician should be concerned to see that pain is relieved, that whatever may give the patient enjoyable days (and nights) is done (perferred foods, cleanliness, comfortable positioning, visits by family or friends, outings), and that no diagnostic or treatment efforts are undertaken that may be unpleasant or painful or that will not contribute to comfort. These guidelines do not eliminate all ambiguity: for example, what should the physician decide when confronted with a new infection such as pneumonia in a patient in whom comfort care is the primary goal? If no treatment is given, the patient will likely have several days of very uncomfortable respiratory distress and may or may not survive. Comfort care in this instance would probably include respiratory therapy to help clear the airway and use of an oral antibiotic, avoiding painful injections or intravenous therapy.

Kane RA, Kane RL: Assessing the Elderly: A Practical Guide to Measurement. Lexington, MA, Lexington Books (DC Heath), 1981.
Loomis MT, Williams TF: Evaluation of care provided to terminally ill patients. Gerontologist 23:493–499, 1983.
Proceedings of NIA Technology Assessment Conference on the Use of Assessment Technology in Evaluating Elderly Patients. J Am Geriatr Soc 31:636; 721, 1983.
Steel RK, Gertman PM, Crescenzi C, Anderson J: Iatrogenic illness on a general medical service at a university hospital. N Engl J Med 304:638–642, 1981.
Steele C, Lucas MJ, Tune LE: An approach to the management of dementia syndromes. Johns Hopkins Med J 151:362–368, 1982.
Verghese A, Berk SL: Bacterial pneumonia in the elderly. Medicine 62:271–285, 1983.
Williams ME, Pannill FC III: Urinary incontinence in the elderly: Physiology, pathophysiology, diagnosis and treatment. Ann Intern Med 97:895–907, 1982.

11. CARE OF DYING PATIENTS AND THEIR FAMILIES

Sylvia A. Lack

Dying patients, as individuals, need to maintain their self-esteem as their dependency on others increases. People need to feel secure in their continued value. Physical distress erodes self-confidence and undermines the ability to make decisions and to give as well as to receive. Good symptom control frees the patient to work on existential and practical matters. Many, regardless of intellectual capability or social class, struggle to answer the question: "What has been the meaning of my life?" Indeed, faced squarely with the fact of death, physicians are forced to consider this question for themselves. The resultant unease may be the reason for the subtle withdrawal perceived by many patients.

THE PHYSICIAN AND DEATH

Physicians mature in their profession through interaction with their patients; patients get well through interchange with their physicians. Dying and the implied loss take their toll on both. It is natural for a physician to feel unhappy when a patient recognizably deteriorates. One way of dealing with the resultant sense of guilt is to work compulsively against the disease until the patient dies. This is clearly beneficial when there is realistic expectation that the disease can be arrested. Many will die in acute care settings during an appropriate battle to maintain life. This chapter does not focus on the management of such patients, but on care for those *dying* with cancer and other chronic, degenerative illness. When death is inevitable, it is counterproductive to continue curative efforts regardless of the consequences for patient comfort.

At the end of life the physician's two principal functions of curing disease and relieving suffering can become increasingly incompatible. For those in whom prognostic indicators show little or no prospect of rehabilitation, the caring physician has to shift gears and concentrate on the patient's immediate well-being. This requires an enlarged perspective, including awareness of the needs of the family and the possibilities of home care. Care of the dying, although analytical, is relaxed, with emphasis on listening, being, and availability. Such care must be the best that skilled nursing and medicine can provide, ideally embodying the organizational characteristics found in the hospice movement (Table 11–1). It keeps abreast of developments while at the same time avoiding ineffective therapy.

AVOIDING INAPPROPRIATE TREATMENT

In the dying patient with irreversible underlying disease, the aim of treatment is to make remaining life comfortable and meaningful. It is no longer to preserve life at all costs. Medical care is a continuum, with cure at one end and comfort care at the other. When cure is no longer possible, disease control and palliation should be considered. When disease escapes control, the emphasis moves to symptom relief and comfort as an end in itself. What may be appropriate treatment when disease is reversible may be ineffective—and thus poor medical care—in the dying. Cardiac resuscitation, artificial ventilation, intravenous fluids, nasogastric tubes, and antibiotics are all primarily measures for use in acute or acute-on-chronic illness. They assist toward recovery of health or a stable state. Their use in the dying is justified only when specifically directed to providing comfort and control of symptoms. The question is not "to

TABLE 11–1. CHARACTERISTICS OF A HOSPICE PROGRAM

1. Coordinated home care—inpatient beds with sufficient administrative autonomy and flexibility to provide intensive personal care.
2. Patient/family regarded as the unit of care.
3. Physician-directed services.
4. Provision of care by an interdisciplinary team.
5. An emphasis on control of symptoms (physical, sociological, psychological, spiritual).
6. Services available on a 24-hour-a-day/7-day-a-week/on-call basis, with emphasis on medical and nursing skills—including at-home availability.
7. Utilization of volunteers as an integral part of the interdisciplinary team.
8. Bereavement follow-up.
9. Structured staff support and communications systems.
10. Patient/family acceptance on the basis of health needs, not ability to pay.

treat or not to treat," but to decide the most appropriate treatment in light of the patient's biologic potential.

Many therapies span the entire spectrum of care from cure to comfort, notably radiation therapy. No particular type of treatment is in itself inappropriate for any category of patient. Instead, the therapeutic aim in any particular patient should be kept clearly in mind when treatment of any kind is employed. Terminal hemorrhage does not mandate blood transfusion, but rather sedation and constant companionship. Terminal penumonia—if symptomatic—may be treated with antitussives and antipyretics. If these fail to control symptoms, antibiotics may be indicated, but the clinical setting must dictate the choice.

COMMUNICATION

The value of good communication cannot be overemphasized. Technical, scientific, and clinical competence are not enough. Those who advocate a conspiracy of silence often convey by action and expression the message they are trying to avoid. It is impossible not to communicate. At a time of increasing uncertainty, the message a patient needs to receive is "You are safe." Only part of this can be said in words:

"One of us will always be available."

"I will be back as often as it takes to get this pain under control."

"Whatever happens, I am going to do all I can to help."

Most of this fundamental communication is nonverbal, transmitted by demonstration and behavior. Normal courtesies are maintained—the handshake, level eye-to-eye contact, a seat taken if at all possible. Greetings include the patient's name and often in this day of fragmented care, a reintroduction of oneself, with a reminder of one's role. Others within hearing range are acknowledged—the neighboring patient and others accompanying the familiar physician.

Once trust is established, a patient will often indicate with a question or statement that he is ready to hear more.

"I don't think I can take this much longer, doctor."

"The wife hopes I'll be home by Christmas? . . ."

"I want to stop chemotherapy; it's not doing me any good."

Total candor is not the only alternative to evasion. No one wants to hear harsh and brutal truths, but almost everyone wants to know what is going on. Words and concepts can be tailored to individual culture, beliefs, fears, frustrations, strengths, and courage. The physician's responsibility is to foster clarity and honesty, but not to force an unwilling patient into realities beyond his capacity to cope psychologically.

PAIN RELIEF

The patient with a diagnosis of cancer frequently waits in a misery of apprehension for the pain to start, but published data suggest that as many as 50 per cent of all cancer patients have no pain at all or negligible discomfort at most. However, 40 per cent do experience severe pain and the remaining 10 per cent suffer pain of a less intense nature. So much can be done to alleviate terminal pain that optimism and determination are justified. A valid base of trust can be maintained in the area of pain management, despite inability to control the disease process itself. The first mild pain should be taken seriously and controlled. This establishes confidence that the physician does have skills to prevent discomfort. This confidence will be a powerful ally if pain becomes troublesome later in the illness.

The goal of effective control is a pain-free patient with normal affect. The very sick patient may doze when external stimuli are minimal but is able to rouse and be alert to friends, family, and surroundings without drug-induced stupor or euphoria. A normal mental state can be sustained through a three-faceted approach as follows:

1. Identification of the primary cause and exacerbating factors.
2. Maintenance of *continuous* pain relief.
3. Ease of administration.

Assessment

Cancer does not preclude other ills; therefore, nonmalignant sources of pain must also be considered. Cystitis, hemorrhoids, toothache, and angina will require specific remedies. The cause of pain, however, is primarily a bedside diagnosis. Extensive investigations are usually not necessary for the terminally ill, and in view of limited life expectancy and vulnerability to pain, treatment is not delayed pending laboratory findings.

Comprehensive management considers all sources of pain, whether they be psychological, spiritual, social, or physical. Emotional responses influence the perception of pain. Chronic, terminal pain can be conceived as a vicious circle: physical pain rouses anxiety; constant anxiety and pain cause insomnia; and pain, anxiety, and insomnia generate depression (Fig. 11–1). Anxiety and depression are part of the long-term nature of pain. These factors lower pain threshold and aggravate the painful sensation. Control will not be achieved unless these components are addressed.

The nature of terminal pain is different from acute pain. Acute pains have a purpose in that they indicate a need for action or hold positive connotations like the birth of a child or healing surgery. For the dying patient new or added pain only proclaims physical deterioration, and an increase in its severity is envisioned.

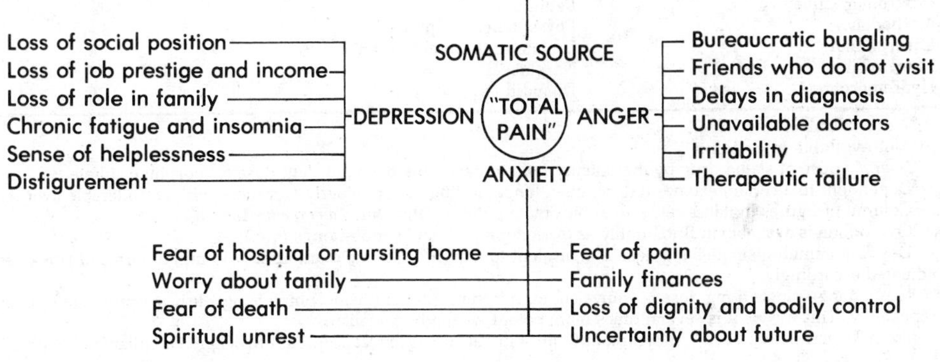

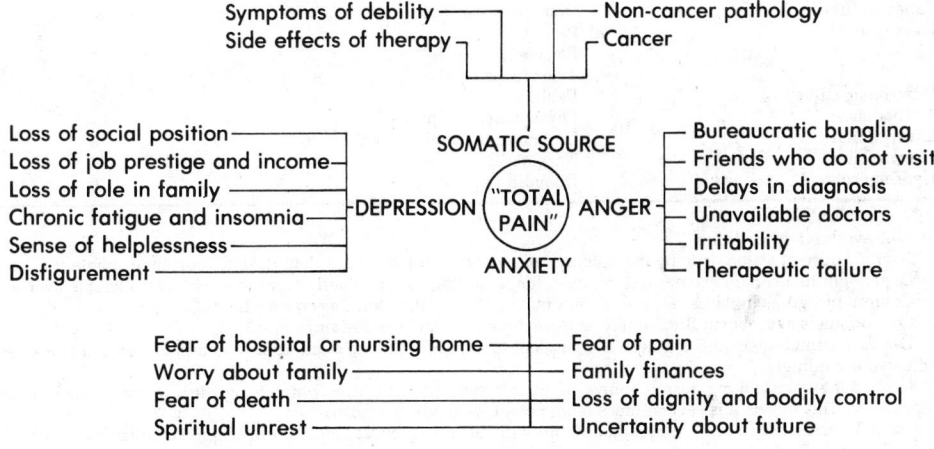

Figure 11–1. Pain is a somatopsychic experience: a diagram indicating some of the many non-physical influences that modify a patient's perception of pain. (From Twycross RG, Lack SA: Symptom Control in Far Advanced Cancer: Pain Relief 1983. Urban and Schwarzenberg/Pitman. With permission.)

Narcotics for Selected Terminal Pain

Pharmacologic control of terminal pain is not usually a matter of exotic new techniques, but the correct use of drugs already known. The aim of treatment is to manage pain so that it will not return. Breakthrough or recurring pain erodes confidence while generating anxiety and fear. Constant pain control is achieved through adequate analgesia given at regular, well-timed intervals. This method uses smaller drug doses, minimizes side effects, and allows the dose to be increased as the disease progresses.

In mild pain aspirin or acetaminophen is used; for moderate pain codeine or dextropropoxyphene; for severe pain morphine is the drug of choice. Useful alternatives are hydromorphone and probably oxycodone, only recently available on its own. Twycross (1977) has shown that there is no clinically observable difference between morphine and heroin when given orally in individually optimized doses at regular intervals.

Meperidine has a two- to three-hour duration of action—rather short for continuous control. Narcotics with longer action are methadone and levorphanol, but these drugs may accumulate in the body, as their half-lives are much longer than their durations of action. In particular, levorphanol accumulation in the older patient manifests clinically by the onset of confusion and restlessness several days after starting regular administration.

Narcotics are used when non-narcotics, used correctly, fail to control pain. Some pains are not narcotic-responsive. Other methods are sought for tension headache, post-herpetic neuralgia, dysesthesia, gastric distention, and muscle spasm. The severity and type of pain guide the choice of analgesic, not the estimate of life expectancy.

Hospice workers have not found narcotic dependence or tolerance to be a practical problem. Addiction, in the popular sense, is rare in patients with no history of drug abuse, despite the widespread use of narcotics for pain control. Drug dependence as defined by the World Health Organization has two components: psychic and physical. Psychic dependence, an overpowering drive to take a drug, occurs in pain patients most commonly after the use of "p.r.n." injections in inadequate dosage. Each request becomes a reminder of the dependence on drugs and the person who administers them. It is preventable by the use of oral narcotics and regular administration. This frees the patient both from the ritual of injections and from continually asking for relief from the presence or threat of pain. With regular analgesia, the self-perpetuating spiral of pain, dependence, and misery is never started. Physical dependence is of little relevance in the patient with limited life expectancy and does not prevent gradual narcotic reduction if the disease goes into remission.

Tolerance is not a problem if the narcotic is precisely adjusted to the degree of pain the patient is experiencing. Patients remain pain-free on the same dose for many weeks or months. With the exception of the first few days, when the pain is being brought under control, the total daily dose does not fluctuate unless disease progression increases nociceptive stimuli.

Optimal Use of Morphine

Common postoperative dosage is not always optimal for terminal pain management. Optimal narcotic doses are determined by titration to effect. Melzack (1979) has confirmed in a double-blind crossover trial that morphine alone in a flavored aqueous solution is clinically equivalent to a Brompton's mixture containing morphine, cocaine, ethyl alcohol, syrup, and chloroform water. Hospices favor an aqueous morphine solution because tighter control can be achieved than with tablets.

An initial dose of morphine for the patient not previously exposed to narcotics may be 5 to 10 mg every four hours by mouth. The sedative effect wears off in two to three days and can be largely avoided by starting with a small dose and increasing gradually. The four-hourly dose is increased at 48-hour intervals by 5-mg increments until control is obtained. If sedation is not a problem, increases can be made more rapidly. If narcotics have been used previously, morphine dosage will be dictated by careful attention to analgesic equivalents (Table 11–2). Once pain is controlled, the dose is stabilized and continued every four hours to prevent recurrence of pain. A double dose at bedtime obviates the 2 a.m. dose in many patients once stability is achieved.

Occasionally pain returns in less than four hours. This problem can be overcome by (1) increasing the regular dose, (2) decreasing the time interval to three hours (never less), or (3) adding a non-narcotic analgesic. Perhaps a trusted favorite from an earlier time, or an antiprostaglandin for bony metastatic pain, will be useful. The correct course of action can be ascertained by asking:

"Does the medicine ever take the pain away completely?"

"Does the pain return before it is time for the next dose of medicine?"

If the answer to the first question is no, then the dose is increased and adjuvant measures adjusted. If the answer to both questions is yes and a judicious increment has been ineffective, then the time interval may be decreased.

TABLE 11–2. STRONG NARCOTIC ANALGESICS: APPROXIMATE ORAL EQUIVALENTS TO MORPHINE SULFATE

Analgesic	Proprietary Name	Potency Ratio with Morphine Sulfate[1]		Duration of Action (Hours)[2]
Pethidine/meperidine	Demerol	1/8	*1/12*[3]	2–3
Dipipanone*	in Diconal	1/2	*1/3*	3–5
Papaveretum	Omnopon, Pantopon	2/3	*1/2*	3–5
Oxycodone†[4]	in Percodan, Percocet, Tylox (capsule)	1	*2/3*	3–5
Dextromoramide*	Palfium	2[5]	*1.5*	2–4
Methadone	Physeptone, Dolophine	3–4[6]	*2–3*	6–8
Levorphanol	Dromoran, Levo-dromoran	5	*3*	4–6
Phenazocine*	Narphen	5	*3*	4–6
Hydromorphone†	Dilaudid	6	*4*	3–4

*Not available in the USA.
†Not available in Britain.
[1]*Multiply* dose of stated drug by the potency ratio to determine the equivalent dose of morphine sulfate.
[2]Dependent to a certain extent on dose, often longer lasting in very elderly and those with considerable liver dysfunction.
[3]Column of figures in italics refers to approximate potency ratio with *diamorphine* (heroin).
[4]Oxycodone is available in Britain only as oxycodone pectinate suppositories (q.v.).
[5]Dextromoramide—single 5 mg dose is equivalent to morphine 15 mg (diamorphine 10 mg) in terms of *peak* effect but is generally shorter acting; overall potency rate adjusted accordingly.
[6]Methadone—single 5 mg dose is equivalent to morphine 7.5 mg (diamorphine 5 mg). It has a prolonged plasma half-life, which leads to accumulation when given repeatedly. This means it is several times more potent when given regularly.
(From Twycross RG, Lack SA: Symptom Control in Far Advanced Cancer: Pain Relief, 1983. Urban and Schwarzenberg/Pitman. With permission.)

TABLE 11–3. PERSISTENT EXCESSIVE DROWSINESS

1. Is the patient still recuperating from prolonged fatigue?
2. If the patient is completely comfortable, reduce the dose and review both drowsiness and pain control.
3. Is the patient on a psychotropic preparation, notably benzodiazepine (e.g., diazepam) or a phenothiazine (e.g., chlorpromazine)? Is it necessary? Can it be reduced or stopped?
4. If the patient is taking a phenothiazine as an antiemetic, can it be changed to haloperidol or metoclopramide?
5. Is the patient more ill than I thought?
6. If the patient is in hepatic or renal failure, try reducing the dose.
7. Is the patient hypoxic because of morphine-exacerbated respiratory failure? (rare)
8. Could the patient have a cerebral secondary lesion, unmasked by the intracranial pressure–elevating effect of morphine?
9. If the patient is not agitated, or if he is cyanotic, consider using dexamphetamine 2.5 or 5 mg each morning. (This is only rarely necessary or appropriate.)

From Twycross RG, Lack SA: Symptom Control in Far Advanced Cancer: Pain Relief, 1983. Urban and Schwarzenberg/Pitman. With permission.

Unwanted effects should receive prompt management. Constipation is so common that a regular narcotic is never prescribed without concomitant attention to the bowels. Stool softeners, peristaltic agents, and small bowel flushers counteract the antiperistaltic narcotic effect. Nausea and vomiting, which are also initiation side effects and are not universal, can be prevented by the use of a piperazine phenothiazine or haloperidol. Persistent sedation is often due to factors other than the morphine (Table 11–3).

General Techniques of Pain Control

Pain control does not begin or end with analgesics; it cannot be achieved by merely writing an order. The therapeutic environment (Table 11–4) is important: light, flowers, art, and, most significantly, caring people. Here the patient is affected by more than drug changes. He is surrounded by a team who are confident that the pain will be under control before long. Peer support comes from other patients who relate their own stories of controlled pain. The patient sees others receive medicine on a regular basis and observes that they are alert and functioning. Diversions such as television, radio, talking books, or physical and occupational therapy turn attention away from pain and onto other subjects. Table 11–5 lists a range of additional pain control methods. Some are seldom effective, but all need consideration. Pain can be avoided by care in moving a pathologically fractured arm or leg. Heat or ice, pillows, and massage all help to ease pain.

Ease of administration is a significant consideration, because it has substantial impact on the patient's way of life. Injections promote dependence on the person administering the drug. Oral administration eliminates local trauma, enables the patient to maintain control over his own drug administration, and helps retain his freedom to choose where to spend his last days.

Insomnia is treated resolutely. Night nurses carry a special responsibility for emotional comfort, for discomfort is often worse at night when the patient is alone with his pain and fear. The cumulative effect of many sleepless, pain-filled nights is a substantial lowering of the pain threshold.

TABLE 11–4. SOME INGREDIENTS OF A THERAPEUTIC ENVIRONMENT FOR THE DYING

- Freedom for pets and children to visit
- Open visiting at all hours of the day and night
- Provision for overnight stays for the family
- Arrangements for patient and friends to eat together
- Provision of edible food at any time when the cancer patient's fickle appetite briefly returns
- Nursing and other care-giving staffing patterns allowing for interdisciplinary conferences
- Provision for even the bedridden patient to have mobility to facilitate trips outside and attendance at parties, religious services, concerts, and the like

TABLE 11–5. ANALGESIC MEASURES FOR THE DYING

Pharmocologic	**Injections**
Antibiotics	Local anesthetic
Anti-inflammatory drugs	Peripheral nerve block
Antiprostaglandins	Autonomic nerve block
Glucocorticosteroids	Intrathecal block
Physical	**Neurosurgery**
Chemical sprays	Peripheral nerve section
Local heat	Cordotomy
Immobilization	Hypophysectomy
Joint compression	**Palliative Surgery**
Electrical stimulation	**Psychological**
Massage	Hypnosis
Irradiation	Relaxation
	Biofeedback

SYMPTOM CONTROL

Physical discomfort looms large in the lives of dying patients, and medicine for the dying must be concerned with smooth sheets, back rubs, relieving constipation, and getting up at night. A person lying in a wet bed is not interested in reassuring words. Patients and families can cope with many emotional crises if they are cared for with common sense and professional skills.

There is never a time when "nothing more can be done." Remedies for all the common problems in terminal disease can be compiled. A problem-oriented approach treats each symptom on its own merit. Thus the patient becomes not Mr. Doe with incurable cancer, but Mr. Doe—the man with severe pain for which we can do a great deal. This enables the physician, as part of the team, to approach the patient with an optimistic, realistic attitude. The limited view of an individual, which can fail to address the complexity of the problems presented by dying, can be overcome by teamwork. Effective teamwork mandates that interdisciplinary personnel gather regularly in conference to work out a coordinated approach.

Inclusion of the family fosters an atmosphere of cooperation and support. If their questions are not answered speedily and satisfactorily, they may stop following their physician's advice and abandon the entire carefully constructed regimen. The attending physician, nurses, and home health aide must also understand the therapy. A visitor's doubts may undermine the positive advantages created by confidence. For the patient, underlying mechanisms are explained in simple terms: "Your shortness of breath is partly due to the illness and partly due to fluid at the base of the right lung. There is some degree of 'waterlogging' throughout the body, particularly in the lungs, and you are slightly anemic—people with your sort of illness often are. I cannot get rid of the underlying tumor—you know that—but this is what we are going to do about the extra fluid. . . ."

The fact that you, the doctor, understand why he, the patient, is having trouble is reassuring. No longer is this condition shrouded in mystery. The doctor understands. Treatment options are discussed with the patient, and, if possible, an immediate course of action is decided upon together. Few things are more demeaning to a person's self-esteem than to be disregarded in discussions concerning treatment. It is hurtful to feel ignored and treated as a nonentity. The dying have a right to be treated for what they usually are: sane, sensible adults. While it is wise not to promise too much, it is important to reassure the patient that the doctor is going to stand by and do all possible to ensure comfort.

Confidence is crucial to successful symptom management. The patient may resist a drug regimen because of a lifelong habit of never giving in or resorting to drugs. Other reasons for resistance may be fear of constipation, addiction, nightmares, and confusion. Once identified through sensitive inquiry, these fears can be dealt with by discussion, education, and control of unwanted effects. In addition to pressing symptoms such as pain, vomiting, and dyspnea, patients may experience a variety of other discomforts. These include dry mouth, altered taste, anorexia, constipation, frequency, pruritus, cough, and insomnia. Because patients tend to be reluctant to bother their doctor about such symptoms, physicians should inquire about them from time to time.

Bedside assessment precedes treatment. Treatment for the same symptom may vary considerably from patient to patient. The treatment of vomiting associated with raised intracranial pressure differs from treatment of vomiting secondary to intestinal obstruction. In the dying symptoms are caused by multiple factors, some treatable and some not. Best results are obtained by aggressively dealing with the treatable elements. Instead of attempting *immediately* to relieve the symptom completely, the physician can wear down the problem a little at a time. It is surprising how much can be achieved with determination and persistence. Although the principal pathologic process may remain unaltered, it is generally possible to relieve symptoms to a considerable extent. Comprehensive treatment is not limited to the use of drugs. Thus, pruritus is relieved in the majority without resorting to antihistaminic drugs. Application of emollient cream to dry, itching skin several times a day and elimination of soap in favor of emulsifying ointment are frequently sufficient.

Clearly defined medical leadership is vital. Frequent contact with specialist colleagues and readiness to consult with others will assist the physician in the search for symptom relief, but the patient should be discouraged from attending a succession of outpatient clinics.

DYING AT HOME

Although home care is not for all, it is a cost-effective alternative that has historic tradition and has proved to be a well-received option in contemporary communities. Physician availability, information about community resources, 24-hour coverage, and education of family members are crucial issues when keeping someone home to die.

Every family must have a sense of security in order to carry on. Most need professional reassurance, and the home visits of a trusted physician are a great boost to morale. Much discomfort, in a terminal setting, can be assessed and alleviated at the bedside, but not over the phone. Moreover, in some states, an at-home pronouncement visit is necessary to avoid legal complications. Bereavement counselling can then begin when the death certificate is put aside and the physician inquires:

"Tell me about the last few hours, how have you managed?"

Reassuring the family that "you did well" will help them to overcome feelings of helplessness and guilt.

Change comes quickly in terminal illness and can be planned for by discussion and practical measures, such as a supply of parenteral essentials kept in the home. Common crises include refusal of medication, impaction, disorientation, new pain, and the onset of incontinence or of coma. All these issues are manageable in the home, but poor preparation precipitates premature inpatient admission. Even the best laid plans can prove inadequate, but families often manage if someone who knows the patient is available at any time of the day or night.

Medication regimens should be kept simple to understand and easy to administer, even at the expense of pharmacologic purity. An impossibly complex schedule will not be followed. Short-acting narcotics such as meperidine are rarely satisfactory at home. Similarly, a two-hourly medication regimen is impossible to maintain for long.

THE LAST TWENTY-FOUR HOURS

Careful assessment is still necessary if the patient is to be kept comfortable. Temporary relief from a painful bedsore can be obtained by the application of a local anesthetic gel, which might not be used when life expectancy is longer. A distended bladder can be relieved by catheterization. The sound of rattling secretions can often be diminished by positioning and scopolamine. Pain will not be troublesome at the very end if control has previously been good. There is no final crescendo of pain. Analgesic requirements may decrease. Patients do, however, experience pain even when comatose. In addition, they may be physically dependent on narcotics. Withdrawal restlessness may mar their peace if narcotics are stopped. For these reasons it is advisable to continue analgesia by suppository or injection when the patient cannot swallow. At one hospice 60 per cent of patients are able to swallow until a few hours before death and need no change in drug administration. Another 25 per cent require one or two narcotic suppositories; only 15 per cent need an injection. Only one fourth of the original daily dose is needed to prevent withdrawal symptoms, so rigid adherence to the previous schedule is not necessary. Morphine every six to eight hours will usually suffice.

Both staff and relatives are informed that, at this late stage, any injection may be the last. This information may allay in *advance* any lingering fears about "killing the patient":

> "She might die just five minutes after you give her the four o'clock injection. How will you feel if that happens? You understand that it would be just a coincidence because she is going to die very soon anyway? We are using injections only to keep her out of pain."

The advent of the modern hospice has done much to raise expectations in both the public and health care professions. We must be wary of replacing one caricature by another—the old image of death as negative and despairing with the new image that "death is beautiful." It does not help to underestimate the problems. Good terminal care is hard work. The very highest standards may be achieved on paper, but this is a futile exercise unless every aspect is tailored to the vagaries of the individual patient and family.

Health and Public Policy Committee, American College of Physicians: Drug therapy for severe, chronic pain in terminal illness. Ann Intern Med 99:870, 1983. *A position paper authoritatively endorsing six principles elaborated by the modern hospice movement over the past 20 years.*

Hinton J: Talking with people about to die. Br Med J 3:25, 1974. *Sixty dying patients comment on their discussions with doctors and nurses, and give their opinions on what degree of truth is desirable. The assumed principle is that the views of dying people count.*

Jacobs S, Ostfeld A: An epidemiological review of the mortality of bereavement. Psychosom Med 39:344, 1977. *Summarizes the literature revealing excess mortality in the newly widowed; heightens, for the clinician's consideration, an awareness of the importance of bereavement as a public health problem.*

Lack SA: Hospice—A concept of care in the final stage of life. Conn Med 43:367, 1979. *Describes hospice as a specialized health care delivery system, emphasizing the essential administrative characteristics of a program organized to meet the needs of the dying and their families.*

Lasagna L: Heroin: A medical me too. N Engl J Med 304:1539, 1981. *A succinct rationale, with good references, emphasizing why improved terminal pain control in the USA does not require the legalization of heroin.*

Marks RM, Sachar EJ: Undertreatment of medical inpatients with narcotic analgesics. Ann Intern Med 78:173, 1973. *A survey of physicians' orders and patient response documenting the authors' belief that the emotional significance of narcotic analgesics appears to interfere with their rational use. Physician education in the proper and adequate use of these drugs is greatly needed.*

Saunders C: Hospice care. Am J Med 65:726, 1978. *The founder traces the origins of the modern hospice movement, correcting some misconceptions in the popular press and defining the position of good terminal management within the mainstream of medicine.*

Twycross RW, Lack SA: Symptom Control in Far Advanced Cancer: Pain Relief, 1983, and Therapeutics in Terminal Cancer, 1984. Urban and Schwarzenberg/Pitman. *More extensive elaboration and detailed discussion of the analytic methods of pain relief and symptom control mentioned in this chapter.*

Part III
PERSONAL HEALTH CARE AND PREVENTIVE MEDICINE

12. PRINCIPLES OF PERSONAL MEDICINE

Stephen B. Hulley

In the early part of this century preventive medicine efforts were focused on infectious disease, the predominant cause of illness and death at the time. The preventive programs included governmental actions such as sanitary control of the water and sewage systems and clinical activities such as immunization (see Ch. 15). In the United States these programs combined with better medical care, improved nutrition, and other factors to largely eradicate death from infectious disease (Table 12–1). These remarkable trends have brought life expectancy to unprecedented heights and have left the noninfectious and chronic diseases as the major causes of death and disability. The result has been the emergence of a new set of preventive medicine strategies focused on the major causes of mortality today: coronary heart disease, cancer, stroke, and injury.

LIFESTYLE INTERVENTION TO PREVENT THE MAJOR CHRONIC DISEASES

The approach to preventing cardiovascular disease and cancer is based on epidemiologic studies that have identified risk factors for these conditions. These risk factors typically involve habitual lifestyles such as diet, exercise, cigarette smoking, and alcohol intake (each of which is addressed in a separate chapter below). As a result, the responsibility for preventing illness has shifted onto the person who must make the lifestyle changes—the patient — and the clinician has assumed the role of health counselor.

Behavior Modification

The process of guiding lifestyle change begins with serving as a model. A physician who has healthy habits and provides an appropriate environment (for example, prohibiting smoking in the waiting room), has set the stage for successful intervention. The *second step* is to explore the individual characteristics of the patient, testing for the presence of risk factors and exploring motivations for changing, and for not changing, unhealthy habits. The *third step* is to provide a clear message about the scientific facts on the determinants of disease, specifying, for example, the precise health consequences of cigarette smoking.

The *fourth step* is to formulate and apply recommendations for change. Behavior modification is an approach to health education that has its origins in the conditioned response research of Pavlov and Skinner. The components include (1) involving the patient as a partner in choosing attainable objectives and in making a firm commitment (written contracts may be helpful); (2) adjusting the environment to promote the desired behavior (by not keeping unhealthy food in the home, for example); (3) giving negative reinforcement for undesired behavior (through criticism or aversive techniques); (4) giving positive reinforcement for desired behavior (through praise or rewards); and (5) involving the family and other social supports. Many clinics include paramedical staff who are trained in specific behavioral techniques, but the personal involvement of physicians in the process is important. It is also helpful to guide the patient's access to other resources for lifestyle changes: providing pamphlets (obtained free from organizations like the American Heart Association) and referral to appropriate books, support groups, and health professionals.

Whatever the intervention approach, the *fifth step* is a sustained effort to follow up on the risk factor levels. Habits are difficult to change, and health counselors need to have the tenacity and imagination to try a variety of approaches over the years. It is important, however, to avoid harassing an unwilling or unsuccessful patient. The best health counselors are sensitive to the preferences of their patients and make careful decisions about when to pursue recommendations for change and when to leave the patient alone.

Implications of Chronic Disease Prevention

If the entire population were fully successful in the lifestyle changes proposed in this second wave of twentieth century preventive medicine efforts, the chief causes of premature death in this country might become far less common. In addition to this further extension of life expectancy, the promise of fully effective lifestyle intervention is the possibility that most people will be able to live their entire lives without major illness or disability.

Speculation of this sort is based in part on the remarkable decline in mortality observed in the United States over the past 15 years (Fig. 12–1). The chief component of the decline is coronary heart disease, which has decreased more rapidly in the United States than in any other nation (2 per cent per year). It seems reasonable to attribute this both to improvements in the management of acute coronary events and to the changes in lifestyle that are occurring in this country. Evidence for the latter may be found in the substantial decline that has occurred in the national prevalence of smoking and of inadequately treated hypertension, the decrease in the mean population level of serum cholesterol, and the widespread efforts to become more physically fit.

OTHER ASPECTS OF PERSONAL HEALTH CARE: INJURIES

The extent and variety of the preventive medicine of today is illustrated by the national objectives in 15 areas of endeavor,

TABLE 12–1. ANNUAL MORTALITY RATES AND YEARS OF LIFE LOST PREMATURELY IN THE UNITED STATES IN 1900 AND IN 1980*

Causes of Death†	1980 Annual Mortality (rate/100,000)	Years of potential life lost before age 65 by persons dying in 1980	1900 Annual Mortality (rate/100,000)
Diseases of the heart	336	1,636,000	137
Malignant neoplasms	184	1,804,000	64
Cerebrovascular disease	75	280,000	107
Injuries	69	4,487,000	83
All others	214	2,199,000	1330
Total	878	10,406,000	1721

*Data are from Center for Environmental Health, CDC, and Last (1980).

†The causes of death are the four most common in 1980. The statistics, which are not age-adjusted, are subject to the usual inaccuracies of death certificate attribution. The top three causes of death in 1900 were pneumonia and influenza (202/100,000), tuberculosis (194/100,000), and diarrhea and enteritis (143/100,000).

formally established in 1979 by the U.S. Department of Health and Human Services. These include the five topics covered in the chapters of this section (smoking, nutrition, physical fitness, alcohol abuse, and immunization), five topics addressed elsewhere in this book (hypertension, sexually transmitted diseases, toxic agents, occupational safety, and infectious disease control), three topics covered by other specialties (family planning, pregnancy and infant health, and dental health), and two miscellaneous topics (accidents, and stress and violence).

These last two topics, the prevention of injuries caused by accidents and violence, have been largely ignored by the medical profession. Because injuries are major causes of death and medical disability, resembling cardiovascular disease and cancer in having risk factors that reveal high risk groups and that are susceptible to intervention, this aspect of preventive medicine will be discussed here in some detail.

The Epidemiology of Injury Due to Accidents

Accidents are the fourth most common cause of death overall in the United States, and for people aged 1 to 45, they are the leading cause of death and disability. One third of all injury deaths are due to automobile accidents and one third to other accidents (the remaining third is evenly divided between suicide and homicide, discussed below). When preventive medicine topics are ranked in order of their contribution to *premature* death (Table 12–1), accidents assume the highest priority of all. In fact, the problem is far larger if nonfatal injuries, many of which cause permanent disability, are included.

The death rate from accidents has declined modestly in the United States since 1950 (Fig. 12–1). Nonmotor vehicle accidents are responsible for this trend. Falls are the commonest cause of accidental death (26 per cent), followed by fire, drowning, and poisoning (each about 10 per cent). The risk of accidental death for males is several times that for females, which is attributed in part to culturally determined behaviors. Nonmotor vehicle accidents are a particularly prominent cause of death among the elderly.

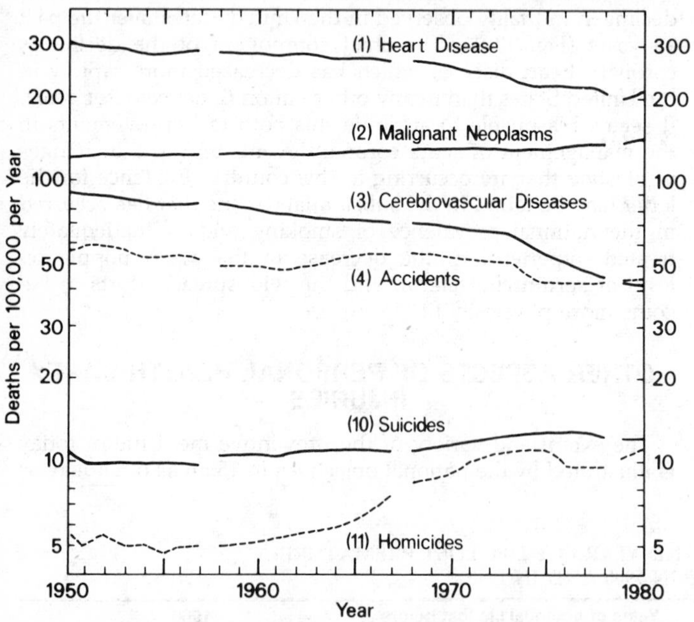

Figure 12–1. Age-adjusted death rate trends from 1950 to 1980 in the United States, plotted on a semi-log scale with current rank order in parentheses. Heart disease and stroke account for most of the 25 per cent decline in overall mortality (not shown) that has been observed over the last 15 years. Accidental death rates have also declined, reflecting a trend in nonmotor vehicle accidents. The small increase in cancer rates is due chiefly to a major rise in lung cancer incidence, outstripping a substantial fall in stomach cancer incidence. Homicide rates, relatively low in 1950, have doubled in recent years. (From DHHS: NCHS Monthly Vital Statistics Report Vol 32, No 4, 1983 [Suppl].)

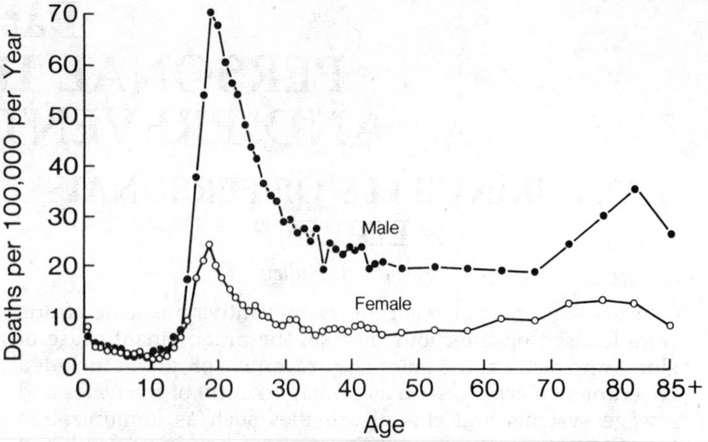

Figure 12–2. Age-specific death rates of motor vehicle occupants in the United States in 1976. The very high rates in 16- to 30-year-old males are a major component of the premature loss of life in this country. (From Haddon W, Baker SP: Injury control. *In* Clark D, MacMahon B (eds.): Preventive and Community Medicine. Boston, Little Brown & Co, 1981, pp 109–140.)

Traffic fatalities decreased by one third in the early 1970's after automobile safety regulations and the 55 MPH national speed limit were instituted, but the benefit has since been lost as average speeds have returned to higher levels and smaller cars have become more prevalent. Deaths due to motor vehicles rise to alarmingly high levels among young adults, particularly males (Fig. 12–2). This is illustrated by the statistic that 1.4 per cent of all 15-year-old boys in the United States die of an injury before age 25.

Prevention of Accidents

Accident prevention has assumed an important role in the practice of medicine only in the field of pediatrics. Perhaps it has not received more attention in internal medicine because the term "accident" connotes an event that has occurred by chance and is therefore unavoidable. This is far from the case; there are many lifestyle risk factors for accidents that are suitable for intervention with various behavioral techniques. The potential for preventing premature death and disability is substantial, and accident prevention advice could become as important in the general practice of medicine as the more familiar interventions on risk factors for cardiovascular disease and cancer.

Advice on preventing *automobile accidents* begins with widely known precepts such as observing the speed limit and using a well-designed seat belt. From the medical viewpoint, patients should be warned when drugs that may impair performance are prescribed, especially those, like diazepam, that may interact with alcohol. But the most important concern is alcohol by itself, which plays a role in more than half of all fatal automobile accidents. The knowledge that a particular patient drinks heavily should prompt a clinician to discuss the danger, not only to that individual, but also to others. Intervention can include counseling on ways to modulate alcohol intake, and on the use of alternate drivers, alternate forms of transportation, or alternate locations for drinking. The alarming accident rate among teenagers can be approached by counseling parents on the rules that they can establish for when and how their teenage children may drive. Society plays an important role in these areas, for example in setting the penalties for drunken driving and for the minimum age for licensing, and physicians can be an important force behind social legislation of this sort.

Injuries due to *falls* are particularly common at the two extremes of the age distribution. Interventions for the elderly include treating diseases that impair mobility and balance (and avoiding drugs that contribute to these problems) and efforts to retard osteoporosis and to prevent hip fracture. Advice can be given on designing an environment that makes tripping unlikely (e.g., by removing loose rugs and using night lights) and that reduces the extent of injury should a fall occur (e.g., through avoiding sharp corners and selecting a home without stairs). The strategies for small children include a different set of environmental control devices (e.g., barriers across upper story windows).

Fire is a source of injury and death that can be made less likely by counseling on such things as the dangers of smoking, the need for properly maintaining electrical and heating equipment, and the usefulness of smoke detectors and fire extinguishers. *Drowning* can be prevented by discussing the need for adequate barriers between small children and all bodies of water, and for instructing children in swimming and water safety rules at an early age. *Poisoning* has become less common with the advent of child-proof drug containers; this source of injury could be further prevented by counseling parents to store cleaning supplies, solvents, and other poisons in a safe place.

The Epidemiology of Injury Due to Violence

The homicide rate in the United States has doubled in recent years and now exceeds 20,000 per year. Homicides usually involve people who know each other, and more than half are carried out with handguns. An extraordinary aspect of the latter statistic is the 100-fold lower rates of homicide by handgun in countries like England, Sweden, and Japan that have strict handgun ownership laws; these countries also have lower overall rates of homicide. Statistics on injury from other forms of violence, including child abuse, wife beating, rape, and assault, are difficult to estimate, but each is undoubtedly far more common than homicide. Suicide rates have also increased in recent years. Almost all forms of violent injury are more common in the male sex and in the socioeconomically disadvantaged.

The Prevention of Injury Due to Violence

The medical profession's role in preventing the death and disability that result from violent behavior begins at an individual level. Violence within the family, such as child abuse, wife beating, or self-destructive activities, can often be discovered in the clinic by sensitive probing, and victims of assault and rape may present themselves for treatment of the injury. Interventions to prevent future episodes often include psychiatric referral, notification of legal and public health authorities (mandatory in some instances), and counseling by the clinician. The appropriate management of such problems is a major challenge to a professional's wisdom, courage, and skill.

The medical profession's most effective avenue for preventing violence may be in guiding the evolution of society and its rules. Doctors are important opinion leaders, and their comments on the medical and epidemiologic facts can help mold legislation directed at such things as handgun control and violence in the media.

Approaches of this sort are probably the only way that the medical profession can have an effect on the most serious preventive medicine issue of our age: the prevention of nuclear war. In addition to their general civic responsibility to express their views on this problem, some physicians take it as a professional responsibility to educate community leaders and acquaintances on medical realities such as the false security of civil defense plans that would be inoperable in the event of nuclear explosions.

SUMMARY

The emergence of noninfectious disease as the predominant cause of death and disability in industrial nations has led to the implication of certain lifestyle factors as causal agents. Among these, cigarette smoking is generally accepted as the single most important modifiable health hazard. At the same time, we now recognize that injuries due to accident and violence are the most important cause of *premature* death and disability, and that they too have lifestyle risk factors. Interventions designed to prevent injury are a useful and neglected focus for preventive medicine.

At an individual level, the clinician's role in preventive medicine includes examining a patient's risk factors, educating the person and listening to preferences for changing (or not changing) lifestyle, implementing the appropriate behavioral interventions, and following up on the progress of these personal health care strategies over the years. In addition, medical professionals have expertise that allows them to contribute usefully to the emergency of social measures dealing with health hazards that range from drunken driving to nuclear war.

Barancik JI, Chatterjee BF, Greene YC, Michenzi EM, Fife D: Northeastern Ohio trauma study: I. Magnitude of the problem. Am J Public Health 73:746, 1983. *Descriptive epidemiology of injury, nonfatal as well as fatal.*

Center for Environmental Health, CDC: Unintentional and intentional injuries—United States. MMWR 31:240–248, 1982. *Recent set of national statistics on injuries.*

Chang RS (ed.): Preventive Health Care. Boston, G K Hall, 1981. *Description of preventive health care, including accident prevention.*

Freis, JR: Aging, natural death, and the compression of morbidity. N Engl J Med. 303:130–135, 1980. *Provocative speculation on the potential ability of lifestyle intervention to postpone chronic disease beyond the normal lifespan of 85 years. See also the response:* N Engl J Med 309:854–855, 1983.

Haddon W, Barker SP: Injury Control. *In* Clark D, MacMahon B (eds.): Preventive and Community Medicine. Boston, Little, Brown & Co., 1981, pp. 109–140. *Comprehensive summary of the epidemiology of all forms of injuries, and of approaches to reducing their frequency and severity.*

Last J M (ed.): Maxcy-Rosenau Public Health and Preventive Medicine. 11th ed. New York, Appleton-Century-Crofts, 1980. *Comprehensive textbook of preventive medicine.*

Levy RI: Declining mortality in coronary heart disease. Arteriosclerosis 1:312–325, 1981. *Review and analysis of secular trends in heart disease; the United States has the most rapid decline of any nation.*

US Department of Health, Education and Welfare: Healthy People: The Surgeon General's Report on Health Promotion and Disease Prevention. DHEW Publ. no. 79-55071, 1979. *Summary of trends in illness and death from 1900 to the present, and of health goals for the future.*

US Department of Health and Human Services: Promoting Health — Preventing Disease: Objectives for the Nation. DHHS, 1980. *Specific objectives for health promotion and protection, to be achieved by 1990, in 15 major categories.*

Wynder EL (ed.): The Book of Health: A Complete Guide to Making Health Last a Lifetime. New York, Franklin Watts, 1981. *Personal health care guide, written for the layman.*

13. THE JUDICIOUS DIET

John P. Kane

The composition of an individual's diet and its relationship to his or her energy needs and to special requirements for growth, repair, or response to stress are among the important variables in the maintenance of health or the advent of disease. In Part XVI of this book, there is an extensive discussion of nutritional requirements for calories, amino acids, essential fatty acids, minerals, and vitamins. Obviously, a judicious diet is one that meets these requirements for the individual. An excess of calories leads to obesity, one of the most prevalent nutritional disorders found in the developed countries of the world. This is discussed in detail in Ch. 216. Undernutrition can also produce serious impairment of health (Ch. 214). Deficits or excesses of other nutrients lead to a wide variety of specific disorders. In this chapter, however, we shall be concerned with variables within what would ordinarily be considered an adequate diet but which may influence the susceptibility of the individual to three major classes of disease: atherosclerosis, hypertension, and cancer.

In few areas relevant to health is there so much misinformation and faddism as in the prevailing public arena concerning diets. Billions of dollars are spent in this major national industry to promote an astonishing variety of nostrums and dietary aberrations alleged to maintain holistic health, vitality, and attractiveness, or to reverse the process of disease. By and large, these programs are ingenious but harmless instruments to defraud the credulous. In some cases, however, they either produce harmful dietary abnormalities or delay the patient's seeking effective medical care. Physicians need to be informed about the dimensions of this cultism in order to be able to advise their patients and to participate effectively in the development of controlling public policy.

DIET AND ARTERIOSCLEROSIS

Lipids, primarily free and esterified cholesterol, constitute a prominent part of early atherosclerotic plaques. In current models of atherogenesis, lipids are thought to be transported into the artery wall by plasma lipoproteins. These lipoproteins include low density lipoproteins (LDL), intermediate density lipoproteins (IDL), and, perhaps to a lesser extent, very low density lipoproteins (VLDL). More extensive descriptions of these lipoproteins and of their metabolism are given in Ch. 183. Elevated levels of LDL and IDL are strongly associated epidemiologically with accelerated atherogenesis. For instance, the risk of coronary heart disease in the United States, where the average level of serum cholesterol in an adult male is approximately 230 mg per deciliter, is several-fold higher than in rural Japan, where the average is about 160 mg per deciliter. The atherogenicity of VLDL is not so strongly supported as that of LDL and IDL in large population studies. Impaired centripetal transport of cholesterol has recently been found in some patients with hypertriglyceridemia, however, suggesting that altered properties of VLDL may indeed contribute to atherogenesis in some individuals. An impressive inverse relationship exists between plasma levels of high density lipoprotein (HDL) cholesterol and risk of coronary heart disease. This presumably reflects the importance of the retrieval mechanisms for cholesterol, which depend upon certain subspecies of HDL.

The risk of coronary heart disease has been shown to correlate with levels of cholesterol in plasma as low as 180 mg per deciliter. The majority of individuals in industrialized western nations would therefore be expected to benefit from reduction of levels of serum cholesterol, reflecting primarily changes in the content of LDL in plasma. The results of several intervention studies tend to support this contention. Increasing the levels of HDL in plasma in order to increase the mobilization and retrieval of cholesterol might be equally attractive, but no studies of the effect of such an intervention on heart disease have yet appeared.

A single pattern of dietary modification is appropriate for individuals with nearly all types of primary hyperlipidemia (excepting only primary chylomicronemia), as well as for those individuals in the population at large who have less striking elevations of levels of atherogenic lipoproteins. The elements of this "universal" diet will be considered individually.

1. *Reduce body weight to the ideal.* This manipulation primarily induces a marked reduction in elevated VLDL levels. It also effects some reduction in LDL cholesterol levels and may increase HDL cholesterol levels slightly.

2. *Decrease the intake of saturated fat.* This change effects a potent and uniform lowering of LDL cholesterol. The typical American diet contains approximately 40 per cent or more of calories as fat (15 per cent saturated fat). Levels of 30 per cent of calories as fat (8 per cent saturated fat) can be achieved easily, and 20 per cent (5 per cent saturated) is attainable with major modifications of food selection. To achieve the 30 per cent level of dietary fat, fat-rich meats, dairy products, and items such as certain baked goods must be restricted. To achieve the 20 per cent level, major substitution of vegetable protein sources for meats must be made.

When the intake of saturated fats is decreased, there are several possible sources of replacement calories: polyunsaturated fats, monounsaturated fats, or carbohydrates. Major substitution with polyunsaturated fat may result in lower levels of HDL cholesterol and of the principal HDL protein, apolipoprotein A-I. Furthermore, polyunsaturated fatty acids are susceptible to hydroperoxidation, which could theoretically lead to generation of free radical chains and perhaps to an enhanced carcinogenesis. Such an effect is probably small if present at all. Since some epidemiologic evidence links total fat intake to cancer (see below), however, substitution of carbohydrates for fat may be more judicious. Monounsaturated fats, abundant in certain vegetable oils such as olive oil, have little effect on LDL levels. Major substitution of carbohydrate for fat is associated with modest elevations of plasma triglyceride levels in the short term, but these levels return to normal after a period of several months. Strict vegetarians tend to have lower levels of both LDL and HDL than individuals on a typical American diet, but the changes in LDL levels are of much greater magnitude. Furthermore, potentially important differences in composition of HDL are seen, with an increased ratio of phospholipid to cholesterol.

3. *Decrease the intake of cholesterol.* Reduction of dietary saturated fats automatically eliminates much cholesterol; however, rich sources such as organ meats and egg yolks should be restricted specifically. The effect of restriction of cholesterol on LDL levels varies widely among individuals. This variation appears to reflect two factors: (a) There is an approximately four-fold difference among individuals in the fraction of dietary cholesterol that is absorbed. (b) There are differences in the degree to which dietary cholesterol is capable of suppressing endogenous cholesterogenesis. Lacking metabolic ward studies on a given patient, it must be presumed that reduction of dietary cholesterol is likely to be of benefit. The typical American diet provides 500 mg or more of cholesterol per day, but an intake of 300 mg per day is relatively easily achieved, and intakes of 100 mg per day can be achieved with more rigorous mixed diets. Strict vegetarian diets contain no cholesterol.

4. *Restrict alcohol.* Alcohol should be limited in all cases to maintain ideal body weight. VLDL secretion is increased dramatically by even limited use of alcohol. Therefore, alcohol should always be eliminated in the diet of individuals with elevated serum triglycerides. Increased alcohol intake may be associated with elevated levels of HDL cholesterol, but it is not yet clear whether this change represents subspecies of HDL that participate in centripetal cholesterol transport. No categorical presumption of beneficial effects of alcohol on HDL can yet be made.

5. *Other factors.* Increased dietary fiber appears to have marginal effect on serum lipoprotein levels. The ingestion of lecithin, which is widely suggested by health food advocates, also lacks significant effect, as do a number of vitamins and minerals that have been similarly recommended.

Individuals following this judicious dietary regimen usually show reductions of 10 to 15 per cent in plasma cholesterol levels on the basis of reduction of saturated fats. An additional reduction of up to 10 per cent may be achieved by restriction of cholesterol. Based on large epidemiologic studies, it can be roughly estimated that at least a two-fold reduction in risk of coronary disease would be expected in the American population if such modifications of lipid levels were uniformly achieved.

DIET AND HYPERTENSION

There is a readily demonstrated relationship between blood pressure and the dietary intake of salt, both in inbred strains of hypertension-prone animals and in many hypertensive humans. A current hypothesis of the underlying mechanism of this relationship is as follows: These animals and humans are thought to be unable to secrete sodium chloride at a normal rate and therefore become somewhat volume expanded. A "natriuretic hormone" is then secreted which affects arterial smooth muscle as well as the kidney, inducing a calcium-for-sodium exchange that critically elevates the intracellular calcium content. The arterial smooth muscle cell is in partial contraction at all times, so this increment of intracellular calcium results in increased tonus. An increased passive sodium leak in the erythrocytes of some hypertensive animals and humans suggests a broad constitutional basis for such exchange effects.

In normotensive individuals, blood pressure is relatively unaffected by dietary intake of salt. Thus, the view is emerging that whereas moderate salt restriction is reasonable for individuals from kindreds in which hypertension occurs and for many hypertensive patients, no broad proscription of salt intake is appropriate for the normotensive population. Patients who tend to become significantly hypertensive in middle age usually have at least moderately elevated blood pressures in young adulthood, which usually allows this discrimination to be made. Most Americans consume 10 to 20 grams of salt daily, but an intake of 4 grams is a reasonable goal for individuals who may be at risk for hypertension.

DIET AND CANCER

The consumption of certain major food components is epidemiologically correlated with an increased incidence of some types of cancer. Although the mechanisms of these associations are still largely unknown, a judicious diet at this time involves changes that would be expected to minimize these risks. A number of components that occur in foods naturally or are formed or added during processing are recognized as mutagens in bacterial test systems (Ames test) or as carcinogens or promoters of carcinogenesis in tests in whole animals. Prudence would dictate elimination of these compounds from human consumption to whatever extent is practicable, because definitive studies demonstrating specific risks of these agents in humans may emerge only slowly.

DIETARY FAT. An increased incidence of cancer of the breast, colon, and prostate is epidemiologically related to a high consumption of total fat. Enhancement of chemical carcinogenesis by dietary fat has also been demonstrated in several animal models. Total fat intake correlates best with carcinogenesis at high levels, but polyunsaturated fats appear to be most important at lower levels of intake. Polyunsaturated fats are substrates for hydroperoxidative reactions initiating free radical chains, and therefore they probably should not constitute a major component of the diet. Reduction of total fat intake, with an increased content of complex carbohydrates, is completely compatible with the "prudent" diet for prevention of arteriosclerotic heart disease. In fact, in multination comparisons coronary heart disease and cancer of the breast show a strong correlation.

FIBER. Carcinogens formed in the bowel may play a major role in development of carcinoma of the colon. It has been suggested that increased fiber in the diet, which would decrease the duration of contact of carcinogens with the mucosa, might reduce the risk of cancer. Only minimal epidemiologic support for this view has been forthcoming, and with the possible exception of pentosans from wheat, fiber has not been proven effective in animal models.

RELATIONSHIP OF CANCER RISK TO LOW LEVELS OF CHOLESTEROL IN PLASMA. An increased risk of cancer has been associated epidemiologically with very low levels of serum cholesterol. Such an association when present is always weak and tends to be present only in the lowest range of cholesterol levels. Further, in nearly 20 prospective population studies, half have shown no such correlation. On the other hand, the correlation of higher levels of cholesterol in plasma with risk of coronary disease is very strong. Thus it appears that dietary modifications directed at lowering the risk of coronary disease should not be abandoned on the premise that a significant increase in the risk of cancer would ensue.

FOOD PREPARATION AND PRESERVATION. Exposure of meats to high temperatures, as in charcoal broiling, may be of importance in oncogenesis because of the formation of compounds with carcinogenic potential. In addition to benzo(a)pyrene, several mutagenic pyrolysates formed from amino acids are recognized. Considerable evidence both from epidemiology and from animal studies has linked components of wood smoke in smoked foods to carcinoma of the gastrointestinal tract. Nitrites, used as preservatives in meats, react with a number of natural amines and even certain medications to form nitrosamines, which are mutagenic. This reaction is favored by low pH; hence it proceeds readily in the stomach. Mutagenesis by nitrosamines is readily demonstrated, and clinical observations tend to link nitrites with carcinogenesis of the stomach and esophagus, at least. Vitamin C inhibits the formation of nitrosamines in vitro. Increased intake of this vitamin by the public may account in part for decreases in the incidence of gastric carcinoma observed in recent years. At the present state of our knowledge, restriction of nitrites and nitrosamines in the diet would appear reasonable. This is complicated by the presence of large amounts of nitrates, which can be reduced to nitrites, in certain vegetables that have been overfertilized by growers. The average American ingests about 75 mg of nitrate, 0.8 mg nitrite, and 1 μg of preformed nitrosamines daily.

NATURALLY OCCURRING CARCINOGENS AND MUTAGENS. Several species of Aspergillus molds produce aflatoxins. These agents are carcinogenic in a number of animals, chiefly causing carcinoma of the liver. Induction of tumors of colon, lung, and kidney has also been observed. Aflatoxins have been linked strongly to hepatocellular carcinoma in humans in Africa and Asia, probably acting in concert with hepatitis B virus. Aflatoxins have been found chiefly in peanuts and grains stored under moist conditions. Efforts to reduce the intake of these agents center on proper storage of foods. Emerging awareness of other naturally occurring mutagens and carcinogens may be expected to lead to an evaluation of their importance in human carcinogenesis. Among these agents are allyl isothiocyanate and the flavonoids quercetin and kaempferol found in many plant sources; hydrazine derivatives found in many mushrooms; safrole of sassafras; the methyl xanthines of coffee, tea, and cocoa; and phorbol esters and pyrrolizidine alkaloids found in herbal teas.

NATURAL INHIBITORS OF CARCINOGENESIS. Some naturally occurring compounds appear to inhibit carcinogenesis by certain agents. Certain indoles found in cruciferous vegetables (broccoli, cabbage, cauliflower, etc.) inhibit the carcinogenicity of benzo(a)pyrene, and substituted isothiocyanates found in these plants inhibit the carcinogenesis induced by polycyclic aromatic hydrocarbons. Higher intakes of retinol and beta carotene have been correlated with reduced risk of cancer in several studies. This effect should be considered unproven, however, until further evidence is brought forth. Selenium, a cofactor in the reduction of hydroperoxides, also may confer resistance to free radical–mediated carcinogenesis.

SUMMARY

Epidemiologic and experimental data are sufficient to support the following recommendations for dietary modifications among the general populace. Caloric intake should be adjusted to achieve and maintain ideal body weight. Fat intake should be reduced to 30 per cent of total calories (8 per cent as saturated fat) or less, and cholesterol intake to 150 mg, or less, per day. Even moderate use of alcohol should be avoided in individuals with hypertriglyceridemia. Complex carbohydrates should be used to make up the caloric deficits resulting from these changes. Individuals with a predisposition to hypertension should limit salt intake to 4 grams per day. Prudence would also suggest reasonable limitation of charcoal-broiled and smoked foods and foods rich in nitrites or nitrates.

Ames BN: Dietary carcinogens and anticarcinogens: Oxygen radicals and degenerative diseases. Science 221:1256–1264, 1983. *A comprehensive review of mutagens and carcinogens in the diet.*

Blaustein MP: Sodium ions, calcium ions, blood pressure regulation and hypertension: A reassessment and a hypothesis. Am J Physiol 232:165–173, 1977. *A review of the underlying mechanisms by which dietary sodium chloride induces hypertension.*

Committee on Diet, Nutrition, and Cancer. Assembly of Life Sciences, National Research Council: Diet, Nutrition and Cancer. National Academic Press, 1982. *A comprehensive evaluation of the roles of dietary components and additives in carcinogenesis.*

Connor WE, Connor SL: The dietary treatment of hyperlipidemia. Med Clin North Am 66:485–518, 1982. *A practical guide to application of dietary principles.*
Havel RJ: Dietary regulation of plasma lipoprotein metabolism in humans. Prog Biochem Pharmacol 19:110–122, 1983. *A discussion of mechanisms underlying dietary effects on lipoproteins.*
Nutrition in cancer causation and prevention. Cancer Research 43 (Suppl):23855–25195, 1983. *A workshop on dietary agents that may cause or prevent cancer.*

14. EXERCISE AND HEALTH

William L. Haskell

The biologic and psychologic benefits ascribed to exercise are extremely diverse and vary substantially with regard to scientific documentation of a causal relationship. Some of these benefits have been definitively established and are achievable by anyone who exercises appropriately. Other benefits, frequently promoted by exercise advocates, usually do not occur, and at times inappropriate advice has been given that has placed patients at undue risk for exercise-caused morbidity or mortality. As with many other areas of health promotion, enthusiasm to help others by encouraging them to exercise can easily outstrip the scientific basis for such actions. While the idea that exercise might promote health is not new, many of the details regarding specific health benefits and exercise requirements are still much debated and under investigation.

EXERCISE AND PHYSICAL WORKING CAPACITY

The most effective method of achieving an increase in physical working capacity or "physical fitness" is through a systematic increase in habitual exercise (exercise training). This increase in capacity is an adaptative response by the body to the stress placed on various tissues and biologic functions by the increased metabolic or physical demands of the exercise. If the appropriate type of exercise is performed at the proper intensity, duration, and frequency, sedentary individuals of all ages will achieve significant improvements in physical working capacity. After training, they will be able to exercise at a greater intensity and for a longer duration than before. Also, at the same submaximal exercise intensity they will experience less fatigue. This increase in functional capacity is due to enhanced metabolic capacity of skeletal muscle, increased capacity for substrate and oxygen delivery to the muscle, and changes in autonomic nervous system regulation during exercise.

Increases in physical working capacity often are equated inappropriately with improvements in health status or disease prevention. This is an important and often difficult distinction to make: that while a very high level of physical fitness usually requires good health, an improvement in fitness does not ensure an increase in resistance to disease or a reduction in clinical manifestations. For example, patients with disorders such as emphysema, diabetes, or hypertension can significantly increase their working capacity through exercise without necessarily changing the severity of their disease or their medical prognosis. Becoming more physically fit and improving health status are interrelated but not synonymous.

HEALTH BENEFITS OF EXERCISE

Most of the health-related benefits of exercise appear to result from the increase in metabolism required to provide the energy needed for skeletal muscle contraction. This increase in demand for energy triggers a number of adaptations designed to enhance the efficiency and capacity of the skeletal muscle to perform work and minimize fatigue. Adaptations also occur in those systems that support the increased energy requirements of skeletal muscle, including the nervous, endocrine, cardiovascular, respiratory, and skeletal systems.

CORONARY HEART DISEASE. The area of greatest scientific inquiry regarding the health benefits of exercise has been its potential role in the prevention of coronary heart disease (CHD). In 1952 J. H. Morris and colleagues published data demonstrating that the conductors on double-decker buses in London developed fewer manifestations of CHD than did the less active bus drivers. Since then it has been repeatedly, but not exclusively, demonstrated that men and women who select more active jobs or leisure-time pursuits tend to experience fewer fatal and nonfatal CHD events. While these studies do not demonstrate a cause and effect relationship, the direction of the association is positive and quite consistent, the magnitude of the differences in CHD events is clinically meaningful, and the amount of exercise performed during leisure-time associated with lower CHD risk is well within the capacity of most clinically healthy adults. As of yet no randomized trial of adequate design has been performed to determine if an increase in exercise by sedentary adults free of clinically evident CHD on entry into the study would significantly reduce future CHD events.

The five controlled clinical trials so far conducted to evaluate the effects of exercise training on recurrent cardiac events in patients following myocardial infarction have yielded statistically negative results. In two of these five studies, the exercise group tended to have fewer events ($p < 0.10 > 0.05$) and in all of the studies the adherence to exercise training was sufficiently poor to raise questions regarding their adequacy as a test of the exercise hypothesis. Thus, no definitive evidence exists to substantiate that an *increase in exercise* will reduce either the primary or secondary occurrence of CHD clinical events.

There are several mechanisms by which exercise might act to reduce CHD risk. Exercise might maintain or increase oxygen supply to the myocardium by decreasing the progression of atherosclerosis, increasing coronary collateralization, or enlarging the diameter of proximal coronary arteries. Only preliminary evidence has been published documenting that any of these changes occur in man. Several studies have demonstrated potentially beneficial blood clotting–fibrinolysis activity and altered plasma lipoprotein profiles following training. These changes might improve the coronary blood flow in some individuals.

In contrast to very little evidence for any exercise-induced increase in myocardial oxygen supply, there is unequivocal evidence that endurance exercise training decreases myocardial oxygen demand. This decrease in demand is achieved primarily by a decrease in heart rate at rest and decreases in heart rate and systolic blood pressure during submaximal exercise. These changes are most likely produced by a modification in central nervous system regulation of cardiovascular function (decreased sympathetic and increased parasympathetic drive) and an increase in blood volume, with little, if any, change occurring in intrinsic myocardial function.

CARBOHYDRATE METABOLISM. A potentially important and often unrecognized health benefit of exercise is its effect on carbohydrate metabolism. During large muscle, dynamic exercise of moderate intensity, the glycogen stored in skeletal muscle is used for the production of energy and becomes partially depleted. For the next 24 to 72 hours this glycogen is replaced by the uptake of glucose from the blood. In addition to this acute effect of increased glucose removal, there also is a more chronic training effect that increases the sensitivity of insulin receptors in skeletal muscle and adipose tissue and thus the rate of glucose removal at any given level of plasma insulin. This "insulin sparing" effect of endurance exercise training probably decreases the long-term insulin production requirements of beta cells and may reduce the risk of insulin deficiency developing with increasing age.

OSTEOPOROSIS. The bone mineral loss that occurs with aging is accelerated by inactivity, especially bed rest. While exercise will not prevent all of this loss, it appears to provide some benefit. For example, in a survey of 59 postmenopausal women, level of habitual activity was one of the major determinants of bone mass as measured by computerized tomography scanning. In the more active women, arm and leg bone mass was greater after accounting for the effects of age, body weight, and calcium intake. Also, when 18 elderly women exercised 3 times per week for 30 minutes each session, an increase in bone mineral content was observed (2.3 per cent), while 12 women who remained sedentary during this time showed a decrease of 3.3 per cent ($p < 0.005$). These experiences support the use of exercise requiring the movement of body weight against gravity as part of a comprehensive program of osteoporosis prevention.

WEIGHT CONTROL. More physically active individuals tend to weigh less than their sedentary counterparts and at any given body weight have a greater muscle mass. Even though calorie consumption frequently goes up when sedentary people substantially increase their exercise, they usually experience some adipose tissue loss. In addition to the increase in calories expended during the exercise, there is some evidence that *resting metabolic rate* is increased for an extended period after exercise, and with a higher percentage of body weight being muscle mass. *Basal metabolic rate* at any given body weight may also increase. For these reasons, exercise, along with proper nutrition, can improve health status by contributing to the maintenance of optimal body composition.

PSYCHOLOGICAL STATUS. Many physically active people state that the major health benefit that keeps them exercising is their improved psychological status. They report less anxiety and depression, more self confidence, and an increased ability to cope with at-home and job-related stress. How frequently such benefits will occur when sedentary people take up exercise is not known, nor is there any understanding of how to design an exercise program to maximize the positive psychological effects. Whether or not a biologic basis rather than just a "situational basis" exists for improvements in psychological status has not been established. Proposed explanations for a biologic basis are the decrease in circulating catecholamines produced by exercise training and/or the acute increase in beta-endorphins that occurs during and following vigorous exercise. Regardless of the mechanism, consideration should be given to getting sedentary people up and away from chronic stress-producing environments and having them participate in an exercise of their choice.

OTHER DISORDERS. There are a number of other situations in which patients with an established disease tend to show some clinical improvement if they exercise properly, but there is no good evidence that exercise prevents these disorders. Diseases included in this category are chronic obstructive lung disease (emphysema and bronchitis), mild or labile hypertension, and intermittent claudication. There are no data supporting the notion that exercise prevents any infectious disease. More active people have a greater morbidity and mortality from accidents than would be the case if they remained sedentary!

A Comment on Safety

When recommending exercise for health promotion, one does battle with the proverbial two-edged sword. Inappropriate exercise literally can pose dangers to limbs and life. The most commonly encountered problem is that of musculoskeletal discomfort or injury due to trauma or overuse. Of more severe consequence, but much less frequent, is the precipitation of a major cardiac event, usually ventricular fibrillation. However, the likelihood is remote that exercise will cause a cardiac arrest in individuals without underlying cardiac disease.

There are many other health risks of exercise, but these usually are limited to individuals with established disease (e.g., diabetes, asthma, or renal failure) or occur with very extended or competitive exercise. The most important of these risks is the development of severe heat injury (Ch. 564). The total prevention of these injuries cannot be achieved if adults are to increase their exercise, but the risks can be reduced by proper medical evaluation, individualized exercise recommendations, and improved public education.

AN EXERCISE PLAN FOR HEALTH

The *type* of exercise that provides the greatest health benefits and permits the greatest increase in energy expenditure with the least fatigue consists of performing rhythmical contractions of large muscles to move the body over a distance or against gravity. Such exercise frequently is referred to as being endurance or "aerobic," since, if it is performed at an intensity that is moderate relative to the person's capacity, most of the resynthesis of high energy compounds in the muscle is performed in the presence of oxygen. Included in this type of exercise is walking, hiking, jogging or running, cycling, cross-country skiing, swimming, active games and sports, selected calisthenics, and vigorous at-home or on-the-job chores. While very specific activities may be required when training for athletic competition, for health purposes any exercise of this type seems to be of benefit if performed frequently enough at the proper intensity.

The exercise-induced changes that contribute to health are achieved when the exercise *intensity* is somewhat greater than that usually performed by the individual. This increased intensity or overload causes adaptations that allow the metabolic needs to the muscles during exercise to be more readily met. While exercise intensities that are even slightly greater than that usually performed will produce changes, the usual recommendation is that exercise for optimizing health should be performed at 50 to 75 per cent of the individual's oxygen transport (aerobic) capacity or at 60 to 85 per cent of maximum achievable heart rate during exercise. Using these guidelines, exercise training heart rates for individuals 30 years of age would range from 114 to 162 beats per minute, whereas at age 60 the range would be from 96 to 137 beats per minute. For most people this recommendation produces a substantial intensity overload, since they usually do not exercise at more than about 45 per cent of their aerobic capacity during everyday activities.

The exercise *duration* to be recommended will depend on the person's health or fitness goals and exercise capacity as well as on the type of exercise being performed. One interpretation of the data available on exercise and health is that people who do even a little bit of exercise on a regular basis are better off than those who do almost nothing. A reasonable goal seems to be an energy expenditure over usual activities of approximately 300 kilocalories per session with a *frequency* of at least every other day. Most clinically healthy adults have the capacity to expend from 400 to 700 kilocalories per hour while performing activity of moderate intensity; thus they can expend 300 kilocalories in 25 to 45 minutes. Activities meeting this goal include walking or jogging 4 kilometers, cycling or swimming for 30 minutes, or playing several sets of singles tennis lasting for 45 minutes. While lower intensity exercise such as walking or gardening will not produce a large increase in exercise capacity, if performed for longer periods or more frequently, it seems to provide many of the health benefits derived from more vigorous exercise (e.g., facilitates weight control, bone mineral retention, etc.).

CONCLUSION

Inactivity does not appear to be the sole cause of any major disease, but a physically active lifestyle improves general health status and retards some of the functional impairments that frequently occur with aging. Success in initiating and maintaining an exercise program is most likely to occur when it is individually designed and takes into account the person's goals, interests, skills, and exercise opportunities, as well as exercise capacity. Instructions should be given to set aside a time for exercise and to fill it with a variety of activities, rather than selecting a single activity as the sole basis for increasing exercise for health purposes. The exercise plan should be convenient to perform, fit within the general lifestyle of the individual, and be considered fun or at least enjoyable. Success at exercise is increased when the individual has acquired the *knowledge* of what is to be done and why, the *confidence* that success can be achieved, and the *patience* to wait for the benefits to accrue.

Clausen JP: Circulatory adjustments to dynamic exercise and effect of physical training in normal subjects and in patients with coronary artery disease. Prog Cardiovasc Dis 28:459, 1976. *Comprehensive yet concise review of acute and chronic cardiovascular responses to exercise.*

Kemmer FW, Berger M: Exercise and diabetes mellitus: Physical activity as a part of daily life and its role in the treatment of diabetic patients. Int J Sports Med 4:77, 1983. *Review of exercise effects on glucose uptake and the benefits and risks of exercise by patients with diabetes.*

Paffenbarger RS, Wing AL, Hyde RT: Physical activity as an index of heart attack in college alumni. Am J Epidemiol 108:161, 1978. *Report of a major study supporting the relationship of sedentary habits to an increased risk of coronary heart disease.*

Ransford CP: A role for amines in the antidepressant effect of exercise: A review. Med Sci Sports Exercise 14:1, 1982. *A review of the effects of exercise on plasma concentrations of catecholamines and beta-endorphins.*

Thompson, JK, Jarvie G, Lahey BB, Cureton KJ: Exercise and obesity: Etiology, physiology and intervention. Psychol Bull 91:35, 1982. *Extensive review of issues regarding use of exercise as an aid in weight control.*

15. IMMUNIZATION

R. Gordon Douglas, Jr.

The major emphasis for immunizations in the United States continues to be immunizations in childhood. Detailed immunization recommendations for the common childhood diseases are best secured from two standard references: the current issue of the Red Book of the American Academy of Pediatrics, and the Collective Immunization Recommendations by the Advisory Committee on Immunization Practices of the U.S. Public Health Service.

It is important to maintain immunizations begun in childhood and to utilize those immunizations primarily intended for adults. The internist must ensure that routine immunizations such as diphtheria-tetanus, influenza, and pneumococcal disease are kept up to date, and that adequate records are maintained. He also must recognize special situations which require less commonly used products or booster doses of common immunizing agents.

Both active and passive immunizing agents are available (Tables 15–1 and 15–2). Active immunization, which is most often carried out in anticipation of exposure to a disease, is achieved by using one of the following as immunogens: inactivated virus or viral protein, live attenuated virus, bacterial protein, or bacterial polysaccharides. Live attenuated virus vaccines are associated with greater and more durable immunity than inactivated viral vaccines, but this is achieved at the expense of greater inherent risks. Bacterial proteins and polysaccharides are effective immunogens, but their protective effect is not lifelong.

Passive immunization, which is used for individuals who have recently been or may soon be exposed to a disease, is achieved by using immune globulin (IG) which contains antibody derived from human blood plasma by cold ethanol frac-

TABLE 15–1. COMMONLY USED ACTIVE IMMUNIZING AGENTS IN ADULTS

Disease	Type of Material	Preparation	Dosage Schedule	Other Uses, Comments
Routine use for all adults:				
Tetanus	Bacterial toxoid	Tetanus toxoid combined with diphtheria toxoid, adult type (Td); tetanus toxoid (T)	IM at least every ten years	Management of wounds
Diphtheria	Bacterial toxoid	Diphtheria toxoid combined with tetanus toxoid, adult type (Td)	IM at least every ten years	Management of contacts of cases of diphtheria
Use in selected populations:				
1. *Elderly persons and persons with chronic disease*				
Influenza	Inactivated virus	Influenza virus vaccine, trivalent	SC annually	Annual immunization of high risk individuals: persons over 65 years of age and persons of any age with chronic disease
Pneumococcal disease	Bacterial polysaccharide	Pneumococcal polysaccharide vaccine	SC once	Immunization of high risk persons over two years of age
2. *Postexposure prophylaxis of animal bites*				
Rabies	Inactivated virus	Human diploid cell rabies vaccine (HDCV)	Five 1-ml doses	Pre-exposure prophylaxis only in special situations
3. *Adolescent and adult females*				
Rubella	Live attenuated virus	Rubella virus vaccine, live	SC once	Adolescent and adult females who are unimmunized or who have no serum antibodies
4. *Adolescent and young adults*				
Measles	Live attenuated virus	Measles live vaccine	SC once	Adolescents and young adults who have not had measles and have no serum antibodies to measles or have not received previous live virus vaccine; postexposure protection
5. *Adolescent and adult males*				
Mumps	Live attenuated virus	Mumps virus vaccine, live	SC once	Prepubertal and adolescent males who have not had mumps or mumps vaccine
6. *Special groups*				
Poliomyelitis	Live attenuated virus	Poliovirus vaccine, live oral, trivalent (oral polio vaccine, OPV)	Three doses	Not for routine use; IPV for primary immunization of special groups of adults; OPV for boosters in special situations; need for routine booster not established
		Poliomyelitis vaccine (inactivated polio vaccine, IPV)	Three doses	
Meningococcal disease	Bacterial polysaccharide	Meningococcal polysaccharide vaccines, Type A, Type C, Types A and C	SC once	Only for special groups or individuals at high risk
Hepatitis B	Inactivated virus	Hepatitis B vaccine	Three doses	Persons at high risk of exposure to hepatitis B

IM = intramuscularly; SC = subcutaneously.

TABLE 15–2. PASSIVE IMMUNIZATIONS FOR ADULTS

Disease	Name of Material	Comments and Use
Hepatitis A	Immune globulin, human (IG)	Protection of household contacts; control of epidemics
Hepatitis B	Immune globulin, human (IG) Hepatitis B immune globulin, human (HBIG)	HBIG for needle stick or mucous membrane contact with HBsAg positive; HBIG for infants born to mothers with HBsAg positive hepatitis; IG for all other contacts
Tetanus	Tetanus immune globulin, human (TIG)	Management of tetanus-prone wounds
Diphtheria	Diphtheria antitoxin, equine	Treatment of established disease; high frequency of reactions to serum of nonhuman origin
Rabies	Rabies immunoglobulin, human (RIG)	Postexposure prophylaxis of animal bites
Herpes zoster	Varicella zoster immune globulin (VZIG)	Persons under 15 years of age with underlying disease who have not had varicella and who are exposed to varicella
Erythroblastosis fetalis	Rh immune globulin (RhIG)	Rh-negative women who give birth to Rh-positive infants or who abort
Rubella	Immune globulin, human (IG)	May modify or suppress symptoms, but does not prevent infection or viremia
Measles	Immune globulin, human (IG)	Prevention or modification of disease in contacts; not for control of epidemics
Botulism	Monovalent E antitoxin, equine Bivalent A and B antitoxin, equine Trivalent A, B, and E antitoxin, equine	Treatment of botulism; trivalent is preferred; most effective is type E
Snakebite	Antivenin, equine (North American coral snake antivenin) Antivenin, equine, Crotalidae, polyvalent	Specific for North American coral snake, *Micrurus fulvius* Effective for viper and pit viper, including rattlesnakes, copperheads, moccasins
Spider bite	Antivenin, equine	Specific for black widow spider, *Latrodectus mactans*, and other members of the genus

tionation. IG contains specified amounts of antibody against diphtheria, measles, one type of poliovirus, hepatitis A, and hepatitis B. Specific immune globulin preparations are also available, e.g., those against varicella zoster, tetanus, rabies, or hepatitis B. They are obtained from donor pools preselected for high antibody content. Human immune globulins are not associated with a risk of transmitting hepatitis A and B. They are much less likely to evoke hypersensitivity reactions than are immune globulins derived from animals. When using animal-derived antitoxins, intradermal testing for hypersensitivity should always precede their administration.

The physician must consider the risks and benefits to an individual patient when administering a vaccine or immunoglobulin. With regard to risks, certain general principles must be kept in mind. Hypersensitivity to any vaccine component is a contraindication to use of that vaccine. This is of most concern with vaccines grown in eggs, such as measles, mumps, and influenza vaccine. This risk may be assessed by history of ability to eat eggs without adverse effects. Although acute hypersensitivity reactions may also be a theoretical problem with vaccines grown in cell cultures, such reactions are very rare. Hypersensitivity to antibiotics (e.g., neomycin) contained in vaccines is another possible risk. However, penicillin is not used in the manufacture of any vaccine, and information concerning specific components of a vaccine is available in the package insert. Persons with acute febrile illness should not be vaccinated until they recover to avoid additive toxicity and possible diminished response.

Patients with altered immunity or household contacts of such persons should not be given live attenuated virus vaccines because of the risk of disseminated disease. In addition, live attenuated virus vaccines should not be given to pregnant women, except in rare circumstances, because of theoretical risk to the fetus.

Persons receiving live attenuated vaccines should not receive immune globulin or hyperimmune globulin simultaneously, since passively acquired antibody can interfere with the response to such vaccines. Children under 12 months of age should not be given measles, mumps, or rubella vaccines because of possible interference with antibody response by maternal antibody. Several vaccines can be given together without loss of efficacy. For example, influenza and pneumococcal vaccines may be given simultaneously (in different sites), and trivalent oral polio vaccine may be given with combined measles-mumps-rubella vaccine without alteration of antibody responses. Patients receiving intermittent immunosuppressive drugs should be given inactivated vaccines between courses of therapy to maximize antibody responses.

TETANUS. Tetanus toxoid is highly effective and provides long-lasting protection. Antitoxins persist at protective levels for ten years or more in individuals who have received a full immunizing series. There are four preparations: tetanus toxoid absorbed (T), tetanus and diphtheria toxoids absorbed (for adult use) (Td), diphtheria and tetanus toxoids and pertussis vaccine (DTP), and diphtheria and tetanus toxoids absorbed (for pediatric use) (DT). The aluminum phosphate absorbed preparations induce more persistent antitoxin titers than fluid forms. DTP and DT are used only for primary immunization and boosters in infants and young children. For all persons over seven years of age, Td is the immunizing preparation of choice because of the increasing frequency of reactions with age to the full dose of diphtheria toxoid contained in DT. T is available for those allergic to diphtheria toxoid. For immunization of individuals not immunized as infants, a series of three doses of Td should be given intramuscularly, the second dose four to eight weeks after the first, and the third, six months to one year after the second. A single booster immunization of Td is recommended for adults every ten years.

Tetanus Prophylaxis in Wound Management. For a clean minor wound, Td is recommended only if the history of tetanus immunization is uncertain, if less than three doses had previously been administered, or if it is more than ten years since the last dose. For all other wounds, Td is indicated unless the patient has received three or more doses of toxoid within five years. In addition, for those with such wounds and incomplete or uncertain vaccine status, 250 units of tetanus immune globulin (TIG) should be considered with Td in separate syringes and at separate sites. Adsorbed Td is preferred over fluid toxoid for administration with TIG because of delayed absorption of the toxoid.

DIPHTHERIA. Diphtheria immunizations significantly decrease the occurrence and severity of clinical disease. Protective levels of antibody persist for at least ten years following a primary series or booster doses of diphtheria toxoid. Diphtheria toxoid is combined with tetanus toxoid and pertussis vaccine (DTP) for use in infants and young children, or with tetanus toxoid (Td), adult type, for use in persons over seven years of age. The diphtheria component in the latter material is only 10 to 25 per cent of that in DTP. A separate diphtheria toxoid is not available in the United States. The primary and booster immunization schedules described for tetanus provide adequate protection against diphtheria.

Diphtheria Immunization for Case Contacts. All asymptomatic, unimmunized household contacts of patients with diphtheria should receive either benzathine penicillin or erythromycin as well as diphtheria toxoid. Since the risk of diphtheria is low in those receiving chemoprophylaxis, diphtheria antitoxin should not be administered. Antitoxin, which is of equine origin, may be useful in therapy of diphtheria. Immediate hypersensitivity reactions occur in 7 per cent and serum sickness in 5 per cent.

INFLUENZA VACCINE. Influenza epidemics can be expected almost every winter. Immunization efforts are aimed at protecting those at greatest risk of serious illness or death. This includes all persons over 65 years of age and persons of any age with chronic underlying diseases. Since 1968, at least 200,000 excess deaths have been attributed to influenza, and excess mortality has been recorded in 75 per cent of winters.

Influenza vaccines are composed of highly purified inactivated virus. Whole virion (whole virus) and subvirion (split virus) preparations are available, the latter prepared by disruption of the membrane with organic solvents. In children, split virus vaccines have been associated with fewer side effects than whole virus vaccines, but in adults the vaccines are comparable. Each year vaccine composition is changed to reflect the most recent serotypes circulating in the United States and worldwide. The vaccine is almost always a bi- or trivalent vaccine containing one or two influenza A virus strains, as well as an influenza B virus strain. The protective efficacy against both influenza A and influenza B is about 70 per cent.

A small percentage of subjects will have local reactions consisting of redness and induration which last one to two days. Fever and other systemic symptoms occur in only 1 to 2 per cent of subjects, begin six to twelve hours after vaccination, and persist for one to two days. Immediate reactions, presumably allergic, are extremely rare after influenza vaccination and probably result from sensitivity to some vaccine component, most likely residual egg protein. Thus, persons with anaphylactic hypersensitivity to eggs should not be given influenza vaccine. In 1976, there was an excess risk of Guillain-Barré syndrome associated with influenza vaccination of approximately 1 case per 100,000 persons vaccinated. Since that time, occurrence of Guillain-Barré syndrome has not been associated with influenza virus vaccine despite widespread use.

PNEUMOCOCCAL DISEASES. Pneumococcal pneumonia, meningitis, otitis media, and bacteremia occur with increased frequency in persons with sickle cell anemia, anatomic or functional asplenia, agammaglobulinemia, multiple myeloma, renal failure, cirrhosis and alcoholism, or basal skull fractures with cerebrospinal rhinorrhea. Persons with diabetes mellitus or chronic cardiorespiratory, hepatic, or renal disease and persons of increased age may also be at increased risk. Vaccine is intended for individuals who are at high risk.

A 14-valent polysaccharide vaccine containing types (Danish) 1, 2, 3, 4, 6A, 7F, 8, 9N, 12F, 14, 18C, 19F, 23F, and 25 is available. These types have been shown to cause 68 per cent of bacteremic pneumococcal disease in the United States. Antibody responses in healthy persons over two years of age are excellent, and the vaccine has been shown to prevent pneumococcal disease. The duration of immunity is unknown. Mild local side effects occur in 50 per cent of subjects. Booster doses should not be given. Influenza and pneumococcal vaccine can be administered in different sites simultaneously without impairment of immune response or enhancement of side effects.

RABIES. ***Postexposure Prophylaxis.*** Postexposure rabies immunization should always include both passively administered antibody and vaccine, except for persons who have previously been immunized with rabies vaccine and have a documented adequate rabies antibody titer.

Rabies vaccine (human diploid) (HDCV) is an inactivated vaccine prepared from rabies virus growth in human diploid cell cultures. Rabies immune globulin, human (RIG) is antirabies gamma globulin concentrated from plasma of hyperimmunized human donors; it contains 150 international units (IU) per milliliter.

Following exposure to animals known or suspected to be rabid, five 1-ml doses of HDCV are given intramuscularly. The first dose is given as soon as possible after exposure, and additional doses are given on days 3, 7, 14, and 28 after the first dose. Serologic testing is no longer recommended following vaccination except for immune-deficient persons, since 99.9 per cent of vaccines have protective antibody levels.

At the time of the bite and concurrent with vaccine, RIG is administered only once at the beginning of antirabies prophylaxis to provide antibodies until the patient responds to vaccination. After about eight days, RIG is unnecessary because antibody response to vaccine has occurred. The recommended dose of RIG is 20 IU per kilogram. If possible, up to half the dose of RIG should be thoroughly infiltrated in the area around the wound, and the rest should be administered intramuscularly. Because RIG may partially suppress active production of antibody, no more than the recommended dose should be given.

Pre-exposure Immunization. Vaccine may be offered to persons in high risk groups such as veterinarians, animal handlers, and laboratory workers. For pre-exposure immunization, three 1-ml injections of HDCV are given intramuscularly, one on each of days 0, 7, and 21 or 28. Serologic testing is no longer required to ascertain response to vaccine except for persons with altered immune status. Booster doses should be given every two years for persons with continuing risk of exposure.

Adverse reactions to HDCV include local pain, erythema, swelling, and itching in about 25 per cent of patients, and mild systemic reactions such as headache, nausea, abdominal pain, muscle aches, and dizziness in about 20 per cent. Rare neurologic reactions have been reported; however, causal relationship has not been established.

RUBELLA. Rubella is a live attenuated vaccine and is recommended for unimmunized prepubertal girls and susceptible adolescent and adult females of childbearing age. Persons working in hospitals and clinics, who, if infected, might transmit rubella to pregnant patients, should be tested and/or immunized against rubella. Because of the theoretical risk to the fetus, females of childbearing age should receive vaccine only if they are not pregnant and must understand that they should not become pregnant for three months after vaccination. Vaccine virus has been recovered from products of conception of aborted women who received vaccine during pregnancy. However, no instance of congenital abnormality has occurred in the offspring of 174 seronegative women who, although vaccinated just prior to or during pregnancy, carried the pregnancy to term. If a woman who has no immunity to rubella is pregnant, vaccine should be administered in the immediate postpartum period prior to discharge from the hospital. Administration of anti-Rho(D) immune globulin or other blood products is not a contraindication to rubella vaccination. Vaccinating susceptible children whose mothers or other household contacts are pregnant does not present a risk. Vaccination after exposure may not prevent illness, but it is not harmful.

Live attenuated rubella virus vaccine is prepared in human diploid cell cultures. It is available as a monovalent vaccine or in combination with measles (MR), or measles and mumps (MMR) vaccines. A single dose of vaccine induces antibodies in more than 95 per cent of susceptibles, and vaccine-induced immunity is protective against clinical illness from natural exposure. Although the duration of immunity is not known, it is expected to be long-term.

Rash and fever are occasional side effects. Arthralgia and transient arthritis, usually involving the small peripheral joints, may occur in up to 40 per cent of subjects. They generally begin two to ten weeks after vaccination, persist for one to three days, and rarely recur. Allergic reactions have not been associated with this vaccine, and it may be safely administered to persons with allergies to eggs, ducks, and feathers.

MEASLES. All adolescents and adults who have not had measles confirmed by a physician, or who do not have laboratory evidence of measles immunity, or who have not been adequately immunized with live measles vaccine when 12 or more months of age should receive vaccine. Persons born prior to 1957 are likely to have been infected naturally and need not be vaccinated. Those vaccinated from 1963 to 1967 may have received inactivated vaccine and should be revaccinated. Persons who received live attenuated vaccine during that period, however, are considered adequately protected. Although established immunity is preferable, live measles vaccine, given within 72 hours of measles exposure, may provide protection.

Live attenuated measles virus vaccine, prepared in chick embryo cell cultures, is available as a monovalent vaccine or in combination with rubella (MR), mumps (MM), or mumps and rubella (MMR). Antibodies which are protective against measles develop in 95 per cent or more of vaccinees. The duration of protective effect, although unknown, appears to be long.

About 5 to 15 per cent of vaccinees will develop fever, beginning about the sixth day after vaccination and lasting up to five days. Transient rashes have been reported rarely. Encephalitis has been reported approximately once for every one million doses administered. No allergic reactions have been associated with the vaccine even among persons with allergies to eggs, chickens, and feathers. Measles vaccine is inactivated by heat and light; it should be stored at 2 to 8° C and protected from light to avoid vaccine failure.

Immune globulin (IG) has been shown to be effective in preventing or modifying measles in a susceptible person exposed less than six days previously. The dose is 0.25 ml per kilogram of body weight. Live measles vaccine can be given after three months. Although effective in individuals, IG should not be used instead of live measles virus vaccine to control epidemics.

MUMPS. Although mumps is generally self-limited, it may be moderately debilitating; and complications involving the central nervous system, including deafness, occur rarely. Orchitis may occur in up to 20 per cent of clinical mumps cases in postpubertal males, but sterility is rare. Susceptible adolescents and adults should be vaccinated against mumps unless otherwise contraindicated. Susceptibility can be determined by documentation of disease by a physician or laboratory or by documented immunization with live mumps vaccine when the subject was 12 months or more of age. Mumps vaccine is not recommended for persons born prior to 1957, because they are likely to have been infected naturally and generally may be considered immune. Many physicians will reserve its use for children approaching puberty and for adolescent and young adult males who have not had mumps. Live attenuated mumps virus vaccine, prepared in chick embryo cell cultures, induces antibodies in over 90 per cent of recipients. The duration of immunity is unknown but is probably long lasting. Side effects are very rare and include allergic reactions, rash, and pruritus. No deaths have been reported.

POLIOMYELITIS. The risk of paralytic poliomyelitis is very small in the United States today, but it is important to maintain immunity of the population to prevent further outbreaks.

Routine primary vaccination of adults in the United States is not necessary. Most adults are already immune by virtue of wild-type poliovirus infection or prior vaccination. Vaccine is recommended in the following adults: laboratory workers handling specimens which may contain polioviruses, health care workers who are in close contact with patients who may be excreting polioviruses, and members of communities or specific population groups with disease caused by wild polioviruses. There are no data to substantiate a harmful effect of vaccine on the fetus, but it is advisable to avoid vaccination during pregnancy if possible. Immunocompromised patients, or household contacts of such patients, should not be given vaccine because of their substantially increased risk of vaccine-associated disease. Inactivated vaccine is safe in such patients, although development of protective immune response does not always occur.

Two types of poliovirus vaccines are currently licensed in the United States: oral polio vaccine (OPV) and inactivated polio vaccine (IPV). Both contain all three poliovirus types. The effectiveness of these vaccines is attested to by the dramatic decline in poliomyelitis since their introduction. For primary immunization of normal adults and young children, OPV is preferred because it induces intestinal immunity, is simple to administer, is well accepted by patients, and results in immunization of some contacts. For children it is usually given beginning at two months of age—an exception to the rule that maternal antibody interferes with development of protective antibody following live attenuated virus vaccines.

For adults who were not previously vaccinated, IPV may be considered because the risk of vaccine-associated paralysis following OPV is slightly higher in adults than in children, although it is exceedingly low in both groups. Three doses of IPV should be given at intervals of one to two months, and a fourth dose at six to twelve months after the third. For those who previously received only one or two doses of vaccine, the remaining required doses of either vaccine, regardless of interval, should be given. For those who have had a complete course, a booster dose of OPV may be given for high risk individuals, but the need for such doses has not been established. Nonimmune parents of infants who are given OPV need not be vaccinated, but there is an exceedingly small risk of OPV-associated paralysis. Therefore, some physicians may wish to give these adults two doses of IPV one month apart or the full series before children receive OPV. If immediate protection is needed, OPV is recommended. IPV has not been associated with serious side effects in the past 20 years.

MENINGOCOCCAL DISEASE. Vaccines against *Neisseria meningitidis* serogroups A, C, Y, and W135 are now available in the United States. Routine vaccination against meningococcal disease is not recommended. The vaccines are reserved to control outbreaks of meningococcal disease caused by one of these serotypes. In the event of an epidemic caused by these serogroups, the population at risk should be identified by some reasonable boundary, and all residents or those at highest risk should be vaccinated. Vaccination should also be considered an adjunct to antibiotic chemoprophylaxis for household contacts of persons with meningococcal disease caused by these serogroups.

Four vaccines are available: monovalent A, monovalent C, bivalent A and C, and multivalent A, C, Y, and W135 combined. They are chemically defined antigens consisting of purified bacterial capsular polysaccharides, each inducing specific serogroup immunity. They have been shown to induce protective antibodies in more than 95 per cent of susceptibles. A single dose of vaccine is sufficient. Local reactions to the vaccine are infrequent and mild, and serious side effects have not been reported.

TYPHOID. Routine administration of typhoid vaccine is no longer recommended for persons in the United States. Selective immunization is indicated for persons with intimate exposure to a documented typhoid carrier such as would occur with continued household contact. There is no reason to use typhoid vaccine for persons in areas of natural disaster such as floods, or in rural summer camps. The adult dosage is 0.5 ml subcutaneously on two occasions, separated by four or more weeks.

OTHER DISEASES FOR WHICH ACTIVE IMMUNIZATIONS ARE AVAILABLE. A number of other vaccines licensed in the United States are used only for laboratory or field personnel working with the infectious agent or for other persons with unusual occupational exposure. These include cholera vaccine, smallpox vaccine, plague vaccine, rabies vaccine, anthrax vaccine, Rocky Mountain spotted fever vaccine, tularemia vaccine, Venezuelan equine encephalitis vaccine, and eastern equine encephalitis vaccine. Live virus vaccines for control of adenovirus types 4, 7, and 21 are available for military but not civilian use. Adenovirus vaccines are not attenuated, but rather produce immunity without disease when introduced into the gastrointestinal tract instead of the respiratory tract, the natural portal of entry.

TUBERCULOSIS. An attenuated strain of *Mycobacterium bovis*, bacille Calmette Guérin (BCG), may be protective against infection with *Mycobacterium tuberculosis.* It is not recommended for general use in this country. It is reserved for uninfected persons living in unavoidable contact with an uncontrolled infected person, or for groups with excessive rates of new infection which cannot be controlled by other measures. Excessive rates have been defined as more than 30 cases per 10,000 population.

HEPATITIS. Hepatitis B vaccine consists of purified inactivated hepatitis B surface antigen (HBsAg) particles obtained from chronic carriers. It is indicated for persons at high risk of exposure to hepatitis B, such as health care workers exposed to blood or blood products, hemodialysis patients, homosexual males, recipients of certain blood products, certain institutionalized individuals, and household or sexual contacts of chronic carriers of HBsAg. Vaccine is administered intramuscularly in three doses at time 0, 1 month, and 6 months. Efficacy is 80 to 95 per cent up to two years after vaccination. Local reactions and low grade fever are mild and infrequent. There is no evidence of association with subsequent development of acquired immunodeficiency syndrome (AIDS), and the vaccine is inactivated by three methods which are effective in inactivating all known viruses. There are no contraindications, and there is no risk to those who are carriers or already immune.

Immune globulin (IG) offers effective protection against the clinical manifestations of hepatitis A. When hepatitis A is suspected, 0.02 ml per kilogram of IG is given intramuscularly to persons with close personal contact who have not had hepatitis A. Usually, this means household but not school, hospital, office, or factory contacts. However, when outbreaks occur that are related to a school or institution, IG may be used to protect contacts. It should be given as early as possible after exposure, but may be given up to two weeks thereafter, and protection will be achieved in approximately 80 to 90 per cent of the contacts.

For hepatitis B, two preparations are available: IG and hepatitis B immunoglobulin (HBIG). IG produced since 1972 contains anti-hepatitis B antibodies. It may reduce the clinical severity of hepatitis B infection when infection is contracted by the percutaneous or oral route with a small viral inoculum. HBIG is prepared from donor pools preselected for high titer of antibody to hepatitis B (titer >1:100,000). It is recommended for acute exposure following a needle contact or a mucous membrane contact with HBsAg-positive blood. The dose is 0.06 ml per kilogram administered as soon as possible but within seven days of exposure, and a second dose administered 25 to 30 days after the first. If HBIG is not available, IG may be given in the same dosage schedule. For infants born to mothers with antigen (HBsAg) positive hepatitis B in the third trimester of pregnancy, HBIG (0.13 ml per kilogram) also is recommended. IG does not prevent maternal transmission. Routine passive immunization is not recommended for high risk groups such as dentists or personnel of hemodialysis units.

VARICELLA. Varicella zoster immune globulin (VZIG) is prepared from pooled plasma containing high titers of antibody to varicella virus, and is intended primarily for susceptible, immunodeficient children after significant exposure to chickenpox or zoster. VZIG is effective in preventing or modifying varicella infection in immunodeficient patients if administered within 96 hours after exposure. Because of the short supply of VZIG, it is distributed through regional blood centers, and its use is restricted to persons with one of the following illnesses or conditions: leukemia or lymphoma, congenital or acquired immunodeficiency, immunosuppressive treatment, or newborns of mothers who had onset of chickenpox less than five days before delivery or within 48 hours after delivery. In addition, exposure to chickenpox or varicella must have been via household contact, playmate contact, hospital contact, or contact between mother and newborn. The recipient should have a negative or unknown prior history of chickenpox and, for most purposes, be less than 15 years of age, since few patients 15 years of age or more are at risk of infection. The recommended dosage of VZIG is one vial for each 10 kg (22 lb) of body weight, up to a maximum of five vials. Thus, it would be advisable to screen immunodeficient children with a negative or unknown history of chickenpox for antibody to varicella zoster virus when first seen or first hospitalized, to avoid unnecessary administration of VZIG.

RH IMMUNE GLOBULIN. Rh immune globulin (RhIG) is effective in preventing erythroblastosis fetalis. RhIG is prepared from donors with high Rh antibody titer. It is recommended for Rh-negative women who give birth to Rh-positive infants or who undergo abortion. A single dose should be given within 72 hours after exposure, be it for delivery or abortion. Immunosuppression is transient, and RhIG may be required for Rh-negative women after each birth or abortion.

BOTULISM. Several preparations of equine antitoxin for passive immunization against *Clostridium botulinum* toxin are available; trivalent containing A, B, and E antitoxins; bivalent A and B; and monovalent E antitoxins. Although the effectiveness of these preparations in treatment is not well established, their use is recommended. The trivalent antitoxin is preferred because of its broader coverage and higher content of antibody. It is available from the Centers for Disease Control. One to three vials of this antiserum should be given intramuscularly as early as possible when botulism is suspected. Twenty per cent of patients will have untoward reactions. Testing for hypersensitivity should always precede its use.

SNAKEBITE. Specific antivenin is effective in neutralizing the systemic effects of snakebite. Two preparations are available: One is polyvalent for snakes of the Crotalidae family, including rattlesnakes, copperheads, moccasins, pit vipers, and vipers; the second is specific for coral snake, *Micrurus fulvius*, bites.

SPIDER BITES. A specific antivenin is highly effective for treatment of systemic effects following bites by the black widow spider, *Latrodectus mactans*, and other members of the genus. The dose is one vial (2.5 ml) intramuscularly.

Anderson LJ, Sikes RK, Langkop CW, et al.: Postexposure trial of human diploid cell strain rabies vaccine. J Infect Dis 142:133, 1980. *Experience with the new human diploid cell rabies vaccine.*

Goodman RA, Orenstein WA, Hinman AR: Vaccination and disease prevention for adults. JAMA 248:1607–1610, 1982. *Recent review of vaccine usage in adults.*

Immunization Practices Advisory Committee, Centers for Disease Control: Inactivated Hepatitis B Virus Vaccine. Recommendation of the Immunization Practices Advisory Committee. Ann Intern Med 97:379–383, 1982.

Immunization Practices Advisory Committee, Centers for Disease Control; General Recommendations on Immunization. Ann Intern Med 98:615–622, 1983. *Definitions, principles, and routine childhood immunization schedules.*

Modlin JF, Herrmann KL, Brandling-Bennett AD, et al.: Risk of congenital abnormality after inadvertent rubella vaccination of pregnant women. N Engl J Med 294:972, 1976. *Follow-up study of women inadvertently given rubella vaccination during pregnancy.*

Seeff LB, Hoofnagle JH: Immunoprophylaxis of viral hepatitis. Gastroenterology 77:161, 1979. *Review of immune globulins in hepatitis.*

16. TOBACCO AND HEALTH

David M. Burns

Cigarette smoking is the largest preventable public health problem currently existing in the United States. An estimated 350,000 deaths per year, one sixth of the total mortality in the United States, occur prematurely secondary to the smoking habits of the American population.

Tobacco use, both oral and smoking, was introduced to European settlers by the American Indian, and tobacco was one of the main cash crops in revolutionary America. With the invention of a cigarette-making machine in the 1880's, a marked shift in tobacco consumption occurred from predominantly pipes, cigars, and chewing tobacco to predominantly cigarettes. Per capita cigarette consumption in the United States increased from 54 in 1900 to a peak of 4336 in 1963. This dramatic switch to cigarette use was followed some 20 to 25 years later by an equally dramatic rise in lung cancer deaths, stimulating some of the early studies that identified the disease risks associated with cigarette smoking. The risks associated with tobacco use appear to be closely related to the amount of smoke inhaled.

Smokers who have used only pipes or cigars tend not to inhale, and therefore the majority of the health risks are correlated with cigarette consumption (Table 16–1).

In the early part of the century cigarette smoking was largely a male phenomenon, but in the late 1930's and early 1940's women began to smoke in large numbers. Currently, smoking habits in young adults are similar for the two sexes. In 1980 approximately one third of American adults were cigarette smokers. This represents a steady decline in smoking prevalence among both men and women. The frequency with which teenagers in the American population are taking up smoking is also declining for both boys and girls.

CIGARETTE SMOKE

Tobacco smoke is a complex mixture of some 4000 individual constituents. The smoke is a combination of pyrolysis and distillation products distributed between a particulate phase and a gas phase. Tar is the total particulate matter of the smoke once the water vapor and nicotine have been removed and contains the bulk of the carcinogenic effect of whole smoke. The gas phase of the smoke has a number of irritating and ciliotoxic agents, as well as high levels of carbon monoxide (1 to 5 per cent). The composition of the smoke varies with the type of tobacco, the processing of the tobacco, the temperature of combustion, and the rate and volume of inhalation, as well as a variety of cigarette design features.

FACTORS DETERMINING RISK

The risks due to cigarette smoking are not evenly spread across the smoking population; they vary with differences in individual smoking habits and the presence of other risk factors. For each of the major diseases associated with smoking, the risk increases with the "dose" of smoke to which an individual has been exposed. The risk increases with increasing number of cigarettes smoked per day, depth of inhalation, and duration of the smoking habit. The risk also increases with the younger age at which regular smoking is begun. The risks due to adolescent and preadolescent smoking may be magnified by a vulnerability of the cardiovascular and respiratory systems during growth and maturation.

A given dose of smoke exposure may interact with other personal characteristics or environmental exposures to greatly magnify the risk of disease. Thus, the risk incurred by cigarette smoking in someone with elevated blood pressure or high levels of asbestos exposure are much larger than the risks for smokers without those characteristics. In addition, the presence of smoking-induced disease in one organ system (e.g., chronic obstructive lung disease) may alter the ability to treat or survive a second disease process (e.g., lung cancer).

TABLE 16–1. INCREASED RISKS FOR CIGARETTE SMOKERS

Cardiovascular Disease
Coronary artery disease
Peripheral vascular disease
Aortic aneurysm
Stroke (at younger ages)
Cancer
Lung
Larynx, oral cavity, esophagus
Bladder, kidney
Pancreas, stomach
Lung Disorders
Cancer (as noted above)
Chronic bronchitis with airflow obstruction
Emphysema
Complications of Pregnancy
Infants—small for gestational age, higher perinatal mortality
Maternal complications—placenta previa, abruptio placenta
Gastrointestinal Complications
Peptic ulcer
Esophageal reflux

CARDIOVASCULAR DISEASE

Approximately half of the excess mortality attributable to cigarette smoking is due to cardiovascular disease. Cigarette smokers have almost twice the risk of nonsmokers of developing a myocardial infarction or dying of coronary heart disease. This relative risk of heart disease is even greater at younger ages, when the incidence of disease would otherwise be very low. The relative risks for sudden death from coronary disease, peripheral vascular disease, and aneurysm of the aorta are even higher. In contrast, cigarette smokers have only a slightly greater risk of developing angina pectoris, and an increased risk of stroke is demonstrable only in smokers at younger ages.

The magnitude of the risk of coronary heart disease associated with cigarette smoking is equivalent to the risks associated with elevated blood pressure or elevated serum cholesterol. The per cent of the population with smoking as a risk factor is substantially larger than the percentage with either elevated blood pressure or elevated serum cholesterol. As a result, *smoking ranks as the largest avoidable cause of coronary heart disease in the American population.*

Cigarette smoking acts as an independent risk factor for coronary heart disease; that is, its effect is not explained by levels of other risk factors. However, when more than one risk factor is present, smoking interacts with the other major risk factors to synergistically increase the risk. Figure 16–1 shows the 10-year incidence of coronary heart disease from the Pooling Project data. The presence of smoking, or of either of the other risk factors, increases the risk by 31 per thousand compared to the risk of someone with none of the risk factors. The presence of a second risk factor in someone who smokes results in an increase in risk of 49 per thousand over the risk when only one risk factor is present, and the addition of a third risk factor increases the risk by 86 per thousand. The actual risk that exists is always greater than the sum of the risks measured independently, suggesting that when multiple risk factors are present they interact to create more disease. This interaction may occur by accelerating the development of atherosclerosis, or it may occur by increasing the likelihood or severity of a myocardial infarction for any given level of atherosclerosis.

Autopsy studies have revealed that smokers have more atherosclerosis than nonsmokers, particularly in the aorta. Smoking a cigarette results in an increase in heart rate and blood pressure, necessitating a greater myocardial oxygen delivery, while the carbon monoxide in the smoke increases the

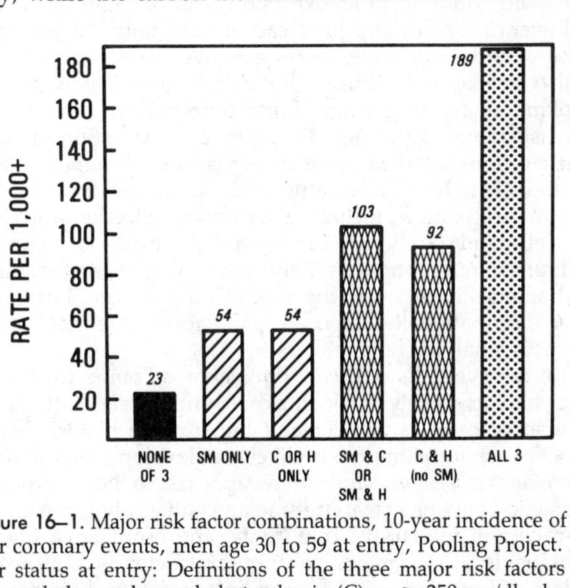

Figure 16–1. Major risk factor combinations, 10-year incidence of first major coronary events, men age 30 to 59 at entry, Pooling Project. Risk factor status at entry: Definitions of the three major risk factors and their symbols are: hypercholesterolemia (C) = ≥ 250 mg/dl; elevated blood pressure (H) = diastolic pressure ≥ 90 mm Hg; cigarette smoking (SM) = any current use of cigarettes at entry.

blood's carboxyhemoglobin level, thus decreasing its oxygen-carrying capacity. Cigarette smoking also increases platelet adhesiveness and lowers the threshold for ventricular fibrillation, and may thereby play a role in the acute events surrounding some thrombotic myocardial infarctions.

Cigarette smokers have also been found to have lower levels of high density lipoproteins, that fraction of blood lipids that is felt to exert a protective effect for coronary heart disease. The mechanism for this effect on blood lipids is unknown, but it provides a theoretical mechanism by which cigarette smoking might exert a synergistic effect on the atherosclerotic process.

For reasons that are poorly understood, cigarette smoking has a more profound effect on the peripheral vascular bed than on the coronary or cerebral vessels. In most series of patients with atherosclerotic peripheral vascular disease, over 90 per cent of the patients are cigarette smokers. The cessation of cigarette smoking is a critical therapeutic intervention in these patients; and in those who fail to quit, there is a higher incidence of amputation and surgical therapy is dramatically less successful.

The risk of coronary heart disease due to smoking is present at all ages beyond 30, but smoking is responsible for a greater proportion of coronary deaths in younger age groups than in older age groups. This risk declines dramatically with the cessation of cigarette smoking. By five years after the last cigarette, the risk in those who had smoked less than one pack per day approximates the risk in lifelong nonsmokers. For those who had smoked more than one pack per day a small residual risk of CHD may persist.

CANCER

Lung cancer is the largest cause of cancer death in men and by the mid 1980's will become the largest cause of cancer death in women, surpassing breast cancer (see Ch. 239). *Approximately 85 per cent of mortality due to lung cancer is causally attributed to cigarette smoking and is therefore potentially preventable.* No other single agent has been examined in as much detail, is more firmly established as a causal agent, or is responsible for more cancer deaths than cigarette smoking.

Cigarette smokers are 10 times more likely to develop lung cancer than nonsmokers. This risk is proportional to the number of cigarettes smoked per day, increasing to 20 to 25 times the risk of the nonsmoker in those who smoke two or more packs of cigarettes per day. Approximately one sixth of those men who continue to smoke two packs of cigarettes per day will eventually develop lung cancer, and only ten per cent of those who develop lung cancer are alive in five years. The risk is also increased in those who inhale more deeply or began smoking at a younger age. Lung cancer death rates begin to increase rapidly after age 35, partly as a reflection of the 20-year lag time between onset of exposure and manifestation of a tumor (Fig. 16–2). Cigarette smoking causes all of the major types of lung cancer, including squamous cell, adenocarcinoma, oat cell, and large cell carcinoma. Asbestos exposure and uranium mining interact synergistically with cigarette smoking to dramatically increase the risk of lung cancer, but even in these occupationally exposed populations the risk of lung cancer is small for nonsmokers.

The relative risks of developing *laryngeal cancer* for the cigarette smoker closely track those of lung cancer, but the total number of cases is smaller and the survival better. Cigarette smokers are five times more likely to develop *cancer of the oral cavity and esophagus,* and there appears to be a synergistic interaction between cigarette smoking and alcohol consumption for cancer of the larynx, oral cavity, and esophagus. Cigarette smoking is also a major contributing factor in *cancers of the bladder, kidney, and pancreas,* and an association between cigarette smoking and *gastric cancer* has been noted. Long-term use of chewing tobacco or snuff has been linked to development of

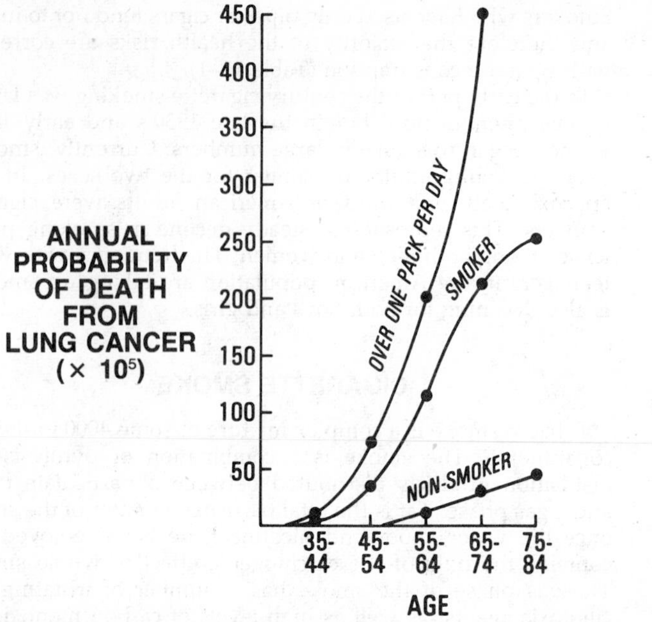

Figure 16–2. Annual death rate from lung cancer in nonsmokers, smokers in general, and those who smoke more than one pack per day.

cancers of the cheek or gum. Overall, tobacco consumption is responsible for approximately 30 per cent of the total United States cancer mortality.

Cigarette smoking induces changes in the respiratory epithelium that progress from hyperplasia to dysplasia and even to carcinoma in situ. These changes probably result from exposure of the respiratory epithelium to the carcinogens in cigarette smoke, predominately the benz-pyrenes and benz-anthracenes. Tobacco smoke contains a variety of tumorigenic agents, including several that can act as complete carcinogens. In addition, tumor initiators, promotors, and co-carcinogens have been identified in smoke. The impact of these tumorigenic agents may be magnified by the ciliotoxic agents in the smoke that interfere with the normal clearance mechanisms of the lung and result in a prolonged retention of the carcinogenic agents in the lung.

Cessation of cigarette smoking results in a lessening of the risk of cancer in comparison with the risk to the continuing smoker. The risk for light smokers approximates the risk of the nonsmoker by 10 to 15 years after cessation. Heavy smokers have a residual two- to three-fold increased risk that is proportional to their lifetime exposure to smoke.

CHRONIC OBSTRUCTIVE PULMONARY DISEASE (COPD)

Cigarette-induced lung injury is characterized by three overlapping syndromes: cough and mucus hypersecretion, bronchitis with airflow obstruction, and emphysema (see Ch. 60). By age 60 most cigarette smokers have changes in the airways and some degree of pathologic emphysema, but only the minority have symptomatic ventilatory limitation. An increased prevalence of cough can be demonstrated in cigarette smokers by the early teens, and abnormalities in the small airways are present in many smokers by early adulthood. However, it is not clear that either of these changes predict those who will eventually go on to develop symptomatic chronic airflow limitation.

Smokers as a group have lower rates of maximal expiratory airflow, and the cigarette smoking habit is the major predictor in a population for the development of COPD. The prevalence of COPD and risk of death from COPD increase with the number of cigarettes smoked per day and the depth of inhalation, as does the prevalence of chronic cough and sputum production, rate of decline in measurements of expiratory airflow, and degree of anatomic emphysema.

In contrast to nonsmokers, the majority of cigarette smokers examined at autopsy have some degree of emphysema and hypertrophic changes of the respiratory epithelium. However, only a minority of cigarette smokers manifest clinically significant airflow obstruction. Those who develop chronic airflow obstruction may be a subset of the smoking population identifiable by a rapidly declining FEV_1 early in the course of disease. In any event, it is rare for symptomatic chronic airflow obstruction to develop in anyone who maintained normal measures of expiratory airflow through age 45.

Cessation of cigarette smoking is of some benefit at all preterminal stages of ventilatory impairment. Changes in the small airways and early declines of FEF_{25-75} may reverse within one year of cessation. Cough and sputum production also lessen, and the annual rate of decline in measures of expiratory airflow moderates and approximates the rate of decline in nonsmokers. These changes are probably related to reversal of the chronic inflammatory changes in the large and small airways and the recovery of ciliary function, as there is no evidence that the emphysematous process is reversible.

The mechanism by which cigarette smoke induces emphysematous lung injury continues to be clarified. Lungs of smokers contain increased numbers of alveolar macrophages and polymorphonuclear leukocytes, probably drawn there as part of the inflammatory response to the irritants in the smoke. These cells produce elastase, which is capable of degrading the structural elements of the lung, resulting in a loss of elastic recoil. This destructive process is normally limited by blood-borne antiproteases. However, cigarette smoke contains a number of oxidants that destroy the function of these protective enzymes, and the result is an imbalance in the protease-antiprotease system favoring degradation and rupture of alveolar walls.

RISKS FOR WOMEN

The early prospective mortality studies, which defined the risks of cigarette smoking for men, suggested that the risks for women were much lower. However, this finding of a lower risk in women is an artifact of the relatively low prevalence of cigarette smoking among women prior to World War II. Moreover, women who did smoke tended to smoke fewer cigarettes per day and to inhale less. We now understand from studies of men and women with comparable smoking habits that there is essentially no protective effect of being female for the risks of developing cancer or chronic lung disease, and that much of the premenopausal difference in cardiovascular risk enjoyed by women disappears in those women who smoke.

In addition to the risks defined for men, women also incur additional risks related to pregnancy and use of oral contraceptives. Infants of smoking mothers are small for their gestational age in weight, length, and head circumference, and they experience a higher perinatal mortality, particularly if other determinants of a high-risk pregnancy are present. The smoking mothers are also at greater risk for the maternal complications of pregnancy, especially placenta previa and abruptio placenta.

Women who smoke and use oral contraceptives are at dramatically increased risk of cardiovascular disease. They are over 30 times more likely to develop a myocardial infarction, and about 20 times more likely to have a subarachnoid hemorrhage, than their nonsmoking peers who do not use oral contraceptives.

INVOLUNTARY SMOKING

The question of the nature of the health risks experienced by the nonsmoker exposed to cigarette smoke–contaminated environments is increasingly being raised because of its public health and legislative implications. Since the constituents of the smoke in the environment are similar to those inhaled by the smoker, the question is not whether these agents can cause disease but rather whether the dose experienced and mode of exposure (low dose but continuous as opposed to high dose and episodic) carries with it a measurable risk.

The majority of nonsmokers express annoyance and experience eye and respiratory tract irritation on exposure to smoke. Individuals with pre-existing disease may become more symptomatic on exposure to smoke, particularly those with allergies, and possibly those with chronic heart and lung disease.

Infants of smoking parents have a higher incidence of bronchitis and pneumonia in the first year of life, and the children of smoking mothers may experience a developmental lag in lung growth.

Some studies have found higher rates of lung cancer and other problems related to active smoking in the nonsmoking wives of smoking husbands. The problems of determining the exposure dose for environmental tobacco smoke and the interaction of smoking behavior with other personal and demographic variables limit the extrapolation of this information to the general public. However, the data do generate a reason for concern and a basis for the recommendation that, where possible, one should avoid prolonged exposure to high levels of environmental tobacco smoke.

LOW TAR AND NICOTINE CIGARETTES

The machine-measured yield of tar and nicotine for the average cigarette smoked by the American population has been steadily declining from a tar yield of 37 mg in 1954 to less than 14 mg in 1982. Unfortunately this decline in tar yield has not been matched by a proportional drop in the disease risks of smoking these cigarettes. Smokers of lower yield cigarettes have a slightly lower risk of lung cancer than smokers of the high yield cigarette, but this benefit disappears if they increase the number of cigarettes they smoke per day. There is also a lower prevalence of cough and phlegm, but probably no major impact on the risk of developing cardiovascular disease or chronic airflow obstruction. There are two major reasons why the decline in machine-measured tar and nicotine yield has not been accompanied by a concomitant reduction in biologic effect: (1) Many smokers may compensate for the decline in yield by increasing the number of cigarettes smoked per day, or by inhaling more deeply, thereby negating any possible reduction in smoke exposure "dose." (2) The machine-measured yield may not corrrespond to the yield when the cigarette is actually smoked. This is particularly true for the very low yield cigarettes that have vents or channels designed into the filter so that the machine draws very little smoke through the filter. These vents can be occluded by the smoker, or the volume of the puff increased, with a resultant dramatic rise in the yield. For these cigarettes, the measured tar and nicotine yields have almost no relation to either actual yield or biologic potency.

An additional concern is the wide variety of flavoring and other additives that have been used to compensate for the decline in tobacco content. These additives are considered trade secrets and may be added to the cigarette without informing the public of their presence and without any review for toxic effects. These additives represent a major gap in the understanding of the disease risks associated with smoking the modern cigarette.

PEPTIC ULCER DISEASE

Cigarette smokers have a greater incidence of gastric and duodenal ulcers and delayed healing of these ulcers. Smoking also relaxes the esophageal sphincter and may contribute to esophageal reflux.

DRUG METABOLISM AND DIAGNOSTIC TESTS

Several of the constituents of tobacco smoke are capable of inducing hepatic microsomal systems, which then alter the metabolism of other drugs. Theophylline, phenacetin, antipyrine, caffeine, and imipramine are metabolized more rapidly by smokers, and adjustment in the dosage may be required with cessation. Smokers have lower blood levels of vitamins C and B_{12}. Hematocrit and hemoglobin levels, as well as carboxyhemoglobin levels, are elevated in smokers; and smoking is one cause of an elevated red cell volume. Smokers also have small alterations in the other diagnostic tests, including a higher leukocyte count, but these differences are not usually clinically significant for an individual patient.

PIPE AND CIGAR SMOKING

Pipe and cigar smokers who have never smoked cigarettes have a lower risk of cardiovascular disease, lung cancer, and chronic airflow obstruction than do cigarette smokers. They have similar risks of cancer of the upper respiratory tract. These differences are due to the tendency of pipe and cigar smokers not to inhale the more irritating smoke of these forms of tobacco. Cigarette smokers who switch to pipes and cigars do tend to inhale, however, and so it is not clear that switching to a pipe or cigars results in a lowering of the risks for the cigarette smoker.

SMOKING BEHAVIOR AND CESSATION

The initiation of regular cigarette smoking occurs almost exclusively during adolescence and early adulthood. The availability of cigarettes and a variety of peer pressures and needs to model adult behavior lead to developing regular smoking behavior, particularly in those adolescents with limited social and academic success. The maintenance of smoking behavior in the adult is conditioned by other factors. The cigarette is used for nonverbal communication, for accentuation of positive feelings, for the reduction of negative feelings, and for coping with stress. An individual may use cigarettes sometimes for stimulation and sometimes for sedation. The result is a pattern of use that builds the cigarette into the way the smoker learns to deal with the world, and the cessation of smoking requires the smoker to give up a major coping mechanism.

Cigarette smoking fulfills all the criteria for an addiction, including a defined withdrawal syndrome. Nicotine almost certainly plays a role in the addictive process, but nicotine alone will not reverse the withdrawal syndrome. Nicotine probably provides a transient pharmacologic stimulus around which the human organism builds a series of psychologic or psychopharmacologic reflexes. These reflexes can be designed to meet the specific needs of an individual, thereby personalizing the cigarette habit. The psychologic and sociologic utility of the smoking behavior may vary qualitatively and quantitatively from individual to individual, and therefore it is not surprising that no single cessation technique will work for all individuals.

The physician can play an important role in cessation. Most smokers say that they would attempt to quit if told to do so by a physician; and, when told, up to one third will actually try to quit. Unfortunately two thirds of current smokers have never been told by their physician either to quit or to reduce the number of cigarettes smoked.

Smoking is a chronic problem and should be approached by the physician as a chronic problem, which requires informing the patient of the risks, urging cessation, and providing continued monitoring of the patient's progress. Simply recommending cessation without subsequent inquiry into the success or failure of the cessation effort implies to the patient that smoking is not a medical problem and that it is not important enough for the doctor to be concerned.

The keys to a successful cessation effort are (1) motivating the patient to quit; (2) helping the patient to understand why he or she smokes; (3) designing an organized approach to the cessation attempt; (4) developing support in the patient's environment for the attempt (especially by the spouse); and (5) continued reinforcement for successful cessation.

A variety of organizations provide organized cessation programs, both in groups and with self-help programs, and these organizations can be located in the telephone directory or by contacting the local heart, lung, or cancer societies. Drug therapy to aid cessation or blunt withdrawal has largely been unsuccessful, but preliminary reports on the use of nicotine chewing gum suggest that its use may modestly improve cessation rates in some groups.

American Heart Association: Report of the ad hoc committee on cigarette smoking and cardiovascular disases. Circulation 57:404A, 1978. *A report of the combined experience of the major CHD incidence studies relating the presence of risk factors to risk of CHD.*

Hammond EC: Smoking in relation to the death rates of one million men and women. *In* Haenszel W (ed.): Epidemiological Approaches to the Study of Cancer and Other Chronic Diseases. National Cancer Institute Monograph no. 19, 1966, pp. 127–204. *The largest prospective mortality study of the causes of death related to smoking. They followed over one million men and women.*

Royal College of Physicians: Smoking or Health. Tunbridge Wells, Kent, Putman Medical, 1977. *A well-written synthesis of smoking and health information*

U.S. Department of Health, Education and Welfare: Smoking and Health: A report of the Surgeon General. DHEW Publication no. (PHS) 79-50066, 1979. *An encyclopedic review of information.*

U.S. Department of Health and Human Services: The Health Consequences of Smoking: The changing cigarette. DHHS Publication no. (PHS) 81-50156, 1981. *A detailed discussion of what is known about low yield cigarettes and the problems associated with them.*

U.S. Department of Health and Human Services: The Health Consequences of Smoking: Cancer. DHHS Publication no. (PHS) 82-50179, 1982. *A review of the evidence on smoking and cancer from the perspective of causality.*

17. ALCOHOL ABUSE AND ALCOHOL-RELATED ILLNESSES

Benjamin Kissin

Alcohol is the oldest psychoactive drug known to man. About 90 million Americans drink alcoholic beverages in one form or another, some occasionally, some moderately but regularly ("social drinkers"), and some heavily ("heavy drinkers"). About 10 million Americans drink enough to cause difficulties in their personal and/or social adjustment ("problem drinkers"). Of these, about 6 million drink sufficiently, over a long time period, to produce the stigmata of alcohol dependence ("alcoholism").

The medical syndromes associated with alcohol abuse fall generally under four major categories: (1) acute alcohol intoxication, (2) alcohol dependence or "alcoholism," (3) acute alcohol withdrawal syndromes, and (4) medical complications. Alcohol abuse, like the abuse of any other psychoactive drug, is the consequence of the action of a specific pharmacologic agent in a specific individual. The clinical syndromes of alcohol abuse derive directly from the pharmacologic effects of ethyl alcohol (ethanol) on body tissues and secondarily from the adaptive responses of the body to excessive exposure to alcohol (tolerance and physical dependence).

PHARMACOLOGY OF ETHANOL

ABSORPTION AND METABOLISM. Ethanol is a colorless liquid usually ingested in a concentration of 5 per cent (beer), 12 per cent (wine), 20 per cent (reinforced wines), or 43 per cent (86 proof whiskey). The distinctive flavor of different alcoholic beverages is a function of the contained congeners (e.g., higher alcohols, aldehydes), as may also be some complications of heavy drinking (e.g., hangovers). However, the major effects of drinking are due to the content of ethanol itself. Ethanol is rapidly absorbed from the stomach and intestines into the bloodstream, thus accounting for its quick pharmacologic action. It is also rapidly metabolized so that a moderate dose will usually clear from the blood in about one hour. Its absorption and metabolic breakdown make ethanol a fast-acting but short-lasting drug.

Ethanol diffuses rapidly into all aqueous compartments of

the body (extracellular and intracellular), so that the blood concentrations of ethanol directly reflect concentrations of the chemical throughout the body. Ethanol concentrations in alveolar air and urine can be utilized to estimate blood concentrations. For nontolerant individuals a blood concentration of 50 mg per deciliter usually results in a sense of relaxation; levels of 150 mg per deciliter, in moderate symptoms of intoxication; and levels of 250 mg per deciliter, in severe symptoms. Higher blood levels (350 mg per deciliter) may result in coma and 500 mg per deciliter, in death.

About 10 per cent of the ethanol in the body is directly eliminated by diffusion through the kidneys or lungs. The rest is metabolized in the liver as illustrated in Figure 17–1. The rate-limiting element in this sequence is hepatic alcohol dehydrogenase, which, in a 70-kg man, can metabolize about 9.0 grams of ethanol (about three fourths of an ounce of whiskey) per hour. This results in a decrease in the blood level of approximately 15 mg per deciliter per hour. Ingestion of ethanol at a greater rate produces cumulatively rising blood levels.

The conversion of NAD to NADH during both phases of the oxidation of ethanol shifts the redox equilibrium and causes several metabolic disturbances. Alcohol dehydrogenase is located almost entirely in the liver. Neutral fat deposition (fatty degeneration of the liver) occurs in about 90 per cent of alcoholics owing to a complex series of metabolic events including increased synthesis. Acetaldehyde dehydrogenase is also concentrated in the liver but is found in other body tissues as well.

Alcohol dehydrogenase occurs in various isoenzyme forms, which metabolize ethanol at different rates. Orientals and American Indians tend to have increased hepatic levels of an atypical isoenzyme, the presence of which is characterized by a more rapid rate of alcohol metabolism and the production of higher levels of acetaldehyde. This is thought to produce the characteristic "Oriental flush," a reaction which occurs in about 80 per cent of genetically Mongoloid individuals.

NEUROPHARMACOLOGY. Ethanol is a powerful depressant of the central nervous system with pharmacologic effects similar to those of ether and chloroform. Ethanol is miscible with fats and rapidly enters cell membranes. It is thought that the neuropharmacologic action of ethanol is exercised through neuronal cell membrane effects (1) upon the activation of calcium ion (Ca^{++}), (2) upon the action of the Na^+ K^+ ATPase pump, or (3) more directly, through the production of increased fluidity.

Because parts of the brain respond differently to ethanol, its behavioral effects may differ from its neuropharmacologic ones; e.g., the depressant effects of ethanol upon inhibitory control centers may paradoxically produce excitatory behavior. Alcohol tends to depress the brain from above downward, first affecting the cortex, then the limbic system and cerebellum, next the reticular formation, and finally the medulla oblongata. Low concentrations of ethanol depress the higher cortical centers, causing increased emotional excitability, decreased mental acuity, and impaired judgment. Moderate levels produce emotional imbalance, slurred speech, and ataxia. High levels produce lethargy, stupor, and coma, and very high levels, death from cardiac and respiratory failure.

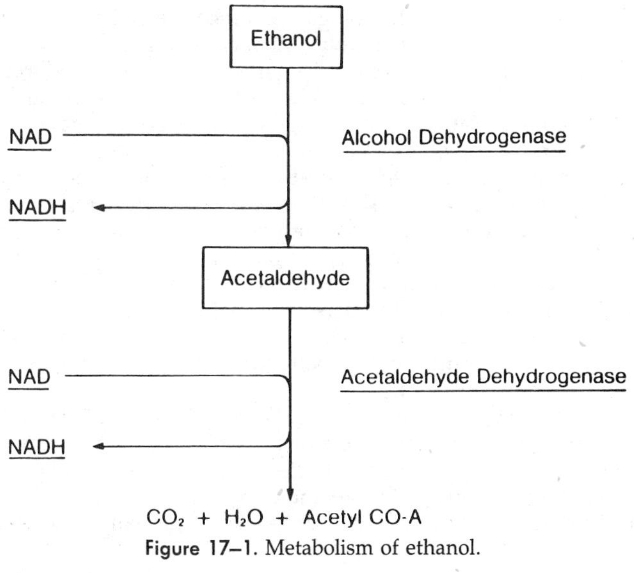

Figure 17–1. Metabolism of ethanol.

In low doses, alcohol acts both as a stimulant (disinhibitor) and as a relaxant; it is widely used for these effects. The drug is also a euphoriant; perhaps the majority of alcoholics drink mainly for this effect. In larger doses, alcohol is a rapidly acting and potent anxiolytic agent and is frequently taken by agitated individuals to obtain relief. The effect is thought to be by sedation of the limbic system.

ACUTE ALCOHOL INTOXICATION

Acute alcohol intoxication occurs infrequently in social drinkers, more frequently in heavy drinkers, and most frequently in problem drinkers and alcoholics. The pattern of aberrant responsiveness is a function of the blood alcohol level (BAL) and of pre-existing tolerance. Alcoholics have a high level of behavioral and physiologic tolerance to ethanol so that they may require blood alcohol levels almost 100 mg per deciliter higher than social drinkers to show comparable impairment. Some alcoholics function adequately with a BAL of 250 mg per deciliter, a concentration at which social drinkers become stuporous.

Acute alcohol intoxication occurs in two stages. In nontolerant individuals, a BAL of about 100 to 200 mg per deciliter will result in disinhibition and hyperexcitability; with a BAL of above 250 mg per deciliter stupor and coma usually ensue. Although these two syndromes are part of a continuum, there is a sufficient change in symptoms at about the level of 200 to 250 mg per deciliter (depending on the tolerance of a given individual) to warrant their separate description.

EXCITATORY STAGE. The social use of alcoholic beverages (as at a party) usually produces a BAL of about 50 mg per deciliter, a sense of relaxation and of well-being. At levels of 75 mg per deciliter, most individuals tend to feel more relaxed and sociable; a few become garrulous or hostile. At about 100 mg per deciliter, signs of ataxia begin. Coordination and judgment may be impaired at the same time that confidence in one's ability increases. At this level, driving may be hazardous; this is reflected in most state laws which define "driving while intoxicated" (DWI) at a BAL of 100 mg per deciliter or higher.

At BALs of about 125 to 150 mg per deciliter, behavioral changes occur which, in general, reflect the underlying personality. Some individuals continue to become more congenial, sociable, and disinhibited; some become hostile and aggressive; and some turn inward and become silent and depressed. Increasing BALs usually continue to be associated with increasing personality-specific responsivities until the more narcotic effects of ethanol begin to manifest themselves at or about the 200 to 250 mg per deciliter level.

In susceptible persons alcohol may precipitate great agitation and acts of violence. To treat this condition one should give intramuscular benzodiazepines in cautiously increasing doses in order to avoid cumulative narcosis with the alcohol (see below). Individuals who show marked depressive reactions while under the influence of alcohol should be given verbal support until the effects wear off. Elevated BALs are found in about 25 per cent of successful suicides.

DEPRESSANT STAGE. When the BAL rises higher than about 200 to 250 mg per deciliter in nontolerant individuals, and to more than about 300 to 350 mg per deciliter in problem drinkers, the individual passes into a depressant syndrome. This condition requires immediate medical care. BALs must be taken and evaluated; a single BAL of 300 mg per deciliter should not be interpreted as contravening treatment, since a reservoir of unabsorbed alcohol may be present in the stomach and small intestine. Gastric gavage and lavage should be undertaken both to reduce this reservoir and to prevent vomiting and pulmonary aspiration. Vital systems must be maintained, with the administration of oxygen, intravenous fluids, and, rarely, ventilatory and circulatory support. Antidotes are ineffective.

HANGOVERS. Ethanol is strongly toxic to both brain and stomach, and its alcohol and aldehyde congeners are even more so, explaining the high incidence of postintoxication malaise, headache, giddiness, tremor, and nausea. These symptoms are generally self-limited and respond readily to antacids and aspirin. More serious symptoms occur in more persistent but not yet fully alcoholic drinkers, in whom the so-called "hangover" may actually be an early withdrawal syndrome.

ALCOHOLISM (Alcohol Dependence)

Alcoholism is a drug-dependence syndrome resulting from the prolonged excessive use of ethanol. It is characterized by (1) a "high risk" individual, (2) the development of self-perpetuating mechanisms producing addiction, (3) a more or less typical clinical course, and (4) specific complications and sequelae. The progressive clinical course is marked by repeated episodes of intoxication followed generally by characteristic withdrawal symptoms. Alcoholism involves major changes in the biologic, psychologic, and social equilibrium of the individual, both in its pathogenesis and in its consequences.

PREDISPOSING FACTORS. Predisposing factors that contribute to susceptibility to alcoholism may be biologic, psychologic, or social.

Goodwin and his coworkers compared two groups of adoptees—one whose biologic fathers were alcoholic, the other whose biologic fathers were nonalcoholic. All adoptees had been separated from their biologic parents before the age of six weeks and placed where possible with nonalcoholic foster parents. Upon reaching adulthood, the incidence of alcoholism in the children of alcoholic biologic parents was four times greater than that in the controls; however, there was equally heavy drinking among the controls as among the probands. These findings suggest that heavy drinking may represent a socially determined pattern as opposed to alcoholism, which may involve a genetic diathesis.

Psychopathology is found more frequently in alcoholics as a group than in nonalcoholics, although it is uncertain which is cause and which effect. The proven occurrence of significant brain damage as a result of prolonged alcoholism lends some weight to the latter argument. However, the reportedly 8 to 10 per cent incidence of major psychoses among alcoholics is significantly higher than the 1 to 2 per cent in the general population. Agitated schizophrenics and manic-depressives not infrequently use alcohol as a means of self-medication. On the other hand, many alcoholics show no evidence of psychologic disturbance prior to the onset of their alcoholism.

Social influences can be the dominant influence in determining the level of drinking. Such factors include sex, ethnicity, religion, nationality, socioeconomic status, occupational subculture, family patterns, and peer pressure. A useful rule for estimating the influence of psychologic and social factors in the development of drug dependence is the "psychosocial" equation. This states that the level of psychopathology in a drug abuser is generally inversely proportional to the acceptability of that form of drug abuse in that individual's subculture. Thus, women alcoholics tend to show more psychopathology than do men, Jewish alcoholics more than Irish, and middle class heroin addicts more than ghetto addicts.

In brief, biologic factors may predispose to the development of physical dependence to ethanol, psychologic factors to the development of psychologic dependence, and social factors to a pattern of increased alcohol ingestion.

THE ADDICTIVE CYCLE. Alcoholism (alcohol dependence, alcohol addiction) is the end result of a series of interacting processes which initiate and then perpetuate heavy drinking. The ingestion of alcohol provides temporary gratification of a need for euphoria or temporary relief from some psychologic or physical tension. However, chronic ethanol ingestion induces psychologic and physiologic processes which increase the desire for more alcohol. A spiral develops in which the substance that satisfies a need increases the need.

The sequence in the elaboration of the addictive cycle in alcoholism is (1) primary psychologic dependence, (2) tolerance, (3) physical dependence, and (4) secondary psychologic dependence.

Psychologic Dependence. The first self-perpetuating mechanism to develop in alcoholism is *primary psychologic dependence*. This reflects behavioral conditioning in which an action and experience that are rewarded, either by pleasure or by the relief of pain and discomfort, will be reinforced by every similar succeeding action and experience. Primary psychologic dependence is the cornerstone of the dependency syndrome to all three classes of psychoactive drugs—the depressants, the stimulants, and the hallucinogens.

This reactivity, together with *secondary psychologic dependence*, is translated clinically into the subjective symptoms of *craving*, symptoms manifested as a continuous preoccupation with thoughts of drinking and with an overwhelming desire for alcohol. Craving is especially strong when reinforced by external stimuli such as a bottle of liquor. With long-term abstinence, there is a decline in the manifestations of primary psychologic dependence, with craving tapering off to a low level after about six months of abstinence and more or less disappearing after about two years. However, craving can be reactivated thereafter by exposure to a strongly stimulating situation, e.g., the bar or tavern previously frequented.

Tolerance. With the continued ingestion of large doses of alcohol (under the influence of psychologic dependence), metabolic changes result in an increased tolerance to ethanol. This is manifested clinically as a decreased responsivity to a given dose of alcohol or as the need to ingest a larger dose in order to obtain a desired effect. Tolerance to ethanol occurs at three different physiologic levels.

1. *Metabolic tolerance* results from the increased efficiency of hepatic enzymes in breaking down ethanol to its metabolic end-products. The effect results partly from an increase in alcohol dehydrogenase activity and partly from the induction of an auxiliary liver microsomal ethanol oxidizing system. These changes increase the metabolic rate only by about 20 per cent.

2. *Physiologic or intracellular tolerance* accounts for the major increase in tolerance to ethanol as evidenced in the behavioral and physiologic resistance of alcoholics to high doses of alcohol. The mechanisms of physiologic tolerance are not well understood but are thought to involve intracellular metabolic changes in the central nervous system. The mechanisms involved in the development of physiologic tolerance to ethanol may be similar to those for barbiturates and other sedatives but different from those for the opiates. Thus, individuals tolerant to ethanol show cross-tolerance to barbiturates and, conversely, those tolerant to barbiturates show increased tolerance to ethanol. Also, withdrawal symptoms from either drug can be relieved by administration of the other.

3. *Behavioral tolerance* is considered to be an overall learning response that enables the person to maintain behavioral function while under the influence of ethanol. As with metabolic tolerance, the contribution of behavioral tolerance to the overall effect is relatively minimal.

Physical Dependence. It is generally believed that the same cellular changes which result in physiologic tolerance are responsible for physical dependence. Neurons develop increased excitability to compensate for the depressant effects of chronic alcohol. If ethanol levels then drop sharply, a marked increase occurs in CNS irritability. The presence of physical dependence on ethanol is expressed by the phenomena of withdrawal.

When a high level of physical dependence develops in alcoholics, withdrawal symptoms become persistent because of the constant rise and fall of the BAL. The alcoholic finds that he is comfortable only while his BAL is rising; a falling BAL is accompanied by distressing withdrawal symptoms. Since quick and effective relief is obtained by alcohol ingestion, withdrawal symptoms become important factors in maintaining drinking behavior. During particularly heavy drinking bouts, severe withdrawal symptoms result whenever the physically dependent alcoholic seeks to stop drinking; this sequence leads to a compulsive pattern of drinking known clinically as *loss of control* or *inability to abstain*.

With prolonged abstinence, physical dependence gradually tapers off at about six months and more or less disappears after about three years. However, as in primary psychologic dependence, physical dependence is rapidly reactivated by ethanol after even years of abstinence and may be re-established after the administration of relatively small doses. This reaction is known as *kindling* and is important in reinitiating addictive drinking.

As a consequence of significant physical dependence and its associated withdrawal symptoms, alcoholics develop a secondary psychologic dependence based on the overlearned experience that continued drinking prevents the uncomfortable experiences of withdrawal. This additional dimension adds to the craving of primary psychologic dependence. Anxiety is activated by β-adrenergic discharges from the brainstem and is associated, through the mechanism of secondary psychologic dependence, with increased craving. Thus, alcoholics who have been abstinent for long periods will characteristically desire alcohol in moments of psychologic stress and may resume their drinking behavior.

CLINICAL COURSE. Some individuals begin as social drinkers and slowly increase their intake, whereas others begin as heavy drinkers and show a strong inclination for alcohol at the very onset. Characteristically, heavy drinking develops in late adolescence, but in certain inner city subcultures it may begin in early adolescence. The early avidity of many future alcoholics suggests the existence of predisposing biologic or psychologic factors.

Depending on the strength of the predisposing factors and of the various processes in the addictive cycle, the individual may progress more or less rapidly from social drinker to heavy drinker to problem drinker to alcoholic, or may stop at any of these levels. A convenient line of demarcation is the development of a strong primary psychologic dependence in problem drinkers and of physical dependence in alcoholics. The distinction between *problem drinking* and *alcoholism* is sometimes difficult to establish clinically because of the similarity in behavioral patterns. It is, however, an important distinction, since problem drinkers have a better prognosis and may require less intensive treatment than physically dependent alcoholics.

A less common clinical variant of alcohol abuse is *episodic drinking*, also known as *dipsomania*. In these cases, the individual may remain abstinent for several months, after which he may indulge in a one- or two-week drinking bout. Similar episodic drinking patterns occur in manic-depressive patients who characteristically drink more heavily during the manic phase.

Problem drinking and alcoholism are progressive syndromes characterized in most instances by repeated episodes of intoxication (in some problem drinkers and in some alcoholics, titration of drinking may conceal such episodes). With the development of physical dependence the tempo of drinking tends to accelerate, and there is increased evidence of physical, psychologic, and social impairment. Besides developing multiple physical ailments, affected individuals tend to become careless in personal appearance, indifferent to family and social responsibilities, and inadequate at work. The addition of these stresses to already overburdened physiologic and psychologic resources tends further to increase drinking behavior.

An early sign of developing alcoholism is *blackouts*. These are episodes of temporary amnesia occurring during periods of intensive drinking. The amnesia is usually for periods of a day or so, but with prolonged drinking may last for up to a week. The syndrome is a characteristic anesthetic effect of alcohol on the brain; it is a precursor to the more chronic forms of brain damage secondary to chronic alcohol abuse.

The acute alcohol withdrawal syndrome occurs episodically after prolonged periods (two to three weeks) of extremely heavy drinking (a fifth of hard liquor daily or its equivalent). It is precipitated either by the cessation of drinking or by a sharp decrease in intake. Many individuals enter treatment for alcoholism after being hospitalized for acute alcohol withdrawal. After a week or so, many of these patients continue to show a low grade withdrawal syndrome characterized by tremulousness, agitation, and insomnia. This constellation has been labeled the *protracted abstinence syndrome;* it may persist to a greater or lesser degree for up to six months. During this period, the individual is particularly susceptible to the effects of alcohol, since the entire addictive cycle is readily reactivated. Hence it is important in detoxifying patients medically during the acute alcohol withdrawal syndrome to be certain that they are adequately detoxified before being discharged.

DIAGNOSIS AND TREATMENT OF ALCOHOL ABUSE. The major aid in the diagnosis of alcohol abuse (problem drinking or alcoholism) is a high index of suspicion. Since alcohol use is so common in our society and since many people occasionally become intoxicated, it is easy to overlook chronic abuse. Denial of heavy drinking is an almost universal response of problem drinkers, so that the matter is often brought up by a husband or wife who becomes aware of the increasing personal and social disruptions. Frequently the physician will be consulted for an alcohol-associated illness such as gastritis. Alternatively, the physician on routine physical may uncover suggestive physical evidence such as hepatomegaly or spider telangiectasia.

The major goal of treatment is to help the patient achieve and maintain total abstinence. The suggestion that treated problem drinkers sometimes may return safely to social drinking has no demonstrated merit and should be discounted. The achievement of abstinence is difficult enough without the interference produced by the reinforcing effects of even small amounts of alcohol. Rehabilitation requires a reconstruction of the individual's physical, psychologic, and social adjustment, to help overcome the long-term dependence, at all three levels, which has been achieved with alcohol. Nor is this a short-term affair. The perpetuating mechanisms of the addictive cycle remain very active during the first six months of abstinence and probably moderately active for the first two or three years of sobriety. The individual in therapy should be encouraged to undertake treatment for at least a two-year period, during which time the necessary changes in physical, psychologic, and social adjustment can occur.

The three most effective treatment modalities for problem drinking and alcoholism are *disulfiram* (Antabuse), *psychotherapy* or counseling, and *Alcoholics Anonymous*. Disulfiram is a slowly excreted, long-acting medication which inhibits the action of acetaldehyde dehydrogenase. Because it is slowly metabolized and slowly excreted, once appropriate blood levels are established by a priming regimen (500 mg daily for one week), each single daily dose of 250 mg will maintain adequate blood levels for the next three or four days. Alcohol in any form is converted by alcohol dehydrogenase to acetaldehyde (see Fig. 17–1) but its further degradation is blocked by disulfiram on acetaldehyde dehydrogenase. The piling up in the blood of acetaldehyde, a highly toxic substance, produces prostrating nausea, vomiting, diffuse flushing, and a shock-like reaction. The emergency treatment for the Antabuse-alcohol reaction consists of intravenous fluids and antihistamines. Most alcoholics who have experienced this reaction are careful not to repeat it, and many achieve and maintain abstinence with this drug.

Psychotherapy or the counseling of individuals who are abusing alcohol is directed (1) toward achieving abstinence and (2) toward accomplishing the changes in psychologic and social adjustment necessary to maintain it. Alcoholics Anonymous (AA), a fraternity of ex-alcoholics, provides the companionship of those who have been able to overcome alcohol addiction; it also offers the strong social support and acceptance which alcoholics so often lack and so desperately need. The greatest chance for success in treating an alcoholic lies with continued supportive counseling by the physician plus the patient's participation in AA.

ACUTE ALCOHOL WITHDRAWAL SYNDROMES

Physically dependent alcoholics who go on a lengthy bout of heavy drinking for a period of one or more weeks will, upon reduction or cessation of alcohol intake, develop *acute alcohol withdrawal syndrome* characterized by cortical (behavioral) and β-adrenergic hyperexcitability. Either pattern may predominate.

DELIRIUM TREMENS. *Delirium tremens* represents the most severe type of acute alcohol withdrawal, with marked symptoms of cortical and brainstem hyperexcitability.

The patient in DTs represents an acute medical emergency, since the untreated mortality rate is about 15 per cent, largely from complications such as pneumonia or acute hepatitis. The patient is characteristically disoriented, agitated, hallucinating, tremulous, and perspiring. His pulse and respirations are rapid, his blood pressure may be high or low, his temperature abnormal. He may complain of severe muscle cramps because of an associated acute myopathy and of generalized paresthesias because of a diffuse polyneuropathy. Patients often have nausea and vomiting caused by acute gastritis. The presence of the gastritis may have induced the reduced alcohol intake and thus precipitated the acute episode.

The course of fully developed DTs usually follows upon alcohol withdrawal or decline by about three to five days, often after a preceding period of increasing restlessness, tremor, and behavioral agitation. A certain percentage follows upon withdrawal seizures. In untreated or inadequately treated cases, confusion and disorientation may last for several weeks. With adequate treatment, most severe symptoms clear within ten days; lesser abstinence symptoms may last for up to six months.

The specific treatment of delirium tremens involves the substitution of a long-acting drug that is cross-tolerant for alcohol. Benzodiazepines are the agents of choice for inducing sedation. Treatment for moderately severe cases consists of chlordiazepoxide, 100 mg orally four times daily the first several days, with gradually tapering doses thereafter. In more severe cases, particularly in those with convulsions, diazepam, 5 to 10 mg intravenously should be used every one to two hours until the condition is stabilized. Fluids, electrolytes, and thiamine, 100 mg, should be given parenterally. A careful search should be made to detect and treat infection. Good nursing care is essential to provide the necessary physical and psychologic support.

WITHDRAWAL CONVULSIONS. In *withdrawal conulsions ("rum fits")* generalized convulsions occur usually singly but sometimes in short runs or even as status epilepticus following a decline in the BAL. Seizures usually occur in the period of 12 to 48 hours after cessation of drinking. Various causative mechanisms have been suggested for withdrawal seizures, including chronic hypocapnia or hypomagnesemia, but none stand as proved. The attacks usually are without focal features, and consistently focal signs deserve further investigation. Otherwise, CT scans of the brain are negative, as are interictal EEG recordings. Treatment consists of stopping the acute convulsion with intravenous diazepam, plus giving a single dilantinizing dose (see Ch. 510) to prevent immediately recurring seizures. Signs of impending delirium tremens emerge postictally in perhaps one third of cases. "Rum fits" occur only on withdrawal from alcohol; prophylactic, chronic treatment with anticonvulsants is useless.

IMPENDING DELIRIUM TREMENS. The most common clinical manifestation of the acute alcohol withdrawal syndrome is *impending dilirium tremens*. Here mild to moderate symptoms of withdrawal are evident, mainly those associated with β-adrenergic brainstem discharge. Mild agitation, vasomotor changes, tremors, and insomnia sometimes respond to the α-adrenergic drug clonidine, an active antagonist to β-adrenergic discharge. However, treatment with cross-tolerant benzodiazepines is both more specific and more effective. A mild case may be controlled with 50 to 75 mg of chlordiazepoxide given orally four times daily for several days. More severe cases will require up to 100 mg of the same drug four times daily for a few days, with gradual tapering off over a period of seven to ten days.

ACUTE ALCOHOLIC HALLUCINOSIS. In *acute alcoholic hallucinosis*, auditory hallucinations dominate the clinical picture as opposed to the more common visual hallucinations seen in delirium tremens. In addition, there is characteristically less clouding of the sensorium, and less agitation and tremulousness. Consequently, the clinical picture looks more like that of an acute schizophrenic episode than like that of alcohol withdrawal, and differential diagnosis may be difficult. However, a history of prolonged heavy drinking, followed by a sudden decrease or cessation, reveals the diagnosis. Treatment is the same as for delirium tremens.

ALCOHOL-RELATED ILLNESSES

Medical conditions secondary to prolonged alcohol abuse fall generally into two categories: (1) nutritional diseases caused by dietary insufficiency and (2) diseases caused by the direct toxic effects of ethanol. Because alcoholic beverages provide 7 calories per gram of ethanol, an individual consuming a fifth of 86 proof liquor daily will derive about 2500 calories from alcohol alone. Under such conditions, most alcoholics consume little other food. Since liquor contains no vitamins, minerals, amino acids, or other essential nutritional elements, alcoholics often show marked nutritional deficiencies. Superimposed on this metabolic insufficiency, the direct toxic effect of ethanol produces further damage. Although the diseases secondary to alcohol abuse are generally categorized as either nutritional or toxic, both effects are probably involved in most cases.

Alcohol-related illnesses can involve all organ systems in the body. These illnesses are discussed under the appropriate headings in other chapters in this text, but some are especially frequent and serious. Table 17–1 indicates alcohol-related illnesses that are due predominantly to the direct toxic effects of prolonged alcohol ingestion and those that are more probably secondary to malnutrition. The effects may be difficult to separate, since most alcoholics are both heavy drinkers and malnourished.

PROGNOSIS

Prognosis in alcoholism is related to the stage and severity of the disease process. Morbidity and mortality can be divided into two major categories: that directly associated with alcohol abuse and that associated with alcohol-related illness.

PROGNOSIS IN THE ALCOHOLISM SYNDROME. Perhaps the most serious consequences of the alcoholism syndrome are deaths related to alcoholic behavior. It has been estimated that 50 per cent of highway fatalities are caused by drunken driving, with half of the victims alcoholic. Twenty-five per cent of

TABLE 17–1. ALCOHOL-RELATED ILLNESSES DUE TO TOXIC AND NUTRITIONAL EFFECTS OF ETHANOL

Organ	Syndromes Due to Toxic Effects	Syndromes Due to Nutritional Effects
Brain	Alcoholic dementia (cortical atrophy)	Wernicke-Korsakoff syndrome (Ch. 482) Cerebellar degeneration Central pontine myelinosis (secondary to electrolyte changes during therapy)
Nerves		Peripheral polyneuropathy (Ch. 525) (thiamine deficiency)
Heart	Alcoholic cardiomyopathy (Ch. 51)	Beriberi heart disease (thiamine deficiency)
Blood	Leukopenia, anemia, thrombocytopenia	Macrocytic hyperchromic anemia (Ch. 135) (folic acid deficiency)
Gastrointestinal tract	Acute and chronic gastritis (Ch. 98) Acute and chronic pancreatitis (Ch. 107) Carcinoma of the head and neck and of the esophagus	Malabsorption syndrome (Ch. 135) (folic acid deficiency)
Liver	Fatty degeneration Acute hepatitis Laennec's cirrhosis	Laennec's cirrhosis (Ch. 125 to 127)
Metabolic	Hyperlipidemia (Ch. 183) Hyperuricemia (exacerbation of gout)	

suicides have a history of prolonged alcoholism. In deaths due to drug overdose, alcohol is the associated agent most commonly found. The combined mortality rates of these three behavioral aberrations, together with those associated with alcohol-related medical illnesses, make alcoholism and its behavioral and medical complications the fourth most common cause of death in the United States after heart disease, strokes, and cancer.

Facts belie the generally negative public opinion about the prognosis of alcoholics. In most industrial alcoholism treatment programs where workers are socially stable and (because of the risk to jobs and pensions) well motivated, recovery rates run at the 70 to 80 per cent level. This remarkably high "cure" rate is probably accounted for mainly by early detection when most of the patients are still problem drinkers and have not yet developed the physical and social stigmata of advanced alcoholism. Once the latter develop, success rates seldom exceed 40 to 50 per cent. Early identification and early intervention remain the most important steps in the treatment of alcoholism.

PROGNOSIS OF ALCOHOL-RELATED MEDICAL ILLNESSES. The prognosis for specific alcohol-related medical illnesses varies with the nature of the illness and with its severity. Practically no alcohol-related medical illness can be cured if the patient continues to abuse alcohol. The major component of the treatment of alcohol-associated medical illness is the treatment of the underlying alcoholism.

Goodwin DW, Erickson CK: Alcoholism and Affective Disorders. New York, Spectrum Press, 1979. *A review of recent work on the clinical and hereditary aspects of alcohol abuse in affective disorders.*

Kissin B: Theory and practice in the treatment of alcoholism. *In* Kissin B, Begleiter H (eds.): The Biology of Alcoholism. Vol 5. New York, Plenum Press, 1977. *A comprehensive review of pathogenetic mechanisms in alcoholism and their relationship to treatment.*

Ludwig A: Why do alcoholics drink? *In* Kissin B, Begleiter H (eds.): The Biology of Alcoholism. Vol 6. New York, Plenum Press, 1983. *On the role of psychologic and physical dependence in perpetuating alcohol drinking behavior.*

Mendelson JH, Mello NK: Biologic concomitants of alcoholism. N Engl J Med 301:912, 1979. *A medical progress article reviewing recent studies dealing with the mechanistic aspects of genetics, metabolism, consequences, behavior, and speculated causes of alcohol addiction.*

Sellers EM, Kalant H: Alcohol intoxication and withdrawal. N Engl J Med 294:757, 1976. *An excellent didactic article dealing with all aspects of acute treatment.*

Thompson WL, John AD, Maddrey WL, et al.: Diazepam and paraldehyde for treatment of severe delirium tremens: A controlled trial. Ann Intern Med 82:175, 1975. *Establishes the clear superiority of diazepam for acute treatment and outlines a clear and effective plan for management.*

18. THE PREVENTIVE HEALTH EXAMINATION

Gary D. Friedman

The primary purpose of preventive health examinations is to maintain or improve health. The rationale is that early detection of disease or of high risk of subsequent disease can lead to treatment or remedial measures that will prevent or postpone morbidity, disability, or mortality.

An "annual physical" for asymptomatic adults was once accepted as good medical practice. In recent years periodic health examinations have become controversial: (1) The costs of a thorough medical history, physical examination, and standard laboratory tests would be enormous if these procedures were annually and universally applied. (2) Many elements of traditional checkups have not been shown to benefit asymptomatic persons. On the other hand, certain simple examination procedures and screening tests can prolong life and prevent disability.

ROUTINE TESTS AND PROCEDURES OF PROVEN OR PROBABLE VALUE IN PREVENTIVE CARE FOR ADULTS. A test is suitable for routine use if it can detect a serious and relatively common disease at an early stage, or at a pre-disease high-risk stage, when treatment or intervention would be more effective. Furthermore, the test should be relatively economical in terms of both money and professional time. A few tests or procedures clearly meet these criteria; a few others are of probable value but less universally accepted. These items are summarized in Table 18–1. The table's designations of "accepted" and "probable" for some of the tests are not agreed on by all authorities.

Routine chest x-rays can now be justified only in settings where tuberculosis is common; they have not proved to be effective in reducing mortality from lung cancer. Although still controversial because of poor sensitivity and specificity, a tonometry test for glaucoma may also be of net benefit. Doubts about tests of probable value revolve primarily around the benefits of treatment as compared to the harm of labeling (e.g., mild asymptomatic diabetes mellitus), the high relative frequency and high cost of evaluating false-positive results (e.g., occult blood in the stool), and the low yield of significant disease in the asymptomatic patient (e.g., palpating the abdomen).

TABLE 18–1. THE PREVENTIVE HEALTH EXAMINATION

Of Accepted Value	Of Probable Value
Medical History of:	
1. Smoking, particularly cigarettes	1. Postmenopausal uterine bleeding
2. Drinking alcohol to excess	2. Immunization status
3. Failure to wear seat belts	3. Use of nonmedicinal drugs other than alcohol
Physical Examination:	
1. Assessment of obesity	1. Search for cancers or precancerous lesions of the skin, mouth and pharynx, thyroid, abdomen, testes, uterus, prostate, and lymph nodes
2. Measurement of blood pressure	
3. Search for cancer or precancerous lesions of the breast and rectum	
Laboratory or Diagnostic Studies:	
1. Mammography in women at least 50 years of age	1. Hemoglobin or hematocrit
2. Sigmoidoscopy for cancer or polyps	2. Test of stool for occult blood
3. Papanicolaou test for cervical cancer	3. Electrocardiogram
4. Serum cholesterol concentration	4. Blood glucose
5. Serological test for latent syphilis and a cervical culture for gonorrhea (in individuals at high risk for venereal disease)	5. Tuberculin skin test (in high-risk groups)

ADDITIONAL BENEFITS OF PREVENTIVE HEALTH APPRAISALS. Detecting disease or abnormalities is not the only benefit of the preventive health examination. Negative findings are also of value in the reassurance they provide to the patient. Reassurance is strongest if the patient has received what he or she perceives to be a thorough examination. In contemplating cuts in the content of routine checkups, physicians and health care planners must weigh the immediate economic gains against the possible decrease in this reassurance if patients perceive the examinations to be abbreviated or cursory.

A lengthy and thorough examination when a patient is first seen permits collection of baseline data that may be useful when symptoms develop later. For example, an electrocardiogram, recorded when the patient is young and healthy, provides a useful benchmark for evaluating electrocardiograms taken later if chest pain or arrhythmia occurs. Also, the additional time spent in obtaining a medical and social history, examining the patient, and discussing the patient's concerns helps to establish a good doctor-patient relationship. Further, certain valuable information can be obtained during a thorough first examination and need not be sought routinely again. A good example is rheumatic heart disease detected by history and cardiac auscultation.

MULTIPHASIC AND SELECTIVE SCREENING. Screening tests aimed at early disease detection are sometimes offered singly, as in special programs to detect tuberculosis, diabetes mellitus, or breast cancer. Clearly it is more economical and efficient to test for several diseases at a single visit than for single diseases at several visits. Multiphasic screening provides several tests comparatively economically at one patient visit and can be used as part of a periodic health examination. Components of health screening or health examinations may be used for some patients and not others, depending on previous findings, risk characteristics, past medical history, or current symptoms of the patient. For example, once a baseline electrocardiogram has been taken, it need not be repeated at each succeeding health examination unless it initially revealed an abnormality or unless cardiovascular symptoms or indicators of high risk occur. This use of screening tests is known as selective or discriminate screening.

FREQUENCY OF EXAMINATIONS. It is not clear how frequently preventive health examinations, either basic or thorough, should be performed. The physician must strike a balance between excessive costs and low yield of too frequent examinations, and the chance that an important and controllable condition will develop and become irreversible if examinations are not provided often enough. Several sets of recommendations have been made recently based on available evidence and "prudent" judgment (see references). A common theme is that the incidence of most disabling and fatal diseases increases with age. Thus, basic examinations containing essential tests such as blood pressure measurement and breast palpation should increase in frequency from once in several years in the patient's twenties to annually in the fifties or sixties and older. As age advances it is advisable to observe the patient for losses in hearing, vision, and mental functioning as well. Even if losses are irreversible, knowledge of these limitations will aid in advising the patient and his or her family. Clearly, in our present state of knowledge, clinical judgment must play an important role both in deciding on the frequency of examinations and in selecting examination components for individual patients based on their age, sex, past medical history, and current risk status.

A health examination is of little value without appropriate follow-up, including treatment of early disease if indicated and counseling to encourage favorable changes in risk factors and a healthier life style.

American Cancer Society: Report on the cancer-related health checkup. CA 30:194–240, 1980. *This is a critical evaluation of methods of early detection of cancer.*

Breslow L, Somers AR: The lifetime health-monitoring program: A practical approach to preventive medicine. N Engl J Med 296:601–660, 1977. *This review of health examinations contains recommendations that emphasize a changing approach for different age groups and the need for cost-effective preventive measures.*

Canadian Task Force on the Periodic Health Examination (Spitzer W, chairman): The periodic health examination. Can Med Assoc J 121:1193–254, 1979. *This is a summary of a thorough review of various components of preventive health examinations and preventive care. The need for a selective rather than routine approach is emphasized.*

Medical Practice Committee, American College of Physicians: Periodic health examination: A guide for designing individualized preventive health care in the asymptomatic patient. Ann Intern Med 95:729–732, 1981. *This review of periodic health examinations provides a diagrammatic summary of recommendations that are viewed as minimal preventive measures to be applied to apparently well asymptomatic individuals at low medical risk.*

Part IV
PRINCIPLES OF DIAGNOSIS

19. CLINICAL APPROACH TO THE PATIENT

William L. Morgan, Jr.

The scientific basis of medical practice is well established, but only recently has the time-honored *art of medicine* come under scientific scrutiny. Medical educators are now beginning to understand how a physician relates to a patient and are introducing new ways to teach noncognitive skills. Data-gathering skills of interviewing and physical examination can be taught with simulated patients or a videotape. Strategies to select and interpret laboratory tests make the diagnosis of disease more scientific. Problem-oriented records have improved the organization and display of medical information. Understanding the role of a physician enables one to adapt such innovations to medical practice. What follows is a description of the abilities needed by a physician to care for a patient.

A task force of the American Board of Internal Medicine studied clinical competence in internal medicine by analyzing the components of the medical encounter (Tables 19–1 and 19–2). Knowledge, skills, and attitudes are the abilities required of a physician caring for a patient. The major tasks involved in solving a medical problem include data gathering, diagnosis, and patient care.

ABILITIES REQUIRED OF A PHYSICIAN

Noncognitive Abilities

Appropriate attitudes, habits, and interpersonal skills are important abilities needed to develop a positive physician-patient relationship. Without effective attitudes and interpersonal skills, and despite keen intellect and medical knowledge, a physician can fail in relating to and caring for a patient. The physician who is motivated primarily by concern for the patient's welfare is more likely to provide the conditions for an effective relationship. The essence of this relationship has never been better stated than in Peabody's classic 1927 article: "One of the essential qualities of the clinician is interest in humanity, for the secret of the care of the patient is caring for the patient."

ATTITUDES AND HABITS. Humanistic qualities, the assumption of responsibility, and continuing scholarship are among the major expectations of a physician. Humanistic qualities include integrity, respect, and compassion for the patient. Moral and ethical values are also essential components of clinical competence. Despite patients' psychological handicaps and failure to comply with treatment, the effective physician is sympathetic and nonjudgmental.

The assumption of full responsibility for the care of a patient is a fundamental requirement of the competent physician. This responsibility includes continuing care despite personal inconvenience and emotional demands of the patient. The physician is committed to doing what is best for the patient, and, when necessary, seeks the help of others.

Continuing scholarship is also an essential requirement of an effective physician. Rapid advances in medical sciences, and the resulting diagnostic and therapeutic innovations, make obsolete yesterday's method of medical practice. Each individual learns to recognize deficiencies in knowledge and adopts a plan to keep up with new information. This plan includes reading journals and texts, attending courses and hospital teaching rounds, and undertaking self-study programs. Continuing scholarship requires self-discipline to set aside personal time on a regular basis. An effective way to learn is to pursue knowledge about the disease at the time one sees a patient with a specific illness.

TABLE 19–1. ABILITIES REQUIRED OF A PHYSICIAN

Noncognitive abilities
- Attitudes and habits
- Interpersonal skills
- Motor and technical skills

Intellectual abilities
- Knowledge
- Organization
- Synthesis
- Clinical judgment

Modified from American Board of Internal Medicine: Clinical competence in internal medicine. Ann Intern Med 90:403, 1979.

TABLE 19–2. TASKS REQUIRED OF A PHYSICIAN

Data gathering
- Medical history
- Physical examination
- Diagnostic studies

Diagnosis or problem definition

Medical care

Modified from American Board of Internal Medicine: Clinical competence in internal medicine. Ann Intern Med 90:403, 1979.

INTERPERSONAL SKILLS. Being able to relate to the patient, to family members, and to others caring for the patient is of particular importance. The ability to communicate well is the basis for effective interpersonal relationships. This communication includes encouraging the patient to share symptoms and personal concerns. One should be aware of nonverbal messages that convey significant information about emotional problems. The physician also has the obligation to transmit information to the patient about the illness itself and about its prognosis and treatment. Competence means communicating well despite intellectual, socioeconomic, and language barriers.

It is a responsibility of the physician to talk with family members, while at the same time respecting patient confidentiality. Knowing with whom to talk and how much to say requires considerable skill. The competent physician also communicates effectively with others caring for the patient. This interpersonal skill includes the ability to present the patient's problem orally and to transmit information through written orders and the written record.

MOTOR AND TECHNICAL SKILLS. Manual skills are necessary in gathering information from the patient as well as in applying specific treatment. Being able to do a well-ordered and accurate physical examination requires effective motor skills. Diagnostic procedures such as biopsies, sampling of body fluids, or endoscopy also depend on motor and technical skills. Examples of treatment involving these skills include performing minor surgery and using machines for life support. Learning new techniques and continuing to practice them are major requirements for maintaining technical competence.

Intellectual Abilities

Disease is a scientific, impersonal term. *Illness* is personalized and refers to disease in a specific patient. Intellectual skills are directed to the understanding, diagnosis, and theoretical management of disease. Noncognitive abilities deal more with the individual. In approaching a medical problem, the physician begins with relevant medical knowledge and synthesizes the information into an integrated concept. Clinical judgment is used to resolve the problem.

To apply medical knowledge to a patient problem, the physician draws on pertinent medical facts from memory, from clinical experience, and from other sources such as journals, textbooks, and experts. An understanding of pathophysiology helps in anticipating the expected course of the disease. Information derived from the patient, together with medical knowledge, is organized into a logical sequence. Synthesis of organized medical knowledge involves integration of medical facts into practical concepts, which are altered as the patient's condition changes or when new information becomes available. Organization and synthesis of information are important in all tasks of a physician, including data gathering, diagnosis, and planning for study and treatment. The highest level of cognitive ability is clinical judgment, where intellectual skills are called upon to solve problems. The physician makes clinical decisions by discriminating between alternative courses of action. Clinical judgment is used to decide what is of greatest benefit to the patient with the least risk and cost.

TASKS REQUIRED OF A PHYSICIAN

When a patient comes for help, the physician follows a logical series of steps, which are called clinical tasks. The physician first obtains the medical history, does a physical examination, and conducts laboratory studies. Based on this information, an initial diagnosis is made upon which definitive medical care is based.

Data Gathering

MEDICAL HISTORY. The most powerful diagnostic tool of the physician is the interview. By this means, one learns the chronological events and the symptoms of the patient's illness. Diagnostic hypotheses are generated and tested as the patient's history unfolds, resulting in the formulation of the most likely diagnoses at the completion of the interview. These hypotheses are extended, confirmed, or refuted by the subsequent physical examination and diagnostic studies.

The interview has considerable importance beyond "history taking" or the gathering of medical facts. It is the principal means of initiating and developing a relationship with the patient. The interview is a shared experience with goals for both participants. For the patient, the goal is alleviation of distress and restoration of health. The patient must be satisfied that the person rendering medical care is not only professionally competent but is also interested in him as an individual. For the physician, the primary objective is to obtain the information needed to understand the illness and to initiate appropriate treatment. This objective is accomplished by demonstrating concern for the patient and by being willing to listen to his personal as well as medical problems. The overt demonstration of concern by the physician will help to build the physician-patient relationship and secure the patient's cooperation.

The most important component of the medical history is the patient's present illness. Here, the interviewer develops a detailed and sequential reconstruction of the symptoms and events contributing to the current illness. The social history is also of considerable importance. The inquiry with interest and empathy into the personal events of the patient's life, while affording the patient time to relate these events, helps to establish a strong physician-patient relationship. Knowledge of the patient's personal circumstances and relationships to others leads to better understanding of his problems and ways of coping with them. More effective planning for the future care of the patient takes place when the limitations imposed on the current life situation are known.

When pursuing information in the interview, the physician begins with open-ended or nondirective questions and concludes with specific questions. Such an approach allows the patient time to respond and to elaborate on his problems. Failure to take time to listen may be interpreted by the patient as a lack of interest on the part of the interviewer and can result in a perfunctory and noninformative interview. To initiate the interview with a series of specific questions may also inhibit the full development of the history. Encouraging the patient to speak freely as the interview proceeds is important, since only the patient can describe what he has been experiencing. On the other hand, the patient does not necessarily understand what the interviewer needs to learn from him. The physician therefore actively pursues the interview in order to develop organization and content. The patient soon learns that events must be dated, sequences established, and symptoms precisely described. Dates and times serve to anchor the history in such a way that relationships between symptoms and events are more clearly understood. Knowledge of disease and clinical syndromes enables the physician to anticipate symptoms the patient does not mention. It is often necessary to intervene in order to clarify terms the patient uses, including medical or quasi-medical terms. Some patients, when asked to tell of their own illnesses, may omit their symptoms altogether and persist in describing only what other doctors said and did. It should be made clear that the interviewer is more interested in learning about the patient's specific symptoms and not the interpretation of those symptoms.

In conducting an effective interview, the physician adapts to the personality of the patient and to limitations imposed by illness. Patients who are especially talkative or who wander from the subject need to be guided back to the pertinent issues. Patients with poverty of associations are encouraged to elaborate on their problems. When an interview becomes primarily a question and answer session, it is likely that the patient is unable to go into detail because of illness or that the interviewer is using poor technique and is therefore missing valuable historical information. In a seriously ill patient, one gives priority to those aspects of the history that appear more relevant to the immediate situation. Other patients, because of the type of disease, may be handicapped in relating their stories. When the interview is limited because of the patient's illness, information is derived from other sources such as family, friends, and previous hospital records. A subsequent interview of the patient at a more opportune time is often valuable.

The appearance and responses of the patient during the interview are diagnostically helpful. The physical examination begins the moment the patient is seen. One studies the patient's appearance, his emotional state, and his physical and mental limitations. Not only is close attention paid to the overt meaning of what is said, but the interviewer is also alert to nonverbal cues. The physician's own feeling of being uncomfortable, uneasy, or unhappy often reflects the attitude of the patient.

The interview, a powerful diagnostic tool, goes far beyond collecting the facts of illness. Through knowledge and experience, the physician delineates subtle symptoms and interrelationships that are often unrecognized by the patient. A skillful interviewer will uncover personal feelings and circumstances underlying the illness. An interview conducted with sensitivity and concern will help to build a strong relationship between the patient and physician.

PHYSICAL EXAMINATION. A general screening examination is conducted following the interview. This examination is influenced by diagnostic hypotheses developed during the interview which direct the physician to do a more detailed study in the area of suspected abnormality.

Consideration for the patient continues during the physical examination. Privacy is provided for dressing and undressing, and the examination is done with appropriate draping. Both the physician and the patient need to be in a comfortable position throughout the examination in order to apply techniques properly. In certain parts of the examination, the physician tells the patient how to cooperate and forewarns him of any uncomfortable impending maneuver. In general, the examination is done in silence except for necessary instructions to the patient. Talking hinders the physician from concentrating fully on possible underlying abnormalities. The examination is carried out with meticulous care, gentleness, and sensitive attention. One avoids comments or facial expressions that can be misinterpreted by the patient as indicating concern or puzzlement. The physician is also alert to signs of patient fatigue or discomfort.

There are two major principles underlying an efficient physical examination. First, the examination is done by regions; second, there is a well-organized order of examination. To be efficient, one approaches regions sequentially, for example, the head, the neck, the posterior thorax and lungs, the anterior thorax and lungs, and the heart. This type of regional approach also takes into account the comfort of the patient by eliminating the need for frequent shifts in position. One begins with a general survey of each region and then focuses on component parts. If no abnormality is found, the examination is brief but comprehensive. If an abnormality is present, it is studied meticulously, using special maneuvers if necessary. One takes advantage of the symmetry of the human body by comparing one side with the other. In this way, subtle changes are recognized. Small differences in the lung examination, for example, are better detected by cross-comparing symmetrical areas of each lung than by examining each lung individually. Following a prescribed order of examination by regions does not imply a lack of flexibility. The examination varies with the condition of the patient and the type of problem present. Evidence of disease in one area alerts the physician to possible related abnormalities in other areas. If the initial physical examination has not been entirely satisfactory, one does not hesitate to return at a later time to recheck findings when circumstances for reexamination may be more favorable.

Observation is an often neglected technique of great importance. Studying the patient and his surroundings yields helpful diagnostic information. By noting what is on the bedside table, for example, one gains insight into the patient's interests and habits and the support of family and friends. Specifically, one looks for reading materials, cigarettes, and the presence of cards or gifts. When beginning to examine each region, the physician pauses to observe. For example, an enlarged thyroid gland will readily be seen when a patient extends his neck slightly and swallows; asymmetry of respiratory motion will be more easily observed from the foot of the bed with the patient on his back; and holding an end of a tongue blade lightly at the cardiac apex will magnify the visible impulse of a left ventricular gallop.

The physician learns to do a comprehensive screening examination. Depending on the condition of the patient, the examination will need to be adapted to special circumstances. The patient may be bed-bound and so ill that the examiner requires assistance with positioning. In an acute emergency where an abbreviated physical examination is carried out with deliberate speed, one simultaneously does a brief interview, obtains laboratory work, and initiates treatment. If the patient has a neurologic problem, a complete neurologic examination is done. Regardless of the problem and the condition of the patient, the physician is considerate, systematic, and logical in approach. One keeps in mind diagnostic possibilities, looks for unsuspected disease, and interrelates abnormal findings that may explain the patient's illness.

DIAGNOSTIC STUDIES. Laboratory tests and diagnostic procedures are obtained following the interview and physical examination. A few initial screening tests are usually done to detect unsuspected common entities, such as anemia, diabetes, or chronic renal disease. Studies are discriminatingly chosen to confirm one's impression and are not used in a routine or excessive way to search for unexpected diagnoses. After considering each of the patient's problems, the physician decides which studies are needed, both to confirm the diagnostic impression and to rule in or out other possibilities. If the prevalence of a problem is low and no effective treatment is available, few diagnostic tests are indicated. Laboratory tests and diagnostic procedures are of value not only to help make the diagnosis, but also to assess the severity, course, and prognosis of the disease and to follow the effect of therapy.

When choosing diagnostic studies, the physician begins with those that yield the most comprehensive information and carry the least risk for the patient. The diagnosis frequently becomes apparent with simple tests; more expensive or potentially hazardous studies may not be required. Laboratory tests are often overemphasized. These tests have limitations in accuracy, and there may be errors and misinterpretation of results. The physician's own clinical findings and judgment take precedence in the interpretation of laboratory data.

Potentially hazardous diagnostic or therapeutic procedures require competence on the part of those doing them. Plans for procedures are discussed with the patient, including possible risks. Time is taken to alleviate patient concern and to interpret the results. In carrying out diagnostic studies and treatment, consultant assistance is often required. The physician in charge of the patient takes into account the expert advice of consultants but continues to supervise overall care and makes the ultimate decisions.

Recent research into clinical decision-making has been helpful in creating a better understanding of the selection and interpretation of diagnostic tests and procedures. Knowledge of the sensitivity and specificity of diagnostic studies leads to their more rational selection. *Sensitivity* is the probability that a test will be positive when the disease is present. *Specificity* is the probability that the test will be negative when the disease is not present. For example, to exclude the possibility of lupus erythematosus, one chooses a sensitive test such as the antinuclear antibody test. The more specific double-stranded DNA antibody test is ordered to confirm the diagnosis.

Diagnosis or Problem Definition

The physician uses the scientific method in clinical problem solving, as does the investigator in conducting an experiment. Clinical information is analyzed to develop working hypotheses that are confirmed or refuted by obtaining further information. Problem solving begins at the time the physician initiates the interview. The symptoms and course of the illness lead to the formulation of several diagnostic hypotheses. These diagnostic possibilities direct further questioning of the patient in order to determine which hypothesis best fits the illness. Hypotheses are repeatedly generated and tested during the interview. As the physician completes the interview and physical examination, one or two possibilities usually become more likely and others less likely. With further information, an attempt is made to explain the patient's presenting illness with a single preliminary diagnosis. This goal is often attainable in young patients but seldom in older ones, in whom multiple diagnoses are usually required. One takes into account the likelihood of the disease process in making a preliminary diagnosis. The most common diseases are considered first, particularly those diseases for which specific treatment is available.

Cognitive or intellectual skills are used in formulating a diagnosis. A physician continually refers to knowledge of medical facts and pathophysiology in analyzing information pertaining to the patient's illness. This analysis consists of collecting information and synthesizing it into integrated concepts compatible with known diseases. Abnormal findings are localized anatomically and are interpreted in terms of their structure and function. Clinical judgment is used to weigh the diagnostic possibilities by assigning values to the data in order to arrive at the most likely conclusion. The experienced clinician is able to apply these intellectual processes rapidly and continually while interviewing the patient.

The written record is used to clarify the physician's diagnostic thinking. When there are several diagnostic possibilities explaining the symptoms and events of the present illness, a differential diagnosis is carried out. For each diagnosis considered, the physician weighs information favoring that possibility against information that makes the diagnosis unlikely. Consideration of alternative possibilities in the differential diagnosis is helpful in directing the physician to select diagnostic studies that confirm or exclude each possible diagnosis. In addition to indicating the most likely diagnosis that explains the present illness, the physician lists in descending order of importance all other active problems affecting the patient. This list includes not only specific diseases, but also such problems as the recent loss of a spouse or exposure to environmental toxins. The physician considers all possible factors in the patient's illness, including psychological stresses and underlying conditions that may alter resistance. The functional impact of the illness in terms of its severity and the degree of resulting disability is also taken into account.

Clinical decisions are influenced by policies determined by tradition, by the medical literature, and by the practice of colleagues. These policies may be based on simplistic or even erroneous reasoning. Greater attention needs to be paid to clinical policies that have been shown to be valid. Ongoing investigation of diagnostic reasoning will eventually lead to better understanding of the ways clinicians solve medical problems. The diagnostic thinking of physicians as they interview simulated patients has been studied, and decision analysis has contributed logic theory to problem solving, including the use of probability and decision trees.

Medical Care

The term *medical care* is used rather than the more authoritative, *patient management*, because it expresses personal concern and responsibility for all of the patient's problems. In caring for a patient, physician attitudes of integrity, respect, and compassion are particularly important, as is the ability to communicate effectively. In addition, the intellectual skills of the physician are necessary attributes. Up-to-date medical knowledge of pharmacologic principles and advances in technology are required. Clinical judgment is used in prescribing drugs, in selecting therapeutic procedures, and in implementing consultant opinions. Knowing when *not* to treat is as important as knowing when to treat. New drugs and procedures are ordered with caution. A full understanding of their potential complications is necessary to be sure that negative side effects do not outweigh possible advantages. To be fully effective, the physician needs the requisite knowledge and skills to treat acute life-threatening illness as well as the supportive staying power to care for the chronically ill patient. One learns to care for patients in a variety of environments: in the office, in the emergency room, in the hospital, by telephone, or when the patient is housebound or in a nursing home.

The care of the patient involves far more than prescribing drugs and completing therapeutic procedures. Attention is paid to the preventive aspects of disease, to the patient's psychological problems, and to conflicts arising from home or place of work. Immunization for infectious disease and advice to avoid smoking and excessive drinking are obvious examples of preventive measures. The patient may need to alter his way of living, if job stress plays a role. Psychiatric or family counseling may help when there are major psychological problems.

Good communication with the patient is required in order to educate him about his illness, its management, and its prevention. A better informed patient will be more motivated to comply with treatment. The ability to communicate well is also needed when dealing with responsible family members and with others caring for the patient. Diabetes mellitus is an excellent example of an illness that requires education and the help of others. The patient needs to understand the disease in order to know why diet is important, why blood sugar levels are high, and why insulin is used. He learns the potential complications and how to prevent them. Nurses help the patient learn to test glucose levels and to use an insulin syringe; dietitians teach a diabetic diet.

In providing excellent care, the competent physician knows how frequently a patient should be seen and how extensive an evaluation is necessary. These decisions require good clinical judgment and a rationale for each action. It is important for the physician to instruct the patient how to obtain medical care at all times, particularly in an acute emergency or when the physician is not available. Above all, the physician demonstrates a continuing personal interest in the patient, is the patient's advocate, and assumes responsibility for all of his health care needs.

THE MEDICAL RECORD

The primary purpose of the medical record is to document the medical experience of the patient. This information is used by those concerned with the patient's current and future care. Legally, it is a public document available to other physicians and to health care providers, to the court by subpoena, and to insurance companies. The medical record varies in format and detail, depending on whether the patient is seen in an ambulatory setting or in the emergency room or is admitted to the hospital.

A major contribution to the organization of the medical record has been the introduction of the problem-oriented method. Of particular importance are the problem list and the problem-oriented progress notes. The medical record of the patient may be organized by combining the traditional format of the history and physical examination with the identification of active problems. If there is a single major problem that is not clearly defined, a formulation is written. The physician gives the reasons for the diagnosis and weighs evidence for and against other diagnostic possibilities. When there are several active problems, these are discussed separately, each with a diagnostic and therapeutic plan.

The problem list is particularly useful when following an ambulatory patient who has chronic illness and multiple problems. A list of active and inactive problems serves as an index to the record. In this way, problems are summarized and can be quickly reviewed. Problem-oriented progress notes help to organize ongoing clinical information. During the course of an illness, they enable one to easily follow individual problems through the record.

Establishment of the scientific basis of the art of medicine will lead to future clarification of each step of the medical encounter between the patient and physician. The expert clinician's resolution of a problem is not easily understood. Research defining the abilities and tasks of a physician will help to eliminate the dichotomy between the art and science of medicine.

American Board of Internal Medicine: Clinical competence in internal medicine. Ann Intern Med 90:402, 1979. *The major components of the medical encounter are analyzed, which include the abilities required of an internist, the tasks performed to solve a medical problem, the medical illness, and the patient.*

Eddy DM: Clinical policies and the quality of clinical practice. N Engl J Med 307:343, 1982. *A description is given of some of the sources of errors and biases in clinical policy-making, with suggested ways to improve the quality of clinical policies.*

Elstein AS, Shulman LS, Sprafka SA: Medical Problem Solving. An Analysis of Clinical Reasoning. Cambridge, Mass., Harvard University Press, 1978. *A detailed, yet readable textbook gives the results of five years of research on medical problem solving and decision making based on the performance of selected internists and students in a variety of experimental situations.*

Griner PF, Mayewski RJ, Mushlin AI, Greenland P: Selection and interpretation of diagnostic tests and procedures. Principles and applications. Ann Intern Med 94 (Part 2):553, 1981. *This is a review of the scientific approach to selecting and interpreting diagnostic tests and procedures. Exercises are included enabling the reader to calculate the likelihood of a given disease, and rational diagnostic strategies are suggested for various diseases.*

Kassirer JP, Gorry GA: Clinical problem solving. A behavioral analysis. Ann Intern Med 89:245, 1978. *Tape-recorded interviews of simulated patients by experienced clinicians are studied to determine how hypothesis generation is used in clinical problem solving.*

Morgan WL, Engel GL: The Clinical Approach to the Patient. Philadelphia, W. B. Saunders Company, 1969. *This is a step-by-step guide to interviewing the patient, organizing the physical examination, and handling clinical information, with particular emphasis on how to relate to the patient.*

Weinstein MC, Fineberg HV: Clinical Decision Analysis. Philadelphia, W. B. Saunders Company, 1980. *A detailed quantitative analysis is given of clinical decision making, which includes the use of decision trees and probabilities and the assigning of values to possible outcomes.*

20. THE USE AND INTERPRETATION OF LABORATORY-DERIVED DATA

James B. Wyngaarden

The basic workup of a patient begins with the acquisition of information. The experienced clinician will insist upon a discerning and sensitive history, a thorough physical examination, and such laboratory tests as may be necessary to evaluate the general health of the patient, to arrive at a specific diagnosis, to assess the functional status of involved organs, or to provide a basis for monitoring effectiveness of therapy.

Until two decades ago only a few laboratory tests were performed routinely in the workup of a patient. When screening was practiced, the panel of tests was usually limited to hemoglobin (or hematocrit) determination, blood cell counts, urinalysis, stool examination for occult blood, and perhaps a chest x-ray and an electrocardiogram, particularly in adults. Additional tests were ordered only when suggested by the clinical assessment. In this setting an attending physician could evaluate the reasoning process that led a resident to order a serum calcium determination, or a serum alkaline phosphatase assay. The ordering of laboratory procedures was a consequence of the intellectual discipline of constructing a logical differential diagnosis, or of the need to monitor the progress of a patient, e.g., one in diabetic ketoacidosis. Thus it was a vital component of the educational process itself.

In 1966 Thiers published a provocative study comparing the results of a screening battery of eleven tests run by an automated multichannel analyzer with those of tests specifically ordered on the same patients by physicians as part of the admission workup. The screening battery detected twice as many abnormal test results as were uncovered by selective ordering. The most common findings were elevated glucose or uric acid concentrations. Ensuing developments were rapid. Ingenious automated analyzers brought an increasing number and variety of tests within the reach of all practitioners. The cost of such a screening battery fell rapidly until soon one could obtain 12 to 18 test results for no more than the cost of three or four selected tests run manually a decade earlier.

The inclusion of a panel of chemical tests or enzyme assays of blood (or urine) became a routine component of a basic medical workup. For more than a decade, medical students and residents have been brought up with a dependency upon such screening batteries of chemical measurements. Only a few hospitals resisted the temptation to institute such screening procedures and continued the traditional practice of letting the intellectual evaluation of the patient determine the indications for further laboratory procedures. The pendulum has now begun to swing back, as the limited utility of large panel testing has become more generally recognized. Only a small number of "screening tests" (history, physical examination, stool guaiac test, and blood pressure measurement) have actually been shown to improve the health outcome of asymptomatic outpatients. Admission screening tests, such as a "Chem 12," complete blood count, or sedimentation rate, have a relatively low yield: fewer than 1 per cent lead to a "new" diagnosis. In fact, fewer than 10 per cent of Chem 12 data are ever used clinically, and as few as 40 per cent of "abnormal" results initiate a follow-up. Furthermore, unnecessary hospitalization has occurred when one laboratory test result of a screening panel was "abnormal" by chance on a statistical basis alone. Whenever 20 procedures are done, whose "normal range" is defined as the central 95 per cent segment, one test result will, on the average, fall outside this range on the basis of chance alone. Statistically, 40 per cent of all Chem 12 panels performed on healthy individuals will result in one "abnormal" result. Repetition of tests showing such aberrant results contributes to the high cost of medical care, but only rarely to the detection of significant dysfunction or disease. As a consequence of this additional experience, some of the larger teaching hospitals have discontinued screening panels. This movement has been accelerated by the exclusion of routine screening procedures from the list of reimbursable expenditures by some third-party payers of medical services.

In order to utilize the results of laboratory tests intelligently (and economically), the physician must be able to evaluate the validity of the test result, understand principles of variation and distribution of values, and integrate the data received from the laboratory with the information acquired from the patient. If the test result deviates from values found in a healthy control population, is the difference trivial, or is it indicative of important dysfunction? Should the test be repeated? How often need a particular measurement be followed up? What additional tests or studies are indicated on the basis of these leads?

The more information the physician has, the more effective the physician should be in caring for the patient. To ensure that this is the result requires knowledge of medical science, clinical judgment, and a profound respect for the limitations of the laboratory. One of the best ways of acquiring the constructively critical attitude so essential to the proper evaluation of laboratory data is to work in a laboratory for a while. There is a paradox in the present pattern of medical education: at a time of increasing reliance upon an expanding array of laboratory tests in the practice of medicine, learning experiences in the laboratory have largely been eliminated from the medical curriculum.

SOME LIMITATIONS OF THE LABORATORY

CRITERIA FOR EVALUATION OF LABORATORY METHODS. A trustworthy laboratory test must pass critical evaluations of analytic specificity, sensitivity, accuracy, and precision.

Specificity refers to the detection of the substance in question and no other. It is doubtful that any test is absolutely specific for the substance being measured. There is always some other substance around that is capable of reacting. In biochemical analyses this limitation is most serious in tests dependent upon color development, less in the case of assays dependent upon degradation of the analyte by purified enzymes, and perhaps least in such procedures as atomic absorption spectroscopy.

Sensitivity refers to the ability of the test to detect the substance in question at the required concentrations, namely, those at which the compound exists in body fluids.

Accuracy refers to the quantitative detection of the correct amount of the substance being measured. This property rests upon both specificity and sensitivity. A test may be accurate in the absence of certain interfering drugs, and only in a certain range of values. It may fail this criterion under other conditions.

Precision embodies *repeatability*, the obtaining of the same result on samples analyzed in replicated fashion, and *reproducibility*, representing quality control over time.

THE "LAW OF ERRORS." Early in the nineteenth century, the German mathematician and physicist, Johann C. F. Gauss, introduced the "law of errors." This law states that in repeated measurements of the *same* object or substance, the random component on the errors will be distributed about the mean as a frequency function. This distribution, which is bell shaped, is often called "normal" or "gaussian." Note that the law applies to repeated measurements of the same item. Its extension to a population of those items is justifiable only under certain circumstances, for not all distributions are bell shaped, and not all bell-shaped distributions are gaussian. The matter of distributions will be discussed further below, when we consider the topic of "normal range" of a biologic variable. First, however, we should emphasize the topic of error, for every laboratory measurement is subject to it.

SOURCES OF ERRORS

These are legion, and include some factors under the control of the clinician, such as the dietary preparation of the patient, and the techniques of collection and handling of samples. Reduction of the error factor to an acceptable minimum requires compulsive attention to every detail of the process.

LABORATORY ERRORS. There is imprecision in every measurement. In tests run by hand, pipetting, timing, reading, and recording errors occur. They are more frequent when technicians are overworked or fatigued. It is common to find greater scatter of results of replicate tests at the end of the day than at the beginning. Technician fatigue can be largely eliminated by automation, but there will always remain the technical limitations of machines and the human error in the preparation of reagents, in the standardization of instruments, and in the copying of test results. The last is not totally avoided by the computer print-out, as even typewriters make misteaks. Quality control varies widely from laboratory to laboratory. Split samples submitted to different laboratories may show surprising disparities in results.

DRUG INTERFERENCE. According to Osler, man is distinguished from all other members of the Animal Kingdom by his desire to take drugs. Since many patients do not regard proprietary pain remedies or vitamins as drugs, the physician may obtain a negative drug history unless questions are appropriately phrased. Drugs have great potential for interference with laboratory tests. High resolution chromatography of urine yields about 300 peaks of ultraviolet absorbing materials. Two hundred and fifty of these disappear if the "normal subject" abstains from salicylates and vitamins for a few days. Salicylates, vitamins, and many other drugs or their metabolites also produce chromogens which interfere with certain analytic methods employed in automated tests, particularly of the urine.

DISTRIBUTIONS OF VALUES

There is widespread belief among medical students and graduate physicians that if the sample of test results from a healthy population is large enough, the distribution will be "normal" (gaussian); that on this assumption one may justifiably determine a mean value ($\bar{x}$) and its standard deviation (s); that the value, $\bar{x} \pm 2s$, will include the central 95 per cent of all measurements; that this segment of the distribution is the "normal range"; and that values which fall outside this range are by definition "abnormal." All of these beliefs are erroneous in most instances. The experimental fact is that for most physiologic variables the distribution is smooth, unimodal, and skewed, and that $\bar{x} \pm 2s$ does not cut off the desired central 95 per cent. Among the distributions of serum calcium, inorganic phosphorus, magnesium, alkaline phosphatase, total proteins, albumin, uric acid, and blood urea, only that of albumin is gaussian. All others are skewed, leptokurtic, or both. The value $\pm$ 2s will cut off many more measurements in one tail of the distribution than the other. The uncritical application of principles of normal distributions in situations in which variables are not normally distributed sometimes leads to values of $\bar{x} - 2s$ that are negative, surely a biologic absurdity.

Once we discard the notion that the distribution of values in healthy persons is gaussian, the question of estimating the mean and standard deviation does not arise. Also, one need not attempt to fit skewed distributions into bell-shaped curves by constructing histograms of logarithms of the data (a technique that has the effect of compressing the skewed tail to disclose a "log-gaussian distribution"), or by constructing plots of cumulative frequencies of values (or log-values) on probability paper (see Fig. 20–1).

These pitfalls can be avoided by use of *nonparametric* methods for estimating the reference range, that is, methods that do not involve any a priori assumption regarding the parental distribution shape except that it is continuous. Two nonparametric methods of normal range estimation are the method of *percentile estimates* with associated nonparametric confidence intervals, and the method of nonparametric *tolerance intervals* which

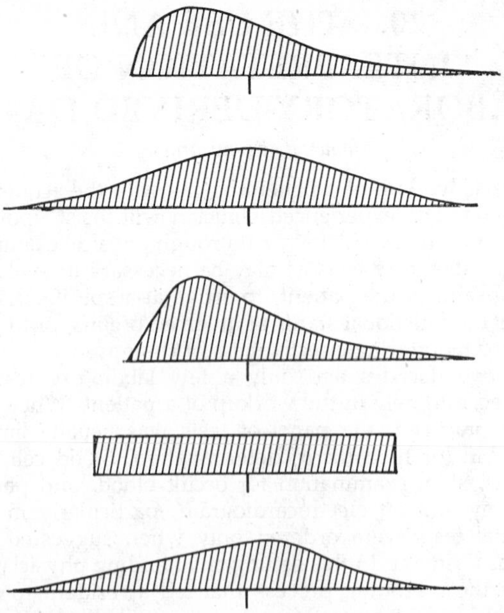

Figure 20–1. Five distributions with the same mean and standard deviation ($\bar{x}$ = 4, s = 2.83). From top to bottom: X_4^2, normal, lognormal, rectangular, and mixture of two normals. (From Elveback LR: Mayo Clinic Proc 47:93, 1972; with permission.)

include a specified proportion of the population with a specified probability.

Physicians are familiar with the percentile method of expressing interindividual variation through the use of pediatric growth charts of height and weight. The method avoids the arbitrary distinction of normal and abnormal. It also removes the aura of precision of the standard deviation. The percentile method appropriately fits the real world of nongaussian distributions.

From every laboratory test for which a good normal-value study has been done, the laboratory can report not only the result but also the percentile corresponding to that result and appropriate to the age and sex of the patient under study. With this information the clinician can appreciate just how common or how unusual the test result is. The percentile method is superior to an arbitrary definition of a normal range, such as $\bar{x} \pm 2s$, even in those few cases in which a distribution is gaussian, for it indicates for each test result the relationship of that result to the healthy population. The percentile method is also superior to the definition of the normal range as the range of all observed values in a healthy sample population, for the latter method seriously underestimates any selected segment, e.g., the central 95 per cent, in small samples, and overestimates it in large samples.

The percentile method does not systematically over- or underestimate any selected range, regardless of sample size. If one wishes to cut off the lowest and highest 2.5 per cent, or 5 per cent, one simply orders all values and finds the value that cuts off the desired percentage of observations at either tail of the distribution. Obvious outlier values are discarded. The complete percentile range is readily defined. No assumptions are required about distribution shape except that it is continuous. From the size of the healthy population represented in the distribution, the confidence limits of a given percentile may be ascertained, with known probability, by reference to standard tables. The method should appeal particularly to clinicians who utilize local norms, which are often based on small samples.

THE "NORMAL RANGE." From this discussion, it is clear that "normal range" is an arbitrary and potentially misleading term. By whatever method it is defined, the normal range will exclude observations of the parental distribution of healthy subjects and will very likely include some values of other distributions. What the clinician desires are cut-off points at either end of a distribution that include nearly all values of healthy individuals in the central segment, and very few values of other distributions, i.e., that the numbers of false-positive and false-negative values are both minimized. Ingrained habits will probably lead us to select the central 95 per cent of the parental distribution as "clinical limits," even though there is no magic in this number. Some clinical investigators advocate use of the central 90 per cent.

The term "normal range" has come in for substantial criticism. The connotation of a sharp demarcation between normal and abnormal values is unfortunate and usually erroneous. A value may fall outside the range, $\bar{x} \pm 2s$, or the central 95 per cent segment, on the basis of chance alone. The present consensus is that laboratory results should be interpreted in relationship to "reference intervals" rather than normal ranges. In most instances the quoted reference intervals for a given laboratory test result are the same as the previously published normal ranges, but the term emphasizes the manner in which such intervals are determined, and avoids an assumption of normality or abnormality of the test result. The newer terminology requires the laboratory to describe what it is using as a reference population to generate the interval values.

Influence of Age. The distributions of values of many plasma constituents vary with age in the apparently healthy population. For example, plasma cholesterol concentrations, mean and 90 per cent limits, are 180 (120 to 240) mg per deciliter in the 20- to 29-year age group, and 245 (160 to 330) mg per deciliter in the 50- to 59-year age group.

Influence of Sex. Distributions in men may differ from those in women. For example, plasma urate concentration values, mean and 90 per cent limits, are 4.9 (2.7 to 7.2) mg per deciliter in men, and 4.0 (2.5 to 6.3) mg per deciliter in premenopausal women. Mean serum calcium values in normal men decline 0.0068 mg per deciliter per year from age 20 to age 80. Those of women show no regression against age. This is an important point in the diagnosis of hyperparathyroidism, which is chiefly a disease of the older age group.

BIOLOGIC RATHER THAN STATISTICAL NORMS. Whether values of serum cholesterol of 325 mg per deciliter in the 50- to 59-year age group are biologically "normal" simply because they fall in the 90 to 95 percentile range can be debated. Epidemiologic studies show that the more serum cholesterol values exceed about 180 mg per deciliter the shorter is the average life expectancy.

Clinical norms of serum cholesterol concentrations should perhaps be defined in terms of age-related values that are neutral, rather than as a 90 percentile range. Such an approach requires a biologic rather than statistical definition. Data are not yet available to set reliable limits in this manner for more than a few substances.

One secure example concerns urate concentration values. An electrolyte solution with the sodium concentration of plasma is saturated with urate at 6.4 to 6.8 mg per deciliter. In addition, proteins of plasma bind urate equivalent to about 4 per cent of the amount in solution. Values above 7.0 (perhaps 7.2) mg per deciliter represent supersaturation and are "abnormal" in that they are associated with increased risk of renal stone and clinical gout. The magnitude of the risk factor increases as urate concentration values increase above 7.0 mg per deciliter. The 95 per cent limits of serum urate values in "healthy" male New Zealand Maoris are 4 to 10 mg per deciliter, and 10 per cent of adult males develop gout. Surely the central 95 per cent of the distribution of serum urate concentrations in this male population cannot be considered "normal," even though the reference interval is appropriately selected by the usual criteria.

DISCONTINUOUS DISTRIBUTIONS. Some traits may be distributed bimodally or trimodally. Such relationships are most likely in families in which there is a monogenetic disease characterized by a chemical abnormality. For example, measurements of galactose-1-phosphate uridyltransferase activity in the families of patients with transferase deficiency galactosemia are distributed trimodally. The effects of two and of one mutant allele

are clearly distinguishable from the normal and from each other. Assay values in the three modes are zero, 7.5 to 13.5 units, and 19.5 to 32 units. The intermediate enzyme assay values are found in subjects who are presumed heterozygotes by pedigree analysis. It is common to hear the term "heterozygote value" applied to an enzyme activity value approximately one half of normal. This practice is justifiable only when assay data are combined with pedigree data, for there may be other reasons for a reduced enzyme assay value that have nothing to do with genetics.

An apparently continuous distribution with marked skewing may at times be dissected into two or even three distribution modes by appropriate clinical and pedigree studies. For example, the distribution of plasma cholesterol concentrations in familial hypercholesterolemia displays marked overlap between subjects who are clinically normal and those who are heterozygotes by pedigree analysis. Similarly, there is considerable overlap between heterozygotes and abnormal homozygotes. Only a complete family pedigree permits adequate definition of the range of values in each distribution mode.

THE PHYSICIAN AND THE LABORATORY TEST RESULT

The tables at the end of this book contain values that define the reference intervals for a large number of substances commonly measured in clinical medicine. They represent the best data currently available, but are subject to all the uncertainties discussed above. In some instances more selective data of an age- and sex-matched control population will need to be consulted by the physician.

Clinical judgment will always be required in the interpretation of laboratory data. For example, a serum BUN concentration of 22 mg per deciliter is not a normal value for a patient on a very low protein diet. Also electrolyte values of sodium 145 mEq per liter, potassium 3.5 mEq per liter, chloride 98 mEq per liter, and CO_2 30 mEq per liter may indicate metabolic alkalosis even though all individual values fall within published reference intervals.

Laboratory tests are critical to the diagnosis of disease and management of patients. The physician must know the limits of reliability and usefulness of each test result in the clinical setting of the individual patient. This is particularly true when all deviant test results have returned to normal but the patient is not improving. It is especially when laboratory data provide little or no help that the patient needs a doctor.

Bryan DJ, Wearne JJ, Viau A, Musser AW, Schoonmaker FW, Thiers RE: Profile of admission chemical data by multichannel automation: An evaluative experiment. Clin Chem 12:137, 1966. *The initial study of screening patients on admission to hospital by a panel of tests run on an automated multichannel analyzer.*

Dales LG, Friedman GD, Collen MF: Evaluating periodic multiphasic health checkups: A controlled trial. J Chronic Dis 32:385, 1979. *Only a limited number of screening tests (history or physical examination, stool test for occult blood, and blood pressure) actually improve health outcome of asymptomatic outpatients.*

Dixon RH, Laszlo J: Utilization of clinical chemistry services by medical house staff. Arch Intern Med 134:1064, 1974. *Less than 10 per cent of data obtained from a panel of 12 tests were used clinically.*

Elveback LR, Guillier CL, Keating FR: Health, normality, and the ghost of Gauss. JAMA 211:69, 1970. *Of eight distributions evaluated, only that of serum albumin was "normal" or gaussian.*

Keating FR, Jones JD, Elveback LR, Randall RV: The relation of age and sex to distribution of values in healthy adults of serum calcium, inorganic phosphorus, magnesium, alkaline phosphatase, total proteins, albumin, and blood urea. J Lab Clin Med 73:825, 1969. *A study of the age- and sex-dependency of several constituents of serum. The downward trend of serum calcium values with age in men is particularly noteworthy.*

Korvin CC, Pearce RH, Stanley J: Admissions screening: Clinical benefits. Ann Intern Med 83:197, 1975. *Admission screening tests have a relatively low benefit. Fewer than 1 per cent lead to new diagnoses of significance to the patient.*

Mainland, D: Remarks on clinical "norms." Clin Chem 17:267, 1971. *An excellent article explaining the use of nonparametric methods for establishing reference intervals.*

Parkerson GR, Eisenson HJ: Association of patient and physician characteristics with follow-up of abnormal laboratory results. J Fam Pract 11:943, 1980. *As few as 40 per cent of abnormal results initiate clinical follow-up.*

21. OVERVIEW OF IMAGING TECHNIQUES AND PROJECTION FOR THE FUTURE

Alexander R. Margulis

HISTORICAL PERSPECTIVE

Radiology has undergone tremendous changes in the post–World War II decades. Progress in technological developments related to medical imaging has been continuously accelerating, making diagnostic radiology one of the most exciting areas of diagnostic medicine during the last few years. Diagnostic imaging has been and continues to be the direct beneficiary of some of the areas of technology that are most heavily subsidized by governments and industry. Space exploration provided miniaturization of imaging equipment components. Extremely high resolution television techniques used for space exploration and photographing of the earth's surface and advances in computers and techniques of storage of information have contributed to the development of digital radiography, highly advanced x-ray CT machines, positron emission tomography, and magnetic resonance imaging. These modalities, although expensive, are eventually cost effective because they significantly reduce invasiveness and permit the performance of many procedures on an outpatient basis. Because of this they have found ready acceptance and have rapidly proliferated, not only in the United States, but throughout the western world and Japan.

PRESENT STATUS OF RADIOLOGIC IMAGING

Conventional Radiography

The term "conventional radiography" is a misnomer today. Equipment that was considered advanced in the early 1970's is today hopelessly obsolete. Although there have been no breakthroughs in x-ray tube design, the generators and controls have become computerized; the television cameras are smaller and more reliable; and the equipment as a whole has grown more functional and often multipurpose. The highly specialized, extremely expensive rooms used in the past for angiography only are changing, particularly in small hospitals, into rooms that can be used for many different procedures, including digital subtraction fluoroscopy (Fig. 21–1). Even conventional darkrooms are being replaced by daylight developing facilities, which save space, time, and personnel. These trends of saving space, time, and personnel will become even more evident in the future as departments of radiology will have to become smaller and more intensively active and will have to serve inpatients and outpatients with the same equipment over longer hours each day.

As computers improve and the capacity to store data increases, the present halide film will be replaced by laser discs or other similar devices that will significantly reduce the size of filing areas and permit rapid and reliable access to images projected on television monitors. Hard copies will be instantly available in multiple formats similar to x-ray computed tomography.

As videotaping improves and better resolution is obtained, fluoroscopic information will be recorded on tape and diagnostic frames will be recorded on multiformatted hard copy as the only record. This will result in reduced radiation exposure and eventually in cost saving.

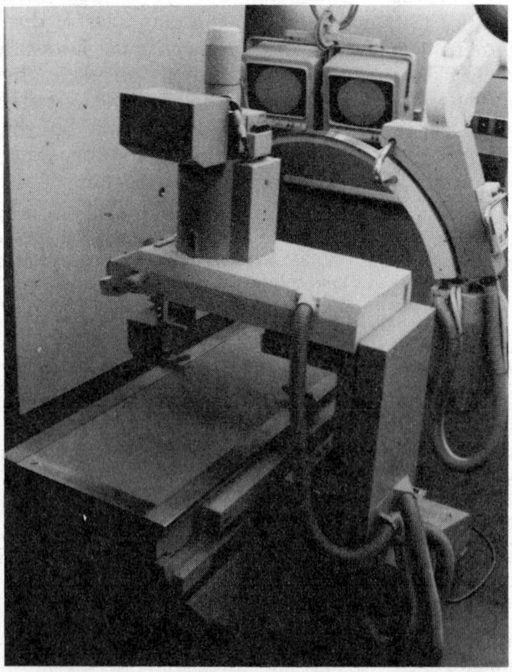

Figure 21–1. Photograph of a bi-plane fluoroscopic and radiographic multipurpose room with digital fluoroscopy. Multiple types of procedures are performed in this room: interventional, angiography, biliary procedures (including gallstone removal), gastrointestinal examinations, myelography, etc. Machines of this type, although expensive, are cost efficient because they are in constant use.

Digital Radiography and Fluoroscopy

Digital subtraction fluoroscopy did not fulfill all the expectations that greeted it when it was introduced at the end of the 1970's. It was expected then that all arteriography would be performed intravenously, noninvasively, with images showing excellent detail. This has not occurred, and angiography still requires that large amounts of iodine-containing contrast media be injected intravenously through catheters advanced into large veins. Even then, owing to breathing or involuntary motion, blurring detracts from the quality of the images. At this time intra-arterial injections of small amounts of contrast medium appear to be the best method for performing digital subtraction angiography (Fig. 21–2). Further improvements in digital subtraction fluoroscopy will probably occur, and eventually it can be expected that most arteriography will be performed with some modification of digital radiography. This is also being facilitated by the continual decrease in price of the equipment.

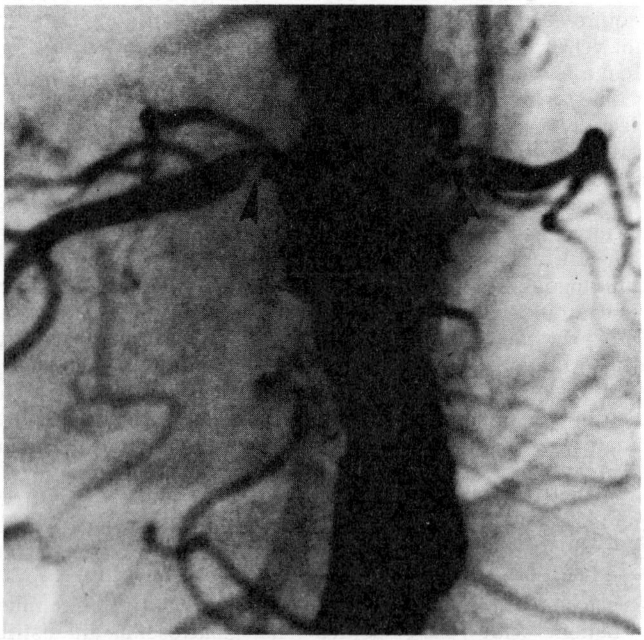

Figure 21–2. Intra-arterial digital subtraction aortogram showing bilateral renal artery stenoses (arrowheads).

Computed Tomography

Computed tomography has become an indispensable diagnostic tool in a modern hospital as well as in sophisticated outpatient centers throughout the United States, Canada, most of Western Europe, and particularly Japan. For the last five years there has been a steady improvement in the quality of images. The speed of scanning, which indirectly also results in better spatial resolution, has come down to one second for conventional CT scanners and is in the 50 msec range for the cine CT scanner, an advanced scanner with no moving parts. Computed tomography is today considered indispensable for the examination of the brain (Fig. 21–3), spine, mediastinum, and chest, as well as the abdomen. It is a tomographic examination in the axial plane, but it also allows redisplay of images in any plane (Fig. 21–4). CT numbers accurately reflect the average density of small tissue volume elements and can be used to identify various tissues, fluids, and lesions. Computed tomography is of great advantage in showing tumors, abscesses, ruptures of organs, and accumulation of fluid, with considerably higher accuracy than any other method up to the introduction of magnetic resonance imaging.

Ultrasonography

Diagnostic ultrasonography uses a pulse echo device to record reflected waves of a sound beam in two dimensions. The resolution of sonographic images is inferior to the image obtained from computed tomography or magnetic resonance. The great advantages of this modality, however, are (1) it is relatively inexpensive, (2) it is rapid, (3) it can produce images in real time, (4) it can obtain images in any plane without revision of format, (5) because of its speed it is ideal for directing certain interventional procedures, (6) no biologic hazards have been demonstrated within the diagnostic range. It does not depend on ionizing radiation. The disadvantages of the method are that (1) it is highly dependent on operator skill, (2) its spatial resolution and resolving power lag behind those of computed tomography and magnetic resonance imaging, and (3) no good contrast media are available at present. In the diagnostic range, ultrasound is of no use in examining the lungs, the brain through the intact skull of an adult, the spine, or areas where there is a great deal of gas. Ultrasound images, however, exceed the quality of CT in asthenic or cachectic individuals. It is currently the method of choice in examining the female pelvis, particularly in obstetrics. An entire field of intrauterine diagnosis of fetal abnormalities by ultrasound has developed, leading also to surgical intrauterine interventions, again guided by ultrasound (Fig. 21–5). Ultrasonography is also of great use in diagnosis of abnormalities of the neonatal brain through the intact skull and in the intraoperative diagnosis of brain abnormalities through open skull flaps.

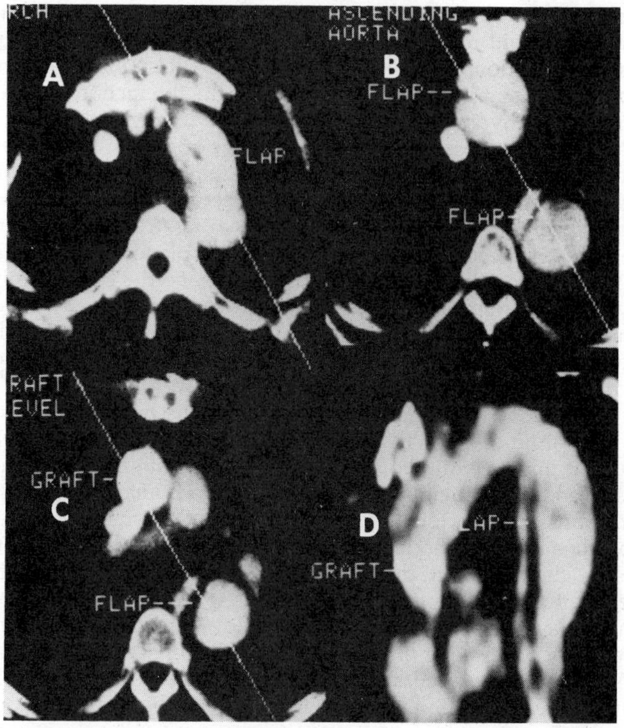

Figure 21–4. Dissecting aneurysm of the descending thoracic aorta demonstrated with exquisite detail on a dynamic computed tomography reformatted along a plane shown by the dotted line on three axial tomograms at different levels and demonstrated in this illustration under A, B, and C. The flap is seen as a vertical dark line on the reformatted image (D). The Teflon graft was introduced a short time before this examination.

Nuclear Magnetic Resonance

Nuclear magnetic resonance is a new imaging modality that has been derived from chemical magnetic resonance. For im-

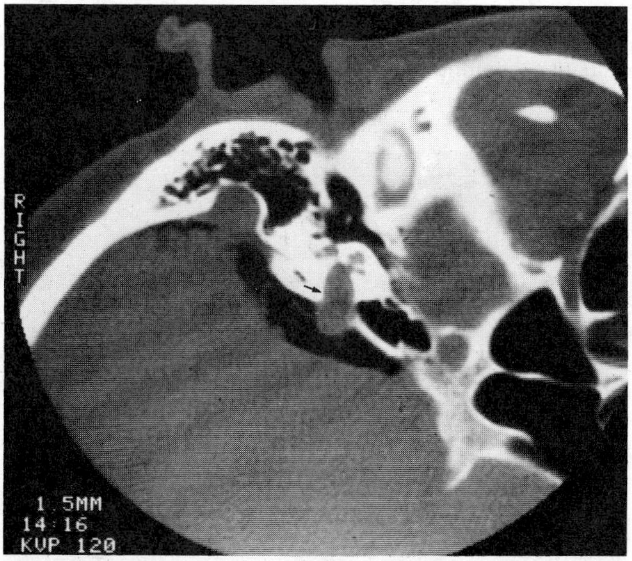

Figure 21–3. High resolution axial view computed tomogram showing an acoustic neuroma widening the internal acoustic meatus. The lesion itself (arrow) is seen with outstanding detail.

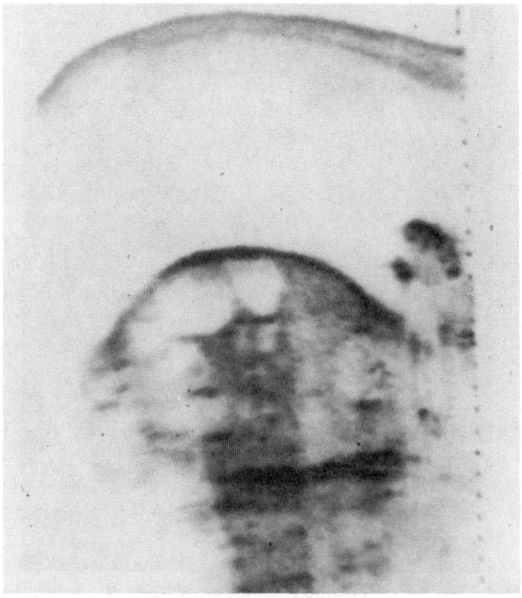

Figure 21–5. Multiple dilated loops of small bowel are demonstrated by ultrasound in this fetus with jejunal atresia.

aging, hydrogen protons give the best images. The strength of the signal will indicate the amount of hydrogen modified by tissue relaxation parameters, T1 and T2. T1, also known as the spin lattice parameter, is dependent on the interaction of other nuclei with hydrogen. T2 depends on the influence of protons on each other. It is also referred to as the spin-spin parameter. The intensity of the signal is also affected by the proton bulk motion effect, which results from the fact that it takes approximately 50 msec for the signal emanating from protons to register. If the protons move through the plane of imaging at a faster rate, the signal will not be recorded. This permits evaluation of speed of flow through blood vessels and visualization of patent blood vessels without contrast media. In addition, the image on NMR is influenced by the technique of acquisition of data. These techniques are so numerous that it is possible to individualize them for given tissue abnormalities and anatomic areas. By applying the right sequence, a great deal of information about the nature of normal and abnormal tissues can be obtained. Magnetic resonance imaging has several further characteristics that are advantages when compared to other imaging modalities. Besides giving information about tissue chemistry and metabolic and biochemical data, magnetic resonance imaging offers superb resolving power. Furthermore, magnetic resonance imaging can provide tomographic sections in any desired plane. By exciting section after section while the remagnetization occurs in the original section, as many as 20 simultaneous sections can be obtained in the time that one section is scanned.

Magnetic resonance imaging is already superior to any other imaging modality in the examination of the brain (Figs. 21–6 and 21–7), spinal cord, cancellous bone, and the male and female pelvic organs (Figs. 21–8 and 21–9). With respiratory and ECG gating, it is providing diagnostic images of the heart (Fig. 21–10) and mediastinum of quality unsurpassed by other modalities. It promises to be as valuable in the examination of the liver and spleen. It already exceeds other techniques in the examination of the kidneys, female breast, and pancreas. Magnetic resonance imaging is of no value in the examination of the bony cortex and does not show calcifications. Further drawbacks are relatively slow scanning (in minutes), the expense of the equipment and siting, the large amounts of space necessary for the facility, and the danger of loose metallic objects flying into the machine. Other disadvantages are the inability to examine patients with pacemakers, large metallic prostheses, prosthetic heart valves made with magnetic materials, or freshly introduced vascular magnetic clips or to study patients who are in need of continuous observation and require life-support systems. Nevertheless, magnetic resonance imaging has so many advantages that most large medical centers will soon have magnetic resonance imagers in addition to their computed tomographic units. If only one can be operated it must be an x-ray computed tomographic unit.

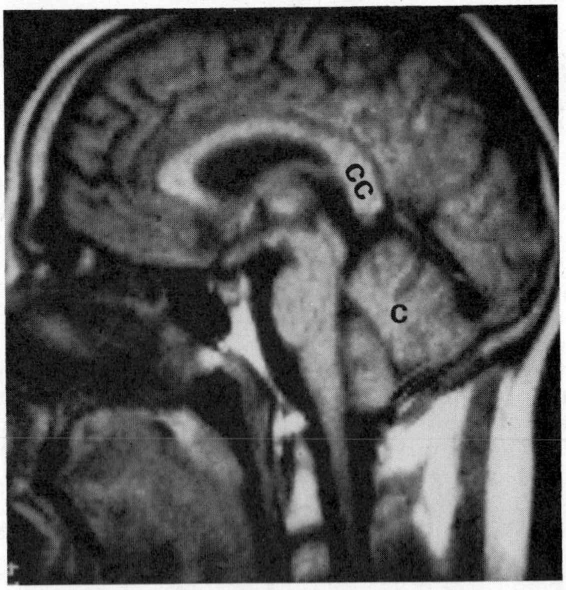

Figure 21–7. Sagittal section through the brain with excellent detail showing all the structures through the mid-section. Notice the beautiful demonstration of the gyri, corpus callosum (cc) and cerebellum (c).

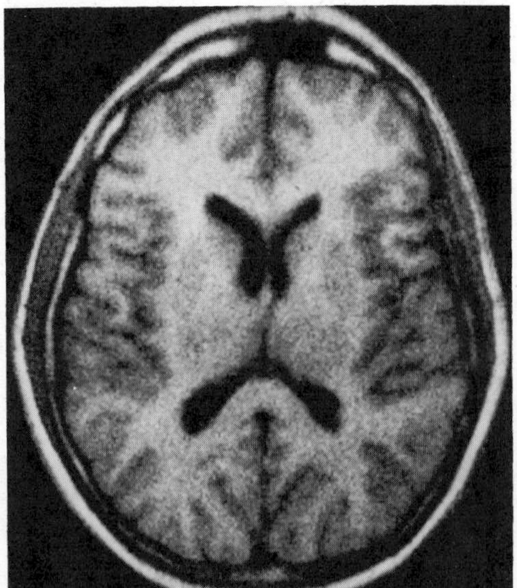

Figure 21–6. Axial section through the normal brain with NMR. Notice the excellent demonstration of the ventricles and gray and white matter.

The Algorithmic Approach

With so many different radiologic modalities, the physician is often in a dilemma as to which examination is indicated and, if several are to be requested, in what order they should be performed. The algorithmic approach offers a logical sequence in which one examination follows the previous one, depending on its results, in order to provide a definitive diagnosis. This approach relies very much on the equipment available as well as on the skills of the operators. It is often linked with local experience and sometimes is tinged with prejudice. The best approach for selecting the proper procedures results from a continuing dialogue between the clinician and radiologist where the two familiarize each other with the newest developments and experiences. A typical example of an algorithm is in the evaluation of jaundice (Ch. 119). When chemical tests indicate

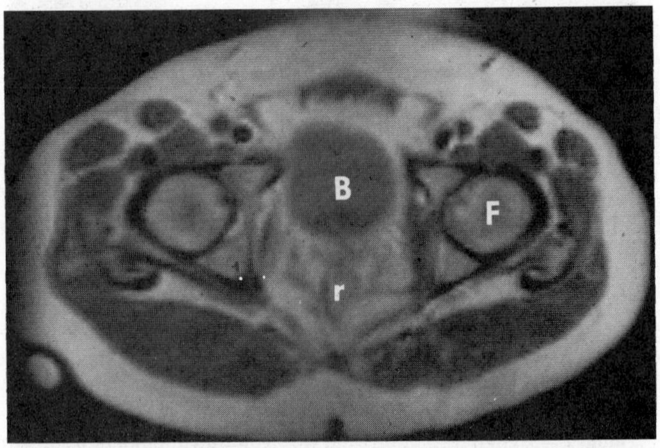

Figure 21–8. Axial NMR section through the pelvis of a male. B, Urinary bladder; r, rectum; F, femoral head.

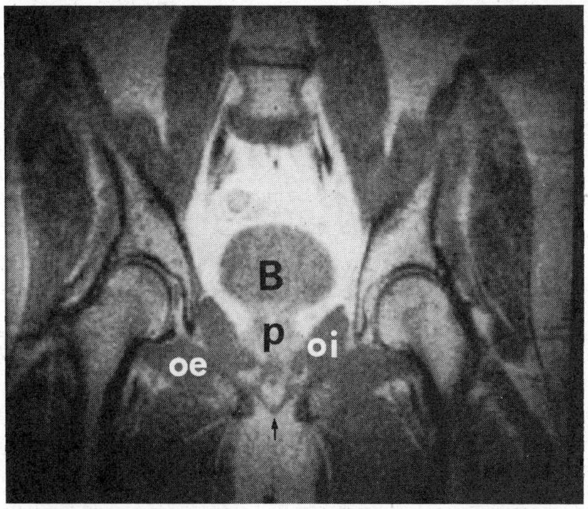

Figure 21–9. Coronal section through the pelvis of the male demonstrated in Figure 21–8. B, Bladder; P, prostate; oi, obturator internus muscle; oe, obturator externus muscle; arrow, bulbus spongiosus.

that the jaundice is most likely due to obstruction, the next procedure is ultrasonography (if that capability exists locally) to determine the width of the biliary tree. If the ducts are dilated, and depending on whether the history suggests tumor or stone, either endoscopic retrograde cholangiography (ERC) or percutaneous transhepatic cholangiography is performed. If a stone is found to be obstructing, sphincterotomy is performed by ERC, and if a tumor is seen, percutaneous transhepatic cholangiography is performed (Fig. 21–11) with drainage through a stent. Computed tomography is then done for staging of the tumor in order to determine whether surgery is indicated and if so whether it is likely to be curative or palliative. For curative surgery, decompression is often valuable. For palliation, an internal stent introduced percutaneously may be all that is necessary. Magnetic resonance imaging has greatly changed many of the previous algorithms as the method is used with increasing frequency in centers that possess such imagers.

Financial Considerations

The cost of radiologic equipment has soared; in most hospitals modern imaging equipment has overwhelmed equipment budgets. The sophistication and expense of the equipment necessitate an organized referral system to prevent duplication

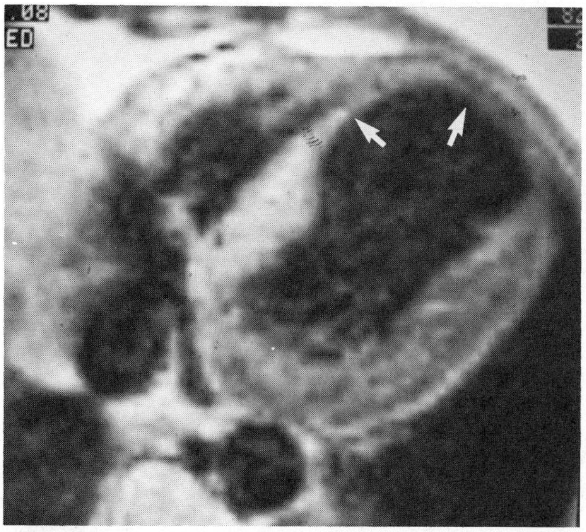

Figure 21–10. Gated (ECG) magnetic resonance image at a transverse level through the left ventricle sharply displays the myocardial walls. In this patient with a prior anteroseptal myocardial infarction, the image shows severe thinning of the anterior septum and anterior wall of the left ventricle (arrows).

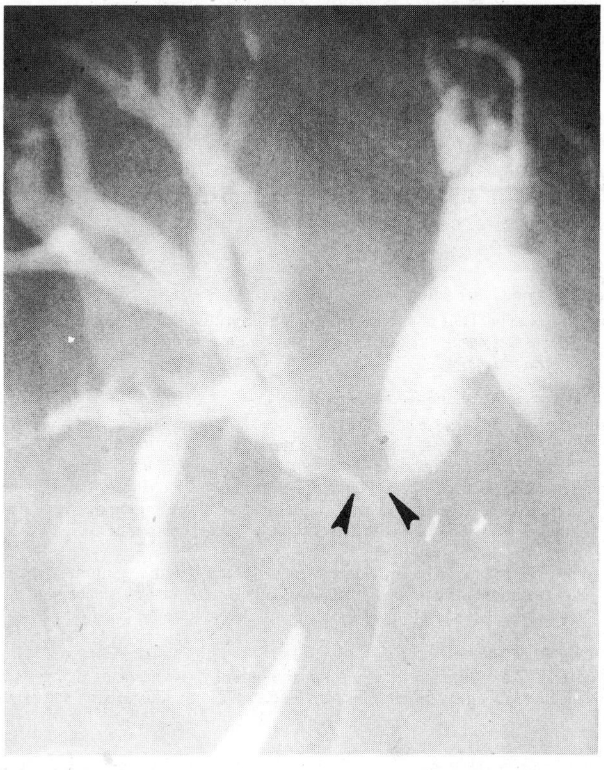

Figure 21–11. Percutaneous transhepatic cholangiogram demonstrates high-grade obstructing lesion of the proximal common hepatic duct involving the ductal bifurcation (arrowheads). Biopsy demonstrated cholangiocarcinoma.

of equipment and to allow utilization of imaging systems to their best advantage. Noninvasive imaging procedures can result in shorter hospital stays, in avoidance of hospitalization altogether, and in almost complete elimination of exploratory surgery. When surgery is necessary, precise preoperative diagnosis shortens the procedure and reduces the number of complications. Properly utilized and properly distributed imaging systems can enhance outpatient diagnostic capabilities, thus shortening hospital stays and greatly reducing the number of acute hospitals needed. The elimination of hospital beds resulting from this technology should eventually lead to enormous cost savings.

FUTURE DEVELOPMENTS IN IMAGING

With the continuous advances in the development of computers and television systems, combining increased versatility and decreased cost, diagnostic imaging can expect to make progress in several new directions. It can be expected that the departments of radiology of the future will become totally computerized, integrating into the hospital's general computer system. This means that images themselves as well as reports will be instantly available on television monitors on wards along with laboratory information and information from medical records and pathology. These systems will be expensive but at the same time will be cost effective, saving on personnel, communication, and duration of hospital stay of the patient. Computers will also help to store data correlating clinical information and allowing the most efficient and most rational algorithmic approaches for reaching the correct diagnosis. Computers will therefore help physicians, surgeons, and radiologists to reach the correct, least invasive, and most time-saving sequence of diagnostic studies. Similarly, artificial intelligence based on clinical experience and previous imaging results will also help select the proper techniques, sequences, and planes of imaging for nuclear magnetic resonance. This again will result not only in improving clinical results but also in making the use of equipment more cost effective and less traumatic for patients.

These remarkable advances in imaging will increasingly attract the interest and collaboration of other physicians (such as internists, neurologists, ophthalmologists, obstetricians, neurosurgeons, and surgeons) with the radiologist in the field of diagnostic imaging in order to optimize progress through the exchange of experience and ideas.

Historical and General References

Grigg ERN: The Trail of the Invisible Light. Springfield, IL, Charles C Thomas, 1965. *An extensive, well-illustrated review of the development of roentgenology from its earliest days.*

Digital Radiography and Fluoroscopy

Crummy AB, Stieghorst MF, Turski PA, et al.: Digital subtraction angiography: Current status and use of intra-arterial injection. Radiology 145:303–307, 1982. *An objective review of the current status of digital angiography.*

Enzmann DR, Djang WT, Riederer SJ, et al.: Low-dose, high-frame-rate versus regular-dose, low-frame-rate digital subtraction angiography. Radiology 146:669–676, 1983. *A clever technical review of two approaches to digital angiography.*

Riederer SJ, Kruger RA: Intravenous digital subtraction: A summary of recent developments. Radiology 147:633–638, 1983. *An extensive summary of multiple approaches with the advantages and disadvantages of each.*

Computed Tomography

Boyd DP: Computerized-transmission tomography of the heart using scanning electron beams. *In* Higgins CA (ed.): CTT of the Heart: Experimental Evaluation and Clinical Application. Mt. Kisco, NY, Futura Publishing Co., 1983. *The author describes an original approach to the generation of scanning an x-ray beam that permits the achievement of cine computed tomography.*

Lee JKT, Sagel SS, Stanley RJ (eds.): Computed Body Tomography. New York, Raven Press, 1982. *A well-illustrated, modern, complete textbook on computed tomography of the body. Particularly good sections on kidney and liver.*

Moss AA, Gamsu G, Genant HK (eds.): Computed Tomography of the Body. Philadelphia, W. B. Saunders Co., 1983. *A large, complete, up-to-date textbook. Particularly good sections on the mediastinum, the digestive tract, and the spine.*

Ultrasonography

Callen PW (ed.): Ultrasonography in Obstetrics and Gynecology. Philadelphia, W. B. Saunders Company, 1983. *A well-illustrated and organized textbook on modern ultrasound applications in the field of obstetrics and gynecology.*

Sarti DA, Sample WF (eds.): Diagnostic Ultrasound. Text and Cases. Boston, G. K. Hall & Co., 1980. *Still the best illustrated book on ultrasonography, with exquisite illustrations.*

Nuclear Magnetic Resonance

Kaufman L, Crooks LE, Margulis AR (eds.): Nuclear Magnetic Resonance in Medicine. New York, Igaku-Shoin, 1981. *A straight, basic approach to the field.*

Margulis AR, Higgins CB, Kaufman L, Crooks LE (eds.): Clinical Magnetic Resonance Imaging. San Francisco, Radiology Research and Education Foundation, 1983. *An illustrated book covering the physics background and clinical applications of magnetic resonance imaging.*

Pykett IL: NMR imaging in medicine. Sci Am 246:78, 1982. *An imaginative, clear, and well-illustrated explanation of the physics and techniques of NMR.*

Economic Data and Benefits

Margulis AR: The Whitehouse lecture: Radiologic imaging: Changing costs, greater benefits. Am J Roentgenol 136:657–665, 1981. *A review of the advantages of modern diagnostic imaging and the need for selectivity in diagnostic approaches.*

Newton DR, Witz S, Norman D, Newton TH: Economic impact of CT scanning on the evaluation of pituitary adenomas. Am J Neurol Radiol 4:57–60, 1983. *A carefully designed study showing the economic benefits of computed tomography in one selected condition where controls were available.*

Part V
PRINCIPLES OF THERAPEUTICS

22. PRINCIPLES OF DRUG THERAPY

Alan S. Nies

Because all patients respond differently to drugs, individualization of drug dosages is required so that therapy will be effective and nontoxic. A basic tenet of clinical pharmacology is that a closer relationship exists between the concentration of drug in the blood and the drug's effect than between drug dose and effect. The relationship between drug concentration and effect has fostered the study of the factors influencing drug movement in the body, a science called pharmacokinetics (Fig. 22–1). Rational drug therapy requires a basic understanding of pharmacokinetic principles that can be applied to patient care. In this way the amount of drug delivered to the target tissue can be controlled within a definable and safe range.

ABSORPTION. When a dose of drug is administered it must first be absorbed into the systemic circulation to produce its effects. The simplest case is that of the drug's being given intravenously, in which absorption is obviously complete and immediate. For all other routes of administration, there will be a delay in drug reaching the circulation and the absorption may be incomplete. Drug absorption is the only part of the pharmacokinetic process directly under the control of the physician and the pharmaceutical industry. Most drugs are absorbed by passive diffusion into the circulation from their site of administration. Since the process of diffusion is dependent upon the concentration of drug in the solution contacting the absorbing surface, the rate of absorption can be influenced by affecting the rate of dissolution of the dosage form. Thus depot intramuscular preparations are available for some drugs (e.g., penicillin, progesterone) that slowly release the active drug into tissue fluids, from which it can be absorbed into the circulation. In this way, drug levels in the blood can be maintained by a continuous absorption process for many hours or many days even though the drug is rapidly eliminated from the body. A similar technique can be used for oral drug administration. Long-acting oral preparations can be formulated for drugs with rapid elimination by producing a dosage form that slowly releases the active drug from a matrix. The duration of sustained absorption from an oral preparation, however, is limited by the gastrointestinal transit time. Drugs that are slowly dissolved and slowly absorbed may be affected by alterations in gut transit time more so than drugs that are rapidly and completely absorbed. An increase in gut motility will lead to a decrease in the extent of absorption of slowly absorbed drugs (such as digoxin), whereas a decrease in motility may actually increase the extent of absorption.

Depending on the drug, absorption can occur from sites other than the gastrointestinal tract, subcutaneous tissue, or muscle. Some lipid-soluble drugs can be absorbed from the skin or through the oral or bronchial mucous membranes. Nitroglycerin can be absorbed both percutaneously and sublingually and illustrates the potential utility of these routes of administration. When given sublingually, nitroglycerin is rapidly absorbed into the systemic circulation and produces a transient effect. When applied to the skin, nitroglycerin has a slow but sustained absorption into the systemic circulation and can produce effects lasting several hours for the ointment or 24 hours with a sustained release patch. The transdermal route of drug administration also can be used for scopolamine and clonidine. However, most drugs cannot be absorbed well from the skin or oral mucous membrane because of the limited surface utilized for absorption and the solubility characteristics of the drug. Occasionally, percutaneous absorption is an unwanted side effect of drugs (e.g., steroids) applied to the skin to produce topical effects.

The sublingual, transbronchial, and percutaneous routes of absorption have the advantage of delivering the drug directly into the systemic circulation as do the standard parenteral methods of drug administration. In contrast, when absorbed by the intestine, the drug enters the portal circulation and is presented to the liver, where a portion of the absorbed drug can be eliminated before reaching the systemic circulation (Fig. 22–1). Thus, nitroglycerin can be absorbed readily from the intestine but is rapidly destroyed by the liver so that only a fraction of the orally administered dose escapes metabolism and reaches the circulation. For this reason, the oral dose of nitroglycerin must be much larger than the sublingual dose required for a given effect. A similar situation exists for propranolol, in which over half of an orally administered dose is removed by the liver prior to reaching the systemic circulation. Hepatic removal during absorption of the drug from the gut is called "first pass" or "presystemic" elimination and, along with poor absorption from the intestine, accounts for the need to give larger oral doses than parenteral doses of some drugs to achieve equivalent pharmacologic effects. "Oral bioavailability"

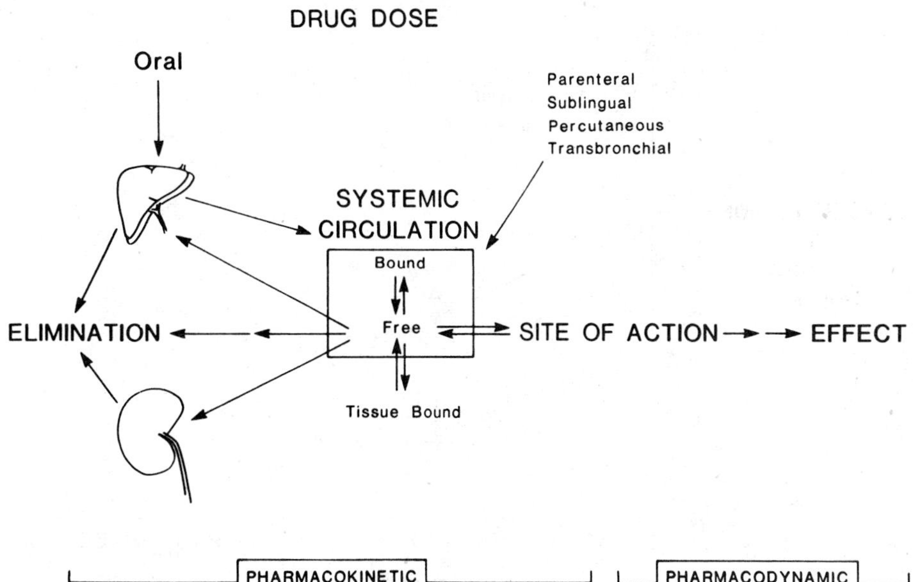

Figure 22–1. Drug movement in the body. The variation in effects following a given dose is related to pharmacokinetic and pharmacodynamic factors.

is the quantitative expression relating the amount of drug reaching the systemic circulation after oral administration to the amount after intravenous administration. Bioavailability, therefore, is reduced not only by poor absorption but also by the hepatic presystemic elimination. For some drugs, such as lidocaine and morphine, the oral bioavailability is sufficiently low to preclude oral administration. For all calculations utilizing the oral dosage, the dosage must be corrected for less than complete bioavailability.

DISTRIBUTION. Once absorbed into the systemic circulation, the drug must distribute throughout the body. If the drug is rapidly administered intravenously, it is first delivered to the well perfused tissues and only more slowly distributed to less well perfused tissues. By measuring drug concentrations in plasma at various times after a drug is administered, a curve can be described from which distribution and elimination can be quantitated. For example, if 100 mg of lidocaine is given as an intravenous bolus to an adult, the curve in Figure 22–2 results. This curve of lidocaine concentration versus time can be separated into an early distribution phase during which the drug rapidly disappears from the circulation and a later elimination phase during which the drug in the blood is in equilibrium with drug in the tissues and is more gradually eliminated from the body (Fig. 22–2). The effects of most drugs are related to the plasma concentration during the elimination phase. However, whether the plasma concentration of the drug during the distribution phase is predictive of drug effects depends on the particular drug. For a drug such as lidocaine that quickly reaches its sites of action, the initial concentrations shortly after a bolus of drug can produce therapeutic antiarrhythmic effects and toxic effects on the heart or brain. On the other hand, digoxin is an example of a drug that requires time to equilibrate or be transported to its receptors. When given intravenously, digoxin does not produce maximal effects for four hours, during which time the blood levels are falling as the drug equilibrates with tissues. After the equilibration period of four hours, digoxin concentrations fall more slowly, and only then does the digoxin concentration correlate with the drug's effects.

Apparent Volume of Distribution. The relationship between the amount of drug in the body and the concentration of drug in the plasma is defined as the "apparent volume of distribution" (V_D) of the drug:

$$V_D = \frac{\text{amount of drug in the body}}{\text{concentration of drug in plasma}}$$

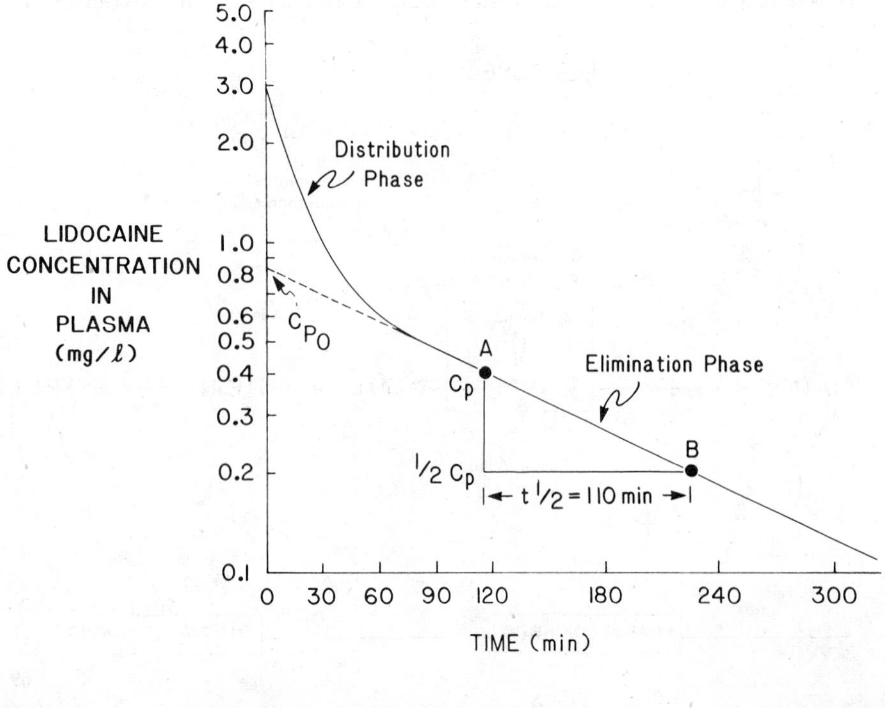

Figure 22–2. Lidocaine concentrations on a log scale plotted against time in minutes following a 100 mg bolus given intravenously to a 70 kg person. The C_{P_0} is the concentration of lidocaine in plasma that would be achieved if the dose was distributed instantaneously to the tissues. C_p at point A is twice the concentration of lidocaine at point B. The time between point A and point B is the half-life (t½).

The V_D is the "apparent" volume needed to contain the entire amount of drug if the drug were everywhere at the same concentration as in the plasma, and it must be determined empirically for each drug. The apparent volume of distribution of a drug during the elimination phase can be determined from a graph of the plasma drug concentration versus time by extrapolating the elimination phase back to zero time giving the C_{P_0} (plasma concentration at time 0), an estimate of the concentration of drug in the plasma that would have been achieved by the intravenous dose of drug if the drug had been distributed throughout the tissues instantaneously. Thus:

$$V_D = \frac{\text{IV dose}}{C_{P_0}}$$

In Figure 22–2, the C_{P_0} for lidocaine is 0.84 mg per liter following a 100 mg dose. The V_D for lidocaine, therefore, is 100 mg ÷ 0.84 mg per liter = 119 liters. The V_D for several drugs are shown in Tables 22–1 and 22–2.

The apparent volume of distribution frequently does not correspond to any given body fluid compartment. For many drugs the V_D is larger than the entire body. For example, digoxin has a V_D of 7 liters per kilogram or about 500 liters in a 70-kg person. When a 0.5 mg dose of digoxin is administered intravenously, it distributes in this "apparent volume" of 500 liters to give a plasma concentration of 1 μg per liter or 1 ng

TABLE 22–1. PHARMACOKINETIC PARAMETERS FOR SOME COMMONLY USED DRUGS

	Cl_r* (ml/min)	Cl_{nr}† (ml/min)	%‡ Nonrenal	V_D (L/kg)	t½ (hours)
Aminoglycosides	70	3	5	0.3	2–3
Carbenicillin	90	8	10	0.13	1
Digitoxin	0	3	100	0.6	165
Digoxin§	110	40	30	7	36
Disopyramide	60	40	40	0.8	6
Lidocaine	60	800	95	1.7	1.7
Lithium	30	0	0	0.6	15
Penicillin G	350	35	10	0.2	0.5
Phenobarbital	1.5	4	70	0.6	86
Procainamide	330	120	30	1.6	3
Quinidine	100	200	65	2.5	7
Theophylline¶	0	55	100	0.5	7

*Cl_r = renal clearance for an adult with normal renal function.
†Cl_{nr} = nonrenal clearance for an adult.
‡Per cent nonrenal is the nonrenal clearance as a percentage of the total clearance.
§The oral bioavailability of digoxin is 65 per cent.
¶Aminophylline is 85 per cent theophylline.

TABLE 22–2. DRUGS SHOWING DOSE-DEPENDENT KINETICS

	Maximal Metabolic Rate	Volume of Distribution
Aspirin	4000 mg/day	0.2–0.6 L/kg*
Ethanol	8000 mg/hour	0.6 L/kg
Phenytoin†	700 mg/day‡	0.6 L/kg

*The volume of distribution of aspirin increases with increasing dose.
†The oral bioavailability of phenytoin is 80 per cent.
‡Some individuals have a lower maximal metabolic rate.

per milliliter. A large apparent volume of distribution is merely an expression of the fact that most of the drug in the body is not in the plasma but is bound to the tissues at a greater concentration than in the plasma. For phenytoin and ethanol the V_D is 0.6 liter per kilogram. Although this figure approximates the value for total body water, it need not be the case that these drugs are distributed only in body water. The V_D is an empirically determined constant that allows one to relate the plasma concentration to the amount of drug in the body and should not be given a physiologic interpretation relating to real body volumes.

LOADING DOSES. One use of the apparent volume of distribution is to calculate the loading dose required to achieve a desired plasma drug concentration. From Figure 22–2 the apparent volume of distribution of lidocaine is 119 liters in a 70-kg person or 1.7 liters per kilogram. In order to rapidly establish a therapeutic plasma lidocaine concentration of 2 mg per liter, a loading dose of 238 mg (desired concentration × V_D) must be given. However, because lidocaine can produce toxic effects during the distribution phase, the entire loading dose cannot be given in a single bolus; to do so would produce lidocaine concentrations during the distribution phase that would exceed the therapeutic levels, potentially resulting in toxicity. The initial high concentrations after a loading dose can be avoided by giving the desired amount of drug in divided doses or as an infusion rather than a bolus. By giving the loading dose more gradually, the clinician can achieve plasma levels of lidocaine that do not exceed the therapeutic range. In addition, the loading of drug into the body can be stopped if early signs of drug toxicity occur. If the drug can be given orally, a loading dose may be given that could cause toxicity if given intravenously. Because of the gradual absorption from the intestine, the drug has time to distribute to the tissues during the absorption process and the very high peak drug concentrations that result from an intravenous bolus do not occur. As an example, the V_D of phenytoin is 0.6 liter per kilogram or 40 liters in a 70-kg adult. To achieve a low therapeutic plasma concentration of 10 mg per liter requires a loading dose of 400 mg. Since phenytoin has an oral bioavailability of 80 to 85 per cent, an oral loading dose of 500 mg will deliver 400 mg to the systemic circulation. The 500 mg of phenytoin can be given safely as a single oral dose even though the 400 mg loading dose given as a bolus intravenously could cause a cardiac arrest. If a patient has an inadequate plasma level, a loading dose can be used to achieve a therapeutic level rapidly. A patient with a phenytoin level of 5 mg per liter can be given a 400 mg phenytoin load (or 500 mg orally) to increase his level by 10 mg per liter to 15 mg per liter.

The estimates of all pharmacokinetic parameters, including the apparent volume of distribution, are derived from an "average" patient and are therefore only first approximations of the doses required in an individual patient. Clinical observations and, in some cases, measured plasma drug concentrations give information to the clinician for proper dosage adjustments.

ELIMINATION. *Drug Clearance.* Once in the circulation, drugs are eliminated from the body by two major processes: hepatic metabolism–biliary excretion and renal filtration–secretion into the urine. With a few important exceptions, the rates of hepatic and renal elimination are directly proportional to the concentration of the drug in the plasma, a process mathematically described as "first order." The pharmacokinetic parameter best describing the efficiency of the elimination processes is drug clearance. Drug clearance is defined as the volume of a fluid (usually plasma or blood) from which all drug is removed per unit of time. Clearance is a familiar term to clinicians discussing renal function. Thus creatinine clearance is the volume of plasma that is completely cleared of creatinine per minute and can be directly determined by relating the rate of creatinine excretion into the urine to the plasma creatinine concentration. Renal drug clearances can be determined in the same way by dividing renal excretory rate of the drug by the plasma drug concentration. Hepatic drug clearance is, by analogy to renal clearance, the volume of blood or plasma entirely cleared of drug by the liver and is therefore the rate of removal of drug by the liver divided by the concentration of drug in blood or plasma. Total body drug clearance (Cl) is the sum of all the individual organ clearances, which consists of renal (Cl_r) and nonrenal (Cl_{nr}) clearances. Total drug clearance is the rate of drug elimination by all processes ($\dot{R}$) divided by the plasma concentration (C_p):

$$Cl = \frac{\dot{R}}{C_p}$$

The clearance of drug by the liver and kidney can be influenced by the blood flow to the clearing organ, the binding of drug to the plasma proteins, and the activity of the processes responsible for drug removal such as hepatic enzyme activity, glomerular filtration rate, and renal secretory processes. In physiologic terms, drug clearance by an organ is the product of organ blood flow ($\dot{Q}$) and the fraction of the drug in the blood extracted on a single passage through the organ (E): $Cl = \dot{Q}E$. The extraction ratio, E, is calculated by dividing the arteriovenous difference in drug concentration ($C_a - C_v$) by the arterial drug concentration (C_a):

$$E = \frac{C_a - C_v}{C_a}$$

Clearance is *independent* of the distribution of drugs in the body (i.e., the V_D), since the eliminating organs "see" and can remove only the drug present in the blood.

Drug Half-Life. Both the clearance and the distribution of drug in the body influence the amount of time necessary to eliminate drug from the body. The proportion of the apparent volume of distribution cleared of drug per unit of time is a constant called the "first order elimination rate constant" or k_e:

$$k_e = \frac{Cl}{V_D}$$

This constant describes the exponential disappearance of drug from the plasma with time during the elimination phase. When plotted on semi-log graph paper, as in Figure 22–2, the exponential elimination phase is a straight line with a slope of k_e. A conceptually more useful term describing the time required to eliminate drug is the drug's elimination half-life ($t\frac{1}{2}$), which is the time required to reduce the plasma concentration of drug (and hence the body load of drug) to half the initial concentration. For drugs with first order elimination, the $t\frac{1}{2}$ is independent of drug concentration. The $t\frac{1}{2}$ is frequently determined graphically as in Figure 22–2, and mathematically the half-life is the natural logarithm of 2 (indicating a reduction of drug concentration by half) divided by the elimination rate constant: $t\frac{1}{2} = \ln 2/k_e = 0.693/k_e$. Since the elimination rate constant is related to both clearance and volume of distribution as independent variables, it can be appreciated that half-life must also be related to these two variables:

$$t\tfrac{1}{2} = \frac{0.693\ V_D}{Cl}$$

As the apparent volume of distribution increases, the half-life is prolonged for any given drug clearance, since a greater "volume" must be cleared of drug; as clearance increases, half-life shortens for any given V_D. A change in half-life frequently is used as an index of a change in efficiency of drug elimination, but this is true only when the apparent volume of distribution is unchanged. Hepatic, renal, and cardiovascular disease not only can decrease drug clearance but also can alter the apparent volume of distribution. Half-life, being affected by both V_D and Cl, may be affected to a greater or lesser extent than drug clearance, and therefore t½ may not indicate the degree of abnormality in drug elimination. For example, patients with congestive heart failure have a 50 per cent reduction in the clearance of lidocaine and may, in addition, have a similarly contracted volume of distribution of the drug. Since both Cl and V_D can be reduced by a similar magnitude, the half-life may be unchanged and not give any clue to the abnormal lidocaine elimination and the need for reduced infusion rates to avoid toxicity.

For exponential or first order drug elimination, an infinite time is required to eliminate drug entirely from the body. Only half the drug is eliminated in the first half-life, half the remaining drug eliminated in the second half-life, and so forth. Thus, by starting with an effective blood level, which we shall call 100 per cent, 50 per cent will be present after one half-life, 25 per cent after two half-lives, 12.5 per cent after three half-lives, 6.25 per cent after four half-lives, and 3.125 per cent after five half-lives, as shown in Figure 22–3 for lidocaine. For practical purposes, most drugs can be considered to be eliminated completely when less than 10 per cent of the effective concentration remains in the body, requiring three to four half-lives. For lidocaine (Fig. 22–3) this time is about six hours.

DRUG ACCUMULATION. When drug is given as a sustained infusion or in repeated doses, drug accumulates in the body until a steady state is achieved at which time the amount of drug being administered is equal to the amount of drug eliminated so that body stores and plasma levels remain constant. The time course of drug accumulation, like the time course of elimination, is determined by the drug's elimination half-life, these processes being mirror images of each other (Fig. 22–3). Thus, accumulation to half the ultimate steady state occurs in one half-life, 75 per cent in two half-lives, 87.5 per cent in three half-lives, and 93.75 per cent in four half-lives. For practical purposes, the steady state is considered achieved when 90 per cent of the ultimate accumulation occurs, requiring three to four half-lives. For drugs with short half-lives, accumulation occurs rapidly and loading doses to achieve immediate therapeutic concentrations may not be necessary. For drugs with long half-lives, accumulation occurs slowly and loading doses are frequently required to achieve a therapeutic effect prior to waiting for full accumulation to occur. Regardless of whether a loading dose is given, the ultimate steady-state concentration achieved depends only on the maintenance dose and drug clearance. The loading dose only allows one to hasten the approach to a therapeutic concentration of drug. Figure 22–3 shows the accumulation of lidocaine to a steady state during a constant intravenous infusion of 3 mg per minute. The ultimate steady-state plasma level is approached with a half-life of 110 minutes. A loading dose would be required to achieve therapeutic concentrations more quickly.

When drug is given intermittently, such as procainamide, illustrated in Figure 22–4, the average concentration approaches steady state with the same time course as during a constant infusion. The more frequently doses are given, the smaller the differences between peak and trough plasma concentrations, and the closer the intermittent dosing approximates an intravenous infusion.

Whenever the drug doses or infusion rates are changed, a new steady state will be achieved. The approach to the new steady state also is dependent on the half-life so that three to four half-lives will be required before the plasma concentrations and body stores of drug are at 90 per cent of the new steady state. Therefore, the effects of a dosage adjustment will not be immediate and will not be fully expressed for a time that is dependent on the drug's half-life.

MAINTENANCE DOSES. Steady state is achieved when the rate of drug administration equals the rate of drug elimination. The rate of drug administration is either the infusion rate (I) or the dose per unit time (D/t), and the rate of drug elimination is the product of drug clearance (Cl) and drug concentration (C_p). Therefore, during a steady-state infusion, $I = ClC_p$, and during intermittent dosing, $D/t = ClC_p$. Note that the steady state concentrations are independent of the distribution of the drug and are solely dependent on drug clearance and the rate of drug administration. The equations for steady state can be used to calculate the infusion rate or the intermittent dose required to achieve a desired plasma concentration, and conversely the plasma concentration at steady state produced by a known infusion rate can be used to calculate drug clearance. For example, in an adult without heart failure or liver disease, the clearance of lidocaine is about 860 ml per minute (Table 22–1). In order to maintain a therapeutic concentration of 3.5 μg per milliliter, an infusion rate of 3 mg per minute must be given: $I = ClC_p$ = 860 ml per minute × 3.5 μg per milliliter = 3000 μg per minute = 3 mg per minute. This is the steady-state value illustrated in Figure 22–3. For procainamide with a clearance of 450 ml per minute, an infusion rate of 2 mg per minute will achieve and maintain a steady-state concentration of 4.4 μg per milliliter: I = 450 ml per minute × 4.4 μg per milliliter = 2 mg per minute. If procainamide is given intermittently, the same average concentration will be achieved if the entire amount of drug infused over a three-hour period (360 mg) is given as a single dose every three hours or half

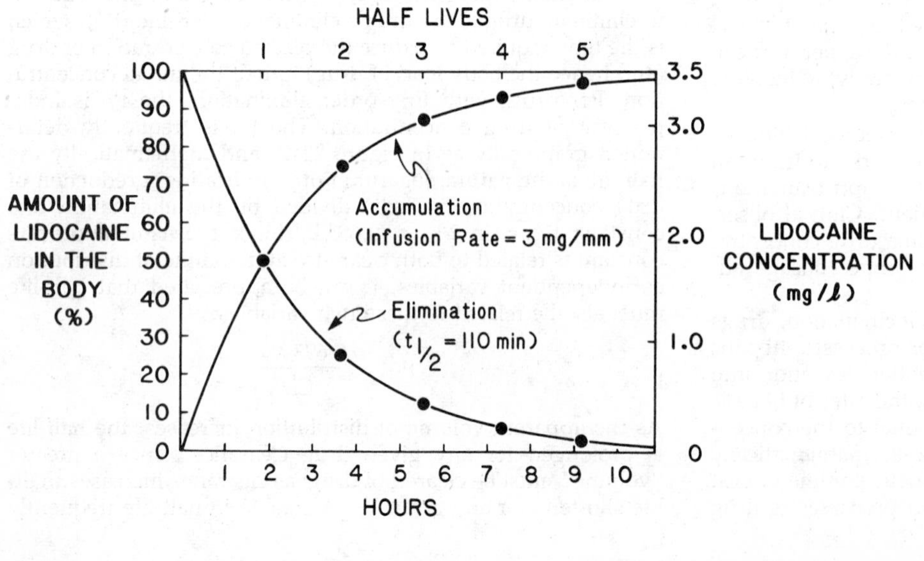

Figure 22–3. The accumulation of lidocaine during an infusion of 3 mg per minute and the elimination of lidocaine after the drug is discontinued. Time is indicated in hours and in half-lives and concentration in milligrams per liter. The amount of lidocaine in the body is the percentage remaining after discontinuation of the drug (elimination curve) or the percentage of the ultimate steady-state value achieved by the chronic infusion (accumulation curve). The two curves are mirror images of each other.

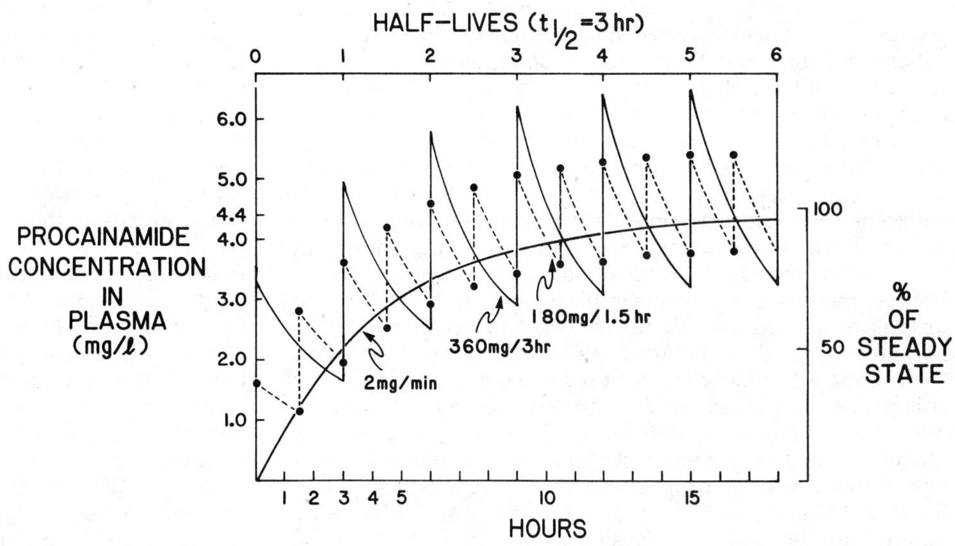

Figure 22–4. The accumulation to steady state of procainamide given as an infusion of 2 mg per minute (smooth curve) or intermittent doses of 180 mg per one and one half hours (dashed line) or 360 mg per three hours (solid line). Regardless of the method of administration, the accumulation follows the same time course and requires three to four half-lives to reach 90 per cent of steady state.

that amount every 90 minutes (Fig. 22–4). Obviously, drug concentrations fluctuate when a drug is given intermittently, and the degree of fluctuation depends on the interval between drug doses, the drug half-life, the route of administration, and the speed of absorption. If a dose is given every half-life, the fluctuation will be at most 100 per cent, that is, the blood levels and body stores will fall to half the initial level by the end of the dosage interval. The dose then boosts the blood level back to the initial value. The dose in this case consists of half the body stores, which is lost during the half-life. If the drug is given more often than the half-life, the fluctuations will be less, with the extreme example being an infusion in which there is no fluctuation. In each case, the drug lost during a dosage interval is replaced by the dose to maintain the steady state. Usually drugs are given at least every half-life to avoid extreme fluctuations of blood levels. Only if very high concentrations are nontoxic or continuously effective plasma levels are not required can a drug be given much less frequently than one half-life. When drugs are given orally, the fluctuations in plasma levels are less than if the same dose is given as a bolus intravenously. Because absorption from the gut occurs gradually over a period of time, the peak concentrations are lower than following intravenous dosing.

DRUG REMOVAL FOLLOWING OVERDOSE. The principles described above can be used to predict the efficacy of hemodialysis or hemoperfusion in removing drug following an overdose. To be a valuable addition to the therapy of overdose, the drug removal process must make a substantial contribution to overall clearance of the drug and the amount of drug removed must be a significant portion of the body load. Consider the case of a digoxin overdose in an adult producing a plasma digoxin level of 8 ng per milliliter. The body load of digoxin is $V_D \times C_p$ or 500 liters × 8 μg per liter = 4 mg. At a clearance of 100 ml per minute with the hemoperfusion apparatus, the rate of drug removal with a C_p of 8 ng per milliliter is $Cl \times C_p$ = 100 ml per minute × 8 ng per milliliter = 800 ng per minute = 48 μg per hour, or only 1 per cent of the body load. Therefore, hemoperfusion cannot be of significant value in reducing the body stores of digoxin. The reason so little drug is removed is related to digoxin's very large V_D of 500 liters so that very little drug is present in the plasma from which it can be cleared. Recently, digoxin antibodies (Fab fragment) have become available in several centers for the experimental treatment of life-threatening digoxin toxicity. These antibodies have such a high affinity for digoxin that the drug is removed from tissue sites, including those areas responsible for toxicity, and becomes bound to the antibody in the plasma. This shift of drug from tissue to plasma results in a reduction of the V_D for digoxin by a factor of 10 or more. Thus not only is toxicity reduced by binding to the antibody, but much more digoxin is present in the plasma, from which it can be cleared either by normal renal excretory processes or, probably, if necessary, by hemoperfusion techniques. In theory this technique could also be applied to other drugs with large V_D.

The other circumstance that limits the benefit to be gained by hemoperfusion is when the drug normally has a very large clearance. The clearance of the tricyclic antidepressants, for instance, is in the range of 1000 ml per minute. If a hemoperfusion apparatus could clear the drug at 100 ml per minute, it would add only 10 per cent to the normal clearance and would therefore not be of substantial value.

DOSE-DEPENDENT PHARMACOKINETICS. For a few drugs, the pharmacokinetics do not follow the rules outlined above, and such drugs are said to have dose-dependent, nonlinear, or saturation kinetics (Table 22–2). For these drugs the amount of drug eliminated is not directly related to the drug concentration (first order), but as the concentration of drug is increased, the relative amount of drug eliminated decreases (i.e., clearance decreases) until a maximal rate of drug metabolism is achieved that is independent of drug concentration, at which point drug elimination is termed zero order. If the amount of drug administered exceeds the maximal metabolic rate for drug elimination, the drug will accumulate indefinitely and very high blood levels will result. Phenytoin is the most important example of a therapeutic agent with dose-dependent kinetics. With phenytoin, clearance is not constant but decreases at increasing dose so that any given increase in dose will result in a disproportionate increase in plasma concentration, and therefore dosage adjustments must be made cautiously. A dose of 300 mg of phenytoin daily may give a plasma level of 8 μg per milliliter, and a dose of 400 mg per day a plasma level of 25 μg per milliliter. Since all patients differ in their ability to eliminate phenytoin, proper dosage adjustments are difficult to predict for an individual patient. In practice, the feedback supplied by plasma concentration measurements (see below) must be used to establish a proper maintenance dose. High dose salicylate therapy also behaves in a dose-dependent manner, as does ethanol.

USE OF PLASMA DRUG CONCENTRATION TO GUIDE THERAPY. The principles outlined above allow the clinician to choose a loading and maintenance dose based on the desired plasma concentration to achieve therapeutic effects without toxicity. The underlying premise is that the concentration of drug in plasma is in equilibrium with drug at the site of action and therefore is a direct reflection of the drug at the target site (Fig. 22–1).

However, the published pharmacokinetic data on which initial dosage recommendations are based are averages for a population and usually need modification for the individual patient. Dosage adjustment is best accomplished when the therapeutic effects of the drug are readily quantifiable. Thus, antihypertensive drugs can be given in a dose sufficient to lower blood pressure, and oral anticoagulants can be given in doses that prolong the prothrombin time into the therapeutic range. With these drugs the desired effect is the appropriate endpoint, and plasma concentrations of the drug are not necessary for dosage adjustment. For many drugs, however, the desired endpoint is difficult to assess clinically, either because there is no readily quantifiable measurement to assess drug effect or because the disease being treated has an intermittent expression so that the clinician cannot be certain that a therapeutic effect has been achieved. Two good examples are epilepsy and sporadic cardiac arrhythmias, in which drug dosage adjustments are difficult to make with precision. Frequently, therefore, patients with sporadic arrhythmias or epilepsy receive doses of drugs based on the average patient, and if these doses are ineffective or toxic, the drug is deemed a failure and the patient is "resistant" or "intolerant" to the therapy, in which case other drugs are tried.

Dosage adjustment can be aided by using the plasma concentration in cases in which there are no other easily quantifiable endpoints by which the drug's therapeutic effects can be gauged. In order for the plasma concentration to have therapeutic meaning, the drug in plasma must be in equilibrium with drug at the site of action and the effects must be reversible. If a drug has irreversible effects, such as the effect of aspirin to inhibit platelet aggregation, the plasma level will not correlate with effect. Fortunately, such situations are uncommon.

The sources of variation in drug effects can be divided into pharmacokinetic and pharmacodynamic factors. Those factors that alter the plasma drug concentration resulting from a given dose are the pharmacokinetic variables—absorption, distribution, and clearance. Those factors that alter the response to a given plasma level are the pharmacodynamic variables. If the pharmacodynamic variation between patients is very large, then plasma drug concentrations will not be a helpful guide for therapy. Fortunately, pharmacokinetic factors account for the major variation between patients for many drugs, and this variability can be minimized with the use of plasma drug level monitoring.

Therapeutic Window. For plasma levels to be a useful guide to therapy, the range of drug concentrations required for optimal therapeutic effects with minimal toxicity must be established. This range is called the "therapeutic window" and is determined experimentally for each drug in a group of patients who are carefully observed for desired and toxic drug effects (Fig. 22–5). The width of the therapeutic window relates to the steepness of the concentration-effect curve and is an index of the pharmacodynamic variability in the population being treated. For procainamide, illustrated in Figure 22–5, the therapeutic window is 4 to 8 mg per liter. The separation between the therapeutic and toxic concentration-effect curves is an index of the toxicity of the drug frequently referred to as the "therapeutic index," which is the toxic dose divided by therapeutic dose. For procainamide the therapeutic index is ~3. With all drugs there is overlap between the therapeutic and toxic ranges. In addition, since the therapeutic window is based on a population of patients, one cannot be certain of the optimal drug concentration for a given patient. Although most patients will achieve a therapeutic effect at some part of the therapeutic range, a few patients require concentrations below or above the range. Similarly, toxicity begins to occur in some patients within the therapeutic window, but the incidence of side effects increases sharply as the therapeutic range is exceeded. Therefore, the plasma concentration cannot be an infallible guide to safe and effective therapy, since it controls only the pharmacokinetic variability and not the pharmacodynamic variability. It is undoubtedly better, however, than the use of a standard dose that allows for no variability.

Table 22–3 lists some drugs for which therapeutic windows have been established. These drugs have several common characteristics: first, their pharmacologic effects are not readily quantifiable; second, they are used for therapy of serious or life-threatening illness so that therapeutic inefficacy cannot be tolerated; and third, their toxicity is serious and the toxic concentration-effect relationship is close to the therapeutic concentration-effect relationship. It should be evident that therapeutic windows are not required for drugs that have a very large therapeutic index and are used for therapy of diseases that do not have serious consequences if undertreated.

Interpretation of Plasma Drug Concentrations. TIMING. Several problems exist in interpretation of plasma drug concentrations. If the blood sample is drawn during the distribution phase shortly after drug administration, the plasma drug concentration will be high, may not reflect drug at the site of action, and certainly will not indicate the steady-state drug concentration. The data on which the therapeutic windows are based are concentrations obtained after the distribution phase and frequently are minimal or trough concentrations. There-

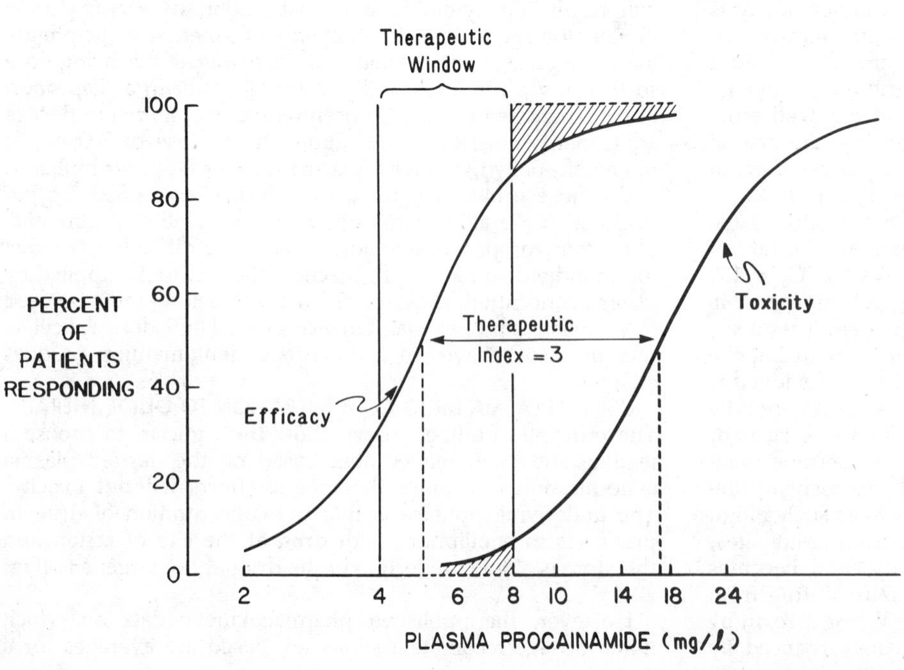

Figure 22–5. Population dose-response curves for the antiarrhythmic and acute toxic effects of procainamide. The therapeutic window is the range encompassing most of the therapeutic dose-effect curve and includes less than 10 per cent of the toxic dose-effect curve. The toxic dose divided by the therapeutic dose is the therapeutic index, here shown for 50 per cent of the population. Individual patients may lie anywhere on these curves.

TABLE 22–3. THERAPEUTIC WINDOWS

Drug	Therapeutic Range
Cardiovascular Drugs:	
Digitoxin	10–25 μg/L
Digoxin	0.8–2 μg/L
Disopyramide	2–6 mg/L
Lidocaine	1.5–5 mg/L
Procainamide	4–8 mg/L
Quinidine	2–6 mg/L
Theophylline	8–20 mg/L
Antiseizure Drugs:	
Carbamazepine	6–12 mg/L
Ethosuximide	40–80 mg/L
Phenobarbital	15–30 mg/L
Phenytoin	10–20 mg/L
Valproic acid	50–100 mg/L
Antibiotics:*	
Amikacin‡	20–40 mg/L
Carbenicillin	100–300 mg/L
Gentamicin‡	5–10 mg/L
Penicillin G†	1–25 mg/L
Tobramycin‡	5–10 mg/L
Others:	
Lithium	0.5–1.5 mEq/L
Nortriptyline	50–150 μg/L
Salicylate	<300 mg/L

*Actual concentration required related to minimal inhibitory concentration for infecting bacterium.
†1 mg of penicillin = 1.6 × 10[6] units.
‡Peak levels.

fore, the best time to draw blood for drug assay is just prior to a dose, during a steady state infusion, or at least four hours after a preceding dose.

PROTEIN BINDING. A second potential problem in interpretation of plasma drug concentration is abnormal binding of drugs to plasma proteins. Many drugs are highly bound (>80 per cent) to plasma protein, and routine assays of plasma for drug concentrations include total (bound plus free) drug. If the fraction bound is constant, then total drug concentration is an accurate index of the free drug concentration that is in equilibrium with the tissues, including the site of action. If binding is altered by other drugs or by disease, then the meaning of a given total concentration of drug will be changed, since a greater proportion of the drug will be unbound. Both liver and kidney disease can alter the protein binding of some drugs (phenytoin, digitoxin, clofibrate, diazoxide, some sulfonamides, valproic acid, and salicylic acid) either by changing the quantity of protein (decreased albumin in liver disease and nephrotic syndrome) or by competition for binding between the drug and endogenous compounds that accumulate in patients with uremia or jaundice. In addition, one drug may compete with another for binding to plasma proteins. Measurement of unbound drug may be required for proper interpretation of the plasma concentration in these circumstances, since if more drug is unbound, the effects or toxicity of any given total plasma concentration will be increased.

Decreased plasma protein binding can also change the kinetics of drug disposition. The volume of distribution will increase because less drug remains in the plasma as the increased free fraction distributes to the tissues. Whether changes in clearance occur with changes in plasma protein binding depends on whether the clearing organ can strip drug from the protein, in which case clearance will not change, since in this circumstance it does not depend on the free drug fraction. However, for many drugs the clearance is restricted to free drug, in which case drug clearance will increase as binding to plasma proteins decreases, since a larger fraction of the total is available for elimination. With these drugs, however, the clearance of *free* drug is unchanged. An unchanged clearance of free drug means that the average plasma free drug concentration will be unchanged at steady state although protein binding is decreased. However, the total drug concentration will decrease because of the increased drug clearance. Since free drug concentration is not changed and free drug determines the effects of most drugs, the daily dose of drug need not be changed. The best studied example is that of phenytoin, which is normally >90 per cent bound to plasma albumin. In patients with uremia, phenytoin binding can decrease to 70 per cent so that the unbound fraction increases from 10 to 30 per cent. As a consequence of the increase in free fraction, the apparent volume of distribution of phenytoin increases and clearance increases. The plasma concentration of total phenytoin falls as a result of the increased clearance, but the average free concentration at steady state is unchanged. A therapeutic phenytoin level with 90 per cent protein binding is 10 to 20 mg per liter, corresponding to an unbound drug concentration of 1 to 2 mg per liter. With 30 per cent unbound the corresponding therapeutic level of total phenytoin would be 3.3 to 6.7 mg per liter to achieve the same free drug concentration. Obviously, if the goal were to attain a total concentration of 10 to 20 mg per liter with 30 per cent unbound phenytoin, toxicity would result, since the free drug concentration would be three-fold higher than therapeutic. The overall pharmacokinetic change resulting from a decrease in phenytoin binding is an unchanged clearance of free drug, an increased clearance of total drug, a lesser increase in the V_D, and a consequent decrease in the half-life to approximately eight hours from the normal 18 to 24 hours. Since the half-life is shortened but the average free drug concentration is unchanged by the change in phenytoin binding, the total daily dose of phenytoin should be the same in patients with renal failure as in patients with normal renal function, but the drug should be given every eight hours instead of every 12 to 24 hours to avoid unwanted large fluctuations in drug level.

ACTIVE METABOLITES. A third pitfall in interpretation of the plasma concentration of some drugs is the presence of unmeasured but active metabolites. Propranolol is metabolized to 4-hydroxypropranolol, which has beta-adrenergic blocking activity. Procainamide is metabolized to N-acetylprocainamide, which has antiarrhythmic activity. The importance of active metabolites depends on their intrinsic activity and the extent to which they accumulate relative to the parent compound. In situations in which an active metabolite accounts for a significant portion of the drug's activity, the metabolite must be measured along with the parent drug for proper interpretation.

PHARMACODYNAMIC CHANGES. A final factor altering the interpretation of plasma levels is a physiologic or pathologic change that alters the response to a given plasma concentration. For instance, a change in serum potassium, magnesium, or calcium concentration will alter the toxic concentration-effect relationship for digoxin such that concentrations not usually associated with adverse effects may now be toxic. These alterations in pharmacodynamics of the drug response emphasize the fact that plasma drug concentrations must be interpreted with other clinical and laboratory data that may influence the response to the drug.

ALTERATIONS OF DRUG DOSES IN DISEASE STATES. ***Renal Disease.*** A decrease in renal function will result in a decreased renal clearance of drugs. Whether a dosage adjustment is required depends on the toxicity of the drug and the relative importance of renal clearance to other pathways for drug clearance. If the drug has significant toxicity and the kidney accounts for most of the drug's elimination, then dosage adjustments must be made in patients with renal disease to avoid toxicity. On the other hand, if the drug is nontoxic, dosage adjustment is less critical even if the drug accumulates in patients with renal failure. For instance, penicillin is cleared >90 per cent by the kidneys, but because it is relatively nontoxic, dosage adjustments are not required for low dose therapy (600,000 to 1,200,000 units per day). However, if massive doses of penicillin are required, then dosage adjustments must be made to avoid penicillin toxicity.

Fortunately, renal drug clearance is closely correlated with the clearance of creatinine even for those drugs that are eliminated by tubular secretion. For this reason, an adjustment of the average drug dose can be calculated from the creatinine clearance. The process is simple: The calculated renal drug clearance is reduced by the same proportion as the reduction from 100 ml per minute in the measured creatinine clearance or the creatinine clearance calculated by the formula:

$$\text{Creatinine Clearance} = \frac{(140 - \text{age}) \times \text{weight (kg)}}{72 \times \text{Serum Creatinine (mg/dl)}}$$

for males, with the creatinine clearance for females being 85 per cent of that for males. If the drug is cleared by nonrenal (usually hepatic) mechanisms as well as by renal mechanisms, only the renal clearance (Cl_r) is adjusted; the nonrenal clearance (Cl_{nr}) remains normal. Assuming that the same average plasma concentration (C_p) is desired in patients with renal failure, the dose is adjusted in direct proportion to the change in total clearance, since $Cl \times C_p$ = dose/time. Renal and nonrenal clearances for some drugs are listed in Table 22–1. Consider as an example of this approach the alteration of digoxin dosage in renal failure. The average renal clearance of digoxin is 110 ml per minute at a creatinine clearance of 100 ml per minute; the nonrenal clearance is 40 ml per minute. If the measured creatinine clearance is 50 ml per minute, or half normal, then the renal clearance of digoxin is reduced by a similar fraction; thus, Cl_r (digoxin) = 55 ml per minute in this patient. If the nonrenal clearance is assumed to be unchanged, the total digoxin clearance is $Cl_{nr} + Cl_r = 40 + 55 = 95$ ml per minute in the patient with a creatinine clearance of 50 ml per minute, versus a total digoxin clearance of 40 + 110 = 150 ml per minute in a patient with normal renal function. The total digoxin clearance is therefore reduced by the fraction $\frac{95}{150}$ and the dose should be adjusted using the same fraction. If the average dose is 0.25 mg per day, this would be decreased to $\frac{95}{150} \times 0.25$ mg = 0.16 mg per day. These calculations can give only a first approximation of the appropriate dose for an individual patient, since they are based on the average dose for the average patient. In practice, the calculated dose or a dose conveniently close to the calculated dose is administered to the patient, and the patient's response and plasma drug concentrations are monitored. With the information provided by either the plasma drug concentrations or clinical observations, the dosage can be adjusted.

If the desired plasma concentration is known, one can calculate the dosage directly from the drug clearance, since dose/t = $Cl \times C_p$. For example, an average procainamide concentration of 5 μg per milliliter is desired in a patient with a creatinine clearance of 50 ml per minute. The total procainamide clearance is $\frac{50}{100} \times 330\ (Cl_r) + 120\ (Cl_{nr}) = 285$ ml per minute. An infusion of 1.4 mg per minute ($Cl \times C_p$) or a dose of 250 mg every three hours will achieve and maintain the desired plasma concentration.

Although drug clearance is the best way to calculate doses for drugs, clearance data are not available for many drugs. For a few drugs, published nomograms are available to guide dosage. It would be preferable, both from a practical and from an intellectual standpoint, to be able to use a more generally applicable method to calculate proper dosage. Two such methods are outlined in the next two paragraphs.

For many drugs, the elimination rate constant (k_e) is known. If the apparent volume of distribution is unchanged in renal disease, then the k_e and Cl are proportional ($k_e = Cl/V_D$) and the change in k_e can be used to adjust the dose in a manner entirely analogous to the use of changes in clearance to adjust dose. Like clearance values, the elimination rate constant can be expressed as the sum of the rate constants for the separate eliminating organs; thus $k_e = k_{renal} + k_{nonrenal}$. Values for k_r and k_{nr} are listed in Table 22–4. To use these values to adjust dosage in renal insufficiency, the procedure is exactly the same as with the clearance calculations used above. Thus, k_e for amikacin in a patient with normal renal function is 0.31, which is made up of $k_r = 0.3$ and a $k_{nr} = 0.01$. The dose alteration in a patient with a creatinine clearance of 25 ml per minute is calculated as follows: The k_r for the patient is $25/100 \times 0.3 = 0.08$. The k_e therefore is $k_r + k_{nr} = 0.08 + 0.01 = 0.09$ versus the normal k_e of 0.31. The dose of amikacin must therefore be reduced to $\frac{0.09}{0.31}$ or 30 per cent of the usual dose per unit time. As can be readily appreciated, the dose of amikacin is reduced almost in proportion to the reduction in creatinine clearance, since the nonrenal elimination is negligible until creatinine clearance is reduced to very low values (i.e., <15 ml per minute). Several other antibiotics are like amikacin in this regard and are in Group A in Table 22–4. For all these drugs, dosage adjustment can be made by multiplying the usual dose by the fraction of the creatinine clearance remaining in the patient. When the patient has essentially no renal function, then the small k_{nr} may be used to calculate doses as illustrated above. For drugs that have nonrenal elimination that is a substantial fraction (e.g., 20 to 50 per cent) of the total elimination, the dosage reduction in renal insufficiency will be less than the reduction in creatinine clearance and can be calculated as illustrated above. These drugs are in Group B. If the nonrenal elimination is greater than 50 per cent of the k_e, then the dosage usually does not need to be adjusted for changes in renal function. In all cases, the calculations adjust only the average dose, and blood level

TABLE 22–4. THE RENAL ELIMINATION RATE CONSTANTS (k_r), NONRENAL ELIMINATION RATE CONSTANTS (k_{nr}), AND PER CENT NONRENAL ELIMINATION IN A NORMAL INDIVIDUAL FOR ANTIMICROBIAL AGENTS

	k_r (per Hour)	k_{nr} (per Hour)	% Nonrenal
Group A (>90% renal)			
Amikacin	0.3	0.01	5
Amoxicillin	0.6	0.1	10
Ampicillin	0.5	0.06	10
Carbenicillin	0.5	0.05	10
Cefazolin	0.3	0.02	5
Cephalexin	0.7	0.03	5
Cephalothin	1.4	0.03	5
Cephradine	0.5	0.05	10
Colistin	0.3	0.02	10
Flucytosine	0.24	0.01	5
Gentamicin	0.3	0.02	5
Kanamycin	0.3	0.01	5
Methicillin	1.2	0.15	10
Penicillin G	1.3	0.1	10
Polymyxin B	0.13	0.02	10
Streptomycin	0.24	0.01	5
Tetracycline	0.07	0.01	10
Ticarcillin	0.6	0.06	10
Tobramycin	0.3	0.01	5
Vancomycin	0.12	0.003	5
Group B (50–80% renal)			
Cephapirin	0.9	0.3	25
Dicloxacillin	0.6	0.6	50
Erythromycin	0.30	0.15	35
Ethambutol	0.09	0.09	50
Isoniazid (slow acetylators)	0.12	0.12	50
Lincomycin	0.1	0.06	40
Nafcillin	0.7	0.5	40
Oxacillin	1.1	0.35	25
Oxytetracycline	0.065	0.015	20
Trimethoprim	0.03	0.03	50
Group C (<50% renal)			
Amphotericin B	0.01	0.02	70
Chloramphenicol	0.02	0.3	80
Clindamycin	0	0.25	100
Doxycycline	0.005	0.03	80
Isoniazid (fast acetylators)	0.1	0.4	80
Minocycline	0	0.06	100
Rifampin	0	0.25	100
Sulfamethoxazole	0.01	0.06	85

determinations are required to make final dosage adjustments. This is particularly true if nonrenal elimination may also be reduced, as in liver or cardiac disease.

A final method for estimating the average dose in patients with renal failure is to use the per cent nonrenal elimination determined in normal individuals. These values are listed in Tables 22–1 and 22–4 and are frequently available for drugs even if clearances or elimination rate constants are not. To use this method, drug clearance as a percentage of normal is plotted against creatinine clearance as in Figure 22–6. A line is drawn to connect the point at 100 per cent drug clearance and 100 ml per minute creatinine clearance with a point on the ordinate corresponding to the per cent nonrenal drug clearance, which is the clearance remaining when creatinine clearance is 0 ml per minute. The per cent drug clearance can then be read directly for any creatinine clearance and the dosage adjusted accordingly. For instance, consider the amikacin example calculated above. Since the per cent nonrenal elimination in a normal individual is ~5 per cent, the clearance values for amikacin fall on the line intersecting the ordinate at 5 per cent in Figure 22–6. The drug clearance as a percentage of normal for a creatinine clearance of 25 ml per minute is ~30 per cent (as indicated by the dotted line), and the dose of this drug in the patient with a creatinine clearance of 25 ml therefore must be 30 per cent normal.

The reduction in dose per unit time can be applied to patient care by giving either the reduced dose at the usual interval or the same dose at a longer interval. By both methods the average plasma level will be the same, but the fluctuations in plasma concentration will be less when the reduced dose is given at the usual intervals.

Loading doses for most drugs used in patients with renal failure need not be adjusted for creatinine clearance. However, since the t½ of renally cleared drugs is prolonged in these patients, drug accumulation during initiation of therapy with maintenance doses will be slower. Because of the slower accumulation, loading doses may be required more frequently in patients with renal failure than in patients with normal renal function in order to rapidly achieve a therapeutic blood concentration. Digoxin, for example, with a half-life of 1.5 days in a patient with normal renal function will accumulate to 90 per cent of steady-state levels in five days (3 to 4 half-lives), and many patients need not be loaded, since this accumulation is sufficiently rapid to produce the desired therapeutic effects. On the other hand, in a patient without renal function, digoxin half-life increases to five days. If the anephric patient is begun on the appropriately reduced maintenance dose of digoxin, accumulation to the same steady-state level will take more than 15 days to occur. In this case, a loading dose may be desired to achieve a more rapid effect without waiting for drug accumulation. However, whether or not a loading dose is given, the ultimate steady-state drug concentration will be the same and, as always, depends only on drug dose and drug clearance.

Some drugs form metabolites that are active or toxic and are eliminated by the kidneys. In patients with renal insufficiency, these metabolites may accumulate and produce effects. As an example, procainamide is in part excreted unchanged and in part metabolized to N-acetylprocainamide, which has antiarrhythmic effects and can produce toxicity. The metabolite may achieve concentrations in renal failure that are many-fold higher than the parent drug and can contribute to the antiarrhythmic effects and toxicity of procainamide. Since the concentration of metabolites is not routinely measured by drug assay laboratories, the plasma concentration of parent drug can be misleading. Drugs with renally excreted active or toxic metabolites include (in addition to procainamide) meperidine, propoxyphene, clofibrate, nitrofurantoin, and nitroprusside. If alternative drugs are available for the treatment of patients with renal insufficiency, it is probably best to avoid those drugs when active or toxic metabolites may accumulate.

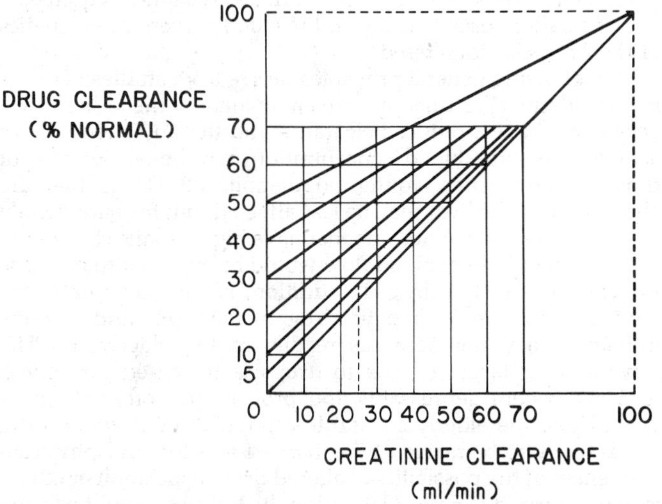

Figure 22–6. A graph of the per cent normal drug clearance plotted against creatinine clearance. When creatinine clearance is zero, the per cent normal drug clearance is the nonrenal clearance determined in individuals with normal renal function. The dose required in patients with renal failure is adjusted by the per cent normal clearance read directly from the graph. The dotted line indicates that at a creatinine clearance of 25 ml per minute the dose of amikacin, which has ~5 per cent nonrenal clearance in normals, must be reduced to 30 per cent of normal. (Modified from Dettli L: Clin Pharmacokinet 1:126, 1976.)

Hepatic Disease. Although many drugs are biotransformed by the liver, no quantitative predictor of the degree of abnormality in drug metabolism is available for patients with liver disease. Severe liver disease can result in a decreased metabolic capacity for a large number of drugs. If the indices of the liver's capacity to form proteins (serum albumin and prothrombin time) are abnormal, then it is probable that drug metabolism will also be abnormal, and the doses of those drugs that are metabolized by the liver should be reduced. Acute liver disease has an inconstant and unpredictable effect on drug metabolism, but in general drug metabolism is not as abnormal as with chronic liver disease.

With chronic liver disease, portacaval anastomoses may develop. Not only will this decrease the blood flow to the liver with consequent reduction in clearance of some drugs, but the portacaval shunting can allow drug absorbed by the gut to pass directly into the systemic circulation and bypass the liver, thereby avoiding the "first pass" or "presystemic" elimination. For those drugs that are largely extracted from the blood by the liver (e.g., propranolol, metoprolol, lidocaine), portacaval shunting will allow a much greater fraction of an orally administered dose to reach the systemic circulation.

Hemodynamic Disorders. Pharmacokinetics can be affected in several ways by disorders of the circulation. Hypotension and poor cardiac output reduce renal blood flow, glomerular filtration rate, and hepatic blood flow. As with primary renal disease, the impairment in renal drug excretion may be estimated by the change in creatinine clearance and dosage adjustments made accordingly. The effects of reduced hepatic blood flow on drug metabolism are highly dependent on the drug. For drugs that are essentially completely cleared from the blood on a single passage through the liver, i.e., when the extraction from blood is close to 100 per cent, a reduction in liver blood flow will reduce hepatic drug clearance proportionately. On the other hand, many drugs that are metabolized are extracted poorly by the liver, and for these drugs a reduction in liver blood flow has relatively little influence on their hepatic clearance. A complicating factor is that circulatory abnormalities also can result in hepatic congestion or tissue hypoxia that can impair hepatocellular function, so that drug metabolism may be reduced during hypotensive states independent of the effects of blood flow on drug delivery to the liver. Therefore, it is difficult to predict in the individual patient the proper dosage of hepatic metabolized drugs in patients with circulatory abnormalities. Certainly a drug such as lidocaine that has a very high hepatic clearance will be cleared less well in congestive heart failure or shock, and the maintenance infusion rates must be reduced by about half in these situations to avoid toxicity.

The distribution of some drugs is also affected by hemodynamic changes. For several drugs with large distribution volumes (lidocaine, quinidine, and procainamide) the apparent volume of distribution is decreased in heart failure and shock, and loading doses should also be reduced to avoid toxic plasma concentrations. However, for theophylline, a drug with a relatively small volume of distribution, the apparent volume of distribution is not changed by heart failure. Since data are not available for most drugs, we advise a conservative approach to loading and maintenance doses of toxic drugs in the setting of congestive heart failure or shock with careful monitoring of the clinical status and plasma levels to guide further dosage adjustments.

USE OF DRUGS IN THE ELDERLY. Elderly persons (over 65 years) comprise about 11 per cent of the United States population, but about 30 per cent of all prescriptions are written for this group of patients. In addition to prescription drugs, 70 per cent of elderly patients regularly use over-the-counter medications, primarily analgesics, compared with only 10 per cent of the general adult population. As an individual ages, changes occur that may affect drug kinetics and drug action. These age-related changes accentuate the normal interindividual variation in drug effects, thus making the elderly the most diverse segment of the adult population in terms of their drug responses. Because of the changes that occur with aging and the large numbers of drugs used in this population, the elderly are highly susceptible to drug interactions as well as to adverse drug effects.

The pharmacokinetic changes that may occur in the elderly are related to changes in body composition as well as to changes in function of pharmacokinetically important organs. The changes in gastrointestinal function that occur with aging are a decrease in gastric acid secretion, a decrease in mucosal absorptive surface of the small bowel by about 30 per cent, and a decrease in splanchnic blood flow by about 40 per cent. In spite of these changes, very few studies have shown much effect of aging on drug absorption. This is probably because most drugs are well absorbed and do not require very much of the small bowel for their absorption. For these drugs, there appears to be a very large reserve for absorption that is not exceeded by the changes that occur in the elderly.

The distribution of drugs may change markedly with aging, probably because lean body mass and total body water decrease as the percentage of total body fat increases. In addition, the plasma concentration of albumin decreases, probably as a result of decreased albumin production by the liver, and this may affect those drugs that are bound to plasma albumin. Alpha$_1$-acid glycoprotein, the major plasma protein that binds basic drugs, is not diminished with aging. Because of the changes in body composition, water-soluble drugs that are not bound to plasma proteins would be expected to have a reduced apparent volume of distribution. However, for lipid-soluble drugs, such as many psychotropic agents, the volume of distribution may be increased, probably because of the increased percentage of body weight as fat. For water-soluble, albumin-bound drugs the changes in distribution with aging are not predictable.

The clearance of many drugs is diminished in the elderly. Both drugs that are metabolized as well as those that are eliminated by the kidneys may have reduced clearance. Cardiac output and blood flow to the kidneys and liver may decrease by 30 to 40 per cent with aging. Glomerular filtration rate may be reduced by as much as 50 per cent in the elderly. Since older persons have a decreased muscle mass, they have a decreased rate of creatinine production. For this reason a reduced creatinine clearance can co-exist with a normal serum creatinine concentration as defined for young healthy adults. As a general rule, one should consider that renal elimination of drugs will be reduced by up to 50 per cent in elderly patients without evidence of renal disease and make dosage adjustments accordingly.

The hepatic clearance of drugs may also be diminished in the elderly, but the interindividual variability in the metabolism of drugs is so large as to preclude any useful predictions for an individual patient without obvious hepatic dysfunction. Both hepatic blood flow and the intrinsic ability of the liver to metabolize some drugs may be reduced. The reduction in hepatic blood flow will influence the elimination of high clearance drugs, such as lidocaine. For low clearance drugs, the hepatic drug metabolizing capacity appears to be most important. Drugs that are metabolized by the hepatic mixed function oxidase system are more likely to be affected than those drugs that are metabolized by conjugation reactions.

The inducibility of hepatic microsomal enzymes may be altered with aging. Evidence from a cross-section of patients comparing smokers with nonsmokers indicated that in a young population, smokers have induced drug metabolism, whereas in the old population, they did not appear to. This implies that smoking may cause induction only in the young and that there may be an impairment in this response in the elderly. Additional studies need to be done to determine whether this is a general phenomenon with inducing agents and aging.

Elimination half-life of many drugs is increased with aging. This is a combination of the effect of changes in the apparent volume of distribution and of changes in metabolic or renal clearance. Frequently, elimination half-life can be prolonged even without changes in drug clearance. This is true with diazepam, which has an increased apparent volume of distribution with no change in metabolic clearance, and this combination of changes produces a prolonged elimination half-life.

The age-related changes that occur with target organ responsiveness are as important as the changes in pharmacokinetics. There is an increased sensitivity to a variety of drugs. The antianxiety agents and sedative hypnotic agents produce greater degrees of depression of central nervous system function in the elderly than in the young even at the same plasma levels. The hypotensive side effects of many psychotropic drugs are greater in the elderly because of reduced functioning of baroreceptor reflexes. Hemorrhage with anticoagulants is more common in the elderly even with good control of the clotting parameters. These changes in pharmacodynamics require the use of smaller doses of drugs in the elderly, even if the kinetics of the drug are not altered.

The following general principles derive from studies of drugs in the elderly: (1) Drugs that are eliminated by the kidneys will very likely have a reduced clearance and the doses required to achieve the same blood concentration may be 50 per cent of those required in a young population. (2) Drugs that are eliminated by the liver may be less affected, but for parenterally given drugs such as lidocaine that have high hepatic clearances, the reduction in liver blood flow would be expected to decrease the clearance of the drug. In addition, some individuals may have a reduction in hepatic drug metabolism, and enzyme induction may not occur as readily in the elderly. (3) The sensitivity of target organs to drugs is increased for central nervous system depressants and probably for other drugs as well. Thus, the elderly constitute a population in whom drug use is likely to be marred by enhanced toxicity, and physician awareness of the possibility of altered drug disposition or effects is mandatory. It is a population in which drugs should be used in the lowest effective doses and only in individuals in whom they are absolutely necessary. That this is not commonly done is indicated by the numbers of drugs taken by elderly individuals, frequently without well-defined endpoints or even well-defined therapeutic indications. Frequent reviews of the patient's drug history, including over-the-counter medications, and discontinuation of those drugs that are not necessary would greatly improve medical care for the elderly population.

Benet LZ (ed.): The Effect of Disease States on Drug Pharmacokinetics. Washington, DC, American Pharmaceutical Association, 1976. *This book contains the proceedings of a symposium held in 1976. Chapters by recognized experts review the effects of disease on pharmacokinetics and the need for individualization of drug dosage.*

Benet LZ, Sheiner LB: Design and optimization of dosage regimens: Pharmacokinetic data. *In* Gilman AG, Goodman LS, Gilman A (eds.): The Pharmacological Basis of Therapeutics. 6th ed. New York, Macmillan, 1980, pp 1675–1737. *This series of tables lists the pharmacokinetic parameters of 98 drugs with references to the literature. This represents the most concise and complete listing currently available.*

Chennavasin P, Brater DC: Nomograms for drug use in renal disease. Clin Pharmacokin 6:193, 1981. *This is a critical review of a variety of published nomograms for determination of creatinine clearance from serum creatinine and for drug dosing in patients with renal disease.*

Dettli L: Drug dosage in renal disease. Clin Pharmacokin 1:126, 1976. *This review of drug elimination in renal disease provides a simple, nomographic approach for adjusting doses and contains most of the data in Table 22–4.*

Gerber JG: Drug usage in the elderly. *In* Schrier RW (ed.): Clinical Internal Medicine in the Aged. Philadelphia, WB Saunders Company, 1982, pp 51–65. *This chapter is an excellent summary of pharmacokinetic principles applied to the elderly patient. The 49 references serve as an entry to the recent literature.*

Reidenberg M: The binding of drugs to plasma proteins and the interpretation of measurements of plasma concentrations of drugs in patients with poor renal function. Am J Med 62:466, 1977. *This review discusses the problems that arise when drug binding to plasma protein is altered by renal disease.*

Wilkinson GR, Shand DG: A physiological approach to hepatic drug clearance. Clin Pharmacol Ther 19:552, 1976. *This article discusses hepatic drug clearance in relation to blood flow, enzyme activity and plasma protein binding. The concepts are valuable for physiologically oriented individuals.*

23. INTERACTIONS BETWEEN DRUGS

Alan S. Nies

Good medical practice frequently demands treatment with multiple drugs for a single disease in an attempt to maximize therapeutic effects and minimize side effects. When one is treating multiple diseases, the number of co-administered drugs increases, as does the possibility of undesirable interactions occurring between the drugs. Entire textbooks have been written to list all of the possible drug interactions. It is obviously impossible for a clinician to remember such lists, and frequently the *clinically important* drug interactions are lost in the midst of large listings of interactions that are based on undocumented case reports, animal experimentation, or theory.

Not all drug interactions that occur are clinically important or even clinically recognized. The reasons for this include the fact that (1) many drugs have such large therapeutic indices that toxicity does not result when there are moderate increases in drug concentration, and thus changes in concentration due to a drug interaction may not be perceived; (2) the disease being treated may not be serious so that a change of drug concentration to less than therapeutic may not be easily recognized; (3) many drugs are given without well-defined therapeutic endpoints, making the drug effect difficult to assess, and therefore changes in drug effect will not be recognized; (4) there is a large intersubject variability due to genetic, environmental, and disease factors that may obscure many drug interactions. These comments are not to imply that drug interactions are not important. Drug interactions will be important if the drug has easily recognizable toxicity and a low therapeutic index such that small changes in amount of drug in the body produce significant toxicity. Second, drug interactions will be recognized and important if the diseases that are being controlled with the drug are serious or potentially fatal if they are undertreated. Third, drug interactions will be recognized if the therapeutic endpoints for the drug are clearly defined or if drug levels are used to maximize therapy for a given drug. Thus major interactions have been reported with anticoagulants and oral hypoglycemics, both of which have easily recognizable toxicity with low therapeutic indices. Drug interactions are reported with antiseizure medication and antiarrhythmic drugs, where not only do the drugs have recognized toxicity, but the diseases being treated become clinically manifest if the amount of drug is inadequate. Drug interactions have also been recognized with cardiac glycosides where blood levels are used to maximize efficacy in some patients.

Clinically important drug interactions are related to either (1) changes in the amount of drug or active metabolite available at the site of action, the so-called pharmacokinetic drug interactions, or (2) changes in drug effect without a change in pharmacokinetics, the pharmacodynamic drug interactions. These latter interactions may result from interactions at a receptor site or from independent actions of two drugs either adding to or counteracting the effects of each other.

PHARMACOKINETIC DRUG INTERACTIONS

These interactions involve the processes of absorption, distribution, renal elimination, and metabolism such that there is a change in the amount of a drug (or an active metabolite) at the site of action. These are the best understood and generally most important drug interactions in clinical medicine. They can be subdivided into those that result in a decreased amount of drug at the site of action and hence a decrease in effect and those that have an increased amount of drug at the site of action and hence an increased effect.

Interactions Resulting in Less Drug Available at the Site of Action

DECREASED ABSORPTION. Since drug absorption generally occurs across the gastrointestinal mucosa by passive diffusion, one drug would not be expected to compete with another for absorption. However, drugs may physically interact in the lumen of the gastrointestinal tract so as to cause decreased absorption. Cholestyramine, a resin used to bind bile acids and to lower serum cholesterol, can also bind a number of other drugs if they are simultaneously present in the gastrointestinal lumen. Thus cholestyramine can diminish the absorption of thyroxin, cardiac glycosides, warfarin, and corticosteroids. It is highly likely that other drugs will also bind to the steroid-binding resins, so that one is advised to view concurrent therapy of these resins with other drugs with caution.

Tetracyclines are potent chelating agents that form insoluble complexes with metal ions such as magnesium, calcium, and aluminum, commonly found in antacids, as well as with iron, with the result that the absorption of tetracycline is reduced. Kaolin used to halt diarrhea will effectively inhibit the absorption of some drugs such as lincomycin and digoxin. In addition, drug products may contain "inert" substances that can interact with other drugs. For instance, para-aminosalicylic acid (PAS) contains bentonite (a kaolin-like substance) that can hamper the absorption of co-administered rifampin.

If a drug is susceptible to degradation at acid pH, anything that delays emptying of the stomach, such as a drug with anticholinergic properties, can result in more degradation of the co-administered acid-sensitive drug, e.g., penicillin G or L-dopa, and thus a decrease in the amount of drug absorbed. Conversely, a drug that speeds gastric emptying, such as metoclopramide, can increase the absorption of acid-unstable drugs. With most other drugs only the time course of absorption is changed so that drug absorption is faster if gastric emptying is enhanced or is slower if gastric emptying is delayed, but the total amount of drug absorbed is unchanged. Whether a change in rate of absorption results in any important clinical effects depends on whether rapid absorption is necessary for drug effect, in which case drug effect will be diminished. Usually, if total absorption is unchanged, then there will not be an important interaction, particularly during chronic administration of drugs.

The pH of the gastrointestinal fluid has little predictable effect on drug absorption. Almost all drugs are absorbed to the greatest extent in the small intestine rather than in the stomach because the major surface area for absorption is in the small intestine. The classic teaching that acidic drugs, such as aspirin, are best absorbed in the stomach at acid pH because less drug is ionized is untrue. Actually, aspirin is more rapidly absorbed from an alkaline medium, since dissolution is enhanced and gastric emptying is speeded.

ALTERED DISTRIBUTION. Some drugs reach their site of action via active transport. In this case, drugs can compete with each other for the transport mechanism, and thus one drug can impair the ability of another to reach its site of action. In order to produce blockade of adrenergic activity, the antihypertensive drugs guanethidine, guanadrel, and bethanidine must be actively transported by an amine transport system into adrenergic neurones. This transport system can be interfered with by tricyclic antidepressants, high doses of phenothiazines, and sympathomimetic amines. Thus coadministration of guanethidine with one of these other compounds will effectively block the antihypertensive effects of guanethidine. This is an undesirable interaction with guanethidine; however, with the antiarrhythmic drug bretylium, sympathetic blockade is an unwanted side effect. Bretylium also gains access to adrenergic neurones via the same amine transport system used by guanethidine. Therapeutic advantage can be taken of a drug interaction that blocks access of bretylium to its antiadrenergic site of action. Thus tricyclic antidepressants or ephedrine will reverse bretylium's sympathetic blocking effects but will not affect the direct antiarrhythmic effects of bretylium.

ENHANCED METABOLISM. Several drugs can increase the ability of the liver to metabolize other drugs. Phenobarbital, other barbiturates, phenytoin, rifampin, glutethimide, griseofulvin, ethanol, phenylbutazone, chronic smoking, certain chlorinated hydrocarbons such as lindane and DDT, carbamazepine, and primidone have all been associated with induction of hepatic microsomal, drug-metabolizing enzymes. The amount of enzyme induction that occurs appears to be under genetic control and so not all individuals experience quantitatively similar effects when taking an inducing agent.

Induction of hepatic metabolizing enzymes can probably affect many drugs. The effects are greatest when the drugs are given orally, because all of the drug must perforce pass through the liver prior to reaching the systemic circulation. Therefore, even for drugs that have a systemic clearance that is largely dependent upon hepatic blood flow, the amount of drug that escapes metabolism on the first pass will be influenced by enzyme-inducing drugs. Some examples of drugs that can have their metabolism induced are oral anticoagulants, quinidine, digitoxin, corticosteroids, low-dose contraceptives, some beta-adrenergic blockers, and theophylline. The induction of corticosteroid metabolism has produced some interesting effects, including (1) inappropriate interpretation of low-dose dexamethasone suppression tests where the enhanced metabolism of dexamethasone produced by enzyme induction resulted in too low a dexamethasone concentration to inhibit normal steroidogenesis; (2) exacerbation of steroid-dependent asthma; and (3) rejection of a renal transplant by individuals who required steroids and received an enzyme-inducing agent.

Frequently the most critical time comes when the inducing agent is discontinued. At this time the drug-metabolizing activity gradually decreases and drug toxicity can occur if dosage adjustments are not made of other co-administered drugs. This phenomenon has been described most frequently with induction of warfarin metabolism and resultant warfarin toxicity when the inducing agent is discontinued.

Interactions Resulting in More Drug Available at the Site of Action

ENHANCED ABSORPTION. In general, absorption is not a common process in which drugs can interact to enhance efficacy. One exception is with acid-unstable drugs and enhanced gastric emptying mentioned above. Another potential interaction is with relatively poorly absorbed drugs, such as digoxin, with which absorption occurs throughout the gastrointestinal tract. With such a drug a decrease in intestinal motility could enhance the degree of absorption by prolonging contact with the absorbing mucosa.

ALTERED DISTRIBUTION. Many drugs are bound to plasma proteins, and drug so bound is not available for action at receptors or for distribution throughout the body. In addition, for many compounds only the free drug is available for metabolism or excretion. The drug bound to plasma protein, therefore, acts as an inactive reservoir of drug in the blood. Since drugs can compete with each other for binding to plasma proteins, a potential for interactions exists. Pure plasma protein binding interactions, however, rarely are clinically significant. The one probable exception to this is the displacement of albumin-bound bilirubin by sulfonamides or salicylates, thus allowing the bilirubin to distribute into the tissues and cause kernicterus in jaundiced infants. With drug/drug interactions, however, when a drug is displaced from plasma protein binding it will very rapidly distribute into the apparent volume of distribution so that the increase in free drug concentration in the plasma is always considerably less than suggested by experiments in vitro. The larger the volume of distribution, the less of an impact a displacement from protein binding will have. Following the immediate displacement and redistribution of the drug, the free fraction generally is readily available for metabolism or excretion and the clearance processes in the body will reduce the free drug concentration to that which existed prior to the protein binding interaction (Fig. 23–1). Therefore the effect of such an interaction will be small, transient, and frequently not recognized clinically. The relationship of free drug to total drug, however, will be changed by such drug interactions, and therefore the interpretation of plasma drug assays that measure total drug in blood may have to be altered (see Ch. 22). Some drugs will interact with other drugs by more than one mechanism, and so interactions at protein-binding sites can coexist with interactions at a metabolic site. These dual drug interactions can be clinically important.

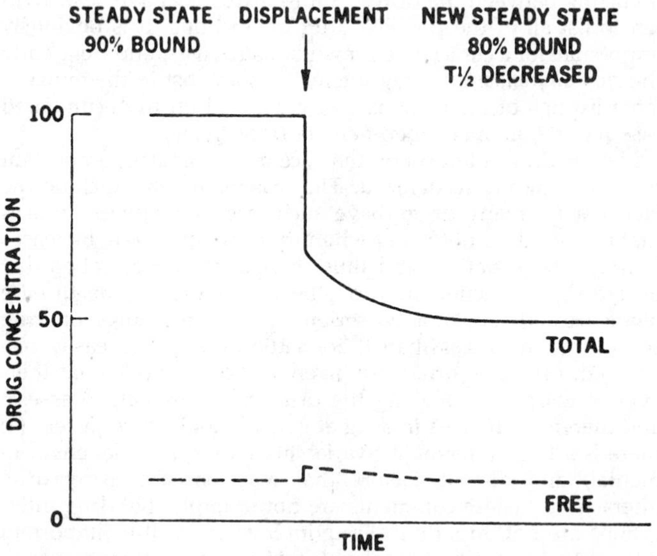

Figure 23–1. The effects of altered plasma drug binding on total and free plasma concentrations of the drug. The drug is assumed to be bound 90 per cent to albumin, not bound to tissues, and to have a V_D of 8.5 L. At the arrow an agent is given that displaces the drug from albumin such that binding is reduced to 80 per cent. The expected changes are an immediate increase in free drug concentration by only 40 per cent, with a fall of total concentration to 70 per cent of the initial value. Since the free drug clearance is not altered by this interaction, a new steady state will be achieved with the same free drug concentration and a reduction of total concentration to 50 per cent. For drugs with larger volumes of distribution, i.e., more tissue binding, the immediate increase of free concentration will be even less than in this example, but the ultimate steady state condition of unchanged free drug concentration and a halving of the concentration of total drug will be the same. (From Shand et al.: Handbook of Experimental Pharmacology. Vol 28, No 3, pp 272–314, 1975, with permission.)

However, it is not the displacement from protein binding that makes these interactions clinically important but rather the alteration of metabolism that does so. These dual drug interactions include interactions of phenylbutazone with warfarin and sulfaphenazole with tolbutamide.

Displacement of drugs from tissue-binding sites has only recently been recognized as a situation for drug interactions. Such an interaction would decrease the apparent volume of distribution of the drug and increase the plasma drug concentration. However, if the dose, plasma drug binding, and drug clearance are not altered, the plasma levels will be only transiently elevated, since steady-state plasma concentrations are independent of the apparent volume of distribution. Thus an interaction resulting in only a displacement from tissue stores would not be easily detected. However, as with displacement interactions from plasma protein, drugs can interact at multiple sites. Thus quinidine will displace digoxin from tissue-binding sites, but the persistent elevation in digoxin plasma concentration that results from the interaction is due to quinidine's ability to reduce the clearance of digoxin.

DECREASED METABOLISM. Inhibition of drug metabolism can have a profound effect on drug disposition, resulting in drug toxicity. Some drugs seem to be rather specific for inhibiting the metabolism of other individual drugs. However, there are a few drugs that can inhibit the metabolism of many drugs. The most commonly used such drug is cimetidine, which can inhibit the metabolism of theophylline, warfarin, diazepam, phenytoin, lidocaine, chlordiazepoxide, propranolol, and probably others. A number of cases of drug toxicity has been reported during concurrent therapy with cimetidine. Other important interactions resulting from decreased metabolism are listed in Table 23–1. The interaction of phenylbutazone and warfarin is a good example of an important interaction with a complex mechanism. Warfarin exists as R and S stereoisomers, with the S isomer being five times more potent an anticoagulant than the R isomer. Since phenylbutazone displaces warfarin from plasma albumin, the normal occurrence would be for warfarin clearance to be increased by the interaction as more free drug becomes available for metabolism. In fact this is true for R warfarin, but the metabolism of the more potent S warfarin is inhibited so that unbound S warfarin accumulates although the total warfarin levels are unchanged or even decreased. It is the increased concentration of unbound S warfarin that results in enhanced anticoagulation.

In addition to inhibition of hepatic drug metabolism via mixed function oxidase, inhibition of metabolism at other enzyme sites can be important. Thus monoamine oxidase inhibitors can inhibit the metabolism of catecholamines and tyramine at multiple sites, allowing for build-up of these substances and the so-called "cheese reaction" due to enhanced catecholamine release with the ingestion of tyramine-containing foods. Allopurinol inhibits xanthine oxidase, which can be important for the metabolism of azathioprine and 6-mercaptopurine as well as for production of uric acid. If allopurinol is given, much less azathioprine or 6-mercaptopurine is needed for equivalent effects. As discussed above, ethanol can induce hepatic microsomal drug-metabolizing enzymes. However, if ethanol is present, it can also act as an inhibitor of drug metabolism. Thus drugs given to an individual who is intoxicated may have an enhanced effect, whereas drugs given to an individual who has been drinking chronically but is no longer intoxicated may have diminished effect.

TABLE 23–1. COMMON DRUGS AND THEIR INHIBITING AGENTS

Metabolism of	Inhibited by
Phenytoin	Isoniazid (in slow acetylators), chloramphenicol, cimetidine, clofibrate, phenylbutazone, disulfiram, sulfaphenazole, dicoumarol
Tolbutamide	Chloramphenicol, phenylbutazone, clofibrate, sulfaphenazole, dicoumarol
Warfarin	Phenylbutazone, alcohol, disulfiram, allopurinol, cimetidine, disopyramide, sulfinpyrazone, trimethoprim-sulfamethoxazole, metronidazole
Azathioprine, 6-mercaptopurine	Allopurinol
Catecholamines, tyramine	Monoamine oxidase inhibitors
Theophylline	Cimetidine, erythromycin, troleandomycin
Phenobarbital	Valproic acid

DIMINISHED RENAL EXCRETION. Some important drug interactions occur when active transport of one drug across the renal tubule is interfered with by another drug. Most of these interactions occur at the acid transport site. Thus probenecid is given to decrease penicillin clearance and thereby increase penicillin blood levels. Phenylbutazone can inhibit the renal clearance of hydroxyhexamide, an active metabolite of acetohexamide, and thereby increase its hypoglycemic effect. Salicylates, phenylbutazone, and probenecid can inhibit the renal elimination of methotrexate and enhance its effect.

Recently it has been shown that quinidine can inhibit the elimination of digoxin into the urine. The exact tubular site at which this interaction occurs is not known, but it is a significant interaction resulting in increased digoxin blood levels and effects. Verapamil probably also interacts with digoxin in the same way by inhibiting renal excretion.

Decreased renal excretion of lithium occurs when proximal tubular reabsorption of the ion is enhanced. Since lithium and sodium are handled similarly in the proximal tubule, anything that results in more proximal tubular sodium reabsorption will also affect lithium in the same way. Thus dietary salt restriction, salt depletion due to diarrhea, and diuretics acting at more distal segments of the nephron can reduce renal lithium excretion, requiring a reduction in lithium dose. Indomethacin also reduces lithium clearance, probably by enhancing proximal tubular reabsorption of the ion.

PHARMACODYNAMIC DRUG INTERACTIONS

There are numerous examples of drugs interacting with each other at receptor sites or having additive effects by acting at separate sites on cells. Thus vitamin K can inhibit the effects of warfarin. Propranolol can interact with epinephrine by blocking the beta-adrenergic receptors and thus allowing the alpha-adrenergic effects of epinephrine to be unopposed, which can result in severe hypertension. Clonidine has been shown to have its antihypertensive effects in man inhibited by tricyclic antidepressants. The mechanism for this is not entirely worked out but might be an interaction at an alpha-adrenergic receptor in the brain.

Examples of drugs producing additive effects are also common, such as the negative cardiac inotropic effects of disopyramide adding to the negative inotropic effects of beta-adrenergic blockers, producing heart failure. Two drugs that may affect the eighth cranial nerve, such as ethacrynic acid and aminoglycosides, may produce additional ototoxicity if given together. Drugs that affect neuromuscular function such as curare will have an enhanced effect if given with aminoglycosides, lincomycin, clindamycin, quinidine, or quinine, which also affect neuromuscular function.

Some drug interactions have not been well characterized, although the interaction is clearly significant. This is true for the interaction of warfarin with clofibrate. Clofibrate has a marked effect to increase the efficacy of warfarin, but there do not appear to be sufficient pharmacokinetic changes to account for this effect even though clofibrate may displace warfarin from plasma protein.

When viewed in perspective, drug interactions are only one of many factors that can alter the response of patients to drugs. Clinicians must be aware of the serious interactions and have well-defined therapeutic goals so that altered amounts or effects of drugs will become evident. The only way to accomplish this is to individualize therapy using effects or plasma drug levels when appropriate. This is particularly important for drugs with low therapeutic indices or during treatment of serious illnesses. Care must be used when a drug regimen is changed in any major way. If an interaction is appreciated, dosage adjustments can be made, and the two drugs often can be used together effectively. Drug interactions are an accepted fact of modern medical practice and should not be ignored, nor should they be overly feared.

Aarons L: Kinetics of drug-drug interactions: Pharmacol Ther 14:321, 1981. *This is a modelling approach to pharmacokinetic interactions that will be of interest to the mathematically oriented physician. The examples used and references cited are current.*

Hansten PD: Drug Interactions. 4th ed. Philadelphia, Lea and Febiger, 1979. *This frequently revised text is a useful compilation of known drug interactions. The interactions listed are referenced, and an estimate of probable clinical significance of the interaction is given.*

McElnay JC, D'Arcy PF: Protein binding displacement interactions and their clinical importance. Drugs 25:495, 1983. *This is a current review that emphasizes the fact that pure binding displacement interactions are unlikely to be of clinical significance.*

Serlin MJ, Breckenridge AM: Drug interactions with warfarin. Drugs 25:610, 1983. *Warfarin is a good model drug to study drug interactions, since its effects are easily measured, and hemorrhage is a readily detectable adverse effect. The several mechanisms of drug interactions affecting warfarin are reviewed with the relevant literature cited.*

Shand DG, Mitchell JR, Oates JA: Pharmacokinetic drug interactions. *In* Gillette JR, Mitchell JR (eds.): Handbook of Experimental Pharmacology, Vol 28, No 3. Concepts in Biochemical Pharmacology. New York, Springer-Verlag, 1975, pp 272–314. *This is a thorough review of pharmacokinetic mechanisms whereby drugs can interact. It is not a complete listing of potential drug interactions, although many illustrative examples for the various mechanisms are given.*

24. ADVERSE REACTIONS TO DRUGS

Alan S. Nies

Although difficult to quantify, there is little doubt that adverse reactions to drugs constitute an inevitable consequence of modern therapeutics. No drug is devoid of the potential to do harm, and benefit vs. risk decisions are made with every decision to start drug therapy. Most ill patients require multiple drugs, and this increases the risk not only of adverse drug reactions but of drug interactions as well. Frequently it is difficult to be certain that an adverse effect is due to an individual drug because of the confounding effects of the underlying disease and the use of multiple drugs.

Studies to determine the incidence of adverse reactions are derived largely from medical services at academic hospitals. The Boston Collaborative Drug Surveillance Program found a 5 per cent incidence of adverse drug reactions, most of which were minor and self-limited. Other studies have estimated a higher incidence, particularly in the very ill patient. In a recent study of complications on a medical ward, adverse drug effects were the largest contributor to iatrogenic events, accounting for 42 per cent of all such occurrences. About 18 per cent of patients admitted to the hospital had an adverse drug effect, and 19 per cent of these were life-threatening or resulted in serious disability. Drugs implicated in such studies include digitalis, theophylline, nitrates, lidocaine, other antiarrhythmics, anticoagulants, benzodiazepines, antihypertensives, and antibiotics.

The recent studies do not indicate that the incidence of adverse drug reactions is decreasing. On the contrary, the risk may be increasing as the number of potent drugs available increases. The studies assessing the incidence of drug problems in an academic medical center cannot be generalized to other therapeutic situations such as outpatient clinics, office practices, or community hospitals. Since one of the major determinants of a drug reaction is how ill the patient is and how many drugs he is receiving, it is likely that adverse drug reactions occur much less commonly in situations outside the large general hospital. Also, it is impossible with present data to make a quantitative statement of risk vs. benefit of medical therapy. It is clear that adverse reactions cannot be completely prevented even under the best of circumstances. Nonetheless, it is reasonable to continue investigation into ways to assess the risk and to reduce both the incidence and severity of these adverse reactions.

MECHANISMS OF ADVERSE DRUG REACTIONS

Unwanted effects of drugs are due to (1) exaggerated responses to the known effects of the drug; (2) immunologic reactions to the drug or its metabolites; and (3) toxic or "idiosyncratic" effects of a drug or its metabolite. The extension of the normal pharmacology accounts for most adverse drug effects. However, since these effects are predictable, they often may be avoided or treated by careful dosage adjustment without necessarily discontinuing drug treatment. The immunologically mediated and toxic adverse effects of drugs are less predictable and may be so severe as to require discontinuation of the offending drug. These latter effects are the least well understood, but mechanisms of some of the toxic drug effects have been discovered. Many reactions initially labelled immunologic may be due to other mechanisms. With time the mechanisms of the "idiosyncratic" drug reactions will be determined so that such reactions may be anticipated or avoided.

EXAGGERATED RESPONSES TO DRUGS

Excessive drug effects result from altered pharmacokinetics or altered target organ response, as have been discussed in the previous chapters. Thus adverse drug effects are more common in the elderly, in patients with abnormal renal or hepatic function, and in patients receiving other drugs that may result in pharmacokinetic or pharmacodynamic interactions. In addition, patients may have genetic abnormalities that make them susceptible to one or another effects of a drug. These genetic differences may be quantitative deviations from the norm or qualitative abnormalities. An example of such quantitative differences is the variability in hepatic drug oxidation that is described by a unimodal frequency distribution. Twin studies have indicated that genetic differences account for much of the variation between individuals in the metabolism of phenytoin, phenylbutazone, warfarin, ethanol, nortriptyline, and salicylate. In addition, several drug metabolic processes are controlled by genes at a single locus such as slow acetylation of isoniazid, some sulfonamides, and procainamide; deficient parahydroxylation of phenytoin; deficient N-glucosidation of amobarbital; and deficient hydrolysis of succinylcholine. The excessive drug effects resulting from the genetically determined slow metabolic processes reflect increased drug available at the site of action.

In addition to these quantitative differences in drug metabolism, there are genetic abnormalities that result in qualitatively different responses to drugs. These reactions are due to known properties of the drug that are usually not important but become markedly exaggerated owing to the genetic defect. Thus individuals with a deficiency of the enzyme activity of glucose-6-phosphate dehydrogenase (G-6PD) are unable to cope with the oxidative stress produced by some drugs, and hemolysis results. Drugs having this effect include primaquine, aspirin, sulfonamides, nitrofurantoin, sulfones, vitamin K, probenecid, quinidine, and quinine. In a similar manner, genetic deficiency of methemoglobin reductase results in inability to maintain hemoglobin in the ferrous form, resulting in methemoglobinemia upon exposure to some oxidizing drugs such as sulfones, sulfonamides, and nitrites. Likewise certain abnormal hemoglobins may be unstable and result in drug-induced hemolysis or methemoglobinemia. Frequently patients with these "pharmacogenetic" syndromes are unaware that there is any abnormality until they are challenged with a drug that produces the adverse effect.

Other genetic defects resulting in adverse drug reactions include the hepatic porphyrias. Individuals with acute intermittent porphyria have a defect in hepatic heme synthesis. When such individuals are given drugs that induce hepatic drug-metabolizing enzymes, the demand for heme increases, and a relative deficiency of heme is produced. As a consequence, there is an increased production of heme precursors that in some unknown way triggers the clinical syndrome of abdominal pain and neuropsychiatric symptoms.

TOXIC AND IMMUNOLOGIC REACTIONS

Adverse drug reactions in these categories are often lumped together because it is frequently difficult to be certain of the etiology of an individual reaction (Table 24–1). Some reactions that previously were considered to be immunologic have been shown to be toxic. The term "idiosyncratic" is often applied to interactions of this type whose etiology is unclear.

Toxic reactions include direct toxic effects of a drug on a target organ, such as the nephrotoxicity and ototoxicity produced by aminoglycosides. In other cases drugs are metabolized to reactive intermediates that can covalently bind to cellular components, often near the site of metabolism, and produce toxicity. This mechanism is well established for the hepatotoxicity produced by overdoses of acetaminophen. During therapeutic use of acetaminophen the small amount of reactive metabolite formed by oxidative metabolism is rapidly detoxified by interacting with reduced glutathione. With overdose, however, the glutathione is depleted, and the reactive metabolite attacks hepatic macromolecules, resulting in liver damage. Other sulfhydryl-containing compounds such as N-acetylcysteine or cysteamine can protect the liver by reducing the amount of toxic metabolite that remains unreacted with a sulfhydryl-containing compound. Other drugs may produce liver disease by somewhat similar mechanisms. Isoniazid-induced hepatitis may result from acetylation to acetyl isoniazid that can be hydrolyzed to acetyl hydrazine, which can be oxidized to a reactive metabolite. There remains considerable controversy regarding the relevance of this theory to the clinical hepatitis that results from isoniazid. It would, however, account for the observation that the incidence of hepatitis seems to be higher in individuals that are fast acetylators and thus form more acetyl hydrazine.

TABLE 24–1. "ALLERGIC" DRUG REACTIONS

Type of Reaction	Example (not inclusive)
Definite Immunologically Mediated Syndromes	
1. Immediate hypersensitivity (IgE-mediated) reactions	Penicillin-induced anaphylaxis Insulin-induced wheal and flare
2. Cytotoxic reactions	Drug-induced destruction of formed elements in the blood: Penicillin-induced hemolytic anemia Quinidine- or quinine-induced thrombocytopenia Phenylbutazone-induced granulocytopenia
3. Immune-complex induced vasculitis	Serum sickness–like reactions to penicillin, sulfonamides, and other drugs presenting as fever, rash, palpable purpura, arthralgia, and/or lymphadenopathy
4. Delayed-hypersensitivity reactions	Contact dermatitis from topically applied drugs
Possible Immunologically Mediated Syndromes but with Unknown Mechanism	
1. Skin rashes of various types	Many drugs and a variety of skin eruptions
2. Fever	Antibiotics, quinidine, methyldopa
3. Pneumonitis	Loeffler's syndrome
4. Lupus erythematosus-like	Procainamide, hydralazine
5. Hepatic dysfunction	Chlorpromazine-induced cholestasis ? Methyldopa-induced hepatitis
6. Renal dysfunction	Interstitial nephritis from methicillin, furosemide, allopurinol
7. Lymphadenopathy	Phenytoin, sulfonamides

Hepatocellular damage, such as that produced by methyldopa or halothane, is frequently felt to be immunologically produced. However, it is entirely possible that reactive metabolites could be important for these as well as a variety of other drugs that produce hepatotoxicity on occasion. The sequence of steps linking the binding of the drug metabolite to the hepatocellular damage is not clear. It is likely that immunologic reactions to the metabolite-macromolecule complex are important in some circumstances, whereas direct cellular damage by as-yet-unknown mechanisms is important for other cases.

Immunologic reactions to drugs probably result from the drug or a reactive metabolite combining with a protein to form an antigenic drug-protein complex that stimulates the immune response. Without such a reaction, most drugs, which have a molecular weight less than 1000, would not be able to elicit an immunologic response. The typical immunologic reaction requires a latent period of 10 to 20 days for stimulation of the production of antibodies and activated immune effector cells that cause the allergic reaction. After the initial exposure, however, the allergic reaction will occur with a much shorter or no latent period after re-exposure to the drug. Drug hypersensitivity can produce mediator release, initiate cell lysis, activate the complement system, or activate cellular hypersensitivity reactions.

The most dramatic allergic reaction is anaphylaxis or IgE-mediated hypersensitivity. Penicillin is the most common drug to produce anaphylaxis, but many other drugs or diagnostic agents (such as Bromsulphalein) can produce this life-threatening reaction. A history of penicillin allergy increases the risk of this reaction occurring, but most (75 per cent) of the 100 to 300 patients dying of penicillin-induced anaphylaxis each year have no history of penicillin allergy. Oral penicillin seems to have a lower incidence of reactions than parenteral penicillin.

Skin testing with penicilloyl polylysine, penicillin G, and penicilloic acid can identify patients at risk for anaphylaxis. Skin tests should be used if there is a history of penicillin allergy and penicillin therapy is felt to be mandatory. Some day it may be common to skin test all patients who are to receive penicillin, but this testing is not currently common practice.

Cytotoxic allergic reactions occur when the drug binds to the surface of a cell and is then attacked by antibody. Penicillin-induced hemolytic anemia is of this type. Immune complexes of drug and antibody may become adsorbed to the cell membrane, resulting in complement-mediated cytotoxicity. Thrombocytopenia and hemolytic anemia due to quinine or quinidine are examples of immune complex–mediated cytotoxicity. Methyldopa-induced Coombs positivity that occurs in up to 20 per cent of patients on therapy for over six months is of unknown etiology but results in antibodies directed at the Rh loci of the red cell. However, the continued presence of the drug is not necessary for the immune reaction to continue, and the Coombs positivity only gradually resolves upon discontinuation of the drug.

Circulating immune complexes of drug and antibody can produce serum sickness characterized by fever, rash, and sometimes lymphadenopathy, arthralgias, and nephritis. This syndrome is a vasculitis produced by deposition of immune complexes in the vasculature with activation of complement. Penicillin, sulfonamides, thiouracil, cholecystographic dyes, phenytoin, and other drugs can cause serum sickness, a term initially used to describe the reactions occurring after the administration of horse serum.

Drug-induced lupus syndromes as caused by procainamide, hydralazine, and isoniazid may be due to circulating immune complexes. In this case the drug or a reactive metabolite may interact with nuclear material to allow formation of antinuclear antibodies. The drug-induced SLE differs from spontaneous lupus by being uncommon in blacks and by only rarely causing nephritis. The acetylator phenotype also is important in drug-induced lupus. Hydralazine-induced lupus is very uncommon in fast acetylators. Procainamide-induced lupus occurs with smaller doses of drugs and at an earlier time after starting the drug in slow acetylators, although fast acetylators are also at risk.

Delayed hypersensitivity accounts for contact dermatitis produced by topically administered drugs. The role of cell-mediated reactions to organ damage, such as pneumonitis, produced by drugs is unknown.

In addition to the well-described immune phenomena outlined above, many other syndromes are attributed to drug allergy. These include a variety of skin rashes, drug fever, pulmonary reactions, hepatocellular or cholestatic reactions, interstitial nephritis, and lymphadenopathy. For most of these reactions, the exact immune mechanism is unknown, and it is possible that some of these reactions are due to direct toxic effects of a drug or metabolite rather than an immune mechanism. One interesting syndrome that is sometimes classified as immune but may involve other mechanisms as well is that of aspirin sensitivity. In some patients this syndrome resembles IgE-mediated allergy with rhinitis, sinusitis, nasal polyps, and asthma. However, other cyclooxygenase inhibitors, such as indomethacin and meclofenamate, also produce asthma in many of these patients, suggesting a possible etiologic role for an arachidonic acid metabolite, such as a leukotriene, rather than an immunologic mechanism. It seems likely that several syndromes of aspirin sensitivity exist, but the exact role of allergy vs. nonallergic mechanisms remains to be determined.

Some adverse drug reactions mimic anaphylactic reactions but are not immune mediated. Such reactions are due to direct release of mediators by drugs and are called anaphylactoid reactions. Reactions to radiocontrast dyes are of this type. The risk of re-exposure to the dye is unpredictable and skin testing is of no value. If re-exposure is absolutely necessary, pretreatment with steroids and antihistamines is the current practice.

RECOGNITION AND IDENTIFICATION

Adverse drug effects must first be suspected to be recognized. In some situations, the adverse effect mimics the illness being treated (for instance, arrhythmias caused by antiarrhythmic drugs or antibiotic-induced fever). In other instances, the reaction is more obviously drug induced, as is the case with characteristic skin rashes or an obvious excessive pharmacologic effect such as anticoagulant-induced bleeding. When an adverse drug effect is suspected, the offending agent should be discontinued. The first confirmation of an adverse reaction is its disappearance with drug withdrawal. In some cases it may be warranted to readminister the putative offending drug cautiously if it is likely that the drug will be required again for therapy. In the case of serious allergic or toxic reactions, however, it may be too dangerous to rechallenge the patient. Tests in vitro are occasionally helpful for drug-induced thrombocytopenia or hemolytic anemia but are not useful for most drug reactions. Skin testing is of value with penicillin, insulin, and horse serum.

Adverse reactions will continue to occur as long as potent drugs are available. Most of the reactions are predictable. The unexpected toxic and immunologic reactions remain a problem that continues to stimulate discussions as to how to detect rare adverse effects. During the process of drug development, reactions occurring less often than 1 per 1000 patients will not be detected. Therefore, the adverse effects of a new drug frequently are not discovered until after marketing. Different systems exist for early detection of drug reactions after marketing. A major mechanism for detection is an early warning that results from anecdotal reports by practicing physicians to pharmaceutical companies, drug regulatory agencies, or most commonly as letters published in general medical journals. Following the first alerts, a verification mechanism is required. It is in this area that much remains to be learned. Postmarketing surveillance of patients taking drugs will not be effective for uncommon drug reactions unless sample sizes of more than 100,000 patients are followed. Surveys of patients with certain diseases to determine the incidence of use of the drug suspected to have caused the illness (case-control study) may be a more efficient way to detect drug-induced illness for rare adverse effects. However, the alert practitioner has been and will continue to be the primary individual who makes the initial important observation that often provides the first clue to an unsuspected adverse drug reaction.

Davies DM (ed.): Textbook of Adverse Drug Reactions. Oxford, Oxford University Press, 1977. *This well-referenced book is organized by specific syndromes, with a discussion of the drugs that may cause the syndrome. General problems of detecting and verifying adverse reactions are also discussed.*

Jick H: The discovery of drug-induced illness. N Engl J Med 296:481, 1977. *This article by the principal investigator of the Boston Collaborative Drug Project discusses ways to discover drug reactions that occur primarily after marketing.*

Mitchell JR, Jollow DJ: Metabolic activation of drugs to toxic substances. Gastroenterology 68:392, 1975. *This is a review of adverse drug reactions that result from metabolism of drugs to reactive metabolites that covalently bind to tissue macromolecules.*

Patterson R, Anderson J: Allergic reactions to drugs and biologic agents. JAMA 248:2637, 1982. *Part of the "primer on allergic and immunologic diseases," this short review outlines the mechanisms of immunologic reactions to drugs. The authors provide relevant references and distinguish between allergic reactions for which the immune mechanisms are established and those that are only conjectured to be immunologically mediated.*

Steel K, Gertman PM, Crescenzi C, Anderson J: Iatrogenic illness on a general medical service at a university hospital. N Engl J Med 304:638, 1981. *This study of a medical service indicates an 18 per cent incidence of iatrogenic illness, of which 42 per cent were drug related.*

Venning GR: Identification of adverse reactions to new drugs. Br Med J 286:199, 289, 365, 458, 544, 1983. *This is a five-part series that describes how the 18 most important unsuspected drug reactions since thalidomide were discovered. The data are derived from physicians and from individuals in drug-regulatory agencies in several countries. The study points to the important role of the practicing physician in making and publicizing the initial observations that led to the discovery of the unsuspected adverse drug reaction.*

25. COMMON POISONINGS

William O. Robertson

DEFINITION. Man's chemical environment was recognized as a threat to his health long before the birth of Christ. Well-documented outbreaks of occupational mercury and lead "poisonings" had been recorded and preventive measures implemented by 200 B.C. The Middle Ages saw arsenic poisoning employed as a political weapon. More recent times have seen increasing recognition of industrial toxins, "accidental poisoning" in childhood, purposeful overdoses in adults, adverse reactions to drugs, and environmental hazards for all of us. The common theme is entrance of an exogenous chemical into an organism and subsequent disruption of its metabolism.The chemical causes themselves have undergone quantitative redefinition now that such ubiquitous substances as table salt and drinking water have been firmly established as being "poisonous." Finally, the host-organism itself has contributed to a better comprehension of the word "poison," as genetic variability has been recognized to determine the impact of a given molecule in such hereditary disorders as phenylketonuria, glucose-6-phosphate dehydrogenase deficiency, and others. As man's understanding of life has expanded, the connotation of poisoning has undergone substantial evolution.

ETIOLOGY. Approximately 1.2 million chemical entities had been identified and coded by 1950; the number had risen to more than 4.3 million by 1976. Between 1965 and 1983, 6.0 million new chemical entities were added. Although not all of these compounds have been marketed, many new organic compounds have appeared in the home and the workplace. For example, available formulations of pesticides have increased forty-fold over the past 30 years. Moreover, manufacturing processes have released additional compounds (e.g., dioxins) into the workplace or the environment with their capabilities of serving as poisons.

New chemical techniques have permitted prompt and complete identification of poisonings, and have uncovered the causes of such diverse entities as Minamata disease (teratogenesis consequent to methyl mercury), an outbreak of ascending paralysis affecting more than 4000 with more than 400 deaths in Iraq (also caused by methyl mercury), the "gray syndrome" in premature infants (caused by chloramphenicol), and an epidemic of angiosarcoma of the liver among industrial workers (caused by vinyl chloride). Nevertheless, many unknowns remain and justify careful monitoring of industry, of the home, and of the environment.

INCIDENCE. Over the past 25 years progressively more reliable data have been gathered about deaths from poisonings, the leading agents and the number of such deaths attributable to each among children less than five years old and among the overall population are given in Table 25–1. Although more than 150,000 cases of childhood poisonings are reported to the National Clearinghouse annually (with more than 125 deaths), many times that number occur as accidental ingestions each year. Among adults precise data are more difficult to retrieve. Incomplete data attest that a minimum of 12,000 deaths occur annually as a result of suicide by poisoning.

EPIDEMIOLOGY. There are significant contrasts in the epidemiology of accidental poisonings among children under five years of age compared with the remainder of the population. With adults, occupational and industrial exposures, suicide gestures or attempts, and homicides depend upon host factors and environmental settings as well as involved chemicals. In contrast, among children under five, host and environmental factors are less variable. In the United States, occurrences peak at 24 to 32 months of age, and more male than female children are involved; poisonings happen most frequently between 11 A.M. and 12 noon or between 5 and 6 P.M., and in places of easiest exposure—the kitchen, the bedroom, and the bathroom. In addition, illness in the family or "life stress situations" increase the likelihood of accidental ingestion.

TABLE 25–1. DEATHS DUE TO POISONINGS IN THE UNITED STATES, 1977, CATEGORIZED BY PROBABLE INTENT*

	Accidental		Suicidal	Undetermined	Homicidal
	Under Five Years of Age	*All Ages*	*All Ages*	*All Ages*	*All Ages*
Medication: total	57	2214	3125	791	
Salicylates and congeners	11	58	73	31	
Sedatives and hypnotics	4	363	847	118	
Psychotropic drugs	9	193	520	85	
Miscellaneous	33	1600	1685	557	
Nondrugs	37	1160	754	277	
Alcohol	0	337			
Petroleum and solvents	12	52			
Pesticides	7	34			
Corrosives	6	17			
Heavy metals	3	21			
Miscellaneous	9	699			
Gases and vapors	35	1596	2608	295	
Carbon monoxide	6	747	2092		
Total	129	4970	6487	1363	42

*From the National Center for Health Statistics, HRA, HEW; Reported in The National Clearinghouse for Poison Control Centers Bulletin, February 1980.

PREVENTION. Avoiding exposure to the toxin is the ultimate precaution; among adults, a variety of approaches have been employed—some with obvious effectiveness, others without. For example, the use of mercury in the felting process of hats has been outlawed since 1941; that source of mercury poisoning has disappeared in the hatting industry. Beryllium has been excluded from fluorescent light bulbs, and that source of exposure no longer exists. Similarly, where arsenic has been eliminated from pesticidal preparations and where naphthylamine has been eliminated from the rubber industry, human illness has been avoided. Some of these steps have resulted from legislative processes; others are the result of voluntary activity on the part of the industry or an aware public.

Among children some approaches have also proved effective; others are without much evidence of success. For example, efforts directed at altering toddlers' personalities in family settings have not proved effective. In contrast, the use of safety caps on medicine bottles had important consequences. For the ten-year period between 1959 and 1969, almost 100 deaths occurred annually from accidental salicylate poisoning in children under five; in 1978, only 12 such deaths were reported. Several variables have been cited as definitely contributory: (1) the manufacturers' voluntary reduction of the number of tablets as well as of the amount of aspirin per bottle; (2) the introduction of a favorable flavor to the "baby aspirin" as an attractive alternative to larger tablets; (3) programs of professional and public education; (4) the appearance of acetaminophen as a rival to aspirin, with its subsequent capture of 25 per cent of the analgesic-antipyretic market; and (5) the mandated use of safety caps or child-resistant containers, which had been documented as effective by Scherz and Stracener in 1969. All have had an impact, but current professional opinion holds that safety caps have contributed approximately 60 per cent of the variance. As safety caps have subsequently been applied to other prescription products and dangerous household items such as petroleum distillates and caustics, their impact has been felt there, also. Unfortunately, safety caps may have a negative effect among the geriatric population, among whom as many as 50 per cent cite them as contributing to their lack of compliance in taking prescribed medications.

Since 1953, more than 500 poison centers have been established across the country. The FDA's National Clearinghouse of Poison Control Centers is intended to serve as the coordinating unit; it also provides technical information to centers. In recent years, several microfiche systems—notably "Poisondex" (Micromedex, Denver)—have been developed to catalogue product information and to outline management approaches; they are capable of storing information on more than 250,000 products in a limited space and in an easily retrievable manner. Moreover, such microfiche systems avoid filing errors and permit updating of information on a quarterly basis. To date computer-based alternatives have not proved as efficient or effective as these microfiche systems.

Over the years the American Association of Poison Control Centers has served to produce educational material aimed at preventing poisoning, to establish standards for the operation of poison centers, to conduct self-assessment examinations for those staffing poison centers, and to implement a nationwide program aimed at regionalizing the poison center network. More recently, the American Academy of Clinical Toxicology and the American Board of Medical Toxicology have been developed to serve as the specialty society and certifying body, respectively, to further the academic and professional goals of physicians involved in such programs.

DIAGNOSIS. The diagnosis of an accidental (or a purposeful) poisoning can be made only if considered; this is particularly true for the small child with unexplained signs or symptoms. Once the possibility of poisoning is entertained, a careful search is made for a container and its label, or for a solid medication form and its drug-identifying imprint; next, the toxic potential of the substance can be verified from existing information or by contacting the nearest poison center. Often the presenting clinical signs and symptoms are so characteristic as to permit diagnosis—i.e., the hyperventilation (following vomiting) of acute salicylism, the extrapyramidal manifestations of phenothiazine reactions. On other occasions, analysis of specimens of body fluids—blood, urine, emesis, gastric contents, or stool—is necessary for diagnosis. As a generalization, "routine toxic screens" have proved to be of relatively little value in the child and are decried by many experts as inaccurate, confusing, and not helpful in the adult. Where the history or the environment provides a lead to the potential toxins, modern technology is proving increasingly useful. In the absence of such leads, helpful results are scarce.

Particularly helpful have been the passage of the Consumer Product Act of 1970 and the Commission Coordinating Safety Packaging Regulations, which have promulgated adequate labeling of hazardous substances across the country. *The label on the container is the single most useful information in accidental poisonings.* In the absence of a label, generic information about ingredients of household, industrial, and pharmaceutical products is available from a poison center or from a particularly useful textbook: Clinical Toxicology of Commercial Products. The information on the prescription bottle or the imprint of the solid medication form (such imprints exist on virtually all tablets and capsules) is equally important and ought to be diligently pursued.

Once the ingested poison has been identified, the problem remains to determine its potential for harm in the particular patient. That potential depends upon the amount ingested, the toxicity of the agent, and a variety of host factors. The amount ingested can sometimes be estimated by observers or by determining the amount of material remaining in the container. The toxicity of a particular poison can be assessed by reference to known data on human experiences, to animal LD50's, and to derivative "minimal lethal doses." One must be particularly cautious about overinterpreting LD50's or animal studies; in many instances the results are not transferable to the human. A toxicity rating has proved useful in estimating the degree of risk to the patient (Table 25–2).

In recent years, toxicologic analysis of body fluids has assumed an increasingly significant role in the diagnosis and management of poisoning, but it remains a relatively small one. Technical developments perfecting chemical analysis by mass spectrophotometry, gas-liquid chromatography, and spin resonance now allow toxic screening for a variety of poisons from minuscule amounts of body fluids. Commercial laboratories as well as a number of hospital, public health, and university laboratories provide qualitative and quantitative analyses for sedatives, narcotics, psychotropics, heavy metals, pesticides, and other compounds, all of which enable a speedy and accurate diagnosis. Nevertheless, such determination (e.g., specifying the type and amount of barbiturate in the blood) often does not alter management of the patient. Thus, in instances of barbiturate overdose, measurements of blood gases and pH prove more effective in coping with the clinical problem than does the quantitative determination of barbiturate level. Notable exceptions occur when specific quantification is critical in deciding on therapy—e.g., the use of acetaminophen blood levels and the Matthews-Rumack nomogram in deciding on the use of its antidote (N-acetylcysteine) before clinical signs or symptoms of illness appear, or the use of the serum salicylate concentration and the Done nomogram in determining the need for therapy in acute salicylate ingestion; and the value of the serum iron concentration along with clinical signs and symptoms in contemplating chelation therapy with desferrioxamine for iron poisoning. So too, identifying the presence of methyl alcohol or ethylene glycol can be critical in therapeutic management. Regardless of these several exceptions, the point remains that historical and physical features are usually paramount. Assisting the physician are a number of texts listed at the end of this chapter.

TABLE 25–2. TOXICITY RATING*

Rating	Probable Lethal Dose	
	mg/kg	*For 70-kg Man*
6—Super toxic	<5	A taste <7 drops
5—Extremely toxic	5–50	7 drops to 1 tsp
4—Very toxic	50–500	1 tsp to 1 oz
3—Moderately toxic	500 mg–5 grams	1 oz to 1 pint
2—Slightly toxic	5–15 grams	1 pint to 1 quart
1—Practically nontoxic	>15 grams	>1 quart

*From Gosselin RE, Hodge HC, Smith RP, Gleason MN: Clinical Toxicity of Commercial Products. Baltimore, Williams & Wilkins Company, 1976.

TREATMENT. Even before the ingested (or inhaled) substance has been identified and its toxic potential determined, first aid measures and supportive care ought to be initiated. Subsequent efforts are directed toward (1) preventing absorption of the substance; (2) curtailing its conversion in the body to its active form, or hastening its conversion to an inactive one; (3) neutralizing or counteracting its clinical effect; and (4) enhancing its excretion from the body. In the majority of instances, instituting measures to enable the patient to tolerate the temporary impact of the toxin and then to recuperate on his or her own remains the most effective course of action and often prevents subsequent poisonings as a result of overzealous treatment.

Supportive Measures. Prompt attention to supportive measures before a crisis has arisen, is, in fact, usually the single most critical element in managing the overdosed patient. The airway must be maintained, ventilation assured, cardiac output sustained, peripheral vascular collapse avoided, convulsions controlled, and hypertension and increased intracranial pressure lowered. Physical and chemical options ought to be carefully reviewed in advance of the patient's arrival if possible. Life support mechanisms can tide the patient over a period of compromised function as a result of anesthesia, an accidental overdose, or the purposeful induction of "barbiturate coma." But those measures must be carefully planned, carried out by skilled personnel, and monitored in detail if optimal benefit is to be achieved.

Prevention of Absorption. This is best accomplished in the conscious child or adult by *induction of emesis* as opposed to gastric lavage. Although gastric lavage has a traditional heritage in emergency medicine, its yield of ingested material falls short of the returns by emesis. Moreover, despite improved emergency transport systems, there are significant time delays in delivering the patient to a health care facility where lavage can be undertaken. During that time, significant absorption takes place. In contrast, efforts to induce vomiting can be initiated in the home—particularly if syrup of ipecac is already available there. If not, it is readily obtained from local pharmacies, 24-hour corner groceries, emergency vehicles, and neighbors. One should administer 15 ml to a child or 15 to 30 ml to an adult together with 200 to 300 ml of fluids—preferably water, soft drinks, or juices—and wait 10 to 15 minutes with an appropriate receptacle for vomiting to occur. If no vomiting ensues in 20 minutes, one should repeat the initial dose of syrup of ipecac and administer more fluids. If no syrup of ipecac is available, one should try gagging the patient but should be prepared for failure; one should then encourage the patient to drink 30 to 45 ml of liquid dishwashing detergents (anionic or nonionic but *not* cationic detergents) together with 240 ml of fluid. If the patient has already arrived in the emergency room, apomorphine can be used. It proves effective in four to five minutes but results in a drowsy patient despite use of naloxone. In all circumstances one should avoid table salt as an emetic agent; its use can compound the problem with acute hypernatremia. One should always avoid emesis in the comatose or convulsing patient, or the patient who has ingested a caustic. Syrup of ipecac proves effective in acute phenothiazine ingestions, but not in the face of chronic overdose; any form of emesis is maximally effective in the first one to one and a half hours after ingestion; seldom is it useful after two to three hours' delay.

Gastric lavage, using a large bore tube and 1000 to 3000 ml of half-strength saline as the rinse, is the only option for the unconscious patient. In patients over two years of age, concomitant use of a cuffed endotracheal tube is indicated to avoid aspiration. Despite the fact that most toxins are absorbed rapidly and thus escape delayed evacuation efforts, on occasion substantial portions of ingested agents have been recovered, especially in suicidal patients who have consumed poisons that delay gastric emptying, slow intestinal motility, or depress overall body function. In those instances attempts at evacuation are recommended, but cannot be expected to be effective in more than one of five patients.

Activated charcoal can be used to complement either of the measures discussed above, but not with syrup of ipecac until after emesis has occurred. The large surface area of charcoal permits significant adsorption of the toxin, precluding its absorption from the gut. Given by mouth or via nasogastric tube in amounts of 5 to 15 times the amount of the ingested toxin, activated charcoal has diminished absorption by as much as 50 per cent with significant therapeutic benefits. Recent pharmacologic research supports the contention that absorption may be prevented by early intervention with charcoal, but equally importantly, finds that excretion of those compounds that are recycled via the gastrointestinal tract can be significantly increased by repetitive oral instillation of activated charcoal.

Cathartics, laxatives, enemas, and *colonic irrigations* are "heroic" measures devoid of evidence of effectiveness; in fact, cathartics increase the rate of absorption of barbiturate.

Inhibition of metabolism of a potential toxin to its active form and conversion to an inactive form are limited options, but, when feasible, they may prove beneficial. For example, methyl alcohol becomes active only after it is converted to formaldehyde and formic acid; administering ethyl alcohol to the patient takes advantage of substrate competition (it is favored over methyl alcohol by the enzymatic processes involved), permitting significant reduction in the rate of metabolism of methyl alcohol, resulting in a diminished amount of formaldehyde and formic acid, which in turn can be more easily scavenged by existent metabolic processes. Currently clinical studies are underway exploring the possible augmentation of enzyme systems—particularly the p-450 cytochrome oxidase pathway—to hasten inactivation of certain toxins.

In other instances, enhancement of enzymatic activity may *activate* a toxin. For example, pretreatment of the pregnant woman and fetal liver with phenobarbital will enhance conjugation of bilirubin, but such pretreatment augments the conversion of carbon tetrachloride to its deleterious metabolite.

Chelating agents also limit the entry of certain toxins into metabolic pathways and augment excretion of the inactivated material. This approach has been particularly useful in poisonings by heavy metals—treatment of arsenic, mercury, and lead with dimercaprol (BAL), D-penicillamine, and edetate (EDTA), respectively. Similarly, desferrioxamine is useful in both acute and chronic iron poisoning.

Specific antidotes to counteract the effects of specific toxins are limited to a few compounds, but when one exists its usefulness is great. Paramount is the example of naloxone, an opiate derivative, which, when administered in adequate amounts (often *considerably more* than the recommended 0.4 mg) to a patient with heroin overdose, results in the patient's sitting up and talking within 20 seconds! Administered to the nonoverdosed patient, naloxone is devoid of any action, thus constituting a unique example of an antagonist drug without any agonist effects. Most other antidotes have agonist as well as antagonist effects. Common examples of such antidotes include atropine for organophosphate and carbamate insecticide poisoning, methylene blue for methemoglobinemia, physostigmine for anticholinergic syndromes (as from tricyclic antidepressants, antihistamines, or atropine), nitrites plus thiosulfate for cyanide ingestion, N-acetylcysteine for acetaminophen overdoses, and diphenhydramine for phenothiazine-induced extrapyramidal reactions.

Enhancing elimination of a toxin can be accomplished by several mechanisms. For example, in carbon monoxide poisoning, use of 100 per cent oxygen by ventilatory mask has both theoretical and practical benefit. In instances of phencyclidine ingestion, continuous gastric lavage, taking advantage of "ion trapping" of the recycled phencyclidine via the gastric mucosa, is reported to be effective. Ion trapping is also employed in acute salicylate poisoning via alkalinization of the urine. In the kidney tubule, free salicylate molecules ionize in the presence of an alkaline medium and are not resorbed, thus being "captured" in the urine and excreted into the bladder. In contrast, amphetamine (a weak base) is captured in the kidney tubule by acidifying the urine with ascorbic acid or ammonium chloride. In general, osmotic diuresis, particularly chemical diuresis with common diuretics (e.g., furosemide), is of little or no benefit in enhancing the excretory processes.

By contrast, *dialysis* and *hemoperfusion* have proved to be effective therapeutic tools, although perhaps not as effective as had been initially believed. For example, a decade ago many patients with barbiturate overdose were subjected to extracorporeal or peritoneal dialysis; today, less than one in 300 such patients is so treated. If renal shutdown has occurred, as in mercury poisoning, dialysis will prove lifesaving, although it is unlikely to augment excretion of the mercury molecule. Exceptions do exist, as in dialysis for ethylene glycol overdoses. Hemoperfusion and lipid dialysis both serve as effective mechanisms in eliminating specific offending substances from the body, e.g., ethchlorvynol. To be effective, a significant proportion of the total body toxin must be present in the blood and must not be tightly bound to serum protein. For many compounds, such as digoxin, tricyclic antidepressants, and phenothiazines, these conditions are not met, and dialysis and hemoperfusion do little to reduce the total body burden of toxin. Knowledge of the "apparent volume of distribution" of a compound permits prediction of the usefulness of dialysis or hemoperfusion.

Occasionally, still other techniques, such as *exchange transfusions* in boric acid or iron poisoning, may be useful. So-called gut lavage, a virtually continuous through-and-through rinse of the bowel via instillation of large amounts of physiologic fluids into the intestine through a nasogastric tube, has been reported effective in paraquat overdoses when no alternatives exist. Careful consideration of the metabolic pathways of the involved substance combined with empiric evidence of previous outcomes serves as the best guide for management.

Treatment of Specific Common Poisonings. In addition to the general principles of treatment discussed above, a few common poisonings warrant specific mention; more details of management are available from standard texts or local poison centers or through physician consultation mechanisms.

Aspirin (salicylate) poisoning formerly accounted for 20 per cent of ingestions among children under five years of age; today, it is responsible for only 1 to 2 per cent. Acute ingestions in excess of 100 mg per kilogram of body weight deserve induction of emesis; aspirin leads to rapid metabolic acidosis in children under four years of age and to initial respiratory alkalosis in the adult. Both groups vomit; this permits early detection and helps in differentiation from acetaminophen ingestion. Alkalinizing the urine proves remarkably effective with the single acute ingestion; one should consult the Done nomogram for prognosis. The administration of intravenous $NaHCO_3$ (3 mEq per kilogram of body weight) to young children usually proves effective in raising urine pH above 7.0. A later second or third dose of approximately half that amount may be necessary to sustain alkalinization of the urine and thereby to promote ionization and reduce reabsorption of salicylate. Urinary elimination of the salicylate moiety removes the cause of the acidosis—a far more effective approach to therapy than treatment of the systemic acidosis itself. In the adult, initial blood pH may be elevated; nonetheless, it is the urine pH that is critical to monitor. In general, additional potassium administration is necessary only for the chronically intoxicated patient or later in the course of acute intoxications in adults. Occasionally dialysis may be warranted, but ordinarily general supportive measures prove sufficient. Chronic overdoses are far less responsive to any specific interventions.

Acetaminophen has captured 30 per cent of today's analgesic-antipyretic market; liquid formulations are being augmented by solid preparation forms, some of which are in "extra strength" dosages. In Britain, acetaminophen has been a particularly popular suicidal substance; management is often complicated by the fact that no significant symptoms may appear until after irreversible liver damage has occurred. If recognized early—preferably less than 12 hours and certainly less than 24 hours after ingestion—determination of the serum level and comparison of it against standards on the Matthews-Rumack nomogram permit an appropriate decision about the possible use of an antidote, either N-acetylcysteine or methionine (both sulfhydryl donors). Both appear to enter into metabolic pathways via glutathione mechanisms and to preclude the formation of an epoxide derivative of acetaminophen which binds covalently to liver macromolecules, resulting in liver cell destruction. An intravenous preparation of the antidote is available that is strongly favored and widely used in Britain. Currently only an oral form is available in the United States, and its use presents difficulties. Of special note is the apparent diminished susceptibility to toxicity in the preadolescent compared with the adult.

Significant overdoses of *anticholinergic substances* in various forms (e.g., atropine, tricyclic antidepressants, antihistamines, phenothiazines, jimson weed) produce fever, flushing, widely dilated pupils, and CNS signs and symptoms varying from somnolence and coma to delirium and seizures. Each of these specific drugs may also produce additional specific symptoms by other mechanisms—e.g., Benadryl occasionally results in extrapyramidal reactions; tricyclic antidepressants cause cardiac arrhythmias. For this class of drugs, physostigmine is available both as a diagnostic agent and as a therapeutic substance for managing seizure. The dose is 0.5 mg administered slowly intravenously for the child under five, and 1 to 2 mg for the adult, repeated as often as necessary to control seizures. In all instances atropine should be immediately available during physostigmine infusion. Tricyclic antidepressant overdoses are now numerically the most serious of prescription medicine hazards. These are best approached by using diazepam (Valium) or phenobarbital to control seizures, by maintaining a blood pH above 7.45 to prevent tachyarrhythmias, and by use of conventional cardiac drugs should arrythmias ensue.

Acute petroleum distillates (hydrocarbons) cause their most significant damage as a function of their initial action on the lungs via aspiration; aspiration is virtually always thought to occur at the time of ingestion or inhalation. Both in laboratory animals and in humans, large amounts of various petroleum distillates have been consumed and retained without development of any signs or symptoms save for odoriferous eructations ("smelly burps") and diarrhea. As a general rule, neither lavage nor induction of emesis is indicated in such ingestions unless some additional toxin (e.g., parathion) has been dissolved in the hydrocarbon. When such is the case, induction of emesis has supplanted gastric lavage as the treatment of choice. When pulmonary aspiration has occurred, supportive measures are introduced; antibiotics and steroids are widely used but without much evidence of effectiveness.

Carbon monoxide (see Ch. 560) ranks high as a contributor to common poisonings, suicides, and accidental deaths. The mechanism of action involves acute interruption of both oxygen transport and oxygen metabolism, with a rapid cessation of life functions. Prompt recognition of exposure and removal of the patient from the contaminated environment are essential. Hastening of excretion of carbon monoxide by administration of oxygen and consideration of hyperbaric oxygen treatment are currently the hallmarks of management.

Caustic compounds, including acids and alkalis, appear to exert their toxic effects largely via alterations of pH and their consequences on the gastrointestinal tract. Experimental evidence suggests that the damage done by alkalis is complete within 30 seconds after exposure; that done by acids may be somewhat slower to appear. Current recommendations of management are avoidance of major efforts to empty the gastrointestinal tract, neutralization of the offending compound by the administration of a protein-containing substance (such as milk), and careful assessment of the esophagus for the possibility of acute burns. This last point frequently necessitates esophagoscopy because the presence or absence of burns in the mouth proves nonpredictive of the status of the esophagus. In addition to concerns about the acute situation—managed by dilatation, steroids, and antibiotics—much interest now focuses on follow-up for 20 to 40 years because of a significantly increased risk of carcinoma of the esophagus.

Cyanide has gained its deserved reputation for toxicity by its ability to inhibit oxygen utilization at the level of the cell via cytochrome oxidase inhibition. Most exposures are occupational; occasional exposures are the result of homicidal efforts, and rare consequences are found subsequent to Laetrile administration or nitroprusside overdose. As soon as cyanide poisoning is suspected, administration of nitrite—via a 3 per cent solution intravenously or amyl nitrite inhalation—is crucial. It converts hemoglobin to methemoglobin, which selectively binds cyanide. This is followed by administration of sodium thiosulfate to convert cyanide to the less toxic thiocyanate. Recent experience in Europe suggests the use of dicobalt edetate may be even more effective.

Drugs of abuse haunt the profession, the emergency room, and our society. Were the offending agent easily identified with certainty—e.g., heroin—the remedy would be obvious—naloxone. Such instances are almost nonexistent; more than 90 per cent of what is bought and sold "on the street" is not what it has been represented to be. Even imprinted capsules have been counterfeited in efforts to "con" the buyer. In other instances the basic ingredient has been "cut" with an inert substance or "laced" with some other psychoactive substance. Enormous geographic variations seem to exist across the country, with phencyclidine ("angel dust," PCP) being particularly popular in Los Angeles and Detroit, Ritalin in Seattle, and heroin and cocaine in New York.

The laboratory may be helpful in instances of opiate overdoses but is of virtually no value for LSD or PCP (see Ch. 481). As a consequence, symptomatic management predominates; the unconscious or convulsing adult may routinely be approached as a potential heroin addict, an alcoholic, or a hypoglycemic individual; the hyperactive, "spacey" patient prompts consideration of PCP, LSD, and related sympathomimetic agents (amphetamine, phenylpropanolamine, etc.), as well as psychosocial decompensation. Supportive measures may include monitoring, restraints, sedatives (diazepam is "customary"), hydration, and ventilatory and cardiac measures. As a generalization, the acute management proves far more successful than treatment of the underlying problem, but efforts ought to be directed at the latter, as it provides the only true solution to the basic problem.

Ethyl alcohol (see Ch. 482) is mentioned here to stress its ubiquity and the epidemiologic point that it is remarkably prevalent as a cause of admission to hospital for children, with both purposeful and accidental ingestions, as well as a cause of birth defects among newborns. Also, ethyl alcohol augments the potential toxicity of a number of other compounds, such as diazepam.

Halogenated hydrocarbons (including chlorinated insecticides such as chlorophenothane, or DDT) serve as a source of a myriad of occupational, industrial, and pharmacologic exposures. Almost invariably lipid soluble, most are readily absorbable by the gastrointestional tract, the respiratory epithelium, or the skin. Fortunately, most are metabolically rather stable compounds within the human organism; thus production of still more hazardous metabolites is minimized. Nonetheless, many of the compounds gain access to fat storage deposits or neural tissue and cause both central and peripheral nervous system symptoms. For some (e.g., 2,3,7,8-tetrachlorodibenzodioxin, or dioxin) there are concerns about long-term toxicity and teratogenicity. Treatment modes include elimination of subsequent exposures, attempts to retrieve unabsorbed quantities from the gastrointestinal tract, and general supportive measures in response to symptoms.

Iron salts ($FeSO_4$, Fe gluconate) represent a hazard confined almost exclusively to children who "accidentally" consume prenatal tablets. To date only three cases of acute poisoning have been reported worldwide in adults. While initial reports of a 50 per cent mortality rate were greatly inflated (instead it hovers at approximately 1 per cent), iron poisoning typifies the problem of the "unsuspected toxin" about which parents, parent surrogates, and physicians may be uninformed. When ingestions are known to exceed 50 to 60 ml per kilogram or when serum levels (taken 3 to 6 hours after ingestion) exceed 400 to 500 micrograms per deciliter, observation and chelation with desferrioxamine ought to be seriously considered, particularly if clinical symptoms such as upper abdominal pain, nausea, and vomiting are present. Management of the acute ingestion calls for prompt gastric emptying and instillation of a 5 per cent solution of sodium bicarbonate into the stomach in an attempt to minimize absorption of the resultant ferrous carbonate compound. More serious overdoses have prompted heroic measures, including surgical extirpation of ingested tablets and attempts at exchange transfusion. To date, studies have documented no serious consequences from ingestion of iron as a component of children's chewable vitamin preparations.

Methanol and *ethylene glycol* present significant problems of metabolic acidosis in clinically poisoned patients. Diagnosis is often considered following discovery of an unexplained anion gap. These compounds both depend upon alcohol dehydrogenase for their metabolism. The current approach to therapy takes advantage of this situation and provides ethanol (5 to 10 grams per hour intravenously) as a competitive inhibitor of toxin metabolism—thus slowing the formation of toxic metabolites, formaldehyde and formic acid from methanol, or glycoaldehyde, glycolic, glyoxylic, and oxalic acids from ethylene glycol, to rates of formation at which these products can be disposed of by ordinary metabolic or excretory pathways. In contrast, for large overdoses hemodialysis may be required to eliminate the offending toxin.

Organophosphate and carbamate insecticides can both prove exquisitely toxic in minute amounts. The mechanism of action involves inhibition of acetylcholine metabolism via cessation of cholinesterase function. Prompt recognition of symptoms secondary to acute exposure can prove lifesaving. Detecting symptoms secondary to acute exposure can prove lifesaving. Detecting symptoms secondary to chronic exposure (e.g., peripheral neuropathy) can serve to eliminate much patient distress and employee unhappiness. In general, acute distress is ushered in via excessive secretions in the upper airway, with respiratory distress, diffuse muscular weakness, nausea, vomiting, and collapse. Treatment requires prompt and repeated administration of large amounts of atropine for both types of poisoning. Pralidoxime (2PAM) is also strongly recommended to assist in the rejuvenation of cholinesterase levels. Introduced in large measure as a "safer" replacement for DDT, these compounds have been responsible for large numbers of acute poisonings but, as far as can be determined, are yet to be implicated in carcinogenicity, teratogenicity, or chronic liver disease.

Paraquat (and its associated congeners) is a particularly popular and effective herbicide. While controversy rages about the consequences of environment exposures, no controversy exists on the issue of acute, purposeful overdoses; they are devastating. Paraquat is a harsh gastrointestinal irritant that also inhibits renal function; its most destructive impact is on the respiratory tract, where it inhibits superoxide dismutase and kills via "oxygen toxicity." Current approaches to therapy favor such dramatic efforts as "gut lavage," with some suggestion that hemoperfusion might be warranted. However, it is uniformly agreed that overdoses are likely to be lethal.

Theophylline and its congeners have been recognized as inducing seizures, cardiac arrhythmias, and occasional deaths in overdose situations. More recently "therapeutic misadventures" have been recognized; inadvertent overdoses, alterations of theophylline metabolism by viral infections and nutritional variations, and the tendency to use theophylline in large quantities for relatively minor illnesses all increase the likelihood of such occurrences. Children seem more resistant to the serious side effects than do adults, but occasionally both groups may have to be considered for hemoperfusion. Peritoneal and extracorporeal hemodialysis have both been reported to be ineffective.

Although ingestions of *plants and plant elements* constitute the single most frequent reason for telephoning poison centers, the overall problem is best put in perspective by Fraser's analysis of Britain's most recent 20-year experience with poisonings:

"Plants are the most overrated poisons of childhood. In earlier decades there were occasional deaths, most caused by the umbelliferae (particularly hemlock water dropwort) and the solanaceae (various nightshades). From 1958 to 1977 there were three deaths, and in one the role of the ingestion in the child's demise is doubtful. The others were caused by hemlock and by *Amanita phalloides* (death cup), both in children aged five and nine. Laburnum is frequently cited as the most toxic and commonly fatal poisonous plant in both children and adults, but there appears to be no report this century of childhood poisoning death. One adult death in unusual circumstances has been recorded."

Chemical hazards have always been a way of life. Today their numbers continue to escalate. As a consequence, the physician is well advised to add poisoning to the differential diagnosis for any unexplained collection of signs or symptoms in a patient of any age. Moreover, unless the physician is confident of the timeliness and completeness of his or her understanding about a specific item, additional consultation is strongly advised.

Arena J: Poisoning: Chemistry, Symptoms and Treatment. Springfield, IL, Charles C Thomas, 1979. *Derived from years of experience and leadership in the poisoning field, this book is well organized, carefully edited, and readable, with a remarkable collection of cases and common sense.*

Doull J, Klassen CD, Amdur MD: Toxicology: The Basic Science of Poisons. 2nd ed. New York, Macmillan, 1980. *This text constitutes the "compleat" basic science approach for the toxicologist. With 42 contributors and critical editing, the final product covers the field from salt to water to radiation.*

Dreisbach RH: Handbook of Poisoning. 11th ed. Los Altos, Calif., Lange Publishing Company, 1983. *This pocket-sized book is both comprehensive and concise. Up-to-date and always helpful to review for omissions in one's approach, it proves particularly valuable to the primary care physician.*

Fraser NC: Accidental poisoning deaths in British children, 1958–77. Br Med J 280:1595, 1980. *An unusually concise and comprehensive review of 20 years' experience.*

Gosselin RE, Hodge HC, Smith RP, Gleason MN: Clinical Toxicology of Commercial Products. 5th ed. Baltimore, Williams & Wilkins Company, 1976. *Long established as the "bible" of the field, this compendium provides a concise overview of poisoning issues, as well as a thorough and well-edited clinical description of approximately 50 generic poisonings. It has a comprehensive listing of trade-name entities and generic items in household and commercial product fields. Authoritative the world over.*

Haddad LM, Winchester JF: Clinical Management of Poisoning and Drug Overdose. Philadelphia, WB Saunders Company, 1983. *A recent book with contri-*

butions chiefly by American experts, this is currently the definitive text for the recognition and clinical management of poisoning.

Proudfoot A: Diagnosis and Management of Poisoning. Oxford, Blackwell Scientific Publications, 1982. *Stemming from the extensive experiences of Edinburgh's Regional Poison Center, this clinically oriented manual ought to prove of special benefit to physicians seeking instantaneous updates on management concepts.*

Journals: Virtually any clinical journal may prove the source of a fascinating case report or a valuable review in the field of poisoning. Lancet, JAMA, N Engl J Med, and the traditional medical and pediatric specialty journals are particularly valuable resources. In the more limited field of clinical toxicology the following are of note: (1) Veterinary and Human Toxicology: The official journal of the American Association of Poison Control Centers and the American Academy of Clinical Toxicology. (2) The American Journal of Emergency Medicine, newly published by W. B. Saunders Company. (3) Clinical Toxicology: A blend of industrial, environmental, and accidental cases appears here, together with results of bench research. (4) Emergency Medicine: A controlled circulation journal particularly noted for "The Toxic Emergency," a monthly contribution of Alan Done.

26. PHARMACOLOGIC PRINCIPLES RELATED TO THE AUTONOMIC NERVOUS SYSTEM

Robert J. Lefkowitz

ORGANIZATION AND PHYSIOLOGY OF THE AUTONOMIC NERVOUS SYSTEM

The autonomic nervous system regulates the functions of smooth muscle, the heart, and glands. It is composed of two major divisions, termed sympathetic and parasympathetic, which are anatomically, physiologically, and biochemically quite distinct. Activation of the sympathetic system leads to the classic "flight or fight" responses of tachycardia, increased force of cardiac contraction, vasoconstriction, mydriasis, bronchodilation, and hyperglycemia. Parasympathetic nervous activity results in a situation better exemplified by "an old man sleeping after dinner," with slow heart rate, noisy respirations (caused by bronchial constriction), meiosis, and saliva running out of the corner of his mouth. Auscultation of the abdomen would reveal loud bowel sounds.

Anatomically, the *sympathetic nervous system* is composed of pathways that originate from neurons with cell bodies in the "thoracolumbar" segments of the spinal cord. These preganglionic neurons synapse in the sympathetic ganglia with postganglionic neurons, which in turn innervate end-organs, including vascular, gastrointestinal, and genitourinary smooth muscle and the heart.

By contrast, the *parasympathetic pathways* originate from neurons that have their cell bodies in the "craniosacral" portions of the neuraxis, including the midbrain, the medulla, and the sacral portions of the spinal cord. Preganglionic fibers synapse in peripheral ganglia that are in general closer to innervated organs than is the case with the sympathetic system.

Communication between neurons in the autonomic nervous system, and between neurons and effector cells, is mediated by chemicals called neurotransmitters. Acetylcholine encodes communication between preganglionic and postganglionic neurons in both the sympathetic and parasympathetic nervous systems. Norepinephrine is generally the neurotransmitter at sympathetic postganglionic nerve endings, whereas acetylcholine is the transmitter at parasympathetic postganglionic nerve endings.

The *adrenal medulla* is anatomically and functionally analogous to the sympathetic ganglia. Its chromaffin cells are innervated by typical preganglionic fibers. The major product of the adrenal medulla is epinephrine, which is secreted into the bloodstream. Epinephrine has many of the same biologic activities as the sympathetic neurotransmitter norepinephrine. Because of the strong analogies and the concerted physiologic functioning of the sympathetic system and the adrenal medulla

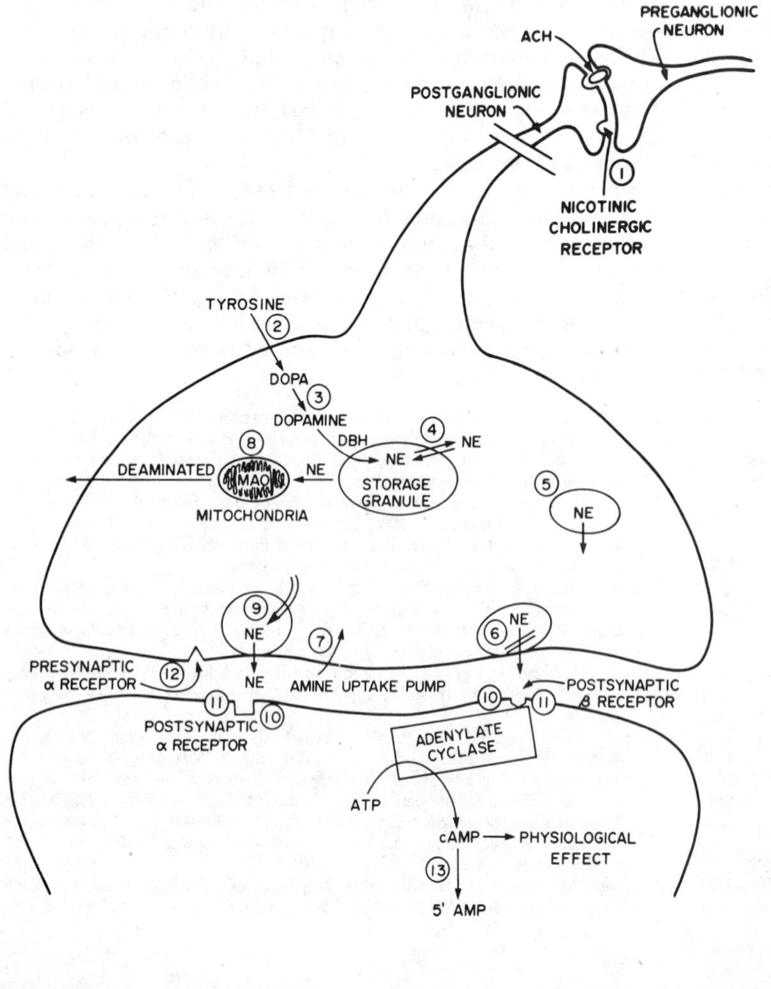

Figure 26–1. Therapeutic interventions in the peripheral adrenergic nervous system. Abbreviations: ACH = acetylcholine; DBH = dopamine beta hydroxylase; DOPA = dihydroxyphenylalanine; NE = norepinephrine; MAO = monoamine oxidase. (1) Competitive antagonism of nicotinic cholinergic receptors on postganglionic neuron in autonomic ganglia, e.g., trimethaphan. (2) Inhibition of transmitter (norepinephrine) synthesis, e.g., alpha methyl-p-tyrosine. (3) Drugs that enter the normal biosynthetic pathway and are transformed into "false neurotransmitters," e.g., alpha-methyldopa→→alpha-methylnorepinephrine. (4) Drugs that prevent the storage of transmitter in granules by inhibiting transport across storage granule membrane, e.g., reserpine. (5) Drugs that deplete transmitter from granules by displacement, e.g., guanethidine. (6) Drugs that inhibit the release of norepinephrine, e.g., bretylium. (7) Drugs that deplete neuronal norepinephrine by blocking the amine transport system of the neuronal membrane, e.g., cocaine or imipramine. Another major mechanism for the termination of norepinephrine action is by metabolism by catechol-o-methyl transferase. (8) Inhibition of metabolic destruction of transmitter, e.g., monoamine oxidase inhibitors. Relation of enzyme inhibition to therapeutic effects not clear, e.g., pargyline. (9) Indirectly acting agonists that displace norepinephrine from storage granules, e.g., tyramine, amphetamine (solely indirect), ephedrine, and metaraminol (also have direct actions). (10) Blockade of postsynaptic alpha receptors (e.g., phentolamine, phenoxybenzamine, prazosin) or beta receptors (propranolol). (11) Agonists that occupy postsynaptic receptors and mimic the effect of the neurotransmitter, e.g., isoproterenol (beta), phenylephrine (alpha). (12) Presynaptic alpha-adrenergic receptors. Although agonists and antagonists that specifically act through these receptors are not in general use, some adverse effects of other drugs, e.g., tachycardia after phentolamine administration, may be due to occupancy of these receptors. (13) Inhibition of breakdown of cyclic AMP by phosphodiesterase, e.g., aminophylline.

in situations such as stress or fright, these two components are often considered a unified "sympathoadrenal system."

NEUROTRANSMITTERS. A great deal is known about the biochemical basis of neurotransmission as mediated by norepinephrine in the sympathetic and acetylcholine in the parasympathetic system. Several discrete processes have been identified and elucidated. These include the mechanisms of (1) biosynthesis of transmitter in nerves, (2) storage of transmitter within granules in sympathetic and parasympathetic nerve endings, (3) release of transmitter at synapses, (4) interaction of transmitter with receptors on effector cells, and (5) termination of transmitter activity by reuptake and/or metabolizing processes.

There is a great diversity of physiologic autonomic effects and, because so much is known about neurotransmitter function, therapeutic interventions that modify autonomic function are among the most rational and important at the physician's disposal. For both the sympathetic and parasympathetic nervous system an understanding of the basic organization and physiology permits predictions of not only therapeutic but also adverse effects of a wide variety of drugs. The purpose of this chapter is to delineate the general principles underlying pharmacologic approaches that modify autonomic nervous system function. Although examples are provided, the reader is referred to other chapters for details of dosage, administration, and specific indications of individual drugs in disease states.

Each of the processes described above, including biosynthesis, uptake and storage in granules, release, receptor binding, and degradation of neurotransmitters, is susceptible to pharmacologic manipulation. A much wider variety of therapeutic interventions is possible in the sympathetic system than in the parasympathetic system, and these are summarized in Figure 26–1.

For the parasympathetic system the major clinical interventions involve drugs that act as agonists or antagonists at postsynaptic muscarinic receptors. Agents are also available which, by inhibiting the destruction of acetylcholine, lead to cholinergic agonist effects at postsynaptic receptors (cholinesterase inhibitors). Botulinus toxin appears to cause neuromuscular blockade by blocking release of acetylcholine from cholinergic nerves.

ADRENERGIC AND CHOLINERGIC RECEPTORS

Of the therapeutic interventions indicated in the figure, the most important relate to drugs that stimulate or block the postsynaptic receptors for adrenergic and cholinergic neurotransmitters. The concept that there are specific receptor molecules that mediate the effects of hormones has been popular throughout most of this century. This hypothesis has gained additional support over the past decade from radioligand binding studies, which have permitted the direct identification of these sites in cells with radioactively labeled drugs. Some of these receptors have been partially or completely purified.

Any discussion about receptors depends on certain essential pharmacologic concepts. Adrenergic receptors are the cellular sites at which catecholamines or related drugs are initially bound. The binding of drugs with adrenergic receptors induces changes in the receptors, which then lead to a series of events in the cell resulting in the characteristic physiologic effects of the drug. Thus adrenergic receptors are recognition sites on the plasma membrane that transduce the interaction of catecholamines with the cell into a physiologic response. Agonist drugs are those capable of inducing a response. A "full" agonist causes a maximal response, whereas a "partial" agonist causes a qualitatively similar response of lesser magnitude. An "antagonist" is a drug that interacts with the receptor but elicits no response on its own. However, by occupying the receptor an antagonist may reduce the effect of an agonist. The "intrinsic activity" of a drug is a measure of its maximal effect. The intrinsic activities of full agonists are defined to be 1.0, whereas those of antagonists are 0. Partial agonists have intrinsic activities greater than 0 but less than 1.

The interaction of a drug with a receptor involves the notion

TABLE 26–1. SOME EXAMPLES OF ADRENERGIC RECEPTOR MEDIATED RESPONSES

$Beta_1$-adrenergic receptors	
	Heart—positive inotropism
	Adipose tissue—lipolysis
$Beta_2$-adrenergic receptors	
	Vascular smooth muscle—relaxation
	Bronchial smooth muscle—relaxation
$Alpha_1$-adrenergic receptors	
	Vascular smooth muscle—contraction
$Alpha_2$-adrenergic receptors	
	Platelets—aggregation
	Presynaptic nerve terminal—inhibition of norepinephrine release

of affinity or potency. Affinity is a measure of the avidity or tightness with which a drug combines with a receptor. The greater the affinity of a drug for a receptor, the lower the concentration of the drug necessary to occupy any specified fraction of the receptors. The affinity of a drug is unrelated to its intrinsic activity. Thus some drugs may have very great affinity for a receptor but virtually no intrinsic activity, e.g., potent antagonists.

ALPHA- AND BETA-ADRENERGIC RECEPTORS. Modern concepts concerning adrenergic receptors, the sites of action of epinephrine and norepinephrine, have their origin in the work of Raymond Ahlquist in 1948. He suggested that there were two main classes of adrenergic receptors, which he termed alpha and beta. This demarcation was based on the relative potencies of several agonist drugs for stimulation of physiologic responses in several tissues. The two major patterns observed were epinephrine>norepinephrine>>isoproterenol (alpha) and isoproterenol>epinephrine>norepinephrine (beta). He suggested that two distinct types of adrenergic receptors (alpha and beta) mediated responses displaying distinct potency series. Virtually all adrenergic responses fell into one or the other category. Table 26–1 lists some typical alpha and beta receptor mediated adrenergic responses.

Although alpha- and beta-adrenergic receptors were originally defined by their agonist potency series, highly specific antagonists were subsequently developed, such as propranolol for the beta-adrenergic receptors and phentolamine for the alpha receptors. Refinements in the classification of adrenergic receptors have occurred over the past three decades with the realization that there are subtypes of both alpha- and beta-adrenergic receptors. For the beta-adrenergic receptors these were originally distinguished based on relative potencies of epinephrine and norepinephrine. Thus at $beta_1$-adrenergic receptors such as those mediating positive inotropic effects in the heart, epinephrine and norepinephrine are of similar potency. By contrast at $beta_2$-adrenergic receptors, such as those found in vascular and bronchial smooth muscle, epinephrine is much more potent than norepinephrine.

$Beta_1$- and $beta_2$-adrenergic receptors both appear to function by mediating stimulation of the plasma membrane bound enzyme adenylate cyclase. The cyclic adenosine monophosphate (cAMP) generated in response to such stimulation leads to phosphorylation of key target proteins by cAMP dependent protein kinases. Alteration in the functioning of such proteins as a result of phosphorylation presumably then leads to the characteristic physiologic or pharmacologic effects of beta-adrenergic drugs.

A number of agonist and antagonist drugs showing preferential selectivity (affinity) for $beta_1$- or $beta_2$-adrenergic receptors are known, and some of these are summarized in Table 26–2. Many drugs show no preference for one or the other receptor subtype. The clinical use of these drugs is discussed below. The beta-adrenergic receptor subtypes in various tissues are listed in Table 26–1.

Alpha-adrenergic receptor subtypes are even more distinct than the beta receptor subtypes, differing not only in pharma-

TABLE 26–2. EXAMPLES OF SOME DRUGS THAT INTERACT WITH ADRENERGIC RECEPTORS

A. Beta-adrenergic agonists
- Not receptor subtype selective ($beta_1$ and $beta_2$)
  - Isoproterenol
  - Epinephrine
- Relatively $beta_1$-adrenergic selective
  - Norepinephrine
  - Dobutamine
- Relatively $beta_2$-adrenergic selective
  - Metaproterenol
  - Isoetharine
  - Salbutamol
  - Terbutaline

B. Beta-adrenergic antagonists
- Not receptor subtype selective ($beta_1$ and $beta_2$)
  - Propranolol
  - Alprenolol
  - Timolol
  - Pindolol
  - Oxprenolol
  - Nadolol
- Relatively $beta_1$ selective
  - Metoprolol
  - Atenolol
- Relatively $beta_2$ selective
  - None clinically available

C. Alpha-adrenergic agonists
- Not receptor subtype selective ($alpha_1$ and $alpha_2$)
  - Epinephrine
  - Norepinephrine
- Relatively $alpha_1$ selective
  - Phenylephrine
  - Methoxamine
- Relatively $alpha_2$ selective
  - Clonidine

D. Alpha-adrenergic antagonists
- Not receptor subtype selective ($alpha_1$ and $alpha_2$)
  - Phentolamine
  - Some ergot alkaloids
- $Alpha_1$ selective
  - Prazosin
- $Alpha_2$ selective
  - None clinically available

cologic specificity but also in biochemical mechanism of action. $Alpha_1$ or typical "postsynaptic" alpha receptors are found, for example, in vascular smooth muscle where they mediate the vasoconstrictor effect of sympathetic nerve stimulation. Pharmacologically such $alpha_1$ receptors are characterized by their very high affinity for certain alpha antagonists such as prazosin and phenoxybenzamine. Typical alpha-adrenergic agonists such as phenylephrine and methoxamine stimulate these $alpha_1$ receptors quite effectively. Although the molecular mechanisms mediating $alpha_1$-adrenergic receptor effects are not clearly understood at present, there is considerable evidence that these may involve changes in calcium concentration.

A second major subclass of alpha-adrenergic receptors, termed $alpha_2$, was originally discovered to play a role in regulating norepinephrine release from nerve terminals. While norepinephrine release from adrenergic nerve terminals is primarily controlled by the rate of firing of the neuron, norepinephrine in an autoinhibitory fashion acts to reduce the amount of norepinephrine released. This effect seems to be mediated by alpha-adrenergic receptors (since it is blocked by classic alpha-adrenergic antagonists) that have distinct pharmacologic characteristics and are possibly located on presynaptic sites on the nerve ending itself. Stimulation of these receptors by norepinephrine in the synaptic cleft serves to reduce the amount of norepinephrine released by subsequent nerve impulses.

In recent years alpha-adrenergic receptors with pharmacologic properties virtually identical to the "presynaptic" receptors described above have been found in a variety of "postsynaptic" locations, e.g., the platelet. In addition there is some evidence that $alpha_2$-adrenergic receptors may play a distinct role in mediating effects on smooth muscle contraction. Because $alpha_2$-adrenergic receptors may be found in both pre- and postsynaptic locations, it seems preferable to use the designations $alpha_1$ and $alpha_2$ rather than the earlier terminology of "presynaptic" and "postsynaptic" alpha receptors. Physiologic effects of $alpha_1$ and $alpha_2$ receptor stimulation are summarized in Table 26–1.

A variety of drugs demonstrate selective affinity for $alpha_2$ receptors. Among agonists the most notable examples are clonidine and related drugs. Yohimbine, a plant alkaloid antagonist, also is somewhat selective for $alpha_2$ receptors. The classic alpha-adrenergic antagonists phentolamine and the ergot alkaloids are not selective and possess comparable affinity for $alpha_1$ and $alpha_2$ receptors. Subtype selectivity of some alpha-adrenergic drugs is listed in Table 26–2.

In several model systems such as the platelet, stimulation of $alpha_2$-adrenergic receptors inhibits the enzyme adenylate cyclase. The resultant reduction in cellular cAMP levels mediates the alpha-adrenergic effect in question—in this case, platelet aggregation. It is not yet known whether adenylate cyclase inhibition is the common biochemical basis of all $alpha_2$-adrenergic effects. $Alpha_1$-adrenergic effects do not seem to involve modification of adenylate cyclase activity.

DOPAMINE RECEPTORS. Catecholamines are also capable of interacting with a third class of receptors termed dopamine receptors. Peripheral dopaminergic receptors are found in the renal and mesenteric vasculature, where they mediate vasodilation. These receptors are characterized by their relatively higher affinity for dopamine than for other catecholamines. Dopamine receptors are also found in certain areas of the brain, such as the corpus striatum. Dopaminergic receptors will not be considered further in this chapter.

RADIOLIGAND BINDING STUDIES. Direct methods are now available to measure adrenergic receptors by radioligand binding techniques. These techniques involve the use of radiolabeled drugs to tag the receptors in whole cell or cell homogenate preparations. Such studies have provided a number of insights of clinical relevance. These methods permit very precise and direct measurement of the affinities of drugs for the various adrenergic receptor subtypes. Such measurements indicate that even for presumably "subtype" selective drugs, the "selectivity" is only relative. Thus a $beta_1$ selective antagonist such as metoprolol has only 10- to 50-fold higher affinity for $beta_1$ receptors in the heart than for $beta_2$ receptors in the lung. As the dose of such a compound is raised, it will occupy increasing numbers of $beta_2$ as well as $beta_1$ receptors; the selectivity therefore is not absolute. Thus, it is not generally possible to block the $beta_1$ receptors in the heart and entirely spare the $beta_2$ receptors in the lung. By contrast, some $alpha_1$ receptor selective antagonists such as prazosin may have as much as 10,000-fold higher affinity for $alpha_1$ than for $alpha_2$ receptors.

Ligand binding studies also suggest that adrenergic receptor subtypes are distinct molecular entities, probably proteins, the pharmacologic properties of which are preserved even through extensive purification. In analogy with isoenzymes, they may represent "isoreceptors," possessing relatively subtle differences in their molecular structures.

Radioligand binding studies have also documented the wide distribution of binding sites throughout the central nervous system that have properties identical to the $beta_1$ and $beta_2$ and $alpha_1$ and $alpha_2$ receptor binding sites present in the peripheral nervous system. In most cases the physiologic role of these "central" adrenergic receptors is not known. It is, however, clear that $alpha_2$-adrenergic receptors in the vasomotor center act to decrease sympathetic outflow and hence sympathetic tone. This is possibly a major site of action of clonidine, an antihypertensive $alpha_2$ agonist.

PHYSIOLOGIC REGULATION OF RECEPTORS. Adrenergic receptors are subject to a wide variety of modulating influences that regulate their numbers and binding properties. For example, chronic exposure of beta receptors to high concentrations of agonists leads to a decrease in the number of beta-adrenergic receptors and a decrease in their efficiency for stimulating adenylate cyclase. The result is a decrease in beta-adrenergic responsiveness often termed *desensitization*. Similar findings have been documented for certain alpha-adrenergic receptors. This may explain the decreased responsiveness of asthmatics to chronically administered beta-agonist bronchodilators. Antagonists do not cause such desensitization effects. Indeed, hypersensitization may occur when receptors are chronically occupied by antagonists. Under such circumstances the number of receptors on cells may increase with the potential for supersensitivity when the antagonist drug is discontinued. (See below for discussion of "propranolol withdrawal syndrome.")

In certain animal models the number of beta receptors may be increased in hyperthyroidism. This provides one possible mechanism for the salutary effect of propranolol in relieving the hyperadrenergic symptoms of hyperthyroidism.

ACETYLCHOLINE RECEPTORS. Most of the principles discussed in relation to receptors for the sympathetic nervous system also apply to receptors for the parasympathetic system. Receptors for acetylcholine appear to be of two major types defined in terms of affinities for interaction with a variety of selective antagonists. The cholinergic receptors present on autonomic effector cells are of one major type termed "muscarinic" cholinergic receptors. These receptors are blocked by muscarinic antagonists such as atropine and stimulated not only by cholinergic agonists such as carbachol but also by drugs that prolong the effect of acetylcholine by blocking its hydrolysis.

The second major type of receptor for acetylcholine is termed "nicotinic" and mediates the effects of the neurotransmitter in autonomic ganglia (sympathetic and parasympathetic) as well as at neuromuscular junctions. The cholinergic receptors of the autonomic ganglion are blocked by antagonists such as hexamethonium or trimethaphan. These nicotinic receptors can be distinguished from the nicotinic receptors of skeletal muscle, which are selectively blocked by antagonists such as decamethonium. Thus there are in effect two subtypes of nicotinic receptors. These are sometimes referred to as N_1 (autonomic ganglia) and N_2 (neuromuscular junction).

The various types of cholinergic receptors have also been studied by ligand binding techniques. The different types of receptors appear to be distinct biochemical entities subject to regulation by excessive stimulation (tolerance or desensitization) as well as other factors.

Nicotinic receptors appear to function by regulating Na^+ conductance and consequent depolarization. By contrast, muscarinic cholinergic receptors may function by inhibiting adenylate cyclase in analogy with the $alpha_2$-adrenergic receptors that inhibit adenylate cyclase in the platelet.

SYMPATHOMIMETIC AMINES

In addition to the various amines that act directly on adrenergic receptors, there are several drugs that appear to act indirectly by causing the release of endogenous catecholamines from nerve terminals. Their pharmacologic effects are therefore similar to those of norepinephrine or epinephrine, i.e., they cause beta-adrenergic stimulation of the heart and alpha-adrenergic mediated vasoconstriction. These drugs include metaraminol, mephentermine, and ephedrine. Since these drugs work by causing secretion of endogenous transmitter, their prolonged use is associated with tachyphylaxis resulting from depletion of transmitter stores.

The most important therapeutic effects of epinephrine and norepinephrine are due to their actions on the heart and smooth muscle. Isoproterenol, epinephrine, and norepinephrine all have strong positive inotropic and chronotropic effects caused by interaction with cardiac beta receptors. In addition, epinephrine and norepinephrine generally have a vasoconstrictor effect (vascular alpha receptors), whereas isoproterenol is a strong and selective vasodilator by virtue of its interaction with vascular $beta_2$ receptors but not with vasoconstrictor alpha receptors. Since epinephrine can also combine with the $beta_2$ receptors, it may also cause vasodilation under certain circumstances. These catecholamines, as well as several related agents such as dopamine and dobutamine, may be used to stabilize the circulation in some forms of shock (see Ch. 43 for details).

Beta-adrenergic sympathomimetic amines may also be used to increase cardiac rate and improve atrioventricular conduction in patients with heart block. Alpha agonists such as metaraminol may be used to elevate blood pressure transiently to revert paroxysmal atrial tachycardia to normal sinus rhythm by provoking a reflex vagal discharge that may slow the heart rate. Their use in such circumstances should always be by slow intravenous infusion with careful monitoring of blood pressure.

The only adrenergic agonist used in the treatment of hypertension is clonidine, a relatively selective $alpha_2$ agonist that appears to have primarily a central nervous system site of action. Rapid discontinuation of antihypertensive treatment with clonidine has occasionally been reported to be associated with marked rebound hypertension. This syndrome may be associated with transient elevations in catecholamine release, and hence alpha-adrenergic antagonists may be of use in its treatment.

A major application of beta-adrenergic agonists is in the treatment of asthma. Epinephrine by injection and isoproterenol by inhalation have long been used to achieve bronchodilation by stimulation of $beta_2$-adrenergic receptors. In recent years a number of $beta_2$ selective agonists have been developed. These include isoetharine, terbutaline, salbutamol, and metaproterenol. These agents have the advantage of causing somewhat less $beta_1$-adrenergic receptor stimulation and hence have less tendency to cause tachycardia for any given level of $beta_2$ stimulation (bronchodilation).

Adverse side effects are often a predictable consequence of the interaction of adrenergic agonists with adrenergic receptors of similar specificity in organs other than those in which specific therapeutic effects are sought. Some examples include tachycardia with bronchodilators and ectopic rhythms after inotropic or vasopressor agents.

ADRENERGIC ANTAGONISTS

BETA-ADRENERGIC BLOCKERS. Beta-adrenergic antagonists are among the most widely used drugs in the practice of medicine. As with adrenergic agonists, both therapeutic and adverse effects of beta-adrenergic antagonists are readily understood in terms of their competitive occupancy of beta-adrenergic receptors. Propranolol is the prototypic example of a beta antagonist. Propranolol and a number of related compounds also possess a direct "membrane stabilizing," "local anesthetic or quinidine-like" effect which gives them additional utility in the treatment of certain arrhythmias. These direct membrane effects can be dissociated from beta blocking properties by the fact that the receptor blocking effects reside largely in the (–) stereoisomer, whereas the membrane effects are present equally in both the (+) and (–) stereoisomers. These membrane effects also appear to require somewhat higher blood concentrations.

Some but not all beta blockers also possess intrinsic sympathomimetic properties; i.e., they have intrinsic activities greater than 0. This means they are weak "partial agonists." Several of the earliest beta-adrenergic antagonists such as dichlorisoproterenol possessed such activity to an extent that markedly limited their therapeutic utility. Propranolol does not possess intrinsic sympathomimetic effects; it is a pure antagonist. Of the commonly used beta blockers only pindolol has significant intrinsic sympathomimetic effects.

Propranolol is readily absorbed from the gastrointestinal tract, but much of the compound is immediately extracted from the portal circulation by the liver. There is marked patient to patient variability in hepatic metabolism, which leads to great differences in plasma drug concentrations at any given dose. An important metabolite of propranolol, 4-OH propranolol, is very active biologically, although it has a shorter half-life. Most of the propranolol in the circulation is bound to plasma proteins.

In normal persons the half-life of propranolol is quite short. At higher doses and with long-term therapy, the half-life may increase. However, many of the therapeutic effects of the drug persist for as long as 24 hours after the last dose. The usual dosage range is 40 to 320 mg per day, with great variations observed in the dose required for optimal effects. Propranolol has generally been administered orally four times daily because of its short half-life. However, especially in the treatment of hypertension, twice a day dosage is adequate. In contrast to the hepatic metabolism and short plasma half-life of propranolol and metoprolol is the renal excretion of largely unchanged drug for atenolol and nadolol. As a result, these drugs are eliminated from the plasma much more slowly, which may permit once-a-day dosage.

It is believed that abrupt withdrawal of propranolol may be followed in some patients by a transient period of "supersensitivity" to catecholamines. This is especially important in patients with ischemic coronary artery disease. This phenomenon has been called the "propranolol withdrawal syndrome" and may be manifest by arrhythmias, angina, and myocardial infarction. The existence of such a syndrome and the possible basis for such supersensitivity is controversial. Experimental work in animals and humans indicates that propranolol therapy may be associated with an increase in beta receptor number in certain tissues. Many physicians prefer to taper the dosage of propranolol rather than to stop it abruptly, especially in patients with coronary artery disease.

Propranolol has equal affinity for $beta_1$- and $beta_2$-adrenergic receptors. The same is true of timolol, alprenolol,* oxprenolol,* and pindolol. In recent years several antagonists have been developed that have relative selectivity for the $beta_1$ receptors in the heart. The first of these, practolol, led to a variety of ocular, dermatologic, and other adverse effects that precluded its use in man. More recently several other agents such as metoprolol, atenolol, and tolamolol* have become available and seem to possess some $beta_1$ selectivity. The indications for and clinical pharmacology of metoprolol are similar to those of propranolol. The potential advantage of such agents is the decreased tendency to provoke bronchospasm in susceptible subjects compared with propranolol (see below). Table 26–3 compares the important properties of several of the β-adrenergic receptor blocking drugs.

There are several major indications for the use of beta-adrenergic antagonist agents. In general, all of the agents have similar activities regardless of selectivity or partial agonism.

Angina. The salutary effect appears to be due primarily to a reduction of myocardial oxygen consumption as a consequence of decreased pulse rate, myocardial contractility, and, in hypertensive patients, blood pressure. Propranolol is one of the mainstays of medical therapy in many patients, and its effects may be additive with those of nitrates.

Hypertension. Beta blockers have become a very important part of antihypertensive therapeutic programs, often being added as a second drug to a diuretic. Despite their proven efficacy, the mode of action of the drugs remains uncertain and may be related to decreased cardiac output, decreased renin release, central nervous system mechanisms, or other effects. These drugs are particularly effective in combination with a peripheral vasodilator such as hydralazine, since the reflex and possibly deleterious cardiac stimulation evoked by the vasodilator is blocked by the beta antagonist. Another positive feature of propranolol as an antihypertensive drug is that it is generally well tolerated, which is important when chronic therapy and patient compliance are required, as in hypertension.

Arrhythmias. Antiarrhythmic effects of beta blockers are the result of both beta receptor blockade and quinidine-like effects. The drug is most useful in situations in which ectopic rhythms caused by excess catecholamines (e.g., pheochromocytoma) or digitalis are involved. (See also Hyperthyroidism, below.) In emergency situations propranolol can be administered intravenously in doses that are a small fraction of the usual oral dose.

Hyperthyroidism. Certain manifestations of hyperthyroidism such as hyperdynamic circulation, palpitations, and tremors mimic a "hyper-beta-adrenergic" state and may reflect alterations in the beta receptors themselves. These symptomatic manifestations are often dramatically improved by beta-adrenergic antagonists. A particular indication is in the circumstance of "thyroid storm" with difficult to control metabolic (e.g., hyperthermia) and cardiovascular (e.g., paroxysmal atrial fibrillation with rapid ventricular response) complications. Digitalis may be particularly ineffective in treating the rapid ventricular response to atrial arrhythmias in such patients, and beta blockers are often uniquely useful. This is one circumstance in which propranolol administration in the presence of congestive heart failure is not contraindicated, since it may reverse the underlying cause (very rapid arrhythmia).

Other Uses. Beta antagonists have also been found useful in circumstances in which ventricular outflow is compromised by hypertrophy and transient increases in cardiac contractility such as hypertrophic cardiomyopathy and tetralogy of Fallot. In addition, propranolol has recently been approved for use in prophylaxis of migraine.

Several other uses, such as benign familial tremor, are promising but currently still under investigation. The beta blocker timolol is used topically for the treatment of open-angle glaucoma.

Beta blockers are also used in the symptomatic treatment of certain of the manifestations of pheochromocytoma. However, they should never be used in the absence of concomitant alpha-adrenergic blockade, since marked hypertension may result.

Side Effects. The adverse effects of beta blockers, like their therapeutic actions, are largely consequences of their competitive occupancy of beta-adrenergic receptors. These include depression of cardiac contractility resulting from loss of normal sympathetic support with precipitation of previously latent or incipient congestive heart failure; worsening or precipitation of high degrees of heart block; and bronchoconstriction caused by blockade of bronchial $beta_2$-adrenergic receptors in susceptible individuals. When bronchoconstriction occurs, the usual beta-agonist bronchodilators may be ineffective owing to the very high affinity of propranolol for beta-adrenergic receptors. In such circumstances drugs, such as aminophylline, which dilate

*Investigational drug for this purpose.

TABLE 26–3. PROPERTIES OF SOME BETA-ADRENERGIC RECEPTOR BLOCKING DRUGS

Drug	Relative Potency (Propranolol = 1)	Relative β_1 Selectivity	Intrinsic Sympathomimetic Activity	Membrane-Stabilizing Activity	Plasma Half-Life (hrs)
Atenolol	1	+	0	0	6-9
Metoprolol	1	+	0	0	3-4
Nadolol	1	0	0	0	14-24
Pindolol	6	0	+	+	3-4
Propranolol	1	0	0	+ +	3.5-6
Timolol	6	0	0	0	3-4

airway smooth muscle without the need for beta receptor interactions are particularly useful.

In diabetics requiring insulin propranolol may, in rare cases, cause or worsen hypoglycemia by interfering with beta-adrenergic mediated hyperglycemic counter-regulatory mechanisms. It may also mask those symptoms of hypoglycemia that are mediated by beta-adrenergic stimulation, such as tachycardia or pupillary dilation. The presence of incipient congestive heart failure, heart block or impaired cardiac conduction, history of bronchoconstriction, or brittle diabetes may represent contraindications to the use of beta-adrenergic antagonists.

Other reported adverse effects with beta blockers include lethargy, depression, lightheadedness, and mild diarrhea. These are all relatively infrequent.

ALPHA-ADRENERGIC ANTAGONISTS. Alpha-adrenergic blockers are used much less frequently than are the beta antagonists. Until recently the two most commonly employed agents have been phentolamine and phenoxybenzamine. Phentolamine is a classic rapidly reversible (i.e., "competitive") antagonist, whereas phenoxybenzamine is an irreversible ("noncompetitive") alpha-adrenergic antagonist. Thus, after occupancy of alpha receptors by phenoxybenzamine, a stable covalent bond forms between the drug and some portion of the receptor by an alkylation mechanism. This may lead to a very prolonged duration of action.

The major indication for these two drugs is in patients with known or suspected pheochromocytoma. As described in Ch. 241, phentolamine may be used in diagnosing pheochromocytoma, in which its injection leads to a marked drop in blood pressure. Both phenoxybenzamine and phentolamine are used to prevent the hypertension of pheochromocytoma, for which they represent highly specific therapy. They are particularly useful in the perioperative period when large fluctuations of serum catecholamines may occur (Ch. 241). Other than in patients with pheochromocytoma, non-subtype selective alpha antagonists such as phentolamine do not appear particularly useful in the treatment of hypertension.

Adverse effects of alpha-antagonists such as phentolamine include nasal stuffiness, orthostatic hypotension, tachycardia, positive inotropic effects, and worsening angina. These effects may be explained, at least in part, by the observation that phentolamine is very potent not only at postsynaptic vascular $alpha_1$ receptors, which mediate smooth muscle contraction, but also at presynaptic $alpha_2$ receptors. Blockade by phentolamine of the $alpha_2$ receptor–mediated autoinhibitory effect of endogenous norepinephrine leads to increased release of norepinephrine in the heart. This increased concentration of norepinephrine causes enhanced stimulation of beta-adrenergic receptors, resulting in positive inotropic and chronotropic effects.

Prazosin is a highly selective $alpha_1$ antagonist that is useful in the treatment of hypertension. It exerts its major antihypertensive effect by reversible blockade of postsynaptic $alpha_1$ receptors. Prazosin is the most potent $alpha_1$ blocking drug currently available. In marked contrast to phentolamine, prazosin is an extremely weak antagonist of $alpha_2$ receptors both in physiologic studies and in direct radioligand binding experiments. This may explain why prazosin is apparently more effective as an antihypertensive agent than non-subtype selective alpha-adrenergic blocking drugs such as phentolamine. The very weak affinity of prazosin for $alpha_2$ receptors presumably accounts not only for its relatively better antihypertensive effect but also in part for the absence of certain adverse effects that are characteristically seen with non-subtype selective alpha blockers (see above). First, tachycardia is uncommon with prazosin. Since it is so weak in blocking $alpha_2$ receptors, enhanced norepinephrine release would not be expected. Second, since enhanced "norepinephrine overflow" from sympathetic nerves does not occur with prazosin, beta-adrenergic stimulation of renin secretion is absent and plasma renin concentrations do not generally rise with prazosin as they do with other alpha-adrenergic antagonists. Also, prazosin would not be expected to block the $alpha_2$ receptors which are conjectured to inhibit renin release.

Another use of prazosin is in the management of patients with severe and intractable congestive heart failure. The beneficial hemodynamic changes are due to a combination of decreased mean arterial pressure (decreased "afterload") and decreased venous tone leading to decreased venous return (decreased "preload") (see Ch. 42).

In addition to the agents discussed above, a number of other drugs not normally thought of as "alpha blockers" have significant alpha-adrenergic antagonist potency. In particular phenothiazines such as chlorpromazine and butyrophenones such as haloperidol are relatively potent alpha blockers. This may explain why hypotension is encountered with these drugs.

CHOLINERGIC DRUGS

ANTAGONISTS. Postganglionic parasympathetic cholinergic receptors are of one major type termed muscarinic. The major clinical muscarinic antagonist is atropine, one of the oldest drugs in medicine. Scopolamine is a closely related alkaloid.

Atropine blocks the effects of the parasympathetic nervous system on smooth muscle, cardiac muscle, and various glandular cells. Because atropine blocks the cardiac actions of the vagus nerve it increases the rate of firing of the sinoatrial node and facilitates conduction through the atrioventricular node. Accordingly atropine can be used in the treatment of atrioventricular block or sinus bradycardia, as for example in the setting of myocardial infarction or after digitalis excess. The drug is generally used intravenously or subcutaneously in such circumstances.

Atropine and less purified preparations of belladonna alkaloids also reduce gastrointestinal motility and gastric secretion and may be useful in symptomatic treatment of peptic ulcer disease.

As with the adrenergic antagonists, adverse effects of atropine are largely extensions of the therapeutic effects of receptor blockade. These include dry mouth, urinary retention, constipation, and blurred vision. Large doses may cause hallucinations, marked agitation, dilated pupils, and dry skin. In cases of severe atropine poisoning anticholinesterases such as physostigmine are quite effective (see below).

CHOLINERGIC AGONISTS. The actions of administered acetylcholine-like drugs are due to their interaction with both muscarinic receptors (parasympathetic effectors) and nicotinic receptors (autonomic ganglia). Because of its rapid inactivation by acetylcholinesterase, acetylcholine itself is not effective systemically. Several synthetic esters of choline are more resistant to hydrolysis and are therefore of greater therapeutic utility. Methacholine (acetyl-beta-methylcholine) and bethanecol have purely muscarinic effects, whereas carbamoylcholine is both nicotinic and muscarinic. Such drugs have limited therapeutic applications. They are used occasionally, for example, in cases of postoperative urinary retention.

ANTICHOLINESTERASES. Inhibition of cholinesterases by inhibitors that bind reversibly to the active site of the enzyme leads to a competitive decrease in the rate of hydrolysis of acetylcholine, thus raising the concentration of the neurotransmitter at nicotinic and muscarinic receptors. Several such drugs are physostigmine, a naturally occurring alkaloid, and the synthetic agents neostigmine, pyridostigmine, and edrophonium. These agents may be used for their nicotinic actions in the treatment of myasthenia gravis (see Ch. 539). Because edrophonium is so short acting, it may be used intravenously to help determine if myasthenia gravis is actually present (marked improvement in symptoms) but is not used therapeutically in this disease. These drugs may also be used for their muscarinic actions to treat paralytic ileus or postoperative urinary retention.

Another application is in the treatment of paroxysmal atrial tachycardia, either alone or in conjunction with carotid sinus massage to stimulate the vagal fibers to the heart. Edrophonium is generally used for this purpose.

Several organophosphorous agents such as diisopropyl fluorophosphate (DFP) and parathion are used in insecticides and are potent *irreversible* inhibitors of cholinesterases. They appear to act by phosphorylation of the active site of the enzyme. Cases of poisoning result from absorption of the agent through the skin or gastrointestinal tract or by inhalation. Symptoms may have a subtle onset with signs of excess cholinergic stimulation, i.e., salivation, hyperhidrosis, pupillary constriction and muscle twitching, and nausea. A relatively specific antidote, pralidoxime, reactivates the enzyme by removing the phosphate group. Atropine is generally used acutely to relieve symptoms.

GANGLIONIC BLOCKERS

Ganglionic blockers competitively antagonize the nicotinic effect of acetylcholine in the autonomic ganglia. They have limited therapeutic applications at present. Because tonic sympathetic nerve outflow to vasculature is reduced after ganglionic blockade, these agents reduce blood pressure. Examples are hexamethonium* and trimethaphan. They are potent drugs and when administered by slow intravenous infusion can be used to titrate the blood pressure in hypertensive emergencies and aortic dissection. As expected, they have a variety of severe side effects that limit their therapeutic utility. These include postural hypotension, ileus, urinary retention, and, at high infusion rates, respiratory arrest.

Frishman WH: Beta-adrenoceptor antagonists: New drugs and new indications. N Engl J Med 305:500, 1981. *A detailed review of the pharmacodynamics and pharmacokinetics of all the commonly available beta blockers.*

Lefkowitz RJ: Clinical physiology of adrenergic receptor regulation. Am J Physiol 234:E43-E47, 1982. *An overview of physiologic and pathophysiologic factors found to regulate adrenergic receptor binding sites.*

Hoffman BB, Lefkowitz RJ: Alpha-adrenergic receptor subtypes. N Engl J Med 302:1390, 1980. *Presents newer concepts concerning alpha$_1$ and alpha$_2$ adrenergic receptor subtypes in the context of therapeutic applications.*

27. ANTIMICROBIAL THERAPY

Lowell S. Young

The advent of antimicrobial therapy represented an historic milestone in the cure and control of many infectious diseases. Invariably fatal infections, like bacterial endocarditis, became treatable for the first time. Subsequently, abundant evidence has accumulated that early treatment of localized bacterial infections may obviate further complications. Two easily cited examples are (1) therapy of acute bacterial otitis media that has resulted in a marked reduction in mastoiditis and (2) prompt treatment of streptococcal sore throat that has led to a dramatic reduction in rheumatic fever and rheumatic heart disease. The greatest progress during the modern era of antimicrobial therapy has been in the treatment of acute bacterial infections, although a few chronic diseases such as tuberculosis have become well controlled. New developments offer promise in controlling viral diseases and parasitic infections that are a major burden on much of mankind. There have been some modest developments in the antifungal area as well. Nonetheless, the initial enthusiasm that greeted the introduction of new agents with antibacterial activitity has been tempered by a more sobering perspective. Antimicrobial agents are not always innocuous to the host, and their widespread usage appears to have fostered increasing drug resistance throughout the world. The growing complexities of antimicrobial therapy appear to be related to the rapid proliferation of agents of several classes, increasing drug resistance, and a greater recognition of interactions between pharmacologic agents, whether or not they have antimicrobial activity.

SOME DEFINITIONS

The terms, *antibiotic, antimicrobic,* and *chemotherapeutic agent* have often been used interchangeably to designate defined chemical substances that possess activity against specific microorganisms. Indeed, the earliest definition of an antibiotic was a substance produced in nature by living microbes that inhibited the growth of other microbial organisms at low concentrations. Viewed in this light, antibiotics seem to be a product of evolution and may confer a selective advantage to the producer in a specific ecosystem. Technically, antibiotics differ from chemotherapeutic agents in that the latter represent the products of chemical synthesis, such as the sulfonamide dyes that were subsequently found to have antibacterial activity. Antibiotics in common use, such as penicillins and aminoglycosides, are derived from natural products but from a functional point of view may be considered interchangeable with chemotherapeutic agents. As the development of new antibacterial agents, has proliferated, restrictive technical terms have become outdated. For instance, new penicillins, cephalosporins, and aminoglycosides contain synthetic or semisynthetic modifications of existing structures that confer potent new biologic activity. The term *antimicrobic* has been proposed to describe all substances with antimicrobial activity whether of natural or synthetic origin, but its acceptance has been variable.

GENERAL PRINCIPLES

The goal of antimicrobial therapy is to kill or inhibit the growth of an infecting pathogen without causing harm to the host. Thus, the basis for such an effect is *selectivity*, whereby the parasite is specifically targeted by virtue of some difference between it and mammalian cells. The first widely used antimicrobial compounds, sulfonamides and penicillins, illustrate very clearly this principle. Sulfonamides are inhibitors of para-amino benzoic acid, an essential requirement for nucleic acid synthesis in many bacteria but not in man. Penicillins and related agents that contain a beta-lactam ring act to disrupt the synthesis of peptidoglycan, which gives the bacterial cell wall its shape and strength. Mammalian cells have no cell wall, making penicillin-type drugs the ideal antibacterial agent in terms of selectivity.

Table 27–1 summarizes the mechanism of action of some of the major groups of antibacterial agents. Unfortunately, the selective action of some important compounds on the infecting microbe is not as specific as with penicillin, and important toxic effects on host cells may be encountered. Some drugs like the sulfonamides merely inhibit the growth of organisms and are *bacteriostatic*. When these agents are used, eradication of an infecting agent depends on host defenses such as phagocytic cells and antibodies. Others, like penicillins and the aminoglycosides, inhibit bacteria at relatively low concentration and at higher (but still usually therapeutic) concentrations can kill them; these are *bactericidal* agents. These designations of a bacteriostatic or bactericidal agent may vary depending on the type of organism: penicillin G is usually bactericidal for gram-positive cocci but is only static against the enterococcus (*Streptococcus faecalis*), while chloramphenicol is usually bacteriostatic even at very high concentrations but can be bactericidal against *Hemophilus influenzae.* Spectrum refers to range of microorganisms affected by a particular agent, which varies from relatively narrow for low doses of penicillin G to quite broad for large doses of the new semisynthetic penicillins. Breadth of spectrum is not necessarily related to mechanism of action.

The interaction between a microbe and therapeutic agent can be complex, and many important variables affect outcome. Intrinsic virulence differs considerably between infecting agents so that the progression of infection ranges from a very indolent tempo to a fulminating course. Host factors influence selection of bactericidal vs. bacteriostatic agents and the breadth of

*Investigational drug for this purpose.

TABLE 27–1. MECHANISM OF ACTION OF ANTIMICROBIAL AGENTS

Agent	Site of Action	Effect	Cidal	Static
Penicillins, Cephalosporins	Cell wall	Inhibit cross-linking of peptidoglycan resulting in spheroplast formation	+	Occasionally
Vancomycin	Cell wall	Block transfer of pentapeptide from cytoplasm to cell membrane	+	Occasionally
Polymyxin B, Colistin	Cytoplasmic membrane	Bind phospholipid and disrupt membrane	+	
Aminoglycosides	Ribosome	Bind to 30S ribosomal subunit, thereby inhibiting attachment of messenger RNA; also affect transfer RNA	+	
Tetracyclines	Ribosome	Bind to 30S subunit and inhibit binding of transfer RNA		+
Chloramphenicol	Ribosome	Bind to 50S subunit and inhibit messenger RNA translation	Occasionally	+
Erythromycin, Clindamycin	Ribosome	Inhibit messenger RNA translation	Occasionally	+
Rifampin	Nucleic acid synthesis	Impaired RNA formation by inhibiting DNA-dependent RNA-polymerase	+	Occasionally
Metronidazole	Nucleic acid synthesis	Damages nucleic acid structure	+	
Sulfonamides	Nucleic acid synthesis	Competitive inhibition of para-amino benzoic acid, thereby blocking formation of thymidine and purines		+

spectrum of therapy. The site of infection influences dose and duration of treatment. The proliferation of therapeutic choices compels the physician to obtain in-depth knowledge of any agent prescribed. Treatment can be guided by laboratory studies, but therapeutic choices must be based on knowledge of antimicrobial spectrum, mode of action, pharmacology, toxicity, and all major factors that affect drug activity.

IDENTIFICATION OF THE INFECTING AGENT

It is highly desirable to have the infecting agent identified prior to initiation of treatment, but in most circumstances culture confirmation and tests in vitro of antimicrobial susceptibility will not be available for at least a day. Clinical decision making is usually based on a perception of probabilities and on simple tests, the most important of which is the Gram stain. Even the latter is not necessary in the case of exudative pharyngitis, because the only treatable bacterial causes of the syndrome are hemolytic streptococci and now, rarely, *Corynebacterium diphtheriae.* Other isolates can usually be ignored and therapy with a penicillin initiated. When only a single infecting organism seems likely, therapy with a narrow-spectrum agent is preferable.

In reality, many infectious processes initially begin as mixed infections: the aspiration of secretions into the lung usually results in the deposition of many types of oral microbes that can lead to pneumonia or lung abscess, or the perforation of an abdominal viscus leads to release of millions of aerobic and anaerobic bacteria into the abdominal cavity. What may survive to be cultured in respiratory secretions or from abdominal drainage may well be the hardiest of bacteria, and not necessarily all of those that were associated with initial infectious morbidity. Not all mixed infectious processes require treatment with broad-spectrum therapy, but the presence of multiple pathogens might explain clinical failure when a mixed infection is being treated and only one component of that infection is being affected by a particular drug regimen.

Initiation of antibiotic therapy prior to obtaining appropriate cultures is perhaps the leading explanation for the failure to document infecting pathogens. On the other hand, the Gram stain or immunofluorescent staining of secretions can still point toward the nature of a process after treatment is started. Irrespective of when it is done, the Gram stain can provide valuable semiquantitative information about predominant pathogens and can help the clinician decide whether a subsequent culture result can actually be relied upon. For instance, the validity of a sample of respiratory secretions is greatly enhanced by the detection of phagocytic cells such as neutrophils or alveolar macrophages. In contrast, presence of squamous epithelial cells should be the basis for rejecting the validity of expectorated sputum, since they reflect oropharyngeal contamination. With regard to quantitative evaluation of a potentially infected body fluid, isolation of greater than 10^5 organisms per milliliter has been accepted as establishing the validity of a urine culture result. However, microscopic examination of uncentrifuged urine may still yield an approximate idea of the degree of infection (any organism seen corresponds with 10^5 bacteria per milliliter), as well as the nature of the infection that is taking place in the urinary tract. Isolation of organisms in pure culture from blood or normally sterile body fluids (like spinal fluid) is an unambiguous laboratory result that establishes an infectious etiology. Occasionally, some bloodstream infections are polymicrobial. Other blood culture isolates may be rejected as contaminants. The latter are usually skin flora like corynebacteria or *Staphylococcus epidermidis.* However, repeated isolation of such organisms from blood culture in association with signs of infection calls for careful clinical assessment. *Staph. epidermidis* and corynebacteria can be valid pathogens in immunosuppressed subjects and patients with prosthetic devices.

SUSCEPTIBILITY, RESISTANCE, AND ANTIBACTERIAL SPECTRA

Appropriate antimicrobial therapy is based on the results of laboratory tests and validated by the clinical effect of treatment. Test results and treatment are not always consistent: Patients who have excellent or intact host defenses may recover from infection irrespective of whether the antibiotic they receive has an effect on the infecting agent. Some important pathogens like Salmonella species are very susceptible in vitro to cephalosporin antibiotics, but clinical efficacy has been poor. Nevertheless, in a serious deep-seated or bloodstream infection, laboratory tests do provide an invaluable guide to the selection or adjustment of therapy. Usually a microbe is considered susceptible to an antibacterial agent if it can be inhibited or killed by a concentration of the drug that is realistically achievable at the site of the infection. The levels of drug that must be achieved in the host will vary depending on the site of infection and could be limited by toxic side effects. A common practice is to set the range of susceptibility at or above realistically achievable blood levels, but there are some notable exceptions. For instance, some agents like nalidixic acid or nitrofurantoin are rapidly excreted in the urine, but only very low blood levels are achieved. Low doses of drugs that are effective for some infections are totally inadequate for deep-seated infections. The best example is the relatively low dose of benzyl penicillin G that is required to cure pneumococcal pneumonia, sometimes less than 100,000 units of penicillin per day, which contrasts with the dose of approximately 20 million units per day that may be necessary to treat pneumococcal endocarditis or meningitis. With aminoglycosides the levels for effective therapy of bloodstream infections have been projected to be in the range of 4 to 6 μg per milliliter of gentamicin or tobramycin, and such concentrations are usually accepted as the upper boundary for susceptibility in vitro. However, it is clear that the peak levels of aminoglycosides like gentamicin and tobramycin are sustained for less than an hour. Nonetheless, that time period seems sufficient to achieve rapid killing of many bacterial strains.

Many methods have been introduced to determine the susceptibility of bacteria to antimicrobials in vitro. They have been best standardized for rapidly growing organisms. The most common involve measuring inhibition of growth in a broth medium or the measurement of growth inhibition around an antibiotic-impregnated disk placed on the surface of agar containing the test strain (disk diffusion test). By varying drug concentrations in a series of test tubes or wells, the broth dilution test yields quantitative data on the drug concentration required to inhibit the organism, the minimum inhibitory concentration, or MIC (usually expressed in micrograms per milliliter). Subcultures of broth media make it possible to determine the concentration of drug that kills the test strain — the minimum bactericidal concentration, or MBC. In the disk diffusion test only growth inhibition can be determined, but the diameter of the zone of inhibition usually correlates inversely with the MIC. The two methods give generally similar results (with the disk test being perhaps somewhat easier to perform) and for most infections susceptibility results based on inhibitory measurements are satisfactory. In treating endocarditis, meningitis, and septicemias occurring in immunocompromised hosts, MBC data on infecting isolates are desirable. Bactericidal activity appears to be a requisite for cure of enterococcal endocarditis, as penicillin G or ampicillin inhibits but does not kill this group of organisms. The phenomenon of "tolerance" has also been observed: a wide discrepancy, 32-fold or more, between MIC and MBC. Some investigators believe that strains of staphylococci isolated from endocarditis or osteomyelitis that prove to be tolerant to penicillins or vancomycin should be treated with the addition of gentamicin or rifampin, but this policy remains controversial.

Table 27–2 summarizes the susceptibilities of clinically important gram-positive and gram-negative bacteria in vitro and indicates agents of choice and alternative therapies. The darkened squares (resistant or not indicated) may include drug-pathogen combinations where clinical evidence fails to support an effect in vitro. Susceptibility testing in vitro is needed because no one agent is predictably effective against all categories of bacteria and because of the increasing incidence and changes in patterns of resistance. There are a few exceptions to this dogma, such as the uniform susceptibility of Group A streptococci to penicillin. On the other hand, relative resistance (intermediate susceptibility) of pneumococci to penicillin G may be increasing, and it is advisable to test blood and CSF isolates.

Antimicrobial resistance may be absolute, in which case increasing the concentration of the agent has no effect, and relative, in which case it may be overcome by dose augmentation. The actual basis and mechanisms of resistance have become a complex field in itself. The simplest approach is to consider (a) the genetic basis for resistance and (b) the actual mechanisms involved. Chromosomal alterations or mutations were the first basis for resistance recognized. These occurred at a relatively predictable rate. Subsequently, a much more common genetic basis has emerged: plasmids or extrachromosomal DNA elements include R-factors or genetic elements that encode for synthesis of enzymes that functionally inactivate or modify antibiotics. The rapid spread of resistance in some hospital and community settings has been related to acquisition of plasmids by the process of conjugation among gram-negative bacilli and transduction by phages among gram-positive cocci. The mechanisms of resistance are summarized in Table 27–3. The most familiar are the beta-lactamases that hydrolyze to varying degrees agents possessing the beta-lactam ring (penicillins, cephalosporins, monobactams). A great variety of these have been described, occurring in both cocci and bacilli and of both a constitutive and inducible nature. The latter poses real problems in laboratory diagnosis, as organisms that are initially thought to be susceptible (like Enterobacter species) may harbor inducible enzymes. Beta-lactamases may be of either chromosomal or plasmid origin and are usually responsible for high level resistance that cannot be overcome by dosage escalation. Inactivation can destroy the usefulness of drugs outside the beta-lactam class. A growing number of R-factor encoded enzymes have been identified that can modify aminoglycosides by the addition of an adenyl, acetyl, or phosphorylating group to hydroxyl or amino groups on the drug structure. These additions create a sterically altered molecule with ablated or reduced antibacterial activity. Conversely, the design of innovative new antimicrobial agents that prove invulnerable to inactivating enzymes involves further modifications of antibiotic structures that can block the access of inactivating enzymes to target sites. In this sense, the development of new aminoglycosides is analogous to the substitutions that protect the beta-lactam ring from hydrolysis and yield the antistaphylococcal penicillins.

One of the most worrisome mechanisms of resistance involves the ability of bacteria to exclude antimicrobial agents from the cell. Aminoglycosides are actively transported into bacteria, but high level, multiresistant strains seem to be impermeable to all aminoglycosides. These appear to arise from chromosomal mutation and are selected by aminoglycoside use. The active transport system for aminoglycosides is oxygen dependent. This probably explains the lack of effect of aminoglycosides versus anaerobic bacteria, since anaerobic conditions impair the activation of the transport system.

Another type of enzymatic resistance is illustrated by organisms that have acquired a plasmid encoded "by-pass" enzyme that subverts the metabolic block of the sulfonamides.

To have an effect, antibiotics that resist hydrolysis or modification must enter the bacterial cell and reach their target site. Target site alteration explains sudden high level streptomycin resistance (30S ribosomal subunit) or erythromycin resistance (50S ribosomal subunit). The basis for these changes appears to be chromosomal mutations. A similar basis is postulated for alterations in penicillin-binding proteins, which can result in both low and high level resistance.

The indiscriminate use of antimicrobial agents generally favors the emergence of resistance. Antibiotics are not mutagens and do not "create" resistant bacteria. Rather, usage selects for strains that are resistant by virtue of chromosomal mutations or spread of plasmids among the bacterial population. Emergence of resistance during treatment is common with some gram-negative rods such as Serratia and Pseudomonas. This phenomenon must be distinguished from superinfection, whereby a new and usually resistant pathogen becomes a secondary invader. Superinfection may be a consequence of prolonged high-dose therapy and may be avoided by use of narrow-spectrum agents in doses that are not excessive.

PHARMACOLOGIC FACTORS

Laboratory conditions for testing antibacterial agents may differ strikingly from conditions in vivo. In clinical situations the rates of growth of bacteria may be slow, thus affecting the rapidity with which cell wall–active drugs can work. More important, blood and tissue concentrations fluctuate with fre-

TABLE 27–2. SUSCEPTIBILITIES OF CERTAIN BACTERIA TO SELECTED ANTIBIOTICS

		SULFONAMIDES	TRIMETHOPRIM/SULFAMETHOXAZOLE	PENICILLIN G/AMPICILLIN	METHICILLIN/NAFCILLIN/OXACILLIN	CARBENICILLIN/TICARCILLIN	AZLOCILLIN/MEZLOCILLIN/PIPERACILLIN	CEPHALOTHIN/CEPHAPIRIN/CEFAZOLIN	CEFUROXIME/CEFAMANDOLE	CEFOXITIN	CEFOTAXIME/CEFTIZOXIME/MOXALACTAM	CEFTAZIDIME/CEFOPERAZONE/CEFSULODIN	GENTAMICIN/TOBRAMYCIN/SISOMICIN	AMIKACIN/NETILMICIN	POLYMIXIN B/COLISTIN	ERYTHROMYCIN	CLINDAMYCIN	TETRACYCLINES	CHLORAMPHENICOL	VANCOMYCIN	RIFAMPIN	ISONIAZID	NALIDIXIC ACID	METRONIDAZOLE
GRAM POSITIVE	Cl. difficile																			1				2
	Cl. perfringens			1	3	3	3	3	3	3	3					2			2	3				2
	Listeria			1		3	3	3	3	3	3					2	3	3	2	3				
	Corynebacterium diphtheriae			1		3	3									1	3	2			2			
	Corynebacteria, other																			1	②			
	Nocardia	1	1	2		3	3	3			3					3		3	3		3			
	Streptococcus			1		3	3	3	3	3	3					2				2				
	Str. faecalis			①		3	3						①			3			3	2				
	Staph. aureus (pen. sens.)			1	3	3	3	3	3	3	3	3				2	3		3	3	3			
	(pen. resis.)				1			2	2	2	3	3	3	3		3	3		3	2	3			
	(meth. resis.)																			1	②			
	M. tuberculosis												3	3							①	①		
GRAM NEGATIVE	Treponema pallidum			1		3	3	3	3							2		2						
	E. coli		3			3	3		3	2	1		1	2	3									
	Klebsiella sp.		2					2	2	2	1		1	1	3									
	Enterobacter		2								3		2	1	3									
	Serratia		2								1		2	1										
	Proteus mirabilis		3	1		3	3	3	3	3	3	3	1	1										
	Providencia												2	1										
	Salmonella		2	1		3	3												1					
	Shigella		1	2																			3	
	Vibrio		2	2														1	3					
	P. aeruginosa					②	1					1	1	1	3									
	Pseudomonas, other																							
	Acinetobacter												2	1										
	Campylobacter															1	3	2	2					
	Legionella		3													1		3			2			
	Hemophilus		2						3		1								1					
	N. gonorrhoeae			1					3	2	2													
	N. meningitidis			1		3	3				3					2			2		3			
	Bacteroides					3	3			2							1		1					1
	Brucella		1															1			②			
	Yersinia		2															1	2					
	Rickettsia																	1	1					

KEY:
- 1 Agent (s) of choice
- 2 Alternative agent
- 3 Usually susceptible
- ☐ (blank box) Variably susceptible
- (shaded box) Resistant or not indictated
- ◯ Use in combination

TABLE 27–3. MECHANISMS OF ANTIBACTERIAL RESISTANCE

Antimicrobial Agent	Mechanisms	Representative Organisms
Beta-lactams (penicillins, cephalosporins, monobactams)	Destruction by beta-lactamase	*Staphylococcus aureus* Enterobacteriaceae *Pseudomonas aeruginosa* *Hemophilus influenzae*
	Alteration of penicillin-binding proteins	*Neisseria gonorrhoeae* *Streptococcus pneumoniae* *Staphylococcus aureus*
	Cell wall impermeability	Enterobacter species *Pseudomonas aeruginosa*
Aminoglycosides	Enzymatic modification by N-acetylation, O-phosphorylation, or N-adenylylation	*Staphylococcus aureus* Enterobacteriaceae *Pseudomonas aeruginosa* *Streptococcus faecalis*
	Membrane transport O_2 dependent	Anaerobes
	Cell wall impermeability	*Pseudomonas aeruginosa* Serratia species *Streptococcus faecalis*
	Altered 30S ribosome (streptomycin)	Enterobacteriaceae
Chloramphenicol	O-acetylation	*Staphylococcus aureus*
	Cell wall impermeability	Enterobacteriaceae *Pseudomonas aeruginosa*
Erythromycin, clindamycin	Alteration of 23S RNA	*Staphylococcus aureus*
Tetracyclines	Decreased permeation plus enhanced removal	Enterobacteriaceae
Sulfonamides	Altered dihydrofolate synthetase	*Staphylococcus aureus* Enterobacteriaceae *Neisseria gonorrhoeae*
Trimethoprim	Altered dihydrofolate synthetase	Enterobacteriaceae
	Cell wall impermeability	*Pseudomonas aeruginosa*
	Alternate enzymatic pathway	Enterococci

quency and method of dosing, and the concentration of drug at the active site of infection may differ from body fluids that are more easily sampled. The distribution of agents even within the same class can vary considerably, as they may be metabolized, inactivated, and eliminated by different pathways. Such factors have a crucial effect on the size of doses, the interval between dosing, and possible drug toxicity. Also, the properties of the infecting agent may affect dosing. After exposure of bacteria to an antibiotic, a certain proportion of the population is killed or inhibited and there may be a significant lag time before multiplication of bacteria resumes after the drug concentration falls. This time interval for regrowth has been called the "post-antibiotic effect." For different organisms and with different antibiotics, there may be varying post-antibiotic effects. Thus, intermittent dosing of agents may be quite feasible if there is rapid killing and a long post-antibiotic effect. Some of the more recalcitrant organisms like Pseudomonas regrow rapidly after exposure to antipseudomonal penicillins, and there is very little post-antibiotic effect. This argues for more frequent or even continuous dosing, but for the great majority of clinical situations the latter has proved impractical and clinical superiority of continuous dosing has not been established.

Table 27–4 summarizes the recommended doses and some pharmacologic data on most of the commonly used agents. Tissue penetration is linked to serum protein binding. The quantity of drug that diffuses into a site of infection is related to the "peak" or maximum serum concentration of free or unbound drug and the duration that the maximum level is maintained. On the other hand, therapeutic outcome does not always correlate with protein-binding affinity, probably because protein binding is usually easily reversible. Lipid solubility of an antibiotic is another factor affecting tissue penetration and influences the ability of an agent to pass through membranes by non-ionic diffusion. Penetration of drug into the spinal fluid is related not only to the drug itself but also to the degree of inflammation in the meninges. Lipid-soluble agents such as chloramphenicol, isoniazid, rifampin, sulfonamides, and metronidazole penetrate spinal fluid well. Aminoglycosides, amphotericin B, and polymyxins do not penetrate well even in the face of inflammation. Penicillins and vancomycin generally penetrate CSF when inflammation is present. Most antibiotics commonly used are excreted primarily through the kidney, but notable exceptions include erythromycin and chloramphenicol. Thus, it may be possible to treat infections of the urinary tract with doses smaller than are required for serious systemic disease, because high urine levels are achieved with most agents. Urine and bile regularly contain higher concentrations of antibiotics than does serum. Penicillins and tetracyclines are concentrated in bile, but aminoglycosides enter bile less well, particularly when liver disease or obstruction is present. Drugs like tetracyclines and clindamycin diffuse readily into bone and have been used successfully in osteomyelitis. Agents that enter prostate tissue well include sulfonamides, trimethoprim, erythromycin, and doxycycline. Some drugs may fail because of pharmacokinetic properties. For instance, amoxicillin is so well absorbed in the small intestine that effective therapeutic levels are usually not achieved in the colon, thereby limiting use for Shigella infections.

Factors besides drug levels per se may limit drug activity. Purulent secretions and high concentrations of calcium and magnesium ions antagonize aminoglycoside activity. Erythromycin and aminoglycosides have markedly diminished activity in acidic environments. Cephalosporins like cephalothin can be metabolized to relatively inactive derivatives, but metabolites of cefotaxime are still quite active.

There is evidence that a high ratio of bactericidal activity in serum (e.g., serum diluted 1:8 or greater possessing a killing effect) against infecting strains is associated with therapeutic success. Such activity may merely reflect the serum concentration required to achieve effective therapy at a site of infection. It should not be assumed that a given dose corrected for weight or body surface area will reliably produce the same levels in all patients. With agents like aminoglycosides that are potentially toxic, therapeutic monitoring is clearly indicated during serious systemic infection. For example, gentamicin peak (postinfusion) levels should exceed 4 μg per milliliter and trough (or "valley") levels should be less than 2 μg per milliliter. Route of administration is important, since orally administered drugs may be poorly absorbed in serious systemic infections. For patients who are in shock, intramuscular or subcutaneous injections should clearly be avoided and all medications should be given intravenously.

TABLE 27–4. DOSAGE, PHARMACOLOGIC FACTORS, AND ADJUSTMENT IN RENAL AND HEPATIC FAILURE

Class/Agent	Dose: Systemic Infection	Dose: Oral	Protein Binding (%)	Normal Serum Half-Life (Hrs)	Dose Adjustment: Hepatic Failure	Dose Adjustment: Renal Failure	Serum Levels Affected by Dialysis
Aminoglycosides							
Amikacin	5–7 mg/kg/q8	—	0	2–3	No	Major	Yes
Gentamicin	1.7 mg/kg/q8	—	0	2–3	No	Major	Yes
Netilmicin	1.7 mg/kg/q8	—	0	2–3	No	Major	Yes
Tobramycin	1.7 mg/kg/q8	—	0	2–3	No	Major	Yes
Antifungal Agents							
Amphotericin B	0.7–1 mg/kg/d	—	90	24	No	No	No
Flucytosine	40 mg/kg/q6	Yes	10	3	No	Major	Yes
Ketoconazole	6 mg/kg/d	Yes	98	8	Avoid	No	No
Miconazole	5 mg/kg/q6–8	—	92	2.2	Avoid	No	No
Antituberculous Agents							
Ethambutol	15 mg/kg/d	Yes	10	1.5	No	Major	Yes
Isoniazid	5 mg/kg/d	Yes	10	3	Yes	Minor	Yes
Rifampin	10 mg/kg/d	Yes	70	3	Yes	Minor	No
Cephalosporins							
Cefaclor	7 mg/kg/q6	Yes	20	1	No	Yes	Yes
Cefamandole	30 mg/kg/q6	—	70	1	No	Yes	Yes
Cefazolin	15 mg/kg/q6	—	80	2	No	Major	Yes
Cefoxitin	30 mg/kg/q6	—	70	0.7	No	Yes	Yes
Cephalothin	30 mg/kg/q6	—	70	0.7	Minor	Yes	Yes
Cephalexin	7 mg/kg/q6	Yes	15	1	No	Yes	Yes
Cefoperazone	30 mg/kg/q8–12	—	90	2	Some	Minor	Yes
Cefotaxime	30 mg/kg/q6	—	50	1.2	Some	Minor	Yes
Cefsulodin†	30 mg/kg/q6–8	—	20	1.6	No	Major	Yes
Ceftizoxime	30 mg/kg/q6–8	—	50	1.3	No	Minor	Yes
Cefatriaxone†	30 mg/kg/q12–24	—	90	8	No	Yes	Yes
Ceftazidime†	30 mg/kg/q8	—	60	2	No	Major	Yes
Moxalactam	30 mg/kg/q8–12	—	50	2	No	Major	Yes
Penicillins							
Amoxicillin	7 mg/kg/q6	Yes	20	1	No	Yes	Yes
Ampicillin	30 mg/kg/q6	Yes	20	1	No	Yes	Yes
Azlocillin	50 mg/kg/q6	—	50	1	Minor	Major	Yes
Carbenicillin	70 mg/kg/q4	—	50	1	Minor	Major	Yes
Cloxacillin	7 mg/kg/q6	Yes	95	0.5	Minor	Minor	Yes
Dicloxacillin	7 mg/kg/q6	Yes	97	0.5	Minor	Minor	No
Methicillin	30 mg/kg/q4–6	—	30	0.5	No	Minor	No
Mezlocillin	50 mg/kg/q6	—	50	1	No	Major	Yes
Nafcillin	30 mg/kg/q4–6	—	90	0.5	Yes	Minor	No
Oxacillin	30 mg/kg/q4–6	—	90	0.5	Yes	Minor	Yes
Penicillin G	0.3–4 million U q4–6h	Yes	60	0.5	No	Yes	Yes
Penicillin V	7 mg/kg/q6	Yes	80	1	No	Minor	Yes
Piperacillin	40 mg/kg/q6	—	50	1	Minor	Major	Yes
Ticarcillin	40 mg/kg/q4–6	—	50	1	Minor	Major	Yes
Tetracycline							
Chlortetracycline	7 mg/kg/q6	Yes	50	5	Avoid	Avoid	No
Demeclocycline	7 mg/kg/q12	Yes	50	10	Avoid	Avoid	Yes
Doxycycline	1.5 mg/kg/q12–24	Yes	90	15–20	No	No	No
Minocycline	3 mg/kg/q12–24	Yes	90	15	Avoid	Avoid	No
Oxytetracycline	7 mg/kg/q6–12	Yes	35	8	Avoid	Avoid	No
Tetracycline HCl	7 mg/kg/q6	Yes	50	7	Avoid	Avoid	No
Sulfonamides							
Sulfadiazine	15 mg/kg/q6	Yes	50	3	Avoid	Major	Yes
Sulfamethoxazole	12 mg/kg/q8	Yes	50	6	Avoid	Major	Yes
Trimethoprim (used with above)	2.3 mg/kg/q8–12	Yes	60	10	No	Major	Yes
Sulfisoxazole	15 mg/kg/q6	Yes	50	6	Avoid	Major	Yes
Other Agents							
Aztreonam†	30 mg/kg/q8	—	60	2.0	No	Major	Yes
Chloramphenicol	7–15 mg/kg/q6	Yes	30	1.5	Some	Minor	Yes
Clindamycin	7 mg/kg/q6	Yes	90	2.5	Some	Minor	No
Colistin	2 mg/kg/q12	—	0	5	No	Avoid	No
Erythromycin	7 mg/kg/q6	Yes	20	1.5	Some	No	No
Metronidazole	15 mg/kg/q6	Yes	20	8	No	No	Yes
Nalidixic Acid	15 mg/kg/q6	Yes	90	1.5	No	Avoid	No
Nitrofurantoin	1 mg/kg/q6	Yes	60	0.3	No	Avoid	No
Polymyxin B	1.5 U/kg/q12	—	0	5	No	Avoid	No
Spectinomycin	30 mg/kg	—	0	2	No	Avoid	No
Vancomycin	7 mg/kg/q6	Yes*	10	6	No	No	No

*Not systemically absorbed.
†Investigational drug in the United States.

MODIFICATION OF DRUG DOSES IN RENAL AND HEPATIC FAILURE

Since the majority of antibiotics are excreted via the kidney, dosage adjustment must be considered in moderate to severe renal failure. Many studies have related serum creatinine level or creatinine clearance to degree of dosage modification, and useful nomograms have been derived that may aid in the calculation of dosage. Table 27–4 indicates the agents affected by renal failure and dialysis. Many of these guidelines have been derived by study of patients who are in the "steady state," i.e., patients in renal failure who are on dialysis programs but who may not be infected. Thus, they may not manifest the hemodynamic instability that is often present in patients with serious systemic infection. In unstable patients, there is no substitute for accurate assays of serum or plasma drug concentrations as a guide to appropriate dosing. While dosage modification is indicated in patients with serious renal failure, the initial doses should probably be the same. The timing of the second dose should probably be based on levels anticipated from nomograms, but peak levels after the end of the second dose and third dose should be monitored in order to calculate the next doses. Increased trough concentrations may help to warn of incipient toxicity. As a general principle, many pharmacologic agents are given every three to four half-lives. In renal failure these half-lives are prolonged many-fold. One strategy is to prolong the interval between maintenance doses, which can result in fairly high "peak" or postinfusion levels and rather prolonged (and occasionally subtherapeutic) troughs. Another strategy is to give more frequent doses but to decrease the size of maintenance doses. Subtherapeutic levels may be avoided by the latter tactic, but the approach could be more nephrotoxic (as in the case of aminoglycoside agents). Dialyzable agents are similarly cleared by peritoneal or extracorporeal hemodialysis. Following dialysis a dose approximately two thirds to three quarters of a maintenance dose should be given, depending upon the degree of removal of the antibiotic by dialysis and the timing of the previous maintenance dose.

Several important antibiotics are metabolized in the liver and are partially excreted in the bile. Agents primarily metabolized by the liver include the sulfonamides, chloramphenicol, and tetracycline. There is usually little reason to alter the dose of penicillin, cephalosporins, and aminoglycosides in patients with liver disease. Even with erythromycin, ethambutol, and clindamycin, there is little evidence that dosage reduction is necessary except in severe hepatic failure. For instance, clindamycin should probably be reduced to half normal doses after two to three days of treatment. Chloramphenicol total dosage should be restricted to 1.5 to 2.0 grams per day (adult) and erythromycin should be reduced to perhaps one half the normal dose after two or three days of treatment. Drugs to be avoided in hepatic failure include sulfonamides and tetracyclines.

COMBINATION ANTIMICROBIAL THERAPY

Use of combinations of antibacterial agents is exceedingly common. The rationale for their use may be summarized as follows: (1) Prior to the identification of pathogens infecting critically ill subjects, combinations offer a broader, more comprehensive antibacterial spectrum than a single agent. No single agent currently available offers comprehensive coverage against all gram-positive and gram-negative organisms of major clinical importance. (2) Use of a drug combination may eradicate an infection that cannot be cured by a single agent, such as the effect of penicillin on enterococci. Addition of an aminoglycoside or a potentiating agent such as rifampin may result in bactericidal activity at a deep-seated focus of infection, as in endocarditis. (3) Combinations are indicated in the treatment of mixed infections, since not all of the pathogens may be susceptible to a single agent. (4) Combinations may decrease the opportunity for emergence of resistance. This has been best documented in tuberculosis. (5) Combinations may interact additively or synergistically against infecting organisms. As a result, there may be an enhancement of antibacterial activity and/or enhanced rate of killing. The latter may lead to more rapid clearing of infection with reduction in duration of therapy. Combinations may permit the use of a lower dosage of one or more components of the regimen, particularly the more toxic component, thereby avoiding undesirable side effects. More rapid killing or greater potency in vivo may be more directly beneficial in patients with impaired host defenses. Some clinical studies suggest an improved clinical response not only when drugs used to treat endocarditis interact synergistically but in sepsis occurring in immunocompromised patients.

The converse of synergism is antagonism between antimicrobial agents. This is best described for combinations of bactericidal plus bacteriostatic agents. Penicillin-type drugs require cell growth to exert their lethal effect. When penicillins are combined with static drugs like tetracycline, only growth inhibition may result. Clinical studies in man indicate poorer results in treatment of pneumococcal meningitis with penicillin plus tetracycline than with penicillin alone.

Empiric therapy is presumptive or "blind" therapy where clinical severity of likely infection dictates that treatment be started. It is not necessarily combination therapy, as some single agents can still be quite effective. Intelligent choices in the absence of microbiologic information can be made based on the clinical syndrome and the likely infecting pathogen. Epidemiologic factors as well as host factors enter into the decision. The setting in which the patient develops infection

TABLE 27–5. INITIAL EMPIRIC THERAPY FOR SERIOUS INFECTION

Syndrome	Qualifying Factors	Recommended Treatment
Septicemia	Immunocompromised Host	
	Neutrophil Count $>500\ \mu l$	Cephalosporin (cefazolin) + aminoglycoside (gentamicin, tobramycin)
	Neutrophil Count $<500\ \mu l$	Azlocillin or piperacillin + aminoglycoside (amikacin, tobramycin)
	Normal Host	
	Urinary source	Ampicillin + gentamicin or 3rd generation cephalosporin
	Biliary source	Ampicillin + gentamicin or 3rd generation cephalosporin
	Abdominal or pelvic source	Aminoglycoside + clindamycin or cefoxitin, or broad-spectrum penicillin
	No source	Oxacillin + gentamicin
	Neonate	
	<48 hrs old	Ampicillin + either cefotaxime or moxalactam
	>48 hrs old	Ampicillin + oxacillin + aminoglycoside
Meningitis	<6 years	Ampicillin + cefotaxime or moxalactam
	>6 years	Ampicillin or penicillin G
Brain Abscess		Penicillin G + cefotaxime or moxalactam + metronidazole
Pneumonia	Community acquired	Ampicillin or penicillin G ± erythromycin
	Post-influenzal	Antistaphylococcal penicillin or cephalosporin
	Post-aspiration	Ampicillin or clindamycin
	Nosocomial	Azlocillin or piperacillin + aminoglycoside, or 3rd generation cephalosporin + aminoglycoside

or a prior exposure or travel history can be of considerable value. Pneumonias contracted outside of the hospital are usually due to streptococci (and pneumococci) and penicillin-sensitive anaerobes. An "atypical" or diffuse pattern raises the likelihood that community-acquired pneumonia will be better treated with erythromycin than penicillin. Infections that occur in the nosocomial setting or in markedly neutropenic patients should always be initially treated with therapy directed against gram-negative bacilli.

Table 27–5 summarizes recommendations for initial empiric therapy by clinical syndrome.

SPECIFIC ANTIMICROBIAL AGENTS

Table 27–2 summarizes recommended choices of antimicrobial agents for specific infecting agents. The organisms are divided into gram-positive and gram-negative isolates, and antimicrobial agents that are similar are grouped together. Clearly, such a table oversimplifies the appropriate choices for various agents. In some situations, there is no clear-cut agent of first choice, and any member of a class may be appropriate. Differences in pharmacology, cost, and side effects might lead to a selection of one agent in preference to another. There is an increasing divergence in antibacterial spectrum among the newer beta-lactam agents, such as the antipseudomonal penicillins and the third-generation cephalosporins. Among the aminoglycosides, anticipated efficacy may be expressed as follows: While gentamicin and tobramycin remain the most widely prescribed, gram-negative bacilli that are resistant to these agents are more likely to be inhibited by netilmicin and amikacin.

Few oral agents are listed in Table 27–2, but it may be inferred that any of the oral anti-staphylococcal agents such as cloxacillin or dicloxacillin could be used to treat mild infections due to penicillinase-producing staphylococci. The spectrum of oral cephalosporins such as cephalexin or cephradine mimics that of cephalothin or cefazolin. In the case of Group A hemolytic streptococci, it would not be necessary to test for susceptibility of these organisms against pencillin G and related penicillins in vitro, since all would be expected to be susceptible. It would, however, be highly desirable if one were to use a penicillin against the Klebsiella species to test that penicillin for susceptibility in vitro; it should probably not be presumed that antibiotics such as piperacillin or mezlocillin will be effective in vitro and in vivo without specific testing. Some agents should always be used in combination to treat serious bloodstream or systemic infections, such as antituberculous therapy (isoniazid plus at least one other agent) or enterococcal sepsis with or without endocarditis (the combination of either a penicillin or vancomycin with an aminoglycoside). Older agents of the aminoglycoside class such as streptomycin or kanamycin are no longer widely used because their activity is more comprehensively covered by newer drugs (gentamicin and amikacin). The exception to this might be in the conventional therapy of *Mycobacterium tuberculosis*, for which streptomycin is still indicated.

Sulfonamides and Sulfa-Containing Combinations

Sulfonamides were the first chemotherapeutic agents to be introduced into wide clinical use. They are bacteriostatic and previously were quite active against many gram-positive and gram-negative organisms. They are, however, no longer among the first choices for serious systemic infections, the exception being *Nocardia asteroides* infections. Sulfonamides remain effective therapy for coliform organisms causing community-acquired urinary tract infections, but they are unreliable against hospital-acquired microorganisms. More commonly used to treat a wide variety of more serious bacterial infections is the fixed combination (1:5) of trimethoprim and sulfamethoxazole. Synergism in vitro against many enteric bacteria can be demonstrated with this combination, yet trimethoprim is a highly active agent itself. A major argument in favor of continued use of the fixed combination is that it may reduce the likelihood of the development of resistance to one component in the pair. Trimethoprim/sulfamethoxazole is usually active against enteric bacteria and *H. influenzae* (including most penicillinase-producing strains), and it has been effective in parasitic infections such as *Pneumocystis carinii* pneumonia. The diffusion of trimethoprim into prostate fluid makes it a useful agent in prostatic infections. Central nervous system penetration is good. The oral preparation is well absorbed, although a parenteral form is available for patients in whom gastrointestinal absorption may be erratic. Occasional side effects include neutropenia and all of the dermal and systemic hypersensitivity reactions that have been well associated with sulfonamides.

Penicillin G and Related Agents

The primary spectrum of penicillin G (benzyl penicillin) is gram-positive, with such organisms as *Streptococcus pyogenes*, *Str. pneumoniae*, and *Str. viridans* remaining exquisitely susceptible. Procaine penicillin is readily administered intramuscularly and because of slow absorption dosing of 600,000 units q12h remains effective therapy for pneumococcal pneumonia. Benzathine penicillin is a long-acting (two to three weeks) agent that is slowly released after I.M. injection and provides therapeutic levels for streptococcal pharyngitis and some forms of syphilis and prophylactic effect against acute rheumatic fever. For oral use in mild respiratory infections, phenoxymethyl penicillin (V) is acid stable and preferable to penicillin G. In large doses penicillin G is still effective against *Neisseria meningitidis*, most *N. gonorrhoeae*, and anaerobic organisms including Clostridium species, but usually not against strains of *Bacteroides fragilis*. Against enterococci, penicillin G or ampicillin should be used in combination with an aminoglycoside such as streptomycin or gentamicin. Ampicillin may be preferable in the treatment of Salmonella, CNS infections due to Hemophilus strains, and *Listeria monocytogenes*. When used in large doses, penicillin G or ampicillin is effective against a few gram-negative organisms, most notably *Proteus mirabilis* (but not other Proteus species). Penicillin G and related penicillins should not be used against the great majority of coagulase-producing staphylococci, most of which now produce beta-lactamases.

Antistaphylococcal Penicillins

The antistaphylococcal penicillins are beta-lactamase–stable and relatively narrow in spectrum. Parenteral preparations include methicillin, nafcillin, and oxacillin. There is little choice among this category of agents in terms of antistaphylococcal activity. There may be some differences in side effects, with methicillin possibly associated with more hypersensitivity nephritis and oxacillin with a greater incidence of abnormal serum elevations of hepatic enzymes. When used in appropriate doses, the central nervous system penetration is probably adequate to treat meningitis. The oral antistaphylococcal agents should not be used to treat serious infections, but mild or moderately severe infections may respond to dicloxacillin or cloxacillin. Combination of antistaphylococcal penicillins with an aminoglycoside or rifampin has been recommended for refractory staphylococcal infections or when the isolates demonstrate tolerance. *Staph. epidermidis* may produce beta-lactamase like most coagulase-positive *Staph. aureus*. However, serious infections like prosthetic valve endocarditis are better treated with vancomycin plus rifampin or an aminoglycoside.

Broad-Spectrum Penicillins

Although ampicillin and amoxicillin are technically classified as broad-spectrum penicillins, the extended spectrum really only includes *Escherichia coli*, *H. influenzae*, Salmonella, and Shigella species. Even then, amoxicillin should not be used orally for Shigella infections because excellent absorption from the upper GI tract results in subtherapeutic levels in the lower gut. Other penicillins like carbenicillin, ticarcillin, mezlocillin, azlocillin, or piperacillin are notable for their activity against

Pseudomonas aeruginosa, most Proteus species, and anaerobic pathogens such as *Bacteroides fragilis.* On a weight basis, carbenicillin and ticarcillin have relatively weak antipseudomonal activity and so must be used in considerably larger doses than most penicillins, in the range of 18 to 30 grams a day for adults (200 to 400 mg per kilogram). The large sodium load given with such doses may aggravate congestive failure and cause electrolyte abnormalities. While these antipseudomonal penicillins are important agents for serious infections, emergence of resistance and variable stability to beta-lactamases has led to the tendency to combine these agents with an aminoglycoside. They are quite active against the coccal organisms that ampicillin usually inhibits, but none of these agents should be used against coagulase-positive staphylococci. Other potential uses of these extended-spectrum penicillins include treatment of infection caused by Acinetobacter species, Listeria, and a variety of anaerobes. Like the antistaphylococcal penicillins, their half-life is relatively short, but protein binding is low. Thus, frequent dosing at 4- to 6-hour intervals is usually necessary. Newer antipseudomonal penicillins such as mezlocillin, azlocillin, or piperacillin are augmented in their antipseudomonal activity, in the case of the latter two approximately 6- to 8-fold by weight in comparison to carbenicillin when organisms are tested at low inoculum concentrations. On the other hand, the tendency has been to use smaller doses of these more potent penicillins in order to avoid the side effects associated with large doses of carbenicillin. The result is that no clear-cut clinical differences have been found between these agents when they are used in combination with aminoglycosides. Some of these newer penicillins, such as mezlocillin and piperacillin, have variable activity against Klebsiella species and must be tested prior to use.

Cephalosporins

Cephalosporins are structurally related to penicillins, yet there are major differences in activity between these agents in vitro and in vivo. The first cephalosporins, such as cephalothin, cephaloridine, and cefazolin, were effective against penicillinase-producing staphylococci as well as pneumococci and streptococci (except enterococci). Additionally, they offered good activity against several important gram-negative pathogens such as *E. coli,* Klebsiella and *Proteus mirabilis.* Despite activity in vitro, they are not effective against Salmonella and Shigella and do not penetrate the blood-brain barrier. The enormous popularity of these agents appears related to a low incidence of side effects, fairly broad coverage against community-acquired respiratory and urinary tract pathogens, and the availability of both oral and parenteral dosing. Nevertheless, these compounds have not been considered the agents of choice for any serious systemic infections. They have been successfully used to treat patients with a history of mild penicillin type reactions, such as rash but not urticaria or anaphylaxis. With the development of newer cephalosporins the principal advantages of these older compounds (often referred to as "the first generation") have been in the prophylactic surgical usage and relatively greater activity against penicillinase-producing *Staph. aureus.*

The so-called "second generation" cephalosporins offer a few improvements over cephalothin and cefazolin. Cefoxitin is a compound with fairly consistent activity against *B. fragilis.* Cefamandole and cefuroxime lack the anaerobic spectrum of cefoxitin but have modestly improved activity against some gram-negative organisms not inhibited by the first generation, such as *H. influenzae* and Enterobacter species. Oral agents include cefaclor, which has greater activity against penicillinase-producing *H. influenzae* than cephalexin.

The newest cephalosporins (often referred to as "third generation"), or structurally related compounds such as moxalactam, a 1-oxy-beta lactam, have markedly enhanced activity against enteric bacteria as well as variable coverage of *P. aeruginosa.* These compounds are stable against the beta-lactamases of *H. influenzae* and *N. gonorrhoeae* and cross the blood-brain barrier in sufficient concentrations to offer effective therapy for gram-negative meningitis (with perhaps the exception of *P. aeruginosa* infection). Among the agents shown to be effective in gram-negative central nervous system infections are cefotaxime, moxalactam, ceftazidime,* and cefatriaxone.* Several of these agents have a much longer half-life than first-generation cephalosporins, permitting dosing intervals of 8 to 12 hours. In the case of one agent, cefatriaxone, once-a-day dosing has been possible in some infections because of an 8-hour half-life. The antipseudomonal activity of these compounds is variable, and clinical data are still lacking to support the claim that these agents may be used as single agents to treat serious systemic pseudomonal infections in immunocompromised hosts. Nonetheless, newer antipseudomonal cephalosporins like cefsulodin and ceftazidime represent some of the most potent antipseudomonal agents introduced into clinical practice, and these compounds appear to be significantly safer than aminoglycosides. Table 27–6 summarizes the relative properties of these agents, as well as selected comments. As a general rule, the increased activity against gram-negative pathogens is also coupled with relatively diminished activity against gram-positive cocci. While the gram-positive, particularly antistaphylococcal, coverage of these agents may be satisfactory for initial therapy, serious staphylococcal disease as well as pneumococcal infection is better and certainly more economically treated with older beta-lactam agents (e.g., oxacillin, penicillin G, respectively). These agents are also not without serious untoward effects, including the triggering of disulfiram reactions, inhibition of platelet adhesiveness, and hypoprothrom-

*Investigational drug in the United States.

TABLE 27–6. THIRD-GENERATION CEPHALOSPORINS AND RELATED COMPOUNDS

Agent	Protein Binding (%)	Peak Serum Levels (μg/ml) After 1 gm I.V.	Half-Life (Hours)	Comments
Aztreoonam	60	50	2	No activity vs. gram-positive organisms.
Cefmenoxime	77	40	1	Weak antipseudomonal activity.
Cefoperazone	90	125	2.1	Primary excretion is biliary with little dose adjustment in renal failure.
Cefotaxime	38	40	1.1	Good CNS penetration but weak antipseudomonal activity.
Cefsulodin	30	65	1.5	Primarily antipseudomonal activity, not much else.
Ceftazidime	20	70	1.9	Potent antipseudomonal activity.
Ceftizoxime	30	75	1.4	Potent gram-negative activity except for Pseudomonas.
Ceftriaxone	85	140	8.0	Very long half-life, good CNS penetration, but poor antipseudomonal activity.
Moxalactam	50	60	2.3	Best anaerobe coverage but associated with coagulopathy.

binemia. In many patients with community-acquired and mild to moderately severe nosocomial infections, third-generation cephalosporins offer the potential of effective single agent therapy. The preliminary results in immunocompromised hosts suggest that these compounds may still be more efficacious when combined with aminoglycosides.

Chloramphenicol

Chloramphenicol is an oral or parenterally administered drug whose spectrum makes it useful for a wide variety of bacterial and rickettsial infections. The antibacterial spectrum includes gram-positive organisms such as streptococci and staphylococci, but the agent has not been considered to be one of the more potent antistaphylococcal compounds. It is usually bacteriostatic except against *H. influenzae*, against which it is bactericidal. Many enteric organisms are inhibited by chloramphenicol, but Pseudomonas strains are usually resistant. Important therapeutic uses include typhoid fever, central nervous system infections, anaerobic infections, intraocular infections, and serious rickettsial infections. Against *B. fragilis*, it remains one of the most useful agents. On the other hand, chloramphenicol has been associated with severe hematologic toxicity. In the great majority of individuals receiving courses in excess of one week of chloramphenicol, there is a dose-dependent inhibition of erythropoiesis. Some patients, estimated at one in 50,000, have developed irreversible aplastic anemia following oral or parenteral dosing. While it remains a highly effective agent in selected situations, there are now a number of very reasonable alternatives to chloramphenicol. The unpredictability of the hematologic toxicity should lead physicians to reserve this agent for serious infections in which there are major indications for avoiding alternative drugs.

The Tetracyclines

Tetracyclines inhibit a wide range of gram-positive and gram-negative bacteria as well as Mycoplasma species, but they are not agents of choice for any serious bacterial infections. Their activity against gram-positive organisms is static and the results do not appear to approach those obtained with bactericidal agents. Gram-negative coverage includes *E. coli* and Klebsiella species, but there are major gaps in their spectrum, including Pseudomonas, Serratia species, and other serious nosocomial pathogens. Tetracycline may be useful in urinary tract infections, rickettsial infections, mycoplasmal infections, and in the prophylaxis or treatment of traveler's diarrhea (caused by toxigenic *E. coli*). Older preparations such as chlorotetracyclines or oxytetracyclines have been supplanted by tetracycline HCl, minocycline, or doxycycline. The latter two preparations have certain pharmacologic advantages, including less frequent dosing, and doxycycline may be used in renal failure.

Erythromycin

This is the most commonly available member of the class of macrolide antibiotics. Traditionally, erythromycin has been regarded as an agent of second choice for streptococcal and staphylococcal infections, to be used in those patients with history of serious penicillin allergy. In this regard, erythromycin remains a useful agent, but its primary appeal in recent years has been its clinical efficacy against several important new causes of infection such as Mycoplasma, Legionella, chlamydia, and Campylobacter species. Against all of these pathogens, erythromycin can be considered the agent of choice. In serious respiratory infections, erythromycin should be administered parenterally, but this use is associated with high incidence of phlebitis. The compound is one of the safest of all antimicrobials, but mild gastrointestinal disturbances are common. Several oral preparations are available, but none seems clinically superior.

Clindamycin and Lincomycin

Clindamycin and lincomycin mimic much of the spectrum of erythromycin. Their major advantage over erythromycin is greater activity against anaerobes, particularly *B. fragilis*. Nonetheless, the antianaerobic spectrum of these compounds is not complete. In the treatment of intra-abdominal infections these agents are usually combined with aminoglycosides for gram-negative coverage. A major problem with clindamycin therapy has been antibiotic-associated diarrhea and pseudomembranous colitis. The incidence and severity of this complication vary, and the problem is not always associated with clindamycin. The development of gastrointestinal symptoms on treatment should be a warning to discontinue use of these agents.

Metronidazole

Metronidazole has long been used for the therapy of trichomoniasis, amebiasis, and giardiasis. Subsequently, it has been found to be a highly effective and bactericidal agent against many anaerobic pathogens, including *B. fragilis*. It is available in both oral and parenteral forms and must be considered the therapy of choice for *B. fragilis* infections involving deep-seated foci such as heart valves and the central nervous system. Many infections involving anaerobes are mixed processes that also involve aerobic organisms. Because it is almost exclusively active against anaerobic pathogens, metronidazole is usually combined with other antimicrobials. The drug must be metabolized to its active form. Its excellent distribution, rapid bactericidal activity, and penetration in "closed spaces" are appealing characteristics, but it also has the potential of inducing disulfiram reactions and potentiating the effects of coumadin. There is concern about metronidazole's carcinogenicity in animals and mutagenicity in bacteria. These effects have not been demonstrated in man, but it seems wise to restrict this agent to use in severe infections.

Rifampin

Rifampin is a semisynthetic derivative of rifamycin B and has been used principally for the therapy of tuberculosis. It is one of the most potent and effective antituberculous agents available, with a spectrum that includes both *M. tuberculosis* and atypical organisms. It has been found to be very active against the wide variety of gram-positive and gram-negative organisms including staphylococci (both coagulase-positive and coagulase-negative) and Legionella species. The compound is one of the few that has been effective in terminating meningococcal carrier state, and it inhibits methicillin-resistant staphylococci. The principal drawback to the use of rifampin is that almost all microbial agents have the ability to develop resistance rapidly. Therefore, even in tuberculosis this drug must be combined with another active agent. It seems useful as an adjunct to other antibacterial agents, such as in combination with antistaphylococcal penicillins to treat "tolerant" strains in endocarditis and meningitis. It inhibits methicillin-resistant staphylococci but is best used with vancomycin. Another potential advantage has been excellent penetration into phagocytic cells. A disadvantage, however, is its potent ability to induce enzymes that decrease the half-life of a number of other pharmacologic agents, including steroids, sulfonylureas, and digitoxin.

Vancomycin

Initially developed during an intense search for agents active against coagulase-producing staphylococci, this agent developed a reputation for efficacy as well as toxicity to the eighth cranial nerve and to renal function. More modern preparations of vancomycin do not appear to be strongly associated with these side effects. Indeed, the compound has been used effectively to treat serious infections in patients with renal failure because it is not significantly excreted by the kidneys; prolonged bactericidal activity results from widely spaced doses. The spectrum includes not only *Staph. aureus*, but *Staph. epidermidis*, *Staph. faecalis* (enterococci), and Corynebacteria species. Vancomycin has not been considered an agent of primary choice for *Staph. aureus*, but is an effective alternative in the penicillin-allergic patient. In prosthetic valve endocarditis caused by *Staph. epidermidis,* it is often considered the agent of choice in combination with rifampin or gentamicin.

Aminoglycosides

Aminoglycosides are rapidly bactericidal against most of the clinically important gram-negative bacilli, including enteric bacteria and *P. aeruginosa.* Most isolates of *Staph. aureus* are also inhibited by aminoglycosides. The initial compounds of this series, like streptomycin, were also shown to be effective against *M. tuberculosis,* and in combination with a penicillin, either streptomycin or gentamicin offers the best available therapy for deep-seated enterococcal infections. Older agents like streptomycin, neomycin, and kanamycin are considerably less useful today because they appear to be relatively more toxic or have been supplanted by agents with greater activity against *P. aeruginosa.* The contemporary aminoglycosides include gentamicin, tobramycin, netilmicin, and amikacin. The latter two compounds offer some advantages in that they are stable to inactivation by some of the plasmid-encoded enzymes that acetylate, adenylate, or phosphorylate the older agents. Thus, amikacin or netilmicin may be preferred to treat infections caused by gentamicin- or tobramycin-resistant strains, but susceptibility testing in vitro is necessary because some isolates may be resistant to all agents within this class. Rapid bactericidal effect and good distribution except for the central nervous system make these highly desirable compounds for the treatment of serious systemic gram-negative infections. Unfortunately, aminoglycosides are toxic to renal function, can cause eighth cranial nerve (both cochlear and vestibular function) and renal damage, and occasionally manifest curare-like effects. Pharmacologically, there is a narrow range between the therapeutic levels achievable by q8-12h dosing and levels that are associated with toxicity. Aminoglycoside therapy should be closely monitored by frequent blood level determinations in treating serious infections, when large doses are used for prolonged courses. These agents are either additive or often synergistic with beta-lactam compounds against pathogens such as *P. aeruginosa,* Serratia sp., and other gram-negative rods. For immunocompromised hosts, aminoglycosides remain an important component of therapy, usually as part of a combination with a beta-lactam agent. Aminoglycosides do not penetrate well into the central nervous system or bone and are not absorbed via the oral route. They are perhaps overused as topical agents and in that setting the rapid emergence of resistance has been documented. For prophylaxis in colonic surgery, older aminoglycosides like neomycin or kanamycin may suffice in regimens that transiently suppress the growth of aerobic bowel flora.

Spectinomycin also belongs to the aminoglycoside class and is used exclusively for the treatment of gonorrhea when penicillin-type agents have failed. Such antigonococcal activity is shared by other members of the class.

Polymyxin, Colistin (Polymyxin E)

Polymyxin B and colistin (polymyxin E) are closely related cationic polypeptide detergents that bind to the lipoproteins of many gram-negative outer cell membranes. They are rapidly bactericidal in vitro, particularly against *P. aeruginosa* and enteric rods except Proteus species and Serratia. These agents are without effect against gram-positive organisms. Resistance has rarely emerged on therapy. Because of poor clinical results and nephrotoxic potential, the use of these compounds has decreased markedly. Lack of clinical efficacy could be due to properties of poor diffusion and rapid binding to tissues.

Urinary Antiseptics

Mandelamine, nitrofurantoin, and nalidixic acid are agents that are only effective in urinary tract infections, and usually as suppressive therapy in chronic infections. Resistance to some of these compounds, particularly nalidixic acid, may emerge rapidly. They may be useful in situations where the goal is suppression rather than a cure because of unremediable anatomic abnormalities. Gastrointestinal side effects have been commonly associated with each of these preparations. Additionally, the optimum antibacterial effect of mandelamine is at urine pH of less than 5.0, so that additional acidification of the urine with acidic substances is required for efficacy.

DURATION OF THERAPY

There are no easy formulas for determining duration of therapy, although a practical guide is treating for two to four days after defervescence and resolution of signs of infection. The site of infection, host factors, the nature and antimicrobial susceptibility of infecting organisms, the severity of infections, and the response to treatment should be taken into consideration. For bloodstream infections not accompanied by endocarditis or bone involvement, 10 to 14 days is a usual course of treatment. Most respiratory infections are adequately treated in the same interval. Uncomplicated meningitis caused by the meningococcus or pneumococcus is probably adequately treated by 7 to 10 days of high-dose parenteral penicillin G. Endocarditis, deep-seated bone infections, and infections involving prostheses require a minimum four- to six-week course of treatment but in some cases more. It is important to remember that signs of inflammation, particularly pulmonary infiltration, may persist long after infecting organisms are killed or contained by host defenses, and delayed resolution of lung infiltrates is not uncommon. On the other hand, deep-seated infections like endocarditis and osteomyelitis may have to be treated for periods long after subsidence of signs of infection. Thus, the decision to continue to stop treatment at the end of an appropriate interval must be based on the thorough clinical examination and careful reasoning. Patients with impaired host defenses may require longer therapy than those individuals who are basically healthy. A single dose of an effective antimicrobial agent may be adequate to cure lower urinary tract infection involving the bladder, but a much longer duration, on the order of several weeks, is required to ensure therapeutic success in treatment of intrarenal infection.

FAILURE TO RESPOND TO TREATMENT

One of the most important clinical dilemmas is the persistence of fever and other manifestations of infection after a course of costly and potentially toxic therapy has been started. At the same time that every component in antimicrobial therapy is being reassessed, an alternative explanation for fever, pain, and inflammation must also be entertained. For instance, tumors or hypersensitivity reactions can incite febrile reactions. Usually, an interval of two to five days is necessary in order to judge the efficacy of treatment. At that point, the following are indicated: (1) Assessing the accuracy of the diagnosis of infection; (2) determining if the drug selection is appropriate, and particularly if the dose and mode of administration are responsible for the lack of success of therapy; and (3) searching for (a) presence of anatomic abnormalities, (b) foreign body, (c) undrained abscess, (d) infarction of tissue, (e) development of superinfection, (f) emergence of resistance, or (g) presence of a simultaneous infectious process that is not being treated by antibacterial therapy. If these are unrevealing, a noninfectious origin of fever or drug reaction should be considered.

In the severely immunosuppressed host, fever and signs of infection may persist despite appropriate therapy. In these patients clinical failure of drug treatment is more realistically regarded as host failure; if any improvement is possible in this difficult situation, it usually correlates with improvement in underlying disease or the immunologic status of the host. If an infection is documented and responds poorly to initially prescribed treatment, then a change to an alternate regimen is indicated. If signs and symptoms progress or new complications appear in spite of seemingly appropriate treatment, a

TABLE 27–7. UNTOWARD EFFECTS OF SOME ANTIMICROBIAL AGENTS

Target	Agent	Mechanism	Manifestation
Endocrine	Ketoconazole	Altered steroid synthesis	Gynecomastia
	Sulfonamides	Block iodine uptake	Goiter
Gastrointestinal	All agents, esp. ampicillin, clindamycin	(1) Altered bowel flora	Diarrhea
		(2) Exotoxin of *Clostridium difficile*	Pseudomembranous colitis
	Isoniazid, rifampin, tetracyclines	Hepatocellular necrosis	Hepatitis
	Neomycin	Villous damage	Malabsorption
Hematologic	Chloramphenicol	(1) Protein synthesis inhibition	Reversible anemia, leukopenia
		(2) Idiosyncratic	Aplastic anemia
	Carbenicillin, others	Inhibition of platelet aggregation	Bleeding
	Moxalactam	Impaired prothrombin synthesis	Bleeding
	Penicillins, many others	Impaired leukopoiesis, thrombopoiesis	Neutropenia, thrombocytopenia
	Sulfonamides	G-6-PD deficiency	Hemolytic anemia
Kidney	Aminoglycosides, polymyxins	Tubular damage	Renal failure
	Amphotericin	Tubular damage	Hypokalemia, renal failure
	Carbenicillin	Na-K exchange	Hypokalemia
	Penicillins	Interstitial nephritis	Renal failure
	Sulfonamides	Tubular crystallization	Renal failure
Nervous System	Aminoglycosides	(1)Damage to hair cells of Corti	Deafness
		(2) Vestibular damage	Vertigo
		(3) Neuromuscular blockade	Respiratory arrest
	Isoniazid	Pyridoxine antagonism	Neuropathy
	Penicillins, cephalosporins	Cortical irritation	Seizures
	Polymyxins	Neuromuscular blockade	Respiratory arrest
Pulmonary	Nitrofurantoin	Interstitial inflammation	Fibrosis
Skin	Tetracyclines	Bind to dermal structures	Photosensitivity
	Penicillins, sulfonamides, tetracyclines, others	Allergic reactions	Rash, serum sickness, erythema multiforme

change in therapy is indicated as well as a search for superinfection or an undiagnosed process such as a viral or fungal infection. One of the greatest clinical dilemmas is presented by the patient in whom drug fever or a hypersensitivity reaction is suspected but in whom discontinuing treatment could be dangerous. In such individuals, it is usually prudent to give alternative medication rather than stop antibacterial therapy.

ANTIBIOTIC TOXICITY AND UNTOWARD REACTIONS

A large proportion of drug reactions are related to antimicrobial agents. As many as 10 per cent of patients receiving penicillins and sulfonamides experience some type of toxic or hypersensitivity reaction. These reactions can be fatal, as in the anaphylaxis associated with penicillin or the aplastic anemia

TABLE 27–8. IMPORTANT ANTIBIOTIC DRUG INTERACTIONS

Antimicrobial Agent	Interacting Drug	Result
Amphotericin B	Curariform drugs	Increased curare-like effect
Aminoglycosides	Neuromuscular blockers (i.e., tubocurarine, pancuronium)	Additive blockade
	Diuretics: ethacrynic acid, furosemide	Increased ototoxicity
	Antibiotics: amphotericin B	Increased nephrotoxicity
	Carbenicillin/ticarcillin (other penicillins)	Inactivation, resulting in reduced activity
Ampicillin/Amoxicillin	Allopurinol	Rash
Cephalosporins (cefamandole, cefoperazone, moxalactam)	Alcohol	Disulfiram reaction
Chloramphenicol	Warfarin	Decreased warfarin metabolism and inhibition of vitamin K–producing gut bacteria, thus increasing prothrombin time
	Phenytoin	Decreased phenytoin metabolism levels
	Oral hypoglycemic agents	Increased hypoglycemia
Isoniazid	Warfarin, phenytoin	Increased risk of toxicity by decreased drug metabolism
	Disulfiram	Psychosis
	Rifampin, para-amino salicylic acid	Additive hepatotoxicity
	Oral contraceptives	Decreased contraceptive effect
Metronidazole	Alcohol	Disulfiram-like reaction (nausea)
	Disulfiram	Psychosis
Nalidixic Acid	Warfarin	Increased prothrombin time
Polymyxins	Curariform drugs	Increased curare-like effect
Rifampin	Warfarin, phenytoin	Decreased warfarin, phenytoin effect
	Isoniazid	Additive hepatotoxicity
	Methadone	Withdrawal symptoms
	Oral contraceptives	Decreased contraceptive effect
	Steroids	Decreased steroid effect
Sulfonamides	Procaine	Decreased sulfonamide effect
	Hypoglycemic agents	Hypoglycemia
	Warfarin, phenytoin	Displace drugs from protein-binding sites causing increased warfarin and phenytoin effects
Tetracyclines	Antacids, oral iron	Decreased tetracycline absorption

due to chloramphenicol. Table 27–7 summarizes some of the major untoward reactions to antibiotics. The majority of toxic reactions are, however, short lived and reversible. Nephrotoxicity secondary to aminoglycosides may be averted by careful therapeutic drug monitoring. A commonly recognized complication of antibiotic therapy is diarrhea and/or pseudomembranous colitis. This is due to bowel overgrowth by *C. difficile,* which elaborates an exotoxin that is responsible for symptoms. Discontinuation of antibiotic therapy will usually lead to resolution of treatment, but some patients require vancomycin.

Besides anaphylaxis, other hypersensitivity reactions include fever, hemolytic anemia, serum sickness, and a wide variety of dermal reactions that include rash and exfoliation. When serious infection is being treated, mild hypersensitivity reactions may be suppressed by a variety of symptomatic medications. Manifestations of hypersensitivity such as rash may fade despite continued treatment, as is common with ampicillin. The decision to continue therapy in the face of such reactions must be based on severity of infection and the lack of reasonable alternatives. Another issue of great clinical importance that is not fully resolved is the potential cross-reactivity between penicillins and cephalosporins. However, the great majority of patients who have only rash following exposure to penicillin, ampicillin, or related penicillins can be safely treated with cephalosporin compounds. The immediate hypersensitivity-type reactions such as anaphylaxis, wheezing, and urticaria should be carefully noted. Patients with a history of immediate reactions to penicillin should not be rechallenged with cephalosporins unless they have life-threatening infections and can be observed under close medical supervision.

MAJOR ANTIBIOTIC DRUG INTERACTIONS

An increasing number of interactions have been reported between antimicrobials, or antimicrobials and other pharmacologic agents that seriously ill patients may be receiving. Some of these are summarized in Table 27–8. Some noteworthy examples include the induction of hepatic enzymes by rifampin, which may hasten the metabolism of other antibiotics or drugs. An unexplored area of drug interactions is that which may involve more than two agents. Penicillins like ampicillin or carbenicillin gradually inactivate aminoglycosides like gentamicin in renal failure, when a long half-life for both types of drugs provides opportunity for complexing between the two classes of agents. While this effect is not apparent when patients have normal renal function, the net effect in patients in renal failure is effectively to lower the levels of circulating aminoglycosides and penicillin.

USE OF TOPICAL ANTIBIOTICS

Topical antibiotics or antiseptics have been commonly applied to burns and open wounds, and they are often incorporated into irrigants. A few studies suggest that topical agents can suppress bacteria in burn wounds and reduce sepsis originating from this source. Some topical antiseptics, such as those that contain iodine, are probably too toxic to inflamed tissues and their local application should be discouraged. Topically applied antibiotics can provide only surface suppression of microbial flora. They also provide ample opportunity for development of resistance, since large numbers of organisms may be present on injured skin. Antibiotics in irrigants may be irritating, may be absorbed in large quantities so as to cause increased toxicity, and may offer little advantage over irrigation per se.

Acar JF, Phillips I, Waldvogel FA: Decision making in aminoglycoside therapy. J Antimicrob Therapy 8(Suppl A), 1981. *Clinically useful symposium covering controversial aspects of aminoglycoside therapy, with emphasis on the issue of antibiotic resistance.*

Appel GB, Neu HC: The nephrotoxicity of antimicrobial agents. N Engl J Med 296:663,722,784, 1977. *Comprehensive review of the subject with practical guidelines for dosage adjustment in renal failure.*

Cunha B (ed.): Symposium on antimicrobial therapy. Med Clin North Am 66:1, 1982. *A modern and practical update on almost all agents used for hospital and outpatient practice.*

Garrod LP, Lambert MP, O'Grady F: Antibiotics and Chemotherapy. London, Churchill-Livingstone, 1981. *Succinct text oriented to microbiologists, but with much information useful to clinicians.*

Gilbert DN, Sanford JP: A clinical perspective of antibiotic therapy: Aminoglycosides versus broad spectrum beta lactams. Rev Infect Dis 5(Suppl 2):S211–S398, 1983. *Deals directly with some of the major controversies involving therapy with the most modern therapeutic agents for serious bacterial infections.*

Neu HC: The new beta lactamase stable cephalosporins. Ann Intern Med 97:408–419, 1982. *Encyclopedic yet clinically relevant review of all agents in this rapidly growing class of antibacterial agents.*

Young LS: Combination or single drug therapy for gram-negative sepsis. *In* Remington JS, Swartz MN (eds.): Current Clinical Topics in Infectious Diseases. New York, McGraw-Hill Book Company, 1982, pp 177–205. *Addresses one of the most widely debated issues in modern antimicrobial therapy.*

28. ANTIVIRAL THERAPY

D. W. Barry

Several effective chemical and biologic antiviral agents are currently available for clinical use, and others will appear within the next few years. This chapter reviews clinical experience with these agents and examines the criteria to be considered before any new therapy is established as safe and effective. Only those agents that have withstood the tests of time and scientific scrutiny will be described.

Although some antiviral agents have been available for over a decade, guidelines governing their use are still in their infancy. Certain fundamental principles of viral infections prevent direct extrapolation from knowledge gained from antibacterial therapy. Viruses are obligate intracellular parasites and must divert normal host cell metabolism into providing the constituents for the reproduction of new viral particles. Thus the effectiveness of any antiviral drug will depend not only on its ability to penetrate mammalian cell membranes but also on its capacity to inhibit viral-directed metabolic functions. Furthermore, the host immune system, including B and T lymphocyte function, macrophages, interferon, and other lymphokines markedly influence the outcome of most viral infections in humans. Because of this variability in viral, cellular, and immune function, basic principles—such as the relationships between the sensitivity of the virus to a drug in vitro, achievable serum levels of the agent, and its ability to cure an infection—are only beginning to be established.

Evaluation of the effectiveness of antiviral agents is difficult because only a few viral infections are consistently fatal or associated with serious morbidity or significant sequelae. The majority of viral infections represent significant medical problems only because of their frequency. In the aggregate they cause significant mortality (influenza), morbidity (herpesvirus), and economic loss (rhinovirus). On an individual basis, most virus infections are self-limited or mild, with virus replication often well past its peak by the time the physician is consulted. Therapeutic intervention will therefore usually occur simultaneously with the rising tide of the body's own defenses, and a "placebo effect" is prominent in mild and self-limited illnesses. Therefore, any study on the effectiveness of an antiviral which is not double blind and placebo controlled in any but the most consistently fatal viral illness must be regarded with skepticism.

CHEMOTHERAPEUTIC AGENTS

Herpesvirus Infections

The most successful example of antiviral chemotherapy has been the treatment of superficial infections of the eye caused by herpesvirus, the most common infectious cause of blindness in the United States. Details of therapy may be found in the ophthalmologic literature, and only certain aspects of the pathophysiology of these viral infections will be discussed here. The reasons for success in the treatment of herpetic keratitis are easily understood. The virus infection occurs in superficial areas only 5 to 7 cells thick, which are easily accessible to the direct instillation of high concentrations of antiviral agents. Because the corneal epithelium is not vascularized and receives its nourishment by simple diffusion, it may be considered an immunologically "privileged" site, and the patient's immune response to infection does not appear to be a complicating variable. In addition, this disease is caused by herpes simplex virus, a virus with substantial differences between its own metabolism and that of the host cell. The majority of the agents found to be effective in the treatment of this illness interfere with viral DNA synthesis. Some, such as trifluorothymidine, idoxuridine, and cytosine arabinoside, are relatively toxic when given systemically because they also interfere with DNA replication in rapidly dividing host cells such as myelocytes and lymphocytes. However, when they are given topically in the eye, only minimal amounts are absorbed. Others, such as adenine arabinoside, acyclovir, and interferon, have much more limited toxicity even when given systemically. The final selection of an anti-herpes keratitis agent will thus depend on such factors as local tolerance, allergic reactions, observed or potential drug resistance, rapidity of healing, depth of corneal ulceration, and the cost of the drug.

IDOXURIDINE. The first effective anti-herpes drug to be developed was idoxuridine, also known as 5-iodo-2′-deoxyuridine or IUDR. It is an analogue of deoxythymidine and is chemically related to trifluorothymidine, which will be discussed later. The mechanism of action of IUDR results in part from its inhibition of thymidine kinase but more significantly by inappropriate incorporation into viral or host cell DNA, forming false base pairs with guanine rather than adenine. First developed in 1959, IUDR showed a wide range of activity in vitro against many DNA viruses. Clinical studies showed that it was extremely effective in the treatment of herpetic keratitis. When given in the usual regimen of one drop of a 0.1 per cent aqueous solution in the affected eye every hour, IUDR will cure 75 to 90 per cent of patients with the milder or "dendritic" form of herpes keratitis. A 0.5 per cent ointment is also available. Unfortunately, IUDR cures a lower percentage (40 to 50 per cent) of patients with the more severe "geographic" ulcers. It appears to be relatively ineffective in patients who have deeper disease involving the corneal stroma or the uveal tract. Some patients are intolerant of or allergic to the drug and develop bothersome edema and erythema of the periorbital tissues. Lack of clinical response as well as resistance in vitro develop fairly rapidly. As with all other antiherpes agents, IUDR does not eradicate "latent" virus when the organism is in a metabolically inactive state and when herpes nucleic acid may be integrated with host cell DNA. Thus, recrudescent infections are common (approximately 50 per cent will recur within two years) and add credence to the pessimism concerning complete cure of herpes infections.

Although this drug provided an effective local treatment for a troublesome disease, comparable success could not be obtained in systemic use. For a number of years IUDR was used to treat herpes encephalitis, a disease with a mortality rate between 50 and 70 per cent, and uncontrolled studies seemed to indicate that the drug was useful in lowering this mortality. Unfortunately, critically controlled studies showed that IUDR was not effective in herpes encephalitis and in fact, because of its significant myelosuppressive effect, it predisposed treated patients to serious superinfection and bleeding. The drug is still used extensively outside the United States for the topical treatment of herpes genital and labial disease as well as cutaneous varicella-zoster infections. Data supporting this use are inconclusive.

ADENINE ARABINOSIDE. Another nucleoside analogue that has been shown to be effective in the treatment of herpetic keratitis is adenine arabinoside, also known as vidarabine, ara-A, or Vira-A. It is phosphorylated intracellularly, and the triphosphate noncompetitively inhibits viral DNA polymerase more efficiently than host cellular DNA polymerase. The 3 per cent ophthalmic ointment applied every three hours has been associated with cure rates of keratitis higher than with IUDR. Like IUDR, it is ineffective against stromal and uveal tract disease. It is also the first drug shown to have some activity in herpes simplex encephalitis, lowering the mortality rate from 70 per cent to approximately 30 to 40 per cent. Some survivors have been left with severe and permanent neurologic residua, and its effectiveness is obvious only in those patients who are not stuporous or comatose when therapy is initiated. Multicenter studies have demonstrated that intravenous ara-A can also significantly reduce the high mortality rate in disseminated neonatal herpes simplex infections if administered early. As with herpes encephalitis, some survivors are left with significant sequelae. Intravenous ara-A has also been shown to produce some clinical improvements, including the prevention of visceral complications, in immunocompromised patients with cutaneous herpes zoster, although the overall clinical improvement was not dramatic. To produce these benefits, the drug must be given within 72 hours of infections, and conflicting data exist showing that clinical benefit is seen only in younger (<35 years of age) or older (>38 years of age) individuals.

Treatment of other viral infections has met with varying success. Ara-A has some beneficial influence on the biochemical markers of chronic active hepatitis, but the degree and permanence of these changes are more impressive when it is given with prolonged courses of interferon. Although active in vitro against variola virus, it was ineffective against clinical smallpox infections. Likewise, it does not appear to be effective in preventing or curing cytomegalovirus pneumonia in patients who have received bone marrow or renal transplants, and its effect on the congenital cytomegalovirus syndrome awaits additional clinical trials.

Ara-A also has a number of significant disadvantages, the first of which is its relative insolubility. Often an adult's daily dose (10 to 15 mg per kilogram intravenously) must be given in 2 or more liters of fluid—a potential hazard in patients with encephalitis, who often have significantly elevated intracranial pressure. In addition, the drug is rapidly deaminated to the relatively ineffective hypoxanthine arabinoside. Because of its insolubility and almost immediate deamination, the drug must be given as a continuous infusion over 12 to 24 hours, a cumbersome dosing schedule to maintain. Maximal levels of less than one fourth to one third of the inhibitory dose in vitro for most herpesviruses are achieved in the serum, an observation which must necessarily engender newer concepts of intracellular micropharmacokinetics in order to explain the apparent clinical activity of the drug. The phosphorylated analogue (Ara-AMP) is considerably more soluble, but clinical trials showed it to be ineffective in herpes encephalitis, possibly because it must be dephosphorylated before it can enter infected cells. At high doses, ara-A suppresses the bone marrow, although considerably less than cytosine arabinoside. Higher dosage regimens have been associated with tremors, hyperexcitability, and seizures. This reaction is more common in patients with compromised renal or hepatic function and is likely the result of higher blood and tissue levels. Like IUDR, it is not effective when applied topically to oral or genital herpetic lesions.

TRIFLURIDINE. Trifluridine, also known as trifluorothymidine, TFT, or Viroptic, is, like IUDR, an analogue of deoxythymidine. It is suitable only for topical use in the treatment of herpetic keratitis (one drop of a 1 per cent solution every two hours) and has not been adequately tested in systemic viral infections because of its toxicity. When given at higher doses intravenously, TFT induces significant bone marrow suppression, but applied topically in the eye, it produces only minimal adverse reactions, primarily mild stinging and burning in a low percentage of patients. Its major advantage is a higher cure rate than that for IUDR, and possibly ara-A, in herpetic keratitis. It is significantly better than IUDR for both dendritic and geographic ulcers and has also proved effective in those cases clinically or virologically resistant to either IUDR or ara-A. The drug has also shown some promise in certain adenovirus infections of the eye. It is not effective when applied topically to cutaneous lesions such as those of herpes genitalis or herpes labialis.

ACYCLOVIR. The next effective anti-herpes agent to be developed was the acyclic nucleoside, 9-(2-hydroxyethoxymethyl)guanine, also known as acyclovir, acycloguanosine, or Zovirax. It is similar in structure to guanosine but only half the ribose ring is present, yielding an "acyclic" structure. This compound has excellent activity in vitro against certain members of the herpesvirus group, and has a unique advantage over other antiviral chemotherapeutic substances currently in use: its selectivity as a substrate for virus-specified thymidine kinase. Normal host cell thymidine kinase does not effectively utilize acyclovir as a substrate. Herpesvirus-specified thymidine kinase converts acyclovir to its monophosphate, which is then transformed by cellular enzymes to di- and triphosphates. The triphosphate is both an inhibitor of and a substrate for herpesvirus-specified DNA polymerase. Its incorporation into viral DNA selectively stops virus replication. The cellular α-DNA polymerase in infected cells is also inhibited by the triphosphate, but only at concentrations severalfold higher than those that inhibit the viral-specified DNA polymerase. Since acyclovir is preferentially taken up and converted to its active form by herpesvirus-infected cells, it has a significantly lower toxic potential for normal, uninfected cells than other antivirals.

Experiments in vitro have shown acyclovir to be effective against herpes simplex Types I and II, varicella-zoster virus, and Epstein-Barr virus, but less potent against cytomegalovirus. Intravenous regimens of 5 to 10 mg per kilogram every eight hours produce peak serum levels of 4 to 15 μg per milliter. If the solubility of the drug (2.5 mg per milliliter at 37°C) is exceeded, either through rapid infusion, poor hydration, or coexistent renal failure, tubular obstruction can occur and lead to usually reversible renal failure. The drug penetrates into the cerebrospinal fluid moderately well (~50 per cent of serum levels) and the inhibitory concentrations for herpes simplex, varicella-zoster, and Epstein-Barr viruses range from ~0.01 to 2 μg per milliliter. Intravenous acyclovir has been shown to be effective in the treatment of mucocutaneous herpes infections and in varicella-zoster infections in normal as well as immunocompromised patients. Its effectiveness in herpes encephalitis, generalized neonatal herpes, and severe mononucleosis awaits the conclusion of ongoing studies. It does not appear to be effective in cytomegalovirus infections. Acyclovir* has limited absorption from the gastrointestinal tract (15 per cent), yet a regimen of 200 to 400 mg every 4 hours has been shown to ameliorate genital herpes infections. Most striking is the fact that 200 mg taken orally 2 to 5 times per day effectively prevents the appearance of recurrent genital lesions. Like IUDR, ara-A, and TFT, it is very effective when applied topically to the lesions of herpes keratitis.

Poxviruses

METHISAZONE. One of the earliest chemotherapeutic agents to demonstrate anti-DNA virus activity was 1-methylisatin-3-thiosemicarbazone, also known as thiosemicarbazone, methisazone, or Marboran.† In the early 1960's, it was found to have a wide antiviral spectrum in vitro, most impressively against variola, the virus that causes smallpox. Several prophylactic studies conducted during that decade showed a reduction in secondary attack rates among household contacts of smallpox cases. Methisazone did not significantly decrease the mortality rate in those who did develop the disease; nor was it effective in acute smallpox infections.

With the worldwide eradication of smallpox over the past two decades, this drug has seen little use. Nevertheless, methisazone is probably effective in treating complications of smallpox vaccination such as vaccinia gangrenosa, vaccinia necrosum, and generalized vaccinia. Although smallpox vaccination has appropriately decreased in frequency over the past decade, some physicians continue to vaccinate for a variety of reasons, including misguided efforts to treat recurrent herpes infections. The drug is an orally administered liquid and is given at a dose of 200 mg per kilogram initially, followed by 50 mg per kilogram every six hours for six to eight doses. The only significant side effects reported are nausea and vomiting, which occur in 10 to 70 per cent of patients.

Influenza

AMANTADINE. One of the most significant advances in anti-RNA virus therapy was the development of amantadine, also known as Symmetrel. A drug with an odd, birdcage-like structure, it was first found to have antiviral activity in the early 1960's. In tissue culture, a broad spectrum of influenza A viruses, but not influenza B viruses, is inhibited by amantadine. Drug resistance can be induced fairly readily in vitro, although the clinical significance of this observation has yet to be established. The gene determining resistance has been linked with that governing the matrix protein. Amantadine appears to inhibit either viral penetration or viral uncoating within the cell by as yet undefined mechanisms. The concentration required to inhibit 50 per cent of the virus in tissue culture (ID_{50}) ranges between 0.1 and 6 μg per milliliter; the ID_{100} is often closer to 25 μg per milliliter. After a single oral dose of 2.5 to 4.0 mg per kilogram (roughly equivalent to the usual adult dose of 200 mg per day) peak serum levels of 0.3 to 0.5 μg per milliliter are attained. Significant concentration (10- to 60-fold) occurs in both mouse and human lung tissue. Amantadine has a very long half-life (20 to 24 hours) and two to three days are required before a steady state is reached. Eventually 90 to 99 per cent is excreted unchanged in the urine, and thus very significant dose reductions must be made in patients with compromised renal function.

Amantadine taken prophylactically provides protection rates against influenza infection in the range of 70 to 90 per cent (similar to that observed following the inoculation of influenza vaccines). At the usual therapeutic and prophylactic dose of 100 mg twice a day, amantadine will induce adverse reactions in 10 per cent or more of recipients. These reactions are generally more frequent and more severe in older individuals, who need most to be protected from influenza. Fortunately, these reactions are generally not severe and consist most often of mild agitation, confusion, mental depression, and insomnia. Adverse reactions are more common or more prominent when the patient is also taking antihistamines. Worsening of congestive heart failure and hypotension have also been observed. Overdosages associated with blood levels above 1.5 μg per milliliter have led to severe central nervous system reactions, including coma and convulsions.

Amantadine also appears to be active against influenza when given orally. This efficacy, however, is more difficult to define, and the difference in the rates of significant clinical improvement between drug- and placebo-treated groups is often marginal. Sophisticated tests, such as those measuring frequency-dependent compliance, have shown that the duration of the diminished pulmonary function that occurs for a number of weeks after influenza may be markedly shortened by the use of amantadine during acute illness. Whether amantadine is effective in the treatment of primary influenza pneumonia has not been established, and early reports have not been encouraging. An analogue, rimantadine, which has been used in some European countries and has been studied in the United States, is reported to have a better therapeutic-toxic ratio than amantadine.

Respiratory Syncytial Virus

RIBAVIRIN. Convincing and consistent results of double-blind, placebo-controlled studies of ribavirin (1-β-D-ribofuranosyl-1,2,4,-triazole-3-carboxamide), also known as Virazole, have

*The oral form of acyclovir is currently not available commercially in the United States.

†Experimental drug available from Burroughs Wellcome Company.

only recently become available. This analogue of guanosine or inosine appears to inhibit inosine monophosphate dehydrogenase and thus interferes with the de novo synthesis of guanine nucleotides necessary for viral replication. It is active against an extremely broad spectrum of RNA and DNA viruses in vitro, although precise levels of sensitivity are quite dependent on the cell substrate employed in the assays. Although clinical studies of ribavirin in herpes and influenza infections have yielded inconclusive or mixed results, the use of continuous or semicontinuous aerosolized ribavirin (20 mg per milliliter in water) for a minimum of 3 days ameliorated the course of respiratory syncytial virus infection in children. Few adverse reactions were noted, although oral dosages of 600 to 1200 mg per day for 5 to 14 days have been associated with reversible depressions in red cell counts and elevations of bilirubin. Ribavirin is also teratogenic in animals, and thus additional experience must be gained before a precise therapeutic index can be determined.

BIOLOGIC AGENTS

INTERFERON. The most prominent and perhaps the most promising biologic agent used for the therapy of virus infections is interferon. This protein, first discovered in 1957 by Isaacs and Lindenmann, has a molecular weight of approximately 20,000. It is a natural compound produced by many types of cells, particularly lymphocytes, in all vertebrate and possibly invertebrate species, but its activity is fairly species specific. In tissue culture, it is effective against a wide variety of viruses if the cells have been treated with interferon before virus is added to the medium. The mechanism of action of interferon is still being elucidated, but it appears to act by interfering with translation functions once the virus has entered the cell. Interferon has an extremely high specific activity of approximately 1 billion units per milligram of protein (1 unit of interferon = the amount required to reduce viral plaques in tissue culture by 50 per cent). It is produced by infecting human lymphocytes, lymphoblasts, or fibroblasts with a virus or exposing them to a chemical inducer. The cells respond by releasing interferon into the medium, and the material is then purified by a number of complex chemical steps. Recently, the gene for interferon production has been inserted in bacteria, allowing for large-scale and efficient production of this complex protein.

Clinical studies have demonstrated the effectiveness of interferon in several viral illnesses. Interferon sprayed intranasally daily attenuates the symptoms associated with experimental rhinovirus infection, and ongoing studies are defining its practical use in the prevention and treatment of the common cold and influenza. When applied topically to the eye, interferon appears effective in the treatment of herpes keratitis. Parenteral interferon can lower or ablate the serum markers of chronic hepatitis B infection. High dose interferon (up to 5.1×10^5 units per kilogram per day) is effective in limiting the severity and progression of both herpes zoster and varicella in immunocompromised patients. The most impressive activity of interferon has occurred in the treatment of infection caused by human papilloma viruses. These agents cause juvenile laryngeal papillomas, which can cause severe and debilitating illness in children, and they also cause genital warts (condyloma accuminata). Daily doses of 1 to 5 million units per square meter of body surface area induce significant lesion reduction or disappearance in the majority of patients. Additional studies will determine the duration or permanence of these remissions. The most common adverse reactions are fever, lassitude, prostration, and hypotension, although tolerance appears to develop and these side effects often diminish as therapy is continued. A number of large molecular weight polymers have also been investigated for their ability to induce endogenous interferon. Some of these compounds have been plagued by chemical instability, severe adverse reactions, and tachyphylaxis.

IMMUNE GLOBULINS. Purified globulins have been used as "postexposure prophylaxis" for viral illnesses for a number of years. Such "prophylaxis" is in reality treatment of the viral infection before it is clinically manifest. Since antibodies cannot enter cells, they are effective only when the virus is circulating in the blood or when the newly formed viruses are spreading through interstitial fluid rather than via direct cell-to-cell contact. Antibodies may also exert their effect by attaching to a cell which has a viral antigen expressed on its surface, allowing complement and/or lymphocytes to destroy the infected cell. Serum prepared from patients convalescing from the illness to be treated, or serum selected to contain high titers of antibody to the virus to be treated, usually produces the best clinical results. The dosage to be given is often expressed in terms of volume (milliliters per kilogram). This is somewhat misleading, because the appropriate dose will be a factor not only of the volume of the serum preparation but also of the concentration of antibody within it. In some instances, this has been standardized.

Human globulin has been shown to be effective in several clinical situations. These include measles, rabies, and hepatitis A and B. Discussion and schedules of globulin therapy are provided under the individual topics. As newer chemical antivirals become available, the importance of these biologicals that do not affect replicating viruses will wane.

Barry DW, Blum MR: Antiviral drugs: Acyclovir. *In* Turner P, Shand DG (eds.): Recent Advances in Clinical Pharmacology. New York, Churchill Livingstone, 1983, pp 57–80. *A review of preclinical and clinical studies of acyclovir.*

Bauer DJ: The Specific Treatment of Virus Diseases. Lancaster, United Kingdom, MTP Press Ltd., 1977. *This book contains an excellent review of the principles of antiviral chemotherapy. Excellent analysis of clinical data relating to methisazone.*

Bean B, Braun C, Balfour HH: Acyclovir therapy for acute herpes zoster. Lancet 2:118, 1982. *Intravenous acyclovir was effective in these normal patients, but crystalluria can occur if infusions are given too rapidly.*

Bryson YJ, et al.: Treatment of first episode of genital herpes simplex virus infection with oral acyclovir. N Engl J Med 308:916, 1983. *This double-blind, placebo-controlled study demonstrated good efficacy with minimal side effects.*

Evans AS (ed.): Viral Infections of Humans. New York, Plenum Medical Book Company, 1976. *The most complete text on the epidemiology, pathophysiology, diagnosis, and therapy of viral infections.*

Galasso GJ, Merigan TC, Buchanan RA (eds.): Antiviral Agents and Viral Diseases of Man. New York, Raven Press, 1979. *This book reflects the status of antiviral chemotherapy in 1979.*

Goepfert H, et al.: Leukocyte interferon in patients with juvenile laryngeal papillomatosis. Ann Otol Rhinol Laryngol 91:431, 1982. *Clear demonstration of the activity of interferon in this viral-induced "proliferative" disease.*

Hall CB, et al.: Aerosolized ribavirin treatment of infants with respiratory syncytial viral infection. N Engl J Med 308:1443, 1983, *Excellent study of a new drug in a difficult disease.*

Heidelberger C, King DH: Trifluorothymidine. Pharmacol Ther 6:427, 1979. *Excellent review of this drug by its originator.*

Hirsch MS, Swartz MN: Antiviral agents. N Engl J Med 302:903, 949, 1980. *This concise review contains up-to-date information on several antivirals, particularly acyclovir and interferon.*

Oxford JS, Drasar FA, Williams JD: Chemotherapy of Herpes Simplex Virus Infections. New York, Academic Press, 1977. *This book thoroughly examines drugs affecting double-stranded DNA virus replication.*

Whitley RJ, et al.: Early vidarabine therapy to control the complications of herpes zoster in immunosuppressed patients. N Engl J Med 307:971–975, 1982. *This article contains the results of a multicenter, double-blind study, which showed the effectiveness of ara-A in herpes zoster.*

Whitley RJ, et al.: Vidarabine therapy of neonatal herpes simplex virus infection. Pediatrics 66:495–501, 1980. *Demonstration of the activity of ara-A in neonatal herpes.*

Whitley RJ, et al.: Adenine arabinoside therapy of biopsy-proven herpes simplex encephalitis. N Engl J Med 297:289, 1977. *This limited study was the basis for the use of ara-A in herpes encephalitis.*

29. GLUCOCORTICOSTEROID THERAPY

Anthony S. Fauci

In 1949, Hench and coworkers reported marked clinical improvement in patients with rheumatoid arthritis treated with cortisone. This proved to be a landmark observation. During the next 30 years glucocorticosteroids became a major factor in the successful chemotherapy of a wide range of diseases, particularly those in which inflammation or immunologically mediated phenomena played a prominent pathophysiologic role. However, these agents have proved to be a mixed blessing, for glucocorticosteroid therapy is also marked by a high incidence of deleterious and often devastating side effects. Perhaps as much as with any therapeutic agents, the use of corticosteroids requires an appreciation of the toxic as well as the beneficial effects of these drugs, since the one is almost invariably associated with the other. An understanding of the mechanisms of action as well as of the advantages and disadvantages of different glucocorticosteroids, and their treatment regimens, is essential for the physician to exercise appropriate clinical judgment in their use.

BIOCHEMISTRY AND PHARMACOLOGY. Glucocorticosteroids are synthesized endogenously by a series of reactions that result in the conversion of cholesterol to cortisol via pregnenolone and progesterone. Approximately 95 per cent of the endogenous cortisol in the circulation is bound to plasma proteins, particularly to a specific corticosteroid-binding globulin (CBG or transcortin); a lesser amount is bound to albumin. Cortisol is rapidly removed from the circulation with a plasma half-life of approximately 90 minutes. Cortisol is rapidly metabolized in a number of tissues, especially the liver. Less than 2 per cent of the cortisol produced is excreted in the urine unchanged. The active moiety of cortisol is the 11-betahydroxyl group. Exogenously administered compounds such as cortisone and prednisone, which are 11-keto compounds, lack glucocorticosteroid activity until they are converted in vivo into the corresponding 11-betahydroxyl compounds cortisol and prednisolone. This reaction occurs chiefly in the liver. Patients with serious impairment of liver function should be given prednisolone instead of prednisone in order to ensure availability of the active compound.

There are a number of synthetic analogues of cortisol in clinical use today. These differ in their plasma half-life, relative anti-inflammatory potency, and salt-retaining potency (Table 29–1). Among the glucocorticosteroid preparations in common use, cortisone and hydrocortisone have the highest sodium-retaining potency. For this reason, these agents are rarely the steroids of choice in situations requiring long-term administration, except when used as replacement therapy in adrenal insufficiency. Certain cortisol analogues such as dexamethasone are much less susceptible than cortisol to metabolic degradation. Thus, their plasma half-lives are longer, contributing to their greater relative anti-inflammatory potency. In general, the greater the plasma half-life of a glucocorticosteroid, the greater is its potency. However, almost invariably associated with greater potency is a greater degree of toxic side effects, including suppression of the hypothalamic-pituitary-adrenal (HPA) axis.

MECHANISMS OF GLUCOCORTICOSTEROID ACTION. Most, if not all, of the cellular and tissue responses to glucocorticosteroids are initiated via the common denominator of an intracellular glucocorticosteroid receptor. Glucocorticosteroid receptors are found in virtually every mammalian tissue. Based on in vitro models, exogenously administered glucocorticosteroids are thought to penetrate the cell membrane and bind with high affinity, but reversibly, to intracellular receptor proteins. The hormone-receptor complex then migrates to the cell nucleus and binds to nuclear protein. The association of the steroid-receptor complex with nuclear DNA modulates gene expression. Specific mRNAs then code for proteins that are thought to be responsible for the expression of the glucocorticosteroid effect. Certain cases of resistance to steroid therapy have been associated with receptor defects, particularly in the refractoriness of some patients with acute lymphoblastic leukemia to glucocorticosteroid therapy.

The effects of glucocorticosteroids subsequent to receptor binding, are exceedingly complex and multifaceted. Glucocorticosteroids are most often administered for their anti-inflammatory and immunosuppressive effects (the use of these agents as tumoricidal drugs in various chemotherapeutic protocols is discussed in Ch. 176). They are also occasionally administered for their ability to stabilize the cardiovascular system, as in hypotensive states arising from sepsis or other causes of cardiovascular collapse. Their efficacy in these latter situations is far less clearly documented than their effectiveness as anti-inflammatory and immunosuppressive agents. It is thought that the efficacy of glucocorticosteroids in clinical shock relates to a vasoconstrictive effect on the capillary bed, either directly or via potentiation of the action of alpha-adrenergic agents. An apparent paradox lies in the fact that glucocorticosteroids cause a decrease in total peripheral vascular resistance in normal humans and in patients in shock. Furthermore, steroids have been employed under certain circumstances as effective vasodilators in low output syndromes. This discrepancy may be explained by the possibility that there is selective vasoconstriction in certain capillary beds with vasodilation in others. Other proposed mechanisms of their efficacy in shock include an increase in cardiac contractility and cardiac output, maintenance of capillary wall integrity, and prevention of tissue breakdown.

Another clinical use of glucocorticosteroids is in the treatment of brain edema, particularly that resulting from brain tumors. The precise mechanisms by which steroids work in this setting are unclear. In situations in which vascular permeability is altered, steroids may act by maintaining vascular integrity, as also postulated in shock. In situations in which brain edema occurs in the presence of an apparently intact vasculature, the mechanisms of steroid effect are even more speculative. However, in these situations the effects are probably related, at least in part, to a decrease in the accumulation of sodium in the tissue edema.

Glucocorticosteroids are also administered therapeutically to ameliorate certain types of hypercalcemia such as that associated with sarcoidosis and certain neoplasms. The therapeutic effect is related to an influence of the steroid on calcium metabolism as well as a redistribution of body calcium.

The mechanisms whereby glucocorticosteroid administration results in anti-inflammatory and immunosuppressive effects are as complex as the inflammatory and immunologic reactions themselves. Glucocorticosteroids cause a rapid (four to six hours after administration) but transient lymphocytopenia and monocytopenia, not by lysis and destruction of cells as in certain animal models, but by a redistribution of cells out of the circulation into other lymphoid compartments, which renders the cells less accessible to sites of inflammation and immune reactivity. In steroid-induced lymphocytopenia, thymus-derived (T) lymphocytes are more markedly depleted than are bone marrow–derived (B) lymphocytes; similarly, within the T cell population, certain subsets of cells are more markedly affected than others. This has potential clinical relevance, since certain immunologically mediated diseases express abnormalities predominantly of specific subpopulations of cells. On the other hand, steroid administration results in a neutrophilia by mobilizing neutrophils from the bone marrow reserve, prolonging the circulating half-life of these cells, and blocking the free migration of these cells out of the circulation into inflammatory and other extravascular sites. One mechanism of this blockage of cell migration is interference with the initial adherence of neutrophils to the microvasculature endothelium prior to the extravascular diapedesis. In addition, steroids may block

TABLE 29–1. COMPARISON OF COMMONLY USED GLUCOCORTICOSTEROID PREPARATIONS

Compound	Equivalent Potency (mg)	Sodium-Retaining Potency	Plasma Half-Life (Minutes)
Cortisone	25	2+	30
Hydrocortisone (cortisol)	20	2+	90
Prednisone	5	1+	60
Prednisolone	5	1+	200
Methylprednisolone	4	0	180
Triamcinolone	4	0	300
Dexamethasone	0.75	0	200

the interaction of various chemotactic factors with neutrophils. Glucocorticosteroid administration also causes a profound eosinopenia. Although the mechanisms of this effect are unknown, the eosinophils are thought to be redistributed out of the circulation similarly to lymphocytes following steroid administration. Furthermore, in vivo and in vitro, glucocorticosteroids interfere with chemotaxis of eosinophils.

Besides affecting the movement and circulatory kinetics of inflammatory and immunologically competent cells, glucocorticosteroids can also have direct effects on their functional capabilities. These include effects on cell activation, proliferation, and differentiation; generation and release of cell products; levels of mediators of inflammation and immune reactions, as well as the response of certain cell types to such mediators; phagocytosis; antigen processing; cytotoxic effector functions; and several others. Various cell types may be selectively sensitive or resistant to the effects of steroids on one or another functional capability. Steroid sensitivity of different cell types also may vary, depending on the stage of activation of the cell. The direct effect of glucocorticosteroids on the functional capability of a cell usually requires higher sustained concentrations of hormone than does their effect on the traffic of the cell.

Of the two major circulating phagocytic cells in man, the monocyte is much more sensitive to direct suppression of its functional capabilities by steroids than is the neutrophil. This has clinically relevant implications, since the monocyte is one of the focal cells in the formation of granulomas, which are quite sensitive to the suppressive effects of glucocorticosteroids. Granulomatous hypersensitivity diseases are generally responsive to steroid therapy, whereas infectious diseases such as tuberculosis and certain fungal diseases which are characterized by granulomatous reactions are prone to exacerbation and relapse during high dose glucocorticosteroid therapy.

Although many antibody and immune complex–mediated diseases are treated with glucocorticosteroids, the antibody-forming cells (B lymphocytes and plasma cells) are relatively resistant to the suppressive effects of these agents. In fact, extremely high doses of drug are required to suppress antibody production by B cells and their progeny. The beneficial effects of steroids in antibody and immune complex–mediated diseases are most likely through indirect effects on the inflammatory response subsequent to the binding of antibody or deposition of immune complexes. At least one of the mechanisms of therapeutic efficacy of glucocorticosteroids in certain of the autoimmune hemolytic anemias and other cytopenias is blockage of the clearance of antibody-coated cells by the reticuloendothelial system.

Glucocorticosteroids are used extensively and beneficially in the treatment of asthma and immediate hypersensitivity allergic conditions. The precise mechanisms for this efficacy are not well understood. Although glucocorticosteroids cause a circulating eosinopenia, the precise role of the eosinophil in allergic and asthmatic reactions is unclear. Glucocorticosteroids have very little effect on serum IgE levels; they also have little effect on the early phase components of immediate hypersensitivity (Type I) immunologic reactions, although they do alter the late phase components. In certain systems, glucocorticosteroids induce an increase in intracellular cyclic adenosine monophosphate (cAMP), which in turn is associated with a decrease in release of certain mediators of inflammation. Corticosteroids also decrease the biosynthesis of certain prostaglandins, most likely by inducing the synthesis of a protein that inhibits the activity of membrane phospholipase A_2. Although corticosteroids do not protect animals against histamine-induced shock, suggesting that these agents do not block histamine release, several days of steroid treatment can decrease the histamine content of certain tissues. Furthermore, corticosteroids inhibit IgE-mediated release of histamine from human basophils after prolonged incubations. Finally, glucocorticosteroids suppress the expression of lymphocyte surface receptors for the Fc portion of IgE as well as the glycosylation of IgE-binding factors.

TREATMENT OF DISEASE STATES WITH GLUCOCORTICOSTEROIDS. A broad range of disease states, some with widely divergent causes and pathophysiologic mechanisms, have been treated effectively with corticosteroids. These include disorders requiring merely physiologic or replacement doses of the hormone, such as adrenal insufficiency, as well as diseases of suspected or proven inflammatory and/or immunologic mediation which require pharmacologic doses of drug. These diseases include the connective tissue disorders, particularly systemic lupus erythematosus, rheumatoid arthritis, acute rheumatic fever, dermatomyositis and polymyositis, and mixed connective tissue disease; several of the vasculitides; the idiopathic nephrotic syndrome; severe asthma; various hypersensitivity and allergic states; prophylaxis and treatment of organ transplant rejection; noninfectious granulomatous diseases such as sarcoidosis; autoimmune hemolytic anemia and the immunologically mediated cytopenias; a wide range of dermatologic and ophthalmologic conditions; and several others. Corticosteroids have proven extremely effective in the amelioration of brain edema, but have been inconsistent in septic shock and as adjunctive therapy to antibiotics in certain infections such as tuberculous meningitis.

From the standpoint of the physician, the critical issue is usually not whether the steroid will have a beneficial effect, but the choice of the most appropriate therapeutic regimen in a given patient at a specific phase of a particular disease.

DESIGN OF GLUCOCORTICOSTEROID THERAPEUTIC REGIMENS. The number of possibilities for different steroid regimens is enormous. To facilitate the proper choice, certain fundamental issues must be addressed. The first and most obvious is whether the disease is serious enough to warrant glucocorticosteroid therapy. A closely related question is whether the disease necessitates long-term administration of the drug for a reasonable therapeutic effect to be realized. For example, in mild asthma that is relatively well controlled on bronchodilators, or rheumatoid arthritis that is well managed on nonsteroidal anti-inflammatory agents, there is little question that administration of glucocorticosteroids would ameliorate symptoms even more. However, the required long-term use of even low doses of steroids militates strongly against their use in such situations. On the other hand, one would not hesitate to administer even massive doses (1 gram of methylprednisolone per dose) for limited periods of time in disorders such as status asthmaticus and acute organ transplant rejection. In clinical situations in which it is generally agreed that glucocorticosteroid therapy will be necessary for more than a brief time, other issues must be addressed by the physician. These include consideration of patient disposition to known toxic side effects of steroid therapy such as diabetes mellitus, peptic ulcer, psychiatric difficulties, osteoporosis (older individuals), exacerbations of underlying infections such as tuberculosis, and other potential hazards. If this is the case, alternative therapeutic regimens or modification of the steroid regimen (alternate-day therapy as opposed to daily therapy) to lessen the incidence of such side effects must be considered.

Local vs. Systemic Therapy. In some clinical situations, local glucocorticosteroid therapy that delivers high concentrations of drug directly to the involved site is much preferable to systemic administration of drug. Typical examples are certain dermatologic conditions such as contact dermatitis, in which steroid-containing creams and ointments can be applied directly to the involved areas. There is generally no need for systemic steroids under these circumstances, since the disease activity is usually sharply localized. However, if a large enough area is exposed to the steroid for a sufficient amount of time, absorption can be great enough to result in systemic effects. Other examples of local administration include topical conjunctival administration of corticosteroids for a variety of ocular conditions as well as steroid enemas for ulcerative proctitis. The latter situation is especially prone to systemic absorption of drug, since denuded mucous membrane is exposed to the hormone.

One of the most important advances in the development of glucocorticosteroid agents has been inhaled aerosol steroids used in the treatment of bronchial asthma. In patients with steroid-dependent asthma, inhalants such as beclomethasone sprayed into the airways via the mouth in doses of two inhalations (100 μg) three to four times per day have allowed a reduction of systemic steroid dosage while controlling symptoms in large numbers of patients.

Type of Agent Employed. Although relatively few glucocorticosteroid preparations are used by clinicians, several factors must be considered in the choice of a steroid agent. A steroid preparation that possesses little or no mineralocorticoid activity is generally preferred in order to avoid the sodium-retaining side effects. Among the commonly used preparations, cortisol (hydrocortisone) has the greatest degree of mineralocorticoid activity. One of the major uses of this agent is in replacement therapy for adrenal insufficiency. Most normal adults secrete about 20 mg of endogenous cortisol per day, and so adults with nearly complete adrenal insufficiency (Addison's disease) require approximately 20 mg of hydrocortisone per day in a single or divided dose. The mineralocorticoid effect is desirable in this situation. In fact, an additional mineralocorticoid (usually fludrocortisone, 0.1 mg per day) is generally administered to the addisonian patient. Hydrocortisone is also indicated in stress situations such as severe trauma and extensive surgical procedures in patients who are or have recently been receiving glucocorticosteroid therapy and may be relatively addisonian (see below).

Among the commonly employed glucocorticosteroids, dexamethasone and methylprednisolone have the least sodium-retaining properties, while prednisone and prednisolone exhibit a slight to moderate degree, significantly less than hydrocortisone (Table 29–1).

Ever since the development of synthetic glucocorticosteroids, great effort has been made to develop agents that are extremely potent and long acting but relatively nontoxic. Unfortunately, as a general rule, there is a correlation between duration of plasma half-life, potency, and toxic side effects. For example, dexamethasone is longer acting, more potent, and associated with greater deleterious side effects than the more commonly used prednisone. From a strictly anti-inflammatory or immunosuppressive standpoint, it would be desirable to administer a high dose of a long-acting agent at frequent intervals for an extended period of time in order to induce and maintain disease remission. However, the toxic side effects of such a regimen render it unacceptable except under the most extraordinary circumstances. In situations such as the chronic connective tissue diseases, it is more appropriate to employ a short-acting agent such as prednisone in a single dose in the morning, or on alternate days. Shorter-acting agents such as prednisone are essential for the construction of long-term regimens that closely mimic the normal diurnal cortisol cycle. What then is the indication for a potent long-acting agent such as dexamethasone? While there are no absolute indications, dexamethasone is generally considered to be the steroid of choice in clinical situations in which sustained high levels of potent glucocorticosteroids are desirable for limited periods of time, as in brain edema.

Dose and Dose Interval of Glucocorticosteroid Administration. BURST OR INTERMITTENT THERAPY. Examples of common, relatively minor ailments for which "burst" or intermittent administration of glucocorticosteroids is employed are poison ivy and poison oak dermatitis. Patients are generally given 60 mg of prednisone for two to three days, followed by rapid tapering of drug by 10 mg decrements over several days until complete discontinuation of therapy. Since the dose is not very large and the duration is short, there is little danger of suppression of the HPA axis or of any of the other complications of long-term steroid therapy (see below). Furthermore, the slight sodium-retaining potential of prednisone is hardly a factor under most circumstances. The burst therapy of high dose dexamethasone for brain edema has been mentioned above. However, there are other situations that call for short periods of "massive" doses of glucocorticosteroid. Some of the most common of these are the treatment of acute organ transplant rejection and the treatment of septic shock. The efficacy of such regimens is clearly documented for organ transplant rejection, in which methylprednisolone is given in doses of several grams per day for a limited time (usually three to five days), followed by conversion to more standard regimens of 60 to 100 mg of prednisone, which is then tapered according to the individual clinical situation. Methylprednisolone is generally employed for the burst therapy because of its relatively low sodium-retaining activity and high potency. Such brief courses of massive dose steroid therapy have also been used in some cases of acute deterioration in certain connective tissue diseases, particularly systemic lupus erythematosus with active nephritis. The efficacy of such an approach is not certain at this time.

DAILY GLUCOCORTICOSTEROID THERAPY. The most commonly employed regimen for inflammatory and immunologically mediated diseases is the administration of prednisone on a daily basis either as a single dose in the morning or in divided doses over the day. A given dose of a relatively short-acting agent such as prednisone is more potent in its anti-inflammatory and immunosuppressive properties when administered in daily divided doses than in a single daily dose. Divided dose therapy is also attended by a greater incidence of complications, particularly suppression of the HPA axis. Administration of the same total amount of drug in a single dose on alternate days provides less of an anti-inflammatory and immunosuppressive effect but also produces significantly fewer toxic side effects than the daily dose regimen. Ideally, a short-acting agent should be administered in a manner that closely mimics the normal diurnal cortisol cycle—namely, peak levels of cortisol early in the morning (6 to 8 A.M.), with tapering off by mid to late afternoon so that the low levels late at night release the pituitary gland from feedback inhibition and permit secretion of adrenocorticotropic hormone (ACTH). The therapeutic aim is to deliver the hormone in a bolus without interrupting the normal feedback mechanisms and thus without disrupting the normal pattern of steroid levels. Persistence of supraphysiologic or pharmacologic levels of hormone late in the day likely accounts for the toxic "tissue" effects and surely accounts for the suppression of the normal HPA cycle seen with daily administration of glucocorticosteroids.

Virtually all therapeutically effective regimens of daily divided dose glucocorticosteroid will have some of these effects. Even single daily doses as low as 15 to 20 mg per day of prednisone will cause both toxic tissue effects and HPA axis suppression. A single dose of dexamethasone will likely have the same deleterious side effects as an equivalent anti-inflammatory dose of prednisone given in divided doses over the day because of its longer plasma half-life. Since most of the complications of glucocorticosteroid therapy are dose, dose interval, and time related, an appropriate guideline in initiating or maintaining glucocorticosteroid therapy in a given patient is to administer the smallest possible dose in the least toxic dose interval over the shortest period of time sufficient to control disease activity. It is inappropriate to initiate steroid therapy in a patient with a flagrantly active inflammatory disease by administering a low dose of a short-acting drug (prednisone) in a single daily dose or on alternate days in order to avoid toxic side effects. It is just as inappropriate to allow a patient whose disease has been put into remission by high doses of divided daily prednisone to remain on that regimen for an inordinate period of time before tapering to a less toxic regimen.

Since the diseases that are treated with glucocorticosteroids are heterogeneous and of varying severity, it is extremely difficult to set strict rules for drug administration. However, there can be general and flexible guidelines. For example, if a patient presents with an inflammatory or hypersensitivity disease that is quite active, one should initiate therapy with prednisone at a dose of at least 1 mg per kilogram per day in up to three divided doses. Although this is a potentially toxic regimen if administered over an extended period of time, it may be essential in order to induce a remission of disease. Initiation with a less aggressive therapeutic regimen may fail to induce a remission of disease while still subjecting the patient to the side effects of the chosen regimen. Once remission has been attained with subjective and objective improvement, attempts should be made to taper to the least toxic regimen, with the ultimate goal of completely discontinuing the drug if possible. A common mistake is to leave the patient on the regimen that induced remission while the toxic side effects go unnoticed for some time. Once clinical remission is induced, the divided daily dose can gradually be consolidated into a single daily dose with administration of the same total dose. If remission is maintained, the daily dose can gradually be tapered while monitoring closely for symptoms of disease exacerbation, adrenal insufficiency, or withdrawal (see below). Tapering is continued until the lowest possible dosage that can maintain remission is reached or until the drug is discontinued. Adjunctive therapy with other agents, such as nonsteroidal anti-inflammatory drugs for connective tissue diseases and disodium cromoglycate or aerosolized steroid in asthma, often facilitates the tapering schedule. Again, the precise schedules for tapering may have to be modified from patient to patient. The advantage of converting from daily divided doses to a single daily dose as opposed to decreasing each of the divided doses is that by arriving at a single dose, the normal diurnal cortisol cycle can be closely mimicked, which will better acclimate the body to the ultimate discontinuation of therapy. One of the most effective regimens for a smooth tapering of glucocorticosteroid therapy is to convert from a daily divided dose to a single daily dose to an alternate-day administration and ultimately to complete discontinuation (see below).

Alternate-Day Glucocorticosteroid Therapy. Many inflammatory diseases can be maintained in clinical remission by alternate-day glucocorticosteroid therapy. The rationale of alternate-day glucocorticosteroid therapy is to deliver at regular intervals (every 48 hours) a dose of a short-acting steroid that will maintain the suppression of disease activity while avoiding the toxic side effects associated with single daily dose or divided daily dose regimens. The drug is administered in a single dose in the morning at a time when the normal endogenous cortisol level is at its peak, with maximal feedback suppression of ACTH secretion already occurring. By evening, the administered drug is no longer present in the circulation and the steroid deprivation will normally signal the HPA axis to secrete ACTH, which in turn will stimulate the secretion of endogenous cortisol the following morning when the patient will not be receiving exogenous hormone. In this way, the normal endogenous cortisol levels will maintain the patient's homeostatic function on the "off" day of exogenous steroid. The following day the drug is again administered, and the pharmacologic effect is apparently sufficient to maintain the disease in clinical remission.

It may be necessary to initiate exogenous hormone therapy on a daily basis or even in divided doses to induce remission of an active inflammatory process. However, once the process is adequately suppressed, doses of steroid as widely spaced as 48 hours may be adequate to prevent the reacceleration and reamplification of the process and so successfully maintain the disease in remission. The suppression of HPA function is directly related to the plasma levels of hormone. Apparently therapeutic effects are not so related.

The logistics of conversion from a daily to an alternate-day steroid regimen are difficult. Two common pitfalls are attempting to accomplish the conversion too rapidly and failing to give a sufficient amount of drug on the "on" day. Although there are no strict rules in the conversion process, one approach has proved successful in a high percentage of patients. If a patient is receiving steroid in a daily divided dose regimen, that dose is first consolidated to a single dose in the morning. Based on the plasma half-life of prednisone, the highest practical single dose that one could administer on an alternate-day basis without suppressing the cortisol cycle on the "off" day is 120 mg. In actual practice, however, 80 to 100 mg is probably maximal. Clearly, a short-acting agent must be used, since administration of a long-acting agent such as dexamethasone on alternate days is intrinsically contradictory. Thus, if a patient is receiving 60 mg of prednisone per day, the daily dose is gradually tapered to 40 or 50 mg per day. At this point, the dose on the ultimate "on" day is immediately doubled to 80 or 100 mg. The dose on the ultimate "off" day is gradually tapered by 5 to 10 mg decrements over several cycles until it reaches 20 mg, and then by 2.5 mg decrements until the patient is receiving no drug that day. The rapidity with which the dosage is tapered on the "off" day varies considerably among patients and depends on the underlying disease, the length of time the patient received daily therapy, and the tolerance of the patient to the tapering process. The judicious use of nonsteroidal anti-inflammatory agents during the tapering process can often prove most helpful. Once the patient has reached a true alternate-day regimen, the dose on the "on" day is maintained for variable periods of time, depending upon individual patient factors, and then it, too, can be tapered to the lowest possible dose required to maintain remission, which may be complete discontinuation of therapy. Although not every patient who requires glucocorticosteroids will be maintained on an alternate-day regimen, such a regimen should be attempted when possible.

ACTH vs. Glucocorticosteroids. The relative merits of using ACTH or glucocorticosteroids in the treatment of various diseases have often been debated. In short, there is no convincing evidence that ACTH is superior to glucocorticosteroids in the treatment of any disease. Furthermore, glucocorticosteroids are preferable to ACTH for a number of reasons. ACTH must be injected, whereas glucocorticosteroids can be administered orally as well as parenterally. The ACTH effect depends on the stimulation of release of variable amounts of cortisol from the adrenal gland, whereas the dose of administered glucocorticosteroid can be precisely controlled. In addition, ACTH stimulates other hormones, such as androgens and mineralocorticoids, which may have undesirable side effects. Also, administration of ACTH may result in hyperpigmentation.

Approach to HPA Axis Suppression. One of the most disputed topics in glucocorticosteroid therapy is the duration of steroid administration that will result in HPA axis suppression. A closely related topic is the duration of HPA axis suppression following cessation of steroid therapy. Reports have been conflicting, and results are variable from patient to patient. It is virtually impossible to identify the shortest period of therapy or the smallest dose at which clinically significant suppression of the HPA axis will occur. The most conservative estimates will be given here.

Patients who have received the equivalent of 30 mg of prednisone per day for more than a week should be considered to have sustained suppression of the HPA axis. This may be asymptomatic except under conditions of severe stress. In patients who have been exposed to high doses of glucocorticosteroids daily over a prolonged period of time, as much as 12 months may be required following cessation of therapy before normal hormonal response to stress returns. If patients who are suspected of HPA axis suppression are to be subjected to severe stress such as a major surgical procedure, they should receive parenteral hydrocortisone in doses of 100 mg every four to six hours during surgery and for several days thereafter, depending on the recovery period.

It is possible to determine the integrity of the HPA axis in a patient who is receiving or who has recently received glucocorticosteroid therapy. The standard test is to administer 50 units of ACTH as a constant intravenous infusion over six to eight hours and measure the resulting rise in plasma cortisol. Alternatively, synthetic ACTH (beta 1-24 ACTH) can be given as a rapid intravenous infusion (250 μg), with measurement of plasma cortisol at 30 minutes and one hour after injection. In patients with normal adrenal glands, plasma cortisol levels should rise to at least 30 μg per milliliter.

Once glucocorticosteroid therapy has been withdrawn, recovery from suppression of the HPA axis is a gradual process, the rate of which varies considerably among patients. There are no proven manipulations to hasten this process. Hypothalamic-pituitary function returns before adrenocortical function. The use of ACTH has not been proved to hasten recovery of HPA function. Conversion to alternate-day steroid therapy prior to withdrawal generally leads to a less symptomatic recovery, but it does not hasten the process. Suppression of the HPA axis can be associated with a diverse array of symptoms (discussed below). Since many of these symptoms may mimic the disease process for which the glucocorticosteroids were originally administered, it is essential for the physician to monitor the patient closely, with appropriate diagnostic measures aimed at determining disease activity as well as integrity of the HPA axis. If the patient manifests HPA axis suppression, reinstitution of glucocorticosteroid therapy with more gradual withdrawal is indicated.

WITHDRAWAL SYNDROMES. Withdrawal from glucocorticosteroid therapy may result in both subjective and objective manifestations of adrenal suppression. Features of the withdrawal syndrome may include lethargy, weakness, anorexia, nausea, fever, arthralgia, orthostatic hypotension with syncope, hypoglycemia, weight loss, and desquamation of the skin. The entire symptom complex may relate to HPA axis suppression, for which replacement therapy is indicated. However, exacerbation of certain underlying diseases may manifest similar symptoms. Furthermore, a number of patients may manifest a physical or psychologic dependence on glucocorticosteroids and yet have neither exacerbation of underlying disease nor suppression of normal HPA function. If the dependence is psychologic, appropriate counseling and encouragement are indicated. However, physical dependence may exist in the face of normal HPA function, since the tissues may have been acclimated to high levels of glucocorticosteroids for such a period of time that, despite "normal" levels of cortisol, the patient experiences symptoms of steroid deprivation. Under these circumstances, reinstitution of physiologic doses of a short-acting drug such as prednisone followed by a more protracted tapering period may be indicated. Finally, certain patients may manifest biochemical evidence of HPA axis suppression without evidence of exacerbation of underlying disease and without symptoms.

COMPLICATIONS OF GLUCOCORTICOSTEROID THERAPY. The major limiting factor in the use of glucocorticosteroid therapy is the wide array of deleterious side effects that may occur in association with these agents (Table 29–2). The frequency and severity of glucocorticosteroid-related complications, although extremely variable among patients, are directly related to the dose, duration, and schedule of therapy. Although all the complications listed in Table 29–2 have been amply documented in patients receiving glucocorticosteroid therapy, the direct cause-effect relationship between drug administration and complications has not been equally convincing for each of the complications. For example, there is a high incidence of spontaneous peptic ulcer in certain diseases that are treated with glucocorticosteroids, particularly rheumatoid arthritis. In addition, other gastrointestinal irritants such as the nonsteroidal anti-inflammatory agents are often administered concomitantly with the steroid. In the absence of adequately controlled studies, it is difficult to determine whether glucocorticosteroids increase the incidence of peptic ulceration. Also, daily administration of steroid is associated with an increase in infectious disease complications. Several diseases that are treated with steroids, such as lymphoid malignancies and systemic lupus erythematosus, have defects of host defense. These act synergistically with the steroid-induced compromise of host defenses to result in an increased incidence of opportunistic infections. On the other hand, patients with asthma who are treated with steroids do not seem to have an increased incidence of infections. This may be related to the otherwise normal host defenses of these patients as well as to the low doses of steroid usually employed. By contrast, osteoporosis and cataracts are commonly and directly related to glucocorticosteroid therapy.

TABLE 29–2. COMPLICATIONS OF GLUCOCORTICOSTEROID THERAPY

Central nervous system	Endocrinologic
Pseudotumor cerebri	Suppression of HPA axis
Psychiatric disorders	Growth failure
Musculoskeletal	Secondary amenorrhea
Osteoporosis with spontaneous fractures	Metabolic
Aseptic necrosis of bone	Hyperglycemia and unmasking of genetic predisposition to diabetes mellitus
Myopathy	Nonketotic hyperosmolar states
Ocular	Hyperlipidemia
Glaucoma	Alterations of fat distribution (typical cushingoid appearance)
Cataracts	Fatty infiltration of the liver
Gastrointestinal	Drug interactions (decreased anticoagulant effect of ethyl biscoumacetate)
Peptic ulceration	Fibroblast inhibition
Intestinal perforation	Inhibition of wound healing
Pancreatitis	Subcutaneous tissue atrophy (striae, purpura, ecchymosis)
Cardiovascular and fluid balance	Suppression of host defenses
Hypertension	Immunosuppression, anergy
Sodium and fluid retention	Effects on phagocyte kinetics and function
Hypokalemic alkalosis	Increased incidence of infections
Hypersensitivity reactions	
Urticaria	
Anaphylaxis	

Questions often arise about the effects of steroid therapy on delayed cutaneous hypersensitivity responses. This effect is variable and dose related. Generally, patients receiving less than 80 mg of prednisone on alternate days have intact delayed cutaneous hypersensitivity. By contrast, patients receiving daily steroid will generally become anergic if the dose is 15 mg of prednisone or greater, with the onset of anergy usually within days after initiation of therapy. Following cessation of therapy, if all other factors involved in delayed hypersensitivity are intact, responses generally return within ten days to two weeks.

Glucocorticosteroids are not considered to increase teratogenic risk among newborns of mothers who receive steroids during pregnancy. However, such infants should be monitored for adrenal insufficiency during the neonatal period. Also, since glucocorticosteroids are excreted in breast milk, inhibition of endogenous steroid production as well as growth suppression can occur in infants who are breast fed by mothers receiving the hormone.

Axelrod L: Glucocorticoid therapy. Medicine 55:39, 1976. *A well-written, comprehensive review article which discusses the scientific basis for many of the practical guidelines in the clinical use of glucocorticosteroids.*

Baxter JD, Rousseau GG: Glucocorticoid Hormone Action. New York, Springer-Verlag, 1979. *An excellent book with comprehensive and sophisticated coverage of basic mechanisms of glucocorticoid action. One of the outstanding works on steroid hormone action, with contributions by recognized leaders in the field.*

Dixon RB, Christy NP: On the various forms of corticosteroid withdrawal syndrome. Am J Med 68:224, 1980. *An excellent, lucidly written discussion of corticosteroid withdrawal syndromes, with use of case presentations as examples.*

Fauci AS: Alternate-day corticosteroid therapy. Am J Med 64:729, 1978. *Concise editorial discussion on usefulness and limitations of alternate-day glucocorticosteroid therapy.*

Fauci AS, Dale DC, Balow JE: Glucocorticosteroid therapy: Mechanisms of action and clinical considerations. Ann Intern Med 84:304, 1976. *An extensive review of mechanisms of action of glucocorticosteroids as they relate to therapeutic efficacy in the treatment of inflammatory and immunologically mediated diseases. Practical outlines of the design and modification of therapeutic regimens.*

Kehrl JH, Fauci AS: The clinical use of glucocorticoids. Ann Allergy 50:2, 1983. *An updated review article on the theoretical and practical aspects of the use of corticosteroids in clinical medicine.*

Thorn GW: Clinical considerations in the use of corticosteroids. N Engl J Med 274:775, 1966. *This superb article remains the classic treatise on the rational use of corticosteroid therapy.*

Part VI
PRINCIPLES OF HUMAN GENETICS

30. HUMAN HEREDITY

James B. Wyngaarden

The appreciation of genetic factors as arbiters of human disease is a relatively recent development in medical history. Scattered references to inheritance of biologic characteristics may be found in the records of several millenia, including the frequently cited Talmudic exemption from circumcision of males born into families of bleeders, but discernible patterns of hereditary transmission were recognized first in the eighteenth and nineteenth centuries. In the 1750's Maupertuis described the autosomal dominant inheritance of polydactyly. The essential features of X-linked inheritance of hemophilia were described in the early 1800's by several writers and the pattern formally outlined by Nasse in 1820. The pattern of inheritance now recognized as autosomal recessive was described by Adams in 1814, and the biologic consequences of consanguinity first reported by Bemiss in 1857. In 1876, Galton introduced the twin method of separating effects of heredity from those of environment; later he initiated quantitative studies of polygenic inheritance.

Genetics as an experimental science owes its origins to Gregor Mendel and his cross-breeding of garden peas, tall and short, yellow seed and green seed, round seed and wrinkled seed. From these studies Mendel derived concepts of dominant and recessive traits, hereditary factors (which we now call *genes*), alternative factors *(alleles)*, true breeding plants with two identical factors *(homozygotes)*, and nontrue breeding plants with alternative factors *(heterozygotes)*. His experiments led to the formulation of laws of *unit inheritance* (that "factors" retain their identity from generation to generation and do not blend in the hybrid), of *segregation* (that two members [alleles] of a single pair of factors [genes] are never found in the same gamete but always segregate), and of *independent assortment* (that members of different pairs of genes [nonalleles] assort to gametes independent of one another). These laws, formulated in 1865, had almost no immediate impact on biologic thought, but they are now cornerstones of genetics. They were rediscovered about 1900 by several workers independently and first applied to human disease by Sir Archibald Garrod in his concept of "inborn errors of metabolism," which he proposed in 1908.

With the emergence of genetics a polemic arose concerning the relative importance of hereditary and environmental factors in the expression of traits and causation of disease. This nature-nurture controversy has been superseded by growing insights into the role of specific environmental factors on the function of specific genes.

Genetics is concerned with the study of hereditary variations. Most of these variations are not harmful; indeed, they confer a distinct biologic advantage by enabling the species to adapt to changing environments. When variations are extreme and impair the health and fitness of the individual, we consider them diseases. These extreme variations are of three principal types: (1) chromosomal aberrations, (2) single-gene differences that exhibit mendelian patterns of inheritance, and (3) polygenic disorders, in which two or more, often multiple, genes each contribute to the characteristic in question. Examples of the first two categories are relatively easy to recognize, and the balance of genetic and environmental influences easy to quantify. Many genetic diseases are dependent upon environmental factors for their expression, e.g., phenylalanine ingestion in phenylketonuria, or milk ingestion in galactosemia. Other hereditary diseases are kept in abeyance by specific environmental factors: scurvy is an inborn error of metabolism (absence of the hepatic enzyme that converts L-gulonolactone to L-ascorbic acid in man, monkey, and guinea pig) kept in remission by vitamin C; metabolic cretinism is foiled in its expression by the administration of thyroid hormone. The greatest difficulty in sorting out the relative importance of genetic and environmental influences is encountered with common diseases. In disorders such as rheumatoid arthritis, essential hypertension, and coronary artery disease, genetic influences are important but hard to identify in specific biochemical terms. Occasionally it is possible to recognize single genes that have a metabolic effect, such as that responsible for one type of hypercholesterolemia, but more often genetic factors are multiple or elusive and still beyond definition.

The pace of genetic advance across the full spectrum of molecular biology to human heredity is currently rapid. The revolution in biology of the past three decades is increasingly molding medical science and practice. As additional genetic mechanisms are disclosed they will illuminate more and more human diseases and from time to time suggest new avenues of therapy.

THE FAMILY HISTORY. A careful family history is indispensable in the assessment and understanding of hereditary disease. The interviewer should ascertain whether anyone in the family has had a condition similar to that of the patient, and whether this condition or any other "runs in the family." Particularly in the case of rare disorders one should inquire whether the parents are related, and, if this is not known, whether they or their families came from the same village or community and whether their forebears may have intermarried. Since some disorders are more common in certain ethnic groups than in others, the ethnic origin of the parents should also be elicited.

The rarer the recessive disorder in a specific population, the greater is the likelihood of parental consanguinity. Tay-Sachs disease is relatively rare in non-Jews, in whom the gene frequency is low, but a high proportion of non-Jewish parents of Tay-Sachs children are consanguineous. By contrast, Tay-Sachs disease is relatively common in Jews of eastern European origin, in whom the gene frequency is relatively high. In parents of Jewish children with Tay-Sachs disease in the United States the frequency of consanguinity is only slightly higher than in the general population.

Certain ethnic backgrounds increase the likelihood of certain diagnostic possibilities while decreasing that of others. Thalassemia is chiefly a disorder of people of the Mediterranean region and of Southeast Asia, familial Mediterranean fever is a disorder of Armenians and Sephardic Jews, acatalasia is a disease of Japanese and Koreans, and gout is very common among the Maori. By contrast, cystic fibrosis is rare in blacks, phenylketonuria is uncommon in Jews, and sickle cell anemia does not occur in Caucasians.

PEDIGREE ANALYSIS. The chief method of study of an inherited disease in man is the observation of its pattern of distribution in kindreds, i.e., of its pedigree pattern. The construction of a pedigree pattern begins with the individual first detected, who is referred to as the proband, index case, or propositus (female = proposita). The pedigree pattern allows one to judge whether the distribution conforms to mendelian principles of segregation and assortment and thus represents single-factor inheritance. Patterns that do not conform to mendelian principles may represent polygenic traits in which a number of genes each contributes a minor effect. Valid pedigrees depend on accurate and extensive information about the kindred. This information is likely to be more reliable when based on observer detection, e.g., direct observation of all family members of several generations for the presence of hypercholesterolemia, than when based on memory, e.g., the recollection of the occurrence of vascular disease in uncles, aunts, and grandparents. Great care must be exercised when very large pedigrees are recorded and analyzed.

MONOGENIC DISORDERS. Disorders caused by single mutant genes show one of four simple (mendelian) patterns of inheritance: (1) autosomal dominant, (2) autosomal recessive, (3) X-linked dominant, or (4) X-linked recessive. Dominant traits are those expressed in the heterozygote (as well as in the homozygote or hemizygote). Recessive traits are those expressed in the homozygotes (or hemizygotes) but silent in the heterozygote. The terms *dominant* and *recessive* refer to the phenotypic expression of the trait, not to the expression of the gene. Thus it is incorrect to speak of a dominant or recessive gene. A gene is either expressed or not expressed. Whether the trait is considered dominant or recessive often depends upon the level of observation. Sickle cell anemia is a recessive trait, i.e., it requires a double dose of the abnormal gene for expression at the clinical level. Nevertheless, the sickle gene is expressed in single dose as well, giving rise to carriers with SA hemoglobin. Recessive traits are often *codominant* when viewed biochemically at the level of the gene product.

With few exceptions, each of the approximately 1600 mendelian diseases is rare. The overall population frequency of monogenic disorders is about 10 per 1000 live births, comprising about 7 per 1000 dominants, about 2.5 per 1000 recessives, and about 0.4 per 1000 X-linked conditions (see Table 30–1).

If a particular disease shows a mendelian pattern of inheritance, its pathogenesis, no matter how complex, must be due to a single abnormal protein molecule. For example, in sickle cell disease, such seemingly unrelated disturbances as hemolytic anemia, painful crises, nephropathy, vascular occlusions, and *Salmonella* osteomyelitis are all physiologic consequences of a single missense mutation (see Fig. 31–2), resulting in a single amino acid substitution in the β-globin chain. When two or more phenotypic characters are controlled by a single gene, that gene is said to have *pleiotropic* effects.

AUTOSOMAL DOMINANT TRAITS. Autosomal genes are those genes situated on chromosomes other than the X or Y. When there are two alleles, A and a, at a locus, three possible genotypes exist: AA, Aa, and aa. Genotypes AA and aa are called *homozygotes;* Aa is a *heterozygote.*

Dominant traits are fully manifest in the presence of a gene in the heterozygous state, i.e., when only one abnormal gene *(mutant allele)* is present and the corresponding partner allele on the homologous chromosome is normal. Figure 30–1 shows a typical pedigree of transmission of an autosomal dominant trait. The following features are characteristic: (1) each affected individual has an affected parent (unless the condition arose by a new mutation in a germ cell that formed the individual); (2) an affected individual will bear, on the average, an equal number of affected and unaffected offspring; (3) males and females will be affected in equal numbers; (4) each sex can transmit the trait to male and female offspring (i.e., male-to-male transmission is possible); (5) normal children of an affected individual will have only normal offspring; and (6) when the trait does not impair viability or reproductive capacity, there will be *vertical* transmission of the trait through successive generations.

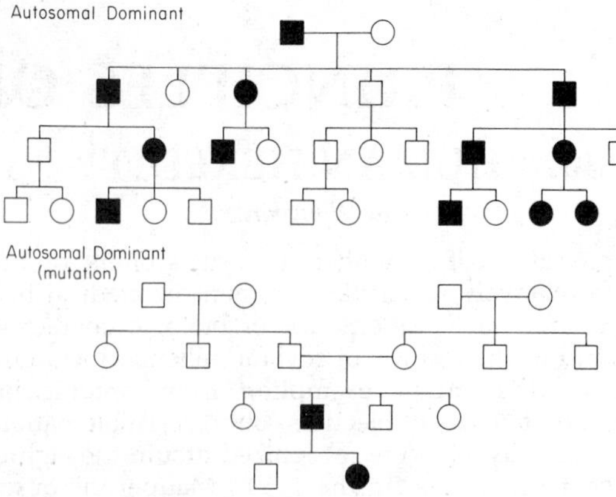

Figure 30–1. Pedigrees of autosomal dominant traits. In the lower pedigree the normal parents of the affected individual suggest the possibility of a new mutation. Solid symbols indicate those affected. (For details see text.)

Most autosomal dominant disorders show two additional characteristics that are not seen in recessive disorders: (1) wide variability in severity, or *expressivity,* and (2) delayed age of onset. Dominant traits in man often exert only mild effects. Occasionally the expression of the abnormal gene is so weak that a generation appears to be skipped because the carrier of the abnormal gene is clinically normal. When this is the case, the trait is said to be *nonpenetrant.* When a dominant gene exists in the homozygous state the effect may be very severe, perhaps lethal. Examples are common in animals in which experimental matings can be constructed, but rare in man, because matings of two affected heterozygotes are exceptional. One example is homozygous familial hypercholesterolemia. Others possibly include achondroplasia and Osler-Weber-Rendu syndrome. Delayed age of onset is seen in disorders such as Huntington's disease and adult polycystic kidney disease. These disorders do not become manifest clinically until adult life, even though the mutant gene has been present since conception.

In every autosomal dominant disease some affected persons owe their disorder to a new mutation rather than to an inherited allele. Since a reasonable estimate of the frequency of mutation is of the order of 5×10^{-6} mutations per gene per generation, and since a dominant trait requires a mutation in only one of the parental gametes, one would expect that about 1 in 100,000 newborn persons would possess a new mutation at any given genetic locus. Many mutations will be silent or will involve a recessive function and not be manifest in a single gene dose. However, others will cause a defective gene product that gives rise to a dominant trait.

The percentage of patients with dominant disorders that represents a new mutation is inversely proportional to the effect of the disease upon *biologic fitness,* i.e., survival to adult life, and reproductive capacity. If a dominant mutation produces early death or absolute infertility, genetic transmission is impossible, and all cases represent new mutations. In tuberous sclerosis, the severe mental retardation reduces biologic fitness to about 20 per cent of normal and the proportion of cases due to new mutations is about 80 per cent. In dominant conditions such as familial hypercholesterolemia in which there is no reduction in biologic fitness, virtually all cases have a family pedigree showing classic vertical transmission.

New mutations appear to be more frequent in the germ cells of fathers of relatively advanced age. Both Marfan's syndrome and achondroplastic dwarfism display such "paternal age ef-

TABLE 30–1. PREVALENCE OF SELECTED MONOGENIC DISORDERS AMONG LIVEBORN INFANTS*

Disorder	Estimated Prevalence
Autosomal dominant	
Familial hypercholesterolemia	1 in 500
Polycystic kidney disease	1 in 1250
Huntington's disease	1 in 2500
Hereditary spherocytosis	1 in 5000
Marfan's syndrome	1 in 20,000
Autosomal recessive	
Sickle cell anemia	1 in 625 (U.S. Blacks)
Cystic fibrosis	1 in 2000 (Caucasians)
Tay-Sachs disease	1 in 3000 (U.S. Jews)
Cystinuria	1 in 7000
Phenylketonuria	1 in 12,000
Mucopolysaccharidoses (all types)	1 in 25,000
Glycogen storage disease (all types)	1 in 50,000
Galactosemia	1 in 57,000
Homocystinuria	1 in 200,000
X-linked	
Duchenne muscular dystrophy	1 in 7000
Hemophilia	1 in 10,000

*Data assembled from Galjaard, Carter, and Motulsky.

fect." Fathers of sporadic cases of both conditions are an average of five to seven years older than the general population of fathers or than fathers who transmit these syndromes because of an inherited mutation. Diagnosis of a new mutation must exclude low expressivity of the trait in the carrier parent and also mistaken paternity.

The molecular basis of most of the more than 900 autosomal dominant disorders is obscure. Because in a dominant disorder expression of the mutation in only 50 per cent of the gene product may be sufficient to cause disease, the mutations are likely to involve two classes of proteins: (1) those that regulate complex metabolic pathways, such as membrane receptors as in familial hypercholesterolemia, and (2) key nonenzymic or structural proteins, such as hemoglobin or collagen, or a membrane protein as in hereditary spherocytosis.

In contrast to recessive disorders, in which an enzyme deficiency is the rule, defective enzymes are only rarely found in dominant disorders. A deficiency of *C1-esterase inhibitor* in hereditary angioedema and of *uroporphyrinogen-1 synthetase* in acute intermittent porphyria are exceptions to this general rule.

AUTOSOMAL RECESSIVE DISORDERS. Autosomal recessive conditions are clinically apparent only in the homozygous state, i.e., when both alleles at a particular genetic locus are mutant alleles. Figure 30–2 shows a typical pedigree of an autosomal recessive trait. The following features are characteristic: (1) the parents are clinically normal; (2) only siblings are affected; (3) males and females are affected in equal proportions; (4) if an affected individual marries a homozygous normal person, none of the children will be affected but all will be heterozygous carriers; (5) if an affected individual marries a heterozygous carrier, one half of the children will be affected, and the pedigree pattern will superficially suggest a dominant trait; (6) if two individuals who are homozygous for the same mutant gene marry, all of their children will be affected; (7) if both parents are heterozygotes, i.e., each a carrier of one mutant allele at the same genetic locus, one fourth of their children will be homozygous affected, one fourth will be homozygous normal, and one half will be heterozygous carriers of the same mutant gene; and (8) the more infrequent the mutant gene is in the population, the greater is the likelihood that the affected individual is the product of consanguine parents.

In actual practice, unless the kinship is very large, the ratio of affected to unaffected sibs is frequently greater than one in four. Inclusion of probands in the enumeration loads the results in favor of the trait. In a sibship of 100 or even 10 the loading factor is not pronounced. However, in all ascertainable one-child sibships the involvement is 100 per cent, in two-child sibships it is 67 per cent (when the fundamental probability is 50 per cent), in three-child sibships it is 57 per cent, and so on. In small sibships a correction must be made for *bias of ascertainment*. The simplest method is to exclude the proband from the calculation, and to determine the proportion of affected children among the remaining sibs.

In most autosomal recessive conditions the clinical presentation tends to be more uniform than in dominant diseases, and the onset is often early in life. Recessive disorders are commonly diagnosed in childhood. Approximately 800 well-established recessive traits have been recognized in man, and in over 250 of these the mutant enzyme or other protein has been identified.

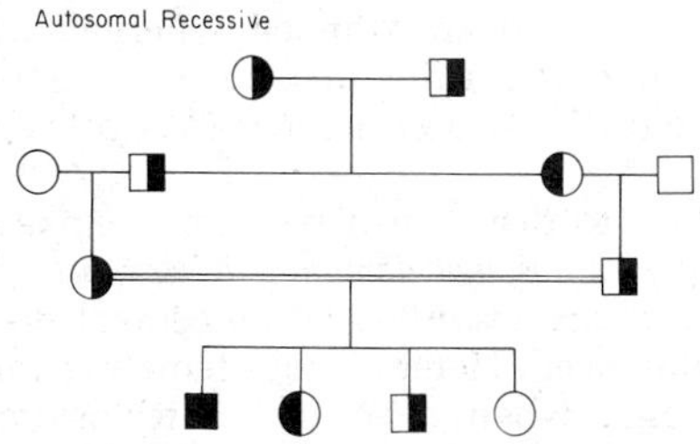

Figure 30–2. Pedigree of autosomal recessive trait. Note: both parents are heterozygous. One sib is affected, two are carriers, and one is normal. Double line (=) indicates that parents are related by descent (first cousins).

A *completely* recessive disease is one in which the heterozygote is clinically normal. When some features of the disease are detectable in the heterozygote, the disease is sometimes said to show *intermediate inheritance*, or to be *incompletely recessive* or *incompletely dominant*. The ambiguity of these terms from classic genetic studies of phenotypes is further emphasized by results of different methods of detection of gene effects. In many instances of completely recessive inheritance, refined biochemical observations enable the recognition of the trait in the clinically normal heterozygote. An example is Tay-Sachs disease, in which clinically normal parents and some sibs can be shown to be heterozygotes by assay of hexosaminidase A in leukocytes. Because of its importance in genetic counseling the detection of healthy heterozygous carriers of genes that in the homozygous state cause overt disease is one of the most significant aspects of medical genetics. Since by definition a dominant trait is one that is detectable in the heterozygous state, Tay-Sachs disease (and many others) is recessive when the clinical phenotype is considered and dominant when the biochemical phenotype is determined.

In pure form a recessive disease requires the inheritance of identical mutant genes from both parents. When the mutant genes are rare, the likelihood that any two unrelated parents are carriers for the same defect is small. Inheritance of two different mutant genes derived from the same locus gives rise to *heteroallelic compounds*. Individuals with Hb SC disease are genetic compounds who have inherited a different abnormal β-globin gene from each parent. Genetic compounds are also known in cystinuria, phenylketonuria, certain of the mucopolysaccharidoses, "homozygous" familial hypercholesterolemia, and several other disorders.

If the parents of a child with a recessive disorder have a common ancestor who carried a mutant gene, then the likelihood that two of the descendants would each have inherited the gene becomes relatively great. The less frequent the gene, the stronger is the likelihood that an affected individual has resulted from a consanguine mating. First cousins share, on the average, one eighth of their genes. When two first cousins marry, an offspring has, on the average, one sixteenth of the loci homozygous for a gene derived from a common ancestor. In general, offspring of first-cousin matings are slightly more likely to have congenital malformations, as well as mental defects and metabolic diseases, than are children born to unrelated parents.

Increased frequency of consanguinity will not be observed if the recessive disease is common. Sickle cell anemia, phenylketonuria, cystic fibrosis, and Tay-Sachs disease are examples in which the carrier (heterozygote) state is frequent in certain populations and in which consanguinity is usually not present in the parents. Increase in consanguinity would also not be expected in dominant or X-linked traits or genetic compounds.

A high percentage of recessive disorders involves abnormalities of enzyme proteins. In most reactions the normal maximal enzyme activity is greatly in excess of catalytic requirements; i.e., the concentration of a substrate is usually maintained at a point well below saturation for the enzyme that metabolizes it. Hence a reduction to 50 per cent of normal activity in a heterozygote does not impair the health of the carrier, whereas a total or near total deficiency may result in a serious inborn error of metabolism. These conditions are discussed in Ch. 32.

X-LINKED INHERITANCE. Diseases or traits that result from genes located on the X chromosome are termed X-linked. Since the female has two X chromosomes, she may be either heterozygous or homozygous for the mutant gene, and the trait may exhibit recessive or dominant expression. The male has only one X chromosome and therefore is *hemizygous* for X-linked traits. Males can be expected to express X-linked traits regardless of their recessive or dominant behavior in the female.

Thus, the terms X-linked dominant or X-linked recessive refer only to expression of the trait in women.

Since males transmit their X chromosome only to daughters, an important feature of X-linked inheritance is the absence of male-to-male transmission. Affected males transmit the trait to all of their daughters and none of their sons.

Since the female carries two X chromosomes in each cell, it might be expected that the concentrations of proteins determined by genes on the X chromosome would be twice that of males who carry only one X chromosome per cell. This is not the case, and the explanation is provided by the process of X-inactivation first proposed by Mary Lyon, and often termed the *Lyon hypothesis.* In all adult female cells only one of the X chromosomes is genetically active. Early in differentiation one of the X chromosomes becomes inactive and forms the *Barr body.* Inactivation is random so that for each cell there is an equal probability that the paternally or maternally derived X chromosome will be inactivated. Once one of the two X chromosomes is inactivated, the same X chromosome remains inactive throughout all subsequent cell divisions. Thus, on the average one half of the cells of a female will express the X chromosome of her father, and one half of her mother: in this respect the normal female is a mosaic. If one of the X chromosomes carries a mutant gene, the probability is that the mutant phenotype will be expressed in one half of her cells. However, this statistical probability may be disturbed in at least two ways: (1) Since inactivation of one of the X chromosomes occurs early in development and is random, some females may by chance have many more cells that carry an active X chromosome derived from one parent than from the other; and (2) if one of the X chromosomes carries a mutant gene that confers a metabolic disadvantage upon cells with that mutation, these cells may survive less frequently during development, and the female offspring may have cells that carry predominantly or exclusively the active X chromosome without the mutation.

Over 115 loci have been identified on the human X chromosome, and several have been mapped to specific regions on the long or the short arm of the chromosome.

X-Linked Dominant Traits. This mode of inheritance (Fig. 30–3) is uncommon. Its characteristic features are as follows: (1) females are affected about twice as often as males, (2) heterozygous females will transmit the trait to both sexes with a frequency of 50 per cent, (3) hemizygous affected males will transmit the trait to all of their daughters and none of their sons, and (4) the expression is more variable and generally less severe in heterozygous females than in hemizygous affected males. Examples of X-linked dominant inheritance include the Xg(a$^+$) blood group, vitamin D–resistant (hypophosphatemic) rickets, and pseudohypoparathyroidism.

Some rare X-linked dominant disorders occur only in the heterozygous female, because the condition is lethal in the hemizygous affected male. Additional characteristics of this form of inheritance are as follows: (1) an affected mother will transmit the trait to one half of her daughters (heterozygotes), and (2) an increased frequency of abortions occurs in affected women, the abortions representing affected male fetuses. Examples of disorders that appear to fit this mode of inheritance include incontinentia pigmenti, focal dermal hypoplasia, orofaciodigital syndrome, and hyperammonemia caused by ornithine transcarbamylase deficiency.

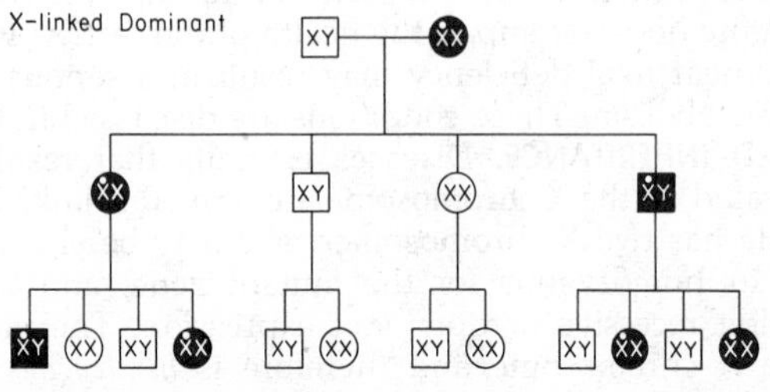

Figure 30–3. Pedigree of dominant X-linked trait. The X chromosome bearing the abnormal gene is designated by a small white dot.

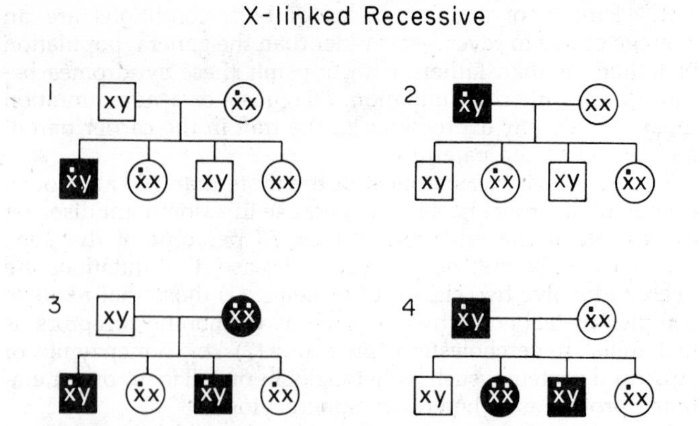

Figure 30–4. Pedigrees of X-linked recessive trait. The X chromosome bearing the abnormal gene is designated by a small dot. Affected individuals are indicated by solid squares (males) and circles (females). Pedigree 1 is commonly observed; pedigree 4 is rare.

X-Linked Recessive Traits. This mode of inheritance (Fig. 30–4) is relatively common. Its characteristic features are as follows: (1) The disorder is fully expressed only in the hemizygous affected male. (2) Heterozygous females are usually normal; occasionally they may exhibit mild features of the disorder; rarely they may be almost as severely affected as the hemizygous affected male (this variability is attributed to the probability that a disproportionate percentage of *normal* X chromosomes of the heterozygous female may have been inactivated early in development [see "Lyon hypothesis," above]). (3) On the average, a heterozygous female will transmit the trait to one half of her sons (hemizygous affected), but the other half will be normal. (4) On the average, one half of daughters of heterozygous female will be carriers and one half will be normal. (5) All daughters of an affected male married to a normal female will be carriers, and no sons of such a union will be affected (no father-to-son transmission). (6) In the rare event of the union of an affected male and a heterozygous female, one half of daughters will be homozygous affected and one half will be heterozygous carriers; one half of sons will be hemizygous affected (maternal inheritance) and one half will be normal. Thus in this situation, one half of all offspring will be affected. (7) If the trait is rare, parents and relatives will be normal except for male relatives in the female line; e.g., on the average, one half of maternal uncles will be affected. This "uncle and nephew" pattern gives rise to an *oblique* pedigree pattern, in contrast to the vertical pattern of autosomal dominant conditions and the horizontal pattern of autosomal recessive conditions.

Examples of X-linked recessive conditions include hemophilia A, Duchenne form of muscular dystrophy, the Lesch-Nyhan syndrome, glucose-6-phosphate dehydrogenase deficiency, and Fabry's disease. In several of these, e.g., Duchenne muscular dystrophy and Fabry's disease, heterozygous females may exhibit mild or even moderately severe forms of the disease. Color blindness is also an X-linked inherited trait, but it is sufficiently frequent (occurring in about 8 per cent of Caucasian males) that the occurrence of homozygous color-blind females is not rare.

It is important to distinguish between X-linked inheritance and *sex-influenced autosomal dominant inheritance.* Baldness and hemochromatosis are examples of autosomal dominant traits that are sex influenced. Heterozygous females express the gene for baldness only when a source of testosterone becomes available (e.g., a masculinizing tumor of the ovary). Heterozygous females rarely develop clinical hemochromatosis because menstruation and pregnancy mitigate the accumulation of iron.

Y-LINKED INHERITANCE. A gene on the Y chromosome will be transmitted through the father to all of his sons and none of his daughters. The only genes currently known to be located on the Y chromosome are those that determine "maleness" and an antigen that influences graft rejection.

POLYGENIC INHERITANCE. Most phenotypic traits are determined by the collaboration of many genes at different loci rather than by single gene effects. Polygenic inheritance is suggested for traits that show continuous variation in the form of a normal distribution curve. Height and intelligence are examples of polygenic traits in which the extremes of the distribution are not necessarily considered abnormal. Parents and offspring, and on average siblings also, have 50 per cent of their genes in common. Second degree relatives share on the average one fourth of all genes $(\frac{1}{2})^2$, and third degree relatives (cousins) share one eighth $(\frac{1}{2})^3$. Thus as the degree of relation becomes more distant, the probability of inheriting the same combination of genes is reduced, and the degree of resemblance is likely to be less.

Many of the common chronic diseases of adults (such as essential hypertension, diabetes mellitus, hyperuricemia, hypercholesterolemia, coronary artery disease, and schizophrenia) and the common birth defects of children (such as cleft palate and lip and congenital heart disease) that tend to run in families fit best into the category of *multifactorial genetic disease.* This category should be suspected when the pedigree of a disease does not support inheritance in a simple dominant or recessive manner. In multifactorial genetic disease there is both a polygenic component and an environmental component of causative factors. In the population at large there are *risk* genes present in low frequency. If in any one individual there is a particularly large number of risk genes, the latent disorder becomes overt. When an individual inherits just the right combination of risk genes, he passes beyond a "risk threshold" at which environmental factors may determine the expression and severity of disease (Fig. 30–5). In order for another family member to develop the same disease, that individual would have to inherit the same or nearly similar combination of genes. The likelihood of such an occurrence is clearly greater in first degree than in more distant relatives. The chances of any relative inheriting the right combination of risk genes also decrease as the number of genes required for the expression of a given trait increases. Elegant and complex mathematical models have been advanced for polygenic-multifactorial disease, but these should not obscure the fact that each of the risk genes must express itself, like any other gene, by way of a specific biochemical product. Eventually the vague concept of genetic susceptibility of polygenic inheritance must yield to the basic premise that genes control the synthesis of specific proteins with specific functions.

The hypothesis of polygenic components in the inheritance of multifactorial disease has been given a potential mechanistic basis by the demonstration that as many as 28 per cent of all gene loci may contain polymorphic alleles that vary among individuals. Such a large degree of variation in normal genes provides a basis for variation in genetic predisposition with which other genetic or environmental factors can interact. To date genetic loci most prominently associated with disease

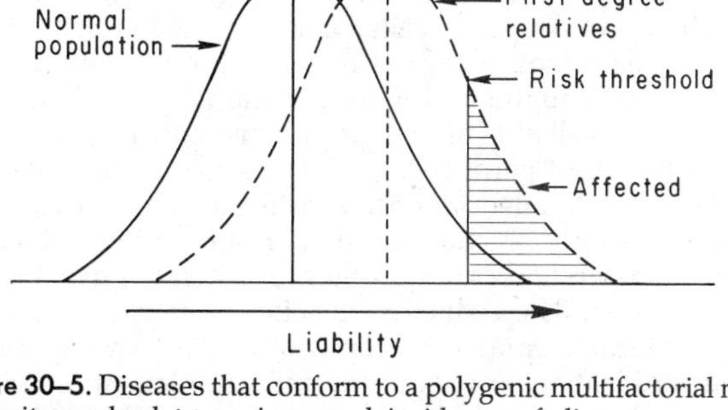

Figure 30–5. Diseases that conform to a polygenic multifactorial model of inheritance lead to an increased incidence of disease among the relatives of affected individuals. This increased incidence is most evident among first degree relatives.

susceptibility are those composing the major histocompatibility (MHC) locus or human leukocyte antigen (HLA) system. The HLA system consists of four distinct but closely linked, highly polymorphic loci situated on the short arm of chromosome 6. These loci as ordered on the chromosome are HLA-A, HLA-C, HLA-B, and HLA-D/DR. The A, B, C, and DR loci are defined serologically; the D locus controls lymphocyte (LD) antigens detectable by the mixed lymphocyte reaction (MLR). The D and DR (D-related) loci are closely linked but may not produce identical antigens. The products of these genes are proteins that are found on the surface of body cells and that enable an individual's immune system to distinguish its own cells (self) from those of someone else (nonself). Each HLA locus in the population consists of multiple alleles, each of which produces an immunologically distinct protein. HLA-A has at least 20 alleles, HLA-B has at least 42, C has at least 8, D has at least 12, and DR has at least 10 identified thus far. The inheritance of certain alleles predisposes to the development of certain diseases, in some instances when the individual is exposed to a particular environmental challenge. For example, the frequency of B27 allele in the white population is approximately 8 per cent. In patients with ankylosing spondylitis the frequency of B27 is over 90 per cent. In Australian aborigines and black Africans the B27 antigen is virtually absent and the frequency of ankylosing spondylitis is sharply reduced. A Caucasian with the B27 antigen is approximately 120 times more likely to develop ankylosing spondylitis than one who does not possess the antigen; the increased liability among Japanese with the B27 antigen is 300 times. Reiter's syndrome may follow an infection of the bowel or urinary tract with *Shigella, Salmonella,* or *Yersinia* organisms. No less than 20 per cent of B27 positive individuals with *Shigella* infections will develop Reiter's syndrome. Other disease associations of the HLA system are discussed in Ch. 436.

Multifactorial or polygenic inheritance must not be confused with genetic heterogeneity. Hypercholesterolemia and hyperuricemia behave as multifactorial traits when viewed at the population level. At the family level, however, it is sometimes possible to identify a single locus that is mainly responsible for the disease in that family. Examples include familial hypercholesterolemia, an autosomal dominant trait present in about 5 per cent of subjects with premature myocardial infarctions, which in single gene dosage produces atherosclerosis in the absence of any extraordinary environmental factor; or hypoxanthine–guanine phosphoribosyltransferase deficiency, an X-linked recessive trait present in about 0.5 per cent of subjects with gout, which in the hemizygous state produces marked purine overproduction without any relationship to obesity or alcohol consumption.

GENE FREQUENCY. The distribution of a mutant gene in the general population may be calculated on the basis of the Hardy-Weinberg equation. If the frequency of a particular gene A is p, then that of its alternative allele is $(1-p) = q$. There will be three genotypes in the population: those who are homozygous AA, those who are heterozygous Aa, and those who are homozygous aa. In a randomly mating population the frequencies of these genotypes will be in the proportion p^2(AA), 2pq(Aa), and q^2(aa). An important consequence of this distribution is that irrespective of the initial frequency of the genes A and a in the population, the proportion of the three genotypes will tend to remain constant in succeeding generations, provided that there is no difference in biologic fitness of any of the genotypes. If there is unequal viability or fertility among the three genotypes, or if mating is not random, the frequency calculations require considerable correction, and in small populations major changes in gene frequency can occur on the basis of chance alone.

If the frequency of a recessive disease in a particular population is known, the frequency of heterozygous carriers and of the abnormal gene can be calculated. Thus for a recessively inherited disease aa (q^2) with a frequency of 1 per 10,000 (e.g., albinism), the frequency of the gene a (q) will be 1 per 100, and that of heterozygous carriers will be $2 \times p \times q = 2 \times 99/100 \times 1/100$ = approximately 1 in 50. Thus, in this particular example there will be 200 clinically unaffected carriers of the abnormal gene for every affected individual. Table 30–1 lists the frequency of several inherited diseases. Cystic fibrosis, a recessively inherited disease, has a prevalence in the white population of about 1 per 2500 (q^2); thus the frequency of the gene (q) is 1 in 50, and of heterozygous carriers is approximately 1 in 25 or 4 per cent of the white population. A similar calculation with respect to sickle cell anemia among United States blacks ($q^2 = 1/625$) yields a frequency of heterozygous carriers of 1 in 12.5, or 8 per cent of the United States black population.

The frequency of most genes in the population is relatively stable. When a gene is rare and severely disadvantageous, the rate of its introduction into a population by spontaneous mutation (see Ch. 31) is balanced by the rate of elimination of the disadvantageous gene by natural selection. The frequency of the disadvantageous gene, however, can be stabilized at a high level if the heterozygotes are slightly favored (increased biologic fitness) and leave a greater number of progeny than either homozygote. When a rare form of a species is present at a frequency that cannot be maintained by recurrent mutation alone, a *balanced polymorphism* is said to exist. Usually this means that the rarer of two allelic forms occurs with a frequency of at least 1 per cent of the population. When this is found, *heterozygote advantage* should be suspected. An example of such a balanced polymorphism is the increased resistance of individuals heterozygous for the sickle cell trait to falciparum malaria. Although persons with sickle cell disease (homozygotes, SS hemoglobin) often die before they can reproduce, and thus remove the sickle cell gene from the population, the prevalence of heterozygotes (SA hemoglobin) may nevertheless reach 40 per cent in certain West African populations. Death from falciparum malaria is much less frequent in carriers of the sickle cell trait than in noncarriers, and thus the heterozygote does have an advantage. Whether the extraordinary frequency of heterozygotes for the sickle gene in West Africa is due entirely to differential mortality or in part to differential fertility is uncertain, but this example suffices to illustrate that the effects of genes can be assessed only in relation to a particular environment. In most instances, however, a distinct advantage for the heterozygote of a polymorphic trait (of which there are many; see Ch. 32) cannot be demonstrated, and the possibility exists that certain polymorphic traits are genetically neutral.

The term *genetic load* has been used to describe the total genetic disability of a population. It comprises both a *mutational load,* based on recurrent mutation of a normal gene to a lethal or sublethal gene, and a *segregational load,* resulting from segregation of the harmful gene from advantaged heterozygotes, as in the example of sickle cell heterozygotes discussed above. Each individual has been estimated to have three to eight genes, which, if homozygous instead of heterozygous, would be lethal. The relative contribution of the segregational and mutational loads to the total genetic load is uncertain.

Carter CO: Monogenic disorders. J Med Genet 14:316, 1977. *An estimate of birth frequencies of selected genetic conditions.*
Cavalli-Sforza LL, Bodmer WF: The Genetics of Human Populations. 2nd ed. San Francisco, W. H. Freeman and Company, 1978. *An authoritative textbook of human genetics.*
Galjaard H: Genetic Metabolic Diseases. Early Diagnosis and Prenatal Analysis. Amsterdam, New York, Oxford, Elsevier/North Holland, Biomedical Press, 1980. *An 850-page book on hereditary disorders, about one third of which is devoted to methods and results of prenatal diagnosis.*
McKusick VA: Human Genetics. 2nd ed. Englewood Cliffs, N.J., Prentice-Hall, 1969. *An excellent introductory survey of human genetics.*
McKusick VA: Mendelian Inheritance in Man. 6th ed. Baltimore, Johns Hopkins University Press, 1983. *A catalogue of autosomal dominant, autosomal recessive, and X-linked phenotypes, with brief descriptions and literature references for each.*
Motulsky AG: Frequency of sickling disorders in U.S. blacks. N Engl J Med 288:31, 1973. *Gives estimated prevalence of all sickling disorders in the population (Hb SS disease, Hb SC disease, and Hb S-β thalassemia).*
Vogel F, Motulsky AG: Human Genetics: Problems and Approaches. Berlin, Springer-Verlag, 1979. *A superb and up-to-date treatment of human genetics.*

31. BIOCHEMICAL GENETICS

James B. Wyngaarden

In 1944 Avery and his associates at the Rockefeller Institute established that the hereditary information in the transforming principle of pneumococci resided in its deoxyribonucleic acid (DNA). From that date onward DNA has been considered the basic material of the gene. In 1953 Watson and Crick proposed a remarkable molecular model for the structure of DNA, consisting of two polynucleotide strands twisted together in a double helix with the purine and pyrimidine bases facing inward and attached to each other, binding the two chains. This model offered a rational structure for replication of DNA and for storage of hereditary information within sequences of purine and pyrimidine bases. This structure has since been established by x-ray crystallography. The genetic code, namely the precise triplet sequences of purine and pyrimidine bases in the structural gene that specify the individual amino acids of a polypeptide chain, was discovered by Nirenberg in 1961.

The amount of DNA in each human cell is sufficient to code for approximately one million polypeptides of average length. Estimates of the number of structural genes in man range from 50,000 to 100,000; large amounts of DNA constitute noncoding sequences whose function is as yet obscure. Only a small number of structural genes have been identified. In the most recent update of his catalogue of *Mendelian Inheritance in Man,* McKusick lists phenotypic variations or diseases of 1637 established genetic loci, thus implying that at least that many genes have undergone mutation so as to cause human disease or polymorphism. The chromosomal location of more than 350 of these genes is now known.

TRANSMISSION OF GENETIC INFORMATION

GENES. The term *gene* was introduced by Johannsen in 1909 to designate the hereditary determinant of a "unit characteristic." The relationship between gene and enzyme was recognized by Garrod in 1908, but first attained clear definition in the one gene–one enzyme hypothesis proposed by Beadle in 1945. A gene is now often defined as a linear segment of DNA that codes for a single polypeptide. A more accurate definition of a gene might relate a segment of DNA to a specific molecule of ribonucleic acid (RNA), because there are genes that specify RNAs that do not code for polypeptides, such as ribosomal and transfer RNAs. The sum of all genes of an individual, i.e., the total genetic endowment, is called the *genome.* The genetic composition of an individual is termed its *genotype.*

CHROMOSOMES. The genes are assembled into lengthy linear arrays that together with certain proteins form rod-shaped structures called *chromosomes.* Normal human nucleated cells, other than germ cells, contain 46 chromosomes, consisting of 23 pairs (diploid state), one of each pair having been derived from each of the individual's parents.

There are two processes by which genetic information is transmitted to daughter cells. During somatic cell division, called *mitosis,* identical copies of each chromosome are transmitted to each daughter cell, thus maintaining a uniform genetic composition in all cells of a single organism. By contrast, during the production of germ cells (ova or spermatozoa) a reductive division occurs, called *meiosis,* with the result that each germ cell contains only 23 chromosomes, representing one copy of each pair of parental chromosomes, one half the usual number (haploid state). The reductive division permits new combinations of chromosomes to occur when ovum and sperm fuse during fertilization to restore the full complement of 46 chromosomes. During meiosis the assortment of chromosomes is random so that each germ cell receives a different combination of maternal and paternal chromosomes. *Independent assortment* of chromosomes into gametes during meiosis results in an enormous diversity among the possible genotypes of the progeny. For each 23 pairs of chromosomes in the gamete, there are 2^{23} possible combinations, and the likelihood that any one set of parents will produce two offspring with identical sets of chromosomes is one in 2^{23} or one in 8.4 million (monozygotic twins excepted).

THE GENE AND PROTEIN SYNTHESIS. In specifying the amino acid sequence of a polypeptide a *structural gene* first transfers its information to a unique type of ribonucleic acid, known as messenger RNA or mRNA. This RNA is complementary to one strand of DNA, and the sequence of purine and pyrimidine bases in the DNA strand determines the base sequence in mRNA, which in turn governs the order of amino acids in the polypeptide. The transfer of information from DNA to RNA involves no change of language (nucleotide →nucleotide) and is called *transcription;* the transfer of information from RNA to polypeptide involves a new language (nucleotide → amino acid) and is called *translation.* These relationships are often referred to as the central dogma of molecular biology. Several RNA animal tumor viruses contain an RNA-dependent DNA polymerase (reverse transcriptase) that uses RNA as a template for synthesis of double-stranded DNA, and thus reverses the familiar direction of information flow. The function of this enzyme remains a question of central biologic importance in the problem of neoplasia. Reverse transcriptase is now widely used in the laboratory to synthesize complementary strands of DNA (called cDNA) from isolated molecules of specific mRNA (see Ch. 33 and 34).

DEOXYRIBONUCLEIC ACID. Deoxyribonucleic acids are linear polymers of deoxyribonucleotides that are formed by phosphodiester linkage between the 5′-phosphate of one nucleotide and the 3′-hydroxyl group of the sugar of the adjacent one. Deoxyribonucleotides consist of a purine or pyrimidine base linked to 2-deoxy-D-ribose-5-phosphate. The phosphate confers on DNA its acidic properties.

The purine bases of DNA are adenine (A) and guanine (G); the pyrimidine bases are thymine (T) and cytosine (C). Native DNA consists of two polynucleotide strands wound around each other. The two strands are held together in part by hydrogen bonding between apposing purine and pyrimidine bases; the sugar-phosphate groups form an external spine. The internal bondings are specific. Adenine always pairs with thymine and guanine with cytosine. Thus, the two chains are not identical but are *complementary* with respect to base pairings, A to T and G to C.

In the replication of DNA during mitosis the parent molecule unwinds and the bases of each strand serve as a template for the synthesis of a new strand of DNA. Thus just prior to cell division the cell has a double complement of DNA and of completed chromosomes. Since each chromosome is now represented four times, this is called the *tetraploid* state. Since both parental strands are conserved in the next generation, each now paired with a newly synthesized complementary partner, replication is termed *semi-conservative.*

In addition to its primary structure, the DNA in eukaryotic (nucleated) cells is organized into a variety of secondary coils and loops under the influence of basic proteins (histones) that bind to DNA. There are about 50 different histone proteins in the cell, some arginine rich, some lysine rich.

RIBONUCLEIC ACID. Ribonucleic acids are also linear polymers of nucleotides, but they differ in important respects from DNA. In RNA the sugar is D-ribose-5-phosphate, and the bases are adenine, guanine, cytosine, and uracil (instead of thymine). In addition, all mammalian RNAs are single stranded.

There are four main types of RNA, distinguishable by characteristic composition, size, functional properties, and cellular location. These are giant or heterogeneous nuclear RNA (hnRNA), messenger RNA (mRNA), ribosomal RNA (rRNA), and transfer RNA (tRNA). At any instant, hnRNA and mRNA constitute 3 to 5 per cent of total cellular RNA, rRNA 80 to 85 per cent, and tRNA 10 to 15 per cent of the total. The roles of each of these RNAs are discussed below.

MESSENGER RNA. The initial product of nuclear gene transcription is a giant molecule of RNA, on the average five to ten times larger than mRNA. The heterogeneous nuclear RNA must be *processed* to form smaller molecules of functional mRNA before the mRNA leaves the nucleus to associate with a ribosome in protein synthesis. The initial synthesis of hnRNA reflects the transcription of the dispersed structural gene (whose segments are called exons) together with intervening segments of noncoding DNA (introns). The function of the introns is not known. Most of the hnRNA remains in the nucleus and is degraded. The biochemical mechanisms of recognition and excision of mRNA segments and of their reassembly into a functional mRNA are not well understood.

The molecules of mRNA vary in size, depending on the length of the polypeptide chain to be synthesized, and range from 300 to 3000 nucleotides in the coding sequence. They also vary in their stability, with half-lives ranging from minutes to many hours. For example, the half-life of globin mRNA is about 14 hours. Since it requires only 10 to 20 seconds to assemble a polypeptide chain, a single molecule of mRNA may participate in the synthesis of many molecules of protein.

THE GENETIC CODE. Because most proteins are composed of 20 different amino acids, and because DNA has only four different nucleotide bases, each codon must contain a minimum of three bases ($4^2 = 16$; $4^3 = 64$). The DNA and RNA triplet codes for each of the 20 amino acids are known (Table 31–1). The 64 different triplets include 61 that have been shown to code for one of the 20 amino acids, and three that function as chain-terminating codons and do not code for any amino acid. The RNA codons for chain termination are UAA, UAG, and UGA. Two codons (AUG and GUG) serve to initiate polypeptide synthesis as well as to insert amino acids and are sometimes designated chain-initiating codons. Since many amino acids have more than one codon, the code is said to be *degenerate.* Each codon, however, is completely specific. Since the same codons code for the same amino acids in all plant, bacterial, viral, and animal systems studied (but see exceptions below, under Mitochondrial DNA), the code is regarded as *universal.* The nucleotide sequences of human genes disclose alternating sequences of coding and noncoding segments. The correspondence of the sequences of DNA and RNA codons in the polynucleotides with the sequence of amino acids in the polypeptides confirms the principle of *colinearity* of the sequential array of the information in the gene and mRNA and the amino acids of the proteins.

MITOCHONDRIAL DNA. A small fraction of cellular DNA is located in the mitochondria and maps as two distinct circular strands. This DNA contains the codes for certain ribosomal and transfer RNAs used by the mitochondria in protein synthesis, e.g., of cytochrome b and cytochrome c oxidases I, II, and III. Mitochondrial DNA lacks intervening sequences or introns. Its codons differ from those of nuclear DNA or of any present-day prokaryotes in a few instances: UGA = tryptophan (not termination), AUA = methionine (not isoleucine), and AGA and AGG = termination (not arginine).

TRANSFER RNA. Amino acids must be "activated" before they can be assembled into polypeptide chains. Activation is accomplished by reaction of the amino acid with ATP to form an amino acid adenylate. The amino acid adenylate then reacts with a molecule of tRNA to form an aminoacyl-tRNA. Both steps are catalyzed by a single enzyme, an aminoacyl-tRNA synthetase, which is specific for the amino acid as well as for the receptor tRNA. Although only a single aminoacyl-tRNA synthetase exists for each of the 20 amino acids commonly found in proteins, there may be several tRNAs for one amino acid. Each amino acid has at least one specific tRNA. tRNAs are transcribed from DNA by RNA polymerase III.

tRNAs are relatively small molecules, each consisting of a single chain of approximately 80 nucleotides, many of whose bases have been modified, e.g., by methylation. Each tRNA is

TABLE 31–1. THE GENETIC CODE

First Nucleotide	Second Nucleotide A or *U*			G or *C*			T or *A*			C or *G*			Third Nucleotide
A	**AAA**	*UUU*	Phe	**AGA**	*UCU*	Ser	**ATA**	*UAU*	Tyr	**ACA**	*UGU*	Cys	A or *U*
or	**AAG**	*UUC*		**AGG**	*UCC*		**ATG**	*UAC*		**ACG**	*UGC*		G or *C*
U	**AAT**	*UUA*	Leu	**AGT**	*UCA*		**ATT**	*UAA*	Stop	**ACT**	*UGA*	Stop	T or *A*
	AAC	*UUG*		**AGC**	*UCG*		**ATC**	*UAG*		**ACC**	*UGG*	Trp	C or *G*
G	**GAA**	*CUU*	Leu	**GGA**	*CCU*	Pro	**GTA**	*CAU*	His	**GCA**	*CGU*	Arg	A or *U*
or	**GAG**	*CUC*		**GGG**	*CCC*		**GTG**	*CAC*		**GCG**	*CGC*		G or *C*
C	**GAT**	*CUA*		**GGT**	*CCA*		**GTT**	*CAA*	Gln	**GCT**	*CGA*		T or *A*
	GAC	*CUG*		**GGC**	*CCG*		**GTC**	*CAG*		**GCC**	*CGG*		C or *G*
T	**TAA**	*AUU*	Ile	**TGA**	*ACU*	Thr	**TTA**	*AAU*	Asn	**TCA**	*AGU*	Ser	A or *U*
or	**TAG**	*AUC*		**TGG**	*ACC*		**TTG**	*AAC*		**TCG**	*AGC*		G or *C*
A	**TAT**	*AUA*		**TGT**	*ACA*		**TTT**	*AAA*	Lys	**TCT**	*AGA*	Arg	T or *A*
	TAC	*AUG*	Met	**TGC**	*ACG*		**TTC**	*AAG*		**TCC**	*AGG*		C or *G*
C	**CAA**	*GUU*	Val	**CGA**	*GCU*	Ala	**CTA**	*GAU*	Asp	**CCA**	*GGU*	Gly	A or *U*
or	**CAG**	*GUC*		**CGG**	*GCC*		**CTG**	*GAC*		**CCG**	*GGC*		G or *C*
G	**CAT**	*GUA*		**CGT**	*GCA*		**CTT**	*GAA*	Glu	**CCT**	*GGA*		T or *A*
	CAC	*GUG*		**CGC**	*GCG*		**CTC**	*GAG*		**CCC**	*GGG*		C or *G*

Note: The DNA codons appear in **boldface** type; the complementary RNA codons are in *italics*. A = adenine, C = cytosine, G = guanine, T = thymine, U = uridine (replaces thymine in RNA). In RNA, adenine is complementary to thymine of DNA, uridine is complementary to adenine of DNA, cytosine is complementary to guanine, and vice versa, "Stop" = punctuation. The amino acids are abbreviated as follows:

Ala = alanine	Gln = glutamine	Leu = leucine	Ser = serine
Arg = arginine	Glu = glutamic acid	Lys = lysine	Thr = threonine
Asn = asparagine	Gly = glycine	Met = methionine	Trp = tryptophan
Asp = aspartic acid	His = histidine	Phe = phenylalanine	Tyr = tyrosine
Cys = cysteine	Ile = isoleucine	Pro = proline	Val = valine

folded into a two-dimensional cloverleaf containing a high frequency of paired bases. The "stem" of the cloverleaf contains a recognition site for an amino acid; the loop opposite the stem contains a recognition site for the specific mRNA codon for that amino acid. Thus, the fidelity of translation is assured by the specific binding of the amino acid to the appropriate tRNA, and by the complementary base pairing of the *anticodon* of the tRNA with the codon of the mRNA.

RIBOSOMES. The template mRNA and the aminoacyl-tRNAs meet on the ribosome, where assembly of polypeptide chains takes place. Ribosomes are cytoplasmic particles composed of about one half protein and one half RNA. In differentiated mammalian cells most of the ribosomes are found in intimate association with membranes of the endoplasmic reticulum. Smaller numbers are present in the nucleus and mitochondria where a limited amount of protein synthesis also takes place. The number of ribosomes per cell is a rather direct function of the rate of cell growth.

The cytoplasmic ribosome in eukaryotic cells has a molecular weight of 4.5 million. It is composed of a small (40S) and a large (60S) subunit. The 40S subunit contains an 18S rRNA molecule of 2000 nucleotide residues and approximately 30 proteins; the 60S subunit contains both a 28S rRNA of 4000 nucleotides and a 5S rRNA of 121 nucleotides, plus approximately 50 different proteins. Ribosomal RNAs have genes that are duplicated and multiply represented in the chromosome. Ribosomal RNAs are transcribed from DNA by RNA polymerase II. Messenger RNA, bearing the instructions for polypeptide synthesis, forms a complex with the smaller ribosomal subunit and with the initiator aminoacyl-tRNA. The larger subunit then attaches to this complex to form a functional ribosome, and the sequential assembly of amino acids into protein can now begin.

PROTEIN SYNTHESIS. The translation of mRNA into a polypeptide occurs in three consecutive phases: initiation, chain elongation, and termination.

Initiation involves formation of a complex of aminoacyl-tRNA and mRNA on the ribosome. The process is complex and involves in addition at least three initiation factors (cytoplasmic proteins) and GTP. In prokaryotes and in mitochondria of eukaryotes initiation is specific for N-formylmethionyl-tRNA, but the eventual protein does not have a terminal N-formylmethionine residue. Thus deformylation takes place before release of the protein from the ribosome. In some proteins the terminal methionine is also removed. In eukaryotic cells, initiation of cytoplasmic protein synthesis also involves methionyl-tRNA, but in this instance the methionine is not formylated.

Once polypeptide chain synthesis has been initiated, continuation of the process requires the attachment of the aminoacyl-tRNA of the second amino acid, as specified by the second codon of the mRNA. Peptidyl synthetase now catalyzes the formation of a peptide bond between the first and second amino acids, and the mRNA then moves along the ribosome so that the third amino acid now comes into position with further elongation of the chain. In like manner the entire polypeptide chain is synthesized from the amino-terminal to carboxy-terminal end. The mRNA has a distinct polarity as it moves along the ribosome, always reading from the 5′ to the 3′ end. When a chain-termination codon (non-sense triplet) is reached, elongation ceases and the polypeptide chain is released from the ribosome.

A single mRNA molecule may move across the surfaces of several ribosomes simultaneously. A cluster of ribosomes attached to a single mRNA strand is called a polyribosome; polyribosomes synthesizing globin chains (MW 17,000) consist, on the average, of four to six ribosomes. A schematic diagram of the genetic control of protein synthesis is shown in Figure 31–1.

MUTATION. Broadly defined, a mutation is a stable, heritable alteration in DNA. Mutations occur approximately once in 10^6 replications per gene. Mutations can involve gross alterations in the structure of a chromosome, such as a duplication or deletion, or the translocation of a portion of one chromosome to another. Disorders resulting from mutations of this type are discussed in Ch. 35.

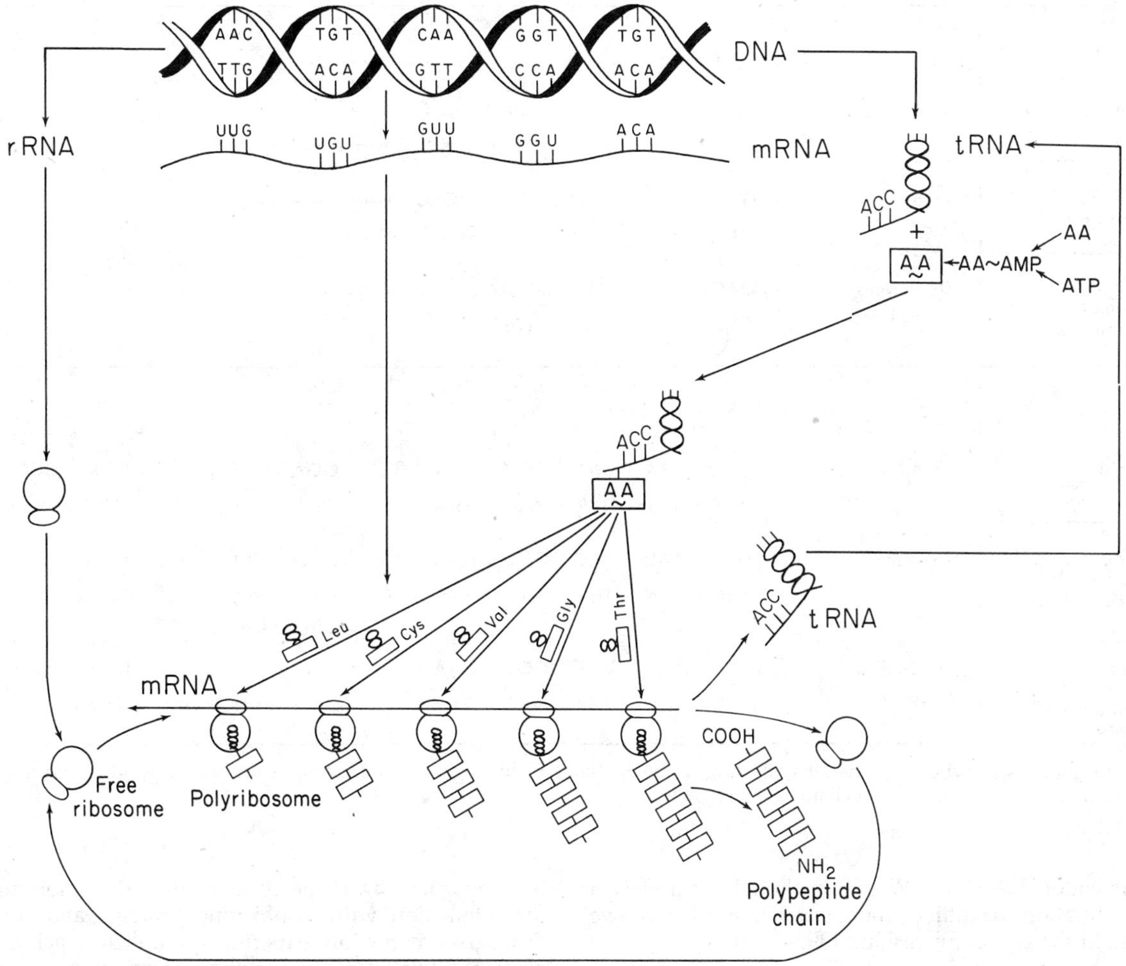

Figure 31–1. Schematic diagram of the genetic control of protein synthesis. A = adenine, T = thymine, G = guanine, C = cytosine, U = uracil. The codons indicated represent code words for the amino acids indicated. The messenger RNA (mRNA) moves across the ribosomes in the direction of the arrow. tRNA = transfer RNA; rRNA = ribosomal RNA. AA = amino acids.

Mutations can also be minute, involving as small a segment of DNA as a single base. When one base is replaced by another, the result is a *point mutation.* Point mutations may be of three types: (1) a *synonymous mutation* (making up about 23 per cent of random point mutations), in which the base substitution results in replacement of one codon by another that codes for the same amino acid, as in a change in DNA from GAA→GAG, both of which code for leucine; (2) a *mis-sense mutation* (73 per cent of point mutations), in which a base replacement changes the codon of one amino acid to that of another, such as AAG →AGG, which results in replacement of a phenylalanine by a serine residue; or (3) a *non-sense mutation* (4 per cent of point mutations, in which the base replacement changes an amino acid codon to one of the terminator codons, such as TTC→ATC, which results in a reading change from lysine to "stop." Following a point mutation there is always a finite chance that a second mutation may occur at the site of the original mutation. If such a mutation corrects the genetic change, it is called a *reversion.*

Deletions or insertions of a single base give rise to *frame-shift mutations* because they alter the reading frame of the genetic code so that every triplet distal to the mutation in the same gene is changed. A frame-shift mutation results in synthesis of a new amino acid sequence beyond the mutation until a stop codon is reached. Frame-shift mutations can be corrected by a second mutation of the opposite type. A single base deletion followed by a single base insertion will restore the original code, and the altered amino acid sequence will be limited to the segment corresponding to the length of coding DNA between the two mutations, unless the first mutation or the frame-shift generates a new stop signal. If the transcribed segment between two mutations is short and does not involve a critical region of the polypeptide, a new protein of normal function may be produced. A second mutation occurring at a new site which corrects the effect of the first, in whole or in part, is called a *suppressor mutation.*

During the meiotic process, homologous chromosomes pair and exchange genetic material by a process called crossing over. If the pairing is not precisely in register along the entire length of the chromosomes, unequal, or *nonhomologous crossing over* occurs and results in deletion of genetic material from one chromosome and duplication in the other. Deletions or insertions can involve segments as small as one or two bases, or as large as major segments of two adjacent genes, or even an array of multiple genes involving thousands of bases.

Examples of almost all of these categories of mutations have been discovered among variant human hemoglobins (Fig. 31–2). For example, sickle cell hemoglobin differs from normal hemoglobin in the replacement of a glutamic acid residue by a valine in the sixth position of the β chain. The mutation results in a replacement of an A by a U in the RNA codon, GAG →GUG. Hb McKees-Rock is a 144 residue β chain variant that lacks the last two C-terminal amino acids tyrosine and histidine, as a result of conversion of a tyrosine codon UAU to

		β Chain
Normal	Hb A	6: GAG ... 144: AAG | 145: UAU | 146: CAC | 147: UAA - GLU - ... - LYS - TYR - HIS (Term)
Mis-sense mutation	Hb S	GUG ... AAG | UAU | CAC | UAA - VAL - ... - LYS - TYR - HIS (Term)
Mutation to premature termination	Hb McKees-Rock	GAG ... AAG | UAA (or G) - GLU - ... - LYS (Term)
		α Chain
Normal	Hb A	138: UCC | 139: AAA | 140: UAC | 141: CGU | 142: UAA | 143: GCU | 144: GGA | 145: GCC | 146: UCG | 147: GUA | 148: GCC - SER - LYS - TYR - ARG (Term)
Deletion in terminator codon → frame shift	Hb Wayne	UCC | AAU (A deleted) | ACC | GUU | AAG | CUG | GAG | CCU | CGG | UAG - SER - ASN - THR - VAL LYS - LEU - GLU - PRO - ARG (Term) (5 additional residues)
Terminator mutation to amino acid codon	Hb Constant Spring	UAC | CGU | 142: CAA ... 173: UGA - TYR - ARG - GLN - (31 additional residues) (Term)

Figure 31–2. Types of mutations affecting α and β chains of hemoglobin. RNA codons and corresponding amino acid residues of hemoglobin chains are shown.

a terminator codon UAA. Hb Wayne is thought to reflect a frame-shift mutation resulting from a deletion of a single adenine base in the codon for residue 139,

$$\overset{139}{\text{-AAA}}\text{-}\overset{140}{\text{UAC}}\text{-}\overset{141}{\text{CGU}}\text{-} \rightarrow \text{-}\overset{139}{\text{AAU}}\text{-}\overset{140}{\text{ACC}}\text{-}\overset{141}{\text{GUU}}\text{-}.$$

Such a deletion could result from unequal crossing over. Two other examples of nonhomologous crossing over are Hb Grady, in which there is an insertion of 3 amino acids between positions 118 and 119 of the α-chain:

$$\overset{115}{\text{ALA}}\text{-}\overset{116}{\text{GLU}}\text{-}\overset{117}{\text{PHE}}\text{-}\overset{118}{\text{THR}}\text{-GLU-PHE-THR-}\overset{119}{\text{PRO}},$$

and the Lepore hemoglobins, in which there is fusion of the δ and β chains, whose genes are contiguous in the DNA polynucleotide sequence. A Lepore hemoglobin has the N-terminal amino acid sequence of the normal δ chain and the C-terminal sequence of the normal β chain.

REGULATION OF GENE ACTION. In mammalian tissues only 10 to 20 per cent of structural genes are transcribed at any time. Different sets of genes are transcribed at different stages of differentiation and in different tissues. One example is hematopoietic cells, which produce first zeta and epsilon, or epsilon and alpha, globin chains (embryonic hemoglobins), then α and γ chains (fetal hemoglobin), then following birth α and β chains (adult hemoglobin) and small amounts of α and δ chains (Hb-A_2). Zeta, ε, and γ chain production is sequentially turned off. The genes for six globin chains are arranged sequentially in the 5′ to 3′ direction on the short arm of chromosome 11: epsilon-2, epsilon-1, G-gamma, A-gamma, delta, and beta. With advancing development of the fetus and infant, the genes nearer the 5′ terminus are switched off and those nearer the 3′ end switched on.

The basis of differential gene action in mammalian cells is poorly understood. For years histones have been considered candidates as regulatory factors in the expression of genetic information, but this is now considered unlikely. Histones appear to cover only about 20 per cent of DNA at random locations, leaving 80 per cent of the DNA molecule available for interaction with nonhistone proteins and nucleic acids. From reconstruction experiments utilizing acidic chromatin proteins isolated from specific organs, it now appears that nonhistone proteins recognize specific sequences in the DNA molecule and that the specificity of gene expression resides in the acidic chromatin proteins, rather than the histones.

Certain hormones have a profound effect on specific gene expression in mammalian systems. Glucocorticoids first bind to a cytoplasmic receptor, and the hormone-receptor complex then enters the nucleus, where it attaches to chromatin and induces specific protein synthesis. Triiodotyrosine, by contrast, binds directly to a nuclear receptor prior to inducing gene expression through an influence upon the activity of DNA-dependent RNA polymerase and the rate of RNA synthesis.

Azacytidine has recently been found to stimulate fetal hemoglobin production in man. This effect may be beneficial in β-thalassemia and sickle-cell disease. The action of azacytidine is so prompt that it may involve an effect on processing of a giant RNA transcript rather than on gene expression.

THE HUMAN GENE MAP. Over 1500 autosomal loci are known, on the basis mainly of characteristic patterns of inheritance of alternative forms of a particular trait. Techniques for assignment of autosomal loci to specific chromosomes began to emerge in about 1970 and developed rapidly thereafter. By late 1983 the chromosomal assignment of over 300 autosomal loci had been determined. In addition over 115 loci are known from pedigree studies to be located on the X chromosome.

Assignment of a locus to a specific chromosome is based on a variety of methods: (1) study of linkage of traits in large families with multiple alleles at two loci (e.g., linkage of ABO blood group and nail-patella syndrome); (2) co-segregation of specific proteins and single chromosomes in clones from somatic cell hybrids (e.g., thymidine kinase segregates with chromosome 17); (3) DNA-RNA annealing in situ (hybridization) (e.g., ribosomal RNAs hybridize to acrocentric chromosomes 13, 14, 15, 21, and 22); (4) deductions from amino acid sequences of proteins (e.g., linkage of δ and β hemoglobin inferred from study of hemoglobin Lepore, a product of the fusion of two loci); (5) deletion mapping (i.e., concurrence of chromosomal deletion and phenotypic evidence of hemizygosity), trisomy mapping (i.e., presence of three alleles in the case of a highly polymorphic locus), or gene dosage effects (i.e, correlation of triplicate state of part or all of a chromosome with 50 per cent excess of a gene product) (e.g., acid phosphatase-1 with chromosome 2 and glutathione reductase with chromosome 8); (6) induction of microscopically detectable chromosomal change by adenovirus; (7) DNA/cDNA molecular hybridization in solution or "Cot analysis" of somatic cell hybrids containing a small number of human chromosomes (e.g., assignment of β-chain of hemoglobin to chromosome 11); and (8) DNA restriction endonuclease techniques (e.g., fine structure of β-globin gene on chromosome 11).

About 60 per cent of gene assignments have been made on the basis of somatic cell hybridization studies (method 2, above), and about 25 per cent of the assignments emerged from study of linkage of traits in families (method 1); about 6 per cent were made independently by both of these methods. The remaining 15 per cent of assignments were made on the basis of one of the other methods listed above (methods 3 to 8).

Some interesting observations have emerged. Structural genes for enzymes that catalyze sequential steps in a metabolic pathway are as a rule not located on the same chromosome. Thus, whereas in bacteria the enzymes for sequential metabolic steps are often determined by linked genes, thus assuring coordinate regulation of activity, the situation in man is quite different. This finding accords with the lack of evidence for coordinate regulation of enzyme activity, or for an operon-like organization of structural genes, in eukaryotic cells. Even the subunits of polymeric proteins may be coded by genes on different chromosomes. The genes for the α chains of hemoglobin are on chromosome 16, whereas that for the β chain is on chromosome 11. Lactate dehydrogenase is an example of an enzymic protein that is constituted by subunits coded by genes on different chromosomes: LDH-A by a gene on chromosome 11, LDH-B by one on chromosome 12.

When the location of a gene is known, physicians can use the concept of gene linkage to predict which individual in a given family will be affected by a given trait. For example, the locus for the gene specifying the Rh blood group factor and the locus for the gene producing one form of the dominant trait, hereditary elliptocytosis, occur in close proximity on chromosome 1. Thus, if a subject with hereditary elliptocytosis transmits the anomaly to an offspring, the offspring will usually inherit the allele that is present at the Rh locus on this chromosome. If the Rh allele on this chromosome happens to be a rare one in the population (such as r′), one can assume that whichever offspring inherits the r′ allele at the Rh locus will also inherit the abnormal allele at the elliptocytosis locus.

The specific chromosomal localizations of the genes for about 35 of the autosomally inherited inborn errors of metabolism are listed in Table 31–2.

TABLE 31–2. METABOLIC DISEASES THAT HAVE BEEN MAPPED TO SPECIFIC AUTOSOMES*

Disease	Chromosome†
Disorders of carbohydrate metabolism	
Glycogen storage disease, Type II (Pompe's disease)	17
Galactosemia	9p
Galactokinase deficiency	17q
Galactose-4-epimerase deficiency	1p
Disorders of amino acid metabolism	
Classic phenylketonuria (phenylalanine hydroxylase deficiency)	1p
Atypical phenylketonuria (dihydropteridine reductase deficiency)	4
Argininosuccinic aciduria	7
Citrullinemia	9
Transcobalamin II deficiency	9q
Tetrahydrofolate methyltransferase deficiency	1
Disorders of lipoprotein and lipid metabolism	
Familial lecithin:cholesterol acyltransferase deficiency	16q
Disorders of lysosomal enzymes	
Mucopolysaccharidosis, Type VI (Maroteaux-Lamy syndrome)	5
Mucopolysaccharidosis, Type VII (β-glucuronidase deficiency)	7
Fucosidosis	1p
Mannosidosis	19
Wolman's disease and cholesteryl ester storage disease	10
Lysosomal acid phosphatase deficiency	11p
Metachromatic leukodystrophy	22q
Sandhoff's disease	5q
Tay-Sachs disease	15q
Generalized gangliosidosis	3
Disorders of steroid metabolism	
Adrenogenital syndrome (steroid 21-hydroxylase deficiency)	6p
Disorders of purine and pyrimidine metabolism	
Adenine phosphoribosyl transferase deficiency	16
Adenosine deaminase deficiency	20q
Nucleoside phosphorylase deficiency	14q
Disorders of metal metabolism	
Hemochromatosis	6p
Disorders of the blood and blood-forming tissues	
Glucosephosphate isomerase deficiency	19
Hexokinase deficiency	10
Triosephosphate isomerase deficiency	12p
Elliptocytosis	1p
Sickle cell anemia and all other β-chain variants	11p
Hemoglobin Constant Spring and all other α-chain variants	16p
α-Thalassemias	16p
β-Thalassemias	11p
Disorders of immune and other defense systems	
C2 deficiency	6p
C4 deficiency	6p

*Modified from McKusick VA: Am J Med 69:267, 1980.
†These numbers indicate the chromosome that carries the particular locus. The chromosome arm is indicated when known: p = short arm; q = long arm.

Inborn Errors of Metabolism in the 1980s. *In* Stanbury JB, Wyngaarden JB, Fredrickson DS, Goldstein JL, Brown MS (eds.): The Metabolic Basis of Inherited Disease. 5th ed. New York, McGraw-Hill Book Company, 1983, pp 3–59. *An introductory chapter on biochemical genetics and the pathogenesis of genetic disease.*

McKusick VA: Mendelian Inheritance in Man. Catalogs of Autosomal Dominant, Autosomal Recessive, and X-Linked Phenotypes. 6th ed. Baltimore, The Johns Hopkins Press, 1983. *Brief descriptions of and references to more than 2800 inherited phenotypes, classified according to patterns of inheritance.*

McKusick VA: The anatomy of the human genome. Am J Med 69:267, 1980. *An excellent discussion of the basis and significance of the assignment of more than 350 genes to specific chromosomes, with a catalogue of assignments up to mid-1980.*

Watson JD: Molecular Biology of the Gene. 3rd ed. New York, Benjamin, 1976. *An authoritative and readable account; superbly illustrated.*

32. INBORN ERRORS OF METABOLISM

James B. Wyngaarden

The inspired concept of inborn errors of metabolism, developed by Archibald Garrod in the first decade of this century, marks the birth of biochemical genetics. Garrod's studies of alcaptonuria, pentosuria, albinism, and cystinuria led to the proposal of a new category of diseases in which a block in a metabolic pathway arises from an inherited deficiency of a specific enzyme. This concept was proved in 1948 when Gibson found a deficiency of NADH-dependent methemoglobin reductase in recessive methemoglobinemia. This was soon followed by the discovery in 1952 by Cori and Cori of a deficiency of glucose-6-phosphatase in von Gierke's disease, in 1953 by Jervis of phenylalanine hydroxylase deficiency in phenylketonuria, and in 1956 by LaDu of homogentisic acid oxidase deficiency in alcaptonuria as originally predicted by Garrod. By 1983 deficiencies of over 200 different enzymes had been associated with hereditary disease. Of even greater importance in the history of genetics was the remarkable insight in Garrod's hypothesis that the primary action of a gene is to control the synthesis of a specific enzyme. Decades later Beadle (1945) independently proposed the one gene–one enzyme hypothesis anticipated by Garrod. With molecular refinement this concept is now often referred to as the one cistron–one polypeptide principle.

In 1949 Pauling, Itano, and associates observed that sickle cell hemoglobin exhibited abnormal electrophoretic behavior and introduced the concept of *molecular disease,* in which a structural alteration in a macromolecule accounted for a specific functional change that was responsible for a disease state. In 1953 Ingram demonstrated the substitution of a single amino acid residue in the β chain of sickle cell hemoglobin, confirming the concept of molecular disease and initiating an ever lengthening series of findings of structural alterations in macromolecules that result from gene mutations. For a time missing enzyme diseases and hemoglobinopathies were thought to represent distinct categories of disease, perhaps representing defects of control and structural genes, respectively. More sensitive techniques have disclosed low levels of residual activity of the deficient enzyme in many inborn errors of metabolism. In some cases the mutation has affected a critical portion of the enzyme, radically reducing its catalytic activity; in others the mutation has rendered the enzyme highly unstable. In the case of erythrocytes that lack a nucleus and cannot continue to synthesize new protein, enzyme lability results in low enzyme activity values in the older cells. In several instances amino acid sequence studies of enzymes have disclosed single amino acid substitutions analogous to the defect in sickle hemoglobin. Thus many inborn errors of metabolism are molecular diseases in which the *primary* defect lies in the genetic specification of the protein.

Although most of the well-defined inborn errors of metabolism are inherited as recessive conditions, in principle any human phenotype showing mendelian genetics must be based on a specific variant or missing protein. Thus not only autosomal and X-linked recessive but also autosomal and X-linked dominant conditions may be expressed through abnormal proteins. Examples in which a mutant protein has been identified include autosomal recessive, alcaptonuria (homogentisic acid oxidase); X-linked recessive, Lesch-Nyhan syndrome (hypoxanthine–guanine phosphoribosyltransferase); autosomal dominant, acute intermittent porphyria (uroporphyrinogen I synthetase). No example of an X-linked dominant condition in which the mutant protein has been identified can be cited as yet. In one condition of this category, vitamin D–resistant (hypophosphatemic) rickets, a defect in phosphate transport is suspected but the membrane carrier has not been identified. The concept of inborn errors of metabolism has broadened considerably since first propounded by Garrod. A reasonable definition would include any condition of clinical significance that shows a mendelian mode of inheritance, but in practice the term is restricted to conditions that have recognizable biochemical manifestations.

A mutant protein that cannot be detected by functional assay may nevertheless retain immunologic reactivity. However, in some instances no protein can be detected by functional or immunologic means. In the terminology of microbial genetics, the former class of mutants is frequently called CRM(+) ("krim" positive) and the latter CRM(−). The presence of CRM(+) material suggests that the genetic defect is due to a mis-sense mutation with a consequent amino acid substitution that destroys the activity but not the antigenicity of the mutant enzyme. In most cases in which mutant enzymes have been studied, cross-reactive material has been detected. However, in the Lesch-Nyhan syndrome only one CRM(+) mutant has been found among 14 studied. At the pseudocholinosterase locus, 17 CRM(+) mutants and 18 CRM(−) mutants have been recognized. A CRM(−) reaction does not prove that no protein is present; the protein may be so altered that both enzyme function and immunologic reactivity have been lost.

Mutation does not necessarily result in loss of enzyme activity. Several examples of increased activity are known. The best examples are three types of phosphoribosylpyrophosphate synthetase overactivity associated with purine overproduction and gout. In one there is a 2.5-fold increase in enzyme activity per molecule; in another, excessive activity is a reflection of diminished affinity for normal intracellular nucleotide inhibitors; in a third, the overactivity results from an increased affinity for ribose 5-phosphate, a substrate of the reaction. All these changes reflect alterations of enzyme structure. Some of the clinical conditions in which an abnormality of a specific protein has been observed are listed in Tables 32–1 and 32–2.

ETIOLOGY. The etiology of an inborn error of metabolism is a mutant gene. If the amino acid sequence of the mutant protein is known, it is possible to deduce the nature of the mutation from the genetic code. The human variant of glucose-6-phosphate dehydrogenase, G6PD Hektoen, differs from normal G6PD in a single amino acid substitution, HIS →TYR. This substitution corresponds to a mutation from GTA(or G) to ATA(or G) in a codon in the structural gene for G6PD. Most of the amino acid sequence information of human mutant proteins has been obtained from studies of red blood cell proteins, such as hemoglobin and G6PD. At least four types of mutations can be discerned by this approach: deletions, duplications, mis-sense mutations, and frame-shift mutations.

Another type of mutation, the non-sense mutation, has also been demonstrated in man, using DNA restriction enzyme analysis and DNA sequencing techniques. The partial nucleotide sequence of β-globin mRNA isolated from a unique patient with homozygous β°-thalassemia disclosed a replacement of an adenine by a uracil in the codon for position 17. This changed the RNA codon from AAG to AUG, a termination codon. As a result a nonfunctional partial β-chain, only 16 amino acids long, was synthesized. Hb McKees-Rock represents another example of mutation of an amino acid codon to a terminator codon, but in this case the β-globin is shortened by only two amino acids and is functional.

DNA cloning techniques permit direct study of the altered DNA sequence in many human mutations, even those that involve genes that code for quantitatively minor proteins, such as most enzymes. These recent developments are discussed in Ch. 33 and 34.

PATHOGENESIS OF GENETIC DISEASE. The consequence of a mutation will depend on the function normally served by the product of the gene. Mutations in genes for rRNA or tRNA would very likely affect protein synthesis generally and might be incompatible with life. No such mutations have been identified in mammalian systems, although they are known in bacteria.

Defects involving nonenzymic protein undoubtedly account for a large number of genetic diseases, but relatively few have been defined biochemically. The hemoglobinopathies are an exception. A few additional examples exist. In one of these, the ZZ variant of α-1-antitrypsin deficiency, two amino acid substitutions (mis-sense mutations) in α-1-antitrypsin lead to the production of a modified protein that is not susceptible to normal post-translational processing. As a consequence carbohydrate residues are not added to the protein in the normal manner, and the defective glycoprotein accumulates in liver cells, possibly because the altered molecule cannot be secreted. Other examples in which a specific mutant protein has been identified, although the precise molecular alteration has not yet been defined, include the abnormal plasma membrane receptor in familial hypercholesterolemia, the abnormal cytoplasmic androgen receptor in the complete form of testicular feminization, an abnormal insulin in familial hyperproinsulinemia, and an abnormal protein called dynein in the microtubules of cilia in Kartagener's syndrome.

The largest number of known inborn errors of metabolism involves deficiencies of enzymes that catalyze discrete steps in

TABLE 32–1. DISORDERS IN WHICH A DEFICIENT ACTIVITY OF A SPECIFIC ENZYME HAS BEEN DEMONSTRATED IN HUMAN BEINGS

Condition	Enzyme with Deficient Activity
Acatalasia	Catalase
Acetyl CoA carboxylase deficiency	Acetyl CoA carboxylase
Acid phosphatase deficiency	Acid phosphatase
Adrenal hyperplasia I	20,21 Desmolase*
Adrenal hyperplasia II	3-β-Hydroxysteroid dehydrogenase*
Adrenal hyperplasia III	21-Hydroxylase*
Adrenal hyperplasia IV	11-β-Hydroxylase*
Adrenal hyperplasia V	17-Hydroxylase*
Albinism	Tyrosinase
Aldosterone deficiency I	18-OH-Dehydrogenase
Alcaptonuria	Homogentisic acid oxidase
Apnea, drug-induced	Pseudocholinesterase
Argininemia	Arginase
Argininosuccinic aciduria	Argininosuccinase
Aspartylglycosaminuria	Special hydrolase (AADG-ase)
Ataxia, intermittent	Pyruvate decarboxylase
Carnosinemia	Carnosinase
Cholesteryl ester deficiency (Norum-Gjone disease)	Lecithin cholesterol acetyltransferase (LCAT)
Citrullinemia	Argininosuccinic acid synthetase
Crigler-Najjar syndrome	Glucuronyl transferase
Cystathioninuria	Cystathionase
2,8-Dihydroxyadenine nephrolithiasis	Adenine phosphoribosyl transferase
Disaccharide intolerance I	Invertase
Disaccharide intolerance II	Invertase, maltase
Disaccharide intolerance III	Lactase
Ehlers-Danlos syndrome, type V	Lysyloxidase
Ehlers-Danlos syndrome, type VI	Collagen lysyl hydroxylase
Ehlers-Danlos syndrome, type VII	Procollagen peptidase
Fabry's disease	α-Galactosidase A
Fanconi's panmyelopathy	Exonuclease*
Farber's lipogranulomatosis	Ceramidase
Formiminotransferase deficiency	Formiminotransferase*
Fructose intolerance	Fructose-1-phosphate aldolase
Fructosuria	Hepatic fructokinase
Fucosidosis	α-L-Fucosidase
Galactokinase deficiency	Galactokinase
Galactose epimerase deficiency	Galactose epimerase
Galactosemia	Galactose-1-phosphate uridyl transferase
Gangliosidosis, G_{M1}, type I or infantile	β-Galactosidase A,B
Gangliosidosis, G_{M1}, type II or juvenile	β-Galactosidase A,B
Gangliosidosis, G_{M2} (Tay-Sachs disease)	Hexosaminidase A
Gangliosidosis, G_{M2}, juvenile	Hexosaminidase A
Gangliosidosis, G_{M2}, adult	Hexosaminidase A
Gangliosidosis, G_{M2} (Sandhoff's disease)	Hexosaminidase A,B
Gangliosidosis, G_{M3}	UDP-N-acetyl-galactosaminyl transferase
Gaucher's disease	Glucocerebrosidase
G6PD deficiency (favism, primaquine sensitivity, etc.)	Glucose-6-phosphate dehydrogenase
Glutathionemia	γ-Glutamyl transferase
Glycogen storage disease I	Glucose-6-phosphatase
Glycogen storage disease II	α-1,4-Glucosidase
Glycogen storage disease III	Amylo-1, 6-glucosidase
Glycogen storage disease IV	Amylo-(1,4 to 1,6)-transglucosidase
Glycogen storage disease V	Muscle phosphorylase
Glycogen storage disease VI	Liver phosphorylase*
Glycogen storage disease VII	Muscle phosphofructokinase
Glycogen storage disease VIII	Liver phosphorylase kinase
Gout, primary	Hypoxanthine-guanine phosphoribosyl transferase
Gout, primary	PP-ribose-P synthetase (increased)
Granulomatous disease	NADPH oxidase
Hemolytic anemia	Adenosine triphosphatase
Hemolytic anemia	Adenylate kinase
Hemolytic anemia	Aldolase A
Hemolytic anemia	Diphosphoglycerate mutase
Hemolytic anemia	γ-Glutamylcysteine synthetase
Hemolytic anemia	Glucose-6-phosphate dehydrogenase
Hemolytic anemia	Glutathione peroxidase
Hemolytic anemia	Glutathione reductase
Hemolytic anemia	Glutathione synthetase
Hemolytic anemia	Hexokinase
Hemolytic anemia	Hexosephosphate isomerase
Hemolytic anemia	6-Phosphogluconate dehydrogenase
Hemolytic anemia	Phosphoglycerate kinase
Hemolytic anemia	Pyrimidine 5′-nucleotidase
Hemolytic anemia	Pyruvate kinase
Hemolytic anemia	Triosephosphate isomerase
Histidinemia	Histidase
Homocystinuria I	Cystathionine synthetase
Homocystinuria II	*N*(5,10)-methylenetetrahydrofolate reductase
2-Hydroxyglutaric aciduria	D-2-Hydroxyglutarate dehydrogenase
β-Hydroxyisovaleric aciduria and methylcrotonyl glycinuria	β-Methylcrotonyl CoA Carboxylase*
Hydroxyprolinemia	Hydroxyproline oxidase
Hyper-β-alaninemia	β-alanine-α-ketoglutarate aminotransferase
Hyperammonemia I	Carbamyl phosphate synthetase
Hyperammonemia II	Ornithine transcarbamylase
Hyperglycinemia, ketotic form	Propionyl CoA carboxylase
Hyperglycinemia, nonketotic form	Glycine formiminotransferase
Hyperlysinemia	Lysine-ketoglutarate reductase
Hyperprolinemia I	Proline oxidase
Hyperprolinemia II	δ-1-Pyrroline-5-carboxylate dehydrogenase*
Hypoglycemia and acidosis	Fructose-1, 6-diphosphatase
Hypophosphatasia	Alkaline phosphatase
Ichthyosis, X-linked	Steroid sulfatase
Immunodeficiency disease	Adenosine deaminase
Immunodeficiency disease	Purine nucleoside phosphorylase
Intestinal lactase deficiency (adult)	Lactase
Isovaleric acidemia	Isovaleryl CoA dehydrogenase
Ketoacidosis, infantile	Succinyl CoA:3-ketoacid CoA-transferase
β-Ketothiolase deficiency	α-Methylacetoacetyl-CoA-β-ketothiolase deficiency
Krabbe's disease	Galactocerebroside β-galactosidase
Lactase deficiency	Lactase
Lactosyl ceramidosis	Lactosyl ceramidase
Leigh's necrotizing encephalomyelopathy	Pyruvate carboxylase
Lesch-Nyhan syndrome	Hypoxanthine-guanine phosphoribosyl transferase
Lipase deficiency, congenital	Lipase (pancreatic)
Lipoprotein lipase deficiency (type I hyperlipoproteinemia)	Lipoprotein lipase
Lysine intolerance	L-Lysine:NAD-oxidoreductase
Male pseudohermaphroditism	Testicular 17,20-desmolase
Male pseudohermaphroditism	Testicular 17-ketosteroid dehydrogenase*
Male pseudohermaphroditism	5α-Reductase*
Mannosidosis	α-Mannosidase
Maple sugar urine disease	Keto acid decarboxylase
Maple syrup urine disease	Dihydrolipoyl dehydrogenase
Metachromatic leukodystrophy I	Arylsulfatase A (sulfatide sulfatase)
Metachromatic leukodystrophy II	Arylsulfatase A, B, C and steroid sulfatase
Methemoglobinemia	NAD-methemoglobin reductase
Methylmalonic aciduria I (vitamin B_{12}-unresponsive)	Methylmalonic CoA mutase

*Inferred from functional deficit. Specific assays not performed.

(*Table continued on following page*)

TABLE 32–1. DISORDERS IN WHICH A DEFICIENT ACTIVITY OF A SPECIFIC ENZYME HAS BEEN DEMONSTRATED IN HUMAN BEINGS *(Continued)*

Condition	Enzyme with Deficient Activity	Condition	Enzyme with Deficient Activity
Methylmalonic aciduria II (vitamin B_{12}-responsive)	5′-Deoxyadenosyl transferase*	Porphyria cutanea tarda	Uroporphyrinogen decarboxylase
Methylmalonic aciduria III	Methylmalonyl-CoA racemase	Porphyria, hereditary copro-	Coproporphyrinogen oxidase*
Mucopolysaccharidosis IH (Hurler's)	α-L-Iduronidase	Porphyria, proto-	Ferrochelatase*
Mucopolysaccharidosis IS (Scheie's)	α-L-Iduronidase	Propionic acidemia	Propionyl CoA carboxylase
Mucopolysaccharidosis II (Hunter's)	Sulfo-iduronidase sulfatase	Pulmonary emphysema, or cirrhosis	α-1-Antitrypsin
Mucopolysaccharidosis IIIA (Sanfilippo's)	Heparan sulfate sulfatase	Pyridoxine-dependent infantile convulsions	Glutamic acid decarboxylase
Mucopolysaccharidosis IIIB (Sanfilippo's)	*N*-acetyl-α-D-glucosaminidase	Pyridoxine-responsive anemia	δ-Aminolevulinic acid synthetase*
Mucopolysaccharidosis IV (Morquio's)	6-Sulfatase*	Pyroglutamic aciduria	Glutathione synthetase
Mucopolysaccharidosis VI (Maroteaux-Lamy)	Arylsulfatase B	Pyruvate carboxylase deficiency	Pyruvate carboxylase
Mucopolysaccharidosis VII	β-Glucuronidase	Pyruvate decarboxylase deficiency	Pyruvate decarboxylase
Myeloperoxidase deficiency with disseminated candidiasis	Myeloperoxidase	Refsum's disease	Phytanic acid α-oxidase
Myopathy	Myoadenylate deaminase	Renal tubular acidosis with deafness	Carbonic anhydrase B
Niemann-Pick disease	Sphingomyelinase	Richner-Hanhart syndrome	Tyrosine aminotransferase
Ornithinemia	Ornithine ketoacid aminotransferase	Rickets, vitamin D dependent	25-Hydroxycholecalciferol 1-hydroxylase*
Orotic aciduria I	Orotidylic pyrophosphorylase and orotidylic decarboxylase	Sarcosinemia	Sarcosine dehydrogenase
Orotic aciduria II	Orotidylic decarboxylase	Sucrase-isomaltase deficiency	Sucrase, isomaltase
Oxalosis I (glycolic aciduria)	2-Oxo-glutarate-glyoxylate carboligase	Sulfite oxidase deficiency	Sulfite oxidase
Oxalosis II (glyceric aciduria)	D-Glyceric dehydrogenase	Thyroid hormonogenesis, defect in, II	Iodide peroxidase
Pentosuria	L-Xylulose reductase	Thyroid hormonogenesis, defect in, IV	Iodotyrosine dehalogenase (deiodinase)
Phenylketonuria	Phenylalanine hydroxylase	Trypsinogen deficiency	Trypsinogen
Phenylketonuria	Dihydropteridine reductase	Tyrosinemia I	Para-hydroxyphenylpyruvate oxidase
Porphyria, acute intermittent	Uroporphyrinogen I synthetase	Tyrosinemia II	Tyrosine transaminase
Porphyria, congenital erythropoietic	Uroporphyrinogen III cosynthetase	Valinemia	Valine transaminase
		Wolman's disease	Acid lipase
		Xanthinuria	Xanthine oxidase
		Xanthinuria	Xanthine oxidase and sulfite oxidase
		Xanthurenic aciduria	Kynureninase
		Xeroderma pigmentosum	DNA-specific endonuclease
		Xylosidase deficiency	Xylosidase

*Inferred from functional deficit. Specific assays not performed.

biosynthetic or catabolic sequences. The consequences of metabolic blocks depend upon the function of the affected sequence and the properties of the affected substrates. In some conditions the disease is manifested by the inability to form a specific product, as in the failure of melanin production in one form of albinism. In others, accumulation of the precursor of a blocked reaction results in toxicity or in a storage disease. In phenylketonuria the block in phenylalanine hydroxylase results in accumulation of phenylalanine and overproduction of toxic phenylketone products. Deficiencies of various catabolic enzymes explain the progressive tissue accumulations in the mucopolysaccharidoses and sphingolipidoses. In some enzyme deficiencies, disease results from failure to modify another protein. For example, in some types of Ehlers-Danlos syndrome collagen polypeptide synthesis is normal but enzymes essential in cross-linking are deficient, with the result that fragile collagen is produced.

TABLE 32–2. DISORDERS IN WHICH A DEFICIENCY OF A PLASMA PROTEIN HAS BEEN DEMONSTRATED IN HUMAN BEINGS

Condition	Plasma Protein
Afibrinogenemia	Fibrinogen
Agammaglobulinemia, X-linked	IgA, IgG
Agammaglobulinemia, selective IgA	IgA
Agammaglobulinemia, selective IgG	IgG
Analbuminemia	Albumin
Atransferrinemia	Transferrin
Complement deficiency states, selective C1q, C1r, C1s, C2, C3, C4, C5, C6, C7, C8	C1q, C1r, C1s, C2, C3, C4, C5, C6, C7, C8
Factor VII deficiency	Factor VII
Factor X (Stuart factor) deficiency	Factor X
Fibrin-stabilizing factor deficiency	Factor XIII
Hageman trait	Factor XII
Hemophilia A	Factor VIII
Hemophilia B	Factor IX
Hereditary angioedema	C1-inhibitor
Hypoprothrombinemia	Factor II
Parahemophilia	Factor V
PTA deficiency	Factor XI

Polymorphism. Many proteins exist in two or more forms in the population. These multiple forms are due to the presence of multiple genes (called *alleles*) at the same genetic locus. If the most common allele at a given locus accounts for fewer than 99 per cent of the alleles in the population, *polymorphism* is said to occur. By definition, when polymorphism exists at a genetic locus, at least 2 per cent of the population must be heterozygous at that locus. Table 32–3 lists selected proteins for which electrophoretically determined polymorphism has been demonstrated. Many of these genetically determined variations in protein structure are unassociated with clinical disease.

Polymorphism appears to be very common. As many as 28 per cent of genetic loci coding for enzyme and other proteins of erythrocytes and serum show multiple alleles in the population, but this figure may be as low as 2 per cent of loci of the more abundant proteins of the cell. An average individual is demonstrably heterozygous at 7 per cent of loci. Since only about one-third of base changes alter the charge of a protein, each individual may actually be heterozygous at as many as 20 per cent of loci.

At most genetic loci (e.g., the gene for β-globin) one standard allele accounts for the vast majority of alleles in the population, and alternative alleles are rare. At other loci, no single allele occurs with sufficient frequency to be designated as standard or normal. The α-chain of haptoglobin, a plasma protein, represents one such extreme example of genetic polymorphism. In this instance all polymorphic forms of haptoglobin appear

TABLE 32–3. PLASMA PROTEINS AND CELLULAR ENZYMES THAT EXHIBIT ELECTROPHORETICALLY DETECTABLE POLYMORPHISMS*

Protein	Locus Name
Plasma proteins	
Haptoglobin (α-chain)	Hp α
Transferrin	Tf
Vitamin D binding protein	Gc (for group-specific component)
Ceruloplasmin	Cp
α-1-Antitrypsin	Pi (for protease inhibitor)
α-1-Acid glycoprotein	Oro (for orosomucoid)
β-2-Glycoprotein I	—
Properdin factor B	Bf
Complement	
Second component	C2
Third component	C3
Fourth component	C4
Sixth component	C6
Enzymes	
Pancreatic amylase	AMY_2
Cholinesterase	E_2
Red blood cell enzyme	
Acid phosphatase 1	ACP_1
Adenosine deaminase	ADA
Adenylate kinase	AK_1
Carbonic anhydrase 2	CA_2
Diaphorase (NADPH-dependent)	DIA_2
Esterase D	ESD
Galactose-1-uridyl transferase	GALT
Glucose-6-phosphate dehydrogenase	Gd
Glutamic pyruvic transaminase	GPT
Glutathione peroxidase	GPX
Glutathione reductase	GSR
Glyoxalase I	GLO
Peptidase A	PEPA
Peptidase C	PEPC
Peptidase D	PEPD
Phosphoglucomutase 1	PGM_1
Phosphoglucomutase 2	PGM_2
Phosphogluconate dehydrogenase	PGD
Uridine monophosphate kinase	UMPK
White blood cell enzymes	
Aconitase (soluble)	$ACON_S$
Cytidine deaminase	CDA
α-L-Fucosidase	αFUC
α-Glucosidase	αGLUC
Glutamic-oxaloacetic transaminase (mitochondrial)	GOT_M
Hexokinase 3	HK_3
Malic enzyme (mitochondrial)	ME_M
Phosphoglucomutase 3	PGM_3

*From Giblett ER: Ann Rev Genet 11:13, 1977.

to function equally in hemoglobin binding. Polymorphisms represent conspicuous examples of human biochemical diversity.

Genetic Heterogeneity. When two or more mutations produce identical or closely similar clinical syndromes, *genetic heterogeneity* is said to exist. In some instances the mutations may be at different loci (*nonallelic* genes), whereas in others they may occur in different portions of the same locus (*allelic* genes). Hemophilia can be caused by a mutation at either of two distinct loci on the X chromosome, one leading to a deficiency of factor VIII (classic hemophilia) and the other to a deficiency of factor IX (Christmas disease). By contrast, the multiple variants of G6PD represent different structural gene mutations at a single locus. A striking example of both allelic and nonallelic heterogeneity is hereditary methemoglobinemia, which can be produced by at least ten different mutations at three distinct loci: two at the locus for the α-chain of hemoglobin, three at the locus for the β-chain, and at least five at the locus for NADH methemoglobin reductase.

In view of the multiple alleles that occur at virtually all genetic loci, persons who appear to be homozygous for a genetic trait may actually have inherited different abnormal alleles from each parent. Such individuals are said to be *genetic compounds*. The clinical syndrome in a genetic compound may be intermediate in severity and manifestations between the syndromes produced by homozygosity for either allele. A classic example is hemoglobin SC disease, which results when an offspring inherits an Hb S gene ($\beta\text{-}6^{glu \rightarrow val}$) from one parent and an Hb C gene ($\beta\text{-}6^{glu \rightarrow lys}$) from the other. Another is the mucopolysaccharide storage disease resulting from inheritance of one gene for Hurler's disease (severe) and one for Scheie's disease (mild). In both these examples the severity is intermediate between the diseases associated with the respective homozygous states. Table 32–4 lists selected inherited diseases for which genetic compounds have been demonstrated.

TREATMENT OF INBORN ERRORS OF METABOLISM. Treatment of the patient with an inherited disorder depends upon accurate diagnosis and an understanding of the pathophysiology of the disease. This understanding includes an appreciation of the interaction of genetic and environmental factors. Well-known examples include phenylketonuria, which predisposes to toxic reactions to dietary phenylalanine; and G6PD deficiency, which predisposes to hemolysis following ingestion of fava beans, during the course of acute viral hepatitis and infectious mononucleosis, or after administration of certain drugs, including aspirin and phenacetin. In such instances control of environmental factors may mitigate or neutralize the effect of the genetic change.

The balance of this chapter will be devoted to a discussion of forms of treatment of value in specific hereditary disorders.

Dietary Restriction of Substrate. Dietary restriction will often reduce the excessive substrate that accumulates behind a metabolic block. A general reduction in protein intake will prevent brain damage in disorders of the urea cycle associated with ammonia intoxication, including argininosuccinicaciduria and citrullinemia. A diet low in phenylalanine is effective in preventing growth and mental retardation in phenylketonuria, if started soon after birth. A fructose-free diet controls the symptoms of hereditary fructose intolerance resulting from deficiency of fructose-1-phosphate aldolase. Similarly, a diet that is virtually galactose free will avert brain damage and cataract formation in children with galactokinase or galactose-1-phosphate uridyl transferase deficiency.

Replacement of the Deficient End-Product. A metabolic block may also result in a critical shortage in the product of the reaction or later products of the sequence. Replacement may alleviate the deficiency state. Goiter resulting from a block in thyroxine production can be treated and cretinism prevented by replacement of thyroid hormone. In the adrenogenital syndromes, corticosteroid administration supplies the missing hormone, corrects the disordered steroidal secretory pattern, and leads to remission of the clinical manifestations. In orotic aciduria, administration of uridine supplies the pyrimidines needed for hematopoietic functions and corrects the macrocytic anemia, and also suppresses orotic acid synthesis and urolithiasis.

TABLE 32–4. INHERITED METABOLIC DISEASES FOR WHICH GENETIC COMPOUNDS HAVE BEEN DEMONSTRATED*

α-1-Antitrypsin deficiency
Cystinosis
Cystinuria
"Homozygous" familial hypercholesterolemia (LDL receptor-internalization defect)
Galactosemia (galactose-1-phosphate uridyl transferase deficiency)
Gaucher's disease (glucocerebrosidase deficiency)
Glucosephosphate isomerase deficiency
Hemoglobin α-chain variants
Hemoglobin β-chain variants
Hurler-Scheie syndrome (α-L-iduronidase deficiency)
Iminoglycinuria
Metachromatic leukodystrophy (cerebroside sulfatase deficiency)
Hereditary methemoglobinemia (NADH dehydrogenase deficiency)
Phenylketonuria (phenylalanine hydroxylase deficiency)
Pseudocholinesterase deficiency
Pyruvate kinase deficiency

*Modified from McKusick VA: Am J Hum Genet 25:446, 1973.

Depletion of Storage Substances. In some hereditary disorders the clinical consequences result from accumulation of stored materials in the tissues, and removal of the excess material may ameliorate the effects of the genetic lesion. Removal of stored copper in Wilson's disease by penicillamine and of excess iron in hemochromatosis by frequent phlebotomy illustrates this approach. Use of uricosuric agents to deplete the body of uric acid in tophaceous gout and of cholestyramine to reduce serum cholesterol levels in familial hypercholesterolemia are additional examples.

Use of Metabolic Inhibitors. When a toxic metabolite accumulates because of a metabolic error, it may be possible to control its production by use of an appropriate metabolic inhibitor. Allopurinol inhibits xanthine oxidase and controls uric acid production in gout and 2,8-dioxyadenine production and renal stone formation in patients with homozygous adenine phosphoribosyltransferase deficiency. Clofibrate, which inhibits synthesis or release of glyceride from the liver, reduces blood lipid levels to normal in type III hyperlipoproteinemia.

Amplification of Enzyme Activity. Many enzyme proteins require cofactors for biologic activity. In some inborn errors the mutation affects the ability of the apoenzyme to combine with its cofactor. In other genetic disorders there is a metabolic defect in the conversion of a precursor vitamin to its active cofactor form. In both situations administration of the appropriate cofactor may increase the catalytic activity of the apoenzyme. Pyridoxine (vitamin B_6) is a cofactor for cystathionine synthetase. In more than one half of patients with homocystinuria caused by deficient synthetase activity, administration of large doses of pyridoxine partially overcomes the block in homocysteine metabolism. Similarly the ketoacidosis of some patients with methylmalonic aciduria is corrected by treatment with pharmacologic doses of vitamin B_{12}, and the clinical and hematologic abnormalities of patients with hereditary dihydrofolate reductase deficiency are corrected by administration of small doses of 5-formyltetrahydrofolate, which bypasses the metabolic block (replacement of deficient end-product).

Phenobarbital and certain other drugs increase production of smooth endoplasmic reticulum and of certain of its enzymes, including NADPH-cytochrome C reductase, cytochrome P-450, and several drug-hydroxylating enzymes. Administration of phenobarbital to patients with unconjugated hyperbilirubinemia in a variant of the Crigler-Najjar syndrome or with Gilbert's syndrome may reduce plasma bilirubin levels following induction of hepatic glucuronyl transferase.

Replacement of Mutant Protein. Direct replacement of the missing protein is an attractive approach to the treatment of recessively inherited diseases. Greater success has been achieved in deficiencies of nonenzymic than of enzymic proteins. Examples include replacement of gamma globulin in agammaglobulinemia, of albumin in analbuminemia, or of factor VIII in hemophilia. In each of these cases, the deficient gene product is a plasma protein. The metabolic and immunologic defects of patients with adenosine deaminase deficiency are transiently corrected by infusion of irradiated erythrocytes containing normal levels of adenosine deaminase.

Much less success has attended efforts to replace missing enzymes that normally function within cells. Enzyme infusions have been attempted in the mucopolysaccharidoses, Gaucher's disease, Tay-Sachs disease, and Pompe's disease, but therapeutic benefits are unproved. The lysosomal storage diseases are perhaps the best candidates for treatment by administration of exogenous enzyme, for cells have highly specific mechanisms for taking up exogenous proteins and delivering them to lysosomes. However, the exogenous protein must bind to a specific recognition site on the plasma membrane of the target cell so that it can be selectively internalized. Enzymes have been coupled covalently to other molecules for which tissues contain receptors, on the theory that in this manner the enzyme might be conveyed to the lysosomes along with the primary ligand. This type of experimental work holds promise for the future.

Modifying the Mutant Protein. Many proteins can be modified by the addition of subgroups. For example, sickle cell hemoglobin can be carbamylated by cyanate at the valine in position 1 of the beta chain, which then blocks the hydrophobic bonding of the normal val-1 to the mutant val-6 of β-globin of Hb S, thereby preventing sickling in vitro. Severe toxic reactions, such as peripheral neuropathy, sharply limit the clinical usefulness of cyanate therapy in patients with sickle cell disease. Nevertheless, this approach holds promise for the future.

Organ Transplantation. Allotransplantation of the organ in which the deficient enzyme is normally synthesized has been attempted in a variety of inherited diseases. The greatest experience has involved renal transplantation, which has been performed in Alport's syndrome, renal amyloidosis, cystinosis, Fabry's disease, Gaucher's disease, oxalosis, and some other conditions. The results in most instances have paralleled those of renal transplantation for other forms of end-stage renal disease. There has been no evidence of reactivation of the renal lesion in patients with Alport's syndrome, or of development of cystinosis or Fabry's disease in the transplanted kidneys. Amyloidosis has recurred in the graft on rare occasions. By contrast severe recurrent oxalosis has developed in a number of transplanted kidneys, and end-stage renal failure resulting from oxalosis is not now considered an indication for renal transplantation. Patients with Fabry's disease have developed measurable levels of the missing enzyme, ceramide trihexosidase, in plasma following renal transplantation, and there have been a few long-term survivals. Nevertheless, renal transplantation in patients with inborn errors of metabolism should be limited to replacement of failed kidneys. Results do not warrant use of renal transplantation primarily for enzyme replacement.

Transplantation of allogenic marrow has successfully corrected a number of immunodeficiency states, including lymphopenic hypogammaglobulinemia (Swiss type), Wiskott-Aldrich syndrome, and severe combined immunodeficiency disease.

Surgical removals also play a role in certain hereditary disorders. Examples include splenectomy in hereditary spherocytosis, and colectomy in preventing neoplastic transformation in polyposis of the colon. Also, surgery offers a quick and permanent cure for polydactyly as well as for certain other dominantly inherited defects.

Genetic Engineering. The use of recombinant DNA technology in the diagnosis and treatment of inborn errors is discussed in Ch. 33.

Giblett ER: Genetic polymorphisms in human blood. Ann Rev Genet 11:13, 1977. *A review of polymorphic protein in blood, including alloantigens of red and white blood cells and plasma proteins, and electrophoretic variants of plasma and cellular components.*

McKusick VA: Phenotypic diversity of human diseases resulting from allelic series. Am J Hum Genet 25:446, 1973. *An analytical review of different disorders that can result from series of mutations involving the same gene.*

Stanbury JB, Wyngaarden JB, Fredrickson DS, Goldstein JL, Brown MS (eds.): The Metabolic Basis of Inherited Disease. 5th ed. New York, McGraw-Hill Book Company, 1983. *Authoritative discussions of all inborn errors of metabolism for which there is a substantial body of metabolic or biochemical information.*

33. EXPECTATIONS FROM RECOMBINANT DNA RESEARCH

W. French Anderson

Over the past ten years a revolution has occurred in DNA research, variously referred to as recombinant DNA technology, genetic engineering, molecular cloning, gene splicing, biotechnology, etc. The new DNA research is beginning to make a major impact on clinical medicine in four major areas: (1) carrier detection and prenatal diagnosis, (2) understanding of the molecular basis of genetic diseases, (3) production of human biological products, and (4) gene therapy. Categories 1 and 2, which are already a reality, are discussed in Ch. 34; categories 3 and 4, which are rapidly approaching, will be examined here.

HUMAN BIOLOGICALS PRODUCED BY BIOTECHNOLOGY

Genetic engineering is currently being used by biotechnology companies to produce large quantities of previously unavailable human biologicals (usually peptides or proteins). What products are being made? Why these products? How are they being made? How good will the products be?

The first three human proteins produced by the new technology are now being studied in clinical trials: insulin, growth hormone (GH), and several of the interferons. In each case, they were chosen because of the importance of the protein in treating specific human disease states (either established: insulin, GH; or postulated: interferons), the commercial market expected for the compound and the ability to apply recombinant DNA techniques to synthesize large quantities of the human protein in bacteria inexpensively.

The Technology

A gene is a sequence of nucleotides in DNA that codes for a product. In order to get a bacterium to produce a human protein, it is necessary to obtain a DNA copy of the protein, in other words, to obtain a piece of double-stranded DNA which carries the precise sequence of nucleotides that code for the protein. This DNA is then inserted into a bacterial plasmid—a circle of naturally occurring nonchromosomal DNA that replicates freely in the cytoplasm of a bacterium. Any gene (bacterial, plant, animal, or human) that is inserted into the plasmid with the correct control signals can, in theory, be transcribed and translated into protein within the bacterium. The synthesized protein can then be purified from the bacterial cells.

There are a number of ways to acquire a human gene suitable for engineered protein production in bacteria. One procedure is to sequence the human protein of interest and then, by using the genetic code, determine the DNA sequence that would give the known amino acid sequence. Then a segment of DNA 12 to 18 nucleotides long is chemically synthesized (longer DNA molecules are very difficult to synthesize and purify) that will be exactly complementary to a portion of the expected sequence of the messenger RNA (mRNA). "Exactly complementary" means that the DNA "probe" will have T (thymine) where the mRNA has an A (adenine), a C (cytosine) where the mRNA has a G (guanine), etc. This DNA probe can be tagged with radioactivity and then be used to find (by hybridization) the desired mRNA in extracts of the appropriate human cells. The mRNA is isolated, purified, and shown to be capable of being translated in vitro to give the predicted human protein. This mRNA is then transcribed into full-length complementary (or copy) DNA, called cDNA, by the enzyme reverse transcriptase. The resulting DNA is an exact code of the mRNA for the human protein. It can now be made double stranded (by the action of other enzymes) and inserted into a bacterial plasmid along with the appropriate control signals.

Several requirements must be met in order to obtain high quantities of human proteins in bacteria. The human gene must be attached within the plasmid to a bacterial control signal that will be switched on at a high level. Several such "promoter" regions are used, including those from the lactose operon, from the bacteriophage lambda, etc. Second, other regulatory signals (for example, a binding site so that the transcribed RNA will attach to and be translated by ribosomes) must be present adjacent to the human gene. Third, any hard-to-handle portion of DNA (for example, nucleotides producing a leader sequence of amino acids or an intervening sequence) should be removed, since bacteria are not equipped to carry out many of the post-transcriptional and post-translational modifications that eukaryotic cells can perform. Requirements such as the addition of sugar groups or the production of hydroxy-amino acids can present a major problem. Fourth, the human protein must be protected from proteinases within the bacterium.

How good are these biologically engineered human proteins? They should be perfectly acceptable for administration to patients. In most cases, they should be pure and contain no infectious contaminants or animal antigenic material. However, unless purified extensively, they might contain clinically relevant amounts of bacterial antigenic substances. In addition, since some products isolated directly from the body have a number of biological compounds bound to them, the clinical effect of a "pure" engineered product (e.g., albumin) might be somewhat different from that of the natural product.

The Next Products

What human biologics are now under development? The next ones being prepared for human trials fall into four broad categories: vaccines, blood components, neurohormones, and diagnostics.

VACCINES. Specific vaccines for influenza, hepatitis, malaria, and other diseases are currently in preparation. This new generation of vaccines should be superior to those in use today. A precise portion of the antigenic surface of a virus or a parasite can be selected and the DNA complement to this moiety prepared. Since a bacterial control signal will transcribe any sequence of DNA attached to it, the DNA coding for just the antigenic site desired can be inserted into bacteria for large scale production of material. Or the DNA could be inserted into, for example, vaccinia in order to take advantage of a well-characterized vaccination agent. It should be possible to prepare highly specific vaccines by this approach.

BLOOD COMPONENTS. Several different types of blood components are being prepared for clinical trials.

Clotting Factors. Factor VIII, von Willebrand factor, and factor IX are under active development. Although the cDNA for factor IX is easiest to prepare technically, the commercial demand is greatest for factor VIII, and, therefore, considerable emphasis is being placed on obtaining a gene copy of factor VIII that can be productively inserted into bacteria.

Albumin. The large demand for albumin as a plasma expander has resulted in a major effort to produce human albumin in bacteria. The advantages of engineered albumin (besides increased availability and decreased cost) should be that there will be no risk of hepatitis or other infectious contamination.

Thrombolytic Agents. Blood clots are a major cause of death and disabling diseases in the United States. Consequently, readily available clot-specific thrombolytic agents would be clinically useful. Biotechnology is being employed to isolate the genes for and to engineer the production of tissue-type and urokinase-type plasminogen activators. These proteins should be superior to the currently available agents, urokinase and streptokinase.

Immune System Agents. Besides the family of interferons that are under active clinical investigation, the interleukins are being prepared for engineered production in bacteria. Major advances in clinical manipulation of the immune system are expected when the genes of the major histocompatibility complex and the immunoglobulin gene families are more fully understood.

NEUROHORMONES. This complex group includes a large number of hormones, various neuropeptides, and the neurotransmitters with their receptors. Insulin and growth hormone are already being tested clinically; peptides from the pro-opiomelanocortin family should be available shortly.

DIAGNOSTICS. Since viruses consist of sequences of DNA or RNA with a coat, diagnostic techniques that would rapidly and accurately identify the presence of specific viruses in body tissues or fluids by using DNA probes are being developed.

OTHER AREAS. Finally, two other areas need to be mentioned. A further understanding of oncogenes and their role in cancer might lead to the development of drugs or antibodies that could be used to inhibit specific steps in the pathway leading from a normal to a malignant cell. Second, the tremendous potential of recombinant DNA research to produce useful new agricultural plants and improved farm animals could have a large effect on the food supply of the world.

GENE THERAPY

By gene therapy is meant the insertion of a normal gene into the appropriate cells of a patient in such a way that the exogenous gene produces a product that will cure, or at least partially offset the abnormalities caused by, the genetic defect. For some genetic conditions (specifically those caused by a single gene mutation that produces a defective product which can be isolated), gene therapy should be a beneficial therapeutic procedure in the future.

Present Capabilities

In recent years genes have been transferred into mammalian cells successfully. Individual cells in tissue culture have been "cured" of genetic defects by insertion of a normal gene. A functional rat growth hormone gene has been microinjected into fertilized mouse eggs; the mice that have grown from these eggs have produced rat growth hormone and are much larger than their normal noninjected siblings. Furthermore, a mouse with a genetic defect in growth hormone production has been partially "cured" by this procedure. In many cases, genes injected into mouse eggs are integrated into the mouse's germ line. Geneticists have successfully carried out very precise gene therapy in *Drosophila* (fruit flies). They have inserted, by means of a eukaryotic transposable (i.e., movable) piece of DNA, a normal eye color gene into adult mutant flies that have defective eye color. The genetic defect is corrected in a number of the fly's offspring.

The Technology of Gene Therapy

It is now possible by the use of recombinant DNA technology to isolate specific normal genes from the DNA of human tissue. A gene can be isolated if it can be recognized, and it can be recognized if the protein product that it makes can be isolated. The defective product in many genetic diseases is a protein (e.g., an enzyme in many of the inborn errors of metabolism; β-globin in sickle cell anemia or Cooley's anemia). In a manner similar to that described above in the section on human biologicals, a DNA probe can be synthesized. With this probe it is possible to locate the gene in human DNA, isolate it, and purify it. The process of isolating and purifying a gene is called "molecular cloning." Any gene can be cloned once a probe for the gene exists.

The cloned gene can be inserted into cells in any one of a number of ways. The three most commonly used techniques are (a) microinjecting directly into a cell's nucleus, (b) forming a calcium phosphate precipitate of the DNA and then incubating tissue culture cells with this precipitate, and (c) inserting the gene into a nonpathogenic virus and infecting cells with this recombinant virus. All three procedures have been used successfully to insert cloned genes into cells growing in tissue culture.

Future Work

Two major obstacles must be overcome in order to carry out successful gene therapy in an animal (or human). First, most cloned genes are unable to function properly when inserted into cells. Second, it is not known how to get the exogenous gene into the appropriate cells inside an animal.

Probes for a large number of human genes, including β-globin, are now available. However, the probes recognize only the coding portion of the gene; they do not recognize the control signals that are necessary for proper functioning of that gene. A great deal of research is now under way attempting to understand what these regulatory regions are and where they are located. Are there any cloned genes that are functional and that make effective amounts of product? There are several such genes, and two have been studied extensively. The first is the thymidine kinase gene of herpes simplex virus. Insertion of the thymidine kinase gene into mutant cells that have no thymidine kinase activity and would otherwise die in selective medium "cures" the cells (i.e., thymidine kinase enzyme is produced in amounts sufficient to replace the product that the defective gene would have made). The second is the metallothionein gene. This gene makes a protein that binds heavy metals and is thought to be involved in zinc homeostasis and resistance to heavy metal toxicity; it is controlled at the transcriptional level by heavy metals and by glucocorticoid hormones. For reasons not yet understood, this gene is active when inserted into a number of different cell types. Just the promoter region for the metallothionein gene (the DNA adjacent to the coding sequence) can be cut out and placed next to any other gene. This recombinant gene can be inserted into cells and will function: the coding sequence will be turned on by the metallothionein promoter. In fact, this is the mechanism whereby the rat growth hormone gene was activated in order to cure growth hormone–deficient mice (see above). Nonetheless, the thymidine kinase and metallothionein genes (and a few others) are the exception. Most cloned genes function poorly or not at all when present in tissue culture cells or in intact animals.

Curing a cell in tissue culture with a functional gene is not the same as curing cells in an intact organism. Bone marrow cells are easy to remove, treat, and reinsert; in addition, they multiply rapidly. But what about brain or liver cells, or cells in the islets of Langerhans? Some genetic diseases may not be treatable, even with a functional gene, because of an inability to get the gene into enough of the affected cells. Furthermore, in tissue culture, growth conditions can be manipulated to kill any cell that loses the gene; thus, the cells maintaining the gene are continually selected. Inside an organism, no such pressure exists. If the selective pressure is removed from tissue culture cells "cured" by gene therapy, the cells gradually lose the gene. Therefore, another important piece of knowledge that must be acquired is how to stabilize a gene once it is in the correct target cell. Even if a functional human β-globin gene now existed and could be inserted into bone marrow stem cells with high efficiency, it is not known how to maintain it there.

The procedure used to cure the growth hormone–deficient mice is not suitable for use in humans. Even though researchers have years of experience, most mouse fertilized eggs that are injected do not develop into mice containing the injected gene. Many eggs are killed by the procedure and others do not incorporate the new DNA for unknown reasons. Furthermore, three out of four eggs that would result from the mating of two carriers would be normal or heterozygous. Therefore, because of the technical uncertainties, the low probability that a given egg would be a homozygous defective, and the ethical objections to experimenting on human zygotes, it is highly unlikely that genes would ever be microinjected into human eggs. Consequently, a delivery system suitable for inserting genes into humans must still be developed.

Risks in Gene Therapy

What about risk? Every procedure carries a potential for harm. It is unknown whether or not the insertion of foreign DNA into a human cell would be detrimental to the cell or, ultimately, the patient. Cells "cured" in tissue culture look normal and appear to grow and divide normally. But these criteria are relatively crude. It is not known whether regulatory pathways in the cells are adversely affected. And, of course, how well such cells would be able to undergo the differentiation processes required in the body (e.g., stem cells to committed erythroid precursors to erythroblasts to RBC's) is uncertain. The mechanisms that regulate cell division are poorly understood. There is concern that alteration of the genetic makeup of a cell might, over time, cause a malignant transformation of the cell. All of these questions should be answered as fully as possible in animals before attempting gene therapy in humans.

Thus, it is generally accepted that three criteria need to be met before it would be ethical to carry out gene therapy in humans. From animal studies it should be shown that (1) the cloned gene can get into, and remain within, the appropriate cells long enough to be helpful; (2) the cloned gene is functional and can make enough product in the animal to be effective; (3) the cloned gene, and the procedure used to insert it, do not cause greater harm than the benefit that is produced. Recently, a mouse mutant has been described that appears to be a close model for the human disease β-thalassemia. This unique mouse line should prove useful for experiments designed to satisfy these three criteria.

Overview

Two classes of disease can be approached by gene therapy. First, correction of a defective gene that produces a circulating factor, e.g., a hormone; second, correction of a defective gene that makes an intracellular product, e.g., hemoglobin, an enzyme, or a structural protein. In the former case the new gene might be effective even if it is inserted into the "wrong" cells, i.e., into cells that do not normally make the factor. The successful gene therapy of the growth hormone–deficient mouse is an example of this type. It is the latter case, however, in which a gene must be inserted directly into the correct cells (and possibly into the correct chromosomal location within the correct cells) that is proving so difficult to accomplish. β-Thalassemia, sickle cell anemia, PKU, and Tay-Sachs disease are examples of this class of disease.

Gene therapy is a procedure with enormous potential. It should, in the future, provide a cure for hereditary diseases caused by a single gene defect. It is even possible that the germ line might be corrected so that the children of a patient will also be free from disease. This would be, indeed, a powerful therapeutic tool. But some claims made about the potential of genetic engineering in humans are highly unlikely. Patients with multigenic diseases, where the genes as well as the intracellular products involved are unknown, will not be candidates for gene therapy for a long time to come, if ever. Likewise, characteristics such as personality and intelligence are probably outside the realm of this technique's potential. Only traits produced by identifiable single genes can be approached by genetic engineering. Of course, if, as now seems the case, some very widespread pathologic conditions (viz., lipid deposition in vessels to produce atherosclerosis) are influenced by identifiable individual genes, then gene therapy might have a far wider application than currently visualized.

The power to cure a genetic defect is an awesome one. But the goal of biomedical research is, and has always been, to alleviate human suffering. Gene therapy is a proper and logical part of that effort.

Anderson WF, Fletcher JC: Gene therapy in human beings: When is it ethical to begin? N Engl J Med 303:1293–1297, 1980. *This article suggests what scientific/medical criteria ought to be met prior to carrying out a gene therapy experiment in humans.*

Gilbert F, Villa-Komaroff L: Useful proteins from recombinant bacteria. Sci Am 242:74–94, 1980. *This is a well-written, easy-to-follow article on the technology of protein production in bacteria.*

Palmiter RD, Brinster RL, Hammer RE, Trumbauer ME, Rosenfeld MG, Birnberg NC, Evans RM: Dramatic growth of mice that develop from eggs microinjected with metallothionein-growth hormone fusion genes. Nature 300:611–615, 1982. *This paper describes the successful insertion of a functioning growth hormone gene, obtained by recombinant DNA techniques, into mice.*

President's Commission for the Study of Ethical Problems in Medicine and Biomedical and Behavioral Research: *Splicing Life.* November, 1982. Washington, DC, US Government Printing Office. *This clearly written report summarizes the scientific and ethical issues surrounding gene therapy in humans.*

Rubin GM, Spradling AC: Genetic transformation of *Drosophila* with transposable element vectors. Science 218:348–353, 1982. *This relatively technical paper describes the elegant gene therapy experiment in which defective eye color was corrected in fruit flies.*

34. CONTRIBUTIONS OF RECOMBINANT DNA RESEARCH TO DIAGNOSIS OF HERITABLE DISEASE

C. Thomas Caskey

Prior to the availability of recombinant DNA techniques, the enormous DNA content of the human genome (5×10^9 base pairs) made chemical analysis of human genes impossible.

Normal and mutant genes can now be compared at single nucleotide levels. The remarkable sensitivity and simplicity of DNA techniques has provided rapid expansion of knowledge about gene structure, regulation, and mutation. At a macroscopic level, localization of genes to chromosomes and their physical relationship (linkage) to each other is establishing a detailed human gene map. This newly acquired knowledge is being applied to diagnosis and prevention of human heritable disease.

MOLECULAR CLONING

The detailed study of man's vast and complex DNA structure required cleaving the DNA molecule into fragments of manageable size. *Restriction endonucleases* provided the means for precise cleavage. These nucleases recognize specific 4–6 base sequences that have symmetry (palindromes). Since there are well over 100 different restriction endonucleases, DNA molecules can be cleaved precisely at a variety of sites, permitting the generation of an infinite number of precisely formed fragments. Since the cleavage of the two DNA strands occurs at opposite ends of a palindrome, each strand is left with a short "sticky" single strand sequence. This "sticky" sequence is critical to formation of new DNA molecules. Since DNA from any two sources cut with the same endonuclease have identical "sticky" sequences, they are readily annealed and joined physically by *DNA ligase.* Thus, restriction endonucleases provide both the method of precise DNA cleavage and means for joining DNA fragments from different sources.

Microbial *cloning* is the method of isolating a single DNA fragment from a large mixture. Two cloning vectors, bacterial *plasmids* and *phage* (virus), have been most used. Each vector is grown on a bacterial cell and can accommodate foreign DNA without interfering with its replication ability. Antibiotic resistance genes of plasmids facilitate the isolation and identification of recombinant plasmids. Foreign DNA cleaved by the endonuclease Pst 1 when inserted into the single Pst 1 site of the plasmid's ampicillin resistance gene acts as a mutation to the resistance gene. Since the plasmid also carried a functional tetracycline resistance gene, the plasmids can be recovered as clones by transfection into sensitive microbes grown on tetracycline-containing media. A single recombinant plasmid molecule gives rise to a microbial colony resistant to tetracycline but sensitive to ampicillin (Fig. 34–1). Thus, a restriction endonuclease DNA fragment is *cloned.* The method provides 10^5 to 10^6 recombinant clones per μg of DNA. The recombinant DNA fragments are usually small (1 to 7,000 base pairs). Bacteriophage λ provides a method for cloning larger DNA fragments (20,000 base pairs) at higher efficiency (10^8 to 10^9 recombinants per μg). The middle portion (20,000 base pairs) of the 40,000 base pair bacteriophage is removed by restriction endonuclease and replaced with foreign DNA. Recombinant bacteriophages are easily identified, since only those that are restored to approximately 40,000 base pair size can be packaged into viral particles, infect microbial cells, and form plaques (Fig. 34–2). Each plaque is the product of infection with a single molecule and thus contains a *clone* of the foreign DNA fragment. The method permits molecular cloning of an individual's genome in 10^6 to 10^7 bacteriophage from μgram quantities of DNA. More recently recombinantly designed cloning vectors that embody the advantage of plasmids and bacteriophage have been developed. These vectors, *cosmids,* clone 40,000 base pair sequences with high efficiency.

The human DNA used in molecular cloning is derived from either nuclear (genomic) or a DNA copy (cDNA) of messenger RNA synthesized in vitro. The strategy differs for isolation of recombinants of individual disease genes. Cloning of β hemoglobin, immunoglobulins, insulin, and growth hormone utilized cDNA cloning, since specialized cells were available where 10 to 90 per cent of the mRNA corresponded to the gene of

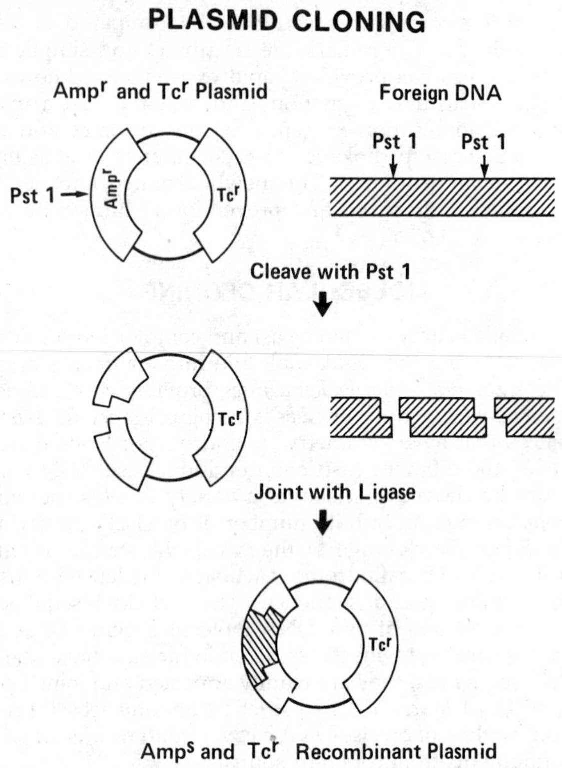

Figure 34–1. Plasmid cloning. The Pst 1 endonuclease fragment of foreign DNA is cloned into the Pst 1 site of the ampicillin gene.

interest. Genomic DNA cloning of purified X-chromosomes was needed for an X recombinant bank. The isolation of oncogenes utilized genomic clones for DNA transfer of the neoplastic trait.

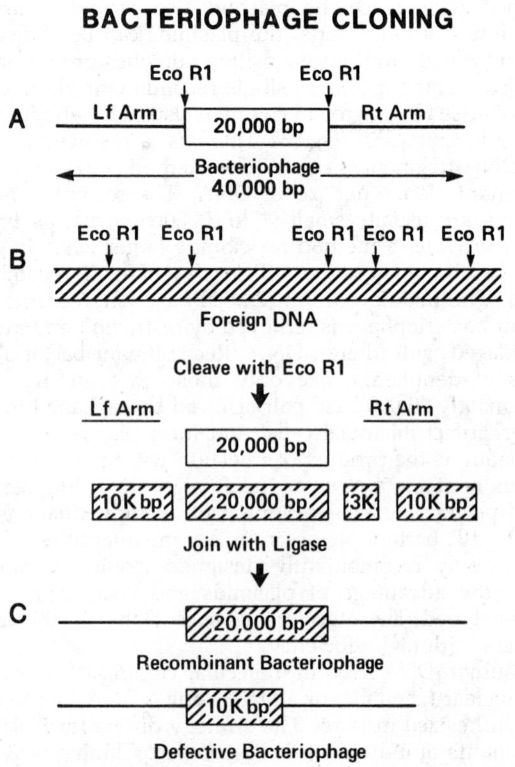

Figure 34–2. Bacteriophage λ cloning. The Eco R1 endonuclease fragment of foreign DNA is cloned into the Eco R1 site of bacteriophage λ.

Each of these methods permits isolation of a small fraction of the human genome (10^6 to 10^7) in a microbial vector. The recombinant is easily amplified to milligram quantities of the gene fragment for detailed chemical study. The simplicity of the methods permits direct comparison of normal and individual patient's disease genes.

GENE STRUCTURE AND MUTATION

The nucleotide structure of genes can be determined by two DNA sequencing techniques developed independently in 1977 by Fred Sanger and Walter Gilbert. DNA sequence comparison of nuclear and mRNA (cDNA) recombinants identified an unusual property of mammalian genes. Mammalian genes are interrupted by intervening DNA sequences (IVS or introns) removed at the level of RNA gene transcripts. In the case of human β globin, two IVS sequences are removed while three protein coding sequences (exons) are joined to form the functional mRNA. The cleavage and rejoining of RNA occurs in the nucleus and is referred to as *splicing*. While β globin's structure is simple, collagen genes are complex because of their many introns. As is clear from recombinant DNA study of cloned β-thalassemia genes, gene splicing mutations can account for disease in man.

Detailed study of the β-thalassemic gene from patients with different classes of molecular defects shows the following defects: transcription defects at 4 sites, translation defects at 10 sites, and RNA splicing defects at 14 sites (Fig. 34–3). One can anticipate that similar detailed knowledge of other disease genes will follow this example. It is already clear that the Lesch-Nyhan syndrome and citrullinemia occur on the basis of mutations in different positions in these genes.

GENETIC MAP AND LINKAGE

Since man's DNA complement can be cloned in entirety, it is theoretically possible to assign these cloned DNA fragments to particular chromosomes and each other (*linkage*). Never has the opportunity been so great to saturate the human genome with defined markers (cloned DNA fragments). Y.W. Kan (1978) discovered that restriction endonucleases could be used to identify natural variation in man's DNA structure for a particular region. He found 70 per cent of the β^S gene on a 13,000 base or 13.0 "kilobase" (kb) DNA restriction fragment, while 95 per cent of the β^A gene was on a 7.6 kb fragment. This variation, referred to as restriction fragment length polymorphism (RFLP), has been shown to occur frequently with other genes and is therefore useful for genetic mapping. It has been estimated that 50 to 100 RFLP's scattered evenly over the human genome would be adequate to determine the linkage association to any human disease gene. The developing gene map of man will enable physicians to identify tightly linked genetic markers to genetic diseases such as Huntington's disease, Duchenne muscular dystrophy, and cystic fibrosis for which no gene product is known.

PRENATAL DIAGNOSIS

An estimated 30,000 patients utilized prenatal diagnosis in the United States in 1983. Inborn errors of metabolism represent 5 per cent of this total. Recombinant DNA methods provide a new approach to their prenatal diagnosis. Since recombinant methods examine the DNA rather than the gene product, amniocytes can be used, avoiding the need for obtaining inaccessible specialized tissues (i.e., blood or liver) by fetoscopy. The risk of pregnancy loss related to amniocentesis is 0.5 per cent, while with fetoscopy it is 5 per cent. Recombinant DNA diagnostic methods have markedly improved the safety of hemoglobinopathy diagnosis, since the need for fetal blood sampling via fetoscopy is eliminated.

A probe is needed for study of mutants of a cloned gene. The probe may be a portion of or the entire normal human gene, or a copy of messenger RNA (cDNA). These recombinant

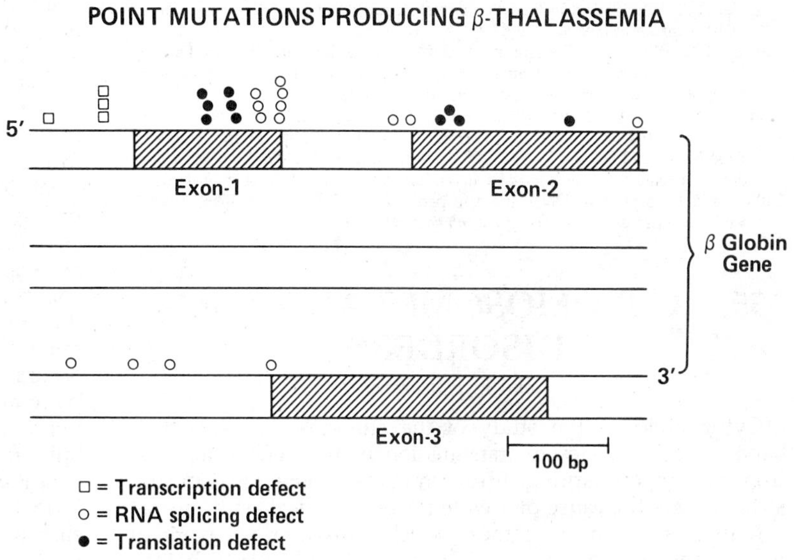

Figure 34–3. Diagrammatic representation of single base (point) mutations resulting in β-thalassemia in man. (Adapted from Orkin SH, Antonarakis SE, Kazazian HH Jr.: Polymorphism and Pathology of the β-Globin Gene, edited by E. B. Brown. New York, Grune & Stratton, 1983, and personal communication.)

probes, made highly radioactive, are able to identify single DNA gene fragments in 10^6 molecules. The gel analysis method developed by Edwin Southern (1977) is used in this detection. DNA is first fragmented for study by restriction endonucleases. With the large number of different endonucleases available, a nuclear gene can be cleaved into a variety of fragments. The DNA fragments are separated by gel electrophoresis, transferred, and immobilized on nitrocellulose filters (blotting). The DNA fragments are detected by molecular hybridization with the radioactive cloned gene probe. Mutations are detected by alteration in the size and number of gene fragments. Analysis requires 1 to 2 μg of nuclear DNA and is completed in 48 hours. Study of disease genes is limited only by the availability of the probe. Recombinant disease probes recently isolated include Lesch-Nyhan, α-1-antitrypsin, phenylketonuria, citrullinemia, adenosine deaminase, HLA, factor IX, and insulin.

Detection of hemoglobinopathy mutations is highly sophisticated and accurate. The prenatal diagnosis of sickle cell disease utilizes knowledge of the gene DNA sequence. Sickle cell anemia involves the point mutation GAGG to GTGG. The restriction enzyme MstII cleaves the β^A gene at this site, since it recognizes GAGG. It does not recognize the β^S sequence GTGG. DNA cleavage of $\beta^S\beta^S$ (sickle cell homozygote) yields 1350 base pair fragments, $\beta^A\beta^A$ (normal homozygote) yields 1150 base pair fragments, while β^{SA} (heterozygote) yields both fragments. Analysis of DNA fragments obtained by restriction endonuclease treatment of amniotic cells therefore establishes accurate diagnosis of the fetus. Another diagnostic approach has broader applicability. Organically synthesized oligonucleotides of 19 bases in length can distinguish between the normal and sickle gene. The mutant single base difference of the two oligonucleotides is positioned in the middle. The difference in the two probes permits melting or dissociation of the inappropriate radioactive probe from the nuclear gene sequence, providing a radioactive probe for its homologous but not heterologous gene. This method successfully identifies the point mutational difference between β^S and β^A genes. Using different oligonucleotides, it is possible to discriminate between the normal and the Mediterranean β^+-thalassemia, which is due to a single base change resulting in aberrant mRNA splicing. Successful discrimination of the M and Z alleles of alpha-1-antitrypsin has also been reported. This method should be amenable to diseases in which amino acid substitution mutations are known but gene structure data are lacking. The oligonucleotide probe method avoids gene cloning and substitutes organic synthesis of gene probes.

Mutations in which all or a portion of the gene has been deleted are readily detected by absence of gene fragments. The gene deletions of $\delta°\beta°$, β^-, and β-thalassemia and some cases of Lesch-Nyhan, factor IX, and growth hormone deficiency are excellent examples.

For some diseases, gene probes are available but knowledge of the precise mutation is not. Genetic linkage methods were first applied to prenatal diagnosis by Y.W. Kan (1978). Restriction endonucleases identify common normal variations in gene structure as restriction fragment length polymorphisms, RFLP. A disease gene can be identified by its linkage association to normal RFLP. Kan utilized the frequent RFLP associated with the β^S gene for this purpose. Additional RFLPs were identified and subsequently successfully applied to prenatal diagnosis of β-thalassemias. This approach has been reported useful to some 100 families. The RFLP approach promises to be applicable to the diagnosis of Lesch-Nyhan syndrome and phenylketonuria where a high frequency of RFLP is reported.

The RFLP linkage method is being applied also to diagnosis of disease genes for which no probe exists. In this circumstance the RFLP is identified with either a probe for a known gene or an "anonymous" gene sequence mapping close to the disease gene. The greater the distance between the RFLP and the disease gene, the more frequent recombinational events dissociate RFLP and disease gene. Anonymous probes that map to the chromosomal region near the disease gene can be used. X chromosome anonymous probes that flank the Duchenne muscular dystrophy gene (Xp21) have loose linkage to the disease gene. In another example, the fragile X chromosome abnormality located at Xq27 is flanked by loose linkage to hypoxanthine-guanine phosphoribosyltransferase and strong linkage to glucose-6-phosphate dehydrogenase. These recombinant DNA probes make it possible to study diseases whose genetic defects are unknown and for which no disease gene probes are available.

The impact of recombinant DNA methods on prenatal diagnosis will continue to increase. In a relatively short period of time recombinant DNA technology has been successfully applied to the task of preventing serious human heritable diseases.

Boehm CD, Antonaykis SE, Phillips JA, Stetten G, Kazazian HW: Prenatal diagnosis using DNA polymorphisms: Report on 95 pregnancies at risk for sickle-cell disease or β thalassemia. N Engl J Med 308:1054–1058, 1983. *The most comprehensive experience of prenatal diagnosis by recombinant DNA methods.*
Botstein D, White RL, Skolnick MH, Davis RW: Construction of a genetic linkage map in man using restriction fragment length polymorphism. Am J Human

Genet 32:314, 1980. *A well-written theoretical paper that describes the recombinant DNA mapping method by RFLP.*
Caskey CT, White RL: Recombinant DNA Applications to Human Disease. Banbury Report 14, Cold Spring Harbor Laboratory, 1983. *A comprehensive series of articles by leading investigators. Well illustrated.*
Conner BJ, Reyes AA, Morin C, Itakura K, Teplitz RJ, Wallace RB: Detection of sickle cell β^S-globin allele by hybridization with synthetic oligonucleotides. Proc Natl Acad Sci 80:278–282, 1983. *The application of synthetic nucleic acids to disease diagnosis, a new approach independent of recombinant DNA methods.*
Miller WL: Recombinant DNA and the pediatrician. J Pediatr 99:1–15, 1981. *A well-illustrated article describing recombinant DNA procedures.*

35. CHROMOSOMES AND THEIR DISORDERS

John L. Hamerton

Cytogenetics is the study of the chromosomes and their behavior as it relates to transmission of the genetic material from parent to offspring. Errors in chromosome behavior and structure are the cause of a wide range of clinical syndromes.

Man has 46 chromosomes, which consist of 22 pairs of homologous chromosomes (identical in regard to morphology and constituent gene loci) and one pair of sex chromosomes (X and Y), one partner of each pair being derived from the mother and one from the father. The genes are arranged along the chromosomes in linear order, each gene having a precise position or *locus.* Genes that have their loci on the same chromosome are said to be *linked,* or more precisely, to be *syntenic.* Alternate forms of a gene that occupy the same locus are called *alleles.* Any one chromosome bears only a single allele at a given locus, although in the population as a whole there may be multiple alleles, any one of which can occupy that specific locus.

The *genotype* of an individual is his individual genetic constitution; the *phenotype* is the expression of the genotype as a morphological, biochemical, physiologic, or clinical trait. The term *genome* refers to the full DNA content of the chromosome set.

CELL DIVISION

The number of chromosomes found in somatic cells is constant and is termed the diploid (2n) number. Each gamete, however, has only half the *diploid* number and is said to be *haploid* (n). In order to maintain this regularity two types of cell division occur: *mitosis,* which is the cell division occurring in somatic tissues during growth and repair, and *meiosis,* which is the specialized form of cell division occurring during the formation of the gametes.

MITOSIS. The function of mitosis is the distribution and maintenance of the continuity of the genetic material in every cell of the body. This process consists of a number of different phases, which results in an equal distribution of the chromosomes to the two daughter cells. Mitosis is part of the cell cycle that has four stages: mitosis or M, G_1, S, and G_2. The G_1 phase follows mitosis, during which RNA and protein synthesis occurs. S is the period during which DNA replication takes place and the DNA content of the cell doubles, and G_2 is the period during which energy requirements for cell division are built up and any repair of errors in DNA synthesis takes place.

MEIOSIS (Fig. 35–1). This process occurs only during the formation of the gametes and results in four daughter cells, each with the haploid number of chromosomes. In males each primary spermatocyte forms four functional spermatids that develop into sperm, while in females each oocyte forms only one ovum, the remaining products of meiosis being nonfunctional polar bodies.

The first division of meiosis consists of an extremely long and complex *prophase* during which DNA replication occurs. This is divided into a number of stages during which crossing over and reassortment of genetic material occur. Initially the chromosomes are apparently single threads that begin to shorten and thicken. This is followed by the commencement of the pairing of homologous chromosomes *(synapsis).* After pairing is completed, the chromosomes continue to shorten and are now known as *bivalents,* which are held together only at specific points *(chiasmata).* At this stage of prophase each homologous chromosome can be seen to be visibly doubled (two chromatids) so that each bivalent, which continues to shorten and thicken, consists of four chromatids.

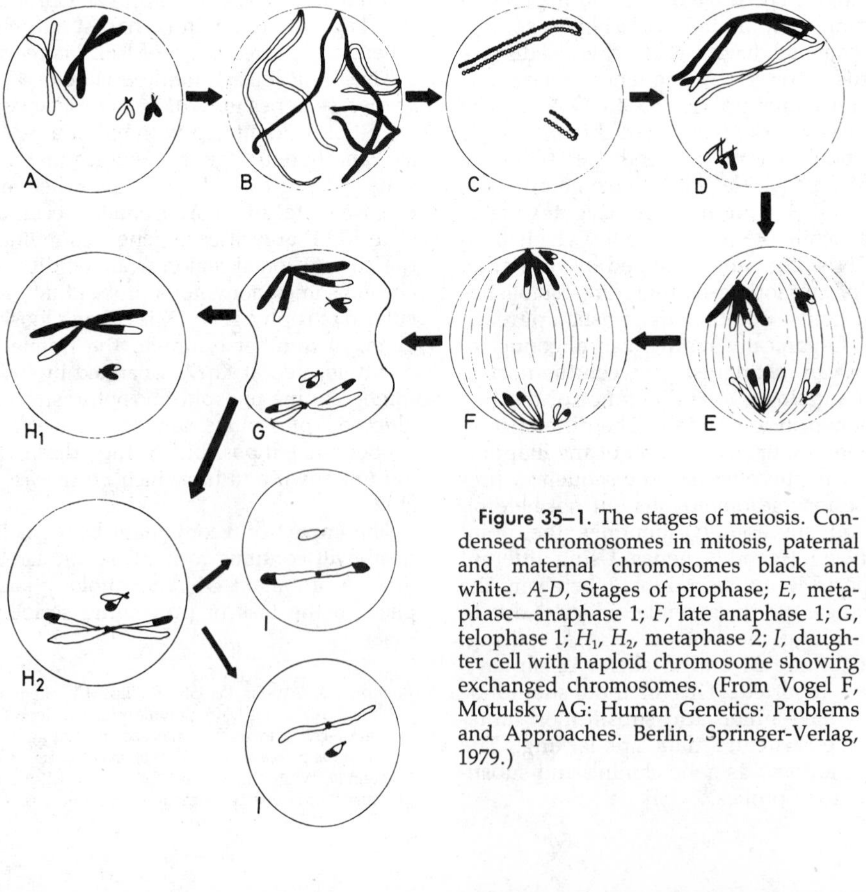

Figure 35–1. The stages of meiosis. Condensed chromosomes in mitosis, paternal and maternal chromosomes black and white. *A-D,* Stages of prophase; *E,* metaphase—anaphase 1; *F,* late anaphase 1; *G,* telophase 1; *H_1, H_2,* metaphase 2; *I,* daughter cell with haploid chromosome showing exchanged chromosomes. (From Vogel F, Motulsky AG: Human Genetics: Problems and Approaches. Berlin, Springer-Verlag, 1979.)

The end of the prophase is marked by the disappearance of the nuclear membrane and the formation of a spindle, heralding entry into *metaphase* of the first meiotic division. The bivalents are arranged on the equatorial plate of the spindle as a result of a series of complex chromosome movements. The homologous centromeres are undivided at this point and lie opposite each other on the equatorial plate (co-orientation). As soon as this process is complete, the paired homologues separate and move to opposite poles *(anaphase).* The cell then proceeds to the second meiotic division. This is essentially a mitotic division in which the chromosomes have already doubled so that there is no need for DNA synthesis. In addition the genetic material has undergone exchange at meiosis I so that the sister chromatids are not genetically identical.

The major consequences of meiosis are threefold: (1) the halving of the chromosome number. (2) the co-orientation of the bivalents on the metaphase plate. This ensures the regular distribution of the chromosomes to the daughter cells. (3) the independent assortment of genetic material that results both from genetic crossing over and from the random assortment of the maternal and paternal homologues to the two daughter cells in meiosis I.

Two processes are fundamental to meiosis: chromosome pairing, which results in formation of the bivalents, and chiasma formation. Chiasmata have two main functions: they are the points on the chromosomes at which genetic crossing over takes place and they serve to maintain bivalent association throughout the prophase and metaphase. Meiosis thus ensures genetic variability as a result of random segregation of the parental homologous chromosomes and the exchange of genetic material by crossing over between nonsister chromatids.

METHODS FOR THE PREPARATION OF CHROMOSOMES

Since nondividing chromosomes cannot be analyzed, dividing cells are required for chromosome analysis. The cell type most commonly used is the mitogenically stimulated peripheral blood lymphocyte. Skin fibroblasts, amniotic fluid cells, and bone marrow cells are also used for special tests. Dividing cells are accumulated at metaphase. Colcemid added to the culture medium toward the end of the culture period is most commonly used to accomplish this. The cells are then subjected to hypotonic treatment, followed by fixation and spreading on microscope slides. The slides are then stained.

Staining techniques may result in either a nonbanded or a banded appearance of the chromosomes. Most laboratories today use one of several banding techniques, since this results in a great deal of additional information. These methods provide a means for the precise identification of an extra or missing chromosome and the precise localization of breakpoints in chromosome rearrangements (Fig. 35–2).

Recent developments have resulted in the expansion of the number of visible bands from between 200 and 300 to between 1000 and 2000. This allows the recognition of small deletions and duplications. Most laboratories today work with chromosomes in which between 400 and 800 bands can be recognized.

HUMAN CHROMOSOME NOMENCLATURE

The 46 human chromosomes consist of three types designated by the position of the centromere or primary constriction. These are metacentric, submetacentric, and acrocentric, depending upon whether the position of the centromere is median, submedian, or terminal. Now that each individual chromosome pair can be recognized, the chromosomes are numbered from 1 to 22 in descending order of length. In the female the two sex chromosomes, designated X chromosomes, are identical, while in the male the two sex chromosomes, designated X and Y, are morphologically different.

Chromosome Variants

This term refers to consistent minor chromosome changes often involving the short arms of the acrocentric chromosomes, the long arm of the Y chromosome, or the constitutive heterochromatin near the centromere of chromosomes 1, 9, and 16. These have little obvious clinical significance but may be useful as genetic markers. They occur much more frequently in the population than do major chromosome abnormalities, and they often segregate in families in a mendelian fashion. Recent studies suggest that about 70 per cent of newborn infants carry one or more variant chromosomes.

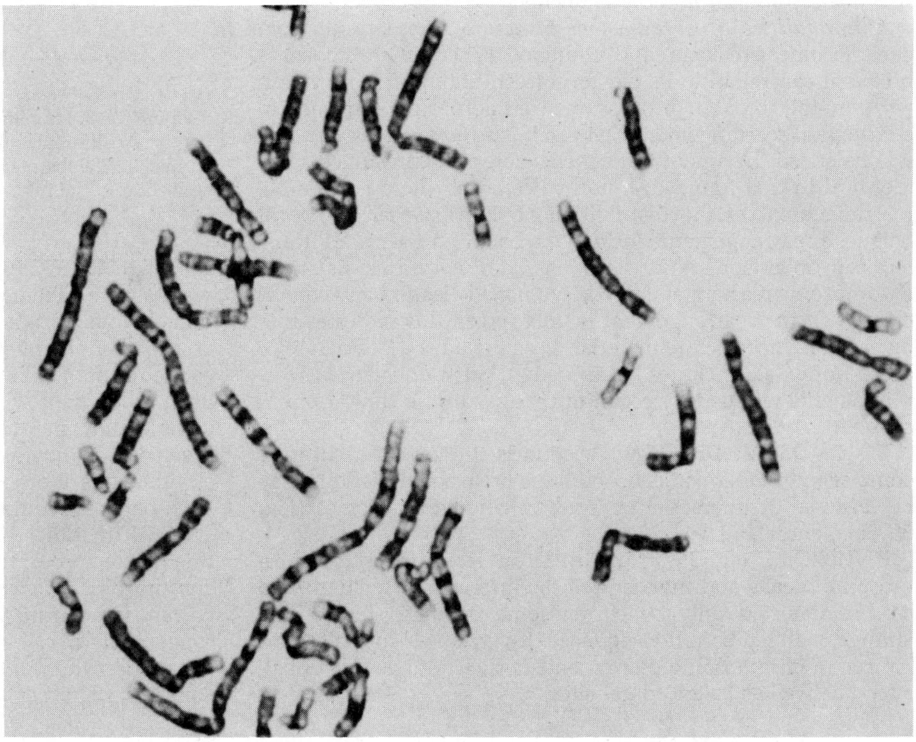

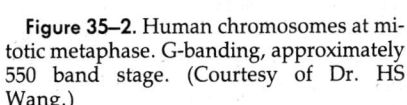

Figure 35–2. Human chromosomes at mitotic metaphase. G-banding, approximately 550 band stage. (Courtesy of Dr. HS Wang.)

Nomenclature

The nomenclature used to describe the chromosomes, chromosome bands, chromosome variants, and chromosome rearrangements is given in detail in ISCN (1978, 1981). A shorthand notation is used to describe the chromosome complement of an individual. In this notation the number of chromosomes is specified first, followed by the listing of the sex chromosomes. Thus a normal female karyotype is designated 46,XX and a normal male karyotype 46,XY. Any deviations from a normal karyotype are written after the sex chromosomes. An individual autosome is referred to by its number, its short arm by the letter "p," and its long arm by the letter "q." A "+" or "−" sign written after the p or q indicates an increase (+) or decrease (−) in the length of the arm. When written before a designated chromosome the sign indicates that the chromosome is extra (+) or missing (−).

Examples: 46,XY,18q− describes a male with 46 chromosomes, including one chromosome 18 whose long arm is diminished in length.

47,XX,+21 describes a female with 47 chromosomes, including an extra chromosome 21 in addition to the 46 chromosomes of the normal karyotype.

A diagrammatic representation of the human chromosome 1 showing differing degrees of chromosome banding is given in Figure 35–3.

CHROMOSOME ABNORMALITIES

Chromosome abnormalities can be divided into two classes: abnormalities of number and those of structure.

Abnormalities of Chromosome Number. These arise from nondisjunction, that is, from *the failure of two homologous chromosomes in the first division of meiosis or of two sister chromatids in mitosis or the second division of meiosis to pass to opposite poles of the cell* (Fig. 35–4). This results in cells with abnormal chromosome numbers. If these cells are gametes, fertilization will result in a zygote with an abnormal chromosome number. If nondisjunction occurs during an early cleavage division of a zygote, then a chromosome mosaic may result. This is an individual with two or more cell lines differing in chromosome complement. Table 35–1 gives examples of chromosome abnormalities resulting from nondisjunction.

Abnormalities of Chromosome Structure. These result from chromosome breakage and reunion. When a chromosome breaks it can rejoin in its old form (restitution) or it can rejoin with another broken chromosome (reunion). Reunion leads to a structural rearrangement that can be *balanced* or *unbalanced*. If it is balanced the amount of genetic material is presumed to be identical to that found in a normal cell, and there is a simple rearrangement of the distribution of this material. Types of balanced rearrangements include the balanced reciprocal translocation, robertsonian translocations, and inversions. Balanced chromosome rearrangements do not usually lead to any clinical change. If the rearrangement is unbalanced this indicates loss or gain of chromosome material. Loss includes a deficiency or a deletion. Gain includes a duplication. Such unbalanced rearrangements will usually result in changes in the clinical phenotype.

CHROMOSOME DELETION. Deletion is the loss of a chromosome segment following chromosome breakage. Deletions may be terminal or interstitial or result in ring chromosomes (Fig. 35–5*a*,*b*, and *e*).

INVERSIONS (Fig. 35–5*c* and *d*). These result from two chromosome breaks and inversion of the intervening segment and can be detected only by chromosome banding studies that show a changed banding sequence. Inversions result in disturbances in chromosome pairing and in the formation of unbalanced as well as balanced gametes.

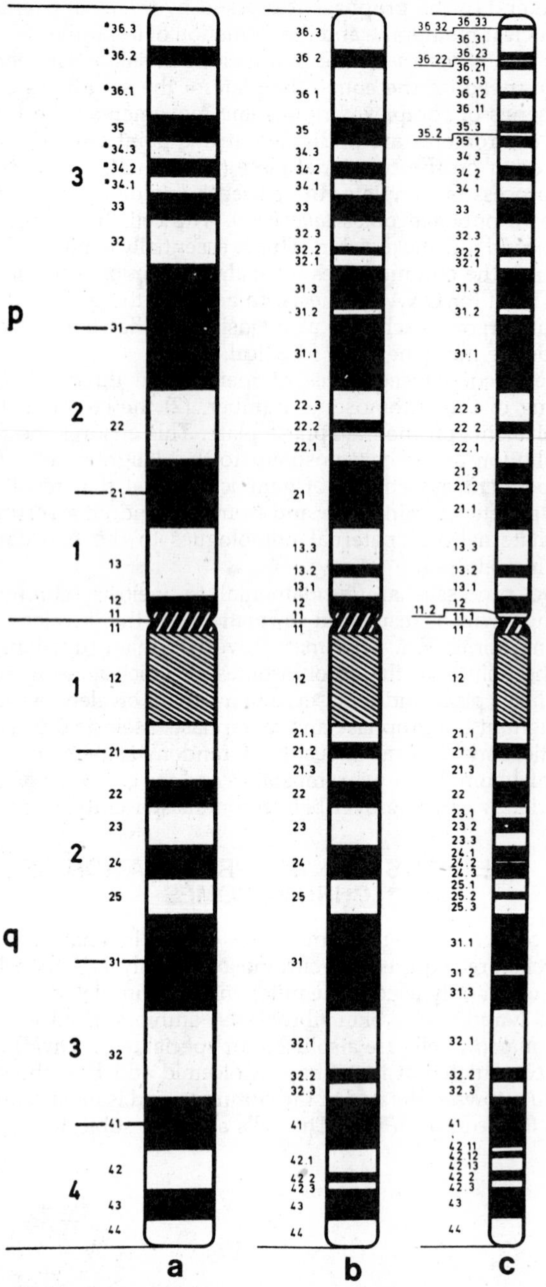

Figure 35–3. Human chromosome 1. Idiogram showing chromosome bands at different resolutions. *a*, Approximately 400 bands; *b*, 550 bands; *c*, 850 bands. The band nomenclature and subdivision are according to the internationally agreed system (ISCN 1981).

BALANCED RECIPROCAL TRANSLOCATION (Fig. 35–6). This results from exchange of chromosome segments between nonhomologous chromosomes. An individual carrying such a rearrangement will have a higher frequency of abnormal gametes as the result of a disturbance in chromosome pairing at meiosis. Such individuals will themselves have a balanced chromosome complement and be clinically normal, but they may have a high risk of having congenitally malformed children and/or spontaneous abortions. Normal children may also be born, and such persons require careful genetic counselling.

ROBERTSONIAN TRANSLOCATION. This is a specific type of unequal reciprocal translocation that occurs between acrocentric chromosomes, resulting in the formation of a new metacentric chromosome from two acrocentric chromosomes. Such rearrangements may be important in the transmission of Down's syndrome when one of the chromosomes involved is chromosome 21, the other usually being chromosome 14.

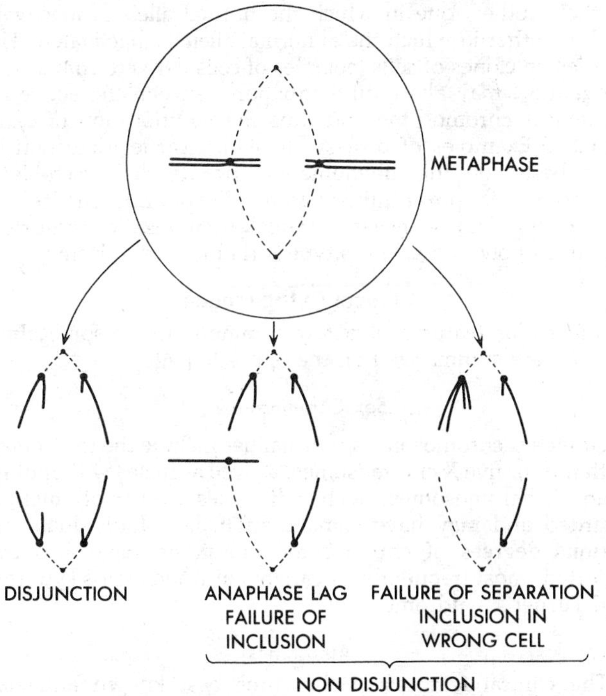

Figure 35–4. Diagram illustrating chromosome disjunction and two types of nondisjunction—anaphase lagging and failure of separation. (From Hamerton JL: Human Cytogenetics, Vol 1. Academic Press, 1971. New York & London.)

POPULATION CYTOGENETICS

Chromosome abnormalities form a significant component of the deleterious genetic load carried by the human population. About 6 per 1000 newborn babies have a major chromosome abnormality that may result in some degree of morbidity or mortality at some time during life. The frequency of the different types of chromosome abnormalities found when large numbers of newborn infants are screened is shown in Table 35–2.

Chromosome abnormalities found among newborn infants at birth are, however, only a very small proportion of the total load of chromosome abnormalities seen at conception. The majority of these are lethal or sublethal and are lost during gestation as either very early abortions or failure of implantation (monosomies, etc.), or as recognized abortions and perinatal deaths. This group includes most trisomies, triploids (3n), and tetraploids (4n). A significant proportion of perinatal and neonatal deaths have been shown to have a major chromosome abnormality. About 50 per cent of all spontaneous abortions have a chromosome abnormality and about 6 per cent of stillbirths and perinatal deaths have been shown to be abnormal.

TABLE 35–1. EXAMPLES OF CHROMOSOME ABNORMALITIES DUE TO NONDISJUNCTION IN MAN

Sex Chromosomes	Autosomes†
47,XXY (Klinefelter's syndrome) *46,XY/47,XXY	21-trisomy (47,XX or XY, +21)
47,XYY	13-trisomy (47,XX or XY, +13)
47,XXX	18-trisomy (47,XX or XY, +18)
45,X (Turner's syndrome) *45,X/46,XX (Ovarian dysgenesis)	21-monosomy (45,XX or XY, −21)

*Examples of chromosome mosaics due to nondisjunction or chromosome loss during an early cleavage division.

†In describing a chromosome abnormality the words "trisomy" and "monosomy" refer simply to an additional or missing chromosome.

In addition to the large amount of data on newborn babies and spontaneous abortions, there are now data on large numbers of mothers who have received amniocentesis for maternal age 35 and over. A recent study of over 50,000 amniocenteses shows that overall about 2 per cent of mid-trimester pregnancies in mothers aged 35 and above have a chromosome abnormality.

SEX CHROMATIN

There are two types of sex chromatin that can be seen in somatic cells: (1) The interphase chromocenter, which represents the genetically inactivated and condensed X chromosome, which is called the X chromatin (sex chromatin, Barr body) and is found in individuals with more than one X chromosome. (2) The smaller, brightly fluorescing chromocenter, which can be seen by fluorescence microscopy after staining with quinacrine. This represents the brightly fluorescent segment of the human Y chromosome and can be seen in all individuals carrying this chromosome. In diploid cells, the number of X chromosomes is always one greater than the maximum number of X chromatin bodies seen and the number of Y chromosomes is equal to the maximum number of fluorescent Y chromatin bodies. Study of the sex chromatin can thus provide a rapid assessment of the numbers of sex chromosomes present in the cells.

Late-replicating X chromosomes can be identified by autoradiography using tritiated thymidine or by the incorporation of 5-bromodeoxyuridine (BUDR) into DNA in place of thymidine, followed by staining with a dye that differentiates between BUDR and thymidine (the Hoechst-BUDR technique). It is now known that the condensed late-replicating X chromosomes are

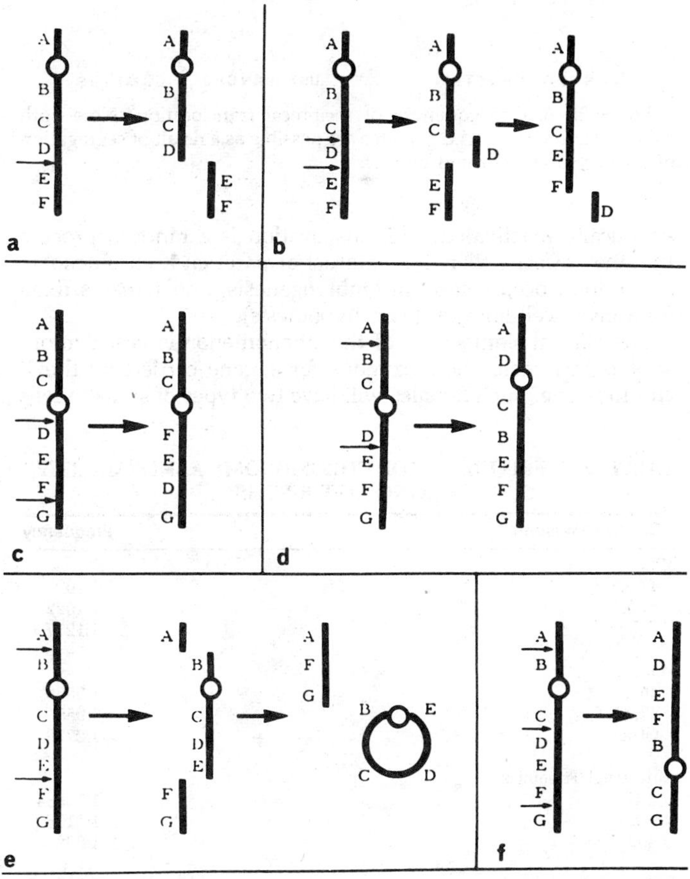

Figure 35–5. Types of chromosome rearrangement: *a*, terminal deletion; *b*, interstitial deletion; *c*, paracentric inversion; *d*, pericentric inversion; *e*, ring chromosome; *f*, segmental shift. (From Hamerton JL: Human Cytogenetics, Vol 1. Academic Press, 1971, New York & London.)

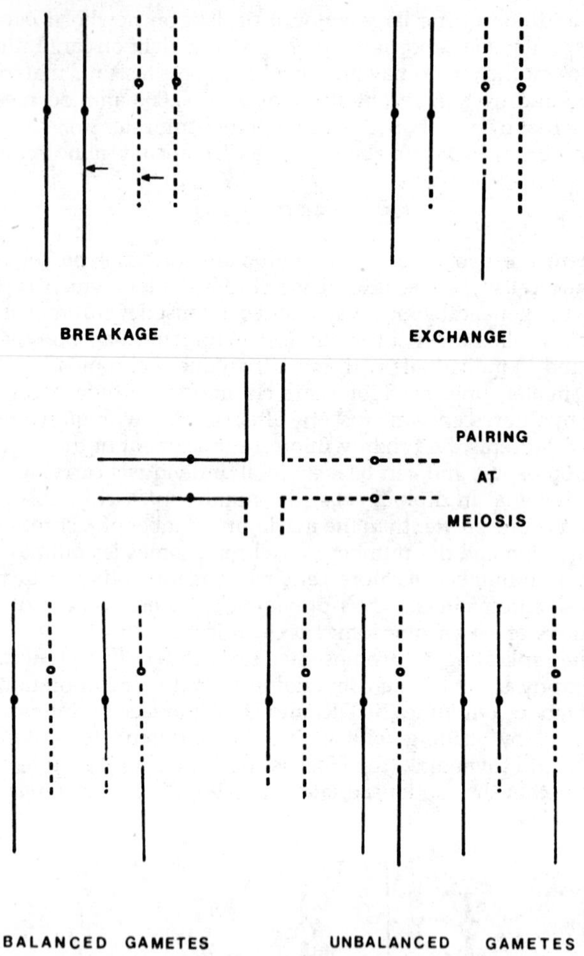

Figure 35–6. Consequences of reciprocal translocation. Note both balanced and unbalanced gametes are possible as a result of segregation of the exchanged chromosomes.

genetically inactivated. This inactivation is a random process that may affect either the maternal or paternal X chromosome at random, occurs early in embryogenesis, and remains fixed for a given cell lineage (Lyon hypothesis).

The clinical significance of this phenomenon is best demonstrated in females heterozygous for a gene carried by the X chromosome. Such females will have two types of somatic cells

TABLE 35–2. FREQUENCY OF CHROMOSOME ABNORMALITIES AMONG LIVE BIRTHS

Sex Chromosomes	Frequency
Male	
47,XYY	1:1022
47,XXY	1:1022
Other	1:1277
Female	
45,X	1:9586
47,XXX	1:958
Other	1:2739
Autosomal Trisomics	
+D	1:18984
+E	1:8136
+G	1:802
Balanced Structural	1:517
Unbalanced Structural	1:1675
Total	1:167

Based on 54,952 babies: 35,779 males, 19,173 females.

in their bodies, one in which the normal allele is inactivated and the other in which the abnormal allele is inactivated. Thus studies on clones of cells (colonies of cells derived from a single progenitor) may allow differentiation between the active and inactive X chromosome and thus the identification of carrier females. Examples of diseases in which carrier detection has been based on this phenomenon include the Lesch-Nyhan syndrome (hypoxanthine-guanine-phosphoribosyltransferase deficiency), Fabry's disease, testicular feminization syndrome, and mucopolysaccharidosis type II (Hunter's syndrome).

Clinical Cytogenetics

The major features of a few common chromosome abnormalities are summarized on the opposite page.

Sex Chromosomes

Other sex chromosome abnormalities include the rare females with four or five X chromosomes, as well as males with multiple X and Y chromosomes. Such individuals are usually mentally retarded and may have somatic anomalies. Individuals with various degrees of chromosome mosaicism have also been reported, most frequently as variants in Klinefelter's syndrome and Turner's syndrome.

Autosomes

The clinical features of the three best known autosomal trisomies are listed on the opposite page.

Other autosomal trisomies surviving to term include trisomies 8, 9, and 22. All other autosomes have been reported as trisomic among spontaneous abortions. The advent of banding techniques has greatly widened the scope of chromosome pathology, and numerous examples of chromosome imbalance resulting from deletion of duplication of chromosome material have been reported. Such chromosome imbalance results in dysmorphic features and often developmental and mental retardation.

INDICATIONS FOR CHROMOSOME STUDY

Chromosome abnormalities form a significant cause of clinical abnormalities, and chromosome studies should be initiated to rule out this etiologic factor in a patient when a recognizable chromosome syndrome is suspected; in patients with two or more unexplained major congenital malformations involving different systems possibly combined with the presence of minor malformations; and in patients with unexplained developmental or mental retardation. Certain cases of abnormal sexual development, leukemia, and certain solid tumors associated with congenital malformations and known to be associated with specific chromosome abnormalities (aniridia, Wilms' tumor, retinoblastoma) require chromosome studies. Chromosome banding is mandatory to identify the chromosome involved as well as to rule out possible structural changes not detectable by other means.

Chromosome Breakage Syndromes

Three diseases are commonly associated with unrepaired chromosome breaks. These are Fanconi's anemia (FA), ataxia-telangiectasia (AT), and Bloom's syndrone (BS). These are so characterized because in addition to their typical clinical features they share the propensity to chromosome breakage that can be seen in cultured cells and that commonly occurs with several times the frequency observed in normal individuals. Each of these diseases is inherited as an autosomal recessive condition. Two of these conditions are associated with congenital malformations (BS and FA), and all three have an increased frequency of malignancy. This may be the consequence of alterations in DNA repair process.

Sister chromatids can be differentially stained by a modification of the Hoechst-BUDR technique. This permits the identification of exchanges between sister chromatids. Such sister chromatid exchanges (SCE) occur with an increased frequency

COMMON CHROMOSOME ABNORMALITIES

Chromosome Complement	Eponym	X Chromatin	Frequency (live births)	Phenotype
Males				
47,XXY	Klinefelter's syndrome	Positive	1:1000	Often tall eunuchoid males with hypogonadism, feminine distribution of hair, gynecomastia, testicular atrophy after puberty with hyalinized tubules, Leydig cell hyperplasia, often low I.Q. May have psychosocial difficulties (see Ch. 234).
47,XYY	—	Negative	1:1000	Often no phenotypic abnormalities; usually tall to very tall. May have psychosocial problems.
Females				
45,X & other variants of the X chromosome and mosaics	Turner's syndrome or ovarian dysgenesis	Negative or positive	1:10,000	These patients have ovarian dysgenesis with webbing of neck, short stature (< 153 cm). Often congenital heart disease, skeletal defects, and renal anomalies. This is Turner's syndrome. Other patients may have ovarian dysgenesis without webbing of the neck and with much less frequent somatic anomalies. Invariably they are of short stature (< 153 cm) (see Ch. 236).
47,XXX	None	Double	1:1000	This is extremely variable. Often no phenotypic abnormalities but may be mentally retarded or may have psychosocial problems. Often fertile although may be infertile.

THREE BEST-KNOWN AUTOSOMAL TRISOMIES

Chromosome Complement	Eponym	Frequency (live births)	Phenotype
21-Trisomy (47,XX,+21 47,XY,+21)	Down's syndrome Mongolism	1:700	Typical, facial appearance, epicanthic folds, oblique palpebral fissures, broad bridge of the nose, protuding tongue, open mouth, square shaped ears, flattened facial profile. Invariable mental retardation, muscular hypotonia, and often congenital heart disease (Fig. 35–7).
18-Trisomy (47,XX,+18 47,XY,+18)	Edwards' syndrome	1:8000	Full-term infants of low birth weight with severe mental and motor retardation. Usually have a prominent occiput, and frequently occurring facial abnormalities including micrognathia, a Grecian nose, low set and malformed ears, cleft lip and palate. Flexion deformities of fingers often severe. Mental retardation is often severe. They are sublethal and survival for more than a few months is rare.
13-Trisomy (47,XX,+13) 47,XY,+13	Patau's syndrome	1:20,000	Usually low birth weight infants of full-term gestation with a typical facial appearance, including a broad nose, hypertelorism, microphthalmia, anophthalmia, often with coloboma, and micrognathia. They are usually microcephalic, ears are low set and malformed, and there is a large broad and bulbous nose. There are often flexion deformities and frequent polydactyly and syndactyly. Survival is usually very short.

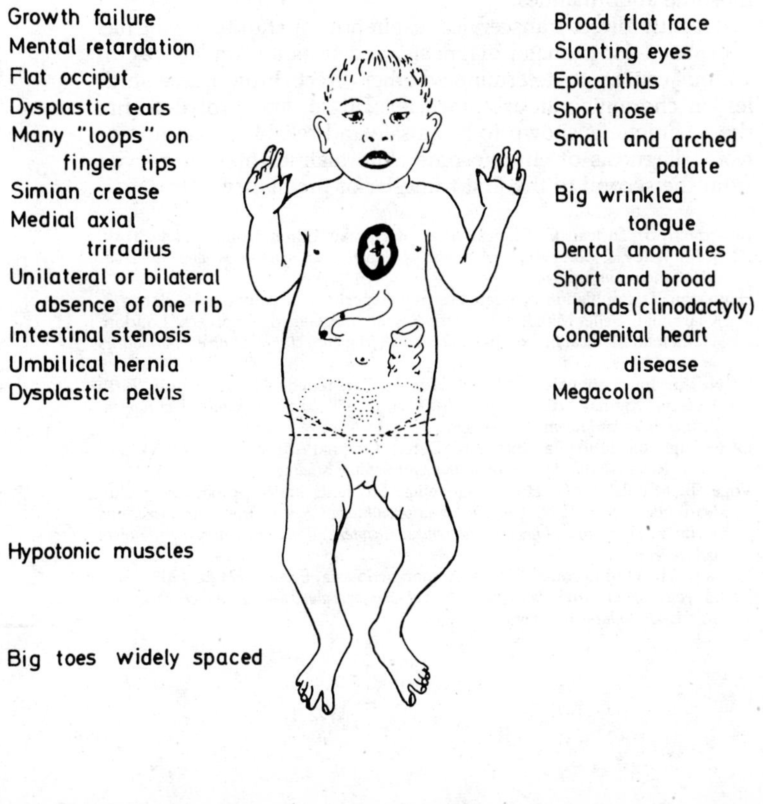

Figure 35–7. Clinical findings in trisomy 21. (From Vogel F, Motulsky AG: Human genetics: Problems and Approaches. Berlin, Springer-Verlag, 1979.)

in BS and in normal individuals may be increased as the result of exposure to chromosome-damaging agents.

Heritable Fragile Sites

Chromosome breakage is usually random; however, some individuals may exhibit breakage or a nonstaining chromosome region (chromosome gap) at a specific site in a significant proportion of metaphases. In many cases such sites may be induced by the use of folate-deficient culture medium, although a few sites are folate-insensitive. These specific sites, known as fragile sites, may represent alterations in the DNA and are often heritable. While most fragile sites are not associated with disease or other clinical problems, the fragile site at Xq28 is known to be associated with one common form of X-linked mental retardation among males.

PRENATAL DIAGNOSIS (AMNIOCENTESIS)

The diagnosis of chromosome abnormalities at mid-trimester gestation is now a routine procedure for certain pregnancies. It involves the aspiration of a small sample of amniotic fluid, culturing of the fetal cells contained in the fluid, and determination of the karyotype of these cells and thus of the fetus. The major indications for the use of this technique for the detection of chromosome abnormalities are: (1) Maternal age—usually offered to all mothers over the age of 35 at the time of delivery. (2) Presence of a parental chromosome abnormality—if one parent is a balanced translocation carrier and particularly if the translocation was detected as the result of the previous birth of a clinically abnormal infant. (3) Previous trisomy—those cases in which the mother has previously had a trisomic infant or possibly where she is known to have had a previous instance of spontaneous abortion in which the abortus was karyotyped and shown to be trisomic.

The safety and reliability of amniocentesis as a diagnostic technique have now been well established by numerous studies, and it is generally accepted that amniocentesis increases the risk of miscarriage by between 1 in 250 and 1 in 500 above the inherent risk for that individual without intervention. Other risks of the test, including fetal and maternal morbidity, are negligible. In competent hands the test has been shown to have a near 100 per cent reliability for the detection of chromosome abnormalities.

Recently direct transcervical aspiration of chorionic villi has been used for prenatal diagnosis, and tests are under way in various centers to determine whether direct chromosome studies on chorionic villi are practicable. If so, and provided that the technique is shown to be as safe and reliable as amniocentesis, diagnosis of chromosome abnormalities may be moved from the second to the first trimester of pregnancy.

DeGrouchy J, Turleau C: Clinical Atlas of Human Chromosomes. New York, John Wiley & Sons, 1977. *A review of chromosomal syndromes with numerous illustrations and references.*

Hamerton JL: Population cytogenetics: A perspective. *In* Adonolfi M, Baron P, Giarnelli F, Seller M (eds.): Pediatric Research: A Genetic Approach. London, Heineman Medical Books, 1982. *Deals with frequency of chromosome abnormalities in populations.*

ISCN: An International System of Human Cytogenetic Nomenclature. Birth Defects Original Article Series, Vol XIV(8), 1978. *The basic handbook of nomenclature rules for human chromosomes.*

ISCN: High Resolution Banding. Birth Defects Original Article Series, Vol XVII(5), 1981. *Rules relating to high resolution chromosome banding.*

Vogel F, Motulsky AG: Human Genetics: Problems and Approaches. Berlin, Springer-Verlag, 1979. *A detailed treatise on human genetics from both a basic and a clinical viewpoint. Numerous references. Chapter 2 deals extensively with human cytogenetics.*

Yunis JJ: The chromosomal basis of human neoplasia. Science 221:227–235, 1983. *A review of our current knowledge about chromosome abnormalities and gene mapping in relation to human tumors.*

36. CONGENITAL MALFORMATIONS

Lewis B. Holmes

INCIDENCE

Two per cent of newborn infants have serious malformations, most of which are compatible with survival. Many additional malformations, such as genitourinary, vertebral, and heart defects, are identified during childhood and the teenage years. Many adults with congenital malformations are unaware of the significance of these problems for their health or the potential significance for their unborn children.

ETIOLOGIES

The recognized causes of malformations include genetic abnormalities, environmental factors, and the combined effects of mutant genes and environmental factors, i.e., multifactorial inheritance (Table 36–1). Multifactorial inheritance is the most common of these etiologies. However, at least 40 per cent of all malformations cannot be explained. One example of a cause that is neither environmental nor genetic is a vascular abnormality. Occlusion of blood vessels during development has been postulated to cause intestinal atresia and hydranencephaly; absence of vessels and abnormal persistence of vessels have been observed in absence of the radius and absence of the tibia.

A few hereditary malformations have been shown to be due to biochemical abnormalities, such as a deficiency of 5α reductase in individuals with pseudovaginal perineoscrotal hypospadias, an autosomal recessive disorder characterized by am-

TABLE 36–1. RECOGNIZED ETIOLOGIES OF MALFORMATIONS PRESENT IN ADULTS

1. Genetic abnormalities	**Example**
a. Single mutant gene	
i. Autosomal dominant trait	polycystic kidney disease, adult type polysyndactyly
ii. Autosomal recessive trait	Mohr's syndrome (oro-facial-digital syndrome, type II)
iii. X-linked dominant trait	telecanthus-hypospadias (BBB) syndrome
iv. X-linked recessive trait	metacarpal 4-5 fusion
b. Chromosome abnormalities	
i. Trisomy of autosomes	Down's syndrome
ii. Interstitial deletion	aniridia-Wilms' tumor
iii. Sex chromosome abnormalities	45,X (Turner's syndrome); 47,XXY (Klinefelter's syndrome)
2. Environmental factors	
a. Uterine factors	amniotic band syndrome
b. Intrauterine infection	congenital rubella syndrome
c. Drugs	fetal hydantoin syndrome
3. Genetic plus environmental factors (multifactorial inheritance)	heart defects
	cleft lip and/or palate
	hypospadias
	pyloric stenosis
	Hirschsprung's disease

biguous genitals. An abnormal alpha-2 chain in type I collagen has been identified in skin fibroblasts from a woman with type I osteogenesis imperfecta, a skeletal dysplasia inherited as an autosomal dominant trait (see Ch. 201).

Persons with malformations due to autosomal dominant disorders are much more likely to survive to the adult years, as their malformations are less severe, in general, than those due to autosomal recessive traits.

In multifactorial inheritance, clinical studies of human and laboratory examples have shown that several genes (including major genes) are involved, as well as environmental factors such as maternal influences, uterine factors, the season of the year, and socioeconomic class. Most individuals with a malformation attributed to multifactorial inheritance are the only affected members of their families. However, the affected individuals have an increased risk of having either affected sibs or affected children. The recurrence risk is usually between 1 and 10 per cent, which is 10 to 40 times greater than the incidence of the malformation in the general population.

About 0.6 per cent of newborn infants have a major chromosome abnormality, but many do not survive to the adult years. Down's syndrome results from the most common trisomy, and survival of most affected newborns to the adult years is now expected. In trisomy 21, the associated chromosome abnormality in 95 per cent of the cases, the extra chromosome comes from the mother 75 per cent of the time. Since women over age 35 now are having a smaller portion of all pregnancies, 80 per cent of the infants with Down's syndrome are being born to women of less than 35 years.

Common sex chromosome abnormalities, such as 47,XYY and 47,XXX, are usually not associated with any congenital malformations. Boys with 47,XXY (Klinefelter's syndrome) may have abnormal physical features that are evident in the teenage years. Girls with the 45,X (Turner's) syndrome are usually recognized in infancy because of associated lymphedema, webbed neck, heart defects, and short stature or in the teenage years because of failure of puberty to occur spontaneously.

CLINICAL RELEVANCE

The following examples illustrate the potential significance of a malformation to the affected adult and his or her children.

Relevance to the Health of the Affected Person

CONGENITAL ABSENCE OF ONE KIDNEY. About 1 in 700 infants has unilateral renal agenesis. Most affected individuals are asymptomatic. However, they have an increased risk of structural malformations of the ureter, such as ureteropelvic junction stricture, and associated infections, hypertension, etc. The affected female may have a bicornuate uterus or absence of the half of the uterus on the same side as the renal aplasia. Affected males may have absence of the vas deferens on the same side. Parents with unilateral renal agenesis have an increased risk of having infants with either the same malformation or bilateral renal agenesis, which is fatal.

BRACHYDACTYLY, TYPE E. Owing to premature closure of epiphyses, persons with this autosomal dominant disorder have short hands and feet with a variable pattern of shortening of the first, fourth, and fifth metacarpals and metatarsals and distal phalanges of the thumb and great toe. They also have a mild to moderate degree of shortness of stature. Severe hypertension is often a problem in the affected teenager and young adult. The cause of the hypertension has not been determined.

BRANCHIO-OTO-RENAL SYNDROME. The person with this autosomal dominant disorder has a pattern of malformations that includes malformed ears, preauricular tags, preauricular sinus, and branchial cleft sinus. The mildly affected adult is often not diagnosed until a more severely affected child is born. The affected adult may have significant hearing loss or renal hypoplasia.

KLIPPEL-FEIL SYNDROME. The person with fusion or hemivertebrae of one or more cervical vertebrae usually has a short neck, limited rotation of the head, a low hairline, and a webbed neck. Common associated problems include hearing loss, heart defects, Sprengel's deformity, and genitourinary anomalies, such as aplasia of mullerian structures. The Klippel-Feil syndrome comprises a heterogeneous group of disorders that includes several patterns of vertebral anomalies, some of which are hereditary.

Relevance to Increased Risk of Having Affected Children

MULTIFACTORIAL INHERITANCE. The adult with one of the common malformations attributed to this process has an increased risk of having an affected child. For malformations that show an altered sex ratio, the sex of the affected parent is important in determining the risk of having an affected child (Table 36–2). In general, the parent of the less frequently affected sex has a greater risk of having affected children. For example, *intestinal aganglionosis* (Hirschsprung's disease) is much more common in males than females, but the affected female has a much greater risk of having affected children (Table 36–2). The risk that an affected parent of either sex will have an affected child is significantly greater than the risk that unaffected parents will have an affected child.

With early surgical closure and better treatment of the associated hydrocephalus and urinary tract infections, males and females with *spina bifida* (myelomeningocele) are surviving to adult years and often have normal intelligence. Both affected males and females may be fertile. The affected adult has an increased risk of about 3 per cent that each child will have a neural tube defect, including myelomeningocele, anencephaly, or encephalocele.

HYPERTELORISM. The mother who has a broad bridge of the nose and hypertelorism* has an increased risk of having severely malformed sons. For example, the female who carries the X-linked gene for the telecanthus-hypospadias (BBB) syndrome will show only hypertelorism, but sons who inherit this gene have a severe malformation syndrome that may include hypertelorism, broad nasal bridge, cleft lip and palate, heart defects, imperforate anus, hypospadias, and mental deficiency. Mothers with the autosomal dominant disorder known as the Opitz-Frias (or G) syndrome also have hypertelorism and a broad bridge of the nose. Their affected sons and daughters have at birth aspiration due to a laryngotracheoesophageal

*Hypertelorism can be determined most precisely from an A-P radiograph that shows an increased bony interorbital distance.

TABLE 36–2. RISK OF AFFECTED CHILDREN FOR PARENT WITH MALFORMATION ATTRIBUTED TO MULTIFACTORIAL INHERITANCE

Malformation	Risk of Affected Child (per cent)	Prevalence of Condition in General Population (per cent)
1. Intestinal aganglionosis (Hirschsprung's disease)	2.0	0.02
2. Hypospadias	6.0	0.8
3. Club foot	1.4	0.13
4. Congenital hip dislocation	4.3	0.8
5. Ventricular septal defect	4.0	0.2
6. Pyloric stenosis	4 (aff. father) 13 (aff. mother)	
7. Cleft palate	6.2	0.3
8. Spina bifida (meningomyelocele)	3.0	0.14

cleft, stridor, and associated malformations such as cleft lip, heart defects, hypospadias (males), and imperforate anus. Unfortunately, the physical feature of broad nasal bridge and hypertelorism is nonspecific and the risk for the woman with no affected children cannot be determined.

MENTAL RETARDATION. There are many causes of mental retardation. The mildly retarded woman without striking physical abnormalities may be a carrier of significant and relatively common genetic abnormalities that give her an increased risk of having severely affected sons. Two examples are the fragile-X syndrome and the Coffin-Lowry syndrome. The fragile-X syndrome is a common cause of mental retardation, mild facial abnormalities, and sometimes macro-orchidism in males. The affected female may show mosaicism for the marker X chromosome, an abnormality of the distal portion of the long arm of the X chromosome that can be identified in cytogenetic studies only if special media and processing are used. The woman who has the X-linked gene for the Coffin-Lowry syndrome shows only mild mental retardation, short stature, short and hyperextensible hands, and tufted distal phalanges. The affected male is much more severely affected, with severe mental deficiency, short stature, stiff joints, coarse facial features, pectus carinatum, and large, soft hands.

PRENATAL DIAGNOSIS

The techniques used most often for diagnosing malformations in the fetus are cell culture of amniocytes removed at 16 to 18 weeks of gestation, assay for alpha-fetoprotein (AFP) in the amniotic fluid and maternal serum, and ultrasound imaging. Parents who have previously had a child with trisomy 21 have a 1 per cent risk of recurrence regardless of the mother's age. To rule out this possibility amniocentesis for chromosome analysis is done at 16 to 18 weeks of pregnancy. For the woman who has previously had a child with anencephaly or spina bifida, prenatal diagnosis includes amniocentesis to measure the level of AFP and ultrasound imaging for hydrocephalus, the cranial defect in anencephaly, and the spinal defect in meningomyelocele. If the level of AFP is elevated, a neural tube defect is confirmed by an increase in the level of acetylcholinesterase in the amniotic fluid. Limb malformations, such as absent radius, ectrodactyly, hydrocephalus, and bilateral renal agenesis, can be investigated with ultrasound imaging. However, the accuracy of this method of prenatal diagnosis is not known.

Prenatal screening for neural tube defects is now available as an option in prenatal care. Serum AFP is measured in the mother at 16 to 18 weeks of pregnancy. AFP is a normal product of the fetal liver that moves from the serum of the fetus into the amniotic fluid through defects in the skin, which are present in anencephaly, meningomyelocele, and omphalocele. The pregnant woman with an elevated serum level of AFP on two occasions should have prenatal studies including amniocentesis for AFP and acetylcholinesterase, and ultrasound imaging. Errors in diagnosis result from incorrect gestational age and alterations in the range of normal values in obese women and in women with diabetes mellitus. Elevations in AFP also occur in twin pregnancies, intrauterine death, and other malformations such as esophageal atresia, omphalocele, and hereditary nephrosis. A skin-covered neural tube defect, such as a lumbar meningocele, will be missed in prenatal screening with serum AFP. In general, prenatal AFP screening is most effective if carried out by individuals who are experienced in identifying the causes of false positive and false negative values, and who educate the parents initially as to the steps involved and the benefits and accuracy of the testing.

FETAL SURGERY

Catheters have been introduced to relieve malformations that cause obstruction of the flow of urine or of cerebrospinal fluid. This approach is experimental. One major problem is to identify an abnormality early enought to permit intervention before the fetus has suffered irreversible damage, such as the lung hypoplasia that is a cause of death in infants with oligohydramnios from urinary tract obstruction. Another problem is that the fetus is whom only hydrocephalus or urinary tract obstruction is visible by ultrasound may have multiple malformations that will be apparent only after birth.

PREVENTION OF MALFORMATION

Pregnant women with several different medical diseases or exposures have an increased risk of having children with birth defects. If informed of this risk before conception or soon after conception, these risks can be either lessened or eliminated. These efforts at prevention require special efforts in education, as most women receive routine prenatal care too late to benefit from counseling. Specific opportunities in prevention include:

CHRONIC ALCOHOLISM. Exposure of the fetus to high maternal levels of alcohol causes growth retardation before and after birth, microcephaly, brain malformations, mental deficiency, a characteristic pattern of craniofacial features, and at times other malformations, such as vertebral anomalies and spina bifida (fetal-alcohol syndrome). These effects correlate best with the level of alcohol consumption before the mother knows she is pregnant. The lower the level of exposure the less the risk of damage to the fetus. If the pregnant woman decreases her alcohol consumption at any time in pregnancy, it is beneficial to the fetus, although a decrease before or soon after conception is the most beneficial.

DIABETES MELLITUS. The woman with insulin-dependent diabetes mellitus is two to three times more likely to have a child with serious malformations than the nondiabetic woman. The malformations include spina bifida, anencephaly, heart defects, vertebral and genitourinary malformations, and multiple malformations. The risk of having a malformed infant correlates inversely with the quality of control of her disease, glucose metabolism in particular, very early in pregnancy. The mother's blood level of hemoglobin A_{1c} indicates the degree of uncontrol during the previous four to six weeks (see Ch. 230). The lower the level of Hgb A_{1c} before or soon after conception, the lower her risk of having a malformed child.

MATERNAL PHENYLKETONURIA (PKU). Children with PKU identified at birth through neonatal screening for metabolic diseases will have normal development and intelligence if the dietary treatment (low phenylalanine, low protein) is begun soon after birth. The diet is usually discontinued in the early school years. However, successfully treated females with PKU who are no longer on the diet have a risk of over 90 per cent that any pregnancy will either end in a spontaneous abortion or result in a child with microcephaly, mental deficiency, and often heart defects as well. The risk of damage to the fetus correlates with the blood level of phenylalanine in the mother. If the woman with PKU resumes the low phenylalanine diet before conception she has a good chance of having a normal child. If the diet is resumed in the first trimester, as soon as she knows she is pregnant, the child is less severely damaged than if no dietary treatment is used during pregnancy. Unfortunately a systematic follow-up of females with PKU has not been carried out in most states to inform them of their risk of having children with serious birth defects.

Bergsma D (ed.): Birth Defect Compendium. 2nd ed. New York, Alan R. Liss, Inc., 1979. *An up-to-date, brief summary on all common birth defects.*

Jacobs PA, Glover TW, Mayer M, Fox P, Gerrard JW, Dunn HG, Herbst DS: X-Linked mental retardation: A study of 7 families. Am J Med Genet 7:471, 1980. *A thorough study of this very common hereditary cause of mental deficiency in affected mlaes and carrier females.*

Lenke RR, Levy HL: Maternal phenylketonuria and hyperphenylalaninemia. N Engl J Med 303:1202, 1980. *The results of an international survery of the teratogenic effect of PKU in the pregnant woman and the attempts at prevention.*

Report of the U.K. Collaborative Study on Alpha-Fetoprotein in Relation to Neural-tube Defects. Amniotic-fluid alpha-fetoprotein measurement in antenatal diagnosis of anencephaly and open spina bifida in early pregnancy. Lancet 2:651, 1979. *A summary of the findings in the U.K. Collaborative Study of using maternal AFP screening to detect fetuses with spina bifida and anencephaly.*

Smith DW: Recognizable Patterns of Human Malformation. 3rd ed. Philadelphia, W. B. Saunders Company, 1982. *A thorough tabulation of recognized malformation syndromes.*

Strobino BR, Kline J, Stein Z: Chemical and physical exposures of parents: Effects on human reproduction and offspring. J Early Hum Develop 1:371, 1978. *A summary of current information on the potential teratogenic effect of many common exposures.*

Temtamy SA, McKusick VA: The Genetics of Hand Malformations. New York, Alan R. Liss, Inc., 1978. *The best source of information on malformations involving arms and legs.*

37. GENETIC COUNSELING

F. Clarke Fraser

Genetic counseling is the process whereby patients and their families are helped to deal with a problem created by the occurrence, or potential occurrence, of a disorder in the family that they think may have a genetic basis. The need for genetic counseling starts with one or more questions. "My child is born with Neverdofit syndrome. What caused it? Will it happen again? Should we stop having children?" "My grandfather has developed Huntington's disease. Might I get it?" "I have fallen in love with my cousin. Would our children all be malformed or mentally retarded?" "I volunteered for a screening program and they say I have the gene for Tay-Sachs disease. What harm will it do?" "I am 35 years old and I read that I should have a test that will make sure my baby will be normal. Should I?"

In many cases the genetic principles underlying the answers to such questions are very simple and should be in the repertoire of every physician. Some cases require more sophisticated calculations or special tests and can be referred to a genetic counselor. The answers may depend not only on genetic principles, but also on complex social and ethical issues that will require several interviews and perhaps the efforts of both the family physician and the genetic counselor to resolve.

DIAGNOSIS

The first step in the counseling process is to confirm, or establish, the diagnosis. This may already have been done, or it may require special tests (karyotype, carrier detection tests, etc.). Do not ignore the family history, which may sometimes be an aid to diagnosis. Genetic heterogeneity (see Ch. 30) may confound the issue and require special tests to be done on the patient or family members. In some cases, a specific diagnosis cannot be reached and the counseling must be done on an "either-or" basis—an unsatisfactory situation, but informed uncertainty is better than erroneous certainty.

ESTABLISHING "P"

Once the diagnosis has been reached, the next step is to derive the probability, P, of the event that concerns the counselee, usually a risk of recurrence. Prerequisite to this is a carefully taken *family history* (see Ch. 30), which will serve not only as the basis for calculating P but also as a screening procedure that may pick up additional warning signals relevant to the counselee (this function applies also to the routine family history taken as part of the workup of any patient). A near relative with a neural tube defect may make the counselee eligible for prenatal diagnosis even though the condition for which she was referred does not. A sib or parent with non-insulin-dependent diabetes mellitus puts the counselee at increased risk for this disease; this raises the question of early detection tests and, where available, preventive measures. The same applies to most common, familial disorders, including hypertension, early coronary disease, the common neoplasms, and the common psychoses.

If the disease is known to have a mendelian basis, P can often be calculated on the basis of the known mode of inheritance (see Ch. 30). In some cases Bayesian algebra can be used to improve the precision of the estimate by using additional family information. For instance, if a man's parent has Huntington's disease, which has a variable age of onset, the man had a 50 per cent chance of inheriting the gene at conception, but the longer he lives, free of the disease, the more likely it is that he did not inherit the gene. Similarly, for a woman who had a 50 per cent chance of inheriting the gene for hemophilia from her mother, the chance that she did inherit it diminishes with each unaffected son she bears. The precise probability can be calculated for the specific family situation. If the necessary calculations tax the mathematical abilities of the physician, a genetic counselor can be consulted.

Diseases that do not fit the mendelian rules of family segregation often fit the expectations for multifactorial inheritance, particularly if they are known to be common (one in 1000 or so), and familial, although this mode of inheritance should not

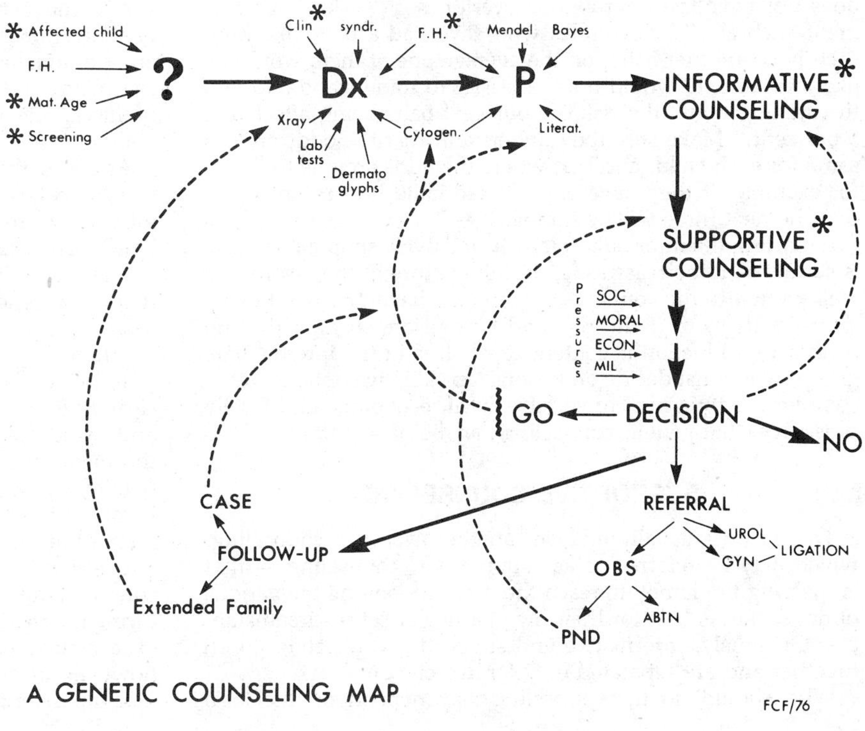

Figure 37–1. Map of the genetic counseling process. It begins with a question, raised by the advent of a child with a ? genetic disorder, other aspect of the family history, etc. There must be a diagnosis (Dx), which may depend on information from clinicians, syndromologists, x-ray studies, laboratory tests, dermatoglyphics, cytogenetics, and the family history (FH). To answer the question usually requires estimating a probability (P), using information from the family history, cytogenetics, the literature, the mendelian principles, and Bayesian calculations. Following informative and supportive counseling (often influenced by social, moral, economic, and family pressures) the counselee may reach a decision either to refrain from reproduction or to go ahead. Both of these may require appropriate referral. If the "GO" decision results in a recurrence, further counseling may be required. Follow-up of the counselee and the extended family may result in reentry into the process. (Reprinted with permission from Nora JJ, Fraser FC: Medical Genetics: Principles and Practice. 2nd ed. Philadelphia, Lea and Febiger, 1981.)

be assumed without evidence. For these conditions the risk increases with the genetic proximity to an affected relative and with the number of affected relatives. Empirical estimates of average risks are available for counselees of varying degrees of relationship to the affected individual, and these can be modified upward or downward, according to the numbers of affected and unaffected relatives, by formulae based on the assumption of polygenic inheritance.

Empirical estimates of risk must also be used for chromosomal disorders. We know the frequencies of liveborn trisomics at various maternal ages (see Ch. 35) and the probability of a recurrence after having had one.

Estimating risks for carriers of balanced chromosomal rearrangements is more difficult. One can derive the theoretical ratios of balanced to unbalanced offspring, but actual segregations are usually not random, and the question of whether theoretically possible unbalanced products will be viable or nonviable complicates the issue. Both segregation ratios and viability will vary with the length and position of the rearranged segments, and it is difficult to obtain enough data for any one rearrangement to derive segregation ratios. The genetic counselor can use a combination of general principles and empirical knowledge to obtain an estimate of the risk but must recognize the uncertainties involved.

Finally, there is the uncomfortably large group of disorders, particularly those involving mental retardation and dysmorphic features, for which the risk of recurrence is unknown. It may be as high as one in four, for an as yet unrecognized autosomal recessive syndrome, or less than 1 per cent for an unrecognized environmental teratogen. Since unrecognized autosomal recessive syndromes will, one hopes, be in the minority (unless there is parental consanguinity), the risk in such cases will average out as low.

INFORMATIVE COUNSELING

Once P has been established as precisely as possible, we pass on to the stage of "informative counseling"—imparting the prognosis, probability of recurrence, and reproductive options to the counselee(s).

The processes by which families reach their reproductive decisions are complex, variable, and not well understood. Odds seem more easily appreciated than percentages, and "chances" does not have the opprobrious overtones of "risks." A statement such as, "if 20 couples who have had a baby like John each have another baby, on the average one of them would be like John and 19 would not," is easier to understand and less threatening than "the risk of your next baby being affected is 5 per cent." Make sure they understand that the odds are the same for each child, and that where the odds are one to three, for example, if they have one affected child it does not mean that the next three will be normal.

Imparting the information may be relatively simple if the risk is so low as to be reassuring, and the nature of the disorder is well known to the counselees, who may have first-hand experience with it, or if the risk and burden are so high that no further reproduction is contemplated. It is in the intermediate group, who must decide on various reproductive options, often complicated by a host of social, ethical, economic, and family pressures, that genetic counseling may be most helpful.

SUPPORTIVE COUNSELING

This process usually involves another aspect of counseling, which may be referred to as "supportive" counseling — that is, helping the family to reach the decision, among the various options, that is best for their own particular set of circumstances. Obviously, informative and supportive counseling go on together and are separated only for didactic purposes.

Who should do the counseling may depend on the local scene. If the physician knows the family best and the genetics is simple, the physician may be the most suitable counselor. If the genetics and the reproductive options are complex, the genetic counselor may be the appropriate resource. Often the two can work together in helping the family to reach an informed and responsible decision.

Parents often tend to ignore the numerical risk and focus on the burden; they may work toward a decision by trying out, in their imagination, various scenarios and selecting the "least-lose" option that they could live with. The risk of recurrence may, in this process, be incorporated into the burden. The "1" in the odds may loom large even if the denominator is quite big, particularly if the counselee is a pessimist. "No matter how big the n is in the 1 in n odds, the 1 never goes away."

The process of deciding may take some time, and the counselees may need several sessions with a counselor, as new issues or questions come up. Throughout this time, the counselor acts as both a source of information and a sounding board, trying to steer an understanding and supportive course between paternalistic directiveness ("with that high a risk, you shouldn't have children") and Olympian detachment ("It's your decision; don't ask me to make it for you.").

REFERRAL

Having reached a decision, the counselee(s) may require referral—for tubal ligation (fallopian or vas deferens), artificial insemination, prenatal diagnosis, or care during the next pregnancy.

PRENATAL DIAGNOSIS

Prenatal diagnosis has changed the face of genetic counseling, since, for a growing number of conditions, it can change odds to certainty. It behooves the physician to know what categories of disorder are eligible, and although he or she cannot be expected to keep up with the latest additions to the list, it is at least possible to establish rapport with a clinical genetics center where this information can be found.

Techniques used in prenatal diagnosis include visualization by ultrasound examination or, less frequently, x-rays. Ultrasonography will detect structural malformations such as anencephaly and overt spina bifida, renal agenesis, polycystic kidney disease, and exomphalos. As techniques improve, the array of detectable defects increases, and it is now possible to detect a remarkable number of disorders, including cleft lip, cleft palate, various heart malformations, microphthalmia, and some types of short-limb dwarfism. In the latter category, x-radiography is an additional aid. Fetoscopy permits direct examination, blood sampling, and even skin or muscle biopsy, although the risk of miscarriage may be as high as 5 per cent, even in experienced hands.

Amniotic fluid can be obtained by amniocentesis at 12 to 14 weeks of gestation, with a risk of fetal damage or induced miscarriage that seems well below 1 per cent in experienced hands. The cells can be cultured for karyotyping or biochemical studies. The fluid can be examined for alpha-fetoprotein, hormones (adrenogenital syndrome), intestinal enzymes (imperforate anus), or other appropriate chemicals. Techniques for chorionic biopsy are now becoming available that will allow examination of cells with the same genotype as the fetus as early as 8 to 10 weeks of gestation, permitting earlier diagnosis and, if necessary, termination of pregnancy. This, along with the increasing array of conditions that can be diagnosed prenatally, will exacerbate the problems, both ethical and practical, involved in deciding what conditions and what circumstances justify the procedure. Genetic counselors tend to be nondirective, assuming that the parents (presumably well-informed and conscientious) are in the best position to balance the burden of caring for an affected child against that of the guilt and suffering of a mid-trimester abortion. They tend to draw the line, however, at prenatal diagnosis for nondiseases, and in particular the determination of sex for reasons of social preference.

The physician's main responsibility would seem to be to ensure that prospective parents at risk are aware that prenatal diagnosis is possible. The desire to practice good preventive medicine may be reinforced by the risk of litigation in cases in which parents have a child affected by some serious condition for which prenatal diagnosis is available, and were not told about it. The main categories of disorders to be kept in mind are:

1. Maternal age: in most centers 35 at the expected time of birth.

2. Neural tube defect in a previous child, in the counselee, or in a first degree relative. The risk of recurrence in a child or sib ranges from 1.5 to 10 per cent, depending on the frequency in the general population, and the risk for a nephew or niece is close to 1 per cent. Neural tube defects in this context include spina bifida occulta if there are multiple vertebral defects or spinal dysraphism. The advisability of maternal serum screening for neural tube defects by alpha-fetoprotein determination is a complex question, which must be answered for each population, depending on the frequency of neural tube defects and the availability of adequate laboratory, amniocentesis, and genetic counseling resources.

3. Chromosomal rearrangement in a parent. Couples who have had two or more spontaneous abortions deserve karyotyping, as about one in 20 will be found to carry a balanced chromosome rearrangement.

4. Sex determination, when the mother is at risk for being a carrier of an X-linked disorder not amenable to prenatal diagnosis.

5. A growing list of inborn errors of metabolism and other mendelian disorders, including the hemoglobinopathies. The dramatic advances in molecular genetics are rapidly expanding the number of such conditions (see Ch. 32 and 34).

6. Structural anomalies detectable by ultrasound, x-radiography, or, possibly, fetoscopy.

In most centers the number of positive diagnoses is about 2 per cent of the total number of cases, and the main benefit is to relieve anxiety and to allow couples who would otherwise refrain from having children, because of their high risk, to go ahead, without fear of the disorder in question.

FOLLOW-UP

The final stage in the genetic counseling process is the follow-up. As with any patient, follow-up is advisable to keep track of the results. The content of the informative counseling should be summarized in a letter, and a telephone call or note a few months later will establish whether the information has been understood, whether new questions have arisen, or whether new circumstances have changed the odds.

It may also be necessary to follow-up the extended family. Often the discovery that a couple is at risk for a genetic disorder means that other family members are at risk, particularly in the case of autosomal dominant and X-linked disorders.

In diseases for which treatment is available, such as Wilson's disease or multiple polyposis of the colon, early detection in high risk relatives is vitally important. Often, it may be possible to test individuals known by pedigree analysis to be at risk, for carrier status. The hemoglobinopathies, G6PD deficiency, Duchenne muscular dystrophy (creatine kinase levels), hemophilia (factor VIII clotting vs. antigenic activity), and Tay-Sachs disease are examples. Cystic fibrosis is not yet on the list.

Good preventive medicine requires that these relatives be informed of their risks. This may require some ingenuity to avoid breaches of confidence. Sometimes a key family member will take on the role of genetic advocate, or an approach through the family doctor may solve the problem. One way or another, one strives to avoid the tragedy of an affected child, born to parents whose family history placed them at increased risk, who bitterly demand "why didn't somebody tell me?"

Bergsma D: Birth Defects Compendium. 2nd ed. New York, Alan R. Liss, 1978. *A useful compilation of descriptive and etiologic data on dysmorphic syndromes and other birth defects.*

Brock DJH: Early diagnosis of fetal defects. Curr Rev Obstet Gynaecol. Edinburgh, Churchill-Livingstone, 1982, p 165. *A review of prenatal diagnosis.*

Capron AM, et al. (eds.): Genetic counselling: Facts, values, and norms. Birth Defects: Original Article Series, XX (2):1–344, 1979. *A multiauthored volume on the concepts, psychology, ethics, and legal issues in genetic counseling.*

Fraser FC: Taking the family history. Am J Med Gen 34:585, 1963. *A discussion of family history taking at various levels from routine office to research.*

Lippman-Hand A, Fraser FC: Genetic counseling — the postcounseling period. II. Making reproductive choices. Am J Med Gen 4:73–87, 1979. *The third in a series of articles on the psychodynamics of genetic counselees.*

McKusick V: Mendelian Inheritance in Man. 6th ed. Baltimore, The Johns Hopkins University Press, 1983. *An exhaustive catalogue of disorders showing mendelian inheritance.*

Nora JJ, Fraser FC: Medical Genetics: Principles and Practice. 2nd ed. Philadelphia, Lea and Febiger, 1981. *A textbook oriented toward physicians.*

Part VII
CARDIOVASCULAR DISEASES

38. APPROACH TO THE PATIENT WITH CARDIOVASCULAR DISEASE

Andrew G. Wallace

This chapter describes an approach to the collection of cardiovascular data, the principles behind certain laboratory tests used to obtain data, and strategies about data acquisition. The objective is to complement the following chapters, which emphasize the data in specific conditions and their use in management decisions.

A textbook of medicine is customarily organized by system. Diseases are presented for each system according to diagnostic categories, and for each category topics such as etiology, pathophysiology, symptoms, physical signs, laboratory data, and treatment are discussed. This approach provides the reader with an integrated picture of diseases that affect the system. The merits of the approach are numerous and outweigh shortcomings; however, there are shortcomings. One is that patients usually do not present to the doctor with an established diagnosis. Another is that textbooks frequently describe a composite of the manifestations of a disease; often patients fail to match this description, either because the description conveys inadequately the continuum of symptoms and signs produced by variable amounts of disease or because the evolution of symptoms and signs over time receives less than optimal attention. Establishing whether or not cardiovascular disease is present is the first objective of a complete evaluation. When disease is present, the diagnosis includes not only a definition of the structural abnormality it produces but also its etiology and severity.

In an effort to exclude cardiovascular disease or to define more precisely structural changes and severity of diseases that are evident from clinical examination, the physician relies on laboratory methods. There are many laboratory methods available that give information about cardiovascular structure and function. Each method has particular conditions for which it is best suited, each has a predictable sensitivity and specificity with respect to particular questions, and among various methods there is an element of redundancy so that essentially the same information can be obtained in more than one way. Laboratory studies vary in cost and risk to the patient. They may give false or misleading information about a condition, especially if interpreted out of context with clinical data. The optimal approach to the patient requires a knowledge of changes in laboratory test results produced by a disease, and also a strategy as to which test and what sequence of studies will help in making the diagnosis and appropriately directing management of the patient.

Making a diagnosis is an important step in defining a clinical problem, but the diagnosis is not an end in itself. Patients within a given diagnostic category typically do not come to common endpoints within a predictable time. This is especially true in common chronic cardiovascular diagnoses such as hypertension, angina pectoris, and mitral stenosis. Prognosis is important to the patient who wants to know what the future holds. Prognosis is important to the doctor who needs to select a therapeutic program. The number of descriptors required to enable a physician to predict outcomes accurately is generally greater than the number needed to make a diagnosis. Large numbers of patients within a diagnostic category are needed to define which descriptors discriminate against certain outcomes. Finally, estimating prognosis is essentially an exercise in the application of probability statistics. The optimal approach to management decisions involves accurate collection of data that contribute to a definition of outcomes, the availability of information on many patients similar to the one being evaluated, and valid systems for assessing the impact of management choices.

COMPONENTS OF THE CARDIOVASCULAR WORKUP

There are five components of the cardiovascular workup: the history, physical examination, electrocardiogram, chest x-rays, and laboratory studies. Patients with heart disease may or may not have symptoms, and they may be referred by one physician to another because of a suspected abnormality in any of the components of the workup. In practice, therefore, the starting point may be anywhere in this scheme. The sequence of acquiring data is less important than a thorough approach to each component.

THE HISTORY. The cardinal symptoms of cardiovascular disease include chest pain, shortness of breath, hemoptysis, palpitation, swelling, faintness or syncope, and cyanosis. *Chest pain* is usually characterized by its location, quality, duration, radiation, and factors that cause, aggravate, or alleviate the symptom. For example, pain caused by coronary artery disease is typically central, is heavy or squeezing, lasts three to ten minutes, may radiate to the arm, neck, or jaw, and is caused by exertion and relieved by rest. Pericardial pain is usually left sided, sharp, and related to breathing and position. Chest wall pain usually has a long duration and can be elicited by pressure over the trigger area. The history is the key to distinguishing among the common causes of chest pain: ischemic heart disease, pericardial disease, pulmonary infarction, aortic aneurysm, chest wall pain, and gastrointestinal disease.

Shortness of breath may occur at rest, only with exertion, or only in certain positions. Shortness of breath resulting from heart failure is more prominent when the patient is supine than when standing, is more evident during exertion than at rest, and correlates with periods of increased weight caused by fluid retention. Pulmonary embolism and pneumonia may cause shortness of breath, but the onset is typically acute. Emphysema causes shortness of breath that is gradual in onset, persistent over long periods of time, and not closely related to position. The history is designed to help distinguish between shortness of breath related to heart failure, pulmonary emboli, intrinsic lung disease, and anxiety. *Hemoptysis* is the production of bloody sputum during coughing. The quantity of blood, its color, and how it is mixed within the sputum (i.e., streaks, clumps, evenly mixed, or pure blood) all are important in distinguishing bronchitis, pulmonary infarction, pulmonary edema, and hemorrhage from a ruptured bronchial vein such as in mitral stenosis. *Palpitation* is an awareness of the heart beating in the chest. This sensation is not unusual in normal subjects when lying in bed or after vigorous exercise. On the other hand, when the sensation has an abrupt onset and termination, or is described as irregular or a skipping sensation, it usually signifies an arrhythmia. *Edema* is swelling in any part of the body as a consequence of excessive fluid retention. Typically, edema is most prominent in the feet, maximal at the end of the day, and less evident in the morning. Local factors may cause or contribute to the site of edema formation. For example, edema of only one leg suggests venous disease confined to the involved leg. Edema that is maximal or confined to the abdomen suggests cirrhosis of the liver or tricuspid insufficiency. Patients who have any cause of edema and who are at bed rest for extended periods of time may accumulate fluid predominantly in the sacral region and posterior aspect of the thighs. *Dizziness* or *syncope* may be a consequence of one of several mechanisms: arrhythmias, obstruction to blood flow, an orthostatic drop in blood pressure, loss of blood volume, or drugs. The history is particularly important in syncope, because abnormal signs are frequently absent. The relation to preceding incidents, associated symptoms such as pain and palpitations, and a history of blood loss or drug use are important to elicit. Other important causes of syncope include cerebrovascular disease, seizures, and hyperventilation. *Cyanosis* is a bluish discoloration of skin or mucous membranes caused by the presence of blood in the capillaries which has more than 4 grams per deciliter of desaturated hemoglobin. This degree of desaturation can occur either as a consequence of poor oxygenation in the lung or shunting (central cyanosis) or from a markedly reduced rate of capillary flow, as in shock or states of vasoconstriction. In these latter conditions left heart blood is adequately oxygenated but becomes desaturated in capillaries owing to stagnation and reduced flow (peripheral cyanosis).

To obtain a good cardiovascular history, remember these two principles: First, let the patient tell the story. Patients will frequently include information that would not come forth in response to a series of directed questions. Gestures used by the patient to describe symptoms and the situations in which they appear are often significant in subsequent management decisions. Second, after hearing the patient's story, ask direct questions to fill in any missing information and to determine the presence or absence of the cardinal symptoms of cardiovascular disease. Pursue each positive response in appropriate detail. Establish the chronology of the history, the severity of symptoms, and whether the course is stable, progressive, or cyclic. Whenever possible, use the patient's words, not your own.

THE PHYSICAL EXAMINATION. There are five parts to the cardiovascular physical examination: physical appearance, venous pressure and pulse, arterial pressure and pulse, precordial movements, and auscultation.

Physical Appearance. The physical appearance of a patient is important for two reasons: it may give clues to a systemic disease that also affects the heart, and it may provide data relevant to the nature and severity of heart disease. Marfan's syndrome involves a typical body habitus and is sometimes associated with mitral and aortic insufficiency and aneurysms of the aorta. Down's syndrome (trisomy 21) is associated with endocardial cushion defects. Bony abnormalities of the upper extremity (especially a fingerized thumb) are associated with atrial septal defect and together constitute the Holt-Oram syndrome. Disturbances of gait may suggest Friedreich's ataxia with associated cardiomyopathy. Acromegaly, disturbances of thyroid function, and rheumatoid arthritis are frequently associated with myocardial, pericardial, or valvular disease. Scleroderma is often associated with a cardiomyopathy. Cyanosis and clubbing are clues to reversal of a shunt in congenital heart disease. A head bob and exaggerated arterial pulsations in the neck suggest increased diastolic run-off, as in aortic insufficiency.

Venous Pressure and Pulse. There are two objectives to examination of the neck veins. The first is to estimate central venous pressure, and the second is to evaluate the wave form of the venous pressure pulse (Fig. 38–1). The examination is a visual one seeking a volume change in the veins. Because the venous system is a low pressure system, neck veins are nearly empty when the patient is sitting up, and they are distended when the patient is lying flat without a pillow. In either position a change in volume synchronous with the heartbeat is usually absent. To examine neck veins ideally, elevate the patient's head to an angle that maximizes the volume change in the veins throughout the cardiac cycle. In the usual patient, the external jugular veins are the most reliable sites to estimate mean venous pressure, but the internal jugular vein is a more reliable source to evaluate venous pulsations. Venous pressure is estimated by identifying the undulating meniscus in the jugular vein, measuring its height in centimeters above the sternal angle of Louis, and adding 5 cm. Normal venous pressure is 5 to 9 cm of H_2O. The "A" wave results from atrial contraction and is exaggerated with right ventricular hypertrophy (reduced compliance), tricuspid stenosis, arrhythmias in which atrial contraction occurs against a closed tricuspid valve

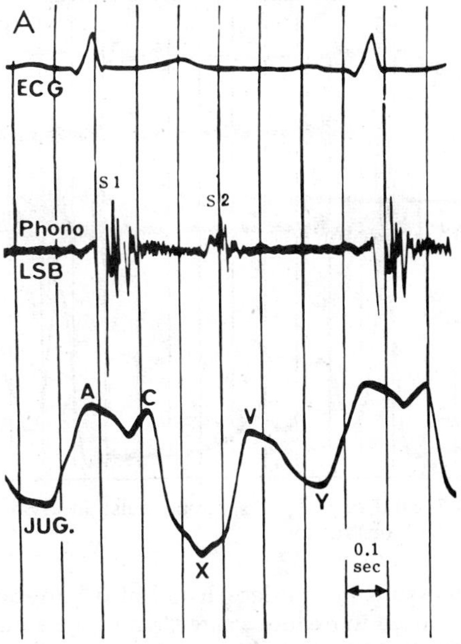

Figure 38–1. Normal jugular venous pulse.

(i.e., cannon waves), and constrictive pericarditis. Obliteration of the "X" descent and a prominent "CV" wave are characteristic of tricuspid insufficiency. Elevated venous pressure with exaggerated "X" and "Y" descents is typical of pericardial constriction.

Arterial Pressure and Pulses. Arterial pulses are examined by palpation with the fingertips. The artery is compressed until it is displaced by the force of the arterial pressure pulse. This sensation of force on the fingertips is related to the amplitude of the pressure pulse, i.e., the difference between systolic and diastolic pressure, and not to pressure or flow per se. The carotid arteries are generally the most valid reflection of cardiac activity because they are centrally located and not influenced importantly by local factors that will affect the amplitude of the radial artery pulse independent of changes in cardiac activity. The amplitude of the carotid pulse is increased with anemia, thyrotoxicosis, and aortic insufficiency. In these conditions stroke volume and the rate of left ventricular ejection are enhanced. The carotid pulse is attenuated in myocardial failure, with rapid heart rates such as atrial fibrillation, and in aortic stenosis. These conditions are characterized by either a reduced stroke volume or a decreased rate of left ventricular ejection, or both. The arterial pulse becomes bifid in certain conditions in which left ventricular ejection is initially very rapid, producing a percussion wave, which is then followed by a tidal wave that represents a reflected pulsation from the periphery (Fig. 38–2). A bifid or bisferious pulse is typically seen in asymmetric septal hypertrophy with obstruction (i.e., hypertrophic subaortic stenosis) and sometimes in aortic valve disease with predominant aortic insufficiency. In addition to examination of the carotid pulse, peripheral arterial pulses should be felt and compared. A diminished or delayed pulse at one site compared with another suggests arterial occlusion. If such a discrepancy is noted, it can be exaggerated by exercising the extremity supplied by the obstructed artery. In patients with claudication arterial pulses are frequently normal at rest, but they become reduced in the affected leg or foot with walking. This happens because at rest the distal arterial bed is constricted, flow in the leg is low, and as a consequence there is little or no gradient across the stenosis. With exercise the distal arterial bed opens up, flow into the leg is limited by the stenosis, and a gradient develops with a marked drop in pressure distal to the stenosis.

Arterial blood pressure should be measured with a cuff of appropriate size. If an elevated blood pressure is obtained in

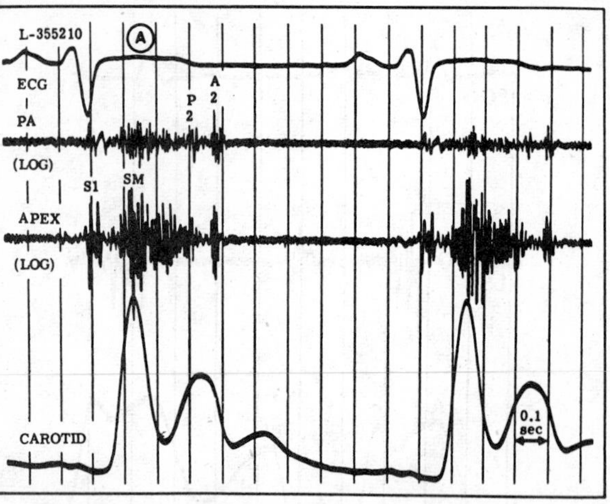

Figure 38–2. Bifid or bisferious carotid pulse in asymmetric septal hypertrophy with obstruction.

the arm, pressure in one leg should also be recorded. This procedure is used to exclude coarctation of the aorta in hypertensive patients. The arterial blood pressure should be recorded in both the supine and the standing positions. If the patient's blood pressure is elevated on the first measurement, several recordings should be obtained. A marked postural drop in arterial pressure suggests either hypovolemia or an inadequate sympathetic vasoconstrictor response. A change of systolic arterial pressure on alternate beats in sinus rhythm is referred to as pulsus alternans (observed in severe myocardial failure), and a change of systolic blood pressure of greater than 10 mm Hg with respiration is referred to as pulsus paradoxus (observed in pericardial tamponade).

Precordial Movements. Precordial movements should be evaluated by inspection and by palpation at the apex, in the left parasternal region, and in the right and left second intercostal spaces. The normal apical impulse is ascribed to left ventricular activity and is seen and felt as a tap of brief duration localized in the fourth or fifth interspace at the midclavicular line. Its distance from the midsternal line should be measured in centimeters and recorded. When the left ventricle is dilated, the impulse is displaced to the left and downward and occupies a larger area. With systolic overloads such as hypertension or aortic stenosis, the impulse is not displaced (in the absence of dilation) but is more forceful and sustained than normal (Fig. 38–3). Right ventricular enlargement typically produces an exaggerated left parasternal early systolic lift or thrust. Dilation of the pulmonary artery or aorta (aneurysm) may produce a systolic pulse or tap in the second left or right intercostal spaces, respectively. In regional myocardial disease or in coronary disease with regional infarction, there is a paradoxical outward systolic movement felt in the third or fourth left intercostal space between the sternum and the nipple. Accentuated heart sounds are often palpable. Gallop sounds are usually palpable when they can be heard and reflect altered ventricular compliance. Palpation of the precordium is directed primarily at assessing ventricular size, ascertaining whether an increase in chamber size is due to dilation or concentric hypertrophy, assessing changes in compliance, and detecting asynchronous contraction of a region of the ventricle caused by a regional disease process.

Auscultation. The first principle of cardiac auscultation is to choose a stethoscope that fits the ears comfortably and has tubing as short as possible. The second principle is to carry out the examination in a room where the ambient noise level is as low as possible. Clinical experience and studies in hearing laboratories have shown that acoustic phenomena of diagnostic importance can be missed even by experienced observers if either of these principles is compromised.

The next important step in auscultation is to remember that you only hear what you listen for. A systematic approach, in which you listen at specific locations and focus on specific sounds and parts of the cardiac cycle, is essential. Devise a mental check list that you move through in stepwise fashion. For example, starting at the apex, ask yourself the following questions: (1) Which is the first and which the second heart sound? (2) What are their relative intensities, and is either accentuated? (3) Is there more than one component to either sound? (4) If there are two components to the first sound, is the extra component an S_4, an ejection click, or splitting? (5) Are there midsystolic or diastolic sounds? (6) Can a murmur be heard in either systole or diastole? Remember that high frequency sounds are best heard with the diaphragm, whereas low frequency sounds are best heard with the bell. Make it a standard part of your examination to listen with the patient supine, in the left lateral position, standing, and after exercise.

In chapters that follow, details of the physical examination in each of the major cardiac disorders will be presented. The point stressed here is the approach to the patient. The examination should be systematic. Abnormal physical findings may be so striking that they cannot be missed; more often, however, they are subtle. Therefore the most reliable approach is a mental check list. Progress through the list in an orderly fashion, and at each step optimize the conditions for eliciting the phenomenon that is sought.

It is rare for a cardiac condition to have only one manifestation on the physical examination. For example, when you see cyanosis you can anticipate certain findings on palpation or auscultation that will help explain it. When you feel an enlarged right ventricle, a palpable first heart sound, and a systolic pulse over the pulmonary artery in a middle-aged person, you can anticipate that auscultation may elicit an opening snap and diastolic rumble. Anticipating the next step is likely to increase the precision of the examination so that less will be missed. Absence of an anticipated finding may redirect tentative conclusions about the diagnosis. Finally, an anticipatory approach encourages synthesis of data as the examiner progresses through the check list. A diagnosis results from a synthesis of data; whether the history and physical examination yield a diagnosis or a definition of the problem that falls short of a diagnosis, synthesis helps define what the next step should be and whether or not that step is necessary.

LABORATORY EXAMINATIONS. Laboratory studies play a central role in the diagnosis of cardiovascular diseases and, even more importantly, in quantifying the severity of these disorders. The paragraphs below are designed to highlight the role of commonly employed laboratory tests in cardiovascular diagnosis. It seems appropriate to discuss briefly the physical or physiologic principles behind these tests, because these principles help clarify the uses and limitations of a particular test.

The X-Ray. Chest roentgenography is the oldest and one of the most useful techniques for imaging the heart. Radiographic

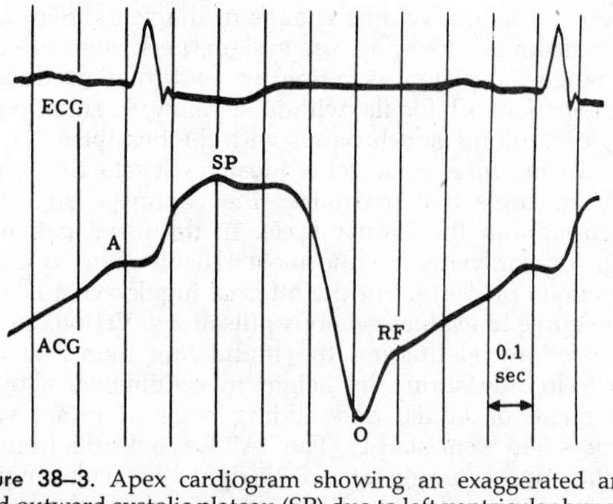

Figure 38–3. Apex cardiogram showing an exaggerated and prolonged outward systolic plateau (SP) due to left ventricular hypertrophy in a patient with aortic stenosis.

examination utilizes x-rays that are a form of electromagnetic energy. In passing through the chest a variable fraction of photons of the x-ray beam is absorbed by body tissues where absorption is determined by the composition of the tissues, their thickness, and the quality of the beam. The photons that emerge from the subject expose a film. The picture created on the film is a superimposition of structures within the chest that absorb x-rays to a variable extent.

The standard radiographic examination of the heart involves a posteroanterior view and a lateral view, usually supplemented by left and right oblique views with barium in the esophagus. Each view is designed to optimize conditions for visualizing various cardiac structures. With appropriate views one can assess the size of individual cardiac chambers, and of the superior vena cava, aorta, and pulmonary artery. The pulmonary vessels can be seen on conventional x-rays, and typical patterns are produced by pulmonary venous engorgement, by increased or decreased pulmonary blood flow, and by pulmonary hypertension. Calcification of valves, the anuli of valves, coronary arteries, and pericardium can be observed (see Ch. 41.1).

In many forms of congenital and acquired heart disease, a diagnosis can be made or strongly suspected on the basis of chest x-rays. In practice, however, x-rays are interpreted together with the history, physical examination, and electrocardiogram. In this context, the most useful role of the x-ray is to confirm structural changes suspected by physical examination, to identify unsuspected structural changes, and to assess the severity of anatomic and physiologic consequences of heart disease. One of the greastest values of the x-ray is for determining the size of cardiovascular structures over time.

The Electrocardiogram. Cardiac muscle is an excitable tissue. On each beat excitation begins at some site in the heart (normally the sinoatrial node), and spreads from cell to cell initially over the atrium, then through the atrioventricular node, and finally to the ventricles. The form of the electrocardiogram at any moment in time is determined by the location, size, and geometry of boundaries between excited and unexcited regions.

Whenever a boundary exists, the voltage difference across the boundary produces an electrical field in the body. The positive side of this boundary can be viewed as a source of current, and the negative side as a sink. Regions on the body surface that face the current source will be on the positive side of the field, whereas those that face the current sink will be on the negative side. Because the location, spatial orientation, and size of the boundary change throughout excitation and recovery, the field changes in strength and orientation. On the body surface the amplitude and sign of the potential change with time. An electrocardiogram is a record of the voltage difference between two points on the body surface with respect to time (see Ch. 41.2).

The electrocardiogram is the most widely used and useful noninvasive cardiac diagnostic technique. Its diagnostic value has developed over the years through (1) correlations with clinical states and pathologic material, (2) physiologic studies designed to establish the relation between the electrocardiogram and normal and abnormal states, and (3) simulation. Analyses of the P wave and the QRS complex, their rate, and their temporal relation to each other provide a definitive approach for recognizing most disturbances of cardiac rhythm. The electrocardiogram gives diagnostic and localizing information about most myocardial infarctions. Criteria have been established for recognizing hypertrophy of the right or left atrium and the right or left ventricle. The electrocardiogram is an important diagnostic aid also in various forms of congenital heart disease. Because it can be obtained repeatedly in the same individual or monitored continuously over days, it is of particular value in assessing pathophysiologic phenomena that change (rhythm, hypertrophy, infarction or ischemia, electrolyte and drug effects).

The Echocardiogram. Echocardiography is a noninvasive technique in which high frequency sound waves are directed into the thoracic cavity and echoes are recorded. Echoes are produced at the interface between tissues of different acoustic impedance (i.e., at the epicardial surface, at the interface of endocardium and blood, and at the interface of structures such as septa and valves and blood). The echoes produced by these structures vary in distance from the transducer throughout the heart cycle, and they vary in distance from each other with respect to time. With appropriate instrumentation and technique, high quality echocardiograms can be obtained in approximately 75 per cent of individuals.

A complete examination should include visualization of the mitral, aortic, tricuspid, and pulmonary valves, and the left atrium, left ventricle, and right ventricle; a sweep from the left ventricle into the aortic root; and assessment of the presence or absence of pericardial fluid.

The importance of echocardiography can be inferred from several observations. An echocardiogram is completely noninvasive, is without risk, and requires approximately 30 minutes. Mitral stenosis can be easily recognized, and the orifice of the stenotic valve can be measured. Aortic stenosis can be easily recognized, and although the orifice size is difficult to measure precisely, a demonstration of cusps that open to the periphery of the aortic root rules out significant aortic stenosis. A pulmonary artery diastolic pressure above 20 mm Hg produces a typical change in the diastolic contour of the pulmonary valve. Echocardiography is probably the most sensitive technique available for recognizing left atrial myxoma, mitral valve prolapse, and asymmetric septal hypertrophy with or without subaortic obstruction. It is the only available technique for visualizing vegetations on the valves in infectious endocarditis. The presence of small amounts of pericardial fluid can be detected, and the volume of fluid can be closely estimated. Although there are limitations to quantitation of ventricular volume and function from echo studies, chamber dimensions and a qualitative assessment of wall motion have proved to be reliable estimates of chamber size and left ventricular function. Images that are diagnostic of certain forms of congenital heart disease have also been reported (see Ch. 41.3).

Radionuclide Studies. Radionuclide studies of the cardiovascular system involve the injection of an isotope into the circulation and subsequent detection of the energy emitted from the isotope by an appropriate external instrument. Isotopes vary in their mode of decay (e.g., emission of electrons or positrons), in their half-life, and in the energy of photons that are liberated as a consequence of decay of the isotope. After variable absorption in body tissues, photons exit from the body and are available for detection. Most detection instruments rely on a thallium-activated sodium iodide crystal, which has the property of giving off electrons when struck by photons. The current generated by this event is then amplified by a photomultiplier tube and used to expose film or to modulate an oscilloscope beam, or, after conversion to a voltage, is stored in a computer.

Radionuclides can be used to label the blood pool and thus produce images of the cardiac chambers throughout the cardiac cycle to estimate chamber volume, ejection fraction, and wall motion. A special application is the construction of time-activity plots over specific regions and the application of indicator dilution principles to locate and quantitate intracardiac shunts. Radionuclides such as potassium-43 and thallium-201 are extracted by normal muscle in proportion to blood flow and can be used to evaluate relative regional myocardial perfusion at rest and during exercise. Technetium-99m phosphate is localized to acutely necrotic myocardium and gives images that are diagnostic of acute infarction (positive images from 12 hours to three to five days after infarction). Theoretically, positron-emitting isotopes can be used for any of the aforementioned applications. A unique application of positron images results from the availability of isotopes of carbon, oxygen, and nitrogen that can be used to label natural metabolites and thus study regional metabolism of ischemic zones noninvasively and sequentially (see Ch. 41.4).

Cardiac Catheterization. Cardiac catheterization provides a method by which the pressure in any or all of the cardiac chambers can be measured with considerable accuracy. Gradients across stenotic valves can be measured, cardiac output and pulmonary blood flow can be estimated, and shunts between the systemic and pulmonary circulation can be localized and quantitated. Contrast agents can be injected to define radiographically the dimensions of the cardiac chambers, to estimate the volume of regurgitation through insufficient valves, and to visualize the anatomy of simple and complex congenital malformations. The aorta and most of its branches, including the coronary arteries, can be selectively catheterized, and deviations from normal anatomy can be defined. The contractile performance of heart muscle can be evaluated, and the adequacy of cardiac output and flow to many individual organs, including the heart, can be deduced from measurement of flow and the arteriovenous difference of several metabolites, including oxygen. Electrode catheters can be used to define the location of conduction delays within the heart, the sequence of excitation, and the mechanism of certain alterations of cardiac rhythm (see Ch. 41.5).

There are many cardiac conditions in which the diagnosis can be established by history, physical examination, and noninvasive tests. The severity of the condition can also be assessed with sufficient clarity to judge that the patient is a surgical candidate. Catheterization in these circumstances is performed primarily to provide the surgeon with anatomic and physiologic detail that will help direct his approach to the patient (e.g., an open or closed approach to mitral stenosis, or which coronary arteries should be bypassed in a patient with angina pectoris). Catheterization may also reveal conditions that are unsuspected on clinical grounds or that cannot be judged quantitatively with the accuracy needed to guide the surgical approach (e.g., the presence of associated anomalous pulmonary venous return in a patient with atrial septal defect or aortic insufficiency in a patient with predominant mitral regurgitation). Catheterization provides information about myocardial function and contributes to the evaluation of surgical risk and the likelihood that correction of a valvular, congenital, or coronary lesion will prolong survival and reduce symptoms.

Another role of cardiac catheterization in patients with known heart disease is to enhance our knowledge of the severity of the condition when there is a discrepancy between symptoms and data obtained from physical examination and noninvasive techniques. One of the most noteworthy examples is the question of whether or not significant mitral stenosis has persisted or recurred in a patient who had mitral commissurotomy with an initially favorable response. On the other hand, patients with hydraulically significant stenosis of the aortic or pulmonary valve or with atrial septal defect may present with clinical signs and electrocardiographic and x-ray findings that indicate the need for surgical correction, and yet there may be few symptoms or none at all.

In certain situations cardiac catheterization is performed as a diagnostic procedure in patients in whom a diagnosis can only be suspected on clinical grounds or to clarify the basis of symptoms or signs of unknown significance. Probably the most frequent example is the adult patient with recurrent chest pain compatible with angina, in whom the electrocardiogram at rest and during exercise fails to provide evidence of myocardial ischemia. When other noncardiac causes of angina-like chest pain have been excluded, coronary artery disease cannot be confirmed or excluded as a basis for the symptoms without coronary arteriography. A normal arteriogram may be useful in directing attention away from the heart. Similarly, the finding of significant coronary artery disease may lead to successful therapy and relief of incapacity.

Despite the usefulness of cardiac catheterization, most cardiac conditions can be recognized and their severity adequately assessed without catheterization. Catheterization requires hospitalization, it is expensive, it causes some discomfort to the patient, and there are risks of arterial injury, embolization, myocardial infarction, reactions to contrast agents, and even death. Fortunately, these occurrences are extremely rare. Catheterization should not be undertaken if significant heart disease can be reasonably excluded on the basis of history and physical examination with or without the use of noninvasive laboratory tests. Similarly, cardiac catheterization is not indicated even in the presence of heart disease if the data obtained will not contribute substantially to decisions about management.

STRATEGIES

When the physician has obtained a thorough history and performed a complete physical examination of the cardiovascular system, the next question is whether or not laboratory studies are indicated and, if so, what tests and in what sequence. The answer to this question is not as straightforward as it might seem. What is important is to have a general strategy and a willingness to adapt that strategy in a manner appropriate to the problem that led the patient to the doctor, or to the findings obtained from the clinical examination. In any situation it is appropriate to pursue studies until a potential problem has been reasonably excluded or until an actual problem has been defined at the level necessary to make a decision about the need for further tests or treatment.

The role of laboratory studies is influenced in part by the age of the patient and the reason for seeking the advice of a doctor. For example, when a teenager is evaluated and the history and physical examination are normal, most doctors would agree that no laboratory studies are indicated. If a same-aged individual is referred to a cardiologist because of a systolic murmur at the base that radiates to the carotid arteries, and the physical examination, x-ray, and electrocardiogram are otherwise normal, an echocardiogram may show a bicuspid aortic valve without evidence of stenosis. This additional information would provide a basis for encouraging athletic participation, and also advice about prophylactic antibiotics and follow-up over the years ahead.

Is there an age at which certain laboratory tests become routine even in the absence of a history of cardiovascular disease or abnormalities on the physical examination? Many physicians would respond to this question in the affirmative. One example is the physician who is oriented toward preventive cardiology and is interested not only in detecting the presence or absence of disease, but also in detecting conditions that may substantially increase the risk of disease in later life. This strategy is invoked by those who advocate measuring serum cholesterol and its distribution between high and low density lipoproteins at least once in early adult life, particularly if there is a family history of premature atherosclerotic disease or hyperlipidemia.

There is another justification for obtaining selected tests on a routine basis in young adults. As patients grow older there is an increased probability that they will develop cardiovascular disease. There is also an increased probability that they will develop conditions that may require surgery. At that stage the consultation of an internist is frequently sought, particularly if the patient is over age 50, and an electrocardiogram and chest x-ray are obtained. If an abnormality is observed, it is useful to have a prior x-ray or electrocardiogram. The availability of one electrocardiogram and chest x-ray at an earlier age when no disease was suspected can be of enormous value in evaluating later records.

When patients present with a history that indicates heart disease or with abnormal physical findings, laboratory tests take on a different role. At one level, certain tests are used to confirm or help interpret an abnormal physical finding. For example, the phonocardiogram can be used to confirm and document the presence and timing of abnormal sounds or murmurs, the apex cardiogram can confirm and document abnormal precordial movements, and external pulse recordings can confirm and document abnormal venous or arterial pulsations. These techniques are useful in teaching and they can be very important when a patient moves from the care of one doctor to another. Echocardiography is probably the most sensitive method to detect mitral valve prolapse, mitral stenosis, pericardial fluid, left atrial myxoma, and asymmetric septal hypertrophy.

The most important point is that laboratory studies should be selected and pursued until the nature and severity of the disease can be established with reasonable certainty. If that can be accomplished with noninvasive methods, then tests of greater expense and potential risk are not necessary. On the other hand, when symptoms or signs suggest a severe disease potentially amenable to surgery, or if significant disease is suspected but cannot be clarified by noninvasive techniques, then catheterization is clearly indicated.

Most forms of heart disease are chronic. The approach of a physician whose focus is on prognosis, management, and follow-up requires more information than is required to make a diagnosis. Furthermore, accurate assessments of severity of disease and the response to management require quantifiable and reproducible descriptors. These considerations never justify the performance of unnecessary tests that subject the patient to a risk of complications. They emphasize, however, that a complete cardiac evaluation very often includes the use of laboratory procedures that exceed the minimal data base required to make a diagnosis.

39. PREVALENCE AND EPIDEMIOLOGY OF CARDIOVASCULAR DISEASE

Robert I. Levy

It is difficult to overemphasize the magnitude of the medical, social, and economic burden of cardiovascular diseases. An estimated 40 million Americans have some form of cardiovascular disease. Each year about 25,000 children are born with congenital heart disease, and of the 6000 of these children who die annually approximately half are less than one year of age. About 70,000 children and 1 million adults have rheumatic heart disease, of whom almost 8,000 die each year. More than 6 million Americans have overt clinical signs of atherosclerosis, primarily of the coronary, cerebral, and peripheral blood vessels. About 35 million Americans (15 per cent of the population of the United States) have hypertension as defined by a blood pressure of 160/95 or higher. Furthermore, the latter two major etiologic processes, atherosclerosis and hypertension, are interactive and result in an estimated 1.5 million heart attacks (of which 750,000 are first events) each year—a rate of 4000 per day or almost three per minute—and 500,000 strokes (of which 400,000 are first events) each year. In 1981, cardiovascular diseases accounted for 989,606 deaths or 49.8 per cent of all deaths in the United States, of which almost 559,000 were due to coronary artery disease (heart attack and sudden death) and 164,000 to cerebrovascular disease (stroke).

The age-adjusted death rate for rheumatic heart disease in the United States declined 69 per cent between 1940 and 1970 and another 38 per cent between 1970 and 1980 to 2.7 deaths per 100,000 population. Although there are few reliable studies of the incidence of rheumatic fever, the data that are available indicate that a significant decrease in both severity and incidence of the disease has occurred in this country since 1940.

The major risk factor for the development of rheumatic fever is a prior throat infection with group A beta-hemolytic streptococci; from 0.3 to 3.0 per cent of individuals so infected develop the disease. Environmental factors have been identified as significant additional risk factors, the most important being overcrowded living conditions. Other risk factors include low socioeconomic status, ethnic status, malnutrition, climate, and geography.

The onset of the downward trend in morbidity and mortality preceded the introduction of antibiotics, although the trend declined more rapidly following the introduction of effective treatment of streptococcal infections. Recurrent attacks of the disease have decreased dramatically following the institution of secondary prevention programs, in which effective drug therapy was utilized to prevent streptococcal infections in subjects who had previously experienced an episode of rheumatic fever. The additional impact of altered environmental factors, such as overcrowding, must be significant.

The prevalence of coronary, cerebrovascular, and hypertensive diseases rises sharply with age. Although 9 per cent of adults under age 45 have hypertension, few have other manifestations of cardiovascular disease. Overt coronary heart disease is present in 8 per cent of males ages 45 to 64 and 15 per cent of males age 65 and over. For females the corresponding rates are 3 per cent and 10 per cent. Cerebrovascular disease, present in 1 per cent of persons ages 45 to 64, is present in 4 per cent age 65 and over. Hypertension is present in at least 52 per cent of women age 65 and over—compared to 44 per cent for men in that age group. In terms of mortality from these diseases, it is from coronary heart disease that mortality is highest. As in prevalence statistics, death rates rise steeply with age, especially after age 35, and for ages under 65 rates for coronary heart disease in men are more than double the rates in women. Death rates for cerebrovascular and hypertensive disease are large in number only after age 65.

Cardiovascular diseases rank second only to respiratory diseases in terms of days of bed disability. They rank first in terms of limitation of activity, Social Security disability, hospital discharges, and total hospital bed days (51 million per year). In terms of economic costs, cardiovascular diseases also rank first among all medical disorders. The estimated economic cost of cardiovascular diseases to the nation in 1979 totaled over $80 billion. Of this amount, $30 billion was related to the direct costs of illness and over $50 billion was due to indirect costs secondary to lost wages and productivity.

In America in 1900, infectious processes, such as pneumonia, influenza, and tuberculosis, reigned as our major health problems. As these disorders were brought under control, cardiovascular disease (especially that of the coronary arteries) became more prevalent and virulent, raising the specter in the late 1940's and 1950's of an "epidemic" of cardiovascular disease and accounting for 55.1 per cent of all deaths in 1962. Over the last 30 years, however, this tide has gradually turned; age-adjusted cardiovascular death rates have been declining slowly since 1950 and more sharply since 1963. In total, since 1950 age-adjusted cardiovascular death rates have decreased by 41.5 per cent. Most significantly, the decline in coronary and cerebrovascular disease mortality rates has been even more precipitous since 1970 (stroke rates down 42 per cent and coronary deaths down 28 per cent between 1970 and 1981). This decline in cardiovascular mortality rates has been observed in both sexes and all age decades from ages 20 to 29 to 70+. In the age range 25 to 44 years, heart disease was the number one cause of death in the 1960's. By 1970 it ranked second, and by 1978 it ranked third behind accidents and cancer. At ages 45 to 54 in 1981, heart disease dropped to second place behind cancer. The decline for all cardiovascular diseases has been so sharp that, despite a growing and aging United States population, cardiovascular disease accounted for fewer than 1 million deaths in 1975 for the first time in a decade and accounted for less than one half of all deaths (in 1981) for the first time in over 30 years. The decline is generally not paralleled in the rest of the world. Since 1969 mortality from coronary heart disease among middle-aged men has increased sharply in Poland, Bulgaria, Yugoslavia, Northern Ireland, Hungary, Sweden, and Switzerland, with lesser increases documented in other countries. In spite of the encouraging trends in the United States, cardiovascular disease remains a problem of staggering proportions, causing almost 50 per cent of all deaths in 1981. The

TABLE 39–1. AGE-ADJUSTED DEATH RATES* FOR MAJOR CARDIOVASCULAR-RENAL DISEASES AND ALL OTHER CAUSES OF DEATH COMBINED—UNITED STATES, DECADES 1900–1980†‡

Year	All Causes	All Causes Except Cardiovascular-Renal Diseases	Cardiovascular-Renal Disease				
			Total	Heart Disease	Cerebro-vascular	Renal	All Other
1900	1778.5	1356.5	422.0	167.3	134.4	97.0	23.3
1910	1578.8	1101.6	477.2	201.7	126.4	107.0	42.1
1920	1423.6	952.2	471.4	203.6	122.6	105.9	39.3
1930	1246.1	754.9	491.2	252.7	106.5	102.5	29.5
1940	1076.1	590.3	485.8	292.7	91.0	79.0	23.1
1950	841.5	401.4	440.1	307.6	88.8	14.5	29.2
1960	760.9	361.6	399.3	286.2	79.7	5.7	27.7
1970	714.3	359.5	354.8	256.8	66.6	6.1	25.3
1980	582.4	323.5	258.9	201.3	40.3	4.7	12.6

*Rate per 100,000 population, age-adjusted to the United States population, 1940.
†Source: Vital Statistics of the United States, National Center for Health Statistics.
‡Comparability ratios were applied to convert these ratios to levels comparable to rates in 1980.

gaps in our knowledge and management of cardiovascular disease thus continue to pose a formidable challenge.

It is hard to attribute the ebb and flow in cardiovascular morbidity and mortality to specific events. It is difficult to differentiate the relative contributions of preventive approaches from those of improved treatment. Clearly, the two major etiologic processes damaging both the heart and the blood vessels are hypertension and atherosclerosis. Both processes are silent but incessant. We now know that hypertension may be present for long periods, as measured by simple blood pressure measurement, without producing signs or symptoms and, similarly, that atherosclerosis develops secretly in focal areas in blood vessels beginning in the first and second decades of life. This secret process may then proceed for two to six decades with no overt signs or symptoms until after two thirds of a vessel's lumen is occluded or the lesion breaks off or vasospasm or hemorrhage occurs. Symptoms appear suddenly in the form of heart attack, sudden death, angina, claudication, or stroke. Because of their ultimately devastating effects on the cardiovascular system, they are now the major subject of cardiovascular disease investigation. As basic researchers seek the cause(s) of arteriosclerosis and hypertension, as well as a better understanding of their basic pathophysiologic effects on the heart and blood vessels, cardiovascular physiologists have sought to develop better invasive (angiography) and noninvasive methods (e.g., echocardiography, nuclear magnetic resonance, nuclear imagery, x-ray densitometry) to diagnose abnormalities of the blood vessels, heart muscle, and heart valves long before signs or symptoms appear. During the past 30 years, cardiovascular epidemiologists have also made important contributions by detecting traits or habits in individuals to identify those who are at increased risk for specific cardiovascular diseases.

Much of the epidemiologic evidence regarding the role of certain personal characteristics ("risk factors") in the occurrence of coronary heart disease derives from several long-term prospective studies of population samples. The Framingham Heart Study is a prototype study in which a general population sample of 5209 residents of the town of Framingham, Massachusetts, has been followed. At their first examination in 1948–1950, these men and women were 30 to 62 years old. Every two years they are re-examined to assess their medical status and to measure the characteristics to be described below. The Tecumseh Study followed a similar design, using all the residents of Tecumseh, Michigan, of whom 8624 participated in the initial examination in 1959. Three subsequent examinations have been completed.

Similar epidemiologic studies were conducted in Albany, using male civil servants aged 39 to 54 years; in Chicago, using male employees of the Chicago Peoples Gas Company aged 40 to 59 years, and another using male employees of Western Electric Company aged 40 to 55 years; and in Evans County, Georgia, using a total community in which one third of the population was black. The Tecumseh, Framingham, and Evans County studies included women as well as men.

A long list of major and minor cardiovascular risk factors have now been enumerated by these studies. They include as major factors *age, male sex, hypertension, cigarette smoking, plasma LDL and HDL cholesterol,* and *diabetes,* and as lesser factors *overweight, sedentary way of life, hardness of water, family history of heart disease before age 65, personality type,* and *stress.*

Prospective epidemiologic studies in other areas have tended to confirm these findings. Most of the other studies have used populations with lower overall rates of heart disease such as Japanese men in Japan, Hawaii, and California, Puerto Rican men, urban and rural men in Yugoslavia, and male civil servants in Israel. The essential features of each of these studies were (1) an effort to obtain a large representative sample of the population, (2) careful assessment of a variety of measurements prior to the onset of clinically overt coronary disease, and (3) complete ascertainment of all cardiac events occurring during the subsequent years of follow-up.

TABLE 39–2. AGE-ADJUSTED DEATH RATES* FOR FOUR SUBGROUPS OF CARDIOVASCULAR DISEASE—UNITED STATES, 1940–1980†‡

Year	Coronary Heart Disease	Hypertensive Disease	Rheumatic Fever and Rheumatic Heart Disease	Congenital Heart Disease
1940	207.2	69.3	20.5	4.8
1945	208.2	59.7	17.1	4.9
1950	226.4	56.0	14.0	4.6
1955	226.0	41.2	11.2	4.3
1960	238.5	29.6	9.7	4.7
1965	237.7	22.4	7.5	4.3
1970‡	228.1	7.9	6.3	3.7
1975‡	172.2	10.5	3.2	3.2
1980	149.4	8.9	2.6	Unknown

*Rate per 100,000 population, age-adjusted to the United States population, 1940.
†Source: Vital Statistics of the United States, National Center for Health Statistics.
‡Comparability ratios were applied to convert these ratios to levels comparable to rates in 1980.

TABLE 39–3. PERCENTAGE OF ALL DEATHS DUE TO CARDIOVASCULAR DISEASES* BY AGE—UNITED STATES, 1962, 1980†

Age	1962	1980
Total	55.1	50.4
Under 25	7.6	7.6
25–44	27.7	17.3
45–64	50.2	41.6
65–74	61.3	51.0
Over 74	71.3	64.1

*Includes congenital heart disease.
†Source: Vital Statistics of the United States, National Center for Health Statistics, and estimates made by the NHLBI.

As a result of such studies there is little doubt of the predictive power of the major cardiovascular risk factors (see accompanying figure). Estimates based on the Framingham Heart Study and national vital statistics indicate that two out of every three coronary events (myocardial infarction, coronary death, or coronary insufficiency) occur in high risk subjects. As detailed in the basic prevalence figures, older age and male sex both are associated with increasing cardiovascular disease. Females seem to have a 15- to 20-year protective buffer before cardiovascular events begin to manifest themselves increasingly in the seventh and eighth decades of life.

Cigarette smoking has clearly been shown to be an independent, potent risk factor for coronary, cerebral, and peripheral vascular disease. Sudden cardiac death, heart attack, angina, claudication, and stroke incidence and prevalence can be related to the number of cigarettes one smokes. The heavier the cigarette smoking history, the higher the risk. Both the nicotine and carbon monoxide inhaled with cigarette smoking have been incriminated as causative factors, but definite understanding of cause and effect still eludes us. Cigar and pipe smoking are not associated with this heightened degree of cardiovascular risk. Furthermore, in contrast to the apparently cumulative relationship of cigarette smoking to lung cancer, a series of prospective and retrospective studies now indicates that if one stops smoking cigarettes, over 90 per cent of the increased cardiovascular risk disappears within two years.

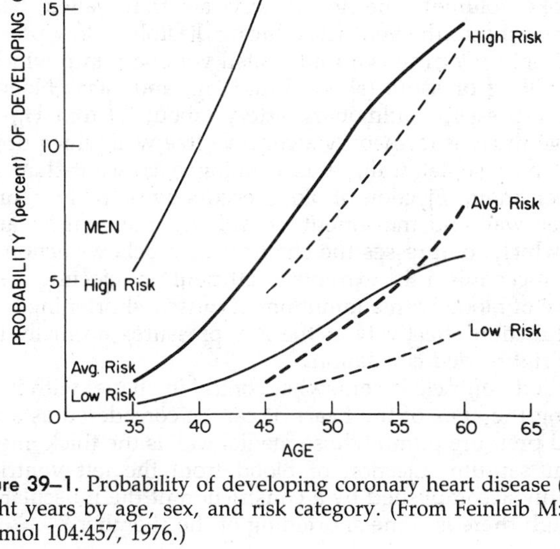

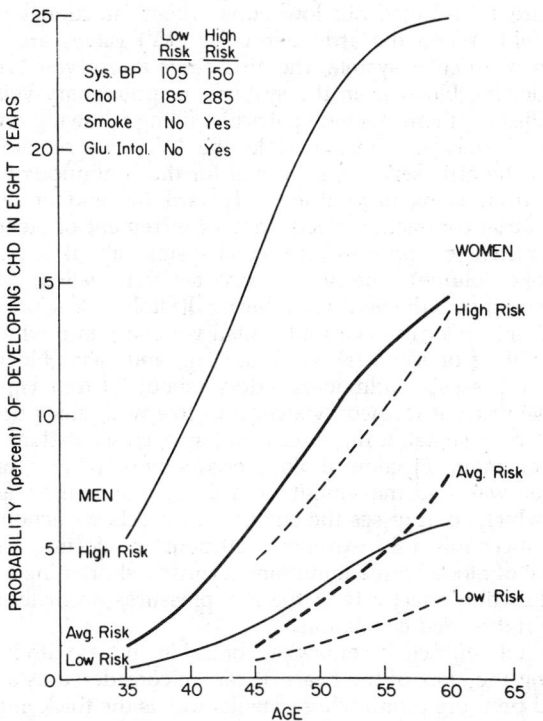

Figure 39–1. Probability of developing coronary heart disease (CHD) in eight years by age, sex, and risk category. (From Feinleib M: Am J Epidemiol 104:457, 1976.)

Hypertension is not only a major direct cause of cardiovascular disease but also appears to greatly accelerate the atherosclerotic process, especially that of the coronary and cerebral vessels. Although we define blood pressures above 160/95 as hypertension, cardiovascular risk begins to increase at considerably lower levels. For example, in a 35-year-old man with a normal blood pressure of 120/80, the risk of mortality over the next 20 years would increase almost two-fold if his pressure were 142/90. That risk increases 2.5 times with a pressure of 152/95.

An elevation of plasma cholesterol levels has long been associated with increased cardiovascular risk. It is now clear that the cholesterol-rich low density lipoproteins (LDL), the major carriers of cholesterol in our blood, are directly and independently associated with cardiovascular risk. Another plasma carrier of cholesterol, high density lipoprotein (HDL) (usually accounting for less than 25 per cent of the total plasma cholesterol) is independently but *inversely* related to cardiovascular risk. Although the biochemical basis of the apparently protective effect of HDL is still speculative, it is clear that the measurement of the plasma levels of HDL and LDL gives more information than the determination of total plasma cholesterol alone. LDL levels are in part genetically determined, although environmental factors, especially diet, appear to have major effects on the plasma levels of this lipoprotein. Diets high in cholesterol and saturated fats increase plasma LDL levels, whereas diets low in cholesterol and saturated fat and/or high in polyunsaturated fat decrease LDL levels. Plasma levels of HDL are much more stable in any given individual and appear to be under stronger genetic control. Cigarette smoking and obesity are associated with lower HDL levels. Exercise and modest ingestion of alcohol appear to raise HDL levels. From the time of adolescence, males have levels of HDL that are 10 to 20 per cent lower than those of females, whereas LDL levels are 10 per cent higher. This sex difference may be explained by the inverse effects of estrogen and testosterone on plasma HDL and LDL levels.

Diabetes is another independent cardiovascular risk factor, with higher levels directly related to the extent of vascular disease. This relationship is true for both the juvenile and adult onset diabetic, and in both groups premature macrovascular disease is the major cause of death. The female diabetic appears to lose all the protective cardiovascular effect usually attributed to the female sex.

Overweight, although associated with increased cardiovascular risk, does not appear to be an independent risk factor for cardiovascular disease. When other associated variables are factored out through multivariate analysis, obesity loses much of its predictive risk power. It appears, rather, to exert its cardiovascular effect through other risk factors. Thus weight gain raises blood pressure, LDL cholesterol, and blood glucose levels and increases sedentary behavior, whereas weight loss lowers each of these variables. Overweight is also associated with lower HDL levels.

The association of sedentary behavior, family history of premature heart disease, water hardness, and personality type with vascular disease risk seems clear cut. However, whether they represent primary or independent risk factors still must be clarified.

Although the existence of the risk factors enumerated above and their predictive value in assessing cardiovascular risk in an individual or group is now firmly established, evidence that modification of risk factors will alter cardiovascular risk is incomplete. Prospective and retrospective analysis leaves little doubt that cessation of cigarette smoking will decrease cardiovascular risk; in fact, it has been suggested that if all Americans stopped smoking, cardiovascular deaths would be reduced by at least 150,000 per year. Little doubt exists of the beneficial effects on many body functions of weight control and regular modest exercise. Therefore, although it has not been firmly established that weight reduction or exercise conditioning will decrease cardiovascular events, these measures are usually recommended. In the case of high blood pressure, there is little doubt that treatment of moderate and severe hypertension will decrease stroke, renal failure, and heart failure; hence we treat hypertension aggressively. Treatment of even mild hypertension reduces stroke and heart attack death. It remains unclear, however, whether treatment of elevated systolic pressure in the elderly is efficacious. Furthermore, the potential preventive benefit of salt restriction and weight control in those at risk for hypertension remains to be proved.

There is little doubt that dietary modifications in cholesterol and saturated fats will reduce levels of LDL cholesterol, and nonhuman primate studies suggest that cholesterol lowering through diet will actually lead to regression of existent atherosclerosis. Furthermore, the results of a recent clinical trial in man provide powerful evidence of the fact that lowering LDL levels lowers the risk of heart attack and heart death. The beneficial effect of lowering blood glucose levels is still being debated.

Conclusive demonstration of the benefit of risk factor modification is of central importance to our current approach to cardiovascular disease. The first clinical signs of cardiovascular disease may also be the last, because one fourth of first heart attacks manifest as sudden death. Epidemiologic evidence shows clearly that after a coronary event, the state of the heart and the degree of damage are more crucial than any of the aforementioned risk factors. There is little doubt therefore that the primary prevention of cardiovascular disease is important. If it can be demonstrated that the basic process of arteriosclerosis and hypertension can be delayed or prevented, either through risk factor modification or by other means, we will clearly have a very cost-effective remedy.

The striking association of the current waning cardiovascular "epidemic" with clear evidence of changing American life styles and habits is very hopeful. Since 1965 the percentage of men who smoke has fallen by 27 per cent, while the percentage of women smokers has decreased by 14 per cent. Between 1963 and 1981, there has been a 35.4 per cent decline in per capita tobacco consumption, a 16 per cent decline in the consumption of fluid milk and cream, a 37.7 per cent decline in butter consumption, a 16.7 per cent decline in egg consumption, a 39.3 per cent decline in the ingestion of animal fats and oils, and a 62.9 per cent increase in the ingestion of vegetable fats and oils. These concomitant changes have been associated with evidence of a 4 to 8 per cent decline in plasma LDL cholesterol levels in the United Staes in the past ten years. Americans are more conscious of the need for exercise. Since 1972, a government-sponsored National High Blood Pressure Education Program has increased by over 8 million the number of adult Americans aware of having hypertension, increased patient visits for hypertension by 50 per cent, and increased by an estimated 6 to 8 million the number of Americans under effective blood pressure control. These life style and habit changes coincide with a declining United States cardiovascular death rate (reinforced by the lack of evidence for a decline in either cardiovascular rates or risk factor status in Europe) and augur a potentially bright future for preventive cardiology.

Five-year findings of the Hypertension, Detection and Follow-up Program: I. Reduction in mortality of persons with high blood pressure, including mild hypertension. JAMA 242:2562, 1979. *Design, methods, and five-year mortality data of the HDFP with detailed tables and graphs. Small but useful reference list of other studies on hypertension.*

Food Consumption, Prices and Expenditures, 1960–1981. Economic Research Service, U.S. Department of Agriculture. Statistical Bulletin No 694, November, 1982. *A compendium of tabulations of per capita consumption data for agricultural products.*

Gordon T, Garcia-Palmieri MR, Kagan A, Kannel WB, Schiffman J: Differences in coronary heart disease in Framingham, Honolulu and Puerto Rico. J Chron Dis 27:329, 1974. *Comparison of differences in coronary heart disease incidence and mortality in three geographically distinct populations. Article explores the relationships of risk factors to coronary heart disease statistics in the three groups.*

Health, United States, 1981. U.S. Department of Health and Human Services, Public Health Service, National Center for Health Statistics, DHHS Pub No (PHS) 82-1232, December, 1981. *DHHS report presenting detailed information on incidence and death rates, health delivery costs, and prevention programs. Extensive tabular data on major diseases. Best single source for overview of nation's health.*

Levy RI, Feinleib M: Risk factors for coronary artery disease and their management. *In* Braunwald E (ed.): Heart Disease: A Textbook of Cardiovascular Medicine. 2nd ed. Philadelphia, W.B. Saunders Company, 1983, pp 1246–1278. *Comprehensive textbook chapter on cardiovascular risk factors, including treatment programs. Exhaustive reference list on all the evidence to date.*

Lipid Research Clinics Coronary Primary Prevention Trial Results: I. Reduction in incidence of coronary heart disease. JAMA 251:351, 1984. *Trial endpoint report on results of ten-year multicenter trial to evaluate effect of cholesterol lowering in man.*

Proceedings of the Conference on the Decline in Coronary Heart Disease Mortality. U. S. Department of Health, Education, and Welfare. Public Health Service. DHEW Pub No (NIH) 79-1610. *Review of all the evidence from a multidisciplinary group of experts. Very useful appendix containing figures and tables in death rates for both cardiovascular and noncardiovascular diseases since 1970.*

Stamler J: Population studies. *In* Levy RI, Rifkind BM, Dennis BH, Ernst ND (eds.): Nutrition, Lipids and Coronary Heart Disease. New York, Raven Press, 1979, pp 25–88. *Exhaustive review of all the epidemiologic evidence on diet, serum lipids, and coronary heart disease. Well documented with tables, figures, and excellent reference list.*

World Health Statistics Annual 1970–1981. World Health Organization. *Vital statistics and population data in tabular form by country.*

40. CIRCULATORY FUNCTION AND CONTROL

William W. Parmley

The normal cardiovascular system has a remarkable capacity to alter its performance. Such adjustments can increase cardiac output three to five times and heart rate two and a half times above basal values. The mechanisms responsible for this reserve capacity have been carefully studied over the years. The purpose of this chapter is to provide a general overview of cardiovascular function. In particular, clinically important concepts will be stressed.

FUNCTIONAL ANATOMY

The normal adult heart (weight approximately 300 grams) is about the size of a person's clenched fist—a gesture, interestingly enough, that the patient with angina pectoris frequently uses to describe the character of his cardiac discomfort. The atria are thin-walled shallow cups whose functional role is three-fold. When the atrioventricular (AV) valves are closed during ventricular systole, the atria serve a reservoir function by collecting blood from the systemic or pulmonary veins. In early diastole there is rapid ventricular filling following opening of the AV valves. In mid-diastole, the AV valves remain open so that the atria serve as a conduit for the continuous flow of blood from veins to ventricles. Toward the end of diastole active atrial contraction ejects another increment of blood into the ventricle just prior to ventricular systole (about 20 per cent of stroke volume). The normal atria are thin walled, because they pump into the ventricles during diastole at low pressure.

The right ventricle is a thin-walled volume pump which has a low filling pressure (about 5 mm Hg) and ejects blood into the low pressure pulmonary artery (about 20 mm Hg). The right ventricle is formed by a concave free wall which opposes the convex septal wall, thus creating a crescent-shaped slit between them. Ejection of blood occurs by both shortening of the free wall and movement toward the interventricular septum, which compresses the chamber by a bellows action. This latter mechanism is extremely efficient in ejecting a large volume of blood with a minimum of muscle shortening but can only function effectively at the low pressures normally found in the right-sided circulation.

The left ventricle is somewhat conical in shape, with its apex forming the apex of the heart. It can be considered as a thick-walled pressure pump whose medial wall is the thick interventricular septum. Ejection of blood from the left ventricle is primarily accomplished by a constriction of the muscular wall, although there is some shortening of the chamber.

The thickness of the ventricular wall is dependent on the relationship between wall stress, intraventricular pressure, and the radius of wall curvature as defined by the Laplace relation:

$$\sigma = \frac{PR}{2h}$$

(σ = wall stress [force/cross-sectional area], P = intraventricular pressure, R = radius of curvature of the wall, and h = wall thickness.) In general, wall stress is relatively constant throughout the heart. Thus the radius of curvature and wall thickness tend to be related. At the apex of the heart where the radius of curvature is short, the wall is thin. By contrast, the free wall of the left ventricle has a longer radius of curvature and a proportionally thicker wall.

Although emphasis is usually placed on a description of the systolic function of the heart, a greater appreciation of the importance of the diastolic properties of the heart has occurred in recent years. A thick hypertrophied ventricle with decreased compliance causes increased resistance to filling. This frequently leads to atrial dilatation and hypertrophy in order to maintain the atrial contribution to ventricular filling. The importance of this contribution is apparent in patients with severe hypertrophy caused, for example, by aortic stenosis or hypertrophic obstructive cardiomyopathy. Loss of an appropriately timed atrial contraction (as with atrial fibrillation) often results in marked exacerbation of left heart failure. In these patients during sinus rhythm, the left ventricular end-diastolic pressure is markedly elevated owing to a large A wave, whereas mean diastolic pressure, which is reflected back through the pulmonary veins into the lungs, is maintained at a lower level. When atrial contribution and the A wave kick are lost, however, there is an increase in mean left atrial and pulmonary venous pressures in an attempt to maintain the same level of end-diastolic pressure and cardiac output. This frequently leads to disabling dyspnea.

CARDIAC PERFORMANCE

We will first consider the factors that alter the performance of the heart and then integrate these factors into the overall function of the intact cardiovascular system. The four most important factors in determining the pump performance of the heart are preload, afterload, contractility, and heart rate.

Preload refers to the initial loading conditions of the heart. In isolated heart muscle, it is defined as the initial resting force stretching the muscle prior to contraction. In the intact heart, it is less easily defined. Estimates of preload include measurements of end-diastolic volume or end-diastolic pressure of the ventricle. In patients, it is often convenient to measure the filling pressures (atrial pressures) of the ventricles as an index of preload. Within limits, as one increases the preload (end-diastolic pressure or volume of the heart), there is an increase in cardiac performance, manifested by an increase in the pressure developed or in the volume of blood ejected. This represents the ascending limb of the familiar Frank-Starling relationship.

This overall relationship is often referred to as a ventricular function curve (Fig. 40–1). Some measure of cardiac performance, such as stroke volume or stroke work (stroke volume × arterial pressure), is plotted as a function of some measure of preload, such as atrial filling pressure or end-diastolic pressure. The concept of the ventricular function curve is important for several reasons. First of all, it allows for a comparison between subjective signs and symptoms and objective measurements. Thus as the level of left atrial pressure rises, the symptoms and signs of pulmonary congestion and edema appear. The ensuing dyspnea is the most common symptom associated with heart failure. The second major symptom complex in heart failure is fatigue resulting from reduced cardiac output. This is related to the vertical axis of the ventricular function curve, because cardiac output is the product of stroke volume and heart rate. This correlation between subjective symptoms and objective measurements is an important conceptual one in evaluating patients with cardiovascular disease.

An important application of preload alteration is exemplified by the therapy of patients with severe acute power failure. In such hypotensive patients, optimization of left ventricular filling pressure will maximize stroke volume or stroke work. The normal left atrial pressure is about 10 mm Hg. The optimal left atrial pressure in critically ill patients appears to be approximately 15 to 20 mm Hg. At higher pressures, there is no further improvement or, in some cases, an actual decline in cardiac performance, whereas the symptoms of pulmonary congestion will increase. In patients who are hypotensive with a very low left ventricular filling pressure, fluid administration is appropriate therapy to raise the filling pressure up to 15 to 20 mm Hg. This therapy is often sufficient to reverse the hypotension and low cardiac output state. An appreciation of preload therefore is of great practical importance in the characterization and management of patients with heart failure.

An important distinction must be made between the right atrial pressure, which represents the filling pressure of the right ventricle, and the left atrial pressure, which is the filling pressure of the left ventricle. Each atrial pressure is related to the functional status of its respective ventricle. In manipulating the volume status of the patients, however, it is far preferable to measure left ventricular filling pressure, because the left ventricle has a more important role in determining arterial pressure and forward cardiac output.

The term *afterload* refers to the load against which the heart must contract. In isolated heart muscle studies, it can be carefully defined as the load resisting shortening as the muscle is stimulated. In the intact heart, it is loosely approximated as the arterial pressure or impedance against which the heart has to work. The effect that afterload has on performance is relatively straightforward. As one increases arterial pressure, the stroke volume will go down because the ventricle has greater difficulty in ejecting blood against a higher load. Conversely, if one can reduce systemic vascular resistance and arterial pressure with vasodilator drugs, one can increase forward stroke volume and cardiac output. One must avoid severe

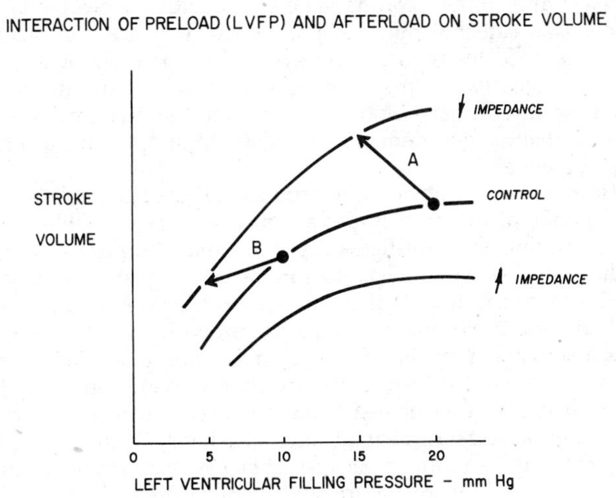

Figure 40–1. Representative ventricular function curves following changes in afterload (impedance). Stroke volume is plotted as a function of left ventricular filling pressure (left atrial pressure). A vasodilator drug such as sodium nitroprusside, which decreases impedance, will shift the ventricular function curve up and to the left. Beginning at a high filling pressure, there will be a decrease in filling pressure and an increase in stroke volume (line A). Beginning at a low filling pressure, nitroprusside will also shift the patient to a new curve, but there may be a reduction in stroke volume (line B) because the patient moves down the ascending limb of the function curve. (From Chatterjee K, Parmley WW: Prog Cardiovasc Dis 29:305, 1977.)

hypotension, however, which will compromise coronary blood flow and therefore reduce cardiac performance. The principle of afterload manipulation is one of the most important new concepts in cardiac therapy within the past decade. Vasodilator therapy for both acute and chronic heart failure is one of the most important adjuncts to more standard forms of therapy.

Changes in preload and afterload are closely related. Thus as the arterial pressure is increased, the ventricle has greater difficulty in ejecting blood and tends to retain more end-diastolic volume, thus increasing its preload. The opposite sequence of events occurs when the afterload is reduced. When one monitors arterial pressure and left atrial pressure simultaneously, particularly in patients with heart failure, the two frequently undergo directionally similar changes.

In terms of a ventricular function curve, vasodilator drugs which reduce both preload and afterload may affect function differently, depending on the initial level of left ventricular filling pressure. As illustrated in Figure 40–1, a vasodilator drug such as sodium nitroprusside, which reduces the resistance (impedance) to aortic ejection, will shift the ventricular function curve upward. Beginning at a high filling pressure (20 mm Hg), there will be both a reduction in filling pressure and an increase in stroke volume (line A, Fig. 40–1). At a normal filling pressure (10 mm Hg), the reduction in filling pressure will move the patient down the ascending limb of the ventricular function curve, and may reduce stroke volume (line B), even though the patient is on a higher curve.

Contractility refers to the vigor of contraction of heart muscle and is best defined in isolated heart muscle as an increased velocity of shortening at a given load. Drugs such as digitalis or the catecholamines increase contractility, whereas hypoxia, ischemia, acidosis, and certain antiarrhythmic drugs or beta-adrenergic blocking agents may reduce contractility. In terms of a ventricular function curve, drugs which increase contractility tend to increase stroke volume or stroke work at a given end-diastolic pressure. With a depression of contractility, the ventricular function curve shifts down and to the right with a reduction in stroke volume at a given left ventricular end-diastolic pressure. Alterations of contractility may not always be beneficial. For example, in patients with coronary artery disease and limited coronary flow, a positive inotropic agent such as a catecholamine will markedly increase contractility and the need for myocardial oxygen. The partially obstructed coronary circulation may not be able to deliver the necessary increase in coronary blood flow. Under these circumstances, myocardial oxygen demand may outstrip supply and produce further ischemia.

Heart rate is an obvious determinant of cardiac performance and is one of the most important mechanisms available to the heart to increase cardiac output (cardiac output = stroke volume × heart rate). The magnitude of the heart rate may be an important indicator of the cardiovascular status of an individual patient. For example, in a patient with acute failure who has a sinus tachycardia of 140, the reduction in stroke volume (downward shift in ventricular function curve) is so great that a marked elevation of heart rate has occurred in an effort to maintain cardiac output at an acceptable level. Of course, stroke volume may be reduced because of low preload (hypovolemia) or because of severe failure with a high preload. It may be necessary to measure the preload to resolve this dilemma. Other factors which raise heart rate must also be considered, including fever, anemia, thyrotoxicosis, and anxiety.

Although the importance of the ascending limb of the Frank-Starling curve is established, there is some question regarding the importance of a descending limb as preload is increased to extremely high levels. In general, studies in isolated heart muscle and whole heart preparations have shown that there is *not* a prominent descending limb. However, in patients with reduced cardiovascular reserve, it is possible to demonstrate a "descending limb" (reduction in cardiac performance and marked increase in preload) by provoking an exercise or afterload stress.

TABLE 40–1. PRESSURES AND VOLUMES IN THE NORMAL HEART

Pressures
- Left-sided
  1. Left atrial pressure (normal mean pressure ≤ 12 mm Hg)
  2. Left ventricular pressure
     a. Peak systolic pressure (wide normal range, usually 100–150 mm Hg in adults)
     b. Left ventricular end-diastolic pressure (normal ≤ 12 mm Hg)
  3. Aorta
     a. Systolic pressure (wide normal range, usually 100–150 mm Hg in adults)
     b. Diastolic pressure (wide normal range, usually 60–100 mm Hg in adults)
- Right-sided
  1. Right atrial pressure (normal mean pressure ≤ 6 mm Hg)
  2. Right ventricular pressure
     a. Peak systolic pressure (normal 15–30 mm Hg)
     b. Right ventricular end-diastolic pressure (normal ≤ 6 mm Hg)
  3. Pulmonary artery
     a. Systolic pressure (normal 15–30 mm Hg)
     b. Diastolic pressure (normal 4–12 mm Hg)

Volumes
- Left-sided (at rest)
  1. Left ventricular end-diastolic volume (normal 70–100 ml/m^2)
  2. Left ventricular end-systolic volume (normal 25–35 ml/m^2)
  3. Stroke volume (wide normal range, usually 40–70 ml/m^2)
  4. Ejection fraction (stroke volume divided by end-diastolic volume (normal 0.55–0.80)

Time-related measurements
  1. Heart rate (wide normal range, usually 60–100 beats/minute)
  2. Cardiac index (2.8–4.2 liters/minute/m^2)

Resistances
  1. Systemic vascular resistance (770–1500 dynes sec cm^{-5})
  2. Pulmonary vascular resistance (20–120 dynes sec cm^{-5})

As quantitative indices of cardiac performance, cardiac pressures and volumes can be measured in the cardiac catheterization laboratory, or in patients in critical care units. For reference, normal pressures, volumes, cardiac output, and vascular resistance are listed in Table 40–1. Volume measurements are normalized for interpatient comparison by dividing by the body surface area (square meters). This latter value is obtained from a standard table, based on height and weight. One useful index of left ventricular function is the ejection fraction, which is defined as stroke volume per end-diastolic volume. A normal ejection fraction is 0.55 or greater. In severe heart failure, ejection fraction may be reduced to less than 0.20.

PERIPHERAL CIRCULATION

The arterial system represents the conduit system for delivery of blood to all parts of the body. Blood pressure remains relatively constant in this system until one reaches the level of the terminal arteries and arterioles. There is about an 80 per cent drop in pressure across this latter network, which is primarily responsible for regulating the peripheral vascular resistance. The subsequent cross-sectional area of the capillaries is enormous so that the relatively large velocity of blood in the aorta (40 to 50 cm per second) is reduced to about 0.07 cm per second in the capillaries.

The venous system is not only responsible for return of blood to the heart, but at any time contains about 75 to 80 per cent of the total blood volume. These larger thin-walled vessels therefore are extremely important in regulating shifts in blood volume between the central and peripheral circulation, depending on their relative constriction or dilatation. Various therapeutic agents can produce important volume shifts. For example, in patients with heart failure, a potent diuretic such as furosemide and sublingual nitroglycerin both produce prompt dilatation of systemic veins, resulting in a redistribution of blood away from the central circulation into the peripheral circulation. This is effective in reducing pulmonary venous and left atrial pressures, thus improving the symptoms of pulmonary congestion.

Cardiac output has an important regional distribution, which may be altered in various pathologic states. For example, the kidney receives a high proportion of cardiac output (approximately 20 per cent), which is necessary for appropriate renal function. Abrupt reductions in cardiac output can compromise renal flow and markedly reduce urine output. Regional circulations, such as the cerebral and coronary circulations, have powerful autoregulatory capabilities so that blood flow can be maintained despite reductions in arterial pressure. Other regional circulations, including the skin and splanchnic bed, are often "sacrificed" during hypotension so that blood may be preferentially shunted to more vital organs.

The primary function of the heart is to pump nutrients and oxygen to all parts of the body. The amount of oxygen delivered to the body is the product of the cardiac output and the arterial-venous oxygen difference. During periods of reduced cardiac output, increased oxygen extraction by peripheral tissues can increase oxygen delivery to the body, although this is a minor compensatory mechanism. The kidneys have a relatively low demand for oxygen so that the arterial-venous oxygen difference across the kidneys is less than in the rest of the body. At the other end of the spectrum, the heart itself tends to extract oxygen nearly completely from the blood delivered through the coronary arteries. Thus an increase in oxygen delivery to the myocardium is accomplished primarily by an increase in coronary flow, rather than by an increase in oxygen extraction.

The capillary system has an enormous total surface area, which facilitates passage of substances into and out of the circulation. Lipid-soluble substances such as O_2 and CO_2 diffuse directly across the capillary walls. Blood flow in capillaries is not uniform and is dependent on the contractile state of the precapillary sphincters. True capillaries have no smooth muscle cells and therefore cannot actively change their cross-sectional area. Ions and small molecules move across the capillary walls at surprising rates, through pore sizes of 40 Å. The primary factor which restrains fluid from leaving the capillaries is the osmotic pressure of the plasma proteins, the most important of which is albumin. The Starling hypothesis states that hydrostatic forces are primarily responsible for fluid movement out of the capillaries, whereas oncotic pressure is primarily responsible for fluid movement back into capillaries. An example of imbalance between these forces is seen in pulmonary edema secondary to an increase in pulmonary venous pressure. Under these circumstances hydrostatic pressure exceeds oncotic pressure, resulting in movement of fluid into the interstitial space and eventually into the alveoli.

INTEGRATED CARDIOVASCULAR FUNCTION

A simplified overview of the circulatory system is diagrammatically illustrated in Figure 40–2. The four factors directly affecting cardiac muscle performance have already been discussed in relation to left ventricular performance. Similar factors apply to right ventricular performance and the pulmonary circulation, although they are not separately shown in Figure 40–2. The discussion to follow will summarize information related to these and other major factors listed in the diagram.

HEART RATE. The heart rate is determined by the frequency of the sinoatrial node impulses, which are related to the rate of depolarization of phase four of their action potential. Heart rate is also markedly affected by the autonomic nervous system. Branches of the sympathetic nerves increase heart rate via norepinephrine release, whereas branches of the vagus nerve decrease heart rate by release of acetylcholine. It appears that the parasympathetic system is the dominant factor in the normal control of heart rate. In individuals who have undergone exercise conditioning and have slow resting heart rates, the initial increase in heart rate during exercise is mediated by a gradual reduction in vagal tone. Only at higher levels of exercise are the sympathetic nerves active in increasing heart rate. On the other hand, in individuals who are not physically conditioned, the sympathetic influence is utilized much sooner in increasing heart rate. Emotional factors have an important influence on heart rate, as is evident during anxiety, fear, or anger. An increase in heart rate also occurs in anticipation of physical exertion before the exercise has been initiated.

Stretch receptors in both the carotid body and aortic arch exert important effects on heart rate. A change in arterial blood pressure alters the frequency of impulses from the baroreceptors to the central nervous system. In general, a drop in arterial pressure induces an acceleration of the heart, whereas an increase in arterial pressure tends to slow the heart. Similarly, externally applied digital pressure on a sensitive carotid body can promptly reduce heart rate. There are a number of other reflex effects mediated through the vagus nerve which may slow heart rate. These include stimulation of the respiratory tract as with intubation, nausea and vomiting, or painful stimuli. On the other hand, an increase in heart rate accompanies any activity in which there is an increase in sympathetic tone or in circulating catecholamines.

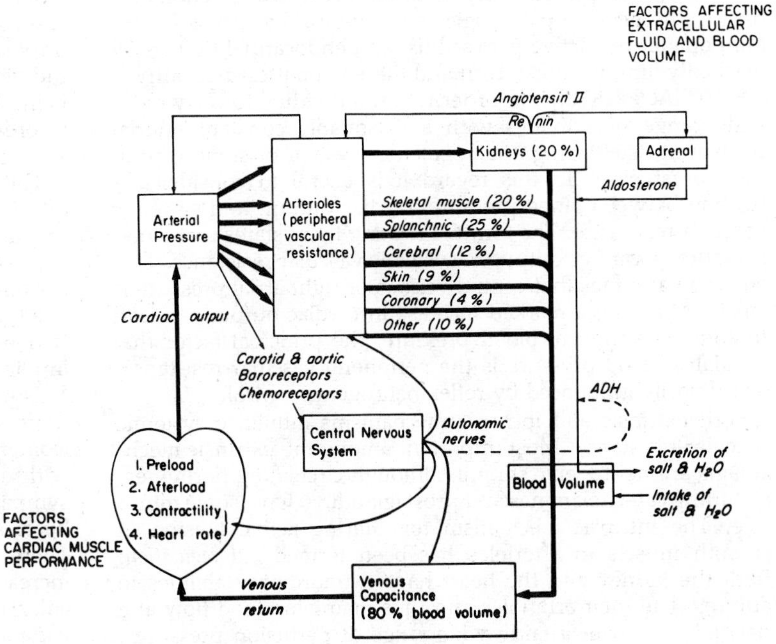

Figure 40–2. Schematic representation of the circulatory system. See text for details.

CARDIAC OUTPUT AND VENOUS RETURN. In general, the cardiac output is normally determined by the peripheral needs of the body. Thus the heart is a relatively passive organ in the circulatory system. It merely pumps out the blood that is returned to it, and cardiac output is determined by the venous return to the heart.

Changes in venous return and cardiac output are largely produced by the altered capacity of the peripheral vascular bed. Both an augmentation of blood volume and a reduction of venous capacitance will tend to augment venous return and raise cardiac output.

Any venoconstriction will improve cardiac filling by slightly elevating the pressure gradient for venous return, thereby displacing blood from the peripheral circulation toward the cardiopulmonary circulation. Since only about 20 per cent of the blood volume is in the arterial system, it is clear that there can be little displacement of blood by constriction of arteries or arterioles.

If one alters heart rate substantially under normal resting conditions, there is usually no change in cardiac output. As the heart rate goes up (as for example by artificial pacing), the stroke volume goes down in a reciprocal manner, and cardiac output remains constant. This further emphasizes the importance of peripheral factors in determining the normal cardiac output. The heart becomes the limiting factor in regulating cardiac output only when it begins to fail. When the diseased heart is unable to pump out all the blood that has returned to it and is unable to supply blood sufficient for the metabolic needs of the body, then a state of heart failure can be said to exist. Under these circumstances, the changes in cardiac output are extremely dependent on myocardial function, which then becomes the limiting factor. Under normal circumstances, however, the heart basically responds to the increased needs of the body and supplies the blood required by the organism at that particular time. Variations in venous return as produced by alteration in posture, activity, or intrathoracic pressure transiently influence cardiac output considerably. When one assumes the upright posture, gravitational forces tend to pool blood in the dependent parts of the body, which may transiently reduce venous return, central blood volume, and diastolic volumes of the heart. The normal changes in intrathoracic pressure which occur with breathing also influence the return of blood to the heart. During inspiration, the negative intrathoracic pressure enhances cardiac filling and stroke volume, whereas the reverse occurs during expiration. Changes in intrapericardial pressure may also markedly affect venous return to the heart in pathologic states. Pericardial effusion with tamponade, restrictive pericarditis, and endocardial fibrosis all markedly limit venous return and thereby limit cardiac output.

ARTERIAL PRESSURE. In order for an individual to carry out a wide range of activities with a reasonably constant arterial pressure, a stabilizing and regulatory system of some magnitude must exist. In this regard it is useful to consider the relation between blood pressure, cardiac output, and systemic vascular resistance. The formula relating them states that blood pressure = cardiac output × systemic vascular resistance. This equation assumes that central venous or right atrial pressure is small. Although a marked increase in cardiac output can lead to some elevation of blood pressure, the principal factor that regulates blood pressure is the peripheral vascular resistance, as primarily influenced by reflex neurogenic control.

Both extrinsic and intrinsic mechanisms influence systemic vascular resistance. Most important among the extrinsic mechanisms are neurogenic stimuli, although circulating hormones, including catecholamines and prostaglandins, have some minor role. The intrinsic mechanism for altering active tension of smooth muscle in arterioles has been termed *autoregulation.* Both the kidney and the heart have extraordinary abilities to autoregulate their arterioles and thus maintain blood flow at a needed level over a fairly wide range of perfusion pressures. This autoregulation is produced by two opposing mechanisms. Stretching of the vascular tissues increases the spontaneous activity of the smooth muscle and thus initiates progressive vasoconstriction. On the other hand, accumulation of tissue metabolites exerts a local vasodilator influence so that the opposing effects of pressure-induced vasoconstriction and metabolite-induced vasodilation tend to maintain flow at a level appropriate to the needs of the tissue. It is also possible that a decrease in oxygen in and of itself may be responsible for vasodilation. One clinically important vascular bed, however, that responds to hypoxia with vasoconstriction is the pulmonary bed, where pulmonary hypertension and pulmonary edema may occur at high altitudes with reduced oxygen content.

Although there are several pressure-sensitive receptors, the best studied baroreceptor involved in blood pressure control is the carotid body, which is located at the junction of the common carotid artery with its internal and external branches. Pressure-sensitive nerve endings in the wall of the receptor alter their discharge rate according to the pressure that is applied. At extremely high pressures the discharge rate is increased, whereas at low pressures the discharge rate from the carotid body is reduced. These impulses pass through the cardiovascular regulatory centers in the medulla, which then alter the relative magnitude of vagal and sympathetic tone. For example, as arterial pressure is increased, the impulses from the carotid body to the cardioregulatory center are also increased. These (1) stimulate the motor nucleus via the vagus to slow heart rate, and (2) inhibit the cardioaccelerator center, which reduces sympathetic tone and peripheral vascular resistance. This latter effect returns blood pressure toward the previous level. Alterations in the sympathetic vasoconstrictor outflow appear to be the most important mechanism for altering or producing changes in peripheral vascular resistance.

Chemoreceptors lying near the carotid bifurcation and in the aortic arch also respond to changes in pH, P_{CO_2} and P_{O_2}. Reduced oxygen, increased CO_2, or lowered pH stimulates the chemoreceptors and leads to an elevation of systemic arterial pressure. A marked reduction in arterial pressure can also make the brainstem ischemic and result in severe peripheral vasoconstriction mediated through the sympathetic nerves. This is presumably an attempt to raise arterial pressure to levels that would relieve the central nervous system ischemia. In general, these latter mechanisms are operative only under extreme conditions and probably are not involved in the normal regulation of arterial pressure.

CARDIOVASCULAR RESPONSE TO STRESS. A major principle related to the evaluation of the cardiovascular system is its response to an imposed stress. Under certain circumstances, resting function may be normal, whereas the response to an imposed stress may be grossly abnormal, thus detecting the individual with reduced cardiovascular reserve. This principle is implicit in history taking when one inquires about shortness of breath, fatigue, chest pain, or other symptoms provoked by exercise and other activities.

The cardiac response to exercise involves the interrelated effect of increased heart rate, catecholamine stimulation, and the utilization of the Frank-Starling mechanism. A treadmill exercise test or other specialized tests are useful in quantitating cardiovascular reserve. Two different stresses that have been used are isotonic and isometric exercise, which represent the two major types of exercise conditioning. Isometric exercise implies little change in the length of exercising skeletal muscles. This would occur during weight lifting or any exertion in which there is little movement of muscles. The usual response to isometric exercise is some degree of peripheral vasoconstriction with an increase in arterial pressure. There is an increase in sympathetic outflow, which increases the contractility of the heart and may result in a slight increase in cardiac output. There is also an increase in heart rate in response to the increased sympathetic tone. In patients with normal cardiovascular reserve, the ventricular function curve therefore shifts generally upward with little change in pulmonary capillary

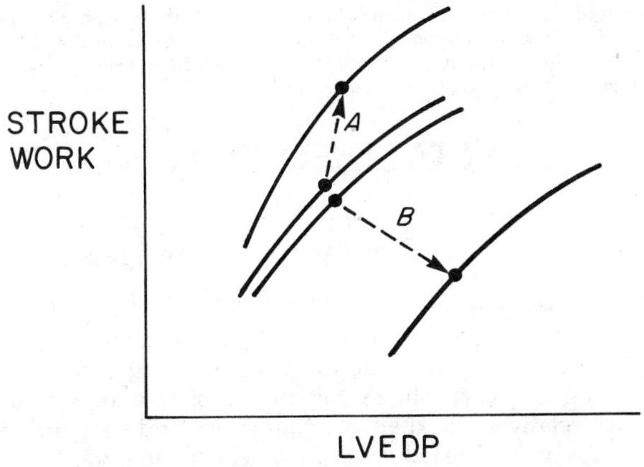

Figure 40–3. Altered ventricular function due to an elevation of arterial pressure produced by handgrip isometric exercise. A normal integrated response (patient A) shows an increase in stroke work with little change in left ventricular end-diastolic pressure (LVEDP). In this case, the increased contractile reserve has overcome the effects of the increased afterload (aortic pressure). The response of patient B indicates a substantial reduction in cardiovascular reserve. Under these circumstances, the marked increase in afterload has reduced the cardiovascular performance and produced a large rise in end-diastolic pressure.

wedge pressure (Fig. 40–3). Patients with poor ventricular reserve, however, may have an adverse response to the increased afterload produced by vasoconstriction. This is characterized by a substantial reduction in stroke volume or stroke work index and a marked rise in left ventricular filling pressure (Fig. 40–3). The response to isometric exercise therefore can be useful in quantitating the cardiovascular reserve of individual patients.

Isotonic exercise implies considerable muscle movement against a constant but low load. This is characteristic of walking, jogging, or running. Those who engage regularly in isotonic exercise programs will "train" their cardiovascular system. This results in a lower resting heart rate with a far greater capacity to increase cardiac output during subsequent exercise. With isotonic exercise, there is a marked reduction in systemic vascular resistance, primarily in the exercising muscles. This improves forward flow and markedly increases cardiac output.

The normal distribution of cardiac output at rest is indicated in Figure 40–2. With exercise, there is a substantial increase in relative and absolute blood flow to the skeletal muscles and skin. There is also an increase in flow through the coronary circulation, but little absolute change in flow to the splanchnic, cerebral, or renal beds.

With the onset of heart failure and a reduced resting cardiac output, there is a reduction in the percentage flow to the renal bed and skin. Exercise during heart failure produces a marked reduction in relative flow to the renal and splanchnic beds, with a greater proportion of flow going to exercising muscles. The absolute increase of flow to skeletal muscle, however, is far less than that found in a normal person during exercise.

Initially, it was assumed that changes in preload (Frank-Starling mechanism) were responsible for the increased cardiac output during exercise. However, most of the changes in cardiac output are mediated by an increase in heart rate. The adrenergic nervous system increases both heart rate and contractility, and leads to peripheral vasodilation. The tachycardia that occurs as a result of the increase in sympathetic tone tends to reduce the cardiac dimensions, and thus to counteract the changes which might occur if the heart were allowed to dilate via the Frank-Starling mechanism. During light or initial exercise, there may be a slight reduction in end-diastolic volume. Because of the increase in contractility of the heart, however, stroke volume tends to remain relatively constant, and the increase in cardiac output is produced primarily by the increase in heart rate. At more profound levels of exercise there may be a slight increase in heart size as the Frank-Starling mechanism is utilized.

BLOOD VOLUME. The magnitude of blood volume is another important factor affecting cardiovascular function. Some of the factors involved in the maintenance of extracellular fluid and blood volume are listed on the right-hand side of Figure 40–2.

An increase in blood volume as might occur by an increased intake of salt and water would increase cardiac output. This, in turn, would tend to increase arterial pressure and renal perfusion and thus increase urine output, which would decrease blood volume back toward normal. Atrial receptors sensitive to dilatation are also responsible for vasodilating reflexes to the kidneys, and reflexes to the central nervous system to diminish the secretion of ADH. Both these factors would tend to increase the output of urine. These volume receptors, however, appear to have only transient effects and are not operative during heart failure with high atrial pressures.

Loss of fluid volume occurs primarily through the kidneys. Sweating, respiratory, and gastrointestinal losses are usually less important, except during extreme conditions. Since approximately 20 per cent of the resting cardiac output passes through the kidneys, they provide an ideal location for regulating salt and water balance. Since this subject is discussed in detail elsewhere, only some of the pertinent factors will be mentioned here.

Reduction in renal perfusion (reduced pressure and flow) is sensed by the juxtaglomerular apparatus, which releases renin. Other factors, such as ischemia and sodium depletion, have also been suggested as stimuli that affect renin release. Overall, the phrase "effective blood volume" is a useful concept to keep in mind. Thus, decreased effective blood volume results in increased renin release, whereas increased effective blood volume turns off the stimulus for renin release. This concept forms the basis for alterations in sodium intake and volume as provocative tests for altering renin levels. Renin promotes the formation of angiotensin I from its precursor in the bloodstream. Angiotensin I is then converted to angiotensin II. Although angiotensin II is a powerful vasoconstrictor substance, this may not be its most important effect on blood pressure. Small subpressor doses of angiotensin II may increase aldosterone secretion, which may be one of its most important roles in regulating blood pressure. Angiotensin is also a potent stimulus for catecholamine release via the central nervous system vasomotor center and from the adrenal medulla.

Aldosterone promotes retention of salt and water. Under normal circumstances, salt and water intake are carefully balanced by their excretion. With congestive heart failure, there is an increased retention of salt and water, which leads to edema formation and increased blood volume. There are usually increased aldosterone levels in severe heart failure secondary to reduced renal perfusion, and probably also owing to decreased metabolism of aldosterone in the liver. It should be recalled that splanchnic flow is often reduced in heart failure, particularly during exercise.

In some patients with severe heart failure, free water excretion may also be severely impaired, and patients may be hyponatremic despite excess body sodium. Under such circumstances, restriction of fluid intake may be necessary to reduce fluid accumulation and reverse the hyponatremia. The potent diuretics available today are usually extremely effective in reversing the excess salt and water retention associated with heart failure. In some cases, excessive diuresis can lead to relative volume depletion and hypovolemia. Although uncommon, it is important to recognize this syndrome, because the associated hypotension and low cardiac output are effectively treated by liberalization of salt and water intake.

CIRCULATORY FAILURE. Heart failure is due to a number of causes, including mechanical or valvular defects, failure of the myocardium (cardiomyopathy), or loss of myocardium (myocardial infarction). In general, as myocardial failure occurs, there is reduction in heart muscle contractility, and the heart becomes the limiting factor in maintaining an appropriate level of cardiac output. In terms of the factors we have discussed, several characteristic alterations occur. First, cardiac output is decreased, and the preload of the heart is generally increased owing to the reduced ability of the heart to eject blood (reduced ejection fraction) and to an increase in circulating blood volume. This may lead to elevated filling pressures on *both* the right and left sides of the heart. Second, there is evidence that the reduction in cardiac output which accompanies heart failure leads to a reflex increase in peripheral vascular resistance in an attempt to maintain arterial blood pressure. This increase in peripheral vascular resistance increases the resistance to ejection and may therefore further reduce cardiac output, resulting in a vicious cycle. The presumed existence of this cycle is supported by the fact that arteriolar dilating drugs such as hydralazine are effective in increasing cardiac output in patients with severe heart failure, with no essential change in arterial pressure, heart rate, or pulmonary capillary wedge pressure. This suggests that systemic vascular resistance may be inappropriately high in heart failure for the level of cardiac output required. Also, the baroreceptor reflex mechanisms are mark edly blunted in congestive heart failure. Thus interventions which reduce arterial pressure do not produce the same reflex increase in heart rate as in the normal individual.

In heart failure, there is a generally heightened sympathetic tone to the peripheral vasculature and to the myocardium in an attempt to maintain cardiovascular compensation. This increased sympathetic tone causes more venoconstriction than in the normal individual, presumably in an attempt to maintain venous return and cardiac output. Heart rate may also be chronically elevated in heart failure in an attempt to maintain cardiac output. Arterial pressure often tends to be somewhat lower in heart failure as the ventricle loses the capacity to generate a normal or high blood pressure. In patients with hypertensive heart failure, however, blood pressure may remain at elevated levels for some time.

A consideration of the aforementioned factors suggests a rationale for the usual interventions employed in the treatment of chronic heart failure. Thus salt restriction and diuretics tend to reduce intravascular volume and reduce preload below the level responsible for dyspnea. Digitalis stimulates the failing myocardium to increase its contractile state and thus improves the ability of the heart to eject blood. An inappropriately high systemic vascular resistance can be treated with arteriolar dilators to reduce the resistance to ejection and thus increase cardiac output. Venodilators, such as nitroglycerin, which predominantly dilate veins can redistribute blood away from the central circulation and also reduce pulmonary capillary wedge pressure.

In summary, the cardiovascular system is a complex, carefully regulated system which has extraordinary capabilities for altering its performance over wide ranges in response to the needs of the body. Usually the cardiac output is determined by the peripheral needs of the body as regulated by changes in venous return. Only when the heart is unable to meet these peripheral needs does a state of "heart failure" occur. At this point, the four factors affecting cardiac muscle performance become important considerations, and their regulation forms the basis of most of our therapeutic interventions in chronic heart failure.

Braunwald E (ed.): Heart Disease: A Textbook of Cardiovascular Medicine. 2nd ed. Philadelphia, W. B. Saunders Company, 1983, Chapters 12–14. *Excellent current review of cardiac performance from the cellular level to the intact heart. Also includes the pathophysiology of heart failure.*

Chatterjee K, Parmley WW: Vasodilator therapy for acute myocardial infarction and chronic congestive heart failure. J Am Coll Cardiol 1:133, 1983. *Overall review of the use of vasodilator drugs in both acute and chronic heart failure.*

Guyton AC: Circulatory Physiology: Cardiac Output and Its Regulation. Philadelphia, W. B. Saunders Company, 1963. *Classic text on the importance of venous return and the relationship between venous return and cardiac output.*

Parmley WW, Talbot L: Heart as a pump. *In* Berne R (ed.): Handbook of Circulation. Baltimore, Waverly Press, 1979, Chapter 11. *Discussion of pump performance and valvular function. Expands on many of the concepts mentioned in this chapter.*

Rushmer RF: Structure and Function of the Cardiovascular System. Philadelphia, W. B. Saunders Company, 1976, Chapters 3–7. *Classic text with excellent illustrations. Focuses on concepts and mechanisms of organ function rather than quantitative aspects of physiologic data.*

41. SPECIALIZED DIAGNOSTIC PROCEDURES

41.1. Radiography of the Heart

Charles E. Putman

The standard posteroanterior (PA) and lateral chest radiographs are the most frequently used imaging procedures in evaluating the heart. The examination is simple to perform and requires relatively inexpensive equipment and very little technical expertise. The advantages of chest radiographs in the evaluation of the cardiac patient are as follows: (1) an experienced observer may detect significant abnormalities not available by other noninvasive methods; (2) recognized abnormalities may be followed, and response to therapy can be documented; and (3) results are easily reproducible, and the radiograph provides a reliable comparative index to changing pathology or alteration of normal cardiovascular function.

TECHNIQUE

There is considerable variation in the configuration of the normal cardiac silhouette. The two most important factors influencing cardiac size and shape are (1) thoracic cavity dimensions and symmetry of the musculoskeletal structure and (2) intrathoracic pulmonary pressure. As the diaphragm descends during normal inspiration, the heart will become smaller and more vertical and conversely during expiration the heart will be larger and more transverse. If the radiograph is exposed during a Valsalva maneuver, there will be a decrease in heart size because of decreased venous return secondary to increased intrathoracic pressure. Variation of technical factors from one examination to another may be responsible for misinterpretation of cardiac dimensions.

INTERPRETATION

To evaluate the cardiovascular status adequately, a systematic approach to reading the standard PA and lateral radiographs is necessary (Figs. 41–1 and 41–2). In addition to evaluating the heart, one should study the great vessels, the pulmonary vascularity, the pleura, the bones, the abdominal viscera, and the extrathoracic structures that may provide useful clues to diagnosis. It is necessary to know which chambers and vascular structures contribute to the cardiac boundaries in the two standard views (Figs. 41–1 to 41–4). When there is suggestive evidence of heart disease, two additional views, the right and left anterior oblique views, may be obtained (Figs. 41–5 and 41–6). These four radiographs are called "the cardiac series" and are usually obtained following the swallowing of barium sulfate to outline and distend the esophagus. Encroachment on the esophageal column by enlarged or displaced cardiac chambers can then be more easily ascertained and the appropriate differential diagnosis facilitated. The value of these views in defining specific cardiac pathology is illustrated in Figures 41–7 to 41–10.

HEART SIZE. Cardiac enlargement is the single most important observation in the suspect cardiac patient, and yet it can be a difficult assessment from the chest radiograph. Various measurements of heart size have been suggested, but the most reliable is a nomogram published by Ungerleider and Gubner. A series of tables indicates predicted normal transverse cardiac diameter for adults of various heights and weights. In actual practice, these tables are rarely used, and instead the cardiothoracic ratio is employed. This measurement is determined by dividing the maximal transverse diameter of the heart by the maximal transverse diameter of the thorax on the PA radiograph. The normal cardiothoracic ratio averages 0.45, but

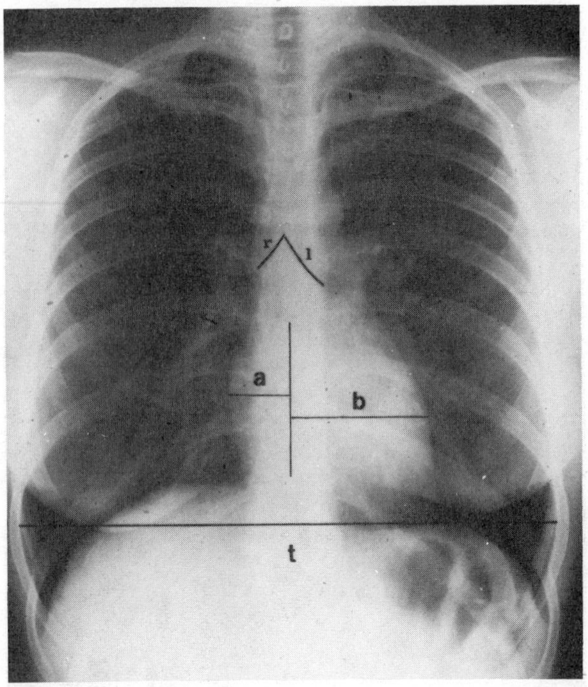

Figure 41–1. Normal PA view. a = transverse diameter of the heart to the right of the midline; b = transverse diameter of the heart to the left of the midline; t = transverse diameter of the thorax; l = lower margin of the left stem bronchus; r = lower margin of the right stem bronchus. The measurements of the right descending pulmonary artery (arrow) are 10 to 15 mm for males and 9 to 14 mm for females. The maximal normal angle between the two bronchi is 75 degrees for adults in deep inspiration. The cardiothoracic ratio = a + b/t.

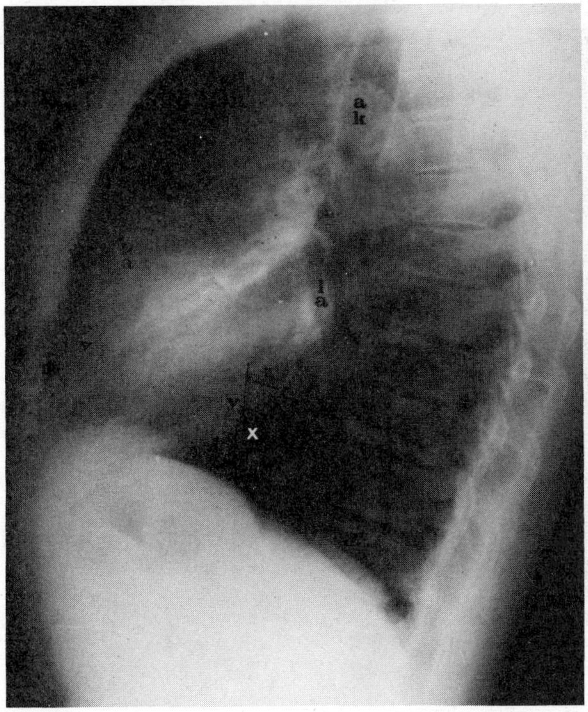

Figure 41–2. Normal lateral view. x = the crossing point between the inferior vena cava and the posterior border of the left ventricle; y = distance from point x, 2 cm cephalad along the inferior vena cava; z = posterior dimension of the left ventricle (according to Hoffman and Rigler), which should be smaller than 1.8 cm. Other abbreviations are as in Figure 41–3. Arrow points to the removal position of the subpericardial fat line (very close to the sternum).

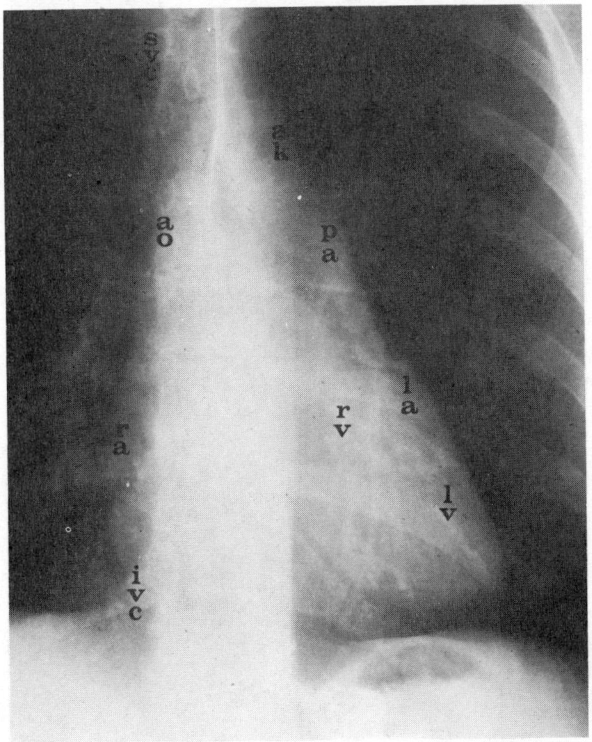

Figure 41–3. PA view of the chest with barium in the esophagus. The major border-forming cardiovascular structures are marked as follows: ak = aortic knob (the arch joining the transverse and descending portions of the thoracic aorta); pa = pulmonary artery (the pulmonary trunk); la = left atrium; lv = left ventricle; rv = right ventricle (left lateral border); ivc = inferior vena cava; ra = right atrium; ao = ascending aorta; svc = superior vena cava.

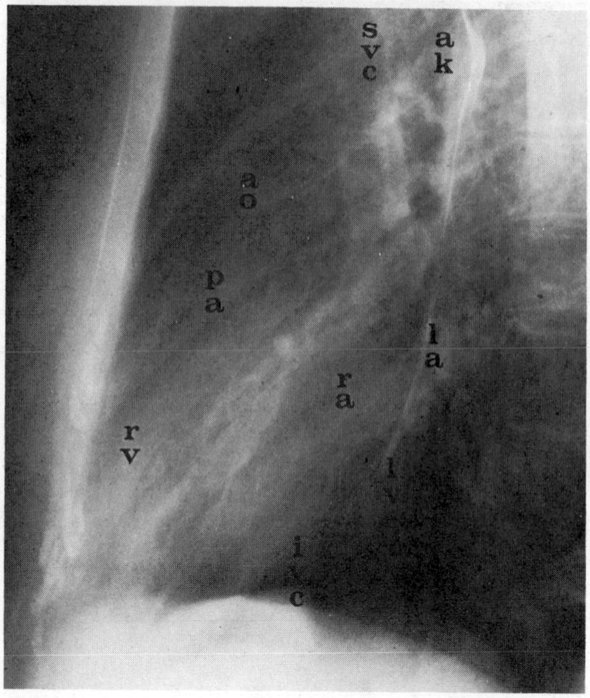

Figure 41–4. Left lateral view of the chest with barium in the esophagus. Abbreviations are as in Figure 41–3.

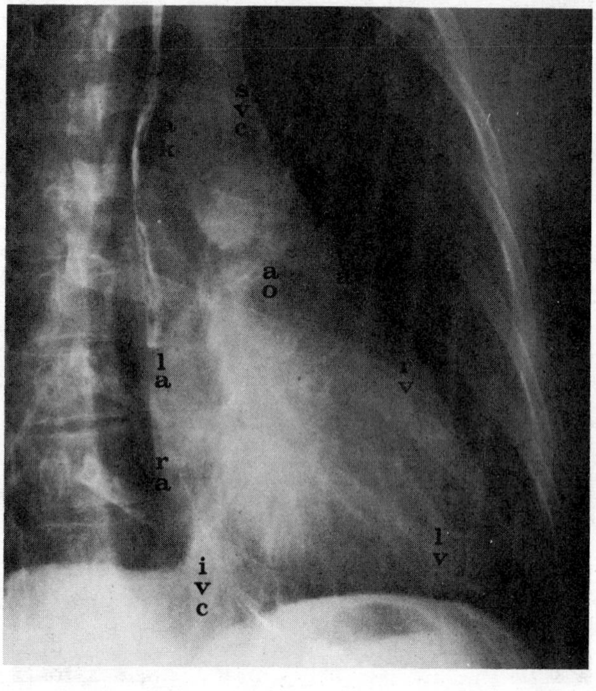

Figure 41–5. Forty-five degree right anterior oblique (RAO) view with barium in the esophagus. Abbreviations are as in Figure 41–3.

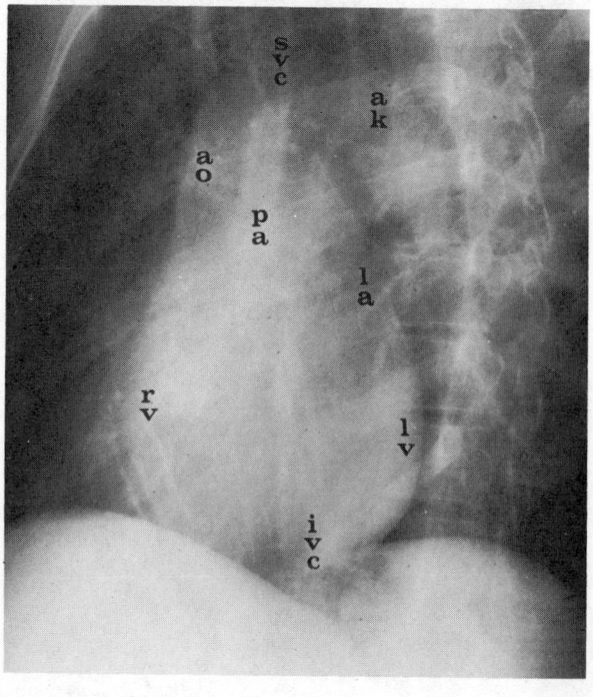

Figure 41–6. Sixty degree left anterior oblique (LAO) view without barium in the esophagus. Abbreviations are as in Figure 41–3.

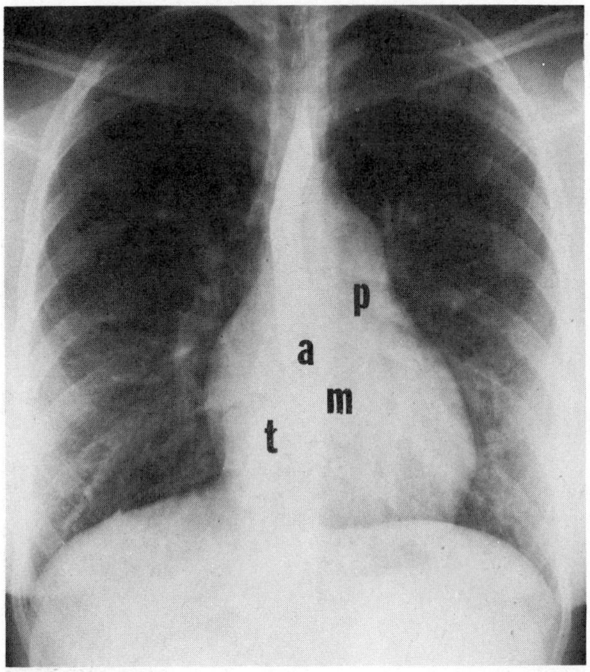

Figure 41–7. PA view of a patient with secundum atrial septal defect showing bilateral increase in pulmonary vascularity, right-sided cardiomegaly, marked dilatation of the pulmonary trunk, and an inconspicuous aortic knob. There is no deviation of the barium-filled esophagus or double density to suggest left atrial enlargement. The four cardiac valve positions are marked as follows: a = aortic valve; m = mitral valve; p = pulmonic valve; t = tricuspid valve.

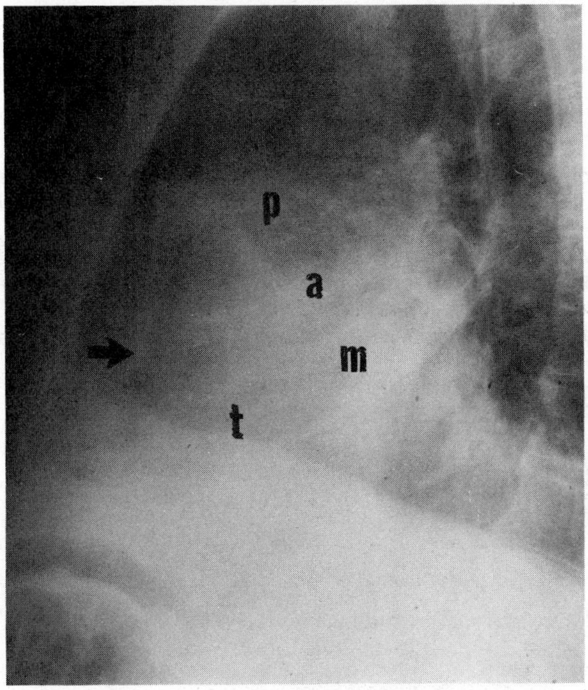

Figure 41–8. Lateral view of a patient with chronic renal failure with a large pericardial effusion showing marked posterior displacement of the subepicardial fat line (arrow). The four valve positions are marked in the same manner as in the PA view (Fig. 41–7).

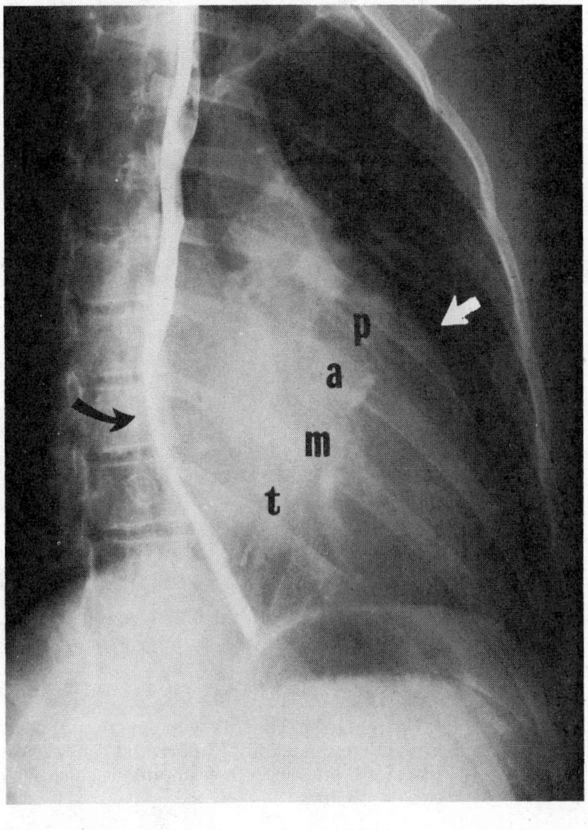

Figure 41–9. RAO view of a patient with mitral stenosis. Note that the barium-filled esophagus is deviated posteriorly by the enlarged left atrium (curved arrow). The right ventricular enlargement presents as an anterior bulge along the upper cardiac border (straight arrow). The four cardiac valve positions in this view are designated as in Figure 41–7.

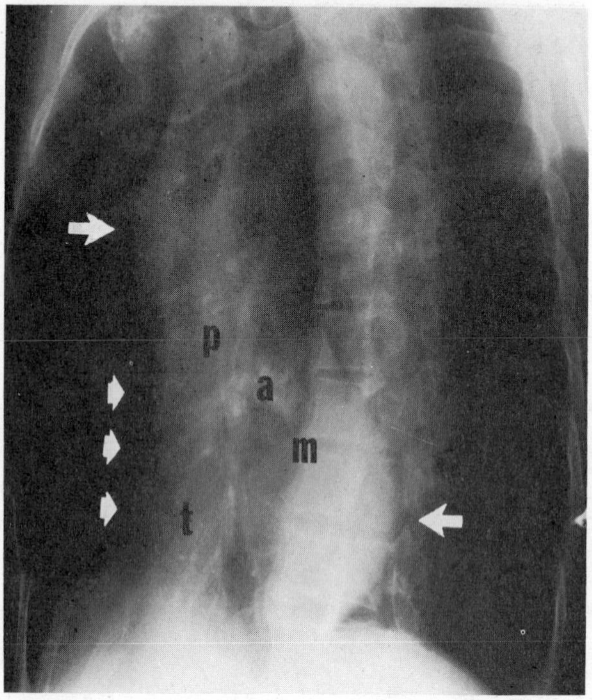

Figure 41–10. LAO view of a patient with cardiac aortic stenosis. The four valve positions are labeled as in Figure 41–7. Heavy aortic valve calcification is visible (a). The upper long arrow points to the post-stenotic dilatation of the ascending aorta. The hypertrophied left ventricle is marked by the lower long arrow posteriorly. The three short arrows point to the left anterior cardiac border formed by the normal right ventricle.

values up to 0.55 may be seen in normal subjects with a greater than average stroke volume. Measurements from the chest radiographs (Figs. 41–1 and 41–2), like other measurements in medicine, are only statistically reliable when applied to subgroups and are therefore less consistent for a given individual. Radiographic cardiac measurements are most meaningful when they can be compared to measurements from previous radiographs of similar quality and technique. Solitary chamber enlargement without cardiomegaly is usually better delineated by the electrocardiogram than by the radiograph.

PULMONARY VESSELS. Following the determination of cardiac size and chamber predominance, an evaluation of the pulmonary vessels allows for a more precise differential diagnosis. There are four basic patterns of abnormal pulmonary circulation

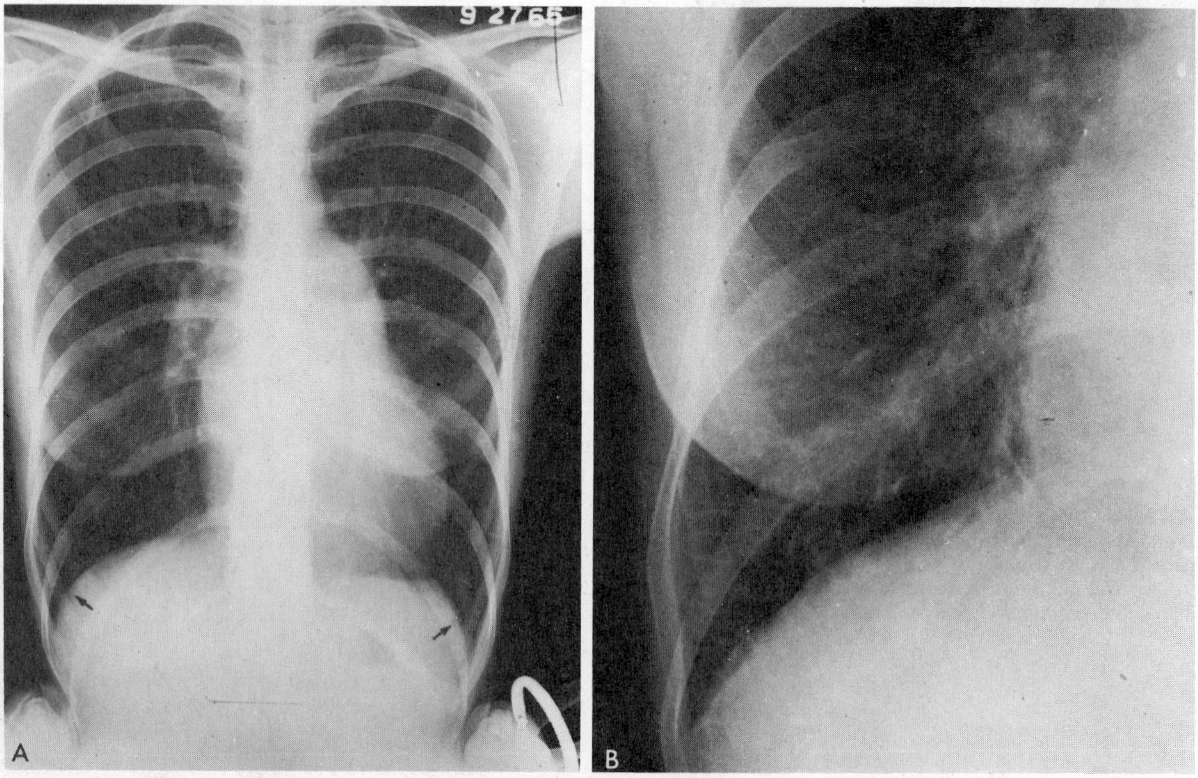

Figure 41–11. Patients with severe mitral stenosis. *A*, PA view shows striking redistribution of pulmonary blood flow. Note dilatation of upper and central vessels and constriction of lower and peripheral vessels. Arrows indicate Kerley's B lines in both costophrenic sulci. *B*, Magnified view of the right lower lung zone, showing multiple distinct Kerley's B lines.

identified by the standard radiograph. Certain groups of diseases may be identified on the basis of (1) decreased flow, (2) increased flow, (3) increased pulmonary resistance, or (4) pulmonary venous hypertension. Each has a specific radiographic pattern that allows for discrimination.

With *decreased pulmonary flow* (e.g., tetralogy of Fallot) there is a decrease in size of the central and peripheral vessels. *Increased pulmonary flow* is indicative of high output states (e.g., hyperthyroidism) or more commonly of left-to-right shunts (e.g., atrial septal defect). With small shunts, no abnormality may be detected by the standard radiograph. Larger shunts cause enlargement and tortuosity of the central and peripheral vessels (Fig. 41–7). Increased pulmonary resistance or *pulmonary arterial hypertension* is identified by dilatation of the central vessels and narrowing or attenuation of the peripheral vessels. *Pulmonary venous hypertension* is a more common hemodynamic state and is usually due to mitral stenosis or left heart failure. In upright man, 60 to 70 per cent of the blood flow normally goes to the lower portion of the chest. This can be appreciated on the standard PA radiograph by visualizing larger vessels at the lung bases than in the upper zones of the lung. Pulmonary venous hypertension produced by increased resistance distal to the pulmonary capillaries causes distention and recruitment of upper lobe vessels because of diversion of blood from the constricted lower zones. Radiographically, this produces an equalization of vascular caliber between the upper and lower lobes. As left heart pressure increases, upper lobe vessels become larger than lower lobe vessels (Fig. 41–11*A*). The ability of the radiograph to detect these subtle changes in left heart pressure is an adequate indication to obtain chest radiographs periodically in patients who are prone to heart failure, e.g., the hypertensive patient.

HEART FAILURE. Other radiologic signs of incipient congestive heart failure may not be so obvious. When the pulmonary venous pressure exceeds 20 mm Hg, fluid will begin to accumulate in the interstitium of the lung. Radiographically, this is detected by the appearance of Kerley's B lines (edema of interlobular septa), which are thin horizontal reticular lines seen most often in the costophrenic angles (Fig. 41–11*B*). Also, the hilar structures may be indistinct and the peripheral vessel margins hazy. As the pulmonary venous pressure exceeds 30 mm Hg, alveolar edema and pleural effusion appear—classic radiographic signs of congestive heart failure.

PERICARDIAL EFFUSION. A large heart does not always imply heart failure but may be indicative of pericardial effusion. A rapidly enlarging cardiac silhouette without evidence of pulmonary venous congestion strongly suggests pericardial fluid accumulation, especially if of the "water-bottle" configuration. A more definitive radiographic sign of pericardial effusion is the inward displacement of the subepicardial fat line (Fig. 41–8; compare with Fig. 41–2).

FLUOROSCOPY. Fluoroscopy, the technique for visualizing the shadows of the radiograph and projecting the image on a recording device such as a television monitor, is a technique commonly applied to evaluate dynamic function of various organ systems. Occasionally it may clarify questionable abnormalities depicted on the standard two- or four-view radiographs of the heart. Pulsation and calcification are better evaluated by fluoroscopy than by static films. Pericardial calcification is curvilinear and is usually seen in the anterior portion of the cardiac shadow. Valvular calcifications are usually seen as multiple dense opacities in the respective valve regions (Figs. 41–10 and 41–12). Myocardial calcification, following myocardial infarction, is linear in distribution and usually occurs at the cardiac apex. Fluoroscopy can reveal faint calcifications in the coronary vessels (Fig. 41–12), which always signify atherosclerosis.

Decrease in cardiac pulsations is suggestive of pericardial effusions, constrictive pericarditis, cardiomyopathy, or generalized cardiac failure. Localized decrease in cardiac motion may be seen in myocardial infarction, and paradoxical movement may be indicative of a ventricular aneurysm. Increased cardiac motion may indicate hyperthyroidism, hypertension, anemia, or aortic insufficiency.

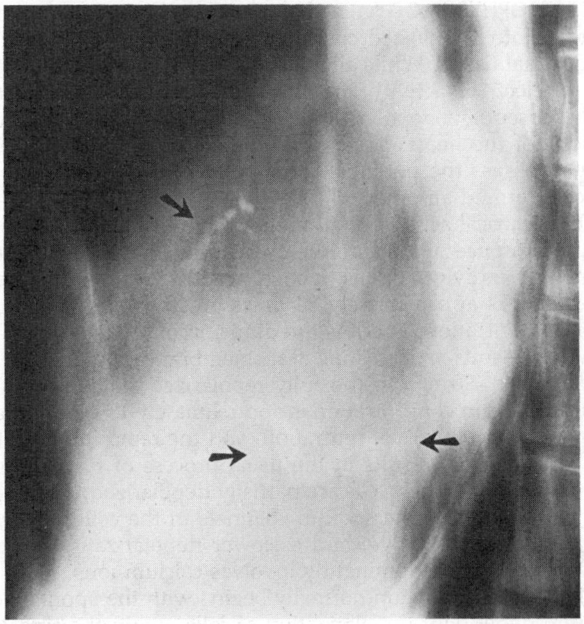

Figure 41–12. Lateral tomogram of a patient with severe calcific mitral stenosis. The heavily calcified mitral valve is indicated by the two opposing arrows. The upper arrow points to a heavily calcified anterior descending coronary artery.

An accurate assessment of the standard radiograph in the evaluation of the suspect or known cardiac patient will depend on an understanding of normal anatomy and physiology, and an appreciation of the reliability and limitations of the radiographic image. Accurate and skillful radiographic interpretation requires a thorough knowledge of the clinical history and physical findings, as well as of radiographic signs.

Chen JT: The plain radiograph in the diagnosis of cardiovascular disease. Radiol Clin North Am. Editor Charles E. Putman, 1984. *This article is the most comprehensive review of the conventional radiograph in evaluation of the cardiovascular system. The bibliography accompanying this paper is current and thorough.*

Colley RN, Capp MP, Lester RG, Meszaros WT, Swischuk LE: Plain Film Diagnosis of Cardiovascular Disease. Syllabus Set 14, Copyright American College of Radiology, 1979. *This is an excellent syllabus and self-evaluation text encompassing all aspects of the interpretation of conventional radiographs. A broad spectrum of cardiac cases is presented, always emphasizing the correlation of the radiographic abnormalities with pertinent clinical, laboratory, and electrocardiographic data.*

41.2. Electrocardiography

Joseph C. Greenfield, Jr.

The electrocardiogram (ECG) is a graphic representation of the electrical activity generated by the heart during the cardiac cycle which is recorded from the body surface. In 1903, Wilhelm Einthoven used a string galvanometer to record the first EKG (Elektrokardiogramm, Ger.). Shortly thereafter, a clinically useful instrument was manufactured by the Cambridge Scientific Instrument Company. Following the pioneering work of Frank N. Wilson and his associates in the development of lead systems in the 1930's, the ECG became standardized. It now consists of 12 leads. The availability of the direct-writing instrument in the 1950's allowed a rapid increase in the routine use of the ECG. The recent use of recorders that obtain three leads simultaneously has markedly improved the diagnostic accuracy and reduced the processing time. At present, the ECG is the most commonly employed noninvasive diagnostic tool in cardiology. Approximately 75 million ECGs are recorded each year in the United States alone.

ELECTROPHYSIOLOGY. Cardiac muscle may be conveniently divided into specialized conducting tissue and nonspecialized myocardial tissue. While all myocardial cells possess the potential for electrical activity, the rate and pattern of depolarization and subsequent repolarization differ markedly in different regions of the heart. Some cells of the specialized conducting tissue possess the potential for spontaneous depolarization, a process termed automaticity.

The electrical activity of all myocardial cells is made possible by the presence of ionic gradients maintained across the membranes of individual cells. The concentration of intracellular potassium is approximately 30 times greater than its extracellular concentration, and it is the diffusion of this ion out of the cell that results in a resting transmembrane potential of approximately −90 mV in the fully repolarized state. The extracellular sodium concentration is approximately 15 times greater than its intracellular concentration, and the rapid influx of this ion into the cells results in the usual process of rapid cellular depolarization. When cells are partially depolarized to less than −55 mV, however, the sodium channels in the cell membrane are no longer operative, and a slower depolarization process may occur that predominantly involves calcium ions.

Myocardial activation normally begins with the spontaneous calcium dependent depolarization of cells within the sinoatrial (SA) node located at the junction of the right atrium and superior vena cava. The impulse then propagates in a wavelike fashion through the atrial myocardium to the atrioventricular (AV) node located in the lower portion of the interatrial septum. Conduction through the AV node primarily involves the calcium dependent process of depolarization and is delayed owing to membrane properties of nodal cells. The membrane properties in the proximal and distal segments of the AV node vary such that conduction in the proximal segment is slow and may occur with decrement, whereas conduction in the distal segment is more rapid.

The impulse is rapidly transmitted through the bundle of His, which then bifurcates into the narrow right bundle branch (RBB) and the fibers which become the left bundle branch (LBB). The LBB divides further into two main collections of fibers forming the anterior (superior) and posterior (inferior) fascicles. The distal portion of the specialized conducting system is a network of smaller fibers termed the Purkinje system, which is responsible for delivering the propagated impulse to the nonspecialized ventricular tissue, resulting in a synchronized myocardial contraction.

LEAD SYSTEMS. Five electrodes are used in the standard ECG lead system. One is placed on each of the four limbs and one at different locations on the anterior chest wall (in instruments that record three leads simultaneously, there are six separate chest electrodes; Table 41–1). The right leg electrode functions as a ground lead. In recording the standard frontal plane limb leads, I, II, and III, the right arm, left arm, and left leg are used as follows: Lead I measures the potential difference between the right arm (−) and the left arm (+). Lead II measures the potential difference between the right arm (−) and the left leg (+). Lead III measures the potential difference between the left arm (−) and the left leg (+). This is the original bipolar lead configuration designed by Einthoven. The other three frontal plane leads, AVR, AVL, and AVF, are constructed using the central terminal of Wilson, which augments the voltage output, hence the prefix AV, and functions as an inactive reference point. The exploring electrode is placed on the right arm (AVR), left arm (AVL), and left leg (AVF), and functions as a positive unipolar lead. The relationship among the six frontal plane leads is shown in Figure 41–13. The six chest leads also function as unipolar leads, using the central terminal as the reference point; the chest leads are the positive electrodes. The spatial relationship between the chest electrodes is illustrated in Figure 41–14. The ECG leads are recorded in sequence, beginning with lead I, II, and III, followed by AVR, AVL, and AVF, and then the chest leads from V1 through V6. In many recently designed instruments, three lead sets are recorded simultaneously. A normal ECG recorded in this manner is illustrated in Figure 41–15.

The ECG is recorded on a paper chart, using a standard paper speed of 25 mm per second. The paper is marked with a vertical light line every millimeter (0.04 second) and a heavy vertical line every 5 mm (0.20 second). The paper also has

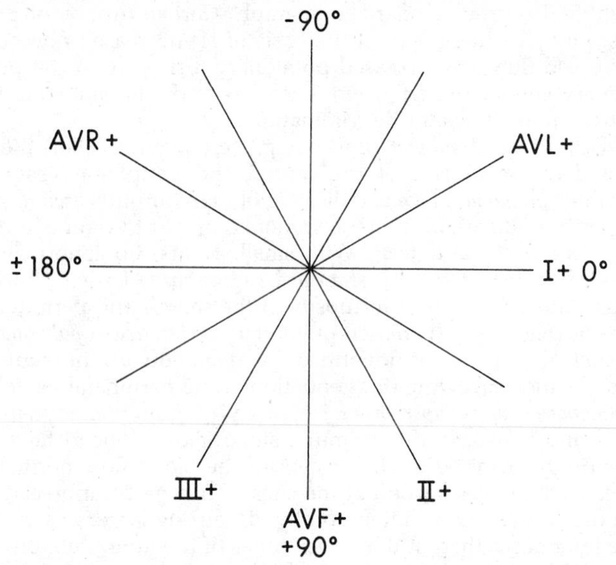

Figure 41–13. The limb leads are used to form a hexaxial reference system for the frontal plane. The axis of each lead is separated by approximately 30 degrees from the axis of the two adjacent leads.

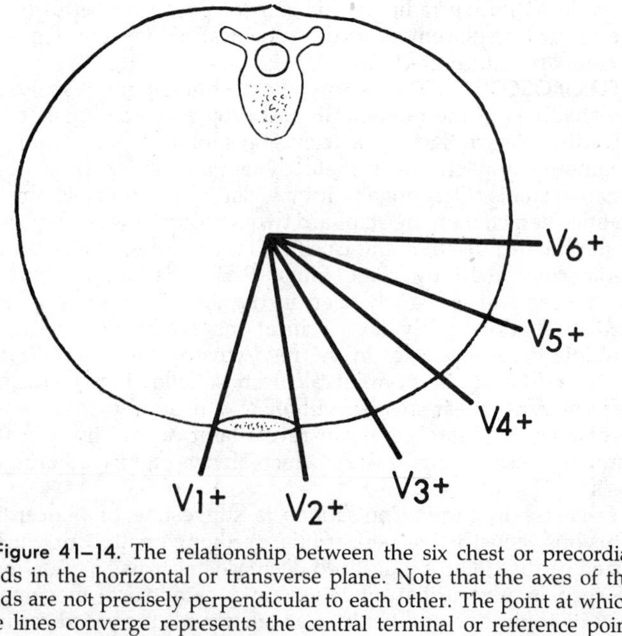

Figure 41–14. The relationship between the six chest or precordial leads in the horizontal or transverse plane. Note that the axes of the leads are not precisely perpendicular to each other. The point at which the lines converge represents the central terminal or reference point for the respective chest electrodes.

TABLE 41–1. POSITION OF CHEST LEADS

V1	Fourth intercostal space (ICS) at the right sternal border
V2	Fourth ICS at the left sternal border
V3	Halfway between V2 and V4
V4	Fifth ICS at the left midclavicular line
V5	Fifth ICS at the anterior axillary line
V6	Fifth ICS at the midaxillary line

When several sequential ECGs are to be obtained, e.g., in the coronary care unit, it is important to mark the location of the chest electrodes to minimize changes in the waveform resulting from variation in electrode placement.

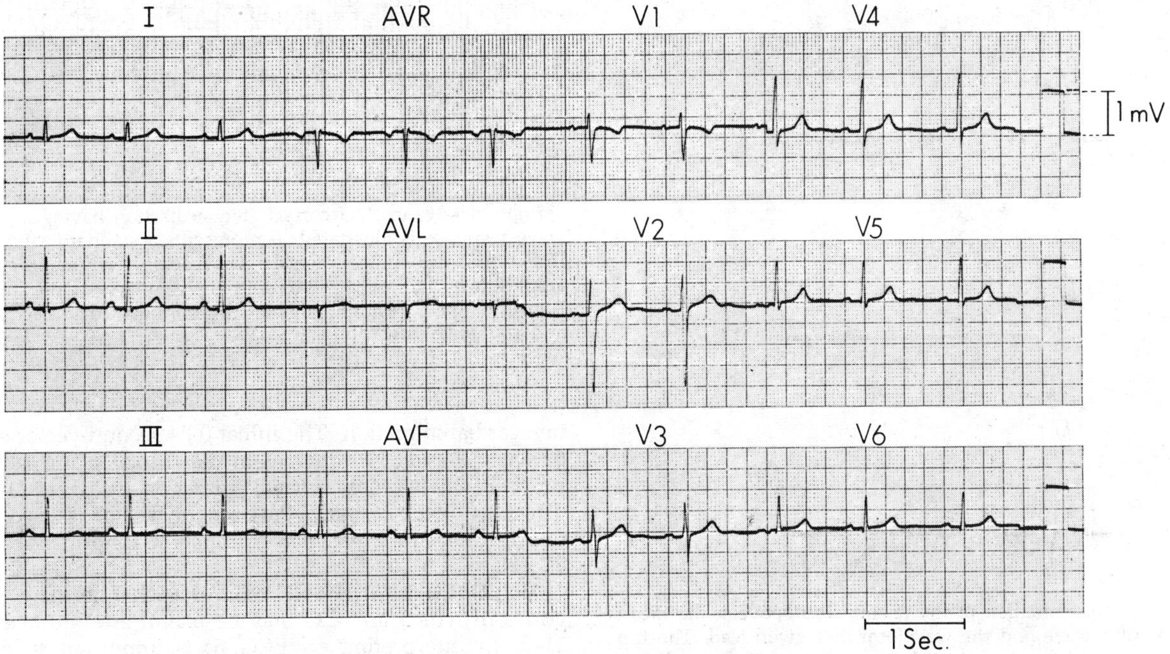

Figure 41–15. Normal electrocardiogram; the three leads in each column or lead set are recorded simultaneously.

horizontal lines separated by 1 mm and a dark horizontal line every 5 mm. Vertical deflection is calibrated in terms of voltage so that 10 mm equals 1.0 millivolt.

WAVEFORMS. The waveforms and intervals of the ECG are shown in Figure 41–16. The P wave is the electrical activity recorded during atrial depolarization and, in the normal ECG, precedes ventricular depolarization. The QRS complex occurs during ventricular depolarization. The Q wave is the initial downward deflection, the R wave is the initial upward, and the S wave the second downward deflection. A second upward deflection or a third downward deflection is defined as R′ or S′, respectively. It is not necessary that a Q, R, and S be present in each lead; e.g., if the entire lead is negative, it is termed a QS wave. The time from the onset of the P wave to the beginning of ventricular depolarization is the P-R interval; normally the range is 0.12 to 0.20 second. The QRS duration is normally less than 0.10 second. The T wave is inscribed during the period of ventricular repolarization. The electrical activity during atrial repolarization is usually masked by the QRS complex. The interval from the end of ventricular depolarization to the beginning of the T wave is termed the S-T segment. The interval from the onset of ventricular depolarization to the end of the T wave is the Q-T interval. This interval is a function of rate. A small deflection following the T wave is the U wave; the origin of this waveform is unknown.

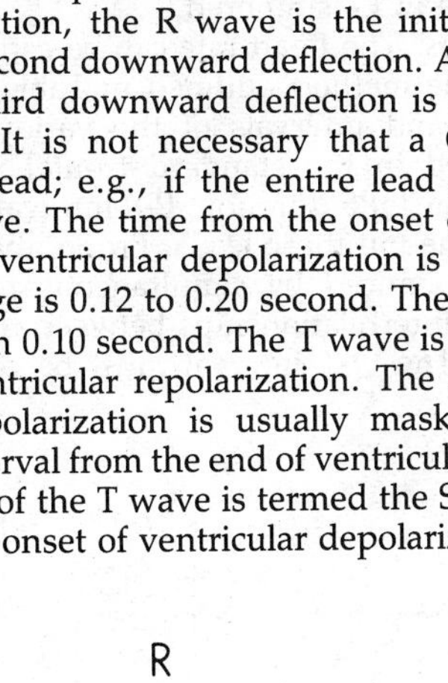

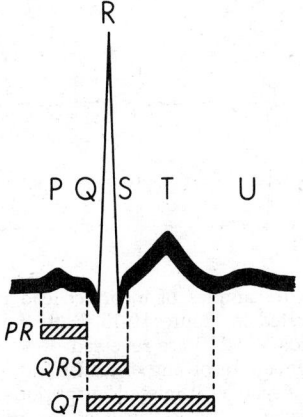

Figure 41–16. The ECG waveforms and intervals (horizontal bars) are illustrated. For description, see text.

LEARNING ELECTROCARDIOGRAPHY. There are two general approaches to learning electrocardiography: (1) the pattern recognition method and (2) the spatial vector approach. In the former, the student memorizes the multiple normal and abnormal waveforms for each lead and gains the necessary expertise through experience in interpreting a large number of ECGs with clinical correlation. This technique is used by all experienced electrocardiographers, and illustrations of this approach are provided in the legends of the figures. In the spatial vector approach, popularized by R. P. Grant, the waveform is reduced to a vector representing the magnitude and direction of the mean electrical forces of P, QRS, and T. Using this technique, the student can quickly learn to define the normal ECG and the major abnormalities. This approach is based on the fact that the magnitude of a wave in any lead is a function of the relationship between the electrical axis of the heart and that lead (Fig. 41–17). From the hexaxial reference system of the six frontal plane leads illustrated in Figure 41–13, the spatial vector approach can be used to obtain the mean frontal plane axis for the normal electrocardiogram (Fig. 41–15). The QRS complex is upright (positive) in lead I; thus the mean axis must be between +90 degrees and –90 degrees—i.e., on the positive side of a line perpendicular to lead I. Since the QRS complex is also positive in leads II and III, the axis must be between +30 and +90 degrees. Since the mean QRS complex is slightly negative in lead AVL, the mean QRS vector is approximately +70 degrees. A similar determination then can be made for P and T waves. In the frontal plane, the mean P vector should be between 0 and +80 degrees, and the mean QRS and T vectors should lie between –30 and +90 degrees. A mean QRS vector more negative than –30 degrees is considered left axis deviation and more positive than +90 degrees is defined as right axis deviation. The angle between the mean QRS and T vectors in the frontal plane should be less than 80 degrees. Application of the spatial vector technique to the transverse plane is somewhat more difficult, since the six precordial leads do not define a precise reference system. An estimate of the vector can be obtained by noting when the waveforms make their transition from a negative to a positive deflection. In a normal

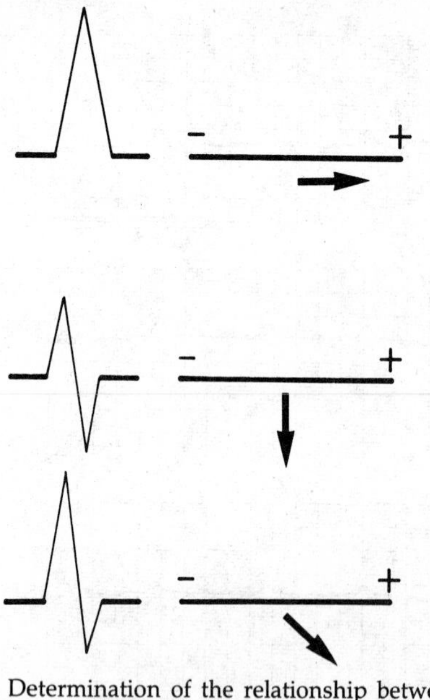

Figure 41–17. Determination of the relationship between the mean electrical axis of a wave and the waveform in a given lead. The top row depicts an entirely positive waveform; thus, the axis is parallel to the lead. In the second row the waveform is biphasic and the summation of the positive and negative parts is zero. In this instance, the mean electrical axis of the wave is perpendicular to the lead. (Note that the arrow could be drawn in the opposite direction and still be perpendicular to the lead.) In the third row, a biphasic waveform is shown in which the majority of the area is positive. The mean electrical axis is roughly at a 45 degree angle to the lead.

ECG, the QRS transition is between V2 and V5, and the T wave makes its transition before the QRS. The next step is to determine the direction of the initial 0.04 second vector of the QRS. It is this portion of the QRS that defines the presence of

TABLE 41–2. DIAGNOSTIC CATEGORIES IN WHICH AN ECG IS USEFUL

Arrhythmias	+ +
Electronic pacemaker function	+ +
Intraventricular conduction disturbances	+ +
Chamber enlargement	
Left and right atrial enlargement	+
Left and right ventricular hypertrophy	+
Myocardial infarction	
Old	+
Acute	+
Myocardial ischemia	+
Pericardial disease	
Pericarditis	±
Pericardial tamponade	±
Electrolyte disturbances	
Hypo- and hyperkalemia	+
Hypo- and hypercalcemia	+
Miscellaneous disorders	
Congenital heart disease	±
Muscular dystrophy	±
Emphysema and/or cor pulmonale	±
Pulmonary emboli	±
Hypothermia	±
Myxedema	±
Drug effects	
Antidysrhythmic drugs (e.g., quinidine)	±
Digitalis	±
Antineoplastic agents (e.g., doxorubicin)	±
Phenothiazine derivatives (e.g., chlorpromazine)	±
Antidepressant drugs (e.g., amitriptyline)	±
Antiparasitic compounds (e.g., emetine)	±

The symbols indicate the necessity for ECG to establish the diagnosis:
+ + ECG is essential for diagnosis.
+ ECG is important for diagnosis.
± ECG may be useful for diagnosis.

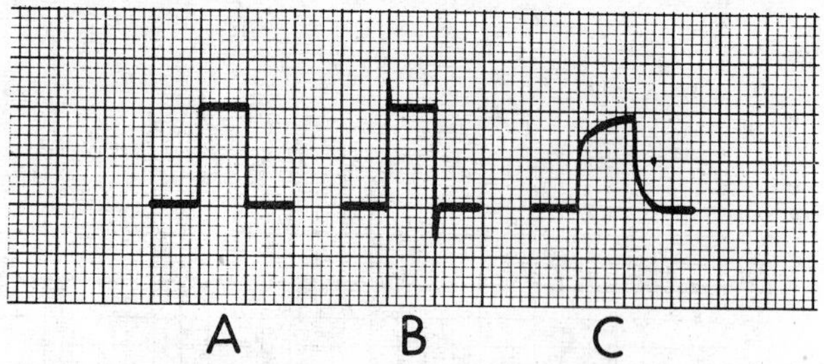

Figure 41–18. In *A*, a correct standardization having a true square wave response is illustrated. *B* represents a standardization obtained from an instrument in which the response is underdamped; the amplitude of the waves will be spuriously enhanced. In *C*, the recorder is overdamped, resulting in both a spuriously decreased amplitude and an increased width of the waveform.

myocardial infarction. The initial 0.04 second vector should lie between 0 and +90 degrees in the frontal plane; outside this range it suggests myocardial infarction (see Fig. 41–20). The direction of the terminal 0.04 second vector is used to aid in the diagnosis of ventricular conduction abnormalities (see Fig. 41–22).

APPROACH TO INTERPRETING AN ECG. The diagnostic categories in which an ECG may be useful are outlined in Table 41–2. In interpreting an ECG, it is important to develop a routine so that each aspect of the recording is carefully analyzed. Since the waveforms of the ECG are influenced to a certain extent by the age and body habitus of the patient, this information should be available to the electrocardiographer. The following eight sequential steps are necessary for proper ECG interpretation.

1. *Quality of the ECG recording.* This includes proper standardization (Fig. 41–18), lead placement (Fig. 41–19), and identification of significant artifact. The student must learn to evaluate the quality of the recording and not interpret an inadequately recorded ECG. Serious misdiagnosis can result if the quality of the ECG is ignored.

2. *Measurements.* The heart rate can be estimated adequately by employing the method outlined in Table 41–3. The amplitude, duration, and intervals of the various waveforms are usually measured in the standard frontal plane limb leads. Abnormality of the QRS duration, P-R interval, and Q-T interval also are determined in these leads. Proper measurement of the waveforms is enhanced by simultaneous recording of three leads, since the interrelationships between the waveforms can be easily seen. The Q-T interval must be corrected for heart

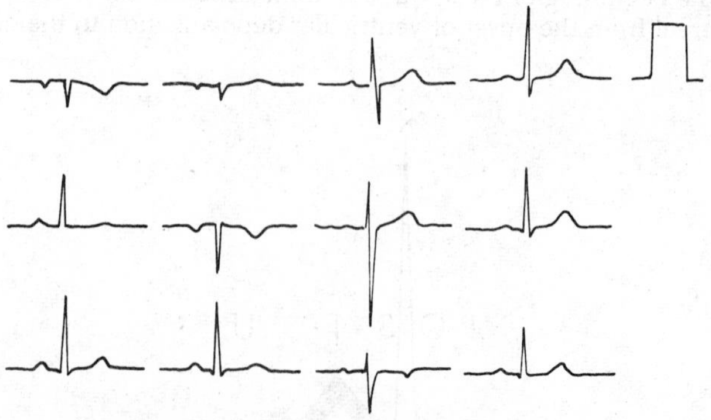

Figure 41–19. Two examples of incorrect lead placement from the same patient illustrated in Figure 41–15. Both the left and right arm leads and chest leads V1, 2, 3 are reversed. Reversal of the arm lead results in a mirror image recording of lead I and is easily recognized, since the P wave is negative. If missed, a spurious diagnosis of lateral wall infarction may be made. Reversal of the right precordial leads may result in an incorrect diagnosis of either right ventricular hypertrophy or posterior wall infarction.

TABLE 41–3. DETERMINATION OF HEART RATE

Interval in Large Boxes Between Two Complexes	Heart Rate (Beats/min)
1	300
2	150
3	100
4	75
5	60
6	50

The ECG recording paper is marked vertically by light lines; every fifth line is heavily marked. The time increment separating two heavy lines (one large box) is 0.20 second. To rapidly determine the rate, note the interval between two complexes and estimate the rate from this table.

rate. The corrected Q-T interval (Q-T$_c$) is given by Bazet's formula:

$$\text{Q-T}_c = \frac{\text{Q-T}}{\sqrt{\text{R-R interval (seconds)}}}$$

and should not exceed 0.44 seconds.

3. *Determination of rhythm.*
4. *Examination of P wave.* Determine if atrial enlargement (see Fig. 41–21) or intra-atrial block is present.
5. *Examination of QRS.* Determine if myocardial infarction (Fig. 41–20), ventricular hypertrophy (Fig. 41–21), or ventricular conduction defect (Fig. 41–22) is present.

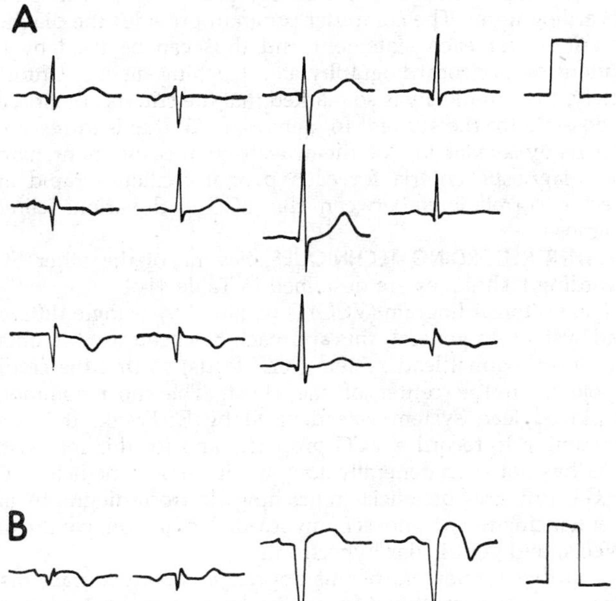

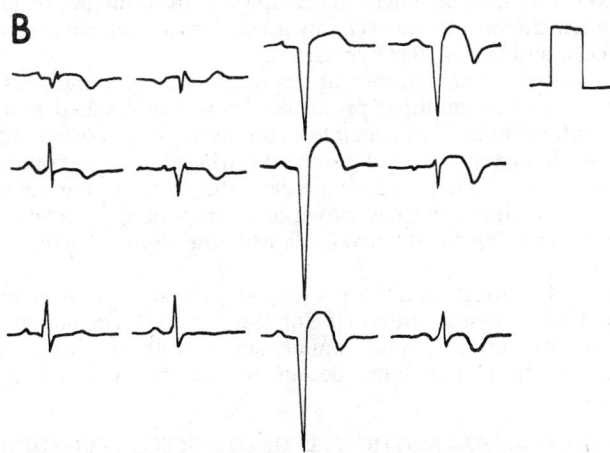

Figure 41–20. The ECG lead sets are recorded in the same sequence as in Figure 41–15. *A*, Inferior and posterior infarction. Note the abnormal superiorly and anteriorly directed initial forces: i.e., significant Q waves in leads II, III, AVF, and a broad R wave in V1. Note the concomitant negative T waves in the same frontal plane leads. *B*, Anterolateral myocardial infarction. The initial forces are posterior and to the right; i.e., extensive Q waves in leads I, AVL, and V1 through V4. Also note the concomitant ST segment elevation and T wave inversion in the precordial leads, indicating that the myocardial infarction is acute.

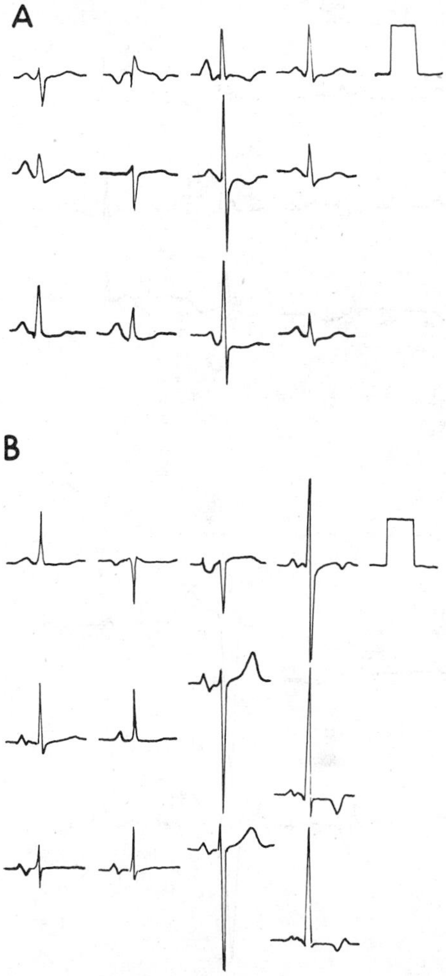

Figure 41–21. *A*, Right ventricular hypertrophy. The mean frontal plane axis is to the right, and there is excessive voltage in the right precordial leads. Also note the tall symmetrical P wave in lead II, indicating right atrial enlargement. *B*, Left ventricular hypertrophy. Note the excessive voltage in the lateral precordial leads and the inverted T waves in the same leads, indicating a strain pattern. The wide biphasic P wave in lead V1 is indicative of left atrial enlargement.

6. *Examination of S-T segment.* Determine if subendocardial (Fig. 41–23) or epicardial (Fig. 41–20) injury is present; abnormal displacement of the S-T segment is defined by convention as injury. The S-T segment is shortened in hypercalcemia and prolonged in hypocalcemia.
7. *Examination of T wave.* Defining the significance of T wave abnormalities is the most difficult aspect of electrocardiography. In general, marked T wave abnormalities that occur either without other ECG abnormalities or with myocardial infarction are defined as ischemic or primary T wave changes (Fig. 41–20). T wave abnormalities that occur with conduction defects or ventricular hypertrophy are spoken of as secondary. The abnormal T wave seen in hypertrophy also has been defined as strain (Fig. 41–21). The T waves also are important in the diagnosis of drug effects and electrolyte abnormalities.
8. *Comparison with patient's previous ECGs.* It is extremely important to compare a new tracing with a previous electrocardiogram for two reasons: (1) although the ECG may still be within the normal range, significant changes may have occurred since the previous record; and (2) a comparison allows the electrocardiographer to date specific abnormalities that may have important therapeutic implications.

COMPUTER INTERPRETATION OF THE ECG. The development of algorithms to process and interpret ECGs has progressed to the point that, at present, there are several acceptable programs

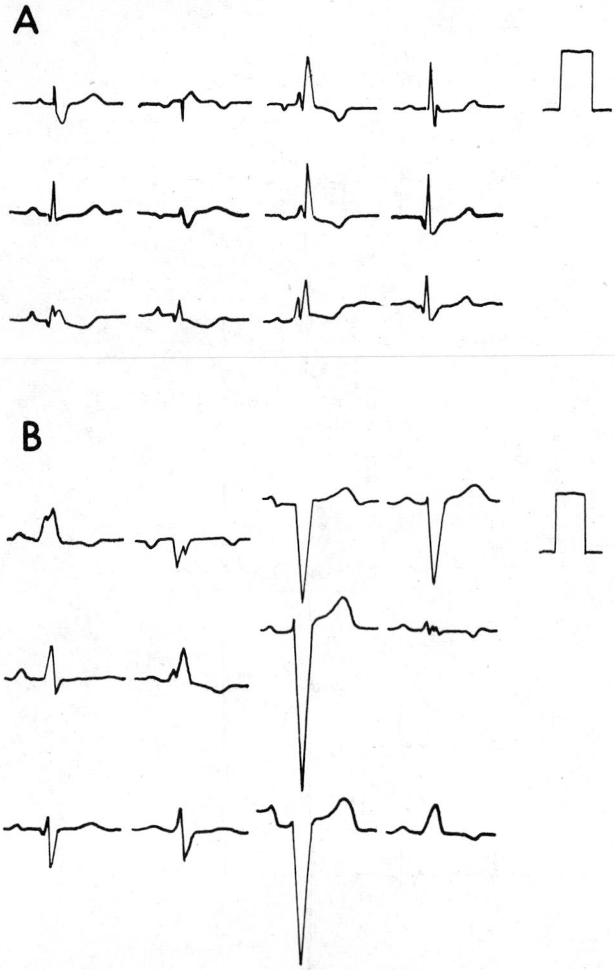

Figure 41–22. *A*, Right bundle branch block. The QRS duration is greater than 0.12 second, and the axis of the terminal 0.04 second of the QRS is to the right and anterior. *B*, Left bundle branch block. The QRS duration is greater than 0.12 second, and the terminal 0.04 second of the QRS is to the left and posterior.

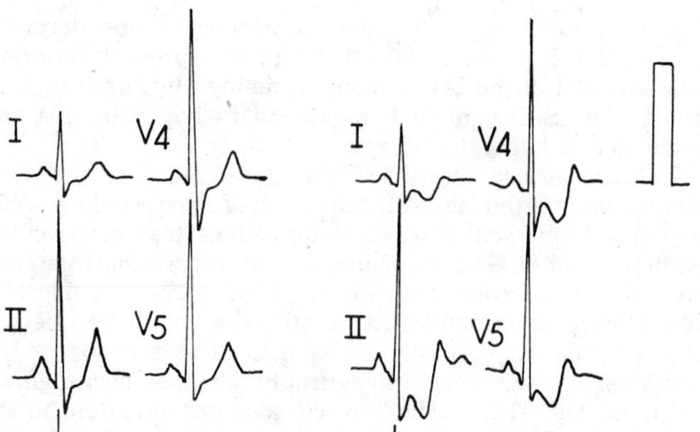

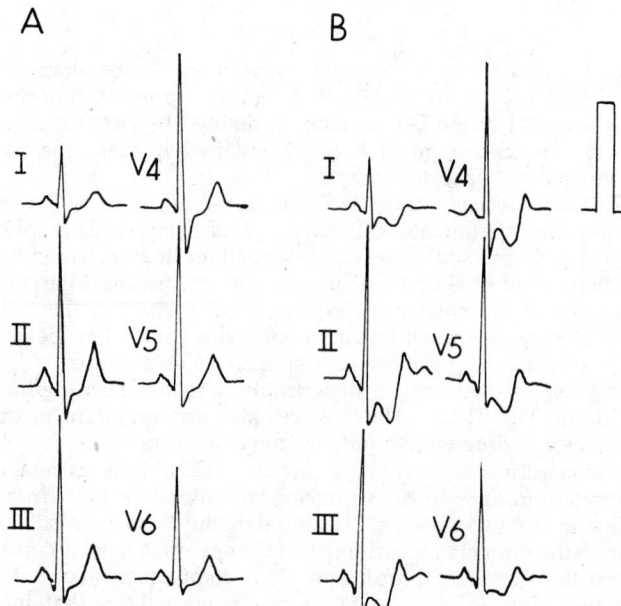

Figure 41–23. Recording obtained prior to *(A)* and during *(B)* an exercise test. Note the depression and downward sloping of the S-T segment wave during exercise. This is a typical pattern of subendocardial injury.

available for routine clinical use. Approximately 10 per cent of the routine ECGs now recorded in the United States are processed by computers. In general these programs reliably separate normal from abnormal ECGs and correctly interpret approximately 85 per cent of abnormal ECGs. Algorithms to compare sequential ECGs from the same patient are not generally available. Thus, at the present state of the art, all computer-interpreted ECGs must also be read by a competent electrocardiographer. Hence, the computer is viewed as an assist device to the electrocardiographer and not as a replacement.

The processing of ECGs by a computer provides a number of advantages: (1) It improves recording techniques. Most of the currently available systems signal the technician as to the quality of the recording. The computer will not accept an ECG with significant artifacts. (2) It speeds processing. The processing time to obtain a diagnosis for each ECG is approximately one minute. Thus, it is quite useful as a screening procedure while awaiting the final interpretation by the electrocardiographer. (3) It assists the electrocardiographer. The algorithm accurately measures the heart rate, amplitude, axis, and duration of the waveforms and the various intervals, as well as listing the diagnostic statements. This preprocessing allows at least a 75 per cent reduction in the time spent by the electrocardiographer in interpreting ECGs. In addition, the program provides a consistent interpretation, eliminating the well-known inter- and intraobserver variabilities found with even the most experienced electrocardiographers. (4) It teaches electrocardiography. The computer program provides the diagnostic criteria for each statement and thus can be used by the student of electrocardiography as a teaching device. Unfortunately, the complexity is so marked that the criteria are virtually impossible for the student to memorize. (5) It aids in research. The ready availability of the waveform measurement matrix and diagnostic criteria for each patient facilitates rapid and specific correlations between the ECG and various clinical diagnoses.

OTHER RECORDING TECHNIQUES. Several of the other ECG recording techniques are described in Table 41–4.

The vectorcardiogram (VCG) is obtained by using a different lead system. In general, this approach has been used to obtain a true orthogonal lead system (XYZ leads) so that the cardiac dipole is in the center of the chest. The most commonly employed lead system was devised by E. Frank. It is time consuming to record a VCG properly, and for this reason the VCG has not been generally accepted in clinical medicine. The VCG is primarily beneficial in teaching electrocardiography and in enhancing the diagnosis of myocardial infarction, conduction defects, and ventricular hypertrophy.

A further refinement of this approach is body surface mapping, in which multiple precordial leads are obtained and a computer is utilized to generate a continuous body surface map of the change in electrical potential during depolarization and repolarization. These techniques are still in the experimental stage, but ultimately may prove to be important in obtaining the maximal information available from the electrical activation of the heart.

The ECG stress test is a widely used physiologic technique designed to assess the ability of the coronary circulation to deliver oxygen at a rate commensurate with the metabolic needs of the myocardium. Because myocardial metabolism is

TABLE 41–4. DIAGNOSTIC USES OF OTHER ECG RECORDING TECHNIQUES

Vectorcardiograms: old myocardial infarction, ventricular hypertrophy, ventricular conduction abnormalities
Body surface mapping: precise definition of instantaneous depolarization and repolarization—primarily experimental at present
Exercise electrocardiography: transient subendocardial or transmural injury
Holter monitoring: arrhythmias, transient subendocardial injury
Transtelephone monitoring: arrhythmias, pacemaker function
His bundle recordings: arrhythmias and conduction defects
Esophageal leads: arrhythmias

almost entirely aerobic, an inadequate increase in coronary flow quickly results in ischemia of the inner layers of the heart. The concomitant S-T segment changes have been empirically defined as subendocardial injury. The characteristic S-T segment response is a flat (square wave) or downward sloping S-T segment of 0.1 mV or greater measured 0.08 second after the end of the QRS complex (Fig. 41–23).

Chou TC, Helm RA: Clinical Vectorcardiography. 2nd ed. New York, Grune & Stratton, 1974. *Complete coverage of vectorcardiography.*

Lipman BS, Massie E, Kleiger RE: Clinical Scalar Electrocardiography. 6th ed. Chicago, Year Book Medical Publishers, 1973. *Excellent general text covering all phases of electrocardiography.*

Marriott HJL: Practical Electrocardiography. 6th ed. Baltimore, Williams & Wilkins, 1977. *A comprehensive description of electrocardiography.*

41.3. Echocardiography

Harvey Feigenbaum

Echocardiography comprises a group of diagnostic procedures in which ultrasound is used to examine the heart. Ultrasound is sound with a frequency above the audible range. The upper limit of audible frequencies is approximately 20,000 cycles per second. The frequency used for echocardiography ranges from 1 million to 7 million cycles per second or 1 to 7 megaHertz. The term echocardiography comes from the fact that a cardiac image is obtained by recording the reflected sound waves or echoes of a beam of ultrasound aimed at the heart. A burst of ultrasound is produced by a transducer, and the sonic waves travel from the transducer much as a light beam from a flashlight. When the ultrasonic beam strikes an interface between two media that have different acoustic properties, such as a difference in density, the ultrasound is reflected and refracted just as when a light beam strikes a reflecting surface such as water. If the reflecting surface is perpendicular to the transducer, some of the reflected ultrasonic waves or echoes will retrace their path and strike the transducer.

If one knows the velocity at which sound travels in the medium being examined and if one knows the time that it takes for a burst of ultrasound to leave the transducer, strike the reflecting object, and return as an echo, one can calculate the distance of the reflecting surface from the transducer. Since the velocity of sound transmission in human soft tissue is known, echocardiographs are calibrated for the velocity of sound in this medium, and distances between reflecting structures and the transducer are automatically indicated on the oscilloscope. Only part of the ultrasonic energy is reflected by any given acoustic interface. The ultrasound that continues through the initial reflecting surface will strike any deeper interfaces and again be reflected back to the transducer. Since the transit time is longer, the deeper interface will be displayed on the oscilloscope as being farther from the transducer. The ultrasound is transmitted in short bursts or ultrasonic pulses at a rate of 1000 per second or more. This rapid sampling rate permits an accurate recording of cardiac motion.

Figure 41–24 demonstrates how one can place an ultrasonic transducer on the surface of the chest and direct it toward the heart. In this example the ultrasonic beam is directed through a small portion of the right ventricle and the mid portion of the left ventricle. The ultrasonic beam initially passes through the chest wall. It then strikes the anterior wall of the right ventricle, the cavity of the right ventricle, the interventricular septum, the cavity of the left ventricle, and then the posterior left ventricular wall. The echocardiogram on the right shows the resultant M-mode recording of such an examination. The term M-mode refers to an ultrasonic recording whereby motion is displayed. The vertical dimension is distance and the horizontal axis is time. Thus, on the M-mode echogram nonmoving structures, such as the chest wall, will be recorded as a band of straight lines, whereas cardiac structures that move will inscribe wavy lines. An electrocardiogram is included on the recording to assist in timing of cardiac motion. The M-mode echocardiogram in Figure 41–24 demonstrates the motion inscribed by the interventricular septum, which is bounded by

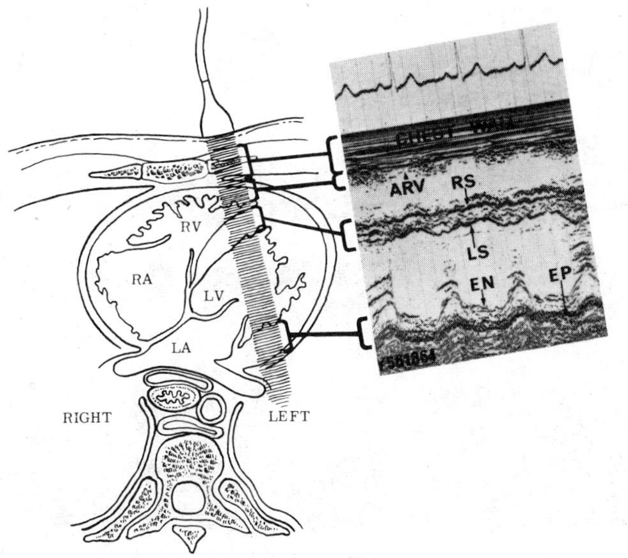

Figure 41–24. Diagrammatic cross-section of the heart with a corresponding echocardiogram showing the path of the ultrasonic beam during an M-mode examination of the left ventricle. ARV = anterior right ventricular wall; RS = right septum; LS = left septum; EN = left ventricular posterior endocardium; EP = left ventricular posterior epicardium. (From Popp RL, Wolfe SB, Hirata T, et al.: Am J Cardiol 24:523, 1969.)

the right septal (RS) and the left septal (LS) echoes, and the posterior left ventricular wall, which is bounded by the left ventricular endocardial (EN) and epicardial (EP) echoes. One can appreciate how the interventricular septum and the posterior left ventricular wall appose each other in systole and move apart during diastole. It is also apparent how one can measure the thickness of the interventricular septum and the posterior left ventricular wall. The blood-filled cavities are relatively homogeneous, and thus one records very few ultrasonic echoes from these spaces.

The ultrasonic beam can be directed to various areas of the heart. A common technique is to tilt the transducer toward the cardiac apex and then, by changing the angle of the transducer, to direct it toward the base of the heart. When one moves the ultrasonic beam in this fashion, an M-mode echocardiogram similar to that diagrammed in Figure 41–25 will be recorded. The section of the echocardiogram indicated by "area two" is comparable to that seen in Figure 41–24. The ultrasonic beam passes through a small portion of the right ventricle and through the body of the left ventricle. Parts of the mitral valve apparatus will be seen during this examination. If the beam is directed toward the apex (area one), one may record echoes from the papillary muscles. No mitral valve echoes will be recorded. As the transducer is directed toward the base of the heart (area three), one sees fairly characteristic echoes from the mitral valve. The anterior mitral leaflet inscribes an M-shaped configuration during diastole. The posterior mitral leaflet moves in an opposite fashion but has a lower amplitude of motion. The two leaflets come together during systole. As the ultrasonic beam moves farther toward the cardiac base (area four), the echo generated by the posterior left ventricular wall gradually merges with that from the posterior left atrial wall. The left ventricular wall moves anteriorly during systole, whereas the left atrial wall remains stationary or moves posteriorly during systole. The interventricular septum merges with the anterior wall of the aorta. The anterior leaflet of the mitral valve is in continuity with the posterior wall of the aorta. The walls of the aorta characteristically move upward or anteriorly in systole and downward in diastole. Between the two aortic walls one sees a box-like configuration formed by the opening of two of

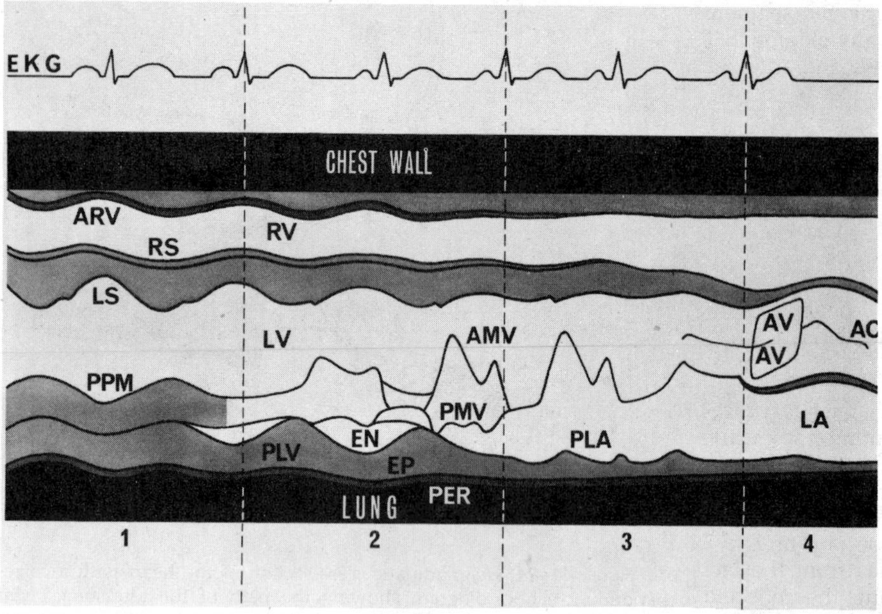

Figure 41–25. Diagrammatic representation of the M-mode echocardiogram as the transducer moves from the apex (position 1) to the base of the heart (position 4). Position 2 corresponds to the echocardiogram noted in Figure 41–24. RV = right ventricle; LV = left ventricle; PPM = posterior papillary muscle; PLV = posterior left ventricular wall; AMV = anterior mitral valve leaflet; PMV = posterior mitral valve leaflet; PER = pericardium; PLA = posterior left atrial wall; AV = aortic valve; AO = aorta; LA = left atrium. Other symbols as in Figure 41–24. (From Feigenbaum H: Prog Cardiovasc Dis 14:531, 1972. By permission.)

the aortic valve leaflets. The two leaflets come together in diastole. Posterior to the aorta is the cavity of the left atrium.

One can change the direction of the ultrasonic beam in order to record the pulmonary valve and the tricuspid valve. The tricuspid valve is medial to the mitral valve; the pulmonary valve is seen by directing the ultrasonic beam superiorly and to the left of the aortic valve. The configuration of the tricuspid valve is similar to that of the mitral valve except that the posterior leaflet of the tricuspid valve is rarely recorded. The configuration of the pulmonary valve is similar to that of the aortic valve; however, it is unusual to be able to record an anterior pulmonary valve leaflet.

The recordings demonstrated in Figures 41–24 and 41–25 are M-mode echocardiograms. This echocardiographic technique was the first to be utilized clinically. Because of the very rapid sampling rate, this type of examination is excellent for recording cardiac motion. Brief or rapid movements of the cardiac walls and valves can be readily appreciated on the M-mode recording. No other diagnostic procedure is as sensitive in recording subtle changes in cardiac motion as is M-mode echocardiography. Many important diagnostic uses depend upon this capability. However, M-mode echocardiography has some deficiencies. The position of the ultrasonic beam is not demonstrated on the tracing, and one does not record useful information from structures that are not perpendicular to the ultrasonic beam. Thus, several areas of the heart, such as the apex and the medial and lateral walls, are difficult to record with M-mode echocardiography. It is also difficult to appreciate the shape of the cardiac structures being examined. For example, a stenotic, domed aortic valve would be missed with M-mode echocardiography.

Two-dimensional echocardiography overcomes most of the deficiencies in M-mode echocardiography. Two-dimensional echocardiography differs from M-mode echocardiography in that the ultrasonic beam is constantly moving or scanning. The ultrasonic beam moves so that one obtains 30 to 60 slices of the heart in a second. The ultrasonic beam can be moved by placing a motor in the probe so that either a single transducer oscillates or multiple transducers rotate. A rotating system requires three or four transducers within the ultrasonic probe. One can also move the ultrasonic beam by electronically steering the wave fronts. This technique utilizes phased array technology and requires a transducer made up of multiple small elements. By controlling the timing with which each small segment of the transducer is fired, one can alter the direction of the ultrasonic beam. Whether one moves the beam electronically or mechanically, the end result is a rapid ultrasonic scan of the heart. Figure 41–26 diagrammatically illustrates a transducer that rapidly moves the ultrasonic beam through an 80- or 90-degree angle. Such a two-dimensional scanner is known as a sector scanner, since the examination produces a pie-shaped sector. It is also possible to use a linear scanner, by means of which the ultrasonic beam moves in a linear fashion and provides a rectangular image of the heart. Unfortunately, the ribs produce technical artifacts with linear scanners. Thus,

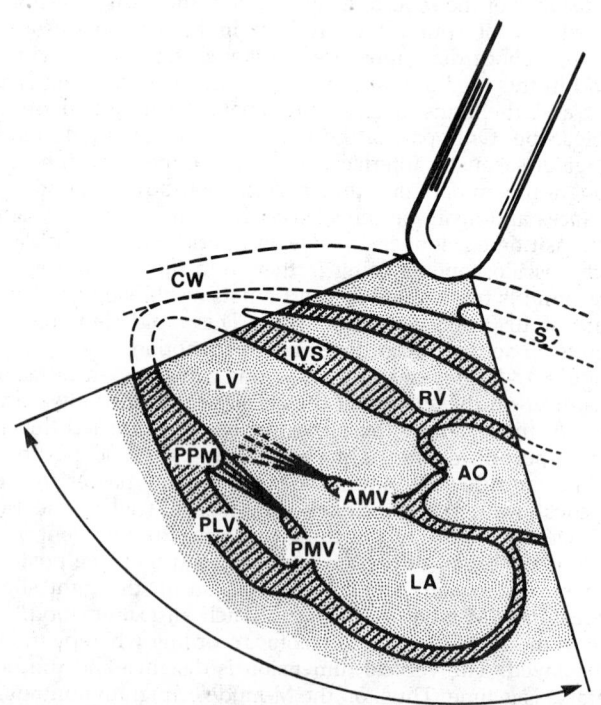

Figure 41–26. Drawing demonstrating how a two-dimensional echocardiographic examination obtains a sector scan between the cardiac apex and the aorta. CW = chest wall; S = sternum; IVS = interventricular septum; other symbols as in Figure 41–25. (From Feigenbaum H: Echocardiography. *In* Braunwald E (ed.): Heart Disease. Philadelphia, W. B. Saunders Company, 1980.)

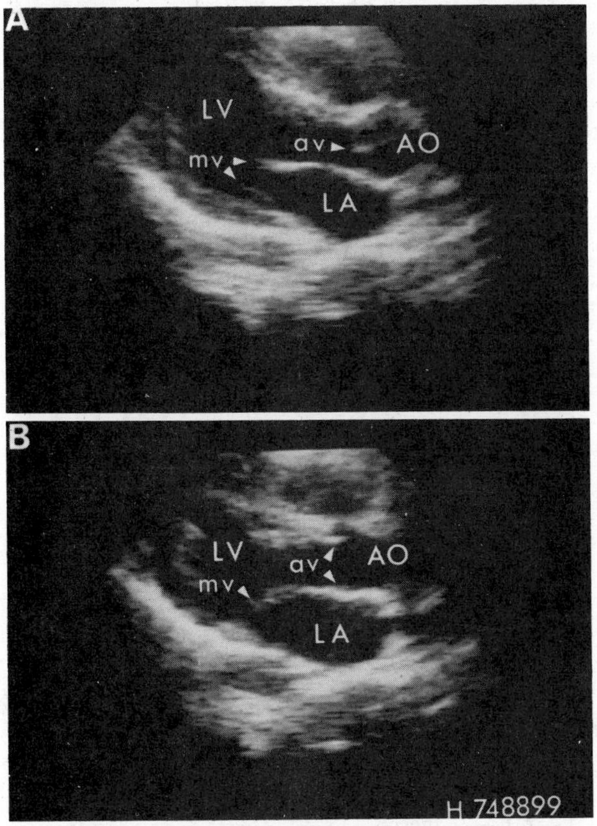

Figure 41–27. Two-dimensional echocardiograms corresponding to the drawing in Figure 41–26. During diastole *(A)* the mitral valve (mv) is open and the aortic valve (av) is closed. With ventricular systole *(B)* the mitral valve is closed and the aortic valve is open. The left ventricular cavity (LV) is smaller during systole *(B)* than in diastole *(A)*. AO = aorta; LA = left atrium.

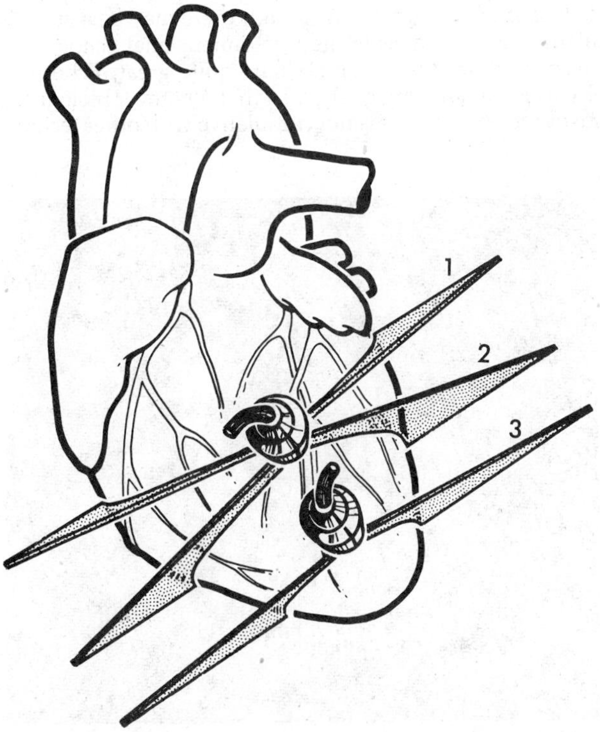

Figure 41–28. Transducer position and examining ultrasonic planes for short-axis examinations of the left ventricle using two-dimensional echocardiography. Examining plane 1 passes through the mitral valve. Plane 2 is through the papillary muscles. Plane 3 is through the left ventricular apex. (From Feigenbaum H: Echocardiography. 3rd ed. Philadelphia, Lea & Febiger, 1980.)

two-dimensional echocardiography is primarily done with sector scanning.

Figure 41–27 demonstrates a two-dimensional echogram of the heart comparable to the examination indicated in Figure 41–26. The echocardiograms in Figure 41–27 are single frames from a videotape recording of the real-time two-dimensional study. The original or real-time examination is displayed on an oscilloscope or television monitor and resembles a cineangiogram. The valve leaflets can be seen opening and closing, and the various cardiac walls are constantly moving on the oscilloscope. Figure 41–27*A* demonstrates the diastolic image in which the mitral valve is open, the left ventricle is relatively large, and the aortic valve is closed. Figure 41–27*B* shows the examination during systole, at which time the mitral valve is closed, the aortic valve is open, and the left ventricular cavity is smaller.

Some of the advantages of two-dimensional echocardiography are as follows: the echograms resemble the true anatomic configuration of the heart, one can identify the shape of the cardiac structures, and one can examine portions of the heart that are not accessible on the M-mode study. It is possible to vary the position and orientation of the sector plane so that one examines the heart in multiple planes or tomograms. Figure 41–28 shows how one can turn the transducer 90 degrees from that used to obtain the echocardiogram in Figure 41–27 and can slice the left ventricle parallel to its short axis. Figure 41–29 demonstrates the resultant short-axis, two-dimensional echograms. Figure 41–29*A* shows the circular left ventricle at the level of the mitral valve. Figure 41–29*B* demonstrates a similar short-axis examination at the level of the papillary muscles. Figure 41–29*C* shows a short-axis two-dimensional examination over the cardiac apex. The medial and lateral walls shown in Figure 41–29 are not recorded with M-mode echocardiography.

A variety of transducer positions and sector planes can be obtained with two-dimensional echocardiography. One of the more important examinations is with the transducer at the cardiac apex (Fig. 41–30). With the transducer in this location one can obtain several views of cardiac structures. One of the more important views is the apical four-chamber view (Plane 1, Fig. 41–30). In the resulting echocardiogram (Fig. 41–31) it is possible to record all four chambers at the same time. The apical four-chamber examination has wide application in echocardiography.

Although echocardiography is usually noninvasive, it is possible to obtain additional diagnostic information by a peripheral venous injection of almost any liquid. Such injections create tiny suspended bubbles of air by a process of cavitation, and these bubbles produce a mass of echoes within the heart. These tiny bubbles do not pass through capillaries. The combination of such injections and echocardiography is known as contrast echocardiography. This technique is particularly helpful in detecting intracardiac shunts and tricuspid regurgitation. Such injections can also be made through catheters in the cardiac catheterization laboratory to obviate or supplement selective angiography. Of course, such a use of echocardiography is no longer noninvasive.

Ultrasound can also provide diagnostic information utilizing the Doppler principle. This principle states that if a sound beam strikes an interface that is moving in the axis of the beam, the motion of that reflecting surface will alter the frequency of the reflected sound. The amount of frequency change is a function of the velocity with which the reflecting object is moving. When dealing with ultrasound the difference in frequency or Doppler shift is in the audible range. Thus, when an ultrasonic beam strikes a reflecting surface which moves, an audible Doppler signal is produced. Doppler ultrasound has been used most extensively by examining moving columns of blood. The reflecting interfaces are red blood cells. The greatest experience has been with the examination of peripheral vessels, using continuous wave ultrasound. More recently, pulsed Doppler has been used for cardiac examinations. Pulsed Dopp-

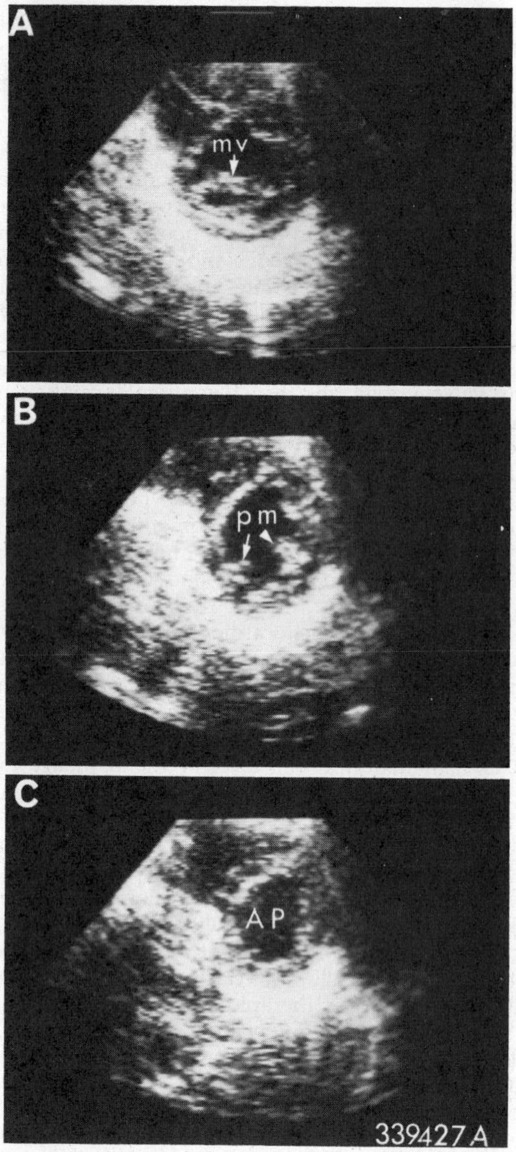

Figure 41–29. Short-axis, two-dimensional echocardiograms of the left ventricle at the level of the mitral valve (mv) *(A)*, the papillary muscles (pm) *(B)*, and the left ventricular apex (AP) *(C)*. (From Feigenbaum H: Echocardiography. 3rd ed. Philadelphia, Lea & Febiger, 1980.)

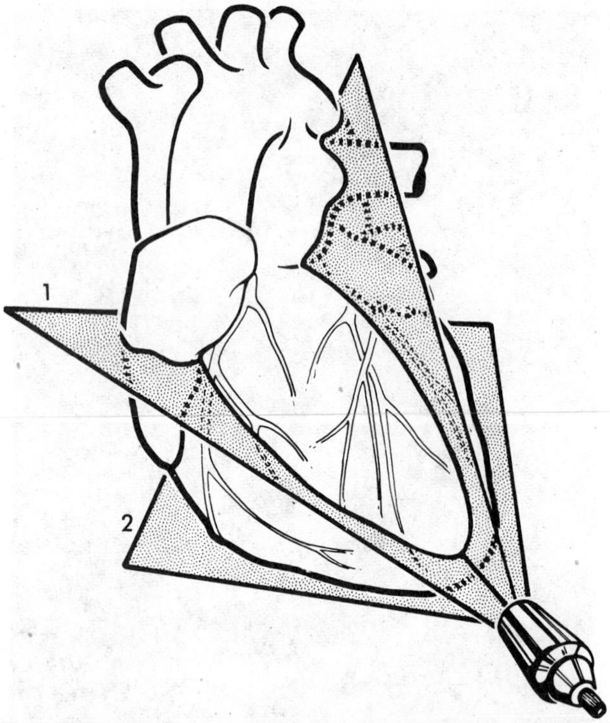

Figure 41–30. Transducer positions and examining planes for apical two-dimensional echocardiograms. Examining plane 1 passes through all four cardiac chambers. Plane 2 passes through the left ventricle and left atrium. (From Feigenbaum H: Echocardiography. 3rd ed. Philadelphia, Lea & Febiger, 1980.)

ler permits one to obtain either an M-mode or a two-dimensional echogram together with the Doppler recording (Fig. 41–32). By gating or positioning the sample volume on the M-mode or two-dimensional image, one can obtain a Doppler recording from various locations within the heart. The Doppler technique can also identify the direction in which the blood is flowing. Figure 41–32 demonstrates how one can place the Doppler sampling gate within the aorta to record the pattern of blood flow above the aortic valve. The spectrum of the Doppler signal is recorded using fast Fourier analysis techniques. The recording gives information concerning the velocity, direction, amplitude, and timing of the blood flow. To calculate the velocity one must know the angle of incidence between the ultrasonic beam and the moving column of red cells. The Doppler recording can also distinguish between laminar flow and turbulent flow that might occur with an intracardiac shunt or with valvular stenosis or insufficiency. With turbulent flow one sees multiple frequencies moving in multiple directions. Doppler echocardiography provides an opportunity to obtain hemodynamic information that complements the imaging techniques of M-mode and two-dimensional echocardiography.

Diagnostic ultrasound obtains its information utilizing reflected rather than transmitted energy. As a result, echocardiography deals in slices or ultrasonic "ice-pick" views of the heart. Radiographic techniques using ionizing radiation usually look at cardiac silhouettes. Although there may be a superficial similarity between a real-time two-dimensional echogram and a cineangiogram, the differences are quite great. Echocardiography uses nonionizing energy, so that whatever biologic effect ultrasound may have, it is not cumulative with other techniques

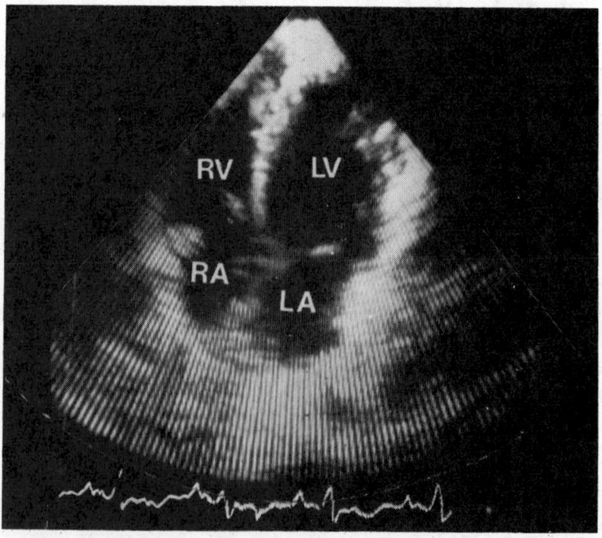

Figure 41–31. Apical, four chamber echocardiogram obtained with examining plane 1 of Figure 41–30. This two-dimensional examination has many diagnostic applications in echocardiography. RV = right ventricle; LV = left ventricle; RA = right atrium; LA = left atrium. (From Feigenbaum H: Echocardiography. *In* Braunwald E (ed.): Heart Disease. Philadelphia, W. B. Saunders Company, 1980.)

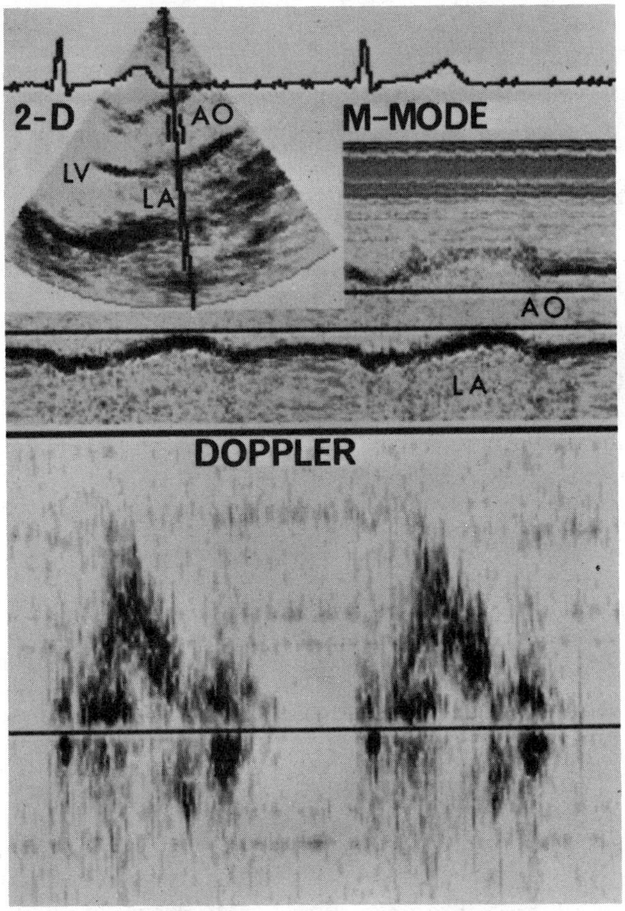

Figure 41–32. Doppler echocardiographic examination with the sample in the root of the aorta (AO). Simultaneous two-dimensional (2-D) and M-mode echocardiograms help to identify the location of the Doppler sampling site. The Doppler recording is a spectral analysis of the audible signal coming from the moving column of blood. LV = left ventricle; LA = left atrium.

which utilize ionizing energy. Thus far the safety of diagnostic ultrasound is extremely good, and no untoward reaction has yet been identified with clinical echocardiography. The ability to obtain frequent serial examinations is one of the virtues of echocardiography.

Bom N, Lancee CT, VanZwieten G, Kloster FE, Roelandt J: Multiscan echocardiography. I. Technical description. Circulation 48:1066, 1973. *A paper describing the use of an electronic linear scanner for examining the heart. This instrument probably was the most influential in popularizing real-time two-dimensional examinations of the heart.*

De Maria AN, Bommer W, Takeda P, Mason DT, Kwan OL, Rasor J: Value and limitations of contrast echocardiography in cardiac diagnosis. Cardiovasc Clin 13:167, 1983. *An article demonstrating the clinical utility of contrast echocardiography.*

Edler I, Gustafson A, Karlefors T, Christensson B: Ultrasound cardiography. Acta Med Scand (Suppl) 370:68, 1961. *A review article describing the early work using ultrasound to examine the heart.*

Feigenbaum H: Echocardiography. 3rd ed. Philadelphia, Lea & Febiger, 1981. *Textbook providing an extensive discussion of echocardiography.*

Feigenbaum H: Echocardiography: An overview. J Am Coll Cardiol 1:216, 1983. *An article presenting the current and future status of echocardiography.*

Pearlman AS: Doppler echocardiography. Int J Cardiol 3:81, 1983. *A review article describing the principles and clinical uses for Doppler echocardiography.*

Popp RL, Rubenson DS, Tucker CR, French JW: Echocardiography: M-mode and two-dimensional. Ann Intern Med 93:844, 1980. *A review article of M-mode and two-dimensional echocardiography.*

Tajik AJ, Seward JB, Hagler DJ, Mair DD, Lie JT: Two-dimensional real-time ultrasonic imaging of the heart and great vessels: Technique image orientation, structure identification, and validation. Mayo Clin Proc 53:271, 1978. *A review article demonstrating the multiple examining planes that one can obtain using two-dimensional echocardiography.*

VonRamm OT, Thurstone FL: Cardiac imaging using a phased array ultrasound system. Circulation 53:258, 1976. *One of the early papers describing the value of phased array sector scanning for examining the heart.*

41.4. Nuclear Cardiology

Barry L. Zaret

Nuclear cardiology is based upon the ability of externally placed instruments to detect, define, and quantify radiation emanating from cardiac structures following injection of a radioisotope. Recently there has been an increasing interest in this relatively new discipline. This interest reflects the growing utility of nuclear procedures for defining pathophysiologic and diagnostic phenomena in cardiac patients. Since these procedures require the intravenous injection of only small quantities of short-lived radioisotopes, they can be safely repeated. The physical properties of the radioisotopes (radionuclides) employed render them suitable for both imaging and biodistribution studies. Changes in cardiac blood volume, myocardial perfusion, and viability can be evaluated.

CARDIAC PERFORMANCE

At present, the major clinical application of nuclear cardiology is in the assessment of cardiac performance. This is achieved with radionuclides that remain within the intravascular space during the period of study, whether that period encompasses 10 to 15 seconds or several hours. Computer technology is critical for making appropriate measurements of both left and right ventricles. Cardiac performance can be assessed in two general ways: during the first pass of the isotope through the central circulation, or following its equilibration in the cardiac blood pool. First-pass radionuclide angiocardiography is completed within 30 seconds following intravenous injection. The raw data are stored for further processing, and then, using computer techniques, regions of interest are selected involving each ventricle. There is temporal and anatomic segregation of the radioactive bolus during its first transit through the central circulation. Thus it is possible to make concomitant measurements of right and left ventricular function without concern that radioactivity present in one ventricle is interfering with the analysis of the other. Analysis of time-activity curves generated from the respective ventricular regions allows determination of ventricular ejection fraction (Fig. 41–33). Count rates emanating from a cardiac chamber are proportional to the volume of the chamber. In addition to analysis of ejection fraction, rates of ventricular filling and emptying, and ventricular volumes, quantitative and qualitative assessments of regional wall motion can be made from the same data (Fig. 41–34). Technetium-99m is administered in

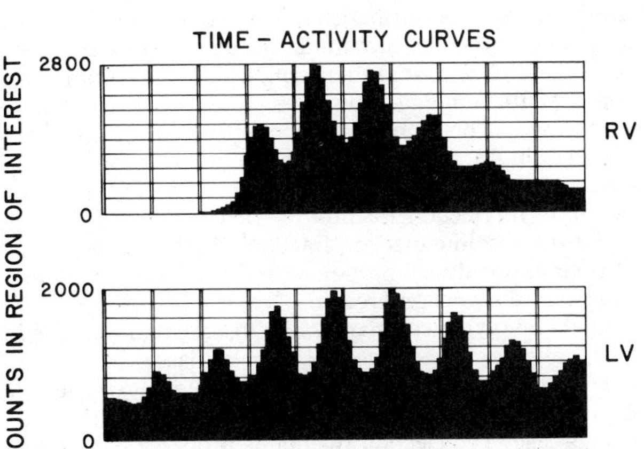

Figure 41–33. Right ventricular (RV) and left ventricular (LV) time-activity curves obtained at 20 frames per second with the computerized multicrystal scintillation camera. Analysis of these time-activity curves allows determination of ventricular ejection fraction. (Reproduced from Berger HJ, et al.: Semin Nucl Med 9:275, 1979.)

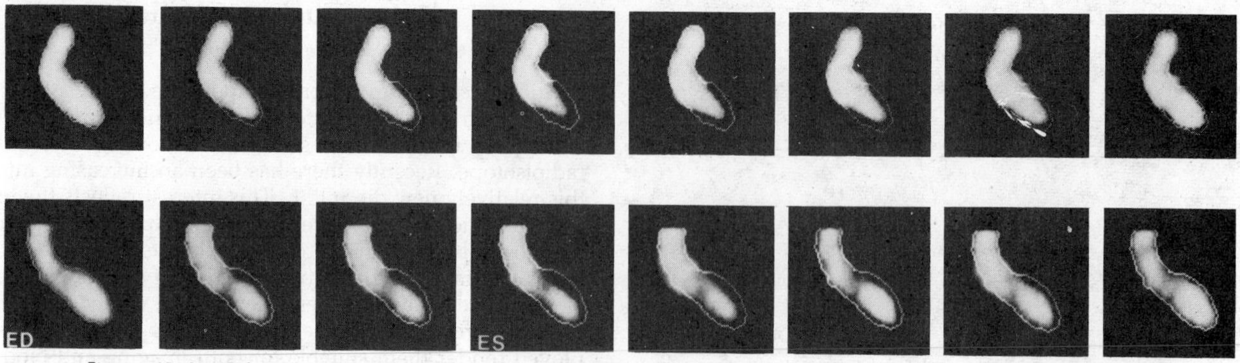

Figure 41–34. Selected serial 50 millisecond left ventricular images obtained throughout the cardiac cycle shown superimposed over the end-diastolic perimeters. The first frame in each series represents end-diastole (ED) and the fourth frame end-systole (ES). The upper row of images was obtained at rest and the lower row during maximal bicycle exercise in a patient with coronary artery disease. The two series are displayed at the same heart rate. Regional wall motion is normal at rest. However, inferoapical hypokinesis is present during exercise. (Reproduced from Berger HJ, et al.: Semin Nucl Med 9:275, 1979.)

various chemical forms or complexes employed. A generator-produced very short-lived radionuclide (gold-195m) also may be used in these studies.

The alternative approach to assessing cardiac performance involves complete equilibration of the radionuclide within the intravascular space. Physiologic signals are introduced which convert the conventional static imaging procedure into a dynamic assessment of cardiac function. To obtain this goal technetium-99m is bound to the patient's own erythrocytes. The technetium-99m label remains evenly distributed throughout the intravascular blood volume for several hours. Using the electrocardiogram as the signal, nuclear data are segregated according to the time of their occurrence within the cardiac cycle. Relationships between the surface electrocardiogram and volumetric changes within the cardiac cycle are employed to develop these dynamic data. The R wave peak corresponds to maximal (end-diastolic) radioactivity. Data are summed over several hundred cardiac cycles, and composite data are quantified and displayed as sequential 20- to 50-millisecond points which together define a representative cardiac cycle. The ventricular volume curve derived from these data is suitable for direct measurement of ejection fraction. The data also may be displayed as a series of images which, when projected in cinematic format, provide a direct visual assessment of the regional contraction patterns of the heart (Fig. 41–35). The same technique may be used to measure ventricular volumes.

Both first-pass and equilibrium techniques can be employed to study cardiac performance under conditions of rest and exercise. Data may be accumulated during either supine or upright bicycle exercise. Often critical data concerning cardiovascular status emerge only when the patient is evaluated during stress. The normal response to exercise involves an augmentation in the pump function of both right and left ventricles. Normal ventricular reserve generally is defined as an increase in ejection fraction of each ventricle of at least 5 per cent (in absolute ejection fraction units), and the presence of normal regional wall motion. Abnormal exercise ventricular reserve may be encountered in a variety of pathophysiologic conditions involving coronary artery disease and intrinsic myocardial, valvular, and congenital heart disease.

The study of cardiac performance employing nuclear techniques has been particularly useful in patients with coronary artery disease. The ejection fraction is probably the single best clinical indicator of global ventricular pump performance. This index is of major prognostic importance in the long-term assessment of patients with coronary artery disease, either immediately following myocardial infarction or in the chronic stable phase of disease. Analysis of the ventricular ejection fraction is based upon radioactivity counts taken over the entire cardiac cycle. It is not dependent upon geometric assumptions concerning ventricular shape or ventricular volume. In coronary artery disease, particularly following myocardial infarction, asymmetric contraction patterns are common. In these ischemic ventricles, cavitary shapes frequently cannot be approximated

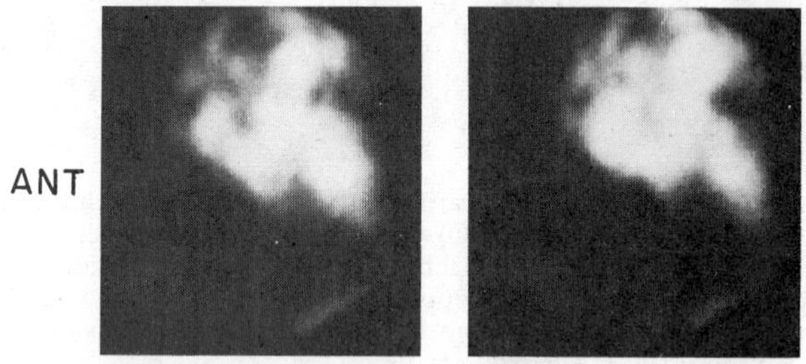

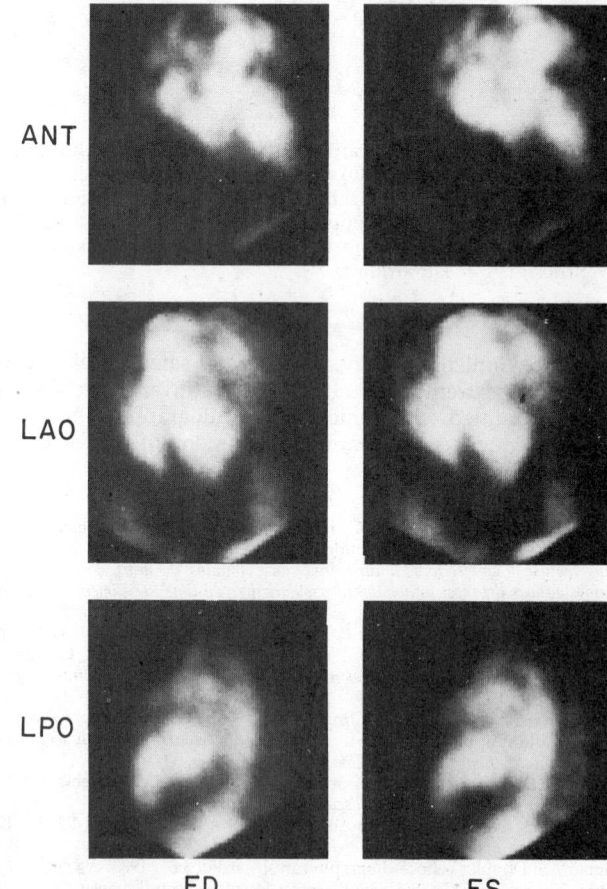

Figure 41–35. Gated cardiac blood pool studies obtained in the anterior (ANT), 45 degree left anterior oblique (LAO), and left posterior oblique (LPO) positions. End-diastolic images (ED) are shown on the left and end-systolic (ES) on the right . Note that radioactivity is present throughout the entire cardiac blood pool. A large anteroapical left ventricular aneurysm is appreciated in all three positions. Note that in the LAO position image the left ventricle is the posterior cardiac structure and the right ventricle the anterior structure. These are separated by the interventricular septum, which is displayed as an area devoid of radioactivity. (Reproduced from Berger HJ, et al.: Radiol Clin North Am 18:441, 1980.)

by idealized geometric models. Using portable equipment, it is possible to study cardiac performance at the bedside of acutely ill patients in coronary and intensive care units. Such studies have demonstrated substantial abnormalities in the functioning of the ischemic left ventricle during the acute phase of myocardial infarction. Abnormalities of both left and right ventricle can be identified. Right ventricular infarction occurring in the course of inferior wall infarction has been identified and further defined. In the patient with coronary artery disease and congestive heart failure, a left ventricular aneurysm amenable to surgery can be differentiated from diffuse left ventricular dysfunction.

Abnormalities of ventricular performance are found in approximately 85 per cent of patients with coronary artery disease studied during exercise stress. Myocardial ischemia is reflected in abnormal ventricular reserve. Abnormal ventricular reserve presents as lack of augmentation or an actual fall of the normal ejection fraction with exercise, or development of regional abnormalities of wall motion. Abnormal responses of the ejection fraction may be encountered in a variety of conditions, but the development of new regional abnormalities of wall motion is quite specific for coronary artery disease.

Radionuclide assessment of ventricular performance may also be employed in the evaluation of patients with valvular disease at rest or exercise. Resting measurements of cardiac function are important preoperative prognostic data and may also be of value in defining the physiologic significance of valvular lesions such as mitral regurgitation. For example, normal left ventricular function in a patient with severe mitral regurgitation would imply a primary valvular problem, whereas severe ventricular dysfunction would suggest that the mitral regurgitation might be secondary to impaired papillary muscle function resulting from diffuse myocardial disease. Assessment of ventricular performance under conditions of hemodynamic stress may help define the advent of irreversible damage in patients with valvular heart disease. This is particularly important in the patient with aortic regurgitation in whom irremediable change in left ventricular function is frequently present by the time valve surgery is considered. This approach is also valuable in the assessment of patients with congenital heart disease involving both left and right ventricles.

Radionuclide studies also have been employed in the evaluation of myocardial function in patients with lung disease. In chronic obstructive pulmonary disease, the major hemodynamic burden falls on the right ventricle. Right ventricular performance can probably be evaluated best with the first-pass radionuclide angiocardiographic technique. Abnormalities in right ventricular performance have been noted at rest and during exercise in patients with chronic obstructive pulmonary disease, and have been related to the degree of impairment in ventilatory performance. Pharmacologic interventions may modify abnormal right ventricular performance.

The techniques for quantitative assessment of ventricular performance have been standardized and validated. This allows utilization of these techniques for long-term studies assessing cardiac therapy, both surgical and medical. A prototype example has been the application of first-pass radionuclide angiocardiography for the serial assessment of ventricular function in patients receiving the antineoplastic agent doxorubicin. Use of this agent has been limited by the frequent development of a drug-induced cardiomyopathy. Serial measurement of cardiac ejection fraction during the course of therapy has led to a set of guidelines of dosage and schedule that help avert cardiotoxicity.

In addition, left-to-right shunts can be detected and quantified during performance of the first-pass radionuclide angiocardiogram. With this technique, a time-activity curve is generated from a region in the lung field. In the presence of a shunt, early recirculation is detected. With additional techniques, the curve can be deconvoluted so that the major components can be assessed individually and quantified, and the pulmonic-systemic blood flow ratios determined. The technique is reliable as long as left ventricular performance is not impaired. In the presence of major left ventricular dysfunction, false-positive results can occur.

MYOCARDIAL PERFUSION IMAGING

Myocardial perfusion imaging utilizes radionuclides which traverse the myocardial capillary system and enter the myocardial cell. The radionuclide employed for these studies is thallium-201. This tracer is considered a potassium analogue, since its distribution generally mirrors that of intracellular potassium. Thallium-201 is produced in the cyclotron and has a physical half-life of approximately 72 hours. The isotope has a relatively low energy spectrum, thereby allowing imaging with conventional scintillation cameras. After intravenous injection it is rapidly extracted and distributed within the myocardium according to regional myocardial blood flow and regional cellular viability. Its accumulation is also dependent upon regional metabolism and factors governing intracellular transport of monovalent cations.

In the resting state the normal myocardial perfusion image demonstrates a homogeneous uptake in the left ventricular wall with a central area of decreased activity corresponding to the left ventricular cavity. In approximately 20 per cent of normal patients there is a region of decreased uptake at the cardiac apex corresponding to a normal anatomic variation of relative thinning of this portion of the left ventricular myocardium. Abnormal image patterns will demonstrate a zone of decreased myocardial perfusion as a region of relatively decreased radionuclide uptake. Images are obtained in multiple positions. This is necessary to confirm the presence of a defect and define its location. The normal right ventricle is not visualized at rest because of its smaller mass compared to that of the left ventricle.

In the resting state abnormalities usually are due to either acute or remote myocardial infarction. However, studies have also demonstrated perfusion defects at rest in patients with unstable angina or coronary spasm (either spontaneous or induced by ergonovine maleate) or, rarely, in patients with severe obstructive coronary disease in the absence of clinical evidence of acute ischemia. Defects are noted with a high degree of sensitivity during the early hours of an acute myocardial infarction. Within the first six hours virtually all infarcts may be identified as perfusion defects. After 24 hours sensitivity falls to 80 to 90 per cent.

In most patients with coronary artery disease without previous infarction, myocardial perfusion patterns appear normal at rest. This is to be expected, since from a pathophysiologic standpoint coronary blood flow is relatively uniform at rest, even in the presence of severe coronary obstruction. The major physiologic abnormality in coronary disease is a diminished coronary vascular reserve under conditions of augmented myocardial oxygen requirement. Therefore to detect perfusion abnormalities in coronary disease it is necessary to study patients under conditions that require increased myocardial blood flow. Most work to date has employed exercise as an appropriate stress. Thallium-201 is injected at peak exercise, and imaging is begun within ten minutes after injection. Since thallium is rapidly extracted by myocardium, it can be injected during the period of maximal heterogeneity of regional myocardial blood flow during exercise. Its distribution within the left ventricular myocardium will reflect this heterogeneity. Comparison of images obtained immediately following exercise with those obtained following a redistribution phase three to four hours after exercise allows definition of transiently ischemic zones (Fig. 41–36). Defects present on exercise but not at redistribution are most consistent with transient ischemia; defects which are unchanged during stress are most consistent with previous infarction and scar; and defects that are present at redistribution but are markedly increased during exercise are most consistent with transient ischemia superimposed upon previous infarction

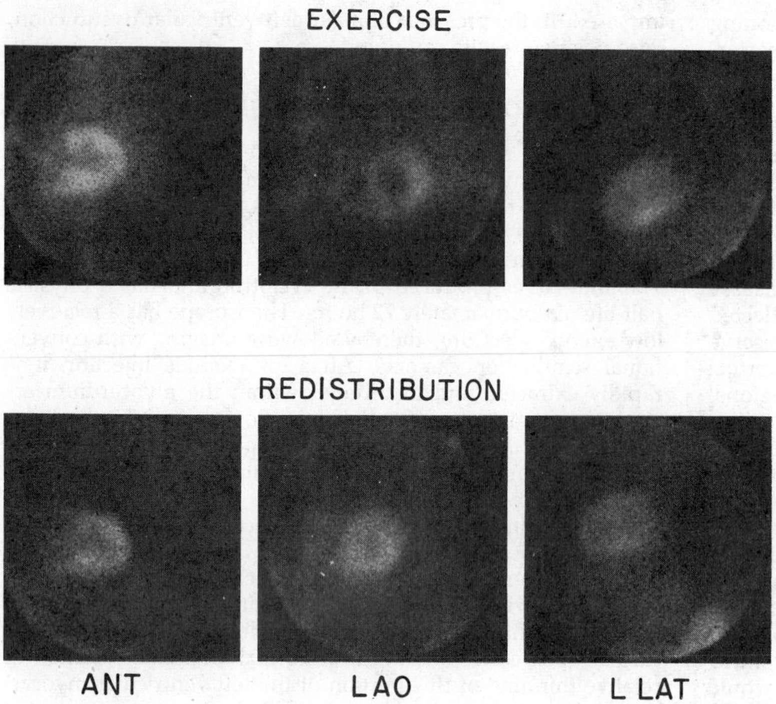

Figure 41–36. Exercise (upper panels) and redistribution (lower panels) thallium-201 myocardial perfusion images in a patient with significant coronary artery disease. Anterior position (ANT) images are shown in the left panels, left anterior oblique (LAO) images in the middle panels, and left lateral (L LAT) images in the right panels. Note a significant perfusion defect present in the anteroseptal wall seen in the LAO image and in the anteroapical wall seen in the L LAT image during exercise, with substantial redistribution and filling in of the perfusion defect on the redistribution images. This study is consistent with transient myocardial ischemia and coronary artery disease involving at least the left anterior descending coronary artery.

and scar. The overall sensitivity of this technique for detecting significant ischemic disease is approximately 80 per cent. The specificity of the technique is excellent. This technique is of greatest value diagnostically in patients with equivocal exercise electrocardiograms, abnormal baseline electrocardiograms, or suspected false-positive or false-negative conventional exercise tests.

An alternative means of stress perfusion imaging involves the injection of the maximal coronary vasodilator dipyridamole. Thallium myocardial distributions following dipyridamole infusion can provide data comparable to those noted with exercise. However, with pharmacologic stress, evaluation is based upon differences in flow without necessarily implying superimposed ischemia, whereas with exercise evaluation is based upon heterogeneity of flow, which generally is associated with concomitant myocardial ischemia.

New technical advances currently are making important contributions to thallium imaging. The first involves quantitative sequential planar imaging, which allows objective definition of the presence of perfusion defects and quantification of regional washout kinetics. Frequently an abnormal region will demonstrate only abnormal radionuclide washout without a visualized exercise perfusion defect. This technique is particularly important diagnostically in defining the extent of coronary disease. The second technique involves tomography. Using a computer and rotating detector(s), the three-dimensional display of radionuclide can be visualized and evaluated in several axes. This technique offers promise in defining lesions that are obscured by overlap of several regions in conventional planar imaging.

INFARCT-AVID IMAGING

The last clinical radionuclide approach to the cardiac patient involves definition of acute myocardial infarction and regions of acute myocardial necrosis. This is performed with "infarct-avid" radiotracers, which bind selectively to regions of acute myocardial necrosis. The agent of choice for this procedure is technetium-99m stannous pyrophosphate. With this technique, acute infarcts are visualized as regions of increased radionuclide uptake. The mechanism of abnormal pyrophosphate accumulation in myocardial necrotic zones appears to be related to regional calcium deposition, as well as binding to denatured proteins within the infarct zone. Pyrophosphate uptake is dependent upon sufficient residual blood flow to allow entry of the radioactive tracer into the zone of myocardial necrosis.

The infarct zone can be imaged within 24 to 48 hours of the onset of infarction. Maximal visualization generally occurs from 48 to 72 hours after the infarct has occurred. Images usually are not positive within the first 24 hours. These results are in direct contrast to patterns seen with thallium-201, with which maximal sensitivity of infarct detection is present in the earliest hours after infarction. Images generally are no longer positive seven to ten days after the infarct. However, some patients maintain persistently positive pyrophosphate images. From the standpoint of diagnosis, pyrophosphate imaging appears to be a sensitive means of detecting acute myocardial infarction as well as extension of the infarct. Sensitivity may be somewhat less in patients with nontransmural as compared to transmural infarction. Pyrophosphate infarct imaging is most valuable in patients presenting several days after infarction when both electrocardiograms and enzyme studies are equivocal or nondiagnostic.

POSITRON TOMOGRAPHY

This technique involves imaging and quantification of the intracardiac distribution of positron-emitting radionuclides. By virtue of the types of radionuclides available and the instrumentation employed, this technique has provided new insight into metabolism and coronary flow. Because of the cost involved and general need for an on-site cyclotron, this technique remains experimental and localized to only a few centers.

Berger HJ, Zaret BL: Nuclear cardiology. N Engl J Med 305:799, 855, 1981. *Relatively comprehensive review of clinical nuclear cardiology with 198 individual references cited.*

Berman DS, Mason DT (eds.): Clinical Nuclear Cardiology. New York, Grune & Stratton, 1981. *An excellent general nuclear cardiology text.*

Freeman LM, Blaufox MD (eds.): Cardiovascular Nuclear Medicine. New York, Grune & Stratton, 1980. *This book represents a compendium of three individual issues of Seminars in Nuclear Medicine. It currently represents a good overall review of the field of nuclear cardiology.*

Strauss HW, Pitt B (eds.): Cardiovascular Nuclear Medicine. St. Louis, C. V. Mosby Company, 1979. *A leading textbook in the field of nuclear cardiology. This book contains 24 individual chapters summarizing the field. In addition to imaging, excellent reviews of radioimmunoassay are given. A balanced presentation is given of all aspects of nuclear imaging.*

41.5. Cardiac Catheterization and Cineangiography

Donald C. Harrison

Cardiac catheterization continues to provide a unique, comprehensive, and quantitative assessment of cardiac structure and function. As facilities have become more widely available and as the risks have decreased, there has been a progressive tendency to employ catheterization in the diagnosis and management of patients with heart disease. With the development of additional techniques such as bedside hemodynamic monitoring, intracardiac electrophysiologic testing, endomyocardial biopsy, and percutaneous transluminal coronary angioplasty, it is increasingly important for the internist to understand the indications, capabilities, and risks of cardiac catheterization.

INDICATIONS FOR CARDIAC CATHETERIZATION. Not all patients with heart disease are candidates for catheterization because of the small but unavoidable risk and moderate patient expense. Only those patients in whom catheterization provides information required for optimal medical or surgical care should be studied. The most common indications are listed in Table 41–5.

Essentially all patients being considered for surgical treatment of congenital, coronary, valvular, or pericardial heart disease should undergo preoperative cardiac catheterization to verify the diagnosis and to exclude unsuspected concomitant cardiac pathology such as significant coronary artery disease in the patient referred for valve replacement.

In some cases, catheterization may be required to determine whether cardiac surgery is necessary. An example would be the patient with mitral stenosis in whom symptoms seem out of proportion to clinical and noninvasive findings and in whom precise hemodynamic measurements facilitate appropriate management. Certain cardiac diseases, such as significant stenosis of the left main coronary artery or severe aortic stenosis, are best treated surgically even when only mild cardiac symptoms are present, and an increasing number of catheterizations are being performed to detect these conditions in patients following noninvasive studies that suggest life-threatening lesions.

Additional indications for cardiac catheterization include evaluation of patients with clinically troublesome but atypical chest pain and assessment of the extent of coronary artery disease in patients about to undergo major surgery for correction of atherosclerotic cerebral or peripheral vascular disease. Catheterization may also be performed to select or evaluate drug therapy in patients with severe hemodynamic or electrophysiologic cardiac dysfunction. Particular use of programmed electrophysiologic stimulation to direct antiarrhythmic drug therapy and select high-risk subjects has increased.

TABLE 41–5. SELECTED INDICATIONS FOR CARDIAC CATHETERIZATION

- Coronary artery disease
  - Angina refractory to medical therapy
  - Unstable angina
  - Noninvasive data suggesting left main coronary stenosis
  - Preoperative evaluation (valve surgery in males over 35 years of age, females over 40 years of age; major vascular surgery in patients with suspected coronary artery disease)
  - After acute infarction (patients under 50 years of age, postinfarction angina, or positive treadmill test at low level exercise)
  - Vasospastic coronary disease
  - Evaluation of strongly positive treadmill-thallium-201 scan in patients with high risk occupations (airline pilots)
- Valvular heart disease
  - Progressive symptoms of congestive heart failure
  - Noninvasive evidence (echocardiography chest x-ray) of worsening cardiac function
  - Aortic stenosis—even minimal symptoms of angina, congestive failure, or exertional syncope
- Congenital heart disease—guided by symptoms and noninvasive studies
- Pericardial disease (effusion, constriction)—elevated right atrial pressure
- Other
  - Percutaneous transluminal coronary angioplasty
  - Electrophysiologic study
  - Endomyocardial biopsy
  - Bedside hemodynamic monitoring

CAPABILITIES OF CARDIAC CATHETERIZATION. All techniques of cardiac catheterization have in common the introduction of tubular radiopaque catheters (outer diameter between 2 and 3 mm) into peripheral arteries or veins and passage of the catheter tip into the heart. Although the brachial cutdown method of vascular access continues to be used, the percutaneous technique developed by Seldinger has found increasing application. In this technique, the desired artery (femoral or axillary) or vein (femoral, antecubital, jugular, or subclavian) is punctured with a specially designed 18 gauge needle inserted under local anesthesia. A flexible metal guide wire is passed through this needle into the vessel lumen and remains in place as the needle is removed. The guide wire can be used to pass a catheter directly into the vessel or to place a short hollow sheath through which the catheter can then be inserted. Using either technique, a series of different catheters can be inserted through the same entry site, enabling pressure measurement, blood sampling, radiographic contrast injection, or such specialized tasks as electrophysiologic recording, endomyocardial biopsy, or percutaneous transluminal coronary angioplasty.

HEMODYNAMIC MEASUREMENTS. Hollow, fluid-filled catheters transmit intracardiac pressures from the catheter tip to an externally located strain gauge which converts these pressures into an electronic signal displayed on a recording device. Pressure transducers have also been miniaturized for direct placement on the tip of catheters. Permanent recordings of pressure traces are scaled in millimeters of mercury relative to a zero reference point (the mid-chest level of the supine patient). By manipulating the catheter where it enters the patient, the operator can direct the catheter tip into various cardiac chambers under fluoroscopic visualization, recording intracavitary pressures from each site. When evaluation of the cardiovascular response to exercise is required, these pressure measurements may be repeated during supine bicycle ergometry. Measurement of intracardiac blood flow or cardiac output may be performed by either the direct Fick or indicator dilution methods and used to evaluate valvular heart disease and to detect intracardiac shunts.

RIGHT HEART CATHETERIZATION. Catheterization of the right heart (right atrium, right ventricle, and pulmonary artery) was initiated by Werner Forssmann in 1929, when he passed a urologic catheter from his antecubital fossa to his right atrium. In the 1940's, this technique was extended to catheterization of the right ventricle and pulmonary artery and to detailed measurements in a variety of cardiac diseases. The utility of right heart catheterization greatly increased in the late 1940's with the application of the pulmonary capillary wedge (or pulmonary artery wedge) pressure, obtained when the catheter tip is advanced peripherally until it occludes a pulmonary artery branch of comparable caliber. While the right atrial pressure (central venous pressure) provides a rough index of intravascular volume status and right ventricular function, the pulmonary capillary wedge pressure reflects the pulmonary venous and left atrial pressure, thereby providing an index of left ventricular filling and function. In the presence of mitral regurgitation, the pulmonary capillary wedge pressure may demonstrate a large systolic "v" wave reflecting the systolic increase in left atrial pressure caused by the flow of regurgitant blood into that chamber. When pericardial effusion or thickening is present, elevation and equalization of diastolic right heart and pulmonary capillary wedge pressures are evidence that pericardial disease is interfering with cardiac function. Although right heart catheterization has declined in importance, it is still required for the measurement of cardiac output, the detection of intracardiac shunts, and the evaluation of primary or secondary right heart dysfunction.

The development in the 1970's of a balloon-tipped catheter

TABLE 41–6. NORMAL RESTING VALUES OF HEMODYNAMIC PARAMETERS

Pressures (in mm Hg)
- Right heart
  - Right atrium (a/v/m) 6/6/4
  - Right ventricle (s/d/ed) 25/0/6
- Pulmonary artery (s/d/m) 25/12/16
  - Pulmonary capillary wedge (a/v/m) 12/12/10
- Left heart
  - Left atrium (a/v/m) 12/12/10
  - Left ventricle (s/d/ed) 120/0/12
  - Aorta (s/d/m) 120/80/93

Flow
- Cardiac index (L/min-M^2) 2.5–3.5
- Cardiac output (L/min) 4–6
- Oxygen consumption (ml O_2/min/M_2) 130 (110–150)
- Arteriovenous oxygen difference (ml O_2/liter blood) 30–50

Resistance (in dyne-sec/cm^5)
- Pulmonary vascular resistance 50–150
- Systemic vascular resistance 800–1200

a = "a" wave.
v = "v" wave.
m = mean.
s = systolic.
d = diastolic.
ed = end-diastolic (post-a wave).

(Swan-Ganz), which can be placed into the pulmonary artery at the bedside without the use of fluoroscopy, has extended right heart catheterization to the intensive care and coronary care units. Once the catheter has been advanced to the pulmonary artery, inflation of the tip balloon causes further advancement into the pulmonary capillary wedge position. The left-sided filling pressure may be monitored by following the pulmonary artery diastolic pressure if it is equal to the pulmonary capillary wedge pressure, as it is in most patients. These measurements of the right and left heart filling pressures and cardiac output by either direct Fick or thermodilution techniques give an ongoing picture of cardiac function in the seriously ill patient, with only minimal risk.

LEFT HEART CATHETERIZATION. Insertion of a catheter into a peripheral artery allows retrograde passage of the catheter to the aortic root, across the aortic valve, and into the left ventricle. When the presence of severe aortic stenosis or a mechanical aortic valve prosthesis prevents retrograde catheterization of the left heart, the left ventricle may be entered by direct percutaneous puncture, or more commonly by the transseptal approach. In transseptal catheterization, a specially shaped catheter is passed from the right atrium to the left atrium by puncture of the interatrial septum in the region of the fossa ovalis. Once in the left atrium, the catheter can be manipulated across the mitral valve into the left ventricle.

Left heart catheterization is essential to the evaluation of mitral and aortic valve dysfunction. Measurement of the left ventricular and aortic pressures allows calculation of the aortic valve area (see below). Measurement of the left atrial (or pulmonary capillary wedge) and left ventricular pressures allows the calculation of the mitral valve area. Left heart catheterization also allows assessment of left ventricular function by measurement of the left ventricular end-diastolic pressure (elevated in left ventricular failure) and measurement of the dP/dt or rate of rise of the early systolic left ventricular pressure (depressed in left ventricular failure). In many laboratories, a special catheter with a miniature strain gauge mounted on the catheter tip is used instead of a fluid-filled catheter, to provide better frequency response in recording the left ventricular pressure and dP/dt.

CARDIAC OUTPUT, VALVE AREA, AND INTRACARDIAC SHUNTS. Measurement of the cardiac output, the amount of blood pumped by the heart in one minute, is an important hemodynamic measurement. This measurement can be performed using the direct Fick principle, in which the pulmonary oxygen

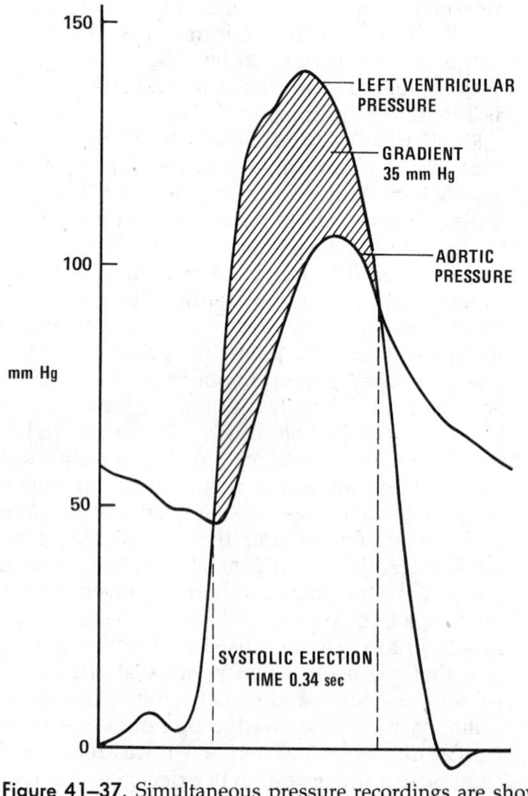

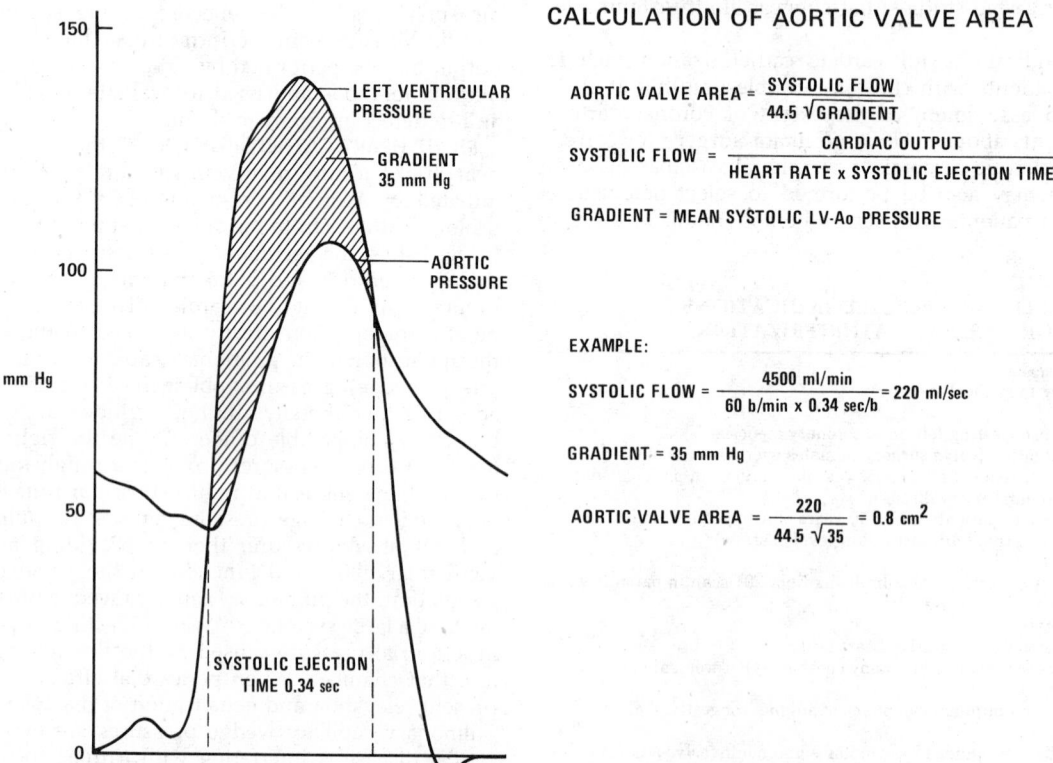

AORTIC STENOSIS: CALCULATION OF AORTIC VALVE AREA

$$\text{AORTIC VALVE AREA} = \frac{\text{SYSTOLIC FLOW}}{44.5\sqrt{\text{GRADIENT}}}$$

$$\text{SYSTOLIC FLOW} = \frac{\text{CARDIAC OUTPUT}}{\text{HEART RATE} \times \text{SYSTOLIC EJECTION TIME}}$$

GRADIENT = MEAN SYSTOLIC LV-Ao PRESSURE

EXAMPLE:

$$\text{SYSTOLIC FLOW} = \frac{4500 \text{ ml/min}}{60 \text{ b/min} \times 0.34 \text{ sec/b}} = 220 \text{ ml/sec}$$

GRADIENT = 35 mm Hg

$$\text{AORTIC VALVE AREA} = \frac{220}{44.5\sqrt{35}} = 0.8 \text{ cm}^2$$

Figure 41–37. Simultaneous pressure recordings are shown from the left ventricle and ascending aorta in a patient with moderately severe aortic stenosis. The Gorlin formula, used to calculate the aortic valve area (orifice), is given at the right of the figure. (LV = left ventricle, Ao = aorta, b/min = beats per minute (heart rate), sec/b = seconds per beat.) The number 44.5 is the constant used for calculating aortic valve area; a different constant (= 38) is used for calculating mitral valve area.

uptake (determined by analysis of expired air) is equated to the product of cardiac output (blood flow through the lungs) and the A-V O_2 difference (the difference in oxygen content between arterial and mixed venous blood).

$$\text{Cardiac output (L/min)} = \frac{\text{Oxygen uptake (ml } O_2\text{/min)}}{\text{A-V } O_2 \text{ difference (ml } O_2\text{/L blood)}}$$

If the oxygen uptake cannot be measured directly, it may be approximated (in the resting patient) as 130 ml O_2 per minute per square meter of body surface area. If the hemoglobin and arterial (A) and pulmonary artery (PA) oxygen saturations are known, the A-V O_2 difference can be calculated:

$$\text{A-V } O_2 \text{ difference (ml } O_2\text{/L blood)} = 13.6 \times \text{hemoglobin (mg/100 ml)} \times (\text{\% sat A} - \text{\% sat PA})$$

Cardiac output may also be measured by the indicator dilution method. A small amount of indocyanine green dye (dye dilution method) or chilled saline (thermodilution method) is injected into the venous circulation, with the downstream concentration of these substances determined by the measurement of dye absorbance or of blood temperature, respectively. The data are processed, usually with the aid of a microcomputer, to determine the amount of blood admixed with the indicator, and hence the cardiac output. The cardiac index is derived by dividing the cardiac output by the body surface area.

Measurement of both the blood flow and the pressure differential (gradient) across a cardiac valve allows determination of the stenotic orifice (valve area) using the Gorlin formula (Fig. 41–37). When the valve in question is regurgitant as well as stenotic, transvalvular flow is greater than reflected by the net forward flow or cardiac output, so that the Gorlin formula tends to underestimate the actual valve area. In this case, greater accuracy may often be obtained by use of the angiographically calculated total left ventricular stroke volume × heart rate (see below) rather than the forward cardiac output.

Determination of the cardiac output is also required for the calculation of the resistance posed by the pulmonary and systemic vascular beds. These resistances are important to the evaluation of congenital and valvular heart disease and to the adjustment of afterload reducing medications in patients with severe left ventricular dysfunction.

$$\text{Pulmonary vascular resistance} = \frac{(\text{Mean PA} - \text{Mean PCW})}{\text{Cardiac output}} \times 80 \; (\text{nl } 50\text{–}150 \; \frac{\text{dyne-sec}}{\text{cm}^5})$$

$$\text{Systemic vascular resistance} = \frac{(\text{Mean Ao} - \text{Mean RA})}{\text{Cardiac output}} \times 80 \; (\text{nl } 800\text{–}1200 \; \frac{\text{dyne-sec}}{\text{cm}^5})$$

When an intracardiac shunt is present (i.e., atrial or ventricular septal defect), the pulmonary and systemic blood flows are no longer equal, but can be individually calculated from the oxygen content of blood samples drawn from the right and left heart chambers (Fig. 41–38). These data allow calculation of the direction, site, and magnitude of an intracardiac shunt. Shunts too small to be detected by this oximetric method may be detected by more sensitive techniques such as angiography (see below). In some laboratories, small boluses of green dye or ascorbic acid are injected into a series of right and left heart chambers to identify a small intracardiac shunt, reflected as

VENTRICULAR SEPTAL DEFECT:
CALCULATION OF INTRACARDIAC SHUNT BY OXIMETRY

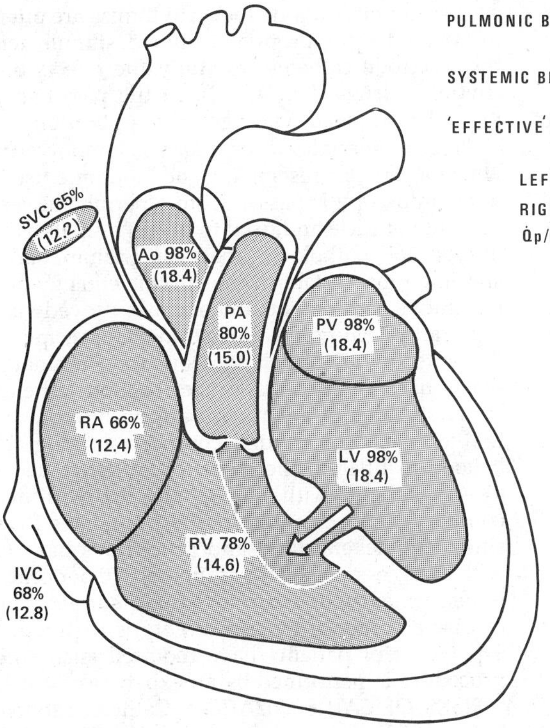

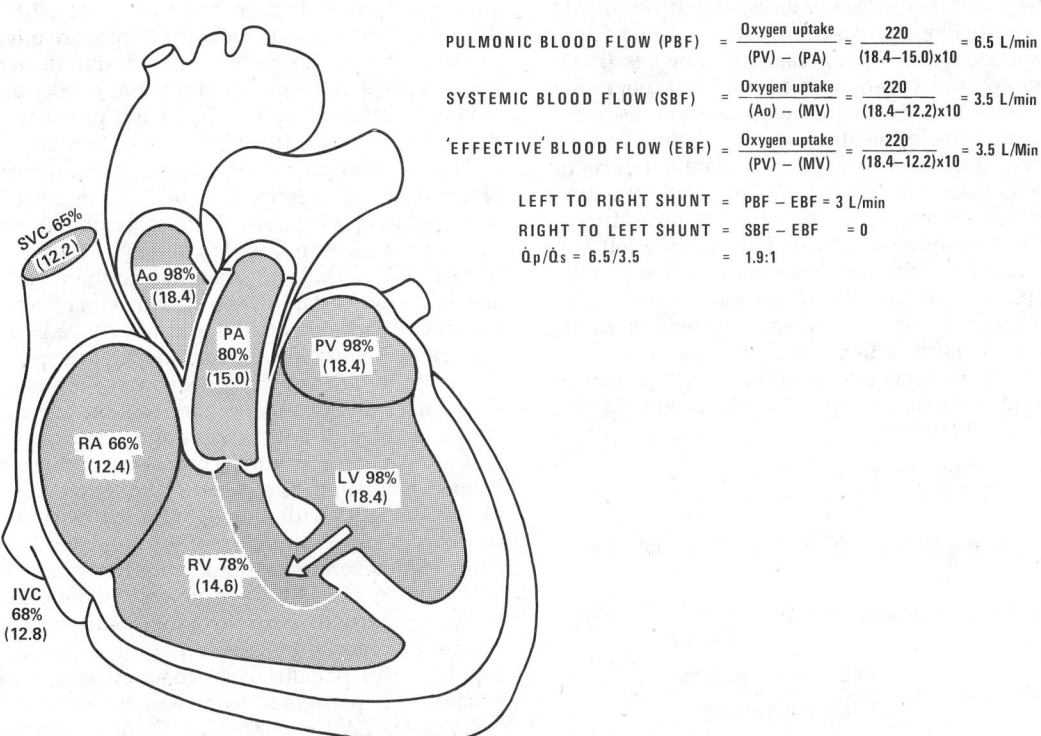

$$\text{PULMONIC BLOOD FLOW (PBF)} = \frac{\text{Oxygen uptake}}{(\text{PV}) - (\text{PA})} = \frac{220}{(18.4-15.0)\text{x}10} = 6.5 \text{ L/min}$$

$$\text{SYSTEMIC BLOOD FLOW (SBF)} = \frac{\text{Oxygen uptake}}{(\text{Ao}) - (\text{MV})} = \frac{220}{(18.4-12.2)\text{x}10} = 3.5 \text{ L/min}$$

$$\text{'EFFECTIVE' BLOOD FLOW (EBF)} = \frac{\text{Oxygen uptake}}{(\text{PV}) - (\text{MV})} = \frac{220}{(18.4-12.2)\text{x}10} = 3.5 \text{ L/Min}$$

LEFT TO RIGHT SHUNT = PBF – EBF = 3 L/min
RIGHT TO LEFT SHUNT = SBF – EBF = 0
$\dot{Q}p/\dot{Q}s$ = 6.5/3.5 = 1.9:1

Figure 41–38. Use of oximetry to define the site, direction, and magnitude of an intracardiac shunt secondary to a ventricular septal defect. Oxygen saturations are shown in per cent saturation for each chamber, and the corresponding oxygen contents (in ml O_2 per 100 ml blood) are shown in parentheses, assuming a hemoglobin concentration of 14 mg per 100 ml. The substantial increase in oxygen content from right atrium to right ventricle localizes the left-to-right shunt to the ventricular level. The formulas at the right illustrate the calculation of pulmonic, systemic, and "effective" blood flow, and their use in calculating the left-to-right and right-to-left shunt flows and the shunt ratio $\dot{Q}p/\dot{Q}s$ (ratio of pulmonic to systemic blood flow). (SVC = superior vena cava, IVC = inferior vena cava, RA = right atrium, RV = right ventricle, PA = pulmonary artery, PV = pulmonary vein, LV = left ventricle, Ao = aorta.) The small discrepancy between RV and PA saturation is due to incomplete blood mixing in the RV.

either the early appearance of indicator in a downstream cardiac chamber or the early recirculation of a fraction of the indicator bolus.

CARDIAC ANGIOGRAPHY. Injection of radiographic contrast material (radiopaque iodinated dyes) through cardiac catheters permits opacification of the cardiac chambers and vessels. The left ventricle and coronary arteries are most frequently studied in this manner. Injections are usually recorded on videotape to allow immediate review in the catheterization laboratory, but are also recorded on high-speed movie film to allow later detailed examination.

Left Ventriculography. Injection of contrast material into the left ventricle, usually a total of 45 ml injected at a rate of 12 ml per second, opacifies the left ventricular cavity and allows observation of the contraction and relaxation of the ventricular wall. Regional damage to the wall resulting from prior myocardial infarction may cause that region to move abnormally during ventricular systole; it may contract less vigorously (hypokinesis), may fail to contract at all (akinesis), or may even move outward during ventricular systole (dyskinesis). The left ventriculogram is usually performed with the patient in the 30 degree right anterior oblique projection (see below), but since no single projection visualizes the entire ventricular wall, it may be repeated in the 60 degree left anterior oblique projection to see the remaining wall segments. Since the projection places the plane of the interventricular septum end-on, it allows visualization of even those ventricular septal defects that are too small to be detected by oximetry.

After correction for radiographic magnification and distortion, analysis of the ventriculogram allows geometric calculation of the end-diastolic and end-systolic ventricular volumes (Dodge formula). The percentage of diastolic volume ejected during systole (ejection fraction) can then be calculated and is one of the most commonly used indices of left ventricular function. While ventriculography is routinely performed during left heart catheterization, two noninvasive techniques (radionuclide angiography and two-dimensional echocardiography) are now alternatives to ventriculography in selected cases.

In addition to assessing left ventricular size and function, left ventriculography is used to detect and quantitate mitral regurgitation. With the patient positioned in the 30 degree right anterior oblique projection, the plane of the atrioventricular valves (mitral and tricuspid) is seen end-on. During left ventriculography, mitral regurgitation allows contrast and blood to pass across this plane from the left ventricle into the left atrium. The more rapid and dense the left atrial opacification, the greater the amount of mitral regurgitation. If the left ventricular stroke volume (end-diastolic minus end-systolic volume) is calculated from quantitative angiography and compared with the forward stroke volume:

$$\frac{\text{Forward cardiac output}}{\text{Heart rate}}$$

two other indices of the severity of mitral regurgitation can be calculated:

$$\text{Regurgitant volume} = \text{Stroke volume} - \text{Forward stroke volume}$$

$$\text{Regurgitant fraction} = \frac{\text{Regurgitant volume}}{\text{Stroke volume}} (\%)$$

Aortic regurgitation may be demonstrated using similar techniques with contrast injection into the ascending aorta and calculations by the above formula.

Coronary Arteriography. Direct injection of contrast material into the coronary arteries has been used since 1959 to allow detailed examination of the human coronary anatomy. In the Sones technique, a single catheter is inserted by brachial arteriotomy and manipulated into first one and then the other coronary artery. In the Judkins technique, catheters shaped to inject either the left or right coronary artery are inserted percutaneously in the femoral artery, using the Seldinger technique. Regardless of which technique is used, each artery must be injected several times (using 3 to 7 ml of contrast per injection), with the patient turned in different positions (projections) relative to the x-ray tube. The use of multiple projections is necessary to visualize all segments of the coronary anatomy, free of foreshortening or concealment by overlapping vessels. The appearance of the coronary arteries in two of the standard projections is illustrated in Figure 41–39. A more recent addition to the standard rotational projections has been the use of cranial and caudal views, in which the x-ray tube is angled toward the patient's head or feet to better visualize the left main coronary artery and the proximal portions of the left anterior descending and circumflex coronary arteries. The location and severity of each stenosis (per cent reduction in vessel diameter) is described. Stenoses of less than 50 per cent reduction in vessel diameter (75 per cent in cross-sectional area) do not generally interfere with coronary artery blood flow. When coronary artery spasm is suspected (Prinzmetal's or variant angina), some centers repeat injection of the coronary arteries after intravenous administration of ergonovine maleate, a drug which may trigger an episode of coronary artery spasm in a susceptible patient. Increases in vascular tone frequently occur in vessels already damaged by atherosclerosis and may contribute to symptoms. This can be documented by the administration of ergonovine.

SPECIAL CATHETERIZATION TECHNIQUES. As experience with cardiac catheterization has increased, specialized techniques have continued to evolve. Intracardiac electrophysiology, developed in the late 1960's, uses catheters equipped with platinum electrodes to record electrical activity from within the heart. These studies are reserved for patients with serious disorders of cardiac conduction or rhythm. Catheters may be positioned in the right atrium, right ventricle, coronary sinus, or left ventricle, or against the septal portion of the tricuspid valve (adjacent to the His bundle), to record the conduction of cardiac depolarization. Tachyrhythmias are often provoked and terminated by appropriately timed stimuli delivered through the electrode catheters to study the effects of various antiarrhythmic drugs (Fig. 41–40). In the past five years this technique has enjoyed wider general application.

Another specialized technique is endomyocardial biopsy, in which a catheter resembling the bioptome used in gastrointestinal endoscopy is passed from a peripheral vessel into the left or right ventricle and used to obtain a small piece of ventricular muscle for pathologic analysis. Examination of the biopsy specimen may establish the specific etiology of a congestive or infiltrative cardiomyopathy and has proved valuable in detecting graft rejection in cardiac transplant recipients.

The technique of percutaneous transluminal coronary angioplasty uses a very small caliber balloon catheter placed within a stenotic area of a coronary artery through a catheter similar to that used for routine coronary arteriography. When the balloon is inflated, the coronary artery stenosis is dilated (Fig. 41–41). Patients with single and a few with multiple proximal coronary stenoses are currently candidates for this procedure; since 1977 several thousand procedures have been performed with a success rate of approximately 70 per cent. The procedure is performed with a cardiovascular surgery team standing by in case emergency bypass surgery is required, but fewer than 5 per cent of patients have required such surgery when the procedure is performed by an experienced cardiologist.

RISKS OF CATHETERIZATION. Catheterization carries a small but real risk of complication or death. The risk depends on the patient's underlying condition and diagnosis, the exact procedure to be performed, and the experience of the operator. Thus the risk of right heart catheterization is only 0.01 per cent, but the average risk of coronary arteriography in experienced centers is 0.1 per cent risk of death and 0.2 per cent risk of major morbidity (myocardial infarction or stroke). Certain clinical conditions such as critical aortic stenosis, severe stenosis of the left main coronary artery, uncontrolled congestive heart

CORONARY ANGIOGRAPHIC ANATOMY: REPRESENTATION IN STANDARD PROJECTIONS

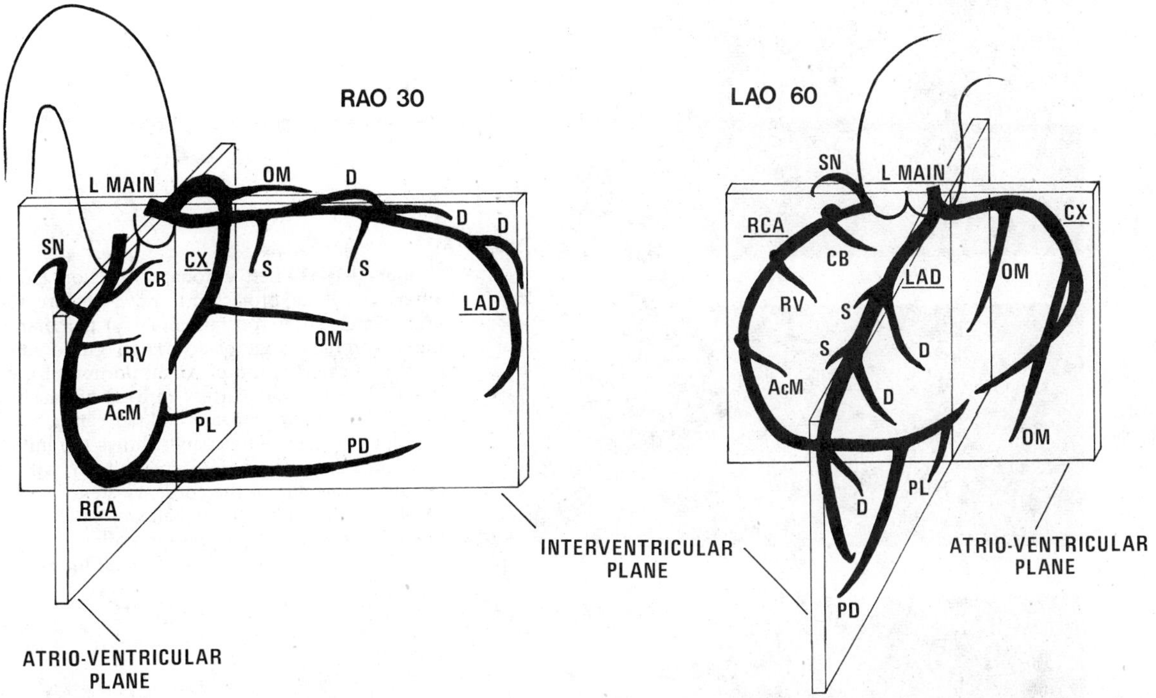

Figure 41–39. The branches of the left and right coronary arteries are shown relative to the atrioventricular and interventricular planes in two standard projections—the 30 degree right anterior oblique and 60 degree left anterior oblique. (L main = left main, LAD = left anterior descending, S = septal, D = diagonal, CX = circumflex, OM = obtuse marginal, RCA = right coronary artery, SN = sinus node branch, CB = conus branch, RV = right ventricular branch, AcM = acute marginal, PD = posterior descending, PL = posterolateral.) Because the PD is supplied by the RCA rather than the Cx, this is a "right dominant" circulation.

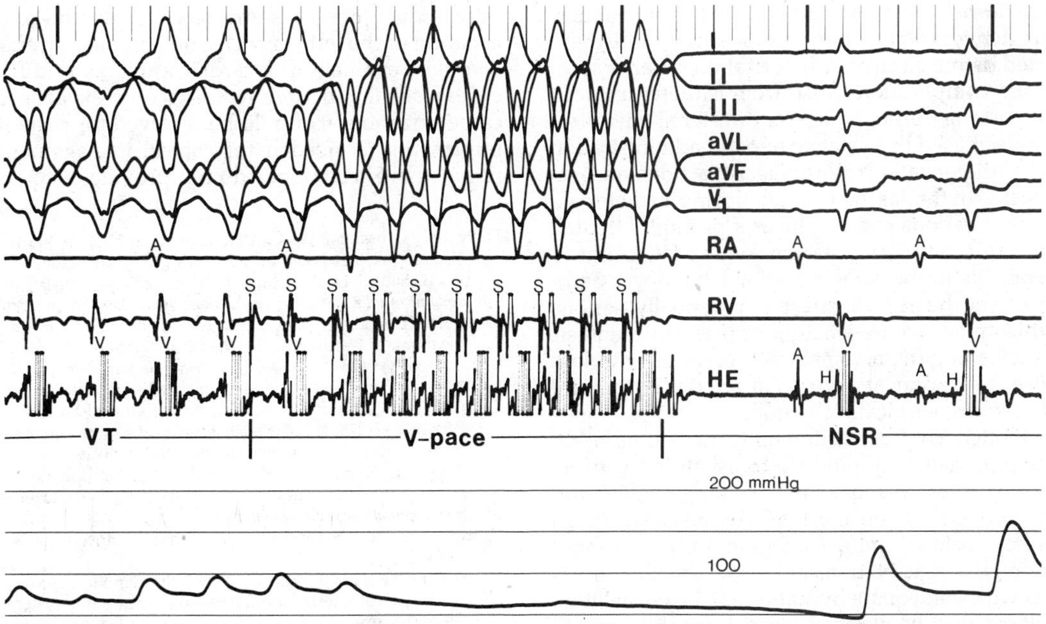

Figure 41–40. Recordings from an intracardiac electrophysiologic study. Surface ECG leads I, II, III, aVL, aVF, and V_1 are displayed with right atrial (RA), right ventricular (RV), and His bundle (HE) intracardiac electrograms. The bold time lines mark one-second intervals. Femoral arterial pressure is recorded at the bottom of the tracing. Sustained ventricular tachycardia (VT) with a rate of 180 beats per minute and complete AV dissociation is present on the left side of the tracing. A burst of rapid ventricular stimuli at 270 beats per minute (V-pace) terminates the tachycardia, and normal sinus rhythm resumes (NSR). Pacing stimuli and atrial, ventricular, and His bundle electrograms are marked by "S," "A," "V," and "H," respectively. (Tracing kindly supplied by Jay W. Mason, M.D., Stanford University.)

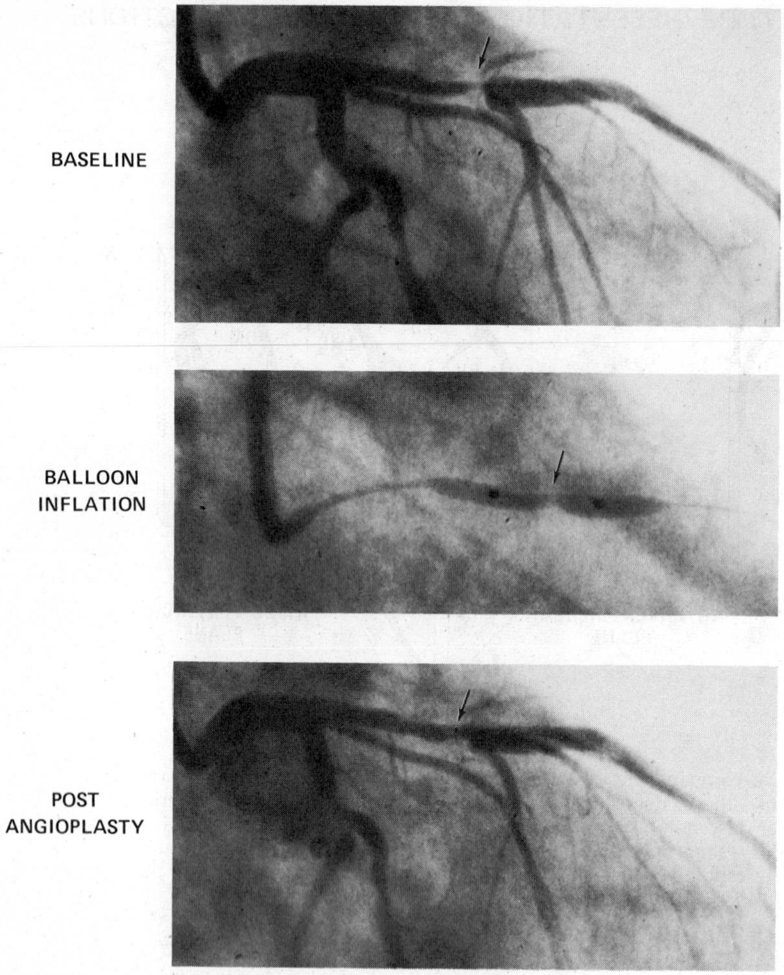

Figure 41–41. Left coronary injection (30 degree right anterior oblique projection) shown before (baseline) and immediately after (postangioplasty) percutaneous transluminal coronary angioplasty. High grade stenosis (80 per cent) is present in the proximal portion of the left anterior descending coronary artery (arrow) at baseline, but is reduced to a "nonsignificant" 40 per cent stenosis following angioplasty. The center panel shows the initial inflation of the contrast-filled angioplasty balloon with a deformity (arrow) at the site of the coronary stenosis. This deformity resolved with subsequent balloon inflations. The patient has been free of angina pectoris after angioplasty despite discontinuation of anti-anginal medications.

failure, and unstable angina pectoris increase the risk of study. Additional avoidable risk factors include electrolyte imbalance, coagulopathy, or dehydration at the time of study, and these should be corrected before elective catheterization is performed.

The most serious complications arise from catheter-induced dissection of the aorta or coronary artery, or arterial embolism (a risk somewhat decreased by systemic heparin administration during left heart catheterization). Vasovagal reactions and severe brady- or tachyrhythmias may occur during catheterization, but do not have serious consequences if promptly treated with appropriate drug, temporary pacemaker, or DC countershock therapy available in the catheterization laboratory. Catheter perforation of the heart is a rare but potentially serious complication, which may require emergency pericardiocentesis or surgery. Local bleeding (hematoma) or thrombosis with loss of the distal pulse may occur at the site of arterial entry, and may occasionally require surgical correction.

The use of iodinated contrast materials carries some additional risk. These materials may produce transient left ventricular dysfunction by their osmotic and volume loads, and negative inotropic effects. When the total contrast load given to the patient is kept below 3 ml per kilogram of body weight per catheterization, the risk of transient renal dysfunction is minimal. Patients with inadequate hydration, diabetes mellitus, or multiple myeloma may be at increased risk for this complication. Allergic or anaphylactoid reactions to contrast material are usually limited to urticaria, but may produce hypotension or bronchospasm in a very small percentage of patients. If any history of allergy to contrast material is obtained during the precatheterization interview, the patient should be premedicated with antihistamines (Benadryl and cimetidine) and high dose steroids.

SUMMARY. Cardiac catheterization, detailed measurement of intracardiac pressures and blood flow, and angiographic visualization of the left ventricle and coronary arteries offer a unique complete evaluation of cardiac anatomy and function. Because of the small but definite risks and expense associated with catheterization, it should be reserved for patients in whom this information is needed for clinical management and in whom noninvasive techniques do not provide adequate data.

Barry BH, Grossman W: Cardiac catheterization. *In* Braunwald E (ed.): Heart Disease: A Textbook of Cardiovascular Medicine. 2nd ed. Philadelphia, W. B. Saunders Company, 1984, pp 279–303. *Update on techniques for hemodynamic study, including calculations of all major cardiovascular parameters.*

Gensini GG: Coronary arteriography. *In* Braunwald E (ed.): Heart Disease: A Textbook of Cardiovascular Medicine. 2nd ed. Philadelphia, W. B. Saunders Company, 1984, pp 304–350. *This chapter describes the technical aspects of cineangiography and discusses its application in patients with heart disease.*

Gensini GG: Coronary Arteriography. Mount Kisco, N.Y., Futura Publishing Company, 1975. *A compilation of techniques of coronary angiography together with extensive examples of the application of the technique.*

Grüntzig AR, Senning A, Siegenthaler W: Non-operative dilation of coronary artery stenosis. N Engl J Med 301:61, 1979. *Initial experience with percutaneous transluminal coronary angioplasty.*

Harrison DC (ed.): Symposium on ventricular arrhythmias—1983. Am J Cardiol 52(6), 1983.

Harrison DC, Ridges JD, Sanders WJ, Alderman EL, Fanton JA: Real time analysis of cardiac catheterization data using a computer system. Circulation 44:709, 1971. *This article validates the use of computer techniques for analysis of hemodynamic data and describes many of the calculations that can be made.*

Mason JW: Techniques for right and left ventricular endomyocardial biopsy. Am J Cardiol 41:887, 1978. *Description of catheter-based methods of cardiac biopsy.*

Sandler H, Dodge HT: The use of single plane angiocardiograms for the calculation of left ventricular volume in man. Am Heart J 75:325, 1968. *Method for quantitative angiography.*

Sones FM Jr, Shirey EK: Cine coronary arteriography. Mod Concepts Cardiovasc Dis 31:735, 1962. *A classic description of cine coronary angiography by the individuals responsible for its introduction in patients with coronary artery disease.*

42. HEART FAILURE

Alfred P. Fishman

The heart is part of an elaborate cardiopulmonary system that is designed to satisfy the metabolic needs of the tissues with respect to oxygen, substrates, and nutrients not only at rest but also during activity. This system includes a sophisticated regulatory apparatus for apportioning the cardiac output according to the physiologic priorities of the moment, e.g., muscular exercise, heat loss, digestion. The same regulatory mechanisms that satisfy physiologic priorities in health also serve to protect vital organs, e.g., the heart and brain, when cardiac output is seriously compromised.

According to its structure and function, the heart may be examined as a pump, as a muscle, or as a component of the cardiopulmonary system. And when one of the two ventricles fails, the consequences may be viewed in the same way. Because of its central role in meeting the needs of the body, and because the pulmonary circulation is lodged between the two ventricles, heart failure not only evokes direct signals that the heart is in trouble, e.g., cardiac dilatation, but also that other organs are not receiving their fair share of blood.

The present chapter will be concerned with heart failure, a final common pathway for many of the diverse etiologies and pathogenic mechanisms that will be discussed subsequently.

GENERAL ASPECTS

In this chapter, the term *heart failure* is used as a synonym for myocardial failure. This approach enables the clinical picture to be related to biochemical, physiologic, and structural changes in the myocardium that culminate in inept performance of the heart as a muscle and as a pump. It also helps to direct medical treatment. This stipulation automatically diverts the discussion from the pathogenesis of syndromes in which the seat of the difficulty is in abnormalities of the heart valves or pericardium or excessive heart rates, each of which can compromise the circulation even though the cardiac muscle is normal.

Disproportion between hemodynamic load and myocardial capacity to cope with it initiates the sequence that culminates in heart failure. In general, the heart tolerates volume overloads better than pressure overloads. For example, *volume* overload of the left ventricle produced by aortic insufficiency may exist for years without causing distress; in contrast, *pressure* overload from aortic stenosis generally elicits signs and symptoms of heart failure much earlier. Sustained overloads are also accommodated better than acute overloads. Thus chronic mitral regurgitation caused by rheumatic heart disease often lasts for years without signs of heart failure, whereas the acute mitral regurgitation produced by a ruptured chorda tendinea is apt to precipitate a disastrous syndrome of heart failure.

The myocardium responds differently to volume and pressure loads. Volume overloads generally elicit dilatation followed by hypertrophy; conversely, pressure overloads characteristically elicit hypertrophy until late in the natural history when dilatation supervenes. Primary myocardial disease generally elicits both dilatation and hypertrophy.

Certain influences and situations often tip the balance of the faltering heart toward overt heart failure. For example, a hot, humid environment increases the work of the heart. Severe anemia may do the same. Fever will do so by increasing heart rate, as will uncontrolled tachycardias of other origin. Clearly, these factors have important therapeutic implications.

Categories of Heart Failure

In the clinic, the type of heart failure is generally categorized according to five features: duration (acute or chronic), initiating mechanisms, the ventricle primarily affected, the clinical syndrome, and the underlying physiologic derangements.

ACUTE VS. CHRONIC HEART FAILURE. Usually the manifestations of heart failure begin insidiously, blurring at the outset with those of the underlying cardiac disorder and continuing gradually into a chronic state. However, the syndrome may also begin precipitously, as after myocardial infarction.

Compensatory adjustments are elicited by both acute and chronic heart failure. These include increase in peripheral vascular resistance, redistribution of blood flow, and increase in erythropoietic activity. But the adaptive mechanisms differ qualitatively, quantitatively, and often in direction. For example, *acute* distention of the left atrium generally promotes a sodium-poor diuresis, whereas *chronic* distention of the left atrium elicits salt and water retention. This distinction between acute and chronic heart failure is relevant to observations on experimental heart failure in animals, which is generally acute in onset and fulminating in course and usually ends abruptly with the death of the animal.

INITIATING MECHANISMS. Each initiating mechanism generally imposes its own distinctive stamp upon the clinical syndrome. Thus the constellation of symptoms and signs originating in rheumatic heart disease differs from that caused by hypertensive heart disease; in turn, both have a different natural history from cor pulmonale. Indeed, even a single etiology, arteriosclerosis, may have distinctly different consequences, depending on the size and location of the vessels that are predominantly affected: progressive narrowing and gradual occlusion of *peripheral* branches of the coronary arteries may be so covert that the characteristic shortness of breath and undue fatigue of left ventricular failure may be misinterpreted as evidence of the general physical decline of advancing age. Conversely, abrupt closure of a major coronary artery, as a consequence of thrombosis superimposed on an arteriosclerotic plaque, may elicit massive myocardial necrosis, followed by extensive myocardial scarring and unremitting heart failure.

LEFT VS. RIGHT HEART FAILURE. Although the ventricles have circumferential muscle and the ventricular septum in common, with rare exception, one ventricle fails before the other. Because of the prevalence of cardiac disorders which overload or damage the left ventricle, e.g., coronary arteriosclerosis and hypertension, heart failure usually begins with the left ventricle. Breathlessness, the key clinical expression of pulmonary congestion and edema, is the most common initial complaint. Conversely, when the right ventricle fails, systemic venous congestion and peripheral edema generally predominate. Left ventricular failure is the most common cause of right ventricular failure, and breathlessness often improves as right ventricular output falls and pulmonary congestion diminishes.

The mechanism by which left ventricular failure causes the right ventricle to fail is not clear. The conventional explanation puts the blame on pulmonary hypertension secondary to left ventricular failure. But the degree of pulmonary hypertension in this circumstance is rarely enough to constitute a formidable burden on the right ventricle. Much more likely as a predominant mechanism is interdependence of the two ventricles, which causes failure of the shared muscle, particularly in the ventricular septum. How often right ventricular failure causes left ventricular failure is still a matter of debate. Resolution of this problem is difficult because of the high frequency of independent and unrelated left ventricular disease in elderly patients with right ventricular failure.

The combination of left and right ventricular failure, in which evidences of systemic and pulmonary venous hypertension predominate, is traditionally referred to as "congestive heart failure." This is a colloquialism that conveys the image of severe physical incapacity, breathlessness, distended neck veins, hepatic engorgement, and troublesome peripheral edema. But it also highlights clinical features that can be measured at the bedside: a high venous pressure, a prolonged circulation time, and a diminished vital capacity, all of which improve as the patient gets better.

BACKWARD VS. FORWARD HEART FAILURE. Somewhat reminiscent of the fable about the blind men and the elephant is the vintage controversy about "backward" versus "forward" heart failure. "Backward failure" calls attention to the damming up of blood in the veins proximal to the failing ventricle and attributes to this venous congestion a critical role in the evolution of the syndrome of heart failure; "forward failure" assigns the same pivotal role to a decrease in cardiac output and hypoperfusion of organs. This distinction has little physiologic validity, because it is inevitable in a closed circuit that the inability of the heart to sustain its output (forward failure) and the pooling of blood on the venous inflow side (backward failure) must go hand in hand. However, this jargon often serves a useful practical purpose in highlighting clinical features.

LOW VS. HIGH OUTPUT FAILURE. Cardiac catheterization in man has made it possible to sort myocardial failure according to the level of the cardiac output. This practice has served at least three purposes: (1) to separate, on clinical and physiologic grounds, a type of myocardial failure ("high output failure") in which the circulation remains vigorous and the extremities remain warm despite venous congestion, edema, and a lower cardiac output than existed prior to the heart failure; (2) to emphasize that the level of the cardiac output and the circulatory adjustments during myocardial failure are, to a large extent, a consequence of the cardiac output that existed prior to heart failure; and (3) to relate etiology and clinical evidences of heart failure to the state of the circulation: the more common causes of heart failure—arteriosclerosis, hypertension, myocardial disease, valvular disease, and pericardial disease—tend to be low output states; less common causes, such as hyperthyroidism, Paget's disease, anemia, beriberi, and arteriovenous fistula, tend to be high output states. But the hemodynamic hallmark of cardiac failure remains the same regardless of the level of cardiac output at rest: an inability of the heart to increase its output (or stroke volume or stroke work) as end-diastolic volume (as well as pressure) is increased (see Preload, below).

The separation into "high" and "low" output failure is concerned with the clinical manifestations, rather than the causes, of myocardial failure. But it is also a hemodynamic reference to which the anatomist and the biochemist can relate the myocardial origins of heart failure. For example, "high output" failure probably has different biochemical bases from "low output" failure. Nor are all types of "low output" or "high output" failure apt to have the same biochemical origins. It is exceedingly unlikely that the "high output" failure of a peripheral arteriovenous fistula has the same anatomic or biochemical beginnings and evolution as the "high output" failure of severe anemia or malnutrition.

CONGESTIVE FAILURE VS. CONGESTED STATE. Overfilling of the circulation, without myocardial failure, is the hallmark of the "congested state." It is now common in intensive care facilities where massive infusions often represent last ditch efforts to combat systemic hypotension. Acutely, it is most often induced by rapid infusions; chronically, it is frequently encountered in severe anemia and in chronic renal insufficiency and less often in Paget's disease or beriberi. In each of these situations, venous hypertension is a consequence of an expanded venous volume and heightened venomotor tone, rather than of heart failure.

In time, persistence of a "hyperkinetic" congested state may cause the heart muscle to fail from overwork. The onset of myocardial failure may then be difficult to detect on clinical grounds, because the hyperkinetic circulation persists and the congestion may be only slightly increased during myocardial failure. Accordingly, the transition from the congested state to congestive heart failure may be difficult to detect on clinical grounds alone. But when heart failure does supervene, cardiac catheterization discloses an inadequate increase in cardiac output for the level of oxygen uptake during exercise as well as a considerable inotropic effect of digitalis. Fortunately, identification of the transition from a "congested state" to "congestive heart failure" is of greater theoretical than practical importance, because therapeutic measures, such as the administration of diuretics and the correction of particular deficiencies, e.g., thiamin in beriberi, are effective in both situations. However, digitalis will exert an important inotropic effect once the myocardium has failed, whereas it is clinically useless when administered to a heart that is coping well with an overfilled circulation.

Subcellular Bases for Contraction

With each beat, the heart develops force and expends energy. Electrical activity at the cell surface activates the contractile machinery. Connecting the electrical activity at the surface and the contractile machinery within the muscle cell is the sarcoplasmic reticulum, which plays a critical role in the release and uptake of calcium during contraction and relaxation.

For the development of the contractile force, heart muscle depends on interactions among contractile proteins, the hypothetical "elastic components" with which they are connected in series, and the constraining bounds within which the contractile elements function. The contractile proteins are contained within sarcomeres, repeating units that compose the individual muscle fibers (myofibrils). Within the sarcomere, the contractile proteins are arranged in two orderly groups of myofilaments, one consisting of myosin, the other predominantly of actin. Holding the contractile apparatus at bay are two modulator proteins, troponin and tropomyosin. Delivery of calcium to troponin from the sarcoplasmic reticulum and sarcolemma sets the contractile process into motion.

To account for changes in the length of heart muscle during contraction and relaxation, the sliding filament hypothesis of Huxley is generally invoked: during contraction, the thin actin filaments slide past the thicker myosin filaments to shorten the sarcomere; the entire muscle cell follows suit. Conversely, during relaxation, the sarcomeres and the muscle cell resume their initial lengths as the original actin-myosin relationships are restored. Nearby mitochondria generate energy for the contractile machinery by oxidative phosphorylation of free fatty acids and glucose supplied by the circulation.

The tension that is developed in cardiac muscle during contraction depends on actin-myosin relationships. Projecting from the myosin filaments are cross-bridges. Before activation, these bridges are not attached to actin filaments. Upon activation, the cross-bridges on the myosin filaments lock into receptor sites on the actin filaments, thereby developing the force that leads to contraction. As the muscle shortens, the cross-bridges disengage and slide along the actin filament, like a pawl on a ratchet, to engage other sites. Depending on the number of cross-bridges that are interlocked at the same time, different tensions will be developed.

Evidence exists that for the sarcomere, as for the whole heart (see Preload, below), the tension developed during contraction is directly related to its initial length. This correspondence implies that, for the whole heart, stretching increases the ability of its individual contractile elements to develop force. Also, since stretching does not affect the rate of interaction of active sites, elongation of cardiac muscle fibers before contraction should not affect the velocity of the subsequent contraction. These considerations underlie many current notions about cardiac contractility. But it is still unclear whether the ultrastructural-physiologic correlations are real or simply models for eliciting a new kind of reflection about an exceedingly complicated problem.

PATHOPHYSIOLOGIC INTERPLAY

Because of their location within the chest, as well as their structure and function, the heart and lungs operate as a functional unit. Moreover, the components of the heart are necessarily interrelated because of the continuity of the muscle that surrounds the ventricular chambers, the ventricular septum that the cardiac chambers share, and the encasing pericardium.

Nonetheless, each ventricle functions as a separate muscular pump supplied by its own booster pump (atrium). The two ventricles empty in unison, simultaneously dispatching their respective contents: the right ventricle sending blood to the lungs for arterialization, the left ventricle sending arterialized blood to the rest of the body for metabolic purposes. In the normal heart, at least 50 per cent of the end-diastolic volume is ejected with each beat. Much of the ejection force is the result of the inherent properties (fiber length and inotropism) of the myocardium. But a wide range of adaptability to the ever-changing metabolic needs of daily life is provided by a superimposed series of extrinsic neurohumoral adjustments which, in daily life, modify and obscure the intrinsic inherent properties of the heart muscle.

Each ventricle is endowed with a finite capacity for stress, strain, and repair. The two ventricles also have somewhat different designs in keeping with their different long-range functions as pumps. The rate of obsolescence of each ventricle depends on the wear and tear to which it is subjected, its supply of nutriments and substrates, and its continuing state of good health. Before birth, both ventricles are taxed equally, because they bear the same pressure loads. After birth, as pulmonary arterial pressure falls, the right ventricular burden decreases and its walls thin. Consequently, other influences remaining equal, the durability of right ventricular performance is destined from birth to exceed that of the left ventricle. The brighter prospects of the right ventricle for longevity in performance are enhanced by the greater vulnerability of the left side of the heart to disease and to disorders in its blood supply.

Assessment of Cardiac Performance

With respect to evaluating cardiac performance, the heart may be regarded from three points of view: as a pump, as a muscle, and as a component of the cardiopulmonary system. Hemodynamic measurements are used to characterize its behavior as a pump: cardiac output, stroke output, stroke work, stroke power, ventricular end-diastolic pressure, ejection fraction, and ventricular end-diastolic volume. To ascertain its behavior as a muscle, principles of muscle mechanics are applied. Its adequacy as a component of the cardiopulmonary system is reflected in the derangements that result from the low cardiac output, the redistribution of blood flow among tissues and organs, organ hypoperfusion, and venous congestion.

Heart as a Pump: Hemodynamics

By the time the heart fails, a variety of mechanisms are operating to bolster its flagging performance. In contrast to the inappropriately low cardiac output, the blood pressure generally remains normal or even increases.

CARDIAC OUTPUT. At each level of activity, in health and disease, a complicated interplay automatically adjusts the extent of shortening of myocardial fibers and, consequently, the stroke volume and the cardiac output. Four principal determinants set the stroke volume: preload (Table 42–1), afterload (ventricular emptying during systole), the inotropic characteristics of the heart, and the coordinated pattern of contraction. A fifth determinant, the heart rate, sets the cardiac output (stroke volume times heart rate). For practical purposes, three of these five principal determinants of cardiac output—preload, afterload, heart rate—are quantifiable. Attempts are currently under way to depict quantitatively the fourth, i.e., the contribution of different regions of the ventricular myocardium to the ejection of blood from the heart. But the fifth, i.e., the inotropic state, remains difficult to assess (Fig. 42–1) except in the extreme, i.e., when the heart is large and evidence exists of venous congestion and organ hypoperfusion.

Relationships among these determinants are not fixed; they play greater or lesser roles, depending on the state of the heart. Thus when the inherent contractility (inotropic state) is impaired, stroke output and cardiac output may be maintained by ventricular dilatation (Frank-Starling mechanism). This flexible arrangement limits the value of cardiac output as a measure

TABLE 42–1. TERMS USED TO DESCRIBE MECHANICAL PERFORMANCE OF THE HEART

Term	Relation to Cardiac Function
Afterload (during ejection)	Force that the ventricle must develop during systole in order to eject the stroke volume. The two major determinants are aortic impedance and left ventricular volume. Afterload is usually expressed as wall stress or wall tension; also, as instantaneous force at some point during ventricular ejection or as mean wall force throughout systole.
Energetics	Generally determined as myocardial oxygen consumption. For any contractile state, the force developed and maintained during contraction represents the major mechanical determinant of oxygen consumption. An increase in myocardial wall force occurs in heart failure as filling pressure increases and the ventricle dilates, thereby increasing the energy cost of contraction (see Fig. 42–2).
Impedance (during ejection)	Instantaneous relationship between rate of change in aortic pressure and aortic blood flow. The aortic input impedance reflects the forces external to the heart that impose a load on the left ventricle, including stiffness of aortic wall. Determined primarily, but not exclusively, by total peripheral vascular resistance to run off from the arterial tree. Normal peripheral resistance is approximately 1500 dynes sec/cm^{-5} or 15 peripheral resistance units.
Inotropic state	A measure of contractility.
Preload	Stretch of myocardial fibers at end-diastole.

of cardiac contractility (inotropic state) to situations in which preload, afterload, and heart rate can be held constant. Unfortunately, this degree of control of loading conditions and heart rate is easier to achieve in the experimental laboratory than in clinical situations.

Indicator-dilution techniques are now widely used for the bedside determination of cardiac output. The normal range in adults at rest is between 2.5 and 3.6 liters per minute per square meter. A decrease in cardiac output at rest represents a late stage in abnormal cardiac performance. Failure to increase cardiac output during exercise occurs much earlier. Thus in normal subjects exercising in a supine position, the increase in cardiac output exceeds 600 ml per minute for each 100 ml increase in oxygen consumption. Lower values indicate abnormal cardiac performance. In heart failure, the arteriovenous difference for oxygen is abnormally wide, resulting almost entirely from the low oxygen content of venous blood returning to the heart rather than from impaired oxygenation in the lungs.

During exercise, heart rate and cardiac output increase as linear functions of oxygen consumption. This is true during both supine and upright exercise, but for any level of exercise the cardiac output is appreciably lower in the upright position. These increases in cardiac output are accomplished principally by acceleration of the heart rate rather than by increase in the stroke volume. In heart failure, cardiac output is even more dependent on heart rate, both at rest and during exercise.

VENTRICULAR END-DIASTOLIC PRESSURE. Inadequate ventricular emptying during systole leads to an increase in the residual volume of blood in the ventricle after systole, and thereby to an increase in end-diastolic ventricular volume. Since end-diastolic ventricular volumes are difficult to measure, end-diastolic ventricular pressures are generally substituted. This practice depends on the premise that a change in pressure is effected by a change in ventricular volume. However, exceptions to this rule do occur: structural changes in the myocardium (fibrosis, edema, hypertrophy, hemorrhage) and pericardial restriction cause end-diastolic pressure to increase without increment in volume, i.e., compliance is decreased. Conversely, in some states of chronic volume overloading of the ventricle,

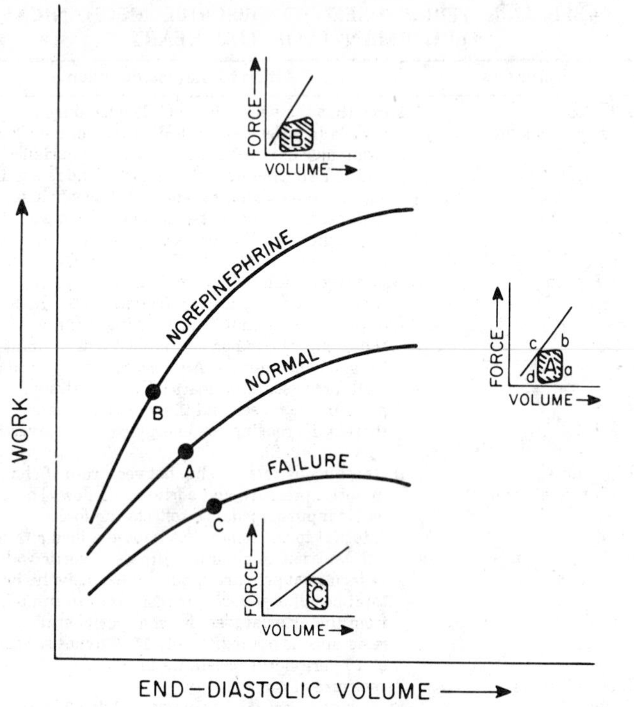

Figure 42–1. The effects of preload and contractility on ventricular function curves. The normal left ventricle increases its stroke output as preload (measured clinically as pulmonary wedge pressure) increases, moving up the ascending limb of the curve until preload reserve is exhausted. In severe heart failure, the ventricular function curve is displaced downward and to the right. The preload reserve is gone, and the heart is operating chronically on the descending limb of the curve. An increase in contractility, as after administering norepinephrine, displaces the curve to the left, i.e., a large stroke output is accomplished at lower filling pressures.

Also shown are work loops per beat corresponding to points B, A, and C on the ventricular function curves. The sloping line in each curve defines the contractility of the particular heart under consideration. On the perimeter of the normal work loop are indicated the following landmarks: a = end diastole; b = opening of aortic valve; c = closure of aortic valve; d = start of filling of heart.

In comparison with the normal heart, the failing heart does just about as much work (total area under curve), at a high filling pressure, but ejects less per beat (d-a). Norepinephrine improves the contractility, so that the end-diastolic volume and pressure decrease whereas the stroke output (d-a) improves greatly. (Based on Weber and Janicki.)

compliance decreases so that large volumes are accommodated at end-diastole without increasing pressure to abnormal levels.

An end-diastolic pressure in the *left* ventricle greater than 12 to 15 mm Hg is abnormal; for the right ventricle, the corresponding upper limit of normal is 10 mm Hg. It is rather simple to estimate the right ventricular end-diastolic pressure by measuring the central venous pressure; the left ventricular end-diastolic pressure is more difficult to estimate because of its inaccessibility. However, in the absence of mitral obstruction or of an increase in pulmonary vascular resistance, pulmonary arterial diastolic pressure provides a useful estimate of left ventricular end-diastolic pressure. Pulmonary wedge pressure is now widely used as a measure of left ventricular end-diastolic pressure.

The performance of the heart depends on two essential components: fiber length (Frank-Starling mechanism) and the inherent contractility (inotropic state) of the muscle. The normal heart is keyed to respond automatically to maintain the cardiac output. The factors that are involved are preload, afterload, contractility, and heart rate. In response to chronic overloading, the heart undergoes dilatation or hypertrophy or a combination of the two.

PRELOAD (THE FRANK-STARLING MECHANISM). According to this mechanism, an increase in end-diastolic volume (preload) is followed by a more forceful contraction that improves ventricular emptying. To assess the Frank-Starling mechanism, only preload should vary, i.e., afterload and heart rate are kept constant for each level of contractility. A distinctive "ventricular performance" curve exists for each state of contractility (Fig. 42–1). Thus the curve for a failing ventricle is depressed and flat so that small stroke volumes are delivered at abnormally high end-diastolic volumes. The high filling pressures are responsible for congestion and edema in the venous beds that lead to the ventricle that has failed.

In the normal heart, the Frank-Starling mechanism operates chiefly to match the stroke outputs of the two ventricles. But in heart failure, this mechanism plays an important part in sustaining the cardiac output.

AFTERLOAD. Afterload refers to the force that the ventricle must develop during systole in order to eject the stroke volume. In principle, it provides a measure of all factors that oppose active shortening of the ventricular fibers. In practice, because of the difficulties of estimating all these factors, impedance is estimated either from the arterial blood pressure or from a calculation of systemic vascular resistance (ratio of blood pressure to flow, expressed in dynes sec/cm^{-5} or in peripheral resistance units).

For clinical purposes, the relationship of blood pressure to cardiac output and peripheral resistance (P/Flow = R) is quite useful. For example, any intervention that causes a large increase in cardiac output without changing systemic blood pressure presumably causes vasodilation, thereby decreasing calculated peripheral vascular resistance, impedance, and afterload (wall force). Accompanying the improved emptying of the left ventricle is a decrease in its filling pressure (measured by pulmonary wedge pressure).

Increasing the afterload on the normal heart (while preload and contractility remain constant) decreases both the degree and speed of wall shortening; reduction in afterload has the opposite effect.

CONTRACTILITY. Increase in sympathetic nervous activity provides the major inotropic effect for the normal heart (in conjunction with increase in heart rate and venous tone). In contrast to the Frank-Starling mechanism, the increase in force and velocity of contraction is accomplished without corresponding increase in fiber length (end-diastolic ventricular volume). Contractility does not limit the performance of the normal heart. In contrast, the failing heart is limited in its myocardial performance as indicated by displacement of the ventricular function curve downward and to the right. An increase in afterload in severe heart failure moves the heart to the descending limb; conversely, improvement in contractility displaces the heart toward the normal curve.

Inotropic State. Clinicians would welcome an objective index of myocardial contractility in which the inotropic state (intrinsic contractility of the muscle) could be measured independent of change in the length of myocardial fibers (Frank-Starling relationship). This would be useful in three different ways: (1) to examine the effects on the myocardium of an acute intervention, such as the administration of digitalis; (2) to determine consecutive changes in the inotropic state of the myocardium in the same individual during the evolution of heart failure and in response to treatment; and (3) to compare the inotropic state in different individuals.

Unfortunately, distinction between the effects of fiber length and of intrinsic contractility is difficult to accomplish for the heart. The main obstacle stems from the strong influence of mechanical loading conditions on hemodynamic measurements. Thus a change in either the preload (length of ventricular fibers at end-diastole) or the afterload (force developed in ventricular muscle during systole) can modify ventricular performance greatly without affecting its intrinsic inotropic state. Another complication is the inability of conventional hemodynamic measurements to take heart size into account, so that comparisons of contractility in hearts of different size are generally unreliable.

EJECTION FRACTION. The fraction of the end-diastolic volume that is ejected per beat is termed the "ejection fraction." It is widely used as a measure of contractility and is estimated angiographically, by radionuclides, or by echocardiography. The normal systolic ejection fraction ranges from 0.56 to 0.78. A reduction in ejection fraction in a patient with normal valves and a dilated ventricle is strong evidence for a depressed inotropic state. That contractility is poor can often be witnessed directly in the pattern of ventricular emptying disclosed by these techniques.

SYSTOLIC TIME INTERVALS. Simultaneous recording of the electrocardiogram, phonocardiogram, and carotid arterial pulse allows indirect bedside appraisal of cardiac function. Unfortunately, these noninvasive techniques do not distinguish between inotropic state and other mechanical determinants of contractility, and their results may be invalidated by disturbances in conduction, valvular disease, and other unanticipated disorders.

Chronic Compensatory Mechanisms

In principle, the heart that is chronically in a state of failure has recourse to four compensatory mechanisms: increased contractility due to sympathetic nervous activity, tachycardia, hypertrophy, and dilatation. Of the four, the increase in sympathetic activity is more of a burden than a blessing, since it increases peripheral vascular resistance without contributing appreciably to the inotropic state of the faltering heart. Sympathetic activity does, however, contribute indirectly to support the cardiac output by reflexly increasing the heart rate.

HEART RATE. Chronic tachycardia is a feature of heart failure. Much of the increase in heart rate stems from cardiac reflexes that are stimulated by distention of the great veins at their junctions with the atria (Bainbridge reflex). However, in terms of energetics, tachycardia is a costly way to run the heart. Indeed, it is possible to produce, or to precipitate, heart failure by inducing tachycardia.

DILATATION. Progressive and persistent dilatation marks the transition between ventricular hypertrophy and failure. For a long while, dilatation may serve as a compensatory mechanism, increasing the contractile force of the heart by way of the Frank-Starling relationship. But dilatation gradually becomes inadequate to maintain stroke output.

Several different mechanisms seem to be involved in the ultimate inability of the dilated heart to maintain its output: (1) slippage and rearrangement of sarcomeres during progressive dilatation; as a result, they neither produce a coordinated contraction nor are properly stretched to enhance contractility as the heart dilates further; (2) high wall tension in accord with the law of Laplace (Fig. 42–2); as the volume of the ventricle increases so that its wall tension for a given pressure in the ventricular cavity during contraction is greater than normal, the myocardial oxygen consumption increases accordingly; (3) protracted maintenance of high wall tension during contraction; in contrast to the normal heart, in which the wall tension decreases in the course of systole, wall tension remains high in the dilated heart; (4) high energy requirements coupled with an inefficient conversion of chemical to mechanical energy; despite the decrease in stroke output, the dilated heart has a higher myocardial oxygen consumption than does the normal heart. Because of these limitations, chronic enlargement is an inefficient and ill-fated mechanism for achieving sustained improvement in cardiac performance.

HYPERTROPHY. Chronic exposure to abnormal pressure and volume loads leads to hypertrophy, i.e., an increase in ventricular mass. This increase in muscle mass takes time to develop. It involves increased protein synthesis in response to mechanical overload or dilatation. The stimulus for hypertrophy may be an increase either in wall force (tension) in accord with the Laplace relationship (Fig. 42–2) or in the energy requirements of a heart that is chronically dilated or operating at high filling pressures.

The pattern of hypertrophy depends on the load. In response to chronic volume overloading, e.g., arteriovenous fistula, the total mass increases as the chamber size enlarges but thickness does not change. This pattern is known as "eccentric" hypertrophy. In contrast, in chronic exposure to increased afterload, e.g., systemic hypertension, the end-diastolic volume remains unchanged, whereas the wall thickens. This pattern is known as "concentric" hypertrophy.

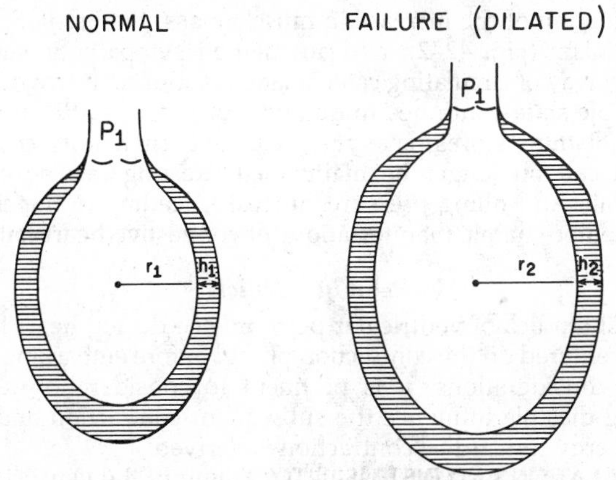

Figure 42–2. Laplace relationship applied to the dilated heart. The tension developed in the wall of the heart during systole (T) is a directional force that is proportional to the product of the mean pressure that the wall is supporting (P) and the mean radius (r). Dilatation of the heart ($r_2 > r_1$) at the same pressure ($P_1 = P_2$) increases wall tension ($T_2 > T_1$). Should the wall become thinner during dilatation, the wall stress would increase as the cross-sectional area of myocardium (h) decreased (equation 2). The use of wall force (equation 3), which is proportional to the pressure and volume of the chamber, eliminates considerations of chamber size and shape and of the thickness of the myocardial wall.

$$\textit{Wall tension} = \text{Force per circumferential length of myocardium} = \frac{P \cdot \pi r^2}{2\pi r} = \frac{P \cdot r}{2} \quad (1)$$

$$\textit{Wall stress} = \text{Force per cross-sectional area of myocardium} = \frac{P \cdot \pi r^2}{2\pi r h} = \frac{P \cdot r}{2h} \quad (2)$$

$$\textit{Wall force} = \text{Pressure} \cdot \text{cross-sectional area of chamber} = P \cdot \pi r^2 \quad (3)$$

Normal ventricular contraction is a smoothly coördinated process by which the ventricular wall moves inward during systole to eject its contents. Abnormal electrical conduction interferes with this smooth performance and with ventricular function. The coordinated mechanism is further disrupted by local disease that causes zones of fibrosis to alternate with normal zones. This disposition of normal and abnormal areas leads to hypertrophy of functioning muscle not only because the geometry of the abnormal ventricle causes it to operate at a mechanical disadvantage but also because normal muscle is obliged to do work, and to expend energy, in moving and stretching damaged muscle or scar upon which it abuts.

Early in hypertrophy, muscle mass and capillary vessels increase proportionately and the contractile properties of the myocardium are preserved. But later, the inotropic behavior becomes abnormal and the capacity of the myocardium to synthesize adrenergic transmitter decreases. Indeed, once hypertrophy begins, the myocardium has been eased on the road to failure.

In the depressed inotropic state associated with hypertrophy, circulatory function is maintained for a long while by the combination of the increase in muscle mass, the Frank-Starling mechanism (Fig. 42–2), and augmented sympathetic stimulation by way of circulating catecholamines. But as the myocardial inotropic state continues to deteriorate, perhaps after intrinsic catecholamine stores have been depleted, circulatory compensation can no longer be maintained. Resting cardiac output then fails and filling pressures increase, leading to the clinical and hemodynamic manifestations of congestive heart failure.

Heart as a Muscle

Most studies of ventricular performance during heart failure have centered on the contraction phase. Before embarking upon these considerations, it is pertinent to consider how events during diastole influence the subsequent contraction and how the energy for cardiac contraction is derived.

RELAXATION AND DISTENSIBILITY. Filling of the ventricle during diastole depends not only on the time available but also on the pattern of relaxation. Relaxation consists of two components: an active one, which promotes relaxation by way of intrinsic mechanisms; and a passive one, arising from extension of the fibers by the inflowing blood. Incomplete relaxation would be expected not only to increase the filling pressure of the heart but also to dissipate energy. In the normal heart, the active and passive components appear to work synergistically to minimize losses in chemical energy. But in heart failure the viscous and elastic properties of the heart muscle seem to change so that there is a diminished resistance to filling (decreased "impedance") and an increased extent of ventricular expansion on filling (increased "compliance"). Thus not only the velocity and duration of relaxation but also changes in the physical properties of the muscle seem involved in heart failure.

ENERGETICS. The heart does work and expends energy during each contraction. For its supply of energy, it depends on aerobic metabolism. Some energy is expended to satisfy its basic oxygen requirements and those of activation. But the bulk of the energy is spent during contraction.

Attempts have been made over the years to dissect physiologically the major determinants of oxygen consumption of the heart. The variables that have been examined are ventricular pressure, volume, work, wall force, and contractile state. The major determinant for any given contractile state has proved to be the force (calculated as the product of ventricular volume and pressure) that is developed in the myocardium at the start of ejection and that continues to the end of systole. At each instant during ejection this wall force is changing. It is the integral of systolic force that relates closely to myocardial oxygen consumption. Other important influences in addition to wall force are heart rate and contractility. In contrast, fiber shortening has negligible effect on myocardial oxygen consumption.

For its contraction, the heart depends on the conversion of the chemical energy of oxidizable substrates into the mechanical energy of muscular contraction. ATP participates in this process as the principal store of energy released by oxidation; its breakdown by myosin ATPase is the principal way by which chemical energy is transformed into mechanical energy. ATP resynthesis in the myocardium is accomplished chiefly through oxidative phosphorylation. The rate of ATP breakdown and the quantity of energy used by the myocardium depend chiefly on the tension that is developed in the myocardial fibers rather than on the degree of shortening or the work done; this developed tension causes the ventricular walls to contract and the blood to be ejected. From a biochemical point of view, the muscle of a ventricle has failed when its generation of free energy, or its utilization of that energy in the process of contraction, is insufficient for the circulatory load which it has to handle.

Unfortunately, the biochemical basis for heart failure is not yet settled. But it is now clear that there are no consistent defects in energy metabolism or in protein synthesis. The investigative focus at present is on excitation-coupling and the role of calcium in the contractile process.

Any physiologic change or pharmacologic intervention will increase myocardial oxygen requirements if it increases either preload or afterload, increases the contractile state of the myocardium, or increases the heart rate. The usual compensatory mechanisms in severe heart failure tend to increase myocardial oxygen requirements by increasing all these parameters: fluid retention increases preload; sympathetic mechanisms increase afterload, contractility, and heart rate. Similarly, the usual interventions employed in heart failure may or may not increase myocardial oxygen requirements further, depending on the balance of changes in the aforementioned determinants in each individual case.

Heart as Component of the Cardiopulmonary System

As the overburdened ventricle fails, it elicits venous hypertension and slowed circulation, and sets into motion peripheral mechanisms to sustain blood pressure and cardiac output.

VENOUS HYPERTENSION. With the onset of failure, the ventricle fails to empty properly during systole so that the volume of blood left in the ventricle after contraction increases, i.e., ejection fraction decreases. An increase in diastolic pressure in the ventricles and in the atrium and veins that lead to the ventricle accompanies the increase in ventricular volume. Several other elements contribute to the venous hypertension: (1) heightened venomotor tone; (2) expansion of the blood volume as a consequence of sodium retention by the kidney; and, on occasion, (3) regurgitation of blood from ventricle to atrium as the atrioventricular valve becomes incompetent either from ventricular dilatation or from improper closure during an arrhythmia.

SLOWED CIRCULATION. The circulation time depends on the cardiac output and the volume of blood interposed between the sites of sampling and injection. Should either ventricle fail, the time for a tracer substance to pass from the site of intravenous injection to the site of detection will be prolonged. For example, in left heart failure, the arm-to-tongue circulation time, measured by using Decholin as a tracer, will be prolonged beyond the normal limits of 10 to 15 seconds; slowing of the tracer in traversing the pulmonary circulation and dilated left heart, as well as excessive dilution of the tracer by the enlarged intervening blood volume, contributes to the delay. Similarly, the arm-to-breath circulation time measured after the intravenous injection of ether will be prolonged in right heart failure. By relating the circulation times to the central venous pressure, it may be possible to establish at the bedside which ventricle has failed. For example, in left heart failure, central venous pressure and ether circulation time will be normal, whereas Decholin time will be prolonged.

PERIPHERAL MECHANISMS TO SUSTAIN CARDIAC OUTPUT AND BLOOD PRESSURE. In order to sustain the cardiac output, to apportion it selectively, and to maintain the systemic arterial blood pressure, a variety of peripheral mechanisms are activated.

Autonomic Nervous System. Normally, a four- or five-fold increase in oxygen consumption elicits a doubling of the cardiac output. When the increase in cardiac output cannot keep pace with the level of activity, distribution of blood flow is altered to defend vital areas, e.g., brain and heart. The autonomic nervous system is deeply involved in this rearrangement of the circulation. It also contributes to activation of the mechanisms for retaining sodium and water.

Peripheral vasoconstriction and tachycardia are the hallmarks of the usual forms of heart failure. Paradoxically, despite a generalized increase in sympathetic nervous activity, norepinephrine stores in the heart muscle are depleted because of defective local synthesis. Consequently, the failing heart, denied local adrenergic support for its inotropic and chronotropic responses, is obliged to rely on norepinephrine delivered to it by the blood from the adrenal medulla and the peripheral vasculature. Pharmacologic agents, such as guanethidine, which further deplete the heart of its cathecholamines, aggravate heart failure. In many respects, the performance of the human heart that has failed resembles that of both the "denervated" heart and the isolated heart-lung preparation that Starling used. The role that the parasympathetic nervous system plays in heart failure is ill defined, but evidence indicates that its contribution to the control of heart rate and baroreceptor activity is impaired.

PERIPHERAL VASOCONSTRICTION. Peripheral arteriolar and venoconstriction, mediated by heightened sympathetic nervous activity, are essential compensatory mechanisms in heart failure. The extent to which accumulation of sodium and water in the arteriolar wall contributes to increased arteriolar resistance is as yet unclear. Selective arteriolar vasoconstriction helps not only to sustain the blood pressure but also to preserve function in critical organs. The pattern of selective vasoconstriction, in turn, influences the cardiac output by determining the total peripheral resistance to cardiac emptying.

Selective venoconstriction promotes venous return by transfer of returning blood to the central veins. Although peripheral venoconstriction may contribute importantly to the increase in central venous pressure, the major determinant is myocardial incompetence in coping with the venous return.

REDISTRIBUTION. In order to maintain oxygen delivery to vital organs (brain and myocardium) during heart failure, blood flow is diverted by heightened sympathetic nervous activity from skin, kidneys, splanchnic viscera, and muscle. At first the redistribution of blood flow among organs occurs during activity or stress, i.e., as cardiac output fails to increase appropriately for the increment in metabolism; later it operates also at rest. The mechanism for diversion is the balance between sympathetic innervation and local metabolism: the circulations to skin, kidney, splanchnic organs, and skeletal muscle are richly innervated, and these viscera have low metabolic rates; sympathetic nervous vasoconstriction easily overrides local metabolites. In contrast, the circulations to brain and myocardium are poor in alpha-adrenergic receptors; these organs, with high oxygen consumption, produce ample metabolic dilators to counterbalance heightened sympathetic activity.

In the normal subject during exercise, as need for heat dissipation increases, cutaneous hyperemia develops. In contrast, the patient in heart failure fails to develop cutaneous hyperemia despite increasing need for heat dissipation. The net effect is that the patient in heart failure, suffering from a low cardiac output during exercise, preserves blood pressure and blood flow to vital organs by paying the penalty of impaired heat loss as well as inadequate blood flow to exercising muscles.

VALSALVA MANEUVER. An abnormal response to the Valsalva maneuver, in which intrathoracic pressure is maintained at approximately 40 mm Hg for 10 to 12 seconds, is a useful test for left heart failure. The autonomic nervous system, operating in conjunction with the expanded volume of blood in the left side of the heart and pulmonary venous system, contributes to the abnormal response. During strain, the normal subject manifests a characteristic decrease in blood pressure and pulse pressure and increase in heart rate; when straining stops, the blood pressure, pulse pressure, and bradycardia "overshoot." In contrast, the patient in left heart failure demonstrates a "square wave response" of blood pressure: at the start of straining, blood pressure increases abruptly, stays high during the maneuver, and drops precipitously to baseline after the maneuver, without overshoot. Throughout the procedure there is little or no change in pulse pressure and no tachycardia. The lack of reflex changes stems from the failure of stroke output or arterial pulse pressure to change during the straining phase, so that no reflex changes are elicited in peripheral vessels.

Salt and Water Retention. As the patient slips into heart failure, the reduction in cardiac output is associated with a decrease in renal blood flow and glomerular filtration rate, and with a redistribution of blood flow within the kidneys. These hemodynamic changes undoubtedly contribute to the sodium and water retention of heart failure, but in different ways and to different degrees according to the stage of heart failure. Early in heart failure, when filtration rate is decreased, much of the sodium retention is attributable to the decrease in the filtered load of sodium presented to the tubules for reabsorption. Later on, humoral factors, predominantly hyperaldosteronism and a group of extra-adrenal, sodium-retaining influences ("factor III") predominate.

The disturbed hemodynamics are importantly involved in activating the renin-angiotensin-aldosterone mechanism by direct effects on the kidney or indirectly via baroreceptors in the distended left atrium. Other reflexes engaged in the intense sympathetic activity of heart failure may also be involved in sodium and water retention. Although pathways for hemodynamic-neurohumoral interplay are not entirely clear, appreciation of the important role of hyperaldosteronism in the genesis of sodium and water retention has provided new approaches to the therapy of heart failure using aldosterone antagonists.

Not only urine but also sweat and saliva are sodium poor. But the underlying mechanisms are different. Antidiuretic hormone is not directly involved in the genesis of the edema of heart failure.

The expansion of the circulating blood volume contributes to sustaining the cardiac output and the perfusion of vital organs. Rarely is the expansion in blood volume marked, usually ranging from 10 to 20 per cent in moderately severe heart failure to 30 to 50 per cent in severe, refractory heart failure. But even modest expansion helps augment the ventricular end-diastolic volume, thereby improving ventricular performance by way of the Frank-Starling principle. Unfortunately, the high end-diastolic volume and pressures promote the formation of edema by raising capillary pressures in the circulation behind the failing ventricle. At a time when circulation blood volume may be increased by 20 per cent, the extravascular fluid volume may have doubled.

EXERCISE TESTING. Based on the concept that the heart has failed as a component of the cardiopulmonary system when it can no longer provide sufficient oxygen to metabolizing tissues to satisfy their metabolic needs, progressive exercise has been used to determine maximum oxygen uptake ("aerobic capacity"). This test involves graded exercise, usually on a treadmill, and can be done noninvasively. The endpoint is generally fatigue, which coincides with maximum oxygen uptake and inability to generate the required cardiac output. This approach is also applicable to the evaluation of new agents for the treatment of heart failure.

CLINICAL MANIFESTATIONS OF HEART FAILURE

The signs and symptoms of heart failure depend on the ventricle that has failed and the duration of the failure. The clinical syndrome of left ventricular failure is dominated by *symptoms* of pulmonary congestion and edema. In contrast, right ventricular failure is dominated by *signs* of systemic venous congestion and peripheral edema. Fatigue and weakness are common in both types of heart failure.

Left Ventricular Failure

Symptoms

Complaints of respiratory discomfort or distress dominate the symptoms of left ventricular failure. They vary with position, stress, and activity. They are often associated with physical signs of disturbances in the lungs or in respiratory control mechanisms.

DYSPNEA. Like pain or anxiety, dyspnea is subjective and difficult to quantify. Because breathing is ordinarily automatic and effortless except after strenuous exertion, the complaint of breathlessness may signify anything from awareness to distress. Dyspnea during modest exertion is usually the first symptom of left heart failure. Usually dyspnea is associated with increased rate of breathing (tachypnea).

The physiologic basis for the sensation of dyspnea remains unclear. Both lungs and the chest muscles may contribute.

Thus interstitial edema in the vicinity of the pulmonary capillaries stimulates juxtacapillary receptors ("J-receptors"), thereby reflexly setting a pattern of rapid, shallow breathing; associated with this abnormal pattern is an increase in the work and oxygen cost of moving the stiff lungs. However, this increased amount of work on the lungs is done in the face of diminished blood flow to the respiratory muscles, a consequence of the diminished cardiac output and redistribution of blood flow. Consequently, the disproportion between work done by the respiratory muscles and the supply of blood delivered to them may contribute to fatigue of the respiratory muscles and to the sensation of dyspnea. Sensory elements within the respiratory muscles may also contribute to respiratory discomfort by registering the disproportion between the inordinate amount of energy that is being spent by muscles and the amount of ventilation that they produce.

Although precise mechanisms for dyspnea remain uncertain, its occurrence in left heart failure clearly depends on the increase in the blood and water content of the lungs at the expense of the air volume. Ventilation increases as the air volume is progressively encroached upon, and, as the minute ventilation approaches the maximal ventilatory capacity, the likelihood of dyspnea increases.

ORTHOPNEA. Progressive, and often urgent, dyspnea that occurs soon after lying flat is designated as orthopnea; it is relieved by sitting up. The physiologic basis for orthopnea is the augmented venous return from the lower extremities and splanchnic bed to the lungs that results from redistribution of gravitational forces in the supine position and the reabsorption of diurnal edema. In the patient with heart disease, orthopnea is reliable evidence of left ventricular failure. In contrast, the dyspnea of chronic lung disease or musculoskeletal disorders is rarely aggravated by lying flat.

The patient learns to avoid respiratory distress at night by supporting head and thorax by two or more pillows. In severe heart failure, orthopnea may force the patient to sleep upright in a chair rather than in bed. In some patients with extensive coronary artery disease and left ventricular failure, orthopnea occurs only in the left lateral position; the mechanism for this is unclear.

Cough and expectoration are common in left heart failure, presumably a consequence of reflexes from the congested lungs and bronchi. The patient may also manifest an orthopneic cough which has the same significance as orthopnea, and is presumably the consequence of venous congestion and edema of the tracheobronchial walls. In some patients, precordial distress may substitute for breathlessness in the supine position. This "nocturnal angina" is also somehow related to the mobilization of water from the tissues to the circulation when the patient goes to bed.

PAROXYSMAL NOCTURNAL DYSPNEA. A bout of urgent respiratory distress, verging on suffocation, may rouse the patient unexpectedly from sleep and cause him to seek relief desperately, either by sitting up or by rushing to the open window to breathe "fresh air." Respiration may be labored and wheezing, hence the designation "cardiac asthma." The episodes represent intolerable aggravation of pulmonary congestion and edema during sleep in the supine position. A combination of dulling of the respiratory center to sensory input from the lungs during sleep and increase in venous return to the lungs makes it possible for pulmonary venous congestion and edema to accumulate to the point of precipitating the frightening episode of breathlessness.

ACUTE PULMONARY EDEMA. In an acute episode of left ventricular failure, such as that which follows myocardial infarction, the inability of the left ventricular myocardium to handle the blood that the competent right ventricle is delivering to it may result in an abrupt increase in pulmonary venous and capillary pressure, followed by flooding of the interstitial spaces and alveoli. If the edema is confined to the interstitial spaces of the lungs, an increase in respiratory frequency because of stiff lungs would be expected to produce alveolar hyperventilation and respiratory alkalosis; conversely, once free fluid enters the terminal bronchioles and mounts the respiratory tree, respiratory acidosis may occur because of imbalances between alveolar ventilation and alveolar blood flow (ventilation-perfusion inhomogeneities).

Pulmonary edema may begin with a cough, with wheezing, or with breathlessness. Often there is a sense of oppression in the chest. At first, except for the abnormal breathing pattern and the evidences of heart disease, there may be few physical signs. In time, as free fluid enters the distal airways, rales become audible, most marked in the dependent parts of the lungs, but extending upward as the attack worsens. In a severe attack, the patient is pale, sweating, cyanotic, obviously gasping for breath, and usually producing frothy sputum which may be blood tinged.

HEMOPTYSIS. Rusty sputum, laden with heart failure cells (alveolar macrophages containing hemosiderin), occurs frequently in severe left heart failure. Frankly bloody sputum is generally a sign of pulmonary infarction. In severe pulmonary edema caused by left ventricular failure, the frothy fluid that pours from the bronchial tree is often pink, i.e., blood tinged, owing to the escape of red cells into the alveoli from the congested minute vessels of the lungs.

CHEYNE-STOKES RESPIRATION. Some patients with severe heart failure display periodic breathing characterized by alternate periods of apnea and hyperventilation. Cyclic changes in arterial blood gas tensions accompany this waxing and waning of the ventilation: during apnea, the arterial P_{O_2} reaches its peak, whereas the arterial P_{CO_2} reaches its nadir. At the same time, alveolar gas tensions are exactly opposite: the alveolar P_{O_2} reaches its peak during hyperpnea; the alveolar P_{CO_2} reaches its nadir during hyperpnea. This discrepancy between arterial and alveolar gas tensions has been attributed to the fact that changes in arterial blood gases *cause* the swings in ventilation, whereas the changes in alveolar gas tension are the *consequences* of the changes in ventilation. The critical role of the arterial blood gases stems from the prolonged circulation time between the lungs and the respiratory centers in the brain. This slowing of the circulation exposes the central respiratory control mechanisms to arterial blood that differs in gaseous composition from that in pulmonary venous blood. In essence, because of slowing of the circulation, negative feedback is delayed. As expected, the longer the circulation time, the longer the cycles of hyperventilation and apnea. The neurologic and cerebrovascular changes of old age predispose to Cheyne-Stokes breathing.

Physical Signs

In addition to being breathless, the patient is generally pale, a bit dusky, and sweaty. His handshake is cold because of peripheral vasoconstriction. The heart rate is rapid and the pulse pressure is narrow, with a modest increase in diastolic blood pressure. If only the left ventricle has failed, the neck veins are not distended.

THE HEART. Enlargement of the heart is usually evident to inspection and palpation of the apical impulse and is confirmed by roentgenologic and radiographic examination. Angina pectoris is not a manifestation of heart failure, nor is palpitation common unless overzealous administration of digitalis and diuretics has occasioned digitalis toxicity. As the left ventricle fails and pulmonary venous pressure increases, pulmonary arterial pressure also increases, and the heart sound attributable to pulmonary valve closure increases in intensity. Also, as the left ventricle dilates, the mitral valve leaflets fail to appose properly, resulting in mild mitral incompetence.

Gallop Rhythm. The advent of a third heart sound during diastole in an adult with heart disease signifies the advent of heart failure. The fixed sequence of the two normal sounds and the abnormal third sound, in conjunction with an increase in heart rate, is responsible for the characteristic cadence of a gallop rhythm. The third heart sound ("S-3 gallop") occurs early in diastole during the state of rapid ventricular filling. This ventricular gallop presumably originates in the vibrations of the ventricular walls as the rapidly inflowing blood is abruptly arrested; this extra sound, normal in young children and in young adults, is generally a reliable sign of ventricular failure in the middle-aged or elderly patient with heart disease.

A gallop rhythm may also originate in the atrial contribution to ventricular filling. This atrial or "S-4 gallop" is not unique for heart failure, because it may reflect diminished ventricular compliance resulting from hypertrophy or ischemia rather than myocardial failure. If a patient with a fourth heart sound develops heart failure, a third sound appears to cause a quadruple rhythm. If the heart rate is rapid or the P-R interval is prolonged, the atrial and ventricular gallop sounds summate ("summation gallop"). In the candidate for heart failure, summation gallop has the same implication as other diastolic gallop rhythms, particularly if it persists as the heart is slowed.

Pulsus Alternans. In patients with heart disease, particularly if the cause is hypertension, cardiomyopathy, or coronary arteriosclerosis, the appearance of alternating strong and weak beats, even though the fundamental rhythm remains regular, heralds the onset of heart failure. This pulsus alternans may be detected by palpation or by sphygmomanometry. It often follows an extrasystole. Rarely is this mechanical alternans associated with electrical alternans. The mechanism for pulsus alternans has been attributed to alternations in fiber length (ventricular end-diastolic volume) or to alternating increase and decrease in the number of contractile units, or to both.

THE LUNGS. A characteristic consequence of interstitial edema and pulmonary venous congestion is tachypnea. As left heart failure progresses, interstitial edema is succeeded by alveolar edema and fluid in the terminal bronchioles, particularly at the lung bases. Accordingly, bilateral basal rales are common in moderate failure of the left ventricle.

Electrocardiogram

Abnormalities in the electrocardiogram arise from the underlying cardiac disorder and from therapeutic agents, e.g., digitalis and diuretics, rather than from heart failure per se.

Radiologic Aspects

The x-ray can be exceedingly helpful in the diagnosis of left ventricular failure. Typically, the cardiac silhouette is enlarged, often assuming telltale configurations that are determined by the underlying disorder. In contrast to the normal, in which pulmonary *arteries* are prominent in the lower lung fields, pulmonary vasculature is prominent at the apices, reflecting pulmonary *venous* hypertension and redistribution of blood flow because of edema and fibrosis at the bases. Enlarged hilar shadows accompany the prominent pulmonary veins in the upper lung fields.

Prominent septal lines, particularly near the costophrenic angles (Kerley's lines), indicate the presence of interstitial edema. The advent of alveolar edema is signaled by a generalized clouding of the lung fields. Pleural effusion may occasionally occur in left heart failure, but is much more apt to occur in biventricular heart failure. Evidence of interstitial and alveolar edema often lessens or disappears when right ventricular failure supervenes. However, hydrothorax generally persists. A widened shadow of the superior vena cava may provide reliable evidence of right ventricular failure and systemic venous congestion.

Pulmonary Function Tests

Traditionally, the course of overt failure of the left ventricle, particularly the response to treatment, has been followed by consecutive determinations of vital capacity. This is an insensitive measure, usually associated with decrease in compliance and occasionally with increase in airway resistance. Earlier in the course of pulmonary edema—presumably when the excess fluid is still confined to the interstitial space around alveoli and terminal airways (less than 2 mm in diameter)—expiratory flow rates at *low lung volumes* are reduced and peripheral airways tend to close prematurely during expiration, trapping gas within the lungs and disturbing the distribution of alveolar gas with respect to pulmonary capillary blood. This has led to a variety of tests (e.g., "closing volumes") which are designed to detect premature closure and resultant maldistribution of air—presumably by interstitial edema—long before compliance falls and total resistance of airways increases. During recovery there is usually a delay before expiratory flow rates and closing volumes return to normal, even though left atrial pressure is again within normal limits. The basis for the persistent abnormalities is presumably the gradual removal of interstitial edema from the vicinity of the small airways and blood vessels.

Associated with the high closing volume is evidence of ventilation-perfusion abnormalities manifested by widening of the alveolar-arterial ΔP_{O_2} and a decrease in arterial P_{O_2} caused by "venous admixture." Nonetheless, arterial oxygen saturation is generally near normal unless independent lung disease is present. Along with the decrease in arterial P_{O_2} is a widening of the arterial-venous difference in O_2 content owing to the increased extraction of oxygen in the tissues. Arterial CO_2 tension remains normal or low unless free fluid enters the terminal airways in the course of pulmonary edema. Abnormally high values for CO_2 tension indicate that considerable free fluid has made its way into the airways.

Right Ventricular Failure

Clinical Manifestations

Isolated failure of the right ventricle is uncommon, generally a consequence of cor pulmonale secondary to intrinsic lung disease. More often, right ventricular failure is a sequel to left ventricular failure. In right ventricular failure, neck veins are distended and fill from below; the engorged liver may be tender to gentle pressure, and compression causes a surge of blood into the neck veins (hepatojugular reflux). In time, when both ventricles have failed, evidence of right ventricular failure may dominate the scene; but continuing dyspnea and rales attest to the persistence of left ventricular failure, and the continuing low cardiac output is manifested by signs of increased sympathetic nervous activity and of organ hypoperfusion.

Weakness may be marked and is occasionally associated with anorexia, weight loss, and malnutrition ("cardiac cachexia"). Not only severe heart failure but also digitalis, diuretics, and electrolyte disturbances are generally involved in the genesis of this cachectic state.

CYANOSIS. Bluish discoloration of the skin and mucous membranes is designated as cyanosis. It is due to an abnormal concentration of reduced hemoglobin (more than 5 grams per 100 ml) in the subpapillary venous plexus of the skin. In right heart failure, the congested venules, containing blood from which considerable oxygen has been extracted because of the slow flow, account for the cyanosis. In left heart failure, cyanosis is usually caused by a complication, e.g., pneumonia, unless overt pulmonary edema is present.

ABNORMAL HEART AND LUNGS. Although the breathlessness of the left ventricular failure may be somewhat relieved by right heart failure, usually some dyspnea persists along with tachypnea and basal rales. Severe right heart failure (and dilatation) may produce tricuspid valvular insufficiency, thereby contributing to systemic venous engorgement. The murmur of tricuspid insufficiency is distinguished from that of mitral insufficiency by its location (lower left border of sternum) and by its tendency to increase during inspiration. Hydrothorax, generally unilateral, is more common than in isolated left ventricular failure.

SYSTEMIC VENOUS CONGESTION. Distention of systemic veins is a hallmark of right heart failure. Several different mechanisms contribute to its genesis: (1) the inability of the failing right ventricle to cope adequately with the venous return; (2) the increase in the quantity of blood contained in the large systemic veins; and (3) increased venomotor tone, resulting from heightened sympathetic nervous activity. The increase in systemic venous pressure underlies the hepatomegaly, splenomegaly, and peripheral edema that characterize right heart failure. Less apparent are the congestion and edema of the gastrointestinal tract that the systemic venous hypertension produces.

Pressure in the superficial jugular vein is a useful index of right atrial pressure and, with experience, may be reliably estimated from the height of the fluid column distending the cervical vein. Normally, the cervical veins are flat in the erect position, whereas in right heart failure they are prominent and distended, usually with a level that pulsates. Functional tricuspid insufficiency, complicating dilatation of the right heart, distorts the normal venous pulse by increasing its *v* wave. Usually superficial venous distention precedes the onset of hepatomegaly and peripheral edema. Occasionally, compression of the abdomen over the liver (hepatojugular reflux) is necessary to display the increased blood volume in the venous system.

LIVER. The liver is usually enlarged and palpable in right heart failure, often in association with mild abdominal discomfort, and generally somewhat tender to compression. In severe right heart failure, particularly if the onset is acute, constraint of the swollen liver by its tight capsule may cause right upper quadrant pain. Tricuspid insufficiency accompanying right ventricular dilatation may cause synchronous pulsations in neck veins and liver. Splenomegaly is uncommon except in prolonged congestion of the liver. Rarely is the enlarged spleen tender from congestion per se.

Early in hepatic congestion, sensitive liver function tests, such as the handling of Bromsulphalein, are apt to be abnormal, and modest increases in the concentrations of cellular enzymes in serum, such as glutamic oxaloacetic transaminase (SGOT), and increases in serum bilirubin are not uncommon. The hyperbilirubinemia consists of a combination of quick- and slow-reacting bilirubin, presumably a consequence of decreased oxygen delivery to the liver arising from hypoperfusion and venous hypertension. But jaundice is uncommon unless hepatic congestion is associated with longstanding pulmonary congestion or with pulmonary infarction.

If cardiac output is severely curtailed and liver congestion is marked and protracted, hypoglycemia may occur, presumably owing to depletion of glycogen stores in the liver and increased formation of lactic acid from glucose because of hypoxia. During physical activity, hepatic blood flow in heart failure decreases further, resulting in a marked decrease in aldosterone breakdown, thereby furthering sodium retention.

Repeated bouts of right heart failure elicit atrophy and necrosis of liver cells in the vicinity of the central veins and stimulate extensive fibrosis ("cardiac cirrhosis"). Many months of reduced hepatic blood flow and high venous pressures are required for this reaction, which may result in a shrunken, fibrotic liver difficult to distinguish from posthepatitic cirrhosis. Hepatic coma is a rare, preterminal complication of severe hepatic congestion and fibrosis.

EXTRACELLULAR FLUID COMPARTMENTS. In normal subjects, the fluid compartments of the body are held remarkably constant as the result of an automatic interplay among *intake* (governed by thirst and appetite), *transcellular exchanges* of fluid and electrolytes (governed by passive and active mechanisms), and *excretion* (regulated mainly by the kidneys). In heart failure, this automatic balance tends to be upset mainly because of inordinate retention of salt and water by the kidneys. The result is an isosmotic expansion of the extracellular fluid in which the circulating blood volume shares. It is conceivable that early in heart failure the conservation of salt and water may serve a useful purpose by expanding the blood volume either to sustain venous return to the failing heart or to relieve the arterial baroreceptors from undue stimulation as the cardiac output fails. But this teleologic explanation does not apply when the myocardium can no longer respond to increased filling pressures and volumes, and the retention of salt and water only aggravates congestion and edema.

The distribution of the excess extracellular fluid varies from patient to patient. In the patient who is up and about, edema accumulates in the feet and ankles under the influence of gravity; in the bedridden patient, the fluid shifts to the sacral region. Low tissue pressure, as around the back of the ankle, predisposes to localization. The level of colloid osmotic pressure and the integrity of the lymphatic system also influence the distribution of the excess fluid.

Subcutaneous Edema. Dependent edema, manifested as swelling of feet or ankles, developing gradually during the day and subsiding by morning, is a characteristic feature of right heart failure. Invariably, it is preceded by systemic venous congestion, but after diuresis subcutaneous edema may linger even though systemic venous hypertension has been relieved by the reduction in venous blood volume. Usually a gain in weight precedes clinical evidence of edema. If edema is allowed to persist, complications such as low-grade cellulitis may occur. The combination of edema and slowed venous flow predisposes to thrombosis and to pulmonary embolism. The massive pitting edema of the lower extremities that was commonly seen before the advent of potent diuretics is now rarely encountered except in instances of gross neglect.

Hydrothorax. It is so uncommon for hydrothorax to complicate isolated failure of the right ventricle, that the association of pleural effusion and cor pulmonale should lead to search for an independent mechanism for the pleural effusion, e.g., pulmonary infarction. On the other hand, it is quite common in combined heart failure (right and left). The pathogenesis of hydrothorax involves impaired removal of water from the pleural space because of high venous pressures in both the pulmonary and systemic circulations, thereby not only compromising transcapillary exchange of water in the pleura but also impeding lymphatic drainage. Hydrothorax contributes to dyspnea not only by encroaching on the air volume but also reflexly, probably by stimuli from lungs and chest wall. Pulmonary infarction may cause pleural effusion in two ways: by direct contiguity of the infarcted area of the lung and the pleural space, or by aggravation of heart failure.

Ascites. Clinically evident excess of free fluid in the abdominal cavity is designated as ascites. It is a late manifestation of right heart failure, generally associated with marked systemic venous hypertension, severe peripheral edema, and hydrothorax. It occurs most frequently in patients with tricuspid valvular disease (or with constrictive pericarditis). Portal and hepatic venous hypertension, coupled with high pressure in the systemic veins draining the peritoneum, seem to be involved in the etiology of ascites; but retention of salt and water is a fundamental prerequisite for ascites to occur. Usually ascites is first noticed by the patient as a gradual increase in abdominal girth. But in severe right heart failure, it may cause anorexia, abdominal discomfort, or pain.

Pericardial Effusion. In severe and persistent heart failure, abnormal quantities of transudate may accumulate in the pericardial sac. Rarely does fluid accumulate to the level of tamponade.

Anasarca. Massive right heart failure may cause excess fluid to accumulate everywhere in the body, most conspicuously in subcutaneous tissues and abdominal and thoracic cavities. Because of the influence of gravity, face and arms are spared until preterminally.

GASTROINTESTINAL TRACT. The bowel wall shares in the systemic venous congestion and edema. These changes rarely interfere with absorption of drugs or foods unless heart failure is extreme. In severe congestive heart failure, anorexia, nausea, and vomiting may occur from reflex, central, or local causes. Occasionally, when right heart failure is severe, a protein-losing enteropathy may develop.

BRAIN. Neurasthenia, headache, and insomnia are common in heart failure. Usually these manifestations are attributed to a combination of a modest diminution of cerebral blood flow and triggering mechanisms, e.g., dyspnea contributing to insomnia. Cerebral manifestations are more frequent when the reduction in cerebral blood flow is superimposed on antecedent cerebrovascular disease, e.g., arteriosclerosis, or personality disorder. Severe heart failure is often associated with irritability, restlessness, and difficulty in fixing attention, particularly in older persons. Preterminally, stupor and coma may develop. The possibility exists that central nervous abnormalities may be enhanced by the delivery to the brain of abnormal products elaborated by remote organs (liver, endocrines, gastrointestinal tract) that suffer deranged metabolism during heart failure as a result of congestion and hypoperfusion.

KIDNEY. Oliguria occurs in both right and left heart failure but is much more striking in the latter. As the heart improves, urinary output increases. The urine is poor in sodium but has a high specific gravity (1.020 to 1.030). Azotemia is common but generally moderate except when intrinsic renal disease is present or after vigorous diuresis. The combination of azotemia and high specific gravity is distinctive for heart failure (and dehydration) and contrasts with the low specific gravity of intrinsic renal disease. Proteinuria is common but rarely severe—usually less than 1 gram per day. A variety of casts accompany the proteinuria. Renal function, as determined by clearance techniques, is only slightly depressed except in severe right failure of long standing.

OTHER MANIFESTATIONS. In severe congestive heart failure, the accumulation of edema may obscure the gradual loss of tissue mass. Often this tissue wasting is associated with *weakness*. In extreme instances, *cachexia* may develop. At this late stage, the patient is usually suffering from anorexia, gastrointestinal upsets, anemia, and electrolyte upsets. Part of the picture undoubtedly stems from organ hypoperfusion and congestion, but often a large contribution has been made by overvigorous use of diuretics and digitalis.

Anxiety. It is not surprising that patients with organic heart disease become anxious. Indeed, anxiety is a regular feature by the time the heart fails. But not always is it an easy matter to distinguish between cardiac complaints as manifestations of anxiety or of the cardiac disorder. Part of the difficulty stems from the nonspecific nature of complaints, such as breathlessness. The difficulty is compounded if the patient misinterprets or exaggerates his symptoms unconsciously. For example, the severely anxious patient may hyperventilate to the point of alkalosis, producing the characteristic lightheadedness, cold hands, and tingling fingers of hypocapnia, reduced cerebral blood flow, and peripheral vasoconstriction, thereby reinforcing his view of the organic nature of his breathlessness. Palpitation is also commonly misinterpreted by the patient suffering from anxiety as a telltale sign of organic heart disease.

The standard approach for the physician is the separate assessment of the organic versus the psychosomatic aspects of the heart disease. Particularly helpful in this regard are excessive or inconsistent complaints for the role of the cardiac disease. Not infrequently, hemodynamic measurements may be required to settle the role of organic heart disease in producing the clinical symptoms.

CLINICAL MANAGEMENT

General Measures

The aim of treatment in heart failure is to arrest and reverse the pathogenic sequence that led to the clinical signs and symptoms. The response to treatment of the more common types of heart failure, i.e., hypertensive and arteriosclerotic, is often dramatic. But each relapse marks another milestone on the road to refractory heart failure, not only by signaling progressive deterioration of the myocardium, but also because intensified and protracted treatment enhances the prospect for eliciting the toxic manifestations of the therapeutic agents.

INCREASING CARDIAC OUTPUT. In most forms of chronic heart failure, the cardiac output can be made to increase by decreasing the cardiac load, by improving myocardial contractility, or by a combination of the two. In the patient with severe bradycardia associated with heart failure, acceleration of the heart rate by cardiac pacing may cure heart failure that would otherwise be refractory. Conversely, severe tachycardia must be arrested if filling times of the ventricles are too greatly curtailed by the abbreviated diastole.

DECREASING THE WORK OF THE HEART. Lightening the cardiac load is prerequisite for the successful treatment of heart failure. The load is always assessed with respect to the state of the myocardium, i.e., a damaged heart may not be able to cope with a blood pressure or volume load that a normal heart handles easily. The aim of treatment is to promote ventricular emptying so that the stroke output of the heart will increase. If successful, the improved cardiac performance reverses the train of clinical manifestations that the low cardiac output had initiated.

The traditional mainstays of cardiotonic therapy are rest, digitalis to improve the inotropic state of the myocardium, and diuretics to reduce the filling pressure of the failing ventricle. Rest is sometimes overlooked as an effective instrument for decreasing the cardiac burden. It must be both physical and mental. For the patient in left ventricular failure, simply sitting upright and breathing more easily is conducive to mental ease. Reassurance is essential to decrease metabolic activity and tachycardia and to relax peripheral vasoconstriction. No amount of reassurance will suffice to relieve a patient experiencing the pangs of severe constipation or urinary retention. Oxygen by nasal catheter (4 to 6 liters per minute) often makes the patient more comfortable even though the degree of arterial hypoxemia is modest, possibly by increasing oxygen delivery to the brain. After recovery from an acute bout of heart failure, a new life style of lessened activity may be required as part of the cardiotonic program. Should reassurance prove inadequate, sedatives or tranquilizers (such as chloral hydrate, 0.5 to 1.0 gram, phenobarbital, 15 to 30 mg, or diazepam, 2 to 10 mg, taken orally three times per day and at bedtime) may be needed to promote mental ease, particularly as the patient improves and grows restless. Narcotics are rarely needed in heart failure unless pulmonary edema has generated intolerable anxiety. Excessive sedation, to the point of immobilizing the patient, enhances the risk of venous thrombosis and embolism, particularly in the elderly.

It is remarkable how often the proper use of rest as the initial step in treatment will promote a vigorous diuresis, slow the heart rate, and relieve dyspnea, thereby allowing a more leisurely use of other cardiotonic agents, such as digitalis and diuretics. On the other hand, if metabolic demands remain high, as during undetected thyrotoxicosis, heart failure may prove refractory to the conventional cardiotonic program until the thyroid overactivity is curtailed.

Acute Pulmonary Edema

Treatment of the acute pulmonary edema of left ventricular failure is begun with the patient in the sitting position, thereby draining the upper portions of his lungs of excess fluid. Meperidine, 50 mg, or morphine, 10 to 15 mg, is administered intravenously for restlessness or dyspnea. These agents seem to act primarily by relieving anxiety and agitation. Morphine is the traditional agent. Most clinicians credit its effectiveness to its role in relaxing the patient and in decreasing tachycardia. However, it also has a central sympatholytic action, thereby causing a decrease in systemic arteriolar resistance and increasing the capacity of the systemic venous system. Unfortunately, distressing side effects, such as nausea, vomiting, and urinary retention, sometimes force recourse to other sedatives. A rapid-acting diuretic, ethacrynic acid or furosemide, is administered intravenously. Even though arterial oxygenation may be near normal, high concentrations of humidified oxygen, 50 to 100 per cent, are frequently used empirically to relieve dyspnea, restlessness, and confusion.

Most initial or mild episodes of pulmonary edema respond quickly to rest, reassurance, morphine, and diuretic. When the prospect of severe and progressive pulmonary edema is likely, attempts are generally instituted to reduce preload or afterload, or both. The drugs that are used are considered subsequently under Unloading Agents. Several other interventions are in common practice: rotating tourniquets on the extremities, phlebotomy (of the order of 200 to 300 ml of blood), or positive pressure breathing which impedes venous return. All three of these interventions have become less popular since the advent of vasodilator therapy. Systemic hypotension is a contraindication to phlebotomy or to positive pressure ventilation.

Digitalis is more essential for supporting the myocardium after the loads on the heart have been lessened than during the acute bout of pulmonary edema. However, a digitalis preparation is usually part of the first wave of therapy in the emergency room. Digitalis (digoxin or deslanoside C, 1.0 mg) may be administered intravenously if the patient has had none during the preceding two weeks. However, the urgency for intravenous injection of digitalis has decreased considerably since the advent of potent, rapid-acting diuretics. An exception to this generalization is the attack of pulmonary edema precipitated by a bout of tachycardia which can be slowed by digitalis, e.g., paroxysmal atrial fibrillation. In this instance, digitalis relieves the heart failure primarily because of its effect on slowing atrioventricular conduction and consequently the ventricular rate, rather than because of its inotropic effect on the heart. In ectopic tachycardias, it may be necessary to resort to DC electroshock in order to restore normal heart action and tolerable heart rates.

Faced with a patient in pulmonary edema, the physician often feels compelled to apply a battery of strenuous measures in rapid succession. Especially for patients in poor condition, this treatment may be worse than the disorder, which is usually self-limited once the upright position has been assumed, mental rest accomplished, and a potent diuretic administered. As soon as the crisis is over, a more conventional cardiotonic program is begun, and a search is made for the cause of the left heart failure as well as for the mechanism that precipitated the episode.

The role of left heart failure in producing high-altitude pulmonary edema is not clear. Prompt recovery usually follows bed rest, descent to lower altitude, and the administration of oxygen.

Drug Interactions

Multiplicity of drugs is the rule in modern therapy. Some drugs are deliberately prescribed in combinations, either to reinforce a desirable therapeutic effect or to avoid an untoward side effect. A familiar example is the combination of digitalis, a potassium-losing diuretic, and potassium supplements for the treatment of heart failure; the dosage of each is individualized to achieve maximal inotropic effect on the heart and to relieve circulatory congestion. But other drugs, such as sleeping pills and anticoagulants that are administered concomitantly for subsidiary or unrelated purposes, may interact and decrease the effectiveness of the cardiotonic program.

There are several ways by which one therapeutic agent can influence the effects of another. Among these are (1) chemical interaction (cholestyramine, a cholesterol-lowering, ion-exchange resin, impedes absorption of digitoxin [and, to a much lesser extent, of digoxin] by binding in the intestine); (2) competition for binding sites on plasma proteins (digitoxin and ethacrynic acid compete for albumin); (3) induction of drug-metabolizing enzymes (phenobarbital and phenylbutazone enhance the metabolism of digitoxin by hepatic microsomal enzymes); and (4) enhanced excretion (polar metabolites of digitoxin are eliminated more rapidly in urine and bile than is digitoxin per se). In conventional dosages, few of these interactions seem to be clinically significant. But they do introduce an element of unpredictability into standard therapeutic programs, and they do urge caution whenever medications are either added to or deleted from a stable therapeutic regimen. Quinidine causes large increments in digoxin levels in serum. The mechanism of action is presumably the displacement of digoxin by quinidine from binding sites in muscle and other tissue, and a reduced renal clearance of digoxin. At the same time, the concentration of digoxin in the myocardium decreases, suggesting an unfavorable combination of increased toxicity and decreased inotropic effect. Large doses of nonsteroidal anti-inflammatory drugs also appreciably increase serum digoxin levels. As a result, the combination of quinidine and digitalis is generally avoided, and caution is urged in using digitalis in patients receiving nonsteroidal anti-inflammatory agents in arthritic disorders.

Related to the concept of drug interaction is the broader concept of drug-biologic interaction, which determines how drugs act. This broader concept includes reactions between the pharmacologic agent and some biologic aspect of the living subject. For example, digitalis effects depend heavily on ion fluxes at ultrastructural membranes; changes in ionic composition and behavior are known to modify the clinical influence of digitalis. Or the physiologic state of the patient may shape the response: acidosis blunts the effectiveness of norepinephrine; the administration of a conventional dose of a ganglionic blocking agent, when sympathetic vasomotor tone is high because of vigorous diuresis and depletion of blood volume, may precipitate circulatory collapse.

The concept of drug-biologic interaction is complicated by individual variability in responsiveness to drugs. Part of this variability is undoubtedly inherited; part is immunologic; most remains to be explained.

Inotropic Agents: Digitalis

As a general rule, heart failure from any cause is an indication for digitalis. However, depending on etiology, in some instances digitalis can be discontinued after clinical recovery. Unfortunately, optimal doses vary from patient to patient and the toxic-therapeutic range is narrow. The situation grows more complicated if preparations of digitalis are switched. Therefore, the physician should master the use of one or two digitalis preparations and always aspire to achieve the minimal effective dose.

GENERAL ASPECTS. Digitalis improves the contractility of the failing myocardium regardless of the type of heart failure, the rate, or the rhythm (Fig. 42–3). After digitalis has been given

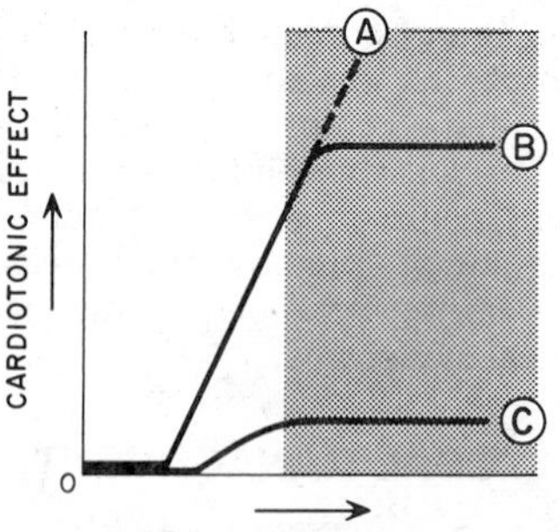

Figure 42–3. Hypothetical effects on contractility elicited by increasing doses (and serum concentrations) of digitalis. Once the inotropic effect of the digitalis preparation begins, it is unlikely that it will continue indefinitely as in A. Instead, it is likely that beyond a certain point the inotropic effects will taper to a plateau despite increasing serum concentration. When this plateau will occur depends on the capability of the heart to respond; a left ventricle that is suffering its first bout of failure is apt to manifest an excellent inotropic response to small increments in serum concentration before the plateau is reached (B). On the other hand, a spent heart that has suffered multiple myocardial infarctions may manifest only a sluggish inotropic response from the start and plateau early despite enormous increments in serum levels of glycoside (C). The shaded area is intended as a reminder of the increasing likelihood of serious arrhythmias as serum glycoside levels continue to increase.

in effective doses and myocardial contractility has increased, the heart shrinks in size, cardiac output increases, end-diastolic volume and pressure decrease, venous pressure normalizes, and evidences of peripheral vasoconstriction, circulatory congestion, and organ hypoperfusion disappear. In the reordering of the circulation that follows relief of congestive heart failure, blood that had been sequestered in the splanchnic venous bed is redirected to the systemic veins by appropriate adjustments in vascular tone, thereby helping to sustain the improved cardiac output.

Molecular Bases. Although the full picture of how digitalis glycosides improve cardiac contractility is not yet clear, they do seem to act by altering surface and intracellular (sarcoplasmic reticulum and mitochondria) membranes so that they release calcium ions more readily. Another manifestation is inhibition of the Na^+-K^+-ATPase activity. However, it is unsettled whether this interference with ATPase, as well as the associated decrease of sodium pumping into the cell, is directly related to the inotropic effect of the glycosides.

Effect on Inotropic State. In low output heart failure, digitalis increases the cardiac output and restores the end-diastolic pressure in the left ventricle to normal. This is a consequence of increased myocardial contractility. A similar effect on contractility occurs in the normal myocardium, but the cardiac output does not increase because of a direct vasoconstricting effect of digitalis on the peripheral resistance vessels. But in low output heart failure in which sympathetic nervous activity is consistently high, restoration of the cardiac output by digitalis reflexly diminishes sympathetic tone, thereby overriding the direct vasoconstricting effects of digitalis on the vessels. These distinctions underscore the unique property of digitalis glycosides as inotropic agents because of their ability to improve myocardial contractility in heart failure without simultaneously eliciting antagonistic effects, such as peripheral vasoconstriction (or tachycardia).

Myocardial Oxygen Consumption. The increase in the strength of contraction produced by the digitalis glycosides increases the oxygen consumption of the myocardium in the normal heart. But this tendency is neutralized in the failing heart which responds to glycosides by shrinking in volume, thereby reducing wall tension and its associated oxygen consumption. Accordingly, the increase in contractility produced in the dilated failing heart is generally accomplished with no increase in myocardial oxygen consumption.

Catecholamine Depletion. Although reduction in cardiac catecholamines is a feature of chronic heart failure, this depletion leaves unaffected the positive inotropic effects of the digitalis glycosides.

Coronary Circulation. In the normal unanesthetized animal, ouabain elicits coronary vasoconstriction. Unfortunately, nothing is known about the behavior of the coronary circulation in response to digitalis during heart failure.

Systemic Circulation. Digitalis elicits an increase in cardiac output, thereby reducing the reflex vasoconstriction of the low output state. But because of the direct constrictor action of cardiac glycosides on vascular smooth muscle, there is apt to be a brief period of increase in systemic arterial pressure, particularly if large doses of cardiac glycosides are administered intravenously.

CHOICE OF DIGITALIS PREPARATION. Five digitalis preparations are in common use today in the United States: digitalis leaf, digoxin, digitoxin, deslanoside (Cedilanid-D), and ouabain. Their basic pharmacologic actions on the heart and their toxic-therapeutic ratios are similar. But they do differ considerably with respect to the rate and degree of absorption from the intestine and both the onset and duration of action.

Digoxin and digitoxin have replaced digitalis leaf for chronic oral administration; ouabain and deslanoside, as well as digoxin, are administered intravenously. Digitoxin is not as satisfactory an intravenous agent, because it is relatively slow in reaching its peak effect. Digitalis leaf is gradually disappearing from use, because it varies in potency, requires bioassay for standardization, and has no therapeutic advantage over digitoxin, its principal constituent.

Traditional practice has relied on a preliminary loading phase to achieve a therapeutic level, followed by maintenance dosage to sustain a balance between intake and elimination. Accordingly, the preset loading dose is administered over a period of one to three days (Table 42–2), providing enough digitalis to load body stores and to compensate for daily elimination. Unless a desperate situation—such as a life-threatening cardiac arrhythmia—calls for acute digitalization, slow digitalization is preferable. Indeed, if there is no hurry, continued administration of the maintenance dose, without a loading dose, has proved to be a practical way to achieve digitalization.

Dosages listed in Table 42–2 are intended to indicate orders of magnitude rather than precise schedules. Dosage is determined individually according to the nature and severity of the heart disease, the clinical setting, the use of other drugs such as potassium-losing diuretics, and continued observation of the patient's response.

Oral Preparations. Digoxin and, less often, digitoxin are the mainstays of chronic oral administration.

DIGOXIN. The maintenance dosage of digoxin is determined by a balance between renal excretion, dose, and absorption. Ordinarily, between 75 and 90 per cent of an oral dose is absorbed. Digoxin is lipid soluble and absorbed from the small intestine by diffusion. Some variation in absorption may occur, depending on the solubility of digoxin molecules in the intestinal fluids. Variability in absorption may also result from different preparations of digoxin. Consequently, once a digoxin preparation from one manufacturer has proved effective, changes should be avoided.

Digoxin is excreted primarily by the kidney, and most of the drug appears unchanged in the urine. When the patient is fully digitalized, the concentration of digoxin in serum is 1 per cent or less of total body stores of digoxin. If renal function is normal, approximately one third of the body stores is eliminated per day; the maintenance dose replenishes this daily loss. The half-life of digoxin in serum is approximately the same in normal subjects and in patients with heart failure,

TABLE 42–2. ADMINISTRATION OF COMMON CARDIAC GLYCOSIDES

	Digitalization			Cardiotonic Effects		Blood Levels	
Preparation	*Loading Dose* (mg/24 hrs)*	*Initial Dose† (mg)*	*Maintenance Dose (mg)*	*Onset of Activity (min)*	*Peak Effect (hrs)*	*Steady-State Therapeutic Level¶ (ng/ml)*	*Half-Life (hrs)*
Digoxin (oral)	2.5	1.0‡	0.25	60–120	1–3	1.5	36
Digitoxin (oral)	1.2	0.75	0.1	30–120	4–6	17	96–144
Deslanoside (IV)	1.6	0.8§	—	10–30	1–2	—	33
(These values are examples to illustrate orders of magnitude.)							

*Total quantity to be administered in 24 hours for therapeutic effect.
†Assuming no prior digitalis during previous two weeks.
‡The initial dose of digoxin by the intravenous route is 0.5 to 1.0 mg. Thereafter, 0.25 mg every 4 to 6 hours is given until the average loading dose is reached.
§When feasible, switch to oral maintenance doses of digoxin or digitoxin.
¶On conventional maintenance doses.

TABLE 42–3. FEATURES OF CARDIAC GLYCOSIDE PREPARATIONS IN COMMON USE

Preparation	Source	Usual Route of Administration*	Gastrointestinal Absorption	Protein Binding†	Principal Route of Elimination
Digoxin	*Digitalis lanata*	Oral	75–90%‡	23%‡	Kidneys
Digitoxin	*Digitalis purpurea*	Oral	90–100%	97%	Liver; kidney for metabolites
Deslanoside	*Digitalis lanata*	Intravenous	Erratic	—	Kidneys
(These values are examples to illustrate orders of magnitude.)					

*All can be administered intravenously.
†Affinity for protein (albumin) determines rate of urinary excretion and persistence in body.
‡Varies according to preparation. Different tablets differ in bioavailability of digoxin.

averaging one and one-half days. The half-life is prolonged in renal failure. The serum level of digoxin in renal insufficiency is directly related to the creatinine clearance and inversely to the concentration of urea nitrogen in the blood (BUN). Formulas have been devised to take these relationships into account, recognizing that, in contrast to the normal daily elimination of one third of body stores of digoxin, the anuric patient eliminates about one seventh. Accordingly, the anuric patient will require one half or less of the usual maintenance dose (see Ch. 22).

Only 5 per cent of digoxin in serum is bound to protein. Its polar structure accounts for the difference between its concentration and that of digitoxin (nonpolar) in the serum (Table 42–3).

Without an initial loading dose, patients receiving digoxin orally reach a steady state in the serum, reflecting equilibrium between body stores, intake, and elimination in about one week. Body stores are related to lean body weight, because digoxin does not accumulate in fat or interstitial fluid. In an adult patient, body stores are generally of the order of 0.01 mg per kilogram of body weight. Rarely are body stores required greater than 0.02 mg per kilogram of body weight. Therefore for a 70-kg patient, digitalization usually requires a minimal dose of approximately 0.7 mg. Should this digitalizing dose be exceeded, the prospects for toxicity will increase accordingly.

The essential features in using digoxin therapeutically are summarized in Table 42–2. Because of its short half-life, a single dose per day will cause a wide swing in serum concentration (and in body stores, including the heart) before the next dose is administered. In practice this swing is often unimportant; but, if desirable, its magnitude may be reduced (and therapeutic control improved) by administering one half the daily dose at 12-hour intervals. Many clinicians use digoxin for intravenous as well as oral administration, because its hemodynamic and biologic properties are comparatively well understood, and dosages are relatively easy to adjust.

Interactions between digoxin and other cardiovascular agents may cause serious clinical problems. Most intensively studied has been the interaction of digoxin and quinidine. The results indicate that co-administration of these two agents has the net effect of increasing the blood level of digoxin and of enhancing its cardiac effects. Therefore, the patient on digoxin maintenance therapy who is given quinidine should concomitantly undergo a decrease in digoxin dosage, e.g., by half, in order to avoid digoxin toxicity.

Interaction is not confined to quinidine. Amiodarone* also increases digoxin concentration in blood. So do verapamil and nifedipine, two popular calcium-channel blocking agents. Certain diuretics, notably spironolactone, are suspected of influencing digoxin levels in blood. Conversely, the addition of vasodilators to the cardiotonic regimen promotes renal elimination of digoxin as cardiac output increases. In essence, each modification of a cardiotonic program that includes digoxin (or other digitalis glycoside) entails the risk of directly or indirectly influencing the level of the cardiac glycoside.

DIGITOXIN. This agent is widely used for chronic administration. It differs importantly from digoxin in its metabolism and its slow rate of elimination; the main route of elimination is by metabolism in the liver, only a small fraction being eliminated by the kidney.

Digitoxin is completely absorbed after oral administration so that oral and intravenous dosages are identical. Body stores and digitalizing doses are approximately the same as with digoxin, but maintenance doses are quite different because of different rates of elimination. Approximately 12 per cent of body stores of digitoxin is eliminated per day in patients with normal renal function. The usual body store is estimated to be of the order of 0.8 mg in a 70-kg adult. Therefore the daily maintenance dose is generally 0.1 mg per day (0.12 × 0.8 mg). Because of its slow dissipation and elimination, serum levels of digitoxin vary less from hour to hour than do digoxin levels. But the drug accumulates insidiously so that maintenance doses established at the onset often prove to be toxic in time.

In contrast to digoxin, digitoxin has a strong avidity for albumin so that 97 per cent in plasma is nondialyzable. This combination is a critical factor in limiting glomerular filtration and excretion of digitoxin by the kidneys. After an oral dose of 1.0 mg, 50 per cent of the inotropic effect is reached in one hour; 85 to 100 per cent is achieved in four hours and sustained for the rest of the day. The average half-life is approximately five days. Digitoxin enters into an enterohepatic cycle. Between 30 and 60 per cent of the 1.0 mg dose is eliminated in the feces and urine, the larger fraction generally in the urine. The remainder is metabolized, primarily to digoxin, which is eliminated in the urine. Digoxin is preferable to digitoxin in renal or hepatic insufficiency.

Intravenous Preparations. As a rule, these are reserved for life-threatening situations. These include acute heart failure complicating a bout of atrial fibrillation with rapid ventricular rate, fulminating pulmonary edema as a complication of left ventricular failure, and the onset of heart failure or a serious arrhythmia during surgery. As a rule, the larger the dose of the glycoside, the more apt it is to create problems, particularly arrhythmias, of its own.

An intravenous bolus of a digitalis preparation may elicit a bout of hypertension, particularly if the dose is large, e.g., 1.0 mg of digoxin. The increase is generally of the order of 20/10 mm Hg, and the effect is generally short lived. But it may suffice to overburden the failing heart and to aggravate the situation until it subsides and is succeeded by the inotropic effect. Hypertension is rarely a problem if the intravenous dose is modest and administered slowly.

DIGOXIN. For rapid digitalization, 0.5 mg is given initially, followed by 0.25 mg every two to four hours as needed, but taking care to avoid exceeding a total dose of 2 mg in 12 hours. As soon as practical, the oral route is substituted for the intravenous route.

DESLANOSIDE. This preparation is identical with digoxin except for the addition of a glucose residue. Its digitalizing effect appears in 10 to 30 minutes after intravenous injection, reaches peak effect in one to two hours, and regresses in 24 hours. For rapid intravenous digitalization, the full 1.6 mg may be given at once, or, preferably, 0.8 mg may be followed by another 0.8 mg, either in four hours or in divided doses, at two- to four-hour intervals for two to three additional doses. Maintenance of digitalization is preferably done by oral digoxin or digitoxin.

*Investigational drug in the United States.

But, if necessary, 0.4 mg may be given intravenously or intramuscularly at 8- to 12-hour intervals.

OUABAIN. This is the traditional digitalis preparation for intravenous use. It is a pure crystalline substance that is unsuitable for oral use because of erratic absorption from the gastrointestinal tract. Its latency after intravenous injection is exceedingly brief (less than five minutes); it is rapidly eliminated so that it is not suitable for maintenance of digitalization. The initial intravenous dose is 0.25 to 0.3 mg, administered slowly. An additional 0.15 or 0.3 mg may be repeated after 24 hours.

Diagnostic Preparations. ACETYLSTROPHANTHIDIN.* This is a partial synthetic which, because of its exceedingly rapid onset of action and dissipation, has been advocated more as a diagnostic test for adequacy of digitalization than as a therapeutic agent for heart failure. In practice, repeated injections of the substance (0.25 mg in 5 ml of glucose and water) are made until toxic or therapeutic effects are observed. Because it is potentially dangerous, other diagnostic tests are being investigated.

GUIDES TO PROPER DOSAGE OF DIGITALIS. In practice, digitalis is used for either its inotropic effect or slowing atrioventricular conduction, or both. Larger quantities are generally required to slow the heart by producing atrioventricular block than to elicit the inotropic effect.

No standard dose exists, and the toxic-therapeutic range is narrow. Older individuals are not only prone to toxic arrhythmias even from very small daily doses but are also apt to have difficulty in complying with instructions. Control of dosage is easier to achieve in the patient with atrial fibrillation than in the patient with normal sinus rhythm: in atrial fibrillation, the drug is given until the heart rate reaches comfortable levels at rest and during mild exercise; whereas in the patient in normal sinus rhythm, the heart rate is a poor therapeutic guide, so that a toxic arrhythmia may develop before optimal slowing is achieved.

DIGITALIS TOXICITY. Digitalis preparations are among the most dangerous, as well as the most useful, of current medications. The incidence of cardiotoxicity is staggering—on the order of 10 to 20 per cent in hospitalized patients receiving conventional doses of digitalis—and mortality from digitalis cardiotoxicity is estimated to run into the thousands per year.

Alertness on the part of the physician can go far in excluding digitalis toxicity: recognizing that certain patients, particularly the elderly and those in renal failure, are at special risk of digitalis toxicity; establishing that no digitalis has been taken for the last two weeks; in the case of a poorly responsive tachycardia, searching for complications, such as hypo- or hyperthyroidism, hypercalcemia, infection, or pulmonary emboli; checking renal function and, if it is impaired, relating drug dosage to degree of renal impairment; using care in administering digitalis intravenously, particularly if digitalis has been taken recently, if the patient is hypoxemic, or if metabolic disturbances are present; avoiding undue reliance on the electrocardiogram as a guide to proper dosage, since it can only disclose toxic effects on conduction and in producing arrhythmias; determining serum levels of the glycoside when toxicity is suspected but keeping in mind that arrhythmias can occur in the face of normal levels; avoiding prophylactic digitalization; and avoiding sudden electrolyte upsets, such as the intravenous admission of calcium-, magnesium-, and potassium-containing solutions.

Digitalis levels in serum often provide valuable information about the likelihood of digitalis toxicity. The usual therapeutic range for digoxin in serum ranges between 0.8 and 2.0 ng per milliliter. But, although levels above 2.0 ng per milliliter are often associated with toxicity, some patients tolerate much higher concentrations. Digoxin levels below 0.8 ng per milliliter are probably not therapeutic. The lack of close correspondence between serum levels of the glycosides and moderate cardiotoxicity in individual patients has kept alive interest in other tests for digitalis toxicity.

Recognition. The electrocardiogram (ECG) is generally the final arbiter of digitalis cardiotoxicity. But three categories of clinical clues direct attention to the electrocardiogram: (1) extracardiac disturbances, such as anorexia, nausea, weight loss, vomiting, diarrhea, visual disturbances, and, much more uncommonly, gynecomastia, psychosis, or abdominal pain; (2) ectopic ventricular rhythms, nonparoxysmal atrioventricular junctional rhythms, atrioventricular dissociation, atrial fibrillation with a ventricular response of less than 50 per minute if associated with ventricular ectopic beats, Mobitz type I atrioventricular block, paroxysmal atrial tachycardia with atrioventricular block, sinoatrial exit block, or sinus arrest; and (3) regularization of the heart rate in the patient with atrial fibrillation while taking maintenance doses of digitalis.

Digitalis cardiotoxicity is primarily a matter of arrhythmias. Almost any cardiac arrhythmia can be produced by digitalis, and the more complicated the arrhythmia in a digitalized patient, the more likely is digitalis toxicity to be the root cause of the problem. Certain disturbances, particularly ventricular premature beats, the Wenckebach phenomenon, and interference dissociation with a reasonable ventricular rate, are not per se evidences of digitalis toxicity. On the other hand, the coincidence of depressed atrioventricular conduction and stimulation of ectopic pacemakers is virtually pathognomonic for digitalis toxicity. This combination accounts for arrhythmias characterized by simultaneous rapid atrial rates and slow ventricular responses, for escape beats, and for nonparoxysmal junctional tachycardia. For example, atrial tachycardia with atrioventricular block, generally precipitated by overzealous administration of potassium-losing diuretics, is characteristic, although not specific, for digitalis toxicity. Even more distinctive is atrioventricular dissociation with junctional rhythm, in which two pacemakers operate independently above and below the intervening area of atrioventricular block. In atrial fibrillation, the advent of serious digitalis toxicity may be signaled by regularization of the ventricular rate because of acceleration of an ectopic focus below a high degree of atrioventricular block.

The usual cause of death in digitalis toxicity is ventricular fibrillation. Rarely does it appear unexpectedly. More often, it is presaged by multifocal premature contractions and runs of ventricular tachycardia. Consequently, premature ventricular beats that appear after digitalis has been started or during maintenance therapy have to be regarded as serious warnings of toxicity, particularly if they are multifocal in origin and if there is bigeminy involving premature beats that are bizarre in appearance. Rarely do ventricular arrhythmias occur without other evidence of digitalis intake, including the characteristic ST-T deformations, disturbances in atrial ventricular conduction, and atrial arrhythmias.

Treatment. The mainstay for treating digitalis cardiotoxicity is to stop the digitalis and to discontinue diuretics that contributed to hypokalemia. There is no specific antidote. Fortunately, most digitalis-induced arrhythmias are arrested by stopping digitalis. Thus junctional rhythms without excessive ventricular rates or evidence of ventricular irritability are generally treated without specific medication or intervention. But if the arrhythmia is characteristic of ventricular irritability or if it has caused hemodynamic upset in the form of hypotension, heart failure, and pulmonary edema, medical intervention is mandatory.

Potassium is the agent of choice for suppressing digitalis-induced automaticity. But because it slows conduction through the myocardium and specialized conduction tissues, thereby potentiating the depression produced by digitalis, it must be used with extreme caution when atrioventricular block is severe. In the latter case, the introduction of a temporary perivenous cardiac pacemaker may prove useful in tiding the patient over the period needed to eliminate the excess digitalis,

*Investigational drug in the United States.

particularly if antiarrhythmic drugs are to be used to suppress ectopic atrial or ventricular beats.

If the arrhythmia has produced no crisis, if renal function is adequate, and if there is no hyperkalemia, potassium salts (4 to 6 grams of potassium chloride per day) may be administered orally. On the other hand, if the situation is deteriorating rapidly because of ectopic beats or uncontrollable tachycardia, potassium salts may be administered intravenously. Continuous electrocardiographic monitoring is mandatory during intravenous administration. The combination of continuous monitoring and careful intravenous titration of the arrhythmia is generally safer than is oral administration. The usual preparation for intravenous use contains 40 mEq of potassium in a 500 ml solution of 5 per cent glucose in water; this is administered slowly, e.g., at a rate of 40 mEq per hour. This may be repeated, if necessary, for up to three doses. Hypotension may limit the amount of potassium that can be given by vein. The electrocardiogram is monitored throughout, recognizing that high plasma concentrations of potassium may per se cause death through cardiac depression, arrhythmias, or arrest. The characteristic changes in the ECG are disappearance of the P wave, widening of the QRS complexes, changes in the S-T segments, and tall, peaked T waves.

Antiarrhythmic drugs which decrease ventricular automaticity by slowing diastolic depolarization, such as procainamide, lidocaine, propranolol, and phenytoin are effective but must be used cautiously. Procainamide is useful when potassium fails to control the arrhythmia or if potassium is contraindicated because of uremia or hyperkalemia. It also has the advantage of sustained action if digitalis toxicity should persist. But it runs the risk of hypotension, depression of contractility, and producing AV block.

Lidocaine (1 to 2 mg per kilogram in one to two minutes by intravenous injection or as continuous infusion) has been used to control premature ventricular beats and ventricular tachycardia resulting from digitalis. It produces an effect within 45 to 90 seconds which is dissipated within 20 minutes. It has the advantage over procainamide of not causing hypotension. Doses less than 750 mg per hour are rarely associated with significant toxic effects, i.e., neurologic disorders and convulsions.

Phenytoin has been advocated for the treatment of digitalis-induced arrhythmias* because it does not depress atrioventricular conduction. It is administered intravenously at a rate of 5 to 10 mg per kilogram over a 5- to 15-minute period. Propranolol, quinidine, bretylium tosylate, and chelating agents such as cholestyramine are also used. Electroconversion by DC shock, which has proved to be remarkably effective in controlling many arrhythmias, is a desperate measure of last resort in digitalis-toxic arrhythmias because of the likelihood of producing uncontrollable paroxysmal ventricular arrhythmias. Digoxin-specific antibodies have been found effective in a few clinics.

BLOOD LEVELS. Determination of serum concentrations of some cardiac glycosides by radioimmunoassay techniques is now available, reliable, accurate, and specific. The usual therapeutic range for digoxin in serum is between 0.8 and 2.0 ng per milliliter. Although levels above 2.0 ng per milliliter are often associated with toxicity, some patients are comfortable with much higher concentrations; conversely, serious arrhythmias can occur despite normal glycoside levels in serum. Digoxin levels below 0.8 ng per milliliter are probably not therapeutic. Although the frequency and severity of toxic effects of digitalis preparations (digoxin, digitoxin) do increase progressively as serum concentrations exceed therapeutic levels, exceptions do occur, especially in the zone between toxic and therapeutic levels. In some instances, the discrepancies between serum concentration and clinical consequences have been attributed to the many physiologic, pathologic, and biochemical influences that can modify the response to a given concentration of glycoside in the serum (and at the site of action): e.g., hypokalemia, acid-base disturbances, hypoxemia, interaction with other drugs, hypoproteinemia, acquisition of tolerance. The exceptions emphasize that serum concentrations must be interpreted in the light of the clinical setting.

Determination of serum concentration of a digitalis glycoside is most useful in patients who are suspected of digitalis toxicity but unable to provide an accurate account of digitalis dosage. It also has a place in guiding dosage in candidates for digitalis toxicity, e.g., heart failure complicated by renal insufficiency or by violent biochemical and physiologic perturbations, as after cardiac surgery. A low serum concentration may indicate that refractory heart failure is a consequence of inadequate dosage.

DIGITALIS IN ACUTE MYOCARDIAL INFARCTION. Utmost caution must be exerted if digitalis is administered for heart failure in the course of acute myocardial infarction, particularly if heart failure is associated with ventricular premature depolarizations. The aim of digitalis in this situation is to improve the contractility of the noninfarcted myocardium. The threat is that ventricular irritability, particularly in the peri-infarcted, ischemic zones, will be enhanced to the point of ectopic foci and uncontrollable ventricular arrhythmias. Another tempering prospect is that any inotropic effects on intact myocardium will be negated by abnormal or paradoxical motions of infarcted and peri-infarcted areas.

These reservations, plus the availability of effective diuretics to clear pulmonary congestion and edema during the first few days of an acute myocardial infarction, encourage extraordinary circumspection in using digitalis during the acute episode. Indeed, some cardiologists no longer consider digitalis to be the agent of choice in this situation, preferring to rely on diuretics and vasodilators, occasionally supplemented by dopamine to tide the patient over the acute crisis. On the other hand, if heart failure persists after the acute crisis—because of either extensive scarring or unremitting hemodynamic overload—digitalis is clearly required because the myocardium has failed globally. Moreover, should atrial fibrillation with a rapid ventricular response complicate acute myocardial infarction early or late in its course, digitalis may be lifesaving. For other supraventricular arrhythmias, which generally require larger doses of digitalis and may even prove refractory, antiarrhythmic agents or electrical conversion are preferable during the phase of increased ventricular irritability.

AMRINONE.† Over the years, efforts to find a safer and more effective inotropic agent than digitalis, or even a reliable alternative, particularly for treating heart failure in the patient with normal sinus rhythm, have proved unrewarding. Among those tried have been the catecholamines, which failed because of their proclivity for inducing arrhythmias, raising systemic arterial blood pressure, and developing tachyphylaxis, as well as the need to administer them intravenously. But recently a new agent, amrinone, a bypyridine derivative, has generated considerable enthusiasm. This agent is a nonglycoside, nonadrenergic inotropic agent that is effective orally as well as after intravenous administration. Its inotropic effect appears to be more powerful than that of the glycosides and it does not cause tachyphylaxis or evoke arrhythmias even in large doses. In experimental heart failure in animals, cardiac output increases while arterial blood pressure remains unchanged and myocardial oxygen consumption falls. To date, the bulk of the evidence in humans is from patients in refractory heart failure who are also taking digitalis, diuretics, and unloading agents. A common side effect (15 per cent) has been a dose-related thrombocytopenia, apparently due to platelet destruction. Another 15 per cent developed drug fever and some manifested gastrointestinal intolerance. A new agent, hopefully of lower toxicity, is milrinone, which is reputed to be much more potent than amrinone so that it can be used in smaller doses. However, the use of this agent is still in its infancy and its toxicity remains to be elucidated.

*This use is not listed in the manufacturer's directive.

†Investigational drug in the United States.

UNLOADING AGENTS (VASODILATOR THERAPY). The idea behind the use of vasodilators in heart failure is to reduce the afterload of a ventricle by relaxing vascular smooth muscle. At first, the use of these agents in heart failure was reserved for those patients who failed to improve despite increasing dosages of digitalis and diuretics. Currently, rules governing the use of these agents have been greatly liberalized (Table 42–4). Nonetheless, their role is still that of adjunct therapy and not as a substitute for a cardiotonic agent, usually digitalis, and diuretics.

Principles. The normal ventricle usually accommodates a change in afterload without much change in cardiac output and stroke volume; if cardiac output does increase, it is because of an increase in heart rate. In contrast, the failing ventricle improves its emptying when afterload is reduced (Fig. 42–4), thereby increasing stroke volume and cardiac output without increasing heart rate. By this tactic, the failing heart responds to a decrease in afterload by shifting its ventricular function curve toward normal even though the inotropic state of the myocardium is unchanged. Thus by reducing afterload the failing heart can increase its output without increasing either preload or contractility. Since contractility, preload, and heart rate are major determinants of myocardial oxygen consumption, the use of agents that reduce afterload in heart failure includes the attractive prospect that better emptying of the ventricle will be achieved while decreasing myocardial oxygen requirements.

As a rule, vasodilators do not exert their effects directly on the heart. Instead, they act—at least predominantly—on vascular smooth muscle. The vascular beds affected may be venous, arterial, or a combination of the two (Table 42–5).

Choice of Vasodilators. Unless otherwise stipulated, the discussion that follows centers on failure of the left ventricle or both ventricles (combined heart failure) but not on right ventricular failure secondary to pulmonary hypertension and cor pulmonale. The effects of vasodilators on the pulmonary circulation are considered in another section.

In choosing the proper vasodilator, a clinical decision has to be made whether the patient would benefit most from a reduction in preload (venous) or afterload (arteriolar) or both.

Venous dilators reduce systemic venous tone and increase the capacity of the systemic venous bed. Because venomotor tone is often high in heart failure and the capacity of the venous bed is large, a considerable shift in blood volume may occur from the systemic to the venous segments of the circulation. In the patient with chronic pulmonary congestion and edema due to abnormally high left atrial pressures, systemic venodilators afford the prospect of providing considerable symptomatic relief as long as the decrease in preload does not jeopardize the cardiac output. The prototype of this group is nitroglycerin.

Arterial dilators are intended to relieve the intense systemic arteriolar vasoconstriction that characterizes left ventricular failure and to promote the normal distribution of the cardiac output. They decrease afterload by reducing systemic arteriolar (and arterial) tone. As a result, stroke volume and, thereby, cardiac output increase, and distribution of blood flow to vital organs, notably brain, kidneys, and heart, improves. Because of the increase in cardiac output, systemic arterial blood pressure generally remains at near-normal levels. However, caution must be exerted to ensure that systemic arterial blood pressure does not decrease inordinately, a likelihood that is particularly threatening in those with impaired contractility and normal preload. The prototype of this group is phentolamine.

Combined venous and arterial dilators decrease both preload and afterload. The actions of this group are a mix of those evoked by venous and arterial vasodilators. For the patient in chronic heart failure, in whom evidence of inadequate organ perfusion coexists with that of high left atrial pressures, these agents afford the prospect of increasing cardiac output and lowering left atrial pressure with little effect on either systemic arterial blood pressure or heart rate. The prototype of this group is nitroprusside.

Probably the most popular vasodilator at present is nitroprusside which, because it is shortlived, can only be given intravenously (Table 42–5). The overall unloading effect of nitroprusside depends on the hemodynamic state of the heart. If the heart is not in failure, nitroprusside has little or no effect on stroke output; left ventricular end-diastolic pressure falls. The unchanged output and the concomitant decrease in filling pressure presumably reflect an equivalent reduction in preload and afterload by the nitroprusside. In contrast, if myocardial function is severely impaired, stroke output increases as left ventricular end-diastolic pressure falls because nitroprusside causes a greater decrease in afterload than in preload. In practical terms, the unloading effect of nitroprusside is most apt to be helpful when the left ventricular end-diastolic pressure is greater than 12 to 15 mm Hg and the cardiac output is low. Unloading of the heart by nitroprusside is not accompanied by a change in heart rate or in contractility. However, as systemic arterial pressure and end-diastolic volume fall, ventricular wall tension decreases and consequently the myocardial oxygen

TABLE 42–4. CURRENT CLINICAL USES OF REDUCTION IN AFTERLOAD

Acute vasodilator therapy
Acute pulmonary edema
Acute myocardial infarction
Particularly with hypertension
With severe heart failure
With cardiogenic shock
With mechanical complication
Mitral regurgitation after ruptured chordae tendineae
Acute aortic regurgitation
Preservation of ischemic myocardium
Acute left ventricular failure due to cardiac overload
Hypertensive crisis
Acute aortic insufficiency
Chronic vasodilator therapy
Hypertension
Chronic myocardial failure
Refractory heart failure in ambulatory patients
Acute heart failure unresponsive to standard cardiotonic and diuretic program

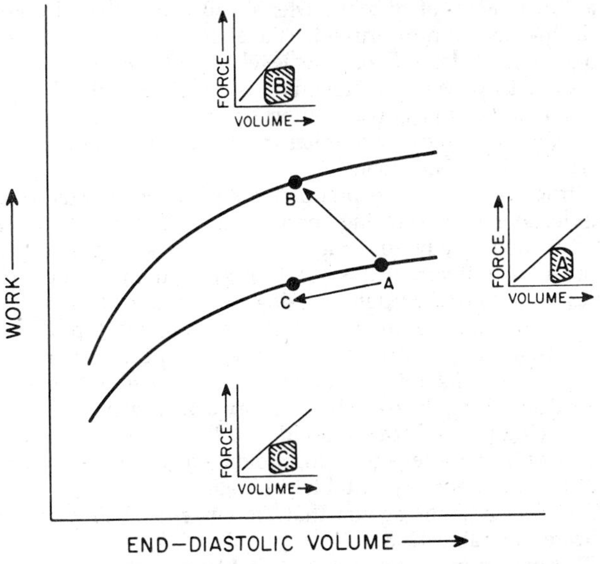

Figure 42–4. Schematic ventricular function curves comparing effects of vasodilator (reduction in afterload) and digitalis (inotropic effect) in heart failure. The administration of a vasodilator in severe heart failure moves the heart to an improved position on the lower curve of impaired contractility (A–C). Digitalis shifts the heart to a curve of improved contractility (A–B). Analysis of work done per beat for points B, A, and C are shown on the left. The landmarks on the work loops are the same as in Figure 42–2.

TABLE 42–5. REPRESENTATIVE VASODILATORS USED TO REDUCE AFTERLOAD IN HEART FAILURE

Agent	Route of Administration	Usual Dosage	Predominant Sites of Action	Predominant Hemodynamic Effects: *Blood Pressure*	*Cardiac Output*	*PA Wedge*	*Heart Rate*	Comment
Sodium nitroprusside	IV	Start with 15 μg/min and increase gradually*; maximum of 400 μg/min; usual, 65 μg/min	A, V†	+	+ +	+ +	0 or +	Hazard of thiocyanate or cyanide toxicity during prolonged therapy or high doses
Phentolamine	IV	Start with 0.1 mg/min*; maximum of 2 mg/min	A, V	+	+ +	+ +	+	Chief effect on arterioles; causes tachycardia
Nitroglycerin	IV Sublingual	5 to 25 μg/min; adjust to response	V	+	+	+ + +	0	Transient (15–30 min); negligible effect on arterioles
Isosorbide dinitrate	Oral Sublingual	20–40 mg 2.5–10 mg	V	+	+	+ + +	0	Same as nitroglycerin but longer (1–4 hrs)
Hydralazine	Oral	50–75 mg q 6 hrs	A	0 or +	+ + +	0 or +	0	Sometimes used in conjunction with venodilator
Prazosin	Oral	5 mg q 8 hrs	A, V	+	+ +	+ +	0 or −	Rapid tolerance to beneficial effects during continued therapy; slow heart rate may be troublesome at start of therapy
Trimethaphan	IV	Start with 2–4 mg/min; decrease, maximum of 6 mg/min	A, V	+	+ +	+ +	0	No reflex increase in heart rate; adjust dose carefully to avoid marked hypotension
Captopril	Oral	Sicker patients require lower starting dose. In hospitalized patients, start with 6.25 or 12.5 mg tid; increase gradually over days. In ambulatory patients, start with 12.5 to 25 mg tid.	A, V	+ +	+ +	+ + +	0	Monitor blood pressure after first dose. Avoid potassium-sparing diuretics. Side effects include hypotension (common), agranulocytosis, nephrotic syndrome, rash.

*Increase every 10 to 15 minutes, using arterial blood pressure and pulmonary wedge pressures as guides. Avoid large fall in systemic blood pressure while pulmonary wedge pressure is returning to about 15 mm Hg.

†A = Arterial bed. V = Venous bed.

requirement falls. Thus in severe heart failure nitroprusside affords the prospect of achieving better emptying of the ventricle while decreasing myocardial oxygen requirements.

The most important threat in using sodium nitroprusside is systemic hypotension, an extension of its therapeutic effect. Because the drug is short-acting, this effect generally subsides spontaneously in minutes. Only uncommonly will a vasoconstrictor be required to restore blood pressure toward normal.

Phentolamine is an alpha-adrenergic blocking agent as well as a direct dilator of systemic arterial and venous blood vessels. As in the case of nitroprusside, the effects of phentolamine on stroke output depend on the level of left ventricular filling pressure. However, phentolamine is chiefly an arteriolar dilator, so that it exerts a greater effect on impedance to ventricular emptying than on preload. It has the disadvantage of increasing heart rate; it is also expensive.

Nitroglycerin exerts its predominant effect on venous smooth muscle, thereby decreasing venous return. It is usually administered sublingually (0.4 mg) but is also occasionally given intravenously (starting dose of 10 μg per minute*) for urgent states of pulmonary edema arising from acute left ventricular failure. For more prolonged effects, it is applied topically, via strips that carry the ointment on one aspect. When given intravenously, its rate of infusion is regulated to lower left ventricular filling pressure (pulmonary artery wedge pressure). In reducing preload, care should be taken to avoid decreasing cardiac output. Other agents for prolonged action are isosorbide dinitrate and pentaerythritol tetranitrate.

Other vasodilator agents that are currently being tried are indicated in Table 42–5.

Captopril merits special notice. It dilates both arterioles and veins. Administration of this agent to patients in chronic heart failure resistant to digitalis and diuretics has shown that captopril can increase cardiac output and decrease pulmonary wedge pressure within two hours of the first dose. This hemodynamic improvement has persisted for months, along with symptomatic improvement, in some patients who have continued to take captopril, digitalis, and diuretics. The drop in systemic blood pressure after the first dose is sometimes threatening. Other adverse effects are agranulocytosis, glomerulopathy, and hyperkalemia. Whether it will prove to be more effective than other oral vasodilator agents, particularly with respect to safety, remains to be settled.

Although vasodilators are conventionally categorized as venous, arterial, or combined, their actions often overlap. Moreover, as indicated above with respect to "forward" and "backward" failure, it is difficult to manipulate afterload in an intact circulation without influencing preload—even in the systemic circulation which is so heavily guarded by automatic regulatory mechanisms. Finally, their dominant effects in any circumstance depend strongly on the state of the heart and circulation. Nonetheless, when used circumspectly, they do contribute to the therapeutic armamentarium for heart failure.

Successful use of vasodilators in heart failure requires awareness of the full hemodynamic consequences of administering a particular agent. Thus, a low output state resulting from systemic vasoconstriction cannot be expected to improve in response to systemic vasodilatation (decrease in afterload) unless venous return to the left ventricle (preload) increases concomitantly. Also, the use of vasodilator therapy to relieve pulmonary edema by decreasing preload has to take into account that acute left ventricular failure generally elicits systemic vasoconstriction as a consequence of the associated renal ischemia and release of renin.

At present, vasodilator agents are used both to unload the overburdened heart acutely and in chronic heart failure. In general, they are reserved for states of heart failure in which the patient remains symptomatic despite adequate digitalis, diuretics, and control of arrhythmias. If successful, vasodilators can be expected to make the patient more comfortable at rest without appreciable increase in exercise performance. They seem to have their greatest potential in patients with severe hemodynamic derangements in whom the control of heart failure by digitalis and diuretics is not optimal.

*Manufacturer's recommended dose: 5 μg per minute.

Four agents are now in vogue: nitrates, hydralazine, prazosin, and captopril. Nitrates (usually isosorbide dinitrate) elicit systemic venodilation, thereby decreasing preload; cardiac output is generally unaffected. Hydralazine decreases arteriolar tone and increases cardiac output, leaving filling pressures unaffected. To date, a combination of nitrate and hydralazine has worked well in most patients, using a little more nitrate if the predominant manifestations are those of pulmonary congestion and edema, and a little more hydralazine if evidences of low cardiac output, e.g., oliguria, predominate. Prazosin decreases both afterload and preload: it decreases arteriolar tone, dilates the systemic venous bed, increases cardiac output, and decreases filling pressures. It has little effect on heart rate. Of these three agents, prazosin has proved easiest to use. However, tolerance is a serious handicap in many patients. Trimazosin* has been introduced as an alternative to prazosin in order to circumvent the problem of tolerance. In some instances captopril has proved more effective than other oral vasodilators.

The use of vasodilators in cardiology extends far beyond heart failure. Its acute uses range from the complications of coronary heart disease (left ventricular failure, pulmonary edema, cardiogenic shock, ventricular septal rupture, mitral regurgitation, preservation of ischemic myocardium) to acute aortic and mitral regurgitation.

Diuretics

Retention of salt and water, followed by expansion of the plasma and the interstitial tissue compartments of the extracellular fluid volume, is a hallmark of congestive heart failure and is responsible for many of its symptoms. Consequently, elimination of the excess salt and water and contraction of the extravascular fluid volume by diuresis are essential for the successful treatment of heart failure.

"DRY" WEIGHT. The use of diuretics entails two separate problems: elimination of excess fluid, and maintenance of edema-free ("dry") weight. In the hospital, where the patient is at rest and salt intake is precisely controlled, low dosages of diuretics may suffice to maintain dry weight. Out of hospital, where the patient is more active and salt intake is not so readily controlled, larger doses may be needed. However, continued use of large doses of diuretics leads to serious derangements in electrolyte balance, often predisposing to digitalis toxicity by way of hypokalemia. Consequently, once the urgent need for brisk diuresis has passed—as during an episode of acute pulmonary edema—the optimal cardiotonic program relies heavily on digitalis and salt restriction and depends on diuretics as an ancillary measure.

SALT AND WATER RESTRICTION. Restriction of sodium intake should be directed not only at sodium chloride per se but also at sodium-containing medications, e.g., antacids. Restriction of water intake is rarely necessary except after the use of potent diuretics which predispose to hyponatremia and water intoxication. In mild heart failure, sodium intake is generally restricted to less than 3 grams per day; in severe congestive heart failure, intake of less than 0.5 gram per day is often needed to promote diuresis and to reduce the blood volume and venous pressure. Overzealous sodium restriction in conjunction with potent sodium-losing diuretics, particularly in the elderly or in others with impaired renal function, may lead to weakness, oliguria, and azotemia.

THE SODIUM CONTROL SYSTEM. The major diuretics increase the rate of sodium excretion by the renal tubule. As indicated previously, the tubule is the end organ of an elaborate control system that is influenced by hemodynamic and neurohumoral mechanisms. For some mysterious reason, the control system seems to be reset in heart failure so that an expanded extracellular fluid volume, usually a stimulus to diuresis, coexists with antidiuresis. Nonetheless, despite this reset, it is possible to modify the handling of sodium by intervening at several different sites in the control system.

*Investigational drug in the United States.

Diuretics interfere with the control system by modifying the reabsorption of sodium, with its accompanying anions and water, by the end organ, the renal tubule (Fig. 42–5). Five distinct categories of diuretics are in common use (Table 42–6). Each affects tubular reabsorption somewhat differently, and each produces its own characteristic abnormalities in electrolyte pattern, hydration, and acid-base balance. These abnormalities represent the pharmacologic consequences of effective drug action. When carried to extremes, or when effects interact, they are responsible for the toxicity of these different diuretics.

THIAZIDES. Because of their effectiveness by mouth, their reliability, and their relative freedom from toxicity, the benzothiadiazine drugs are usually the diuretics of choice in cardiac edema. The prototypes of this group are chlorothiazide and hydrochlorothiazide (Table 42–7). *Acute* administration promotes the urinary excretion of sodium, chloride, and potassium without consistent change in urinary pH or bicarbonate excretion. The predominant diuretic effect (natriuresis and chloruresis) has been localized to inhibition of sodium absorption in the distal nephron (Fig. 42–5). Although there is also a carbonic anhydrase–inhibiting effect, it is generally insignificant until large daily doses are reached (of the order of 2000 mg per day). Kaliuresis depends on an increase in the quantity of sodium delivered to the distal nephron. Intravenous administration of chlorothiazide is uricosuric, whereas chronic administration results in hyperuricemia. The mechanisms responsible for the paradoxical uric acid effects are still unclear.

Hypokalemia is particularly apt to arise after intensive diuresis with thiazides or after prolonged thiazide therapy. Supplementary doses of potassium may then be required. Several generalizations have proved useful as practical guides to therapy. Acute hypokalemia that is modest in degree is managed by diet; if diet fails to correct the hypokalemia, supplementary doses of potassium may be required. Potassium chloride is generally the agent of choice for oral supplementation, because hypochloremic metabolic alkalosis usually accompanies di-

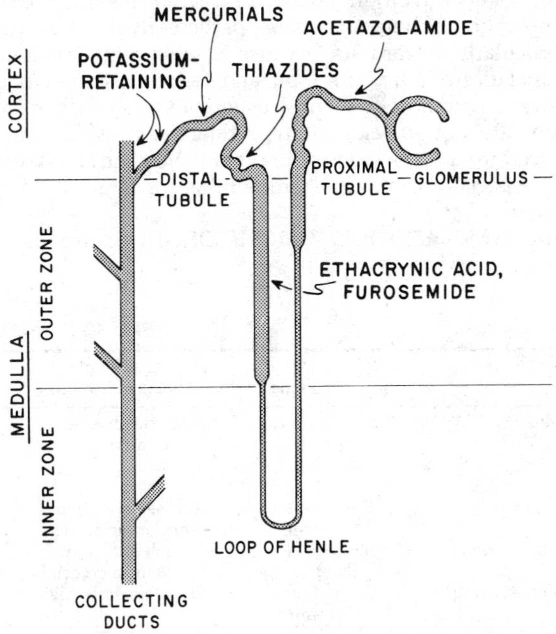

Figure 42–5. Schematic representation of a nephron, indicating predominant sites of action of the five groups of diuretics. Carbonic anhydrase inhibitors exert predominant effects on the proximal tubule. The potassium-retaining diuretics affect the distal nephron. The major diuretic effect of the thiazides is at a site of urine dilution in the cortical portion of the ascending limb of the loop of Henle. Ethacrynic acid, furosemide, and the organomercurials act chiefly on the loop of Henle, affecting both the diluting and concentrating segments to achieve potent diuretic effects.

TABLE 42–6. DIURETIC AGENTS IN HEART FAILURE

	Effect on Kidney		Effect on Electrolytes			
Type of Diuretic	*Principal Site of Action*	*Mechanism*	*In Urine*	*In Blood*	**Toxic Manifestations**	**Special Features**
Thiazides (chloruretic sulfonamides)	Ascending limb of loop of Henle; distal tubule	Interference with dilution of urine	Increased excretion of Na, Cl, K	Hypochloremic alkalosis; hypokalemia	Nausea; vomiting; skin rashes; hyperuricemia; hypercalcemia; hyperglycemia; azotemia	Loss of effectiveness and hypokalemia are common on continued administration
Ethacrynic acid*	Ascending limb of loop of Henle; distal tubule; probably proximal tubule	Interference with dilution and concentration of urine	Increased excretion of Na, Cl, HCO_3, K, H	Hypochloremic alkalosis; hypokalemia; hyponatremia	Hypotension; contraction alkalosis; hyperuricemia; hypercalcemia; azotemia; hyperglycemia; hearing loss	Causes renal vasodilatation; effective in renal insufficiency, systemic acidosis or alkalosis; potent diuresis often followed by rebound
Organo-mercurials	Proximal and/or distal tubule	Decrease of isosmotic reabsorption	Increased excretion of Na, Cl, H	Hypochloremic alkalosis	Mercury intoxication; sudden death (after IV injection); occasional agranulocytosis	Inactivated by hypochloremic alkalosis; hazardous in oliguria
Potassium-sparing†	Distal tubule	Aldosterone antagonism for Na-K exchange	Decreased excretion of K and H; slight increase in Na, Cl, HCO_3	Hyperkalemia	Generally nontoxic; GI upset; gynecomastia; rare agranulocytosis	Synergistic with thiazides and ethacrynic acid; avoid in renal insufficiency and in hyperkalemia
Carbonic anhydrase inhibitors	Proximal tubule	Inhibition of enzyme involved in acidification of urine	Increased excretion of Na, K, HCO_3; decrease in H	Hyperchloremic acidosis; hypokalemia	Generally nontoxic; mild GI and mental upsets; occasional sulfonamide idiosyncrasy	Not very potent and loses effectiveness in a few days

*Furosemide (Lasix), a nonthiazide sulfonamide, has practically the same indications and effects despite its different chemical structure.
†Spironolactone (Aldactone) operates as a competitive inhibitor of endogenous aldosterone; triamterene and amiloride are noncompetitive inhibitors and produce the characteristic effects on the urine even though aldosterone is absent.

uretic-induced hypokalemia. For severe hypokalemia, intravenous infusions are used. To prevent hypokalemia during chronic administration of potassium-losing diuretics, aldosterone inhibitors are useful.

Certain precautions merit attention. Potassium salts administered orally cause gastric irritation. This side effect is generally tolerable, especially in the hospital, where potassium chloride can be safely given in liquid form after meals. Prolonged administration of potassium salts, particularly if enteric coated, is particularly hazardous because of the high incidence of intestinal ulceration, perforation, and peritonitis, often followed by intestinal stenosis and obstruction. Excessive doses of potassium are apt to lead to hyperkalemia. This likelihood is enhanced in older persons who often have slight renal impairment, especially if an aldosterone inhibitor is given concomitantly.

ETHACRYNIC ACID AND FUROSEMIDE. These are the most potent natriuretic agents currently available. They are quite different chemically. Furosemide is a sulfonamide–anthranilic acid derivative related to the thiazide diuretics, whereas ethacrynic acid is a ketone derivative of aryloxyacetic acid (Table 42–7). Like the thiazides, they are effective orally and are rapid acting. They exert powerful diuretic effects by inhibiting both the renal diluting and concentrating mechanisms in the ascending limb of the loop of Henle (Fig. 42–5). Ethacrynic acid is without appreciable effect on carbonic anhydrase, whereas furosemide elicits modest anti–carbonic anhydrase activity. Ethacrynic acid appears to relax vascular smooth muscle by a direct effect. Although this effect could contribute importantly to unloading the failing heart, it is difficult to dissociate from the diuretic effect per se.

Ethacrynic acid, administered orally, exerts its effects in 30 minutes and continues to act for six to eight hours; administered intravenously, it acts within a few minutes, reaching its peak

TABLE 42–7. ADMINISTRATION OF DIURETICS

	Example	Relevant Chemical Structure	Preferred Route of Administration	Usual Range of Daily Dosage	Suggested Pattern of Administration
Thiazides	Chlorothiazide (Diuril)	Benzothiadiazine derivative	Oral	500 mg × 2–4	Standard type of diuretic to start treatment; few days on, few days off to avoid refractoriness and serious electrolyte disturbances
Ethacrynic acid*	Ethacrynic acid (Edecrin)	Ketone derivative of aryloxyacetic acid	Oral or IV*	50 mg × 2–3	Reserve for serious or refractory edema
Organomercurials	Mersalyl and theophylline	Theophylline plus organic mercurial	IM	2 ml	Adjunct diuretic or for moderately rapid response in hospital
Potassium-sparing†	Triamterene (Dyrenium)	Pteridine derivative	Oral	200 mg	Continuous administration in conjunction with more potent potassium-losing diuretics; do not use with potassium supplements
Carbonic anhydrase inhibitors	Acetazolamide (Diamox)	Sulfanilamide derivative	Oral	250 mg × 4–6	Episodic as booster diuretic; useful before injection of organomercurial for chloride-retaining effect

*Furosemide and ethacrynic acid may be given intravenously as well as by mouth. For ordinary use, however, furosemide is administered as a single oral dose in the morning. In an urgent situation (pulmonary edema), furosemide, as well as ethacrynic acid, may be administered intravenously (50 mg). Intravenous administration should not be done at less than six-hour intervals.
†Spironolactone (Aldactone), 75 to 100 mg per day, is commonly used as a potassium-sparing diuretic. In refractory heart failure doses of 100 to 600 mg per day have proved helpful.

activity in one hour. Both agents elicit a marked increase in urine flow containing large quantities of sodium and chloride (of the order of 20 to 30 per cent of the filtered load). Kaliuresis is appreciable. In conventional doses, neither drug consistently increases bicarbonate secretion or modifies urine pH. But chronic administration of ethacrynic acid promotes hydrogen loss in a bicarbonate-free urine, i.e., produces metabolic alkalosis.

A cardinal virtue of these agents (in contrast with thiazides and carbonic anhydrase inhibitors) is their lack of effect on filtration rate or renal plasma flow unless sodium depletion occurs. At peak effect, both agents decrease renal vascular resistance.

Ethacrynic acid and furosemide are effective despite gross electrolyte disturbances and hypoalbuminemia. If pushed, either may cause hyponatremia, volume depletion, fall in blood pressure, fall in urine volume, azotemia, and water retention. Because of the upsets in the electrolyte concentrations which they induce, other diuretics are preferred for maintenance treatment. They are most valuable in three situations: in acute pulmonary edema (25 to 50 mg intravenously), in severe or refractory heart failure, or when renal function is impaired (because they increase renal blood flow). Both agents produce "contraction alkalosis," i.e., an increase in plasma bicarbonate consequent to the decrease in extracellular fluid volume that follows excretion of a large volume of bicarbonate-poor urine. The metabolic alkalosis that follows hydrogen depletion and "contraction" predisposes to alveolar hypoventilation through its depressant effects on respiratory control mechanisms.

BUMETANIDE. This is a new "loop" diuretic similar to furosemide and ethacrynic acid in its actions. It seems to be as effective as furosemide and sometimes works when furosemide fails. The usual oral dose is 0.5 to 2.0 mg taken as a single dose, but supplements can be taken every four hours up to a total daily dose of 10 mg. Because experience with this agent is not as large as with furosemide, its safety is not as well established.

ORGANOMERCURIAL DIURETICS. Until the advent of potent oral diuretics, the organomercurials, generally a combination of an organic mercurial and theophylline, were the diuretic agents of choice in heart failure. Now they are rarely used and generally reserved for parenteral administration in hospital.

ALDOSTERONE ANTAGONISTS. A characteristic feature of chronic heart failure is high circulating levels of renin and aldosterone. Aldosterone enhances sodium reabsorption. Water follows passively. Aldosterone also increases potassium excretion. In heart failure, hyperaldosteronism causes continuing sodium retention, whereas potassium excretion remains normal, i.e., no hypokalemia.

Aldosterone antagonists interfere with these actions, causing potassium retention and sodium excretion. Three agents are available: spironolactone, triamterene, and amiloride (MK-870). Spironolactone is most popular; amiloride is not yet available for general use. Although all three act by competing for receptor sites in the distal tubule, the intimate mechanisms involved in electrolyte secretion may be different. The major site of action of spironolactone is in the distal tubule, in the region of the aldosterone-stimulated secretion of hydrogen and potassium. It is a specific competitive inhibitor of aldosterone and has no action if aldosterone is absent. It promotes natriuresis, water loss, and potassium retention by depressing aldosterone-dependent sodium-potassium exchange in the distal tubule. It is effective only in the presence of high levels of mineralocorticoid activity; it is devoid of effect after adrenalectomy. Conversely, triamterene (Table 42–7) and amiloride are noncompetitive agents that inhibit potassium and hydrogen ion excretion even if aldosterone is absent. Their mechanism of action is unclear. Although these natriuretic agents are far less potent than the thiazides, ethacrynic acid, furosemides, and the organomercurials, they have the extraordinary advantage for prolonged use of continuing effectiveness, minor electrolyte derangements, and the virtual absence of toxicity as long as hyperkalemia is avoided. These agents are unique in that, in contrast to the thiazides, ethacrynic acid, furosemide, and bumetanide, they do not lose effectiveness in a few days nor do they cause violent electrolyte upheavals.

Spironolactone is expensive but effective. Oral doses, ranging from 100 to 400 mg per day, are well tolerated for months. A few days may elapse before its action becomes apparent. It is used primarily to potentiate the effects of the more powerful diuretics, particularly if potassium depletion is a serious consideration.

CARBONIC ANHYDRASE INHIBITORS. These agents are effective by mouth. They elicit an increase in excretion of bicarbonate, sodium, and potassium and an increase in urine pH. The most striking increments are in bicarbonate and potassium. By interfering with carbonic anhydrase activity in the kidney, they inhibit hydrogen ion secretion primarily in the proximal and distal portions of the nephron, exerting lesser effects on the loop of Henle, i.e., little effect on urinary diluting or concentrating mechanisms.

The prototype of this group is acetazolamide (Table 42–7). It is a weak diuretic and loses its effectiveness as hyperchloremic metabolic acidosis develops because of diminished hydrogen ion excretion (usually in 48 hours). Like ammonium chloride, this class of diuretics is particularly valuable in patients with high serum bicarbonate, as occurs in cor pulmonale or metabolic alkalosis. They are valuable in preparing for a mercurial diuresis because of the hyperchloremic acidosis that they produce. This group also enhances natriuresis produced by thiazides, ethacrynic acid, and furosemide. A contraindication for its use is severe acidosis, as from renal failure or hepatic insufficiency.

SPECIAL DIURETICS. This is a miscellaneous group of agents that are used with extreme caution and under special conditions. For example, osmotic diuretics such as mannitol and albumin, which expand the circulating blood volume, have the potential for increasing the renal blood flow and for blocking the reabsorption of sodium and water at the proximal tubule. However, in heart failure they entail the risk of circulatory overload and pulmonary edema.

COMBINATIONS. There are two main reasons for introducing a combination of diuretics into a cardiotonic program: to avoid serious electrolyte upsets that occur if the powerful primary diuretics are administered without pause, in large dosage, for long periods; and to stimulate diuresis when the prevailing cardiotonic program no longer suffices to prevent edema. In either case, the net diuretic effect of the combination will be determined by a wide variety of influences: the respective sites of action on the renal tubule of each agent, the extent of competitive inhibition at common receptor sites, the dose-response curves of the individual drugs, strategic timing of the administration of one agent with respect to the other, and the acid-base and electrolyte balances at the time the agents are given.

A currently popular duo of diuretics is a potassium-sparing agent (triamterene or spironolactone) that is taken daily and a thiazide that is taken intermittently (e.g., for four days of each week). In time, the thiazide may be succeeded by ethacrynic acid or ethacrynic acid may be given sporadically as needed to sustain the edema-free state. On occasion, particularly in the hospital, a mercurial diuretic (after prior acidification) may prove helpful in overcoming a resistant state of edema. In contrast to the foregoing, other combinations hold little promise for success. Thus the combined use of acetazolamide and a mercurial diuretic is not apt to be effective, because, by preventing acidification of the urine, the carbonic anhydrase inhibitor is apt to block, rather than to enhance, the diuretic effect of the mercurial.

The same general principles govern the use of combinations of diuretics in the treatment of refractory edema. This troublesome state is now relatively uncommon because of the advent of powerful primary diuretics, particularly furosemide and ethacrynic acid, coupled with a better understanding of the sites of action of the auxiliary diuretics. On the other hand, refractory edema may again become tractable by reversing electrolyte and acid-base imbalances that have been produced by unremitting administration of the primary diuretics for long periods. As a working principle, resistance to diuresis is overcome by deliberate selection of agents that act on different parts of the tubule. This approach presupposes that digitalis dosage is optimal. On occasion, aminophylline, by its inotropic effect, may reinforce the diuretic action of a thiazide or ethacrynic acid. Clearly, many opportunities exist for the physician to devise original sequences and combinations of diuretics. However, a restraining influence is imposed by the complicated interplay between the diuretic agents themselves and with the deranged internal environment that generally is a feature of the refractory state.

REFRACTORY EDEMA. This is a state of edema that resists conventional cardiotonic and diuretic measures. Before embarking on an endless train of drug combinations, the physician should search carefully for a complication or an underlying disorder that has been overlooked: a surgically correctable disorder, such as mitral stenosis or constrictive pericarditis; a medical disorder, including hyperthyroidism, anemia, pulmonary emboli, bacterial endocarditis, persistent infection, and arrhythmias; inappropriate or excessive diuretic therapy that elicits serious disturbances in blood volume and electrolyte composition, digitalis toxicity, and water intoxication; physical overactivity; excessive salt intake and renal disease; sodium-containing medicaments, such as antacids, or agents such as reserpine, propranolol, and guanethidine which depress the myocardium to the point of failure.

COMPLICATIONS. A variety of disturbances may complicate effective diuretic therapy. These include hypotension and vascular collapse from rapid, massive diuresis; sodium depletion, usually the consequence of prolonged and effective diuretic therapy in conjunction with excessive water intake; hypokalemia from uninterrupted use of diuretics, predisposing to digitalis toxicity; hyperkalemia from injudicious administration of aldosterone antagonists and potassium supplements; metabolic alkalosis, either from a massive excretion of a bicarbonate-poor urine or from a combination of increased hydrogen ion excretion in the urine and alveolar hypoventilation as produced by ethacrynic acid or potassium depletion; and hyperuricemia after prolonged administration of small doses of the thiazides, ethacrynic acid, and furosemide, which share an inhibiting effect on uric acid excretion. In predisposed individuals, the hyperuricemia of prolonged diuretic therapy may precipitate an episode of gout. The thiazides, and occasionally furosemide, may precipitate diabetes which is rarely severe.

GENERAL COMMENTS. In treating heart failure, rarely is there a desperate need to restore everything to normal at once by vigorous diuresis. The temptation to restore the patient immediately to dry weight and to free him of breathlessness and congestion must be tempered by the penalty of dehydration and severe electrolyte disturbances. The more leisurely the diuretic therapy, the more durable and tolerable the relief.

The ability of potent diuretics to elicit dramatic diuresis has led to their abuse. Thus without direct inotropic effect on the heart, a single injection of ethacrynic acid can effect a decrease in blood volume, a decrease in intracardiac filling pressures, an increase in cardiac output, and clear edema. But ethacrynic acid is rarely advisable as the mainstay of therapy unless edema is refractory and less drastic measures have proved ineffective. Only when coupled with a full cardiotonic program can judicious control of heart failure be maintained, particularly if the underlying heart disease is progressive and severe complications of diuretic therapy are to be avoided.

SURGICAL THERAPY OF REFRACTORY HEART FAILURE. Attempts are under way in several medical centers to provide temporary respite for the heart in acute refractory failure that is judged to be reversible, e.g., after myocardial infarction. The common feature of the different approaches is to unload the heart for hours to days while it is recuperating. The most popular devices are (1) venoarterial bypass, which assists the heart by diverting blood to a pump that returns it to the arterial tree, and (2) counterpulsation, which operates in synchrony with the heartbeat to adjust the aortic blood pressure by rhythmically changing either the volume of blood in the aorta (using an external pump) or the capacity of the aorta (using an internal balloon). All methods aim to reduce the external work of the heart and the tension that it develops during systole and to decrease myocardial oxygen consumption at the same time as coronary arterial perfusion is improved. Technical problems have restricted the use of these appliances in man to biding time in desperate situations, e.g., in cardiogenic shock. As yet, there are very few long-term survivors.

Cardiac replacement and the development of an artificial heart to assist or replace the failing heart are also being pursued as last measures for refractory heart failure. Experience with cardiac replacement began more than ten years ago. Since then, results have improved considerably. Morbidity, particularly during the first few months after replacement, is high. Those who survive the first three months have a survival rate of up to 80 per cent at one year; thereafter, the number of survivors decreases at a rate of about 5 per cent per year. Many practical problems handicap the wider use of cardiac transplantation. These range from limited donor supply, continuing threat of rejection of the graft, and infection in the immunosuppressed host, to the high cost of the procedure and the difficulty in obtaining reimbursement from insurance companies.

The artificial heart program currently has the greatest promise as an assist device for the left ventricle. This modality is still experimental, has no long-term survivors, and is handicapped by incompatibilities between blood and artificial materials that compose the synthetic heart.

Fishman AP (ed.): Heart Failure. Washington, DC, Hemisphere, 1978. *An up-to-date account of current interests in heart failure. Particular emphasis is placed on pathophysiology.*

Kramer BL, Massie BM, Topic N: Controlled trial of captopril in chronic heart failure: A rest and exercise hemodynamic study. Circulation 67:807–816, 1983. *Captopril administered to 16 ambulatory patients in chronic heart failure who were stable on digoxin and diuretics proved to be an effective adjunctive agent for long-term therapy. The next three papers in the same issue, dealing with isosorbide dinitrate and two new agents (MDL 17,043 and propylbutyldopamine), suggest that this capability may not be unique for captopril.*

LeJemtel TH, Keung E, Ribner HS, Matsumoto M, Davis R, Schwartz W, Alousi AA, Davolos DD, Sonnenblick EH: Amrinone: A new non-glycoside, non-adrenergic cardiotonic agent effective in the treatment of intractable myocardial failure in man. Circulation 59:1098, 1979. *A useful introduction to a new inotropic agent that is currently generating a great deal of interest as an alternative to digitalis glycosides.*

Massie B, Ports T, Chatterjee K, Parmley W, Ostland J, O'Young J, Haughom F: Long-term vasodilator therapy for heart failure: Clinical response and its relationship to hemodynamic measurements. Circulation 63:269–278, 1981. *Effects of chronic vasodilator therapy for refractory congestive heart failure in 56 patients treated with hydralazine, usually in combination with long-acting nitrates, for 3 to 30 months (mean of 13 months). Many improved clinically, and early hemodynamic measurements correlated well in predicting the outcome of therapy.*

Walsh WF, Greenberg BH: Results of long-term vasodilator therapy in patients with refractory heart failure. Circulation 64:499–505, 1981. *Compare with paper by Massie et al. (see above) for perspective. Effects of chronic vasodilator therapy for refractory heart failure in 34 patients with hydralazine and long-acting nitrates. Emphasizes that about one half of patients with refractory congestive heart failure either do not improve on chronic vasodilator therapy or discontinue it because of side effects. Of those who continue therapy (about half of those started), half have sustained clinical benefit (about one fourth of those started). The prognosis for patients in refractory heart failure remains poor whether maintained on vasodilators or on more conventional therapy alone. Early hemodynamic improvement after vasodilator (hydralazine) is not necessarily predictive of long-term clinical improvement.*

Weber KT, Janicki JS, Fishman AP: Respiratory gas exchange during exercise in the noninvasive evaluation of the severity of chronic cardiac failure. *In* Braunwald E, Mock MB, Watson JT (eds.): Congestive Heart Failure: Current Research and Clinical Applications. New York, Grune & Stratton, 1982, pp 221–235. *Noninvasive monitoring of external gas exchange during graded exercise and determination of maximum oxygen uptake is useful for the objective assessment of the severity of heart failure and the effectiveness of cardiovascular agents used in therapy.*

Weber KT, Kinasewitz GT, Janicki JS, Fishman AP: Oxygen utilization and ventilation during exercise in patients with chronic cardiac failure. Circulation 65:1213–1223, 1982. *Exercise intolerance in chronic congestive heart failure is due primarily to inadequate oxygen transport to the working muscles. This conclusion is supported by progressive increases in blood lactate concentration and oxygen extraction during submaximal and maximal exercise (plateau in oxygen uptake).*

43. SHOCK

*François M. Abboud**

Shock is a complex clinical syndrome that demands vigilant medical attention, careful hemodynamic monitoring, and thorough understanding of the basic principles of circulatory control and of the pharmacology of cardiac and vasoactive drugs. This chapter covers the basic principles of *circulatory control* as they relate to the shock syndrome, the *cellular mechanisms* involved in the pathogenesis of shock, and the *therapy* of shock.

DEFINITION. The common denominator in shock, regardless of cause, is a failure of the circulatory system to deliver the chemical substances necessary for cellular survival and to remove the waste products of cellular metabolism. This leads to cellular membrane dysfunction, abnormal cellular metabolism, and eventually cellular death.

CAUSES. Table 43–1 lists the most common clinical situations associated with decreased cardiac output, hypotension, decreased tissue perfusion, capillary endothelial injury, and cellular damage.

TABLE 43–1. CAUSES OF SHOCK AND INITIATING MECHANISMS

I. **Decreased intravascular volume**
  A. Acute hemorrhage (e.g., gastrointestinal bleeding, retroperitoneal bleeding, ruptured aortic aneurysm, hemoptysis, hemothorax, trauma)
  B. Excessive fluid loss
    1. Vomiting (intestinal or pyloric obstruction)
    2. Severe diarrhea, sweating, and dehydration
    3. Excessive urine (e.g., diabetes mellitus, diabetes insipidus, excessive diuretics, diuretic phase of acute renal failure)
    4. Peritonitis, pancreatitis, splanchnic ischemia, intestinal obstruction, and gangrene
    5. Trauma and extensive muscle injury
    6. Burns
  C. Vasodilatation (relative hypovolemia)
    1. Neurogenic: drug induced (e.g., anesthesia, ganglionic and adrenergic blockers, overdoses such as barbiturates, poisons); nervous system damage (e.g., spinal cord injury, cerebral vascular accident, severe dysautonomia)
    2. Metabolic, toxic, or humoral vasodilatation: septicemia (gram-negative endotoxemia or gram-positive bacteremia); acute adrenal insufficiency, anaphylactic reaction

II. **Cardiac**
  A. Acute myocardial infarction
  B. Myocarditis, myocardial depression (hypoxia, acidosis, septic shock, myocardial depressant factors [MDF], drugs, hypoglycemia), severe low output failure
  C. Acute valvular insufficiency, myocardial rupture, septal perforation
  D. Arrhythmias: severe bradycardia, tachycardia, and fibrillation
  E. Mechanical compression or obstruction
    1. Pericardial effusion or tamponade
    2. Positive pressure ventilation, tension pneumothorax
    3. Pulmonary embolism
    4. Ball-valve thrombus or atrial myxoma

III. **Microcirculatory endothelial injury and aggregation of corpuscles**
  A. Anaphylaxis
  B. Disseminated intravascular coagulation
  C. Burns, septic shock, trauma

IV. **Cellular membrane injury**
  A. Septic shock
  B. Anaphylaxis
  C. Ischemia, prolonged hypoxia, pancreatitis, tissue injury

CLINICAL PICTURE. The classic clinical presentation is one of a patient who is hypotensive (with a systolic blood pressure of 90 mm Hg or less); is hyperventilating; has cold, clammy, cyanotic skin; has a tachycardia with a thready pulse; and has a dulled sensorium ranging from agitation to stupor or coma. The patient is frequently oliguric, with a urinary output of less than 20 ml per hour.

This clinical picture may not always be present, and it is the recognition of the subtle or early presentation of shock that may be crucial. Although a patient may have a "normal" blood pressure (i.e., 110/70), this may actually represent "relative hypotension" if the patient has a history of hypertension. Early shock may be indicated only by unexplained agitation or tachycardia in the absence of cardiovascular collapse. Some patients with septic shock may initially present with warm hyperperfused extremities (so-called warm shock) due to abnormal peripheral vasodilatation.

Frequently, the physical findings follow a progressive pattern as shock evolves from the early compensated phase to the advanced stages (Table 43–2). This basic clinical picture is present in addition to the signs and symptoms of the underlying precipitating disease, e.g., severe chest pain of acute myocardial infarction or dissecting aneurysm, visible bleeding, burn, peritonitis, sepsis, or trauma.

PATHOPHYSIOLOGY AND STAGES OF SHOCK. The basic elements in the pathogenesis of shock as they relate to the stages of the syndrome and the types of shock are portrayed in Figure 43–1.

Stage I: Compensated. Hypotension may be caused either by a fall in cardiac output or by vasodilatation. The fall in cardiac output and hypotension trigger effective compensatory mechanisms, which restore arterial pressure and blood flow to the more vital organs such as brain and heart. Symptoms and signs are minimal, and appropriate intervention is most effective.

Stage II: Decompensated. Here the compensatory mechanisms to maintain perfusion of vital organs are maximal but insufficient. The evidence of decreased cerebral perfusion may be apparent from the mental state of the patient; decreased renal perfusion may reduce urinary output, and patients with coronary artery disease may begin to suffer from myocardial ischemia. The external appearance of the patient also reflects excessive sympathetic discharge, with cyanosis, coldness, and clamminess of the skin. The majority of patients are seen in this phase, and rapid aggressive intervention to restore cardiac output and perfusion of the tissues may reverse the shock syndrome.

Stage III: Irreversible. Excessive and prolonged reduction of tissue perfusion leads to significant alterations in cellular membrane function, aggregation of blood corpuscles, and "sludging" in the capillaries. The vasoconstriction which has taken place in the less vital organs in order to maintain blood pressure is now excessive and has reduced flow to such an extent that cellular damage occurs.

Arterial pressure continues to fall progressively to a critical level at which the perfusion of vital organs is reduced. Critical impairment of renal perfusion leads to acute tubular necrosis. Ischemia of the gastrointestinal tract leads to necrotic damage of the mucosa and absorption into the circulation of bacteria and toxic bacterial products, which have detrimental effects on other organs and may lead to generalized endothelial damage with disseminated intravascular coagulation. Bacterial toxins react with neutrophils and cause the release of vasodilator polypeptides, which contribute to the fall in arterial pressure. The severe acidosis resulting from anaerobic metabolism also contributes to vasodilatation. The decreased perfusion pressure of the coronary vessels, particularly in patients with coronary disease, results in reduction of myocardial perfusion, which in turn decreases myocardial contractility and creates a vicious

TABLE 43–2. CLINICAL FINDINGS AT VARIOUS STAGES OF SHOCK

Stages	I Compensated*	II Decompensated	III Irreversible
Arterial blood pressure	N or ↓	↓	↓↓
Heart rate	↑	↑↑	↑↑ → ↓↓
Pulse pressure	↓	↓↓	↓↓
Cardiac output	↓	↓↓	↓↓↓
Respiratory rate	N	↑	↑↑ → ↓↓
Mental status	Anxiety	Obtunded	Coma
Urinary output	N or ↓	↓↓	Anuria
Skin	Cool	Mottled	Cold, cyanotic

*N = no change

*The author acknowledges the assistance of David W. Ferguson in the revision of this chapter.

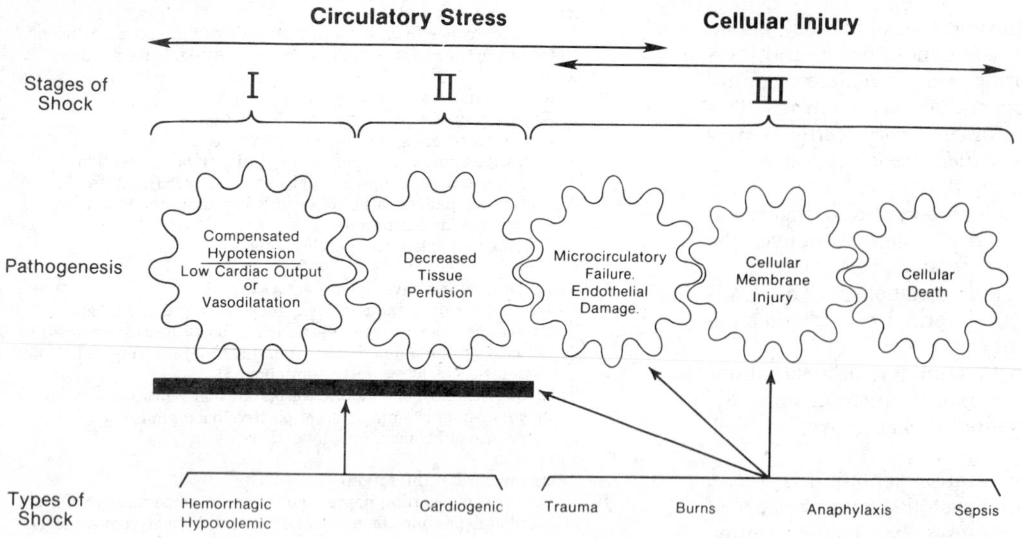

Figure 43–1. Pathophysiology of shock.

circle as the decreased contractility causes further decrements in arterial blood pressure. Similarly, reduction in perfusion pressure and ischemia of the central nervous system impair reflex neurogenic circulatory adjustments which help in maintaining arterial pressure. Damage to the capillary endothelium leads to loss of fluid and proteins through the capillaries, with exacerbation of hypovolemia and hypotension. Damage to cellular membranes from ischemia leads to the leak of lysosomal enzymes and intracellular ions, to the progressive reduction in high energy phosphate reserves, and to cellular destruction.

CIRCULATORY CONTROL IN SHOCK

Major Determinants of Tissue Perfusion

The major determinants of hemodynamics and tissue perfusion are listed in Table 43–3. The perfusion of any organ depends upon the systemic arterial pressure (which is the driving force for blood to flow through all organs), the resistance offered by the vasculature of that organ, and the patency of nutritional capillaries. Systemic arterial pressure is in turn determined by cardiac output and the resistance of the total vascular tree. Vascular resistance is predominantly a function of the radius or caliber of blood vessels. Vascular caliber is influenced by neurogenic, humoral, and myogenic factors that regulate the tone of vascular smooth muscle. Thus blood flow to any one organ depends on cardiac function and on vascular muscle tone and caliber in all the arterial tree as well as in the organ itself. The determinant of exchange of substrates and metabolites with the tissues is the microcirculation. A patent nutritional capillary network is the critical interface between the circulation and the cell.

This discussion deals with cardiac, vascular, and microcirculatory factors.

CARDIAC FACTORS. Cardiac output is the product of heart rate and stroke volume. A rate of 70 beats per minute and a stroke volume of 70 ml per beat give a cardiac output of approximately 5 liters per minute, an amount more than sufficient to deliver 250 ml of oxygen per minute to all the tissues. This consumption of oxygen reflects metabolic needs at rest. A drop in cardiac output below 2 liters per minute per square meter is an indication of severe shock.

Heart Rate. Tachycardia usually increases cardiac output, but a marked increase in heart rate may limit cardiac diastolic filling time and result in a low cardiac output and arterial blood pressure. For example, ventricular tachycardia or rapid atrial fibrillation in a patient with recent myocardial infarction causes a reduction in cardiac output and arterial pressure which, if uncorrected, could result in cardiogenic shock. Immediate treatment to restore heart rate is essential. In considering the treatment of tachycardia in shock, one has to be cautious in avoiding treatment of a "compensatory tachycardia" often seen in patients with fever, anemia, sepsis, hemorrhage, or severe hypovolemia. Tachycardia is often an appropriate reflex circulatory adjustment to maintain cardiac output.

Extreme bradycardia may also cause a low output and hypotension. Sinus bradycardia and atrioventricular block are often seen immediately following myocardial infarction and should be reversed if they contribute to hypotension. Severe bradycardia is also seen in the "common faint" syndrome or vasovagal syncope; the patient usually falls to the horizontal position and recovers spontaneously.

Stroke Volume. A decrease in stroke volume may be caused by (1) a decrease in cardiac filling, (2) a decrease in myocardial contractility, or (3) an increased afterload (Fig. 43–2).

DECREASE IN CARDIAC FILLING PRESSURE. The amount of blood filling the ventricles at the end of diastole is the "preload" and it regulates the subsequent contraction and stroke volume (Starling's law of the heart). Although there are many factors that determine filling pressure, such as the rate and duration of filling, ventricular compliance, and venous tone, a most important determinant is total blood volume. Reduction in blood volume may be either absolute or relative to the capacity of the vascular tree. Absolute reductions in blood volume are apparent when blood or fluids are lost, causing a hypovolemic state leading to hypovolemic shock. This is seen in hemorrhage (either external or internal bleeding), excessive vomiting, diarrhea, burns, renal loss of fluids such as in diabetes mellitus or diabetes insipidus, excessive diuresis, and excessive perspiration without fluid replacement. Internal losses of fluid occur in peritonitis, intestinal obstruction with extravasation of fluid, splanchnic ischemia with bowel necrosis and gangrene, fractures with extensive muscle trauma, hemothorax, and hemoperitoneum.

Relative decreases in blood volume occur when there is loss of vascular tone because of the administration of anesthetics or ganglion blockers, after spinal cord injury, and in patients with neuropathy or autonomic insufficiency. Pooling of blood thus results in a decrease in filling pressure. Compression of the heart may also prevent its filling, as is seen during pericardial tamponade, in tension pneumothorax, or in the superior vena caval syndrome. Mechanical obstruction to blood flow may cause hypotension and shock in patients with atrial myxoma, a ball-valve thrombus, or pulmonary embolism.

DECREASE IN MYOCARDIAL CONTRACTILITY. Reduced contractility of the heart (negative inotropic effect) is the primary cause of shock after myocardial infarction, and it is a complicating factor in the late phases of any shock. There are many factors that contribute to it.

TABLE 43–3. MAJOR DETERMINANTS OF HEMODYNAMICS AND TISSUE PERFUSION

I. Systemic arterial pressure
- A. Total vascular resistance
  - 1. Total arteriolar resistance, vascular muscle tone
    - a. Tissue metabolism
    - b. Neurohumoral factors, toxins
  - 2. Viscosity of blood
- B. Cardiac output
  - 1. Heart rate
  - 2. Stroke volume
    - a. Cardiac filling pressure (preload)
      - i. Venous (vascular) tone
      - ii. Blood volume (total and central)
        - Capillary hydrostatic pressure: post-precapillary resistance
        - Capillary permeability
        - Oncotic pressure, plasma proteins
      - iii. Posture
      - iv. Atrial contraction
      - v. Diastolic filling time (heart rate)
      - vi. Mechanical obstruction (e.g., pericardial tamponade, pulmonary embolus)
    - b. Myocardial contractility
      - i. Arterial blood pH, Po_2
      - ii. Myocardial O_2 supply:
        - Increase supply:
          - ↑ Diastolic arterial pressure (norepinephrine, dopamine)
          - Capillary diffusion
          - Coronary dilatation (nitroglycerin, dopamine, metabolites)
        - Decrease supply:
          - ↓ Diastolic arterial pressure (isoproterenol, vasodilators)
          - Coronary artery disease, myocardial infarction
          - Hypoxia, anemia
      - iii. Myocardial O_2 demand
        - Increase demand:
          - ↑ Cardiac size (pulmonary wedge pressure)
          - ↑ Afterload (systolic arterial pressure, impedance)
          - ↑ Contractility (norepinephrine, dopamine, isoproterenol) and heart rate
        - Decrease demand:
          - ↓ Cardiac size
            - { Digitalis, ↑ ejection fraction
            - Venodilatation (nitroprusside, nitroglycerin, phentolamine)
            - Diuretics }
          - ↓ Afterload, impedance (vasodilators)
          - ↓ Contractility and heart rate
      - iv. Humoral factors
        - Catecholamines
        - Myocardial depressant factors
      - v. Drugs
        - Increase norepinephrine, dopamine, isoproterenol, digitalis
        - Decrease propranolol, anesthetics
    - c. Afterload
      - i. Arterial blood pressure, vascular impedance
      - ii. End-diastolic cardiac wall tension
      - iii. Severe aortic stenosis

II. Organ vascular resistance
- A. Occlusive arterial disease
- B. Local arteriolar resistance
- C. Local venular resistance
- D. Viscosity of blood

III. Patency of nutritional capillaries
- A. Precapillary sphincter tone
- B. Intracapillary aggregation of corpuscles
- C. Capillary endothelial integrity

Hypoxia. Hypoxia resulting from ventilation-perfusion abnormalities of the lung occurs in shock and has several effects on the circulation. A direct, vascular effect causes vasodilatation in organs such as the heart and brain. Hypoxia also activates chemoreceptors, causing a sympathetic vasoconstrictor response in vessels of skeletal muscle, skin, and the splanchnic bed, thus permitting the redistribution of blood to the vital organs with higher oxygen demand. When the central nervous system is hypoxic and ischemic, a significant sympathetic discharge also takes place. Despite these and other compensatory adjustments, myocardial performance is impaired in the presence of decreased arterial Po_2. The severity of arterial hypoxia is often a reflection of the extent of myocardial damage following myocardial infarction. It is an important, potentially reversible cause of depression of myocardial contractility.

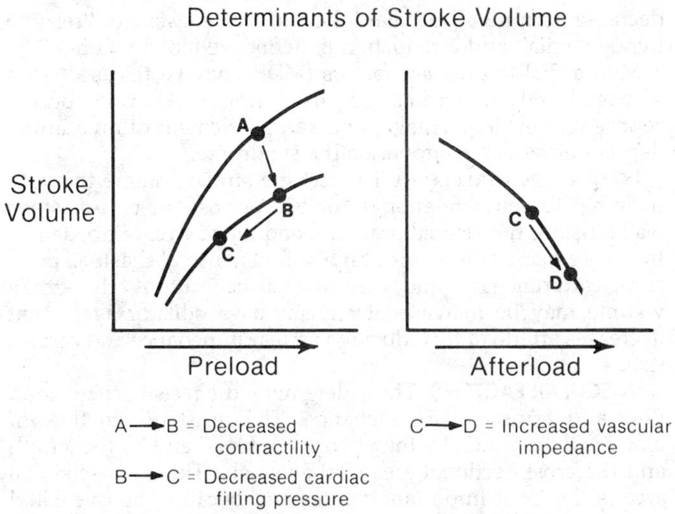

Figure 43–2. Determinants of stroke volume.

Acidosis. Acidosis results from anaerobic metabolism with release of lactate, from decreased renal perfusion with accumulation of organic acids, and possibly from hypoventilation of certain pulmonary segments, leading to respiratory acidosis. Acidosis reduces myocardial contractility and the vasoconstrictor response to various neurohumoral factors.

Myocardial Ischemia and Perfusion Pressure. Myocardial performance depends on perfusion of the ischemic myocardium, which is determined to a great extent by the level of arterial diastolic pressure. The fall in arterial pressure during hemorrhagic or hypovolemic shock in patients with coronary artery disease may complicate the syndrome by causing myocardial ischemia. Restoration of arterial pressure is critical to preservation of myocardial function. In the presence of coronary artery disease, the resistance to flow is due largely to structural changes in the vessel wall, and the degree of vasomotor tone is minimal because of excessive accumulation of vasodilator metabolites downstream from the site of coronary narrowing and in the region of ischemia. Thus arterial pressure becomes the determinant of perfusion of the ischemic segment through collateral vessels or across a narrowing or a plaque.

Increased Myocardial Oxygen Demand Relative to Supply. Although oxygen supply to the ischemic myocardium is increased by increasing arterial pressure, hypertension is detrimental, as it increases myocardial work and oxygen demand. Conversely, hypotension decreases myocardial work and oxygen needs, but it also reduces myocardial perfusion as mentioned above. Judicious restoration of arterial pressure is necessary.

Increased cardiac size is associated with greater myocardial oxygen consumption as myocardial wall tension increases. Reductions in preload, cardiac size, and oxygen demand may be achieved with appropriate venodilator and diuretic therapy. Drugs such as isoproterenol might increase myocardial oxygen demand out of proportion to the associated increase in coronary flow and would have a detrimental effect. Conversely, propranolol decreases myocardial oxygen demand and could be protective, but its myocardial depressant action in patients with cardiogenic shock would be a hazardous complication.

Other Factors That Depress Contractility. Drugs may depress cardiac output by a direct effect on the myocardium such as might occur with the barbiturates or, more frequently, by suppression of the adrenergic drive to the myocardium by such agents as propranolol, ganglion-blocking drugs, catecholamine depleters such as reserpine or guanethidine, or high spinal anesthetics, or by such conditions as spinal cord injury or an intracranial lesion involving the medullary centers. These interventions not only depress myocardial contraction but also decrease peripheral vascular tone and create a state of "relative hypovolemia" and a reduction in "effective blood volume."

Myocardial depressant factors (MDF) may be released from damaged cells in various organs during shock from burns, septicemia, or hemorrhage, and add an element of myocardial depression which compounds the syndrome.

INCREASE IN AFTERLOAD. To eject the stroke volume the ventricle has to generate enough force to oppose the end-diastolic wall tension, the arterial pressure, and the vascular impedance. In severe heart failure with high ventricular end-diastolic pressure, cardiomegaly, and very low cardiac output, the stroke volume may be increased by giving a vasodilator agent that decreases afterload by reducing vascular impedance and cardiac size.

VASCULAR FACTORS. These determine the resistance to blood flow and transcapillary exchange. The resistance to flow of blood is determined by the viscosity of blood and by the length and the cross-sectional area of the vessels. The cross-sectional area is the most important component, because the calculated resistance is inversely proportional to the fourth power of the radius of the vessels. The radius is in turn determined by the tone of vascular smooth muscle in the wall of the vessels. The vascular smooth muscle tone is modulated by neurogenic influences mediated primarily through the sympathoadrenal system and by circulating humoral and local metabolic factors.

Neurogenic Control. The sympathoadrenal discharge to the circulatory system is regulated by medullary neurons in the vasomotor center. The activity of these neurons is modulated by afferent neural impulses originating in various receptors located in strategic areas around the body. Important among these receptors are the arterial and cardiac baroreceptors, the chemoreceptors, the somatic receptors in skeletal muscle, and the thermal receptors. Activity originating in various parts of the central nervous system (cerebellum, fastigial and vestibular nuclei, and hypothalamus) also impinges upon the vasomotor center to modulate its output. Activation of cardiac sensory afferent receptors, particularly those in the left ventricle during stretch of the myocardium, inhibits sympathoadrenal activity. The severe bradycardia and hypotension often seen following myocardial infarction, especially inferior wall infarction, can be ascribed to dyskinesis of the infarcted ventricle. Conversely, reduction in the stretch of these ventricular receptors during hypovolemia and hemorrhage releases the sympathoadrenal efferent activity to cause reflex tachycardia and vasoconstriction, to restore arterial blood pressure, and to release renin. The arterial baroreceptors, activated by a rise in blood pressure, suppress sympathoadrenal tone; conversely, during hypotension they increase sympathoadrenal drive and restore arterial pressure.

Severe hypoxia, often associated with shock from any cause, activates the chemoreceptor reflex and causes an increase in sympathoadrenal drive. The reduction of central or cardiopulmonary blood volume and arterial pressure during hemorrhage activates the cardiopulmonary reflex and the arterial baroreceptor reflex simultaneously, and the two reflexes are synergistic with respect to the final sympathetic efferent activity. Similarly, the combined activation of the arterial baroreceptor reflex by hypotension and the chemoreceptor reflex by hypoxia results in a significant synergistic effect on the ventilatory response as well as the circulatory sympathetic drive.

On the other hand, there may be situations in which the reflex responses have opposite effects. This may occur, for example, when cardiac receptors are activated following acute myocardial infarction by the dyskinetic bulge of the left ventricle, while the arterial baroreceptors are unloaded because of hypotension. In the experimental preparation the inhibitory influence of the bulging left ventricular wall on the sympathetic outflow predominates and overrides the arterial baroreflex, preventing vasoconstriction and thus causing a decrease in the afterload of the damaged left ventricle. Teleologically, this effect may be beneficial, as it will tend to decrease left ventricular work following its acute insult.

There have been few studies of the effects of endotoxin on neurocirculatory reflexes. An increase in baroreceptor activity for any level of arterial blood pressure has been reported in endotoxemia, a situation which would tend to inhibit sympathoadrenal tone, and might explain in part, if confirmed, the decreased vascular resistance often seen in septic shock.

Humoral Factors. The release of hormones such as renin, vasopressin, steroids, prostaglandins, and kinins is partly mediated through the sympathoadrenal system and cardiovascular mechanoreceptors and partly through direct and indirect cellular effects of toxins, ischemia, and antigens in various organs. These hormones have direct cardiovascular and renal effects and indirect effects on central or peripheral adrenergic transmission.

RENIN-ANGIOTENSIN. A fall in arterial blood pressure or an increase in sympathoadrenal sympathetic discharge to the kidney causes the release of renin. The resulting formation of angiotensin causes peripheral vasoconstriction, maintains arterial pressure, stimulates the release of aldosterone to retain sodium and water, and has an intrarenal effect on tubular sodium reabsorption which also permits greater sodium and water retention and preserves blood volume during hypotensive states.

VASOPRESSIN. This important constrictor hormone is released from the posterior pituitary primarily in response to changes in osmolality, and may also play a role in the circulatory control in shock. Its release may be significantly reduced by stretch of the left atrial receptors during hypervolemia or by stretch of the arterial baroreceptor during hypertension; conversely, during hemorrhage and systemic hypotension, or when patients are on cardiopulmonary bypass, the blood levels of vasopressin increase significantly. Recent observations suggest that thirst and the release of vasopressin may be induced by a central nervous system action of angiotensin.

KININS. A variety of potent vasodilator polypeptides are formed by the action of certain proteolytic enzymes on plasma protein precursors. The substance bradykinin serves as the prototype for this class of endogenous peptides. Their major physiologic role may be the local regulation of blood flow and function of such organs as the salivary gland, pancreas, and kidney. In pathophysiologic states, kinins are believed to play a part in the hyperemia associated with inflammation and as vasodilators in hypotension produced by anaphylactic reactions and anaphylactic shock. Renal kinins may cause diuresis and natriuresis.

SEROTONIN AND HISTAMINE. Serotonin released from platelets and histamine released from mast cells during anaphylaxis or during complement activation in shock may play an important role in regulating local vascular tone and capillary permeability.

PROSTACYCLIN AND THROMBOXANE A_2. Prostaglandins may be released in various organs during periods of ischemia and may contribute to the reactive hyperemia and vasodilatation. The prostaglandin endoperoxides formed in platelets and in blood vessels are pivotal in the synthesis of two potent substances with opposing effects on the formation of thrombi. Prostacyclin, a powerful vasodilator and inhibitor of platelet aggregation, is synthesized in the vascular wall, mostly in the endothelial layers, from endoperoxides. In the platelets, however, endoperoxides are converted to thromboxane A_2, which causes vasoconstriction and platelet aggregation. In shock, damage to endothelial cells may inhibit synthesis of prostacyclin; in addition, platelets may release thromboxane A_2, causing intravascular platelet aggregation, clumping, and vasoconstriction.

ENDORPHINS. The endogenous opiate β-endorphin and pituitary adrenocorticotropin are stored in the pituitary gland and secreted concomitantly under stress. Recent preliminary studies in endotoxin (*E. coli*) shock in rats and dogs and in hemorrhagic shock indicate that the administration of a specific opiate antagonist, naloxone, rapidly reversed the hypotension primarily through a positive inotropic effect on the heart. The site of primary action of naloxone is not known, since there are opiate receptors in the central nervous system which could modulate autonomic control of cardiovascular function as well as in the gastrointestinal tract, adrenals, kidney, and heart. Naloxone has minimal cardiovascular effects in the absence of shock. It seems possible, since endotoxins release ACTH from the pituitary (probably through activation of hypothalamic releasing factors), that β-endorphins also are released and contribute directly or indirectly to myocardial depression in shock. The beneficial effect of synthetic steroids in experimental shock and the sensitivity of adrenalectomized animals to shock may be caused in part by suppression or release of β-endorphins, respectively.

Local Autoregulatory Adjustment of Blood Vessels. Blood vessels have an intrinsic ability to regulate vascular tone and thereby maintain blood flow to the organ over a wide range of perfusion pressures. This property is referred to as the autoregulatory capacity for blood flow and is independent of systemic neurogenic influences or humoral factors. Different vascular beds vary with respect to their ability to maintain blood flow. The cerebral, coronary, and renal circulations are most potent. Thus during a fall in arterial pressure, vasodilatation of the cerebral, coronary, and renal vasculatures maintains blood flow and oxygen delivery to the brain and heart as well as sodium and water balance. Although a myogenic response intrinsic to the smooth muscle may explain the phenomenon, accumulation of tissue metabolites following a transient period of ischemia may also cause vasodilatation and restore blood flow. The specific mediator of metabolic vasodilatation is not known, but it is likely that a combination of changes in oxygen, carbon dioxide, hydrogen ion, and other cations, in osmolality, in the amount of adenosine compounds, and in Krebs cycle intermediates and other metabolites released in the immediate environment of blood vessels contributes to adjustments in vascular tone.

MICROCIRCULATION AND TRANSCAPILLARY EXCHANGE. Perhaps the most critical aspect of the pathogenesis of the shock syndrome takes place at the level of the microcirculation. The delivery of a significant amount of blood to an organ does not ascertain that all the segments of that organ and all capillaries are perfused appropriately.

Intraorgan Blood Flow Distribution. Adequate tissue perfusion depends on blood flow through vascular channels in which diffusion between the blood and tissues can occur. These are referred to as nutritional capillaries, as contrasted with nonnutritional vessels that do not permit capillary exchange. The latter are also referred to as arteriovenous shunts, although there may be little anatomic evidence for the existence of such shunts. An example of the importance of the intraorgan redistribution of blood flow is observed in myocardial infarction, in which an increase in coronary blood flow may not increase perfusion to the infarcted segment. Under some circumstances a coronary vasodilator might redistribute flow away from the ischemic into the nonischemic regions.

Similarly, intraorgan blood flow distribution may be critical in the kidney. Acute tubular necrosis associated with shock may reflect a reduction in glomerular filtration in the outer cortex because of a localized increase in vascular resistance in this region and a selective reduction in blood flow. Interventions that alter total renal blood flow can produce significant redistribution of flow within the kidney; for example, renal vasoconstriction following adrenergic discharge tends to shunt blood away from the outer cortex, whereas renal vasodilators such as furosemide shunt blood toward the outer cortical nephrons.

Pre- and Postcapillary Resistance. The *precapillary sphincters* regulate the patency of nutritional or "exchange" capillaries. The tone of those sphincters may be modulated by neurohumoral factors which contribute to the circulatory adjustments in shock. The metabolic products at the local tissue level are important determinants of the patency of these sphincters, which regulate the total capillary surface area and in turn determine the intravascular-extracellular fluid and solute exchange. The capillary hydrostatic force driving fluid out of the capillaries into the extracellular space is dependent on the ratio of the post- to the precapillary resistances. In hypovolemic or hemorrhagic shock, the fall in arterial pressure causes activation of the sympathoadrenal system, constriction of the precapillary resistance vessels, and a fall in capillary hydrostatic pressure, facilitating the movement of fluids from the extracellular into the intravascular space. This partially restores intravascular volume. Hematocrit and viscosity of blood and plasma oncotic pressure fall. The decline in plasma oncotic pressure may be partially corrected by rapid synthesis of new proteins; but as the hypotension persists and ischemia is prolonged, the vasoconstrictor response of the precapillary resistance vessels becomes less pronounced because of tissue acidosis but the resistance of *postcapillary* vessels (venules) increases, a situation in which more fluid is lost from the vascular to the interstitial space. Thus, *venular resistance* and the reactivity of venules to the various vasoactive agents involved in the shock syndrome become important. The venules may even be *relatively* more reactive than the precapillary resistance vessels to catecholamines which activate constrictor alpha receptors. This differential effect in favor of postcapillary vasoconstriction also increases further hydrostatic pressure and intravascular fluid loss. The administration of alpha blockers in this situation might reverse this detrimental imbalance between post- and precapillary resistance. The ratio of post- to precapillary resistance and the consequent hydrostatic pressure may vary significantly from organ to organ as well as during the various stages of shock, and it is difficult to propose a specific uniform course of management directed at a reversal of that particular state, although one might consider the administration of a venodilating drug in late stages of shock, in which the failure of the microcirculation is a predominant factor.

Capillary Permeability and Oncotic Pressure. The colloidal osmotic pressure is a major determinant of the intravascular volume. Albumin (molecular weight, 69,000) is the main osmotically active protein in plasma. The balance between the colloidal osmotic pressure and the capillary hydrostatic pressure determines the balance between the intravascular and extracellular fluid spaces. A significant degree of hypovolemia and hemoconcentration may take place either because of excessive capillary hydrostatic pressure from an increase in the ratio of post- to precapillary resistance or because of a reduction in plasma protein and consequently reduction of plasma oncotic pressure. Significant reduction in serum albumin not only lowers oncotic pressure but also increases the hydraulic conductivity of capillaries, thus facilitating the loss of intravascular fluid. Reduction of plasma protein occurs as the result of increased capillary permeability and loss of plasma protein from the intravascular to the extracellular space. The balance between oncotic and hydrostatic pressures is also an important determinant of the level of pulmonary edema and is critical in the management of the shock lung syndrome. Plasma oncotic pressure should be restored through careful selection of the type of fluid to be used in volume replacement. Fluids containing crystalloids may be undesirable, as these further decrease the oncotic pressure. On the other hand, administration of blood or colloids may be more appropriate to reduce pulmonary edema if pulmonary venous (or wedge) pressure is low. If there is increased vascular permeability in the lung because of damage to pulmonary capillaries, only a fall in hydrostatic pressure reduces pulmonary interstitial fluid. Positive end-expiratory pressure or an increase in oncotic pressure do not help.

Shock resulting from increased vascular permeability, such as anaphylactic shock or snake venom poisoning, is characterized by a dramatic reduction of plasma volume. Hematocrit rises sharply and oncotic pressure drops. This increase in capillary permeability may be partly related to the release of histamine from macrophages or the release of other metabolites or humoral factors which alter endothelial permeability.

Intravascular Hemagglutination and "Blood Sludging." The erythrocytes, leukocytes, and platelets undergo agglutination to a variable degree in association with the shock syndromes in thermal burn, sepsis, trauma, and perhaps even hemorrhage. These aggregates may cause obstruction of capillaries as well as arterioles. The precipitating events are numerous. They may include platelet aggregation by catecholamines; damage to endothelial lining of small blood vessels and capillaries with subsequent fibrin deposition and accumulation of microthrombi; hypoxia increasing the rigidity of red cells; and release of vasoactive peptides and anaphylatoxins as a result of complement activation, which may in turn have an effect on permeability of endothelial cells and tone of precapillary sphincters, leading to further reduction in tissue perfusion and tissue damage.

Disseminated intravascular coagulation is a syndrome often seen in shock, particularly from gram-negative septicemia. The syndrome causes renal cortical necrosis, generalized ischemic damage of multiple organs, consumption of coagulation factors, and bleeding, and may contribute also to the pathogenesis of the shock lung.

Shock Lung. Pathologic studies of the lungs in patients dying from the shock syndrome may reveal marked capillary dilatation, pulmonary edema, alveolar hemorrhages, massive pulmonary vascular congestion and hyaline membrane formation, atelectasis, superimposed bronchial pneumonia, and, if the patient survives for weeks or months after the initial injury, pulmonary fibrosis. Shock affects the lung by producing endothelial damage in the vast capillary bed or precapillary arterioles. Microaggregates of platelets, polymorphonuclear leukocytes, and red cells block capillaries, destroy capillary endothelial cells by releasing hydrolytic enzymes and/or superoxide radicals, and eventually cause the increased capillary permeability that is responsible for the pulmonary interstitial edema seen in shock. The trigger for aggregation of neutrophils in the lung is not clear. Complement is a likely candidate; C5A produced with the activation of complement may cause white cells to aggregate in the lung. In the balance of forces responsible for interstitial fluid in the lung, one must keep in mind the role of lymphatic drainage. Lymph flow is greatly increased in the very early stages of shock, and patients dying in hemorrhagic shock may have a widely distended pulmonary lymphatic system filled with proteinaceous material.

The decrease in pulmonary blood flow may also interfere with the production of surfactant. Lack of surfactant reduces the patency of alveoli and perpetuates leakage of fluid across pulmonary arterioles. Pulmonary venular constriction in response to tissue hypoxia may also contribute to pulmonary capillary congestion. It is also possible that with cerebral ischemia and hypoxia, neurogenic influences on the lung may cause a differential increase in venular resistance and increase capillary hydrostatic pressure and permeability. During *Pseudomonas* infusions in animals, there may be a direct effect of the endotoxin on capillary permeability, although sometimes a delayed response suggests an immune reaction with release of serotonin, contributing to the pulmonary edema. Regardless of its cause, the damage to the pulmonary capillary endothelium in shock perpetuates both the resistance to blood flow and systemic hypoxia and accelerates cellular death.

CELLULAR AND BIOCHEMICAL FACTORS IN SHOCK

OXYGEN-Hb AFFINITY. Arterial blood with normal hemoglobin and oxygen saturation of 90 per cent at a Po_2 of 100 mm Hg carries close to 20 ml of O_2 per deciliter to the tissues. The mixed venous blood has an oxygen saturation of 75 per cent at a Po_2 of 40 mm Hg and contains 15 ml of O_2 per deciliter. The normal arteriovenous oxygen difference is 5 ml per deciliter. The extraction of oxygen from Hb by the tissues is not complete and depends to a large extent on the affinity of O_2 to Hb, i.e., the shape of the oxygen dissociation curve. Hydrogen ion (Bohr effect), carbon dioxide, and 2,3-diphosphoglyceric acid (2,3-DPG) cause greater dissociation of O_2 from Hb because of their preferential affinity for reduced hemoglobin. 2,3-DPG concentration in red cells results from a side reaction of glycolysis and increases during anemia, hypoxia, and acidosis. A drop in hemoglobin, hypoxia, and acidosis may thus be partly compensated for by a shift of the O_2 dissociation curve to the right, favoring greater delivery of O_2 to the tissues at the same Po_2. This compensatory mechanism, in addition to the increase in cardiac output, provides for better oxygenation as extraction of O_2 from the O_2 reserve in venous blood increases. In certain tissues, however, such as the myocardium, extraction of O_2 at rest is already large, and any additional oxygen demand or a decrease in oxygen-Hb dissociation such as in alkalosis requires greater delivery of O_2, i.e., higher coronary blood flow.

In shock, the pH, carbon dioxide, and 2,3-DPG levels are changing, and one cannot calculate oxygen extraction from values of Po_2 because the shape of the O_2 dissociation curve cannot be predicted accurately. It is preferable to measure O_2 content or saturation of venous and arterial blood; if saturation is lower than predicted from values of Po_2, one can deduce that there is a shift of the dissociation curve to the right, and vice versa. Overzealous correction of acidosis with bicarbonate may, through the Bohr effect on Hb affinity for O_2, actually reduce O_2 delivery to the tissues. Hypophosphatemia reported during hyperalimentation may decrease 2,3-DPG and O_2 delivery.

CELLULAR STRUCTURE AND FUNCTION IN SHOCK. Survival of aerobic cells depends on the availability of substrates and oxygen to the mitochondria, which provide most of the high energy phosphate needs of the cell and utilize most of the available oxygen in the process. During oxidative phosphorylation, 36 moles of adenosine triphosphate (ATP) are produced per mole of glucose, whereas in the anaerobic state, glycolysis provides only two ATP molecules during the breakdown of one glucose molecule. Synthesis of ATP from adenosine diphosphate (ADP) is associated with the most active state of respiration in mitochondria (state 3 respiration) and is determined by the cell energy demands. In addition to oxidative phosphorylation and ATP synthesis, the mitochondria bind and accumulate calcium. This function determines calcium availability for other intracellular organelles and thereby regulates biochemical processes or contractile events, as in cardiac or vascular muscle.

Two processes may lead to cellular death. One is a marked inhibition of the electron transport system caused by severe ischemia or anoxia or by the administration of cyanide or actinomycin A. This process leads to depletion of ATP, and the electron microscopic appearance of the cells undergoing that type of death does not show any calcium phosphate accumulation in the mitochondria, presumably because of inhibition of the energy-dependent calcium transport mechanism. The other type of cell death is initiated by an injury to the cell membrane caused by activation of complement, or by antigen-antibody reaction, or by the administration of certain polyenes, such as amphotericin B, or certain bacterial or microbiologic products, such as the phospholipases or antitoxin. This type of cellular membrane damage is generally characterized by the precipitation of calcium phosphate in the mitochondria, presumably because active processes requiring ATP are preserved until late stages and calcium can be transported into the mitochondria.

Several structural changes take place in cellular membranes in shock. The earliest manifestation consists of swelling of the cell associated with an increase in intracellular sodium and clumping of nuclear chromatin, followed by dilatation of the endoplasmic reticulum. In this phase the cell membrane is unstable, and "blebs" may appear at the surface. The mitochondria will then begin to swell, and electron-dense clumps of flocculent material will appear within them. As the swelling of the mitochondria continues, Ca^{++} may or may not accumulate in them, depending on the type of cellular damage. The process of cell death becomes irreversible, lysosomes begin to disappear from the cell, and finally the cell is converted to a mass of debris, with large inclusions resembling myelin.

One can relate the sequence of structural changes in the cellular membranes to specific biochemical changes. Initially there is probably an increase in cellular permeability for sodium and water causing cellular swelling, followed by increased sodium-potassium ATPase activity in an attempt to drive sodium out of the cell. Increased membrane ATPase activity might eventually lead to the depletion of ATP and cyclic AMP, the latter leading to alteration of the cellular response to insulin, glucagon, catecholamines, and other hormones. For example, the effect of insulin on glucose uptake in muscle of animals that have been subjected to hemorrhagic shock is reduced. The unresponsiveness to insulin in the peripheral tissues may be one of the reasons for hyperglycemia of injured individuals. There is also a decrease in ATP, particularly in the liver in early shock and in most other organs in late shock. It is difficult to determine the critical level of ATP that is necessary for cellular function, but it is believed that as long as there is ADP and oxygen, and substrate is provided, ATP generation can be resumed within minutes as long as mitochondrial structure is preserved. The organs that are most seriously affected in the process of shock include, in descending order, the liver, kidneys, muscle, and lung.

MITOCHONDRIAL FUNCTION. Hypoxia may reduce the rate of ATP synthesis by mitochondria, but it does not cause significant damage to mitochondrial membrane functions unless it is severe, sustained, or associated with ischemia, which also reduces the availability of other substrates. In fact, an adaptation to hypoxia appears to take place such that when mitochondria are isolated from animal tissues after the animals have been exposed to brief periods of hypoxia (at Po_2 of 30 to 40 mm Hg), their capacity to respire and synthesize ATP in vitro is even enhanced. In contrast to hypoxia, hemorrhagic and endotoxin shock reduce calcium transport by mitochondrial membranes, particularly in the organs that become ischemic; state 3 respiratory activity and ATP synthesis and mitochondrial ATPase activity are inhibited, and finally mitochondrial damage ensues. The mechanism by which ischemia and endotoxins induce mitochondrial damage is not known. Whether such mitochondrial changes are the direct effects of deprivation of vital substrates or are secondary to the release of lysosomal enzymes, changes in intracellular pH, or other changes in cellular ionic environment with accumulation of metabolites is not apparent.

Glucocorticoids may exert a protective effect on mitochondrial function in endotoxemia in rats. Very large doses of glucocorticoids completely protect the mitochondria when rats are given an LD 60 dose of endotoxin. The protective effect is not apparent, however, when a dose of LD 90 is given. One may summarize the mitochondrial effects by saying that hypoxia by itself triggers some adaptive mechanisms which tend to increase respiratory activity if oxygen and ADP become available, but ischemia and endotoxemia can induce significant mitochondrial damage which heralds cellular death.

THE LYSOSOMAL THEORY. Lysosomes are cytoplasmic granules which contain a variety of potent hydrolytic enzymes bound in a latent form in a relatively impermeable membrane. These enzymes are capable of hydrolyzing a wide variety of both natural and synthetic substances and can digest all intra- and extracellular macromolecules if they are released from their membranes. When released from the organelles, either inside or outside the cell, as a consequence of certain forms of cellular injury, they may contribute to the pathogenesis or the propagation and perpetuation of shock. They are most active at an acid pH, which would make them potentially more destructive in the setting of hypoxia and shock.

Numerous morphologic and biochemical observations implicate the lysosomal enzymes in the perpetuation of shock, but at this time the evidence for their primary involvement is not convincing. In organs such as liver, spleen, and intestine, the lysosomes enlarge and lose their granules during the early phases of shock. This is associated with a decrease in the total activity of lysosomal hydrolases in tissues and a corresponding increase in activity in the soluble fraction of the tissue homogenate. This indicates a loss of lysosomal membrane integrity in vivo. The lysosomes obtained from animals in shock demonstrate an enhanced release of enzymes in vitro. A reduction in lysosomal membrane integrity has also been observed in animals after the administration of endotoxin. In several animal studies the levels of hydrolases found in blood, lymph, or serum seem to correlate with severity of shock.

The appearance of a *myocardial depressant factor* or factors (MDF) in shock, although still controversial, may be an indirect manifestation of the effect of lysosomal enzymes. In experimentally induced pancreatitis and in a variety of other shock states, plasma MDF activity closely parallels lysosomal hydrolases in the plasma. It has been suggested that pancreatic ischemia associated with shock results in the release of lysosomal and other enzymes within the pancreas, which act on an endogenous substrate to yield a peptide with low molecular weight and MDF activity, which is then released into the circulation. The resulting myocardial depression maintains the state of low cardiac output and sustains shock.

Another indication of the involvement of MDF has been the reproducibility of the shock syndrome with infusion of lysosomal hydrolases in animals. These animals demonstrate the hypotension, circulatory collapse, and pathologic changes in the tissues that are seen in experimental forms of shock.

Other suggestive evidence of the involvement of MDF has been the responsiveness of certain animals in shock to large amounts of corticosteroids. In vitro, corticosteroids stabilize the lysosomal membranes and prevent their lysis. Treatment with steroids has been shown to suppress circulating serum levels of lysosomal hydrolases in a variety of shock states.

Endotoxemia is associated with increased levels of serum hydrolases, but in vitro the endotoxins do not increase the lysis of lysosome. It has been suggested that endotoxins may cause the formation of a lysosomal releasing factor, LRF, through activation of the alternative as well as the classic complement pathways. Activation of complement in fresh human serum has been found to generate a factor (LRF) which stimulates human polymorphonuclear leukocytes to release their lysosomal enzymes. This factor has many of the properties of human C5a, a complement component known to have chemotactic and anaphylatoxin activities.

COMPLEMENT ACTIVATION IN SHOCK. The complement system consists of a series of discrete plasma proteins which are present as inactive precursors until they are activated by highly specific biochemical reactions, some of which involve limited proteolytic cleavage. Numerous components have been isolated and characterized. The activity of the immune system may depend on "complements," which may be the primary humoral mediators of antigen-antibody reactions. Not all antigen-antibody reactions depend on complements. For example, the anaphylactic shock seen after penicillin or pollen antigens involving the IgE antibodies does not include complement. IgE immunoglobulins may act directly on cells to release histamine, slow reactive substance, and eosinophil chemotactic factor. In contrast, many other antigen-antibody reactions, particularly those involving the IgG and IgM immunoglobulins, which can also evoke an acute anaphylactic reaction, depend on complement. The various types of complements are designated numerically, and from a functional standpoint one could think of these various proteins as having a *recognition*, an *activation*, or a *cellular attack* function. The recognition function is carried out by three proteins forming a macromolecular complex in the plasma, which attaches itself to the membrane surface of a target cell with the appropriate antibody. The activation mechanism is triggered primarily by the antigen-antibody complex (classic pathway), but it may also be triggered by bacterial or fungal mucopolysaccharides without the participation of any immunoglobulins (alternative pathway). Regardless of pathways of activation, the results in terms of generation of various effectors, anaphylatoxins, or direct cellular damage are the same. Activation of complement causes the release of several low molecular weight vasoactive peptides from the complement molecules by cleavage, and these in turn have significant biologic effects. For example, during the activation of C2, a cleavage product occurs which has kinin-like activity, which then can significantly influence capillary permeability. Two other activation peptides, C3a and C5a, release histamine from mast cells, have chemotactic activity, and constrict vascular smooth muscle. Another fragment, C3b, acts as an opsonin and facilitates phagocytosis. Polymorphonuclear leukocytes may be attracted chemotactically through activation of esterases on their surface and may release their lysosomal enzymes if the concentration of the complement reaction product C5a is large enough. Platelets may have an increase in their procoagulant activity, and endothelial cells may contract. In addition to the direct and indirect effects of the fragments of activated complement on cells, their aggregation as decamolecular complexes on the surface of the cell membranes causes cellular destruction. The expressions of all these effects are increased capillary permeability; increased leukocyte accumulation and infiltration, such as is sometimes observed in glomerulitis; release of lysosomal enzymes, which could cause necrotizing vasculitis; and intravascular coagulation factors, which would induce the Shwartzman reaction, thrombocytopenia, and other manifestations of microcirculatory collapse and intravascular plugging seen in prolonged shock and in endotoxemia.

Although the side effects of complement activation in shock are detrimental, leading to cellular death, the fundamental biologic activities of the complement components are beneficial in enhancing phagocytosis and mediating the inflammatory response to local infection or irritation, in the vital neutralizing of viruses, and, finally, in modulating the immune response.

TREATMENT OF SHOCK

GENERAL PRINCIPLES. There are five main goals in the management of the patient in shock: (1) rapid recognition of the shock state, (2) correction of the initiating insult (e.g., pericardiocentesis, defibrillation, hemostasis, antibiotics), (3) correction of the secondary consequences of the shock state (e.g., acidosis, hypoxemia, disseminated intravascular coagulation), (4) maintenance of the function of vital organs (e.g., cardiac output, arterial pressure, urinary output), and (5) identification and correction of aggravating factors. All five goals are approached simultaneously. The prognosis of a patient in shock is determined by the etiology of the shock state (e.g., hypovolemic traumatic shock in a young, healthy adult carries a mortality of less than 20 per cent in many centers, while cardiogenic shock due to massive anterior infarct carries a mortality of more than 70 per cent even in the most aggressive medical center), by the duration of shock and consequent secondary organ dysfunction, and by the speed of recognition and appropriateness of medical intervention.

A key element in the patient in shock is hemodynamic monitoring.

PATIENT MONITORING. Management of the patient in shock requires accurate and serial measurements of heart rate and rhythm, respiratory rate and adequacy of gas exchange, systemic blood pressure and cardiac filling pressures, cardiac output and tissue perfusion indices, and end-organ function (mental status, urine output, liver function, etc.).

1. *The electrocardiogram* permits serial assessment of cardiac rate and rhythm and promptly detects serious arrhythmias such as premature ventricular beats, ventricular tachycardia or fibrillation, high degree heart block, serious sinus bradycardia, and atrial arrhythmias. In addition, serial 12-lead ECG's may allow an indirect assessment of the severity of myocardial ischemia.

2. *Arterial blood gases and pH.* These should also be monitored routinely. Correction of acidosis and hypoxia are essential elements in the management of the early phases of shock.

3. *Central venous and Swan-Ganz catheters.* The monitoring of central venous pressure provides an index of the status of absolute and relative blood volume and of the need for fluid replacement. The catheter should be inserted through the antecubital or external jugular vein; only if the physician is experienced should it be introduced through the subclavian or the internal jugular vein. Central venous pressure obtained with the catheter advanced to the superior vena cava is normally between 5 and 8 mm Hg, but it should be elevated to 10 mm Hg if one is to expect an adequate cardiac output in patients in shock. Central venous pressure reflects the filling pressure of the right ventricle and hence is an adequate indicator of cardiac filling pressure *only* in patients who have no underlying cardiac or pulmonary disease and are not on a mechanical ventilator. The central venous pressure is probably adequate only for the initial management of young adults suffering from traumatic hypovolemic shock. In the patient with known or suspected cardiac or pulmonary disease, or in whom management includes the use of positive-pressure ventilation, state of the art management requires the use of a Swan-Ganz catheter to measure pulmonary capillary wedge pressure as an indicator of left ventricular filling pressure. In addition, the Swan-Ganz catheter allows serial assessment of cardiac output and provides a route for serial oximetric studies.

The filling pressure of the left ventricle can be estimated from measurement of the "pulmonary capillary wedge" pressure with a Swan-Ganz balloon-tip catheter. A triple lumen thermodilution catheter is introduced intravenously with or without fluoroscopy but with electrocardiographic monitoring. Its tip is advanced to the pulmonary artery; the balloon is inflated with air, and it can be floated to a wedge position in one of the pulmonary arteries. The recorded pressure downstream from the inflated balloon is the "pulmonary capillary wedge" pressure, and the appearance of the left atrial pressure wave form on the oscilloscope confirms the position of the catheter tip. The wedge pressure reflects left ventricular end-diastolic pressure, but a discrepancy between the two may occur if there is severe mitral stenosis or left atrial tumors. If for some reason one is unable to get the wedge pressure, the pulmonary artery diastolic pressure may be a useful index of the wedge pressure.

The double lumen Swan-Ganz catheter has been modified to include an extra lumen that allows measurement of right ventricular end-diastolic pressure simultaneously with the wedge pressure. Another modification includes a temperature sensor device at the tip that allows the detection of changes in temperature following injection of cold dextrose in the right atrium, and the temperature dilution curve obtained with the temperature sensor provides an estimate of cardiac output. A further modification of the Swan-Ganz catheter includes an electrical lead to allow the continuous monitoring of intracardiac electrocardiogram.

While the Swan-Ganz catheter is expensive, and complications may accompany its use (such as arrhythmias, sepsis, or pulmonary infarction), nevertheless, it is a very important tool for monitoring patients with severe shock and for providing an important data base for judicious administration of fluids and sympathomimetic amines. One can suspect pulmonary infarction as a complication of Swan-Ganz catheterization if the pulmonary artery pressure rises. The catheter should probably be removed within 48 hours after its insertion to avoid sepsis or pulmonary infarction, and should not be left continuously in the "wedged" position. The normal wedge pressure is 12 mm Hg, but it should be raised to 15 to 20 mm Hg in shock unless pulmonary capillary permeability is increased and there is pulmonary edema. The wedge pressure should be maintained at the lowest level that provides for adequate organ perfusion.

A discrepancy between right atrial and left atrial pressures may occur in patients with acute myocardial infarction, sepsis, or trauma when a high left atrial or pulmonary capillary wedge pressure may be accompanied by a low right atrial pressure, and under those circumstances monitoring right atrial pressure alone may lead to excessive administration of fluids. Conversely, patients with pulmonary disease, pulmonary embolism, pulmonary hypertension, and right ventricular infarction have relatively high levels of right atrial pressure compared to the pulmonary capillary wedge pressure, and the avoidance of fluids under those circumstances may deprive the patient of important therapy. In addition to providing information on pressure, the triple lumen Swan-Ganz catheter provides proximal and distal ports for sampling of right atrial and pulmonary arterial blood for oximetry to rule out a left to right intracardiac shunt. The sampling of "mixed venous" (pulmonary arterial) and systemic arterial blood to measure the oxygen content allows the estimation of cardiac output, since output equals oxygen consumption divided by the arteriovenous oxygen difference. The use of a thermodilution catheter permits serial direct measurements of cardiac output by the thermodilution technique. At least three consecutive samples of thermodilution curves with less than 10 per cent variance should be averaged.

4. *Urinary catheter*. This allows the routine hourly measurement of urinary output. A decline in urinary output to less than 20 ml per hour is an indication of the inadequacy of arterial pressure and renal perfusion. It is a sensitive index of the progress of the shock syndrome and reflects the effectiveness of management. The most frequent cause of oliguria in shock is hypovolemia. Fluid deficits are often underestimated, particularly in the presence of sepsis. If oliguria persists despite adequate administration of fluid and elevated wedge pressure, diuretic therapy may be necessary to avoid acute renal tubular necrosis which complicates prolonged hypotension.

5. *Arterial catheterization for arterial pressure monitoring*. Patients with severe or persistent hypotension and shock in whom it is difficult to measure blood pressure with the sphygmomanometer are candidates for intra-arterial pressure monitoring. There is often a discrepancy between the intra-arterial pressure measurements and the cuff pressure. There may be a low or even no recordable arterial pressure by the cuff technique when intra-arterial pressure by cannulation is normal or even at times slightly elevated. This discrepancy may result from severe peripheral vasoconstriction and low output and pulse pressure. Since the sphygmomanometric measurement of arterial pressure in shock may be erroneously low, it is advisable to palpate the femoral artery in the groin to get a better index of the strength of the pulse pressure in this more proximal large artery and to introduce an arterial cannula for monitoring arterial pressure before administering vasopressors or resorting to counterpulsation. An arterial cannula also allows the frequent determination of blood gases and pH. The radial, brachial, or femoral arteries may be cannulated. We prefer to cannulate the radial artery, if possible, as this site has the lowest complication rate. Brachial or femoral arterial cannulation is preferred in patients who are severely hypotensive, who are on large doses of vasoactive drugs, who are markedly vasoconstricted, and in whom the radial artery is difficult to palpate.

6. *Cardiac output*. Measurement of cardiac output by thermal or dye dilution techniques is used for management of selected patients or for the evaluation of new therapeutic regimens. The mixed venous blood oxygen content may be used as an index of total body perfusion. Within certain limitations, one can estimate the effectiveness of total body perfusion and delivery of oxygen to the tissues by monitoring the oxygen content of mixed venous or pulmonary arterial blood. The assumptions are that the total body oxygen consumption is constant or does not change drastically and that the arterial oxygen content is high and does not vary significantly. An arteriovenous oxygen difference of 6 ml per deciliter or more indicates poor tissue perfusion.

MANAGEMENT. *General Measures.* Management consists of primary therapy, directed at the underlying insult, and secondary therapy, directed at the consequences of the shock state. Patients in shock may be in pain, apprehensive, and frightened. They should be reassured and put in a horizontal position with the legs slightly elevated, unless this position is uncomfortable or causes shortness of breath. In that case, they should be allowed to be in the most comfortable position. Pain should be relieved with morphine sulfate intravenously, preferably in small repeated doses of 2 to 5 mg; if side effects occur, such as hypotension, cold clammy skin, bradycardia, nausea, and vomiting, atropine may cause some relief. Another analgesic, meperidine, 50 to 100 mg, may be given intravenously. Intravenous fluid and monitoring of various functions should begin promptly to guide further therapy. Oxygen, norepinephrine, or dopamine may be initiated while the cause of shock is determined. Reversible factors which decrease cardiac output and cause hypotension should be corrected promptly (i.e., tension pneumothorax, marked acidosis or alkalosis, cardiac tamponade).

Correction of Hypovolemia. Hypovolemia may occur in any type of shock whether or not it is associated with external signs of blood or fluid loss. If there is no evidence of actual fluid or blood loss, there may be a significant shift of fluid from the intravascular to the extracellular space because of increased capillary permeability and endothelial damage. This may occur in any vascular bed, but more specifically in the splanchnic and the pulmonary vasculature. Fluid may also shift intracellularly because of changes in cellular membrane permeability with increased intracellular sodium and water in any shock syndrome associated with decreased tissue perfusion. Fluid replacement is essential for the restoration of cardiac output. Without an adequate filling pressure, there will not be an adequate cardiac output. The administration of potent cardiotonic drugs in the presence of hypovolemia and low cardiac filling pressure may be ineffective and may potentially aggravate the clinical condition rather than improve it. On the other hand, these drugs increase cardiac output significantly if left ventricular end-diastolic pressure and volume are adequate.

If the patient has cardiogenic shock or if there are signs of pulmonary congestion or edema, one should insert a Swan-Ganz balloon catheter into the pulmonary artery or pulmonary arterial wedge position for measurements of the pulmonary artery diastolic pressure or the pulmonary capillary wedge pressure. If the pulmonary artery diastolic or pulmonary artery wedge pressure is less than 15 mm Hg, one should give 100 ml of Ringer's lactate, saline, or dextran every 10 to 15 minutes. If perfusion improves and wedge pressure remains less than 15 mm Hg, one should continue infusion at the same rate, trying to achieve a pressure between 15 and 20 mm Hg. If perfusion of the tissues is unchanged or worse, if wedge pressure increases above 20 mm Hg, or if there are signs of pulmonary congestion, one should stop volume expansion. Improvement in tissue perfusion is evaluated by examining the degree of cyanosis, clamminess of the skin, the level of arterial blood pressure, and urinary output, as well as the sensorium and alertness of the patient, blood gases, and pH.

If a Swan-Ganz catheter is not available or if pulmonary artery diastolic pressure or wedge pressure cannot be obtained, the insertion of a central venous catheter is a helpful guide for administration of fluids. If the central venous pressure is less than 10 mm Hg, one should expand volume until arterial pressure and tissue perfusion return to satisfactory levels, central venous pressure is between 10 and 15 mm Hg, or pulmonary congestion develops. The central venous or pulmonary capillary wedge pressures should be measured with careful reference to a constant point marked on the chest at the level of the right atrium or the phlebostatic axis. Patients who are on respirators or are receiving positive pressure assistance or positive pressure ventilation will have an abnormally elevated pressure. Under those circumstances, the filling pressure should be recorded at the time the respirator is transiently disconnected.

Treatment for hemorrhagic hypotension is with blood replacement; but while waiting for typing and cross-matching, the patient should be given saline or Ringer's lactate. The effects of these fluids are transient, because the crystalloids will rapidly leave the intravascular space. A more effective treatment might include colloids that stay longer in the circulation and increase oncotic pressure. This is particularly important when patients have manifestations of the shock lung syndrome, when extensive endothelial damage and interstitial edema are suspected, or when patients are chronically ill or malnourished and have hypoalbuminemia. Under those circumstances, dextran or mannitol, albumin or plasma would expand blood volume. The excretion of dextran or mannitol by the kidney will increase oncotic pressure in Bowman's capsule and create a favorable hydrostatic-oncotic pressure gradient across the glomerulus, facilitating filtration even at low arterial pressure. If arterial pressure is not rapidly restored or oliguria persists despite the administration of diuretics such as furosemide in conjunction with fluid replacement, then there might be danger of overexpansion of plasma volume and accentuation of the pulmonary edema.

The development of pulmonary edema is closely correlated with the gradient between plasma oncotic and pulmonary artery wedge pressure, which reflects the capillary hydrostatic pressure in the lung. Plasma oncotic pressure of normal adults is approximately 25 mm Hg, whereas pulmonary wedge pressure is 10 to 12 mm Hg. Capillary filtration takes place normally in the lung despite a low hydrostatic and a relatively high oncotic pressure, because of the equally high interstitial oncotic pressure in the lung. Plasma oncotic pressure may fluctuate. After 12 hours of bed rest, for example, it declines markedly. If oncotic pressure remains significantly higher (>8 mm Hg) than pulmonary capillary hydrostatic pressure, the risk of pulmonary edema is negligible; but if oncotic pressure is only 1 to 3 mm Hg higher than pulmonary wedge pressure, the patient is at high risk for pulmonary edema.

Types of Fluid. The isotonic saline solution contains 140 mEq of sodium and 140 mEq of chloride, whereas Ringer's lactate solution has 130 mEq of sodium, 4 mEq of potassium, 108 mEq of chloride, and 28 mEq of lactate. Lactate and acetate are converted to bicarbonate and maintain the alkalinity of the blood. When large volumes of fluid are administered, isotonic saline causes a dilution acidosis, which can be avoided if Ringer's lactate is used.

Human serum albumin comes in two concentrations, 5 grams per deciliter, which is the usual dose used, or 25 grams per deciliter salt-poor albumin. The 25 grams per deciliter is necessary only in the presence of severe hypoalbuminemia. An alternative is purified plasma protein, which is free of hepatitis virus contamination but has some contamination with vasoactive substances, causing the Food and Drug Administration to express concern about its use. Both albumin and purified plasma protein are expensive. They cost between $70 and $300 per 500 ml and represent a significant strain on blood donor programs. They should not be used indiscriminately.

There are two types of dextran: dextran 40 with 40,000 molecular weight, and dextran 70 with approximately 70,000 molecular weight. Dextran 70 comes in a 6 per cent solution, and dextran 40 comes in a 10 per cent solution. The dextran solutions maintain intravascular volume for several hours; but if given in amounts exceeding 1 liter, they may cause serious side effects, including platelet dysfunction and abnormalities in bleeding and coagulation, the nature of which are not clearly defined, and occasional anaphylactoid reactions. Approximately 5 per cent of patients receiving dextran have had such reactions, but very few of these are fatal. It should probably be avoided in patients with hypofibrinogenemia and bleeding dyscrasias.

With dextran 40 there is an incidence of acute renal failure, presumably because the rapid filtration of the low molecular weight dextran into the urine is accompanied by maximal reabsorption of the filtered salt and water, leading to a high intratubular concentration with an increase in intratubular viscosity and possibly physical occlusion of the renal tubule by dextran precipitates. This does not seem to occur with dextran 70 because it is filtered at a much slower rate owing to its molecular size.

Another colloid is hydroxyethyl starch or hetastarch, which maintains volume expansion almost twice as long as dextran and has fewer side effects. It interferes minimally with coagulation, it has a very mild anaphylactoid effect, and its cost is one fifth that of albumin. New synthetic oxygen-carrying compounds are currently under investigation for use in the setting of acute hemorrhagic shock.

Correction of Hypoxia. Oxygenation of the patient and interpretation of serial blood gases requires the use of high-flow O_2 delivery systems, where the delivery system supplies all the inspired mixture of oxygen and air. The currently used high flow systems include intubation with mechanical ventilation or T-tube devices, or tight fitting face masks making use of the Venturi principle. These systems deliver a fixed inspired oxygen concentration (FIO_2), allow careful titration of O_2 as a drug, and permit the calculation of alveolar-arterial O_2 gradients that require a constant FIO_2. Low flow systems (such as nasal prongs or simple face masks) do *not* deliver the entire inspired gas mixture and hence the FIO_2 varies with the rate and depth of ventilation. While more comfortable, these low flow systems are much less accurate.

Adequacy of the airway should be assessed in any patient in shock. If the patient is obtunded and cannot protect his airway, intubation with a cuffed endotracheal tube is essential. Occasionally the use of positive pressure respirators to improve gas exchange has been necessary. Positive pressure ventilation may simultaneously decrease the venous return by increasing intrathoracic pressure, and thereby perpetuate and aggravate a low output state. Also, 100 per cent oxygen by mask may lead to toxic changes in the lung if continued more than a few hours. Thus when a respirator is required, the preferred approach is to select an FIO_2 of 50 per cent, and to increase the FIO_2 and employ positive pressure only if needed to achieve a PO_2 of about 70 mm Hg.

Correction of Acidosis. If the arterial blood pH is less than 7.3 and respiratory acidosis has been ruled out, it is advisable to give 1 vial of sodium bicarbonate intravenously (44.6 mEq). If the arterial blood pH is less than 7.2, 2 vials intravenously may be administered and values repeated for further therapy in 15 to 30 minutes. Overcorrection of acidosis to alkalosis may decrease oxygen delivery to tissues by shifting the oxyhemoglobin dissociation curve to the left. Serial assessment of arterial blood gases permits careful titration of $NaHCO_3$.

Treatment of Arrhythmias. Arrhythmias, particularly after myocardial infarction, may limit cardiac output and perpetuate shock.

Sustained ventricular tachycardia may be treated first with intravenous lidocaine in a bolus of 50 to 100 mg; if there is associated hypotension or any evidence of hemodynamic deterioration, electroshock should be used immediately. Ventricular fibrillation should be treated immediately with electroshock. If the first or second shock is unsuccessful, the patient must receive closed chest massage, mouth-to-mouth respiration, and possibly intravenous sodium bicarbonate before again attempting electrocardioversion. In patients who fail to respond to adequate doses of lidocaine and have recurrent refractory ventricular fibrillation or tachycardia, bretylium tosylate in a bolus dose of 5 mg per kilogram of body weight is the next preferred agent.

Accelerated idioventricular rhythm is seen frequently in patients with myocardial infarction, particularly in those with diaphragmatic infarction. The rate is slightly faster than sinus rhythm, and a period of sinus bradycardia seems to favor the development of this arrhythmia. This is usually a benign rhythm and does not require therapy unless it degenerates into rapid ventricular tachycardia.

Supraventricular arrhythmias (atrial tachycardias, flutter, fibrillation, or junctional rhythms) should generally be treated with digoxin; but if the rhythm persists or there is an associated hypotension or hemodynamic deterioration, electroshock therapy should be utilized immediately. Sinus bradycardia, if severe (less than 40 beats per minute), can contribute to hypotension. It is commonly associated with inferior infarction, and, if accompanied by frequent premature ventricular beats, restoration of a more rapid sinus rhythm can eliminate them. Atropine is most effective intravenously in doses of 0.4 mg up to 1 or even 2 mg. If bradycardia persists and hypotension or other signs of hypoperfusion are evident, electrical pacing should be instituted.

Conduction disturbances such as atrioventricular block carry a variable prognosis. The conduction disturbance that occurs with inferior infarction has a better prognosis. It generally occurs early, is associated with sinus bradycardia, and may be caused by a temporary reflex increase in vagal tone to the conduction system or by atrioventricular nodal ischemia with only localized necrosis of this discrete structure. In anterior wall infarction heart block is related to ischemic damage of the three fascicles of the conduction system, which results from a more extensive degree of necrosis and is associated with higher mortality. Patients with inferior infarction benefit from temporary electrical pacing if they do not respond to atropine, whereas those with anteroseptal infarction generally require a permanent pacemaker.

Treatment of Sepsis. Both gram-negative and gram-positive organisms have been associated with septic shock (see Ch. 256). In gram-negative septicemia, *E. coli* is the predominant organism, and infections with *Klebsiella-Aerobacter* (enterobacter) groups are not uncommon; endotoxin is an important factor in the pathogenesis of this syndrome. Gram-positive infections without endotoxemia, such as in pneumococcal pneumonia, *Staphylococcus aureus,* or streptococcal bacteremia, may cause shock. Chronic alcoholism is a common associated illness among these patients. The toxic shock syndrome, a complication of *S. aureus* infection most commonly associated with tampon usage in women, is discussed in Ch. 270.

The characteristic hemodynamic abnormality in septic shock (whether gram-positive or gram-negative) is a marked decrease in peripheral vascular resistance; cardiac output may be increased, normal, or decreased. In contrast, in cardiogenic shock cardiac output is low and peripheral resistance is normal, increased, or occasionally decreased, and in hypovolemic shock cardiac output is low and peripheral resistance is increased. The treatment of septic shock includes the aggressive treatment of the infection with antibiotics and drainage of any abscesses. Although cardiac output may be normal or high, it may be insufficient to meet metabolic needs of the tissues. An absolute or relative decrease in intravascular volume requires fluid administration. Crystalloids or colloids are given to restore and raise central venous pressure to levels of 10 to 15 mm Hg or pulmonary wedge pressure to 20 mm Hg. In these patients who have marked peripheral vasodilation in the face of arterial hypotension, a potent peripheral vasoconstricting agent such as norepinephrine may be the agent of choice if correction of intravascular volume fails to provide adequate arterial blood pressure.

Use of Steroids. Corticosteroids are used by most physicians in very large doses early in the treatment of shock. Their beneficial effect appears to be related primarily to their action on cellular membranes. Steroids interact with biomembranes and probably become incorporated within their bilayer structures. A stabilizing effect on biomembranes has been demonstrated in vitro in studies of lysosomes isolated from animals treated with these agents. These lysosomes acquire a resistance to lysis in vitro. Apparently this beneficial action of corticosteroids is not related to their glucocorticoid properties. For example, testosterone is another potent membrane stabilizing agent. The reason for the continued question concerning the effectiveness of corticosteroids is that the consequences of membrane stabilization by corticosteroids in vivo are not really known. Experimental studies in animals subjected to septic, endotoxin, or hemorrhagic shock indicate improved survival with administration of corticosteroids. In shock, considerable damage to the microcirculation may be attributed to membrane interactions between platelets, polymorphonuclear leukocytes, and endothelium. Activation by the bacteria of the alternative complement pathway with the release of various peptides may favor platelet aggregation with endothelium and leukocytes, clot formation, and obstruction of the microcirculation. Corticosteroids may prevent these membrane interactions in vivo. Steroids may also prevent the pituitary release of β-endorphins, which may cause myocardial depression. Animals pretreated with cortisone or naloxone (β-endorphin antagonist) exhibit an impressive resistance to endotoxin-mediated shock. Nevertheless the use of corticosteroids in doses of 30 mg per kilogram of methylprednisolone as early as possible in patients with septicemia and hypotension might be justifiable, based on extensive experimental work. The extension of the use of corticosteroids to patients with cardiogenic shock is unwise. There is evidence that malignant arrhythmias develop after the administration of corticosteroids to such patients, and the incidence of ventricular aneurysms may be increased.

It is claimed that corticosteroids have significant cardiovascular effects with possible alpha receptor blocking activities, but pharmacologic studies indicate that the steroids have little if any significant direct cardiovascular action; they may augment the action of catecholamines, but they do not block alpha receptors.

Use of Sympathomimetic Amines. These drugs are used to increase cardiac output through their cardiotonic effect, and to redistribute blood flow to vital organs by their selective vasoconstricting action; by virtue of these two effects, they raise arterial pressure and allow the perfusion of ischemic regions, particularly in the myocardium, through collateral vessels. There are two potential problems with their use. If arterial pressure is elevated significantly, the hypertension may be detrimental, as it increases myocardial work and oxygen demand. Thus judicious elevation of arterial pressure to levels between 110 and 120 mm Hg systolic pressure would be reasonable. One cannot predict the optimal arterial pressure necessary to perfuse the coronaries in any particular patient because one does not know the severity of coronary disease and its extent, or the extent of myocardial reserve that would allow the heart to cope with a slight increase in afterload induced by the rising arterial pressure. Nevertheless, hypotension, particularly following myocardial infarction, should be corrected and arterial pressure maintained. The second potential problem with use of these drugs is their vasoconstricting effect; however, some vasoconstriction can be beneficial if it occurs in nonvital organs and if it is associated with increased cardiac output. This combination of effects raises arterial pressure and improves perfusion of vital organs. Therefore the proper use of sympathomimetic amines in shock requires a thorough knowledge of their cardiovascular effects. They have a structure similar to that of the natural adrenergic neurotransmitter norepinephrine and activate adrenergic receptors in various cells. Their action depends upon their affinity for various types of adrenergic receptors (see Ch. 26).

ADRENERGIC RECEPTORS. The adrenergic receptors may be classified as alpha or beta receptors with respect to their cardiovascular action. The alpha receptors are predominantly in blood vessels and mediate vasoconstriction. The beta receptors are present in the blood vessels as well as the myocardium. Activation of the beta-1 receptors in the myocardium causes an increase in myocardial contractility and in heart rate, whereas activation of beta-2 receptors in blood vessels causes vasodilatation. The same catecholamine may activate both alpha and beta receptors, depending on the dose and the organ in which it is acting (Table 43–4). The sympathomimetic amines that are available clinically include norepinephrine, epinephrine, do-

TABLE 43–4. ADRENERGIC RECEPTORS

Receptor Type	Site	Action
Beta-1	Myocardium	↑ Atrial and ventricular contraction
	Sinoatrial node	↑ Heart rate
	Atrioventricular	↑ Atrioventricular conduction
Beta-2	Arterioles	Vasodilation
	Lung	Bronchial dilation
Alpha	Arterioles	Vasoconstriction
	Venules	
	Veins	

pamine, isoproterenol, phenylephrine, and dobutamine. The relative actions and potencies of these agents are summarized in Tables 43–5 and 43–6.

NOREPINEPHRINE. Norepinephrine increases myocardial contractility by activating beta-1 receptors and thus may increase cardiac output. In blood vessels it activates primarily alpha or vasoconstricting receptors. The magnitude of its effect on alpha receptors varies from one organ to another. It is a very potent vasoconstrictor in skin, muscle, and splanchnic beds, whereas in the coronary vessels it activates the beta-2 receptors as well as the alpha receptors; and because there is a paucity of alpha receptors in the coronary vessels in contrast to other vascular beds, the drug causes vasodilatation of the coronaries.

It offers several distinct advantages in the treatment of shock. It increases cardiac output and redistributes blood flow away from the extremities and toward the heart and brain and increases arterial pressure, which in turn increases coronary flow to ischemic myocardium. It should be administered intravenously through an indwelling catheter to avoid the risk of extravasation, which results in necrosis of subcutaneous tissues. Two ampules of Levophed (4 mg base per ampule) may be dissolved in 500 ml glucose and water and an infusion started at a very low rate to determine the smallest dose necessary to maintain arterial pressure between 100 and 120 mm Hg, which should provide adequate perfusion to the heart, brain, and kidney (unless the patient was hypertensive or has extensive arteriosclerotic disease). A dose of 4 μg per minute may occasionally be adequate; however, many patients require up to 40 μg per minute; and in general if such doses are necessary to maintain pressure, prognosis is poor. An average dose would be between 10 and 15 μg per minute. If hypoxia, hypovolemia, and acidosis have been corrected, the lack of response to norepinephrine is probably an indication of significant myocardial damage. Norepinephrine may be the preferred agent in the management of profound hypotensive septic shock.

DOPAMINE. This is a naturally occurring precursor of norepinephrine. Its cardiovascular effect depends on its dose. When given in low concentrations, 2 to 5 μg per kilogram per minute, it has a vasodilator action in the renal and mesenteric vessels, with only slight dilatation of cerebral and coronary vessels. The dilator effect is mediated through beta-2 receptors and through specific dopaminergic receptors. In doses of 5 to 10 μg per kilogram per minute, it increases myocardial contractility and cardiac output through the activation of beta-1 receptors. In larger doses of >20 μg per kilogram per minute, it causes vasoconstriction through activation of alpha-adrenergic receptors of arteries and veins in most vascular beds. Thus this drug may redistribute blood flow away from the extremities and toward the kidney, gut, heart, and brain; however, it may be necessary to give large doses to maintain arterial pressure and coronary blood flow, particularly following myocardial infarction; these large doses tend to oppose the beneficial vasodilator effects in some vascular beds. Dopamine may cause nausea and vomiting and increased cardiac irritability in some patients.

TABLE 43–5. RELATIVE ADRENERGIC POTENCIES

Amine	Alpha (Vascular)	Beta-1 (Cardiac)	Beta-2 (Vascular)
Norephinephrine	++++	+++	+
Epinephrine	+++	++++	++
Dopamine	++	++++	++
Isoproterenol	0	++++	++++
Phenylephrine	++++	0	0
Dobutamine	+	++++	++

TABLE 43–6. RELATIVE INITIAL HEMODYNAMIC EFFECTS

A mine	Heart Rate	Arterial Pressure	Cardiac Output	Systemic Resistance
Norepinephrine	↑	↑↑	↑→	↑↑
Epinephrine	↑	↑	↑	↑→
Dopamine	↑	↑	↑	↑→
Isoproterenol	↑	↓→	↑↑	↓
Phenylephrine	→	↑	→↓	↑↑
Dobutamine	→	→	↑	→

EPINEPHRINE. Epinephrine is released from the adrenal gland; it activates myocardial beta-1 receptors and vasoconstrictor alpha receptors in most vessels except in skeletal muscle and coronary vessels, where it activates beta-2 receptors when administered in low doses. It increases cardiac output, but redistributes flow away from the kidney and splanchnic circulations toward skeletal muscle. Given in a dose range from 2 to 30 μg per minute intravenously, its effect on the redistribution flow is not optimal, and its effect on arterial pressure is only modest because of its vasodilator effect in skeletal muscle.

ISOPROTERENOL. Isoproterenol is a synthetic sympathomimetic amine which activates primarily vascular beta-2 receptors, causing vasodilatation, and myocardial beta-1 receptors, increasing cardiac output. The magnitude of the vasodilator effect of isoproterenol varies in different vascular beds, depending on the density of beta-2 receptors and the affinity of the drug for them. The major vasodilator action of isoproterenol is in skeletal muscle beds.

This drug is not recommended in either cardiogenic or septic shock. In hemorrhagic shock, burns, or trauma the major line of treatment should be blood or fluid replacement. In cardiogenic shock, isoproterenol significantly increases myocardial oxygen requirement, and, despite the increase in coronary flow, the ischemic region of the myocardium may be hypoperfused as indicated by increased lactate production. In contrast, the administration of norepinephrine tends to decrease lactate production by the heart. Dopamine is also beneficial if arterial pressure is maintained. The use of isoproterenol should probably be limited to the treatment of complete heart block in an attempt to maintain an idioventricular rhythm until more definitive therapy can be carried out. The usual dose of isoproterenol is 0.5 to 4 μg per minute.

DOBUTAMINE. Dobutamine is a synthetic sympathomimetic amine that has predominant beta-1 activity. In contrast to dopamine, dobutamine has much less alpha-vasoconstricting activity but equal positive inotropic effects. Thus, in equal inotropic doses, dobutamine tends to lower the pulmonary capillary wedge pressure while dopamine tends to increase it. Dobutamine is also reported to have a lower incidence of cardiac arrhythmias. In experimental models of canine infarction, the administration of dobutamine results in significantly smaller infarcts as compared to dopamine, possibly owing to the intracardiac release of norepinephrine produced by dopamine. Thus, especially in the setting of acute myocardial infarction with low output but no significant hypotension, dobutamine may be a preferred agent over dopamine for improvement in the cardiac output.

One can summarize the use of sympathomimetic amines by saying that the goal is to attain an arterial pressure adequate to perfuse the kidney, the ischemic myocardial segment, and the brain without overloading the left ventricle. The drug used should redistribute blood flow toward the more vital organs and away from skin and muscle for the optimal utilization of the limited cardiac output in shock. Finally, the drug should also have an inotropic action, and drugs such as methoxamine and phenylephrine, which only cause arterial vasoconstriction by activating alpha receptors without stimulating the heart, should be avoided. With these goals in mind, norepinephrine, dopamine, and dobutamine should be chosen in the management of shock.

Vasodilator Therapy in Shock. The beneficial effects of vasodilator therapy are (1) to decrease myocardial oxygen demands by decreasing preload or cardiac filling pressure and cardiac size and decreasing afterload by decreasing arterial pressure and arterial impedance, and (2) to dilate microcirculatory vessels.

The effectiveness of vasodilators (nitroprusside, nitroglycerin, phentolamine, or hydralazine) is impressive in the acutely failing heart following myocardial infarction without shock and with an elevated left ventricular end-diastolic pressure or capillary wedge pressure above 20 or 25 mm Hg; but the presence of *hypotension* should be a contraindication to the use of this therapy alone. Under those circumstances one may have to use a vasodilator drug along with norepinephrine or dopamine.

REDUCTION IN PRELOAD. One can reduce oxygen demand of the myocardium by decreasing cardiac volume in patients who have a high filling pressure. Reduction in cardiac size decreases myocardial wall tension, which is a major determinant of myocardial oxygen requirements. It may be achieved by administration of diuretics or venodilator drugs, which reduce filling pressure by pooling blood in the peripheral veins. The goal of "venodilator therapy" is to decrease preload and cardiac size and not to decrease arterial blood pressure. This effect is desirable as long as cardiac filling pressure does not drop excessively, causing a drop in cardiac output. In some patients with severe pulmonary congestion and high cardiac filling pressure with systemic arterial hypotension, it might be necessary to combine the vasodilator therapy with another drug that will cause selective arteriolar vasoconstriction in certain organs and will increase peripheral vascular resistance and raise and maintain arterial pressure, such as dopamine or norepinephrine.

REDUCTION IN AFTERLOAD. This is a beneficial effect of the vasodilators, because it will decrease the arterial impedance against which the left ventricle ejects its blood; thus ejection fraction may improve. This is desirable as long as it is not associated with a significant reduction in systemic arterial diastolic pressure, particularly in patients who are normotensive or have borderline hypotension. The dose of the vasodilator drug must be adjusted so that it will not cause a significant reduction in diastolic arterial pressure. Any drop in arterial pressure by more than 10 mm Hg should be avoided, and the diastolic pressure should certainly not be allowed to decrease below 65 mm Hg. Reduction in afterload is ideal in patients with chronic severe congestive failure with high filling pressure, pulmonary congestion, and low cardiac output, but without a significant reduction in arterial pressure. Patients with cardiomyopathy but without coronary artery disease may be the best candidates for this therapy.

Neither a vasodilator alone nor propranolol, which also reduces myocardial oxygen demand, has a place in the management of cardiogenic hypotension following myocardial infarction. The elimination of the cardiotonic effect of the normal sympathetic drive by propranolol may significantly impair cardiac output and precipitate failure. If the patient has continuing pain and *a normal or elevated blood pressure,* despite the administration of narcotics, morphine or meperidine, and nitroglycerin, the administration of propranolol might then be considered.

MICROCIRCULATORY VASOCONSTRICTION AND ALPHA RECEPTOR BLOCKERS. In some patients, despite prolonged administration of dopamine or norepinephrine, tissue perfusion is not improved. The reasons may be that the myocardial infarction or the cellular damage is extensive. It is also possible that constriction of microcirculatory vessels may be preventing the perfusion of exchange capillaries. The alpha receptor blocker phentolamine has a specific effect on the vasoconstricting alpha receptors and does not block the beta receptors in the myocardium. Thus the cardiotonic effect of sympathomimetic amines is not prevented, yet vasoconstricting effects at the microcirculatory level are antagonized. Phentolamine has a greater inhibitory effect on alpha receptors in venules and veins than in arterioles, and its dilator action may therefore be greater in veins than in arterioles. This effect calls for a note of caution, because rapid relaxation of large veins may abruptly lower cardiac filling pressure if the patient is hypovolemic. For this reason, it is essential to ascertain that the patient has received adequate amounts of fluid before giving phentolamine.

In this setting of shock with high circulating catecholamines and after prolonged infusions of high concentrations of norepinephrine and dopamine and with persisting evidence of decreased tissue perfusion, the use of the alpha receptor blocker phentolamine offers several theoretical advantages over other vasodilators based on animal work. It dilates venules to decrease capillary hydrostatic pressure and opens up precapillary sphincters, which allow perfusion of nutritional capillaries. Other vasodilators may have a negligible effect on veins and venules, and although they increase blood flow, they do not necessarily increase perfusion of the microcirculation. Unfortunately there are no clinical studies that confirm the beneficial effects of phentolamine* in that stage of shock, which in general carries a poor prognosis. An initial dose of 2 mg given intravenously, followed by 5 mg, should be attempted, with careful monitoring of the intra-arterial and central venous pressures to ascertain that the patient is not hypovolemic and does not have a decreased effective blood volume. If hypotension results from this small dose, more rapid fluid replacement will be necessary before adding phentolamine. Phentolamine may be added to the intravenous fluid containing norepinephrine. One or 2 ampules of phentolamine (5 mg per ampule) may be added for each ampule of norepinephrine in the intravenous fluid. If given alone, 4 ampules in 500 ml or 40 μg per milliliter is a reasonable concentration, and the usual dose is between 20 and 80 μg per minute.

NITROPRUSSIDE. This is a very effective vasodilator drug that causes relaxation of veins to decrease preload and some relaxation of arterioles to decrease arterial impedance. It may be started intravenously at a dose of 16 μg per minute and increased to 200 μg per minute with constant monitoring of arterial pressure. Occasionally larger doses have been necessary.

NITROGLYCERIN. This is also a very effective vasodilator with predominant effects on the venous system and lesser effects on the arteriolar resistance vessels. When given as an intravenous infusion of 15 to 100 μg per minute, it reduces preload and is useful in congestive heart failure complicating acute myocardial infarction, particularly when the wedge pressure is high and the arterial pressure is normal. Intravenous nitroglycerin may also cause coronary vasodilatation and improve subendocardial flow.

In the presence of cardiogenic shock with arterial hypotension and an elevated pulmonary artery wedge pressure, the combination of intravenous nitroglycerin and dopamine may be appropriate.

Other vasodilator drugs, such as hydralazine, which primarily exert an action on the arterioles, would not be very effective in reducing cardiac size and myocardial oxygen demand, and may be detrimental in causing a significant reduction in arterial blood pressure.

DIGITALIS. It is advisable not to use digitalis in patients in cardiogenic shock due to acute myocardial infarction even if there is evidence of pulmonary congestion and an elevated pulmonary artery wedge pressure. In the setting of acute

*Experimental drug for this purpose.

myocardial infarction it may increase myocardial irritability. In addition, the renal excretion of digoxin may be impaired because of decreased renal perfusion and arterial blood pressure.

Surgical Treatment in Cardiogenic Shock. Intra-aortic balloon counterpulsation may be beneficial in cardiogenic shock. The balloon is introduced into the aorta at the end of a catheter inserted through the femoral artery via surgical cutdown or percutaneously via the Seldinger technique. It is inflated during early diastole and is collapsed during systole. This sequence decreases afterload during ejection and increases coronary perfusion pressure and coronary flow during diastole. Improvement of the hemodynamic status has been observed, but because a large number of patients with myocardial infarction and shock have extensive coronary artery disease, the long-term survival is still disappointing. The balloon counterpulsation appears to be of greatest potential benefit in the support of patients who have seriously compromised hemodynamics after myocardial infarction, are refractory to medical management, and are candidates for a surgical procedure. This mechanical assistance sustains the hemodynamics during cardiac catheterization and coronary arteriography in preparation for surgery. Emergency revascularization surgery or infarctectomy, which has been carried out in some centers, has not been uniformly encouraging. Two complications of myocardial infarction require surgical intervention and carry a reasonable prognosis; these are ruptured papillary muscle and interventricular septal perforation. In both, there is decreased ejection from the left ventricle and a fall in arterial pressure. Attempts to increase systemic arterial pressure with drugs exaggerate the regurgitation or the left to right shunt. In these circumstances, the selective lowering of arterial systolic pressure with intra-aortic balloon counterpulsation is ideal, as it will facilitate ejection and reduce mitral regurgitation or left to right shunt. A significant reduction in afterload and vasodilatation may also be achieved with drugs such as nitroprusside or nitroglycerin, but the associated fall in diastolic pressure may extend the myocardial ischemia. Surgical management, as soon as it is feasible and safe, should be the course to pursue. Severe papillary muscle dysfunction or papillary muscle rupture (the posterior more frequently than the anterior) may cause significant left ventricular failure, and the surgical replacement of the mitral valve has been satisfactory, particularly in patients with good myocardial function. Patients with a perforation of the ventricular septum have congestive failure in association with the sudden appearance of a pansystolic murmur, often accompanied by a thrill. Clinically, it is often impossible to differentiate this condition from a ruptured papillary muscle. The demonstration of a left to right shunt by cardiac catheterization or radionuclide angiography confirms the diagnosis. Rupture of the septum should be treated surgically, preferably six to eight weeks after infarction, so that the margins of the defect can have sufficient scar tissue to permit surgical closure with relative ease.

Abboud FM, et al.: Reflex control of the peripheral circulation. Prog Cardiovasc Dis 18:371, 1976. *This is a review of the factors that regulate peripheral vascular resistance (neural, humoral, local, and metabolic). The characteristic behavior of different vascular beds and various vascular segments is described. The role of cardiac sensory receptors, arterial baroreceptors, and chemoreceptors in the reflex control of the circulation is also described. Circulatory adjustments to various stressful conditions, including hypotension, acute myocardial infarction, and hypoxia, in animals and in man are discussed.*

Berne R: The coronary circulation. *In* The Handbook of Physiology, Section 2: The Cardiovascular System. Bethesda, American Physiological Society, 1979, pp 873–952. *This is a thorough review of the factors that regulate coronary blood flow, with emphasis on the potential metabolic determinants and interplay between local metabolic control and neurogenic control.*

Braunwald E (ed.): Protection of the ischemic myocardium. Circulation 53 (Suppl I), 1976. *Proceedings of a symposium held in September 1975. Several important concepts related to cellular mechanisms of ischemia and infarction and assessment of interventions designed to reduce myocardial ischemia damage were emphasized. For example:* Williamson JR, et al.: Contribution of tissue acidosis to ischemic injury in the perfused rat heart, pp 3–14. *The authors demonstrate that the effects of ischemia on myocardial contractility are similar to those of acidosis. Lowering of intracellular pH reduces the rate of energy production relative to the rate of energy demand. They suggest, however, that the reduction in contractility with either acidosis or ischemia is not a result of a defective energy metabolism but is due to alteration of the calcium cycle of the heart. AM Katz had suggested earlier that intracellular acidosis causes a displacement of calcium ion bound to troponin during systole, which results in failure of activation of the actin-myosin interaction and impaired contractility.* Trump BF, et al.: Studies on the subcellular pathophysiology of ischemia, pp 17–26. *The authors review the mitochondrial changes which occur during ischemia as well as the plasma membrane changes.* Maroko PR, Braunwald E: Effects of metabolic and pharmacologic interventions of myocardial infarct size following coronary occlusion, pp 162–168. *This article emphasizes the fact that the protection of ischemic myocardium requires an adequate perfusion pressure and stresses the importance of the collateral circulation and the possibility of a coronary steal syndrome when certain vasodilators are administered. The importance of the relationship between myocardial oxygen demand and supply for the viability of the myocardium is stressed. A number of hemodynamic, pharmacologic, and metabolic interventions are found to change the extent of acute ischemic injury of the myocardium.*

Chaudry IH: Cellular mechanisms in shock and ischemia and their correction. Am J Physiol (Regulatory Integrative Comparative Physiology 14) 245:R117, 1983. *This is a review that deals specifically with cellular and subcellular alterations in shock. The potential mechanisms responsible for mitochondrial abnormalities, for alterations in cellular nucleotide levels, for the reduction in transmembrane potential, and for the increase in sodium-potassium ATPase activity are discussed. The depression of the reticuloendothelial system phagocytic activity and the release of lysosomal enzymes are also mentioned. The therapeutic attempts to restore cellular integrity by providing specific substrates are reviewed briefly, with emphasis on the proven effectiveness of ATP $MgCl_2$ as an adjunct therapy in restoring cellular function and improving survival rates in experimental shock.*

Goldberg LI: Dopamine—clinical uses of an endogenous catecholamine. N Engl J Med 291:707, 1974. *This is a review of the cardiovascular and renal actions of dopamine, of its hemodynamic effects in man, and its effectiveness in the treatment of shock. The action of dopamine is contrasted with that of other sympathomimetic amines. A regimen for its use in shock and its adverse effects are described.*

Lefer AM, Schumer W (eds.): Molecular and Cellular Aspects of Shock and Trauma. New York, Alan R. Liss Inc, 1983. *This volume represents the proceedings of a USA-Japan Binational Conference on this topic held in June, 1982. New concepts in cellular and metabolic aspects of shock and their therapeutic implications were reviewed. Following are brief comments on some of the articles:*

Ozawa K: Biological significance of mitochondrial redox potential in shock and multiple organ failure—Redox theory, pp 39–66. *In shock, the lowering of oxygen availability in the electron transport chain induces a marked decrease in mitochondrial $NAD^+/NADH$ ratio, the mitochondrial redox potential. When the mitochondrial redox state is reduced, the capability of mitochondria to produce energy with glucose through the Krebs cycle is decreased.*

Lefer AM: Pharmacologic and surgical modulation of myocardial depressant factor (MDF) formation and action during shock, pp 111–123, *This is a review of the chemical properties and the formation as well as the pathophysiology of MDF. There are no specific antagonists to MDF, and the author reviews the means of prevention of its formation and some of the pharmacologic approaches to counteracting its action.*

Goldfarb RD, Glenn TM: Regulation of lysosomal membrane stabilization via cyclic nucleotides and prostaglandins—the effects of steroid and indomethacine, pp 147–166. *The authors review data that suggest a significant change in the integrity of myocardial lysosomes during myocardial ischemia and propose that intramyocardial lysosome stability can be positively correlated with myocardial cyclic AMP/cyclic GMP ratio. Furthermore, intramyocardial cyclic AMP concentration was negatively correlated with prostaglandin A and E concentrations. In that study, indomethacin treatment decreased myocardial prostaglandin A and E concentration approximately 60 per cent following coronary arterial ligation. One might conclude that myocardial infarction induces synthesis and release of prostaglandins, which, in turn, induce alterations in intramyocardial cyclic nucleotide ratio such that release of lysosomal enzymes is promoted.*

Holaday JW: Endorphins in shock and spinal injury: Therapeutic effects of naloxone and thyrotropin-releasing hormone, pp 167–184. *The author presents data that indicate that the endorphin system is involved in the etiology of shock as well as spinal cord injury. The therapeutic effectiveness of naloxone is reviewed and appears to be stereospecific, dose-related, and mediated at neuroeffector sites within the central nervous system. The adverse side effects of naloxone are the intensification of traumatic pain and the blockade of morphine analgesia. In an attempt to avoid this adverse side effect, thyrotropin-releasing factor was used to reverse the cardiovascular effects of endorphin without altering their analgesic activity, and the results are promising.*

In a section of the monograph entitled Therapeutics of Shock and Trauma *(pp 199–322), several authors review different approaches considered at the experimental stage. These include the use of dibutyryl cyclic AMP; a comparison of methylprednisolone and hydrocortisone in the treatment of shock patients (double blind study suggesting that methylprednisolone may have a more beneficial effect); the use of calcium channel blockers in the treatment of shock, particularly after myocardial infarction, which may have a direct cellular effect that could be beneficial independently of changes in perfusion; the use of the antiproteolytic enzyme, aprotinin, in endotoxin shock, which preserves the phagocytic function of the reticuloendothelial system (aprotinin antagonizes serine endopeptidases and thus prevents the conversion of prekallikrein to kallikrein and consequently the conversion of kininogen to kinin) and protects the integrity of the capillaries and prevents aggregation of leukocytes in endotoxin shock.*

Nishijima H, et al: Hemodynamic and metabolic studies on shock associated with gram-negative bacteremia. Medicine 52:287, 1973. *Detailed hemodynamic res-*

piratory and metabolic studies are presented on a group of 32 patients in whom shock was associated with gram-negative bacteremia. Survival rate of the patients who had a normal or high cardiac output was significantly better than that of patients in whom cardiac output was reduced. A reduction in cardiac output associated with a relatively small AV difference of oxygen gave an especially poor prognosis. Decreased plasma volume or total blood volume, increased arterial blood concentrations of lactate with metabolic acidosis, and high venous oxygen content were observed in patients who died. These data point to a peripheral defect in perfusion associated with hypovolemia and eventually myocardial depression as the hemodynamic mechanisms accounting for septic shock.

The Cell in Shock. Proceedings of a Symposium on Recent Research Developments and Current Clinical Practice in Shock. The Upjohn Company, April, 1976. *Several important concepts are reviewed. For example:* Baue AE: Mitochondrial function in shock, pp 11–15. *This article reviews Dr. Baue's research on the cellular events which may take place during shock and ischemia. A sequence of cellular membrane damage, mitochondrial dysfunction, and lysosomal breakdown is discussed.* Trump BF: The role of cellular membrane systems in shock, pp 16–19. *This is a detailed analysis of the sequential structural changes that occur in cells in shock correlated with biochemical changes.* Goldstein IM: Lysosomes and their relation to the cell in shock, pp 30–34. *The potential role of lysosomal enzymes in cellular destruction in endotoxin shock is reviewed. The mechanisms of lysosomal enzyme release from human leukocytes, microtubule assembly, and membrane fusion induced by a component of complement (C5a/chemotaxis cytochalasin B/C AMP:cGMP antagonism) are reviewed. A lysosomal releasing factor, or LRF, sharing many of the components of human C5a, appears to stimulate human polymorphonuclear leukocytes to selectively release lysosomal enzymes.* Müller-Eberhard HJ: The significance of complement activity in shock, pp 35–38. *This is a brief review of the complement system, its activation, and its role in the release of vasoactive peptide, which may contribute to the syndrome of shock.*

The Organ in Shock. Proceedings of the Second Symposium on Recent Research Developments and Current Clinical Practice in Shock. The Upjohn Company, April, 1977. *The following are brief comments on some of the articles:* Mela LM: Oxygen's role in health and shock, pp 8–15. *Dr. Mela reviews the membrane alterations induced by ischemic cell injury which are characteristically different in each organ, reflecting the particular organ's most delicately balanced plasma membrane functions. The author emphasizes that hypoxia alone does not induce inhibition in mitochondrial activity, whereas ischemia does.* Ayres, SM: The shock lung, pp 24–31. *The role of lymphatics, capillary permeability, and AV shunts in the pathogenesis of the shock lung syndrome is reviewed, and the structural and functional changes in the lungs are discussed.* Mueller HS: The heart and oxygen transport, pp 38–49. *This is a review of the treatment of coronary shock in patients with acute myocardial infarction. A careful survey of the hemodynamic changes and of survival in response to various catecholamines, and intra-aortic balloon counterpulsation, is described. Emphasis is placed on the early recognition and aggressive management of patients with incipient ventricular failure to improve survival rate. Caution regarding the use of vasodilators in patients who have low systolic blood pressures is expressed, and potential use of intra-aortic balloon counterpulsation coupled with an aggressive work-up and surgical approach to severe cardiogenic shock unresponsive to medical management is discussed.*

Ziegler EJ, McCutchan JA, Fierer J, Glauser MP, Sadoff JD, Douglas H, Braude AI: Treatment of gram-negative bacteremia and shock with human antiserum to a mutant *Escherichia coli*. N Engl J Med 307:1225, 1982. *This is a randomized controlled trial of human J5 antiserum in patients with gram-negative bacteremia and shock. The antiserum was prepared by vaccinating healthy men with heat-killed* E. coli *J5 mutant, which lacks lipopolysaccharide-oligosaccharide side chains so that the core (which is nearly identical to that of most other gram-negative bacteria) is exposed for antibody formation. The antiserum reduced death substantially.*

44. CONGENITAL HEART DISEASE

Samuel Kaplan

Congenital diseases of the heart occur in about 8 to 10 of 1000 live births. The spectrum of severity varies widely. One fourth to one third are symptomatic in the first year of life, frequently as neonates. In others, such as in patients with a functionally normal bicuspid aortic valve, the lesion may remain silent throughout life or until complications occur during adult life. With the development of palliative or radical surgical treatment another large group has evolved who were treated during infancy or childhood and who have reached adult life. Accordingly, adults with congenital heart disease fall into several groups: some have anomalies with a natural history for long survival, others have had successful palliative or "curative" surgery in childhood, and still others have had lesions that were mild in childhood but have increased in severity in adult life (e.g., aortic stenosis).

Etiology

The cause is usually unknown in individual patients. The etiology of congenital heart disease is thought to be multifactorial, primarily due to an interaction between genetic predisposition and intrauterine environmental factors. It is estimated that congenital heart disease is associated with chromosomal abnormalities in 5 per cent of cases, and with single mutant genes and environmental factors in 3 per cent each (Table 44–1). Among *chromosomal abnormalities* the incidence of congenital heart disease is about 50 per cent in trisomy 21 (Down's syndrome), 95 per cent in trisomy 18, 90 per cent in trisomy 13, and 35 per cent in Turner's (XO) syndrome (Table 44–1). Among *single mutant gene* disorders (autosomal dominant or recessive or X-linked phenotypes), the more frequent syndromes in which the heart is involved are hypertrophic cardiomyopathy and the syndromes of Noonan and Holt-Oram (Table 44–1). Numerous *environmental factors* have been implicated in congenital heart disease. Women who contract rubella during the first trimester of pregnancy may give birth to infants with pulmonic stenosis (especially pulmonary artery branch stenosis), persistent patent ductus arteriosus, and less often other defects. Other viral illnesses have also been implicated, but the evidence that they produce congenital heart disease is not as strong. These include cytomegalovirus, coxsackievirus, and herpesvirus. Among drugs whose use during pregnancy has been implicated in congenital heart disease are the anticonvulsants, especially phenytoin and trimethadione, and lithium salts (with an apparent predilection for atrioventricular valve disease, especially Ebstein's malformation of the tricuspid valve), progesterone, warfarin, and amphetamines. The offspring of diabetic women are at greater risk for a variety of congenital heart diseases. Patent ductus arteriosus is more frequent in children born at high altitudes. It is estimated that about one half of the offspring of alcoholic mothers have congenital heart disease, usually left to right shunts.

Counseling

Parents of children with congenital heart disease are concerned about the cause of the malformation and about the possibility of recurrence in future pregnancies. This concern is greatest when the child is first born or the baby succumbs during the neonatal period. An explanation should be offered about the known causes of congenital heart disease and guilt feelings allayed. Parents should be advised that the prevalence of congenital heart disease in a second infant is 2 to 5 per cent. Although this figure is higher than in the general population, it is still quite low and parents should be supported if they decide to have another child. When congenital heart disease has recurred in two siblings, the prevalence is higher in a third pregnancy (estimated to be 20 to 25 per cent). Many girls with congenital heart disease who had corrective surgery during childhood have reached an age when pregnancy is being considered. The prevalence of congenital heart disease in their children is 2 to 5 per cent.

Fetal and Neonatal Circulations

The physiologic effects of congenital heart disease can be considerably modified by the dramatic circulatory adjustments at birth. In the fetus, oxygenated blood from the placenta flows through the umbilical vein and through the ductus venosus into the inferior vena cava. This blood then mixes with that returning to the heart from the caudal part of the body and enters the right atrium from the inferior vena cava. This relatively oxygenated blood flows preferentially across the foramen ovale to the left atrium and is ejected from the left ventricle into the ascending aorta. Thus, the important coronary and cerebral circulations in the fetus are perfused with blood having a higher Po_2. Desaturated superior vena caval blood enters the right atrium and flows preferentially into the right ventricle. This blood is ejected into the pulmonary artery, flows preferentially through the ductus arteriosus into the descending aorta to the placenta (via the umbilical arteries), and also perfuses the caudal part of the body. Pulmonary circulation is limited in the fetal unexpanded lungs because of high pulmonary vascular resistance produced by thick-walled pulmonary

TABLE 44–1. CARDIOVASCULAR INVOLVEMENT IN SYNDROMES

Syndrome	**Autosomal Chromosomal Abnormalities** *Major Noncardiac Features*	*Major Cardiovascular Anomalies*
Trisomy 21 (Down's)	Hypotonia, flat facies, slanted palpebral fissures, small ears	VSD, ECD, ASD, PDA
Trisomy 18	Clenched hand, short sternum, low arch dermal ridge patterning on fingertips	VSD, PDA, PS
Trisomy 13	Defects of eye, nose, lip, skin, and forebrain, polydactyly	VSD, DORV, PDA, ASD
Deletions		
4p−	Hypertelorism, broad or beaked nose, microcephaly, low set simple ears	VSD, AS, PDA
5p−	Cat cry in infancy, microcephaly, downward slant of palpebral fissures	VSD, PDA, AS
13q−	Microcephaly with high nasal bridge, eye defect, thumb hypoplasia	VSD
18q−	Midface hypoplasia, prominent antehelix, whorl digital pattern	VSD
Sex chromosomes		
XO	Short female, broad chest, congenital lymphedema, web neck	Coarct, AS, ASD
XXY	Small testicles, tall stature	TOF, Ebstein
XXXXY	Hypogonadism, limited elbow pronation, low dermal ridge count	PDA, ASD
XXXXX	Upward slant to palpebral fissures, small hands, clinodactyly of fifth finger	PDA
Heritable and possibly heritable		
Aase	Triphalangeal thumb, congenital anemia	ASD, VSD
Apert's	Craniosynostosis, midfacial hypoplasia, syndactyly, broad distal phalanx of thumb and big toe	VSD
Asplenia	Bilateral visceral right-sidedness	ECD, SV, anomalous venous return, etc.
Cat-eye	Coloboma of iris, anal atresia	Septal defects, TAPVR, TOF
Carpenter's	Acrocephaly, polydactyly, syndactyly, lateral displacement of inner canthi	PDA, VSD, PS, TGV
Cerebro-costo-mandibular	Rib gap with small thorax, micrognathia	VSD
CHARGE	*C*oloboma, *h*eart disease, *a*tresia choanae, *r*etarded growth and development, *g*enital and *e*ar anomalies	TOF, PDA, DORV, VSD, ASD, right aortic arch
Cockayne's	Senile-like appearance, retinal degeneration, impaired hearing, photosensitive skin	Premature atherosclerosis
Congenital hypertrophic cardiomyopathy		CM
Conradi's	Chondrodysplasia punctata	VSD, PDA
Cornelia de Lange's	Short stature, synophrys, micromelia	VSD, PDA
Crouzon's	Shallow orbits, premature craniosynostosis, maxillary hypoplasia	PDA, Coarct
Cutis laxa	Lax skin, hernias	Pulmonary hypertension, PBS
DiGeorge's	Developmental defects of the parathyroids, thymus, or great vessels	Truncus, IAA, VSD, PDA, TOF
Ellis-van Creveld	Short distal extremities, polydactyly, nail hypoplasia	ASD, single atrium
Familial deafness		Arrhythmias, sudden death
Forney's	Short stature, skeletal defects, conductive deafness	MR
Goldenhar's	Hemifacial microsomia	VSD, PDA, TOF, Coarct
Holt-Oram	Upper limb defect, narrow shoulders	ASD, PDA, VSD, Coarct
Jervell-Lange-Nielsen		Prolonged QT, sudden death
Kartagener's	Sinusitis, bronchitis, situs inversus	Dextrocardia
Laurence-Moon-Biedl	Retinal pigmentation, obesity, polydactyly	PDA, PS, aortic cusp anomaly
LEOPARD	Lentigines, hypertelorism, deafness, etc.	PS, EKG abnormalities, aortic valve dysplasia
Marfucci's	Enchondromatosis, hemangiomata	Hemangiomas
Meckel-Gruber	Encephalocele, polydactyly, polycystic kidneys	Septal defects, PDA, Coarct, PS
Mucopolysaccharidoses		
Maroteaux-Lamy	Coarse facies, stiff joints, cloudy corneas, deficiency of arylsulfatase B	AI
Morquio's	Mild coarse facies, severe kyphosis, cloudy corneas, deficiency of 6 sulfo-N-acetyl hexosaminidine sulfatase	AI
Pseudohurler	Coarse facies, stiff joints, clear corneas, deficiency of alpha-L-iduronidase	AI
Scheie's	Broad mouth, full lips, early corneal opacity, normal mentality	AI
Neurofibromatosis	Multiple neurofibromata, cafe-au-lait spots, bone lesions	PS, Pheo, Coarct
Neurologic and muscular diseases		
Friedreich's ataxia	Progressive ataxia, skeletal deformities	CM
Muscular dystrophy	Gradual muscle fiber degeneration	CM
Myotonic dystrophy	Hypotonia, developmental delay, myotonia	Arrhythmias, CM
Refsum's	Ataxia, polyneuritis, phytanic acid accumulation	Arrhythmias, sudden death
Riley-Day	Autonomic instability, insensitivity to pain	Episodic hypertension, postural hypotension
Noonan's	Short stature, web neck, pectus excavatum, cryptorchidism	PS, PBS, PDA, ASD, TOF, AS, Coarct, CM
Pierre-Robin	Micrognathia, glossoptosis, cleft soft palate	PDA, PFO, ASD
Polysplenia	Bilateral visceral left-sidedness	ASD, ECD, etc.
Progeria	Senile-like appearance, alopecia, fat atrophy, skeletal dysplasia	Atherosclerosis
Rendu-Osler-Weber	Multiple telangiectasias	AV fistulas
Romano-Ward		Long QT interval
Rubinstein-Taybi	Short stature, broad thumbs and toes, slanted palpebral fissures, hypoplastic maxillae	VSD, PDA
Scimitar	Lung hypoplasia, anomalous arterial supply and venous drainage (right lung)	RV hypoplasia, dextrocardia, VSD, PDA, TOF, Coarct
Seckel's	Severe short stature, microcephaly, prominent nose	VSD, PDA
Shprintzen's	Cleft palate, prominent nose, long face, learning disabilities	VSD, right aortic arch, TOF
Smith-Lemli-Opitz	Anteverted nostrils, ptosis, syndactyly, hypospadias, cryptorchidism	VSD, PDA, TOF, ECD, Coarct
TAR	*T*hrombocytopenia, *a*bsent *r*adius	TOF, ASD
Treacher-Collins	Malar hypoplasia with downslanting palpebral fissures, defect of lower lid, malformation of external ear	VSD, ASD, PDA
Tuberous sclerosis	Skin nodules, seizures, phakomata, bone lesions	Rhabdomyomata of heart
VACTERL	*V*ertebral anomalies, *a*nal atresia, *c*ardiac *t*racheo-*e*sophageal fistula, *r*enal dysplasia, *l*imb anomaly	VSD

TABLE 44–1. CARDIOVASCULAR INVOLVEMENT IN SYNDROMES *(Continued)*

Syndrome	**Autosomal Chromosomal Abnormalities** *Major Noncardiac Features*	*Major Cardiovascular Anomalies*
von Hippel-Lindau	Retinal angiomata, cerebellar hemangioblastoma	Hemangioma
Waardenburg's	Lateral displacement of medial canthi, partial albinism, deafness	VSD
Weill-Marchesani	Brachydactyly, spherophakia	PDA
Werner's	Senile-like appearance, cataract, thin skin	Vascular sclerosis
Williams's	Prominent lips, hoarse voice	Supravalvar AS, PBS
Zellweger's	Hypotonia, high forehead, flat facies, hepatomegaly	PDA, septal defects
Inborn Errors of Metabolism		
Alcaptonuria	Black discoloration of mesenchymal tissues and urine	Atherosclerosis
Homocystinuria	Subluxation of lens, malar flush, osteoporosis	Aortic dilatation, thrombosis
Pompe's	Hypotonia, large tongue, hepatosplenomegaly	Glycogen storage disease of the heart, CM
Connective tissue disorders		
Arterial calcification in infancy		Coronary calcinosis
Ehler-Danlos	Skin and joint hyperextensibility, poor wound healing	MVP, dilatation of the aorta, AI
Marfan's	Arachnodactyly with hyperextensibility, lens subluxation	MI, aortic dilatation
Osteogenesis imperfecta	Fragile bones, blue sclerae, hyperextensibility	AI
Pseudoxanthoma elasticum	Cutaneous and mucosal lesions	

AI = aortic incompetence
AS = aortic stenosis
ASD = atrial septal defect
CM = cardiomyopathy
Coarct = coarctation
DORV = double outlet right ventricle
ECD = endocardial cushion defect
IAA = interrupted aortic arch
IVC = inferior vena cava
MR = mitral regurgitation
PA = pulmonary artery
PBS = pulmonary branch stenosis
PDA = patent ductus arteriosus
PFO = patent foramen ovale
Pheo = pheochromocytoma
PS = pulmonic stenosis
PV = pulmonary valve
QT = QT interval of electrocardiogram
SV = single ventricle
TAPVR = total anomalous pulmonary venous return
TGV = transposition great vessels
TOF = tetralogy of Fallot
VSD = ventricular septal defect

arteries and arterioles that are surrounded by fluid-containing airways.

Adaptation to extrauterine life is associated with dramatic changes in the fetal circulation. Many of these changes occur shortly after birth, but some may be delayed for hours or even days. The immediate change is transfer of the function of gas exchange from the placenta to the lungs, which are expanded during the initiation of breathing. Features that characterize circulatory changes after birth include the following: (1) A marked fall in pulmonary vascular resistance as pulmonary vessels enlarge and dilate in response to the increased oxygen tension to which they are exposed. Also, extravascular pressure is reduced as fetal fluid in the airways is replaced by air. As pulmonary arterial pressure falls, pulmonary blood flow increases markedly. (2) A rise in systemic vascular resistance with elimination of the low resistance placental circulation. (3) An abrupt rise in pulmonary blood flow, resulting in a rise of left atrial volume and pressure; this facilitates functional closure of the foramen ovale. (4) Functional constriction of the ductus arteriosus in response to the effects of vasoactive substances and an elevated arterial P_{O_2}. Some of the above changes may not be complete during the first few days of life. For example, (1) the pulmonary arteries and arterioles still respond vigorously to hypoxemia, hypercapnia, and acidemia by vasoconstriction, (2) right to left shunting may persist temporarily across the foramen ovale, (3) delayed closure of the ductus arteriosus may allow left to right shunting (especially in prematures) or bidirectional shunting, (4) newborns have an unusual tolerance for a low arterial P_{O_2}, and (5) there is interference with delivery of oxygen to the tissues if there is a high percentage of fetal hemoglobin; cardiac output is increased under these circumstances for proper oxygen delivery to the tissues.

Circulatory Shunts

MAGNITUDE AND DIRECTION. Factors that determine the magnitude and direction of intra- and extracardiac shunts are the size of the defect, pressure differences between the cardiac chambers or vessels, and resistance to ejection produced by outflow obstruction, as well as the ratio of systemic to pulmonary vascular resistance. Since normal systemic vascular pressures and resistances greatly exceed those in the pulmonary circuit, flow across small defects (such as ventricular septal defects) is from left to right but is limited in magnitude by the small opening. When the defect is large and nonrestrictive, peak systolic pressures in the ventricles are virtually identical, so that the direction and magnitude of flow are regulated by outflow resistance. If systemic vascular resistance significantly exceeds that in the pulmonary circuit with large defects (in the absence of pulmonic stenosis), torrential left to right shunts are present. The magnitude of the shunt is decreased as pulmonary vascular resistance approaches that in the systemic circuit, and it is bidirectional or right to left with continued increase of pulmonary resistance. When severe pulmonic stenosis is present, resistance to right ventricular ejection virtually equalizes peak systolic pressures in both ventricles so that flow across ventricular defects is right to left or bidirectional. A major determinant of direction and magnitude of shunting at the atrial level is the diastolic distensibility of the ventricles. Flow, frequently torrential, is from left to right, since the thin-walled right ventricle is easily filled even though atrial pressures are equal and low.

PULMONARY BLOOD FLOW AND SYSTEMIC DESATURATION. Right to left shunts are characteristically associated with arterial oxygen desaturation. However, the degree of desaturation is determined by pulmonary blood flow and not the magnitude of right to left shunt. When effective pulmonary blood flow is markedly reduced (as in tetralogy of Fallot), systemic venous blood is ejected preferentially through the ventricular septal defect into the left ventricle and aorta, so that arterial oxygen saturation is severely reduced and cyanosis is obvious. On the other hand, right to left shunts may be associated with torrential pulmonary blood flow (as in transposition of the great arteries with ventricular septal defect). In this situation pulmonary venous blood is almost fully saturated so that systemic arterial saturation is nearly normal. Cyanosis is not easily appreciated in the latter group of patients, but they suffer from volume loading and failure of the left ventricle.

ARTERIAL HYPOXEMIA. *Cyanosis,* a dusky purple color of the skin but especially the mucous membranes and nail beds, is due to reduced hemoglobin in the arterial blood from right to left shunts. Clinical cyanosis may not be evident until the arterial oxygen saturation is below 85 per cent (normal 94 to 98 per cent). *Clubbing* of fingers and toes is common, especially when arterial hypoxemia is marked. This sign may appear in childhood (beyond the age of one year) and is progressive. When arterial oxygen saturation returns to normal (at rest and during exercise), as occurs after surgical correction, clubbing regresses and even severe forms disappear within two to three years after operation.

Polycythemia with elevated hemoglobin and hematocrit levels results from adaptation of the hemopoietic system to the anoxic stimulus. This compensatory mechanism increases arterial oxygen content. When the hematocrit exceeds 65 to 70 per cent, blood viscosity increases so that the patient is at risk for intravascular thrombosis. Thrombi may develop in any organ system but are more frequent in the cerebral circulation (generally in the dural sinuses and cerebral veins) and pulmonary arteries. Dehydration increases the risk of intravascular thrombosis. Headaches are common in severely polycythemic patients (see Eisenmenger Syndrome, p 241). The combination of iron deficiency anemia and polycythemia is not well tolerated and may result in increasing dyspnea and heart failure. There is greater risk for intravascular thrombosis, and iron therapy is required even though this results in a further elevation of hematocrit. Severely polycythemic patients have a delicate balance between intravascular thrombosis and bleeding from coagulation defects. The more frequent abnormalities associated with a bleeding diathesis are a combination of thrombocytopenia, accelerated fibrinolysis, hypofibrinogenemia, prolonged prothrombin time, and prolonged partial thromboplastin time. These laboratory test results should be evaluated cautiously, since many are influenced by variations in technique (especially in polycythemic blood with a small plasma volume) that may result in falsely abnormal findings. Nevertheless they should be undertaken in patients who are to undergo elective cardiac or noncardiac surgery.

Hypoxic ("blue") spells occur primarily in infants with hypoxemia, especially when the underlying defect is tetralogy of Fallot. These spells consist of a sudden onset of dyspnea, restlessness, increased cyanosis, gasping respirations, and syncope. They are associated with a further decrease of arterial P_{O_2} and a reduction of an already compromised pulmonary blood flow. These frightening episodes are treated by placing the child in a knee-chest position and by administering oxygen and intravenous bicarbonate if acidemia develops. The frequency and severity of these episodes can be reduced by oral propranolol. However, surgical treatment is generally indicated to increase pulmonary blood flow and thus relieve the hypoxemia.

Squatting is common in children with hypoxemia (especially tetralogy of Fallot), who may assume a squatting position to relieve dyspnea associated with exertion. Physical activity is normally resumed within a few minutes. Squatting decreases the magnitude of right to left shunt by increasing systemic vascular resistance and pulmonary blood flow. Adults seldom squat because they know the limitation of their exercise tolerance and discontinue physical activity before arterial P_{O_2} is significantly decreased.

BRAIN ABSCESS AND PARADOXIC EMBOLUS. Brain abscess occurs in older children and adults. Predisposing factors include previous occlusive microcirculatory disease from thrombosis or emboli. Clinical recognition may be difficult because the onset is insidious, symptoms are vague, and fever is low grade. In others, the onset is more acute, with headache, seizures, and localized neurologic signs that are dependent on the size and site of the abscess and the presence of increased intracranial pressure. The diagnosis is established with computed axial tomography. Treatment is with antibiotic therapy, generally followed by surgical drainage. In patients with right to left shunts, venous blood bypasses the lungs so that emboli arising from systemic veins enter the systemic circulation directly to occlude an artery anywhere in the body, especially the brain. This complication is rare.

PULMONARY HYPERTENSION. This complication, common in congenital heart disease, results from increased pulmonary blood flow and/or resistance. Torrential pulmonary blood flow (as in secundum atrial septal defects) can be accommodated by the pulmonary circulation without increase in pressure. Pulmonary hypertension develops frequently in the presence of large defects at the ventricular level or communications between the aorta and pulmonary arteries. In infants and small children with these defects, "hyperkinetic" pulmonary hypertension is present. This term refers to a vasoactive pulmonary bed that undergoes vasodilation in response to oxygen or tolazoline. These agents reduce the level of pulmonary arterial pressure by pulmonary vasodilation even though pulmonary blood flow increases. Hyperkinetic pulmonary hypertension is uncommon in adults but is seen in some with secundum atrial septal defects. Generally pulmonary vascular disease is present in adults, so that pulmonary vascular resistance is greatly increased even when pulmonary blood flow is not excessive (see Eisenmenger Syndrome, p 241). The status of the pulmonary vascular bed determines the clinical picture, prognosis, and feasibility of surgical treatment of intra- and extracardiac shunts. The goal of management is to prevent the development of severe pulmonary vascular changes by surgical ablation of the shunt. This implies serial measurements of pulmonary and systemic pressures and resistances, especially in infants and toddlers with large ventricular or aortopulmonary defects.

SHUNT LESIONS

Atrial Septal Defect

Atrial septal defects occur more frequently in females and are designated according to their site in the septum. The most common are in the region of the fossa ovalis (*ostium secundum defect*) and are among the most prevalent congenital cardiac anomalies in adults. A less frequent variety (*sinus venosus defect*) occupies the upper part of the atrial septum and is closely related to the entry of the superior vena cava. This structure receives one or more anomalously draining pulmonary veins, usually from the right lung. (The *ostium primum defect* is discussed under Endocardial Cushion Defect, p 230.)

The principal factors that determine the magnitude of the left to right shunt are the size of the defect, the relative compliance of the cardiac chambers, and the vascular resistances in the pulmonary and systemic circulations. If the defect is moderate or large (>2 cm in diameter in an adult), the greater distensibility of the right atrium and ventricle and the low pulmonary vascular resistance allow a torrential left to right shunt. On the other hand, in infancy the relatively thick and less compliant right ventricle limits the magnitude of left to right shunts. Large defects with torrential left to right shunts produce right atrial and ventricular enlargement, which encroaches on the left-sided chambers. Pulmonary pressures and resistances are generally normal. In the unusual instances in which they are elevated, the pulmonary circulation remains vasoactive, so that pressures and resistances return to normal after surgical ablation of the shunt. Those with severe pulmonary vascular disease are described under Eisenmenger Syndrome (p 241).

DIAGNOSIS. Although symptoms are trivial and physical signs subtle, the diagnosis is usually made during childhood. However, many escape detection in the first decade of life and are recognized in later years only because of effort dyspnea and fatigue. Superimposed coronary artery disease or systemic hypertension can cause the left ventricle to be less distensible, favoring the development or worsening of these symptoms because of a further increase in left to right shunt and right volume overload. In some instances the presence of the defect is first appreciated when pulmonary hypertension develops with persistence of a torrential left to right shunt. The advent of atrial arrhythmias, fibrillation, flutter, or paroxysms of supraventricular tachycardia is not well tolerated. These events increase in frequency beyond the fourth decade. Some patients with an uncomplicated atrial septal defect are recognized for the first time because of an abnormal "routine" chest roentgenogram.

In children failure to gain weight is common but by no means the rule. The characteristic physical appearance is that of a thin child with nearly normal height and a gracile habitus. Generally adults have a normal physical appearance but again some are thin and gracile. The jugular venous pulse shows "a" and "v" waves of equal heights because the atria are in free communication. Dominant "a" waves suggest the presence of pulmonary hypertension, and dominant "v" waves are associated with tricuspid regurgitation. Right ventricular volume overload results in an easily palpable left parasternal lift. The importance of this sign cannot be overemphasized and in some the dilated pulmonary artery is palpated in the second left interspace. The soft ejection systolic murmur, seldom accompanied by a thrill, is best heard at the upper left sternal edge and is produced by increased blood flow into the pulmonary artery. The murmur, especially a loud one, is widely transmitted to the chest anteriorly and posteriorly, especially in slightly built patients. The murmur is preceded by an accentuated first heart sound and sometimes by a pulmonic ejection sound. The auscultatory hallmark is the easily audible, widely split second heart sound. This split is virtually fixed in all phases of respiration and during the Valsalva maneuver. When the defect is large, a mid-diastolic murmur is audible at the lower left sternal edge and is produced by torrential flow across the tricuspid valve. An early diastolic murmur of pulmonary regurgitation may accompany pulmonary hypertension, but this is rare.

The *electrocardiogram* shows right axis deviation and right ventricular hypertrophy (generally rsR^1 in right precordial leads). This pattern is due to terminal depolarization of the hypertrophied right ventricular outflow tract. Less frequent findings include tall P waves (because of right atrial enlargement), complete right bundle branch block, a prolonged P-R interval, and Wolff-Parkinson-White syndrome. Supraventricular arrhythmias may be detected in untreated adults or many years after surgical closure of the defect. These consist of atrial fibrillation or flutter, paroxysmal atrial tachycardia, and multiple premature atrial contractions. Left axis deviation usually denotes the presence of an ostium primum atrial defect but is seen occasionally in secundum defects. Another rare finding is a normal electrocardiogram.

The *chest roentgenogram* is often distinctive, especially in adults. Varying degrees of cardiac enlargement are due to dilatation of the right atrium and ventricle, which displaces the normal or relatively small left-sided chambers posteriorly. The large pulmonary trunk contrasts with the smaller aortic knob, which is especially notable on the posteroanterior view. The primary branches of the pulmonary artery are enlarged and the vascularity increased toward the periphery of both lung fields.

Echocardiography not only is diagnostic but also is useful in excluding other suspected anomalies. In uncomplicated secundum atrial defects the right ventricular end-diastolic dimension is increased and the ventricular septal motion is flat or paradoxical. Real-time two-dimensional echocardiograms define the location and size of the defect and also confirm the significant enlargement of the right atrium. The deformity of the ventricular septum resulting from right ventricular volume overload is recognized, and its encroachment into the left ventricular cavity is visualized. Flow disturbance across the interatrial septum can be detected by measurements based on the Doppler principle. The pulmonary and aortic flows can be estimated by two-dimensional echo and Doppler techniques, and the difference between these flows represents the shunt volume. *Mitral valve prolapse* may be associated with secundum atrial septal defects and in many instances the suspicion is raised by the echocardiogram. Since various criteria are used for the echo diagnosis of mitral valve prolapse, caution should be exercised in the diagnosis of combined atrial septal defect and mitral valve prolapse. It is probable that the association has been overestimated.

There is an ongoing debate about whether *cardiac catheterization* is indicated in all patients. Physical examination supplemented by the electrocardiogram and chest roentgenogram usually suggests the diagnosis. This can be confirmed by visualizing the site of the defect by echocardiography and estimating the pulmonary-systemic flow ratio. However, this view is not held universally and some prefer to confirm the shunt by demonstration of a step-up in oxygen concentration between the vena cava and the right atrium, to define the site of entry of pulmonary veins, and to measure the level of pulmonary arterial pressure and resistance. The study should be undertaken in the adult in whom pulmonary hypertension or coexisting coronary artery disease is suspected.

NATURAL HISTORY. The vast majority of secundum atrial septal defects are recognized and treated surgically during childhood or adolescence. Spontaneous closure does occur, but this is usually prior to the age of about three years. Although life expectancy is shortened, adult survival is the rule and some live to an advanced age. Pregnancy is usually well tolerated, especially in women who were asymptomatic prior to pregnancy.

COMPLICATIONS. After the age of 40 years complications are frequent, and most patients who survive beyond the age of 60 years show symptoms of effort dyspnea and fatigue. Death may be unrelated to the defect, but when a relationship exists cardiac failure is the most common cause. Heart failure may be due to right ventricular failure alone or may be intensified by a dilated tricuspid valve ring with resultant incompetence. The prevalence of atrial arrhythmias increases after the fourth decade and may precipitate heart failure, especially when the ventricular response is rapid in the presence of a large shunt. Coronary artery disease or systemic hypertension may result in a less distensible left ventricle, which favors an increase in left to right shunting. Pulmonary hypertension may be due to the high pulmonary blood flow or may progress to a state in which pulmonary and systemic vascular resistances are virtually identical and the shunt is abolished or reversed (see Eisenmenger Syndrome, p 241). Infective endocarditis is rare in isolated lesions.

TREATMENT. Treatment is surgical ablation of the shunt, especially when the pulmonary systemic flow ratio exceeds 2:1. This is preferably accomplished between the ages of about 3 and 4 years, when the surgical risk is minimal. In these young patients the right ventricular dimension returns to normal. Surgical treatment in older children and adolescents usually improves the size of the right-sided chambers, but they may not return to normal. When the operation is performed in adults, patchy fibrosis of the chronically volume-loaded right ventricle persists, as does some degree of right ventricular dilatation. These residua may explain the blunted chronotropic response during exercise, with resultant decreased cardiac output and decreased working capacity. Nevertheless, patients in the fifth, sixth, or even seventh decade with high pulmonary blood flow and low resistance benefit from surgical repair, which can be done with a comparatively low risk. Defects in older patients can be closed surgically at an acceptable risk despite moderate pulmonary hypertension and cardiac failure, provided there is still a significant left to right shunt. Operation is contraindicated when pulmonary vascular resistance is greatly elevated so that the shunt is abolished or reversed. Late-onset arrhythmias occur in fewer than 5 per cent, 10 to 20 years after surgery. The commonest are atrial flutter, atrial fibrillation, paroxysmal supraventricular tachycardia, and frequent premature atrial contractions. Less frequent arrhythmias are sick sinus syndrome, junctional tachycardia, and complete heart block.

Lutembacher's Syndrome

This condition consists of a secundum atrial septal defect with acquired mitral stenosis. Obstruction to left ventricular inflow aggravates the left to right shunt across the atrial septum. Atrial fibrillation is common. A prominent jugular "a" wave is visible because left atrial pressure is transmitted to the right atrium and the systemic venous return. Physical findings resemble those described under secundum atrial septal defects. Auscultatory findings of mitral stenosis are present but may not be obvious. The echocardiogram is diagnostic in that signs of mitral stenosis are superimposed on right ventricular volume overload. Patients with this condition derive great symptomatic relief after intracardiac repair.

Endocardial Cushion Defect

The embryonic endocardial cushions contribute to the development of the mitral and tricuspid valves and to the growth and convergence of the atrial and ventricular septum. Maldevelopment during this stage of cardiac morphogenesis results in varying degrees of complex malformations involving the atrioventricular valves and the atrial and ventricular septa. The *ostium primum defect* is situated in the lower portion of the atrial septum overlying both the mitral and tricuspid valves. A cleft in the anterior leaflet to the mitral valve is usual, and the tricuspid valve is frequently thickened but otherwise normal. The ventricular septum is intact functionally. *Common atrioventricular canal* (complete endocardial cushion defect) consists of a common defect of both the intra-atrial and intraventricular septa with a single atrioventricular valve. This valve, common to both ventricles, has an anterior and posterior leaflet with a lateral leaflet in each ventricle. This anomaly is relatively common in patients with Down's syndrome. *Transitional forms* are intermediate between atrioventricular canal and ostium primum defects.

OSTIUM PRIMUM DEFECTS. Ostium primum defects may be associated with recurrent lower respiratory tract infections with or without congestive heart failure during infancy and early childhood. However, the majority are asymptomatic and are recognized because of the murmur of mitral incompetence. In others, the degree of mitral regurgitation is trivial. The physical signs resemble those of ostium secundum defects with superimposed mitral regurgitation. The electrocardiogram is distinctive in that there is a superior counterclockwise frontal plane axis (left axis deviation), varying degrees of right ventricular hypertrophy (rsR^1 is common), and sometimes voltage criteria for left ventricular hypertrophy because of mitral regurgitation. The chest radiograph simulates an ostium secundum atrial septal defect. The echocardiogram is also characteristic, showing enlargement of both right ventricle and right atrium, a low lying atrial septal defect, and a cleft in the anterior mitral leaflet. The mitral valve apparatus is displaced so that the anterior mitral leaflet encroaches upon the left ventricular outflow. Cardiac catheterization demonstrates the left to right atrial shunt, the level of pulmonary arterial pressure, and the degree of mitral valve incompetence. Left ventriculography shows the characteristic "goose-neck" deformity produced by the abnormal position of the mitral valve. Surgical treatment is advised during infancy or childhood with the purpose of obliterating the left to right shunt and alleviating mitral valve incompetence. In adult life, many years after surgery, atrial arrhythmias may occur as described under secundum atrial septal defect. In addition, a small number of patients have progressive mitral valve incompetence that may require mitral valve replacement.

COMPLETE ATRIOVENTRICULAR CANAL. Congestive cardiac failure, significant elevation of pulmonary artery pressures, and resistances and intercurrent pulmonary infections are common during infancy. At that time surgical treatment is undertaken to attempt to prevent progression of these complications. Without treatment, survival of these patients to adolescence and adult life is usually associated with the development of severe pulmonary vascular disease (see Eisenmenger Syndrome, p 241) or congenital obstruction to right ventricular outflow, which limits pulmonary blood flow.

Ventricular Septal Defect

The commonest form of congenital heart disease is an isolated ventricular septal defect. Perimembranous defects are the most frequent; when viewed from the left ventricle the defect is immediately below the aortic valve, and when viewed from the right ventricle it is below the crista supraventricularis and closely related to the tricuspid valve. Less frequently, the defects occur in the subpulmonic (supracristal) region, in the inflow portion of the right ventricle (posterior), or in the midseptal or apical area of the muscle, where they are frequently multiple. The magnitude of the shunt depends on the size of the defect and status of the pulmonary vascular bed. A small defect limits the size of the left to right shunt so that cardiac chambers are normal in size and pulmonary arterial pressures and resistances remain within normal limits. Large defects are associated with a marked increase in pulmonary blood flow, as well as varying degrees of elevation of pulmonary arterial pressures and resistance. In these instances pulmonary vascular disease may be progressive, so that systemic and pulmonary vascular resistances are virtually equal (Eisenmenger syndrome). In the neonatal period a large nonrestrictive ventricular septal defect may not be easily appreciated because pulmonary vascular resistance remains high, which limits the left to right shunt. However, within a few weeks signs of the defect are present because a fall in pulmonary vascular resistance is associated with left to right shunting.

SMALL VENTRICULAR SEPTAL DEFECTS. A small defect produces a prominent pansystolic murmur heard best at the lower left sternal edge in a patient who is otherwise normal. Spontaneous closure of the defect is frequent, especially in the first year of life, and is estimated to occur in more than one half of instances. If the defect does not close spontaneously within the first three years of life, it is likely that the clinical condition will remain unchanged. These patients are generally asymptomatic and have a normal heart size. A systolic thrill may be palpable at the lower left sternal edge and is accompanied by a harsh, loud pansystolic murmur that is widely distributed but loudest at the site of the thrill. The electrocardiogram and chest roentgenogram are normal. Generally these defects are too small to be visualized by two-dimensional echocardiograms, although turbulence is recorded in the right ventricle by the Doppler principle, especially the outflow. It is now believed that spontaneous closure of a small ventricular septal defect occurs in early adult life. This notion is based on the fact that congenital ventricular septal defects are seldom seen in older adults. The mechanism of spontaneous closure is not clearly established, and it has been suggested that a small aneurysm develops at the site of the defect and protrudes into the right ventricle and the tip of the aneurysm gets progressively smaller until it ultimately closes. Another mechanism is closure of the defect by a part of the tricuspid valve leaflet. This can be recognized clinically by a change in the auscultatory findings in that the intensity and length of the murmur decrease and the thrill disappears. Sometimes the development of an ejection click, presumably related to the ventricular septal aneurysm, heralds a course that in a few years is associated with complete disappearance of all abnormal auscultatory findings when the defect is completely closed. Uncomplicated small ventricular septal defects do not require surgical closure and the only treatment is prophylaxis against infective endocarditis.

LARGE VENTRICULAR SEPTAL DEFECTS. Large defects with unrestricted flow from the left to the right ventricle and into the pulmonary vascular bed are common in early life and rare in adults. These defects are associated with increased pulmonary vascular pressure and resistance. Furthermore, volume loading of the left heart may lead to superimposed left ventricular failure. Symptoms are present during infancy, especially between the ages of two and six months, and are produced by congestive cardiac failure, poor physical development, and recurrent pulmonary infections. These infants may respond to anticongestive measures with improvement of signs of congestive heart failure and pulmonary hypertension. If this improvement is maintained, especially beyond the age of one year, the defect frequently decreases in size, with continuing clinical improvement. However, in a significant number response to therapy is not maintained, physical development remains poor, and signs of pulmonary hypertension persist. In these instances surgical closure of the defect is indicated, since the mortality rate from surgery is acceptably low and soon after operation there is a growth spurt when heart failure and pulmonary hypertension regress.

Clinical improvement in some babies with a large ventricular septal defect may be due to the development of *acquired pulmonic stenosis,* which limits pulmonary blood flow. Generally, right ventricular outflow tract obstruction is due to infundibular hypertrophy and is progressive. During infancy or early childhood the clinical course changes in that signs of heart failure improve and heart size decreases because pulmonary blood flow is limited by the pulmonic stenosis. Right ventricular pressure rises to approximately that of the left ventricle, with resultant right to left shunting and cyanosis. The clinical picture resembles that of tetralogy of Fallot (p 233).

VENTRICULAR SEPTAL DEFECT WITH AORTIC REGURGITATION. The ventricular septal defect is usually small or moderate in size and its presence is known from infancy. During childhood or adolescence aortic valve regurgitation occurs because of prolapse of the right, or at times, the noncoronary cusp. The clinical picture is extremely variable, from the asymptomatic child with a small left to right shunt and trivial aortic regurgitation to the symptomatic young adult with congestive cardiac failure, angina pectoris, massive cardiomegaly, and florid aortic regurgitation. The latter patient requires surgical closure of the defect and relief of aortic regurgitation; this generally requires aortic valve replacement. The asymptomatic patient with mild regurgitation needs to be observed closely. Some believe that closure of the ventricular defect will prevent further prolapse of the aortic valve. Others recommend simultaneous aortic valvuloplasty prior to the development of significant valvular regurgitation and left ventricular dysfunction.

VENTRICULAR SEPTAL DEFECT WITH LEFT VENTRICULAR–RIGHT ATRIAL SHUNT. The membranous ventricular septum (atrioventricular septum) is divided by the insertions of the tricuspid valve and the mitral valve. The insertion of the tricuspid valve is below that of the mitral. Thus, this area is common to the right atrium and left ventricle, and a defect in this area allows shunting from the left ventricle directly into the right atrium. In others the defect is below the tricuspid valve and is associated with an abnormal tricuspid septal leaflet. The physical signs simulate those of an isolated small to moderate ventricular septal defect. If the shunt is above the tricuspid valve, cardiac catheterization demonstrates a left to right shunt at the atrial level which may be confused with an atrial septal defect; this issue is resolved by the fact that the physical signs are not compatible with an atrial septal defect and left ventriculography demonstrates direct opacification of the right atrium from the left ventricle. This condition should be treated surgically.

OTHER DEFECTS ASSOCIATED WITH VENTRICULAR SEPTAL DEFECTS. ***Patent Ductus Arteriosus.*** In some instances the murmurs of both lesions are audible, so that a continuous murmur is present at the upper left sternal edge and a holosystolic murmur is heard at the lower left sternal edge. However, in many patients both murmurs may not be discernible and the physical findings are dominated by either the ventricular defect or the patent ductus arteriosus. Real-time echocardiography combined with the Doppler technique is helpful in the diagnosis in that there is evidence of shunting at the ventricular level as well as visualization of the patent ductus arteriosus. Left ventriculography demonstrates the ventricular septal defect, and aortography is necessary to confirm the associated ductus arteriosus if this structure is not entered directly by the catheter from the pulmonary artery.

Secundum Atrial Septal Defect. In patients with a ventricular septal defect and an ostium secundum atrial septal defect, the clinical picture is usually dominated by the ventricular defect. This combination of defects is more likely to be present during infancy and may result in torrential pulmonary blood flow, pulmonary hypertension, and congestive heart failure. The defects are recognized by real-time echocardiography and if uncontrolled by medical measures are both treated surgically during the same procedure.

Coarctation of the Aorta. Signs of coarctation of the aorta usually dominate, and sometimes the signs of ventricular septal defect are erroneously attributed to the collateral circulation associated with coarctation.

Communications Between the Aorta and Pulmonary Arteries

PATENT DUCTUS ARTERIOSUS. During fetal life most of the pulmonary arterial blood flows through the ductus arteriosus to the descending aorta for oxygenation in the placenta. Physiologic occlusion soon after birth is due to a number of factors, including the marked increase in arterial oxygen tension that accompanies the onset of ventilation and changes in the metabolism of vasoactive substances, especially prostaglandins. In the normal baby anatomic closure is generally complete several weeks after birth. Persistent patency of the ductus arteriosus is more frequent in females, in premature babies, in infants born at high altitude, and in infants whose first trimester of intrauterine life is complicated by maternal rubella. The aortic end of the ductus is opposite the origin of the left subclavian artery and the vessel enters the pulmonary artery, usually at its bifurcation.

The hemodynamic effects of a patent ductus arteriosus depend on the size of the communication, the length of the ductus, and the resistance relationships between the systemic and pulmonary circulations. Generally, the flow through the ductus is small to moderate so that pulmonary arterial pressures and resistances remain normal. These patients usually are asymptomatic, and the only abnormal physical sign is a typical continuous murmur. This murmur, sometimes accompanied by a thrill, is heard best at the upper left sternal edge, rises to a peak in late systole, continues without interruption through the second sound, and wanes during the course of diastole. Larger shunts with a significant aortic runoff result in a wide pulse pressure and a "waterhammer" or bounding arterial pulse. The left atrium and ventricle enlarge to accommodate the increased pulmonary blood flow, and this is recognized by a lateral and downward displacement of the apical impulse, which is lifting in character. The typical continuous murmur is still present, but in addition an apical mid-diastolic murmur may be audible because of increased flow across the mitral valve. In mature infants and sometimes older children congestive cardiac failure may supervene. When pulmonary arterial pressure and resistance rise to systemic levels, flow across the ductus is limited. In patients with pulmonary hypertension effort dyspnea is common, the wide pulse pressure disappears, and right ventricular enlargement is prominent. The auscultatory findings are dominated by those produced by pulmonary hypertension in that the typical continuous murmur disappears and is replaced by a short systolic murmur frequently preceded by an ejection click, a booming second heart sound due to loud pulmonary valve closure, and sometimes an early diastolic murmur of pulmonary valve incompetence. Occasionally the shunt through the ductus is reversed so that the descending aorta is perfused with desaturated pulmonary arterial blood. This results in cyanotic lower extremities with clubbing of the toes and normal color and shape of the fingers and fingernails.

The *electrocardiographic findings* depend on the hemodynamic consequences. The electrocardiogram is normal when the ductus is small. Moderate or large flows result in left ventricular hypertrophy associated with increased R wave voltage in the left precordial and inferior leads, and with tall, peaked T waves that may flatten or become inverted as left ventricular volume overload increases. In the presence of severe pulmonary hypertension right ventricular hypertrophy dominates. The *chest roentgenogram* is normal if the flow is small. With larger flows the heart is enlarged because of left atrial and left ventricular prominence, the pulmonary arterial trunk and aorta are enlarged, and there is pulmonary plethora. With the development of severe pulmonary hypertension, heart size decreases, there is prominence of the right ventricle and especially the main pulmonary artery, and the size of the aorta may not be increased. In older patients calcification of the ductus may be present. The *echocardiogram* defines and identifies the degree of chamber enlargement and visualizes the ductus. Evidence of continuous flow is recorded using the Doppler technique from the ductus arteriosus and the major pulmonary arteries.

Generally patency of the ductus arteriosus is recognized during childhood because of the presence of a typical murmur. *Surgical correction* is advisable by division of the ductus. In the adult with a large left to right shunt and normal pulmonary vascular resistance surgery is also advised. Extensive calcification of the ductus increases the surgical risk, but surgery should still be advised if the shunt is large. Occasionally, an adult is seen with a small, hemodynamically insignificant patent ductus. The decision of surgical treatment for these patients must take into account that they are at risk for infective endocarditis, but on the other hand they may remain asymptomatic and some may experience spontaneous closure of the defect. Thus individual judgment is required in these patients.

In very low birth weight infants (weighing less than 1500 grams), persistent patency of the ductus arteriosus is common. The left to right shunt increases the severity of respiratory distress syndrome. Generally, these babies are treated with oxygen (to maintain a PaO_2 between 50 and 70 torr), fluid restriction, diuretic therapy, and correction of anemia. Positive pressure ventilation or continuous positive airway pressure may be required. If these measures fail, manipulation of the ductus arteriosus is undertaken to decrease the left to right shunt. This may be accomplished by prostaglandin synthesis inhibitors (indomethacin) or surgical ligation.

AORTIC-PULMONARY SEPTAL DEFECT. This rare anomaly consists of a communication between the ascending aorta and the pulmonary arterial trunk. The defect is generally large and associated with a torrential pulmonary blood flow and pulmonary hypertension. Symptoms are usual during infancy and childhood and consist of those produced by congestive cardiac failure. In the absence of severe pulmonary hypertension the signs are dominated by a wide pulse pressure, cardiomegaly, a systolic murmur at the left and right upper sternal edges, and occasionally a continuous murmur. The electrocardiogram generally shows biventricular hypertrophy, although isolated left or right dominance may be present. Roentgenographic examination of the chest defines the degree of cardiomegaly and shows prominence of the pulmonary artery and ascending aorta, as well as pulmonary plethora. The echocardiogram is helpful in defining the presence to two semilunar valves (which excludes the diagnosis of truncus arteriosus) and shows a normal relationship of a large aorta and pulmonary artery. The diagnosis is confirmed by aortography, with injection of contrast into the root of the aorta and/or left ventricle; these studies identify the anomaly. The hemodynamic effects are measured at the same time by cardiac catheterization. These defects usually require surgical correction.

TRUNCUS ARTERIOSUS. A single arterial trunk supplies the systemic, pulmonary, and coronary circulations. Both ventricles eject blood through a ventricular septal defect into the single trunk. The number of semilunar valve cusps varies from two to six and in most patients pulmonary arteries arise from the ascending portion of the truncus proximal to the origin of the innominate artery. When the major source of pulmonary blood flow is from the bronchial arteries or other vessels from the descending thoracic aorta, the condition is considered to be pulmonary atresia with ventricular septal defect (previously known as truncus arteriosus type IV or pseudotruncus arteriosus).

In the majority the pulmonary blood flow, pressure, and resistance are greatly increased, so that signs of heart failure appear in infancy. Cyanosis is minimal or absent. The heart is usually enlarged, the precordium is hyperdynamic, a systolic ejection murmur sometimes preceded by a click is audible along the left sternal edge, and the second heart sound is loud and generally single, although it may be split. Occasional patients survive infancy because of the development of severe pulmonary vascular disease which limits pulmonary blood flow. The clinical picture in these patients simulates that of the Eisenmenger syndrome. Incompetence of the truncal valve or less frequently stenosis of this valve may complicate the picture at any age. The diagnosis is confirmed by cardiac catheterization and angiocardiography. Since rapid deterioration is frequent during infancy, surgical treatment is advised, at which time the ventricular septal defect is closed, the pulmonary arteries are detached from the truncus, and a tubular conduit is inserted from the right ventricle to the pulmonary arteries.

Communication Shunts Between the Aortic Root and the Right Heart

CORONARY ARTERIAL FISTULA. A fistulous branch, most frequently from the right coronary artery, enters the right atrium or right ventricle and occasionally the pulmonary trunk. The right coronary artery becomes massively dilated. Although the volume of shunt from the coronary artery to the right heart is variable, it is usually small. The diagnosis is suspected when an atypically located continuous precordial murmur is heard. Since the shunt is frequently small, the electrocardiogram and chest x-ray are normal. Studies using the Doppler technique will demonstrate the site of entry of the fistula in that a continuous murmur is present at this site. The diagnosis is confirmed with an aortic root injection of contrast material that demonstrates the large tortuous right coronary artery and its site of entry into the right heart. Surgical treatment is advised because the risk is low, blood flow in the right coronary artery is channeled in the proper direction, and the risk of endocarditis is eliminated.

CONGENITAL ANEURYSMS OF THE SINUSES OF VALSALVA. The usual aneurysm involves the right or noncoronary sinus, which begins as a blind pouch or diverticulum. The aneurysms may remain as unruptured diverticula but usually enter the right ventricle or right atrium. Patients with these aneurysms are generally asymptomatic and the left to right shunt is small. The diagnosis is suspected because of an atypically located continuous murmur and confirmed by injection of contrast material into the ascending aorta, which outlines the abnormality. Surgical treatment is advisable even in asymptomatic patients. Acute rupture of a large aneurysm in a previously healthy young adult produces a dramatic clinical picture. This is characterized by sudden onset of dyspnea, chest pain, brisk arterial pulses, and a loud continuous murmur. Cardiac failure with pulmonary edema supervenes rapidly. The electrocardiogram shows left or combined ventricular hypertrophy. The chest x-ray shows cardiomegaly with prominent vascular markings due to pulmonary arterial overcirculation and prominent pulmonary veins and signs of pulmonary edema. The diagnosis is confirmed by two-dimensional echocardiography and Doppler methods, supplemented by cardiac catheterization and aortography. Surgical correction is urgently indicated in acute rupture.

ANOMALOUS ORIGIN OF THE LEFT CORONARY ARTERY FROM THE PULMONARY TRUNK. The right coronary artery originates normally from the aorta, and the left coronary artery receives blood from intercoronary anastomoses so that blood flow in the left coronary artery drains *into* the pulmonary trunk. Thus, left ventricular myocardial perfusion is significantly compromised. Generally symptoms are present within the first few months of life because of myocardial infarction, congestive cardiac failure, and mitral valve incompetence due to papillary muscle dysfunction. Surgical treatment to re-establish normal perfusion of the left coronary artery from the aorta is advised if there is failure of medical therapy. In those who improve with anticongestive medication, surgical therapy can be postponed for one to three years when the risk of surgery is small. About 15 per cent of patients with this anomaly reach adult life because of exuberant intercoronary anastomoses, which may produce a continuous murmur. The electrocardiogram is important because signs of anterior and anterolateral myocardial infarction are present in a relatively young person. The chest x-ray shows cardiomegaly with dominance of the left ventricle. The origin of the left coronary artery from the aorta cannot be demonstrated by real-time echocardiography. The diagnosis is confirmed by selective right coronary arteriography, which demonstrates the dilated right coronary artery, the intercoronary anastomoses, and opacification of the left coronary artery from these anastomoses as it enters the pulmonary artery. Reconstitution of normal coronary flow from the aorta to the left coronary artery is advised, although in many instances fibrosis of the left ventricle has resulted in permanent damage to ventricular function.

Pulmonary Arteriovenous Fistula

Fistulous communications between the pulmonary arteries and pulmonary veins may be multiple, small, and diffuse in both lungs or large and relatively localized. Hereditary hemorrhagic telangiectasia (Rendu-Osler-Weber syndrome) with angiomata of the buccal and nasal mucous membranes, gastrointestinal tract, and liver is present in about one half of patients or other members of their family. Desaturated pulmonary arterial blood flows through the fistula and enters the pulmonary vein without oxygenation. When total flow across the fistulous communications is significant, left atrial and left ventricular blood is desaturated, resulting in cyanosis and digital clubbing. Pulmonary arterial pressure remains normal because the flow across the fistula is at low pressure and resistance; cardiomegaly is unusual and heart failure uncommon. Hemoptysis may occur and is sometimes massive. Recurrent epistaxes and gastrointestinal bleeding are features of hereditary hemorrhagic telangiectasia. Transitory central nervous symptoms, including dizziness, vertigo, speech disturbances, visual aberrations, motor weakness, and convulsions, may result from paradoxic emboli, cerebral thromboses, or abscess. Findings on auscultation of the chest may be normal; in others soft systolic or continuous murmurs are audible anywhere in the chest. The electrocardiogram is usually normal. Roentgenographic examination of the chest shows the presence of large fistulas only. Selective pulmonary arteriography is diagnostic and visualizes the site, extent, and distribution of the fistulas. Large localized fistulous communications are treated surgically by lobectomy or wedge resection. Smaller communications may be obliterated by embolization; these emboli are introduced selectively through a strategically placed catheter in the branch of the pulmonary artery that feeds the fistula. Successful treatment is usually followed by disappearance of symptoms, although in some there is postoperative growth of small previously unrecognized fistulas and recurrence of symptoms.

OBSTRUCTIVE LESIONS WITH OR WITHOUT SHUNTS

Tetralogy of Fallot

The tetralogy of Fallot comprises a combination of four defects consisting of (1) right ventricular outflow tract obstruction (pulmonic stenosis), (2) ventricular septal defect, (3) overriding of the aorta above the ventricular defect, and (4) right ventricular hypertrophy. The pulmonic stenosis is usually a combination of obstruction at the valve as well as in the right ventricular outflow. The pulmonary arterial trunk may be short and smaller than normal and there may be branch stenosis. The pulmonary valve is often bicuspid, may have a small ring, and occasionally is the only site of obstruction. Infundibular stenosis is produced by hypertrophy of the crista supraventricularis. Occasionally, right ventricular outflow is completely obstructed (pulmonary atresia) and pulmonary blood flow is maintained by a patent ductus arteriosus and/or collateral flow via bronchial arteries. The ventricular septal defect is generally large, approximating the size of the aortic orifice, and is related to the right and posterior aortic cusps. The ascending aorta is displaced anteriorly (dextraposed) and the aortic arch is to the right in about 20 per cent.

The severity of right ventricular outflow tract obstruction determines the hemodynamics and therefore the clinical picture. In the presence of severe obstruction, pulmonary blood flow is decreased and blood is shunted from the right ventricle across the ventricular defect into the aorta. This right to left shunt results in systemic hypoxemia manifested as marked cyanosis, digital clubbing, and polycythemia. When obstruction to right ventricular outflow and a ventricular septal defect coexist without right to left shunting, the condition is known as acyanotic tetralogy of Fallot.

In severe cases, *cyanosis* is present from birth. In others, this finding is present in infancy, generally before the first birthday. The absence of cyanosis in the neonatal period is related to maintenance of pulmonary blood flow via a patent ductus arteriosus, which closes spontaneously in the first few months of life. Cyanosis increases in intensity progressively during the first years and is associated with poor physical development. *Dyspnea* with exertion is usual. Toddlers play actively for a short time and rest by assuming a squatting position for the relief of dyspnea; others sit or lie down and then are able to resume physical activity within a few minutes. *Paroxysmal dyspneic attacks* (anoxic blue spells) may be a major problem during the first two years of life (see p 228).

Physical examination confirms the presence of delayed growth and development, cyanosis, and clubbing. Characteristically, the heart size is normal but the apical impulse is tapping owing to right ventricular hypertrophy. The systolic murmur, sometimes accompanied by a thrill, is produced by the right ventricular outflow tract obstruction. Auscultatory findings are variable; the systolic murmur, which is loudest at the upper left sternal edge but is widely transmitted, may be ejection in type or pansystolic. The murmur is less intense when the obstruction is severe. Aortic blood flow is increased, and this may result in an early ejection click. The second heart sound is single, produced by aortic valve closure, and pulmonary valve closure is generally inaudible. In rare instances a systolic and diastolic murmur may be audible in any part of the chest, anteriorly or posteriorly, and is produced by bronchial collateral flow to the lung or rarely by a patent ductus arteriosus. This auscultatory finding is frequent with pulmonary atresia.

Roentgenographically the heart size is normal, with a rounded elevated cardiac apex likened to a wooden shoe (coeur en sabot). There is a concavity in the region of the main pulmonary artery, and the pulmonary vasculature is diminished. The aorta is large and arches to the right in 20 per cent. The *electrocardiogram* shows right axis deviation and right ventricular hypertrophy. Sometimes the P wave is tall and peaked. *Echocardiography* demonstrates the major intracardiac abnormalities. Real-time examinations show the large ventricular septal defect, the degree of aortic override, and the thick right ventricle; the right ventricular outflow tract obstruction may be visualized or inferred from Doppler turbulence in this area. The echocardiogram also helps to distinguish tetralogy of Fallot from other anomalies that may closely simulate this condition, namely double outlet right ventricle with pulmonic stenosis, arterial transposition with pulmonic stenosis and ventricular septal defect, and a group of complex cardiac malformations consisting primarily of single ventricle and pulmonic stenosis.

These abnormalities are also excluded by *cardiac catheterization and angiocardiography,* and these tests are essential prior to planning surgical management. Cardiac catheterization confirms that the peak systolic pressures in both ventricles are virtually identical and that there is a significant gradient across the right ventricular outflow. The degree and direction of shunting at the ventricular level are also demonstrated so that the shunt may be exclusively right to left or bidirectional. Arterial oxygen saturation is decreased and at rest is usually between 75 and 85 per cent. Selective right ventriculography identifies the site or sites of right ventricular outflow tract obstruction, the narrowed pulmonary valve ring, the presence of abnormalities of the pulmonary arterial trunk, and any stenoses of the pulmonary arterial branches. In patients with pulmonary atresia the anatomy of pulmonary blood flow is complex. Although there may not be filling of the main pulmonary artery a central confluence of left and right intrapulmonary arteries may be present. Left ventriculography shows the position and size of the ventricular septal defect and the presence of an overriding aorta. In a few instances, a large coronary artery courses over the right ventricular outflow; preservation of this artery during surgical repair is essential. *Surgical treatment* is usually advised during infancy or childhood. The type of surgical procedure and its timing are still controversial. Infants with severe anoxemia in the first few months of life are frequently treated with a systemic to pulmonary arterial shunt to augment pulmonary arterial blood flow. Beyond the age of one to two years correction of the defect is advised, at which time any previous systemic to pulmonary shunt is taken down. Older children should have surgical correction of the anomaly because they are generally symptomatic. In all groups surgical correction is more difficult when there is severe deformity of the right ventricular outflow, including a small pulmonary valve ring. The surgical procedure consists of closure of the ventricular septal defect and relief of obstruction by infundibular resection and/or pulmonary valvotomy. Right ventricular outflow may need to be enlarged by an outflow patch that may cross the pulmonary valve ring.

Ebstein's Anomaly of the Tricuspid Valve

This abnormality consists of an abnormal tricuspid valve that is displaced into the right ventricular cavity so that portions of the valve leaflet are attached to the right ventricular wall rather than to the atrioventricular ring. The portion of the right ventricle proximal to the tricuspid valve is thin, functions as an extension of the right atrium, and is known as "atrialized right ventricle." Leaflets of the tricuspid valve are generally redundant and frequently incompetent. The right atrium is large and an atrial septal defect or patent foramen ovale may be present. Increased right atrial pressure, as from tricuspid regurgitation, results in a right to left shunt across the atrial septum and cyanosis of varying degrees. Pulmonary blood flow is decreased.

Some patients succumb during infancy because of anoxemia. However, Ebstein's anomaly in adults varies considerably in severity, so that many patients have active and productive lives, but survival beyond age 50 years is unusual. Symptoms vary in intensity, and with mild anomalies the only complaint is fatigue. Cardiac arrhythmias are frequent and generally supraventricular, the commonest being attacks of paroxysmal atrial tachycardia. The precordium is quiet to palpation. Auscultation reveals a systolic murmur, sometimes accompanied by a thrill over most of the anterior left chest, and third and fourth heart sounds are audible, resulting in triple or quadruple rhythms. A diastolic murmur is frequent, appears to be superficial, and may mimic a pericardial friction rub. Other auscultatory findings include multiple systolic ejection clicks and an opening snap of the tricuspid valve. The *electrocardiogram* shows right bundle branch block, tall and/or broad P waves, and a prolonged PR interval. Wolff-Parkinson-White syndrome (usually type B) is present in some. *Roentgenographic examination* shows a variable heart size; in extreme instances massive cardiomegaly is present because of great enlargement of the right atrium. The outflow portion of the right ventricle is sometimes visible in the region usually occupied by the pulmonary artery in the posteroanterior view. The pulmonary vasculature is normal to decreased, and the aorta small. The *echocardiogram* shows significant delay in tricuspid valve closure and an increased amplitude of motion of the tricuspid valve. The large right atrium and the displaced tricuspid valve can also be visualized. Surgical treatment should be advised in symptomatic patients, especially those with progressive cyanosis. Therapy consists of tricuspid valvuloplasty or valve replacement and ablation of the anomalous pathways between the atrium and ventricle in patients with Wolff-Parkinson-White syndrome and supraventricular tachycardia.

Tricuspid Atresia

In this condition there is no communication between the right atrium and right ventricle so that the entire systemic venous return enters the left heart through a defect in the intra-atrial septum. The left ventricle ejects blood into the normally related aorta and pulmonary arteries. If these vessels are transposed, the aorta arises from a hypoplastic right ventricle that fills from a ventricular septal defect. These patients have a marked increase in pulmonary blood flow and pressure so that heart failure and minimal cyanosis are common in infancy. Survival usually depends upon pulmonary arterial banding to limit pulmonary arterial flow. When the great arteries are normally related, the right ventricle can be minute and associated with marked pulmonic stenosis or atresia. In these patients pulmonary blood flow is derived from a patent ductus arteriosus or collateral bronchial flow. In other instances the left ventricle ejects its blood through a ventricular septal defect into a small right ventricle and then into the pulmonary artery.

Symptoms are usual during infancy and with decreased pulmonary blood flow consist of cyanosis, anoxemia, and poor physical development. Minimal cardiac enlargement is present and the systolic ejection murmur along the left sternal edge is nonspecific. Left axis deviation with left ventricular hypertrophy are usual, and these *electrocardiographic findings* in the presence of cyanosis suggest the diagnosis. *Roentgenograms* of the chest show pulmonary undercirculation but are otherwise nonspecific. The *echocardiogram* confirms absence of the tricuspid valve, delineates the size of the small right ventricle, confirms the presence of a large left ventricle, and identifies the presence or absence of transposition of the great arteries. Most infants with decreased pulmonary blood flow require enlargement of the intra-atrial septal defect to ensure easy communication between the two atria as well as a systemic to pulmonary shunt. In later years more radical surgery is undertaken when the Fontan principle is applied, with anastomosis of the right atrium to the pulmonary artery and closure of the intra-atrial septal defect. This procedure effectively separates pulmonary and systemic blood flows, abolishes cyanosis, and improves exercise tolerance. A similar procedure is also used in patients who had pulmonary arterial banding during infancy.

Single Ventricle

Atrial blood empties through two separate atrioventricular valves or a common valve into a single ventricle from which the aorta and pulmonary artery arise. Associated cardiac abnormalities are present, but their nature varies considerably. The most frequent ones are transposition of the great arteries, pulmonic stenosis, and aortic origin from a rudimentary outlet chamber. The clinical picture depends on the nature of the associated anomalies. If pulmonic stenosis is severe, cyanosis and anoxemia dominate. In the absence of pulmonic stenosis pulmonary blood flow and vascular resistance are increased. The clinical picture is then dominated by congestive heart failure. Although these malformations are complex, surgical palliation is undertaken. In the presence of pulmonic stenosis the blood flow is increased with a systemic pulmonary shunt. On the other hand, high pulmonary blood flow is treated with a pulmonary arterial band. In later years, the Fontan principle is applied when surgical connection is established between the right atrium and pulmonary artery, and the atria are partitioned so that systemic venous return flows into the pulmonary artery and pulmonary venous return is ejected from the single ventricle into the aorta.

Inflow Obstruction to the Left Ventricle

Conditions of inflow obstruction are grouped together, since they result in high pulmonary venous pressure with potential pulmonary edema. The lesions may occur anywhere from the insertion of the pulmonary veins into the left atrium to the area of the mitral valve. They are extremely rare abnormalities. *Pulmonary vein stenoses* at their site of entry into the left atrium are difficult to treat surgically or by balloon angioplasty. *Cor triatriatum* consists of a diaphragmatic partition of the left atrium. The upper portion receives the pulmonary veins, and the distal portion communicates with the mitral valve or through an atrial septal defect into the right atrium. The opening in the diaphragm is generally small so that symptoms are present in early life. The condition is surgically correctable by excision of the diaphragm and closure of associated atrial septal defects. *A supravalvular ring* above the mitral valve produces a similar clinical picture. *Congenital mitral stenosis* may be due to marked abnormality of the mitral valve apparatus, which includes fused, thickened mitral valve leaflets with short chordae, or the valve may have a parachute deformity in which the leaflets are also abnormal but the chordae converge and insert into a single papillary muscle.

Hypoplastic Left Heart Syndrome

Varying degrees of underdevelopment of the left side of the heart coexist, including marked underdevelopment of the left ventricle and atrium, and stenosis or atresia of the aortic and mitral orifices with hypoplasia of the ascending aorta. This complex malformation is a significant cause of cardiovascular death in the neonatal period. Attempts at surgical management have been undertaken but have not been standardized.

OBSTRUCTIVE AND REGURGITANT LESIONS

Pulmonary Stenosis with Intact Ventricular Septum

Obstruction to right ventricular outflow can be valvular, subvalvular, supravalvular, or a combination of obstructions at these sites. Valvular obstruction, the most common variety, results from varying degrees of commissural fusion so that the deformed valve appears domelike. Dysplastic thick valve leaflets are less common and may accompany Noonan's syndrome. Isolated subvalvular obstruction usually accompanies severe valvular stenosis, is due to infundibular hypertrophy, and occasionally is seen as an isolated abnormality with a normal pulmonic valve. Pulmonary arterial branch stenosis may be isolated or may occur at multiple sites and may be associated with supravalvular stenosis. These peripheral lesions are a feature of congenital rubella.

The hemodynamic consequences of valvular pulmonic stenosis are produced by the severity of obstruction. When the right ventricular outflow gradient is between 50 and 80 mm Hg the obstruction is considered to be moderate; pressures below and above that range are considered mild and severe, respectively. Pulmonary arterial pressure is normal or low. The arterial oxygen saturation is normal except when the obstruction is severe (sometimes with suprasystemic right ventricular pressure). Poor right ventricular compliance with or without an increase in right ventricular end-diastolic pressure increases right atrial pressure and may result in right to left shunting across the intra-atrial septum.

Symptoms are usually absent when the obstruction is mild or moderate, but when it is severe, effort dyspnea may be present. The physique is frequently normal and some patients appear robust. When the stenosis is *mild* the venous pressure is normal and the heart is not enlarged. A systolic murmur of varying intensity with midsystolic peaking is heard best at the upper left sternal edge and is preceded by a pulmonic ejection click. The second heart sound may be normal, but the pulmonary component is frequently delayed and of normal intensity. The electrocardiogram is normal or shows signs of minimal right ventricular hypertrophy. The chest *roentgenogram* shows prominence of the pulmonary arterial trunk because of post-stenotic dilatation, but the heart size and pulmonary vasculature are normal. Real-time echocardiography shows the domed stenotic valve. When the severity of pulmonic stenosis is *moderate* the venous pressure may be normal or slightly elevated, with a prominent "a" wave in the jugular pulse. A right ventricular parasternal lift is palpable and may be accompanied by a systolic thrill at the upper left sternal edge. The systolic murmur, frequently preceded by an ejection sound, is accentuated in late systole. The second heart sound is split with a delayed and diminished pulmonary component. Electrocardiographic evidence of right ventricular hypertrophy is usual, sometimes with a prominent spiked P wave. The chest roentgenogram shows a normal or mildly enlarged heart, prominence of the pulmonary arterial trunk, and normal pulmonary vasculature. The abnormal valve is visualized by real-time echograms.

In *severe* pulmonic stenosis cyanosis may be present, owing to a small cardiac output or a right to left shunt across the intra-atrial septum. A large presystolic "a" wave is usual in the jugular venous pulse and the increased venous pressure may be transmitted to the liver, resulting in a presystolic pulsation. The heart is moderately or greatly enlarged, with a conspicuous parasternal right ventricular lift. The systolic ejection murmur is usually loud, frequently accompaned by a thrill, and audible maximally at the upper left sternal edge, but it may radiate widely over the entire precordium and into the neck and back. The murmur is accentuated in late systole, frequently encompasses the aortic component of the second heart sound, and may be preceded by an ejection sound. The pulmonary component of the second heart sound is either inaudible or soft and very late. The electrocardiogram shows gross right ventricular hypertrophy with tall P waves attributed to right atrial enlargement. The chest roentgenogram confirms the cardiac enlargement, prominence of the right ventricle and atrium, post-stenotic dilatation of the pulmonary artery, and pulmonary vasculature that is either normal or decreased. The echocardiogram demonstrates systolic doming of the stenotic leaflets into the dilated pulmonary arterial trunk. In the presence of significant obstruction, the right ventricular wall is thick, the right atrium is enlarged, and the intra-atrial septum bows toward the left. It may be possible to quantify the degree of obstruction by correlating maximal Doppler shift with transvalvular peak pressure gradients.

Cardiac catheterization demonstrates the pressure gradient across the pulmonic valve and determines the degree of severity. Selective right ventriculography visualizes the site and nature of the obstruction. During ventricular systole contrast material is seen as a jet through the domed stenotic valve. Subvalvular hypertrophy, which may intensify the obstruction, is also demonstrated by this method.

The clinical course of patients with mild obstruction is usually good and progression of the severity of the disease is unusual, especially in adolescence and adult life. Many with moderate obstruction also do well, although their progress needs to be evaluated at regular intervals, especially during childhood. Progression of the obstruction is detected clinically by the change in character of the murmur, which becomes accentuated in late systole. Also, the width of the splitting of the second heart sound increases as the right ventricular pressure rises. These signs are associated with an increase in the severity of the electrocardiographic signs of right ventricular hypertrophy.

Two options are now available for treatment of moderate to severe obstruction. These consist of surgical valvotomy or balloon valvuloplasty. There is a long experience with surgical treatment, and it is known that children with isolated pulmonic stenosis generally do extremely well for many years after valvotomy. This is due to immediate decrease in right ventricular pressure after valvotomy. Pulmonary valve incompetence after surgery is usually mild, presents as a short early diastolic murmur, and is generally of no clinical significance. Recurrence of obstruction after surgery is extremely rare. The results of surgery in adults with severe obstruction may not be uniformly good. Right ventricular dysfunction may persist despite relief of the gradient, and this has been attributed to a poorly compliant right ventricle due to persistent hypertrophy and fibrosis. Pulmonary valvuloplasty for valvular stenosis has been introduced recently and is accomplished by a balloon catheter inserted percutaneously. Patients who have had this new form of treatment are at present being observed to determine whether the initial reduction of gradient is maintained over many years. This method is attractive because it obviates thoracotomy and open heart surgery.

Biscuspid Aortic Valve

This condition is frequent and is said to occur in about 2 per cent of the population. The valve consists of two commissures and two cusps, one of which is generally larger. The bicuspid aortic valve may have normal function so that there is no systolic gradient across the valve and during diastole the valve remains competent. This normal function may continue throughout life and the bicuspid valve may be found only incidentally at necropsy. In others, abnormality of the aortic valve can be suspected during examination of teenagers or young adults. These findings relate to minor degrees of valvular obstruction and/or incompetence. The auscultatory findings consist of short soft systolic murmurs heard at the upper right sternal edge that simulate innocent brachiocephalic systolic murmurs. However, the presence of an early aortic ejection click, which precedes the murmur, excludes an innocent murmur. In others, the systolic murmur may be followed by a short, high-pitched early diastolic murmur of aortic incompetence. The diagnosis may be confirmed by echocardiography that demonstrates the presence of only two aortic leaflets.

The natural course of bicuspid aortic valves is variable. In some, the valve may function normally for many decades and produce no abnormal clinical signs. In others the valve leaflets become thickened, fibrotic, and calcified, so that clear signs of aortic stenosis of varying severity develop during early or mid-adult life. In others, there is eversion or prolapse of one of the aortic cusps, resulting in progressive aortic regurgitation that can become severe. A bicuspid aortic valve is particularly susceptible to infective endocarditis, which may convert a benign lesion into one associated with acute severe aortic regurgitation.

Congenital Valvular Aortic Stenosis

This lesion, which is more common in males, is associated with thickening of the aortic valve leaflets and fusion of the commissures to varying degrees. In others, the valve appears to be bicuspid, although remnants of complete fusion of one of the commissures may be recognizable. Unicuspid valves are less frequent. In adults, heavy calcification of the valve may distort the leaflets in such a way that the original leaflets are no longer discernible. In young patients, associated abnormalities include coarctation of the aorta and ventricular septal defect.

In rare instances critical aortic valvular stenosis is present in the neonatal period or in early infancy. These patients present with signs of heart failure and require urgent valvotomy to relieve the obstruction. Children and young adolescents, however, are frequently asymptomatic. In others, especially older patients, symptoms consist of effort intolerance, angina pectoris, dizziness, and syncope. These symptoms generally denote the presence of severe obstruction. The pulse pressure is narrowed and in adults the pulse has a slow rise and a sustained peak with a slow collapse if the obstruction is severe (anacrotic pulse). The heart size is normal when the stenosis is mild, but a heaving left ventricular apical impulse with cardiomegaly indicates the presence of left ventricular enlargement. Thrills are palpable when the stenotic murmur is loud. This murmur is preceded by an ejection sound that is present if the valve leaflets are mobile and is produced by the abrupt opening of the dome-shaped stenotic valve. Marked calcification impairs valve mobility so that the ejection sound may be inaudible. This ejection click is heard best at the apex but is also audible along the left sternal edge and at the base. The systolic murmur that is initiated by the click is harsh, coarse, and rasping, especially when its intensity is grade III/VI or louder. Loud murmurs that peak in late systole suggest that the obstruction is severe, but this sign is extremely variable so that the murmur may peak much earlier in systole even when stenosis is marked. In others with severe aortic stenosis and complicating left ventricular failure the murmur may be unimpressive and mid-systolic in timing. The murmur of aortic stenosis is best heard in the second right interspace, with radiation to the suprasternal notch and over both carotids, especially the right. The murmur is also transmitted down the left and right sternal edges and toward the apex. In some instances the murmur is maximal at the apex or at the lower left sternal edge. The second heart sound is normal if the valve is not calcified, even in the presence of significant obstruction. However, severe stenosis may result in prolonged left ventricular ejection time so that the second heart sound is split paradoxically, with aortic valve closure following that of the pulmonary valve. Mild aortic regurgitation may be present and is recognized by an early, short, high-pitched diastolic murmur. A fourth heart sound is audible in severe obstruction, but this sign is not reliable after the age of about 40 years.

The *electrocardiogram* is normal when obstruction is mild. It may also be normal when severe stenosis is present but usually there are signs of left ventricular hypertrophy as evident by increased R-wave voltage in left precordial and/or inferior leads. ST segmental depression with T-wave inversion is associated with severe obstruction. The early repolarization syndrome is a normal variant in adolescents and young adults and should not be confused with signs of left ventricular hypertrophy. *Roentgenograms* of the chest are normal in the presence of mild disease. With more severe degrees of obstruction left ventricular enlargement occurs and is associated with a prominent ascending aorta due to post-stenotic dilatation. Valvular calcification is common, especially in adults. *Echocardiograms* identify the abnormal aortic valve and are also helpful in estimating the severity of obstruction, especially when obtained sequentially. Systolic doming of the valve is visible, the size of the valve ring can be measured, and the dilated aortic root is identified. The number of valve cusps can be recognized and the degree of their separation during systole is significantly limited when obstruction is severe. The extent of valvular calcification is also identified and the degree of left ventricular hypertrophy is indicated by a thickened free wall and septum. The M-mode echogram shows multiple diastolic echoes of the aortic valve. In the absence of heart failure the left ventricle is hypercontractile so that the shortening fraction is increased. The Doppler method records systolic turbulence in the ascending aorta, and aortic valve regurgitation into the outflow tract of the left ventricle. Indirect estimation of severity has been used, especially in children and adolescents. This estimation is based on the hypothesis that wall stress is directly related to left ventricular peak systolic pressure and cavity size but inversely related to wall thickness. Left ventricular peak systolic pressure is calculated from the left ventricular wall thickness in end-systole multiplied by a constant of 225 and divided by the left ventricular internal dimension at end-systole. The difference between this figure and the systolic blood pressure obtained by cuff measurement is the estimated gradient. This method is not used in older patients, especially in the presence of coronary artery disease or left ventricular failure. *Graded exercise testing* has also been used to estimate the severity of the disease, especially in children and adolescents. When the obstruction is moderate or severe, ST segmental depression may be induced, the normal rise of systolic pressure is blunted, and stroke volume is decreased. *Cardiac catheterization and angiography* are undertaken in patients who have clinical signs and evidence from noninvasive evaluation that the obstruction is significant. The measurement of the gradient across the valve establishes the severity of obstruction when cardiac output is normal.

These studies also indicate the presence or absence of left ventricular dysfunction. Ascending aortography or left ventriculography identify the anatomic abnormality of the aortic valve. Coronary arteriography is also indicated, especially in older patients or when the valve is heavily calcified.

TREATMENT. In asymptomatic patients, especially children and adolescents with obstruction, the major risk is that of infective endocarditis, and prophylactic measures with suitable antibiotics are indicated at the time of risk. It is probably unwise to allow these patients to participate in competitive sports. Surgical treatment is indicated when the obstruction is severe, as judged by a systolic gradient of 70 mm Hg or more or a calculated effective aortic orifice less than 0.5 cm^2 per square meter of body surface area. Because of the risk of sudden death in children and adolescents with critical stenosis, surgery is advised even if the patient is asymptomatic. In young patients aortic valvotomy is the preferred procedure, because relief of the gradient may last for many years. Trivial aortic incompetence may occur after valvotomy and can progress many years after operation. In adults who have had a previous valvotomy with recurrence of obstruction or have critical stenosis without previous surgery, aortic valve replacement is usually undertaken.

Subvalvular Aortic Stenosis (Discrete)

Obstruction to left ventricular outflow is produced by a fibrous membrane situated just below the aortic valve. The membrane is a collar-like structure extending from the intraventricular septum and involving the anterior mitral leaflet. The high velocity jet of blood flowing through the obstructed area during ventricular systole impinges on the aortic valve, which results in fibrous thickening and incompetence of the valve. The clinical picture simulates that of valvular aortic stenosis with important exceptions. An aortic ejection sound is usually absent and the murmur occupies the whole of systole. In childhood this condition is frequently mistaken for a ventricular septal defect or mitral incompetence. Mild forms of obstruction may coexist with other lesions, especially a ventricular septal defect. This obstruction may be unrecognized at the time of surgical closure of the ventricular septal defect and the obstruction may progress over the ensuing years. A useful differential sign is the presence of an early diastolic murmur of aortic valve incompetence, which is a common finding when the obstruction is moderate or severe. Laboratory findings simulate those described under valvular aortic stenosis. However, the real-time echocardiogram is diagnostic in that the discrete membrane is visualized. Cardiac catheterization and angiocardiography are undertaken to measure the severity of obstruction and to outline the membrane by left ventriculography or aortography if the aortic valve is incompetent. Indications for surgery are liberalized, since continued damage to the aortic valve should be prevented. Excision of the membrane gives immediate good results, but complications include damage to the anterior mitral leaflet with resultant regurgitation or conduction abnormalities, including complete heart block from trauma to the intraventricular septum. Furthermore, there may be recurrence of obstruction from regrowth of the membrane.

A rarer form of subaortic stenosis is a long, narrow fibromuscular channel frequently associated with hypoplasia of the aortic ring. This disease is more frequent in childhood and is difficult to treat surgically because relief of obstruction may require enlargement of the aortic valve ring. In extreme cases a valve-bearing conduit is inserted between the left ventricle and the aorta.

Hypertrophic Cardiomyopathy

See Ch. 51.

Supravalvular Aortic Stenosis

The obstruction may be localized to a segmental hourglass-shaped narrowing immediately above the aortic sinuses. Beyond the area of obstruction the aorta may be normal in diameter or show varying degrees of tubular hypoplasia, frequently involving the ascending aorta but occasionally extending for a varying length along the course of the aorta, even to its bifurcation. Aortic valve leaflets may be thickened, with resultant mild aortic regurgitation. During systole the aortic valve leaflets may impinge upon the orifices of the coronary arteries so that coronary flow is impaired; this may be further aggravated by the coronary arteries themselves, which can be enlarged and tortuous but have a narrow lumen. Supravalvular aortic stenosis is frequently associated with the *Williams syndrome,* consisting of atypical facies (broad prominent forehead, flattened bridge of the nose, epicanthal folds, and long upper lip), mild mental retardation, and a low-pitched voice; children with this syndrome are particularly friendly and converse easily. In the absence of Williams syndrome, supravalvular aortic stenosis occurs sporadically and is sometimes familial. In the latter, pulmonary arterial branch stenosis may coexist. Carotid and brachial arterial pulses may be asymmetric, with more conspicuous pulses on the right side. This finding has been attributed to preferential flow into the innominate artery. Other components of the clinical picture simualte those described under valvular aortic stenosis. Echocardiography visualizes the ascending aorta, identifies the area of obstruction, and defines the degree of aortic hypoplasia. Cardiac catheterization and angiocardiography determine the severity of the obstruction, visualize the anatomy of the aorta and the obstruction, and demonstrate severity of pulmonary arterial branch stenosis, if present. Surgical treatment to relieve the obstruction is advised when the gradient is severe. However, surgical treatment is complicated, especially when the transverse and thoracic aortae are markedly hypoplastic.

Coarctation of the Aorta

Narrowing of the aortic lumen may occur at isolated or multiple sites in the aorta. By far the commonest site of discrete obstruction is just distal to the origin of the left subclavian artery. The lesion is more frequent in males and is also seen in patients with Turner's (XO) syndrome. Associated cardiac malformations are frequent, the commonest being a bicuspid aortic valve, congenital aortic stenosis with or without incompetence, ventricular septal defect, and lesions of the mitral valve with or without valvular regurgitation. Extensive collateralization usually develops, especially from branches of the subclavian, internal mammary, superior intercostal, and axillary arteries. These vessels join the intercostal arteries of the descending aorta and inferior epigastric branches of the femoral arteries, which allow channels for arterial blood to bypass the area of coarctation. These collateral vessels can become enormously enlarged and tortuous by early adult life.

Symptoms and signs may develop during the neonatal period or infancy and are dominated by congestive cardiac failure and pulmonary hypertension, and, especially in the neonate, rapidly progress to a state of cardiogenic shock. In preparation for surgical treatment of the neonate, patency of the ductus arteriosus is maintained by infusions of prostaglandin E_1.

Children and young adults are generally asymptomatic. However, hypertension may develop in the arteries above the coarctation and may be associated with epistaxis and throbbing headaches. Other symptoms include leg fatigue, complaints of cold extremities, and occasionally intermittent claudication. Beyond the second decade coarctation may be discovered by the finding of brachial arterial hypertension during routine physical examination. The methods of presentation in adults include infective endocarditis, usually involving the aortic valve, and rupture of the aorta or dissecting aneurysm may occur especially in the 20's and 30's. The site of rupture is either in the proximal aorta or in an aneurysm in the area of coarctation. Cerebral vascular disease with resultant cerebral hemorrhage or infarction may result from complications of hypertension or from the rupture of an aneurysm, usually of the circle of Willis. Hypertension and associated atherosclerosis of the coronary circulation may result in congestive cardiac failure, sometimes preceded by acute myocardial infarction. Pregnancy is usually well tolerated, especially if hypertension is controlled. However, the risk of aortic rupture is increased especially toward the end of the third trimester.

Classic signs of aortic coarctation are the disparity in pulsations and blood pressures of the arms and legs. The bounding pulses of the arms and carotid vessels contrast with the weak, delayed, or absent femoral and/or distal arterial pulses in the legs. Also, the blood pressure in the arms exceeds that in the legs. This applies especially to the systolic reading, and there is a further rise of systolic blood pressure in response to exercise. If the systolic arterial pressure in the right arm exceeds that of the left arm by more than 30 mm Hg, the left subclavian artery is involved in the coarctation. Collateral arterial circulation may be visible but is usually palpable, especially in the back, at the angles of the scapulae and in the axillae. Murmurs are variable in location, quality, and intensity. The usual is a precordial midsystolic murmur heard best at the left sternal edge, but it may be loudest in the back between the scapulae. Additional systolic or sometimes continuous murmurs are audible over the anterior or posterior chest and are produced by flow through the large, tortuous collateral arteries. The *electrocardiogram* is usually normal during childhood and adolescence. In adults, varying degrees of left ventricular hypertrophy are present. *Roentgenographic* examinations during childhood may not be striking. However, prominence of the left ventricle occurs thereafter and during adult life. The heart may be moderately enlarged. Notching of the inferior border of the ribs from collateral vessels is common. This may be unilateral if one of the subclavian arteries arises below the area of coarctation. Post-stenotic dilatation of the descending aorta is usual and is demonstrated by a barium esophagogram, and the prominent left subclavian artery produces a shadow in the left mediastinum. Real-time *echocardiography* visualizes the area of coarctation, the large left subclavian artery, post-stenotic dilatation of the descending aorta, and associated intracardiac anomalies, especially those of the aortic valve. These associated anomalies are confirmed by cardiac catheterization and selective left ventriculography and angiography. Coarctectomy is advised, preferably in early childhood between ages three and five years.

Pulmonary Valvular Regurgitation

Isolated congenital pulmonary valve regurgitation is rare and seldom produces symptoms; an early diastolic murmur at the upper left sternal edge is the only abnormal sign. However, pulmonary valvular regurgitation may accompany other conditions such as those associated with severe pulmonary hypertension or after surgical transection of the pulmonary valve ring for the treatment of severe obstruction of the right ventricular outflow.

Absence of Pulmonic Valve

Absence of the pulmonic valve is a congenital anomaly in which pulmonary valve leaflets are virtually absent. Although the lesion may be isolated it is usually associated with other defects, especially tetralogy of Fallot or isolated ventricular septal defect. In infancy the pulmonary arteries may be dilated, and large aneurysms of the major trunks compress the bronchi; this is not well tolerated and is frequently lethal. Surgical treatment is difficult.

Vascular Rings and Other Aortic Arch Anomalies

The more common anomalies are double aortic arch, right aortic arch with left ligamentum arteriosum, origin of the right subclavian artery from the thoracic aorta distal to the left subclavian artery, anomalous origin of the innominate or left carotid arteries, and anomalous left pulmonary artery which arises from the elongated pulmonary trunk and courses between the trachea and the esophagus. The clinical picture is extremely variable and in many instances there are no symptoms. Tracheal compression, especially during infancy, produces respiratory distress with wheezing and a brassy cough. Dysphagia may occur in older patients. Surgery is advised in symptomatic patients to relieve the tracheal and esophageal compression.

THE TRANSPOSITIONS

Transposition of the Great Arteries

In this condition the aorta arises from the right ventricle and the pulmonary artery from the left ventricle. Systemic venous return is to the right atrium and pulmonary venous return is to the left atrium. Systemic venous blood flows through the tricuspid valve into the right ventricle and is ejected into the aorta. Pulmonary venous blood flows from the left atrium through the mitral valve into the left ventricle and is ejected into the pulmonary artery. Thus, the circulations are parallel. Survival is dependent on mixture of blood through the foramen ovale, a ventricular septal defect, or patency of the ductus arteriosus. This condition is a common malformation that occurs predominantly in males, with symptoms in the neonatal period or soon thereafter.

ISOLATED "SIMPLE" TRANSPOSITION OF THE GREAT ARTERIES. In this malformation the ventricular septum is intact. Mixing of systemic and pulmonary blood occurs primarily from bidirectional shunting across the foramen ovale. This condition produces symptoms and signs of anoxemia in the neonate, is suspected in an otherwise normal neonate who is cyanotic and tachypneic, and is verified by echocardiography that demonstrates the abnormal origin of the great arteries, as well as the fact that the aorta is usually anterior to the pulmonary artery. Emergency balloon atrial septostomy that ruptures the foramen ovale allows greater mixing at the atrial level and decompresses the left atrium. Generally, these babies do well for many months, until surgical treatment is undertaken, usually between the ages of 6 and 12 months. Currently there is debate as to the preferred method of surgical treatment. There has been greater experience with intra-atrial redirection of venous return so that systemic venous blood flows into the left ventricle and is ejected out the pulmonary artery; pulmonary venous return flows through the tricuspid valve and is pumped by the right ventricle into the aorta. Immediate results are excellent, but concern has been expressed about late onset of supraventricular arrhythmias and about right ventricular failure and pulmonary edema, since this ventricle is ejecting blood into the aorta. Because of the concern about long-term right ventricular function, the arterial switch operation was developed whereby the origins of the great arteries are transected and the pulmonary artery is connected to the stump of the vessel arising from the right ventricle and the aorta to the left ventricle with implantation of the coronary arteries into the new aorta. This procedure cannot be undertaken if left ventricular pressure is low, as occurs in simple transposition, so that the left ventricle is "prepared" by pulmonary arterial banding in the neonatal period.

TRANSPOSITION OF THE GREAT ARTERIES WITH VENTRICULAR SEPTAL DEFECT. When the septal defect is small the clinical picture is similar to that of simple transposition, and many of these small defects close spontaneously. If the ventricular septal defect is large and nonrestrictive, significant mixing of blood occurs and symptoms are frequently delayed until the baby is a few months old. The clinical picture is dominated by signs of congestive cardiac failure with minimal cyanosis. In the untreated state there is progressive pulmonary hypertension with severe pulmonary vascular disease. Treatment is required during infancy and a number of options are available for surgical treatment. The greatest experience has been with a staged procedure. Pulmonary arterial banding is done during infancy to restrict pulmonary blood flow and prevent the onset of pulmonary vascular disease. In later years, usually during childhood, the second stage is undertaken when the pulmonary artery is debanded and transected, the ventricular septal defect is closed so that the left ventricle ejects blood into the aorta, and a conduit is placed from the right ventricle to the transected pulmonary artery *(Rastelli procedure)*. When the ventricular septal defect is subpulmonic *(Taussig-Bing anomaly)*, the ventricular septal defect may be closed and venous return redirected as described under simple transposition of the great arteries. The third option consists of the arterial switch operation as described above.

TRANSPOSITION OF THE GREAT ARTERIES WITH PULMONIC STENOSIS. The importance of this condition is that it may closely simulate the clinical picture produced by tetralogy of Fallot. The condition generally requires an aortic pulmonary shunt during infancy to increase pulmonary blood flow and relieve the symptoms of anoxemia. In later years the Rastelli procedure is undertaken.

Double Outlet Right Ventricle

In this malformation both the pulmonary artery and the aorta arise from the right ventricle, and the only outlet from the left ventricle is a ventricular septal defect. The clinical picture simulates a large, uncomplicated ventricular septal defect with pulmonary hypertension. The echocardiogram is diagnostic in that there is discontinuity between the anterior mitral leaflet and the aorta, since the latter structure arises from the right ventricle. Uncontrollable heart failure and pulmonary hypertension are frequent during infancy so that pulmonary arterial banding is usually required. In later years, generally during childhood, the Rastelli operation is advised. Double outlet right ventricle may be complicated by the development of pulmonic stenosis when the condition simulates that described under tetralogy of Fallot.

Corrected Transposition (L Transposition of the Great Arteries)

This condition consists of *ventricular inversion* and transposition of the great arteries. Systemic venous blood enters a normal right atrium, flows through a mitral valve into the left ventricle, and is ejected into the pulmonary artery. Pulmonary venous blood flows from the left atrium through a tricuspid valve into the right ventricle and is ejected into the aorta. If the condition is uncomplicated, blood flow and hemodynamics are normal. However, associated anomalies are usual, such as ventricular septal defect, pulmonary stenosis, left atrioventricular valve (tricuspid) anomalies including an Ebstein-like malformation of this valve, and atrioventricular conduction abnormalities—frequently complete atrioventricular block. The clinical picture is dominated by the associated lesions. The chest x-ray may suggest the abnormal origin of the great arteries in that the ascending aorta occupies the upper left border of the cardiac silhouette in the posteroanterior view. Since ventricular inversion is present, the electrocardiogram may show absent q waves in leads I and V6, initial q waves in 3, AVF, and VI, and prominent T waves in the right precordial leads. During surgical treatment the bundle of His may be injured because it is located abnormally, so that complete heart block may occur. In others, significant regurgitation via the Ebstein-like tricuspid valve requires valve replacement.

Anomalous Pulmonary Venous Connection

The anomalous pulmonary venous return may be partial or total. *Partial anomalous pulmonary venous return* simulates the clinical picture produced by a secundum atrial septal defect. In fact, one of these forms is the sinus venosus defect (see p 228).

TOTAL ANOMALOUS PULMONARY VENOUS CONNECTION. The site of entry of the pulmonary veins may be supradiaphragmatic (into a left superior vena cava or vertical vein, coronary sinus, right superior vena cava, or right atrium) or infradiaphragmatic (portal vein, hepatic veins, or inferior vena cava). Thus, there is no connection between the pulmonary vein and the left atrium. Generally the pulmonary veins converge to form a single trunk which then enters the systemic venous circulation. Varying degrees of pulmonary venous obstruction are present

and depend on the length of the common pulmonary venous trunk before its entry into the systemic vein as well as localized areas of obstruction.

The clinical picture is variable. In some instances, especially those of infradiaphragmatic connection, pulmonary edema and cyanosis are present in the neonatal period or soon thereafter. When there is a large intra-atrial communication and obstruction to pulmonary venous return is moderate, symptoms occur in later infancy and the clinical picture is dominated by congestive cardiac failure. When pulmonary venous obstruction is absent and there is a large communication between the right and left atria, symptoms may be delayed until early childhood and very occasionally adolescence. The clinical picture of these patients simulates those produced by a large left to right shunt at the atrial level.

The *electrocardiogram* reflects the hemodynamic state so that symptomatic infants have marked right ventricular hypertrophy with prominent P waves. Chest *roentgenograms* in neonates with pulmonary venous obstruction are characterized by pulmonary edema with a normal heart size. In older infants the heart is large and pulmonary overcirculation evident. In older children with pulmonary venous connection to the left superior vena cava the cardiac silhouette has the appearance of a snowman or figure 8. The supracardiac shadow is produced by marked dilatation of the left superior vena cava, innominate vein, and right superior vena cava. The *echocardiogram* shows signs of right volume overload and sometimes a common venous trunk is visualized, especially if it lies directly behind the left atrium. *Cardiac catheterization* demonstrates the severity of pulmonary hypertension, and pulmonary arteriograms show return of contrast material to the pulmonary veins and their anomalous site of insertion into the systemic venous system. Surgical treatment is indicated when the common pulmonary venous trunk is anastomosed to the left atrium, the atrial septal defect closed, and the anomalous connection to the systemic venous system obliterated. Results of surgical treatment have been good, with greatest risk in symptomatic neonates.

CARDIAC MALPOSITION

Knowledge of the position of the heart as well as the location (situs) of abdominal viscera aids in defining the nature of these anomalies. X-ray of the abdomen helps identify abdominal situs by localizing the position of the stomach bubble and other abdominal structures, but many viscera cannot be visualized by this method alone. Generally atrial and visceral situs are related; if the viscera are normally located the atria have a normal position. In abdominal situs inversus the left atrium is usually to the right and the right atrium to the left. Location of the atria is further and more accurately assessed by evaluation of the tracheobronchial air column on chest x-ray. A normal tracheobronchial tree with an epiarterial bronchus on the right indicates normal atrial situs, and this finding is independent of the position of the heart.

Dextrocardia

The heart is in the right chest and the cardiac apex points to the right. Associated abdominal situs inversus (mirror-image dextrocardia) in adults is usually associated with a normally functioning heart. However, poorly motile cilia may result in sinusitis and bronchiectasis (Kartagener's syndrome). Dextrocardia may be discovered by physical examination when the heart sounds are more clear in the right chest or accidentally on a routine chest film. The electrocardiogram demonstrates the mirror image so that the P, QRS, and T are inverted in lead 1; aVR and aVL are the reverse of normal and the right precordial leads resemble those usually recorded from the left chest. *Isolated dextrocardia* with abdominal viscera in normal position (situs solitus) is invariably associated with various combinations of severe cardiac malformations, the commonest being ventricular inversion, single ventricle, pulmonic stenosis, abnormalities of the atrioventricular valves, and anomalies of systemic and pulmonary venous return.

Isolated Levocardia

Isolated levocardia is accompanied by varying degrees of anomalous position of abdominal viscera (heterotaxia) so that situs inversus is partial or complete. Severe cardiac malformations are usual, including various combinations of anomalies of systemic and pulmonary venous return, common atrioventricular canal, pulmonary stenosis or atresia, defects of the atrial and ventricular septa, and single ventricle.

Mesocardia

Mesocardia is the term used when the heart is centrally located in the chest or the cardiac silhouette on x-ray is toward the right chest. The cardiac anatomy is normal with normal relationships of the cardiac chambers, venous return, and origin of the great arteries. Cardiac malformations are usually absent.

Asplenia Syndrome

This condition is characterized by absence of the spleen, undefinable situs of the abdominal viscera (situs ambiguus), bilateral *right-sidedness,* and complex severe cardiac malformations. Bilateral right-sidedness is identified by bilateral trilobed lungs with bilateral epiarterial bronchi. In the majority the liver is located centrally so that the liver edge is palpable across the entire upper abdomen. The stomach is located on the right in about half the patients, and varying degrees of malrotation of the small bowel are present. Both atria have the morphological characteristics of the right atrium. Common cardiovascular anomalies include total anomalous pulmonary venous connection, transposition of the great arteries, pulmonic stenosis or atresia, complete atrioventricular canal, single ventricle, and dextrocardia. The condition is suspected in a deeply cyanotic male infant with dextrocardia and a centrally placed liver. Howell-Jolly and Heinz bodies in the peripheral red blood cells are suggestive of asplenia, but these findings are not conclusive. Infants with asplenia are susceptible to severe intercurrent infections so that continued antibiotic prophylaxis has been suggested as a preventive measure. Aortopulmonary shunts during infancy are indicated when severe anoxemia is present due to pulmonic stenosis, and right atrial–pulmonary shunts (Fontan) are advised in later years.

Polysplenia Syndrome

The features of this condition are multiple splenic masses (two or more), ambiguous abdominal situs, and *bilateral left sidedness;* while cardiovascular abnormalities are frequent they are generally not as complex as in the asplenia syndrome. The lungs are bilobed and epiarterial bronchi are absent. The liver is frequently located centrally in the upper abdomen and the stomach is right- or left-sided. Malrotation of the bowel is common. Both atria have the morphologic features of the left atrium. The hepatic segment of the inferior vena cava is frequently absent so that systemic venous return is by way of the azygos vein. The cardiac apex points to the left in the majority. Pulmonary venous return may be normal, arterial transposition is present in only a minority, and pulmonic stenosis is unusual. The cardiac malformations are generally associated with left to right shunts at atrial or ventricular levels.

THE ADULT WITH "UNCURED" CONGENITAL HEART DISEASE

Strategies of management of symptomatic patients with congenital heart disease have changed recently so that the majority are treated during infancy or early childhood. A large group of adolescents and adults now exists who have trivial lesions, have remained asymptomatic, and have lived a normal life style. Other patients have anomalies that are silent until adult life. Palliative surgery may have been undertaken in another group who have remained relatively well and have now approached adult life. Another cohort of patients who may not have had surgical treatment during early life, develop progressive pulmonary hypertension during childhood, and in adult life their lesions are associated with severe pulmonary vascular disease. This section discusses these groups of patients.

VENTRICULAR SEPTAL DEFECTS. A significant number of patients seen in pediatric cardiac clinics have trivial shunts across a small ventricular septal defect. They remain asymptomatic throughout the growing years and as adults the only abnormal physical sign is a long harsh systolic murmur, which may be accompanied by a thrill and is heard best at the lower left sternal edge. It is unusual to see such patients beyond the age of 40 years so that it has been assumed that many of these defects close spontaneously. While the defect remains these patients are at risk to develop infective endocarditis and occasionally aortic regurgitation or discrete subaortic stenosis.

VALVULAR PULMONIC STENOSIS. Generally asymptomatic children with mild pulmonic stenosis (resting peak right ventricular pressure less than one-half systolic systemic pressure) do not require surgical treatment. There is no consensus about the course of untreated mild to moderate pulmonic stenosis. The generally held belief, however, is that progressive increase in severity is unusual, especially if the patient is beyond the age of 12 years. This optimistic view also applies to those who had a valvotomy during childhood which relieved the obstruction. Restriction of physicial activity is not required, pregnancy is well tolerated, and, although infective endocarditis of the pulmonic valve is not common, prophylaxis is advisable at the time of risk for this complication.

AORTIC VALVE DISEASE. A functionally normal bicuspid aortic valve and mild congenital aortic stenosis are discussed on page 252.

CONGENITAL COMPLETE HEART BLOCK. Fetal echocardiography may be prompted by the recognition of intrauterine bradycardia, and this test unmasks the presence of complete atrioventricular (AV) block. This study is especially important during pregnancy of mothers with connective tissue disease, such as systemic lupus erythematosus, since the offspring are at greater risk for complete AV block. It is suggested that antinuclear antibodies of the IgG category cross the placenta and damage the fetal conduction system. This occurs in mothers whose disease is active but also when there are no overt clinical manifestations and only positive serologic evidence is present. In about 70 per cent of children with complete AV block the lesion is isolated, and the remainder have associated complex cardiac malformations, such as ventricular inversion or single ventricle. Familial complete AV block is well recognized. Adolescents and adults with isolated congenital complete AV block are usually asymptomatic, but it is not possible to predict episodes of syncope. The pulse rate is inappropriately slow for age. The large stroke volume and vasodilatation produce jerky pulses, systolic hypertension, and cardiomegaly. Cannon waves may be visible in the jugular venous pulse. The first heart sound varies in intensity and may be followed by a nonspecific systolic ejection murmur. The diagnosis is confirmed by the electrocardiogram, in which there is no constant relationship between the P waves and QRS complexes. Usually the QRS is of normal duration, which suggests that the site of the lesion is above the bundle of His. Marked ventricular slowing may be recorded by continuous, 24-hour electrocardiographic monitoring, especially during sleep. It is not known whether there is any relationship between the slow ventricular rates during sleep and the prognosis. Since patients with congenital complete AV block have been observed in late adult life, there is a generally held view that the prognosis is good. However, the lesion is not benign, in that complications may occur at any time and are not predictable. Syncope is an indication for implantation of a permanent pacemaker. Decisions about treatment in asymptomatic patients are more difficult. The demonstration of ventricular tachycardia or fibrilla tion during continuous electrocardiographic monitoring or graded exercise testing is an indication for pacemaker implantation. There remains a group of asymptomatic patients in whom treatment is not standardized, including those with premature ventricular contractions during and after exercise, extreme nocturnal bradycardia, and ventricular depolarization initiated from a focus low in the bundle of His.

EISENMENGER SYNDROME. This syndrome is associated with marked elevation of pulmonar vascular resistance with reversed or bidirectional shunt, which is intracardiac or between the aorta and pulmonary arteries. Thus, pulmonary vascular disease is the hallmark of this syndrome and the site of the shunt is incidental. Medial hypertrophy of pulmonary arteries and arterioles is present and is associated with cellular, fibrotic, and fibroelastic intimal reactions, and in more severe forms plexiform lesions encroach into the lumen of the vessel. These changes in the pulmonary vascular bed are directly related to pulmonary arterial pressure. Extension of muscle into the peripheral arteries occurs when pulmonary hypertesion is still associated with increased pulmonary blood flow. With progressive vascular disease, a reduction in the number of small arteries may precede obliterative pulmonary vascular disease.

Historically these patients are frequently symptomatic during infancy and early childhood because of congestive cardiac failure, poor physical development, and recurrent lower respiratory tract infections. As pulmonary vascular resistance rises, the left to right shunt decreases so that symptoms improve. These children may lead nearly normal lives, but their stamina is limited and mild exertional cyanosis is evident. In early adult life there is progressive anoxemia with intensification of cyanosis, digital clubbing may be extreme, and polycythemia increases. Progressive decrease in effort tolerance develops over many years, culminating in congestive cardiac failure in early or mid-adult life. Other symptoms include hemoptysis, angina pectoris attributed to right ventricular ischemia, syncope, and palpitations from premature atrial or ventricular contractions. Jugular venous pressure is increased, with a prominent "v" wave in the presence of complicating tricuspid valve regurgitation. Hepatomegaly and marked dependent edema with ascites are usual with heart failure. The heart size is increased to a variable extent, greatest when there are shunts at the atrial level and when there is complicating tricuspid and/or pulmonary valve incompetence. The precordium is active with a right ventricular heave along the left sternal edge. Pulmonary arterial pulsations and the second heart sound may be palpable at the upper left sternal edge. The systolic murmur varies in intensity and is frequently initiated by a pulmonic ejection click. The second heart sound is booming, single, or narrowly split in ventricular shunts, but wide, fixed splitting may be audible in isolated atrial shunts. Signs of pulmonary and/or tricuspid valve regurgitation are superimposed when there is dilatation of these valve rings secondary to pulmonary hypertension or right ventricular failure. The *electrocardiogram* shows marked right ventricular or biventricular hypertrophy with prominent P waves. Complete right bundle branch block may be present, especially when the shunt is at the atrial level. In others the electrocardiogram is influenced by the underlying anomaly (e.g., single ventricle, ventricular inversion, etc.). The *chest roentgenogram* confirms the degree of cardiomegaly. The pulmonary trunk is enlarged with prominence of the primary divisions, which diminish in caliber in the peripheral branches. The *echocardiogram* helps to identify the anatomy of the underlying intracardiac or extracardiac malformation. *Cardiac catheterization* is undertaken when the diagnosis cannot be established by clinical findings and noninvasive studies. One of the purposes of catheterization is to determine whether the pulmonary vascular bed is vasoactive, as indicated by a fall in pulmonary artery pressure and resistance during the breathing of 100 per cent oxygen. Another major indication is to exclude the presence of left ventricular inflow lesions, which result in elevation of pulmonary venous pressure and secondary pulmonary hypertension. Angiocardiography carries a small increased risk because the contrast medium may produce a fall in systemic vascular resistance and increased right to left shunting with a further fall in systemic arterial saturation.

Polycythemia may become extreme, and when the hematocrit exceeds 70 per cent excruciating headaches may occur. These are difficult to treat but do respond to repeated venesection. This treatment should not be undertaken lightly, since reduction of red cell count and blood volume is not tolerated. Heart rate and blood pressure are monitored during the procedure. Small aliquots of blood (± 30 ml) are removed and immediately replaced with a similar volume of fresh frozen plasma or human albumin. Repeated venesection results in iron deficiency anemia so that daily oral iron replacement is essential. The usual goal is to reduce the hematocrit to between 55 and 60 per cent. *Hemoptysis* occurs from rupture of pulmonary vessels or is due to pulmonary arterial thrombosis or embolism. This symptom is usually limited to adult life, blood loss is not excessive, and symptomatic treatment is all that is needed. However, hemoptysis can be life threatening if associated with hypotension, an increase in the degree of hypoxemia, and the development of acidemia. Long-term anticoagulation is not indicated. *Syncope and sudden death* cannot be predicted, but patients with Eisenmenger syndrome between the ages of about 20 and 40 years are at risk. The mechanism is not clear but has been attributed to arrhythmias, probably ventricular tachyarrhythmias, which result in hypotension and an increase in right to left shunting. *Pregnancy* is not well tolerated and sudden death has been reported during the third trimester or in the postpartum period.

Treatment. Surgical treatment of the cardiac anomaly is contraindicated because these patients succumb to the effects of pulmonary vascular disease. Palliation has been successful in the presence of transposition of the great arteries, ventricular septal deffect, and severe pulmonary vascular disease; the procedure involves redirection of the venous return (as described under transposition of the great arteries), but the ventricular defect is not closed. The experience with transplantation of the heart and lungs is still small and follow-up is short, but this therapy is being watched with interest, since patients with progressive symptoms are at great risk of dying. Drugs have been used to attempt to manipulate pulmonary and systemic vascular resistance to reduce the right to left shunt; generally the results have been disappointing.

COMPLEX CARDIAC MALFORMATIONS. When pulmonic stenosis is an important part of the anomaly, surgical aortopulmonary shunting is undertaken during infancy or childhood to alleviate hypoxemia. In others with torrential pulmonary blood flow and pulmonary hypertension, pulmonary arterial banding is undertaken in infancy to prevent progressive pulmonary vascular disease. Many have now reached adolescence or adult life with normal or low pulmonary vascular resistance. These patients are candidates for operation using the Fontan principle (direct anastomosis of the right atrium to the pulmonary artery).

THE ADULT WITH SURGICALLY "CURED" CONGENITAL HEART DISEASE

Surgical treatment for extracardiac anomalies has been undertaken for four decades, and 30 years have elapsed since the introduction of surgical procedures for intracardiac congenital malformations. Immediate results after operation continue to be excellent, even dramatic, but it is now recognized that complications may develop many years after surgery.

INTRA-ATRIAL SURGERY. Many anomalies may be treated by an approach through the right atrium. These include atrial septal defects of all types, endocardial cushion defects, transposition of the great arteries, and total anomalous pulmonary venous connection. Frequently isolated ventricular septal defects are closed surgically transatrially and the defect (especially the more common perimembranous defect) is approached through the tricuspid valve and the shunt obliterated. Persistent *conduction disturbances* may occur immediately after operation or appear for the first time many years later. These consist of supraventricular arrhythmias (atrial flutter or fibrillation, paroxysmal supraventricular tachycardia, and junctional rhythm), sick sinus syndrome, or varying degrees of atrioventricular block. These rhythm disturbances occur even when there is complete anatomic correction of the abnormality. The treatment of these abnormalities in conduction is similar to the treatment of these arrhythmias of any cause. The *function of the right ventricle* and competence of the tricuspid valve have also been of concern especially in transposition of the great arteries (see p 238).

INTRAVENTRICULAR SURGERY. Right ventriculotomy is the approach used in most patients who require intraventricular surgery. The more common lesions treated this way include some forms of ventricular septal defect, tetralogy of Fallot with or without pulmonary atresia, and various forms of transposition of the great arteries. Some of these complications may be reduced in future years, since earlier operation is being advised, especially in some patients with tetralogy of Fallot.

Conduction Disturbances. Permanent complete heart block from intraoperative trauma to the conduction system has decreased to a point where it is no longer a major problem soon after operation. *Bifascicular block* (left anterior hemiblock with complete right bundle branch block) may occur from intraoperative trauma to the bundle of His and its branches. These patients usually remain well for many years after operation, but the conduction abnormality may progress to complete AV block. Bifascicular block does not require treatment. *Sudden unexpected cardiac arrest* may occur many years after operation. While this catastrophe may occasionally occur from complete AV block, more frequent mechanisms are ventricular tachyarrhythmias and deterioration into ventricular fibrillation. The risk of ventricular tachycardia is higher in patients who have multiple unifocal or multifocal premature ventricular contractions at rest. Bursts of ventricular tachyarrhythmia may be recorded during 24-hour electrocardiographic recording or unmasked during or immediately after graded exercise testing. While these arrhythmias may occur in patients who have had adequate relief of right ventricular outflow tract obstruction and in whom the ventricular defect is closed, there appears to be greater risk when residual defects are present, such as severe pulmonic stenosis, persistent large shunts across the ventricular septum, and right ventricular aneurysms. Significant residual defects should be treated by reoperation, and the ventricular arrhythmia may be abolished by excision of arrhythmogenic right ventricular aneurysms. Medical treatment of the ventricular tachycardia is indicated and although there is a choice of many drugs, phenytoin (Dilantin) has been used with particular success.

Reconstruction of the Right Ventricular Outflow Tract. Treatment of extreme forms of tetralogy of Fallot, especially pulmonary atresia, and many forms of transposition of the great arteries with pulmonic stenosis or previous arterial banding, requires a prosthesis to establish continuity between the right ventricle and the pulmonary artery. During the last decade the most frequently used prosthesis consisted of a Dacron tube with an aortic valve bearing a porcine heterograft. The durability of this prosthesis is unpredictable, since recurrence of obstruction may occur anywhere along its length from narrowing of the anastomotic sites or from development of an exuberant neointima that encroaches on the lumen of the Dacron tube. Others have used fresh human aortic homografts. A durable, long-lasting prosthesis is still being sought.

Congenital Aortic Stenosis. See p 252.

Valvular Pulmonic Stenosis. See p 256.

Coarctation of the Aorta. It is now common practice to advise surgical treatment of coarctation of the aorta in pre-school years. One of the reasons for earlier operation is the notion that late-onset complications will be reduced. These complications in adult life have been related to recurrence of hypertension, progressive atherosclerosis, myocardial infarction, and cerebral vascular accidents. It is therefore advisable that patients who have had previous coarctation therapy be followed carefully so that treatment can be instituted, especially for hypertension, prior to the onset of some of these complications.

Adams FH, Emmanouilides GC: Moss' Heart Disease in Infants, Children and Adolescents. 3rd ed. Baltimore, Williams and Wilkins, 1983. *The standard comprehensive text on all aspects of congenital heart disease.*

Fontan F, Deville C, Quaegebeur J, Ottenkamp J, Sourdille N, Choussat A, Brom GA: Repair of tricuspid atresia in 100 patients. J Thorac Cardiovasc Surg 85:647, 1983. *Evolution of the principles for treatment of tricuspid atresia. These principles are also applicable to many complex cardiac malformations.*

Garson A, Nihill MR, McNamara DG, Cooley DA: Status of the adult and adolescent after repair of tetralogy of Fallot. Circulation 59:1232, 1979. *Long-term results are evaluated with emphasis on complications in the adult.*

Garson A: The Electrocardiogram in Infants and Children. Philadelphia, Lea and Febiger, 1983. *A text for the novice as well as the experienced clinician.*

Giuliani ER, Fuster V, Brandenberg RO, Mair DD: Ebstein's anomaly. Mayo Clin Proc 54:163, 1979. *Clinical features and natural history are reviewed in a lucid manner.*

Goldberg SJ, Allen HD, Sahn DJ: Pediatric and Adolescent Echocardiography. 2nd ed. Chicago, Year Book Medical Publishers, 1980. *A comprehensive handbook describing the M-mode, two-dimensional, and Doppler features of congenital cardiac malformations.*

Kirklin JW, Karp RB: The Tetralogy of Fallot: From a Surgical Viewpoint. Philadelphia, WB Saunders Company, 1970. *This is a classic monograph. Others have elaborated on the text, but basic ideas have not changed.*

Krongrad E: Prognosis for patients with congenital heart disease and postoperative intraventricular conduction defects. Circulation 57:867, 1978. *A useful guide to mechanisms, prognosis, and treatment.*

Liberthson RR, Boucher CA, Strauss HW, Dinsmore RE, McKusick KA, Pohost GM: Right ventricular function in adult atrial septal defect. Am J Cardiol 57:56, 1981. *This preoperative and postoperative assessment has important clinical applications relative to the effects of preoperative right ventricular dysfunction and pulmonary hypertension on the expected result from operation.*

Meyer RA: Echocardiography. *In* Adams FH, Emmanouilides GC (eds.): Moss' Heart Disease in Infants, Children and Adolescents. 3rd ed. Baltimore, Williams and Wilkins, 1983, pp 58–82. *Up-to-date, concise, and well-illusrated. Discusses anatomic features as well as cardiac performance.*

Perloff JK: The Clinical Recognition of Congenital Heart Disease. 2nd ed. Philadelphia, WB Saunders Company, 1978. *A book that focuses on the anatomic and physiologic derangements in congenital heart disease, setting the stage for an understanding of the history, physical signs, electrocardiogram, chest x-ray, and echocardiogram. All age groups are dealt with.*

Perloff JK: Late postoperative concerns in adults with congenital heart disease. *In* Engle MA (ed.): Pediatric Cardiovascular Disease. Philadelphia, FA Davis Company, 1981. *A paper dealing with long-term residua and sequelae after operation for congenital heart disease.*

Rabinovitch M: Pulmonary hypertension. *In* Adams FH, Emmanouilides GC (eds.): Moss' Heart Disease in Infants, Children and Adolescents. 3rd ed. Baltimore, Williams and Wilkins, 1983, pp 669–692. *Up-to-date information on quantitative structural analysis of the pulmonary vascular bed in congenital heart disease.*

Roberts WC: Congenital Heart Disease in Adults. 2nd ed. Philadelphia, FA Davis Company, 1984. *The specific focus is on adults with congenital heart disease. Natural history and surgical treatment are considered.*

Rudolph AM: Changes in the circulation after birth. Their importance in congenital heart disease. Circulation 41:343, 1970. *A basic paper describing the dramatic circulatory changes at and shortly after birth and the impact of these changes on congenital heart disease.*

45. VALVULAR HEART DISEASE

Charles E. Rackley

The clinical manifestations of valvular heart disease result from either stenosis or incompetence of cardiac valves, or both. These mechanical disturbances lead to either pressure or volume overload on the adjacent chambers. The most common cardiac chamber affected by valvular heart disease is the left ventricle, which compensates for chronic pressure or volume overload with dilatation and hypertrophy. Oxygen requirements of the myocardium are related to the increased mechanical work and hypertrophy of the myocardium. In the late stage of valvular heart disease, myocardial decompensation, a reduction in cardiac output, and coronary perfusion may impair oxygen delivery even though myocardial oxygen demands remain high.

The prevalence of various etiologies of valvular heart disease has changed in recent years. Although rheumatic heart disease remains prevalent in temperate climates of the world, control of streptococcal infections has significantly reduced the incidence of rheumatic fever and subsequent rheumatic heart disease in the United States. Mitral valve prolapse is today the most common valvular abnormality. Mitral regurgitation due to dilatation of the left ventricle is a common secondary form of valvular incompetence. A congenitally bicuspid aortic valve is the most frequent cause of aortic stenosis, and calcific stenosis of the aortic valve is now recognized more frequently in the aging adult. Aortic regurgitation can be caused by structural defects in the aortic wall such as cystic medionecrosis as well as by chronic hypertension and gradual aortic valve incompetence. Finally, with the technical skill and accomplishments of cardiac surgery, patients with prosthetic valves are now living longer, and thus the prosthetic cardiac valve can eventually become another source for valvular dysfunction.

The initial evidence of valvular heart disease is often a cardiac murmur on routine physical examination in patients without symptoms. Cardiac enlargement and cardiac symptoms generally occur late in the course of valvular heart disease. However, even late manifestations such as heart failure can be the initial presentation if a cardiac murmur has been previously unrecognized.

The approach to the medical assessment of the patient with valvular heart disease begins with the traditional history. Symptoms may be related to pulmonary congestion either during exercise or at rest. Disturbances in rhythm and reduction in myocardial perfusion may create palpitations or chest discomfort. Although pulmonary edema may be the presenting manifestation of valvular heart disease, symptoms are a late expression of the process and indicate a decline in cardiac compensatory mechanisms and myocardial contractility.

The physical exam is essential for detection of abnormalities. Valvular heart disease usually presents with cardiac murmurs; also, abnormalities in peripheral arterial and venous pulsations can reflect valvular incompetence or stenosis, or impaired left ventricular function. The clinical exam is also important for follow-up and for assessment of cardiac deterioration as the cause of heart failure or pulmonary edema.

Noninvasive studies in valvular heart disease always include x-rays of the chest for cardiac and pulmonary assessment and the electrocardiogram for evidence of chamber enlargement. In recent years, these techniques have been supplemented by echocardiography for anatomic delineation of valves, chambers, and wall motion, and by exercise tests for assessment of cardiac reserve and symptom development and for correlation with other circulatory alterations. Radionuclide studies have also contributed to assessment of cardiac function, chamber size, and valve incompetence in selected patients.

Cardiac catheterization remains an important technique to evaluate patients with valvular heart disease. Recognition of the abnormality affecting one or more of the cardiac valves, assessment of the overload imposed on the affected heart chambers, evaluation of left ventricular function, detection of unsuspected cardiac lesions, and finally anatomic visualization of the coronary arteries constitute important indications for cardiac catheterization. In patients with prosthetic valve replacements, the development of new murmurs, aggravation of heart failure, or suspected endocarditis are additional reasons for cardiac catheterization.

GENERAL APPROACH TO THE PATIENT WITH VALVULAR HEART DISEASE

History

Since the patient with valvular heart disease often presents for medical evaluation with a history of a heart murmur, specific inquiry should be directed to the first recognition of the murmur and any possible influences on previous health. A murmur may have been recognized at birth or in early infancy and a comment made by the pediatrician to the parents. Detection may have been made in childhood during the usual pediatric examination or preschool physical. In the teenage years, individuals may be examined prior to physical education programs, athletics, preparation for college, entry into the armed forces, or marriage. Females may be examined during pregnancy and males and females with the purchase of life insurance.

Appraisal of the physical activity status from childhood and adolescence to adulthood is important to detect limitations in the individual. In childhood and adolescence, physical activity is generally unrestrained even though advice by parents and physicians may be to the contrary. Interrogation should cover usual household activities, hobbies, sports, and conditioning programs.

The earliest mention to the patient of an enlarged heart is important, whether detected by physical examination or chest x-ray, and previous records should be obtained for confirmation. Previous routine electrocardiograms should be reviewed. Unexplained medical illnesses should be carefully queried for the possibility of bacterial endocarditis with prolonged fever, night sweats, or embolic phenomena.

The initial onset of dyspnea or fatigue should be carefully characterized—specifically the time, activity, patient's response, and recurrence. Whether avoidance of exertional activity is voluntary or involuntary is important, since it may have been suggested by the physician when a heart murmur was first detected. Specific inquiry for chest discomfort, palpitations, fluid retention, and syncope is necessary. Previous medical care, changes in lifestyle, therapy, and the symptomatic response are historically important. If the patient has undergone cardiac surgery, careful description of symptoms prior to surgery, the postoperative course for three to six months, and comparison of newly developed symptoms become essential for clinical evaluation.

The family history is useful for additional evidence of congenital cardiac lesions, rheumatic heart disease, heritable disorders of connective tissue such as Marfan's syndrome, and mitral valve prolapse. Finally, certain forms of cardiomyopathy and related murmurs can occur in family members.

Physical Examination

Although evaluation of the patient with valvular disease requires attention to the vascular system and heart, a complete examination should be performed in the standard manner. This begins with particular attention to the vital signs. Fever should raise the possibility of bacterial endocarditis or a recurrence of rheumatic fever. Palpation of a peripheral artery may alert the examiner to an abnormality of the amplitude, upstroke, or duration of the peripheral pulse. A wide pulse amplitude should suggest incompetence of the aortic valve, but a brisk upstroke can be observed in hypertrophic subaortic stenosis or mitral regurgitation. Any peripheral left to right shunt will also increase the amplitude of the pulse. A delayed upstroke is characteristic of stenosis of the aortic valve, but severe mitral stenosis may reduce the amplitude of the pulse as well. Measurement of the blood pressure can further confirm the peripheral vascular abnormalities in valvular disease. A widening of the difference between systolic and diastolic pressures is characteristic of incompetence of the aortic valve. Narrowing of the systolic and diastolic pressure difference similarly suggests obstruction of the aortic valve. However, myocardial failure from any cause can also result in a narrowed pressure difference. The general appearance of the patient may suggest certain valvular abnormalities such as severe mitral stenosis (facial plethora and congestion) or Marfan's syndrome (typical body habitus). Skin changes may be associated with heritable disorders of connective tissue. Head bobbing indicates severe aortic incompetence. Ophthalmologic exam may reveal abnormalities in the lens and elongation of the globe in Marfan's syndrome. Pulsations of the retinal arterioles with aortic incompetence can be visualized, as well as the boat-shaped hemorrhages or Roth's spots in bacterial endocarditis.

The venous pressure can be estimated best in the sitting position. Any distention above the head of the clavicle represents increased central venous pressure. For accurate detection of pulse waves in the neck veins, simultaneous cardiac auscultation should be performed for identification of the first heart sound. Any movement of the neck veins prior to or simultaneous with the first heart sound represents an A wave or atrial contraction. Exaggerated A waves suggest restriction to right ventricular filling, which can be caused by tricuspid stenosis or hypertrophy of the right ventricle. An exaggerated V wave indicates incompetence of the tricuspid valve and is a more sustained rise in the venous pulse than the sharp A wave upstroke. Many patients with evidence of fluid retention in the extremities due to valvular heart disease will exhibit some degree of tricuspid regurgitation which can be appreciated from the V wave.

The cardiac exam should be performed in the traditional sequence of inspection, palpation, percussion, and auscultation. Precordial movements in the area of the left ventricular apical impulse as well as along the left sternal border and the base of the heart should be noted. Palpation at the apex, the left sternal border, and the base of the heart should recognize a shock or palpable heart sound, a thrill or palpable heart murmur, and evidence of right or left ventricular enlargement. Palpation is important, not only in the recumbent but also in the sitting position, particularly in searching for the palpable murmur or thrill of aortic stenosis in the right second interspace. Palpation is best performed with the palm of the hand rather than the tips of the fingers. Although percussion of the heart is denigrated by some as being inaccurate, significant cardiac enlargement can be recognized by finding extension of the left border of dullness beyond the estimated midclavicular line. Dullness to the right of the sternum is abnormal and suggests the possibility of displacement or enlargement of the right heart or dilatation of the ascending aorta.

The method of auscultation should be orderly and repetitious from one patient to the other. Identifying the first heart sound, by simultaneous palpation of the carotid pulse, is frequently helpful when the heart rate exceeds 100. The first heart sound should be characterized as to its intensity and whether one or two components are present. Increased intensity of the first heart sound should suggest the possibility of mitral stenosis but can occur with thyrotoxicosis or any shortening of the PR interval on the electrocardiogram. If two components are present one must differentiate physiologic splitting from an atrial gallop followed by a single first heart sound, or the first heart sound followed by an ejection click. Atrial gallops are low-pitched sounds, heard best with the bell of the stethoscope in the left lateral decubitus position, and are common in coronary artery disease, hypertension, and cardiomyopathies. An ejection click should raise the possibility of mitral valve prolapse but can also occur with a bicuspid aortic valve or dilatation of the ascending aorta. The second sound is usually single at the apex. Sounds immediately following the second heart sound at the apex include the opening snap of mitral stenosis and the protodiastolic ventricular gallop, generally a hallmark of a failing left ventricle.

After description of the first and second sounds at the apex, systole should be examined for the presence, timing, and character of any murmur. Systolic murmurs at the apex suggest either turbulence of flow across the aortic valve or regurgitation across the mitral valve. Onset with the first heart sound is helpful in differentiating mitral from aortic murmurs. However, the murmur of the mitral valve prolapse can occur in mid- or late systole. Finally, differentiation of functional systolic murmurs from those generated by abnormal turbulence requires an arbitrary designation based on the intensity of the murmur and associated auscultatory abnormalities. Diastolic murmurs are abnormal and are produced by incompetence of the aortic valve or stenosis of the mitral valve.

Similar maneuvers and the same auscultatory procedures as for first sound, second sound, systole, and diastole should be repeated along the left sternal border and the aortic and pulmonic areas. Murmurs heard along the lower left sternal border may reflect tricuspid valve abnormalities and are influenced by respiration. Aortic and pulmonic murmurs are most prominent at the base of the heart. Auscultatory maneuvers should be performed in the recumbent and the sitting positions. To complete a thorough cardiac auscultatory exam, a mild form of exercise should be induced, such as sit-ups in bed or hopping on one foot to increase the heart rate. The diastolic rumble of mitral stenosis may become audible for the first time.

Examination of peripheral pulses should include the presence and equality of radial, femoral, and dependent pulses in the feet. Disparity between upper and lower extremity pulses should raise the possibility of a bicuspid aortic valve with coarctation of the aorta. The abdominal examination should evaluate liver size and tenderness, presence of ascites, and transmitted abdominal murmurs. Attention should be given to the lower extremities for the presence of edema as well as calf tenderness. Evidence of focal neurologic deficits should suggest embolization from thrombus formation or infection of the valves. A thorough neurologic examination can be helpful in future assessment of the patient should complications occur in the subsequent course of valvular heart disease or after prosthetic valve replacement.

Laboratory Studies

Electrocardiogram

The electrocardiogram is useful in the assessment of valvular heart disease in the recognition of atrial and ventricular enlargement. Left atrial enlargement as seen in mitral stenosis can be recognized by prominence and increased duration of the P wave in inferior leads 2,3, and AVL, as well as of the P terminal force in lead V_1. Left ventricular hypertrophy can be recognized by an increase in voltage as well as accompanying ST-T wave segment changes. The hypertrophy can be secondary to the pressure overload of aortic stenosis or to the volume overload of aortic or mitral regurgitation. Right axis deviation of the QRS complex suggests right ventricular hypertrophy in response to pulmonary hypertension. Atrial fibrillation often accompanies any degree of left atrial enlargement due to mitral stenosis and/or regurgitation. Conduction disturbances such as bundle branch block and complete heart block can develop in the course of valvular heart disease.

Chest X-Ray

Changes in the pulmonary vasculature as well as cardiac chambers can be evaluated by the standard chest films. Pulmonary venous hypertension leads to prominence of the veins, often with redistribution toward the apices of the lungs. Enlargement of the hilar vessels as well as a conspicuous main pulmonary artery along the left sternal border may indicate pulmonary hypertension. Cardiac chamber enlargement can be assessed from different views. Although the cardiothoracic ratio is not a sensitive measure of left ventricular enlargement, a ratio greater than 50 per cent correlates with an abnormal increase in the end-diastolic volume of the left ventricle. Left atrial enlargement can be recognized by the double contour along the right sternal border as well as elevation of the left mainstem bronchus and straightening of the left cardiac border. Right ventricular dilatation can be recognized from the lateral view by encroachment of the cardiac silhouette on the sternum. Both right ventricular and right atrial enlargement can be suspected when the cardiac shadow protrudes beyond the sternum to the right. Additional oblique and angulated views can further assess chamber enlargement of the atria and ventricles.

Echocardiography

Echocardiography in valvular heart disease can frequently provide a reliable estimate of chamber size, wall thickness, and ejection fraction. Valvular anatomy and motion can be defined and provide a basis for confirming mitral valve prolapse, atrial myxomas, and mitral stenosis (Fig. 45–1). In aortic stenosis the number of cusps can sometimes be recognized, along with calcification of the valves. Fluttering of the mitral leaflets during diastole from regurgitant flow across the aortic valve can be recognized. The characteristic motion of the stenotic mitral valve may also be attended by echoes from any calcification. One of the most frequent and significant contributions of echocardiography is the detection of mitral valve prolapse with the characteristic late systolic movement of the posterior leaflet. Mitral valve prolapse can involve both leaflets. Left atrial myxomas produce a classic echocardiogram with multiple echoes and motion across the mitral valve. Bacterial endocarditis of either the aortic or the mitral valve can sometimes be detected with echocardiography.

Cardiac Catheterization

Cardiac catheterization in valvular heart disease remains the most definitive procedure to complete the cardiac evaluation. Objectives for cardiac catheterization are (1) to identify the underlying valve lesion, (2) to assess ventricular function, (3) to evaluate the anatomy of the coronary arteries, (4) to recognize any additional cardiac lesions, and (5) to assess the integrity of prosthetic heart valves. Since the morbidity and mortality of cardiac catheterization have significantly decreased with improvement in technical skills and equipment in recent years, this procedure can be offered initially to provide definitive diagnostic, prognostic, and therapeutic information on valvular heart disease. Another application of cardiac catheterization is to provide a basis of calibration in the individual patient for noninvasive technologies such as echocardiography and radionuclide angiography. Thus, after the initial catheterization assessment of valvular and cardiac function, the patient with valvular heart disease can often be followed with noninvasive tests. Cardiac catheterization should not necessarily be withheld or delayed in the patient with valvular heart disease until surgery is contemplated.

The crucial hemodynamic measurement in catheterization of patients with mitral stenosis is the gradient across the mitral valve. However, many patients with mitral stenosis experience their initial symptoms with exertion, and therefore it is important to exercise these patients if the resting mitral gradient is minimal. In addition to measuring the gradient, an accurate determination of cardiac output is important for calculation of the valve orifice size using the Gorlin formula. In mitral regurgitation, the essential procedure is demonstration and quantitation of regurgitation across the mitral valve during systole. This is shown angiographically with the injection of contrast into the left ventricle and regurgitation back into the left atrium. The right anterior oblique position is optimal for recognition of the mitral valve apparatus, as well as the size of the left atrium. In aortic stenosis, like mitral stenosis, the important measurement is the gradient across the aortic valve during systole. This is obtained with a pull-back catheter recording from the left ventricular chamber into the aorta. Aortic regurgitation is confirmed and quantified by aortic root injection of contrast material with streaming into the left ventricle during angiography. Lesions of the pulmonic and tricus-

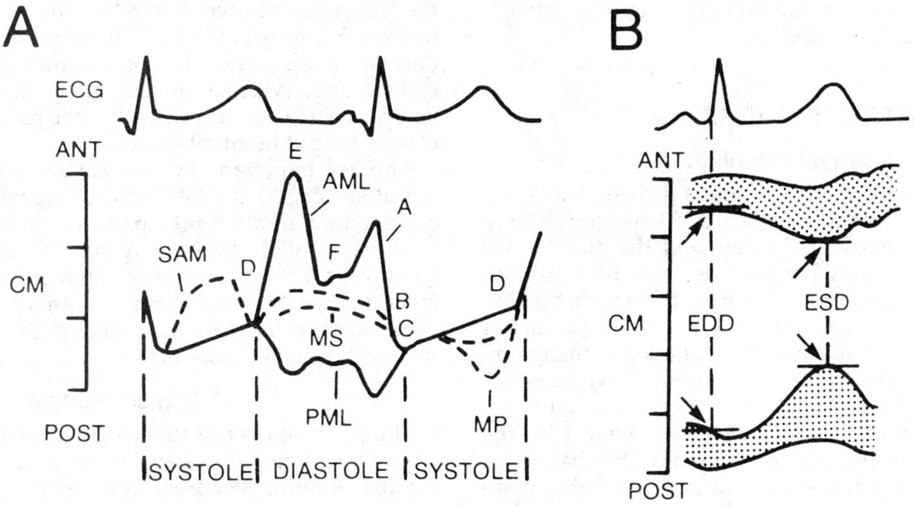

Figure 45–1. *A,* Characteristic normal and abnormal motions of the mitral valve. Simplified diagrammatic echocardiogram of the motions of normal mitral valve as obtained by M-mode echocardiography. AML = anterior mitral leaflet; PML = posterior mitral leaflet; ECG = simultaneously recorded electrocardiogram. The scale is in centimeters from anterior (ANT) to posterior (POST). In the normal tracing (solid lines) during left ventricular systole the two leaflets are normally closed and there is a gradual anterior motion, as the whole heart moves forward during ventricular ejection. With the onset of diastole (D) the leaflets open rapidly in opposite directions, and during early rapid ventricular filling the anterior leaflet rapidly reaches its most forward position (E). The anterior leaflet then moves back to a partially closed position as rapid filling diminishes (E to F slope), and a brief period of slow filling or diastasis is shown, followed by another rapid opening of both leaflets resulting from late rapid filling during atrial contraction, which reaches a peak at point A. With atrial relaxation the leaflets again close. The onset of mechanical ventricular contraction sometimes causes a notch (not shown) at point B, and is then followed by closure of the mitral valve at point C.

Abnormal mitral valve motions are indicated by dashed lines. In the typical patient with severe mitral stenosis (MS), the abnormalities are represented by the dashed lines during diastole. Both the anterior and posterior mitral leaflets move anteriorly during diastole; the forward excursion of the anterior leaflet to the E point is much reduced, and its E to F slope illustrates marked systolic anterior movement (SAM) of the anterior mitral leaflet. In some instances this motion may cause the anterior leaflet to touch the hypertrophied interventricular septum during systole, thereby leading to obstruction in the left ventricular outflow tract. Mitral valve prolapse (MP) occurs during left ventricular systole, as illustrated in the right-hand systolic period. Typically, the leaflets move posteriorly during the latter half of systole, the motion often being most marked in the posterior leaflet, as shown. Occasionally, the posterior movement is holosystolic.

B, Diagram of left ventricular septal and posterior walls by M-mode echocardiography. EDD = end-diastolic diameter (measured from the onset of the QRS complex, vertical dashed line). ESD = end-systolic diameter.

$$\text{Fractional shortening} = \frac{\text{EDD} - \text{ESD}}{\text{EDD}}$$

pid valves are more often associated with congenital heart disease and require appropriate angiographic injection sites. Right ventricular injection is often difficult, and tricuspid regurgitation is confirmed with difficulty at cardiac catheterization. In addition to specific valve assessment, information on left ventricular function with angiographic measurements of chamber size, ejection fraction, wall thickness, mass, and wall motion can be obtained with quantitative angiography. Wall motion abnormalities can be examined and quantitated in patients with coexistent coronary artery disease. The coronary arteries should be visualized in any patient with valvular disease above the age of 40 years.

Since additional valvular disease often coexists with mitral or aortic disease, catheterization should be directed at recognizing clinically unsuspected lesions. In the presence of severe mitral stenosis the murmur of aortic stenosis may be minimal or inaudible, and therefore a pull-back pressure recording should be obtained from the left ventricle into the aorta. In aortic valve lesions or any form of left ventricular dilatation, secondary mitral regurgitation may occur and therefore a left ventricular angiogram is important to evaluate the competence of the mitral valve. Finally, in the presence of prosthetic heart valves the clinical assessment, including auscultation and use of noninvasive techniques, may not accurately detect paravalvular leaks, thrombus, or infection of the valves. Angiography becomes particularly useful in assessing the function of the prosthetic valves.

The general consequences of stenotic and regurgitant valvular lesions are summarized in Figure 45–2.

MITRAL STENOSIS

Etiology and Pathology

The predominant cause of mitral stenosis is rheumatic fever, which remains a prevalent cardiovascular disease in the temperate climates of the world. Calcification of the mitral valve annulus occurs in the elderly but does not present significant hemodynamic obstruction. Unusual causes of mitral obstruction may be space-occupying lesions, such as left atrial myxoma, or thrombus formation. A characteristic pathologic change in rheumatic fever is scarring, particularly at the valve margins. This also extends into the chordae, with shortening and fusion. Eventually calcification of the valve develops, along with the fibrotic and destructive changes. In addition to the changes in the mitral valve there are also significant pathologic abnormalities in the lungs, with thickening of the pulmonary veins, capillaries, and arteries with intimal and medial proliferation. There is also fibrosis and often hemosiderosis in the pulmonary parenchyma. All of these changes are the result of chronic pulmonary hypertension. In the patient with advanced mitral stenosis accompanied by severe pulmonary hypertension, there will also be right ventricular hypertrophy and fibrosis. With longstanding severe mitral stenosis, areas of atrophy have been described in the left ventricular myocardium.

Physiology

The hemodynamic changes and the alterations in cardiac function in mitral stenosis result from obstruction to blood flow through the mitral valve orifice into the left ventricle during diastole. The normal cross-sectional area of the mitral valve orifice ranges from 4 to 6 sq cm. Turbulence with impairment of diastolic flow occurs when the valve orifice is reduced below 2 sq cm.

The average age for acute rheumatic fever is around 10 to 12 years, and generally there is a subsequent 10-year period before a murmur of mitral stenosis may be detected. Another 10 to 12 years is usually required after detection of the murmur before symptoms develop that are caused by impaired diastolic filling of the left ventricle and subsequent left atrial pulmonary venous hypertension. Initially exercise, increased cardiac output, fever, or tachycardia may be necessary to produce the murmur when there is only moderate mitral stenosis of between 1.5 and 2 sq cm. Thus, patients may be free of symptoms at rest and notice dyspnea only during conditions that increase cardiac demands and require commensurate increases in diastolic filling of the left ventricle.

With progressive reduction in mitral orifice size, a diastolic gradient develops between the left atrium and the left ventricle even under resting conditions. This gradient results in fixed elevation of left atrial and pulmonary venous pressures, and minimal effort or exercise may further exaggerate these abnormalities. Constant pulmonary venous hypertension will be transmitted to the pulmonary capillary bed, which in the course of longstanding mitral stenosis undergoes proliferation and capillary thickening. Thus, in the second stage of the hemodynamic development of mitral stenosis the patients may exhibit a diastolic murmur and significant pulmonary hypertension.

The most advanced stage of the physiologic alterations occurs with moderate to severe pulmonary hypertension due to further reduction in mitral orifice size below 1.0 sq cm. Left atrial and pulmonary hypertension have become significant and fixed, and the pulmonary capillary pressure often exceeds 20 to 25 mm Hg. This leads to significant pulmonary arterial hypertension, pressure overload on the right ventricle, and compensatory hypertrophy of the right ventricle. With the chronic nature of mitral stenosis, this condition can lead to elevations of pulmonary arterial pressure approaching those of the systemic circulation. The resting cardiac output can be maintained until the late stages of severe mitral stenosis and pulmonary hypertension. However, exercise will not produce a normal or nearly normal increase in cardiac output owing to the impaired diastolic filling. With severe pulmonary hypertension and right ventricular failure, there is a further reduction even in resting cardiac output in mitral stenosis.

Another important hemodynamic complication in chronic mitral stenosis is the left atrial enlargement due to sustained elevation of left atrial pressures. This creates the circumstance in which atrial fibrillation may initially occur on an intermittent basis but eventually becomes chronic. Atrial fibrillation, by its increased ventricular response, can aggravate the hemodynamic abnormalities by increasing the heart rate and reducing the diastolic filling period.

Clinical Features

Mitral stenosis tends to affect females more than males, and often symptoms first develop at ages 25 to 30. However, significant mitral stenosis can develop in early childhood, and severe hemodynamic impairment can be present by the age of 10 to 12 years. Dyspnea is secondary to pulmonary venous hypertension and congestion. The initial clinical symptoms are often precipitated by increased exertional demands on the left ventricle, such as exercise, febrile conditions, or sudden increases in heart rate. Paroxysmal atrial fibrillation can precipitate symptoms by increasing the heart rate and reducing the diastolic filling period, leading to pulmonary venous congestion. As stenosis progresses, patients may have dyspnea with minimal effort. However, the compensatory changes in pulmonary capillary thickening due to chronic pulmonary hypertension and longstanding mitral stenosis tend to protect the lungs from extravasation of fluid even with severe elevations of pulmonary pressure.

Another clinical manifestation of mitral stenosis can be systemic embolization due to underlying atrial fibrillation, either paroxysmal or chronic. Left atrial thrombus can develop from the stagnation of blood after loss of atrial contraction. Thus, an embolic event in a young female should always raise the possibility of underlying mitral stenosis. A systemic embolus can be the first manifestation of initial mitral stenosis. Females can become symptomatic during the second trimester of pregnancy, when there are significant increases in blood volume and further elevation of the left atrial and pulmonary venous pressures. As the blood volume begins to stabilize or diminish in the third trimester, the symptoms may be somewhat less.

Additional pulmonary symptoms include cough due to left atrial enlargement and infringement on the mainstem bronchus. Hemoptysis results from rupture of small vessels in the bronchi due to the longstanding pulmonary venous hypertension. Rarely the hemoptysis can be sufficiently massive to require emergency intervention. Finally, bacterial endocarditis can develop at any stage of the illness with mitral stenosis.

Physical Findings

On physical examination in a patient with severe mitral stenosis, the peripheral pulse and blood pressure may reflect the reduced stroke volume by a diminished pulse pressure and narrowing of the systolic and diastolic pressure difference. Patients with longstanding mitral stenosis develop typical facies with fluid congestion of the cheeks. Neck vein distention in the sitting position suggests right ventricular failure with secondary tricuspid regurgitation. If tricuspid stenosis coexists with the mitral stenosis, a prominent A wave may be observed in the neck. Findings in the lungs will vary from clear breath sounds to the fine rales of left ventricular failure. The precordium may display activity along the left sternal border, suggesting pulmonary hypertension and right ventricular enlargement. On palpation at the apex the first heart sound may be sufficiently accentuated to be felt. Occasionally the diastolic rumble can be palpated at the apex. A prominent pulmonic second sound with severe pulmonary hypertension can also be detected by the hand as well as the right ventricular lift along the left sternal border. In the early stages of mitral stenosis, percussion may reveal normal cardiac dimensions. As the left atrium enlarges, dullness may persist laterally in the third interspace. With right ventricular hypertrophy and dilatation, the left ventricular apical impulse may be displaced laterally and superiorly. If the right cardiac border is percussed to the right of the sternum, right ventricular enlargement is usually present.

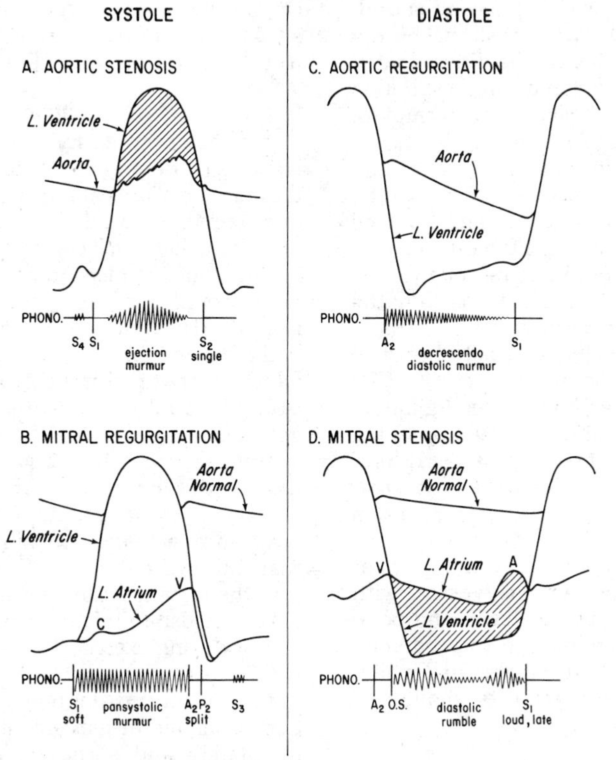

Figure 45–2. Diagrams of pressure tracings and phonocardiograms in valvular heart disease. The left-hand panels illustrate systole; the right-hand panels, diastole.

A, Pressure tracings in the aorta and left ventricle in aortic stenosis. The shaded area indicates the pressure gradient between left ventricle and aorta. The presystolic (A wave) in the left ventricle correlates with the atrial diastolic gallop (S_4) on the phonocardiogram (Phono). The murmur follows the time course of the pressure gradient during ventricular ejection, and the prolonged left ventricular ejection time results in a single second heart sound (S_2).

B, Pressure tracings in the aorta, left ventricle, and left atrium in mitral regurgitation. (Similar events occur in the right atrium, jugular venous pulse, and right ventricle in tricuspid regurgitation.) A prominent V wave is visible in the left atrium, and the pansystolic murmur on the phonocardiogram persists as long as there is a pressure gradient from left ventricle to left atrium across the leaking mitral valve. The A_2P_2 interval is more widely split than normal because of a shortened left ventricular ejection time in severe mitral regurgitation. The rapid filling wave in the left ventricle and left atrium is often accompanied by a ventricular diastolic gallop (S_3).

C, Pressure tracings in the aorta and left ventricle in aortic regurgitation. There is a widened arterial pulse pressure with a rapidly falling aortic diastolic pressure. On the phonocardiogram the decrescendo diastolic murmur follows the time course of the diminishing diastolic pressure gradient from the aorta to the left ventricle across the leaking aortic valve.

D, Pressure tracings in the aorta, left ventricle, and left atrium in mitral stenosis. (Similar events occur in the right atrium, jugular venous pulse, and right ventricle in tricuspid stenosis.) The left atrial pressure is elevated and the pressure gradient between left atrium and left ventricle during diastole is indicated by the shaded area. The slow fall in left atrial pressure after the V wave (slow Y descent) indicates obstruction to left atrial emptying, and the prominent A wave of left atrial contraction is not transmitted to the ventricle. The dumbbell-shaped diastolic rumble of mitral stenosis in the presence of normal sinus rhythm follows the time course of the pressure gradient, which is greatest early and again late in diastole. An increase or a decrease in the height of the left atrial pressure will move the mitral opening snap (O.S.) closer to or farther from, respectively, the aortic closure sound (A_2); similarly a higher left atrial pressure will result in a later and louder first heart sound (S_1).

Characteristic auscultatory findings are the accentuated first sound at the apex, an opening snap following the second heart sound, and an early mid-diastolic rumble at the apex. The opening snap can vary from 0.04 to 0.10 second after the second sound at the apex. The shorter intervals indicate more severe stenosis. The opening snap is high pitched and best detected in the left lateral decubitus position. It can be transmitted to the base of the heart and sometimes into the suprasternal notch. Since the pulmonic second sound can be accentuated and split, gradual inching from the pulmonic area to the apex is useful in differentiating the split pulmonic second sound from an opening snap at the apex. The diastolic rumble at the apex is characteristically low pitched following the opening snap. If normal sinus rhythm is preserved there is presystolic accentuation attributed to atrial contraction. Rarely the presystolic accentuation can occur even in the presence of atrial fibrillation, but generally it disappears with the onset of the arrhythmia and loss of atrial contractility. In addition to the splitting and accentuation of the pulmonic second sound, there may be a systolic murmur at the lower left sternal border representing tricuspid regurgitation. This can be differentiated from mitral regurgitation by its accentuation during inspiration and by the large V wave in the neck. Since the murmur of mitral stenosis may be faint or inaudible in the early stages, exercise should be induced during the initial physical examination by sit-ups or hops on one foot to increase the heart rate. Auscultation of the apex should be performed in the left lateral decubitus position. The diastolic murmur of pulmonic insufficiency along the left sternal border should also be sought.

Mitral stenosis is often accompanied by some degree of mitral regurgitation owing to the fibrotic or calcified valve. Thus, a holosystolic murmur of varying intensity is usually heard at the apex and may radiate into the axilla or into the back. The intensity of the first sound is reduced with mitral regurgitation; this may help in deciding whether mitral stenosis or mitral insufficiency is the dominant lesion. Timing of the early protodiastolic third sound as an opening snap or a ventricular gallop is also helpful in differentiating the predominant lesion of the valve.

If tricuspid insufficiency is severe, there will be enlargement and pulsation of the liver. Splenomegaly may occur with bacterial endocarditis or after acute rheumatic fever, and occasionally in congestive failure. Fluid retention in the abdomen and lower extremities indicates right ventricular failure. Finally, evidence of thrombophlebitis in the extremities should be recognized.

Laboratory Studies

Electrocardiogram

The characteristic changes on the electrocardiogram reflect left atrial enlargement and right ventricular hypertrophy due to pulmonary hypertension. Left atrial enlargement produces prolongation of the P wave and characteristic notching that can be easily observed in inferior leads 2, 3, and AVF. Also, the P terminal force in lead V_1 will be negative and at least 1 mm in amplitude, with significant left atrial enlargement. Even after the onset of atrial fibrillation the coarse fibrillatory waves correlate with significant left atrial enlargement. A vertical QRS complex or right axis deviation indicates pulmonary hypertension and right ventricular hypertrophy. Increased amplitude of the R wave in V_1 can be additional evidence of right ventricular hypertrophy. Any electrocardiographic evidence of left ventricular hypertrophy should raise the suspicion of underlying mitral regurgitation or coexisting aortic valve disease.

Chest X-Ray

Evaluation of the chest film should seek evidence of left atrial enlargement and pulmonary venous and arterial hypertension. Enlargement of the left atrium will initially produce a double contour along the right cardiac silhouette as the left atrium enlarges both posteriorly and to the right. Also, there may be elevation of the left mainstem bronchus and straightening of the left cardiac border due to an enlarged left atrial appendage and chamber. With sustained pulmonary venous hypertension, there is redistribution of the venous pattern and blood flow to the apices of the lung. Finally, with significant hypertension, there will be prominence of the hilar arteries, which taper abruptly in the peripheral areas. There may be Kerley's B lines due to fibrosis and lymphatic engorgement of interlobular septa, seen as transverse linear densities about 1 cm in length and located at the lung bases laterally above the diaphragm. Pleural effusion is a manifestation of combined ventricular failure.

Echocardiogram

The echocardiographic features of mitral stenosis are diagnostic from the characteristic motion of the mitral valve, which resembles a square wave during diastole. Calcification will produce additional echoes from the stenotic mitral valve. Dimensions of the left atrium as well as left ventricular function can be assessed. Enlargement of the right ventricle can also be suspected from the echocardiogram. A left atrial myxoma or a thrombus will produce multiple echoes during diastolic filling.

Cardiac Catheterization

A necessary measurement for the confirmation of mitral stenosis is the pressure gradient across the mitral valve during diastole. Pressures are measured by a direct left atrial recording or a pulmonary capillary wedge recording simultaneously with that of the left ventricle, both at rest and after induced exercise. A simultaneous measurement of the forward cardiac output is necessary if the orifice size is calculated using the Gorlin formula. This hydraulic formula is based on the diastolic flow and the simultaneous pressure gradient across the mitral valve, which correlate with the anatomic orifice size. In patients with isolated mitral stenosis, the gradient across the mitral valve generally ranges from 5 to 20 mm Hg. In individuals without symptoms, the mitral valve area ranges from 1.5 to 2 sq cm; in those with symptoms on unusual activity, valve size is between 1.0 and 1.5 sq cm; and in patients who have marked limitations of physical activity, the mitral valve orifice size is usually less than 1.0 sq cm.

Catheterization can be useful not only to confirm the diagnosis but also to relate severity of symptoms to the gradient at rest or during exercise. Occasionally a minimal gradient at rest will increase markedly with exercise, with resultant pulmonary hypertension and symptoms of heart failure. In addition to the hemodynamic measurements, coexistent lesions of mitral regurgitation and aortic stenosis should be evaluated. Aortic stenosis may be completely obscured by the reduced diastolic filling of the left ventricle, with little turbulence across the aortic valve during systole. Other associated lesions such as atrial septal defects are sometimes confused with mitral stenosis, since the auscultatory findings can be very similar. Finally, in patients above the age of 40 years, visualization of the coronary arteries is important to detect coexistent disease.

Differential Diagnosis

Several cardiac conditions can be confused with the early symptoms and physical findings of mitral stenosis. Primary pulmonary hypertension in young women can produce dyspnea and an accentuated pulmonary second sound but lacks the auscultatory and hemodynamic findings of mitral stenosis. Left atrial myxoma can produce sudden dyspnea or syncope with a diastolic rumble across the valve, but usually this finding is not hemodynamically significant. Finally, an atrial septal defect can produce similar auscultatory events such as accentuated first sound, a possible opening snap, and diastolic rumble. The accentuated first sound in atrial septal defect is due to tricuspid valve closure. The opening snap can be confused with the wide fixed splitting of the pulmonic second sound, and the diastolic rumble can be created by the large diastolic flow across the tricuspid valve.

Medical Treatment

Since mitral stenosis creates a mechanical obstruction to filling of the left ventricle and results in pulmonary venous engorgement, medical therapy can be directed only at reducing the recurrence of rheumatic fever, dental prophylaxis for bacterial endocarditis, control of atrial fibrillation and the ventricular response, and anticoagulation for thromboembolic phenomena. The patients probably should continue on rheumatic fever prophylaxis until the age of 25 years (30 years in females).

Dental prophylaxis should be a standard maneuver throughout life in patients with a stenotic or prosthetic mitral valve. For dental procedures, tonsillectomy, and bronchoscopy, an adult should receive 600,000 units of procaine penicillin G mixed with 1,000,000 units of aqueous crystalline penicillin G intramuscularly 30 to 60 minutes prior to the procedure, and this should be followed by 500 mg penicillin V orally every 6 hours for 8 doses. If the individual is allergic to penicillin, he should receive erythromycin 1 gram orally 1 to 2 hours prior to the procedure and then 500 mg every 6 hours for 8 doses. In individuals with prosthetic mitral valves, intramuscular penicillin as previously described plus streptomycin 1 gram IM should be administered 30 to 60 minutes before the procedure and then followed by penicillin V 500 mg orally every 6 hours for 8 doses. For gastrointestinal and genitourinary surgery, instrumentation and surgery of infected tissues, 2,000,000 units of aqueous penicillin G IM or IV or 1 gram ampicillin IM or IV plus gentamicin 1.5 mg per kilogram (not to exceed 80 mg) IM or IV, or streptomycin 1 gram IM should be given 30 to 60 minutes before the procedure. If gentamicin is used, it should be repeated every 8 hours for 2 additional doses or if streptomycin is used, every 12 hours for 2 additional doses. If the individual is allergic to penicillin, vancomycin plus streptomycin should be employed. In children, appropriately reduced dosages for each of these programs should be used.

Atrial fibrillation can be intermittent and often aggravates or precipitates symptoms of pulmonary congestion. Digitalis should be administered to control the ventricular response. Anticoagulation should be considered on a chronic basis in all patients with mitral stenosis and atrial fibrillation. An attempt at cardioversion should be considered early in the course and especially if the patient develops pulmonary edema. Ideally the patient should be anticoagulated electively two weeks prior to cardioversion. Quinidine should be started two days before the elective procedure and if digitalis has been administered, this may be discontinued one day prior to the cardioversion. If successful, the patient should remain on long-term anticoagulation and quinidine therapy. In thromboembolic phenomena from the left atrium in patients with mitral stenosis, anticoagulation is indicated. For acute embolization to the extremities or abdomen, surgical embolectomy may be beneficial.

Surgical Treatment

Since patients may survive for several years with mitral stenosis, the decision for surgery is based on development of symptoms of pulmonary congestion during activity or at rest or a voluntary restriction of activity to prevent such symptoms. In addition to dyspnea and pulmonary congestion, recurrent atrial fibrillation with aggravation of pulmonary congestion, thromboembolic phenomena, or hemoptysis can also be indications for surgery.

Mitral commissurotomy remains the procedure of choice with a pliable mitral valve without calcification or mitral regurgitation and carries an operative mortality of less than 1 per cent. This procedure should be considered particularly for the young female who has become pregnant, and occasionally commissurotomy is warranted before the development of significant symptoms. The patients often benefit for 5 to 20 years after a commissurotomy. If the symptoms recur at a later time, total mitral valve replacement should be considered.

Mitral valve replacement carries an operative mortality of 2 to 3 per cent. The type of mitral valve inserted depends on the age of the patient, as well as the circumstances for anticoagulation in the young female still wishing to have children. A porcine valve can be inserted without the need for chronic anticoagulation but may require replacement after 7 to 10 years. If the patient's own valve is calcified or if the patient has had a previous commissurotomy and is beyond the childbearing years, a prosthetic device is preferred. However, if there persists a contraindication to anticoagulation, the porcine valve can still be used in later life.

Anticoagulation and dental prophylaxis will be needed in patients with a prosthetic valve. If atrial fibrillation persists and the ventricular response is rapid, digitalis may have to be administered. The long-term complications of prosthetic mitral valves such as thrombus formation, infection, and mechanical dysfunction are estimated to occur at rates of 1 or 2 per cent per year.

The long-term complications of a mechanical mitral valve are thromboembolism (3 per cent per year), valve dysfunction, and endocarditis.

MITRAL REGURGITATION

Etiology and Pathologic Findings

Although for many years rheumatic heart disease was considered the principal cause of mitral regurgitation, other diseases and their complications now account for a majority of cases (Table 45–1). Mitral valve prolapse has become the leading cause of mitral regurgitation. Coronary artery disease with its impairment of wall motion and papillary muscle function often produces mitral valve incompetence. Left ventricular dilatation in any condition affecting the myocardium and producing a volume overload can displace the mitral valve apparatus so that the valves are not competent during systole. Connective tissue disorders can also result in redundancy of the mitral valve. Papillary muscle dysfunction can result not only from coronary disease but also from other infiltrative diseases as well as endocardial and inflammatory disorders. Congenital heart disease, such as partial AV canal, corrected transposition of great arteries, and isolated cleft of the mitral valve can be associated with mitral regurgitation.

Acute mitral regurgitation can also be produced by conditions that suddenly disrupt the normal function of the mitral valve apparatus. Ruptured mitral valve chordae can result from endocarditis, mitral valve prolapse, or trauma or can occur spontaneously. Acute myocardial infarction can rupture the papillary muscle. Perforation of the mitral valve leaflet can develop with bacterial endocarditis. This acute disturbances of mitral valve function can be imposed on chronic mitral regurgitation as well.

Physiology

Incompetence of the mitral valve during systolic ejection permits regurgitation of blood into the left atrium and pulmonary veins. The hemodynamic abnormalities of the left ventricle

TABLE 45–1. MECHANISMS OF CHRONIC AND ACUTE MITRAL REGURGITATION

Chronic Mechanisms
Rheumatic fever
Mitral valve prolapse
Coronary artery disease
Left ventricular dilatation
Calcified mitral annulus
Heritable disorders of connective tissue
Papillary muscle dysfunction
Congenital heart disease
Acute Mechanisms
Rupture of chordae
Rupture of papillary muscle
Perforation of leaflet

and the left atrium are influenced by the chronic or acute nature of the mitral regurgitation, as well as by pre-existing conditions of left ventricular function. In chronic mitral regurgitation, a volume overload is imposed on the left ventricle, and the amount of the regurgitant volume will determine the increase in the end-diastolic volume. The pressure abnormality is the development of a prominent V wave in the left atrium. Under normal conditions, the V wave reflects left atrial filling from the pulmonary venous inflow. The distensibility of the left atrium and the pulmonary veins, as well as the increase in compliant properties of the overloaded left ventricle, permits rapid diastolic filling in mitral regurgitation. Therefore, the left ventricular end-diastolic pressure and the mean left atrial pressure remain within or near the normal range in chronic mitral regurgitation.

The additional mechanical work imposed on the left ventricle in mitral regurgitation is caused by the increase in end-diastolic volume required to maintain the forward cardiac output. The volume overload increases the preload on the left ventricle. The large left ventricular stroke volume is partly ejected into a low impedance area of the left atrium and the pulmonary veins. The duration of systole may be shortened. These factors minimize the increased myocardial oxygen consumption, although left ventricular hypertrophy does accompany the volume-overloaded ventricle.

In chronic mitral regurgitation the total left ventricular stroke volume is large, and thus this condition causes a state of high cardiac output. Eventually,there is a decline in the contractile properties of the left ventricular myocardium, and this decline causes an increase in the end-systolic volume. Although the left ventricular stroke volume remains high when the myocardial inotropic state begins to decline, the ability of the ventricle to dilate further is impaired and the end-diastolic pressure begins to rise abnormally. The ejection fraction begins to fall and may be reduced below the normal range in the early stage of left ventricular decompensation. In this manner, mitral regurgitation leads to a form of high-output heart failure, since the total output of the left ventricle may remain markedly elevated despite a significant decline in the peripheral cardiac output. On rare occasions, deterioration of left ventricular function in mitral regurgitation is attended by significant enlargement of the left atrium such that the ventricular end-diastolic and left atrial pressures remain normal. This situation is sometimes termed the "giant left atrium" syndrome.

In mitral valve prolapse, the regurgitant volume is generally small. Regurgitation can occur in mid- and late systole or throughout the entire systolic phase. The click is produced by the sudden deceleration of blood beneath the prolapsed leaflet, with possible increased tension on the chordae. Generally, the end-diastolic pressure, volume, and left ventricular mass remain within the normal range in mitral valve prolapse, but deterioration in the course of the disorder can lead to significant regurgitation and volume overload on the left ventricle.

In coronary artery disease, mitral regurgitation is usually caused by abnormalities of posterior wall motion and the affected posterior papillary muscle. Lesions are usually found in the right coronary artery and often in the left circumflex artery as well. Ischemia of the papillary muscle has been proposed as a mechanism, but this usually involves the posterior wall also. Once the size of the abnormally contracting segment of the left ventricle exceeds 17 per cent of the total surface area, there will be compensatory dilatation of the ventricle that can further aggravate the mitral regurgitation.

Severe dilatation of the left ventricle from either primary volume overload or secondary myocardial decompensation will eventually create mitral regurgitation. The dilatation of the left ventricular chamber displaces the papillary muscles so that during systole the fixed length of the chordae does not permit adequate coaptation of the mitral valve. Since most of these conditions of ventricular dilatation are associated with significant depression of the contractile state, the hemodynamic abnormalities of the left ventricle reflect primarily those of myocardial failure even though the regurgitation does impose an additional load on the ventricle.

In acute mitral regurgitation, a pressure overload may be imposed on the left atrium and pulmonary veins along with the regurgitant volume from the left ventricle. This acute disturbance is usually accompanied by minimal dilatation of the left ventricular chamber, and the V wave in the left atrium may be as high as 60 to 70 mm Hg. The result is usually the development of acute pulmonary edema.

Clinical Features

In mitral regurgitation caused by a primary defect in the mitral apparatus, patients develop significant cardiomegaly but preserve exercise tolerance and often remain symptom free for long periods of time. Since pulmonary venous hypertension and congestion are not features of mitral regurgitation, fatigue due to a reduced forward cardiac output is a more frequent initial symptom than dyspnea. Gradual impairment of the contractile state of the myocardium leads to further increases in both left ventricular end-systolic and end-diastolic volumes and subsequently to elevations in the filling pressure. Thus, fatigue, limitations on physical exertion, and eventually dyspnea develop as symptoms. Atrial fibrillation is also common when the left atrium enlarges and may create bothersome palpitations as well as aggravate symptoms of heart failure.

In mitral valve prolapse, symptoms are generally unrelated to the mitral regurgitation but more commonly are palpitations, chest discomfort, fatigue, and anxiety. Although palpitations are a very common complaint, monitoring may not confirm underlying rhythm disturbances. The chest discomfort may be indistinguishable from angina pectoris. Almost two thirds of the patients with mitral valve prolapse are female, and there can be a familial incidence of the syndrome.

In coronary artery disease, the mitral regurgitation is usually accompanied by symptoms of impaired left ventricular function, such as dyspnea, fatigue, and orthopnea. This condition is sometimes designated as the ischemic cardiomyopathy syndrome.

In other conditions producing severe ventricular dilatation and secondary mitral regurgitation, the symptoms are primarily those of left ventricular decompensation, which are dyspnea and fluid retention. In the acute syndromes of mitral regurgitation, pulmonary edema is the usual presentation due to both pressure and volume overload of the left atrium and pulmonary venous system.

Physical Examination

Patients with chronic mitral regurgitation can present quite differently from those individuals who develop sudden regurgitation across the valve. In chronic mitral regurgitation the peripheral pulse is sometimes rapid in upstroke and of short duration, similar to the wide pulse pressure in aortic regurgitation. This pulse abnormality is due to a shortened systolic ejection time of the left ventricular stroke volume into the systemic circulation, since a large volume of blood is regurgitated into the low-pressure left atrial system. The neck veins reveal abnormalities only if right ventricular failure has developed. The lungs remain clear unless heart failure has developed on a chronic basis.

Inspection of the precordium may reveal a diffuse hyperdynamic apical impulse displaced laterally and inferiorly due to ventricular dilatation. Palpation of the apical impulse confirms the hyperdynamic motion secondary to volume overload of the left ventricle. Auscultation will reveal a diminution of the first heart sound followed by the characteristic holosystolic murmur, which begins immediately with onset of the first sound and persists until the second heart sound. The murmur often radiates into the axilla and back as well as along the left sternal border. There may be splitting of the second sound at the apex due to the abbreviated period of left ventricular systole. A protodiastolic or ventricular gallop is often audible, and this may be followed by an early diastolic rumble due to the large rapid inflow of blood from the left atrium. In the presence of a large left ventricle and prominent systolic murmur, the third heart sound may be comparable to the physiologic third sound induced by an accelerated early diastolic filling. However, when the mitral regurgitation murmur becomes less intense, the third sound may indicate myocardial failure and depression of the contractile state. Only in the late stages of mitral regurgitation with severe left ventricular failure or coexisting mitral stenosis will the pulmonic second sound become accentuated.

In mitral valve prolapse, inspection and palpation of the precordium are unremarkable. The first heart sound at the apex is usually preserved, followed first by a systolic click that may occur in early, mid-, or late systole and then by a systolic murmur that usually persists until the second sound. The systolic murmur may be holosystolic in about 10 per cent of the patients. Maneuvers that increase the afterload of the left ventricle will delay the onset of the click and the murmur, whereas reductions in left ventricular diastolic volume will cause the click and the murmur to migrate toward the first heart sound.

When mitral regurgitation is associated with depression of the contractile state of the left ventricle, such as in coronary artery disease and idiopathic cardiomyopathies, the ventricle is dilated and hypertrophied. The mitral murmur may be mid-, late, or holosystolic. Under these circumstances, the mitral regurgitant murmur is usually Grade II or less and accompanied by a ventricular gallop.

In acute mitral regurgitation due to rupture of the mitral valve apparatus, cardiac dimensions are normal unless there has been pre-existing cardiomegaly. The murmur tends to be much harsher, Grade III or IV, and may be accompanied by a palpable thrill at the apex or lateral to the third left interspace. Rarely the murmur and thrill can be felt in the primary aortic area owing to the regurgitant jet across the mitral valve striking the atrial septum and transmitting vibrations into the aorta. If the mitral regurgitation is rheumatic in nature, associated mitral stenosis or aortic valve disease is generally present. In hypertrophic cardiomyopathies there may be an audible murmur across the infundibular outflow tract similar to that of aortic valve stenosis as well as the murmur of mitral regurgitation.

In the remainder of the physical examination of mitral regurgitation the pulses should be examined for patency in all extremities, particularly if the basis is coronary artery disease. Evidence for hepatic enlargement and fluid retention occurs when there is accompanying right ventricular failure.

Laboratory Studies

Electrocardiogram

The electrocardiogram should be examined for evidence of left ventricular dilatation and hypertrophy. A left ventricular volume overload pattern of increased voltage amplitude and tall T waves is sometimes seen in the precordial leads. Left atrial enlargement causes prominence of the P terminal force in V_1, which is negative when chamber enlargement becomes significant. Atrial fibrillation eventually accompanies left atrial enlargement. If coronary artery disease is involved in the production of mitral regurgitation, evidence for previous infarction with persistent Q waves should be sought.

Chest X-Ray

The chest x-ray should be examined for changes in the pulmonary venous pattern as well as for size and shape of cardiac chambers. Left ventricular enlargement due to the volume overload can be assessed by the cardiothoracic ratio. Left atrial enlargement will cause a double contour along the right sternal border and elevation of the left mainstem bronchus as in mitral stenosis. The pulmonary venous pattern may show no abnormalities until heart failure and venous congestion have developed.

Echocardiogram

The echocardiogram can provide helpful information on the anatomy of the mitral valve apparatus as well as left ventricular chamber dimensions and function. The echocardiogram is diagnostic in mitral valve prolapse, since the late systolic motion of the posterior or both leaflets can be accurately detected by this procedure. Rarely the flail mitral leaflet caused by chordal rupture can be identified in prolapse or other acute conditions. Secondary causes of mitral regurgitation can be assessed from the end-diastolic and systolic dimensions and function of the left ventricle. When the mitral regurgitation is acute in onset, a flail leaflet or a nidus of infection with bacterial endocarditis can be detected by the echocardiogram. In hypertrophic cardiomyopathies, the characteristic motion of the anterior septal leaflet as well as the asymmetric increase in septal wall thickness can be diagnostic.

Cardiac Catheterization

The primary diagnostic finding is regurgitation of contrast material from the left ventricle into the left atrium, which is best seen in the right anterior oblique position at angiography. Although angiography will not always define the mechanism, prolapse of the mitral valve can often be observed on angiography with ballooning of the leaflet into the left atrium. Ventricular function can be accurately evaluated with chamber dimensions, calculation of the ejection fraction, and left ventricular mass. Coronary artery disease is confirmed with accompanying coronary arteriography. This is also useful in excluding underlying coronary disease as the mechanism when failure has developed. A prominent V wave is detected in the pulmonary capillary wedge pressure or the left atrium. In acute mitral regurgitation, dimensions of the left ventricle and the left atrium are normal, but the V wave can rise to 60 or 70 mm Hg in the left atrium and the capillary system. Cardiac catheterization is also useful in identifying coexistent lesions of the aortic valve. The assessment of the contractile state is important in all causes of mitral regurgitation because the ejection fraction may be spuriously elevated or maintained higher than under other conditions affecting the left ventricle due to the regurgitation into the low impedance zone. Estimation of the contractile state from the end-systolic pressure volume has proved useful.

Differential Diagnosis

The holosystolic murmur usually identifies mitral regurgitation, but the mechanism may not be apparent. When the murmur is not holosystolic, conditions such as aortic stenosis may be entertained. In calcific aortic stenosis of the elderly, the murmur sometimes is more prominent at the apex than at the aortic area and can be confused with mitral regurgitation. A ventricular septal defect produces a harsh holosystolic murmur with palpable vibrations at the lower left sternal border but radiates to the right of the sternum.

Medical Treatment

In the early asymptomatic phase of mitral regurgitation, dental prophylaxis is warranted. Owing to the variable causes, rheumatic fever prophylaxis may not be indicated. In mitral valve prolapse, palpitations may respond to a beta-blocking agent. Dental prophylaxis as described for mitral stenosis should be administered to these patients as well. For the chest discomfort, nitrates or calcium-blocking agents sometimes relieve the symptoms even though coronary anatomy is normal.

If atrial fibrillation develops with mitral regurgitation, medications to slow the ventricular response or stabilize irritability can be useful. The development of heart failure requires the usual treatment with diuretics and inotropic agents and should prompt considerations for surgery. In recent years, afterload-reducing agents have also been useful in various forms of mitral regurgitation. Nitrates and a variety of antihypertensive agents have been found to maintain the forward stroke volume. These are particularly helpful once severe mitral regurgitation has developed.

Surgical Considerations

Since the operative mortality for mitral valve replacement in regurgitant lesions may be slightly higher than the 2 or 3 per cent in mitral stenosis, surgery is generally delayed until patients develop symptoms of dyspnea or congestion. Replacement of the valve and the subsequent postoperative course must be weighed against the level of the contractile state of the ventricle. When the ejection fraction falls below 20 per cent, there is an increase in postoperative morbidity, and mortality with mitral valve replacement may reach 24 per cent. The selection of a porcine over a prosthetic valve rests with the age of the patient as well as with the underlying condition and consideration for anticoagulation. However, prosthetic valves remain most likely to develop thrombus material in the mitral valve position, so anticoagulation must be maintained. Any contraindication to anticoagulation would warrant a porcine valve. Fluoroscopy at the time of replacement is also important, to be repeated in subsequent periods for any complications that prosthetic valves may develop. For preoperative functional classes I through III, there is a yearly mortality rate of 3 per cent over a 10-year follow-up period. The incidence of thromboembolism in mechanical valves with anticoagulation is 3 per cent per year.

AORTIC STENOSIS

Etiology and Pathology

The conditions of the aortic valve that result in significant stenosis are the congenitally bicuspid valve, rheumatic fever, and calcification of the valve in the aging patient. The bicuspid valve functions as two cusps, but invariably there is a raphe in one of the cusps, which indicates failure of the commissure to develop. Although the bicuspid valve initially is not stenotic, fibrosis and thickening lead to eventual narrowing and calcification. The rheumatic valve progressively scars at the margin of the leaflet, and there is eventual fusion of the commissures with ultimate calcification. In approximately 50 per cent of adults with aortic stenosis the valve will be bicuspid, but with extreme fibrosis and calcification pathologic examination may not be able to differentiate between the bicuspid and tricuspid valves. In the calcified valve of the aging patient, the calcium deposits develop in the sinuses but the margins of the leaflets remain uninvolved. This calcification may extend into the annulus.

In the course of any of the conditions producing hemodynamic stenosis of the aortic valve with systolic hypertension in the left ventricle, there is concentric hypertrophy. As myocardial failure develops, the ventricle will dilate. There is usually fibrosis in the hypertrophied myocardium as well.

Pathologic Physiology

Obstruction of the aortic valve produces an elevated left ventricular systolic pressure. Pressure overload on the left ventricle stimulates hypertrophy without dilatation. Left ventricular wall stress or the force per unit of cross-sectional area of myocardium is related directly to cavitary pressure, to the chamber radius cubed (r^3), and inversely to wall thickness. Thus, doubling of cavitary pressure produces a much greater increase in wall stress than doubling of volume. Also, to the extent that myocardial hypertrophy causes an increase in wall thickness, wall stress will be reduced for any given cavitary pressure and volume. In the early phases of aortic stenosis, the wall stress is maintained within the normal range due to concentric hypertrophy of the myocardium and a resulting increase in thickness. The ejection fraction remains normal even though the left ventricular end-diastolic pressure may be significantly elevated. This elevation in the end-diastolic pressure is due to hypertrophy or fibrosis and the resulting decrease of compliance of the ventricle.

Although gradual reduction in the orifice size of the aortic valve will produce turbulence and the characteristic murmur of aortic stenosis, narrowing of 50 or 60 per cent is required before a pressure gradient develops. The hemodynamic obstruction results in a narrowing of the systemic arterial pressure, with a tendency toward a decline in the diastolic pressure as well. These hemodynamic alterations can reduce coronary perfusion. Myocardial oxygen consumption is increased owing to the elevation of the systolic pressure in the left ventricle as well as to the increase in the mass of the left ventricular myocardium. Thus, the conditions are created by significant aortic stenosis to increase myocardial oxygen demands while simultaneously reducing the oxygen supply. These circumstances lead to subendocardial ischemia. Eventually there is a decline in the inotropic state of the myocardium, a reduction in the ejection fraction, dilatation of the left ventricle, and elevation of the left ventricular filling pressure, which is reflected back into the pulmonary venous and capillary system.

The increased myocardial oxygen demands in aortic stenosis associated with the relative underperfusion of the subendocardial myocardium can produce the clinical symptoms of arrhythmia and chest pain, and even sudden death. In adults with aortic stenosis, there may also be coexisting coronary artery disease that can further contribute to myocardial ischemia.

Clinical Features

Symptoms and Clinical Course

The characteristic symptoms of aortic stenosis are chest pain, syncope, and heart failure. A significant gradient across the aortic valve can be present for several years before the patient develops symptoms. In children with congenital aortic stenosis a severe gradient may exist prior to the development of symptoms, while in adults the development of symptoms is attended by a significant mortality in only a few years.

The chest discomfort is usually exertional in nature and indistinguishable from that of ischemic heart disease. Furthermore, significant anatomic coronary artery disease will be present in 50 per cent of adults above the age of 40 years with aortic stenosis whether or not they have angina. Syncope may be the first symptom in aortic stenosis and is probably related to the same mechanism that produces chest pain, a critical reduction in myocardial oxygen supply with increased demands. Orthostatic syncope may develop when the cardiac output is unable to increase with the abrupt assumption of the upright position. Exertional syncope may develop when vasodilatation due to exercise is unaccompanied by an increase in cardiac output. Arrhythmias due to the ischemia may also contribute to syncope and sudden death. Approximately 15 per cent of patients with aortic stenosis at postmortem have died suddenly.

Life expectancy after the development of heart failure in aortic stenosis is often less than two years, whereas patients with angina may survive an average of five years. Life expectancy in aortic stenosis with syncope ranges from two to more than five years. Finally, patients with aortic stenosis are also susceptible to bacterial endocarditis. With calcification of the valve, hemolytic anemia due to destruction of red cells can become a complicating feature.

Physical Examination

Abnormalities on the physical examination in aortic stenosis are a decrease in pulse pressure with a delay of systolic ejection, a diamond-shaped crescendo-decrescendo murmur, and left ventricular hypertrophy. The peripheral pulse reveals the typical diminished pulse amplitude, the delay in upstroke, and the prolongation of the ejection phase (pulsus tardus et parvus). The blood pressure is narrowed, with a tendency toward a gradual decline in the diastolic pressure as well. The carotid arteries transmit the harsh murmurs from the aortic valve, sometimes with a palpable thrill. Neck veins are not abnormally distended unless right ventricular failure has developed. Lung fields remain clear until the onset of heart failure and congestion.

Cardiac examination may reveal no visible abnormalities of chest wall activity, since the heart dimensions do not become increased with concentric hypertrophy. However, on palpitation the apical impulse of the pressure overloaded ventricle will be sustained, although localized. As dilatation develops, there may be a downward and lateral displacement with a more diffuse apical impulse. The most important physical finding is the detection of palpable vibrations over the primary aortic area, which can be brought out with the patient in the sitting position during full expiration. Appreciation of the thrill in aortic stenosis correlates with a gradient across the valve of more than 40 mm Hg. Findings of the heart size on percussion remain within normal limits until failure and dilatation have developed.

On auscultation, the first sound at the apex is usually preserved with normal intensity. Often an atrial gallop is present. Sometimes with a bicuspid aortic valve, an ejection click may be audible along the left sternal border. The aortic second sound is often diminished except in calcific aortic stenosis of the elderly. The characteristic murmur is the diamond-shaped ejection murmur that develops after the first sound, peaks in mid- or late systole, and disappears completely before the second heart sound. If an ejection click is present, the murmur will begin immediately after the click, and this can be confusing if the click is erroneously identified as the first heart sound. Although the murmur is heard over the precordium, the intensity is loudest along the left sternal border and over the primary aortic area. Sometimes, in the elderly patient with calcific aortic stenosis, the musical quality of the murmur is loudest at the apex and aortic stenosis is confused with mitral regurgitation owing solely to the location of the murmur. Often a faint diastolic flow murmur of aortic incompetence can be heard along the left sternal border, since the severely stenotic valve may not close completely during diastole.

Laboratory Studies

Electrocardiogram

The major finding is left ventricular hypertrophy. The pressure overload produces significant changes in the amplitude of the QRS complex and the characteristic ST-T depression of left ventricular hypertrophy. Left axis deviation may develop with marked hypertrophy as well as conduction disturbances of bundle branch block. In severe aortic stenosis there may be slight enlargement of the left atrium, and the P terminal force may become negative in V_1. With significant hypertrophy and underlying fibrosis small Q waves may be seen in the precordial leads.

Chest X-Ray

The cardiac silhouette often remains unimpressive during the initial phases, since the hypertrophy does not increase the cardiothoracic ratio. There may be slight post-stenotic dilatation and prominence of the ascending aorta. Calcification in the aortic valve is difficult to discern on the plain film but can be readily appreciated on cardiac fluoroscopy. As heart failure develops and dilatation of the ventricle occurs, there will be a significant increase in heart size along with congestion of the pulmonary vessels. Since a bicuspid aortic valve is sometimes associated with coarctation of the aorta, rib notching should always be sought on the chest film in the patient with aortic stenosis.

Echocardiogram

The echocardiogram can be useful in aortic stenosis in identifying thickening of the aortic leaflets, determining the number of leaflets present, detecting calcification of the valve, and measuring left ventricular wall thickness. Cross-sectional echocardiography permits estimation of the size of the aortic orifice. The dimensions of the left ventricle and wall thickness indicate the magnitude of hypertrophy.

Cardiac Catheterization

Aortic stenosis is confirmed by a gradient across the aortic valve measured during pull-back of the catheter from the left ventricle to the aorta. Aortic orifice size bears a direct relationship to flow and an indirect relationship to the square root of the gradient. Therefore, a decline in cardiac output will be associated with a major reduction in the pressure gradient across the valve, and if the gradient alone is used as a measure of aortic stenosis, the valve size will be underestimated in situations in which there is a reduction in cardiac output.

The normal aortic orifice size is 2.5 to 3 sq cm. Mild stenosis develops when the orifice size is reduced to 0.75 to 1.5 sq cm. Moderate stenosis is associated with an orifice size of 0.5 to 0.75 sq cm, and stenosis is severe when aortic size is less than 0.5 sq cm. Surgery is usually advised when the aortic valve gradient is greater than 50 mm Hg or the valve area is less than 0.8 sq cm. Left ventricular angiography is helpful in assessing chamber size, ejection fraction, and ventricular function and in determining the presence of mitral regurgitation. Since coronary artery disease may be present in 50 per cent of patients with aortic stenosis with or without chest pain, coronary arteriography should be performed in all adults with aortic stenosis.

Differential Diagnosis

Valvular aortic stenosis has to be differentiated from congenital forms of both supra- and infravalvular stenosis in children. In hypertrophic subaortic stenosis the systolic ejection murmur is similar to that of valvular aortic stenosis, but the peripheral pulse displays a hyperdynamic rapid upstroke and bisferious or double-notched pulse, rather than a delayed upstroke as in valvular aortic stenosis. In acute mitral regurgitation with rupture of a chorda or papillary muscle, the regurgitant jet may be transmitted from the left atrial wall into the aorta, and the murmur is audible over the primary aortic area and accompanied by a palpable thrill. Close attention to the aortic area murmur will reveal that it is holosystolic rather than the diamond-shaped murmur of valvular aortic stenosis. Finally, in significant aortic regurgitation, there is invariably a systolic murmur caused by turbulence across the aortic valve during ejection, but a gradient is usually not present.

Medical Therapy

In the asymptomatic patient with aortic stenosis, dental prophylaxis with antibiotics is indicated to reduce the likelihood of bacterial endocarditis. Prophylaxis as outlined under mitral stenosis should also be given during other invasive procedures, which include studies of the genitourinary and lower gastrointestinal tract. If the patient with aortic stenosis develops an arrhythmia or supraventricular tachycardia, digitalis and an antiarrhythmic drug may be necessary to slow the ventricular response, since such conditions can depress the hemodynamic function of the left ventricle. The development of chest pain warrants consideration of cardiac catheterization to evaluate underlying coronary disease. The use of nitrates in valvular aortic stenosis should be undertaken with great caution, since the arterial systolic pressure may fall and a compensatory increase in cardiac output may be prevented by the stenosis. Since life expectancy after the development of symptoms in aortic stenosis is generally short with medical treatment, the development of chest pain, syncope, or heart failure warrants catheterization, coronary arteriography, and consideration of surgery.

Surgical Treatment

The operative mortality for aortic valve replacement is 2 or 3 per cent and rises to 5 per cent if coronary bypass is also performed. In children with aortic stenosis, surgery may be considered before the development of symptoms if the pressure gradient is high, since annuloplasty can sometimes be performed. Even if the patient has developed heart failure, surgery should be considered, since ventricular function can sometimes improve following prosthetic valve replacement. The prosthetic valve will require long-term anticoagulation, but the porcine valve, which does not require anticoagulation, may deteriorate in 5 to 10 years. In the elderly patient, a porcine heterograft may be preferred to avoid anticoagulation. If indicated, coronary bypass surgery should be performed at the time of aortic valve replacement. The ten-year survival of combined aortic valve replacement and coronary revascularization approaches 55 per cent. Late cardiac events include reoperation, a neurologic event, myocardial infarction, congestive heart failure, endocarditis, bleeding, and thromboembolism, and these occur at a rate of 6 per cent per year.

AORTIC REGURGITATION

Etiology and Pathology

Conditions causing incompetence of the aortic valve include intrinsic disease in the aortic cusps and primary disease of the ascending aorta. Some of these diseases are chronic in nature; others acutely impair the competence of the valve (Table 45–2). Rheumatic fever remains a significant cause of aortic incompetence and is attended by scarring and fibrosis of the valve margins. The bicuspid aortic valve is predominantly stenotic, but incompetence can also develop with scarring and calcification. An aneurysm of the sinus of Valsalva may be associated with a ventricular septal defect. Myxomatous degeneration of the aortic valve cusp can lead to incompetence with the characteristic findings on pathologic examination. Longstanding hypertension as well as arteriosclerosis can be associated with scarring of the aortic valve and mild incompetence. Acute conditions that can disrupt the aortic valve include bacterial endocarditis, which can perforate the leaflets. Rarely with acute rheumatic fever, retraction of the leaflets produces acute aortic regurgitation.

The conditions and diseases that affect the ascending aorta and produce aortic valve incompetence include syphilis, heritable disorders of connective tissue, several arthritic diseases, and cystic medionecrosis of the aorta. In syphilis the granulomatous scarring process can result in calcification of the aorta, extreme dilatation, and ostial narrowing of the coronary arteries. Myxomatous degeneration of the aortic valve occurs in Marfan's syndrome. Arthritic conditions, notably ankylosing spondylitis, rheumatoid arthritis, and Reiter's syndrome, can produce changes in the ascending aorta with secondary aortic regurgitation. Cystic medionecrosis of the aorta can produce dilatation of the ascending aorta even to an aneurysmal degree with secondary aortic regurgitation. Acute aortic regurgitation can result from dissection of the ascending aorta in Marfan's syndrome and from cystic medionecrosis of the aorta.

TABLE 45–2. MECHANISMS OF CHRONIC AND ACUTE AORTIC REGURGITATION

Chronic Mechanisms
Rheumatic fever
Syphilis
Heritable disorders of connective tissue
Marfan's syndrome
Osteogenesis imperfecta
Arthritic diseases
Ankylosing spondylitis
Reiter's syndrome
Rheumatoid arthritis
Cystic medionecrosis of aorta
Sinus of Valsalva aneurysm
Hypertension
Arteriosclerosis
Myxomatous degeneration of valve
Acute Mechanisms
Dissection of aorta
Bacterial endocarditis
Rheumatic fever

Pathologic Physiology

The principal hemodynamic disturbances imposed on cardiac function by aortic incompetence are volume overload of the left ventricle and reduced diastolic perfusion of the coronary arteries. In the early phases of volume overload the end-diastolic pressure is normal or only slightly elevated. As volume overload increases it raises end-diastolic pressure and produces dilatation of the ventricular chamber by slippage of myocardial fibers as well as by sarcomere replication and secondary hypertrophy. The increase in end-diastolic volume thus permits a large left ventricular stroke volume to be achieved with a normal ejection fraction of greater than 50 per cent.

Since the increased left ventricular stroke volume is ejected into a high-impedance area of the systemic circulation, there is usually an associated elevation in the systolic pressure. Even though wall stress may be maintained within the normal range by hypertrophy, the myocardial oxygen demands are significantly increased. The decline in aortic diastolic pressure and the regurgitation of blood into the left ventricle can reduce coronary blood flow. Thus, conditions for subendocardial myocardial ischemia develop in patients with chronic aortic regurgitation.

Although the volume overload can be tolerated for several years, eventually there is a decline in the inotropic state of the myocardium. The ejection fraction falls and thus further dilatation is required to maintain the effective forward stroke volume. The deteriorating inotropic state and the limits of the dilatation-hypertrophy mechanism lead to abnormal elevations of the left ventricular filling pressure and to pulmonary venous and capillary congestion.

In acute aortic regurgitation, the regurgitant volume may be imposed on a normal end-diastolic volume. Under these circumstances there is a marked elevation in the left ventricular filling pressure, since the dilatation mechanism is unable to accommodate these changes in a brief period of time. With rapid flow from the aorta the mitral valve may close prematurely and the aortic diastolic blowing murmur may persist beyond the diminished first heart sound.

Clinical Course and Physical Findings

Clinical Course

The volume overload imposed by aortic regurgitation is well tolerated over a period of time. Even though there may not be restriction of cardiac performance, patients may be aware of prominent precordial activity. Pulsatile carotid arteries may occasionally cause discomfort. Unusual sweating patterns over the body and vague abdominal discomfort are other symptoms. Clinical follow-up of patients with aortic regurgitation has demonstrated that a pulse pressure greater than 140/40 mm Hg and left ventricular enlargement demonstrated by electrocardiogram or chest x-ray are associated with accelerated development of angina, heart failure, or sudden death in one to two years. With the onset of impaired left ventricular contractility and pulmonary venous hypertension, dyspnea, orthopnea, and paroxysmal nocturnal dyspnea develop. Exertional chest pain can also result from relative myocardial ischemia. Tachyarrhythmias may impair ventricular function, but the shortening of the diastolic filling period can be beneficial in terms of reducing the degree of aortic regurgitation.

In patients developing acute aortic regurgitation, pulmonary edema is a prompt complication. These patients often describe the severe pain of aortic dissection as well. These symptoms are frequently misinterpreted as representing an acute myocardial infarction.

Physical Examination

The physical findings in aortic regurgitation reflect the increased left ventricular stroke volume and the rapid diastolic run-off into the left ventricle. The peripheral pulse reveals a widened amplitude with a bounding "water hammer" character. Additional findings include head bobbing, pulsation of retinal arterioles, bounding carotid pulses with transmitted systolic and diastolic murmurs, pistol shot sounds over the femoral arteries, a to-and-fro murmur over the femoral artery with slight compression by the stethoscope, and capillary pulsations in the nail beds. The lungs are usually clear until heart failure develops. In Marfan's syndrome the patient may present with long thin extremities, a high arched palate, pectus excavatum, and skeletal changes in the feet with a high arch. In Marie Strumpell arthritis there may be kyphosis of the spine as well as the skeletal abnormalities of rheumatoid arthritis.

Cardiac examination often reveals an apical impulse that is displaced downward and laterally and is hyperdynamic owing to the volume overload. Palpation confirms a hyperdynamic impulse that occupies more than one interspace. A palpable diastolic thrill along the left or the right sternal border suggests acute disruption of the aortic valve or the ascending aorta with a vibrating membrane in the diastolic flow of blood. Percussion confirms enlargement of the left ventricle, and heart size may achieve the largest proportion found in any of the valvular abnormalities. Percussion to the right of the sternum suggests aneurysmal dilatation of the ascending aorta. On auscultation, the first heart sound is usually preserved. There may be a holosystolic murmur at the apex due to secondary mitral dilation from ventricular enlargement. The typical murmur of aortic regurgitation is a high-pitched diastolic blow following the second sound, heard best along the left sternal border and in the primary aortic area. In the early phases of the condition, the murmur may be brought out only in the sitting position during full expiration. As the regurgitation becomes more severe, there may be impingement on the mitral valve during diastolic flow, and the typical rumble of the Austin Flint murmur may be audible at the apex. A prominent murmur of aortic regurgitation to the right of the sternum suggests aneurysmal dilatation of the ascending aorta. With heart failure a ventricular gallop is audible.

In acute aortic regurgitation, the diastolic murmur may assume vibratory or musical qualities due to a prolapsed aortic valve or to vibration of the intima of the aorta during diastolic flow. The remaining findings on physical examination may reflect heart failure with peripheral edema, ascites, and hepatic congestion.

Laboratory Studies

Electrocardiogram

The changes on the electrocardiogram are those of left ventricular hypertrophy with increased voltage amplitude and the ST-T wave changes of the strain pattern.

Chest X-Ray

Cardiomegaly is usually present in aortic regurgitation and the increase in heart size reflects the dilatation of the ventricle. If there is involvement of the ascending aorta, it will be prominent. Calcification of the ascending aorta should suggest the possibility of underlying syphilis. Calcium in the aortic valve or in the annulus can best be appreciated with fluoroscopy. Pulmonary congestion and vascular prominence are present with left ventricular failure.

Echocardiogram

The echocardiogram may record aortic valve abnormalities but is more helpful in assessing the dimensions of the ascending aorta and of the annulus. Vibrations of the anterior mitral leaflet can be appreciated when the Austin Flint murmur is present. Left ventricular chamber dimensions can be used to assess overall mechanical function, and wall thickness can help estimate the degree of hypertrophy. Postoperative follow-up of heart size in aortic regurgitation has disclosed that valve replacement performed before the end-systolic dimension exceeds 55 mm is associated with a reduction of heart size, whereas valve replacement performed when this figure has been exceeded is followed by irreversible dilatation and failure.

Cardiac Catheterization

The procedure to confirm aortic regurgitation is aortic root injection. The regurgitant jet into the left ventricle will be identified, and the anatomy of the aortic valve, perforation, prolapse of a cusp, size of the ascending aorta, and possible recent or chronic dissection will be defined. Left ventricular dimensions, volume, and ejection fraction will indicate the functional state of the left ventricle. Coronary arteriography is also useful, since there may be a coexisting coronary artery disease in the adult.

Differential Diagnosis

Pulmonic insufficiency due to pulmonary hypertension can produce a diastolic blow along the left sternal border. The assessment of the pulsatile characteristics of aortic regurgitation can help differentiate between incompetence of the pulmonic and aortic valves. There may be coexisting aortic stenosis with a systolic murmur reflecting the relatively large left ventricular stroke volume, and rarely a systolic thrill will accompany severe aortic regurgitation without evidence of a gradient across the aortic valve. In systemic hypertension, the tambour qualities of the aortic second sound can sometimes suggest the faint murmur of aortic regurgitation, and the level of the diastolic pressure may be helpful in differentiating these entities.

Medical Therapy

In patients with aortic regurgitation, dental prophylaxis is usually indicated. Even in asymptomatic patients, ventricular dilatation as measured by an end-systolic dimension of 55 mm by echocardiography may indicate the approach of irreversible cardiac decompensation. Patients with a systolic pressure greater than 140 mm Hg and a diastolic pressure less than 40 mm Hg and left ventricular enlargement by electrocardiogram and chest x-ray are at risk for accelerated development of angina, heart failure, and sudden death. Patients in these two categories can be identified for surgery before irreversible or accelerated deterioration of left ventricular function has developed. Clinical heart failure can be initially managed with digitalis and diuretics. Afterload-reducing agents are also beneficial.

Surgical Therapy

Even in patients with symptoms and with significant left ventricular enlargement, valve replacement can be undertaken with mortality of less than 3 to 5 per cent. Mitral valve replacement may also be necessary if rheumatic mitral regurgitation coexists, and the operative mortality becomes 5 to 10 per cent. If a prosthetic valve is required, anticoagulation will be necessary in the future.

TRICUSPID STENOSIS

Rheumatic fever is the most common cause of stenosis of the tricuspid valve, and this condition is almost invariably associated with involvement of the left-sided valves by the same disease. Rare conditions such as a carcinoid tumor, endocardial fibroelastosis, and right atrial myxoma may cause stenosis or obstruction of the tricuspid valve. The stenosis leads to right atrial hypertension and an elevated venous pressure. Stenosis of the tricuspid valve may serve as a protective mechanism for the pulmonary vascular bed in patients with mitral stenosis. The symptoms of tricuspid stenosis are dyspnea and fatigue, but the pulmonary symptoms of mitral stenosis can diminish with the development of significant stenosis of the tricuspid valve. Pulsations of the neck veins as well as peripheral edema may also develop. On examination there is a prominent and sometimes giant A wave in the neck veins. A diastolic murmur is heard along the left lower sternal border and is usually presystolic if the patient is in sinus rhythm or midsystolic in atrial fibrillation. The murmur increases prominently with inspiration, but an opening snap is rarely heard. Evidence for pulmonary hypertension and right ventricular hypertrophy should be absent on the physical examination.

The electrocardiographic finding is the typical tall tented P wave in leads II, III, and AVF, and absence of right ventricular hypertrophy. The chest x-ray should reveal a large right atrium without prominence of the pulmonary arteries. At catheterization, documentation of a gradient across the tricuspid valve requires simultaneous catheters in the right atrium and right ventricle, since respiratory variations will render a pull-back pressure with a single catheter inaccurate. Treatment usually consists of antibiotic coverage and if surgery is performed for left heart lesions, correction of the tricuspid lesion can also be undertaken.

TRICUSPID INSUFFICIENCY

Tricuspid insufficiency is most commonly secondary to right ventricular dilatation and hypertrophy. Rarely, isolated tricuspid regurgitation can result from bacterial endocarditis, trauma, prolapse, or congenital heart disease such as atrial septal defect or Ebstein's anomaly. Symptoms of tricuspid regurgitation are usually those of pulmonary congestion and peripheral edema.

On physical examination, atrial fibrillation is commonly present and there is a large V wave in the neck veins. The murmur is holosystolic along the left sternal border and prominently increases with inspiration. The electrocardiogram may reveal atrial fibrillation without other features. The chest film will demonstrate a prominent right atrium and right ventricle. The echocardiogram is sometimes useful in documenting prolapse of one of the tricuspid leaflets as well as a site of bacterial infection. Therapy usually consists of treatment of conditions leading to the right ventricular failure. If surgery is performed for left-sided lesions, the tricuspid valve can be inspected. Generally the leaflets are found to be anatomically normal, and an annuloplasty can be performed. The operative mortality for tricuspid valve replacement along with mitral and aortic prostheses remains high at 20 per cent.

PULMONIC REGURGITATION

Regurgitation of the pulmonic valve is almost invariably secondary to severe pulmonary hypertension, which can be caused by mitral stenosis, chronic lung disease, or pulmonary emboli. Inflammatory diseases and endocarditis can sometimes render the pulmonic valve incompetent, and previous surgery for congenital heart disease may create pulmonic regurgitation. Regurgitation across the valve produces a right ventricular flow pattern. The murmur is typically a high-pitched diastolic blow along the left sternal border similar to aortic regurgitation. The electrocardiogram reveals no useful changes, but the chest x-ray will often demonstrate a prominent pulmonary artery. Cardiac catheterization may be necessary to exclude aortic regurgitation as a cause of the diastolic murmur. Treatment consists of management of the pulmonary hypertension with medical agents (see Ch. 46).

PULMONIC STENOSIS

Stenotic lesions of the pulmonary valve are almost always caused by congenital malformations. Rarely hypertrophic subaortic stenosis can involve the right side of the heart with obstruction of the right ventricular outflow tract.

Mitral Valve Disease

Rackley CE, Edwards JE, Karp RB, Kirklin JW: Mitral valve disease. *In* Hurst JW (Ed.): The Heart. 5th ed. New York, McGraw Hill Book Company, 1982, p 892.

Rapaport E: Natural history of aortic and mitral valve disease. Am J Cardiol 35:221, 1975. *A 10-year follow-up of the stenotic and regurgitant lesions of the aortic and mitral valves.*

Wood P: An appreciation of mitral stenosis. Br Heart J 1:1051, 1954. *A classic description of this disorder.*

Aortic Valve Disease

Rackley CE, Edwards JE, Karp RB, Kirklin JW: Aortic valve disease. *In* Hurst JW (Ed.): The Heart. 5th ed. New York, McGraw Hill Book Company, 1982, p 863.

Spagnuolo M, Kloth H, Taranta A, Doyle E, Pasternack B: Natural history of rheumatic aortic regurgitation: Criteria predictive of death, congestive heart failure, and angina in young patients. Circulation 44:368, 1971. *Useful clinical prognostic features in aortic regurgitation.*

Wood P: Aortic stenosis. Am J Cardiol 1:553, 1958. *A classic description of aortic stenosis.*

Valve Surgery

Fioretti P, Roelandt J, Bos RJ, Meltzer RS, van Hoogenhuijze D, Serruys PW, Nauta J, Hugenholtz PG: Echocardiography and chronic aortic insufficiency: Is valve replacement too late when left ventricular end systolic dimension reaches 55 mm? Circulation 67:216, 1983. *A clinical consideration for early aortic valve replacement.*

Kirklin JW, Pacifico AC: Surgery for required valvular heart disease. N Engl J Med 288:133, 1973. *A useful authoritative clinical review.*

Lytle BW, Cosgrove DM, Loop FD, Taylor PC, Gill CC, Golding LAR, Goormastic M, Groves LK: Replacement of aortic valve combined with myocardial revascularization: Determinants of early and late risk for 500 patients, 1967 and 1981. Circulation 68:1149, 1983. *A long-term follow-up of combined aortic valve replacement and coronary artery bypass surgery.*

Schuler G, Peterson KL, Johnson A, Francęs G, Dennish G, Utley J, Dailu PO, Ashburn W, Ross J Jr: Temporal response of left ventricular performance to mitral valve surgery. Circulation 59:1218, 1979. *Quantitative ventricular changes following mitral valve replacement.*

Williams JB, Karp RB, Kirklin JW, Kouchoukos NT, Pacifico AC, Zorn GL Jr, Blackstone EH, Brown RN, Piantadoso S, Bradley EL: Considerations in selection and management of patients undergoing valve replacement with glutaraldehyde-fixed porcine bioprostheses. Ann Thorac Surg 30:247, 1980. *A helpful guide in heterograft valve selections.*

46. PULMONARY HYPERTENSION

Alfred P. Fishman

The pulmonary circulation is a highly distensible, low-resistance vascular bed interposed between the systemic veins and the systemic arteries. Its major function is gas exchange with ambient air. It differs from the circulation to other organs in that it is perfused by the entire output of the right ventricle (the cardiac output) and from the systemic circulation in that it lacks elaborate mechanisms for regulating blood pressure. Because of its large capacity, its great distensibility, and its low resistance, the pulmonary circulation is not prone to become hypertensive. When pulmonary hypertension does occur, it is usually secondary to cardiac or pulmonary disease. Only on rare occasion is "primary" or "unexplained" pulmonary hypertension encountered. Nonetheless, although uncommon, "primary" pulmonary hypertension is of considerable theoretical interest for the understanding of the clinical picture, natural history, and management of uncomplicated pulmonary hypertension.

The normal pulmonary hemodynamics of adults residing at sea level and at altitude are indicated in Table 46–1. Because of the passive nature of the pulmonary vascular bed, the pulmonary arterial pressure—particularly in hypertensive states—must be assessed with respect to the pulmonary blood

TABLE 46–1. REPRESENTATIVE VALUES AT REST FOR THE NORMAL PULMONARY CIRCULATION AT SEA LEVEL AND AT ALTITUDE

	Sea Level	14,900 ft
Pulmonary arterial pressure (mm Hg (systolic/diastolic, mean)	20/12,15	38/14,25
Cardiac output (liters/min)	6.0	6.0
Cardiac index (liters min/m² BSA)	3.1	3.1
Left atrial pressure (mm Hg)	5	5
Pulmonary vascular resistance (R units*)	0.1†	0.2

*R units express calculated resistance in terms of $\frac{\text{mm Hg}}{\text{ml/sec}}$ To convert to C.G.S. units (dynes · sec · cm^{-5}), the value in R units is multiplied by 1328.

†Based on the data in this table, at sea level, $R = \frac{15 - 5}{6000/60} = 0.1$ R units

flow (cardiac output). For a cardiac output of 5 to 6 liters per minute, the normal pulmonary arterial pressure at sea level is about 20 mm Hg systolic and 12 mm Hg diastolic, with a mean of about 15 mm Hg; the same level of blood flow is associated with higher pressures at altitude. Pulmonary arterial pressures also tend to increase somewhat with age.

Pulmonary hypertension is a colloquialism for pulmonary *arterial* hypertension. Unless otherwise stipulated, the term refers to *chronic* pulmonary hypertension. Acute pulmonary hypertension occurs most often clinically as a result of pulmonary embolism or the adult respiratory distress syndrome. This chapter will be confined to the chronic states.

Criteria for pulmonary hypertension depend on the altitude: in the resting individual at sea level, a *mean* pulmonary arterial pressure greater than 19 to 20 mm Hg establishes the diagnosis; the corresponding limit at altitude is higher: at about 15,000 feet, a *mean* pulmonary arterial pressure greater than 25 mm Hg signifies pulmonary hypertension. Pulmonary hypertension is important primarily as a burden for the right ventricle. Thus mild pulmonary hypertension is clinically insignificant because it can be well tolerated by the right ventricle for a lifetime. However, mild pulmonary hypertension at rest generally signifies higher levels during exercise or upon exposure to a pulmonary vasoconstricting stimulus, e.g., hypoxia. Not infrequently, pulmonary hypertension remains subclinical until an explanation is sought for unanticipated right ventricular failure. This is so because the normal right ventricle can handle comfortably a moderate afterload; e.g., it can generate systolic pressures of about 50 mm Hg. It can also cope with heavier work loads if allowed time to hypertrophy. However, when inordinate loads are imposed, e.g., pulmonary arterial pressures approximating systemic arterial pressures, it is destined to fail. Moreover, at high levels, hazards other than ventricular failure often supervene, including a propensity to syncope, precordial pain, and sudden death.

Pulmonary *venous* hypertension is a different entity with respect to etiology, pathogenesis, clinical manifestations, and management. It is said to exist when pulmonary venous or left atrial pressure exceeds 12 mm Hg; this limit applies to altitude as well as to sea level. In the normal pulmonary circulation an acute increase in pulmonary venous pressure to the range of 20 to 30 mm Hg increases the risk of pulmonary edema. The same levels are less threatening when sustained chronically, as in mitral valve disease, presumably by thickening of the walls of the fluid-exchanging vessels in the lungs. However, in these individuals, a further increment in venous pressure—as by exercise or infusions—topples them into pulmonary edema.

THE NORMAL PULMONARY CIRCULATION

Structure

In the normal adult, the small muscular arteries and arterioles constitute the "resistance" vessels. In the adult at sea level, these vessels are thin-walled and sparsely equipped with muscle; in the fetus and in the native resident at altitude, the muscle is thicker and more extensive. In contrast to the pulmonary circulation, the normal bronchial circulation is minute but capable of undergoing remarkable proliferation in congenital heart disease and in pulmonary disorders involving local suppuration and fibrosis.

Hemodynamics

Because of the low resistance and high distensibility of the pulmonary vascular bed and the pulsatile nature of pulmonary blood pressure, the large pulmonary blood flow is accomplished by only a small drop in mean pressure between the pulmonary artery and the left atrium (Table 46–1). The mean pressure difference is ordinarily about 5 to 10 mm Hg.

Calculated pulmonary vascular resistance has become a popular tool for assessing the state of the normal and abnormal pulmonary circulation and for detecting pulmonary vasoconstriction or vasodilation. Unfortunately, interpretation in terms of vasomotor activity can be clouded by passive changes that occur when pulmonary vascular blood pressures, or flow, or both are changing. For example, exercise normally elicits a passive decrease in resistance due to distention of open vessels and recruitment of vessels that were previously closed. Also, clinical short-cuts, such as the substitution of pulmonary arterial pressure for the pressure drop between pulmonary artery and left atrium, deprive the calculation of any physiologic meaning, although it may still suffice in pulmonary hypertensive states as an empirical tool. Finally, since the calculation involves a ratio, interpretation in terms of clinical significance can become highly subjective. For example, a decrease in calculated pulmonary resistance involving a drop in pulmonary arterial pressure in conjunction with an increase in cardiac output (while heart rate and left atrial and systemic blood pressures remain unchanged) would seem preferable for the welfare and favorable prognosis of a patient to the same decrease in resistance brought about by an increase in cardiac output, an unchanged pulmonary arterial pressure, and tachycardia.

A large increase in cardiac output, i.e., three times that at rest, increases pulmonary arterial pressure in the normal lung by only a few millimeters of mercury. But after restriction of the pulmonary vascular bed by disease or surgery, lesser increments in pulmonary blood flow elicit more striking increases in pulmonary arterial pressure.

The role of increase in the pulmonary blood volume is much more subtle and less susceptible to measurement. The normal pulmonary blood volume is about 500 ml, approximately 100 ml of which is in the pulmonary capillaries. Expansion of the pulmonary blood volume limits the distensibility of the pulmonary circulation and decreases the capability for avoiding sizable increments in pulmonary arterial pressure by recruiting new vessels. The pulmonary blood volume expands as cardiac output increases and during systemic vasoconstriction.

Although autonomic nerves supply the pulmonary vascular tree, they are far less effective in mediating vasoconstriction or vasodilation than are local stimuli. Indeed, hypoxia acting within the lungs is the most powerful mechanism for eliciting pulmonary vasoconstriction, particularly if reinforced by a concomitant acidosis. The mechanism by which hypoxia exerts its local pressor effect is unknown. Hypercapnia also exerts a pressor effect, presumably by way of the local acidosis that it generates.

CLINICAL MANIFESTATIONS

As indicated above, most cases of pulmonary hypertension are secondary (Table 46–2). As a rule, in these pulmonary hypertensive states, the clinical picture is dominated by the

TABLE 46–2. CLASSIFICATION OF CHRONIC PULMONARY (ARTERIAL) HYPERTENSION

I. **Secondary**
   A. Cardiac Disease
      1. Acquired disorders of the left side of the heart causing pulmonary venous hypertension
         Left ventricular failure
         Mitral valve disease
         Left atrial myxoma
         Decrease in left ventricular compliance
      2. Congenital heart disease
         Pre-tricuspid
         Post-tricuspid
   B. Occlusive Pulmonary Vascular Disease
   C. Respiratory Disorders
      1. Interstitial fibrosis
      2. Obstructive airways disease
      3. Combined fibrosis, emphysema, and chronic bronchitis
      4. Alveolar hypoventilation despite normal lungs
      5. Adult respiratory distress syndrome
      6. Multiple systemic diseases

II. **Primary**

signs and symptoms of the underlying disease, which also shapes the natural history, prognosis, and response to treatment. The clinical entity of "primary pulmonary hypertension," in which the heart and lungs are not etiologically related to the pulmonary hypertension, is described subsequently.

SECONDARY PULMONARY HYPERTENSION

As causes of secondary pulmonary hypertension, heart or lung diseases dominate in numbers. Less impressive in number but of great clinical importance because of the potential for prevention and cure on the one hand and catastrophe on the other is pulmonary thromboembolic disease. Heart disease exerts its effects by increasing pulmonary blood flow or pulmonary venous pressure. In contrast, lung disease and thromboembolic disease cause pulmonary hypertension by increasing resistance to blood flow, albeit by different mechanisms.

Cardiac Disease

Acquired disorders of the left side of the heart and certain types of congenital heart disease often lead to pulmonary hypertension.

ACQUIRED DISORDERS OF THE LEFT SIDE OF THE HEART. Left ventricular failure is the outstanding cause of pulmonary hypertension. It is also the most common cause of right ventricular failure. Rarely is the level of pulmonary hypertension sufficient to account for the right ventricular failure. The discrepancy is usually attributed to concomitant failure of the muscle in the ventricular septum.

Myocardial disorders and lesions of the mitral and aortic valves are the more common left ventricular disorders leading to pulmonary hypertension. Occasional instances also occur of constrictive pericarditis, which compromises primarily the compliance of the left ventricle, thereby increasing its end-diastolic pressure. All cause pulmonary arterial hypertension by first raising pulmonary venous pressure, which, in turn, gradually evokes (1) occlusive intimal and medial changes in pulmonary *precapillary* vessels as well as in pulmonary venules and veins; (2) perivascular interstitial edema, which not only contributes directly to the increase in resistance to blood flow but also indirectly by stimulating perivascular fibrosis; under the influence of gravity, the vascular and perivascular changes are most marked in the dependent portions of the lungs; and (3) occlusion of small pulmonary vessels by emboli or thrombi; especially in states of slowed systemic blood flow, emboli are much more apt to arise from thrombi in the veins of the extremities than from the right side of the heart. Depending on the reversibility of the vascular and perivascular lesions, surgical relief of the pulmonary venous hypertension, as by mitral valve commissurotomy or replacement, generally, but not invariably, reduces the pulmonary arterial pressure.

CONGENITAL HEART DISEASE. At term, pulmonary arterial pressure approximates aortic pressure and is generally about 70/40, with a mean of 50 mm Hg. After birth, the combination of closure of the ductus arteriosus and pulmonary vasodilation causes pulmonary arterial pressure to fall rapidly to about one half of systemic levels. Thereafter, a gradual drop usually brings pulmonary arterial pressures to normal adult values in one to four weeks.

Congenital defects that produce left to right shunting of blood within the heart or between the great vessels are commonly associated with pulmonary arterial hypertension. But acute left to right shunts per se do not produce appreciable pulmonary hypertension in normal lungs unless flow is massive, i.e., at least three times greater than normal. Therefore, even though the increase in pulmonary blood flow produced by the left to right shunt is often the cardinal initiating element in this type of pulmonary hypertension, important contributing factors are the degree of arterial hypoxemia and the duration of the hemodynamic abnormalities. The interplay of these mechanisms leads to occlusive pulmonary vascular changes that, depending on the congenital defect, preferentially damage pulmonary vascular intima or media and inflict different degrees of pulmonary vascular injury. Not infrequently, as the hemodynamic abnormalities persist, the anatomic changes in the pulmonary resistance vessels take over as the dominant mechanism in sustaining the pulmonary hypertension and in determining its reversibility.

It was noted above that the pulmonary vascular lesions in pulmonary arterial hypertension are somewhat variable. However, sustained increases in pulmonary arterial pressure and arterial hypoxemia are generally associated with medial hypertrophy, whereas large pulmonary blood flows usually elicit intimal proliferation. Once pulmonary hypertension becomes chronic, distinctions between pressure and flow effects on the vascular wall tend to blur. In addition, as the pulmonary hypertension approaches systemic levels, various consequences of necrotizing arteritis supervene, including plexiform and angiomatoid lesions. Congenital defects in which pulmonary hypertension persists from birth also seem to interfere with the normal involution of the pulmonary resistance vessels so that the characteristic thin-walled resistance vessels of the normal adult lung fail to evolve. To complicate matters further, atherosclerotic lesions in the pulmonary hypertensive circulation and local thrombi or emboli add a final hypertensive element to the occlusive pulmonary vascular processes.

Important differences exist with respect to the natural history of pulmonary hypertension caused by "pre-tricuspid" congenital defects (e.g., secundum atrial septal defect) on the one hand and "post-tricuspid" congenital defects (e.g., ventricular septal defect) on the other. These are described elsewhere in this volume.

Occlusive Pulmonary Vascular Disease

The causes of secondary pulmonary hypertension due to occlusive vascular disease vary with geography. In the United States and Europe, extensive obliteration of the pulmonary arterial tree by pulmonary emboli is a common cause. In other parts of the world, other etiologies predominate. Thus, in Egypt, where schistosomiasis is endemic, pulmonary vascular disease caused by mechanical obstruction and hypersensitivity reactions is not uncommon. Elsewhere, filariasis is considered to be an important cause of pulmonary hypertension. In the United States, sickle-cell disease, the most common cause of pulmonary vascular thrombosis, rarely causes pulmonary hypertension. Several types of cancer, notably choriocarcinoma, can embolize the pulmonary circulation after the tumor has invaded the liver or the inferior vena cava.

Another important, but less common, cause of obliterative pulmonary vascular disease is the connective tissue disorders, such as systemic lupus erythematosus. Although it is generally held on morphologic grounds that connective tissue disorders of the lungs favor large, rather than small, vessels, recent improvements in the sensitivity and diversity of serologic testing for autoimmune disorders have lent credence to the proposition that connective tissue disorders may affect the small pulmonary vessels more often than previously believed.

The common denominator in pulmonary hypertension due to chronic obliterative pulmonary vascular disease is amputation and occlusion of large segments of the pulmonary circulation, abetted by pulmonary vasoconstriction largely attributable to systemic arterial hypoxemia. Early in the course of embolic pulmonary vascular disease, systemic arterial hypoxemia is mild and contributes little to the pulmonary arterial hypertension. Preterminally, however, as the right ventricle fails, the role of the "anatomic venous admixture," or "shunt," increases considerably as the O_2 content of blood returning to the lung decreases because of the slowed circulation and greater O_2 extraction in peripheral tissues.

In patients who have chronic pulmonary hypertension secondary to pulmonary emboli, two different types of pathogenetic sequence can usually be identified: (1) *clinically detectable* thromboembolic disease originating in systemic veins that is either progressive, overlooked, or neglected, and (2) a syndrome of "multiple pulmonary emboli" that is covert and mimics primary pulmonary hypertension in its clinical expression and natural history. In the latter type, precapillary vessels throughout the lung are partially or totally occluded by organized clots. Since the lesions are microscopic, only lung biopsy or autopsy can distinguish multiple pulmonary emboli from primary pulmonary hypertension. Although the possibility exists that the multiple pulmonary "emboli" are in reality multiple pulmonary thrombi secondary to widespread endothelial damage, by the time that the nature of the disorder is recognized, scarring has occurred and the practical implications for management are identical and no different from that of primary pulmonary hypertension.

Usually management involves antithrombotic therapy, occasionally supplemented by surgical elimination of the veins from which the emboli originate. Much less amenable to medical or surgical interventions are the covert multiple pulmonary emboli, in which the source and occurrence of pulmonary emboli are inapparent during life.

Tachypnea is a hallmark of pulmonary emboli. It persists during sleep and is generally associated with tachycardia. This pattern of rapid, shallow breathing is indistinguishable from that arising from stiffened lungs of any cause, e.g., interstitial pulmonary edema. And, by analogy with pulmonary interstitial edema, vagal afferent impulses arising from juxtacapillary (J) receptors and irritant receptors are generally believed to be responsible. The result of the rapid, shallow breathing is alveolar and dead space hyperventilation that, in turn, decreases the P_{CO_2} in arterial blood and alveolar gas and widens the alveolar-arterial difference in P_{O_2}. Indeed, the combination of arterial hypoxemia, hypocapnia, and a widened alveolar-arterial gradient for P_{O_2} suggests pulmonary emboli.

Since there is no obstructive disease of the airways to cloud the clinical picture, right ventricular enlargement secondary to pulmonary hypertension is manifested in pure form (see Primary Pulmonary Hypertension).

The "gold standard" for detecting pulmonary emboli is selective, high-resolution pulmonary angiography. However, even this paragon is not perfect, especially in detecting multiple pulmonary emboli of minute vessels. More expedient, but far less certain, are lung scans that have great consistency when normal in excluding pulmonary emboli and, when abnormal, in pinpointing areas of the lungs to be explored by selective angiography. By the time that the characteristic chest radiograph of pulmonary hypertension has evolved, angiography and lung scans are rarely of much help in distinguishing healed multiple pulmonary emboli from primary pulmonary hypertension. But, on occasion, they do settle the issue by disclosing one or more organized clots in the pulmonary arterial tree. Right-sided heart catheterization is often done to determine the level of the pulmonary arterial hypertension, to confirm that pulmonary wedge pressures are normal, to assess the state of right ventricular performance, and to test the efficacy of pulmonary vasodilator agents.

Once pulmonary hypertension has been established in the patient with thromboembolic disease, it is generally irreversible. Therefore, preventive measures, directed at the source of emboli, hold more promise than treatment. The medical and surgical approaches to thromboembolic disease are described elsewhere in this volume.

As symptomatic measures, oxygen-enriched inspired mixtures are often helpful in relieving breathlessness, in enhancing cerebration, in relieving arterial hypoxemia, and, thereby, in decreasing the level of pulmonary hypertension. However, unless arterial hypoxemia is marked, the drop in pulmonary arterial pressure during O_2 breathing is rarely striking, and it is usually unclear whether the slight relief in pulmonary arterial pressure is due to a decrease in cardiac output or to pulmonary vasodilation. Almost invariably, once the diagnosis is entertained or established, anticoagulation is initiated even if a search for the sources of emboli proves fruitless. The investigation and treatment are rarely more than gestures, because the pulmonary disease is usually too far advanced for impressive improvement to occur or for the downhill course of the disease to be arrested. Pulmonary vasodilators have not proved to be a reliable form of therapy.

Other forms of secondary obliterative pulmonary vascular disease are usually equally difficult to manage unless a reversible component can be identified, as in a collagen disorder that responds to steroids. The lessons learned from pulmonary embolic disease are the importance of prevention and early intervention to control or eliminate the systemic venous (rarely cardiac) source of clots to the lungs.

Respiratory Disorders

Respiratory disorders elicit pulmonary hypertension in different ways: widespread interstitial fibrosis and/or inflammation in the vicinity of the minute pulmonary vessels, by encroaching upon vascular lumens, thereby limiting their distensibility and amputating peripheral segments of the pulmonary vascular tree; obstructive airways disease by causing arterial hypoxemia; conglomerate fibrosis, emphysema, and chronic bronchitis by a combination—in varying proportions—of distorting, encasing, and occluding large segments of the pulmonary vascular tree and promoting vasoconstriction of the pulmonary resistance vessels by inducing alveolar hypoxia and arterial hypoxemia.

INTERSTITIAL FIBROSIS. Familiar examples of this category are sarcoidosis, asbestosis, and radiation fibrosis. Lymphangitic spread of carcinoma within the lungs can produce the same functional effect.

The clinical picture is generally dominated by dyspnea and tachypnea; cough is rarely a prominent feature. The chest radiograph is particularly diagnostic in disclosing a widespread pattern that is consistent with either interstitial fibrosis or infiltration, or both. Corticosteroids are usually the main hope in therapy, often in conjunction with enriched oxygen mixtures. Oxygen therapy holds little promise for relieving pulmonary hypertension unless appreciable arterial hypoxemia is present at rest.

OBSTRUCTIVE AIRWAYS DISEASE. Chronic bronchitis and emphysema ("chronic obstructive lung disease, or COPD") is the most common cause of pulmonary hypertension and cor pulmonale. Even though chronic bronchitis and emphysema generally coexist, it is the chronic bronchitis that is predominantly responsible for the alveolar hypoxia and the low P_{O_2}, high P_{CO_2}, and resultant low pH that lead to pulmonary hypertension. Emphysema per se probably does predispose to pulmonary hypertension by amputating segments of the pulmonary vascular bed. But emphysema does not cause pulmonary hypertension, even when rarefaction of the lungs is extensive, because ventilation-perfusion relationships are not severely deranged as in chronic bronchitis. Cystic fibrosis provides another illustration of the importance of chronic obstructive airways disease in evoking pulmonary hypertension. Here, as in chronic bronchitis, the basic mechanism is persistent alveolar hypoxia, arterial hypoxemia, and, to a lesser extent, respiratory acidosis resulting from ventilation-perfusion abnormalities.

The indiscriminate use of "COPD" to designate the spectrum of obstructive airways disease, without distinguishing between predominant bronchitis and predominant emphysema, tends to promote ambiguity with respect to perceptions of the natural history of this group of diseases. In essence, pulmonary hypertension (often leading to cor pulmonale) is encountered in two different settings: episodically in the "pink puffer" during an acute respiratory infection and chronically in the "blue bloater," with periodic exacerbations during an acute respiratory infection. In the "blue bloater" the course of the pulmonary hypertension is inexorably progressive. It is noteworthy that in the patient first seen during a bout of respiratory failure, clinical distinction between a "pink puffer" and a "blue bloater" is often impossible. However, after recovery from the acute episode, distinction is usually quite simple.

One of the cardinal signs of pulmonary hypertension is right ventricular enlargement. However, recognition of right ventricular enlargement may be difficult in obstructive airways disease because of hyperinflation and cardiac rotation. Right ventricular failure often is accompanied by striking cyanosis, unexplained drowsiness or inappropriate behavior, distended neck veins, warm hands, suffused conjunctivas, hepatomegaly, and edema of the extremities. Right ventricular gallops (S_3 and S_4) are generally present, and the murmur of tricuspid insufficiency can often be elicited. Not only is the liver generally displaced downward by the low diaphragm, but it is also enlarged and tender to gentle pressure over the abdomen. Hepatomegaly is invariably associated with distended neck veins and often with peripheral edema. Once suspicion is raised that the clinical picture of right ventricular failure stems from ventilation-perfusion abnormalities, an arterial blood sample will confirm that the P_{O_2} is low ($P_{O_2} < 40$ to 50 torr), the P_{CO_2} is high ($P_{CO_2} >$ 50 torr), and respiratory acidosis is present. Such arterial blood gas tensions are rare in left ventricular failure unless the patient is in frank pulmonary edema. The chest radiograph is often more helpful in detecting right ventricular enlargement retrospectively than during right ventricular failure.

Electrocardiographic evidence of right ventricular enlargement is also often equivocal in patients with bronchitis and emphysema because of rotation and displacement of the heart, widened distances between electrodes and the cardiac surface, and the predominance of dilation over hypertrophy in the cardiac enlargement. Indeed, if right ventricular enlargement is apparent, it can be assumed that the degree of cardiomegaly is severe.

Because of these limitations, it is not surprising that standard electrocardiographic criteria for right ventricular enlargement apply in about only one third of patients with chronic bronchitis and emphysema who have right ventricular hypertrophy at autopsy. Consecutive changes in the electrocardiogram are often more useful than a single electrocardiogram in detecting right ventricular overload due to pulmonary hypertension. As the arterial P_{O_2} drops to distinctly subnormal levels (e.g., below 60 to 70 torr while awake), T waves tend to become inverted, biphasic, or flat in the right precordial leads (V_1 to V_3), the mean electrical axis of the QRS shifts 30 degrees or more to the right of the patient's usual axis, ST segments become depressed in leads II, III, and aVF, and right bundle branch block (incomplete or complete) often appears. These changes tend to reverse as arterial oxygenation improves.

In the patient with bronchitis and/or emphysema in whom pulmonary hypertension has been elicited or aggravated by a bout of bronchitis or pneumonia, the goal of therapy is to maintain tolerable levels of arterial oxygenation while waiting for the upper respiratory infection to subside. If the pulmonary hypertension is acute, modest enrichment of inspired air with oxygen, as by 28 per cent O_2 delivered by a Venturi mask, generally suffices to relieve arterial hypoxemia and to restore pulmonary arterial pressures toward normal. Considerable improvement may also be accomplished even in the individual who has chronic pulmonary hypertension by sustained (virtually continuous) breathing of O_2-enriched air that restores arterial P_{O_2} to nearly normal values.

Once the right ventricle has failed, cardiotonic agents must be used cautiously because of the threat of arrhythmias posed by arterial hypoxemia and respiratory acidosis. Moreover, after adequate oxygenation has been achieved, the need for digitalis and diuretics often decreases, since the hemodynamic burden on the right ventricle (i.e., the pulmonary arterial hypertension) decreases. Even though each episode of acute hypoxia and acidosis seems to elicit about the same increment in pulmonary arterial pressure, each bout of pulmonary hypertension appears to leave behind a slightly higher level of pulmonary hypertension after recovery.

Arterial blood gas composition is the therapeutic compass to the control of pulmonary hypertension in obstructive airways disease. The degree of hypoxia is usually underestimated by conventional practice for blood sampling, since hypoxemia is regularly more marked during sleep than during waking hours. In managing ambulatory patients, serial determinations of the hematocrit may serve as a practical clue to the occurrence of covert arterial hypoxemia. However, once right ventricular failure has set in, there is no substitute for determining arterial P_{O_2} and P_{CO_2} as a guide to therapy. Ensuring the return of arterial oxygenation toward normal is much more vital than is the administration of cardiotonic measures. When respiratory infection has triggered the episode of pulmonary hypertension, a vital strategy for achieving a lasting improvement in arterial oxygenation is the administration of an appropriate antibiotic. While awaiting the salutary effects of antibiotic therapy, attention is paid to hydration, to postural drainage, and to adequate alveolar ventilation. The management of respiratory acidosis is described elsewhere in this volume.

Phlebotomy was once popular as an ancillary measure because of the prospect that increased blood viscosity contributes importantly to the pulmonary hypertension. This practice has fallen into disuse. Polycythemia is rarely severe enough to be a serious problem in cor pulmonale that is associated with bronchitis and emphysema.

Vasodilators have recently been tried in various types of secondary pulmonary hypertension, including that due to obstructive airways disease. The agents tried are the same as those outlined for primary pulmonary hypertension and their efficacy is far less impressive or predictable. To date, the most reliable approach to pulmonary vasodilation in obstructive arterial hypoxemia is enriching inspired air with oxygen.

CONGLOMERATE FIBROSIS, EMPHYSEMA, AND CHRONIC BRONCHITIS. Pulmonary hypertension is uncommon in uncomplicated silicosis or tuberculosis. However, it is not uncommon in the shrunken, distorted lung brought about by silicosis, anthrosilicosis, or longstanding smouldering tuberculosis. These disorders can cause pulmonary hypertension by producing conglomerate, massive fibrosis, distorting adjacent parenchyma, shrinking lobes, and evoking chronic bronchitis. The likelihood of pulmonary hypertension (and cor pulmonale) is enhanced by chronic pleurisy, fibrothorax, or excisional surgery, which exert their effects by a combination of anatomic restriction of the vascular bed and disturbances in gas exchange. Of all of these derangements, the disturbances in gas exchange are most susceptible to relief. Although these combinations are generally complicated, the principles of management are those outlined above for obstructive airways disease. Unfortunately, therapeutic triumphs are uncommon, because of the fixed anatomic changes.

ALVEOLAR HYPOVENTILATION IN PATIENTS WITH NORMAL LUNGS. In those individuals who develop net alveolar hypoventilation even though their lungs are normal, as in those with ventilation-perfusion abnormalities, the common pathogenetic denominators are alveolar hypoxia and arterial hypoxemia, often reinforced by respiratory acidosis. The global alveolar hypoventilation in individuals with normal lungs generally originates in either an inadequate ventilatory drive in subtle upper airways obstruction, as in the sleep apnea syndromes, or in an ineffective chest bellows. Among the disorders associated with global alveolar hypoventilation are residual paralyses of respiratory muscles, unresponsive respiratory "centers," kyphoscoliosis, and extreme obesity. The corresponding clinical syndromes are considered elsewhere in this volume.

The clinical manifestations are determined by the etiology and pathogenesis; the occurrence of pulmonary hypertension depends on the development of alveolar hypoxia sufficient to evoke arterial hypoxemia. Early in the disorder, when arterial hypoxemia (and hypercapnia) is minimal, cyanosis may appear only during exercise, as the ventilation fails to keep pace with the increased metabolic demand. Alternatively, as in the sleep apnea syndromes, arterial hypoxemia and hypercapnia may become appreciable only during sleep. Regardless of the underlying cause, an upper respiratory infection often topples the subject into acute respiratory failure and severe pulmonary hypertension.

For the patient in combined respiratory and cardiac (right ventricular) failure, the highest priority is to improve oxygenation. Success with this strategy results in a decrease in pulmonary arterial pressures, thereby relieving the overburdened right ventricle. Recently, potent but short-acting pulmonary vasodilators, such as prostacyclin, have been advocated for urgent relief of right ventricular overload. But, in this category of patients, pharmacologic therapy is rarely needed because of the efficiency of the oxygen therapy in promoting pulmonary vasodilation.

ADULT RESPIRATORY DISTRESS SYNDROME. In this disorder, pulmonary hypertension is quite common, occasionally in conjunction with pulmonary venous hypertension secondary to fluid overload but more often as a consequence of mechanical influences exerted by pulmonary edema and atelectasis operating in conjunction with respiratory acidosis. This concomitant disorder requires no special treatment, since it follows the course of the illness, decreasing spontaneously as the patient recovers.

MULTIPLE SYSTEM DISEASES. Pulmonary hypertension is occasionally caused by the pulmonary arterial lesions of collagen vascular diseases, notably lupus erythematosus, scleroderma, and dermatomyositis. However, the most common cause of pulmonary hypertension in systemic disorders is sarcoidosis, not only because this disorder is more prevalent than the collagen vascular disorders but also because of the proclivity of the parenchymal lesions for the vicinity of the small pulmonary arteries and arterioles.

PRIMARY (UNEXPLAINED) PULMONARY HYPERTENSION

Definition

Primary pulmonary hypertension is a synonym for "unexplained" pulmonary arterial hypertension. It is also a diagnosis of exclusion. As a rule, pulmonary veno-occlusive disease (see below) is not included under the rubric of primary pulmonary hypertension because, although unexplained in etiology, its pathologic features and pathogenetic mechanisms are different and usually quite distinctive.

The clinical diagnosis of primary pulmonary hypertension rests on three different types of evidence: (1) clinical, radiographic, and electrocardiographic manifestations of pulmonary hypertension, (2) demonstration by right heart catheterization of the typical hemodynamic constellation of abnormally high pulmonary arterial pressures and pulmonary vascular resistance in association with a normal pulmonary wedge pressure and a nearly normal cardiac output, and (3) inability to attribute the pulmonary hypertension to a disorder of the heart, lungs, or systemic circulation.

With respect to corroborating the clinical diagnosis, the pathologist is most helpful in proving that the cause of the pulmonary hypertension is as obscure after death as it was during life. Unfortunately, the idea of a pathognomonic vascular lesion—notably the "plexiform" lesion—has not been rewarding on three accounts: (1) primary pulmonary hypertension seems to be the final common pathway for multiple unknown etiologies; (2) the vascular lesions have been shown by biopsy and at autopsy to be quite heterogeneous; and (3) plexiform lesions probably represent a healed pulmonary arteritis and are diagnostic of one type of primary pulmonary hypertension if other causes of plexiform lesions can be excluded.

GENERAL FEATURES. Primary pulmonary hypertension is an uncommon disorder and, at autopsy, is responsible for about 1 per cent of all causes of cor pulmonale. A total of about 1000 cases have been reported.

After puberty, females predominate, most strikingly between 10 and 40 years of age. Before puberty, no sex difference is discernible. Consequently, the paradigmatic patient with primary pulmonary hypertension is a young woman in the prime of life without discernible cause for symptoms. This fact is sometimes useful in the clinical differentiation between primary pulmonary hypertension and pulmonary thromboembolic disease, which, unless preceded by a predisposing disease, trauma, or intervention, favors men, particularly in their later years.

Until recently, virtually all reports of primary pulmonary hypertension dealt with sporadic cases. About 25 families have now been identified in which the disease seems to be hereditary. The question has been raised whether detailed histories would demonstrate that some sporadic cases are actually familial.

Over the years, evidence has accumulated that primary pulmonary hypertension may be the end result of diverse etiologies, ranging from incomplete involution of the fetal circulation to autoimmunity, diet, and drugs (Table 46–3). The diversity of potential causes complicates management. In addition, they confuse descriptions of natural history. Thus, although the paradigm cited above indicates death within two to three years, several instances now exist of much longer life spans. Moreover, occasional instances are known of regression of the disease, most notably during the subsidence of the epidemic of primary pulmonary hypertension associated with the ingestion of the anorectic agent Aminorex in Europe between 1967 and 1970.

Pathology

The seat of the disease is the small pulmonary arteries (between 40 and 100 μ in diameter). The obliterative lesions

TABLE 46–3. SUGGESTED ETIOLOGIES FOR PRIMARY PULMONARY HYPERTENSION

Etiology	Comment
Autoimmune mechanisms	Especially in young women, associated with Raynaud's phenomenon and collagen diseases, such as disseminated lupus erythematosus, rheumatoid arthritis, progressive systemic sclerosis, polyarteritis nodosa, and dermatomyositis.
Persistence of fetal pulmonary vascular bed	A distinct syndrome in neonatal life that is questionably related to the adult syndrome.
Dietary pulmonary hypertension	Suggested by an outbreak of primary pulmonary hypertension related to an anorectic agent, Aminorex. Only 2% of those who ingested the drug developed pulmonary hypertension, suggesting individual predisposition. Pulmonary hypertension (with different vascular lesions) also produced experimentally by ingesting seeds of leguminous plant *Crotalaria spectabilis*.
Sustained vasoconstriction	A classic suggestion which is difficult to accept as initiating mechanism; more likely a contributing factor.
Combined portal and pulmonary hypertension	Common denominator suggested by occurrence of pulmonary hypertension in some patients with hepatic cirrhosis. Also related to mechanism of dietary pulmonary hypertension.
Multiple pulmonary emboli	Once considered to be the major cause of primary pulmonary hypertension. May still be difficult to distinguish on clinical grounds but can almost always be distinguished morphologically.
Familial pulmonary hypertension	Although familial instances do occur, and individual susceptibility has been demonstrated in some instances, the connecting links between inherited defect or predisposition and clinical disease are unclear.

are diverse, affecting one or more layers of the small muscular arteries and arterioles. In some instances, medial hypertrophy predominates; in others, combinations of inflammation and fibrosis coexist. The "classic" picture of concentric intimal fibrosis, necrotizing arteritis, and plexiform lesions encountered in the Aminorex epidemic is far from the rule. Pathologists can usually distinguish with confidence the obliterated vessels of primary pulmonary hypertension from those of multiple pulmonary emboli. An important basis for this distinction is the *concentric* pattern of the fibroelastosis that obliterates the vascular lumens in primary pulmonary hypertension and the *eccentric* fibroelastosis that follows organization of venous clots after pulmonary embolization. But these differences are not absolute.

Pathophysiology

The hemodynamic hallmarks of primary pulmonary hypertension studied at rest are well known: a high pulmonary arterial pressure in association with a nearly normal cardiac output and a normal left atrial (pulmonary wedge) pressure. As a result of this constellation, calculated pulmonary vascular resistance is high, generally leading to the logical conclusion that the resistance vessels, i.e., the small muscular arteries and arterioles, are the predominant sites of vascular obstruction. During exercise, as cardiac output increases, pulmonary arterial pressures increase; the increments in pressure in the pulmonary hypertensive circuit are generally much more striking than in the normotensive pulmonary circulation.

Most protocols using pulmonary vasodilators currently center on the response to rest and exercise. Several clinical and hemodynamic changes are sought as desirable endpoints:

1. Improvement in exercise tolerance. This increase in physical capacity is usually accompanied by an increase in cardiac output and presumably improved distribution of blood flow to peripheral organs and tissues.
2. A decrease in the level of pulmonary arterial hypertension, both at rest and during exercise.
3. A decrease in calculated pulmonary vascular resistance. Although this goal is often attained in acute experiments, its clinical value is doubtful unless an increase in cardiac output (with minimal increase in heart rate) occurs in conjunction with a decrease in pulmonary arterial pressure.
4. Agents that relax pulmonary vessels also usually cause vasodilation if they gain access to the systemic circulation, thereby unloading the left ventricle and calling into play the systemic baroreceptors. As a result, pulmonary blood volume and pressure may fall even though systemic arterial pressures remain virtually unchanged.

It remains to be learned if pulmonary vasodilation will promote long-term survival, even though there now seems to be little doubt that an increase in cardiac output, and the accompanying redistribution of systemic blood flow, can provide symptomatic relief.

Clinical Picture

In its early stages, the disease is difficult to recognize. In the sporadic case, the first clue is often an abnormal chest radiograph or electrocardiograph indicative of right ventricular hypertrophy. Initial complaints, particularly easy fatiguability and chest discomfort, are often dismissed except during the course of an epidemic, as that associated with Aminorex, or in familial pulmonary hypertension. Direct determination of pulmonary circulatory pressures by cardiac catheterization is currently the only way to prove the diagnosis.

When the disease is advanced, dyspnea, particularly during exercise, is common. Many patients are tachypneic and complain of nondescript chest pain as well as breathlessness. Other common symptoms are weakness, fatigue, and effort syncope. In time, right-sided heart failure develops. On rare occasion, an enlarged pulmonary artery causes hoarseness because of compression of the left recurrent laryngeal nerve.

Patients with severe pulmonary hypertension seem prone to sudden death. Thus, death has occurred unexpectedly during normal activities, cardiac catheterization, and surgical procedures, and after the administration of barbiturates or anesthetic agents. The mechanisms for sudden death are not clear.

On physical examination, there is no evidence of primary pulmonary hypertension or cardiac disease. The jugular venous pulse usually shows a prominent "a" wave. Right ventricular hypertrophy causes a cardiac thrust along the left sternal border, and a distinct impulse is palpable over the region of the main pulmonary artery. The pulmonic component of the second sound is markedly accentuated, the second heart sound is narrowly split, and an ejection click is heard in the pulmonic area. Often a fourth heart sound emanating from the hypertrophied right ventricle is heard at the lower left sternal border. In some patients an ejection murmur is audible at the pulmonic area; as pulmonary arterial pressures approximate systemic arterial levels, the murmur of pulmonary valvular insufficiency often appears.

Right ventricular failure is accompanied by jugular venous distention and a gallop (S_3); inspiration intensifies the gallop. The liver becomes enlarged and tender and a hepatojugular reflux can be elicited; in time dilation of the failing right ventricle leads to tricuspid insufficiency manifested by a holosystolic murmur, best heard in the fourth interspace to the left of the sternum, which increases in intensity during inspiration. The liver develops expansile pulsations synchronous with the heart beat. Hydrothorax and ascites are uncommon even in the face of hepatomegaly and peripheral edema.

In the early stage, the chest radiograph is generally normal. Later it shows cardiac enlargement in association with enlargement of the pulmonary trunk while the peripheral pulmonary arterial branches are attenuated; the lung fields appear oligemic. Although fullness of the central pulmonary arterial trunks and peripheral "pruning" are distinctive, appearances vary somewhat from patient to patient in accord with the level and pace of the pulmonary hypertension and the age of the patient. The electrocardiogram almost always shows some evidence of right ventricular enlargement and usually of right atrial enlargement. Radiographic evidence of right ventricular enlargement usually becomes overt only late in the course of the pulmonary hypertension.

Lung scans and angiography help to exclude multiple pulmonary emboli. Rarely do these procedures prove to be more enlightening than the standard chest radiograph.

The results of cardiac catheterization are consistent with diffuse obliterative disease of the pulmonary arterial tree: pulmonary arterial hypertension is associated with a normal pulmonary wedge pressure and a normal, or nearly normal, cardiac output (see Pathophysiology). Cardiac catheterization is most valuable in excluding known causes of pulmonary arterial hypertension and in screening the response of the pulmonary circulation to vasodilator agents.

Diagnosis

The diagnosis of primary pulmonary hypertension rests on two pillars: (1) the detection of pulmonary hypertension, and (2) exclusion of known causes of high pulmonary arterial pressure. The history is of utmost importance. Before categorizing pulmonary hypertension as "primary" or "unexplained," due regard must be paid to the predilection of primary pulmonary hypertension for young women, its occasional familial occurrence, associated signs and symptoms of connective tissue disorders (e.g., Raynaud's phenomenon), and, above all, the likelihood of pulmonary thromboembolism. Pulmonary function tests are useful in excluding diffuse pulmonary disorders, particularly interstitial fibrosis and granuloma. The value of cardiac catheterization in eliminating acquired or congenital heart disease has been indicated above. But even after these procedures, distinction is often not possible, particularly between primary pulmonary hypertension and pulmonary arterial hypertension secondary to multiple pulmonary emboli. Theoretically, this distinction is of great importance because of the possibility of intervening therapeutically in thromboembolic disease by using anticoagulants, inferior vena caval or common femoral vein ligation, or even pulmonary embolectomy. Unfortunately, by the time pulmonary hypertension is recognized, the anatomic lesions are generally so far advanced that the likelihood of arresting or reversing the obliterative pulmonary vascular disease in either disorder is exceedingly slim.

Treatment

GENERAL FEATURES. The aim of treatment in primary pulmonary hypertension is to decrease pulmonary arterial pressure, preferably in conjunction with an increase in cardiac output. By this combination, the afterload on the right ventricle will decrease and organ blood flow will improve. In recent years, attempts have been made to identify pulmonary vasodilators that, by decreasing pulmonary vascular resistance, will provide symptomatic relief and prolong life.

To aid in pursuing this goal, the National Heart, Lung, and Blood Institute has established a national registry by which experiences with the disease and with the use of pharmacologic agents can be shared. To date, about 100 patients have satisfied the criteria for inclusion in the registry. Although the data have not yet been analyzed in detail, enough information is already on hand to underscore the difficulties in evaluating therapy: (1) The natural history of primary pulmonary hypertension is inconsistent, probably in keeping with the diverse etiologies that can elicit pulmonary hypertension. (2) Instances are being reported of long-term survival without vasodilator therapy. (3) Unless documented by morphologic studies, i.e., lung biopsy or autopsy, secondary pulmonary hypertension—notably multiple pulmonary emboli and less often vasculitis—can masquerade clinically as primary pulmonary hypertension. (4) All vasodilators, except those destroyed during a single pulmonary circulation (currently acetylcholine and prostacyclin), cannot be administered so that they act solely on the pulmonary circulation; as a corollary, all run the risk of troublesome side effects on the heart and systemic circulation. (5) For both acute and chronic administration, optimal therapeutic doses are difficult to establish. (6) Criteria for efficacy in acute studies are inconsistent; many rely almost entirely on a drop in calculated pulmonary vascular resistance even though pulmonary arterial pressure usually remains unchanged and the work of the right ventricle increases. (7) Symptomatic improvement after the acute administration of a presumed pulmonary vasodilator is most closely related to an increase in cardiac output. (8) The acute response to a pulmonary vasodilator is not a reliable predictor of the chronic response. Because of these reservations, optimism for the use of pulmonary vasodilators in primary pulmonary hypertension remains cautious. The ideal would still be prevention (as in thromboembolic disease) or treatment according to etiology (e.g., corticosteroids for interstitial granulomas due to sarcoidosis).

Despite these general caveats and uncertainties, pulmonary vasodilator therapy continues to be tried in the hope that individual patients will respond. The pulmonary vasodilators currently in use are summarized in Table 46–4. Not shown are acetylcholine and prostacyclin, both of which have been used to assess the potential for pulmonary vasodilation. Although promising as agents for testing and for acute reduction of right ventricular overloading, neither is as yet available for chronic administration. Nor is oxygen listed, since it is only apt to cause pulmonary vasodilation if arterial hypoxemia coexists with pulmonary hypertension.

DIRECTLY ACTING DRUGS. Three agents in this category are currently used for acute administration: nitroprusside, hydralazine, and diazoxide.

Nitroprusside. Nitroprusside elicits vasodilation in both arteries and veins. It is ideal for acute testing, but cannot be administered chronically. Sublingual nitroglycerin has been tried for chronic administration of a nitrate. However, its effectiveness as a chronic pulmonary vasodilator has not been documented. Instead, when nitroprusside given intravenously does produce pulmonary vasodilation, oral therapy with long-acting nitrates is usually begun, using a combination of isosorbide dinitrate, which primarily causes venodilatation, and hydralazine, an alpha-adrenergic blocker, which acts primarily on the arterial resistance vessels (arterioles). The effectiveness of the isosorbide in this combination is conjectural.

Hydralazine. This agent is currently very much in vogue. It exerts its vasodilator effect predominantly on vascular smooth muscle, much more on arterioles than on veins. It also increases cardiac output, both by a positive inotropic effect and by tachycardia; the latter seems to originate centrally as well as peripherally in response to the drop in systemic arterial pressure that the drug produces. When used in the treatment of systemic hypertension, the incidence of side effects is high but many can be avoided, or eliminated, by concurrent administration of a beta-adrenergic antagonist, e.g., propranolol. Although experience with this agent in treating primary pulmonary hypertension is limited, enthusiasm is high.

Side effects have not been reported despite its high potential for evoking circulatory upsets. Noteworthy is the observation that during chronic hydralazine therapy, pulmonary arterial pressure remains high even though pulmonary vascular resistance drops, both at rest and during exercise, and even though the patients feel better and can do more. The basis for the sustained pulmonary hypertension is the concomitant increase in cardiac output. Unexplained is the increase in oxygen consumption during hydralazine therapy, possibly related to cutaneous vasodilatation and heat loss, a property that hydralazine shares with other cutaneous vasodilators.

Diazoxide. Diazoxide is closely related to the thiazide diuretics and is a direct vasodilator, evoking a secondary increase in cardiac output as it dilates the pulmonary resistance vessels. It acts quickly, affecting primarily the precapillary resistance vessels. In contrast to thiazide diuretics, diazoxide causes salt and water retention, often to a marked degree. Although relatively safe when used for short periods of time, prolonged use entails the risks of systemic hypertension and hyperglycemia. Individual case reports indicate that this agent decreases pulmonary arterial pressure, both at rest and during exercise, in conjunction with a considerable increase in cardiac output and an unchanged heart rate. A high incidence of side effects has dampened the initial enthusiasm for this agent.

DRUGS ACTING ON ADRENERGIC RECEPTORS. Two agents in this broad category are now quite popular: isoproterenol and phentolamine.

Isoproterenol. Isoproterenol is a powerful sympathomimetic amine that acts on beta receptors everywhere, leaving alpha receptors virtually unaffected. Its predominant effects are on the heart and the smooth muscle of vessels and bronchi. Intravenous administration raises the cardiac output because of the chronotropic and inotropic effects of the drug coupled with the increase in venous return effected by peripheral vasodilation. Sublingual or oral administration is unreliable. Its effectiveness as a pulmonary vasodilator has been remarkably unpredictable and inconsistent.

Phentolamine. Phentolamine (Regitine) in doses of 100 to 200 mg per day acts primarily on vascular smooth muscle to cause vasodilation; this direct effect is supplemented by a modest degree of blockade of sympathetic nervous activity and of antagonism to circulating catecholamines; higher doses elicit the full picture of alpha-adrenergic blockade, including marked gastrointestinal side effects. Its use has not been uniformly successful.

Quinazoline Derivatives. Prazosin also acts predominantly as an alpha-adrenergic blocking agent on vascular smooth muscle. It resembles nitroprusside in its effects on the systemic arterial and venous circulations. However, it has been reported to become increasingly ineffective during prolonged adminis-

TABLE 46-4. SOME VASODILATOR DRUGS CURRENTLY USED IN THE MANAGEMENT OF PRIMARY PULMONARY HYPERTENSION*

	Mechanism of Action	Acute Testing	Usual Maintenance Therapy	Major Side Effects; Comments
Nitroprusside	Directly on vascular smooth muscle; relaxes both systemic arteries and veins.	10 μg/min IV, increasing by 10 μg/min every 4 min until systemic systolic < 95 torr or PA systolic > 10 torr over control (max 60 μg/min).	Hydralazine 10 mg every 6 h increasing up to 50 mg every 6 h, + isosorbide dinitrate 10 mg every 6 h increasing up to 50 mg every 6 h.	Systemic vasodilation and hypotension, cyanide toxicity at high concentrations. Half-life of a few minutes.
Hydralazine	Directly on vascular smooth muscle; greater dilator effect on arterioles than on veins; myocardial stimulant.	10 mg IV repeated once after 10 min. Resting hemodynamics followed by exercise 20 min later.	Hydralazine, start with 10 mg every 6 h, increase to 50–75 mg every 6 h.	Flushing, nasal congestion, conjunctivitis, CNS stimulation, drug fever, muscle cramps. Lupus-like syndrome at doses of 200–400 mg/day. Side effects lessened by gradual increase in dosage. Surprisingly few side effects reported as yet in treating primary pulmonary hypertension.
Diazoxide	Probably directly on vascular smooth muscle; greater dilator effect on arterioles than on veins; may antagonize action of calcium.	Sequence of IV doses by rapid injection; 50 mg, 100 mg, 200 mg, and 300 mg. Hemodynamics repeated 5 min after each dose. The sequence is stopped if PA systolic > 5 torr over control.	Diazoxide 100 mg bid increasing to 100 mg tid.	Systemic vasodilation and hypotension, hyperglycemia with prolonged use, salt and water retention. Very limited experience to date.
Isoproterenol	Beta-adrenergic agonist. Relaxes vascular smooth muscle when tone is high; increases venous return to heart; positive inotropic and chronotropic effects.	1 μg/min IV and increasing by 1 μg/min until heart rate > 120/min or PA systolic > 10 torr over control, up to maximum dose of 5 μg/min.	Isoproterenol (sublingual) 10 mg every 4 h increasing up to 20 mg every 3 h. Terbutaline 5 mg tid.	Palpitation, tachycardia, flushing, cardiac arrhythmias exceedingly common.
Phentolamine	Alpha-adrenergic blocker; dilates both systemic arterioles and large veins; positive inotropic effect.	0.5 mg/min IV to a maximum of 10 mg.	Phentolamine 25 mg every 6 h increasing to 50 mg every 3 h while awake. Phenoxybenzamine 10 mg daily increasing by 10 mg every 4 days to a maximum of 40 mg daily. Prazosin 2 mg tid increasing up to 5 mg tid.	Tachycardia, cardiac arrhythmias, angina. GI stimulation.
Verapamil	Interferes with calcium fluxes in vascular smooth muscle.	0.1 mg/kg given at 1 mg/min IV.	Verapamil 80 mg tid.	Systemic vasodilation and hypotension, negative inotropic and chronotropic effects, gastric intolerance, CNS disturbances, pruritus, galactorrhea. Limited experience to date but gradually being succeeded by nifedipine.
Nifedipine	Interferes with calcium fluxes in vascular smooth muscle.	10 mg sublingually repeated once after 15 min. Exercise 15 min later.	Nifedipine 50 mg bid.	Systemic vasodilation and hypotension; flushing, dysesthesias, peripheral edema. Little experience to date.
Captopril	Inhibition of angiotensin I converting enzyme.	6 mg IV in single dose.†	Captopril, 12.5 to 50 mg, tid.	Systemic vasodilation and hypotension; proteinuria, neutropenia, agranulocytosis and myeloid hypoplasia; urticaria and angioedema; dysgeusia. Very limited experience to date.

*Based on a table developed by a working group as part of suggested protocols for use by centers for primary pulmonary hypertension, recently established by the National Heart, Lung, and Blood Institute. Members of this working group were Drs. Edward H. Bergofsky (chairman), Michael Beaven, Alfred P. Fishman, Michael Heymann, John T. Reeves, Lynne M. Reid, and Marvin A. Sackner. (Reprinted with permission from Fishman AP (ed.): Update: Pulmonary Diseases and Disorders. New York, McGraw-Hill Book Company, 1982.)

†IV form of captopril is investigational only at this time.

tration. Trimazosin,* another quinazoline derivative, presumably has the advantage of not eliciting tachyphylaxis. However, no reports have yet appeared of its use in pulmonary hypertension.

DRUGS THAT BLOCK CALCIUM TRANSPORT. The designation *calcium blocker* or *calcium antagonist* refers to a heterogeneous group of agents of different structural, pharmacologic, and electrophysiologic properties. The agents currently receiving the most clinical attention as potential pulmonary vasodilators are verapamil, nifedipine, and diltiazem. Of the three, nifedipine is the agent for choice for primary pulmonary hypertension, succeeding verapamil, which as an undesirable negative inotropic effect.

Nifedipine. Nifedipine is a synthetic agent that is unrelated to other vasoactive or cardiotonic drugs. It is a potent, long-acting systemic vasodilator that has grown increasingly popular for the treatment of coronary vasospasm. No myocardial depressant effects have been demonstrated, nor does it seem to

*Investigational drug.

possess antiarrhythmic properties. In practice, it has been used uneventfully in conjunction with a beta-receptor blocking agent to manage angina. However, experience with this drug in the treatment of primary pulmonary hypertension is still meager.

DRUGS THAT INTERFERE WITH THE CONVERSION OF ANGIOTENSIN I TO ANGIOTENSIN II. The pulmonary pressor response elicited by administering angiotensin II to animals is blocked by administering saralasin acetate (I-Sar-8-Ala-angiotensin II acetate), a competitive inhibitor of angiotensin II. This agent does not block the pressor response to acute hypoxia, suggesting that it operates differently from the calcium blockers. Preliminary trials have raised the possibility that inhibitors of the angiotensin-converting enzyme might be effective in relieving pulmonary hypertension arising from increased pulmonary vascular tone.

Captopril. Captopril is an inhibitor of the converting enzyme for angiotensin (and bradykinin). It can exert its effects in a variety of ways—inhibiting the formation of angiotensin II, decreasing the formation of kinins, or interfering with the formation of vasodilator prostaglandins and prostacyclin.

Prognosis

The diagnosis of primary pulmonary hypertension carries with it a poor prognosis. Although death usually occurs within a few years after the onset of symptoms, instances of long-term survival do occur. Exceptions to the rule of a short and fatal course were also reported in the Aminorex epidemic in patients in whom the drug was stopped. At present, there is no specific treatment for primary pulmonary hypertension. Pulmonary vasodilators have, in some patients, improved exercise tolerance and the quality of life but have not yet been shown to prolong life. Neither anticoagulants nor corticosteroids have been of value. The cause of death is generally right ventricular failure. In some patients, sudden death terminates the illness.

PULMONARY VENO-OCCLUSIVE DISEASE

In a few patients with unexplained pulmonary arterial hypertension the disease appears to originate in progressive obstruction of pulmonary veins. Characteristically, anatomic lesions in the pulmonary veins predominate, but pulmonary arteries and arterioles are also involved. The etiology is unknown, but the obstructive venous lesions seem attributable to thrombosis after local injury, possibly secondary to a viral infection.

When the pulmonary hypertension is suspected to originate distal to the pulmonary capillary bed, mitral valve disease or myocardial dysfunction, or even left atrial myxoma, has the greater likelihood of being the cause than does primary pulmonary venous obstruction. More esoteric etiologies for the pulmonary venous hypertension to be excluded are congenital atresia of pulmonary veins and coexistent phlebitis of systemic and pulmonary veins.

Predominantly children and young adults are affected, but the age range has been from infancy to 48 years. There seems to be no sex difference. Although hints exist of possibly related familial cardiac disorders, the patients are too few to do more than raise suspicion of a familial or common environmental cause.

Clinical suspicion of this disorder generally arises when a patient with congested and edematous lungs, consistent with occult mitral valvular disease or left ventricular failure, proves to have a normal mitral valve and left ventricle. However, this stereotype is not always encountered and some patients have carried the diagnosis of primary pulmonary arterial hypertension until autopsy disclosed the characteristic pulmonary venous lesions.

The cardinal signs are dyspnea and fatigue on exertion in conjunction with evidence of pulmonary hypertension, particularly radiologic evidence of postcapillary pulmonary hypertension without evidence of an increase in left atrial pressure. Pleural effusions are common. Cyanosis, syncope, hemoptysis, and finger clubbing have been inconsistent findings.

Cardiac catheterization discloses a high pulmonary arterial pressure, often with a normal pulmonary wedge pressure. The low wedge pressure has been attributed to discontinuities and channels of high resistance between the pulmonary capillaries and the pulmonary and bronchial venous channels so that wedging interrupts all sources of flow distal to the area blocked by the catheter. A few lung biopsies have been done during life.

Both lungs are involved, but the venous lesions may be more marked in one region than in another. As a rule, the pulmonary arteries as well as the pulmonary veins are affected, but the lesions are different. Most striking are the morphologic changes in the pulmonary veins and venules, which are narrowed or occluded by fibrous tissue; up to 95 per cent of the veins and venules may be affected, but complete occlusion is uncommon. Bronchial veins and bronchopulmonary anastomoses share in the occlusive process. Hypertrophy in the walls of the pulmonary arteries may be also quite striking, whereas the pulmonary capillary bed is generally unaffected. Thrombi in the pulmonary arteries are common. The lungs show congestion, edema, and focal fibrosis, which may become extensive.

Management has been disappointing, since the lesions are generally irreversible. The usual duration after recognition ranges from a few weeks in infants to several years in adults, with seven the maximum.

Camerini F, Albert E, Klugman S, Salvi A: Primary pulmonary hypertension: Effects of nifedipine. Br. Heart J 44:352, 1980. *A typical case report illustrating the clinical improvement that often follows chronic administration of nifedipine. The acute catheterization study also disclosed a frequent pattern of response: increase in cardiac output and virtually unchanged pulmonary and systemic arterial pressures.*

Case Records of the Massachusetts General Hospital (Case 38-1981). N Engl J Med 305:685, 1981. *Illustrating the approach to differential diagnosis in the patient with pulmonary arterial hypertension secondary to recurrent pulmonary emboli.*

Fishman AP: Dynamics of the pulmonary circulation. *In* Hamilton WF, Dow P (eds.): Handbook of Physiology. Circulation. Vol. 2. Washington DC, American Physiological Society, 1963, pp 1667–1743. *A comprehensive survey of the regulation of the pulmonary circulation, useful as a background for considerations of pulmonary hypertension. Particular attention is paid to the concepts of pulmonary vascular resistance, pulmonary wedge pressures, and identification of vasomotor activity.*

Fishman AP: Pulmonary thromboembolism: Pathophysiology and clinical features. *In* Fishman AP (ed.): Pulmonary Diseases and Disorders. New York, McGraw-Hill Book Company, 1980, pp 809–826. *A succinct account of pulmonary thromboembolic disease that calls special attention to the category of multiple pulmonary emboli.*

Fishman AP, Pietra GG: Primary pulmonary hypertension. Ann Rev Med 31:421, 1980. *A review of current understanding of primary pulmonary hypertension with special emphasis on etiology. Comprehensive bibliography.*

Rubin LJ, Peter RH: Oral hydralazine therapy for primary pulmonary hypertension. N Engl J Med 302:69, 1980. *Hydralazine taken orally (50 mg q 6 h) by four patients increased cardiac output and exercise tolerance, leaving pulmonary arterial pressure unchanged; heart rate increased in all. Although calculated vascular resistance fell in each instance, the hemodynamic burden of the right ventricle was unchanged. Clinical improvement was probably related to increased cardiac output.*

Ruskin JN, Hutter AM Jr: Primary pulmonary hypertension treated with oral phentolamine. Ann Intern Med 90:772, 1979. *Detailed description of one patient in whom phentolamine by mouth caused clinical and hemodynamic improvement. Illustrates standard protocols, at rest and during exercise.*

Trell E: Benign, idiopathic pulmonary hypertension. Acta Med Scand 193:137, 1973. *Two cases of unusually long duration of idiopathic pulmonary hypertension (about 27 and 40 years, respectively) are presented and discussed with respect to others reported in the literature. No autopsy or biopsy findings.*

Voelkel N, Reeves JT: Primary pulmonary hypertension. *In* Moser KM (ed.): Pulmonary Vascular Diseases. New York, Marcel Dekker, 1979, pp 573–628. *Excellent clinical and physiologic review of current understanding of primary pulmonary hypertension against a background of a large personal experience with both this disorder and the pulmonary hypertension of high altitude.*

Wagenvoort CA, Wagenvoort N: Pathology of Pulmonary Hypertension. New York, John Wiley & Sons, 1977. *Splendid morphologic treatise on primary pulmonary hypertension based on years of collecting pathologic material, careful analysis, and intriguing extrapolations from morbid anatomy to etiology and clinical syndromes.*

47. ARTERIAL HYPERTENSION

C. T. Dollery

DEFINITION

A wide range of blood pressure values is found among human populations. The values are not normally distributed, and there is a skew toward higher ones. The distribution of blood pressure readings (Fig. 47–1) has no natural break separating normality from abnormality, so the definition of what constitutes hypertension is empirical. Much effort has been expended, probably needlessly, in trying to define hypertension. Several different operational definitions are possible. Very high values of blood pressure—above 230 systolic and 130 diastolic mm Hg—are associated with a high probability that the individual will develop left ventricular failure or accelerated hypertension and thus present with a clinical illness that can be termed hypertension. Below this level of pressure most patients are not ill, but there is an increasing incidence of some symptoms such as morning headache with pressure from approximately 170 systolic and 110 diastolic mm Hg upward. However, the usual problem for an individual with a blood pressure in the upper part of the distribution range is not the development of symptoms resulting from the blood pressure but the sudden and apparently unpredictable catastrophe of a myocardial infarction or a cerebrovascular accident. Several prospective epidemiologic studies of human populations have shown that the risk of such a catastrophe increases with the level of systolic pressures, although the slope becomes steeper at higher levels. The situation is somewhat different with diastolic pressure, for which the slope is flat until the pressure exceeds approximately 90 mm Hg (Fig. 47–2). Possibly the most useful definition of hypertension for the physician would be that level of pressure above which treatment has been shown to be beneficial. At present this cut-off is about 160/95 mm Hg, but clinical trials are in progress that may require it to be modified.

Thus the main clinical importance of hypertension is not that it is a disease in the usual sense but that it is the most important single factor that enables a physician to make a prediction about the future risk of vascular disease, and that furthermore it is a risk that can be reduced by lowering the blood pressure.

MEASUREMENT OF BLOOD PRESSURE

Before measuring the pressure make sure that the patient is seated or lying comfortably and note the position in which the pressure is taken. Make sure the arm is supported so that the patient is not having to carry out isometric exercise while the reading is taken. If an adult arm is very large a wider than normal cuff will be needed and if the patient is a child a narrower cuff should be used. It is worth asking the patient if he or she has had a cup of coffee or a cigarette recently, as these can raise the pressure appreciably.

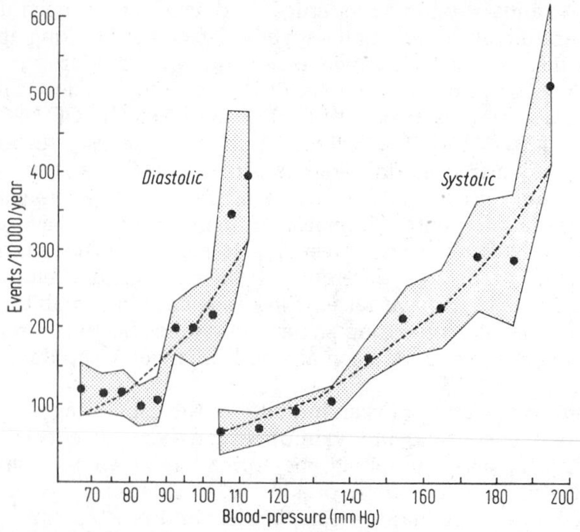

Figure 47–2. Annual incidence of cardiovascular events at Framingham over 18 years of follow-up, by level of blood-pressure, all ages, mean of male and female rates. (From Anderson TW: Lancet 2:1140, 1978. Reproduced with permission.)

The sphygmomanometer column is calibrated in 10- and 2-mm divisions. Most physicians show a strong preference for numbers ending in zero and record the blood pressure only to the nearest 10 mm Hg. As decisions about patient management may be altered by differences in diastolic pressure of this magnitude, it is much preferable to read the instrument to the nearest 2 mm Hg. It is also important to deflate the cuff slowly when taking blood pressure. Rapid deflation may bring about a considerable difference in the pressure in the cuff and that indicated by the column because of the inertia of the mercury. Furthermore, it is almost impossible to read the column accurately if the meniscus is rushing past the calibration points.

It is useful to make a rough check of the systolic pressure by palpation during inflation and to start deflation from 20 mm Hg above the systolic value. This avoids the problem of errors caused by "silent zones" during deflation, which can cause the observer to fail to record the true (and much higher) level of systolic pressure. As the column falls, the silence is broken by a faint but distinctive tapping sound in time with the pulse. This is phase 1 of the sounds described by Korotkoff and corresponds to the systolic pressure. Less skilled observers usually record this value more accurately than the diastolic pressure, which has a less clear-cut endpoint. During further deflation the quality of the sound changes. At first it grows louder and has a roaring quality and then it becomes abruptly

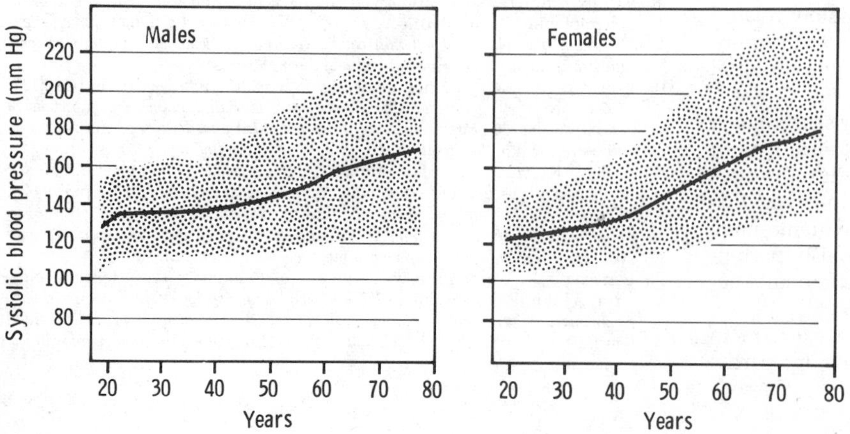

Figure 47–1. Median systolic blood pressure with 5 per cent and 95 per cent limits in male and female inhabitants of Bergen, Norway, over the whole span of age found in an adult population sample. (From Boe et al.: Acta Med Scand (Suppl 321)157:1–252, 1957.)

muffled. The point of muffling is the fourth phase, and the disappearance of sound, which usually occurs soon afterward, is the fifth phase. The true diastolic pressure lies between the fourth and fifth phase sounds but, as it is usually closer to the fifth, it is now official policy to record this as the diastolic blood pressure. Some individuals may have a diastolic pressure that is difficult or impossible to record precisely because the sound fades gradually without a clear point of muffling or disappearance. This is a particular problem if the peripheral circulation is dilated after exercise or under the action of a vasodilator drug. Under such circumstances the systolic pressure is more reproducible but is more variable with anxiety and exercise, and it is probably for this reason that many clinicians still prefer to base their decisions upon the diastolic reading.

The blood pressure varies widely with mood and activity. A patient seen for the first time is usually more anxious than on the second or third visit to the same doctor and clinic. It is common to find a fall of 10 mm Hg in systolic pressure from the first visit to the second, and about 4 mm Hg from the second to the third. A blood pressure taken at the beginning of a consultation is almost always higher than one taken near its end. There has been much debate as to which, if any, of these is the most representative. The blood pressure taken on the first visit without any special preparation is often termed "casual" blood pressure. It probably corresponds most nearly to those used in epidemiologic surveys. The blood pressure recorded under conditions of rest, tranquillity, and even sedation is sometimes referred to as the "basal" blood pressure. As there is no generally accepted preparation for recording a "basal" reading, it cannot be precisely defined. There is evidence that a series of readings taken over the waking day provides a better prediction of prognosis than a single casual one, but portable equipment to provide such readings is expensive and not generally used.

Reading the mercury column of the sphygmomanometer is prone to systematic bias as well as digit preference and boundary avoidance. For exact work such as therapeutic trials and epidemiologic surveys it is usual to employ an instrument that has provision for concealing the mercury columns, which are stopped by pressing a switch (The London School of Hygiene Sphygmomanometer), or for incorporating a device to "muddle" the zero by up to 80 mm Hg (Hawksley sphygmomanometer), so that the observer cannot anticipate any particular pressure level. The zero offset can only be read after the systolic and diastolic pressures have been recorded.

EPIDEMIOLOGY

Many factors affect the blood pressure of an individual within a population or may cause differences between populations. Study of these factors may yield information about pathogenesis and suggest possible preventive measures.

Age and Sex

Blood pressure tends to rise throughout life, although the rate of rise varies at different ages. There is a relatively rapid rise from the low values of the neonate to the higher values of a child and young adult. The upward trend is slower between the ages of 20 and 45 years in both men and women; it then resumes an upward march, the systolic pressure rising at an average rate of 0.5 to 1.0 mm Hg each year until the seventh decade is reached. Values in older people are affected by differential mortality of those with higher pressures, and population means tend to level out or even fall in extreme old age. Women have slightly lower pressures than men in the third and fourth decades and slightly higher ones thereafter. The rate of rise of pressure is not uniform within a population, and the range of pressures found widens as age advances. The rate of rise varies widely between individuals and they tend to maintain the same relative position in the distribution curve, a phenomenon known as tracking. Individuals who ultimately develop pressure levels requiring treatment may lie in the upper part of the distribution as young as the age of one year.

Race and Environment

Studies of the distribution of blood pressure values have been carried out in many countries of the world, and almost all populations show a progressive rise in pressure with age and a distribution of values resembling in varying degrees that found in Western Europe and the United States. Although the pattern is similar, the proportion falling into higher pressure categories shows some interesting geographical and racial variations. Black people in West and East Africa, the West Indies, and the United States have a similar proportion of higher values to those found in whites, and in some samples significantly more. The proportion of individuals with higher values appears to be somewhat lower in population samples from the Indian subcontinent.

Some communities have been found in which the blood pressure shows little increase with age and the distribution curve lacks the upward skew of higher values found in Caucasians. Such communities include nomads in East Africa, bushmen in Southern Africa, and the inhabitants of some Pacific islands such as Pukapuka in the Northern Cook Islands.

There is conclusive evidence that blood pressure is heritable, but wide divergencies of opinion exist concerning the proportion of the blood pressure variability in populations that is genetically controlled. Estimates of the genetic contribution to variation in systolic blood pressure range from as high as 82 per cent to as low as 30 per cent. The evidence of a major genetic contribution comes from several sources. Blood pressures of parents and their natural children are highly significantly correlated (r0.3), whereas those of adopted children are not. There is a much lower correlation of spouse blood pressures than of family members who are genetically related. The correlation of blood pressures in monozygotic twins (0.55) is higher than that in dizygotic twins (0.25). It was once contended that blood pressure distribution in populations was bimodal and controlled by a single gene. The error arose because of digit preference for blood pressures ending in zero and boundary avoidance of pressures around 150 mm Hg systolic. It is now generally agreed that blood pressure is unimodally distributed and must be controlled by more than one gene. How many genes are important and what they control are still doubt.

Extremes of body weight and salt intake can alter blood pressure, so that differences in body weight and salt intake found between races probably exercise some influence on the range of blood pressures that prevail among them. There is also the question of how much urban and social pressures may contribute to the elevation of arterial pressure. The evidence here is conflicting. Some studies of rural populations have demonstrated pressures as high as, or even higher than, those of genetically similar people living in crowded conditions in cities. A group with one of the highest proportions of high blood pressure values ever reported is black people living in rural Georgia in the United States. Yet studies of Pacific islanders have suggested that groups in closer contact with modern society have higher pressure values than those found in communities from which they migrated. The practical implication of these results is that, with the possible exception of obesity and salt intake, no factor has yet been identified that can be utilized in a program to prevent high blood pressure.

Body Weight

Many epidemiologic studies have demonstrated a positive correlation between body weight and both systolic and diastolic blood pressure. The correlation is strongest among young and middle-aged adults. Prospective studies suggest that weight gain is associated with a significant rise in blood pressure in those initially normotensive and, conversely, that weight loss lessens the chance of developing hypertension in those who were normotensive at the outset. There is also epidemiologic evidence that loss of weight among individuals who are hypertensive lowers blood pressure. Clinical studies have been conflicting in that loss of weight does not always lower blood pressure, and it has been argued that when it does so reduced sodium intake may be as important as reduced total calorie intake and body mass.

The improved nutrition of many countries that has resulted from developments in agriculture and in food distribution and processing may increase the number of individuals who are overweight, who have a high salt intake, and who are hypertensive and glucose intolerant. The prevention of obesity is a worthwhile objective in relation to several other health problems besides hypertension, but few attempts have been made to persuade the population to restrict their food intake.

Salt Intake

One of the earliest effective methods of lowering the blood pressure was the rice diet introduced by Kempner, which owed it efficacy to its very low content of sodium chloride. Unfortunately, few patients were willing to persist with this tasteless and monotonous regimen, and such an extreme reduction of salt intake would be impractical as a preventive measure. Even the word salary is a reminder that the Roman legionaries were partly paid in salt, and the craving for this substance is deep seated in man and animals. Several studies have been made both within and between communities to establish how far variability in blood pressure is due to salt intake. Variations between communities are difficult to interpret because of genetic differences, but it has been established that the range of salt intake found within individual western countries does not appear to be a major influence upon individual levels of blood pressure. However, the spread of convenience foods high in salt is a worrying trend. Individuals who consume large quantities of such foods may have salt intakes in excess of 250 mEq per day. Reduction of salt intake to approximately 100 mEq daily usually brings about a 3 to 5 mm Hg fall in diastolic blood pressure. Interesting selective breeding experiments have been carried out in a rat colony at Brookhaven in which it has proved possible to breed a strain of animal that readily develops severe hypertension when given a high salt intake. Another strain was bred from the same original stock that was highly resistant to the blood pressure–elevating effect of a high salt intake. There is little information about the range of responsiveness to changes in salt intake among humans with normal renal function, although the sensitivity to salt of patients with advanced renal failure is well known.

RISK FACTORS FOR PREDICTING VASCULAR DISEASE

Physicians are accustomed to making predictions about the likely future course of an illness to recovery or death. The use of risk factors to predict the future likelihood of developing an illness is no more than an extension of the same principle. The first to make extensive use of this concept were the life insurance companies, who recognized that factors such as high blood pressure, overweight, and proteinuria increased the probability of their having to pay out the proceeds of a policy, and they learned to adjust their premiums accordingly. As a result of prospective epidemiologic studies such as those carried out in Framingham, Massachusetts, by the National Institutes of Health, it has been possible to study whole populations and to calculate correlation coefficients for many factors that have predictive power in relation to the risk of developing vascular disease. The concept is a most important one to grasp, because it alters radically the clinical management of a patient with a given level of pressure, depending upon the burden of associated factors of risk. It is also important to grasp the difference between absolute risk and relative risk. A young man with a systolic blood pressure of 160 mm Hg has two and one-half times the chance of dying compared with a standard risk. In an older man the ratio is slightly lower. But as older men who are not hypertensive have a much higher chance than younger men of suffering a stroke or myocardial infarction, the absolute risk for the older man is much greater.

The most important factors for predicting the future risk of myocardial infarction are level of blood pressure and cigarette smoking habit. Blood lipids are an important predictor in younger people but less so in the elderly. Blood pressure and cigarette smoking are overwhelmingly the most important treatable factors. Other important factors include the presence of both voltage and T wave signs of left ventricular hypertrophy, glucose intolerance, and obesity. In absolute terms, age and sex are most important because the incidence of morbidity and mortality from vascular disease increases sharply as age advances, but the incidence at younger ages is less in women than in men. Simple computer programs have been constructed that make it possible to calculate the relative risk by providing information about these risk factors, and their importance is illustrated by two case histories for a man of 45 years who has a systolic pressure of 170 mm Hg with and without a high risk category in other respects (Table 47–1). Recent studies have shown that the combination of heavy cigarette smoking and an elevated blood pressure carries a particularly high risk of vascular disease. A further illustration is given in Figure 47–3, which shows histograms of risk of developing coronary disease at various levels of systolic pressure from 105 to 195 mm Hg as the burden of other risk factors increases. It can be seen that the risk associated with the lower blood pressures in someone with a full load of other factors is greater than that of someone in the highest pressure category who is free of other risk factors.

The concept of risk factors is very important, but it has certain limitations. The demonstration of a correlation with predictive power does not by any means prove that there is a cause-and-effect relationship. It cannot be assumed that reduction of a risk factor will automatically bring about a proportional, or indeed any, reduction in risk. However, if a risk factor can be diminished without any obvious countervailing disadvantage, it is a matter of common sense to try to reduce it while awaiting the scientific evidence. This argument applies especially strongly to reduction of cigarette use and blood pressure. The value of reducing lipids is a matter that has caused great controversy. In epidemiologic surveys low density lipoproteins are associated with increased risk of vascular disease and high density lipoproteins have a protective action. Measures that reduce blood lipids may not automatically reduce the amount of lipid in atheromatous lesions of the arterial wall. Primary prevention trials with lipid-lowering drugs have been negative and one, with clofibrate, showed an increased mortality in the treated group.

TABLE 47–1. EFFECT OF ASSOCIATED RISK FACTORS UPON OUTCOME IN HYPERTENSION*

	Case I	Case II
Age	45 years	45 years
Sex	Male	Male
Systolic blood pressure	170 mm Hg	170 mm Hg
Cigarette smoker	Yes	No
Serum cholesterol	260 mg/100 ml	185 mg/100 ml
Glucose intolerance	Yes	No
Left ventricular hypertrophy on the ECG	Yes	No
Relative risk compared with age/sex average	7.15	0.78
Patient's risk of developing cardiovascular disease over eight years	54.1	6.33
Average risk for this age and sex group over eight years	8.0	8.0

*Based upon data from the Framingham Survey (program by courtesy of Dr. R. H. Roberts, Ciba-Geigy, Summit, N.J.).

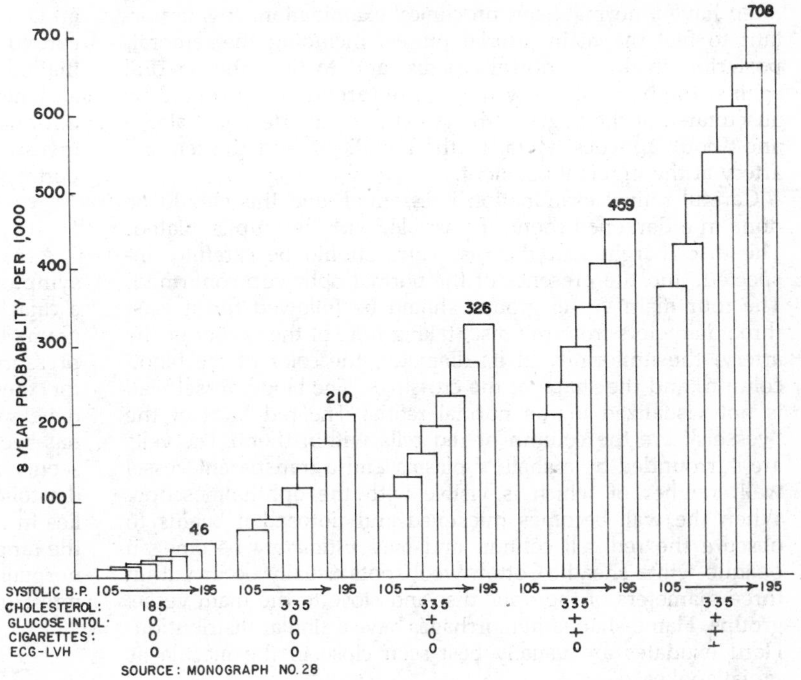

Figure 47–3. Risk of cardiovascular death according to systolic blood pressure at specified levels of other risk factors in 40-year-old men in Framingham, Mass. (By permission of Dr. W. B. Kannel.)

CAUSES OF DEATH IN HYPERTENSION

The main cause of death in hypertensive individuals is from damage to blood vessels in vital organs, causing myocardial infarction, stroke, peripheral vascular disease, and renal failure. The only causes of death that relate directly to the level of pressure at the time are accelerated hypertension, cerebral hemorrhage, heart failure, and (possibly) dissecting aneurysm. Myocardial infarction is by far the most important and accounts for over half the deaths.

A number of prospective studies, such as that carried out at Framingham, have demonstrated the steep gradient of risk with levels of blood pressure for each of these causes of death. Comparing normotensive individuals with those having a pressure exceeding 160 systolic and 95 diastolic mm Hg, the gradients were three-fold for coronary disease and peripheral vascular disease, four-fold for congestive heart failure, and seven-fold for stroke. The increase in risk with level of blood pressure is most striking for stroke deaths. In the age group 40 to 49 years the risk of stroke is ten times higher in individuals with a diastolic pressure exceeding 104 mm Hg than in those in whom it is below 85 mm Hg.

These data also highlight a problem when the control of blood pressure is used as a public health measure to decrease the incidence of stroke and coronary disease. The risk is much greater at high pressure levels, but the number of individuals involved is relatively small. Individuals with modest elevations of blood pressure are so much more numerous that they account for a large fraction of the hypertension-related morbidity and mortality, although at present many of them would probably not be considered for treatment.

CLINICAL MANIFESTATIONS

The assessment of the patient with hypertension has three main objectives: to ascertain the extent of organ damage that has already resulted from the high pressure, to detect any treatable cause, and to define and, when possible, to reduce the factors that determine a high risk of cardiovascular disease. Information relevant to these three factors can be obtained from the history, physical examination, and laboratory investigations.

The Extent of Organ Damage

Patients with severe hypertension may present to the physician with symptoms, although most patients with mild to moderate hypertension have no symptoms directly referable to the disease. Common symptoms include headache, dyspnea, giddiness, and blurred vision. The relationship of headache to hypertension has caused much confusion. Most headaches, including those in the majority of patients with high blood pressure, bear no relationship to the level of blood pressure. However, patients with diastolic pressures exceeding about 110 mm Hg, especially younger patients, often complain of morning headaches similar to those seen in patients with other causes of raised intracranial pressure. These headaches are related to the level of blood pressure. Breathlessness and/or a slow walking pace are also common symptoms at higher pressure levels, but many patients with these complaints also have ischemic heart disease. The complaint of giddiness or unsteadiness is common in patients with untreated hypertension, although rather similar complaints may arise as a result of reducing the pressure to a point where cerebral perfusion is impaired. Blurred vision usually indicates the presence of cotton wool spots and/or macular edema, but also arises as a result of a branch retinal vein occlusion, which is more common in hypertensives than in normotensive people. There is a change in the normal diurnal rhythm of urine flow in many patients with hypertension, and they may complain of nocturia even though there is little other evidence of impaired renal function. Hypertension also commonly presents as a result of ischemia that has resulted from altheromatous narrowing or occlusion of an artery in the brain, heart, or lower limbs. Unfortunately, some patients with hypertension have already suffered such severe damage to the function of the brain or myocardium as to make the value of treatment debatable.

Clinical examination is focused mainly upon the cardiovascular system and the brain. Patients with severe hypertension usually have an apex beat that is displaced to the left and that has a forceful sustained character. They frequently also have an atrial sound. In patients with very severe hypertension there may also be signs of left ventricular failure, basal crepitations in the lungs, a third heart sound, pulsus alternans, or congestive heart failure with a raised jugular venous pressure and peripheral edema. Patients with mild to moderate hypertension often have a normal heart on clinical examination. It is important to feel the main arterial pulses, including the femoral, posterior tibial, and dorsalis pedis, and to time the femoral against the brachial artery pulse. The carotid artery should be auscultated at the angle of the jaw, the renal artery just above and about 2 inches lateral to the umbilicus, and the femoral artery at the inguinal ligament.

Careful retinal examination is essential, and this should be done in a darkened room, if possible, with the pupils dilated. The disc margin and the disc color should be carefully inspected, and the presence of the normal optic cup confirmed. The four main vessel groups should be followed for at least three diameters from the disc, taking note of the caliber of the artery, the uniformity of its diameter, the color of the blood column, and the shape of the crossings. The blood vessel wall is not visualized in the normal retina. The red lines of the "vessels" are the column of red cells within them. The cells are surrounded by a shell of plasma and a transparent vessel wall, neither of which is visible with the ophthalmoscope. When the wall becomes thickened and fibrosed it begins to obscure the red cell column and may ultimately become an opaque white sheath. Cotton wool spots usually occur within three diameters of the optic disc and close to the main vessel groups. Flame-shaped hemorrhages have a similar distribution. Hard exudates are usually best seen close to the macula as radial spokes.

The most important investigations designed to assess organ involvement are the ECG, the chest radiograph, and tests of renal function, particularly the serum creatinine concentration. The ECG should be carefully examined. Common findings are an increased voltage, left axis deviation, and flattening of inversion of the T waves in leads 1, aVL, and V_{4-6}. The chest radiograph may confirm the clinical assessment of left ventricular enlargement but is often normal. There is frequently some evidence of aortic disease such as dilatation or tortuosity with unfolding of the thoracic aorta. The degree of renal impairment varies, but some reduction of glomerular filtration rate is present in most patients with severe hypertension, although usually only to about 65 ml per minute if the patient is not in the accelerated phase. Mild and moderate hypertension usually leaves renal function unimpaired.

Detection of Treatable Causes

There has been much controversy about the extent to which it is desirable to investigate patients for etiologic factors that may be treatable by surgery. The three main classes of treatable causes are excess catecholamine production from a tumor of the chromaffin tissue; excess mineralocorticoid production from the adrenal, e.g., Cushing's syndrome or hyperaldosteronism; and vascular obstruction such as coarctation of the aorta or renal artery stenosis. Causes of renal disease other than arterial disease are less important, because they less commonly lead to cure of hypertension.

The basic screening investigation of pheochromocytoma is the urinary vanillylmandelic acid (VMA), which some clinics measure in all hypertensive patients. It should certainly be measured in patients with a suggestive history of fluctuant severe hypertension. The simplest screen for mineralocorticoid excess is measurement of serum potassium and sodium concentrations. There is debate about the extent to which it is necessary to search for renal artery disease if there are no suggestive features such as resistance to treatment or rapid onset of a high pressure level. Availability of renal artery dilatation with balloon catheters has rekindled interest in the detection of renal artery stenosis, but it remains a relatively rare cause of hypertension in unselected series.

Evaluation of Risk

Many of the basic data for evaluating risk will have been derived from the patient's history. This includes date of birth, sex, previous vascular episodes, family history of hypertension and vascular disease, and history of renal disease or diabetes. An assessment of tobacco and alcohol intake should be made and, in women, use of the contraceptive pill should be recorded. These findings will be reinforced by the clinical examination and in particular by the blood pressure, body weight and height, and urinalysis for protein and sugar. The only information of value in prediction of risk to be derived from investigations is the ECG for evidence of left ventricular hypertrophy and/or ischemia and fractionation of the blood lipids.

Case Finding

As most patients with elevated levels of blood pressure are symptomless, the only practical way of detecting them before a catastrophe occurs is to conduct an active case-finding program. This means that every physician ought to take the blood pressure of every patient he sees, whatever the primary reason for the consultation. Several attempts have been made to develop rules about the frequency of rescreening if the pressure has been taken in the past. Based upon epidemiologic data, it seems reasonable to rescreen after ten years if the initial diastolic pressure is less than 80 mm Hg, after five years if it lies in the range of 80 to 89 mm Hg, and every year if it is in the range of 90 to 99 mm Hg. Higher pressures than this would normally be treated, as would some in the range of 90 to 99 mm Hg.

CLINICAL SYNDROMES OF HYPERTENSION

High blood pressure can present clinically in a wide variety of ways. Before treatment of mild to moderate hypertension became widespread, patients frequently presented with accelerated hypertension, left ventricular failure, or cerebral hemorrhage. A few patients still slip through the net of case-finding programs and suffer these catastrophes prior to initiation of antihypertensive therapy, but these are less common than they used to be. The clinical presentation of hypertension is now most commonly as part of the spectrum of risk factors in a patient who has suffered a stroke or a myocardial infarction or as a chance finding during clinical examination for another purpose.

Malignant or Accelerated Hypertension

The patient with malignant hypertension is almost always ill with symptoms such as morning headaches, blurred vision, dyspnea, and/or symptoms of uremia. Such patients are commonly in their fourth, fifth, or sixth decade of life. Their blood pressure is almost always above 110 mm Hg diastolic in adults and frequently much higher, with diastolic pressures in the range of 130 to 170 mm Hg being commonplace. Clinical examination usually reveals an enlarged left ventricle and early signs of pulmonary edema. The retinal finding of cotton wool spots and/or papilledema is essential to make the diagnosis. Investigation usually shows some degree of renal impairment with raised blood urea and serum creatinine values. The serum potassium concentration is often reduced. The blood film may show evidence of intravascular coagulation of "microangiopathic hemolytic anemia" with circulating red cell fragments and fibrin degradation products. The platelet count may be reduced. Irrespective of whether the underlying cause is renal, there is likely to be proteinuria and microscopic hematuria. The characteristic pathologic change of accelerated hypertension is fibrinoid necrosis of small arterioles. Accelerated hypertension is rare in elderly people, even though high pressure levels are common. Conversely, younger patients, especially children, may develop the retinal features of accelerated hypertension at lower levels of pressure than is the case in adults.

Accelerated hypertension is a medical emergency because it causes progressive damage to the blood vessels in vital organs, particularly the kidney. Such a patient is also in severe danger of suffering cerebral hemorrhage. When the diagnosis is made, a patient should be admitted to hospital at once for blood pressure reduction.

RETINOPATHY IN ACCELERATED HYPERTENSION. The diagnosis of malignant or accelerated hypertension is based clinically upon the retinal finding of cotton wool spots, linear hemorrhages, and papilledema, and its pathologic hallmark is the presence of fibrinoid necrosis in the arterioles of many organs, particularly the kidney. The retinal changes in accelerated hypertension are all direct consequences of the pressure elevation. As the pressure rises, the arterioles constrict and thus maintain an approximately normal pressure in the distal arterioles and the capillaries. If the pressure rises to a very high level, particularly if it does so quickly, the arterioles may not be able to withstand the high level pressure and begin to give way. The result is that a much higher pressure than usual is applied to the proximal ends of capillaries. In the retina the high pressure capillaries fed directly from the arterioles lie amid the nerve fibers; when hemorrhage takes place from the capillaries, its spread is confined by the nerve fibers so that it has a linear or flame-shaped appearance. A general transudation of fluid as a result of the disturbed Starling pressure equilibrium in the capillary leads to the formation of a grayish retinal edema. The walls of some arterioles that have given way in the face of the high pressure become disrupted, allowing the insudation of plasma through the endothelial cells into the wall. The plasma penetration is often accompanied by cellular elements such as platelets and red cells. This stage can be recognized on a fluorescence angiogram of the retina by the presence of multiple leaking points on small arterioles. The swelling and disruption of the arteriolar wall as a result of the penetration of plasma may obstruct the lumen and lead to downstream ischemia. Interruption of axoplasmic flow through this region causes the accumulation of organelles with swelling of the axon and formation of the visible cotton wool spot. Pathologic examination of the wall of the arteriole at this stage shows necrosis of myofibrillae in smooth muscle cells, penetration of plasma, and precipitation of fibrin. This is the appearance that pathologists term "fibrinoid necrosis." The term is descriptive of the appearances but misleading in terms of the pathophysiology, because the deposition of fibrin has little or nothing to do with the causation of the lesion. Autoregulatory failure in the vessels of the nerve head causes swelling, engorgement of the capillaries, transudation of fluid, and sometimes also formation of cotton wool spots on the nerve head itself. Keith, Wagener and Barker (1939) described the presence of hemorrhages and exudates as the third grade of retinopathy and papilledema as the fourth. As they have the same basic pathogenetic mechanisms, it seems best to describe both as accelerated hypertension. Hard exudates are not present in the earlier stage of the development of hypertensive retinopathy, but they appear soon after cotton wool spots and papilledema are established and are often arranged in radial spokes from the macula, giving the appearance of a star or fan. Hard exudates are fine, punctate, shiny deposits of lipid in the deep layers of the retina and are readily distinguished with the ophthalmoscope from the larger, more diffuse white cotton wool spot with blurred edges that lies in the nerve fiber layer. Eventually the intra-axonal debris in cotton wool spots aggregates into dense masses that have a superficial resemblance to a cell nucleus. The swollen axon containing its pseudonucleus is sometimes referred to as a cytoid body. As cotton wool spots clear, they can take on a punctate appearance that may be confused with hard exudates. The punctate white areas are the cytoid bodies.

Hypertensive Encephalopathy

Hypertensive encephalopathy is the cerebral counterpart of retinal cotton wool spots. It often occurs in patients who also have the retinal features of accelerated hypertension, but these are not always present.

Patients usually present clinically with a very high level of pressure and increasingly severe headaches. These sometimes progress to general impairment of higher functions and eventually to stupor. Focal and usually transient neurologic signs may develop in the course of the illness. Investigation shows generalized swelling of the brain substance, and animal studies have demonstrated leakage of plasma from arterioles. The diagnosis is a most important one to make accurately, because the patient's condition will improve rapidly if the blood pressure is reduced to a level at which cerebrovascular autoregulation is once again possible.

There is a resemblance between hypertensive encephalopathy and other syndromes in brain autoregulatory failure such as high altitude cerebral edema or carbon dioxide narcosis, although these less commonly manifest focal neurologic signs.

Hypertension in Pregnancy

A raised arterial pressure during pregnancy usually leads to impaired placental function and a small baby. There is an increased risk of intrauterine death and increased neonatal mortality because of prematurity. Toxemia of pregnancy is characterized by a rise in blood pressure from 28 weeks' gestation onward, with edema and proteinuria. The most feared complication is progression to severe hypertension with convulsions and coma. Eclamptic convulsions are essentially hypertensive encephalopathic attacks occurring in a previously normotensive young woman who has suffered a rapid rise in blood pressure. They should not occur in women who have received proper antenatal care and control of blood pressure. Toxemia is hypertension provoked by pregnancy, but many women who have mild hypertension become pregnant or may be first found to be hypertensive when they consult a physician at about 8 to 12 weeks of pregnancy for antenatal care. In the past there was a different approach to treatment in a pregnant hypertensive than in the nonpregnant female with high blood pressure. This view is now changing, and most internists and obstetricians use the same methods of management in pregnancy as at other times but aim to achieve particularly accurate control of pressure during the pregnancy. There is evidence that effective antihypertensive therapy reduces fetal loss during pregnancy, and the aim should be to keep the pressure below 130 systolic and 85 diastolic mm Hg if possible. The main drugs used to control blood pressure are methyldopa and beta-adrenergic blockers. There has been concern that antihypertensive drugs might damage development of the fetal nervous system by interfering with catecholamine pathways, but studies of babies whose mothers have been treated for hypertension with these drugs are reassuring. There has been debate about the use of beta-adrenergic blocking drugs because they obscure the interpretation of fetal bradycardia and may increase the incidence of the respiratory distress syndrome but a recent clinical trial has been reassuring.

Cerebral Hemorrhage

Abrupt onset of major neurologic signs, sometimes accompanied by severe headache and progressing rapidly to loss of consciousness, usually signifies the onset of intracranial bleeding in a hypertensive patient. The bleeding may occur into the subarachnoid space from a berry aneurysm, but the common source in hypertensive patients appears to be the minute arterial aneurysms on the striate arteries on the base of the brain, first described by Charcot and Bouchard in France over 100 years ago. These aneurysms are rare in individuals who have a normal blood pressure. Their pathogenesis has not been completely elucidated, but there may be areas of high-pressure autoregulatory failure on the thin-walled cerebral vessels. The hemorrhage usually begins in the substance of the brain but may rupture into the ventricular system. Once intracranial bleeding has reached the subarachnoid space, the prognosis is very poor. Small hemorrhages have a better prognosis and can be difficult to differentiate clinically from the cerebral infarction caused by vascular occlusion. They are readily distinguished by computerized axial tomography.

Hypertensive Left Ventricular Failure

The presence of a high systemic arterial pressure increases the afterload of the left ventricle, and in consequence the ventricle hypertrophies. As the pressure rises to a very high level, the ventricles dilate and eventually fail, and the patient then presents with pulmonary edema. This may range in severity from a patient who is asphyxiating with airways full of white or pink froth to mild dyspnea on exertion or occasional attacks of noctural dyspnea. In older people with hypertension the clinical presentation of pulmonary edema is frequently precipitated by the onset of atrial fibrillation or by ischemic heart disease. If pulmonary edema is caused by a high blood pressure, the clinical improvement as a result of pressure reduction can be almost miraculous in its rapidity.

"Benign Essential" Hypertension

Patients with an elevated pressure who are not in the accelerated phase are often described as having benign essential hypertension. The term "benign" is inappropriate, as an elevated blood pressure always carries some risk. Although no cause can be identified in most individuals with high pressure, the use of the word "essential" to describe it adds nothing, and it too is best avoided. What then are the clinical features of hypertension which is not in the accelerated phase? They are rarely dramatic. The elevated level of pressure is often the only clinical finding of note. A mild degree of left ventricular hypertrophy may be identified clinically or by means of the electrocardiogram. Vascular damage may be evident either from its consequences on the heart or brain or by loss of pulses or arterial bruits.

RETINOPATHY IN "BENIGN" HYPERTENSION. Keith, Wagener and Barker applied the terms grade I and grade II retinopathy to the retinal changes found in hypertensive patients who are not in the accelerated phase. The main features which they described include narrowing of the arterioles, often with caliber irregularity, and nicking of the veins at the crossing. The appearance of the arteriolar wall changed so that it became shinier and more irregular, whereas the color of the underlying blood columns was partly concealed so that it took on a coppery or silvery hue. Narrowing of the retinal vessels is due to vasoconstriction. All the other changes represent thickening of the vessel wall as a result of muscle hypertrophy and fibrous replacement. The problem with these features is that none of them is by itself characteristic of hypertension. Elderly people who are normotensive may show all of them. They are still of clinical value if the patient is young but of little use in drawing conclusions about the severity of hypertension in the elderly. Recording of these features is very prone to observer error, and attempts to standardize the recording of the diameter of the arteries by comparing them with the nearby veins have foundered on the variability of the branching pattern of the retinal vessels. The presence of these features does not add much to the knowledge of the patient in most cases.

MECHANISMS

The systemic arterial pressure must be maintained at a level that permits the brain and eyes to function and allows pressure filtration in the kidneys and perfusion of the coronary arteries. It is not surprising that this most vital function is defended by several different control systems that prevent its falling too low. The blood pressure must also be prevented from rising too high, because vascular damage might result. Four control systems play the major part in maintaining the blood pressure between these limits. These are the arterial baroreflex, the regulation of body fluid volume, the renin-angiotensin system, and vascular autoregulation. All these mechanisms participate in blood pressure regulation in normotension and in hypertension. It is uncertain how far derangement of any one of them plays a role in the pathogenesis of hypertension.

The Arterial Baroreflex

The main concentration of pressure sensors lies in the carotid sinus, although there are others in the aorta and the wall of the left ventricle. These sensors continually monitor the level of arterial pressure, and their rate of firing changes between systole and diastole. They form the afferent limb of the fastest responding blood pressure regulating system. Sensory impulses from the baroreceptors are relayed and processed in the brainstem. Norepinephrine- and epinephrine-containing fibers around the nucleus of the solitary tract play an important part in regulating the gain of the baroreflex. The efferent fibers proceed through sympathetic adrenergic nerves to the heart and blood vessels and through vagal cholinergic fibers. A sudden rise in pressure causes baroreflex discharge, which results in vagally mediated cardiac slowing and vasodilatation with decreased sympathetic tone. The result is to lower the blood pressure, although not all the way to the prestimulus level. A sudden fall in pressure diminishes the rate of firing and causes sympathetic stimulation of the rate and force of cardiac contraction and constriction of peripheral arterioles and veins. The result is partly to restore the level of blood pressure. Denervation of the carotid sinus in animals causes extreme lability of blood pressure, which is sometimes termed neurogenic hypertension. However, the rise in arterial pressure is not usually very great except when the animal is stimulated, and the characteristic is more of extreme instability than sustained elevation of pressure.

It is important to realize that the baroreflex arc is not simply a fixed feedback loop such as might be found in an audio frequency amplifier. Depending upon the physiologic circumstances, the response to the same level of blood pressure can be quite different. A blood pressure of 85 systolic and 55 diastolic mm Hg caused by bleeding would cause an intense sympathetic discharge and tachycardia. The same level of pressure during deep sleep would be accompanied by the normal bradycardia of the sleeping subject. A pressure of 200 systolic and 100 diastolic mm Hg is readily achieved during heavy exercise and is accompanied by tachycardia. The same pressure brought about by infusion of norepinephrine would cause extreme cardiac slowing mediated by the baroreflex. The pressure is the same, but the interpretation at CNS level is completely different.

If the pressure remains elevated, the baroreflex begins to regulate at the new level within 24 to 48 hours. The ability of the baroreflex to reset so quickly argues against its playing an important role in long-term pressure regulation. Baroreflex function in patients with hypertension appears to be intact and not to differ qualitatively from that found in normotensives.

The effector side of the baroreflex is via the autonomic nervous system. Vagal impulses can slow the heart while, conversely, sympathetic stimulation can constrict arteries and veins and stimulate cardiac contractility and rate. The importance of this side of the reflex is seen in the postural hypotension suffered by many patients in whom it is inhibited by ganglion-blocking or adrenergic neuron-blocking drugs. The baroreflex is not the only control system that uses the adrenergic nerves to raise blood pressure. The rise in pressure that occurs with fear, anxiety, pain, or mental activity is also mediated by increasing cardiac output or peripheral resistance through these pathways. One possible mechanism for long-term elevation of blood pressure would be excessive central nervous system–mediated stimulation of adrenergic nerves. Evidence for this possibility has been sought by comparing the level of blood pressure at rest with the plasma concentration of the adrenergic neurotransmitter norepinephrine. There is evidence for a wider spread of norepinephrine levels in plasma in hypertensives, about 40 per cent of them being higher than those found in healthy normotensive volunteers, but the higher values reported in patients are, at least in part, due to increased sympathetic activity caused by anxiety at the time of sampling. The best evidence implicating increased sympathetic activity lies in the elevated heart rate and cardiac output reported in many younger patients with mild hypertension. However, only in rare situations, such as virus infections involving the hindbrain, or in patients with high intracranial pressures is it possible to be sure that the blood pressure has been raised by the brain.

Fluid Volume

If the body is severely depleted of salt and water, the blood pressure falls; if it is overloaded, the pressure rises. The mechanisms involved are complex and have been discussed cogently by Guyton. Changes in fluid volume alter the distention of the venous system and change the venous return to the heart. If the cardiac filling pressure rises, so does the cardiac output; if it falls the output also falls. The short-term effects of cardiac output changes upon blood pressure are buffered by the baroreflex, but in the longer term changes in tissue perfusion that are inappropriate to metabolic requirements lead to autoregulatory changes in the peripheral resistance and thus to changes in the blood pressure. If the kidneys are intact, a rise in pressure leads to a diuresis and a fall in pressure to conservation of salt and water. Thus the feedback loop is closed, and Guyton has claimed that this system, unlike the baroreflex, has infinite gain so that it can exactly restore the previous level of pressure.

Pathologic changes that alter the pressure threshold at which the kidneys excrete salt and water will alter the level of systemic arterial pressure. At one extreme a complete lack of kidneys should lead to a great sensitivity to changes in volume, and this has proved to be the case. Relatively small increases in salt and water intake in nephrectomized individuals cause a large increase in blood pressure. This type of hypertension is sometimes termed "renoprival." Other mechanisms such as the lack of a renal depressor substance may also play a part in the abnormal pressure regulation. If excretory function is diminished, the blood pressure will become responsive to an abnormally high sodium load. Mineralocorticoid excess will cause the kidney to retain salt at a pressure level at which it would normally be excreted and thereby raise the arterial pressure. Anything that increases the pressure gradient between the aorta and the glomeruli will tend to raise the systemic arterial pressure as renal retention of salt and water endeavors to restore the preobstruction renal perfusion pressure. This will apply to obstruction of the main renal arteries and of the arterial branches within the kidney. An experimental analogy is the one-kidney Goldblatt model. Here one kidney has been removed and the other has an arterial clip upon it. The renin levels are low, and the pressure gradient across the renal artery appears to be the important factor in causing the hypertension through the salt and water retention that results from diminished perfusion pressure applied to the clipped kidney.

Renin and Angiotensin

Renin is an enzyme released from the kidney which splits a decapeptide from a plasma globulin substrate. This decapeptide, angiotensin I, has little pharmacologic activity, but a dipeptide residue is removed by a converting enzyme located in the lung and other tissues, to form an octapeptide, angiotensin II. Until the discovery of thromboxane A_2, this was the most potent vasoconstrictor agent known. Angiotensin II has a direct action upon blood vessels, but it is also an important physiologic stimulant of aldosterone secretion from the adrenal gland.

Standing or salt depletion raises renin output, and recumbency and salt loading reduce it. In conditions of primary mineralocorticoid excess the renin falls to a low value. Four mechanisms have been identified that control the release of renin from the kidney. The first mechanism is the renal barostat, which senses changes in renal perfusion pressure and releases renin when the pressure falls; the second mechanism is the short feedback loop of plasma angiotensin II levels upon renin release. If angiotensin effects are blocked with its competitive antagonist saralasin, renin levels rise rapidly. The third mechanism is mediated by beta-adrenergic receptors in the kidney which release renin when they are stimulated, and the fourth mechanism depends upon sensing tubular concentrations of sodium.

The importance of angiotensin II in maintaining blood pressure at any particular time depends upon the level of sodium intake. In a sodium-replete individual inhibition of angiotensin II has little effect upon blood pressure; but if the same person is salt-depleted, the result of inhibition may be a substantial fall. There is good evidence that angiotensin II is the cause of the blood pressure elevation in the experimental two-kidney Goldblatt hypertension and in human hypertension caused by renal artery stenosis. In the two-kidney Goldblatt model one kidney is clipped and the other is not. Thus the unclipped kidney should be able to prevent a rise in pressure due to salt and water retention resulting from the pressure gradient across the clipped artery. In the first phase of this form of hypertension the blood pressure rises and so do the plasma renin and angiotensin. Infusion of the competitive angiotensin II antagonist saralasin causes a prompt fall to a normal level of pressure. However, in experimental hypertension and probably also in human hypertension the pressure continues to rise in the second phase, whereas the renin subsides almost to normal.

Discovery of the converting enzyme (ACE) inhibitors, typified by captopril, has necessitated a revision of the role assigned to the renin-angiotensin system in blood pressure regulation. ACE inhibitors prevent the conversion of the decapeptide angiotensin I to the active octapeptide angiotensin II. They can lower blood pressure in patients with a high, normal, or low renin, although the reduction is greatest in the high renin patients. There has been an intensive search for other possible explanations of the hypotensive action, including effects upon ACE in brain, kidney, and vascular walls and inhibition of the pulmonary breakdown of bradykinin, which has a vasodilator action. Present evidence suggests that prevention of the conversion of A-I to A-II is the main action.

The role of angiotensin II in the causation of human hypertension remains to be elucidated in full, but there is no evidence that it is an important etiologic factor in "benign" hypertension. The situation is different in accelerated hypertension. The renin levels are often high because of the multiple small areas of ischemia downstream to zones of arteriolar necrosis. Elevated angiotensin II contributes to the vicious circle of high pressure in these patients and, by stimulating aldosterone production, often causes secondary hyperaldosteronism.

Vascular Autoregulation

In many tissues, of which the brain is the best example, a change in perfusion pressure does not cause a corresponding change in tissue perfusion. Instead the vascular resistance is adjusted by local mechanisms to keep perfusion roughly constant over a wide range of arterial pressures. This phenomenon is known as "vascular autoregulation." If flow changes rather than pressure, autoregulation will diminish the vascular resistance in response to a reduction in flow and raise it in response to an increase. Thus changes in cardiac output that are inappropriate to metabolic demand should produce corresponding changes in blood pressure. This is probably an important mechanism in the causation of the hypertension that accompanies salt and water overload, but it is uncertain how significant it is in other circumstances.

Circulatory Dynamics

The level of the systemic arterial pressure is set by the match between cardiac output and peripheral vascular resistance. Elevation of blood pressure could result from either or both. In the early stages of hypertension some patients have a raised cardiac output and some a raised peripheral resistance, but in the majority of patients with established hypertension the cardiac output is normal and peripheral resistance is raised. In the later stages of severe hypertension the cardiac output is often less than normal and the peripheral resistance is greatly increased. Thus in looking for factors that maintain hypertension, it seems most profitable to concentrate upon those that raise the peripheral resistance.

Elevation of the arterial pressure causes many changes in the cardiovascular system. A high level of pressure stimulates hypertrophy of the vessel wall and increases the thickness of the smooth muscle coat. These changes probably account for the moderately enhanced sensitivity to pressor stimuli in patients with established or early hypertension. Such stimuli include exposure to cold, fear, mental arithmetic, and so forth. A greater thickness of muscle means that the change in vessel caliber for a given degree of fiber shortening will be greater. Hypertrophy of the vessel wall also raises the minimum vascular resistance of tissues such as the human forearm under conditions of maximal vasodilatation.

Besides the hypertrophic changes, other structural changes take place in the arteries. Some of the muscle in the thickened wall is replaced by fibrous tissue. The most important vascular change is that the deposition of atheroma is increased by the presence of hypertension. The reason is not known, but it is a change manifest in pulmonary hypertension as well as systemic hypertension. As the predominant causes of death in hypertension patients are stroke and myocardial infarction, the significance of accelerated formation of atheroma cannot be denied, but the mechanism is uncertain.

The cardiac muscle also hypertrophies and, if pressure elevation is extreme, the cavity of the ventricle dilates. Local imbalance between metabolic demand and perfusion within the increased muscle mass may lead to relative ischemia and areas of fibrosis. These may lead to ineffective contraction that, combined with the dilated chamber and the afterload of the high pressure, will eventually bring about heart failure.

The regulation of plasma volume is altered in hypertension. Some patients have a relatively contracted plasma volume with a high hematocrit, probably because of the increased capillary pressure. There is a marked diurnal variation of plasma volume, with the value almost 10 per cent lower in the morning than in the evening in hypertensive subjects. An infused sodium load is excreted more rapidly by hypertensive patients than by normotensive controls.

ETIOLOGY

In most diseases the need to establish a diagnosis is paramount because the prognosis and the treatment given may be entirely different, depending upon which of the possible alternatives is the cause of the illness. The position with hypertension is different. There are very few causes of hypertension that are life threatening other than by their effect upon the blood pressure. The most important condition in this category is renal failure, but this is usually readily detected clinically or by the use of a biochemical screen at presentation. Only coarctation of the aorta and a pheochromocytoma are sufficiently serious in themselves as well as through the pressure elevation they cause to make it essential that they be diagnosed at once. Although it is desirable to make a diagnosis of renal artery stenosis or primary hyperaldosteronism, if present, some delay will not usually cause harm to the patients if the pressure has been controlled with drugs in the meantime. Thus the diagnostic problem in a patient with hypertension is how to detect as large a proportion as possible of the rare treatable causes without exposing millions of patients without such factors to unnecessary and uncomfortable investigations. The answer is to use screening tests and to be willing to reconsider the diagnosis in treated patients if the clinical course is atypical.

Obstruction or Loss of Elasticity in the Large Arteries

COARCTATION OF AORTA (see Ch. 44). Routine palpation of the femoral pulses with simultaneous timing against the radial is part of the basic clinical examination of a patient with hypertension. Other clinical features, such as a wide pulse pressure in the arteries fed by the aorta proximal to the coarctation, confirm the diagnosis that has been made. Occasionally the diagnosis is first made radiologically by direct visualization of the coarctation or of rib notching on a routine chest radiograph. Operative treatment is indicated if it is technically feasible.

SYSTOLIC HYPERTENSION. Many elderly patients present with considerable elevation of the systolic pressure while having a relatively normal diastolic pressure. A typical pressure might be 200 systolic and 80 diastolic mm Hg in such an individual. The principal factors governing the magnitude of the pulse pressure are the stroke volume and acceleration of the blood from the left ventricle and the elasticity of the large arteries, particularly the aorta. Factors that increase the stroke volume, such as bradycardia, aortic incompetence, anemia, and anxiety, may all lead to an increase in systolic pressure with a normal or low diastolic pressure. In the elderly the most common cause is not an increase in stroke volume but a loss of elastic compliance of the large arteries. Epidemiologic studies have shown that such patients have an increased risk of cardiovascular morbidity and mortality even if their diastolic pressure is relatively low. However, it is not clear whether this cardiovascular disease is a cause or consequence of the systolic hypertension. It may be that the presence of a systolic hypertension is itself a marker of arterial disease and the level of systolic pressure has no other significance. There is no evidence as to whether reduction of systolic hypertension with a normal diastolic pressure conveys any advantage to the patient.

Hypertension Associated with Catecholamine Excess

PHEOCHROMOCYTOMA (see Ch. 241). Pheochromocytoma is a very rare cause of hypertension. Larger tumors can be suspected clinically in half to two thirds of the patients. Pounding palpitations and/or headaches, paroxysmal skin color changes, tremor, sweating, agitation, glycosuria, and hypermetabolism may all point to the likelihood of this diagnosis. However, in patients with small tumors, who form the majority now diagnosed, these features are not conspicuous and the diagnosis is often first suspected from a routine urinary VMA.

Rarely patients may know that pressure over the tumor area can provoke an attack. A very rare but striking example is the precipitation of a paroxysm by micturition in a patient with pheochromocytoma of the bladder. In some patients there are only occasional spikes of hypertension, or even of hypotension, whereas in others there may be a sustained elevation in the blood pressure. There is sometimes marked orthostatic hypotension in the absence of the use of drugs with a postural effect.

It is common practice to measure the urinary VMA as a screening test to detect pheochromocytoma in all hypertensive patients irrespective of clinical suspicions. A single estimate is about 80 per cent reliable in detecting a pheochromocytoma, but many slightly elevated values occur as false positives. Once firmly suspected, the diagnosis should be confirmed by further measurements of the urinary VMA and of metanephrines or catecholamines. Other causes of increased sympathetic activity such as left ventricular failure and myocardial infarction should be ruled out. Increasingly the measurements of plasma norepinephrine are being used to make and confirm the diagnosis of pheochromocytoma. False-positive elevations caused by anxiety can be excluded by a suppression test using a ganglion-blocking drug such as pentolinium or the centrally acting drug clonidine to inhibit neurally mediated release while leaving autonomous production by a tumor unaffected. Tumors can usually be localized by a CAT scan or, in difficult cases, by segmental venous sampling with measurement of plasma norepinephrine.

MONOAMINE OXIDASE INHIBITORS: INTERACTION WITH TYRAMINE. Patients taking drugs that inhibit the monoamine oxidase in the gut wall and in the body at large may develop paroxysmal hypertension if they consume food or drink containing tyramine or medicines such as cold cures that contain pressor amines such as phenylpropanolamine. Tyramine and phenylpropanolamine are both capable of releasing norepinephrine from adrenergic nerve endings. Normally the amounts of these releasing agents that penetrate into the body are small because of metabolism by monoamine oxidase in the gut wall. If this enzyme is inhibited, larger amounts reach the systemic circulation where the adrenergic nerve endings release an excessive amount of norepinephrine because of the local inhibition of monoamine oxidase. The result can be a catastrophic increase in circulating norepinephrine, causing a very high blood pressure with a risk of cerebral hemorrhage or paroxysmal cardiac arrhythmia.

CLONIDINE WITHDRAWAL. The imidazoline clonidine is an effective antihypertensive agent. It acts centrally as an alpha-adrenoceptor agonist and causes a decrease in the sympathetic outflow by stimulating a brainstem inhibitory system. If treatment with the drug is suddenly withdrawn patients may develop a syndrome of catecholamine excess 16 to 48 hours later which closely resembles a pheochromocytoma. Some patients complain of anxiety, tremor, palpitations, and insomnia with severe headache. Both plasma and urinary catecholamines can reach high levels. The precise mechanism underlying this reaction has not yet been determined, but sympathetic efferent activity is greatly increased. The blood pressure can be controlled by restarting clonidine or by use of alpha-adrenergic blocking agents.

MANAGEMENT OF CATECHOLAMINE EXCESS HYPERTENSION. The long-term treatment of hypertension associated with gross excess of circulating catecholamines is to treat the cause. However, in the short term the blood pressure and cardiac rhythm disturbances, if present, must be controlled. Alpha-adrenergic blocking drugs such as injections of phentolamine should be used to control the immediate rise in pressure; oral agents, such as phenoxybenzamine, that alkylate the alpha receptor can be used in longer term treatment. Tachycardia or tachyarrhythmias can be controlled by use of beta receptor blocking agents, such as propranolol. Patients with a pheochromocytoma should always be prepared for surgery by pharmacologic control of hypertension and cardiac arrhythmias.

RENAL HYPERTENSION

All forms of chronic renal disease may be associated with an increased incidence of hypertension. This is true of chronic glomerulonephritis due to immune complex deposition, chronic pyelonephritis due to infection, vascular lesions such as occur in polyarteritis nodosa and lupus erythematosus, and in the main renal arteries due to congenital bands, intimal fibroplasia, and atheroma. Renal carcinoma can cause hypertension, as can polycystic disease, although isolated renal cysts rarely do so. Obstructive uropathies, analgesic abuse, and renal calculi can also cause hypertension. Acute renal failure resulting from glomerulonephritis or tubular necrosis can cause rapid elevation of blood pressure, especially in fluid-overloaded patients.

There are two main reasons for making an accurate diagnosis of renal hypertension. The first is that the renal or urologic condition that has caused the hypertension may itself require treatment, e.g., infection, stone, obstruction, tumor. Of the conditions that fall into this category, infection is the most important. Pyelonephritis is an important cause of renal damage and hypertension, especially in children. Its numerical importance in relation to adult hypertension is difficult to establish because of the difficulty of proving a diagnosis of chronic pyelonephritis.

The relationship between bacilluria and hypertension is disputed, but there is an increased incidence of hypertension in patients whose urograms show segmental "pyelonephritic scars." There are vascular lesions in the vicinity of these scars, and there seems little doubt that the scars are ischemic in origin. Such lesions can be caused by hypertensive changes in the vessels without any infection, and it is not clear how far infection of the renal parenchyma can cause vascular lesions and initiate hypertension in a previously normotensive individual. But in children with vesicoureteral reflux, urinary infection, renal scars, and hypertension, there seems little doubt that reflux and infection start the whole process.

The second reason for investigating a patient to determine if hypertension has a renal cause is the possibility of treating renovascular disease. Cure of hypertension also resulted from nephrectomy in several types of unilateral renal disease, including pyelonephritis, hydronephrosis, and tumor, but such operations are rarely undertaken with treatment of hypertension as the main aim because success rates are low.

SALT AND WATER OVERLOAD HYPERTENSION. Patients without kidneys or those in terminal renal failure with very low values of glomerular filtration are extremely sensitive to changes in salt and water balance. The plasma renin and angiotensin II levels are usually low (although they may be higher than appropriate to the exchangeable body sodium) unless the patient has entered the accelerated phase of hypertension. This form of hypertension can usually be managed successfully by restriction of salt and water intake and elimination of excess by dialysis. The body weight is often a better guide to progress than the sphygmomanometer.

RENIN-DEPENDENT HYPERTENSION. The extent to which renin contributes to control of blood pressure in the majority of patients with hypertension is controversial. Renin concentrations in plasma cannot be interpreted without knowledge of the 24-hour urine sodium or the exchangeable body sodium. Sensitivity to the pressor effects of angiotensin II is also critically dependent upon sodium homeostasis. Salt overload greatly increases sensitivity to angiotensin II, whereas salt depletion reduces it. Patients with untreated Addison's disease have hypotension accompanied by very high levels of renin and angiotensin. The spread of renin values is wider among hypertensives than normotensives, and those subjects with values above and below the normal range, related to sodium intake, are often called "high renin" and "low renin" hypertensives. The view that renin itself may be a factor causing damage to blood vessels has not been confirmed. As plasma renin falls with age and the risk of vascular disease increases, a negative association has been proposed based upon epidemiologic studies. Renin contributes to the elevation of blood pressure in accelerated hypertension and causes it in renal disease associated with ischemia. Many types of renal disease can be associated with localized areas of ischemia, but the most important is renal artery obstruction caused by medial fibroplasia or atheromatous disease. The detection of these conditions has given rise to much controversy on the grounds of prevalence, costs, and results of surgery.

RENAL ARTERY STENOSIS. There are no reliable figures for the incidence of renal artery stenosis in the community. It may cause 3 to 5 per cent of severe hypertension treated in hospital but less than 1 per cent of the mild hypertension now being treated in the community.

There are few clinical features that help in making a diagnosis. Suspicion should be aroused by severe hypertension in a patient under 35 years old, or sudden increase in severity in an older patient. Rarely an attack of flank pain may point to a renal artery embolus, and a bruit above and radiating laterally from the umbilicus may be helpful. Unfortunately many of the bruits heard over the abdominal aorta do not originate in the renal arteries. The most common means of diagnosis is an intravenous urogram. Typical features include one kidney more than 1.5 cm shorter than the other, delay in appearance of the nephrogram on the ischemic side, and delay in emptying on that side because of the low flow of concentrated urine. The most reliable means of confirming the diagnosis is an angiogram of the abdominal aorta and renal arteries, but this should only be done if there are features suggesting renal artery stenosis. Many centers have abandoned routine urography in asymptomatic hypertensive patients with normal renal function. Ultrasound provides a reliable noninvasive method of estimating renal size. When the diagnosis of renal artery stenosis has been confirmed anatomically, it is desirable to establish whether the elevation of blood pressure is due to excess renin production. The methods used currently include measurement of renin concentration in blood drawn from an artery and both renal veins. The difference should exceed 1.5 to 2 times, and the nonstenosed kidney has its production of renin suppressed.

The invention of the Grunzig balloon catheter, which permits transarterial dilatation of renal artery stenosis, has revolutionized the approach to this condition. Result rates vary with the skill of the operator and the pathology but are particularly good in patients with fibromuscular hyperplasia. The procedure can be repeated. The only serious complication is tearing the renal artery, which necessitates immediate surgery. Very tight stenoses are difficult to dilate, but in these patients the kidney is usually so shrunken that its function cannot be restored.

A special situation may arise in patients with renal failure and bilateral renal artery obstruction, in whom dilatation or surgery can sometimes improve overall renal function. Captopril and other ACE inhibitors are now the first choice for treating severe renin-dependent hypertension.

MINERALOCORTICOID EXCESS HYPERTENSION. Mineralocorticoids, both natural and synthetic, can cause retention of salt and water and resultant hypertension. Thus hypertension is a common complication of Cushing's syndrome, both natural and iatrogenic. The contraceptive pill is capable of causing elevation of blood pressure, and there are worrying indications that this may be progressive over several years. The elevation each year is an apparently trivial 1.5 to 2.0 mm Hg rise in diastolic pressure, but the cumulative effect over several years can begin to be significant in epidemiologic terms in relation to the incidence of stroke and myocardial infarction. Blood pressure elevation may also result from the salt-retaining effects of carbenoxolone sodium given to treat gastric ulcer.

Among these factors the contraceptive pill gives rise to by far the greatest difficulty because of the extent of its use. Severe hypertension in users of the pill is very uncommon, although accelerated hypertension has been reported. More commonly a woman who has used the pill for several years develops a pressure level which is on the threshold of an indication for treatment. There is no certain method of establishing whether the pill is responsible short of stopping it for six weeks or substituting another method. Progestogen-only contraceptive pills appear to be free of a blood pressure–elevating effect and are the best alternative for hypertensive patients.

Endogenous mineralocorticoid excess can also pose difficult problems of detection and treatment. Cushing's syndrome or congenital adrenal hyperplasia as a cause of hypertension can usually be diagnosed clinically, although patients with an ACTH-producing malignant tumor may present with hypertension and severe hypokalemia without much other evidence of Cushing's syndrome. The main problem is the diagnosis of primary hyperaldosteronism. Some patients give a history that suggests potassium depletion with muscle weakness and edema, but most do not. The presence of hypokalemia is a useful guide if the patient has not received a thiazide diuretic, but most patients have been treated with these agents before they get to a hospital clinic. If potassium depletion is severe and the serum sodium is high, the diagnosis is very likely to be hyperaldosteronism, and it can be confirmed by measuring plasma or urinary aldosterone and plasma renin. A patient with primary hyperaldosteronism has an increased production of aldosterone with a suppressed plasma renin. A trial of treatment with the aldosterone antagonist spironolactone predicts fairly accurately the eventual response of both blood pressure and serum potassium concentration to operative removal of an adrenal tumor. Primary hyperaldosteronism can be caused by an adrenal adenoma or by diffuse "micronodular" hyperplasia. A few patients have been described with hypertension secondary to primary hyperaldosteronism who had a normal serum potassium level some or all of the time. These patients are impossible to diagnose without full investigation of aldosterone and renin, and this does not appear justified as a routine procedure for the very low yield of treatable cases likely to result. Newer diagnostic methods such as CT scans and ultrasound are helpful in localizing a suspected tumor.

TREATMENT

The proportion of hypertensive patients in the community who might benefit from pressure reduction and who have a surgically remediable cause is very small, probably less than 1 per cent of those requiring treatment. Intelligent management of long-term drug treatment is the main challenge for the physician who treats hypertensive patients. As the average severity of disease in patients treated has declined, the emphasis has shifted from blood pressure reduction at all costs to finding regimens that combine efficacy with convenience and a low burden of symptoms.

Reduction of Risk

The aim of patient management in hypertension is to reduce the likelihood of cardiovascular complications, and the approach adopted depends upon the level of blood pressure and the burden of associated risk factors. If the blood pressure is very high, this is the dominant consideration, and other considerations can be deferred until the pressure has been reduced. However, in many patients with only moderate elevation of pressure, other factors such as cigarette smoking may be of comparable significance to the blood pressure. Careful assessment is required to decide which factors should receive the most attention. A patient who is told to stop smoking, to lose 20 pounds in weight, and to take pills to lower blood pressure is likely to find the task so difficult that he will end up doing none of them. Failure to comply with the physician's advice is the most common cause of treatment failure, and strategies must be developed to try to improve compliance. A close relationship between the patient and a single physician is a significant factor. A patient who knows, likes, and trusts his physician is more likely to take his advice irrespective of its quality. That advice should be simple and unequivocal.

The drug regimen should consist of as few different drugs and tablets as possible, and regimens that require doses to be taken during the working day should be avoided. The patient should know the name and purpose of each tablet, when to take them, and how many to take. The very fact that the doctor takes an interest in the drugs reinforces their importance in the eyes of a patient. A hastily written prescription handed over without an explanation may have the contrary effect. Patients often find it helpful to purchase a small metal pillbox and to count their tablets for the next day into it just before they go to bed. If the box is empty again by the next evening, the patient will know he has taken exactly the right amount. If the patient is elderly or confused, a family member can be enlisted to help count out the tablets and make sure they have been consumed. A wife or husband often seems more concerned about the outcome of therapy than the patient does.

Despite these measures to improve compliance with advice, some patients will drop out from treatment and attendance at follow-up. Few will do so by deliberate rejection of therapy, which is their right. In most cases it is more a matter of oversight. A well-run clinic should have a system to detect nonattendance and to issue reminders. A special register for hypertensive patients is the best arrangement.

Antihypertensive Drugs

In most countries there are many different antihypertensive drugs available, and the range of choice may seem bewildering. If the drugs are categorized in terms of their main pharmacologic action, much of this confusion disappears, and the choice of a particular drug within a group is of less importance than the correct choice of the main action. The main groups of drugs used to lower blood pressure are diuretics, beta-blocking drugs, angiotensin-converting enzyme inhibitors, vasodilators, alpha-

TABLE 47–2. DRUGS AND DOSES USED TO TREAT HIGH BLOOD PRESSURE

Type of Action	Drug Name	Dose Range in General Use (mg per day)
Diuretic	Bendroflumethazide	2.5–10
	Hydrochlorothiazide	12.5–100
	Chlorthalidone	12.5–50
	Polythiazide	0.5–2
Beta-adrenergic blocker	Propranolol	40–480
	Oxprenolol	40–480
	Atenolol	25–100
	Metoprolol	200–600
Centrally acting alpha agonist	Methyldopa	500–2000
	Clonidine	0.3–1.0
Vasodilator	Hydralazine	50–200
	Minoxidil	5–40
Converting enzyme inhibitor	Captopril	25–150
	Enalapril*	5–40
Calcium slow-channel blocker	Nifedipine	30–60
	Verapamil	80–480
Alpha receptor antagonist	Prazosin†	0.5–15
Norepinephrine-depleting agents	Reserpine	0.1–0.25
Adrenergic neuron-blocking drug	Guanethidine†	10–100

*Investigational drug.
†Special care is needed to avoid postural hypotension. Start with a low dose.
See manufacturers' data sheets for full prescribing information and contraindications.

adrenergic antagonists, and centrally acting sympathetic inhibitors (Table 47–2). Drugs that blockade autonomic ganglia and adrenergic neurons are now used infrequently.

DIURETICS. Most of the diuretics used to treat hypertension are related to chlorothiazide and, despite differences in activity per unit weight and duration of action, are of similar efficacy. It is more convenient for the patient to use a diuretic with a long duration of action for hypertension because a sudden diuresis is an inconvenience. All diuretics of this type cause depletion of salt and water with a loss of extracellular and plasma fluid volume. During long-term treatment these changes in volume are less marked, but the blood pressure reduction is maintained. There is a reduction of peripheral vascular resistance without alteration in the cardiac output. The dose response curve is flat, which is an advantage, as it permits use of a single fixed low dose in most patients. The precise mechanism of action in reducing peripheral resistance is not well defined but probably depends upon changes in the fluid and ionic content of the blood vessel wall. The main advantage of the thiazides and related diuretics is that they cause few symptoms in most patients, although they can cause impotence in men. Serious toxicity is rare. The main long-term concern with thiazide diuretics has been in respect of their metabolic effects, e.g., potassium depletion, hyperuricemia, glucose intolerance, and reduction of urinary calcium excretion. Some reduction of serum potassium almost always occurs, the magnitude depending upon the dose. Thiazides increase the incidence of ventricular ectopic beats and hypokalemia may be the explanation. The serum potassium concentration can be maintained by concurrent administration of potassium-retaining diuretics (amiloride, triamterene, or sprionolactone). Potassium supplements also reduce the fall in serum potassium, but the doses required to maintain a normal serum potassium are high.

Reduction of urate clearance and elevation of serum urate values are also almost invariable accompaniments of treatment with thiazide diuretics. Use of a diuretic occasionally precipitates an acute attack of gout, and the mild hyperuricemia of prolonged diuretic therapy increases the long-term incidence of acute gouty arthritis. Routine use of allopurinol or probenecid does not appear to be necessary, unless the patient develops gout or the serum urate concentration is very high.

A potentially more serious problem is a slow deterioration of glucose tolerance among patients treated with thiazides. Decreased glucose tolerance is much more likely if it is already abnormal, such as in patients with obesity. At present there is not sufficient evidence to seek to restrict the use of thiazides, but administration for very long periods should be accompanied by occasional urine testing for sugar. There is also a moderate increase in serum lipid concentrations during treatment with thiazides, but the significance of this in relation to cardiovascular risk factors is not clear. As the dose-response curve for the hypotensive effect of diuretics is relatively flat and that for the unwanted metabolic effects is steeper, it is sensible to limit the dose of diuretic used in patients with normal renal function (e.g., 12.5 to 25 mg hydrochlorothiazide).

BETA-ADRENERGIC RECEPTOR BLOCKING DRUGS. Beta-adrenergic receptors are widely distributed in the heart, lungs, blood vessels, and metabolic and endocrine systems. Beta-adrenergic receptor blocking drugs cause competitive blockade of the action of norepinephrine and other beta receptor agonists. Their main cardiovascular action is to reduce the rate and force of cardiac contraction and thus lower the cardiac output. They also blockade bronchial beta receptors and may precipitate asthma in susceptible individuals. Among the many other consequences of beta receptor blockade are inhibition of sympathetically mediated renin release from the kidney and inhibition of sympathetically mediated mobilization of muscle glycogen. Some beta receptor–blocking drugs readily penetrate the central nervous system, and central sites of action have been postulated.

The mechanism of the hypotensive action of beta receptor blocking drugs is still disputed among four main hypotheses. These are reduction of cardiac output, inhibition of renin release, a central action upon sympathetic receptors, and a peripheral action upon a beta receptor on the presynaptic surface of the adrenergic nerve endings. Reduction of cardiac output with loss of the full baroreflex-mediated compensatory increase in peripheral resistance seems the most likely of these explanations. Low concentrations of propranolol will cause maximal inhibition of renin release, but higher concentrations are required for an optimal effect upon blood pressure.

Beta-adrenergic blocking drugs do not cause a large and immediate fall in blood pressure such as can be seen with a drug that blocks sympathetic transmission elsewhere, at the alpha receptor or the sympathetic nerve ending, for example. However, the blood pressure begins to fall in two to four hours after a large dose, and most of the hypotensive effect is manifest within two or three days. In mild hypertension the fall in pressure achieved is comparable to that obtained with diuretics, but in more severe hypertension results comparable to those with methyldopa and guanethidine have been obtained. The reduction in pressure is similar in the lying and standing positions, and the normal rise in pressure on exercise is much reduced. Beta receptor–blocking drugs are less effective than diuretics in older patients.

The main contraindications to the use of beta-blocking drugs are a history of asthma or wheezing and the presence of cardiac conduction defects or a history of heart failure. Beta-blocking drugs should be used with great care, if at all, in unstable diabetics on insulin or sulfonylureas.

Beta-adrenergic blocking drugs cause many symptoms, but few of them are disabling. Reduction of cardiac output may cause cold extremities in cold weather and may worsen intermittent claudication in patients with obstructive disease of their leg arteries. Central nervous system side effects include a feeling of "muzziness," an exactly descriptive English word that seems to have no American equivalent, vivid dreams, and insomnia. Some patients on high doses may suffer daytime visual hallucinations. Serious toxicity has been very rare, but one beta-adrenergic blocking drug, practolol, had to be withdrawn from use because it caused a dry eye, progressing in some cases to perforation of the anterior chamber, a psoriasiform skin rash, and peritoneal fibrosis. This toxicity was apparently unique to practolol.

Besides competitive beta receptor blockade, these drugs may possess in varying degree three other pharmacologic properties. These are beta-1 selectivity, membrane effects, and partial agonist activity. Beta-1 selective agents appear to be just as effective in lowering the blood pressure as nonselective ones. Their main advantage is a lesser degree of blockade of bronchial beta receptors and thus a lesser likelihood of precipitating asthma and a greater ease of treating it with beta receptor agonists if it occurs. Unfortunately the degree of selectivity for the beta-1 receptors is insufficient to avoid a substantial degree of bronchial beta-2 blockade at higher doses. Partial agonist activity means the ability to stimulate as well as blockade the beta receptors; it is sometimes referred to as "intrinsic sympathomimetic activity," or ISA. The consequence of partial agonist activity is less slowing of the resting heart rate. Claims have been made that drugs with partial agonist activity are less likely to precipitate heart failure or asthma and cause a lower incidence of cold extremities. The evidence to support these claims, particularly the first two, is slender. Membrane activity does not contribute to the hypotensive effect of beta blockers.

Several trials have shown that beta adrenergic–blocking drugs reduce mortality for up to three years after a myocardial infarction. As myocardial infarction is the leading cause of death in treated hypertension, it is of great importance to know whether the same is true of patients who are on beta blocking therapy for hypertension when they suffer an infarct. Trials are in progress that may answer this question. Long-term use of beta-adrenergic blocking drugs elevates serum triglycerides and lowers the concentration of high density lipoproteins. In theory this could have a long-term adverse effect upon atheromatous vascular disease.

Angiotensin-Converting Enzyme (ACE) Inhibitors

Drugs of this class inhibit the peptidyl dipeptidase that removes a dipeptide from angiotensin I to convert it into the active form, angiotensin II. ACE inhibitors are noteworthy for their very low incidence of pharmacodynamic side effects, although the only agent generally available, captopril, has caused appreciable toxicity (skin rash, loss of taste, proteinuria, agranulocytosis).

ACE inhibitors reduce the blood pressure in patients of all grades of severity and renin status but are most effective in patients who have a high renin level or who are slightly salt depleted by diuretics or a sodium-restricted diet. Severly salt-depleted patients may suffer severe hypotension when treated with ACE inhibitors.

Early studies with captopril used high doses in patients with very severe hypertension, some of whom had collagen vascular disease or renal impairment, and the incidence of toxic effects was high enough to be disturbing. Recent studies have used lower doses in patients with mild hypertension with a considerable reduction of toxicity. Captopril toxicity resembles that of penicillamine, another sulfhydryl-containing compound. ACE inhibitors without the -SH group are under development and appear to be free of this type of toxicity, e.g., enalapril.

The feeling of well-being in patients treated with ACE inhibitors is probably not a specific euphoriant effect but more an absence of unpleasant symptoms caused by alternative drugs. This favorable experience contrasts with most other antihypertensive drugs and may lead to a considerable extension of the use of ACE inhibitors.

VASODILATORS. As the main hemodynamic abnormality in hypertension is an increased peripheral vascular resistance, use of a drug that directly dilates arteries might appear to be the most logical approach to treatment. Hydralazine and minoxidil are the most widely used drugs in this class, although use of calcium slow-channel blocking agents such as nifedipine and verapamil is rapidly increasing.

Parenteral administration of hydralazine leads to dilatation of arteriolar beds, with flushing of the skin, a fall in pressure, stimulation of the baroreflex, and a reflex increase in heart rate and force. If the patient has ischemic heart disease, the resultant increase in left ventricular work can precipitate angina or even myocardial infarction. Concurrent use of a beta-adrenergic blocking drug prevents most of the increase in heart rate caused by vasodilators, and this combination is widely used in oral therapy.

The main problem with hydralazine is its toxicity if the dose is increased above 200 mg daily. Even if the dose is kept down to this level, about 1.5 per cent of patients develop a drug-induced lupus syndrome with arthralgia, muscle pains, fever, and skin rashes. Those affected by this syndrome are predominantly Caucasian females who are slow acetylators and of HLA group Drw-4. As in other drug-induced lupus syndromes, the DNA binding is normal. If the acetylator phenotype is known to be fast, it is possible to increase the hydralazine dose to 300 mg daily without undue risk of drug-induced lupus. Because of the limitation on dosage imposed by its toxicity, hydralazine is only a moderately effective hypotensive agent and is usually the third step in combinations with a beta-adrenergic blocking drug and a diuretic.

Nifedipine and verapamil dilate arterioles by inhibiting calcium transport through slow channels in smooth muscle cell membranes. In higher doses they cause flushing, tachycardia, and a sensation of dizziness. They also cause fluid retention but to a smaller extent than some other vasodilators (e.g., minoxidil). Verapamil slows conduction in the N region of the AV node, and concurrent administration with a beta blocking drug is generally held to be unwise. However, both drugs appear to be free of serious toxicity, and they are gradually superseding hydralazine in combinations with beta-blocking drugs and diuretics. Unlike hydralazine, calcium slow-channel blocking drugs are also effective as sole therapy in some patients with mild hypertension.

Minoxidil has a special place in the therapy of patients with hypertension that responds poorly to other drugs. It is a powerful vasodilator but has prominent side effects. The main problems associated with minoxidil therapy are fluid retention, which requires high doses of a loop diuretic in some cases, and increased growth of lanugo hair on the face, torso, and limbs.

CENTRALLY ACTING DRUGS. The level of efferent sympathetic activity is controlled by the brain. Drugs such as methyldopa and clonidine diminish the flow of impulses in peripheral sympathetic nerves as a result of a direct stimulant action upon alpha-2 receptors in the brainstem. Methyldopa must be transformed into methylnorepinephrine to exert this effect, but clonidine is an alpha receptor agonist in its own right. Stimulation of alpha-2 receptors in the brain potentiates the vasodepressor baroreflex. Reduction of sympathetic activity is manifest by lowering the plasma norepinephrine concentration and reduced amounts of catecholamine metabolites in the urine. As the baroreflex remains intact, postural adjustments of pressure can still be made, although there is sometimes a degree of fall in pressure on standing. The main problem of this type of action is that stimulation of brain alpha receptors also causes sedation and reduction in the flow of saliva. These are troublesome side effects for some patients, especially in the early days of therapy or after an increase in dose. Apart from its central nervous system side effects, the main concern with methyldopa has been with its toxicity. Ten to 30 per cent of patients given the drug develop a positive response to a direct antiglobulin test on their red cells, depending upon the dose used. A very small proportion of these will go on to develop an autoimmune hemolytic anemia. Mild diarrhea is a common symptom. A less common problem is the development of a maculopapular skin rash. Rarer forms of toxicity include a drug-induced fever, usually manifest in the first 14 days of therapy, and a hepatitic type of liver damage. However, the drug has been very widely used and is effective, and problems with toxicity have necessitated withdrawal in only a small proportion of patients.

Clonidine has a similar action and side-effect profile to methyldopa except that it causes constipation rather than diarrhea. The main concern with the drug has been a syndrome of sympathetic hyperactivity with tachycardia, high blood pressure, tremor, sweating, and insomnia that occur in some patients if the drug is stopped suddenly. Blood pressure may begin to rise within 16 to 24 hours of cessation of therapy.

ADRENERGIC NEURON-BLOCKING DRUGS. These drugs—examples include guanethidine, bethanidine,* and debrisoquine*—are concentrated in adrenergic nerve endings by the amine pump and, once they achieve a high enough concentration, blockade transmission by preventing norepinephrine release. They are effective hypotensive agents, but interfere more severely than other agents with normal blood pressure regulation. There is often a substantial fall in blood pressure on standing and after exercise. Ejaculation during sexual intercourse in the male may be inhibited. Because of these problems these drugs are now less often used. Tricyclic antidepressants, which blockade the amine pump in adrenergic nerve endings, interfere with the hypotensive effect of adrenergic neuron-blocking drugs.

ALPHA-ADRENERGIC RECEPTOR-BLOCKING DRUGS. The alpha-adrenergic receptor-blocking drugs phentolamine and phenoxybenzamine have been known for some years and are used to treat hypertension caused by excess circulating catecholamines. Prazosin has an alpha receptor-blocking action that is selective for the post-junctional alpha-1 receptor. It is a powerful hypotensive agent without serious toxic effects. However, prazosin is prone to cause postural hypotension, especially with the first dose unless this is kept low. Another common consequence of alpha-adrenergic blockade is impotence in the male.

COMBINED DRUG TREATMENT OF HYPERTENSION. The main groups of antihypertensive drugs lower the blood pressure by somewhat different mechanisms; if more than one type of action is used at the same time, the result is often an additive effect. As unwanted side effects are often related to the dose of one particular drug, this opens the possibility that drug combinations can be used to achieve the same or greater fall in pressure with fewer side effects. A second possibility is that the effect of the use of two drugs might be greater than the addition of the two individual actions because of a synergistic action of the combination. The most widely used combination is that of a diuretic with a beta-adrenergic blocker. A vasodilator is often added as a third step (Table 47–3). Other widely used two-drug combinations are a centrally acting drug, an alpha-adrenergic blocking drug, and an ACE inhibitor with a diuretic.

Concern about the long-term metabolic effects of diuretics has led to use of lower doses, e.g., 12.5 or 25 mg of hydrochlorothiazide rather than 50 or 100 mg. Increasingly, beta-adrenergic blocking drugs are the first choice. Whichever is the first step, the other is normally the second. If beta-adrenergic blocking drugs are contraindicated or not well tolerated, an ACE inhibitor, a centrally acting drug, or an alpha blocking drug is the best alternative. In severe cases requiring three drugs, nifedipine or verapamil can be added. Minoxidil remains useful in the most difficult patients.

EMERGENCY REDUCTION OF BLOOD PRESSURE. There are only a few circumstances in which it is necessary to reduce the blood pressure rapidly. These include hypertensive left ventricular failure, hypertensive encephalopathy, including eclampsia, and accelerated hypertension. Other situations such as intracranial bleeding and dissecting aneurysm need careful evaluation before a decision is reached. Sudden reduction of blood pressure may be dangerous and it is almost never necessary to reduce the level abruptly to 120 systolic and 80 diastolic mm Hg or below. Reduction to a level that relieves the immediate crisis (e.g., 160/100 mm Hg) is all that is necessary; fine adjustment can more safely be done later with oral therapy.

There are many methods of lowering the blood pressure quickly. If an immediate action is needed an intravenous bolus injection of diazoxide or an infusion pump–controlled administration of sodium nitroprusside is effective in most cases. The

*Investigational drug.

TABLE 47–3. BLOOD PRESSURE RESPONSE TO COMBINED DRUG THERAPY*

Regimen	Fall in Pressure from Placebo (mm Hg)
Diuretic alone	21/11
Beta-adrenergic blocker alone	26/16
Diuretic + beta-adrenergic blocker	34/20
Diuretic + beta-adrenergic blocker + vasodilator	46/26

*Figures taken from Wilcox and Mitchell: Br Med J 2:547, 1977.

patient must be carefully monitored with frequent readings of blood pressure, and baseline investigations such as an ECG and plasma electrolytes should be taken, if possible, before lowering the pressure. If reduction within a few hours is the objective, a small oral dose of verapamil or nifedipine is usually effective.

STOPPING HYPOTENSIVE THERAPY. Once drug treatment of hypertension has begun, it can rarely be stopped. Both patient and doctor should understand the long-term nature of the course they have taken. If the drugs are stopped, the subsequent course of the blood pressure is variable. It may return to pretreatment levels within a few days, but more commonly it slowly rises over a few weeks or months. Withdrawal of treatment is usually considered in three circumstances: extreme old age, intercurrent illness, and surgery. If the main reason for treating hypertension is to prevent a late risk of myocardial infarction or stroke, there is little point in continuing it in a patient who is terminally ill. Old age of itself is not a reason for stopping therapy, but extreme senility is. There is usually no need to interrupt therapy for a surgical operation, but it is essential that the anesthesiologist be aware of current therapy.

Clonidine should never be stopped suddenly because of the abrupt rise in pressure that may result. Sudden withdrawal of beta-adrenergic blocking drugs is also inadvisable. Beta-receptor numbers increase during chronic blockade, and there is a period of increased sensitivity to endogenous sympathetic stimulation if treatment is stopped abruptly. Worsening of angina pectoris and even a myocardial infarction may occur.

THERAPEUTIC CHOICES. Three main considerations govern the choice of antihypertensive drugs for a particular patient: simplicity, tolerability, and efficacy. Absent from this list is one important consideration, the prediction of individual drug response.

As some patients do not respond well to one drug but do to another, it would be advantageous if an accurate prediction could be made to avoid the delays of trial and error. Some progress has been made in making predictions. There is evidence that hypertensives who have a low plasma renin respond less well than other patients to beta-adrenergic blocking drugs and ACE inhibitors but are responsive to diuretics. A higher proportion of black patients than Caucasians have a low plasma renin. Elderly hypertensives are more responsive to diuretics than to beta-adrenergic blockade.

Some side effects are more acceptable to one type of patient than to another. Younger men are less likely to accept drug-related problems with erection or ejaculation with diuretics, alpha receptor–blocking drugs, or adrenergic neuron-blocking drugs. Patients who work outside in cold weather may find cold limbs caused by beta-adrenergic blockade particularly trying. Dry mouth and sedation are likely to be troublesome side effects for a patient who has to participate in business meetings.

Thus a degree of intelligent anticipation of both efficacy and side effects is possible, but a large component of empiricism remains. There is little evidence about the predictability of response to drug combinations, and it may be that the "catch-all" philosophy of two- or three-drug combination therapy may reduce the need to find the optimal single drug.

The ideal treatment for hypertension would be a once-for-all intervention that permanently lowered blood pressure. Long-term daily administration of hypotensive agents—effective but inconvenient—is all that we have to offer at present. Two measures may simplify the patient's regimen. The first is to use drugs with a long duration of action to avoid the necessity of a midday drug dose, and when possible to give the drugs only once a day. The second is to be prepared to use combined drug preparations when the mutual efficacy and safety of the components has been well proven. However, the availability of newer drugs with low symptom profiles and high efficacy such as some of the newer angiotensin-converting enzyme inhibitors and calcium slow-channel blocking drugs may revive interest in single drug regimens.

Blood pressure should be reduced as close to normal as symptoms will allow. There is very little evidence that relates blood pressure levels on treatment to outcome, but it seems reasonable to aim to reduce the systolic pressure to below 150 mm Hg and the diastolic to below 90 mm Hg. Unfortunately there are still many patients in whom drug side effects preclude administration of high enough doses to reach this target.

PROGNOSIS

In patients with accelerated hypertension and left ventricular failure the results of treatment are so dramatically beneficial that a controlled clinical trial was never considered necessary to establish them. Improvement in pulmonary edema is often evident within seconds of lowering the blood pressure, although full resolution may take much longer. The retinopathy of accelerated hypertension ceases to progress within two or three days of pressure reduction, and those lesions that appear after pressure reduction were probably already in process of formation at the time treatment began. All the features of accelerated hypertensive retinopathy will eventually regress in periods varying from 6 to 12 weeks for the cotton wool spots, linear hemorrhages, and papilledema, to up to a year or more for the macular star figure of hard exudate. Renal function ceases to deteriorate at a rapid rate, and in patients with an abrupt onset of accelerated hypertension, there may be some improvement in glomerular filtration. The survival of patients with accelerated hypertension is greatly improved by treatment although still dominated by the extent of deterioration of renal function at the time of diagnosis. Patients with severe impairment of renal function tend to continue to deteriorate despite pressure control. The availability of renal dialysis and transplant programs has become the main consideration in the long-term survival of these patients. However, the five-year survival of patients with accelerated hypertension under treatment is now 35 to 50 per cent without the help of renal support, which compares with only 1 to 5 per cent prior to the introduction of antihypertensive therapy. Accelerated hypertension should be looked upon as a preventable condition, and the widespread introduction of treatment for mild to moderate hypertension is leading to a rapid decrease in the number of patients with accelerated hypertension who are being diagnosed.

The great majority of patients with elevated blood pressure are not in the accelerated phase, and the benefits of treatment are less obvious in the short term. Some symptoms, such as headache in the morning, are relieved by blood pressure reduction, but the loss of some symptoms is often roughly balanced by the gain of others that are due to the drugs. The only objective signs of improvement may be a reduction in voltage and regression of repolarization abnormalities in the electrocardiogram. Retinal vascular changes such as caliber irregularity and crossing changes rarely show much difference when the pressure is lowered. However, if the rise in pressure has been recent and rapid and the retina shows a uniform narrowing of the retinal arteries, there may be some dilatation when the pressure is lowered.

The benefits of treatment of this type of hypertension had to be established by controlled clinical trials. These include the Veterans Administration trials, which provide the best evidence of the efficacy of treatment in severe hypertension, and the Australian National Blood Pressure Study and the United States Hypertension Detection and Follow-up Program, which are of particular value with regard to less severe hypertension. Taken together, these studies have shown clear evidence of the benefit of treatment for patients of both sexes under 65 years old who have levels of diastolic pressure of about 100 mm Hg or more. Deaths resulting from cerebral hemorrhage and heart failure are all much less frequent in the treated groups. The effects upon myocardial infarction are less and in most instances not statistically significant.

The Hypertension Detection and Follow-up Program showed a statistically significant reduction in cardiovascular morbidity and mortality in the group of patients treated in special clinics compared with those referred for customary medical care. There was also a significant reduction in mortality from noncardiovascular causes, for which no ready explanation is apparent. Enthusiasm generated by this trial result has been tempered by the negative results obtained in the multiple risk factor intervention trial (MRFIT). Some analysts of the MRFIT trial have even suggested that treatment of hypertension in patients with ECG abnormalities might have had an adverse effect.

Two major areas of doubt remain concerning the efficacy of hypotensive therapy. The first concerns the benefit of treatment in the great majority of hypertensive patients whose casual pressure lies in the range 90 to 100 mm Hg. A placebo-controlled trial is in progress in the United Kingdom to try to answer this question. Until the results are available in 1985 it seems reasonable to treat those patients with mild hypertension who have a particularly high burden of risk factors, but not to treat those who lie in a relatively low-risk group. The second question concerns the effects of treatment upon different types of cardiovascular pathology, especially that leading to myocardial infarction. The majority of deaths in patients with mild to moderate hypertension occur as a result of myocardial infarction. None of the individual clinical trials thus far carried out has shown a significant reduction in morbidity or mortality from myocardial infarction, although the pooled results of several trials suggest that there may have been a reduction. Whether the advent of new types of drug such as ACE inhibitors and calcium antagonists will alter the picture remains to be seen. Each successful clinical trial renders the ethics of the next one slightly more difficult to justify, yet it would seem unwise to assume that new types of drugs are safe and effective without exposing them to the crucible of a large scale outcome trial. Lowering blood pressure is easy; preventing atheromatous vascular disease associated with hypertension is not.

Anderson TW: Re-examination of some of the Framingham blood pressure data. Lancet 2:1139, 1978.

Dollery CT: Adrenergic drugs in the treatment of hypertension. Br Med Bull 29:158, 1973.

Genest J, Koiw E, Kuchel O (eds.): Hypertension. New York, McGraw-Hill Book Company, 1983.

Hypertension Detection and Follow-up Program Cooperative Group. JAMA 242:2562, 1979.

Keith NM, Wagener HP, Barker NW: Some different types of essential hypertension: Their course and prognosis. Am J Med Sci 197:332, 1939.

Multiple Risk Factor Intervention Trial Research Group. Multiple risk factor intervention trial. JAMA 248:1465, 1982.

Sackett DL, Haynes RB (eds.): Compliance with Therapeutic Regimens. Baltimore, Johns Hopkins University Press, 1976.

Stamler R, Pullman RN: The Epidemiology of Hypertension. New York, Grune & Stratton, 1967.

Veterans Administration Cooperative Study Group on antihypertensive agents. JAMA 202:1028, 1957, and 213:1143, 1970.

48. ATHEROSCLEROSIS

Harvey Wolinsky

HISTORY. The antiquity of atherosclerosis has been established from studies of Egyptian mummies. The term *atheroma,* derived from the Greek word for porridge, was first used in the context of arterial disease in 1904, when Marchand coined the term *atherosclerosis.* This disease is lipid rich, as contrasted with *arteriosclerosis,* an older and more general term for thickening and stiffening of the vessel wall. Arteriosclerotic involvement of a blood vessel wall tends to be concentric and diffuse, whereas atherosclerotic lesions are more eccentric and focal. The interrelation among coronary disease, myocardial damage, and clinical syndromes was first appreciated in the latter part of the nineteenth century. Following the proposal by Herrick in 1918, a connection between clinically detected nonlethal heart damage and atherosclerotic coronary disease gained acceptance.

PATHOLOGY. Atherosclerosis tends to involve large and medium-sized arteries. Most commonly affected are the aorta and the iliac, femoral, coronary, and cerebral arteries. Clinical symptoms occur because the atherosclerotic plaque reduces blood flow through the involved artery and compromises tissue or organ function distal to it. Ischemia or necrosis of the perfused tissue results in characteristic clinical syndromes, and myocardial infarction and sudden death are common fatal outcomes.

By the time it is large enough to cause symptoms, the atherosclerotic plaque is a complicated mixture of three components: (1) cells, mostly smooth muscle in origin, (2) connective tissue (elastin, collagen, glycosaminoglycans), often concentrated as a "cap" on the lesion, and (3) lipid deposits, both intra- and extracellular, representing complex aggregates of cholesteryl ester, cholesterol, triglyceride, and phospholipids. Cell necrosis contributes to the gruel-like nature of the lesion. Calcification is often present in advanced lesions, and hemorrhage from small ingrowing vessels frequently occurs. A slowly progressive increase in the plaque mass is usually responsible for its clinical sequelae. Sudden symptoms can be provoked by transient or progressive deposition of platelet clumps or thrombus on the irregular luminal surface, rupture of the plaque and release of its components, hemorrhage into a plaque, dissection of blood into the wall, and perhaps spasm.

Clinical events in middle age that are associated with the advanced plaque represent the culmination of decades of slow growth of the lesion beginning in childhood. In the first decade of life, blood vessels undergo structural remodeling, which mainly involves the intima. This takes the form of concentric fibromuscular intimal thickening and development of intimal cushions at branch sites. In all human populations studied, this thickening develops progressively throughout life. However, in populations with a predilection for development of atherosclerosis, this arteriosclerotic thickening is well developed long before lipid deposition is prominent. Enhanced intimal thickening of certain artery segments, especially in the male, also predicts patterns of subsequent atherosclerotic lesions. In human societies not vulnerable to atherosclerosis, this concentric intimal thickening, even when prominent, does not in itself compromise blood flow.

Upon this matrix, lipid accumulates in the form of *fatty streaks* in all populations. These yellow, soft, raised lesions may be transient, but their prevalence increases to a peak in the third decade of life. Microscopically, these consist largely of smooth muscle cells in the intimal layer that are filled with lipid deposits, mainly cholesterol and cholesteryl ester. In populations prone to atherosclerotic vascular disease, *plaques,* as described above, begin to be seen in the third decade and become more numerous with time in common disease sites, such as the proximal coronary vessels. The *fibrous plaque* is grayish white, focal, and raised and microscopically consists of a prominent extracellular matrix, with less prominence of visible lipid (although by biochemical analysis the lipid content is high). It is thought that these lesions usually develop from fatty streaks. The forces required for this transformation are not well understood, but hypertension seems to be one such stimulus. The further accumulation of cells, connective tissue, and fat over decades results in the severe lesions so often found at autopsy to provide the "explanation" for a clinical event.

LOCALIZATION. Although tending to occur in large elastic and muscular arteries, the distribution of atherosclerosis is far from uniform. The aorta is heavily involved, particularly in its abdominal portion. The large caliber of this vessel makes it an uncommon site for occlusive symptoms, although it may be a source of embolic clot or plaque material to peripheral branches. Atheromas are most common in the proximal coronary tree, although lesions occur peripherally as well. Curiously, lesions occur in the extramural portions of the coronary blood vessels and not in those segments which are intramural and surrounded by muscle. The renal arteries, even when arising from a heavily diseased abdominal aorta, are frequently spared of disease despite having a caliber similar to that of the main coronary arteries.

Arteries of the lower extremities have much more atherosclerosis than those of the upper limbs. The distribution patterns may be focal and proximal or diffuse. Clinical symptoms rarely arise from isolated lesions because of the rich collateral blood supply. The major hazard to patients with peripheral vascular disease, even when symptomatic, is the likelihood of concurrent coronary artery disease.

The vertebral or carotid vessels may develop patchy lesions which present clinically with neurologic deficits. Particularly likely sites are the proximal portions of these arteries or the carotid bifurcation. Predisposed intracranial sites are the basilar artery, the middle cerebral artery, and the carotid artery as it angulates in the region of the carotid siphon.

Atherosclerosis of the smaller muscular arteries is especially common in individuals who use cigarettes or have glucose intolerance. Basement membrane abnormalities that frequently occur in small blood vessels of diabetics could also contribute to vascular insufficiency in these individuals.

The low-pressure venous system and pulmonary arteries are infrequent sites of atherosclerosis except under circumstances of increased intravascular pressure, as occurs in pulmonary hypertension.

RISK FACTORS. The concept of risk factors for atherosclerosis derives from epidemiologic studies. A profile of risk can be obtained from the frequency with which specific characteristics and chemical values are associated with occurrence of certain clinical events in a given population. The epidemiologist points out associations; he can neither determine mechanism nor be certain of a direct interaction between a particular characteristic and the presence of disease. The value of these constructs, however, is that they identify high-risk populations in which "reduction" of risk factors can be attempted, and they suggest potentially fruitful areas of investigation to elucidate mechanisms of pathogenesis. Possible links between known risk factors and aspects of cellular involvement in atherogenesis are summarized under Pathogenesis, below.

Risk is a continuous gradient throughout the entire range of observed values, habits, or characteristics for virtually every risk factor. For example, an increasing risk of occurrence of a cerebrovascular event attends increasing blood pressure, even within the "normotensive" range of pressures. It is only within the "hypertensive" range, however, that the degree of risk is generally thought to justify intervention.

Age. The risk of myocardial infarction increases with age regardless of sex. Little is known about this factor, although it is assumed that it represents duration of exposure to other factors. For example, several epidemiologic studies have shown that subgroups of teenagers attain levels of blood pressure and serum lipids characteristic of the general adult population.

Sex. A 10- to 15-year lag in extent of atherosclerosis of the coronary, cerebral, and peripheral vasculature and its sequelae is seen in women compared to men until approximately 50 years of age. After that point, which roughly corresponds to the menopause, the rates of disease in both sexes are more nearly similar. This may represent increased risk in women or decreased risk in men owing to early elimination of high-risk males. Acceleration of vascular disease in younger individuals with diabetes mellitus blurs the usual sex differences.

Blood Pressure. A systolic blood pressure of greater than 160 mm Hg or a diastolic of greater than 95 mm Hg carries a five-fold increased risk of coronary heart disease compared to normotensive levels. Hypertension is the strongest risk factor overall for clinical disease in individuals older than 45 years; it is especially predictive of atherosclerotic brain infarction. (In the absence of uniform autopsy reporting, this designation may include pure hemorrhagic stroke as well as atherosclerotic sequelae.) A striking effect of blood pressure reduction on the incidence of stroke in individuals with diastolic pressures of 105 to 115 mm Hg is seen after a three-year period of treatment. Treatment of milder hypertension, with diastolic pressures of 90 to 104 mm Hg, also reduces mortality from stroke and myocardial infarction. Treatment is beneficial to survivors of a first myocardial infarction as well.

Hyperlipidemia. Another major risk factor is the presence of elevated circulating blood lipids—cholesterol and triglyceride. The problem may be broken into two components: (1) generally elevated lipid levels in industrialized populations compared to agricultural societies, and (2) identification of high-risk individuals with high lipid levels within a given population range. The increased levels found in entire populations seem largely due to diet, although genetic factors may play a role. Increased intakes of saturated fat, refined sugar, and total calories by a sedentary population seem of major importance.

Using ultracentrifugal and electrophoretic techniques, four major lipoprotein classes have been identified as carriers of lipid in plasma (see Ch. 183). *Chylomicrons* are the largest particles, contain the most lipid (mainly triglyceride) and least protein (1 to 2 per cent by weight), and are normally found in the circulation only shortly after meals. In the fasting state, *very low density lipoproteins* (VLDL) carry most circulating triglycerides as well as lesser amounts of cholesterol and cholesteryl ester. *Low-density lipoproteins* (LDL) are derived from metabolism of VLDL and carry most of the serum cholesterol and cholesteryl ester. *High-density lipoproteins* (HDL), the smallest particles, contain the most protein (50 per cent by weight); phospholipid and cholesterol account for about 45 per cent and 35 per cent, respectively, of the lipid. HDL are involved in the esterification of free cholesterol released into plasma from the tissues. Whole plasma triglyceride accurately reflects VLDL levels and total plasma cholesterol generally reflects LDL-cholesterol levels in man, although this latter relationship is not as consistent (see below).

The three most common electrophoretic patterns of serum lipoproteins in individuals with premature atherosclerotic vascular disease are increased LDL or Type IIa (elevated cholesterol, normal triglyceride), increased VLDL and LDL or Type IIb (elevated cholesterol, elevated triglyceride), and increased VLDL or Type IV (normal or slightly increased cholesterol, elevated triglyceride). These three patterns appear with about equal frequency in survivors of an acute myocardial infarction below age 60. About one third of all such individuals will have these patterns, and familial distributions of each have been demonstrated. Whereas Types IIa and IV show autosomal dominant inheritance, the inheritance of Type IIb is not yet completely defined. However, when Type IIb is found in a proband, familial expressions may include elevations of cholesterol or triglyceride or both. To screen for the most common disorders, therefore, measurement of total plasma cholesterol and triglyceride provides the same detection of risk as do more complicated lipoprotein pattern analyses. In adults under age 55, a value of plasma cholesterol greater than 250 mg per deciliter or fasting triglyceride greater than 200 mg per deciliter indicates the need for further investigation (see Ch. 183).

Current knowledge about lipoprotein metabolism does not permit a clear-cut assessment of the precise roles of various lipoproteins in the clinical definition of risk for unselected populations. However, prospective epidemiologic studies show a positive correlation between plasma cholesterol levels (particularly LDL) and risk of clinical atherosclerotic events. This relationship is evident under age 50, but not in older age groups. Increasing plasma VLDL (triglyceride) levels seem to add risk to a given plasma LDL (cholesterol) level. Triglyceride levels alone, however, are less strongly related to clinical atherosclerotic events. The risk associated with triglyceride, seen more clearly in women, is eliminated when obesity or glucose intolerance is taken into account and may therefore not be an independent variable. The risk of coronary heart disease is inversely related to the level of HDL cholesterol. The emergence of HDL as an important protective factor has complicated the use of total plasma cholesterol to assess risk. Since this measurement requires isolated HDL and LDL, the total cholesterol level alone is less informative. HDL levels are significantly higher in women than in men at all age levels, are reduced by the presence of diabetes mellitus, are increased by regular exercise (e.g., jogging), and are not predictably related to levels of LDL in the same individual. Therefore a plasma lipid profile of total cholesterol, HDL cholesterol, and fasting triglyceride may be the best predictor of coronary disease.

Cigarette Smoking. Increased risk of atherosclerotic vascular disease manifested by stroke, myocardial infarction, and intermittent claudication is seen in male smokers compared to nonsmokers; in female smokers, the occurrence of intermittent claudication is increased. By age 45, the excess risk in males approaches 70 per cent. The increased incidence of atherosclerosis found in smokers at autopsy correlates with the degree of previous smoking activity. In addition to atheromatous changes in larger coronary blood vessels, small intramyocardial arteries show increased diffuse fibromuscular intimal thickening. These changes are related in degree to numbers of cigarettes smoked, and cigar and pipe smokers have impressive increases over nonsmokers as well.

Sudden death is the most frequent clinical event associated with cigarette smoking. Cessation of smoking promptly and sharply reduces the risk of this event; benefit extends even to survivors of a first myocardial infarction. Increased levels of carboxyhemoglobin in smokers, of whom about 15 per cent regularly achieve levels of carboxyhemoglobin of 5 per cent or more, may be responsible. Men in the age group of 30 to 69 years who achieve this level of carboxyhemoglobin show a 20-fold increased prevalence of atherosclerotic vascular disease events (myocardial infarction, angina pectoris, intermittent claudication) compared to nonsmokers or smokers with levels of 3 per cent or less. A narrowed coronary artery may be unable to deliver the 20 per cent increase in blood flow required to offset the decreased availability of oxygen from blood containing 5 per cent carboxyhemoglobin. Indeed, a lower threshold for angina pectoris occurs in cardiac patients in whom comparable levels of carboxyhemoglobin have been experimentally achieved.

Glucose Intolerance. Glucose intolerance, defined as a casual blood glucose of 120 mg per deciliter or more or the presence of glucose in the urine, acts independently of other commonly associated risk factors, namely, triglyceride elevation, obesity, and hypertension. It is somewhat more important in women than in men. The excess risk associated with glucose intolerance may be 100 per cent. Intermittent claudication is the cardiovascular symptom most associated with glucose intolerance. If associated with a fasting plasma triglyceride level of greater than 150 mg per deciliter, a marked synergistic effect of diabetes mellitus on development of angiographically demonstrable, diffuse coronary disease is found. The contribution to this process of basement membrane abnormalities in the small coronary branches in diabetics is not known.

Obesity. Obesity, particularly at 20 per cent or more above ideal weight, carries significantly increased risk. Associated risk factors, including hypertension, hyperlipidemia, and diabetes mellitus, contribute to this risk. However, obesity of greater than 10 per cent above ideal weight has recently been demonstrated to be an independent predictor of disease, particularly in those under age 50. Thus, multiple salutary effects of weight reduction make it a prime focus of intervention.

Physical Activity. It is difficult to separate the risk of this variable from confounding factors. Sedentary individuals have many other risk factors as well. Epidemiologic studies show that only heavy physical work, of the type done in rural communities or by the most active dockworkers, is associated with decreased risk of myocardial infarction and sudden death. The remarkable decrease in sudden death in these groups suggests that exercised myocardium may be less vulnerable to a fatal ischemic event. Exercise tolerance can be improved in individuals with coronary artery disease through a program of regular, moderate exercise.

Personality Factors. A suspicion has long been held that angina pectoris and sudden death are strongly associated with emotional stress or anxiety. The Type A pattern of behavior (enhanced aggressiveness, ambitiousness, competitive drive, and chronic sense of time urgency) is frequently associated with many other risk factors, and the converse Type B is less closely associated. A prospective study by the Western Collaborative Group showed that even after removal of associated risk components, Type A behavior, determined from interviews, had a residual two-fold risk of clinical coronary heart disease over the Type B personality type. The possible metabolic, genetic, and other components of this behavior pattern have not been identified, nor has behavior modification been convincingly shown to be feasible or effective in modifying risk.

Genetic Factors. Familial inheritance patterns of hyperlipidemia, hypertension, and diabetes mellitus are well known. Segregation of behavioral factors within families, including tobacco smoking, obesity, and perhaps physical activity, is also seen. These associations may provide the physician the best opportunities to detect clusters of risk factors and to attempt preventive measures.

Other. A host of other variables associated with cardiac risk have been enumerated, but in sum they appear to contribute only a minor portion of risk. Included among many others are lung vital capacity, serum uric acid level, blood group type, and mineral salt content of local drinking water. Moderate alcohol consumption seems to be associated with decreased risk of myocardial infarction, perhaps through a positive effect on HDL:LDL ratios. Electrocardiographic evidence for left ventricular hypertrophy carries about a three-fold risk for new coronary artery disease, independent of other variables, including blood pressure.

Unknown. All known risk factors taken together account for approximately 50 per cent of the risk of an individual's developing coronary heart disease in the United States. Important risk determinants remain to be discovered. For example, little has been said about the contribution made by inherent properties of vascular tissue, genetic or otherwise, to cardiovascular disease. Each risk factor must ultimately be expressed at the tissue or cellular level if it is in fact related to the development of atherosclerosis.

PATHOGENESIS. Atherosclerosis is undoubtedly multifactorial in origin and progression. The sharp contrast between the frequent suddenness of clinical events and the slow progressiveness of vascular lesions suggests that different factors are responsible for each. Autopsy studies of advanced lesions generated the classic theories which invoked processes of vascular injury, lipid infiltration, thrombosis, and hemorrhage. These terms are now being incorporated into concepts more consonant with newer knowledge of cell biology. Vascular tissue is increasingly appreciated to be a dynamic responsive organ system of great complexity, rather than a simple conduit with limited responses. The normal blood vessel is a tightly organized, highly regulated, and closely integrated fibrocellular system. The two major cell types found in blood vessel walls are smooth muscle cells and endothelial cells. Each has characteristic and diverse metabolic capabilities. Endothelium seems to be important in determining the rate of entrance of circulating materials, including lipoproteins, into the blood vessel wall and in maintaining the nonthrombogenicity of the vascular surface; prostacyclin may be responsible for this latter property. Smooth muscle cells elaborate the extensive connective tissue matrix of the arterial wall and metabolize those circulating plasma components which gain entrance to the vessel wall. When atherosclerosis occurs there is smooth muscle cell proliferation, connective tissue deposition, and lipid accumulation.

Alteration in the functional or structural barrier presented by the endothelial cell-lining layer is thought to be an early event in the pathogenesis of atherosclerosis. Local turbulence or shear force generated by blood flowing at high pressure could determine the susceptibility of certain sites to disruption of the surface layer. Two major consequences of endothelial loss would be increased thrombogenicity of the denuded sites and increased entrance of circulating lipoproteins and other plasma components into the blood vessel wall. Platelet adhesion and aggregation quickly occur on the exposed region; another prostaglandin, thromboxane A_2, is involved in this reaction. Platelets contain a mitogen which can stimulate smooth muscle cell proliferation in vitro; LDL itself might stimulate cell proliferation. Evidence that cells in each human atherosclerotic plaque tend to be monoclonal raises the possibility that selective growth advantage or even neoplastic transformation of certain cells could contribute to this aspect of plaque growth. Experimentally produced atherosclerotic lesions are polyclonal, so that this issue is far from resolved.

Increased connective tissue synthesis is closely linked to cell proliferation whether studied in intact blood vessels or in isolated cell systems. Specific stimuli at the cellular level for increased synthesis of connective tissue proteins have not been identified, although hypertension in particular seems to promote fibrosis and estradiol given experimentally seems to retard it. Circulating lipoprotein, particularly LDL, can be detected immunologically in very low concentrations in normal human blood vessels. With loss of endothelial integrity, it is presumed that an increased influx of this lipoprotein results in progressive accumulation of lipid by two mechanisms. In more advanced lesions binding to excessive extracellular matrix might occur. In early lesions the metabolic capacity of the vascular smooth muscle cell to cope with the incoming lipid may be compromised. The ability of the cell to maintain balance among internalization and catabolism of complex lipoproteins (including hydrolysis of cholesteryl ester to free cholesterol and fatty acid) and synthesis of lipid may determine its susceptibility to intracellular lipid accumulation. In the sense that ingress of substrate may exceed egress of product, lipid accumulation can be thought of as a subtle form of storage disease in the muscle cell, which becomes a repository of slowly permeant cholesteryl ester and other lipids. "Risk factors" may exert an influence on this influx-efflux balance. For example, relationships among LDL and HDL levels and risk of disease may derive in part from the putative role attributed to LDL of carrying cholesterol to the cell and to HDL of carrying cholesterol away from the cell. Influences of sex, age, and exercise as risk factors might stem, at least in part, from associated changes in levels of these lipoproteins. The increased vascular permeability seen with hypertension could lead to increased influx of lipoprotein into the cell, and diabetes mellitus may reduce efflux from the cell.

Active areas of inquiry in current research include plasma membrane receptors, endocytosis, lysosomal function and intracellular lipoprotein metabolism, and the nature of lipid transfer between isolated lipoprotein fractions and the cell. A phenotypic hypercholesterolemia with monogenic inheritance is associated with a specific deficiency of surface receptors for LDL molecules in cultured cells. Absence of the normal function of these receptors in regulating intracellular cholesterol synthesis results in hypercholesterolemia. The mechanisms by which this deficiency is translated into a marked predisposition to lipid accumulation by vascular cells and by which other "risk factors" exert their effects at the cellular level are yet to be identified.

TREATMENT, REGRESSION, AND PREVENTION. Current treatment of clinical atherosclerotic complications revolves around coronary care units, replacement of diseased vascular segments with prosthetic or natural grafts, use of antiarrhythmic agents, anticoagulants, and plasma lipid lowering agents, and even heart transplantation. Remarkable as these accomplishments are, they are addressed to the late stages of a disease process for which prevention is clearly the best goal. Extreme manipulation of diets that result in great reductions in serum lipid levels and regression of established lesions in nonhuman primates are not usually possible in man. Although an occasional study suggests that progression of atherosclerotic lesions may be slowed or arrested by stringent diet control in man, results are not conclusive. The clinician might therefore encourage a "prudent" course that involves moderation of intake of cholesterol and saturated fat. This approach, together with reduction of elevated blood pressure and cigarette use, both of proved benefit, and control of obesity and other risk factors, reflects the best information now available for the prevention of atherosclerosis.

Fowler S, Wolinsky H: Lysosomes in vascular smooth muscle cells. *In* Bohr D, Somlyo AP, Sparks HV (Eds.): Vascular Smooth Muscle. Handbook on the Cardiovascular System. Washington, DC, American Physiological Society, 1980, p 133. *Summary of one specialized area of investigation into the cell biology of vascular tissue.*

Goldstein JL, Brown MS: Lipoprotein receptors: Genetic defense against atherosclerosis. Clin Res 30:417, 1982. *Implications of the receptor for human disease.*

Kannel WB, Castelli WP, Gordon T: Cholesterol in the prediction of atherosclerotic disease. Ann Intern Med 90:85, 1979. *Clinical evaluation and importance of serum lipids.*

Nerem R: Arterial fluid dynamics and interactions with the vessel walls. *In* Schwartz CJ, Werthessen NT, Wolf S (Eds.): Structure and Function of the Circulation. Vol 2. New York, Plenum Press, 1981, p 719. *Thorough analysis of hemodynamic factors and atherogenesis.*

Ross R: Atherosclerosis: A problem of the biology of arterial wall cells and their interactions with blood components. Arteriosclerosis 1:293, 1981. *Progress in identification of cells in the plaque and mechanisms of lesion growth.*

Solberg LA, Strong JP: Risk factors and atherosclerotic lesions: A review of autopsy studies. Arteriosclerosis 3:187, 1983. *The link between arterial pathology and risk factors.*

Vane JR, Bunting S, Moncada S: Prostacyclin in physiology and pathophysiology. Int Rev Exp Pathol 23:161, 1982. *Current status of prostaglandins and vascular disease.*

49. DISORDERS OF CORONARY ARTERIES

49.1. Angina Pectoris

James T. Willerson

Angina pectoris is the clinical term used to describe chest pain resulting from a relative oxygen deficiency in heart muscle. Angina occurs when oxygen demand exceeds oxygen supply. Most individuals with angina pectoris have underlying atherosclerotic coronary artery disease, but angina may also develop in some patients with ventricular hypertrophy, left ventricular outflow obstruction, severe aortic regurgitation, cardiomyopathy, or dilated ventricles, in whom coronary artery disease is not present. The explanation for angina developing in these circumstances is that under certain conditions even normal coronary arteries may not adequately supply hypertrophied, dilated, or failing heart muscle with oxygen. Normal individuals do not develop angina, probably because the heart is protected from an important imbalance in oxygen delivery by factors that limit physical activity, such as dyspnea and fatigue.

The predisposing pathologic alteration in coronary arteries ordinarily responsible for angina is atherosclerosis. Severe narrowing of the lumen of coronary arteries results in a decreased ability to deliver oxygen to areas supplied by the involved vessels. Consequently, under conditions of exercise, cold exposure, or emotional stress, or after eating, angina may develop. This is most easily understood by recalling that the primary determinants of oxygen demand in the heart are heart rate, contractile state, and wall tension. Emphasis upon relative oxygen demand makes it easier to understand why some individuals with valvular and subvalvular aortic stenosis and others with ventricular hypertrophy develop angina even in the absence of coronary artery disease. Systolic pressure development is relatively costly in terms of oxygen utilization, and, together with ventricular hypertrophy and increased wall tension, is the most likely explanation for angina in patients with valvular aortic stenosis without coronary artery disease. Angina developing in individuals with marked pulmonary hypertension may be the result of increased right ventricular pressure load.

Angina pectoris may also develop in individuals with severe volume overload of the ventricle, including aortic regurgitation or mitral regurgitation. "Volume work" results in a smaller increase in oxygen demand than "pressure work" until important cardiac dilatation occurs. At this point, increased oxygen demand may not be met because of reduced diastolic coronary perfusion pressure. The presence of angina pectoris in patients with aortic regurgitation is ordinarily an ominous prognostic sign.

Angina may also occur because of extracardiac influences. In particular, severe anemia or carbon monoxide exposure limits the capacity of the blood to carry or release oxygen and may result in angina under conditions that the subject would otherwise tolerate well. Increases in systemic arterial pressure and consequent dilatation of the heart may result in angina pectoris. Increases in heart rate or contractile state, such as occur with hyperthyroidism, with pheochromocytoma, or with exogenous administration or endogenous release of catecholamine, all may result in angina pectoris.

Primary decreases in oxygen delivery, such as occur with coronary arterial spasm or with transient platelet aggregation, may also result in angina pectoris. There is current suspicion that coronary spasm and platelet aggregation may interact with intrinsic narrowing in coronary luminal diameter to produce angina. Under these circumstances there is no association between the symptoms and exertion, and the majority of the anginal episodes occur at rest. These patients have little change in heart rate or blood pressure prior to the onset of pain, or the pain occurs first and is followed only later by an increase in blood pressure or heart rate. Continuous electrocardiographic monitoring may document transient S-T segment change with the onset of pain, usually S-T segment elevation indicating transmural ischemia, but sometimes S-T depression when subendocardial ischemia occurs.

PATHOPHYSIOLOGY. Angina occurs most commonly in circumstances in which regional myocardial oxygen demand exceeds oxygen availability. This occurs when myocardial oxygen demand is increased by (1) an increase in intramyocardial systolic tension resulting from increases in blood pressure, cold exposure, congestive heart failure, ventricular hypertrophy, or left ventricular outflow obstruction; increases in intramyocardial systolic tension are directly proportional to blood pressure and the radius of the ventricle ("Laplace rule"); (2) an increase in heart rate, such as occurs with exercise or emotion; and (3) an increase in the contractile state of the myocardium, such as occurs during physical effort, with catecholamine administration, with fright, or with the use of certain pharmacologic interventions that increase inotropy and myocardial oxygen demand more than they increase myocardial oxygen delivery. Rest generally relieves angina that occurs with effort, emotion, or exercise. Nitroglycerin also relieves angina, typically within three to five minutes. The beneficial effect of nitroglycerin is related to its ability to dilate medium-sized penetrating coronary vessels (and occasionally epicardial vessels) and thus improve coronary blood flow and its distribution. An additional factor is the action of nitroglycerin to dilate systemic veins so that it decreases venous return to the heart and ventricular end-diastolic volume, thereby reducing wall tension and oxygen demand.

CLINICAL DIAGNOSIS. Angina is typically described as a substernal or left precordial chest pain that is perceived as a "tightness" or "heaviness," "like a weight on my chest," or as "a pressure." The pain may radiate into the neck and often radiates down the ulnar aspect of the left arm. It is typically produced by effort, exercise, emotion, or cold exposure, or after eating a large meal; it is relieved by rest or nitroglycerin. As mentioned earlier, it may also occur at rest, as an expression of coronary artery spasm or of platelet aggregation at sites of severe coronary arterial stenosis. Some patients do not describe their angina in typical terms, but refer to it as "a hurt," "a little pain," or "a sharp pain." Others note the pain in atypical locations, including the jaw, the teeth, the forearm, or only in the back. Some describe their angina as beginning in the epigastric region and radiating up into the chest. Finally, some patients have "silent" angina, i.e., they have no pain despite the fact that heart failure or acute myocardial infarction occurs. Ten to 20 per cent of patients with diabetes mellitus have "silent" angina and acute myocardial infarcts. Many patients after cardiac transplantation also do not perceive angina even though coronary artery atherosclerosis recurs in the coronary arteries of the transplanted heart.

Left or right ventricular dysfunction may develop even with transient anginal episodes. This explains the dyspnea or orthopnea, paroxysmal nocturnal dyspnea, tachycardia, and alterations in blood pressure, including hypotension, that occur with some episodes of angina. Further, some patients develop transient murmurs of mitral or tricuspid regurgitation because of papillary muscle dysfunction occurring as a consequence of the ischemic process. Typically, left ventricular end-diastolic pressure rises during angina; this is a consequence of a reduction in compliance and, in some instances, possibly of "incomplete relaxation." Palpation of the precordium during an episode of angina may disclose an ectopic impulse. Auscultation may reveal a third heart sound and rales, or a murmur of mitral or tricuspid insufficiency. Occasionally, patients develop paradoxical splitting of their second heart sound. The murmur of papillary muscle dysfunction reflects mild to moderate mitral regurgitation and is classically a mid to late systolic murmur, but may be holosystolic.

Many noncardiac problems also result in chest pain, including peptic ulcer disease, pancreatitis, cholecystitis, esophageal reflux or spasm, and primary pulmonary abnormalities such as pneumonia, pulmonary embolism with infarction, atelectasis, and spontaneous pneumothorax. Other causes of chest pain that must be differentiated from angina pectoris are the pain of dissecting aortic aneurysm, musculoskeletal chest pain, and the pain that occurs with herpes zoster of the chest, which may develop before skin lesions occur.

CLINICAL CLASSIFICATION OF ANGINAL SYNDROMES. Table 49–1 lists the various coronary artery syndromes that should receive specific attention. Segregating of patients with coronary artery disease into the various anginal syndromes is useful diagnostically, therapeutically, and prognostically. Patients with stable angina pectoris have angina with effort or exercise or during other conditions in which myocardial oxygen demand is increased. This occurs in a predictable manner and is usually relieved promptly by rest or nitroglycerin.

Increasingly frequent angina with chest pain produced by less effort or provocation and occurring in a crescendo pattern is generally termed "unstable angina pectoris." Individuals with unstable angina pectoris may also have pain at rest, and the pain may last for longer periods of time and be more difficult to relieve. Unstable angina is considered a medical emergency by most physicians and warrants hospitalization and study of the patient for acute myocardial infarction. Pain relief occurs following complete bed rest in 90 per cent of these patients. Patients who continue to have pain at bed rest are given nitrates. Those thought not to have coronary artery spasm as the cause for their chest pain often receive a beta blocker such as propranolol. If pain relief does not occur with bed rest and the use of appropriate drugs, the risk of subsequent myocardial infarction, sudden death, or important ventricular arrhythmias is increased. In those believed to have coronary artery spasm, i.e., those having chest pain at rest with transient S-T segment deviation during the episode of pain and without preceding increases in heart rate or blood pressure, calcium antagonists such as nifedipine, verapamil, or diltiazem may be used instead of propranolol. Coronary arteriography is generally recommended in patients with unstable angina pectoris once the pain is controlled and a myocardial infarct is excluded. This approach is recommended because 15 per cent of patients with this syndrome have significant main left coronary artery disease warranting surgery and 10 per cent have no angiographic evidence of the disease. Thus, in 25 per cent of these patients, the angiographic findings help to provide a therapeutic approach. In the remaining patients, the location and extent of coronary artery disease are prognostically helpful.

Acute coronary insufficiency or the "intermediate coronary syndrome" is characterized by a more prolonged episode of pain than is typical of stable angina pectoris. Ordinarily, patients experience pain that lasts 15 to 30 minutes and may be associated with some diaphoresis and nausea. These patients generally come to the hospital concerned that the pain has lasted a longer period of time and is more severe than is typical of their usual angina. Every effort is made to rule out an acute myocardial infarct with serial electrocardiograms and enzyme determinations and, at our institution, with myocardial scintigraphic techniques, including "infarct avid" myocardial scintigraphy (technetium-99m stannous pyrophosphate myocardial scintigrams). "Cold spot" myocardial scintigraphy (thallium-201 scintigrams) may also be used for this purpose. Those patients without infarcts are placed on an appropriate medical regimen. Subsequently, exercise testing is usually conducted: submaximal exercise tests within seven to ten days after an infarct is excluded and angina is controlled, followed several weeks later by a more vigorous exercise test. Patients with continuing angina despite a good medical regimen undergo coronary arteriography and, when appropriate, coronary artery revascularization.

Variant angina pectoris ("Prinzmetal's angina") is defined as chest pain at rest in association with S-T segment deviation (ordinarily S-T segment elevation, but S-T segment depression may also occur, depending on the size of the coronary vessel in which spasm occurs) without preceding increase in heart rate or blood pressure. The mechanism of variant angina is coronary artery spasm, shown by coronary arteriography to involve large and medium-sized vessels with transmural myocardial blood flow distribution. As the chest pain disappears, the S-T segment deviation resolves, in association with relief of the coronary spasm. Many more episodes of S-T segment deviation occur than of chest pain, and so continuous recording of multilead electrocardiograms is recommended for patients with this abnormality. In those circumstances in which the coronary artery spasm is prolonged, acute myocardial infarction, important ventricular arrhythmias, heart block, or sudden death may develop. Prinzmetal's angina is generally treated with nitrate vasodilators and, more recently, with calcium antagonists, including nifedipine, verapamil, or diltiazem. Calcium antagonists appear to be uniquely successful in reducing the frequency of episodes of coronary artery spasm. Direct coronary artery surgery has not been as successful in these

TABLE 49–1. ANGINAL SYNDROMES OF PATIENTS WITH CORONARY ARTERY DISEASE

Stable angina pectoris
Unstable angina pectoris
Acute coronary insufficiency
Variant angina pectoris ("Prinzmetal's angina")
Acute myocardial infarction

patients as in those with more typical angina pectoris, although it is used in patients with important underlying coronary artery disease in whom one cannot obtain symptomatic relief of the angina. One report (Bertrand, 1980) suggests that plexectomy coupled with coronary artery revascularization may be more successful than coronary revascularization by itself. Ten to 20 per cent of patients with Prinzmetal's angina have normal coronary arteries; this further emphasizes the role of spasm in the pathophysiology of variant angina. The most common arteriographic pattern is significant single vessel disease involving the proximal portion of either the right or left anterior descending coronary artery. However, any pattern of coronary artery disease may be seen. Although variant angina pectoris attributable to coronary spasm occurs as a specific syndrome, there is also speculation that spasm may be a factor in more patients with stable angina pectoris than previously realized.

It is not clear which pathophysiologic factors are most important in the conversion of stable angina to the various anginal syndromes mentioned above. Current interest centers on the role of platelet aggregability, coronary artery spasm, hemorrhage into atherosclerotic plaques, and increases in local vascular concentrations of thromboxane or relative decreases in prostacyclin concentration at the site of coronary arterial intimal injury and/or atherosclerotic plaque.

DIAGNOSTIC TESTS. An association of the chest pain with exercise, effort, and emotion and of relief with rest or nitroglycerin is presumptive evidence that the chest pain represents angina pectoris. Additionally, certain diagnostic maneuvers, such as carotid sinus pressure or the Valsalva maneuver, help to determine the etiology of chest pain. Both these maneuvers slow the heart rate and reduce the blood pressure as a consequence of increased vagal and reduced sympathetic tone.

One may also use certain tests to provoke angina. In particular, exercise testing on a bicycle or on a treadmill is often used for this purpose. The patient exercises at graded loads, starting from low and progressing to higher ones. Blood pressure and heart rate are monitored throughout and multilead electrocardiograms are obtained prior to, during, and toward the end of each exercise load (continuous multilead monitoring of the electrocardiogram is preferable). An exercise test result is positive if associated with S-T segment deviation of 1 mm or greater, flat or downsloping, 0.08 second after the S-T junction. There are both false-positive and false-negative exercise test results, however. Particularly in women, false-positive results occur in up to 20 or 30 per cent of patients. False-positive results may also occur with electrolyte abnormalities, in those taking digoxin, in those with ventricular hypertrophy, conduction abnormalities (including left or right bundle branch block), or S-T–T wave abnormalities prior to the onset of exercise. Additionally, in some patients with important coronary artery disease, diagnostic ECG changes do not occur with stress. The incidence of false-negative results with adequate exercise tests and multilead ECG analysis is at least 10 to 15 per cent.

Additions to the standard exercise ECG include the use of radionuclides in association with the exercise. One approach uses a myocardial perfusion agent such as thallium-201, which is injected at the peak of exercise. Myocardial scintigraphic images are obtained immediately thereafter. Regions of relative perfusion deficit observed during exercise which are normal at rest are highly suggestive of obstructive coronary disease.

An alternative approach is to label the patient's own red blood cells in vivo with technetium-99m pertechnetate or to inject intravenously a radionuclide such as technetium-labeled albumin or technetium pertechnetate at the peak of exercise. With either approach, one may measure global and segmental ventricular performance at rest and at exercise and determine directly whether alterations in regional wall motion, ventricular volumes, or global ejection fraction occur. In most normal individuals, ventricular ejection fraction should increase with exercise, but in those with important coronary artery disease, and particularly those with multivessel disease, the ventricular ejection fraction either does not change or decreases. Similarly, with important coronary artery disease, end-systolic volumes increase rather than decrease, and segmental wall motion abnormalities may develop.

CORONARY ARTERIOGRAPHY. Coronary arteriography is the most reliable diagnostic test currently available to detect anatomically important coronary atherosclerosis, considered to be present when at least 50 per cent luminal diameter narrowing of a coronary artery exists, and to estimate the extent of such disease. Many, however, feel that a better definition is luminal diameter narrowing equal to or greater than 70 per cent. Resting coronary blood flow is not decreased, but effort coronary blood flow may be reduced by coronary artery luminal narrowing of 50 per cent. Resting coronary blood flow may be reduced by narrowing of greater than 70 per cent.

A small population of patients, probably less than 1 per cent of those with angina, have normal coronary arteriograms but objective evidence of myocardial ischemia by ECG criteria and by lactate production during rapid pacing. This syndrome occurs most commonly in females.

Indications for coronary arteriography in patients with angina vary. A widely accepted clinical indication is the presence of limiting angina on a good medical regimen. However, some also use coronary arteriography to evaluate young patients (those less than 40 years of age) who have had previous acute myocardial infarcts. Others use coronary arteriography and left ventricular catheterization to evaluate the cause of congestive heart failure in patients in whom the etiology is not clear. Radionuclide ventriculography and echocardiography may also be used for this purpose, especially to characterize regional and global ventricular function, to exclude sizable ventricular aneurysms, to identify valvular regurgitation and estimate its severity, and to detect shunt lesions. Coronary arteriography may also be used to help resolve the etiology of undiagnosed chest pain that is limiting or frightening for the individual. In general, however, coronary arteriography is reserved for patients selected as potential candidates for coronary artery surgery because of symptomatic angina pectoris.

MANAGEMENT. The therapeutic approach to patients with angina pectoris can be "medical" or "surgical," i.e., coronary artery revascularization. Often, however, these are not in fact separate, since many patients continue to take long-acting nitrates, propranolol, a calcium antagonist, or combinations of these agents following coronary artery revascularization. Also, one does everything possible to correct underlying risk factors such as smoking, overweight, systemic arterial hypertension, hypercholesterolemia, major stress, and emotional conflicts, and to encourage proper amounts of exercise.

Patients with angina pectoris should be encouraged to carry nitroglycerin with them. Nitroglycerin should be taken when angina develops in order to prevent it from becoming severe; if one nitroglycerin tablet is ineffective, a second should be taken. In addition, the patient should sit or lie down in order to help relieve the pain. If the angina is not relieved by 2 or 3 nitroglycerin tablets and rest, the individual should go to the hospital for further evaluation, specifically to exclude the possibility that he is having an acute myocardial infarct. Nitroglycerin may also be taken prophylactically prior to engaging in activities the individual knows will produce angina, i.e., prior to physical effort, sexual intercourse, or an emotional experience that cannot be avoided. Nitroglycerin tablets should be replaced every 6 to 12 months, since they deteriorate. One needs to be certain that important reductions in blood pressure or increases in heart rate do not occur following the administration of nitroglycerin, since under these circumstances coronary flow to the vulnerable myocardium may actually decrease.

Long-acting nitrates may also be used. The effectiveness, proper dosage, and route of administration are subjects of controversy. However, isosorbide dinitrate may be taken sublingually or orally and it exerts an effect similar to that of nitroglycerin for 40 to 60 minutes after its administration. Nitroglycerin ointment is also an effective long-acting agent in most patients. It is generally applied to a small area of the chest as a thin film.

The second major group of agents used to control angina consists of beta-adrenergic blocking drugs. Propranolol is the most commonly used agent at present. Beta-adrenergic blockers decrease heart rate and blood pressure responses to exercise and reduce the frequency of angina. They also decrease the inotropic response to exercise in normal hearts but may actually increase global and segmental contractility for any particular exercise load in those with important coronary artery disease. The most common contraindications to the use of propranolol are congestive heart failure, extreme bradycardia, bronchospastic lung disease, i.e., asthma, a tendency toward hypoglycemia, and insulin-requiring diabetes. Second or third degree heart block is also a contraindication to the use of propranolol. More specific beta blockers (such as metoprolol) that exert their effect on heart rate and blood pressure rather than on bronchial dilatation are alternatives. However, at higher dosages, the more specific beta-adrenergic blockers behave in a manner similar to propranolol. The use of calcium antagonists, such as nifedipine, verapamil, or diltiazem, is gaining in popularity. These agents reduce "slow channel calcium transport" and specifically reduce the transport of calcium from the extracellular to the intracellular spaces. This effect results in a reduction in contractility and in coronary vascular resistance. These agents appear to be effective in treating patients with vasospastic angina ("Prinzmetal's angina"), but they are also useful in treating those with stable angina pectoris. Some calcium antagonists will decrease contractility and alter atrioventricular conduction (verapamil and diltiazem), so they must be used with caution in patients with congestive heart failure, bradycardia, or conduction blocks, but they do not augment bronchoconstriction and thus may be of particular benefit as an alternative to propranolol for those with bronchospasm and chronic lung disease. Nifedipine does not alter contractility or AV conduction.

Many patients are given long-acting nitrates and beta blockers or calcium antagonists concomitantly. Continuing angina at low levels of effort is generally considered an indication for coronary arteriography and possibly coronary artery revascularization.

Avoidance of cigarette smoking by patients with angina should be emphasized. The nicotine in cigarettes increases heart rate and blood pressure, and the carbon monoxide that is inhaled may result in a shift in the oxyhemoglobin dissociation curve, making oxygen less available at the tissue level. Nicotine may also result in direct constriction of coronary vessels. Carefully supervised and individually developed physical training and exercise programs are also appropriate for patients with stable angina. The major benefit of training appears to be to improve the hemodynamic response to exercise, including reducing heart rate and blood pressure changes for any given exercise load. Whether exercise programs increase collateral coronary blood flow is controversial.

PROGNOSIS. There is extreme variance in the symptoms and progression of the disease in the individual patient. In some, angina may remain stable for many years. However, approximately 25 per cent of men and 12 per cent of women with angina can expect a myocardial infarct within five years. In the population over 55 years of age, the general five-year survival rate is 75 per cent for those with stable angina pectoris.

The prognosis of patients with chronic ischemic heart disease is related directly to the location and extent of the coronary artery disease. Patients with three vessel coronary disease have an expected annual mortality of 6 to 8 per cent; if they also have damage to their hearts (i.e., previous myocardial infarct), the mortality rate is increased. On the other hand, patients with single vessel coronary artery disease have an annual mortality rate on medical therapy of approximately 3 to 4 per cent. Patients with main left coronary artery disease equal to or greater than 70 per cent luminal diameter narrowing have a prognosis similar to those with three vessel coronary disease. In fact, most patients with left main coronary disease also have extensive additional coronary disease. Coronary artery surgery with complete coronary artery revascularization relieves chest pain in the majority of patients with angina pectoris either completely or largely for months to years. In a few individuals, angina is not relieved by coronary artery revascularization, usually because of clotted grafts, incomplete revascularization, or important vascular disease beyond the site of graft insertion. However, although coronary artery revascularization reduces morbidity, it is not clear that it improves longevity except in patients with main left coronary artery disease.

DIRECT CORONARY ARTERY SURGERY. Large groups of patients now have undergone direct coronary artery surgery in the form of saphenous vein or internal mammary artery bypass grafting occasionally associated with coronary endarterectomy (see Ch. 49.4). These surgical procedures result in relief or reduction in the frequency of angina for months to years after the procedure in the majority of patients. For patients with important left main coronary disease, improved survival has been documented following coronary artery surgery. The most optimistic results from coronary artery surgery are obtained (1) in patients with "limiting angina" on a medical regimen but without congestive heart failure or significant left ventricular dysfunction; (2) in those with important proximal coronary artery narrowing but with good distal vessels; and (3) in those in whom the most important obstructing lesions can be corrected completely with coronary revascularization.

Graft occlusion during the first year varies from 10 to 12 per cent. Only a small additional percentage of grafts occlude during the second and third years following the procedure. However, coronary artery surgery is a palliative procedure, and most patients will redevelop angina months to years after the procedure. The most common reason for redevelopment of angina is progression of the intrinsic coronary artery disease. Incomplete revascularization may also be a cause for persistent angina or angina that develops soon after surgery. Graft occlusion and inadequate revascularization with inadequate increases in blood flow are additional reasons for less than favorable results.

Grafted vessels develop atherosclerosis in some individuals over time. This occurs most commonly in those with important hypercholesterolemia, in patients with diabetes mellitus, and in those with important distal vascular disease so that coronary graft flow is relatively sluggish. Native coronary arteries proximal to the site of insertion of coronary artery bypass grafts may develop an accelerated pattern of atherosclerosis following coronary artery surgery.

There is a risk of perioperative myocardial infarction, but the frequency with which this occurs is controversial. If the electrocardiogram is used to document the frequency of perioperative infarction, estimates run from 1 to 10 per cent. However, if myocardial scintigraphic techniques are used, the incidence is approximately twice as high. This discrepancy probably reflects subendocardial infarction not detected by the electrocardiogram.

While the subjective relief of angina is impressive following coronary artery revascularization, some patients also have objective improvement in ventricular function, both at rest and during exercise.

CORONARY ARTERY ANGIOPLASTY. Grüntzig has advocated the use of direct coronary artery dilatation with a balloon catheter for proximal coronary artery lesions in some patients. This procedure provides a means to increase luminal diameter size in selected patients. Moreover, important complications occur relatively infrequently, although it has been stressed that this procedure should be performed only with facilities available for direct coronary artery surgery should that be necessary. This procedure is utilized to dilate a proximal and important coronary arterial stenosis.

Braunwald E: Coronary artery surgery at the crossroads. N Engl J Med 297:661E, 1977. *A review of the results and implications of coronary artery surgery.*

Brensike JF, Levy RI, Kelsey SF, et al.: Effects of therapy with cholestyramine on progression of coronary arteriosclerosis: Results of the NHLBI Type II Coronary Intervention Study. Circulation 69:313, 1984. *A beneficial effect from lowering serum cholesterol values on progression of coronary arteriosclerosis is suggested by these data.*

Brown MS, Goldstein JL: Receptor-mediated control of cholesterol metabolism. Science 191:150, 1976. *This study provides very important insight into cellular mechanisms involved in the metabolism of cholesterol.*

Folts JD, Crowell EB, Rowe GG: Platelet aggregation in partially obstructed vessels and its elimination with aspirin. Circulation 54:365, 1976. *This study suggests that intermittent platelet aggregation can decrease coronary blood flow in narrowed canine coronary arteries.*

Grüntzig AR: Transluminal dilatation of coronary artery stenosis. Lancet 1:263, 1978. *A description of transluminal dilatation of coronary arteries.*

Hillis LD, Braunwald E: Coronary artery spasm. N Engl J Med 299:695, 1978. *An elegant and detailed review of coronary artery spasm.*

Hillis LD, Braunwald E: Myocardial ischemia. N Engl J Med 296:971, 1977. *A thorough review of myocardial ischemia.*

Holloway DH: Systolic murmur developing after myocardial ischemia or infarction: Differential diagnosis. JAMA 191:888, 1965. *The title is self-explanatory.*

Roberts WC: The coronary arteries and left ventricle in clinically isolated angina pectoris: A necropsy analysis. Circulation 54:388, 1976. *Postmortem findings as regards coronary artery disease and ventriculographic abnormalities in patients with angina pectoris.*

Ross R, Glomset JA: The pathogenesis of atherosclerosis. N Engl J Med 295:369, 1976. *An elegant review of the pathogenesis of coronary atherosclerosis.*

Swan HJC, Ganz WD, Forrester JS, et al.: Catheterization of the heart in man with the use of a flow-directed balloon-tipped catheter. N Engl J Med 283:447, 1970. *The original description of the techniques and uses of the Swan-Ganz catheter for measuring pulmonary artery and pulmonary capillary wedge pressures.*

Truett J, Cornfield J, Kannel WB: A multivariate analysis of the risk of coronary heart disease in Framingham. J Chronic Dis 20:511, 1967. *Detailed analysis of risk factors involved in the acquisition of coronary artery disease.*

Weisfeldt ML: Angina. *In* Willerson JT, Sanders CA (eds.): Clinical Cardiology. New York, Grune & Stratton, 1977, pp 337–346. *A thorough review of angina.*

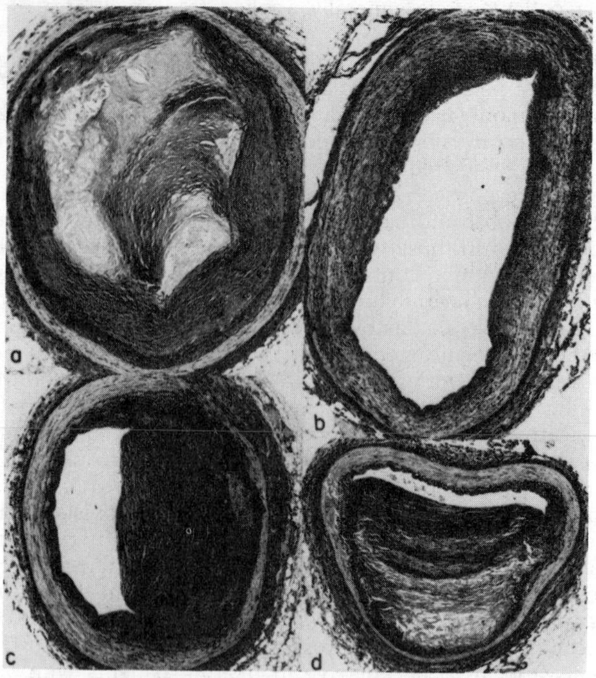

Figure 49–1. Sections of coronary arteries at sites of maximal narrowing in a 54-year-old woman who died suddenly at home. She had angina pectoris. *a,* Right coronary artery 3 cm from the aortic ostium. The lumen is more than 90 per cent obstructed. *b,* Left main coronary artery. *c,* Left circumflex coronary artery in the first 1 cm. *d,* Left anterior descending coronary artery 3 cm from the bifurcation of the left main coronary artery. These sections demonstrate the extent of coronary artery disease that may be present in an individual patient. (From Roberts WC: Circulation 48:1161, 1973. Reproduced by permission of The American Heart Association, Inc.)

49.2. Acute Myocardial Infarction

James T. Willerson

Myocardial infarction is the term used to describe irreversible cellular injury and necrosis occurring as a consequence of prolonged ischemia. Infarction may occur secondary to coronary occlusion, major reduction in blood flow to certain regions of heart muscle, or an insufficient increase in coronary blood flow relative to regional oxygen demand during periods of severe stress. In almost every instance, some degree of narrowing of coronary artery luminal diameter resulting from coronary atherosclerosis exists, but there are exceptions. Acute myocardial infarcts may also result from coronary artery dissection, coronary emboli, coronary artery spasm, vasculitis, anomalous origin of one of the coronary arteries from the pulmonary artery, and congenital coronary arteriovenous fistula.

The pathogenesis of coronary atherosclerosis is considered in detail in Ch. 48 and in brief in Ch. 49.1.

RISK FACTORS FOR CORONARY HEART DISEASE. Several epidemiologic studies have established that hyperlipidemia, especially hypercholesterolemia, constitutes a major risk factor predisposing to the development of premature atherosclerosis. Approximately one third of survivors of acute myocardial infarction at an age less than 60 years have some form of hyperlipidemia, defined as serum cholesterol and/or triglyceride levels above the ninety-fifth percentile for the control population. Other factors associated with an increased risk of development of coronary atherosclerotic disease include systemic arterial hypertension, smoking, lack of regular physical activity, and emotional stress. Risk factors are discussed more extensively in Ch. 39 and 48.

MECHANISMS OF ACUTE MYOCARDIAL INFARCTION. Acute myocardial infarction occurs primarily in patients with significant coronary artery disease (Fig. 49–1). In such patients, the primary determinants of vulnerability to acute myocardial infarction include (1) prolonged increases in myocardial oxygen demand under conditions in which increases in oxygen delivery cannot occur because of significant coronary artery disease (included are prolonged and marked increases in heart rate, contractility, and myocardial wall tension) or (2) primary decreases in oxygen delivery to the myocardium. The latter may be caused by (a) coronary artery thrombosis, (b) coronary artery spasm, (c) hemorrhage into an atherosclerotic plaque, and (d) systemic arterial hypotension (coronary artery perfusion is dependent on mean and diastolic aortic blood pressure).

Numerous clinicopathologic studies of patients with fatal ischemic heart disease have attempted to define the pathogenesis of acute myocardial infarction and other ischemic heart disease syndromes. Controversy persists, however, regarding the frequency and significance of various coronary arterial lesions, including acute coronary thrombi in patients with acute myocardial infarcts. A new dimension has been raised with the evidence that coronary artery spasm may act as a pathophysiologic factor in patients with angina pectoris and acute myocardial infarction.

The variation in clinical and pathologic findings in patients with acute ischemic heart disease (and in particular, acute myocardial infarcts) has resulted in differing interpretations of the role of acute thrombosis and other acute occlusive coronary arterial lesions in the genesis of the various syndromes of coronary heart disease. Several studies suggest that coronary thrombi develop independently of acute myocardial infarction or as purely secondary phenomena relatively late after infarction.

An important observation which appeared to favor a secondary role for coronary thrombosis in acute myocardial infarction was the low incidence of thrombi in cases of sudden cardiac death. However, sudden cardiac death syndromes and acute myocardial infarction are usually separate entities with differing pathogenesis, since the majority of patients resuscitated from sudden death do not develop evidence of important myocardial infarction. Sudden cardiac death appears to result from a primary ventricular arrhythmia, usually ventricular tachycardia or fibrillation, produced by an acute ischemic event but not involving major coronary thrombosis, or it develops from ventricular ectopy occurring against a background of chronic coronary artery disease but not necessarily triggered by acute myocardial ischemia.

Postmortem studies and clinicopathologic correlations have shown (1) a strong association between acute coronary artery occlusion and regional myocardial infarcts, especially transmural infarcts; (2) a spatial relationship in most instances between infarct location and an acute occlusion in the artery supplying the infarcted area; (3) a chronologic relationship, within the limits of the histologic method, between the age of the thrombus and the age of the infarct; (4) a lack of uniformity in the severity of atherosclerosis, including distal disease in arteries developing thrombi; and (5) frequent association of coronary thrombi with focal arterial lesions, plaque rupture, or hemorrhage—lesions which likely predispose to thrombus formation. In experimental animals, radiofibrinogen becomes incorporated into thrombi formed prior to injection of the tracer. In most human thrombi, a radionegative central core can be demonstrated suggesting initial thrombus formation prior to injection of the tracer.

In a clinicopathologic study of 100 episodes of acute ischemic heart disease, the prevalence of acute coronary occlusion was 61 per cent (57 in situ thrombi, 2 thromboemboli, and 2 isolated plaque hemorrhages), including 90 per cent for transmural infarcts, 35 per cent for subendocardial infarcts, and 11 per cent for multifocal microinfarcts associated with clinical acute coronary insufficiency syndromes (Buja and Willerson). The prevalence of plaque erosion or rupture with coronary thrombus formation was 68 per cent for infarcts of age three weeks or less, but decreased to 20 per cent with older infarcts, probably because organization and healing made identification of these lesions more difficult. Others, using serial section techniques, have described a higher prevalence (usually over 90 per cent) of plaque erosion and rupture associated with major plaque hemorrhage and acute coronary thrombosis. Potential causative factors for plaque rupture include hemodynamic trauma, inflammatory or chemical injury to coronary artery endothelium and subendothelial tissue, increased intraplaque pressure resulting from infiltration of blood or other mechanisms, and coronary vasospasm. Oliva (1977) has described arteriographic evidence of coronary artery spasm in 6 of 15 patients with acute myocardial infarcts. However, the frequency and role of spasm in the sequence of coronary artery wall damage, acute coronary occlusion, and the development or evolution of acute myocardial infarcts remain uncertain. Factors to be considered in this speculative sequence include prostaglandins (thromboxane A_2 and prostacyclin), platelet aggregation, local increase of catecholamines, autonomic neural influences, and local alterations in clotting or fibrinolytic systems.

Although acute myocardial infarction has a variable pathogenesis, several clinical observations suggest an important role for acute coronary occlusion in the genesis of many infarcts. Pertinent clinical observations include (1) a high prevalence of hemodynamic alterations such as heart failure, shock, or aortic stenosis predisposing to reduced coronary perfusion in patients with infarction unassociated with coronary thrombi and (2) a low prevalence of such predisposing hemodynamic factors in patients with infarction associated with coronary thrombi. Relatively small infarcts without cardiogenic shock and larger infarcts with cardiogenic shock have a similarly high incidence of coronary thrombi. Clinicopathologic correlates appear to negate the argument that formation of coronary thrombi can be explained on the basis of a generalized impairment in coronary perfusion following the onset of acute myocardial infarction.

It also seems plausible that coronary thrombosis may develop without plaque disruption in severely stenotic coronary arteries. Experimental studies in canine models show increased coronary vascular resistance and reduced reflow in the necrotic or severely damaged subendocardium after 90 to 120 minutes of coronary artery occlusion. Coronary collateral flow may sometimes compensate for acute coronary thrombosis so that no important myocardial necrosis results. It seems likely that variations in the extent of generalized coronary atherosclerosis and of coronary collateral flow may influence the extent and location of acute infarction subsequent to an acute coronary thrombosis.

RECOGNITION OF ACUTE MYOCARDIAL INFARCTS. ***History.*** The history is of the utmost importance in the recognition of acute myocardial infarction. Typically, the chest pain is severe and usually lasts until the patient receives analgesic medication from a physician. The pain is ordinarily described as being substernal or left precordial, as a "heaviness" or "tightness," or "like a weight on my chest," and is often associated with nausea and diaphoresis. The chest pain may radiate to the back, the neck, the jaw, or the left arm, particularly down its ulnar aspect. Occasionally, the pain may exist only in the back, the jaw, the left arm, or the neck. Chest pain in patients with acute myocardial infarcts generally lasts longer than 30 minutes and is typically the most severe pain an individual has experienced. Many patients with acute myocardial infarcts have unstable angina pectoris for hours to days prior to their acute myocardial infarcts; by contrast, 10 to 20 per cent of patients with acute myocardial infarction have "silent," i.e., painless, infarcts. Painless infarction is noted with special frequency in diabetic patients.

Physical Examination. GENERAL. Patients with small myocardial infarcts, particularly subendocardial infarcts, may not have any detectable abnormalities on physical examination. At the other extreme, patients with more than 40 per cent irreversible cellular damage to the left ventricle often develop severe left ventricular failure with pulmonary edema and possibly cardiogenic shock.

INSPECTION AND PALPATION. The findings depend on the extent of the myocardial damage. Most patients are in obvious discomfort. They are often diaphoretic, pale, and extremely anxious. Those with extensive damage develop a reduction in systemic arterial blood pressure ranging from mild to severe. Cardiogenic shock is defined as hypotension resulting from extensive myocardial damage, with evidence of inadequate systemic perfusion, such as cool skin, mental confusion, and oliguria. Patients with extensive myocardial necrosis may also have an alternating force of their pulse ("pulsus alternans"). Most patients have frequent ventricular premature beats.

Patients with second or third degree atrioventricular block may have intermittent "cannon" A waves in their jugular venous pulse. Patients with atrial fibrillation lack an "A" wave and have an irregularly irregular pulse. Patients with right ventricular failure have an increased jugular venous pressure, right upper quadrant tenderness when acute hepatic congestion develops, and possibly ascites and peripheral and/or sacral edema.

AUSCULTATION. Fourth heart sounds are almost invariably heard, and the heart sounds are usually soft. When the mitral valve apparatus is damaged, a murmur of mitral insufficiency may be audible. These murmurs have variable auscultatory characteristics and may occur in mid to late systole or be holosystolic. Acute mitral insufficiency occurs most commonly in patients with inferior, lateral, or subendocardial myocardial infarcts. Patients with inferior myocardial infarcts and structural damage to the tricuspid valve may develop tricuspid insufficiency. Rupture of the interventricular septum occurs most commonly in patients with acute anterior myocardial infarcts. Murmurs resulting from ventricular septal defects are located along the lower left sternal border and are holosystolic. They may radiate toward the cardiac apex. Acute interventricular septal defects are often associated with a systolic thrill along the left sternal border. The distinction between a holosystolic murmur caused by acute mitral insufficiency and a ruptured septum is not always clear by physical examination.

Third heart sounds occur in patients with ventricular filling pressures of 15 mm Hg or greater (ventricular failure) or in those with at least moderately severe mitral insufficiency. The second heart sound is paradoxically split in some patients with left ventricular failure, in some with left bundle branch block, and in some during chest pain. The pulmonic closure sound is increased in intensity in patients with pulmonary hypertension resulting from left ventricular failure. Pericardial friction rubs are detected in less than 10 per cent of patients with acute transmural myocardial infarcts. Patients with audible pericardial friction rubs are ordinarily those with the largest transmural infarcts. If large pericardial effusions develop, heart sounds may be distant and the jugular venous pressure is elevated. Cardiac tamponade results in shock, pulsus paradoxus, distant heart sounds, and an elevated jugular venous pressure. Bibasilar or more extensive moist rales develop in patients with left ventricular failure. Pulmonary edema occurs with extensive myocardial infarction and in patients with myocardial ischemia superimposed on extensive previous myocardial infarction. Evidence of reduced peripheral perfusion accompanied by clear lungs and an elevated jugular venous pressure should raise the question of right ventricular infarction.

Electrocardiographic Diagnosis. The electrocardiogram (ECG) provides an excellent means for recognition of transmural acute myocardial infarction (Figs. 49–2 to 49–4). The characteristic sequence of ECG alterations with transmural infarction is as follows: (1) the initial development of prominent peaked T waves in the ECG leads representing sites of epicardial injury; (2) the development of hyperacute S-T segment elevation; (3) the development of significant Q waves, i.e., of 0.04 second in duration, and/or loss of >30 per cent of the amplitude of the R wave (Fig. 49–2). The rate of evolution of these ECG changes is variable; they may occur in minutes or may be delayed for several hours. Some patients with acute myocardial infarcts have relatively normal electrocardiograms in the first few hours after the event. Problems in using the ECG to identify acute myocardial infarction are as follows: (1) in patients with left bundle branch block, acute anterior myocardial infarcts are not recognized by the ECG; (2) in patients with previous transmural infarction, recognition of new injury can be difficult; and (3) in individuals in whom rapid ECG evolution occurs, it may not be possible to differentiate old from new myocardial infarction. S-T segment elevation may also occur (1) with normal early repolarization (Fig. 49–3); (2) with transient myocardial ischemia, as in Prinzmetal's angina or with ischemia in an area of previous myocardial damage; (3) in some individuals with chronic ventricular aneurysms; (4) transiently, following electrical cardioversion; (5) in the anterior precordial ECG leads in patients with left bundle branch block; (6) in patients with left ventricular hypertrophy; and (7) in some patients with hyperkalemia.

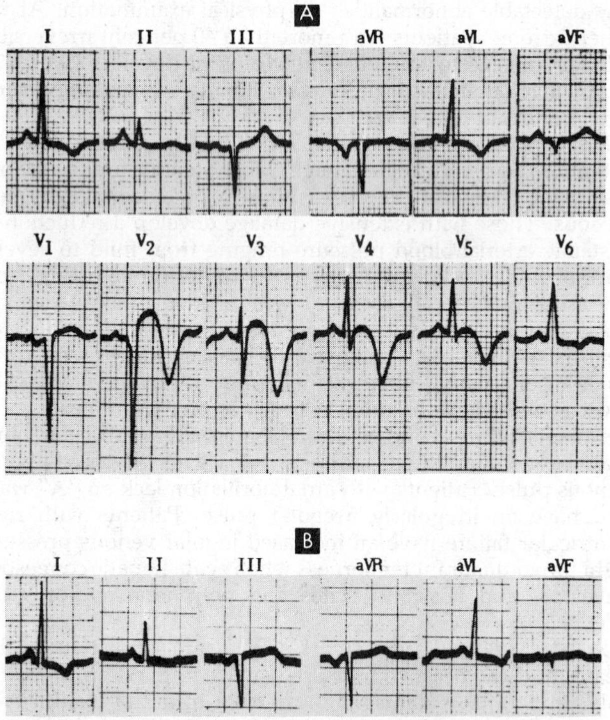

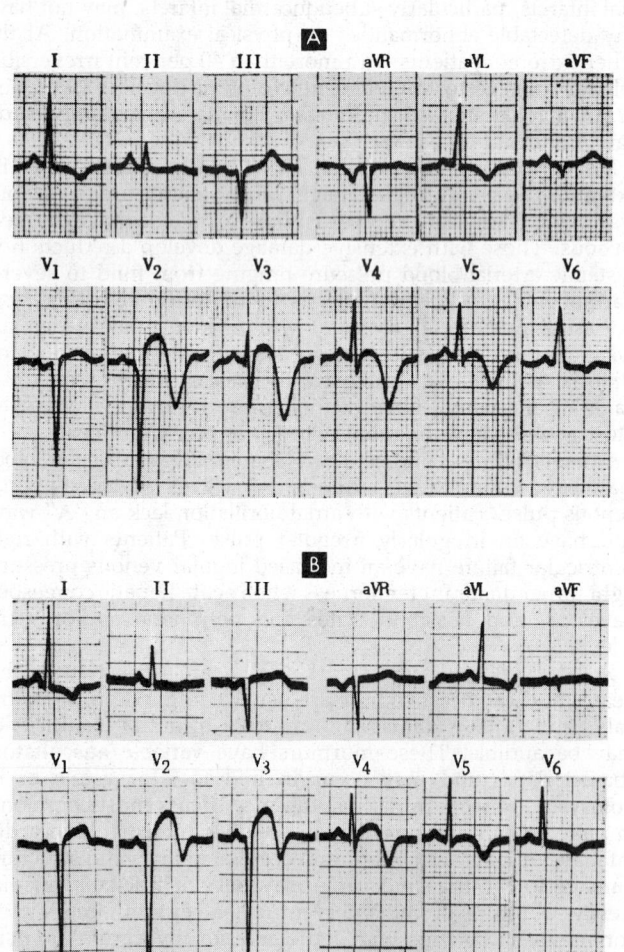

Figure 49–2. Acute anteroseptal myocardial infarction. Panel *A* was obtained on the day of hospitalization and demonstrates inverted T waves in V_2 through V_5 and a Q wave in V_2. Panel *B* was obtained three days later and shows further evolutionary changes compatible with an acute anteroseptal myocardial infarction. (Reproduced by permission from Lipman BS, Massie E, Kleiger RE: Clinical Scalar Electrocardiography. 6th ed. Chicago, Year Book Medical Publishers, 1979.)

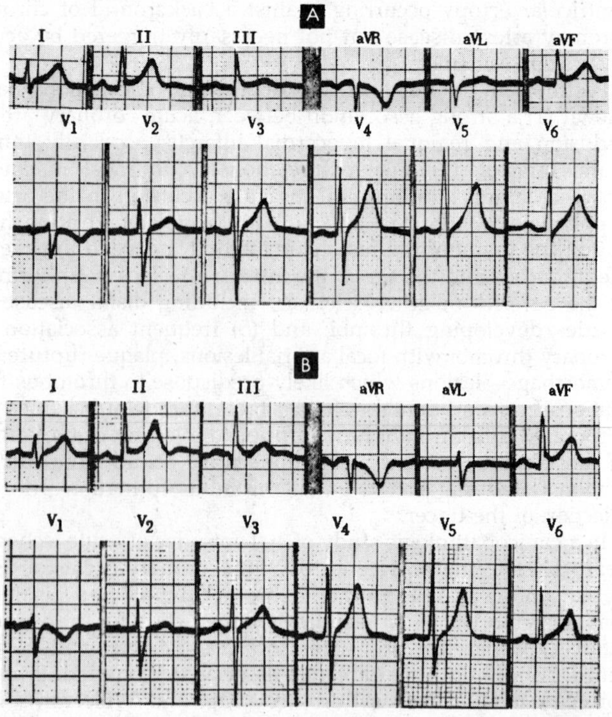

Figure 49–3. Normal early repolarization. The electrocardiograms obtained in panels *A* and *B* were taken two weeks apart in a patient without heart disease. The ST elevation in leads II, III, and AVF represent normal early repolarization. (Reproduced by permission from Lipman BS, Massie E, Kleiger RE: Clinical Scalar Electrocardiography. 6th ed. Chicago, Year Book Medical Publishers, 1979.)

In contrast to the usefulness of the ECG in the recognition of transmural myocardial infarcts, the ECG does not allow one to recognize acute nontransmural myocardial infarction (subendocardial infarction) with certainty. The ECG demonstrates S-T depression and T wave inversion with nontransmural myocardial infarction; the only evolution is a return to baseline. Unfortunately, subendocardial ischemia, ventricular hypertrophy, rapid heart rates, emotional influences, electrolyte alterations, and the use of certain medications, including cardiac glycosides, may produce the same ECG changes. Indeed, bizarre T wave alterations occur even in patients with intracerebral hemorrhage. The only useful rule in the ECG recognition

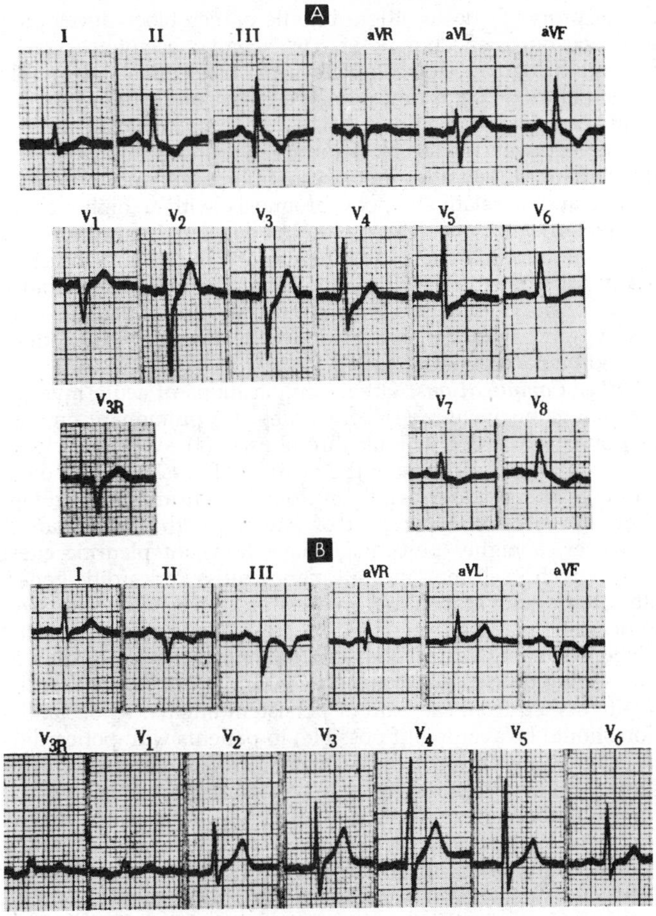

Figure 49–4. A true posterior myocardial infarct (panel *B*). Panel *A* contains the ECG of a middle-aged male eight hours following the onset of severe chest pain. Panel *B* demonstrates the ECG 72 hours later, at which time prominent R waves have developed in precordial leads V_1 and V_2. Panel *B* also demonstrates an acute inferior transmural myocardial infarct.

of nontransmural myocardial infarction is that the deeper the S-T segment depression and the longer it lasts, the more likely the presence of acute subendocardial myocardial infarction.

Serum Enzyme Changes. Currently, the preferred enzymatic technique is the measurement of creatine kinase (CK) and in particular, the "myocardial specific" CK-MB isoenzyme measured by spectrophotometric, fluorometric, or radioimmunoassay technique. CK-MB increases in the sera of patients approximately two hours after acute myocardial infarction, peaks at 10 to 12 hours, and often returns to normal within 24 hours after the event. Radioimmunoassay measurement of alterations in serum myoglobin concentration allows slightly earlier recognition of acute myocardial infarction, but at present there is no means to distinguish myoglobin release from the heart and skeletal muscle when both are injured. Radioimmunoassay measurement of alterations in the serum concentration of the light chain of myosin may also allow a relatively early and precise recognition of acute myocardial infarction, but extensive clinical studies have not yet been reported. In the past, serial serum measurements of glutamic oxalacetic transaminase (SGOT) or of lactic dehydrogenase (LDH) or of the LDH isoenzymes have been used to recognize acute myocardial infarction.

Myocardial Scintigraphy. The use of radionuclide myocardial scintigraphic techniques to recognize acute myocardial infarction has gained in popularity (see Ch. 41.4). These techniques allow one to see the region(s) of acute myocardial infarction (infarct-avid imaging techniques) or to identify areas of severely decreased myocardial perfusion ("cold spot" imaging techniques). The prototype infarct-avid imaging agent is technetium-99m stannous pyrophosphate. This agent accumulates in irreversibly damaged myocardium one to five days after infarction; its sensitivity in the detection of acute infarction of 3 grams or larger is greater than 90 per cent. Thallium-201 (Tl-201) is the "cold spot" imaging agent of choice. When used within 24 hours after acute infarction, its sensitivity is approximately 90 per cent. The extent of the initial Tl-201 defect after acute myocardial infarction appears to have prognostic significance. Finally, one may employ technetium-labeled red blood cells to evaluate the impact of acute myocardial infarction on regional and global ventricular function, using "dynamic myocardial scintigraphy." This technique allows one to measure or identify ventricular ejection-fraction, ventricular volumes, regional wall motion, left to right shunts (i.e., ventricular septal defects), ventricular aneurysms, and valvular insufficiency, including mitral or tricuspid regurgitation.

DIFFERENTIAL DIAGNOSIS. The differential diagnosis of acute myocardial infarction theoretically includes every cause of chest pain, cardiac arrhythmias, and heart failure. Important diagnostic considerations are (1) acute coronary insufficiency, (2) unstable angina pectoris, (3) Prinzmetal's angina, and (4) dissecting aortic aneurysm. Less common as difficult diagnoses to exclude, but still sometimes important to differentiate, are (1) peptic ulcer disease, (2) pancreatitis, (3) cholecystitis, (4) pulmonary embolic disease, (5) spontaneous pneumothorax, (6) pericarditis, and (7) pneumonitis. Careful attention to the history and physical examination and the proper use of relevant blood tests, electrocardiograms, and myocardial scintigraphy usually allow one to make the proper diagnosis.

COMPLICATIONS OF ACUTE MYOCARDIAL INFARCTS. ***Mechanical Complications.*** Patients with cardiogenic shock as a consequence of extensive left ventricular damage occurring with acute myocardial infarction have a poor prognosis. Cardiac assistance devices such as intra-aortic balloon counterpulsation have reduced mortality slightly in patients with acute myocardial infarcts and cardiogenic shock, particularly when coupled with coronary artery revascularization or ventricular aneurysmectomy. However, the extent of myocardial damage is generally so severe that a majority of these patients still succumb.

An important complication of acute myocardial infarction is infarct extension or expansion. Approximately 20 per cent of patients extend their myocardial infarcts within the first five days following myocardial infarction. The incidence is slightly higher for those with anterior transmural infarcts, and the consequences of infarct extension for patients in this group are more serious. The incidence of infarct extension is approximately twice as high when assessed by laboratory methods as by clinical symptoms alone. Infarct expansion may be associated with worsening ventricular function and increased morbidity and mortality.

Other mechanical problems that may complicate acute myocardial infarction include papillary muscle dysfunction or rupture with consequent acute mitral regurgitation or the development of a ventricular septal defect. Rupture of an entire papillary muscle is ordinarily fatal within minutes to hours owing to massive mitral regurgitation, which results in severe left ventricular failure and cardiogenic shock. Rupture of one head of a papillary muscle may be tolerated for longer periods of time, allowing clinical evaluation and occasionally surgical correction. Partial or complete rupture of a papillary muscle occurs in less than 5 per cent of patients with acute infarction. Dysfunction of a papillary muscle occurs more commonly when ischemia or infarction of the papillary muscle prevents proper coaptation of the mitral leaflets, causing mitral regurgitation. Patients with papillary muscle dysfunction generally have milder left ventricular failure and are responsive to medical intervention. Acute mitral regurgitation occurs most commonly in patients with inferior, lateral, or subendocardial infarcts. Patients who develop acute mitral insufficiency usually do so within one to seven days after acute myocardial infarction and present with a new murmur which is loudest at the apex or along the left sternal border.

Rupture of a portion of the ventricular septum is usually associated with a holosystolic murmur and systolic thrill along the left sternal border. Ventricular septal defects develop in about 1 per cent of acute myocardial infarcts, and often result in right and left ventricular failure. They may occur within hours or as late as 10 to 12 days following infarction. If ventricular failure is severe, one may consider emergency surgical correction even though surgical mortality rates are highest within the first month after myocardial infarction. "Afterload reduction," using intra-aortic balloon counterpulsation or pharmacologic means, or both, may benefit patients with ventricular septal defects or mitral regurgitation occurring acutely after myocardial infarction.

Ventricular aneurysms usually develop within hours of myocardial infarction and enlarge over subsequent weeks or months. If sizable, they may result in congestive heart failure. They may also be associated with ventricular arrhythmias or with mural thrombosis and systemic embolization. Significant endocardial clots can be demonstrated in at least 50 per cent of autopsied patients with ventricular aneurysms.

Right ventricular infarction develops occasionally in patients with inferoposterior myocardial infarction. Occasionally, right ventricular involvement may be sufficient to give rise to systemic hypotension with low pulmonary capillary wedge and left ventricular filling pressures. Alternatively, extensive right ventricular infarction may simulate a large pericardial effusion and cardiac tamponade. Recognition is important, since proper therapy includes fluid administration, which is not usually employed in the hypotensive patient with a dominant left ventricular infarct. Right ventricular infarction may also lead to tricuspid valvular insufficiency secondary to papillary muscle dysfunction.

Arrhythmias and Heart Block. More than 90 per cent of patients develop ventricular premature beats in the first 72 hours after acute myocardial infarction. Ventricular premature beats are suppressed by pharmacologic intervention in most patients. However, in those with large infarcts, they may be difficult to suppress, and death may occur because of medically refractory arrhythmias.

Various types of atrioventricular block and intraventricular block may occur as a consequence of acute myocardial infarction. First degree heart block is common with acute inferior infarction, and as an isolated finding it is not a cause for concern. Second degree heart block of the Mobitz I type ("Wenckebach block") also occurs following acute inferior infarction. It is usually transient and even if it progresses to complete heart block, it is usually only temporary. Temporary pacemaker insertion is indicated in patients with Mobitz I block who have slow ventricular rates resulting in syncope, congestive heart failure, angina pectoris, or ventricular arrhythmias. Mobitz II heart block occurs most often as a consequence of anterior myocardial infarction. The level of block is located below the atrioventricular junction within the ventricle. Mobitz II block should be treated with a pacemaker as soon as it is recognized. Permanent pacing is indicated in such patients at a later date.

Complete heart block may develop abruptly or follow either of the two forms of second degree heart block described above. Complete heart block complicating acute anterior myocardial infarction is often permanent, and usually requires permanent pacing. Complete heart block after inferior myocardial infarction is ordinarily only transient and temporary ventricular pacing almost always suffices.

Acute left bundle branch block ordinarily develops as a consequence of a large anterior myocardial infarction. The risk of complete heart block in patients who develop left bundle branch block with acute infarction is between 40 and 60 per cent, and many physicians elect to insert a temporary pacemaker prophylactically. Right bundle branch block developing acutely is not a reflection of infarct size and does not necessarily indicate a high risk of complete heart block. Bilateral bundle branch block (left axis deviation and right bundle branch block, right axis deviation and right bundle branch block, or first degree atrioventricular block and left bundle branch block) developing acutely after myocardial infarction indicates a large infarct and a relatively poor prognosis with a high risk of complete heart block. These patterns develop most commonly with anterior infarction, and temporary pacers are inserted. Many patients who develop acute bilateral bundle branch block die as a consequence of a low output state. Those patients who survive and who develop evidence of atrioventricular block should be paced permanently.

Other Complications. Other complications of acute myocardial infarction include (1) pericarditis, (2) pulmonary emboli, (3) lower extremity venous thrombosis, (4) systemic arterial embolization, (5) rupture of the heart, (6) Dressler's syndrome, and (7) the "shoulder-hand syndrome." Pericarditis is evident clinically in 7 to 15 per cent of patients with acute infarcts. However, a higher percentage have transient pleuritic chest pain, which itself may indicate pericarditis. Pericarditis generally occurs with transmural infarcts of at least moderate size. Pericarditis may be recognized by auscultation of a pericardial friction rub, but the majority of patients with pericarditis in this setting do not have rubs. The pain of pericarditis must be distinguished from the pain of persistent angina. Anticoagulation should be avoided (if possible) in patients with pericarditis in order to minimize the risk of hemorrhagic pericardial effusion. Pulmonary embolism is treated with heparinization followed by longer-term anticoagulation; lower extremity venous thrombosis is treated similarly. Systemic embolization generally occurs from a mural thrombus developing in the damaged left ventricle, and when it occurs systemic anticoagulation is indicated. Rupture of the heart occurs one to ten days following infarction and is the cause of death in 2 to 15 per cent of fatal cases. Rupture is most common in patients with systemic arterial hypertension and following an initial anterior infarct. The classic clinical clue indicating myocardial rupture is "electromechanical dissociation," in which electrical activity persists without detectable blood pressure or pulse. When rupture occurs, death is ordinarily so rapid that surgical intervention is not possible. An occasional patient, however, may develop a slow leak of blood into the pericardial space, and clotting of blood may serve to compress and partially seal the tear in the heart. This may allow emergency pericardiocentesis and an attempt at surgical repair. Untreated survivors of a sealed-off rupture typically develop "false aneurysms" of the left ventricle. Dressler's syndrome is characterized by pericarditis and pericardial effusion, pleural effusion, and often fever two weeks to nine months after myocardial infarction. The etiology of this syndrome is not clear. It is treated with aspirin or indomethacin. If these agents are unsuccessful, steroids usually relieve the chest pain, suppress the fever, and result in the ultimate disappearance of the effusions. The "shoulder-hand syndrome" is extremely rare, but consists of the development of pain and stiffness in the left shoulder or hand, and vasomotor changes sometimes associated with muscle atrophy. Typically, it occurs several weeks to months after the infarct. It is believed that the prolonged immobilization and bed rest used in patients with acute myocardial infarction in the past may have been responsible for the development of this problem.

ESTIMATION OF INFARCT SIZE. Accurate measurements of the extent of reversible and irreversible cellular damage are needed. Such measurements must be relatively noninvasive, ideally should be applicable early in the patient's clinical course, should be capable of being repeated with reasonable frequency, should provide measurements of the extent of damage with various types of infarcts, and should be available generally. No perfect measurement of infarct size or of the extent of ischemic damage exists presently, but there are many promising developments. Included in such a list are (1) enzymatic indices of infarct size, including most importantly measurement of creatine kinase enzyme release from the heart; (2) electrocardiographic estimates of the extent of ischemic injury, including precordial electrocardiographic mapping to identify the extent of QRS alterations; (3) scintigraphic measurements of infarct size, including infarct-avid and "cold spot" techniques (see above); and (4) dynamic myocardial scintigraphy to estimate abnormalities of global and segmental ventricular function, using either first pass or equilibrium studies. Each of these techniques has its limitations, but each also provides important information concerning location or relative size of infarcts. For the scintigraphic measurements, it is necessary to develop three-dimensional estimates of the extent of myocardial damage; such methodologic advances are occurring presently, and in the near future tomographic cameras that may be used with gamma emitting radionuclides will become generally available.

EVALUATION OF VENTRICULAR FUNCTION IN PATIENTS WITH MYOCARDIAL INFARCTS. Invasive and noninvasive techniques have been developed to allow more precise characterization of ventricular function in patients with reduced systemic arterial blood pressure and uncertain left ventricular functional status in order to assess the need for volume replacement, diuresis, or inotropic support. The Swan-Ganz catheter allows measurement of left ventricular filling pressure without entering a systemic artery or the left ventricle. This balloon-tipped, flow-directed catheter may be placed in the pulmonary artery from a systemic vein. One positions the Swan-Ganz catheter in the pulmonary artery, either with the aid of fluoroscopy or with continuous pressure monitoring to identify the characteristic right atrial, right ventricular, and pulmonary artery pressures. Once the catheter is in the pulmonary artery, the balloon is partly inflated, allowing the measurement of pulmonary capillary wedge pressure. In the absence of mitral valve disease, the mean pulmonary capillary wedge pressure is equivalent to the left ventricular end-diastolic or filling pressure. Measurements of left ventricular filling pressure with the Swan-Ganz catheter will differentiate between hypotension because of hypovolemia and hypotension because of left ventricular failure. Cardiac output may also be measured. Patients with acute myocardial infarctions with shock should have an indwelling arterial cannula inserted to allow accurate measurement of arterial pressure and moment-to-moment monitoring of pressure changes.

Noninvasive assessments of left and right ventricular function following acute myocardial infarction may also be made, using either dynamic myocardial scintigraphy or echocardiography. Both methodologies allow one to measure ventricular ejection fraction, ventricular dimensions or volumes, and segmental wall motion. Two-dimensional rather than M-mode echocardiography must be used to measure ventricular ejection fraction and end-systolic dimension accurately in patients with ischemic heart disease.

PROGNOSIS. Most patients with acute myocardial infarction have an uncomplicated course. Some patients, however, develop life-threatening complications during the first one to two weeks and others die (Table 49–2). In the early 1970's, 50 per cent or more of patients died prior to reaching the hospital; these deaths were due to ventricular arrhythmias developing in the initial seconds or minutes following the onset of chest pain. Optimal emergency ambulance systems have achieved a 25 to 30 per cent reduction in the incidence of death prior to hospitalization in patients with acute myocardial infarction and sudden cardiac arrest syndromes.

TABLE 49–2. POTENTIAL LIFE-THREATENING COMPLICATIONS OF ACUTE MYOCARDIAL INFARCTION

Ventricular arrhythmias (ventricular tachycardia, ventricular fibrillation or asystole)
Extremely rapid atrial arrhythmias in association with extensive myocardial infarction (atrial flutter or atrial fibrillation)
Heart block (second or third degree types)
Marked bradycardia
Loss of atrial contribution to cardiac contraction (atrioventricular junctional rhythm)
Infarction ≧ 40 per cent of left ventricle
Extensive right ventricular infarction
Acute ventricular septal defects
Acute and severe mitral regurgitation
Severe pulmonary edema
Rupture of the heart
Systemic and/or pulmonary emboli

Overall mortality in patients with acute myocardial infarction who reach the hospital ranges from 3 to 30 per cent, depending upon the population studied. In general, patients with anterior infarction have a higher mortality than patients with inferior infarction; this appears to be related to greater loss of left ventricular muscle with anterior infarcts.

Patients can be divided into groups with differing prognoses on the basis of initial hemodynamic measurements. Those without left ventricular failure and with a mean systolic arterial pressure of greater than 110 mm Hg, an average cardiac index greater than 2.5 liters per minute per square meter, and a normal pulmonary capillary wedge pressure (or pulmonary artery diastolic pressure) have relatively low mortality rates, i.e., approximately 3 to 12 per cent. If death occurs in patients in this group, it is generally from a ventricular arrhythmia, from later infarct extension, or from a mechanical complication such as myocardial, septal, or papillary muscle rupture. Patients with cardiogenic shock, including hypotension with systolic arterial pressures less than 90 mm Hg, with decreased peripheral perfusion without a reversible cause, and with reduced mean cardiac index (less than 2.0 liters per minute per square meter), and an increased pulmonary capillary wedge or pulmonary diastolic pressure (greater than 25 mm Hg), have a mortality rate of greater than 80 per cent. Those with clinical evidence of left ventricular failure and a normal or elevated systemic arterial pressure have an expected mortality rate of 5 to 30 per cent.

Long-term mortality following recovery from an initial myocardial infarct is related to the presence of ventricular arrhythmias, the extent of myocardial damage, and the age of the patient. In general, if the patient is less than 50 years of age at the time of the initial infarct, the yearly mortality rate is approximately 5 per cent. If the patient is older than 50 years of age, the mortality rate is approximately doubled. If a patient survives one year following infarction, there is a 75 per cent chance he will survive five years; if he survives five years following infarction, there is approximately a 50 per cent chance he will live 15 years.

In-hospital and immediate post-hospital discharge complications are related to infarct size. When more than 40 per cent of the left ventricular muscle mass is irreversibly damaged, one can expect "power failure" complications, including cardiogenic shock, congestive heart failure, and medically refractory ventricular arrhythmias. Patients with small infarcts (irrespective of the location) are less likely to experience such complications. However, a strategically located small infarct may result in heart block, the acute development of a ventricular septal defect, or papillary muscle dysfunction or rupture resulting in acute mitral insufficiency. In addition, patients with multiple small infarcts may ultimately develop cardiogenic shock, medically refractory heart failure, or medically refractory arrhythmias as a consequence of the cumulative muscle loss. Even small infarcts may be associated with important ventricular arrhythmias, and there is therefore a need for continuous electrocardiographic monitoring for at least three or four days following acute myocardial infarction irrespective of infarct size. This approach was made practical by advances in the 1950's and 1960's in ECG monitoring and in the electrical and pharmacologic conversion of ventricular arrhythmias.

Accurate predictors of longer-term prognosis in patients with acute myocardial infarction are needed. Such predictors should be helpful at the time of hospital admission, during the hospitalization, and following hospital discharge. Ideally, one should be able to identify patients at high risk for death or complications from extensive pump damage within the first few minutes to hours following hospital admission, as well as those most at risk for sudden death, recurrent myocardial infarction, persistent heart failure, or new ischemic events following hospital discharge. Considerable progress has been made in the development of such prognostic indices. Specifically, serum creatine kinase measurements are prognostically important in that patients with the largest infarcts are those most likely to experience cardiogenic shock, refractory congestive failure, or refractory ventricular arrhythmias, but several hours to a few days are required to complete such measurements.

"Cold spot" thallium-201 myocardial scintigraphy is valuable at the time of hospital admission for assessing the extent of the myocardial perfusion defect. Those patients with the largest perfusion defects have a poor prognosis during hospitalization and a higher mortality rate in the short-term follow-up. Similarly, those patients with the most extensive ventricular function abnormalities as detected by dynamic scintigraphy and patients with large anterior infarcts by technetium-99m stannous pyrophosphate scintigraphy are those who develop "pump failure" and important ventricular arrhythmias. Patients with anterior transmural myocardial infarction who extend their infarct size in hospital also have increased mortality and morbidity. Finally, patients with ventricular ejection fractions below 30 per cent and important ventricular ectopic beats at the time of hospital discharge and patients with severe global and segmental ventricular dysfunction on exercise testing at the time of hospital discharge also have a relatively poor prognosis. Persistently abnormal technetium-99m stannous pyrophosphate myocardial scintigrams several months following myocardial infarction may indicate chronic ischemic injury.

TREATMENT. Patients with proven or suspected acute myocardial infarction should be admitted to a coronary care unit, where their heart rate and rhythm are monitored continuously. The major contribution of coronary care units has been to provide an environment for surveillance for important arrhythmias and a capability to treat promptly "malignant ventricular ectopy." More than 90 per cent of patients with acute myocardial infarction have ventricular ectopy, which often requires pharmacologic suppression. Since many of the important complications of acute myocardial infarction occur in the first 96 hours after the event, it is advisable to keep patients in a coronary care unit for this period. Complete bed rest is recommended for this interval, and emotional stimulation and strenuous physical effort are to be avoided. Persistent angina during the initial 48 hours after the infarct is treated with opiates, usually intravenous morphine or meperidine. Thereafter, long- and short-acting nitrates are used to treat recurrent angina. Propranolol is also added in maximally tolerated doses if angina recurs after the initial 48 hours and persists at either rest or minimal effort. Angina that recurs frequently at minimal activity despite long-acting nitrates and propranolol is often treated with a constant intravenous infusion of nitroglycerin. If this is unsuccessful, intra-aortic balloon counterpulsation may be used for temporary control of the angina. However, if this aggressive effort is required to control angina, one also prepares the patient for coronary arteriography and probable coronary artery revascularization within hours to a few days after insertion of the intra-aortic balloon. Two points of caution regarding persistent or recurrent angina at rest or minimal effort in patients with acute myocardial infarction are indicated, however. One does need to determine that intermittent coronary spasm is not responsible for angina occurring at rest. This may be accomplished by obtaining 24-hour multilead ECG monitoring, allowing identification of S-T segment shifts with and without anginal episodes. Such findings unassociated with preceding alteration in blood pressure or heart rate are presumptive evidence of coronary artery spasm and/or platelet aggregation at the site(s) of a severely narrowed coronary artery causing further phasic reductions in coronary blood flow. Recurrent coronary spasm is treated with nitrates and calcium antagonists, such as verapamil, diltiazem, or nifedipine rather than with a beta blocker such as propranolol. One also needs to be certain that recurrent chest pain after myocardial infarction is not due to pericarditis (which is treated with indomethacin or salicylates) or to some noncardiac problem such as atelectasis, pneumonia, pulmonary embolic disease, pancreatitis, peptic ulcer disease, cholecystitis, or emotion.

During the initial few hours after acute myocardial infarction, oxygen is usually administered by face mask or nasal cannula. Vital signs are checked frequently, chest pain is relieved with opiates, and sedatives are provided as necessary. Reassurance that the chest pain will be relieved and that survival will most likely occur is important. Specific complications of the acute myocardial infarction are recognized, using the clinical criteria described earlier and using methods described in more detail later in this chapter. Anticoagulants are not administered uniformly to patients with acute myocardial infarction. Some physicians use low dose heparin or warfarin to prevent the post–myocardial infarction complications related to prolonged bed rest and restricted activity. However, there is no convincing evidence that anticoagulants prevent recurrent myocardial infarction or specific ischemic complications of the infarction. Anticoagulants are contraindicated in the very elderly, in patients with severe hypertension, bleeding diatheses, or peptic ulcer disease, and in patients who develop pericarditis. Anticoagulants administered to patients with pericarditis complicating acute myocardial infarction may result in the development of hemorrhagic, large pericardial effusions and pericardial tamponade.

Smoking is prohibited in the coronary care unit, and one attempts to convince the patient to discontinue smoking altogether. The patient with an uncomplicated myocardial infarction is allowed to use a bedside commode, but those with shock, severe heart failure, or frequent and recurrent angina use a Foley catheter or bedpan. Stool softeners and laxatives are administered to prevent fecal impaction and to prevent the patient from straining to defecate.

Patients are allowed regular diets depending on their special needs, with the following exceptions: extremes of hot or cold beverages are avoided in the first two or three days, salt restriction is provided for those with important heart failure, low cholesterol diets are often used, and certain calorie and carbohydrate restrictions are provided for obese and diabetic patients, respectively. Diabetic patients receiving insulin are treated with regular insulin for the initial several days after their infarct.

Patients with uncomplicated myocardial infarction are usually discharged from the coronary care unit after four days to an "intermediate care" or "step down" unit. Such areas should be able to monitor heart rate and rhythm for several additional days. Most physicians begin a gradual rehabilitation program that encourages patients to be up in a chair several times a day beginning on approximately day four or five and to walk in their rooms and short distances in the hall outside their rooms by six to eight days after myocardial infarction. Patients with complications such as severe congestive heart failure, shock, important arrhythmias, or recurrent angina at rest or low levels of effort remain in the coronary care unit until they are stable.

Some physicians recommend relatively early discharge from the hospital, even by seven or eight days after the event for patients with uncomplicated myocardial infarctions. Other physicians feel that 12 to 14 days in the hospital are indicated even for those with uncomplicated myocardial infarctions. Patients with complicated myocardial infarctions remain in the hospital for at least 14 days and, depending on the severity of their complications, for as long as three to four weeks. Once at home, patients are gradually rehabilitated so that by four to six weeks they return to work and to a more normal life style. Resumption of sexual activity and mild exercise is allowed at approximately four weeks after myocardial infarction for asymptomatic patients. Angina that develops with minimal to moderate effort requires medical therapy with long-acting nitrates and, when appropriate, with a beta blocker or a calcium antagonist. Patients who continue to have symptoms at moderate or less effort on good medical regimens should undergo coronary arteriography and have coronary artery revascularization considered. Patients, with their physicians' help, should also be encouraged to correct all risk factors, including overweight, hypercholesterolemia, cigarette smoking, sedentary activity, and emotionally difficult circumstances. They should also be encouraged to get appropriate amounts of exercise in the future, but the exact type, duration, and level of effort should be guided by a responsible physician. Three recent studies have demonstrated that the beta-adrenergic antagonists timolol, metoprolol, and propranolol reduce mortality in selected patients with uncomplicated myocardial infarction when administered beginning soon after the myocardial infarction and continued for periods ranging from 90 days to 3 years. In addition, timolol has been shown to reduce the risk of reinfarction after myocardial infarction. More work is needed to identify specific patients most likely to benefit from beta blocker therapy, but it does appear that beta-adrenergic blockers have the potential to reduce mortality in selected patients with uncomplicated myocardial infarction.

Protection of Ischemic Myocardium and Containment of Infarct Size. There has been considerable interest in the possibility that one may limit infarct size with pharmacologic or physiologic interventions that reduce myocardial oxygen demand, increase myocardial oxygen delivery (increase coronary blood flow), reduce inflammatory processes, reduce or retard lysosomal enzyme release, or alter metabolism or calcium influx in such a way as to prevent cell death. In experimental animals, pharmacologic interventions that increase coronary blood flow to the ischemically injured tissue (particularly the subendocardial region) and those that reduce oxygen demands (particularly to the subendocardial region) have been effective in reducing the enzymatic, ECG, and morphologic indices of the size of experimentally induced myocardial infarction. Containment of infarct size depends on pharmacologic intervention within the first six hours after infarction. Beyond that time, some interventions are less successful or ineffective. In experimental animals, certain interventions may increase infarct size. This group includes those interventions that (1) increase myocardial oxygen demand, (2) divert coronary blood flow from the ischemic tissue, (3) reduce systemic arterial pressure and thereby coronary perfusion pressure, (4) alter myocardial metabolism in a detrimental manner, or (5) primarily decrease oxygen availability. In particular, the administration of isoproterenol or the development of hypotension, hypoglycemia, hypoxemia, and rapid heart rates results in an increase in infarct size in experimental animal models. Some of the interventions capable of limiting infarct size in experimental animal models are listed in Table 49–3.

TABLE 49–3. INTERVENTIONS CAPABLE OF LIMITING INFARCT SIZE IN EXPERIMENTAL ANIMAL MODELS

1. Interventions that reduce myocardial oxygen demand and myocardial work
   a. Beta blockers (propranolol)
   b. Calcium antagonists (nifedipine, verapamil, or diltiazem)
   c. Circulatory assistance (intra-aortic balloon counterpulsation)
2. Interventions that increase coronary blood flow to the damaged myocardium
   a. Nitrates (nitroglycerin)
   b. Calcium antagonists
   c. Hyperosmotic agents (hypertonic mannitol)*
   d. Hyaluronidase
   e. Corticosteroids
   f. Circulatory assistance
3. Agents that decrease inflammation, alter immunologic mechanisms, stabilize lysosomal membranes, and/or directly protect myocardial cells and sarcolemmal membranes
   a. Hyaluronidase
   b. Corticosteroids†
   c. Hypertonic agents (hypertonic mannitol)*
   d. Glucose, potassium, and insulin
   e. Cobra venom
   f. Calcium antagonists
   g. Chlorpromazine
   h. Anti-inflammatory agents (ibuprofen)

*Effective for approximately one hour after experimental coronary occlusion when serum osmolality is increased by 30 to 40 mOsm.

†Given in modest dosage and only once or twice.

Whether pharmacologic or physiologic interventions are capable of limiting infarct size in patients with acute myocardial infarction is at present unknown, but this possibility is receiving considerable attention. There are data suggesting that the administration of glucose, potassium, and insulin, the use of noninvasive circulatory assistance, and the administration of hyaluronidase are capable of limiting infarct size in patients. However, randomized, controlled double-blind studies of large numbers of patients are needed.

Coronary Artery Revascularization and Pharmacologic Dissolution of Coronary Thrombi. There is interest both in acute coronary artery revascularization and in pharmacologic intervention to lyse coronary thrombi in patients with acute myocardial infarcts as a means to limit infarct size. However, in experimental animals, release of a coronary artery occlusion following acute myocardial infarction may *limit* or fail to influence the extent of the infarct, depending on time factors. If release is accomplished within two hours of temporary coronary artery occlusion, one may achieve a reduction in infarct size as shown by improved regional function, reduced enzymatic indices of infarct size, and a reduction in the extent of damage as detected by morphologic evaluation. However, if release is performed after four hours, one may not find evidence for a reduction in ischemic damage and protection of regional ventricular function. In addition, "reperfusion arrhythmias" and extensive hemorrhagic infarction are well described following release of temporary coronary artery occlusion; both may occur with coronary occlusions as short as 40 to 60 minutes followed by reperfusion in experimental animals. Therefore extreme caution is indicated in patients with acute myocardial infarction, since late interventions could be harmful. The possibility that reperfusion following thrombolytic therapy within the initial 4 to 6 hours after the event improves or protects global and segmental ventricular function in patients with acute transmural myocardial infarcts is being extensively evaluated at the present time.

Indications for Coronary Artery Revascularization Following Acute Myocardial Infarction. There are several well-established indications for coronary artery revascularization following acute myocardial infarcts. Medically refractory angina following a myocardial infarct is one. However, one must be certain that recurrent chest pain after myocardial infarction is angina pectoris. If chest pain recurs frequently at rest or minimal effort or if angina pectoris is persistent, medical therapy is indicated; if that is unsuccessful, coronary artery surgery should be considered. Medical therapy includes nitrates; beta-blocking agents (when the recurrent chest pain is not thought to be due to coronary artery spasm); calcium antagonists (especially when there are relative contraindications to the use of beta-adrenergic blockers or when coronary artery spasm is present); circulatory assistance, including intra-aortic balloon counterpulsation in those patients with otherwise medically refractory angina; appropriate reduction in blood pressure if elevated; and sedation when indicated. However, with severe and recurrent or refractory angina pectoris after myocardial infarction, coronary arteriography and coronary artery revascularization should be considered. In some patients, such radical intervention is necessary within a few days after myocardial infarction, and in others recurrent chest pain develops weeks to months following the event. Relative risks of coronary artery revascularization are higher within the first month following infarction; but when absolutely necessary, surgery can be accomplished safely as early as a few days to one month after the coronary event.

Brown MS, Goldstein JL: Familial hypercholesterolemia. A genetic defect in the low-density lipoprotein receptor. N Engl J Med 294:1386, 1976. *A thorough review of the pathogenesis of this particular lipid abnormality.*

Brown MS, Goldstein JL: Receptor-mediated control of cholesterol metabolism. Science 191:150, 1976. *Detailed description of the cellular metabolism of cholesterol.*

Buja LM, Willerson JT: Clinicopathologic correlates of acute ischemic heart disease syndromes. Am J Cardiol 47:343, 1981. *Detailed postmortem pathophysiologic correlates of anatomic and clinical relationships.*

Corbett J, Dehmer GJ, Lewis SE, et al.: The prognostic value of submaximal exercise testing with radionuclide ventriculography following acute myocardial infarction. Circulation 64:535, 1981. *This study demonstrates the prognostic value of submaximal exercise testing coupled with dynamic myocardial scintigraphy in predicting prognosis for patients after their myocardial infarcts.*

Friedberg CK, Horn H: Acute myocardial infarction not due to coronary artery occlusion. JAMA 112:1675, 1939. *The title is self-explanatory.*

Gibson RS, Watson DD, Craddock GB, et al.: Prediction of cardiac events after uncomplicated myocardial infarction: A prospective study comparing predischarge exercise thallium-201 scintigraphy and coronary angiography. Circulation 68:321, 1984. *Thallium-201 myocardial scintigraphy with submaximal exercise at hospital discharge following myocardial infarction may be used to identify patients at risk for future ischemic heart disease complications.*

Hutchins GM, Bulkley BH: Infarct expansion versus extension: Two different complications of acute myocardial infarction. Am J Cardiol 41:1127, 1978. *The concept of "infarct expansion" is described.*

Maroko PR, Kjekshus JK, Sobel BE, et al.: Factors influencing infarct size following experimental coronary artery occlusion. Circulation 43:67, 1971. *The innovative study that emphasized that various pharmacologic interventions may either extend or limit the size of experimental myocardial infarcts.*

Maseri A, L'Abbate A, Baroldi G, et al.: Coronary vasospasm as a possible cause of myocardial infarction: A conclusion derived from the study of "preinfarction" angina. N Engl J Med 299:1271, 1978. *An interesting suggestion that coronary artery spasm may play a role in the pathogenesis of acute myocardial infarcts.*

Norwegian Multicenter Study Group: Timolol-induced reduction in mortality and reinfarction in patients surviving acute myocardial infarction. N Engl J Med 304:801, 1981.

Page DL, Caulfield JB, Kastor JA, DeSanctis RW, Sanders CA: Myocardial changes associated with cardiogenic shock. N Engl J Med 285:133, 1971. *Detailed postmortem analyses that show that "pump failure" consequences of myocardial infarcts occur when 40 per cent or more of the left ventricular muscle mass is irreversibly damaged.*

Pearson TA, Kramer EC, Solez K, Heptinstall RH: The human atherosclerotic plaque. Am J Pathol 86:657, 1977. *Detailed analysis of the characteristics of the human atherosclerotic plaque.*

Pitt B, Strauss HW: Current concepts: Evaluation of ventricular function by radioisotope technics. N Engl J Med 296:1097, 1977. *A thorough review of myocardial scintigraphic techniques.*

Roberts WC: Does thrombosis play a major role in the development of symptom-producing atherosclerotic plaques? Circulation 48:1161, 1973. *The title is self-explanatory.*

Ross R, Glomset JA: The pathogenesis of atherosclerosis. N Engl J Med 295:369, 1976. *A thorough analysis and suggested scheme to explain the pathogenesis of atherosclerosis.*

Rothkopf M, Boerner J, Stone M, et al.: Detection of myocardial infarction extension by CK-B radioimmunoassay. Circulation 59:268, 1979. *The frequency with which in-hospital extension of acute myocardial infarcts occurs is described in this study.*

Sobel BE, Bresnahan GF, Shell WE, Yoder RD: Estimation of infarct size in man and its relation to prognosis. Circulation 46:640, 1972. *The use of serial serum measurements of creatine kinase to estimate infarct size is described.*

Swan HJC, Ganz W, Forrester J, Marcus H, Diamond G, Chonette D: Catheterization of the heart in men with the use of a flow-directed balloon-tipped catheter. N Engl J Med 283:447, 1970. *The description of the development of the Swan-Ganz catheter.*

Trahern CA, Gere JB, Krauth GH, et al.: Clinical assessment of serum myosin light chains in the diagnosis of acute myocardial infarction. Am J Cardiol 41:641, 1978. *The use of serum measurements of the light chain of myosin to recognize acute myocardial infarcts is described.*

Wackers FJ, Busemann S, Samson G, et al.: Value and limitations of thallium-201 scintigraphy in the acute phase of myocardial infarction. N Engl J Med 295:1, 1975. *A description of the advantages and limitations of a "cold spot" imaging technique, thallium-201 myocardial scintigraphy, in infarct recognition.*

Weisfeldt ML, Flaherty JT: Myocardial infarction. *In* Willerson JT, Sanders CA (eds.): Clinical Cardiology. New York, Grune & Stratton, 1977, pp 346–369. *A thorough review of all aspects of acute myocardial infarction.*

Willerson JT, Parkey RW, Bonte FJ, Meyer SL, Atkins JM, Stokely EM: Technetium stannous pyrophosphate myocardial scintigrams in patients with chest pain of varying etiology. Circulation 51:1046, 1975. *The application and usefulness of an infarct-avid myocardial imaging technique, technetium-99m stannous pyrophosphate, in the recognition of acute myocardial infarcts is described.*

49.3. Sudden Cardiac Death

James T. Willerson

DEFINITION AND FREQUENCY. The definition of *sudden cardiac death* used in this chapter is the sudden cessation of effective cardiac contraction resulting from ventricular tachycardia–fibrillation or asystole. Sudden cardiac death claims approximately 1200 lives daily in the United States. It is the leading cause of death among men between the ages of 20 and 60, and approximately 25 per cent of patients dying suddenly have had no previously recognized symptoms of heart disease. Sudden cardiac death among women is approximately one fourth as frequent as among men.

ETIOLOGY AND PATHOGENESIS. Important data regarding the individual who suffers sudden cardiac death come from the Seattle Heart Watch study. During a six-year period of 1710 episodes of ventricular fibrillation, there were 346 long-term survivors. Cobb has shown that most instances of sudden cardiac death are not related to identifiable acute myocardial infarcts, which were detected by electrocardiography in only 19 per cent of patients hospitalized after resuscitation from ventricular fibrillation. Nevertheless, the majority of individuals resuscitated have extensive coronary artery disease, including 75 per cent with multivessel involvement. In addition, patients experiencing cardiac arrest without concomitant acute myocardial infarcts have a considerably higher incidence of recurrent sudden death in the next two years than do those with acute infarcts. The annual recurrence rate is approximately 30 per cent for those without acute infarcts.

It seems likely that the most critical etiologic factor is electrophysiologic instability related to chronic ischemic heart disease, to cellular damage associated with cardiomyopathy, or to chronic severe valvular heart disease. Since the frequency of recurrence of sudden death is high in those with chronic ischemic heart disease without acute infarcts, it is important to protect such patients with antiarrhythmic agents and, when appropriate, also with coronary artery revascularization.

Most patients with sudden death have chronic ischemic heart disease or chronic myocardial scarring and ventricular dysfunction. However, sudden death from ventricular arrhythmias occurs in some individuals with mitral valve prolapse, in some with left ventricular outflow obstruction, including valvular aortic stenosis and asymmetric septal hypertrophy, and in some with hereditary prolongation of the Q-T interval with or without associated deafness. Sudden death also occurs in individuals with various cardiomyopathies, in those with chronic valvular insufficiency and myocardial dilatation and/or hypertrophy, in those with cardiac tamponade, in some young athletes while they are exercising, and in an occasional individual suddenly aroused or frightened by an external event. Sudden death from a ventricular arrhythmia may also occur in the Wolff-Parkinson-White syndrome, in those with advanced atrioventricular block without pacemakers, or with diffuse conduction system disease ("sick sinus syndrome"), and in severe electrolyte alterations, including hypokalemia, hyperkalemia, and hypercalcemia. Drug overdose, particularly with cardiac glycosides, may also be a cause for sudden cardiac death. Additional causes for sudden death or death within a few hours that do not initially involve the heart include intracerebral or subarachnoid hemorrhage, pulmonary emboli, severe drug overdose, hypoxia associated with chronic obstructive lung disease or lung injury, dissecting aortic aneurysms, and rupture of an aortic aneurysm.

In order to reduce the frequency and risk of sudden death in susceptible individuals, at least two additional developments are needed: (1) better means to identify those at risk and (2) better understanding of mechanisms involved in ventricular tachycardia or fibrillation in susceptible patients. Although most patients who experience sudden death have heart disease, the risk factors for atherosclerosis do not singly or in combination identify a subset of patients prone to sudden death. The mechanism of sudden death is ordinarily ventricular fibrillation.

IDENTIFICATION OF HIGH-RISK PATIENTS. In patients with acute infarction, certain types of ventricular premature beats are considered precursors of ventricular fibrillation. In coronary care units, more than seven ventricular premature beats per minute, multiform ventricular premature beats, ventricular premature beats occurring on or close to the apex of the T wave, and runs of two or more ventricular premature beats are considered potential harbingers of ventricular tachycardia or fibrillation. These "malignant ventricular premature beats" are ordinarily suppressed by pharmacologic agents such as xylocaine. However, some patients with acute myocardial infarcts have ventricular tachycardia or fibrillation without precursor ventricular arrhythmias. Moreover, there is a relationship between recurrent ventricular tachycardia or fibrillation and the overall size of myocardial infarcts such that patients with large infarcts may have recurrent ventricular (and supraventricular) arrhythmias.

In patients with chronic ischemic heart disease, only advanced grades or complex ventricular premature beats predict sudden cardiac death. The frequency of sudden death and of ventricular premature complexes increases with age. In addition, the frequency of ventricular premature beats increases in relationship to the extent of ventricular damage from earlier myocardial infarcts. Ventricular ectopic activity is more frequent and more complex in patients with multivessel coronary artery disease than in those with only single vessel involvement. Therefore, a knowledge of the extent of coronary disease and of ventricular dysfunction may be useful in predicting sudden death. Patients with a left ventricular ejection function <40 per cent and (a) frequent ventricular premature beats (≧ 10/minute) and/or (b) complex ventricular premature beats have a several fold increased risk of sudden death in the initial six months after myocardial infarction. An increased risk has also been claimed for patients demonstrating repetitive ventricular beating following ventricular stimulation. Dynamic myocardial scintigraphic characterization of ventricular function at rest and during submaximal exercise in patients with acute infarction prior to hospital discharge may identify those most at risk for important additional ischemic events. Increasing in popularity are techniques that determine the efficacy of a particular antiarrhythmic regimen prior to hospital discharge in patients at risk. Such approaches include electrophysiologic studies in a cardiac catheterization laboratory, which test individual vulnerability for sustained ventricular arrhythmias while on and off selected antiarrhythmic regimens. This approach is important because merely administering an antiarrhythmic agent to a patient with the hope of preventing fatalities is often not successful. Schaffer and Cobb (1975) reported that 73 per cent of 64 patients with recurrent ventricular fibrillation were receiving antiarrhythmic therapy at the time of sudden death. This emphasizes the need to select and optimize antiarrhythmic therapy for the individual patient. It is also important to realize that antiarrhythmic agents, particularly quinidine and pronestyl, given in excess or given in normal doses to the patient with a prolonged QT interval, may cause life-threatening ventricular arrhythmias, including a ventricular tachycardia known as "torsade de pointes."

PREVENTION OF SUDDEN DEATH. It is critically important that we develop an improved understanding of mechanisms that initiate and sustain life-threatening ventricular arrhythmias in patients in diverse clinical settings. Unanswered questions include the following: Does platelet aggregation play a role in sudden death in those with ischemic heart disease in the absence of identifiable acute myocardial infarction? Are the important ventricular arrhythmias that develop with acute myocardial ischemia related primarily to re-entrant mechanisms or to increased ventricular automaticity resulting in part from variations in regional concentrations of potassium or catecholamines, from alterations in autonomic nervous system activity, from alterations in adrenergic receptor numbers or affinity, or from local accumulation of phospholipid degradation products, e.g., lysophosphatidyl choline? It is important to determine why some individuals with chronic congestive heart failure and others with chronic cardiomegaly and ventricular dysfunction are at risk of sudden death from ventricular arrhythmias. It is not clear at present whether increased triglyceride uptake and the inability of injured myocardial cells to metabolize long chain fatty acids contribute to the ventricular arrhythmias of ischemic heart disease. Specific myocardial cellular mechanisms associated with increased risk of ventricular arrhythmias need to be elucidated, as does the role of psychologic stress in the initiation of ventricular arrhythmias in man.

Extensive efforts are being made to develop more effective means of correcting recurrent and life-threatening ventricular arrhythmias. New antiarrhythmic agents are being developed and tested, but still unavailable is one or more agents with (a) marked efficacy against ventricular and supraventricular arrhythmias, (b) few or no important side effects, and (c) the need for relatively infrequent administration, i.e., once per day. In addition, surgical resection of ventricular sites of ectopic impulse formation has been utilized following epicardial and endocardial "activation mapping." Clinical experience has also emphasized the value of aggressive treatment of "malignant" ventricular arrhythmias with procainamide. Improved control of ventricular arrhythmias is achieved with doses sufficient either to correct the arrhythmia or to produce QRS and/or QT widening (≦25 per cent) or other side effects, at which time the dosage is reduced or another antiarrhythmic agent is chosen. Mirowski has developed an implantable automatic defibrillator for use by the patient to convert his own tachyrhythmia. This device is potentially important, allowing conversion of ventricular arrhythmias when adequate control is not provided by antiarrhythmic agents. Implantable programmable pacemakers capable of sensing and correcting ventricular tachyrhythmias by rapid and brief pacing have also been developed. Thus, methodologic advances are making available increasingly powerful means of preventing sudden cardiac death in patients documented as being at risk.

Bigger JT, Jr., Fleiss JL, Kleiger R, et al.: The relationships among ventricular arrhythmias, left ventricular dysfunction, and mortality in the 2 years after myocardial infarction. Circulation 69:250, 1984. *A thorough review of these relationships.*

Calvert A, Lown B, Gorlin R: Ventricular premature beats and anatomically defined coronary heart disease. Am J Cardiol 39:627, 1977. *A review of these relationships.*

Cobb LA, Baun RS, Alvarez H III, Schaffer WA: Resuscitation from out-of-hospital ventricular fibrillation: 4 year follow-up. Circulation 51, 52: Suppl III:III–223, 1975. *A follow-up of patients following resuscitation from sudden death.*

Doyle JT, Kannel WB, McNamara RM, Quickenton P, Gordon T: Factors related to the suddenness of death from coronary disease: Combined Albany-Framingham Studies. Am J Cardiol 37:1073, 1976. *An epidemiologic study of factors involved in sudden death.*

Horowitz LN, Harken AH, Kastor JA, Josephson ME: Ventricular resection guided by epicardial and endocardial mapping for treatment of recurrent ventricular tachycardia. N Engl J Med 302:589, 1980. *Aggressive but effective surgical techniques for abolishing ventricular rhythm disturbances are described.*

Kannel WB, Doyle JT, McNamara PM, Quickenton P, Gordon T: Precursors of sudden coronary death. Factors related to incidence of sudden death. Circulation 51:606, 1975. *A review of risk factors related to sudden death.*

Lie KI, Wellens HJ, van Capelle FJ, et al.: Lidocaine in the prevention of primary ventricular fibrillation. N Engl J Med 291:1324, 1974. *A description of the usefulness of lidocaine in suppressing ventricular arrhythmias.*

Lown B: Sudden cardiac death: The major challenge confronting contemporary cardiology. Am J Cardiol 43:313, 1979. *A thorough review of this subject.*

Mason JW, Winkle RA: Electrode-catheter arrhythmia induction in the selection and assessment of antiarrhythmic drug therapy for recurrent ventricular tachycardia. Circulation 58:971, 1978. *A description of an invasive technique for establishing the efficacy of antiarrhythmic agents.*

Mirowski M, Reid PR, Mower MM, et al.: Termination of malignant ventricular arrhythmias in man with an implanted defibrillator. N Engl J Med 303:322, 1980. *The development of an implantable defibrillator is described.*

Ruberman W, Weinblatt E, Goldberg JD, Frank CW, Shapiro S: Ventricular premature beats and mortality after myocardial infarction. N Engl J Med 297:750, 1977. *A review of the relationship between premature ventricular beats and death with myocardial infarction.*

The Anturane Reinfarction Trial Research Group: Sulfinpyrazone in the prevention of cardiac death after myocardial infarction. N Engl J Med 298:289, 1978. *A cooperative trial that obtained data suggesting that Anturane is capable of reducing the frequency of sudden death in the first few months after myocardial infarcts.*

Willerson JT: Prevention and control of ventricular arrhythmias. N Engl J Med 303:332, 1980 (editorial). *A review of the prevention and control of sudden death.*

49.4. Surgical Treatment of Coronary Artery Disease

David C. Sabiston, Jr.

The development of coronary artery bypass grafts (CABG) has made a remarkable impact upon the management of ischemic heart disease. Significant numbers of patients with symptomatic coronary disease have undergone this procedure, and it is currently the most common operation performed in cardiac surgery. Complete relief of anginal pain is achieved in more than two thirds of patients following CABG, and the procedure increases the life span in certain groups of patients. For such lesions as significant stenosis of the left main coronary artery, the life expectancy is greatly improved, and therefore CABG is routinely recommended for patients with this lesion, as well as most patients with triple vessel disease for a similar reason (Fig. 49–5).

The *natural history* of coronary atherosclerosis is of considerable importance in selection of the appropriate therapeutic approach, and a number of factors are of significance in evaluating the prognosis. These factors include the number of coronary arteries involved, the severity and extent of the atherosclerotic lesions, the status of left ventricular performance, and the presence of associated cardiac disorders such as a valvular lesion or a ventricular aneurysm. The prognosis of patients with angina pectoris is adversely affected by certain factors, including a familial history of coronary disease, cigarette smoking, hypertension, diabetes, and obesity.

The overall mortality for patients with angina pectoris was formerly thought to approximate 5 per cent annually, although in more recent reports the prognosis has become more favorable. For example, in the Coronary Artery Surgery Study (CASS), a randomized multicenter evaluation sponsored by the NIHLB (1975–1979) provided an objective evaluation of patients with Class I and II angina who were less than 65 years of age, had not had a history of congestive heart failure or previous CABG, and had an ejection fraction of greater than 35 per cent. In that series, the annual mortality for single-, double-, and triple-vessel disease was 1.1, 0.6, and 1.2 per cent, respectively, and comparable figures for the surgical group were 0.8, 0.8, and 1.2 per cent. However, it should be emphasized that this group represents a subset of the more favorable patients (Mock et al.). These data for *medically* treated patients have also been confirmed by others (Pryor et al.). The improved results with medical management are probably due to greater intensification of medical therapy such as beta blockers and nitrates, and more recently through the use of calcium channel blockers. Moreover, patients have become more aware of the signficance of the basic risk factors in coronary artery disease, and attention to these has probably had a positive effect. However, if one considers those patients in the larger part of the study including Class III and IV angina, there were less favorable rates of survival, with the four-year survival rate for one-vessel, two-vessel, and three-vessel disease being approximately 92, 84, and 68 per cent. This would represent an "annual mortality" of some 2, 4, and 8 per cent. Therefore, considerable attention should be given the *specific characteristics* of each patient in evaluating his total risk, whether managed medically or surgically (CASS). The results of the CASS study are somewhat at variance with the European Coronary Surgery Study Group (Varnauskas). This study of randomized patients convincingly demonstrated that coronary bypass, if technically feasible, was significantly superior to medical treatment, with a survival of 95 per cent in patients with three-vessel disease in the surgical group, compared with 81 per cent in those treated medically.

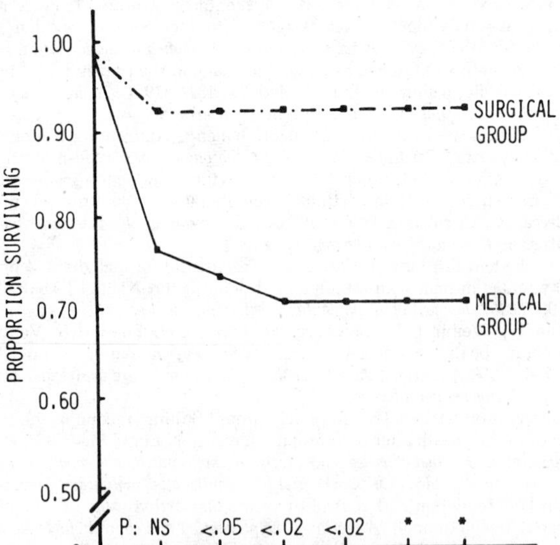

Figure 49–5. Accumulative survival rates of 83 patients with significant lesions of the left main coronary artery, who were randomly allocated into medical or surgical treatment groups in 1972, 1973, and 1974. There were 41 patients in the medical group and 42 patients in the surgical group. (From Takaro T, Hultgren HN, Lipton MJ, Detre KM, and Participants in the Study Group: Circulation [Suppl 3] 54:107, 1976.)

SELECTION OF PATIENTS FOR SURGICAL THERAPY. Although it is difficult to state precisely the number of patients who are appropriate candidates for myocardial revascularization, it is generally estimated that some 25 per cent of patients with angina pectoris do not obtain satisfactory pain relief by pharmacologic means alone. In addition, the annual mortality in medically treated series in certain groups is sufficiently high to warrant CABG for this reason. The most common indication for CABG is *relief of anginal pain.* Myocardial revascularization is also indicated for other manifestations of ischemic heart disease, including refractory cardiac dysrhythmias, preinfarction angina, and congestive heart failure in the presence of a ventricular aneurysm.

The role of noninvasive radionuclide angiocardiography in selection of patients for CABG has expanded greatly in the past several years. This rapid, safe, and relatively simple technique makes possible the determination of a number of factors for the objective evaluation of ventricular function, including end-systolic and end-diastolic ventricular volumes, ejection fraction, cardiac output, and left ventricular wall motion. These parameters may be determined both *at rest* and *during exercise.* Patients with significant coronary artery disease may have essentially normal values at rest, but deterioration of cardiac function can often be documented during exercise. Thallium and technetium scans, which demonstrate ischemia during exertion, and ventricular function studies, which may demonstrate a deterioration of ejection fraction and local abnormalities of wall motion, enhance the ability to recognize ischemia by noninvasive techniques. Such studies have been quite helpful in screening those patients who require coronary arteriography and cardiac catheterization for more complete evaluation of cardiac function and the choice of medical versus surgical therapy (Jones RH, et al.).

Coronary arteriography is essential in the selection of patients for CABG. The diseased vessels to be grafted should have a reasonable lumen, and whenever possible the distal runoff should indicate a patent peripheral coronary bed. A coronary artery suitable for anastomosis should have a diameter of at least 1 mm. If extensive intrinsic disease is present in the distal coronary arteries, the postoperative result is apt to be unsatisfactory. Fortunately, in 80 per cent or more of patients with symptomatic coronary disease the anatomy is appropriate for direct aortocoronary grafts. The majority of surgical candidates have several significant lesions in the proximal portions of the major coronary arteries. In patients with *complete* occlusion of a proximal coronary artery, arteriography may not demonstrate a distal patent coronary artery by way of collateral channels even though a patent vessel may be present. Experience both at the time of operation and in postmortem studies has indicated that at the time of coronary arteriography the collateral circulation may be inadequate to opacify the vessel distal to a complete occlusion.

Both cardiac catheterization and noninvasive radionuclide arteriography provide helpful data for assessment of ventricular function. Certain features are apt to be associated with an *increased* surgical risk; these include cardiomegaly, a low ejection fraction (below 25 per cent), an increased left ventricular volume, a large arteriovenous oxygen difference (greater than 6 volumes per cent), and, to a lesser extent, an elevated left ventricular end-diastolic pressure. However, the presence of any one or a combination of these abnormalities does not necessarily represent a contraindication to operation or to a successful postoperative result.

Left ventricular *aneurysms* may follow myocardial infarction and are hazardous both for the paradoxical dilatation which occurs during systole, producing cardiac inefficiency, and as a source of systemic arterial emboli. These aneurysms may also be the site of electrical instability and cause refractory dysrhythmias.

Patients with impending myocardial infarction (preinfarction or unstable angina) may be candidates for urgent CABG. Although many patients with unstable angina can be managed by intensive pharmacologic therapy, CABG may be preferable if the anginal pain cannot be rapidly controlled.

In a recent study of 100 consecutive patients with atypical angina on the Coronary Care Unit, relief of anginal pain could not be obtained despite the use of intravenous nitroglycerin, propranolol, and nifedipine. Therefore, CABG was undertaken. In this group, 52 had a myocardial infarction (6 hours to 30 days prior to operation) and 75 had serious disease as evidenced by either left main or three-vessel disease or an injection fraction less than 45 per cent. The operative mortality in this group was only 4 per cent, indicating that the procedure can be undertaken even in severely ill patients with expectation of outstanding results (Rankin et al.).

Interest continues in an effort to reduce the mortality of *acute* myocardial infarction associated with intractable *shock*. An immediate CABG has been performed in selected patients, often combined with resection of a portion of the left ventricle for either severe dyskinesia or aneurysm formation. The intra-aortic balloon pump for diastolic augmentation is usually employed simultaneously.

Acute myocardial infarction may be associated with several complications that are often best managed by surgical means. An acquired ventricular septal defect (VSD) occurs in 1 to 2 per cent of patients following myocardial *infarction*. The prognosis is poor, with the survival being only 20 per cent at two months if operation is not done. Surgical closure is indicated in nearly all patients. When the cardiovascular status permits, it is preferable to allow the infarct to heal as much as possible, so that the edges of the defect become fibrotic and enable a better operative repair. Intractable cardiac failure often follows the development of postinfarction VSD, and early or even urgent operation may become necessary. *Multiple* VSDs are present in approximately a third of patients and should be carefully sought at operation. The defects are generally closed with a plastic prosthesis, and CABG may be necessary to provide adequate coronary blood flow. If early operation is mandatory, the results are less favorable than in those patients who are able to survive for several weeks and undergo an elective operative procedure.

SURGICAL PROCEDURES. For most patients undergoing CABG, an *autologous vein* is anastomosed between the ascending aorta and the coronary artery distal to the obstruction. The saphenous vein from the thigh or leg is usually chosen, and the vessel is reversed to permit flow in the direction of open valves. Extracorporeal circulation is used to ensure a quiet heart and to permit a careful coronary arterial anastomosis to be performed. Moderate total body hypothermia is used in conjunction with extracorporeal circulation, and generally the temperature of the heart is further lowered by infusion of a potassium solution at 4° C to produce cardioplegia. In order to maintain a myocardial temperature of 10 to 15° C, cold saline or ice slush is usually introduced to surround the heart. The objective of the intracoronary injection of potassium solution is to eliminate cardiac contraction totally and, together with hypothermia, to reduce myocardial metabolism to a very low level. Cardioplegic solution produces a flaccid and motionless heart that enhances the ease of the operative procedure. Meticulous attention to detail is essential in performing the anastomosis if a good postoperative result is to be obtained. The use of very fine, monofilament sutures, often placed with the use of magnifying lenses, has been helpful in achieving long-term patency in these small vessels. Comparative data also show that *all* major coronary arteries with significant stenoses should be grafted. In addition, branches of the primary vessels are also frequently bypassed beyond significant stenoses.

POSTOPERATIVE MANAGEMENT. A number of postoperative problems may arise in patients following myocardial revascularization and require prompt diagnosis and immediate therapy. Adequate oxygenation is essential, and the endotracheal tube is generally left in place for assurance of adequate ventilation by the respirator until it is apparent that early postoperative complications have not developed. The effectiveness of the ventilatory support should be assessed by blood gas measurements, including PO_2, PCO_2, and pH. The cardiac output should be maintained at a normal level by continuous monitoring of central venous pressure, systemic arterial pressure, the electrocardiogram, and urinary output. Determinations of cardiac output are also important, especially if doubt exists concerning the circulatory status. Should a *low cardiac output syndrome* develop postoperatively, dopamine, dobutamine, and other agents should be employed as necessary with careful and continuous monitoring. In many patients pulmonary artery diastolic pressure is continuously monitored during the early postoperative period, and a direct reading of left atrial pressure through an indwelling catheter placed at operation may be helpful, particularly in patients with poor left ventricular function. Cardiac dysrhythmias are common and may require the use of appropriate drugs, pacing, or electrical cardioversion.

Myocardial infarction following CABG is usually reported in the range of 5 to 10 per cent. The incidence is largely dependent upon the sensitivity of the tests employed for diagnosis. For example, when CPK-MB isoenzyme activity is determined, the incidence of intraoperative and perioperative myocardial infarction is higher, since it is very sensitive. This contrasts with an incidence of less than 10 per cent if new Q waves are used. Moreover, in most patients in whom perioperative infarction occurs, the clinical manifestations are minimal and the diagnosis is made primarily upon ECG and enzymatic changes. It is relatively unusual for such patients to experience the signs and symptoms of a clinical myocardial infarction in the characteristic sense. In fact, in the majority of these patients, the infarction might well be unrecognized were it not for the changes in serum enzymes and in the ECG.

RESULTS. The operative mortality has fallen considerably in the last several years and is currently in the range of 1 to 2 per cent for patients with *uncomplicated* angina pectoris. The mortality is higher in those patients with severe left ventricular dysfunction, ventricular aneurysms, or associated valvular disease.

RELIEF OF PAIN. In nearly all series, an excellent symptomatic response is obtained and in some two thirds of patients the angina is *completely* relieved with no further medication being required, and much improvement occurs in an additional 25 per cent. With the passage of time, progressive pathologic changes may occur in some of the vessels, both in the native coronary arteries and in the inserted grafts. Such changes may be responsible for reappearance of symptoms. When these are present, further clinical evaluation, including coronary arteriography, is indicated.

GRAFT PATENCY. The patency rate of venous grafts during the first year following operation approximates 90 per cent. Later, intimal fibrosis may occur in the vein graft and reduce its caliber or produce complete obstruction. The graft may also thrombose, and this is generally the cause of *early* graft failure. In addition, technical features at the site of the anastomosis, such as kinking of the graft, can produce obstruction. A distinctive fibrous proliferation that occurs in these grafts is a common cause of occlusion. The basic atherosclerotic process may progress in the coronary arteries. In one series followed one to four years postoperatively with repeat arteriography, 55 per cent of the original lesions *proximal* to the graft progressed. In this series, 14 per cent of the ungrafted vessels showed progression of atherosclerosis (McLaughlin et al.).

REOPERATION. If symptoms recur following myocardial revascularization, reoperation may be indicated. While the technical procedure is somewhat more difficult, nevertheless favorable results can be predicted in the majority of such patients. In one series of 1000 consecutive patients undergoing reoperation for CABG, the surgical mortality declined from 5 per cent early in the series to 2 per cent at present, and during the same period the number of grafts added at the second operation increased from 1.4 to 2.3 (Loop et al.). The five-year actuarial survival for patients was 89 per cent and was affected by the extent of disease and preoperative level of ventricular performance.

PERCUTANEOUS TRANSLUMINAL CORONARY ANGIOPLASTY. Percutaneous transluminal coronary angioplasty (PTCA) was first performed in 1977, and more procedures are being done each year. A recent analysis by a center that does large numbers of both CABG and PTCA indicates an appropriate role for both depending upon the indications. PTCA may be indicated in patients with early clinical manifestations, especially single-vessel disease, and particularly those who have good left ventricular function. There is an intermediate group in which it has not been definitely decided which of the two techniques is preferable. For patients with multiple-vessel disease, especially those with compromised left ventricular function, CABG appears preferable (Jones EL, et al.).

RESULTS OF MEDICAL VERSUS SURGICAL MANAGEMENT IN RANDOMIZED STUDIES. The conclusion reached from nearly all studies involving left main coronary disease indicates longer survival in surgical patients than in those managed medically. For patients with triple-vessel disease, the European Cooperative Study indicated improved survival in those patients managed surgically, whereas the conclusion drawn from the CASS Study was that there is no statistical difference in survival (Class I and II) between the two types of therapy. Other groups have provided evidence that surgical management of both double- and triple-vessel disease provides greater longevity than medical therapy alone (Hurst et al.). Further evaluation and more updated randomized trials will be likely to provide more definitive data on this issue.

Austen WG, McEnany MT: The role of surgery in the treatment of patients with complications of acute myocardial infarction. World J Surg 2:709, 1978. *This is a thorough review of the complications of acute myocardial infarction amenable to surgical therapy. Rupture of the interventricular septum, acute mitral regurgitation, severe dysrhythmias, and the management of intractable shock following acute myocardial infarction are all discussed in detail.*

CASS Principal Investigators and their Associates: Coronary artery surgery study (CASS): A randomized trial of coronary artery bypass surgery survival data. Circulation 68:939, 1983. *The CASS study includes a multicenter patient registry and randomized control clinical trial in patients with stable ischemic heart disease assigned to either medical or surgical management. The group as a whole was low risk from the point of view of annual mortality, and the survival in the surgical group for single-, double-, and triple-vessel disease was essentially the same as that in the medically managed group.*

Hurst JW, King SB III, Logue RB, Hatcher CR Jr, Jones EL, Craver JM, Douglas JS Jr, Franch RH, Dorney ER, Cobbs BW Jr, Robinson PH, Clements SD Jr, Kaplan JA, Bradford JM: Value of coronary bypass surgery. Controversies in cardiology: Part I. Am J Cardiol 42:308, 1978. *This is a very comprehensive review of published data concerning the relative roles of medical and surgical treatment of angina pectoris. The authors conclude that the data support the concept that, compared with modern medical therapy, properly performed coronary bypass procedures appear to prolong the life of patients with left main, triple-, or double-vessel coronary artery disease.*

Jones EL, Craver JM, Guyton RA, Bone DK, Hatcher CR Jr: Trends in the treatment of coronary disease today. Selective use of PTCA and bypass surgery. Ann Surg 197:728, 1983. *This is an updated review of the selection and treatment of patients for revascularization by percutaneous transluminal coronary angioplasty as contrasted with coronary artery bypass grafts. More percutaneous angioplasties are performed in this institution than in any other in the United States at this time, and their data demonstrate that both PTCA and CABG may be accomplished with a low perioperative complication rate and low hospital mortality. The indications for each approach are reviewed.*

Jones RH, Floyd RD, Austin EH, Sabiston DC Jr: The role of radionuclide angiocardiography in the preoperative prediction of pain relief and prolonged survival following coronary artery bypass grafting. Ann Surg 197:743, 1983. *In this study, the authors evaluate the usefulness of radionuclide angiocardiography in the selection and prognosis of a group of patients with coronary artery disease. Calculations comparing the maximal potential increase in survival and complete pain relief, using multiple criteria known to provide prognostic information, identified the exercise response on RNA as the single most important variable for selection of therapy.*

Loop FD, Lytle BW, Gill CC, Golding LAR, Cosgrove DM, Taylor PC: Trends in selection and results of coronary artery reoperations. Ann Thorac Surg 36:380, 1983. *This is the largest series yet reported of patients undergoing reoperation for myocardial revascularization. Emphasis is placed upon the fact that the mortality is now relatively low, despite the technical difficulties encountered in some of these procedures, and in addition the results are quite favorable.*

McLaughlin PR, Berman ND, Morton BC, McLoughlin MJ, Aldridge HE, Adelman AG, Goldman BS, Trimble AS, Morch JE: Saphenous vein bypass grafting. Changes in native circulation and collaterals. Circulation (Suppl 1) 51–52:66, 1975. *This is a carefully performed study of the continuing changes that occur in the coronary circulation after an initial diagnosis of stenotic atherosclerotic coronary disease. It emphasizes the need for continuing attention directed toward prevention of the basic process in addition to surgical therapy.*

Mock MB, Ringqvist I, Fisher LD, David KB, Chaitman BR, Kouchoukos NT, Kaiser GC, Alderman E, Ryan TJ, Russell RO Jr, Mullin S, Fray D, Killip T III, and Participants in the Coronary Artery Surgery Study: Survival of medically treated patients in the coronary artery surgery study (CASS) registry. Circulation 66:562, 1982. *This is an evaluation of the impact on survival of anatomic extent of obstructive coronary disease and of left ventricular performance. The four-year survival of medically treated patients with no significant obstructive disease was 97 per cent, in contrast to 92, 84, and 68 per cent in patients with one-, two-, and three-vessel disease, respectively. The presence of left main coronary disease decreased survival. Patients with good left ventricular function had survivals of 94, 91, and 79 per cent for one-, two-, and three-vessel disease, respectively, compared with those with poor left ventricular function, in whom the survival at four years was 67, 61, and 42 per cent, respectively, for one-, two-, and three-vessel disease.*

Pryor DB, Harrell FE Jr, Lee KL, Califf RM, Rosati RA: An improving prognosis over time in medically treated patients with coronary artery disease. Am J Cardiol 52:444, 1983. *This study emphasizes that the national mortality from coronary heart disease has decreased during the past decade. This decrease cannot be explained only by the fact that less ill patients are being evaluated, but is due at least in part to the decrease of coronary heart disease mortality in the past decade.*

Rankin JS, Newton JR, Califf RM, Jones RH, Wechsler AS, Oldham HN, Wolfe WG, Lowe JE: Management of medically refractory unstable angina. Circulation, in press. *A unique series of seriously ill patients, all on the Coronary Care Unit with refractory unstable angina, in whom coronary artery bypass procedures were performed with unusually high survival rates.*

Sabiston DC Jr: The coronary circulation. The William F. Rienhoff, Jr, Lecture. Johns Hopkins Med J 134:314, 1974. *A review of the anatomic, physiologic, and pathologic aspects of the coronary circulation. The data presented are based upon experimental and clinical findings in the normal and pathologic coronary circulation and their relationships to the surgical management of coronary artery disease.*

Varnauskas E: Prospective randomized study of coronary artery bypass surgery in stable angina pectoris: A progress report on survival. Circulation 65:11–67, 1982. *This is the report of the European Coronary Surgery Study Group reporting a four-year randomized study in patients treated either surgically or medically. This study showed an increase in the survival time in patients with three-vessel disease managed surgically in whom a technically feasible coronary artery bypass was possible.*

50. CARDIAC ARRHYTHMIAS

John J. Gallagher

The sinoatrial (SA) node is normally the dominant cardiac pacemaker because it has the most rapid inherent rate of discharge (i.e., highest degree of automaticity). Impulses arising regularly in the sinus node at the rate of 60 to 100 per minute result in atrial contraction followed by ventricular contraction. The heart rate is primarily related to the metabolic activity of the body, and a linear relationship exists between heart rate and oxygen consumption. Optimal hemodynamic function is achieved when atrial contractions are coupled at a critical interval to ventricular contractions as a result of the orderly transmission of the sinus node impulse to the ventricles over specialized conducting tissue (i.e., atrioventricular [AV] node, bundle of His, bundle branches, and subendocardial Purkinje networks).

Deviations from this normal order of events may occur, resulting in an *arrhythmia*. These may include abnormalities in rate or regularity of the heart beat and also any situation in which the sequence of a normal atrial activation coupled at a physiologic interval to normal ventricular activation is disturbed whether or not rate or rhythm is disturbed.

ANATOMY OF THE CONDUCTION SYSTEM. Pacemaker function normally resides in the sinus node, which is situated on the anterolateral margin of the junction of the superior vena cava and the right atrium. The sinus node is a tapering cylindrical structure 15 × 3 × 2 mm in size, and surrounds the sinus node artery, which arises from either the proximal 3 cm of the right coronary artery (60 per cent) or the left circumflex coronary artery (40 per cent). Controversy surrounds the anatomic and electrophysiologic data which propose the existence of pathways between the SA node and AV node (i.e., anterior, middle, and posterior internodal pathways). These portions of the atria undoubtedly play some role in the transmission of the impulse from the sinus node to the AV node. What is unclear is whether they do so in the sense of specialized conducting tissues or simply represent apparent preferential routes of conduction owing to the anatomic grouping of fibers in these areas.

Normally the ordinary or so-called working myocardial cells of the atria and ventricles are linked to each other in only one site: the AV junctional area. In this region, cells histologically distinct from ordinary working myocardial cells permit electrical activity to pass between atria and ventricles, which are otherwise electrically insulated from each other by connective tissue and fat. Atrial muscle fibers are intimately related to the atrioventricular node, which lies in the base of the interatrial septum just above the tricuspid annulus, 1 to 2 cm anterior to the orifice of the coronary sinus. The AV node receives important contributions from the left as well as the right side of the atrial septum. Conduction velocity within the AV node is slow (0.05 meter per second), compared to that of ordinary myocardium (0.8 to 1.0 meter per second) or His-Purkinje tissue (1 to 3 meters per second), resulting in physiologic AV delay reflected in the normal P-R interval. Microscopically the AV node is characterized by small diameter fibers with a loosely arranged interweaving architecture. The AV node is supplied in 90 per cent of cases by the posterior descending coronary artery, accounting for the frequent association of conduction disturbances in the AV node with diaphragmatic myocardial infarction; in the remaining cases the AV node receives its blood supply from the left circumflex coronary artery.

The bundle of His emerges from the anteroinferior border of the AV node and penetrates the central fibrous body, which represents a confluence of connective tissue in the region of the aortic, tricuspid, and mitral valve rings. The penetrating portion of the bundle of His is enveloped by connective tissue of the fibrous body and then courses forward along the membranous interventricular septum to the top of the muscular interventricular septum. The His bundle is approximately 15 mm long from its origin to its branching point and constitutes the only normal connection between atria and ventricles. Because of its intimate relationship to the cardiac skeleton, including the mitral and aortic valve, degenerative changes in these areas can readily lead to AV block.

The branching portion of the bundle of His begins with the emergence of the His bundle from the central fibrous body. The left bundle branch cascades as a sheet of fibers onto the left side of the interventricular septum. The configuration of these fibers is somewhat variable. It has been clinically useful to consider the left bundle branch as being composed of two major fascicles—the left anterior and left posterior fascicles—although anatomically no such discrete subdivisions can be identified. Indeed, extensive interconnections exist between these two groups, constituting what might be considered the septal division of the left bundle branch. After giving rise to the left bundle branch, the branching portion of the bundle of His continues as the right bundle branch. Both bundle branch systems subdivide extensively, ultimately forming the lacy networks on the endocardial surfaces of both ventricles known as the Purkinje system. The His bundle derives its blood supply from two sources, the AV nodal artery and the first septal perforator of the left anterior descending branch of the left coronary artery. In 50 per cent of cases, the right bundle branch has a two-fold blood supply: the AV nodal artery and the first septal perforator of the left anterior descending coronary artery; in the other 50 per cent, the right bundle branch derives its blood from a single source, the first septal perforator of the left anterior descending coronary artery. The anterior fascicle of the left bundle branch has the same blood supply as the right bundle branch, accounting for the frequent association of right bundle branch block with left anterior fascicular block during acute myocardial infarction involving the septum. Finally, the left posterior fascicle derives its blood supply from the AV nodal artery in 50 per cent of cases; in the remainder, it has a dual blood supply: the first septal perforator of the left anterior descending and the AV nodal artery.

INTRACARDIAC RECORDINGS. The potentials generated by the specialized conducting tissues are small, and many of the specific events underlying impulse formation and conduction are not discernible on routine surface electrocardiographic leads. Thus the potentials of the sinus node cannot be recorded on the body surface but can be inferred by observing the inscription of P waves on the standard electrocardiogram. Similarly, the events of AV conduction can be inferred by observing the relationship of atrial muscle depolarization (P waves) to ventricular muscle depolarization (QRS complex).

With the introduction of electrode catheter techniques, routine intracavitary recordings of the specialized conducting tissues of the human heart became possible. Briefly, the technique of His bundle recording consists of the percutaneous introduction of an electrode catheter into a femoral vein with advancement of the catheter under fluoroscopic and electrocardiographic control into the heart. The catheter passes up the inferior vena cava and across the tricuspid valve into the right ventricle, from which it is slowly withdrawn while recording electrograms which are greatly amplified and filtered (Fig. 50–1). Because of the proximity of the His bundle to the tricuspid annulus, electrical activity arising from the His bundle can be directly recorded. An electrode catheter lying across the tricuspid annulus in the region of the His bundle in fact records three separate electrical events (Fig. 50–2): an atrial electrogram arising in the low interatrial septum (A), the His bundle deflection itself (H), and ventricular activity arising in the high interventricular septum (V). Thus the recording of the His bundle electrogram readily permits the dissection of the P-R interval into intervals corresponding to conduction in the atrium (P-A interval; normal range, 25 to 45 msec), the AV node (A-H interval; normal range, 60 to 130 msec), and the His-Purkinje system (H-V interval; normal range, 30 to 55 msec).

His bundle recordings can usually be obtained within five to ten minutes after catheter introduction and remain stable for prolonged periods of time. As with any venous catheterization, potential risks include the induction of serious cardiac arrhythmias, cardiac perforation, local bleeding, infection, and thrombophlebitis. Special care must be exercised in recording His bundle activity in patients with complete left bundle branch block because inadvertent trauma to the right bundle branch may result in transient complete heart block.

APPLICATIONS OF INTRACARDIAC RECORDINGS. The ability to record directly the activity of the His bundle provides a method to localize disorders of impulse formation or conduction to above (i.e., supraventricular) or below (i.e., ventricular) the level of the His bundle. The prognostic importance of these observations will be further discussed later in this chapter. When a ventricular complex is preceded by a His bundle deflection at an interval equal to or greater than the H-V interval present during sinus rhythm, a site of origin proximal to or in the His bundle is suggested (i.e., supraventricular). Conversely, absence of a His deflection before a ventricular complex, or a His bundle deflection that precedes the ventricular complex by a value significantly less than normal, suggests a ventricular origin. Representative examples are shown in Figures 50–3 and 50–4.

Figure 50–3 demonstrates intracardiac recordings obtained

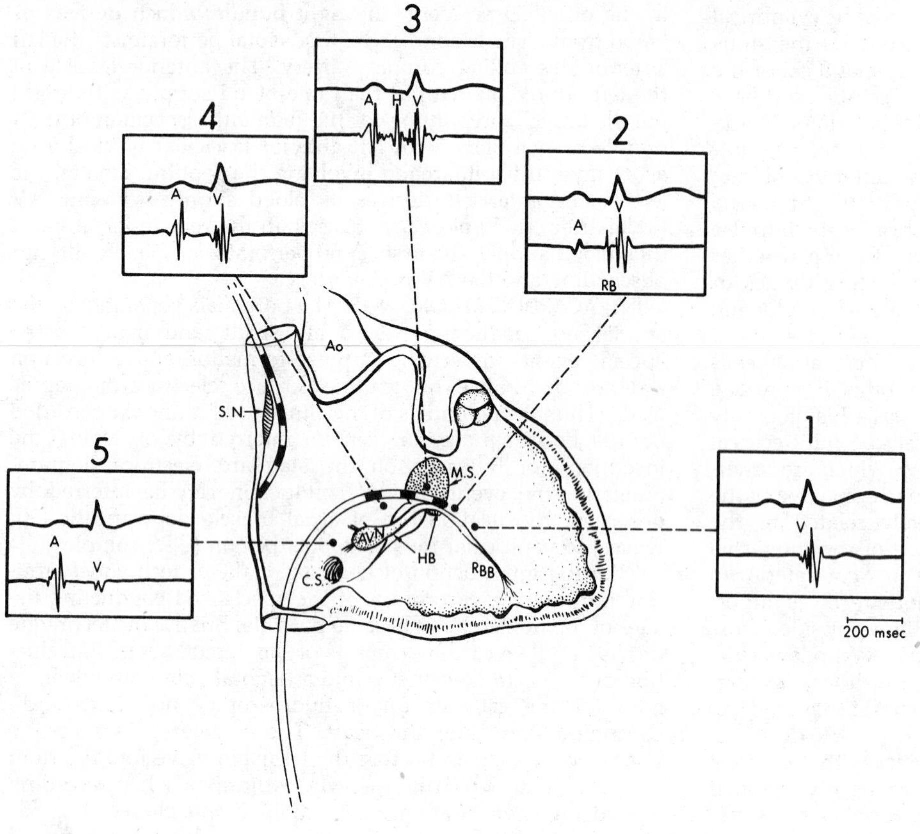

Figure 50–1. Technique of His bundle recording. A cutaway view of the heart, demonstrating the electrode catheter lying across the tricuspid valve. The intracavitary electrograms obtained during progressive withdrawal of the catheter are shown in panels 1 to 5. Also shown is a quadripolar electrode catheter positioned in the high right lateral atrium, adjacent to the junction of the superior vena cava with the right atrium. SN = sinus node; CS = orifice of the coronary sinus; AVN = atrioventricular node; HB = His bundle; MS = membranous septum; RBB = right bundle branch; A = atrial electrogram; H = His bundle electrogram; V = ventricular electrogram; Ao = aorta. (Reprinted, with permission, from Gallagher JJ, et al.: *In* Grossman W [Ed.]: Cardiac Catheterization and Angiography. Philadelphia, Lea & Febiger, 1974, p 215.)

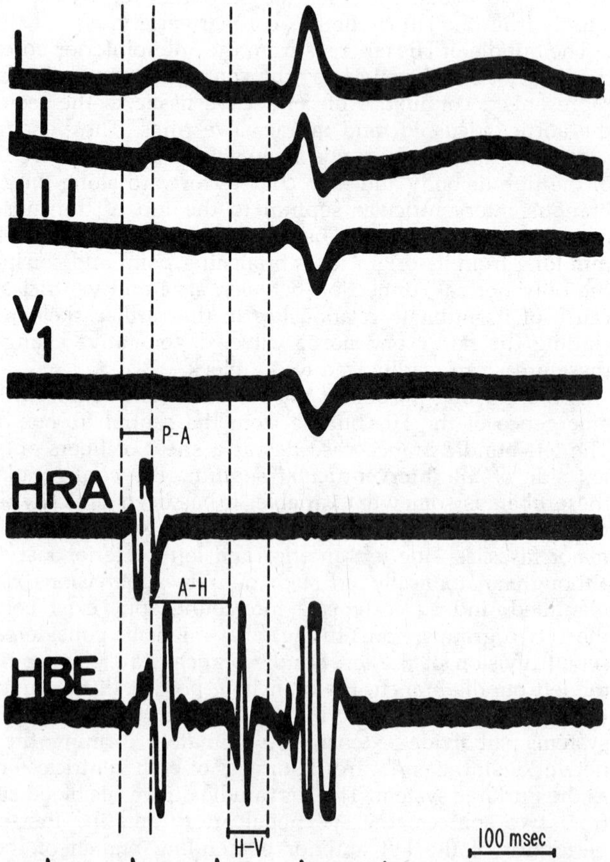

Figure 50–2. His bundle recording. Recordings from top to bottom are ECG leads I to III, precordial lead V_1, a high right atrial electrogram (HRA), His bundle electrogram (HBE), and time lines at 10 and 100 msec. The P-A, A-H, and H-V intervals are demonstrated.

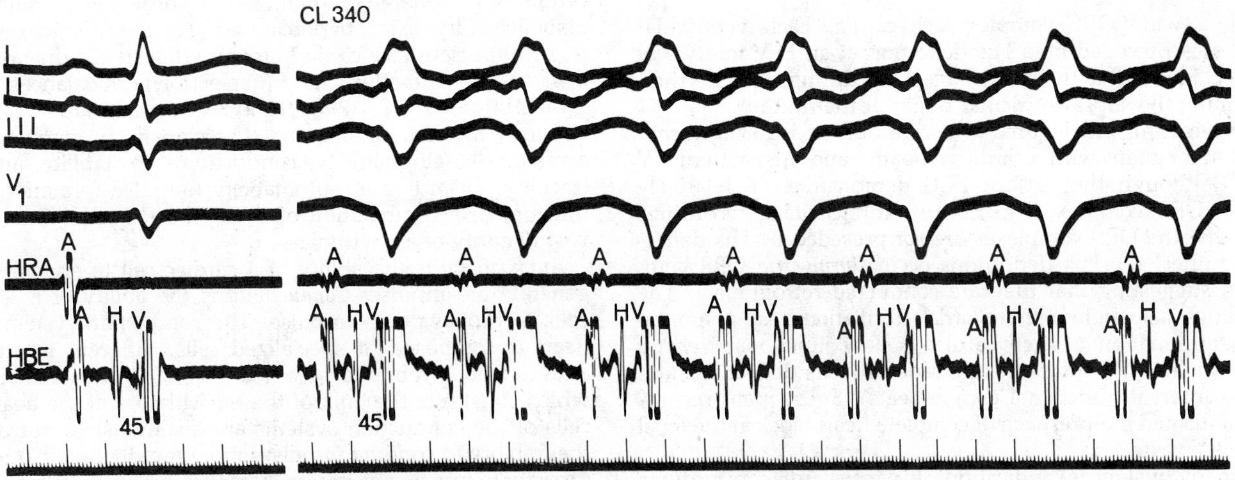

Figure 50–3. His bundle recordings during a wide QRS complex tachycardia. The panel to the left shows baseline tracings obtained during sinus rhythm in patients prone to recurrent wide QRS complex tachycardia. Note the normal sequence of atrial activation proceeding from the high right atrium (HRA) to the low interatrial septum recorded on the HBE tracing. The surface QRS complex is normal and is preceded by a His deflection at a normal interval of 45 msec. The panel to the right was obtained during a spontaneous episode of wide QRS complex tachycardia. The surface ECG leads suggest the presence of left bundle branch block aberration. Each ventricular complex is preceded by a His deflection at an H-V interval of 45 msec, confirming a supraventricular origin. In addition, note the reversal of the sequence of activation of the atria.

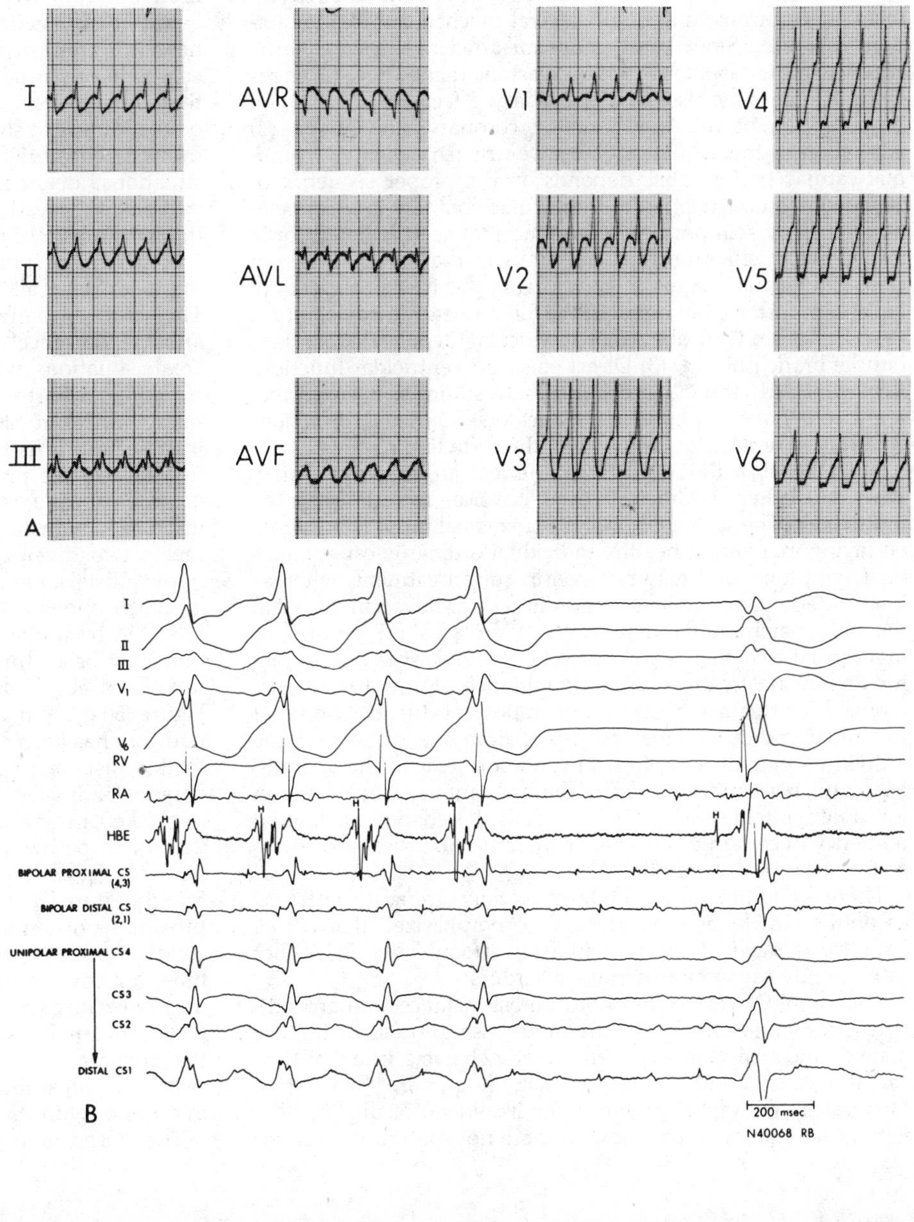

Figure 50–4. His bundle recordings during tachycardia of unknown etiology. *A* demonstrates a 12 lead electrocardiogram during a rapid tachycardia associated with relatively narrow QRS complexes. There is no discernible atrial activity evident on the tracing. *B*, Intracavitary recordings obtained during the tachycardia shown in *A*. The recordings from top to bottom are standard ECG leads I to III, V_1, V_6, bipolar electrograms from the right ventricle (RV), the right atrium (RA), the region of the His bundle (HBE), and recordings of the medial and lateral left atrium via the coronary sinus; the unipolar recordings of the coronary sinus electrode are shown in the bottom four tracings. During the tachycardia, the His bundle deflection is inscribed after the onset of the surface QRS complex, suggesting a retrograde origin of the deflection. After four beats of tachycardia, spontaneous termination occurs, followed by a junctional escape beat. The junctional escape beat is preceded by a His bundle deflection at an interval of 70 msec. Note that despite the regularity of the tachycardia, atrial fibrillation is evident on the tracings obtained from the right atrium, the atrial septum, and the left atrium. The tracings thus demonstrate the presence of ventricular tachycardia. See text for discussion.

during a wide QRS complex tachycardia. Each ventricular complex is preceded by a His deflection at an H-V interval of 45 msec, identical to the interval recorded during sinus rhythm, confirming the supraventricular origin of the rhythm.

The recordings in Figure 50–4 were obtained during tachycardia in a patient with a cardiomyopathy and intermittent AV block. Although the surface ECG demonstrates a relatively narrow QRS complex (Fig. 50–4*A*), intracavitary recordings show that the QRS complexes are *not* preceded by His deflections; rather, the His deflections occur *during* the QRS complexes, suggesting that they are conducted retrogradely. The recordings also demonstrate atrial fibrillation. After spontaneous termination of tachycardia, a slow junctional rhythm appears with QRS complexes preceded by His deflections at a normal interval (junctional escape beats). Subsequent recordings confirmed the presence of complete heart block at the level of the AV node.

In many instances, indications for intracardiac recordings clearly overlap areas where clinical judgment alone might suffice. However, in patients with atypical patterns of conduction delay and block, His bundle recordings may define the site of pathology. Electrophysiologic studies combining intracardiac recording with pacing can be used to induce many types of tachycardia so that their mechanism can be elucidated and therapeutic interventions tried under controlled circumstances.

HEMODYNAMIC CONSEQUENCES OF ARRHYTHMIAS. Arrhythmias affect cardiac output by several mechanisms: (1) Alterations in rate. Slow rates cause insufficient forward flow, whereas rapid rates encroach on diastolic filling time. Changes in heart rate may also have secondary effects on the oxygen consumption of the heart and on coronary blood flow. (2) Alteration in the sequence of atrioventricular activation. Optimal cardiac performance depends on the proper sequence of atrial contraction relative to ventricular contraction. This relationship is most important in the abnormal heart, where proper timing may augment cardiac output by as much as 30 to 40 per cent. The precise sequence of ventricular activation appears to be less important, but again in the failing heart, cardiac output may be lower with abnormal ventricular depolarization (i.e., bundle branch block). (3) Direct effect on ventricular function. Recurrent arrhythmias, notably those resulting in tachycardia, appear to have a depressant effect on ventricular function, which may outlast the duration of the arrhythmia.

ARRHYTHMIAS IN CONTEXT. The effect an arrhythmia may have is further modified by the physical condition of the individual patient. For example, paroxysmal atrial tachycardia occurring in a young healthy individual ordinarily causes minimal symptoms and may not even require treatment, whereas in an elderly patient with a compromised cardiovascular system the same arrhythmia may cause symptoms of cerebral or myocardial ischemia, shock, or congestive heart failure calling for immediate treatment. The importance of any arrhythmia, its need for treatment, and, more important, the exact type of treatment indicated must be assessed in the context of the individual patient, his physical condition *prior* to the arrhythmia, and his condition *during* the arrhythmia. Consideration for treatment may also be reasonably based on the known tendency of certain prodromal arrhythmias to progress to more serious cardiac arrhythmias.

There is an unfortunate tendency to view cardiac arrhythmias as entities in themselves. It must be emphasized that *not all arrhythmias should be treated;* indeed, attempts to do so not infrequently cause more serious disorders.

ETIOLOGY OF ARRHYTHMIAS. In most instances, an arrhythmia is a manifestation of some more basic process or disease state. Some arrhythmias are sufficiently characteristic that they themselves shed light on their etiology (e.g., paroxysmal atrial tachycardia with block suggests the likelihood of digitalis toxicity). Many arrhythmias, however, are not specific and call for a systematic assessment of the patient. This will include a careful search for (1) primary cardiovascular disorders, either central or peripheral; (2) pulmonary disorders (e.g., pulmonary embolism, hypoxia, hypercapnia); (3) autonomic disorders (e.g., hypersensitive carotid sinus); (4) systemic disorders; (5) drug-related side effects; and (6) electrolyte imbalances.

MECHANISMS OF ARRHYTHMIAS. Normal cardiac function depends on certain inherent characteristic properties of the cardiac cells: automaticity, conductivity, excitability, and contractility. Disorders of automaticity (impulse formation), conduction, or a combination of these two form the basis of the vast majority of arrhythmias.

Automaticity is the ability of a cardiac cell to spontaneously generate an impulse. *Conductivity* is the ability of a series of cells to propagate an impulse. The conduction system of the heart is composed of specialized cells, different in structure and function from the so-called "working myocardial cells" which constitute the bulk of the musculature of the heart. The cells of the conduction systems are distinguished not only by their ability to conduct impulses more rapidly but also by their capacity to function as pacemakers that initiate impulses, which in turn activate the myocardium. Automaticity normally resides in the specialized conducting tissues of the heart where a hierarchy exists, dominated by the cells of the sinus node. Under abnormal conditions, *ectopic* pacemakers can emerge which usurp control of the cardiac rhythm. Similarly, the failure of the normal sinus pacemaker to depolarize may lead to the appearance of an "escape" subsidiary pacemaker.

After electrical discharge, a pacemaker cell, conducting fiber, or myocardial "working cell" requires a finite period of recovery before it can again be depolarized. This period of responsiveness is termed *refractoriness.* Such unresponsiveness may be complete or partial. If a propagated impulse encounters tissue that is completely refractory, *block* of further propagation may occur, leading to slowing of the heart beat. If partially refractory tissue is encountered, conduction *delay* may occur. In certain situations, disorders of conduction (delay and/or block) can paradoxically lead to an abnormally rapid cardiac rhythm by the mechanism of *re-entry* (Fig. 50–5).

A variety of potential routes of divergence of the cardiac impulse exist at all levels of the heart during normal conduction. The ability of many cardiac fibers to conduct in both directions and the presence of cross-connections between cardiac fibers create situations in which conduction can occur in a functionally closed loop. Fortunately, there is uniformity of conduction and refractoriness at each "level" of the heart (i.e., atria, atrioventricular node, His-Purkinje system), resulting in uniform direction of impulse propagation. This normal sequence of events is schematically represented in Figure 50–5*A,* in which an impulse conducting through a proximal common pathway meets two divergent pathways (alpha and beta) converging upon a distal common pathway. Uniform depolarization results in synchronous activation of both divergent pathways and is followed by uniform recovery. This pattern of uniform activation may be disturbed by pathologic processes as well as by functional abnormalities that accompany premature beats. In Figure 50–5*B,* an area of depressed conduction in the beta pathway has been schematically represented as a stippled zone. In this instance, the propagating impulse encounters two divergent pathways with different properties. Thus the impulse is blocked in one pathway (beta), and passes slowly through the other pathway (alpha) to the distal common pathway, where it enters the beta pathway retrogradely. In Figure 50–5*C,* the impulse has arrived in the previously depolarized proximal portion of the beta pathway. As a result of the conduction delay in the alpha pathway, the beta pathway has time to recover from its state of refractoriness and the impulse may re-excite or re-enter this area, giving rise to a new impulse. In this manner a sustained re-entry can occur (Fig. 50–5*D*). If the circulating wavefront exits from the closed loop with each cycle, the surrounding cardiac tissue will also be depolarized in cadence with the loop.

The closed loop of re-entry may be formed by anatomic or

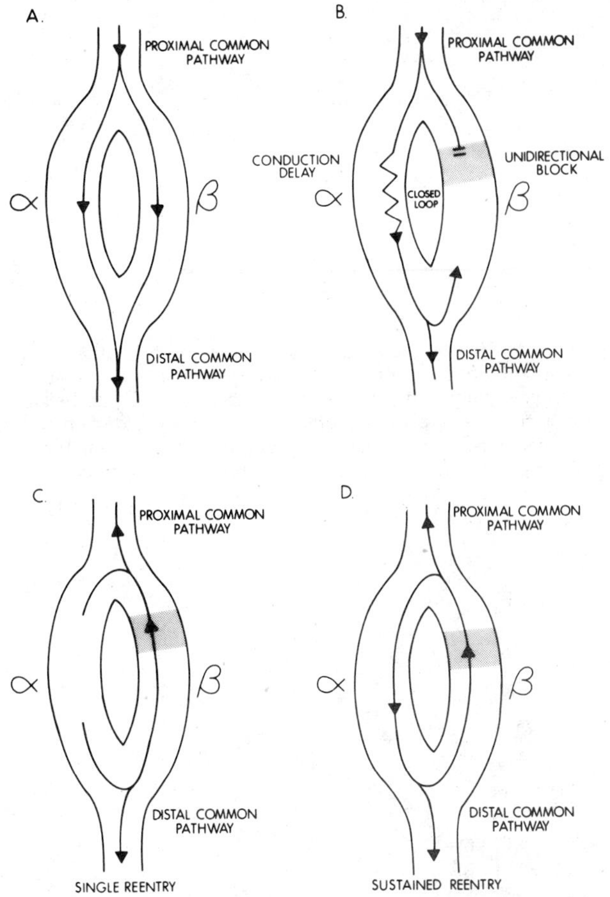

Figure 50–5. Diagrammatic representation of re-entry. A theoretical re-entry circuit is illustrated, consisting of a proximal common pathway, two divergent limbs (alpha and beta pathways), and a distal common pathway. The requisite conditions of re-entry are shown and consist of a closed loop, conduction delay, and unidirectional block. See text for discussion.

functional elements in normal cardiac structures or may be comprised in part by an accessory pathway. The latter situation is encountered in the group of disorders known as the pre-excitation syndromes (see below). Regardless of the location of the closed loop, the requirements for re-entry to occur are in general the same as those depicted in Figure 50–5*B*: a closed loop, conduction delay, and an area of unidirectional block.

The actual mechanism involved in any given cardiac arrhythmia has a variety of diagnostic and therapeutic implications; some of these will be discussed later in this chapter.

CLASSIFICATION OF ARRHYTHMIAS. Arrhythmias are commonly classified by either their mechanisms (e.g., automaticity versus re-entry) or their site of origin (e.g., supraventricular versus ventricular). Unfortunately there is a considerable amount of overlap in the mechanisms of clinical arrhythmias. Thus an abnormality of conduction delay may be required to perpetuate re-entry, which in turn can result in a rapid heart rate, while a similar disorder of conduction may result in block of transmission of impulses from the atria to the ventricles, resulting in a slow rate. Classification of arrhythmias by their site of origin presumes that the location of the arrhythmia is already known. Since the rate and regularity of the heart beat are customarily assessed in the general physical examination of every patient, it seems logical to use the pulse as a means of classifying arrhythmias, since this type of classification allows a logical pursuit of the cause of the arrhythmia in any given patient. For this reason, arrhythmias will be arbitrarily divided into those resulting in tachycardia (ventricular rate greater than 100 per minute) or bradycardia (ventricular rate less than 60 per minute).

Before proceeding to a discussion of tachycardias and bradycardias, the subject of isolated ectopic beats must be considered briefly. Ectopic beats are found in both health and disease and are important because they may mimic more significant cardiac arrhythmias and at times may herald the onset of a serious cardiac arrhythmia.

ECTOPIC BEATS. Ectopic beats include all impulses arising outside the sinus node. We are concerned here primarily with premature beats arising anywhere in the atria, atrioventricular junction, or ventricles. The mechanism of such isolated premature beats is not known with certainty and they may be observed in the presence or absence of heart disease. In general the tendency to have premature beats at any "level" of the heart is aggravated by fatigue, emotion, alcohol, caffeine, and smoking. The presence of three consecutive premature beats satisfies the conventional definition of an ectopic tachycardia.

Atrial Premature Beats. Atrial premature beats, also known as premature atrial contractions or atrial extrasystoles, are premature impulses arising from ectopic foci situated anywhere in the atria. They may precede the onset of the atrial fibrillation, ectopic atrial tachycardia (especially in the setting of digitalis toxicity), or a sustained re-entrant tachycardia arising at some other location. They are particularly common in conditions associated with distention of the atria such as congestive heart failure and are also commonly observed in the course of myocardial infarction. The majority of patients are unaware of atrial premature beats when they occur, although some may complain of a sensation of skipping of the heart beat or palpitations resulting from the pause and more forceful contraction of the overfilled ventricles which follow a premature beat.

Electrocardiographically, atrial premature beats are manifest as P waves, which may differ in a marked or subtle way from the sinus P wave. Early premature atrial beats may fail to conduct (i.e., block) owing to physiologic refractoriness at some level of the conduction system. Such early blocked beats may be manifested only by a subtle deformity in the S-T segment or T wave of the preceding conducted beat (Fig. 50–6).

Nonconducted atrial premature beats (1) reset the sinus node and/or (2) influence conduction of a subsequent sinus beat. Thus, premature atrial beats can prematurely depolarize the sinus node, causing a reset of the sinus cycle, which is reflected in the pause that follows. Most often the sum of the pre- and the postextrasystolic P-P intervals is less than twice two sinus

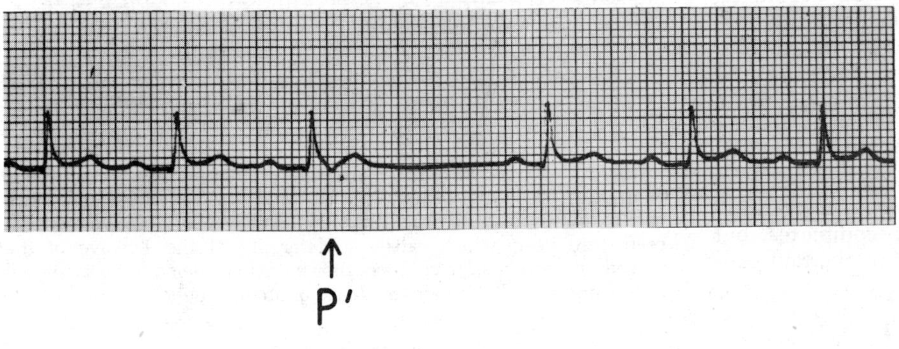

Figure 50–6. Blocked atrial premature beat mimicking a sinus pause. Following three normal sinus beats, a sudden pause occurs. Careful examination of the S-T segment of the third sinus beat reveals a deformity resulting from the presence of a nonconducted atrial premature beat (P').

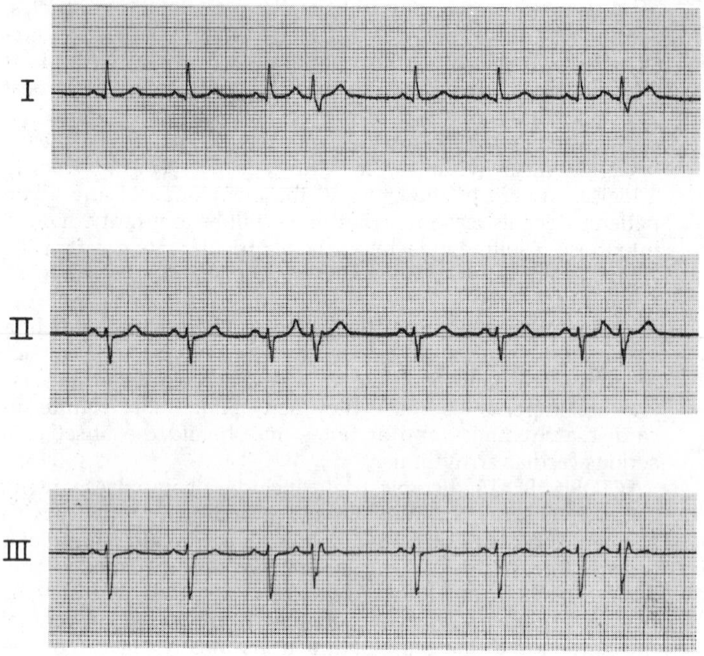

Figure 50–7. Conducted atrial premature beats. Following three normal sinus beats, a premature extrasystole is noted with a QRS morphology suggestive of ventricular aberration. Careful examination of the T wave of the preceding sinus beat demonstrates a deformity (best seen in lead II) owing to an atrial premature beat. Following three more sinus beats, the process is repeated.

cycles and is said to be noncompensatory. Even if an early premature atrial beat is not conducted, it may alter recovery of the AV node and result in prolongation of the P-R interval of the next conducted sinus beat. This latter phenomenon is known as "concealed conduction."

Most premature atrial beats fall in the relatively refractory period of the AV conduction system, resulting in prolongation of the P-R interval. If the premature beat enters the His-Purkinje system during its refractory period, the sequence of ventricular activation may be altered, resulting in *aberrant* conduction. The premature atrial beat in this instance may conduct with a wide QRS complex because of asynchronous spread through the incompletely recovered structures of the specialized conduction system (Fig. 50–7). The recovery period of the specialized conducting tissues of the right ventricle outlasts that of the left ventricle; as a result right bundle branch block is the most frequently encountered form of aberration. If the preceding atrial premature beat is unrecognized, the resulting wide QRS complex may be misdiagnosed as a ventricular premature beat (see below) (Fig. 50–8).

In general mild sedation and elimination of the precipitating factor are all that are necessary for treatment of atrial premature beats. When atrial premature beats are associated with more serious cardiac arrhythmias, they may be suppressed by treatment with quinidine sulfate or disopyramide phosphate.

Premature AV Junctional Beats. Premature AV junctional beats are much less common than atrial or ventricular premature beats either in health or disease. Because of their site of origin, premature beats arising in the junction can spread simultaneously toward the atria and the ventricles. Depending on the degree of delay or block encountered in either direction, the atria may be activated before, simultaneously with, or after the ventricles. A variety of conduction disturbances may be mimicked by the presence of premature junctional beats owing to the phenomenon of concealed conduction. Patients exhibiting unusual combinations of first, second, or third degree heart block (see below) should have long rhythm strips recorded for evidence of conducted junctional extrasystoles. These are almost invariably associated with normal QRS complexes, but when sufficiently premature they may result in aberrant conduction.

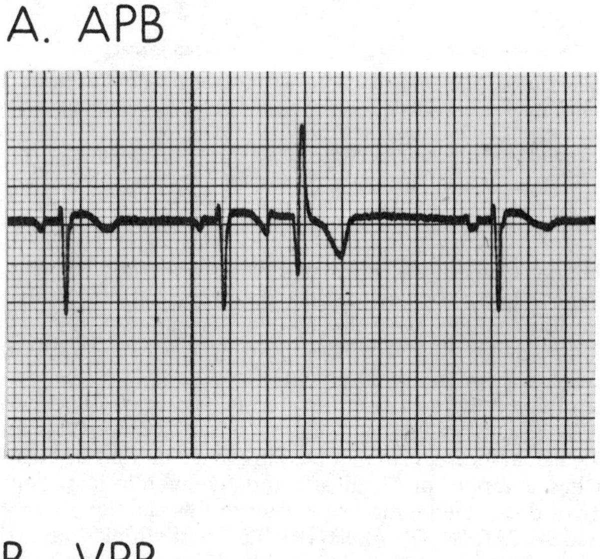

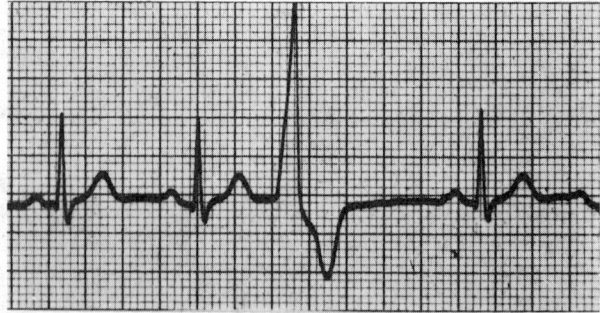

Figure 50–8. Comparison of an atrial premature beat (APB) and a ventricular premature beat (VPB). In *A* and *B*, a wide QRS premature beat follows two sinus beats. In *A* this extrasystole is due to an atrial premature beat, which causes a deformity of the T wave of the preceding sinus beat. In contrast, the ventricular premature beat shown in *B* is not preceded by any evidence of atrial activity.

The treatment of premature AV junctional beats is essentially the same as for atrial premature beats. Digitalis toxicity should always be suspected.

Ventricular Premature Beats. Ventricular premature beats are the most common form of arrhythmia in patients with or without heart disease. Patients with no evidence of heart disease have been followed with persistent ventricular premature beats for many years. They are extremely frequent in the setting of acute myocardial infarction, being noted in up to 80 per cent of such patients. Excess digitalis is a common cause of premature ventricular beats, especially when hypokalemia is present.

Electrocardiographically, ventricular premature beats are characterized by wide (greater than 0.14 second), occasionally bizarre QRS complexes without preceding P waves (Fig. 50–8). They often have a fairly constant coupling interval relative to the preceding sinus beat. Ventricular premature beats that occur near the peak of descending limb of the T wave are said to occur during the "vulnerable period" of the ventricles and constitute a risk for developing ventricular tachycardia and fibrillation (the R-on-T phenomenon). In the setting of acute ischemia, however, late ventricular premature beats have proved to be equally malignant. Most ventricular premature beats do not disturb the sinus rhythm and are therefore followed by a fully compensatory pause. Some ventricular premature beats conduct retrogradely to the atria, inscribing retrograde P waves on the S-T segment. Such beats are frequently followed by pauses that are less than compensatory. Ventricular premature beats with a long QRS duration (greater than 0.16 second) or associated with fragmented morphology have been said to be indicative of underlying heart disease.

The treatment of premature ventricular beats is again primarily directed to the underlying condition. The associated symptoms and frequency of the extrasystoles should be taken into account. Digitalis excess and hypokalemia should be corrected when present. Ventricular premature beats occurring in the setting of acute myocardial infarction require antiarrhythmic therapy. Intravenous lidocaine is the treatment of choice in acute situations. Regardless of the underlying condition, antiarrhythmic therapy also appears desirable when ventricular extrasystoles demonstrate the R-on-T phenomenon, are multifocal, or appear in salvos. Long-term oral therapy with quinidine sulfate, procainamide, or disopyramide phosphate is usually effective in reducing the frequency of extrasystoles, although complete suppression is the exception rather than the rule. If these agents fail, propranolol can be tried.

TACHYCARDIA

GENERAL APPROACH TO THE PATIENT WITH TACHYCARDIA. In almost any situation short of a cardiac arrest, an electrocardiographic machine will be available and can be connected to the patient. Clearly, if the patient is pulseless and in cardiovascular collapse, cardiopulmonary resuscitation is indicated. If on the other hand the patient is reasonably stable (i.e., no chest pain, no congestive failure, neurologically intact), then the physician should consider that a small amount of time spent establishing the level of origin and mechanism of tachycardia may have profound prognostic and therapeutic importance to the patient. Such an assessment requires information concerning (1) the rate, regularity, and morphology of the atrial activity; (2) the rate, regularity, and QRS morphology of ventricular activity; (3) the relationship of atrial and ventricular activity; (4) the response to carotid sinus massage (when indicated); and (5) if possible, observations concerning the mode of onset and termination of tachycardia. Some of these findings will be evident on physical examination, while others will require electrocardiographic recordings and possibly additional esophageal or intra-atrial leads. Long rhythm strips are always advisable, with leads which optimally demonstrate P waves such as lead II or V_1.

CLINICAL EXAMINATION. If the patient is in urgent need of treatment of tachycardia, it is useful to consider the availability of cardioversion equipment on arrival. A good intravenous route should be present. Some initial stabilization may be obtained by raising the legs to increase the venous return. Specific attention during physical examination should be directed to examination of the jugular venous pulse, the arterial pulse, and the intensity of the first heart sound. If the cardiac rhythm is irregular, the first sound will usually vary in intensity; a constant first sound in the setting of an irregular heart beat should suggest the possibility of mitral stenosis. In the presence of a regular cardiac rhythm, variation of the first sound suggests atrioventricular dissociation. Examination of the neck veins may demonstrate flutter waves or the presence of cannon waves, suggesting either a junctional or ventricular tachycardia with a ventriculoatrial dissociation. The arterial pulse may similarly reflect atrioventricular dissociation if variable intensity of the pulse amplitude is felt; clearly these must be distinguished from pulsus alternans and pulsus paradoxus.

THE ELECTROCARDIOGRAM. The presence of atrial activity on the electrocardiogram may not always be evident on the surface tracings, and in some cases it may be necessary to determine the atrial activity by a more invasive means. Classically, Lewis leads were used if examination of the routine electrocardiographic leads failed to demonstrate evidence of atrial activity. A Lewis lead can be recorded by taking the right and left arm leads of the electrocardiographic machine and placing them at either end of the sternum while recording lead I (the leg leads must be attached). However, such recordings not infrequently fail to detect atrial activity, and furthermore they impair one's ability to record other body surface leads simultaneously. The esophageal lead has solved these problems. In the past many esophageal leads were large, mechanically bulky, and difficult to pass. Not infrequently they proved therapeutic in that tachycardia terminated on introduction of the lead because of gagging. A discarded permanent transvenous pacing electrode lead is ideally suited for use as an esophageal lead. Such a lead is soft and flexible and easily passed through the nasopharynx. The patient should be lying down with his head pushed slightly forward on his chest. The lead is lubricated and passed through the nose and the patient encouraged to swallow frequently during its passage. Once the lead is passed successfully down the esophagus, it is connected by a single alligator clip to the V_1 precordial lead of the standard electrocardiographic machine (Fig. 50–9). This also requires that the remaining leads be hooked up to the arms and legs in the usual manner. The esophageal lead can also be attached to a precordial monitoring lead for more prolonged periods of rhythm analysis. The use of a three-channel electrocardiographic machine allows one to record the esophageal lead simultaneously with two other precordial leads (Fig. 50–10). In addition it is helpful to use a machine with variable gain and paper speed. If the esophageal lead fails to demonstrate evidence of atrial activity, flow-directed transvenous electrodes can be advanced to the atrium under electrocardiographic control and used to record intra-atrial potentials.

Some rhythms will defy any attempt to categorize them on the basis of the aforementioned observations. Such rhythms include ventricular tachycardia in which persistent 1:1 retrograde conduction is present. The use of a vagal maneuver may dissociate atrial from ventricular activity. Even with all the maneuvers described, it may still be necessary to resort to intracardiac recordings of the conduction system in conjunction with stimulation techniques in selected cases.

THE USE OF CAROTID SINUS MASSAGE. Carotid sinus massage is a simple maneuver useful in the evaluation of tachycardia. As a precaution, the carotid should be auscultated for a bruit and carotid massage not performed over a vessel with a bruit. An electrocardiogram should be hooked up to the patient, although in urgent situations a stethoscope may be used to auscultate the chest during carotid massage. One should be prepared for overdrive suppression following termination of

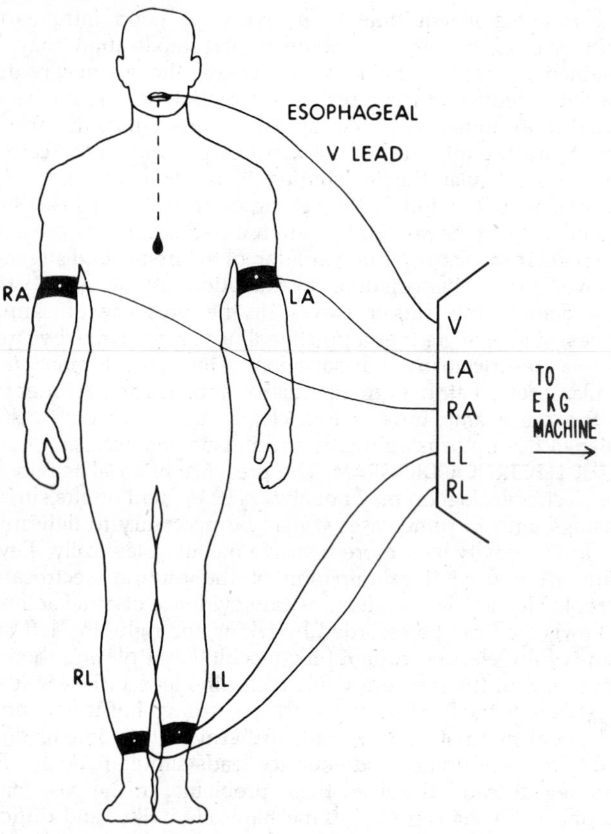

Figure 50–9. Connections for recording an esophageal electrogram. A 12 lead electrocardiographic machine is diagrammatically shown with the conventional electrode placements for limb leads. The precordial V lead is shown attached to an esophageal lead for recording a unipolar esophageal electrogram.

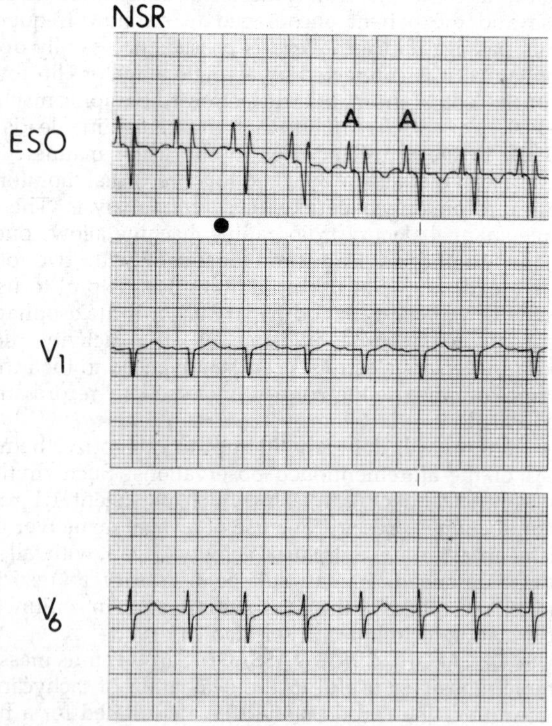

Figure 50–10. Representative esophageal electrogram recorded during sinus rhythm. A representative strip from a 12 lead electrocardiographic machine is shown with recordings from the esophageal lead (ESO), and standard precordial leads V_1, V_6. Note the prominent atrial electrogram (A) recorded on the esophageal lead.

the tachycardia by carotid massage. Ventricular fibrillation has been induced by carotid massage, hence the utility of access to a cardioversion machine.

The patient should be positioned flat with his neck extended by placing a small pillow under the shoulders. The effectiveness of the massage can be enhanced by elevating the feet and increasing blood pressure. The head should be turned away from the side being massaged. The massage should be performed at the bifurcation of the carotid just below the angle of the jaw, on one side at a time. One should begin with slight pressure because a hypersensitive reflex may be present in some patients. The duration of the massage should never exceed five seconds. If carotid massage is ineffective, it may be useful to repeat it after the administration of edrophonium chloride.* To guard against oversensitivity, an initial dose of 2 mg is given intravenously. If no untoward response is noted, the remaining 8 mg is given.

SINUS TACHYCARDIA. Sinus tachycardia in the adult is a regular tachycardia occurring at rates of 100 to 180 per minute. The rhythm is usually associated with a gradual onset and offset. Normally sinus tachycardia represents a physiologic response to exercise, anxiety, stress, emotion, fever, congestive heart failure, volume depletion, and hypotension. Vagolytic drugs such as atropine can also cause sinus tachycardia. There is a tendency for the sinus rate to vary with changes in posture or activity, more so than in the case of ectopic atrial pacemakers. Carotid sinus massage generally slows the sinus rates slightly, with a gradual increase in rate to the original level on termination of the massage.

Electrocardiographically, sinus tachycardia is distinguished by the presence of P waves of sinus contour preceding each QRS (Fig. 50–11). Because the increase of the sinus rate is frequently mediated by increased sympathetic activity, the P-R interval during sinus tachycardia is typically normal or slightly decreased. The maximal rate of sinus tachycardia is usually 180, and rates in excess of 200 per minute are distinctively unusual. Sinus tachycardia must be distinguished from two other entities, sinus node re-entry and sinus arrhythmia. Sinus node re-entry is an unusual cause of tachycardia. Since this rhythm arises in the region of the sinus node, the P wave is indistinguishable from the normal sinus P wave. The rhythm is recognized by its abrupt onset and termination, characteristic of re-entrant rhythms, and rarely exceeds 150 per minute. Sinus arrhythmia on the other hand refers to the normal physiologic waxing and waning of the sinus rate with respiration, with the maximal rate noted at the end of inspiration. These normal respiratory changes are believed to result from vagal reflexes and are most prominent in children and young adults. The phenomenon of sinus arrhythmia may become exaggerated with heart disease and mimic various atrial arrhythmias, but more commonly it is conspicuous by its absence in the presence of congestive heart failure.

Treatment of sinus tachycardia is again directed toward the underlying etiology. Digitalis is ineffective in slowing the heart rate unless the tachycardia is related to underlying congestive heart failure.

ECTOPIC ATRIAL TACHYCARDIA. Ectopic atrial tachycardia is associated with atrial rates of 150 to 220 per minute and is usually accompanied by some degree of atrioventricular block. Digitalis toxicity accounts for perhaps three fourths of all observed cases, especially in the setting of hypokalemia. Ectopic atrial tachycardia is also typically observed in patients with chronic obstructive lung disease or in patients with advanced pathology of the atria, but the rhythm may occur in otherwise normal patients.

Electrocardiographically (Fig. 50–12), the configuration of the P wave is different from that of the sinus beats. When associated with digitalis toxicity, small bizarre spiked P waves which vary in amplitude are observed. Partial atrioventricular block is generally present, and carotid massage results in a decrease in ventricular rate owing to an increase in the degree of atrioven-

*Experimental drug for this purpose.

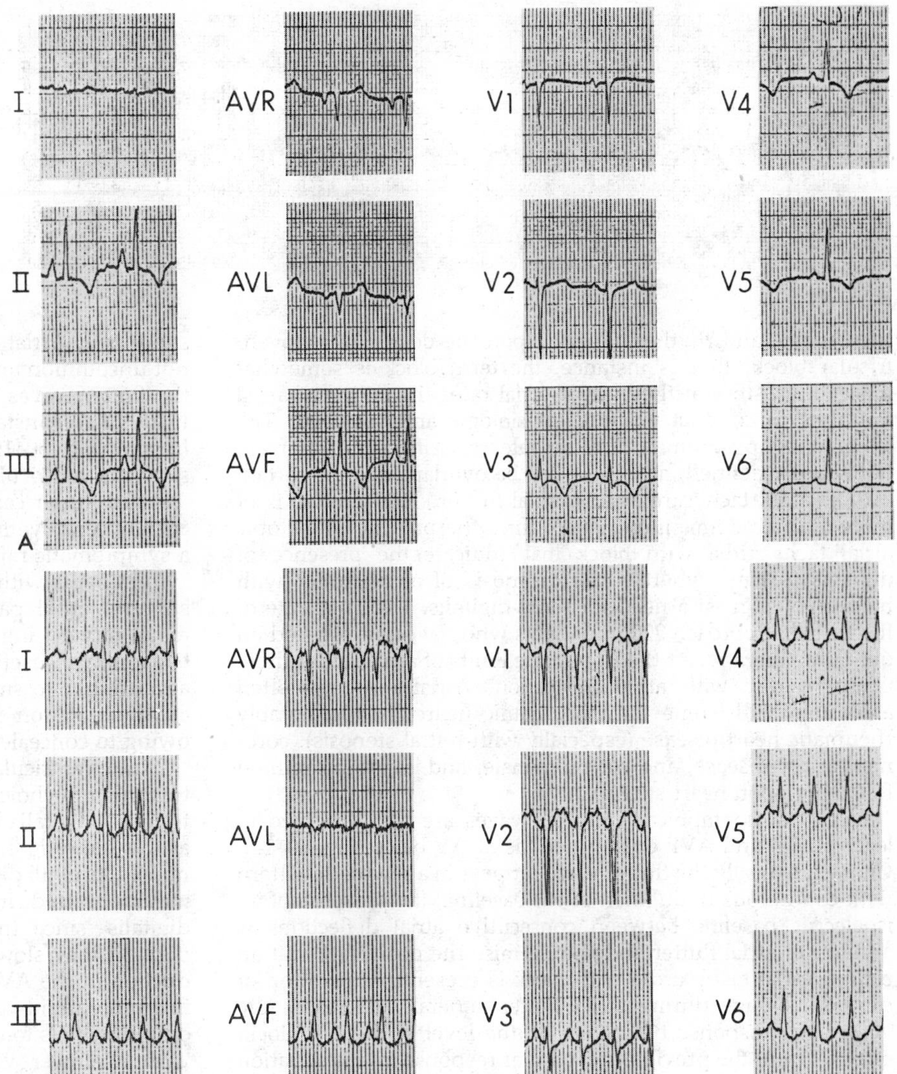

Figure 50–11. Sinus tachycardia. *A*, A 12 lead electrocardiogram recorded in a patient subject to recurrent supraventricular tachycardia. *B*, A 12 lead electrocardiogram recorded during a paroxysm of tachycardia in the same patient as in *A*. Note the distinctive features of sinus tachycardia: the P wave during tachycardia is identical to that observed in sinus rhythm, and the P-R interval is essentially unchanged. This tachycardia was due to self-administered catecholamines.

tricular block. The slowing of the ventricular response achieved by carotid massage may reveal the presence of underlying ventricular irritability, further supporting the possibility of digitalis toxicity. In contrast to atrial flutter (see below), the baseline between P waves remains isoelectric. When three or more separate P wave morphologies can be recognized during the tachycardia, the rhythm is termed multifocal atrial tachycardia (MAT) (Fig. 50–13). It is frequently associated with chronic obstructive lung disease or atrial disease.

The treatment of ectopic atrial tachycardia related to digitalis toxicity requires withdrawal of digitalis. Ectopic atrial tachycardia occurring in patients with chronic obstructive lung disease is extremely refractory to treatment and requires that therapy be directed toward reversing the pulmonary abnormalities. Attempts at treatment of ectopic atrial tachycardia with digitalis in the setting of chronic lung disease frequently result in digitalis toxicity. Therapy in extremely refractory cases can be directed toward blocking conduction in the AV node by the use of beta blockers. Although beta blockers such as propranolol are generally contraindicated in patients with chronic obstructive disease (because they cause bronchospasm), newer types of beta-blocking agents are becoming available which have either minimal effect on the lungs (e.g., atenolol) or at least less marked effects than propranolol (e.g., metoprolol). Ectopic atrial tachycardias from other causes may be suppressed with quinidine sulfate, procainamide, or disopyramide phosphate, or an attempt may be made to increase AV block by the use of digitalis and propranolol.

ATRIAL FLUTTER. Atrial flutter is characterized by a rapid regular atrial rate between 220 and 360 per minute. The ven-

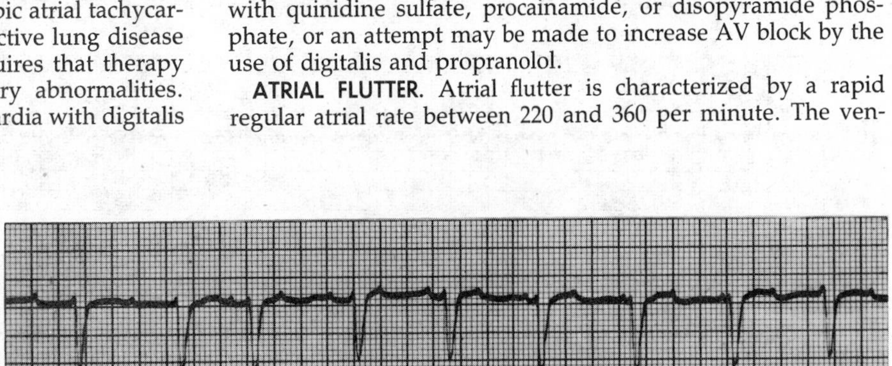

Figure 50–12. Atrial tachycardia with block due to digitalis toxicity. Atrial tachycardia at a rate of 150 per minute is present with varying AV block, a finding that should immediately suggest the presence of digitalis toxicity.

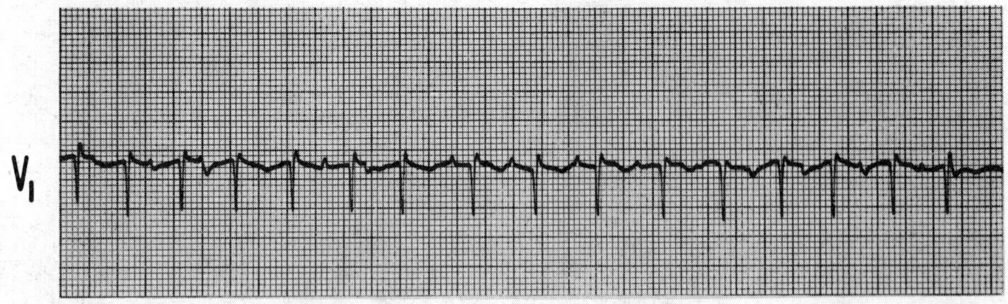

Figure 50–13. Multifocal atrial tachycardia (MAT). This rhythm strip demonstrates the criteria for multifocal atrial tachycardia, namely, the presence of a rapid atrial tachycardia with at least three different morphologies of the P waves. This patient had severe chronic obstructive lung disease.

tricular rate and rhythm depend upon the degree of atrioventricular block. In this instance, the term block is somewhat misleading, since at these rapid atrial rates the failure of atrial impulses to conduct is quite physiologic and expected. The lower and upper limits of atrial rates classified as flutter are not sharply defined, and there can be overlap between certain ectopic atrial tachycardias and atrial flutter. This overlap is of more than academic importance, since the presence of ectopic atrial tachycardia with block may indicate the presence of digitalis toxicity, whereas the diagnosis of atrial flutter with block may suggest a need for more digitalis. The atrial rate of flutter may approach 220 in patients who have been started on quinidine therapy. At the upper rate limits of atrial flutter there is an overlap with atrial fibrillation. Atrial flutter is often associated with some form of organic heart disease, notably rheumatic heart disease (especially with mitral stenosis), coronary artery disease, and cor pulmonale, and is not uncommon following open heart surgery.

Electrocardiographically, flutter waves are best observed in leads II, III, and AVF during periods of AV block (Fig. 50–14). Characteristically the flutter waves appear in a sawtooth pattern with continuous undulation of the baseline; the presence of an isoelectric baseline between consecutive atrial deflections is atypical of atrial flutter and should raise the possibility that an ectopic atrial tachycardia with block is present. Application of carotid massage during atrial flutter generally decreases the ventricular response by increasing the level of the AV block. The return to the previous ventricular response in this situation is not gradual but occurs in stepwise fashion. Occasionally carotid massage during atrial flutter will cause a transition into atrial fibrillation, and rarely the atrial flutter may terminate. A 1:1 relation between the atrial and ventricular rate during flutter is rare except in patients who have been treated with quinidine sulfate prior to digitalization or in patients with a pre-excitation syndrome. Atrial flutter with a 2:1 atrioventricular response is not uncommon and can be difficult to diagnose because one of the flutter waves is buried in the QRS complex (Fig. 50–15*A*). In this latter instance, an esophageal lead can be particularly helpful (Fig. 50–15*B*), especially when carotid massage fails to slow the ventricular response.

Atrial flutter can be effectively treated by low energy direct current cardioversion, and this is the treatment of choice when a symptomatic rapid ventricular response is present.

In patients with recurring atrial flutter following open heart surgery, atrial pacing by means of an electrode catheter or temporary pacing wires implanted at the time of surgery can be extremely useful. Rapid atrial pacing can either convert the atrial flutter to sinus rhythm or precipitate the appearance of atrial fibrillation with a slowing of the ventricular response owing to concealed conduction.

If the ventricular response is not excessive, digitalis is the treatment of choice for atrial flutter. By shortening atrial refractoriness, digitalis may convert atrial flutter to atrial fibrillation; at the same time, digitalis acts to slow conduction in the AV node. Once full digitalization is accomplished, quinidine sulfate may be started. It is always advisable to begin treatment with digitalis, since therapy with quinidine in a patient not on digitalis may slow the atrial flutter rate while enhancing conduction in the AV node (owing to a vagolytic effect), resulting in a more rapid ventricular response. If the use of digitalis and quinidine fails to convert atrial flutter to either atrial fibrillation with a slower ventricular response or sinus rhythm, it is inadvisable to proceed to cardioversion because of the possibility of precipitating more serious ventricular dysrhythmias in the presence of digitalis. In this latter instance, intravenous propranolol may be of use in slowing the ventricular response; this is also an excellent situation in which to use rapid atrial pacing with a temporary pacing electrode catheter.

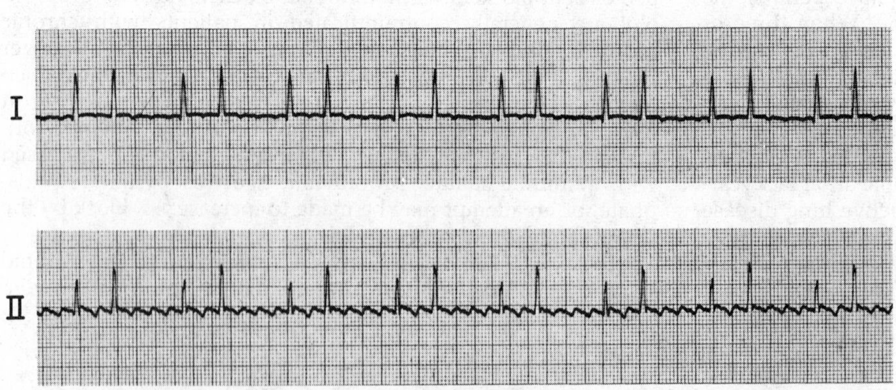

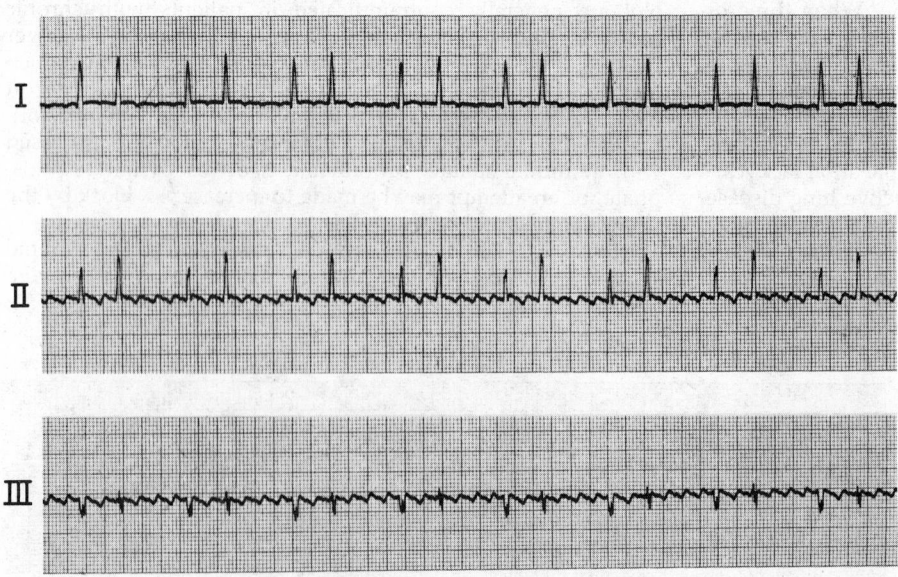

Figure 50–14. Atrial flutter with varying AV block. This electrocardiogram, recorded during a period of varying AV block induced by a vagal maneuver, demonstrates the characteristic "sawtooth" appearance of P waves during atrial flutter.

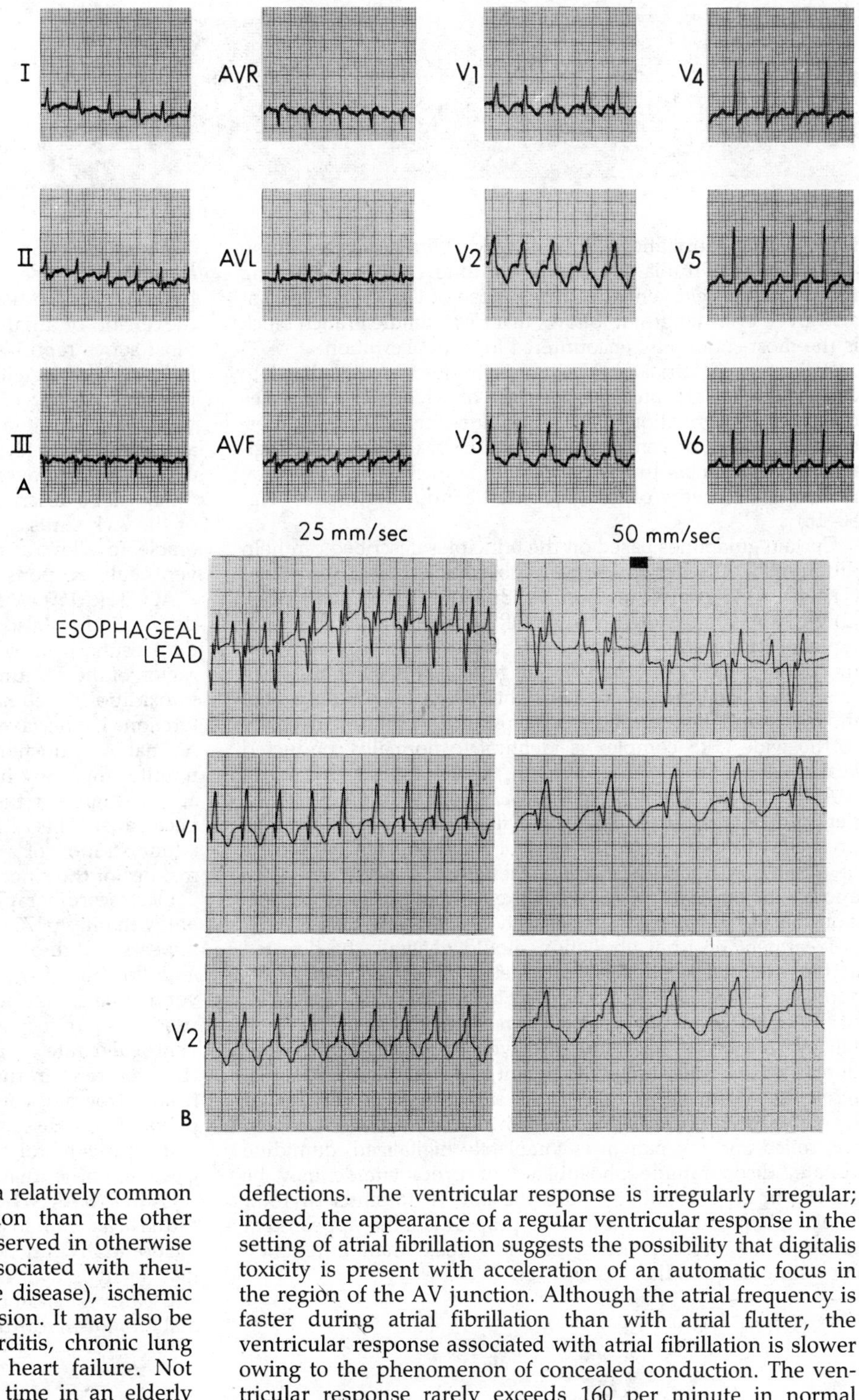

Figure 50–15. Atrial flutter with persistent 2:1 AV block. In *A*, a 12 lead electrocardiogram demonstrates a regular supraventricular tachycardia associated with a ventricular response of 167 per minute. Persistent right bundle branch block is present. In *B*, an esophageal lead recorded simultaneously with V_1 and V_2 demonstrates atrial flutter at a rate of 334 per minute. Although in retrospect one of the flutter waves can be identified midway between the two QRS complexes in *A*, the second flutter wave is buried in the QRS complex and can only be identified on the esophageal lead.

ATRIAL FIBRILLATION. Atrial fibrillation is a relatively common arrhythmia and considerably more common than the other forms of atrial arrhythmias. It has been observed in otherwise normal subjects but is most frequently associated with rheumatic heart disease (especially mitral valve disease), ischemic heart disease, thyrotoxicosis, and hypertension. It may also be associated with atrial septal defect, pericarditis, chronic lung disease, cardiomyopathy, and congestive heart failure. Not uncommonly, it may appear for the first time in an elderly patient hospitalized with a febrile illness such as pneumonia.

Atrial fibrillation can precipitate congestive heart failure by depriving the heart of an effective atrial contraction as well as by bombarding the atrioventricular junction with rapid and irregular impulses, resulting in a rapid irregular ventricular response. Atrial fibrillation also predisposes to both pulmonary and peripheral emboli. Approximately 30 per cent of patients with longstanding atrial fibrillation (especially in association with mitral valve disease) will experience at least one embolic episode.

Electrocardiographically, atrial fibrillation is distinguished by disorganized atrial activity with an approximate frequency of 400 to 650 per minute. No discrete P waves can be identified, and atrial activity manifests itself only as uneven irregular deflections. The ventricular response is irregularly irregular; indeed, the appearance of a regular ventricular response in the setting of atrial fibrillation suggests the possibility that digitalis toxicity is present with acceleration of an automatic focus in the region of the AV junction. Although the atrial frequency is faster during atrial fibrillation than with atrial flutter, the ventricular response associated with atrial fibrillation is slower owing to the phenomenon of concealed conduction. The ventricular response rarely exceeds 160 per minute in normal subjects (Fig. 50–16).

The presence of irregularly irregular ventricular responses during atrial fibrillation promotes the appearance of aberrantly conducted beats. This phenomenon can best be understood by recalling a few features of the basic electrophysiology of the heart. In general, the recovery time or refractoriness of cardiac tissue is directly proportional to the duration of the preceding cycle or R-R interval. Thus longer cycle lengths are followed by longer periods of refractoriness. It follows that a supraventricular beat is more likely to encounter refractoriness and be conducted aberrantly if it occurs early after a long preceding R-R interval. The association of aberration with "long-short" sequences in R-R intervals has been called the "Ashman phenomenon." The irregularity of ventricular responses character-

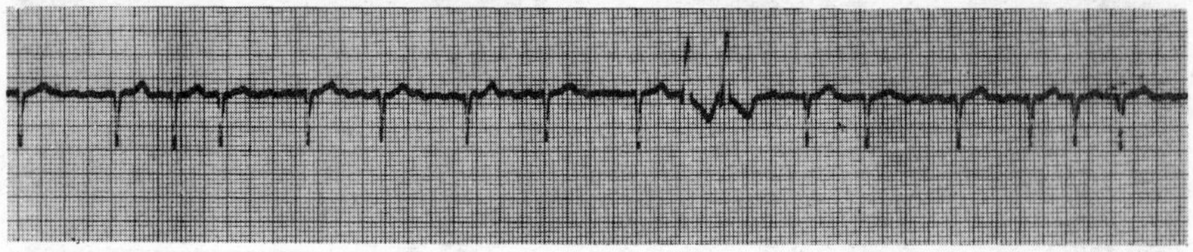

Figure 50–16. Ventricular aberration during atrial fibrillation. An irregularly irregular ventricular response is present. Two wide QRS complexes are observed following a long-short sequence. These beats are most likely supraventricular impulses associated with aberrant conduction. See text for discussion.

istic of atrial fibrillation explains why aberration is common with this arrhythmia. The recovery time of the conducting tissues of the *right* ventricle *exceeds* those of the left ventricle at any given cycle length; it follows that *right* bundle branch block is the most commonly encountered form of aberration.

Patients with atrial fibrillation are frequently digitalized to control their heart rate. The presence of wide QRS complexes during atrial fibrillation in these patients thus raises the differential diagnosis of ventricular premature beats caused by digitalis toxicity versus functional bundle branch block caused by incomplete recovery of the specialized conducting tissues (Fig. 50–16).

Certain guidelines based on the principles described can help differentiate these two entities. Aberration is favored when (1) wide QRS complexes occur with "long-short" sequences, (2) the appearance of the wide QRS complex conforms to a typical configuration of functional aberration (a triphasic rSR′ morphology in V_1 is especially suggestive of aberration, since this is the usual morphology of right bundle branch block, the most common variety of aberration), and (3) the initial vector of the wide QRS complex is identical to normally conducted beats.

As mentioned above, a ventricular response in excess of 160 per minute associated with atrial fibrillation is unusual; the presence of a ventricular response of 200 or greater in a setting of atrial fibrillation (especially when this is associated with anomalous-appearing QRS complexes) should raise the suspicion that some variety of pre-excitation is present.

Treatment of atrial fibrillation should generally be directed at the underlying etiology, provided that the ventricular response is not causing hemodynamic compromise. If a suspicion of pre-excitation exists (ventricular rate greater than 200), digitalis should be avoided and cardioversion carried out expeditiously. If the situation is less urgent, digitalis can be administered intravenously or orally until slowing of the ventricular response has occurred. Once the ventricular response has been controlled and the patient is completely digitalized, quinidine sulfate, disopyramide phosphate,* or procainamide may be started in an attempt to return the patient to sinus rhythm. The combination of quinidine and propranolol has appeared at times to be more effective and less toxic than a regimen consisting of quinidine alone.

*Experimental drug for this purpose.

If atrial fibrillation has been longstanding or associated with advanced disease of the atria, conversion is less likely to be longlasting. The use of anticoagulants prior to attempted cardioversion of atrial fibrillation has remained controversial, but most series report a 2 per cent incidence of peripheral emboli following conversion to sinus rhythm. In patients with a previous history of emboli or in patients with known mitral valve disease, it appears judicious to institute a course of anticoagulation for at least three to six weeks prior to any attempt at cardioversion.

As will be described later, atrial fibrillation may be one aspect of the sick sinus syndrome. In such patients, it may be preferable to allow atrial fibrillation to persist with a controlled ventricular response.

ACCELERATED AV JUNCTIONAL RHYTHM. Accelerated AV junctional rhythm (also called nonparoxysmal AV nodal tachycardia) results from conditions that enhance automaticity in the region of the AV junction and is most commonly due to digitalis intoxication, rheumatic fever, or diaphragmatic myocardial infarction. If one takes into account that the *inherent* rate of the normal AV junctional pacemakers ranges from 40 to 60 per minute, then any intrinsic rhythm arising in the AV junction at a rate greater than 60 per minute represents an enhanced pacemaker. This arrhythmia can also be observed following the administration of atropine in patients with underlying abnormalities of the sinus node.

Electrocardiographically, a regular ventricular rhythm is present with rates of 70 to 140 per minute. This arrhythmia generally appears and disappears through a process of gradual speeding and slowing of the junctional pacemaker. An increase in the ventricular rate is noted on exercise, and carotid sinus massage produces no response or results in gradual slowing of the ventricular rate. A normal QRS complex is the rule. Since the rhythm arises in the AV junction, atrial activation may result from retrograde conduction from the AV junction or be independent (AV dissociation) (Fig. 50–17).

It is unusual for enhanced AV junctional rhythms to require treatment other than that indicated for the underlying disorder.

PAROXYSMAL ATRIAL TACHYCARDIA. Paroxysmal atrial tachycardia is a common arrhythmia referred to by a variety of terms, including AV junctional tachycardia, paroxysmal supraventricular tachycardia, reciprocating supraventricular tachycardia, and paroxysmal nodal tachycardia. The popular term paroxysmal atrial tachycardia is in fact a misnomer, since the tachycar-

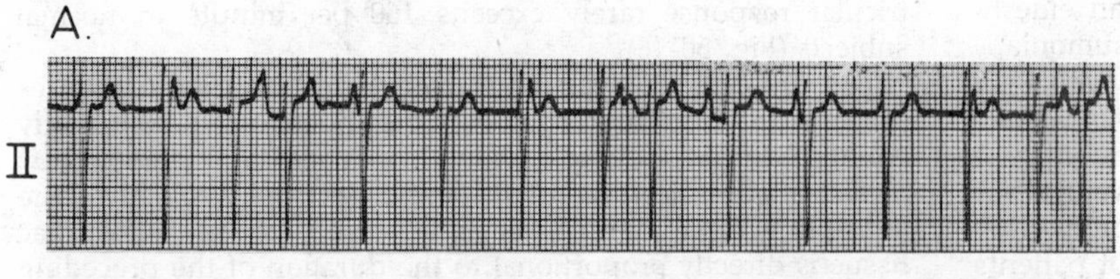

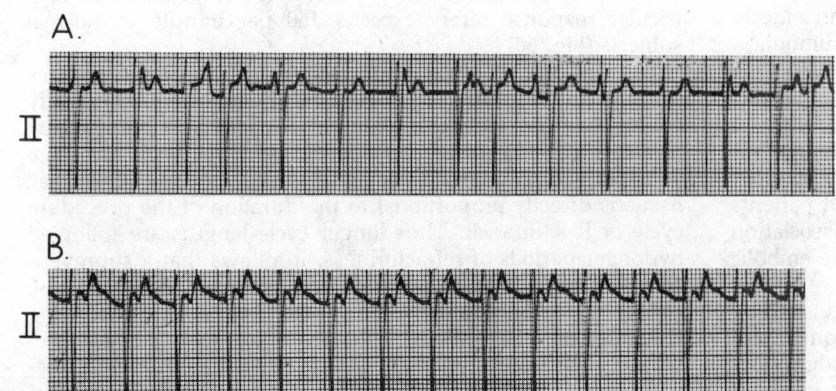

Figure 50–17. Nonparoxysmal junctional tachycardia due to digitalis toxicity. In *A*, a narrow QRS tachycardia is present at 107 per minute. Sinus P waves are present at a slower rate of 96 per minute with occasional capture beats. In *B*, the junctional rate has increased to 125 per minute and is now associated with 1:1 retrograde conduction to the atrium. Note the absence of P wave activity preceding junctional beats in *A* and *B*.

dia usually does not arise in the atrium. The arrhythmia of true atrial origin has been previously discussed under Ectopic Atrial Tachycardia. Of all the terms used, AV junctional tachycardia seems preferable, since it focuses attention on the region of the AV junction, which is an essential link in the re-entry loop regardless of the underlying mechanism. Although a variety of potential mechanisms exist for AV junctional tachycardia, the two most common include re-entry confined to the region of the AV node and re-entry utilizing an accessory pathway between the ventricles and the atria. Because much of the description of AV junctional tachycardia must be related to the pre-excitation syndromes, discussion of the mechanisms of this arrhythmia is best considered as a unit and will be deferred until consideration of the pre-excitation syndromes (see below).

ACCELERATED IDIOVENTRICULAR RHYTHM. The inherent rate of an idioventricular pacemaker (located distal to the His bundle) is approximately 30 to 40 per minute. When such a focus is observed at a rate greater than this, it is referred to as an accelerated idioventricular rhythm. Accelerated idioventricular rhythms are commonly observed with rates of 60 to 120 per minute, with the average rate being approximately 100 per minute, bordering on the rate criteria for clinical tachycardia. Most commonly, this arrhythmia is observed in the setting of diaphragmatic myocardial infarction, digitalis toxicity, complete heart block, and hypokalemia.

Electrocardiographically, the QRS complexes are wide, greater than 0.14 second in duration, and bizarre in appearance, as is the case with all ventricular pacemakers. The rate of the ectopic pacemaker is frequently close to the prevailing sinus rate, accounting for the presence of frequent *fusion* beats (Fig. 50–18). Fusion beats are complexes that appear somewhat intermediate between completely normal sinus beats and the wide bizarre ventricular complexes. Fusion beats have particular significance because they suggest that activation of the ventricle arises in part from a supraventricular impulse with varying contribution to the activation by a ventricular impulse. Accelerated idioventricular rhythms generally emerge late in the cardiac cycle, frequently in the form of a fusion beat. Brief periods of isorhythmic dissociation (see later discussion) may be observed.

Accelerated idioventricular rhythms rarely require treatment unless the resulting dissociation compromises hemodynamic function, in which case small doses of atropine will usually speed the sinus rates sufficiently to suppress the rhythm. Rarely, accelerated idioventricular rhythms have been associated with more rapid ventricular arrhythmias.

VENTRICULAR TACHYCARDIA. The presence of three or more ectopic ventricular beats (arising below the level of the His bundle) at a rate in excess of 100 per minute constitutes ventricular tachycardia. Ventricular tachycardia invariably occurs at a rate in excess of 120 per minute and most often occurs in the range of 150 to 210 per minute. Ventricular tachycardia is usually associated with organic heart disease, with common etiologies including acute myocardial infarction, chronic ischemic heart disease (at times associated with a ventricular aneurysm), cardiomyopathy, and rheumatic heart disease. It may also be observed with prolapse of the mitral valve and digitalis toxicity. Ventricular tachycardia has been reported in some young patients with no evidence of heart disease. Numerous drugs have also been incriminated in the genesis of ventricular tachycardia.

The clinical presentation of a patient in ventricular tachycardia is entirely related to the rate of tachycardia and the underlying hemodynamic condition of the heart. Electrocardiographically, wide QRS complexes, which are frequently bizarre, occur regularly at rates in excess of 120 per minute. The paroxysm of tachycardia frequently is initiated by a premature ventricular beat. It is important to differentiate this arrhythmia from a supraventricular tachycardia associated with functional aberration (Figs. 50–19 and 50–20). The differentiation of supraventricular tachycardia with aberration from ventricular tachycardia can frequently be made on the basis of the electrocardiogram alone. A QRS duration exceeding 0.14 second is suggestive of a ventricular origin of tachycardia; left axis deviation in the frontal plane is also suggestive of a ventricular origin. Certain QRS configurations observed in lead V_1 are helpful; thus, the presence of a "classic" triphasic pattern (i.e., rsR') in V_1 is highly suggestive of a supraventricular origin. Ventricular tachycardia is generally associated with a regular rhythm; the presence of an irregular tachycardia with wide QRS complexes associated with a rate in excess of 200 per minute should arouse suspicion of atrial fibrillation with conduction over an anomalous accessory pathway. The presence of capture beats with normal QRS complexes or fusion beats with intermediate QRS morphology resulting from conduction of dissociated atrial activity during tachycardia strongly favors the presence of ventricular tachycardia, but unfortunately these findings are uncommon, occurring primarily in cases of slow ventricular tachycardia (Fig. 50–21). The presence of AV dissociation during tachycardia is an extremely helpful finding. If the ventricular rate of a wide QRS tachycardia is greater than the atrial rate, ventricular tachycardia is almost invariably present. This should prompt an exhaustive search for the P wave in the electrocardiogram as well as evidence on physical examination of atrioventricular dissociation. If no atrial activity is observed, esophageal recording can be used to find the nature of atrial activity (Fig. 50–19). Carotid sinus massage usually has no effect on the ventricular rate of ventricular tachycardia but may permit dissociation of atrial activity when 1:1 VA conduction is present. Rarely, carotid sinus massage results in termination of documented ventricular tachycardia. The mechanism of this termi-

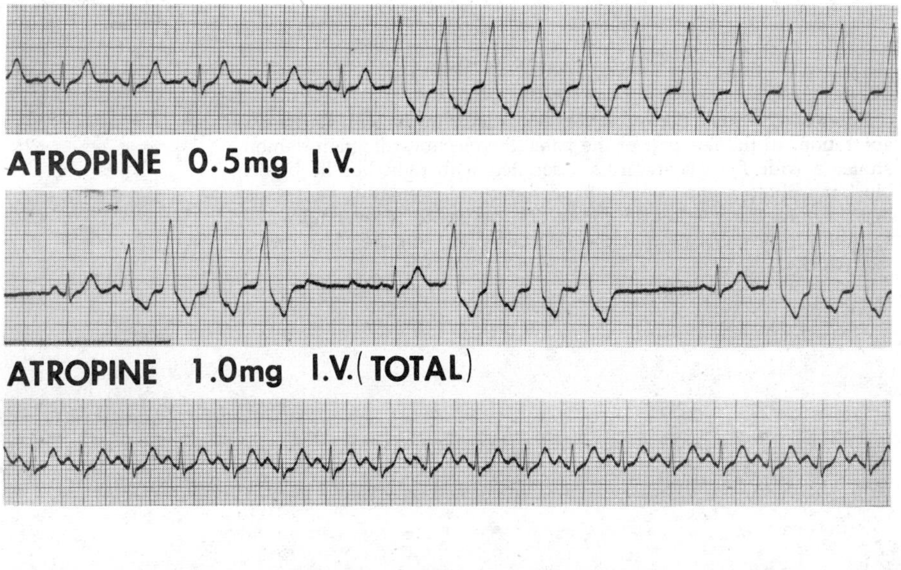

Figure 50–18. Accelerated idioventricular rhythm. In the top panel, sinus rhythm is interrupted by a wide QRS tachycardia, which emerges in late diastole. The deformity on the S-T segment of the wide QRS complexes is probably due to retrograde P wave activity. In the middle panel, 0.5 mg of atropine has been administered intravenously. Sinus rhythm is again interrupted by wide QRS tachycardia emerging in late diastole. Note that the first episode of tachycardia is introduced by a ventricular complex that is intermediate in morphology between the sinus complex and the wide QRS complex of the sustained rhythm. This beat is a fusion beat. The bottom panel was recorded after the administration of a total of 1.0 mg of atropine intravenously. The sinus rate has now increased to 130 per minute and has completely suppressed the accelerated idioventricular rhythm.

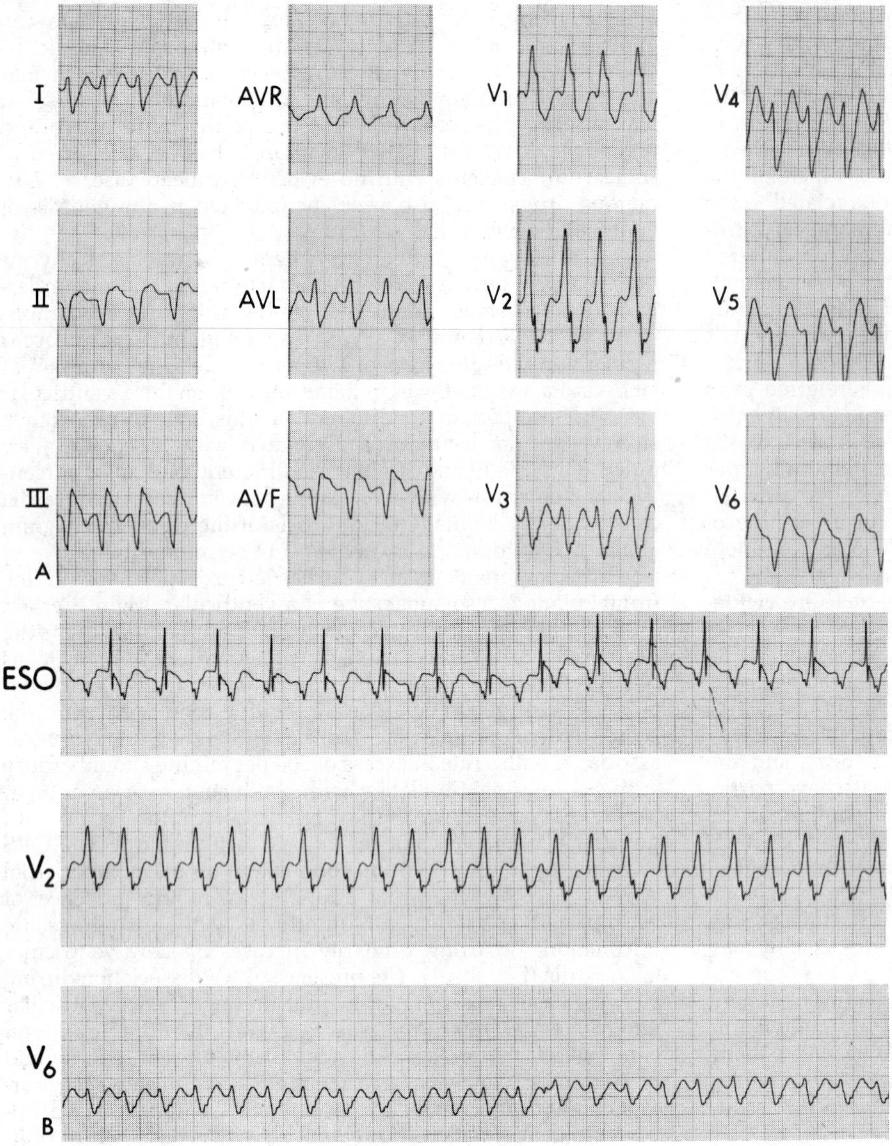

Figure 50–19. Ventricular tachycardia. *A* is a 12 lead electrocardiogram recorded during a wide QRS complex tachycardia of 150 per minute in a patient with ischemic heart disease. The QRS demonstrates a qR morphology in V_1 and a superiorly directed axis suggesting ventricular tachycardia. No discrete P wave activity can be observed. The S-T segment in V_2 suggests retrograde P wave activity, but the amplitude is too large for atrial activity. *B* demonstrates an esophageal recording obtained during the same tachycardia as *A* and documents the presence of sinus tachycardia at a rate of 100 per minute and complete ventriculoatrial dissociation.

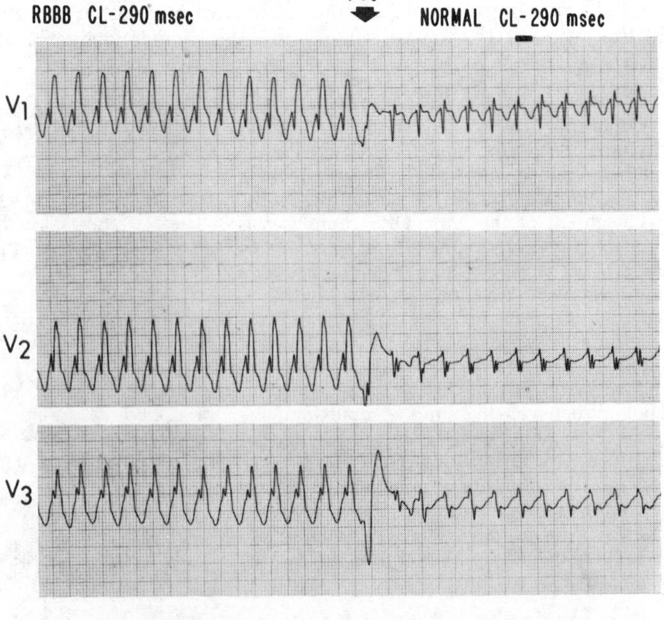

Figure 50–20. Sustained supraventricular tachycardia with ventricular aberration. In the left part of the panel the electrocardiogram demonstrates a wide QRS tachycardia associated with right bundle branch block morphology at a rate of 207 per minute. A premature ventricular beat permits the specialized conducting tissues to recover normally, resulting in normalization of the QRS complex with the same rate of tachycardia.

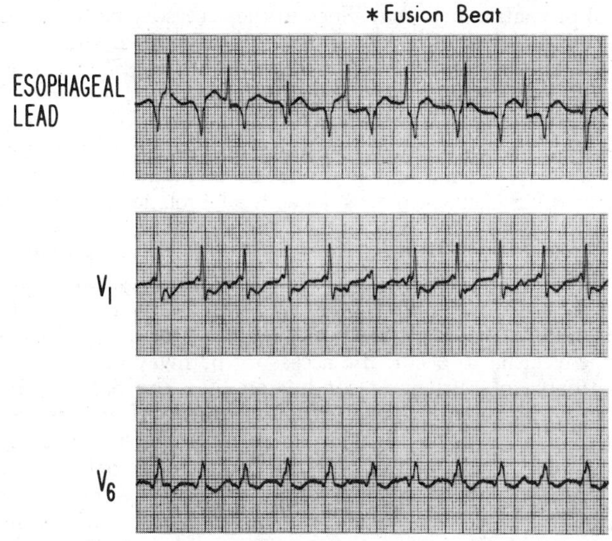

Figure 50–21. Fusion beats during ventricular tachycardia. Recordings are shown from an esophageal lead and standard precordial leads V_1 and V_6 during a wide QRS tachycardia at a rate of 120 per minute. The esophageal lead demonstrates atrial activity at a rate of 86 per minute. After five ventricular complexes, a QRS complex is noted which appears more normal in configuration. Note that this fusion beat is preceded by atrial activity.

nation has been ascribed to a reflex inhibition of sympathetic nervous activity, but this phenomenon should be considered rare.

The choice of therapy for ventricular tachycardia depends largely on the setting in which the tachycardia is observed. If immediate restoration to sinus rhythm is desirable because of hemodynamic considerations, low energy direct current cardioversion is the treatment of choice unless digitalis toxicity is suspected. Intravenous lidocaine is quite effective in suppressing the arrhythmia in most cases. Intravenous procainamide is also useful in terminating an acute attack. Long-term suppression of ventricular tachycardia can be accomplished by the administration of quinidine sulfate, procainamide, or disopyramide phosphate. Propranolol and phenytoin may also be useful. In general, refractory cases require a combination of drugs. Patients with recurring ventricular tachycardia in the setting of a slow basic heart rate may require ventricular pacing at a more rapid rate to effect suppression.

VENTRICULAR FIBRILLATION. Ventricular fibrillation consists of disorganized, chaotic activity on the surface electrocardiogram. Unless immediately cardioverted, it is a terminal rhythm. Bretylium may be effective in allowing sinus rhythm to be restored by cardioversion when the latter alone has proved unsuccessful.

TORSADES DE POINTES. Torsades de pointes (Fig. 50–22) refers to a particular type of ventricular tachycardia–fibrillation, the recognition of which has important therapeutic implications. Patients prone to this type of arrhythmia frequently exhibit prolongation of the Q-T interval during sinus rhythm. Recognized causes of torsades de pointes include slow cardiac rhythm owing to high grade AV block or SA block, electrolyte deficiencies such as hypokalemia or hypomagnesemia, congenital Q-T syndromes with or without deafness, and drugs including quinidine, disopyramide, procainamide, and various psychotropic agents such as phenothiazines and tricyclic antidepressants. Clinically, attacks of the rhythm may be brief and self-terminated and may be a cause of syncope. Some cases, however, progress to typical ventricular fibrillation resulting in death. The onset of the tachycardia is somewhat unusual; whereas ventricular tachycardia frequently follows an early premature ventricular beat which falls on the T wave, in torsades de pointes the initiating extrasystole is usually late.

Electrocardiographically, the appearance of this arrhythmia is distinctive, consisting of paroxysms of tachycardia in which the QRS axis undulates over runs of 5 to 20 beats, resulting in twisting of the points of the QRS complexes around an imaginary isoelectric line.

Treatment is generally directed toward the underlying cause. In cases in which the arrhythmia is recurring, immediate therapy consists somewhat paradoxically of the infusion of isoproterenol to shorten repolarization and to make recovery of the ventricles more uniform. Overdrive atrial or ventricular pacing at rates from 120 to 150 per minute is a convenient way to stabilize this rhythm until the underlying factors can receive attention. In some patients, therapy with propranolol may be indicated, provided that a slow basic rate was not contributory to the appearance of the rhythm. Left stellate ganglionectomy has been advocated as a potential mode of treatment.

THE PRE-EXCITATION SYNDROME. The term pre-excitation refers to a variety of situations whereby an accessory pathway "bypasses" some portion of the normal conduction system, with two important consequences: (1) The presence of such an accessory pathway may allow the normal physiologic delaying mechanism of the AV node to be bypassed, and (2) the presence of a parallel conduction system at some level of the heart provides a route for re-entry. The most common variety of pre-excitation is found in the Wolff-Parkinson-White syndrome resulting from an accessory atrioventricular pathway (the so-called bundle of Kent). The QRS complex in patients with an accessory AV pathway results from fusion of impulses reaching the ventricle over the normal conduction system and over the accessory pathway (Fig. 50–23). The result is an abbreviated P-R interval (owing to bypass of the physiologic delay of the AV node) and a wide anomalous QRS complex (owing to eccentric depolarization initiated in the ventricle by the accessory pathway). The abnormal initial forces arising from the "pre-excited area" constitute the delta wave, and this varies according to the degree of pre-excitation. The vector of the delta wave is determined by the location of the accessory pathway. Unless recognized, such abnormal initial forces may lead to an erroneous diagnosis of previous myocardial infarction (Fig. 50–24).

The designation "syndrome" arises from the fact that patients with accessory pathways are subject to recurring palpitations resulting from mechanisms to be described below. These are of two general varieties. The first is paroxysmal atrial tachycardia (AV junctional tachycardia), alluded to above. The second is atrial fibrillation associated with a rapid ventricular response, at times resulting in ventricular fibrillation.

The mechanism of AV junctional tachycardia can be briefly summarized by referring to Figure 50–23. As an example, an

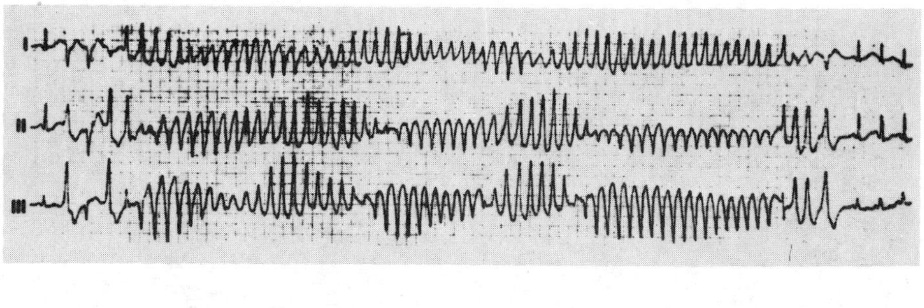

Figure 50–22. Torsades de pointes. Sinus rhythm associated with a long Q-T interval is present at the beginning and at the end of this rhythm strip. Sinus rhythm is interrupted by a rapid wide QRS tachycardia. Note that during the tachycardia, the direction of the points of the QRS complex appear to revolve around an imaginary isoelectric line. (From Krikler DM, Curry PVL: Br Heart J 38:118, 1976. With permission of the British Heart Journal and authors.)

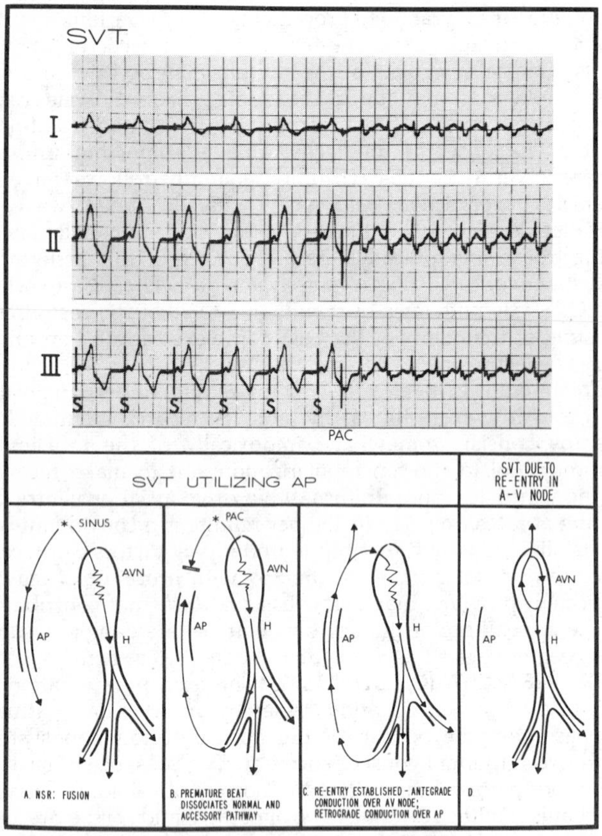

Figure 50–23. Mechanism of supraventricular tachycardia utilizing an accessory pathway. The upper panel demonstrates an electrocardiogram recorded in a patient with Wolff-Parkinson-White syndrome during straight atrial pacing and the introduction of a premature atrial beat. The first five beats are preceded by a stimulus artifact (S); a short P-R interval and a wide QRS complex indicate the presence of pre-excitation. Following the introduction of a premature beat, a narrow QRS tachycardia is initiated. The events underlying this supraventricular tachycardia are diagrammatically shown in the lower panels. During sinus rhythm *(A)*, fusion is present owing to conduction over the AV node (AVN) and the accessory pathway (AP). In *B*, a premature atrial contraction (PAC) blocks in the accessory pathway and conducts with delay over the AV node, thus dissociating the activity of the normal and accessory pathways. In *C*, the impulse conducting through the ventricle travels retrograde over the accessory pathway and re-enters the atrium, establishing a tachycardia. *D* demonstrates schematically the re-entry circuit underlying supraventricular tachycardia resulting from re-entry confined to the AV node.

atrial premature beat may block in the accessory pathway, and be conducted after delay in the AV node over the normal conduction system to the ventricles (normal QRS). After activation reaches the base of the ventricle (terminal portion of the QRS complex), it can return *retrograde* over the accessory pathway to the atrium. The analogy of this type of re-entry to that shown schematically in Figure 50–5 should be obvious. A narrow QRS tachycardia ensues with a 1:1 relationship between ventricles and atria but, notably, one in which the P wave *follows* the QRS complex. Reversal of this re-entry circuit is rarely observed. An examination of the re-entry loop reveals that it is not necessary for the accessory pathway to conduct antegradely (i.e., from atrium to ventricle) for this mechanism of tachycardia to occur; the accessory pathway only needs to be capable of retrograde conduction (i.e., the pathway may have unidirectional block). The phenomenon of unidirectional block has been recognized for some time, and recent studies have sought evidence of this phenomenon in patients with recurrent supraventricular tachycardia with no evidence of pre-excitation. In referral series, the incidence with which such concealed accessory pathways constitute the underlying mechanism of tachycardia ranges from 20 to 40 per cent. This mechanism of AV junctional tachycardia must be distinguished from conventional re-entry in the AV node (Fig. 50–23*D*). In the latter case, re-entry is confined to the AV node. Because of its location, re-entry in the AV node can spread toward the atria and ventricles simultaneously. Theoretically, since both atria and ventricles are "bystanders," they can bear any time relationship to each other, even to the point of dissociation. In point of fact, there is usually a consistent 1:1 relationship between the atria and ventricles, and, typically, both depolarize almost simultaneously, accounting for superimposition of the P wave on the QRS complex.

Supraventricular tachycardia resulting from one of these two mechanisms accounts for the most common forms of paroxysmal tachycardia encountered in children and young adults. Although congenital in the case of an accessory pathway, tachycardia can appear at any age, presumably because the initiation of re-entry generally requires an ectopic beat from the atria, AV junction, or ventricles; the latter events increase in frequency with age.

Clinically, AV junctional tachycardias are generally well tolerated in the absence of associated heart disease. The presence of angina accompanying tachycardia is rare provided that the heart rate is less than 170 per minute, and should raise the suspicion that coronary artery disease is also present. A post-tachycardia diuresis may follow a paroxysm of tachycardia resulting from a stretch reflex in the atrial wall. Regardless of the mechanism, tachycardia characteristically occurs with sudden onset and sudden offset. During the actual paroxysm, both mechanisms of tachycardia can be associated either with normal QRS complexes or with functional aberration. As previously

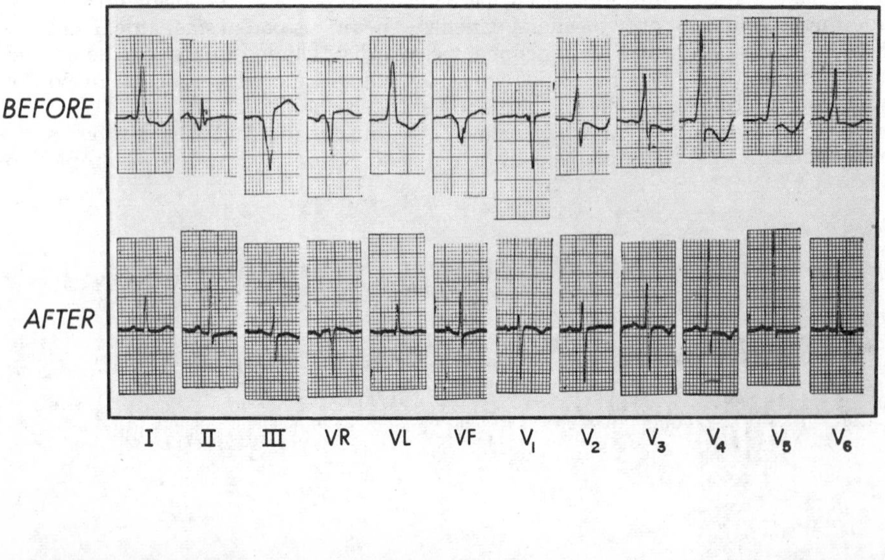

Figure 50–24. Electrocardiogram in a patient with Wolff-Parkinson-White syndrome before and after surgical division of the accessory pathway. Note that prior to division of the accessory pathway, a short P-R interval and a wide QRS complex are present. After surgical division of the accessory pathway, the P-R interval as well as the QRS complex becomes normal.

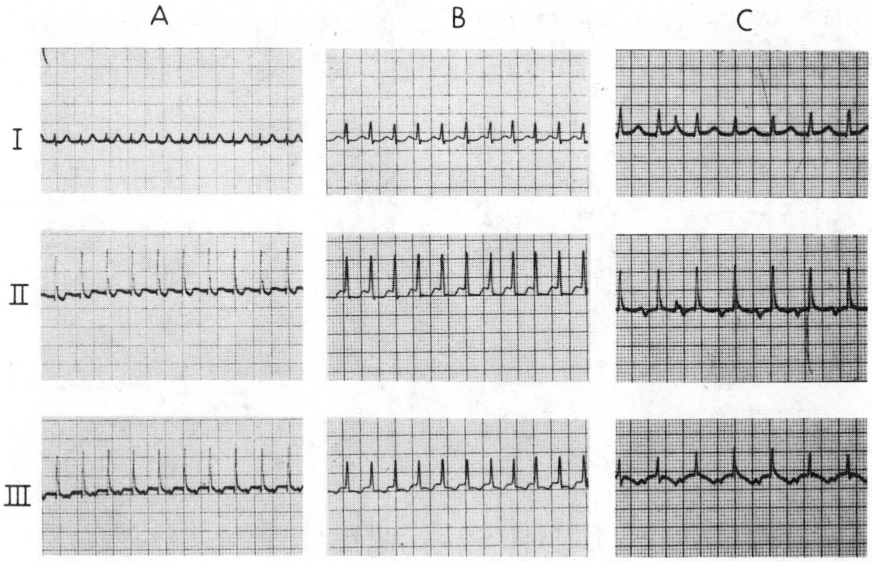

Figure 50–25. Diagnostic significance of the relation of the P wave and QRS complex in various types of supraventricular tachycardia. *A* was recorded during supraventricular tachycardia in a patient with a concealed accessory pathway between the ventricles and atria. Retrograde P waves can be observed following each QRS complex in III. This close relation of a retrograde P wave to a preceding QRS complex is characteristic and should suggest the possibility of concealed accessory pathway. *B* is a tracing reported during supraventricular tachycardia caused by re-entry in the AV node. No retrograde P wave activity can be identified because the atria and ventricles are depolarized simultaneously owing to re-entry in the AV node. In *C*, there is a 1:1 relationship between the P wave and the QRS. The P wave is closer to the succeeding QRS complex. The differential of this tachycardia includes an ectopic atrial tachycardia with antegrade conduction to the ventricle, an atypical form of re-entry in the AV node and the so-called "permanent form of junctional reciprocating tachycardia," a tachycardia which utilizes an accessory AV node for retrograde conduction. Careful observation of the P wave in relation to the QRS complex allows supraventricular tachycardias to be readily classified into certain diagnostic categories.

mentioned, a 1:1 relationship of atria and ventricles is typical, but the position of the P wave relative to the QRS complex provides insight into the underlying mechanism (Fig. 50–25). Carotid sinus massage during an episode of tachycardia may have no effect or may result in prompt termination of tachycardia. Examination of the ECG during the period of enhanced vagal tone which accompanies the termination of tachycardia by carotid massage may unmask evidence of antegrade pre-excitation (i.e., delta wave). The question of whether or not an accessory pathway is involved is more than academic, not only because the medical management may differ but also because surgical techniques are available to make division of the accessory pathway possible, thus relieving the patient of the need for further drug therapy.

The treatment of AV junctional tachycardias can be divided into acute and chronic management. Acutely, such maneuvers as carotid sinus massage and the Valsalva maneuver should be performed with the patient recumbent and legs elevated. If these prove ineffective, edrophonium chloride, 10 mg intravenously, can be administered as previously noted to enhance the vagal effect.† Intravenous verapamil is exceptionally effective in terminating these tachycardias. Phenylephrine, 0.5 to 1.0 mg, can be administered slowly intravenously over two to three minutes with termination of tachycardia mediated by a vagal baroreceptor reflex from the resulting hypertension. When hemodynamic collapse accompanies tachycardia, transvenous pacing or direct current cardioversion can be used. Intravenous propranolol (0.1 mg per kilogram given at a rate of 1.0 mg every two minutes) or digitalis can also be effective in terminating a paroxysm, although it is preferable to avoid digitalis in patients known to have pre-excitation (see below).

Chronic management of AV junctional tachycardia is directed toward abolishing the premature beats that initiate re-entry (quinidine sulfate, disopyramide phosphate, procainamide) as well as modifying the "weak link" in the re-entry circuit so as to prevent re-entry from occurring. The latter objective can be satisfied by attempting to block the AV node with digitalis or propranolol or by attempting to prolong refractoriness and delay conduction in the accessory pathway (if present) by administering quinidine sulfate, disopyramide phosphate,* or procainamide.

The second major arrhythmia related to the pre-excitation syndromes occurs in the setting of atrial fibrillation. Assuming that the accessory pathway is capable of conducting antegrade from atrium to ventricle, rapid impulses arising in the fibrillating atria can propagate to the ventricles over the accessory pathway, resulting in a rapid irregular ventricular response associated with bizarre QRS complexes (Fig. 50–26). Occasionally, this can terminate in ventricular fibrillation, accounting for reports of sudden death in the pre-excitation syndromes. Therapy in this instance must be directed toward preventing the atrial fibrillation or by blocking antegrade conduction over the accessory pathway. Happily both objectives are achieved by the administration of quinidine sulfate, disopyramide phosphate, or procainamide. Propranolol notably has no effect on conduction in the accessory pathway. In some patients, digitalis can shorten refractoriness and speed conduction in the accessory pathway, resulting in a more rapid ventricular response. The use of digitalis is therefore inadvisable in patients with known pre-excitation unless their accessory pathway is known to be incapable of conducting rapidly during atrial fibrillation. Finally, in patients refractory to conventional management, surgical interruption of the accessory pathway may be successful.

BRADYCARDIA

Bradycardia is said to be present when the heart rate is less than 60 per minute and can result from an abnormality of impulse formation, impulse propagation, or both. The presence or absence of symptoms is an important qualifier to any condition in which bradycardia is present. Nevertheless, it is important to note at the outset that often the presence of symptoms is appreciated only in retrospect once the bradycardia has been corrected by removing the causal factor or by the institution of artificial pacing. This phenomenon is especially common in the elderly, in whom such vague and insidious symptoms as confusion or early dementia may clear once a normal ventricular response is restored.

SINUS BRADYCARDIA. Sinus bradycardia is defined as a sinus rate of less than 60 per minute and is an expected normal finding in young healthy adults and athletes. It is difficult to ascribe an absolute cutoff for a rate that can be considered clearly pathologic. The actual rate must be interpreted as appropriate or inappropriate, considering the circumstances in which it is observed. Thus, sinus bradycardia that persists in

*Experimental drug for this purpose.
†This use is not listed in the manufacturer's directive.

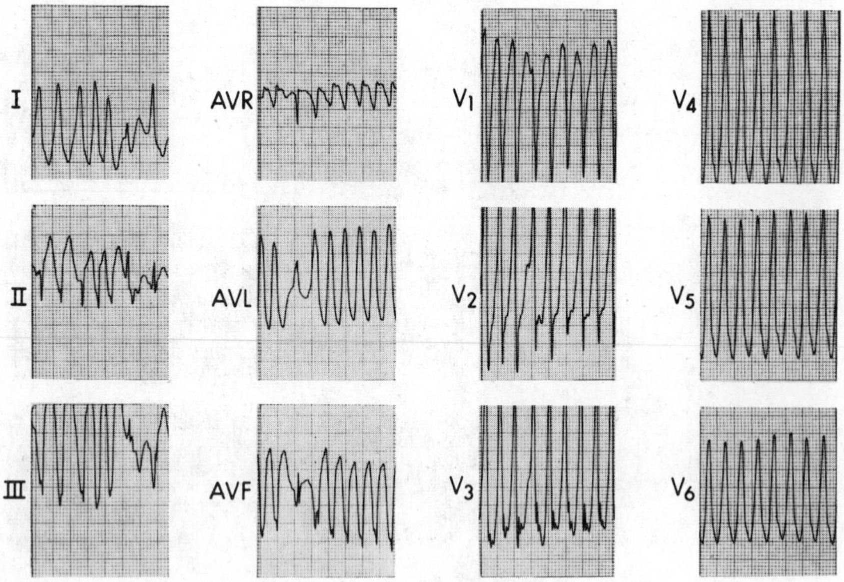

Figure 50–26. Atrial fibrillation in the Wolff-Parkinson-White syndrome. The electrocardiogram demonstrates the irregularly irregular response associated with anomalous-appearing QRS complexes resulting from atrial fibrillation with rapid conduction over the accessory pathway to the ventricle.

the presence of congestive heart failure, pain, or exercise or following the administration of atropine or isoproterenol may be considered abnormal. Sinus bradycardia normally accompanies the administration of such drugs as propranolol, morphine, and reserpine. In normal patients, digitalis does not normally slow the sinus rate. Sinus bradycardia is a common finding early in the course of a diaphragmatic infarction. Other, more unusual causes of sinus bradycardia include various infectious diseases, myxedema, increased intracranial pressure, obstructive jaundice, and hypothermia.

In general, sinus bradycardia does not require treatment. Bradycardia accompanied by hypotension or evidence of low cardiac output can be treated by *cautious* administration of small (i.e., 0.4 mg) incremental doses of atropine intravenously. If there is any suggestion that symptoms such as congestive heart failure, presyncope or syncope, poor exercise tolerance, or cerebral symptoms are due to a persistent inappropriately slow rate, a trial of temporary pacing should be strongly considered.

SICK SINUS SYNDROME. The term sick sinus syndrome refers to a constellation of electrocardiographic findings, all of which have in common dysfunction of the sinus node. The term as such is misleading because it gives undue importance to the role of the sinus node per se in the pathogenesis of the various abnormalities observed. In many instances, for example, it is more probable that a global atrial disease process is present, which somewhat incidentally involves the sinus node. Nevertheless for didactic purposes the term is useful, since the dysfunction of the sinus node plays a prominent role in the clinical presentation. The following abnormalities are generally encompassed by the sick sinus syndrome: (1) persistent inappropriate sinus bradycardia; (2) sinoatrial (SA) block; (3) SA arrest with no appearance of escape rhythm from the atrium, junction, or ventricle; and (4) "bradycardia-tachycardia" syndrome, in which bursts of ectopic atrial tachycardia or atrial fibrillation alternate with inappropriate suppression of the sinus node as well as subsidiary pacemaker activity. In addition, some workers include persistent atrial fibrillation associated with a slow ventricular response in the absence of medication, as well as those cases in which cardioversion of atrial fibrillation is followed by prolonged asystole.

SA block is said to be present when impulses fail to emerge or emerge only after a delay from the sinus node. An attempt has been made to classify such conduction disorders in the sinus node in a fashion analogous to the classification used for atrioventricular block. Clearly it is impossible to recognize simple delay in emergence of impulses from the sinus node (first degree SA block) on a standard electrocardiogram. However, second degree SA block may be recognized by periodic failure of a sinus impulse (P wave) to appear (Fig. 50–27), or there may be some evidence of decrease in the P-P intervals prior to the missing P wave. SA block is an uncommon finding and usually suggests the presence of structural disease or drug toxicity. Digitalis and quinidine are both potent causes of SA block. Although vagal stimulation can precipitate SA block, more often some underlying process such as ischemia, inflammation, or a degenerative process is present.

Electrocardiographically, SA block is recognized by the absence of expected sinus P waves. In the case of a single dropped P wave, the interval encompassing the dropped P wave is twice the basic sinus interval. In some instances of second degree SA block, the P-P intervals may gradually shorten prior to disappearance of a P wave, and such variation in the sinus cycle may be misinterpreted as sinus arrhythmia. As with any instance of sinus pause, it is important to examine the electrocardiogram for evidence of blocked atrial premature beats obscured by other deflections on the electrocardiogram. For example, sinus bradycardia can be easily mimicked by the presence of persistent atrial bigeminy, in which the coupled atrial premature beat is always blocked.

The bradycardia-tachycardia syndrome is manifested by periods of ectopic atrial tachycardia or atrial fibrillation, followed by marked depression of the sinus node and subsidiary pace-

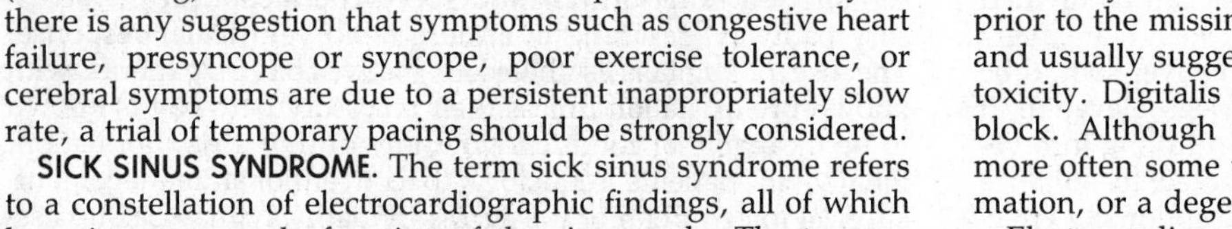

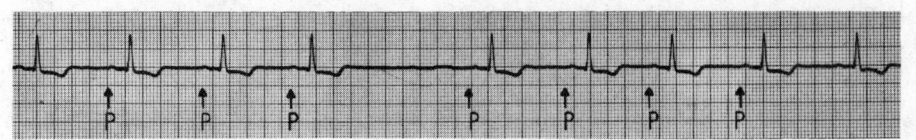

Figure 50–27. Sinus node exit block. Following four normal sinus beats there is an abrupt pause. Careful examination demonstrates the presence of regular P waves as indicated by the arrows. The pause is due to failure of the expected sinus beat to exit from the region of the sinus node.

makers. This is an important entity to recognize, because attempts at suppressing the tachyrhythmia will invariably aggravate the bradyrhythmia (Fig. 50–28). The same etiologies described for SA block apply to the sick sinus syndrome. The abnormality in this instance is not confined primarily to the sinus node or even the atrial muscle; invasive studies often demonstrate that additional abnormalities of impulse formation and conduction exist in the AV node and His-Purkinje system.

Treatment of the various electrocardiographic abnormalities observed in the sick sinus syndrome is not indicated unless symptoms are present. If a reversible cause is identified, the offending agent is removed if possible. If symptoms can be related to the bradycardia, implantation of a permanent pacemaker is indicated. In the case of bradycardia-tachycardia syndrome, a pacemaker implantation allows the use of antiarrhythmic agents for control of the tachyrhythmia without further compromising the ventricular response. When the cardiac output is compromised in diseased hearts by the loss of effective atrial contraction, "physiologic pacing," utilizing an AV sequential pacemaker, should be considered (see below). Atrial pacing in this instance may also effectively suppress the tendency to develop atrial fibrillation. In patients with recurrent alternation between tachycardia and bradycardia, embolic episodes constitute a significant cause of long-term morbidity, and in this situation long-term anticoagulation may be advisable.

JUNCTIONAL RHYTHM. Junctional rhythm should not be considered a cause of bradycardia but rather can usually be ascribed to failure of impulse formation or conduction at a higher level. Junctional rhythm can also be observed in the setting of digitalis toxicity. Electrocardiographically, the ventricular complexes are associated with normal QRS complexes recurring at a rate of 40 to 60 per minute. Retrograde capture of the atrium may be manifested by a retrograde P wave following the QRS complex. Treatment is indicated only if warranted by the underlying cause.

ATRIOVENTRICULAR BLOCK. Since the discovery that certain types of conduction disturbances can warn of impending progression to complete heart block, attention has focused on electrocardiographic signs that might be used prognostically to identify patients at risk for this. Unfortunately, the traditional didactic approach to the problem has settled into a routine of cataloguing conduction disturbances by simple conduction ratios. Thus, atrioventricular (AV) block is divided into first degree (all impulses propagate to the ventricle with delay), second degree (some impulses fail to propagate to the ventricle), and third degree block (no atrial impulses propagate to the ventricle). Such a classification is clearly oversimplified and fails to take advantage of other important information registered on the ECG. A more physiologic approach suggests the need for additional modifiers. The ultimate objective of electrocardiographic analyses of conduction disturbances is to identify

patients at risk for the development of hemodynamic collapse owing to (1) progression of their conduction disturbance and (2) failure to develop a subsidiary escape rhythm, distal to the site of block, capable of sustaining an adequate cardiac output. Thus the key points that emerge are the site of block and the adequacy of escape rhythms that arise distal to the site of block. Conduction disturbances can be divided into those that occur proximal to the His bundle (primarily in the AV node) and those that occur distal to the His bundle. Conduction disorders within the His bundle itself (intra-Hisian) are reasonably uncommon. Both of these levels of the conduction system have somewhat distinctive properties of impulse formation and conduction that should be kept in mind as one searches the ECG for points of localizing value. In general, conduction disorders in the AV node are accompanied by obvious changes in conduction time during periods of unstable conduction, whereas the His-Purkinje system usually behaves in an all-or-none fashion, with only small variations in the conduction time of propagated beats. Exceptions are encountered; thus when conduction in the AV node is already severely stressed (i.e., long P-R interval), block may precipitously appear in the face of a sudden vagal stimulus; similarly, severely diseased tissues in the His-Purkinje system may exhibit characteristics of conduction that are suggestive of the decremental conduction observed in the AV node.

Perhaps more important than the behavior or the site of block is the behavior of the subsidiary escape pacemakers available distal to the site of block. Pacemakers in the region of the AV node or His bundle generally fire at 40 to 60 per minute, are associated with a normal QRS in the absence of other disease, and are stable reliable pacemakers; in contrast, escape rhythms from the distal His-Purkinje system fire at 20 to 40 per minute, are associated with wide QRS complexes of bizarre morphology, and are capricious in their behavior. In the case of block in the AV node, both the conducted beats and escape rhythms are usually associated with normal QRS complexes, while in the case of more distal conduction disorders, conducted beats typically exhibit evidence of distal disease (i.e., bundle branch block). The "company it keeps" can add important modifiers to the profile of a given conduction disorder if attention is directed to the functional behavior of the level of block, the state of conducting tissues distal to the His bundle as manifested by the morphology of conducted beats, and the probable site of origin of the subsidiary escape rhythm (as shown by the rate and morphology).

Conduction delay or even block is physiologic under certain circumstances. This *normal* function of the conduction system prevents an excessive number of impulses from arriving in the

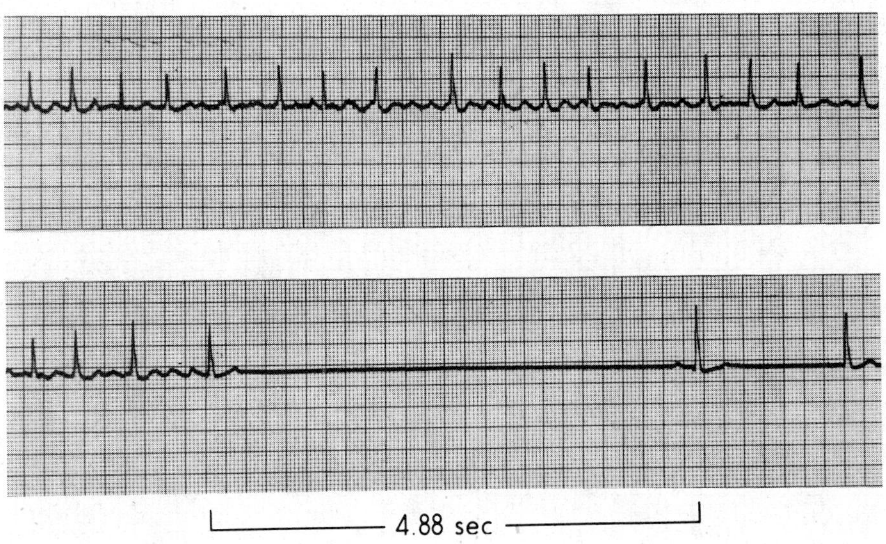

Figure 50–28. Bradycardia-tachycardia syndrome. Atrial fibrillation with an irregularly irregular ventricular response is initially present. In the lower tracing, atrial fibrillation spontaneously terminates and is followed by asystole for 4.88 seconds.

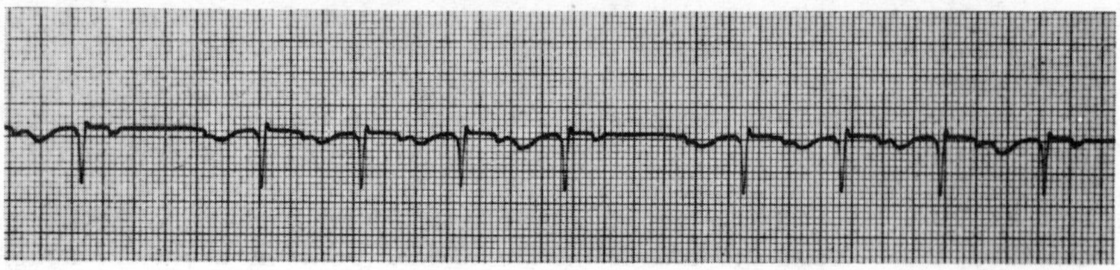

Figure 50–29. Type I second degree (Wenckebach) AV block. Note the presence of regular P-P intervals. The QRS morphology of the conducted beats is normal. The P-R interval gradually prolongs over four cycles, and the fifth P wave is nonconducted. The next conducted beat has a P-R interval significantly shorter than the last conducted beat of the Wenckebach cycle.

ventricle and also prevents any single impulse from arriving in the ventricle during its vulnerable period. At times, the dividing line between the physiologic and pathologic is ill defined; misdiagnosis invariably results when one attempts to classify every situation according to such simple criteria as the conduction ratio. A more realistic approach takes all the available information into account. Attention should be paid to the atrial rate at which a given conduction disturbance appears (is block physiologic and expected?), the rate and morphology of the ventricular response (is bundle branch block present, suggesting distal disease?), the nature of the conduction pattern between the atria and the ventricles (are large fluctuations in conduction intervals present, suggesting that delay or block is occurring in the AV node, or are the fluctuations small or absent, suggesting block in the His-Purkinje system?). After consideration of these factors, a final appropriate question to ask is: considering the atrial rate, the ventricular rate, and the underlying behavior of the AV conducting tissues, should conduction have been expected? (Or phrased another way, is block really present?) All the aforementioned observations should of course be interpreted in the context of the circumstances during which they were observed (e.g., was abnormal vagal tone present?).

With these considerations in mind, one may take an "enlightened look" at the classification of heart block.

First degree heart block is said to be present when the P-R interval is greater than 0.20 second. If the QRS is normal, the delay is invariably in the AV node. If the QRS is wide, delay may be present at one of multiple levels, including the atrium, the AV node, and the His-Purkinje system. His bundle recordings are necessary to localize exactly the level of delay, but no definitive therapy is indicated in any event on the basis of this isolated finding.

Second degree heart block is said to be present when some atrial impulses fail to propagate to the ventricle. Two varieties are distinguished: type I (Wenckebach) and type II (Mobitz). With type I second degree AV block, the QRS is typically normal; the P-R interval undergoes gradual prolongation prior to block of an atrial impulse. Importantly, the P-R interval of the first conducted beat following the pause exhibits marked abbreviation when compared to the last conducted beat prior to the blocked P wave (Fig. 50–29). This type of block is nearly always localized to the AV node and is observed in most cases as a transient phenomenon such as with a diaphragmatic myocardial infarction. This type of block infrequently progresses, and when it does a stable subsidiary escape rhythm is anticipated. Therapy is usually conservative and dictated by the ventricular response. A second variety of second degree block, type II (Mobitz), is typically associated with bundle branch block of the conducted beats. Conduction failure occurs in an "all or none" fashion (i.e., P waves block suddenly and unexpectedly). Care must be taken to ensure that the P-P is regular (Fig. 50–30). Type II second degree AV block is an uncommon but ominous finding because progression to complete heart block is likely. The site of block is in the His-Purkinje system, and the subsidiary escape pacemaker in this instance is likely to be a slow, unstable idioventricular pacemaker. This type of block is usually due to diffuse degenerative processes involving the His-Purkinje system but can be observed in the course of anteroseptal infarction. Pacing is always indicated.

A variety of second degree AV block not included in the definitions above is that of *2:1 AV block*. This type of block should be thought of as uncommitted, and the probable site of block should be judged by the "company it keeps." Thus if the QRS complex is wide and periods of sustained conduction followed by sudden block are observed, a distal site of block is probable. If the 2:1 block is interspersed with periods of typical type I Wenckebach cycles and the QRS is narrow, block at the level of the AV node is probable. In any event, therapy is again dictated by the ventricular response. When fixed 2:1 AV block is present, it is useful to attempt to disturb this ratio by mild exercise or by administering a small dose of atropine. Persistent 2:1 block with a wide QRS complex evident in the conducted beats requires His bundle recording for accurate localization, but even without these data pacemaker implantation may be indicated if the resultant ventricular response is too slow.

Finally, *third degree heart block* is said to be present when no atrial impulse propagates to the ventricles. Again, if the QRS complex of the escape rhythm is narrow and occurring at a rate of 40 to 60 per minute, block in the AV node is probable, although block within the His bundle has been described. Congenital heart block may present in this way. If, on the other hand, the QRS is wide and associated with a rate less than 40, block is likely to be distally located and pacing should be instituted because of the capricious behavior of the subsidiary pacemaker in such settings (Figs. 50–31 and 50–32).

The failure to observe ventricular capture should not be taken as synonymous with AV block. Care must be taken to ensure that conduction might reasonably have been expected, before concluding it has failed. This dilemma usually arises in the setting of digitalis toxicity (Fig. 50–33), in which the combination of an enhanced junctional or an enhanced idioventricular

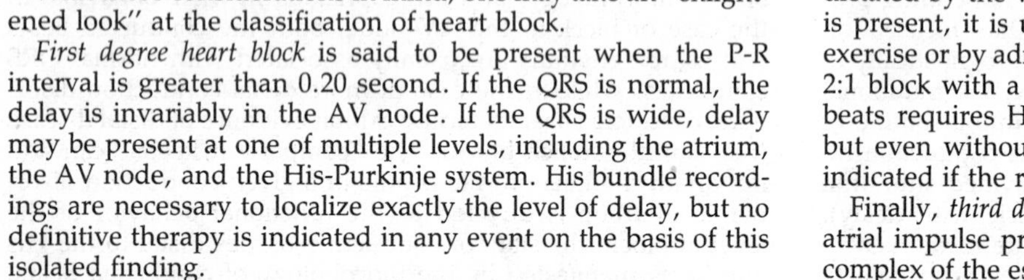

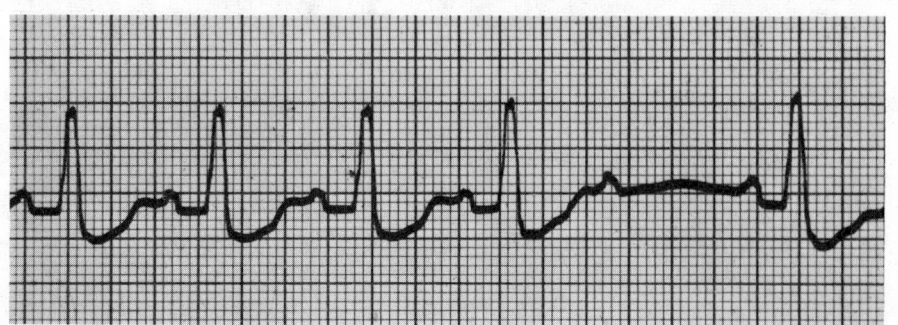

Figure 50–30. Type II (Mobitz) second degree AV block. Note the presence of regular P-P intervals. The QRS morphology of the conducted beats is wide, indicating bundle branch block. The P-R interval is constant during the first four cycles. The fifth P wave suddenly and unexpectedly fails to conduct. The P-R interval remains constant prior to the sudden unexpected failure of the P wave to conduct. The next conducted complex has the same P-R interval as the other conducted beats.

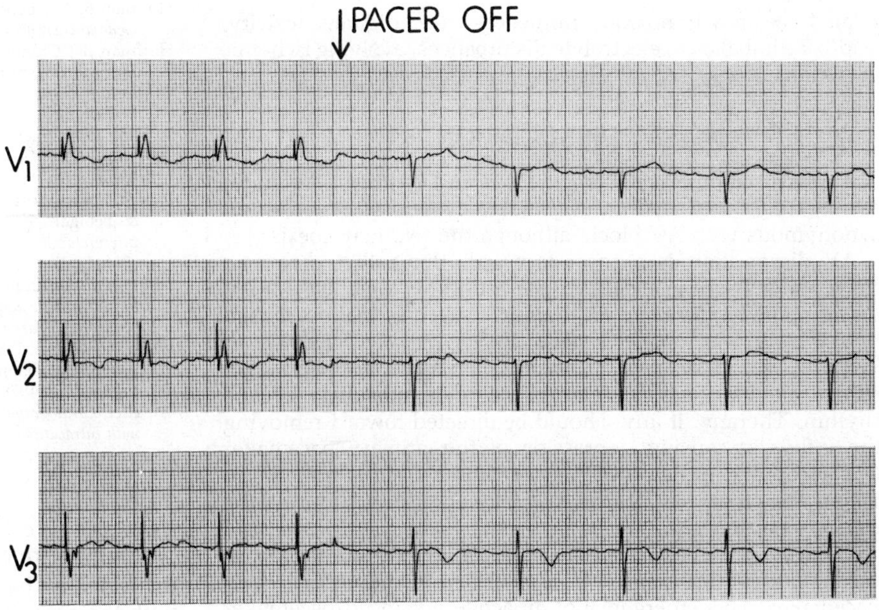

Figure 50–31. Demonstration of the escape rhythm in a patient with third degree block at the level of the AV node. Careful examination of the baseline demonstrates the presence of underlying atrial flutter at a rate of 300 per minute. The first four complexes are due to activation of the ventricles by an artificial ventricular pacemaker. The pacemaker is then turned off, and a narrow QRS escape rhythm promptly appears at a rate of 53 per minute. The slow regular ventricular response in the face of underlying atrial flutter suggests the presence of complete heart block, which was documented by further electrophysiologic study.

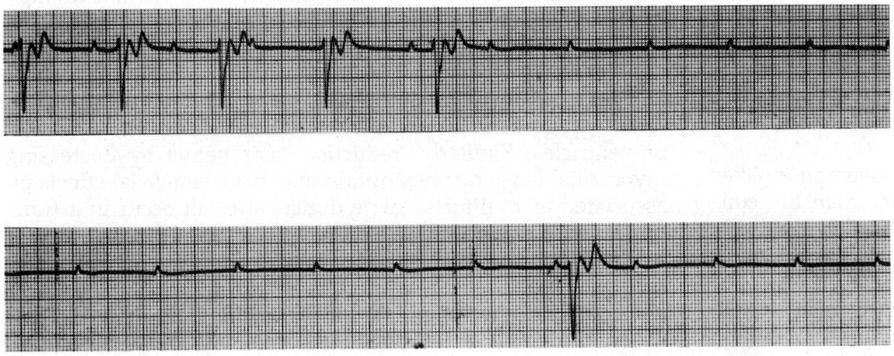

Figure 50–32. Behavior of the escape rhythm in a case of third degree AV block occurring in the His-Purkinje system. In this continuous strip, third degree heart block is present. The ventricular complexes occur at a rate of 52 per minute and are associated with a wide QRS complex. The ventricular escape rhythm gradually slows and then abruptly disappears, resulting in a prolonged episode of ventricular asystole.

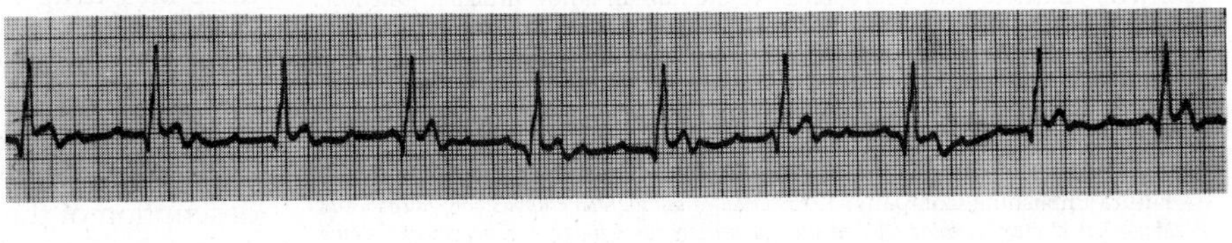

Figure 50–33. Complete AV dissociation with an atrial tachycardia and accelerated idioventricular focus due to digitalis toxicity. Discrete atrial activity is observed at a rate of 167 per minute and completely dissociated from a wide QRS ventricular rhythm at a rate of 56 per minute. Sinus rhythm returned upon termination of digitalis and normalization of the serum potassium level.

focus in concert with a minor degree of conduction abnormality can result in complete AV dissociation (see below). Therefore, when the inherent rate of the observed subsidiary pacemaker (in cases of apparent complete heart block) is greater than expected (taking into account the presumptive location of the escape rhythm), one should strongly suspect that dissociation *without* block is present.

The terminal rhythm of patients with complete heart block experiencing sudden death is not necessarily asystole, as one might expect; in approximately half of cases, ventricular tachycardia–fibrillation is the terminal event. Considering the diffuse nature of disease present in the ventricles of such patients, the presence of ventricular irritability, especially in the setting of a slow heart rate, is perhaps not unexpected.

Pacemaker therapy (see below) is indicated on a temporary or permanent basis in any case of second or third degree AV block, in which the ventricular response is incapable of sustaining an appropriate cardiac output, as well as in those circumstances described above in which progression to a state of block with a slow ventricular response appears likely.

Acutely, AV block can be treated by a trial of incremental doses of atropine sulfate, up to 2.0 mg intravenously. If no response occurs and immediate pacing is unavailable, isoproterenol in doses of 0.5 to 4.0 μg per minute can be administered intravenously. The appearance of ventricular irritability, excessive peripheral vasodilation resulting in hypotension, or angina indicates the need to decrease the rate of drug administration.

Temporary pacing may be of value in cases of AV block

related to known noxious influences (i.e., digitalis toxicity, acid-base imbalance, electrolyte disturbances, evolving ischemic episode).

AV DISSOCIATION

AV dissociation exists when the atria and ventricles are under the control of two separate pacemakers. AV dissociation is not synonymous with AV block, although the two may coexist.

AV dissociation is a secondary arrhythmia that occurs in three general settings: (1) AV dissociation by "default," (2) AV dissociation by "usurpation," and (3) AV dissociation caused by AV block.

AV dissociation by "default" occurs when a primary pacemaker slows, allowing passive emergence of a subsidiary escape rhythm. Therapy, if any, should be directed toward removing the influence causing depression of the primary pacemaker (e.g., stopping propranolol) or speeding the sinus node (e.g., giving atropine). No attempt should be made to suppress the escape rhythm itself.

AV dissociation by "usurpation" occurs when a pacemaker in the AV junction or ventricles competes with the normal sinus pacemaker. This emergence of an active enhanced pacemaker may be due to digitalis toxicity, hypokalemia, or ischemia. Accelerated junctional and accelerated idioventricular rhythms are common examples. When the two pacemakers have similar rates, isorhythmic AV dissociation is said to be present, and long rhythm strips may be required to demonstrate coincidental relationship of atria to ventricles (Fig. 50–34). Therapy is directed toward removing the offending drug or correcting the underlying abnormality. Suppression with antiarrhythmic agents should be considered only if the subsidiary focus is rapid.

In the setting of incomplete AV block, a subsidiary pacemaker may emerge because its inherent rate is faster than the conducted rhythm, resulting in *AV dissociation caused by AV block.* This escape rhythm in turn may further impair AV conduction by the phenomenon of concealed retrograde conduction into the area of block. When any doubt exists concerning the degree of AV block in cases of AV dissociation, therapy should be directed toward the underlying block by discontinuing responsible drugs or correcting electrolyte disorders. Pacing may be indicated on a temporary basis if indicated by the hemodynamic status. Therapy should *not* be directed toward suppression of the escape rhythm, which may be life supporting.

Becker AE, Anderson RH: Morphology of the human atrioventricular junction. *In* Wellens HJJ, Lie KI, Janse MJ (eds.): The Conduction System of the Heart. Philadelphia, Lea & Febiger, 1976, pp 263–286. *In-depth, well-illustrated chapter dealing with the normal anatomy of the atrioventricular junction.*

Bellet A: Clinical Disorders of the Heart Beat. Philadelphia, Lea & Febiger, 1971. *Detailed encyclopedic textbook of electrocardiography.*

Cranefield PF: The Conduction of the Cardiac Impulse. Mount Kisco, N.Y., Futura Publishing Company, 1975. *Detailed monograph emphasizing normal and abnormal electrophysiology based on microelectrode techniques. Concept of "slow" channel ion transport heavily emphasized.*

Gallagher JJ, Damato AN: Technique of recording His bundle activity in man. *In* Grossman W (ed.): Cardiac Catheterization and Angiography. Philadelphia, Lea & Febiger, 1974, pp 213–232. *A "how-to" guide to the technique and application of intracardiac recordings.*

Gallagher JJ, Pritchett ELC, Sealy WC, Kasell J, Wallace AG: The preexcitation syndromes. Prog Cardiovasc Dis 20:285, 1978. *Review article dealing with the basis of the WPW syndrome and its variants. Rationale for medical, pacemaker, or surgical treatment is presented.*

Hackel DB: Anatomy and pathology of the cardiac conducting system. *In* Edwards JE, Lev M, Abell MA (eds.): The Heart. Baltimore, Williams & Wilkins Company, 1974, pp 232–247. *A concise description of the normal anatomy and pathology of the conduction system.*

Harvey WP, Ronan JA: Bedside diagnosis of arrhythmias. Prog Cardiovasc Dis 8:419, 1966. *Excellent article which correlates bedside physical findings with various cardiac arrhythmias.*

Hoffman B: The genesis of cardiac arrhythmias. Prog Cardiovasc Dis 8:319, 1966. *General treatment of the genesis of cardiac arrhythmias.*

Hoffman BF, Cranefield PF: Electrophysiology of the Heart. Mount Kisco, N.Y., Futura Publishing Company, 1976. *Reprinted edition of the first major work on basic electrophysiology. The monograph emphasizes the use of microelectrodes and still stands as a classic work in the field.*

Marriott HJL: Practical Electrocardiography. Baltimore, Williams & Wilkins Company, 1977. *A concise textbook of electrocardiography which provides a working knowledge of the electrocardiogram with a minimum of theoretical considerations.*

Pick A, Langendorf R: Interpretation of Complex Arrhythmias. Philadelphia, Lea & Febiger, 1979. *Monograph which provides a guide to the exploration and interpretation of complex arrhythmias. Requires knowledge of the fundamentals of electrocardiography.*

Smith WM, Gallagher JJ: Les torsades de pointes. Ann Intern Med 93:578, 1980. *Review article detailing the characteristics of congenital and acquired long Q-T syndromes. Various modes of therapy are stressed.*

Wellens HJJ, Bar FWHM, Lie KH: The value of the electrocardiogram in the differential diagnosis of a tachycardia with a widened QRS complex. Am J Med 64:27, 1978. *Excellent article which provides more detailed criteria for the electrocardiographic diagnosis of ventricular tachycardia, based on correlative studies with intracardiac recordings.*

ANTIARRHYTHMIC DRUGS

INTRODUCTION. Appropriate treatment of a cardiac arrhythmia must be based on an adequate diagnosis and formulated with the context of the arrhythmia in mind. Treatment should always begin with an effort to correct reversible abnormalities that may be present; not only may such abnormalities play a primary role in the genesis of the arrhythmia under treatment, but their continued presence may make antiarrhythmic therapy ineffective. Before focusing on the *direct* pharmacologic treatment of arrhythmias, one should not overlook indirect measures of therapy. Thus, such factors as blood volume and preload and afterload may require treatment by diuretic or afterload-reducing agents in an effort to decrease stretch of the atria and/or ventricles. Similarly, reduction of ischemia by decreasing myocardial oxygen consumption may have beneficial effects on associated arrhythmias. Arrhythmias after all occur in a functional-anatomic setting under the influence of a large variety of dynamic extrinsic and local factors. The underlying factors of most cardiac arrhythmias are not static (or else most arrhythmias would be incessant). In this light, the day-to-day variability in control of arrhythmia so commonly seen clinically is perhaps not so surprising.

For the majority of available antiarrhythmic drugs, the toxic-therapeutic ratio is rather narrow. The aim of therapy is to achieve an adequate level of drug in the body tissues with minimal daily fluctuations and minimal toxicity. The proper dose of a drug for an individual arrhythmia in an individual patient cannot be precisely anticipated except to say that dosage should be enough but not too much. Suggested regimens are intended as guidelines for initial therapy to be modified by continued feedback from the clinical situation.

PHARMACOKINETICS. Space limitations preclude a detailed description of the pharmacokinetics of available antiarrhythmic agents. Some are discussed in Ch. 22.

The majority of antiarrhythmic drugs are eliminated by first order kinetic processes; i.e., the rate of elimination is directly proportional to the amount in the body and thus the drug disappears in an exponential fashion. Once a total loading body dose is achieved, one attempts to maintain balance of intake and loss by giving approximately half the total body loading dose every half-life of the drug with suitable adjustments made for absorptive loss and presystemic metabolism. With drugs eliminated by first order kinetic processes, steady state is generally reached in four to five half-lives of the drug regardless

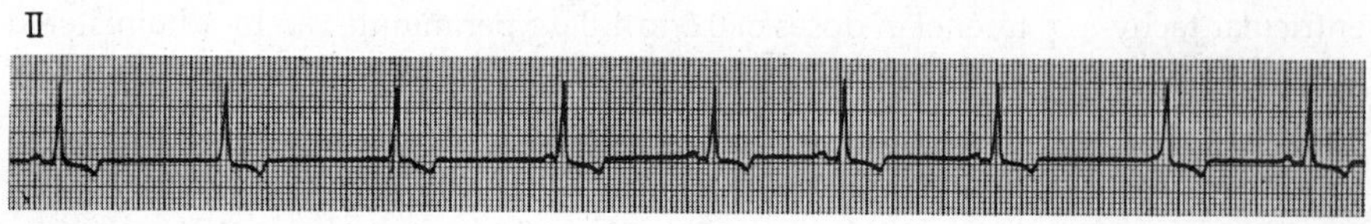

Figure 50–34. Isorhythmic AV dissociation. In this rhythm strip, atrial and ventricular activity is dissociated but the atrial and ventricular rates are strikingly similar.

of whether one is initiating treatment, changing the dosage, or discontinuing therapy.

The total body loading dose is determined by the desired therapeutic level and the volume of distribution of the drug. In general the size of body compartments varies in proportion to the size of the individual. Important contractions in the functional size of certain body compartments result from low output states (e.g., shock, congestive heart failure) and may require a decrease in the maintenance dose by one third to one half. Therefore, the therapeutic level must be individualized for the patient and his arrhythmia.

The half-life of a drug is determined largely by the route and rate of its metabolism and/or elimination. The extent to which metabolism-excretion is impaired by disease states will greatly alter the half-life of the drug and thus the dosing schedule in any individual patient.

Plasma levels are useful during therapy; patient compliance and adequacy of intake are ensured, effective levels can be defined, and accumulation of potentially toxic levels of drug can be detected. Drug levels should be viewed as relative guidelines, taking into account the wide variability of individual response. Furthermore, drug levels do not usually reflect the antiarrhythmic activity or toxic side effects of metabolites that may be present.

With this general introduction, the standard antiarrhythmic agents currently available in the United States will be briefly described, taking into account their indications, routes of metabolism-excretion, half-life, dosage schedule, range of therapeutic plasma levels, electrocardiographic effects, and toxic side effects.

DIGOXIN. The clinical use of digitalis for the treatment of dropsy was first described by William Withering in 1785. Its use in heart failure is discussed in Ch. 42. In addition to its positive inotropic effect, digitalis has several important electrophysiologic effects which qualify it as an antiarrhythmic agent. Although a variety of digitalis preparations exist, digoxin is the most popular cardiac glycoside and the one that will be emphasized in this presentation.

Digoxin exerts a centrally mediated vagal action on the heart. Direct effects include a slowing of conduction in the AV node, prolongation of refractoriness in the AV node, and a decrease in refractoriness of atrial tissue. All these effects in concert have important implications for the treatment of supraventricular tachycardia, especially atrial flutter-fibrillation. By decreasing the refractoriness of atrial tissues, atrial flutter can be converted to atrial fibrillation, which results in slowing of the ventricular response by the phenomenon of concealed conduction. Atrial fibrillation is also more likely to convert to sinus rhythm spontaneously than atrial flutter. By slowing conduction and prolonging refractoriness in the AV node, digitalis impairs the ability of impulses to propagate rapidly through the AV node in transit to the ventricle. Thus it not only attenuates the ventricular response during atrial fibrillation but is also useful for supraventricular tachycardias that conduct to the ventricles by the AV node (i.e., junctional reciprocating tachycardia). The ability of digoxin to decrease the refractoriness of atrial tissue accounts for its ability to speed the ventricular response during atrial fibrillation with conduction over an accessory pathway (see Pre-excitation Syndromes, above) owing to the functional similarity of many types of accessory pathways to atrial tissue. Digoxin also increases automaticity, resulting in the appearance of enhanced atrial and junctional foci in the presence of digitalis toxicity.

Digoxin is almost completely absorbed (70 to 90 per cent) and is excreted by the kidneys without undergoing biotransformation. The half-life of the drug is 36 to 48 hours. The intravenous loading dose of digoxin is approximately 1.0 mg, whereas the oral loading dose is approximately 1.5 mg. The rate of administration is generally determined by clinical necessity, but it is desirable if possible to administer the drug in divided doses over a 24-hour period. The oral maintenance dose of digoxin ranges from 0.125 to 0.5 mg daily. When therapy is less urgent, full digitalization can be accomplished in six to seven days by initiating therapy with a maintenance dose without administering a loading dose. The therapeutic level in general ranges from 1 to 2 ng per milliliter.

Another popular preparation of digitalis that has a longer action is digitoxin. Digitoxin undergoes an enterohepatic cycle with renal excretion of the metabolites. The half-life ranges from four to six days. The oral loading dose is 0.7 to 1.2 mg administered over 24 hours with a maintenance dose of 0.1 mg daily.

Digoxin does not affect the sinus rate in normal subjects. However, slowing of sinus tachycardia may be observed in patients with congestive heart failure being treated with digitalis, and sinus node dysfunction may appear in patients with underlying sick sinus syndrome. The P-R interval may be slightly prolonged by digoxin. No changes are expected in the QRS complex. The Q-T interval may be slightly shortened, and scooping of the S-T segment is expected. Toxic reactions to digitalis are common. Digitalis can cause *any* arrhythmia, a fact that should be kept in mind in evaluating arrhythmias occurring in patients on digitalis therapy. Gastrointestinal symptoms of toxicity include anorexia, nausea, vomiting, diarrhea, abdominal pain, and bloating. Toxic central nervous system effects include fatigue, weakness, psychic disturbances, and disorders of color vision. Electrocardiographically, digitalis toxicity may be manifested by enhanced impulse formation, especially in the region of the junction, but also in the atrium or ventricle. First degree AV block, type I second degree (Wenckebach) block, and third degree AV block may be encountered. Atrial tachycardia with block, ventricular tachycardia, and SA block are other manifestations.

QUINIDINE. Quinidine is an alkaloid derived from the bark of the cinchona tree and is frequently used for the long-term oral treatment of atrial and ventricular arrhythmias. Quinidine appears to have little effect on normal automaticity but depresses automaticity arising in abnormal cells. The latter can result in depression of subsidiary escape rhythms in patients with heart block. Quinidine has a number of actions that make it useful for the treatment of re-entrant rhythms. It increases the threshold of excitability in atrial and ventricular tissue. In general it slows conduction and prolongs refractoriness in most cardiac tissues; however, because of a vagolytic action, conduction in the AV node is enhanced. All these actions combine to make quinidine an effective agent for the treatment of a variety of supraventricular and ventricular arrhythmias. Quinidine can be used to suppress atrial and ventricular premature beats, which are often the initiating mechanism of tachyrhythmias. Quinidine has been used to revert atrial flutter and atrial fibrillation to sinus rhythm, although with the advent of cardioversion this application has become less frequent. More often, quinidine is used to maintain sinus rhythm once conversion has been achieved by cardioversion. Certain precautions must be observed if quinidine is to be used to convert atrial fibrillation or atrial flutter to sinus rhythm. Because it is capable of slowing the rate of atrial flutter while enhancing conduction in the AV node, quinidine administration can paradoxically cause an *increase* in the ventricular response, occasionally leading to atrial flutter with 1:1 AV conduction. Because of this, no patient with atrial flutter-fibrillation should be given quinidine before being digitalized. The one exception to this rule is in the case of the Wolff-Parkinson-White syndrome. Quinidine prolongs refractoriness and slows conduction of accessory pathways and thus can be used for treating the rapid ventricular response that attends atrial fibrillation in patients with WPW syndrome.

Intravenous use of quinidine is not recommended because of an alpha-adrenergic blocking property that can cause vasodilatation, resulting in hypotension. Oral quinidine is approximately 80 per cent bioavailable and should be taken on an empty stomach. Concomitant administration of antacids may interfere with its absorption. It is largely metabolized in the liver, although 10 to 40 per cent is excreted unchanged in the urine. The presence of an alkaline urine impairs renal excretion. The use of phenytoin (diphenylhydantoin) decreases the half-life of quinidine by approximately 50 per cent. Quinidine also prolongs the prothrombin time when administered with warfarin compounds. The half-life of quinidine is five to nine hours. The therapeutic level ranges from 2 to 6 μg per milliliter, and this is achieved by administering oral quinidine sulfate, 200 to 600 mg every six hours (mean, 400 mg). Toxic effects are common with levels greater than 10 μg per milliliter. A longer-acting form of quinidine, quinidine gluconate, is available and can be administered in doses of 300 to 600 mg every eight to twelve hours.

Electrocardiographically, quinidine can prolong the duration of the QRS complex and the Q-T interval. Widening of the QRS complex by 25 per cent should be viewed with concern, and an increase of 50 per cent should prompt discontinuation of the drug. Quinidine has been administered safely to patients with bundle branch block but should be avoided in patients with evidence of second or third degree atrioventricular block.

Quinidine has a nonspecific myocardial depressant action common to all so-called membrane-active antiarrhythmic drugs. It should thus be used cautiously in patients suffering from congestive heart failure.

It has been recently shown that the administration of quinidine to patients digitalized with digoxin can raise the plasma concentration of digoxin two-fold owing to displacement of digoxin from tissue-binding sites and a decrease in renal clearance of digoxin. These phenomena have *not* been observed with digitoxin.

Adverse effects of quinidine most commonly include diarrhea, nausea, and vomiting. Some patients experience inordinate prolongation of the Q-T interval. This situation can lead to episodes of ventricular tachycardia and ventricular fibrillation of the torsades de pointes variety, accounting for so-called quinidine syncope. Because of this it is advisable to initiate therapy with quinidine while the patient is under observation and to discontinue the drug if excessive prolongation of the Q-T interval occurs. Other adverse effects of quinidine include tinnitus, hearing impairment, vertigo, diplopia, confusion, rash, headache, and fever. Occasionally, thrombocytopenia can develop weeks or months after initiating therapy owing to an immune mechanism.

PROCAINAMIDE. The indications for procainamide are markedly similar to those described above for quinidine sulfate. Procainamide appears to be more effective on ventricular arrhythmias than on atrial arrhythmias. Unlike quinidine, procainamide has no alpha-blocking effect and has a much weaker vagolytic effect.

The pharmacokinetic properties of procainamide make it difficult to establish effective dosage regimens. Procainamide has a short half-life of two to four hours, and 40 to 70 per cent is excreted unchanged by the kidney. The acetylated metabolite, N-acetyl-procainamide or NAPA, has electrophysiologic effects and toxicity similar to quinidine and has a somewhat longer half-life than procainamide.

Procainamide is well tolerated intravenously. A loading dose of 10 to 12 mg per kilogram is generally administered at the rate of 25 mg per minute. Maintenance is achieved by continuous infusion at 1 to 5 mg per minute. The usual oral dose is 250 to 750 mg every three to four hours because of the short elimination half-life of 3.5 hours. A sustained release form is available, permitting dosing every six to eight hours. Therapeutic blood levels range from 4 to 10 μg per milliliter. Procainamide is partly eliminated by the kidneys and partly acetylated by the liver to N-acetyl procainamide, which has antiarrhythmic action and is almost entirely excreted by the kidneys. The half-life of this metabolite in patients with normal renal function is six to eight hours, and effective plasma levels range from 2 to 22 μg per milliliter.

The electrocardiographic side effects of procainamide are similar to those described for quinidine, and the same precautions are necessary. Marked prolongation of the Q-T interval and torsades de pointes have been rarely reported with procainamide.

Adverse effects of procainamide include gastrointestinal symptoms of nausea, vomiting, and anorexia but rarely diarrhea. Central nervous system side effects can be encountered. A systemic lupus erythematosus–like syndrome has been described in association with procainamide. Unlike typical SLE, the syndrome induced by procainamide spares the brain and kidney and there is no predilection for females. Nonetheless, fever, arthralgia, and pericarditis with hemorrhagic effusion have been observed. Seventy-five per cent of patients on procainamide therapy will develop antinuclear antibodies (ANA), but only one third of these will develop the SLE syndrome. The latter is more common in patients who are slow acetylators of the drug.

DISOPYRAMIDE. Disopyramide phosphate was approved in 1978 by the Food and Drug Administration for the long-term oral treatment of ventricular arrhythmias. Although it has been less extensively studied than quinidine or procainamide, available information suggests that its antiarrhythmic spectrum and mechanism of action are quite similar to those of quinidine and procainamide.

Disopyramide is absorbed and is approximately 80 per cent bioavailable. Fifty per cent of the drug is excreted unchanged in the urine, with the remainder undergoing metabolism in the liver. The half-life of disopyramide is six to nine hours. The usual oral dose is 100 to 300 mg administered every six hours, and the therapeutic level is 2 to 5 μg per milliliter.

The electrocardiographic side effects of disopyramide are comparable to those described for quinidine and procainamide.

Disopyramide has prominent anticholinergic side effects, which result in dry mouth, blurred vision, constipation, and urinary hesitancy. The drug must be used with extreme caution in patients with prostatic hypertrophy and is relatively contraindicated in patients with glaucoma. Clinically, the severity of anticholinergic side effects may spontaneously decrease after administration of the drug for two weeks. Marked prolongation of the Q-T interval associated with torsades de pointes has been reported in a few patients, suggesting that the drug is comparable to quinidine in this respect. The most serious adverse side effect of disopyramide is its negative inotropic effect. This appears to be much more prominent than that encountered with either quinidine or procainamide. Low cardiac output has been reported, resulting in cardiogenic shock and death. This complication has almost invariably occurred in patients with severely impaired myocardial contractility. Patients with a history of congestive heart failure or elderly patients with significant ischemic heart disease should be carefully monitored during administration of disopyramide, and increases in dosage should be undertaken extremely cautiously, allowing five half-lives for equilibration before increasing the dose.

LIDOCAINE. Lidocaine is a popular antiarrhythmic drug whose use is confined almost entirely to the intravenous treatment of ventricular arrhythmias and has no significant interactions with the autonomic nervous system. Lidocaine has some effect on certain abnormal forms of automaticity, but it is most noted for its ability to abolish ventricular re-entry. The drug has minimal effect on atrial tissue and does not affect the atrial rate in atrial flutter or fibrillation. A few isolated reports indicated that lidocaine might be useful in suppressing conduction over accessory pathways during atrial fibrillation in patients with pre-excitation. However, in the majority of such patients, lidocaine has no effect on the accessory pathway, and in a few case reports has actually accelerated conduction over the accessory pathway.

Lidocaine undergoes extensive metabolism during its first pass through the liver. This drug is eliminated by the liver, suggesting the need to decrease dosage in the presence of liver disease or decreased perfusion of the liver. Lidocaine is almost invariably administered intravenously. An initial bolus of 1 mg per kilogram is given, followed in ten minutes by a repeat bolus. After the second bolus is given, a maintenence infusion of 1 to 5 mg per minute (mean, 2 mg) is begun. The rate of administration is generally decreased in patients with heart failure or with low output or shock. The use of intramuscular lidocaine in doses of 4 to 5 mg per kilogram has been described for emergency use outside the hospital and results in a therapeutic level in 15 minutes lasting up to 90 minutes. The half-life of lidocaine is approximately one and a half hours, and the therapeutic level ranges from 0.5 to 5.0 μg per milliliter.

Lidocaine has minimal electrocardiographic effects, although it has been reported to aggravate pre-existing conduction defects in the His-Purkinje system. The adverse side effects of lidocaine primarily involve the central nervous system. Symptoms of dizziness, paresthesias, confusion, agitation, muscle tremor, and frank seizure have been described and generally occur at levels in excess of 5.0 μg per milliliter. Lidocaine has minimal hemodynamic effects but can depress ventricular function.

PHENYTOIN (DIPHENYLHYDANTOIN).* Phenytoin is an anticonvulsant drug that has electrophysiologic effects somewhat similar to those of lidocaine. It has limited efficacy against atrial and ventricular arrhythmias in man except when these have been due to digitalis intoxication. Phenytoin shortens the refractory period and reduces automaticity in both atrial and His-Purkinje tissue. It is effective in abolishing abnormal automaticity in Purkinje fibers made toxic by digitalis, accounting for its efficacy in the treatment of digitalis-toxic arrhythmias in man.

Phenytoin undergoes erratic absorption from the gastrointestinal tract and is extensively bound to serum albumin in the blood. It is metabolized in the liver, with only 5 per cent being excreted unchanged. The drug is unusual in that the enzymes that metabolize phenytoin conform to first-order kinetics up to the point at which they are saturated; thereafter, only a fixed amount of drug is eliminated per unit time. This latter feature can predispose patients to drug toxicity, often sudden in onset, once enzyme saturation occurs. The half-life of phenytoin is 15 to 36 hours.

The usual method of intravenous administration is to give repeated doses of 100 mg intravenously every five minutes until the arrhythmia has terminated, 1.0 gram has been administered, or adverse side effects such as hypotension are encountered. Phenytoin is solubilized in a vehicle with a markedly alkaline pH and readily causes phlebitis. The vehicle also causes hypotension, so intravenous therapy should be given with *extreme caution*. When therapy is initiated on an oral basis, an initial loading dose of 1 gram is given the first day. The maintenance dose is 300 to 400 mg daily. The therapeutic level ranges from 10 to 18 μg per milliliter, and toxic side effects usually occur with levels in excess of 20 μg per milliliter.

Phenytoin has little or no effect on a standard electrocardiogram. Adverse side effects are primarily confined to the central nervous system and include drowsiness, nystagmus, ataxia, and vertigo. Hypotension accompanies rapid intravenous infusion. Long-term administration can lead to enlargement of gingiva. When phenytoin is administered concomitantly with quinidine, it can decrease the half-life of quinidine sulfate by 50 per cent. Phenytoin also has some important interactions with a number of other drugs. Its metabolism is increased by phenobarbital and inhibited by warfarin or isoniazid.

PROPRANOLOL. Propranolol is an antiarrhythmic drug whose effect is mediated by blockade of the beta-adrenergic stimulating actions of catecholamines on the heart. Many of the pharmacologic properties can therefore be anticipated by assuming blockade of catecholamine effect. Sinus slowing is commonly observed. Propranolol slows conduction and prolongs refractoriness in the AV node, making it a useful drug for a variety of supraventricular arrhythmias. It has been used in combination with digoxin to slow the ventricular response in patients with atrial fibrillation and an uncontrolled ventricular response. It is important to note that propranolol does not exert any effect on the accessory pathway of patients with atrial fibrillation and is not useful for slowing the ventricular response in such patients. Propranolol is effective in decreasing the incidence of arrhythmias that appear in the setting of increased sympathetic tone. It has also been used for arrhythmias related to hyperthyroidism, exercise-related arrhythmias, ventricular arrhythmias related to the prolonged Q-T syndrome, and those related to mitral valve prolapse.

Propranolol is well absorbed from the gastrointestinal tract but undergoes extensive metabolism on its first pass through the liver. Only about 20 to 50 per cent of the oral dose is bioavailable; the half-life of propranolol is three to six hours.

Propranolol can be administered intravenously in a dose of 0.5 mg per minute until a total of 0.1 mg per kilogram has been administered. This type of administration should be avoided in patients with known ventricular dysfunction, evidence of sick sinus syndrome, or conduction disturbances. The usual oral dose of propranolol is 20 to 80 mg administered every six hours, although in resistant cases of ventricular arrhythmias up to 1 gram per day in divided doses every six hours has been used with success. The therapeutic level ranges from 20 to 100 ng per milliliter.

Propranolol has minimal effects on the electrocardiogram. Sinus bradycardia and slight prolongation of the P-R interval may be observed. Propranolol has a prominent negative inotropic effect and can result in severe hypotension, left ventricular failure, and cardiogenic shock in patients with left ventricular dysfunction. These side effects are especially likely following intravenous use. Because of its effect on the atrioventricular node, propranolol has been observed to cause heart block and asystole and should be avoided in patients with conduction system abnormalities whenever possible. Propranolol can cause pulmonary vasoconstriction in patients with asthma or obstructive lung disease; in these settings, drugs with less prominent effects on the beta receptors in the lung should be used such as metoprolol or atenolol. Propranolol should be avoided if possible in insulin-dependent diabetics because of its ability to mask symptoms of hypoglycemia. Sudden withdrawal of propranolol in patients with ischemic heart disease has led to increasing angina, acute myocardial infarction, and cardiac arrhythmias. In such patients, withdrawal of propranolol should be gradual over a period of one week.

VERAPAMIL. Verapamil is a parenteral antiarrhythmic agent that appears to mediate its effect by interfering with movement of calcium through the so-called "slow channel." The slow channel assumes considerable importance in the region of the sinus node and AV node, and not surprisingly verapamil exerts a potent effect on the sinus node as well as the AV node. Indeed, intravenous verapamil is so effective in the treatment of paroxysmal AV junctional tachycardias that it has become the treatment of choice in acute situations in almost all countries having access to this drug.

The use of verapamil is confined almost solely to intravenous use because of poor bioavailability with oral administration owing to presystemic metabolism in the liver. There is little information available concerning the pharmacokinetics of the drug, but the half-life is said to be approximately two hours. The usual intravenous dose is 5 to 10 mg given slowly intravenously.

The effect of verapamil on calcium results in a prominent negative inotropic effect. It appears advisable to avoid verapamil in patients who are taking other negative inotropic agents, especially propranolol, disopyramide, and quinidine. Verapamil must also be avoided in patients with sick sinus syndrome, in whom its use can result in bradycardia and asystole. Because of its prominent effect on the AV node, it can cause heart block in patients with underlying abnormalities in the AV node.

*Investigational drug for this purpose.

BRETYLIUM. Bretylium, originally developed as an antihypertensive agent, has recently been discovered to have significant antiarrhythmic action. Intravenous bretylium results initially in a release of catecholamines followed by sympathetic blockade. Since these actions are quite comparable to those of guanethidine, which does not possess antiarrhythmic activity, it is probable that bretylium mediates its effects by additional mechanisms. Bretylium prolongs the refractoriness of tissues in the His-Purkinje system as well as the ventricles. It is currently used for the emergency treatment of life-threatening ventricular tachycardia and ventricular fibrillation that has been resistant to drug treatment. A number of reports attest to the ability of bretylium to permit conversion of refractory ventricular fibrillation when DC cardioversion has failed.

Bretylium is eliminated by the kidneys and has a half-life of approximately 8 hours. The usual intravenous dose is 5 mg per kilogram given every six hours. Oral bretylium is available on an investigational basis but has poor bioavailability, and long-term oral administration of bretylium is limited by significant side effects. The therapeutic level is 0.5 to 1.5 mg per liter.

Following the initial administration of bretylium, transient increases in heart rate and blood pressure occur owing to the release of catecholamines. The most prominent adverse side effect is postural hypotension. Nausea and vomiting have been observed following parenteral administration. Chronic oral administration of bretylium has resulted in the onset of parotid gland pain, especially at times of increased salivation.

AMIODARONE. Amiodarone is an experimental antiarrhythmic agent that was introduced in Europe in 1968 and has been evaluated extensively in the United States over the past five years. It is of interest because of a unique mode of action, probably related either to cardioselective blockade of T_4 conversion to T_3 or to blockade of the nuclear T_3 receptor. Amiodarone is effective in 75 to 80 per cent of supraventricular and ventricular arrhythmias refractory to usual antiarrhythmic agents. However, significant side effects limit its long-term use, and it must be discontinued in 20 to 25 per cent of patients because of these side effects. For this reason amiodarone has not yet been approved by the FDA for general use in the United States.

Bigger JT, Giardina EGV: Rational use of antiarrhythmic drugs alone and in combination. Cardiovasc Clin 6:103, 1974. *Particularities of combining antiarrhythmic drugs are discussed.*

Hager WD, Fenster P, Mayersohn M, Perrier D, Graves P, Marcus FI, Goldman S: Digoxin-quinidine interaction: Pharmacokinetic evaluation. N Engl J Med 300:1238, 1979. *New information concerning the interaction of a commonly prescribed drug combination.*

Harrison DC, Meffin PJ, Winkle RA: Clinical pharmacokinetics of antiarrhythmic drugs. Prog Cardiovasc Dis 20:217, 1978. *Oriented toward use of antiarrhythmic drugs with strong emphasis on pharmacokinetic principles.*

Heger JJ, Prystowsky EN, Zipes DP: Clinical efficacy of amiodarone in ventricular tachycardia and ventricular fibrillation. Am Heart J 106:887, 1983.

Lucchesi BR: Antiarrhythmic drugs. *In* Antonaccio M (Ed.): Cardiovascular Pharmacology. New York, Raven Press, 1977, p 269. *Comprehensive discussion of the clinical use of conventional antiarrhythmic agents in a precise synopsis form.*

Zipes DP, Troup PJ: New antiarrhythmic agents. Am J Cardiol 41:1005, 1978. *Up-to-date information on new antiarrhythmic agents available on investigational basis.*

PACEMAKERS

A pacing system consists of an electronic device that generates stimuli (pulse generator) for delivery to the endocardium or myocardium by electrodes (pacing leads). The system may be used on a temporary basis when reversible factors are present or can be permanently implanted. A variety of systems are available, which differ according to the chamber(s) paced (i.e., atrium and/or ventricle), the type of lead placement (i.e., transvenous, transmediastinal), the type of pulse generator used (i.e., demand or asynchronous, programmable), and the sensing and pacing modality used (i.e., unipolar or bipolar).

The specific indications for pacing have been described above. In general these can be divided into applications relating to tachyrhythmias or bradyrhythmias.

The most common type of pacing system is that of a demand ventricular pacemaker (Fig. 50–35), which senses spontaneous ventricular activity and, failing to detect activity after a certain set interval, delivers a stimulus to the ventricle.

More recently, dual-chambered devices capable of sensing and pacing both atria and ventricles have been developed which attempt to restore the electrical activity of the heart to a more physiologic state whereby each atrial contraction (spontaneous or paced) is followed at an appropriate P-R interval by a ventricular contraction (spontaneous or paced) (Fig. 50–36).

Pacing systems have also been developed for the treatment of tachyrhythmias, including supraventricular and ventricular tachycardia of the re-entrant variety. These systems provide impulses which are delivered in a programmed or random fashion in an attempt to cause refractoriness in some limb of the re-entry circuit leading to termination of re-entry. To date these devices have been largely limited to the treatment of supraventricular tachycardia. One such device consists of a radiofrequency pulse generator, which is implanted subcutaneously and powered by an external transmitter activated by the patient. The transmitter provides radiofrequency energy, which is converted to stimuli by the implanted receiver and delivered to the pacing lead. Attempts to apply similar pacing systems to the treatment of ventricular tachycardia has occasionally led to acceleration of the underlying ventricular tachycardia, making this an undesirable system for out-of-hospital use by the patient.

A number of recent improvements have increased the reliability of pacing systems and have broadened the capability of and thus indications for cardiac pacing. Transvenous electrodes are no longer subject to a high rate of displacement owing to the development of "tined leads," which anchor the lead more securely to the endocardial surface. The development of polyurethane leads has resulted in a marked decrease in lead size and greater ease of lead placement. Percutaneous introducers have been developed which simplify entry into the venous system. All the developments have led to a progressive return to transvenous pacing systems. Transvenous systems can be implanted under local anesthesia with minimal risks and are preferred in elderly patients or in patients with poor cardiorespiratory function, in whom the risk of anesthesia or a thoracic procedure is undesirable. Direct placement of electrodes on the ventricles can also be achieved by a transmediastinal exposure which does not enter the pleural cavities. The development of direct screw-in myocardial leads has made this particular approach attractive for implantation of a stable lead system, but this approach carries a slightly higher risk than the transvenous approach, and late threshold rises have been experienced.

Pulse generators have been made substantially smaller and the longevity of a typical lithium iodide source can be anticipated to be seven to ten years. The development of external programming now makes it possible to change noninvasively many of the pulse generator parameters (e.g., rate, pulse width,

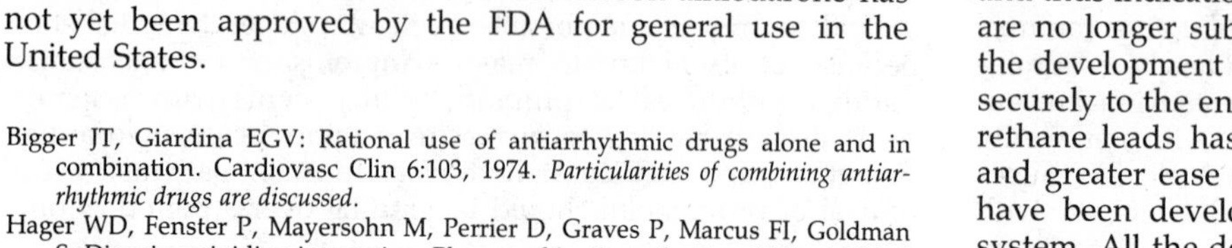

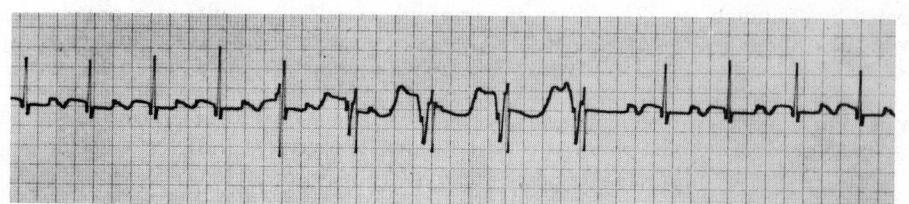

Figure 50–35. Demand ventricular pacemaker. Sinus rhythm is initially present with a long P-R interval and a narrow QRS complex, suggesting delay in the AV node. The fifth P wave fails to conduct, and a pause results. Following a programmed interval, the ventricular pacemaker begins to fire until AV conduction resumes.

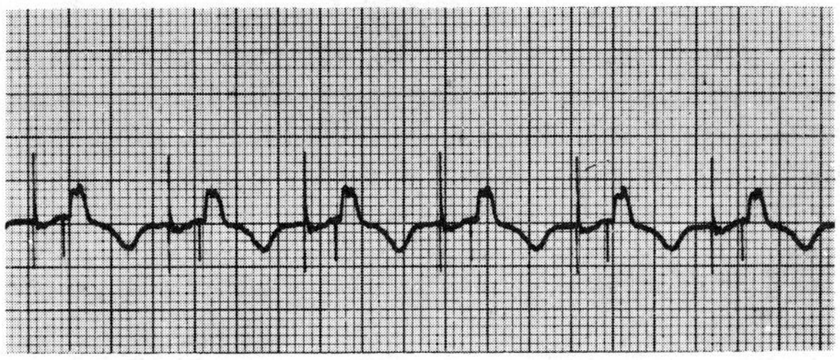

Figure 50–36. AV sequential pacemaker. Note that two varieties of stimulus artifact are present, one preceding the P wave and one preceding the QRS complex. Both atria and ventricle are under the control of artificial pacing, and the P-R interval is itself controlled by the pacemaker.

sensing characteristics). The increased sophistication of pacing devices has also led to greater expense and higher incidence of technical malfunctions. At present it is not clear whether the majority of patients will require the advanced technology offered by these new pacing devices.

Complications of pacemakers are largely determined by the route of lead placement. Thus the transvenous route has been associated with cardiac perforations, arrhythmias on lead insertion, infection, thrombosis, emboli, and lead displacement. Transmediastinal lead placement carries with it the risk of general anesthesia, bleeding, infection, compromise of respiratory mechanics in the postoperative period, and late threshold rises associated with the use of traumatic myocardial leads. With both routes of implantation the pulse generator may be subject to erosion through the skin if the pacemaker pouch is too superficial or excessively manipulated by the patient. Many of the previous complications of pacemakers such as inappropriate acceleration of the pacing rate (i.e., runaway pacemaker) have been eliminated by technical advances. Pacemaker interference has been largely eliminated by shielding of the pulse generator case and modification of the sensing circuit, but inhibition of the pacing system or reversion to fixed rate pacing can still occur when patients are in close proximity to large telephone transformers, microwave devices, diathermy, cautery, intense magnetic fields such as those that may be encountered during radiation therapy and near anti-theft devices, and close proximity to certain types of motors and razors. Unipolar pacemakers may be inhibited by local myopotentials generated by skeletal muscles near the pacemaker pouch. All these complications, however, remain rare.

All pacing devices require careful follow-up. To this end, transtelephonic monitoring devices have been developed, which permit patients to transmit the pulse width and rate of firing of the implanted pacemaker over the telephone. Such electronic monitoring enables the early detection of predictable changes in the rate and pulse width of the implanted generator, heralding the development of critical battery depletion.

CARDIOVERSION

The technique of direct current (DC) cardioversion to convert atrial and ventricular arrhythmias was first described by Lown in 1962 and is now an accepted method for treatment on an emergency or elective basis. A slow rising, underdamped wave form 2.5 msec in duration is delivered to the heart by discharging a charged capacitor across externally placed thoracic paddles, resulting in global depolarization of the cardiac cells. The technique is especially effective for the treatment of re-entrant rhythms (i.e., atrial flutter, atrial fibrillation, most varieties of ventricular tachycardia and fibrillation, and reciprocating supraventricular tachycardia) but is ineffective in achieving permanent cessation of a tachyrhythmia when the underlying mechanism is that of enhanced automaticity. A state of enhanced vagal tone, which is relatively constant at all energy levels, frequently appears after cardioversion and results from stimulation of thoracic parasympathetic nerves. Cardioversion also results in a sympathomimetic effect, caused by local release of catecholamines; this effect seems to be proportional to the energy level used. Because autonomic tone fluctuates following a cardioversion, the mechanism of a cardiac arrhythmia cannot be accurately judged based on its response to cardioversion. Experimental manipulation of autonomic tone has been shown to induce as well as abolish automatic rhythms; in addition, in vitro sustained tachyrhythmias resulting from delayed afterdepolarizations in a single cell can be terminated by single stimuli. The varying degrees of vagal and sympathetic stimulation also explain certain brady- and tachyrhythmias that may be observed following successful cardioversion.

TECHNIQUE OF CARDIOVERSION. Patients undergoing elective cardioversion should abstain from food or drink for eight to twelve hours prior to the procedure. Digoxin should be withheld for 24 to 36 hours prior to cardioversion, and longer-acting preparations such as digitoxin should be withheld for five to seven days. The patient should be brought to the laboratory with a good intravenous route established and should lie down on a firm surface which will facilitate cardiac resuscitation should this be necessary. Dentures, if present, should be removed prior to sedation. Patients should be sedated with diazepam in doses of 5 to 10 mg administered intravenously every three to five minutes until they become somnolent and lose the ability to count backwards. Amnesia of the cardioversion may be achieved with doses of 15 to 20 mg intravenously, but considerably higher dosages (i.e., 40 to 60 mg) may be necessary in patients who chronically ingest sedatives or alcohol. In such patients, an anesthesiologist should be consulted. Respiratory depression can occur with these dosages of diazepam, and the physician should be prepared to assist respiration if necessary. For conversion of all arrhythmias other than ventricular fibrillation, the R-synchronous mode of the cardioversion apparatus should be utilized. Care should be taken to ensure that the stimulus will be delivered within 20 msec of the R-wave. Most modern cardioversion machines permit one to monitor exactly where during the QRS the shock will occur before actually delivering one. Paddles should be approximately 9 cm in diameter and well covered with a conductive paste to reduce skin resistance. Whenever possible the anteroposterior configuration should be used, with the back paddle being placed just beneath the tip of the left scapula and the front paddle placed just below the manubrium of the sternum.

Certain tachyrhythmias, such as atrial flutter and certain varieties of ventricular tachycardia, will revert with low energy discharges in the range of 50 watt-seconds. While it is desirable to use the minimal energy required, ineffective low-energy discharges invariably arouse the patient, requiring further sedation and recurrent shock to be used. Unless some specific contraindication exists, it has been our practice generally to begin conversion in such situations with 100 watt-seconds. In the case of atrial fibrillation, attempts at conversion begin at a level of 200 watt-seconds. Lidocaine should be available at all times and administered if any evidence of ventricular irritability appears following cardioversion. Similarly, atropine should be administered if bradyrhythmia is observed following conversion. In the case of unsuccessful cardioversion, it is important to document the events that follow the delivery of the shock. In some instances, cardioversion of the tachyrhythmia is achieved only to be followed by immediate recurrence of the arrhythmia. Many modern cardioversion devices are equipped with a feature that enables the baseline to be immediately reset following delivery of the shock, allowing such phenomena to be documented. If reversion of the tachyrhythmias is observed, further attempts at cardioversion should be deferred until antiarrhythmic therapy is administered.

Following cardioversion, a steroid cream should be applied to the site of paddle application to minimize erythema. Using the dosage of diazepam suggested, most patients will have amnesia of the conversion and will be reasonably alert and stable within 20 minutes.

SPECIFIC INDICATIONS FOR CARDIOVERSION. Cardioversion may be indicated for the emergency treatment of any tachyrhythmia that compromises hemodynamics, provided that excess levels of digitalis are not present. When discrete QRS complexes can be seen during the tachyrhythmia, it is advisable to use the R-synchronous mode of conversion, which ensures that discharge will occur 20 msec after the R wave, thus avoiding the vulnerable period of the T wave, which could lead to ventricular fibrillation. Cardioversion is also useful for the elective treatment of certain arrhythmias that are difficult to treat medically but quite sensitive to cardioversion (i.e., atrial flutter). Atrial fibrillation represents a particularly common tachyrhythmia for which cardioversion is frequently utilized, and deserves some further comment. Quinidine sulfate should generally be started 24 to 36 hours prior to the procedure. Approximately 15 to 20 per cent of patients may be expected to revert just from the institution of quinidine. In patients who are intolerant of quinidine, disopyramide phosphate or procainamide may be useful alternatives. Embolic phenomena can be anticipated in 1 to 3 per cent of all patients undergoing cardioversion for atrial fibrillation. Although the role of anticoagulants has remained somewhat controversial, it is generally agreed that anticoagulation should be administered for three to six weeks if there is a previous history of emboli or if the patient has a prosthetic heart valve or markedly enlarged left atrium, or is in moderate congestive heart failure. Most studies indicate that the likelihood of successful conversion to and maintenance of sinus rhythm is directly related to the duration of atrial fibrillation prior to attempted conversion. Thus when atrial fibrillation has been present for more than one year prior to conversion, 90 per cent of patients will revert to atrial fibrillation at the end of one year, compared with 65 per cent of patients in whom atrial fibrillation was present for less than one year. Most reported series of long-term quinidine maintenance show a higher percentage of patients remaining in sinus rhythm at the end of a year. If quinidine cannot be tolerated, disopyramide phosphate or procainamide should be considered.

CONTRAINDICATIONS TO CARDIOVERSION. Cardioversion should not be employed in situations in which it is likely that the tachyrhythmia will immediately recur or in situations in which attempts at cardioversion may lead to more serious arrhythmias. Thus cardioversion should be avoided in the following situations: (1) longstanding atrial fibrillation (i.e., greater than one year), (2) less than six weeks following open heart surgery, (3) following recent embolic episodes (should receive three to six weeks of anticoagulation), (4) suspected digitalis toxicity, (5) markedly enlarged left atrium, (6) sick sinus syndrome, (7) uncorrected hyperthyroidism, (8) pulmonary disease with uncorrected hypoxia or hypercapnia, (9) arrhythmias secondary to continued alcohol ingestion, and (10) active inflammatory conditions of the heart (e.g., pericarditis).

COMPLICATIONS OF CARDIOVERSION. In the vast majority of cases, cardioversion can be carried out uneventfully if the precautions indicated above are taken. Failure to synchronize the shock with the R wave may result in the R-on-T phenomenon, leading to ventricular fibrillation. Asystole or severe bradycardia may result in patients with underlying sinus node dysfunction. Complex ventricular arrhythmias may appear after cardioversion, especially in patients on digitalis. The ability of cardioversion to damage myocardium has been demonstrated in animals, resulting in release of the cardiac-specific isoenzyme (MB) of creatinine phosphokinase. Although the release of CPK-MB in man is unusual, repeated cardioversions, especially with high energy levels, can lead to a cardiomyopathy. There is greater concern for this development in children, whose chest wall impedance is less than that in adults. Occasionally, worsening of congestive heart failure or frank pulmonary edema may develop within hours of cardioversion. A variety of causes have been postulated, including left atrial paralysis and primary left ventricular dysfunction secondary to the effects of cardioversion. In most cases, improvement of hemodynamic function lags behind the conversion to sinus rhythm, and maximal benefit may not be appreciated until days or weeks following cardioversion.

Ewy G: Cardiac arrest and resuscitation: Defibrillators and defibrillation. *In* Harvey P (Ed.): Current Problems in Cardiology, Vol. II, No. 11. Chicago, Year Book Publishers, 1978. *Monograph which explores the "physics" of cardioversion.*

Lown B, Amarasigham R, Neuman J, Berkovitz B: The use of synchronized direct current countershock in the treatment of cardiac arrhythmias. J Clin Invest 41:1381, 1962. *Classic paper detailing the use of direct current cardioversion.*

SURGICAL TREATMENT OF ARRHYTHMIAS

A variety of surgical interventions have evolved for the treatment of intractable or life-threatening arrhythmias unresponsive to conventional pharmacologic or pacemaker therapy. These include procedures relating to (1) supraventricular and junctional tachyrhythmias, (2) ventricular arrhythmias, and (3) arrhythmias associated with the pre-excitation syndromes. The therapeutic alternatives include ablation of the site or origin of arrhythmia (excision or destruction in situ), modification of the milieu of the site of origin (e.g., autonomic manipulation, revascularization), or interruption of a link in the re-entry pathway (i.e., accessory pathway).

Isolated cases have been reported in which an ectopic focus in the atrium was directly ablated. For supraventricular arrhythmias arising above the level of the bundle of His, indirect therapy is available in the form of interruption of the normal conduction system, thereby protecting the ventricles from inappropriate rate responses. This technique requires implantation of a permanent pacemaker.

When an accessory pathway that participates in the mechanism of an arrhythmia can be demonstrated, more definitive therapy is available in the form of direct ablation of the accessory pathway. Catheter electrode techniques are now available which permit one to document and localize the presence of an accessory pathway preoperatively. Intraoperatively, cardiac mapping of the atria and ventricles is used to demonstrate the location of the accessory pathway. Substantial advances have been achieved in surgical techniques in the last decade, and it is now feasible to interrupt accessory pathways with a high degree of success in patients with refractory disabling or life-threatening arrhythmias related to pre-excitation syndromes.

The underlying mechanism of most ventricular arrhythmias is poorly understood and probably differs according to the associated disease process. A variety of therapeutic interventions have been empirically introduced in the past and a relatively high failure rate reported with most. Such interventions include cardiac sympathectomy, limited resection of cardiac tissue, and revascularization. In the past few years several new promising techniques have become available. In general these require extensive preoperative and intraoperative electrophysiologic studies to define more precisely the nature of the mechanism and the site of origin of the arrhythmia. Direct cardiac mapping is utilized during a sustained episode of tachyrhythmia to localize precisely the site of origin. Based on this localization, such techniques as simple ventriculotomy, encircling endocardial ventriculotomy, and subendocardial resection have been developed for the treatment of ventricular arrhythmias not only secondary to cardiomyopathy but also related to ischemic heart disease.

The life-threatening nature of ventricular tachycardia and its occasional failure to respond to preventive pharmacologic approaches have led several groups to develop direct surgical approaches to the problem. Conventional aneurysmectomy guided by electrophysiologic mapping has improved both the short- and long-term outlook for these patients. Various techniques to ablate (cryothermic) or resect endocardium beneath areas of infarction, guided by endocardial mapping, have also proven effective. The total number of reported cases of direct surgical treatment of ventricular tachycardia now exceeds 100, with a 12-month survival rate of 65 to 85 per cent. One of the most significant recent developments is the implantable defibrillator. Although the guidelines for its use and long-term results remain to be clarified, early results appear very promising.

Anderson KP, Mason JW: Surgical management of ventricular tachycardia. Clin Cardiol 6:415, 1983.
Gallagher JJ: Surgical treatment of arrhythmias: Current status and future directions. Am J Cardiol 41:1035, 1978. *Overview of the surgical treatment of all varieties of cardiac arrhythmias: supraventricular, junctional, and ventricular.*
Gallagher JJ, Cox JL: Editorial: Status of surgery for ventricular arrhythmias. Circulation 60:1440, 1979. *Current information concerning the status of new innovative surgical procedures for the treatment of ventricular tachycardia.*

51. DISEASES OF THE MYOCARDIUM

Victor S. Behar

Myocardial failure may occur as the result of primary myocardial disease or secondary to hyperkinetic states or valvular or ischemic heart disease. The following chapters will deal with the primary myocardial diseases in which the basic pathology specifically involves the myocardium, thereby differentiating them from those caused by abnormalities of other cardiac structures. Much of the ambiguity surrounding the generalized term of cardiomyopathy stems from the inability of our predecessors to arrive at an etiologic diagnosis in patients with ill-defined heart disease. This frequently led them to the use of such terms as chronic myocarditis, idiopathic myocardial hypertrophy, and idiopathic cardiomyopathy, to name a few. In many of the underdeveloped parts of the world, primary myocardial disease may account for 15 per cent or more of the patients with clinical heart disease. It has been estimated that in the United States, however, fewer than 1 per cent of cardiac deaths are due to primary myocardial disease. This may be an underestimate because of the difficulty in recognizing the disease as well as the tendency to attribute its etiology to a more common process such as coronary atherosclerosis.

The presentation and clinical course of patients with a cardiomyopathy are variable. The onset may frequently be silent and accompany an infectious disease with the development of a myocarditis manifest only by nonspecific electrocardiographic changes. These patients usually do not suffer any cardiac disability, and the persistence of the electrocardiographic abnormalities is variable. Although complete recovery is common with this type of presentation, patients may develop asymptomatic cardiomegaly, frequent bouts of congestive heart failure, systemic or pulmonary emboli, or rapid deterioration and sudden death.

The symptoms of a cardiomyopathy are not unlike those of other forms of heart disease. Weakness, fatigue, and dyspnea on exertion are the most frequent manifestations and are due to a low cardiac output. The signs and symptoms of right ventricular failure may occur soon after the development of left ventricular failure, and the combination appears to be more common than in other forms of heart disease. Although uncommon, chest pain may be suggestive of angina in character or due to an associated pericarditis. Right upper quadrant pain caused by congestive hepatomegaly is much more likely to occur and can be especially distressing during acute right ventricular decompensation. Palpitations are frequent and may be due to extrasystoles or arrhythmias, especially in acute myocarditis, alcoholic cardiomyopathy, or the familial cardiomyopathies.

The diagnosis of primary myocardial disease should be suspected in the young, normotensive individual with cardiomegaly or congestive heart failure in the absence of a prior history of congenital, valvular, or ischemic heart disease. The electrocardiogram characteristically demonstrates left ventricular hypertrophy, arrhythmias, or conduction defects. Because of the lack of etiologic information in the majority of these patients, it has proved useful to classify them by their pathophysiology into congestive, hypertrophic, and restrictive types. The causes of cardiomyopathy are diverse, as shown in Table 51–1. In the

TABLE 51–1. CLASSIFICATION OF CARDIOMYOPATHIES

Type	Etiology	Pathophysiology	Laboratory Findings
Congestive	I. Infective a. Viral b. Bacterial c. Parasitic 2. Metabolic a. Puerperal b. Endocrine c. Hemochromatosis d. Beriberi e. Amyloid 3. Heredofamilial neuromuscular diseases 4. Systemic diseases a. Collagen vascular b. Sarcoid 5. Toxic a. Alcohol b. Heavy metals c. Drugs 6. Hypersensitivity reactions a. Serum sickness b. Postvaccinal 7. Radiation	Cardiac dilatation and systolic pump failure of the left ventricle; with progressive congestive failure there may be mitral and tricuspid regurgitation	X-ray: cardiomegaly and pulmonary congestion; ECG: conduction abnormalities and Q waves simulating myocardial infarction
Hypertrophic	1. Familial: Transmitted as dominant trait with the clinical marker of asymmetric septal hypertrophy by echocardiogram 2. Sporadic	Ventricular hypertrophy with or without outflow tract obstruction; the hypertrophy may reduce compliance and lead to diastolic failure of the ventricle with impaired filling; pump function is usually maintained until late in the disease	X-ray: concentric left ventricular hypertrophy; ECG: left ventricular hypertrophy, Q waves simulating myocardial infarction; echocardiogram: asymmetric septal hypertrophy (ASH), systolic anterior movement of the anterior mitral leaflet (SAM)
Restrictive	1. Amyloidosis 2. Endomyocardial fibrosis (African type) 3. Löffler's fibroplastic eosinophilic endocarditis	Pump function and heart size may be normal with reduced ventricular compliance simulating constrictive pericarditis	X-ray: mild or no cardiomegaly or pulmonary congestion; ECG: low voltage, conduction disturbances, and arrhythmias

presence of an entity with a known predilection for involvement of the heart, appropriate noninvasive diagnostic studies should be performed in order to demonstrate subclinical involvement. These studies should routinely include a chest x-ray and electrocardiogram and, when appropriate, Holter monitoring, treadmill exercise testing, echocardiography, and radionuclide angiocardiography. Cardiac catheterization and contrast angiography may be necessary to differentiate a primary myocardial process from constrictive pericarditis or ischemic cardiomyopathy. Endomyocardial biopsy via a bioptome introduced through a cardiac catheter should be reserved for special indications such as the necessity to document the presence of an acute and reversible process, differentiation of primary from secondary cardiomyopathy, documentation of the presence and severity of drug toxicity, i.e., doxorubicin, and homograft rejection. Infiltrative cardiomyopathies such as amyloidosis, hemosiderosis, and glycogen storage disease may be diagnosed more readily in tissues obtained from other sites.

Fuster V, Gersh BJ, Giuliani ER, Tajik AJ, Brandenberg RO, Frye RL: The natural history of idiopathic dilated cardiomyopathy. Am J Cardiol 47:525, 1981. *A follow-up study of 104 patients with idiopathic dilated cardiomyopathy documented by cardiac catheterization. An excellent discussion of their etiologic, clinical, and hemodynamic features, as well as a description of their clinical course of prognosis.*

Goodwin JF: Clarification of the cardiomyopathies. Mod Concepts Cardiovasc Dis 41:41, 1972. *A general clinical and pathophysiologic review of congestive, hypertrophic, and obliterative cardiomyopathies.*

Oakley CM: Clinical recognition of the cardiomyopathies. Circ Res 35 (Suppl II):II-152, 1974. *A summary of the author's experience in 300 patients with a large spectrum of cardiomyopathies.*

Perloff JK: The cardiomyopathies—current perspectives. Circulation 44:942, 1971. *A review of primary myocardial disease with a discussion of its recognition, pathophysiology, etiology, natural history, and treatment.*

Stapleton JF, Segal JP, Harvey WP: Clinical pathways of cardiomyopathy. Circ Res 35 (Suppl II):II-168, 1974. *An interesting discussion of the natural history of cardiomyopathy highlighted by brief case histories.*

ASYMMETRIC SEPTAL HYPERTROPHY

In recent years, asymmetric septal hypertrophy (ASH) has been identified as the unifying characteristic of the elusive disease which has been called idiopathic hypertrophic subaortic stenosis (IHSS), hypertrophic obstructive cardiomyopathy (HOCM), and muscular subaortic stenosis (MSS). Early accounts of this abnormality described marked hypertrophy of the left ventricular outflow tract with obstruction to ventricular ejection, leading ultimately to generalized ventricular hypertrophy. Our understanding of this disease progressed most rapidly with the advent of cardiac catheterization and echocardiography as diagnostic and research tools. These techniques have provided documentation of the unique clinical, physiologic, and pathologic characteristics of ASH. It was soon appreciated that patients with similar symptoms and physical findings may fall along a spectrum of hemodynamic abnormalities, ranging from severe resting gradients to gradients only with provocative maneuvers or to total absence of outflow tract obstruction. The confusion in this dynamic entity was greatly alleviated by the observation that the asymmetric septal hypertrophy, so readily seen at autopsy, can be visualized noninvasively during life through the use of echocardiography. The echocardiographic demonstration of a septal to posterior free wall ratio of 1.3 or greater provides a clinical marker for identifying patients with ASH independent of the existence of outflow tract obstruction (Fig. 51–1). Although IHSS was originally felt to exist in both sporadic and familial forms, documentation of the latter was possible in only about 30 per cent of cases. The presence of asymmetric septal hypertrophy by echocardiogram throughout the entire spectrum of the disease provides a unique opportunity to study its pattern of inheritance. Such studies in first degree relatives of propositi illustrated that ASH is a genetic disease in almost all patients and is inherited as an autosomal dominant trait with a high degree of penetrance.

The most common clinical manifestations in symptomatic patients include dyspnea, angina, presyncope, syncope, paroxysmal nocturnal dyspnea, and palpitations. These symptoms bear a striking resemblance to those occurring in valvular aortic stenosis. However, in valvular aortic stenosis, syncope is associated with severe aortic valvular gradients, whereas patients with ASH and syncope frequently have little or no outflow tract gradients at rest. In addition, syncope in ASH is often postural in nature or produced after the cessation of exercise, whereas in valvular aortic stenosis syncope usually occurs during the actual performance of exercise.

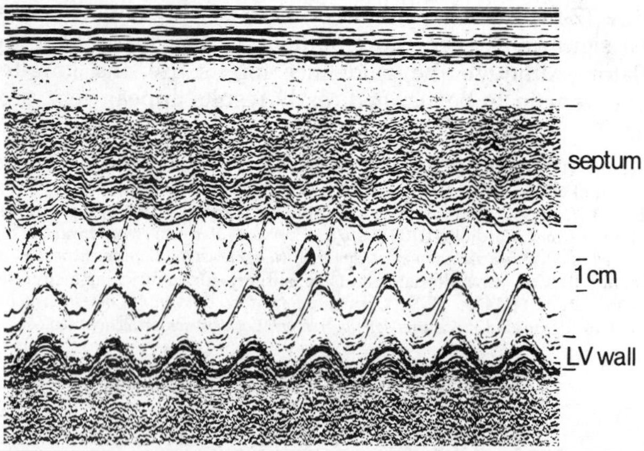

Figure 51–1. Time motion echocardiogram of the left ventricle in idiopathic hypertrophic subaortic stenosis. The septal thickness is markedly increased, and the septal to posterior free wall ratio is abnormal at 3.5. In addition, the arrow identifies anterior motion of the anterior leaflet of the mitral valve during ventricular systole. The apposition of the septum and anterior mitral leaflet is responsible for the outflow tract obstruction.

On physical examination, a large "a" wave may be seen in the jugular venous pulse owing to reduced distensibility of the right ventricle. The carotid arterial pulse is brisk and bifid in contour with a rapid initial rise followed by a mid-systolic dip and late systolic rise. This bisferious character of the pulse is most prominent in the presence of outflow tract obstruction. The heart is usually enlarged with a double apical impulse owing to presystolic expansion during atrial contraction. On auscultation, there is usually a loud atrial gallop. A parasternal thrill is frequently palpable and accompanies a holosystolic or systolic ejection murmur of variable intensity best heard at the left sternal border and apex. The second heart sound is usually normal but may be single or paradoxically split. A diastolic murmur is uncommon. A ventricular gallop may also be present at the apex. The variable intensity of the outflow tract murmur is due to its dependence upon the dimensions of the outflow tract and consequently the degree of obstruction during ventricular systole. Widening of the outflow tract with reduced obstruction occurs with an increase in end-diastolic volume, an increase in distending pressure during systole, or a decrease in the inotropic state of the myocardium. Increased obstruction occurs with opposite hemodynamic conditions. Because of these effects, the murmur classically increases in intensity during the Valsalva maneuver or upon assumption of the upright position; the murmur will decrease in intensity during leg raising and may completely disappear during squatting. Inhalation of amyl nitrite markedly increases the intensity of the murmur and outflow tract obstruction by its ability to decrease blood pressure and increase heart rate, as well as to increase the level of myocardial contractility. Other provocative maneuvers which increase outflow obstruction include postextrasystolic potentiation of the beat following a premature ventricular contraction, digitalis, nitroglycerin, isoproterenol, and exercise. Methoxamine or phenylephrine infusion and hypervolemia increase the dimensions of the outflow tract, thereby reducing or obliterating the gradient.

The electrocardiogram usually shows normal sinus rhythm and left ventricular hypertrophy. The occurrence of atrial fibrillation is an ominous sign because of the dependence of diastolic filling on atrial contraction. A short P-R interval, either with or without a delta wave and QRS prolongation characteristic of the Wolff-Parkinson-White syndrome, is not uncommon. Large Q waves may occur in more than half the patients, simulating a previous myocardial infarction. This has been attributed to abnormal septal depolarization.

The chest x-ray shows left ventricular enlargement, and to a lesser extent, left atrial enlargement. The aorta is usually not dilated, and the absence of aortic valvular calcification is helpful in excluding fixed valvular stenosis.

At cardiac catheterization, a resting gradient is frequently present within the left ventricular outflow tract or can be elicited with provocative maneuvers as described above. The gradient is labile and may vary on a beat-to-beat basis as well as during serial observations. Elevation of the left ventricular end-diastolic pressure is common. The angiocardiogram demonstrates marked thickening of the ventricular septum and left ventricular free wall. The papillary muscles are large and distort the shape of the ventricle, producing an hourglass configuration. Mitral regurgitation is common and is probably related to the altered geometry of the ventricle rather than deformity of the leaflets themselves. Systolic anterior motion of the anterior mitral leaflet is common and is thought to produce the outflow tract obstruction by its apposition to the hypertrophied septum. Systolic anterior motion of the anterior mitral leaflet may also be demonstrated by echocardiography (Fig. 51–1) and correlates well with the presence of obstruction, on a beat-to-beat basis as well as during longitudinal studies and following surgery.

In patients with obstruction, the basic pathologic abnormality is thought to reside only in the asymmetric septum. The ventricular free wall is thickened but has a similar configuration to the chamber in patients with valvular aortic stenosis, suggesting that free wall hypertrophy is secondary to obstruction. Ultrastructural studies show bizarre cell-to-cell and intracellular abnormalities in the septum, with only rare cellular changes in the free wall. In nonobstructive patients, however, there are similar septal changes but a nonuniform distribution of free wall thickening associated with many disorganized and bizarre cells. This is interpreted as evidence that unlike obstructive ASH, in which the defect is localized to the septum, the functional impairment in nonobstructive ASH is due to a diffuse expression of the genetic defect.

Although the echocardiographic finding of asymmetric septal hypertrophy and the histologic observations of myocardial fiber disarray are important morphologic features of this cardiomyopathy, they are not pathognomonic. ASH has been demonstrated in the normally developing heart and in the newborn. In addition, an abnormal septal to free wall ratio has been observed in approximately 20 per cent of patients with congenital heart disease primarily involving the right heart. Although a minor degree of ASH has been found in adult hearts with acquired right ventricular hypertrophy as well as in patients with coronary artery disease, the septal to free wall ratio on the echocardiogram generally does not exceed 1:3. The absence of ASH in first degree relatives of these patients indicates that this disproportionate septal hypertrophy does not represent genetically transmitted ASH. Focal zones of myocardial fiber disarray have also been observed in the normal heart and occur at the junction of the septum and free wall, as well as in the right ventricular infundibulum. Severe fiber disorganization has been found in congenital defects, characterized by hypertrophied ventricles, obliterated cavities, and outflow tract atresia, such as pulmonic atresia or the tetralogy of Fallot. These severe histologic abnormalities have not been found in acquired heart disease with right, left, or biventricular hypertrophy.

Another form of outflow tract obstruction, tunnel subaortic stenosis, may share some of the characteristics of this cardiomyopathy. Tunnel subaortic stenosis is characterized by a fibromuscular tubular narrowing whose dimensions remain unchanged throughout the cardiac cycle. In addition to this abnormality of the outflow tract, the aortic anulus may be abnormally small and there may be other cardiovascular defects as well. Tunnel subaortic stenosis is a distinct entity, and although ASH, systolic anterior motion of the anterior mitral leaflet, and disorganization of myocardial fibers may be present, these findings are uncommon.

Relatively few patients with ASH are symptomatic. In the presence of symptoms the echocardiogram can be used to substantiate the diagnosis, and a trial of propranolol should then be attempted. Drugs such as nitroglycerin, digitalis, and diuretics should be avoided except for control of atrial fibrillation or the symptoms of congestive heart failure. As an important adjunct to therapy, patients should be taught to avoid the rapid assumption of the upright position, the Valsalva maneuver, and paroxysms of coughing. In some patients who do not respond to beta-receptor blockade, verapamil has been demonstrated to be an alternative drug. Verapamil* is usually administered in a hospital setting at a dose of 80 mg every eight hours, and if tolerated for 48 hours, increased to 120 mg every eight hours. Patients refractory to this standard dose have received as much as 720 mg† per day in divided doses. Although the mechanism of its effect is unknown, it has been demonstrated to reduce the outflow tract obstruction when administered acutely and to improve exercise capacity and symptoms when administered during long-term therapy. However, caution must be exercised in its use. Hemodynamic complications including pulmonary congestion, hypotension, and death have been reported to occur in 12 per cent and adverse electrophysiologic effects in 13 per cent of patients. Because of this, verapamil is not recommended in patients with an elevated pulmonary capillary wedge pressure, a history of congestive heart failure, sick sinus syndrome, or significant atrioventricular junctional disease without an implanted pacemaker. Approximately 10 to 15 per cent of symptomatic patients will not respond to medical therapy and will require surgery. Cardiac catheterization should be performed prior to surgery to document the severity of the resting or inducible gradient. The surgical procedure is that of left ventriculomyotomy and myectomy, which is performed through a vertical aortotomy during cardiopulmonary bypass. Excellent symptomatic improvement has been reported in these patients with respect to dyspnea, angina, and syncope, but the amelioration of congestive heart failure has been somewhat disappointing. Postoperative hemodynamic studies in patients with obstruction at rest preoperatively have demonstrated complete abolition of the resting gradient in 90 per cent of patients, with the remainder having residual gradients of 25 mm Hg or less. Although mitral valve replacement has been advocated for the treatment of IHSS at some medical centers, the consensus suggests that valve replacement is not necessary even in the presence of significant mitral regurgitation, which has been found to regress clinically following left ventriculomyotomy and myectomy.

Patients with tunnel subaortic stenosis, on the other hand, have a uniformly poor prognosis and high incidence of sudden death during adolescence. Surgical therapy for this form of outflow tract obstruction has been ineffective in reducing the gradient or changing the prognosis. The factors responsible for the poor surgical result remain elusive, although the presence of a small aortic anulus and other cardiovascular defects undoubtedly plays a role.

Braunwald E, Lambrew CT, Rockoff SD, Ross J Jr, Morrow AG: Idiopathic hypertrophic subaortic stenosis. Circulation 30 (Suppl IV):IV-3, 1964. *A detailed description of the clinical, hemodynamic, and angiographic findings in 64 patients with idiopathic hypertrophic subaortic stenosis. This is a classic study of the disease.*

Bulkley BH, Weisfeldt ML, Hutchings GM: Asymmetric septal hypertrophy and myocardial fiber disarray. Features of normal, developing, and malformed hearts. Circulation 56:292, 1977. *A morphologic study of asymmetric septal hypertrophy and myocardial fiber disarray in the normal developing heart, normal hearts of children and adults, and patients with a variety of cardiac diseases.*

Clark CE, Henry WL, Epstein SE: Familial prevalence and genetic transmission of idiopathic hypertrophic subaortic stenosis. N Engl J Med 289:709, 1973. *An echocardiographic study in 30 families of patients with idiopathic hypertrophic subaortic stenosis. Asymmetric septal hypertrophy was demonstrated to be transmitted as an autosomal dominant trait.*

---

*This use is not listed in the manufacturer's directive.
†May exceed the recommended dose.

Epstein SE, Rosing DR: Verapamil: Its potential for causing serious complications in patients with hypertrophic cardiomyopathy. Circulation 64:437, 1981. *A review of the complications encountered with the use of verapamil in patients with hypertrophic cardiomyopathy, with recommendations as to its use.*

Henry WL, Clark CE, Epstein SE: Asymmetric septal hypertrophy. Circulation 47:225, 1973. *A study of the sensitivity and specificity of asymmetric septal hypertrophy in idiopathic hypertrophic subaortic stenosis.*

Henry WL, Clark CE, Roberts WC, Morrow AG, Epstein SE: Differences in distribution of myocardial abnormalities in patients with obstructive and nonobstructive asymmetric septal hypertrophy (echo and gross anatomic findings). Circulation 50:447, 1974. *A description of the gross morphologic features of idiopathic hypertrophic subaortic stenosis determined by ultrasound and necropsy as they relate to the pathophysiology of obstructive and nonobstructive asymmetric septal hypertrophy.*

Maron BJ, Ferrans VJ, Henry WL, Clark CE, Redwood DR, Roberts WC, Morrow AG, Epstein SE: Differences in distribution of myocardial abnormalities in patients with obstructive and nonobstructive asymmetric septal hypertrophy. Circulation 50:436, 1974. *A light and electron microscopic study demonstrating the morphologic distribution of the myocardial cellular abnormalities and how they may relate to the pathophysiology of obstructive and nonobstructive asymmetric septal hypertrophy.*

Maron BJ, Merrill WH, Freier PA, Kent KM, Epstein SE, Morrow AG: Long-term clinical course and symptomatic status of patients after operation for hypertrophic subaortic stenosis. Circulation 57:1205, 1978. *A follow-up of 124 patients who underwent surgery between 1960 and 1975. The clinical response to surgery and predictors of late postoperative mortality were analyzed.*

Maron BJ, Redwood DR, Roberts WC, Henry WH, Morrow AG, Epstein SE: Tunnel subaortic stenosis. Circulation 54:404, 1976. *A comprehensive report of an interesting part of the spectrum of outflow tract obstruction. The clinical echocardiographic, hemodynamic, angiographic, surgical, and necropsy findings are described.*

Maron BJ, Roberts WC, Epstein SE: Sudden death in hypertrophic cardiomyopathy: A profile of 78 patients. Circulation 65:1388, 1982. *A comparison of the clinical, hemodynamic, and therapeutic characteristics of patients with HCM and sudden death with a matched group of controls. The study re-affirms the absence of a clinical or morphologic descriptor for predicting sudden death in these patients except for a predilection for those less than 30 years old, a family history of premature death, and asymptomatic ventricular tachycardia during ambulatory monitoring.*

McKenna W, Deanfield J, Faruqui A, England D, Oakley C, Goodwin J: Prognosis in hypertrophic cardiomyopathy: Role of age, and clinical, electrocardiographic and hemodynamic features. Am J Cardiol 47:532, 1981. *A retrospective analysis of the medical course in 254 patients followed for a mean of 6 years.*

Rosing DR, Condit JR, Maron BJ, Kent KM, Leon MB, Bonow RO, Lipson LC, Epstein SE: Verapamil therapy: A new approach to the pharmacologic treatment of hypertrophic cardiomyopathy: III. Effects of long-term administration. Am J Cardiol 48:545, 1981. *A report on the long-term use of verapamil in 78 patients with hypertrophic cardiomyopathy. The improvement in symptoms as well as the response to treadmill exercise is detailed, in addition to a discussion on its adverse effects.*

FAMILIAL CARDIOMYOPATHY

Although the term familial cardiomyopathy suggests a single disease entity, it more likely encompasses a variety of clinical and pathologic conditions. Included in this broad category are familial cardiomyopathy, asymmetric septal hypertrophy with or without obstruction, endocardial fibroelastosis, glycogen storage disease, Hunter's and Hurler's syndromes, and the heredofamilial neuromyopathic diseases.

FAMILIAL CARDIOMYOPATHY. Evans proposed the term familial cardiomyopathy in 1949 when he described three cases of heart disease in a single family. Clinically, the patients had palpitations, presyncope, congestive heart failure, or sudden death. Physical examination showed cardiomegaly and signs of left ventricular failure. The electrocardiogram showed extrasystoles, arrhythmias, and conduction abnormalities. At autopsy, there was generalized myocardial fibrosis and hypertrophy of the remaining myocardium. In addition, mural thrombi were present. The prognosis in young patients was worse than in adults, and death occurred from progressive congestive heart failure or was sudden. In recent years, the most frequent form of familial cardiomyopathy seen clinically is *asymmetric septal hypertrophy (ASH),* either with or without left ventricular outflow obstruction (see above).

ENDOCARDIAL FIBROELASTOSIS. Endocardial fibroelastosis is an obscure disease of unknown cause which may occur as an isolated lesion or in association with other cardiac anomalies. It is thought to be transmitted as an autosomal recessive trait. Endocardial fibroelastosis occurs in infancy and has no predilection for sex or race. The symptoms are usually dyspnea, orthopnea, wheezing, cyanosis, and failure to thrive. The course may be acute with rapid deterioration due to heart failure and death in several weeks, or chronic with remissions and exacerbations. Ninety per cent of patients are dead within one year because of heart failure, emboli, arrhythmias, or infection. The electrocardiogram shows left ventricular hypertrophy and, to a lesser extent, low voltage and conduction abnormalities. At autopsy, there is cardiomegaly with endocardial fibroelastosis involving all chambers, especially the left side of the heart. Grossly, the endocardium appears thickened, smooth, and porcelain white. The heart valves may be thickened and sclerotic in half the cases. The microscopic findings show increased amounts of endocardial ground substance with dense accumulation of elastic tissue and collagen at the junction with the subendocardium. Signs of inflammation and fibrous scarring of the myocardium are conspicuously absent. In addition, there is a periarterial adventitial hyperelastosis. The group of patients with associated cardiac anomalies may have aortic stenosis, mitral stenosis, coarctation of the aorta, ventricular septal defect, or the hypoplastic left heart syndrome. Although a genetic cause has been proposed, other suggested causes include maternal infection, fetal endocarditis, anoxia, or mechanical factors resulting from pressure or volume overload. Factor described an eight-month-old infant with primary endocardial fibroelastosis that had pathologic changes consistent with a primary viral myocarditis.

POMPE'S DISEASE. This severe form of glycogen storage disease, also known as Type II glycogenosis, is characterized by the generalized deposition of normal glycogen in the tissues and severe cardiomegaly. The defect is a deficiency of α-1,4-glucosidase and is transmitted as an autosomal recessive trait. Clinically, the infant appears cretinoid with an enlarged tongue and has marked muscular hypotonicity and cardiomegaly. Hypoglycemia, ketosis, and hyperlipidemia do not occur, as in other types of glycogen storage disease. Tissue damage is thought to be due to progressive replacement by glycogen. The electrocardiogram shows left ventricular hypertrophy, and pathologically the interventricular septum is particularly involved and may produce outflow tract obstruction. Microscopic examination reveals glycogen-filled lysosomes.

HURLER'S SYNDROME AND HUNTER'S SYNDROME. Both of these mucopolysaccharidoses may be associated with a cardiomyopathy. Hurler's syndrome is transmitted as an autosomal recessive trait and Hunter's syndrome by an X-linked gene. Hurler's syndrome is differentiated from Hunter's syndrome by its more severe clinical manifestations. They are characterized by the deposition of dermatan sulfate and heparan sulfate within cells and connective tissues. The cardiomegaly is generalized with involvement of the heart valves as well as the endocardium. In addition, there is intimal proliferation in the coronary arteries. Death is primarily due to congestive heart failure.

FABRY'S DISEASE. This is a sex-linked disorder characterized by deficient activity of α-galactosidase A. Males are primarily affected by this disorder, which results in the deposition of glycosphingolipids (chiefly globotriaosylceramide) in the walls of blood vessels, myocardium, and nerves. There is progressive cardiomegaly and death from left ventricular failure.

HEREDOFAMILIAL NEUROMYOPATHIC DISEASES. The nonmyotonic muscular dystrophies are frequently complicated by a cardiomyopathy. It is most common in the classic, rapidly progressive, sex-linked Duchenne's pseudohypertrophic form, which affects males in the first five years of life. The cardiomyopathy occurs in as many as 50 per cent of patients. The symptoms of heart failure are unusual in these patients because of their markedly diminished activity. On physical examination, it is common to hear atrial and ventricular gallop sounds as well as the murmur of mitral regurgitation. Cardiac chamber abnormalities are difficult to interpret by chest x-ray because of the severe thoracic abnormalities which are present. Cardiac involvement is most readily detected by the electrocardiogram. These changes include tall R waves in leads V_1 and V_3R, with an increased R/S ratio in V_1 together with deep Q waves in the standard limb leads and lateral precordial leads. Identical changes have been observed in female carriers of the dystrophy, who have also been demonstrated to have creatine kinase abnormalities. In addition, the electrocardiogram shows labile sinus tachycardia, premature atrial and ventricular extrasystoles, and atrial or ventricular tachycardia. Postmortem studies show selective scarring of the posterobasal left ventricle and the posteromedial papillary muscle. Noninflammatory degenerative changes have also been described in the arteries supplying the sinoatrial and atrioventricular nodes with sparing of the larger epicardial vessels.

Slowly progressive Duchenne's dystrophy (sex-linked recessive), limb-girdle dystrophy of Erb (autosomal recessive), and fascioscapulohumeral dystrophy of Dejerine and Landouzy (autosomal dominant) may also be associated with a cardiomyopathy, in decreasing order of frequency.

The electrocardiogram is the most sensitive indicator of cardiac involvement in *myotonic muscular dystrophy*, and is abnormal in over half the patients. The electrocardiographic changes include sinus bradycardia, intraventricular and atrioventricular conduction disturbances, left axis deviation, low voltage, and supraventricular tachycardias. The conduction abnormalities may progress to complete heart block with Stokes-Adams attacks and sudden death. At autopsy, there is myocardial fibrosis and fatty infiltration.

The cardiac symptoms in *Friedreich's ataxia* include congestive heart failure and, less commonly, chest pain. The heart is clinically involved in 30 to 50 per cent of patients, although electrocardiographic changes may be present in as many as 90 per cent. These changes include sinus tachycardia, supraventricular tachycardias, and T wave inversion primarily involving leads I, II, AVF, and V_3 to V_6. In addition, left and right ventricular hypertrophy have been observed. Family members with the disease often show similar electrocardiographic changes. At autopsy, the heart demonstrates myocardial fiber hypertrophy, interstitial fibrosis, focal degeneration, and occasionally active necrosis. The coronary arteries may show atheromatous changes, and there is frequently medial degeneration and intimal hyperplasia in the small intramural vessels. Death is due to congestive heart failure or cor pulmonale secondary to the severe thoracic deformities.

Factor, SM: Endocardial fibroelastosis: Myocardial and vascular alterations associated with viral-like nuclear particles. Am Heart J 96:791, 1978. *First report of EFE linking a viral myocarditis to the human disease.*

Griggs RC: Hypertrophy and cardiomyopathy in the neuromuscular diseases. Cir Res 35 (Suppl II):II–145, 1974. *A general review of factors which produce hypertrophy in skeletal muscle with special reference to neuropathic and myopathic disorders. Interrelationships between cardiomyopathies and skeletal muscle disease are discussed.*

Perloff JK: Cardiomyopathy associated with heredofamilial neuromyopathic diseases. Mod Concepts Cardiovasc Dis 40:23, 1971. *A summary of the cardiovascular manifestations of Friedreich's ataxia, myotonic muscular dystrophy, and progressive muscular dystrophy.*

Still WJS: Endocardial fibroelastosis. Am Heart J 61:579, 1961. *An editorial review of the pathogenesis of endocardial fibroelastosis.*

INFLAMMATORY OR INFECTIVE CARDIOMYOPATHY (Myocarditis)

The ubiquitous nature of myocarditis in a variety of infectious diseases makes it important to recognize. Myocarditis may be associated with viral, bacterial, rickettsial, parasitic, fungal, or spirochetal disease, although with varying degrees of documentation. Myocarditis also may occur secondary to a systemic process such as a hypersensitivity reaction or connective tissue disease. The true incidence of myocarditis in the population is impossible to ascertain. Focal or diffuse myocarditis has been found to be relatively common in routine autopsy cases, ranging from 3.4 to 9.3 per cent. In addition, as many as one third of patients with common infectious diseases may have electrocardiographic abnormalities suggesting myocardial involvement. From these observations, it appears that myocarditis is most often silent and not accompanied by overt ventricular dysfunction. It has been postulated, however, that chronic cardiomyopathy may be a late manifestation of an acute myocarditis. It is well documented, for example, that such diseases as acute rheumatic carditis, Chagas' disease, and toxoplasmosis may progress to a stage of chronic fibrosis. Further credence is given to this postulate from observations that the incidence and severity of experimental myocarditis are increased by hypoxia, exercise, or concomitant exposure to bacterial toxins. In addition, treatment of experimental myocarditis with steroids may lead to diffuse myocardial abnormalities rather than focal lesions. One may speculate that factors such as these may select out patients with "silent" myocarditis to develop more extensive disease over time, leading ultimately to an "idiopathic" cardiomyopathy.

Myocarditis is frequently unrecognized either because of its subclinical nature or because of the severity of associated conditions. When symptomatic, the patient may complain of fever, palpitations, pleuropericardial pain, dyspnea, edema, or fatigue, or may die suddenly. The physical examination shows biventricular failure, including elevated venous pressure, cardiomegaly, soft first heart sound, ventricular gallop, mitral and tricuspid regurgitation, pulmonary rales, and congestive hepatomegaly. A pericardial friction rub is heard in the presence of an associated pericarditis. The electrocardiogram may show atrial and ventricular extrasystoles, arrhythmias, conduction disturbances, and ST-T wave abnormalities. Measurement of cardiac isoenzyme activities may be helpful in differentiating cardiac involvement from passive hepatic congestion.

Specific treatment is indicated for such conditions as rickettsial or *Mycoplasma pneumoniae* infections. The management of congestive heart failure includes digitalis, diuretics, salt restriction, and afterload reduction as described in Ch. 42. Short-acting digitalis preparations are recommended because of the propensity of these patients to develop digitalis toxicity. In addition, patients should be placed at bed rest and administered oxygen, if hypoxic, to reduce the deleterious effects of activity and hypoxia observed in experimental myocarditis. Lidocaine, quinidine, or procainamide may be necessary to control arrhythmias, but propranolol should be used with caution because of its negative inotropic effect. Although steroids may be of great benefit in acute rheumatic carditis, they should be used only as a last resort for infectious myocarditis because of the potential of more widespread myocardial disease as shown in the experimental model. A report describing ten patients with the sudden onset of congestive heart failure and cardiomegaly is of particular interest in this regard. All underwent transvenous endomyocardial biopsy because of the recent onset of symptoms, and were found to have diffuse lymphocytic infiltrates within the myocardium or striking infiltration of IgG. Treatment was instituted with prednisone at an initial dose of 50 to 100 mg per day and/or azathioprine,* 100 to 150 mg per day, with complete disappearance of symptoms and hemodynamic abnormalities, as well as complete resolution of the histologic changes, in five patients. Four others had no further progression of their symptoms, whereas the remaining patient became worse. Although this report appears promising, prospective studies and longer follow-up are necessary before one can recommend such an invasive approach.

VIRAL MYOCARDITIS. Myocarditis with or without pericarditis is frequently caused by Group B coxsackieviruses, and less often by Group A coxsackieviruses. The only clinical manifestation may be electrocardiographic changes. Less commonly, cardiac enlargement and decreased exercise tolerance may occur. Idiopathic benign pericarditis, which is frequently associated with myocarditis, is increasingly felt to represent coxsackievirus B disease.

Myocardial damage by a virus may result from its myocytolytic effect, through direct cellular invasion and multiplication, or by an immunologic process. Studies of coxsackievirus B-3 infection in mice by Wong et al. demonstrated that this cytotoxic effect is mediated by sensitized T lymphocytes without a significant role being played by B cells and macrophages. In T cell–deficient animals there was a marked reduction in tissue injury despite the abundance of B-3 coxsackievirus. Microscop-

*This use is not listed in the manufacturer's directive.

ically, interstitial edema, round cell infiltration, loss of striations, and areas of necrosis are found. The newborn infant is particularly susceptible to viral myocarditis, which may be rapidly progressive, leading to congestive heart failure and death. In the adult, complete healing usually occurs, but chronic fibrosis may ensue. Although it has not been possible to isolate a virus in the chronic stage of the disease, studies in mice have shown continued inflammation and fibrosis well after disappearance of the virus from the myocardium. Through fluorescent antibody techniques, viral antigens have been identified in human cardiomyopathies, suggesting the possibility of a chronic, active process. Appropriate laboratory studies must be carried out during the acute or subacute stages in order to define the specific offending agent. These include viral isolation from pharynx and feces by tissue culture, and analysis of paired sera for type-specific IgM neutralizing or hemagglutination-inhibiting antibodies.

Poliomyelitis is frequently accompanied by myocarditis as manifest by conduction abnormalities and ST-T wave changes on the electrocardiogram. The significance of these changes is difficult to ascertain, however, as they may be due to concomitant brainstem disease, metabolic imbalance, or hypoxia. Cardiovascular collapse is a frequent cause of death in patients with bulbar poliomyelitis. The myocarditis is significantly more severe in these patients than in those dying of other polio-related causes. The myocardial lesions range from perivascular inflammation to diffuse myocardial involvement with edema, loss of striations, and fragmentation of myocardial cells. In addition, these patients appear to have more extensive involvement of the reticular substance in the medulla. A combination of vasoconstriction, mediated by the medullary lesion in bulbar poliomyelitis, and the extensive myocarditis may be responsible for the acute heart failure with pulmonary edema and cardiogenic shock.

Many other viruses have been implicated in the production of myocarditis. These include measles, mumps, *Mycoplasma pneumoniae,* influenza, rabies, varicella, choriomeningitis, and infectious mononucleosis. Treatment of viral myocarditis is largely supportive and symptomatic. Since it appears that steroids may be responsible for more widespread inflammation during the early intracellular viral infection, they should be withheld initially and added later to inhibit the chronic inflammatory process. The efficacy of steroids in limiting chronic inflammation and subsequent fibrosis is still controversial.

BACTERIAL MYOCARDITIS. Primary bacterial invasion of the myocardium is rare. It remains a grave complication, however, of bacterial endocarditis and may account for ventricular dysfunction because of myocardial microabscess formation. Later, during the reparative stage, ventricular dysfunction may result from chronic myocardial damage. The organisms most commonly involved are streptococci and staphylococci.

DIPHTHERITIC MYOCARDITIS. Myocarditis is an ominous complication of *Corynebacterium diphtheriae* infection and accounts for the majority of deaths. The protein exotoxin, responsible for many of the clinical manifestations of the disease, is thought to interfere with the synthesis of polypeptide chains by inhibiting the transfer of amino acids from soluble RNA. In the myocardium, the oxidation of long-chain fatty acids is inhibited with resultant accumulation of triglycerides.

In a large compilation of patients with diphtheria, the overall mortality rate has been reported as 11 per cent, whereas in those with an associated myocarditis the mortality rate may be as high as 60 per cent. The electrocardiogram is a sensitive histotoxic indicator of myocardial involvement and is abnormal in 20 to 40 per cent of patients by the second week of the disease. Clinically evident myocarditis, however, occurs in less than 10 per cent of cases. The prognosis for patients with P-R interval prolongation and T wave changes is excellent. Conduction disturbances which occur later in the illness have a poor prognosis, with reported mortality rates of 50 per cent for bundle branch block and 100 per cent for patients with complete heart block. Causes of death include congestive heart failure and arrhythmias. At autopsy, the hearts are dilated and flabby. Histologic examination reveals interstitial edema, fibrinoid degeneration and necrosis, and focal infiltrates of inflammatory cells. The treatment for diphtheria is prevention by immunization, antitoxin, and symptomatic therapy for the complications caused by myocarditis.

TOXOPLASMA MYOCARDITIS. *Toxoplasma gondii* is a protozoan which infects humans as both a congenital and an acquired disease. The prevalence of *Toxoplasma* infection is highest in women of childbearing age and approaches 90 per cent in some areas of the world. The congenital form is thought to arise by transmission in utero and frequently results in abortion, premature birth, or neonatal death. Maternal infection in the first trimester of pregnancy is most likely to cause fetal infection with resultant central nervous system damage. Myocarditis is not prominent in congenital toxoplasmosis. The mode of transmission is unclear for the acquired form, but the ingestion of poorly cooked meat and unpasteurized milk and exposure to cat excrement have been implicated. In the adult, the disease is usually subclinical or mild and self-limiting. It is common for several members of the same family to be infected. Lethal disseminated toxoplasmosis may occur, however, and myocarditis or pericarditis is frequent in this situation. The disseminated form usually occurs in debilitated patients receiving cancer chemotherapy, irradiation, or steroids. The myocarditis is characterized pathologically by scattered areas of focal necrosis and inflammation. Intracellular organisms without surrounding inflammation are frequently observed in the myocardium, whereas other areas show severe inflammatory foci in the absence of the protozoan. The antemortem diagnosis is difficult and depends on the demonstration of the organism in tissue by animal inoculation or positive serologic tests. The latter include the Sabin-Feldman methylene blue dye test, hemagglutination, and fluorescent antibody tests. Leak and Meghji have reported that routine serologic screening of patients presenting with a variety of arrhythmias (especially atrial fibrillation, ventricular arrhythmias, and heart block), atypical chest pain, and congestive heart failure in the absence of any of the common forms of heart disease will yield a sizable population of patients with evidence of chronic or latent toxoplasmic infection. They reported 18 cases in a span of two years and suggested that toxoplasmic myocarditis may represent a relatively common form of cardiomyopathy. The treatment of choice is combined pyrimethamine and sulfonamides, which act synergistically against the organism, as well as the tetracyclines, which have proved successful in both experimental and clinical studies. Since toxoplasmic myocarditis is usually a chronic infection, treatment is frequently unsatisfactory and relapses are not uncommon. The latter may occur at times of stable, rising, or falling serologic titers. At present, prevention is the best therapy available and should include care in the handling of cat litter, hand washing after handling uncooked meat, and more complete cooking of meat.

TRICHINOSIS. Although trichinosis is thought to be the most common helminthic infestation in man, the majority of patients are asymptomatic. Neurologic and myocardial involvement account for the fatalities. Symptoms of encephalitis begin during the stage of larval dissemination during the second week; more localizing neurologic signs begin during the encystment stage in the third week. Myocardial involvement, characterized by retrosternal chest pain, tachycardia, dyspnea, and congestive failure, usually begins after the third week. The electrocardiogram reveals nonspecific ST-T wave changes, conduction abnormalities, and extrasystoles. The majority of patients recover, but when death occurs it is usually between the fourth and eighth week. At autopsy, cardiomegaly, scattered areas of myocardial necrosis, and inflammatory infiltrates are found. Steroids appear to be beneficial for both the neurologic and cardiac complications.

AMERICAN TRYPANOSOMIASIS. Chagas' disease is produced by a protozoan, *Trypanosoma cruzi,* which is harbored by hematophagous insects common in South and Central America. Although less than 1 per cent of infected individuals develop the acute form of Chagas' disease, approximately 30 per cent will develop chronic chagasic myocarditis 20 years after the initial infection. Acute Chagas' disease has a mortality rate of 1 per cent, largely resulting from myocarditis or meningoencephalitis, whereas approximately 20 per cent of those with the chronic myocarditis die within two years of diagnosis. Most cases of acute chagasic myocarditis are self-limited, and most patients recover with only transient cardiomegaly and minor electrocardiographic abnormalities. In patients with fatal cases, however, there is rapid deterioration due to congestive heart failure secondary to a panmyocarditis. Parasites are present in variable numbers within myocardial fibers, and there is extensive interstitial inflammation, necrosis, and hyaline degeneration. Toxic as well as immunoallergic mechanisms have been postulated. Chronic chagasic myocarditis manifests itself most commonly as a congestive cardiomyopathy and less often with restrictive signs and symptoms simulating constrictive pericarditis. An apical aneurysm of distended thinned myocardium is a characteristic lesion of Chagas' disease. The electrocardiogram classically shows right bundle branch block and S-T segment changes compatible with acute infarction. Right bundle branch block occurs in as many as 60 per cent of patients and is frequently associated with left anterior hemiblock, whereas left bundle branch block is rare. Premature ventricular contractions are common, as are ST-T wave changes and Q waves mimicking myocardial infarction. The diagnosis is made by demonstrating the organism in the patient's blood, culture, complement fixation test, or xenodiagnosis. Treatment is directed toward control of the arrhythmias and congestive heart failure.

GIANT CELL MYOCARDITIS. Idiopathic giant cell myocarditis is an uncommon disease of unknown cause that may present clinically as congestive heart failure, arrhythmias, or sudden death. All ages may be affected, and there is no predominance of either sex. Proposed causes include viral infection, autoimmune disease, and sarcoidosis. Histologically, there is interstitial edema with scattered areas of granulomatous lesions associated with fibrosis, multinucleated giant cells, plasma cells, lymphocytes, histiocytes, and fragments of degenerating myocardial fibers. In areas of myocardial necrosis, multinucleated giant cells are rare and polymorphonuclear cells are common. No other organs are involved. These observations by light microscopy and electron microscopy suggest that the process involves an unusual form of myocardial degeneration in which the multinucleated giant cells are myogenic in origin. The initiating cause of this degeneration is unknown, but of interest is the association with other diseases, including thymoma, myositis, thyroiditis, and systemic lupus erythematosus. There is no specific therapy, and the reports of results with steroids are conflicting.

Abelmann WH: Myocarditis. N Engl J Med 275:832, 944, 1966. *General review of the etiology, clinical presentation, and treatment of acute myocarditis.*

Gleason TH, Hamlin WB: Disseminated toxoplasmosis in the compromised host. Arch Intern Med 134:1059, 1974. *A clinical study of five patients with lethal disseminated toxoplasmosis. The importance of the patient's underlying disease and its treatment is stressed. Guidelines for diagnosis and treatment are described.*

Gray DF, Morse BS, Phillips WF: Trichinosis with neurologic and cardiac involvement. Ann Intern Med 57:230, 1962. *A report of three cases and a review of the literature. The life cycle of* T. spiralis *and the natural history of human trichinosis are discussed with special attention to the cardiac and neurologic manifestations.*

Hirschman SZ, Hammer GS: Coxsackie virus myopericarditis. Am J Cardiol 34:224, 1974. *A review article of the microbiology and epidemiology of coxsackieviruses as well as a description of their clinical manifestations, diagnosis, and therapy.*

Leak D, Meghji M: Toxoplasmic infection in cardiac disease. Am J Cardiol 43:841, 1979. *The authors describe their experience with 18 patients who were found to have toxoplasmic myocarditis during a two-year study period. All were identified by routine toxoplasmic antibody studies when no other form of heart disease was identified.*

Mason JW, Billingham ME, Ricci DR: Treatment of acute inflammatory myocarditis assisted by endomyocardial biopsy. Am J Cardiol 45:1037, 1980. *A provocative report of ten patients with acute inflammatory myocarditis or myocardial infiltration with IgG treated with immunosuppressive therapy. Recommendations for diagnosis and treatment are proposed.*

O'Connell JB, Robinson JA, Henkin RE, Gunnar RM: Immunosuppressive therapy in patients with congestive cardiomyopathy and myocardial uptake of gallium-67. Circulation 64:780, 1981. *This study describes the clinical usefulness of gallium-67 myocardial imaging as an indicator of myocardial inflammation and as an index of the clinical response to immunosuppressive therapy.*

Pyun KS, Kim YH, Katzenstein RE, Kikkawa Y: Giant cell myocarditis. Arch Pathol 90:181, 1970. *A case report of a patient with giant cell myocarditis and a general review of the possible etiologic factors.*

Wong CY, Woodruff JJ, Woodruff JF: Generation of cytotoxic T lymphocytes during Coxsackie virus B-3 infection. J Immunol 118:1165, 1977. *Studies in mice which demonstrate that the cytotoxic spleen cells responsible for lysis of fibroblasts and myocardial cells infected with coxsackievirus B-3 are thymus-derived lymphocytes (T cells). The relationship between this cell-mediated immunity and heart disease is discussed.*

NUTRITIONAL CARDIOMYOPATHY

Nutritional deficiencies have been known to produce as well as contribute to heart disease in virtually all parts of the world, although most commonly in the underdeveloped countries. In most instances, the precise cause remains unknown, and multiple factors no doubt exist.

Two identifiable forms of nutritional heart disease have been described in Africans. *Bantu hypokinetic heart disease* occurs in the adult Bantu with a poor nutritional background. The diet of those afflicted is primarily composed of carbohydrate and lacks protein and essential amino acids. No single food factor or vitamin has been identified. The patient has cardiomegaly and recurrent episodes of congestive heart failure. The circulation is described as "hypokinetic," and the cardiac output is usually between 1 and 2 liters per minute. In the early stages, the disease is reversible by the intake of a balanced diet. Without dietary therapy, the heart failure becomes intractable to conventional therapy and death is frequently sudden. At autopsy, there is cirrhosis of the liver with histologic features of hemochromatosis or cytosiderosis. The heart is dilated and hypertrophied, with mural thrombi seen on gross examination. Microscopically, there is interstitial edema and scattered areas of fibrosis, which at times may be extensive. Hemosiderin is not seen in the heart.

The second form of nutritional African heart disease is *kwashiorkor*, which is produced by a protein deficiency in infancy. The infant appears markedly cachectic with hepatomegaly and edema. With cardiovascular involvement, venous distention, decreased pulse pressure, cold extremities, and peripheral cyanosis occur. The heart is characteristically small both on chest x-ray and at autopsy. The histologic appearance is nonspecific. The electrocardiogram shows low voltage, and arrhythmias are uncommon. The Q-T interval is prolonged, and there are broad, deep ST-T wave changes. The severity of these findings is of prognostic value; they frequently revert to normal following adequate protein intake. Death is often sudden and unexplained.

Beriberi is the most common cause of nutritional heart disease in the world. The criteria for beriberi heart disease have been broadened since its first description in the Orient. The classic description was that of a hyperkinetic circulation with bounding and pistol shot pulses, predominant right heart failure with venous engorgement, flushing of the skin with peripheral vasodilation, and syncope or shock. In the Occidental form, there is usually biventricular failure, and the hyperkinetic aspects are masked or absent. The common denominator, however, is the low nutritional intake of vitamin B_1 (thiamine) and a high carbohydrate diet. The polished rice diet in the Orient accounts for this combination, whereas in the Western countries the disease occurs primarily in chronic alcoholics. It is an uncommon form of heart disease in alcoholics, however, but it may complicate the course and treatment of other organic types of heart disease. The electrocardiogram shows low voltage, nonspecific ST-T wave changes, and prolongation of the Q-T interval. Conduction disturbances and arrhythmias are uncommon. Pathologically, the heart is markedly dilated, especially the right ventricle, and hypertrophied. Mural thrombi are not uncommon and may result in emboli. The histologic changes are nonspecific and include interstitial edema and hydropic degeneration, especially in the subendocardial myocardium.

The clinical diagnosis can be made in the presence of cardiomegaly, edema, increased venous pressure, peripheral neuritis or pellagra, and dietary deficiency of three months or greater. The hemodynamic abnormalities of high cardiac output, low arteriovenous oxygen difference, and low peripheral vascular resistance return toward normal both acutely and chronically following the administration of thiamine. Digitalis and diuretics have also proved useful for the control of congestive heart failure.

Potassium deficiency produces characteristic abnormalities on the electrocardiogram. These include prolongation of the Q-T interval, depressed S-T segments, flattening of the T wave, and the appearance of large U waves. Prolonged hypokalemia in animals fed a diet deficient in potassium or made hypokalemic by the administration of desoxycorticosterone acetate has been shown to produce typical histologic changes in the kidneys as well as the heart. Similar histologic changes have been observed in humans with chronic steatorrhea following prolonged periods of hypokalemia. The myocarditis of potassium deficiency is characterized by an early focal infiltration of polymorphonuclear neutrophils surrounding normal myocardial fibers, and later by loss of muscle striations, necrosis, influx of inflammatory cells, and bands of fibrosis. Treatment is, of course, early potassium replacement in order to prevent the development of permanent changes and fibrosis.

ALCOHOLIC CARDIOMYOPATHY. This is a well-known clinical entity characterized by congestive heart failure in the absence of a known cause for heart disease other than the presence of alcoholism. The dietary state of these patients is usually adequate, and there is no deficiency of thiamine or other essential nutrients. The clinical recognition of cardiomyopathy in patients with chronic alcoholism is usually not difficult and can be documented by hemodynamic abnormalities of ventricular function both invasively and noninvasively. With these techniques, patients with an alcoholic fatty liver in the absence of clinical evidence of cardiac involvement may also have significant depression of ventricular function. Studies in noncardiac chronic alcoholics reveal that the depressed resting level of ventricular function may be further depressed by the acute ingestion of ethanol in a moderate dose, but not following a low dose. However, normal subjects receiving a similar low dose, which produces nonintoxicating ethanol blood levels, showed significant transient depression of ventricular performance. These findings suggest that there is a myocardial adaptation to chronic alcohol use in which the threshold for myocardial depression is increased. Metabolic studies in animals and man during acute ingestion of ethanol in intoxicating amounts show a rise in the myocardial respiratory quotient followed by a return to control levels in 90 minutes. This is accompanied by a decrease in myocardial free fatty acid extraction and an increase in triglyceride uptake. Transient myocardial injury following ethanol administration has been demonstrated by an efflux of ions and transaminase in coronary sinus blood. It is therefore apparent that chronic ingestion of alcohol adversely affects the heart and that these changes are reversible prior to development of the overt cardiomyopathy of alcoholism.

The clinical manifestations are palpitations, secondary to extrasystoles and arrhythmias, followed by the symptoms of congestive heart failure and thromboembolic episodes. On physical examination, a resting tachycardia, cardiomegaly, atrial and ventricular gallop sounds, and the murmurs of mitral or tricuspid regurgitation are found. Other common signs of heart failure include venous distention, hepatomegaly, and edema. These signs of a hypokinetic circulation are readily differentiated from the hyperkinetic circulation of beriberi. The electrocardiogram shows distinctive T wave changes described as spinous (peaked), dimpled (shallow notch in Q-T segment), and cloven (cleft at summit of low T wave). The T waves may later become inverted, falsely suggesting coronary disease. In addition, there may be left ventricular hypertrophy, conduction disturbances, S-T segment depression, pathologic Q waves, and arrhythmias, including premature atrial and ventricular systoles as well as atrial fibrillation. The chest x-ray reveals cardiomegaly and pulmonary congestion.

At autopsy, there is marked cardiomegaly with both dilatation and hypertrophy. Mural thrombi are common. Histologic study shows hypertrophy of the myocardial fibers, increased glycogen and neutral lipid, interstitial edema, necrosis, and fibrosis. Electron microscopic studies of tissue obtained by endomyocardial biopsy following acute infusion of ethanol show severe alterations of myocardial cellular organelles. These changes include mitochondrial swelling with loss of its cristae and swelling of the sarcoplasmic reticulum.

In the natural course of alcoholic cardiomyopathy the three-year mortality rate exceeds 40 per cent after the development of symptoms. The prognosis is significantly better in those patients with a shorter duration of symptoms and those who are able to abstain from further alcohol ingestion. Prolonged bed rest has not substantially improved the long-term response to conventional therapy, which is largely supportive and symptomatic.

COBALT-BEER CARDIOMYOPATHY. In August, 1965, a bizarre cardiomyopathy became manifest in Quebec City, affecting heavy beer drinkers who were primarily males over the age of 25. The illness was fulminating with biventricular failure associated with polycythemia, low cardiac output, cyanosis, cardiomegaly, gallop rhythm, pericardial effusion, cardiogenic shock, and severe lactic acidosis. A similar disease occurred in Minneapolis and Omaha, as well as in several other cities throughout the world. The electrocardiogram in these patients showed sinus tachycardia, whereas arrhythmias were rare. A rightward shift of the P wave and QRS complex was observed, as were large Q waves simulating anterior myocardial infarction. The chest x-ray revealed cardiomegaly and signs of pericardial effusion. Serum glutamic oxaloacetic transaminase, lactic dehydrogenase, and creatine kinase were markedly elevated. The mortality rate was 40 to 45 per cent. At autopsy, electron microscopic studies of the heart showed dissolution of myofibrils, with loss of myofibrillar proteins and replacement by glycogen; abnormal and shrunken mitochondria, which contained large intramitochondrial vacuoles; and dilatation of the sarcoplasmic reticulum, with formation of large vesicles. The sarcolemma appeared to be intact. The thyroid gland demonstrated follicular hyperplasia and little or no colloid. These changes in the thyroid gland were an important clue in the final identification of cobalt as the toxic agent. Because of the extensive use of detergents in washing glassware, beer poured into glasses with residual detergent was unable to maintain its foam. Cobalt chloride was added to the beer in order to stabilize the foam. The metabolic action of cobalt is to block the oxidation of pyruvate to acetyl-CoA and α-ketoglutarate to succinyl-CoA without affecting the synthesis of glycogen and triglyceride. The relative toxicity of cobalt on the heart is complicated by other factors such as duration of ethanol intake, dietary protein, thiamine deficiency, and pre-existing heart disease. Although the majority of survivors had a satisfactory recovery, residual electrocardiographic changes and chronic heart failure were not unusual. Since the removal of cobalt from beer, no additional cases have been reported.

Ahmed SS, Levinson GE, Regan TJ: Depression of myocardial contractility with low doses of ethanol in normal man. Circulation 48:378, 1973. *Noninvasive studies in normal subjects which demonstrate the depressant effect of nonintoxicating dosages of alcohol on left ventricular function.*

Akbarian M, Yankopoulos NA, Abelmann WH: Hemodynamic studies in beriberi heart disease. Am J Med 41:197, 1966. *Detailed hemodynamic studies in four male alcoholic patients with beriberi heart disease before and after thiamine therapy.*

Demakis JG, Proskey A, Rahimtoola SH, Jamil M, Sutton GC, Rosen KM, Gunnar RM, Tobin JR: The natural course of alcoholic cardiomyopathy. Ann Intern Med 80:293, 1974. *A prospective follow-up study of 57 patients with alcoholic cardiomyopathy demonstrating improvement in 26 per cent, deterioration in 53 per cent, and no change in 21 per cent. The best results were related to abstinence from alcohol and a short duration of symptoms.*

Higginson J, Gillanders AD, Murray JF: The heart in chronic malnutrition. Br Heart J 14:213, 1952. *The authors describe the clinical and pathologic features in 12 patients with a chronic nutritional form of heart disease prevalent in the South African Bantu. In addition there is a pertinent discussion of the differential diagnosis.*

McAllen PM: Myocardial changes occurring in potassium deficiency. Br Heart J 17:5, 1955. *A report of the clinical, laboratory, and pathologic findings in two patients with prolonged potassium deficiency.*

Morin YC, Foley AR, Martineau G, Roussel J: Quebec beer-drinkers' cardiomyopathy: 48 cases. Can Med Assoc J 97:881, 1967. *A fascinating description of an "epidemic" of heart failure in patients ingesting a particular beer with a cobalt additive used to improve the stability of the foam. The clinical, hemodynamic, and pathologic findings are reported.*

Regan TJ, Levinson GE, Oldewurtel HA, Frank MJ, Weisse AB, Moschos CB: Ventricular function in noncardiacs with alcoholic fatty liver: Role of ethanol in the production of cardiomyopathy. J Clin Invest 48:397, 1969. *Studies of left ventricular function in alcoholic patients before and after two dosage levels of alcohol and during chronic alcohol ingestion.*

Smythe PM, Swanepoel A: The heart in kwashiorkor. Br Med J 1:67, 1962. *A clinical report of 98 patients with kwashiorkor, including one-year follow-up data in 16 and necropsy data in 24. Factors predisposing patients to congestive heart failure and sudden death are discussed.*

CARDIAC AMYLOIDOSIS

Cardiac amyloidosis is a disease of unknown cause characterized by the widespread tissue deposition of an amorphous hyaline-like substance. The disease is uncommon under age 40 and affects the sexes equally. The prevalence of amyloidosis in the general population is not known. Although patients with multiple myeloma may have an incidence of amyloidosis as high as 15 per cent, it occurs in less than 1 per cent of unselected cases at autopsy. The relationship of amyloidosis to the aging process is of particular interest, as it has been found in as many as 90 per cent of patients dying of senile dementia when specifically looked for in brain, heart, or pancreas.

Amyloidosis presents clinically most often with renal involvement, especially the nephrotic syndrome, congestive heart failure, carpal tunnel syndrome, sprue, peripheral neuropathy, or orthostatic hypotension. The most common symptoms are fatigue, weight loss, edema, dyspnea, and, to a lesser extent, hoarseness, paresthesias, or the carpal tunnel syndrome. Although the edema may be produced by either the nephrotic syndrome or congestive heart failure, the presence of dizziness, syncope, and orthostatic hypotension should suggest cardiac amyloidosis.

On physical examination hepatomegaly, splenomegaly, and macroglossia are usually found, the last being more common in patients with multiple myeloma. In addition, there may be lymphadenopathy, especially in the submandibular region, purpura, and skin lesions. The cardiac manifestations may simulate constrictive pericarditis because of impaired ventricular filling during diastole and include an elevated jugular venous pressure with a rapid "y" descent and an early diastolic filling sound. However, if the left heart is more severely involved, the signs of left heart failure may predominate.

The electrocardiogram shows low voltage, which may falsely suggest constrictive pericarditis, as well as Q wave abnormalities, which may be misinterpreted as old myocardial infarction. Supraventricular arrhythmias are frequently seen, as well as the entire spectrum of conduction abnormalities. Patients with cardiac amyloidosis are particularly susceptible to digitalis-induced arrhythmias, possibly because of the infiltration of amyloid in the perivascular region of the sinoatrial node.

Pathologically, the heart is increased in size and firm in consistency. Nodular lesions may be seen in the endocardium, valves, and pericardium. Histologic examination reveals diffuse interstitial infiltration of amyloid within the myocardium and in the blood vessels. Amyloid is identified by its distinctive green birefringence when stained with Congo red and examined under a polarizing microscope.

The clinical diagnosis is proved by tissue biopsy from the rectum in over 80 per cent of patients, and in more than 90 per cent when tissue is obtained from the kidney, carpal tunnel, or liver, making it essentially unnecessary to resort to endomyocardial biopsy. Two-year survival for patients with primary amyloidosis is 35 per cent, but only 10 per cent for those with amyloidosis associated with multiple myeloma. Congestive heart failure is the most common cause of death, and sudden death, presumably from arrhythmias, is also frequent.

Buerger L, Braunstein H: Senile cardiac amyloidosis. Am J Med 28:357, 1960. *The pathologic features of senile amyloid heart disease are described for two study periods (1941–1944 and 1953–1956). The paucity of clinical and laboratory findings and the absence of predisposing factors are discussed.*

James TN: Pathology of the cardiac conduction system in amyloidosis. Ann Intern Med 65:28, 1966. *The author reports on the cardiac pathology in five patients dying with amyloidosis and documented cardiac arrhythmias or abnormalities of conduction. Particular attention was directed toward the sinus node and atrioventricular node which were sectioned subserially.*

Kyle RA, Bayrd ED: Amyloidosis: Review of 236 cases. Medicine 54:271, 1975. *An excellent review of the Mayo Clinic experience in 236 ptients with amyloidosis between 1960 and 1972. The excellent presentation of the clinical, laboratory, and pathologic data is complimented by complete follow-up information permitting clinicopathologic correlations and analysis of survival curves.*

Meaney E, Shabetai R, Bhargava V, Shearer M, Weidner C, Mangiardi LM, Smalling R, Peterson K: Cardiac amyloidosis, constrictive pericarditis and restrictive cardiomyopathy. Am J Cardiol 38:547, 1976. *An excellent review of the clinical and hemodynamic characteristics of restrictive cardiomyopathies in comparison with constrictive pericarditis.*

OTHER CARDIOMYOPATHIES

ENDOMYOCARDIAL FIBROSIS. Endomyocardial fibrosis has been reported to be responsible for approximately 15 per cent of the cardiac deaths from heart failure in Uganda. The disease has also been reported in Sri Lanka and Sudan. No known cause has been defined, although increased consumption of African plantain, which is rich in serotonin, has been implicated, as well as persistence of the infantile form of fibroelastosis, hypersensitivity reactions, and inflammation caused by viral or parasitic disease. Both sexes and all age groups are affected. The manifestations are progressive biventricular failure with dyspnea, edema, ascites, and pain from hepatic congestion. Mitral regurgitation is common, and tricuspid regurgitation may occur in the presence of right ventricular failure. The signs of a restrictive cardiomyopathy are usually dominant both on physical examination and at cardiac catheterization, falsely suggesting constrictive pericarditis. The frequent occurrence of pulmonary hypertension, however, is strong evidence against constriction.

At autopsy, all chambers may show the endocardial and myocardial changes, but the ventricles are more severely involved. Microscopically, the endocardium demonstrates the presence of an acellular, hyalinized, fibrous tissue. These changes, together with granulation tissue, extend into the inner one third of the myocardium. Mural thrombi are common despite the infrequent history of systemic emboli. There is no specific treatment for endomyocardial fibrosis other than the symptomatic management of congestive heart failure.

LÖFFLER'S FIBROPLASTIC ENDOCARDITIS. In 1936, Löffler reported a series of patients with progressive and refractory heart failure who had a febrile illness associated with a persistent eosinophilia and multiple systemic emboli (see also Ch. 54). The mode of onset may be either acute, with abdominal, cerebral, or respiratory symptoms, or insidious, with a gradual decrease in exercise tolerance and the clinical picture of a restrictive cardiomyopathy simulating constrictive pericarditis. Mitral regurgitation is common, but murmurs of mitral stenosis and tricuspid regurgitation may also be heard. The electrocardiogram demonstrates low voltage with nonspecific S-T segment and T wave abnormalities. The chest x-ray shows pulmonary congestion and infiltrates as well as pleural effusions.

The acute phase of the disease is characterized by an eosinophilic arteritis involving the heart and other organs. In the late stages of the disease, the heart is enlarged and there is a leathery, graying-white thickening of the endocardium which involves all chambers. The fibrosis extends into the myocardium as well as the papillary muscles and chordae tendineae, with resultant mitral and tricuspid valvular incompetence.

It has been suggested that eosinophilic leukemia, cardiovascular collagenosis, and Löffler's endocarditis with eosinophilia are all manifestations of the hypereosinophilic syndrome with differing degrees of organ involvement. The prognosis for these patients is grave, with a reported average survival of nine months and a three-year survival of 12 per cent. In a series of patients reported by Parrillo et al., prednisone therapy produced a good response in 38 per cent, partial response in 31 per cent, and poor response in 31 per cent of patients. The initial dose of prednisone was 60 mg per day for one week, followed by 60 mg every other day for one year, at which time the drug was reduced to a maintenance level. Patients with angioedema, elevated IgE, or a prolonged eosinopenic response to a challenge dose of prednisone had the best response to steroid therapy. In addition, hydroxyurea, an inhibitor of DNA synthesis, was effective in 75 per cent of patients when administered in a dosage of 1 to 2 grams daily, and is considered the drug of choice in steroid-unresponsive patients.

SARCOIDOSIS. Although clinical manifestations of cardiac involvement are unusual in sarcoidosis, postmortem studies have demonstrated parenchymal cardiac involvement in 20 per cent of cases. The patients with cardiac symptoms are frequently young or middle aged, with equal prevalence in males and females. There is almost always a known history of sarcoidosis. The clinical manifestations are most often palpitations, presyncope, or syncope; chest pain and congestive heart failure occur less often. Congestive heart failure is primarily due to cor pulmonale and not to direct myocardial involvement. The electrocardiogram demonstrates a high incidence of atrioventricular block, bundle branch block, ventricular ectopic beats, and ventricular tachycardia and fibrillation. Worsening of the arrhythmias has been noted during exercise testing. Death frequently occurs within six months of the onset of cardiac symptoms, and 75 per cent of patients are dead within two years. The cause of death is unexplained and sudden in approximately two thirds of patients. Arrhythmias and complete heart block, which occur in 30 per cent of patients, must, of course, be implicated. At autopsy, the typical lesion is a noncaseating granulomatous follicle composed of epithelioid cells and giant cells of the Langerhans type surrounded by a narrow zone of lymphocytes. Although many organs are involved, the lungs are frequently most severely affected, with progressive fibrosis leading to cor pulmonale. The myocardial lesions most often involve the left ventricle and the upper posterior part of the interventricular septum. The histologic lesions are variable but may be categorized as exudative, granulomatous, granulomatous plus fibrotic, and predominantly fibrotic. Although treatment is frequently disappointing, improvement in the recurrent arrhythmias has been observed with prednisone alone or in various combinations with procainamide, quinidine, and propranolol.

PERIPARTUM CARDIOMYOPATHY (PUERPERAL MYOCARDITIS). Peripartum cardiomyopathy is characterized by congestive heart failure in the last month of pregnancy or within five months of delivery in the absence of any pre-existing form of heart disease. The incidence is highest in multiparous blacks and is more common with increasing age, poor nutrition and prenatal care, toxemia, and multiple births. The onset of left ventricular failure occurs most often within the first three months post partum. The electrocardiogram may show left ventricular hypertrophy with inverted T waves, low voltage, and nonspecific ST-T wave abnormalities. The chest x-ray demonstrates cardiomegaly and pulmonary venous congestion.

Although the early prognosis is good, significant cardiac disability and death may ensue. The patients segregate into low risk and high risk groups, according to changes in heart size. In as many as 50 per cent of patients, heart size may return to normal within six months. In these patients, the persistence of gallop sounds, recurrence of heart failure, or recurrence of postpartum failure following subsequent pregnancies is rare. In the patients with persistent cardiomegaly, however, chronic heart failure and pulmonary or systemic emboli are common. Furthermore, in this poor risk group, subsequent pregnancies frequently result in worsening of symptoms and death. Long-term survival for these patients is approximately 15 per cent in five years.

Myocardial biopsy obtained within three months of the onset of heart failure shows myocardial hypertrophy and varying degrees of fibrosis. At autopsy, the heart is dilated and appears hypertrophied. Mural thrombi are common and frequently result in emboli. Histologically, there is myocardial hypertrophy, fibrosis, interstitial edema, and focal accumulation of lymphocytes.

No specific form of therapy is indicated other than the management of congestive heart failure. The risk of subsequent pregnancies is substantial, and the likelihood of carrying the pregnancy to term is reduced.

RADIATION MYOCARDITIS. Cardiac injury is clinically apparent in approximately 5 per cent of patients receiving 4000 rads or more in the form of either orthovoltage or supervoltage. Patients receiving larger amounts of radiation, as in those undergoing retreatment therapy for Hodgkin's disease, have a much higher incidence of carditis. In the large series of patients treated at Stanford, 50 per cent of those receiving more than 6000 rads developed carditis, which in some cases was a severe pancarditis. Radiation heart disease is most commonly manifest in the form of pericardial disease, including acute pericarditis, chronic effusion, or chronic constrictive pericarditis. Less commonly, myocardial fibrosis may accompany pericarditis and has been observed to produce conduction disturbances, including bundle branch block and varying degrees of heart block, as well as ventricular dysfunction and mitral regurgitation. Of particular interest is the controversy that radiation injury produces premature coronary atherosclerosis. Indeed, there are many autopsy reports of patients dying in the second or third decade with extensive coronary artery disease and myocardial infarctions following radiation therapy. In addition to these clinical observations, there are experimental data that the changes induced in the dog aorta by radiation are very similar to those which occur during the normal aging process. Other studies in atherogenic animal models further substantiate the clinical observation in that more severe atheromatous lesions occur following exposure to high dose radiation. The microcirculation has also been shown to participate in the process of myocardial damage from radiation. Immediately following exposure, there is an acute and transient inflammatory exudate in all cardiac tissues. After a latent period, however, a focal cytoplasmic degeneration occurs in the endothelial cells of myocardial capillaries, followed by a proliferation of these cells in an apparent attempt to form new capillaries. Ischemia and diffuse myocardial fibrosis result from this gradual loss of the microcirculation.

With the advent of megavoltage therapy and innovative rotational techniques, more effective tumor doses can now be delivered and survival significantly prolonged. As a byproduct of this, however, the treatment of thoracic malignancy also results in more radiation to the heart, and because of the longer survival there is greater opportunity for the delayed effects of myocardial damage to occur. It is important to recognize that although acute pericarditis may occur during the period of radiation treatment itself, it is more likely that the signs and symptoms of cardiac damage will occur after a variable latent period, frequently years.

DRUG-INDUCED MYOCARDITIS. Doxorubicin (Adriamycin), which closely resembles its parent compound daunorubicin, has been observed to produce cardiotoxicity during the treatment of far-advanced cancer. The cardiotoxicity is manifest as electrocardiographic changes or congestive heart failure. The electrocardiographic abnormalities occur in approximately 10 per cent of patients and include sinus tachycardia, ST-T wave changes, and premature ventricular contractions. These changes are reversible in 48 per cent, progressive in 15 per cent, and stable in 38 per cent of patients. Histologic evidence of cardiotoxicity is dose related and was found by Bristow and coworkers in over 90 per cent of biopsy specimens taken from patients who had received a cumulative dose greater than 240 mg per square meter. There was considerable variability, however, in the drug dosage to produce a cardiomyopathic effect, with degenerative changes observed at a dose as low as 45 mg per square meter and normal biopsy material obtained from a patient who had received 400 mg per square meter. Noninvasive measures of left ventricular function did not correlate well with the degree of morphologic changes seen on the biopsy material or with the symptoms of congestive heart failure. Furthermore the ratio of the pre-ejection period to left ventricular ejection time did not become abnormal until a dose of 400 mg per square meter had been exceeded. These changes in ventricular function may be reversible, but the recovery time is directly related to the cumulative dose.

Clinically manifest congestive heart failure has been observed from 0 to 231 days after the last dose of doxorubicin, with a mean duration of 33 days. The prognosis after the development of symptoms is poor, with a mortality rate of 60 per cent and death occurring within three weeks of the onset of symptoms. In a retrospectively conducted cooperative study of 3941 patients receiving doxorubicin, Von Hoff et al. found an incidence of congestive heart failure of 2.2 per cent. They found a continuum of increasing risk for the development of heart failure as the total dose of drug increased, with a relatively abrupt increase in risk at 550 mg per square meter. The lowest risk occurred in patients on a weekly schedule as opposed to those receiving a single dose repeated every three weeks or those receiving three consecutive daily doses repeated every three weeks. No difference in risk was noted between the latter two schedules. In addition, increasing age was statistically related to an increased risk of drug-induced heart failure. Although heart failure was more likely to develop in patients with a prior history of heart disease or hypertension, this difference was not statistically significant. Other studies have suggested that the risk of doxorubicin-induced heart failure is increased in patients who have previously received mediastinal radiotherapy or concomitant cyclophosphamide administration. Race, sex, tumor type, or performance status did not appear to be related to doxorubicin cardiotoxicity.

Other drugs which may produce electrocardiographic changes or toxicity include the tricyclic antidepressants, phenothiazines, and emetine.

Bristow MR, Mason JW, Bilingham ME, Daniels JR: Doxorubicin cardiomyopathy: Evaluation by phonocardiography, endomyocardial biopsy, and cardiac catheterization. Ann Intern Med 88:168, 1978. *A correlative study of clinical descriptors, endomyocardial biopsy material, and noninvasive measures of left ventricular function in 33 patients receiving varying dosages of doxorubicin.*

Cohn KE, Stewart JR, Fajardo LF, Hancock EW: Heart disease following radiation. Medicine 46:281, 1967. *The authors report on the incidence of acute pericarditis, chronic pericardial effusion, chronic constrictive pericarditis, cardiomyopathy, and myocardial infarction in 21 patients undergoing radiation treatment of malignant neoplasms.*

Demakis JG, Rahimtoola SH, Sutton GC, Meadows WR, Szanto PB, Tobin JR, Gunnar RM: Natural course of peripartum cardiomyopathy. Circulation 44:1053, 1971. *A clinicopathologic study of 27 patients with peripartum cardiomyopathy followed up to 21 years from the onset of symptoms. Risk factors for the development of heart failure and prognostic indicators for late morbidity and mortality are discussed.*

Fajardo LF, Stewart JR: Pathogenesis of radiation-induced myocardial fibrosis. Lab Invest 29:244, 1973. *A pathophysiologic study of radiation-induced myocarditis in rabbits, using both light and electron microscopy. In addition, capillary endothelial cell injury and subsequent proliferation were studied by means of radioautographs after the injection of tritiated thymidine.*

Lefrak EA, Pitha J, Rosenheim S, Gottlieb JA: A clinicopathologic analysis of Adriamycin cardiotoxicity. Cancer 32:302, 1973. *The authors present two case reports of patients dying after the administration of doxorubicin with detailed histopathologic studies. In addition they review their clinical experience in 399 patients receiving the drug in an attempt to determine factors related to its cardiotoxicity.*

Matsui Y, Iwai K, Tachibana T, Fruie T, Shigematsu N, Izumimoto M: Clinicopathologic study on fatal myocardial sarcoidosis. Ann NY Acad Sci 278:455, 1976. *The clinical and electrocardiographic findings as well as the mode of death are reported for 42 patients with myocardial sarcoidosis studied at postmortem examination. The distribution of cardiac lesions is discussed, and a histologic classification is presented.*

Parillo JE, Fauci AS, Wolff SM: Therapy of the hypereosinophilic syndrome. Ann Intern Med 89:167, 1978. *A prospective study of the hypereosinophilic syndrome in 26 patients followed from 3 months to 9 years. Survival curves, prognostic factors, and therapy are discussed.*

Stein E, Stimmel B, Siltzbach LE: Clinical course of cardiac sarcoidosis. Ann NY Acad Sci 278:470, 1976. *A report of the clinical presentation, electrocardiographic changes, and therapy in 15 patients with cardiac sarcoidosis followed for an average of 40.2 months. The effectiveness of various antiarrhythmic drug combinations is presented with recommendations for the evaluation of arrhythmias and their treatment.*

Von Hoff DD, Layard MW, Basa P, Davis, HL Jr, Von Hoff AL, Rozencweig M, Muggia FM: Risk factors for doxorubicin-induced congestive heart failure. Ann Intern Med 91:710, 1979. *The report of a clinical cooperative study based upon the information compiled from a total of 4018 patients who had received doxorubicin therapy. The importance of cumulative dose and three different drug schedules is discussed, together with other descriptors of risk for heart failure.*

52. DISORDERS OF THE PERICARDIUM

Robert E. Whalen

Claudius Galen first noted and named the pericardium in the second century A.D. The function of the pericardium has been a matter of conjecture. Its role as a structure that allows smooth, frictionless motion of the heart in relation to other mediastinal structures, its role as a barrier to infection or inflammation arising in other thoracic organs, and its role in preventing limitation or excessive inflow and outflow of blood to and from the heart have been hypothesized but not proved. Patients who have undergone pericardiectomy, who have had their pericardium left open after cardiac surgery, or who have been born without a pericardium have not shown the deleterious effects that might be predicted from speculation and experimental studies.

Diseases of the pericardium typically present in one or more of three clinical forms: acute pericarditis, pericardial effusion, and pericardial constriction. Pericardial involvement may progress from inflammation to effusion and then constriction, or it may present as effusion or constriction without clinical evidence of preceding inflammation.

The pericardium may be the site of a variety of inflammatory, neoplastic, and congenital disorders. The incidence of such disorders, which are listed in the accompanying table, has changed markedly over the past several decades. This change stems from four major factors: the introduction of antibiotics, which has significantly decreased the incidence of bacterial involvement of the pericardium; the increasing clinical awareness of the involvement of the pericardium in various connective tissue diseases; the marked increase in the postpericardiotomy syndrome accompanying the advent of modern cardiac surgery; and the growing recognition of acute and delayed signs of pericardial involvement associated with myocardial infarction.

ACUTE PERICARDITIS

By far the most common initial manifestation of pericardial disease is acute pericarditis. This condition may be due to diverse causes. In many cases the same etiologic factors may persist over long periods of time and thus produce a recurrent, subacute, or chronic disorder.

ETIOLOGY. ***Nonspecific "Benign" or Idiopathic Pericarditis.*** This is perhaps the most common type of acute pericarditis in adults. The term benign should probably not be applied to this entity, because the symptomatology is certainly not benign and the disease can be accompanied by acute pericardial effusion or lead to chronic constriction. For many years this syndrome has been attributed to either a viral agent or a hypersensitivity reaction, but there has been no effective proof of this. Typically the syndrome occurs in late adolescence and early adulthood. It is often preceded by an upper respiratory infection days to several weeks before fever and precordial pain bring the patient to medical attention. The syndrome usually lasts one to several weeks, during which time the patient is mildly febrile and has varying degrees of precordial pain. Occasionally pericardial effusion may appear early, and sometimes it is the first sign of the syndrome. Although the acute symptoms may subside after

TABLE 52–1. ETIOLOGY OF DISORDERS OF THE PERICARDIUM

- I. Inflammatory
  - A. Acute pericarditis
    - 1. Nonspecific "benign" or idiopathic
    - 2. Infections
      - a. Viral
      - b. Bacterial
      - c. Tuberculous
      - d. Fungal
      - e. Others
    - 3. Myocardial infarction
      - a. Acute myocardial infarction
      - b. Postmyocardial infarction
    - 4. Postpericardiotomy or thoracotomy
    - 5. Post-traumatic
    - 6. Connective tissue disorders
    - 7. Allergic and hypersensitivity disorders
    - 8. Metabolic disorders
    - 9. Physical or chemical agents
  - B. Chronic pericarditis (virtually all of the above)
- II. Neoplastic disease
  - A. Benign
  - B. Malignant
    - 1. Primary
    - 2. Secondary
- III. Congenital lesions of the pericardium
  - A. Pericardial cysts and diverticula
  - B. Partial or complete absence of the pericardium
- IV. Disease of diverse or uknown etiology

a brief time, the patient may be left with easy fatigability for several months. This may reflect the fact that in virtually all cases of acute pericarditis there is some inflammatory response in the subepicardial myocardium, and there may be a greater degree of myocarditis than is recognized clinically. Exacerbations of the syndrome, particularly of precordial pain, are not rare and may occur sporadically for several months to years after the initial attack. The development of constrictive pericarditis is extremely rare.

TREATMENT. In most cases bed rest and analgesics will produce relief of symptoms in one to two weeks. If these measures fail, various nonsteroidal anti-inflammatory agents, such as aspirin and indomethacin, have been effective. In patients with unusually severe and prolonged pain, adrenal corticosteroid hormone therapy may be indicated, but this should be undertaken only if bacterial infection can be reasonably excluded.

Infectious Pericarditis. Infections of proved etiology account for a significant number of cases of pericarditis. Various *viral agents* have long been suspected as causes for "idiopathic nonspecific" pericarditis. However, even with careful viral isolation studies, only a small percentage of cases have been demonstrated to be associated with viral infection of the pericardium or myocardium. The most common viral agent is coxsackievirus Type B; rarely, coxsackievirus Type A is the agent. Pericarditis has been reported to be due to Type A echovirus, mumps, and infectious mononucleosis. Although it has been suggested that diffuse myalgias, rubelliform rashes, and lymphadenopathy are more common in viral pericarditis than in idiopathic pericarditis, there have been insufficient viral studies in patients labeled as having idiopathic pericarditis to warrant this as being a diagnostic feature for separating the two entities, if indeed they are truly separate. The clinical course, physical findings, and method of treatment in proven cases of viral pericarditis are not significantly different from those discussed under Nonspecific "Benign" or Idiopathic Pericarditis.

Bacterial infections of the pericardium may arise by direct extension of infection from foci in the thorax such as pneumonia or empyema. Less frequently bacterial pericarditis is caused by a septicemia which is initiated from a distant site of infection. The emergence of antibiotic-resistant strains of staphylococci, particularly in the hospital, has served to increase the frequency of this organism as a causative agent in relation to other previously classic bacterial causes for pericarditis. The susceptibility of the pneumococcus to penicillin has almost completely eliminated this organism as a cause for bacterial pericarditis, and cases are seldom seen unless treatment has been long delayed and the patient has empyema. A large number of other types of organisms have been implicated in the development of pericarditis, including the meningococcus, gonococcus, *Hemophilus influenzae,* and streptococcal organisms. Although gram-negative organisms are a relatively rare cause for acute pericarditis, their frequency has increased because of the development of antibiotic-resistant strains, particularly in patients having complications after cardiac surgery and in patients on immunosuppressive therapy for malignancies. Bacterial pericarditis rarely is the initial sign of infection and often appears only as a late complication of either untreated or poorly controlled bacterial infection. When it does appear, it may present with the classic signs of acute pericarditis and may eventuate in a pericardial effusion or constriction. However, the classic signs of acute pericarditis are present in probably less than half of patients with bacterial pericarditis, and therefore the diagnosis should not be discarded because of the absence of clinical signs of acute pericarditis. Once the diagnosis is suspected, diagnostic studies must be initiated immediately, for time is of the essence if the infection is to be successfully treated. If suspicion is sufficient and diagnostic pericardial fluid cannot be obtained by pericardiocentesis, an exploratory thoracotomy should be performed promptly. If the diagnosis is not established either by pericardiocentesis or by exploratory thoracotomy, a pericardiectomy or a pleuropericardial window procedure should be performed.

Although *tuberculous* involvement of the pericardium might justifiably be considered with the bacterial forms of pericarditis, it has earned a place of its own because of its prevalence in earlier decades and its propensity to produce constrictive pericarditis. Tuberculous pericarditis occurs predominantly in males, particularly in blacks, who have approximately ten times the incidence of the disease found in whites. Although tuberculous pericarditis may be the only evidence of the infection, it probably arises as a secondary manifestation of the disease rather than as a primary focus. Approximately half the patients with tuberculous pericarditis have evidence of previous or concurrent infection of the lung. In the acute phase it cannot be differentiated from other forms of infectious pericarditis. In the chronic phase it may have an insidious onset characterized by systemic symptoms such as low grade fever and weakness. In the chronic form the progressive constrictive process may be its predominant manifestation. The disease must be considered in any patient presenting with acute pericarditis, pericardial effusion, or constriction. The diagnosis may sometimes be made by examination and culture of the pericardial fluid, although this is difficult unless large volumes of pericardial fluid can be obtained. The diagnosis is more likely to be made by suitable pathologic examination and culture of pericardium obtained at surgery.

TREATMENT. Evidence of old or active tuberculosis by chest x-ray or the presence of a positive tuberculin skin test in a patient who had a previous negative skin test not only heightens the likelihood of the diagnosis but should raise the question that antituberculous therapy should be started on clinical grounds alone. The effects of progressive tuberculous involvement of the pericardium are so devastating and the institution of antituberculous therapy is of such relatively low morbidity that on some occasions the clinician will feel forced to treat pericarditis of unknown cause as though it might be tuberculous. When the diagnosis is likely on clinical grounds but cannot be proved by culture or pathologic studies, a more conservative approach with a combination of isoniazid and rifampin or ethambutol for 18 months, along with continued follow-up to be certain that there is no progression, may be indicated. If the index of suspicion is great and pericardiocentesis has not demonstrated an organism, a pericardiectomy, both to establish a diagnosis and to prevent future constriction, is frequently employed. When the diagnosis is established, triple therapy with isoniazid, streptomycin, and rifampin or ethambutol is indicated for 18 to 24 months. If the diagnosis has been made and antituberculous therapy has not eliminated signs of effusion or constriction in several months, a pericardiectomy should be performed.

Various *fungal disorders,* including histoplasmosis, coccidioidomycosis, actinomycosis, and nocardiosis, have been reported as etiologic agents in the development of pericarditis. Although these represent an extremely small number of cases, the possibility should be considered in patients who are especially susceptible to fungal infections, particularly those with lymphomas and leukemia and those who are undergoing immunosuppressant therapy for other systemic diseases. *Parasites* represent a very small but definite class of etiologic agents in the development of pericarditis. Infection with *Entamoeba histolytica* has been reported to produce pericarditis by hematogenous spread to the pericardium or by rupture of a hepatic cyst into the pericardial space. Although *Echinococcus* is a rare cause of pericarditis, over 100 cases of such involvement have been reported in the literature. Pericardial infection almost inevitably stems from initial invasion and cyst formation in the myocardium with rupture into the pericardial space.

Myocardial Infarction. Pericarditis associated with myocardial infarction may take two forms, and on occasion it may be difficult to be certain whether one is dealing with a late-appearing *acute pericarditis* or an early appearance of *postmyocardial infarction pericarditis.* Acute inflammation of the pericardium frequently accompanies acute myocardial infarction, particularly if it is transmural. The clinical recognition of this, such as the development of typical pericardial pain and a pericardial friction rub, is directly related to the frequency with which the patient is examined. With repetitive examination, signs may be recognized in at least two thirds of patients rather than the 20 per cent previously reported. The symptoms usually occur between the second and fifth days and rarely after the tenth day. The syndrome is thought to be due to an inflammatory response in the subepicardial region of the infarcted myocardium with some extension of inflammation to contiguous areas of the epicardium. It is almost invariably a self-limited process and requires only analgesics or a nonsteroidal anti-inflammatory agent to control the symptoms. A pericardial effusion rarely presents a problem unless the patient has been anticoagulated. A second form of pericardial involvement occurs from several weeks to several months after an acute myocardial infarction. This so-called *postmyocardial infarction pericarditis,* or *Dressler's syndrome,* is characterized by the onset of typical pericardial pain, particularly precipitated by changes in position or cough. It may be accompanied by fever and significant pericardial effusion. There may be a friction rub and systemic symptoms such as malaise and myalgias. The major differential diagnosis in such patients is the possibility of a recurrence of myocardial infarction, but the almost consistent complaint of accentuation of symptoms by changes in body position, coughing, and inspiration, along with the presence of a pericardial rub without evidence of further infarction by ECG, serves to alert the clinician to the correct diagnosis.

TREATMENT. The syndrome is usually self-limited and can be treated with analgesics or nonsteroidal anti-inflammatory agents, but on occasion the syndrome may become so repetitive that it is necessary to rely on a tapering course of corticosteroid hormone therapy.

The Postpericardiotomy Syndrome. This has become a commonly recognized form of pericarditis. Although the incidence of the syndrome is reported to be approximately 10 per cent among patients undergoing cardiac surgery, it is undoubtedly higher than this, particularly if minor manifestations of the syndrome are taken into account. The exact cause of the syndrome is not understood. It has been suggested that a common denominator which ties together the pericarditis following myocardial infarction, cardiac surgery, and trauma to the pericardium is blood in the pericardium, which produces an inflammatory response. However, the presence of blood in the pericardium is not mandatory for the development of the syndrome, and recent evidence suggests that there may be a viral agent involved, perhaps arising from infection carried in the multiple transfusions often associated with cardiac surgery. Actual entrance into the pericardium at surgery is not a necessity for the development of the syndrome, because it has been reported after thoracic surgery for pulmonary resection and repair of a hiatus hernia. The syndrome may occur as early as a week postoperatively, but frequently will not manifest itself until several weeks or months after surgery. Although the typical findings of acute pericarditis, such as fever, substernal chest pain, and a pericardial rub, usually are associated with the syndrome, it may appear with only one of these manifestations. Fever, typical ECG changes, and even an elevation of sedimentation rate may not accompany the syndrome, and thus the absence of these abnormalities should not be used as evidence against the diagnosis of the postpericardiotomy syndrome. It is frequently accompanied by a diffuse pleural reaction and associated small pleural effusions. Although the development of pericarditis several weeks postoperatively always raises the specter of a complicating postoperative bacterial pericarditis, the syndrome is almost invariably due to the postpericardiotomy syndrome rather than actual bacterial infection.

Post-traumatic Pericarditis. Pericarditis may develop after both penetrating and nonpenetrating injury to the chest. The syndrome may appear early after a penetrating wound, and under these circumstances there is always concern that it may be due to bacterial infection of the pericardial space. The syndrome tends to occur weeks or even months after blunt trauma to the chest such as a steering wheel injury. Under these circumstances the concern about bacterial infection is less, and one can move quickly with anti-inflammatory agents to suppress the symptoms.

Connective Tissue Disorders. These have become commonly recognized causes of pericarditis. In childhood the most common cause may be acute rheumatic fever. However, in the adult, pericarditis is a relatively rare manifestation of acute rheumatic fever. In adults connective tissue disorders, such as systemic lupus erythematosus, rheumatoid arthritis, periarteritis, and, less frequently, scleroderma, are much more likely causes of pericarditis. Pericarditis may be the first sign of systemic lupus erythematosus and may precede other manifestations by months. It may be associated with a rapidly accumulating effusion, which may present such a predominant and life-threatening clinical picture that other signs of the disease do not gain attention until the symptoms of pericarditis and effusion are controlled. Pericardial involvement has been noted in up to 40 per cent of documented cases of systemic lupus erythematosus. The diagnosis can be reasonably inferred when LE cells and anti-DNA antibodies are detectable in the blood. Steroid therapy is almost invariably necessary to control the symptoms of pericarditis. Clinical signs of typical acute pericarditis may be seen in approximately 3 per cent of patients with rheumatoid arthritis, even though autopsy series indicate that at least 10 per cent of patients with rheumatoid arthritis have an inflammatory response in the pericardium. Small pericardial effusions may be detected in as many as one third of patients with rheumatoid arthritis. Pericarditis is most commonly seen in patients with active rheumatoid disease, particularly those with rheumatoid nodules and markedly elevated titers of rheumatoid factor in serum. The pericarditis is seldom severe, but on rare occasions it can be accompanied by significant effusion. Examination of the pericardial fluid reveals a characteristic marked decrease in the concentration of glucose and elevated LDH enzyme levels as well as increased globulins and decreased complement values. Large round or oval multinucleated cells have been noted in the fluid and are thought by some to be pathognomonic of the disease. These "RA" cells contain cytoplasmic inclusion bodies thought to represent phagocytized rheumatoid factor complex. Other connective tissue disorders, such as periarteritis nodosa and scleroderma, as well as giant cell arteritis, have been reported to be associated with pericarditis less commonly. In particular, scleroderma more frequently involves the myocardium and is a rare cause of pericarditis.

Allergic and Hypersensitivity Disorders. Serum sickness, giant urticaria, and allergic responses to penicillin have been associated with pericarditis. In addition to penicillin, other drugs, including phenytoin, hydralazine, and procainamide, have been implicated in the development of pericarditis. With the renewed emphasis on prevention of cardiac arrhythmias following myocardial infarction and the consequent increased use of procainamide, a lupus-like syndrome involving the pericardium has been more frequently recognized after prolonged use of this drug.

Metabolic Disorders. Uremia and myxedema may provoke pericardial reactions. It has been long recognized that pericarditis, frequently with hemorrhagic pericardial effusions, may occur in the terminal phase of uremia; but before the advent of life-prolonging dialysis programs the incidence of this complication was relatively low. As many as 15 per cent of patients on dialysis programs may develop pericarditis, often with effusion. The etiology of uremic pericarditis is not well understood. It may develop in patients well controlled with dialysis, but more frequent dialysis may lead to a remission in the pericarditis and pericardial effusion.

Cardiomegaly is not uncommon in hypothyroidism. In almost all cases the increase in cardiac silhouette is due primarily to pericardial effusion. Effusions usually develop slowly and may become quite large with a minimum of symptoms. Hemodynamic embarrassment is rare. The condition responds promptly to thyroid replacement therapy.

Physical or Chemical Agents. The recent popularization of high dose radiation therapy for lymphomatous disease in the mediastinum has disclosed that the pericardium is more susceptible to radiation injury than had previously been thought. Acute pericarditis, pericardial effusion, and constriction have all been reported to follow high dose radiation to the mediastinum. This entity now is recognized as an uncommon but definite complication of radiation therapy, and congestive heart failure may result from either pericardial effusion or constriction, even as a late complication of therapy.

CLINICAL MANIFESTATIONS. The hallmark of acute pericarditis is the development of substernal chest pain, which is usually sharp and knife-like but may be a dull or oppressive sensation. The pain frequently is referred or radiates to other areas of the chest, particularly the left supraclavicular region. It may also be referred to the neck and shoulders, which may lead to an initial false impression that the symptom is primarily musculoskeletal in origin rather than due to acute pericarditis. Deep inspiration, rotation of the trunk, and coughing usually will precipitate the pain. Many patients find that it is accentuated and virtually intolerable when they lie on the back or the left side, but the pain can be partially alleviated by sitting up and leaning forward. Fever usually accompanies or initiates the pain and is often associated with other systemic symptoms, such as malaise, fatigue, and myalgias.

A characteristic physical finding in acute pericarditis is a pericardial friction rub. This leathery or scratchy sound may be heard over any portion of the anterior precordium, but it is most frequently heard low along the left sternal border. It may consist of one, two, or three components, presumably depending upon the extent of inflammatory involvement of the pericardium. When there is only a single component to the rub, it is usually confined to systole and may mimic a systolic cardiac murmur. Changes in the intensity and quality of the isolated systolic rub produced by variations in respiration and positions during auscultation will help differentiate a rub from a cardiac murmur. More commonly the pericardial rub has two or three components. When two components are heard, they occur during systole and diastole and are due to the rubbing of the inflamed epicardial surface against the parietal pericardial surface during systole and diastole. The presence of a third component to the rub, which is common, will eliminate any confusion as to whether the rub is due to an intracardiac murmur or pericardial inflammation. The third component is due to atrial contraction and occurs in the presystolic phase of the cardiac cycle. Frequently a rub may have a variable number of components, depending upon the position in which the patient is examined. Acute pericarditis is often accompanied by cardiac arrhythmias, which may be intermittent. However, arrhythmias are uncommon in uncomplicated idiopathic or viral pericarditis. They are usually evidence of the presence of another underlying process, such as myocardial infarction, collagen disease, or bacterial infection. The vast majority of arrhythmias are supraventricular arrhythmias, including frequent premature atrial contractions, paroxysmal atrial tachycardia, fibrillation, and flutter. This has been attributed to irritation and involvement of the sinus node, which lies close to the epicardial surface of the heart.

LABORATORY FINDINGS. Acute pericarditis is usually accompanied by a leukocytosis and an elevation in sedimentation rate, but these are by no means invariable. Chest x-ray may show a slight increase in cardiac size owing to either inflammatory thickening of the pericardium or a small pericardial effusion. In addition, there may be evidence of pleural involvement characterized by small pleural effusions. Pulmonary infiltrates also are common. The electrocardiogram usually shows a typical pattern of S-T segment elevation without changes in the QRS morphology. The S-T segment elevation may last for weeks at a time, and frequently the elevation will show evolutionary changes with T wave inversion several days to weeks after the onset of the S-T segment changes. These electrocardiographic changes may be isolated to only several leads and are due to involvement of the subepicardial myocardium rather than involvement of the pericardium itself, since the pericardium is electrically silent. Serum levels of enzymes such as glutamic-oxaloacetic transaminase (SGOT) and lactic dehydrogenase (LDH) may be moderately elevated because there is inflammatory involvement of the subepicardial portion of the myocardium. Cardiac isoenzyme changes, including the presence of CPK-MB and LDH-1 greater than LDH-2 configurations, are less frequent but have been noted. The echocardiogram may show thickening of the pericardium and will often show a variable amount of pericardial effusion, as there is an almost inevitable increase in fluid in the pericardial space above the 25 to 35 ml normally present in the cavity.

DIFFERENTIAL DIAGNOSIS. When acute pericarditis presents in a young patient with sudden onset of sharp or grating substernal pain accentuated by changes in position and partially relieved by sitting up, plus a characteristic multicomponent rub and S-T segment elevation, the diagnosis is relatively simple. However, frequently the condition does not present in such a classic fashion. In such cases it is necessary to entertain other diagnoses, including acute myocardial infarction, pleurisy with or without pneumonia, pulmonary embolization, dissection of the aorta, pneumothorax, mediastinal emphysema, or an abdominal source for the complaint. Examination of serial electrocardiograms and serum cardiac isoenzyme levels will usually establish whether the primary process is due to myocardial infarction or pericarditis alone. The rub accompanying pleurisy which may raise the possibility of pericarditis is clearly related to and accentuated by the respiratory cycle and is usually heard diffusely over the chest or frequently in the lateral portions of the chest rather than in the precordial area. Pulmonary embolization may mimic pericarditis; but when further studies, such as serial chest x-rays, lung scans, and, if necessary, pulmonary arteriograms, are obtained, the differentiation becomes clear. Dissecting aortic aneurysm may simulate pericarditis and on occasion may actually be a cause for pericarditis owing to rupture of the base of the aorta, with a leak of blood into the pericardium which provokes a pericardial inflammatory reaction. However, the pain of dissection is usually more severe and unremitting than that of pericarditis and is usually noted in the intrascapular area, which is uncommon in pericarditis. Pneumothorax can be differentiated from pericarditis by physical examination, which indicates absent breath sounds on the affected side if it is a large pneumothorax and by chest x-ray if it is not discernible by physical examination. Intra-abdominal events may produce pain that suggests acute pericarditis. Acute cholecystitis with referral of pain to the supraclavicular area must be considered. Pancreatitis and splenic infarction can also produce a confusing picture suggestive of pericarditis. When there is inflammatory involvement of the diaphragm, the pain may be referred to the left supraclavicular area, a favorite site for the referral of the pain of acute pericarditis, and there may be an associated small pleural effusion as well as nonspecific T wave changes.

PERICARDIAL EFFUSION

PATHOPHYSIOLOGY. Pericardial effusion, the accumulation of serous or serosanguineous fluid in excess of the normal 25 to 35 ml of lymphatic fluid in the pericardial space, may present in either acute or chronic form. It may be the first sign of acute pericarditis, and its severe hemodynamic consequences may actually obscure the classic signs of the underlying pericarditis. Although chronic pericardial effusion may be accompanied by a pericardial rub, the insidious development of this condition without other evidence of pericardial involvement may simulate progressive heart failure and, unless readily recognized, may lead to death, even though it is an easily treatable condition. An understanding of the pathophysiology of pericardial effusion and tamponade makes the physical findings of this disorder more obvious and understandable. The circulatory effects of pericardial effusion and tamponade are directly related to the rate at which the effusion develops. The sudden development of a pericardial effusion of several hundred milliliters of fluid may provoke profound hemodynamic changes, whereas the more gradual development of pericardial effusion may be almost asymptomatic despite accumulations of several liters of fluid. The primary cause for the clinical and hemodynamic signs of pericardial effusion and tamponade is the accumulation of fluid in the pericardium sufficient to prevent adequate filling of the cardiac chambers. Since venous inflow to the heart is markedly decreased, there is accumulation of blood in the venous system that is reflected in marked jugular venous distention and hepatic engorgement. If the process is chronic, there is usually peripheral edema as well. Jugular venous distention is usually unchanged or decreased by deep inspiration. The striking increase in jugular venous distention with inspiration (Kussmaul's sign), which is frequently seen in constrictive pericarditis, is rarely seen in pericardial effusion because the expected increase in venous inflow into the right heart during inspiration is still preserved.

CARDIAC TAMPONADE. The most severe complication of a pericardial effusion, no matter what its cause, is the development of cardiac tamponade. Cardiac tamponade is a classic example of the vicious circle process in medicine. Accumulation of fluid in the relatively nondistensible pericardium initially limits cardiac filling and therefore cardiac output. As cardiac output declines, arterial pressure and coronary artery filling decrease. Coronary flow and thus myocardial function are further compromised by tachycardia and external pressure on the superficially lying coronary arteries. Eventually this decline in cardiac filling, decrease in cardiac output, fall in arterial and coronary artery filling pressure, and decreased coronary flow lead to severe myocardial ischemia, which initiates an even greater decline in myocardial function. Unless this cycle of events is contravened by elimination of the effusion, a fatal outcome is certain.

CLINICAL MANIFESTATIONS. Dyspnea, tachycardia, distended jugular veins, cyanosis, varying degrees of consciousness, and a rapid, thready pulse with a frequently palpable decrease in the force of the peripheral pulse during inspiration warn of the presence of pericardial effusion. Examination of the lung fields may elicit Ewart's or Pins' sign, characterized by increased dullness, increased fremitis, and bronchial breath sounds at the base of the lung below the angle of the left scapula. These findings are believed to be due to compression of the lower lobe of the left lung by the distended pericardial sac. In large pericardial effusions percussion over the lower half of the sternum will reveal dullness caused by the underlying fluid in the pericardial sac, whereas under normal circumstances percussion over this region produces a resonant note. This sign may be obscured when there is obvious deformity of the anterior chest wall or emphysema, and it may be falsely present when there is marked obesity or right ventricular hypertrophy. Examination of the heart may reveal a quiet precordium with no palpable cardiac activity, but this is by no means the rule, and frequently significant pericardial effusions may be present with quite a distinct cardiac apex impulse. On auscultation the heart sounds may be normal or muffled, and there is often a pericardial rub even though the effusion may be a chronic one.

A characteristic of a pericardial effusion is the presence of an abnormal paradoxical pulse. The paradoxical pulse is actually an exaggeration of a normal physiologic response. It is detected by determining the systolic blood pressure during inspiration and expiration. During normal inspiration the capacity of the lung to accept blood volume is increased, and there is a decrease in venous return as well as filling pressure in the left heart. Thus, left ventricular stroke volume falls, as does systolic blood pressure. During tamponade left ventricular filling may be further compromised by displacement of the ventricular septum posteriorly, resulting from excessive filling of the right ventricle during inspiration while right-sided filling pressures are elevated. The normal variation in systolic blood pressure between inspiration and expiration is in the range of 8 to 10 mm Hg. In the case of a pericardial effusion the systolic pressure may decline during inspiration to a point at which it is undetectable. In severe cases of pericardial effusion, this can be observed by simply palpating the peripheral pulse and noting a decrease in volume or complete absence of the pulse during inspiration. This is also a frequent accompaniment of chronic obstructive lung disease and cannot be used as a pathognomonic sign of pericardial effusion alone.

LABORATORY FINDINGS. The electrocardiogram may appear entirely normal, show generalized low voltage, reveal S-T segment elevation with or without T wave inversion, or demonstrate complete electrical alternans, which is characterized by a decrease in the size of the P, QRS, and T waves with alternate beats. Chest x-ray may show a normal-sized heart if the pericardial effusion is acute; but even in this situation, if previous chest x-rays are available, it will be apparent that there has been an increase in cardiac silhouette size.

In less acute situations the cardiac shadow may slowly enlarge and assume a pear shape. The normal contour of the left heart border may become straightened, and there may be a convex bulging of the right cardiophrenic junction. Signs of pulmonary congestion are variable. Cardiac fluoroscopy is suggestive but not definitive for the diagnosis if there is markedly decreased or no discernible cardiac pulsation and the epicardial fat line lies significantly inside the border of the presumed cardiac shadow. Further radiographic evidence of a pericardial effusion can be sought by placing a catheter in the right atrium and noting that the catheter tip cannot be passed to the lateral border of the cardiac shadow, indicating that there is either a significant effusion or pericardial thickening. This can be further confirmed by injection of contrast media, which will outline the chamber size in relation to the total cardiac shadow. Since the development of echocardiography these invasive catheterization techniques are seldom warranted, because even small pericardial effusions can be detected with a high degree of accuracy with the echocardiogram. However, in rare cases in which the pericardial effusion is loculated, particularly in the space anterior to the heart, angiographic studies may be necessary.

TREATMENT: PERICARDIOCENTESIS. The ultimate proof of the diagnosis of pericardial effusion and also an often mandatory procedure to provide relief from cardiac tamponade is pericardiocentesis. This is accomplished by inserting a medium-sized needle high in the epigastrium in the angle formed between the left border of the xiphoid process and the lower left rib cage. After suitable local anesthesia, the exploring metal needle is connected by an insulated wire to the V lead electrode of the ECG. The needle is slowly advanced upward and slightly posterior in a line toward the medial third of the right clavicle. While the needle is being advanced, the electrocardiogram should be continuously monitored. Contact with the epicardium will be signaled by the development of marked S-T segment elevation on the ECG record. This procedure not only helps prevent puncture of the heart but also provides confidence that one has not perforated the heart if a frankly bloody pericardial effusion is encountered. In acute cases of tamponade such as can occur with aortic dissection or cardiac trauma, it may be impossible to ascertain whether one is draining the pericardial space or actually removing blood directly from a cardiac chamber. This quandary can usually be eliminated by making certain that there has been no evidence of a current of injury on the recorded V lead of the ECG. Once fluid is obtained by aspiration, it should be examined microscopically for the number and type of cells present and the presence of bacteria. The fluid should also undergo cytologic examination, be submitted for bacterial and tuberculous culture, and be analyzed for sugar and protein content, as well as LDH enzyme and rheumatoid factor if clinically indicated.

PERICARDIAL CONSTRICTION

PATHOPHYSIOLOGY. Constrictive pericarditis may be the last step in the process initiated by acute pericarditis and followed by a pericardial effusion. However, in many cases it develops insidiously without any previous evidence of pericardial disease, and its first manifestations are those suggestive of heart failure. The pericardium can become thickened, fibrosed, and eventually calcified in a remarkably short time. There are well-documented cases of this whole process occurring in less than six months after the onset of bacterial or tuberculous disease involving the pericardium. The fundamental anatomic derangement that leads to the ultimate symptomatology of constrictive pericarditis is obstruction or constriction of either the cardiac chambers or the orifices of the great veins entering the heart. The constrictive process can be localized to isolated chambers of the heart and even small areas of the pericardium surrounding these chambers. Cases of localized constriction in the region of the outflow tract of the right ventricle have simulated subpulmonic stenosis. Isolated adhesions and constriction of the posterior portion of the epicardium have led to severe left ventricular dysfunction. The fundamental pathophysiologic process is one of inexorable decrease in cardiac filling, with consequent venous pooling in the periphery and decline in cardiac output. The process may be so slow that the onset of new symptoms is almost unrecognized by the patient and his physician. If the constriction is prolonged and generalized enough, there may be necrosis of myocardial tissue, and even eventual relief of the constriction will not eliminate symptoms of heart failure because of residual myocardial damage.

Pericardial effusion and constriction may coexist, leading to the term "subacute effusive-constrictive pericarditis." If pericardiocentesis with removal of adequate amounts of fluid fails to correct the signs of cardiac compression, the possibility of an underlying process of fibrotic constriction in addition to effusion must be considered. Computerized tomographic imaging of the heart may demonstrate the thickened constricting pericardium as well as the effusion. This is an indication for thoracotomy and pericardial stripping.

CLINICAL MANIFESTATIONS. The classic clinical picture of constrictive pericarditis is an emaciated patient with obvious venous distention in the neck, a potbellied appearance caused by ascites, and spindly, wasted, and often edematous extremities. The patient may be overtly dyspneic at rest or may complain only of dyspnea on exertion. Careful examination of the neck veins will demonstrate a prominent "Y" descent which corresponds with sudden brief right ventricular filling. Examination of the heart may reveal a quiet precordium with no palpable apical impulse, although this is by no means the rule. The heart sounds may be muffled, and frequently there is a prominent third heart sound occurring 0.09 to 0.12 second after the aortic closure sound. This so-called "pericardial knock" can easily be confused with the S_3 gallop associated with congestive heart failure. Atrial fibrillation is frequently encountered in the late stages of the disease. Hemodynamic deterioration of a patient with rapid atrial fibrillation who has been given digitalis on the presumption that he has congestive heart failure should alert the clinician to the possibility of constrictive pericarditis. Administration of digitalis to the patient with rapid atrial fibrillation and heart failure should relieve signs of failure. However, the patient with constrictive pericarditis may be dependent for an effective cardiac output on a relatively rapid ventricular rate. When this ventricular rate is lowered by digitalis in a patient with atrial fibrillation and constriction, the patient is unable to increase ventricular filling and generate a greater stroke volume to maintain a normal cardiac output. Thus, hemodynamic deterioration rather than improvement ensues.

LABORATORY FINDINGS. The electrocardiogram is almost invariably abnormal, with a decrease in QRS voltage, nonspecific S-T and T wave changes, and an irregular contour to the P waves. Chest x-ray will usually show a heart of smaller than expected or even normal size despite the evidence of severe hemodynamic derangement. However, this is not invariable, and the diagnosis should not be discarded if the cardiac size is large, because much of this enlargement may be due to a markedly thickened pericardium. A characteristic of pericardial constriction is the presence of calcium in the pericardium, but this may not be seen on the standard chest x-ray because of technical factors. Thus if it is suspected, overpenetrated x-rays of the heart in different views should be obtained. Careful fluoroscopy with image intensification will demonstrate calcification in over 75 per cent of cases of constrictive pericarditis. Echocardiography may play an important role in alerting the unsuspecting clinician that he is dealing with constrictive pericarditis rather than advanced heart failure. An echocardiogram that demonstrates a thickened pericardium, small ventricular chamber size, and increased atrial chamber size should raise the possibility of constrictive pericarditis. Cardiac catheterization provides a series of typical findings, but they are not absolutely diagnostic of constrictive pericarditis. The right atrial pressure may be seen to rise with inspiration, which is analogous to Kussmaul's sign seen in the jugular veins; the right atrial pressure tracing shows a typical "M or W" shape; and the right ventricular pressure demonstrates a so-called early diastolic dip and a late diastolic shoulder. The early diastolic dip conforms to the early rapid filling of the ventricle and is coincident with the sharp "Y" descent seen in the jugular venous pulse. There is a generalized equalization of all end-diastolic pressures in the chambers of the heart as well as in the pulmonary artery. Although these findings are typical, exactly the same findings can be observed in patients with cardiomyopathies, and thus their presence or absence should not be the sole determining factor as to whether or not a patient should undergo an exploratory thoracotomy. In occasional patients with subclinical constriction, these hemodynamic findings become evident only after the patient has received a rapid infusion of saline.

Angiography is frequently helpful in demonstrating that the cardiac chamber is markedly smaller than might be surmised from the total cardiac contour. Furthermore, an unusual downward tugging of the bifurcation of the opacified main pulmonary artery during systole has been noted and is presumably due to the flexible uninvolved pulmonary artery actually being tugged back toward the heart by the contracting ventricles that are encased in an immobile pericardial sac. Results of liver function studies are almost invariably abnormal, and there may be hypoalbuminemia on the basis of both hepatic disease and a protein-losing enteropathy.

TREATMENT. The definitive treatment for constrictive pericarditis is a pericardiectomy. If delayed too long, the constrictive process may be so advanced that adequate stripping, particularly of the epicardial portion of the pericardium, cannot be accomplished, or there may have been such advanced degeneration of myocardial muscle that postoperative results are less than satisfactory. Isolated epicardial constriction may not be apparent until the epicardium is actually dissected away from the myocardium itself. Constrictive epicarditis has become a more frequent entity as a complication of aorto–coronary artery bypass graft surgery. The development of signs of constriction after such surgery should alert the clinician to this possibility. The prognosis for recovery from constrictive pericarditis is a function of the age of the patient, the severity of the fibrotic process, and the degree to which the patient's general medical condition has deteriorated before the pericardiectomy is performed. With the lowering of the operative mortality for pericardiectomy to less than 5 per cent, particularly if done early, there is a general tendency now to operate at the first suggestion of constriction, particularly if the patient is known to have had a bacterial or tuberculous pericardial infection in the past.

NEOPLASTIC DISEASES

The pericardium may be the site of primary or metastatic tumors. Primary tumors are rare and may be generally classified into mesotheliomas, which encompass tumors that have previously been classified as fibromas and sarcomas, vascular tumors such as hemangiomas and lymphangiomas, pericardial cysts, lipomas, and tumors of heterotopic tissue such as bronchial cysts, teratomas, and dermoids. The pericardium is not a rare location for metastatic tumors. Metastatic tumors from the lung in men and the breast in women are the most common types encountered. Lymphomatous disease, particularly Hodgkin's disease, also may involve the pericardium. Occasionally involvement of the pericardium and its attendant restriction, either by tumor mass or effusion, may be the first sign of a malignancy. Pericardial effusion, which is often bloody, can be found with even small-sized tumors and a small number of metastases.

CONGENITAL LESIONS OF THE PERICARDIUM

Congenital true pericardial cysts may be celomic, lymphangiomatous, bronchial, or teratomatous. These seldom produce significant clinical symptoms and usually come to light when a routine chest x-ray is obtained. The major problem they present is that of differentiation from a mediastinal tumor. They may gradually increase in size and necessitate an exploratory thoracotomy to rule out malignant disease. In addition to true congenital pericardial cysts, a diverticulum of the pericardium may occur. The diverticulum appears as a sharply outlined semicircular or oval area protruding from the cardiac silhouette, usually in the region of the right lower portion of the cardiac shadow. Such diverticula cannot be differentiated from a pericardial cyst without exploratory thoracotomy.

There may be a congenital complete or, less frequently, partial absence of the pericardium. When the defect is a partial one, it occurs on the left side of the pericardium in two thirds of the cases and is seen most frequently in males. The defect should be suspected when the left atrial appendage appears disproportionately prominent on chest x-ray. The diagnosis can be confirmed by inducing a pneumothorax which demonstrates a pneumopericardium in addition to the pneumothorax.

DISEASES OF DIVERSE UNKNOWN CAUSE

In addition to the conditions discussed previously, the pericardium may be the site of involvement in a variety of other diseases. *Familial Mediterranean fever,* which involves various serous membranes, may also involve the pericardium. Although *sarcoidosis* more frequently involves the myocardium, granulomas can be found in the pericardium. *Hydropericardium,* which is an excessive accumulation of transudate in the pericardial cavity, may occur in conjunction with advanced cardiac or renal failure, as well as in association with inflammatory or malignant diseases which may obstruct lymphatic drainage from the pericardium. A *chylous pericardial effusion* may develop following traumatic rupture or obstruction of the thoracic duct by a primary or metastatic malignancy. The pericardial fluid is milky white or brownish yellow, contains fat globules which can be visualized under the light microscope, and has markedly elevated triglyceride levels. *Cholesterol pericarditis,* which is characterized by an elevated level of cholesterol in the pericardial effusion and frequently by the appearance of a shiny or scintillating gold paint quality to the effusion, has been thought in the past to be a separate clinical entity. However, cholesterol pericarditis has been associated with a variety of disease states. Approximately one fourth of the cases reported have been associated with hypothyroidism. It is now thought that it is a manifestation of prolonged pericardial effusion with impairment of absorption of cholesterol from the chronically inflamed or scarred pericardium. There is subsequent gradual accumulation of large amounts of cholesterol crystals which give the effusion its unique appearance.

Bush CA, Stang JM, Wooley CF, Kilman JW: Occult constrictive pericardial disease: Diagnosis by rapid volume expansion and correction by pericardiectomy. Circulation 56:924, 1977. *The authors describe 19 patients with symptoms suggestive of constrictive pericardial disease but normal resting hemodynamics at cardiac catheterization. One liter of intravenous normal saline given over a six- to eight-minute period produced the typical hemodynamic signs of constriction. Eleven of the patients underwent pericardiectomy when the diagnosis was confirmed and have had clinical improvement.*

Cortes FM: The Pericardium and Its Disorders. Springfield, Ill., Charles C Thomas, 1970. *This is an excellent monograph describing the various conditions which affect the pericardium.*

Dressler W: The postmyocardial infarction syndrome. A report on forty-four cases. Arch Intern Med 103:28, 1959. *In this article the author summarizes his experience in 44 cases of pericarditis following a myocardial infarction. He emphasizes the difference in this syndrome from the acute pericarditis of myocardial infarction and estimates that the syndrome occurs in from 3 to 4 per cent of all myocardial infarctions.*

Feigenbaum H: Pericardial disease. *In* Echocardiography. Philadelphia, Lea & Febiger, 1981, p 478. *In this standard textbook the author outlines the signs of pericardial disease, particularly emphasizing the echocardiographic features of pericardial effusion.*

Hancock EW: Subacute effusive-constrictive pericarditis. Circulation 43:183, 1971. *The author describes 13 patients in whom relief of pericardial effusion did not eliminate the symptoms of cardiac compression. Four of the 13 patients progressed from a stage of effusion plus constriction to a noneffusive constrictive pericarditis.*

Koontz CH, Ray CG: The role of coxsackie Group B virus infection in sporadic myopericarditis. Am Heart J 82:750, 1971. *The author reports on 45 patients with myopericarditis who underwent examination for neutralizing antibody titers to coxsackievirus B in acute and convalescent serum after the illness. Twenty of the 45 patients had significant antibody titers to coxsackievirus B antigens.*

Reedy P, Leon D, Shaver J: Pericardial Disease. New York, Raven Press, 1982. *In addition to an excellent exposition of the histology of the pericardium, this book contains the most up-to-date experimental and clinical studies concerning the physiology and pathophysiology of the normal pericardium, pericardial tamponade, and constriction.*

53. DISEASES OF THE AORTA

Noble O. Fowler

The aorta begins just superior to the aortic valve and ends at its bifurcation opposite the fourth lumbar vertebra. A pathologic process which involves both the aorta and its branches may obstruct these branches and thereby call attention to aortic disease. For example, obstruction of a coronary artery at its origin by aortic intimal disease may produce the pain of myocardial ischemia (angina pectoris). Takayasu's arteritis and syphilitic aortitis may represent examples of this mechanism.

Aortic arch disease can lead to the *aortic arch syndrome.* In this syndrome (see below), obstruction of the orifice of the innominate or left common carotid artery can cause symptoms of cerebral ischemia or visual disturbance. Narrowing of the orifice of the innominate artery or left subclavian artery may cause ischemia of the upper extremities or syncope because of the "subclavian steal" syndrome. Thus patients with aortic atherosclerosis or Takayasu's arteritis may have attacks of syncope, transient pain, or transient monocular blindness with use of that arm with impaired blood supply. Occlusion of the mesenteric arteries may lead to bowel ischemia with postprandial abdominal angina, or even to infarction of the bowel. Occlusion of a renal artery may lead to systemic hypertension through the Goldblatt mechanism: increased renin production by the affected kidney activates an alpha$_2$ globulin in plasma to angiotensin. Obstructive disease of the aorta may lead to absence or diminution of pulse in the carotid arteries, the subclavian and brachial arteries, or the femoral arteries. Extensive aortic intimal atherosclerosis may lead to cholesterol emboli or atheroembolism, which may cause transient cerebral ischemic attacks (TIA), renal insufficiency, pancreatitis, or cyanosis of one or more toes. Cholesterol emboli to the retinal arteries may be visualized by ophthalmoscopy.

Aortic disease may come to attention in other ways. When the aortic lumen is narrowed by disease, murmurs may be produced. Supravalvular aortic stenosis, aortic coarctation, and dissecting hematoma of the aorta each may produce a systolic murmur which is loudest downstream from the site of narrowing. On the other hand, when the aortic lumen is enlarged by aneurysm formation, the aneurysm may be appreciated by physical examination of the abdomen or chest; but more often it is detected because it produces pain, because it compresses other vital structures, or because it begins to leak, thereby causing bleeding and shock.

Many times aortic disease is discovered or evaluated more precisely by roentgenograms. Much of the thoracic aorta can be studied by roentgenograms of the chest without the use of contrast media. Although the sinuses of Valsalva are usually lost within the cardiac shadow, when the walls of an aneurysm are calcified, it may be possible to identify the aneurysm precisely by plain radiograms, even though it is in the aortic sinuses. Both the thoracic aorta and the abdominal aorta are better evaluated by contrast media. Newer noninvasive methods of studying the aorta include echocardiography, computed tomography, and intravenous digital subtraction angiography. At present only the ascending thoracic aorta and the abdominal aorta can be studied accurately by echocardiography. In adults the remainder of the thoracic aorta lies too deep within the chest for good echocardiographic evaluation. CT scanning with intravenous contrast medium enhancement is often used in place of invasive aortography when aortic aneurysm or other disease of the aorta is suspected. Intravenous digital subtraction angiography may also be of value.

CONGENITAL DISEASES OF THE AORTA

Congenital diseases of the aorta are not rare in children. They are rather uncommon problems in adult life and only a few will be considered here (see Ch. 44).

COARCTATION OF THE ABDOMINAL AORTA. In addition to coarctation of the aorta at the usual site just distal to the left subclavian artery, coarctation may occur in the abdominal aorta. This lesion may be congenital, or it may be associated with Takayasu's syndrome (see p. 352). Coarctation of the abdominal aorta may involve the celiac axis or the mesenteric arteries. There may be associated hypertension because of the renal arterial involvement. Abdominal aortic coarctation is more common in women, whereas thoracic aortic coarctation is more common in men.

CONGENITAL AORTIC ANEURYSM. Congenital aortic aneurysms of the sinus of Valsalva involve either the right or noncoronary sinus in 90 per cent of instances. Those of the right aortic sinus usually project into the right ventricle, and those of the noncoronary sinus, into the right atrium. Aortic sinus aneurysms are difficult to see on plain roentgenogram of the chest unless they are calcified. They are recognizable, however, by echocardiography and by aortography. These aneurysms tend to rupture eventually, usually into the right atrium or ventricle where they produce a continuous shunt. The continuous shunt is associated with a continuous systolic and diastolic murmur, widening of the systemic arterial pulse pressure, and a tendency to heart failure. These conditions may be corrected surgically. The murmur of an aortic sinus aneurysm which has ruptured into the right heart resembles that of a patent ductus arteriosus except that it tends to be louder in the fourth and fifth left intercostal spaces near the sternum. The systemic arterial pulse pressure tends to be increased. It is said that these congenital aortic sinus aneurysms tend to rupture into the heart, whereas acquired syphilitic aneurysms in the same location tend to rupture into the pericardial sac. A similar condition is that of aortico–left ventricular tunnel, in which there is a long tubular communication between the aortic sinus and the left ventricle. The unperforated aortic sinus aneurysm is usually asymptomatic but may cause cardiac conduction disturbances, myocardial ischemia due to coronary occlusion, or pulmonary stenosis or tricuspid insufficiency (Bulkley et al.).

Another congenital condition is that of aberrant right subclavian artery. It is said to occur in one of 200 individuals. In this condition the right subclavian artery is the last major branch of the aortic arch, rather than arising from the innominate artery as it does normally. It then passes behind the esophagus to reach the right arm. As a result the blood pressure may be lower in the right arm than in the left; the pulse may be absent in the right upper extremity. Dysphagia may result from pressure of the aberrant artery on the esophagus. Barium esophagram shows an oblique compression of the posterior esophagus by the aberrant artery. Aortography shows the condition more clearly. Rarely the aberrant right subclavian artery may be associated with coarctation of the aorta proximal to the left subclavian artery; then arterial pulses tend to be feeble or absent in both upper and lower extremities.

Bulkley BH, Hutchins GM, Ross RS: Aortic sinus of Valsalva aneurysms simulating primary right-sided valvular disease. Circulation 52:696, 1975. *A report of pathologic study of five patients with aortic sinus of Valsalva aneurysm. The aneurysm produced tricuspid incompetence in two patients and right ventricular outflow tract obstruction in three.*

HEREDOFAMILIAL DISEASES OF THE AORTA

A number of heredofamilial disorders of connective tissue may be associated with diseases of the aorta and its branches (McKusick). These conditions most commonly cause weakening of the aortic wall and aneurysms, but at times there is occlusive aortic disease owing to thrombosis.

MARFAN'S SYNDROME. Marfan's syndrome (arachnodactyly) is a heredofamilial disorder of connective tissue which affects the blood vessels, the osseous skeleton, and the ligaments (see Ch. 199). The principal cardiovascular manifestations are in the ascending aorta. The aortic lesion is cystic medial necrosis. The second most common cardiovascular abnormality involves the mitral valve. Occasionally, the tricuspid valve or the pulmonary artery is affected. Smaller arteries are usually not involved. The aortic lesion characteristically produces either sinus of Valsalva aneurysm or aneurysm in the ascending aorta above the sinuses. Its principal complications are dissecting aneurysm of the aorta, rupture of the aorta, and aortic insufficiency. Abdominal aortic aneurysm is rare. Mitral prolapse and mitral insufficiency may occur.

EHLERS-DANLOS SYNDROME (CUTIS HYPERELASTICA). Dissecting aortic aneurysm is a recognized complication. Spontaneous rupture of the aorta or aortic rupture following slight trauma may occur (see Ch. 200).

HOMOCYSTINURIA. Homocystinuria has some features in common with Marfan's syndrome (see Ch. 199). Ectopia lentis and disease of the aorta may occur in either condition. In homocystinuria more commonly there is occlusive disease of systemic arteries and veins. The coronary arteries may be occluded. Thrombosis of the terminal aorta may occur. The elastic pattern of the aortic media is abnormal. It is uncertain whether aortic aneurysm is an essential part of this disease.

OSTEOGENESIS IMPERFECTA. With osteogenesis imperfecta, deafness, fragilitas ossium, and blue sclerae are common (see Ch. 201). A dilated aortic root and aortic insufficiency are also common. Mitral insufficiency is also a frequent cardiovascular manifestation.

MUCOPOLYSACCHARIDOSES. In these disorders, including Hurler's syndrome, Hunter's syndrome, and others, there may be ballooned storage cells in the aorta. The principal involvement is of the aortic valve and coronary arteries. Aortic dilation and the aortic arch syndrome (see Ch. 198) have been described.

PSEUDOXANTHOMA ELASTICUM. Thrombosis of the terminal aorta has been described, but its relationship to pseudoxanthoma elasticum is uncertain. Thrombotic occlusion involving coronary arteries and those of the extremities is a recognized complication. The iliac and femoral arteries may be smaller than normal. Thus impaired pulsations in the lower extremities may cause confusion with coarctation of the aorta (see Ch. 202).

McKusick VA: Heritable Disorders of Connective Tissue. 4th ed. St. Louis, C. V. Mosby Company, 1972. *This is an 878-page book, presented in 15 chapters, on the major varieties of heritable connective tissue disease, written by an outstanding authority. Emphasis is placed upon the cardiovascular aspects of these diseases and their natural history. There are extensive references.*

EFFECTS OF AGING UPON THE AORTA

Arteriosclerosis affects the aorta more commonly in "advanced" than in primitive societies. The process tends to be progressively more severe as one proceeds down the descending aorta, unlike syphilitic aortitis, which is more pronounced in the ascending aorta just superior to the aortic valve. Arteriosclerosis may cause elongation or dilation of the aorta, producing an irregularity observed on chest radiogram. Commonly, in older patients one sees a calcific deposit in the aortic knob (arch). Roentgen evidence of aortic atherosclerosis includes calcification of the knob, increase in the width of the aorta, and unusual tortuosity or uncoiling. These changes are not seen in normal persons under the age of 30 years and in only 2.5 per cent of individuals under the age of 40 years (Felson). Extensive aortic intimal atherosclerosis may lead to ulcerative lesions with cholesterol deposits and to emboli. These emboli may consist of cholesterol or may arise from thrombi. Emboli in the renal arteries may cause hypertension; peripheral emboli may cause impairment of femoral blood flow. Cholesterol emboli arising from the ascending aorta or aortic arch may cause retinal ischemia and myocardial or cerebral infarction. Arteriosclerotic aortic aneurysms are most common in the abdominal aorta just inferior to the renal arteries but may occur also in the thoracic aorta and in the abdominal aorta above the origin of the renal arteries. Aortic arteriosclerosis causes loss of elasticity with decreased compliance during left ventricular ejection. Thus left ventricular work may rise with aging, contributing to a decrease of circulatory reserve with age.

Felson B: Chest Roentgenology. Philadelphia, W. B. Saunders Company, 1973. *This is a 574-page book presented in 15 chapters by one of the nation's leading teachers of clinical radiology. The style is informal and the reading is easy. There are numerous excellent illustrations.*

Smith MC, Ghose MK, Henry AR: The clinical spectrum of renal cholesterol embolization. Am J Med 71:174, 1981. *A brief review of the problem of cholesterol embolism, with 47 references.*

INCREASED AORTIC DIMENSIONS

The aorta may increase in length or diameter or both. Increase in length usually reflects arteriosclerotic changes with aging. Increase in length may cause an irregular margin, apparent widening, kinking, tortuosity, or buckling. Increased diameter of the aorta may be generalized, as in hypertensive disease, or localized. Localized increase of dimension may be called *ectasia* when of minor degree but more commonly is called *aneurysm.* Aneurysms of the aorta may be saccular or fusiform.

Aortic aneurysms are discussed in detail under the headings of the individual causative diseases. However, it is useful to summarize the relation of the location of an aneurysm to its etiology. Aortic aneurysms may be classified by etiology into congenital and acquired groups (DeBakey and Noon). By location, they are classified as follows: (1) ascending aorta, (2) aortic arch, (3) descending thoracic aorta, and (4) thoracoabdominal aorta. Aortic sinus aneurysms are most commonly congenital but may be due to Marfan's syndrome, syphilis, or infective endocarditis. Ascending aortic aneurysms are most commonly due to atherosclerosis, Marfan's syndrome, aortic dissection, or cystic medial necrosis without the other features of Marfan's syndrome. They may also be caused by syphilis, bacterial infection (mycotic), or trauma. Aortic arch aneurysms are most often due to atherosclerosis or dissection. They may be caused by trauma, infection, or syphilis. An aneurysm of the descending thoracic aorta may be caused by syphilis, arteriosclerosis, or dissection (Carlson et al., 1983). An aneurysm at the beginning of the descending aorta may be caused by trauma. Aneurysms of the abdominal aorta are most often caused by arteriosclerosis but may be the result of syphilis or the extension of aortic dissection from the thoracic aorta.

Other diseases may cause aortic aneurysms, which are usually smaller than those enumerated above and in varying sites. Septicemia or tuberculosis may cause mycotic aneurysms. Relapsing polychondritis may be associated with aneurysm of either the thoracic or the abdominal aorta. Localized aortic aneurysms often occur with Takayasu's aortitis and with giant cell aortitis. Rarely, they may occur with Kawasaki disease.

Aortic aneurysms are uncommon in children, but they may be congenital (sinus of Valsalva), traumatic, associated with aortic coarctation or Marfan's syndrome, or mycotic.

ARTERIOSCLEROTIC AORTIC ANEURYSM. Arteriosclerotic aneurysms of the aorta, most common in the abdominal aorta, usually originate below the renal arteries. They are most common in men over the age of 50 years. One study reported an autopsy incidence of 1.8 per cent. Probably more than 95 per cent of abdominal aortic aneurysms are of arteriosclerotic origin. These aneurysms are most often discovered by physical or roentgen examination of an asymptomatic patient. However, they may be discovered when the patient has pain—the pain may be in the back or the epigastrium, or may radiate to the flanks. Unfortunately, the first evidence of aneurysm may be that of rupture attended by severe and persistent pain and shock. Persistent abdominal pain of lesser severity may precede the more severe pain of aortic rupture.

ABDOMINAL AORTIC ANEURYSMS. Abdominal aortic aneurysms may be diagnosed by physical examination. However, in obese or muscular patients or in those with small aneurysms, detection by physical examination is difficult. Abdominal aneurysm may also be diagnosed in error. One must determine that there is actual increase in the width of the aorta and not merely a prominent aortic pulsation, which is common as a normal finding, especially in thin women with lax abdominal walls and lumbar lordosis. This often leads to the diagnosis of aneurysm by physical examination where none exists—"students' aneurysm." A prominent aortic pulsation may be due to an uncoiling of the aorta resulting from atherosclerosis or to aortic insufficiency or to a high output state producing an increased pulse pressure in the absence of aneurysm. Another pitfall in diagnosis is that a tumor overlying the aorta, such as pancreatic neoplasm, may appear to have an intrinsic pulsation and thus be mistaken for an aneurysm. Abdominal aneurysms may lead to ureteral obstruction with hydronephrosis. These aneurysms may also lead to consumption coagulopathy with diminished circulating platelets, reduced serum fibrinogen, and prolonged prothrombin time. Cholesterol emboli to the smaller arteries of the feet and toes, leading to digital cyanosis and coldness, may suggest an aortic arteriosclerotic aneurysm. Rupture into the inferior vena cava may produce an arteriovenous fistula with a loud continuous abdominal murmur.

Diagnosis. Roentgenograms of the abdomen may show calcification in the walls of the aneurysm. It is important to have lateral and oblique views in addition to anteroposterior views. Aortic wall calcification per se does not signify an aneurysm unless there is definite increase in the diameter of the aorta. The psoas shadow may be obliterated when rupture has occurred. Ultrasound scanning and radionuclide angiography may be useful in the diagnosis of abdominal aortic aneurysms. Computed tomography is also of value. Aortography with radiopaque contrast medium or ultrasound scanning is the diagnostic method of choice. Some consider abdominal ultrasound examination to be the current preferred method.

Prognosis. The prognosis of patients with abdominal arteriosclerotic aneurysms is generally poor, with only a small percentage of patients surviving for five years or more. The outlook is better when the lesion is less than 7.5 cm in diameter. However, it is difficult to know the true prognosis. In a review of 24,000 consecutive autopsies at the Massachusetts General Hospital, Darling and colleagues concluded that operative repair should be considered even when aneurysms were as small as 4 cm in diameter. Most patients who are operated upon and most patients who have been followed without operation were originally discovered because they had symptoms. The prognosis might conceivably be more favorable in patients who are asymptomatic. Many unoperated patients had a poor prognosis because operation was considered inadvisable owing to an associated severe illness.

Surgical Treatment. Once the diagnosis of abdominal aortic aneurysm is made, surgical replacement of the aneurysm is generally recommended even though the patient is asymptomatic. If the patient is having pain in relation to the aneurysm, replacement should be considered as an emergency. Surgical removal with insertion of a synthetic aortic graft of woven Dacron is the usual operative procedure. Aortic homografts are no longer used because they tend to rupture at the line of anastomosis. However, late rupture at the suture line may be a problem even with synthetic grafts (Thompson et al.). There are two groups of patients in whom surgical resection might not be recommended. One is composed of those who are asymptomatic with aneurysms under 6 cm in diameter; the other group consists of patients who have some other life-threatening disease or who are very old and debilitated. Among the contraindications to resection are intractable heart failure, advanced renal failure, metastatic neoplasm, unstable angina pectoris or recent cardiac infarction, advanced cerebrovascular disease, and severe pulmonary insufficiency. The reported in-hospital mortality rate of elective abdominal aneurysm resection in several large series is 3.5 to 9.5 per cent. It is greatly increased when there is severe cardiorenal disease or advanced age. A study of 68 late deaths among 176 survivors of operative repair found that acute cardiac infarction caused 23 and cerebrovascular accidents caused 11 (Gardner et al.). The signs, symptoms, and treatment of thoracic aortic aneurysms are discussed below.

Bergan JJ, Yao JST: Modern management of abdominal aortic aneurysms. Surg Clin North Am 54:175, 1974. *A summary of the natural history, surgical indications, techniques, and operative complications of abdominal aortic aneurysms. Seven studies of natural history of unoperated aneurysms and eleven studies of operative results are presented in tabular form.*

Bottsford JE, Beardon RC, Bottsford JG: A ten year community hospital experience with abdominal aortic aneurysms. J So Carolina Med Assoc 79:57, 1983. *A ten-year experience with 116 cases. Sixty-six were operated upon. For elective operations, the mortality rate was 5.6 per cent.*

Carlson DE, Karp RB, Kouchoukos NT: Surgical treatment of aneurysms of the descending aorta. Ann Thorac Surg 35:58, 1983. *In this series of 85 patients, 39 were due to arteriosclerosis, 35 to chronic dissection, and 11 were post-traumatic.*

Darling RC, Messina CR, Brewster DC, et al.: Autopsy study of unoperated abdominal aortic aneurysm: The case for early resection. Circulation 56:Suppl II-161, 1977. *A review of 24,000 consecutive autopsies performed at the Massachusetts General Hospital between 1952 and 1975. Four hundred and seventy-three patients died with unoperated abdominal aortic aneurysm. Rupture of the aneurysm was common even in those between 4 and 7 cm in diameter.*

DeBakey ME, Beall AC, Mattox KL: Surgical treatment of diseases of the aorta and major arteries. *In* Hurst JW, Logue RB, Schlant RC, Wenger NK (eds.): The Heart. Arteries and Veins. 4th ed. New York, McGraw-Hill Book Company, 1978, pp 1917–1934. *This is a textbook chapter of 17 pages, written by one of the nation's most experienced surgical teams in the treatment of vascular disease. Surgical techniques, immediate operative results, and long-term operative results in more than 10,000 patients treated at Baylor University are presented.*

DeBakey ME, Noon GP: Aneurysms of the thoracic aorta. Mod Concepts Cardiovasc Dis 44:53, 1975. *This is a brief summary (6 pages) of the experiences at Baylor University with thoracic aortic aneurysms. Classification, incidence, clinical features, diagnosis, clinical course, treatment, and prognosis are succinctly described.*

Gardner RJ, Gardner NL, Tarnay TJ, et al.: The surgical experience and a one to sixteen year followup of 272 abdominal aortic aneurysms. Am J Surg 135:226, 1978. *This study, from West Virginia University Medical Center, reviews the surgical experience with 277 patients with abdominal aortic aneurysm. One hundred and ninety-three patients had intact aneurysms, and 84 had ruptured aneurysms. The operative mortality was 8.8 per cent for patients with intact aneurysms and 66.7 per cent for those with ruptured aneurysms.*

Thompson WM, Johnsrude IS, Jackson DC, et al.: Late complications of abdominal aortic reconstructive surgery; roentgen evaluation. Ann Surg 185:326, 1977. *This is a review made at Duke University of 636 patients who underwent reconstructive procedures upon the abdominal aorta and/or iliac arteries between 1969 and 1974; 8.5 per cent of patients developed late complications, including occlusion (the most common), stenosis, false aneurysm, enteric fistula, and infection.*

TRAUMATIC AORTIC DISEASE

The aorta may be damaged by nonpenetrating or penetrating trauma. Trauma is most likely to affect that part just beyond the origin of the left subclavian artery (aortic isthmus) (Fig. 53–1). In one series of 284 cases (Finkelmeier et al.), 94 per cent were at the aortic isthmus, 3 per cent just above the aortic valve, and 3 per cent in the aortic arch. When rapid movement of the body is followed by a sudden deceleration, as in a fall or auto accident, differential rates of acceleration are greatest in the isthmus area because the aortic arch is relatively fixed by the root vessels. The aorta may be lacerated or may rupture with either complete or partial transection. Extravasation of blood, tamponaded by the mediastinal structures, may lead to a false aneurysm (pseudoaneurysm). Patients with nonpenetrating aortic trauma may have little or no external evidence of chest injury. Shortly after decelerative-type injury, the patient may be in shock with a rapidly developing hemothorax—most commonly on the left side. Anuria and paraplegia, absence of femoral arterial pulse, and cold, pale lower extremities are common. Arterial hypertension may be present as well. A chest radiogram may show widening of the mediastinum. A possible sequel is chronic traumatic aortic aneurysm, which may rupture days or years after the original injury.The diagnosis is made by aortography; the treatment is surgical removal, usually with a graft replacement.

Finkelmeier BA, Mentzer RM Jr, Kaiser DL, et al.: Chronic traumatic thoracic aneurysm. J Thorac Cardiovasc Surg 84:257, 1982. *A large series of 401 cases of chronic traumatic aortic aneurysm is described. Forty-two per cent of patients developed signs or symptoms of aneurysm expansion within five years of injury. Of 60 not operated upon, 20 died of the aortic lesion. Over 300 patients underwent operative repair with an immediate mortality rate of 4.6 per cent (120 references).*

SYPHILITIC AORTITIS AND SYPHILITIC HEART DISEASE

Syphilitic aortitis is the principal cardiovascular manifestation of syphilis. Syphilis does not ordinarily affect the cardiac valves, although the aortic valve commissures may be separated. Rarely, it may affect the myocardium. It may affect the coronary arteries more often, but usually only the proximal few centimeters of these vessels are involved. Syphilitic aortitis may be complicated by aortic insufficiency, angina pectoris, and aortic aneurysm. Syphilitic aortitis is usually recognized 10 to 30 years after the initial primary chancre, but occasionally only a few years after the original infection. The disease produces aortic medial destruction with necrosis of smooth muscle and elastic tissue and periarterial inflammation with lymphocyte cuffing of the vasa vasorum. There is also intimal wrinkling with

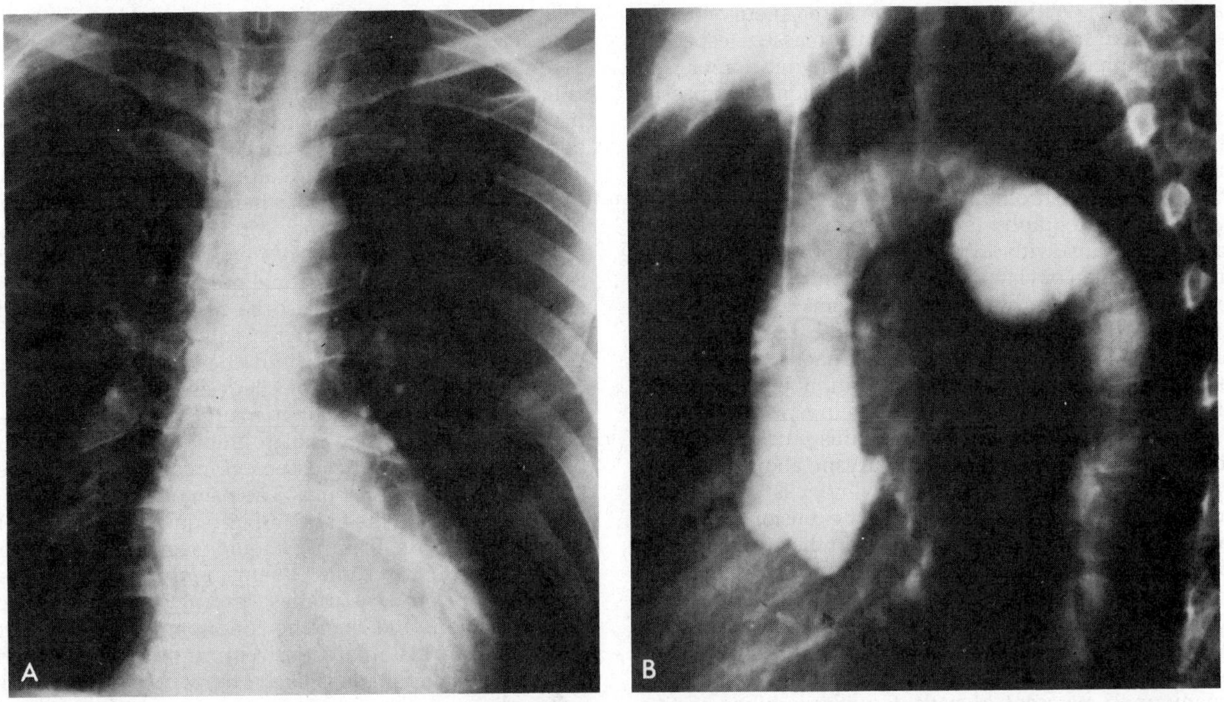

Figure 53–1. Traumatic aortic aneurysm just distal to the subclavian artery. *A,* This posteroanterior roentgenogram demonstrates calcification in the aneurysm, which appears in the region of the aortic knob. *B,* Aortogram demonstrating opacification of the aneurysm, which lies just beyond the subclavian artery. (From Fowler NO: Cardiac Diagnosis and Treatment, 3rd ed., 1980. With permission of Harper & Row, Publishers, Inc.)

treebark formation and a tendency to narrow the orifice of the coronary arteries and to dilate the aortic root. Innominate artery aneurysm may occur, but more distal arterial aneurysms are unusual. The syphilitic process, unlike arteriosclerosis, is usually more intense in the aortic root than in the distal aorta. Congenital syphilis seldom produces aortitis. Because of the delay in clinical manifestations, patients with syphilitic aortitis are ordinarily more than 30 years of age when recognized clinically and are usually over 50 years of age when syphilitic aneurysms are recognized. Uncomplicated syphilitic aortitis ordinarily produces no symptoms and may be recognized only at the autopsy table. It produces dilation and perhaps calcification in the ascending aorta. The latter may be detected radiologically (Fig. 53–2).

SYPHILITIC AORTIC ANEURYSM. Aneurysms occur in 10 to 40 per cent of patients with syphilitic aortitis. Syphilitic aneurysms, once the most common cause of thoracic aneurysms, are much less common than a few decades ago. Nearly half occur in the ascending aorta, 30 to 40 per cent in the arch, and 15 per cent in the descending thoracic aorta. Syphilitic aortic aneurysms may occur in the abdominal aorta but are distinctly uncommon there, especially if there is no syphilitic aneurysm in the thoracic aorta. With ascending aortic aneurysm, aortic insufficiency is often present; rarely, there is a visible pulsatile mass in the first and second right intercostal spaces with exaggerated pulsations of the right sternoclavicular joint or in the episternal notch. Chest pain, the most common symptom, may occur owing to rib, sternal, or vertebral erosion. The pain is usually substernal, in the dorsal spine, or at the side of the chest. Increasing intensity of pain is usually an ominous sign associated with impending rupture. A chest radiogram may demonstrate erosion of ribs and sternum by the aneurysm. Respiratory difficulty may indicate that the aneurysm is in the arch of the aorta; there may be a tracheal tug; hoarseness and a brassy cough suggest recurrent laryngeal nerve paralysis. There may be Horner's syndrome with ptosis, miosis, and decreased sweating on the left side of the face. There may be superior vena caval obstruction with distended nonpulsatile jugular veins, dyspnea, and collateral venous circulation over the thorax. Today, however, more than 95 per cent of superior caval obstruction is caused by malignant tumors. Aortic arch aneurysm may produce compression of the left mainstem bronchus, with atelectasis of the left lung or of the left lower lobe. Hemoptysis suggests tracheal or bronchial ulceration. Hematemesis may indicate rupture into the esophagus. In the descending thoracic aorta, rarely the aneurysm may present as a pulsatile mass medial to, or inferior to, the angle of the left scapula. In these cases, vertebral erosion may occur. Cardiac enlargement does not occur because of aneurysm alone.

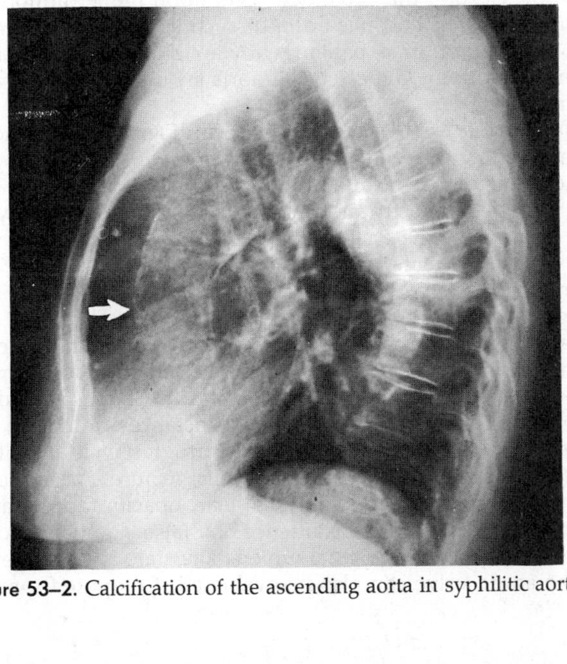

Figure 53–2. Calcification of the ascending aorta in syphilitic aortitis.

Radiologic studies are helpful in diagnosing thoracic aneurysm of any cause. Calcification limited to the ascending aorta suggests syphilitic aortitis but may occur with other varieties of aortitis, healed dissection, and arteriosclerosis. A mass continuous with the aorta with calcification in its wall is very likely an aneurysm. Without calcification aortic aneurysm must be distinguished from other mediastinal masses, especially tumors of lymph nodes, dermoid cysts, thymic tumor, and substernal thyroid gland. Evaluation of pulsations of a mass by fluoroscopy is virtually worthless; pulsatory movements transmitted into contiguous tumors are indistinguishable from those of intrinsic pulsations of the aorta. Conversely, aneurysms which are lined with thrombus may fail to show visible pulsations. Contrast aortography is the precise way of settling the diagnosis. CT scans with intravenous contrast medium enhancement will often obviate the need for contrast aortography.

Course and Prognosis. Syphilitic aneurysms tend to rupture eventually. The rupture may take place into the right or left pleural space, into the trachea or esophagus, or into the pulmonary artery, where it produces a continuous murmur like that of patent ductus arteriosus. The aneurysm may rupture into the right heart, producing a continuous murmur like that described under Congenital Aortic Aneurysm, above. Laplace's law states that tension in walls of a cylinder is equal to the product of pressure times radius. Hence the tension in the wall of an aortic aneurysm is greater than that in the adjacent aorta. Surgical resection of syphilitic aneurysms is recommended when feasible and when the patient does not suffer from some other disease which materially limits life expectancy.

Serologic studies of patients suspected of syphilitic aortitis may be misleading. The Kahn serologic test may be negative in as many as 23 per cent of patients with syphilitic aortitis. The VDRL test is said to be positive in 98 to 99 per cent of such patients but may be negative in patients over 65 years of age. The *Treponema pallidum* immobilization test may be positive when the VDRL test is negative and is especially useful when the patient is over 65 years of age or has had antisyphilitic therapy.

Antisyphilitic Treatment. The Venereal Disease Control Advisory Committee recommended that patients who have cardiovascular syphilis receive benzathine penicillin, 2.4 million units intramuscularly weekly for three successive weeks, or aqueous procaine penicillin, 600,000 units intramuscularly daily for 15 days. Such therapy may not allay the progression of syphilitic aortitis or aneurysm, as the weakened aortic wall continues to expand despite the absence of active infection.

Jaffe HW: The laboratory diagnosis of syphilis. Ann Intern Med 83:846, 1975. *A brief review of laboratory tests for syphilis. The several tests are discussed with regard to their sensitivity and specificity in the various stages of acquired syphilis and the several forms of congenital syphilis.*

Syphilis: Recommended Treatment Schedules, 1976. Center for Disease Control, Atlanta, Georgia. Ann Intern Med 85:94, 1976. *This is a brief summary of the recommendations of the Venereal Disease Control Advisory Committee of the Center for Disease Control, Atlanta, Georgia. Treatment schedules for early syphilis, late syphilis, syphilis during pregnancy, and congenital syphilis are described.*

DISSECTING ANEURYSM OF THE AORTA

Dissecting aneurysm of the aorta is also called dissecting hematoma of the aorta. According to Wolfe and Moran, there are at least 2000 new cases of dissecting aneurysm each year in the United States. The disease tends to occur in certain settings. It is most common in men of middle age with hypertension, but is also found in Marfan's syndrome, cystic medial necrosis, or coarctation of the aorta and seems more common in pregnancy. The relationship of dissecting aneurysm to pregnancy is discussed in a recent article (Am J Med, 1983). Dissecting aneurysm may occur in certain heritable disorders of connective tissue, including Ehlers-Danlos syndrome, and has been described as a complication of relapsing polychondritis. The prevalence of aortic dissection is increased in patients with bicuspid aortic valves (Roberts).

Ordinarily the dissection begins with an aortic intimal tear, followed by a dissecting channel in the media, followed by reentry from the intima back into the aortic lumen or rupture through the adventitia. Thus a double-barreled aorta may be produced. Approximately 50 per cent of aortic dissections begin in the ascending aorta, 30 per cent in the aortic arch, and 20 per cent in the descending aorta. Dissecting aneurysm may be related to trauma, especially that produced by an angiographic catheter or aortic balloon catheter striking an arteriosclerotic plaque in the aorta. Aortocoronary bypass grafting may be complicated by dissecting aneurysm. A dissecting aneurysm may extend proximally to the aortic valve area, thus causing aortic valvular insufficiency; it may surround the coronary arteries, producing myocardial infarction; it may extend along the carotid sheath to cause hemiplegia. It may involve the blood supply to the spinal cord, leading to paraplegia and anesthesia below the level of involvement. It may involve the renal artery, thus aggravating pre-existing arterial hypertension. Hypertension may also be aggravated by carotid artery involvement when it interferes with the carotid sinus baroreceptor response. Rupture into the pericardium may lead to cardiac tamponade and rapid demise.

HISTORY. Most dissecting aneurysms are associated with chest pain, which may radiate into the abdomen or into the back. The pain of aortic dissection must be distinguished from that of myocardial ischemia. The pain of ischemic heart disease seldom radiates to the back and infrequently extends below the diaphragm; those features should suggest the possibility of aortic dissection. In some patients, a proximal aortic dissection involves the coronary arteries, leading to cardiac infarction as a complication, and then the condition may masquerade as a case of myocardial infarction. With rupture into the pericardial sac, cardiac tamponade is likely, but with gradual leak into the pericardial sac, the patient may appear to have unexplained pericarditis. The sudden appearance of aortic insufficiency should raise the possibility of dissecting aneurysm even when pain is absent. Hemiplegia, paraplegia, or syncope may be the presenting features, as may the aortic arch syndrome (see next section). The prevalence of pain is believed to be about 70 per cent. Occasional patients appear with aortic insufficiency, a large heart, and heart failure without a history of an acute episode of aortic dissection.

PHYSICAL FINDINGS. The patient is often hypertensive and often complains of chest pain; commonly, the patient is a man between the ages of 40 and 60 years. When the process involves the orifices of the femoral arteries or arteries to the head and neck, asymmetrical arterial pulses may be found. Although abnormal peripheral arterial pulses were found in 13 of 18 cases in one series of patients with aortic dissection, most series find the minority of patients to have significant differences of pulse and blood pressure in the arms, legs, or carotid arteries. Possibly 25 per cent of patients develop aortic insufficiency. Either sternoclavicular joint may transmit an abnormal pulsation. Unilateral distention of the left external jugular vein results from pressure of the expanded aorta upon the left innominate vein. This sign is not specific for dissecting aneurysm, however, and may occur in a patient with an elongated and kinked arteriosclerotic or hypertensive aorta in the absence of aneurysm.

LABORATORY STUDIES. The electrocardiogram may be normal or may show left ventricular hypertrophy. It may show evidence of acute pericarditis. In approximately one case in six of one series, the electrocardiogram showed changes of myocardial infarction. The chest roentgenogram is very important in the study of patients, especially if there are serial studies. Rapid change in the width of the aorta, especially the aortic arch, suggests dissection or mediastinal bleeding. The chest radiogram may show changes virtually specific for dissection by demonstrating a separation of more than a few millimeters between a calcified intimal plaque and the external border of the aorta. However, the majority of instances cannot be diagnosed from plain roentgenogram; aortography is usually required (Fig. 53–3). The aortographic features of dissecting hematoma are evidence of intimal tear, opacification of a false channel, and the indirect evidence of a false channel produced by narrowing of the original lumen. The state and competence of the aortic valve can also be evaluated. Computed tomogra-

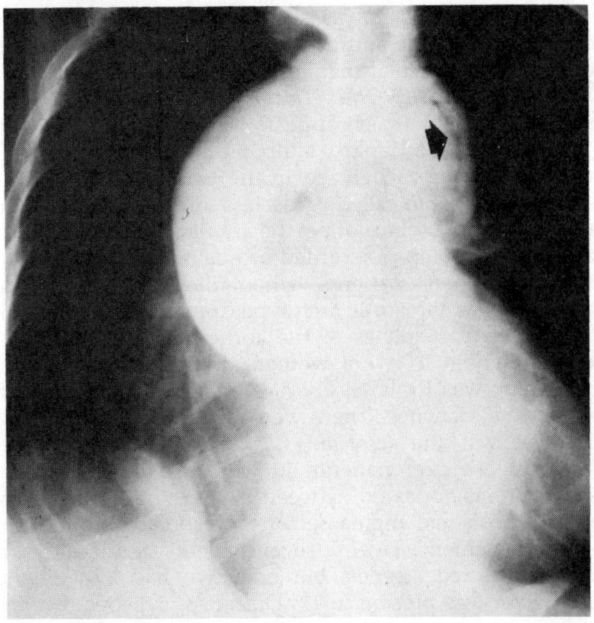

Figure 53–3. Aortogram: dissecting aneurysm. The arrow indicates line of separation between true and false channels. (Courtesy of Dr. Harold Spitz.)

phy with contrast enhancement is a useful noninvasive method. When the process involves the ascending aorta, echocardiography may be of value in showing thickening of the aortic wall, aortic root dilation, and a double aortic lumen.

The diagnosis requires a high index of suspicion. A patient thought to have myocardial infarction should be suspected of dissecting aortic aneurysm if the pain radiates to the back or into the abdomen, if the electrocardiogram shows no change or changes of pericarditis, and if the serum enzyme values (especially the MB fraction of creatine phosphokinase) remain normal. Aortic dissection should be considered when there is aortic insufficiency of recent onset or if there are impaired arterial pulses in the neck or extremities. Changes in aortic contour demonstrated by serial roentgenograms are highly suggestive. The diagnosis may be proved in most cases by aortography. Uncommonly, the aortogram does not show specific changes and the diagnosis can only be suspected from the unusual thickening of the aortic wall.

In one series (Slater and DeSanctis), syncope with aortic dissection was usually caused by cardiac tamponade. Dissection involving the proximal ascending aorta differed from distal dissection involving the descending thoracic aorta. In 53 patients with proximal dissection, the patients were younger and had a higher incidence of Marfan's syndrome or cystic medial necrosis. Anterior chest pain, pulse deficit, neurologic compromise, aortic insufficiency, and congestive heart failure were more common. With distal dissection, back pain, hypertension, and atherosclerosis were more common. Chest radiograms almost always showed an abnormal aortic contour, although aortography was necessary to be certain of the diagnosis.

PROGNOSIS. The prognosis is poor in aortic dissecting aneurysm. If untreated, approximately 20 per cent of patients die within 24 hours and 37 per cent in 48 hours. A small percentage of patients, probably less than 10 per cent, live for a year and may survive with chronic or even severe aortic insufficiency. Rarely, a dissection in the descending aorta may re-enter the original lumen, producing a double-barreled aorta, which may allow survival for years. With surgical resection of the diseased segment and aortic graft replacement, as many as 75 per cent may survive. At Stanford, the operative mortality was 29 per cent in 125 patients. Of those who survived operation, 76 per cent lived five years or more (Miller et al.). The prognosis is better for either medical or surgical treatment when the dissection begins distal to the aortic arch. In this group, 50 per cent may survive the first three weeks even without modern therapy.

TREATMENT. Treatment may be either surgical or medical. Surgical management usually consists of resection of the involved segment and replacement with a prosthetic graft. Operative management is especially to be considered in the following circumstances: (1) when there is leaking from the dissection, which most commonly takes place into the left hemithorax or pericardium; (2) when the ascending aorta or arch is involved; (3) when the cerebral circulation is compromised but not to a degree incompatible with recovery; (4) with severe heart failure caused by aortic regurgitation; (5) when there is evidence of continued dissection; (6) when pain and blood pressure cannot be controlled; and (7) when hypertension is absent.

Initial medical management is suggested when the process is limited to the descending aorta, except when there is continued pain, evidence of bleeding, or extension of the dissection. Medical management involves control of hypertension and administration of drugs to lessen the systolic ejection force of the heart. Hypertension is treated with trimethaphan (Arfonad) or with oral or intravenous alpha methyldopa. Wolfe and Moran favor intravenous sodium nitroprusside as the initial agent. The systolic blood pressure is reduced to 100 to 120 mm Hg. Along with these antihypertensive agents, oral propranolol, 10 to 40 mg four times daily, is given to reduce the velocity of left ventricular ejection. In one series, 17 of 33 patients treated medically survived, and in another, 10 of 12. In the Peter Bent Brigham Hospital series, 26 of 31 patients with aortic dissection had contraindications to medical therapy; 17 of 22 did well after surgical correction. When dissection was limited to the descending aorta, none of 14 patients had contraindications to medical therapy, which was successful in each instance.

Medical management may be considered when the process is more than two weeks old. Resection of the dissected area, followed by grafting, may be done later when the condition of the patient is stabilized. Progressive enlargement of the aneurysm is an indication for surgical repair in patients who have received medical therapy. The majority can be brought through the acute phase of the illness alive. However, the long-term outlook in medically treated patients is uncertain, and many will do better with surgical treatment once the condition has stabilized. Long-term antihypertensive therapy should be considered, if indicated.

Clinicopathologic Conference: Chest pain, collapse, and death in late pregnancy. Am J Med 75:691, 1983.

Heiberg E, Wolverson M, Sundaram M, et al.: CT findings in thoracic aortic dissection. Am J Roentgenol 136:13, 1981. *A review of 13 cases studied by CT scanning. CT scanning will often render aortography unnecessary in patients suspected of dissecting aortic aneurysm.*

Miller DC, Stinson EB, Oyer PE, et al.: Operative treatment of aortic dissections. J Thorac Cardiovasc Surg 78:365, 1979. *This paper reviews operative treatment and results in 125 patients with aortic dissecting aneurysm at Stanford University over a 16-year period between 1963 and 1979. The overall operative mortality rate was 29 per cent; the death rate was 37 per cent in those with acute dissection and 17 per cent in those with chronic dissection. Late postoperative course and complications are presented.*

Roberts WC: Aortic dissection: Anatomy, consequences, and causes. Am Heart J 101:195, 1981. *A timely review of the etiologic background and complications of aortic dissection. The roles of hypertension, bicuspid aortic valve, and iatrogenic trauma are emphasized. Atherosclerosis and syphilis are considered unlikely causes (56 references).*

Slater EE, DeSanctis RW: The clinical recognition of dissecting aortic aneurysm. Am J Med 60:625, 1976. *This paper presents clinical, radiologic, and laboratory findings in 124 patients with aortic dissecting aneurysm who were studied at the Massachusetts General Hospital. The authors point out differences in age, predisposing disease, and clinical features between ascending aortic or proximal dissection and descending aortic or distal dissection.*

Wheat MW: Acute dissection of the aorta. *In* McGoon DC (ed.): Cardiac Surgery. Cardiovasc Clin, Vol 12, 1982. *A concise review of the current status of medical and surgical therapy of aortic dissection.*

Wolfe WG, Moran JF: Editorial. The evolution of medical and surgical management of acute aortic dissection. Circulation 56:503, 1977. *This editorial briefly reviews experiences at various centers with the medical and surgical treatments of aortic dissecting aneurysm, with 27 references. The authors give their recommendations for medical management and indicate their criteria for early operative management of acute dissecting aortic aneurysm.*

MISCELLANEOUS FORMS OF AORTITIS AND THE AORTIC ARCH SYNDROME

The aorta may be affected by a number of inflammatory processes in addition to those previously described. The aorta may be involved by septicemia or by inflammation of contiguous structures. Aortitis may be a part of a generalized disorder of connective tissue. The process may encroach upon the origin of the aortic arch vessels. Blood supply to the areas supplied by these vessels, namely, the innominate artery, the left common carotid artery, and the left subclavian artery, may be impaired. This syndrome is called the *aortic arch syndrome.* Thus one may find cerebral ischemia, syncope, visual difficulties, claudication during exercise of the upper extremities, impairment of the pulse in the upper extremities, or intermittent claudication of the jaw muscles with chewing. The aortic arch syndrome may be produced by Takayasu's syndrome, by syphilis, by arteriosclerosis, by giant cell arteritis, or by dissecting aneurysm. The aorta may be involved by tuberculosis, usually as a result of inflammation of continuous tuberculous lymph nodes. Septicemia may lead to mycotic aneurysm of the aorta. Mycotic aneurysm of the aorta is reviewed by Ewart et al. This may be a complication of infectious endocarditis. Relapsing polychondritis may lead to aortic involvement, and aortic aneurysms occur fairly frequently in this condition. The aneurysms may involve both the thoracic and abdominal aorta. The aorta may be involved by idiopathic aortitis, a process which resembles syphilis anatomically, but there is no serologic or bacteriologic evidence of syphilis. This process may lead to calcification of the ascending aorta and perhaps of the aortic and mitral valves. The aorta may be involved in rheumatic fever and in rheumatoid disease (Heggtveit et al.). Giant cell aortitis may occur in 10 to 15 per cent of all cases of temporal arteritis. It may lead to the aortic arch syndrome, aortic incompetence, dissecting aneurysm, or, rarely, to aortic aneurysm. In ankylosing spondylitis, 5 to 10 per cent of patients develop a proximal aortitis closely resembling syphilitic aortitis. Aortic regurgitation often occurs. The disease affects men nine times as often as women. Kawasaki's mucocutaneous lymph node syndrome may cause aortitis, but coronary artery involvement is the principal vascular manifestation.

TAKAYASU'S SYNDROME. Takayasu's arteritis is a form of aortic involvement which appears to be much more common in females and in Japan, although increasing numbers of patients are being recognized in the United States. This syndrome has also been called "pulseless disease," but since there are other diseases which affect the arterial pulses similarly, this term should be either discarded or qualified. Nakao and associates reviewed 84 patients, whom they divided into three types. One was the aortic arch type (they usually had stenosis or occlusion of branches of the aortic arch). Forty-seven patients, of whom 41 were women, were in this group. The second type was the *extensive type,* which involved the entire aorta and its branches. There were 27 cases in this group. The third type was the *descending thoracic and abdominal type,* in which there were ten patients. In over three fourths of patients first symptoms appeared between the ages of 11 and 29 years. Eleven patients had angina pectoris, presumably from coronary artery involvement. Twenty-seven patients had localized pain over the affected arteries, but only two had loss of arterial pulse. Fever was present in 17. Dizziness, syncope, headache, and impaired vision with claudication in the upper or lower extremities were common. Thirty-four of 75 had slight anemia, and 46 of 76 had an increased erythrocyte sedimentation rate. Aortographic studies were essential in confirming the diagnosis. In some, aortography showed localized aneurysms in each of the three types. Six of 15 of the *extensive type* showed coarctation of the abdominal aorta, and eight of nine of the *descending thoracic and abdominal aortic type* showed abdominal aortic coarctation. Both types frequently showed narrowing of the lumen of the renal or mesenteric arteries (Fig. 53–4), and some showed femoral artery occlusion.

The patients commonly complained of arthralgia; carditis and high fever were not present. Six of the patients in this report died; three died of left-sided heart failure, one had angina and pericarditis, and two died suddenly. Two died less than a year after onset of symptoms; two, in one to four years; and two, 20 to 29 years after the onset of symptoms. Ishikawa's report emphasized pulmonary artery involvement, which occurred in

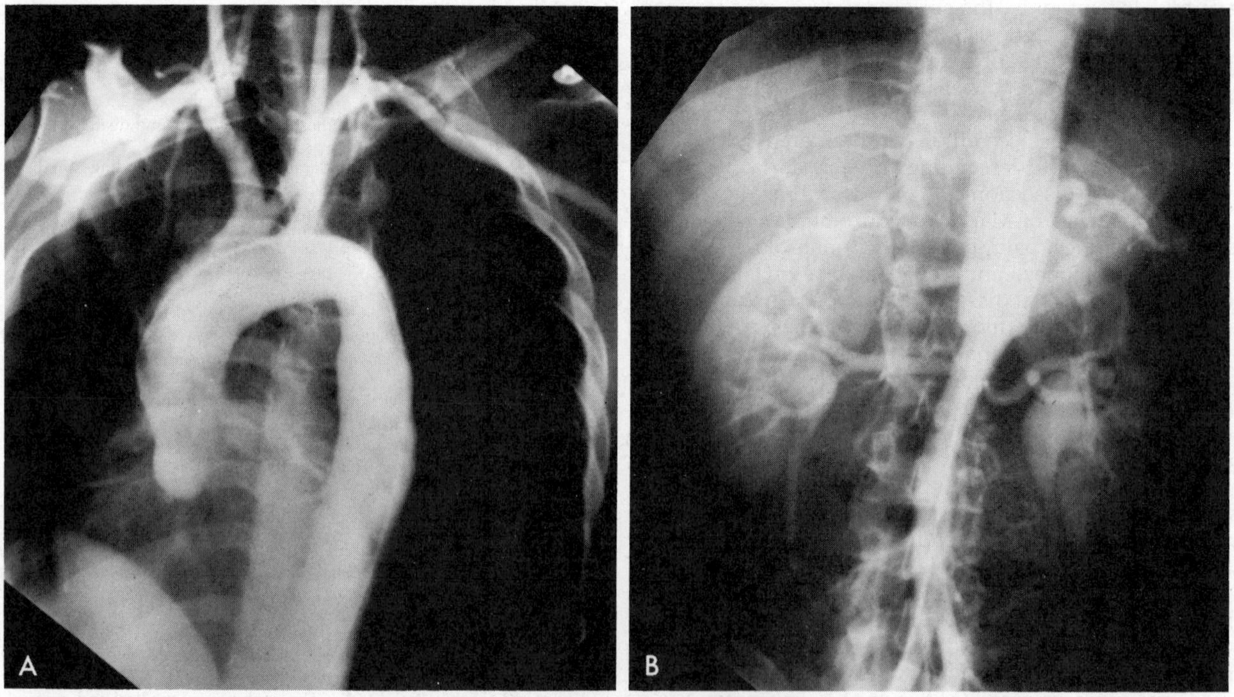

Figure 53–4. Takayasu's aortitis in a 26-year-old black man. Thoracic *(A)* and abdominal *(B)* aortograms show dilation, irregularity, and wall thickening extending from the proximal descending thoracic aorta to the abdominal aorta a few centimeters above the renal arteries. *A,* The cervical branches of the aortic arch are normal. *B,* There is a 30 per cent narrowing of the left main renal artery. The picture is consistent with Takayasu's arteritis. (Courtesy of Dr. Harold Spitz.)

19 of 43 patients studied. Lower thoracic and abdominal aortic aneurysms may occur. Coronary artery aneurysms and thrombotic coronary occlusion are described.

Pathologic Lesions. Takayasu's disease is a segmental panaortitis, or panarteritis, characterized by cicatrization of all layers of involved arteries and dense bands of medial inflammatory cells. In advanced stages, the arteries become thick-walled, rigid tubes, followed by luminal obliteration caused by superimposed thrombosis. There may be occlusive narrowing of the coronary ostia. The fibrous mural thickening exceeds that usually seen in other forms of aortic disease.

Treatment. Twenty-nine of Nakao's patients received adrenal corticosteroids; of these, 18 had remissions and 11 had no suppression of the inflammatory findings. Anticoagulants were thought helpful in only one of 12 patients in whom they were used. Although a few of the patients had increased antistreptolysin "O" serologic titers or positive rheumatoid factor tests, none met the clinical criteria for either rheumatoid arthritis or acute rheumatic fever.

Cipriano PR, Alonso DR, Baltaxe HA, et al.: Multiple aortic aneurysms in relapsing polychondritis. Am J Cardiol 37:1097, 1976. *This is a case report of a patient with relapsing polychondritis and both thoracic and abdominal aortic aneurysms. The medical literature was searched. A summary of the ten known cases with relapsing polychondritis and aortic aneurysm is presented in tabular form.*

Ewart JM, Burke ML, Bunt TJ: Spontaneous abdominal aortic infections. Am Surg 49:37, 1983. *A review of 34 survivors of mycotic abdominal aortic aneurysm (81 references).*

Heggtveit HS, Hennigar GR, Morrione TG: Panaortitis. Am J Pathol 42:151, 1963. *This paper presents ten cases of panaortitis gathered from 11,500 necropsy examinations. The authors differentiate these ten cases from syphilitic aortitis and from Takayasu's disease. The clinical and anatomic features of the ten cases are presented in two tables.*

Ishikawa K: Natural history and classification of occlusive thromboaortopathy (Takayasu's disease). Circulation 57:27, 1978. *This paper presents a study of 54 Japanese patients with Takayasu's disease. Retinopathy, pulmonary arterial involvement, aortic regurgitation, aortic aneurysm, and secondary hypertension are discussed as features of the disease. Renovascular hypertension may occur.*

Nakao K, Ikeda M, Kimata S, et al.: Takayasu's aortitis. Clinical report of eighty four cases and immunological studies of seven cases. Circulation 35:1141, 1967. *This paper presents a study of the manifestations of Takayasu's arteritis of the aorta in 84 Japanese patients, of whom 54 had aortographic examination. The cases were divided into three types: (1) arch type (47 cases); (2) extensive type, with involvement of entire aorta and its branches (27 cases); and (3) descending thoracic and abdominal type (10 cases). Only 12 patients were male. The first symptoms occurred between 11 and 48 years of age.*

Radford DJ, Sondheimer HM, Williams GJ, et al.: Mucocutaneous lymph node syndrome with coronary artery aneurysm. Am J Dis Child 130:596, 1976. *This paper describes 16 cases of mucocutaneous lymph node syndrome (Kawasaki's disease) seen in a Hawaiian hospital. The disease occurs principally in children of Oriental origin but is now being recognized in the USA. Autopsies have shown generalized arteritis, especially of the coronary arteries, with aneurysmal dilatation and extensive thrombosis of these vessels. Aortitis may occur.*

AORTIC OCCLUSION SYNDROMES

Occlusion of the terminal aorta at its bifurcation may be produced by traumatic severance, by acute aortic dissection, by arteriosclerotic thrombosis, or suddenly by embolism. The predisposing causes of emboli are most commonly atrial fibrillation, infective endocarditis, myocardial infarction, cardiomyopathy, prosthetic heart valves, ventricular or aortic aneurysm, and rheumatic mitral disease. Gradual occlusion of the terminal aorta is often well tolerated without gangrene of the lower extremities, although the patient may have pain in the hips and thighs with exercise, and the male may suffer from impotence (Leriche's syndrome). Sudden occlusion of the aorta at its bifurcation is poorly tolerated, and immediate surgical treatment is needed. Patients with this condition suffer from pain (but pain may be absent in as many as 50 per cent of instances), loss of the femoral pulses, coldness, pallor, and often ensuing gangrene of the lower extremities. Weakness or paralysis of the lower limbs, loss of deep tendon reflexes, and impairment or loss of sensation are usually present. Two patients seen at the Cincinnati General Hospital were referred to neurologists because of sudden paraplegia. The diagnosis was originally overlooked because of failure to examine the femoral pulses. The superficial veins of the lower extremities are usually collapsed. The diagnosis is made clinically and confirmed by aortography. With acute embolism, embolectomy is necessary to prevent massive fatal gangrene of the lower extremities and pelvis. With chronic aortic thrombotic occlusion at the bifurcation, a synthetic bypass graft is used to bridge the obstructed area, provided that the iliac and femoral arterial vascular beds are adequate. Endarterectomy may be employed alone when the process is localized, or combined with bypass grafting when the process is more extensive. A single case treated successfully by nonsurgical angioplasty is reported.

Juergens JL, Fairbairn JR II, Spittell JA Jr: Allen-Barker-Hines Peripheral Vascular Diseases. 5th ed. Philadelphia, W. B. Saunders Company, 1980. *This revision of the Allen, Barker, and Hines classic textbook from the Mayo Clinic is the leader in its field. It deals not only with diseases of arteries, veins, and lymphatics but also with pulmonary embolism, cerebrovascular diseases, and diseases of the aorta. The material is well-organized and presented, and can be recommended for the medical student and medical specialist alike. It is adequately referenced for further reading.*

Stubbs DH, Kasulke RJ, Kapsch DN, et al.: Populations with the Leriche syndrome. Surgery 89:612, 1981. *Total infrarenal aortic occlusion occurs in 4 to 10 per cent of patients requiring arterial reconstruction or bypass of the distal aorta. This review presents 20 cases, 11 with normal distal vessels who were younger and did well with operation. The nine with distal vessel disease were older, had been symptomatic longer, and had a less satisfactory operative result (30 references).*

54. VASCULAR DISEASES OF THE LIMBS

Hermes A. Kontos

VASCULAR DISEASES OF THE LIMBS DUE TO ABNORMAL RESPONSES OF VASCULAR SMOOTH MUSCLE

Raynaud's Phenomenon and Disease

DEFINITION. Raynaud's phenomenon is a syndrome manifested by attacks of pallor and cyanosis of the digits in response to cold or to emotion. When the disorder is primary, it is called Raynaud's disease; when it is secondary to another disease or recognizable cause, it is called Raynaud's phenomenon.

ETIOLOGY AND INCIDENCE. Raynaud's disease is the most common cause of Raynaud's phenomenon, accounting for 60 per cent of the patients with this disorder. The cause of Raynaud's disease is unknown. Although it can begin at any age, it becomes clinically manifest most commonly between the ages of 20 and 40 years. Raynaud's disease is much more common in women than in men. Two theories have been advanced to explain its occurrence. Raynaud believed that it is caused by increased sympathetic nerve activity. Lewis discovered that attacks of Raynaud's phenomenon could be induced after interruption of the sympathetic nerves. He concluded that the cause of the disorder was a fault in the arterial wall that rendered the vessels hyperresponsive to the vasoconstrictive effects of cold. He ascribed the vasospastic attacks to spasm of the digital arteries as a result of this hypersensitivity. In his view, increased sympathetic activity could, under certain circumstances, contribute to the development of the attack by constricting smaller vessels, thereby reducing further the level of blood flow. Little is known about the defect in the vessel wall, which renders the vessel hypersensitive to cold. Assay values for monoamine oxidase activity of biopsy material from digital arteries from two patients with Raynaud's disease were low. It was suggested that this deficiency allows catecholamines to achieve a higher level than normal and causes the vasospastic attacks. Subsequent evidence, however, did not support this hypothesis. The circulation of the digits of patients with Raynaud's disease is not hypersensitive to infused norepinephrine. Also, determination of the arteriovenous concentration differences of norepinephrine and epinephrine across the hand showed that there was no excessive release of catecholamines from the hands of patients with Raynaud's disease.

In a recent study, 26 per cent of patients with variant type of angina pectoris, a disorder caused by spasm of the coronary arteries, were found to have migraine and 24 per cent were found to have Raynaud's phenomenon. This suggested the possibility that in some patients with Raynaud's phenomenon, we may be dealing with a generalized defect that predisposes arteries in many regions to vasospasm. An association of Raynaud's phenomenon with idiopathic pulmonary hypertension has also been reported. It is unlikely, however, that this has any bearing on the etiology of Raynaud's disease. It is more likely that the cause of Raynaud's attacks in patients with idiopathic pulmonary hypertension is a very high level of peripheral vascular tone secondary to the severe reduction in cardiac output.

Secondary Raynaud's phenomenon is observed frequently as a manifestation of the following groups of diseases: (1) Occlusive arterial disease, such as thromboangiitis obliterans, arteriosclerosis obliterans, or arterial obstruction as a result of embolism. In the presence of arterial obstruction in these disorders, vasoconstrictive stimuli that normally do not cause clinical manifestations result in more severe reductions in blood flow and may cause Raynaud's phenomenon. (2) Connective tissue diseases, including rheumatoid arthritis, systemic lupus erythematosus, and, particularly, scleroderma. The incidence of Raynaud's phenomenon in scleroderma is about 90 per cent. A distinctive syndrome consisting of calcinosis, Raynaud's phenomenon, abnormal esophageal motility, sclerodactyly, and telangiectasia (CREST syndrome) is recognized. Raynaud's phenomenon may be the presenting manifestation in connective tissue diseases and may precede the appearance of other manifestations by several years. The presence of abnormal nailfold capillaries in patients with Raynaud's phenomenon has predictive value for the future development of scleroderma. Structural changes in the vessel wall that limit flow and increase the sensitivity to vasoconstrictive influences appear to account for the frequent occurrence of Raynaud's phenomenon in these diseases. (3) Repetitive minor trauma to the digits, as might occur from various occupations. Raynaud's phenomenon from this cause is seen in typists, pianists, and pneumatic hammer operators. The mechanism of Raynaud's phenomenon seems to be similar to that seen in connective tissue disorders. (4) Neurogenic lesions, such as thoracic outlet compression syndromes (cervical rib, scalenus anticus muscle, hyperabduction syndrome), carpal tunnel syndromes, sympathetic causalgia, and disorders of the spinal cord, such as syringomyelia. In these diseases, Raynaud's phenomenon is caused by irritation of sympathetic nerves, and consequent neurogenic vasoconstriction. (5) Administration of certain drugs, such as ergotamine and methysergide, or exposure to chemicals, such as polyvinyl chloride, or in ergotism. These agents cause vascular smooth muscle contraction and thereby induce decreases in blood flow. Raynaud's phenomenon occurs in 3 to 6 per cent of patients taking beta-adrenergic receptor blocking drugs. Propranolol is the main offender. These drugs block a beta-adrenergic vasodilative mechanism in the digits and may also enhance the vasoconstrictive effects of norepinephrine. (6) Intravascular coagulation of the blood or aggregation of blood elements, as seen in cryoglobulinemia or in the presence of cold agglutinins. The intravascular aggregation or coagulation of blood elements obstructs the vessels and causes ischemia.

PATHOPHYSIOLOGY. The pallor during the attack of Raynaud's phenomenon is explained by intense vasoconstriction or spasm of the digital arteries. This results in severe reduction in blood flow. In a later stage of the attack, as the vasoconstriction becomes less severe, blood flow reduction is less pronounced, allowing some filling of the capillaries and veins with blood whose hemoglobin becomes markedly deoxygenated. This accounts for the cyanosis. Upon rewarming, cyanosis is replaced by an intense red color associated with reactive hyperemia. Between attacks, blood flow to the digits is usually reduced, especially in patients who have trophic changes, but may be normal in some patients. In those patients without trophic changes, blood flow to the hand during maximum vasodilation is the same as in normal individuals, but it is severely reduced in those with trophic changes, a reflection of structural changes in the blood vessels.

PATHOLOGY. In the early stages of the disease, the digital blood vessels are histologically normal. In longstanding cases, the intima becomes thickened, and the media may be hypertrophied. In severe progressive cases, complete obstruction from thrombosis may occur, and gangrene of the tips of the digits may ensue.

CLINICAL MANIFESTATIONS. The onset of Raynaud's disease is usually gradual. The patient notices an occasional mild and short-lasting attack during winter. Over succeeding years, the severity and duration of the attacks may increase. A wide variation in severity is present. Most commonly the attacks are provoked by exposure to cold. In some patients, attacks are also precipitated by emotion. The attacks may be terminated by rewarming or they may abate spontaneously. Between attacks, in a warm environment, the patient is asymptomatic and physical examination shows no abnormalities. Some patients, however, complain of chronically cold hands and feet, and they may have cold fingers with cyanosis on examination, a reflection of a reduced level of blood flow. In a typical attack of Raynaud's phenomenon, the digits become pale. Usually, all digits are affected symmetrically. The pallor is sharply demarcated at the level of the metacarpophalangeal joints, a reflection of the fact that the ischemia is caused mainly by spasm of the digital arteries. At a later stage during the attack, pallor is replaced by cyanosis. The patient may have feelings of coldness, numbness, and occasionally pain. Upon rewarming, the cyanosis is replaced by intense redness, and the patient may feel tingling or throbbing. Most commonly, only the hands are affected. Frequently, both hands and feet are affected. Rarely, the nose, cheeks, ears, and chin are affected also.

Atypical attacks are not infrequent. In these, the involvement of the digits may be asymmetrical, with only one or two digits being affected. In some cases, only a portion of the digit is affected. In these instances, the most severely affected portion of the digit is the most distal one. Thus, one may see pallor of the fingertip or of the terminal phalanx of one digit. In other cases, more than one phalanx may be involved. This pattern is the result of the spasm of the digital artery, which leads to the most severe reduction in blood flow in the most distal portions of the digit.

In severe, progressive cases, trophic changes may occur after a few years of involvement. The hair may disappear from the dorsal aspect of the digits. The nails grow more slowly and become brittle and deformed. The skin becomes atrophic, thin, and tight (sclerodactyly). Ulcerations may develop at the fingertips or around the nail bed. These heal slowly and may become infected. They are extremely painful, especially at night. When they heal, they leave small characteristic pitted scars.

DIAGNOSIS. The diagnosis of Raynaud's phenomenon can usually be made on the basis of the history of vasospastic attacks in the digits, precipitated by cold and relieved by warming. In atypical cases or when the patient's description of the attack is not sufficiently clear, provocation of an attack may be helpful. This may be done by immersing the hands in water at a temperature of 10 to 15°C. Whole-body exposure to cold is more successful in provoking attacks. A negative result does not exclude Raynaud's phenomenon.

In typical cases, Raynaud's phenomenon is easily distinguished from acrocyanosis, but when involvement is atypical, the differentiation may be more difficult. Distinguishing features include the following: The color changes in Raynaud's phenomenon are episodic, while in acrocyanosis they are sustained. Pallor is not a prominent feature of acrocyanosis. Cyanosis is the more typical color change, while in Raynaud's disease digital pallor is characteristic. In Raynaud's disease, only the digits are involved, while in acrocyanosis the color changes usually involve the whole hand or foot and sometimes even more proximal portions of the limbs. In Raynaud's disease the skin of the palms is usually dry, while in acrocyanosis it is wet and clammy with sweat. Finally, acrocyanosis rarely causes trophic changes and ulcerations.

Obstruction of major arteries from arteriosclerosis, angiitis, embolism, or thrombosis may lead to color changes in the digits which simulate Raynaud's phenomenon. The distinction is made by the demonstration of changes in arterial pulses and by the fact that the color changes in these disorders are likely to be confined to one limb rather than symmetrical. Arteriography, which demonstrates the arterial lesion, is helpful. However, secondary Raynaud's phenomenon may be superimposed upon any of these diseases. In Raynaud's phenomenon, Doppler velocity studies show patent arteries and sharply peaked blood flow velocity patterns in the digits. Arteriography shows normalcy of the major arteries and diffuse spasm of the digital arteries.

The distinction of Raynaud's disease from secondary Raynaud's phenomenon is based mainly on the exclusion of disorders that are known to cause secondary Raynaud's phenomenon. The exclusion of obstructive arterial disease is discussed above. Connective tissue disorders, particularly scleroderma, are excluded by the absence of arthralgias or arthritis, alterations of esophageal motility, and the absence of a pulmonary oxygen diffusion defect. The presence of a normal sedimentation rate and the absence of circulating autoantibodies, such as antinuclear antibodies, provide additional reassurance. A careful occupational history is necessary to exclude Raynaud's phenomenon secondary to minor repetitive trauma. A history of drug ingestion or exposure to chemicals is helpful in identifying drug-induced Raynaud's phenomenon. Neurologic disorders can be recognized by their somatic neurologic manifestations. Thoracic outlet compression syndromes can be excluded by the appropriate maneuvers, which are designed to bring about compression of nerves and obstruction of blood vessels at the thoracic outlet. The presence of intravascular agglutination or coagulation of the blood elements may be suspected if in the presence of cyanosis the blood cannot be expelled from vessels by pressure, and when there are isolated areas of redness as the attack abates during rewarming. Confirmation is obtained by demonstrating the cold agglutinins or cryoglobulins in the patient's blood.

PROGNOSIS. The prognosis of patients with Raynaud's disease is good. There is no mortality associated with the disease and morbidity is low; it is generally limited to loss of portions of digits as a result of ulcerations. In approximately 50 per cent of patients with Raynaud's disease, the disorder improves and may disappear completely after several years. In only a fraction of 1 per cent of the patients is amputation necessary. Approximately 15 per cent of patients with Raynaud's disease eventually develop a connective tissue disorder, particularly scleroderma.

The prognosis in secondary Raynaud's phenomenon depends on the course of the primary disorder. In scleroderma, the prognosis is unsatisfactory, particularly when the disease has caused digital ulcerations. In advanced cases of scleroderma, the external pressure from the changes in the skin becomes very high, with resultant compression of the vessels, and the structural changes in the vessel wall further limit blood flow. Under these conditions, treatment becomes ineffectual, and persistent ulcerations requiring eventual amputation are common.

TREATMENT. Patients with mild or moderately severe Raynaud's disease without ulcerations or other trophic changes do not require drug therapy. Reassurance and protective measures against cold exposure usually suffice. These patients should limit the duration of exposure to cold to the extent possible. They should wear heavy clothing, protecting not only the hands and feet, but also their face and trunk, especially when there is a cold wind; this is important because cold exposure of other portions of the body may reflexly induce vasoconstriction in the digits and precipitate Raynaud's phenomenon. When prolonged exposure to cold is unavoidable, the use of electrically powered or solid fuel–powered hand and foot warmers is advisable. The patients should be taught to recognize and terminate attacks by returning promptly to a warm environment, placing their hands in warm water, or using a warm-air hair blower to warm their hands rapidly. Smoking causes cutaneous vasoconstriction; therefore, tobacco smoking is contraindicated in Raynaud's phenomenon. The use of induced vasodilation by placing the hands in warm water (43°C) has been reported to raise skin temperature and minimize the severity of attacks of Raynaud's phenomenon. Biofeedback to teach patients to raise their skin temperature voluntarily has been shown to limit the duration and frequency of vasospastic attacks, but its effect is nonspecific, because it is also seen in control patients who receive no such treatment, and in those in whom biofeedback is used to teach them to relax.

Drug therapy should be used in severe cases of Raynaud's disease and phenomenon, particularly in those who have trophic changes. The aim of drug therapy is to induce vascular smooth muscle relaxation, thereby raising resting blood flow and limiting the degree of ischemia during attacks. In this manner, the severity and duration of attacks may be minimized. Several types of agents have been used to achieve this result. (1) Calcium antagonists. There are several well-controlled double blind studies in which nifedipine* was found to be effective in the treatment of Raynaud's disease. The drug is administered at a dose of 10 to 20 mg, three or four times daily. Verapamil was found to be less effective. (2) Drugs that interfere with the function of the adrenergic nervous system, such as reserpine,* guanethidine,* or alpha methyldopa.* Reserpine is the best studied of these drugs. It should be administered by mouth in doses of 0.1 to 0.5 mg daily. In cases where ulcerations have developed, it may be given intra-arterially in a dose of 0.5 to 1 mg dissolved in saline and administered into the brachial artery by slow infusion over several minutes. These drugs have also been administered by means of tourniquet-controlled intravenous injection (Bier block). The administration by the last two routes gives a much higher local concentration and largely avoids systemic side effects. (3) Drugs that cause alpha-adrenergic receptor blockade, such as phenoxybenzamine* and prazosin.* Tolazoline, a drug that also blocks alpha-adrenergic receptors but also has a direct relaxing effect on vascular small muscle has also been used for the same purpose. (4) Drugs that relax vascular smooth muscle by direct action. In a controlled trial, nitroglycerin ointment has been found effective in Raynaud's disease. It should be noted that vasodilators given intravenously may not have the same effect on cutaneous blood vessels, because the local relaxant action of the drugs may be counteracted by reflex vasoconstriction secondary to changes in blood pressure. There are reports that prostaglandin E_1* (PGE_1) or prostacyclin (PGI_2) administered intravenously has a beneficial effect in patients with Raynaud's phenomenon. These drugs can be given by constant intravenous infusion in a dose of 6 to 10 ng per kilogram per minute for a few hours, or for up to three days. It is reported that the beneficial effect outlasts this therapy by several weeks. (5) A novel but effective way of inducing vasodilation in the digits is via the iatrogenic induction of hyperthyroidism by the administration of triiodothyronine,* 75 μg daily. The resultant hypermetabolism elicits the normal thermoregulatory reflex and causes cutaneous vasodilation. The combination of triiodothyronine and reserpine has been found to be most effective.

Preganglionic sympathectomy to eliminate vasoconstrictor tone may have a beneficial immediate result, but the long-term results from this type of surgery are disappointing. It seems that an equally satisfactory result can be achieved by the use of drugs and that the duration of benefit is limited by regeneration of the nerves. If sympathectomy is contemplated, it is advisable to try sympathetic blockade with local anesthetics to verify a beneficial result. A recently devised technique that

*Investigational drug for this purpose.

involves surgical stripping of the palmar and digital arteries to bring about a local sympathectomy may also be tried, but its results have not been fully evaluated.

Coffman JD, Davis WT: Vasospastic diseases: A review. Prog Cardiovasc Dis 18:123, 1975. *A comprehensive, well-referenced review of vasospastic diseases.*

Cohen RA, Coffman JD: β-adrenergic vasodilator mechanism in the finger. Circ Res 49:1196, 1981. *Demonstration of a beta-adrenergic, humorally activated, vasodilative mechanism in the AV anastomoses of the human finger. Blockade of this mechanism may explain the occurrence of Raynaud's phenomenon in patients taking beta-adrenergic receptor blocking drugs.*

Harper FE, Maricq HR, Turner RE, Lidman RW, Leroy EC: A prospective study of Raynaud's phenomenon and early connective tissue disease. Am J Med 72:883, 1982. *This study of capillaries of the nailfold shows that the presence of capillary abnormalities in patients with Raynaud's phenomenon may have predictive value for the future development of scleroderma.*

Kontos HA, Wasserman AJ: Effect of reserpine in Raynaud's phenomenon. Circulation 39:259, 1969. *An analysis of the effects of reserpine given intra-arterially and orally on hand blood flow in patients with Raynaud's disease. It also contains evidence against the hypothesis that defective catecholamine metabolism may account for Raynaud's disease. Beneficial results from oral administration of reserpine are also presented.*

Miller D, Waters DD, Warnica W, Szlachcic J, Kreeft J, Théroux P: Is variant angina the coronary manifestation of a generalized vasospastic disorder? N Engl J Med 304:763, 1981. *Provocative study showing high incidence of migraine and Raynaud's phenomenon in patients with variant angina, suggesting the possibility that we may be dealing with a generalized vasospastic disorder.*

Smith CD, McKendry RJR: Controlled trial of nifedipine in the treatment of Raynaud's phenomenon. Lancet 2:1299, 1982. *Controlled trial showing beneficial results from nifedipine in Raynaud's phenomenon.*

Acrocyanosis

DEFINITION. Acrocyanosis is a rare disorder characterized by persistent cyanosis of the skin of the hands and, less commonly, of the feet associated with reduced skin temperature.

ETIOLOGY. Acrocyanosis, in contrast to Raynaud's phenomenon, is a primary disorder. Its cause is unknown. It is much more common in women than in men. The onset of the disease is usually in young adults or middle-aged persons. The high incidence of the disease among patients with psychiatric disorders is of unknown significance.

PATHOPHYSIOLOGY. The smaller precapillary vessels (arterioles) are abnormally constricted in acrocyanosis, causing reduction in blood flow and accounting for cyanosis and reduced skin temperature. The veins are secondarily dilated, perhaps because of the effects of ischemia. This constriction of the arterioles occurs under normal environmental conditions and becomes more pronounced on exposure to cold because of increased sensitivity of these vessels to the effects of cold. An important feature of acrocyanosis is the reduced venous tone. No venous obstruction is present. These features can be demonstrated by elevating the involved limb and eliminating the blue color or intensifying the blue color by placing the limb in a dependent position and overfilling the veins.

CLINICAL MANIFESTATIONS. Patients with acrocyanosis have persistent blue discoloration of the hands. Less commonly, the feet are also involved. In some cases, the blue color extends to more proximal portions of the limbs. The skin is cold, and the palms are wet and clammy from sweat. No pallor is usually present. In some cases, there may be spots of pallor surrounded by confluent cyanosis. The blue color is intensified by exposure to cold, and it is converted into purplish or red color by exposure to heat. There are few accompanying symptoms. The patient has feelings of coldness and, occasionally, numbness. Ulcerations and other trophic changes are distinctly unusual. Patients with acrocyanosis seek medical advice either because they are frightened by the occurrence of the cyanosis or because the cyanosis is cosmetically unappealing.

DIAGNOSIS. The distinction between acrocyanosis and Raynaud's phenomenon is discussed above in the section on Raynaud's phenomenon. Differentiation from cyanosis secondary to arterial obstruction can be made on the basis of normal pulses, by the bilateral and symmetrical occurrence of acrocyanosis and, if necessary, by the angiographic verification of absence of obstruction. The limitation of the cyanosis to the hands and feet, the improvement in a warm environment, and the absence of reduced arterial blood saturation distinguish acrocyanosis from generalized, systemic cyanosis.

TREATMENT. Since acrocyanosis is a benign disease that causes few symptoms and no serious morbidity, no drug therapy is usually required. Reassurance and protection from cold usually suffice. In some cases, cosmetic considerations or unusually severe symptoms may necessitate drug therapy. In these cases, the same drugs that are useful in Raynaud's phenomenon may be tried.

Lewis T, Landis EM: Observations upon the vascular mechanism in acrocyanosis. Heart 15:229, 1930. *Classic description of the clinical features of acrocyanosis. Evidence is presented showing that the disease is the result of an abnormal responsiveness of the smaller blood vessels.*

Livedo Reticularis

DEFINITION. Livedo reticularis is a reticular, bluish discoloration of the skin of the extremities which produces a lacy, irregular appearance outlining central areas of normal-appearing skin.

ETIOLOGY. The etiology of livedo reticularis is not known.

INCIDENCE. The disorder usually begins in young individuals before age 20 to 30 years. It is equally common in men and women but tends to be symptomatic more often in women.

PATHOLOGY. Proliferative lesions of the arterioles of the skin with perivascular infiltration have been described. In some cases, there may be thrombosis of arterioles with obstructions of the lumen leading to cutaneous infarction and ulceration. Similar changes are seen in the veins.

PATHOPHYSIOLOGY. The mechanism of livedo reticularis is presumed to be similar to that of acrocyanosis, namely, constriction of arterioles followed by stasis and dilation of capillaries and veins. The latter are filled with blood having desaturated hemoglobin and give the bluish discoloration to the skin. The reticular appearance of livedo reticularis is due to the anatomical arrangement of the affected vessels. It is believed that the bluish areas represent the arborizations of peripheral capillaries from central penetrating arterioles. Blood flow is faster in the central regions closer to the penetrating arteriole, while the more distant areas have lower flow with consequent stasis and cyanosis.

CLINICAL MANIFESTATIONS. The patients seek medical attention for cosmetic reasons or because they are frightened by the appearance of the bluish discoloration. The lower extremities are involved more often than the upper extremities. The patient usually has no symptoms. In some cases, there may be paresthesias or a feeling of coldness. The bluish discoloration becomes more intense on exposure to cold and may disappear in a warm environment. Ulcerations occur rarely; when they do, they appear in the winter months, and they heal in the summer.

TREATMENT. In most cases, no treatment is required. Protection from cold and abstinence from tobacco are useful. In severe cases, drugs useful in the treatment of Raynaud's phenomenon such as nifedipine and reserpine may be tried.

Feldaker M, Hines EA, Kierland RR: Livedo reticularis with ulcerations. Circulation 13:196, 1956. *Report of the clinical and pathologic features of 18 patients with livedo reticularis with ulcerations. A brief review of the earlier literature is included.*

Erythromelalgia (Erythermalgia)

DEFINITION. Erythromelalgia is a disorder manifested by episodes of erythema accompanied by increased skin temperature and by pain involving the feet and, less commonly, the hands.

ETIOLOGY. Erythromelalgia may be primary or it may be secondary to other disorders. These include obstructive arterial disease, polycythemia, and hypertension. There is no sex predilection, and the disease may occur at any age. It is occasionally hereditary.

PATHOPHYSIOLOGY. The symptoms of erythromelalgia are critically dependent on skin temperature. Rise in skin temperature above a certain level causes the manifestations. In each person this critical point is fairly constant. Vasodilation and consequent hyperemia are the usual causes of the rise in skin temperature that initiates the symptoms. However, an increased blood flow is not essential, as shown by the fact that after local heating initiates the disorder by raising the skin temperature above the critical level, the symptoms may continue even though blood flow is reduced to zero by inflating a cuff to a pressure level above systolic blood pressure. These features suggest that the cause of the disorder is abnormal sensitivity of the cutaneous pain fibers to heat or tension from the dilated blood vessels.

CLINICAL MANIFESTATIONS. The onset of the disease is gradual. With progression, the frequency and duration of the attacks become more pronounced. Finally, symptoms may become frequent or almost continuous and cause total disability. The patient, during an attack, complains of burning pain, usually in the feet and, less commonly, in the hands. Occasionally, more proximal portions of the limb may also be affected. Most commonly, the pain is located in the balls of the feet and in the tips of the toes and in the corresponding parts of the hands. The pain is aggravated by placing the involved limbs in a dependent position and ameliorated by elevating the limbs. Exposure to heat aggravates the disorder, while cold provides relief. Trophic changes, ulcerations, and gangrene are rare.

DIAGNOSIS. Peripheral neuropathy may cause burning pain simulating the pain of erythromelalgia. The pain may be accompanied by cutaneous vasodilation. The detection of the associated sensory and motor manifestations of peripheral neuropathy should help distinguish this condition from erythromelalgia. Arteriosclerosis obliterans or thromboangiitis obliterans may also produce localized burning pain and redness. The alterations in the arterial pulses and the absence of high skin temperature distinguish these conditions from erythromelalgia. Vascular damage from prolonged exposure to cold, as after frostbite, may simulate the manifestations of erythromelalgia. In these cases, the condition is more persistent and the history of cold exposure should help make the distinction possible.

TREATMENT. Avoidance of exposure to heat, particularly dry heat, prevents attacks of eyrthromelalgia. Should an attack occur, elevation of the extremity and application of cold may terminate the attack. Aspirin 0.5 gram orally relieves the pain in many cases. The response is sometimes so striking that it is of diagnostic value. Vasoconstrictive agents, such as methysergide or epinephrine, or beta-adrenergic blocking agents, such as propranolol, have been reported to be effective in some patients. In secondary cases, treatment of the primary disorder may alleviate the attacks.

Babb RR, Alarçon-Segovia D, Fairbairn JF: Erythermalgia: Review of 51 cases. Circulation 29:136, 1964. *Description of the features of primary and secondary erythromelalgia based on a study of a large number of patients.*

Lewis T: Clinical observations and experiments relating to burning pain in the extremities, and to so-called "erythromelalgia" in particular. Clin Sci 1:175, 1933. *A classic paper with detailed clinical descriptions of the manifestations of erythromelalgia. The paper also presents clinical investigations pertinent to the pathogenesis of the disease.*

VASCULAR DISEASES OF THE LIMBS CAUSED BY DAMAGE DUE TO COLD

Immersion Foot (Trench Foot)

DEFINITION. Immersion foot refers to the syndrome characterized by vascular damage resulting from prolonged exposure of the extremities to cold and dampness.

ETIOLOGY. Trench foot is seen following exposure to a cold environment while wearing wet socks or wet footwear for prolonged periods of time, usually several days. Trench foot has usually followed exposures to cold around 0°C. Dependency of limbs and immobility, as well as conditions that lead to general debility (lack of sleep and starvation), are contributory factors. The condition has been described primarily in soldiers at war.

Immersion foot has been described in survivors of shipwrecks, who were compelled to sit in crowded small craft for prolonged periods of time, and were exposed to a wet and cold environment that additionally caused immobility. Maceration of the skin with sea water and secondary infection also play a role in causing this condition.

PATHOPHYSIOLOGY. This condition results from vascular injury. The initial effect of a cold environment is to cause vasoconstriction. Loss of heat is facilitated by moisture. The resultant ischemia causes tissue and vascular injury with increased endothelial permeability to protein. There is extensive extravasation of protein and edema. As a result of the loss of fluid from the vessels, there may be increased hematocrit, sludging, and further aggravation of ischemia.

PATHOLOGY. Little is known about the earliest pathologic change in the blood vessels in immersion foot. Most of the available information was obtained from advanced cases with extensive vascular injury and gangrene. In these cases, the small arteries exhibit periarterial fibrosis and thickening and they may be occluded. The veins show perivenous fibrosis, inflammatory reaction, and hemorrhage. The nerves may also be affected. In cases of immersion foot at relatively high temperatures, hyperhydration of the plantar stratum corneum may be the only finding.

CLINICAL MANIFESTATIONS. Three successive stages, each with distinct clinical manifestations, are recognized. During exposure to the wet, cold environment, there is vasoconstriction. The involved extremity becomes pale and cool, and the patient has paresthesias and a feeling of coldness. A second hyperemic stage follows. The patients are observed most commonly during this stage, because this is the time when they seek attention. The involved extremity is red, hot, and edematous. There may be pain or paresthesias. The swelling may be aggravated by heat and by placing the limb in a dependent position. Subsequently, blebs appear in the affected limb. They are filled with serous or hemorrhagic fluid. Hemorrhages may occur into the skin and subcutaneous tissue. This stage may persist for several days. In severe cases, gangrene may supervene. The condition may be complicated by the development of lymphangitis, cellulitis, and thrombophlebitis. Mild cases or those treated early may recover after this second hyperemic phase. In other cases, a third late vasospastic phase occurs in which there is increased sensitivity to cold and typical secondary Raynaud's phenomenon, with excessive sweating. The patient has coldness, pain, and paresthesias of the lower extremities. This phase may persist for years.

TREATMENT. If the patient is seen in the initial vasoconstrictive phase, bed rest with the extremity in the horizontal position and a warm environment are necessary. During the hyperemic phase, the extremity should be placed at heart level and should be kept cool to diminish the development of edema. Local care to keep the foot dry and clean should be instituted to avoid infection. Control of pain may require analgesics or narcotics. Sympathectomy may be helpful in the hyperemic stage and also in preventing the late vasospastic phenomena.

Abramson DI, Lerner D, Shumacker HB, Hick FK: Clinical picture and treatment of the later stage of trench foot. Am Heart J 32:52, 1946. *Clinical report based on study of 633 patients with trench foot. Emphasis is placed on the late sequelae of the disorder.*

Frostbite

DEFINITION. Frostbite results from exposure of a limb to very low temperatures, which cause freezing of the tissues and consequent vascular injury.

ETIOLOGY. In most cases, frostbite occurred during prolonged exposure to temperatures below 0°C. In addition to the severity of the cold and duration of exposure, other environmental factors play a role, such as high wind and humidity. Predisposing factors include the presence of vascular disease, inadequate clothing, lack of acclimatization, and factors that lead to general debility.

PATHOPHYSIOLOGY. Tissue damage results from a combination of freezing of the tissues and ischemia, as a result of the cold-induced vasoconstriction. Freezing causes water crystal formation in cells, and dehydration. Vasoconstriction due to the direct or reflex effects of cold leads to reduced blood flow and stasis. Endothelial damage with increased permeability to protein ensues, causes edema, and further contributes to stasis and eventual thrombosis.

PATHOLOGY. The vessels are affected with endothelial swelling and vacuolization and with proliferative changes. Subsequently there is some inflammatory reaction and atrophic changes in the skin.

CLINICAL MANIFESTATION. Initially, the patient notices a prickling sensation followed by numbness. The skin becomes bloodless and appears white and cold. This is followed by redness, swelling, and increased temperature. Blisters may form 24 to 48 hours after thawing. They are filled with either serous yellow fluid or hemorrhagic fluid. There may be hemorrhages under the nail beds. Necrosis and gangrene may supervene. The subsequent course may be similar to what is seen in sudden arterial occlusion followed by severe ischemia and gangrene. Spontaneous amputation may require several weeks or months. After an attack of frostbite, the affected extremities may remain sensitive to cold for a period of time or permanently, and secondary Raynaud's phenomenon may be manifest.

TREATMENT. Frostbite should be treated with immediate rewarming. If frostbite affects deep tissues, rewarming should be done with water at 40 to 44°C. Muscular exercise of the involved limb or massage should be avoided, because they tend to increase edema and pain. If pain is severe, it should be treated with analgesics or narcotics as required. After the tissues have thawed, the exposed parts should remain at room temperature. Vesicles should be left untouched, and the limb should be left exposed, without dressings. Antibiotic therapy should be used if infection is present. Sympathectomy has been reported to be beneficial in the initial stages as well as in preventing the delayed sequelae of frostbite.

Washburn B: Frostbite. N Engl J Med 266:974, 1962. *Comprehensive consideration of the clinical features, pathology, diagnosis, prevention, and treatment of frostbite.*

Chilblain (Pernio)

DEFINITION. Chilblain is an inflammatory condition of the skin of the extremities induced by cold and characterized by erythema, itching, and ulceration.

ETIOLOGY AND INCIDENCE. The cause of chilblain is unknown. It is more common in cold, damp climates. The condition is much more common in England than it is in the United States. Women are affected more commonly than men. In most patients, the disease begins before the age of 20 years.

PATHOLOGY. In chronic cases, the lesions consist of angiitis with intimal proliferation, thickening of the arterial wall, and perivascular infiltration with lymphocytes and polymorphonuclear leukocytes. There may be necrosis of the adipose tissue and chronic inflammatory infiltrates in the subcutaneous tissue.

CLINICAL MANIFESTATIONS. Both acute and chronic forms of the disease are recognized. The typical patient is a young woman who in the winter notices bluish-red discoloration and edema of the skin of the lower limbs associated with burning and warmth. The lesions are persistent and are associated with itching. They generally last from 7 to 10 days and then clear up, sometimes leaving residual pigmentation of the skin. In severe cases, the lesions may become hemorrhagic or blebs may appear. Infection may supervene.

With repeated exposure to cold, susceptible persons may develop chronic lesions. These are erythematous, ulcerative, and hemorrhagic lesions that begin as raised erythematous areas 0.5 to 1 cm in diameter. These lesions are then transformed into blebs and finally ulcerate. Healing occurs in the summer, leaving a permanently pigmented region.

DIAGNOSIS. Acute chilblain is distinguished from other forms of dermatitis by its characteristic distribution and by its relationship to cold. Chronic chilblain needs to be distinguished from erythema induratum and erythema nodosum. Erythema induratum of Bazin is caused by *Mycobacterium tuberculosis.* If the infection is active, the differential diagnosis may be made by the microscopic demonstration or culture of bacteria. Erythema induratum affects the upper part of the legs more frequently than the lower part. The lesions are more nodular, deeper, and infiltrative. They are also more permanent, while those of chronic chilblain clear up in the summer. Erythema nodosum is a more acute process, and it is usually associated with a systemic reaction, consisting of fever, malaise, and arthralgias. There is no seasonal association.

TREATMENT. In mild cases, protection from cold, local application of anti-inflammatory ointments, avoidance of scratching, and cessation of smoking are usually sufficient. In more severe cases, drugs that have been found useful in the treatment of Raynaud's phenomenon, such as reserpine, may be effective.

Eskell J: Reserpine in the treatment of chilblains. Practitioner 189:792, 1962. *Report of a controlled clinical trial of reserpine in patients with chilblain showing excellent benefit.*

Lynn RB: Chilblains. Surg Gynecol Obstet 99:720, 1954. *Concise description of the clinical and pathologic features of chilblain.*

VASCULAR DISEASES OF THE LIMBS DUE TO ORGANIC ARTERIAL OBSTRUCTION

Arteriosclerosis Obliterans

DEFINITION. Arteriosclerosis obliterans consists of segmental arteriosclerotic narrowing or obstruction of the lumen in the arteries supplying the limbs.

ETIOLOGY AND INCIDENCE. The etiology of arteriosclerosis in general is discussed in another chapter (see Ch. 48).

Arteriosclerosis obliterans is the commonest cause of arterial obstructive disease of the extremities. The disease becomes clinically manifest usually between the ages of 50 and 70. It is unusual in individuals younger than 30 years of age. Men are affected more often than women. The lower limbs are involved much more frequently than the upper limbs. The most commonly affected vessel is the superficial femoral artery. The distal aorta and its bifurcation into the two iliac arteries and the popliteal artery are the next most frequent sites of involvement. The presence of diabetes mellitus influences arteriosclerosis obliterans in a number of important ways. In diabetics, arteriosclerosis obliterans is likely to be more progressive. This is reflected in a much higher incidence of intermittent claudication in diabetics. The disease affects arterial vessels of smaller caliber and more distally located vessels more frequently than in nondiabetics. The incidence of involvement of vessels below the knee with arteriosclerosis obliterans in diabetics is considerably higher than in nondiabetics.

PATHOLOGY. The lesions of arteriosclerosis obliterans are typical atheromatous plaques involving the intima of the arteries. As a rule, there is superimposed thrombus formation. The media of the vessels shows degenerative changes. Calcification of the media is frequent and may take the form of a ringlike arrangement as in Mönckeberg's sclerosis. Medial calcification is twice as frequent in diabetics as in nondiabetics. These arteriosclerotic lesions are segmental, and they are typically multiple. Weakening of the media may give rise to aneurysmal dilation of the involved artery. Such arteriosclerotic aneurysms are most common in the popliteal fossa or in the femoral artery below the inguinal ligament. They may be filled with thrombi.

PATHOPHYSIOLOGY. The arterial obstruction or narrowing causes reduction in blood flow during exercise or at rest. Clinical symptoms are caused by the consequent ischemia. The most important feature of the stenosis in determining the occurrence of ischemia is the cross-sectional area of the stenotic segment. Because the vascular bed of the extremities generally has a high resting vascular tone and, therefore, a large capacity for vasodilation, a moderate degree of stenosis can be compensated fully by downstream dilation. Stenoses that decrease the cross-sectional area of the vessel by less than 75 per cent do not usually affect resting blood flow. When the prevailing flow rates are high, as in exercise, decreases of 60 per cent or more of the cross-sectional area of the vessel are required before a reduction in flow occurs. Vasodilation in response to ischemia is the result of the action of local mechanisms. These include myogenic mechanisms related to reduction in intravascular pressure or metabolic mechanisms due to release of vasodilative metabolites from the ischemic tissues. These local mechanisms compete with neurogenic mechanisms that, when activated, cause vasoconstriction. Increased sympathetic activity, as from exposure to cold, may, therefore, induce ischemia in the presence of an arterial obstructing lesion.

The presence or absence of ischemia in the face of severe arterial stenosis or obstruction is frequently determined by the degree of development of collateral circulation. Some of these collateral vessels are present in the normal limb but are not used until the obstruction takes place. They open up immediately after an acute arterial occlusion. Others take several weeks or months to become fully developed. Little is known about the responsiveness of collateral vessels. They are subject to neurogenic vasoconstriction from the action of adrenergic nerves. They dilate in response to increased blood pressure, so that an increased pressure will result in improved collateral blood flow through these vessels.

CLINICAL MANIFESTATIONS. The symptoms of arteriosclerosis obliterans are intermittent claudication, rest pain, and trophic changes in the involved limb. Intermittent claudication denotes pain that develops in a limb on exercise and disappears when the patient rests. The pain is usually described as a cramp or a tightness or as severe fatigue of the exercising muscles. The amount of exercise necessary to induce the pain is usually constant for any given patient. The pain is usually bilateral but may be unilateral. In some patients, the pain disappears by slowing the pace of walking without complete cessation of exercise. The location of the pain is distal to the arterial obstruction. The most frequently affected muscles are those of the calf, because these muscles are the ones that do most of the work during exercise and because of the high frequency with which the femoral artery is involved. The muscles of the lower part of the back, the buttocks, the thigh, and the foot may also be affected.

Rest pain occurs when a pronounced reduction in resting blood flow is present. It is a sign of severe disease. The pain may be localized to one or more toes, or it may have a stocking-type distribution. The character of the pain is usually burning or gnawing. It is generally worse at night. It is improved by placing the limb in a dependent position and by cooling. There may be associated symptoms, such as feelings of coldness and numbness, together with cyanosis or pallor of the extremity.

Examination of the patient with clinically manifest arteriosclerosis obliterans discloses reduced or absent arterial pulses distal to the obstruction. There may be bruits audible over the aorta or its branches. These may be systolic, or they may be continuous. In advanced cases, examination may reveal signs of ischemia. The skin temperature may be abnormally low, or there may be pallor or cyanosis. Ischemic damage may cause persistent reddish or reddish-blue discoloration. There may be trophic changes, including a dry, scaly, and shiny atrophic skin. The hair may disappear, and the toenails may become brittle, ridged, and deformed. There may be ulcerations or gangrene. The ischemic ulcers are usually at pressure points, and they may be inflamed and painful.

Leriche's syndrome refers to isolated aortoiliac disease, which produces a fairly characteristic clinical picture. There is intermittent claudication of the low back, buttocks, and thigh or calf muscles. There is atrophy of the limbs and pallor of the skin of the feet and legs. Impotence may also be present. Arterial pulses in the legs are absent; they may be present but weak in the femoral arteries. Systolic bruits may be audible over the femoral arteries and lower abdomen.

Arteriosclerotic aneurysms may occur. The presence of a pulsatile, expansible mass in the popliteal fossa or in the femoral artery below the inguinal ligament indicates the presence of aneurysms. These may cause symptoms by pressure on adjacent structures and, occasionally, by either embolism of peripheral vessels or by hemorrhage into the tissues.

DIAGNOSIS. The diagnostic approach to the patient with arteriosclerosis obliterans should be directed at establishing the site of the arterial obstruction, its severity, the degree of ischemia, and the adequacy of the collateral circulation. The examination of the arterial pulses by palpation and the presence of bruits by auscultation usually suffice to determine the presence and site of arterial obstruction. Trophic changes and alterations in skin color and temperature indicate the presence of ischemia. The latter, as well as the adequacy of the collateral circulation, can be further ascertained by determining the blood pressure at the ankle at rest and during exercise. Several tests may be helpful. With the patient in a warm environment, so that vasoconstrictor tone is low, the leg is raised at a 45 degree angle while the patient is supine. The color of the plantar surface of the foot is observed. Pallor during this test is indicative of severe arterial insufficiency. Venous and capillary filling times can be measured when the patient goes from the recumbent to the sitting position. Ordinarily, delay in flushing by more than 20 to 30 seconds indicates inadequate collateral circulation. The systolic blood pressure in the dorsalis pedis or posterior tibial arteries can be determined with the use of a Doppler velocitometer at rest as well as during exercise. Ordinarily, this pressure should not be lower than 90 per cent of the level of systolic pressure in the brachial artery. In the presence of severe ischemia, pressures may fall to very low levels. As a rule, pressures less than 30 mm Hg indicate ischemia of sufficient severity to cause gangrene.

The confirmation of the presence of arterial obstruction is carried out by arteriography which is essential to establish the exact anatomy of the arterial vessels and to determine the advisability of surgery.

Arterial embolism is usually distinguishable from arteriosclerosis obliterans because of the sudden onset of the ischemic manifestations and the usually unilateral involvement. Intermittent claudication may occur in severe anemia, venous disease, and in muscle phosphorylase deficiency (McArdle's syndrome). These conditions are distinguished from arteriosclerosis obliterans by the presence of normal pulses. Ergotamine or methysergide toxicity may cause severe vasospasm, which may affect the large arteries and cause diminution of pulses. The history of drug ingestion may help distinguish these from arteriosclerosis obliterans. In difficult cases, angiography shows the generalized vasospasm and absence of segmental obstructions. A number of conditions of nonvascular nature, such as arthritis and lumbar disc disorders, may cause pain in the limbs that may be confused with intermittent claudication. The presence of normal pulses and other manifestations of these diseases distinguishes them from arteriosclerotic obliterans. In diabetics, ulcerations may be present as a result of diabetic neuropathy. The distinction of the cause of these ulcers may be difficult in the presence of associated arteriosclerosis obliterans.

TREATMENT. Patients with arteriosclerosis obliterans without evidence of ischemia should be treated medically. Limitation of physical activity, avoidance of tobacco smoking (which causes vasoconstriction), and a regular exercise program are advisable. The treatment of hyperlipidemia, if present, may prevent development of new arteriosclerotic lesions. The control of diabetes, if present, is required. Patients should maintain the skin of the affected limbs clean, dry, and soft, and protect it from cold and trauma. Infections and trauma should be attended to promptly. There is no evidence that vasodilative drugs are effective in the treatment of arteriosclerosis obliterans. In fact, they may be harmful under certain circumstances by lowering arterial blood pressure and reducing collateral blood flow, or by diverting blood to proximal healthy areas, thereby reducing the perfusion pressure in the more distal portions of the limb.

Surgical treatment is advisable when evidence of ischemia is present, or if intermittent claudication seriously interferes with the patient's activities. Surgery is aimed at restoring the continuity of the arterial circulation beyond the segmental obstruction or stenosis of the artery, which is responsible for the reduction in blood flow. This involves either endarterectomy or a bypass operation. Bypass is performed by either a vein graft obtained from the saphenous vein or by synthetic material. Vein grafts are preferred because of the lower incidence of thrombosis. It is essential that the presence of patent vessels below the obstruction be ascertained before the grafting procedure is carried out. A variety of connections is possible. Axillofemoral or femorofemoral grafts for aortoiliac disease have been successful. The larger the size of the vessels grafted, the higher the rate of successful restoration of blood flow.

Percutaneous transluminal angioplasty has been recently introduced for the treatment of arteriosclerosis obliterans. In this technique, the segmental stenosis or obstruction is dilated by inflating suddenly a balloon introduced into the artery at the site of the lesion by percutaneous catheterization. The initial results show a high incidence of successful dilation of the stenosis and good long-term rates of patency of the dilated vessels. Angioplasty is more successful in larger vessels, when the stenotic segment is relatively short and when the vessel is not completely, or almost completely, occluded. The technique is simple, has low morbidity, and is less costly than surgery.

If the anatomy of the disease makes surgery impossible and ischemic manifestations are present, bed rest is essential. The affected extremity should be kept in a slightly dependent position at 20 to 30 degrees below horizontal, and direct application of heat should be avoided. The limb is best kept warm by placing it under a cradle, under which the temperature is regulated below 38°C. Analgesics or narcotics may be required to control pain. Ulcers should be kept clean with warm saline soaks and should undergo debridement. Appropriate antibiotics should be used if infection is present. It has been reported that the intra-arterial administration of PGE_1* in patients with gangrene or ulceration in whom surgery was not possible was beneficial in avoiding amputation. Amputation may be necessary to arrest advancing gangrene. The level of amputation is chosen by the presence of warm, viable tissue having normal color.

Long-term anticoagulants are of questionable value. Fibrinolytic therapy with intravenous streptokinase is reported to be helpful in a few patients with recent onset of the disease.

Preganglionic lumbar sympathectomy may be performed as an acute intervention to treat ischemic manifestations of arteriosclerosis obliterans. Before surgery, it must be demonstrated that the interruption of sympathetic nerves is likely to cause improvement in the circulation of the limb. This is done by inducing temporary sympathetic blockade with local anesthetics. This is essential, especially in diabetics in whom peripheral neuropathy may have already produced spontaneous sympathectomy. Sympathectomy does not influence the long-term progress of intermittent claudication.

PROGNOSIS. Arteriosclerosis obliterans in the absence of diabetes is a slowly progressive disease. No significant deterioration may be detected for several years. In the presence of diabetes, the disease tends to progress more rapidly, and the prognosis is less satisfactory. The location of obstructing lesions also influences the prognosis. When the lesions are in larger arteries, the probability of successful surgical intervention or percutaneous angioplasty is higher, and the prognosis is better. Frequently, arteriosclerosis obliterans is only one of the manifestations of a generalized arteriosclerotic process. Mortality results from arteriosclerotic involvement of other vascular beds, such as the coronary or the cerebral circulation, with death from myocardial infarction or stroke.

Coffman JD: Intermittent claudication and rest pain. Physiologic concepts and therapeutic approaches. Prog Cardiovasc Dis 22:53, 1979. *A comprehensive, well-referenced consideration of the clinical features, diagnosis, and treatment of arteriosclerosis obliterans.*

Coffman JD: Vasodilator drugs in peripheral vascular disease. N Engl J Med 300:713, 1979. *A critical evaluation of vasodilative drugs in arteriosclerosis obliterans.*

Freiman DB, Spence R, Gatenby R, Gertner M, Roberts B, Berkowitz HD, Ring EJ, Oleaga JA: Transluminal angioplasty of the iliac and femoral arteries: Follow-up results with anticoagulation. Radiology 141:347, 1981. *Transluminal angioplasty for the treatment of obstructive disease of the iliac and femoral arteries. Excellent results are reported in 192 patients.*

Schadt DC, Hines EA, Juergens JL, Barker NW: Chronic atherosclerotic occlusion of the femoral artery. JAMA 175:937, 1961. *A long-term follow-up study showing slow progression of arteriosclerosis obliterans.*

Thromboangiitis Obliterans (Buerger's Disease)

DEFINITION. Thromboangiitis obliterans is an obstructive arterial disease caused by segmental inflammatory and proliferative lesions of the medium and small arteries and veins of the limbs.

ETIOLOGY. The cause of thromboangiitis obliterans is unknown. There is a very strong association with tobacco smoking, particularly cigarette smoking. Almost all patients with this disease are moderate or heavy smokers. Because of a high incidence of cutaneous hypersensitivity to intradermally injected tobacco products, it was suggested that the disorder may represent a hypersensitivity reaction to tobacco. A high prevalence of HLA-A9 and HLA-B5 antigens in affected persons led to the suggestion that a specific phenotype may be susceptible to precipitation of the disease by exposure to tobacco. The possibility that this disease may be caused by autoimmune factors was strengthened recently in a study of cellular and humoral immune responses of 39 patients with thromboangiitis obliterans. Lymphocytes from 77 per cent of these patients exhibited cellular sensitivity to human Type I and Type III collagen, both of which are constituents of the vascular wall. In addition, approximately 50 per cent of the patients had significant levels of anticollagen antibodies in their blood. In contrast, normal controls and patients with arteriosclerosis obliterans had considerably lower levels of cellular sensitivity to collagen and no circulating anticollagen antibodies.

INCIDENCE. Thromboangiitis obliterans is a disease mostly of young males. The disease begins most frequently between the ages of 20 and 40 years, and the ratio of men to women affected varies from 9:1 to as high as 75:1. There is a high prevalence of the disorder in Israel, in the Orient, and in India as compared with the United States and Western Europe, suggesting the possibility of a genetic predisposition. The disease has been occasionally reported to occur in familial form.

PATHOLOGY. The disease affects small and medium size arteries and veins in segmental fashion. The diseased portions of the vessels are separated by unaffected areas. Acute lesions are manifested by proliferation of the intima and thrombosis. There is inflammatory infiltration with polymorphonuclear leukocytes, lymphocytes, and giant cells of all coats of the artery or vein, extending into the thrombus. The media remains intact. Calcium deposition or cholesterol deposition does not occur. These lesions are distinguished from those of arteriosclerosis obliterans because of the more cellular thrombus, the preservation of the media, and the inflammatory infiltration of all coats of the vessel. Destruction of the media with fibrosis and calcification and atheromatous changes are not seen. Older lesions become less cellular and eventually they may be transformed into a dense scar. Typically, in any one vessel, lesions of varying ages are seen. This is the result of the development of new lesions in crops separated by quiescent periods.

CLINICAL MANIFESTATIONS. The typical patient with thromboangiitis obliterans is a young man who smokes cigarettes heavily, has manifestations of ischemia of the extremities and either evidence of superficial thrombophlebitis or a history of thrombophlebitis. Common presenting complaints are Raynaud's phenomenon with digital ulcerations or pain from

*Investigational drug for this purpose.

ischemia. Pain in thromboangiitis obliterans may be of several types. The most frequent type is rest pain in one or more digits. This pain may be accompanied by manifestations of ischemia, such as color changes or temperature changes of the skin. This type of pain may be a forerunner of impending ulceration or gangrene. In the presence of these trophic lesions there may be localized pain that is aching in character and is more severe at night. Another type of pain may occur along the course of the inflamed blood vessels. Ischemic neuropathy may result and cause a paroxysmal shocklike pain, which may follow the distribution of sensory nerves. Paresthesias may be an accompaniment of this type of pain. Typical intermittent claudication occurs commonly in the lower extremities. It is most often seen in the arch of the foot because of the involvement of the vessels of the leg and sparing of the femoral and iliac arteries. Some patients have intermittent claudication of the muscles of the forearm or hand. Sensitivity to cold with complaints of coldness and paresthesias and the development of secondary Raynaud's phenomenon are common. Migratory superficial thrombophlebitis is manifested by the development of inflamed, tender, red segments of the superficial veins which subside over a period of several weeks.

Physical examination discloses impaired arterial pulsations. The abnormal pulses are in the more distal portions of the limbs such as the radial, ulnar, dorsalis pedis, and posterior tibial arteries. The more proximal arteries are normal, a finding that contrasts with arteriosclerosis obliterans. There may be cyanosis or pallor, or persistent redness in the digits and associated changes in temperature may be noted. Postural changes in color are also common. Gangrene or ulcerations of the digits are commonly seen. They may be present in both the upper and lower extremities. Edema of the foot is common. Occasional patients have involvement of visceral arteries with stenosis or occlusion of mesenteric, coronary, cerebral, or renal arteries and manifestations of ischemia of these organs.

DIAGNOSIS. The diagnosis of thromboangiitis obliterans should be entertained when there is evidence of ischemia of the extremities from arterial occlusive disease in association with migratory superficial thrombophlebitis. The age and sex of the individual and the involvement of the upper extremities are additional helpful characteristics. Arteriography may be helpful in disclosing segmental multiple occlusions of the medium size and small arteries associated with collateral vessel visualization. The larger arteries are generally spared, a finding that also helps distinguish this disorder from arteriosclerosis obliterans. Final confirmation may be obtained only from biopsy material of an early lesion and the histologic demonstration of the characteristic inflammatory and proliferative lesion of the disease.

PROGNOSIS. Thromboangiitis obliterans is not usually life-threatening except in rare individuals in whom the visceral arteries are involved. The disease, however, results in disability and amputation of the extremities in a high percentage of cases. It is generally more rapidly progressive than arteriosclerosis obliterans, especially in individuals who refuse to stop smoking.

TREATMENT. Cessation of tobacco smoking is essential. Continuation of smoking results in a progressive course. If the patient stops smoking, new lesions do not develop or they develop more rarely. The approach to the patient with thromboangiitis obliterans is generally the same as that of patients with advanced arteriosclerosis obliterans. It consists of conservative measures, including protection from cold, local care in the event of ulceration or gangrene, and eventually amputation, if these lesions occur. Sympathectomy is tried frequently and may be effective, at least temporarily, if vasospasm is a prominent feature. Vasodilative drug therapy can be tried in cases of Raynaud's phenomenon with ulcerations, but its effectiveness is questionable.

Adar R, Papa MZ, Halpern Z, Mozes M, Soshan S, Sofer B, Zinger H, Dayan M, Mozes E: Cellular sensitivity to collagen in thromboangiitis obliterans. N Engl J Med 308:1113, 1983. *An important study showing high incidence of cellular sensitivity to collagen, and the presence of circulating anticollagen antibodies in patients with thromboangiitis obliterans. The results have profound implications concerning the etiology of the disease and offer possible means of differentiating it from arteriosclerosis obliterans.*

McKusick VA, Harris WS, Ottesen OE, Goodman RM, Shelley WM, Bloodwell RD: Buerger's disease: A distinct clinical and pathologic entity. JAMA 181:5, 1962. *A concise and thoughtful consideration of the clinical features, arteriographic findings, and histopathology of 30 cases with Buerger's disease.*

Sudden Arterial Occlusion

DEFINITION. Sudden arterial occlusion may result from obstruction of an artery of the extremity by embolism or by thrombosis in situ. The clinical manifestations are the result of the consequent ischemia.

ETIOLOGY. Sudden arterial thrombosis occurs in about 10 per cent of the cases of arteriosclerosis obliterans. The condition is rare in thromboangiitis obliterans. Polyarteritis nodosa is a rare cause of sudden arterial thrombosis. Acute arterial thrombosis may occur in conditions in which the coagulability of the blood is increased in the presence of normal vessels, such as in polycythemia vera or in cryoglobulinemia. Rarely, arterial thrombosis may occur in the presence of normal vessels in infections such as septicemia, pneumonia, peritonitis, tuberculosis, ulcerative colitis, and other debilitating diseases. Trauma from penetrating wounds as from arterial puncture or catheterization may cause arterial occlusion.

Fragments of thrombus from another source in the blood stream which break away and occlude an artery are the major causes of arterial embolism. The heart is the most frequent source of emboli in this syndrome. Emboli may arise from thrombi in the left atrium in the presence of atrial fibrillation or in the presence of mitral valve disease, usually mitral stenosis. Emboli may also arise from mural thrombi from a myocardial infarction or in the presence of a cardiomyopathy. Septic emboli may arise from vegetations from the mitral or aortic valves in the presence of bacterial endocarditis. Less commonly, emboli may arise from an arteriosclerotic plaque in more proximal parts of the arterial tree or from aneurysms. In rare cases, the embolus may arise from the venous side and enter the arterial tree via a patent foramen ovale (paradoxical embolism). More rarely, the embolus consists of calcium fragments from a calcified valve leaflet, cholesterol crystals from an arteriosclerotic plaque, or foreign materials such as a bullet.

PATHOLOGY. The structure of emboli that arise from thrombi in the heart or from aneurysms is the same as that of the parent thrombi. Emboli lodge in an artery and obstruct the vessel. There may be extension of the thrombus distally by further clotting of the blood. The fate of the embolus varies. In some cases it may become organized and finally be recanalized, and in other cases it may become fragmented and the fragments may lodge in more distal vessels.

PATHOPHYSIOLOGY. The sudden arterial occlusion causes reduction of blood flow to the more distal portions of the limb and consequent ischemia. There have been suggestions that vasoactive agents released from the emboli, such as serotonin from platelets, may cause contraction of vascular smooth muscle in more distal portions of the vascular tree and result in vasospasm that further aggravates ischemia. The severity and extent of ischemia depend on the size of the vessel occluded and on the extent of collateral circulation. The larger the occluded vessel, the more likely it is that severe ischemia would result.

CLINICAL MANIFESTATIONS. Sudden arterial occlusion causes the abrupt onset of severe pain accompanied by manifestations of ischemia in about half the patients. In the remainder, the onset is gradual with either mild pain or numbness and paresthesias. Pain is present in about 75 per cent of the cases. There may be muscular weakness or outright paralysis. A saddle embolus of the aortic bifurcation causes abdominal pain, nausea, and vomiting and may result in a shocklike state.

Examination of the patient discloses diminished or absent pulses distal to the occlusion. Evidence of ischemia is present with low skin temperature and either pallor or cyanosis or a combination of the two. If the occluded artery is superficial, the site of lodgement of the embolus may be identified as a tender region. The subsequent course of the condition depends on the adequacy of the collateral circulation. If this is adequate, gradual improvement occurs. Otherwise, gangrene supervenes.

DIAGNOSIS. The diagnosis of sudden arterial occlusion is usually relatively easy in the patient who has the acute onset of pain and ischemia of an extremity. If the cause of the occlusion is an embolus, its source may be evident. Rarely, patients with acute thrombophlebitis of the iliac and femoral veins may have feeble or absent arterial pulses and show manifestations resembling those of ischemia from an arterial embolus. In these cases, the demonstration of the feeble pulse and the presence of distended veins and pronounced edema help make the differentiation possible.

PROGNOSIS. The outcome of acute arterial obstruction depends on the size of the vessel affected, the age of the patient, the extent of the collateral circulation, and the timing of therapeutic intervention. When a large artery is occluded, the prognosis is poor without surgical treatment. In older patients with pre-existing arterial occlusive disease, the prognosis is poor because of obstruction of multiple vessels including collateral vessels.

TREATMENT. Urgent embolectomy is the preferred method of treatment when a large artery is occluded, such as with a saddle embolus at the bifurcation of the aorta. When smaller vessels are occluded, conservative medical treatment should be tried first. The patient should be placed at rest. The limb should be placed in a slightly dependent position under a cradle whose temperature is controlled at 30 to 35°C. Anticoagulation with heparin should be started as soon as possible to prevent extension of the thrombus and to prevent formation of additional emboli. If vasospasm is prominent, lumbar sympathectomy may be tried to reduce vasomotor tone and improve blood flow to the limb. Thrombolytic therapy with intravenous streptokinase results in lysis of the thrombus and patency of the occluded artery in about one third of the cases. It should be followed by anticoagulation.

When a patient is treated by conservative medical measures, he should be followed closely for evidence of deterioration. If this occurs, immediate surgical intervention and embolectomy should be attempted. The results of embolectomy depend, to a large extent, on the timing of intervention. Therefore, surgery should not be delayed longer than a few hours. If therapy fails, gangrene may supervene and amputation may become necessary.

Haimovici H: Peripheral arterial embolism. Angiology 1:20, 1950. *Detailed consideration of the clinical features of embolism of the arteries of the limbs based on study of 330 cases.*

Hargrove WC, Barker CF, Berkowitz HD, Perloff LJ, McLean G, Freiman D, Ring EJ, Roberts B: Treatment of acute peripheral arterial and graft thromboses with low-dose streptokinase. Surgery 92:981, 1982. *A report of good results from the use of intra-arterial streptokinase for the treatment of acute arterial thrombosis.*

Hinton RC, Kistler JP, Fallon JT, Friedlich AL, Fisher CM: Influence of etiology of atrial fibrillation on incidence of systemic embolism. Am J Cardiol 40:509, 1977. *A study of the pathology of arterial embolism in 333 patients with atrial fibrillation. The paper emphasizes that the risk of embolism is independent of the cause of atrial fibrillation.*

VASCULAR DISEASES OF THE LIMBS DUE TO ABNORMAL COMMUNICATION BETWEEN ARTERIES AND VEINS

Arteriovenous Fistula

DEFINITION. Arteriovenous fistula is an abnormal direct communication between an artery and a vein.

ETIOLOGY. Arteriovenous fistulas in the limbs may be congenital or acquired. Congenital fistulas are usually multiple; acquired ones are usually single. The most common type is iatrogenic, created to carry out renal dialysis. Other causes of acquired arteriovenous fistulas are trauma from penetrating wounds or in the course of surgery.

PATHOPHYSIOLOGY. The low resistance of the direct communication between artery and vein results in a high arterial inflow into the vein, with a resultant increase in venous pressure. The elevated venous pressure causes engorgement of the vein and distention and may lead to the production of varicose veins. In the region of the fistula, blood flow is high, while more distal portions are deprived of capillary blood flow and may show ischemia and trophic changes.

Large fistulas cause a reduction in systemic vascular resistance and impose a burden on the heart because of the associated increase in cardiac output. Total blood volume may be increased. Left ventricular failure may eventually result.

PATHOLOGY. In the region of the fistula the veins become thickened while the artery undergoes thinning and loss of elastic and muscular fibers in the media.

CLINICAL MANIFESTATIONS. The patient may be totally asymptomatic and the discovery of the fistula may be accidental. In other cases, there may be pain in the location of the fistula, edema, varicosities, and asymmetry in the size of the limbs. In some cases, the presenting symptoms may be those of cardiac decompensation with dyspnea on exertion, palpitations, and orthopnea. Examination of the involved limb reveals tortuous, dilated, superficial veins and venous pulsation at the site of the fistula. The temperature of the skin may be high while distal portions of the limb may show ischemic changes. A bruit or a thrill may be heard over the fistula during systole. At other times, a continuous bruit may be present. The extremity may be swollen or the girth of the limb may be increased because of hypertrophy of the soft tissues. Temporary compression of the artery proximal to the fistula causes immediate increase in systemic vascular resistance and leads to reflex decrease in heart rate (Branham's sign), a change that may be helpful diagnostically.

DIAGNOSIS. When the fistula is superficial and large, the diagnosis can be made easily. If this is not possible from the physical examination, arteriography should be attempted for a definitive diagnosis. The oxygen saturation of the venous blood from the involved limb is higher than that of its contralateral part, and this comparison may be helpful in making the diagnosis.

TREATMENT. Surgical intervention with closure of the fistula and re-establishment of the continuity of the involved artery and vein is the treatment of choice. If this type of complete restoration is not possible, ligation of the artery or vein or both may be necessary, but this may lead to arterial or venous insufficiency of the limb. In some cases, the fistula involves an anomalous artery. In this case, the ligation of the artery and the obstruction of the veins by the injection of sclerosing solutions may give a satisfactory result. It may not be practical to treat surgically patients with multiple fistulas. In these cases, conservative measures consisting of local care, relief of pain, and wearing of elastic bandages may be helpful. If the fistula is inoperable and cardiac decompensation is present or threatened, amputation may be necessary.

Nickerson JL, Elkin DC, Warren JV: The effect of temporary occlusion of arteriovenous fistulas on heart rate, stroke volume, and cardiac output. J Clin Invest 30:215, 1951. *A classic study of the systemic hemodynamic effects of arteriovenous fistulas in a large number of patients.*

Rossi P, Carillo FJ, Alfidi RJ, Ruzicka FF: Iatrogenic arteriovenous fistulas. Radiology 111:47, 1974. *A comprehensive review of 154 cases of iatrogenic arteriovenous fistulas. The paper provides a good review of the literature.*

Glomus Tumor (Glomangioma)

DEFINITION. Glomangioma or glomus tumor is a benign tumor of the glomus body.

PATHOLOGY. The glomus tumor is an encapsulated structure consisting of a hypertrophied arteriovenous anastomosis. The tumor varies in size from 0.5 to 2.5 cm in diameter. It can be found in various parts of the upper and lower extremities but is most frequently located in the nail beds.

CLINICAL MANIFESTATIONS. The most common symptom is severe burning pain in the location of the tumor. The pain may precede the appearance of the tumor. Pain may occur spontaneously or it may be precipitated by exposure to heat or cold. Occasionally, the tumor is exquisitely sensitive to touch and even the slightest pressure from contact with clothing may cause severe pain. Severe disability and atrophy of the limb from disuse may occur secondary to fear by the patient of using the extremity because of the pain. Examination of the involved area shows a reddish, purplish, or bluish mass that is sharply demarcated from the surrounding tissues. At times, the tumor may not be easily visible or palpable. In this case, pressure with the head of a pin may help identify the location of the tumor. When it is located under the nail bed, the nail and the phalanx may be visibly deformed, thereby giving a clue as to the location of the tumor.

TREATMENT. The glomus tumor is a benign tumor. Surgical excision results in complete relief without recurrence.

Cooke SAR: Misleading features in the clinical diagnosis of the peripheral glomus tumour. Br J Surg 58:602, 1971. *The clinical manifestations of glomus tumor are described based on the study of 24 cases.*

DISEASES OF THE VEINS OF THE LIMBS

Thrombophlebitis

DEFINITION. Thrombophlebitis refers to venous thrombosis with or without accompanying inflammation of the venous wall.

PATHOLOGY. Thrombi in veins are of the red variety. They consist mostly of red cells with a few platelets held together with fibrin. They propagate in the direction of the blood stream by extension of the thrombotic process. They attach to the wall of the vein at one end, while the more proximal end floats freely into the lumen of the vessel. This is the portion that is commonly broken off and travels to the lungs. Varying degrees of inflammatory reaction of the venous wall may be present. Venous thrombosis may exist in the absence of inflammation, as is the case in some patients with malignancy. This is referred to as "phlebothrombosis." In most cases, however, inflammation and thrombosis coexist. The disorder may start as a pure thrombotic process, and inflammation usually occurs secondary to the presence of the thrombus.

INCIDENCE. Thrombophlebitis is a common disorder. It is more common in women than in men. All races seem to be affected equally, at least in civilized countries. The incidence of the disease increases with advancing age. The disease is very common in hospitalized patients. Approximately one third of the patients over age 40 undergoing major surgery or after an acute myocardial infarction develop thrombophlebitis. The incidence is even higher after certain operations such as repair of hip fractures or prostatectomy. Patients with thrombotic strokes have an equally high incidence of thrombophlebitis. This occurs almost exclusively in the paralyzed limb.

PATHOGENESIS. Venous stasis, injury to the venous wall, and a hypercoagulable state are the three main factors that lead to venous thrombosis. In most cases, more than one of these factors are present, and their effect may be cumulative. The combination of venous stasis and changes in the clotting mechanism of the blood accounts for the increased incidence of thrombophlebitis in pregnancy and during administration of oral contraceptives. Venous stasis is the major factor in the development of thrombophlebitis in patients with heart disease, in paralyzed patients, in patients undergoing major surgery, in those that have varicose veins, and in healthy individuals after long trips. Increased viscosity, leading to stasis, and alterations in the clotting factors of the blood account for the high incidence in polycythemia vera. Patients with a rare familial decrease in antithrombin III are susceptible to thrombophlebitis. Injury to the venous wall may result from administration of certain vasoconstrictive or chemotherapeutic agents, or it may result from infectious agents. Patients with malignancies may have migrating thrombophlebitis, which has been attributed to low grade activation of intravascular coagulation. A migratory type of thrombophlebitis is also present in patients with thromboangiitis obliterans.

CLINICAL MANIFESTATIONS. About half of the patients with thrombophlebitis are asymptomatic. The first manifestation of thrombophlebitis may be the occurrence of pulmonary embolism. Pain in the region of the thrombosed veins at rest or only during exercise and edema distal to the obstructed veins are the usual symptoms of thrombophlebitis. Examination of the patient may disclose several helpful manifestations. Edema or pitting of the malleolar fossa may be present and may cause loss of the normal concavity of that portion of the leg. There may be a difference between the two legs in the circumference of the calf. A difference in maximal circumference in excess of 1.4 cm in men and 1.2 cm in women is highly suspicious. The temperature of the skin may be increased as a result of the inflammatory reaction, and palpation may disclose the thrombosed veins in the calf or in the popliteal fossa. An inflamed vein may be apparent as a red, tender cord. There may be tenderness to palpation. Increased resistance or pain on voluntary dorsiflexion of the foot (Homans' sign) may be present. A useful sign is the presence of tenderness on inflation of a blood pressure cuff around the calf. Most normal individuals tolerate this without pain up to pressures of 160 to 180 mm Hg.

Thrombosis of the iliac and femoral veins usually presents with a characteristic clinical picture consisting of rapidly advancing swelling of the entire limb. The thrombosed vein may be evident as a tender cord if it extends below the inguinal ligament. Collateral distended veins may be present in the upper part of the thigh. In some cases, secondary ischemia may occur as a result of the very high venous pressure that impedes arterial inflow. Cyanosis of the toes and even gangrene may occur under these circumstances.

Thrombosis of the subclavian vein may result in swelling of the upper extremity, and collateral veins may be present. In axillary thrombosis, a similar clinical picture occurs; the thrombosed vein may be felt in the axilla. A history of walking on crutches or sleeping in a sitting position on a bench with the arms behind the backrest may be helpful. Thrombosis of the superior vena cava causes increased venous pressure in the neck and face with distention of the neck veins in the upper part of the chest.

In septic thrombophlebitis, the manifestations are similar to those with simple, noninfected thrombophlebitis, except that there may be systemic manifestations of infection, such as fever, chills, and leukocytosis. In cases where septic phlebitis begins from infected needles or catheters, an inflamed tender cord may appear at the site of the venipuncture or insertion of the catheter.

DIAGNOSIS. Ileofemoral thrombophlebitis is usually easily recognized by the rapid swelling of the entire limb, the presence of engorged collateral veins in the thigh, and the presence of signs of inflammation such as increased skin temperature.

In contrast, in the majority of cases of calf thrombophlebitis, the clinical picture is not sufficiently distinctive to allow diagnosis with a high degree of confidence. Confirmation of the diagnosis can be provided by resorting to one or more of a number of diagnostic tests. The most commonly employed tests are the following:

Venography. Venography is generally accepted as one of the most accurate means of making the diagnosis of thrombophlebitis. The test involves the injection of a contrast medium into the venous system, which has been previously emptied of blood by gravity. The test relies on finding a filling defect or a sharp cutoff indicating the presence of occluding thrombus in the vein. The test may result in inflammatory reaction followed by thrombosis in a few cases. It is sensitive and highly specific. However, even in cases with a typical clinical picture it may be negative.

Radioisotope-labelled Fibrinogen. This test consists of intravenous administration of fibrinogen labelled with ^{125}I and the subsequent incorporation of the radioactive material into the thrombus. The accumulation of radioactivity is detected by external counting. This test detects an active thrombophlebitis; it may be negative in cases where the active process has stopped, but thrombi exist in the veins. The reliability of the test depends on the location of the thrombus. It is of little use in detecting pelvic thrombi because of the high background due to the bladder and iliac arteries. It is most useful in detecting thrombosis of the calf. Another disadvantage is that it requires one or two days for a sufficient number of counts to build into the thrombosed vein for detection. This test is, therefore, most useful in longitudinal screening of high risk populations.

Ultrasonography. This test utilizes the Doppler principle to detect venous obstruction. Thus, during various maneuvers that alter venous flow, such as deep inspiration, Valsalva maneuver, or leg compression, the ultrasonogram may be able to detect the presence of obstructed veins. The disadvantages of the technique are that a high degree of stenosis is necessary for the test result to be abnormal and that it does not distinguish between occlusion from external pressure and occlusion by thrombus. Also, the result may be negative if an effective collateral circulation has developed. The test is most sensitive for thrombosis of the veins above the knee.

Impedance Plethysmography. This test detects alterations in blood volume of the extremities by detecting changes in the electrical impedance of the tissues. The test is carried out during respiratory maneuvers or during alterations in blood flow by occluding the limb with a pneumatic pressure cuff. Like ultrasonography, this test requires significant proximal obstruction for positive results. The reported sensitivity and specificity of the test are high (over 90 per cent). The choice of tests to be performed depends to a large extent on their availability. If all are available, it is preferable to use first ultrasonography and impedance plethysmography and resort to venography only if the results of these are inconclusive. The radioactive fibrinogen test should be reserved for screening of patients at high risk.

DIFFERENTIAL DIAGNOSIS. A number of conditions that cause localized pain or edema in the lower extremities may be confused with thrombophlebitis. A ruptured popliteal synovial membrane or cyst (Baker's cyst) may simulate most of the manifestations of thrombophlebitis. The diagnosis can be suspected if there is a history or physical findings of arthritis of the knee joint. The diagnosis may be confirmed by an arthrogram revealing the entry of dye from the joint into the calf muscles. Rupture of the calf muscles may cause pain, tenderness, and edema and may simulate thrombophlebitis. The diagnosis can be made from the history of strenuous or unusual exercise, the presence of ecchymosis from extravasated blood, and the palpation of a hematoma. Sometimes the patient reports that he has heard a snap during the activity when the pain first occurred. The differential diagnosis is important because anticoagulants are contraindicated in this condition. A severe muscle cramp may cause pain and swelling for a considerable period of time. Other manifestations of thrombophlebitis are, however, lacking in this situation. The pain of a lumbar disc may be localized in the calf. There are no other manifestations of thrombophlebitis, however, and there may be neurologic findings to identify the cause of the pain. Lymphedema is recognized by its slower and gradual onset and the absence of signs of inflammation and of collateral veins. Finally, cellulitis may be confused with superficial thrombophlebitis.

COMPLICATIONS. Pulmonary embolism is a frequent and serious complication of thrombophlebitis. About 80 to 90 per cent of pulmonary emboli arise in the deep veins of the lower limbs. Although thrombophlebitis may begin frequently in the veins of the calf, it is only when the thrombosis extends above the knee that serious pulmonary embolism occurs.

About 5 per cent of patients with thrombophlebitis develop venous insufficiency with stasis dermatitis (postphlebitic syndrome). This is more likely to occur in those with more proximal venous obstruction. A rare complication of iliofemoral thrombophlebitis is venous claudication, in which the patient develops pain on exercise which is relieved by rest, as is seen typically in arterial occlusive disease.

PROPHYLAXIS. Prophylactic therapy against thrombophlebitis should be attempted in high risk patients. The exact regimen used must take into consideration the risk of thrombophlebitis and consequent pulmonary embolism and the potential risk of hemorrhagic complications from the prophylactic therapy. Low dose heparin is currently the most commonly used prophylactic technique against thrombophlebitis. For surgical patients, this consists of administration of 5,000 units of heparin subcutaneously two hours before surgery and then every 8 or 12 hours until the patient is ambulatory. This method has been shown to be effective in reducing the incidence of thrombophlebitis and pulmonary embolism in patients subjected to a variety of surgical procedures. It has also been found effective in reducing the incidence of thrombophlebitis in patients following acute myocardial infarction, but it is not known whether or not there is also a reduction in the incidence of pulmonary embolism. Low dose heparin has been shown to be ineffective in patients undergoing surgery for hip fracture and hip replacement, and its effectiveness has not been established in urologic procedures. Warfarin and other similar drugs have been shown to be effective in protecting patients from thromboembolism during a variety of surgical techniques. Low molecular weight dextran given to surgical patients on the day of surgery and at suitable intervals thereafter has been reported in most cases to give favorable results. There is a risk of fluid overload, and, to a lesser extent, hemorrhagic complications. This method can be used in instances where there is a high risk of bleeding from anticoagulants. Drugs that interfere with platelet aggregation, such as aspirin and other nonsteroidal anti-inflammatory agents, have not been shown convincingly to be effective as prophylactic agents. In patients in whom anticoagulation is contraindicated, such as patients with neurosurgical procedures, it is prudent to use conservative means of prophylaxis. These include early ambulation, elastic stockings, and external periodic calf compression. The external compression devices have been reported to be effective. There are no risks associated with their use; the only negative aspect is low patient acceptance during prolonged use, because they are uncomfortable or cumbersome.

TREATMENT. Anticoagulation is not necessary for the treatment of superficial thrombophlebitis. Local measures, sometimes coupled with administration of anti-inflammatory drugs, such as indomethacin, suffice to bring about healing and relief of symptoms.

Full anticoagulation is the preferred treatment for deep vein thrombophlebitis. Heparin is preferred for initiation of treatment because of its immediate action, while the action of warfarin-type drugs may not become fully effective for a considerable period of time. Heparin inhibits coagulation by binding and activation of antithrombin III, an inhibitor of activated factor X. Heparin is best administered by constant infusion. Initially a bolus of 5,000 units is given intravenously, followed by constant infusion of 750 to 1,000 units per hour. The dose is adjusted by monitoring the activated partial thromboplastin time (APTT) so that a level about two times the normal control is achieved. APTT is checked 4 to 6 hours after the initial bolus and once a day thereafter. An alternative method is intermittent intravenous administration of 5,000 to 10,000 units every 4 to 6 hours. If no suitable veins are found, heparin may be administered subcutaneously in a dose of 15,000 to 30,000 units every 12 hours. After five days of heparin therapy, oral warfarin at a dose of 10 to 15 mg daily is started until the one-stage prothrombin time (PT) is one and one half to two times the normal level. Subsequently, a daily maintenance dose is administered to maintain the PT at the desired level. Warfarin brings about anticoagulation by decreasing the level of factors II, VII, IX, and X. Many drugs interact with warfarin. Some of them potentiate its action and others inhibit it. If the patient requires other drug therapy while on warfarin, each drug should be carefully screened for potential interaction. If bleeding occurs in the course of heparin therapy, its effect can be counteracted by administration of 1 mg of protamine per 100 units of heparin. If bleeding develops in the course of warfarin treatment, the patient should receive vitamin K_1 intramuscularly to reduce PT to the therapeutic range (0.25 to 1.0 mg usually suffices). If bleeding is serious, blood or fresh frozen plasma may be necessary.

In patients in whom anticoagulation is contraindicated, simple measures—elevation of the extremity and local heat—should be used. When the risk of pulmonary embolism is low, as is the case when thrombophlebitis involves the calf, these measures suffice. In patients with thrombophlebitis extending above the knee, in whom the risk of pulmonary embolism is high, implantation of an inferior vena caval filter or ligation of the inferior vena cava may also be considered.

Bed rest should be continued until local signs of inflammation, including tenderness and edema, subside. After 7 to 15 days the patient is allowed to walk wearing elastic stockings. If no discomfort occurs, resumption of full activity is allowed one to two weeks later. The duration of anticoagulation is largely arbitrary. Six weeks' to three months' anticoagulation is usually advised.

Thrombolysis with fibrinolytic agents, such as streptokinase or urokinase, given intravenously for two or three days followed by anticoagulation with heparin, is a recently used technique for the treatment of thrombophlebitis. These agents act by causing activation of plasminogen to plasmin, thereby causing dissolution of the thrombus. At present, this technique should be reserved for serious cases of iliofemoral or subclavian vein thrombophlebitis.

Coon WW: Epidemiology of venous thromboembolism. Ann Surg 186:149, 1977. *A detailed, well-referenced consideration of the epidemiology of venous thrombosis.*

Koch-Weser J, Sellers EM: Drug interactions with coumarin anticoagulants (second of two parts). N Engl J Med 285:547, 1971. *A detailed consideration of the interactions of coumarin anticoagulants with other drugs.*

Moser KM, Fedullo PF: Venous thromboembolism, three simple decisions (part 1). Chest 83:117, 1983. *A practical, well-reasoned approach to the prophylaxis and treatment for venous thrombosis is presented.*

Mudge M, Hughes LE: The long term sequelae of deep vein thrombosis. J Surg 65:692, 1978. *A report of long-term follow-up of patients who had evidence of venous thrombosis after surgery. The sequelae of venous thrombosis are described.*

Painter TD: Thrombophlebitis: Diagnostic techniques. Angiology 31:386, 1980. *Comprehensive consideration of the diagnostic techniques for venous thrombosis.*

Sharma GVRK, Cella G, Parisi AF, Sasahara AA: Thrombolytic therapy. N Engl J Med 306:1268, 1982. *Detailed consideration of the use of streptokinase and urokinase in vascular thrombosis.*

Wessler S, Gitel SN: Low-dose heparin: Is the risk worth the benefit? Am Heart J 98:94, 1979. *A review of the use of low-dose heparin for prophylaxis against venous thrombosis.*

Varicose Veins

DEFINITION. Varicose veins are prominent, abnormally distended, and tortuous veins.

INCIDENCE. Varicose veins are common. Approximately 20 per cent of adults develop the disorder. A familial history is present in 15 per cent of patients. They are more common in women than in men by a factor of 5 to 1. Most women date the onset of varicose veins from the time of pregnancy. The veins of the lower extremities are most frequently affected, because of the effects of gravity on venous pressure.

ETIOLOGY. Congenitally absent or defective valves are a recognized cause of varicose veins in early life. Varicose veins may develop secondary to sustained elevations of venous pressure from obstruction of the veins. The cause of the obstruction may be thrombosis secondary to thrombophlebitis or external pressure, as is the case in pregnancy, ascites, and tumors. In most affected individuals, no clearly identifiable cause or precipitating factor can be found. The possibility of a genetically determined structural defect in the venous wall has been suggested. Individuals with varicose veins in the lower extremities have been found to have increased venous distensibility and reduced amounts of collagen and hexosamine in the wall of unaffected veins. In the face of such a generalized defect, a sustained elevation in venous pressure from the effects of gravity in the lower extremities or from other factors may lead to stretching of the wall and, finally, to incompetence of the valves and overdistention of the veins. An association of varicose veins with hemorrhoids and diverticulosis of the bowel suggests the possibility that increased intra-abdominal pressure during bowel movements may play a role in their pathogenesis.

CLINICAL MANIFESTATIONS. Most patients are asymptomatic, especially in the early stages of the disease. They may seek attention because the dilated tortuous varicosities are cosmetically unappealing. In some cases, aching in the lower extremities and edema, especially after prolonged standing or exercise, may be present. The edema usually subsides overnight. When the communicating veins are incompetent, symptoms are more common. Prolonged venous insufficiency leads to the development of the postphlebitic syndrome with sustained edema, induration, and fibrosis. Eventually, trophic changes with brownish discoloration of the skin and ulceration may result. Ulcers usually occur above the medial malleolus. An incompetent communicating vein may be identified in the vicinity of the ulcer. The arterial pulses are normal, and no evidence of ischemia is present.

DIAGNOSIS. Clinical inspection suffices to make the diagnosis. The Trendelenburg test can identify the presence of defective valves and incompetent communicating veins. With the patient recumbent, the leg is elevated to empty the veins, and a tourniquet is then applied to occlude the superficial veins. The patient is instructed to resume the erect position, and the tourniquet is released. If the venous valves are incompetent, the veins immediately become distended as a result of the back flow. If two tourniquets are applied, the distention of the veins in the intervening portion of the limb identifies the presence of incompetent communicating veins. The patency of the deep venous system can be examined by venography. It is prudent to exclude other causes of edema, such as congestive heart failure and renal disease.

PROGNOSIS. The prognosis of uncomplicated superficial varicose veins is excellent. The postphlebitic syndrome, once established, is usually progressive and resistant to treatment.

TREATMENT. Simple measures usually suffice to treat uncomplicated varicose veins. These consist of frequent periods of rest with elevation of the limbs, external pressure with elastic stockings or bandages, and avoidance of obstruction of the veins by garments, such as girdles. In more severe or advanced cases, ligation and stripping of the saphenous veins or injection of sclerosing solutions may become necessary to prevent the postphlebitis syndrome. An injection/compression technique in which the sclerosing solution is injected into a vein emptied of blood, followed by compression by external pressure, is simple, cheap, and effective. It is widely used in Europe. When stasis ulcers are present, local care with warm, wet dressings is necessary. If infection is present, local and systemic antibiotics may be administered. If considerable fibrosis is present, it may be necessary to excise the entire area and carry out skin grafting to eliminate ulceration.

Beresford SAA, Chant ADB, Jones HO, Pachaud D, Weddell JM: Varicose veins: A comparison of surgery and injection/compression sclerotherapy. Lancet 1:921, 1978. *A five-year follow-up comparing the effects of surgery and injection/compression sclerotherapy for varicose veins.*

Hobbs JT: The treatment of venous disorders: A comprehensive review of current practice in the management of varicose veins and post-thrombotic syndrome. Philadelphia, J. B. Lippincott Company, 1977. *A well-written, comprehensive consideration of the clinical features, diagnosis, and treatment of varicose veins and post-thrombotic syndromes.*

DISEASES OF THE LYMPHATIC VESSELS OF THE LIMBS

Lymphangitis

DEFINITION. Lymphangitis is an inflammation of the lymphatic vessels. It is usually of bacterial origin.

ETIOLOGY. In most cases the responsible infective agent is the hemolytic Streptococcus or *Staphylococcus aureus*, coagulase-positive. The bacteria gain access to the lymphatics via local trauma or from ulcerations. In many instances no identifiable portal of entry can be found. Infection spreads from the lymphatics to the regional lymph nodes.

PATHOLOGY. Various stages of inflammation are found in the subcutaneous tissue and regional lymph nodes.

CLINICAL MANIFESTATIONS. The local manifestations of lymphangitis consist of a red streak that appears at the site of initial entry of the infective organism and extends to the regional lymph nodes. The latter are swollen and tender. There may be a surrounding area of cellulitis with redness and warmth of the skin and local tenderness and edema. The systemic accompaniments of infection, including malaise, headache, nausea, vomiting, chills, and fever, may be present and may constitute the presenting manifestations.

DIAGNOSIS. The local manifestations of lymphangitis and the accompanying systemic reaction are usually sufficiently characteristic to make the diagnosis. Leukocytosis with predominance of polymorphonuclear leukocytes may be present. Confirmation is obtained by culturing the organism from the portal of entry or from the subcutaneous tissues. Acute lymphangitis may be difficult to distinguish from a generalized cellulitis or from thrombophlebitis.

PROGNOSIS. With treatment the prognosis is good when one is dealing with an initial attack in an otherwise normal limb. In the case of recurrent attacks, lymphedema may develop and residual increase in the girth of the limb may occur.

TREATMENT. This consists of systemic administration of the appropriate antibiotics. In addition, surgical drainage of the focus of infection is important. Supportive measures, including rest and elevation of the infected limb and local warm, wet dressings, are also helpful. The use of elastic support hose may be necessary for a period of several weeks after attack to prevent the production of lymphedema. In recurrent cases, the causes of secondary lymphedema should be sought and excluded.

Schinger A, Martin WJ, Spittell JA: Acute lymphangitis and cellulitis. Minnesota Med 48:191, 1965. *Concise consideration of the clinical features, diagnosis, and treatment of lymphangitis.*

Lymphedema

DEFINITION. Lymphedema refers to edema from accumulation of lymph secondary to obstruction to its flow.

ETIOLOGY AND INCIDENCE. Lymphedema can be primary or secondary. Several forms of primary lymphedema are recognized. The most frequent type is simple congenital lymphedema, which is not familial and is present at birth. A congenital familial form (Milroy's disease) is inherited as an autosomal dominant trait. Another hereditary form is associated with Noonan's syndrome in about 15 per cent of cases. Lymphedema praecox becomes manifest in puberty and is associated with congenital hypoplasia of the lymphatics. A late form may become manifest in middle age.

Secondary lymphedema results most commonly from traumatic interference with lymphatics and lymph nodes. Commonly, secondary lymphedema results from surgical removal of lymph nodes and from fibrosis secondary to radiation following surgery for cancer. Lymphomas or metastatic carcinoma involving the lymph nodes may also cause obstruction to the flow of lymph and lymphedema. Filaria infection in the tropics is a cause of secondary lymphedema.

Primary lymphedema is more common in women. Most cases are manifest at birth or become apparent before age 40. A syndrome characterized by yellow nails, recurrent pleural effusion, and lymphedema is believed to be secondary to multiple lymphatic abnormalities in the areas involved. A familial syndrome consisting of recurrent intrahepatic cholestasis and lymphedema is probably due to defective hepatic lymphatic vessels as well as those in the extremity.

PATHOLOGY. In cases of congenital lymphedema there is absence or hypoplasia of the lymphatic vessels. In secondary lymphedema there are numerous small, irregular lymphatics together with tortuous and sometimes greatly enlarged varicose lymphatic vessels.

CLINICAL MANIFESTATIONS. Typically, lymphedema begins gradually with an enlargement of the involved limb without other manifestations. The swollen extremity is soft and pitting. The edema subsides at night. With time, the skin becomes thickened and cannot be raised into a fold and the edema becomes more persistent. The lower extremities are involved most often. In about half the patients the edema is unilateral. Superimposed lymphangitis and cellulitis may occur, and in longstanding cases lymphangiosarcoma may develop.

PROGNOSIS. Primary lymphedema is usually a slowly progressive disorder, not easily amenable to treatment. The prognosis of secondary lymphedema depends on the cause. In cases where it is due to infection it can be effectively managed by treating the latter.

TREATMENT. In primary lymphedema this is aimed at keeping the limb as free of edema as possible to prevent fibrosis and secondary infection. Frequent elevation of the limb, the use of elastic stockings, and the administration of diuretics may be useful. In cases not controlled by these simple measures, benzopyrones have been reported to be useful. These drugs break down protein by activating macrophages; hence, they reduce viscosity and facilitate the flow of lymph. Surgery may be tried in advanced cases to remove subcutaneous tissue and to induce new lymph vessel formation. Anastomosis of small lymphatic vessels with veins by microsurgery has been reported to give good results in some cases.

Allen EV, Ghormley RK: Lymphedema of the extremities: Etiology, classification and treatment; report of 300 cases. Ann Intern Med 9:516, 1935. *Comprehensive consideration of the clinical features of primary and secondary lymphedema in a large series of cases.*

O'Brien BM, Shafiroff BB: Microlymphaticovenous and resectional surgery in obstructive lymphedema. World J Surg 3:3, 1979. *A report of good results from the application of this relatively new technique for the treatment of lymphedema.*

Pillar NB: Lymphoedema, macrophages and benzopyrones. Lymphology 13:109, 1980. *Discussion of the role of macrophages in lymphedema. The effectiveness of benzopyrones in this disease is ascribed to activation of macrophages.*

55. TUMORS OF THE HEART

Robert E. Whalen

The heart can be the site of a host of primary as well as metastatic tumors. Almost every type of malignant tumor has been found in metastatic form in the heart, but by far the most frequent types are melanomas, leukemia, and lymphomas. Although metastatic tumors of the heart are more frequent than previously realized, they seldom play a significant role in the patient's course. A large variety of primary tumors of the heart has been described, including myxomas, lipomas, fibromas, hemangiomas, lymphangiomas, mesotheliomas, and sarcomas, including rhabdomyosarcomas.

The *cardiac myxoma* is the most frequent and also clinically the most significant primary tumor of the heart, for its discovery and treatment can be lifesaving. Myxomas can arise from the endocardial surface of any of the cardiac chambers, but 95 per cent of them arise in the atria, with at least 75 per cent of these arising in the left atrium. The classic location for a myxoma is the region of the fossa ovalis in the left atrium. Bilateral atrial myxomas have been reported. Myxomas occur from youth to old age, but are most frequent in the middle years. In most series there is a higher incidence among females. They usually present in one or more of three typical ways. The most frequent presentation, which is due to enlargement of the tumor within the cardiac chamber, involves progressive decrease in exercise tolerance, increased dyspnea on exertion, and pulmonary or peripheral edema. Occasionally syncope may be a presenting symptom, but presyncope with changes in position or physical activity is more common. Next, the first sign of a myxoma may be occlusion of a major artery with fragments of the myxoma or thrombus previously lodged on the surface of the intracardiac myxoma. Cerebrovascular accidents and sudden ischemia to limbs from this mechanism often herald the presence of a myxoma. The least frequent manifestation of a myxoma is the development of systemic symptoms which may simulate acute rheumatic fever, bacterial endocarditis, systemic lupus erythematosus, or a fever of unknown etiology.

Myxomas are almost always accompanied by a systolic regurgitant heart murmur, owing to incompetence of either the tricuspid or the mitral valve produced by distortion of the valve leaflets. Less frequently the murmur of tricuspid or mitral stenosis may be the most prominent feature because of obstruction of either one of these orifices. The intensity of the murmurs may vary markedly with changes in position. A hallmark of the myxoma, frequently detected by auscultation, is a third heart sound which varies in time after the second heart sound. This "tumor plop" is due to the acceleration of the tumor mass through the atrioventricular valve and often its impact against the ventricular wall. The presence of any of the aforementioned manifestations in the setting of a normal cardiothoracic ratio, particularly with atrial prominence by chest x-ray, should raise suspicion of a myxoma. The electrocardiogram may show atrial hypertrophy. The presence of a variable third heart sound by phonocardiography, the presence of either an elevated sedimentation rate or increased gamma globulin level, and the variable indentation of the barium-filled esophagus during systole under fluoroscopic observation should enhance suspicion.

The diagnosis of an atrial myxoma is best confirmed by echocardiography, which provides a characteristic picture of the tumor mass as it moves from the atrium to the ventricle during diastole. Angiocardiography is seldom necessary. The life-threatening nature of a cardiac myxoma, the ease with which the diagnosis can be made by echocardiography, and the success of open heart surgery in eliminating the condition emphasize the importance of having a high index of suspicion when seeing a patient with symptoms suggestive of heart failure but with a normal heart size.

Fine G: Neoplasms of the pericardium and heart. *In* Gould SE (ed.): Pathology of the Heart and Blood Vessels. Springfield, Ill., Charles C Thomas, 1968, p 851. *This is a comprehensive classification and description of the many tumors that may involve the heart and pericardium.*

Hardin NJ, Wilson JM, Gray GF, Gay WA: Experience with primary tumors of the heart: Clinical and pathological study of seventeen cases. Johns Hopkins Med J 134:141, 1974. *A review of the clinical and pathologic features of 17 patients with primary tumors of the heart.*

Johnson ML, Sieker HO, Behar VS, Whalen RE: Echocardiographic diagnosis of a left atrial myxoma found attached to the free left atrial wall. J Clin Ultrasound 1:75, 1973. *This report emphasizes the echocardiographic features of atrial myxoma with a discussion of possible false-positive and false-negative echocardiographic findings.*

Peters MN, Hall RJ, Cooley DA, Leachman RD, Garcia E: The clinical syndrome of atrial myxoma. JAMA 230:695, 1974. *A review of the clinical course of 17 patients with atrial myxoma.*

Selzer A, Sakai FJ, Popper RW: Protean clinical manifestations of primary tumors of the heart. Am J Med 52:9, 1972. *A review of the signs and symptoms encountered in 13 patients with primary tumors of the heart, emphasizing the wide spectrum of clinical presentation.*

Part VIII
RESPIRATORY DISEASES

56. INTRODUCTION

John F. Murray

Respiration includes all the processes that contribute to O_2 uptake and CO_2 elimination. The lungs are the major organs of gas exchange, but the nose, oropharynx, extrapulmonary airways, brain, spinal cord, nerves, thoracic cage, respiratory muscles, lymph nodes and vessels, and cardiovascular system are also involved. Thus respiratory diseases, literally interpreted, include a large variety of abnormalities arising in all the different structures concerned with gas exchange. In general, a more limited definition applies, and respiratory diseases are considered to include disturbances of the air passages, lungs, pleura, chest wall, muscles of respiration, and mediastinum (excluding the heart, systemic vessels, and esophagus).

Acute respiratory diseases are probably the most common afflictions of mankind and are responsible for more absences from school and work than any other type of illness. Chronic respiratory diseases, particularly emphysema and bronchitis, are second only to cardiovascular diseases as causes of disability payments. Cancer of the lung kills more persons each year than any other kind of malignancy. Because of the remarkable incidence of these and other respiratory diseases, it is important that all physicians, not just internists and chest specialists, be well versed in the clinical manifestations and methods of diagnosis, treatment, and prevention of the most common disorders. The material concerned with respiratory diseases here and elsewhere in the book is intended as a primer of necessary knowledge with which to recognize and to treat the major respiratory diseases; additional information is available in the references cited at the end of each chapter.

Patients with respiratory disease often seek medical attention because they have at least one of three cardinal manifestations: *cough* (including its derivative hemoptysis), *chest pain,* and *dyspnea.* These are nonspecific and sometimes trivial abnormalities, but the frequency with which they are associated with serious underlying thoracic disease means that the complaints must always be considered carefully and often become the focus of diagnostic evaluations. Because of the clinical importance of cough, chest pain, and dyspnea, the mechanisms, special features, and diagnostic approach to each symptom are briefly reviewed in the following pages. Further information can be found under the headings of the specific diseases in which the sensations occur.

COUGH

Normal persons seldom cough; their scant bronchial secretions, although constantly being produced, are imperceptibly carried up the tracheobronchial system by the action of cilia and, after reaching the pharynx, swallowed. Coughing is an essential defense mechanism that protects the airways from the adverse effects of inhaled noxious substances and also serves to clear them of retained secretions. Coughing, therefore, indicates an abnormality, but one that may be transient and unimportant or one that may indicate the presence of severe intrathoracic disease.

MECHANISM. Coughing may be produced voluntarily, but more often it results from reflex stimulation. Extrathoracic cough receptors are located in the nose, oropharynx, larynx, and upper trachea. Intrathoracic rapidly adapting irritant receptors, which cause cough, are located in the lower trachea and large central bronchi, which are the air passages from which coughing is effective in clearing secretions or removing foreign material. Depending on which cough receptors are activated, afferent stimuli travel to the brain via the trigeminal, glossopharyngeal, superior laryngeal, or vagus nerves. Efferent pathways include the recurrent laryngeal nerves, to cause closure of the glottis, and the corticospinal tract and peripheral nerves, to cause contraction of the thoracic and abdominal musculature. The cough reflex begins with a deep breath followed by glottic closure, relaxation of the diaphragm, and contraction of the expiratory muscles. Collectively, these acts generate a positive pressure within the thorax, which is suddenly released when the glottis opens. During cough, the *volume*-rate of flow out of the lungs (liters per second) is only slightly greater than or the same as it is during a forced expiratory maneuver, a fact that is not always appreciated. However, because the positive pressure in the pleural space is higher than the luminal pressure in the trachea and central bronchi, a pressure difference is created that causes the posterior membranous portion of the airway walls to fold inward and nearly to obliterate the lumen. By this means, the *linear* velocity of air flow through the narrowed channels (centimeters per second) is markedly increased and a shearing force is created that dislodges secretions and particles from the mucosal surface.

PRODUCTIVE COUGH. The daily quantity of bronchial secretions produced by a normal person is not known, but it is sufficiently small to be removed by mucociliary action alone, and coughing and expectoration are not required. Secretions can accumulate in the tracheobronchial system in the presence of one or more of the following abnormalities: excessive production, altered physical properties, and deficient clearance. Thus, productive cough, which clears retained secretions from the airways, is an important defense mechanism and one of the hallmarks of acute and chronic inflammatory conditions of the lungs and airways. One of the major efforts of respiratory therapists is to employ physical maneuvers that enhance the removal of retained secretions. Patients who are unconscious, intubated, or for other reasons cannot cough must have their tracheobronchial secretions removed by suctioning to prevent the complications of atelectasis and/or bronchopulmonary infection.

NONPRODUCTIVE COUGH. In addition to the cough that serves an expectoration function, another type of cough—an irritative phenomenon—is encountered frequently. The stimulus may be mechanical, chemical, thermal, or inflammatory, including reactions from infection. There is increasing evidence that alteration of the surface epithelium of the major airways, into which the terminal filaments of irritant receptors are inserted, exposes the receptors more directly or somehow sensitizes them to the effects of stimulants; the cough reflex thus becomes hyperreactive, and coughing occurs in response to ordinarily innocuous stimuli. Such nonproductive cough serves no useful purpose. Indeed, the repetitious scouring of the mucosa may cause mechanical trauma and aggravate the injury that sensitized the receptors in the first place, resulting in a vicious circle.

COMPLICATIONS. Coughing seems to perpetuate coughing, perhaps through the cycle noted above. Paroxysms of coughing, as in pertussis, may terminate in vomiting, which seems to break the cycle. Paroxysmal attacks may also terminate in syncope. The mechanism of *cough syncope* is uncertain, but the effects of increased intrathoracic pressure on venous return and cardiac output and possibly the accompanying respiratory alkalosis are believed to play a role. At times, severe coughing attacks have continued to the point of utter exhaustion. The muscular force developed during coughing may be sufficient to cause occasional fractures of ribs *(cough fractures)* and even compression fractures of vertebral bodies.

DIAGNOSTIC APPROACH. It is difficult to generalize about a condition as common but as varied as coughing. Obviously, many episodes of coughing are innocent and transient. The essential first step in evaluating a patient complaining of cough is to obtain a thorough history with particular attention to the following aspects: (1) acute or chronic, (2) productive or nonproductive, (3) character, (4) time relationships, (5) type and quantity of sputum, and (6) associated features.

An acute cough is usually associated with viral laryngotracheobronchitis but may signify other bronchopulmonary infections. Less commonly, acute episodes of coughing may be the chief manifestation of the inhalation of various immunologic or irritative substances. A chronic cough is the diagnostic hallmark of chronic bronchitis but also occurs in tuberculosis, bronchiectasis, and bronchogenic carcinoma. The frequency with which chronic bronchitis and bronchogenic carcinoma coexist, both being a complication of cigarette smoking, has led to the important axiom that *any change in the character or pattern of a chronic cough warrants immediate diagnostic evaluation, with special attention directed toward the detection of bronchogenic carcinoma.* Chronic persistent cough may be the sole symptom of patients with bronchial asthma.

A productive cough usually implies an underlying inflammatory process, often infectious, whereas a nonproductive cough signifies a mechanical or other irritative stimulus. The character of the cough may be described as "brassy" from major airways involvement or "barking" or "croupy" from laryngeal disease. Paroxysmal coughing with "whoops" is characteristic of pertussis. A cough that occurs mainly at night may accompany congestive cardiac failure; one occurring at meals suggests esophagogastric disease, such as hiatal hernia or diverticulum; and the cough of severe bronchitis or bronchiectasis is often worse upon awakening because of pooling of secretions during sleep. Each of these patterns tends to recur repeatedly under similar circumstances.

A description of the secretions produced in association with cough is diagnostically useful. Foul-smelling sputum indicates anaerobic infection, as in lung abscess or necrotizing pneumonia. Abundant frothy saliva-like sputum is a well known but rare symptom of bronchoalveolar carcinoma. Pink foamy sputum, which is often voluminous, indicates pulmonary edema. In pneumococcal pneumonia, the classic rust-colored or "prune juice"–colored sputum may be observed. The chronic production of copious purulent sputum with intermittent blood streaking, especially on change of postures, is an important clue to bronchiectasis.

The associated features of coughing episodes are of considerable clinical importance: wheezing—a disorder with obstruction to air flow such as asthma; stridor—involvement of the pharynx–larynx–extrathoracic trachea; fever and chills—acute infection; weakness and weight loss—tuberculosis or other chronic infection or malignancy; and recurrent pneumonias—bronchiectasis, foreign body, or obstructing tumor. In view of the importance of cigarette smoking in the pathogenesis of cough, a careful smoking history is crucial to the evaluation of cough.

Physical examination may reveal signs of pulmonary involvement that provide clues to the specific diagnosis. Regardless of the presence or absence of physical findings, evaluation of significant cough entails roentgenographic examination of the chest. When indicated, simple pulmonary function tests will demonstrate abnormalities of air flow and/or lung volumes. In patients whose routine spirometric tests are normal, bronchial provocation studies are indicated. Appropriate studies of sputum, especially culture and cytology, are often the easiest and most direct way of establishing a diagnosis. Additional diagnostic refinements are described in Ch. 58.

TREATMENT. The ideal treatment of cough is elimination of its underlying cause. This is possible in most kinds of bronchopulmonary infections by suitable antimicrobial treatment of the responsible microorganism. Cessation of cigarette smoking nearly always eliminates the cough of chronic bronchitis. Disabling, irritative nonproductive cough may be suppressed by an antitussive drug such as codeine, 15 mg every six hours. In contrast, productive cough should not be suppressed because retention of secretions impairs the distribution of inspired air, which worsens gas exchange, and promotes the development of atelectasis and secondary infection. Adequate hydration, not overhydration, is traditionally recommended, although its effect on pulmonary secretions is difficult to substantiate. Expectorants and ultrasonic aerosols have not been shown to be beneficial. When secretions are difficult to raise because of their physical properties and/or ineffective coughing, respiratory physical therapy with postural drainage and percussion may be helpful and a trial is warranted.

HEMOPTYSIS

Regardless of whether the sputum is grossly bloody or merely blood streaked, the expectoration of any blood whatsoever denotes hemoptysis. Patients with chronic bronchitis may produce faintly blood-tinged sputum from time to time, but apart from this exception every patient with hemoptysis deserves a thorough diagnostic work-up. A substantial proportion of all patients who expectorate bloody sputum have a serious disease; approximate figures indicate bronchogenic carcinoma 20 to 30 per cent; bronchiectasis 20 to 30 per cent; bronchitis 10 to 20 per cent; and other inflammatory disorders, including tuberculosis, 10 to 20 per cent. Other conditions that may present with hemoptysis include pulmonary embolism, mitral stenosis, pulmonary arteriovenous fistula, and Goodpasture's syndrome. All series include an appreciable number (5 to 15 per cent) of undiagnosed cases despite complete investigation.

DIAGNOSTIC APPROACH. The amount of expectorated blood may vary widely, from slight streaking of sputum to massive exsanguinating hemorrhage. The patient may not be aware of the pulmonary origin of his bleeding and often states that the blood "welled up" in his throat. For this reason, patients with true hemoptysis may seek the services of an otolaryngologist. Although it is always wise to examine the nasopharynx thoroughly, it is rare that hemoptysis is due to lesions in that portion of the respiratory tract.

Bleeding of esophageal, gastric, or duodenal origin may be confused with bleeding from the respiratory tract. Hematemesis can usually be differentiated from hemoptysis by the presence of symptoms of gastrointestinal involvement such as nausea and vomiting, a history of peptic ulcer disease or alcoholism, or signs of cirrhosis. Prompt endoscopy will settle the issue in doubtful cases.

Historical and physical examinations may provide clues to the underlying cause of hemoptysis but are seldom diagnostic. Chest roentgenograms, which should be obtained in all patients complaining of hemoptysis, may reveal evidence of old or new inflammatory lesions, probable malignancies, or vascular abnormalities. At times, the underlying lesion may be obscured by the densities caused by the presence of blood itself. Once the bleeding has stopped, however, intra-alveolar blood usually clears within a week so that delayed roentgenographic examinations are often helpful. Routine laboratory evaluation should include a complete blood count and tests to exclude a coagulopathy.

Virtually every patient with significant hemoptysis should be bronchoscoped to determine the site of bleeding and its cause. Even if the cause cannot be ascertained during the initial examination, it is important to determine from which bronchus the blood is coming; this is absolutely necessary in patients bleeding massively who are being considered for surgery, but it is also extremely difficult because the tracheobronchial system contains so much blood that it is frequently impossible to identify a bleeding point. The fiberoptic bronchoscope is often used in patients with hemoptysis, but many experts prefer the rigid scope because its larger lumen permits easier aspiration of blood and, when necessary, control of bleeding by packing.

If surgical treatment is a consideration, the origin of the bleeding must be identified each time hemoptysis occurs. Even if a lesion is obvious on chest roentgenographic examination, the patient may be bleeding from an occult site. Similarly, even if a source of blood has been identified on a previous occasion, the blood may come from a different abnormality next time.

TREATMENT. Fortunately, intrapulmonary bleeding usually stops spontaneously. Until it does, the patient should be kept with the affected lung, from which the bleeding is occurring, in the dependent position; the airways should be kept free of blood—coughing may suffice but suction may be necessary; and strong sedatives, which abolish cough, should be avoided. A thoracic surgeon should be notified about the problem, and an endotracheal tube and suction apparatus must be ready at the bedside. If massive bleeding suddenly occurs, the tube can be inserted blindly into the right main bronchus and the balloon inflated to separate the two lungs and keep the blood confined to one of them. If circumstances permit, it is even better to put a balloon catheter, under bronchoscopic guidance, into a lobar or segmental bronchus to isolate the blood to as small a region of lung as possible. Blood transfusions are given according to the usual clinical guidelines of quantity of blood lost, hematocrit, blood pressure, pulse rate, and urine output.

After the bleeding stops, the patient should be investigated as outlined to determine the cause of the hemorrhage as well as the extent and severity of the underlying disease(s). Then, in consultation with a thoracic surgeon, a rational decision can be made concerning the need for and likelihood of success of an operation. Ordinarily, localized lesions (e.g., bronchial adenoma or sequestration) are resected and generalized lesions (e.g., widespread bronchiectasis or multiple fistulas) are left alone. However, there is considerable clinical ground between these two extremes and each patient must be considered individually.

An even more difficult problem is the selection of patients with "massive" hemoptysis for emergency pulmonary resection, usually lobectomy but occasionally pneumonectomy. Part of the problem lies in defining what actually constitutes "life-threatening" hemorrhage. Emergency resection in the presence of bleeding from relatively localized, chronic conditions (e.g., broncholithiasis) produces good results; in contrast, in patients hemorrhaging from acute parenchymal infections (e.g., lung abscess), there is a high incidence of postoperative complications. Patients who bleed massively from bronchogenic carcinomas or extensive benign lesions that are nonresectable are particularly difficult; a new method of bronchial or intercostal arterial catheterization and embolization with Gelfoam to occlude the bleeding site has been tried with some success in these patients.

CHEST PAIN

Various types of chest pain are extremely common. Chest pain is one of the most frequent symptoms that cause the sufferer to seek medical attention. Because there is no clear relationship between the intensity of the discomfort and the importance of its underlying cause, all complaints of chest pain must be considered carefully. Pain that is virtually diagnostic because of its typical pattern of onset, location, and relation to effort and to respiratory movements is found in pleurisy, intercostal neuritis, costochondral disease, and disorders of the chest wall. The location and character of pain from myocardial ischemia are also characteristic but may be simulated by the pain of acute and chronic pulmonary hypertension. Occasionally, chest pain is elusive and difficult to diagnose, but it must always be taken seriously. A *meticulous history* is essential in evaluating chest pain. From the patient's story alone, a differential diagnosis can be formulated that serves as the basis for subsequent examinations.

MECHANISM. The anatomy, physiology, and biochemistry of pain in the body are reviewed in Ch. 476. Chest pain is no different from other types in that receptors and afferent pathways transmit a stimulus to the central nervous system where that stimulus is perceived as pain. However, the capacity of various intrathoracic structures to serve as a source of pain differs. The lung parenchyma and the visceral pleura covering it are insensitive to ordinarily painful stimuli. In contrast, pain often accompanies involvement of the parietal pleura, the major airways, the chest wall, the diaphragm, or the mediastinal structures, including the heart. The mechanism of pain in myocardial ischemia is unknown, but the actuating event is clearly an imbalance between myocardial oxygen supply and demand. The pain of pericarditis may be in part related to involvement of the adjacent pleura, thus accounting for the striking respiratory component of what is primarily a cardiac disease. Pain in the esophagus is provoked by stimulation of receptors from acid reflux or muscle spasm.

PLEURAL PAIN. Pleurisy, or acute inflammation of the pleural surfaces, usually causes chest pain that has several distinctive features. The pain is restricted in distribution rather than diffuse, is nearly always on one side or the other, and tends to be distributed along the intercostal nerve zones. Pain from diaphragmatic pleurisy is often referred to the shoulder and side of the neck. The most striking and important characteristic of pleural pain is its clear relationship to respiratory movements. The pain may be variously described as "achy," "sharp," "burning," or simply a "catch," but whatever its designation, it is typically worsened by taking a deep breath, and coughing or sneezing causes intense distress. Patients with pleurisy frequently also complain of dyspnea because the aggravation of their pain during inspiration makes them conscious of every breath. Movement of the trunk, including bending, stooping, or even turning in bed, increases pleural pain, and patients usually find and remain in the position in which movements of the affected region are most restricted.

The rapidity of development of pleural pain provides a clue to its cause. An immediate onset attends pulmonary embolism or spontaneous pneumothorax; a slower but still acute onset over a few hours, especially with fever and cough, accompanies pneumonia; finally, a gradual onset over days or even weeks, often associated with features of chronic illness such as weakness and weight loss, suggests tuberculosis or malignancy.

INTERCOSTAL NEURITIS. The distribution and superficial and knifelike quality of the pain of intercostal neuritis may resemble pleural pain. Similarly, the pain of intercostal neuritis is worsened by vigorous respiratory movements such as coughing, sneezing, and straining but, unlike pleurisy, not by ordinary breathing. A neuritic origin may be suggested by the presence of lancinating or electric shock sensations unrelated to movements, and hyperalgesia or anesthesia over the distribution of the affected intercostal nerve provides further confirmatory evidence.

COSTOCHONDRAL DISEASE. Pain localized to the costosternal cartilaginous junctions may be confused with other, more serious causes of chest pain. The discomfort is usually described as dull with a gnawing, aching quality; there is little if any relationship to respiratory or other movements, although the pain may be most noticeable when the patient is lying in bed at night. The diagnostic key lies in the fact that there is tenderness to palpation that is clearly localized to one or more of the costal cartilages. There may be redness, swelling, and enlargement of the costal bridges *(Tietze's syndrome)*, but the frequency of these is overemphasized. The most common sites of costosternal perichondritis are the second, third, and fourth cartilages, but any part of the large and complex cartilaginous shield along the central and lower portions of the anterior thoracic cage may be involved.

DISORDERS OF THE CHEST WALL. The system of joints, muscles, and fasciae involved in movements of the thoracic wall is complex. Because these structures are in constant motion throughout a person's life, it is surprising that "rheumatic" pains of the chest do not occur more frequently than they do. Fibrositis of the muscle-bone attachments may simultaneously involve the chest wall and other parts of the skeleton. Similarly, spondylitis of the thoracic spine may have its rib cage component, and many less definable skeletal disorders may produce discomfort in the chest. Localized pain in the thoracic cage may be related to unusually severe exercise or motion of the involved area. At times, the abnormality appears to be spontaneous, although even in these cases it is possible that pain was delayed in onset after either injury to the muscles of the chest wall or fractures of ribs during minor trauma or an unnoticed episode of coughing.

PULMONARY HYPERTENSION. The pain of pulmonary hypertension may simulate the pain of myocardial ischemia in its substernal location, its pattern of radiation, and its crushing or constricting quality. This type of pain may occur in patients with acute pulmonary hypertension from multiple and/or massive pulmonary emboli or in patients with chronic pulmonary hypertension from vasculitis or mitral stenosis. The mechanism of the pain is unknown, but it is believed to differ in the acute and chronic varieties. In the former it is related to sudden distention of the main pulmonary artery and stimulation of mechanoreceptors, and in the latter to an imbalance between the oxygen supplied to and utilized by the pressure-overloaded right ventricle. Although substernal pain related to the sudden onset of pulmonary hypertension is a well recognized complication of pulmonary embolism, more commonly emboli cause pain in the lateral part of the chest that is typically pleuritic in character whether or not they produce pulmonary infarction.

MYOCARDIAL ISCHEMIA. Among the most important types of chest pain is that of myocardial ischemia, which is usually caused by coronary artery atherosclerosis (see Ch. 49). These attacks are provoked by an imbalance, which may be transient or permanent, between the supply of and demand for oxygen by the ventricular myocardium. Ischemic pain spans a continuum of severity from angina pectoris on the one hand to myocardial infarction on the other. Typical anginal pain is induced by exercise, heavy meals, and emotional upsets; the pain is usually described as a substernal "pressure," "constriction," or "squeezing" that, when intense, may radiate to the neck or down the ulnar aspect of one or both arms. Variant or Prinzmetal's anginal pain is similar in location and quality to typical angina pectoris but occurs in cycles at rest rather than during stressful episodes. Both typical and variant types of angina pectoris are relieved by coronary vasodilatory drugs such as nitroglycerin. Typical angina also decreases with rest or removing the inciting stress. In contrast, the pain of myocardial infarction, although similar in location and character to anginal pain, is usually of greater intensity and duration, is not alleviated by rest or by nitroglycerin, may require large doses of opiates, and is often accompanied by diaphoresis, nausea, hypotension, and arrhythmias. Although patients are often short of breath during attacks of myocardial ischemia, and myocardial infarction may induce severe pulmonary edema, the pain itself is neither related to breathing nor affected by respiratory movements.

OTHER SOURCES. Pericarditis causes pain that is usually pleuritic in nature but may be steady and substernal; dissecting aneurysm of the aorta is associated with severe unremitting anterior chest pain that often radiates through to the back or into the abdomen; and a deep substernal pain may result from esophageal reflux or spasm or from spontaneous mediastinal emphysema. Finally, psychogenic disorders may be associated with various forms of chest pain, the most common of which is a substernal tightness or aching sensation that may last from 30 minutes to several days. The pain may vary somewhat in intensity from time to time, and the ancillary features of myocardial infarction and a respiratory component are absent.

DIAGNOSTIC APPROACH. The approach to the general problem of the diagnosis of chest pain varies according to how seriously ill the patient is when first seen. Patients with acute chest pain who are gravely ill, as evidenced by hypotension, intense dyspnea, profuse diaphoresis, agitation, and restlessness, are usually evaluated first in the emergency room. The chief diagnostic considerations in this common clinical complex are myocardial infarction, pulmonary embolism, and dissecting aneurysm; less likely possibilities are tension pneumothorax, pericardial tamponade, and ruptured esophagus. An initial tentative diagnosis can usually be made from the results of careful historical and physical examinations, supplemented by an electrocardiogram and chest roentgenograms. Except when the electrocardiogram reveals clear evidence of acute myocardial ischemia, definitive diagnosis depends on the results of later studies such as ventilation-perfusion lung scans, pulmonary angiography, aortography, serial enzyme determinations, and coronary artery catheterization.

Patients with less severe chest pain may present during an episode of pain or afterward. Again, a detailed history of the character and behavior of the pain provides the best guide for the selection of subsequent diagnostic studies. Most patients will require an electrocardiogram, ideally taken during an episode of pain, and chest roentgenograms; then, based on the results of these examinations, diagnostic evaluation proceeds as needed for the particular entities under consideration.

TREATMENT. The treatment of chest pain depends on its cause. Anginal pain responds to coronary artery vasodilator drugs, whereas myocardial infarction usually requires opiates, often in large doses. Pleural pain responds to analgesics, given as required. However, pleurisy in association with pneumonia may be alleviated by anti-inflammatory drugs such as indomethacin; in refractory cases, intercostal nerve block is needed. For costochondral and other types of chest wall pain, mild analgesia, reassurance, and time usually suffice; rapid relief can be obtained, when necessary, by injection of local anesthetic agents into the involved area.

DYSPNEA

When healthy persons undertake a steadily increasing amount of physical activity, they will eventually become aware of their breathing; the exercise required to provoke this sensation depends on their physical fitness. If they increase the level of activity even further, the awareness will increase as the sensation becomes progressively more unpleasant; if they stop exercising, the feeling will quickly disappear. The sensation experienced by normal subjects during physical exertion is aptly described as "shortness of breath" but not as dyspnea. The term dyspnea implies that the awareness is disproportionate to the stimulus and, moreover, that the sensation is abnormally uncomfortable. Many patients will describe their breathing discomfort as "breathlessness," but many others will complain only of "tightness," "choking," "inability to take a deep breath," "suffocating," and, simply "can't get enough air." Thus dyspnea is difficult to define precisely and it is impossible to quantify. As with the evaluation of chest pain, a thorough history is required to explore all the vagaries of this elusive symptom.

MECHANISM. It is impossible to find a common mechanism for what appears to be the same or similar sensation of difficulty in breathing that may occur in respiratory, cardiac, erythropoietic, metabolic, and psychogenic disorders. Dyspnea in patients with respiratory diseases is believed to have a reflex origin and thus must begin with stimulation of receptors in one or more of the organs concerned with breathing. There are three types of intrapulmonary receptors (stretch, irritant, and C-fibers, which include the J- and probably other receptors), each of which has its afferent pathway to the central nervous system in the vagus nerve. There are also receptors in the muscles and tendons that participate in breathing. The theory of "length-tension inappropriateness" postulates that misalignment of muscle spindles in the respiratory musculature serves as the genesis of dyspnea. However, the exact location of the receptors has never been proved, and the central nervous system ramifications of the signals, whatever their origin, are also poorly understood. The prevailing belief is that multiple pathways are involved.

PATTERNS. Dyspnea occurs with many underlying conditions and in several different patterns. Some of these are sufficiently characteristic to warrant separate designations. Episodes of breathlessness that wake patients from a sound sleep are called *paroxysmal nocturnal dyspnea;* these are most often observed in patients with chronic left ventricular failure but may also occur in patients with chronic pulmonary diseases because of pooling of secretions, gravity-induced decreases in lung volumes, or sleep-induced increases in air flow resistance. *Orthopnea,* or the onset or worsening of dyspnea on assuming the supine position, like paroxysmal nocturnal dyspnea, is found in patients with heart disease and occasionally in patients with chronic lung disease. The inability to assume the supine position (instant orthopnea) is particularly characteristic of the rare condition of paralysis of both hemidiaphragms. *Platypnea* denotes dyspnea that occurs in the upright position and *trepopnea* the even rarer form of dyspnea that develops in either the right or left lateral decubitus position. Both the terms *hyperpnea,* an increase in minute volume, and *hyperventilation,* an increase in alveolar ventilation in excess of carbon dioxide production, indicate that ventilation is increased above normal. However, neither term carries any implication about the presence or absence of dyspnea.

DIAGNOSTIC APPROACH. The differential diagnosis of the dyspneic patient begins with a careful history. In patients with chronic respiratory or cardiac disease, dyspnea initially develops only during physical activity, and the amount of exertion required to provoke the symptom relates in a general way to the severity of the underlying condition. Sudden episodes of dyspnea, unrelated to physical activity, typically occur with pulmonary embolism, spontaneous pneumothorax, and anxiety; the acute attacks in each of these disorders characteristically remit, but bouts of breathlessness may recur with varying severity.

The results of historical and physical examinations, routine blood tests, electrocardiography, and chest roentgenography nearly always indicate whether the dyspneic patient is suffering from a respiratory, cardiac, hematologic, renal, or hepatic abnormality. Special diagnostic studies are often then required to determine what specific kind of disease is present. Measurements of lung volumes, expiratory flow rates, and diffusing capacity, studies during exercise, and noninvasive tests of cardiac function are particularly valuable in three difficult clinical situations: (1) differentiating between dyspnea of cardiac and pulmonary origin and, if abnormalities of both systems coexist, as is often the case, estimating the severity of each; (2) identifying the presence of either pulmonary vascular obstructive disease or diffuse pulmonary infiltrative disorders in dyspneic patients whose routine studies, including chest roentgenograms, are normal; and (3) helping to establish, by ruling out significant cardiorespiratory abnormalities, that dyspnea in a given patient is psychogenic in origin (a diagnosis that is always tenuous).

TREATMENT. Unlike cough, for which there are effective antitussives, and pain, for which there are powerful analgesics, there is no category of medications for relief of dyspnea. Cure or alleviation of dyspnea depends on recognizing its origin and treating the basic abnormality. In acute reversible conditions, the dyspnea subsides along with improvement of its underlying cause. In chronic cardiac and pulmonary disorders, sufficient physical exertion will continue to provoke dyspnea, but even in these conditions rehabilitation programs can be used to enable patients to increase their physical activity up to the maximum of the limits imposed by their disease.

CONCLUSION

This introduction to the three most common and important symptoms of *all* diseases of the respiratory system is meant to supplement the material presented not only in the remainder of Part VIII but also elsewhere in the book. Acute infections of the upper and lower respiratory tract caused by viruses, bacteria, fungi, protozoa, and helminths are discussed in Parts XIX and XX. Systemic diseases in which the lungs may be involved are also discussed elsewhere: Wegener's granulomatosis (Ch. 452), eosinophilic syndromes (Ch. 162), and the "collagen diseases" (Ch. 440 to 466). Various abnormalities of the pulmonary circulation, exclusive of pulmonary embolism, and pulmonary edema, an important disorder (not disease) of the lungs, are discussed chiefly in Part VII.

Gold W: Dyspnea. *In* Blacklow RS (ed.): Signs and Symptoms. 6th ed. Philadelphia, J. B. Lippincott Company, 1979. *Good review of the pathophysiology of dyspnea.*

Gong H Jr, Salvatierra C: Clinical efficacy of early and delayed fiberoptic bronchoscopy in patients with hemoptysis. Am Rev Respir Dis 124:221, 1981. *A nice review of the pros and cons of early and delayed bronchoscopy for hemoptysis, but few patients with persistent massive bleeding were included. Good references.*

Hinshaw HC, Murray JF: Diseases of the Chest. 4th ed. Philadelphia, W. B. Saunders Company, 1980. *First five chapters review clinical history, physical examination, and diagnostic methods used in evaluating patients with lung disease.*

Irwin RS, Corrao WM, Pratter MR: Chronic persistent cough in the adult: The spectrum and frequency of causes and successful outcome of specific therapy. Am Rev Respir Dis 123:413, 1981. *An up-to-date review of the diagnosis and treatment of chronic persistent cough.*

Wasserman K: Dyspnea on exertion: Is it the heart or the lungs? JAMA 248:2039, 1982. *A brief review of the physiology of exercise and how these principles can be used to define the clinical origin of dyspnea.*

57. RESPIRATORY STRUCTURE AND FUNCTION

John F. Murray

Respiration can be defined as "those processes concerned with gas exchange between an organism and its environment." This definition, which emphasizes that the chief function of the respiratory system is *gas exchange,* is sufficiently comprehensive to apply to all animals, ranging from simple one-celled protozoa to infinitely more complex mammals. In human beings, the basic processes leading to gas exchange, or the uptake of O_2 and the elimination of CO_2, are usually separated into four functional subdivisions:

1. *Ventilation*—the movement of air from outside to inside the body and the distribution of air within the tracheobronchial system to the gas exchange units of the lungs.
2. *Diffusion*—the movement of O_2 and CO_2 across the alveolar-capillary membrane between the gas in alveolar spaces and the blood in pulmonary capillaries.
3. *Perfusion*—the flow of mixed venous blood through the pulmonary arterial circulation, distribution of the blood to the capillaries of the gas exchange units, and removal of the blood from the lungs through pulmonary veins.
4. *Control of breathing*—the regulation of ventilation, usually in accordance with changing metabolic demands.

VENTILATION

Air moves from outside the body into the gas exchange units of the lung because contraction of the muscles of respiration normally generates sufficient force to expand the lungs and chest wall and to overcome the resistance and inertia in the system. Accordingly, the volume of gas that reaches the individual gas exchange units is determined by the mechanical properties of the lung parenchyma, airways, and chest wall, and by the force provided by the muscles of respiration (or by a mechanical ventilator).

The amount of air that enters the lung with each breath is called the *tidal volume.* When the lungs are fully expanded, the amount of gas they contain is called the *total lung capacity.* The maximal volume of gas that a person can exhale from total lung capacity is called the *vital capacity,* and the amount of gas remaining in the lungs at the end of maximal expiration is called the *residual volume.* Another important static lung volume is the *functional residual capacity,* which is the volume of gas in the lungs at the end of a normal breath. The relationships among these different lung volumes, which vary in different disorders and which will be frequently referred to, are shown in Figure 57–1.

Static Properties

Both the lungs and chest wall are elastic structures. This means that they can be distended and, when the distending force is removed, they recoil back to their resting volumes. Although the lungs and chest wall are similar in this respect, they differ considerably in their respective resting volumes when there is no expanding force.

The elastic properties of isolated lungs are shown by the dashed line in Figure 57–1. The slope of the line, or the change in volume (ΔV) for a given change in pressure (ΔP), is known as the compliance of the lung. This curve demonstrates that (1) the lungs collapse almost completely when there is no distending pressure, (2) the slope of the volume-pressure curve is relatively steep at low lung volumes (i.e., as the lungs are beginning to inflate, their compliance is high), and (3) at high lung volumes, the curve flattens (compliance decreases) so that little increase in volume results from a large increase in pressure. The elastic forces of the lungs originate within the tissues that are being stretched, particularly those containing elastin and collagen, and from the surface tension of the film of *surfactant* that lines the air-liquid interface of alveolar spaces. The static properties of the isolated chest wall (including the diaphragm and abdominal contents that must be displaced during breathing) are shown by the dotted line in Figure 57–1. The chest wall is a compressible and distensible structure that contains an appreciable volume in its resting state. To decrease the volume of the thorax, a force must be applied to overcome the tendency of the chest wall to resist compression and recoil back to its resting position. Conversely, to increase the volume of the thorax, the applied force must overcome the elastic forces in the chest wall that also cause it to recoil back to its resting position.

It is useful conceptually to consider the behavior of the lung and chest wall separately, but obviously they function together. Because their action is coupled by the pleural pressure that keeps the lung expanded against the chest wall, the lungs and chest wall ordinarily change their volumes by exactly the same amount. Thus the pressures required to change the volume of the respiratory system are obtained by simply adding the separate pressures necessary to inflate the lungs and chest wall to a given volume. The solid line in Figure 57–1 indicates the pressure that must be produced by contraction of the respiratory muscles, or by a mechanical ventilator, to inflate or deflate both the lungs and chest wall. Figure 57–1 also shows that functional residual capacity is the volume at which the inward recoil force of the lung is equal and opposite to the outward recoil force of the chest wall; in other words, functional residual capacity is that volume at which the net force of the respiratory system is zero.

During inspiration, the force developed by the contracting muscles of inspiration meets progressively increasing (inward) recoil forces from the combined expansion of the lungs and chest wall. Furthermore, because shortening muscle fibers generate progressively less force, inspiration finally ceases at that volume (total lung capacity) at which the weakening inspiratory muscle forces can no longer overcome the increasing forces required to expand the lungs and chest wall. Similarly, during expiration, the net force developed by the contracting muscles of expiration meets progressively increasing (outward) recoil forces from the chest wall. In children and young adults, expiration ceases at that volume (residual volume) at which the decreasing expiratory muscle forces can no longer overcome the increasing forces required to compress the chest wall. In older persons, residual volume is governed mainly by factors that regulate the caliber and patency of peripheral airways; thus even though the expiratory muscles are capable of further compression of the thorax, emptying is prevented by airway closure and trapping of gas in the lungs.

Vital capacity, or the volume between total lung capacity and residual volume, is determined by the factors that influence maximum inspiration and expiration, i.e., the balance of forces generated by the muscles of respiration and by the mechanical properties of the lungs and chest wall combined. Changes in these variables explain the characteristic changes in lung volumes that occur in patients with the respiratory disorders discussed in subsequent chapters.

Lung volumes also vary among healthy persons according to their age, sex, and physical structure (especially height). Because body build varies slightly from one ethnic group to another, it is important to have normal data that pertain to the population being studied. Measured volumes are usually expressed as both the observed value and the percentage of the predicted mean value for a normal subject of the same age, sex, and height. Measured values should not be considered abnormal unless they are clearly outside the range of values likely to be found in normal persons (100 per cent ± 20 per cent for vital capacity and 100 per cent ± 25 per cent for total lung capacity, residual volume, and functional residual capacity).

Vital capacity is easily measured with a spirometer or one of a variety of commercially available recording systems. Most spirometers can also be used to determine rates of expiratory airflow (see Dynamic Properties, below), but they do not measure total lung capacity, functional residual capacity, or residual volume.

To measure *all* the gas in the lungs at any of these volumes, one of two basically different methods must be used: either dilution or washout of an inert gas or whole body plethysmography. Functional residual capacity is usually determined because it is the normal end-expiratory lung volume and thus is an easy volume for subjects to maintain during the breathing test. After measuring functional residual capacity, residual volume is derived by subtracting expiratory reserve volume,

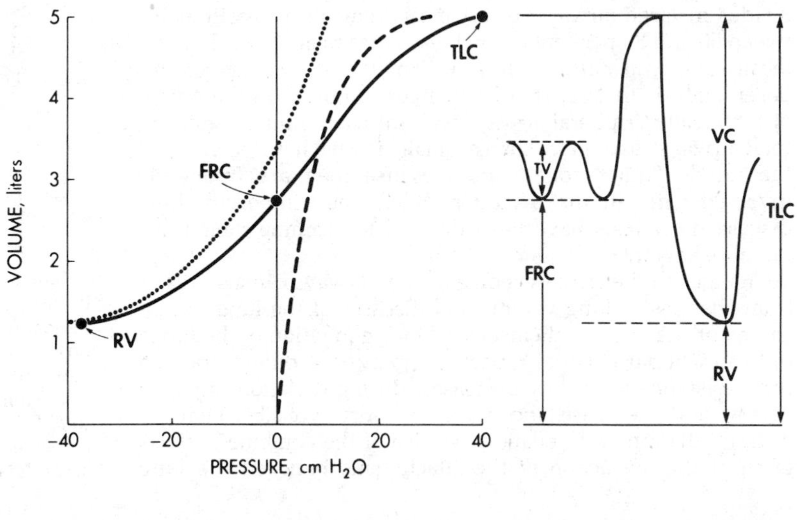

Figure 57–1. Schematic representation of the volume-pressure relationships of the chest wall (dotted line), lungs (dashed line), and chest wall and lungs combined (solid line). Total lung capacity (TLC) occurs when the lungs are fully expanded, and residual volume (RV) is the amount of gas remaining in the lungs at the end of a maximal expiration. Functional residual capacity (FRC) occurs at that volume at which the recoil pressures of the chest wall and lung are equal and opposite (i.e., the distending pressure = 0 cm H_2O). On the right is a spirometric tracing (volume-time) of the breathing maneuvers of the person whose pressure-volume curves are on the left. TV = tidal volume; VC = vital capacity.

and total lung capacity is obtained by adding vital capacity to the residual volume.

Gas dilution or washout involves measurement of the volume and concentration of an inert gas such as nitrogen (N_2), neon (Ne), or helium (He). These methods measure the amount of gas that communicates freely with the airways during the breathing maneuver; dilution or washout techniques do not detect gas trapped beyond closed (or very narrowed) airways and in poorly communicating regions, like bullae.

Body plethysmography involves placing the subject in the plethysmograph, a large airtight box resembling a telephone booth, and having him breathe through a mouthpiece in which a shutter can be closed to stop the flow of air. When the subject attempts to pant against the closed shutter, the volume of the thorax and gas in the lungs expands and contracts, which changes the pressure measured inside the mouthpiece. Movement of the thorax also changes the pressure in the box by compressing and expanding the gas surrounding the subject. From application of Boyle's law, which states that the pressure times the volume of a gas is constant if temperature remains the same, the volume of gas in the thorax can be calculated. The body plethysmograph measures all the gas present during the breathing maneuver, including that in freely communicating air-spaces and any that may be trapped behind poorly communicating airways or in closed spaces (pneumothorax).

In normal subjects, measurements of functional residual capacity by dilution (or washout) and plethysmographic techniques are virtually identical. In contrast, in patients with airways obstruction or bullous disease, the communicating volume may be considerably less than the plethysmographic volume and the difference is a measure of the noncommunicating (sometimes called trapped) volume.

Dynamic Properties

To cause air to flow from outside the body into the gas exchange units, a muscular (or other mechanical) force must be exerted to overcome not only the elastic recoil properties of the lungs and chest wall but also their resistive and inertial properties. In contrast to distensibility, which is not affected by the rate of movement, the forces required to offset resistance and inertia are markedly influenced by the velocity of airflow. Except in a few patients (e.g., those with severe obesity), inertial forces are ordinarily small and usually ignored; thus only those factors affecting airways resistance need be considered in detail.

Resistance to airflow is affected chiefly by the caliber of the air passages. Although the diameter of each successive generation of airways decreases, the combined total cross-sectional area at any level increases steadily throughout the tracheobronchial tree from the main bronchi to the peripheral airways. This means that airways resistance progressively decreases and that most of the resistance of the human tracheobronchial tree resides in large airways: direct measurements reveal that between 50 and 80 per cent of total resistance to airflow originates in airways *greater than* 2 mm in diameter. A corollary of this observation is that substantial changes can occur in the caliber of the small peripheral airways without having much effect on total airways resistance. Hence, small airways have been called the lung's "quiet zone," and because they are frequently involved early in the evolution of clinically important lung disease, new tests have been devised to examine their functional behavior.

Changes in the cross-sectional area of airways can also result from changes in lung volume and diseases of the lung parenchyma or the airways themselves. During inflation of the lungs from functional residual capacity, airways are pulled open so that resistance to airflow decreases; during deflation, airways narrow and their resistance increases. Airway caliber changes during inflation and deflation because of the combined effects of the tethering action of the attachments between the lung parenchyma and the smallest airways and the distending effect of pleural pressure on larger airways. Elastic recoil of the lung, which governs the pull of the attachments and the magnitude of pleural pressure, affects the size of all airways. It follows that when elastic recoil is decreased, as in patients with emphysema, airways are narrowed and resistance is increased; this mechanism accounts for much of the airflow obstruction found in patients with emphysema.

Airway narrowing can also result from bronchospasm, edema of the mucosal lining, and secretions within the lumen. Also, changes in the viscosity and density of the inspired gas affect airways resistance, and gas mixtures of different densities are sometimes used to study the dynamic properties of the tracheobronchial system.

Resistance to airflow can be measured in a body plethysmograph; however, this procedure has limited clinical usefulness. Fortunately, the important dynamic properties of the respiratory system can be assessed by several readily available tests of airways function. The simplest and most widely used of these is the forced expiratory volume in one second (FEV_1), expressed as a ratio of the forced vital capacity (FVC), or FEV_1/FVC (Fig. 57–2). To perform the FVC maneuver, the subject inhales fully and then exhales as rapidly and completely as possible. In normal persons, the FVC equals the vital capacity from a slow or nonexpulsive maneuver, but in patients with airways obstruction, vigorous expiration may cause airways to narrow and close prematurely so that the FVC may be less than the vital capacity; the magnitude of the difference between the two values is an indication of the amount of air trapped behind compressed airways. The FEV_1/FVC decreases with age in normal persons after reaching adulthood and is usually higher in women than in men at all ages.

Additional measurements of airways behavior besides the FEV_1 can be obtained from the tracing obtained during the FVC maneuver (Fig. 57–2): several derivatives of time such as the $FEV_{0.5}$ and FEV_3 (the subscript denoting the number of seconds after beginning expiration at which the expired volume is measured), the maximal expiratory flow rate (MEFR or often $MEFR_{200-1200\ ml}$, indicating that the flow rate was measured between expired volumes of 200 and 1200 ml), and the maximal mid-expiratory flow rate (MMFR or often $MMFR_{25-75\%}$, indicating that the rate was measured between expired volumes of 25 and 75 per cent of the FVC). None of these has any particular advantage over the FEV_1 except that the MMFR is less depend-

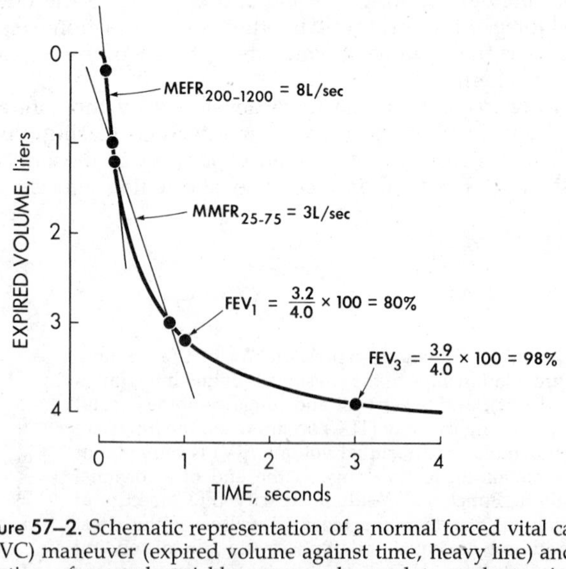

Figure 57–2. Schematic representation of a normal forced vital capacity (FVC) maneuver (expired volume against time, heavy line) and the derivation of several variables commonly used to evaluate airways obstruction. $MEFR_{200-1200}$ = maximal expiratory flow rate, measured between expired volumes of 200 and 1200 ml; $MMER_{25-75}$ = maximal mid-expiratory flow rate, measured between 25 and 75 per cent of the total FVC; FEV_1 = forced expiratory volume in one second, expressed as percentage of total FVC; FEV_3 = forced expiratory volume in three seconds, expressed as percentage of total FVC.

ent on the effort exerted by the subject than the other variables and reflects the flow properties of small as well as large airways.

Another way of examining the events during an FVC maneuver is by recording flow against volume instead of volume against time, which provides a maximal expiratory flow–volume curve (Fig. 57–3). From these records, maximal flow rates at any given fraction of the expired vital capacity, usually 50 per cent ($\dot{V}max_{50}$) or 75 per cent ($\dot{V}max_{75}$), can be determined and reported as the percentage of the predicted values for a subject of the same age, sex, and body size. The early portion of the maximal expiratory flow–volume curve, which includes peak flow, is determined by the effort exerted by the subject and is thus called the effort-*dependent* segment; the later portion is less influenced by effort and is called the effort-*independent* segment or that part of the curve during which expiratory airflow limitation occurs. Additional effort does not increase expiratory airflow (i.e., maximal velocity is limited), because the transmural pressure and the cross-sectional area of the compressible airways are affected just enough to offset the increased applied pressure causing the flow. Because events recorded in the effort-independent portion of the flow-volume curve require less cooperation and understanding by the subject, they are more reproducible than those in the effort-dependent portion.

Maximal expiratory flow-volume curves can also be recorded after a few breaths of 79 per cent He and 21 per cent O_2 (He-O_2) as well as after breathing room air (79 per cent N_2 and 21 per cent O_2). In normal persons, the two curves differ from each other because He is a less dense but more viscous gas than N_2. Thus higher flow rates are achieved with He-O_2 during the early and mid portions of expiration in which turbulence and convective acceleration (both density-dependent phenomena) occur; later, when slow laminar flow develops, viscous effects prevail and the He-O_2 curve is identical with or even lower than the room air curve. In general, in normal subjects, flow rates are higher with He-O_2 than with room air throughout most of expiration; appreciable differences in flows are evident at 50 per cent ($\Delta\dot{V}max_{50}$) and 75 per cent ($\Delta\dot{V}max_{75}$) of the expired vital capacity, and the volume at which the two curves intersect ($Viso_{\dot{V}}$) is close to residual volume.

In the presence of narrowing of peripheral airways, turbulence and convective acceleration are less prominent, so the He-O_2 curve is nearer to the room air curve than it should be; this means that $\Delta\dot{V}max_{50}$ and $\Delta\dot{V}max_{75}$ decrease and $Viso_{\dot{V}}$

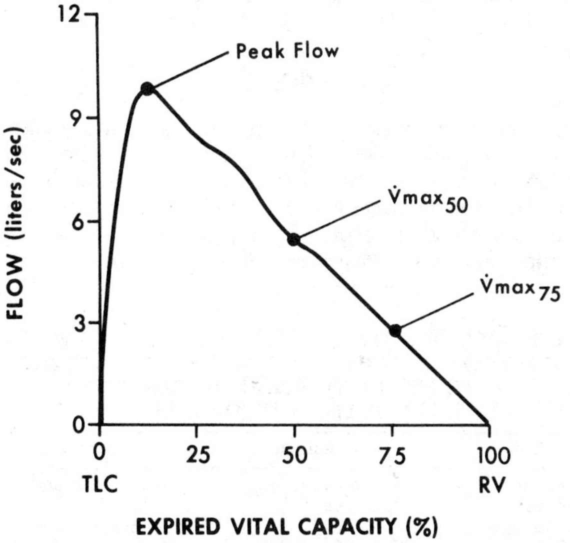

Figure 57–3. Typical forced expiratory flow-volume tracing of a normal adult man showing points of peak flow, maximal flow at 50 per cent expired vital capacity ($\dot{V}max_{50}$) and maximal flow at 75 per cent expired vital capacity ($\dot{V}max_{75}$). TLC = total lung capacity; RV = residual volume. (From Smith LH, Thier SO: Pathophysiology: The Biological Principles of Disease. Philadelphia, W. B. Saunders Company, 1981.)

increases. Comparison of maximal expiratory flow–volume curves obtained while breathing room air and He-O_2 seems to be one of the most sensitive tests for demonstrating structural abnormalities that are located in the small airways of the lungs; however, the value of these tests in detecting patients who will subsequently develop chronic bronchitis and emphysema remains to be proved.

Distribution of Ventilation

During the movement of air from outside the body into the lungs during inhalation, the airstream is partitioned as it flows through the tracheobronchial to the terminal respiratory units where gas exchange takes place. Even in healthy persons ventilation is not distributed uniformly, and marked derangements may develop in patients with lung disease.

The unevenness of ventilation found in normal subjects results from the vertical gradient of pleural pressure between the uppermost and lowermost parts of the lungs. The origins of the vertical gradient in different mammals are complex and include the weight of the lungs, their attachments at the hilum, and the shape and effects of the chest wall and abdominal contents; in humans, the weight of the lungs is the most important determinant. Because of the gradient in the pressure surrounding the lungs, alveoli are larger at the top than at the bottom, and there are regional differences in the distribution of inspired ventilation.

When breathing slowly from functional residual capacity, more inspired air is distributed to the dependent regions of the lungs than to the superior regions because the differences in pleural pressure cause the two regions to function on different segments of the same volume-pressure curve. Because the *change* in intrapleural pressure during quiet breathing is the same throughout the pleural space, the lower regions inflate more than the upper regions because they are operating on a steeper part of the curve and thus receive more volume for the same pressure change. When inspiration continues to total lung capacity, alveoli at the top and bottom of the lungs inflate to nearly the same size because both regions are functioning on the flat portion of the volume-pressure curve even though the pleural pressure difference persists. When the rate of inspiratory airflow increases, as during exercise, the distribution of ventilation becomes more uniform than it is at rest.

During expiration, pleural pressure surrounding the most dependent portion of each lung becomes positive; this causes airways in that region to close. As expiration continues, airway closure progresses from the lowermost regions up the lungs involving more and more airways. Regional differences in the distribution of ventilation can be examined by the test of closing volume (Fig. 57–4). After labeling alveolar gas by one of two methods (bolus or resident gas techniques), gas concentration measured at the mouth during the subsequent exhalation varies according to the sequence of regional emptying and occurs in four phases. Phase 1 reflects the composition of gas from the tracheobronchial system and contains none of the label; the concentration rapidly rises during Phase 2 as alveoli containing the label begin to empty; a near-plateau is evident in Phase 3 as alveoli throughout the entire lung deflate; finally, the plateau terminates abruptly with a steep rise in concentration during Phase 4. Closing volume is the junction between Phases 3 and 4 and is that volume at which airways in the dependent regions of the lung begin to close; accordingly, the rising concentration of the label in the subsequent expirate indicates the progressively increasing contributions from the preferentially labeled alveoli in the upper regions of the lung.

Because an increase in closing volume reflects premature closure or narrowing of airways, an increase in closing volume occurs in patients with lung disorders in which the caliber of peripheral airways is decreased from either decreased elastic recoil (e.g., in emphysema) or abnormalities of the airways themselves (e.g., in bronchitis or asthma). Furthermore, in-

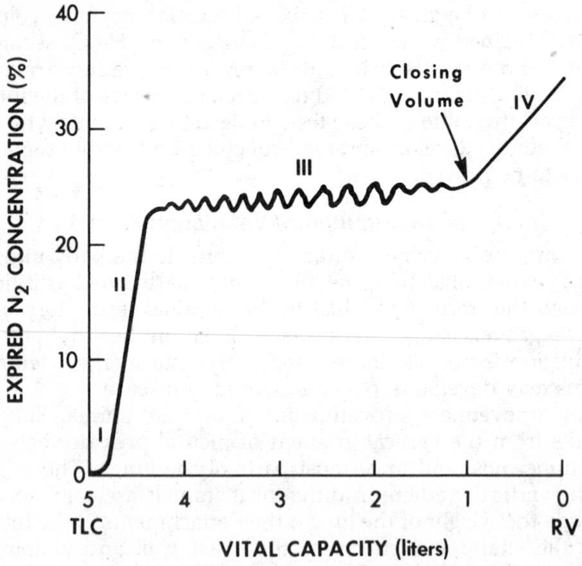

Figure 57–4. Representative tracing of expired nitrogen (N_2) concentration after taking a single breath of 100 per cent oxygen. An explanation of the four numbered phases (I, II, III, IV) is provided in the text. TLC = total lung capacity; RV = residual volume. (From Smith LH, Thier SO: Pathophysiology: The Biological Principles of Disease. Philadelphia, W. B. Saunders Company, 1981.)

creases in closing volume have been detected in asymptomatic patients, usually smokers, and may be an early manifestation of lung disease. In addition, the slope of Phase 3 is useful because it provides a sensitive measure of the adequacy of the distribution of ventilation. Well ventilated units fill and empty more completely and rapidly than poorly ventilated units; this means that the concentration of the label will be lower in the better ventilated regions that empty early during exhalation than in the poorly ventilated regions. Thus the more uneven the distribution of ventilation within the lung, the steeper the slope of Phase 3.

Other tests of the distribution of ventilation utilize the gamma ray–emitting properties of certain radioactive gases, chiefly ^{133}Xe, which are nontoxic and can be detected after inhalation in low concentrations by external counters. The distribution of ventilation can be assessed during a breath hold at end-inspiration after a single breath of ^{133}Xe or at intervals during its elimination by normal breathing after the lung has been labeled uniformly by rebreathing ^{133}Xe from a closed system.

Abnormalities of Ventilation

Lung diseases that cause abnormalities of ventilation are usually divided into two different categories: restrictive and obstructive ventilatory disorders. This classification is not completely satisfactory because it ignores the fact that disturbances of the distribution of ventilation are the earliest and by far the most common abnormality of ventilation and can occur in the absence of manifestations of coexisting obstructive or restrictive disorders.

DISTURBANCES OF DISTRIBUTION. Whenever a disease process involves the lung parenchyma or airways unevenly, abnormalities in the distribution of ventilation are likely to occur because more inspired gas will reach the normal regions of the lung compared with the regions distal to the sites of bronchial narrowing, or the regions in which the distensibility is impaired. Whether these functional changes can be detected depends on the extent and severity of the disease and the sensitivity of the test being used. The slope of Phase 3 of the closing volume maneuver is the most commonly used test for detecting early abnormalities in the distribution of ventilation. Frequency dependence of compliance is an extremely sensitive test for distribution of ventilation but is seldom used owing to its technical complexities.

RESTRICTIVE VENTILATORY DISORDERS. The term *restrictive ventilatory disorder* denotes a pattern of abnormalities in lung function. The word "restrictive" is employed to indicate a restriction of or limitation to the amount of gas within the lungs. Thus restrictive ventilatory disorders are characterized by reductions in lung volumes (Table 57–1). The hallmark of restriction is a decreased vital capacity, but because this change also occurs in obstructive ventilatory disorders, it is important to exclude the presence of airways obstruction (see Obstructive Ventilatory Disorders, below) or demonstrate the presence of reductions in other lung volumes, particularly total lung capacity.

Many components of the lung, chest wall, and respiratory control system determine the amount of gas that can be breathed into the lungs. Accordingly, restrictive ventilatory disorders can develop in diseases that (1) affect the chest wall or respiratory muscles (pectus excavatum, myasthenia gravis), (2) cause infiltrations in the lung parenchyma or air spaces (diffuse interstitial fibrosis, pulmonary edema), (3) involve the pleura (pleural thickening), (4) occupy space within the thorax (tumors, effusions, cardiac enlargement), and (5) occur after lung resection (pneumonectomy).

OBSTRUCTIVE VENTILATORY DISORDERS. The term *obstructive ventilatory disorder* denotes the constellation of abnormalities that results from limitation of expiratory airflow, regardless of its cause. Because the functional disturbances depend on the presence of increased airways resistance, obstructive ventilatory disorders are detected mainly by tests of the behavior of the respiratory system under dynamic conditions (Table 57–1). The FEV_1/FVC test is the most widely used, but tests of maximal flow-volume relationships are being used increasingly in the *early* diagnosis of airways obstruction, especially when the obstruction is situated in peripheral airways.

Obstructive ventilatory disorders are found in patients with asthma, bronchitis, emphysema, advanced bronchiectasis, or other diseases that cause narrowing of the tracheobronchial system. When the term "obstructive" was originally employed, it was not possible to differentiate among these various entities, so they were lumped together in the nonspecific category of chronic obstructive pulmonary disease. Now, however, it is possible by means of specialized tests of lung function to sort out the various diseases that cause airways obstruction, even when they coexist; the characteristic features of asthma, chronic bronchitis, and emphysema are described in subsequent chapters.

DIFFUSION

Diffusion can be defined as the movement of molecules from a region of higher to one of lower concentration; accordingly, diffusion tends to eliminate differences in concentration within the various regions accessible to the molecules. Diffusion is a passive process that results from the kinetic motion of the molecules, and no extra energy is required. In the lung, O_2

TABLE 57–1. CHARACTERISTIC CHANGES IN LUNG VOLUMES AND TESTS OF AIRWAYS RESISTANCE IN PATIENTS WITH RESTRICTIVE AND OBSTRUCTIVE VENTILATORY DISORDERS*

Test	Restrictive	Obstructive
Vital capacity	Decreased	Decreased or normal
Residual volume	Decreased	Increased
Total lung capacity	Decreased	Normal or increased
RV/TLC	Normal or slightly increased	Markedly increased
FEV_1/FVC	Normal or increased	Decreased
MMFR	Normal or decreased	Decreased
Slope of phase 3	Normal or increased	Increased

*Abbreviations: RV/TLC = residual volume to total lung capacity ratio; FEV_1/FVC = forced expiratory volume in one second to forced vital capacity ratio; MMFR = maximum mid-expiratory flow rate.

moves by diffusion from alveolar gas into pulmonary capillary blood; similarly, in the tissues, O_2 moves by diffusion from capillary blood in peripheral tissues into neighboring cells. Carbon dioxide also moves by diffusion but usually in the direction opposite to that of O_2. Both O_2 and CO_2 undergo chemical reactions in the bloodstream at the start and finish of their journeys between the lungs and the peripheral tissues; O_2 reacts solely with hemoglobin, and CO_2 reacts in part with hemoglobin and in part to form bicarbonate.

Diffusing Capacity

The diffusing capacity of the lung for any gas indicates the quantity of that gas that diffuses across the alveolar-capillary membrane per unit time in response to the difference in mean pressures of the gas within the alveolus and pulmonary capillary. Most inert gases (e.g., N_2) diffuse across the air-blood barrier so rapidly that the amount taken up by the lung is not detectably limited by the diffusibility of the gas and the properties of the lung and blood but is determined solely by the solubility of the gas and the volume of tissue and blood into which it can dissolve. This phenomenon enables use of highly soluble gases like acetylene, dimethyl ether, or nitrous oxide to measure lung tissue volume and pulmonary capillary blood flow.

The only two gases that measure the diffusing capacity of the lungs are O_2 and CO. Because of their unique ability to combine with hemoglobin, both have to diffuse across the alveolar-capillary membrane in large quantities to saturate the available hemoglobin at the gas pressure prevailing in the alveoli. Thus it may not be possible for complete equilibrium to occur before the hemoglobin-containing red blood cells leave the pulmonary capillaries and gas transfer ceases. Of the two gases, CO is much more widely used for the measurement of diffusing capacity than O_2 because of the ease and convenience of applying the various CO tests and because CO uptake is always diffusion limited. In contrast, O_2 uptake is not limited by diffusion (i.e., is not a test of diffusing capacity) in normal subjects except during heavy exercise or while breathing low concentrations of O_2.

Two general types of tests using CO are available that involve either a breath-holding maneuver (single breath method) or continuous rebreathing (steady state methods). These two methods yield systematically different results, largely because neither technique summarizes accurately the events taking place in the 100,000 gas exchange units of the lung, in each of which P_{CO} varies according to the ventilation and blood flow to the unit. Despite this shortcoming, measurements of the diffusing capacity of the lung have provided useful empirical information concerning the function of the lung in healthy persons and patients with lung diseases.

The quantity of CO that will diffuse in a known period of time from alveolar gas into capillary blood and combine with hemoglobin in response to a given pressure difference between gas and blood depends on (1) the solubility and diffusibility of CO in each layer of the air-blood barrier, (2) the surface area and thickness of the barrier, and (3) the rate of the chemical reaction between CO and hemoglobin within red blood cells. Because the solubility and diffusibility of CO are physical characteristics that presumably do not change under ordinary circumstances, the two chief components of diffusing capacity are the area and thickness of the alveolar-capillary membrane available for diffusion (D_M) and the pulmonary capillary blood volume (V_C), both of which can be derived by performing several measurements of diffusing capacity ($D_{L_{CO}}$) with the subject breathing gas mixtures of different concentrations of CO and O_2.

Normal values for CO-diffusing capacity depend chiefly on the person's lung volume and therefore closely correlate with body size, especially height. Approximately half the total resistance to diffusion of CO from alveolar gas to capillary blood resides in the membrane compartment and the other half in the chemical reaction that takes place in the pulmonary capillary blood volume. Accordingly, changes in the hemoglobin concentration have a calculable effect on total CO diffusion that should be taken into account when establishing the predicted "normal" value for a patient with anemia or polycythemia.

Diffusing capacity is normally higher in the supine than the erect posture because position changes V_C, and at high compared with low lung volumes because inflation recruits alveolar-capillary surface. When blood flow to the lung increases, as in muscular exercise, V_C also increases owing to recruitment of previously nonperfused capillaries and dilatation of others; these phenomena account for the progressive increase in $D_{L_{CO}}$ during increasingly strenuous levels of exercise. Similarly, the elevated pulmonary arterial pressures encountered in persons who live at high altitudes also recruit capillaries, increase V_C, and cause an increase in "normal" $D_{L_{CO}}$. For unexplained reasons (possibly genetic), natives of high altitudes have higher $D_{L_{CO}}$ values than sojourners fully acclimatized to the same altitude.

Abnormalities of CO-Diffusing Capacity

Based on the physiologic principles that govern the diffusion of CO, it can be inferred that $D_{L_{CO}}$ may increase or decrease in patients with various cardiopulmonary disorders that affect V_C, D_M, or both. When tests of diffusing capacity were first used to study patients with various forms of lung disease, it was assumed that abnormalities of gas transfer would result from thickening of the air-blood barrier by a pathologic process that lengthened the pathway for diffusion of gases; this concept led to the formulation of what became widely known as the *alveolar-capillary block syndrome*. The "block" meant that the distance CO molecules had to travel from gas to blood was increased and, in turn, that extra time was required for diffusion to reach equilibrium across the air-blood barrier. Now it is known that the importance of alveolar-capillary block has been greatly exaggerated because a decreased diffusing capacity is not a satisfactory cause for arterial hypoxia, especially in patients at rest; when a low P_{O_2} occurs, it is nearly always attributable to a ventilation-perfusion abnormality, or less often to a right-to-left shunt.

Pulmonary vascular disorders, such as pulmonary emboli and pulmonary vasculitis, that affect (directly or indirectly) the pulmonary capillary bed decrease D_L through a decrease in V_C. Similarly, $D_{L_{CO}}$ is reduced because of decreases in V_C in patients with infiltrative disorders of the interalveolar septum that obliterate or destroy capillaries. This is the usual mechanism underlying reduction of $D_{L_{CO}}$ in patients with sarcoidosis, diffuse interstitial fibrosis, berylliosis, or collagen diseases of the lung.

Changes in D_M account for a decreased $D_{L_{CO}}$ in patients with diseases in which some form of intra-alveolar filling process has occurred and the air-to-blood diffusion pathway is actually lengthened: pneumonia, pulmonary edema, alveolar proteinosis. A decrease in both D_M and V_C produces a low $D_{L_{CO}}$ in patients with disorders associated with removal or destruction of lung tissue, such as resectional surgery or emphysema.

An increase in $D_{L_{CO}}$ results occasionally from an increase in V_C secondary to hemodynamic changes in the pulmonary circulation: an increase in pulmonary arterial or left atrial pressures or an increase in pulmonary blood flow. The $D_{L_{CO}}$ is sometimes increased in patients with bronchial asthma during an attack, but the cause of this change is not known.

PERFUSION

The pulmonary circulation delivers blood in a thin film to the gas exchange units so that O_2 uptake and CO_2 elimination can occur. The physiologic determinants of pulmonary blood flow are analogous to those of ventilation in that the total volumes of ventilation and blood flow must be adequate to meet metabolic needs, and the distribution of both must be such that proportionate amounts of inspired fresh air and incoming mixed venous blood are delivered to individual gas exchange units. Ventilatory volume is controlled by the factors that regulate breathing (see below), whereas the volume of blood flowing through the lungs is determined mainly by the extrapulmonary mechanisms that govern cardiac output.

Distribution of Pulmonary Blood Flow

Pulmonary blood flow is not distributed uniformly throughout the lungs but is normally greatest in the dependent regions where pulmonary arterial pressure is highest and, conversely, is least in the superior regions where pulmonary arterial pressure is lowest. In the upright subject under resting conditions, the apices of the lungs are barely perfused and considerably more blood flows, even allowing for differences in the amount of lung tissue, to the basilar regions. The presence of nonuniform blood flow, which is not matched by comparable changes in ventilation, leads to important differences between regions of the lung in their defense capabilities and efficiency of gas exchange.

Regional blood flow is also governed by local factors, the most important of which is vasoconstriction secondary to alveolar hypoxia. As a consequence, blood flow is redistributed away from poorly ventilated gas exchange units and the matching of ventilation and perfusion is preserved.

Distribution of pulmonary blood flow can readily be measured by injecting radioactive substances, such as ^{125}I-albumin aggregates or ^{133}Xe dissolved in saline, and then detecting their location in the lung with an external counter system. Abnormalities in the volume and distribution of pulmonary blood flow may result from diseases that involve the blood vessels themselves (emboli, vasculitis, emphysema), from compression of blood vessels (tumors, cysts), or from vasoconstriction of blood vessels (alveolar hypoxia secondary to local abnormality of ventilation).

Other Functions

The pulmonary circulation has important functions besides providing blood flow for continuous gas exchange: (1) it acts as a filter of virtually the entire venous drainage; (2) it supplies substrates for the nutrition and metabolic needs of the lung, including the synthesis of surfactant; (3) it serves as a reservoir of blood for the left ventricle; (4) it affects endocrine function by modifying the pharmacologic properties of a variety of circulating substances; and (5) it provides a large surface area for the absorption and filtration of liquids and solutes.

CONTROL OF BREATHING

The respiratory system must maintain gas exchange during periods of stress, such as exercise and other forms of increased metabolic needs. The O_2 consumption may increase more than ten-fold from rest to strenuous exercise; over this range, arterial PO_2 remains remarkably constant. The correspondence between the volume of ventilation and the demands for O_2 uptake and CO_2 elimination results from the responsiveness of three reasonably well-characterized receptor systems that interact to regulate breathing in normal persons and patients with a variety of disease states: (1) receptors in the airways and lung parenchyma, (2) peripheral chemoreceptors, and (3) central chemoreceptors. Nerve impulse traffic from these receptors is integrated and modulated in the medulla with impulses arising from higher centers in the brain. The medulla can be viewed as the main headquarters for initiating, processing, and relaying messages concerning breathing to other parts of the body via nervous pathways. Some of the resulting medullary neural activity may reach the cerebral cortex and evoke conscious perception of breathing (i.e., the symptom of dyspnea); other impulses may travel through efferent pathways in the autonomic nervous system to the lungs and other organs; still other impulses may descend in the spinal cord to be processed with afferent impulses from peripheral nerves at different cord segments before finally being transmitted to the muscles of respiration and other effectors.

Abnormalities of Control of Breathing

Variations, usually increases, in the rate and depth of breathing occur in patients with many common clinical disturbances such as fever, metabolic diseases, or psychiatric disorders. Several frequently used drugs (e.g., aspirin, antidepressants, and alcohol) also affect ventilation. *Hyperventilation* occurs when ventilation increases out of proportion to CO_2 production and arterial PCO_2 decreases; *hypoventilation* is the converse. *Hyperpnea* signifies an increase in the rate and depth of breathing, such as occurs during exercise, but carries no implication concerning arterial PCO_2 values. It should be emphasized that a decrease in the O_2 pressure (PO_2) of arterial blood has several causes. In contrast, the pressure of CO_2 (PCO_2) is governed simply by the relationship between CO_2 production ($\dot{V}CO_2$) and CO_2 elimination by alveolar ventilation ($\dot{V}alv$):

$$PCO_2 = k\dot{V}CO_2/\dot{V}alv.$$

Because alveolar ventilation normally changes to keep pace with CO_2 production, for practical purposes abnormal arterial PCO_2 values can always be interpreted as indicating hyper- or hypoventilation.

Abnormalities of the control of breathing can result from excitation of intrapulmonary receptors (pulmonary embolism, pneumonia, asthma), depression of peripheral chemoreceptors (natives of high altitudes, sedative drugs, severe chronic bronchitis), stimulation of peripheral chemoreceptors (drugs such as doxapram), depression of central chemoreceptors (sedative drugs, obesity, myxedema, neurologic disorders), and stimulation of central chemoreceptors (drugs such as aspirin, irritative neurologic lesions). Special tests of the ventilatory response to breathing gas mixtures with increased CO_2 or decreased O_2 and a test that determines the pressure developed during the first 0.1 second of breathing against a closed mouthpiece ($P_{0.1}$) help in defining the physiologic derangements among these disorders.

GAS EXCHANGE

The end product of respiration is gas exchange, which in human beings consists of maintaining the values for PO_2 and PCO_2 in arterial blood within normal limits. As stated previously, respiration consists of ventilation, including the distribution of inspired air throughout the tracheobronchial system, diffusion, blood flow, including the distribution of mixed venous blood throughout pulmonary capillaries, and the control of breathing. Each of these contributes in a unique way to gas exchange such that an impairment in one process cannot be compensated for by improvement in another.

Ambient air consists primarily of N_2 and O_2 with varying amounts of water vapor. As air is inhaled, it is warmed to body temperature and fully saturated with water vapor (PH_2O 37° C = 47 mm Hg); the addition of water vapor has the effect of diluting the inspired mixture of N_2 and O_2 and reduces their respective pressures proportionately. During gas exchange in the alveoli, more O_2 is removed than CO_2 is added; this causes the volume of each respiratory unit to decrease slightly and raises the concentration and pressure of N_2 slightly. When ventilation and perfusion are each uniformly distributed to various units (Fig. 57–5), "ideal" conditions for gas exchange exist and there is no difference between the PO_2 values in (mean) alveolar gas and arterial blood. The alveolar-arterial PO_2 difference is an important measure of the uniformity of matching of ventilation and perfusion. The difference is derived from a direct measurement of the arterial PO_2, which is subtracted from alveolar PO_2 (PA_{O_2}) calculated according to the following equation:

$$PA_{O_2} = PI_{O_2} - PA_{CO_2}\left[FI_{O_2} + \frac{1 - FI_{O_2}}{R}\right]$$

were $P_{I_{O_2}}$ = P_{O_2} of inspired gas, $P_{A_{CO_2}}$ = alveolar P_{CO_2} (usually assumed to equal arterial P_{CO_2}), $F_{I_{O_2}}$ = fractional concentration of O_2 in inspired gas, and R = respiratory exchange ratio (often assumed to equal 0.8).

However, gas exchange in healthy lungs is not perfect because there is a small (5 to 10 mm Hg) alveolar-arterial P_{O_2} difference, which occurs because of the normal presence of a slight nonuniformity in the distribution of ventilation with respect to perfusion and a small right-to-left shunt. It is also noteworthy that the sum of the pressures of the individual gases in mixed venous blood is less than the total atmospheric pressure. Because the tissues and spaces of the body are in approximate equilibrium with venous blood, these structures are also subatmospheric. The "suction" serves to keep the lung expanded against the chest wall and to cause the reabsorption of gas from tissue spaces (e.g., a pneumothorax).

Abnormal Gas Exchange

Measurements of arterial P_{O_2} and P_{CO_2} and calculations of the alveolar-arterial P_{O_2} difference are reliable guides to the overall adequacy of respiration. In determining whether or not an abnormality is present, it must be remembered that normal values for P_{O_2}, but not P_{CO_2}, vary with age and that both P_{O_2} and P_{CO_2} are influenced by the altitude at which the subject is living. There are five physiologic mechanisms known to cause arterial hypoxia, defined as a decrease below normal of arterial P_{O_2}: (1) hypoventilation, (2) decreased diffusion, (3) ventilation-perfusion imbalance, (4) right-to-left shunting of blood, and (5) breathing air (or a gas mixture) with a low P_{O_2}. Except for a few uncommon clinical examples, such as breathing air with its P_{O_2} reduced by combustion of O_2 and addition of smoke or suffocation, item 5 can be ignored. Items 1 to 4 can be separated, at least for practical clinical purposes, by analyzing the values from a given blood specimen and a few easy tests.

HYPOVENTILATION. The simplest disturbance of gas exchange occurs when not enough fresh air is breathed into alveolar spaces to raise pulmonary capillary P_{O_2} to normal levels and to allow CO_2 to leave the bloodstream. Although arterial P_{CO_2} may theoretically increase in patients with other disturbances of gas exchange (ventilation-perfusion abnormalities and right-to-left shunts), for clinical purposes an elevated value should be interpreted as indicating alveolar hypoventilation.

Pure hypoventilation is a relatively uncommon clinical event. When it is found, depression of the central nervous system resulting from anesthetic agents or other sedative drugs is the usual cause. More commonly, hypoventilation occurs in association with other disturbances of oxygenation. When these coexist, they can be recognized by the fact that the decrease in arterial P_{O_2} is more than can be accounted for by the increase in arterial P_{CO_2}.

IMPAIRED DIFFUSION. Decreased diffusion, from either loss of pulmonary capillaries or thickening of the air-blood barrier, does not usually cause important alveolar-arterial P_{O_2} differences *at rest*. Thus abnormalities of diffusion can be ignored in patients with arterial hypoxia whose blood specimens are obtained while they are resting. In contrast, impaired diffusion is one of the two major causes of severely worsening hypoxia

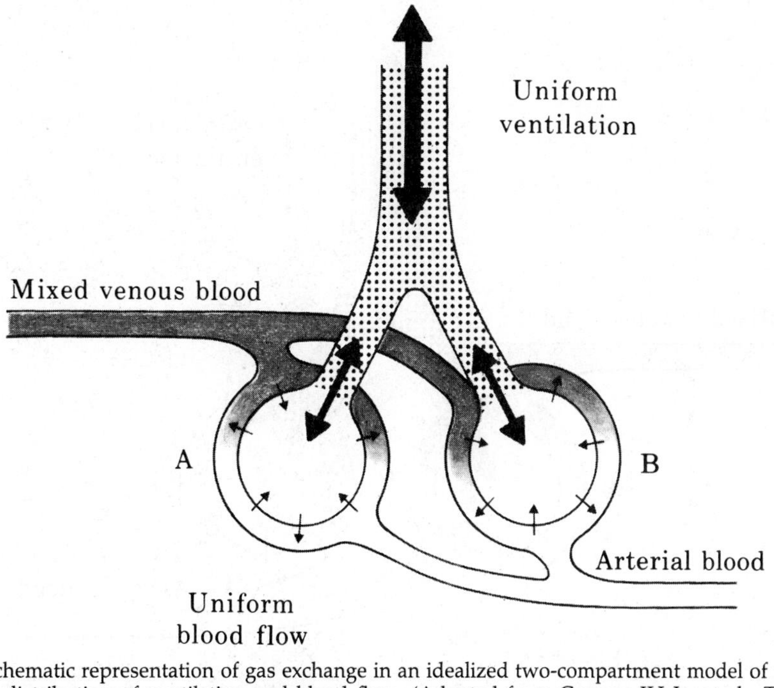

Figure 57–5. Schematic representation of gas exchange in an idealized two-compartment model of the lung in which there is uniform distribution of ventilation and blood flow. (Adapted from Comroe JH Jr, et al.: The Lung: Clinical Physiology and Pulmonary Function Tests. 2nd ed. Chicago, Year Book Medical Publishers, 1962. Reprinted by permission from the authors and Year Book Publisher, Inc.)

	A	*B*	*A + B*	*Units*
Alveolar ventilation	2.4	2.4	4.8	L/min
Pulmonary blood flow	3.0	3.0	6.0	L/min
Ventilation-perfusion ratio	0.8	0.8	0.8	
Mixed venous P_{O_2}	40	40	40	mm Hg
Mixed venous S_{O_2}	75	75	75	per cent
Mixed venous P_{CO_2}	46	46	46	mm Hg
Alveolar P_{O_2}	101	101	101	mm Hg
Arterial P_{O_2}	101	101	101	mm Hg
Arterial S_{O_2}	97.5	97.5	97.5	per cent
Arterial P_{CO_2}	40	40	40	mm Hg
Alveolar-arterial P_{O_2} difference	0	0	0	mm Hg

during exercise (right-to-left shunting of blood is the other). Regardless of the cause of the diffusing impairment, under resting conditions there is sufficient time to allow gas transfer to reach equilibrium between gas and blood. However, during exercise, cardiac output and the velocity of blood flow through pulmonary capillaries increase; thus the time for gas transfer is reduced and alveolar–end-capillary Po_2 differences may occur.

VENTILATION-PERFUSION MISMATCHING. Because the distributions of inspired air and pulmonary blood flow in normal lungs are neither uniform nor proportionate to each other, a slight ventilation-perfusion imbalance exists in healthy persons. Moreover, increased (above normal) mismatching of ventilation and perfusion is by far the most common cause of arterial hypoxia encountered clinically. Virtually all forms of lung disease are associated with a detectable ventilation-perfusion abnormality.

When a unit is underventilated relative to its perfusion (i.e., has a low ventilation-perfusion ratio), O_2 uptake by that unit must decrease so that the Po_2 of its end-capillary blood is lower than normal; Pco_2 tends to increase but cannot rise above the value in mixed venous blood (Fig. 57–6). Thus the process affects values for Po_2 more than Pco_2. Furthermore, in those units that are overventilated owing to a redistribution of inspired air, the high ventilation-perfusion ratio causes Po_2 to increase and Pco_2 to decrease. But there is an important difference in the effects of these changes in pressures on the actual quantities (contents) of O_2 and CO_2 in the capillary blood leaving units with high ventilation-perfusion ratios. Given the shapes of the respective dissociation curves, O_2 content is not appreciably increased but CO_2 content is decreased. Thus increasing ventilation with respect to perfusion in some regions corrects the tendency to CO_2 retention that would otherwise exist but does not correct the hypoxia caused by low ventilation-perfusion relationships in other units. Another invariable consequence of a ventilation-perfusion abnormality is an increase in the alveolar-arterial Po_2 difference.

RIGHT-TO-LEFT SHUNTING. A small right-to-left shunt of blood is found in normal persons, and shunts of considerable magnitude may occur in patients with pulmonary disease. A right-to-left shunt may be visualized as a pathway(s) through which mixed venous blood flows from the right to the left side of the heart without having contacted functioning gas exchange units along the way. Thus there is a continuous admixture of venous blood with arterialized blood that has come from normal pathways in the lungs. Arterial hypoxia and an increased alveolar-arterial Po_2 difference occur that vary in severity with the magnitude of the shunt and its O_2 content. Right-to-left shunts occur through intracardiac communications in patients with congenital heart disease. In patients with lung disease, although shunts may be extremely large, they seldom occur through abnormal vascular channels such as pulmonary arteriovenous fistulas; instead, they are caused by blood perfusing normal vessels in regions of lung that are atelectatic or in which alveoli are filled with edema fluid, pus, or blood; in either case, because gas transfer is impossible, a shunt occurs.

The consequences of a right-to-left shunt are similar to those of a ventilation-perfusion imbalance owing to basic similarities between the two disturbances. A shunt can be viewed as an extreme ventilation-perfusion abnormality in which there is perfusion but *no* ventilation at all. It is impossible to differentiate between a ventilation-perfusion disturbance and a right-

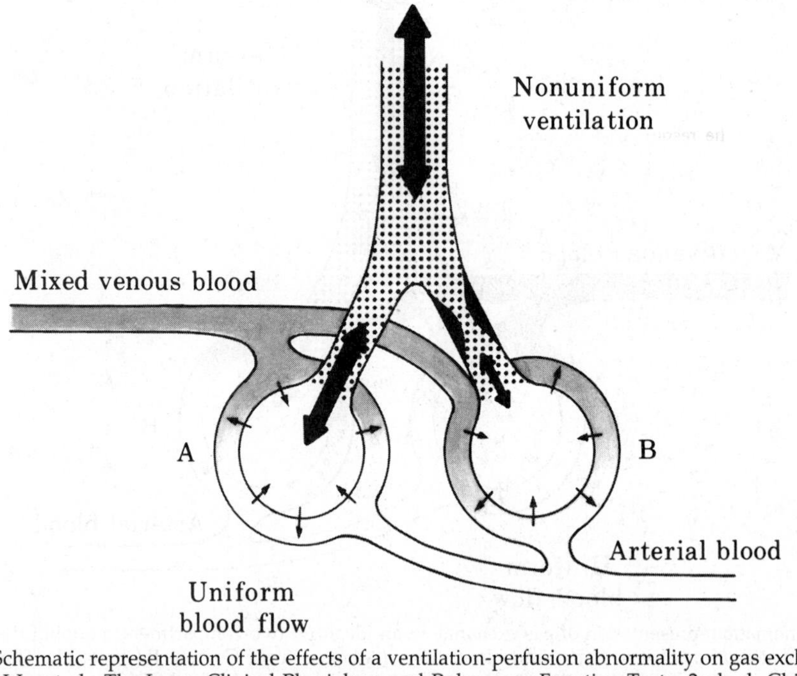

Figure 57–6. Schematic representation of the effects of a ventilation-perfusion abnormality on gas exchange. (Adapted from Comroe JH Jr, et al.: The Lung: Clinical Physiology and Pulmonary Function Tests. 2nd ed. Chicago, Year Book Medical Publishers, 1962. Reprinted by permission from the authors and Year Book Publisher, Inc.)

	A	*B*	*A + B*	*Units*
Alveolar ventilation	3.6	1.2	4.8	L/min
Pulmonary blood flow	3.0	3.0	6.0	L/min
Ventilation-perfusion ratio	1.2	0.4	0.8	
Mixed venous Po_2	40	40	40	mm Hg
Mixed venous So_2	75	75	75	per cent
Mixed venous Pco_2	46	46	46	mm Hg
Alveolar Po_2	114	77	106	mm Hg
Arterial Po_2	114	77	89	mm Hg
Arterial So_2	98.2	95.4	96.8	per cent
Arterial Pco_2	36	45	40	mm Hg
Alveolar-arterial Po_2 difference	0	0	17	mm Hg

to-left shunt while the subject is breathing ambient air; therefore the effects of both are combined and designated as venous admixture or a "shunt-like" effect. The two causes of hypoxia can be separated by giving the patient 100 per cent O_2 to breathe and measuring arterial Po_2 after all the N_2 has been washed out of the lungs. When a ventilation-perfusion abnormality exists, the N_2 is replaced by O_2 and all the blood perfusing the lungs equilibrates at a high Po_2 (approximately 600 mm Hg); in this way 100 per cent O_2 is said to "correct" a ventilation-perfusion disturbance. In contrast, in the presence of a right-to-left shunt, the admixture of mixed venous blood continues despite breathing 100 per cent O_2 and arterial hypoxia persists. In fact, the alveolar-arterial Po_2 difference in patients with a right-to-left shunt is higher during breathing of 100 per cent O_2 compared with room air, whereas the opposite occurs in patients with ventilation-perfusion inequalities.

Significance of Arterial Blood Gas Values

The availability of accurate rapid analyzers for measuring Po_2, Pco_2, and pH has been one of the major clinical advances of the last 25 years. Virtually the entire therapeutic approach to patients with acute and chronic respiratory failure is dictated by the presence and magnitude of blood gas and pH abnormalities (see Ch. 70). Every physician should know the mechanisms of arterial hypoxia and how to differentiate them, because it is important clinically whether a patient's hypoxia results from hypoventilation, impaired diffusion, ventilation-perfusion mismatching, or right-to-left shunting. Evaluating the course and prognosis of the lung disease, determining the need for and outcome of therapy, and assessing disability, operability, and the limits of resection in patients considered for pulmonary surgery all depend to some extent on the findings of blood gas analysis. Thus all physicians who care for patients must become familiar with the technique of arterial puncture and must know how to interpret the results of blood gas analysis.

Cotes JE: Lung Function. 4th ed. Philadelphia, J. B. Lippincott Company, 1979. *Good textbook of pulmonary physiology.*

Derenne J-P, Macklem PT, Roussos CH: The respiratory muscles: Mechanics, control and pathophysiology. Am Rev Respir Dis 118:119, 373, 581, 1978. *Detailed, three-part review of all you need to know about the respiratory muscles; 443 references.*

Hughes JMB: Editorial review. Pulmonary gas exchange. Clin Sci 58:119, 1980. *Good overview of normal and abnormal gas exchange.*

Murray JF: The Normal Lung: The Basis for Diagnosis and Treatment of Pulmonary Disease. Philadelphia, W. B. Saunders Company, 1976. *Review of normal anatomy, pulmonary physiology, and structure-function correlations.*

Sampson MG, Grassino A: Neuromechanical properties in obese patients during carbon dioxide breathing. Am J Med 75:81, 1983. *Elegant study using the latest techniques that explains abnormal pulmonary function findings in massive obesity.*

Tisi GM: Preoperative evaluation of pulmonary function. Validity, indications, and benefits. Am Rev Respir Dis 119:293, 1979. *Good review of indications for, types of tests used in, and value of preoperative functional evaluation; 113 references.*

Wanner A: Interpretation of pulmonary function tests. *In* Sackner MA (ed.): Diagnostic Techniques in Pulmonary Disease. Part 1. New York, Marcel Dekker, Inc., 1980, 353 pgs. *A thorough review of the clinical usefulness of pulmonary function testing in adults.*

Wilson TA, Hyatt RE, Rodarte JR: The mechanisms that limit expiratory airflow. Lung 158:193, 1980. *A review of the latest theories and models to explain expiratory airflow limitation. For the mathematically inclined only.*

58. SPECIAL DIAGNOSTIC PROCEDURES IN PULMONARY DISEASE

Gordon L. Snider

Pulmonary disease comes to light because the patient has respiratory symptoms, because the physician finds abnormalities on physical examination, or because a chest roentgenogram has disclosed an abnormal shadow. With the data in hand from the history and physical examination, chest film (see below), and basic blood and urine laboratory tests, the physician must choose among a broad array of special procedures in order to establish a diagnosis and develop a plan of management. Clinical pulmonary function testing is discussed in Ch. 57. This chapter will review the special diagnostic procedures applicable to pulmonary disease, with comments on when they are to be used and on their limitations.

THE CHEST ROENTGENOGRAM

STANDARD VIEWS. The chest roentgenogram can detect abnormalities in the asymptomatic patient with a normal physical examination of the chest. Even in the presence of respiratory symptoms, the chest roentgenogram may be abnormal when the physical examination is nonrevealing. On the other hand, the full inspiration chest roentgenogram provides no dynamic information, and crackles denoting parenchymal disease or wheezes indicating bronchial disease may be present when the lung fields appear normal in the roentgenogram. Complete evaluation of the respiratory system in the individual who is symptomatic, or who is suspected on other grounds of having pulmonary disease, must include both a physical examination and a chest roentgenogram.

The standard projections are the posteroanterior (PA) and lateral views of the chest. The PA view is taken in full inspiration with the patient's anterior chest wall against the film and the scapulae rotated anterolaterally; the x-ray tube is about 2 meters from the patient so that divergence of the x-ray beam is minimal and the images of the heart and any pulmonary lesions are not magnified. The lateral chest film exposes to view portions of the lungs obscured in the PA view by the heart, the mediastinal structures, and the leaflets of the diaphragm. Precise localization of a lesion usually requires display in both the PA and lateral projections.

The pulmonary parenchyma has two major components: (1) the respiratory tissues are strikingly radiolucent because they are more than 90 per cent air at total lung capacity; and (2) the pulmonary vessels present as a branching pattern of denser shadows gradually tapering from the hilum to the periphery but normally seen in a film of good quality to within 1 cm of the edge of the lung. The air columns in lobar and smaller bronchi are not usually seen except adjacent to the lung roots. Variations in density of the lung fields are caused not just by disease processes but also by differences in the depth of respiration and the technical factors of positioning the patient, x-ray exposure, and processing of the film.

Parenchymal abnormalities may be manifest by either an increase or a decrease in roentgenographic density. Diseases which cause an increase in density may be classified into predominant air-space disease, predominant interstitial disease, or shadows due to atelectasis. Air-space consolidation is characterized by poorly marginated densities, often patchy in distribution, and with a tendency to coalesce. Shadows of the air-filled bronchi may become visible in contrast to the consolidated lung tissue surrounding them, an appearance known as an air bronchogram. Densities abutting pleural surfaces, including the fissures, are sharply marginated, a property which aids in their localization. The volume of affected lung is normal or even increased. Bacterial pneumonia and pulmonary edema are examples of air-space consolidation.

Processes which predominantly affect the parenchymal interstitium, such as viral pneumonia and chemical injury of the lung, tend to give rise to linear or lacy patterns of abnormal shadows. The processes are widespread but often uneven in intensity and may be accompanied by some degree of alveolar exudation. Fibrosis with incorporation of alveoli into the interstitium causes loss of lung volume.

Atelectasis is a state in which lung tissue is shrunken and airless. The process may be due to bronchial obstruction, to compression of lung by air or fluid in the pleural space, to pulmonary fibrosis, or to alveolar collapse from impaired surfactant activity. The volume of lung affected may vary from less than a segment to an entire lung. Loss of volume may be evidenced on the roentgenogram by shifting of the interlobar fissures, the chest wall, or mediastinal structures toward the atelectatic region.

Dense, circumscribed shadows may result from neoplasms, inflammatory processes, or fluid-filled cysts. These shadows may be well or poorly marginated and single or multiple, and may range in size from less than 1 cm to densities which almost fill a hemithorax. It is common to refer to large solitary circumscribed shadows as mass lesions. Central radiolucencies representing necrosis and cavitation may be seen in circumscribed lesions.

There are a number of parenchymal processes which give rise to a focal or widespread decrease in roentgen density. In emphysema (see Ch. 60), the destruction of lung parenchyma results in increased transradiancy and attenuation of the vascular pattern. When the process is very severe locally, bullae may be evident as localized radiolucent zones partially or completely surrounded by arcuate hairline shadows. Increased transradiancy of lung parenchyma is also observed in conditions in which there is high-grade obstruction of the distal airways with pulmonary overdistention, as in severe asthma (see Ch. 59) and obliterative bronchiolitis (see Ch. 60). A decrease in the amount of blood in relation to tissue is also noted in congenital or acquired narrowing or obstruction of the pulmonary arteries.

Some disease processes show predilections for particular zones of the lung. For example, postprimary tuberculosis occurs most frequently in the apical-posterior segments of the upper lobes; pulmonary embolism and infarction favor the lower lobes. These preferential localizations, although not always rationally explained, are often helpful in differential diagnosis.

Pleural fluid causes an increase in roentgenographic density; the different types of fluid are not roentgenographically distinguishable. A small amount of free fluid in the subcostal pleural space presents as obliteration of the costophrenic angle; larger amounts of fluid present as homogeneous basilar densities with an upper border which is concave. Pleural fluid may occasionally present atypically with a border which is convex upward, mimicking an elevated hemidiaphragm—a so-called infrapulmonary effusion. Fluid may also be loculated in the interlobar fissures, in the subcostal pleura, or paramediastinally. Such shadows usually present as sharply marginated, homogeneous, ovoid densities. The pleura may also be the site of fibrous thickening, calcification, or neoplastic processes.

Pneumothorax is identified by the presence of a radiolucent zone without vascular markings which subtends part or all of the subcostal parietal pleura. In massive pneumothorax, the underlying lung may be completely collapsed and the mediastinum is shifted to the contralateral side. With lesser degrees of pneumothorax, the lung will be variably aerated and the sharp margin of the visceral pleura can be identified, separating the pneumothorax on one side and the slightly denser lung on the other. If fluid accompanies the pneumothorax, its upper border is horizontal, presenting as an air-fluid level.

FLUOROSCOPY. Fluoroscopy permits inspection of the chest during motion and is useful for establishing the diagnosis of diaphragmatic paralysis, for localizing circumscribed dense shadows in preparation for further roentgenographic study, or for guiding placement of a needle, a bronchial brush, or a biopsy forceps. The extent of diaphragmatic excursion during deep breathing is readily determined; paradoxical upward movement of the hemidiaphragm during an inspiratory sniff or downward movement during cough helps confirm the suspicion of paralysis.

INSPIRATION-EXPIRATION VIEWS. Films taken a few moments apart in full inspiration and full expiration provide a record of the respiratory system at total lung capacity and at residual volume. An expiration film is useful for confirming the presence of a small pneumothorax; the air in the pleural space shows an apparent increase in size and air leaves the underlying lung, making it more dense and enhancing contrast with the pneumothorax. Inspiration-expiration films are also useful for the demonstration of unilateral or focal obstruction of airways, whether by foreign body or tumor in the large airways or by generalized disease of the small airways. In the expiratory film, the parenchyma beyond the involved airways will empty poorly and the mediastinum will shift away from the involved lung.

SPECIAL VIEWS AND TECHNIQUES. Special views should generally be ordered only after consultation with the radiologist. The lordotic projection throws the images of the clavicles and anterior ends of the first ribs upward, thus bringing the structures in the apical-posterior segments of the upper lobes into clear view. This projection is useful when tuberculosis is suspected; it may more clearly show small nodular shadows due to granulomatous disease and may occasionally show a cavity which is not seen in the plain PA film; however, the lordotic view may conceal a lesion in the anterior segment of the upper lobe.

Portable films are views taken at the bedside in seriously ill patients. The views are anteroposterior (AP) in projection with the patient "upright" at an angle of 45 to 80 degrees. The tube-film distance is about 4 feet, resulting in magnification of the heart shadow. These films have more limitations in diagnostic potential than standard PA films but are frequently necessary.

Lateral decubitus views are made with the patient lying on one side with the x-ray beam oriented in a horizontal plane. This technique is of great value in the identification of small pleural effusions which are free in the subcostal pleural space. Comparison of the lateral decubitus and PA films reveals the appearance in the former of a dense shadow along the lateral chest wall due to fluid which has flowed from above the diaphragm in response to the effects of gravity. Less than 100 ml of fluid may be identified, and the presence of fluid with an atypical presentation may be readily shown. The technique may also be used to confirm the presence of air-fluid levels in the thorax and for demonstrating whether a structure that appears within a cavity is really an intracavitary, freely moving body such as a mycetoma (fungus ball).

Comparison of current PA and lateral views with old films often yields information of signal importance. A solitary pulmonary nodule may be shown to have been present and unchanging for years or alternatively to have appeared in the recent past. It may become obvious that an air-fluid level in the lung represents an infected bulla rather than a lung abscess. Few diagnostic procedures will as richly repay the physician's efforts as an assiduous search for old chest roentgenograms.

Special views for study of the bones are often helpful. Rib films in suspected fracture and spine films in the evaluation of chest pain are examples. Contrast studies of the esophagus and stomach are valuable in studying mediastinal masses and diaphragmatic hernias as well as in the detection of disorders of esophageal function such as achalasia or intrinsic disorders of these organs.

COMPUTED TOMOGRAPHIC SCANNING. Computed tomographic (CT) scanning provides a transverse image of a thin "slice" of the thorax. A thin beam of x-rays passes through the thorax, and the change in the attenuation of the x-rays is measured by a series of detectors. A computer reconstructs a pictorial image which represents the differential absorption of the x-ray beam through the chest. Newer equipment completes a single scan in two to ten seconds, a time which permits breath-holding. The examination is usually performed in the supine position, but prone and lateral recumbent projections can also be utilized. The contrast of mediastinal blood vessels can be enhanced, readily marking their identity, by intravenous infusion of a small amount of an iodinated material.

The method is unique in imaging the mediastinal structures, embedded as they are in a radiolucent matrix of fatty areolar tissue. CT scanning is the method of choice for staging the mediastinum in bronchogenic carcinoma. The absence of lymph nodes >1.5 cm in diameter indicates that the probability of metastatic disease in nodes is low (<8%). Larger lymph nodes should be sampled for histologic study by CT-directed mediastinoscopy or anterior mediastinotomy. Abnormal masses are readily seen; hilar enlargement caused by enlarged vessels is easily distinguished from that caused by lymphadenopathy by means of vascular contrast enhancement. Collections of fat can be unequivocally identified by the characteristic, computer-generated attenuation number. The method is more sensitive than linear tomography in screening for small nodular shadows, such as metastatic neoplasm, and is of unique value in detecting focal areas of pleural thickening and differentiating them from peripheral pulmonary lesions; CT is sensitive in detecting calcification and is useful in studying solitary pulmonary nodules (see accompanying figure). The technique is also used for identifying pulmonary lesions in areas which are ordinarily poorly seen in conventional roentgenograms or tomograms such as the lung adjacent to mediastinal structures, including the paravertebral areas (especially at the thoracoabdominal junction) and the posterior costophrenic sulci. Lesions in the parenchyma which are obscured by complex pleural or parenchymal shadows are well shown; the method is therefore useful in evaluating suppurative processes that involve both the pleura and lung parenchyma. Bronchiectasis may be diagnosed by CT scanning especially when the ectatic bronchi are surrounded by nonaerated lung parenchyma.

LINEAR TOMOGRAPHY. Tomography is a technique in which films are exposed while the x-ray tube and the film move proportionally in opposite directions. The effect is to allow selective visualization of a predetermined layer of tissue to the exclusion of structures lying superficial or deep to this layer. In essence, the image is that of a thin "slice" of lung. The procedure provides more precise delineation of lesions visible on plain films but obscured by overlying densities, and it may resolve lesions not seen on plain films. Identification of cavities, detection of calcification in nodules, and visualization of nodular tumor metastases not visible in plain films are examples of its uses. However, the widespread availability of CT scanning of the thorax, with its further resolving power, has largely supplanted linear tomography.

BRONCHOGRAPHY. Bronchograms are made by taking a roentgenogram of the chest after the surface of the bronchial mucosa is coated by a contrast medium. The procedure is most often carried out after topical anesthesia of the bronchial tree but may be performed under general anesthesia. The contrast medium is usually oily propyliodone, although other contrast media have been used. Bronchography is readily performed by injecting the contrast medium through a fiberoptic bronchoscope.

Bronchography is most useful for the diagnosis of bronchiectasis, although it is sometimes of value in investigating segmental bronchial obstruction when the nature of the obstructing process is not readily apparent from bronchoscopy or tomography. The procedure is used on occasion for the study of air-filled or solid densities within the thorax such as intralobar sequestration.

The performance of a bronchogram causes transient impairment of ventilatory and gas exchange function, with the amount of function loss dependent upon the amount of bronchographic medium used and the presence of a bronchoconstrictor response to the local anesthetic or bronchographic medium, as in asthma. Needless to say, in patients with pulmonary insufficiency, a bronchogram can precipitate acute respiratory failure. As with any diagnostic procedure, the risks must be weighed against the benefits.

ANGIOGRAPHY. ***Pulmonary Angiography.*** Pulmonary angiography is the making of a sequential series of chest roentgenograms, following the rapid injection of a contrast medium into the pulmonary arterial circulation. Visualization is best if the injection is made through a catheter positioned in the pulmonary artery. More selective pulmonary angiograms can be made by injection into the right or left main pulmonary arteries or even into smaller branches. Although most information is obtained from a study of the opacified pulmonary arteries, the contrast medium is also usually followed as it passes through the capillary circulation of the lung into the pulmonary veins; the pulmonary angiogram also gives information about vascular transit times and the presence of anomalous vascular communications.

Pulmonary angiography is most frequently used for the diagnosis of pulmonary embolism and is the most accurate test for that entity. The presence of pulmonary emboli is revealed by the demonstration of areas of vascular cut-off or intravascular filling defects (see Ch. 65).

A less frequent but nevertheless important use of pulmonary angiography is the demonstration of oligemic areas in patients with unilateral hyperlucent lungs or in patients with giant bullous emphysema who are being considered for surgical therapy. In the latter group, pulmonary angiography usefully identifies lung which is being compressed by the giant bullae. Pulmonary angiography is also useful for demonstrating congenital anomalies of the pulmonary vascular tree such as agenesis or hypoplasia of a pulmonary artery, stenosis of peripheral pulmonary vessels, idiopathic dilation of the pulmonary artery, and arteriovenous malformation of the lungs, including pulmonary venous varix. Pulmonary angiography may be used to determine whether an enlarged hilum is due to a dilated pulmonary artery or to lymphadenopathy.

In general, the procedure is well tolerated even by seriously ill patients. However, there is a decidedly increased risk of cardiopulmonary arrest when this test is performed in patients with severe pulmonary hypertension. If, in this circumstance, the physician decides that the procedure still must be done, the amount of contrast medium injected should be sharply decreased and consideration given to carrying out several small, selective injections.

Aortography. Aortography, best carried out by direct catheterization of the aorta by a percutaneously inserted catheter, is useful for the diagnosis of aneurysm of the aorta and the differentiation of dilations and distortions of the great vessels from other mediastinal masses. The procedure should also be performed prior to exploratory thoracotomy in a patient who may have intralobar sequestration of the lung in order to identify the anomalous aortic vessel which often supplies such a sequestration.

Superior Vena Cava Angiography. The superior vena cava is opacified by the injection of contrast medium into a catheter which has been passed into the vessel or into one of its large tributaries. The technique is useful in the investigation of obstruction of the superior vena cava, especially with incomplete manifestations of the superior vena cava syndrome; angiographic confirmation of complete obstruction of the superior vena cava is not necessary.

Bronchial Arteriography. The bronchial arterial circulation can be opacified by the injection of contrast medium through a catheter which has been passed through the aorta directly into one of the bronchial arteries. Bronchial arteriography carries the risk of spinal cord injury if contrast medium is injected into a vessel communicating with the anterior spinal artery. Its main use is in preparation for bronchial arterial embolization, which is being used to control life-threatening hemoptysis.

Felson B: Chest Roentgenology. Philadelphia, W. B. Saunders Company, 1973. *Although it is pre-CT, this is still the best book to use for a sound introduction to interpreting the plain chest radiograph.*

Fraser RG, Paré JAP: Diagnosis of Diseases of the Chest. 2nd ed. Philadelphia, W. B. Saunders Company, 1978–79. *Superb radiographic illustrations make this encyclopedic text of pulmonary disease useful for reference.*

Pugatch RD, Faling LJ, Robbins AM, Spira R: CT diagnosis of benign mediastinal abnormalities. Am J Roentgenol 134:685, 1980. *Forty-nine benign mediastinal abnormalities are analyzed. Specific diagnoses established by CT include 14 cases of local or diffuse fat deposition, five cysts, and six anomalies or aneurysms of great vessels. CT is advocated for initial evaluation of most patients with radiographic evidence of mediastinal abnormality.*

Pugatch RD, Faling LJ: Computed tomography of the thorax: A status report. Chest 80:618, 1981.

Brown LR, Muhm JR: Computed tomography of the thorax; current perspectives. Chest 83:806, 1983.

These two papers provide reasonably current, critical reviews of the use of CT scanning of the thorax, and they provide an entry into the literature on this rapidly evolving topic.

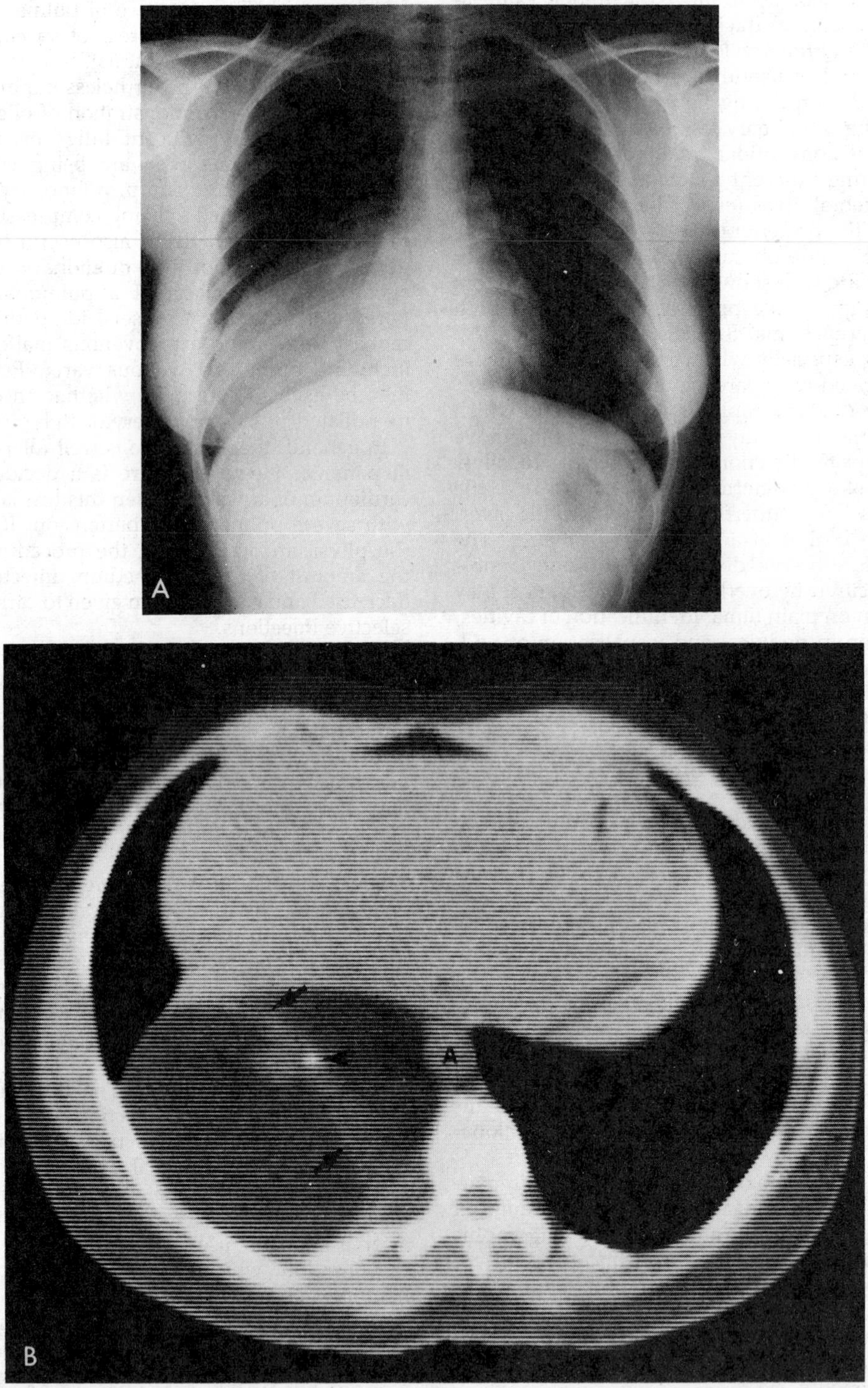

Figure 58–1. A sharply marginated mass fills the lower hemithorax in the frontal radiograph *(A)* of this 24-year-old woman with grippal symptoms. The clearly seen right heart border suggests that the lesion is posterior, and there is a lower thoracic scoliosis to the left. A computed tomographic scan *(B)* made just below the dome of the diaphragm reveals the mass, contiguous with the prevertebral and para-aortic tissues, extending from the mediastinum into the right hemithorax; the aorta is labeled. *A,* Attenuation values of most of the mass are those of fat; the eccentric nodule (arrowhead) reveals a high attenuation value typical for calcified tissue, and the broad band of tissue crossing the mass (two arrows) has intermediate attenuation values. Thoracotomy confirmed the preoperative diagnosis of dermoid tumor. (Case courtesy of Dr. Robert D. Pugatch.)

RADIONUCLIDE IMAGING

In a relatively few years, radionuclide lung scanning has come into widespread use. The procedure is most often carried out with the gamma scintillation camera coupled to a digital computer system and cathode ray display; photographs of the display are made for permanent records. Lung scanning is most often used for the diagnosis of pulmonary embolism; however, the technique is also used for the evaluation of regional lung function and for imaging of the superior vena cava.

The lung perfusion scan is based on the following considerations. There are billions of arterioles and capillaries in the lung which are less than 30 μm in diameter. Following the injection of about 50,000 microspheres of radioactive human serum albumin of 30 μm diameter, a small proportion of these vessels will be blocked temporarily by the particles. Because the density of the microspheres is comparable to that of red blood cells, their distribution throughout the lungs will be determined by the distribution of pulmonary arterial blood flow. External imaging of the radioactivity within the lung can be carried out in six projections: the anterior, posterior, both lateral, and both posterior oblique projections. Foci of the lung with impaired arteriolar and capillary perfusion will be disclosed as areas partially or completely devoid of radioactivity. Vessels occluded by emboli will thus be revealed as fairly sharply defined segmental or lobar defects. However, areas of parenchymal pulmonary infiltration caused by pneumonia, fibrosis, or tumor will also show as impaired zones of perfusion; the presence of such areas can, of course, be detected by a study of the plain chest roentgenogram. Emphysematous lung or areas where there is impaired perfusion due to focal increase in intra-alveolar pressure, as in asthma, will also appear as areas of impaired perfusion. Such perfusion defects are usually nonsegmental in nature and are vague in outline. This latter class of perfusion defects is not readily detectable from a study of the plain chest roentgenogram.

Regional ventilation can be determined by imaging with a scintillation camera, the initial distribution and subsequent washout of air mixed with a radioactive gas, ^{133}xenon. Imaging after an initial period of breathing the gas to equilibration reveals "cold" areas of lung which may be aerated (as seen in the chest films) but not communicating with the bronchial tree. Study of images done at regular intervals during washout of the ^{133}Xe permits estimation of total and regional rates of ventilation. The normal lung is cleared of xenon at the end of about three minutes of breathing air. The perfusion scan, of course, gives information regarding regional perfusion. Regional ventilation and perfusion relations may be assessed visually or by processing of the information with the computer. The two lungs may be studied separately to give information comparable to that obtained by differential bronchospirometry but without the need for using an invasive technique. The computer may also be programmed to provide the ventilation-perfusion relationships of more limited zones of the lung such as the upper, middle, and lower lung zones of each of the lungs separately.

A negative perfusion lung scintigram of good technical quality excludes the diagnosis of angiographically detectable pulmonary embolism. In pulmonary embolism without infarction, perfusion of the embolized area is profoundly impaired, with minimal impairment of ventilation; in emphysema both regional perfusion and ventilation are impaired. Consequently, the combination of impaired perfusion with maintained ventilation permits improved accuracy in the diagnosis of pulmonary embolism (see Ch. 65).

Regional ventilation and perfusion relationships are also useful in the evaluation of unilateral hyperlucent lung and in more precise evaluation of the localized severity of emphysema than is possible in the plain chest roentgenogram.

^{67}Gallium citrate, a radioisotope with a half-life of 78 hours which emits gamma rays, concentrates in rapidly dividing cells. Thus the radioisotope will appear in rapidly growing tumors and in inflammatory lesions. Although this technique has been used to detect occult mediastinal metastases in patients with known bronchogenic carcinoma, all tumors do not take up the isotope with equal avidity, and CT scanning is a superior procedure for mediastinal staging. Its use in establishing the activity of such diseases as idiopathic interstitial pulmonary fibrosis and sarcoidosis of the lungs is still under exploration.

Moser KM: Pulmonary embolism. State of the art. Am Rev Respir Dis 115:829, 1977.

Rosenow EC III, Osmundson PJ, Brown ML: Pulmonary embolism. Mayo Clin Proc 56:161, 1981.

Two excellent, comprehensive reviews. Provide a good entry into the literature on venous thrombosis as well as into pulmonary embolism.

ULTRASONOGRAPHY

Ultrasound is the term applied to a class of mechanical pressure waves that can be propagated through liquids and solids and which, for medical use, have a frequency of oscillation between 1 and 20 MHz. A high frequency sound wave is emitted from a transducer which is applied to the patient's skin. A portion of the wave is reflected back to the transducer as it passes through the tissues being scanned. An image is produced on a cathode ray tube for immediate viewing or is photographed for producing permanent records. Ultrasonography can be applied in a variety of different modes which permit localization of the depth of visualized structures, show the rate of motion of structures such as the diaphragm and heart valves, or generate cross-sectional images which can show outlines of solid viscera such as the liver, large blood vessels, and solid or cystic masses.

Ultrasound waves do not penetrate far into the aerated lung, and the technique is therefore applicable only in pleural or juxtamediastinal disease. Ultrasonography has proved to be helpful in the evaluation of pleural opacities, especially in the localization and identification of loculated pleural effusions. Pleural effusion, whether serous, sanguineous, or purulent, presents as an echo-free space. Consolidated lung conducts sound but, unlike pleural fluid, produces numerous echoes. Pleural fibrosis behaves similarly to consolidated lung and can thus be differentiated from pleural fluid. Subdiaphragmatic fluid collections are often clearly identified. Ultrasonography is useful for determining the site of thoracentesis and may be used to determine the depth to which the needle or a chest tube must be inserted in order to drain a pleural loculation. In most circumstances, ultrasonography is superior to fluoroscopy or chest roentgenography in assisting in the diagnosis and management of loculated pleural effusion. Its use is unnecessary in uncomplicated pleural effusion.

Matalon TA, Neiman HL, Mintzer RA: Noncardiac chest sonography; the state of the art. Chest 83:675, 1983. *An up-to-date, nicely illustrated short review of the use of ultrasound in the localization of pleural fluid and its differentiation from pleural fibrosis. Identification of subdiaphragmatic fluid collections is also stressed.*

SKIN AND SEROLOGIC TESTS

Skin and serologic tests are of value in the investigation of many viral, bacterial, and fungal diseases of the lungs as well as in the investigation of hypersensitivity lung diseases. Skin tests may be divided into three broad categories: immediate or wheal-and-flare reactions, immune complex or Arthus-type reactions, and delayed or tuberculin-type reactions.

IMMEDIATE SKIN REACTIONS. Immediate, wheal-and-flare or Type I skin reactions result from the release of chemical mediators from IgE-sensitized basophils and mast cells which have contacted a specific antigen. Solutions for skin testing are made from extracts of material which are inhaled or ingested, and which may be causing symptoms, such as the pollens of trees, grasses and weeds, house dust, animal danders, mold spores, or foods. Dilutions may also be made from insect venoms and animal sera. These tests are most safely performed by applying the test solutions to scratches or pricks and demonstrating a wheal-and-flare reaction, which is usually obvious within 15 to 20 minutes after the test is performed and which is greater than the reaction produced by a simultaneously applied test diluent. Intradermal tests may be done with 0.02 ml amounts of solution when scratch tests have been negative. As with any laboratory test the results of skin tests must be interpreted in their clinical context. These tests are used to indicate the atopic nature of asthma and nasal symptoms and to guide the use of specific therapy such as hyposensitization and cromolyn.

The presence of antigen-specific serum IgE may also be detected by the *radioallergosorbent test.* In this test an insoluble polymer-antigen conjugate is mixed with the serum to be tested. IgE specific for the antigen present in the serum will attach to the conjugate. The quantity of antigen-specific IgE in the serum is quantified by adding ^{125}I-labeled anti-IgE antibody and measuring the amount of radioactivity taken up by the conjugate.

Bronchial inhalational challenge may be carried out by using graded doses of a highly dilute extract of the allergen to be tested. Development of airways obstruction is demonstrated by serial measurements of airways resistance or indices derived from the forced expiratory spirogram or flow volume loop.

IMMUNE COMPLEX SKIN REACTIONS. Skin test reactions manifest by an erythematous, edematous area developing about six hours after the intradermal injection of the test solution are known as Type III or immune complex reactions. They are believed to result from the deposition of a soluble circulating antigen-antibody (immune) complex in the vessels or tissues. Both wheal-and-flare and immune complex reactions may occur following the same skin test material, as with aspergillus antigen solutions. Except for aspergillosis, this type of skin test reaction has limited clinical use.

DELAYED SKIN REACTIONS. Delayed, tuberculin-type hypersensitivity or Type IV reactions are believed to be caused by activation of sensitized lymphocytes after contact with antigen. An inflammatory reaction results from direct cytotoxicity or from the release of lymphokines. A positive reaction is manifest by an area of induration occurring 48 hours or more after the injection of an appropriate test solution.

The intracutaneous or Mantoux test is the "gold standard" of delayed-type hypersensitivity testing in tuberculosis; 0.1 ml of stabilized solution of PPD-tuberculin containing 5 tuberculin units is injected intradermally into the skin of the forearm. The test is read on the second or third day after injection: 10 mm or more of induration is interpreted as a positive reaction indicating infection with *Mycobacterium tuberculosis*, with or without associated disease. Induration of 5 to 9 mm diameter is interpreted as doubtful (such reactions can result from either infection with *M. tuberculosis* or one of the nontuberculous mycobacteria), and the test must be interpreted in clinical context and may have to be repeated; 0 to 4 mm induration is interpreted as a negative reaction, representing either no evidence of infection with *M. tuberculosis* or low grade sensitivity caused by nontuberculous mycobacterial infection. A weakly positive (doubtful) reaction may be boosted or increased in size when a repeat tuberculin test is done one or more weeks after the first. This approach is also recommended when the tuberculin test is being used for surveillance of an "at-risk" population, such as nurses, so that spurious tuberculin skin-test conversions will not be diagnosed. Multiple puncture tests, such as the tine test, should be used only for screening, and positive reactions should be confirmed by an intradermal test.

A positive tuberculin skin test indicates that infection has occurred at some time in the past. In a child the possibility of recent conversion of the tuberculin test is great, and a positive skin test is generally taken to indicate the presence of active primary tuberculosis. Conversion of a negative to a positive skin test in an adult has the same connotation.

Skin testing materials are available for studying patients who may have coccidioidomycosis (coccidioidin, spherulin) and histoplasmosis (histoplasmin); 0.1 ml of a 1:100 dilution is given intradermally, and induration of 5 mm or greater is interpreted as a positive reaction. As with the tuberculin reaction, the test may take several weeks after infection to become positive, is often negative in severe or disseminated disease, and may be falsely negative when there is cutaneous anergy as in advanced age or severe febrile illnesses, especially those due to viruses. The state of skin reactivity may be established by testing with a common antigen such as mumps or *Trichophyton.* Skin tests for blastomycosis, cryptococcosis, nocardiosis, and actinomycosis are not clinically useful. The histoplasmin skin test often causes a rise in histoplasmin complement-fixing titer and is often negative in early or disseminated disease and so is also of very limited clinical usefulness.

SEROLOGIC TESTS. Serologic tests demonstrate the presence of specific antibodies in the patient's serum by measuring agglutination, precipitating, complement-fixation, or other reactions. The specificity and sensitivity of these tests vary, and the experience of a particular laboratory with a particular test must generally be known to permit the most useful interpretation. The tests must always be interpreted in the light of the full clinical picture, and the results must often be considered confirmatory or supportive rather than diagnostic.

In acute viral, mycoplasmal, and rickettsial infections, the occurrence of recent infection must generally be documented by showing a rise in titer to the antigen occurring over time (10 to 21 days). A single positive test may indicate nothing more than infection in the distant past. Thus these tests are often of most value in identifying the nature of an epidemic in a community rather than being of help in the diagnosis and treatment of the acutely ill patient.

Nonspecific cold agglutination antibodies are found in about half the patients with *Mycoplasma pneumoniae* infections, and a rising titer of cold agglutinins in an appropriate clinical setting is strong evidence for the presence of this disease.

Precipitin reactions are positive during the early weeks of histoplasmosis and coccidioidomycosis and then wane. Complement-fixation (CF) tests then become positive. In coccidioidomycosis a rising CF titer, especially above 1:64, presages dissemination. In histoplasmosis, complement-fixing antibodies tend to disappear with dissemination. The coccidioidin skin test does not affect the coccidioidin CF test, but the histoplasmin skin test tends to cause a rise in histoplasmin CF titer. Serologic tests for blastomycosis are not useful.

Precipitin tests for aspergillosis tend to be positive in patients with invasive aspergillosis and aspergilloma and in many patients with allergic bronchopulmonary aspergillosis; serum IgE and aspergillus-specific IgE levels are also elevated in the last entity.

Cryptococcal antigen in blood, or especially spinal fluid, is helpful in establishing the diagnosis of infection with *Cryptococcus neoformans* and in following the course of treatment; as the patient improves, antigen levels tend to fall and antibodies to the Cryptococcus are detectable in increasing titer. These tests have had little application in uncomplicated pulmonary cryptococcosis.

In autoimmune disorders, antibodies may develop to various components of the individual's own cells (see Ch. 427). These antibodies may be specific for components of the nucleus or of the cytoplasm of the cells. One of the most widely used of these is the antinuclear antibody test. The demonstration of the lupus erythematosus cell is also dependent upon this type of immune disorder.

Serologic tests have proved to be disappointing in the diagnosis of hypersensitivity lung disease. Although precipitin antibodies to the agent in question are often demonstrated in patients with these diseases, they are also frequently found in persons who have had inhalational exposure to the causative organic dusts but who have not developed any illness. The tests thus have a confirmatory rather than a pathognomonic role in diagnosis.

Diagnostic Standards and Classification of Tuberculosis and Other Mycobacterial Diseases. New York, American Lung Association, 1981. *Includes a clear, brief review of the techniques, reading, method of interpretation, and significance of the tuberculin skin test.*

Emmons CW, Binford CH, Utz JP, Kwon-Chung KJ: Medical Mycology. 3rd ed. Philadelphia, Lea & Febiger, 1977. *An outstanding text, always useful for reference on the various aspects of mycology.*

Thompson NJ, Glassroth JL, Snider DE Jr, Farer LS: The booster phenomenon in serial tuberculin testing. Am Rev Respir Dis 119:587, 1979. *Boosted reactions occur in weakly tuberculin skin test positive individuals who are tested a second time one or more weeks after an initial tuberculin skin test. This phenomenon may be used to help determine the significance of a doubtful test. Duplicate tests one week apart may be used to distinguish boosted from converted skin tests when serial tuberculin skin testing is used for control of tuberculosis.*

EXAMINATION OF THE SPUTUM

COLLECTION OF THE SPECIMEN. The tracheobronchial glands and goblet cells produce about 100 ml of secretion per day. Virtually all this material is swallowed after being carried to the oropharynx by the mucociliary elevator. Expectoration of bronchial secretions represents an abnormal state, and much information can be garnered by a study of sputum using microscopic and cultural methods. In patients with acute or chronic pulmonary disease who are not expectorating sputum, a specimen may be obtained by passing a suction catheter through the nose into the trachea (the nasotracheal specimen), or sputum production may be induced by having the patient inhale an ultrasonically generated aerosol of physiologic saline for 15 minutes. An aerosol of hypertonic sodium chloride solution heated to near body temperature may also be used for this purpose. When cultural studies are to be carried out for organisms such as *M. tuberculosis* or pathogenic fungi, which can withstand an acid milieu, a specimen of lower respiratory secretions can generally be obtained by early morning aspiration of gastric contents. However, specimens obtained in this way do not have a higher yield than induced sputa.

Since expectorated sputum is always contaminated by mouth flora, anaerobic cultures require a special technique such as transtracheal aspiration. Transtracheal aspiration is performed under local anesthesia by inserting a 14-gauge, thin-walled needle through the cricothyroid membrane into the lumen of the trachea. A sterile plastic catheter is threaded through the needle into the trachea, and secretions are aspirated; if necessary, a few milliliters of sterile saline are instilled to provoke cough. Transtracheal aspiration has been complicated by infection, mediastinal and subcutaneous emphysema, pneumothorax, hemoptysis, acute ventilatory failure, and sudden death; the presence of a coagulopathy contraindicates its performance. Specimens for microscopic and cultural studies may also be collected via the fiberoptic bronchoscope. Special occluded-tip, telescoping, catheter-brush systems are necessary to avoid contamination with oral anaerobes of specimens to be cultured; such precautions are not needed for mycobacterial and fungal cultures. These procedures have little to offer in previously well persons with community-acquired pneumonia or when the etiology seems clear cut, as in anaerobic lung abscess. These collection techniques are of most use in patients who cannot raise sputum and whose risk of unusual infection is high.

INSPECTION. Inspection of sputum with the naked eye serves to distinguish mucoid from mucopurulent sputum and discloses the presence of blood, black pigment as in anthracosis, or stones and gravel as in broncholithiasis. The viscosity of the sputum and the presence of plugs or casts of the bronchi can be ascertained.

MICROSCOPIC EXAMINATION. A fleck of sputum, carefully chosen because it is opaque, is placed on a microscope slide. This is spread out under a coverslip and, after scanning with the low power lens, is examined with the oil-immersion lens with the condenser racked down and the diaphragm adjusted to give a quasi-darkfield effect (Fig. 58–2). In such a preparation eosinophils can be recognized by their large, brightly refractile granules and a bilobed nucleus. The granules of neutrophils

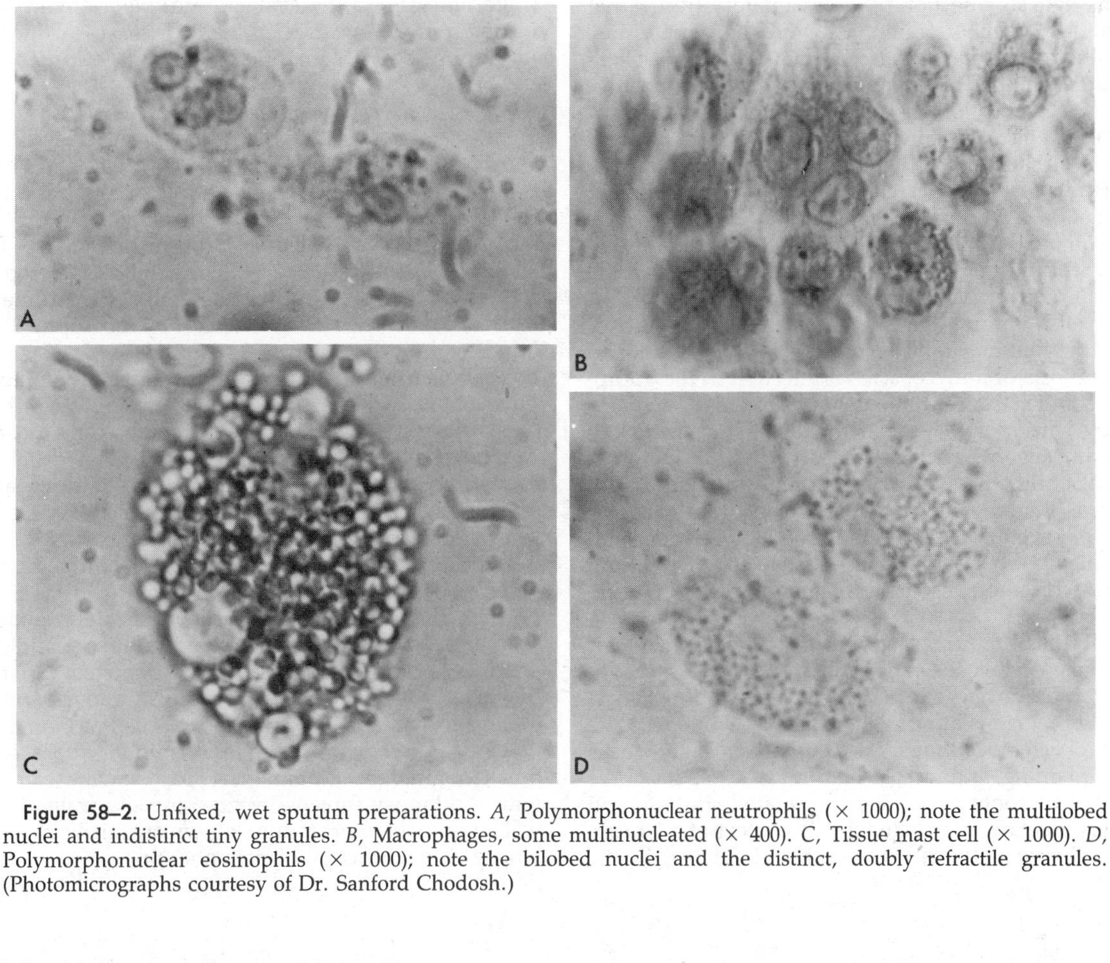

Figure 58–2. Unfixed, wet sputum preparations. *A*, Polymorphonuclear neutrophils (× 1000); note the multilobed nuclei and indistinct tiny granules. *B*, Macrophages, some multinucleated (× 400). *C*, Tissue mast cell (× 1000). *D*, Polymorphonuclear eosinophils (× 1000); note the bilobed nuclei and the distinct, doubly refractile granules. (Photomicrographs courtesy of Dr. Sanford Chodosh.)

are smaller and often display brownian motion; these cells have multilobed nuclei. The numbers of cells present indicate whether grossly observed purulence of the sputum is due to eosinophils or neutrophils. The presence of more than 20 per cent eosinophils suggests the presence of atopic disease. Macrophages are larger, are rounded, and often contain granular and pigmented inclusions. These cells come only from the lower respiratory tract and are observed in large numbers in the quiescent phases of chronic bronchitis. In lipoid pneumonia, clear lipid droplets abound in their cytoplasm. Hemosiderin-laden macrophages are observed in chronic left ventricular failure and in idiopathic hemosiderosis.

Charcot-Leyden crystals, which are elongated, rhomboid, needle-like shapes varying from 10 to 400 μm in length, are derived from the granules of eosinophils and have the same significance. Fungi such as the budding forms of candida, the septate hyphae characteristic of aspergillus, and the endospore-filled spherules of coccidioidomycosis can be recognized. Detection of fungi may be improved by clearing the specimen with potassium hydroxide.

The presence of squamous epithelial cells identifies contamination with oral secretions, indicating that further microscopic and cultural examination should not be carried out on that portion of the specimen. Study of the morphologic variants of bronchial-epithelial cells by this method is of little clinical value.

The smear may be stained with Gram's stain for evaluation of staining characteristics and morphology of bacterial flora. Squamous epithelial cells are easily identified, and areas near such cells should be avoided or another smear made. The morphology of bacteria often permits tentative identification such as the flame-shaped, gram-positive diplococci that denote the pneumococcus or the clumped, rounded, gram-positive cocci of the staphylococcus; the fine gram-negative rod of *Hemophilus influenzae* can usually be differentiated from the plump, sometimes encapsulated gram-negative rod that is *Klebsiella pneumoniae*. The predominance of large numbers of one organism suggests infection of the respiratory tract rather than colonization. Sheets of gram-negative rods, to the virtual exclusion of other organisms, suggest a gram-negative bacillary infection; a large number of gram-negative and gram-positive organisms of great morphologic variability suggests the possibility of a mixed anaerobic infection. The Gram's stain is of little value by itself, but is often helpful in establishing a clinical diagnosis when its results are carefully integrated with all other clinical information. Although cultures of sputum provide the most accurate qualitative information, integration of the sputum Gram's stain with cultural data provides the best easily available estimate of quantitative bacteriology of the respiratory tract.

Examination of a sputum smear stained by the acid-fast or Ziehl-Neelsen method may quickly identify acid-fast bacilli and lead to the diagnosis of a mycobacterial infection in the appropriate clinical setting. Concentration of sputum with low bacillary counts by smear of the sediment after solubilization of mucus by adding agents such as N-acetyl-cysteine increases the sensitivity of both the smear and cultural techniques and, when sputum is scanty, may be applied to sputum collected over a period of several days. Mycobacteria may be seen with even more sensitivity but somewhat less specificity in sputum smears stained with fluorochrome dyes and examined by ultraviolet microscopy.

SPUTUM CULTURES. Cultures of sputum may be made for pyogenic organisms, mycobacteria, and fungi; drug susceptibility testing can be carried out on the pyogens and mycobacteria. Reports on pyogens are usually available within 24 to 72 hours, but mycobacterial cultures take from three to eight weeks from time of planting and fungal cultures take about three weeks. Mouth flora contaminate all expectorated sputum, and cultural studies must be interpreted in the context of a Gram's stain and the clinical findings. Positive blood cultures in the appropriate clinical setting provide the most powerful evidence of the etiology of bacterial pneumonia.

When dealing with an exacerbation of a chronic bronchopulmonary process, it is appropriate to start antibiotic therapy for the most commonly found organisms (*D. pneumoniae* or *H. influenzae*) without doing a culture, provided that the Gram's stain does not show predominance of some other organism.

Cultures for mycobacteria done on concentrated specimens are much more sensitive diagnostically than microscopic examination, and accuracy improves as multiple cultures, up to five in number, are performed. Cultures are also required for precise identification of mycobacteria.

SPUTUM CYTOLOGY. Smears are prepared for cytologic examination either by ethanol-ether fixation of a freshly expectorated specimen or by homogenization and concentration of a specimen previously expectorated into a fixative solution. Staining is carried out by the Papanicolaou method. Tumor cells can be identified in as high a proportion as 90 per cent of central tumors and a lower proportion of midzonal tumors. Cytologic study is of little value in diagnosing peripheral tumors. Diagnostic yield increases with the examination of multiple specimens, but there is little increase in the rate of return after five specimens have been examined. In many instances, the cytologist can accurately identify the histologic type of the tumor. Positive sputum cytology can result from neoplasms in the nasopharynx, larynx, mouth, and esophagus, a fact that is of special importance when the chest roentgenogram is negative.

Bartlett JG: Diagnostic accuracy of transtracheal aspiration bacteriologic studies. Am Rev Respir Dis 115:777, 1977. *An analysis of 488 patients. In 23 patients with bacteremic pneumonia the same organism was also recovered in the transtracheal aspirate. The overall incidence of false-negative cultures was 1 per cent and of false-positive cultures 21 per cent.*

Epstein RL: Constituents of sputum: A simple method. Ann Intern Med 77:259, 1972. *Nicely describes technique of wet-preparation microscopic study of sputum cells and illustrates the cellular constituents found in the common disease states.*

EXAMINATION OF PLEURAL FLUID

The examination of pleural fluid is often an important procedure in the diagnosis of chest diseases. The technique of thoracentesis and the evaluation of pleural fluid are described in detail in the chapter entitled "Diseases of the Pleura, Mediastinum, Diaphragm, and Chest Wall" (Ch. 69).

BRONCHOSCOPY

Bronchoscopy is the inspection of the lumen of the tracheobronchial tree with a lighted optical system or endoscope. The rigid bronchoscope, a hollow metal tube with a blunted tip, and a system for providing light at its end, has been largely superseded by the flexible fiberoptic bronchoscope except for the removal of foreign bodies. In these instruments, light is carried to the tip of the device by fiberoptic light-carrying bundles and the image is returned to the eye through an objective lens and fiberoptic bundle. Aspiration may be carried out directly through this channel, or suction catheters, bronchial brushes, and various types of biopsy and grasping forceps can be passed through the channel. The distal end of the bronchoscope can be angulated to facilitate visualization and entry of various portions of the bronchial tree by moving a lever at the proximal end of the instrument.

The flexible fiberoptic bronchoscope can be passed through either the nose or the mouth with the neck in its normal position. Inspection of the tracheobronchial tree down to subsegmental bronchi or beyond is readily possible. Cytologic specimens can be collected on the bronchial brush, and fragments of bronchial wall can be readily removed with the biopsy forceps for histologic examination. Brush or biopsy forceps can be passed directly into solid lesions under fluoroscopic control. Small fragments of pulmonary parenchyma can be obtained with the biopsy forceps by grasping the walls of distal, thin-walled bronchi, a procedure known as transbronchoscopic lung biopsy. Bronchoscopy of patients who are receiving mechanically assisted ventilation is carried out by passing the instrument through either the endotracheal or tracheostomy tube. Special adapters are used to maintain assisted ventilation during the procedure.

Bronchoscopy is a major tool in evaluating patients with suspect bronchogenic carcinoma who present with hemoptysis or a shadow in the chest film that suggests bronchial obstruction or a mass lesion. The method is of greatest value in central and mid-zonal lesions. Although the flexible bronchoscope can be used for foreign body removal, the rigid bronchoscope is much more versatile for this purpose. Bronchoscopy can be used therapeutically for aspirating secretions, but since the aspiration channel is small and the method cannot be applied at frequent intervals, it is of limited value.

Flexible fiberoptic bronchoscopy is not innocuous. Asthmatic patients may have an adverse reaction to the local anesthetic agent; mild hypoxemia is a regular accompaniment of the procedure and may be hazardous in patients with underlying lung disease. Life-threatening hemorrhage may complicate bronchial wall or transbronchoscopic lung biopsy. Fever may occur without a parenchymal pulmonary infiltration, and pneumonia may be a complication of bronchoscopy, especially in elderly individuals with obstructing bronchial lesions.

As with any diagnostic procedure, the risks of the procedure should be weighed against the benefits, and alternative methods for diagnosis should be considered. Thus, if precise anatomic information regarding the presence of an endobronchial tumor is not necessary, sputum cytology should be considered first for tumor diagnosis. In the elderly, seriously ill individual with a large peripheral tumor, cytologic examination of a specimen obtained by percutaneous fine-needle aspiration may entail a lower risk than bronchoscopy.

Stradling P: Diagnostic Bronchoscopy. 4th ed. New York, Churchill Livingstone, 1981. *A good discussion of techniques, complications, and excellent illustrations of bronchoscopic findings.*

BIOPSY TECHNIQUES

LYMPH NODE BIOPSY. Biopsy of palpable superficial lymph nodes is generally helpful in evaluating pulmonary disease that is part of a systemic process or when primary tumor of the lung has spread outside the confines of the thorax.

MEDIASTINOSCOPY. Mediastinoscopy is performed under general anesthesia, using an endotracheal tube. An incision is made in the suprasternal notch, and the mediastinoscope, a metal tube with light carried to its beveled end, is inserted via the tissue planes adjacent to the trachea as far as the carina. Anterior mediastinal, right paratracheal, and even subcarinal lymph nodes may be seen and biopsied. The left paratracheal area is more difficult to approach because of the presence of the aortic arch. This procedure has almost 100 per cent yield in granulomatous disease such as sarcoidosis and, as noted earlier in this chapter, is useful in staging patients with bronchogenic carcinoma.

PLEURAL BIOPSY. Biopsy of the parietal pleura using the side-cutting Cope or Abrams needles is of major importance in the diagnosis of pleural effusion. In patients who do not have an obvious explanation for pleural effusion, biopsy should be considered at the time of the initial thoracentesis. The Abrams needle has the advantage that large pieces of tissue can be obtained with a very low risk of inducing a pneumothorax, and several biopsies tangential to the needle puncture can be obtained with a single insertion of the needle. The Cope needle produces smaller pieces of tissue than the Abrams needle. Pleural biopsy yields a diagnosis in a high proportion of patients with pleural carcinomatosis; mesothelioma is difficult to diagnose from needle biopsy material. Granulomatous inflammation, sometimes with acid-fast bacilli seen in special stains, is commonly observed in tuberculous pleural effusion.

The major risk of pleural biopsy is bleeding due to injury of the intercostal artery, and biopsy should never be performed on the cephalad side of the intercostal puncture wound. The procedure should obviously not be performed on patients with a coagulopathy. Because of the focal nature of pleural disease, a second or third biopsy is often performed if the first biopsy has failed to yield diagnostic information. Consideration should always be given to culturing a piece of tissue as well as to histologic examination, because the yield of positive cultures for *M. tuberculosis* is much higher from tissue than from pleural fluid. Pleuroscopy and biopsy of an abnormality visualized with a fiberoptic endoscope may at times yield a diagnosis when blind biopsy does not.

LUNG BIOPSY. In instances in which simpler diagnostic studies have not been fruitful, consideration should be given to obtaining lung tissue for laboratory diagnosis. The approach to sampling lung tissue for cytologic, histologic, or bacteriologic diagnosis varies, depending on whether the patient has a diffuse pulmonary lesion or has a circumscribed and presumably solid lesion.

The endoscopic approach to solid lesions by the means of the fluoroscopically guided biopsy forceps or brush has been referred to above. Material for cytologic examination can often be obtained by fine needle aspiration of the mass lesion carried out under fluoroscopic control. If the lesion is not adherent to the pleura, pneumothorax may result, requiring the insertion of a chest tube. When the lesion is adherent to the chest wall, core biopsy with a cutting needle, obtaining material for both cytologic and histologic examination, is probably a preferable procedure. Percutaneous methods are useful when surgical therapy is contraindicated and proof of diagnosis is required to plan nonoperative therapy. Needle aspiration does not often provide the etiology of non-neoplastic nodular densities.

Diffuse pulmonary lesions may be approached by transbronchoscopic lung biopsy. This method should be particularly considered when the differential diagnosis includes lesions which can be readily diagnosed by the pathologist on small amounts of tissue. Included in this category are granulomatous and neoplastic lesions and the suspected presence of infectious agents readily identified histologically, such as *Pneumocystis carinii*, aspergillus, or one of the obligatory pathogenic fungi. The procedure is less helpful in diagnosing lymphoma than carcinoma and is of limited value in the diagnosis of chronic interstitial fibrosis in which the histology of small amounts of tissue is nonspecific and there is a serious sampling problem. In the latter circumstance, open lung biopsy performed through a short intercostal incision permits biopsy of a larger portion of lung, often from two sites, and provides enough tissue for a variety of histologic, cultural, and immunopathologic examinations. Core biopsy, using the high speed air-powered biopsy drill or one of the core biopsy needles, has been applied to diffuse pulmonary lesions; but except in the hands of the most highly skilled and experienced operators, it carries more hazard than either transbronchoscopic or open lung biopsy.

Gaensler EA, Carrington CB: Open biopsy for chronic diffuse infiltrative lung disease: Clinical, roentgenographic and physiological correlations in 502 patients. Ann Thorac Surg 30:411 1980. *An excellent review of open biopsy procedures and comparison with "closed" biopsy techniques.*

Rossiter SJ, Miller DC, Churg AM, Carrington CB, Monk JBD: Open lung biopsy in the immunosuppressed patient. J Thorac Cardiovasc Surg 77:338, 1979. *Compares open and closed biopsy techniques.*

Westcott JL: Direct percutaneous needle aspiration of localized pulmonary lesions: Results in 422 patients. Radiology 137:31, 1980. *This paper reports the outstanding results of one of the most skilled practitioners of this technique. Twenty-gauge needles were used with a high rate of accuracy, especially for malignancy. Minor hemoptysis occurred in 8 per cent and pneumothorax in 27 per cent of procedures.*

Zvala DC, Schoell JE: Ultrathin needle aspiration of the lung in infectious and malignant disease. Am Rev Respir Dis 123:125, 1981. *Reports a greater than 90 per cent diagnostic yield from localized neoplasms and 42 per cent diagnostic yield from infected cavities, using 24 to 25 gauge needles. Provides a good entry to the literature on this topic.*

MISCELLANEOUS PROCEDURES

THE ELECTROCARDIOGRAM. Electrocardiographic changes occur in only a small proportion of patients with pulmonary embolism, but the procedure is noninvasive and inexpensive and should therefore be regularly used when this diagnosis is suspected. The changes are transient so that serial examination is helpful; P pulmonale, right bundle branch block, right axis deviation, and supraventricular arrhythmias are most frequently seen (see Ch. 50). Electrocardiographic evidence of right ventricular hypertrophy correlates quite well with the degree of pulmonary hypertension and cor pulmonale in patients with disorders causing restriction of the vascular bed of the lung. The electrocardiogram is a less sensitive indicator of right ventricular enlargement in patients whose cor pulmonale is due to chronic bronchitis and emphysema (see Ch. 60). The changes of myocardial ischemia may be helpful in discerning the etiology of chest pain, and those of ischemia and left ventricular hypertrophy may be helpful in patients with acute cardiogenic pulmonary edema, especially when the presentation is atypical (see Ch. 42).

EXTRAPULMONARY RADIONUCLIDE IMAGING. Scintiscanning of the neck and mediastinum after administration of radioiodine is useful in the evaluation of an upper mediastinal mass which may be substernal goiter (see Ch. 228). Liver scans are useful in detecting bacterial or amebic abscess of the liver but are neither very sensitive nor specific in detecting metastatic bronchogenic carcinoma, and the technique should not be routinely used in the preoperative evaluation of patients with this neoplasm (see Ch. 68). Bone scans after ^{99m}technetium-labeled polyphosphate often can detect metastatic carcinoma before lesions are roentgenographically visible; however, focal injury to bone from any cause may cause increased concentration of radionuclide, and some highly lytic lesions may not be revealed by this method (see Part XVIII).

TESTS OF MUSCLE FUNCTION. Disorders of the muscular system may involve the muscles of the respiratory system and be suspected because of loss of vital and total lung capacities. Brief reversal of the impaired vital capacity after administration of the short-acting anticholinesterase edrophonium supports the diagnosis of myasthenia gravis (see Ch. 539). Electromyography may be helpful in establishing this diagnosis as well as that of other neurologic or muscular disorders (see Ch. 471). Elevation of serum creatine phosphokinase and aldolase levels is helpful in the diagnosis of polymyositis or dermatomyositis (see Ch. 454).

SPECIAL TESTS. Sweat chloride concentrations above 60 mEq per liter in the absence of adrenal insufficiency or nephrogenic diabetes insipidus support the diagnosis of cystic fibrosis; 95 per cent of adult males with this disorder have azoospermia (see Ch. 64). Patients with Kartagener's syndrome (situs inversus, sinusitis, and bronchiectasis) and the closely allied immotile cilia syndrome have ultrastructurally identifiable abnormalities of their cilia which can be detected in nasal or bronchial mucosal biopsies; in males with these disorders, motility of sperm is markedly impaired. In homozygous alpha$_1$ antitrypsin deficiency, serum alpha$_1$ globulin and serum trypsin inhibitory capacity levels are markedly decreased.

59. ASTHMA

Ronald P. Daniele

DEFINITION AND PREVALENCE. Asthma is a disorder that is characterized by increased responsiveness of the trachea and bronchi to various stimuli, resulting in widespread narrowing of the airways. These changes are reversible either spontaneously or as a result of therapy. The currently accepted definition does not specify a cause or causes, identify unique clinical or pathologic features, or mention immunologic mechanisms. It does describe, however, the fundamental abnormality that is common to all asthmatic patients—reversible hyperresponsiveness of tracheobronchial smooth muscle.

Most asthmatic patients are diagnosed by a triad of episodic symptoms: wheezing, cough, and dyspnea. Characteristically, these signs and symptoms are highly variable in severity and duration. They may run the gamut from being completely absent for days, months, and even years to being protracted and unresponsive to outpatient therapy (status asthmaticus).

Asthma may afflict as many as 5 per cent of the population in the United States. In over half the cases it is diagnosed between ages 2 and 17 years, and in this group it is the leading cause of disease and disability. About one third of asthmatic patients are first diagnosed after 30 years of age.

CLASSIFICATION. Patients with asthma may be separated into two clinical groups, extrinsic and intrinsic (Table 59–1). Extrinsic asthma is characterized by childhood onset, seasonal variation, and a well-defined allergic history to a variety of inhaled allergens (atopy). The extrinsic form accounts for less than 10 per cent of all patients. Intrinsic asthma usually begins after the age of 30 and tends to be perennial and more severe; status asthmaticus is more common in this group. By definition, in intrinsic asthma an allergic etiology cannot be identified. More than 80 per cent of asthmatic patients have clinical features that are common to both groups, but for purposes of discussion each will be discussed separately.

PATHOLOGY. Most descriptions of the pathologic features of asthma come from patients dying in status asthmaticus. In these cases, the lungs are markedly distended and fail to collapse owing to the occlusion of most bronchi by thick, tenacious plugs of mucus, which often extend to the terminal bronchioles. Histopathologic hallmarks include bronchial smooth muscle hypertrophy, mucosal edema, thickening of the basement membrane, and inflammatory cells in submucosal tissue, particularly eosinophils. The lung parenchyma is remarkably spared with no evidence of fibrosis or destruction of the alveolar septa. Unexpectedly, similar abnormalities have been found in asthmatic patients dying from other causes who were presumably symptom free prior to death. The presence of mucous plugs in the small airways (less than 2 mm) of these patients may explain some of the persistent functional abnormalities (reduced mid-maximum expiratory flow rate [MMF] and increased alveolar-arterial difference for P_{O_2}) found even in asymptomatic patients.

PATHOPHYSIOLOGY OF EXTRINSIC ASTHMA. In extrinsic asthma, the sequence of events after sensitization leading to the pathologic features described above is shown in Figure 59–1. Inhaled allergens interact with specific IgE antibodies that are fixed to mast cells which line the tracheobronchial tree. Mast cells (and possibly basophils) that are sensitized with IgE are primed to respond to specific allergens when cell-bound IgE is bridged by divalent allergen. This membrane event signals mast cells to secrete a variety of mediators by two processes. First, preformed mediators contained in metachromatic granules of mast cells are released by a process of exocytosis. Important examples of preformed mediators include histamine, eosinophilic factors of anaphylaxis (ECF-A), and neutrophil chemotactic factor (NCF). In the second process, unstored mediators such as slow-reacting substance of anaphylaxis (SRS-A) (also called the leukotrienes), platelet activating factors (PAF), and possibly prostaglandins (PG) are synthesized and secreted by mast cells within minutes after antigen stimulation. Some of the properties and functional characteristics of

TABLE 59–1. CLASSIFICATION OF ASTHMATIC PATIENTS

Extrinsic*	Intrinsic*
Known external allergens	No known external allergens
Positive immediate skin tests	Negative skin tests
IgE raised in 50–60% of subjects	IgE normal or low
Onset usually in childhood or early adult life	Onset usually (but not invariably) in older adults
Intermittent asthma	More continuous asthma
Other allergies (hay fever and eczema) often present (54%)	Other allergies uncommon (7%)
Family history of multiple allergies (asthma, hay fever, eczema) common (50%)	Family history of multiple allergies less common (20%)

*Blood and sputum eosinophilia common in *both* groups.

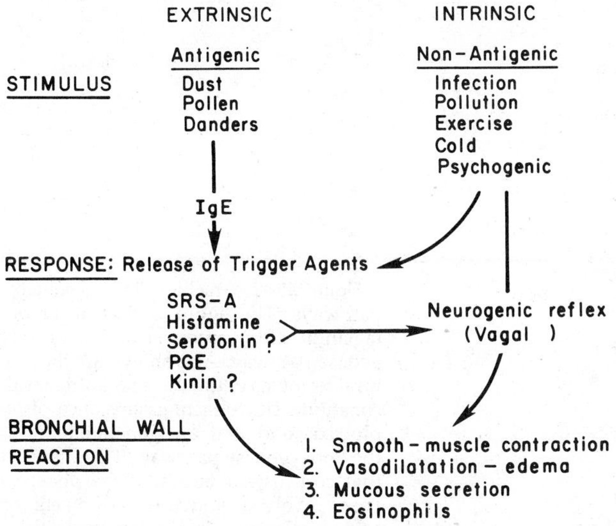

Figure 59–1. Dual pathways involved in the pathogenesis of bronchial constriction. (From Fishman AP [ed.]: Pulmonary Diseases and Disorders. New York, McGraw-Hill Book Company, 1980.)

these mediators are summarized in Table 59–2. For a more extensive discussion of mast cell structure and function, the reader is referred to Ch. 438.

Two advances have extended our knowledge on the role of mediators in asthma: The elucidation of the arachidonic acid metabolic pathways, and the characterization and synthesis of SRS-A, which proved to be a group of compounds called leukotrienes. Leukotrienes as well as prostaglandins are synthesized from the 20-carbon unsaturated fatty acid, arachidonic acid (Fig. 59–2). Arachidonic acid is derived from cell membrane phospholipids by the action of phospholipases and may be converted by cyclooxygenase to prostaglandins and thromboxanes. A second pathway that is catalyzed by 5-lipoxygenase leads to the formation of monohydroxyeicosatetraenoic acids (5-HPETE) and then to an unstable intermediate, leukotriene A_4 (LTA_4). LTA_4 may then be converted to leukotriene B_4, a potent chemotactic factor for eosinophils and neutrophils. Alternatively, LTA_4 may be transformed by several cell types (mononuclear cells and basophils) into leukotriene C_4 by the enzymatic addition of glutathione (S-glutamylcysteinylglycine). Leukotriene C_4 may undergo further conversion to leukotriene D_4 (S-cysteinylglycine) by enzymatic removal of glutamine and then by removal of glycine to leukotriene E_4 (S-cysteine). SRS-A is composed of the cysteinyl-containing leukotrienes (LTC_4, LTD_4, and LTE_4), of which LTD_4 is the most potent bronchoconstrictor (Table 59–2). The leukotrienes are a thousand times more potent on a molar basis than histamine or prostaglandin $F_{2\alpha}$ and exert their effect predominantly in the small or distal airways. In asthmatic patients, allergens induce the release of leukotriene C_4, D_4, and E_4 from the lung tissue in amounts that correlate well with their capacity to induce bronchial contraction.

Secretion of primary mediators described in Table 59–2 apparently initiates the release of secondary mediators, such as serotonin, prostaglandins, and possibly kinins. Serotonin constricts bronchial smooth muscle directly but may also induce bronchoconstriction by stimulating irritant receptors (see below). Prostaglandins of the E series (PGE_1 and PGE_2) are potent dilators of airways and blood vessels; those of the F series constrict bronchi and blood vessels. Although the lung is a major site for their production, the cell types involved are not defined.

The effects of these mediators may be viewed as two waves of an inflammatory response: The first is an immediate serous transudation caused by increased capillary permeability. The second occurs hours to days after antigen stimulation and involves the accumulation of inflammatory cells, primarily eosinophils, platelets, and neutrophils in the bronchial submucosa.

The role of the eosinophil in the atopic response may be to provide a counterpoise to the cascade of inflammatory mediators initiated by mast cells and other inflammatory cells. The eosinophil rapidly secretes at least three types of inhibitory substances: histaminase, arylsulfatase, and phospholipase D. Histaminase oxidatively deaminates histamine; arylsulfatase B inactivates some of the leukotrienes, and phospholipase D appears to degrade one form of the platelet activating factors. Thus, the eosinophil appears to play a role in the *intercellular* control mechanisms of the allergic inflammatory response.

The eosinophil, however, may also inflict injury. Granular constituents derived from the eosinophil, especially major basic protein, and the secretion of oxygen-free radicals, can injure bronchial epithelial cells, rendering the mucosa more permeable to allergens and possibly lowering the threshold of underlying irritant receptors.

Mast Cell Receptors—Intracellular Regulation. As shown in Figure 59–3, secretion by mast cells and basophils is regulated by two classes of membrane receptors: those which activate

TABLE 59–2. MEDIATORS IN THE ATOPIC INFLAMMATORY RESPONSE

Mediator	Molecular Characteristics	Source	Function
Histamine	β-imidazolylethylamine MW = 111	Mast cells, basophils, preformed and stored in granules	Increases vascular permeability, bronchial smooth muscle contraction (H1 type) ↑ cyclic AMP in mast cells (H2 type) ↑ mucous secretion
Slow-reacting substance of anaphylaxis (SRS-A) Leukotrienes C_4 (LTC_4) LTD_4 LTE_4	Polyunsaturated substituted C-20 fatty acids MW ≃ 625 ≃ 500 ≃ 425	Mast cells, neutrophils, mononuclears, lung cells? (not preformed)	Increases vascular permeability, bronchial smooth muscle contraction
Eosinophil chemotactic factors of anaphylaxis (ECF-A)	Tetrapeptides (Val/Ala-Gly-Ser-Glu), MW ≃ 360–390, and acid peptides	Mast cells, basophils, preformed and stored in granules	Attracts eosinophils
Neutrophil chemotactic factor (NCF)	Structure ? MW > 750,000	Mast cells, basophils, lung tissue, preformed and stored	Attracts neutrophils
Platelet-aggregating factors (PAF)	Phospholipids 1-0-alkyl-2-acetyl-sn-glyceryl-3-phosphorylcholine MW ≃ 520–550	Neutrophils, ? mass cells, basophils, other lung cells? (not preformed)	Aggregates platelets and release of other mediators (serotonin, PG)
Prostaglandins (PG)	Polyunsaturated C-20 fatty acids, MW ≃ 350	Mast cells, basophils, platelets, other lung cells? (not preformed)	↑ cyclic AMP PGE_1, PGE_2—dilate smooth muscle $PGF_{\alpha 2}$—contracts smooth muscle Release of PG is probably stimulated by other mediators

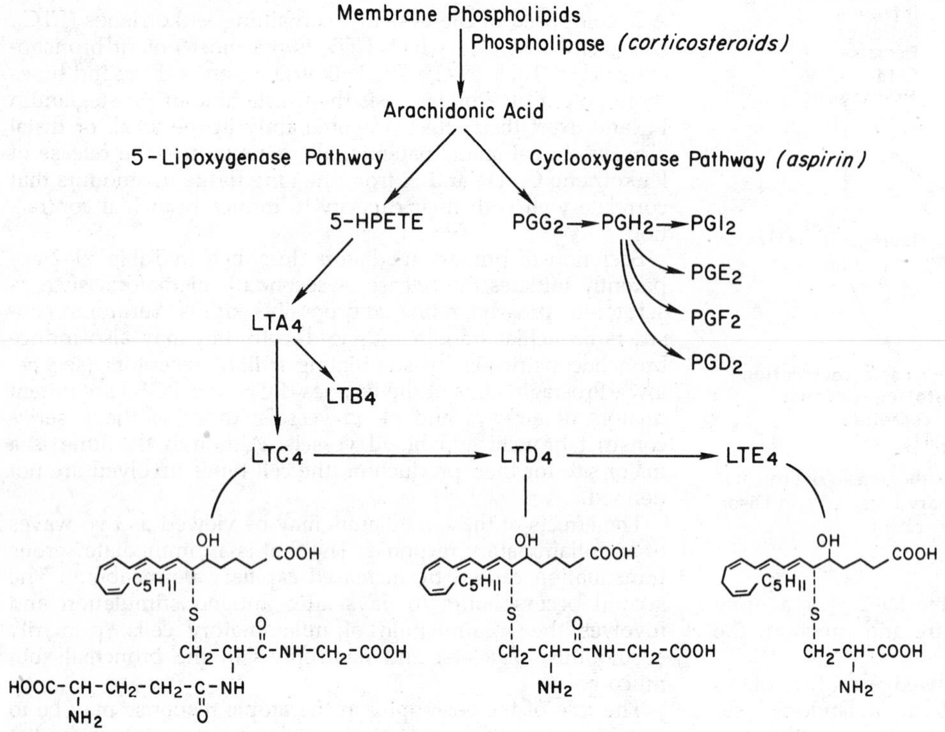

Figure 59–2. Arachidonic acid metabolic pathways. The figure depicts major prostaglandin (PG) products of the cyclooxygenase pathway. Also shown are the structural formulas of the three leukotrienes that constitute slow-reacting substance of anaphylaxis and that are generated through the lipoxygenase pathway. It is noteworthy that corticosteroids inhibit the phospholipases involved in synthesis of arachidonic acid. Not shown in the figure are thromboxanes that are derived from PGH2.

adenylate cyclase to produce cyclic adenosine-3′,5′-monophosphate (cyclic AMP); and those which stimulate guanylate cyclase to form cyclic guanosine-3′,5′-monophosphate (cyclic GMP).

The transient increase of cytoplasmic cyclic AMP inhibits the release of histamine, SRS-A, and other mediators. The best studied receptor that activates adenylate cyclase is the beta receptor. Drugs that are beta agonists (isoproterenol > epinephrine > norepinephrine) correlate both in dose and rank order of potency with the levels of cyclic AMP they induce in isolated leukocytes and lung fragments. The increased level of cyclic AMP is transient because it is rapidly degraded by another cytoplasmic enzyme, phosphodiesterase. Methylxanthine drugs, such as aminophylline, are potent competitive inhibitors of phosphodiesterase and thus tend to sustain intracellular levels of cyclic AMP.

Two additional receptors have also been shown to stimulate adenylate cyclase: histamine (H_2 type) and prostaglandin (PGE) receptors. These receptors provide some evidence for a negative feedback control mechanism for mast cells and basophils. Such receptors would allow a cell to "perceive" the levels of histamine (and other mediators) secreted by itself and other cells, activate the synthesis of cyclic AMP, and thereby limit further mediator release. A similar role may exist for the prostaglandin receptor.

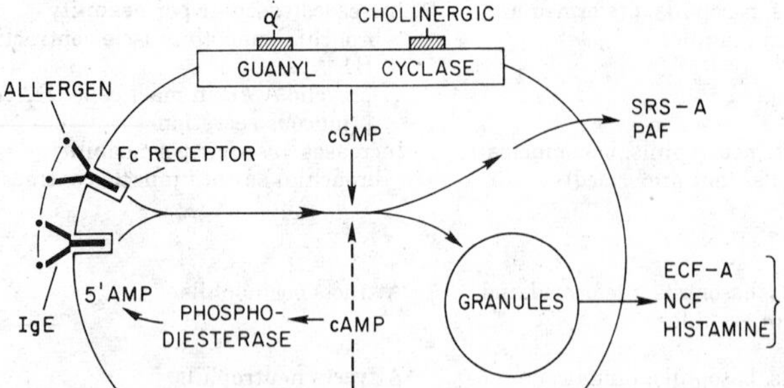

Figure 59–3. Membrane receptor interactions involving allergen-IgE and agonists that result in the stimulation of cyclic AMP or cyclic GMP and modulation of mediator release from mast cells and basophils. (From Fishman AP [ed.]: Pulmonary Diseases and Disorders. New York, McGraw-Hill Book Company, 1980.)

In contrast, guanylate cyclase stimulates the formation of cyclic GMP, which enhances mediator release. Less is known about the location of this enzyme and its associated receptors. However, a cholinergic receptor has been identified whereby acetylcholine stimulates the production of cyclic GMP.

According to a current hypothesis, the balance between the inhibitory (cyclic AMP) and excitatory (cyclic GMP) messenger molecules regulates mediator release. It has been proposed that asthma results from a partial blockade of beta receptor, leading to an imbalance of these regulatory molecules.

The elucidation of the mechanisms of mediator release in asthma has greatly extended our understanding of bronchospasm and provides a more rational basis for therapy. Nevertheless, most attacks of asthma are not precipitated by allergens.

INTRINSIC ASTHMA—PATHOPHYSIOLOGIC MECHANISMS. In intrinsic asthma, reversible airways obstruction is caused by a variety of stimuli that are nonantigenic and seemingly unrelated. Nonetheless, as shown in Figure 59–1, these stimuli lead to pathologic lesions similar to those seen in extrinsic asthma.

According to one hypothesis, intrinsic asthma represents an abnormality of the parasympathetic nervous system. Bronchospasm is provoked when certain agents stimulate rapidly adapting irritant receptors which are located in the subepithelial region of the tracheobronchial tree (Fig. 59–4). Impulses from these receptors are carried by the afferent vagal fibers; the reflex arc is completed by efferent vagal fibers, which innervate bronchial smooth muscle and cause bronchoconstriction. In the asthmatic patient, it is proposed that there is a lowered threshold for stimulation of these irritant receptors. Similarly, disturbances in parasympathetic function have been invoked to explain the abnormalities in mucus secretion and production. In certain patients, for example, cough and bronchospasm induced by nonspecific irritants and even allergens may be relieved or abolished by atropine. The presence of abnormal

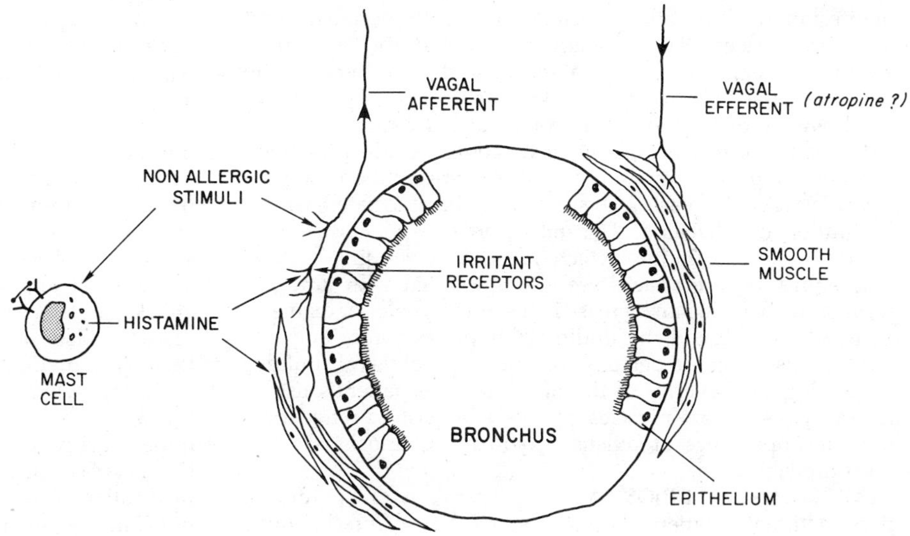

Figure 59–4. Possible interactions between mediators and neurogenic reflexes in the elicitation of bronchial smooth muscle contraction in asthma. Also indicated in the figure is one potential site of action for anticholinergic drugs in asthma.

neurogenic responses does not exclude involvement of mediator release in the allergic phenomenon.

Interaction of Mediator and Neurogenic Mechanisms. Any unifying concept of the pathogenesis of asthma must reconcile the evidence implicating mediator release on the one hand and autonomic or neurogenic dysfunction on the other. Such an hypothesis must also take into account that most patients do not have primarily extrinsic or intrinsic forms of asthma but a mixture of the two, and that most attacks are provoked by nonspecific stimuli, even in atopic patients. But how does extrinsic or atopic asthma relate to abnormalities in neurogenic discharge?

Several schemes may link these two hypotheses (Fig. 59–4). Nonspecific stimuli may excite irritant receptors leading to bronchospasm by way of efferent vagal pathways. Allergen-antibody complexes may stimulate mast cells, releasing mediators that might have a direct action on smooth muscle as well as an indirect effect by stimulating irritant receptors and thereby producing bronchospasm. Alternatively, both nonspecific irritants and allergen-antibody interaction might stimulate mediator release from mast cells. Certain mediators, such as histamine and serotonin, are potent stimulants of irritant receptors. By such a scheme, stimuli may induce bronchospasm by direct action of mediators on smooth muscle or by indirect action that operates via neurogenic reflexes, or by both mechanisms.

Nonallergic Provocative Stimuli. One of the most important nonspecific irritants is *respiratory tract infection*, particularly by viral agents. Both lower and upper respiratory infections may initiate or aggravate bronchospasm. This is not due to a hypersensitivity to the infecting agents, but is thought to result from the capacity of viral agents to lower the threshold for stimulation of irritant receptors.

Airborne pollutants may play a role in the pathogenesis of asthma. In "Tokyo-Yokohama asthma" and in "New Orleans asthma," a high density of air pollutants was found to have initiated or aggravated wheezing and dyspnea in asthmatic patients as well as in certain previously asymptomatic individuals who were later shown to have *hyperirritable* airways. Air pollutants (e.g., ozone) are thought to increase hyperreactivity of bronchial smooth muscle by stimulating irritant receptors in the tracheobronchial tree.

It is now appreciated that a variety of *occupational dusts and fumes* may provoke asthmatic attacks in susceptible individuals. The onset of wheezing, cough, or dyspnea may be related to the working hours. More commonly, however, symptoms are not closely linked to occupation but may be delayed for several hours until after the patient has left the work place. Important diagnostic clues include a cyclic pattern in which symptom-free periods occur during weekends or vacations. Both allergic and irritant stimuli are thought to be involved in occupational asthma. A more extensive discussion of occupational asthma is contained in Ch. 559.

In some patients, *hyperpnea, laughing*, or *exercise* may also induce bronchoconstriction. Moreover, the inhalation of *cold air* may initiate or intensify bronchospasm. The underlying mechanism whereby bronchospasm is induced by such diverse ventilatory maneuvers appears to involve heat transfer from the respiratory tree. When all other variables are controlled, the major determinant is the volume of air that is to be warmed and humidified on inspiration. Heat and water loss occur as the minute ventilation increases in response to exercise. This loss is independent of whether the minute ventilation is voluntary or is the result of exercise. Moreover, when conditions of temperature and humidity are controlled, the nature of the exercise is not crucial. Cromolyn or β-2 drugs or both may blunt or prevent symptoms when given by inhalation prior to exercise. Measures that humidify and warm inhaled air, such as cold weather masks, are also helpful. Whether these stimuli cause mediator release or act through irritant receptors is unsettled.

In about 10 per cent of asthmatic patients, a peculiar triad exists of *bronchospasm, nasal polyps, and sensitivity to aspirin.* Ingestion of aspirin, indomethacin, aminopyrine, or yellow food additives (e.g., tartrazine yellow) may induce severe bronchospasm, urticaria, and even hypotension. Interestingly, these patients are sensitive to acetylsalicylic acid but not to sodium salicylate. The reaction is not immunologic but appears related to an abnormality in prostaglandin metabolism which is unmasked by these drugs. The arachidonic acid pathways may provide a clue to this abnormality (Fig. 59–2). In certain asthmatic patients, ingestion of aspirin or indomethacin, known inhibitors of cyclooxygenase, may divert arachidonic metabolism toward the lipoxygenase pathway and the production of spasmogenic leukotrienes.

Least understood are the *psychologic factors* that influence the asthmatic patient. It is thought that emotional stress influences bronchomotor tone, rendering it more susceptible to irritant and allergic stimuli.

Bronchospasm is usually induced by nonspecific stimuli that presumably involve nonimmunologic pathways. Allergic asthma also has a background of hyperreactivity to nonspecific stimuli, and this abnormality may persist long after atopy disappears.

CLINICAL MANIFESTATIONS. In most patients, an asthma attack begins with a nonproductive cough and wheezing, usually followed by a tightness in the chest and dyspnea. In a minority of patients, cough may be the most conspicuous and even sole manifestation of the attack. Attacks frequently occur at night and during sleep. They usually do not last for more than several hours and resolve spontaneously or with therapy. The end of an attack is often heralded by a change to a productive cough with expectoration of mucous plugs and casts.

Physical findings of airway obstruction include prolonged expiration and wheezing in both phases of respiration. In more severe attacks, increasing dyspnea may be associated with a diminution of wheezing. This may lead to a silent chest, an especially serious finding which suggests impending respiratory failure. Severe attacks are also associated with lung hyperinflation, causing an increase in the anteroposterior diameter of the chest wall and the finding of hyperresonance and low diaphragms on chest percussion. Important physical findings in gauging the severity of the attack are the patient's use of accessory respiratory muscles, sternocleidomastoid retractions, and the appearance of pulsus paradoxus. Cyanosis is a late and unreliable sign.

LABORATORY FINDINGS. A wet preparation of sputum of many asthmatic patients contains spiral casts (Curschmann's spirals), eosinophils, and Charcot-Leyden crystals. The presence of sputum and blood eosinophilia is suggestive of the diagnosis of asthma but does not distinguish between extrinsic and intrinsic types.

Arterial blood gases should be obtained only in patients experiencing severe asthmatic attacks or prolonged attacks that are unresponsive to bronchodilator therapy. Hypoxemia is invariably present during an acute attack and, when mild to moderately severe, is usually associated with a decrease in the arterial P_{CO_2} and an increase in arterial pH. Hypocapnia and respiratory alkalosis are due to increased alveolar ventilation. Respiration may be stimulated by increased chemical drive (when Pa_{O_2} is less than 60 torr), but neurogenic reflexes (irritant and stretch receptors) are probably more important. Determination of arterial blood gases is important for two reasons. First, the degree of hypoxemia generally reflects the degree of mismatching of ventilation to perfusion ($\dot{V}/\dot{Q}$) and thus gives some objective measure of the severity of airways disease. Second, a *normal* or increased Pa_{CO_2} signals severe airway obstruction and impending respiratory failure.

Chest roentgenograms may demonstrate lung hyperinflation, usually without parenchymal infiltrates. However, in patients with severe disease, roentgenograms should be scrutinized for (1) infiltrates suggesting a respiratory infection; (2) atelectasis or collapse of a segment or lobe, implicating mucous plugging of a bronchus; and (3) the presence of pneumothorax or pneumomediastinum.

Pulmonary function tests are important in assessing the severity of an attack and the response to bronchodilator therapy and in providing objective information about the resolution of disease. Pulmonary function tests may also be used to define hyperirritable airways in an asymptomatic asthma patient by provoking increases in airway resistance with aerosolized doses of histamine or methacholine, which would have no effect in normal individuals. Pulmonary function tests may also identify patients with exercise-induced asthma.

During the acute attack, airway narrowing decreases the forced expiratory volume in one second (FEV_1), the maximal mid-expiratory flow rates (MMF), and the peak expiratory flow rates. When the FEV_1 is less than 25 per cent of predicted (e.g., <1.0 L), it is often accompanied by other signs of severe disease (e.g., pulsus paradoxus). All lung volumes are affected in an acute attack. There is a decrease in vital capacity (VC), with large increases in residual volume (RV), functional residual capacity (FRC), and total lung capacity (TLC). The peak expiratory flow rate (PEFR) is a particularly useful measurement because it is easy to perform repeatedly and does not require the patient to do the entire forced expiratory maneuver. The devices available for such measurements are small and convenient and may be kept in the home so that patients can produce daily records of their airway function.

Signs and symptoms are not entirely reliable in assessing the severity of an asthma attack or the optimal response to therapy. For example, in patients whose symptoms remit and signs of wheezing disappear, FEV_1's may be 40 to 60 per cent of normal and residual volumes greater than 200 per cent of predicted. Moreover, in patients whose attack has resolved for weeks or months, maximal mid-expiratory flow rates may remain abnormal. The latter test emphasizes that the peripheral airways (less than 2 mm in diameter) are "silent" zones where considerable airway disease and obstruction may exist without signs or symptoms. These considerations have important therapeutic and clinical implications because the tendency for asthmatic attacks to recur seems to depend on the degree of residual disease. Also, a subpopulation of patients may have disease that exists predominantly in peripheral airways.

During symptom-free periods, skin tests or specific serum IgE antibodies (RAST test) may be useful in demonstrating hypersensitivity to suspected allergens. The use of RAST avoids the risk of sensitization or anaphylaxis and the need to interrupt medication. When compared to skin testing, however, it does not improve on specificity or sensitivity. Moreover, a positive skin test does not necessarily mean that exposure to the same allergen will produce respiratory symptoms. Newer inhalational tests may be more precise in identifying offending agents, including those that are implicated in occupational asthma. Use of these tests should be restricted to atypical patients in whom usual approaches are insufficient to establish a causative role for inhaled antigens.

DIFFERENTIAL DIAGNOSIS. Recurrent bronchospasm may occur in other diseases such as congestive heart failure, pulmonary embolism, and chronic bronchitis (see Ch. 60). There is usually little difficulty in distinguishing bronchospasm of congestive heart failure, since it is associated with other signs of underlying cardiac dysfunction. Distinguishing features of recurrent pulmonary emboli include pleural pain and effusions, signs of venous disease in the lower extremities, and characteristic findings on radioisotope lung scans and arteriography. Episodic and reversible wheezing may occur in patients with chronic bronchitis. In these patients, however, a persistent and productive cough exists in a setting of hyperirritable airways. Bronchospasm usually responds to bronchodilator therapy.

TREATMENT. Management of the asthmatic patient may be divided into two phases: treatment of the acute episode and maintenance therapy. The major classes of drugs will be reviewed as a background for recommendations on their optimal use in the treatment of asthma.

Sympathomimetic Drugs. *Epinephrine* has direct beta-adrenergic action but also stimulates alpha receptors. Its usefulness is limited by its actions on the heart, its restrictive use by inhalational and parenteral administration, and its short duration of action. Epinephrine is used in the treatment of acute asthmatic attacks and for this purpose is usually given in adults subcutaneously (0.2 to 0.5 ml of a 1 to 1000 solution). Tolerance develops after repeated use.

Isoproterenol has a potent selective beta-adrenergic effect. It is not absorbed orally, it has a relatively short duration of action, and certain patients may become refractory to its effects. Isoproterenol is usually administered by inhalation.

There are two types of beta-adrenergic receptors: β-1 agonists are cardiac stimulants (e.g., tachycardia); β-2 agonists relax bronchial smooth muscle and blood vessels with little effect on the heart. The potential for selective β-2 activity has led to the generation of new beta agonists with minimal or reduced cardiac side effects. These include the resorcinols such as *metaproterenol* and *terbutaline*. The advantages of these agents are rapid onset of action, the potential for oral administration, and longer duration of action. Both agents are available in the United States for parenteral, oral, and aerosol administration. Skeletal muscle tremors are the main side effect. Newer agents with similar advantages but apparently even greater β-2 selectivity are now available in the United States (e.g., *albuterol*). The use of β-2 agents will probably replace the use of older, less specific drugs such as ephedrine.

The administration of β-2 drugs, such as albuterol, has a number of advantages when used by the inhalational as compared to the oral route. These include a rapid onset of action, fewer systemic side effects (skeletal muscle tremors), and preservation of β-2 selectivity. When given by mouth, β-2 drugs have a longer duration of action, but lose β-2 selectivity.

Methylxanthines. Methylxanthines are believed to cause smooth muscle relaxation by their action on the cytoplasmic enzyme phosphodiesterase. The separate site of action of this drug in elevating cytoplasmic cyclic AMP raises the possibility that methylxanthines may be additive or even synergistic with sympathomimetic drugs in inducing bronchodilatation. The recommended therapeutic concentration of *theophylline* in plasma is between 10 and 20 μg per milliliter. Because of considerable variation in metabolism of the drug, maintenance doses may range between 500 and 5000* mg per day. Thus, when theophylline preparations are used alone, blood levels should be determined to establish the proper dosage. When levels exceed 20 μg per milliliter, anorexia, nausea and gastrointestinal upset, and central nervous system irritability may occur. Newer timed-release preparations show promise of achieving more stable blood levels, reducing side effects, and permitting twice a day administration. Patients with congestive heart failure and liver disease usually require lower maintenance dosages; smokers may require higher doses.

Corticosteroids. Why corticosteroids are so effective in the treatment of asthma remains unclear. They stabilize cellular lysosomal membranes, reduce cellular stores of histamine and SRS-A, and restore the responsiveness of leukocytes and airway smooth muscle to beta agonists. Interestingly, corticosteroids do not inhibit the release of mediators or influence their effect on target cells. Their main action may be to inhibit the late cellular inflammatory response. Nonetheless, steroids are important therapeutic agents in patients whose symptoms cannot be controlled with optimal combinations of bronchodilator therapy or whose disease becomes progressively severe and life threatening.

The onset of action, whether the drug is given intravenously or orally, occurs at about six hours. Thus, patients whose disease is severe enough to require intravenous steroids should continue to receive optimal doses of bronchodilator therapy. Patients who require maintenance steroid therapy should receive a short-acting drug, such as *prednisone*, in a single morning dose, and the course of therapy should be as short as possible to reduce pituitary adrenal suppression. Alternate-day administration is preferable, and the dose should be tapered as rapidly as possible. Patients receiving corticosteroid therapy should be monitored for complications such as ulcer disease, reactivation of tuberculosis, hypertension, diabetes, and cataracts.

Some synthetic steroids, such as *beclomethasone diproprionate*, can be delivered by inhalation. When doses remain below 400 μg (eight puffs daily), there is minimal if any systemic absorption. Side effects include oropharyngeal candidiasis and exacerbation of rhinitis, nasal polyposis, and atopic dermatitis. Inhaled steroids are usually used to withdraw patients from long-term systemic steroids. In this situation, it is important to watch for signs of adrenal insufficiency. Inhaled steroids are used to prevent asthmatic symptoms; they should not be used to treat acute attacks.

The Cromones. *Disodium cromoglycate* is believed to reduce the release of chemical mediators by its action on the mast cell or basophil membrane. It is not a bronchodilator, and it does not have anti-inflammatory or antihistaminic effects. Thus, it is a prophylactic drug and is not to be used during an acute asthmatic attack. In fact, inhalation of the dry powder may initiate or aggravate bronchospasm. Response or failure of response to cromolyn sodium is unpredictable. For example, not only patients with extrinsic asthma but also a significant number of patients with mixed or intrinsic asthma, particularly those with exercise-induced bronchospasm, may benefit from the drug. In patients who respond to the drug, it may be possible to reduce or eliminate the use of corticosteroids. Because of its low frequency of toxicity and side effects, a trial of therapy with cromolyn sodium should be carried out in patients with moderate to severe asthma in whom conventional bronchodilator therapy has been inadequate. Proper evaluation of the drug requires a four- to eight-week course of therapy.

Anticholinergic Agents. Atropine is one of the oldest treatments in asthma but has been all but abandoned because of its untoward side effects. Interest, however, has been rekindled in atropine-like drugs because of new insights into neurogenic mechanisms involving the vagal reflexes (Fig. 59–4) and the development of a congener of atropine *(ipratropium)*, which is a nonabsorbable aerosol and remarkably free of side effects. Although still an investigational drug in the United States, ipratropium appears to benefit asthmatic patients whose predominant symptom is chronic bronchitis or cough.

Calcium Antagonists. Another group of investigational drugs are the calcium antagonists. The translocation of calcium from the external medium or cell stores into the cytosol is a fundamental signal in the stimulation of mast cell and mucous gland secretion and smooth muscle contraction. With the aim of blocking this signal, calcium antagonists (*verapamil* and *nifedipine*) have been given by mouth or inhalation to asthmatic patients to alleviate bronchoconstriction. Some benefit has been achieved in patients with exercise-induced asthma, but the exact role of these agents in the management of asthma is unclear.

Management of the Acute Asthmatic Attack. There is no simple recipe for the management of the asthmatic patient. Each therapeutic program must be tailored to the patient. The following comments are meant to be general guidelines.

For patients with mild attacks, one drug may suffice. Therapy may begin with a theophylline preparation or a β-2 sympathomimetic amine or both. Theophylline may be started at dosages (200 mg) that produce few or no side effects. If this is inadequate, the addition of a beta-sympathomimetic amine, terbutaline (2.5 mg) or metaproterenol (10 mg), may be effective with relatively low doses of theophylline. There is an additive effect when a beta-adrenergic agent is combined with theophylline. Thus, when used together, therapeutic doses and side effects of either agent may be reduced.

In the treatment of asthma, therapy should be guided by objective evidence (e.g., pulmonary function tests) rather than relying solely on the resolution of symptoms or signs. The measurement of the FEV_1 is appropriate in patients with large airway disease; the MMF may be more important in patients with predominantly small airway disease.

If asthma persists or becomes progressively more severe, then the patient is best managed in the hospital. Aminophylline may then be given by continuous intravenous infusion. The initial recommended dosage for adult patients is a loading dose of 5.6 mg per kilogram given over 15 to 30 minutes, followed by a continuous infusion of 0.9 mg per kilogram per hour for smokers, 0.6 mg per kilogram per hour for nonsmokers, and 0.3 mg per kilogram per hour for severely ill patients (e.g., congestive heart failure, pneumonia, and liver disease). Maintenance doses must also be reduced (≃ 0.3 mg per kilogram per hour) for patients taking certain drugs, such as cimetidine or triacetyloleandomycin, which interfere with hepatic microsomal enzymes. After 36 hours, theophylline levels should be measured. If patients have recently received theophylline, then the loading dose should be decreased (50 to 75 per cent) or eliminated to avoid toxic levels and a continuous infusion begun. Patients should also receive controlled oxygen therapy and physiotherapy to relieve bronchial secretions. Fluids are given by mouth or intravenous infusion to correct dehydration if present. Electrolyte imbalance, particularly hypokalemia, should be corrected. Tranquilizers and sedatives must be avoided.

*Exceeds manufacturer's maximum recommended dose.

If the patient remains unresponsive or the attack becomes more severe, then corticosteroids should be given intravenously with continuation of full dosages of bronchodilator therapy. The correct dosage for intravenous corticosteroids is unsettled. One regimen recommends 1000 mg of hydrocortisone initially, followed by 4 mg per kilogram every four hours. When clinical signs and objective evidence indicate that the patient is responding to therapy, usually after 48 to 72 hours, then steroids may be converted to oral preparations. Sixty mg of prednisone may be started as a single morning dose. If the patient continues to improve, it may be reduced by 5 mg every third or fourth day.

In some patients it may not be possible to withdraw steroids. In this situation, the following approaches may be tried: maintenance with the lowest possible dose given on alternate days, a trial of cromolyn therapy, or conversion to aerosolized steroids. It is important that the latter two agents should be started only after there has been an optimal therapeutic response for the acute attack.

Long-Term Management. Maintenance therapy should be based on similar clinical and objective criteria as in treating the acute attack. For example, outpatient spirograms should be used routinely in following the patient. Also, the patient should be convinced as to the chronicity of the disease and dissuaded from adjusting or stopping medication when symptoms abate. Asthma should not be treated symptomatically.

It is also important to identify specific precipitating or triggering factors, including allergic and nonallergic stimuli. A thorough history may allow elimination of offending agents from the environment or occupation. Other underlying conditions such as chronic sinusitis should be carefully evaluated (e.g., sinus roentgenograms). The successful medical or surgical treatment of chronic sinusitis may have a dramatic impact on the treatment of asthma.

Immunotherapy with extracts of allergens may benefit certain allergic patients. This form of therapy, however, is just beginning to be established on firm scientific grounds.

PROGNOSIS. There are about 9 million patients with asthma in the United States, and several thousand deaths per year are attributable to the disease. Statistics concerning the long-term prognosis of asthma are as variable as the disease. For example, the percentage of childhood asthma reported to persist until adult life varies from 26 to 78 per cent. Also, it is generally held, without good data, that adult asthma improves or disappears with age. Taken together, the evidence supports Osler's adage that "asthmatics pant their way into old age."

Boushey HA, Holtzman MJ, Sheller JR, Nadel JA: State of the art: Bronchial hyperreactivity. Am Rev Respir Dis 121:389, 1980. *A review of bronchial hyperreactivity. Discusses mechanisms of hyperreactivity as well as methods of assessment. It also contains an extensive bibliography on the subject.*

Daniele RP: Pathophysiologic mechanisms in asthma. *In* Fishman AP (eds.): Pulmonary Diseases and Disorders. New York, McGraw-Hill Book Company, 1979, pp 567–576. *A more detailed account of the pathophysiologic mechanisms in asthma.*

Farr RS: Asthma in adults: The ambulatory patient. Hosp Pract 13:113, 1978. *This review emphasizes the clinical aspects of asthma; it also contains key references on the same subject.*

Lichtenstein LM, Austen KF, Simon AS (eds.): Asthma: Physiology, Immunopharmacology, and Treatment. New York, Academic Press, 1978. *Reviews the basic mechanisms of physiology and immunopharmacology in asthma by authorities in the field; the text is especially useful for those interested in current research.*

McFadden ER Jr: Respiratory heat and water exchange; Physiological and clinical implications. J Appl Physiol 54:331, 1983. *This review contains a detailed description of the physiologic features of heat exchange within the respiratory tract. It also relates this phenomenon to other aspects of airway function, especially exercise-induced asthma.*

McFadden ER Jr, Feldman NT: Asthma: Pathophysiology and clinical correlates. Med Clin North Am 61:1229, 1977. *A review which summarizes the correlations between clinical manifestations and pulmonary function abnormalities.*

Webb-Johnson DC, Andrews JL Jr: Bronchodilator therapy. N Engl J Med 297:476, 758, 1977. *A summary on the treatment of asthma. Contains details on drug preparations and their doses.*

Weissmann G: The eicosanoids of asthma. N Engl J Med 308:454, 1983. *This is a concise and current summary of the arachidonic acid metabolic pathways. It emphasizes how the compounds known as slow-reacting substance of anaphylaxis, or leukotrienes, are generated within the lung, and their potential role in bronchial contraction.*

Williams MH: Beclomethasone dipropanate. Ann Intern Med 95:464, 1981. *This survey identifies the current indications, efficacy, and side effects of topical steroids that are used in the therapy of bronchial asthma. It also contains a complete bibliography.*

60. CHRONIC AIRWAYS DISEASES

Benjamin Burrows

Chronic Bronchitis and Emphysema

The present discussion deals with chronic generalized airways disorders which are not the direct result of an underlying "specific" bronchopulmonary disease. It includes chronic bronchitis, chronic bronchitis–associated reversible airways obstruction (asthmatic bronchitis), emphysema, and chronic obstructive pulmonary disease.

INTRODUCTION

DEFINITIONS OF TERMS AND INTERRELATIONSHIPS OF DIAGNOSTIC ENTITIES. As seen in Figure 60–1, the bronchopulmonary system may respond in different ways when exposed to irritants or allergens. The type of response depends on the nature and severity of the exposure and on host susceptibility.

Chronic, relatively low-grade exposure to bronchial irritants in a subject without hyperreactive airways results in stimulation of mucus secretion, reduction in bronchial ciliary activity, and impaired resistance to bronchial infection. In the present discussion, the resulting syndrome, characterized primarily by chronic productive cough, is called *simple chronic bronchitis.*

In subjects with hyperreactive or "twitchy" airways, exposure to a variety of provocative factors can lead to bronchospasm (i.e., constriction of bronchial smooth muscles, often accompanied by edema of bronchial walls and abnormal mucus production). Recurrent episodes of bronchospasm of sufficient severity to lead to symptoms are called *asthma.*

Classic "asthma" with episodic symptoms is discussed in Ch. 59. It is impossible, however, totally to disregard broncho-

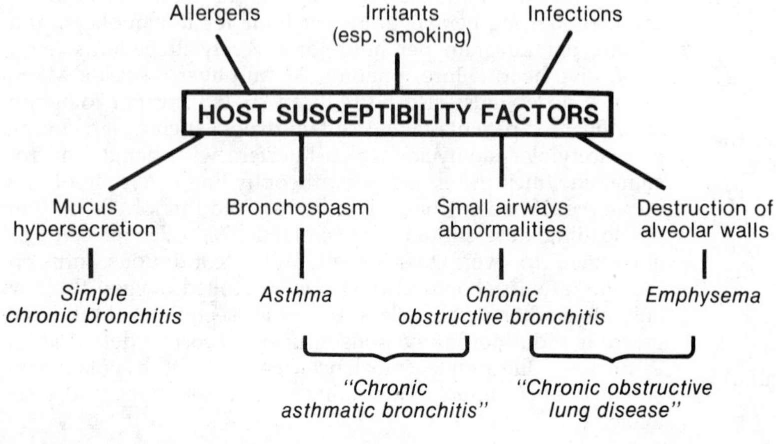

Figure 60–1. Provocative factors and the bronchopulmonary reactions they produce, depending in part on host susceptibility factors.

spasm in the present discussion, since some degree of reversible airways obstruction so often accompanies other reactions to inhaled noxious agents which will be discussed. Indeed, chronic bronchitis with episodic airways obstruction is a very common clinical entity. It is sometimes called *asthmatic bronchitis* and may be difficult to distinguish from classic asthma. The term *chronic asthmatic bronchitis* is used when there is significant persistent obstruction in a patient whose major problem is episodic bronchospasm.

In a relatively small proportion of subjects, chronic exposure to bronchial irritants results in severe irreversible narrowing of airways, a condition called *chronic obstructive bronchitis.* Much of the obstruction is in airways less than 2 mm in diameter, including bronchioles as well as bronchi, and the term "*small airways disease*" has been introduced to emphasize this point. There would seem little use, however, in delineating this as a separate disease.

Finally, the lung may respond to noxious stimuli by developing *emphysema,* a condition characterized by dilatation of air spaces distal to the terminal bronchiole with destruction of their walls. Emphysematous changes reduce the elastic recoil of the lung, allowing excessive airways collapse on expiration and leading to an irreversible obstructive problem.

The definitions of the aforementioned terms are in no way mutually exclusive. Most patients with emphysema have a chronic productive cough at some stage of their illness, allowing a secondary diagnosis of simple chronic bronchitis. Some obliteration of small airways generally accompanies emphysema, and without elaborate tests it may be difficult to determine the relative importance of chronic obstructive bronchitis and emphysema in a severe irreversible airways obstructive disorder. This has led to the use of general terms such as *chronic obstructive pulmonary (or lung) disease* (abbreviated COPD) to describe this clinical syndrome.

In practice, one generally applies the single diagnostic term which best describes the patient's major problem. But this must not limit one's therapeutic efforts. Therapy should be directed at all features of the patient's disease, not simply at those which determine the primary diagnosis.

The term *chronic bronchitis,* unqualified, has been used in various ways by different authors, sometimes referring to a simple smoker's cough and at other times (especially in the British literature) to severe COPD. In view of its ambiguity, it will be used in the present discussion only when qualified as "simple," "obstructive," or "asthmatic."

PATHOPHYSIOLOGY OF AIRWAYS OBSTRUCTION. In clinical practice, airways obstruction is synonymous with slowing of forced expiration. As discussed in Ch. 57, determinants of the speed of forced expiration include the intrinsic resistance of the airways, the recoil of the lungs, and the compressibility of the airways. A high airways resistance, low lung recoil, or excessive collapsibility of airways will lead to a reduction in maximum expiratory flow ($\dot{V}max$).

The presence of airways obstruction is generally determined by finding a low FEV_1/FVC ratio and the severity of the airflow obstruction is assessed by the amount of reduction in the FEV_1 itself. In some laboratories, the average flow over the middle half of a forced expiration ($FEF_{25-75\%}$) is used instead of the FEV_1.

In recent years, actual $\dot{V}max$ values have often been measured (Fig. 60–2). These are commonly determined at 50 per cent or 75 per cent of the forced expired volume ($\dot{V}max_{50\%}$ or $\dot{V}max_{75\%}$, respectively*).

The $\dot{V}max_{75\%}$ appears more sensitive than the FEV_1 for detecting subclinical airways dysfunction and has become popular in epidemiologic studies. However, the FEV_1 is more widely used in clinical practice, since it is easily measured, is highly reproducible, has a relatively narrow normal range, and tends to reflect the clinical severity of disease.

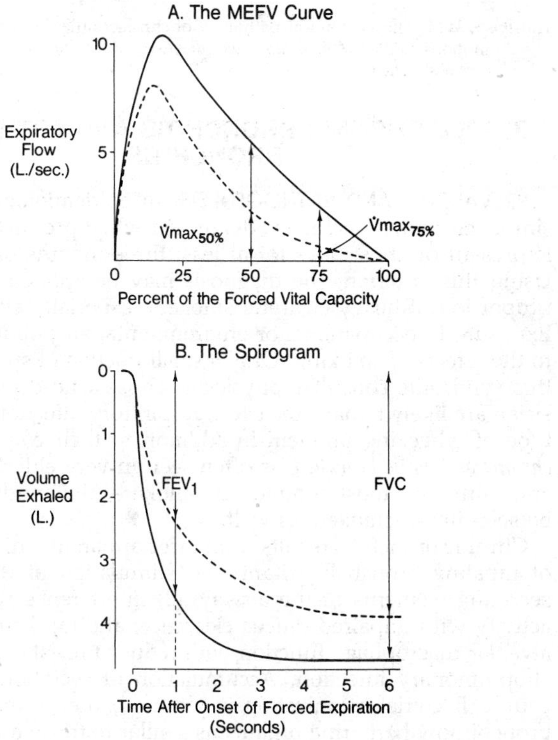

Figure 60–2. Solid lines are used to show a normal maximum expiratory flow-volume (MEFV) in *A* and a normal spirogram in *B.* Broken lines indicate typical curves for a patient with mild airways obstruction. Measurements of the forced vital capacity (FVC), the forced expiratory volume at one second (FEV_1), and forced flow rates at 50 per cent and 75 per cent of the FVC ($\dot{V}_{max50\%}$ and $\dot{V}_{max75\%}$) are depicted as vertical lines.

As discussed in Ch. 57, airways obstructive disorders may lead to a variety of other physiologic abnormalities. Mismatching of ventilation and perfusion may cause increased venous admixture and hypoxemia. It may also lead to an increased physiologic dead space which requires an increase in overall ventilation if hypercapnia is to be avoided. When the airways obstruction is severe enough or when the drive to breathe is diminished, CO_2 retention is likely to occur.

Obstructed airways tend to close prematurely during a maximum exhalation, leading to trapping of air and an increase in residual volume. In emphysema the total lung capacity is also increased. As might be expected, the pulmonary diffusing capacity measurement is almost always reduced in emphysema. It gives variable results in chronic obstructive bronchitis.

The small airways have a very large total cross-sectional diameter, and extensive changes in this "quiet zone" of the lung are required to produce a discernible effect on measurements such as the FEV_1. More sensitive tests are needed to detect mild small airways abnormalities. Many new tests have been proposed, including measurements of $\dot{V}max$ late in forced expiration, "closing volume," "helium response of the MEFV curve," and "frequency dependence of compliance." Although these tests may prove useful for detecting subclinical disease and in research studies, their specificity for small airways abnormalities is doubtful and they have no proved clinical application.

Burrows B: An overview of obstructive lung diseases. Med Clin North Am 65:455, 1981. *This is the lead article of an 11-chapter symposium on obstructive lung diseases. The entire symposium is recommended reading and an excellent source of original references.*

Fishman AP: The spectrum of chronic obstructive disease of the airways. *In* Fishman AP (ed.): Pulmonary Diseases and Disorders, New York, McGraw-Hill Book Company, 1980, pp 458-469. *A concise, clearly written description of the different types of airways obstructive disorders and how they overlap.*

*There is considerable confusion in use of these symbols. It has been recommended that $\dot{V}max_{50\%}$ and $\dot{V}max_{75\%}$ be expressed as $FEF_{50\%}$ and $FEF_{75\%}$, respectively. Also, the $\dot{V}max_{75\%}$ as defined herein is sometimes reported as $\dot{V}max_{25\%}$, the 25% then referring to the portion of the FVC remaining when the flow measurement is made.

Thurlbeck WM: The anatomical pathology of chronic airflow obstruction. Curr Pulmonol 4:1, 1982. *A good, up-to-date discussion of the pathology associated with airways obstruction.*

SIMPLE CHRONIC BRONCHITIS AND ASTHMATIC BRONCHITIS

PREVALENCE AND PATHOGENESIS. In epidemiologic studies, simple chronic bronchitis is diagnosed when productive cough is present on most days for at least three months of the year. Using this criterion, the diagnosis may be applied to a large proportion of heavy cigarette smokers, especially after age 45. Exposure to occupational or environmental air pollutants adds to the effects of smoking. Only a small fraction of subjects with this syndrome consult a physician. Those who do see a physician are likely to have recurrent respiratory infections or some type of wheezing problem in addition to their cough. Severe *chronic asthmatic bronchitis* is often seen in very elderly subjects and, although most common in smokers, the syndrome may be seen in nonsmokers as well.

Chronic bronchitis results from three apparently direct effects of inhaling bronchial irritants: (1) stimulation of the mucus-secreting elements of the airway; (2) interference with ciliary activity with impaired mucus clearance; and (3) disturbance of alveolar macrophage function with reduced resistance to bronchopulmonary infection. Accumulation of secretions leads to cough. Bacterial colonization is common, the normally sterile bronchi now harboring organisms similar to those found in the nasopharynx.

The mechanisms underlying the reversible airways obstruction observed in many of these patients remain obscure. In a few instances, retention of secretions appears to be a major contributor. In most cases, however, patients appear to have a subacute or even persistent bronchospasm which resembles that seen in asthma. It is unclear, however, to what extent the immunologic factors identified in asthma are contributing to the reversible airways obstruction and to what extent mast cell mediators are involved in the reaction.

PATHOLOGY. The most characteristic finding is hypertrophy of mucous glands and goblet cells. In addition, one finds retained bronchial secretions and variable degrees of inflammatory change in the bronchial walls. Even in the absence of clinically significant obstruction, careful studies may show narrowing or obliteration of some small airways and scattered centrilobular emphysema. Similar small airways and emphysematous changes are noted in asymptomatic smokers, however, and it is uncertain that they are related to simple chronic bronchitis except through their common association with cigarette use.

CLINICAL MANIFESTATIONS. In mild disease, *cough* is noted primarily on arising or after smoking the first cigarette of the day, is productive of a small quantity of mucoid sputum, and is present most regularly during the winter months. As the disorder becomes more severe, cough tends to recur throughout the day, symptoms persist throughout the year, larger volumes of sputum are raised, and increasingly severe paroxysms of cough are noted. *Wheezing* is common at the end of a severe coughing spell, probably representing cough-induced bronchospasm. Wheezing may also occur on reclining. This type of wheeze is probably a direct result of retained secretions, as it is often relieved by cough.

Periodic exacerbations of symptoms occur, often accompanied by purulence of the sputum. Most such episodes appear to follow viral respiratory infections, and purulence of the sputum is regarded as evidence of bacterial overgrowth. Cultures generally show the normal nasopharyngeal flora, although *H. influenzae* and *S. pneumoniae* are often present as well. These organisms probably represent secondary invaders rather than primary causes of the exacerbations. Varying degrees of bronchospasm may occur during exacerbations, and there is no clear distinction between such episodes and asthma. *Blood-streaked sputum* occurs occasionally, but repeated or severe hemoptysis should lead one to suspect a more serious disease than simple chronic bronchitis.

With further progression of the disorder, the sputum may become chronically purulent. The term *mucopurulent bronchitis* is sometimes applied to this stage of illness. Sputum cultures may now reveal drug-resistant organisms such as *P. aeruginosa;* this is especially likely to occur if the patient has received a variety of antibiotics.

Physical examination may be entirely normal in mild disease. Later, scattered wheezes and variable coarse crackles are heard. These may clear or change location after cough. A wheeze or paroxysm of coughing is often induced by a forced expiratory effort.

When reversible airways obstruction is present, wheezing and slowing of forced expiration may be prominent features and the patient may closely resemble the typical asthmatic subject.

LABORATORY FINDINGS. In uncomplicated cases, blood counts and differential smear are normal, as is the chest radiograph. Sputum examination shows variable numbers of leukocytes and a mixed flora of organisms, as already noted. Spirometry may be within normal limits but often shows slight slowing of forced expiration. In *chronic asthmatic bronchitis*, there may be quite severe functional abnormalities even between episodic exacerbations.

More severe functional abnormalities are noted during episodes of bronchospasm, and in patients with asthmatic bronchitis eosinophilia of blood and sputum may be noted.

COURSE AND PROGNOSIS. Patients with simple chronic bronchitis often show considerable fluctuation in symptoms. Cough and sputum production worsen with increased cigarette use, during inclement weather, and following acute respiratory infections. In mild cases, symptoms usually disappear completely with cessation of smoking. Although simple chronic bronchitis is often associated with slight reduction in ventilatory function, at least one prospective study has failed to show that smokers with chronic productive cough have a significantly greater rate of decline in lung function than asymptomatic smokers. A diagnosis of simple chronic bronchitis does not imply that the patient will inevitably develop progressive disabling respiratory insufficiency.

Very little is known about the long-term course of asthmatic bronchitis. Many patients show an excellent initial response to therapy and may be kept relatively asymptomatic for many years. Others appear to require increasing amounts of medication to prevent bronchospasm, and at least a few appear to progress to irreversible airways obstruction (COPD) despite optimal medical management.

DIFFERENTIAL DIAGNOSIS. The diagnosis is justified when there is persistent cough which cannot be ascribed to a parenchymal lung disease, a disorder of the upper respiratory tract, a specific endobronchial disease, or an allergic reaction of the airway. Thus a chest radiograph is required to exclude a parenchymal lesion. A careful examination of the upper airway is indicated, and one must exclude physical findings which might indicate a localized airways disorder (such as a persistent localized wheeze). In children or in young adults with severe symptoms, cystic fibrosis must also be excluded (see Ch. 64). Symptoms of chronic bronchitis may also be associated with one of the immotile cilia syndromes (see Ch. 63).

One should be cautious in diagnosing simple chronic bronchitis in the absence of an obvious source of chronic bronchial irritation. In a nonsmoker, in a patient whose history suggests an association between symptoms and exposure to allergens, or in a patient with episodes of wheezing dyspnea, one should check for eosinophilia in the sputum and blood. High eosinophil levels suggest the diagnosis of asthmatic bronchitis, which may respond to bronchodilator or corticosteroid therapy.

Repeated or severe hemoptysis, or physical findings suggesting localized disease, may call for bronchoscopy and even bronchography to rule out an endobronchial lesion or localized bronchiectasis, but these procedures are not indicated in the routine case. Spirometry should be carried out to determine the degree of associated ventilatory impairment.

There may be a problem in distinguishing severe mucopurulent bronchitis from bronchiectasis. Mild diffuse cylindrical dilatation of bronchi is noted in many severe bronchitics. Recurrent hemoptysis, repeated pneumonias in the same lung region, or areas of honeycombing on chest radiographs suggest that there may be areas of frank saccular bronchiectasis. Bronchography is required for accurate diagnosis but is usually indicated only if resection of the bronchiectatic areas would be considered. Otherwise, there is little difference in the therapy of mucopurulent bronchitis and bronchiectasis.

TREATMENT. Removal of the provocative factors (usually cigarettes) is of primary importance and may totally relieve the condition. When symptoms persist despite maximal efforts to avoid bronchial irritants or are severe enough to require more immediate relief, the following measures are employed:

Antibiotic Therapy. Noneosinophilic purulent sputum is regarded as evidence of infection and is treated with a seven- to ten-day course of sulfamethoxazole-trimethoprim, one tablet twice a day, or of tetracycline or ampicillin, 1 gram daily in divided doses. If the sputum fails to clear, further antibiotic therapy should be determined by sputum culture and sensitivity. Successive doses of different antibiotics should be avoided, however, because they tend to lead to a resistant flora. Failure of therapy is more often related to poor drainage of bronchial secretions than to inadequate antibacterial agents.

Very severe exacerbations of disease generally respond better to ampicillin or cephalothin than to tetracycline, and it is reasonable to use these agents as initial therapy when the specific infecting organism is unknown. (Penicillin has proved inappropriate therapy for severe purulent exacerbations of bronchitis.) When resistant organisms are cultured from the sputum, the antibiotic regimen may have to be adjusted in accord with drug susceptibility studies.

Bronchodilator Agents. Bronchodilator medications are the mainstays of therapy for control of any reversible component in COPD and for management of bronchospasm associated with simple chronic bronchitis. They are also useful adjuncts to bronchial hygiene treatments, as described below. Both of the main classes of bronchodilators, beta-adrenergic agonists and methylxanthines, are useful to relieve existing bronchospasm and to prevent recurrent attacks. The principles and details for the therapeutic use of these agents for relief of bronchospasm are the same as those for asthma, described in Ch. 59.

Adrenocortical Hormones. The use of corticosteroids in asthmatic bronchitis is justified when significant airways obstruction persists or recurs frequently despite maximal bronchodilator therapy. In the ambulant patient, drugs are given in moderate doses (e.g., 20 to 40 mg of prednisone per day) for a few days and rapidly tapered to the lowest level compatible with sustained improvement. In many cases, improvement is rapid and the medication may be discontinued totally within five to seven days. Occasional relapses are then treated by repeated short "bursts" of steroids. In some patients, however, symptoms recur when the steroid dose falls below a certain level. One must then taper slowly to the lowest dose compatible with patient comfort and reasonably normal ventilatory function. If possible, maintenance steroids should be administered as a single dose given on alternate days.

Once a maintenance dose has been reached, an attempt should be made to replace some or all of the oral corticosteroid with an inhaled poorly absorbed preparation such as beclomethasone. This agent is supplied in a pressurized container, and the standard dose is two inhalations (100 μg) four times a day. This generally replaces 7.5 to 10 mg per day of oral prednisone and produces no discernible systemic side effects. Some patients require premedication with an inhaled bronchodilator to ameliorate irritation from the beclomethasone aerosol.

In the steroid-dependent patient who has received oral medication for many months or years, systemic medication must be discontinued very slowly (over several months) to avoid adrenal insufficiency. Nasal symptoms, previously suppressed with oral medications, may exacerbate, requiring reinstitution of oral medications. In some subjects (up to 30 per cent in some series) oropharyngeal candidiasis occurs. Fortunately, this responds promptly to specific therapy and rarely requires discontinuation of inhaled steroids.

Bronchial Hygiene Measures. The objective of these measures is to clear retained bronchial secretions. The most important steps are deep breathing followed by deliberate coughing. This may be made more effective by positioning the patient so that the most affected lung regions are in a superior position (postural drainage). In some subjects, chest percussion and vibration further increase sputum production.

Premedication with an inhaled bronchodilator may greatly improve the patient's tolerance of bronchial hygiene measures and increase their effectiveness. This may be followed by inhalation of bland mist in an attempt to loosen secretions. It has been difficult to show objective effects from bland mist therapy, but some patients are convinced of its beneficial effects. Treatments are usually prescribed twice daily for ambulant patients and more often during exacerbations. Patients vary in their reactions to such therapy. Only those measures which prove effective for the individual patient should be continued, as the full program is time consuming and uncomfortable.

All patients should be encouraged to keep well hydrated to avoid inspissation of secretions. In acute exacerbations, this may require intravenous fluids. The usefulness of expectorant medications is questionable. Some authorities recommend 10 to 12 drops of a saturated solution of potassium iodide three times a day. This does seem to be effective in some patients, but it is associated with a high rate of side effects, some of which can be severe. Cough syrups and lozenges may help relieve a "tickle" in the throat but have little effect on the viscosity of bronchial secretions. Cough sedatives are generally contraindicated. They should be used only for acute episodes of severe nonproductive cough.

Treatment of Severe Exacerbations. Severe exacerbations of asthmatic bronchitis with severe airways obstruction are life-threatening events. They are treated in the same manner as status asthmaticus, discussed in Ch. 59. These patients, however, may require even greater attention to bronchial hygiene measures to assist in clearing of secretions than does the usual classic asthmatic.

Burrows B: Irreversible airways obstruction and asthma. Pract Cardiol 8:69, 1982. *This article presents in more detail the author's views concerning the overlap of reversible and irreversible airways obstructive diseases.*

Burrows B, Lebowitz MD, Barbee RA, Knudson RJ, Halonen M: Interactions of smoking and immunological factors in relationship to airways obstruction. Chest 84:657, 1983. *This paper presents new evidence that chronic asthmatic bronchitis may result from an interaction of the irritant effects of smoking and immunologic factors.*

Sachs FL: Chronic bronchitis. Clin Chest Med 2:79, 1981. *This paper reviews briefly the role of infection in chronic bronchitis and the management of this aspect of the disease.*

Scientific Basis of In-hospital Respiratory Therapy. Conference Proceedings. Am Rev Respir Dis 122:No 5, Part 2, Nov 1980. *This conference report represents an in-depth review of what is actually known about the usefulness of respiratory therapy procedures.*

Weinberger M, Hendeles L, Ahrens R: Pharmacological management of reversible airways obstruction. Med Clin North Am 65:579, 1981. *A good review of the use of bronchodilators and steroids in asthma and asthmatic bronchitis, with an extensive reference list.*

CHRONIC OBSTRUCTIVE BRONCHITIS AND EMPHYSEMA
(Chronic Obstructive Pulmonary Disease)

PREVALENCE AND PATHOGENESIS. Chronic obstructive pulmonary disease (COPD) is a major cause of disability in older subjects, ranking behind heart diseases and schizophrenia in United States Social Security statistics. It is also an increasingly important cause of mortality. The disease is usually first diagnosed between ages 55 and 65. It is much more common in men than in women, but this may reflect, at least in part, the different smoking habits of the sexes earlier in the century.

Smoking. As already noted, COPD results from some combination of chronic obstructive bronchitis and pulmonary emphysema. Both disorders are closely related to cigarette smoking. The intrinsic airways disease is generally considered a direct consequence of bronchial irritation in a susceptible individual. Emphysema probably results from the effect of proteolytic enzymes on lung tissue. When there is a very severe congenital deficiency of serum antiproteolytic activity, emphysema is likely to develop by age 40 if the subject smokes and by age 60 if he does not. Without such a severe deficiency (which accounts for only 0.5 to 2 per cent of COPD), the development of emphysema depends on prolonged exposure to noxious irritants, usually cigarette smoke. Presumably, such exposure leads to reduction in lung defense mechanisms, low grade inflammatory changes in the lung parenchyma, and release of sufficient leukocytic proteases to overwhelm the body's antiproteolytic mechanisms.

Epidemiologic studies reveal a close relationship between cigarette smoking and slowing of forced exhalation. Whereas the average nonsmoking adult shows a rate of decline in FEV_1 of 20 to 25 ml per year of age, the average heavy smoker shows a decline of 40 to 45 ml per year. The excess rate of decline appears to cease if smoking is discontinued. But this average effect of cigarettes is not sufficient to explain the much more severe impairment of FEV_1 noted in clinically significant COPD. Presumably there are subjects who are especially susceptible to the effects of smoking. There is great interest in identifying factors which cause a minority of smokers to develop clinically significant COPD. Respiratory disorders in childhood and intercurrent respiratory infections may be contributory factors. Genetic factors may also play a role.

The generally accepted concept of the early, preclinical history of COPD is that susceptible subjects who smoke show a very excessive rate of decline in lung function throughout adult life. According to this concept, the subject who will later develop COPD should be recognizable by age 40 because he will already show a mild ventilatory abnormality. This has led to some enthusiasm for screening of young to middle-aged adults in order to detect early COPD. There is no direct evidence, however, that the individual who will later develop severe disabling disease can be identified reliably by any physiologic test applied early in life.

Alpha$_1$-Antitrypsin Deficiency. There are a few families in whom a deficiency of serum antiproteolytic activity is associated with a susceptibility to COPD. The serum's trypsin inhibitory capacity is determined by the *p*rotease *i*nhibitor or "Pi" phenotype of the subject. A normal individual has two M genes (Pi phenotype MM). Severe deficiency of alpha$_1$ globulin, which contains most of the serum's antiproteolytic (antitrypsin) activity, occurs when there are only Z genes. This is found in approximately 1:4000 of the population. It is associated with hepatitis in infancy as well as emphysema in middle age. A heterozygotic state (phenotype MZ) is much more common, occurring in 3 to 5 per cent of the population. It is associated with moderate reduction in serum antiproteolytic activity. In some families, such an MZ phenotype appears to be associated with an increased tendency to COPD. On the other hand, general population studies have failed to show any overall tendency for MZ subjects to develop an excess of respiratory disease or for respiratory disorders to be related to the level of serum trypsin inhibitory capacity except in PiZ subjects. A variety of other Pi genes have been identified (of which S is the most common), but only the Z gene is clearly associated with COPD. The hepatic manifestations of alpha$_1$-antitrypsin deficiency are discussed in Ch. 124.

PATHOLOGY. The basic defect in emphysema is destruction of alveolar walls, leading to a reduced number of enlarged air spaces. This is often most severe in the central portion of the lobule (centrilobular emphysema), but it may occur uniformly throughout the acinus (panacinar emphysema). Both types of change may occur in the same lung, and severe centrilobular changes may progress to a point at which the process appears to involve the entire acinus.

Changes in the large airways characteristic of simple chronic bronchitis vary considerably in severity. But there are usually widespread abnormalities in small bronchi and bronchioles, including inflammation in and around air passages with narrowing of their lumens, mucous impaction, and obliterative changes. The extent of the abnormalities in small airways is not obvious on casual examination of the lung and can be quantified only by morphometric studies.

CLINICAL MANIFESTATIONS. Dyspnea is the most common chief complaint, but some patients first see a physician because of cough, wheezing, recurrent respiratory infections, or even weakness or weight loss. The dyspnea is usually described as insidious in onset and progressive. Some patients, however, are aware of shortness of breath only during exacerbations of disease and give a history more suggestive of asthma than COPD. Others date their chronic symptoms from an acute respiratory infection.

Most patients admit to some cough and expectoration, but often this consists only of clearing a small quantity of mucus from the chest shortly after awakening. Other patients complain of more severe cough and more copious, sometimes purulent sputum.

Physical findings are extremely variable and depend to some extent on the stage of the disease. In relatively early illness (FEV_1 above 1.0 liter), the examination is often normal except for slowing of forced expiration. Rhonchi may be present or the chest may be unusually quiet on auscultation. Other physical findings occur with increasing frequency as the disease progresses. There may be gross overinflation with low diaphragms and a decreased area of cardiac dullness. Labored breathing, sometimes through pursed lips, may be present after slight exertion or even at rest. The patient may assume a stooped posture, tend to lean on his elbows when sitting, and use accessory muscles of respiration. Cyanosis may be present, and slight dependent edema is common.

Evidences of cor pulmonale generally appear only in advanced stages of illness when the FEV_1 is below 1 liter, but the severity of cardiac complications is quite variable. Pulmonary hypertension and cor pulmonale in COPD are more closely related to the severity of hypoxemia than to the degree of ventilatory impairment and are generally noted only when the resting arterial Po_2 is below 45 torr. Occasionally, patients first seek medical attention at this stage of illness, their major presenting features being those of heart failure secondary to cor pulmonale.

The variability in findings in patients with COPD is explained, at least in part, by differences in the severity of their emphysema and their intrinsic airway disease. Occasionally, relatively distinctive syndromes can be distinguished which relate to the underlying pathology. These have been called the emphysematous (Type A) and bronchial (Type B) types of COPD (Table 60–1). Since typical Type A patients often hyperventilate, thereby maintaining reasonably normal arterial oxygen tensions, they have been described as "pink puffers." Cyanosis and congestive heart failure are more common in Type B disease, and patients with these features have been called "blue bloaters." It should be recognized, however, that these clinical types represent extremes of a spectrum of presentations. Most patients display a mixture of findings, especially if followed over a period of time. It is far more important to distinguish the largely reversible chronic asthmatic bronchitic patient from the patient with irreversible COPD than to be concerned with the type of irreversible disease.

Disordered breathing during sleep, which is common in COPD patients, may also lead to the "blue bloater" syndrome.

LABORATORY FINDINGS. Except for some erythrocytosis in

severely hypoxemic patients, the routine blood count and differential are normal. The finding of eosinophilia should lead one to suspect that there is a reversible (asthmatic-bronchitic) component to the disease.

The chest radiograph may be entirely normal early in the disease, or it may reveal only the residua of previous inflammatory changes. With severe emphysema, marked overinflation is noted with flattening of the diaphragms, increased retrosternal space, and regional attenuation of vessels. In some cases, there are frank bullae demarcated by hairline margins. COPD should never be diagnosed solely on the basis of the appearance of the radiograph. Radiographs which appear typical of the disease may occur in subjects with perfectly normal lung function.

The most characteristic feature of COPD is persistent reduction in forced expiratory flow rates. The residual volume is increased, as is the residual volume : total lung capacity ratio. Nonuniformity of ventilation and some mismatch of ventilation and perfusion are generally noted, but the severity of physiologic shunting and hypoxemia varies greatly from case to case. Most other pulmonary function abnormalities are also variable and depend to some extent on the relative severity of the emphysema and intrinsic airways disease. For example, a very low diffusing capacity and a frankly increased total lung capacity suggest that there is extensive emphysema.

Isotopic lung scans show the uneven ventilation and perfusion. Areas of diminished perfusion may even be mistaken for pulmonary emboli, and lung scans must be interpreted cautiously in patients with any chronic pulmonary disease.

The electrocardiogram is often normal, especially early in the disease. Later, one may find some right axis shift and a delayed transition of the QRS complexes across the precordial leads. Peaked P waves ("P pulmonale") may be noted, especially during exacerbations of disease. These changes, although characteristic of severe COPD, are not well correlated with pulmonary hypertension or cor pulmonale. The most reliable indication of the latter condition is the presence of R waves over the right precordium.

COURSE AND PROGNOSIS. The initial response to therapy is variable and depends on the degree of bronchospasm associated with the disease. Some patients show considerable initial symptomatic and physiologic improvement. After this, the disease tends to progress slowly, with an average decline in FEV_1 between 50 and 75 ml per year. The rate of loss of function can be assessed only after several years of follow-up, however, because the variability in FEV_1 may exceed its true annual decline. Almost all symptoms also tend to worsen slowly. Cough and sputum production are exceptions. These often improve, especially if the patient stops smoking.

As a rule, patients note dyspnea on moderate exertion when the FEV_1 is between 1.2 and 1.5 liters, become limited to relatively sedentary activity when the FEV_1 is near 1 liter, and become invalided as the FEV_1 approaches 500 ml. Chronic hypercapnia, severe hypoxemia, and cor pulmonale are usually noted only when the FEV_1 is below 1 liter. Median survival is approximately ten years when the FEV_1 exceeds 1.2 liters, is near five years when the FEV_1 is 1.0, and approaches two years when the FEV_1 is less than 700 ml, but there is considerable variability around these median survivals, some patients living 12 to 15 years despite a very low initial FEV_1. Rapid heart rate at rest, severe blood gas abnormalities, or evidences of cor pulmonale are poor prognostic signs. Longevity is reduced in patients residing at altitudes in excess of 3500 feet.

Many patients show periodic exacerbations of their disease characterized by increased cough and dyspnea. These exacerbations often follow acute respiratory infections and are associated with variable degrees of bronchospasm. In patients with severe COPD, such exacerbations are life threatening, leading to acute respiratory failure and to heart failure secondary to cor pulmonale.

DIFFERENTIAL DIAGNOSIS. There are three criteria for the diagnosis of COPD: (1) there must be slowing of forced expiration, and the reduction of FEV_1 must be disproportionate to any reduction in FVC (i.e., both the per cent predicted FEV_1 and the FEV_1/FVC ratio must be reduced); (2) the expiratory slowing must persist despite prolonged and intensive medical therapy; and (3) specific bronchopulmonary diseases which might explain the physiologic abnormalities must be excluded. Failure to demonstrate extensive parenchymal disease on chest radiograph and an absence of any signs of upper airway obstruction (e.g., stridor, neck mass, or narrowing of the upper airway on chest radiogram) are generally considered sufficient for the last criterion. It is more difficult to exclude reversibility of the disease. This is discussed further under Treatment.

Determining the relative importance of intrinsic airways changes and emphysema may also present a challenge, but attenuation of vascular markings and increased transradiancy of the lung are usually noted on the chest radiograph if the emphysema is severe. A well-preserved diffusing capacity suggests that extensive emphysema is not present. The esophageal balloon measurements required to measure the elastic properties of the lung (the best guide to the severity of emphysema) are rarely justified for clinical evaluation.

A homozygotic $alpha_1$-antitrypsin deficiency should be suspected when there is a family history of emphysema or when

TABLE 60–1. FEATURES OF THE EMPHYSEMATOUS AND BRONCHIAL TYPES OF COPD

	Emphysematous (Type A)	Bronchial (Type B)
Clinical features		
Dyspnea	Insidious onset, slowly progressive	Often noted first only during chest infections
Sputum	Usually scant and mucoid	Often copious and purulent
Weight loss	Often marked	Usually slight or absent
Chronic cor pulmonale with heart failure	Infrequent until terminal stages of the disease	Common
Chest examination	Quiet chest (except slight wheeze at end expiration), marked hyperinflation	Noisy chest, slight hyperinflation
Chest radiograph	Hyperlucent, overinflated lung; often regional attenuation of vessels	Often evidence of old inflammatory disease
Physiologic tests		
Total lung capacity	Increased	Normal or slightly decreased
Residual volume	Markedly increased	Moderately increased
Lung compliance, static	Increased	Near normal
Lung compliance, dynamic	Normal or slightly low	Very low
Lung recoil	Markedly reduced	Variable
Inspiratory airways resistance	Normal	Increased
Diffusing capacity	Markedly reduced	Variable
Arterial P_{O_2}	Slight reduction at rest; usually falls with exertion	Often very low at rest; variable change with exertion
Arterial P_{CO_2}	Usually normal or low	Often chronically elevated
Resting pulmonary artery pressure	Normal or slightly elevated at rest; increases with exertion	Often markedly elevated at rest
Cardiac output	Often low	Usually near normal

there is an early age of onset of an emphysematous type of COPD, especially if the patient is a nonsmoker or is female, or when the radiograph reveals a bilateral basilar distribution of the emphysematous changes. The diagnosis is confirmed by almost complete absence of alpha$_1$ globulin, by very low serum trypsin inhibitory capacity, and, most definitively, by demonstration of the pattern of a pure Z phenotype on crossed immunoelectrophoresis of the serum.

TREATMENT. The goals of therapy of COPD are as follows: (1) relief of any reversible component of the airways obstruction; (2) control of cough and bronchial secretions; (3) elimination and prevention of bronchopulmonary infection; (4) increase in exercise tolerance to the limits imposed by the patient's permanent physiologic impairment; (5) control of remediable complications of the disease, including cardiovascular problems and excessive hypoxemia; (6) avoidance of factors which may aggravate the disease such as inhaled irritants, sedatives and narcotics, or unnecessary surgery; and (7) relief of depression and anxiety which often accompany the disorder.

A comprehensive therapeutic program can ameliorate symptoms, reduce the frequency of hospital admission, prevent premature death, and allow patients to lead more active and more satisfying lives. Most patients with severe COPD show a slow progression of ventilatory impairment despite treatment but this should not lead to therapeutic nihilism.

The usefulness of a team approach to therapy of COPD (e.g., a formal rehabilitation program) has been well demonstrated. However, good results can be obtained by a dedicated individual physician, perhaps assisted by an office nurse to help patients with bronchial hygiene and physical therapy measures.

Initial Treatment. One cannot predict accurately the degree of reversibility of the airways obstruction when the patient is first seen, and all patients should be regarded as having potentially reversible disease. Bronchodilators should be given to tolerance, as described in the therapy of asthmatic bronchitis and asthma. Smoking should be eliminated or minimized and other sources of bronchial irritants avoided. Bronchial hygiene measures and, when appropriate, antibiotics should be used, as outlined in the therapy of simple chronic bronchitis. If signs of congestive heart failure are present, diuretics should be prescribed. Pneumovax and yearly influenza vaccine are recommended.

The appropriateness of this regimen should be evaluated after its effects on symptoms and ventilatory tests have been observed. Therapy may have to be adjusted to minimize side effects, and apparently useless measures (such as postural drainage which leads to no sputum production or symptomatic relief) should be discontinued. The physician must then decide if the possibility of further reversibility of the disease is sufficiently great to justify a three- to four-week trial of corticosteroids.

The following features suggest potential reversibility of the disease and indicate that a trial of steroids is worthwhile in a patient with apparent COPD: (1) improvement in FEV$_1$ of greater than 20 per cent after inhalation of a bronchodilator; (2) similar degree of improvement in FEV$_1$ over several weeks of intensive bronchodilator therapy; (3) history of considerable fluctuation in severity of symptoms or of acute attacks of wheezing dyspnea not precipitated by exertion; (4) prominent wheeze or noisy chest on physical examination; (5) chest radiograph which appears normal except for hyperinflation; (6) eosinophilia of the blood or sputum; (7) evidences of atopy, such as a history of hay fever, positive allergy skin tests, or high serum IgE level; (8) associated vasomotor rhinitis or nasal polyps; or (9) normal pulmonary diffusing capacity measurement.

Corticosteroids are given in moderate doses (e.g., 20 to 40 mg per day of prednisone) for three to four weeks, and their effectiveness is assessed by changes in spirometric tests. Full doses of bronchodilators are maintained during this trial period. If significant improvement in FEV$_1$ is not observed, steroids should be discontinued gradually over one to two weeks. If improvement does occur, medications should be tapered to the smallest possible maintenance dose, as described in the therapy of asthmatic bronchitis.

Maintenance Therapy. Even if no objective improvement is obtained with bronchodilator drugs, maintenance doses of theophyllines, in conjunction with beta-adrenergic drugs, are usually advised to prevent episodes of superimposed bronchospasm. Adrenergic aerosols may also be used regularly, prior to exposure to known bronchial irritants, for treatment of acute attacks of dyspnea, or as part of a bronchial hygiene program. In patients who show significant improvement with bronchodilators or with adrenocortical hormones, these drugs should be maintained as described in the therapy of asthmatic bronchitis. Those measures described for the treatment of simple chronic bronchitis are fully applicable to patients with COPD who suffer from productive cough, recurrent bronchopulmonary infection, or retained secretions. Certain other types of treatment are more uniquely applicable to COPD.

PHYSICAL THERAPY. Unless contraindicated by a cardiac disorder, a program of gradually increasing exercise (usually graded walking) should be prescribed. Exercise does not improve lung function but it does train skeletal muscles to function more efficiently, thereby increasing exercise tolerance. For very severely disabled patients, exercise therapy may have to be initiated by a trained physical therapist, but in the usual case an appropriate program can be recommended directly to the patient by his physician. Patients with severe exertional hypoxemia may need supplemental oxygen during exercise, and it is advisable to obtain arterial blood gas at rest and after exercise before embarking on a vigorous exercise program in patients with an FEV$_1$ below 1 liter.

"Breathing exercises" are sometimes recommended in the hope of encouraging diaphragmatic breathing. It is doubtful, however, that one can alter the patient's usual breathing pattern. More realistically, one can teach the patient that dyspnea per se is not harmful, that slow deep breathing relieves dyspnea more quickly than rapid shallow "panic breathing," and that breath holding during exertion is to be avoided. Mechanical devices, such as emphysema belts and IPPB machines, are of no proven value, but training of inspiratory muscles by breathing against a graded resistor is now recommended by many authorities.

OXYGEN THERAPY. There are clear indications for home oxygen therapy in some patients with COPD. Low flow oxygen by nasal cannula may be employed during exercise in patients with severe exertional hypoxemia (Pa_{O_2} <40 torr) who show an increase in their exercise tolerance with supplemental O_2.

Both quality of life and longevity are improved with continuous administration of low flow oxygen when there is severe persistent arterial hypoxemia at rest (Pa_{O_2} <55 torr or a Pa_{O_2} of 55 to 60 torr plus secondary signs of hypoxemia). Continuous therapy produces better results than previously recommended regimens, in which oxygen was given for 12 to 15 hours each day. The proper oxygen dose is one which raises the Pa_{O_2} to 60 to 80 torr, usually 1 to 3 liters per minute by nasal prongs. Before prescribing continuous O_2 therapy one should be sure that all other therapeutic measures have been exhausted and that frank hypoxemia persists despite complete recovery from an exacerbation of disease.

Oxygen should not be used to treat episodes of dyspnea. Patients become habituated to this form of therapy, adding to their invalidism.

ENVIRONMENTAL CONTROL. A move to a lower altitude is certainly justified for patients living at altitudes above 4000 feet. (All patients with severe COPD should be advised to avoid high altitudes, and those with severe hypoxemia may require supplemental oxygen when traveling by air.) A change in residence may also be indicated for patients residing in areas of very heavy air pollution.

Many patients consider moving to escape a cold winter climate. Some find relief in warm humid regions, whereas others prefer dry warm desert climates. There is no evidence that the overall course of the disease is altered by a move to either type of area. A decision to relocate in a more salubrious climate should be made only after weighing the possible symptomatic relief against the social and economic hardships of the move. The specific area is best chosen on the basis of a trial period to assess both symptomatic relief and the patient's fondness for the locale.

TREATMENT OF EDEMA AND COR PULMONALE. Pedal edema is common even in the absence of other evidence of congestive heart failure and is usually readily controlled with small doses of diuretics. Recurrent or chronic congestive failure secondary to cor pulmonale is a more difficult problem. In addition to the usual therapy for heart failure (using digitalis with great care), phlebotomies may be needed to maintain the hematocrit below 56, and all treatments may fail unless hypoxemia is controlled with oxygen therapy.

TREATMENT OF HYPERCAPNIA. Chronic hypercapnia is common in late stages of the disease. It requires no specific therapy but does indicate the need to monitor blood gases closely during exacerbations of the disease and to avoid totally the use of sedatives, tranquilizers, or narcotics. There is no justification for respiratory stimulants or mechanical assistance to ventilation in patients with chronic stable hypercapnia.

SURGICAL THERAPY. A few patients with very large bullae which compress relatively normal lung may be benefited by bullectomy. However, the selection of suitable operative candidates requires careful and detailed preoperative evaluation.

SUPPORTIVE MEASURES. It is essential that patients understand the nature of their disease, the significance of symptoms which may develop (e.g., purulent sputum), the possible side effects of medications, and the goals of therapy. Provision must be made for prompt treatment of exacerbations. Most importantly, patients must be encouraged to live active and interesting lives within the limits imposed by their respiratory impairment and within the constraints imposed by any therapeutic measures which are employed. Occupational therapy and vocational rehabilitation are useful for some patients.

Treatment of Exacerbations. Mild symptomatic exacerbations, often associated with infection, are treated with more vigorous application of the measures mentioned above. Antibiotics, increased bronchodilators, and even a course of steroids are often indicated. Blood gases should be monitored and cardiovascular status assessed. Severe hypoxemia, increasing arterial carbon dioxide tension, or evidence of congestive heart failure dictates immediate hospitalization. The management of acute respiratory failure and heart failure from cor pulmonale is discussed in Ch. 70 and 42, respectively. Patients with refractory bronchospasm superimposed on their COPD should receive the same type of management as patients with status asthmaticus, as described in the therapy of asthma.

Bloom J, Burrows B: Diseases associated with airflow limitation. Curr Pulmonol 5:255, 1983. *This is an up-to-date review of the recent literature on airways obstructive diseases with an extensive bibliography.*

Burrows B: Value of annual spirometric examination of smokers. Pract Cardiol 9:143, 1983. *While noting the potential usefulness of routine office spirometry, this paper points out the potential problems and limitations of the procedure.*

De Marco FJ Jr, Wynne JW, Block AJ, Boysen PG, Taasan VC: Oxygen desaturation during sleep as a determinant of the "blue and bloated" syndrome. Chest 79:621, 1981. *One of several papers by this group of investigators proposing that sleep-related breathing disorders are important in COPD patients.*

Higgins MW, Keller JB: Estimating your patients' risk of COPD. J Respir Dis 4:97, 1983. *This paper discusses the use of routine spirometric testing to detect subjects who are at high risk of developing clinically significant airways obstructive disease.*

Hudson LD, Pierson DJ: Comprehensive respiratory care for patients with chronic obstructive pulmonary disease. Med Clin North Am 65:629, 1981. *This is a brief but good review of the principles involved in managing patients with chronic airflow obstruction.*

Nocturnal Oxygen Therapy Trial Group: Continuous or nocturnal oxygen therapy in hypoxemic chronic obstructive lung disease. Ann Intern Med 93:391, 1980. *A report of a collaborative study showing the superiority of continuous oxygen supplementation.*

Localized Airway Obstruction

Localized obstruction to air flow may result from extrinsic compression of airways, from diseases of the airways themselves, or from intraluminal obstructions. Signs and symptoms depend on whether the lesion is above or below the tracheal bifurcation, on whether the obstruction is complete or partial, and on whether the obstruction is fixed or variable.

OBSTRUCTION ABOVE THE TRACHEAL BIFURCATION

PARTIAL OBSTRUCTION. The characteristic finding in partial obstruction above the tracheal carina is stridor, often accompanied by inspiratory retraction of the intercostal spaces. Slowing of air flow is noted on both forced inspiration and forced expiration, and the MEFV curve may have a characteristic appearance. The spirometric findings depend on the site and nature of the obstruction, as seen in Figure 60–3. With severe obstruction, adequate overall ventilation may not be maintained, resulting in hypercapnia and hypoxemia.

Diseases intrinsic to the airways which may lead to partial obstruction include enlarged tonsils and adenoids (especially in young children); neoplasms of the hypopharynx, larynx, vocal cords, or trachea; stenosing lesions secondary to trauma; bilateral vocal cord paralysis; laryngeal edema or spasm; and inflammatory lesions of the pharynx (as in peritonsillar abscess), larynx (as in croup), or trachea (as in diphtheria). Extrinsic compression of the larynx or trachea may occur secondary to enlarged thyroid, paratracheal neoplasm, or, rarely, mediastinal infection. If the primary cause of the obstruction cannot be eliminated, an artificial airway, tracheostomy, or surgical repair is indicated.

COMPLETE OBSTRUCTION. Unless promptly relieved, complete obstruction above the tracheal carina leads to rapid asphyxiation. The presentation is pathognomonic with lack of air flow at the mouth despite inspiratory efforts and inspiratory retraction of the intercostal spaces. Acute obstruction is most commonly caused by aspiration of poorly chewed food. This emergency is treated by a sharp blow on the back. If this fails to dislodge the offending agent, one applies forceful pressure to the epigastrium, using the *Heimlich maneuver.*

Episodic complete obstruction of the upper airway occurs during sleep in some obese individuals owing to falling back of the glossopharyngeal structures. It may also occur in subjects with local abnormalities in the hypopharynx. This causes frequent awakening, troubled sleeping, and somnolence. The resulting clinical picture can be confused with the pickwickian syndrome and represents one form of sleep apnea, which is discussed in more detail in Ch. 472.5.

OBSTRUCTION BELOW THE TRACHEAL BIFURCATION

PARTIAL OBSTRUCTION. Characteristically, this results in a localized expiratory wheeze over the site of obstruction and hyperinflation of the distal lung. It is most commonly caused by a primary neoplasm which grows into or compresses an airway, but it may result from acute or chronic inflammatory lesions of the bronchi, aspiration of foreign bodies, compression of bronchi from enlarged hilar lymph nodes, or mucous plugs. Since airflow from the remaining lung is unimpaired, spirometry may be relatively normal, but other tests will reveal evidence of nonuniformity of ventilation. The area of diminished airflow may be detected by ventilation scans. Definitive diagnosis generally depends on bronchoscopy, and treatment is directed at the underlying disease.

Partial bronchial obstruction impairs clearance of secretions from the distal lung, leading to infection and even abscess formation. Recurrent infections in the same area of lung, slow clearing of pneumonia, or lung abscess should make one suspect partial obstruction of the bronchus leading to the affected region.

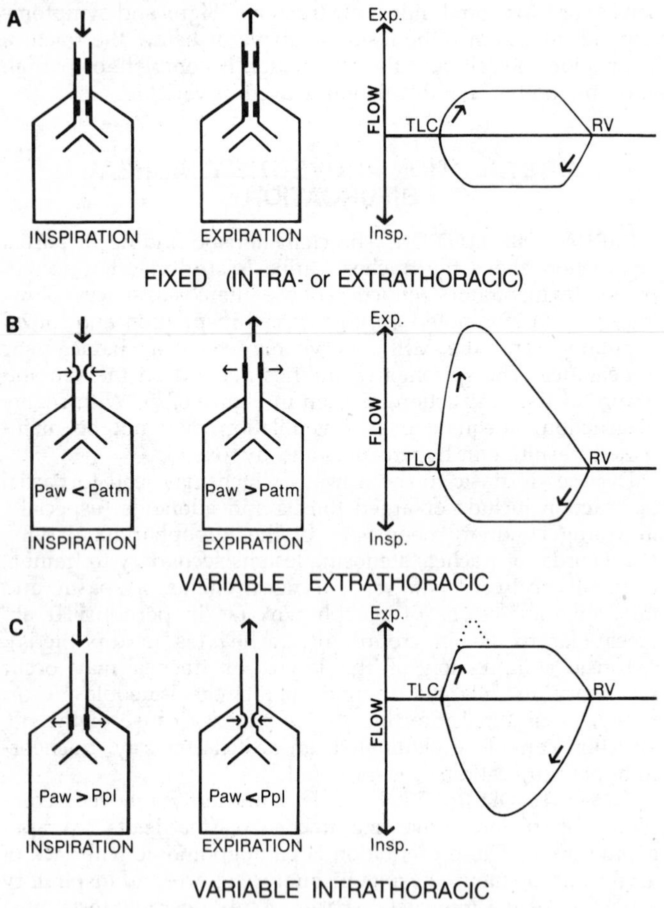

Figure 60–3. Airways obstruction above the carina may produce characteristic flow-volume abnormalities, depending on the type and site of obstruction. *A*, If the obstruction is fixed, both inspiratory and expiratory flows will be decreased whether the obstruction is intrathoracic or extrathoracic (for purposes of illustration, obstruction is shown in both locations). *B*, When a variable obstruction is extrathoracic in location, the airway narrows during inspiration when airway pressure (Paw) is less than atmospheric (Patm) and only inspiratory flow is diminished. *C*, When a variable obstruction is intrathoracic in location, airway pressure is less than pleural pressure (Ppl) during expiration, and only expiratory flow is diminished. (Reproduced with permission from Burrows B, et al: Respiratory Disorders—A Pathophysiologic Approach, 2nd ed. Copyright © 1983 by Year Book Medical Publishers, Inc., Chicago.)

COMPLETE OBSTRUCTION. Air in the lung distal to a complete obstruction is absorbed into the bloodstream, leading to collapse of the affected region, a condition called "obstructive atelectasis." Its features are discussed under Atelectasis in Ch. 61. Any of the disorders mentioned above as causes of partial obstruction may progress to the point of complete occlusion of a bronchus and lead to obstructive atelectasis.

Heimlich HJ: A life-saving maneuver to prevent food-choking. JAMA 234:398, 1975. *The original report on a now standard method to remove aspirated food from the airway.*

Loughlin GM, Taussig LM: Upper airway obstruction. Sem Respir Med 1:131, 1979. *This is an excellent review of upper airways obstructive disorders in infants and children.*

Miller RD: Obstructing lesions of the larynx and trachea: Clinical and pathophysiologic aspects. *In* Fishman AP (ed.): Pulmonary Diseases and Disorders. New York, McGraw-Hill Book Company, 1980, pp 490-502. *An excellent review of the causes, consequences, and treatment of tracheolaryngeal obstruction.*

61. ABNORMALITIES OF LUNG AERATION

Benjamin Burrows

LOCALIZED HYPOAERATION (ATELECTASIS)

Atelectasis refers to diminished aeration of the lung. It is a feature of many bronchopulmonary diseases, and several types of atelectasis have been described. When total airlessness of a portion of the lung occurs, blood traversing the region fails to participate in gas exchange and behaves as if it were being shunted directly from the right to the left side of the heart. Thus total atelectasis leads to an "anatomic-like" or "absolute" shunt. Unlike the "physiologic" or "relative" shunt noted in most bronchopulmonary diseases, the "absolute shunt" produced by atelectasis is not fully corrected by inhalation of 100 per cent oxygen.

TYPES OF ATELECTASIS AND THEIR PATHOGENESIS. When there is complete obstruction of an airway distal to the tracheal bifurcation, air in the lung behind the obstruction is gradually absorbed into the bloodstream, leading to complete collapse over a period of a few hours, a condition called *obstructive atelectasis*. The rate of collapse is limited by the poor solubility of nitrogen and is much more rapid in an oxygen-filled than in an air-filled lung. Thus high inspired oxygen tensions encourage the development of atelectasis behind obstructing mucous plugs.

Atelectasis may also occur when the recoil of a local area of the lung is greatly increased by fibrotic changes. This results in shrinkage of the involved region rather than total airlessness and is called *contraction atelectasis*.

When widespread alveolar instability occurs in the respiratory distress syndromes (in newborns owing to a surfactant abnormality), *patchy atelectasis* may develop throughout the lung.

A portion of the lung may be allowed to decrease in volume when the intrapleural pressure is elevated as a result of a large pneumothorax, pleural effusion, or other space-occupying lesion in the thorax. This has been called "compression atelectasis" but is more properly termed *relaxation atelectasis*, because it occurs as a result of the lungs' own tendency to recoil when distending forces are relaxed. With marked relaxation atelectasis, small airways in the affected region collapse, and any air remaining distally is removed by the bloodstream.

Finally, a condition called *plate-like atelectasis* may be noted on a chest radiograph. Its pathologic significance is uncertain. The horizontal radiopaque streaks which characterize the condition occur most often at the bases of the lung. They are associated with poor aeration of the lung and are commonly seen when the diaphragm is elevated or when the patient has been unable to breathe deeply for a prolonged period.

CLINICAL MANIFESTATIONS. The clinical and physiologic consequences of atelectasis depend on the extent and chronicity of the process. Sudden collapse of a large portion of the lung may cause severe dyspnea and profound hypoxemia. Over a period of hours, blood flow through the nonventilated lung diminishes, and both symptoms and hypoxemia become less severe. The acute picture is apt to be noted when obstructive atelectasis develops rapidly from retained secretions (as occurs occasionally in the postoperative period) or from aspiration of a foreign body. When the obstruction develops slowly, as is usually the case with bronchial neoplasms, there may be few or no symptoms and only minimal hypoxemia.

Physical findings depend on the type of atelectasis. With relaxation atelectasis, the findings are those of the underlying condition (e.g., pneumothorax or pleural effusion). In patchy atelectasis, findings are those of the respiratory distress syndrome, which is discussed in Ch. 70. Plate-like atelectasis is not associated with any distinctive physical findings and is basically a radiographic interpretation. With contraction or obstructive atelectasis, physical findings depend on the amount of lung involved. If the atelectatic area is sufficiently large, the trachea and mediastinum are deviated to the affected side, the diaphragm is raised, and the entire hemithorax may be smaller and show less respiratory motion than the unaffected side.

DIAGNOSIS AND TREATMENT. The presence of atelectasis is confirmed radiographically. If the appearance suggests an obstructive type of disease, bronchoscopy is needed to determine its specific etiology. Occasionally, it is possible to remove the occluding material through the bronchoscope. Obstructive atelectasis in a patient who is not severely ill always should raise the question of a bronchogenic neoplasm.

In nonobstructive types of atelectasis, treatment is directed at the underlying cause of the disorder.

THE RIGHT MIDDLE LOBE SYNDROME. In relaxation atelectasis, the lung is usually restored to normal when it is allowed to reexpand (as with relief of a large pneumothorax). With obstructive atelectasis, however, secondary infection is common, leading to fibrosis, abscess formation, and localized bronchiectasis. Thus after prolonged collapse, the affected lung may fail to reexpand normally when the obstruction is relieved. This is commonly noted when the right middle lobe bronchus has been compressed by large hilar lymph nodes in primary tuberculosis or other granulomatous lung diseases. When the lymph nodes finally decrease in size, the affected lung may fail to reexpand fully. It often shows bronchiectatic changes and becomes the site of recurrent or chronic infection. This has been called the *right middle lobe syndrome.* Less commonly, the same sequence of events occurs in other lung regions. When recurrent pneumonia, chronic suppuration, or hemoptysis occurs, the involved lung may have to be resected.

Acres JC, Kryger MH: Clinical significance of pulmonary function tests: Upper airway obstruction. Chest 80:207, 1981. *A good description of the physiologic diagnosis of upper airway obstruction using the flow-volume loop.*

Albo RJ, Grimes OF: The middle lobe syndrome; a clinical study. Dis Chest 50:509, 1966. *A good description of a common clinical entity.*

Sackner MA: Bronchofiberoscopy. Am Rev Respir Dis 111:62, 1975. *A good state of the art review of various uses of fiberoptic bronchoscopy for both therapeutic and diagnostic indications.*

LOCALIZED HYPERAERATION

A partial bronchial obstruction may lead to overinflation of the affected lung. Increased aeration is also seen in emphysematous lung regions, and pockets of air may be noted within abscesses or cavities. These conditions are discussed elsewhere. The present discussion is limited to bullous lesions, blebs, cysts, and the so-called unilateral hyperlucent lung.

BLEBS AND BULLAE. Small subpleural collections of air, called blebs, are commonly found in otherwise normal lungs. They are of clinical importance only if they rupture and lead to spontaneous pneumothorax. They are not visible radiographically.

Bullae are larger air spaces involving the substance of the lung and associated with some destruction of lung tissue. There is no clear distinction between severe localized emphysema leading to the formation of a large air space and a bulla. Indeed, bullae frequently occur in patients with chronic obstructive emphysema. Bullae may also occur, however, in subjects who do not have diffuse emphysema or any generalized airways obstructive disorder. They are often multiple and occur most commonly in the apices. Pathologically, they are distinguished from cysts by a lack of an endothelial lining. Their radiographic appearance is different as well. Bullae have very thin "hairline margins" and, in contrast to cysts, are usually somewhat irregular in shape, are often trabeculated, and rarely contain fluid.

Small bullae are of little functional significance unless they rupture and lead to a pneumothorax. Rarely do they become infected. They do become clinically important, however, when they enlarge sufficiently to compromise the function of the remaining normal lung and produce dyspnea.

The major problem then is to determine whether bullae observed radiographically are in themselves a cause of dyspnea or whether they are simply one feature of a diffuse pulmonary emphysema. Bullectomy is indicated in the former but rarely in the latter case. Extensive studies may be needed to make this distinction, including angiograms to assess the state of the remaining lung. In general, however, bullae that occupy less than half a hemithorax are rarely associated with dyspnea or significant functional impairment unless there is a concomitant generalized airways obstructive disease. Even with very large bullae, severe expiratory slowing is uncommon unless there is diffuse disease. The ideal candidate for surgery is a patient with bullae that fill most of a hemithorax, who has moderate to severe dyspnea, but who shows relatively mild slowing of forced expiration.

Diminished breath sounds and a tympanitic percussion note may be noted over very large bullae, but usually the diagnosis is made radiographically. One must be careful not to mistake the radiolucency caused by a very large bulla for a pneumothorax.

BRONCHOGENIC CYSTS. Bronchogenic cysts are congenital malformations, distinguished from bullae by their epithelial lining. They may occur either within the lung parenchyma or in the mediastinum. They are usually filled with mucoid material. Mediastinal cysts present as paratracheal, hilar, or paraesophageal masses on the chest radiograph. Parenchymal lesions, when fluid filled, present as nodular lesions and are most commonly found in the lower lobes. Although large cysts may lead to serious respiratory problems in young children, in adults most do not cause significant symptoms. They are usually discovered as an incidental finding on a routine radiograph. Mediastinal cysts must be distinguished from other causes of mediastinal masses. Filled parenchymal cysts fall into the differential diagnosis of the solitary pulmonary nodule. Since definitive diagnosis is usually impossible without resection, many of these lesions come to diagnostic thoracotomy.

Bronchogenic cysts present as abnormalities in lung aeration only when they have some bronchial communication. They may then appear as air spaces, although they are usually at least partially fluid filled. Such lesions are of concern primarily when they become infected, a relatively uncommon event which may require excision of the lesion after treatment with antibiotics. Air-containing cysts are readily distinguished from bullae by their regular outline, lack of trabeculation, and the presence of a fluid level. There may be greater difficulty in distinguishing them from thin-walled cavities secondary to granulomatous infections.

Intralobar *bronchopulmonary sequestration* may be associated with cystic lesions. This disorder results from early abnormal budding of the embryonic tracheobronchial tree. The affected lung is nonfunctional and most frequently located in the posterior aspects of the lung bases. Such abnormal areas present as opacities on the radiograph. Air-containing cystic lesions occur only if there is communication with a bronchus. As with ordinary cysts, the major danger in bronchopulmonary sequestration is secondary infection. In the absence of infection, the lesions usually do not cause symptoms and are discovered on a routine radiograph. In contrast to simple cysts, however, the diagnosis can often be established by an aortogram which reveals an abnormal vascular supply to the lesions. Some sequestrations are supplied by arteries which originate below the diaphragm. The only known treatment is surgical excision.

THE UNILATERAL HYPERLUCENT LUNG. This relatively rare disorder (Swyer-James or Macleod's syndrome) is generally discovered radiographically. Vascular markings in one lung are diminished, leading to increased transradiancy of one hemithorax. Usually there is no accompanying hyperinflation of the affected lung. Pathologically, there is extensive bronchitis and bronchiolitis of the involved lung. Productive cough is generally present, and some patients complain of dyspnea and occasional hemoptysis.

Bronchoscopy shows the absence of obstruction of the main bronchi. Bronchograms reveal dilatation and irregularity of the small airways. Angiograms reveal that the pulmonary artery is patent, distinguishing the condition from atresia or stenosis of a pulmonary artery. Lung scans reveal diminished perfusion and ventilation of the affected side. Lung function studies are quite variable but usually do not show a severe degree of expiratory slowing.

Treatment generally consists only of management of infection, and resection is not indicated.

Boushy SF, Kohen R, Billig DM, Heiman MJ: Bullous emphysema: Clinical, roentgenologic and physiologic study of 49 patients. Dis Chest 54:327, 1968. *A good description of the range of manifestations seen with pulmonary bullae.*

Hamilton CR Jr, Ballinger WF II, Cader G: The unilateral hyperlucent lung syndrome. Bull Johns Hopkins Hosp 123:222, 1968. *A good review of this unusual syndrome.*

Heithoff KB, Sane SM, Williams HJ, Jarvis CJ, Carter J, Kane P, Brennom W: Bronchopulmonary foregut malformations: A unifying etiological concept. Am J Roentgenol 126:46, 1976. *Probably the most comprehensive and systematic recent review of these congenital abnormalities of the lung.*

Pride NB, Barter CE, Hugh-Jones P: The ventilation of bullae and the effect of their removal on thoracic gas volumes and tests of overall pulmonary function. Am Rev Respir Dis 107:83, 1973. *A well done study on the effects of bullectomy.*

62. INTERSTITIAL LUNG DISEASE

Ronald G. Crystal

General Description

The interstitial lung diseases (ILD) are a heterogenous group of diffuse, noninfectious, nonmalignant inflammatory disorders of the lower respiratory tract. The term "interstitial lung disease" refers to the fact that the interstitium of the alveolar walls is thickened, usually by fibrosis. While this is true, the ILD are also characterized by derangements of the epithelial and endothelial cells of the alveolar walls and, in many cases, of the small airways and/or blood vessels of the lung parenchyma.

The list of ILD includes at least 180 disorders, approximately 135 of known etiology and 45 of unknown etiology, each identifiable by a combination of clinical, laboratory, and morphologic features. The natural history of these disorders is generally one of slowly progressive loss of the functional alveolar-capillary units, often eventuating in respiratory insufficiency and death. Because of their insidious nature and the nonspecificity of the accompanying symptoms such as dyspnea on exertion or a nonproductive cough, the ILD often go undiagnosed and untreated until large numbers of alveolar-capillary units become scarred and irrevocably lost.

These disorders are inflammatory diseases; the bulk of the damage to the lung parenchyma is caused by activated inflammatory cells that have accumulated in the alveolar structures. The diagnosis, staging, and treatment of the ILD require defining the character and intensity of the inflammation in the lung and the derangements of the alveolar structures caused by the inflammation.

Anatomy

The lower respiratory tract is composed of alveoli, grapelike units branching off the terminal bronchioles, and the vascular network of pulmonary arterioles, capillaries, and venules that bring blood to and from the lung (Fig. 62–1). The walls of the alveoli are lined by a single layer of epithelial cells resting on a

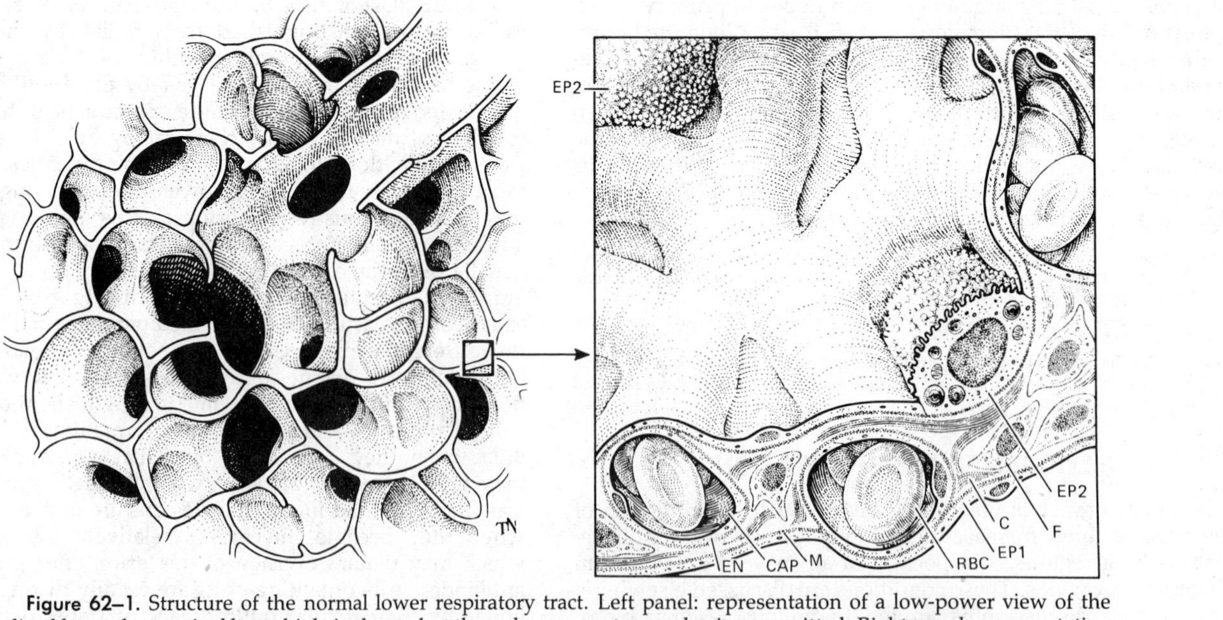

Figure 62–1. Structure of the normal lower respiratory tract. Left panel: representation of a low-power view of the distal lung; the terminal bronchiole is shown but the pulmonary artery and vein are omitted. Right panel: representation of a high-power view of an alveolus; the cut surface demonstrates the type I (EP1) and type II (EP2) epithelial cells, endothelial cells (EN), basement membranes (M), red blood cells (RBC) in the capillaries (CAP), fibroblasts (F), and connective tissue (C). Inflammatory cells are not shown. (Reprinted with permission from Crystal RG, Bitterman PB, Rennard SI, Hance AJ, Keogh BA: Interstitial lung diseases of unknown cause: Disorders characterized by chronic inflammation of the lower respiratory tract. N Engl J Med 310:154, 1984.)

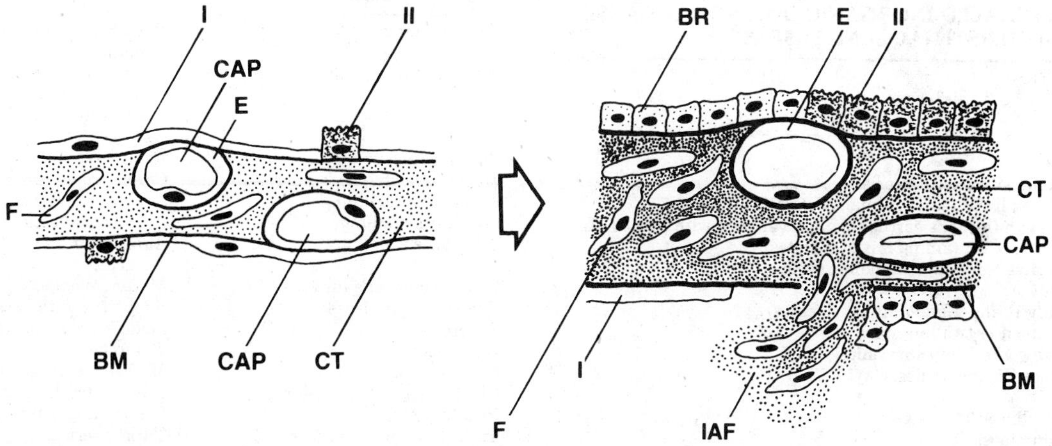

Figure 62–2. Typical form of derangement of the alveolar structures in the interstitial lung disorders. Left: Schematic of a cut surface of the normal alveolar wall. Right: Schematic of a similar view of the alveolar wall in a typical interstitial lung disease. I = type I epithelial cell; II = type II epithelial cell; E = endothelial cell; F = fibroblast; BM = basement membrane; CAP = capillary; CT = connective tissue; BR = bronchiolar cells; IAF = intra-alveolar fibrosis. In interstitial lung disease, the type I cells are injured, leaving denuded basement membrane; in some areas, the interstitial contents protrude into the airspace, causing intra-alveolar fibrosis. Note that some of the injured type I cells have been replaced by the type II cells and bronchiolar cells that have migrated down from airways. Capillaries are injured, the basement membranes are thickened, and the density of connective tissue is increased.

thin, continuous basement membrane. Ninety-five per cent of the alveolar surface is covered by type I epithelial cells, with the remainder by type II epithelial cells, the cell that produces the surface-active material that prevents alveolar collapse. Underneath the epithelial basement membrane is the alveolar interstitium, a region containing fibroblasts and supporting connective tissue matrix composed of collagen, elastic fibers, proteoglycans, and various glycoproteins. The pulmonary capillaries form a branching network of tubes lined by a single layer of endothelial cells resting on their own basement membrane. The capillaries weave through the interstitium such that the capillary basement membrane often abuts the epithelial basement membrane beneath the type I epithelial cells. It is at these sites that air and blood are in closest approximation and where gas exchange takes place.

The normal alveolar wall is thin (5 to 10 μm wide) compared to the space occupied by air (200 to 300 μm). In the ILD, the walls are thickened severalfold and the space for air is correspondingly less. The epithelial surface is often altered: flat type I epithelial cells are lost and the surface is repopulated with cuboidal cells derived from proliferating type II cells and bronchiolar cells migrating down from the terminal airways (Fig. 62–2). Alveolar capillary endothelial cells are usually injured and lost. The interstitium is thickened with edema and proliferation of interstitial fibroblasts and accumulation of connective tissue products secreted by the fibroblasts, particularly collagen. The interstitium is scarred and fibrotic—hence the term "fibrotic lung disease" is often used synonymously with the term "interstitial lung disease." In the more aggressive ILD, there are breaks in the epithelial basement membrane through which the interstitial contents protrude; this often expands into intra-alveolar fibrotic masses called "intra-alveolar buds." As these diseases progress, the alveolar-capillary units become less distinguishable, and the lung parenchyma takes on the appearance of "end-stage lung" characterized by masses of fibrotic tissue interspaced with cystic areas representing the remnants of alveoli and dilated terminal bronchioles.

Epidemiology

Approximately two thirds of all cases of ILD are of unknown etiology (Table 62–1). It is estimated that the ILD of unknown etiology are responsible for more than 10,000 hospital admissions in the United States per year and have a prevalence of approximately 5 to 10 cases per 100,000 of the population. The most common ILD of unknown etiology are idiopathic pulmonary fibrosis (IPF), chronic ILD associated with the collagen-vascular disorders, and sarcoidosis. Much less common are histiocytosis-X, Goodpasture's syndrome, chronic eosinophilic pneumonia, idiopathic pulmonary hemosiderosis, and the ILD associated with the pulmonary vasculitides. The other ILD of unknown etiology are very rare, with far fewer than 1000 cases of each reported in the world literature.

For approximately one third of patients with ILD a specific etiologic agent can be identified. These diseases are most commonly due to the inhalation of inorganic dusts, particularly

TABLE 62–1. INTERSTITIAL LUNG DISEASES (ILD) OF UNKNOWN ETIOLOGY*

• Idiopathic Pulmonary Fibrosis (IPF)	ILD Associated with Pulmonary Airway Disease
• Sarcoidosis	Bronchocentric granulomatosis
• ILD Associated with the Collagen-Vascular Disorders	Bronchopulmonary aspergillosis
Rheumatoid arthritis	Lymphangioleiomyomatosis
Progressive systemic sclerosis	Alveolar Proteinosis
Systemic lupus erythematosus	ILD Associated with Liver Disease
Polymyositis/dermatomyositis	Chronic active hepatitis
Sjögren's syndrome	Primary biliary cirrhosis
Mixed connective tissue disease	ILD Associated with Bowel Disease
Ankylosing spondylitis	Whipple's disease
Histiocytosis-X	Ulcerative colitis
Goodpasture's Syndrome	Crohn's disease
Idiopathic Pulmonary Hemosiderosis	Weber-Christian Disease
Chronic Eosinophilic Pneumonia	Amyloidosis
Lymphocytic Infiltrative Disorders	Hypereosinophilic Syndrome
Immunoblastic lymphadenopathy	Pulmonary Veno-occlusive Disease
Lymphocytic interstitial pneumonitis	ILD Caused by Failure of Other Organs
ILD Associated with Pulmonary Vasculitides	Chronic left ventricular failure
Wegener's granulomatosis	Chronic left-to-right intracardiac shunt
Lymphomatoid granulomatosis	Chronic renal disease with uremia
Churg-Strauss syndrome	Graft-versus-Host Disease
Systemic necrotizing vasculitides ("overlap" vasculitides)	Recovery Phase of Adult Respiratory Distress Syndrome
Hypersensitivity vasculitis	
Inherited Disorders	
Familial pulmonary fibrosis	
Neurofibromatosis	
Tuberous sclerosis	
Hermansky-Pudlak syndrome	
Niemann-Pick disease	
Gaucher's disease	

*Disorders indicated with "•" are the most common ILD of unknown etiology.

TABLE 62–2. INHALED INORGANIC DUSTS THAT CAUSE INTERSTITIAL LUNG DISEASE*†

Silica (variants of SiO_2)
- ● Crystalline silica ("silicosis")
- Amorphous

Silicates
- ● Asbestos ("asbestosis")
- Talc (hydrated Mg silicates; "talcosis")
- Kaolin (china clay, hydrated aluminum silicate)
- Diatomaceous earth (Fuller's earth, aluminum silicate with Fe and Mg)
- Nepheline (hard rock containing mixed silicates)
- Aluminum silicates (sericite, sillimanite, zeolite)
- Portland cement
- Mica (principally K and Mg aluminum silicates)

Carbon (with or without crystalline silica)
- ● Coal dust ("coal worker's pneumoconiosis")
- Graphite ("carbon pneumoconiosis")

Metals
- Beryllium ("berylliosis")
- Aluminum ("aluminosis")
  - Powdered aluminum ("aluminum lung")
  - Bauxite (aluminum oxide; "Shaver's disease")
- Barium (powder of baryte or $BaSO_4$; "baritosis")
- Iron ("siderosis")
- Tin ("stannosis")
- Antimony (oxides and alloys)
- Mixed dusts
  - Hematite (mixed dusts of iron oxide, silica and silicates; "siderosilicosis")
  - Mixed dusts of silver and iron oxide; "arygrosiderosis")
- Hard metals
  - Titanium oxide
  - Tungsten, titanium, hafnium, niobium, cobalt, and vanadium carbides
  - Cadmium

Rare earths (cerium, scandium, yttrium, lanthanum)

$CuSO_4$ neutralized with hydrated lime (Bordeaux mixture; "vineyard sprayer's lung")

*The most common inorganic dust–induced interstitial lung diseases are indicated with "●".

†Disorders given a specific name are indicated in quotes in parentheses; others are referred as "(name of the dust) pneumoconiosis."

crystalline silica and silicates such as asbestosis (Table 62–2), the hypersensitivity pneumonitides (diseases caused by the repeated inhalation of organic dust; Table 62–3), and the drug-induced ILD (Table 62–4). Much less frequent are the ILD resulting from paraquat, radiation, the sequelae of known infectious agents, and the inhalation of gases, aerosols, chemical dusts, fumes, and vapors (Table 62–5).

Differential Diagnosis

The initial problem in assessing ILD is to differentiate it from the infectious and malignant disorders that may also present with symptoms of respiratory deficiency and a diffuse pattern on the chest radiograph. This requires (1) a detailed workup for possible lung infections, particularly mycobacterial and fungal agents and, in immune-compromised patients, opportunistic infections; and (2) evaluation of specimens from the lower respiratory tract for the presence of malignant cells.

The diagnosis of a specific ILD is made by a combination of historical, physical exam, blood, urine, roentgenographic, physiologic, scintigraphic, and bronchoscopic criteria. In addition, unless an agent of known etiology is apparent (e.g., long-term asbestos exposure), it is mandatory to evaluate the disease by morphologic means, usually by open lung biopsy. The only exception to this rule is where the ILD is in clear association with a systemic disorder (e.g., a collagen-vascular disease, Goodpasture's syndrome) in which the diagnosis can be made by evaluation of organs other than the lung.

Pathogenesis

The ILD are inflammatory disorders in which most of the derangements of the alveolar walls, including the fibrosis, are mediated by the accumulated inflammatory and immune effector cells. The inflammation, usually referred to as the "alveolitis" of the disease, not only involves the alveoli, but often involves the walls of small airways and sometimes the pulmonary blood vessels. The critical importance of the alveolitis is simply stated: although dysfunction of the alveolar-capillary units causes the symptoms and impairment of the patient, it is the alveolitis that causes the injury and fibrosis that deranges these units, resulting in their dysfunction and eventual loss (Fig. 62–3).

TABLE 62–3. INHALED ORGANIC DUSTS THAT CAUSE INTERSTITIAL LUNG DISEASE

Disorder	Causative Agent*
Farmer's lung	*M. faeni, T. vulgaris, A. fumigatus, T. candidus*
Humidifier lung, air conditioner lung	*T. vulgaris, T. candidus,* thermotolerant bacteria, protozoa, penicillium species, *Naegleria gruberi*
Pigeon breeder's disease	Avian proteins
Maple bark stripper's lung	*Cryptostroma corticale*
Cheese worker's lung	*A. clavatus, Penicillium caseii*
Malt worker's lung	*A. clavatus, A. fumigatus*
Sequoiosis	*Aureobasidium pullulans,* Graphium species
Paprika splitter's lung	*Mucor stolonifer*
Wheat weevil disease	*Sitophilus granarius*
Suberosis	*Penicillium frequentans*
Bagassosis	*T. sacchari*
Mushroom worker's lung	*M. faeni, T. vulgaris*
Chicken handler's disease	Chicken feathers and serum
Pituitary snuff lung	Porcine and bovine proteins
Turkey handler's disease	Turkey serum
Duck fever	Duck feathers
Wood-pulp worker's disease	Alternaria species
Sauna-taker's disease	Aureobasidium species
Detergent worker's lung	*Bacillus subtilis*
Lycoperdonosis	*Lycoperdon bovista*
Rodent handler's disease	Serum and urine constituents
Dry rot disease	*Merulius lacrymans*
Wood-dust worker's lung	Unknown
Coffee worker's lung	Unknown
Furrier's lung	Unknown
New Guinea lung	*Saccharomonospora irridis*
Coptic disease (mummy unwrapper's disease)	Antigens associated with mummy wrappings
"Summer type" disease	*Cryptococcus neoformans*
	†Cephalosporium species
	†*Streptomyces albus*
	†*Bacillus subtilis*

*M. = Micropolyspora; T. = Thermoactinomyces; A. = Aspergillus.

†Hypersensitivity pneumonitis has been described in association with these agents, but no common name has been given to the disorder.

TABLE 62–4. DRUGS THAT CAUSE INTERSTITIAL LUNG DISEASE

Antineoplastic Agents	Cardiovascular Drugs	Anti-inflammatory Agents
Azathioprine	Hydralazine	Gold salts
Bleomycin	Procainamide	Phenylbutazone
Cyclophosphamide	Beta blockers (propranolol, practolol, pindolol, acebutolol)	Beclomethasone
Methotrexate	Tocainide	Naproxen
Nitrosoureas	Amiodarone	**Oral Hypoglycemic Agents**
Carmustine (BCNU)	Reserpine	Chlorpropamide
Semustine (methyl-CCNU)	**Central Nervous System Drugs**	Tolbutamide
Chlorozotocin (DCNU)	Phenytoin	Tolazamide
Melphalan	Carbamazepine	**Miscellaneous**
Chlorambucil	Chlorpromazine	Penicillamine
6-Mercaptopurine	Imipramine	Allopurinol
6-Thioguanine	Amitriptyline	Cromolyn sodium
Mitomycin C	**Ganglionic Blocking Agents**	Hydrochlorothiazide
Procarbazine	Mecamylamine	Mineral oil
Uracil mustard	Hexamethonium	Intravenous drugs containing particulate material
Zinostatin	Pentolinium	Silicon used for tissue augmentation
Antibiotics		
Nitrofurantoin		
Penicillins		
Sulfonamides		
Erythromycin		
Tetracycline		
Isoniazid		
para-Aminosalicylic acid		
Niridazole		

TABLE 62–5. OTHER AGENTS KNOWN TO CAUSE INTERSTITIAL LUNG DISEASE

Paraquat
Radiation
Sequela of Known Infectious Agents
Bacteria
Mycobacteria
Fungi
Viruses
Mycoplasma
Legionella pneumophila
Parasites
Inhaled Agents Other Than Inorganic or Organic Dusts
Gases
Oxygen
Oxides of nitrogen
Chlorine gas
Sulfur dioxide
Aerosols
Aspiration pneumonia
Fats
Oils
Pyrethrum (a natural insecticide)
Toluene diisocyanate
Pauli's reagent (sodium diazobenzene sulfate)
Chemical dusts
Synthetic fibers (Orlon, polyesters, nylon, acrylic)
Bakelite
Vinyl chloride, polyvinyl chloride powder
Fumes
Oxides of Zn, Cu, Mn, Cd, Fe, Mg, Ni, Se, Sn, Sb, V, and brass
Diphenylmethane diisocyanate
Trimellitic anhydride
Vapors
Hydrocarbons
Mercury
Thermosetting resins

INITIATION OF THE ALVEOLITIS. Although it is not clear what initiates the inflammation in the ILD of unknown etiology, many of the processes that maintain the alveolitis are understood. For example, in idiopathic pulmonary fibrosis, alveolar macrophages, activated by immune complexes, release neutrophil-specific chemotactic factors that attract blood neutrophils to the lung. In contrast, in sarcoidosis, activated lung T lymphocytes release a monocyte-specific chemotactic factor that modulates the accumulation of blood monocytes in the alveolar structures.

For the disorders of known etiology, the causative agent most commonly activates the inflammatory cells that are normally present, which, in turn, propagate the alveolitis. For example, asbestos fibers can induce the normal alveolar macrophages to recruit neutrophils. Alternatively, the causative agent may directly injure the alveolar walls to produce alveolitis. For example, bleomycin, an antineoplastic drug, can injure lung parenchyma cells and by unknown mechanisms induce the formation of an alveolitis.

CHARACTER OF THE ALVEOLITIS. The inflammatory component of the ILD is defined by the number, type, and state of activation of the effector cells comprising the alveolitis. The differences in the form and extent of injury and fibrosis of these disorders are defined by the sum of these characteristics.

In the normal lung there are approximately 80 inflammatory cells per alveolus. Most (greater than 90 per cent) are alveolar macrophages, phagocytic cells derived from blood monocytes. The remainder are lymphocytes, mostly T cells, but with a small number of B cells. Polymorphonuclear leukocytes are rare in the normal lung, although small numbers do accumulate with a long history of cigarette smoking. As a general rule, alveolar macrophages and T and B lymphocytes are not activated in the normal lung. Immunoglobulins are present in the normal lower respiratory tract (IgG $>$ IgA $>>$ IgM), as are most complement components. Macromolecules that defend against inflammatory injury, including antiproteases and antioxidants, are also present.

Active, untreated ILD are generally characterized by a marked increase in the number of inflammatory cells in the alveolar walls and on the alveolar epithelial surface. Commonly, this increase in numbers of effector cells is also characterized by a shift in their relative proportions. Different patterns of alveolitis are generally referred to by the cell types that are most abundant. For example, when the inflammation is dominated by neutrophils and macrophages it is referred to as a neutrophil-macrophage alveolitis. The alveolitis patterns most frequently observed in ILD are a macrophage-dominant alveolitis, a lymphocyte-macrophage alveolitis, and a neutrophil-macrophage alveolitis. Eosinophils play a role in the alveolitis of many ILD but rarely dominate it. Subcategories of the common alveolitis patterns have also been described. For example, the granulomatous lung disorders, sarcoidosis and berylliosis, are characterized by a T helper–cell macrophage alveolitis, while chronic hypersensitivity pneumonitis is usually characterized by a T suppressor/cytotoxic–cell macrophage alveolitis, sometimes including neutrophils.

In addition to the numbers and types of inflammatory cells present, the consequences of the alveolitis critically depend on

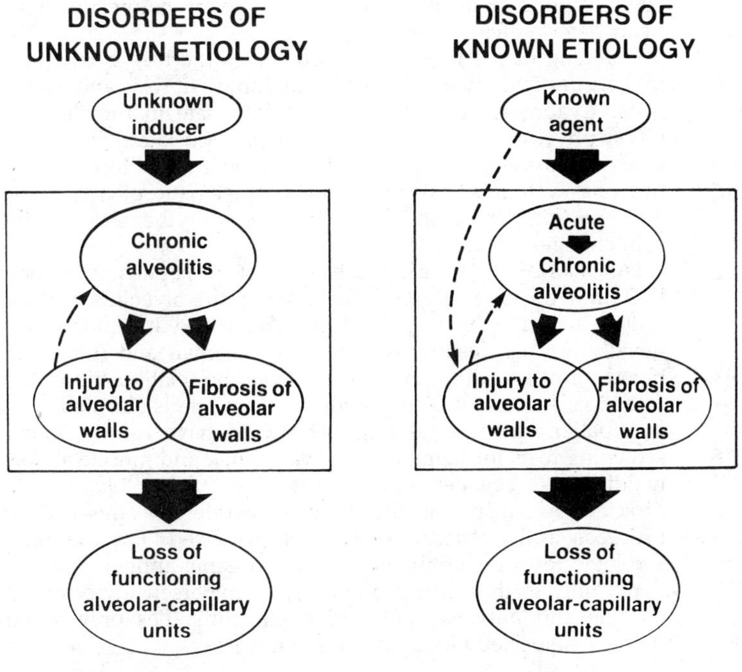

Figure 62–3. Pathogenesis of the interstitial lung diseases of unknown and known etiology. In both groups, the inflammation (alveolitis) is responsible for the bulk of the injury and fibrosis of the alveolar walls. In the disorders of unknown etiology the alveolitis is chronic and usually precedes the injury. In some disorders, the injured wall components may accelerate the alveolitis by recruiting additional inflammatory cells. In the disorders of known etiology, the causative agent initiates an acute alveolitis that may become chronic. Alternatively, the causative agent may directly damage the alveolar structures, which, in turn, initiates and/or accelerates the alveolitis.

the state of activation of these cells. The simple presence of the inflammatory cells in the alveolar structures is not damaging other than through the distortion they induce within the alveolar walls. When activated, however, the inflammatory cells injure the alveolar walls, particularly the sensitive type I epithelial cells and capillary endothelial cells. If the alveolitis is self limiting, or if it is suppressed by therapy before the injury becomes too severe, the architecture of the lower respiratory tract can be re-established and normal lung function restored. If, however, the injury is extensive, with fibroblast proliferation and collagen deposition, the normal architecture of the affected alveolar-capillary units can never be fully re-established. Therapeutic success in treating ILD means suppression of the alveolitis and thus prevention of further loss of alveolar-capillary units. The activation of the inflammatory cells is most important to suppress. For example, in pulmonary sarcoidosis, if T helper cells are prevented from releasing mediators that attract and activate mononuclear phagocytes, granuloma formation will be halted.

INJURY, REPAIR, AND FIBROSIS. The type of injury, the extent of repair, and the formation of fibrosis are dictated by the characteristics of the alveolitis. The neutrophil is the most damaging of all inflammatory cells by virtue of its highly reactive oxygen metabolites that are toxic to the parenchymal cells and its connective tissue–specific proteases that can damage the interstitial collagens and basement membranes. Injury to the epithelial basement membrane has profound consequences because the epithelial cells no longer have a surface upon which to migrate, making it impossible to reconstruct a normal alveolar surface. The eosinophil can also injure lung parenchymal cells and connective tissue, but on a per cell basis it is far less potent than the neutrophil. The type of injury mediated by lymphocytes is less well understood, but T helper lymphocytes likely direct the process of granuloma formation.

Activated human alveolar macrophages release toxic oxidants, are cytotoxic to normal lung parenchymal cells, and secrete connective tissue–specific proteases, albeit to a lesser extent than neutrophils. The macrophage in the ILD has the ability to mediate fibrosis of the alveolar walls. While this process may serve a useful purpose (e.g., to maintain the backbone structure of the injured alveolar wall), the fibrosis causes physiologic problems because it alters the mechanical properties of the lung parenchyma. The fundamental problem in the development of the fibrosis is the accumulation of fibroblasts in the alveolar walls. Since fibroblasts are major producers of collagen, the consequence of an increase in fibroblast numbers is an accumulation of collagen in the alveolar interstitium. As a result, the alveolar wall is thickened and scarred and has decreased compliance. The macrophage mediates the accumulation of fibroblasts by releasing two mediators, fibronectin and alveolar macrophage–derived growth factor. Fibronectin, a 440,000 dalton glycoprotein, attracts fibroblasts, attaches them to the extracellular matrix, and stimulates them to enter the cell cycle. The alveolar macrophage–derived growth factor, an 18,000 dalton protein, induces the fibronectin-primed fibroblasts to continue through the cell cycle and proliferate.

Clinical Features

HISTORY. Occasional patients are detected as having ILD because a routine chest radiograph is noted to be abnormal, but most come to medical attention because of symptoms related to the chest. All ILD are characterized by abnormalities in the transfer of oxygen from air to blood secondary to slowly progressive derangement and fibrosis of the lower respiratory tract. The initial symptoms are those of insufficient oxygen transfer such as *fatigue* and *breathlessness with exertion*. These symptoms are often initially denied by the patient or are attributed to being "out of shape" or "overweight" or to a prior chest infection, usually a viral syndrome. As the disease progresses, the dyspnea becomes more apparent and eventually is felt at rest. In contrast to cardiac-induced dyspnea, paroxysmal nocturnal dyspnea and orthopnea are rare, as are platypnea and trepopnea. Nonproductive cough, pleuritic pain, and hemoptysis are less common presenting complaints. Early in the disease, chest pain is rare, although later, when pulmonary hypertension develops, substernal discomfort may be noted.

The history also plays an important role in the diagnosis of the type of interstitial disease. Since a large number of agents cause ILD, a careful exposure history is essential in order to determine not only the agents to which the patient has been exposed, but also the circumstances, intensity, and duration of exposure. Exposure to agents that cause ILD may be found in nonclassic situations. For example, silicosis has been described in workers involved in the manufacture of pencils, furniture, and tombstones; talcosis in the manufacture of rubber condoms; and hypersensitivity pneumonitis in office buildings where the offending organic antigen was located in the air conditioning system.

The lack of a history of exposure to a known agent that causes interstitial disease is very important to diagnosing the ILD of unknown etiology. For example, pulmonary sarcoidosis is very difficult to separate from berylliosis unless there is a clear negative history of beryllium exposure. Likewise, idiopathic pulmonary fibrosis is difficult to diagnose if an exposure history is unavailable or if there is a clear history of exposure to one or more agents that cause ILD. Many ILD of unknown etiology are associated with other diseases, such as the collagen-vascular disorders, primary biliary cirrhosis, and Wegener's granulomatosis, which may be suspected from the history.

PHYSICAL EXAMINATION. Most patients with ILD have fine, crackling inspiratory and expiratory rales, heard best at the posterior lung bases. These rales have a characteristic sound, described as "Velcro-like" (i.e., the sound of unwrapping a blood pressure cuff) or like the sound of rubbing hair together. Coarse rales, wheezing, and rhonchi are occasionally heard. As the disease progresses, these patients may be tachypneic at rest but unlike emphysema victims, they do not use the accessory muscles of respiration and do not assume the posture of placing their hands on their thighs to "fix" the upper body to assist in respiration.

Early in the disease, examination of the heart is normal. Later, an accentuated P_2 reflects mild pulmonary hypertension. Eventually, obvious evidence of pulmonary hypertension is noted, including a right ventricular heave. Patients with ILD rarely develop frank right-sided failure with liver enlargement and peripheral edema, presumably because they die from the complications of insufficient oxygen delivery before the right heart deteriorates.

Clubbing of the fingers and sometimes the toes is common in ILD, particularly in idiopathic pulmonary fibrosis and asbestosis. Cyanosis occurs, but usually very late in the disease. Other physical findings in ILD are those associated with problems with oxygen transport (e.g., left ventricular failure, central nervous system signs) and those characteristic of associated diseases (e.g., the rash of systemic lupus erythematosus, the skin changes of scleroderma).

LABORATORY STUDIES. No blood test is diagnostic for one ILD, and the intensity and character of the alveolitis are not reflected in the blood. The hemoglobin and hematocrit are usually normal despite associated hypoxemia, and the white blood count and differential usually bear no relationship to the alveolitis. In most ILD, the sedimentation rate is elevated.

A patient with suspected ILD should have routine blood screening tests for hematologic, liver, renal, and muscle abnormalities and collagen-vascular disorders. Other blood tests directed toward specific diseases may be ordered as the workup proceeds and a specific disease is suspected. For example, serologic tests for antibodies against organic antigens are ordered only in the context of suspected hypersensitivity pneumonitis and antibasement membrane antibodies only when there is suspected Goodpasture's syndrome.

Rheumatoid factor and antinuclear antibodies are occasionally present in low titer and do not necessarily indicate the presence of an underlying collagen-vascular disorder. Plasma immunoglobulins may be elevated, but this finding is usually nonspecific. Except in those circumstances in which the disease is systemic (e.g., sarcoidosis, a collagen-vascular disorder), the other screening blood studies are generally normal.

The EKG is usually normal in ILD except for evidence of pulmonary hypertension. As the loss of alveolar-capillary units progresses, the EKG demonstrates a pattern of right atrial and ventricular strain. The hypoxemia of ILD may exacerbate coexisting coronary heart disease, evoking arrhythmias and evidence of coronary insufficiency, particularly with exercise.

RADIOGRAPHIC STUDIES. The posterior-anterior and lateral chest film play a major role in establishing the diagnosis of ILD, although 5 to 10 per cent of patients with biopsy-proven disease have a normal chest film. A ground-glass pattern may be seen early in the disease. More typically, the chest radiograph demonstrates a diffuse, finely nodular, reticular, or reticulonodular pattern usually more prominent at the bases. As the disease evolves, the pattern becomes coarser, with cystic areas appearing, and finally, a honeycomb pattern. Initially the pulmonary arteries appear normal, but in the later stages of ILD evidence of pulmonary hypertension may be present.

A definitive diagnosis of a specific ILD can never be made by the chest radiograph alone. However, certain radiographic patterns are characteristic of specific diseases or groups of diseases and thus are very helpful in establishing a diagnosis. For example, some ILD are also characterized by hilar and/or paratracheal lymph node enlargement, while others manifest pleural disease.

Except for rare circumstances, radiographic studies other than the routine chest film have little use in the evaluation of ILD. Oblique films, tomography, bronchography, or angiography are occasionally used to evaluate localized lesions on a background of ILD but usually are difficult to interpret. At present, computerized axial tomographic (CT) scans of the chest are not used in the evaluation of these patients except in the circumstance where questionable pleural lesions are being evaluated.

PULMONARY FUNCTION TESTS. The classic physiologic alterations in ILD include reduced lung volumes (vital capacity, total lung capacity), reduced diffusing capacity, and normal airway function (as evidenced by a normal ratio of forced expiratory volume in 1 second to forced vital capacity). In some ILD, more sensitive tests such as flow-volume curves and maximum flow–static recoil curves can detect mild limitation of airflow. Measurement of static lung compliance demonstrates decreased lung volumes for a given transpulmonary pressure, and an increased maximal transpulmonary pressure, i.e., very high negative pressures (relative to the atmosphere), must be generated to open the fibrotic alveoli.

Arterial blood gases typically show mild hypoxemia; CO_2 retention is rare even late in the course of the disease. Patients with ILD tend to hyperventilate and have a reduced P_{CO_2} and compensated respiratory alkalosis, mostly as a result of an increase in respiratory rate. The drive to hyperventilate is not due to hypoxemia or abnormalities in acid-base status but rather to the subjective sense of dyspnea, probably from an increased stimulation of the respiratory center from neural signals arising in the deranged lung parenchyma. With exercise, the arterial P_{O_2} drops, while P_{CO_2} remains constant. The loss of alveolar-capillary bed in ILD and hence the limitation of cardiac output seriously impair oxygen delivery and thereby markedly limit the exercise tolerance of these patients. This leads to their propensity to suffer hypoxic damage to vital organs. The arterial pH is usually normal in ILD, but it can fall with exercise as a consequence of oxygen deprivation of muscles, which then resort to anaerobic metabolism.

At rest, the hypoxemia of ILD results from abnormal matching of pulmonary ventilation and perfusion. With exercise, however, an apparent "diffusion block" also contributes. It was originally thought that this resulted from a limited O_2 diffusion through the thickened alveolar walls, but it is now recognized to be due to red blood cells passing through the functioning pulmonary capillaries too rapidly to permit full saturation of hemoglobin. In rare instances, some of the hypoxemia of ILD results from shunts, either in the lung parenchyma or through a patent foramen ovale.

The loss of pulmonary capillary bed in ILD is associated with pulmonary hypertension, first with exercise only and later at rest. The pulmonary hypertension likely results from mechanical reasons (e.g., the loss of pulmonary capillary bed) and not from hypoxia-induced vasoconstriction or from local mediators. Right ventricular end-diastolic pressure rises late in the disease, but this rarely leads to frank right-sided failure.

SCINTIGRAPHIC STUDIES. Conventional ventilation and perfusion scans usually demonstrate diffuse abnormalities. The perfusion scans show multiple subsegmental areas of impaired perfusion. The normal, upright individual has limited blood flow to the upper lobes at rest. The perfusion scan in ILD, however, shows a redistribution of perfusion to the upper lobes resulting from the loss of pulmonary capillary bed and developing pulmonary hypertension. The ventilation scan shows multiple subsegmental areas of reduced ventilation. Comparison of the perfusion and ventilation scans demonstrates numerous areas of ventilation and perfusion mismatch. The presence of numerous perfusion defects limits the usefulness of these techniques in evaluation of patients with ILD with suspected pulmonary emboli. In such circumstances, pulmonary angiography is mandatory.

Gallium-67 scans are used to evaluate the alveolitis of ILD. Whereas the normal lung parenchyma takes up little gallium-67, ILD with an active alveolitis demonstrate positive gallium-67 lung scans with either a diffuse or patchy pattern. A high density of activated alveolar macrophages is thought to play a major role in the lung uptake of gallium-67 in these patients.

BRONCHOSCOPIC STUDIES. Most patients with suspected ILD are evaluated by fiberoptic bronchoscopy to rule out neoplastic or infectious disease. In selected patients (see below), transbronchial biopsy can be carried out at the same time.

The technique of bronchoalveolar lavage is used to sample the inflammatory cells comprising the alveolitis. To accomplish this, the bronchoscope is wedged into a distal bronchus and aliquots of sterile saline are used to recover the inflammatory cells and epithelial lining fluid of the lower respiratory tract. In normal individuals, 90 per cent or more of the recovered cells demonstrate alveolar macrophages, with the remainder being lymphocytes (almost all T lymphocytes). Polymorphonuclear leukocytes are normally very rare. In patients with ILD, the pattern of alveolitis is reflected by the cells recovered by lavage. For example, in pulmonary sarcoidosis, the proportions of T cells may be 20 to 60 per cent, while in idiopathic pulmonary fibrosis, the proportion of neutrophils is greater than 10 per cent. The diagnostic usefulness of bronchoalveolar lavage has not been established, but it can help to orient the clinician to the category of alveolitis that is present. Furthermore, because alveolar macrophages are phagocytic and ingest foreign materials present in the lung parenchyma, bronchoalveolar lavage can also be used to help diagnose specific agents that cause ILD, including inorganic dust diseases.

BIOPSY. The diagnosis of many ILD depends upon pathologic studies of lung parenchyma. The method of choice is the open lung biopsy, usually performed in the right middle lobe or lingula in an area of "average" disease as judged by the chest film. Transbronchial biopsy through the fiberoptic bronchoscope is useful for diagnosing sarcoidosis, but for most other ILD the samples are too small for a definitive diagnosis to be made.

Staging and Therapy

A patient with ILD should be evaluated to assess the contribution of the disease to his functional impairment. The activity of the disease process should be independently assessed. Once both are known, rational decisions can be made concerning prognosis and therapy.

ASSESSMENT OF IMPAIRMENT. The consequences of ILD are assessed by history, chest radiograph, and lung function testing. A careful history of the patient's sensation of breathlessness, combined with an estimate of exercise tolerance, allows a rough estimate of lung injury. The chest radiograph is somewhat more objective, and comparison with prior films helps to determine if the disease has become more extensive. Pulmonary function tests are the most accurate means to assess impairment. Of the tests routinely available, vital capacity, total lung capacity, diffusing capacity, and arterial Po_2 most accurately gauge the loss of functioning alveolar-capillary units. Measurements of the changes in Po_2 with exercise and of static compliance are more sensitive indicators of disease, but these tests are more difficult to perform and are not widely available.

ASSESSMENT OF ACTIVITY. Alveolitis is confined to the lower respiratory tract, so that its character or extent is difficult to measure directly. Circulating immune complexes and angiotensin-converting enzyme have been suggested as measures of the alveolitis in idiopathic pulmonary fibrosis and sarcoidosis, respectively, but neither test is very sensitive or specific. Likewise, attempts to correlate the chest radiograph or lung function tests with morphologic evidence of the alveolitis have been disappointing, and thus neither can be used to evaluate accurately the alveolitis.

Open lung biopsy, bronchoalveolar lavage, and *gallium-67 scanning* are the best present methods to stage alveolitis. Open biopsy is the most accurate method but is very rarely performed more than once in the course of the disease. Bronchoalveolar lavage and gallium-67 scanning are both sensitive to and specific for the alveolitis, but neither has been fully validated for routine clinical use. At this time, bronchoalveolar lavage is most useful for evaluating the intensity of the neutrophil, eosinophil, and lymphocyte components of the alveolitis and gallium-67 scanning for the macrophage component.

THERAPY. The principal aim of therapy in ILD is to suppress the alveolitis. For the ILD of unknown etiology, the conventional approach is to treat with oral corticosteroids, usually prednisone. Relatively high doses are used (1 mg per kilogram daily) for one to two months followed by tapering doses over two to three months to maintenance levels (0.25 mg per kilogram daily), which are continued for varying periods of time. The corticosteroids are generally given once daily; it is not known if alternate-day regimens are equally effective. There has never been a large controlled trial of corticosteroids in any ILD, but some patients with ILD respond to corticosteroids in a fashion that cannot be explained by spontaneous remission. "Successful" therapy does not necessarily mean improvement in pulmonary function, chest radiograph, or subjective symptoms, since severely damaged alveoli are lost forever. In this context, successful suppression of the alveolitis usually means no further loss of alveoli. If improvement does occur, it likely results from suppression of the contribution of the inflammation itself to the derangements of the alveolar structures.

If the disease stabilizes, the corticosteroids are usually tapered. If the deterioration restarts after a period of quiescence, corticosteroids are often restarted, but their efficacy under these circumstances is limited. A variety of cytotoxic and other anti-inflammatory drugs has also been used in the treatment of the ILD of unknown etiology, but there has been no controlled series to demonstrate their efficacy.

For the ILD of known etiology, the initial treatment is to remove exposure to the causative agent. If the inflammation persists months after removal from the known agent, the patients are usually treated in a similar fashion to ILD of unknown etiology. The exception to this rule is in most of the pneumoconioses, for which no therapy is used.

In all ILD, attention should be given to prompt treatment of lung infections. Bronchodilators are sometimes used in mid to late course in these diseases to help mobilize secretions. Oxygen therapy, particularly with exercise, is often used as the patient reaches the late stage of ILD, but its efficacy in increasing the life span of these patients is unproven.

INTERSTITIAL LUNG DISEASES OF UNKNOWN ETIOLOGY

The ILD of unknown etiology represent two thirds of all cases of ILD. Although of unknown etiology, each represents a specific entity with distinct features (Table 62–1). The best understood ILD of unknown etiology are idiopathic pulmonary fibrosis and sarcoidosis.

Idiopathic Pulmonary Fibrosis (IPF)

CLINICAL MANIFESTATIONS. IPF is the "classic" fibrotic lung disease characterized by a neutrophil-alveolar macrophage alveolitis and progressive scarring of alveolar-capillary units. In the past IPF was sometimes called the Hamman-Rich syndrome, but this designation is not generally used now. Typically, IPF presents in middle age, but all age groups can be affected. The sex distribution is equal. Patients present with dyspnea on exertion and/or a dry cough, often following a viral illness. Fever is rare. Physical examination demonstrates dry, bibasilar rales, often associated with clubbing of the fingers and sometimes of the toes. The chest radiograph typically shows a diffuse reticulonodular infiltrate most prominent at the bases without hilar or pleural abnormalities. Some patients have various "autoimmune" abnormalities that likely represent nonspecific epiphenomena. Circulating immune complexes are common. Pulmonary function tests are typical for ILD, with reduced volumes and diffusing capacity. Routine tests of airflow are normal, but sensitive tests reveal mild airflow limitation, an observation that correlates with morphologic evidence of narrowing of small airways. Patients with IPF have mild resting hypoxemia that drops significantly with physical activity. Typically, a resting Po_2 of 80 torr will fall to 50 torr with exercise equivalent to walking up one flight of stairs. Ventilation and perfusion studies reveal diffuse patchy abnormalities with mismatching of air and blood. The gallium-67 scan usually shows a diffuse uptake of isotope throughout the lung parenchyma, and bronchoalveolar lavage reveals an alveolitis pattern dominated by neutrophils and macrophages, with fewer numbers of lymphocytes and eosinophils. The epithelial lining fluid

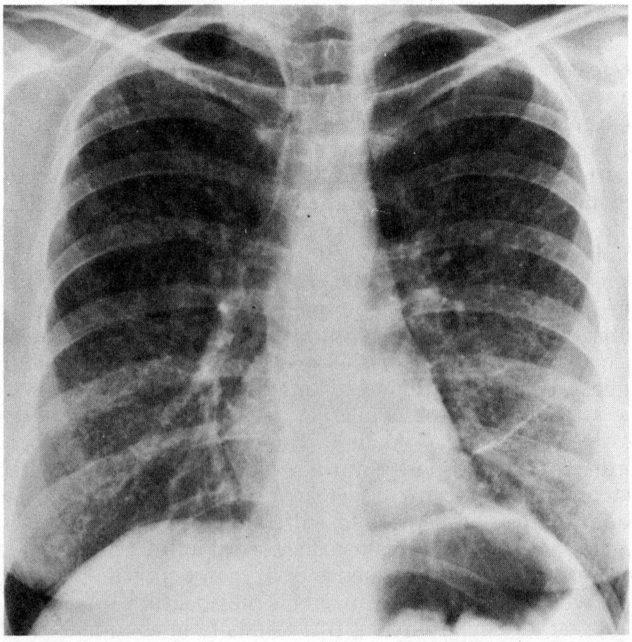

Figure 62–4. Chest x-ray of a patient with idiopathic pulmonary fibrosis, typical of the x-ray findings of many interstitial lung diseases. There is a diffuse reticulonodular infiltrate throughout the lung fields, most prominent at the bases. The heart and pleura are normal.

of the lower respiratory tract contains elevated levels of IgG, immune complexes, and neutrophil products, including collagenase and myeloperoxidase. Open lung biopsy shows a diffuse alveolitis that is patchy in its intensity. There is marked derangement of the alveolar walls, including denudation of the epithelial basement membranes, replacement of the type I epithelial cells by type II epithelial cells and bronchiolar cells, loss of capillaries, and expansion of the interstitium with edema, increased fibroblast numbers, and masses of deranged collagen fibers. The epithelial basement membranes have holes through which the interstitial fibrosis extends into the airspaces.

The clinical course of IPF is characterized by progressive loss of alveolar-capillary units, with eventual respiratory failure and death an average of five years after the onset of symptoms. Occasional patients have a rapidly progressive course; others may live for ten or more years. IPF is associated with a higher-than-expected incidence of lung carcinoma, myocardial infarction, and pulmonary embolism.

DIFFERENTIAL DIAGNOSIS. Although the term "IPF" suggests that the diagnosis is one of exclusion, its features are so characteristic that the diagnosis is usually not difficult. Most confusion comes in separating ILD associated with the collagen-vascular disorders, which are systemic diseases, whereas IPF is compartmentalized to the lung. A negative history of exposure to known causes of ILD is mandatory to make the diagnosis of IPF. An open lung biopsy is also necessary, but the diagnosis of IPF cannot be made using morphologic criteria alone. While the biopsy features of IPF fit the morphologic categories of "usual interstitial pneumonitis (UIP)," "desquamative interstitial pneumonitis (DIP)," or more commonly, a mixture of UIP and DIP, these features are not specific for IPF and can be found in other ILD of both known and unknown etiology.

PATHOGENESIS. IPF likely results from uncontrolled inflammatory processes that ensue after any of a variety of insults to the lower respiratory tract of susceptible individuals. There is likely an inherited susceptibility to this disease, but specific links to histocompatibility loci have not been made. The neutrophil-macrophage–dominated alveolitis, the first known manifestation of IPF, may be driven by immune complexes of unknown origin formed within the lower respiratory tract. The immune complexes are probably associated with enhanced lung B cell immunoglobulin production, with at least some of the immunoglobulins directed against local self antigens. These immune complexes activate alveolar macrophages to release neutrophil-specific chemotactic factors that continuously recruit neutrophils to the alveolar structures. The neutrophils damage the alveolar walls by releasing toxic oxygen radicals and proteases. IPF macrophages spontaneously release fibronectin and alveolar macrophage–derived growth factor and thus expand the numbers of fibroblasts, resulting in fibrosis of the alveolar walls.

STAGING AND THERAPY. The degree of lung damage in IPF is followed by history, chest radiograph, and pulmonary function testing. The intensity of the alveolitis of IPF is gauged by gallium-67 scanning and bronchoalveolar lavage, with particular emphasis placed on the intensity of the neutrophil component of the alveolitis. Conventional therapy is use of corticosteroids, usually as lifelong therapy. Approximately 10 to 20 per cent of IPF patients improve with corticosteroids, particularly if the disease is detected early before the alveolitis causes significant abnormalities. The second line of therapy is either the addition of massive doses of methylprednisolone sodium succinate (Solu-Medrol) (2 grams IV once weekly) or oral cyclophosphamide (1.5 mg per kilogram daily). Either approach helps suppress the alveolitis, but their long-term efficacy is unknown.

Sarcoidosis (Ch. 67)

Sarcoidosis is a multisystem granulomatous disease of unknown etiology characterized in affected organs by a T helper lymphocyte-mononuclear phagocyte inflammatory process, noncaseating granulomata, and derangement of normal tissue

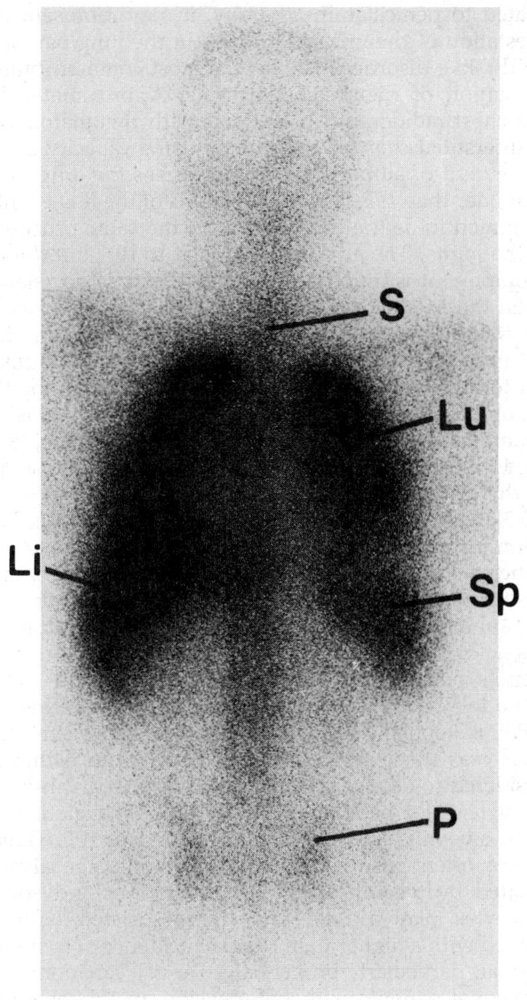

Figure 62–5. Gallium-67 scan of a patient with sarcoidosis. There is diffuse uptake of the isotope throughout the lung parenchyma (Lu). Structures that normally take up gallium-67 are also seen including the spine (S), liver (Li), spleen (Sp), and pelvis (P).

architecture. While most organs can be affected by sarcoidosis, the lower respiratory tract is the site that most commonly causes morbidity and mortality. Pulmonary sarcoidosis is characterized by sharply circumscribed granulomata in the alveolar, bronchial, and vascular walls, composed of tightly packed cells derived from the mononuclear phagocyte system. In addition, the alveolar walls are deranged in a fashion similar to IPF, but much less so. Significant interstitial fibrosis occurs in 20 to 25 per cent of patients. Sarcoidosis is described in detail in Ch. 67 and will not be discussed further here.

ILD Associated with the Collagen-Vascular Disorders

All collagen-vascular disorders are associated with ILD. In most cases the collagen-vascular disorder is apparent before lung involvement is noted, but occasionally the ILD develops first and the other characteristic systemic signs and symptoms appear later. In either case, these disorders are frequently confused with IPF.

RHEUMATOID ARTHRITIS (Ch. 444). The ILD associated with rheumatoid arthritis include (1) an IPF-like disorder, (2) Caplan's syndrome (rheumatoid arthritis associated with coal-worker's pneumoconiosis), (3) pulmonary parenchymal rheumatoid nodules, (4) pulmonary arteritis, and (5) apical fibrobullous disease. A few patients with rheumatoid arthritis have been described with dyspnea, severe irreversible airway obstruction with hyperinflation, and morphologic evidence of obliterative bronchiolitis. While some of this terminal airway disease may be related to penicillamine therapy, it may represent another manifestation of rheumatoid arthritis in the lung parenchyma.

The IPF-like disorder is by far the most common pulmonary manifestation of rheumatoid arthritis. Approximately 25 per cent of chest radiographs of patients with rheumatoid arthritis show interstitial changes and the diffusing capacity is reduced in 50 per cent of all patients. In most cases the lung disease is much milder than IPF. The pathogenesis of the ILD is unknown but assumed to be the consequence of the same processes that affect the joints. The alveolitis is similar to IPF, but the neutrophil component is much less evident. There is no relationship between the extent of disease and the titer of the rheumatoid factor. Most cases of ILD associated with rheumatoid arthritis do not need to be treated. If treatment is instituted, guidelines similar to those for IPF are used. Gold salts, a common therapy for rheumatoid arthritis, also can induce ILD. There is no way to distinguish between gold salt and rheumatoid arthritis-induced ILD, except that the gold-induced disease may reverse when the drug is discontinued.

PROGRESSIVE SYSTEMIC SCLEROSIS (PSS) (Ch. 548). The most common form of ILD associated with PSS is similar to IPF. The incidence of ILD among patients with PSS is very high; at autopsy, morphologic changes are found in 90 per cent and radiographic evidence of ILD is found in 30 to 40 per cent of patients. PSS patients with the CREST syndrome (calcinosis, Raynaud's phenomenon, esophageal involvement, sclerodactyly, and telangiectasia) rarely develop ILD. The ILD associated with PSS is generally indolent, but if it becomes symptomatic, the four-year survival rate is about 50 per cent. Although PSS is considered to be a connective tissue disorder with fibrosis as its main feature, patients with the ILD associated with PSS have an alveolitis, albeit milder than that of IPF. Gallium-67 scans are often positive. For most patients, the alveolitis is dominated by macrophages, but neutrophils and sometimes lymphocytes play a role. The ILD associated with PSS is associated with a higher than normal incidence of bronchogenic carcinoma, particularly bronchoalveolar cell carcinoma.

Occasional patients with PSS develop an ILD characterized by pulmonary hypertension with relatively less disease of the alveolar-capillary units. Morphologically, there is thickening of the pulmonary arteries with fibrosis and some inflammation. Many of these patients develop rapidly progressive respiratory failure.

The pathogenesis of the ILD associated with PSS is unknown. The therapeutic guidelines are unclear, although patients with progressive disease usually are treated in a similar fashion to those with IPF. Penicillamine has been suggested as an alternative therapy, but its efficacy is unproven.

SYSTEMIC LUPUS ERYTHEMATOSUS (SLE) (Ch. 447). The common manifestations of SLE in the lung include pleurisy with or without effusion, atelectasis, or acute pneumonitis. Less frequently, SLE manifests as uremic pulmonary edema, diaphragmatic dysfunction, parenchymal hemorrhage, or chronic ILD. Most cases of chronic ILD have pulmonary features similar to IPF, together with the systemic findings of SLE. Rarely, ILD associated with SLE can also present with a lymphocytic alveolitis similar to Sjögren's syndrome, a disorder similar to idiopathic pulmonary hemosiderosis, or a hypersensitivity vasculitis–like picture. Together, the incidence of acute and chronic pulmonary involvement in SLE is less than 20 per cent of all cases of SLE, and chronic ILD occurs in less than 5 per cent. Chronic ILD can appear insidiously or follow the acute pneumonitis of SLE, a severe illness characterized by fever, tachypnea, radiographic evidence of patchy or diffuse infiltrates, and hypoxemia. The pathogenesis of the ILD associated with SLE is thought to result from the deposition of circulating immune complexes in the alveolar walls. Therapy is usually with corticosteroids, but specific treatment guidelines have not been established. SLE can be associated with pulmonary infections, and this must be distinguished from ILD before corticosteroid therapy is started.

POLYMYOSITIS/DERMATOMYOSITIS (Ch. 454). The incidence of ILD in polymyositis/dermatomyositis is 5 to 10 per cent. Of all the collagen-vascular disorders, a higher proportion of patients who develop the ILD associated with polymyositis/dermatomyositis develop the ILD before the other systemic manifestations of the disease. The ILD is similar to IPF, but its pathogenesis is unclear. Patients are usually treated with corticosteroids, but methotrexate has been suggested as alternative therapy.

SJÖGREN'S SYNDROME (Ch. 449). Approximately 3 per cent of patients with Sjögren's syndrome develop ILD that manifests as either a mild IPF-like disease or, more commonly, a disorder with a lymphocyte-dominant alveolitis, similar to the lymphocytic infiltration of other organs in these patients. This lymphocytic form of ILD can be mild to severe and can undergo transformation to a lymphocytic malignancy, an event that is invariably fatal. Therapy of either ILD associated with Sjögren's is controversial; hence corticosteroids, immunosuppressive agents, and no therapy have all been advocated.

MIXED CONNECTIVE TISSUE DISEASE (Ch. 448). Up to 80 per cent of patients with this systemic disorder have ILD. The lung disease is usually IPF-like. Pulmonary hypertension is common and can occur without significant parenchymal involvement. Therapy is usually with corticosteroids with or without cytotoxic agents.

ANKYLOSING SPONDYLITIS (Ch. 445). Lung disease, manifested as chest wall restriction and upper lobe fibrobullous disease, occurs in about 1 per cent of patients with ankylosing spondylitis. Most patients are asymptomatic, but colonization with organisms such as Aspergillus or atypical mycobacteria is common, and hemoptysis and pneumothorax occur in the late stages of the disease. While HLA-B27 is strongly associated with ankylosing spondylitis, it is not common in those patients with the associated ILD. The morphology of the ILD is IPF-like together with localized destruction of alveolar walls and bullae. There is no known therapy.

Histiocytosis-X (Ch. 161)

Histiocytosis-X (HX), also called "primary pulmonary histiocytosis" and "eosinophilic granuloma," is a fibrotic-destructive disorder of the lower respiratory tract associated with an intense mononuclear phagocyte-dominant alveolitis. HX is grouped with the other proliferative disorders of the mononuclear phagocyte system, such as Letterer-Siwe and Hand-Schüller-Christian disease. In adults, HX is primarily a lung disease, although bone, skin, and central nervous system manifestations do occur. At least 50 per cent of all patients have chronic symptoms, and the disease is often fatal. More than 1000 cases have been reported; most new patients are 20 to 40 years of age and there is an equal sex distribution. Almost all patients with HX have been cigarette smokers.

HX presents with a nonproductive cough, dyspnea on exertion, or chest pain. Spontaneous pneumothorax occurs in 10 per cent of cases; fever, weight loss, hemoptysis, and wheezing are occasionally noted. Bone involvement is present in a minority of patients. Posterior pituitary involvement with diabetes insipidus is unusual, as are skin lesions. Physical examination commonly reveals decreased breath sounds and rales. The chest radiograph shows upper and midzone small irregular nodules superimposed on a delicate cystic pattern. The costophrenic angles are usually clear, and the pleura and hila are normal. Pulmonary function tests show a mixed restrictive-obstructive pattern with reduced lung volumes, reduced diffusing capacity, airflow limitation, and hypoxemia that worsens with exercise.

Definitive diagnosis is made by open lung biopsy. The disease is focal but poorly demarcated. There are sites of intense alveolitis dominated by alveolar macrophages and Langerhan's cells. Gallium-67 scans are usually negative. Bronchoalveolar lavage reveals a macrophage-dominant alveolitis, and the Langerhan's cells can be detected in lavage by ultrastructure and the T6 monoclonal antibody. The pathogenesis and treatment of this rare entity are discussed in Ch. 161.

Goodpasture's Syndrome (Ch. 80)

This disorder is characterized by diffuse pulmonary hemorrhage, ILD, glomerulonephritis, and circulating antiglomerular basement membrane (anti-GBM) and antialveolar basement membrane (anti-ABM) antibodies. It is assumed that the anti-GBM and anti-ABM antibodies are identical and cross-react with identical components in the kidney and lung basement membranes. Goodpasture's syndrome can be mimicked by systemic SLE, Wegener's granulomatosis, and the systemic necrotizing vasculitides. In the appropriate clinical setting, the diagnosis of Goodpasture's syndrome is straightforward but does require (1) demonstration of the circulating antibodies, (2) characteristic linear deposits of immunoglobulin along the glomerular basement membrane, and (3) demonstration that the antibodies (either those circulating or those eluted from the kidney) are specific. It is usually not necessary to obtain lung tissue to make the diagnosis, but the diagnosis can be confirmed by histologic and immunofluorescence study of lung tissue obtained by transbronchial biopsy.

Almost all of the antibasement membrane antibodies in Goodpasture's syndrome are IgG, but IgA, anti-GBM, and anti-ABM antibodies have been described in the setting of pulmonary hemorrhage and glomerulonephritis. The basement membrane antigen(s) against which the antibodies are directed is thought to be a portion of type IV (basement membrane) collagen that is somehow unmasked in the kidney and lung.

Goodpasture's syndrome occurs mostly in young men. In most cases, evidence of alveolar hemorrhage precedes the clinical evidence of renal disease. Hemoptysis occurs in almost all cases, tends to be recurrent, and occasionally is massive and life-threatening. In such cases, death is from "drowning." Anemia is almost always present. The chest radiograph reveals interstitial and alveolar infiltrates. The patchy infiltrates due to the hemorrhage often clear, but the interstitial markings, reflecting chronic ILD, often remain. Histologic findings include alveolar hemorrhage, hemosiderin-laden macrophages, focal areas of alveolitis, and interstitial fibrosis. Linear deposits of IgG can be detected in the alveolar walls.

Spontaneous remissions of Goodpasture's syndrome can occur but are rare. Therapy generally consists of corticosteroids, cytotoxic agents, and plasmapheresis.

Idiopathic Pulmonary Hemosiderosis (IPH)

IPH is a rare disorder of unknown cause characterized by alveolar hemorrhage, iron deficiency anemia, transient parenchymal infiltrates on the chest radiograph, and ILD. The disease is most common in individuals less than 20 years of age, but adult cases are seen. The disease is occasionally found in families, but a genetic basis has not been proven. IPH is compartmentalized in the lung and must be distinguished from Goodpasture's, Wegener's, SLE, and the vasculitides.

IPH presents with repetitive acute episodes of dyspnea, cough with hemoptysis, and fever. Iron deficiency anemia is common. The chest radiographs associated with these acute episodes reveal transient infiltrates, a miliary pattern, or massive confluent shadows. On this background of intermittent episodes, a chronic ILD develops with increasing dyspnea, rales, clubbing, and pulmonary hypertension. While the childhood form of the disease is aggressive, with a mean survival of about three years, adult IPH tends to be more insidious. Lung function tests are typical for ILD, but the diffusing capacity may be falsely high due to increased uptake of the carbon monoxide (used as the test gas) by free hemoglobin in the lung parenchyma. Hemosiderin-laden macrophages in sputum or lavage fluid suggest prior parenchymal hemorrhage. In the appropriate clinical setting, when there are no detectable anti-GBM antibodies, a definitive diagnosis of IPH can be made with an open lung biopsy revealing focal hemorrhage, a macrophage-dominant alveolitis with hemosiderin-positive macrophages, and typical findings of ILD. Corticosteroids are generally used to treat the acute episodes and the chronic ILD, but there is no evidence as to their efficacy. Breaks in alveolar wall elastic fibers and basement membranes have been described in IPH, but it is not known whether these changes are primary or secondary.

Chronic Eosinophilic Pneumonia (CEP)

CEP is a chronic ILD characterized by cough, dyspnea, malaise, fever, night sweats, weight loss, variable degrees of blood eosinophilia, and a chest film revealing peripheral, nonsegmental, nonmigratory infiltrates. Hilar adenopathy rarely occurs. Asthma accompanies CEP in 50 to 60 per cent of cases. High proportions of eosinophils are sometimes recovered in sputum or by lavage. A very high sedimentation rate is common, and elevated levels of IgE during acute episodes have been described. The histologic findings of CEP include a diffuse alveolitis dominated by eosinophils and macrophages with fewer numbers of neutrophils and lymphocytes. Eosinophilic abscesses, multinucleated giant cells, angiitis of small pulmonary vessels, and interstitial fibrosis are common.

Although the stimulus to the accumulation of the eosinophils in the lung is unknown, the eosinophil can damage the cells and matrix of the alveolar walls through its release of toxic oxygen radicals, collagenase, and major basic protein, a highly charged polypeptide associated with the eosinophil granules.

An open lung biopsy is required to make a definitive diagnosis. However, because CEP usually responds dramatically to corticosteroids, a tentative diagnosis is often made on clinical grounds only without biopsy confirmation and corticosteroid therapy is instituted. In some patients, the disease is only partly suppressed by corticosteroids, and long-term treatment is required.

Lymphocytic Infiltrative Disorders

This is a group of rare, diffuse ILD characterized by infiltration of the alveolar structures by cells of the lymphocyte series. Most patients present with cough and dyspnea, occasionally with fever. All of the lymphocyte infiltrative disorders of lung can progress to frank lymphoma.

Immunoblastic lymphadenopathy (also called angioimmunoblastic lymphadenopathy) is a systemic disorder, usually of elderly individuals, characterized by generalized lymphadenopathy, hepatosplenomegaly, and variable amounts of ILD. The disease has no known etiology, but associations with drugs have been reported, including antibiotics and phenytoin. A skin rash is observed in one third of cases; there may be a coexistent collagen-vascular disorder or hemolytic anemia. There are polyclonal increases in serum immunoglobulins. The alveolar structures exhibit a pleomorphic alveolitis representing all levels of lymphocyte differentiation. Diagnosis is usually made by lymph node biopsy. The disease can remit spontaneously, but patients die from either progressive respiratory failure, infection, or malignancy. There is a variable response to therapy with corticosteroids and/or cytotoxic agents.

Lymphocytic interstitial pneumonitis is limited to the lung. The signs and symptoms are typical for an insidious, slowly progressive ILD. It is most common in women in their 40's, but it is observed in males and all age groups. The chest radiograph characteristically shows diffuse reticulonodular infiltrates. Most patients have dysproteinemias. Hyper- and hypogammaglobulinemia have been described, and an association with Sjögren's syndrome is common. The diagnosis is made by an open lung biopsy revealing diffuse parenchymal infiltration with mature lymphocytes, plasma cells, and immunoblasts. Granulomas are sometimes observed. Because the infiltrating cells may form germinal centers, the disease is sometimes called "pseudolymphoma." The prognosis of lymphocytic interstitial pneumonitis is variable, and some patients progress to end-stage lung disease or lymphoma. Treatment is with corticosteroids and/or immunosuppressive agents.

ILD Associated with Pulmonary Vasculitis

Many of the systemic vasculitides result in ILD as a consequence of a pulmonary vasculitis causing a secondary alveolitis and derangements of the alveolar structures.

Wegener's granulomatosis is a granulomatous vasculitis of the upper and lower respiratory tracts and glomerulonephritis (Ch. 452). There is a limited form of the disease without clinically apparent renal disease. All patients have pulmonary involvement, but only one third have symptoms related to the lungs. Airway involvement is common. The parenchymal lung disease can appear as discrete nodules and/or diffuse ILD; either can undergo necrosis and cavity formation. Hemoptysis, cough, sputum production, dyspnea, and pleuritic pain are common. Lung function tests reveal a mixed restrictive-obstructive pattern. Diagnosis is usually made by open lung biopsy. Untreated disease is usually fatal, but with cyclophosphamide therapy long-term survival is the rule.

Lymphomatoid granulomatosis is a systemic vasculitis involving the lung, skin, central nervous system, and kidneys. The lung is always affected, but involvement of other organs is variable. In the lung, the walls of the blood vessels are infiltrated with typical and atypical lymphocytes together with some granulomata, and there is associated ILD. A mild form of lymphomatoid granulomatosis has been described ("benign lymphocytic angiitis and granulomatosis"). The disease is most common in middle age. There are multiple, fleeting nodular densities on the chest film; occasionally there are diffuse infiltrates. Death is usually due to parenchymal destruction with sepsis and occasionally due to massive hemoptysis. The diagnosis is usually established by biopsy of the lung or skin. The lung disease often responds to corticosteroids and cyclophosphamide, but the central nervous system lesions do not. Lymphoma occurs in about 10 per cent of cases.

The *Churg-Strauss syndrome* ("allergic angiitis and granulomatosis") (Ch. 450) is a form of systemic necrotizing vasculitis that almost always involves the lung, unlike classic polyarteritis nodosa, which rarely does. The pulmonary manifestations, consisting of asthma and diffuse infiltrates, often precede systemic involvement by one or two years. An allergic history is common. An elevated sedimentation rate and total eosinophil count are common. The systemic vasculitis involves skin, heart, and gastrointestinal tract. Diagnosis is made by open lung biopsy, which shows a granulomatous vasculitis with eosinophilic infiltration, a secondary diffuse alveolitis, interstitial granulomata, and fibrosis. Treatment is the same as for the other pulmonary vasculitides.

"Hypersensitivity vasculitis" represents a heterogenous group of vasculitides whose development is thought to be related to sensitization to exogenous (e.g., drugs) or endogenous (e.g., serum proteins) antigens. Skin involvement is most common; most cases do not involve the lung. When they do there is a small vessel polymorphonuclear leukocyte vasculitis with fibrinoid necrosis and secondary ILD. Diagnosis is usually made by skin biopsy, and the disorder is often self limiting. A similar disorder can occur in association with mixed cryoglobulinemia or Henoch-Schönlein purpura.

Inherited Disorders

There is a small group of rare ILD that are clearly inherited. Almost all are autosomal dominant disorders, although the autosomal recessive disorders Hermansky-Pudlak syndrome, Niemann-Pick disease, and Gaucher's disease may rarely be associated with interstitial lung disease.

FAMILIAL PULMONARY FIBROSIS. This is a chronic, usually fatal autosomal dominant disorder identical to IPF. Symptoms usually begin in the fifth or sixth decade, but the disease can be manifested earlier. Some of the asymptomatic children of affected family members have evidence of a mild alveolitis yet with normal lung function, suggesting that the disease begins with an alveolitis.

NEUROFIBROMATOSIS (Ch. 492). Von Recklinghausen's disease is an autosomal dominant disorder characterized by pigmented skin lesions and neurofibromas of the peripheral and central nervous system. In 10 to 20 per cent of adult cases there is a coexisting ILD and/or bullous lung disease. The ILD has histologic features similar to IPF, but it is not known whether it responds to similar therapies.

TUBEROUS SCLEROSIS (Ch. 492). This is a hamartomatous autosomal dominant disorder involving the central nervous system, skin, kidneys, eyes, bones, heart, and, in 1 per cent of patients, the lungs. Although the hamartomatous "tumors" are composed of various cell types in most affected organs, in the lung they are composed only of smooth muscle cells. The interstitial deposits of smooth muscle cells cause ILD together with parenchymal destruction. Unlike most ILD, there is little alveolitis. The chest radiograph shows diffuse infiltrates and honeycombing, and lung function tests show a mixed pattern with a dominant obstructive pattern. Pneumothorax is common. There is no known therapy.

ILD Associated with Pulmonary Airway Disease

This term refers to disorders in which the ILD is likely secondary to a primary airway disease. It is unclear if there are many such diseases or only one. The characteristic lesions are necrotic granulomas in the bronchial walls, with the bronchiolar lumens filled with palisading epithelioid cells, cellular debris, and polymorphonuclear leukocytes. There are usually a diffuse alveolitis and nongranulomatous ILD. Approximately one third have asthma, blood eosinophilia, mucus plugging, fungal hyphae identifiable in the airways, and positive sputum cultures for Aspergillus organisms. These patients are usually referred to as having *"bronchopulmonary aspergillosis"* (see Ch. 373). It is unclear, however, whether the fungus is a primary cause of the disease or represents a secondary process.

The remaining two thirds of patients, referred to as having *"bronchocentric granulomatosis,"* do not have asthma, microscopic evidence of fungi, or blood eosinophilia. The disease can present in an insidious manner or as an acute febrile illness. The chest film usually shows nodular or mass lesions; diffuse infiltrates are seen in about 20 per cent of cases. Lung function tests demonstrate a mixed obstructive-restrictive pattern. Corticosteroids are usually the therapy of choice.

Lymphangioleiomyomatosis

This is a rare disease of women, usually of childbearing age, characterized by the proliferation of benign but atypical smooth muscle cells in walls of the lymphatics of the lower respiratory tract, pleura, mediastinum, and retroperitoneum. Although it is an ILD characterized by thickening and derangements of the alveolar walls, there is very little inflammation present. Eventual destruction of the alveolar walls is common. The clinical findings include dyspnea, recurrent unilateral or bilateral chylous pleural effusions, pneumothorax, hemoptysis, and occasionally peritoneal chylous effusions. The chest radiograph has a characteristic reticulonodular pattern on a background of diffuse cystic changes, similar to that seen in histiocytosis-X. Lung function tests reveal a mixed obstructive-restrictive pattern. An open lung biopsy is required to make the diagnosis. It has been theorized that the disease results from an abnormal response to estrogens, and thus oophorectomy, progesterone, and tamoxifen therapy have all been tried in these patients. There is no proven efficacy of such therapies, and the disease is invariably fatal, usually within 10 years of diagnosis.

Alveolar Proteinosis

In this disorder the alveoli are filled with a periodic acid–Schiff (PAS) positive lipid and protein-rich granular material. There may be an accompanying mononuclear cell alveolitis, alveolar wall derangement, and interstitial fibrosis. Although of unknown etiology, alveolar proteinosis can be associated with silicosis, hematologic malignancies, bronchogenic cyst, and mycobacterial and fungal diseases of the lung. Why this material accumulates in the alveoli is unknown but is speculated to result from the breakdown of cells in the lower respiratory tract, from the overproduction of substances normally secreted into the alveolar spaces (e.g., surfactant), from increased transudation of plasma proteins, or from decreased alveolar clearance mechanisms.

The disease usually begins insidiously with dyspnea as the initial symptom. The chest radiograph has a characteristic diffuse, finely nodular alveolar filling pattern. Lung function tests show decreased lung volumes and diffusing capacity. There is usually hypoxemia secondary to pulmonary blood shunting by filled alveoli. Open lung biopsy is usually required for the diagnosis. However, in the appropriate clinical setting, bronchoalveolar lavage recovery of the typical material, together with transbronchial biopsy evidence of alveoli filled with PAS-positive material, is usually diagnostic. Alveolar proteinosis can be fatal but can also spontaneously resolve. The recommended therapy is massive whole lung lavage under general anesthesia. Corticosteroid therapy has no proven use and may lead to the development of opportunistic infections.

Miscellaneous Other ILD of Unknown Etiology

There are several other ILD of unknown etiology that are reasonably well defined but so rare that there is little information available concerning their pathogenesis and no apparent guidelines relating to their staging and therapy. These are included by list in Table 62–1 but will not be discussed individually here.

INTERSTITIAL LUNG DISEASE OF KNOWN ETIOLOGY

There are approximately 135 agents known to cause ILD, but together they are responsible for only one third of all cases of ILD. In terms of numbers of patients that come to medical attention, the most important agents are crystalline silica, asbestos, coal dust, organic dusts of the Micropolyspora and Thermoactinomyces families and those derived from avian proteins, some antineoplastic drugs, nitrofurantoin, and hyperoxia.

Inhaled Inorganic Dusts

ILD resulting from the chronic inhalation of an inorganic dust is called a "pneumoconiosis" (see Table 62–2). The most common are silicosis, asbestosis, and coal worker's pneumoconiosis.

There are several important principles relevant to understanding the pneumoconioses. (1) The dusts themselves cause little damage to the lung parenchyma; it is the inflammatory response to the dusts that causes the loss of functional alveolar-capillary units. (2) A number of defense mechanisms prevent such dusts from reaching the alveoli, and others remove most dusts that might reach the lower respiratory tract. Just because an individual has been exposed to an inorganic dust does not mean that the dust has necessarily caused ILD. (3) Abnormalities on a chest radiograph consistent with exposure to an inorganic dust do not prove that the individual has a functionally significant ILD. (4) These chronic disorders result from the inhalation of inorganic dusts over many years; i.e., history of a brief exposure sometime in the past is not sufficient evidence to implicate a particular dust. (5) No known therapy has proven efficacy for any pneumoconiosis; current "treatment" for all pneumoconiosis is permanent removal from inhalation of the causative agent. (6) Many individuals exposed to inorganic dusts also have a history of chronic cigarette smoking; this must be taken into account when evaluating these patients. (7) Physical evidence of the inorganic dust in the lung is useful but not critical in making the diagnosis of a common pneumoconiosis (silicosis, asbestosis, coal worker's pneumoconiosis) as long as the chronic exposure history is very clear and unambiguous. For the other inorganic dusts, however, biopsy evidence is required to make a definitive diagnosis. (8) While the miners and millers of these inorganic dusts represent the "classic" exposure situations, inorganic dust materials are widely used in manufacturing. A careful occupational history is required or the exposure history may be missed. *Coal worker's pneumoconiosis, silicosis, asbestosis,* and *berylliosis* are described in Ch. 559 on Occupational Lung Disease.

Inhaled Organic Dusts (see also Ch. 559)

The repeated inhalation of certain organic dusts causes a granulomatous ILD called *"hypersensitivity pneumonitis"* or *"extrinsic allergic alveolitis."* The term "hypersensitivity pneumonitis" is reserved for those ILD caused by organic dusts derived from living sources. A large number of organic dusts have been implicated (Table 62–3), but the most common are the thermophilic organisms of the Micropolyspora and Thermoactinomyces groups and those derived from avian proteins.

The nomenclature relating to hypersensitivity pneumonitis is confusing because the "name" of the disease usually refers to the situation of exposure (e.g., "maple bark stripper's disease," "humidifier lung") even though the organic dusts causing different "diseases" may be identical. For example, *Thermoactinomyces vulgaris* can cause "farmer's lung," "humidifier lung," and "mushroom worker's lung." The most common exposure situations are farmers exposed to moldy hay, individuals exposed to organic antigens growing in humidifiers and air conditioners, and bird breeders, particularly those raising pigeons. The other exposure situations are varied and the list is ever expanding (Table 62–3).

Classically, four to six hours after inhalation of the antigen, a sensitized individual develops acute symptoms of hypersensitivity pneumonitis, including fever, cough, dyspnea, and malaise. The chest film at this time shows diffuse parenchymal infiltrates, and lung function tests demonstrate decreased lung volumes, decreased diffusing capacity, mild airflow limitation, and hypoxemia. If the individual is removed from the antigen exposure there is gradual improvement in symptoms, the chest film, and lung function tests over a 24-hour period. If the exposures are few, there are few sequelae other than the acute episodes. However, in some individuals, for unknown reasons, repetitive exposure leads to a chronic ILD characterized by lymphocyte-macrophage alveolitis occasionally mixed with neutrophils, injury to the alveolar walls, granulomata, and interstitial and intra-alveolar fibrosis. Rarely, the chronic form develops in an insidious manner without the acute episodes.

The diagnosis of hypersensitivity pneumonitis is made in the context of a history of exposure to a known causative antigen, the presence of ILD, the presence of antigen-specific antibodies in the blood, and an open lung biopsy demonstrating the characteristic morphology. The gallium-67 scan is usually positive, and bronchoalveolar lavage shows a lymphocyte-macrophage alveolitis, mixed with neutrophils when the exposure has been recent. When the history is typical, a biopsy is not necessary to make the diagnosis, but there must be a clear demonstration of the acute symptoms four to six hours after inhalation of the antigen.

The mechanisms by which sensitization to these organic dusts causes either the acute or chronic disease are unknown. T lymphocytes, the majority of which have suppressor/cytotoxic surface markers, are associated with the alveolitis. The T cells in the lung and blood are sensitized to the offending antigen. Besides the circulating antigen-specific immunoglobulins, there are increased levels of IgG and IgM in the lower respiratory tract. However, there is no evidence that the immunoglobulins play a role in the pathogenesis of the disease, and immune complexes have not been convincingly demonstrated in the lower respiratory tract. One of the confusing aspects of this disease is that, although many exposed individuals become sensitized to the organic antigen (as manifest by the presence of antigen-specific antibodies in the blood), only a very small proportion will develop either the acute or chronic symptoms of hypersensitivity pneumonitis.

The prognosis of chronic hypersensitivity pneumonitis is not clear. In those with farmer's lung, there is a 10 per cent mortality over six years, with an additional 30 per cent having significant functional impairment. Management of hypersensitivity pneumonitis is directed toward removing the patient from the source of antigen and suppressing the alveolitis, usually with corticosteroids.

Drug-Induced ILD

Drug-induced ILD are disorders in which the lower respiratory tract is structurally and/or functionally deranged as a result of a pharmacologic agent. The list of drugs reported to cause ILD is large (Table 62–4) and includes acute, subacute, and chronic ILD. Drug-induced ILD can be serious and sometimes fatal, but they are usually effectively treated simply by recognizing the disorder and discontinuing the responsible drug.

It is generally assumed that many of the drug-induced ILD are "hypersensitivity" reactions, but proof of an immune basis for these diseases is circumstantial at best. In many cases, it is thought that the drug injures the lung parenchyma in some fashion to initiate an alveolitis that propagates the injury.

Typically, the acute and subacute forms of drug-induced ILD present with respiratory decompensation following a prodrome of fever and cough. At this time there are usually increased heart and respiratory rates, dry rales, and, occasionally, cyanosis. The chest radiograph shows a patchy or diffuse reticulonodular infiltrate that can be confused with pulmonary edema. Pleural effusions are common. Blood studies often show eosinophilia and arterial hypoxemia and hypocarbia. Lung function tests are typical for ILD, and the gallium-67 scan is often positive. Open lung biopsy demonstrates parenchymal cell injury, edema of the alveolar wall, fibrin in the air spaces, and a patchy lymphocyte-macrophage alveolitis, sometimes mixed with neutrophils and/or eosinophils. In many cases, the course is rapidly downhill, requiring mechanical ventilation and oxygen administration. The disease is usually reversible if the drug is discontinued but can be fatal if this is not done early in the course.

One major area of confusion in conceptualizing and categorizing the drug-induced ILD disorders has resulted from the use of the term "pulmonary infiltration with eosinophilia (PIE) syndrome" to describe patients receiving drugs who develop an acute or subacute disorder characterized by blood eosinophilia and parenchymal infiltrates on the chest film. However, the PIE syndrome is far from diagnostic as a drug-induced ILD. Many nondrug-associated ILD of both known (e.g., acute beryllium-induced disease) and unknown etiology (e.g., IPF, sarcoidosis) can be associated with blood eosinophilia, and tropical eosinophilia presents in an identical manner. In addition, there is no evidence that the blood eosinophilia has any relevance to the pathogenesis of the disease in the lung. Thus, most clinicians have abandoned the concept of the "PIE syndrome" and simply think of these disorders as part of the spectrum of ILD in which the presence of blood eosinophilia is a helpful, but not definitive, clue to the diagnosis.

The chronic form of drug-induced ILD is much more insidious and difficult to associate with a drug as the etiologic agent. Fever is less common, and patients usually present with typical ILD. Occasionally there is blood eosinophilia. The gallium-67 scan is usually positive. Open lung biopsy usually shows a lymphocyte-macrophage alveolitis with mixed numbers of polymorphonuclear leukocytes. The derangements are IPF-like, but there often is a greater amount of intra-alveolar fibrosis. Unlike the acute and subacute forms of the drug-induced ILD, the chronic form often persists after the drug is discontinued. The reasons why this occurs are not clear, but it is likely that the injury to the parenchyma has been sufficient to establish a chronic alveolitis that propagates the disorder in the absence of the initial stimulus. In such cases, therapeutic strategies are directed toward suppressing the alveolitis, usually with corticosteroids.

ANTINEOPLASTIC AGENTS. *Bleomycin*-induced disease is common; up to 10 per cent of patients receiving bleomycin develop some ILD and 1 per cent die from the ILD. Toxicity from this agent occurs in both acute and chronic forms and is potentiated by concomitant therapy with oxygen or irradiation. *Busulfan* lung disease occurs in 2 to 3 per cent of those receiving the drug. The disease is chronic, usually takes at least one year of therapy before it appears, and usually does not respond to withdrawal of the drug or to corticosteroids. *Methotrexate*-induced ILD can appear in acute or chronic form. Leucovorin or corticosteroids are not protective, but recovery is common once the drug is stopped. There are increasing numbers of reports of ILD induced by the *nitrosoureas*, including carmustine, lomustine, and semustine. The incidence of toxicity is about 1 per cent and occurs two months to three years after initiation of therapy. *Procarbazine* causes an acute ILD with pleural effusions, peripheral eosinophilia, and an eosinophilic alveolitis. Although *cyclophosphamide* is used to treat many ILD of unknown etiology, it can rarely cause acute or chronic ILD. Several other antineoplastic agents are reported to cause ILD but very rarely.

ANTIBIOTICS. ILD induced by *nitrofurantoin* is a common adverse drug reaction, occurring in both acute and chronic forms. The acute form, five to ten times more frequent than the chronic form, occurs in sensitized individuals within one month of reinstituting treatment. The disease almost always clears when the drug is discontinued. The chronic disease occurs following 6 to 12 months of therapy. Approximately 60 per cent have positive antinuclear antibodies. The prognosis is good once the drug is stopped, but permanent loss of lung function is common, and approximately 10 per cent die from the disease. The ILD caused by other antibiotics are also mostly acute disorders and are very rare.

CARDIOVASCULAR DRUGS. *Hydralazine* and *procainamide* induce an acute ILD similar to that associated with systemic lupus erythematosus (SLE). In contrast to spontaneously occurring SLE, which is common in blacks and females, both occur more commonly in whites and affect a significant number of males. Most affected individuals have serum antinuclear antibodies. The disease usually disappears when the drug is stopped. Other drugs that can cause a similar syndrome include isoniazid, phenytoin, and allopurinol. The beta-blockers can cause chronic ILD, but rarely. The disease is insidious and IPF-like but often associated with fibrosis elsewhere in the body.

OTHER DRUGS. *Gold salts* can induce ILD after one to six months of therapy and can be difficult to distinguish from the ILD associated with rheumatoid arthritis. The disease is thought to represent a hypersensitivity reaction. *Mineral oil*–induced ILD, sometimes called "lipoid pneumonia," results from the aspiration of mineral oil used as nose drops or ingested as a laxative. The open lung biopsy demonstrates a typical picture of lymphoid cells, lipid-laden macrophages, and fibrosis. With the appropriate history, however, the diagnosis can be made by recovering lipid-laden macrophages by bronchoalveolar lavage. The intravenous use of drugs meant for oral use can cause ILD by virtue of the presence of particulate material in the drugs, including talc, starch, maltose, or quinine. The disease is usually chronic and characterized by foreign-body granulomatous reactions affecting pulmonary capillaries.

Many other drugs are known to cause acute and/or chronic ILD, and the list is ever expanding. Because these disorders are all potentially curable if the drug is stopped, it is critical to have a high index of suspicion of drug-induced disease whenever confronted by a patient with ILD.

Other Agents Known to Cause ILD

Beyond inorganic dusts, organic dusts, and drugs, the most important known causes of ILD are paraquat, radiation, the sequela of prior infectious processes, hyperoxia, and chronic aspiration pneumonia. The others are very rare and mostly represent anecdotal case reports (see Table 62–5).

PARAQUAT. Poisoning with the herbicide paraquat can occur with oral, parenteral, aerosol, or dermal exposure. Paraquat is available in granules, aerosols, and liquid concentrates; ingestion of the liquid either by accident or by suicidal intent is the most common means of paraquat poisoning. Paraquat is an extremely potent cause of parenchymal derangement and fibrosis and consequent respiratory insufficiency. As little as one teaspoon of the concentrate can be fatal. The disease is usually acute, but chronic cases have been described. In the acute cases, dyspnea, fever, fatigue, and gastrointestinal complaints follow one to five days after poisoning. Mouth, pharyngeal, and esophageal ulcerations are common following oral ingestion. Diffuse radiographic changes of ILD are quickly followed by rapidly progressive respiratory failure, usually requiring ventilatory support. Open lung biopsy reveals a neutrophil-macrophage alveolitis and alveolar wall derangements typical of ILD, but very severe. In addition to interstitial fibrosis, intra-alveolar fibrosis is common. In these acute cases, there is a rough correlation between plasma levels of paraquat and survival. If the plasma paraquat concentration eight hours after ingestion is greater than 1200 μg per liter, death is inevitable. In addition to these acute cases, intermittent skin exposure may be hazardous for agricultural workers and lead to a chronic ILD.

Paraquat causes ILD by virtue of its propensity to be taken up by parenchymal cells of the lower respiratory tract where it generates toxic oxygen radicals sufficient to severely damage the normal parenchymal components. There is a secondary alveolitis that further injures the parenchyma and mediates the development of fibrosis. Treatment of paraquat poisoning is mostly supportive. Attempts should be made to remove the paraquat (gastric lavage with bentonite, Fuller's earth, or charcoal, followed by charcoal hemoperfusion). Since hyperoxia accelerates paraquat-induced injury, oxygen concentrations should be kept as low as possible. Antioxidant therapy (e.g., vitamin E) has been suggested, but its efficacy is unknown. In chronic cases, corticosteroids are usually used to suppress the alveolitis.

RADIATION. ILD resulting from thoracic irradiation is a common sequela of radiotherapy of breast, lung, or esophageal carcinoma and lymphoma and is potentiated by the concomitant use of antineoplastic drugs known to cause ILD. Radiation-induced lung disease is described in Ch. 562.

SEQUELA OF KNOWN INFECTIOUS AGENTS. All types of infections of the lower respiratory tract may occasionally result in significant injury and fibrosis. Usually, the ILD remains localized to the site of infection and does not progress after eradication of the infectious agent. A typical example is the localized upper lobe scars left by mycobacterial infection. ILD has been described following mycoplasma infection as well as Legionella pneumonia, and there are scattered reports of viral infections causing a progressive ILD. Tropical eosinophilia due to chronic microfilarial infestation is an acute ILD (see Ch. 416) and can evolve into a chronic ILD.

INHALED AGENTS OTHER THAN INORGANIC OR ORGANIC DUSTS. These agents include gases, aerosols, chemical dusts, fumes, and vapors. Most are rare causes of ILD, and there is little information available concerning pathogenesis, clinical course, staging, or therapy. Most are acute disorders that reverse when the agent is removed unless significant injury to the parenchyma has occurred.

The most common gas causing ILD is *oxygen*. The inhalation of high concentrations of oxygen over several days often causes parenchymal lung damage, particularly in the setting of acute respiratory failure in the intensive care situation (see Ch. 70). Oxygen toxicity can also be chronic. In contrast, the inhalation of gases such as the oxides of nitrogen, chlorine gas, and sulfur dioxide almost always cause only acute injury; if the patient survives the initial insult and respiratory failure, there are rarely any sequelae.

Aerosols are particles of liquid suspended in a gas. The most

common examples of ILD due to aerosol inhalation are the acute and chronic ILD resulting from aspiration of gastric contents (see Ch. 560) and the aspiration of mineral oil. Exposure to aerosols of cooking oils, pyrethrum (a neutral insecticide used in commercial and household products), and toluene diisocyanate has also been implicated as a cause of ILD.

ILD due to the inhalation of chemical dusts such as synthetic fibers, bakelite, and vinyl chloride and polyvinyl chloride powder are probably hypersensitivity type disorders similar to those associated with the repeated inhalation of organic dusts from living sources. Little is known about the clinical course of these disorders. ILD have also followed the inhalation of various fumes and vapors (Table 62–5).

Crystal RG, Bitterman PB, Rennard SI, Hance AJ, Keogh BA: Interstitial lung diseases of unknown cause: Disorders characterized by chronic inflammation of the lower respiratory tract. N Engl J Med 310:154, 235, 1984. *The most recent review of the interstitial lung disorders of unknown etiology.*

Crystal RG, Gadek JE, Ferrans VJ, Fulmer JD, Line BR, Hunninghake GW: Interstitial lung disease: Current concepts of pathogenesis, staging, and therapy. Am J Med 70:542–568, 1981. *Overviews the current concepts of the pathogenesis of the interstitial lung disorders and emphasizes the current approaches to staging and therapy.*

Davis WB, Crystal RG: Chronic interstitial lung disease. *In* Simmons DH (ed.): Current Pulmonology, Vol V. New York, John Wiley and Sons, 1984, pp 347–473. *Reviews the recent observations in each of the interstitial lung disorders.*

Fanburg BL (ed.): Sarcoidosis and Other Granulomatous Diseases of the Lung. New York, Marcel Dekker, 1983. *A good general review of sarcoidosis.*

Hunninghake GW, Fauci AS: Pulmonary involvement in the collagen vascular diseases. Am Rev Respir Dis 119:471–503, 1979. *A detailed review of the interstitial lung disorders associated with the collagen vascular diseases.*

Hunninghake GW, Gadek JE, Kawanami O, Ferrans VJ, Crystal RG: Inflammatory and immune processes in the human lung in health and disease: Evaluation of bronchoalveolar lavage. Am J Pathol 97:149–206, 1979. *Details the technique and use of bronchoalveolar lavage in the evaluation of inflammatory disorders of the lower respiratory tract.*

Katzenstein AL, Askin FB: Surgical Pathology of Non-neoplastic Lung Disease. Philadelphia, W. B. Saunders Company, 1982. *The most recent text detailing the morphologic findings in the interstitial lung disorders.*

Keogh BA, Crystal RG: Alveolitis: The key to the interstitial lung disorders. Thorax 37:1–10, 1982. *Summarizes the importance of alveolitis in the interstitial disorders.*

Morgan WKC, Seaton A: Occupational Lung Diseases. Philadelphia, W. B. Saunders Company, 1975. *Although written in 1975, it is the best overall text available detailing the interstitial lung disorders resulting from the inhalation of inorganic dusts.*

Rennard SI, Crystal RG: Collagen in the lung in health and disease. *In* Jayson MIV, Weiss JB (eds.): Collagen in Health and Disease. Edinburgh, Churchill Livingstone, 1982, pp 424–444. *Summarizes the role of connective tissue in the lung in normals and patients with interstitial lung disease.*

Schoenberger CI, Crystal RG: Drug induced lung disease. *In* Isselbacher KJ, Adams RD, Braunwald E, Martin JB, Petersdorf RG, Wilson JD (eds.): Harrison's Principles of Internal Medicine. Update IV, New York, McGraw-Hill Book Company, 1983, pp 49–74. *Details the pathogenesis and clinical findings in all of the drug-induced interstitial lung disorders.*

63. LUNG ABSCESS

John G. Bartlett

DEFINITION. Lung abscess literally means a collection of pus within a destroyed portion of the lung; thus there are numerous possible causes of such a lesion (Table 63–1). As used clinically, however, the term lung abscess refers to a pulmonary infection with parenchymal necrosis, generally caused by bacteria other than mycobacteria. Lung abscesses are usually solitary, but occasionally multiple discrete lesions are observed. Numerous small abscesses confined to a given region of the lung are properly referred to as necrotizing pneumonia, a condition sometimes also called pulmonary gangrene. "Primary" lung abscess is an obsolete term because virtually all of these are now believed to be secondary to aspiration. The term "putrid" lung abscess indicates that the sputum of a patient with an abscess has a foul odor and that the abscess is almost certainly caused by anaerobic bacteria. Because they share a common pathogenesis, there is considerable overlap among aspiration pneumonia, lung abscess, and necrotizing pneumonia, and each of these may lead to and coexist with an empyema (a collection of pus within the pleural space).

ETIOLOGY. As indicated in Table 63–1, many different underlying processes can lead to the formation of a lung abscess. By far the most important are necrotizing pulmonary infections and, of these, anaerobic bacteria are responsible for the majority. These organisms account for essentially all "putrid" lung abscesses, and nearly all that have been classified as "nonspecific" or "primary." Most of these infections involve multiple bacterial species, which may include aerobic organisms as well as streptococci. The dominant bacteria are *Fusobacterium nucleatum, Bacteroides melaninogenicus, B. asaccharolyticus, B. ruminicola,* peptostreptococcus, peptococcus, and microaerophilic streptococci.

Pneumonia, particularly cases caused by *Staphylococcus aureus* and *Klebsiella pneumoniae,* may also be complicated by abscess formation. Less frequent but well-documented agents of lung abscess include *Streptococcus pyogenes* (group A beta hemolytic streptococci), *S. pneumoniae* (especially type 3), *Streptococcus milleri, Hemophilus influenzae* (type B), *Pseudomonas aeruginosa, Pseudomonas mallei* (glanders), *Pseudomonas pseudomallei* (melioidosis), *Actinomyces* (actinomycosis), *Legionella, Nocardia, Paragonimus westermani* (lung fluke), and *Entamoeba histolytica* (amebiasis). Enteric gram-negative bacilli other than *K. pneumoniae* may cause lung abscess, but this occurs almost exclusively in debilitated patients with severe associated medical-surgical conditions. Necrotizing alveolitis is a separate entity diagnosed by microscopic examination and usually caused by *Pseudomonas aeruginosa;* sometimes these microabscesses coalesce to form radiographically detectable cavities.

INCIDENCE AND PREVALENCE. The incidence of primary lung abscess has decreased substantially since the prechemotherapeutic era. Nevertheless, most large academic centers encounter 10 to 30 cases annually.

EPIDEMIOLOGY. Most lung abscesses, and nearly all involving anaerobic bacteria, involve the normal flora of the oropharynx. Abscesses involving *S. aureus* or gram-negative bacilli are more likely to be nosocomial in origin. Amebic lung abscess results from the direct extension of an hepatic abscess through the diaphragm into the lung. *Nocardia* causes lung abscess almost exclusively in immunocompromised hosts, especially in recipients of corticosteroids. Septic pulmonary emboli commonly lead to multiple solitary abscesses in noncontiguous sites and are usually caused by *S. aureus,* anaerobic bacteria, or *P. aeruginosa;* hematogenous abscesses are most often found in intravenous drug abusers or in hospitalized patients with infected indwelling cannulas. Lung abscess due to the lung fluke, *Paragonimus westermani,* is most frequently acquired in the Far East or Indonesia.

PATHOGENESIS. The formation of an anaerobic lung abscess nearly always involves two coexisting abnormalities: (1) periodontal sepsis such as gingivitis or pyorrhea, which provides the inoculum, and (2) aspiration, which provides access to the lung parenchyma. The usual causes for aspiration are those that compromise consciousness and the gag reflex, such as alcoholism, drug addiction, general anesthesia, seizure disorder, sedative use, or neurologic disorders. Other factors predisposing to aspiration include dysphagia resulting from esophageal disorders or neurologic deficits; disruption of the usual mechanical barriers as with nasogastric intubation, tracheostomy, or nasogastric feeding tubes; or pharyngeal anesthesia as seen with dental procedures or surgery involving the upper airway. Most healthy persons periodically aspirate small inocula from the upper airways, but these are readily cleared by the normal cough reflex and other pulmonary defense mechanisms without deleterious consequences. Patients who develop aspiration pneumonia and lung abscesses presumably do so because of the relatively large inocula of bacteria and failure of the usual protective mechanisms.

The initial lesion is pneumonitis, or "aspiration pneumonia," that typically involves dependent pulmonary segments, e.g., those favored by gravitational flow. The dependent pulmonary segments most likely to be involved in patients who aspirate in the recumbent position are the superior segments of the lower lobes or posterior segments of the upper lobes. Aspiration in the upright or semi-upright position favors involvement of the basilar segments of the lower lobes. Patients who have a defined period of known or probable aspiration demonstrate with sequential x-rays that 7 to 14 days are usually required for the appearance of a typical air-fluid level on chest x-ray.

CLINICAL MANIFESTATIONS. Patients with anaerobic abscesses tend to have indolent symptomatology with medical complaints dating for two or more weeks before presentation. The usual symptoms are fever, malaise, cough, sputum production, and pleuritic pain. The frequent observation of weight loss and anemia provides testimony to the chronicity of the infection. There may be "chilliness," but frank rigors are rare and their presence suggests organisms other than anaerobes. The cough often becomes more productive at the time of cavitation; there may be hemoptysis, and it is at this time that the patient is most likely to note the onset of putrid discharge. Putrid sputum, which is considered diagnostic of anaerobic infection, is found in 60 per cent of patients with a confirmed anaerobic etiology. Many patients will also note an unusually noxious taste to the sputum. Most patients have a history of compromised consciousness or other risk factors for aspiration, and many have gingival crevice disease. Nevertheless, about 10 per cent of patients with anaerobic lung abscess have no identifiable predisposing condition. Occasional patients with anaerobic lung abscesses are edentulous; the incidence of underlying bronchogenic neoplasms seems particularly high in this group. Patients with lung abscesses due to *S. aureus,* gram-negative bacilli, and amebae usually have a more fulminant course, with the precipitous onset of symptoms. Other features that may be noted in this group include chills, the lack of putrid discharge, and the absence of the usual associated findings. The physical findings in the early phases of disease are those of pneumonia, with or without a pleural effusion. At a later stage there may be amphoric or cavernous breath sounds, pleural effusions are common, and approximately 25 per cent of patients have an associated empyema.

DIAGNOSIS. The diagnosis of lung abscess is usually established with a chest radiograph showing a parenchymal infiltrate with a cavity containing an air-fluid level (Fig. 63–1). The differential diagnosis of this roentgenographic finding is included in Table 63–1. Certain roentgenographic features may provide clues to the presence of an infected cyst, bulla, or sequestration. Massive pulmonary fibrosis with necrosis from occupational exposure is usually distinctive. A loculated empyema with an air-fluid level secondary to a bronchopleural fistula or gas-producing bacteria may be particularly difficult to differentiate from a lung abscess adjacent to the chest wall. This distinction, which has important therapeutic implications, is now greatly facilitated by the use of computerized tomography.

Because the signs, symptoms, and roentgenographic appearance of lung abscesses secondary to infection are remarkably similar, great care needs to be taken to identify microorganisms for which specific treatment is available. However, studies for an etiologic agent are often hampered by the limitations of bacteriologic analysis of expectorated sputum. These specimens are useful in detecting mycobacteria, pathogenic fungi, and parasites, and they may be used for cytologic studies. However, routine aerobic cultures often give erroneous results, and they are not valid for meaningful culture due to the universal presence in oral secretions of anaerobes that contaminate the specimen during passage through the upper airways. Blood cultures are useful, primarily for patients with infections involving *S. aureus* or gram-negative bacilli, but most patients with anaerobic abscesses do not have bacteremia. Pleural fluid is a valuable culture source for both aerobic and anaerobic bacteria in any patient with an empyema; accordingly, in patients with a roentgenographically detectable pleural effusion, thoracentesis should be performed before treatment is begun. For most patients with anaerobic pulmonary infections

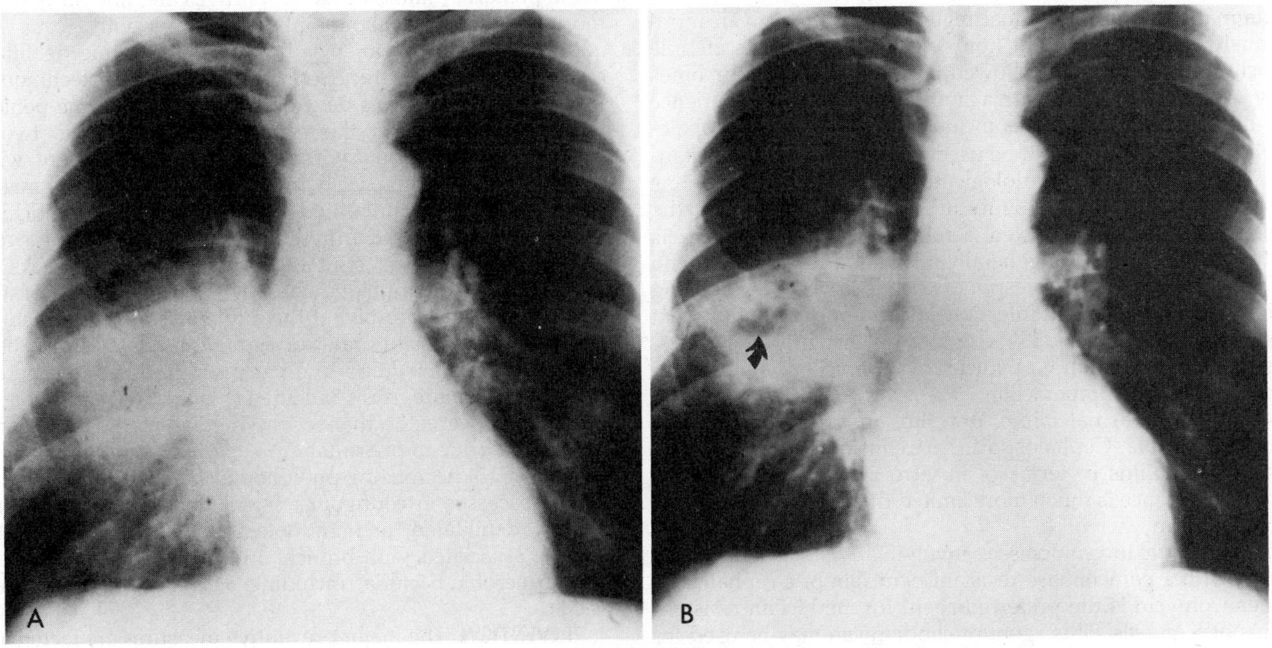

Figure 63–1. Chest x-rays of a 55-year-old alcoholic man. The first film *(A)* shows pneumonitis involving the superior segment of the right lower lobe, a common segment for aspiration pneumonia. The second x-ray *(B)*, taken one week later, shows cavitation with an air-fluid level as indicated by the arrow. A transtracheal aspirate yielded *F. nucleatum*, *B. melaninogenicus*, and anaerobic streptococci. The final diagnosis was aspiration pneumonia with progression to lung disease due to anaerobic bacteria.

restricted to the pulmonary parenchyma, the preferred specimen source to establish the etiologic diagnosis is a transtracheal aspiration performed prior to the institution of antibiotic treatment. This is an invasive diagnostic technique that should be restricted to clinical situations in which technical expertise is available, there are good microbiologic resources, the severity of the illness justifies the risk incurred, and there are no patient contraindications. Most patients with good clinical evidence of an aspiration-related lung abscess, particularly those associated with putrid sputum, do not require transtracheal aspiration, since they may be treated empirically. Prompt bronchoscopy, which used to be performed routinely in patients with lung abscesses, is now restricted to patients who fail to respond to antibiotic treatment or to those in whom an obstructing tumor or foreign body is suspected. Bronchoscopy specimens collected and processed with the usual microbiologic techniques are of little more value than expectorated sputum. The use of a special double-lumen catheter with a distal occluding plug, combined

TABLE 63–1. CLASSIFICATION OF LUNG ABSCESS

I. Necrotizing infections
  A. Pyogenic bacteria *(Staphylococcus aureus, Klebsiella,* mixed anaerobes, *Nocardia asteroides)*
  B. Mycobacteria *(Mycobacterium tuberculosis, M. kansasii,* and *M. avium-intracellulare)*
  C. Fungi *(Coccidioides immitis, Histoplasma capsulatum)*
  D. Parasites *(Entamoeba histolytica, Paragonimus westermani)*
II. Cavitary infarction
  A. Bland embolism
  B. Septic embolism *(Staphylococcus aureus, Candida)*
  C. Vasculitis (Wegener's granulomatosis, periarteritis)
III. Cavitary malignancy
  A. Bronchogenic carcinoma
  B. Lymphoma
  C. Metastatic malignancies
IV. Other
  A. Infected cysts, bullae, or sequestration
  B. Necrotic conglomerate lesions (silicosis, coal miner's pneumoconiosis)

Adapted from Hirschmann JV, Murray JF: Pulmonary and lung abscess. *In* Petersdorf RG, et al. (eds.): Harrison's Principles of Internal Medicine. 10th ed. New York, McGraw-Hill, p 1532.

with quantitative cultures, improves the diagnostic accuracy of bronchoscopy aspirates, although the experience with this technique in patients with lung abscess is limited.

TREATMENT. Obviously, treatment of lung abscess will depend on the underlying cause. For those due to infection, the most important facets of the treatment program are the administration of appropriate antibiotics and adequate drainage of any associated empyema. Physiotherapy with postural drainage should be utilized when possible; however, this must be done with considerable caution in patients with large lung abscesses because of the possibility of spillage of purulent contents with extensive involvement of other lobes.

The drugs of choice for the treatment of abscesses caused by aerobic pyogenic microorganisms, *M. tuberculosis*, fungi, and *Entamoeba histolytica* are reviewed in detail elsewhere in this volume. For aspiration-related lung abscess involving anaerobic bacteria, penicillin has traditionally been regarded as the favored drug on the basis of its long, well-established track record. There is considerable variation in the dosage recommendations, but most authorities recommend penicillin G in doses of 10 to 20 million units per day. This is continued until the patient is afebrile and clinically improved, at which time treatment is changed to intramuscular or oral penicillin using penicillin G, penicillin V, or ampicillin in doses of 500 to 750 mg four times daily. Some authorities suggest a total duration of treatment of three to six weeks, while others base this decision on findings with serial radiographs. In the latter instance, treatment is continued until the chest radiograph changes have cleared or there is only a small stable residual lesion. This commonly requires two to four months or longer but may be necessary to prevent relapses.

Clindamycin is the major alternative to penicillin. This agent is active against most penicillin-resistant anaerobes that are found in 20 to 25 per cent of cases, including many or most strains of *B. melaninogenicus, B. fragilis, B. ruminicola,* and *B. ureolyticum*. Some regard clindamycin as the preferred agent for all lung abscesses due to anaerobic bacteria; others advocate it only for patients who fail to respond to penicillin, have a contraindication to penicillin, or have a serious infection with a fulminant course. The usual regimen is 600 mg given intravenously every six to eight hours until the patient is afebrile and clinically improved, followed by 300 mg orally four times daily. Alternative agents with a limited but favorable experience for anaerobic lung abscesses include tetracycline and cephalosporins. These drugs could be used in extenuating circumstances, such as unusual bacteriologic findings or contraindications to both penicillin and clindamycin. The necessity to treat the aerobic component of mixed aerobic-anaerobic infections is controversial, but this is generally advocated for patients who are seriously ill or fail to respond to clindamycin. In selecting regimens for these mixed infections, it is important to note that most penicillins are equally effective against oral anaerobes. This includes penicillin G, penicillin V, ampicillin, amoxicillin, carbenicillin, and piperacillin. However, antistaphylococcal penicillins, such as nafcillin or oxacillin, are considered inferior and unacceptable. Cephalosporins are considered nearly equivalent to penicillins in terms of in vitro activity, although the clinical experience is much more limited than it is with penicillin or clindamycin.

Patients with lung abscesses involving *S. aureus* should be treated with a penicillinase-resistant penicillin or a cephalosporin. Vancomycin is the preferred agent for methicillin-resistant strains of *S. aureus*. This agent or clindamycin may be used for patients with a contraindication to beta-lactam antibiotics. Penicillin G is the preferred agent for infections involving group A beta-streptococcal infection. Antibiotic selection for infections involving gram-negative bacilli requires in vitro sensitivity data. This usually consists of an aminoglycoside combined with an expanded spectrum penicillin such as ticarcillin for *P. aeruginosa* or an aminoglycoside combined with a cephalosporin for *Enterobacteriaceae*. Sulfonamides are preferred agents for *Nocardia* infections.

The expected response to antimicrobial agents is subjective improvement with decreased fever within 3 to 7 days and elimination of fever within 7 to 14 days. The putrid odor of the sputum, when initially present, usually resolves in three to ten days. Radiographic response is delayed; in fact there is often extension of the infiltrate and increased cavity size or new cavity formation during the first one or two weeks. However, radiographic evidence of progression after two weeks of treatment usually indicates inadequate response. Chest radiographs should be followed at two- to three-week intervals with the expectation that infiltrates will clear and that there will be a small residual scar or a thin-walled cyst. Compliance to long-term oral regimens of antibiotics among outpatients may be a problem, particularly in the patient population most likely to develop primary lung abscesses.

Bronchoscopy is indicated after a week or two of hospitalization and treatment in patients with an atypical presentation and in those who fail to respond to recommended antimicrobial regimens. The major purpose of the procedure is to detect underlying lesions, such as bronchogenic neoplasms, bronchostenosis, or a foreign body, but it may also be used to facilitate drainage. Other considerations in patients who fail to respond include alternative etiologic agents, the use of alternative antibiotics, and the possibility of an empyema requiring drainage. Nearly all patients respond to antibiotics and do not require surgery. The major indications for surgery are uncontrollable or life-threatening hemorrhage or a lung abscess that proves absolutely refractory to medical treatment. Medical failures are most common in patients with an obstructed bronchus, those with extremely large abscesses, those with abscesses that have been present for an extended period before the institution of treatment, and those with infections involving certain bacteria such as gram-negative bacilli. The usual surgical procedure is lobectomy. Patients with an inadequate pulmonary reserve may undergo wedge resection or an external drainage procedure.

PROGNOSIS. The natural course of lung abscesses was best studied in the prechemotherapeutic era. Treatment at that time was nearly equally divided between conservative management using postural drainage and supportive care, and surgery. The mortality rate was about 33 per cent in both groups. An additional third of patients developed a chronic debilitating disease or suffered recurrent symptoms. The technique of resectional surgery was developed at about the time penicillin became available and the relative merits of these two approaches as the primary therapeutic modality were widely debated. During the past two decades, however, the majority of patients have been treated with antibiotics alone, including those with "delayed closure" (i.e., the persistence of a cavity demonstrated by a chest radiograph at four to six weeks after the initiation of antibiotic therapy), because most of these cavities eventually resolve if the antibiotics are continued long enough. The mortality rate for aspiration-related lung abscess is currently reported at 5 to 6 per cent. Findings that herald a relatively poor prognosis include (1) large cavity size, particularly cavities greater than 6 cm in diameter, (2) prolonged symptoms prior to presentation, especially symptoms for over six weeks, (3) necrotizing pneumonia characterized by multiple small abscesses in contiguous segments, (4) patients who are elderly, debilitated, or immunologically compromised, (5) abscesses associated with bronchial obstruction, and (6) abscess due to aerobic bacteria, including *S. aureus* or gram-negative bacilli.

PREVENTION. The major preventive measures are factors used to reduce the incidence or magnitude of aspiration, appropriate care of periodontal disease, early treatment of pneumonia, and adequate courses of antimicrobials to prevent relapses.

Bartlett JG: Lung abscess. Johns Hopkins Med J 150:141, 1982. *The literature is reviewed, including a summary of bacteriologic studies, treatment guidelines, and prognosis.*

Bartlett JG, Gorbach SL, Tally FP, Finegold SM: Bacteriology and treatment of primary lung abscess. Am Rev Resp Dis 109:510, 1974. *The authors report their experience with lung abscesses using transtracheal aspiration to define the infecting flora.*

Hagan JL, Hardy JD: Lung abscess revisited. A survey of 184 cases. Ann Surg 197:755, 1983. *Update on the surgical point of view concerning lung abscess; 11 per cent were operated on.*

Levison ME, Manguar CT, Lorber B, Abrutyn E, Pesanti EL, Levy RS, MacGregor RR, Schwartz AR: Clindamycin compared with penicillin for the treatment of anaerobic lung abscesses. Ann Intern Med 98:466, 1983. *Results of a prospective, randomized multicenter study suggests clindamycin is superior to penicillin in the treatment of putrid lung abscesses.*

Stark DD, Federle MP, Goodman PC, Podrasky AE, Webb WR: Differentiating lung abscess and empyema: Radiography and computed tomography. Am J Roentgenol 141:163, 1983. *Nice demonstration that computed tomography is extremely useful in this important differential diagnosis.*

64. BRONCHIECTASIS AND CYSTIC FIBROSIS

John G. Bartlett

64.1. Bronchiectasis

DEFINITION. Bronchiectasis is an anatomic diagnosis implying irreversible dilatation of the proximal and medium-sized bronchi due to destruction of the elastic and muscular components of the bronchial wall. Clinical expression of the disease reflects hypersecretion of mucus and chronic or recurrent infections.

ETIOLOGY. The ultimate cause of bronchiectasis is nearly always a necrotizing infection that involves the walls of conducting airways. It is doubtful if "congenital" bronchiectasis exists, although certain congenital lesions such as cul-de-sacs and bronchomalacia predispose to secondary infection that may lead to bronchiectasis. Similarly, bronchial obstruction from tumors, foreign bodies, stenosis, or external compression favors the development of bronchiectasis by impairing mucociliary clearance and thus enhancing the development of infection.

In the past, acute pyogenic bacterial infections of the lung were important precursors of bronchiectasis, especially when associated with bronchial obstruction, delayed or ineffective treatment, slow resolution, or parenchymal necrosis. These are much less common now than in the preantimicrobial era, although suppurative pneumonias are still major causes of bronchiectasis in the developing countries of the world. Immunization, where available, has reduced the incidence of bronchiectasis as a complication of measles, pertussis, and influenza. Pulmonary tuberculosis also used to be an important cause of bronchiectasis because of the frequency with which it caused necrosis from endobronchial involvement, bronchial obstruction from contiguous lymph node enlargement, and distortion of the airways from parenchymal scarring.

Today in North America and much of Europe, bronchiectasis is less likely to be caused by an inadequately treated primary pulmonary pyogenic infection or tuberculosis; it is more likely to be associated with an underlying systemic disorder such as hypogammaglobulinemia, the immotile cilia syndrome (which includes Kartagener's syndrome), and cystic fibrosis. Characteristic features of Kartagener's syndrome are dextrocardia, situs inversus, sinusitis, and bronchiectasis. The partial or complete absence of dynein arms of cilia is responsible for immotile sperm in males and delayed mucociliary transport in the lower airways, which presumably causes chronic pulmonary disease. The mechanism of bronchiectasis in cystic fibrosis is unknown but probably includes bronchial obstruction secondary to tenacious secretions and the inevitable development of infection with *Staphylococcus aureus* and *Pseudomonas aeruginosa,* both necrotizing organisms.

An unusual type of bronchiectasis in proximal airways occurs in patients with allergic bronchopulmonary aspergillosis. The pathogenesis is unknown but may involve secondary bacterial infection and/or direct (mechanical or toxic) effects of the fungus on the bronchial wall.

PATHOGENESIS AND PATHOLOGY. Major contributing factors to the development of bronchiectasis are systemic disorders and/or local obstruction that favor the development of prolonged infection. Resected bronchiectatic segments show dilated lumens filled with suppurative material and inflamed, often necrotic, mucosal surfaces. The infection extends into the bronchial wall, disrupting smooth muscle and elastic tissue. The ciliated columnar epithelium is replaced by nonciliated cuboidal cells or fibrous tissue, resulting in localized dilatation or saccules. These changes promote further stasis, infection, and eventually traction as a result of peribronchial scarring. Depending on the gross appearance of the dilated segment, bronchiectatic changes are classified as cylindrical, varicose, or saccular. Cylindrical bronchiectasis is mild bronchial dilatation with mucous plugging that is usually managed conservatively. Varicose bronchiectasis is a more advanced stage characterized by moderate dilatation and distortion of bronchi that resemble varicose veins. The most advanced form is cystic or saccular bronchiectasis, which usually involves proximal (central) bronchi. The most common sites of involvement are the posterior basilar segments of the lower lobes, presumably due to the lack of gravitational drainage. The middle lobe of the right lung is also predisposed owing to angulation of the lobar bronchus at its take-off and the presence of peribronchial lymph nodes at the origin, which may be involved in a number of pathologic processes. Upper lobe bronchiectasis is most commonly secondary to tuberculosis or lung abscess.

CLINICAL MANIFESTATIONS. The classic form of bronchiectasis was described in the preantibiotic era, when it usually occurred in children or young adults after a bout of necrotizing pneumonia and was characterized by copious amounts of putrid sputum, emaciation, severe secondary parenchymal infections, repeated episodes of hemoptysis, clubbing of the digits, and reduced life expectancy. This presentation is now seldom seen and bronchiectasis is more likely to be a manifestation of a systemic disorder than of a local pulmonary process. The usual symptoms in the present era are chronic cough, purulent sputum production, hemoptysis, and recurrent bouts of pneumonia. The cough may be especially disturbing when the patient is in the recumbent position, since secretions tend to pool in the larger bronchi. The recurrent pulmonary infections usually involve the same pulmonary segment or lobe when the disease is localized. Exertional dyspnea, fatigue, and malaise may be noted in patients with extensive disease. The most characteristic finding on physical examination is persistent, moist, coarse rales over the area involved. Only occasional patients exhibit clubbing, and secondary amyloidosis is now extremely rare.

DIAGNOSIS. Bronchiectasis should be suspected in patients who have chronic sputum production, often with hemoptysis, that is not otherwise explained and those with recurrent pneumonias, particularly when there is involvement of the same segment or lobe. Major alternative diagnostic considerations in patients with chronic cough and sputum production are chronic bronchitis, tuberculosis, and chronic lung abscess. Plain chest roentgenograms in patients with bronchiectasis may be normal or show only coarse lung markings. In more advanced cases, the diagnosis may be made from the presence of multiple cystic lesions with or without fluid levels. Bronchography will establish the diagnosis, determine the extent of involvement, and describe the distribution of lesions, but it is indicated only in patients who are potential candidates for surgery. Bronchography should not be performed until at least three months after any pulmonary infection, since reversible changes in the bronchi that are similar to those of bronchiectasis may occur during this period. Bronchoscopy is useful for detecting certain associated conditions that cause obstruction, such as tumors, strictures, or foreign bodies, and for identifying the location of bleeding. Roentgenograms of the paranasal sinuses demonstrate sinusitis in up to 40 per cent of patients with bronchiectasis. Appropriate studies should be taken to document an immune deficiency disease, cystic fibrosis, or the immotile cilia syndrome when other clinical features suggest these conditions.

TREATMENT. The anatomic defects are irreversible, so that medical therapy is directed against controlling symptoms and preventing progression. Basic supportive measures include postural drainage to mobilize secretions, hydration, bronchodilators for patients with bronchospasm, discontinuation of smoking, and treatment of associated sinusitis. Antimicrobials are indicated for infectious exacerbations manifested by increased purulent sputum production, progressive dyspnea, fever, and hemoptysis. Available evidence suggests that the most common causes of superimposed infections in patients without cystic fibrosis (see Ch. 64.2) are *Hemophilus influenzae, Streptococcus pneumoniae,* and anaerobes. Ampicillin is an appropriate drug for empiric use, and tetracycline should suffice in patients who have a contraindication to penicillins. Surgery, once a mainstay of treatment, is seldom indicated because patients with mild symptoms usually respond to medical therapy and those with severe symptoms usually have extensive disease with involvement of multiple segments that precludes complete resection. Factors to consider when surgery is contemplated are the age of the patient, the extent and distribution of disease, associated bronchitis, and pulmonary reserve. The major indication for resectional surgery is localized disease that does not respond to medical treatment, particularly in young patients with profuse sputum, fetid breath, severe cough, or recurrent bouts of pneumonia that impair their ability to live a normal life. In these cases, segmental resection or lobectomy may be curative. A rare indication for surgery is massive hemoptysis resulting from an aneurysmal vascular deformity in a bronchiectatic cavity. Embolization of bronchial arteries is warranted in hemorrhaging patients who cannot tolerate pulmonary resection.

PROGNOSIS. Progression within involved segments is common, but extension to previously normal segments is unusual unless the underlying disease is a generalized process such as cystic fibrosis, bronchial asthma, the immotile cilia syndrome, or agammaglobulinemia, i.e., conditions that predispose the entire bronchial system. Judicious use of antibiotics may effectively control symptoms, minimize disability, and obviate any need for surgery. Resection may be curative in those few patients with localized disease complicated by persistent or debilitating symptoms. Patients with advanced, bilateral disease have severe symptoms and are not surgical candidates, but may do relatively well with good medical therapy.

Davis PB, Hubbard VS, McCoy K, Taussig LM: Familial bronchiectasis. J Pediatr 102:177, 1983. *Nice review of the various familial syndromes that lead to recurrent infections and bronchiectasis; 67 references.*

Ellis DA, Thornley PE, Wightman AJ, Walker M, Chalmers J, Crofton JW: Present outlook in bronchiectasis: Clinical and social study and review of factors influencing prognosis. Thorax 36:659, 1981. *Good perspective of bronchiectasis in the "modern era."*

Rivera M, Nicotra MB: *Pseudomonas aeruginosa* mucoid strain. Its significance in adult chest diseases. Am Rev Respir Dis 126:833, 1982. *Useful evidence that when this organism is cultured from the sputum of an adult, bronchiectasis is present.*

64.2. Cystic Fibrosis: The Adolescent and Adult Patient*

DEFINITION. Cystic fibrosis (CF) is a genetic disorder of eccrine and exocrine gland function that is characterized by abnormally viscid secretions from mucous glands leading to chronic pulmonary disease, pancreatic insufficiency, and elevated levels of sweat sodium and chloride, along with other manifestations (Table 64–1). First described in 1936, it is probably the most common lethal genetic disease of the white population in the United States.

PREVALENCE. Cystic fibrosis is transmitted as an autosomal recessive trait. The carrier rate of the abnormal gene is about 5 per cent in Caucasians, resulting in a prevalence of the homozygous state of 1 per 1,600 to 2,000 Caucasian (compared to 1 per 17,000 black) births. Homozygotes for the CF gene have almost all of the clinical features of the disease, but heterozygotes are clinically normal. The disease is recognized in most patients prior to adolescence; rarely the diagnosis may not be made until the third or fourth decade of life.

PATHOGENESIS. The unknown primary biologic defect presumably leads secondarily to the changes in the physical characteristics of mucus in cystic fibrosis, which in turn lead to obstruction and dilatation of glands and their ducts. No primary abnormalities of the mucoproteins secreted, of ciliary function, or of host defenses (including cell-mediated, humoral, and secretory immunity) have been demonstrated. Thus, the reason for the obstruction of glands caused by abnormal mucous clearance remains unknown.

Although morphologically normal, the sweat glands in CF have defective tubular reabsorption of electrolytes and/or water, resulting in a striking increase in the levels of sodium and chloride in the sweat. This is not thought to play an important role in disease expression. Similar abnormalities have not been found in the secretions of other glands with the exception of the submaxillary salivary glands.

*We express our appreciation to Christopher J.L. Newth, M.B., for his useful criticisms and suggestions about this chapter.

CLINICAL MANIFESTATIONS. Meconium ileus at birth, which occurs in about 10 to 15 per cent of CF patients, is the earliest common manifestation. The major medical problems encountered in adolescents or young adults with cystic fibrosis are disorders of the tracheobronchial tree, the pancreas, and the gastrointestinal tract (Table 64–2). There are no abnormalities in the respiratory tract at birth; the earliest changes are hypertrophy of bronchial glands and metaplasia of goblet cells. The pulmonary problems increase and dominate the clinical picture as the patient gets older, while problems with malabsorption seem to decline.

Chronic pulmonary disease characterized by chest deformity, clubbing, and bronchiectasis is present in 97 per cent of adults with homozygous cystic fibrosis and is the major cause of morbidity and mortality. Pulmonary function tests show mixed obstructive and restrictive disease, with the obstructive element being dominant in most patients. The serial measurement of FEF_{25-75} appears to be the most sensitive index of pulmonary decline. A sudden change, particularly in female adolescents, is a very serious sign. The respiratory disease is characterized by recurrent flare-ups of chronic bacterial bronchitis and bronchopneumonia, terminating in respiratory failure and death. The recurrent and chronic bacterial infection is due primarily to mucoid strains of *Pseudomonas aeruginosa*. *Staphylococcus aureus,* which is present in about 50 per cent of adult patients, is rarely implicated in acute pulmonary complications. *Pseudomonas cepacia* occurs in the sputum of 5 to 10 per cent of patients with cystic fibrosis and is associated with a more rapid decline in pulmonary function. In adults with cystic fibrosis, minor hemoptysis occurs in 60 per cent, massive hemoptysis in 7 per cent, and pneumothorax in 16 per cent. Half of the adults with this disease have nasal polyps, but usually with no obstructive symptoms from them. Over 70 per cent of patients die with cor pulmonale; the appearance of right ventricular failure usually means death within two years.

Pancreatic exocrine insufficiency occurs in 85 to 90 per cent of patients with CF. This results in deficient enzymatic hydrolysis of nutrients, particularly fats (Ch. 103). Protein is better tolerated, and the salivary amylase allows normal carbohydrate metabolism. Malabsorption of fat may be associated with deficiencies in essential fatty acids such as linoleic acid and the fat-soluble vitamins (A, D, E, K). Pancreatic function may decline with age in those patients born without malabsorption. Patients

TABLE 64–1. CLINICAL MANIFESTATIONS OF CYSTIC FIBROSIS

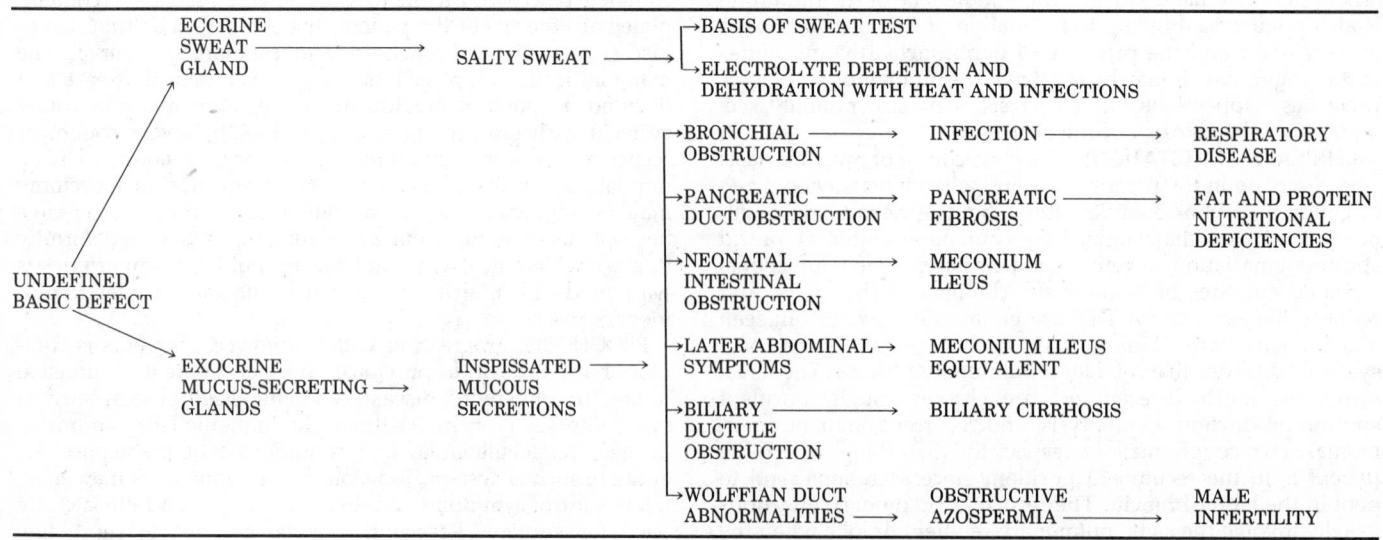

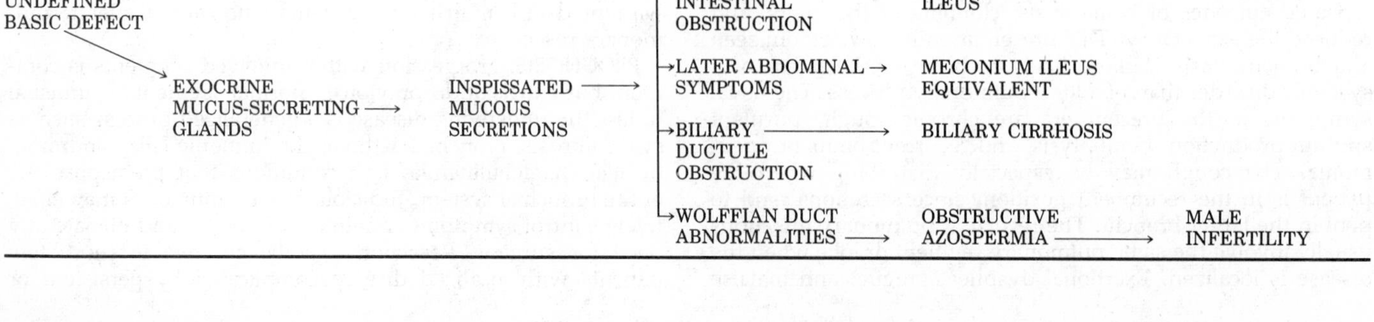

TABLE 64–2. CLINICAL MANIFESTATIONS OF CYSTIC FIBROSIS IN ADOLESCENTS AND ADULTS*

Clinical Feature	Percentage
Pulmonary disease	97
Hemoptysis	60
Pneumothorax	16
Nasal polyps	48
Cirrhosis	5
Heat prostration	5
Intestinal obstruction	21
Meconium ileus equivalent	24
Intussusception	5
Pancreatic insufficiency	95
Glucosuria	8

*Modified from di Sant'Agnese PA, Davis PB: Cystic fibrosis in adults. Am J Med 66:121, 1979.

with residual pancreatic exocrine function tend to have better pulmonary function and probably a better prognosis.

Cystic fibrosis may also affect the small bowel, liver, bile ducts, and male reproductive organs. Intestinal obstruction secondary to meconium ileus is seen at birth. Later intestinal obstruction, or "meconium ileus equivalent," occurs in about 20 per cent of older patients and is presumably related to inspissation of mucofeculent material in the distal small bowel, especially in the ileocecal area. Patchy biliary cirrhosis may result in hepatic enlargement and rarely may progress to severe portal hypertension with varices. The incidence of cholelithiasis is increased due to lithogenic bile rich in cholesterol. Diabetes mellitus occurs in about 10 per cent of adults, associated with decreased levels of insulin and glucagon. The diabetes is relatively easy to control and ketoacidosis is rare. Puberty, skeletal maturity, and the pubertal growth spurt are delayed in the majority of adolescents. Males are infertile due to absence of the vasa deferentia function and the females, although able to conceive despite an abnormal cervical mucus, frequently develop secondary amenorrhea as they deteriorate clinically.

DIAGNOSIS. Cystic fibrosis is diagnosed in nearly 80 per cent of patients in the first three years of life. However, the diagnosis should be suspected in any adolescent or young adult presenting with chronic bronchopulmonary disease and pancreatic insufficiency. For diagnosing CF, a quantitative pilocarpine iontophoresis sweat test should be performed in a laboratory with established expertise. At least 50 mg of sweat should be collected and the results should be confirmed with a second test. Elevated sweat sodium and chloride concentrations, exceeding 60 mEq per liter in children and 70 mEq per liter in adults, are diagnostic of CF.

No screening tests are available for detecting the heterozygous state. Prenatal tests are available for the homozygous condition, but their reliability has not yet been established. In the first four to six weeks of life, when it is difficult to obtain sufficient sweat for testing, high serum concentrations of immunoreactive trypsin may prove to be diagnostic and can be used for routine newborn screening.

TREATMENT. An increasingly large number of patients with cystic fibrosis survive into adulthood, and an additional small number of patients with previously undiagnosed cystic fibrosis will be identified in young adulthood. The major source of morbidity in later life is pulmonary disease. Vigorous pulmonary toilet is basic, and good bronchial clearance can be obtained with a combination of chest physical therapy, active coughing, and exercise. Patients should be encouraged to pursue any form of exercise within their capacity. About 50 per cent of adult patients have bronchial hyper-reactivity with significant variability of air flow rates. Aerosols of bronchodilators in normal saline are sometimes partially effective. In occasional cases, air flow can be improved by oral corticosteroids without any evidence of worsening of the bronchopulmonary infection.

Antimicrobial agents are particularly important in the therapy of CF lung disease. Chronic antistaphylococcal therapy can be given orally for years without evidence of drug resistance or complications. Antipseudomonal agents are essential for acute exacerbations of bronchial infections and intermittent bouts of pneumonia. These infections generally remain localized in the lungs; bacteremia, empyema, and extrapulmonary spread are unusual. The initial treatment of *Pseudomonas aeruginosa* in adolescents and adults is most commonly with the combination of tobramycin and ticarcillin. Subsequent modification should be based on the results of sputum cultures and in vitro sensitivity tests. When the acute or the chronic bronchopulmonary exacerbation is due to *Pseudomonas cepacia*, the antimicrobial choice is usually extremely limited.

Most patients with pancreatic insufficiency can be maintained on a normal diet with supplemental pancreatic enzymes. The preferred agents are enteric-coated microsphere pancreatic enzyme preparations, such as Pancrease and Cotazym-S, given in doses of three to five capsules per meal. The concomitant use of sodium bicarbonate or H_2-receptor antagonists (cimetidine, ranitidine) may also improve the fat and protein absorption, since the efficacy of pancreatic enzymes is markedly increased at higher intraluminal pH levels. The treatment of malabsorption is more extensively discussed in Ch. 103.

"Meconium ileus equivalent" can usually be treated with enemas or nasogastric suction. Surgery is necessary on rare occasions. The administration of substantial amounts of pancreatic enzymes may reduce the frequency of this complication of intestinal obstruction. The lithogenicity of the bile can be reversed with appropriate pancreatic enzyme replacement. No treatment is available for the hepatic or vas deferens abnormalities. Nocturnal oxygen therapy is being evaluated to determine if prevention of sleeping arterial oxygen desaturation decreases cardiopulmonary morbidity and prolongs survival. The psychosocial aspects of this disease are formidable, and where possible patients should be cared for by special units so that their manifold problems can be dealt with by staff experienced in their management.

PROGNOSIS. About half of the patients with cystic fibrosis in the United States live to be 20 years of age. However, in areas where patients are cared for by special units, such as those supported by the Cystic Fibrosis Foundation and NIH, 50 per cent may survive to at least 25 years of age, with males doing much better than females.

Factors associated with a better prognosis in cystic fibrosis are the male sex, maintenance of appropriate weight, single system (gastrointestinal or pulmonary) involvement at presentation, and a normal chest radiograph within the first year of presentation. Additional good prognostic factors are likely to be the presence of pancreatic function and the absence of *Pseudomonas cepacia*. Early diagnosis of cystic fibrosis has not been shown to influence the long-term survival of these patients.

di Sant'Agnese PA, Davis PB: Cystic fibrosis in adults. Am J Med 66:121, 1979. *An excellent review of the clinical aspects of CF as the disease is seen by the internist in the adolescent and adult patient.*

Kuzemko JA: Evolution of lung disease in cystic fibrosis. Lancet 1:448, 1983. *This article describes an interesting hypothesis that circulating pancreatic proteases may play a role in lung injury in CF, to be followed by superinfections with bacteria and/or viruses.*

Moss AJ: The cardiovascular system in cystic fibrosis. Pediatrics 70:728, 1982. *An extensive review, with 135 references, concerning the cardiovascular findings in CF, with special emphasis on the importance of cor pulmonale as a complication.*

Teffer RS, Skatrud JB, Dempsey JA: Ventilation and oxygenation changes during sleep in cystic fibrosis. Chest 84:388, 1983. *A recent study of the abnormal ventilation and resulting arterial oxygen desaturation of patients with CF during sleep, with the conclusion that hypoventilation during REM sleep is an important contributing factor.*

Wilcken B, Brown ARD, Urwin R, Brown DA: Cystic fibrosis screening by dried blood spot trypsin assay: Results in 75,000 newborn infants. J Pediatr 102:383, 1983. *An extensive Australian study that documents the validity of measuring immunoreactive trypsin by a blood spot method as a screening technique for newborns.*

65. PULMONARY EMBOLISM

James E. Wilson III

DEFINITION. Pulmonary embolism is the impaction of a dislodged thrombus or other particulate matter in the pulmonary vascular bed. Pulmonary infarction is necrosis of lung parenchyma caused by interference with its blood supply. Because the lung has a dual blood supply, most pulmonary emboli do not lead to infarction.

ETIOLOGY. The predisposing factors can be grouped in the manner originally suggested by Virchow in 1856: *stasis, vein injury,* and *hypercoagulability.* Stasis occurs with immobilization, obesity, varicose veins, congestive heart failure, and pregnancy. Vein injury occurs with surgery, trauma, and burns. The exact definition of hypercoagulability is controversial; in a broad sense it is an altered state of the coagulation system predisposing to the development of thrombus. Hypercoagulability may exist with carcinoma, polycythemia rubra vera, hemolytic anemia, splenectomy with thrombocytosis, homocystinuria, and perhaps use of oral contraceptives. Recurrent venous thromboembolism is known to occur with abnormalities of platelets, of the coagulation cascade, and of spontaneous fibrinolysis. Some patients have been reported to have increased platelet adhesiveness and decreased platelet survival. Increased venous thrombosis has occurred in association with large increases in factor V or VIII, abnormal fibrinogens, and antithrombin III deficiency. Recurrent venous thromboembolism has also been associated with both a decrease in plasminogen activator in venous endothelium and a decrease in the release of plasminogen activator with various stimuli. Increased inhibitors of plasmin or plasminogen activators as well as abnormal plasminogens are relatively rare predisposing factors. The relative frequency with which these abnormalities of platelet function, coagulation, and fibrinolysis account for recurrent venous thromboembolism is unknown. For a patient to develop pulmonary embolism without an obvious precipitating cause is a relatively ominous sign that recurrence is likely to happen. Thrombophlebitis is discussed in greater detail in Ch. 54.

Pulmonary emboli usually come from the deep veins of the lower extremities. Nevertheless, pelvic veins or the right heart may be occasional sources of emboli as well. Many patients with angiographically proven pulmonary emboli have negative venograms in the lower extremities, which may indicate either that the entire thrombus has embolized or that other venous systems are involved.

INCIDENCE AND PREVALENCE. Pulmonary embolism is a serious and difficult medical problem that is particularly common in immobilized or hospitalized patients. Pulmonary embolism is estimated to be the sole cause of death in 100,000 patients and a major contributing cause of death in another 100,000 patients in the United States each year, and as such is the third most frequent cause of death in the United States. Pulmonary embolism may not be suspected. Thirty-three per cent of deaths occur within one hour, before the diagnosis can be made and therapy instituted. Sixty per cent of deaths occur in patients in whom the diagnosis was not suspected at all. Only 7 per cent of the deaths occur in patients in whom the diagnosis was suspected and therapy was instituted. On the other hand, pulmonary embolism may be erroneously diagnosed and treated. Unfortunately current therapy has significant associated morbidity and mortality, and in addition an inaccurate diagnosis needlessly burdens a patient with fear of sudden death and difficulties in obtaining employment or insurance. Therefore, an accurate diagnosis is critical in confirming or excluding pulmonary embolism.

MECHANISMS OF DISEASE. Embolization of a branch of the pulmonary artery obstructs blood flow to a ventilated region of lung, increasing wasted ventilation. The increase in minute ventilation that is required to achieve the same alveolar ventilation may contribute to the sensation of *dyspnea.*

Hypoxemia commonly occurs with pulmonary embolism. In humans with angiographically proven emboli the hypoxemia seen while breathing room air can be accounted for by the amount of true shunting measured by the 100 per cent oxygen technique. A recent study utilizing the technique of multiple gases with different solubilities has confirmed shunting as the sole cause of hypoxemia in two patients with acute pulmonary embolism proven angiographically. The hypoxemia can be temporarily reversed if a breath as large as 80 per cent of the predicted inspiratory capacity is taken. The return of hypoxemia within 15 minutes suggests a mechanical instability of the lung that promotes multiple areas of microatelectasis. If there is no other underlying heart or lung disease, pulmonary embolism (unless massive) rarely leads to an arterial oxygen tension below 55 mm Hg. Even with massive pulmonary embolism the arterial Po_2 can be deceptively normal. In the setting of a low cardiac output, pulmonary capillary blood flow tends to go to the areas with best ventilation, which have the least resistance to perfusion. Hypoxemia may become worse with measures that increase blood flow to poorly ventilated regions.

Death or *shock* caused by pulmonary embolism occurs as a general rule only with massive emboli occluding well over 50 per cent of the pulmonary vascular bed, but this rule does not apply to patients with pre-existing heart and lung disease. In some patients without known pre-existing heart or lung disease, pulmonary hypertension with acute pulmonary embolism appears to be disproportionate to the degree of occlusion of the pulmonary vascular bed. This suggests that pulmonary vasoconstriction may occur with pulmonary embolism. Even with active pulmonary vasoconstriction, mean pulmonary arterial pressure does not exceed 40 mm Hg in a formerly healthy person who has sustained an acute embolus. The right heart is a volume pump, not a pressure pump, and with an acute increase in afterload the right ventricle dilates and produces tricuspid regurgitation. A mean pulmonary artery pressure of 50 mm Hg or more suggests right ventricular hypertrophy secondary to recurrent pulmonary embolism over a long period of time or some other underlying disease.

PATHOLOGY. Pulmonary emboli are usually multiple and bilateral, and are found predominantly in the lower lobes, especially on the right side. The distribution is undoubtedly related to normal regional blood flow in the upright position. Only about one in ten pulmonary emboli causes a pulmonary infarction. Since pulmonary emboli are usually multiple, at least half the subjects with pulmonary emboli have a complete or incomplete infarct. Infection and left heart failure contribute to the likelihood of pulmonary infarction, but infarcts also occur frequently in patients without previous infection, heart disease, or lung disease.

Microscopically a pulmonary infarct shows coagulative necrosis of alveolar walls and alveoli full of erythrocytes with little inflammatory response. Radiographically this type of true infarct produces an infiltrate that lasts more than a week and heals, leaving a linear scar. An incomplete infarct has extravasation of erythrocytes into alveoli without necrosis of alveolar wall and produces an infiltrate on radiographs that usually clears in two to four days without a residual scar.

The development of a pulmonary infarct is related to the degree of occlusion of the embolized vessel and the rapidity with which adequate systemic bronchial collateral flow increases in the days following the occlusion in the pulmonary circulation.

CLINICAL MANIFESTATIONS. There are at least three distinct clinical syndromes of acute pulmonary embolism. *Massive pulmonary embolism* involving lobar or larger vessels is more likely to present as sudden *syncope, central chest pain,* or *dyspnea.* The dyspnea can be surprisingly minor. On examination one is likely to find hypotension and signs of right ventricular overload such as distended jugular veins, hepatojugular reflux, right ventricular heave, increased pulmonic component of the second heart sound, a right-sided gallop rhythm, and a murmur of tricuspid insufficiency. The right-sided gallop rhythm and the tricuspid insufficiency murmur both increase with inspiration and diminish or disappear with a Valsalva maneuver.

In the syndrome of *medium-sized pulmonary embolism* involving mainly segmental and subsegmental branches of the pulmonary artery, the patient is more likely to experience *pleuritic chest pain* and *hemoptysis*. The patient is unlikely to have syncope or hypotension unless there is pre-existing heart or lung disease with minimal reserve. On examination cardiovascular findings are less prominent, and pulmonary findings, such as *pleural friction rub*, findings of *consolidation*, or findings of a *pleural effusion*, are more common. The typical findings of lung parenchymal consolidation, such as increased tactile fremitus, dullness to percussion, loud tubular breath sounds, egophony, and increased whispered pectoriloquy, are frequently modified by the presence of a pleural effusion. Over a pleural effusion there is decreased tactile fremitus, flatness to percussion, and diminished breath sounds. Intercostal tenderness over the effusion is common and may suggest an empyema. With infarction there may be fever, leukocytosis, and mild icterus. If there is no infarction, there may be no physical findings. Audible wheezing is uncommon and occurs in no more than 15 per cent of patients.

Microembolization of the lungs with very small fibrin clots, platelet aggregates, aggregates of polymorphonuclear leukocytes, and perhaps particulate matter from dead tissue can all result in the sequence of clinical, physiologic, and roentgenographic abnormalities known as the adult respiratory distress syndrome (see Ch. 71). Factors are released that increase capillary permeability and lead to pulmonary edema, causing stiff lungs with poor ability to oxygenate blood.

Medium-sized pulmonary emboli can at times be relatively asymptomatic and recur over several months or years, leading to cor pulmonale with severe pulmonary hypertension and right heart failure. Whether cor pulmonale can result from recurrent very small emboli is controversial. Distinguishing recurrent small pulmonary emboli from primary pulmonary hypertension is difficult and requires an open lung biopsy. A familial occurrence or association with Raynaud's phenomenon favors primary pulmonary hypertension. The pulmonary hypertension usually does not improve with anticoagulation unless medium-sized pulmonary emboli can be detected with pulmonary angiography.

DIAGNOSIS. History and physical examination cannot adequately confirm or exclude acute pulmonary embolism, but several factors, if present, make the diagnosis unlikely: (1) no reasonable precipitating cause; (2) recurrent chest pain in the same location; (3) hemoptysis of more than 5 ml of blood without an infiltrate on chest radiograph; (4) recurrent hemoptysis; (5) temperature greater than 39°C; (6) pericardial as well as pleural friction rub; and (7) systemic hypotension without elevated neck vein pressure.

The clinical diagnosis of pulmonary embolism is frequently incorrect. When the clinical diagnosis of pulmonary embolism is made, no emboli are found at autopsy in two thirds of the patients; when emboli are found at autopsy, the diagnosis had not been suspected in two thirds of the patients. In patients clinically suspected of having the disorder, pulmonary angiography fails to demonstrate pulmonary emboli in 50 to 60 per cent. However, these studies did not record how strongly the diagnosis of pulmonary embolism was suspected. The clinical diagnosis is more accurate if three categories—high, intermediate, and low probability—are considered (see below).

The *differential diagnosis* of massive pulmonary embolism includes conditions that are associated with acute central chest pain and/or hypotension such as acute myocardial infarction, dissecting aortic aneurysm, severe left heart failure, and ruptured esophagus. Acute embolization of medium-sized pulmonary vessels without infarction can easily be confused with the hyperventilation syndrome, asthma, extrinsic allergic alveolitis, pleurodynia caused by coxsackievirus B, or serositis associated with connective tissue diseases. Acute pulmonary embolism with infarction frequently resembles lobar pneumonia, mucous plugging of a bronchus, lung cancer with postobstructive pneumonia, empyema, or tuberculous pleural effusion.

DIAGNOSTIC AIDS. ***Enzymes.*** Serum levels of enzymes such as lactic dehydrogenase, glutamic oxaloacetic transaminase, and creatine kinase are of no benefit in the diagnosis of pulmonary embolism.

Soluble Fibrin Complexes and Fibrin Degradation Products. Soluble fibrin complexes can indicate recent thrombin generation, and fibrin degradation products reflect recent plasmin generation. When pulmonary embolism is occurring, either thrombin generation or plasmin generation or both are likely to be occurring. Only about 3 per cent of patients with angiographically proven pulmonary embolism have both tests negative. Patients with positive angiograms have both tests positive 55 to 75 per cent of the time. Other conditions that can be confused with pulmonary embolism have both tests positive less than 10 per cent of the time. Thus finding both tests negative is strong evidence against the diagnosis of pulmonary embolism, whereas finding both tests positive adds strength to the diagnosis.

Arterial Blood Gases. About 85 per cent of patients with pulmonary embolism have a Pa_{O_2} on room air of less than 80 mm Hg. If the Pa_{O_2} is normal, pulmonary embolism is less likely than if the Pa_{O_2} were abnormal. Because of the frequent association of hyperventilation, which raises PA_{O_2} and lowers Pa_{CO_2}, the alveolar-arterial Po_2 differences (Aa_{DO_2}) is more likely to be abnormal than the values for arterial Po_2 alone. Unfortunately, most of the conditions with which pulmonary embolism is confused also have arterial hypoxemia or widening of the Aa_{DO_2}.

Electrocardiogram. With moderate-sized pulmonary emboli, the electrocardiogram usually shows only tachycardia or nonspecific findings. In massive pulmonary embolism, evidence of right axis deviation, right heart strain, or right bundle branch block pattern is frequently present. These changes may be transient and disappear within a few hours.

Pleural Fluid. The pleural effusion associated with pulmonary embolism may be an exudate or transudate, and there are no diagnostic pleural fluid findings in pulmonary embolism. Sixty-five per cent of the effusions are grossly bloody, and these are usually associated with infiltrates seen on the chest radiograph. Other than trauma or malignant neoplasm, there are very few other causes of grossly bloody pleural effusion. The major value of a thoracentesis is to exclude an empyema.

Chest Radiograph (Fig. 65–1A). Even though only about 10 per cent of pulmonary emboli produce infarction in autopsy studies, most patients have multiple pulmonary emboli, and therefore it is rare for a patient to have a normal chest radiograph. A totally normal chest radiograph is found with pulmonary embolism about 10 per cent of the time. Up to 75 per cent of patients with pulmonary emboli have an infiltrate. A pleural effusion is found in 45 per cent. Infiltrate and effusion can occur together or separately. Pleural effusions resulting from pulmonary emboli are very rarely bilateral even though the pulmonary emboli are usually bilateral. Other radiographic findings are elevation of the hemidiaphragm, areas of plate-like atelectasis, and occasionally areas of oligemia. Dilatation of the pulmonary artery, azygos vein, or superior vena cava can occur.

Perfusion Lung Scans. Perfusion lung scans are performed by the intravenous injection of technetium 99m-labeled macroaggregates of albumin, which diffusely embolize about 1 out of 1000 pulmonary capillaries. Images are obtained by measuring the gamma emission pattern from these trapped particles, whose distribution should accurately reflect pulmonary blood flow. The normal lung shows a homogeneous pattern of radio-

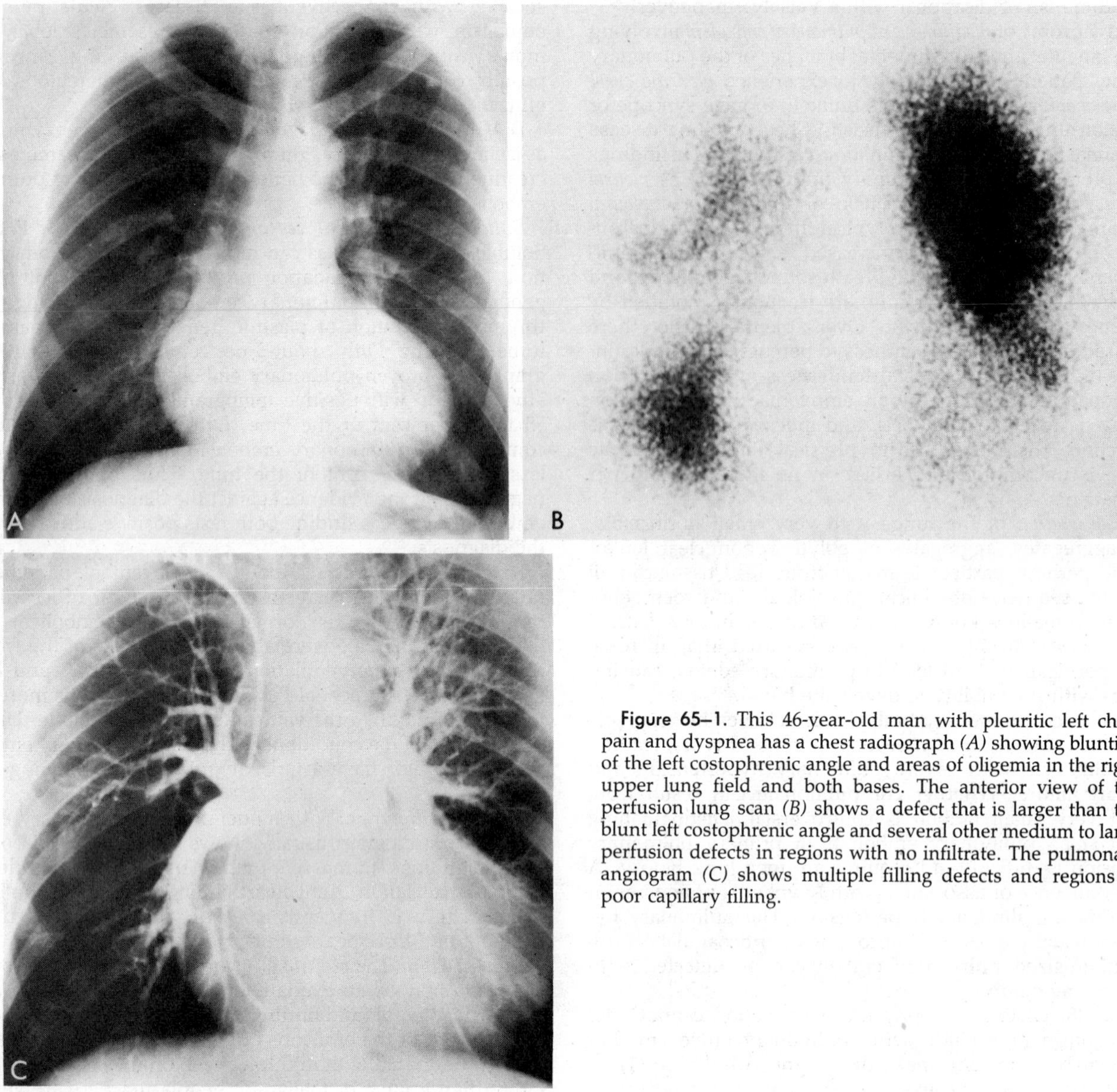

Figure 65–1. This 46-year-old man with pleuritic left chest pain and dyspnea has a chest radiograph *(A)* showing blunting of the left costophrenic angle and areas of oligemia in the right upper lung field and both bases. The anterior view of the perfusion lung scan *(B)* shows a defect that is larger than the blunt left costophrenic angle and several other medium to large perfusion defects in regions with no infiltrate. The pulmonary angiogram *(C)* shows multiple filling defects and regions of poor capillary filling.

activity with sharp margins which coincide with the topography of the lung. Multiple views from different projections are obtained to help confirm that a suspicious filling defect within the center of one view causes a concavity on the periphery of another appropriate view. *A good quality normal perfusion lung scan virtually eliminates the diagnosis of pulmonary embolism.* In experimental animal studies the ability of perfusion lung scans to detect small completely occlusive emboli 2.5 mm in diameter or less is better than for pulmonary angiography. Pulmonary angiography can detect small elongated emboli that do not completely occlude a vessel better than can perfusion lung scans. However, pulmonary emboli are usually multiple and bilateral, and both types of defects are generally present if the patient has pulmonary embolism.

Perfusion lung scans have adequate sensitivity. The problem is specificity. Any condition that causes a radiographic density within the lung fields or causes regional obstruction to ventilation can cause a perfusion lung scan defect. In general, the larger the defects, the sharper and the more multiple they are, and the greater the probability of pulmonary embolism. Some argue that the only usefulness of a perfusion lung scan is to exclude pulmonary embolism if the scan is normal, since pulmonary angiography must be performed if the perfusion lung scan has any abnormality and pulmonary embolism is suspected. Others are willing to use perfusion lung scan information combined with clinical probability or ^{133}Xe ventilation scans in the appropriate setting (see below). The perfusion lung scan always has to be interpreted in connection with a current chest radiograph, since almost any process causing a radiographic infiltrate results in a compensatory decrease in local perfusion. The chest radiographic findings along with the perfusion scan defects can be used to estimate the probability of pulmonary embolism independently of clinical information. Low probability patterns include (1) single or multiple small defects that are less than one fourth of a segment in size (about 3 or 4 cm in diameter) and usually have vague margins and (2) a perfusion defect that is substantially smaller than a radiographic infiltrate. Patterns of high probability for pulmonary embolism include two or more medium-sized defects or one large defect that is larger than a segment in size (Fig. 65–1*B*). All these defects must be either in an area of no radiographic abnormality or substantially larger than an infiltrate in the region of the defect. Any other findings, such as a single moderate-sized defect or defects that are the same size as is the radiographic density, fall into an intermediate probability category. Using these criteria, in the author's experience, pulmonary angiography confirms acute pulmonary embolism in 78, 38, and 10 per cent of high, intermediate, and low probability perfusion scans, respectively.

Perfusion Lung Scan Plus Clinical Assessment. A useful technique in the clinical diagnosis is to weigh the estimated probability of pulmonary embolism as high, intermediate, or low, similar to perfusion scan interpretations. The more important factors for judging the clinical probability of pulmonary embolism as high or low are shown in Table 65–1. Patients with intermediate clinical probability of pulmonary embolism are those who do not fit many of the criteria for high or low and frequently have another reasonable cause for their findings, such as postoperative atelectasis or pneumonia. In the author's experience the frequency of positive pulmonary angiograms associated with clinical probability assessments of high, intermediate, and low are 70 per cent, 45 per cent, and 10 per cent, respectively. Other published data are 78 per cent, 58 per cent, and 33 per cent, respectively. If the clinical assessment is made independently of the evaluation of the perfusion lung scan, the two sources of information can be combined by Bayes' theorem. Without going into the mathematics, a high probability perfusion scan is more likely to correctly identify pulmonary embolism and less likely to be falsely positive in a population of patients with a 70 per cent prevalence of pulmonary embolism than in a population with a 45 per cent or 10 per cent prevalence. Thus, if the clinical probability of pulmonary embolism is judged high and the perfusion scan pattern is also high probability, the overall probability of pulmonary embolism is raised to over 90 per cent. Similarly, if the clinical and the perfusion scan probabilities are both low, the overall probability of pulmonary embolism is less than 1 per cent. Other combinations of clinical likelihood and perfusion scan patterns do not adequately confirm or exclude pulmonary embolism, and pulmonary angiography is needed.

Perfusion Lung Scan Plus Ventilation Scan. Ventilation scans are expected to be normal or mismatched in the regions of perfusion defects due to pulmonary emboli and abnormal or matched in the regions of perfusion defects secondary to obstructive airways disease. However, recent studies show that ventilation scans with ^{127}Xe are frequently abnormal in regions with pulmonary emboli associated with large perfusion defects. Using ^{133}Xe, ventilation scans often have delayed washout in regions with small infiltrates on the chest radiograph. The ventilation scan may appear normal in regions with small perfusion defects due to obstructive airways disease because of the fact that ^{99m}Tc macro aggregates of albumin can detect a smaller perfusion defect than the lower energy gamma rays from ^{133}Xe can detect a ventilation defect. Thus, ventilation scans cannot reliably accomplish the thing that would be most helpful—to identify perfusion defects due to causes other than pulmonary emboli.

Perfusion Scan Plus Venography. In the setting of clinical suspicion of pulmonary embolism and a perfusion scan abnormality compatible with pulmonary emboli, a positive venogram confirms the diagnosis of venous thromboembolism. However, a negative venogram does not exclude pulmonary embolism, and pulmonary angiography is indicated when the diagnosis is uncertain. Venograms can be positive despite negative pulmonary angiograms. This suggests that perfusion scans can at times detect small emboli that are missed by pulmonary angiography, a fact already known from animal studies with artificial emboli. In the author's opinion, the combination of a clinical impression that pulmonary embolism is unlikely and a low probability perfusion scan adequately excludes pulmonary emboli, but in other settings both venography and pulmonary angiography may be necessary to adequately exclude pulmonary embolism. Satisfactory diagnostic endpoints are summarized in Table 65–2.

TABLE 65–1. CRITERIA FOR THE CLINICAL DIAGNOSIS OF PULMONARY EMBOLISM

Clinical Findings	Likelihood of Pulmonary Embolism High	Low
Reasonable precipitating cause	Yes	No
Typical symptoms and signs	Several	Few
$Pa_{O_2} < 80$ mm Hg	Yes	No
FDP and SFC*	Both positive	Both negative
Chest x-ray	Abnormal	Normal

*FDP = Fibrin degradation products; SFC = soluble fibrin complexes.

TABLE 65–2. ACCEPTABLE DIAGNOSTIC ENDPOINTS WITHOUT PULMONARY ANGIOGRAPHY

A. Pulmonary embolism is excluded
  1. Normal perfusion scan
  2. Low probability perfusion scan with
    a. low estimate of clinical likelihood of pulmonary embolisms or
    b. normal chest radiograph

B. Pulmonary embolism is confirmed
  High probability perfusion scan with
    a. high clinical likelihood or
    b. normal ventilation scan or
    c. positive venogram or impedance plethysmography

Pulmonary Angiography. Many patients (perhaps 50 per cent) suspected of having pulmonary embolism cannot have the diagnosis adequately confirmed or excluded by the criteria outlined above. Pulmonary angiography is the only alternative method now available to confirm or exclude emboli in these patients. Although not a perfect diagnostic tool, pulmonary angiography is considered the final denominator in the diagnosis of pulmonary embolus short of autopsy examination, since it supplies direct anatomic information about the pulmonary blood vessels.

In general the pulmonary angiogram may, within its powers of resolution, demonstrate three types of abnormalities in the pulmonary vasculature of patients with pulmonary emboli (Fig. 65–1C): (1) filling defects in the arterial system outlined by the radiopaque contrast material, (2) actual occlusions of pulmonary arterial vessels leading the abrupt "cutoffs," and (3) areas of segmental hypoperfusion in the lung. Standard pulmonary angiograms frequently miss small, completely occlusive emboli 2.5 mm in diameter or less, even though they can reliably detect more elongated nonocclusive emboli down to 1 mm in diameter. Because of this, standard pulmonary angiography gives equivocal results as much as 25 per cent of the time, probably even more often in the situations that lead to equivocal perfusion lung scans. These equivocal angiograms can usually be resolved if some augmentation technique is used, such as balloon-occlusion angiography, or magnification roentgenography with subselective injections, utilizing a small focal spot. Most authorities agree that *a negative pulmonary angiogram, utilizing augmentation techniques, reliably excludes pulmonary embolism.*

Other useful information can be obtained at the time of pulmonary angiography. The wedge pressure may indicate left heart failure rather than pulmonary embolism. The distance between the catheter tip and the cardiac silhouette may disclose a significant pericardial effusion. The degree of pulmonary hypertension gives information about the duration of pulmonary embolization. Acute pulmonary embolization rarely produces mean pulmonary artery pressures of 40 mm Hg because of the acute development of tricuspid insufficiency. Higher pressures suggest recurrent pulmonary embolism.

The benefits of confirming or excluding pulmonary emboli with as much reliability as is possible generally outweigh the small risk and morbidity (4 to 10 per cent) of pulmonary angiography: urticaria, a rare anaphylactic reaction, fever, wound hematomas, or arrhythmias. The arrhythmias are usually premature atrial or ventricular contractions or a right bundle branch block pattern and resolve spontaneously. Deaths, which have been reported as high as 0.4 per cent in a large series, largely occurred in the past from perforation of the right ventricle when stiffer catheters were being used.

Pulmonary angiography is dangerous in the face of severe pulmonary hypertension. Cardiac arrest frequently occurs. In these circumstances, if an angiogram is considered essential, a subselective injection should be done.

TREATMENT. ***Anticoagulation with Heparin.*** Without anticoagulation, recurrence rates of pulmonary embolism are between 30 and 50 per cent and up to half the recurrences are fatal. Therefore, a rapidly acting anticoagulant, intravenous heparin, is commonly utilized initially for ten days while starting an oral anticoagulant such as warfarin on the fifth day. Intermittent intravenous heparin has been reported to be associated with significantly more major bleeding complications (around 15 per cent) than has continuous intravenous heparin (around 1 per cent). Whether these differences are due to the method of administration or the total daily dose is not clear, since larger doses of heparin are required to keep an activated partial thromboplastin time (APTT) or a Lee-White clotting time in the range of 1.5 to 2.5 times normal by the intermittent route (approximately 36,000 units per day) than by the continuous route (approximately 25,000 units per day). However, a more recent study, which was restricted to patients with objective diagnostic tests confirming pulmonary embolism or deep venous thrombosis, has found a significantly higher recurrence rate with continuous heparin (27 per cent) than with intermittent heparin (3 per cent).

There are several important factors associated with increased risk for bleeding complications during therapy with intermittent heparin: (1) age greater than 60 years, (2) abnormal prothrombin time, APTT, or platelet count, (3) uremia, (4) alcoholic liver disease, (5) recent surgery (within two weeks), (6) previous gastrointestinal bleeding within six months, (7) severe systemic hypertension with diastolic pressure greater than 110, or (8) massive pulmonary embolism with severe pulmonary hypertension. If a patient with a risk factor for bleeding is to be treated with intermittent heparin, it is wise to use a lower dose and to keep the APTT or Lee-White clotting time no more than 1.5 times normal just before the next dose is due. If continuous heparin is used, larger doses should probably be used to push the activated APTT or Lee-White clotting time closer to 2.5 times normal. Higher doses may reduce the recurrence rate with continuous heparin but unfortunately will likely produce more major bleeding complications. Continuous heparin in an average dose of 33,000 units per day has been reported to have a major bleeding complication rate of 15 per cent.

Thrombolytic Therapy. In general, thrombolytic therapy is indicated only for pulmonary embolism massive enough to threaten life or to leave the patient with inadequate pulmonary reserve. Most pulmonary emboli lyse spontaneously to a large extent within two weeks, and anticoagulation therapy is adequate. Larger or massive emboli may require several months to lyse completely. On the other hand, the pulmonary capillary bed may be more fully restored with thrombolytic therapy than with heparin therapy. Thrombolytic therapy is more effective if the embolus is acute (symptoms less than 48 hours) and if it does not obstruct the vessel in which it is lodged. Thrombolytic therapy must not be utilized unless the diagnosis of massive pulmonary embolism is firmly established, preferably by angiography, and the risk factors for serious bleeding are fully assessed. The only absolute contraindications to thrombolytic therapy are (1) increased risk of intracranial bleeding such as a stroke within two months and (2) active bleeding. Relative contraindications include situations in which there are protective hemostatic plugs formed within the past two weeks such as with surgery, trauma, childbirth, biopsy in an inaccessible site, or external cardiac massage. If the benefit is potentially life saving, of course, this outweighs a relative contraindication to thrombolytic therapy.

Two agents are available for thrombolytic therapy, urokinase and streptokinase. Urokinase directly converts plasminogen to plasmin. It is not antigenic but is ten times more expensive than streptokinase. Streptokinase combines with plasminogen, and the streptokinase-plasminogen complex serves as the activator to convert other free plasminogen molecules to plasmin. It is antigenic in man and cross-reacts with antistreptococcal antibodies. A standard loading dose of 250,000 units of streptokinase given over 30 minutes is sufficient in over 90 per cent of patients, and is followed by a maintenance infusion of 100,000 units per hour for 24 hours. With urokinase the standard loading dose is 2000 CTA units per pound of body weight intravenously over ten minutes, followed by 2000 CTA units per pound of body weight per hour for 12 to 24 hours. Attempts to control the dose of thrombolytic therapy with laboratory tests have not helped avoid bleeding complications or improved the results of lysis.

A national cooperative study has compared urokinase followed by heparin with heparin alone in the treatment of angiographically proven pulmonary embolism. Within 24 hours urokinase resulted in significantly lower mean pulmonary artery pressures and total pulmonary resistance than did heparin and also gave significantly more improvement in the degree of lysis as judged by pulmonary angiography. By the fourteenth day the degree of lysis was virtually identical. The mortality rate was low with both forms of treatment and was not significantly different. However, in both massive embolism and in patients who were in shock with pulmonary emboli, the degree of lysis seen on repeated angiograms at 24 hours was impressively more with urokinase than with heparin. In a single small randomized prospective trial comparing heparin and thrombolytic therapy in life-threatening pulmonary embolism no significant difference in mortality was found, but patients treated with streptokinase had significantly more improvement in hemodynamics and degree of clot lysis (on repeat pulmonary angiography) than did patients treated with heparin alone. Thrombolytic therapy may produce lysis rapidly enough to allow some patients to survive who would have died without this additional treatment. When pulmonary embolism is extremely massive and angiograms show no capillary filling in more than 70 per cent of the pulmonary vascular bed, the drug may not be able to reach the emboli to cause lysis rapidly enough. Under these circumstances pulmonary embolectomy may be the only choice.

In the national cooperative trials, major bleeding complications with urokinase or streptokinase varied from 13 to 27 per cent. In subsequent experience, when invasive procedures have been more carefully avoided, major bleeding complications have been very infrequent. If major bleeding occurs, the thrombolytic therapy should be stopped and whole blood transfusion should be given. Epsilon-aminocaproic acid, an inhibitor of plasminogen activator, is needed very infrequently.

Pulmonary Embolectomy. Most patients with massive pulmonary embolism warrant a trial with thrombolytic therapy before pulmonary embolectomy is attempted. If there is a contraindication to or failure of thrombolytic therapy, the criteria for a pulmonary embolectomy should be (1) angiographic proof of obstruction of greater than 50 per cent of the pulmonary vascular bed with emboli that can be reached in the main, right, or left pulmonary artery; (2) hypotension persisting despite maximal medical therapy; and (3) evidence of decreased function of vital organs such as the brain or kidney. Pulmonary embolectomy, when performed as an extreme emergency, has a mortality rate of over 60 per cent. When embolectomy is performed as a semi-emergency according to the aforementioned guidelines, the mortality rate is closer to 25 per cent.

General Supportive Measures. Some patients require support of their deteriorating cardiovascular system by a continuous isoproterenol infusion and increased intravenous fluids to improve right-sided filling pressures. Isoproterenol, which has been shown to increase cardiac output and decrease pulmonary vascular resistance in massive pulmonary embolism, should be used cautiously at a rate of 0.5 to 5.0 μg per minute. In animal studies with experimental pulmonary emboli large enough to produce severe pulmonary hypertension, prostacyclin infusion has produced significantly increased cardiac output and Pa_{O_2}

and decreased pulmonary artery pressure, pulmonary vascular resistance, and dead space ventilation. The findings are best explained by reversal of pulmonary vasoconstriction. The effects of prostacyclin infusion in human pulmonary embolism have not been reported, but some improvement has been seen with hydralazine infusion. If the patient has a severe hypoxemia, intubation and ventilation with large tidal volumes as well as increased inspired oxygen tension may dramatically correct the hypoxemia.

Vena Cava Interruption. Anticoagulation is effective treatment for most pulmonary emboli, and vena cava interruption is rarely needed. The accepted indications are (1) an absolute contraindication to anticoagulation, (2) major bleeding or recurrence of embolism on effective anticoagulation, (3) recurrent pulmonary embolism leading to severe pulmonary hypertension, and (4) septic pulmonary emboli from an infected focus in the lower extremities or pelvis. Vena cava clips are usually recommended for the first two indications, and vena cava ligations are usually recommended for recurrent emboli or septic emboli. However, for septic emboli at times the combination of an effective antibiotic combined with cautious heparinization proves adequate. In severely ill patients, particularly those with congestive heart failure, the mortality rate with surgery for clips or ligation is prohibitive. Under these circumstances an umbrella inserted by means of a cutdown on the internal jugular vein or a filter introduced from the femoral vein into the vena cava may be used. Vena cava interruption procedures appear relatively effective for preventing death from massive embolism. However, large collateral channels develop, and eventual recurrence is not uncommon.

Long-Term Therapy. There are no randomized prospective trials comparing long-term anticoagulation with no anticoagulation following ten days of heparin therapy for pulmonary embolism. The best estimates are that oral anticoagulation produces its maximal benefit within the first six weeks, but is probably worthwhile for at least three months. Whether long-term anticoagulative regimens that are effective following acute deep venous thrombosis will be effective following acute pulmonary embolism is unknown. After 10 days of continuous intravenous heparin therapy of acute deep venous thrombosis, the following treatment regimens are effective with minimal bleeding complications: (1) Subcutaneous heparin every 12 hours with dose tailored to prolong APTT to 1.5 times normal six hours after injection. (2) Less intense oral warfarin with therapeutic goal of a simplastin prothrombin time of about 15 seconds with a control of 12 seconds. Oral anticoagulation with warfarin and the usual therapeutic goal of simplastin prothrombin time of about 20 seconds with control of 12 seconds is very effective in preventing recurrence of deep venous thrombosis but has major bleeding complications of about 4 to 12 per cent despite the best control possible. Low dose subcutaneous heparin in a dose of 5000 units every 12 hours following 10 days of continuing intravenous heparin for deep venous thrombosis has almost no bleeding complications but is associated with a recurrence rate of about 25 per cent. In recurrent deep venous thrombosis, low dose subcutaneous heparin and conventional oral anticoagulation with warfarin are frequently ineffective, with recurrence rates of over 25 per cent. In these patients antiplatelet drugs with aspirin* 1200 mg per day and dipyridamole* 100 mg per day significantly reduce recurrences. Whether the antiplatelet drug would be effective in recurrent pulmonary embolism despite oral anticoagulation is unknown.

PROGNOSIS. Most patients even with massive pulmonary embolism and hypotension will survive if given nothing but anticoagulation therapy. Considering all patients in whom pulmonary embolism is diagnosed and treated, the overall mortality rate is about 8 per cent. Factors that can be asssociated with massive pulmonary embolism and indicate a worse prognosis are hypotension (25 per cent mortality rate), a pulmonary angiogram showing absent capillary filling in over 70 per cent of the pulmonary vascular bed (33 per cent mortality rate), a concurrent cardiac arrest (45 per cent mortality rate), and severe elevations of right-sided pressures (as high as 90 per cent mortality rate).

The late prognosis for patients who survive initial treatment for pulmonary embolism is very good. Chronic cor pulmonale is rare. Overall recurrence rate is about 10 per cent, but patients rarely die because of the recurrence. Recurrence rate is less if there was a reversible precipitating cause, and is higher if the patient had already had a previous episode.

PREVENTION. Low dose subcutaneous heparin (5000 units twice per day) significantly reduces the incidence of deep venous thrombosis and deaths from pulmonary embolism associated with major surgery. Low dose heparin also appears to be effective following myocardial infarction, but not after operations that are more traumatic such as total hip replacement. Patients undergoing major surgery who are at high risk for developing venous thromboembolism should receive low dose heparin prophylactically. The high risk factors include age over 40 years, malignancy, marked obesity, varicose veins, and history of previous deep venous thrombosis or pulmonary embolism.

Bates ER, Crevey BJ, Sprague ER, Pitt B: Oral hydralazine therapy for acute pulmonary embolism and low output state. Arch Intern Med 141:1537, 1981. *A case report of dramatic decrease in PVR and increase in cardiac index following oral hydralazine in acute massive pulmonary embolism.*

Bregman RM, Wilson JE III, Hillis D, Christensen EE, et al.: Clinical assessment and ventilation imaging in the diagnosis of pulmonary embolism. Manuscript submitted. *Shows accuracy of clinical diagnosis of pulmonary embolism when guidelines are used to separate patients with high and low probability of pulmonary embolism. Shows that ventilation scans with* ^{133}*Xe frequently show delayed washout from regions with an incomplete pulmonary infarct and a small infiltrate due to angiographically proven pulmonary emboli. Shows that in prospective patients 75 per cent of patients with positive pulmonary angiograms had an infiltrate on the routine chest radiograph.*

D'Alonzo GE, Bowes JS, DeHart P, Dantzler DR: The mechanisms of abnormal gas exchange in acute massive pulmonary embolism. Am Rev Respir Dis 128:170, 1983. *Utilizes the technique of multiple inert gas elimination to confirm that the major cause of hypoxemia in acute pulmonary embolism in humans is true shunting.*

Hull R, Hirsh J, Jay R, Carter C, et al.: Different intensities of oral anticoagulation therapy in the treatment of proximal-vein thrombosis. N Engl J Med 307:1676, 1982. *Contains references for low dose and tailored dose subcutaneous heparin for long-term treatment of deep venous thrombosis. Shows the effectiveness and safety of low intensity therapy with warfarin.*

Hull RD, Hirsh J, Carter CJ, Jay RM, et al.: Pulmonary angiography, ventilation lung scanning and venography for clinically suspected pulmonary embolism with abnormal perfusion lung scan. Ann Intern Med 98:891, 1983. *Shows the accuracy of clinical diagnosis when stratified into high, intermediate and low probability. Shows that venograms are negative 30 per cent of the time with angiographically proven emboli. Shows that venograms are frequently abnormal when pulmonary angiograms are normal in setting of suspected emboli. Ventilation scans with* ^{127}*Xe show poor washout in large perfusion defect due to pulmonary emboli.*

Wilson JE III: Pulmonary embolism: Diagnosis and treatment. Clin Note Respir Dis 19:3 and 20:3, 1981. *Contains a complete set of references for the views expressed in this chapter except for references listed below.*

Wilson JE III, Bregman RM, Parkey RW: Heparin therapy in venous thromboembolism. Am J Med 70:808, 1981. *Demonstrates that continuous heparin therapy in acute pulmonary embolism and deep venous thrombosis is associated with a high recurrence rate. Shows that intermittent intravenous heparin is safe if there is no pre-existing risk factor for bleeding.*

66. FAT EMBOLISM SYNDROME

James E. Wilson III

Fat embolism of the lungs results from the impaction of particulate fat globules in the pulmonary circulation. After long bone fractures most patients develop fat embolism, but most do not develop the fat embolism syndrome, which includes the presence of at least one of three major symptoms: respiratory insufficiency, cerebral symptoms, or petechiae. For example, microscopic fat emboli can be detected in the femoral vein draining the operative site in virtually all patients undergoing a total hip replacement, but none of the patients develop the fat embolism syndrome. With fractures of the pelvis or long bones in the legs only 2 per cent of patients develop the overt fat embolism syndrome, but approximately half develop tran-

*Investigational use.

sient hypoxemia, often with thrombocytopenia, suggesting a subclinical fat embolism syndrome.

PATHOGENESIS. The pathogenesis of the fat embolism syndrome may be more complicated than the simple physical occlusion of arterioles by fat globules released from marrow. It may relate to the hydrolysis of the triglycerides by lipoprotein lipase, releasing free fatty acids which are considerably more toxic to the endothelium than the triglycerides themselves. The concentration of free fatty acids may be higher in the immediate vicinity of fat globules obstructing pulmonary arterioles or capillaries, producing additional chemical injury, complicated by platelet and fibrin thromboses.

Since many patients with fractures develop fat emboli, why do only a few develop the fat embolism syndrome? There is evidence that patients who develop the syndrome are constitutionally different from people with similar degrees of trauma who do not; they have significant abnormalities of carbohydrate and lipid metabolism and of coagulation, increased capillary fragility, and abnormal neurohumoral regulation in response to exercise stress. In particular, they have a higher incidence of elevated blood sugar or diabetic history and significantly higher levels of beta lipoproteins. Both the diabetic state and familial elevations of beta lipoproteins have been shown to be associated with abnormalities of platelet aggregation.

CLINICAL FEATURES. In the typical patient with the fat embolism syndrome *tachycardia* of 140 beats per minute, *tachypnea* of 30 to 40 breaths per minute, and *fever* up to 39°C are noted two or three days after a fracture. The patient may or may not appear cyanotic, rales may be heard, and *petechiae* are common, particularly around the axillary folds, the neck and upper chest, and the conjunctivae or optic fundi. The patient often develops restlessness or increasing irritability, which may progress to *delirium* or coma. Not every patient has all these findings. A reasonable approach to the diagnosis is to insist on one major feature and four minor features, along with demonstration of fat macroglobulinemia and hypoxemia.

The major features of the fat embolism syndrome are (1) respiratory insufficiency, (2) cerebral involvement, and (3) petechial rash. The minor features are (1) pyrexia, (2) tachycardia, (3) retinal changes, (4) jaundice, (5) renal changes, (6) anemia, (7) thrombocytopenia, and (8) elevated sedimentation rate. Fat globules can be demonstrated in venous blood with a cryostat technique or by filtering serum through an 8 micron Millipore filter and staining the filter for fat with a Sudan IV stain. In 100 patients with the fat embolism syndrome, the initial findings on admission were cerebral symptoms (usually drowsiness or confusion), 34 per cent; tachycardia and pyrexia, 29 per cent; respiratory dysfunction with dyspnea, tachypnea, or hemoptysis, 20 per cent; and petechial rash, 17 per cent. Recovery was complete in 77 patients and partial in seven. Sixteen patients died, eight from the fat embolism syndrome and eight from the trauma itself.

Three different syndromes of fat embolism have been described: (1) In the hyperacute response, death is due to systemic embolization of the brain or coronary arteries. (2) In the classic response, roentgenographic findings in the chest are variable, ranging from a normal pattern or patchy densities to linear streaks radiating out from the hilar region. About a third of the patients show frank pulmonary edema, yet their hypoxemia may be fully corrected by increasing the fraction of inspired oxygen to 40 per cent. Mild abnormalities of the prothrombin time and activated partial thromboplastin time (APTT) and platelet counts occur. (3) The third syndrome is the adult respiratory distress syndrome. These patients have acute pulmonary edema demonstrated radiographically and require an increase in FI_{O_2} to 60 per cent to correct hypoxemia. They have evidence of disseminated intravascular coagulation with thrombocytopenia, prolonged prothrombin time and APTT, lowered fibrinogin concentration, and elevations of fibrin degradation products. At autopsy, intra-alveolar hemorrhage, infiltration of macrophages and mononuclear cells, and platelet and fibrin aggregation within multiple capillaries and arterioles are found.

TREATMENT. The most important aspect of treatment is oxygen therapy. If more than 50 per cent oxygen is required, intubation of the patient is advisable so that positive end-expiratory pressure (PEEP) can be used. An optimal level of PEEP can usually be found that allows greater delivery of oxygen to the tissues at a lower inspired oxygen tension than without PEEP. Early treatment with corticosteroids, although unproved, may be beneficial. For example, when massive doses of methylprednisolone (30 mg per kilogram intravenously at eight-hour intervals) are used prophylactically in patients at high risk for fat embolism syndrome, there is significant improvement in the arterial oxygen tension and prevention of abnormalities of coagulation tests and platelet counts.

PROGNOSIS. The prognosis for the fat embolism syndrome is better than for most causes of the adult respiratory distress syndrome. In fat embolism syndrome the mortality rate is about 8 per cent, compared to about a 50 per cent mortality rate for most other causes of the adult respiratory distress syndrome.

Avikainen V, Willman K, Rokkanen P: Stress hormones, lipids, and factors of hemostasis in trauma patients with and without fat embolism syndrome. A comparative study at least one year after severe trauma. J Trauma 20:148, 1980. *This study shows reasons why some patients with severe trauma develop the fat embolism syndrome and others do not.*

Curtis AM, Knowles GD, Putnam CE, et al.: The three syndromes of fat embolism: Pulmonary manifestations. Yale J Biol Med 52:149, 1979. *In this study three syndromes of fat embolism are described.*

Gurd AR, Wilson RI: The fat embolism syndrome. J Bone Joint Surg 56B:408, 1974. *A reasonable standardized approach to the diagnosis is presented. Method for detecting fat macroglobules in venous blood is described.*

67. SARCOIDOSIS

D. Geraint James

DEFINITION. Sarcoidosis is a multisystem disorder of unknown etiology most commonly affecting young adults and presenting most frequently with bilateral hilar lymphadenopathy, pulmonary infiltration, and ocular and skin lesions. The diagnosis is established most securely when well-recognized clinicoradiographic findings are supported by histologic evidence of widespread epithelioid cell granulomas in more than one system. Markers of activity of the disease include a positive Kveim-Siltzbach skin test, an elevated level of serum angiotensin-converting enzyme (SACE), hypercalciuria and hypercalcemia, intrathoracic uptake of radioactive gallium, and abnormal cytology of bronchoalveolar lavage fluid.

The course and prognosis of the disorder correlate with the mode of onset; an acute onset usually heralds a self-limiting course with spontaneous resolution while an insidious onset may be followed by relentless progressive fibrosis.

Corticosteroids relieve symptoms, suppress granuloma formation (including the Kveim-Siltzbach skin test), normalize raised SACE levels, and neutralize gallium uptake.

ETIOLOGY. The cause remains unknown despite an extensive search to uncover an infective agent, an immunologic upset, an allergic mechanism, or a specific diathesis. Hypotheses therefore abound.

Infection. Sarcoidosis was long regarded as an odd form of tuberculosis, but there are crucial differences. Attempts have been made to detect granulomagenic components of various mycobacteria in sarcoid tissue without consistent success. Many claims have been made for infection due to fungi, viruses, and bacteria, but their occasional presence seems coincidental rather than causal.

Immunologic Derangement. Sarcoidosis is a lymphoproliferative disorder with evidence of depression of delayed-type hypersensitivity, activated thymus-mediated (T_4) helper cells, hyper-reactive B cells, and frequent circulating immune complexes. Could this be a background factor providing an infective agent or other antigenic insult with a salubrious soil? The immunologic abnormalities will be described further, below. Although sarcoidosis is characterized by multiple immunologic abnormalities, in general patients with this disease are not "immunocompromised hosts." In the absence of steroid therapy they are not at increased risk for the development of unusual fungal, mycobacterial, viral, or parasitic infections. It is true the mycetomas of *Aspergillus* are found not infrequently in the lungs of patients with advanced sarcoid lung disease, but the fungus does not disseminate as invasive aspergillosis.

Hypersensitivity. Claims have been made for such diverse regional contributory factors as pine pollen, peanut dust, clay eating, and chewing pine pitch. Beryllium and zirconium are known to produce sarcoid granulomas in sensitized individuals. Local environmental factors should not be overlooked, for they may provide the final of several provoking factors in a multicausal disorder.

Predisposition. Hormonal factors play some part, for erythema nodosum due to sarcoidosis commonly occurs in women in the childbearing years of life, during early pregnancy, and also in women taking the oral contraceptive pill.

Sarcoid arthritis and erythema nodosum are most likely to occur in persons who are HLA-B8, AI, CW7, and DR3. This predisposition is associated with a short course and good prognosis, whereas HLA-B13 is more likely to be associated with chronicity of the disease.

IMMUNOPATHOLOGY. ***Granuloma Formation.*** The sarcoid granuloma is a battleground between antigen and the cellular and humoral defenses of the body. Macrophages are stimulated by the antigenic attack and eventually coalesce into giant cells and epithelioid cell granulomas (Fig. 67–1, also Fig. 148–8). T helper cells are mobilized to this point of activity and cooperate with macrophages leading to B cell overactivity. Activated T_4 helper cells secrete interleukin-2, which leads to a clonal proliferation of the same T_4 cells to augment their presence at sites of activity (Fig. 67–1). This phenomenon does not include blood T lymphocytes and hence the relative anergy away from sites of activity. The T cells provide various lymphokines and the B cells produce immunoglobulins. The enzymes secreted by the granuloma include angiotensin-converting enzyme, lysozyme, glucuronidase, collagenase, and elastase. Calcitriol, the active form of vitamin D, may be formed in the granuloma as well. With aging, the granulomas are infiltrated by fibroblasts, and early fibrosis is recognized by increasing deposition of intracellular reticulin, which is gradually replaced by collagen. This in turn is transformed into structureless eosinophilic hyaline material.

Macrophages. At least three different types of macrophages collectively make up about two thirds of the cell population in the sarcoid granuloma. The periphery contains a large number of antigen-presenting interdigitating cells similar to those found in the lymph node paracortex and at the corticomedullary junction of the thymus. The center of the granuloma consists of epithelioid and giant cells, which are derived from macrophages. The third type, tissue histiocytes, are occasionally seen more diffusely distributed in the granuloma and not even restricted to the granuloma itself. There is evidence of synergism between the interdigitating cells and suppressor-cytotoxic T cells in the periphery of the granuloma and between the epithelioid cells with helper T cells in its center. It is possible that this cellular configuration may be important in the pathogenesis of sarcoidosis and other granulomatous diseases.

Lymphokines. The antigen-stimulated, activated macrophage, bearing cell-surface HLA DR^+ gene products, produces interleukin-1, which in turn activates T_4 helper-inducer cells to produce interleukin-2 (Fig. 67–1). This glycoprotein lymphokine is the T-cell growth factor that signals clonal proliferation in the lungs. It does not stimulate blood T lymphocytes. The

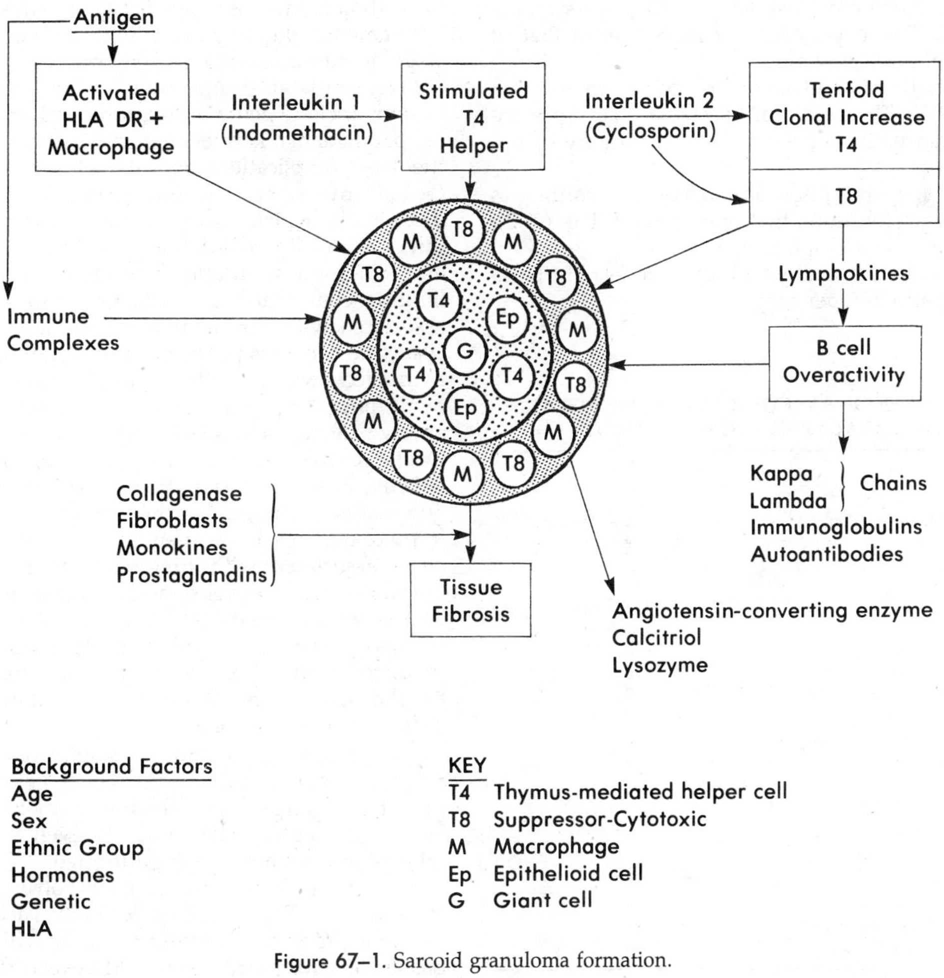

Figure 67–1. Sarcoid granuloma formation.

action of interleukin-1 on the T lymphocyte may call into play a prostaglandin-induced feedback mechanism that is inhibited by prostaglandin inhibitors. Interleukin-2 production is inhibited by Cyclosporin A. Several other soluble and secretory products play an important role in inhibiting macrophage migration away from the sarcoid battleground. These cellular relationships are of obvious importance in our slowly developing knowledge of the immunopathology of sarcoidosis.

EPIDEMIOLOGY. Although distributed worldwide, sarcoidosis occurs most frequently in sophisticated communities. Whenever tuberculosis and/or leprosy are rampant, sarcoidosis is in eclipse, but as they are brought under control sarcoidosis will become more evident. It has a similar prevalence in the Western World and Eastern Europe.

Sarcoidosis is ten times more frequent in American blacks than in the white population. It is a very common disorder in the black population of the Caribbean, particularly when they migrate to Europe. Likewise it is common in Puerto Ricans living in New York. Is this due to genetic predisposition or environmental factors confronting susceptible individuals migrating from a rural to an urban community? Is the breeding ground for sarcoidosis in his native environment or in the sophisticated new world to which he adapts? It may be a bit of both worlds.

Sarcoidosis is also becoming more evident in the black populations of Africa. Sarcoidosis is frequently seen in the white population of Scandinavia and Ireland and throughout Europe. It is well recognized in Japan, probably because they have a special commission searching for it. It is extremely rare in the rest of Asia, possibly because it is obscured by the presence of tuberculosis.

CLINICAL FEATURES. Some of the clinical features of 818 patients with clinical and histologic evidence of sarcoidosis attending the Royal Northern Hospital, London, are summarized in Table 67–1. This experience is comparable to that of other centers throughout the world.

Intrathoracic. Intrathoracic involvement occurs in fully 88 per cent of patients with sarcoidosis (Table 67–1). Approximately half of sarcoid patients present with respiratory symptoms.

It is customary to stage intrathoracic sarcoidosis according to the chest x-ray changes found on first presentation (Fig. 67–2):

Stage 0—Clear chest radiograph (14 per cent)

Stage 1—Hilar lymphadenopathy with or without right paratracheal adenopathy (65 per cent)

Stage 2—Hilar lymphadenopathy associated with pulmonary infiltration (22 per cent)

Stage 3—Pulmonary infiltration without hilar adenopathy (13 per cent)

This is a crude classification with much overlapping. Lung biopsy may unexpectedly reveal sarcoid granulomas in Stages 0 and 1. Stage 3 may be an indivisible radiologic mixture of irreversible fibrosis and reversible granulomas. Allowing for many shortcomings, this staging is simple and, most important, it is recognized and understood throughout the world. Some centers make refinements, such as adding Stage 4; this suggests an even more advanced stage than 3, with more irreversible fibrosis and perhaps evidence of complicating cor pulmonale. The prevalence of these radiographic findings at the time of diagnosis and their prognosis is shown in Table 67–2.

Sarcoidosis is a restrictive lung disease with abnormal gas exchange; its pathophysiology is similar to that of other interstitial lung disease, with decreased lung compliance and decreased lung volumes and capacities as the main features. There is diminished carbon monoxide diffusing capacity and increased alveolar-arterial oxygen gradient. The latter may cause hypoxemia at rest and this worsens with exercise. These tests are helpful in defining the functional impairment and in monitoring progress. However, quite often they do not correlate with the symptoms or signs, with the stage of chest x-ray abnormality, or with the immunologic upset. More rarely sarcoidosis may lead to airways obstruction as well as to restrictive disease and reductions in diffusing capacity.

The paucity of symptoms despite widespread radiographic changes distinguishes sarcoidosis from other interstitial lung diseases. Cough is an infrequent feature, and wheezing or bronchospasm points to segmental bronchial narrowing. Breathlessness suggests irreversible chronic fibrotic disease, and hemoptysis also indicates this late stage with secondary *Aspergillus* infection or cavitation or both. Pleurisy, pleural effusions, and finger clubbing are sufficiently infrequent that they should raise the possibility of an alternative diagnosis. Spontaneous pneumothorax is a rare complication of the late stage of chronic fibrotic sarcoidosis.

Eyes. Slit-lamp examination of the eyes should be routine. Lesions include acute and chronic iridocyclitis, choroidoretinitis, papilledema, keratoconjunctivitis, conjunctival follicles, and the late complications of cataract and secondary glaucoma. Ocular involvement is one manifestation of a multisystem disorder in which there are many clinical associations often interwoven into well-defined patterns of disease. Acute iritis, erythema nodosum, and hilar adenopathy have a benign self-limiting course and a satisfactory outcome. Lupus pernio is associated with chronic uveitis, pulmonary fibrosis, and bone cysts; the course is persistent and troublesome. Keratoconjunctivitis sicca, with or without parotid and lacrimal gland enlargement, mimics Sjögren's syndrome. Parotid gland enlargement, anterior uveitis, and facial palsy constitute *Heerfordt's syndrome.* Ocular sarcoidosis is discussed more extensively in Ch. 544.

Skin. *Erythema nodosum* is associated with bilateral hilar lymphadenopathy, polyarthralgia, and occasionally acute iritis. It predominates in women of the childbearing years and is often associated with pregnancy or lactation, suggesting a hormonal factor in its genesis. Transient circulating immune complexes may be detectable in this phase of sarcoidosis.

Lupus pernio is a chronic persistent violaceous lesion with a predilection for nose, cheeks, and ears. It reflects chronic fibrotic sarcoidosis. It develops insidiously and progresses indolently over the years.

Other skin lesions include persistent plaques, maculopapular eruptions, scars, and keloids. These keloids may be found at the sites of surgery, earpiercing, tattooing, repeated venesection in the antecubital fossa, or even where tuberculin and other skin tests have been performed.

Neurosarcoidosis. Sarcoidosis involves the nervous system in about 4 to 7 per cent of patients. Facial palsy is the most frequent presentation either alone or with other cranial nerve palsies or with papilledema. Other features include peripheral

TABLE 67–1. FEATURES OF SARCOIDOSIS IN THE ROYAL NORTHERN HOSPITAL SERIES OF 818 PATIENTS

Feature	Per Cent
Female	61
Presentation before age 40	74
Intrathoracic	88
Ocular	27
Skin lesions	
Erythema nodosum	34
Lupus pernio	4
Other skin lesions	14
Parotid enlargement	6
Splenomegaly	12
Hepatomegaly	10
Lymphadenopathy	27
Nervous system	9
Bone	3
Heart	3
Kidney	1
Upper respiratory tract	6
Hyperglobulinemia	31
Hypercalcemia	18
Skin tests	
Positive Kveim-Siltzbach	84
Negative tuberculin	70

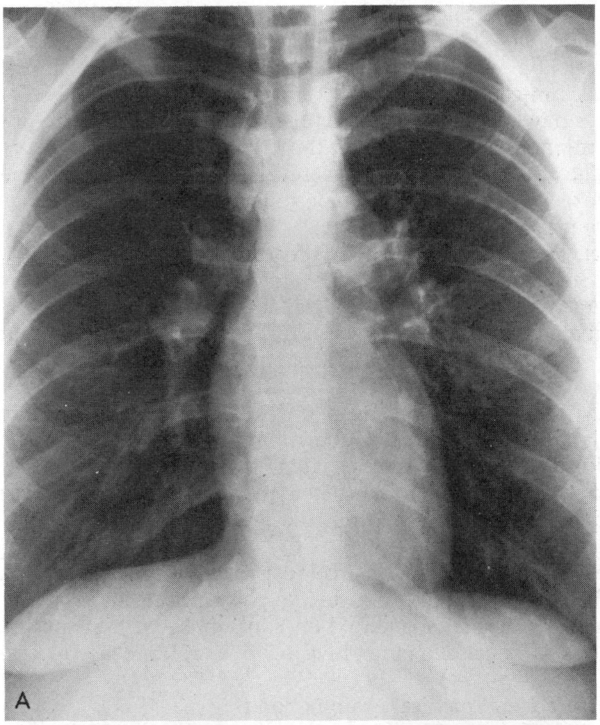

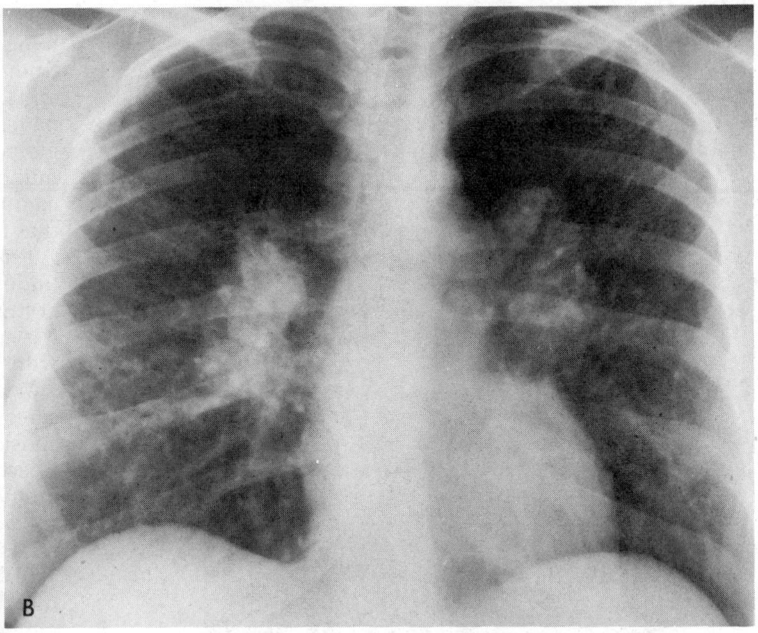

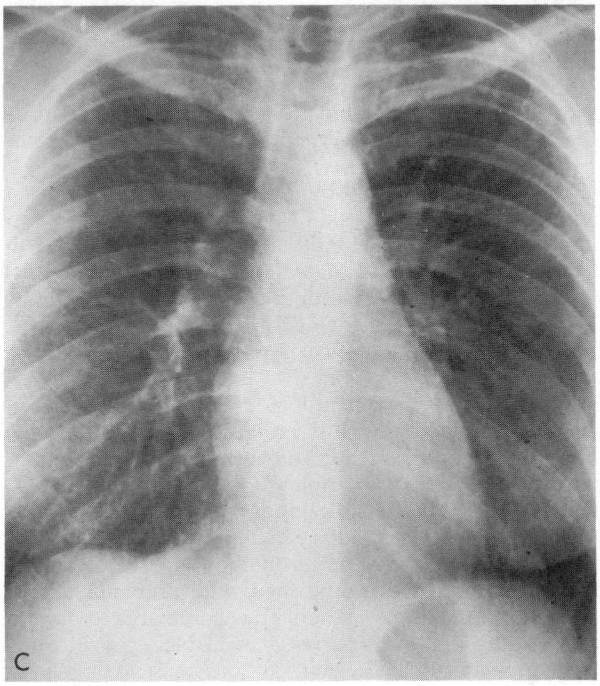

Figure 67–2. Chest radiographic stages of sarcoidosis. *A*, Stage I pulmonary sarcoidosis: Asymptomatic 24-year-old woman. A frontal chest radiograph shows moderate to marked bilateral hilar adenopathy. Enlarged right paratracheal and aortopulmonic window lymph nodes are also demonstrated. The lungs are normal. *B*, Stage II pulmonary sarcoidosis: 29-year-old woman with uveitis and skin lesions. A frontal chest radiograph shows marked bilateral hilar and mediastinal lymphadenopathy. The lungs are diffusely abnormal with a nodular and coarse linear pattern of disease. *C*, Stage III pulmonary sarcoidosis: 34-year-old black woman four years after a diagnosis of pulmonary sarcoidosis has been made. On a frontal radiograph the lungs are diffusely abnormal with a pattern of small, ill-defined nodules, indicative of pulmonary granulomas. Adenopathy is not present. (Courtesy of Gordon Gamsu, M.D., Department of Radiology, University of California, San Francisco.)

neuropathy, myopathy, meningitis, space-occupying lesions, epilepsy, cerebellar ataxia, hypopituitarism, and diabetes insipidus. Space-occupying granulomas and granulomatous meningitis may be associated with increased intracranial pressure and/or seizures. Lumbar puncture will often reveal CSF pleocytosis, increased protein, and, rarely, low glucose. Neurosarcoidosis has a mortality of 10 per cent, which is more than twice the overall mortality of sarcoidosis. The response to corticosteroids is more likely to occur in younger patients with an explosive onset of meningitis associated with erythema nodosum than in those with a space-occupying intracranial mass, chronic skin lesions, chronic uveitis, or pulmonary fibrosis.

TABLE 67–2. CHEST X-RAY CHANGES IN SARCOIDOSIS (ROYAL NORTHERN HOSPITAL SERIES OF 818 PATIENTS)

Stage at Presentation	Per Cent	Resolution of Abnormalities (per cent)
0	14	No abnormalities by definition
1	65	59
2	22	39
3	13	38

The Heart. Myocardial sarcoidosis is difficult to recognize clinically, although granulomas are found in the heart in about 20 to 25 per cent of all patients dying of sarcoidosis. It should be considered if a patient with florid multisystem sarcoidosis develops bundle branch block, arrhythmias, congestive cardiac failure, pericarditis, or clinical evidence of cardiomyopathy. Sudden death without previous evidence of a heart lesion may

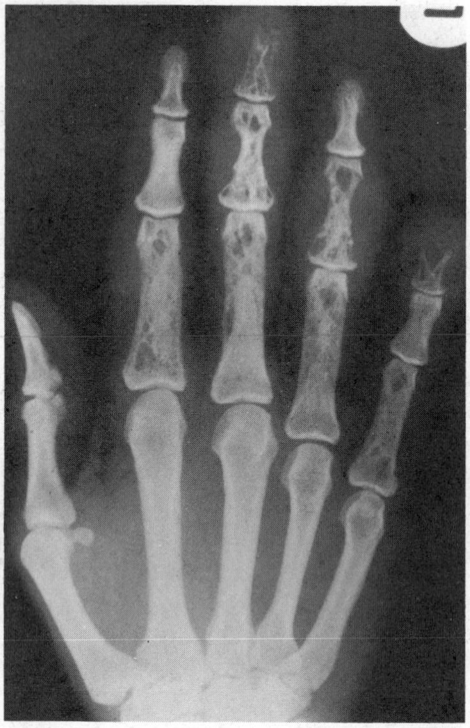

Figure 67–3. Sarcoidosis of bone. The hands show many areas of bone destruction with marked soft tissue swelling but with no periosteal reactions visible.

occur, particularly in patients over 40 years of age. Macroscopic changes are most evident in the posterior part of the ventricular septum. Microscopy discloses granulomas or fibrous tissue or an admixture. The most frequent cause of heart disease in sarcoidosis is probably cor pulmonale secondary to chronic lung disease.

Musculoskeletal. *Bone sarcoidosis,* the hallmark of chronic fibrotic sarcoidosis, occurs in 3 to 4 per cent of patients. It is most frequent in hands (Fig. 67–3) and feet, but rarely it involves temporal or frontal bone, the hard palate, and nasal cartilage. It is associated with soft tissue swelling, joint stiffness, and pain. There is no correlation between bone involvement and abnormal calcium metabolism.

Joint involvement reflected by polyarthralgia is experienced by one half of patients with erythema nodosum. It commonly occurs during the two weeks preceding or following the onset of erythema nodosum. It may occur up to six weeks before the appearance of the telltale eruption, and it is then most often mistakenly called rheumatic fever because of flitting joint pains, fever, sweating, and an elevated sedimentation rate (Ch. 556). Polyarthralgia subsides spontaneously in the course of one month; a nonsteroidal anti-inflammatory agent provides symptomatic relief. Chronic arthritis with joint stiffness, pain, and soft tissue swelling of hands and feet, is commonly associated with lupus pernio and bone cysts.

Muscle disease runs an independent course from bone disease but may be just as troublesome. It comprises acute polymyositis, chronic myopathy, muscle nodules, contractures, and atrophy.

Kidney. Renal involvement is diagnosed during life in only about 1 per cent of patients but is found in up to 20 per cent of patients by renal biopsy and necropsy studies. Three kinds of renal involvement have been described: (1) direct granulomatous involvement, (2) nephrocalcinosis and/or kidney stones, and (3) glomerulonephritis. Extensive granulomatous involvement may rarely produce marked interstitial nephritis and parenchymal destruction with modest proteinuria, nonspecific cylindruria, and sterile pyuria. This usually responds to glucocorticoid therapy. Patients with sarcoidosis have altered metabolism of vitamin D, to be described later, which often leads to enhanced absorption of intestinal calcium. Even in the absence of hypercalcemia there is often persistent absorptive hypercalciuria. These abnormalities may lead to renal failure from calcium nephropathy associated with nephrocalcinosis and calcium-containing kidney stones. Recently a number of patients have been described with sarcoidosis associated with glomerulonephritis, including the nephrotic syndrome. Immunofluorescence studies have revealed glomerular immune complexes, and the spectrum of lesions found closely resembles that found in lupus nephritis.

Fever. Fever is not a particular feature of sarcoidosis, except under certain circumstances. It almost always accompanies erythema nodosum, polyarthralgia, and hilar adenopathy, and it is equally self-limiting. It frequently occurs in the black patient with considerable hepatic involvement.

When fever is a prominent feature in a patient in whom sarcoid granulomas have been uncovered, then the primary consideration is to exclude tuberculosis, reticulosis, or fungal infection. When fever is associated with hepatic granulomas but no other features of multisystem sarcoidosis, then one must consider hepatic granulomatous disease (granulomatous hepatitis).

CLINICAL MANAGEMENT. Sarcoidosis usually presents during the 20 to 40 years age group to the chest physician, ophthalmologist, or dermatologist. When confronted with suspected sarcoidosis, the following investigative routine is recommended:

1. Full general medical examination (Fig. 67–4).
2. Slit lamp examination of the eyes, for otherwise silent lesions may be overlooked.
3. Chest radiography.
4. Serum calcium level, which is elevated in up to 20 per cent. It is also preferable to do routine 24-hour urine calcium levels, for hypercalciuria may occur despite normal serum calcium levels.
5. Histologic confirmation by fiberoptic bronchoscopy or biopsy of lymph node, skin, liver, minor salivary gland, nasal mucosa, gum, or muscle, or Kveim-Siltzbach skin test using a carefully validated antigen.
6. Serum angiotensin-converting enzyme, which offers a monitor of progress of the disease.
7. Tuberculin skin test, which is negative in two thirds of patients.
8. Special situations may include fluorescein angiography for suspected posterior uveitis, radioactive thallium for evidence of myocardial involvement, or CT scanning for neurosarcoidosis, for example.

CRITERIA OF ACTIVITY. In clinical practice, a method is needed to follow the activity of sarcoidosis in a given patient as a guide to prognosis and therapy. Such a method should be specific and reliable, reproducible around the world, preferably cheap, and sufficiently easy to permit serial measurements to monitor progress. No such method is currently available. As a substitute other measures are utilized. First, the progress of the clinical manifestations of the disease in the individual patient may be followed, including changes in the chest x-ray. Chemical changes include hypercalcemia and hypercalciuria or elevation of angiotensin convertase. Abnormalities in pulmonary function tests, as described earlier, may be particularly useful to follow. There are four methods to determine activity of sarcoidosis that are useful: (1) measurement of serum angiotensin–converting enzyme activity, (2) radioactive gallium scanning of the lung, (3) examination of cellular and humoral components obtained by bronchoalveolar lavage, and (4) the Kveim-Siltzbach skin test.

Serum Angiotensin Converting Enzyme (SACE). SACE is an enzyme normally found in the endothelial cells of pulmonary capillaries. It is also abnormally synthesized and released by some cellular element of sarcoid granulomas, quite possibly the macrophage or epithelioid cell. SACE is elevated in about 60 per cent of patients with active sarcoidosis, and levels tend to

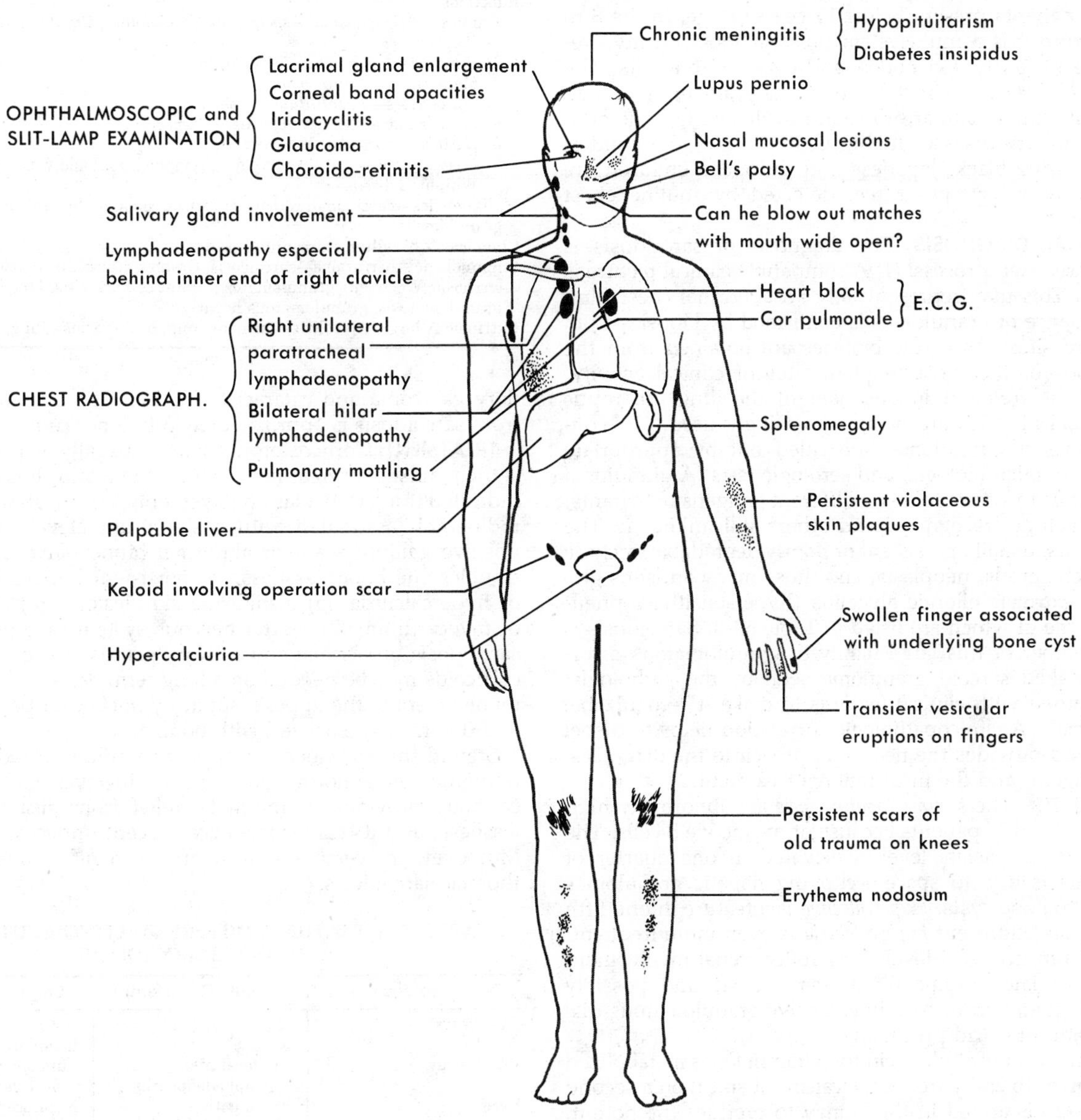

Figure 67–4. Clinical examination of a patient with suspected sarcoidosis.

return toward normal with spontaneous or glucocorticoid-induced remissions. SACE is also associated with a false-positive rate of about 10 per cent, however, and therefore is not a good diagnostic test. Its true value is to monitor progress of known sarcoidosis. In this respect it is a more sensitive index of activity of epithelioid cell granulomas than the chest radiograph. Its introduction should reduce the number of chest radiographs done, particularly since many are unnecessary. It is an invaluable monitor in pregnancy.

Radioactive Gallium Scanning. The activated macrophages in granulomas avidly accumulate gallium and delineate the extent of granulomatous involvement in lungs and hilar lymph nodes. Gallium is taken up by liver, spleen, and bone in the normal person, so it is not helpful in detecting granulomas in the abdominal viscera or in the central nervous system. Lung uptake is crudely measured by comparison with the density of liver uptake. Radioactive gallium is also taken up by protein of inflammatory exudates, so it is not specific for sarcoidosis. Positive scans are found in asbestosis, silicosis, fibrosing alveolitis, cancer, bleomycin lung, and lymphomas. Its value, like SACE, is as a monitor of progress. Its drawback is its cost, which would be prohibitive in many centers.

Bronchoalveolar Lavage (BAL). Bronchopulmonary lavage with about 100 to 300 ml of fluid provides specimens that can be measured for alveolar macrophages, lymphocytes, T and B cells, angiotensin-converting enzyme, lysozyme, protein, complement, and immunoglobulins. The more active the pulmonary disorder, the richer the yield and the more interesting the differential diagnosis. Findings differ in various interstitial lung disorders. At present this is a research procedure confined to centers, but it seems to offer promise of more widespread utilization in the future.

PREGNANCY. Sarcoidosis is not a contraindication to pregnancy. In fact, most patients improve and are able to abandon steroid therapy during the second trimester. Chest radiography is unnecessary until after delivery and also inadvisable during pregnancy. After delivery there is sometimes a relapse and recurrence of sarcoidosis during the first six months after parturition, so a chest radiograph should be done within six months of childbirth. During pregnancy, vitamin preparations containing vitamin D should be used sparingly because of the excessive activation of vitamin D in sarcoidosis. It is also worth checking the serum calcium levels during pregnancy. Progress of sarcoidosis during pregnancy and after delivery is best monitored by serum angiotensin-converting enzyme levels.

CHILDHOOD. Sarcoidosis is infrequent in childhood; only 4 per cent of patients present below 15 years of age. In the 8 to 15 years group it is a multisystem presentation with involvement of the lungs, lymph nodes, and eyes, as in adults. The picture is a different one in children aged 4 years and younger; they present with a rash, arthritis, and uveitis without demonstrable pulmonary disease. In the United States the child is most likely to be black. Japanese and European children are more likely to be symptom-free, detected by routine chest radiography.

DIFFERENTIAL DIAGNOSIS. The diagnosis of sarcoidosis is usually a three-step process: (1) A compatible clinical picture is established. This may represent only an abnormal chest film. (2) The presence of granulomas is confirmed by biopsies from one or more sites. As a rule biopsies are obtained from the most obvious or the most frequent sites of clinical activity. Because of the frequent involvement of the lung, fiberoptic transbronchial biopsies are being increasingly used. (3) Nonsarcoid causes of granulomas are ruled out by appropriate histochemical, microbiologic, and serologic tests. A granuloma is a nonspecific response to many different antigens or irritants, some of which are recognized and others still unknown. The inciting agents, usually persistent or poorly degradable, include infections, chemicals, neoplasia, and those many antigens giving rise to extrinsic allergic alveolitis (hypersensitivity pneumonitis), some of which are listed in Table 67–3. Sarcoidosis is but one member of this large family of granulomatous disorders. The naked sarcoid granuloma seen by the pathologist must be clothed with clinical features to make it recognizable to the clinician. A clinicopathologic correlation helps to dispel confusion and provides the nearest approach to the diagnosis, the causal agent, and the most rational treatment.

BIOCHEMISTRY. The *serum globulin levels* are abnormally high in about one third of patients because of overactive B cells. The *serum alkaline phosphatase* level is elevated in one quarter of patients; this is due to space-occupying hepatic granulomas rather than to bone cysts. *Hypercalcemia* is a feature in one fifth of patients, and transient *hypercalciuria* is even more frequent. Elevated serum uric acid levels may reflect renal involvement at a stage of late chronic fibrotic sarcoidosis and possibly increased degradation of cells in extensive granulomatous disease, releasing uric acid precursors.

The natural form of cholecalciferol (vitamin D_3) is metabolized first in the liver to 25-hydroxycholecalciferol and then a second hydroxy group is added in the kidney to produce the potent, highly active 1,25-dihydroxycholecalciferol (calcitriol) (see Ch. 244). Calcitriol causes increased intestinal calcium absorption and in excess leads to hypercalcemia and hypercalciuria. For reasons that are unclear, patients with sarcoidosis tend to have excessive conversion of 25-hydroxycholecalciferol to 1,25-hydroxycholecalciferol. In sarcoidosis, this enhanced synthesis can be induced by sunlight; it is reversed by steroid therapy. Calcitriol levels correlate with hypercalciuria rather than with hypercalcemia or with parathormone levels (which tend to be secondarily suppressed). There may be extrarenal generation of calcitriol in sarcoid tissue itself, and particularly in activated macrophages, since the abnormality has been shown to persist following bilateral nephrectomy in a patient with sarcoidosis.

COURSE AND PROGNOSIS. There are two distinct forms of sarcoidosis—acute and chronic—with clear-cut differences in onset, natural history, course, prognosis, and response to treatment (Table 67–4). Acute sarcoidosis has a high incidence of spontaneous remission. Chronic sarcoidosis has an insidious onset and a persistent or relapsing chronic fibrotic course with certain well-defined complications. They are pulmonary fibrosis followed by cor pulmonale and both respiratory and cardiac failure. Death may also occur from central nervous system involvement. Abnormal calcium metabolism may lead to nephrocalcinosis and renal failure. Myocardial sarcoidosis may cause sudden death. Chronic uveitis may be complicated by secondary glaucoma and cataract formation. The overall death rate from sarcoidosis is approximately 3 to 5 per cent.

TABLE 67–3. A CLASSIFICATION OF GRANULOMATOUS DISORDERS (A PARTIAL LISTING)

Infections
1. Fungi—*Histoplasma, Aspergillus, Coccidioides, Cryptococcus, Blastomyces*
2. Protozoa—*Leishmania, Toxoplasma*
3. Metazoa—*Toxocara, Schistosoma*
4. Spirochetes—*T. pallidum*
5. Mycobacteria—*M. tuberculosis, M. leprae*
6. Bacteria—*Brucella, Yersinia*
7. Miscellaneous—cat scratch fever, lymphogranuloma venereum, Whipple's disease

Malignancies—carcinoma, reticulum cell sarcoma, malignant nasal granuloma

Chemicals—beryllium, zirconium, starch

Immunologic Aberrations—sarcoidosis, Crohn's disease, primary biliary cirrhosis, Wegener's granulomatosis, giant cell arteritis, lymphomatoid granulomatosis, granulomatous hepatitis

Extrinsic Allergic Alveolitis—farmer's lung, bird fancier's lung, etc.

TREATMENT. Corticosteroid therapy, usually as prednisolone, is the mainstay of treatment around the world. It is particularly indicated for (1) ocular involvement, (2) an abnormal chest radiograph associated with a significant elevation of SACE, positive gallium scan, or abnormal bronchoalveolar fluid, (3) troublesome breathlessness, (4) persistent hypercalcemia and/or hypercalciuria, (5) disfiguring skin lesions, (6) involvement of myocardium, (7) central nervous system sarcoidosis, or (8) sarcoidosis of lacrimal and salivary glands. More rarely glucocorticoids may be needed on a long-term basis for troublesome involvement of the upper respiratory tract or for pain, swelling, and deformity associated with bone cysts.

Steroid therapy does not appear to influence radiologic resolution of the abnormal chest x-ray. However, steroid therapy certainly provides symptomatic relief from disabling breathlessness, and its earlier use may prevent unnecessary fibrosis. Moreover, it overcomes most of the manifestations of extrathoracic sarcoidosis.

TABLE 67–4. FEATURES DIFFERENTIATING ACUTE FROM CHRONIC SARCOIDOSIS

Sarcoidosis	Acute (Transient)	Chronic (Persistent)
Age (years)	< 30	> 40
Onset	Abrupt	Insidious
Chest x-ray	Bilateral hilar lymphadenopathy	Pulmonary infiltration/fibrosis
Eyes	Acute iritis, conjunctivitis, conjunctival nodules	Keratoconjunctivitis, chronic uveitis, glaucoma, cataract
Skin	Erythema nodosum, vesicles, maculopapular rash	Lupus pernio, plaques, scars, keloids
Parotitis Lymphadenopathy Splenomegaly Bell's palsy	Usually transient	Sometimes permanent
Bone cysts	No	Yes
Histology	Epithelioid and giant cells	Hyaline fibrosis Interstitial pneumonitis
Calcium metabolism	Hypercalcemia, hypercalciuria	Nephrocalcinosis
Kveim-Siltzbach test	Positive	May be negative
Tuberculin test	Negative	±
Gallium-67 uptake	High	Low
Angiotensin-converting enzyme	High	May be raised
Serum lysozyme	Increased	May be increased
Alveolitis as judged by bronchoalveolar lavage	High intensity	Low intensity
Spontaneous remission	Frequent	Rare
Steroid therapy	Abortive effect	Symptomatic relief
Alternative drugs	Oxyphenbutazone	Chloroquine: Potaba methotrexate
Recurrence after steroid therapy	Rare	Frequent
Prognosis	Good	Poor

Treatment of ocular involvement requires special consideration. The inflamed iris is rested by local atropine eye drops to maintain a dilated pupil. Topical corticosteroid eye drops applied frequently during the day and corticosteroid eye ointment at night may be sufficient to control anterior uveitis. If there is no substantial improvement in one week, then a local subconjunctival injection of triamcinolone is helpful. Oral prednisolone (40 mg daily for three months) is indicated if local treatment does not lead to a rapid response or if ophthalmoscopy reveals posterior uveitis. A raised intraocular pressure on local steroid eye drops is a signal to switch to fluoromethalone eye drops, which are least likely to cause a rise in pressure, and also to consider Timoptic eye drops, which will return the intraocular pressure to normal.

ALTERNATIVE REGIMENS. Steroid therapy may be contraindicated or may need reinforcement. Alternative drugs include indomethacin and oxyphenbutazone for acute exudative disease and methotrexate and chloroquine for chronic fibrotic persistent sarcoidosis. Once-weekly methotrexate is most helpful in overcoming chronic skin lesions, including lupus pernio.

Cyclosporin A is a fungal metabolite with interesting immunosuppressant properties. It acts selectively on T helper cells, interfering with interleukin-2 production and thereby preventing organ rejection. It exerts profound effects on experimental epithelioid cell granulomas, preventing the formation of the granulomas or the development of caseous necrosis. Its value in sarcoidosis is being assessed.

Brown JK, Ludmer P: New and old concepts in sarcoidosis. Medical Staff Conference, University of California, San Francisco. West J Med 138:546, 1983. *This is a brief but excellent general review of current concepts of pathogenesis, diagnosis, and treatment of sarcoidosis.*

Crystal RG, Roberts MC, Hunninghake GW, Cadek JE, Fulmer JD, Line BR: Pulmonary sarcoid: A disease characterized and perpetuated by activated lung T-lymphocytes. Ann Intern Med 94:73, 1981.

James DG, Jones Williams W: Immunology of sarcoidosis. Am J Med 72:5, 1982. *A review of immunology.*

James DG, Jones Williams W: Sarcoidosis and Other Granulomatous Disorders. Philadelphia, W. B. Saunders Company, 1984. *A new textbook.*

James DG, Neville E, Siltzbach LE, Turiaf J, et al.: A worldwide review of sarcoidosis. Ann NY Acad Sci 278:321, 1976. *A bird's eye view of sarcoidosis around the world.*

Mason RS, Frankel T, Chan Y-L, Lissner D, Posen S: Vitamin D conversion by sarcoid lymph node homogenate. Ann Intern Med 100:59, 1984. *This interesting study documents the synthesis of calcitriol by tissue preparations from sarcoid nodes.*

Mishra BB, Poulter LW, Janossy G, James DG: The distribution of macrophage and lymphocyte subsets in the sarcoid and Kveim test granulomas. Clin Exp Immunol 54:705, 1983.

Modlin RL, Hofman FM, Meyer RP, Sharma OP, Taylor CR, Rea TH: In situ demonstration of T-lymphocyte subsets in granulomatous inflammation. Clin Exp Immunol 51:430, 1983.

Pinkston P, Bitterman PB, Crystal RG: Spontaneous release of interleukin-2 by lung T-lymphocytes in active pulmonary sarcoidosis. N Engl J Med 308:793, 1983.

Studdy P, Bird R, James DG, Sherlock S: Serum angiotensin-converting enzyme in sarcoidosis and other granulomatous disorders. Lancet 2:1331, 1978.

68. NEOPLASMS OF THE LUNG

Leo F. Black

The lung may be the site of many types of neoplasms. Primary and metastatic malignancies involving the lung are common clinical problems. The classification of primary lung neoplasms by the World Health Organization is shown in Table 68–1. Groups I through V constitute approximately 90 per cent of the primary lung neoplasms and are commonly designated bronchogenic carcinomas. Benign tumors such as hamartomas, lipomas, and papillomas occur infrequently compared with malignant tumors.

TABLE 68–1. WORLD HEALTH ORGANIZATION CLASSIFICATION OF PRIMARY LUNG NEOPLASMS

I.	Epidermoid carcinomas	
II.	Small cell anaplastic carcinomas	
	1. Fusiform cell type	
	2. Polygonal cell type	
	3. Lymphocyte-like ("oat-cell") type	
	4. Others	
III.	Adenocarcinomas	
	1. Bronchogenic	
	a. Acinar	with or without mucin formation
	b. Papillary	with or without mucin formation
	2. Bronchiolo-alveolar	
IV.	Large cell carcinomas	
	1. Solid tumors with mucin-like content	
	2. Solid tumors without mucin-like content	
	3. Giant cell carcinomas	
	4. "Clear" cell carcinomas	
V.	Combined epidermoid and adenocarcinomas	
VI.	Carcinoid tumors	
VII.	Bronchial gland tumors	
	1. Cylindromas	
	2. Mucoepidermoid tumors	
	3. Others	
VIII.	Papillary tumors of the surface epithelium	
	1. Epidermoid	
	2. Epidermoid with goblet cells	
	3. Others	
IX.	"Mixed" tumors and carcinosarcomas	
X.	Sarcomas	
XI.	Unclassified	
XII.	Mesotheliomas	
	1. Localized	
	2. Diffuse	
XIII.	Melanomas	

BRONCHOGENIC CARCINOMA

DEFINITION. Lung cancer is now the leading cause of cancer deaths in men and is the second leading cause of cancer deaths in women, after cancer of the breast. Bronchogenic carcinoma occurs most frequently between the ages of 45 and 75 years, and there is a male-to-female preponderance of about 2.3:1. The incidence of the various histologic types of bronchogenic carcinoma varies in several reported series. Adenocarcinoma is now the most common cell type of bronchogenic carcinoma with an incidence of 30 per cent. The incidence of squamous or epidermoid carcinoma is 25 to 30 per cent, small cell carcinoma 20 to 25 per cent, and large cell carcinoma 10 to 20 per cent.

ETIOLOGY AND PATHOGENESIS. The major known factor in the development of bronchogenic carcinoma is the inhalation of carcinogenic pollutants, especially tobacco smoke, by susceptible hosts. Epidermoid and small cell anaplastic carcinomas have been most closely associated with cigarette smoking. Three principal types of changes related to smoking have been described in the respiratory epithelium: a loss of cilia, an increase in the number of cell rows, and the presence of atypical cells. Each of these three changes increases with increased amounts of cigarette smoking. Epithelial lesions are much more frequent in cigarette smokers than in pipe and cigar smokers. Eventually, the columnar epithelial lining is replaced by metaplastic squamous epithelium. Subsequently, atypical proliferation, dysplasia, and carcinoma develop. When carcinomatous change is present and located above the basement membrane, the lesion is referred to as carcinoma in situ. Invasive epidermoid carcinoma is the end result of this progression. Ex-smokers have fewer hyperplastic epithelial cells and also fewer cells with atypical nuclei than do current smokers. The number of such cells decreases progressively as the number of years of nonsmoking increases, although they do not reach the level seen in never-smokers. In parallel the incidence of bronchogenic carcinoma decreases in ex-smokers compared with current smokers, although not reaching the incidence level in never-smokers.

Host factors must be important in the development of this disease, since many smokers do not develop lung cancer. Indeed, there is a significant excess mortality from lung cancer among relatives of patients with lung cancer that cannot be accounted for by smoking. There appears to be a synergistic interaction between the familial and smoking factors, the nature of which has not been determined.

Lung cancer occurs more frequently in association with certain other environmental exposures. Higher mortality rates from lung cancer occur in heavily industrialized areas, where air pollution is characterized by elevated concentrations of benzo*(a)*pyrene and other polynuclear aromatic hydrocarbons. The incidence of lung cancer is increased in both smoking and nonsmoking asbestos workers. The effects of smoking and asbestos exposure appear to be multiplicative rather than additive, since the incidence of carcinoma is much higher in people exposed to both risk factors than in those exposed to either risk factor alone. The relative risk for the development of cancer also depends on the type of exposure and the type of asbestos fiber involved.

Workers in uranium mines have an increased incidence of lung cancer which cannot be explained solely by smoking. The histologic types of these cancers are mainly epidermoid and small cell anaplastic carcinomas. An increased incidence of lung cancer has been reported in male workers exposed to chloromethyl methyl ether. Most were smokers, but some had never smoked. These tumors were predominantly small cell anaplastic carcinomas. Other occupations in which an increased incidence of lung cancer has been reported include those in which workers are exposed to chromium, arsenic, nickel, and mustard gas.

Lung cancer, especially adenocarcinoma, may develop in areas of pulmonary fibrosis or scars. Such lesions may result from proliferating epithelial changes that are sometimes associated with chronic inflammation in the pulmonary parenchyma.

CLINICAL MANIFESTATIONS. The clinical manifestations of bronchogenic carcinoma may be related to the primary lesion, extension of the tumor beyond the lung parenchyma, distant metastasis, and syndromes produced by systemic nonmetastatic effects of the neoplasm (Table 68–2). Many patients with lung cancer are asymptomatic when the pulmonary lesion is discovered.

Symptoms Due to the Primary Lesion. *Cough* is a common symptom of lung cancer, and it may be a particularly troublesome symptom when the lesion is located near the carina. In smokers a change in the character of a chronic cough may signal the development of the new lesion. *Sputum production* commonly accompanies the cough. The amount is generally small. Profuse expectoration may at times result from the presence of a diffuse bronchiolo-alveolar cell carcinoma, but even with this tumor large amounts of sputum are unusual. *Hemoptysis* occurs frequently owing to ulceration of the primary bronchial lesion. Usually, this is in the form of blood streaking of the sputum. Occasionally, the bleeding is more vigorous, as small blood vessels are eroded by the tumor. Massive hemoptysis leading to death occasionally occurs in advanced disease when the neoplasm erodes into a large blood vessel. *Dyspnea* may result from the primary tumor, an associated disease, or a combination of both. When lung function is otherwise normal, dyspnea may develop when the neoplasm involves a main bronchus and compromises ventilation to one lung or when it has spread extensively within the thorax. Frequently, patients have associated chronic obstructive pulmonary disease, and this process is a factor in the development or worsening of dyspnea. The onset of dyspnea may be associated with the development of a *pleural effusion* resulting from the neoplasm, and at times this occurs when the primary neoplasm is small but has spread extensively to the pleural space. Rarely, a primary lung neoplasm may be associated with the development of a pneumothorax, leading to an acute episode of dyspnea.

Fever and chills resulting from pneumonitis may occur secondary to a bronchogenic carcinoma. The tumor may produce partial or complete bronchial obstruction, leading to an obstructive pneumonitis or atelectasis. Any patient with recurrent pneumonitis or an unresolved pneumonitis should be evaluated for the possibility of a bronchial neoplasm. *Loss of weight* is a frequent symptom of bronchogenic carcinoma but generally occurs with more extensive disease beyond the time when the neoplasm is limited to the lung parenchyma. *Wheezing* occasionally may be the primary complaint of the patient when the primary bronchial lesion has narrowed a major airway to the degree that air flow and removal of secretions are impaired.

Symptoms Due to Local Extension. *Chest pain* may be due to pleural involvement by the tumor or to direct involvement of the ribs and chest wall (Fig. 68–1). The pain may have pleuritic qualities or may be dull and boring in character. *Dysphagia* may result from invasion or compression of the esophagus by a tumor that has spread into the mediastinum. *Hoarseness* is usually due to involvement of the recurrent laryngeal nerve owing to extension of a tumor from the left lung. *Superior vena caval compression or obstruction* results from mediastinal extension of a tumor. This produces edema of the face, neck, and upper extremities, along with a dilated superficial venous pattern in these areas. Some of these patients complain of headache and dizziness or vertigo. Neoplasms at the extreme apex of the

TABLE 68–2. CLINICAL MANIFESTATIONS OF CARCINOMA OF THE LUNG

1. *Due to primary lesion*	
Cough	Fever and chills
Sputum production	Loss of weight
Hemoptysis	Wheezing
Dyspnea	
2. *Due to local extension*	
Chest pain	Pancoast's syndrome
Dysphagia	Pericardial effusion
Hoarseness	Pleural effusion
Superior vena caval compression	
3. *Due to metastases*	
Involvement of liver, brain, and bone most often symptomatic	
4. *Due to paraneoplastic syndromes*	
Endocrine—Cushing's syndrome, hypercalcemia, inappropriate ADH secretion, gynecomastia	
Neuromuscular—dementia, neuropathy, subacute cerebellar degeneration, myasthenia, myopathy	
Dermatologic—acanthosis nigricans	
Hematologic—anemia, leukocytosis, eosinophilia, thrombocytopenia	
Miscellaneous—hypertrophic pulmonary osteoarthropathy, marantic endocarditis, thrombophlebitis (Trousseau's syndrome)	

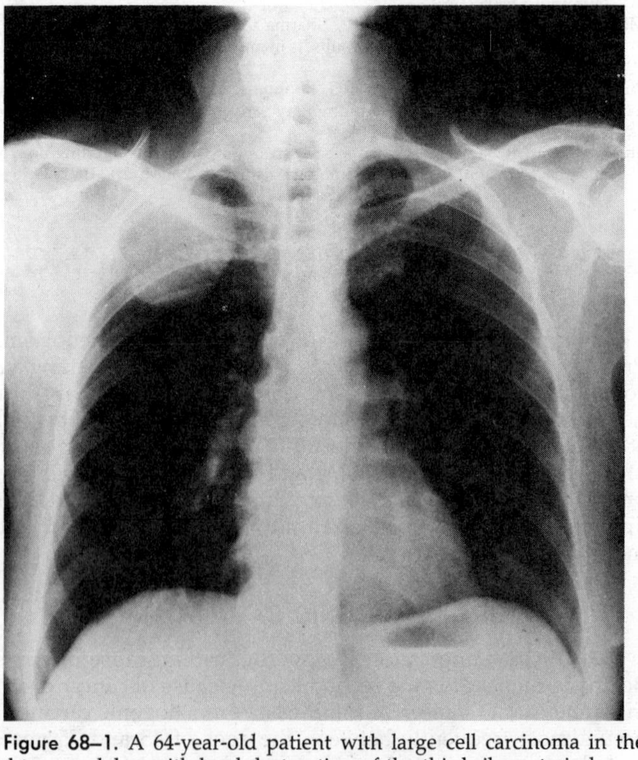

Figure 68–1. A 64-year-old patient with large cell carcinoma in the right upper lobe, with local destruction of the third rib posteriorly.

lung may invade contiguous structures, producing *Pancoast's syndrome.* In this condition, pain is the most common initial complaint. This pain may be felt in the shoulder, scapular or interscapular area, upper anterior chest, arm, neck, or axilla. Other components of the syndrome include ipsilateral Horner's syndrome, muscle weakness of the upper extremity, and sensory disturbances in the upper extremity. The pain is due to neoplastic involvement of the pleura, ribs, spinal column, and brachial plexus. Horner's syndrome results from tumor extension into the inferior cervical sympathetic ganglion. The upper extremity weakness and sensory disturbances result from involvement of the inferior trunk of the brachial plexus or the eighth cervical and first and second thoracic nerves. Occasionally, such patients complain of hoarseness, which is due to tumor invasion of the right laryngeal nerve, which normally passes around the right subclavian artery in this area.

Metastasis. Metastasis is common with bronchogenic carcinoma and the most frequent extrapulmonary sites are mediastinal and prescalene lymph nodes, liver, brain, bone, and adrenals. A wide variety of symptoms may result. *Bone pain* may result from osseous metastasis, especially to the ribs, spinal column, and pelvis. *Headache, cranial nerve palsy, monoparalysis, hemiplegia,* and various other neurologic symptoms may result from metastasis to the central nervous system. *Lymphadenopathy,* especially in the supraclavicular and cervical areas, is common, and occasionally this finding is the first abnormality noted by the patient. *Anorexia, epigastric distress, and jaundice* may result from hepatic metastasis.

Systemic Effects. A wide variety of syndromes have been noted in patients with lung cancer from systemic effects of the neoplasm unrelated to metastases. These syndromes may involve many systems, including endocrine, neuromuscular, dermatologic, connective tissue, hematologic, and vascular abnormalities. They are described in detail in Part XIV. In some of these conditions, hormone or hormone-like secretion by the primary neoplasm has been demonstrated. In lung cancer the most commonly encountered endocrine syndromes are *inappropriate antidiuretic hormone secretion, Cushing's syndrome,* and *gynecomastia.* Small cell anaplastic carcinoma especially is associated with the development of these syndromes, suggesting hormone overproduction. Small cell anaplastic carcinoma may be derived from malignant change in the Kulchitsky or K-type cell in the basal layer of the bronchial epithelium. These cells may be of neural crest derivation and may have the potential for secreting many different chemical mediators.

Hypercalcemia associated with lung cancer may be due to metastatic destruction of bone, ectopic formation of parathyroid hormone, or formation by the tumor of an osteolytic substance other than parathyroid hormone. Hypercalcemia may be accompanied by such symptoms as nausea, vomiting, lethargy, polydipsia, polyuria, and mental confusion. The most common cell type of lung cancer associated with this finding is epidermoid carcinoma. Depending on the type of radioimmunoassay utilized, 20 to 70 per cent of tumors that cause hypercalcemia do so by producing ectopic parathyroid hormone. The serum phosphorus level varies, depending on the presence or absence of azotemia, but generally in nonazotemic patients the level is decreased. Removal of the primary lung tumor may lead to prompt return of the serum calcium and phosphorus levels to normal. Recurrence of the tumor may lead to a return of the electrolyte abnormalities.

Hypertrophic pulmonary osteoarthropathy may be associated with various neoplasms, but it is most commonly associated with bronchogenic carcinoma. This syndrome occurs frequently with large localized fibrous mesotheliomas of the pleura and may occur with metastatic tumors to the lung from the breast, uterus, and prostate. The syndrome consists of a symmetric proliferating subperiosteal osteitis with subperiosteal new bone formation. This process most commonly involves the distal long bones of the arms and legs. The ankles, knees, and wrists may show chronic synovitis, effusion, pannus formation, and cartilage erosion. This produces arthralgias, limitation of motion, and tenderness on palpation. The circumference of the limbs may be increased, and at times severe edema of the legs may be noted. Hypertrophic pulmonary osteoarthropathy is almost always associated with *digital clubbing,* but the latter frequently occurs alone. The symptoms from this syndrome may precede, occur simultaneously with, or follow the development of symptoms related to the lung tumor. Removal of the lung tumor produces relief of symptoms, and in some cases vagotomy alone relieves symptoms. Bone changes may gradually revert to normal after resection of the tumor.

A number of *neurologic syndromes* that are not due to metastasis have been associated with lung cancer (see Ch. 174). The cause of these syndromes is unknown. These may be due to immunologic reaction, infection resulting from altered immunity, or toxin production by the tumor. The neurologic symptoms may antedate discovery of the tumor by several years, may occur at the same time as symptoms from the tumor, or may develop after resection of the tumor. There is no correlation between the neurologic symptoms, the size of the tumor, and the presence or absence of metastases. The neurologic symptoms may occur when the lung tumor is curable, but the neurologic manifestations generally do not change after resection of the tumor. The lung cancer is frequently of small cell anaplastic type, but the syndromes have been associated with all types of bronchogenic carcinoma. The neural and neuromuscular syndromes include *corticocerebellar degeneration, spinocerebellar degeneration, peripheral neuropathy, myasthenia,* and *myopathy.*

Thrombophlebitis, when it is recurrent or migratory and without apparent cause and when it is resistant to treatment with anticoagulants and involves unusual sites, suggests the possibility of an underlying neoplasm, which may include carcinoma of the lung.

Nonbacterial thrombotic endocarditis (marantic endocarditis) may occur with lung neoplasms, especially with bronchiolo-alveolar cell carcinomas and adenocarcinomas. Vegetations occur most frequently on the mitral valve, but they may occur on the aortic valve alone or on both the aortic and mitral valves. These lesions may result in embolization to the brain or the myocardium.

DIAGNOSIS. The diagnosis of bronchogenic carcinoma is generally established by some combination of clinical history, physical examination, thoracic roentgenogram, sputum cytologic examination, bronchoscopic examination, biopsy of involved structures, and thoracotomy. The many symptoms that bronchogenic carcinoma may produce have been described, and most of them are not specific for carcinoma. Physical examination of the chest may reveal a localized wheeze caused by bronchial obstruction, dullness to percussion and decreased breath sounds caused by presence of a pleural effusion, or other abnormalities such as rhonchi and expiratory slowing. However, in many patients, examination of the chest reveals no abnormalities. A complete physical examination is very important because it may reveal, for example, evidence of mediastinal spread of the tumor producing the signs of superior vena caval obstruction, as well as evidence of distant metastasis to supraclavicular or cervical lymph nodes or to the liver, with resultant hepatomegaly. Such findings are important in guiding the subsequent workup and evaluation of the patient.

The *thoracic roentgenogram* may reveal the presence of the neoplasm, give clues as to the histologic cell type of the neoplasm, and provide information on the extent of the neoplasm within the thorax. Epidermoid carcinomas most frequently present as hilar or perihilar masses, although they also may present as peripheral nodules. At times, the thoracic roentgenogram reveals obstructive hyperlucency, obstructive pneumonitis, or atelectasis that is secondary to the intrabronchial tumor. Cavitation has been reported to occur in about 7 per cent of patients with epidermoid carcinomas. The cavity may be thick walled and contain an air-fluid level, thereby resembling a lung abscess. The cavitation may be central or eccentric. Small cell anaplastic carcinoma generally presents as a hilar or perihilar mass, frequently with mediastinal widening. There may be associated obstructive pneumonitis or loss of lung volume. Large cell carcinoma appears most commonly as a peripheral mass. Cavitation may occur with this tumor, and the cavity usually appears to have a thick wall. Adenocarcinoma usually appears as a peripheral mass, and rarely it may also undergo cavity formation. Bronchiolo-alveolar cell carcinoma may present as single or multiple nodules or as diffuse lobar infiltrates. At times, one can recognize radiolucent spaces within the nodules. The margins of the nodules in alveolar cell carcinoma may be less sharply defined and less dense than nodules of metastatic tumor, and this may aid in the differential diagnosis of multiple pulmonary nodules.

The thoracic roentgenogram also may demonstrate hilar and mediastinal lymph node involvement (Fig. 68–2), pleural effusion caused by the tumor, rib metastasis, elevation of a hemidiaphragm, tracheal compression or distortion, and pericardial effusion. Special roentgenographic studies may be helpful. Bilateral decubitus thoracic roentgenograms may demonstrate small amounts of pleural fluid that are not apparent on routine films. Tomograms of pulmonary nodules are helpful if they demonstrate central calcification suggestive of a granuloma or stippled calcification suggestive of a hamartoma. Eccentric calcification does not necessarily indicate a benign process because the calcium may have been engulfed by an enlarging neoplasm. Whole-lung tomograms and computed tomographic scans may be helpful in differentiating a primary lung cancer and a metastatic lesion from a previously resected cancer elsewhere in the body. If these tests reveal multiple lesions, which may not be apparent on routine films, the diagnosis of metastatic disease is favored. Pulmonary nodules must be at least 1 cm in diameter before they can be detected on the routine thoracic roentgenogram. Lesions even larger than this may be hidden by overlying bone structures, the diaphragm, and the heart and great vessels.

Cytologic studies of the sputum are very helpful in establishing the diagnosis of bronchogenic carcinoma. The frequency of positive results in patients with lung cancer depends on the number and types of specimens examined and the location of the neoplasms. Centrally located lesions may be positive in about two thirds of cases, whereas peripheral lesions are positive in about one third or fewer of cases. Epidermoid and small cell anaplastic carcinomas that are central in location are most frequently associated with positive cytologic examinations. Bronchiolo-alveolar carcinoma, when present as a diffuse lesion rather than as a discrete nodule, can also be identified frequently by this means. Sputum for examination may be collected as a one-day spontaneous specimen, a three-day pooled spontaneous specimen, or an induced sputum specimen. The three-day pooled specimen is superior to the one-day spontaneous specimen and has a similar percentage of positivity to induced sputum specimens. The induced sputum technique is of greatest value in patients who cannot expectorate spontaneously. Experienced cytologists can be very accurate in providing information regarding the cell type in epidermoid and small cell carcinomas and adenocarcinomas. The sputum cytologic examination and the thoracic roentgenogram have been shown to be complementary in several studies. The thoracic roentgenogram is especially valuable in detecting early peripheral lesions, whereas sputum cytologic examination is more helpful in detecting early central lesions. False-positive sputum cytologic examinations are unusual but can occur with such illnesses as acute pulmonary infections and pulmonary infarctions.

Bronchoscopic examination is an important technique in the diagnosis and localization of bronchogenic carcinoma. The bronchofiberscope enables close examination of the segmental and subsegmental bronchi in the upper lobes, which was not possible with previous instruments. A definitive diagnosis frequently can be established by direct visualization and biopsy of the lesion. Bronchial washings also may be obtained for cytologic examination. In addition, brushing of a peripheral lesion under fluoroscopic guidance may yield the diagnosis when direct biopsy is not possible. Hematoporphyrin derivative in combination with a bronchoscopic fluorescence detection system has recently been utilized to detect and localize radiographically occult early squamous cell carcinoma.

Lung cancer may spread extensively within the thorax and

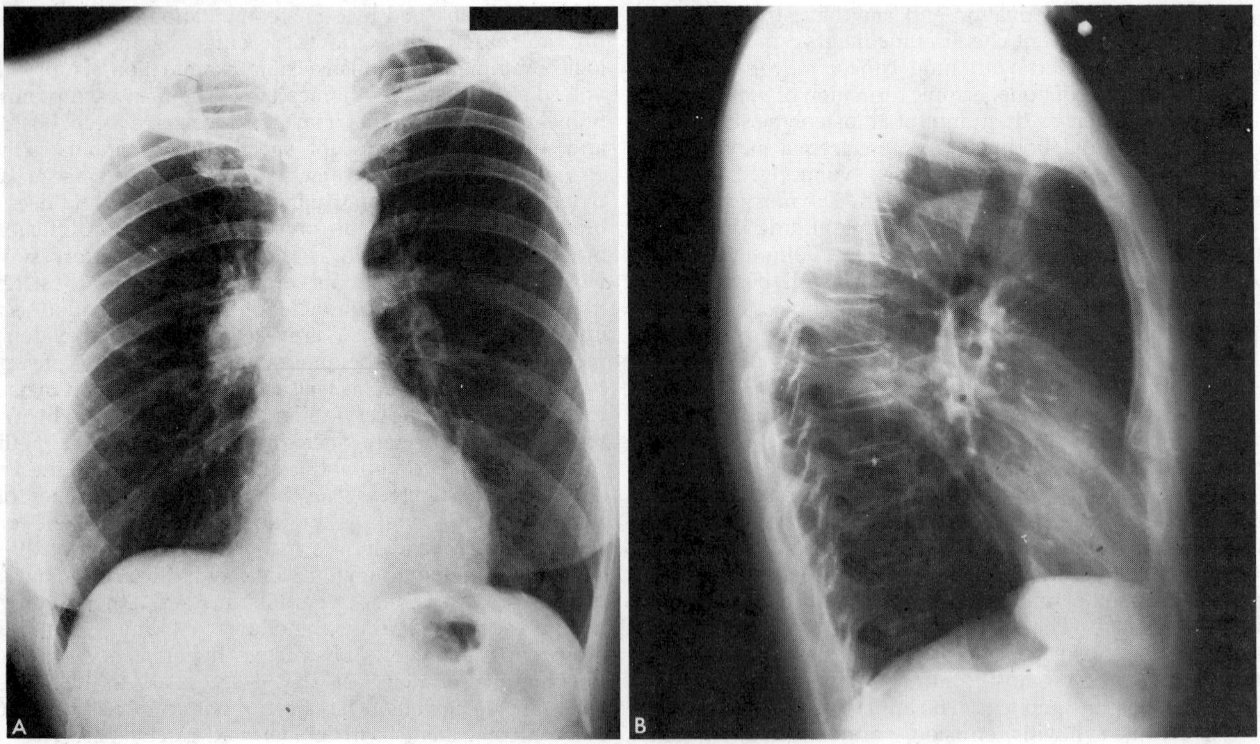

Figure 68–2. A 71-year-old patient with large cell carcinoma of the superior segment of right lower lobe with metastases to the right paratracheal lymph nodes.

metastasize widely throughout the body. The extent of local spread and distant metastases must be documented to determine prognosis and to plan therapy. The evaluation of the extent of the disease should be based on clinical history, physical examination, and standard blood chemical tests. Multiorgan scans in the absence of symptoms, physical findings, and abnormal blood chemistries are generally not helpful and have a significant rate of false positivity. *Biopsy of enlarged cervical and supraclavicular nodes* will establish the presence of extrathoracic metastasis. Liver metastasis is common, and when clinically suspected it may be detected by *liver function tests* and *isotope scans. Liver biopsy* may be indicated. *Bone roentgenograms* and *bone isotope scans* in patients with bone pain may demonstrate metastasis. Most metastatic lesions from lung cancer are osteolytic. The brain is a frequent site of metastatic disease, and when neurologic symptoms are present, this involvement can be documented by *neurologic examination* and *computed tomographic studies.* Mediastinoscopy may be indicated to demonstrate metastasis to mediastinal nodes. It is indicated in patients with proven or suspected bronchogenic carcinoma who have hilar or mediastinal lymphadenopathy in the thoracic roentgenogram. Some authorities also recommend this procedure for patients with peripheral lesions greater than 2 or 3 cm in diameter with or without radiographic evidence of hilar or mediastinal lymphadenopathy. Mediastinal metastasis from epidermoid carcinoma is not necessarily an absolute contraindication to resection, since five-year survivals up to 34 per cent have been reported for this group. However, the presence of mediastinal metastasis from lung cancer of other cell types is a poor prognostic sign and usually indicates unresectability. Pleural effusion may be due either to direct tumor involvement of the pleura or to lymphatic obstruction by the tumor, or may be secondary to obstructive pneumonitis. Generally, the effusion is an exudate with a protein concentration that is greater than 3 grams per deciliter. Frequently, it is bloody or serosanguineous. *Cytologic examination of the pleural fluid or pathologic examination of material obtained by needle biopsy of the pleura* usually will establish the cause for the effusion. Some patients present with single nodules in the lung, and for various reasons they may not be suitable candidates for thoracotomy. The diagnosis of lung cancer in these patients frequently can be made by *cytologic examination of transthoracic needle aspirates.* The procedure is carried out under fluoroscopic guidance.

STAGING OF BRONCHOGENIC CARCINOMA. A method for staging lung cancer, proposed by the American Joint Committee for Cancer Staging and End-Results Reporting (Table 68–3), is based on an estimate of the anatomic extent of the disease. In this system, the letter T describes the extent of the primary tumor, the letter N describes the presence or absence of regional lymph node involvement, and the letter M describes the presence or absence of distant metastases. Utilizing this system, a clinical-diagnostic stage for all patients can be determined after the initial examination. If the patient undergoes thoracotomy, a surgical-evaluative stage or a postsurgical treatment–pathologic stage may be determined. A re-treatment stage may be assigned if the cancer recurs after treatment. Small cell anaplastic carcinoma is generally staged as either limited or extensive. Limited disease refers to a tumor confined to one hemithorax and ipsilateral hilar, mediastinal, and supraclavicular lymph nodes. Extensive disease indicates more widespread intrathoracic or extrathoracic metastasis.

TREATMENT AND PROGNOSIS. ***Surgery.*** *Surgery* remains the most effective therapy for bronchogenic carcinoma. One exception is in the patients with small cell anaplastic carcinoma where treatment consists of chemotherapy and radiation therapy. For Stages I and II bronchogenic carcinomas, surgical resection is recommended. Some Stage III carcinomas are resectable if the extent of the disease is such that all the cancer can be excised. This may be true for some peripheral lesions that directly involve the chest wall in which the entire disease can be removed en bloc. Overall, the prognosis for all patients with lung cancer is poor. For the last 20 years the five-year survival rate for all stages of bronchogenic carcinoma has been

Table 68–3. TNM CLASSIFICATION FOR STAGING OF BRONCHOGENIC CARCINOMA

Primary tumor (T)	
T_0:	No evidence of primary tumor
T_x:	Tumor proved by malignant cells in bronchopulmonary secretions but not visualized roentgenographically or bronchoscopically
T_{IS}:	Carcinoma in situ
T_1:	Tumor is 3.0 cm or less in greatest diameter without bronchoscopic evidence of invasion proximal to a lobar bronchus
T_2:	Tumor greater than 3.0 cm in greatest diameter or any tumor invading visceral pleura or with atelectasis or obstructive pneumonitis extending to the hilum; bronchoscopically, the tumor must be at least 2.0 cm distal to the carina; there must be no pleural effusion, and any atelectasis or obstructive pneumonitis must involve less than the entire lung
T_3:	Tumor of any size with intrathoracic spread or demonstrable bronchoscopically to involve main bronchus less than 2.0 cm distal to the carina or associated with pleural effusion, atelectasis, or obstructive pneumonitis of an entire lung
Regional lymph node involvement (N)	
N_0:	Negative regional nodes
N_1:	Positive peribronchial or ipsilateral hilar nodes
N_2:	Positive mediastinal nodes
Distant metastasis (M)	
M_0:	No known metastasis
M_1:	Distant metastasis
Stage grouping	
Occult carcinoma—$T_xN_0M_0$	
Stage 1—$T_{IS}N_0M_0$, $T_1N_0M_0$, $T_1N_1M_0$, $T_2N_0M_0$	
Stage 2—$T_2N_1M_0$	
Stage 3—T_3 with any N or M, N_2 with any T or M, M_1 with any T or N	

about 9 per cent. The size and extent of the primary lesion are important determinants of survival. Relatively high five-year survival rates of about 70 per cent have been reported for patients with carcinoma in situ or minimally invasive carcinoma. Patients with peripheral lesions 4 cm or less in diameter also have improved survival rates. In one study of 193 patients with peripheral lesions of this type, resection for cure was carried out in 182 patients or 94 per cent of the group. The operative mortality was 7 per cent. Of patients who survived surgery, the five-year survival rate was 51 per cent. In this study, 49 per cent of the lesions were adenocarcinomas, 21 per cent were large cell carcinomas, 18 per cent were epidermoid carcinomas, 10 per cent were bronchiolo-alveolar cell carcinomas, and 2 per cent were small cell anaplastic carcinomas. The survival rates for patients with adenocarcinoma, epidermoid carcinoma, and large cell carcinoma were similar. The survival rate for those with bronchiolo-alveolar carcinoma was higher. Other studies have reported five-year survival rates of 50 to 80 per cent for patients with localized bronchiolo-alveolar cell carcinomas. Patients with the diffuse variety of bronchiolo-alveolar cell carcinoma have a uniformly poor prognosis. Further evidence of the importance of the extent of disease, based on the stage of the disease determined by the method previously discussed, is apparent from reported five-year survival rates following curative resection for bronchogenic carcinoma of 50 per cent for postsurgical Stage I, 30 per cent for postsurgical Stage II, and 15 per cent for postsurgical Stage III. Thus improvement in survival of patients with lung cancer probably will come from earlier diagnosis of the neoplasm, at least until chemotherapy or other forms of treatment become more effective.

When a patient presents with a lesion that is compatible with a bronchogenic carcinoma, it is important to determine whether the patient is a surgical candidate. Surgery may not be feasible because of spread of the primary tumor or because of associated diseases. The tumor is generally considered to be inoperable if there is widespread mediastinal lymph node metastasis, superior vena caval obstruction, neoplastic pleural involvement, or evidence of distant metastasis. Evaluation of general health is important, especially in relation to the presence of chronic obstructive pulmonary disease. When such disease is present, one must estimate the pulmonary function that the patient would have after the operation. In evaluating this, it is important to consider the extent of the contemplated surgery (lobectomy or pneumonectomy) and whether the tumor is significantly impairing pulmonary function preoperatively. For example, in a patient with a tumor occluding a mainstem bronchus, the results of pulmonary function tests before operation probably closely reflect what the patient will be able to do after the operation. However, a patient with a small peripheral lesion will undoubtedly lose functioning lung in the course of the operation. Patients with reduction of 50 per cent in the forced vital capacity, the one-second forced expiratory volume (expressed as a percentage of the forced vital capacity), maximal voluntary ventilation, and diffusing capacity for carbon monoxide are high-risk patients, but many can successfully undergo surgery. Additional studies, such as isotope perfusion scans, to evaluate the pulmonary capillary bed may help the clinician determine whether a patient can tolerate surgery in selected instances. With modern methods of intensive respiratory care, it is often surprising how well resectional surgery is tolerated.

Radiation. *Radiation therapy* may be considered for Stages I and II bronchogenic carcinoma when surgical treatment is contraindicated. This form of therapy may also be considered for Stage III neoplasms when the disease is limited to the involved hemithorax and ipsilateral supraclavicular lymph nodes and when surgical treatment is not possible. Preoperative radiation to lung cancers has not increased survival rates in general. Preoperative radiotherapy to superior sulcus tumors has been advocated in some studies. Patients with advanced lung cancer frequently may receive palliation with radiotherapy. Bone pain, superior vena caval obstruction, pleural effusion, brachial plexus involvement, and hemoptysis may be controlled in as many as 75 per cent of the patients. When radiation therapy is considered for limited disease in patients with pulmonary insufficiency, it is important to realize that the radiation therapy will damage the adjacent lung tissue and thereby further impair lung function.

Chemotherapy. *Chemotherapy* is superior to radiotherapy, and chemotherapy plus radiotherapy is superior to radiotherapy alone for patients with small cell anaplastic carcinoma. Combinations of chemotherapeutic agents are more effective than the use of single drugs. A variety of active drugs including vincristine, cyclophosphamide, VP-16, doxorubicin, cis-platinum, methotrexate, procarbazine, and CCNU have been used in various combinations.

For patients with small cell anaplastic carcinoma, treatment involves the administration of a combination of three or more drugs. Thoracic radiation and prophylactic brain radiation have been given in some studies, the latter especially when the primary lesion has shown a good response to chemotherapy. If a complete response has been obtained, chemotherapy is usually discontinued after 9 to 12 months of treatment. If a complete response is not obtained, the patients are generally continued on the chemotherapeutic agents until there is evidence of tumor progression, at which time therapy is changed to a different combination of drugs. With advanced disease, radiotherapy may be a useful treatment for symptomatic metastatic lesions or for the primary pulmonary lesion.

With treatment, about 90 per cent of patients will obtain a partial or complete remission. About 40 to 50 per cent of the patients with limited disease will obtain a complete remission, while 20 to 30 per cent of patients with extensive disease obtain complete remission. Of the complete responders, small numbers of patients have now survived without disease for periods of two years or more. The median survival of all patients with limited disease is about 14 to 18 months and for patients with extensive disease it is about 10 months.

Immunotherapy. *Immunotherapy*, based on studies that suggest that cellular immunity is impaired in patients with lung cancer, is currently being evaluated in a variety of experimental clinical studies.

General Measures. In spite of the poor prognosis for most patients with advanced lung cancer, much can be done to alleviate their distress. Judicious use of analgesics and narcotics, together with appropriate radiotherapy, will control pain in many patients. Occasionally, neurosurgical procedures are necessary for symptomatic relief. Antibiotics for symptoms of obstructive pneumonitis, and bronchodilator therapy for dyspnea resulting from or aggravated by accompanying chronic obstructive pulmonary disease, are helpful. Occasionally, oxygen therapy at home aids in relieving dyspnea. Recurrent pleural effusion may be benefited by intercostal tube drainage with the instillation of sclerosing agents, such as tetracycline. Neodymium:YAG laser therapy has recently been utilized to produce temporary relief of tracheobronchial obstruction due to malignant disease.

Auerbach O, Stout AP, Hammond EC, Garfinkel L: Changes in bronchial epithelium in relation to sex, age, residence, smoking and pneumonia. N Engl J Med 267:111, 1962. *A comprehensive study of the effects of smoking habits on the bronchial epithelium, including comparison with the epithelial changes seen in nonsmokers.*

Bone RC, Balk R: Staging of bronchogenic carcinoma. Chest 82:473, 1982. *A brief, clear review of staging, diagnostic tests, and operability in lung cancer.*

Byrd RB, Carr DT, Miller WE, Payne WS, Woolner LB: Radiographic abnormalities in carcinoma of the lung as related to histological cell type. Thorax 24:573, 1969. *A detailed study of the radiographic abnormalities in 600 patients with bronchogenic carcinoma classified according to histologic cell type.*

Cox JD, Yesner RA: Adenocarcinoma of the lung: Recent results from the Veterans Administration Lung Group. Am Rev Respir Dis 120:1025, 1979. *This study illustrates some important differences in the clinical course of patients with adenocarcinoma of the lung compared to other types of lung cancer. It also provides evidence that adenocarcinoma is becoming the most prevalent type of primary lung cancer.*

Koh HK, Prout MN: The efficient workup of suspected lung cancer. Arch Intern Med 142:966, 1982. *A concise review of this subject, with an extensive bibliography covering a variety of diagnostic tests and procedures.*

Lung Cancer. *In* Clark, RL (ed.): The Cancer Bulletin 32(3):75–124. Houston, Medical Arts Publishing Foundation, 1980. *A comprehensive review of lung cancer including etiology, classification, roentgenographic appearance, diagnosis, and treatment. Excellent references are provided for each area.*

Mittman C, Bruderman I: Lung cancer: To operate or not? Am Rev Respir Dis 116:477, 1977. *An excellent review article summarizing information regarding classification of lung cancer and the clinical and laboratory evaluation of patients with lung cancer. An extensive bibliography is presented.*

Mountain CF, Carr DT, Anderson WAD: A system for the clinical staging of lung cancer. Am J Roentgenol 120:130, 1974. *A detailed description of the TNM system for staging lung cancer. Survival curves based on this type of classification are presented.*

Nathanson L, Hall TC: Lung tumors: How they produce their syndromes. Ann NY Acad Sci 230:367, 1974. *An excellent review of the paraneoplastic syndromes with a discussion of the possible mechanisms responsible for the syndrome.*

Rubenstein I, Baum GL, Kalter Y, Pauzner Y, Lieberman Y, Bubis J: The influence of cell type and lymph node metastases on survival of patients with carcinoma of the lung undergoing thoracotomy. Am Rev Respir Dis 119:253, 1979. *A recent study of the five year survival rates of patients with lung cancer undergoing thoracotomy.*

Symposium on Lung Cancer. Chest 71:624, 1977. *An excellent series of papers dealing with diagnostic methods, staging, immunology, and patterns of survival in lung cancer.*

Vincent RG, Pickren JW, Lane WW, Bross I, Takita H, Houten L, Gutierrez AC, Rzepka T: The changing histopathology of lung cancer—a review of 1682 cases. Cancer 39:1647, 1977. *An extensive review of the histopathology of lung cancer occurring in patients at a major medical center, suggesting that the prevalence of adenocarcinoma is increasing.*

CARCINOID TUMORS

The term "bronchial adenoma" has been used in the past to describe slow-growing intrabronchial lesions that subsequently have been subdivided into three distinct pathologic entities: bronchial carcinoids, cylindromas, and mucoepidermoid tumors. Because these tumors have different biologic courses, as well as different histologic features, they should be considered as separate entities rather than under the broad category of bronchial adenoma. True bronchial adenomas of bronchial gland origin are extremely rare. All forms of carcinoid tumors, including bronchial carcinoids, are discussed in Ch. 242.

PRIMARY LYMPHOMA OF THE LUNG

The major discussions of lymphomas are to be found in Ch. 157 to 160. The lung and intrathoracic lymph nodes may be the primary sites of Hodgkin's disease and non-Hodgkin's lymphoma. Pseudolymphoma and lymphocytic interstitial pneumonitis are additional entities that may lead to difficulties in establishing a diagnosis.

The clinical manifestations produced by Hodgkin's disease and non-Hodgkin's lymphoma are variable, depending on the extent of the disease. Fever, cough, dyspnea, pleuritic pain, and loss of weight are frequent.

With Hodgkin's disease, the thoracic roentgenogram may reveal a solitary mass that may cavitate, an area of parenchymal consolidation, pleural effusion, or obstructive pneumonitis or atelectasis resulting from bronchial occlusion. Mediastinal lymph node enlargement is common. The anterior mediastinal nodes are often involved, a finding that is rare in sarcoidosis and may be helpful in the differential diagnosis of mediastinal adenopathy. Direct parenchymal invasion via the lymphatic vessels may occur and produce a pattern of diffuse linear infiltration on the thoracic roentgenogram. Non-Hodgkin's lymphoma may produce similar roentgenographic patterns. When this disease is primary in the lung, the most common pattern is that of a homogeneous mass within the lung parenchyma with or without hilar and mediastinal lymph node enlargement. Bronchial obstruction rarely occurs, and cavitation in the parenchymal mass is uncommon. Lesions caused by non-Hodgkin's lymphoma may seem to progress very slowly on serial thoracic roentgenograms.

Pseudolymphoma and lymphocytic interstitial pneumonitis are lymphoproliferative disorders that are incompletely understood at present. The pathologic changes are similar in both, with the pseudolymphoma presenting as a nodular lesion and lymphocytic interstitial pneumonitis presenting as a diffuse infiltrate. Pathologically, these lesions may be very difficult to distinguish from a well-differentiated malignant lymphoma of the lymphocytic type. In fact, some patients who were considered to have pseudolymphoma or lymphocytic interstitial pneumonitis initially have developed true malignant lymphoma. Involvement of the hilar or mediastinal lymph nodes in a patient in whom the differentiation is difficult points strongly toward the diagnosis of a malignant lymphoma.

Diagnosis of intrathoracic lymphoproliferative disease depends on obtaining tissue for pathologic examination. Bronchoscopy and cytologic studies of the sputum and bronchial washings are generally not helpful. Occasionally, bronchoscopic biopsy of an endobronchial lesion will be diagnostic in Hodgkin's disease. Transbronchoscopic lung biopsy, mediastinoscopy, mediastinotomy, and thoracotomy are employed to establish the diagnosis when the disease is limited to the thorax.

Hodgkin's disease and non-Hodgkin's lymphoma are treated with radiation therapy and chemotherapy. Surgical resection of non-Hodgkin's lymphoma localized to the lung parenchyma has been carried out at the time of thoracotomy for diagnosis, with radiotherapy given postoperatively in many patients. These studies report a five-year survival of about 45 per cent. Pseudolymphoma of the lung is generally resected when surgical exploration is carried out to obtain the diagnosis. The proper therapy for lymphocytic interstitial pneumonitis has not been established. Some clinicians have treated these patients with immunosuppressive drugs.

Greenberg SD, Heisler JG, Gyorkey F, Jenkins DE: Pulmonary lymphoma versus pseudolymphoma: A perplexing problem. South Med J 65:775, 1972. *An excellent discussion of the histologic characteristics of these two conditions and the problems in differentiating between them.*

Heitzman ER, Markarian B, De Lise CT: Lymphoproliferative disorders of the thorax. Semin Roentgenol 10:73, 1975. *A description of the continuum of lymphoproliferative disorders that involve the lung, with emphasis on the radiologic appearance of these diseases.*

UNCOMMON PRIMARY LUNG MALIGNANCIES

Cylindromas or adenoid cystic carcinomas derive from the mucous glands of the bronchial epithelium. Most are located in the trachea or main bronchi. There is an equal sex incidence, and the age range at the time of diagnosis has been reported to be between 30 and 65 years. Cylindroma is the second most common tumor of the trachea (the most common being epidermoid carcinoma). It produces its symptoms by bronchial irritation and obstruction. Bronchoscopic examination reveals a polypoid infiltrative tumor that partially or completely obstructs the airway and may bleed easily. Treatment is surgical resection. The prognosis must be guarded because of the tendency for distant metastasis to develop ultimately.

Mucoepidermoid tumors are rare structures of mucous gland origin, occurring in the age range of 40 to 55 years. On bronchoscopic examination, they present as polypoid masses with a smooth surface. Treatment is surgical resection, and the prognosis is better with these than with adenoid cystic carcinomas.

Carcinosarcoma is a rare entity that has both malignant epithelial and sarcomatous elements. It may present as a peripheral parenchymal mass or as an endobronchial lesion with bronchial obstruction. Treatment is surgical resection.

Pulmonary blastoma probably is a malignancy of primitive mesodermal cells capable of producing both epithelial and stromal components. It tends to arise in the peripheral portion of the lung. Treatment is surgical resection, and the prognosis is poor.

Primary sarcomas of the lung are rare and include fibrosarcomas, leiomyosarcomas, hemangiopericytomas, and osteosarcomas. Treatment is surgical excision.

Nascimento AG, Unni KK, Bernatz PE: Sarcomas of the lung. Mayo Clin Proc 57:355, 1982. *A concise review of the clinical, roentgenographic, histologic, and surgical features of these rare tumors.*

Payne WS, Ellis FH Jr, Woolner LB, Moersch HJ: The surgical treatment of cylindroma (adenoid cystic carcinoma) and muco-epidermoid tumors of the bronchus. J Thorac Cardiovasc Surg 38:709, 1959. *This is an excellent study of the symptoms, treatment, and survival of patients with these unusual tumors.*

METASTATIC NEOPLASMS OF THE LUNG

The lung is a frequent location of metastases from carcinomas and sarcomas. These lesions may have several different patterns on the thoracic roentgenogram, patterns which may provide clues to aid in the search for the primary lesion if it is not apparent. *Solitary metastatic lesions to the lung* commonly originate from carcinomas of the colon, rectum, breast, kidney, testis, and cervix and from melanomas. Osteogenic and synovial cell sarcomas may produce this pattern. *Diffuse hematogenous metastasis* may appear as multiple micronodular shadows or large masses on the thoracic roentgenogram. Nodules may be of one size, suggesting one shower of tumor emboli, or may vary in size, suggesting tumor embolization at different times. A fine micronodular pattern is suggestive of metastasis from thyroid, renal, or trophoblastic tumors or from bone sarcomas. Rarely, diffuse hematogenous metastasis may produce a clinical pattern of cor pulmonale, with the thoracic roentgenogram revealing large hilar vessels but no parenchymal infiltration or nodules. *Diffuse lymphatic metastasis* may develop owing to involvement of the bronchomediastinal lymph nodes, with retrograde spread through the pulmonary lymphatics, or to vascular metastasis, with invasion of the peripheral lymphatic vessels and spread toward the hilar regions. Tumors that frequently present these findings are carcinomas from the breast, stomach, pancreas, thyroid, larynx, and lung. The roentgenographic pattern is one of increased linear and reticulonodular markings throughout the lung. *Cavitation* in metastatic lesions is suggestive of an epidermoid carcinoma from the head and neck regions and female reproductive organs, of a carcinoma of the colon, or of a metastatic sarcoma. *Calcification* in metastatic lesions is suggestive of an osteogenic sarcoma or a chondrosarcoma. *Pleural effusions* may be produced by metastasis from almost any primary neoplasm. *Pneumothorax* may be due to metastatic lesions, especially from bone, or to synovial cell sarcomas.

Cytologic examination of the sputum may be positive in as many as 50 per cent of patients with lung metastasis, depending on the extent of the disease. Bronchoscopy with biopsy of endobronchial lesions due to metastasis is occasionally helpful in renal, pancreatic, and adrenal carcinomas and malignant melanoma.

Surgical resection should be considered for solitary metastases to the lung. Five-year survival rates of 20 to 40 per cent have been reported, depending on the cell type of the original tumor. The resection should be conservative, and the primary neoplasm should be controlled. There should be no other evidence of metastatic disease. It has been suggested that a patient with a presumed solitary metastasis should be observed three months to see if additional lesions develop before proceeding with surgery. In some situations (patients with metastatic osteogenic sarcomas), multiple lung resections have been performed, with good results. It is important to remember that a solitary nodule in a patient with a previous malignancy may be a new primary lung malignancy.

McCormack PM, Bains MS, Beattie EJ Jr, Martini N: Pulmonary resection in metastatic carcinoma. Chest 73:163, 1978. *The results of a study of 188 patients who underwent thoracotomy for resection of metastatic carcinoma are presented, along with the criteria for surgical treatment of such metastases.*

BENIGN TUMORS OF THE LUNG

In comparison with malignant neoplasms of the lung, benign tumors are uncommon. They present as solitary nodules in asymptomatic persons or as endobronchial lesions. In the latter instance, they may produce cough, hemoptysis, dyspnea, and recurrent pneumonitis, depending on size and location. The *hamartoma*, the most common benign lung neoplasm, is composed of tissues normally present in the lung, but these elements are unorganized, and include fat, epithelial tissue, fibrous tissue, and cartilage. These tumors are usually not diagnosed until adulthood, and there is a 2:1 or 3:1 male predominance. Most of them are peripheral and present as a solitary lung nodule. There may be calcification in the lesion, and sometimes this has the characteristic stippled or "popcorn" appearance. About 10 per cent of hamartomas are endobronchial. Treatment is surgical excision, and the prognosis is excellent.

Papillomas are most often encountered as laryngeal tumors in children. They may involve the trachea and bronchi. Histologically, they are composed of vascular connective tissue covered by stratified squamous epithelium. They may be of viral cause. In an unusual situation in which multiple papillomas extend throughout many bronchi, the clinical course may be characterized by repeated pneumonitis, atelectasis, bronchiectasis, and chronic pulmonary infection. Management is difficult and includes repeated bronchoscopic removal of the tumors if possible. Malignant change has been reported.

Granular cell myoblastomas are rare benign tumors usually found in the walls of the large bronchi. They may present as a mass lesion on the thoracic roentgenogram or with symptoms suggestive of a bronchial obstructing lesion. Treatment is surgical resection. Other uncommon benign lung tumors include *lipomas*, *fibromas*, *leiomyomas*, *chondromas*, and *hemangiomas*.

Arrigoni MG, Woolner LB, Bernatz PE, Miller WE, Fontana RS: Benign tumors of the lung: A ten-year surgical experience. J Thorac Cardiovasc Surg 60:589, 1970. *An excellent review of 130 patients who had benign tumors of the lung. Symptoms of the patients, radiographic features, and pathologic findings are discussed.*

THE SOLITARY NODULE

The clinician frequently encounters a patient who has a solitary nodule on the thoracic roentgenogram. A solitary nodule is generally defined as a localized round or ovoid mass surrounded by normal lung parenchyma. The patient is usually asymptomatic. The clinical problem relates to the fact that while these nodules often are benign, a significant percentage represent lung cancer, which has a higher resectability rate and long-term survival when detected as small nodules. From a study of five reported series of patients with solitary pulmonary nodules, 54 per cent of the nodules were granulomas, 28 per cent were bronchogenic carcinomas, 7 per cent were hamartomas, 4 per cent were metastatic tumors, 2 per cent were bronchial adenomas, and the remainder represented a variety of benign conditions.

Proper management of a solitary nodule in an individual patient depends on a variety of factors. *Age* is important in that bronchogenic carcinoma is very unusual below 35 years. Nodules in people younger than this may generally be carefully followed by serial thoracic roentgenograms, and surgical resection undertaken only if enlargement is demonstrated. There is an increase in the incidence of lung cancer with increasing age over 35 years, with the incidence reported to be 40 to 70 per cent in patients over 50 years, depending on the selection criteria used. *Geographic residence* of the patient must be considered because of the frequent occurrence of benign granulomas resulting from histoplasmosis in the Midwest and coccidioidomycosis in the Southwest. *Previous thoracic roentgenograms* are very important. If a solitary nodule can be documented to be unchanged in size over two years, it is almost always benign. Growth of the lesion, even very slow growth, is a matter of concern. Adenocarcinoma or bronchoalveolar carcinoma may grow only very slowly in some patients.

The presence and type of *calcification* in a solitary nodule can frequently be very helpful. Demonstration by tomography of a dense central nidus of calcification or laminated calcification almost always indicates that the lesion is a granuloma. Diffuse irregular nodular ("popcorn") calcification is highly suggestive of a hamartoma. Eccentric flecks of calcium in a lesion do not exclude carcinoma, because tumors may engulf calcium as they grow. Recent studies have employed computed tomographic scanning to evaluate more closely the density of small lesions in an effort to separate benign from malignant nodules, but the results are not conclusive at this time.

The *size* of the nodule is another important factor, because the likelihood of malignancy increases directly with size. Lesions above 2.5 cm are highly suspicious for malignancy. The relationship of *cigarette smoking* to lung cancer is clear, and the more an individual has smoked, the greater is the probability that the lung nodule represents a bronchogenic carcinoma.

If a patient is over 35 years of age, has an uncalcified lung nodule, and old thoracic roentgenograms are not available for comparison, additional diagnostic studies must be considered. *Sputum cytologic examination* is generally not likely to be positive in patients with small peripheral carcinomas. The larger the carcinoma, the more likely the sputum examination will be positive. *Fiberbronchoscopy* with localized washings and brushing under fluoroscopic guidance has been advocated in the evaluation of these patients. Here again the size of the lesion is important. In peripheral tumors less than 2.5 cm in diameter, the incidence of positive findings by this technique is probably less than 25 per cent. *Transthoracic needle aspiration* of solitary nodules has been carried out by some groups with a reported success rate of 80 to 90 per cent in diagnosing malignant lesions. A problem with this technique is to know how secure one can be that a lesion is truly benign if the aspiration cytology is negative.

Although a small proportion of resected malignant lung nodules are metastases, the overwhelming majority are primary bronchogenic carcinomas. If a patient with a solitary lung nodule has no complaints relative to other organ systems, a diagnostic workup for a primary lesion outside the lung is not indicated.

In a patient with an uncalcified nodule of unknown duration, the possibility of malignancy is increasingly greater with increased age, increased size, and a history of cigarette smoking. If the diagnostic tests described above are positive for malignancy, surgical resection must be considered. Surgical resection of the lesion may be preceded by mediastinoscopy if the lesion is 2 to 3 cm or larger to ensure the absence of mediastinal metastasis that might preclude resection. Surgical resection must also be considered if diagnostic tests are negative unless the benign nature of the process has been established histologically. Prior to surgical resection, the clinician must also consider such factors as the patient's respiratory reserve and general health, because a variety of factors may cause the physician to choose a course of careful observation rather than immediate resection.

Lillington G: The solitary pulmonary nodule—1974. Am Rev Respir Dis 110:699, 1974. *A concise review of the diagnostic evaluation of patients with solitary nodules.*

Siegelman SS, Stitik FP, Summer WR: Management of the patient with a localized pulmonary lesion. *In* Siegelman SS, Stitik FP, Summer WR (eds.): Pulmonary System—Practical Approaches to Pulmonary Diagnosis. New York, Grune & Stratton, 1979, pp 339-358. *An excellent review of reported studies in patients with solitary nodules, important factors to consider in patient management, and an outlined approach to the individual problem. This book also contains excellent chapters on other aspects of pulmonary diagnosis, including bronchoscopy, mediastinoscopy, and lung biopsy.*

69. DISEASES OF THE PLEURA, MEDIASTINUM, DIAPHRAGM, AND CHEST WALL

Jerome S. Brody

THE PLEURA

ANATOMY AND PHYSIOLOGY. The pleura is composed of a single layer of mesothelial cells supported by a sparse network of connective tissue, vessels, and lymphatics. The parietal pleura covers the surface of the chest wall, diaphragm, and mediastinum, from which it separates with ease. It receives its blood supply from the systemic circulation and contains sensory nerve endings. The visceral pleura covers and adheres to the entire surface of both lungs. It receives its blood supply from the low pressure pulmonary circulation and contains no sensory nerve fibers. Either pleural surface can be the site of a primary disease process; pleural disease, however, is most often an extension of, or a reflection of, disease that arises elsewhere.

The visceral and parietal pleural surfaces are separated by a potential space that is filled with 10 to 30 ml of fluid, which spreads out in a layer several angstroms thick. This serous fluid has a protein concentration of less than 2 grams per deciliter and a pH and glucose concentration similar to those of blood. The fluid in the pleural space turns over at a rate of 35 to 75 per cent per hour in a fashion dependent in part on Starling forces similar to those governing interstitial fluid exchange. Hydrostatic pressures are systemic in the parietal pleura (30 cm H_2O), pulmonary in the visceral pleura (10 cm H_2O), and subatmospheric in the pleural space itself (–5 cm H_2O at end expiration in normals). Colloid oncotic pressure results in pressure gradients of 25 cm H_2O from pleural space to each pleural surface. The net result of these forces is an inflow pressure gradient of 5 to 10 cm H_2O from parietal pleura to pleural space and an outflow pressure gradient of 5 to 10 cm H_2O from pleural space to visceral pleura. Augmenting this outflow pressure gradient are factors other than Starling forces such as pulmonary lymphatic flow, the relatively greater vascular bed in the visceral pleura, and the increased number of microvilli on visceral pleura mesothelial cells, all of which favor movement of fluid out of the pleural space.

The major forces involved in pleural fluid movement can help explain why fluid may accumulate in the pleural space. Excess hydrostatic forces or decreased oncotic pressures produce filtrates across intact capillary walls and result in protein-poor transudates. Breakdown of the normal formation-resorption mechanism because of damage to pleural capillaries (e.g., produced by inflammation) or blocking of lymphatics results in protein-rich exudates.

DIAGNOSTIC PROCEDURES. ***History and Physical Examination.*** Pleural pain and dyspnea are the symptoms most frequently associated with pleural disease, although considerable pleural disease can occur in the absence of symptoms. Pleural pain is usually unilateral, arising from irritation or inflammation of the parietal rather than visceral pleura. Because nerve fibers of the parietal pleura are derived from intercostal nerves, the pain may be referred to the abdomen, neck, or shoulder. Pleuritic pain is usually unilateral, sharp, and accentuated by deep breathing, coughing, or movement of the chest cage. The patient may find relief by splinting the area of involvement. Pleural pain often disappears once pleural effusion develops.

A collection of pleural fluid may produce respiratory dysfunction by compressing normal lung tissue and creating ventilation-perfusion mismatches, or by flattening the diaphragm and placing it at a mechanical disadvantage. These effects produce dyspnea in patients with otherwise normal lung function but may precipitate respiratory failure in patients with underlying lung disease.

The physical examination in pleural disease varies considerably, depending on the nature of the accompanying lung or systemic disease. Patients usually have rapid, shallow respirations, impaired chest wall motion (splinting), intercostal tenderness, and decreased breath sounds over the affected area. A pleural friction rub is the characteristic physical sign, but it is often entirely absent or audible for only 24 to 48 hours after the onset of the pain. Impaired percussion note, absent tactile fremitus, decreased or absent breath sounds, and E to A change of the spoken voice (egobronchophony) at the upper border of the fluid are frequent signs of pleural effusion.

Radiologic Examination. Up to 300 ml of pleural fluid may fail to be seen on the posteroanterior chest film. However, as little as 150 ml can be seen in a lateral decubitus film. Early signs of fluid accumulation include blunting and medial displacement of the normally sharp costophrenic angle and widening of the shadow between the gas-containing stomach and lower margin of the left lung. Larger volumes of fluid track up the pleural space, outlining the pleural fissures and producing a concave shadow with its highest margin along the pleural surface. Large amounts of pleural fluid may accumulate in the area between the lung base and diaphragm (subpulmonic effusion), producing the radiologic appearance of an elevated hemidiaphragm. In patients with small or subpulmonic effusions, bilateral decubitus roentgenograms will often reveal the presence of free pleural fluid and allow visualization of underlying lung tissue. Collections of pleural air and fluid (hydro-, pyo-, or hemopneumothorax) usually produce horizontal rather than concave areas of fluid. Loculated pockets of pleural fluid, pleural-based tumors, and parenchymal disease are often difficult to localize and define anatomically. Ultrasonic studies and computed tomography have provided more precise anatomic definition of pleural and contiguous parenchymal abnormalities.

Thoracentesis. Removal of pleural fluid serves both diagnostic and therapeutic functions. Diagnostic thoracentesis should be performed when the cause of the effusion is uncertain. Therapeutic thoracentesis should be performed when the effusion is producing symptoms or when infection is present within the pleural space. The patient is usually placed in a sitting position; the area of fluid is defined by physical examination; and, using sterile techniques, the fluid is removed. Diagnostic thoracentesis requires relatively small amounts of material, which may be obtained through a small gauge needle. Therapeutic thoracentesis usually involves removing large amounts of fluid. However, no more than 1000 to 1500 ml of fluid should be removed at one time, since re-expansion pulmonary edema may occur as the fluid compressing the underlying lung is removed. Although pleural fluid can be classified as either transudative or exudative, the difference between transudate and exudate is relative and serves only to suggest likely categories of disease.

Transudates (Table 69–1) are defined by (1) a total protein content less than 3.0 grams per deciliter (or with a pleural fluid to serum protein ratio of less than 0.5) and (2) a lactic dehydrogenase (LDH) level of less than 200 units per milliliter (or a pleural to serum LDH level of less than 0.6). Such fluids usually have white blood cell counts less than 1000 per cubic millimeter. Transudates are usually seen in congestive heart failure or

TABLE 69–1. CHARACTERISTICS OF PLEURAL FLUID TRANSUDATES

	Absolute Value	Pleural Fluid: Serum Ratio
Protein	<3.0 grams/dl	<0.5
Glucose	>60 mg/dl	1.0
WBC	<1000	—
LDH	<200 IU/L	<0.6

hypoalbuminemia, or with movement of peritoneal fluid into the pleural space.

Exudates (Table 69–2) are most frequently produced by infection or malignancy. As there is overlap in these categories, white cell counts and differentials, acid-fast and Gram's stains, aerobic and anaerobic cultures, and cytologic analysis of fluid should be included in all studies of pleural fluid. A predominance of polymorphonuclear leukocytes is most compatible with bacterial infection, while a predominance of lymphocytes, particularly with a paucity of mesothelial cells, suggests tuberculosis. Lymphomas and lymphatic leukemias producing pleural disease also produce lymphocytic effusions. Pleural fluid eosinophilia is a nonspecific finding usually associated with effusions of long duration. Blood-tinged (serosanguineous) fluid may be produced by as few as 5000 red blood cells per cubic millimeter. Malignancy, trauma, and pulmonary infarction are the most frequent causes of bloody pleural effusion, although congestive heart failure and infection can produce serosanguineous effusions. Substantial amounts of pleural fluid with a high hematocrit (>10 per cent) nearly always indicate trauma, a neoplasm that has bled into the pleural space, or a vascular abnormality. A variety of special diagnostic studies can be performed on pleural fluid, and these studies will be mentioned under discussion of specific disease entities.

Pleural Biopsy. Needle biopsy of the pleura with a hook type needle (Cope or Abrams needle) is indicated in exudative effusions when the diagnosis is uncertain. Pleural biopsy provides a specific tissue diagnosis most frequently in tuberculosis and malignancy. Histologic examination with acid-fast stains and culture of pleural tissue adds significantly to the diagnostic evaluation of tuberculous effusions. In each instance, pleural implants may be patchy so that diagnostic yield increases with repeat biopsies. Biopsy is usually reserved for those patients who have sufficient pleural fluid to separate safely visceral and parietal pleura. In patients with small or loculated effusions, localization of the fluid with ultrasound can increase the yield and safety of pleural biopsy.

Exploration of the Pleura. In 5 to 10 per cent of cases, a diagnosis cannot be established on the initial evaluation. In most instances, if one waits, the effusion will either not recur or its cause will become evident. The alternative approach, surgical exploration of the pleura, will usually provide the diagnosis. However, even in some of these patients the diagnosis will not be established. In most of these cases the effusion will not recur, although in 25 per cent the cause will prove to be a malignancy. An alternative to surgery is exploration of the pleura through a thoracoscope inserted percutaneously under general anesthesia. Experience with this approach has been limited in this country.

TABLE 69–2. EVALUATION OF PLEURAL FLUID EXUDATES

Test	Disease(s)
pH (<7.20)	Infection, malignancy, rheumatoid arthritis
Glucose (<60 mg/dl)	Infection, malignancy, rheumatoid arthritis
Amylase (>200 units/dl)	Pancreatic disease, malignancy, esophageal rupture
Rheumatoid factor, ANA, LE cells	Collagen-vascular disease
Complement (decreased)	Lupus erythematosus, rheumatoid arthritis
Biopsy (+)	Malignancy, tuberculosis
RBC (>5000/μl)	Pulmonary embolus, malignancy, trauma

PLEURAL INFLAMMATION AND EFFUSION. ***Pleural Transudates (Simple Hydrothorax).*** The most common cause of pleural transudates is congestive heart failure. Left ventricular failure increases hydrostatic pressure in visceral pleural vessels, thereby diminishing reabsorption. Right ventricular failure increases parietal pleural and central venous pressures, thereby increasing transudation and decreasing lymphatic reabsorption. Pleural effusions are often a manifestation of biventricular failure. Pleural effusion resulting from cardiac disease is most often bilateral and usually larger on the right side. If unilateral, right-sided effusions are most frequent. On rare occasions, effusions are localized within fissures, simulating lung masses that vanish as congestive heart failure regresses (phantom tumors). Chronic effusions from cardiac causes may increase their protein concentration such that the fluid may appear exudative. Hypoalbuminemia of any cause may produce transudative pleural effusions; these are usually bilateral and associated with fluid accumulation elsewhere in the body. Intra-abdominal disease may also produce large transudative hydrothoraces. Pleural effusions occur in 5 to 10 per cent of patients with cirrhosis of the liver. In these patients, ascites is usually evident, but massive effusions may appear with little or no demonstrable ascites. In this setting, peritoneal fluid appears to traverse the diaphragm either through lymphatics or through minor channels between muscle fibers in the diaphragm. The effusions are usually right sided but may be bilateral or left sided. A similar mechanism is thought to be responsible for all the pleural fluid that appears following peritoneal dialysis.

Tuberculosis. Localized tuberculosis of the pleura occurs in most patients with pulmonary tuberculosis but is usually clinically inapparent. Pleural tuberculosis may be the first manifestation of primary infection, producing a febrile illness with serous fluid and often no evidence of parenchymal disease. The effusion in this setting results from hypersensitivity to tubercular protein in pleural tubercles. The acute illness usually subsides, even if untreated, although a few such patients develop progressive primary tuberculosis. The purified protein derivative is usually positive, but skin test conversion may not yet have occurred. Patients with pleural manifestations of primary infection have a high risk of future disease, as two thirds develop clinically apparent tuberculosis within the succeeding five years. A second form of pleural tuberculosis occurs when parenchymal disease, usually reinfection tuberculosis, extends into the pleural space, producing a tuberculous empyema. Diagnosis in this case is relatively simple, since the patient will have a positive tuberculin skin test, evidence of parenchymal disease, and often positive sputum smears. Pleural fluid is exudative and usually reveals lymphocytosis; occasionally a predominance of polymorphonuclear leukocytes may be found initially. Acid-fast bacilli are rarely seen in pleural fluid, but histologic examination for granulomas and culture of material obtained at biopsy, together with culture of pleural fluid, yields the diagnosis in 80 to 90 per cent of cases. When uncertain, the pleural biopsy and purified protein derivative skin test should be repeated and the patient treated for tuberculosis until culture results are available. Treatment of all types of pleural tuberculosis is with standard antibiotic regimens (see Ch. 298), although tube drainage of tuberculous empyema may be necessary.

Pleural Effusions with Pneumonia. Inflammation of adjacent pleura occurs in most patients with pneumonia whatever the cause. The extent of pleural inflammation in bacterial pneumonia varies widely. There may be minor inflammation producing pleural pain with no clinically detectable fluid, exudative effusions containing inflammatory cells but no bacteria (parapneumonic or sympathetic effusion), or large collections of purulent fluid containing numerous bacteria (empyema). Antibiotics are usually sufficient for treating parapneumonic effusions, with thoracentesis being reserved for diagnosis or for relieving dyspnea.

Empyema tends to occur in bacterial diseases associated with tissue necrosis, e.g., infections with anaerobes, staphylococci, and gram-negative organisms. Gram's stains and aerobic and anaerobic cultures of pleural fluid are mandatory, although Gram's stains of sputum and the clinical picture are often the best initial means of identifying the infecting organism. Empyema fluid should be completely removed either by one to three thoracenteses, using a large bore venous catheter, or by closed tube drainage. Appropriate systemic antibiotics are also required. Since bacteria are not always seen on Gram's stain, thick purulent fluid with more than 100,000 cells per cubic millimeter or fluid with pH values less than or equal to 7.20 should be treated as a presumptive empyema with drainage. In some instances, placement of the tube or catheter will require ultrasound or computed tomography to locate loculated effusions. Occasionally an empyema will be associated with air in the pleural space resulting from tissue necrosis, infection with a gas-forming organism, or communication of the bronchial tree with the pleural space (bronchopleural fistula). Tube drainage and adequate antibiotic coverage will result in closure of most such fistulas. Untreated, however, they can communicate with skin (bronchopleurocutaneous fistula) and require surgical therapy (open drainage with rib resection, decortication, myoplasty involving insertion of flaps of skin or intercostal muscles into the empyema space, or occasionally thoracoplasty). Surgery, however, should be postponed until prolonged drainage and antibiotic therapy have failed.

Pleural involvement by nonbacterial, nontuberculous infections is uncommon. Viral and mycoplasmal pneumonias rarely produce pleural symptoms. Fungal disease is also not characterized by pleural disease except in coccidioidomycosis, in which a hypersensitivity pleuritis over frank empyema can occur.

Pulmonary Embolus and Infarction. Pulmonary embolus frequently produces pleural disease, with more than half of patients having detectable effusions. These effusions are usually exudates which often contain blood, although occasionally transudates may be found. Unless repeated embolization occurs, the effusion disappears with time and requires no treatment. Pulmonary embolus is discussed in detail in Ch. 65.

Hemothorax. Frank blood in the pleural space (pleural fluid hematocrit greater than 25 per cent of peripheral blood hematocrit) may be associated with either blunt or penetrating chest trauma, but may also result from spontaneous pneumothorax, hematologic disorders, and pleural malignancies. Left-sided hemothorax, particularly when associated with a widened superior mediastinum, may indicate dissection or rupture of the aorta. Pleural blood often does not clot and can be removed by thoracentesis. Small amounts of blood are readily reabsorbed via the lymphatics, but large collections should be removed by tube drainage. Persistent pleural bleeding requires surgical intervention.

Chylothorax. The leakage of thoracic duct lymph or chyle into the pleural space is most frequently due to *trauma* but may be due to *granulomatous disease* or to invasion of the thoracic duct by *tumor*. Lymphomas are most commonly implicated, although mediastinal involvement from any carcinoma can produce a chylothorax. The symptoms of chylothorax are those of the underlying lesion unless the chylothorax is large enough to produce pulmonary symptoms. Since chyle collects within the posterior mediastinum following trauma, the chylothorax does not appear until the mediastinal pleura ruptures, often days after the trauma. The chylous fluid is a milky exudate and, if allowed to stand, a creamy layer forms on top. The lipid content of the fluid is high, as manifested microscopically by sudanophilic fat droplets and a high concentration of neutral fat and fatty acids. Cholesterol content is low, and the fluid contains few cells. Initial therapy is conservative with repeated thoracenteses or tube drainage. Most cases involving trauma require surgical intervention and ligation of the thoracic duct at the site of the rupture. Radiation therapy may be of benefit in some cases when chylothorax is due to malignancy. *Pseudochylothorax* or cholesterol effusion, a milky effusion with high cholesterol and low neutral lipid and fatty acid content, is seen in patients who have longstanding pleural effusions and is often associated with large numbers of degenerating leukocytes and the presence of cholesterol crystals. Treatment is usually not required, but occasionally pleural decortication may be indicated.

Miscellaneous Disorders. *Systemic lupus erythematosus* (SLE) and *rheumatoid arthritis* are frequently associated with pleuritis and pleural effusion. Pleural abnormalities may be the first manifestation of each of these diseases, but most often pleural changes occur after the diagnosis has been established.

SLE may have pleural involvement in over 70 per cent of patients. Sometimes transient episodes of pleuritic pain are the only manifestation, but pleural effusions are seen in up to 50 per cent of cases. They may be the only radiographic abnormality, or there may be associated nonspecific parenchymal infiltrates. The effusions are usually exudates containing varying numbers of leukocytes. Lower than normal concentrations of hemolytic complement and its C3 and C4 components are present, and classic LE cells may be found in the fluid.

Rheumatoid arthritis may result in pleural effusions in approximately 5 per cent of patients. The effusion may be associated with rheumatoid lung disease, but most often it occurs in the absence of other pulmonary changes. The effusions are exudates, often with a predominance of lymphocytes, often have a low pH, and usually contain extremely low concentrations of glucose (less than 15 mg per deciliter and in some cases less than 5 mg per deciliter). Rheumatoid factor may be present, but this is a nonspecific finding. Pleural biopsy may reveal typical rheumatoid nodules and occasionally palisades of histiocytes, similar to those in rheumatoid nodules, appear in the fluid. In contrast to SLE effusions, rheumatoid pleural effusions may persist for weeks or months and may require repeated thoracenteses.

Subdiaphragmatic abscess resulting from hepatic disease, gastrointestinal perforations, or prior surgery may be associated with pleuritic chest pain, fever, and abdominal findings. Elevation of a hemidiaphragm on the affected side and impaired diaphragmatic motion are characteristic. Exudative pleural effusions, occasionally containing bacteria, and basilar pneumonias are frequent. Treatment includes surgical drainage of the abscess and antibiotics.

Pancreatitis or pancreatic pseudocysts may be associated with pleural effusions, most often on the left side, although a significant number are bilateral. Effusions usually are not large. They are exudates, may be blood tinged, and contain levels of amylase that exceed those in serum. Effusions may be due to irritation and inflammation of the diaphragmatic pleura, extension of fluid through diaphragmatic lymphatics, or actual communication of a pseudocyst with the pleural space. The effusion will subside with treatment of the pancreatic problem. Acute pancreatitis may also be a cause of the adult respiratory distress syndrome (ARDS).

Meig's syndrome is the association of ascites, benign fibroma, or other ovarian tumors and frequently massive and recurrent pleural effusions. The effusion is usually a transudate but may be exudative or serosanguineous. Removal of the tumor relieves the ascites and effusion. The mechanism for the formation of pleural and peritoneal fluid has not been completely explained. The diagnosis should be considered in women with pleural effusion of obscure origin, especially if there is evidence of concurrent ascites and pelvic disease.

Uremia is associated with a polyserositis which may include the pleural space. The effusions are exudates and often contain varying amounts of blood. At least half the effusions are asymptomatic. Effusions resolve with treatment of the uremia, but repeated thoracenteses may be necessary to control symptoms.

Asbestosis is frequently associated with pleural disease (see Ch. 559). Asbestos is the main cause of pleural plaques, which often appear along diaphragmatic and pericardial pleura. These plaques often calcify 20 to 40 years after exposure and bear no direct relation to amount of asbestos exposure. They cause no functional impairment and do not lead to mesotheliomas. Pleural fibrosis is seen in 10 to 20 per cent of asbestos workers. It is usually bilateral, is not associated with interstitial fibrosis, and may in rare instances lead to functional impairment. Pleural effusion from asbestos is often bilateral, may be recurrent, is an exudate, and is often serosanguineous. There is no direct relation between duration or intensity of exposure and pleural effusions. In contrast to other complications of asbestosis, the latency for pleural effusions is less than 20 years from the initial exposure. Other rare causes of pleural effusions are sarcoidosis, myxedema, hypersensitivity reactions, hepatitis, and amebiasis.

NEOPLASMS OF THE PLEURA. ***Metastatic Tumors.*** Involvement of pleura by malignancies arising elsewhere is common. In middle and older age groups, metastatic disease (through either pleural implants or mediastinal lymphatic obstruction) accounts for 30 to 40 per cent of pleural effusions. Carcinoma of the lung and breast are the neoplasms that most commonly involve the pleura, although virtually any neoplasm may be implicated. Involvement of pleura is considered a sign of inoperability in bronchogenic carcinomas other than superior sulcus tumors. Malignant pleural fluid is usually exudative and may contain blood. Pleural fluid cytology is positive in 20 to 25 per cent of cases, and pleural biopsy provides a diagnosis of malignancy in an additional 25 to 40 per cent of cases. The course of malignant pleural effusions usually involves reaccumulation of fluid despite repeated thoracenteses. Under such circumstances, treatment is aimed at obliterating the pleural space with tube drainage or with one of a number of irritating substances. Intrapleural tetracycline is the present drug of choice, since it produces pleural symphysis in the majority of cases with no systemic and few local side effects. For best results, 1000 mg of the drug is introduced through a chest tube, is left in the pleural space for 24 hours, and then is drained as the pleural surfaces are approximated by suction applied to the tube.

Mesothelioma. Mesotheliomas, the main primary pleural tumor, may be benign or malignant. Benign mesotheliomas are rare, have the histologic appearance of a fibroma, and generally present as a localized tumor mass. They usually arise from visceral pleura and may reach a rather large size, compressing normal lung and thereby causing symptoms. Parietal pleural lesions may be pedunculated. In either case, benign mesotheliomas appear on roentgenogram as smooth lobulated masses along the pleural surface. Hypertrophic pulmonary osteoarthropathy and clubbing are particularly common in patients with benign mesothelioma. Treatment involves surgical removal. Malignant mesotheliomas are related to asbestos exposure in 80 to 90 per cent of cases, although the dose relationship is a weak one. Smoking is not a factor. These tumors are diffuse and infiltrate the pleura widely, often completely encasing the lung. Symptoms of cough, chest pain, and dyspnea are frequent late in the disease, as are bloody pleural effusions. Although the diagnosis of a malignancy is made readily by the demonstration of malignant cells either in pleural fluid or from a pleural biopsy, distinguishing mesothelioma pathologically from metastatic disease on small tissue samples can be difficult. Prognosis is poor, with median survivals on the order of one year. Surgery is not possible, and radiation and chemotherapy have been largely unsuccessful to date.

Pneumothorax. A pneumothorax is an accumulation of gas within the pleural space. Gas may appear in the pleural space as a result of (1) perforation of the visceral pleura and entry of gas from the lung; (2) penetration of the chest wall, diaphragm, mediastinum, or esophagus; or (3) gas generated by microorganisms in an empyema. Spontaneous rupture of pleura and entry of air from the lung may occur in the absence of known disease (simple pneumothorax) or may occur as a result of parenchymal lung disease (secondary pneumothorax).

Simple spontaneous pneumothorax occurs most commonly in previously healthy men 20 to 40 years of age and is due to rupture of subpleural blebs that appear at the apex of the lung. The cause of these blebs and their predominance in men is not known. The right side is more frequently involved than the left, and recurrence is frequent (30 per cent on the same side, 10 per cent on the opposite side). The clinical presentation involves sudden onset of chest pain with dyspnea appearing in proportion to the size of the pneumothorax. The precipitating event is usually not clear, although some occur during vigorous effort, particularly with rapid large swings in intrathoracic pressure. The pneumothorax may vary in size from minor, being visible only on an expiratory film, to 100 per cent of the hemithorax being filled with air producing collapse of the lung. Small amounts of pleural fluid are present in 25 per cent of simple pneumothoraces. Tension pneumothorax (produced by increasing positive pressures in the hemithorax through a "ball-valve" air leak) is rare but can shift the mediastinum and compromise circulation. Treatment of a simple pneumothorax depends on its size. Small pneumothoraces occupying less than 25 per cent of the hemithorax in asymptomatic individuals can be treated on an outpatient basis without removing the air, since they will reabsorb over a period of seven to ten days. Larger pneumothoraces may be treated by removing air through a small catheter, and pneumothoraces of over 50 per cent or those associated with lung collapse should be treated with a chest tube initially connected to suction and, once the lung is expanded, placed under water seal drainage. The tube should be left in place for two to four days. For recurrent simple pneumothoraces, surgical obliteration of the apical pleural space (scarification, abrasion, or even decortication in certain circumstances) should be undertaken at the time of the second or third episode. Tension pneumothorax requires immediate decompression of the involved side with insertion of a large bore needle through an intercostal space.

Secondary or complicated pneumothorax occurs as a result of trauma or as a result of some other pulmonary disease. Widespread emphysema is the most common pulmonary process producing secondary pneumothorax. Pneumothorax may complicate pulmonary infection by rupture of infected material into the pleural space (pyopneumothorax). Less common pulmonary diseases associated with pneumothorax are bronchial asthma, staphylococcal pneumatoceles, and advanced pulmonary fibrosis. Eosinophilic granuloma is an interstitial disease that is characteristically associated with spontaneous pneumothorax. Pneumothorax may also appear as a complication of mechanical ventilation when high intrathoracic pressures are utilized. In contrast to simple or primary pneumothorax, in which dyspnea and evidence of ventilatory compromise are unusual unless the pneumothorax is large, relatively small pneumothoraces may produce severe respiratory symptoms when superimposed on pre-existing pulmonary disease. Thus, treatment of patients with secondary pneumothorax is more aggressive, with thoracotomy tube drainage being employed more frequently. Persistent pleural leaks (bronchopleural fistulas) and tension pneumothorax are also more frequent with secondary pneumothorax, particularly in those patients who develop a pneumothorax while on mechanical ventilation.

Black LF: The pleural space and pleural fluid. Mayo Clin Proc 47:493, 1972. *An excellent discussion of the physiology of normal and abnormal pleural fluid formation. Not much has been added since this article was published.*

Chernow B, Sahn SA: Carcinomatous involvement of the pleura: An analysis of 96 cases. Am J Med 63:695, 1977. *Defines prevalence, presentation, and prognosis of metastatic disease to the pleura. Diagnostic features of carcinomatous fluid are discussed, and frequency of pleural disease as the first manifestation of malignancy is emphasized.*

Epler GR, McLoud TC, Gaensler EA: Prevalence and incidence of benign asbestos pleural effusion in a working population. JAMA 247:617, 1982. *Puts asbestos pleural effusion in perspective. Reviews diagnostic criteria and epidemiology and emphasizes early onset of pleural effusion as a complication of asbestos exposure.*

Light RW, MacGregor MI, Luchsinger PC, Ball WC Jr: Pleural effusions: The diagnostic separation of transudates and exudates. Ann Intern Med 77:507,

1972. *The "classic" paper which separates transudates and exudates on the basis of pleural fluid to serum ratios of protein and LDH.*

Lowell JR: Pleural Effusions: A Comprehensive Review. Baltimore, University Park Press, 1977. *A thorough review of the causes and treatment of various types of pleural effusion. Reference list is exhaustive.*

Ryan CJ, Rodgers RF, Unni KK, and Hepper NGG: The outcome of patients with pleural effusion of indeterminate cause at thoracotomy. Mayo Clin Proc 56:145, 1981. *An interesting study of the natural history of pleural effusions that could not be diagnosed at thoracotomy.*

Taryle DA, Lakshminarayan S, Sahn SA: Pleural mesotheliomas—an analysis of 18 cases and review of the literature. Medicine 55:153, 1976. *A detailed analysis of mesotheliomas from their own institution and from the literature. This disease of increasing importance has a poor prognosis.*

THE MEDIASTINUM

ANATOMY. The mediastinum is the anatomic space that lies in the mid-thorax. It separates the two pleural cavities and is defined by the diaphragm below and the suprasternal thoracic outlet above. The mediastinum contains several vital structures contiguous to one another in a relatively small space. Thus, abnormalities within the mediastinum, regardless of their cause, can produce a number of serious symptoms. It is convenient for clinical purposes to divide the mediastinum into *anterior, middle,* and *posterior* areas. The anterior mediastinal compartment is bounded posteriorly by the pericardium, ascending aorta, and brachial cephalic vessels and anteriorly by the sternum. This compartment contains the thymus gland, substernal extensions of the thyroid and parathyroid glands, blood vessels, pericardium, and lymph nodes. The middle mediastinal compartment extends from the posterior limit of the anterior compartment to the anterior border of the vertebral bodies. The middle mediastinum contains the heart, great vessels, trachea, main bronchi, esophagus, and phrenic and vagus nerves. The posterior mediastinum extends from the anterior surface of the vertebral bodies to the dorsal chest wall. This compartment contains the vertebral bodies, the descending thoracic aorta, the esophagus, the thoracic duct, the azygous and the hemiazygous veins, the lower portion of the vagus nerve plus the sympathetic chains, and a posterior group of mediastinal nodes.

SIGNS AND SYMPTOMS. *Chest pain, cough, hoarseness,* and *dyspnea* are the most common complaints. Less common symptoms are *stridor, dysphagia,* and *Horner's syndrome.* However, most patients with mediastinal masses are asymptomatic. Occasionally, specific syndromes are associated with primary lesions of the mediastinum. Nearly half of all thymomas are associated with myasthenia gravis (see Ch. 539). Mesotheliomas, fibrosarcomas, and occasional teratomas have been associated with hypoglycemia. Parathyroid tumors may present with hypercalcemia. Neurogenic tumors may result in pressure against the spinal cord, causing a variety of symptoms. Because of the crowding within the normal mediastinum of a large number of structures, more than one organ is likely to be affected by a given disorder. Signs and symptoms of mediastinal disorders are thus nonspecific. The physical findings of mediastinal air or inflammation are specific and discussed below. Physical findings in a patient with a mediastinal mass, however, are unusual unless the mass is large or impinges on a vital structure. Rarely, the mass may be so large that the pleural cavity is obliterated, leading to findings consistent with pleural effusion. Occasionally, a mediastinal tumor may produce superior vena caval obstruction with typical signs of facial edema, dilated neck veins over the thorax, and edema of the upper extremities. A mass can also erode into the trachea, esophagus, or great vessels with life-threatening sequelae.

DIAGNOSIS. Radiographic studies are the most helpful procedures in evaluating patients with mediastinal disorders. A large percentage of such lesions are first detected on routine chest roentgenograms (Fig. 69–1*A*). Computed tomography (CT) has dramatically improved visualization and definition of mediastinal structures and will replace routine tomography in time (Fig. 69–1*B*). The angiographic definition of great vessels and barium esophagograms are often of considerable value in defining mediastinal lesions.

In those patients in whom specific diagnoses cannot be established by radiographic methods, surgical approaches to obtaining tissue for histologic diagnosis are necessary. Anterior and some middle mediastinal lesions can be approached through mediastinoscopy or mediastonotomy. Both procedures provide lymph nodes for histologic and cultural examination without the need for major surgery. Thoracotomy is necessary when tissue from middle and posterior mediastinal lesions is

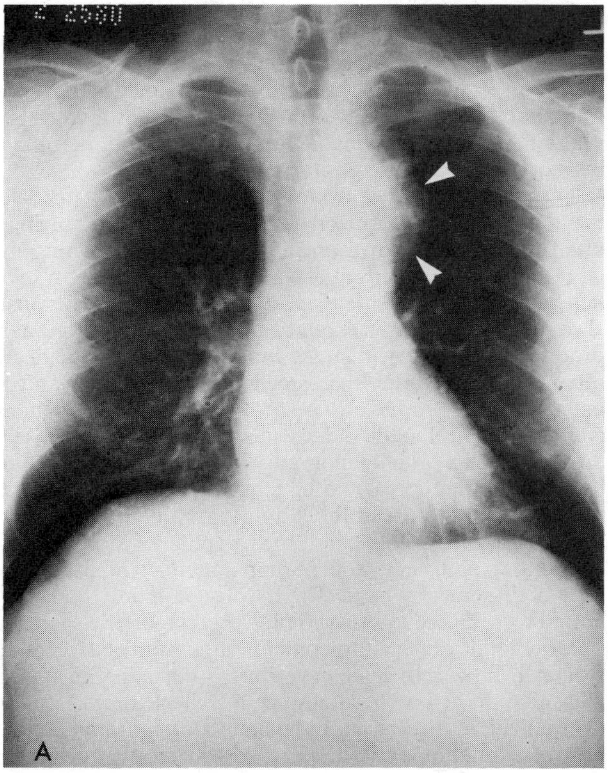

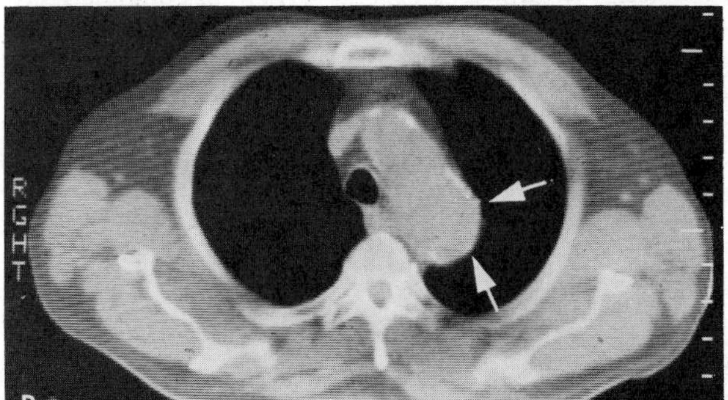

Figure 69–1. *A,* Posteroanterior chest roentgenogram of 61-year-old man with mass noted adjacent to aortic arch (arrows). On lateral film the mass projected posteriorly. There was a history of an automobile accident 17 years previously. *B,* CT scan shows large mass projecting from the aorta (arrows). Dense calcium can be seen in the wall of this post-traumatic aortic aneurysm, which enhanced with injection of a small bolus of contrast medium (film not shown).

required. Thoracotomy not only provides the opportunity for tissue diagnosis but also allows drainage or definitive resection of specific lesions.

SPECIFIC DISEASES. ***Infections.*** Acute mediastinitis is rare and most often results from endoscopy, surgery, or trauma to the esophagus. Fever, chest pain, widening of the mediastinal shadow by x-ray, and a history of trauma or manipulation of the esophagus suggest the diagnosis. X-ray studies with contrast material may demonstrate esophageal perforation. Complicating pleural effusions are occasionally observed and, if untreated, often develop into an empyema. Repair of the esophageal perforation, surgical drainage of mediastinal abscesses, and antibiotic therapy should be employed. Chronic fibrosing mediastinitis caused by extension of granulomatous disease (especially histoplasmosis) from mediastinal lymph nodes is rare but may cause severe irreversible mediastinal fibrosis with superior vena caval obstruction.

Pneumomediastinum. Air may enter the mediastinum either as a result of a tear in the esophagus or tracheobronchial tree or because of the dissection of air from ruptured alveoli along the peribronchovascular sheath. Rupture of the esophagus usually is associated with instrumentation or trauma. Pneumomediastinum from alveolar rupture may occur spontaneously in individuals with no underlying lung disease or may be a complication of severe diffuse disease or artificial ventilation. In many cases of pneumomediastinum, air will rupture through the mediastinal pleura producing an associated pneumothorax which may be bilateral. The air may dissect into the subcutaneous tissues of the neck and produce generalized subcutaneous emphysema. In children, the air may collect within the mediastinum, compressing the great vessels. Patients with pneumomediastinum may be asymptomatic or at times may develop substernal chest pain indistinguishable from that of myocardial infarction. Physical examination may reveal subcutaneous emphysema in the neck, and auscultation often reveals a mediastinal crunch, a crackling sound synchronous with cardiac systole, best heard over the left sternal border when the patient is upright *(Hamman's sign)*. A lateral chest roentgenogram is most effective in demonstrating air in the mediastinum. A simple, spontaneous pneumomediastinum usually subsides without treatment. When pneumomediastinum is severe, complicates airway or esophageal rupture, or involves compression of great vessels, surgical drainage and vigorous treatment of the underlying disease are required.

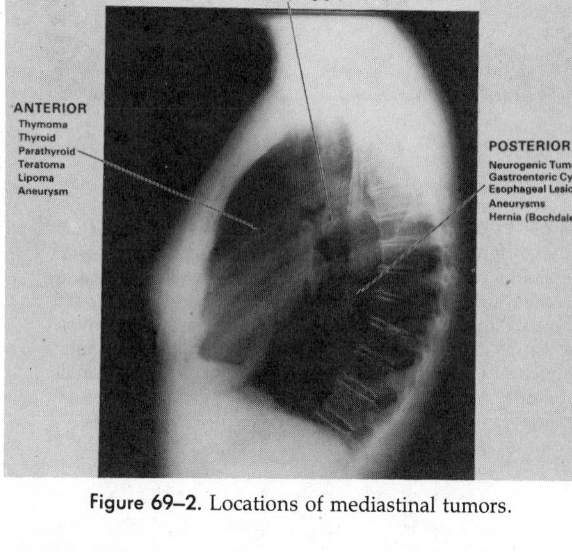

Figure 69–2. Locations of mediastinal tumors.

Tumors. Tumors of the mediastinum are the most common major disorder of this region. In young adults they are often primary in the mediastinum and benign; in older adults they are often malignant and metastatic. Figure 69–2 lists the usual position of common mediastinal tumors. Of primary mediastinal tumors, approximately 20 per cent represent cysts, 20 per cent are neurogenic, 20 per cent are thymomas, 10 per cent are lymphomas, 10 per cent are teratomas, and the remainder are of miscellaneous origin. As noted above, most mediastinal tumors are asymptomatic, but when symptoms do arise they are the result of compression of vital structures within the mediastinum and usually represent malignant lesions. Surgical removal is the treatment of choice of most benign mediastinal tumors, even if asymptomatic, to prevent obstructive symptoms and potential malignant changes. Most malignant tumors are inoperable, although some, such as small cell carcinoma or lymphoma, may respond to radiation therapy or chemotherapy.

Benjamin SP, McCormack LJ, Effler DB, Groves LK: Primary tumors of the mediastinum. Chest 62:297, 1972. *A review of nonvascular mediastinal tumors. Many patients were asymptomatic, with masses being discovered on routine roentgenograms.*

Brown LR, Muhn JR: Computed tomography of the thorax: Current perspectives. Chest 83:806, 1983. *An excellent state-of-the-art review of the role that CT scanning plays in diagnosis of mediastinal and other thoracic diseases.*

Fraser RG, Paré JAP: Diagnosis of Diseases of the Chest. 2nd ed. Philadelphia, W. B. Saunders Company, 1979. *Excellent review of differential diagnosis and roentgenographic characteristics of mediastinal masses.*

Pugatch RD, Faling LJ, Robbins AH, Spira R: CT diagnosis of benign mediastinal abnormalities. Am J Roentgenol 134:685, 1980. *Makes case for computed axial tomography as the initial procedure and most productive tool for evaluation of mediastinal abnormalities detected on plain chest roentgenogram. Excellent pictures and definition of mediastinal anatomy.*

THE DIAPHRAGM

The diaphragm is an airtight sheet of muscle and tendon lined by parietal pleura on one side and peritoneal membrane on the other. Its muscle fibers arise from the lower ribs and thoracic vertebrae and converge and insert into the margins of the crescentic central tendon. There is a hiatus for each of the principal structures that pass from thorax to abdomen. Motor and sensory fibers reach the diaphragm via the phrenic nerves, with separate innervation to the right and left halves. The diaphragm is the principal muscle of respiration. Diaphragmatic contraction tends to displace abdominal contents downward and to raise the ribs upward and outward, thus creating the negative intrapleural pressure of inspiration.

DIAPHRAGMATIC HERNIAS. Herniation of abdominal or retroperitoneal structures may occur through congenitally weak or incompletely fused areas of the diaphragm, may result from traumatic rupture, or may occur through the esophageal hiatus. The latter accounts for over three fourths of all diaphragmatic hernias and is considered in Ch. 97.

Hernias posteriorly through the foramina of Bochdalek are the most common form of hernia in infancy, occurring more often on the left than the right. The hernial opening may be large because of a virtual absence of the diaphragm owing to failure of its posterolateral portion to close. In this instance, abdominal viscera may extend freely into the left pleural space, producing respiratory distress and requiring immediate surgical repair. When the defect is small, the peritoneum and pleura usually fuse, producing a sac that contains the herniated contents. In adults, the defect is usually small and is discovered on routine chest roentgenogram. The defect is usually posterolateral, and the hernial contents usually contain retroperitoneal fat or the upper pole of the kidney or, rarely, the spleen.

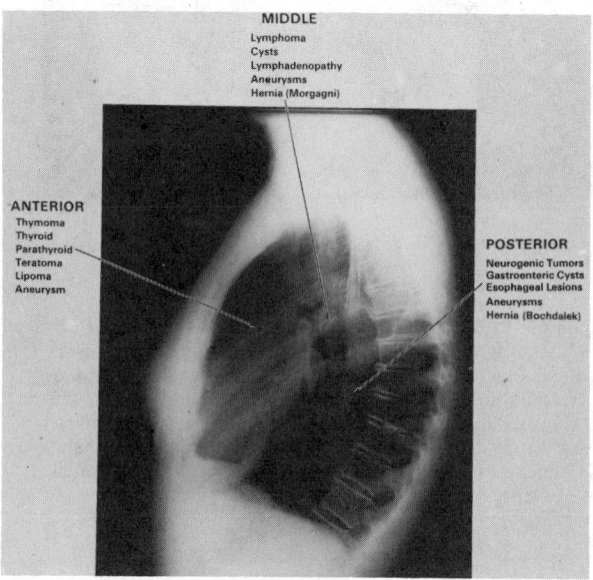

Hernias anteriorly through the foramina of Morgagni are rare and tend to occur in the obese or in patients who have increased intra-abdominal pressure. The hernia commonly presents as an anterior, rounded density in the region of the right cardiophrenic angle. It usually contains omentum, but occasionally stomach, bowel, or liver may appear when hernias are large. Auscultation of borborygmi over the chest, radioisotope scans of the liver, routine gastrointestinal contrast films, and induction of a pneumoperitoneum followed by an upright film of the abdomen may all be useful diagnostic procedures. Therapy of both types of hernias may not be needed, especially when old films demonstrate that the abnormality has been present for a long time. Occasionally surgery is necessary for diagnosis or to relieve strangulation of hernia sac contents.

Traumatic hernias of the diaphragm may result from direct injury to the diaphragm or indirectly from severe abdominal compression. Signs and symptoms may occur immediately owing to extension of abdominal contents into the pleural space with resultant strangulation. More often, a latent period, which may extend for several years, intervenes before either respiratory or abdominal symptoms develop. Diagnosis is accomplished roentgenographically, and treatment is surgical.

DISORDERS OF DIAPHRAGMATIC MOTION. A variety of structural and functional abnormalities interfere with the ability of the diaphragm to develop inspiratory muscle strength. The resulting impairment of diaphragmatic function may be involved in many forms of respiratory failure.

Hiccup. Hiccup or singultus is a common disturbance produced by spasm of the diaphragm followed by sudden closure of the glottis during an inspiratory effort. A characteristic sound is produced as the glottis closes, and discomfort may be experienced as thoracic pressure is lowered by continued contraction of the diaphragm. Hiccup is usually of short duration but may persist for days or weeks. Hiccup is most often of unknown cause, presumably resulting from functional gastrointestinal disturbances. Occasionally, hiccups are a sign of serious disease, such as central nervous system disorders (encephalitis, tumor), uremia, herpes zoster, and pleural or abdominal processes that invade or irritate the diaphragm. Prolonged hiccups are sometimes thought to be psychogenic in origin. Hiccups usually subside spontaneously or when the initiating disease has been successfully treated. In persistent, debilitating hiccups, local anesthesia or actual crushing of one of the phrenic nerves may be required (crushing theoretically produces paralysis of only several months, but permanent paralysis is frequent).

Diaphragmatic Flutter. This is a rare disorder in which rapid rhythmic contractions of the diaphragm occur at a rate of 1 to 8 per second, lasting for seconds or as long as weeks or months. The contractions produce a cogwheel type of respiration and, when frequent, may hamper gas exchange. They are not accompanied by an inspiratory sound, and one or both diaphragms may be affected. Etiology is unclear, although psychogenic causes, central nervous system disease, and diseases which might irritate the diaphragm or phrenic nerve have been implicated. Treatment is similar to that for hiccup.

Diaphragmatic Paralysis. Interruption of the phrenic nerve anywhere from its origin in the C_3–C_5 nerve roots to its entry into the diaphragm produces diaphragmatic paralysis. Unilateral paralysis is frequently associated with invasion of the phrenic nerve by tumor (usually metastatic bronchogenic carcinoma). Paralysis has also been reported in various neurologic disorders such as poliomyelitis and herpes zoster. In an occasional patient, unilateral paralysis appears to be idiopathic. The paralyzed diaphragmatic leaf is not only nonfunctional but elevated, reducing lung volume on the side of paralysis. Diagnosis is made fluoroscopically by observing paradoxical diaphragmatic motion on sniff and cough. Unilateral paralysis is usually asymptomatic and rarely requires treatment. Bilateral paralysis may occur in association with various myopathies and with high transections of the spinal cord. Respiratory symptoms and arterial blood gases are worse in the supine position, since abdominal contents displace the passive diaphragm upward into the thorax. With bilateral paralysis, fluoroscopy of the diaphragm is less conclusive as a bilaterally flaccid diaphragm may drop with rib cage expansion. The diagnosis can be suspected at the bedside by observing inward, instead of outward, motion of the abdomen on inspiration. The diagnosis can be confirmed by recording muscle action potentials or by measuring esophageal and gastric (transdiaphragmatic) pressures on inspiration. Electrical stimulation of the phrenic nerve with measurement of conduction time may be helpful in diagnosing peripheral neuropathy. The hypoventilation of bilateral paralysis often produces respiratory failure. The hypoventilation of bilateral phrenic nerve paralysis can be treated by ventilating the patient on an intermittent or continuous schedule or by implanting and pacing phrenic nerve electrodes.

Eventration. Diaphragm eventration is a localized elevation of the diaphragm resulting from impaired muscle development or local muscle weakness. The diaphragm muscle is either absent or atrophic in the area of eventration. The elevation is usually on the right side of the anteromedial portion of the diaphragm. It most often appears in middle-aged, obese patients. The condition is usually asymptomatic, being recognized on routine chest roentgenograms. It must be differentiated from neoplasms, paralysis, and hernias and rarely requires surgical treatment.

Derene J-PH, Macklem PT, Roussos CH: The respiratory muscles: Mechanics, control and pathophysiology. Am Rev Respir Dis 118:119, 373, 581, 1978. *A detailed and often complex review of the physiology of the respiratory muscles, of which the diaphragm is number one. Not easy reading but excellent physiology.*

Loh L, Goldman M, Davis JN: The assessment of the diaphragm function. Medicine 56:165, 1977. *A clear and easy-to-read review of diaphragm function and its importance clinically. Reference is made (Quart J Med 45:87, 1976) to the role of diaphragm function in respiratory failure.*

THE CHEST WALL

The chest bellows serves to move air in and out of the lungs and is made up of the bony thoracic case and the various muscles of respiration.

The neuromuscular–chest cage system is a major determinant of ventilatory patterns and of static and dynamic lung volumes. Disease of this system may influence total alveolar ventilation and ventilation-perfusion relationships and thus be responsible for hypoxemia or hypercapnia. Disorders of chest bellows function may be classified into two broad categories according to whether they result from impairment of the neuromuscular apparatus or from impairment of mechanical properties of the chest wall. The former are discussed as individual diseases in Part XXIII. Only the latter group will be discussed here.

KYPHOSCOLIOSIS. This deformity of the chest wall is due to a combination of posterior angulation (kyphosis) and lateral angulation and rotation (scoliosis) of the spine. Scoliosis is categorized as to the right or left according to the direction of the convexity of the primary curvature. Idiopathic scoliosis is more frequently to the right in the thorax with a compensatory left curvature in the lumbar region.

The severity of scoliosis may be quantified by measuring the angle between upper and lower portions of spinal curve on a roentgenogram. Greater angles signify more severe deformity and imply greater respiratory impairment. In thoracic kyphoscoliosis the rib cage is distorted so that on the convex side of the spine the ribs are widely separated and rotation of the spine angulates them posteriorly, producing the kyphotic hump. On the concave side, the ribs are crowded and displaced anteriorly. Because of the kyphosis and loss of thoracic height, the lower anterior chest wall tends to bulge forward. Although mild degrees of kyphoscoliosis are common, severe distortion of the chest cage is unusual. Kyphoscoliosis usually begins in childhood but becomes more prominent during the rapid growth years of adolescence. In most cases (80 per cent) there is no discernible etiology; neurologic disorders that influence chest wall muscles and congenital abnormalities account for a small percentage of cases.

Patients are usually asymptomatic in early life. When kyphoscoliosis is severe (greater angle than 90 degrees) or when patients develop pulmonary infections (as a result of locally impaired bronchial clearance mechanisms), dyspnea appears. In these instances, gradual progression, respiratory failure, and cor pulmonale occur with death in the fourth through sixth decade. Patients with mild or moderate kyphoscoliosis (angle less than 50 degrees) who remain free of respiratory infections may have normal life expectancy.

Depending upon the degree of kyphoscoliosis, static lung volumes are reduced with preservation of residual volume; chest wall compliance is reduced, with lung compliance being slightly reduced or normal. Airflow rates are usually reduced only in proportion to the reduction of vital capacity. Studies of regional lung function tend to show variable shifts of ventilation and perfusion owing to the chest wall deformity. Arterial blood gases are also variable. Many patients have mild hypoxemia, secondary to ventilation-perfusion mismatch, but severe hypoxemia and hypercapnia occur only late in the disease and are most commonly associated with superimposed infection.

A variety of methods have been used to restore normal curvature or prevent progressive curvature of the spine. These include surgery, plaster casts, and various types of traction. With most, the cosmetic effect is greater than the physiologic effect, although they may prevent progression of curvature, particularly in those patients with idiopathic kyphoscoliosis. Efforts should be made to prevent airways disease; the patient should discontinue smoking, and respiratory infections should be treated early and vigorously. In patients with severe disease, episodic use of intermittent positive pressure breathing has been found to increase transiently functional residual capacity and total thoracic compliance and may be of value in ambulatory management. Episodes of acute respiratory failure, usually associated with respiratory infections, may require intubation and assisted ventilation. In some patients with chronic respiratory failure, night time ventilatory assistance may be sufficient to control symptoms. Home oxygen should be used in those patients with severe hypoxemia.

PECTUS EXCAVATUM. This is a congenital deformity of the lower portion of the sternum with symmetric bowing of the anterior ribs. The defect, which is often familial, is thought to be due to a short central tendon of the diaphragm. When the deformity is severe, the heart and mediastinal structures are displaced laterally, but significant functional impairment is rare. Surgical correction is not necessary and is done only for cosmetic purposes.

ANKYLOSING SPONDYLITIS. This disease is characterized by fusion of costotransverse and vertebral joints and may also involve sternomanubrial and clavicular joints (see Ch. 445). The chest cage tends to be fixed in an inspiratory position, with the result that vital capacity is decreased while residual volume and functional residual capacity are increased. Although a small number of patients develop idiopathic upper lobe fibrosis, in most patients gas exchange is normal and respiratory disease is unusual.

FLAIL CHEST. Trauma to the chest that produces multiple anterior rib fractures may lead to instability of a large area of the anterior chest wall. This occurs most commonly in motor vehicle accidents or following cardiopulmonary resuscitation. Paradoxical motion occurs during respiration, with the injured area moving opposite the remainder of the chest wall. Hypoxemia is common in flail chest, although alveolar hypoventilation with hypercapnia is rare. Hypoxemia is most often the result of diminished lung compliance and ventilation-perfusion mismatch. Artificial ventilation with volume ventilators is not necessary in many cases. Aggressive supportive care with attention to maintaining adequate oxygenation and clearance of airway secretions is the best approach to therapy.

Bergofsky EH: Respiratory failure in disorders of the thoracic cage. Am Rev Respir Dis 119:643, 1979. *A detailed clinical and physiologic review of the chest cage and its disorders. Contains an extensive list of references. Easy reading and "state of the art" for this topic.*

Kafer ER: Idiopathic scoliosis: Gas exchange and the age dependence of arterial blood gases. J Clin Invest 58:825, 1976. *A detailed study of the physiologic consequences of scoliosis and the importance of angle of deformity and age as they affect gas exchange.*

Sharkford SR, Smith DE, Zarins CK, et al.: The management of flail chest. Am J Surg 132:759, 1976. *A retrospective review of personal cases and of the literature, establishing that not all patients with flail chest need to be intubated and ventilated.*

70. RESPIRATORY FAILURE

John F. Murray

INTRODUCTION

Adequate respiration consists of the uptake of sufficient amounts of O_2 and the elimination of sufficient amounts of CO_2 to maintain PO_2 and PCO_2 in arterial blood at their respective normal values. It follows that *respiratory failure* is associated with disturbances in the exchange of O_2 and CO_2 between gas in alveoli and blood in pulmonary capillaries and that these abnormalities must be reflected by changes in the PO_2 and PCO_2 in arterial blood. Thus respiratory failure is defined as a condition in which arterial PO_2 is below the normal range (excluding hypoxemia from intracardiac right-to-left shunting of blood) or arterial PCO_2 is above the normal range (excluding respiratory compensation for metabolic alkalosis). This definition, which is physiologically precise as well as clinically applicable, implies that the diagnosis of respiratory failure depends chiefly on laboratory analysis of arterial blood and not on clinical findings.

Respiratory failure is not a disease but a disorder of function that can be caused by a variety of conditions that affect the lungs; in some instances, the lungs are completely normal (e.g., overdose of sedative drugs). Respiratory failure is analogous to heart failure and renal failure, both of which represent the consequences of impaired normal function resulting from numerous disparate diseases.

Respiratory failure is traditionally divided into acute and chronic varieties, depending on the time it takes for the abnormalities in gas exchange to occur. This arbitrary classification does not take into account the common clinical occurrence of an acute worsening of arterial PO_2 and PCO_2 in a patient who already has chronic respiratory failure as a result of some underlying disorder. However, the distinction between acute and chronic respiratory failure has important etiologic and therapeutic connotations and will be referred to frequently.

PATHOPHYSIOLOGY OF RESPIRATORY FAILURE

In human beings, respiration has been subdivided into four functional processes: *ventilation, diffusion, perfusion*, and *control of breathing*. Each of these contributes uniquely to the maintenance of normal values of PO_2 and PCO_2 in arterial blood. Therefore, abnormalities in any one of the four processes, if sufficiently severe, will cause respiratory failure; furthermore, in many common respiratory disorders, multiple abnormalities coexist.

Normal Gas Exchange

The physiology of normal gas exchange is described in Ch. 57 and will not be reviewed here. However, understanding what is meant by normal is important, because arterial PO_2 varies with age, and both arterial PO_2 and PCO_2 vary according to the altitude (i.e., the prevailing barometric pressure) at which the person happens to be when the blood specimen is obtained and to the extent of acclimatization. The normal range includes the biologic variabilities among individuals and the analytic variations inherent in the measurements. Because the diagnosis of respiratory failure should be made in the laboratory and not at the bedside, the physician's ability to establish the diagnosis depends on the accuracy of the laboratory tests used to measure PO_2 and PCO_2. Normal mean arterial PO_2 (Pa_{O_2}) values in subjects 20 years of age or older can be calculated from the regression equation $Pa_{O_2} = 100.1 - 0.323$ (age in years). The normal range of variation is $\pm$ 5 mm Hg from the mean value. Arterial PCO_2 does not vary with age and is normally within the range of 40 $\pm$ 5 mm Hg in healthy persons at sea level. Values of PO_2 *below* or PCO_2 *above* normal limits indicate the presence of respiratory failure.

Abnormal Gas Exchange

The pathophysiology of abnormal gas exchange is also discussed in Ch. 57. Hypoventilation, impaired diffusion, ventilation-perfusion mismatching, right-to-left shunting of blood, and breathing air with a low P_{O_2} all cause arterial hypoxia (a decrease below normal of P_{O_2}); in contrast, for practical purposes only hypoventilation causes arterial hypercapnia (an increase above normal of P_{CO_2}). In view of the therapeutic importance of recognizing the abnormal mechanism(s) leading to a patient's respiratory failure, each will be reviewed briefly.

HYPOVENTILATION. Alveolar hypoventilation is present when the arterial P_{CO_2} is increased. Furthermore, as arterial P_{CO_2} increases, P_{O_2} decreases *except* when the patient is breathing gas with an enriched concentration of O_2. Because arterial P_{O_2} and P_{CO_2} change in opposite directions by nearly the same amount during hypoventilation, the contribution of hypoventilation to the patient's arterial hypoxia can be readily assessed. (In a 60-year-old person, for example, if P_{O_2} = 50 mm Hg and P_{CO_2} = 70 mm Hg, both have changed from their normal values by the same amount [30 mm Hg] and "pure" hypoventilation is present; in contrast, if P_{O_2} = 30 mm Hg and P_{CO_2} = 70 mm Hg, the change from normal of P_{CO_2} does not account for the entire change in P_{O_2}; therefore, some other cause in addition to hypoxia from hypoventilation must be present.) Arterial hypoxia from alveolar hypoventilation is not associated with an increased alveolar-arterial P_{O_2} difference and is "corrected" by breathing 100 per cent O_2.

IMPAIRED DIFFUSION. Abnormalities of diffusion do not cause arterial hypoxia in persons at rest unless they are extremely severe. Although these occur in occasional patients with respiratory failure, for practical purposes the possible contributions of an abnormality of diffusion to a given patient's arterial hypoxia can be ignored except during exercise or at high altitude. This practice is permissible because diffusion disturbances, even when marked, cause only relatively small increases in the patient's alveolar-arterial P_{O_2} difference, and this abnormality, if it exists, is readily corrected by adding small amounts of O_2 to the inspired air.

VENTILATION-PERFUSION IMBALANCE. When gas exchange units receive more blood flow than ventilation, arterial hypoxia results. Mismatching of ventilation-perfusion is by far the most common cause of arterial hypoxia and can be recognized by giving the patient 100 per cent O_2 to breathe; this causes the alveolar-arterial P_{O_2} difference from pure mismatching that is present while the patient breathes room air to decrease and arterial P_{O_2} to increase to normal values (>550 mm Hg). The importance of breathing 100 per cent O_2 is shown in Figure 70–1; in the presence of a severe ventilation-perfusion disturbance (σ = 2.0 in the figure), even an $F_{I_{O_2}}$ of 0.8 fails to raise P_{O_2} to normal values but 1.0 does. Although a "pure" ventilation-perfusion inequality can lead to CO_2 retention, this is an uncommon cause of hypercapnia because as arterial P_{CO_2} tends to increase, it stimulates peripheral and central chemoreceptors and increases ventilation; this, in turn, reduces P_{CO_2} back to normal values but, owing to the shape of the oxyhemoglobin dissociation curve, does not correct the hypoxia.

RIGHT-TO-LEFT SHUNTS. Shunts of blood from right to left may occur through abnormal anatomic communications in the lung (e.g., pulmonary arteriovenous fistula) but much more frequently by perfusion of lung units that are completely unventilated because they are either collapsed (atelectasis) or filled with fluid (pulmonary edema, pneumonia, alveolar proteinosis). Regardless of the cause, an alveolar-arterial P_{O_2} difference results that increases when the patient breathes 100 per cent O_2 compared with the value obtained while breathing room air. For reasons similar to those occurring in patients with ventilation-perfusion imbalances, CO_2 retention seldom occurs in patients with right-to-left shunts.

DECREASED INSPIRED P_{O_2}. Expected values of arterial P_{O_2} are corrected for the influence of decreasing barometric pressure; strictly speaking, therefore, the effects of altitude on inspired P_{O_2} and the resulting decreased arterial P_{O_2} are not an abnormal cause of hypoxia, even though the hypoxia may be severe and dangerous. Occasionally, pathologic hypoxia occurs when ambient P_{O_2} is reduced because of combustion of O_2 or because of dilution by some other gas. However, this phenomenon is not

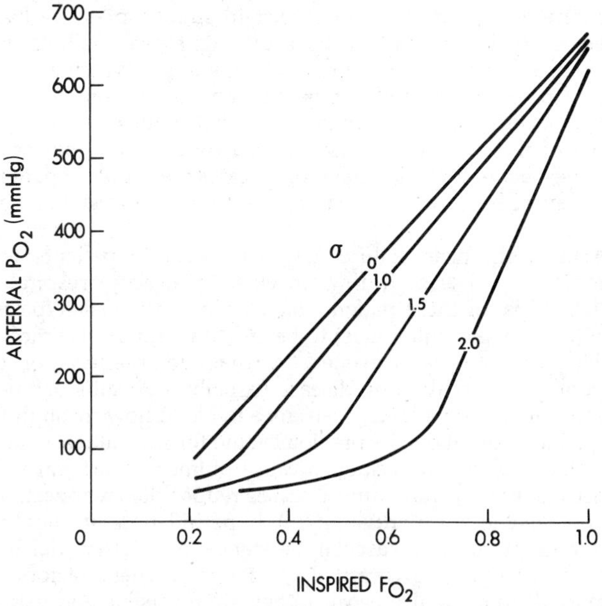

Figure 70–1. Graph showing the effects of changing inspired O_2 concentration (F_{O_2}) on arterial P_{O_2} in the presence of varying amounts of ventilation-perfusion inequality. When ventilation and perfusion are evenly matched (σ = 0), the relationship between inspired F_{O_2} and arterial P_{O_2} is linear. As ventilation-perfusion inequalities worsen (σ = 1.0 to 2.0), the effect of breathing a given F_{O_2} is progressively less. (Modified from West JB, Wagner PD: Bioengineering Aspects of the Lung. New York, Marcel Dekker, Inc., 1977. Reprinted with permission of the authors and publisher.)

of importance when interpreting the results of analysis of arterial blood specimens obtained in the hospital or clinic.

HYPERCAPNIA. In contrast to arterial hypoxia, which may result from five different pathophysiologic derangements, arterial hypercapnia can always be interpreted as signifying alveolar hypoventilation. This is true because arterial P_{CO_2} (Pa_{CO_2}) is governed by the relationship between CO_2 production ($\dot{V}_{CO_2}$) and alveolar ventilation ($\dot{V}_A$); $Pa_{CO_2} = k\dot{V}_{CO_2}/\dot{V}_A$. Normally, however, even when CO_2 production increases markedly, alveolar ventilation increases proportionately and arterial P_{CO_2} is maintained within narrow limits. Thus an increase in arterial P_{CO_2} can always be viewed as respiratory failure in the sense that alveolar ventilation is inadequate to eliminate all the CO_2 being produced at that time. Severe ventilation-perfusion imbalances and right-to-left shunts can produce CO_2 retention, but this is uncommon because, as already emphasized, alveolar ventilation increases and corrects the disturbance.

An increase or decrease in P_{CO_2} in the blood has a direct effect on the amount of carbonic acid in the blood and a reciprocal effect on pH. Acute changes in P_{CO_2} have a more profound effect on pH than chronic changes owing to differences in plasma bicarbonate. With acute increases or decreases in P_{CO_2}, there is little change in bicarbonate level and a considerable change in pH; after three to five days of sustained changes in P_{CO_2}, renal compensation has increased plasma bicarbonate in hypercapnia and decreased it in hypocapnia, both tending to restore pH toward normal. Many patients with respiratory failure have mixed respiratory and nonrespiratory acid-base disturbances. Knowledge of the time course of a patient's problem as well as the magnitude of changes in plasma bicarbonate is extremely useful in providing the necessary understanding for appropriate treatment of all components of the disorder.

Right Heart Failure

Acute respiratory failure can cause acute right heart failure (acute cor pulmonale). The normal right ventricle is not a good pressure generator and cannot sustain sudden pressure loads over 40 to 50 mm Hg. Thus acute right heart failure may develop in any condition in which pulmonary vascular resistance increases abruptly; this happens most commonly in patients with multiple pulmonary emboli with obstruction of much of the pulmonary vascular bed (usually >60 per cent). At times, acute cor pulmonale complicates the course of patients with severe bronchial asthma or other forms of marked airways obstruction.

Acute right heart failure may also occur in patients with chronic lung disease during an episode of acute respiratory failure. Most of these patients have right ventricular hypertrophy (chronic cor pulmonale) to begin with, and a subclinical or stable condition is worsened by the added effects of the superimposed acute lung disease (usually bronchitis or pneumonia). In these patients, resistance to blood flow through the lungs increases above its previous value for several reasons: (1) alveolar hypoxia and acidemia cause pulmonary arterial vasoconstriction; (2) certain lung diseases reduce the cross-sectional area available for perfusion; (3) hyperinflation of the lung increases pulmonary vascular resistance; and (4) arterial hypoxia may depress myocardial contractility. These factors are important to recognize because they are reversible and usually respond well to appropriate treatment of the intercurrent acute disorder.

CAUSES OF RESPIRATORY FAILURE

Because respiratory failure is defined as the presence of arterial hypoxia with or without hypercapnia, it is obvious that a large variety of disorders are capable of producing these abnormalities. For convenience, the multiple causes of respiratory failure can be classified, depending on which component of the respiratory system is involved. Because most of these disorders characteristically cause either acute or chronic respiratory failure, they can be subdivided further into these categories.

Diseases Causing Airways Obstruction

ACUTE. Obstruction may result from acute diseases that involve any portion of the upper and lower airways. The presence of respiratory failure depends on the magnitude and extent of the narrowing. Obstruction of the *extra*thoracic airway (nasopharynx, larynx, extrathoracic portion of the trachea) usually causes stridor, a characteristic alteration of breathing that is associated with harsh, high-pitched respiratory noises that are louder and more pronounced during inspiration than expiration. In contrast, obstruction of the *intra*thoracic airways causes wheezing, an abnormality of breathing in which expiration is louder and longer than inspiration.

Obstruction of the upper airways can result from (1) inflammation-induced swelling of the mucosa secondary to infections, allergic reactions, and, less commonly, thermal or mechanical injuries and (2) impaction of foreign bodies or, occasionally, tumors. Acute obstruction of the upper airways is particularly likely to develop in infants and young children who have smaller and hence more vulnerable upper passages than older children and adults.

Acute obstruction of the lower airways is usually caused by swelling of the mucosa, secretions in the lumen, or bronchospasm. Accordingly, bronchial asthma, infections, bronchiolitis, and the inhalation of chemicals (such as nitrogen dioxide in silo-filler's disease) are important causes of acute respiratory failure.

CHRONIC. Diffuse obstruction may result from disorders originating in large bronchi (bronchiectasis), small bronchi (bronchitis), or the lung parenchyma (emphysema). These abnormalities characteristically progress gradually and lead to chronic respiratory failure. Of considerable importance are the intercurrent episodes of acute disease, usually pneumonia or bronchitis, that complicate the underlying disorder and often worsen the severity of existing respiratory failure.

Diseases Causing Parenchymal Infiltration

ACUTE. The most common cause of acute infiltration of the parenchyma is pneumonia, which usually has an infectious origin but occasionally is caused by inhalation or aspiration of a toxic chemical. Whether acute respiratory failure develops depends on the extent and severity of the disease. Immunologic reactions from drugs, migrating parasites, or leukoagglutinins are uncommon causes of acute respiratory failure but are important because of their special therapeutic requirements.

CHRONIC. There are over 100 different conditions that can cause chronic diffuse parenchymal infiltration. When severe, any of these can cause chronic respiratory failure. As in patients with chronic airways obstruction, patients with chronic infiltrative diseases may have intercurrent episodes of bronchopulmonary infection that cause acute worsening of their underlying respiratory status.

Diseases Causing Pulmonary Edema

CARDIOGENIC. Pulmonary edema in patients with heart disease may be acute or chronic in onset; both varieties are caused by an increase in the hydrostatic pressure within pulmonary capillaries. Pulmonary edema may follow an acute myocardial infarction or acute left ventricular failure of any cause (hypertensive crises, arrhythmias), or it may be precipitated in patients with valvular or other forms of chronic heart disease by sudden changes in their cardiorespiratory status (from arrhythmias, hypoxemia, or increased systemic blood pressure). Chronic pulmonary edema is found in patients with chronic, usually refractory, heart failure, but even in these patients the amount of edema increases and decreases according to changing hemodynamics and therapy.

NONCARDIOGENIC. It has long been recognized that acute pulmonary edema can accompany certain conditions that do not involve the heart. The basic pathophysiologic abnormality in most of these disorders appears to be an increased permeability of the pulmonary capillary endothelium, but other forms of pulmonary edema (high altitude pulmonary edema, reexpansion pulmonary edema) also occur. Pulmonary edema resulting from increased permeability is an important and apparently steadily increasing cause of acute respiratory failure, especially in patients who are hospitalized with serious medical or surgical illnesses that initially do not involve the lungs. After a latent period of 6 to 24 hours, these patients develop progressive arterial hypoxia, decreased compliance, and extensive roentgenographic infiltrations; in fatal cases, the lungs are found to be nearly airless, intensely congested, and filled with a proteinaceous edema fluid that also contains large numbers of red blood cells; occasionally, hyaline membranes are found. This constellation of clinical, physiologic, and pathologic events is now known as the *adult respiratory distress syndrome* and has been reported as a complication of many apparently unrelated conditions (Table 70–1). The feature common to all these disorders is the presence of diffuse injury to the alveolar-capillary membrane. Once damage has occurred, probably by many different pathways, and the permeability of the membrane is increased, pulmonary edema follows; thus the clinical, physiologic, and pathologic manifestations are similar, regardless of the cause of the injury. The adult respiratory distress syndrome is described at greater length in Ch. 71.

Pulmonary Vascular Diseases

ACUTE. Pulmonary embolism is usually accompanied by a decreased arterial P_{O_2} and P_{CO_2}, the latter reflecting the hyperventilation that nearly always occurs. Pulmonary embolism is also an important cause of worsening respiratory failure in patients with underlying chronic lung disease. Fat emboli and emboli from platelet-fibrin aggregates can cause marked hypoxia by increasing the permeability of the alveolar-capillary membrane and producing severe pulmonary edema.

CHRONIC. Pulmonary vasculitis and recurrent thromboem-

TABLE 70–1. PARTIAL LIST OF CONDITIONS THAT HAVE BEEN ASSOCIATED WITH THE ADULT RESPIRATORY DISTRESS SYNDROME

Shock of any etiology	Inhaled toxins
Infections	O_2 (high concentrations)
Gram-negative sepsis	Smoke
Viral pneumonia	Corrosive chemicals (NO_2, Cl_2, NH_3, phosgene, cadmium)
Bacterial pneumonia	Hematologic disorders
Trauma	Intravascular coagulation
Fat emboli	Massive blood transfusion
Lung contusion	Metabolic disorders
Nonthoracic trauma (including head injury)	Pancreatitis
Liquid aspiration	Uremia
Gastric juice	Paraquat ingestion
Fresh and salt water (drowning)	Miscellaneous
Hydrocarbon fluids	Increased intracranial pressure (including seizures)
Drug overdose	Eclampsia
Heroin	Postcardioversion
Methadone	Radiation pneumonitis
Propoxyphene	Postcardiopulmonary bypass
Barbiturates	
Colchicine	

bolism are not common conditions and, when present, usually do not cause respiratory failure until the late stages of the disease. Recurrent thromboembolism occurs in intravenous drug abusers and in patients with chronic peripheral venous thrombi, sickle cell anemia, and schistosomiasis. Pulmonary vasculitis occurs in patients with scleroderma, other collagen diseases, and primary pulmonary hypertension.

Diseases of the Chest Wall and Pleura

ACUTE. The most important cause of sudden respiratory failure from acute disorders involving the thoracic cage is injury to the chest wall. Segmental fractures of several ribs or fractures of ribs on both sides of the sternum can result in a flail chest. Besides the impairment of ventilatory function that results from the unstable chest wall, gas exchange abnormalities are often compounded by contusion of the lung underneath the site of injury. Spontaneous or traumatic pneumothorax is an important cause of acute respiratory failure, which may be severe and which often afflicts otherwise healthy persons.

CHRONIC. Severe idiopathic or acquired kyphoscoliosis can cause chronic respiratory failure, which is often associated with cor pulmonale. Patients with massive pleural effusion(s) or with thickened, constrictive pleural layer(s) may also have chronic respiratory failure.

Disorders of the Neuromuscular System

Disorders of the neuromuscular system are classified into which part of the effector system is involved, i.e., the brain, neuronal pathways, or muscles of respiration, rather than into acute and chronic varieties. Patients with these disorders often have normal lungs; respiratory failure occurs from lack of ventilation.

BRAIN DISORDERS. Probably the most common cause of respiratory failure from impaired function of the central nervous system comes from the use of sedative drugs or anesthetic agents. Suppression of ventilatory drive from opiates, barbiturates, psychic depressants, alcohol, and a variety of sedative drugs results in hypoxia and hypercapnia that may be life threatening. Ventilatory stimuli can also be depressed by many diseases of the central nervous system, including vascular diseases, tumors, and infections.

SPINAL CORD AND PERIPHERAL NERVE DISORDERS. Injuries to the cervical or high thoracic spinal cord may produce immediate respiratory failure from paralysis of the muscles of respiration. Loss of anterior horn cell function in patients with poliomyelitis was an important cause of acute and chronic respiratory failure but is seldom encountered now because of the widespread use of vaccination. Polyneuritis, whether postinfectious (Guillain-Barré syndrome) or toxic, is an uncommon but important cause of respiratory failure in view of its inherent reversibility.

MUSCULAR DISORDERS. The final effectors in the system that controls breathing are the skeletal muscles of respiration. When these muscles are involved by generalized myopathies, such as muscular dystrophy or myasthenia gravis, respiratory failure results. Respiratory failure in patients with myasthenia gravis occurs during myasthenic or cholinergic crises. In contrast, respiratory failure in patients with muscular dystrophy is nearly always chronic and related to an advanced stage in the progression of the disease.

SLEEP APNEA. Brief periods of apnea occur in normal persons during deep sleep. Much more prolonged episodes associated with severe hypoxia have been documented in patients with massive obesity, chronic mountain sickness, enlarged tonsils, and many other disorders. Apnea results from either failure of ventilatory drive or obstruction of the upper airway. Severe sleep apnea can cause chronic respiratory failure, cor pulmonale, psychosis, and pathologic daytime sleepiness, a condition sometimes called the pickwickian syndrome, with somewhat dubious literary authenticity. Sleep apnea is discussed at greater length in Ch. 472.

CLINICAL MANIFESTATIONS

Given the great variety of disorders that can cause respiratory failure, it is obvious that the clinical manifestations in a given patient depend in large part on which underlying disease he or she has; these are dealt with elsewhere in this book. When respiratory failure ensues and if the blood gas disturbances are sufficiently severe, the signs and symptoms of hypoxia, and possible hypercapnia, become superimposed upon the signs and symptoms of the underlying disease. It should be emphasized that the clinical manifestations of hypoxia and hypercapnia are nonspecific and usually occur late in the evolution of the clinical problem. This statement underscores the earlier axiom that the diagnosis of respiratory failure is made in the laboratory and not at the bedside.

Hypoxia

The signs and symptoms of acute hypoxia are chiefly caused by abnormalities in central nervous system and cardiovascular function. Characteristic features are impaired judgment and motor instability, a clinical picture closely resembling acute alcoholism. As hypoxia worsens, the brainstem is affected and death results from depression of the medullary respiratory centers. The initial cardiovascular effects of acute hypoxia are tachycardia and increased blood pressure; when hypoxia is very severe, bradycardia, myocardial depression, and shock ensue. Recognizable cyanosis of the lips, mucous membranes, and nail beds usually occurs when the concentration of reduced hemoglobin in the capillaries is >5 grams per deciliter Accordingly, cyanosis can result from decreases in either arterial Po_2 or blood flow. In patients with lung disease, cyanosis cannot be detected by most physicians until arterial Po_2 is <50 mm Hg; some observers cannot recognize cyanosis unless arterial Po_2 is <40 mm Hg!

In patients with chronic hypoxia, the central nervous system manifestations are drowsiness, inattentiveness, apathy, fatigue, and delayed reaction time. The chronic cardiovascular effects are often minimal, but pulmonary hypertension or even cor pulmonale with signs of right heart failure may be detected on clinical examination. One of the hallmarks of chronic hypoxia is erythrocytosis, which may cause noticeable plethora and changes in the hemoglobin concentration, hematocrit ratio, or red blood cell count. However, the increase in red blood cell mass in many patients with chronic hypoxia is masked by an almost proportionate increase in plasma volume; in these patients, the usual peripheral blood indices of the red blood cell production (hemoglobin, hematocrit) do not reveal the full extent of the erythropoietic response.

Hypercapnia

The physiologic consequences of hypercapnia depend not only on the amount of excess CO_2 in the body but also on the rate at which retention develops. Increases in P_{CO_2} from acute respiratory failure lead to a constellation of progressive disturbances of central nervous system function: apprehension, confusion, drowsiness, coma, and death. The vascular responses represent a mixture of vasoconstriction, from generalized sympathetic activity, and vasodilation, from local accumulation of CO_2; thus the cardiovascular abnormalities are variable and depend on whether vasoconstrictor or vasodilator influences predominate. There are usually tachycardia and sweating, but blood pressure may be high, low, or normal.

In contrast, if P_{CO_2} increases slowly, compensation takes place and the clinical consequences may be minimal at values of arterial P_{CO_2} that would cause death if reached suddenly. There are numerous patients with arterial P_{CO_2} values over 100 mm Hg who are ambulatory and at times living active lives, although most breathe supplementary O_2 to prevent life-threatening hypoxia. Patients with hypercapnia from chronic respiratory failure frequently complain of headaches and drowsiness; these symptoms are probably attributable to the potent cerebral vasodilating effect of excess CO_2. In addition, patients with chronic hypercapnia may have papilledema, muscular twitching, coarse myoclonic jerky motions, and asterixis. At times, the neurologic findings simulate those of a brain tumor.

TREATMENT OF ACUTE RESPIRATORY FAILURE

The time course of worsening abnormalities varies in patients with acute respiratory failure from almost instantaneous (flail chest, pulmonary embolism) to a gradual crescendo during a period of several hours or even days (respiratory tract infections, bronchial asthma). The demands for treatment and the speed with which it must be provided obviously differ from one patient to another. It is difficult to generalize about such an extremely variable clinical condition, but the principles of treatment of acute respiratory failure are as follows: *first,* establish an airway, administer O_2, and maintain adequate alveolar ventilation; *second,* identify and treat the underlying condition and monitor the patient's progress carefully.

Establish an Airway

The upper airway tends to be occluded in unconscious patients because of relaxation of the oropharyngeal muscles and tongue and the presence of saliva, vomitus, and other secretions. When respiratory arrest occurs away from medical facilities, clear all material from the oropharynx and place the victim on his or her back with the head tilted backward as far as possible and extend the jaw forward. Sometimes these simple maneuvers are all that is required to enable breathing to resume spontaneously. If it does not, start mouth-to-mouth breathing; after three or four quick full breaths without allowing time for deflation to occur, maintain deep breaths once every five seconds until the emergency is over.

An airway can be established by three different methods: an oropharyngeal tube, an endotracheal tube passed via the nose or mouth, and a tracheostomy. Selection of the procedure depends on available facilities and personnel and on the site and severity of the obstruction.

OROPHARYNGEAL AIRWAY. An oropharyngeal airway is valuable in unconscious patients who are breathing spontaneously (e.g., during recovery from general anesthesia, after a cerebrovascular accident). An oropharyngeal airway is also useful in patients who are apneic during emergency resuscitation but who are receiving some form of assisted ventilation (mouth-to-mouth respiration, bag-mask system). Although an oropharyngeal tube is commonly used in these clinical circumstances, its role must be viewed as temporary, either while the patient is waking up or until an endotracheal tube can be inserted.

ENDOTRACHEAL TUBE. The preferred method of establishing an airway in most emergencies is with an endotracheal tube. Once inserted, the tube is used to remove secretions and to provide ventilation. Endotracheal tubes can usually be passed quickly through the nose or, at times, through the mouth into the trachea by an experienced person; the airway is then sealed by inflating a balloon near the tip of the tube. Endotracheal tubes should be used in nearly all patients with acute respiratory failure severe enough to require control of their airways.

TRACHEOSTOMY. Emergency tracheostomy was formerly the only way of quickly establishing an airway in patients with acute respiratory failure. Now, emergency tracheostomy is contraindicated except in one clinical situation: acute obstruction of upper airways (e.g., from foreign bodies, trauma, or inflammation). Otherwise, intubation with an endotracheal tube is the treatment of choice for acute respiratory failure. Tracheostomy, if needed, can be performed at a later time in the operating room under ideal conditions. There is virtually no mortality and very little morbidity with an elective tracheostomy, in contrast to the high incidence of complications associated with emergency tracheostomy performed at the bedside.

The decision to convert a satisfactory endotracheal intubation to a tracheostomy is not an easy one and must be individualized in each case. The availability of tubes of inert plastic with low pressure cuffs permits endotracheal tubes to be used for weeks rather than days without prohibitive injury; the main mechanical difference between endotracheal and tracheostomy tubes is the trauma to the vocal cords from the former and problems related to the stoma in the latter. The usual reasons for performing a tracheostomy in a patient with a satisfactory endotracheal tube are (1) failure to control secretions (sometimes it is difficult to suction the lungs adequately, especially the left side, through a long endotracheal tube) and (2) the need for prolonged (i.e., several weeks) intubation for assisted ventilation and/or removal of secretions (these circumstances are uncommon but occur particularly in patients with neuromuscular disease and chest wall injuries).

The presence of a tube and its cuff in the airways can cause necrosis of the mucosa of the trachea; at times the entire airway wall may be eroded with penetration of the esophagus (tracheoesophageal fistula) or a neighboring blood vessel (innominate artery), causing severe hemorrhage. Delayed complications after extubation are caused by damage to the trachea or larynx from the tube or cuff; injury to the vocal cords merely impairs phonation, but serious and life-threatening obstruction to airflow can result from stenosis or malacia of the tracheal wall. These complications should be considered and evaluated in any patient who complains of persisting hoarseness or who develops breathlessness or stridor at any time after endotracheal intubation.

HUMIDIFICATION. Insertion of an endotracheal or tracheostomy tube bypasses the normal source of humidification of the inspired air. When this occurs and unhumidified air or gas mixture is breathed, the result is drying of the mucosa and impairment of mucociliary clearance. Thus as long as the upper airway is bypassed, patients must receive air or a mixture of O_2 that is fully saturated with water vapor at their body temperature. This is easily accomplished if the patient is being ventilated with most commercial ventilators that have heated humidifiers in the circuit. If the patient is breathing spontaneously, humidified gas can be delivered through a T-piece connected to the endotracheal or tracheostomy tube. When proper humidification is carried out, remember that there is *no* insensible water loss through the respiratory tract when evaluating the patient's daily fluid balance.

Administer Oxygen

Acute respiratory failure, by definition, includes decreased arterial P_{O_2}. When respiratory failure is severe, death results from the central nervous system or cardiovascular consequences of hypoxia. During emergencies, supplementary O_2 is given without worrying about the concentration being used; in general, the higher the concentration of O_2, the better. After the patient's emergency condition has stabilized, attention is directed to administering O_2 in the lowest possible concentration required to correct the hypoxia. Any more O_2 than required to raise arterial Po_2 to a safe level exposes the patient to the direct toxicity of O_2 on the lung parenchyma and other undesirable effects: suppression of alveolar macrophage function and mucociliary clearance. In patients with chronic obstructive pulmonary disease, especially those with chronic hypercapnia, the administration of O_2 is likely to worsen the CO_2 retention. The further increase in Pco_2 can be explained in part by suppression of pre-existing hypoxic ventilatory drive; the remaining increase can be accounted for through the effects of O_2 on the matching of ventilation and perfusion and the Haldane effect. In general, the higher the inspired O_2 concentration, the greater the CO_2 retention; this observation underlies the use of "low-flow" O_2 for these patients as described below under Treatment of Chronic Respiratory Failure.

The usual goal of O_2 therapy in acute respiratory failure is to raise arterial Po_2 to between 60 and 80 mm Hg. Because these values lie on the flat portion of the oxyhemoglobin dissociation curve, most of the available hemoglobin is saturated with O_2; raising arterial Po_2 values even higher adds very little additional O_2 to the blood and may require increases in alveolar Po_2 concentrations to toxic levels. At times, especially when the mechanism of arterial hypoxia is right-to-left shunting of blood, arterial Po_2 may be considerably less than 60 mm Hg even with the patient breathing 100 per cent O_2. When this occurs, other maneuvers such as addition of end-expiratory pressure are required to raise arterial Po_2 and to allow a reduction in inspired O_2 concentration.

There are several ways of giving supplementary O_2 to a patient. Which method is chosen depends on the cause and severity of the arterial hypoxia and convenience to the patient. It is important to emphasize that no method can be relied upon to produce a certain increase in arterial Po_2; the response depends on which physiologic mechanism(s) is responsible for the hypoxia. Thus it is always advisable to monitor the effects of O_2 administration by serial analyses of arterial blood.

NASAL CANNULAS OR PRONGS. The concentration of O_2 in the inspired air can be enriched by nasal cannulas, catheters, or prongs. These devices work well even when patients breathe through their mouths. However, because of the drying effects of unhumidified O_2 on the nasal mucous membranes, if >3 to 5 liters per minute is needed to achieve satisfactory arterial oxygenation, other methods of administration are advisable.

VENTURI MASKS. These masks work on the principle of entrainment of a fixed proportion of air that mixes with the O_2 being supplied and results in a constant inspired concentration: 24, 28, 35, or 40 per cent O_2. Although a properly used Venturi mask ensures that the inspired O_2 concentration is constant, the effects on arterial Po_2 vary considerably from one patient to another. The mask is somewhat uncomfortable and must be removed for eating and drinking. Because of these disadvantages and high cost, other simpler and cheaper methods usually suffice to deliver relatively low (21 to 41 per cent) concentrations of O_2.

RESERVOIR MASKS. When high concentrations of O_2 (40 to 80 per cent) are needed in patients who are not intubated, reservoir masks are used. To ensure optimal efficiency of operation, the masks must be tight fitting to avoid leaks; because this often causes discomfort, it is difficult to deliver high concentrations of O_2 by reservoir masks for long periods.

OTHER METHODS. Most of the recently developed mechanical ventilators have regulators that can be set to deliver an inspired O_2 concentration that ranges from 21 to 100 per cent. One of the best ways of ensuring that patients actually receive high concentrations of O_2 (60 to 100 per cent) is to use a mechanical ventilator connected to an endotracheal or tracheostomy tube.

Maintain Alveolar Ventilation

Emergency resuscitation after respiratory arrest requires ventilation by mouth-to-mouth respiration or a bag and mask device. As soon as possible thereafter, if the patient does not resume spontaneous breathing, intubation and ventilation by a mechanical ventilator are indicated. Similar considerations apply to patients with acute respiratory failure whose breathing is insufficient to maintain adequate gas exchange. The main indications for mechanical ventilation are ventilatory failure, shown by an elevated or rising Pco_2, or severe refractory hypoxia, shown by a low Po_2 that cannot be corrected without high concentrations of O_2 and often end-expiratory pressure. Special indications include the need to produce alkalosis, as in head injuries and certain drug overdoses, or to stabilize the thorax, as in traumatic injuries that result in flail chest.

MECHANICAL VENTILATION. Two types of mechanical ventilators can be used to provide assisted ventilation: pressure ventilators, in which a certain (adjustable) airway pressure is reached by the machine during each breathing cycle, or volume ventilators, in which a constant (adjustable) tidal volume is delivered to the patient with each breath. Most commercially available ventilators of both types can be set either to cycle automatically or to assist breathing once it is initiated by the patient. Most instruments also provide means of controlling inspiratory and expiratory flow rates. Pressure ventilators were widely used for many years, but almost all hospitals now use volume ventilators, which are more versatile and more reliable.

END-EXPIRATORY PRESSURE. Mechanical ventilators ordinarily raise airway pressure during inspiration and allow it to fall to zero (atmospheric) pressure during expiration; this pattern of assisted ventilation is known as intermittent positive pressure ventilation, or IPPV. At times, it is desirable to add positive pressure to the airway during expiration as well as inspiration to hold the lung at a higher end-expiratory lung volume (functional residual capacity) than it would reach at zero end-expiratory pressure; this pattern of assisted ventilation is known as continuous positive pressure ventilation, or CPPV. Keeping the lung at a high end-expiratory lung volume prevents closure of alveoli and airways during expiration and often improves arterial Po_2 considerably. Positive end-expiratory pressure (or PEEP) is most useful in patients with the conditions that cause the adult respiratory distress syndrome (Table 70–1).

Although end-expiratory pressure usually results in an improvement in arterial Po_2 and O_2 content, it may also decrease cardiac output by impairing venous return. Accordingly, the actual delivery of O_2 to the tissues of the body may decrease. Thus it is important to monitor both the respiratory and circulatory responses to end-expiratory pressure to determine the optimal amount of pressure and the need for additional therapeutic interventions. Another common and serious hazard of end-expiratory pressure is its tendency to cause spontaneous pneumothorax and pneumomediastinum.

Identify and Treat the Underlying Condition

Acute respiratory failure always has a precipitating cause. Consequently, the cause of the condition should be identified as soon as possible after emergency measures have been started and the patient's condition has stabilized. Usually, the diagnosis can be established easily by a thorough history and physical examination, analysis of the blood and urine, and chest roentgenogram. Helpful auxiliary tests include those that evaluate central nervous system or cardiac function, those that determine the presence of drugs or poisons in the body, and bacteriologic study of secretions and blood.

Treatment obviously depends on the underlying cause, and the reader is referred to the appropriate chapters of this book for information about the therapy of specific pulmonary and other disorders that lead to acute respiratory failure. In all patients with acute respiratory failure, careful attention should be paid to fluid balance. Overhydration is a frequent and serious complication that can usually be avoided by careful attention to fluid replacement and monitoring of pulmonary capillary (wedge) pressure.

Many patients cared for in intensive care units are nutritionally depleted at the time of admission or become so soon afterward. Because morbidity and mortality are closely linked to nutritional status, it is important that this be assessed and, when necessary, treated by appropriate enteral or parenteral supplementation.

Monitor the Patient's Progress

The need for monitoring varies from patient to patient according to the response to initial treatment. If the disorder is readily reversible (e.g., bronchial asthma), the patient may respond sufficiently to go home shortly after being seen and treated. Other less rapidly responding conditions causing acute respiratory failure often require hospital care, and seriously ill patients are best treated in special acute care facilities (intensive care units) when available. Intensive care units provide an institutional focus of trained personnel and special equipment for the care of critically ill patients.

All seriously ill patients should have frequent measurements of blood pressure, constant monitoring of heart rate, careful recording of fluid intake and output, and determination of weight daily. Arterial blood gas analysis should be performed as often as needed but usually at least once daily. Special studies include measurement of cardiac output and placement of a Swan-Ganz catheter in the pulmonary artery for determination of pulmonary arterial and wedge pressures and sampling of mixed venous blood; this information is very helpful in guiding fluid replacement and ventilator adjustments, including levels of end-expiratory pressure. In general, wedge pressure values should be maintained in the normal range (5 to 10 mm Hg) and not allowed to increase above 10 mm Hg, especially in patients with the adult respiratory distress syndrome. Less reliance is being placed now, compared to previous years, on values of mixed venous Po_2 as a guide to oxygen delivery, especially in disorders such as sepsis and the adult respiratory distress syndrome. Attention is currently directed at improving oxygen delivery by increasing cardiac output through pharmacologic means or by increasing oxygen content through transfusions of packed red blood cells.

TREATMENT OF CHRONIC RESPIRATORY FAILURE

Patients with chronic lung disease often have sufficient alterations in their arterial Po_2 and Pco_2 values that they are said to be in chronic respiratory failure. Therapeutic regimens for these patients, whose disease is relatively stable, are delivered mainly on an outpatient basis and are designed to meet two objectives: (1) preventing or minimizing the number and severity of the intercurrent complications that would otherwise occur and (2) treating maximally all reversible elements of the underlying disorder. Many of the specific remedies are used for both purposes, and the approaches to preventive and maintenance therapy for patients with the most common chronic lung diseases, asthma, bronchitis, and emphysema, are discussed in Ch. 59 and 60.

Despite emphasis on preventing intercurrent complications, these attacks continue to plague the lives of patients with chronic lung disease. Acute episodes of bronchopulmonary infection, pneumothorax, pulmonary embolism, surgical procedures, and misuse of sedatives all add their effects to those of the underlying lung disease and frequently produce serious disturbances of blood gases. These episodes are potentially life threatening, are usually associated with prolonged morbidity, and frequently require hospitalization. The principles of therapy are to maintain oxygenation while treating all new, presumably reversible, elements of the disease in an effort to restore the patient to his or her former state of health.

Oxygen

Patients with chronic obstructive lung disease and superimposed episodes of acute respiratory failure nearly always have severe hypoxia from a combination of hypoventilation and ventilation-perfusion mismatching. Typical arterial blood values are Po_2 of approximately 30 mm Hg, Pco_2 of 70 mm Hg, and pH of 7.30. Neither the hypercapnia nor the acidemia is life threatening, but the hypoxia is potentially fatal. Thus treatment is directed mainly at alleviating the disturbance in oxygenation; the changes in Pco_2 and pH will return to the ordinary values for that patient as the acute condition improves. In view of the possibility that O_2 therapy may depress ventilation further by withdrawing the hypoxic stimulus to breathe and worsening the matching of ventilation and perfusion, O_2 is given initially in low concentrations (1 to 3 liters per minute). The goal is to raise Po_2 to satisfactory levels (50 to 60 mm Hg) without depressing ventilation to the extent that unacceptable increases in Pco_2 and decreases in pH (particularly) occur.

The O_2 is usually started at 2 liters per minute, and an arterial blood specimen is analyzed 15 to 30 minutes later to determine the patient's response. Depending on the Po_2 value, the flow of O_2 can be adjusted. If hypoventilation and acidemia result from too much O_2 (e.g., Po_2 80 mm Hg, Pco_2 80 mm Hg, and pH 7.25), the supplementary O_2 should *not* be discontinued but the flow rate should be decreased. The Po_2 decreases much faster than the stimulus to breathe returns, and cardiac arrest or other serious complications of hypoxia may result.

Intubation-Assisted Ventilation

Low-flow O_2 given in the manner described provides satisfactory relief of hypoxia in nearly all instances. Although the goal of low-flow O_2 is an arterial Po_2 of 50 to 60 mm Hg, at times one has to be satisfied with 40 to 50 mm Hg. When oxygenation cannot be achieved without intolerable hypercapnia and acidemia, the decision whether to intubate and ventilate the patient must be made. Experience with intubation and mechanical ventilation in this group of patients has been extremely unrewarding, particularly because of the prolonged need for assisted ventilation once intubation is performed and the poor prognosis for lengthy survival and return to useful life after recovery from the acute episode. Although each case must be considered individually, in general, patients with chronic obstructive pulmonary disease who develop superimposed acute respiratory failure should not be intubated. The major exception to this axiom is the need for ventilator support during the postoperative period. Doxapram (see Respiratory Stimulants, below) often allows administration of "extra" O_2 without depressing ventilatory drive.

Bronchodilators

Most intercurrent episodes of acute respiratory failure in patients with chronic obstructive pulmonary disease are associated with increased airways resistance from the presence of secretions, edema of the mucosa, and bronchospasm. Because it is impossible to discriminate among these, bronchodilator drugs are always included in the treatment regimen to take advantage of the reversibility of whatever element of bronchospasm is present.

When patients seek medical attention for intercurrent attacks, they frequently have already tried—and failed to respond to—oral and aerosolized bronchodilators. In this circumstance, intravenous aminophylline is the initial drug of choice. Aminophylline can be injected slowly in 250-mg or 500-mg boluses, or, if the patient has been hospitalized and prolonged treatment is envisioned, by a loading dose (5.6 mg per kilogram of body weight) and constant sustaining infusion (0.9 mg per kilogram of body weight per hour). These dosages should be reduced in patients who have been receiving aminophylline, who are elderly, or, especially, who have liver disease or heart failure. It is advisable to determine the aminophylline plasma level at the outset in those who have been taking the drug and 24 to 36 hours after the constant infusion regimen has been started to ensure that values are in the therapeutic range (10 to 20 μg per milliliter) and to avoid toxicity.

Selective β-2 sympathomimetic drugs, usually administered by aerosol, are another mainstay of treatment. Because aerosolized drugs fail to penetrate effectively throughout the tracheobronchial system in the presence of airways secretions and severe narrowing, they are given more frequently than normal, usually at 1- or 2-hour intervals.

The indications for and dosage of corticosteroids in this clinical setting are controversial, although there is an increasing tendency to use these drugs in virtually all patients with asthma or chronic obstructive lung disease whose exacerbation is severe enough to warrant hospitalization. Either methylprednisolone, 60 mg, or hydrocortisone, 100 mg, intravenously every six hours is indicated. Much higher doses of corticosteroids (e.g., methylprednisolone, 15 mg per kilogram of body weight per day in divided doses) have been recommended, but there is no evidence to suggest that these are more efficacious in this clinical setting than the lower doses recommended above.

Antimicrobials

Infections are the most frequent and important cause of acute respiratory failure in patients with chronic underlying lung disease. Intercurrent attacks usually begin as a typical cold, with rhinitis, pharyngitis, and headaches. Shortly afterward, lower respiratory involvement appears with increasing cough, sputum production, purulence, wheezing, and breathlessness. These episodes occur several times a year in most patients with chronic obstructive pulmonary disease. (It should be noted that fever, leukocytosis, and new roentgenographic infiltrations are uncommon in this syndrome). When airway infection is present, the sputum is not only purulent but usually contains numerous microorganisms detectable by Gram's stain of the secretions. Sputum cultures, however, often fail to reveal pathogenic bacteria, although at times *Streptococcus pneumoniae* and/or *Hemophilus influenzae* may be grown. Regardless of the presence or absence of identifiable pathogens, oral treatment with ampicillin (250 to 500 mg every six hours), a combined preparation of trimethoprim-sulfamethoxazole (160 mg and 800 mg, respectively, every 12 hours), or tetracycline (250 to 500 mg every six hours) frequently results in decreased volume of sputum, thinning of the secretions, change in sputum appearance from purulent to mucoid, and improvement in blood gases.

When pneumonia is present, signified by the presence of new infiltration(s) on the chest roentgenogram, Gram's stain of the sputum is likely to show one bacterial species predominating, and the initial selection of antimicrobials should cover this organism. Therapy can be revised, if necessary, when the results of the sputum cultures are available.

Control of Secretions

Many patients complain of thick tenacious sputum that is troublesome to clear. Although it seems desirable to attempt to alter the character of these secretions to facilitate their removal, there is no clear evidence that it is possible to do so by pharmacologic means. Iodides, enzymes, detergents, and acetylcysteine, administered orally or by aerosol, have been tried extensively, but none has been shown convincingly to be effective. Moreover, each has potential toxic side effects. Similarly, mist tents and ultrasonic nebulizers, once widely used, are seldom employed today. The best way to control secretions is to control infection with antimicrobials and to ensure adequate (but not excessive) hydration by the administration of intravenous fluids.

Patients with troublesome sputum retention may require intermittent nasotracheal suction to control the volume of secretions. Manual or mechanical percussion serves to loosen secretions and enhances their removal in patients who have retained sputum in their airways. Respiratory physical therapy, especially when carried out by a skilled therapist, may result in an increase in arterial P_{O_2} related to the improvement in the distribution of ventilation from clearance of sputum.

Treatment of Heart Failure

Cor pulmonale is an inevitable complication of severe chronic lung disease. Right ventricular hypertrophy followed by heart failure occurs secondary to the increased work load imposed on the ventricle by the changes in the pulmonary circulation from the effects of lung disease. Resistance to blood flow through the lungs increases when pulmonary blood vessels are destroyed (as in emphysema), obstructed (as in pulmonary thromboembolism), narrowed (from vasoconstriction), or compressed (breathing at high lung volumes), or the blood is unusually viscous (polycythemia). Patients whose cor pulmonale is well compensated or even inapparent while their chronic lung disease is stable often develop acute right heart failure during intercurrent attacks of acute respiratory failure. Peripheral edema, increased venous pressure, and an enlarged, painful liver are important clues to the presence of acute cardiac decompensation.

Most patients with right heart failure from cor pulmonale, even if severe, have a satisfactory diuresis when put to bed, given O_2 and treated appropriately for their underlying lung disease. Diuretics may make patients feel more comfortable by diminishing peripheral edema and hepatic and gastrointestinal congestion faster than spontaneous diuresis; but if used, the drugs should be administered orally in low doses. Intravenous ethacrynic acid or furosemide can cause excessive renal loss of Cl^- that worsens existing acid-base disturbances and depletes intravascular volume sufficiently to decrease cardiac output and blood pressure. A particularly dangerous situation occurs in patients who already have coexisting nonrespiratory (metabolic) alkalosis often from Cl^--losing diuretics, in addition to their hypercapnia from chronic respiratory failure; when the measures designed to improve ventilation lower arterial P_{CO_2} the nonrespiratory alkalosis becomes "unmasked" and arterial pH becomes markedly alkaline. When this occurs, the patients can develop cardiac arrhythmias, become comatose, or manifest convulsive seizures or other focal neurologic abnormalities.

If an element of pulmonary edema or pulmonary vascular congestion is present from left heart failure, this may also respond to diuretics. Whether left heart failure can occur secondary to purely right-sided disease is controversial. Of greater importance are coexisting causes of left-sided involvement (e.g., valvular disease, coronary atherosclerosis); furthermore, chronic hypoxia and severe polycythemia may impair left ventricular as well as right ventricular function.

Present evidence indicates that digitalis preparations are not beneficial in patients with cor pulmonale. Also, the use of digitalis is hazardous in patients with chronic respiratory failure owing to the sudden shifts in acid-base balance and electrolyte concentrations that may occur in these patients. Therefore digitalis drugs should be used only in patients with digitalis-responsive arrhythmias or coexisting left heart failure.

Respiratory Stimulants

With few exceptions, respiratory stimulants are obsolete. Nikethamide, picrotoxin, and ethamivan have been replaced by other less hazardous and more efficient methods of maintaining ventilation. Doxapram, a drug that works by stimulating carotid chemoreceptors rather than neurons in the brain, appears to be much safer than centrally acting stimulants. The chief use of doxapram is to minimize or prevent the depression of ventilation, with consequent increase in P_{CO_2} and decrease in pH, that occurs in some hypoxic patients with hypercapnia who are given O_2 to breathe.

Sedation

All sedative drugs should be avoided in patients with chronic lung disease and intercurrent acute respiratory failure, including diazepam (Valium) and chlordiazepoxide (Librium), which can suppress ventilation. Exceptions to this cardinal rule are made from time to time, but usually only when the patient is being mechanically ventilated and sedation is required to enable breathing synchronous with the machine.

Postoperative Complications

Patients with chronic respiratory failure are high-risk operative candidates. Moreover, the closer the surgical incision to the thorax, the higher the incidence of postoperative complications. Despite this caveat, it is safe to say that virtually *all* patients who have respiratory failure can safely undergo *non*-thoracic surgery or *nonresectional* thoracic surgery. Postoperative complications can be anticipated and often prevented by attention to the general principles of care outlined in this chapter. Close observation and monitoring are usually required, and these can best be carried out in an intensive care unit.

Aubier M, Murciano D, Milic-Emili J, Touaty E, Daghfous J, Pariente R, Derenne JP: Effects of the administration of O_2 on ventilation and blood gases in patients with chronic obstructive pulmonary disease during acute respiratory failure. Am Rev Respir Dis 122:747, 1980. *Nice study that explains and discusses why P_{CO_2} increases in patients with chronic obstructive pulmonary diseases when given supplementary O_2 to breathe.*

Bergofsky EH: Respiratory failure in disorders of the thoracic cage. Am Rev Respir Dis 119:643, 1979. *Comprehensive review of the pathophysiology of respiratory failure in kyphoscoliosis, obesity, and other disorders of the thoracic cage; 143 references.*

Martin L: Respiratory failure. Med Clin North Am 61:1369, 1977. *Emphasizes physiologic basis of diagnosis and treatment.*

Moser KM, Shibel EM, Beamon AJ: Acute respiratory failure in obstructive lung disease. Long-term survival after treatment in an intensive care unit. JAMA 225:705, 1973. *Documents poor prognosis.*

Nocturnal Oxygen Therapy Group: Continuous or nocturnal oxygen therapy in hypoxemic chronic obstructive lung disease: A clinical trial. Ann Intern Med 93:391, 1980. *Useful report of the controlled trial that has provided the standards for current administration of O_2 in chronic respiratory failure.*

Roussos C, Macklem PT: The respiratory muscles. N Engl J Med 307:786, 1982. *A classic new review concerning the contribution of respiratory muscles to respiratory failure, including how to recognize and treat this condition.*

Tate RM, Repine JE: Neutrophils and the adult respiratory distress syndrome. Am Rev Respir Dis 128:552, 1983. *Good review of the pathogenesis of acute lung injury with emphasis on the neutrophil. 136 references.*

Part IX
CRITICAL CARE MEDICINE

71. CRITICAL CARE MEDICINE

Philip C. Hopewell

Specialized hospital units for patients with severe illnesses were first utilized in the early 1950's for patients with poliomyelitis who required artificial ventilation. Now various types of critical care units are to be found in more than 80 per cent of hospitals in the United States having more than 200 beds. Life-threatening illnesses demand intensive medical care that is peculiar to these units and that depends upon a unique body of knowledge. The specialty that has evolved is known as critical care medicine.

The practice of critical care medicine involves virtually all areas in general internal medicine. Severe illness represents one end of a spectrum of pathophysiologic derangement that shades into less severe illness related to the same organ systems. The same basic diagnostic and therapeutic principles therefore apply. A wide variety of clinical problems are commonly encountered in critical care units, many of which are discussed in other chapters. This section will focus on areas in critical care medicine that are not extensively described elsewhere in this text and on the aspects of medical care that are unique to critical care units.

In the critically ill patient, perhaps more than in any other setting, the interdependence of organ systems must remain in sharp focus. Limited attention to one component of the illness, even if that component is predominant, will frequently yield a therapeutic approach that is detrimental to the patient as a whole. Not uncommonly, management of the critically ill patient presents extremely difficult dilemmas. For example, treatment directed toward reducing the pulmonary capillary wedge pressure in patients with the adult respiratory distress syndrome may adversely affect renal and central nervous system perfusion. Conversely, increasing the pulmonary artery wedge pressure to optimize cardiac output in a patient with ischemic heart disease may result in noncardiogenic pulmonary edema if there has been a pre-existing acute diffuse lung injury. Bronchodilating agents may increase cardiac irritability and therefore cause significant arrhythmias, particularly in the presence of hypoxemia or acid base disturbances or both. Nephrotoxic antimicrobial agents may be essential in the treatment of sepsis in a patient with pre-existing or acute renal disease. The physician who is primarily responsible for the care of a gravely ill patient must often synthesize an overall diagnostic and treatment strategy that incorporates the views of various consultants with a more narrow focus and reconcile the conflicting effects of their recommendations.

ATTRIBUTES OF A CRITICAL CARE UNIT

A critical care unit is defined by its ability to provide the environment, facilities, and personnel for the care of severely ill patients. The important features required of such a unit are listed in Table 71–1.

Critical care units may have a general orientation, treating all types of severely ill patients, or be more specialized, accepting only specific categories of patients as defined by the type of illness (for example, burn units), organ system involved (coronary and acute neurologic care units), specialty service designation (medical and surgical units), or patient age (neonatal intensive care units). In addition to the basic attributes listed in Table 71–1, specialized units provide medical personnel specifically skilled in the area of care provided by the unit and have available particular forms of technology with applications generally limited to the category of patients accepted by the unit.

TABLE 71–1. UNIQUE FEATURES OF CRITICAL CARE UNITS

1. High nurse-to-patient ratio
2. Ready accessibility of physicians
3. Ability to provide invasive hemodynamic monitoring
4. Availability of respiratory support techniques
5. Ability to provide supervised continuous intravenous infusions of pharmacologic agents

Critical care units usually need administrative policies and procedures that differ from those of standard hospital units. Because of the gravity of illness of their patients, critical care units require clear delineation of administrative and medical lines of authority and responsibility. Likewise, there must be at least general guidelines for admission and discharge of patients, specifically described nursing roles, standing orders, and a program of continuing staff education. The existence of such policies reduces the apparent ambiguity often inherent in the difficult environment of a critical care unit and enables prompt decision making.

National Institutes of Health. Consensus development of conference on critical care medicine. Crit Care Med 11:466, 1983. *This report summarizes the discussions of a large consensus development group that addressed issues of critical care unit utilization, organization, training of personnel, and research needs.*

GENERAL PRINCIPLES OF ASSESSMENT OF SEVERE RESPIRATORY DYSFUNCTION

The discussion in this section will focus on the techniques of assessment generally applicable to severely ill patients in whom it usually is neither possible nor desirable to perform elaborate comprehensive assessments of pulmonary function. Patients often cannot cooperate, and measurements made under unsteady conditions are generally inaccurate. The basic components of normal respiratory function are discussed in Ch. 57 and the characteristic abnormalities of various types of lung disorders in other chapters of Part VIII.

Nonspecific Indicators of Severity

Respiratory rate is perhaps the simplest measurement that can be made. Although influenced by many factors, the respiratory rate provides a general indication of cardiorespiratory function and may be the first clue to impending or early respiratory failure. In addition, periodic counting of respiratory rate serves as a simple monitoring technique.

The degree of pulsus paradoxus correlates with the forced expiratory volume in 1 sec (FEV_1) in patients with acute airways obstruction and therefore may indicate the severity of airways narrowing. Similarly, the presence of suprasternal, supraclavicular, and intercostal space retractions also correlates roughly with the degree of airways obstruction.

The mental status of the patient is an important, albeit even more nonspecific, indicator of the status of cardiorespiratory function. Behavioral alterations may reflect changes in the partial pressure of oxygen (Pa_{O_2}) and carbon dioxide (Pa_{CO_2}) in arterial blood.

Measurements of Lung Function

The lung function studies applicable in severely ill patients are rather limited. Depending on the type and severity of illness and the patient's ability to cooperate, one may measure vital capacity (VC), maximal inspiratory pressure (MIP), timed forced expiratory volume, and peak expiratory flow rate (PEFR).

The vital capacity is the maximal volume of air that can be slowly exhaled after maximal inspiration and as such provides an indication of the patient's ventilatory capability (Fig. 57–2). The VC is influenced by the respiratory neuromuscular system, the chest wall, the elastic properties of the lung, and the caliber of the airways. It cannot therefore be used to identify specific abnormalities. Nevertheless, it is particularly helpful in assessing and following patients with neuromuscular illnesses and in evaluating patients being mechanically ventilated to determine if it is feasible to consider weaning from the ventilator. A minimal acceptable VC is 10 to 15 ml per kilogram of body weight.

The maximal inspiratory pressure is somewhat analogous to the VC in the information that it provides and the factors by which it is influenced. However, the ability to generate an acceptable inspiratory pressure, less (more negative) than −20 cm H_2O, does not necessarily imply that the VC will be acceptable.

The timed forced expiratory volume, which is usually expressed as the forced expiratory volume in 1 second (FEV_1) over the forced vital capacity (FVC), measures the severity of airways obstruction in patients with asthma or chronic airways obstruction. The measurement may not be possible in patients with severe airways obstruction who have marked tachypnea. However, it does provide the best objective indicator of the degree of airways obstruction and, when measured serially, the response to therapy. Absolute FEV_1 values of less than .75 liter or less than 25 per cent of the predicted value are commonly associated with increased Pa_{CO_2} values and hence are indicative of severe obstruction.

Peak expiratory flow rate provides information similar to the FEV_1 in patients with airways obstruction. It has the distinct advantage of not requiring a full inhalation followed by a full forced exhalation, a maneuver that may actually worsen airways obstruction. The PEFR is measured by having the patient slowly inhale and then blow a short forced puff through the flowmeter, a maneuver similar to a cough. Values below 60 liters per minute are indicative of severe obstruction.

Arterial Blood Gas and pH Measurements

The Pa_{O_2}, Pa_{CO_2}, *and arterial pH* provide the most informative indication of integrated cardiorespiratory function. These values are not particularly sensitive to early cardiorespiratory abnormalities and are not specific for the kind of abnormality present, but they provide crucial information in patients with severe dysfunction. The mechanisms of normal gas exchange and its abnormalities are discussed in Ch. 57. This section will focus on the interpretation of arterial blood gas and pH values in the assessment of severely ill patients and how these interpretations can be used to ascertain the pathophysiology and indicate the proper approach to treatment.

HYPOXEMIA. Clinically significant reductions in Pa_{O_2} can result from *hypoventilation, mismatching of ventilation to perfusion,* and *shunting*. It is important to determine which of these mechanisms is operative in a given patient.

Hypoventilation as the cause of hypoxemia implies that the lung itself is normal and that the only necessary therapeutic goal is improved ventilation. This type of hypoxemia is characterized by a normal alveolar-to-arterial Po_2 difference ($P(A\text{-}a)_{O_2}$). The $P(A\text{-}a)_{O_2}$ can be determined by using the alveolar gas equation (Equation 5) to calculate PA_{O_2} and by measuring Pa_{O_2}. In patients breathing room air, the difference should not be greater than 10 mm Hg, and with an increased fractional concentration of oxygen in inspired gas (FI_{O_2}) sufficient to cause a PA_{O_2} of 200 mm Hg or greater, the $P(A\text{-}a)_{O_2}$ should not be greater than 40 mm Hg.

Ventilation-perfusion mismatching and *shunting* can be distinguished by measuring the response to administration of 100 per cent oxygen. The Pa_{O_2} will increase normally to values of nearly 600 mm Hg if the hypoxemia is due purely to mismatching, whereas with a shunt the increase may be markedly reduced depending on the magnitude of the shunt flow. Figure 71–1 shows the relationship between Pa_{O_2} and FI_{O_2} with different shunt fractions, and Figure 71–2 demonstrates the effect of increasing amounts of mismatching of ventilation to perfusion on Pa_{O_2} with different FI_{O_2} values. The percentage of cardiac output that is shunted can be calculated using Equation 10. The approach to treatment varies considerably, depending on whether the hypoxemia is caused by shunting or ventilation-perfusion mismatching. Mechanical ventilation is much more likely to be necessary in the former situation, whereas conservative management may be sufficient in the latter.

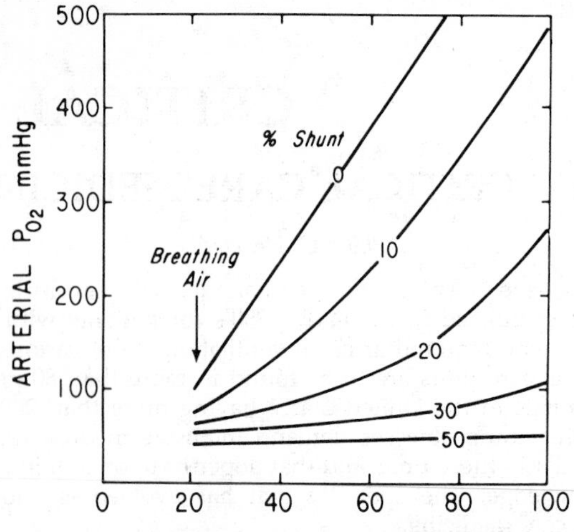

Figure 71–1. The relationship of Pa_{O_2} to FI_{O_2} with increasing amounts of shunt. Note that with 30 per cent of the cardiac output being shunted there is only a slight increase in Pa_{O_2} with increasing FI_{O_2} and with 50 per cent shunting, there is no increase in Pa_{O_2}. (From West JR: Pulmonary Pathophysiology: The Essentials. Copyright 1977, Baltimore, The Williams and Wilkins Company.)

It is also important to know the period of time during which the hypoxemia developed in a given patient. Blood gas criteria per se will not provide this information; however, it can be inferred that the patient is chronically hypoxic if secondary polycythemia or right heart failure or both are present. The absence of these findings, however, does not exclude chronic hypoxemia.

HYPERCAPNIA. Hypercapnia is caused only by alveolar hypoventilation. The amount of alveolar ventilation necessary to eliminate carbon dioxide and maintain a normal Pa_{CO_2} will vary depending on carbon dioxide production in accordance with Equation 1. Alveolar ventilation will in turn be influenced by the amount of wasted ventilation as shown in Equation 4.

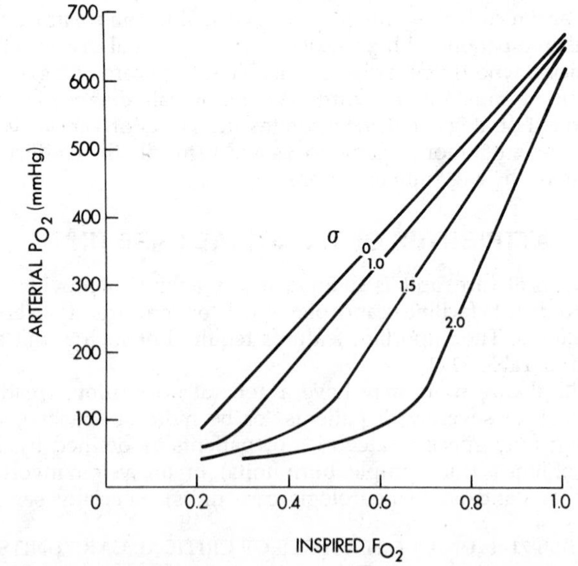

Figure 71–2. The relationship of Pa_{O_2} to FI_{O_2} with increasing amounts of ventilation to perfusion mismatching (σ = standard deviation of log normal distribution of ventilation and perfusion). Note that even with marked mismatching the Pa_{O_2} increases to nearly normal values with a very high FI_{O_2}. (From West JR: Pulmonary Pathophysiology: The Essentials. Copyright 1977, Baltimore, The Williams and Wilkins Company.)

Thus, alveolar hypoventilation can occur because of increased production of carbon dioxide or increased wasted ventilation or both.

The relationship between Pa_{CO_2} and blood bicarbonate concentration determines the arterial pH as indicated by the Henderson-Hasselbalch equation (Equation 13). The relationship between Pa_{CO_2} and arterial pH varies, however, depending on the time during which the Pa_{CO_2} has been increased and its rate of increase. Thus, by examining the relationships among Pa_{CO_2}, arterial pH, and $[HCO_3^-]$, the acuteness or chronicity of the carbon dioxide elevation can be inferred. Acute increases in Pa_{CO_2} are accompanied by only small increases in $[HCO_3^-]$ and arterial pH changes in a nearly linear fashion with Pa_{CO_2}. There is approximately a 0.0075 pH unit change in the opposite direction for every 1 mm Hg change in Pa_{CO_2}. Thus, an acute rise in Pa_{CO_2} from 40 mm Hg to 60 mm Hg would be expected to cause a decrease in arterial pH to 7.25. Over a period of one to three days, however, renal bicarbonate retention causes the $[HCO_3^-]$ to increase and buffer the arterial pH change. Thus, for a given change in Pa_{CO_2} the change in arterial pH is much less than when the change occurs acutely. These relationships are shown in Figure 71–3. Obviously the therapeutic implication of an acute as opposed to a chronic change in Pa_{CO_2} makes this an important distinction.

CHANGES IN pH. Respiratory acidosis has already been discussed; however, metabolic acidosis and metabolic and respiratory alkalosis also are of significance in patients with serious respiratory dysfunction. One of the several causes of metabolic acidosis is an imbalance between oxygen delivery and metabolic oxygen needs, leading to anaerobic metabolism and lactic acid production. In patients with severe respiratory disorders, this imbalance may occur because the work of breathing increases the demand for oxygen in the presence of hypoxia caused by the lung disease. Metabolic acidosis in this setting is a particularly ominous finding, suggesting that rapid deterioration is imminent and that prompt therapeutic interventions are necessary.

Both respiratory and metabolic alkalosis have important nonrespiratory effects in critically ill patients. Alkalosis predisposes to arrhythmias, decreases cardiac output, and reduces the seizure threshold. Hypocapnia per se with or without alkalosis reduces cerebral blood flow and may depress the level of consciousness. For these reasons alkalosis should be recognized as an important acid-base disturbance and corrective measures should be taken.

Calculations of Respiratory Variables

A number of equations and calculations are helpful in the assessment of respiratory function. Only brief descriptions of the physiologic principles involved with the equations will be presented in this section.

Representative normal values for selected cardiorespiratory variables are listed in Table 71–2.

EQUATIONS RELATED TO VENTILATION. Arterial P_{CO_2} is related directly to carbon dioxide production ($\dot{V}_{CO_2}$ in milliliters per minute) and inversely to alveolar ventilation ($\dot{V}_A$ in liters per minute) as follows:

$$Pa_{CO_2} = K\frac{\dot{V}_{CO_2}}{\dot{V}_A} \qquad (1)$$

where K is a constant.

The $\dot{V}_A$ is the difference between the tidal volume (V_T in liters) and the wasted or dead space ventilation (V_D) multiplied by the respiratory rate (F in breaths per minute).

$$\dot{V}_A = (V_T - V_D) \times F \qquad (2)$$

Total minute ventilation ($\dot{V}_E$ in liters per minute) is the product of V_T and F.

$$\dot{V}_E = V_T \times F \qquad (3)$$

From these three equations it can be seen that the factors determining the Pa_{CO_2} are V_T, V_D, F, and $\dot{V}_{CO_2}$.

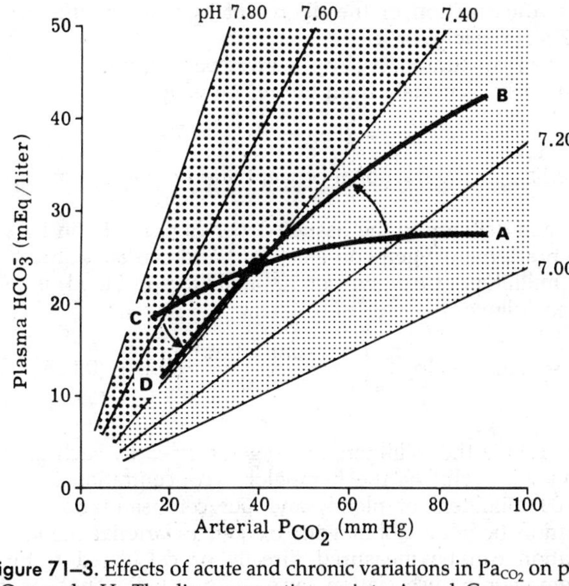

Figure 71–3. Effects of acute and chronic variations in Pa_{CO_2} on plasma HCO_3^- and pH. The line connecting points A and C represents the effects of an acute change in Pa_{CO_2} to a value above or below 40 mm Hg. Renal compensation over time results in a shift of the relationship to that represented by the line connecting points B and D as is indicated by the arrows. (From Murray JF: The Normal Lung. Philadelphia, W. B. Saunders Company, 1976.)

The volume of wasted ventilation can be calculated from a modification of the Bohr equation:

$$V_D = \frac{(Pa_{CO_2} - Pe_{CO_2})}{Pa_{CO_2}} \times V_T \qquad (4)$$

where Pe_{CO_2} = the partial pressure of carbon dioxide in expired air. The V_D so derived is commonly expressed as a ratio of V_T. Normal values are from 0.30 to 0.35.

EQUATIONS RELATED TO OXYGENATION. The partial pressure of oxygen in the alveolus (PA_{O_2}) can be calculated from the *alveolar gas equation* as follows:

$$PA_{O_2} = FI_{O_2}(P_B - 47) - Pa_{CO_2}/R \qquad (5)$$

where R = the respiratory exchange ratio ($\dot{V}_{CO_2}/\dot{V}_{O_2}$), P_B = barometric pressure, and 47 = the partial pressure of water vapor in mm Hg in fully saturated air at body temperature. The value for R is usually assumed to be 0.8. Having calculated the PA_{O_2}, the $P(A\text{-}a)_{O_2}$ can then be determined, enabling a more

TABLE 71–2. REPRESENTATIVE NORMAL VALUES FOR SELECTED RESPIRATORY AND HEMODYNAMIC VARIABLES

	Normal
Pa_{O_2}	95 mm Hg
Pa_{CO_2}	40 mm Hg
pH (arterial)	7.40
$P(A\text{-}a)_{O_2}$	<10 mm Hg
O_2 saturation	98%
Ca_{O_2}	19.8 ml/100 ml
$P\bar{v}_{O_2}$	40 mm Hg
$\dot{V}_{O_2}$	240 ml/min
$\dot{V}_{CO_2}$	192 ml/min
R	0.8
Respiratory rate	12
$\dot{V}_E$	6 L/min
V_D	150 ml
V_T	450 ml
V_D/V_T	.33
$\dot{Q}_T$	5 L/min
$\dot{Q}_S/\dot{Q}_T$	<7%
PVR	50–150 dyne sec/cm^5
SVR	800–1200 dyne sec/cm^5
$C\bar{v}_{O_2}$	14.6 ml/100 ml

precise quantitation of the degree of hypoxemia and mechanisms responsible for it.

Oxygen consumption ($\dot{V}O_2$ in liters per minute) can be estimated fairly accurately from the relationship

$$\dot{V}O_2 = (FI_{O_2} - FE_{O_2}) \times \dot{V}E \tag{6}$$

where FE_{O_2} = the fractional concentration of oxygen in expired air.

Oxygen delivery to the tissues depends not only on Pa_{O_2} but also on arterial oxygen content (Ca_{O_2}) and cardiac output. The Ca_{O_2} (milliliters of oxygen per 100 milliliters of blood) is calculated as follows:

$$Ca_{O_2} = 1.34 \times [Hb] \times \left(\frac{\text{per cent saturation}}{100}\right) + (0.003 \times Pa_{O_2}) \tag{7}$$

where 1.34 is the milliliters of oxygen carried by each gram of hemoglobin, [Hb] = the hemoglobin concentration in grams per 100 milliliters of blood, and per cent saturation = the saturation of hemoglobin with oxygen in arterial blood. The saturation can be measured directly or calculated from the oxyhemoglobin dissociation curve (Fig. 71–4). The constant 0.003, is the amount of dissolved (unbound) oxygen in blood in milliliters per mm Hg Pa_{O_2}.

Systemic oxygen transport (SO_2T) in milliliters per minute is calculated as follows:

$$SO_2T = Ca_{O_2} \times \dot{Q}T \tag{8}$$

where $\dot{Q}T$ = cardiac output in liters per minute.

Thus, it can be seen that oxygen delivery to the tissues depends not only on Pa_{O_2} but on [Hb] and $\dot{Q}T$ as well. In evaluating and managing patients with severe respiratory dysfunction, all of these factors need to be taken into account.

The balance between oxygen supply and systemic oxygen demands can be evaluated by calculating the difference between Ca_{O_2} and the content of oxygen in mixed venous blood ($C\bar{v}_{O_2}$). The $C\bar{v}_{O_2}$ is calculated in the same manner as the Ca_{O_2} (Equation 7) but using the oxyhemoglobin saturation value in mixed venous (pulmonary artery) blood.

Using the $\dot{V}O_2$ and the $C(a\text{-}\bar{v})_{O_2}$, the cardiac output can be calculated according to the Fick Principle:

$$\dot{Q}T = \frac{\dot{V}O_2}{C(a\text{-}\bar{v})_{O_2}}. \tag{9}$$

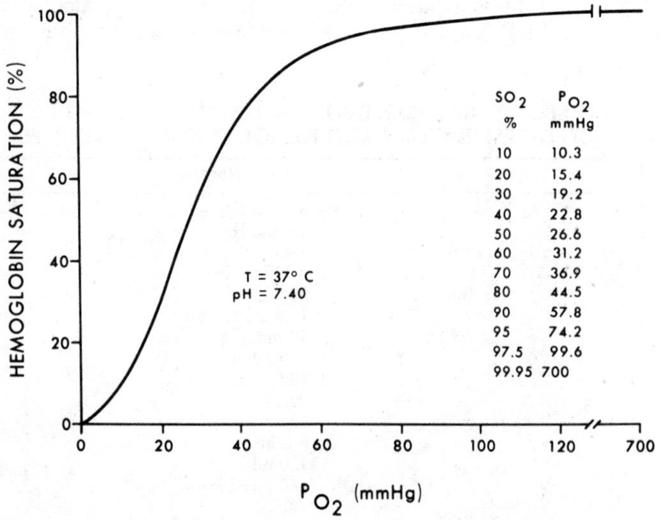

Figure 71–4. Relationship of per cent hemoglobin saturation to Pa_{O_2} in man at 37° C and pH 7.40. Note that there is very little increase in hemoglobin saturation for increases in Pa_{O_2} above 60 mm Hg. (From Murray JF: The Normal Lung. Philadelphia, W. B. Saunders Company, 1976.)

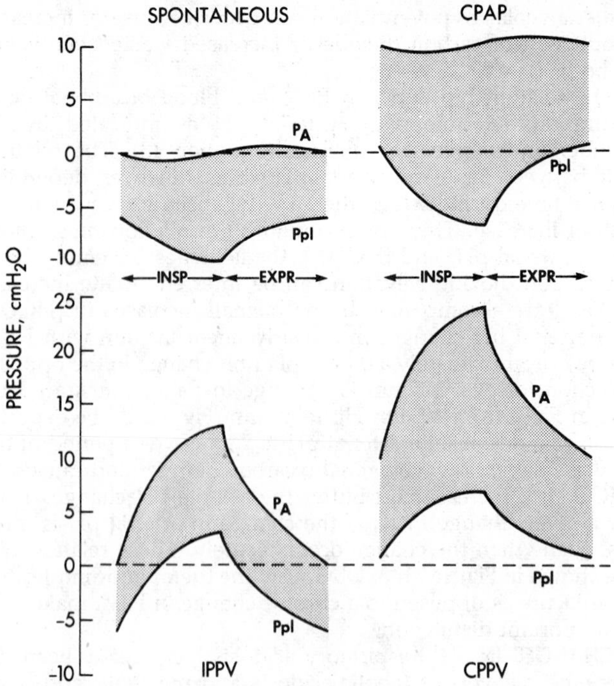

Figure 71–5. Schematic representations of airway and pleural pressures with spontaneous respiration, spontaneous respiration with continuous positive airway pressure (CPAP) intermittent positive pressure ventilation (IPPV), and continuous positive pressure ventilation (CPPV). Note that with CPAP and CPPV, the pressure gradient between the airway and the pleural space is increased compared to spontaneous respiration and IPPV, respectively. (From Hinshaw HC, Murray JF (eds): Diseases of the Chest. Philadelphia, W. B. Saunders Company, 1980.)

The contribution of right-to-left shunting of blood to hypoxemia can be quantitated in patients receiving an FI_{O_2} of 1.0 using the following shunt equation:

$$\frac{\dot{Q}S}{\dot{Q}T} = \frac{Cc'_{O_2} - Ca_{O_2}}{Cc'_{O_2} - C\bar{v}_{O_2}} \tag{10}$$

where $\dot{Q}S$ = the volume of shunted blood, Cc'_{O_2} = an approximation of end capillary blood oxygen content, assuming the Pc'_{O_2} to be the same as PA_{O_2} and calculating the Cc'_{O_2} on the basis of this assumption.

The effect of the per cent shunt on Pa_{O_2} as calculated from this equation is shown in Figure 71–1. This figure illustrates the lack of responsiveness of Pa_{O_2} to increases in FI_{O_2} (PA_{O_2}) once the $\dot{Q}S/\dot{Q}T$ exceeds 30 per cent.

ACID-BASE RELATIONSHIPS. The essential relationships among the factors controlling arterial blood pH are described in the Henderson-Hasselbalch equation:

$$pH = pK + \log \frac{[HCO_3^-]}{[H_2CO_3]} \tag{11}$$

where pK, the dissociation constant, = 6.1 for plasma at 37° C. Because

$$[H_2CO_3] = Pa_{CO_2} \times 0.0301 \tag{12}$$

where 0.0301 is the solubility constant of carbon dioxide in plasma at 37°, Equation 11 can be substituted as follows:

$$pH = 6.1 + \frac{\log [HCO_3^-]}{Pa_{CO_2} \times 0.0301}. \tag{13}$$

The relationships among these variables under acute and chronic conditions are shown in Fig. 71–3.

LUNG MECHANICS. The stiffness of the lung and chest wall—that is, its resistance to inflation—is termed the *compliance of the respiratory system* (CRS). In patients being mechanically ventilated it is expressed by the following formula:

$$C_{RS} = V_T/P_{plateau} - P_{EE} \quad (14)$$

where V_T is the tidal volume delivered by the ventilator, Pplateau is the inspiratory plateau pressure (see Fig. 71–5) and P_{EE} is the end expiratory pressure read from the manometer of the ventilator. The effect of airways resistance can be included in the measurement by using the peak inspiratory pressure (Ppeak) rather than Pplateau. This is termed the *effective compliance* (Ceff).

$$C_{eff} = V_T/P_{peak} - P_{EE} \quad (15)$$

Assuming that the compliance of the chest wall is stable, changes in C_{RS} reflect changes in lung mechanical properties, whereas changes in Ceff may indicate changes in airways resistance (if inspiratory flow is unchanged) as well as lung compliance.

Murray JF: The Normal Lung. Philadelphia, W. B. Saunders Company, 1976. *A concise review of normal lung function that provides the basis for an understanding of pulmonary pathophysiology.*

TECHNIQUES OF RESPIRATORY SUPPORT

External Devices for Administering Oxygen

Supplemental oxygen must frequently be administered by external devices in patients with any cardiorespiratory disorder that results in hypoxemia. The decision to use an external device as opposed to an endotracheal tube depends on the amount of oxygen needed and the potential consequences of failure to provide oxygen should the external device come off. Generally speaking, it is not prudent to rely on external devices for patients with hypoxemia severe enough to require an $F_{I_{O_2}}$ of 0.5 and who could be expected to suffer major consequences should the device not be positioned properly.

A variety of types of delivery systems can be used to provide supplemental oxygen. The choice of a particular method depends on four factors: (1) the amount of oxygen needed, (2) the need for precise control of $F_{I_{O_2}}$, (3) the need for humidification, and (4) the patient's comfort. *Nasal prongs* are the simplest and most comfortable delivery device. However, the $F_{I_{O_2}}$ provided cannot be reliably quantitated and humidification is poor. *Open face masks or face tents* provide a high flow of well-humidified, premixed air and oxygen with a moderately reliable $F_{I_{O_2}}$ usually set by a Venturi device in a humidifier/mixer. *Tight-fitting face masks* provide higher yet generally imprecise concentrations of oxygen. As with nasal prongs, humidification is minimal. The same sort of tight mask fitted with a nonrebreathing valve and a reservoir bag can be used to provide even higher concentrations of oxygen, perhaps up to an $F_{I_{O_2}}$ of 0.7 for short periods, but it is generally uncomfortable and the oxygen is poorly humidified. The $F_{I_{O_2}}$ is controlled much more precisely by the Venturi mask, which uses a calibrated Venturi device in the delivery line to provide high flows of gas containing 24, 28, 35, or 40 per cent oxygen. This sort of mask is used for patients with chronic airways obstruction and hypoventilation in whom there is concern that uncontrolled high oxygen concentrations will cause further hypoventilation by reducing ventilatory drive. For short periods of time, very high oxygen concentrations can be delivered by a tight-fitting anesthesia mask either strapped to the patient or held in place by hand. Obviously, this is not practical for long-term oxygen administration.

Ventilatory Assist Devices

A wide variety of devices can be used to provide ventilatory assistance without resorting to an endotracheal airway and mechanical ventilation. Generally, these devices are of limited usefulness; however, under proper circumstances, some may be quite helpful. Simple ventilators provide intermittent positive pressure ventilation via a mouthpiece but only transiently increase alveolar ventilation and, at least for this purpose, are of little value. External negative pressure devices such as the cuirass ventilator, which fits over the chest wall and augments ventilation by lowering the pressure around the chest causing it to expand, may be of value in patients with chronic neuromuscular diseases. Other ventilatory assist devices including the rocking bed and surgically implanted phrenic nerve pacemakers are of little general applicability.

Artificial Airways and Airway Management

When it is necessary, mechanical ventilation is best provided at least initially through an endotracheal tube passed through the mouth or nose. The oral route has the advantage of being more easily utilized under emergency circumstances, whereas the nasal route is better suited for long-term needs. Tracheostomy should be reserved for patients who will need long-term mechanical ventilation or who cannot tolerate either a nasal or an oral tube. The endotracheal tube should be fitted with a bonded high volume, low pressure cuff that will occlude the trachea around the tube, enabling positive pressure mechanical ventilation and preventing aspiration of oropharyngeal contents. Care should be taken to avoid overinflation of the cuff, which predisposes to pressure necrosis of the adjacent tracheal mucosa and to the development of a tracheoesophageal fistula or subsequent tracheal stenosis.

Semielective tube placement in a spontaneously ventilating patient may be accomplished via the nose without direct visualization of the vocal cords; however, direct visualization may be necessary to guide the tube into the larynx. In apneic patients the oral route with direct visualization of the vocal cords must be used. Placement of the tube over a fiberoptic bronchoscope may be helpful in difficult intubations. In any case intubation should be performed only by persons experienced with the procedure who are familiar with the often necessary pharmacologic adjuncts, such as intravenous anesthetics and muscle-relaxing agents.

Immediately after the tube is placed, the lungs should be auscultated to determine if air is entering both hemithoraces. Because of the relatively obtuse angle of the right main bronchus, positioning of the tip of the tube in this airway is quite common. If the tube seems to be in good position, it should be taped securely in place. The position should then be confirmed by a chest radiograph. The tip of the tube should be midway between the thoracic inlet, indicated by the sternoclavicular joints, and the carina.

Complete responsibility for an endotracheal or tracheostomy tube rests with the persons caring for the patient. The patient can no longer humidify inspired air, cough effectively, or defend the lower airways against airborne microorganisms. Perhaps more important, the patient cannot call for help or unblock the tube should it become obstructed. For all of these reasons, in addition to the gravity of the illness for which the tube was placed, patients with artificial airways should nearly always be managed in a critical care unit.

Nasal or, in occasional circumstances, oral endotracheal tubes can be left in place with no absolute time limit in patients who continue to require mechanical ventilation or airway protection. Tracheostomy may be necessary, however, because of complications, such as infection or soft tissue necrosis in the upper air passages including the nose. Occasionally, tracheostomy facilitates removal of secretions more effectively than does an endotracheal tube. In addition, patients may find a tracheostomy more comfortable and may be able to eat and talk with a tracheostomy tube in place.

Endotracheal and tracheostomy tubes bypass the normal humidifying mechanisms in the upper airway; all inspired gas must therefore be fully humidified. Removal of pulmonary secretions using a suction catheter with sterile technique should be performed at regular intervals as determined by the volume of secretions present. All gas delivery circuits in direct communication with the airway should be sterile when connected and changed at least at 48-hour intervals.

Definitive indications for endotracheal intubation that apply

TABLE 71–3. INDICATIONS FOR ENDOTRACHEAL INTUBATION

1. Need for an $FI_{O_2} > 0.5$ to maintain adequate oxygenation
2. Progressive hypoventilation with respiratory acidosis not responding to conservative management
3. Apnea
4. Loss of airway protective mechanisms
5. Inability to clear secretions
6. Need for heavy sedation or paralysis to control patient for diagnostic or therapeutic interventions

to all situations are difficult to determine. Nevertheless, the criteria listed in Table 71–3 seem generally applicable. The decision to perform endotracheal intubation is often based on more subjective criteria and/or observation of the patient's course during a period of time. In each of the listed situations, the potential reversibility of the patient's underlying disorder must be taken into account in determining if intubation is indicated.

Mechanical Ventilation

INDICATIONS. As with endotracheal intubation, the indications for mechanical ventilation are not always easily definable. In general terms, however, mechanical ventilation is clearly necessary in the following situations: (1) progressive hypoxemia that is unresponsive to treatment of its underlying causes and in which external devices cannot provide a sufficiently high FI_{O_2} and (2) progressive hypoventilation with respiratory acidosis that is unresponsive to treatment of the underlying disorder. Less clear indications include: (1) "prophylactic" mechanical ventilation in patients in whom respiratory failure is anticipated, such as after thoracic or upper abdominal surgery and (2) patients who are barely maintaining adequate gas exchange at the expense of expending energy on the considerable work of breathing. Finally, mechanical ventilation is occasionally necessary in patients who require general anesthesia or heavy sedation to allow diagnostic or therapeutic intervention.

TYPES OF MECHANICAL VENTILATORS. The most important variable used to categorize mechanical ventilators is the mechanism determining the point at which the changeover from the inspiratory phase to the expiratory phase takes place (Fig. 71–5). This point may be determined by the volume of gas delivered *(volume-cycled)*, the airway pressure achieved *(pressure-cycled)*, or the elapsed time of inspiration *(time-cycled)*. Both time-cycled and pressure-cycled ventilators have the disadvantage of not necessarily delivering a constant tidal volume. For this reason volume-cycled ventilators are most commonly used. Many ventilators, however, have options that allow the device to be pressure- or time-cycled in addition to a volume-cycling mode.

FEATURES OF MECHANICAL VENTILATORS. Mechanical ventilators must have certain essential features in order to provide adequate ventilatory support in different patients with different types of respiratory disorders. Chief among these is the ability to deliver a wide range of tidal volumes (100 to 2000 ml), with an adjustable respiratory frequency (5 to 60) and an accurate adjustable FI_{O_2} (0.21 to 1.0). Additional important features include controls for adjusting the inspiration-expiration ratio (or the inspiratory flow rate) and the inspiratory pressure limit. The device should be capable of operating in an assist (patient-triggered) mode, a controlled (machine-triggered) mode, and an assist-control combination mode. The ventilator must be equipped with devices that monitor exhaled tidal volume, inspiratory pressure, the temperature of the inspiratory gas and FI_{O_2} and have battery-operated alarms that signal loss of exhaled tidal volume, excessive inspiratory pressure, and reduction in FI_{O_2}.

Preferably, ventilators should also have built-in controls for adjusting positive end-expiratory pressure (PEEP), for allowing intermittent mandatory ventilation (IMV), and for providing continuous positive airway pressure (CPAP) in spontaneously breathing patients.

PATTERNS OF VENTILATORY SUPPORT. Two basic patterns of ventilatory support may be employed in the management of patients with respiratory failure: (1) *intermittent positive pressure ventilation* (IPPV) and *intermittent mandatory ventilation* (IMV). The fluctuations in airway pressure that characterize these patterns are shown in Figure 71–5. The obvious difference is that there is no allowance for spontaneous ventilation with IPPV, whereas with IMV a portion of the patient's ventilation is spontaneous. The use of one or the other of these two patterns is often a matter of the physician's personal preference; however, some guidelines can be provided.

IPPV is clearly indicated in patients who have no spontaneous ventilation, who have severe pain with respiration and/or an unstable chest wall, or in whom the work of breathing represents a significant energy drain.

IMV offers the advantage of maintaining the condition of the respiratory muscles, and for this reason may be useful in patients who do not have chronic processes with pre-existing deconditioned muscles. In addition, patients may find IMV more comfortable than IPPV. Intermittent mandatory ventilation is also useful for patients who have significant reductions of cardiac output with mechanical ventilation, especially with PEEP, in that it may allow greater amounts of PEEP to be used. In patients who are not capable of synchronizing their inspiratory efforts with the ventilator and have a chaotic ventilatory pattern, IMV may allow adequate ventilation without the need for sedation or muscle relaxing agents. It may also be a useful weaning technique in some situations.

POSITIVE END-EXPIRATORY PRESSURE (PEEP). PEEP increases the mean distending pressure across the walls of the airways and alveoli and thereby increases the volume of gas in the lung. This effect is beneficial in disorders characterized by pulmonary edema (usually noncardiogenic in origin) with consequent loss of functioning gas exchange units because of fluid filling or atelectasis. Positive end expiratory pressure tends to re-expand collapsed units and allow gas exchange to take place, thereby reducing intrapulmonary shunting of blood and improving Pa_{O_2}. PEEP can be added to IPPV to produce continuous positive pressure ventilation (CPPV) or to IMV. In addition, it can be used in spontaneously ventilating patients to produce CPAP or expiratory positive airway pressure (EPAP).

Positive end-expiratory pressure is not beneficial and in fact may be harmful in patients with other types of respiratory failure, especially those failures caused by airways obstruction wherein the lung is already overinflated. In such cases further increases in lung volume may be hazardous. This dictum applies not only to CPPV but also to IMV with PEEP and to CPAP and EPAP.

The conventional levels of PEEP range from 3 cm H_2O to 20 cm H_2O. Higher levels are occasionally used with IMV, but the indications for and the value of high levels of PEEP remain to be defined.

CONSIDERATIONS IN INITIATING MECHANICAL VENTILATION. Once it is decided to initiate mechanical ventilation, a series of nearly equally important decisions should be made (Table 71–4). Much of the decision making is influenced by the pathophysiology of the underlying disorder for which mechanical ventilation is necessary.

VENTILATOR EMERGENCIES. Patients who are being mechanically ventilated are subject to a variety of potentially disastrous

TABLE 71–4. DECISIONS IN INITIATING MECHANICAL VENTILATION

Type of ventilator
Pattern of ventilation (IPPV vs. IMV)
Mode (assist, control, or assist/control)
Tidal volume
Frequency
FI_{O_2}
Inspiration:expiration ratio
End-expiratory pressure (PEEP vs. no PEEP)

events that can occur suddenly and may be related either to the underlying disorder that made mechanical ventilation necessary or to malfunction of the ventilator or artificial airway. Such occurrences may rapidly be fatal. It is important that persons caring for critically ill patients develop a routine for assessment and management of these situations. The first indication that a problem is developing is usually that the patient is no longer being adequately ventilated as manifested by patient distress, by the high pressure limit or low V_T, by sounding of the ventilator alarm, or by sudden hemodynamic changes in the patient.

When the high pressure limit is exceeded, problems that should be suspected include obstruction of the endotracheal or tracheostomy tube, obstruction in the patient's airways, or pneumothorax. Occasionally, migration of the tip of the tube into a mainstem bronchus (usually the right) will cause the high pressure limit to be exceeded, but this is usually not so dramatic an occurrence. Less commonly, obstruction of the artificial airway may result from overinflation of the cuff with subsequent tube compression or herniation of the cuff over the tip of the tube.

When the high pressure limit is exceeded and the patient is not being ventilated, the first step is to disconnect the patient from the ventilator and begin hand ventilation with an anesthesia bag using an $F_{I_{O_2}}$ of 1.0. At nearly the same time as bagging begins, the artificial airway should be checked for position and for evidence of external obstruction such as kinking between the ventilator tubing connection and the nose or mouth or in the hypopharynx. If there is no external obstruction, the tube position seems correct, and compression of the bag is still difficult, the next step is to pass a suction catheter through the airway to check its patency and to remove mucus plugs or blood clots that may be causing the obstruction. If the obstruction is not removed, the tube cuff should be deflated to determine if it is causing the problem.

Assuming that the suction catheter can be passed, failure of these maneuvers to relieve the apparent obstruction indicates that the problem is within the patient and may be caused by major airway obstruction that was not removed by suctioning, sudden severe and more peripheral airways obstruction, or pneumothorax. The problem can usually be ascertained by a rapid physical examination of the chest. Tracheal obstruction is manifested by the finding of no or markedly reduced entry of air into the lungs. Mainstem bronchial obstruction is indicated by the absence of entry of air into the lung distal to the obstruction, causing a rocking motion of the chest with the affected side not expanding with inspiration and the unobstructed side being overinflated. Peripheral airways obstruction may be suspected from the patient's history and is usually indicated by wheezing, although with severe bronchoconstriction there may be little air movement and thus little or no wheezing. Pneumothorax in a patient being mechanically ventilated usually becomes a tension pneumothorax, characterized by difficulty with ventilation, reduction in arterial blood pressure, and an increase in central venous pressure. Examination of the chest shows no entry of air on the affected side, but, in contrast to the findings of mainstem bronchial obstruction, the affected side is hyperinflated and hyper-resonant to percussion. If the clinical situation allows, a chest roentgenogram can aid in a definitive diagnosis; however, a chest film showing a large tension pneumothorax may be viewed as being analogous to a 12 lead electrocardiogram in a patient with asystole.

Management of each of these situations is obviously different. Vigorous chest physical therapy and suctioning of the airway usually will remove obstructing mucus plugs or clots. Occasionally emergency fiberoptic bronchoscopy may be necessary. Tension pneumothorax requires prompt intervention to reduce the intrathoracic pressure. In an emergency situation a 14 gauge needle can be placed in the second anterior intercostal space. This will serve to relieve the tension with prompt restoration of the hemodynamic status and ability to ventilate the patient. After the needle is inserted, a chest tube should always be placed. Even if the diagnosis of pneumothorax was mistaken, a chest tube must be placed because of the high probability of lung puncture with the needle.

When the patient is suddenly not receiving adequate ventilation, but the high pressure limit is not being exceeded, the problems that should be considered are leaks in the ventilator tubing or around the cuff of the artificial airway, ventilator malfunction, or a tracheoesophageal fistula. Again, the first step is to disconnect the ventilator and begin manual ventilation with an $F_{I_{O_2}}$ of 1.0. At the same time, the position of the tube and the inflation of the cuff of the endotracheal or tracheostomy tube should be checked. If the external pilot balloon is deflated, more air should be added. Leaks around the cuff may be caused by breaks in the cuff itself or in the external pilot balloon, or by enlargement of the trachea at the site of the cuff because of pressure on the tracheal wall. Occasionally, an endotracheal tube may be positioned too high in the airway with the cuff at the level of the vocal cords or higher, causing air to leak around the cuff. If the cuff itself is leaking, the tube must be replaced. With some kinds of tubes, the outer pilot balloon may be replaced, if defective, without changing the tube. If the leak is occurring because of tracheal enlargement, the problem may be solved by adding air to the cuff or by changing the level of the cuff within the trachea. If air is added, care should be taken not to exceed a measured intracuff pressure of 20 mm Hg.

Tracheal dilatation is often the precursor of a much more serious problem, formation of a tracheoesophageal fistula. This usually can be prevented by maintaining intracuff pressures of less than 20 mm Hg. When a fistula does develop, however, it is usually catastrophic. Patients with fistulas can sometimes be managed temporarily by placing the tube at a lower level in the trachea with the cuff below the fistula. Definitive management is surgical correction of the fistula.

WEANING FROM MECHANICAL VENTILATION. Patients being mechanically ventilated should be evaluated frequently to determine if their lung function has improved sufficiently to allow weaning from the ventilator and subsequent removal of the endotracheal tube. Factors other than the condition of the lungs play an important role in determining if the patient is ready to be weaned and in the outcome of the weaning process (Table 71–5).

The techniques and the rapidity of weaning vary considerably depending on the nature of the underlying disorders that caused the need for mechanical ventilation. There are some basic criteria that are generally applicable in determining if it is feasible to initiate weaning. First, the patient should be awake and fairly alert. Lung function should be adequate as indicated by the ability of the patient to generate a VC of greater than 10 ml per kilogram of body weight. This ability may also be inferred by the generation of a maximum inspiratory pressure of less (more negative) than -20 cm H_2O. In addition, the patient should not require an $F_{I_{O_2}}$ of greater than 0.5. Additional criteria that may be useful include a resting minute ventilation of less than 10 liters, the ability to double this volume voluntarily, a $P(A\text{-}a)_{O_2}$ less than 350 mm Hg and a V_D/V_T of less than 0.55.

In patients who meet these criteria, weaning can commence. The techniques used include progressive lengthening of periods of spontaneous ventilation with the endotracheal tube attached to a "T-piece," a similar arrangement but with CPAP and IMV with a progressive reduction in the number of breaths delivered

TABLE 71–5. NONPULMONARY FACTORS THAT AFFECT WEANING FROM MECHANICAL VENTILATION

Cardiac function
Nutritional status
Electrolyte balance
Fluid balance
Pain
Mental status

by the ventilator. Patients whose lungs were previously normal and who have required only a short period of mechanical ventilation usually can be weaned and extubated quickly. The process is often much longer in patients with chronic airways obstruction who have required a long period of ventilatory support.

Caldwell SL, Sullivan KN: On tubes, techniques and procedures. *In* Burton GG, Gee GM, Hodgkin JE (eds.): Respiratory Care. Philadelphia, J. B. Lippincott Company, 1977, pp 501–523. *Provides a technical yet practical discussion of endotracheal and tracheostomy tubes.*

Gong H Jr, Tierney DF: Respiratory distress syndrome: Use of positive end-expiratory pressure and outcome. *In* Simmons DH (ed.): Current Pulmonology. Vol. 2. Boston, Houghton-Mifflin Professional Publishers, 1980, pp 103–134. *Presents a comprehensive review of the effects of PEEP in patients with ARDS.*

Lanken PM: Weaning from mechanical ventilation. *In* Fishman AP (ed.): Update: Pulmonary Diseases and Disorders. New York, McGraw-Hill Book Company, 1982, pp 366–386. *Presents a comprehensive well-referenced discussion of weaning. Reviews the basic pathophysiology of respiratory failure, criteria for weaning, and weaning techniques.*

Luce JM, Pierson DJ, Hudson LD: Intermittent mandatory ventilation. Chest 76:678, 1981. *An up-to-date review of the physiology and uses of IMV.*

Mushin WW, Rendell-Baker L, Thompson PW, Mapleson WW: Automatic Ventilation of the Lungs. 3rd ed. Oxford, Blackwell Scientific Publications, 1980. *The most comprehensive single-source reference on mechanical ventilation and ventilators that exists. Provides detailed technical information on nearly every commercially available positive-pressure mechanical ventilator.*

Rattenborg CC: Clinical Use of Mechanical Ventilation. Chicago, Year Book Medical Publishers, 1981. *Describes approaches to the use of mechanical ventilation in a variety of clinical situations.*

Rizk NW, Murray JF: PEEP in pulmonary edema. Am J Med 72:381, 1982. *A concise updating of thinking concerning the effects of PEEP on lung fluid balance.*

Snider GL, Rinaldo JE: Oxygen therapy in medical patients hospitalized outside the intensive care unit. Am Rev Respir Dis 122(2):29, 1980. *A good description of available methods for providing supplemental oxygen with a discussion of the pros and cons of different techniques.*

PATHOPHYSIOLOGY, ASSESSMENT, AND CRITICAL CARE MANAGEMENT OF SPECIFIC FORMS OF RESPIRATORY FAILURE

The causes of respiratory failure may be categorized by the component of the respiratory system primarily involved and by the time course of the process. Life threatening or fatal respiratory failure may occur as the result of processes involving the respiratory neuromuscular system, the chest wall, the extrathoracic and intrathoracic airways, the lung parenchyma, and the pulmonary vasculature. Each of these produces respiratory failure by a different basic pathophysiologic mechanism and entails different approaches to treatment. In many instances, however, there is a mixture of the mechanisms that are causing respiratory failure. For example, fatigue of the respiratory muscles may be the final event precipitating full-blown respiratory failure in patients with other primary lung disorders. Thus, although the basic approach to management is determined by the major underlying pathophysiologic mechanism, a variety of secondary approaches may be called for as well.

Central Nervous System, Peripheral Nervous System, and Muscular Causes of Respiratory Failure

Processes such as sedative hypnotic drug overdose and brain injuries and infections can reduce or abolish central respiratory drive, resulting in respiratory failure that is characterized predominantly by hypoventilation. The airways and lung parenchyma are unaffected except by atelectasis, which may occur because of a lack of periodic hyperinflations (sighs). Once ventilation is provided, gas exchange is normal unless atelectasis has occurred. The same pathophysiologic pattern can result from high cervical spinal cord injuries, peripheral nervous system disorders such as Guillain-Barré syndrome, or muscular disorders such as myasthenia gravis.

Use of critical care in these instances is dictated by the requirement for careful observation and/or for ventilatory support. Generally ventilatory support is indicated for patients in this category who have hypoventilation that does not respond to initial conservative management.

Measurements of Pa_{CO_2}, Pa_{O_2}, and arterial pH in comatose or sedated patients provide a direct indication of alveolar ventilation and also inferential information on the status of the lung parenchyma. In patients with spinal cord injury or neuromuscular disease measurement of arterial blood gas tensions and pH are similarly useful, but gas exchange may be well preserved until there is a marked reduction in ventilatory capability. Serial measurements of VC and maximal inspiratory pressure are therefore of value in predicting the likelihood of hypoventilation and the need for ventilatory support. In persons with normal ventilatory control mechanisms, hypoventilation does not occur with a VC of greater than 1 liter. Once the ventilatory capability is reduced to this degree, however, any further decrease is likely to be associated with a sudden increase in Pa_{CO_2}. Similarly, decreases in maximal inspiratory force to less than 20 cm H_2O are indicative of a critical reduction in ventilatory capability and the imminent possibility of hypoventilation. Apart from the direct respiratory consequences of these processes, critical care may be required to provide adequate airway protection and, in the case of drug overdose, to treat other toxic effects such as hemodynamic instability.

The pathophysiologic manifestations in this group of disorders are nearly identical, so that the approach to respiratory support of existing or imminent hypoventilation is the same. An oral or nasal endotracheal tube should be used to provide mechanical ventilation, preferably with a volume-limited ventilator. An initial tidal volume of 10 ml per kilogram of body weight is used in the control mode for apneic patients or in the assist/control mode for patients capable of initiating breaths. The ventilator frequency should be 8 to 10 breaths per minute with an inspiration:expiration ratio of 1:3. The appropriateness of this level of alveolar ventilation must be checked by measuring Pa_{CO_2}, Pa_{O_2}, and arterial pH approximately 10 minutes after initiating mechanical ventilation.

If the gas exchange abnormality is purely hypoventilation, use of supplemental oxygen should not be necessary. However, this is rarely the case. It is good practice to initiate mechanical ventilation using an FI_{O_2} of 1.0; after the initial measurement of Pa_{O_2}, FI_{O_2} should be adjusted downward. PEEP is generally not necessary in this category of illness but may be beneficial in preventing collapse or in re-expanding existing atelectatic areas of the lungs, complications not infrequent in patients with neurologic or muscular disorders.

Weaning from mechanical ventilation and the decision to remove the endotracheal tube should be made in accordance with the guidelines discussed previously. Generally, the weaning and extubation of drug-overdosed patients who do not have complications proceeds quite rapidly once they are awake. Patients with chronic neuromuscular disorders present much more of a problem and may require long-term ventilatory support.

Respiratory Failure Caused by Chest Wall Abnormalities

The most frequently encountered cause of this type of respiratory failure is traumatic injury to the chest wall with consequent rib fractures. This is associated with pain that inhibits full lung inflation, with atelectasis, and occasionally with hypoventilation. Multiple ribs fractured in multiple places, in addition to causing pain, can interfere with lung inflation because of the loss of chest wall rigidity and subsequent paradoxic motion of the involved area, so-called *flail chest.* Atelectasis, hypoxemia, and hypoventilation in severe cases characterize the pathophysiologic picture. In addition, the underlying lung is frequently contused, which adds to the abnormalities of gas exchange. Chronic deformities of the chest wall or marked pleural disease also can result in respiratory failure, although in these situations the pathophysiologic alterations are more complex than in injuries to the chest wall and often involve parenchymal and vascular abnormalities as well.

The primary mode of assessment is measurement of arterial

blood gas tensions. The basic indications for placement of an endotracheal tube are an inability to maintain adequate oxygenation with external oxygen delivery devices and significant increases in Pa_{CO_2}. The need for ventilatory support may be anticipated in patients who require large doses of narcotic agents to control their pain.

The pattern of mechanical ventilation utilized in this group of patients is much the same as that described for patients with neuromuscular disorders. However, because of the greater likelihood of involvement of the lung parenchyma with atelectasis and hemorrhage, a higher VT (12 to 15 ml per kilogram) and PEEP may be beneficial. The use of PEEP also helps to correct or prevent atelectasis and to stabilize the injured chest wall.

Weaning from mechanical ventilation does not necessarily have to await full stabilization of the chest wall, which can take weeks. Standard criteria can be used as the basis for making decisions concerning weaning and removal of the endotracheal tube.

Respiratory Failure Caused by Airways Obstruction

Impediments in the proximal portion of the airways (e.g., hypopharynx, larynx, and trachea) or generalized narrowing of the peripheral airways can severely obstruct air flow. With proximal obstruction hypoventilation is the major pathophysiologic abnormality. Gas exchange is normal once the obstruction is removed or bypassed. Similarly, hypoventilation is the hallmark of respiratory failure associated with diffuse airways obstruction (i.e., asthma, chronic bronchitis, and emphysema); however, the hypoventilation is invariably associated with hypoxemia due largely to ventilation-perfusion mismatching.

In this latter group of disorders, the primary abnormality is an increased resistance to air flow resulting from intrinsic narrowing of the airways or loss of airway tethering forces, or both. Regardless of the mechanism, the results are hypoxemia caused by mismatching of ventilation and perfusion and hypoventilation resulting from the airways obstruction itself plus fatigue of the respiratory muscles.

Measurements of air flow rates and arterial blood gas tensions are helpful in evaluating the severity of obstruction of air flow, and serial measurements describe the course of the episode and enable quantitation of response to treatment. The interpretation of a given set of values varies considerably depending on the time over which the abnormalities develop and their rate of change.

In patients with asthma or chronic airways obstruction, Pa_{CO_2} begins to increase when the FEV_1 is reduced to 750 ml or less, or approximately 25 per cent of its predicted value. With further reductions below the predicted value, Pa_{CO_2} tends to increase rapidly. Increased Pa_{CO_2} values occurring in association with FEV_1s of greater than 750 to 1000 ml may be the result of reduced ventilatory drive or increased production of carbon dioxide in a patient with a limited ability to increase the alveolar ventilation. As previously described, the distinction between acute and chronic hypoventilation can be determined by analyzing the relationships among Pa_{CO_2}, arterial pH, and $[HCO_3^-]$. Acute hypoventilation obviously dictates a more prompt response than chronic partially compensated respiratory acidosis.

The presence of metabolic acidosis is a more ominous finding than pure respiratory acidosis in the setting of airways obstruction. It implies a failure of the oxygen delivery system to provide sufficient amounts of oxygen to meet the demands imposed by the increased work of breathing. Such a situation cannot exist in steady state, and unless these patients rapidly improve, their condition will rapidly deteriorate.

Although hypoxemia invariably is present in patients with severe airways obstruction, the degree of reduction in Pa_{O_2} is generally in itself not sufficient to require respiratory support other than supplemental oxygen via external devices.

One cannot definitively state criteria for placement of an endotracheal tube and use of mechanical ventilation in patients with severe airways obstruction. Arterial blood gas and pH values at a single point in time showing marked acute respiratory acidosis or respiratory plus metabolic acidosis may be sufficient information on which to base the decision to provide mechanical ventilation. More commonly, however, it is necessary to evaluate the patient during a period of time while maximum conservative therapy is being administered and to evaluate the response to therapy. If the blood gas values are worsening or not improving in spite of maximum treatment, mechanical ventilation is the next logical step. In addition to the objective evaluation provided by arterial blood gas and pH measurements, subjective assessments are also of value. Patients who are confused, somnolent, or uncooperative may require ventilatory support because their mental status may indicate an end organ effect of the blood gas abnormalities and because the patients cannot cooperate with conservative management.

Severe airways obstruction presents a difficult situation in which to apply mechanical ventilation. There is the need to allow adequate exhalation time in the presence of marked expiratory air flow slowing, but also slow inspiratory flows are desirable to optimize the distribution of ventilation and to minimize the airways pressure required to deliver the set VT. To accomplish these goals, at least early in the course of mechanical ventilation, it is often necessary to sedate the patient to effect a slow respiratory frequency, which results in an appropriate inspiration:expiration ratio. The VT should be approximately 10 ml per kilogram and the FI_{O_2} adjusted to provide an adequate Pa_{O_2}. As the airways obstruction improves, the need for sedation will decrease. In initiating mechanical ventilation in patients with chronic hypoventilation, it is important not to reduce the Pa_{CO_2} rapidly because it will result in uncompensated metabolic alkalosis. The minute ventilation should be set to reduce the Pa_{CO_2} gradually, allowing the arterial pH to go no higher than 7.50. Positive end-expiratory pressure should not be used in patients with airways obstruction because it will further distend the already overinflated lungs.

Weaning patients with airways obstruction from mechanical ventilation also may present a difficult problem. Patients with asthma may be weaned and extubated quickly. However, patients with chronic airways obstruction may at best have marginal lung function with persistent retention of carbon dioxide. Generally speaking, the arterial blood gas pattern that is estimated to exist when the patient is "well" should be approximated while mechanical ventilation is still being used. Ideally, weaning can then proceed using previously described indicators. In many instances, however, patients with chronic airways obstruction never meet the objective criteria for weaning and extubation. When this occurs, the decisions in weaning and extubation are based on subjective criteria, such as level of alertness, patient cooperation, and prognosis. These factors obviously cannot be quantitated. Once the patient has demonstrated the ability to ventilate spontaneously for 30 to 60 minutes, the endotracheal tube should be removed.

It is important to try to determine which patients with chronic airways obstruction have a component of reversible respiratory dysfunction and which patients have simply reached the end stage of their disease. Although chronic mechanical ventilation is occasionally used to maintain life in a patient with end-stage chronic airways obstruction, the decision to pursue this course should be carefully considered by the patient, the family, and the physician, preferably before the patient is placed on a mechanical ventilator.

Disorders of the Lung Parenchyma Causing Respiratory Failure

Disorders of the lung parenchyma can be divided into those that predominantly involve the interstitium and those that involve the alveolar air spaces. Accumulations of fluid in alveoli can be caused by cardiogenic pulmonary edema (left ventricular failure or mitral stenosis) or diffuse injury to the lung causing noncardiogenic pulmonary edema (adult respiratory distress syndrome [ARDS]). A list of the conditions that have been associated with ARDS is provided in Ch. 70.

Both cardiogenic and noncardiogenic pulmonary edema may cause respiratory failure that is characterized by hypoxemia caused by right-to-left intrapulmonary shunting of blood and ventilation-perfusion mismatching. In severe cases retention of carbon dioxide can occur. Although mechanical ventilation may be required in both forms of pulmonary edema, other therapeutic interventions and response to treatment are quite different. This section will focus on pulmonary edema resulting from an increase in the permeability of the alveolar-capillary membrane. Cardiogenic pulmonary edema is discussed in Ch. 42.

ADULT RESPIRATORY DISTRESS SYNDROME (ARDS). A constellation of clinical, radiographic, and pathophysiologic findings that result from diffuse injury to the lung parenchyma define ARDS. The characteristics of the syndrome are (1) hypoxemia due to intrapulmonary shunting of blood, (2) increased lung stiffness (or decreased compliance), and (3) presence of diffuse infiltration on the chest roentgenogram. The common abnormality that accounts for these features is an increase in the permeability of the endothelium of the pulmonary capillary and the epithelium of the alveolar wall. This allows fluid to leak from the capillary into the alveolus even though the hydrostatic pressure within the capillary is normal; hence, noncardiogenic pulmonary edema results.

The injury to the lung that results in ARDS may be delivered via the airways or via the circulation. In many instances (e.g., aspiration of gastric juice and diffuse pneumonia), the mechanism by which the injury occurs is easily understood. However, in others (e.g., sepsis and pancreatitis), the mechanism is obscure and remains so despite vigorous investigative efforts.

Regardless of the type or mechanism of injury, both the pathophysiologic and the pathologic abnormalities are uniform. Grossly, the lung is edematous and hemorrhagic. Microscopic examination reveals intra-alveolar collections of proteinaceous fluid, red blood cells, and often inflammatory cells. Microthrombi or white blood cell aggregates may occasionally be seen in small vessels. After 24 to 48 hours, hyaline membranes line the inner aspects of alveoli and alveolar ducts. These membranes are formed by fibrin that has escaped through the leaking capillaries. Subsequently, as repair of the injury occurs, fibrosis may ensue although this is not an invariable consequence.

The pathophysiologic alterations affect lung volume, mechanical properties on the lung, and gas exchange. Reductions in VC and functional residual capacity (FRC) are characteristic of ARDS and are caused in part by fluid replacing alveolar air. As previously noted, one of the hallmarks of ARDS is the increased stiffness of the lung. This results not only from fluid in the alveoli but probably also from interaction between extravasated protein and surfactant, which increase surface forces at the air-liquid interface. The work of breathing considerably increases because of these effects on lung volume and lung compliance. The major and most frequent gas exchange abnormality is *hypoxemia.* This again is related predominantly to alveolar filling with fluid, causing these units to be the sites of shunting. In other less involved portions of the lung, ventilation-perfusion mismatching occurs and contributes to the hypoxemia.

In severe forms of ARDS as the process evolves from injury to repair the gas exchange abnormalities also evolve. Lung fibrosis may result in obliteration of capillaries and coalescence of air spaces to produce an increased VD/VT with overall alveolar hypoventilation, as indicated by an increased Pa_{CO_2}.

Definite abnormalities of gas exchange are seen only when the process has advanced to the stage of alveolar flooding. Thus, such measurements of blood gas tensions are relatively insensitive in assessing the lung injury. Nevertheless, patients who either have or are at risk of developing ARDS should be carefully observed and Pa_{O_2}, Pa_{CO_2} and arterial pH should be measured frequently. Early in the course, the critical variable is the Pa_{O_2}. Because patients frequently hyperventilate at this stage, the $P(A\text{-}a)_{O_2}$ should be calculated to provide an accurate index of the course of the process. The occurrence of either respiratory or metabolic acidosis in this setting is an ominous finding. In addition to blood gas tensions, it is usually necessary to measure the pulmonary artery wedge pressure both to determine if there is a contribution of cardiogenic pulmonary edema to the process and to serve as a guide for fluid management.

Patients who have fully developed ARDS invariably require mechanical ventilation. The determination of when to intervene with ventilatory support in patients who are at risk of developing ARDS or who have minor abnormalities of pulmonary function that suggest early ARDS may be quite difficult. The occurrence of edema and consequent loss of lung volume tends to be a self-perpetuating cycle, so that it is generally better to provide mechanical ventilation earlier rather than later.

When mechanical ventilation is undertaken, VT of 12 to 15 ml per kilogram of body weight should be used. Volumes of this magnitude are more effective in preventing or reversing atelectasis. In addition, use of PEEP has a well-documented role in the management of patients with ARDS. The beneficial effect of this pattern of ventilation is mainly attributable to the increase in FRC that it produces. By maintaining a continuously positive distending pressure across the walls of alveoli and airways, PEEP re-establishes their patency allowing gas exchange to resume in these units. Thus, shunting is decreased and Pa_{O_2} is improved.

Use of PEEP is not without hazards: (1) The increase in intrathoracic pressure caused by PEEP may reduce cardiac output. This appears to occur predominantly because of a reduction in venous inflow to the right side of the heart. It is therefore important to assess carefully the effects of PEEP not only on Pa_{O_2} but also on system oxygen transport by measuring cardiac output after PEEP is applied and after changes in PEEP. (2) The second potential complication of PEEP is the occurrence of pneumothorax. This seems more likely to occur later in the course of ARDS as architectural rearrangements take place in the lung that weaken its structure.

The application of PEEP may decrease Pa_{O_2} in situations in which there is considerable regional variation in the distribution of lung pathology. This results from shifting blood flow away from the more normal portions of the lung to the more abnormal portions and thereby increasing shunting.

Appropriate use of intravenous fluids is an important component of the management of ARDS. Pulmonary capillary permeability is increased and the regulatory mechanisms that normally tend to protect the lung from fluid overload are impaired. The prevailing capillary hydrostatic pressure therefore assumes an enhanced importance. Thus, administration of fluid, which increases the capillary hydrostatic pressure, tends to increase the amount of water in the lung. The relationship between capillary hydrostatic pressure and lung water content is shown schematically in Figure 71–6.

On the other hand, adequate pulmonary and systemic perfusion may also be important in preventing lung damage, and systemic perfusion is clearly important in maintaining renal, cardiac, and central nervous system functions. Thus, the effects of fluid administration should be carefully monitored with clear endpoints in mind. Rather than using systemic arterial pressure or central venous pressure alone to guide treatment, indexes of end-organ perfusion, such as urine output or mental functioning, should also be monitored. Frequently, at least early in the course of the process, a Swan-Ganz pulmonary artery catheter may be extremely helpful. Sufficient fluid should be administered to maintain perfusion of critical organs with as little effect as possible on the pulmonary artery wedge pressure.

Crystalloid solutions are probably preferable to colloid solutions, at least early in the course of the process when the increase in capillary permeability is most marked. At present

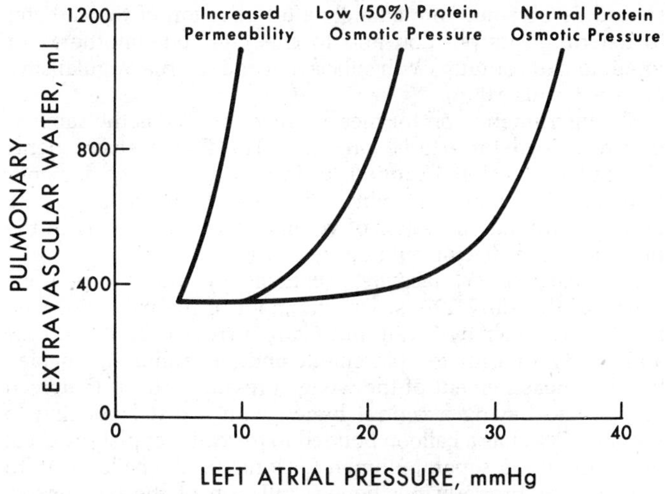

Figure 71–6. Schematic representation of the relationship of pulmonary extravascular water volume and left atrial or pulmonary artery wedge pressure. Curve at right represents the relationships when both capillary permeability and plasma protein osmotic pressures are normal; middle curve represents normal permeability but a reduction in plasma protein osmotic pressure of 50 per cent; left curve shows relationship when permeability of the capillaries is increased. (From Hopewell PC, Murray JF: Adult respiratory distress syndrome. *In* Moser KM, Spragg RG (eds.): Respiratory Emergencies, 2nd ed. St. Louis, The C. V. Mosby Company, 1982.)

there are not sufficient clinical data to support the use of corticosteroids in the treatment of patients who either have or are at risk of developing ARDS.

Pulmonary Vascular Diseases

The major effects of pulmonary vascular obstruction are circulatory rather than respiratory. Nevertheless, both acute pulmonary embolism and chronic pulmonary vasculitis are commonly associated with hypoxemia. In the former it is thought to be caused by microatelectasis producing right-to-left shunting. In the latter, the gas exchange abnormalities probably relate to pulmonary parenchymal abnormalities adjacent to vascular inflammation and result from a mixture of shunting and ventilation-perfusion mismatching.

Both the assessment and the management of the respiratory abnormalities caused by pulmonary vascular disease are directed toward the vascular process itself. Rarely is mechanical ventilation necessary solely because of gas exchange abnormalities caused by pulmonary vascular disease. However, small and occasionally large pulmonary emboli may occur in patients with other respiratory illnesses, thus compounding their cardiorespiratory abnormalities.

Bell RC, Coalson JJ, Smith JD, Johanson WG Jr: Multiple organ system failure and infection in adult respiratory distress syndrome. Ann Intern Med 99:293, 1983. *A prospective study evaluating the role of multiple organ system failure and infection in patients with ARDS. The overall survival rate was 26.2 per cent and was significantly worse in patients who developed central nervous system, gastrointestinal, renal, endocrine, or coagulation disorders and in patients who had infections.*

Hopewell PC, Miller WT: Respiratory failure in status asthmaticus. Clin Chest Med. In press. *Presents a review of the pathophysiology, assessment, and management of severe asthma.*

Hopewell PC, Murray JF: Adult respiratory distress syndrome. *In* Moses KM and Spragg RG (eds.): Respiratory Emergencies. 2nd ed. St. Louis, C. V. Mosby Company, 1982. *A comprehensive review of pathogenesis, pathophysiology, pathology, and management of ARDS.*

Jay SJ, Waldemar GJ, Pierce AK: Respiratory complications of overdose with sedative drugs. Am Rev Respir Dis 112:591, 1975. *Categorizes the specific pulmonary problems associated with sedative drug overdose and reviews management.*

Prewitt RM, Matthay MA, Ghignone M: Hemodynamic management in the adult respiratory distress syndrome. Clin Chest Med 4:251, 1983. *Discusses the important cardiopulmonary interactions in ARDS and optimal management strategies.*

Rinaldo JE, Rogers RM: Adult respiratory distress syndrome: Changing concepts of lung injury and repair. N Engl J Med 306:900, 1982. *An excellent review of ARDS emphasizing the mechanisms by which the lung injury might occur.*

Shackford SR, Smith DE, Zarins CK, Rice CL, Vigilio RW: The management of flail chest. Am J Surg 132:759, 1976. *Discusses the criteria for the use of mechanical ventilation in patients with flail chest.*

CRITICAL CARE MONITORING

A critical care unit is unique in its ability to provide continuous and often invasive measurements of respiratory and hemodynamic status in severely ill patients. Such monitoring enables early detection of changes in the patient's condition and provides information that both directs therapy and assists in evaluating the response to treatment. The complexity of monitoring systems varies considerably, ranging from simple electrocardiographic monitoring with only a real-time screen display to automated "closed loop" systems wherein the monitored data, through a computer program, serve to regulate intravenous infusions of fluids and drugs. Usually, the kind of system employed relates to the kinds of patients being cared for in the unit.

Respiratory Monitoring

As a minimum, respiratory monitoring should consist of measurement of respiratory rate and periodic (sometimes no more often than daily) measurement of Pa_{O_2}, Pa_{CO_2}, and arterial pH. Respiratory rate can be measured and recorded automatically in nonintubated patients using impedance devices to which alarms can be attached. Both respiratory rate and V_T can be monitored in intubated, spontaneously breathing patients using a pneumotachograph and appropriate alarms.

In patients who are being mechanically ventilated, monitoring of respiratory rate, exhaled V_T, and airway pressure is essential. Additional monitoring techniques are available but do not yet have a demonstrated role. These include breath by breath measurements of respiratory system compliance and volume-pressure and volume-flow relationships. In addition, multiplexed mass spectrometer-based systems are available for measurement of $F_{I_{O_2}}$ and exhaled carbon dioxide and oxygen. These systems may provide early indications of changes in Pa_{CO_2}, but their usefulness and general applicability remain to be determined.

The transcutaneous P_{O_2} and P_{CO_2} that are indirect reflections of Pa_{O_2} and Pa_{CO_2} can be measured continuously using heated skin electrodes. Measurement of transcutaneous P_{O_2} in infants has proved to be a helpful monitoring technique, but the value of this measurement in adults is uncertain.

The ear oximeter is another noninvasive monitoring device that measures and records oxyhemoglobin saturation. This technique has proved to be useful in a variety of clinical situations, including weaning from mechanical ventilation and evaluating oxygenation during sleep and during procedures such as bronchoscopy.

Indwelling catheter electrodes for continuous intra-arterial measurement of Pa_{O_2}, Pa_{CO_2}, and arterial pH have been used but still have important technical limitations. More recently, a fiberoptic pulmonary artery catheter for continuous measurement of oxyhemoglobin saturation in mixed venous blood has been developed but does not have a defined role as yet.

Hemodynamic Monitoring

Most critical care units have the basic capacity to monitor and record heart rate and rhythm (usually with a built-in memory and recall capability), venous pressure, pulmonary arterial pressure, and systemic arterial pressure. In addition, many units have the instruments necessary for measurement of cardiac output.

Electrocardiographic monitoring is clearly of value in patients with specific cardiac disorders such as acute myocardial infarction or cardiac arrhythmia. This form of assessment is also essential in patients with any illness severe enough to require critical care. Abnormalities in heart rate or rhythm may signal the worsening of a respiratory condition, electrolyte abnormalities, or a variety of other noncardiac problems. Ideally, the system should have a built-in memory and should be able to display frequency and kinds of arrhythmias occurring in a given period of time. Both high-rate and low-rate alarms are necessary to complete the system.

Systemic arterial pressure monitoring by a continuous technique is of obvious value: (1) Assuming it is performed with accurate and properly calibrated transducers and amplifiers, the measurement is more accurate than that obtained with a blood pressure cuff. (2) Changes are immediately detected and therefore allow beat by beat assessment of the effects of such maneuvers as changes in ventilatory pattern or infusion of vasoactive drugs. (3) Continuous measurement of the blood pressure decreases the amount of time necessary for staff members to spend with the patient. (4) An arterial catheter provides ready access to arterial blood for measurement of blood gases.

Each of these advantages has a corollary disadvantage, however. If the equipment is not properly calibrated, an inaccurate reading may be obtained that may result in inappropriate decisions. Beat to beat variations in blood pressure may not warrant specific intervention. In many instances it is better for the nurse to be at the patient's bedside rather than watching a monitor screen. Finally, the presence of an arterial catheter may encourage withdrawal of more blood than is necessary for measurement of blood gases.

The advantages and disadvantages of arterial pressure monitoring must be taken into account in deciding when arterial catheter placement is indicated. In additon to the problems just listed, there are specific complications of arterial catheterization, which are discussed below (see Complications of Hemodynamic Monitoring, Systemic Arterial Pressure).

Given these considerations, the basic indication for monitoring arterial blood pressure is the presence or anticipation of hemodynamic instability as a result of either the disease process or the therapeutic intervention. In patients who require frequent measurement of arterial blood gases, insertion of an arterial catheter may be indicated to provide access to arterial blood.

The usual technique of monitoring systemic arterial pressure is to insert percutaneously a Teflon catheter into an accessible artery. The radial artery of the nondominant hand is usually the vessel of choice. The Allen's test should be performed to determine the patency of the palmar arterial arch before insertion of the catheter. The femoral artery is the second choice for placement. The brachial artery and dorsalis pedis artery have also been used.

The catheter is connected via a stopcock to a rigid connecting tube that in turn is attached to a transducer. Commonly, a device that continuously flushes the catheter with a small volume of heparinized solution is also connected to the catheter.

Central venous pressure monitoring by a continuous technique is useful in quantitating and following the course of right ventricular failure, right ventricular infarction, tricuspid regurgitation, and cardiac tamponade. In addition, it is useful in evaluating the intravascular volume status of patients who have no pulmonary or cardiac disease.

Under normal circumstances, central venous pressure (CVP) is equivalent to right atrial and right ventricular diastolic pressures and bears a more or less constant relationship to the pulmonary wedge pressure (pulmonary artery wedge pressure [PPAW] = CVP + 6 mm Hg). However, if cardiac or pulmonary disease is present, the CVP does not reflect the left atrial filling pressure (pulmonary artery wedge pressure). In fact, the CVP may provide misleading information leading to erroneous therapeutic decisions.

To monitor CVP a catheter is inserted percutaneously into either the subclavian or the external or internal jugular vein. An antecubital vein may also be used for catheter insertion either percutaneously or via a cutdown. Care should be taken to avoid passing the catheter into the right ventricle where it can cause ventricular arrhythmias. A chest roentgenogram should be obtained immediately after insertion of the catheter to determine its position and to check for pneumothorax or pneumomediastinum (with subclavian and internal jugular sites of catheter insertion).

The instrumentation for measurement of CVP is the same as that described for arterial pressure. The CVP measurements should be interpreted cautiously. In patients who have significant hemodynamic instability, the CVP should not be relied on as an accurate indicator of volume status, especially in the presence of cardiac or pulmonary disease.

Pulmonary arterial pressure monitoring in critical care units began in the early 1970's. Development of the balloon-tipped flotation catheter by Swan and Ganz increased both the ease and safety of catheter placement and, in addition, enabled bedside measurement of the wedge pressure. This catheter, in addition to having a central lumen with a distal opening to measure PPA, has a balloon bonded to the catheter just proximal to the tip and a separate lumen for inflating the balloon. With the catheter properly positioned, inflation of the balloon occludes the vessel in which the tip resides, stopping blood flow and allowing measurement of the pulmonary artery wedge pressure. In addition to the basic single lumen No. 5 F catheter there are a variety of modifications. The most versatile version is a No. 7 F size that has, in addition to the distal lumen, a proximal lumen for measurement of CVP and a thermistor near the tip that allows measurement of cardiac output using the thermal dilution technique.

Thus, the Swan-Ganz pulmonary artery catheter provides measurement of PPA, PPAW, CVP, and cardiac output. In addition, blood can be sampled from the pulmonary artery for measurement of oxygen content. The indications for monitoring PPA are listed in Table 71–6.

It is important to recognize the limitations of monitoring PPA. First, because of the effects of oscillations in pleural pressure on the measured intravascular pressure, the values are extremely difficult to determine in persons who are breathing rapidly. Second, the values are altered by PEEP; an accurate absolute value cannot be obtained in a patient in whom PEEP is being used. The measurement has a relative value, however, that can be used comparatively to evaluate a therapeutic maneuver unless the catheter is positioned in a portion of the lung in which alveolar pressure is greater than pulmonary venous pressure alone or PPA and pulmonary venous pressure (an unlikely occurrence). If this occurs, the reading of pulmonary artery wedge pressure will reflect alveolar pressure rather than left atrial pressure. Finally, pulmonary artery wedge pressure will not reflect the left ventricular filling pressure in the presence of mitral stenosis or pulmonary venous obstruction.

To obtain the maximal amount of information from the procedure, a recording of the wave form and pressures should be made as the catheter passes from the superior vena cava to the right atrium, right ventricle, and pulmonary artery. Figure 71–7 shows the normal wave forms encountered during passage of the catheter. Specific abnormal patterns may be seen in patients with tricuspid regurgitation or cardiac tamponade and constriction.

Insertion of the catheter is via the same choice of routes described for insertion of the catheter for measuring CVP. The instrumentation is also the same. The procedure must be performed with continuous electrocardiographic monitoring to allow identification of ventricular arrhythmias induced by the

TABLE 71–6. INDICATIONS FOR PULMONARY ARTERIAL PRESSURE MONITORING

1. To help distinguish cardiogenic from noncardiogenic pulmonary edema.
2. To provide information in the differential diagnosis of hypotension.
3. To assist in determining the cause of hypoxemia.
4. To characterize the patterns of abnormal cardiac function after myocardial infarction.
5. To monitor the effects of various therapeutic interventions such as vasoactive agents, intravenous fluids, diuretics, digitalis, and CPPV.

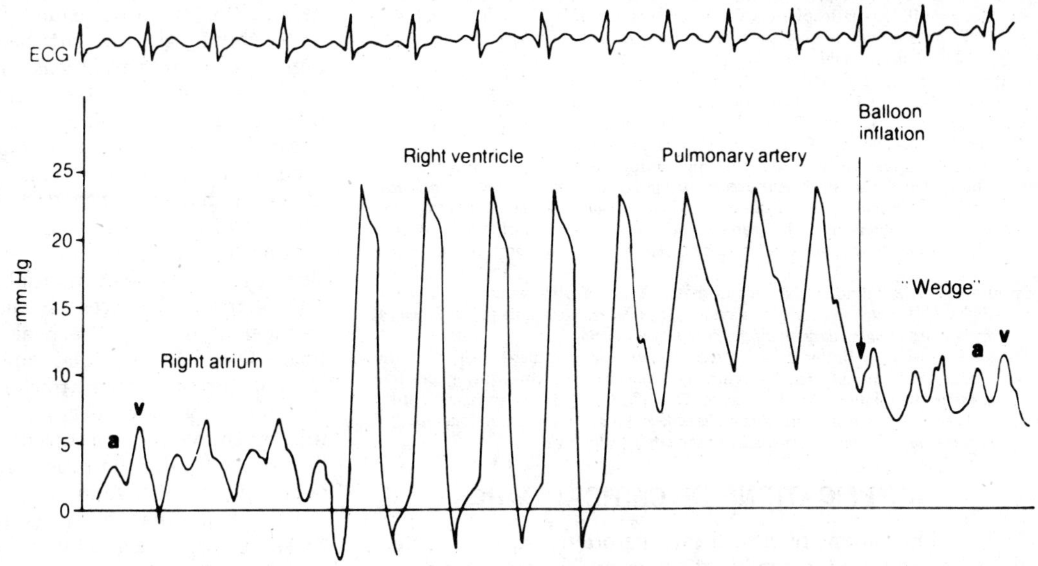

Figure 71–7. Tracing of pressures during passage of a Swan-Ganz catheter from the internal jugular vein into the pulmonary artery. Pressures and wave form are normal. (From Matthay MA: Invasive hemodynamic monitoring in critically ill patients. Clin Chest Med 4:233, 1983.)

catheter passing through the right ventricle. Because of the possibility of ventricular arrhythmias, lidocaine for immediate intravenous administration must be available. The catheter should be positioned so that a pulmonary artery wedge pressure tracing is seen with 1 ml of air in the balloon (for a No. 7 F catheter with a 1.5 ml capacity balloon). The catheter should then be secured in that position and a chest roentgenogram taken to confirm and record the position and to check for pneumothorax. The PPA tracing should be monitored continuously to detect distal migration and permanent wedging of the catheter, which may cause pulmonary infarction.

Measurements of cardiac output can be obtained easily and routinely using the thermistor-equipped Swan-Ganz catheter. Such measurements complement the pressure measurements described earlier and enable nearly complete characterization of the hemodynamic status of the severely ill patient.

The instrumentation required to perform thermal dilution determinations includes, in addition to the Swan-Ganz catheter, a cardiac output computer that processes the indicator-dilution measurements and calculates cardiac output. Such measurements are not without error, but, using standard techniques, the results are of acceptable accuracy.

Patterns of hemodynamic abnormalities are often of value. Using the systemic and pulmonary arterial pressure, CVP, and cardiac output, the resistance across the pulmonary and systemic vascular beds can be calculated as follows:

$$\text{PVR} = \frac{\overline{\text{PPA}} - \overline{\text{PPAW}} \times 80}{\dot{\text{Q}}\text{T}}$$

$$\text{SVR} = \frac{\overline{\text{PSA}} - \overline{\text{PRA}} \times 80}{\dot{\text{Q}}\text{T}}$$

where PVR = pulmonary vascular resistance, SVR = systemic vascular resistance, $\overline{\text{PPAW}}$ = mean pulmonary artery wedge pressure, $\overline{\text{PSA}}$ = mean systemic arterial pressure, $\overline{\text{PRA}}$ = mean right atrial pressure. Normal values are 50 to 150 dyne-sec per centimeter^5 for PVR and 800 to 1200 dyne-sec per centimeter^5 for SVR.

Using these calculated variables plus the measured vascular pressures and cardiac output, patterns of hemodynamic abnormalities can be determined. Table 71–7 shows the hemodynamic patterns characteristic of the problems most frequently encountered in a critical care unit.

TABLE 71–7. PATTERNS OF HEMODYNAMIC ABNORMALITIES IN SEVERELY ILL PATIENTS

Situation	$\overline{\text{PSA}}$	$\overline{\text{PRA}}$	$\overline{\text{PPA}}$	$\overline{\text{PPAW}}$	$C(a-\bar{v})_{O_2}$	$\dot{Q}T$	PVR	SVR	$P\bar{v}_{O_2}$
Hypovolemic Shock	↓	↓	↓	↓	↑	↓	↑	↑	↓
Septic Shock	↓	↓	↓	↓	↓	↑	↓	↓	↑
Cardiogenic Shock	↓	↑	↑	↑	↑	↓	↑	↑	↓
Pulmonary Embolism	↓	↑	↑	→↓	↑	↓	↑	↑	↓
Airways Obstruction	→	→↑	↑	→	→	→	↑	→	→
Right Ventricular Infarct	↓	↑	→	↓→↑	↑	↓	→	→↑	→↓
Cardiac Tamponade	↓	↑	↑	↑	↑	↓	→	↑	↓
End Stage Liver Disease	↓	→↓	→↓	→↓	↓	↑	→	↓	↑

$\overline{\text{PSA}}$–mean systemic arterial pressure
$\overline{\text{PRA}}$–mean right atrial or central venous pressure
$\overline{\text{PPA}}$–mean pulmonary arterial pressure
$\overline{\text{PPAW}}$–mean pulmonary arterial wedge pressure
$C(a-\bar{v})_{O_2}$–arteriovenous O_2 content difference
$\dot{Q}T$–cardiac output
PVR–pulmonary vascular resistance
SVR–systemic vascular resistance
$P\bar{v}_{O_2}$–mixed venous P_{O_2}

Fallat RJ, Osborn JJ: Patient monitoring techniques. *In* Burton GG, Gee GN, Hodgkin JE (eds.): Respiratory Care. Philadelphia, J. B. Lippincott Company, 1977, pp 950–965. *A comprehensive review of available techniques for respiratory and hemodynamic monitoring.*

Fragen RJ: Arterial catheterization and maintenance of indwelling arterial lines. *In* Beal JM (ed.): Critical Care for Surgical Patients. New York, The Macmillan Company, 1982, pp 73–89. *A brief but complete review of techniques and complications of intra-arterial blood pressure monitoring.*

Matthay MA: Invasive hemodynamic monitoring in critically ill patients. Clin Chest Med 4:233, 1983. *An excellent comprehensive review of indications, techniques, interpretation, and pitfalls of hemodynamic monitoring in critical care units.*

Osborn JJ: Computers in critical care medicine: Promises and pitfalls. Crit Care Med 10:807, 1982. *Discusses the current state of use of computers in critical care units.*

Sprung CL: The Pulmonary Artery Catheter. Baltimore, University Park Press, 1983. *A thorough review of indications, techniques, complications, and clinical applications of pulmonary artery pressure measurements.*

Tooker J, Huseby J, Butler J: The effect of Swan-Ganz catheter height on the wedge pressure-left atrial pressure relationship in edema during positive pressure ventilation. Am Rev Respir Dis 117:721, 1978. *An experimental study that demonstrated that positioning of the catheter tip in the upper lung zones resulted in wedge pressure measurements that were artefactually high.*

COMPLICATIONS OF CRITICAL CARE

The complications of critical care are often difficult to detect and separate from the complications of the illnesses that necessitated the care. Iatrogenic diseases uniquely associated with the technology that constitutes critical care clearly cause significant morbidity and occasionally death, however.

Some complications are straightforward and clearly related to an intervention taking place in a critical care unit, such as ventricular tachycardia occurring during the passage of a Swan-Ganz catheter through the right ventricle. The cause of other untoward events is less easy to discover. For example, cardiac arrhythmias or gastrointestinal hemorrhage are common in patients in critical care units but are not necessarily caused by the sort of care rendered in the unit. Confounding the issue further are errors in management that, because they occur in severely ill patients, may have much graver consequences than the same error would have in a less sick patient on a medical ward.

In addition to patient-related complications, the critical care environment takes its toll on the personnel who work there. The psychologic effects of working under what often are high-pressure conditions can result in nurse or physician "burnout." Moreover, personnel in the unit may be at greater risk for certain organic diseases.

The kinds of complications to which patients are prone relate to the kind of illness they have and to the diagnostic and therapeutic interventions carried out. Respiratory support has its unique complications as does hemodynamic support and monitoring.

Complications of Respiratory Support

Oxygen therapy administered by external devices may be associated with the following adverse effects: (1) discomfort related to the device or to administration of dry gas, (2) fires, and (3) hypoventilation because of uncontrolled administration of oxygen in patients who need a precisely controlled $F_{I_{O_2}}$. The first of these is not of great consequence and usually is easily managed by changing the device or improving the humidification. Fires related to oxygen delivery equipment may be catastrophic for the patient but fortunately are uncommon and generally preventable by prohibiting smoking where oxygen is being used. The last complication may be related to the wrong choice of an oxygen delivery device or to using too high a concentration of oxygen. It may also be unavoidable because of the pathophysiology underlying the disease. In any case, severe hypoventilation may be prevented by close observation of such patients and measurement of arterial blood gas tensions early in the course of oxygen administration.

Artificial airways may be associated with a number of complications. The placement of an endotracheal tube may cause immediate injury to the structures through which the tube passes—nose, hypopharynx, larynx, or trachea. The tube may be improperly positioned either at the time of placement or as a result of subsequent migration. This can result in the tube being either too low, usually in the right mainstem bronchus, or too high, with the cuff being at the level of the larynx or higher, causing an air leak around the cuff with inadequate ventilation. These problems may be minimized by the use of a tube that is easily visible on a roentgenogram and by taking a chest film immediately after placement or adjustment of the tube. In addition, daily chest roentgenograms should be obtained in patients with endotracheal tubes in place and the position of the tube noted.

Long-term problems from endotracheal tubes include necrosis of the nasal alae or internal nasal structures, sinus infection, retropharyngeal abscess formation, vocal cord damage, and tracheal injury. The tracheal injury may take the form of a tracheoesophageal fistula, which usually develops at the site of the cuff, or subsequent tracheal stenosis, also at the cuff site, that may not become apparent for several months after the tube is removed. Vocal cord or laryngeal injury may be apparent immediately after the tube is removed or may slowly progress over a period of several months.

The proper use of tubes with high compliance and low pressure cuffs has greatly reduced the risk of injury at the cuff site. To reduce the risk still further, the pressures in the cuff should be checked periodically and kept below 20 mm Hg. The probability of injury at the other sites may be minimized by careful taping and stabilization of the tube, use of an appropriate-sized tube and careful intubation technique. The tape holding the tube should be changed daily and the nose (if a nasal tube is used) inspected for areas of skin breakdown or necrosis.

Tracheostomy, because it bypasses the upper airway, avoids the problems associated with a tube passing through the aforementioned structures. However, tracheostomy itself has its own unique complications that more than offset its advantages. Early problems include hemorrhage, mediastinal and subcutaneous emphysema, and malpositioning of the tube. Subsequently, soft tissue infection, late hemorrhage, and tracheal stenosis may occur either at the site where the tube cuff impinged on the tracheal wall or, more commonly, at the site of the opening into the trachea. The overall frequency of complications, particularly the occurrence of tracheal stenosis, appears to be greater with tracheostomy than with endotracheal tubes. The frequency of tracheostomy complications can be reduced by careful operative techniques, use of tubes with low-pressure cuffs, effective stabilization of the tube, and meticulous wound care.

Obstruction of either endotracheal or trachesotomy tubes may occur as a result of inspissated secretions or blood clots. This problem may be prevented by adequate humidification of the inspired gas mixture and by frequent suctioning through the tube.

Both endotracheal and tracheostomy tubes are associated with an increased risk of *pulmonary infection.* The presence of the tube considerably compromises the normal mechanisms by which the airways rid themselves of potentially infecting agents. In addition, hospitalized patients, particularly those in critical care units, are much more likely to have colonization of the airways with organisms that are more pathogenic than those usually present. Both aerobic gram-negative organisms and staphylococci tend to replace the normal oropharyngeal flora in critically ill patients. The distinction between airway colonization with these organisms and true pulmonary infection may be quite difficult. Patients with endotracheal or tracheostomy tubes in place should have daily Gram's stains (not cultures) of aspirated sputum. Infection is often heralded by an increasing number of organisms and polymorphonuclear leukocytes present in the sputum with a subsequent increase in abnormalities on the chest roentgenogram and the appearance of or increase in fever. The finding of organisms per se in the sputum should not in itself be interpreted as indicating infection.

Mechanical ventilation may be associated with complications apart from the artificial airway, for example *overventilation* and *underventilation, reduction in cardiac output,* and *pneumothorax* and/or *pneumomediastinum*. Use of the guidelines for mechanical ventilation discussed in Ch. 70 will minimize the likelihood of either overventilation or underventilation. Nevertheless, Pa_{O_2}, Pa_{CO_2}, and arterial pH must be determined shortly after mechanical ventilation is initiated and after changes in either ventilator settings or the patient's condition. The ventilator can then be further adjusted if necessary.

The mechanisms by which mechanical ventilation and particularly CPPV reduce cardiac output have been widely debated. Although the cause is probably multifactorial, the major effect seems to be a reduction of right ventricular inflow caused by decreased transmural right ventricular filling pressure. This effect is particularly evident in patients who are hypovolemic and may be offset by volume replacement. High levels of PEEP usually reduce cardiac output in normovolemic as well as hypovolemic patients. When cardiac output is reduced by PEEP, its beneficial effects must be weighed against the potential deleterious effects of further administration of intravenous fluids. In evaluating the usefulness of PEEP in a given patient, the overall effect on systemic oxygen transport should be measured and PEEP adjusted to yield the optimal balance between Pa_{O_2} and cardiac output.

Lung rupture with subsequent pneumothorax or pneumomediastinum probably relates to the increased transmural distending pressure in airways and alveoli. This pressure results in less distention of abnormal alveoli and relative overdistention of the more normal alveoli that can predispose them to rupture. For this reason as well as to minimize the effects of pressure on cardiac output, the minimal amount of PEEP that is consistent with optimal oxygen transport should be used. Peak airway pressure can be lowered by using inspiratory flows that are as slow as possible while still maintaining an appropriate inspiration:expiration ratio.

Oxygen toxicity is not a complication of mechanical ventilation per se but usually occurs in patients who are being mechanically ventilated with gas mixtures containing high concentrations of oxygen (see Ch. 560). Although it is not clearly determined, the threshold for clinically significant oxygen toxicity seems to be approximately 0.6 atmospheres, the important variable being PI_{O_2} rather than FI_{O_2}. Histologic changes in the lung that are compatible with oxygen toxicity have been noted in persons receiving lower concentrations of oxygen for long periods of time, but the clinical significance of these observations appears to be minimal.

The clinical syndromes produced by hyperoxia include tracheobronchitis, ARDS, and bronchopulmonary dysplasia. *Tracheobronchitis* is usually acute, manifested by substernal chest pain and nonproductive cough occurring after 12 to 24 hours of breathing oxygen at 1 atmosphere. The time course of *ARDS caused by oxygen* is not well defined and probably varies, being influenced by other factors in addition to the FI_{O_2}. *Bronchopulmonary dysplasia* probably does not occur in adults but is common in neonates given high concentrations of oxygen.

The diagnosis of oxygen toxicity is extremely difficult to establish. Patients who require high oxygen concentrations already have sufficient clinical, physiologic, radiographic, and histologic abnormalities to obscure any additional changes caused by oxygen. Thus, at present the diagnosis is usually presumptive.

The prevention of oxygen toxicity rests with the general principle of using as low an inspired oxygen concentration as possible that provides the patient with adequate systemic oxygen transport. From the oxyhemoglobin dissociation curve (Fig. 71–4) it is apparent that at a Pa_{O_2} of 60 mm Hg, hemoglobin is nearly fully saturated. Further increases in Pa_{O_2} add little to oxygen transport. Thus, a Pa_{O_2} of 60 mm Hg, in general, should be regarded as satisfactory. In patients with ARDS the use of PEEP as previously described will often allow reduction of the FI_{O_2}. At present, there are no proved biochemical approaches to the prevention of oxygen toxicity, although several theoretically attractive possibilities exist.

Complications of Hemodynamic Monitoring

There are primarily three types of problems associated with hemodynamic monitoring: local complications associated with vascular access, passage and final positioning of the catheter, and inappropriate decision making based on inaccurate data or misinterpretation of information from the monitoring device. The last complications can best be prevented by proper maintenance of equipment and accurate and frequent calibration checks. As a general rule, monitoring data that are not consistent with the clinical situation or on which crucial therapeutic decisions hinge should not be accepted until the system has been thoroughly checked, zeroed, and calibrated.

SYSTEMIC ARTERIAL PRESSURE. The most frequent complication of systemic arterial blood pressure monitoring is formation of a hematoma at the site of the arterial puncture. This may be prevented or minimized by careful insertion technique, manual application of pressure immediately after insertion, and use of a pressure dressing, with care taken not to compromise distal circulation. Actual laceration of the vessel may require surgical repair.

Peripheral nerve damage may result from direct injury at the time of insertion or from a hematoma. Prevention involves careful insertion technique and measures to reduce the likelihood of formation of a hematoma.

Ischemia distal to the site of catheter insertion may result from arterial obstruction by the catheter itself, because of a clot forming around the catheter or because of embolization from clots on the tip of the catheter. Use of the appropriate-sized catheter will reduce the likelihood of obstruction of flow. Newer materials such as polyamine resins and Teflon are minimally thrombogenic and decrease the risk of a clot forming around the catheter. Also, continuous flush devices that deliver a small constant volume of heparinized solution greatly decrease clotting at the catheter tip or in the lumen.

Local infection at the site of insertion of a percutaneous arterial catheter or in the vessel itself is less common than with venous catheters but nevertheless may be a problem. This risk can be minimized by careful asepsis at the time of catheter insertion, sterile dressings changed daily, and prompt discontinuation of the catheter when it is no longer needed or serving its intended purpose.

CENTRAL VENOUS PRESSURE. The complications of central venous pressure monitoring include problems related to venous access, air embolism, infection, and venous thrombosis. When the subclavian or internal jugular vein is used for venous access, important complications include pneumothorax, hydrothorax, hemothorax, mediastinal hematoma, and subclavian or carotid artery puncture. If the left internal jugular or subclavian vein is used, the thoracic duct may be damaged, resulting in lymph fistula or chylothorax. Brachial nerve injury also may result from attempted subclavian vein catheterization. When an antecubital cutdown is used for central venous catheter placement, the brachial artery or median nerve may be injured. With each of these approaches local or intravascular infection or both and venous thrombosis may occur. If insertion is via a needle, withdrawal of the catheter through the needle may shear the catheter and create embolism of a foreign body.

Prevention of all of these complications is best approached through the use of meticulous insertion technique and maintenance of asepsis. Catheters placed and maintained with strict aseptic technique may be kept in place for long periods of time. However, under standard conditions in severely ill patients, they should not be left in place for more than 48 to 72 hours. A chest roentgenogram should be obtained promptly after catheter placement to look for evidence of pneumothorax or pleural fluid and to check the catheter position. Catheters that have entered the right ventricle should be withdrawn into the superior vena cava.

PULMONARY ARTERY PRESSURE. All of the complications attendant to central venous pressure monitoring may also occur with a pulmonary artery catheter. In addition, problems occur that are unique to this form of hemodynamic monitoring. The most common complication is a disturbance of cardiac rhythm or conduction or both. Premature ventricular contractions occur quite commonly as the catheter passes through the right ventricle. These generally are self-limited, at least with prompt catheter passage, but may occasionally require intravenous administration of 50 to 75 mg of lidocaine. Sustained ventricular tachycardia and ventricular fibrillation may also occur.

The frequency of ventricular arrhythmias can be minimized by using the full balloon inflation volume for the size catheter being placed and attempting rapid passage through the right ventricle. Guide wires and central venous catheters should not be advanced into the ventricle. Electrocardiographic monitoring with a visual display and audible signal should always be used during insertion. If ventricular arrhythmias occur, the catheter should promptly be withdrawn from the ventricle. Finally, intravenous lidocaine, a defibrillator, and resuscitation equipment should be immediately available.

During catheter insertion and occasionally after placement, right bundle branch block can develop. This usually does not present a problem unless there was a pre-existing left bundle branch block. In patients with left bundle branch block who need a pulmonary artery catheter passed, it may be advisable to first place a temporary transvenous pacemaker.

Intrapulmonary complications of Swan-Ganz catheters include pulmonary infarction and pulmonary artery rupture. Pulmonary infarction occurs because the tip of the catheter has migrated into and obstructed a peripheral vessel or because of clot propagation at the catheter tip. These can be avoided by continuously monitoring the pulmonary artery pressure to look for a "permanent wedge" pressure tracing. If this is noted, the catheter should be withdrawn to a point where the pulmonary artery wedge pressure appears only after the balloon is inflated with 1 ml of air. Clot propagation is minimized by using the continuous flow device described previously. The likelihood of rupture of the pulmonary artery is also decreased by ensuring that the catheter is positioned properly in a more proximal vessel.

Psychologic Consequences of Critical Care

CONSEQUENCES FOR THE PATIENT. The patient-related psychologic consequences of critical care are difficult to define and quantitate. In many instances what might appear as disordered behavior in a critically ill patient in fact represents an appropriate response to a genuinely threatening situation. In others the behavior is an organic effect of the illness itself; for example, patients with chronic airways obstruction and hypoxemia have been found to have well-defined behavioral alterations. It is only logical to assume, however, that an environment so foreign and so frightening as a critical care unit that operates totally independent of and without concern for any biologic rhythm could in and of itself produce significant psychologic disturbances, especially when superimposed on the effects of critical illness. Pain and discomfort, sensory deprivation—often with beeps, hisses, and buzzes as the major input—erratic and interrupted sleep patterns, immobilization, and total dependence on others are certainly capable of contributing to clouding of consciousness, perceptual distortion, behavioral confusion, and delusional experiences.

Because of the difficulty in identifying and quantitating the psychologic consequences of critical care, specific preventive measures are not so clearly definable as with other complications. However, standard approaches in critical care management of patients should be geared to providing a milieu that is least likely to generate the factors previously cited as contributing to psychiatric syndromes. Patients should be treated as cognizant, intelligent human beings by all staff. Every attempt should be made to incorporate the patient into discussions regarding care. A patient, even one who appears to be comatose, should not be treated as an inanimate object around which an esoteric discussion is held. Monitoring equipment should not be used as a substitute for interpersonal contact. The equipment used and procedures performed should be carefully explained to the patient. Insofar as possible, the day-night sleep cycle should be maintained. Providing the patient with a calendar serves to create or maintain a correct time orientation. A television set in the room may provide more "normal" sensory input serving to override the barrage of alarms and noises from ventilators and other sources. A liberal visiting policy allows needed "outside world" contact and helps to maintain contact with a familiar frame of reference. Sedative drugs and narcotics should be used only for specific indications such as for adequate pain relief. Benzodiazepines (such as Valium) and occasionally haloperidol (Haldol) can be extremely helpful in managing the psychiatric syndromes that do not respond to supportive treatment. Perhaps more important than all of these is the establishment of a pattern of behavior and interaction on the part of the critical care staff that fosters patient trust and confidence.

CONSEQUENCES FOR THE STAFF. Critical care staff members are also subject to the psychologic effects associated with providing care to severely ill patients. A variety of factors have been identified as contributing to the stress on critical care personnel, especially the nursing staff. First, the work is physically demanding and tiring. Second, patients, families, and physicians are emotionally demanding; emotional fatigue becomes superimposed on physical fatigue. The responsibilities are great and the performance expectations high while quite commonly the level of responsibility is not matched by decision-making authority. Such authority is vested in physicians who may have considerably less experience and expertise in critical care than the nurses. Nurses see what they may consider to be errors being made or patients getting worse and they are powerless to intervene in a meaningful way. These sorts of conflicts compound the already heightened emotional tension almost invariably present in critical care units. In addition, there is the genuine sorrow, distress, and sometimes guilt that accompanies deaths occurring in the unit.

The important consequences of these factors are that patient care may be compromised and that the turnover of unit personnel is high. Prevention of these sorts of situations is not easy. Many of the problems are inherent in the job. However, provision of clearly defined administrative guidelines describing the lines of authority and responsibility may minimize the conflicts. Likewise, having standard policies that are developed and agreed upon by the nursing and physician staff members provides support for independent nursing action. Nursing administrative policies also have considerable influence on the emotional well-being of the staff. Staffing ratios, hours worked per shift, and work breaks all are important factors that can be manipulated to reduce stress among the critical care staff. Finally, it is important that there be a single physician in charge of the unit through whom "official" communication between the nursing and medical staff takes place and to whom members of each group can present their problems and complaints. This physician, working in concert with the head nurse, can develop mechanisms for dealing with the various stressful situations either as they arise or preferably before they occur.

Fisher AB: Oxygen therapy: Side effects and toxicity. Am Rev Respir Dis. 122:61, 1980. *A concise review of what is known about oxygen toxicity. Discusses approaches to prevention.*

Kieley WF, Procci WR: Psychiatric aspects of critical care. *In* Zschoche DA (ed.): Comprehensive Review of Critical Care. St. Louis, C. V. Mosby Company, 1981, pp 107–114. *A review of the kinds of psychiatric disorders commonly seen in critically ill patients with a discussion of specific approaches to management.*

Mitchell SE, Clark RA: Complications of central venous catheterization. Am J Roentgenol 133:467, 1979. *Discusses the complications of central venous catheterization using the internal jugular or subclavian approaches. Reviews the anatomy and emphasizes the radiographic findings that indicate problems.*

Spring CL: Complications of pulmonary artery catheterization. *In* Spring CL (ed.): The Pulmonary Artery Catheter. Baltimore, University Park Press, 1983, pp 73–101. *An extensively referenced discussion of the complications occurring with Swan-Ganz pulmonary artery catheters. Presents the mechanisms by which the complications occur and the means for their prevention.*

Stauffer JL, Olson DE, Petty TL: Complications and consequences of endotracheal intubation and tracheostomy. Am J Med 70:65, 1981. *A prospective study of 150 patients requiring either endotracheal intubation or tracheostomy because of critical illness. Points out that, although the frequency of complications was similar with the two artificial airways, the complications of tracheostomy were much more likely to be severe than those associated with endotracheal tubes.*

Steel K, Gertman PK, Crescenzi C, Anderson J: Iatrogenic illness on a general medical service at a university hospital. N Engl J Med 304:638, 1981. *Presents a systematic review of complication occurring because of hospitalization in a university hospital and identifies factors associated with high risk of iatrogenic disease.*

Zwillich CW, Pierson DJ, Creagh CE, Sutton FD, Petty TL: Complications of assisted ventilation: A prospective study of 354 consecutive episodes. Am J Med. 57:161, 1974. *Describes the total spectrum of complications associated with mechanical ventilation. Also presents data on survival in different categories of patients.*

SOCIAL AND ETHICAL ISSUES IN CRITICAL CARE

Indications for and Value of Critical Care

Although defining the value of critical care and its indications would not seem to pertain to a discussion of social and ethical issues, this is, in fact, the topic area in which such considerations are most appropriate. The kinds of technology used and techniques involved in critical care are rather easily described in a straightforward scientific manner. The ends achieved by these interventions are not so clearly defined. If the relationship was strictly one between science and health or between medical practice and the patient's well-being, the discussion would be simple. Unfortunately, medical practice and the patient's well-being are not clearly and directly related when the connection is through the medium of a critical care unit. Critical care is very expensive in the consumption of public resources, and its indications and values are poorly defined. The uses of critical care have therefore become a matter involving serious ethical and public policy considerations.

Critical care units have been utilized more or less in their present form for approximately 20 years, yet their contribution to health has not been quantitated. Studies of patients suspected of having a myocardial infarction have suggested that if there are no early (initial 2 hours in one study and 24 hours in the second) indications of complications, management in a coronary care unit does not offer any advantage over management in a general ward or at home. Unfortunately, no such studies exist for the usual category of patients admitted to a general critical care unit. The available data generally describe features of patients admitted to general critical care units and construct evaluative indexes that can be correlated with prognosis. In theory, patients for whom the index indicates a poor prognosis should not be admitted to a critical care unit because it is highly unlikely that all of the interventions available will produce a favorable result. In practice, most physicians caring for a gravely ill patient want the patient to have every opportunity to survive and will request that critical care be provided almost regardless of ultimate prognosis. This is a dilemma that to date has not been solved.

Some categories of patients such as those with end-stage malignancies or those who are very old should clearly not be treated in critical care units. Mentally competent adults who do not wish to undergo the potential rigors of critical care and so inform their physicians should not be admitted to such a unit. On the other hand, patients with significant cardiac arrhythmias, drug-overdosed patients, patients with reversible neuromuscular diseases, those with severe asthma, and victims of multiple trauma, in general, definitely benefit from critical care.

Death rates in critical care units vary considerably depending on the type of unit and the severity of illness for patients admitted. The apparent overall mortality ranges from approximately 10 per cent to 30 per cent. The mortality is higher if patients have a chronic disease. Patients who require mechanical ventilation do much less well than the group as a whole. In one study the need for mechanical ventilation for 48 hours, independent of the reasons for ventilation, was associated with an in-hospital mortality rate of 64 per cent, a one-year mortality rate of 70 per cent and a three-year mortality rate of 72 per cent. In another study of patients with acute respiratory failure the mortality rate for those who required mechanical ventilation with an $F_{I_{O_2}}$ of 0.5 or greater for more than 24 hours was 66 per cent; patients who required an $F_{I_{O_2}}$ of 1.0 with a PEEP of 5 cm H_2O or more for 2 hours or an $F_{I_{O_2}}$ of 0.6 and a PEEP of 5 cm H_2O for 12 hours or more had a mortality rate of 92 per cent.

Unfortunately, with the data available, physicians are not able to predict reliably who will benefit from critical care and who will not. For this reason much of the decision making regarding who should be admitted to a critical care unit will in the future probably be conditioned by social (i.e., public policy) and ethical considerations rather than by scientific analyses.

Specific Ethical Issues

The basic precepts of medical ethics are discussed in Ch. 5. In this section specific concerns that arise in critical care are addressed.

THE INFLUENCE OF PATIENT WISHES ON THE CARE GIVEN. The autonomy of a mentally competent patient must be respected. If he indicates that a specific intervention such as endotracheal intubation, mechanical ventilation, or cardiopulmonary resuscitation is not to be used, it should not be used. The concern with the patient's competence, however, often clouds the issue and makes the decision less than clear-cut. The physician charged with the care of the patient must thoroughly review the process by which the decision was made with the patient and, when appropriate, with the patient's family. If there is a question in the physician's mind as to the competence of the patient, consultation should be sought.

"DO NOT RESUSCITATE" ORDERS. Orders not to initiate cardiopulmonary resuscitation (CPR) may be written at the request of patients as just discussed or may be initiated by physicians caring for patients when to the best of the physician's knowledge CPR is an intervention that will not be successful in the broad sense of restoring meaningful life. Such decisions must, however, be discussed with the patient and, when appropriate, with the family. The order should then be written in standard fashion in the order sheet and a note describing the basis for the order and the discussions that took place with the patient and family should be included in the chart. These orders should be reviewed at least daily because circumstances may change. Such orders clarify the ambiguity that surrounds the decisions concerning critical care for a patient with an irreversible illness and relieve the nurse or uninvolved physicians from the responsibility of deciding not to initiate CPR in such a patient.

So-called "no code" patients may still benefit from critical care. Treating airways obstruction, heart failure, metabolic abnormalities, or arrhythmias may at least temporarily improve the patient's condition, making the existence of "do not resuscitate" orders a moot point.

TERMINATION OF LIFE SUPPORT SYSTEMS. Supportive measures may be discontinued when there is no hope for recovery. Continuation of such measures serves only to prolong the process of dying. Defining the hopeless situation, however, may be difficult. The most straightforward instance is that of brain death. Brain death has been defined by several sets of unambiguous medical criteria (see Ch. 472). The American Bar Association and a number of states have adopted the broader concept that "for all legal purposes a human body with irreversible cessation of brain function, according to usual and customary standards of medical practice, shall be considered dead."

Various prognostic indicators have been developed to allow

prediction of the likelihood of recovery after severe brain insults. These provide guidance in instances in which all criteria for brain death are not present.

Black PMcL: Brain death. N Engl J Med 299:338 and 393, 1978. *An extensive review of all aspects of brain death including legal considerations.*
Chassin MR: Costs and outcome of medical intensive care. Med Care 20:165, 1982. *In addition to discussing costs and outcomes in critical care, this report describes the growth of critical care units in the United States.*
Cohen CB: Ethical problems of intensive care. Anesthesiology 47:217, 1977. *An extensive review and analysis of ethical considerations arising in critical care units.*
Detsky AS, Stricker SL, Mulley AG, Thibault GE: Prognosis, survival, and the expenditure of hospital resources for patients in an intensive care unit. N Engl J Med 305:667, 1981. *A study in which physicians were asked to estimate prognosis at the time of admission of a patient to a medical critical care unit and then examine the relationship between this prognosis and outcome.*
Hill JD, Hampton JR, Mitchell JRA: A randomized trial of home-versus-hospital management for patients with suspected myocardial infarction. Lancet 1:837, 1978. *A report of the only well-designed prospective randomized study of the value of critical care (in this case, coronary care). Demonstrated that if the myocardial infarction was not complicated, hospital care offered no clear advantage over home care.*
Levy DE, Bates D, Caronna JJ, Cartlidge NEF, Knill-Jones RP, Lapinski RH, Singer BH, Shaw DA, Plum F: Prognosis in nontraumatic coma. Ann Intern Med 94:293, 1981. *Presents the results of a prospective study of 500 patients with nontraumatic coma. Identifies factors that allow early identification of patients in whom recovery is very unlikely.*
Lo B, Jonsen AR: Clinical decisions to limit treatment. Ann Intern Med 94:764, 1980. *An analysis of the reasons presented for limiting care. The authors conclude that it is valid to limit care when a competent patient so desires and when treatment would be futile.*
Miles SH, Crawford R, Schultz AL: The do-not-resuscitate order in a teaching hospital. Ann Intern Med 96:660, 1982. *The authors present a policy for implementing a "do not resuscitate" order and discuss the ethical, legal, and practical issues involved.*
Robin ED: A critical look at critical care. Crit Care Med 11:144, 1983. *A provocative discussion of the role of critical care in modern medical care. Presents a plea for objective evaluation of the indications and value of critical care.*
Schmidt CD, Elliott CG, Carmelli D, Jensen RL, Cengiz M, Schmidt JC, Tolman ED, Clemmer TP: Prolonged mechanical ventilation for respiratory failure: a cost benefit analysis. Crit Care Med 11:407, 1983. *Defines the cost and benefits associated with prolonged (48 hours or more) mechanical ventilation primarily in medical patients.*
Wallace-Barnhill G, Roth MD, Briggs BA, Bastron DR, Barrocas A: Medical, legal and ethical issues in critical care. Crit Care Med 10:57, 1982. *This article summarizes the existing legislation concerning definitions of death and termination of life support.*

CARDIOPULMONARY RESUSCITATION

Cardiopulmonary resuscitation is the supportive and sometimes definitive treatment applied to persons in whom, for whatever reason, effective cardiac and ventilatory activity have stopped. The situations in which this catastrophic event may occur unexpectedly include primary cardiac arrhythmias, arrhythmias associated with myocardial infarction, drowning, electrocution, acute upper airways obstruction, drug intoxication, and accidental trauma. In addition, cardiorespiratory arrest may result from a variety of underlying disease processes that reduce myocardial oxygen delivery or are associated with marked electrolyte or acid-base disturbances.

There are no data on the annual number of cardiorespiratory arrests occurring in this country. It is estimated, however, that more than one million persons have myocardial infarctions each year and that 650,000 persons die annually of coronary artery disease (Ch. 49). About 350,000 of these deaths take place out of the hospital, usually within two hours of the onset of symptoms. These data have suggested that for CPR to be truly effective it should be applied in the community at large rather than being limited to an in-hospital technique. For this reason, beginning in 1973 a standard program for training lay persons in basic life support was developed and implemented throughout the country. As of 1980 over 12 million persons in the United States had received this training. A second more advanced program in advanced cardiac life support was implemented in 1975.

In some communities more than 40 per cent of patients with documented ventricular fibrillation occurring out of the hospital have been resuscitated and in some subgroups survival has been as high as 60 to 80 per cent. These rates of success are generally attributed to the intervention of trained bystanders in initiating CPR and maintaining support until paramedical personnel arrive. The rate of survival following in-hospital cardiac arrest is much lower, ranging from 5 to 20 per cent. Different subgroups have markedly different rates, however. In one series patients with evidence of cardiac failure prior to the arrest had only a 2 per cent likelihood of survival and renal failure was associated with 3 per cent survival rate. Only 4 per cent of patients who were homebound before hospitalization in which the cardiac arrest occurred survived. On the other hand 27 per cent of patients who were active before entering the hospital survived.

Pathophysiology of Cardiorespiratory Arrest

SYSTEMIC EFFECTS. Cardiorespiratory arrest results in the cessation of effective delivery of oxygen to body tissues. The immediate effects are the same as those described in the discussion of shock (Ch. 43). Catecholamine release results in peripheral vasoconstriction in an attempt to preserve blood flow to the brain and heart at the expense of cutaneous, muscle, and renal blood flow. Without oxygen tissue metabolic processes become anaerobic with production of lactic acid, a by-product of anaerobic glycolysis, resulting in systemic metabolic acidosis. The amount of acidosis is determined largely by the balance between oxygen supply and oxygen demand. Thus, hypothermic patients, such as near-drowning victims, because of reduced oxygen needs have less lactate production and less tissue damage. Because there is no circulation or the circulation is much reduced, the lactic acid is not cleared from the tissues. As the hydrogen ion concentration increases, the effectiveness of catecholamines rapidly decreases, resulting in full vasodilation that abolishes the major mechanisms by which the blood volume is preferentially distributed to the brain and the heart. Irreversible damage to these critical organs ensues.

The critical determinants of the outcome of a cardiorespiratory arrest and resuscitation attempts are: (1) the reversibility of the abnormality leading to the cessation of effective cardiac output and (2) the success of the CPR in providing sufficient oxygen to the brain to prevent permanent damage.

CEREBRAL EFFECTS. Oxygen consumption by the brain ranges from 3 to 5 ml per minute per 100 grams of tissue during normal consciousness and cerebral blood flow (CBF) averages 50 to 60 ml per minute per 100 grams of tissue. Aerobic metabolism can be supported by as little as 0.21 ml of oxygen per minute per 100 grams of tissue. Experimentally, CBF carrying a normal amount of oxygen can be reduced to 16 to 18 ml per minute per 100 grams of tissue before electroencephalographic evidence of injury is seen. The determinants of CBF are the mean systemic arterial pressure ($\overline{PSA}$), the cerebrovascular resistance (CVR), and the intracranial pressure (ICP), which determines cerebral venous pressure. Thus,

$$CBF = \frac{\overline{PSA} - ICP}{CVR}.$$

Under normal circumstances, CBF increases with increases in Pa_{CO_2} and with hypoxemia (below Pa_{O_2} 50 mm Hg) because of decreases in CVR.

Sudden cessation of blood flow to the brain, as occurs with cardiorespiratory arrest, results in unconsciousness within 10 seconds. Cerebral glycolysis is stimulated seven-fold, but endogenous stores of glucose are inadequate to maintain cellular viability for more than a few minutes. When brain adenosine triphosphate is reduced to 20 per cent of basal levels, which occurs within five minutes of cessation of effective CBF, lactate production ceases and irreversible neuronal damage results. Because oxygen utilization is nonuniform within the brain, some areas such as the frontal and temporal cortexes are more susceptible to ischemia than areas of lower metabolic activity. Restoration of cerebral perfusion after a period of no flow may result in transient increases in ICP, perhaps causing focal hypoperfusion and further ischemic injury.

CARDIAC EFFECTS. Myocardial oxygen consumption ranges from 8 to 10 ml of oxygen per minute per 100 grams of tissue for basal needs in the normally beating, nonischemic heart and 4 to 5 ml of oxygen per minute per 100 grams of tissue during ventricular fibrillation. Assuming normal Ca_{O_2} and an extraction of oxygen of 75 per cent, a myocardial blood flow of approximately 60 ml per minute per 100 grams of tissue would be required to meet oxygen needs in normal sinus rhythm. In ventricular fibrillation this figure would be 25 ml per minute per 100 grams of tissue. Myocardial blood flow (MBF) is determined by the $\overline{PSA}$, the coronary venous sinus pressure approximated by the mean right atrial pressure ($\overline{PRA}$), and the coronary vascular resistance CVR, as follows:

$$MBF = \frac{\overline{PSA} - \overline{PRA}}{CVR}.$$

Coronary flow normally occurs during diastole when the aortic valve is closed. Thus, maintenance of coronary perfusion during CPR requires that the aortic valve close normally, that $\overline{PSA}$ remain elevated above $\overline{PRA}$, and that time for coronary filling be allowed. Coronary vascular resistance is likely to be minimal during ventricular fibrillation or asystole; however, in the presence of coronary artery disease, resistance and therefore flow will be nonuniform and probably cause regional ischemia and perhaps infarction. Fortunately, myocardial oxygen needs should also be low.

EFFECTS ON RESPIRATORY MUSCLES. Under normal circumstances the oxygen consumption of the respiratory muscles, primarily the diaphragm, is less than 5 per cent of total body oxygen consumption. However, as the work of breathing increases because of cardiac or pulmonary disorders or metabolic acidosis the oxygen needs of the respiratory muscles increase. In cardiogenic shock the respiratory muscles may become the most metabolically active tissues in the body. Because the oxygen need is increasing at a time when supply is decreasing, the ability of these muscles to maintain their work level may be impaired and hypoventilation may ensue.

Fatigue of the diaphragm may play an important role in augmenting the factors that lead to cardiorespiratory arrest. This suggests also that restoration of respiratory muscle function is an important goal in CPR. Restoration of function depends on improvement in muscle blood flow, which is determined by $\overline{PSA}$, $\overline{PRA}$, and muscle vascular resistance (MVR):

$$MRF = \frac{\overline{PSA} - \overline{PRA}}{MVR}.$$

Furthermore, the oxygen needs of the respiratory muscles can be greatly reduced by effective mechanical ventilation.

RENAL EFFECTS. Renal blood flow suffers from the preferential redistribution of cardiac output to the brain and heart when hypotension occurs. Under baseline conditions, renal blood flow is approximately 25 per cent of the normal resting cardiac output and oxygen consumption is 9 to 10 ml of oxygen per minute per 100 grams of tissue. Although autoregulation of renal perfusion tends to maintain blood flow over a wide range of perfusion pressures, in shock the flow is markedly reduced. This may result in cellular injury and acute renal failure even if circulation is properly restored.

Administering Cardiopulmonary Resuscitation

IMMEDIATE INTERVENTIONS. The immediate sequence of events that should be undertaken by the person who first encounters a victim of a cardiorespiratory arrest is listed in Table 71–8. The mechanisms for providing the necessary support will, of course, vary depending on the training of the person or persons on the scene and whether or not the arrest occurs within a hospital.

TABLE 71–8. IMMEDIATE SEQUENCE OF EVENTS IN CPR

Establish unresponsiveness
Call for help
Position victim
Open airway
Check for foreign body in airway
Institute mouth-to-mouth breathing
Check for pulse
Initiate closed chest compression

Artificial Ventilation. An important determinant of success in CPR is the provision of adequate ventilation. The first step is to open the airway and assure its patency. The most common cause of obstruction is the tongue. This may be corrected simply by tilting the head backward and lifting the chin or lower jaw forward. Mouth-to-mouth ventilation can then be applied unless there is a foreign body obstructing the airway.

A resuscitator's exhaled air may provide an FI_{O_2} of approximately 0.17 during mouth-to-mouth ventilation and carbon dioxide will be eliminated because of passive lung deflation. Commonly, however, gas exchange within the lungs is not normal and significant hypoxemia develops. For this reason supplemental oxygen should be administered as soon as it is available. Both oxygen administration and ventilation can be accomplished via a tight-fitting face mask and ventilation bag, preferably one capable of delivering an FI_{O_2} of 1.0. Endotracheal intubation provides the most reliable closed system of oxygen administration and also protects the airway against the aspiration of gastric contents.

Closed Chest Compression. Closed chest compression should be administered to patients who do not have a palpable pulse. The patient should be supine and on a firm surface. Sufficient pressure should be applied to the lower half of the sternum to depress it 4 to 5 cm in most adults and 2 cm in children. The pressure should be relaxed after each compression, allowing the sternum to return to its relaxed position. The recommended compression-to-relaxation ratio is 50:50 and the rate of compressions should be about one per second. The adequacy of closed chest compression should be determined by attempting to palpate a carotid or femoral pulse produced by the compression.

The mechanism by which closed chest compression causes blood to circulate is not clear. The original concept was that by compressing the chest the heart was squeezed between the sternum and the vertebral column, producing a mechanical systole in which right and left ventricular pressures exceed pulmonary artery and aortic pressures, respectively, causing forward blood flow. Release of the pressure caused diastolic filling of the ventricles due to the gradient between the peripheral venous system and the intrathoracic structures.

More recent data suggest that it is the total intrathoracic pressure that causes forward blood flow rather than cardiac compression. For example, cough in itself has sustained cardiac output and consciousness in patients with ventricular fibrillation. A variety of experimental studies are consistent with this contention.

INTERMEDIATE INTERVENTIONS. The arrival of persons with more advanced training and equipment marks the second or intermediate phase of CPR. Electrocardiographic monitoring enables proper application of direct current countershock for defibrillation or conversion of ventricular tachycardia. A current of 200 to 400 watt-seconds should be used for ventricular fibrillation and 25 to 50 watt-seconds for ventricular tachycardias. The current given should be increased if there is no response to the initial shock. In patients with ventricular fibrillation, epinephrine should be administered routinely either intravenously or via an endotracheal tube before countershock is applied. Epinephrine enhances myocardial contractility, constricts peripheral vasculature, and lowers the defibrillation threshold. This combination of effects operates to improve cerebral and cardiac perfusion and to increase the likelihood of defibrillation occurring. Standard doses are 0.5 to 1.0 mg or 5 to 10 ml of a 1:10,000 dilution. The dose can be repeated at approximately five-minute intervals. Calcium chloride also improves myocardial contractility and ventricular automaticity but should not be administered to aid defibrillation until epinephrine has been tried and failed. Calcium may also be effective in severe hypotension associated with electromechanical dissociation. The usual dose of calcium chloride is 5 ml of a 10 per cent solution (5 to 7 mg per kilogram). This can be repeated at 10-minute intervals.

Lidocaine is the initial drug of choice to suppress ventricular ectopy in the setting of cardiorespiratory arrest. The usual dose is approximately 1 mg per kilogram (50 to 75 mg) given intravenously as a bolus injection. A second bolus dose may be given in 10 minutes. This is then followed by a continuous intravenous infusion of 1 to 4 mg per minute. Other agents that may be useful for ventricular arrhythmias not responsive to lidocaine include bretylium tosylate, procainamide, and verapamil. The doses and uses of these drugs are discussed in Ch. 50.

Atropine sulfate is useful in treating sinus bradycardia or complete heart block because it increases the rate of discharge of the sinus node and improves atrioventricular conduction. The usual dose of atropine sulfate is 0.5 mg administered intravenously and repeated at 5-minute intervals until the desired rate is achieved or a total dose of 2 mg is given.

Isoproterenol may also be used to treat hemodynamically significant bradycardia resulting from heart block that is refractory to atropine. Caution should be exercised in the use of both of these agents in that myocardial oxygen requirements increase with increases in heart rate. Thus, ischemia may be worsened by increasing heart rate above that necessary to provide an adequate cardiac output.

The metabolic acidosis that accompanies cardiorespiratory arrest can interfere with the actions of both endogenous and exogenous catecholamines. The arterial pH value at which this occurs is thought to be approximately 7.25. For this reason sodium bicarbonate should be administered to most patients undergoing CPR. Ideally administration of $NaHCO_3$ should be guided by measurements of arterial pH; however, often this is not possible. Empiric treatment using 1 mEq per kilogram can be administered as the initial dose followed by 0.5 mEq per kilogram every 10 minutes for the duration of the arrest.

INTERVENTIONS AFTER INITIAL RECOVERY. All patients who have been resuscitated successfully should be transferred as quickly as possible to a critical care unit. As a minimum, electrocardiographic monitoring should be provided. The need for invasive hemodynamic monitoring depends on the causes and consequences of the cardiorespiratory arrest. Often, at least transiently, it is necessary to provide mechanical ventilation. This allows rest and functional recovery of the respiratory muscles and minimizes total oxygen needs. The major determinant of return of brain function is the adequacy of cerebral perfusion during the period of cardiac arrest. Subsequently, after recovery of cardiac function, all factors that influence oxygen delivery to the brain should be evaluated and made normal where possible. Measures to prevent elevation in intracranial pressure (ICP) such as keeping the patient's head elevated, controlling arterial pH and Pa_{CO_2}, and treating seizures and agitation should be undertaken. The effectiveness of measures designed to minimize brain damage including the use of barbiturates, calcium channel-blocking agents, and hypothermia remains to be proven.

REASONS FOR FAILURE. Obviously, not all persons who sustain cardiac arrest can or should be resuscitated. Often the process leading to the arrest is irreversible or the resulting cardiac injury is so severe that it precludes successful resuscitation. In some instances, however, reversible factors may play a major role in the failure of CPR to restore an adequate cardiac output. These factors include severe electrolyte and acid-base disturbances, inadequate oxygenation or ventilation because of faulty technique, hypovolemia, pneumothorax (especially tension pneumothorax), and cardiac tamponade. Abnormalities of electrolyte and acid-base balance as well as inadequate oxygenation and/or ventilation usually manifest themselves as an inability to restore an adequate cardiac rate and rhythm. Hypovolemia, tension pneumothorax, and cardiac tamponade usually cause electromechanical dissociation in which the rate and rhythm of the heart are satisfactory but the cardiac output is inadequate. When electromechanical dissociation is detected, the initial response should be to administer epinephrine, and if this is unsuccessful, to give calcium chloride. Failure of both of these agents to increase cardiac output should prompt an immediate evaluation for mechanical factors that may be preventing adequate blood flow. If such factors are detected, pericardiocentesis, chest tube placement, or volume replacement may be lifesaving.

American Medical Association. Standards and guidelines for cardiopulmonary resuscitation (CPR) and emergency cardiac care. JAMA 244:453, 1980. *This is the basic reference source describing CPR.*

Bedell SE, Delbanco TL, Cook EF, Epstein FH: Survival after cardiopulmonary resuscitation in the hospital. N Engl J Med 309:569, 1983. *Reviews the results of in-hospital CPR and describes factors associated with prognosis.*

Cobb LA, Hallstrom AP, Thompson RG, Mandel LP, Copass MK: Community cardiopulmonary resuscitation. Annu Rev Med 31:453, 1980. *Reviews the results of a very active community based program for CPR.*

Eisenberg MS, Hallstrom AP, Bergner L: Long-term survival after out of hospital cardiac arrest. N Engl J Med 306:1340, 1982. *Presents data concerning survival after out-of-hospital CPR and identifies factors that relate to outcome.*

Luce JM, Cary JM, Ross BK, Culver BH, Butler J: New developments in cardiopulmonary resuscitation. JAMA 244:1366, 1980. *Discusses the theories of the mechanisms for blood flow during CPR.*

Luce JM, Ross BK, O'Quin RJ, Culver BH, Sivarajan M, Amory DW, Niskanen RA, Alferness CA, Kirk WL, Pierson LR, Butler J: Regional blood flow during cardiopulmonary resuscitation in dogs using simultaneous and nonsimultaneous compression and ventilation. Circulation 67:258, 1983. *An experimental study of the factors influencing organ blood flow in two forms of CPR.*

Part X
RENAL DISEASES

72. APPROACH TO THE PATIENT WITH RENAL DISEASE

Thomas E. Andreoli

This chapter provides a general overview of the signs and symptoms that represent the cardinal findings in patients with diseases of the kidney or urinary tract and formulates a relatively simple classification for considering these disorders. The signs and symptoms associated with renal disease are quite variable and depend, among other things, on the nature and severity of the disease process, the acuteness or chronicity of the disease, and the presence or absence of associated systemic disease. The first manifestation of severe renal failure may be the random detection of an abnormality on urinalysis. Alternatively, a striking presenting complaint, for example hematuria, may point to an ominous lesion such as a renal neoplasm or may be the presenting manifestation of a relatively mild, self-limited disorder such as cystitis.

An analysis of the signs and symptoms of renal disease in terms of the structural and functional characteristics of the kidneys and urinary tract affords a rational and useful approach for integrating a series of clinical and laboratory data into the formulation of diagnostic and therapeutic strategies for renal disorders. Accordingly, this chapter begins with a brief consideration of the cardinal functions of the kidney. A more detailed consideration of renal physiology is presented in Chapter 73. Subsequently the cardinal urinary abnormalities of renal disease are described, since urinalysis represents the single most common laboratory study utilized in evaluating patients for disorders of the kidney or urinary tract. The third section of this chapter enumerates briefly the primary findings in the more common syndromes involving the kidneys and urinary tract, and the fourth section describes the consequences of complete or nearly complete failure of renal function, that is, the uremic syndrome. Finally, the last section considers the relationship between the adaptive response to a reduction in nephron mass and the potential contribution of one of these adaptive responses, renal hyperfiltration, to the pathogenesis of progressive renal disease.

CARDINAL ELEMENTS OF RENAL FUNCTION

URINE FORMATION. The kidneys maintain constancy of the volume and composition of body fluids by forming urine whose composition is ultimately determined by the dietary intake of solute and water and by the rate and kind of metabolic transformation of endogenous and exogenous carbohydrates, proteins, lipids, and nucleic acids. The kidneys also serve as the major route for the excretion of a large number of drugs. The formation of urine serves two purposes: a *regulatory* function, that is, the maintenance of a constant volume and composition for body fluids; and an *excretory* function, that is, elimination of endogenous and exogenous metabolic end-products.

Urine is formed by a sequence of five events:

1. The glomerulus filters approximately 180 liters of extracellular fluid daily across glomerular capillaries and the visceral epithelium of Bowman's capsule, using as a driving force the mean arterial pressure. The glomerular capillary endothelium and basement membrane and the visceral epithelium of Bowman's capsule are freely permeable to water and solutes of relatively low molecular weight (that is, under 6,000 to 8,000 daltons), moderately permeable to large molecular weight species such as myoglobin (molecular weight, approximately 16,000 daltons), and virtually impermeable to macromolecules such as albumin. Filtration is also influenced by molecular charge as well as size. The result is an isotonic, virtually protein-free filtrate whose daily volume is more than ten-fold greater than the volume of extracellular fluid (ECF).

2. The proximal tubule isotonically reabsorbs approximately two thirds of the glomerular filtrate. In the process certain alterations in the composition of tubular fluid are produced by specialized transport mechanisms: the preferential absorption of sodium with bicarbonate rather than chloride; the virtually complete absorption of organic solutes such as glucose and amino acids; and the absorption of organic acids such as uric acid and other nonamino acids in early segments of the proximal nephron, followed by secretion of these acids into tubular fluid in the late proximal nephron. Thus the volume of tubular fluid delivered to the loop of Henle is approximately one third of the volume of glomerular filtrate, has a sodium concentration equal to that of plasma and a bicarbonate concentration about 10 per cent of that in plasma, and contains little or no glucose or amino acids.

3. The loop of Henle dissociates the absorption of sodium and water. The descending limb of Henle passively abstracts water into the hypertonic medullary interstitium, concentrating the tubular fluid. Conversely, the water-impermeable thick ascending limb of Henle actively absorbs approximately 25 per cent of filtered sodium chloride but little water. As a result, about 18 liters of tubular fluid enter the distal convoluted tubule daily. This fluid, which is approximately 10 per cent of the initial glomerular filtrate, is almost maximally dilute, having an osmolality of approximately 50 mOsm per kilogram of H_2O.

4. The distal convoluted tubule primarily absorbs sodium under the influence of aldosterone and secretes protons, ammonia, and potassium. Aldosterone regulates sodium absorption in this nephron segment.

5. The collecting duct system regulates the osmolality of urine. When antidiuretic hormone (ADH) is present, water is absorbed across the collecting duct and tubular fluid equilibrates osmotically with the hypertonic medullary interstitium; when ADH is absent, the water permeability of collecting ducts is at a minimum and a dilute urine is excreted.

THE KIDNEY AS AN ENDOCRINE RECEPTOR. Among many hormones that regulate renal function, three are of particular importance: parathyroid hormone (PTH), aldosterone, and antidiuretic hormone (ADH). PTH enhances the absorption of calcium and magnesium and inhibits the absorption of phosphate and bicarbonate in the proximal tubule by increasing intracellular cyclic 3′,5′-adenosine monophosphate (cAMP). PTH also stimulates the renal conversion of 25-hydroxycholecalciferol, the major metabolite of vitamin D_3, to 1,25-dihydroxycholecalciferol, which is the major biologically active form of vitamin D_3 (Ch. 244).

Aldosterone and other mineralocorticoids stimulate the rate of sodium absorption in the distal nephron. Aldosterone also increases the rate of net potassium secretion and net proton secretion (and consequently, the rate of bicarbonate regeneration) by the distal nephron.

ADH promotes the formation of a hypertonic urine both by increasing the rate of salt absorption in the thick ascending limb of Henle and by increasing the water permeability of the collecting duct system. Both actions are mediated by ADH-dependent increases in cytosolic cAMP in those renal tubular segments.

THE KIDNEY AS AN ENDOCRINE ORGAN. The kidney plays a major role in prostaglandin production, in the operation of the kallikrein-kinin system, and in the degradation of low molecular weight proteins. The kidney is also the major site for the synthesis of erythropoietin and of renin. Erythropoietin is a glycoprotein produced by renal enzymatic action on a circulating precursor of hepatic origin. The principal action of erythropoietin is to stimulate the rate of red blood cell production by the bone marrow.

Renin is secreted by the granular cells of the juxtaglomerular apparatus in response to reductions in renal perfusion pressure or in effective circulating volume. Renin increases the rate of conversion of angiotensinogen to angiotensin I, which in turn is a precursor of angiotensin II. In turn, angiotensin II is a potent vasoconstrictor agent and a strong stimulus to thirst and to aldosterone production. Thus, the kidney, by way of renin production, plays a central role in the volume repletion reaction.

URINARY MANIFESTATIONS OF RENAL DISEASE (Ch. 75)

Urinary abnormalities are among the major findings in most forms of renal disease; urinalysis is one of the major laboratory studies used in the diagnosis of renal disease. This section considers the nature and significance of the more common urinary abnormalities in disorders of the kidneys and urinary tract.

HEMATURIA. Hematuria is a specific indicator of an abnormality in the kidneys or urinary tract but is a nonspecific indicator of any particular form of renal disease. Hematuria of itself is not painful; however, the passage of blood clots along the ureter or urethra may produce renal colic or dysuria, respectively. In general, hematuria occurs in the following disorders: (1) Systemic disorders such as the hemoglobinopathies, coagulation disorders, sepsis, and, rarely, severe congestive heart failure. Hematuria may also occur following severe exercise. (2) Inflammatory and necrotizing glomerular diseases. Hematuria also occurs in certain types of interstitial nephritis, particularly those that are acute, and in renal infarction. (3) Diseases characterized by disruption of the normal structure of the kidneys or urinary tract, as in neoplasms, urolithiasis, trauma, or cystic disease of the kidney. (4) Irritative or inflammatory disorders of the kidneys, ureter, or lower urinary tract, as in pyelonephritis or lower urinary tract infection.

Because hematuria is a relatively nonspecific indicator of renal disease, an assessment of the origin of hematuria requires a careful history and physical examination as well as a laboratory evaluation, including urinalysis in particular. The presence of red blood cell casts indicates, by definition, that the hematuria is of renal parenchymal origin. Red blood cell casts are seen most commonly in acute glomerular diseases but do not exclude the presence of a systemic disorder, such as a coagulopathy, or of a tubular derangement. Proteinuria in combination with hematuria is a classic indicator of parenchymal renal disease; massive proteinuria (in excess of 3.0 grams per 24 hours) in combination with hematuria is typically, but not exclusively, a characteristic of glomerular disease.

Isolated, painless hematuria in the absence of associated urinary abnormalities such as red cell casts or proteinuria or of systemic disease or obvious entities such as urolithiasis or urinary tract infection generally requires more detailed studies such as renal ultrasonography, CT scanning, arteriography, or renal biopsy. The intent of such studies is the detection of either occult glomerular or interstitial disease or of renal tumors or cysts.

Isolated hematuria may occur in association with entirely normal renal imaging studies, a normal renal biopsy, and negligible proteinuria. This condition, which occurs most frequently in children and is often termed *benign recurrent hematuria of childhood*, is characterized by recurrent bouts of microscopic and gross hematuria. To date, there is no evidence that this disorder, when accompanied by normal glomerular architecture and negative glomerular immunofluorescence, leads to progressive renal disease.

PROTEINURIA. The normal daily rate of urinary protein excretion averages less than 150 milligrams per 24 hours. In certain instances, notably fever, severe congestive heart failure, and severe exercise, the rate of urinary protein excretion may be increased transiently in the absence of intrinsic renal disease. Furthermore, in young individuals, so-called "postural" proteinuria, defined as transient or consistent proteinuria in the upright but not recumbent positions, may occur in the absence of histologically detectable lesions on renal biopsy; the long-term outlook in such individuals appears to be excellent.

However, persistent proteinuria, occurring in both the recumbent and upright position and exceeding 750 mg per 24 hours, is a specific indicator of parenchymal renal disease. Proteinuria of less than 2.0 grams per 24 hours occurs commonly either in interstitial or in glomerular disease, but when in excess of 3.0 to 3.5 grams per 24 hours usually indicates glomerular disease and, more specifically, the nephrotic syndrome. However, massive proteinuria may also occur in severe congestive heart failure, in accelerated hypertension, and rarely in acute allergic interstitial nephritis.

URINARY LEUKOCYTES, CASTS, AND BACTERIA. The excretion of leukocytes in the urine is generally defined as *pyuria* when more than five to ten white blood cells per high power field are found in centrifuged samples of the urinary sediment. However, pyuria is not a specific finding for bacterial infection of the urinary tract but rather is indicative of an inflammatory process within the kidneys or urinary tract. When leukocyte casts are also found, renal parenchymal inflammation is usually present.

Cylinduria, the presence of tubular urinary casts, is traditionally regarded as evidence of renal parenchymal injury, but no single type of cast is explicitly diagnostic of any specific disease entity. Red cell casts are most often indicative of glomerular injury, whereas white cell casts are suggestive of parenchymal inflammation. The specific significance of granular, epithelial, hyaline, or fatty casts is not always clear.

The matrix of most urinary casts is composed mainly of Tamm-Horsfall glycoprotein derived from the renal tubular epithelium. Casts originate within the renal parenchyma, and the usual urinary cast is probably formed within the distal nephron. So-called "broad" casts are formed within the region of the collecting duct or dilated nephron segments. The presence of abnormal urinary casts is generally indicative of altered renal structure or function, or both, but it is not necessarily true that their number and type are indicative of the extent of injury.

Significant *bacteriuria* indicates bacterial colonization of urine. The presence of bacteria in freshly collected, clean-voided urine specimens generally correlates closely with bacterial counts in excess of 100,000 organisms per milliliter of urine, and a Gram's stain of the urinary sediment of a similarly collected specimen is generally helpful in identifying whether the offending organism is gram-positive or gram-negative.

MISCELLANEOUS URINARY FINDINGS. *Urinary cytologic studies* are ordinarily not a part of the routine urinalysis. However, an evaluation of urinary cytology, done conveniently by a Wright's stain of the urinary sediment, is a useful diagnostic test for transitional cell tumors of the renal pelvis or ureter. Similarly, cytologic examination of bladder washings may be helpful in the diagnosis of bladder neoplasia (Ch. 92).

Pneumaturia, the passage of urine mixed with air, can occur in the presence of fistula tracts from either the bowel or the vagina into the bladder. These tracts may follow surgical procedures, pelvic infections, or inflammatory bowel disease. A plain film of the abdomen may also indicate the presence of air in the urinary bladder.

THE MAJOR RENAL SYNDROMES

Renal disorders are often nonspecific in their manifestations, as hematuria, azotemia, hypertension, or metabolic acidosis, for example. The interpretation of a group of findings obtained by history, physical examination, and routine laboratory stud-

TABLE 72–1. THE PRERENAL (HYPOPERFUSION) SYNDROMES

Class of Disorder	Major Findings
Reduced Effective Circulating Volume	Oliguria Azotemia Reduced fractional sodium excretion Elevated plasma renin Normotension
Occlusive Renal Artery Disease	Hypertension Elevated plasma renin Azotemia: with severe, bilateral disease or an affected solitary kidney

ies, however, may be used to describe some of the more common syndromes and disorders affecting the kidneys and urinary tract, which are briefly described below.

THE PRERENAL SYNDROMES. The major classes of prerenal disorders are (1) renal hypoperfusion secondary to a reduction in effective circulating volume, and (2) renal ischemia because of occlusive disease in one or both renal arteries. Both sets of disorders are associated with hyperreninemia, but the clinical manifestations of the two diseases differ significantly (Table 72–1).

Renal hypoperfusion secondary to a *reduction in effective circulating volume* may occur in association with true volume contraction; an increase in vascular capacitance, as in sepsis; sequestration of fluid in interstitial compartments, as in ascites and the hepatorenal syndrome; or an inability to transfer fluid from the venous to the arterial limbs of the circulation, as in severe congestive heart failure, constrictive pericarditis, or pericardial tamponade. In any of these instances, when the effective circulating volume is sufficiently reduced, the kidneys are hypoperfused, the glomerular filtration rate is reduced, and renin is released. This results in oliguria, an elevation in serum BUN and creatinine concentrations, and a reduced fractional excretion rate for sodium (that is, generally less than 1 per cent). Although plasma renin levels are elevated, the patients are ordinarily normotensive, presumably because the effective circulating volume is decreased.

Renal ischemia produced by *occlusive disease* of the renal arteries results in renin release from the ischemic kidney without a reduction in effective circulating volume and consequently is manifested primarily as hypertension, since pressor activity is elevated while filling of the arterial tree is normal or only slightly reduced. If the renal arterial occlusive disease is limited to one kidney and the contralateral kidney retains normal function, azotemia is absent. However, if the hypertension results in injury to the unaffected kidney, azotemia may ensue. When both renal arteries are involved, azotemia occurs when renal ischemia is sufficiently severe that renal autoregulatory mechanisms are inadequate to maintain an adequate glomerular filtration rate.

THE RENAL PARENCHYMAL SYNDROMES. ***Acute Glomerular Disorders.*** GLOMERULONEPHRITIS AND THE NEPHROTIC SYNDROME (Ch. 80). Two major types of disorders affect the glomerulus: (1) the *acute nephritic syndrome*, characterized mainly by inflammatory and/or necrotizing lesions within glomeruli, and (2) the *nephrotic syndrome*, a predominantly noninflammatory derangement of the glomeruli characterized by an abnormal "leakiness" of the glomeruli to albumin and other macromolecules. This disorder may arise in association with systemic lupus erythematosus, as a consequence of autoimmune renal disease, in combination with inflammatory renal lesions such as membranoproliferative glomerulonephritis, in association with neoplasia or exogenous toxins, and for unknown reasons.

The acute nephritic syndrome may result from systemic diseases such as disseminated vasculitis, autoimmune renal disorders such as postinfectious glomerulonephritis, as a consequence of accelerated hypertension, or from other unknown causes, for example, idiopathic rapidly progressive glomerulonephritis. While the general histologic characteristic of these disorders is glomerular inflammation, the extent of renal inflammation may be quite variable for a given disease. For example, in Henoch-Schönlein purpura with hematuria and red blood cell casts, the renal lesion may vary from a mild focal nephritis to a fulminant necrosis of glomerular tufts. Furthermore, while there is a reasonable degree of correlation between the extent of glomerular injury and the severity of the clinical syndrome, the correlation is not entirely satisfactory. The etiologic, histologic, and clinical characteristics of the glomerulonephritic and nephrotic syndromes overlap to a considerable degree: (1) A given disease process, for example systemic lupus erythematosus, may produce a mild, focal glomerulonephritis with hematuria, mild proteinuria but no azotemia; a diffuse proliferative glomerulonephritis with hematuria, proteinuria, and severe renal failure; or membranous nephropathy characterized by a relatively pure nephrotic syndrome. (2) Glomerular lesions may evolve; for example, Goodpasture's syndrome can begin as a mild, focal nephritis and progress to a diffuse, necrotic glomerulonephritis. (3) The extent of glomerular injury, as viewed on renal biopsy, correlates generally but inexactly with the severity of the clinical picture. (4) A given pathogenic mechanism, for example immune complex disease, may in some instances result in acute glomerulonephritis and in other cases in a pure nephrotic syndrome. (5) In certain disorders such as membranoproliferative nephritis, both a nephritic picture and a nephrotic picture may coexist simultaneously.

These diverse glomerular disorders can be somewhat arbitrarily classified by four major patterns that may be defined by the initial presentation of the patient (Table 72–2).

THE MILD ACUTE GLOMERULONEPHRITIS SYNDROMES. In this class of glomerular inflammation, glomerular blood flow is sufficient to maintain the glomerular filtration at a normal or near normal rate. Mild acute glomerulonephritis is characterized by hematuria, red cell casts, modest proteinuria, minimal azotemia, and mild or no edema. Because renal perfusion is not severely compromised, hypertension and/or salt retention are generally absent. In general, this pattern is observed most commonly with mild, focal glomerular lesions, particularly the focal nephritis seen in systemic lupus erythematosus and in the Henoch-Schönlein syndrome of children.

THE DIFFUSE ACUTE GLOMERULONEPHRITIS SYNDROMES. These glomerulonephritic syndromes are usually characterized by diffuse glomerular inflammation and/or necrosis sufficiently severe that hematuria and proteinuria are accompanied by a

TABLE 72–2. THE MAJOR GLOMERULAR SYNDROMES

Class of Disorder	Major Derangement	Major Findings
1. Mild Acute Glomerulonephritis	Mild glomerular inflammation	Hematuria, proteinuria Absent or mild azotemia Absent or mild edema
2. Severe Acute Glomerulonephritis	Extensive glomerular inflammation Renal ischemia Primary tubular sodium acquisitiveness	Hematuria, proteinuria Azotemia Plasma volume expansion Hypertension Edema Circulatory overload (if severe)
3. Pure Nephrotic Syndrome	Glomerular protein leak	Massive proteinuria Reduced plasma oncotic pressure Anasarca Normotensive Sensitive to diuretics
4. Mixed Disorders	1 plus 3 or 2 plus 3	Hematuria Massive proteinuria Azotemia (variable) Hypertension (variable) Edema

reduction in filtration rate and, consequently, azotemia of varying degrees. Simultaneously, for reasons that are not well understood, the proximal nephron becomes remarkably salt-acquisitive. Thus if dietary intake is not curtailed, there is also plasma volume expansion.

Sodium acquisitiveness in acute glomerulonephritis is considerably greater than that expected solely from the reduction in glomerular filtration rate. Plasma albumin is generally normal, so that a significant fraction of retained sodium remains in the vascular compartment and may result in hypertension, plasma volume dilution, circulatory overload, congestive heart failure, and a suppression of plasma renin activity.

The diffuse, or severe, acute glomerulonephritis syndromes are usually seen in association with diffusely proliferative or necrotic glomerular lesions, particularly in the more severe forms of diffuse proliferative lupus nephritis, Goodpasture's syndrome, postinfectious glomerulonephritis, and rapidly progressive glomerulonephritis.

NEPHROTIC SYNDROME. In the pure nephrotic syndrome the glomerular filtration barrier is abnormally permeable to macromolecules, so that massive proteinuria occurs even though the filtration rate may be normal. This large urinary loss of protein contributes to the characteristic hypoalbuminemia in such patients; furthermore, the development of hypercholesterolemia correlates closely with the degree of hypoalbuminemia.

Nephrotic patients are usually salt-acquisitive and edematous. In the nephrotic syndromes the reduced plasma oncotic pressure leads to translocation of fluid to the interstitium, a reduced effective circulating volume, and a secondary sodium acquisitiveness and edema. Patients with the pure nephrotic syndrome often are normotensive, rarely develop circulatory overload, and frequently have elevated plasma renin activities. As further evidence for a reduced effective circulating volume, severely nephrotic patients may have postural hypotension even in the presence of anasarca and may have hemoconcentration and renal hypoperfusion with attendant azotemia following excessive diuretic use.

The pure nephrotic syndrome is seen most commonly in the nil lesion of childhood, in idiopathic membranous nephropathy, in the membranous nephropathy accompanying systemic lupus erythematosus and carcinoma (particularly of the colon), and in amyloidosis. The nephrotic syndrome also occurs following exposure to certain toxins. A common form of nephrotic syndrome of this type, seen with increasing frequency in modern society, is heroin nephropathy characterized by focal glomerular sclerosis on renal biopsy and, in clinical terms, as a nephrotic syndrome with mild to moderate—but progressive—azotemia.

The Interstitial Nephritis Syndromes (Ch. 81.1). In the interstitial nephritis syndromes, the primary abnormality is damage to the tubulointerstitial system of the kidney with secondary glomerular damage. Thus renal tubular function tends to be deranged disproportionately to reductions in glomerular filtration rate.

Generalized tubulointerstitial disorders often damage the juxtaglomerular apparatus and therefore tend to impair renin production. As a consequence of hyporeninemia, aldosterone production is curtailed. The combination of a reduced rate of aldosterone secretion from the adrenal cortex, coupled with damage to the distal nephron, generally results in hyporeninemia, hypoaldosteronism, modest degrees of salt wasting, hyperkalemia, and hyperchloremic metabolic acidosis. These abnormalities, which resemble those of Addison's disease, occur even when the glomerular filtration rate is only modestly reduced. In contrast to Addison's disease, however, mineralocorticoids are usually ineffective in treating these abnormalities unless high doses are used.

Urinary abnormalities such as hematuria and proteinuria are usually but not always relatively modest in patients with tubulointerstitial disease, in comparison to patients with glomerular disease. Three general classes of tubulointerstitial diseases can be defined:

1. *Chronic tubulointerstitial disease* may occur as a consequence of any one of a large number of diseases that produce chronic damage to the renal interstitium: chronic hypertension, with progressive ischemia to the renal interstitium; diabetes mellitus, where microvascular disease within the kidney effects the same end result; occlusive disease of smaller renal vessels, as in sickle cell disease; chronic pyelonephritis; gout; and exogenous toxins, notably illicit alcohol containing lead, and analgesic abuse, particularly the combination of phenacetin and aspirin. Chronic interstitial disease is generally detected in individuals who have modest degrees of sodium wasting, hyperkalemia, metabolic acidosis, and an acid urine. These abnormalities may occur even when only mild degrees of azotemia exist. The plasma renin activity is generally reduced, as are rates of aldosterone secretion. Most commonly, hematuria and significant proteinuria are not characteristic of chronic interstitial disease.

2. *Acute allergic interstitial disease* occurs when patients are treated with antibiotics, notably penicillin and related drugs, or with nonsteroidal anti-inflammatory agents. In addition to producing electrolyte abnormalities similar to those described above for chronic interstitial nephritis, acute allergic interstitial nephritis may severely reduce glomerular filtration and be associated with marked hematuria and proteinuria, and with oliguria. There is often eosinophilia and eosinophils may be present in the urine. Since penicillin and related antibiotics and nonsteroidal anti-inflammatory agents are commonly used, acute allergic interstitial nephritis should always be considered in the differential diagnosis of oliguria that develops in hospitalized patients.

Oliguria and azotemia associated with acute allergic interstitial nephritis may be difficult to differentiate from that of acute tubular necrosis. In this setting an electrolyte pattern of hyperkalemic, hyperchloremic metabolic acidosis, a reduced plasma renin activity and rates of aldosterone secretion, an elevated fractional excretion rate for sodium, eosinophilia, and the presence of eosinophils in the urine would strongly suggest acute allergic interstitial nephritis. Since these latter findings are not universally seen, a renal biopsy may be required to make this differential diagnosis.

3. *Acute pyelonephritis*, a form of acute interstitial nephritis due to bacterial invasion of the kidney, usually produces a septic picture with fever, flank pain, leukocytosis, and dysuria (Ch. 85). Factors that predispose to acute pyelonephritis are often present, such as diabetes mellitus, obstructive uropathy, prior instrumentation of the urinary tract, or bacterial endocarditis with septic renal emboli. The electrolyte changes in acute pyelonephritis may include the combination of azotemia; hyperkalemic, hyperchloremic metabolic acidosis; and suppressed plasma renin activity with a reduced rate of aldosterone secretion. However, the most useful clues to the presence of acute pyelonephritis include a septic picture, costovertebral angle tenderness, pyuria, leukocyte casts, the presence of bacteria in unspun samples of urine, and positive urine cultures.

Isolated Tubular Defects (Ch. 83). In addition to the tubular derangements secondary to diffuse tubulointerstitial disease, a number of specific defects of tubular function, either congenital or acquired, may manifest themselves primarily by selective abnormalities of tubular function.

PROXIMAL TUBULAR DEFECTS. The normal proximal tubule isotonically absorbs sodium and preferentially absorbs bicarbonate, glucose, amino acids, and phosphate. A variety of proximal tubular defects, occurring alone or in combination, may therefore occur.

Renal glycosuria occurs when the glucose threshold of the proximal nephron is reduced. *Renal phosphate wasting* results when the rate of proximal absorption of phosphate is reduced. Similarly *aminoaciduria* may result from tubular defects that are either generalized or specific. Finally, the rate of bicarbonate absorption by the proximal nephron may be reduced, resulting in profound bicarbonate wasting, a syndrome entitled *proximal renal tubular acidosis* (Ch. 83.2).

Renal phosphate wasting, renal glycosuria, renal aminoaciduria, and proximal renal tubular acidosis occurring simultaneously constitute the Fanconi syndrome (Ch. 85.5). These proximal tubular defects may be congenital; they may also occur in association with heavy metal poisoning of the proximal nephron, notably by copper in Wilson's disease, following exposure to toxic agents such as maleic acid, and in the gammopathies.

Isolated proximal tubular defects often carry an excellent prognosis. However, in certain instances such as cystinosis a reduction in total renal mass may also occur leading to azotemia. In proximal renal tubular acidosis, the degree of bicarbonate wasting and the resulting hyperchloremic metabolic acidosis may stunt the growth of children afflicted with the disorder, as well as result in profound hypokalemia.

POSSIBLE LOOP OF HENLE DEFECT. The pathogenesis of *Bartter's syndrome* has not been elucidated (Ch. 83.5). Yet it appears that many of the findings of Bartter's syndrome, including profound salt wasting, potassium wasting, and compensatory hypertrophy of the juxtaglomerular apparatus with hyperreninemia, may be the result of a salt-absorptive defect in the thick ascending limb. Most commonly, a clinical syndrome resembling Bartter's syndrome occurs because of surreptitious ingestion of furosemide or furosemide-like diuretics.

DISTAL TUBULAR DEFECTS. *Distal, gradient-limited renal tubular acidosis* represents a specific defect of the distal nephron (Ch. 83.2). In this disorder the distal nephron is abnormally permeable to protons and cannot therefore maintain an adequately acid urine. In contrast to patients who have tubulointerstitial disease, the classic electrolyte abnormalities in distal, gradient-limited renal tubular acidosis include a tendency to salt wasting, hyperchloremic metabolic acidosis, a urine that is relatively alkaline with respect to arterial pH, and profound hypokalemia. The hypokalemia of distal, gradient-limited renal tubular acidosis is probably a consequence of aldosterone release in response to salt depletion. In contrast to proximal renal tubular acidosis or to the hyperkalemic, hyperchloremic renal tubular acidosis of diffuse tubulointerstitial disease, gradient-limited distal renal tubular acidosis is frequently associated with severe nephrocalcinosis, renal calculi, renal infection, and progressive destruction of renal mass.

Distal, gradient-limited renal tubular acidosis may occur congenitally. The disorder may also occur as a consequence of exposure to exogenous agents, notably amphotericin B and lithium, and in association with the gammopathies.

COLLECTING DUCT DEFECTS. The unique tubular defect of the collecting duct is nephrogenic diabetes insipidus (NDI) in which the collecting duct is refractory to the action of ADH (Ch. 226). Consequently, these patients are consistently polyuric, even when large amounts of ADH are administered. The disorder may occur congenitally; in association with certain systemic disorders, such as Sjögren's syndrome and sarcoidosis; and as a result of lithium intoxication or exposure to the antibiotic demethylchlortetracycline.

In short, these specific tubular defects differ from those observed in generalized tubulointerstitial disease because of their specificity, and because, in the absence of complicating factors and with appropriate therapy, renal insufficiency need not ensue. A more detailed discussion of these tubular disorders is presented in Ch. 83.

The Renal Calculus Syndromes. The origin and composition of renal calculi are described in Ch. 89; most renal calculi contain either magnesium-ammonium-phosphate, calcium oxalate, uric acid, a combination of calcium oxalate and uric acid, or cystine as their main crystalloids. Of these, all but uric acid stones are radiopaque.

Renal calculi may be asymptomatic and detected only on routine radiographic examination of the kidney, especially isolated calculi that do not move down the urinary tract and staghorn calculi lodged within the renal pelvis. Calculi may obstruct urine flow and consequently lead to pyelonephritis. Therefore, in any patient in whom pyelonephritis is suspected, a careful radiographic and urologic examination for renal calculi is mandatory. *Renal colic* refers to the passage of a renal calculus from the renal pelvis into the ureter characterized by exquisite pain, generally beginning in the flank and radiating into the groin. Patients almost always describe renal colic as the worst pain that they have ever experienced. Renal colic is invariably accompanied by hematuria, unless the calculus is lodged within a ureter and produces complete unilateral obstruction to urine flow. Under these circumstances, the urine voided by the patient represents red cell–free urine from the unaffected kidney.

Kidney stones are among the more common renal disorders. It is generally prudent, particularly in patients with multiple renal calculi or with a family history of renal calculi, to evaluate the patient for potential underlying causes for stone formation (for example, gout, absorptive hypercalciuria, cystinuria, distal, gradient-limited renal tubular acidosis, or primary hyperparathyroidism). The presence of nephrocalcinosis should alert the physician to the possibility of distal, gradient-limited renal tubular acidosis or to primary hyperparathyroidism.

The patient with renal colic also warrants an evaluation for obstructive uropathy on the affected side and for urinary tract infection. These approaches generally involve culture of the urine, plain films of the abdomen, and, when indicated, ultrasonography of the kidneys, excretory urography, evaluation of parathyroid function, and evaluation for an absorptive hypercalciuric state.

Renal Cystic Disease (Ch. 90). There are three major forms of renal cystic disease: single or multiple cysts, polycystic kidney disease, and microcystic disease of the renal medulla. The clinical characteristics, significance, and clinical presentations of these three kinds of renal cysts vary significantly. There is no evidence that either true simple cysts, multiple simple cysts, or polycystic kidney disease progresses to renal neoplasia.

Isolated simple cysts, either single or multiple, form sporadically for unknown reasons within the renal parenchyma, generally within the renal cortex. Single cysts in particular usually cause no symptoms; they are generally detected in one of two circumstances: episodes of renal trauma that provoke cyst rupture and hematuria, or on routine excretory urography. The true simple, single cyst (in contrast to the cystic neoplasm, see below) is innocuous and needs no therapy. *Multiple, simple cysts* probably represent an extension of the process described above and are also similarly innocuous unless they encroach on renal parenchyma. Multiple simple cysts should be distinguished from polycystic kidney disease, a disorder with a more ominous prognosis. These two forms of multicystic disease can be distinguished by excretory urography; in individuals with multiple simple cysts, the overall size of the kidney is normal and the calyceal system is not elongated and only minimally distorted.

Adult polycystic kidney disease is a form of nephropathy that is generally inherited by autosomal dominance with incomplete penetrance. If a parent has polycystic kidney disease, approximately one half of the progeny will ultimately develop the disorder, although the time at which polycystic kidney disease becomes manifest is highly variable.

Polycystic kidney disease may present with recurrent bouts of hematuria, renal colic, hypertension, or urinary tract infection because of intrarenal obstruction due to cysts. Many patients with polycystic kidney disease develop renal failure, although the rate and extent of development of renal failure depend on the degree of penetrance of the autosomal dominant trait.

Three factors distinguish between patients with polycystic kidney disease and those with multiple, simple cysts: (1) A positive family history consistent with an autosomal dominant trait. (2) Enlargement of the kidneys, generally detected as a pole-to-pole diameter in excess of 15 to 17 cm, and a cortical thickness in excess of 3 cm. (3) Elongation and deformation of the calyceal structure from the progressive enlargement of the parenchymal cysts.

Microcystic kidney disease of the renal medulla, a disorder of children generally inherited as a recessive trait, is characterized by progressive disruption and destruction of the renal medullary architecture by multiple cysts. The disease is generally detected when young children complain of fatigue and are noted to have mild degrees of proteinuria, anemia, and mild azotemia. The clinical course is characterized by an inordinantly high requirement for salt intake in order to maintain blood pressure and an adequate filtration rate; and by stunted growth due to chronic illness, to uremia, and to excessive urinary calcium losses. Nephrons are gradually destroyed, usually with progression to end-stage renal disease before the age of 30.

Renal Neoplasia (Ch. 92). Two major classes of renal tumors occur in adults: *renal cell carcinomas* (sometimes called hypernephromas), which originate in the renal cortex, and *transitional cell tumors* of the renal pelvis. Hypernephromas are versatile tumors and are often difficult to diagnose. Many patients present simply with painless hematuria. However, hypernephromas also produce a number of unusual syndromes, the detection of whose significance taxes the skill of the physician. These include polycythemia, presumably due to excessive erythropoietin production; hypertension, presumably because the neoplasm acts as the equivalent of an arteriovenous fistula and results in renin release by the affected kidney; fever of unknown origin; and hypercalcemia, presumably because of ectopic release of parathyroid hormone (see Table 92–3).

The approach to evaluating individuals with renal cortical masses suspected of being hypernephromas includes the distinction between simple renal cysts; solid hypernephromas; hypernephromas with central necrosis, which may resemble cysts; and hamartomas, either isolated or in association with adenoma sebaceum. The algorithm presented in Figure 92–1 provides a rational approach to the evaluation of these various disorders.

Transitional cell tumors of the renal pelvis commonly present as hematuria, which may be painless or accompanied by renal colic if clots are passed. The systemic manifestations described for hypernephroma are uncommonly found in transitional cell tumors. A careful examination of urine cytology, done conveniently on the wards by a Wright's stain of the urinary sediment, may provide a useful diagnostic clue to the presence of these tumors.

Acute Renal Failure (Ch. 77). Acute renal failure refers either to the sudden cessation of urine flow or to sudden oliguria. Acute renal failure caused by acute glomerular disorders is generally evident from the findings described above for the acute glomerulonephritic syndromes. The general approach to the differential diagnosis of individuals with acute renal failure, particularly in hospitalized patients, involves the distinction among three major classes of disorders: (1) the prerenal hypoperfusion syndromes indicated in Table 72–1; (2) intrarenal syndromes, especially acute tubular necrosis and acute allergic interstitial nephritis; and (3) postrenal syndromes, that is, oligoanuria resulting from urinary tract obstruction.

The general approach to these patients involves the following cardinal maneuvers: (1) An assessment of circulatory dynamics to exclude the possibility of reduced effective circulating volume as a cause of oliguria and azotemia. (2) A careful history to assess possible antecedent hypotension or exposure to nephrotoxic agents, coupled with a measurement of the fractional excretion of sodium, to evaluate the possibility of acute tubular necrosis; and a diligent search for therapy with penicillin and related antibiotics, eosinophilia, or urinary eosinophils, which might point to acute allergic interstitial nephritis. (3) Renal ultrasonography to exclude the possibility of obstruction of both kidneys, or obstruction of a solitary kidney, as in an individual with renal agenesis or with renal transplantation. These maneuvers are generally helpful in distinguishing between prerenal, intrarenal, and postrenal causes of oliguria. Invasive hemodynamic monitoring, coupled with a fluid challenge, may still be required to exclude rigorously the possibility of oliguria due to a reduced effective circulating volume. A percutaneous renal biopsy may be indicated to distinguish between acute tubular necrosis and acute allergic interstitial nephritis. This distinction may be particularly important if agents suspected of causing acute allergic interstitial nephritis—such as penicillin or related agents—are considered mandatory for the treatment of life-threatening infections. Renal ultrasonography has greatly reduced the need for retrograde ureteral catheterization as a means for excluding obstructive uropathy.

THE POSTRENAL SYNDROMES (Ch. 82). The postrenal syndromes result from obstruction of urine flow at various loci in the urinary tract from the renal papillae to the urethral meatus. Azotemia and oliguria occur in urinary tract obstruction only when the urinary tract is obstructed bilaterally or when obstruction exists in a sole functioning kidney. The degree of azotemia depends upon the extent of the obstruction; partial obstruction may produce only moderate degrees of azotemia, while complete obstruction of the urinary tract obviously produces anuria. Obstruction of urine flow can irreversibly damage the kidneys. If the obstruction is partial or nearly complete, renal function may be preserved for as long as four to five weeks following the onset of obstruction. Obstructive uropathy also carries with it the possible complication of urinary tract infection.

Bilateral ureteral obstruction most frequently occurs at three major sites: (1) the *ureteropelvic junction,* where the obstruction is generally due to scar formation or, less commonly, to renal vessels crossing the ureter; (2) the site where the ureters cross the *pelvic brim*—neoplasms are the primary cause of such obstruction, particularly extensive carcinoma of the cervix; (3) the *ureterovesical junction,* because of either neoplasm or scar formation. Less commonly, other disorders such as *retroperitoneal fibrosis* or disseminated retroperitoneal lymphoma may cause bilateral ureteral obstruction between the ureterovesical junction and where the ureters cross the pelvic brim. The probability of renal calculi causing bilateral ureteral obstruction is small unless one kidney is already nonfunctional and a stone obstructs the outflow of urine from the other kidney. Prostatic enlargement is a common cause of partial or complete obstruction to urine outflow. In contrast to patients with ureteral obstruction, the urinary bladder distends and often results in overflow urinary incontinence. The patient may therefore present with azotemia secondary to a profound reduction in glomerular filtration and yet have significant volumes of urine flow.

Urinary tract obstruction represents a potentially remediable cause of renal failure; every attempt should be made to exclude obstructive uropathy in individuals who are oliguric or anuric. Renal ultrasonography has simplified this task greatly, since it noninvasively detects whether or not the renal calyces are dilated and the ureters narrow, as occurs in ureteropelvic junction obstruction; or whether the ureters and renal calyces are both dilated, as occurs in ureterovesical obstruction or urethral obstruction.

RENAL FAILURE: THE UREMIC SYNDROME (Ch. 78)

The uremic syndrome occurs when the functional renal mass is reduced sufficiently that the kidney is no longer able to carry out excretory functions, functions relating to the regulation of the volume and composition of body fluids, functions as an endocrine receptor, and functions as an endocrine organ. The manifestations of *acute* uremia may differ from those of *chronic* uremia, but these differences relate more to the rate of development of renal failure than to fundamental differences in pathophysiology.

Uremia is in part a syndrome of "autointoxication." While the chemical agents responsible for this autointoxication have not been clearly identified, uremic syndromes may be ameliorated by dialysis (which generally removes molecules having molecular weights less than 1,000 to 2,000 daltons), and severe protein restriction may minimize the rate of development of the uremic symptoms. Thus it is plausible to presume that the retention of the end products of protein metabolism, reflected primarily by the BUN and serum creatinine levels as well as by other factors such as acidosis, are responsible for many of the manifestations of the uremic syndrome.

Uremic symptoms that relate primarily to a reduction in glomerular filtration rate begin to occur when the GFR is reduced below 5 to 10 per cent of normal. The primary findings include central nervous system symptoms ranging from lethargy and confusion to coma and seizures; a bleeding tendency, due at least in part to interference with adequate platelet function; peripheral neuropathy, which is most evident in individuals with long-standing rather than acute uremia; intense pruritus; and asthenia.

In uremia the major electrolyte alterations include hypocalcemia, presumably due to the inability to form 1,25-dihydroxycholecalciferol as renal mass is reduced and to hyperphosphatemia; hyperphosphatemia resulting from a reduction in glomerular filtration rate; and metabolic acidosis, which results from a reduction in the renal excretion of "fixed" acids (that is, incompletely combusted organic acids; and sulfate and phosphate, which represent the end products of protein and nucleic acid metabolism, respectively).

The occurrence of hyperkalemia among uremic individuals is variable and depends on a number of factors, including the rate of potassium intake, the rate of tissue catabolism, and the rate at which renal failure has evolved. In general, patients in whom the uremic syndrome evolves acutely do not develop adaptive mechanisms (both renal and extrarenal) for potassium elimination and are therefore more prone to develop hyperkalemia. In contrast, individuals who approach end-stage renal disease gradually may often be normokalemic even when the glomerular filtration rate is less than 5 per cent of normal. Two factors may account for this phenomenon: (1) the development of renal disease is accompanied by asthenia and anorexia so that dietary intake of potassium may be minimized; and (2) both renal and extrarenal mechanisms for more efficient potassium excretion are gradually developed.

Uremia, whether acute or chronic, is a catabolic disorder. In individuals with acute renal failure, even extensive hyperalimentation fails to prevent the loss of approximately 0.5 to 1.0 pound daily. In individuals with chronic renal failure, weight loss is more gradual and less easily perceived by patients. But in both acute and chronic renal failure, asthenia and loss of lean body mass are inevitable sequelae.

As the functional renal mass is diminished, erythropoietin production is also reduced. Thus patients with either acute or chronic renal failure inevitably develop anemia. Acute renal failure is characterized by a relative preservation of the hematocrit but only in its earliest stages. Within two weeks of the onset of acute renal failure, the combination of diminished erythrocyte production and an accelerated rate of red cell destruction invariably reduces the hematocrit level to the range of 20 to 25 per cent. Similar hematocrits are found in patients with chronic renal failure, particularly prior to dialysis therapy. Polycystic kidney disease represents an exception in that profound reductions of glomerular filtration rate may occur coincident with the maintenance of an hematocrit well in excess of 30 per cent. Presumably, the large renal mass of polycystic kidney disease produces sufficient erythropoietin to maintain an adequate hematocrit.

Two symptoms of uremia are seen commonly in individuals with chronic renal failure but are rare in acute uremia: *peripheral neuropathy* and *renal osteodystrophy.* Peripheral neuropathy almost never develops in individuals with acute renal failure but is common in individuals with long-standing uremia who have not been treated with dialysis. Individuals with acute renal failure do not develop significant bone disease. In contrast, individuals with chronic, severe reductions in glomerular filtration rate and in functional renal mass often have significant bone disease, termed renal osteodystrophy (Ch. 248). At least four factors may contribute to the complex bone disorders in uremia: (1) The synthesis of 1,25-hydroxycholecalciferol in the kidney is reduced with consequent diminished calcium absorption from the gut. (2) The calcium malabsorption leads to secondary hyperparathyroidism, which mobilizes calcium from bone in an attempt to maintain a normal level of serum ionized calcium and in the process produces osteitis fibrosa (Ch. 246). (3) Bone calcium is exchanged for retained protons in buffering the metabolic acidosis of chronic renal failure with partial maintenance of acid-base homeostasis, but at the expense of progressive dissolution of bone. (4) The uremic state impairs protein synthesis in bone and with this the formation of osteoid.

In short, the uremic syndrome results from varying impairment in the ability of the kidney to meet all of its normal metabolic and physiologic obligations: to regulate the volume and composition of body fluids, to excrete the end products of metabolism, to serve as an endocrine receptor, and to serve as an endocrine organ. Within that framework the particular manifestations of uremia in any given patient will depend largely on the rate at which kidney failure has occurred, the severity of the renal failure (that is, the extent to which residual nephron mass is able to maintain homeostasis), and the homeostatic stresses to which the individual is subjected.

ADAPTATION TO RENAL INJURY AND THE PATHOGENESIS OF PROGRESSIVE RENAL FAILURE

There are two added characteristics of nearly all forms of chronic renal disease that warrant particular consideration. First, nephron loss may be accompanied by *adaptive functional changes* in residual nephrons which tend to minimize the effects of reducing the functional nephron mass on the chemical composition of blood. This point of view, espoused by Bricker and colleagues, is generally termed the *intact nephron hypothesis* and considers that, in chronic renal disease, the function of residual nephrons may be normal or supranormal. Among the cardinal adaptive characteristics described by the intact nephron hypothesis have been an increased glomerular filtration rate per nephron with elevated serum BUN concentrations or increased rates of protein feeding, and an increase in the rate of phosphate excretion per nephron mediated through secondary hyperparathyroidism, such that, in chronic renal failure, serum phosphate levels do not rise until the glomerular filtration rate is reduced to about 30 per cent of normal.

Second, Bricker recognized that such adaptive responses might ultimately be harmful to the kidney or other organs and termed this aspect of the intact nephron hypothesis the "trade-off postulate": for example, the maintenance of relatively normal serum calcium and phosphate concentrations in a setting of modest reductions in glomerular filtration rate (that is, to 30 to 40 per cent of normal) by secondary hyperparathyroidism is achieved at the expense of bone dissolution. Likewise, the recent observations of Brenner and colleagues have provided evidence that increases in protein intake lead to glomerular hyperperfusion and that the elevated glomerular filtration rate produced by this hyperperfusion can result in progressive glomerular sclerosis. Thus, in principle, glomerular hyperperfusion produced by a protein intake that is large in relation to the residual nephron mass could contribute to the progression of chronic renal disease. A corollary to this hypothesis is the possibility that dietary protein restriction early in the course of chronic renal failure might ameliorate the rate of progression of renal disease.

Brenner BM: Hemodynamically mediated glomerular injury and the progressive nature of kidney disease. Kidney Int 23:647, 1983. *A detailed analysis of the relation between glomerular hyperfiltration and progressive renal damage.*

Bricker NS, Shapiro RJ, Shapiro MS: Physiology and pathology of electrolyte metabolism in chronic renal disease. *In* Seldin DW, Giebisch GH (eds.):

Physiology and Pathology of Electrolyte Metabolism. New York, Plenum Press. In press. *A summary of the arguments for the intact nephron hypothesis.*
Culpepper RM, Andreoli TE: The pathophysiology of the glomerulonephropathies. *In* Stollerman GH (ed.): Adv Intern Med 28:161, 1982. *A thorough review of the etiology, pathogenesis, and clinical manifestations of glomerular disorders.*
Earle DP: Clinical Evaluation. *In* Earle DP (ed.): Manual of Clinical Nephrology. Philadelphia, W. B. Saunders Company, 1982. *A valuable clinical approach to the evaluation of physical findings and laboratory tests in patients with renal disease.*

73. STRUCTURE AND FUNCTION OF THE KIDNEYS

Saulo Klahr

This chapter reviews the structure and function of the normal mammalian kidney as a framework for understanding the derangements that occur with kidney disease.

Renal Structure

The kidneys are paired organs located retroperitoneally along each side of the vertebral column. Their upper and lower poles lie opposite the twelfth thoracic and third lumbar vertebrae, respectively. Because of the presence of the liver, the right kidney is generally inferior to the left. Each adult kidney weighs 130 to 170 grams and measures about 12 by 6 by 3 cm. Located on the medial surface of the kidney is a slit, the hilus, through which pass a renal artery and vein, lymphatics, a nerve plexus, and the *renal pelvis,* which subdivides into the *three major calices* and subsequently into eight or more *minor calices.* A coronal section of the kidney reveals two distinct regions: a dark inner region, the medulla, and a paler outer region, the cortex. The *renal medulla* is composed generally of 12 to 18 conical masses, the *pyramids.* The base of each pyramid is located on the corticomedullary boundary, and the apex extends toward the renal pelvis forming the *papilla,* which projects into the minor calix. Each papilla is perforated by the distal end of 15 or more *terminal collecting ducts* (of Bellini). The *renal cortex,* about 1 cm in thickness, covers the base of the pyramids and extends medially between the individual pyramids to form the renal columns (of Bertin).

BLOOD SUPPLY

Generally, each kidney is supplied by a single artery originating from the aorta at the level of the first lumbar vertebra. This artery generally divides into two branches (anterior and posterior) before entering the renal sinus. The anterior branch gives rise to upper, middle, and lower branches *(lobar arteries).* As these arteries enter the renal parenchyma they form the *interlobar arteries* that course toward the cortex along the lateral borders of the medullary pyramids. The interlobar arteries then run across the base of the renal medulla, forming the *arcuate arteries.* The *interlobular arteries,* branching at right angles from the arcuate vessels, course through the cortex to the periphery. They give rise to *afferent arterioles,* each of which ends in a fine capillary bed known as a glomerulus. Thus, the glomerulus is supplied by a single afferent arteriole and drained, in turn, by an *efferent arteriole,* which emerges at the glomerular vascular pole and immediately ramifies into numerous peritubular capillaries which surround the tubular segments of the cortex. The *vasa recta,* which extend medially into the medulla, are the capillaries that originate from efferent arterioles of juxtamedullary glomeruli.

The venous system follows the same pattern as the arterial system, with the capillaries forming venules which unite into interlobular, arcuate, lobular, and ultimately renal veins. Each renal vein drains into the inferior vena cava.

THE NEPHRON

The nephron is the functional unit of the kidney. There are approximately 1,200,000 nephrons in each human kidney. Each is composed of a malpighian corpuscle (the *glomerulus* and *Bowman's capsule*) and its attached *tubule.* The tubule contains several distinct anatomic and functional segments: proximal tubule, loop of Henle, distal convoluted tubule, and cortical collecting tubule. The latter structures join to form the collecting ducts, which traverse the medulla and terminate at the tip of the papilla. There are two distinct populations of nephrons in the human kidney: those with glomeruli located in the outer cortex *(superficial nephrons)* and those with glomeruli situated near the corticomedullary junction *(juxtamedullary nephrons).* The superficial nephrons, which constitute about 85 per cent of the total nephron population, have short loops of Henle that frequently do not penetrate the medulla. The juxtamedullary nephrons have long loops of Henle that extend into the inner medulla and are in close apposition to the vasa recta.

GLOMERULUS. The glomerulus (Fig. 73–1) is a network of capillaries originating from the afferent arteriole. After dividing into four to eight lobules to form the glomerular tuft, the capillaries rejoin to form the efferent arteriole, which leaves the glomerulus at the vascular pole. The glomerular tuft is surrounded by *Bowman's capsule,* which is an extension of the basement membrane and connective tissue of the proximal tubule. The *urinary* or *Bowman's space* separates the capsule from the glomerular tuft. Bowman's capsule contains a single layer of squamous cells *(parietal epithelial cells),* which undergo an abrupt transition to taller columnar cells typical of the proximal tubule at the urinary pole of the glomerulus. In the glomerular tuft there are three distinct cell types (endothelial, mesangial, and epithelial), a capillary wall (basement membrane), and an interstitial or supporting region (mesangium).

Capillary Wall. The capillary wall contains endothelial cells, a basement membrane, and epithelial cells (see Fig. 73–1). The *endothelial cells* line the capillary lumen. Their nuclei lie adjacent to the mesangium, and their cytoplasm is attenuated along the circumference of the capillary. Fenestrae or pores (approximate diameter 700 Å, covered by thin diaphragms are present in the attenuated endothelium. In certain diseases (toxemia of pregnancy, acute poststreptococcal glomerulonephritis) the capillary lumen may be occluded owing to cytoplasmic swelling of the endothelial cells. The *basement membrane,* a structure with an average thickness in the adult of 3200 Å, contains three distinct areas: a central electron-dense *lamina densa* and, on either side, a *lamina rara externa* and *lamina rara interna* (see Fig. 73–1). The major constituents of the basement membrane are collagen and glycoprotein. Thickening of this structure, resulting from deposition of immune complexes or other materials, is seen in a number of glomerular diseases. The *visceral epithelial cells,* or *podocytes,* are the largest of the glomerular cells. Extending from the body of the podocyte are primary processes, from which individual *foot processes,* or *pedicels,* project to come into contact with the lamina rara externa of the basement membrane. Between the foot processes is a space (*filtration slit* or *slit pore*) 250 to 400 Å wide, which is covered by a thin membrane, the *filtration slit diaphragm,* which is located approximately 600 Å from the basement membrane. This slit diaphragm is a zipper-like structure composed of rectangular pores (40 to 140 Å in a cross-section). The estimated total area of these pores is approximately 3 per cent of the total surface area of the glomerular capillaries. In renal diseases characterized by proteinuria the pedicels of the podocytes are replaced by a continuous band of cytoplasm adjacent to the lamina rara externa (fusion of foot processes).

The Mesangium. The mesangium is the interstitial portion of the glomerular lobules and is composed of *mesangial cells* (axial or intercapillary) and *mesangial matrix.* The latter is a homogeneous fibrillary material containing mucopolysaccharides and glycoprotein. The mesangial cells, which have phagocytic properties, resemble smooth muscle cells, contain myosin, and usually do not communicate directly with the vascular space. The mesangium is unique in that entry of a substance into the space does not require passage through a capillary basement membrane. In human glomerulonephritis, immune deposits are found in the mesangium, often exclusively.

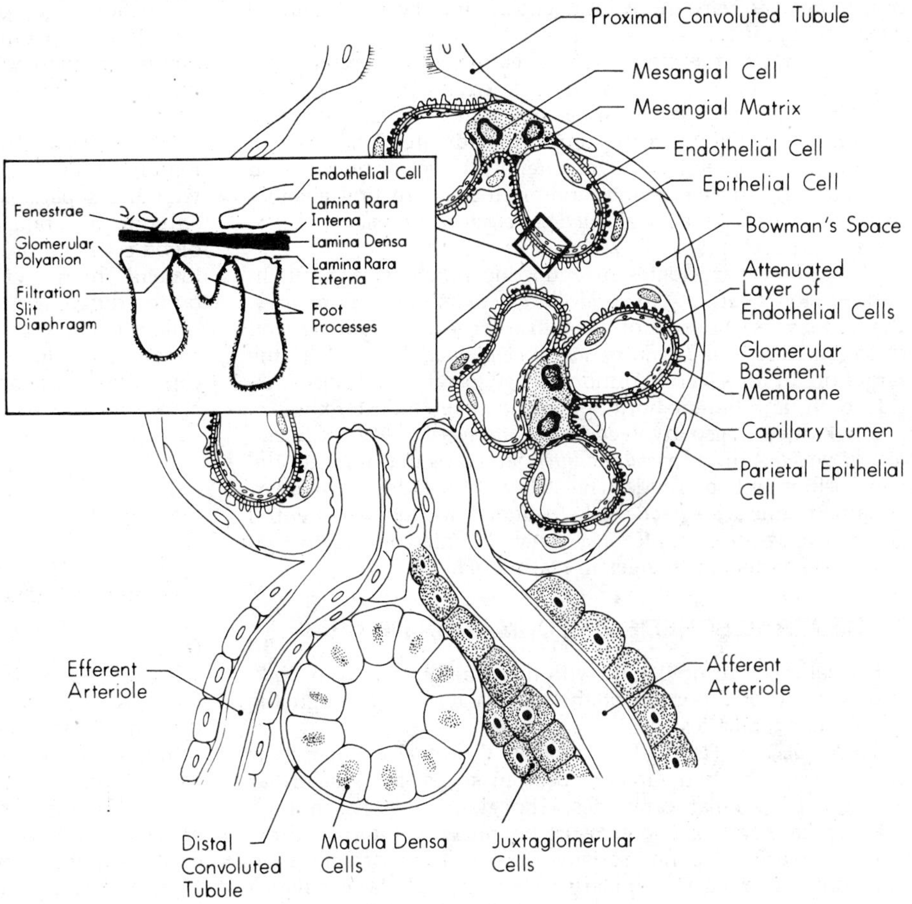

Figure 73–1. Schematic representation of the glomerulus, illustrating the three major types of cells (endothelial, epithelial, and mesangial) and the close relationship of the distal convoluted tubule to afferent and efferent arterioles ("juxtaglomerular apparatus"). Notice that there is no basement membrane interposed between the mesangium and the lumen of the capillaries. The inset shows a magnified view of the capillary wall, illustrating the gaps between the endothelial cells (fenestrae), the three layers of the basement membrane, and the foot processes of the epithelial cells. For more details see text.

THE TUBULE. The renal tubule is composed of distinct anatomic and functional segments: The *proximal convoluted tubule*, the *pars recta* or *straight portion* of the proximal tubule, the *thin descending* and *ascending limbs of Henle's loop*, the *thick ascending limb of Henle's loop*, the *distal convoluted tubule*, the *cortical collecting tubule*, and the *medullary collecting duct*. These segments differ in their location, length, diameter, characteristics of the lining epithelium, including number and size of mitochondria, appearance of intercellular channels, presence of luminal microvilli (brush border), and complexity of basal infoldings. The functional differences among nephron segments are described below.

JUXTAGLOMERULAR APPARATUS. The juxtaglomerular apparatus is a region near the glomerular vascular pole in which the *distal convoluted tubule* and the *afferent* and *efferent arterioles* come into juxtaposition. Here, the cells of the distal tubule become smaller and more numerous *(macula densa)*, and cells derived from the afferent arteriole *(juxtaglomerular cells)* are present between the distal tubule and the vascular pole (Fig. 73–1). These cells may be granular (containing renin) or agranular. Adrenergic nerve endings have been demonstrated in the juxtaglomerular region.

INTERSTITIUM

The interstitial connective tissue of the kidney is scant and consists primarily of *reticular fibers* and *interstitial cells*. It is more prominent in the medulla than in the cortex. In addition to capillaries, the interstitium contains *lymphatics* and *motor* and *sensory nerves*. In interstitial disease this region may be infiltrated by white blood cells and contain increased amounts of connective tissue.

Normal Renal Function

The principal functions of the kidney are summarized in Table 73–1. The kidneys have a central role in the *maintenance of volume and ionic composition of body fluids* (homeostasis). This function is accomplished by regulation of the rate of excretion of water and/or ions. Regulation entails feedback mechanisms which involve participation of the nervous system, the endocrine system, or both. Some of the homeostatic functions of the kidney are concerned with the balance of water, sodium, chloride, potassium, magnesium, phosphate, and hydrogen ions. The large changes in urine volume and composition, which occur in response to alterations in the diet, reflect the adaptability of the kidney to the requirements of homeostasis. There is no fixed normal volume or composition of the urine. Normal homeostatic renal function is defined by the capacity

TABLE 73–1. PRINCIPAL FUNCTIONS OF THE KIDNEY

1. Maintenance of volume and ionic composition of body fluids (homeostasis)
2. Excretion of metabolic waste products—e.g., urea, uric acid, creatinine
3. Detoxification and elimination of toxins, drugs, and their metabolites
4. Endocrine regulation of extracellular fluid volume and blood pressure
   a. Renin-angiotensin system
   b. Renal prostaglandins
   c. Renal kallikrein-kinin system
5. Control of red blood cell mass: erythropoietin
6. Endocrine control of mineral metabolism: formation of 1,25-dihydroxycholecalciferol and 24,25-dihydroxycholecalciferol
7. Degradation and catabolism of peptide hormones: insulin, glucagon, parathyroid hormone, calcitonin, growth hormone, etc.
8. Catabolism of small molecular weight proteins: light chains, β-2 microglobulin
9. Metabolic interconversions: gluconeogenesis, lipid metabolism

of the organ to vary the volume and composition of the urine over a wide range.

The kidney is the main route of elimination of fixed (nonvolatile) metabolic waste products *(excretory function).* These substances usually serve no biologic function, and some of them are potentially toxic. Examples include urea (end-product of protein metabolism), uric acid (end-product of nucleic acid metabolism), and creatinine (end-product of creatine metabolism). The kidney also *eliminates exogenous chemicals (drugs, toxins)* and their metabolites.

The kidney participates in endocrine functions as well. In addition to its capacity to *metabolize and excrete certain hormones,* the kidney is the site of *production* of *renin, erythropoietin, prostaglandins, 1,25-dihydroxycholecalciferol,* and *kinins.* It is the target organ for several hormones (e.g., parathyroid hormone, calcitonin, antidiuretic hormone, angiotensin, aldosterone).

The kidney is also involved in the *catabolism of small molecular weight proteins* and in *metabolic interconversions* that regulate the composition of body fluids. The ability of the kidney to convert certain organic acids (lactic, α-ketoglutaric) to glucose (a neutral substance) is an example of a metabolic interconversion that minimizes potential changes in plasma pH.

GENERAL SCHEME OF FORMATION OF URINE

Formation of urine begins with the ultrafiltration into Bowman's space of a portion of the plasma flowing through the glomerular capillaries.

RENAL BLOOD FLOW. Functionally, the renal circulation is characterized by two capillary beds in series: the glomerular and the peritubular capillaries. The glomerulus has a high intracapillary hydrostatic pressure because it is interposed between two arterioles, i.e., resistive vessels. Therefore, filtration is favored. The second capillary system (peritubular capillaries in the cortex, vasa recta in the medulla) is a high flow, low pressure system which acts as a reservoir for tubular reabsorption and secretion.

The kidneys receive 20 to 25 per cent of the cardiac output, or approximately 1.1 liters of blood per minute. In subjects with a physiologic hematocrit of 45 per cent, total renal plasma flow is about 600 ml per minute. Cortical blood flow is about 75 per cent and medullary blood flow 25 per cent of total renal blood flow. Only 1 per cent of the renal blood flow reaches the papilla. As blood flows through the glomerular capillaries, hydrostatic forces translocate about 20 per cent of the plasma volume (120 ml per minute) across the capillary wall into Bowman's space (glomerular filtration). The ratio of glomerular filtration rate (GFR) to renal plasma flow is called the *filtration fraction.*

Autoregulation generally maintains renal blood flow relatively constant even in the face of wide variations (80 to 180 mm Hg) in perfusion pressure (i.e., mean pressure in the renal artery). This is achieved by changes in renal vascular resistance proportional to changes in perfusion pressure. Since the afferent and efferent arterioles determine renal vascular resistance, changes in arteriolar resistance will alter renal blood flow. When blood pressure falls below 80 or rises above 180 mm Hg, autoregulation is no longer operative and renal blood flow changes in proportion to pressure. Although the events underlying autoregulation are not fully understood, the phenomenon does not depend on renal nerves or on vasopressor substances in the systemic circulation. The afferent arteriole appears to have the intrinsic ability to sense transmural pressure and adjust wall tension to keep resistance proportional to pressure. One main effect of autoregulation of renal blood flow is the maintenance of a constant GFR despite altered perfusion pressure. Although the kidneys are innervated by adrenergic nerve fibers, renal sympathetic tone probably does not play a significant role in regulating renal blood flow under basal conditions. Thus, denervation or α- or β-adrenergic blockers do not alter renal blood flow. However, augmented sympathetic activity (e.g., fright, pain, exercise, norepinephrine, congestive heart failure) increases renal vascular resistance and reduces renal blood flow. Both afferent and efferent arterioles contract, but GFR falls less than renal blood flow, suggesting that catecholamines exert their major effect at the efferent arteriole. Renal blood flow is increased by substances inducing fever (pyrogenic reaction).

GLOMERULAR FILTRATION RATE. The initial step in the formation of urine (ultrafiltration) occurs across the glomerular wall and separates the plasma water and its nonprotein constituents (crystalloids), which enter Bowman's space, from the blood cells and protein (colloids), which remain in the capillary lumen. The rate of glomerular ultrafiltration (GFR) is governed by the differences between transcapillary hydrostatic (ΔP) and colloid osmotic pressures (ΔΠ). GFR is influenced also by the filtration coefficient (K_f), which is a function of both total capillary surface area and the permeability per unit of surface area. Thus:

$$GFR = K_f\,(\Delta P - \Delta\Pi) \text{ or } GFR = K_f\,[(P_{GC} - P_{BS}) - \Pi_{GC}]$$

The difference in hydrostatic pressure (ΔP) between glomerular capillaries (P_{GC}) and Bowman's space (P_{BS}) favors filtration, whereas the colloid osmotic pressure inside the capillaries (Π_{GC}) opposes it. (The colloid osmotic pressure in Bowman's space is normally negligible and can be disregarded.) Hydrostatic pressure (P_{GC}) remains relatively constant along glomerular capillaries; however, the colloid osmotic pressure (Π_{GC}) undergoes a large progressive increase because filtration of "protein-free fluid" results in an increase of protein concentration along the capillary lumen. Hence, the mean effective pressure for ultrafiltration ($\Delta P - \Delta\Pi$) decreases along the glomerular capillary as ΔΠ increases. In rats with surface glomeruli, the rise in glomerular capillary Π, as a function of length, is such that effective ultrafiltration pressure becomes zero before the end of the capillary. In other words, *filtration pressure equilibrium* ($P_{GC} = \Pi_{GC} + P_{BS}$) occurs, and filtration ceases before the end of the glomerular capillary. This fact makes GFR highly dependent on the flow rate of plasma entering the glomerulus, because at high flow rates, a slower rise in colloid osmotic pressure (Π_{GC}) occurs. Thus, glomerular filtration takes place across a greater length of the capillary. Hence, increased plasma flow tends to elevate GFR, whereas decreased plasma flow may cause a fall in GFR. As noted previously, renal blood flow and GFR are autoregulated within a wide range of renal arterial pressure. When perfusion pressure falls, the resistance of the afferent arteriole decreases. Thus, glomerular plasma flow and GFR are maintained. Below 80 to 90 mm Hg, renal plasma flow and GFR vary directly with arterial pressure, and the GFR ceases when the pressure falls below 50 mm Hg.

At a physiologic GFR of 120 ml per minute, the filtration rate per nephron (assuming 2,400,000 nephrons in both kidneys) would be 50 nanoliters per minute. However, just as superficial and juxtamedullary nephrons differ anatomically, they also appear to differ functionally. The larger juxtamedullary glomeruli have filtration rates that are about twice as high as the superficial ones. Single nephron GFR probably is progressively lower in successively more superficial glomeruli. The physiologic implications of this extensive heterogeneity are not clear, although it has been suggested that redistribution of intrarenal blood flow toward deeper nephrons is associated with salt retention, and may contribute to edema in hepatic disease and congestive heart failure.

Alterations by disease states of any of the primary determinants discussed above may modify GFR. Thus, GFR can fall as a result of (1) decreased hydrostatic pressure in glomerular capillaries (marked hypotension); (2) increased hydrostatic pressure in Bowman's space (intratubular or urinary tract obstruction); (3) elevated glomerular plasma oncotic pressure as a consequence of increased concentration of proteins in the systemic circulation (dehydration: vomiting, diarrhea); (4) decreased renal blood flow (glomerular plasma flow), which may lead to filtration equilibrium at a more proximal region along the glomerular capillary, and hence may decrease the total surface area of capillary available for filtration (e.g., congestive heart failure, hepatic disease); or (5) a decrease in the filtration coefficient (K_f) owing to a fall in permeability or to a reduction in total surface area available for filtration (intrinsic renal disease: certain nephrotoxins, acute or chronic glomerulonephritis).

Permselectivity of the Glomerular Capillary Wall. The glomerular capillary wall is highly permeable to small solutes and water. Molecules the size of inulin (molecular weight 5200) or smaller are present in the glomerular filtrate at the same concentration as in plasma water. Constituents with increasing *molecular size* exhibit progressively decreasing concentration in the filtrate. For example, albumin (molecular weight 69,000) is filtered to a very limited degree. However, plasma proteins with molecular sizes smaller than albumin are filtered at least to some degree.

In addition to molecular size, *molecular configuration, deformability,* and *net electric charge* influence the filtration of macromolecules across the glomerular capillary wall. Negatively charged dextrans, of comparable size to albumin (a polyanion), have a clearance similar to albumin (less than 1 per cent that of inulin). In contrast, uncharged (neutral) dextran molecules of the same size as albumin are filtered at a much greater rate (20 per cent the rate of inulin), and filtration of cationic (positively charged) dextrans is even greater. Therefore, at constant molecular size, negative charge of the solute restricts and positive charge accelerates its filtration, suggesting that, phenomenologically, glomerular filtration occurs through pores with negative charges. Recently, a negatively charged glycoprotein *("glomerular polyanion")*, predominantly found lining the foot processes of the epithelial cells, has been identified. Loss of these negative charges, in certain glomerular diseases, may lead to increased filtration of albumin.

HOMEOSTATIC AND EXCRETORY FUNCTIONS OF THE KIDNEY

The formation of urine begins with the elaboration of a protein-free plasma ultrafiltrate across the glomerular capillaries *(glomerular filtration).* As this ultrafiltrate flows through the renal tubule, solutes and water are reabsorbed from lumen to blood *(reabsorption).* Other solutes are secreted into the tubular lumen from the blood *(secretion).* In some cases, both processes (reabsorption and secretion) affect a given substance, permitting flexible regulation of its excretion. Quantitatively, about 170 liters of fluid is ultrafiltered daily, of which less than 1 liter to more than 10 liters may be excreted as urine, depending on the water balance of the individual. Large amounts of filtered sodium, chloride, calcium, magnesium, and phosphate are reabsorbed, with the quantity remaining in the final urine varying according to the dietary intake of each one of these solutes. Substances such as glucose, amino acids, and bicarbonate are almost completely reabsorbed and, under physiologic conditions, do not appear in the urine. The contribution of tubular transport to homeostasis is discussed in more detail below.

TUBULAR TRANSPORT. The renal tubule can be divided functionally into three major segments: (1) the proximal tubule, (2) the loop of Henle, and (3) the distal nephron. Although there are physiologic and morphologic subdivisions of these segments, it is possible to ascribe a general function to each. The proximal tubule reabsorbs, rather nonselectively, a large fraction (two thirds) of the glomerular filtrate. The loop of Henle has unique water and solute transport properties and serves to establish a hyperosmolar medullary interstitium that influences the ultimate concentration or dilution of the urine. The distal nephron is the site of fine regulation of water and electrolyte excretion and appears to be the main target of hormones that control these processes. Since the tubule segments are arranged in series, the function of any segment depends not only on its own intrinsic transport characteristics but also on the volume and composition of the fluid delivered to it from the previous segment.

Proximal Tubule. The proximal tubule reabsorbs sodium, several other solutes, and water at a high rate. Active sodium reabsorption and hydrogen ion secretion are the essential processes to which transport of chloride, several organic solutes, and water is coupled by a variety of mechanisms. Fluid transport is isosmotic, so that concentration gradients of solute across the wall are small. Functionally, the proximal tubule can be divided into three segments:

INITIAL PORTION OF THE CONVOLUTED SEGMENT. Sodium reabsorption in this portion occurs through cells and intercellular spaces. Transcellular reabsorption of sodium is active, generating a small transtubular electrical potential (1 to 5 millivolts, lumen negative) (Fig. 73–2). It requires entry of sodium across luminal (brush border) membranes and extrusion of sodium across basolateral membranes. Entry of sodium across luminal membranes is passive and occurs (1) by diffusion, (2) coupled to the transport of other solutes (e.g., glucose, amino acids, phosphate), and (3) in exchange with H^+ secreted from cell to lumen. Sodium extrusion from cells into the intercellular spaces and across the basolateral membrane is an active (energy-requiring) process which is accomplished by the sodium-potassium pump (Na^+–K^+ ATPase). Transport of sodium into the intercellular channels increases the concentration of solute in these spaces and creates an osmotic pressure gradient favoring the flow of water from lumen to intercellular spaces across the tight junctions that connect, toward the lumen, the lateral boundaries of the epithelial cells. The osmotic flow of water carries salt with it (solvent drag) and leads to bulk reabsorption of sodium.

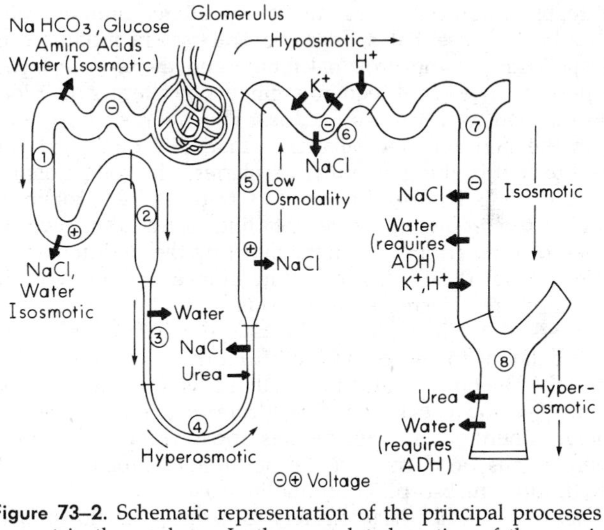

Figure 73–2. Schematic representation of the principal processes of transport in the nephron. In the convoluted portion of the proximal tubule (1) salt and water are reabsorbed at high rates, in isotonic proportions. Bulk reabsorption of most of the filtrate (65 to 70 per cent) and virtually complete reabsorption of glucose, amino acids, and bicarbonate take place in this segment. In the pars recta (2) organic acids are secreted and continuous reabsorption of sodium chloride takes place. The loop of Henle comprises three segments: the thin descending (3) and ascending (4) limbs and the thick ascending limb (5). The fluid becomes hyperosmotic, because of water abstraction, as it flows toward the bend of the loop and hyposmotic, because of sodium chloride reabsorption, as it flows toward the distal convoluted tubule (6). Active sodium reabsorption occurs in the distal convoluted tubule and in the cortical collecting tubule (7). This latter segment is water impermeable in the absence of ADH, and the reabsorption of sodium in this segment is increased by aldosterone. The collecting duct (8) allows equilibration of water with the hyperosmotic interstitium when ADH is present. For further details see text. (Adapted from figure by A Iselin, from Burg MB: Hosp Pract 13:99, 1978. Reproduced with permission.)

Preferential reabsorption of bicarbonate resulting from H^+ secretion occurs in this segment, with bicarbonate concentration falling and chloride concentration increasing to an equivalent degree as the fluid flows along this segment of the tubule. The reabsorption of glucose and amino acids is active, is coupled to sodium transport, and is essentially complete in this segment. Some permeant solutes, such as urea, are partially reabsorbed by a passive mechanism because of the increase in their luminal concentration as water is absorbed.

DISTAL TWO THIRDS OF THE CONVOLUTED SEGMENT. The luminal fluid of the last two thirds of the convoluted tubule is characterized by a low concentration of bicarbonate and by the absence of glucose and amino acids. The tubular fluid remains isosmotic with plasma and has the same concentration of sodium as does the filtrate. The concentration of chloride in the lumen, however, exceeds the concentration of chloride in the peritubular capillary. This concentration gradient for chloride favors its diffusion out of the lumen generating a lumen-positive potential (which is in the order of 1 to 3 mV). In experiments in vitro in which luminal and peritubular fluids have identical compositions, active sodium transport occurs. Therefore, sodium reabsorption in this segment occurs by (1) active transport, (2) passive flow (because of the positive luminal potential), and (3) solvent drag.

STRAIGHT SEGMENT (PARS RECTA). This segment is the main site of secretion of organic acids (penicillin, uric acid). Its rate of sodium and fluid transport is slower, and its capacity for glucose and amino acid reabsorption is minimal when compared to that of the convoluted segments. The potential of the lumen is positive, and sodium and chloride are transported by the same mechanisms as in the last two thirds of the proximal convoluted tubule.

Modulation of Reabsorption by the Proximal Tubule. Proximal reabsorption conserves most of the filtered fluid and all of a number of essential solutes. Several factors modulate the transport rate at the proximal tubule and therefore influence the performance of subsequent segments by altering their load.

TRANSTUBULAR PHYSICAL FACTORS. The hydrostatic pressure (P) in the peritubular capillaries is markedly decreased compared to that in the glomerular capillaries. The colloid osmotic pressure (Π) is increased owing to filtration of a "protein-free fluid" at the glomeruli. These "Starling forces" thus favor the uptake of fluid (from the interstitium) by the peritubular capillaries. When Π falls or P rises, the uptake of fluid by peritubular capillaries decreases. This leads to fluid accumulation in the interstitium, increased hydrostatic pressure in this space, and a delay in the egress of fluid from the lateral intercellular channels. The limiting junctions of these channels become more permeable, and backflux of fluid (from intercellular spaces to tubular lumen) occurs, thus diminishing net fluid reabsorption. When P falls or Π rises in the peritubular capillaries, as in dehydration, reabsorption of fluid increases.

Glomerular tubular balance refers to a direct relationship between GFR and the prevailing rates of proximal tubular reabsorption and has been ascribed to changes in Π in the peritubular circulation which result from changes in GFR (increases in GFR and hence in filtration fraction lead to a greater protein concentration and increases in Π in the efferent arterioles and peritubular capillaries; a decrease in GFR has the opposite effect). Thus, when GFR increases, a greater amount of fluid is delivered to the proximal tubule; however, the resulting rise in peritubular Π leads to a proportional increase in the reabsorption of fluid in this segment so that the percentage of the filtrate reabsorbed in the proximal tubule remains constant. An alternative mechanism accounting for glomerular tubular balance is a link between fluid reabsorption in the proximal tubule and flow rates of tubular fluid. Increases in GFR, and hence in proximal tubular flow, augment reabsorption; decreases in GFR and in flow decrease reabsorption.

EFFECTS OF HORMONES ON SODIUM REABSORPTION BY THE PROXIMAL TUBULE. Parathyroid hormone reduces sodium and fluid reabsorption in the proximal tubule; catecholamines may stimulate fluid reabsorption in this segment. However, the physiologic significance of these observations has not been established.

Loop of Henle. The loop of Henle, which is interposed between the proximal and distal tubules, is a hairpin-shaped structure extending into the renal medulla (Fig. 73–2). Under physiologic conditions it reabsorbs about 25 per cent of the filtered sodium and chloride and 15 per cent of the filtered water. In consequence, the isotonic fluid entering Henle's loop becomes hypotonic to plasma before entering the distal tubule.

The maintenance of water balance requires the excretion of urine of varied tonicity. The formation of a dilute (hypotonic to plasma) or concentrated (hypertonic to plasma) urine takes place by means of a *countercurrent system* that involves not only the loops of Henle but also the distal tubule, the collecting ducts, and the blood vessels supplying these segments. The excretion of a hypertonic urine involves two basic steps: (1) creation of a hypertonic medullary interstitium and (2) osmotic equilibration of the fluid that enters the medullary collecting duct with the hypertonic interstitium. Antidiuretic hormone (ADH) is required in this latter process. Hypotonic urine is excreted when the fluid which enters the medullary collecting duct does not equilibrate with the hypertonic interstitium owing to low levels or absence of ADH. Only the juxtamedullary nephrons contribute significantly to the production of medullary hypertonicity. However, the fluid from both superficial and deep nephrons drains into the collecting ducts and reaches osmotic equilibrium with the interstitium in the presence of ADH.

In normal human subjects the maximal osmolality of urine that can be achieved is around 1200 mOsm per kilogram. Since the tubular fluid reaches this osmolality by equilibration with the medullary interstitium, it follows that the interstitium must have a similar osmolality. *Countercurrent multiplication* is the process by which the interstitial osmolality is increased from 285 mOsm per kilogram in the cortex (the same osmolality as plasma) to 1200 mOsm per kilogram in the papillary tip. The thin descending and ascending limbs of juxtamedullary nephrons lie in close proximity to each other in the medulla. Flow through them is countercurrent. Fluid obtained from thin ascending limbs has a lower osmolality than fluid obtained from thin descending limbs at comparable levels in the papilla. This is due to functional differences. Whereas the descending limb is highly permeable to water, slightly permeable to urea, and highly impermeable to sodium, the ascending limb is highly permeable to sodium, moderately permeable to urea, and impermeable to water. In normal mammals, the medullary interstitium is hyperosmotic owing to the accumulation of high concentrations of both urea and sodium chloride (see below). This composition and the properties of the two segments of the loop result in quite specific transport processes. The isotonic fluid delivered from the proximal tubule becomes progressively hypertonic as it traverses the thin descending limb owing to net water flow from lumen to interstitium. The highest osmolality of the luminal fluid is achieved at the tip of the loop. This hyperosmolar fluid becomes diluted progressively as it flows up the thin ascending limb, owing to the movement of sodium without water from the lumen to the interstitium. Urea present in the interstitium diffuses inward. However, since the permeability of this segment to sodium chloride is greater than to urea, the net effect is a greater exit of sodium chloride than urea entry, resulting in net addition of solute to the interstitial fluid. In addition, since the thin ascending limb is impermeable to water, the fluid is diluted (hypotonic) with respect to the interstitial fluid at the same level. The thick ascending limb of the loop reabsorbs sodium chloride actively. This segment is essentially impermeable to water, even when ADH is present; therefore, salt transport from lumen to interstitial fluid decreases the osmolality of the luminal fluid and increases the osmolality of the interstitium. This increased osmolality of the outer medullary interstitium promotes the exit of water from the thin descending limb. The function of the thick ascending limb accounts for the countercurrent multiplication that occurs in the renal medulla. Although analysis of the electrochemical gradient (Fig. 73–2) might suggest active chloride transport, there is strong evidence that sodium transport is primary and active and that chloride is moved across the luminal membrane in cotransport with sodium as neutral sodium chloride. The amount of urea present in the fluid of the thick ascending limb is higher than in the fluid entering the thin descending limb. This is due to water abstraction, in excess of urea, out of the latter segment and net urea entry (recycled from the collecting duct) into the thin ascending and descending limbs of Henle's loop.

Urea and sodium chloride contribute most of the 1200 mOsm per kilogram of solute present at the papillary tip during antidiuresis. Antidiuretic hormone plays a critical role in this high interstitial urea concentration. In the cortical collecting duct ADH increases water but not urea permeability. This results, as water is lost from the tubular fluid, in a rise in concentration of urea in the tubular lumen. In the medullary collecting duct, ADH enhances the permeabilities of both water and urea. As water leaves the collecting duct, urea concentration increases further and urea enters the interstitium; it then enters the thin descending (very little) and ascending limbs, increasing the amount of urea in the tubular fluid (see above). The net result is that both urinary and medullary urea concentrations are maintained at high levels in the presence of ADH (antidiuresis).

The fluid emerging from the loop of Henle is virtually always hyposmotic (about 150 mOsm per kilogram) compared to plasma, regardless of the final urine osmolality. With low or absent ADH the luminal fluid in the cortical collecting duct does not equilibrate with the isosmotic cortical interstitium or in the medullary collecting duct with the hypertonic medulla. Hence, the volume of fluid delivered to the tip of the collecting duct is increased and its osmolality decreased compared to plasma. The osmolality of this fluid can be further decreased to as low as 30 mOsm per kilogram by the reabsorption of solute in excess of water in distal tubule and cortical and medullary collecting ducts (see below).

Since the maximal urine osmolality cannot exceed that in the interstitium, the ability to conserve water by excreting a highly concentrated urine is reduced when the hypertonicity of the medullary interstitium is decreased. This may be due to reduced papillary urea accumulation such as occurs in protein malnutrition, as a consequence of decreased urea production, or due to reduced interstitial sodium chloride accumulation (use of loop diuretics, hypercalcemia). Reduced levels or absence of ADH (diabetes insipidus) or unresponsiveness of the collecting duct to the action of ADH (nephrogenic diabetes insipidus) may prevent equilibration of the fluid in the collecting duct with the hypertonic interstitium, leading to an impairment in water conservation.

Distal Nephron (Distal Convoluted Tubule, Cortical Collecting Tubule, and Medullary Collecting Duct). The distal nephron accomplishes the final and delicate adjustments in the reabsorption of water, sodium, chloride, phosphate, and calcium in response to the hormones aldosterone, ADH, and parathyroid hormone.

The *distal convoluted tubule* is defined anatomically as the segment which extends from the macula densa to the site of transition from homogeneous cells to a mixture of dark and light cells (typical of the collecting duct). The distal convoluted tubule is essentially impermeable to water and unresponsive to ADH. Sodium chloride is reabsorbed at a slower rate than in the proximal tubule or in the loop, but against large concentration gradients. The rate of reabsorption is proportional to the load. The transtubular electrical potential, lumen negative, is related to the reabsorption of sodium and varies from −10 in the initial portion to −45 mV in the distal portion. Most of the reabsorption of sodium chloride occurs transcellularly. Potassium is secreted in this segment from peritubular capillary into the lumen (see below). Acidification of the luminal fluid in the distal tubule has been attributed to an active H^+ transport mechanism located at the luminal membrane.

The *cortical collecting tubule* extends from the end of the distal tubule to the corticomedullary junction. Under basal conditions, water permeability is negligible in this segment. It is increased markedly by ADH. Sodium chloride is actively reabsorbed at this level; therefore, in the absence of ADH the luminal fluid osmolality falls further. When ADH is present the luminal fluid equilibrates with the cortical interstitial fluid and becomes isosmotic with plasma; at the same time, luminal urea concentrations rise (see above). The transtubular electrical potential is about 35 mV, lumen negative; it is related to active reabsorption of sodium and is highly dependent on the levels of mineralocorticoids which increase sodium reabsorption. Potassium and hydrogen are secreted in this segment. Aldosterone increases sodium reabsorption as well as potassium and H^+ secretion in this portion of the nephron (Fig. 73–2).

The *medullary collecting duct* starts at the corticomedullary junction and ends on the surface of the papilla. Water and urea permeabilities are low in the absence of ADH. Continuous sodium chloride reabsorption at this level, in the absence of ADH, results in a further drop in urine osmolality. ADH increases water and urea permeability and allows the equilibration of the luminal osmolality with that of the hypertonic interstitium.

To recapitulate, in the proximal tubule salt and water are transported at high rates, in isotonic proportions. Bulk reabsorption of most of the filtrate (65 to 70 per cent) and virtually complete reabsorption of "metabolically useful" solutes (glucose, amino acids, bicarbonate) take place in this segment. The *loop of Henle* comprises three segments with strikingly different properties of active transport and permeability of water and solute. Because of these properties, the medullary interstitium is made hyperosmolar and acts as the driving force for final water reabsorption. The loop reabsorbs additional sodium chloride (about 25 per cent of that filtered) and water (about 15 per cent of the filtrate) and leaves about 10 per cent of the sodium and 15 per cent of the water to be reabsorbed in the last segments of the tubule.

The distal convoluted tubule and the collecting tubule can establish large sodium gradients between fluid in the lumen and in the peritubular capillary. The collecting ducts, water impermeable in the absence of ADH, become permeable to water in response to the hormone. It is in these segments that the final volume and osmolality of the urine are determined. Salt transport occurs at a slower rate than in the preceding segments but against large concentration gradients. The final regulation of salt excretion takes place in these segments, under the influence of aldosterone. Potassium and H^+ excretion are regulated also in these segments.

ROLE OF THE KIDNEY IN SODIUM CHLORIDE HOMEOSTASIS. Normally the kidney regulates sodium balance (and hence extracellular fluid volume) in a very efficient manner. The daily intake of sodium varies considerably. In the Western world the average diet contains about 170 mEq per 24 hours. About 98 per cent of this amount is excreted in the urine. However, even when the normal daily excretion of sodium is 165 to 170 mEq per day, i.e., sufficient to maintain sodium balance on a relatively high sodium intake, less than 1 per cent of the amount of sodium filtered (140 mEq per liter × 170 liters = 23,800 mEq per day) is excreted in the urine. Thus, maintenance of sodium homeostasis is primarily a function of the renal tubule and reabsorption of filtered sodium; changes in GFR appear to be quantitatively less important. Thus, (1) sizable increases in GFR, not accompanied by ECF volume expansion, do not result in a marked natriuresis because of glomerular tubular balance (see above), and (2) the natriuresis of ECF volume expansion occurs under experimental conditions in which GFR is maintained constant or even decreased experimentally. When a normal subject increases the intake of salt, urine sodium excretion increases progressively, reaching, in three to four days, a steady-state level equal to and offsetting intake. During the interval of adjustment, positive sodium balance occurs, with an accompanying retention of water and consequent gain in body weight. When salt intake is suddenly reduced, the opposite effects are observed. Sodium excretion decreases, reaching a level equal to intake within three to five days with a reduction in total body water and body weight.

Several physiologic mechanisms ordinarily control sodium reabsorption by the kidney to maintain the sodium content of the extracellular fluid (ECF). Changes in sodium mass are not sensed as such, but secondarily as changes in ECF volume. Total ECF volume changes are sensed through their effects on circulatory dynamics ("effective arterial blood volume"). The determinants of effective arterial blood volume are (1) the degree of filling of the arterial tree, which depends in large part on cardiac output, and (2) peripheral vascular resistance, which depends on the compliance of the peripheral vessels and the magnitude of the arterial runoff. Decreases in effective volume (dehydration, hemorrhage, venodilation, venous pooling) lead to renal retention of salt. Increases in effective volume (saline administration, excessive salt intake) lead to a rise in salt excretion by the kidney.

Factors Which Influence the Tubular Reabsorption of Sodium. Alterations in effective arterial volume affect handling of sodium by the kidney through the renin-angiotensin-aldosterone system, the sympathetic nervous system, and other less well-defined factors. The last category probably includes changes in intrarenal hydrostatic and oncotic pressures (so-called physical factors), a natriuretic (or salt-losing) hormone, and possibly the distribution of blood flow within the kidneys (Fig. 73–3).

Role of Physical Factors in the Reabsorption of Sodium. A fall in effective arterial blood volume (dehydration, hemorrhage) and the consequent decline in blood pressure decrease renal perfusion. In response to reductions in renal perfusion pressure, glomerular plasma flow decreases more than does glomerular capillary hydrostatic pressure, resulting in a fall in GFR which is proportionally less than the decline in renal plasma flow. This disparity is due to a greater vasoconstriction of efferent compared to afferent arterioles in response to increased levels of catecholamines and angiotensin II in the circulation. The lesser fall in GFR compared to renal plasma flow increases filtration fraction and hence the concentration of protein in the efferent arterioles and peritubular capillaries. In addition, vasoconstriction of the efferent arteriole results in a fall in hydrostatic pressure (P) in the peritubular capillaries. The increase in Π and the decrease in P in the peritubular capillaries augment sodium and water reabsorption along the proximal segments of the nephron. Thus, in response to contraction of effective arterial volume, the glomerular and peritubular microcirculation act in concert to minimize fluid losses by both lowering GFR and augmenting salt and water reabsorption by the tubules (Fig. 73–3).

Expansion of the ECF volume elicits opposite effects. The increase in renal perfusion pressure leads to not only a rise in GFR but also a proportionally greater rise in renal plasma flow; consequently filtration fraction falls. The net effect is a decrease in peritubular protein concentration and hence in Π, with a decrease in reabsorption of fluid by peritubular capillaries. The importance of such physical factors in the normal control of sodium and water reabsorption is not exactly clear. Since alterations in Π and P in the peritubular capillaries influence fluid reabsorption mainly, if not exclusively, in the proximal tubule, it is likely that changes in physical factors are important only when fluid balance deficits or gains are very large (as, for example, with severe hemorrhage or marked expansion of the ECF volume). Whether significant changes in proximal reabsorption occur in response to more modest alterations in fluid balance (as might result, for example, in response to a diet very low or very high in sodium chloride) remains uncertain.

Redistribution of Blood Flow. Another mechanism potentially altering sodium excretion is redistribution of blood flow. It has been suggested that certain nephrons, those with superficially placed glomeruli, have less capacity to reabsorb sodium than others. If so, at any given total GFR, the relative amounts of fluid filtered by the two different nephron populations would be an important determinant of sodium excretion. Redistribu-

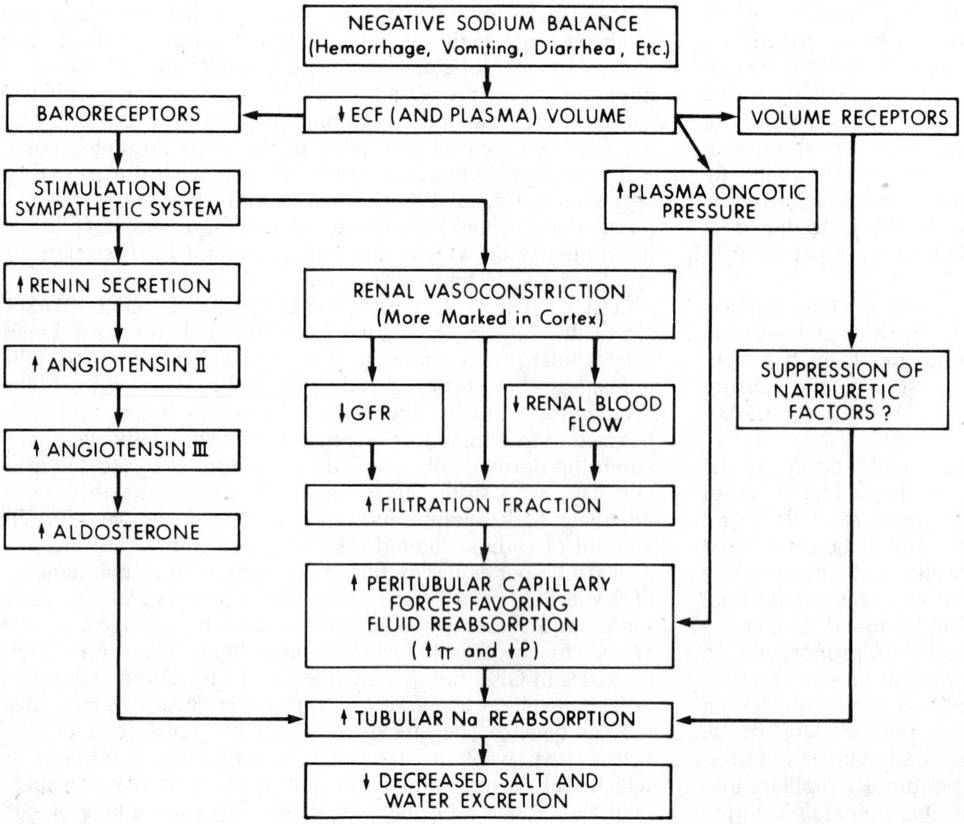

Figure 73–3. Mechanisms responsible for increased sodium reabsorption in the renal tubule in response to a negative sodium balance. These mechanisms and the accompanying stimulation of thirst and antidiuretic hormone secretion tend to restore the extracellular fluid (ECF) volume. The arrows indicate a decrease (↓) or an increase (↑). Oncotic pressure and hydrostatic pressure in peritubular capillaries are indicated by Π and P, respectively.

tion of GFR toward the "high reabsorption nephrons" (juxtamedullary nephrons) would be associated with decreased sodium excretion because of the greater capacity of these nephrons to reabsorb sodium. Despite the attractiveness of this theory, evidence favoring it is scanty.

RENIN-ANGIOTENSIN-ALDOSTERONE. Sodium balance is controlled also by *mineralocorticoid hormones, mainly aldosterone*. Only a small but significant fraction (some 2 per cent) of the filtered sodium is under hormonal control. Yet loss or gain of an amount of sodium equivalent to 2 per cent of the filtered load (about 500 mEq per day) has profound effects on sodium balance. Aldosterone increases sodium reabsorption in the distal tubule and collecting duct. Lack of aldosterone leads to loss of sodium in the urine. The factors controlling aldosterone secretion include (1) plasma concentration of sodium, (2) plasma concentration of potassium, (3) adrenocorticotropic hormone (ACTH), and (4) angiotensin. Circulating levels of angiotensin are increased by hemorrhage, dietary salt restriction, changes in distribution of blood and fluids (venous pooling and edema forming states), and other states of increased secretion of renin. *Renin* is a proteolytic enzyme secreted by the granular cells of the juxtaglomerular apparatus. The mechanisms controlling its release are not fully understood, but seem to depend on (1) changes in renal perfusion pressure, (2) factors reflecting the rate of delivery of sodium or chloride to the macula densa, and (3) activity of the renal sympathetic nerves. When perfusion pressure or the delivery of sodium falls, or the activity of the sympathetic nerves increases, the release of renin is enhanced. Renin acts on a substrate in plasma, *angiotensinogen,* to form *angiotensin I* (a decapeptide). *Converting enzyme* splits two amino acids from angiotensin I to form *angiotensin II* (an octapeptide). The latter is a potent hormone, central to the regulation of salt and water balance. It produces vasoconstriction and stimulates the secretion of aldosterone, thirst, and the renal reabsorption of sodium. Another split product of angiotensin, *angiotensin III* (a heptapeptide), also increases aldosterone secretion from the zona glomerulosa of the adrenal.

OTHER HORMONAL AGENTS. Cortisol, estrogen, growth hormone, and insulin all can enhance sodium reabsorption. Glucagon, progesterone, and parathyroid hormone can decrease it. It is almost certain that when circulating levels of these hormones are elevated (as, for example, estrogen during pregnancy), significant influences occur on sodium reabsorption and thereby excretion. However, there is no evidence that any of them, unlike the factors described previously, are controlled specifically as part of the homeostatic regulation of sodium balance. Of great interest is the possible role played by intrarenally produced substances such as *prostaglandins* and *kinins.* These agents are potent vasodilators and may reduce sodium reabsorption, by altering regional intrarenal vascular resistance or by direct actions on the tubular cells. Their levels change with alterations of sodium balance, but it is not yet clear how extensively they participate in the renal regulation of sodium excretion.

The existence of a natriuretic, or salt-losing, hormone has not yet been established. However, it has been suggested that such a hormone is released when ECF volume is expanded and that it acts upon the proximal tubule and collecting ducts to inhibit sodium reabsorption.

RENAL NERVES. The renal sympathetic nerves play a prominent role in sodium homeostasis by modulating (1) secretion of aldosterone via the renin-angiotensin system, (2) intrarenal physical factors, (3) the reabsorptive activity of the tubular cells themselves, and (4) GFR. Yet, because of the many other known (and potential) factors involved, a transplanted and, therefore, denervated kidney maintains sodium homeostasis quite well.

RENAL REGULATION OF WATER EXCRETION. The capacity to regulate renal excretion of water, independent of solute excretion, maintains the osmolality of body fluids within narrow limits despite wide variations in intake of water. Roughly 170 liters of water is filtered daily. Of this amount, less than 2 liters, or about 1 per cent of the amount filtered, is excreted. Except for setting an upper limit for the amount of water that can be excreted per unit time, GFR is not involved in the regulation of water excretion. This upper limit assumes importance only when GFR is profoundly reduced as in acute renal failure or advanced chronic renal disease.

The tubule is the major site for renal regulation of water excretion. Net absorption of water occurs all along the nephron and is due to passive diffusion of water down its concentration gradient into a region of higher osmolality. In the proximal tubule, this gradient is established by the active transport of sodium into the basolateral and intercellular spaces. About two thirds of the filtered water is reabsorbed isosmotically in the proximal tubule. Reabsorption of water in this segment is intimately related to the reabsorption of sodium. When the luminal fluid reaches the end of the proximal tubule, the direct relationship between water and sodium reabsorption is lost. Since water reabsorption in the remaining segments of the nephron is to a large extent independent of the reabsorption of solute, the process is referred to frequently as the reabsorption of solute-free water, or simply *free water.*

The reabsorption of free water is dependent largely on interrelationships among four factors: (1) the concentration of solute in the interstitium through which the renal tubule passes, (2) the concentration of solute in the tubular fluid, (3) the permeability of the renal tubule to water and solute, and (4) the circulating levels of ADH. About 15 per cent of the filtered water enters the distal tubule. A variable fraction of this water is reabsorbed by the distal tubules and collecting ducts. Absorption of this final fraction is controlled by antidiuretic hormone (ADH), which serves as the main regulator of the osmolality of body fluids. ADH is synthesized by nerve cells in the hypothalamus and liberated from their terminals in the posterior lobe and pituitary stalk. The major stimulus for the secretion of ADH into the circulation is an increase in plasma osmolality, mediated by osmoreceptors which are exquisitely sensitive to changes in osmolality. The feedback system they provide helps to maintain the tonicity of plasma within a standard deviation of ± 2 mOsm per kilogram (a change of less than 1 per cent). Although changes in osmolality are the most sensitive and therefore the primary regulators of ADH release, alterations in ECF volume can modulate and sometimes override the effects of tonicity. However, secretion of ADH is not increased unless volume loss is greater than 10 per cent. Baroreceptor stimulation appears to mediate the increase in ADH secretion resulting from volume contraction. This effect is potentiated by elevated levels of circulating catecholamines which act directly on these receptors. Angiotensin II, prostaglandins, and nicotine may also affect ADH release through activation of arterial baroreceptors. When a surfeit of body water develops, ADH release is inhibited and a dilute urine is excreted; when a water deficit is present, free water is reabsorbed and the urine becomes concentrated by mechanisms discussed previously.

The human kidney can dilute urine ten-fold with respect to plasma (to about 30 mOsm per kilogram) but can concentrate it only to a maximum of four-fold with respect to plasma (to about 1200 mOsm per kilogram). The daily volume of urine depends on the intake of fluid and can be varied from 600 ml to over 24 liters. When a large load of water is ingested, the following events occur: (1) the osmolar concentration (osmolality) of plasma falls; (2) over the next 15 to 20 minutes ADH levels fall, and as a consequence the flow rate of urine increases, reaching a maximum in 45 to 60 minutes. The maximal increase in urine flow occurs when free water excretion is about 15 per cent of GFR.

ROLE OF THE KIDNEY IN THE PRESERVATION OF POTASSIUM BALANCE. Total body potassium approximates 3500 mEq; the ECF contains 50 to 70 mEq. The remainder is intracellular. Extracellular fluid potassium concentration is about 3.5 to 4.5

mEq per liter. Intracellular potassium is some 40 times higher, at 160 mEq per liter. The ratio of intracellular to extracellular concentrations of potassium is the principal determinant of the membrane potential in excitable tissues. The distribution of potassium between ECF and ICF is influenced by several factors, including acid-base balance and circulating levels of insulin and catecholamines. Acidosis decreases intracellular potassium, and alkalosis favors the movement of potassium from the ECF into the cells.

The daily intake of potassium ranges from 50 to 150 mEq. Most of the potassium ingested is absorbed (less than 10 mEq is excreted in the stool); thus, maintenance of balance requires the daily renal excretion of an amount of potassium identical to that absorbed from the gut. Under physiologic conditions, approximately 70 per cent of the potassium filtered is reabsorbed in the proximal tubule (Fig. 73–4). The loop of Henle reabsorbs the remaining 20 to 30 per cent. Distal segments of the nephron can both reabsorb and secrete potassium. The balance between distal reabsorption and secretion determines the net urinary excretion of this cation. On a normal diet (100 mEq per day) the kidneys excrete approximately 90 mEq of potassium per day. The potassium that appears in the urine is secreted in the distal tubule and collecting duct. The secretion of potassium is influenced by the potassium concentration in renal tubular cells and by the magnitude of the electrochemical gradient between cell interior and tubular lumen (see below). The rate of renal potassium excretion can vary considerably in response to changes in potassium intake. If potassium intake is increased acutely, renal excretion of potassium can rise more than ten-fold. About 50 per cent of the amount administered appears in the urine within 12 hours. The renal response to potassium deprivation is sluggish. Excretion falls to levels of 10 to 15 mEq per 24 hours only after 7 to 14 days of a potassium-free diet. During this interval a deficit of as much as 200 mEq of potassium may be incurred. In adults with increased catabolism (infections, surgery), the renal excretion of potassium may exceed the amount ingested.

Potassium excretion is affected by changes in the *levels of mineralocorticoids,* particularly *aldosterone; alterations in acid-base balance;* and changes in *flow rate* and *sodium reabsorption* in the distal tubule. Urinary excretion of potassium depends on its rate of secretion by the distal tubule. Increased net secretory rates of potassium in this segment could be due to (1) increased active uptake by the peritubular membrane leading to increased cell potassium concentration and increased passive leak across the luminal membrane, (2) increased permeability of the luminal membrane to potassium, (3) decreased active reabsorption of potassium by the luminal membrane, or (4) decreased electrical potential difference across the luminal membrane.

A high concentration of potassium in distal tubular cells is established and maintained through the action of a Na^+–K^+ exchange pump located in the peritubular membrane. Potassium uptake via this pump is stimulated by high plasma levels of potassium, alkalosis, aldosterone, and increased sodium reabsorption. All factors which raise cell potassium (increased peritubular pump activity, dehydration) favor its diffusion into the lumen. If the cellular potassium concentration falls (potassium deprivation, acidosis, dilution of body fluids), the rate of potassium translocation into the lumen falls and may be less than the potassium uptake across the luminal membrane. Under these conditions, net reabsorption of potassium may replace net potassium secretion.

The difference in electrical potential across the entire distal tubular cell is established by the active reabsorption of sodium and is about 50 mV (lumen negative to peritubular fluid). The cell interior is negative (–70 mV) in relation to the peritubular capillary. Thus, the luminal membrane potential difference is about 20 mV (cell negative to lumen). This electrical profile favors a greater leak of potassium across the luminal membrane than across the peritubular membrane. Thus, potassium is pumped into distal tubular cells and then leaks across the luminal membrane into the tubular lumen. Such passive translocation of potassium from the cell into the lumen depends not only on the electrical potential difference across the luminal membrane but also on the chemical concentration gradient. A decrease in luminal membrane potential difference (increased lumen electronegativity) or factors that increase cellular potassium or lower luminal potassium have been shown to augment potassium secretion.

Augmented sodium reabsorption in the distal tubule increases lumen electronegativity, which favors potassium secretion from the cell interior into the tubular fluid. Hence, increased distal sodium reabsorption will favor potassium excretion. For example, diuretic administration increases sodium delivery distally, which, in turn, increases potassium excretion, particularly in patients with secondary aldosteronism. Hyperkalemia increases potassium excretion by two mechanisms: it stimulates aldosterone secretion directly, and it also enhances renal secretion, presumably via increased cell content of potassium. Alkalosis enhances and acidosis depresses potassium secretion, probably by inducing corresponding changes in renal cell potassium. The rates of *distal tubular flow* also influence potassium excretion, presumably because of the rapid dissipation of the concentration of potassium in the tubular lumen at higher flow rates. Fast flow rates increase and slow flow rates decrease potassium excretion.

ROLE OF THE KIDNEY IN ACID-BASE BALANCE. The pH of the

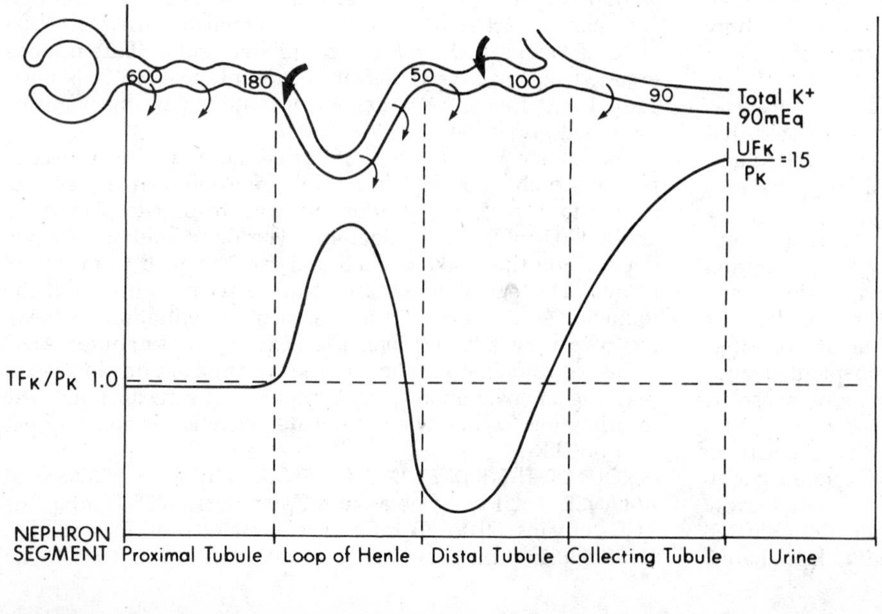

Figure 73–4. Tubular sites of potassium secretion (◆) and reabsorption (←). The numbers within the figure indicate the approximate amount of total potassium (in mEq per 24 hours) at the beginning and end of each nephron segment and in the urine. The curve shows the changes in potassium concentration in the tubular fluid expressed as a ratio of potassium in the tubular fluid or urine to potassium in plasma. (Adapted from Sullivan LP, Grantham JJ: Physiology of the Kidney. 2nd ed. Philadelphia, Lea and Febiger, 1982.)

extracellular fluid is maintained near 7.40 under a wide variety of physiologic conditions, despite the daily production of approximately 15,000 mmol of CO_2 (potential carbonic acid) and 50 to 100 mEq of nonvolatile acids. Buffers present in body fluids minimize the change in pH that would otherwise occur. The lungs excrete the CO_2 and the kidneys excrete the H^+ from the so-called nonvolatile acids. With usual rates of CO_2 production, alveolar ventilation maintains the P_{CO_2} of blood at approximately 40 mm Hg—i.e., 1.2 mmol of dissolved CO_2 per liter of plasma. Acidosis potentially resulting from the production of nonvolatile acids is prevented through buffering, mainly by bicarbonate. The continuous titration of nonvolatile acids by bicarbonate would deplete the body stores of this buffer, unless the bicarbonate consumed were replenished. The kidney maintains plasma pH in a physiologic range by regulating the concentration of plasma bicarbonate. This is accomplished by the excretion in the urine of 50 to 100 mEq of hydrogen ion in the form of ammonium (NH_4^+) and titratable acid (the amount of alkali required to titrate the urine to the pH of plasma). Disodium phosphate (Na_2HPO_4) present in the filtrate is converted to NaH_2PO_4, which accounts for most of the titratable acid excreted in the urine. Net excretion of acid (titratable acid + ammonium excretion − bicarbonate excretion) equals the daily production of nonvolatile acids under physiologic conditions. Both the *reclamation* of filtered bicarbonate and the *regeneration* of bicarbonate depend on the secretion of H^+ from the tubular cells into the lumen. The secreted H^+ is generated within the tubular cells by the *carbonic anhydrase*–catalyzed hydration of CO_2 to H_2CO_3, which immediately dissociates into H^+ and HCO_3^-. The H^+ is secreted into the tubular fluid, and the bicarbonate, concomitantly produced intracellularly, enters the peritubular capillary. Thus, H^+ secretion results in addition of bicarbonate to plasma. When the H^+ secreted into the lumen combines with filtered bicarbonate, it forms H_2CO_3, which quickly dissociates to CO_2 and H_2O. As a consequence, a bicarbonate disappears from the lumen, and the net effect is bicarbonate reabsorption (reclamation).

At a physiologic GFR of 170 liters per day and a plasma bicarbonate of 24 mEq per liter, the reabsorption of over 4000 mEq of bicarbonate requires the secretion of an equivalent amount of H^+, whereas the excretion of net acid requires the secretion of 50 to 100 mEq of H^+ daily (Table 73–2). The process of bicarbonate reclamation operates to reabsorb all the filtered bicarbonate below a critical serum concentration, the *bicarbonate threshold concentration,* which in adult man is normally about 24 mEq per liter, essentially identical to the concentration of bicarbonate in plasma. When plasma bicarbonate concentration rises above this threshold, renal reclamation is incomplete and the excess bicarbonate escapes into the urine, enabling the plasma bicarbonate concentration to return to the threshold level. Under physiologic conditions the virtually complete reabsorption of bicarbonate serves to preserve bicarbonate stores but does not replace the bicarbonate consumed in the buffering of nonvolatile acids. If the secreted H^+ combines with buffers, such as HPO_4^- or NH_3, a new bicarbonate ion (de novo synthesis) is added to the peritubular capillary blood. This results in replacement of the bicarbonate consumed in buffering the daily acid load (Table 73–2).

In the steady state, the net amount of H^+ excreted is equal to the H^+ load, about 50 to 100 mEq per day. At times, net acid excretion is absent or has a negative value. This occurs after ingestion of an alkaline load (bicarbonate or substances that can be metabolized to bicarbonate). Ammonium excretion accounts for two thirds and titratable acid for one third of the urinary excretion of acid. When the daily H^+ load increases (e.g., increased catabolism, infection), the rise in acid excretion by the kidney is usually due to increased ammonium excretion. Ammonia (NH_3), produced within the renal tubular cells from glutamine, diffuses into the peritubular capillary or lumen down its concentration gradient. In the lumen it combines with H^+ to form NH_4^+. As noted, each mole of NH_4^+ excreted will result in the de novo generation of 1 mole of bicarbonate. Thus, when metabolic acidosis develops and the need for regenerating bicarbonate increases, synthesis of ammonia and NH_4^+ excretion usually increase.

TABLE 73–2. ROLE OF THE KIDNEY IN ACID-BASE BALANCE

Function	mEq/24 hrs
1. Reabsorption of filtered bicarbonate ("reclamation")	≅ 4000
2. Generation of new bicarbonate (net excretion of acid)	50–100
a. Ammonium excretion	35–65
b. Titratable acid excretion	15–35

Hydrogen secretion occurs in both proximal and distal segments of the nephron. As the concentration of bicarbonate in the lumen decreases, the concentration of H^+ increases, and as a result a limitation is imposed on the net rate of H^+ secretion. The maximal H^+ gradient achievable between cell and collecting duct lumen is about 800:1 (luminal fluid pH of 4.5).

Factors That Regulate the Renal Secretion of Hydrogen Ions. The major factors that influence the renal secretion of H^+ are (1) *effective circulating volume,* (2) *arterial pH and* P_{CO_2}, (3) *plasma concentration of potassium,* and (4) *mineralocorticoids (aldosterone).*

EFFECTIVE CIRCULATING VOLUME. Hydrogen ion secretion is increased by volume depletion (increased sodium reabsorption) and diminished by ECF volume expansion. Hydrogen secretion is stimulated also when significant amounts of nonreabsorbable anions, i.e., sulfate ions, are present in the distal nephron and when sodium reabsorption is enhanced by any mechanism. Thus, the effective circulating volume of the ECF and the amounts of nonreabsorbable anion accompanying sodium through the distal nephron are important determinants of renal H^+ secretion.

ARTERIAL PH AND P_{CO_2}. Net acid excretion is increased with acidosis and decreased with alkalosis. Acidosis, resulting from a decrease in the plasma concentration of bicarbonate (metabolic acidosis) or induced by an elevation in P_{CO_2} (respiratory acidosis), augments H^+ excretion and increases the renal synthesis of bicarbonate. Metabolic alkalosis (increased plasma bicarbonate) or respiratory alkalosis (decreased P_{CO_2}) has the opposite effects. The effects of arterial pH on net acid excretion are most likely mediated by changes in renal tubular cell pH. Elevations in arterial P_{CO_2} increase bicarbonate reabsorption, and a fall in arterial P_{CO_2} reduces bicarbonate reabsorption.

PLASMA POTASSIUM CONCENTRATION. Hypokalemia increases and hyperkalemia decreases bicarbonate reabsorption. These effects are due to changes in intracellular H^+ concentration induced by cation shifts between the ICF and the ECF. In hypokalemia, potassium leaves the cell and is replaced by H^+ and sodium. The increase in intracellular H^+ concentration (intracellular acidosis) leads to the enhanced H^+ secretion and bicarbonate reabsorption associated with potassium depletion. The opposite occurs with hyperkalemia.

ALDOSTERONE. Aldosterone stimulates secretion of both potassium and hydrogen in the distal nephron. Excess of aldosterone may cause metabolic alkalosis, and its deficiency may lead to metabolic acidosis by decreasing H^+ excretion.

ROLE OF THE KIDNEY IN MINERAL HOMEOSTASIS. The kidney regulates the homeostasis of minerals not only by modifying the excretion of phosphate, calcium, and magnesium (see below) but also by influencing the metabolism of vitamin D. Vitamin D_3 (cholecalciferol) is metabolized to 25(OH) cholecalciferol in the liver and subsequently to a number of dihydroxylated derivatives by the kidney. Of these derivatives, $1,25(OH)_2D_3$ and $24,25(OH)_2D_3$ appear to be the most significant biologically. The $1,25(OH)_2D_3$ is the calcemic hormone produced in the kidney in response to hypophosphatemia or elevated levels of parathyroid hormone (when hypocalcemia occurs), and $24,25(OH)_2D_3$ is produced preferentially when balance of minerals is normal. The $1,25(OH)_2D_3$ increases absorption of calcium and phosphate from the gut as well as mineral mobilization from bone. The role of $24,25(OH)_2D_3$ is less well defined; it seems to promote bone mineralization and suppress parathyroid hormone release.

REGULATION OF PHOSPHORUS METABOLISM. The kidneys play a major role in maintaining the serum phosphorus concentration within narrow limits, about 3.0 to 4.5 mg per deciliter in adults. On an average diet, 1 gram of phosphorus is ingested daily, of which 700 mg is absorbed and the rest is excreted in the stool. The kidneys filter about 7 grams of phosphorus daily, of which 6.3 grams (90 per cent) is reabsorbed and 700 mg is excreted in the urine. As serum phosphorus and filtered load of phosphorus rise, the capacity to reabsorb phosphorus increases until a transport maximum (Tm) for phosphorus reabsorption is reached when serum phosphorus concentrations are between 6 and 9 mg per deciliter. Under physiologic conditions, about 70 per cent of the filtered phosphorus is reabsorbed in the proximal tubule and 10 to 15 per cent in the distal tubule and collecting ducts; thus, 5 to 20 per cent of the filtered phosphorus is excreted in the urine. In other words, the tubular reabsorption of phosphate (TRP) ranges normally from 80 to 95 per cent.

Numerous factors (the major ones being dietary phosphorus load and the serum levels of parathyroid hormone) affect the reabsorption of phosphorus. Phosphorus reabsorption approaches 100 per cent in patients fed a very low phosphorus diet. In contrast, patients ingesting 2 to 3 grams of phosphorus daily can excrete 60 to 70 per cent of this amount in the urine. Changes in phosphorus intake affect phosphorus excretion directly and also by altering the levels of ionized calcium that modify the release of parathyroid hormone. Parathyroid hormone (via stimulation of production of cyclic AMP by tubular cells) decreases phosphorus reabsorption in both proximal and distal segments of the nephron. An excess of parathyroid hormone may increase fractional excretion of phosphorus from a basal value of 10 per cent to 30 per cent or more. In the absence of parathyroid hormone the tubular capacity to reabsorb phosphorus is increased. Additional factors affect phosphorus reabsorption by the kidney. Volume expansion of the ECF, calcitonin, glucocorticoids, metabolic acidosis or alkalosis, and glycosuria increase urinary phosphorus excretion. On the other hand, administration of growth hormone and respiratory acidosis decrease phosphorus excretion. The influence of vitamin D and its metabolites on phosphorus reabsorption by the kidney is not clear, since divergent results have been obtained by several different groups of investigators.

RENAL REGULATION OF CALCIUM METABOLISM. Serum calcium concentrations in man are maintained between 9 and 10 mg per deciliter despite wide variations in dietary calcium intake. Total serum calcium consists of ultrafilterable calcium (approximately 60 per cent of the total) and calcium bound to protein, primarily albumin. The ultrafilterable fraction includes both the ionized calcium (50 per cent of the total) and calcium complexed to citrate, bicarbonate, and phosphate, which represents 10 per cent of total serum calcium. Serum calcium levels are maintained relatively constant through modification of calcium absorption from the gastrointestinal tract, changes in renal calcium excretion, and mobilization of calcium from bone.

Approximately 1000 mg of calcium is ingested daily in the diet. About 800 mg appears in the stool (from unabsorbed dietary calcium and intestinal secretion) and 200 mg in the urine. The percentage of dietary calcium absorbed from the intestine increases when calcium intake is low and decreases when it is high. Parathyroid hormone and vitamin D participate in these adaptations. Thus, in patients fed a low calcium diet, the development of mild and transient hypocalcemia increases the release of parathyroid hormone, which augments the renal conversion of $25(OH)D_3$ to $1,25(OH)_2D_3$. This latter compound increases intestinal calcium absorption and mobilizes calcium from bone, synergistically with parathyroid hormone. Thus, serum calcium returns toward normal. On the other hand, in patients fed a high calcium diet, the mild hypercalcemia that may occur suppresses the release of parathyroid hormone, leading to decreased activity of the renal 1-hydroxylase enzyme and the preferential production of $24,25(OH)_2D_3$. This metabolite is less efficient than $1,25(OH)_2D_3$ in promoting calcium absorption from the intestine and in mobilizing calcium from the skeleton.

The kidneys filter approximately 10 grams of calcium per day, but usually less than 200 mg appears in the urine. Thus over 98 per cent of the filtered load is reabsorbed. Calcium reabsorption occurs throughout the nephron, and parallels to some degree the reabsorption of sodium. Approximately 55 per cent of the filtered calcium is reabsorbed in the proximal tubule, 20 to 30 per cent in the loop of Henle, 10 to 15 per cent in the distal tubule, and 2 to 8 per cent in the terminal nephron, including the collecting duct. Most maneuvers that decrease sodium and fluid reabsorption in the proximal tubule (infusion of saline, administration of acetazolamide, or mild to moderate hypercalcemia) decrease calcium reabsorption in this segment as well. The reabsorption of calcium in the loop of Henle also parallels sodium reabsorption. It is only distal to the loop of Henle that calcium and sodium are influenced separately and independently.

Parathyroid hormone stimulates the renal absorption of calcium and decreases urinary calcium excretion. Acute parathyroidectomy increases calcium excretion despite a fall in total serum calcium and hence in the filtered load of calcium. However, the degree of calciuria declines when the plasma concentration of calcium falls below 7 mg per deciliter. Pharmacologic doses of vitamin D usually increase intestinal absorption of calcium and bone resorption, leading to increases in serum calcium, the filtered load of calcium, and urinary calcium excretion. Metabolic acidosis or phosphate depletion produces hypercalciuria. Both furosemide and ethacrynic acid inhibit sodium and calcium transport in the thick ascending limb of Henle's loop and increase calcium excretion. Chronic administration of thiazides results in natriuresis and hypocalciuria. This effect may be due to contraction of ECF volume and increased calcium reabsorption in the proximal segments. In addition, thiazides may potentiate the effect of parathyroid hormone on calcium reabsorption in the distal segment.

RENAL REGULATION OF MAGNESIUM METABOLISM. Total body magnesium is approximately 2000 mEq (or 25 grams). About 60 per cent of total body magnesium is found in bone. Another 20 per cent is present in muscle. Only a small fraction (about 1 per cent) is present in the ECF. The normal plasma concentration of magnesium in humans is 1.7 to 2.2 mg per deciliter, of which 80 per cent is ultrafilterable and the remainder protein bound. Most of the ultrafilterable magnesium is ionized. Roughly 300 mg or 25 mEq of magnesium is ingested daily in the diet. About two thirds of this amount appears in the stool and one third is eliminated in the urine. The kidney filters about 2 grams of magnesium daily, and approximately 100 mg (5 per cent) appears in the urine; thus, 95 per cent of the filtered magnesium is reabsorbed. Renal excretion of magnesium can be reduced to less than 0.5 per cent of the filtered load during magnesium deprivation. On the other hand, during infusion of magnesium or among patients with advanced chronic renal insufficiency the kidney can excrete 40 to 70 per cent of the filtered magnesium. The proximal tubules reabsorb about 20 to 30 per cent of the filtered magnesium, with 50 to 60 per cent being reabsorbed in the loop of Henle. Expansion of the ECF volume, produced by infusion of saline or chronic administration of mineralocorticoids, reduces the reabsorption of magnesium. Diets deficient in magnesium or the administration of parathyroid hormone enhance the reabsorption of magnesium in the thick ascending limb of Henle's loop. Infusions of calcium, ingestion of alcohol, administration of glucose, diets containing large amounts of magnesium, and diuretics such as furosemide or ethacrynic acid increase the urinary excretion of magnesium.

OTHER NONEXCRETORY FUNCTIONS OF THE KIDNEY

In addition to its role in the secretion of renin and the metabolism of vitamin D already discussed, the kidney has several other nonexcretory functions.

REGULATION OF THE RED BLOOD CELL MASS. *Erythropoietin* promotes the differentiation, proliferation, and maturation of red blood cell precursors in the bone marrow. The site of synthesis of this glycoprotein within the kidney has not been clearly defined, but the juxtaglomerular cells have been implicated. The stimulus to increased erythropoietin production by the kidney appears to be decreased renal oxygen tension or decreased renal perfusion (anemia, hypoxia, renal ischemia) or circulatory alterations induced by vasoconstrictors such as norepinephrine, angiotensin, or vasopressin. Increased erythropoietin levels may be seen in association with renal artery stenosis, renal cysts, renal cell carcinoma, and hydronephrosis and after renal transplantation. Production of erythropoietin decreases with hyperoxia or an excess red blood cell volume.

RENAL METABOLISM OF PLASMA PROTEINS AND PEPTIDE HORMONES. The kidney is an important catabolic site for low molecular weight proteins (less than 50,000) but not for proteins with a molecular weight exceeding 68,000 (e.g., albumin, immunoglobulins).

Low molecular weight proteins are filterable. In the absence of tubular reabsorption they would be excreted quantitatively in the urine. Reabsorption of proteins or their catabolic products by the kidney prevents their loss in the urine, thereby conserving nutritionally important components. The proteins catabolized by the kidney are broken down to amino acids or polypeptides prior to return into the renal venous blood. The kidney, therefore, contributes to the regulation of their concentrations in plasma and precludes extensive loss of protein components in the urine.

In some patients with abnormalities of renal tubular function, low molecular weight proteins may appear in the urine in the absence of albumin owing to decreased tubular reabsorption. Conversely, in patients with reduced GFR the fractional catabolic rate of low molecular weight proteins (lysozyme, ribonuclease, beta-2 microglobulins, insulin, proinsulin, gastrin, glucagon, parathyroid hormone, Bence Jones protein, retinol binding protein, and growth hormone) is decreased and their levels in plasma are elevated.

Insulin, parathyroid hormone, and glucagon are catabolized by the kidney by filtration and subsequent tubular reabsorption as well as by peritubular uptake.

The catabolism of albumin, immunoglobulins, and larger plasma proteins is relatively low, with the kidney accounting for less than 5 per cent of their fractional and catabolic rate, unless the nephrotic syndrome is present, in which case albumin catabolism could be significantly increased owing to both urinary losses and increased tubular degradation.

THE KALLIKREIN-KININ SYSTEM. Kallikrein is a peptidase produced in various tissues, including the kidney, which acts on a specific substrate (kininogen) to split off a peptide, kinin. The kinin is destroyed by plasma and tissue peptidases (kininases). Kinins are potent vasodilators. The renal kallikrein-kinin system may constitute a local hormonal mechanism involved in the regulation of renal blood flow and sodium excretion. Renal kallikrein is probably produced by the cortex and excreted into the urine. It acts on a kininogen substrate to produce the potent vasodilator decapeptide (kallidin). Kallikrein excretion is augmented by reduced sodium intake. In contrast, high sodium intake decreases it. Administration of mineralocorticoids increases the excretion of kallikrein, and the increased kallikrein excretion of a low salt diet is blocked by aldosterone antagonists (spironolactones). However, the role of the renal kallikrein system in sodium homeostasis is not yet established.

RENAL PROSTAGLANDINS. The prostaglandins are 20 carbon unsaturated fatty acids. Both vasodilator prostaglandins (PGE_2, prostacyclin, or PGI_2) and vasoconstrictor substances (thromboxanes) are synthesized in renal cortex (by arteries and glomeruli) and medulla (by interstitial and collecting duct cells) from free arachidonic acid, released from phospholipids. Renal prostaglandins may play a role in control of blood flow and in sodium and water excretion. They affect renin secretion as well. Their synthesis is stimulated by bradykinin, angiotensin II, ADH, and catecholamines. The latter substances are vasoconstrictors that tend to diminish renal plasma flow. Therefore when constrictor stimuli are operative, renal prostaglandin production may increase, resulting in maintenance of renal blood flow.

Two other pathways of arachidonic acid metabolism have been described recently in the kidney: (1) an NADPH-dependent monooxygenase pathway which leads to the formation of 19 and 20 hydroxy eicosatetranoic acid (19-HETE and 20-HETE), 19 keto-arachidonic acid, and 1,20-dicarboxylic acid; and (2) a calcium-dependent lipoxygenase pathway with synthesis of 15-HETE, 12-HETE, and leukotrienes. The physiologic or pathophysiologic importance of these pathways is unknown, but it should be remembered that the HETE's are potent chemotactic compounds and, therefore, may play a role in inflammatory glomerular disease.

Brenner BM, Ichikawa I, Deen WM: Glomerular filtration. *In* Brenner BM, Rector JC (eds.): The Kidney. 2nd ed. Philadelphia, W.B. Saunders Company, 1981, pp 289–327. *An excellent chapter written by a group of investigators responsible for most of the recent advances in our understanding of glomerular physiology.*

Burg MB: The nephron in transport of sodium, amino acids, and glucose. Hosp Pract 13:99, 1978. *An extremely well written account of the transport functions of the renal tubule.*

Dunn MJ: Renal prostaglandins. *In* Klahr S, Massry SG (eds.): Contemporary Nephrology. Volume II. New York, Plenum Publishing Company, 1983, pp. 145–192. *This chapter updates, in a lucid manner, most of the relevant information of the last two years in the area of renal prostaglandins.*

Klahr S, Peck WA: Cyclic nucleotides in bone and mineral metabolism. II. Cyclic nucleotides and the renal regulation of mineral metabolism. *In* Greengard P, Robison AG (eds.): Advances in Cyclic Nucleotide Research. Vol. 13. New York, Raven Press, 1980, pp 133–180. *A detailed review of the regulation of phosphate, calcium, and magnesium by the kidney. Numerous references.*

Stein JH: Hormones and the kidney. Hosp Pract 14:91, 1979. *An excellent article on the role of the kidney as an endocrine organ.*

Tisher CC: Anatomy of the kidney. *In* Brenner BM, Rector JC (eds.): The Kidney. 2nd ed. Philadelphia, W. B. Saunders Company, 1981, pp 1–75. *An authoritative and up-to-date review of kidney structure.*

Valtin H: Renal Function. Mechanisms Preserving Fluid and Solute Balance in Health. 2nd ed. Boston, Little, Brown and Co., 1983. *This book presents the essential elements in renal, fluid, and electrolyte physiology, which every medical student should master.*

74. MECHANISMS OF RENAL INJURY

Richard J. Glassock

The mechanisms of renal parenchymal injury are complex and diverse. They embrace abnormal immunologic processes, disturbances in coagulation, infection, biochemical and metabolic perturbations, vascular disorders, mechanical obstruction to urine flow, neoplasia, and trauma. Each mechanism may interact with another to produce disease. Various segments of the nephron, the interstitium, or the vascular tree may be the principal target of these disturbances. The clinical expression of renal injury, e.g., acute renal failure, nephrotic syndrome, hypertension, will at least in part depend upon the primary locus of injury as well as the tempo of the pathogenetic process itself. Perhaps the best understood and most thoroughly investigated of the mechanisms of renal injury are those which involve aberrant immunologic processes.

IMMUNE-MEDIATED INJURY

The majority of the glomerulonephritides are thought to be the result of immunologic processes. This conclusion is primarily based on the finding of deposits of immunoglobulin (Ig) and/or complement (C) during immunofluorescence studies of renal tissue. The importance of immunologic mechanisms in tubulointerstitial disease is also being increasingly appreciated. Several different mechanisms are recognized.

ANTI-TISSUE ANTIBODY–MEDIATED DISEASES. ***Anti-glomerular Basement Membrane Antibody Disease.*** In this circumstance, antibody, usually of the IgG class, is directed toward a *native insoluble* glomerular basement membrane (GBM) antigen believed to be a noncollagenous glycopeptide component of GBM. This antigen is uniformly and continuously distributed along the capillary wall. The antibody is usually host derived (autoantibody), but rarely the antibody may be of exogenous origin. This mechanism has been well studied in experimental animals (nephrotoxic serum nephritis). The binding of circulating antibody to the GBM antigen in situ gives rise to a "linear" pattern of deposited IgG upon immunofluorescence study of diseased renal tissue (Figs. 74–1*A* and 74–2*A*). "Linear" deposits of IgG may also occur in diseases in which anti-GBM antibody production and deposition have not yet been firmly established. For example, "linear" deposits of IgG, often accompanied by deposits of albumin in a similar distribution, frequently occur in diabetic glomerulopathy. Recovery of tissue-specific antibody activity in eluates of diseased renal tissue is a definitive test for the antibody nature of "linear" IgG deposits. As further proof, circulating anti-GBM antibodies may be detectable using indirect immunofluorescence or radioimmunoassay techniques.

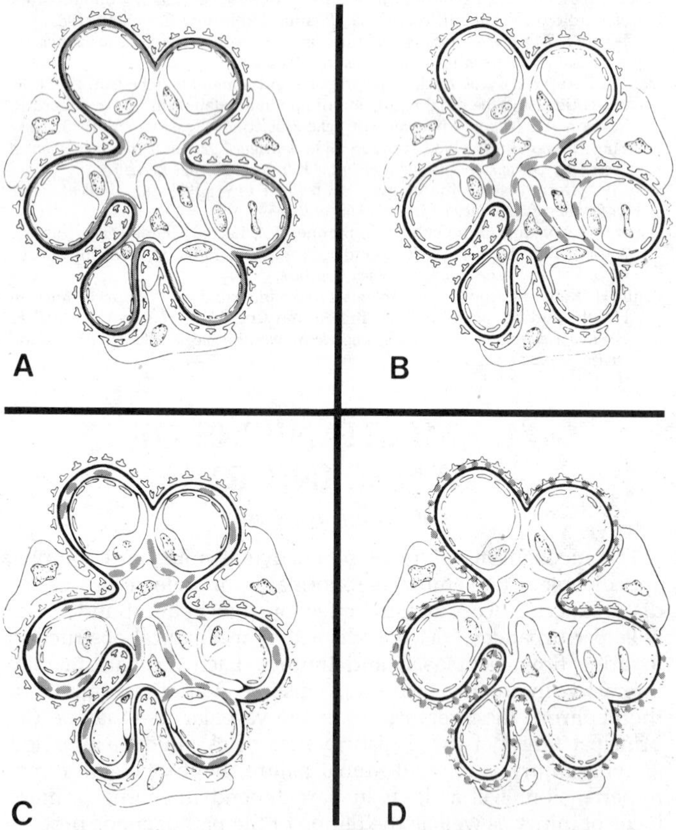

Figure 74–1. Diagrammatic representation of the pattern of immunoglobulin (Ig) deposits (by immunofluorescence) and/or electron-dense deposits (by electron microscopy) in immunologically induced glomerular disease (stippled area = immune deposit). *A, Linear* deposits of Ig along glomerular capillary walls as observed in antiglomerular basement membrane antibody disease. *B, Granular* mesangial deposits as observed in circulating or in situ immune complex–mediated disease. *C, Granular mesangial and subendothelial* deposits as observed in circulating or in situ immune complex disease. *D, Granular subepithelial* deposits as described in an in situ immune complex disease (fixed or planted glomerular antigen).

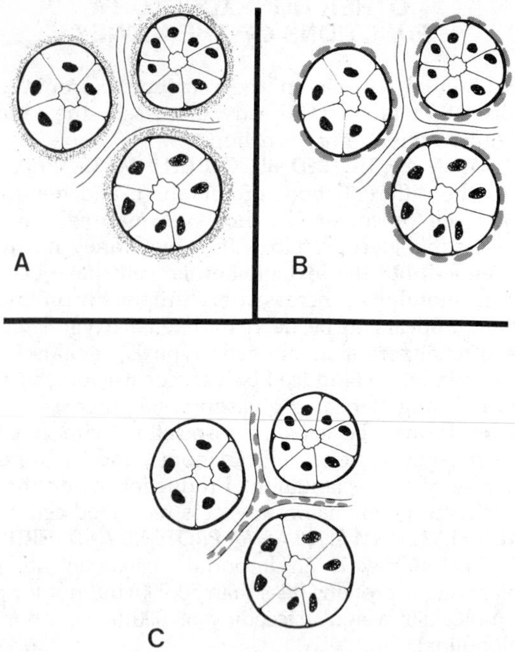

Figure 74–2. Diagrammatic representation of the patterns of immunoglobulin (Ig) deposits (by immunofluorescence) and/or electron-dense deposits (by electron microscopy) in immunologically induced tubulointerstitial disease (stippled area = immune deposit). *A, Linear* tubular basement membrane deposits as observed in antitubular basement membrane antibody–mediated nephritis. *B, Granular* tubular basement membrane deposited as observed in circulating or in situ immune complex disease. *C, Granular* peritubular capillary deposits as observed in circulating or in situ immune complex disease.

Anti-GBM antibody–mediated glomerulonephritis is uncommon, and the morphologic and clinical expression of disease varies widely. At one extreme, the glomerular lesions are explosive, consisting of extensive extracapillary proliferation (crescents), accompanied by rapidly progressive renal failure and at times by pulmonary hemorrhage (Goodpasture's syndrome). At the other end of the spectrum, very mild renal disease, sometimes detectable only by renal biopsy and immunopathologic study, may be the only manifestation of anti-GBM antibody formation. The explanation for the variation in clinical and morphologic findings is obscure. Circulating levels of antibody do not correlate well with the severity or nature of the clinical or morphologic findings. The factors that initiate antibody production are poorly understood, but susceptibility is linked to the major histocompatibility gene complex.

The classic C sequence is frequently activated via the recognition by C1q of the in situ–formed complex of anti-GBM antibody with the native tissue antigen. C activation leads to the generation of biologically active fragments with phlogistic, chemotactic, permeability-promoting, and vasoactive properties. Polymorphonuclear leukocytes and monocytes may be attracted to the sites of antibody deposition via C or Fc receptors and result in local basement membrane and cellular disruption. Sequential activation of the terminal C components may also lead to cytolysis of endothelial cells and exposure of the collagen matrix of GBM, thus resulting in localized platelet aggregation and fibrin formation. Focal disruption of the glomerular capillary wall with leakage of monocytes and fibrinogen into Bowman's space may underlie the development of crescentic disease.

Anti-tubular Basement Membrane Antibody Disease. The binding of antibody to the intrinsic antigens of tubular basement membranes (TBM) may also result in renal disease in a fashion similar to anti-GBM antibody disease. "Linear" TBM deposits of Ig may frequently be found in association with "linear" GBM deposits or in an isolated form, thus indicating that TBM contains antigens that are not necessarily shared by GBM. Circulating antibody to TBM may be found, and eluates of renal tissue have been shown to contain anti-TBM antibody activity.

The binding of antibody to TBM may elicit both acute and chronic progressive forms of tubulointerstitial nephritis. Significant mononuclear (macrophage) infiltration is often observed in such lesions. Anti-TBM antibody–mediated disease in man is relatively uncommon. Examples include the acute hypersensitivity interstitial nephritis following methicillin administration as well as other drugs and rare instances of idiopathic chronic tubulointerstitial nephritis.

Antibody to Other Native Insoluble Constituents of Glomerular or Tubular Structures. The concept of anti-tissue antibody disease has been broadened considerably by an intensive exploration in experimental models of the possible role of antigens other than the noncollagen glycopeptide GBM or TBM antigens. It is possible, even likely, that a variety of antigens exist in normal glomerular and tubular structures (e.g., basement membrane, epithelial cells, mesangium) and that an autoantibody to these antigens can lead to disease under appropriate circumstances. If these antigens are not uniformly distributed along GBM or TBM, the pattern of Ig deposition may differ substantially from that of the classic "linear" deposits found when antibody is directed to the principal GBM or TBM glycopeptide. Studies in experimental models have clearly shown that irregular or "granular" (see below) deposits of Ig within glomerular structures can arise from the in situ reaction of circulating antibody and such native glomerular antigens (Figs. 74–1*B*, *C*, *D*; 74–2*B*, *C*). Although well established in animal models, bona fide instances of this mechanism in human disease remain uncommon.

Antibody to Altered Tissue Antigens. Another form of immunologically mediated renal injury, also currently better understood in experimental animal models than in man, is that which arises when an antigen, normally extrinsic to the kidney, is bound to basement membrane or other renal structures by biochemical or immunologic reactions. The anionic nature of the biochemical constituents of the glomerular capillary wall is an important factor in the glomerular localization of these extrinsic, soluble antigens. Once bound to tissue, this antigen then serves as a focus for a host-derived immune response, one that may be directed to the bound or "planted" antigen itself, rather than to the native renal structures. Theoretically at least, native antigens that are not normally exposed to the circulation may also be uncovered by tissue injury and thus evoke a systemic antibody response. Examples of antigens that may bind to tissue include certain plant lectins, DNA, aggregated proteins, cationic macromolecules, chemically reactive drugs, and heterologous anti-GBM antibodies. Similarly, rheumatoid factor and anti-idiotypic antibody may bind to autologous Ig in glomerular immune deposits. This mechanism may account for human diseases in which Ig deposits are noted in glomerular or tubular basement membranes in the absence of circulating immune complexes or antibody to native renal antigens (Figs. 74–1*D*, 74–2*B*, *C*).

CIRCULATING IMMUNE COMPLEX–MEDIATED DISEASES. ***Glomerular Disease.*** In this category, glomerular and vascular structures of the kidney are damaged largely as a result of the deposition of circulating, *soluble* antigen-antibody complexes having no necessary immunochemical relationship to renal structures. Such immune aggregates may be formed by the reaction of antibody with any of a wide variety of soluble circulating antigens of exogenous or endogenous (autologous) origin (Table 74–1). This form of immunologic renal injury is much more common than that mediated by anti-tissue antibodies.

In order to generate soluble immune complexes, these antigens must be intrinsically immunogenic or acquire immunogenicity by an alteration in structure or binding to a carrier protein. Furthermore, the antigen must gain access to the circulation and remain for a period of time sufficient for reaction with antibody as it is formed and secreted. Immune complexes formed with multivalent antigens in *antibody excess* develop an extensive interconnecting lattice network and become essentially insoluble particulate material. Thus they readily undergo phagocytosis by the mononuclear-phagocyte system and are not available for deposition in the glomeruli or vessels of the kidney. Immune complexes formed at *equivalence or in slight antigen excess* tend to be of intermediate size, remain in solution, and localize in glomeruli and vessels. Immune complexes formed in *large antigen excess* tend to be quite small and very soluble, and to remain in the circulation for protracted periods of time with little avidity for tissue localization.

TABLE 74–1. AGENTS IMPLICATED IN HUMAN CIRCULATING IMMUNE COMPLEX–MEDIATED RENAL DISEASE

Antigens	Clinical Syndrome(s)
Exogenous	
Therapeutic agents	
Organic gold; inorganic, organic and elemental mercury, penicillamine; captopril; foreign serum proteins	Serum sickness, nephrotic syndrome
Infectious disease	
Bacteria: nephritogenic streptococci, staphylococci, *Klebsiella, Salmonella, T. pallidum, Corynebacterium, P. acnes*	Acute nephritis, nephrotic syndrome
Viruses: hepatitis B, measles, Epstein-Barr, oncornavirus (retrovirus)	Vasculitis, acute nephritis, systemic lupus erythematosus (?)
Parasites: *P. malariae, Schistosoma mansoni, Toxoplasma gondii*	Nephrotic syndrome, acute nephritis
Endogenous	
Nuclear antigens (e.g., DNA)	Systemic lupus erythematosus
Thyroglobulin	Acute neprhritis with thyroiditis
Tumor-associated antigen (e.g., carcinoembryonic antigen)	Nephrotic syndrome with malignancy of colon, breast, stomach, lung; melanoma
Immunoglobulins	Cryoimmunoglobulinemia, leukemia
Erythrocyte stroma	Glomerulonephritis and autoerythrocyte sensitization

The mechanism for glomerular or vascular deposition of circulating immune complexes is not completely understood. It may involve several important factors that are intrinsic to the immune complex itself, e.g., size, Ig class, charge, and capability to fix C and induce the liberation of permeability factors such as histamine. Other factors are renal in origin, e.g., intraglomerular pressures and flow, Fc and C receptors, and the ionic charge of the basement membrane. Circulating immune complexes may localize in various locations within the glomeruli, including the mesangium, between the endothelial cells and the GBM, within the basement membrane proper, and at the interface between visceral epithelial cells and the GBM. The precise explanation for differences in the site of deposition is not yet well understood. The size of immune complexes (a function of their antigen-antibody composition) and properties of the glomerular capillary wall itself appear to be important.

Immunofluorescent microscopy of renal tissue from patients with circulating immune complex–mediated disease reveals discontinuous, "granular" deposits (Figs. 74–1*B*, *C* and 74–2*B*, *C*) of Ig that are often accompanied by C components. The deposits also contain the relevant exogenous or endogenous antigen. This "granular" deposition of Ig and C is often taken as the hallmark of immune complex deposition, but, as previously noted, circulating antibody forming an immune complex in situ by reacting with a native insoluble or an extrinsic slanted antigen can also produce this pattern of Ig deposition. Once deposited within the glomeruli, immune complexes exist in dynamic equilibrium with circulating antigen and antibody. For example, if additional antigen is administered after an immune complex has been deposited, its solubility may be affected in such a way that the size of the deposited immune complex may decrease. Contrariwise, the size of immune complex deposits may increase further if additional antibody is administered.

Glomerular deposition of immune complexes will be relatively short lived and the disease will be potentially reversible if the source of the antigen is limited. This is best exemplified experimentally and clinically by acute serum sickness resulting from the parenteral administration of foreign (heterologous) serum protein antigens (tetanus antitoxin, snake antivenom). Initially, the administered serum proteins will equilibrate with the intra- and extravascular spaces and undergo slow metabolic degradation. Subsequently, as antibody formation and secretion begin, circulating immune complexes will be formed and the serum protein antigens will be removed from the circulation at an accelerated rate. As a balance is achieved between the amount of antigen and antibody, immune complexes will be formed and deposited in various structures, including the glomeruli, blood vessels, joints, heart valves, lung, and spleen. Serum C levels will transiently decrease. Only a very small fraction of the resultant complexes will deposit within the glomerular structures and provoke an acute inflammatory reaction. The level of circulating immune complexes will decrease as all the administered antigen is removed from the circulation and not replenished by additional injections. As antibody excess develops, the immune complexes will be increasingly removed by the mononuclear phagocyte system. Ultimately, the inflammation will subside as the deposited immune complexes are removed by phagocytosis and metabolism. Both infiltrating polymorphonuclear leukocytes and monocytes participate in the removal of immune complexes from glomerular deposits.

If antigen is administered repeatedly or if it is capable of replication (e.g., a bacterial, viral, protozoal, or autologous tissue antigen), circulating immune complexes will be maintained at a persistent but variable level. Chronic disease may develop as a function of the size and nature of the antigen, the rate of its entrance into the circulation, the availability of antibody, and the propensity of a given complex to localize in a particular area of the glomerulus. Nearly every recognized form of altered glomerular morphology can occur as a result of such chronic, immune complex–mediated disease. When the load of circulating immune complexes is great and the capacity of the mononuclear phagocyte system has been exhausted, severe glomerular destructive lesions may result. When the immune complex load is small or intermittent and the size of immune complexes favors glomerular capillary wall localization, a slowly progressive chronic disease may ensue. Substantial amounts of immune complexes may be deposited in a variety of glomerular structures without evoking a clinically recognizable renal disease. Humoral and cellular mediator systems similar to those described for anti-GBM antibody disease may be involved in tissue injury. Monocyte infiltration of the glomerulus is an important mediator of injury.

Tubulointerstitial Disease. The tubulointerstitial areas of the kidney may be involved in immune complex–mediated disease. Granular deposits of Ig and C components may be found along and within the TBM or peritubular capillaries in a variety of diseases. In most instances, similar granular deposits are found in the glomerular capillaries, but tubule-associated deposits of Ig alone can occur occasionally. It is not well understood whether TBM and peritubular capillary deposits occur as a result of "spillover" from the glomerular circulation or because of the diffusion of antigens from the tubule cells toward the circulation with a resultant interaction with circulating antibody and local formation of immune complexes in situ.

COMPLEMENT ACTIVATION–ASSOCIATED GLOMERULONEPHRITIS. In recent years a new group of glomerular disorders has been defined largely on the basis of association with prominent or isolated glomerular deposition of C3 or abnormalities of circulating levels of complement components, or both. Although the precise pathogenetic relationship of these phenomena to tissue injury has not been well established, it seems appropriate to consider them under the category of immunologically mediated glomerular diseases. The morphologic lesion typically associated with C activation is *membranoproliferative glomerulonephritis* (MPGN). This lesion is characterized by proliferation of mesangial cells with thickening of the peripheral capillary wall owing to the interposition of mesangial cells. Under some circumstances, MPGN may be associated with glomerular C3 deposition without immunoglobulin deposition. Isolated C3 deposition may also occur in the absence of deposits of early-acting C components such as C1q, C4, and C2, thus suggesting involvement of the alternative pathway of C activation. In many cases isolated glomerular C3 deposition is accompanied by a distinct reduction of the plasma C3 level, with normal levels of C1q and C4, abnormal circulating levels of breakdown products of C3 and factors of the alternative pathway, increased C3 turnover, decreased C3 synthesis, and the presence of a circulating factor capable of cleaving native C3 in vitro (C3 nephritic factor or NF). Such NF is now known to be an autoantibody to the C3 convertase enzyme of the alternative pathway. Many but not all cases revealing this pattern of complement abnormalities demonstrate a unique ultrastructural lesion, consisting of transformation of the renal basement membranes into an extremely electron-dense structure (dense deposit disease).

Since it has proved difficult to demonstrate experimentally that prolonged activation of C via the alternative pathway per se leads to glomerular damage, the demonstrable C abnormalities may be an epiphenomenon of a more basic but as yet obscure pathogenetic mechanism. Perhaps a pre-existing deficiency of C components may lead to defective mechanisms for processing potentially immunogenic environmental agents and thus predispose to the development of an immune complex–mediated renal disease. Such an explanation, however, could not account for the absence of immunoglobulin deposits in many of these lesions. Furthermore, several of the C components are determined by genes of the major histocompatibility complex (MHC) on chromosome 6. It is possible that the C abnormalities may be associated with certain genes in the immune response region of the MHC. This may predispose to aberrant immune responses to a variety of environmental or autologous tissue antigens.

CELL-MEDIATED IMMUNITY. The role of cell-mediated immunity (CMI) is well established in the rejection of human renal allografts, which serves as the prototype for this mechanism of renal injury. In allograft rejection, a subclass of T cells (cytotoxic T cells) specifically sensitized to tissue alloantigens of the donor interacts to result in tissue damage. Insofar as other glomerular, vascular, and tubulointerstitial diseases are concerned, a *primary* role of CMI is far from established. Nonetheless, largely as a result of work with experimental animals, it seems likely that many renal parenchymal diseases have a component of cell-mediated injury. In vitro studies have demonstrated such cell-mediated immunity to a variety of normal or altered tissue antigens in renal disease. These in vitro studies cannot be used to prove cause and effect relationships. Infiltration of the renal parenchyma by lymphocytes and monocytes cannot be taken as an index of involvement of CMI, as similar infiltrates may be observed in lesions unquestionably induced by humoral or nonimmune mechanisms. However, certain tubulointerstitial diseases in man have prominent morphologic hallmarks of CMI and occur in the absence of other signs of humoral immunity. Monocytes infiltrating damaged glomeruli have potentially injurious effects.

It is possible that the structure and function of the kidney might be altered by cell-mediated processes without a direct cell-tissue interaction. Lymphocytes and monocytes are known to exert profound effects on the function of other cells and organs by virtue of their ability to secrete biologically active materials known as *lymphokines* and *monokines*. These substances exert potent cellular effects such as activation of proliferation, cell aggregation, fibrogenesis, inhibition of growth, and cytotoxicity. It is tempting to speculate that such secretory products may produce structural or functional glomerular alterations under some circumstances.

A possible candidate for the involvement of cell-mediated immunity in glomerular disease is the *minimal change lesion* category of idiopathic nephrotic syndrome. This disorder is characterized by recurring episodes of heavy proteinuria. It is characterized morphologically by optically normal or minimally altered glomeruli, absence of Ig and C deposits, and diffuse effacement of the epithelial cell foot processes. An identical lesion may be found in Hodgkin's disease. A variety of studies have demonstrated in vitro abnormalities in CMI in the minimal change lesion. Lymphocytes may secrete permeability-promoting factors. Although these observations have led to some speculations, proof of a pivotal role of CMI in the pathogenesis of this disorder is lacking.

COAGULATION-INDUCED INJURY

A role of intrarenal vascular coagulation in renal disease is suggested by several lines of evidence: (1) the histochemical, ultrastructural, or immunofluorescent demonstration of proteins related to fibrinogen or fibrin (fibrin-related antigens, FRA) within the diseased glomeruli or vascular structures; (2) production of renal lesions by the induction of intravascular coagulation; (3) accelerated turnover of fibrinogen and/or platelets; (4) accumulation of fibrin or fibrinogen degradation products (FDP) in the serum and/or increased excretion of FDP in the urine in renal disease; and (5) a beneficial effect of pharmacologic agents affecting coagulation on the morphology or clinical expression of renal diseases.

Much of the evidence supporting a pathogenic role for coagulation in renal disease has been generated from studies of the Shwartzman-Sanarelli phenomenon in animals. This phenomenon is induced by giving two injections of bacterial endotoxin 18 hours apart. The first injection primes the animal, and the second injection is followed by massive disseminated intravascular coagulation (DIC) with extensive thrombosis in the vascular tree and the glomerular capillary bed. Under some circumstances DIC may occur with a single injection of endotoxin (e.g., in pregnant and corticosteroid-treated animals). It is presumed that endotoxin disrupts the endothelial surfaces and leads to the activation of clotting factors and platelet aggregation. Endotoxin may also diminish glomerular fibrinolytic activity. The Shwartzman-Sanarelli reaction is polymorphonuclear leukocyte dependent but it does not require a fully active C system. Vasoconstriction plays a role in the development of renal lesions, because adrenergic blockade and inhibition of angiotensin are protective. Low grade or intermittent intravascular coagulation may result in the development of morphologic glomerular lesions which encompass the entire spectrum seen in glomerulonephritis, with the possible exception of membranous glomerulopathy.

Extensive interrelationships exist between coagulation, the immune system, and complement. The activation of factor XII (Hageman factor) also induces fibrinolysis, kinin generation, and activation of the first component of complement (C1). Plasmin generated in the process of fibrinolysis may also cleave C3 into C3b and C3a and thus initiate late-acting complement component activation via the alternative pathway. Antigen-antibody complexes that have fixed C1q or contain bacterial antigens can directly activate factor XII and thus initiate the intrinsic pathway of coagulation. Immune complexes may interact with basophils and platelets and lead to the aggregation and release of potentially inflammatory substances that facilitate the tissue localization of immune complexes. The fixation of antibodies on the glomerular basement membrane or the deposition of immune complexes in the glomerular capillary bed may disrupt the endothelial surface and expose the collagenous matrix of GBM to the circulation, leading to factor XII activation or platelet aggregation.

The use of anticoagulants in experimental immunologic glomerular disease has led to conflicting results. Early studies employing mild forms of nephritis indicated a beneficial effect;

however, more recent studies have indicated that anticoagulants (heparin or warfarin) have little effect in severe anti-GBM– and immune complex–mediated nephritis. Ancrod, a product of the pit viper venom which leads to fibrinogen lysis, seems to lead to better preservation of renal function in experimental anti-GBM– and immune complex–mediated glomerulonephritis. The interaction of infiltrating monocytes and localized coagulation within Bowman's spaces is a likely mechanism for the development of extracapillary proliferative (crescentic) glomerulonephritis.

The features of a number of disorders do indicate that intrarenal vascular coagulation may play a dominant role in their genesis. Examples include the hemolytic-uremic syndrome (childhood, adult, and postpartum forms), thrombotic thrombocytopenic purpura, and hyperacute or accelerated renal allograft rejection. Intrarenal vascular coagulation may also be involved in the renal injury observed in scleroderma, malignant hypertension, acute renal failure (acute tubular necrosis), and toxemia of pregnancy.

TOXIN-MEDIATED INJURY

Toxic nephropathy may be defined as a renal alteration produced by a chemical or biologic product or its metabolites. In the broadest sense, the term encompasses toxins of exogenous origin (e.g., lead, mercury, antibiotics), the toxic effect of abnormal concentrations of endogenous metabolites (e.g., oxalate, myoglobin, hemoglobin, uric acid), and the damaging effects of physical agents (e.g., x-ray, heat). A classification of the major nephrotoxins is given in Table 74–2. The major mechanisms of toxin-induced injury include (1) direct cellular toxicity, including cell necrosis and interference with normal metabolic function; (2) obstruction to urine flow owing to intraluminal crystallization or precipitation; (3) deposition of crystalline material in tubulointerstitial areas, leading to chronic inflammation; and (4) alteration of the renal macro- and microcirculation, including formation of glomerular ultrafiltrate. In addition, certain agents exert their toxic effect via hypersensitivity mechanisms, as discussed above.

Certain properties of the kidneys render them particularly vulnerable to toxic injury—namely, a high blood flow–tissue mass ratio, an extensive endothelial surface area, a countercurrent mechanism for urine concentration leading to a high medullary solute concentration, transcellular transport, alterations in pH and ionic composition in the distal nephron, ionic charge of GBM and tubular lumina, and the ultrafiltering capacity of the glomerular capillary wall. These properties play an important role in determining the distribution of lesions

TABLE 74–2. CLASSIFICATION OF MAJOR NEPHROTOXINS

Exogenous
Metals
Mercury, gold, silver, arsenic, lead, cadmium, uranium, lithium salts
Solvents
Carbon tetrachloride and other halogenated hydrocarbons, ethylene glycol
Diagnostic agents
Iodinated x-ray contrast media
Therapeutic agents
Antimicrobials (aminoglycosides, amphotericin B, sulfonamides)
Analgesics (phenacetin, aspirin)
Anesthetics (methoxyflurane)
Hormones (vitamin D)
Antineoplastics (methotrexate, cis-platinum, cyclophosphamide)
X-irradiation
Miscellaneous
Elemental phosphorus, venoms, mushrooms, fluoride
Endogenous
Uric acid
Oxalate
Pigments (myoglobin, hemoglobin)
Bence Jones protein
Hormones (e.g., parathyroid hormone)

seen after toxin exposure. Acute renal failure and chronic tubulointerstitial nephritis are common manifestations of toxin-mediated injury.

Several illustrative examples of toxic nephropathy may be cited. Excessive consumption of analgesic compounds leads to necrotizing lesions initially confined to the renal papilla. The concentration of analgesics and metabolites in the lumina and interstitium of the papilla is increased by the countercurrent multiplication system. The relatively anaerobic environment of the deeper zones of the medulla and papilla contributes to their vulnerability in this form of toxic nephropathy. Uric acid may crystallize in the distal nephron under conditions of high concentration and low pH. Such aggregates may lead to intranephronal obstruction and renal injury. High concentrations of urate or oxalate salts in the interstitial areas lead to crystallization and inflammatory changes. Some toxic agents, including nephrotoxic antimicrobials, halogenated hydrocarbons, and heavy metals, lead to a disturbance in formation of glomerular ultrafiltrate, in addition to exerting direct toxic effects on the tubule cells. The propensity for direct tubular cell injury of some of these compounds may be related to binding to cell membrane constituents or interference with intracellular metabolic machinery (e.g., mitochondrial injury). Enhanced entry of calcuim into intracellular pools may represent a final common pathway of cell injury in toxic- and ischemia-induced tubular cell necrosis.

INFECTION-MEDIATED INJURY

Infections of the kidney and urinary tract lead to renal injury in a variety of ways. Direct invasion of renal tissue by organisms and the release of endotoxins or exotoxins result in direct tissue damage. The calling forth of cellular elements of inflammation leads to the localization of infection and to the formation of abscesses which may enlarge and compress adjacent renal tissue. Localized release of proteases and other enzymes by the invading leukocytes may lead to the disruption of normal renal architecture, alterations of the renal microcirculation, and frank tissue necrosis. Vascular lesions induced by acute infections may ultimately lead to chronic ischemic changes. Urinary tract infection may interfere with normal urinary flow dynamics, thus predisposing to the stagnation of urine and stone formation. The integrity of the vesicoureteral valve may be altered by infection, thus leading to a free reflux of bladder urine and a high ureteric pressure during voiding, with pressure-induced changes in the calyceal architecture (see below). Certain infections, primarily tuberculosis, are noted for their tendency to produce stenosis and obstruction in the upper urinary tract. Furthermore, some organisms (*Proteus* species) may degrade urinary urea into ammonia and CO_2, leading to a chronically elevated urinary pH and ammonia concentration. This alteration in urine composition predisposes to crystallization of magnesium–ammonium phosphate stones (struvite or infection stones), which may subsequently aggregate into casts of the caliceal system (staghorn calculi) and lead to significant degrees of obstruction and renal parenchymal damage. Infection of the urinary tract may lead to interference with certain specialized functions of the kidney, most notably the ability to excrete maximally concentrated urine following water deprivation. Chronic bacterial infection of the urinary tract in the absence of associated disease (such as diabetes mellitus, analgesic abuse, or outflow obstruction) seldom leads to progressive parenchymal disease.

Remote infection of a viral, bacterial, protozoal, or helminthic nature (e.g., visceral abscesses, infective endocarditis, chronic hepatitis B, malaria, or toxoplasmosis) may result in renal damage indirectly by the formation of circulating immune complexes. These may deposit in the glomerular and vascular structures to evoke an array of morphologic changes and clinical syndromes.

HEREDITARY, BIOCHEMICAL, AND METABOLIC INJURY

Disordered biochemical and metabolic processes may lead to renal injury. These abnormalities may be the result of defective or excessive synthesis of a normal or abnormal structural component of renal tissue, the abnormal accumulation of metabolites in the kidney, or defects in the tubular transport or renal excretion of endogenous metabolites. Such alterations are frequently observed in the heredofamilial renal diseases. For example, *diabetes mellitus* is commonly complicated by progressive renal disease. These lesions are the consequence of the abnormal diabetic milieu, at least in part. The biochemical counterpart of the structural change seen in diabetic glomerular disease, i.e., increased thickness of the capillary basement membrane and increased production of mesangial matrix, is unknown. *Alport's syndrome* (hereditary nephritis and deafness) may be another example of a biochemical lesion specifically affecting the structure and function of basement membranes. In this disease, renal basement membranes display a variety of ultrastructural lesions, perhaps as a result of abnormal GBM synthesis or degradation.

Excessive accumulation of normal metabolites in the kidneys may at times result in damage. *Fabry's disease*, an X-linked lipid storage disease resulting from a generalized deficiency of ceramide trihexosidase (α-galactosidase A), leads to the deposition of a glycosphingolipid in the endothelial wall of vessels and in the epithelial cells of glomeruli. Deposition of *amyloid* in glomeruli may be another example of accumulation of an abnormal substance leading to disease. In *cystinosis*, the amino acid cystine accumulates in cells of the mononuclear-phagocyte system and the proximal tubule and in leukocytes. Such storage, or an independent but associated defect, leads to an anatomic lesion of the proximal tubule and disturbance of many functions of the proximal tubule such as glucose, phosphate, uric acid, and amino acid reabsorption.

Disordered transport of amino acids may lead to renal injury. For example, defective transport of cystine and basic amino acids in kidneys and intestines may lead to excessive excretion of poorly soluble cystine in the urine. Cystine crystalluria ensues and may ultimately be associated with urinary obstruction, infection, and renal parenchymal damage. In disorders of uric acid metabolism, salts of uric acid may accumulate in the interstitium of the kidney and provoke chronic interstitial nephritis or uric acid may crystallize within the tubule and cause obstruction.

Excessive excretion of the products of endocrine glands may result in renal damage from time to time. For example, nephrocalcinosis not uncommonly complicates primary hyperparathyroidism. Excessive elaboration of ACTH may lead to serious renal potassium wastage and kaliopenic nephropathy.

Although the mechanisms responsible for *cystic diseases* of the kidney are still largely unknown, they constitute an important group of hereditary disorders of the kidney and as such are likely to be the result of some biochemical defect. *Polycystic kidney disease* occurs in two forms. The adult form, transmitted as an autosomal dominant trait, is usually recognized in the fourth or fifth decade of life. The childhood form, transmitted as an autosomal recessive trait, is usually recognized in infancy. In adult polycystic kidney disease, the cysts are variable in size and involve the medullary collecting ducts and the cortical convoluted tubules. Cystic changes in the liver and pancreas and aneurysms of the cerebral circulation are associated abnormalities. In the childhood form, fusiform dilatation of the distal nephron occurs, leading to a relatively uniform array of cysts. Associated lesions include periportal hepatic fibrosis and biliary duct ectasia. Cysts chiefly involving the medulla are seen in the relatively benign *medullary sponge kidney*, in which cystic ectasia is present only at the tip of the papilla. By contrast, *medullary cystic disease*, occurring as either an autosomal dominant or recessive trait, pursues a relentlessly progressive course. In the latter disorder cysts are present throughout the medulla and at the cortical medullary junction, in association with progressive interstitial fibrosis and tubular atrophy of the outer cortex.

VASCULAR INJURY

Lesions of the renal circulation which lead to impairment of blood flow to renal tissue, if slowly developing and incomplete, may result in ischemic atrophy of the renal parenchyma and progressive interstitial and glomerular sclerosis. If they are rapid and complete, then tissue necrosis (e.g., acute tubular necrosis, infarction) develops. Such lesions may occur at any level of the renal circulation and may be bilateral or unilateral. They may be the result of an inflammatory disturbance (frequently immunologic or infectious in nature), the result of intrarenal vascular coagulation, secondary to embolization by clot or atheromatous debris, or due to poorly understood mechanisms often associated with chronically elevated arterial pressure and leading to endothelial proliferation, muscular hypertrophy, and luminal obliteration. *Functional* alterations in the renal microcirculation may underlie acute renal failure associated with toxin exposure or ischemic episodes. Weakening of the wall of vessels because of damage to elastic lamina may predispose to aneurysm formation. Impaired blood flow may also be due to alterations in the rheologic properties of blood (e.g., sickle cell disease, hyperviscosity) and not to intrinsic vascular disease. Sickle cell disease and trait may be associated with renal injury primarily because of chronic or recurring disturbance of the renal circulation, principally in the medulla. The erythrocytes containing S hemoglobin may undergo sickle transformation during passage through the relatively hypoxic and hyperosmolar environment of the medulla, thus leading to a disturbance in the medullary circulation and to the impairment of the function of the deeper nephrons largely responsible for maximal urinary concentrating ability. At times the disturbance in the medullary circulation may be so severe as to lead to papillary necrosis.

OBSTRUCTIVE INJURY

Any process which impedes the normal flow of urine has the potential of inflicting renal injury. Intrarenal obstruction may occur consequent to crystallization or precipitation of urinary solutes (e.g., uric acid, Bence Jones proteins) or from extrinsic compression (e.g., edema, cysts). Extrarenal obstruction may be unilateral or bilateral and may develop at any site from the pelvocalyceal system to the tip of the urethra. Such obstruction may be consequent to a variety of conditions intrinsic (e.g., tumors, stones) or extrinsic (e.g., retroperitoneal fibrosis) to the urinary tract.

If obstruction to urine flow is abrupt, complete, and proximal to the ureterovesical junction, the formation of glomerular ultrafiltrate will practically cease, and pressures within the nephron usually will not rise above the difference between intraglomerular hydraulic pressure and the systemic oncotic pressure. Permanent injury will not occur if such obstruction is relieved promptly and infection is absent. Longstanding obstruction leads to tubular atrophy and interstitial fibrosis with irreversible loss of renal function.

Slowly developing partial obstruction leads to progressive dilatation of the urinary tract and, depending upon the compliance of the system, less transmission of elevated pressure to the nephron. Nonetheless, chronic partial obstruction leads to defects in specific functions of the kidney, such as urinary concentrating ability and acidification. Progressive dilatation of the pelvocalyceal system and complicating infection ultimately lead to a loss of renal parenchyma. These changes begin in the deeper cortical nephrons and extend later to the outer cortex.

NEOPLASTIC INJURY

Under many circumstances the mechanism of neoplasm-induced renal injury is direct and obvious. Thus primary renal neoplasms (e.g., renal cell carcinoma) destroy parenchyma by direct invasion, interference with blood supply, or compression of adjacent normal tissue. Neoplasms originating at distant sites (metastatic carcinoma, lymphoma, leukemia) may also involve and damage renal tissue. Obstruction to urine flow may result from tumors originating at any site in the urinary tract.

Renal injury consequent to neoplastic disease may also be less obvious and indirect. Thus renal disease may result from the excessive elaboration by tumors of substances capable of inflicting tissue injury (e.g., parathyroid hormone, Bence Jones protein, precursors of uric acid). As previously noted, antibody responses to tumor-associated antigens may also lead to formation of potentially damaging circulating immune complexes.

Cotran RS, Penington JE: Urinary tract infection, pyelonephritis and reflux nephropathy. *In* Brenner B, Rector F (eds.): The Kidney. 2nd ed. Philadelphia, W. B. Saunders Company, 1981, pp 1571–1632. *A broad overview of mechanisms of urinary tract infection–induced renal injury.*

Heptinstall RH: Pathology of the Kidney, 3rd ed. Boston, Little, Brown, & Co., 1983. *The definitive text on the pathologic manifestations of renal injury by diverse mechanisms. A classic work by an internationally recognized expert.*

Kincaid-Smith P: The Kidney: A Clinico-Pathological Study. Oxford, Blackwell, 1975, pp 205–259. *An excellent overview of the role of coagulation and vascular injury in pathogenesis of renal disease.*

Leaf A, Cheung JY, Mills JW, Bonventre JV. Nature of the insult in acute renal failure. *In* Brenner B, Lazarus M (eds.): Acute Renal Failure. Philadelphia, W. B. Saunders Company, 1983, pp 2–20. *An excellent and comprehensive review of the fundamental aspects of ischemic injury to the kidney.*

Mudge G, Duggin GG (eds.): Drug effects on the kidney. Kidney Int 18:539–713, 1980. *A collection of papers dealing with various aspects of drug-related toxic effects on the kidney.*

Rieselbach RE, Garnick MB (eds.): Cancer and the Kidney. Philadelphia, Lea and Febiger, 1982. *The definitive text on cancer-related renal injury.*

Wilson CB, Dixon FJ: The renal response to immunologic injury. *In* Brenner B, Rector F (eds.): The Kidney. 2nd ed. Philadelphia, W. B. Saunders Company, 1981, pp 1237–1350. *A definitive review of the immunologic mechanisms of renal injury.*

Wright FS, Howards SS: Obstructive injury. *In* Brenner B, Rector F (eds.): The Kidney. 2nd ed. Philadelphia, W. B. Saunders Company, 1981, pp 2000–2044. *A detailed review of the fundamental aspects of renal injury consequent to urinary tract obstruction.*

75. INVESTIGATIONS OF RENAL FUNCTION

Vincent W. Dennis

Specific methods are available to assess the functional integrity of the glomerular ultrafiltration barrier, the presence of urogenital inflammation, the overall rate of glomerular filtration, the ability to dilute, concentrate or acidify urine, and the ability to conserve or to excrete specific solutes. Measurements of certain values in blood and urine may identify the presence of abnormalities in renal function and may occasionally diagnose specific etiologies, but a final diagnosis usually requires direct or indirect visualization of the kidneys and urogenital system or morphologic examination of renal tissue.

PROTEINURIA. Increased urinary excretion of protein is one of the most common and most easily detected signs of renal disease. The normal excretion rate of urinary protein is less than 150 mg per 24 hours for adults, but values as high as 300 mg per 24 hours may occur in apparently healthy adolescents. The normal composition of urinary protein includes about 40 per cent albumin, 40 per cent tissue proteins originating from renal and other urogenital tissues, 15 per cent immunoglobulins and their fragments, and 5 per cent other plasma proteins. Abnormalities may occur in both the quantity and the composition of urinary proteins.

Historically, the detection of increased amounts of urinary protein relied on the formation of a coagulum or turbidity upon exposure of urine to heat or to strong acid. Now urinary protein is usually detected by a colorimetric test ("dipstick test"), which depends on the ability of proteins, especially albumin, to alter the color reaction of a pH-sensitive dye. Such qualitative tests may detect protein concentrations as low as 15 mg per deciliter and result in a positive test if a normal amount of protein is

TABLE 75–1. MECHANISMS OF PROTEINURIA (> 150 mg per 24 hours)

1. Overflow proteinuria	
	Light-chains of immunoglobulins (Bence Jones)
	Myoglobin
	Hemoglobin
2. Increased glomerular permeability	
	Selective pattern; mostly albumin
	Nonselective pattern; albumin plus higher molecular weight proteins
3. Tubular proteinuria	
	Beta-2-microglobulin
	Other plasma proteins < 20,000 daltons
4. Altered renal hemodynamics	
	Exercise, fever, seizures, vasoactive drugs, etc.

present in a concentrated volume of urine. Conversely, abnormal rates of protein excretion may remain undetected in large volumes of dilute urine. It is therefore important to have some estimate of the degree of urine concentration when considering the significance of a positive qualitative test for protein. A positive qualitative test for urinary protein usually warrants more accurate measurement of the absolute protein excretion rate per 24 hours and, if elevated, consideration of the full range of factors that alter the amount and composition of urinary protein. Proteinuria usually results from: (1) elevated plasma concentration of normal or abnormal proteins, (2) increased glomerular permeability, (3) decreased tubular reabsorption of normally filtered proteins, and (4) alterations in renal hemodynamics (Table 75–1).

Overflow Proteinuria. Changes in plasma protein concentrations may alter the rates of protein excretion by both the normal and the abnormal kidney. This type of proteinuria may occur from the presence in plasma of increased concentrations of proteins not normally present in significant amounts. Examples include light-chain immunoglobulin fragments such as Bence Jones protein associated with plasma cell disorders (see Ch. 163) or myoglobin associated with rhabdomyolysis. The presence of increased concentrations of abnormal proteins in either plasma or urine may be confirmed by electrophoresis. Changes in the concentration of normal plasma proteins may also influence passage across the *abnormal* glomerular capillary wall. For example, increases or decreases in the plasma concentration of albumin may increase or decrease its rate of urinary excretion without necessarily indicating improvement or worsening of the renal conditions that led to proteinuria.

Increased Glomerular Permeability. The glomerular capillary wall consists of capillary endothelium, basement membrane, visceral epithelium, and mesangium. Each of these four anatomic components contributes directly or indirectly to the formation and maintenance of the functional ultrafiltration barrier that limits the passage of proteins into the urinary space. The glomerular capillary wall restricts the passage of plasma proteins according to their size (steric hindrance) and surface charge (electrostatic hindrance). Specifically, the glomerular capillary wall restricts, to increasing degrees, molecules of increasing size. Also, at any given molecular size, negative charges on the glomerular capillary basement membrane hinder the passage of negatively charged molecules more than positively charged molecules.

A number of systemic and primary renal diseases may affect one or more glomerular structures and thereby increase the effective permeability of the glomerular capillary wall to proteins. Under these conditions, the degree of proteinuria may range from 0.2 to greater than 20 grams per 24 hours. Proteinuria that exceeds about 3 to 5 grams of normal plasma protein per 24 hours provides direct evidence of increased effective permeability of the glomerular capillary wall, since these amounts exceed those that may be filtered by the normal glomerulus and reabsorbed by the renal tubules. Such massive losses of plasma proteins may be responsible for changes in plasma oncotic pressure and thereby set in motion the events that are manifest clinically as the nephrotic syndrome (see Ch. 80).

Because of its low molecular weight and its dominance among plasma proteins, albumin is typically the major urinary protein in this type of proteinuria. However, the relative proportion of albumin in the urine, even if corrected for changes in its proportion in plasma, is lower in some forms of renal diseases than in others. *Selective proteinuria* refers to the ability of the glomerulus to retain higher molecular weight proteins despite increased filtration of low molecular weight proteins. A highly selective proteinuria therefore consists almost exclusively of increased excretion of albumin, whereas a poorly selective proteinuria contains proportionately greater amounts of higher molecular weight proteins and is generally associated with severe disruption of the glomerular capillary wall. This selectivity may be attributed to the glomerulus only if the composition of urinary proteins is not affected significantly by downstream events such as tubular reabsorption. This requirement is presumably met with levels of proteinuria that exceed 3 to 5 grams per 24 hours, but the selectivity pattern of lesser amounts of proteinuria may be significantly influenced by tubular reabsorption. To define glomerular selectivity requires measurements of the relative clearances of specific proteins with increasing molecular weights such as albumin (69,000), transferrin (90,000), gamma globulin (150,000), and alpha-2-glycoprotein (820,000). Although attractive in theory and potentially useful as an index of the severity of glomerular damage, the techniques required to characterize the selectivity of proteinuria are generally too laborious and too imprecise to have achieved widespread clinical applicability. Nevertheless, heavy proteinuria characterized by the dominance of albumin and the absence of higher molecular weight globulins is typical of minimal change or nil lesion (see Ch. 80), whereas the detection of a nonselective pattern is highly suggestive of the presence of some other form of otherwise undefined glomerular disease.

Tubular Proteinuria. Many polypeptides and low molecular weight proteins normally present in plasma are filtered freely at the glomerulus and are reabsorbed by the tubules. Examples include polypeptide hormones such as insulin, glucagon, and parathyroid hormone and plasma proteins smaller than 20,000 daltons. Once filtered, these proteins are absorbed by specific endocytic processes that bind and engulf the filtered proteins. The presence of tubular disorders, especially injuries that result from various antibiotics or heavy metals (see Ch. 81), may be associated with increased urinary excretion of low molecular weight proteins and relatively slight increases in the excretion of albumin (*tubular proteinuria*). This pattern is in marked contrast to the predominance of albumin in the urine of patients with glomerular disorders. Patients characterized clinically as having tubulointerstitial rather than glomerular diseases have increased urine protein excretion (generally less than 2 grams per 24 hours) and increased renal clearance of beta-2-microglobulin, especially relative to albumin. The presence of increased clearance of beta-2-microglobulin, which can be measured by a relatively simple, commercially available radioimmunoassay, suggests impaired function of the renal tubule such as might occur after exposure to heavy metals or to certain antibiotics. Beta-2-microglobulinuria is less likely to occur in those disease processes such as diabetes mellitus that cause proteinuria via effects on glomerular permeability. The clinical significance of tubular proteinuria is unclear at this time because there is still insufficient documentation of correlations between tubular proteinuria and detailed functional, biochemical, and morphologic descriptions of the underlying diseases in which it has been observed.

Proteinuria from Altered Renal Hemodynamics. Changes in protein excretion rate may also occur in response to changes in renal hemodynamics. Exercise, major motor seizures, change to the standing position, fever, and vasoactive agents such as renin, angiotensin, and norepinephrine increase urine protein excretion by mechanisms that seem related to reductions in renal blood flow. Changes in renal blood flow may alter urine protein excretion in normal subjects as well as in those with abnormal rates of protein excretion. The mechanisms by which changes in renal hemodynamics might increase protein excretion include local increases in protein concentration within the glomerular capillary, increased effective permeability of the glomerular capillary wall, increased transglomerular hydrostatic pressure, or increased effective filtration area. Hemodynamic increases in urine protein excretion are generally transient or additive to other causes of proteinuria.

LEUKOCYTURIA. The urinary leukocyte excretion rate in apparently healthy individuals ranges between 0 and 300,000 leukocytes per hour; rates greater than 400,000 per hour are generally regarded as abnormal. If appropriate cleansing precautions are used, there is no difference in leukocyte excretion rates between apparently healthy males and females or between urine samples obtained from suprapubic puncture and midstream urine.

In practice, leukocyte excretion rates are estimated indirectly by microscopic examination of urinary sediment resuspended after centrifugation of approximately 10 ml of urine. Abnormal leukocyturia probably exists when more than five white blood cells occur per high-power field. However, about 20 per cent of urine specimens from patients excreting more than 400,000 white blood cells per hour may demonstrate fewer than five leukocytes per high-power field. The indirect method thus underestimates the prevalence of abnormal leukocyturia, although increased numbers of white blood cells per high-power field appear to correspond well to increased rates of leukocyte excretion.

The disintegration of urinary leukocytes is accelerated in the presence of dilute, alkaline urine maintained at or near body temperature. Conversely, leukocytes are preserved in acid, concentrated urine that is refrigerated or maintained at room temperature. Coexistent proteinuria may also help preserve urinary leukocytes. Leukocyturia results frequently from urinary tract infection (see Ch. 85) but may also indicate other causes of inflammation such as tubulointerstitial diseases (see Ch. 81).

HEMATURIA. The detection of hematuria is aided by the widespread use of the multifunctional "dipstick," which includes a section impregnated with orthotolidine. The test is sufficiently sensitive to detect the equivalent of greater than 10,000 red blood cells per milliliter of urine but is negative in normal individuals despite the wide range of red blood cell excretion rates. A positive orthotolidine test may also occur in the presence of free hemoglobin or myoglobin in urine. Free hemoglobin in the urine generally results from the lysis of red blood cells in the urine, but may also reflect free hemoglobin in the plasma. When indicated, this question can be resolved by direct measurements of plasma hemoglobin and haptoglobin concentrations. Myoglobin in the urine is detected by the differential precipitation of hemoglobin with ammonium sulfate, by spectrophotometry of the ferricyanide derivatives of hemoglobin and myoglobin, by the co-migration on paper electrophoresis of myoglobin with hemoglobin C, or, preferably, by direct immunoassay of myoglobin in plasma or urine.

As with leukocytes, the presence of red blood cells in urine is quantified in terms of red blood cells per high-power field and is normally 0 to 1 in males but may be slightly higher in females. Nevertheless, the persistent presence in males or females of even small numbers of red blood cells in urine is cause for concern and may indicate the presence of a coagulopathy, hemoglobinopathy, renal parenchymal disease, tumor, trauma, or inflammation anywhere along the renal and urinary tract. Hematuria accompanied by proteinuria generally indicates renal parenchymal disease.

GLOMERULAR FILTRATION RATE. Measurements of glomerular filtration rate are used clinically largely as estimates of the mass of functional renal tissue or of the number of functioning nephrons. To be useful in the measure of glomerular filtration rate, a substance should be filtered freely at the glomerulus and not secreted, reabsorbed, catabolized, or synthesized by the kidney. The substance should be harmless, inexpensive, and easy to administer and measure accurately. A number of exogenous substances fulfill some of these requirements, but there is no ideal material of endogenous origin. Overall, however, the most useful indicators of glomerular filtration rate are measurements of *creatinine clearance* and *plasma creatinine concentration*. Figure 75–1 shows the idealized relationship between creatinine clearance and plasma creatinine concentration. The curve is a rectangular hyperbola. It reflects the mathematical reality that values on the vertical axis are determined by the reciprocals of values on the horizontal axis, since the formula for creatinine clearance includes the plasma creatinine concentration in the denominator. To the extent that creatinine clearance and glomerular filtration rate are equivalent, the same ideal relationship applies between glomerular filtration rate and plasma creatinine concentration. Deviations from this ideal occur, however.

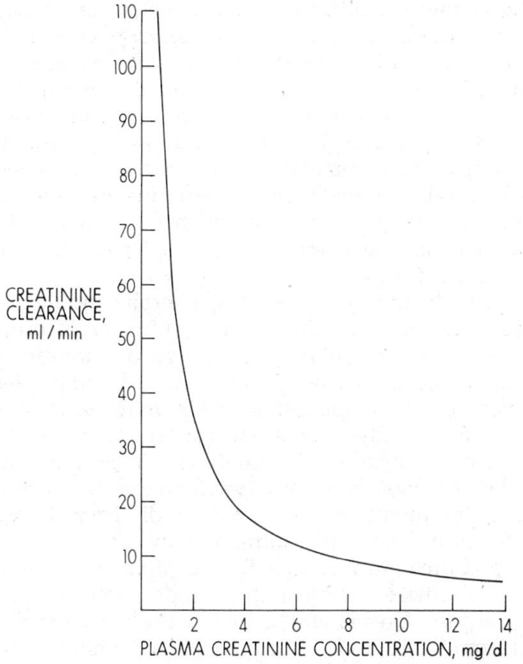

Figure 75–1. Idealized relationship between creatinine clearance and plasma creatinine concentration. To the extent that creatinine clearance is an accurate measure of glomerular filtration rate, the figure has more meaning biologically if viewed on its side, since the plasma creatinine concentration is determined by the glomerular filtration rate.

Creatinine is an end-product of creatine metabolism. Its endogenous production averages about 15 mg per kilogram of body weight per day, correlates with muscle mass, and tends to be constant for a given individual. Creatinine is filtered freely at the glomerulus and is secreted by the proximal tubule to an extent that may increase with elevated plasma concentration. The excretion rate of creatinine thus reflects the combined effects of filtration and secretion, and normally the clearance of creatinine exceeds the glomerular filtration rate. In practice, however, automated measurements of plasma creatinine concentration include a significant and variable component of noncreatinine chromogen that is not excreted in the urine. This overestimate offsets in part the error introduced by the renal secretion of creatinine. Endogenous creatinine clearances thus correlate well with clearances of exogenous inulin, at least in the normal range.

In the presence of renal failure, however, plasma creatinine concentration rises much more so than that of noncreatinine chromogens, and thus measurements of plasma creatinine concentration approach the true creatinine concentration. Moreover, in the presence of moderate degrees of renal failure, the secretory component of creatinine excretion may increase until the glomerular filtration rate falls below about 10 ml per minute. For these reasons, in the presence of moderate renal failure the clearance of creatinine tends to overestimate the glomerular filtration rate. In advanced renal failure (glomerular filtration rate less than 10 ml per minute), creatinine clearance again approximates the glomerular filtration rate. Despite these shortcomings, measurements of plasma creatinine concentration and clearance of endogenous creatinine are useful indices of filtration rate largely because of the ease with which repeated observations may be made in individual patients along the course of their disease.

The most accurate measures of glomerular filtration rate in man are obtained with the use of a number of exogenous substances such as inulin or a variety of radioisotopically labeled compounds such as ^{125}I-iothalamate. Standard clearance techniques for these measurements require infusion of the compound to a steady-state plasma concentration and then the timed collection of urine. Alternatively, single injection clearance techniques have been described for a variety of isotopically labeled compounds that are cleared rapidly from the vascular compartment by glomerular filtration only.

The blood urea nitrogen (BUN) concentration is an imperfect quantitative indicator of renal filtration despite its frequent use for this purpose. Urea is synthesized by the liver from ammonia derived from the catabolism of proteins and amino acids. Urea production is therefore variable and is influenced by hepatic as well as dietary conditions. At the kidneys, urea is filtered, reabsorbed, and secreted. Reabsorption dominates, but the rate of reabsorption varies with the degree of hydration. Those conditions, such as dehydration, that tend to increase the renal reabsorption of volume also increase the reabsorption of urea. Accordingly, blood urea nitrogen concentration may increase without any abnormality in renal function. Conversely, in the presence of renal excretory failure and reduced filtration rate, the blood urea nitrogen concentration may be influenced significantly by the degree of dietary protein intake. For these reasons, measurement of plasma creatinine concentration provides a more reliable index of renal filtration rate than the BUN.

RENAL CONCENTRATING AND DILUTING ABILITY. The total solute concentration of urine is generally assessed clinically by measurement of urinary specific gravity, which relates the weight of a unit volume of urine to an equal volume of water. Because of its simplicity, this technique has persisted despite well-recognized deficiencies. Errors of technique relate primarily to poor calibration of the hygrometer, but even in the absence of faulty technique the specific gravity of urine provides only a rough indication of urine osmolality. For example, urines that contain high concentrations of urea have lower specific gravities than expected for their osmolality, and urines that contain higher density solutes, such as glucose, iodinated contrast material, or protein, have higher specific gravities relative to their osmolalities. Within these limitations, however, there is a useful correlation between the specific gravity and osmolality of urine such that urinary osmolality in milliosmoles per kilogram of water may be estimated as 40 times the increase in specific gravity of urine above the value of water, which is 1.000. Thus, urine with a specific gravity of 1.007 would have an estimated osmolality of 280 mOsm, similar to that of plasma, and urine with a specific gravity of 1.020 would be distinctly concentrated with an estimated osmolality of 800 mOsm. Nonetheless, measurements of urine specific gravity represent only crude estimates of osmolality, and, when indicated, accurate and precise measurements of urine osmolality may be made easily and inexpensively by measurement of freezing-point depression in a cryoscopic osmometer.

Maximal urine concentrating ability is measured by restricting fluid intake until the patient loses a minimum of 3 per cent or a maximum of 5 per cent body weight, or until three consecutive urine specimens show no further increase in osmolality. These results are usually achieved within 16 hours of fluid restriction but may occur much earlier in patients with severe inability to conserve water. Once either one of these end-points is achieved, additional information may be obtained by the subcutaneous administration of 5 units of aqueous vasopressin to determine if any further increase in urine osmolality can be achieved. Normal subjects achieve maximal urine osmolality of 1000 ± 200 (SD) mOsm without further change after vasopressin. Patients who have complete or incomplete defects in antidiuretic hormone secretion, nephrogenic diabetes insipidus, or psychogenic polydipsia will have abnormal and distinctive patterns of response.

Maximum diluting capacity of the kidney is assessed by the rapid administration of 1200 ml of water by mouth to a fasting subject. The osmolality of three hourly urine specimens is measured and should achieve values lower than 80 mOsm or specific gravity of 1.002. Measurements of the rate or extent of excretion of the administered water are quite variable and are not generally useful. Both maximal diluting and maximal concentrating ability of the kidney may be impaired by diuretics, especially potent loop diuretics such as furosemide and ethacrynic acid, and by diuretic states such as glucosuria.

ACIDIFICATION CAPACITY. The urine is normally more acid than body fluids because of the endogenous production and renal excretion of nonvolatile acids derived primarily from sulfate and phosphate contained in dietary protein. Even at low pH, however, the amount of acid excreted as free hydrogen ion is negligible, and most hydrogen ion is excreted in the form of ammonium or titratable acids. For these reasons, the pH of a random specimen of urine provides only limited information about renal function and essentially no reliable information about the systemic acid-base status. The urinary pH does, however, affect the amount of acid that is excreted as ammonium or as titratable acids, and thus information about the acidification capacity of the kidney can be obtained from measurements of the lowest pH that occurs in response to spontaneous or induced metabolic acidosis.

Assessment of the renal acidification capacity is accomplished by the *ammonium chloride tolerance test.* The basis of this test is to induce mild metabolic acidosis by the administration of ammonium chloride by mouth and to measure the maximal depression in urinary pH, maximal excretion rate of ammonium and titratable acid, and the percentage of excretion of the administered hydrogen ion equivalent. Because the purpose of the ammonium chloride is to induce metabolic acidosis, its administration is not necessary if acidosis is present spontaneously. Indications for the ammonium chloride test are generally restricted to those conditions, usually suspected abnormalities in tubular function, that are not associated with other than mild reductions in glomerular filtration rate. Ammonium chloride, 0.1 gram per kilogram, is administered by mouth, and urine is collected hourly for six to eight hours. A normal response is to achieve a urinary pH of 5.4 or less and to excrete at least 30 per cent of the administered hydrogen ion equivalent. An abnormal response consists of failure to acidify the urine below pH 5.4 despite a measured reduction in arterial pH. This indicates a defect in maximal acidification capacity. The ammonium chloride tolerance test is not generally performed in patients with renal insufficiency, but, if performed, these patients usually achieve reduction in the urinary pH below 5.4, although there is reduced excretion of ammonium and titratable acid.

URINARY ELECTROLYTES. Measurements of urinary sodium, potassium, and chloride may provide important information but only in a limited set of clinical circumstances. Two types of measurements are made. The absolute daily excretion of sodium, potassium, or chloride (milliequivalents per day) is derived from the electrolyte concentration of a 24-hour collection of urine. Such measurements provide quantification of the daily intake of these electrolytes provided that two requirements are met. First, total body weight must be constant to indicate that overall intake equals output. Second, electrolyte excretion must be limited to the urine, and losses via the gastrointestinal tract or skin must be negligible. Under these conditions, the daily excretion of sodium, potassium, or chloride will reflect the dietary intake, but this information has only limited clinical value.

On the other hand, measurement of the *concentration* of sodium, potassium, or chloride in a random urine sample may provide information of importance in certain circumstances such as the evaluation of hyponatremia, acute oliguria, volume depletion, hypokalemia, and metabolic alkalosis. In the evaluation of hyponatremia, a urinary sodium concentration less than 10 mEq per liter indicates the presence of reduced effective extracellular volume with an appropriate increase in mineralocorticoid and ADH activity that leads to the renal retention of sodium and solute-free water. Higher urinary sodium concentrations indicate significant renal losses of sodium such as might occur from diuretics or, less commonly, from mineralocorticoid or glucocorticoid insufficiency or with volume expansion from the inappropriate secretion of ADH. Similarly, in the evaluation of patients with reduced extracellular volume, urinary sodium concentrations greater than 10 to 20 mEq per liter indicate that the kidney is participating in the loss of sodium and volume, perhaps because of renal or adrenal insufficiency, whereas urinary sodium concentrations less than 5 to 10 mEq per liter indicate that losses of sodium and volume are occurring via extrarenal routes.

In the setting of acute oliguria, urine sodium concentration greater than 20 to 40 mEq per liter occurs frequently with acute renal failure or incomplete obstruction, whereas urine sodium concentrations are generally less than 20 mEq per liter in the presence of severe volume depletion (prerenal azotemia), acute glomerulonephritis, congestive heart failure, the hepatorenal syndrome, and acute transplant rejection (Ch. 79.2). As is often the case, however, these values may be modified by many factors, including the administration of diuretics, and urine sodium concentrations are not generally regarded as sufficiently discriminatory to be useful in the differential diagnosis of acute oliguria.

The urine potassium concentration may be useful in the evaluation of unexplained hypokalemia. In the presence of hypokalemia, urine potassium concentrations greater than 20 mEq per liter indicate significant renal losses such as might occur from diuretics or increased mineralocorticoid activity. Urine potassium concentrations less than 10 mEq per liter indicate that the hypokalemia may be related to gastrointestinal losses such as may occur from the surreptitious use of laxatives or may indicate changes in plasma potassium concentration without potassium deficits such as may occur with hypokalemic periodic paralysis (see Ch. 538).

Urine chloride concentrations provide important information in the evaluation of metabolic alkalosis. Persistent metabolic alkalosis results most often from the depletion of chloride via the gastrointestinal tract or urine. In the presence of metabolic alkalosis, urine chloride concentrations greater than 10 mEq per liter suggest the presence of diuretic-induced increases in chloride excretion, severe depletion of potassium, Bartter's syndrome, or increased adrenocortical hormone activity. On the other hand, urine chloride concentrations less than 10 mEq per liter point to losses of chloride via extrarenal routes, usually vomiting, and indicate further that the metabolic alkalosis is likely to respond to replacement of volume and chloride.

The interpretation of measurements of urinary electrolytes is difficult in the presence of any recent exposure to diuretics or in the presence of diuretic states such as occur with glucosuria or from the administration of mannitol. In the absence of these circumstances measurements of urinary electrolytes may provide simple and inexpensive means to identify the source of important electrolyte abnormalities.

IMAGING OF THE KIDNEYS AND UROGENITAL TRACT

Imaging techniques of importance in the evaluation of renal abnormalities include roentgenography, ultrasonography, and radionuclide studies. These techniques are used (1) to visualize the number, size, and location of the kidneys; (2) to identify the presence and site of obstruction; (3) to detect and to characterize mass lesions; (4) to visualize renal arteries and veins; and (5) to guide percutaneous diagnostic and therapeutic interventions such as biopsy and nephrostomy. The choice of a technique is based on its relative simplicity, its safety, its potential to yield results that for a particular suspected disorder are neither falsely positive (lack of specificity) nor falsely negative (lack of sensitivity), and its potential to provide additional information not already available from previous studies.

ROENTGENOGRAPHIC STUDIES. The most simple radiologic study of the kidneys and urogenital system is the plain roentgenogram of the kidneys, ureter, and bladder (KUB), which will often reveal abnormal calcifications and may reveal renal size if not obscured by overlying bowel. If indicated, tomography may be necessary to determine the renal outlines.

Excretory Urogram. The excretory urogram, also known as the intravenous pyelogram or IVP, is the standard radiologic method to detect anatomic abnormalities of the kidneys and ureters and to evaluate patients with renal abnormalities. The basic excretory urogram is performed by the intravenous injection of iodinated contrast material, which is filtered at the glomerulus and concentrated within the tubular lumens and collecting system by the renal reabsorption of volume. Visualization of the contrast material within the renal parenchyma yields a *nephrogram,* and visualization within the major collecting system yields a *pyelogram.* Each of these phases is dependent on the amount of radiocontrast material that is delivered to the kidneys and filtered and also on the degree of extraction of volume that concentrates the dye within the parenchyma and collecting system. Modern radiocontrast materials are not secreted. In view of these mechanisms, it is useful to limit hydration prior to an excretory urogram in an effort to increase the intrarenal concentration of the contrast material. In some patients, however, especially those with renal insufficiency, restriction of fluid intake prior to an excretory urogram appears to increase the rate of adverse reaction and is now deemed more harmful than beneficial.

A nephrogram normally appears within one to three minutes after injection of the contrast material. The nephrogram provides an opportunity to determine the number of kidneys, their size and configuration, and the possible presence of inhomogeneous areas or filling defects. In addition, the symmetric and timely appearance of nephrograms bilaterally provides qualitative information on the relative blood flow and filtration rate of each kidney. The pyelogram phase occurs within five minutes after the injection of dye as the nephrogram fades (Fig. 75–2*A*). Aided if necessary by abdominal compression over the ureters, this phase allows visualization of the calyceal system, ureters, and bladder and provides opportunities to detect abnormalities in shape, size, or drainage that might result from intrinsic defects or from extrinsic compression. The presence of abnormalities in either filtration or concentration of the dye such as occur with vascular or outflow obstructions may result in marked delays in the onset of both the nephrogram and pyelogram phases, as well as subsequent persistence of these phases once they occur. Accordingly, when indicated, nonvisualization of specific areas should be re-examined with later films.

Retrograde Pyelography. Retrograde pyelography is the direct injection of radiocontrast material into the ureter and upper urinary tract. The approach to this area is achieved via insertion of a ureteral catheter under direct visualization through cystoscopy. Some form of anesthesia may be required. Although retrograde pyelography was used frequently to assess renal size and to evaluate the possibility of ureteral obstruction in patients who presented with advanced renal failure, these questions are now resolved more readily with high-dose intravenous pyelography and with ultrasonography. Retrograde

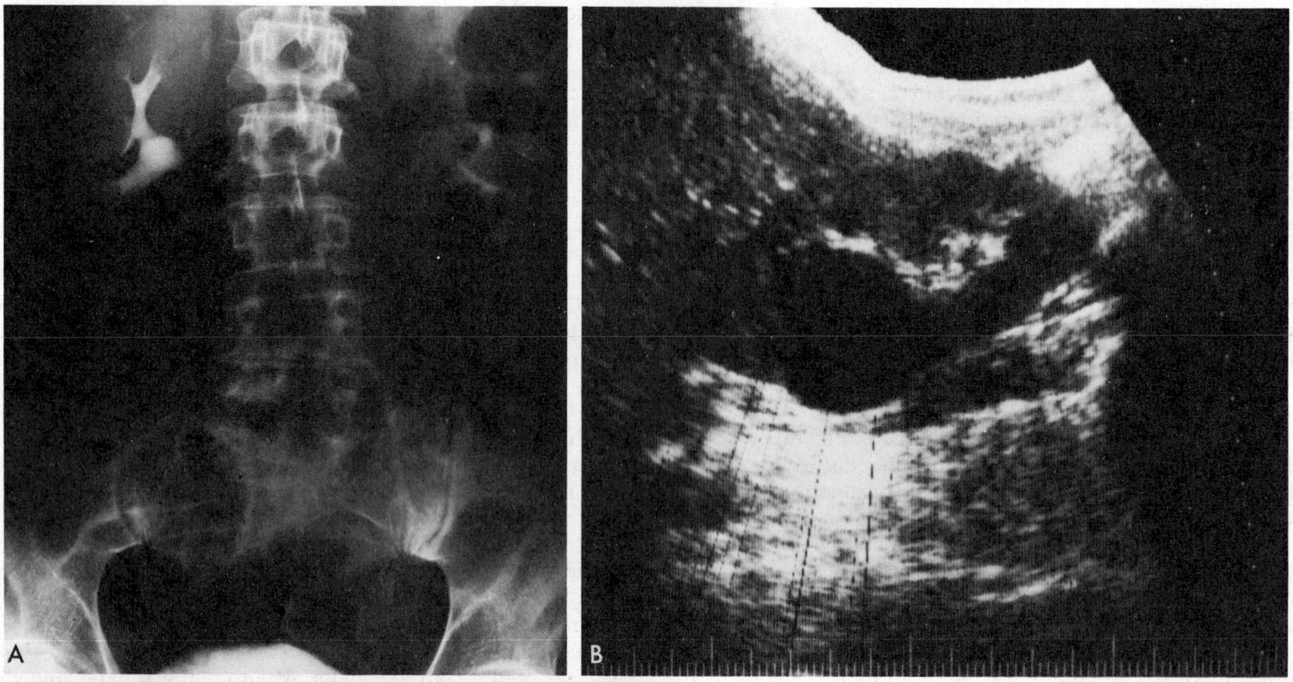

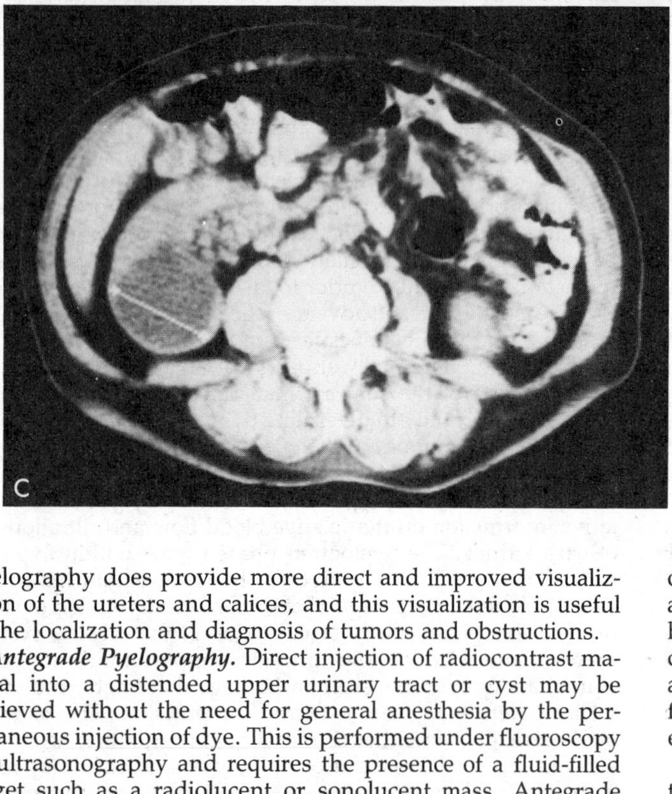

Figure 75–2. *A*, Pyelographic phase of a standard intravenous urogram. The right kidney is visualized well. It is normal except for stretching and splaying of the calices in the middle portion of the kidney. The terminal ureter on the left is bifid. *B*, Ultrasonograph of the right kidney from the patient shown in *A*. There is a single, large nonechogenic mass; through transmission is enhanced as revealed by increased echogenicity beyond the mass. These are sonographic characteristics of the renal cyst. *C*, Computed tomography of the abdomen of the same patient. The orientation is looking upward from toes to head. The right kidney is visualized at this level, but only a small portion of the left kidney is shown. There is a large, well-demarcated, homogenous mass (white diagonal) in the right kidney that has the density of water rather than tissue. This is characteristic of a renal cyst.

pyelography does provide more direct and improved visualization of the ureters and calices, and this visualization is useful in the localization and diagnosis of tumors and obstructions.

Antegrade Pyelography. Direct injection of radiocontrast material into a distended upper urinary tract or cyst may be achieved without the need for general anesthesia by the percutaneous injection of dye. This is performed under fluoroscopy or ultrasonography and requires the presence of a fluid-filled target such as a radiolucent or sonolucent mass. Antegrade pyelography may be useful to distinguish cysts from hydronephrosis.

Interventional Percutaneous Pyeloureteral Techniques. The combination of visualizing techniques such as roentgenographic fluoroscopy or ultrasonography and the availability of percutaneous catheters allows placement of a catheter in the renal pelvis, calices, or perirenal space if these spaces are distended by abnormal collections of fluid. Percutaneous catheter placement allows drainage and irrigation of pyonephrosis, abscesses, and obstructions, and placement of temporary nephrostomy catheters.

Renal Arteriography and Venography. The renal vasculature is visualized with radiocontrast material injected via a catheter introduced usually through the femoral vessels. Renal arteriography is performed most often to evaluate possible renal arterial stenosis as a cause or aggravating factor in systemic hypertension and to evaluate renal mass lesions. In general, cystic mass lesions are devoid of vasculature and may stretch and distort normal renal vessels and calices. Solid tumors are frequently vascular with irregular and erratic vessels that fill early as a blush of contrast material.

Renal venography is limited largely to searches for renal vein thrombosis and venous extension of renal cell carcinoma. Because renal venography requires the injection of dye against usually heavy renal venous outflow, turbulence may on occasion distort the distribution of dye and give the appearance of an intravascular filling defect. For this reason, renal venography is sometimes performed with intra-arterial infusion of epinephrine to reduce renal blood flow.

Digital Subtraction Angiography. Digital subtraction angiography uses high-quality image intensifiers and video camera recordings to visualize major arterial vessels following the rapid intravenous injection of radiocontrast material. Standard x-ray sources are used to produce sequential images at rates of about one per second beginning at the time of injection of radiocontrast material into a central or peripheral vein. Images are intensified electronically, displayed on a video camera, digitized, and stored on magnetic tape in a memory system. Images obtained prior to the arrival of radiocontrast material at a particular vascular region are subtracted electronically from the subsequent images to enhance the contrast between vessels and other tissues. With regard to the detection of renal vascular diseases, digital subtraction angiography has an overall accuracy of about 70 to 80 per cent compared with conventional arteriography. Technically successful studies are generally sensitive enough to detect significant renal vascular lesions, but false-positive results may be as frequent as 20 to 30 per cent. Because digital subtraction angiography does not require an arteriotomy, it can be performed without hospitalization at considerably less cost than direct arteriography.

Computed Tomography. Computed tomography represents a sophisticated extension of roentgenography and may be performed with or without contrast material. Its usefulness in the evaluation of renal abnormalities consists primarily in its application as a tertiary mode after excretory urograms and ultrasonography to detect and localize mass lesions. Computed tomography may detect cystic masses as small as 0.5 cm in diameter, but the sensitivity is less for noncalcific solid masses (Fig. 75–2C). Computed tomography is also useful to detect and evaluate obstruction and dilatation of the major collecting system in patients allergic to iodinated contrast material or for whom ultrasonography is inconclusive for technical reasons such as interference by bone, calcifications, or gas.

Adverse Effects of Urography. Two types of adverse effects should be considered in relation to the performance of excretory urograms, angiograms, or computed tomography with intravenous contrast material. First, any exposure to radiation is associated with a finite, statistical risk of permanent alteration in DNA. Depending on the question being asked, alternative modes of visualization such as ultrasonography might be considered in certain circumstances, especially those that involve pregnancy or those that may require repeated examinations over time.

The second type of adverse effect of excretory urography relates to toxic reactions to the iodinated contrast material. The overall incidence of adverse reactions to intravenous contrast is about 5 per cent for the general population and about 10 per cent for those with any allergies. The most common reactions involve nausea or urticaria; about 10 per cent of reactions will involve life-threatening events such as hypotension, laryngeal edema, or cardiac arrhythmias.

Excretory urography is a remarkably safe procedure, especially when performed in essentially healthy individuals. Not unexpectedly, excretory urography is less safe in individuals who are less healthy. Patients with diabetes mellitus and associated renal abnormalities are at increased risk to develop additional renal injury from excretory urography. Increases in plasma creatinine concentration may occur in as many as 75 per cent of diabetics with pre-existing renal disease, although for the most part the injury is mild and reversible. On the other hand, more severe renal failure has an approximate incidence of two episodes in 1000 urograms performed in diabetics with pre-existing renal disease as compared to no observed episodes in more than 100,000 procedures done at the same institution in nondiabetic patients. This high incidence of aggravation of renal injury in diabetics who undergo excretory urography is unexplained but warrants avoidance of the procedure in this population whenever possible and consideration of alternative means of visualization such as ultrasonography, radionuclide excretion studies, or, in selected instances, computed tomography without radiocontrast material.

Renal function may also deteriorate more frequently following excretory urography in patients with advanced age, marked dehydration, hyperuricemia, proteinuria, and pre-existing azotemia. Perhaps based on one or more of these factors, patients with multiple myeloma are at increased risk to develop adverse reactions to radiocontrast material. Appropriate precautions are indicated: consideration of alternative modes of visualization, attention to optimal hydration, and use of the minimal amount of contrast material consistent with an adequate examination.

The incidence of acute renal failure occurring in association with major angiography (renal, cerebral, abdominal, or peripheral) is variable and uncertain but not insignificant. The typical patient who undergoes major angiography may be expected to have coexisting factors such as advanced age, diabetes mellitus, pre-existing renal disease, and atherosclerotic vascular disease, which may increase the risk of complications.

ULTRASONOGRAPHY. Ultrasonography represents a major advance in the noninvasive visualization of the kidneys and genitourinary system. The acoustic impedance of a tissue to ultrasonic waves is the product of its density and the velocity of sound in that tissue. Accordingly, significant differences in acoustic impedance occur among tissues that differ in their content of water, fat, collagen, minerals, and other solids, and interfaces between these tissues will reflect portions of the sound energy back to the transmitting transducer. These reflections are recorded as electrical signals and may be visualized by various display modes. The brightness modulation or B-mode displays echoes as bright dots plotted along the vertical and horizontal axes of an oscilloscope at positions corresponding to their point of origin in the area being scanned and, through so-called gray-scale processing, in degrees of brightness that correspond to their amplitude (Fig. 75–2*B*). So-called "real-time" imaging or sonofluoroscopy, produces repetitive scans that give the impression of a continuous image. The resolution provided by currently available units is generally inferior to that of standard B-mode scans, although technical advances in this area are rapid.

Sonography can usually allow delineation of the renal outlines and measurement of the longitudinal and transverse dimensions. Difficulties may arise from overlying ribs that may obscure the upper poles or from similarities in the acoustic impedance of perirenal fat and renal cortex such that the renal margins are poorly defined. The structures within the renal parenchyma are sufficiently similar that few intrarenal echoes are produced except by the vascular and calyceal structures of the renal pelvis. Advanced gray-scale examination of the kidney may permit identification of the cortex, medulla, arcuate vessels, and renal pyramids. The ureters are not normally visualized unless distended.

The primary applications of ultrasonography to the evaluation of renal abnormalities include assessment of renal size, especially in the presence of severe renal failure, evaluation of mass lesions detected by excretory urography, examination of the perinephric area, and detection and grading of hydronephrosis. Renal ultrasonography may serve as the primary imaging procedure for patients with unexplained acute renal failure, for diabetics and other individuals at higher risks for adverse reactions to contrast material, in the presence of pregnancy, and to diagnose suspected polycystic kidney disease.

Evaluation of Renal Mass Lesions. Ultrasonography is used widely and effectively in the evaluation of renal mass lesions detected by excretory urography. Fluid-filled cysts as small as 1 to 2 cm in diameter may be detected, but reliable detection and evaluation of consistency generally require lesions greater than 2.5 to 3.0 cm. The primary application of ultrasonography is to describe the ultrasonographic characteristics of mass lesions according to three patterns: cystic, solid, or complex. Cystic lesions are free of internal echoes, have smooth, sharply defined margins, and cause accentuation of echoes from their far wall (Fig. 75–2*B*). Solid lesions have less distinct margins because of attenuation of the signal by solid tissue and also demonstrate internal echoes related to vessels, connective tissue, or hemorrhage. Complex lesions represent features of both patterns. Because of the inherent limitations of the technique, ultrasonographically defined lesions should be described simply as having the *characteristics* of cysts or solids. Physically solid lesions that may appear on ultrasonography as cysts include melanomas, lymphomas, and certain metastases. Localized areas of hydronephrosis may also appear as cysts.

Renal ultrasonography is most nearly diagnostic in adult polycystic kidney disease and severe hydronephrosis. In other instances, ultrasonography should be regarded as informative rather than diagnostic. In the evaluation of renal mass lesions, combinations of ultrasonography, computed tomography (Fig. 75–2C), and arteriography may distinguish between benign cysts and potentially malignant solid tumors with remarkable accuracy. Clinical judgment will still be needed to decide whether even a 90 to 95 per cent level of accuracy is sufficient in an individual instance or whether surgery is indicated to obtain a definite diagnosis.

RADIONUCLIDE SCINTILLATION IMAGING. Radionuclide imaging has not achieved a major role in the evaluation of the kidneys and urinary tract. Two advantages of these techniques, however, make them useful in special circumstances. First, radionuclide imaging does not require the injection of radiocontrast material. Second, radionuclide studies are relatively simple and rapid and may be performed repeatedly at intervals of 24 to 48 hours. For these reasons, radionuclide imaging has perhaps its greatest application in the evaluation of patients at high risk for adverse reaction to radiocontrast material and in the evaluation of patients in the period immediately after renal transplantation. Otherwise, these techniques have few advantages over more direct radiologic and ultrasonographic methods.

With regard to the kidneys, radionuclide imaging techniques involve the intravenous injection of an agent labeled with a radionuclide that emits gamma radiation. Use of a scintillation camera allows the performance of dynamic studies that monitor the passage of a radiopharmaceutical agent through the vascular, renal parenchymal, and urinary tract compartments. Static studies examine the local accumulation of radionuclide activity. At present, radiopharmaceuticals of value in studies of the kidney contain either ^{131}I or ^{99m}Tc (technetium).

Static Imaging. Static imaging of the kidney consists of the administration of a radiopharmaceutical agent, usually ^{99m}Tc-glucoheptonate, that accumulates within the renal parenchyma and persists for several hours. Static imaging provides information on the location, size, and contour of functional renal tissue and may reveal areas of inhomogeneity or filling defects.

Dynamic Imaging. Dynamic scintillation imaging consists of the intravenous injection of a radiopharmaceutical agent and the visualization of its course through the vascular, renal parenchymal, and urinary collecting system by external monitoring of regional radioactivity with a scintillation camera. The time-course of the appearance and disappearance of radioactivity is recorded in intervals as brief as one second. The radiopharmaceuticals used most frequently include ^{131}I-orthoiodohippurate, which is excreted by secretion with only a small component of filtration, and ^{99m}Tc-diethylenetriamine pentacetic acid (DTPA), which is excreted by filtration only. Thus, although the delivery of both radiopharmaceuticals to the kidneys is dependent on intact renal blood flow, the renal excretion of DTPA requires intact filtration, whereas the excretion of orthoiodohippurate may occur in the presence of reduced filtration but intact tubular function.

The time-activity data observed for the passage of either radionuclide generally delineate three discrete phases. The vascular phase is the first 15 to 60 seconds after injection and consists of a rapid increase in radioactivity in the region viewed by the scintillation camera. The second phase occurs over the next three to five minutes and consists of slower accumulation of regional radioactivity. The third, or excretory, phase refers to the decrease in activity that occurs as the radionuclide is excreted from the region of interest. Unilateral or bilateral disturbances in renal blood flow, renal filtration, renal tubular function, or excretion cause disturbances in the various phases of this renogram. Although some efforts have been made to provide quantification of the various phases, interpretation of renograms still depends for the most part on the recognition of patterns in the scintillation displays. Dynamic imaging is especially useful for comparing excretory function between the right and left kidneys when renal dysfunction is asymmetric, such as may occur with congenital, vascular, or urologic disorders.

RENAL BIOPSY

Biopsy of the renal parenchyma by either the percutaneous or open technique is useful (1) to define the morphologic expression of primary renal diseases, (2) to determine the type and extent of renal involvement by systemic diseases, and (3) to diagnose systemic diseases. The performance of renal biopsy is seldom necessary to *diagnose* systemic diseases, however, because diseases such as systemic lupus erythematosus, multiple myeloma, and diabetes mellitus, which may have typical but seldom diagnostic morphologic patterns, are diagnosed more readily by other means. Systemic lupus erythematosus, diabetes mellitus, thrombotic thrombocytopenic purpura, Wegener's granulomatosis, and amyloidosis may on occasion display pathognomonic features on renal biopsy, but of these diseases only amyloidosis is likely to require renal biopsy for diagnosis.

Renal biopsy is performed most frequently via the percutaneous technique. The indications for percutaneous biopsy are listed in Table 75–2; the contraindications are the presence of a single kidney, bleeding disorders, and uncontrolled hypertension. In experienced hands, percutaneous renal biopsy is a safe and effective technique that should provide sufficient tissue in more than 90 per cent of the attempts. Complications occur in 5 to 10 per cent of the attempts, and the most frequent complication is gross hematuria that usually resolves uneventfully in 24 to 48 hours. The formation of a perirenal hematoma may on occasion require surgical evacuation. Microscopic hematuria occurs very frequently and is not generally considered as a complication. Complications that occur less frequently include persistent bleeding, formation of arteriovenous fistula, aggravation of hypertension, and inadvertent biopsy of nonrenal tissue such as muscle, liver, pancreas, spleen, or small bowel. Although fluoroscopy and ultrasonography may on occasion be useful or even necessary to localize the kidney for biopsy, it is not clear that these added maneuvers diminish the occurrence of complications or notably improve the rate of success. Complications of percutaneous renal biopsy occur more often in younger patients and in those with hypertension or small, diseased kidneys. Because hemorrhagic complications of percutaneous renal biopsy are the most common, the patient should be advised to refrain from strenuous exercises, especially lifting, and from contact sports for at least two weeks after biopsy.

The information obtained from a renal biopsy depends on the quality of tissue examination. Tissue should be examined by light microscopy, immunofluorescence microscopy, and, on occasion, electron microscopy. Accurate morphologic definition of possible primary renal disease or of the type and extent of renal involvement by systemic disease is often essential prior

TABLE 75–2. INDICATIONS FOR RENAL BIOPSY

Presumptive presence of glomerular disease
Heavy proteinuria (> 3 to 5 grams per 24 hours)
Nephrotic syndrome
Acute nephritic syndrome
Proteinuria with hematuria
Renal involvement by systemic disease
Connective tissue disease
Vasculitis
Amyloidosis
Suspected Goodpasture's disease
Unexplained acute renal failure
Persistent acute renal failure (beyond two to four weeks)
Renal transplantation
Acute rejection
Chronic rejection
Recurrence of original disease

to therapeutic decisions that might involve the use of life-threatening immunosuppressive therapy and to inform the physician and patient as to the expected natural history of any renal abnormality. Moreover, for those renal disorders that may be treated ultimately by renal transplantation, knowledge of the nature of the original renal disease is important to predictions of whether that disease is likely to recur in the transplanted kidney.

Buonocore E, Meaney TF, Borkowski GP, Pavlicek W, Gallagher J: Digital subtraction angiography of the abdominal aorta and renal arteries. Radiology 139:281, 1981. *Along with some early results from a comparison between conventional and digital subtraction angiography, there are some useful insights into relevant technology and procedures.*

Doolan PD, Alpen EL, Thiel GB: A clinical appraisal of the plasma concentration and endogenous clearance of creatine. Am J Med 32:65, 1962. *This article provides careful and critical assessments of creatinine as a marker of glomerular filtration rate in the normal as well as diseased state.*

Diaz-Buxo JA, Wagoner RD, Hattery RR, Palumbo PF: Acute renal failure after excretory urography in diabetic patients. Ann Intern Med 83:155, 1975. *This brief report alerts us to the increased risks of urography in diabetic patients.*

Hilson AJW, Maisey MN, Brown CB, Ogg CS, Bewick MS: Dynamic renal transplant imaging with Tc-99m DTPA (Sn) supplemented by a transplant perfusion index in the management of renal transplants. J Nucl Med 19:994, 1978. *This provides examples of the usefulness of radionuclide studies in differentiating causes of renal failure in the transplant population. Data from 955 studies in 152 patients are summarized.*

Kaye AD, Pollack HM: Diagnostic imaging approach to the patient with obstructive uropathy. Semin Nephrol 2:55, 1982. *This article reviews the range of techniques available to visualize the kidney and genitourinary tract. It also provides examples of abnormal findings.*

Narins RG, Jones ER, Strom MC, Rudnick MR, Bastl CP: Diagnostic strategies in disorders of fluid, electrolytes and acid-base homeostasis. Am J Med 72:496, 1982. *The graphics and text of this article provide useful insights into common clinical disorders.*

Rutherford WE, Blondin J, Miller JP, Greenwalt AS, Vavra JD: Chronic progressive renal disease: Rate of change of serum creatinine concentration. Kidney Int 11:672, 1977. *An interesting concept is advanced. Data from 63 patients provide simple mathematical models that may describe the orderly rate of progression of different types of renal disease.*

Scheibel W, Talner LB: Gray scale ultrasound and the genitourinary tract. Radiol Clin North Am 17:281, 1979. *This review of clinical applications of ultrasonography is one of many useful articles in an issue devoted to the physics and applications of ultrasound.*

Schrier RW: Water metabolism. Kidney Int 10:1, 1976. *This entire issue reviews the physiology of water with emphasis on clinical disorders. It represents the most thorough and compact collection of information.*

Shehadi WH: Contrast media adverse reactions: Occurrence, recurrence, and distribution patterns. Radiology 143:11, 1982. *This is one of a series of articles that summarizes information obtained from a collaborative survey of more than 300,000 radiocontrast studies done in 45 institutions. Variables that may affect the incidence of reactions are considered.*

76. DISORDERS OF FLUID VOLUME, ELECTROLYTE, AND ACID-BASE BALANCE

Thomas E. Andreoli

Electrolyte abnormalities, including disorders of acid-base homeostasis, disturbances in osmoregulation, and derangements in the volume and/or distribution of body fluids, need not be isolated entities. Rather, these disorders generally occur as manifestations of underlying illnesses. In turn, fluid and electrolyte abnormalities, of themselves, produce systemic derangements. This chapter begins with principles that are generally applicable to analyzing clinical derangements of fluid and electrolyte balance. The subsequent sections consider particular disorders of fluid and electrolyte balance.

A striking characteristic of body fluid homeostasis is the fact that, in health, the volume and composition of the body fluid compartments remain remarkably constant despite wide daily variations in solute and water intake, or in the face of significant environmental fluctuations. While all of the factors regulating fluid and electrolyte homeostasis are not yet understood, many fluid and electrolyte disorders can be analyzed in terms of integrated responses that involve four key variables: *sensor* elements, *effector* elements, *input* parameters, and *output* parameters.

ACKNOWLEDGMENT: I acknowledge the dialogue and constructive suggestions provided by Steven C. Hebert, M.D., Assistant Professor of Internal Medicine, University of Texas Medical School, Houston, in the preparation of this chapter.

A frame of reference for considering the relations among these four variables is presented in Figure 76–1. The major body fluid compartments—intravascular, interstitial, and intracellular—are interconnected. The solid line at the top of each compartment indicates normality, with respect to either volume or concentration. The shaded areas above and below the line of normality indicate the acceptable physiologic variations in the volume or composition of these compartments. This range of variation is remarkably small. In normal individuals, for example, body water osmolality or blood hydrogen ion concentration varies by less than 1 to 2 per cent.

When the volume or composition of body fluids varies beyond these acceptable limits, *sensor* elements are activated. The sensing element illustrated in Figure 76–1 has been placed in the vascular compartment because, with few exceptions, stimuli that trigger homeostatic responses to changes in fluid and electrolyte balance generally result, either directly or indirectly, from changes in plasma volume or composition. In general, activation of sensor elements results in afferent stimuli (the solid arrows in Fig. 76–1) that trigger *effector* mechanisms; the latter activate homeostatic responses that modulate both *input* and *output*. Negative feedback systems (the dashed arrows in Fig. 76–1) set the limits of these responses by deactivating the effectors. Thus disturbances in homeostasis result in an integrated response that involves changes in both intake and output parameters.

In health, the functional capacities of the mechanisms regulating water and electrolyte balance are so large that man can vary the intake of solutes and water over a wide range without developing perceptible metabolic disturbances. But when these mechanisms are impaired, the limits between which solute and water intake can be varied become narrower.

This concept is illustrated schematically in Figure 76–2. The safe range, or the range over which homeostasis is maintained, is bounded at the lower level by the minimum physiologic requirement and at the upper level by the maximum physiologic tolerance. These limits become progressively narrowed in disease. As the degree of functional impairment progresses, minimum requirements often tend to increase while maximum tolerances tend to decrease. For example, salt intake in normal individuals can vary from approximately 10 mEq per day to several hundred milliequivalents per day without affecting volume homeostasis. However, in the presence of chronic renal disease, the minimum requirement rises and the maximum tolerance decreases, so that dietary salt intake must be kept within a much narrower range if ECF volume depletion or volume overload is to be avoided.

Volume Disorders

PHYSIOLOGIC CONSIDERATIONS

Protection of extracellular fluid volume is the most fundamental characteristic of fluid and electrolyte homeostasis. When significant degrees of volume contraction and electrolyte disturbances occur simultaneously, the response invariably involves volume conservation even at the expense of aggravating the electrolyte disorder.

It is useful in this context to state the concept of *effective circulating volume*. The latter cannot be defined in an absolute sense. In operational terms, effective circulating volume may be viewed as adequate filling of the arterial tree, that is, an arterial flow rate that is sufficient to maintain adequate perfusion of body tissues. The mechanisms regulating volume balance respond primarily to changes in the effective circulating volume.

The Body Fluid Compartments

In healthy adults, body water comprises approximately 60 per cent of body weight and exists in two compartments: the

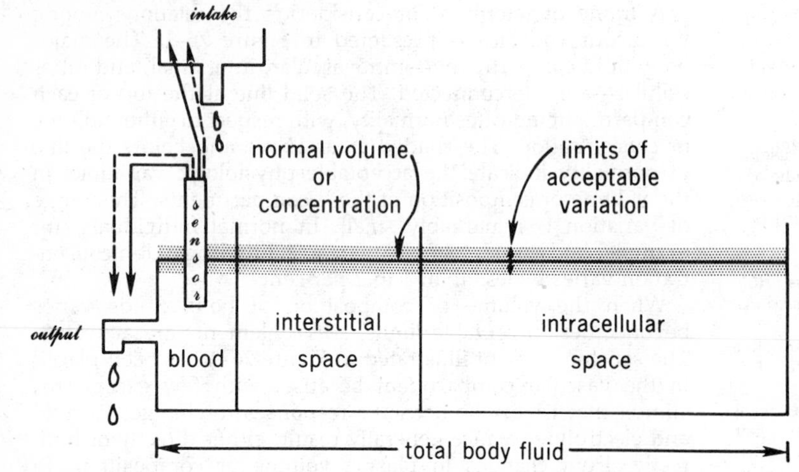

Figure 76–1. Frame of reference for analyzing the integrated homeostatic response in terms of the relations among *sensor* elements, *effector* elements, *input* elements, and *output* elements. The solid line at the top of each body fluid compartment indicates normality, and the shaded areas above and below the line indicate the acceptable physiologic variation. The solid arrows from the *sensor* to either *intake* or *output* represent afferent stimuli that trigger *effector* mechanisms; the dashed arrows represent negative feedback systems that limit the responses.

intracellular compartment fluid (ICF) comprises two thirds of body water, or 40 per cent of body weight; the extracellular compartment fluid (ECF) comprises the remaining one third of total body water; and total blood volume, that is, plasma plus formed elements, constitutes one third of the total ECF volume. This "rule of thirds" for the body fluid compartments is useful in the assessment of most clinically encountered fluid and electrolyte disorders. Thus in a healthy 70 kg man, total body water comprises about 40 liters, of which 25 liters are intracellular. The functional extracellular fluid volume is 15 liters, 5 liters of which is blood; and since the normal hematocrit is 40 to 45 per cent, total plasma volume is approximately 2.75 to 3.0 liters.

More than 95 per cent of total body sodium is extracellular, and sodium and its associated anions, primarily chloride and bicarbonate, constitute the principal solutes of the ECF. Albumin and other macromolecules present in plasma are restricted to the vascular bed and constitute 5 per cent of plasma volume, so that plasma is about 95 per cent water. Since capillaries are freely permeable to water and small solutes, interstitial fluid is a protein-poor, but not entirely protein-free, ultrafiltrate of plasma.

Potassium is the principal cation of intracellular fluid, and nearly 98 per cent of total body potassium is intracellular. The principal anions of intracellular fluid vary among different cells.

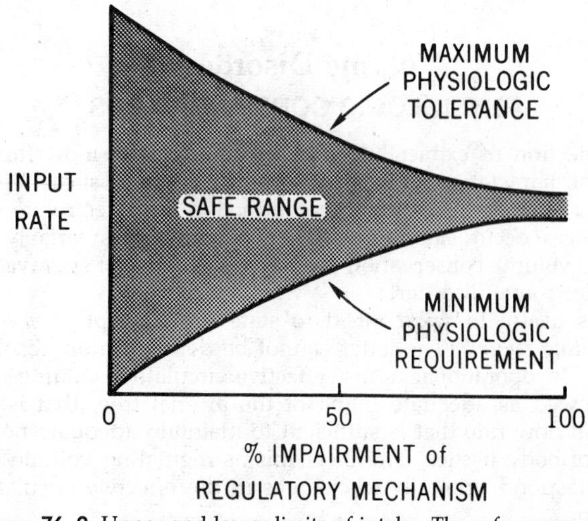

Figure 76–2. Upper and lower limits of intake. The safe range, or the range over which homeostasis is maintained, is bounded at the upper level by the maximum physiologic tolerance and at the lower level by the minimum physiologic requirement. Impairment of the regulating mechanism by disease narrows the safe range.

In muscle cells, they include phosphate, sulfate, and negatively charged macromolecules; and in red blood cells, the latter anions together with chloride and bicarbonate.

Regulation of Fluid Transfer Among Compartments

The transfer of fluid between vascular and interstitial compartments occurs at the capillary level and is governed by the balance between hydrostatic pressure gradients and plasma oncotic pressure gradients. This relation may be stated by the familiar Starling equation:

$$J_v = K_f\,(\Delta P - \Delta\pi)$$

where J_v is rate of fluid transfer between vascular and interstitial compartments, K_f is the water permeability of the capillary bed, ΔP is the hydrostatic pressure difference between capillary and interstitium, and $\Delta\pi$ is the oncotic pressure difference between capillary and interstitial fluids. Under normal circumstances, interstitial tissue pressure is low and the ΔP term in the Starling equation represents the vascular hydrostatic pressure gradient from arteriolar to venular ends of a capillary. Since interstitial fluid is protein-poor, the $\Delta\pi$ term in the Starling equation is given by the oncotic pressure of plasma proteins, principally albumin; 5 grams of albumin per 100 ml of plasma exert an oncotic pressure of about 15 mm Hg.

Regulation of External Fluid Balance

A 2 to 3 per cent decrease in extracellular fluid volume, which amounts to loss of 40 to 60 mEq of sodium, results in virtual elimination of sodium from the urine. Since there are 2500 to 3000 mEq of exchangeable sodium in the ECF, this trivial sodium loss attests to the sensitivity of the systems for renal sodium conservation.

However, a 2 to 3 per cent reduction in extracellular fluid volume, even when acute, produces negligible changes in systemic hemodynamic factors such as the heart rate, blood pressure, postural changes in blood pressure, systemic vascular resistance, and pulmonary capillary wedge pressure. Thus, in practical terms, we may consider that, in a patient with functionally intact kidneys, the renal sodium repletion response provides a uniquely sensitive index to early, modest reductions in effective circulating volume. Figure 76–3 provides a schematic summary of the renal volume repletion response. The separate details of this integrated mechanism are presented below. But it will be noted that this response includes renal sodium avidity, renal water avidity with relatively severe volume contraction, and vasoconstrictive events referable to the autonomic venous system; hence we use the term "integrated volume response."

SENSORS AND EFFECTORS. Changes in effective ECF volume that exceed acceptable physiologic limits are sensed by baro-

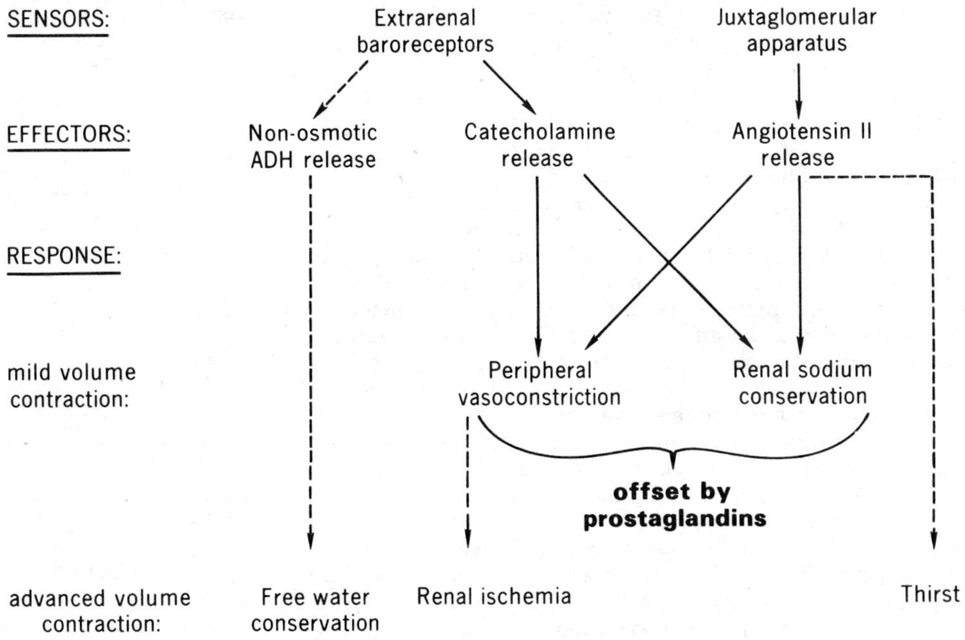

Figure 76–3. The volume repletion reaction. The integrated operation of the sensor and effector mechanisms protecting effective circulating volume is shown. The solid arrows indicate mechanisms activated when volume depletion is modest; the dashed arrows indicate mechanisms activated with severe volume depletion. Note the overlapping effects of angiotensin II and catecholamines, and the antagonisms of prostaglandins for the vasoconstrictive effects of angiotensin II and catecholamines.

receptors located in both the high- and low-pressure regions of the circulation. The low-pressure baroreceptors are located primarily in the left atrium and in major thoracic veins, while the arterial high-pressure baroreceptors are located in the carotid body and aortic arch. Both sets of baroreceptors respond to pressure and stretch stimuli associated with changes in effective circulating volume. Activation of these extrarenal baroreceptors by relatively slight reductions in effective circulating volume results in increased sympathetic nerve activity and in rises in plasma catecholamine activity.

This effector response raises blood pressure by increasing arteriolar resistance and heart rate while simultaneously decreasing venous capacitance. Increases in arteriolar resistance also reduce capillary hydrostatic pressure and therefore promote fluid transfer from interstitial fluid to the vascular compartment. Finally, adrenergic nerve terminals are also in direct contact with proximal renal tubular epithelial cells. Direct stimulation of these sympathetic nerves can increase proximal sodium absorption without affecting either renal hemodynamics or glomerular filtration rate.

A second effector mechanism for the volume repletion response that is activated by stimulation of extrarenal baroreceptors is release of antidiuretic hormone (ADH). When blood volume is isotonically contracted by more than 8 to 10 per cent, afferent stimuli carried by the ninth and tenth cranial nerves result in nonosmotic ADH release by the neurohypophysis, even to the extent of producing dilutional hyponatremia. Thus water conservation is a component of the volume repletion mechanism. While sympathetic effector mechanisms are activated by small reductions in effective circulating volume, nonosmotic ADH release requires an 8 to 10 per cent blood volume depletion. In other words, the sensitivities of these two extrarenal baroreceptor-activated effector mechanisms are quite different. Likewise, activation of the effector system for renal sodium avidity requires the loss of only about 100 ml of ECF, while as noted above, volume-mediated ADH release requires blood volume depletion of approximately 500 ml, that is, as indicated above, about 10 per cent of blood volume.

In addition to these multiple extrarenal baroreceptors, the renal juxtaglomerular apparatus serves as an intrarenal baroreceptor system. Sympathetic nerve stimulation, reductions in afferent arteriolar blood pressure, or reduction in the rates of distal tubular sodium delivery enhance renin release by the juxtaglomerular apparatus. Renal renin release into plasma accelerates the formation of angiotensin II according to the following general scheme:

Renin Substrate
↓ renin
Angiotensin I
↓ pulmonary converting enzyme
Angiotensin II
↓ circulating angiotensinase
Angiotensin III

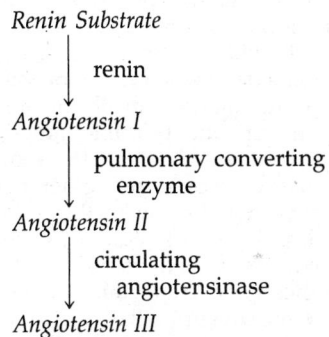

The octapeptide angiotensin II has three major effects. It is a potent pressor agent: on a molar basis, angiotensin II is a more potent vasoconstrictor than norepinephrine. Second, angiotensin II is the major stimulus to aldosterone secretion and consequently is a key factor modulating sodium conservation. Finally, angiotensin II is a potent stimulus to thirst. The heptapeptide angiotensin III is also a potent vasoconstrictor but is not as potent a stimulator of aldosterone secretion as is angiotensin II; angiotensin III also stimulates thirst.

INTAKE AND OUTPUT ELEMENTS. The kidneys respond to slight reductions in effective circulating volume by increasing the rate of proximal tubular sodium absorption without disturbing either glomerular filtration rate or osmoregulatory mechanisms. Under normal circumstances, approximately 70 per cent of filtered sodium is absorbed by the proximal nephron. So long as euvolemia persists, the fractional rate of proximal sodium absorption remains constant when the glomerular filtration rate is varied; this constant relation is referred to as *glomerulotubular balance*.

A number of factors modulate glomerulotubular balance in association with changes in effective circulating volume; in empirical terms, this modulation includes a down-setting of glomerular tubular balance in volume-expanded states and an increase in the rate of fractional proximal sodium absorption when filling of the arterial tree is impaired. Among these, the hemodynamic regulation of oncotic pressure in peritubular capillaries seems to have a dominant role. At relatively low concentrations, angiotensin II has a vasoconstricting effect on efferent but not afferent glomerular arterioles. Therefore this agent, by increasing glomerular filtration fraction, can increase peritubular capillary oncotic pressure and thereby enhance proximal tubular rates of sodium absorption. At high concentrations, angiotensin II, like norepinephrine, produces afferent glomerular arteriolar constriction, which results in reductions in glomerular filtration rate and in renal ischemia.

The kidney responds to modest sodium depletion by increasing the rate of tubular sodium absorption without altering glomerular filtration rate. Glomerulotubular balance is reset upward, so that a greater fraction of glomerular filtrate is absorbed in the proximal nephron; both direct stimulation of renal nerves and the effect of angiotensin II on efferent glomerular arterioles contribute in part to this resetting of glomerulotubular balance. Angiotensin II also provides a second mechanism for renal sodium conservation by increasing the rate of aldosterone secretion, which enhances sodium absorption in the terminal regions of the distal tubule. Finally, increased sodium absorption by more terminal portions of the collecting duct may also be part of the volume repletion reaction. When volume contraction becomes severe, the vasoconstrictive effects of high levels of norepinephrine and angiotensin II tend to reduce both the glomerular filtration rate and the rate of renal sodium excretion.

Conversely, prostaglandins, particularly of the E series, are potent renal vasodilators, and in most instances are also natriuretic, although it is not yet established whether the natriuretic effect of prostaglandins is due to changes in renal hemodynamics or to a direct inhibition of tubular sodium absorption. Thus prostaglandin-mediated renal vasodilation plays a major role in protecting the kidneys from ischemia in circumstances such as volume depletion, when levels of the vasoconstrictor agents, angiotensin II, and norepinephrine are increased.

An important therapeutic principle follows from a consideration of the renal vasodilatory effects of prostaglandin. Specifically, the use of aspirin and other nonsteroidal anti-inflammatory agents should be avoided in circumstances characterized by a high degree of sodium avidity, that is, by a reduction in effective circulating volume. These agents inhibit protaglandin synthesis and thus reduce the rate of prostaglandin production. Consequently, the use of aspirin or other nonsteroidal anti-inflammatory agents will increase the rate of development of renal ischemia, and hence azotemia, in sodium-avid states.

THE VOLUME REPLETION REACTION. When considered in an overall context, two features of the volume repletion reaction illustrated in Figure 76–3 are noteworthy. First, redundant mechanisms protect effective circulating volume. Angiotensin II release and catecholamine release produce overlapping results: each agent affects both the peripheral vasculature and renal sodium conservation. On the other hand, prostaglandins, because of their renal vasodilatory effects, tend to minimize renal ischemia and to promote natriuresis.

Second, the magnitude of the volume repletion reaction varies depending on the degree of volume contraction. In modestly volume-contracted states, peripheral vasoconstriction and renal sodium conservation occur, but renal blood flow, glomerular filtration rate, and osmoregulation are unaffected. When volume contraction becomes advanced, nonosmotic ADH release and angiotensin II–mediated thirst, coupled with reductions in the rate of salt delivery to the loop of Henle, result in hyponatremia. Finally, when catecholamine release and angiotensin II release become sufficiently great that renal blood flow is compromised beyond autoregulatory limits, prerenal azotemia ensues.

VOLUME DEPLETION

DEFINITION. In true hypovolemia total body water, functional ECF volume, and ICF volume are reduced. This occurs when the rate of salt and water intake is less than the combined rates of renal plus extrarenal volume losses. In chronic volume-contracted states, input and output may be equal.

TABLE 76–1. MAJOR CAUSES OF VOLUME DEPLETION

Renal Losses	Extrarenal Losses
Effector Loss (Hormonal Deficit)	**Hemorrhage**
Pituitary diabetes insipidus	**Cutaneous Losses**
Aldosterone insufficiency	Sweating
Addison's disease	Burns
Hyporeninemic hypoaldosteronism	
Interstitial nephritis	**Gastrointestinal Losses**
Output Loss (Renal Deficits)	Vomiting
Specific tubular nephropathies	Diarrheal disorders
Renal tubular acidosis	Gastrointestinal fistulas
Proximal	Tube drainage
Distal, gradient-limited	
Bartter's syndrome	
Nephrogenic diabetes insipidus	
Diuretic abuse	
Post-obstructive diuresis	
Excessive filtration of nonelectrolytes	
Osmotic diuresis	
Generalized renal disease	
Chronic renal failure	

ETIOLOGY AND PATHOGENESIS. Three major groups of diseases, occurring individually or in combination, account for most clinically encountered states of true volume contraction. Table 76–1 summarizes these three sets of disorders, and the more common specific diseases in each group. First, renal losses of salt or water may occur because of a loss of effector hormones that regulate renal salt and water conservation. Second, renal salt and water losses may occur either because of intrinsic renal disease or because abnormally high rates of nonelectrolyte excretion impair renal salt and water conservation. Finally, true volume contraction may occur because of extrarenal losses of body fluids, as in hemorrhage, burns, and diarrhea.

Effector Loss. Volume contraction can occur whenever there is loss of ADH or aldosterone, namely, the cardinal effector hormones regulating renal water and sodium conservation, respectively. Untreated *diabetes insipidus*, either pituitary or nephrogenic, produces profound volume contraction and hypertonic encephalopathy in patients denied free access to water. Approximately 10 per cent of the glomerular filtrate, or about 18 liters daily, reaches the early distal convoluted tubule. Under normal circumstances, this fluid is hypotonic and, so long as ADH is present, is concentrated by osmotic equilibration with the hypertonic renal medullary interstitium. In diabetes insipidus, a large fraction of hypotonic tubular fluid may escape reabsorption and appear in the urine. Thus the obligatory loss of solute-free water in diabetes insipidus may be as high as 10 to 18 liters daily. Both forms of diabetes insipidus are discussed in detail in Ch. 225.

Addison's disease may impair aldosterone production and hence lead to renal sodium wasting. A second major cause of aldosterone lack occurs in *hyporeninemic hypoaldosteronism,* which may accompany interstitial renal disease. Disorders that damage the renal interstitium, such as hypertension, diabetes mellitus, gout, sickle cell disease, chronic ingestion of lead-containing illicit alcohol, and analgesic abuse, can suppress the ability of the juxtaglomerular apparatus to produce renin. In turn, the low rate of renin secretion results in low rates of aldosterone secretion. Thus hyporeninemic hyperaldosteronism represents a disorder in which intrinsic renal disease, namely interstitial nephritis, and effector lack, namely impaired aldosterone production, contribute simultaneously to renal salt wasting, hyperkalemia, and metabolic acidosis. It is not yet known whether interstitial nephritis associated with hyporeninemic hypoaldosteronism is also accompanied by defects in aldosterone biosynthesis. The latter has been inferred because hyperkalemia, which is a potent stimulus to aldosterone secretion, fails to enhance rates of aldosterone secretion in patients with hyporeninemic hypoaldosteronism.

Output Loss. A number of kinds of disorders impairing renal tubular sodium or water conservation may also lead to volume contraction. For convenience, these derangements may be grouped into three classes.

First, there are various tubular nephropathies characterized by specific deficits in salt or water absorption. As mentioned above, nephrogenic diabetes insipidus and interstitial renal disease may produce water or sodium wasting, respectively. Because interstitial renal disease often results in hyperchloremic, hyperkalemic metabolic acidosis, the term "renal tubular acidosis, type IV" is often applied to this disorder. However, the general term "renal tubular acidosis" also includes other sodium-wasting disorders accompanied by hyperchloremic acidosis, such as proximal tubular acidosis, a specific proximal defect in bicarbonate reabsorption, and gradient-limited distal renal tubular acidosis, a specific defect in distal tubular sodium bicarbonate regeneration (Ch. 83.2).

Alternatively, Bartter's syndrome is a specific tubular nephropathy that results in failure of sodium chloride absorption by distal regions of the nephron; the disorder is accompanied by excessive production of prostaglandins by the renal medullary interstitium, and is characterized by sodium chloride wasting, juxtaglomerular hyperplasia, high renin levels, and secondary hyperaldosteronism; the latter results in hypokalemic metabolic alkalosis (Ch. 83.5).

Inhibition of tubular sodium absorptive processes due to *chronic diuretic abuse* may also lead to salt wasting, volume contraction, and specific metabolic acid-base abnormalities. These abnormalities are discussed in connection with Table 76–4 (see below). Diuretics such as furosemide and thiazides may produce serum electrolyte changes indistinguishable from those of Bartter's syndrome.

Profound but reversible defects in tubular salt and water absorption may occur during *post-obstructive diuresis*, that is, shortly after relief of partial or complete urinary tract obstruction. Salt and water losses may also occur in the *diuretic phase* of acute tubular necrosis. However, profound salt and water losses associated with the diuretic phase of acute tubular necrosis are seen uncommonly if extracellular fluid volume is carefully controlled during oliguric acute tubular necrosis.

Third, glomerular filtration of large amounts of nonelectrolytes may produce volume deficits by overwhelming renal tubular reabsorptive capacity for salt and water; in this instance, water losses predominate so that hypernatremia generally occurs. This phenomenon, termed *osmotic diuresis* or *solute diuresis*, occurs in diabetic ketoacidosis, hyperglycemic hyperosmolar coma, or hyperalimentation with large glucose loads in chronically debilitated patients; in burns, where there are abnormally high rates of urea production; and during mannitol or glycerol administration to patients with central nervous system disorders requiring reductions of intracranial pressure.

Finally, in *chronic renal failure* of any cause, there is an obligatory loss of sodium. As indicated in Figure 76–2, chronic renal failure of any cause is associated with a significant increase in the minimum physiologic requirement for maintaining sodium balance. The extent of obligatory sodium loss in chronic renal failure is most pronounced in cystic renal diseases, notably medullary cystic disease and polycystic kidney disease.

Extrarenal Losses. Three classes of extrarenal losses account for the remaining major causes of true volume contraction. Simple dehydration may result from increased insensible water loss in *excessive sweating* due to high ambient temperatures or to fever. Because sweat usually contains less than 50 mEq per liter of sodium, the ICF and the ECF share the water loss, and body water osmolality rises while ECF volume loss is modest. Second, *burns* allow the loss of large amounts of plasma and interstitial fluid through affected areas and therefore can lead rapidly to profound ECF losses.

Finally, gastrointestinal volume losses are extremely common and occur when any portion of the 8 to 10 liters of normal gastrointestinal secretions is lost. This circumstance occurs most commonly in secretory rather than inflammatory diarrheas (Ch. 102). Volume depletion is most commonly the consequence of vomiting, gastric drainage, or diarrhea but may occur with any type of bowel fistula. Loss of hydrochloric acid from the stomach may produce metabolic alkalosis, while loss of sodium bicarbonate from pancreatic secretions lost through the lower gastrointestinal tract, as in diarrhea, may produce metabolic acidosis.

CLINICAL MANIFESTATIONS. The clinical findings in states of true volume contraction are referable both to underfilling of the arterial tree and to the renal and hemodynamic responses to this underfilling. In mild or partially compensated volume contraction, particularly when the latter has occurred gradually, the patient may exhibit nothing more than mild postural giddiness, postural tachycardia, and weakness. In more advanced stages of volume depletion, particularly those occurring acutely, there may be recumbent hypotension, tachycardia, and a reduced urine volume. Finally, when volume contraction is severe, the combination of profound fluid loss and increased sympathetic activity produces circulatory collapse characterized by oliguria, a nondetectable blood pressure (except by Doppler studies), recumbent tachycardia, and cold extremities. In short, mild to severe volume contraction may range from minimal symptoms to life-threatening circulatory collapse.

Importantly, the lack of physical findings does not exclude the presence of mild to moderate volume contraction in a given patient. In carefully controlled comparisons of blood volume and hemodynamic variables in postoperative patients, Lazrove and colleagues found that 7 to 10 per cent blood volume losses were frequently accompanied by normal vital signs and by only slight decreases in the central venous pressure or the pulmonary capillary wedge pressure.

Skin turgor and the moistness of mucous membranes are valuable indices to the volume of body water in infants but are unreliable in adults. In young adults, reductions in skin turgor do not occur unless profound volume contraction is present, and normal loss of skin elasticity makes skin turgor difficult to assess in older patients. Likewise, mouth breathing and other factors affect the oral mucosa independently of external volume balances.

The signs and symptoms of volume contraction, regardless of cause, are referable to a reduction in effective circulating volume. Consequently, the clinical findings in volume contraction depend primarily on the interplay among four major factors: (1) the magnitude of the volume loss; (2) the rate of volume loss; (3) the nature of the fluid loss, that is, whether the fluid loss is primarily water, a combined sodium plus water loss, or a blood loss; and (4) the responsiveness of the vasculature to volume reduction. Some simple considerations can serve to illustrate these relations.

The clinical manifestations of volume contraction are obviously related intimately to the volume and rate of fluid loss. For example, an acute gastrointestinal hemorrhage of one liter of blood can easily result in oliguria coupled with the signs and symptoms of circulatory collapse while the hematocrit remains constant. In other words, the hemorrhage is sufficiently acute that fluid flux from the interstitial to the vascular bed makes a negligible contribution to expanding the vascular bed. However, the same amount of gastrointestinal blood loss occurring more slowly, for example, over a one-day period, permits a partial transfer of fluid from the interstitium to the vascular bed and consequently a fall in hematocrit; but since the effective circulating volume is at least partially restored by this fluid shift, the volume of urine flow and the hemodynamic response to volume contraction may be minimally affected.

Second, the kind of fluid loss significantly affects the clinical findings in volume contraction. Consider, for example, a one liter loss of different kinds of body fluids in a 70 kg man having a total body water of 40 liters and a hematocrit of 45 per cent. The acute loss of one liter of predominantly solute-free water, as in diabetes insipidus, would produce a 2.5 per cent reduction in blood volume; urine flow and systemic hemodynamics would thus be minimally affected. The acute loss of one liter of predominantly extracellular fluid, as in a burned patient, would produce a 6.6 per cent reduction in blood volume, since sodium is confined to the ECF; in this circumstance, modest oliguria and recumbent tachycardia would ensue. Lastly, the acute loss of one liter of blood by hemorrhage would reduce blood volume by 20 per cent, thus resulting in profound oliguria and near-circulatory collapse.

Finally, peripheral vasoconstriction and tachycardia represent important physiologic responses to volume losses. Consequently, the signs and symptoms of volume contraction, even of modest degree, may be amplified appreciably in patients with diminished myocardial reserve or reduced sympathetic nervous system function. The former occurs commonly in cardiomyopathies of any cause or in pericardial tamponade or pericardial constriction. The latter occurs commonly in patients subjected to prolonged bedrest, in diabetic patients with autonomic neuropathy, and as a consequence of therapy with certain antihypertensive drugs, notably alpha-methyldopa and guanethidine.

DIAGNOSIS. The pulse, blood pressure, and changes of these variables with position, together with a clinical estimate of the venous pressure and skin temperature, provide an initial assessment of circulatory dynamics. Because these findings may be inconclusive in moderate degrees of volume contraction, invasive hemodynamic monitoring may be required in critically ill patients who are hemodynamically unstable. In such patients, the central venous pressure may correlate poorly with cardiac output and with pulmonary vascular volume. Measurement of the pulmonary capillary wedge pressure with a Swan-Ganz (flow-directed) catheter may therefore be required (Ch. 71).

However, even the pulmonary capillary wedge pressure may remain within normal limits when blood volume has been reduced by 5 to 10 per cent. Consequently, a fluid challenge may be useful in the evaluation of critically ill patients in whom a volume deficit is thought to be a contributory factor to a reduced cardiac output. A convenient way of achieving this goal is to administer 500 ml of normal saline over 1 to 3 hours and to measure the change in the pulmonary capillary wedge pressure or the cardiac output, as estimated by thermal dilution.

The cardinal laboratory findings associated with volume contraction follow directly from the volume repletion mechanism summarized in Figure 76–3. The initial renal responses to a decrease in effective circulating blood volume result in a fall in urine volume and in a reduction in sodium excretion. Severe degrees of volume contraction also produce filtration rate reductions and pre-renal azotemia.

The urinary sodium concentration and the fraction of filtered sodium excreted in the urine, denoted as FE_{Na}, are clinically useful indices to renal sodium avidity. The FE_{Na} is calculated as the urine-to-plasma sodium concentration ratio divided by the urine-to-plasma creatinine concentration ratio. In the volume-contracted state, the urinary sodium concentration is generally less than 10 mEq per liter and the FE_{Na} is less than 1 per cent, while in acute tubular necrosis, the urinary sodium concentration is greater than 40 mEq per liter and the FE_{Na} is greater than 1 per cent. These indices are useful in the differential diagnosis between acute oliguric tubular necrosis and volume contraction associated with pre-renal azotemia, with certain notable exceptions.

The urinary sodium indices are not reliable determinants of volume contraction when there is obligatory renal sodium wasting, as in interstitial nephritis. When volume contraction is due to the renal losses listed in Table 76–1 (except for diabetes insipidus), the urinary sodium concentration and the FE_{Na} may both be elevated even when volume losses are large enough to produce azotemia. The urinary sodium excretion may also be elevated in volume contraction due to upper gastrointestinal losses associated with vomiting or gastric drainage. This occurs during early metabolic alkalosis if the filtered load of bicarbonate exceeds the renal tubular reabsorptive capacity for bicarbonate. During this interval, the urinary chloride concentration is a more reliable index of renal salt avidity. Finally, antecedent diuretic therapy may invalidate FE_{Na} measurements.

TREATMENT. The major goal of the treatment of volume contraction is to expand the effective circulating volume by replacing fluid deficits. The type of fluid, the route and rate of fluid administration, and the total amount of fluid to be given will vary with the particular circumstance. For example, a mild, nonpersisting upper gastrointestinal hemorrhage may be treated appropriately by infusion of normal saline, while a major, persisting upper gastrointestinal hemorrhage will generally require replacement with whole blood.

The degree to which a given volume of crystalloid solution expands the effective circulating volume depends on solution composition. If glucose metabolism is normal, the infusion of 5 per cent glucose in water (D5W) is equivalent to administering solute-free water that distributes uniformly in total body water. Since less than 10 per cent of total body water is in the intravascular compartment, infusion of 1 liter of 5 per cent dextrose in water expands the intravascular volume by 75 to 100 ml, that is, by about 2 per cent.

Solutions containing sodium as the principal solute preferentially expand the extracellular fluid volume. Infusion of one liter of a normal saline solution can be expected to increase blood volume by about 300 ml, or about 6 per cent; the remaining portion is distributed in the interstitial compartment. Hypotonic sodium-containing salt solutions have an effect on intravascular volume expansion that is intermediate between that of 5 per cent dextrose in water and normal saline.

Colloid-containing solutions, such as iso-oncotic albumin solutions and plasma, preferentially expand the intravascular compartment, since large molecules like albumin are mainly restricted to the intravascular space. Finally, blood, which contains formed elements, is the most potent expander of the intravascular space. A unit of packed red blood cells will remain entirely in the vascular bed. A unit of whole blood having a hematocrit of 45 per cent will retain all formed elements in the vascular bed; of the remaining 55 per cent volume of that unit, more than 40 per cent of the plasma will also remain in the vascular bed because of the oncotic effect of plasma proteins.

Three other factors concerning fluid replacement therapy warrant consideration. First, when large volumes of glucose-containing solutions are given rapidly, an increase in plasma glucose concentration which results in glycosuria produces an obligate renal loss of sodium and water that aggravates volume losses. Second, iso-oncotic albumin solutions are effective in expanding intravascular volume rapidly. However, the half-life of infused albumin in critically ill patients is only 4 to 6 hours, and the cost of an iso-oncotic albumin solution is approximately 90 times greater than that of an equal volume of normal saline. For these reasons, the use of iso-oncotic albumin solutions should be limited to hemodynamically unstable patients in whom rapid intravascular expansion is critical.

Finally, because volume contraction is associated with vasoconstriction in both the venous and arterial circuits, transient changes in the pulmonary capillary wedge pressure may not reflect accurately the volume status of the patient. During volume expansion, the wedge pressure rises and subsequently falls. The initial pressure elevation is due to fluid infusion into a vasoconstricted, low capacity vascular bed and should not be misinterpreted to indicate adequacy of volume repletion. The subsequent reduction in wedge pressure coincides with decreases in arterial resistance coupled with increases in venous capacitance.

CIRCULATORY COMPROMISE WITHOUT TRUE VOLUME CONTRACTION

DEFINITION. In the previous section, we considered those disorders characterized by inadequate filling of the arterial tree which occurred because of fluid losses to the external environment. Clearly, the cardinal signs and symptoms of these disorders are referable to responses accompanying the integrated volume repletion reaction (Fig. 76–3). There are also disorders in which inadequate arterial filling occurs in the absence of external fluid losses. The signs and symptoms of these disorders mimic closely those that characterize true volume contraction.

ETIOLOGY AND PATHOGENESIS. Table 76–2 lists three commonly encountered classes of derangements that may present clinically with tachycardia, acute hypotension, oliguria, azotemia, and a reduced FE_{Na}. These disorders can be termed "non–volume contracted circulatory compromise," with the understanding that the term "non–volume contracted" refers to the absence of body fluid losses to the external environment.

Impaired Cardiac Output. A profound collapse of cardiac output, referable to acute myocardial infarction with pump failure (cardiogenic shock) or to acute pericardial tamponade, may clearly result in circulatory collapse. In this instance, failure to fill the arterial tree and to maintain an effective circulatory volume occurs because the heart fails to translocate blood adequately from venous to arterial beds.

Increased Vascular Capacitance. Circulatory collapse and its attendant signs and symptoms will occur when there is a sudden increase in the capacitance of the vascular bed, most notably in the venous part of the circulation. This kind of increase in ratio of vascular capacitance to vascular volume occurs most commonly in sepsis but may also be seen in circumstances in which peripheral vasodilators, particularly those having a postarteriolar locus of action, are administered injudiciously.

Vascular-Interstitial Fluid Shifts. Profound hypotension, tachycardia, progressive oliguria, and azotemia are also encountered when there is a rapid translocation of fluid from vascular to interstitial compartments, presumably because of a sudden, profound increase in the permeability characteristics of peripheral capillaries. Some common derangements of this type include infarction of the small or large intestine, extensive tissue trauma, acute pancreatitis, and rhabdomyolysis. An analogous mechanism, namely a marked increase in the permeability of pulmonary capillaries, is also presumed to account for the formation of noncardiogenic pulmonary edema in the adult respiratory distress syndrome (Ch. 71).

DIAGNOSIS AND THERAPY. The diagnosis and therapy of acute myocardial infarction with circulatory collapse, and of acute pericardial tamponade, are considered in detail in Section VII of this book. It is, however, worth citing certain factors particularly germane to the management of fluid therapy in such patients. In individuals affected either by right ventricular infarction or by pericardial tamponade, maintenance of adequate filling of the systemic arterial tree depends critically on maintaining a relatively high venous preload to the right heart. Attempts at volume contraction in patients with right ventricular infarcts or pericardial tamponade may increase appreciably systemic hypotension. Thus treatment of these disorders generally requires concomitant hemodynamic monitoring with a flow-directed Swan-Ganz catheter to avoid excessive preload to the left heart.

In patients with left ventricular infarction and systemic hypotension, particular attention should be directed to excluding the possibility that antecedent true volume depletion, for example with prolonged diuretic therapy and salt restriction prior to the myocardial infarction, may be a significant contributor to what otherwise might be mistaken for true cardiogenic shock. The combined findings of acute left ventricular infarction, systemic arterial hypotension, a reduced pulmonary capillary wedge pressure, and an antecedent history of prolonged diuretic therapy, when taken together, indicate that improved systemic hemodynamics may be achieved by cautious attempts at volume expansion carried out in combination with serial measurements of the cardiac output and the pulmonary capillary wedge pressure.

TABLE 76–2. CIRCULATORY COMPROMISE WITHOUT EXTERNAL FLUID LOSSES

Impaired Cardiac Output
Acute myocardial infarction
Pericardial tamponade
Increased Vascular Capacitance
Septic shock
Vascular → Interstitial Fluid Shifts
Acute pancreatitis
Bowel infarction
Rhabdomyolysis
Noncardiogenic pulmonary edema

The distinction between hypotension as being due either to true volume contraction or to an increase in the capacitance/volume ratio of the vascular bed, as occurs in sepsis, is often difficult. This distinction is particularly difficult in individuals who have been on intensive care units for prolonged periods of time and may have an innately high risk for developing sepsis, such as the cancer patient treated with potent chemotherapeutic agents. A useful clue to the presence of septic circulatory collapse is the combined occurrence of warm extremities coupled with hypotension and oliguria, since true hypovolemia, particularly when advanced, is ordinarily accompanied by profound peripheral vasoconstriction and hence cool and often cyanotic extremities.

True hypovolemia and sepsis may also coexist. In such a circumstance, invasive hemodynamic monitoring may be helpful. Both in true hypovolemia and in sepsis, the pulmonary capillary wedge pressure is reduced; however, in septic circulatory collapse the calculated systemic vascular resistance falls because of peripheral vasodilation, whereas in true hypovolemia peripheral vasoconstriction ordinarily raises the systemic vascular resistance. The diagnosis of disorders producing rapid transfer of fluids from the vascular bed to the interstitium, such as trauma, acute pancreatitis, or rhabdomyolysis, is generally evident from a clinical appraisal.

The treatment of patients with sepsis and an increased vascular capacitance/volume ratio, as well as those individuals with rapid vascular to interstitial fluid shifts, has as a mainstay the administration of sufficient sodium-containing fluids, generally isotonic saline, to permit adequate filling of the arterial tree. However, it should be recognized that, in the absence of external fluid losses, such therapy necessarily expands total body water, particularly in the vascular and interstitial compartments. Consequently, during recovery from the underlying disorder, care must be taken to avoid unnecessary expansion of the vascular bed, and consequently the risk of volume-mediated cardiac decompensation.

VOLUME EXCESS

DEFINITION. Volume-expanded states are characterized by an increase in total body water that is accompanied, in most but not all circumstances, by an increase in total body sodium. Total body salt and water may be increased, while the effective circulating volume is decreased. In other words, certain volume-expanded states are characterized by dissociation between total body salt and water and the effective circulating volume.

ETIOLOGY AND PATHOGENESIS. Volume expansion occurs whenever the rate of salt or water intake exceeds the rate of renal plus extrarenal losses; in chronic volume expansion, the external salt and water balance may be normal. A convenient way of considering volume-expanded states is to view them in the context of three different classes of physiologic explanations. Table 76–3 presents such a classification; the discussion that follows is based on this classification.

Disturbances in Starling Forces. The most common diseases encountered in which both volume expansion and edema occur are those disorders in which derangements in the Starling forces regulating fluid transfer between capillaries and interstitium tend to promote expansion of the interstitial compartment at the expense of the effective circulating volume. Consequently, renal sodium retention and edema occur. By definition, this group of disorders is characterized by increases in capillary hydrostatic pressure, by decreases in capillary oncotic pressure, or by a combination of these two factors.

Four groups include most edematous states characterized by abnormal Starling forces (Table 76–3): (1) The systemic venous pressure may be increased because of primary cardiac disorders, such as right heart failure or constrictive pericarditis. (2) Local elevations in pulmonary or systemic venous pressure may occur as in left heart failure, vena cava obstruction, or portal vein obstruction. (3) A reduction in plasma oncotic pressure, and consequently a net increase in the tendency for fluid transudation from capillaries to interstitium, accounts plausibly for edema formation in the nephrotic syndrome. (4) A combination of these factors may be responsible for edema formation. For example, both hypoalbuminemia and portal hypertension are major contributory factors to the development of ascites in hepatic cirrhosis (Ch. 125).

Plasma renin activity and aldosterone concentrations in these disorders tend to be elevated, although the results also tend to be variable. In advanced cases of disorders characterized by local or systemic venous pressure increases, most notably in severe congestive heart failure and in cirrhosis, hyponatremia may occur; this finding represents an ominous prognostic sign. Finally, edema formation due to such derangements of Starling forces may result in the "third space" phenomenon, namely, the sequestration of large volumes of interstitial fluid in regions such as the pleural or peritoneal cavities.

Primary Hormonal (Effector) Excess. Disorders characterized by effector excess include those hormonal disturbances in which there is unregulated production of mineralocorticoids or of ADH. The volume expansion that occurs in states of mineralocorticoid excess, such as primary hyperaldosteronism, is due to sodium retention, and is accompanied by a primary, preferential expansion of the ECF and consequently by hypertension. The serum sodium is generally normal. In the syndrome of inappropriate ADH production (SIADH), primary water retention occurs. Consequently, the volume expansion involves both the ICF and the ECF; dilutional hyponatremia is the hallmark of SIADH, while hypertension is uncommon. Edema is not characteristic in either of these two disorders. Instead, patients with primary aldosteronism or SIADH reach a volume-expanded steady state in which output equals input.

Primary Renal Sodium Retention. Abnormal renal sodium retention may also occur when the effective circulating volume is normal and there is no effector excess. Acute glomerulonephritis is an example of a disorder in which unidentified renal mechanisms are primarily responsible for edema formation. Patients with acute glomerulonephritis retain salt and water and become hypertensive without reductions in glomerular filtration rate or in effective circulating volume. Furthermore, sodium retention and edema develop when plasma renin activity and aldosterone concentration are normal or reduced and when the serum albumin concentration is normal. Thus, the renal tubule may be abnormally avid for sodium in acute glomerulonephritis. Congestive heart failure may occur as a secondary consequence of the volume expansion.

TABLE 76–3. DISORDERS OF VOLUME EXCESS

Disturbed Starling Forces
(Reduced effective circulating volume; edema formation)
Systemic venous pressure increases
Right heart failure
Constrictive pericarditis
Local venous pressure increases
Left heart failure
Vena cava obstruction
Portal vein obstruction
Reduced oncotic pressure
Nephrotic syndrome
Combined disorders
Cirrhosis
Primary Hormone Excess
(Increased effective circulating volume)
Primary aldosteronism
Cushing's syndrome
SIADH
Primary Renal Sodium Retention
(Increased effective circulating volume)
Acute glomerulonephritis

DIAGNOSIS AND TREATMENT. The recognition and management of volume-expanded states depend on proper identification and treatment of the underlying disorder. However, it is appropriate to cite certain general principles of therapy. Clearly, the cornerstones of therapy in volume-expanded states characterized by sodium expansion rather than primary water retention (as in SIADH) include salt restriction and diuretics. Consequently, Table 76–4 provides a summary of some of the major diuretics used commonly, and certain of their properties; for convenience, these drugs have been classified according to their sites of action in the nephron. Since osmotic diuretics and mercurial diuretics are uncommonly used in current clinical practice, these agents have been omitted from Table 76–4.

Proximal Diuretics. The cardinal example of a proximal tubular diuretic is acetazolamide, a carbonic anhydrase inhibitor that blocks proximal reabsorption of sodium bicarbonate by inhibiting apical Na^+/H^+ exchange. Consequently, prolonged use of acetazolamide may lead to hyperchloremic acidosis, in contrast to all other diuretics that act at loci prior to the late distal nephron. Metolazone is a congener of the thiazide class of diuretics that blocks sodium chloride absorption at two or more nephron sites by an unknown mechanism. Specifically, in addition to an action on the early distal tubule, it has been inferred that metolazone also inhibits proximal tubular sodium chloride absorption, since the major locus for phosphate absorption is in the proximal nephron, and the phosphaturia accompanying metolazone administration exceeds considerably that observed with other thiazide class diuretics.

Loop Diuretics. Loop diuretics such as ethacrynic acid and furosemide produce diuresis by inhibiting the coupled entry of Na^+, Cl^-, and K^+ across apical plasma membranes in the thick

TABLE 76–4. CHARACTERISTICS OF COMMONLY USED DIURETICS

Diuretic	Primary Effect	Secondary Effect	Complications
Proximal Diuretics			
Acetazolamide	↓ Na^+/H^+ exchange	↑ K^+ loss, ↑ HCO_3^- loss	hypokalemic, hyperchloremic acidosis
Metolazone	↓ Na^+ absorption	↑ K^+ loss, ↑ Cl^- loss	hypokalemic alkalosis
Loop Diuretics			
Furosemide, Ethacrynic acid	↓ Na^+:K^+:$2Cl^-$ absorption	↑ K^+ loss, ↑ H^+ secretion	hypokalemic alkalosis
Early Distal Diuretics			
Thiazide, Metolazone	↓ Na^+ absorption	↑ K^+ loss, ↑ H^+ secretion	hypokalemic alkalosis
Late Distal Diuretics			
Aldosterone antagonists			
Spironolactone			
Nonaldosterone antagonists			
Triamterene, Amiloride	↓ Na^+ absorption	↓ K^+ loss, ↓ H^+ secretion	hyperkalemic acidosis

ascending limb of Henle. The latter is responsible for the reabsorption of approximately 25 per cent of filtered sodium; and the dose-response characteristics of these diuretic agents, so far as natriuresis is concerned, are considerably more linear than all other currently used diuretics. Consequently, the loop diuretics are, for practical purposes, the most potent diuretics currently available; therefore these drugs are commonly referred to as "high-ceiling" diuretics.

Early Distal Tubule Diuretics. Early distal tubule diuretics, such as thiazide and metolazone, interfere primarily with sodium absorption, and secondarily with chloride absorption, in the earliest segments of the distal convoluted tubule. The thiazide diuretics appear to exert their effect by blocking sodium entry from tubular fluid across apical plasma membranes into distal tubular cells.

It will be noticed that, with the exception of acetazolamide (which impairs bicarbonate absorption), hypokalemia and metabolic alkalosis may complicate the administration of proximal diuretics, loop diuretics, and early distal tubular diuretics. This occurs because, in practical terms, the rate of sodium delivery to terminal distal tubular regions, where a significant fraction of potassium and proton secretion occur, is a major factor promoting these latter two processes. Consequently, an increased delivery of salt to the late distal nephron, occasioned by inhibition of sodium reabsorption in either the proximal tubule, the ascending limb of Henle, or the early distal tubule, leads to accelerated rates of proton and potassium secretion, and consequently to hypokalemia and metabolic alkalosis.

Late Distal Nephron Diuretics. Finally, there is a group of agents that inhibit sodium absorption in terminal regions of the distal tubule and concomitantly suppress indirectly potassium secretion and proton secretion. Thus the prolonged use of such agents leads to hyperkalemia coupled with hyperchloremic metabolic acidosis. One such agent is spironolactone, which competes with aldosterone; the primary use of this agent is restricted to conditions of aldosterone excess, either primary or secondary. Alternatively, both triamterene and amiloride operate independently of aldosterone. These agents block directly sodium uptake by late distal tubular cells and concomitantly suppress indirectly both potassium and proton secretion. Accordingly, hyperkalemic, hyperchloremic metabolic acidosis may complicate the injudicious use of either spironolactone, triamterene, or amiloride.

Given the availability of potent diuretics, one factor common to the treatment of certain disorders with reduced effective circulating volumes and expanded ECF volumes merits particular consideration. A major factor in edema formation in such patients is an increase in the Starling forces promoting fluid translocation from the vascular to interstitial spaces. Consequently, when potent diuretics are administered to patients with portal hypertension or with hypoalbuminemia, urinary sodium excretion may exceed the rate at which salt and water are transferred from the interstitium to the vascular bed. As a result, vigorous diuretic therapy in these patients may result in volume contraction, reduced salt delivery to diluting segments, nonosmotic ADH release, and consequently hyponatremia. In advanced cases of diuretic abuse, hypotension, hemoconcentration, and azotemia also occur.

Finally, a similar effect may occur in volume-expanded patients, particularly those exhibiting a third-space effect and having significant hypoalbuminemia, if relatively large volumes of ascitic fluid are removed by paracentesis. In this circumstance, the transudation of fluid from the vascular space to the interstitial space may result in circulatory collapse.

Brenner BM, Badr KF, Schor N, Ichikawa I: Hormonal influences on glomerular filtration. Mineral Electrolyte Metab 4:49–56, 1980. *A brief discussion of the effect of hormones on the glomerular filtration rate, especially the interactions of prostaglandins and angiotensin II.*

Currie MG, et al.: Purification and sequence analysis of bioactive atrial peptides (atriopeptins). Science 223:67, 1984. *The isolation of a natriuretic factor from cardiac atria which may be released in relation to atrial baroreceptor stimulation.*

Haber E: The role of renin in normal and pathological cardiovascular homeostasis. Circulation 54:849–861, 1976. *An excellent review of the physiology of the renin-angiotensin system and the role of angiotensin II in maintenance of blood pressure during ECF volume depletion.*

Hauser CJ, Shoemaker WC: Volume therapy. Part I: Diagnosis of hypovolemia. Hosp Physician 38–41, September, 1980. *A concise, easy-to-read discussion of the physiology of volume depletion and the use of hemodynamic monitoring in the diagnosis of ECF volume depletion.*

Hauser CJ, Shoemaker WC: Volume therapy. Part II: Treatment of hypovolemia. Hosp Physician 38–45, October, 1980. *An easy-to-read review of the efficacy of various parenteral fluids in increasing ECF and blood volume and the effects on hemodynamics of the various fluid therapies.*

Levy M: The pathophysiology of sodium balance. Hosp Prac 95–106, November, 1978. *A good general review of the physiology of sodium homeostasis and the pathophysiology of the major depletion and retention states.*

Lifschitz MD, Stein JH: Hormonal regulation of renal salt excretion. Semin Nephrol 3:196–204, 1983. *A topical review of sodium excretion and its modulation by hormones.*

Smith HW: Salt and water volume receptors. Am J Med 23:623–651, 1957. *A critical review of the state of knowledge concerning volume receptors prior to 1960; a classic.*

Thier SO: The Kidney. Diuretics. *In* Smith LH, Thier SO (eds.): Pathophysiology. Philadelphia, W. B. Saunders Company, 1985, in press.

Osmolality Disturbances

PHYSIOLOGIC CONSIDERATIONS

In normal individuals, the serum osmolality is virtually constant from day to day, and the serum sodium concentration is an accurate index to body water osmolality. In fact, the normal range for serum sodium concentrations or for serum osmolalities in populations of healthy individuals depends on small differences in body water osmolality among individuals, rather than on variations in body water osmolality in a given individual. Because cell membranes are freely permeable to water, the fact that the serum osmolality is constant also means that the ratio of solute to water in all body fluid compartments is constant. Since cell membrane cation pumps, such as membrane-bound sodium plus potassium adenosine triphosphatase ($Na^+ + K^+$)–ATPase, maintain cellular cation content at a constant level, these considerations indicate that one of the cardinal functions of osmoregulation is to maintain cell volume at a constant level.

It is useful in this context to define the concept of "effective ECF osmolality," since the osmoregulatory mechanisms that adjust water balance in normal individuals are determined primarily by changes in cell volume that result from variations in effective ECF osmolality. In dilutional states, the measured and effective ECF osmolalities are approximately equal, since ECF dilution also produces ICF dilution and, at least acutely, cell swelling. Osmoregulatory mechanisms are activated when ECF hypertonicity is due to a solute that is excluded from cells and therefore produces, at least acutely, cell shrinkage; in this case, the measured and effective ECF osmolalities are approximately equal. However, if the ECF osmolality is increased by solutes, such as urea, which penetrate cell membranes readily, acute cell shrinkage does not occur and osmoregulatory mechanisms are not activated; in this case, the measured ECF osmolality is greater than the effective ECF osmolality.

In practical terms, the serum osmolality may be calculated from the formula:

$$\text{osmolality} = 2[\text{Na}^+] + \frac{[\text{glucose}]}{18} + \frac{[\text{BUN}]}{2.8}$$

where the glucose and blood urea nitrogen (BUN) concentrations are expressed as milligrams per deciliter, and the serum sodium concentration is expressed as milliequivalents per liter. Under normal circumstances, glucose contributes 5.5 mOsm per kilogram of H_2O and urea contributes 2 to 6 mOsm per kilogram of H_2O to the serum osmolality. When hyperglycemia occurs, the effective ECF osmolality rises because glucose entry into cells is limited. When azotemia occurs, the effective ECF osmolality does not rise because urea enters cells readily.

Cell Volume Regulation

Starling forces regulate fluid transfer between the ICF and the ECF; however, because plasma membranes can tolerate negligibly small hydrostatic gradients, the operational Starling forces between ICF and ECF are almost entirely osmotic. Significant changes in cell volume, particularly in the central nervous system, are by themselves potentially lethal. Moreover, the development of hydrostatic pressure gradients between cells and the ECF can lead to cell lysis. Thus the goals of fluid transport between the ECF and ICF are to maintain constancy of cell volume and a negligible hydrostatic pressure gradient between cells and the ECF. Since cell membranes are freely permeable to water, the latter two goals are achieved when the ECF osmolality is normal and intracellular and extracellular osmolalities are identical.

Since cell membranes are partially permeable to sodium and potassium, there is a tendency for sodium to leak into cells and for potassium to leak out of cells. Because impermeant macromolecules account for a large fraction of intracellular anions, passive sodium and potassium movements tend toward a Donnan distribution in which total intracellular cations would exceed total interstitial cations, in precise analogy to the way in which total plasma water cations exceed total interstitial cations. If these passive cation movements across cell membranes were unopposed, osmotic water movement into cells would tend to produce cell lysis. Consequently, active transport mechanisms are required to balance intracellular and interstitial cation concentrations.

Specifically, both sodium leakage from the ECF into cells and potassium leakage out of cells into the ECF are counterbalanced exactly by active outward sodium transport coupled to active inward potassium transport. These active transport events maintain the intracellular cation (and therefore osmolar) content equal to that of extracellular fluid, and also maintain the predominant extracellular and intracellular distributions of sodium and potassium, respectively. Thus, because cellular cation pumps balance cellular cation leaks, cells are *operationally* impermeable to sodium and to potassium. Active sodium efflux coupled to active potassium influx is mediated by membrane-bound ($Na^+ + K^+$)–ATPase, and the activity of these cellular cation pumps accounts for more than 50 per cent of the basal caloric consumption. It is thought that the cellular swelling seen in debilitated states (often referred to as the "sick cell syndrome") is the result of impairment of these cellular cation pumps.

Cation transport mediated by ($Na^+ + K^+$)–ATPase is the major factor regulating cell volume when the effective ECF osmolality is normal. When the effective ECF osmolality is increased or decreased, additional processes are required to maintain the constancy of cell volume. These auxiliary mechanisms are of particular importance in minimizing potentially lethal changes in brain volume because of osmotic water shifts into or out of brain cells.

In chronic hypotonic disorders, cell swelling is offset by the loss of potassium chloride from cells. This potassium chloride efflux mechanism appears to be activated by small increases in cell volume produced by ECF dilution. In chronic hypernatremia, brain shrinkage is minimized by the accumulation of additional solutes within brain cells. These latter solutes, often called "idiogenic osmoles," include amino acids and other unidentified solutes. The mechanisms by which cells accumulate intracellular solutes are not understood, but they appear to be activated by small decreases in brain cell volume produced by extracellular fluid hypertonicity. As will be discussed in the section on Treatment, these auxiliary transport processes affect significantly the therapeutic approach to patients with osmoregulatory failure.

The Water Repletion Reaction

The key elements regulating water balance are summarized in Figure 76–4. The solid lines indicate osmoregulatory mechanisms that, as indicated above, maintain constancy of cell volume. When the effective circulating volume is reduced by more than 10 per cent, volume-mediated stimuli participate in the regulation of water balance. These pathways are indicated by the dashed lines in Figure 76–4. It will be recognized that the water repletion reaction shares many elements in common with the volume repletion reaction presented in Figure 76–3.

SENSORS AND EFFECTORS. Three kinds of *sensor* elements adjust water balance. Two of these, osmoreceptors and the thirst center, respond to small changes in effective ECF osmolality, while baroreceptors respond to changes in effective circulating volume. The osmoreceptors are situated in the supraoptic and paraventricular nuclei of the hypothalamus, while the thirst center is in another region of the anterior hypothalamus. As little as a 2 per cent increase in effective ECF osmolality produced by solutes such as sodium chloride, but not urea, cause shrinkage of osmoreceptor cells and thirst center cells. In turn the osmoreceptors stimulate the release of the *effector* hormone ADH from storage sites in the posterior pituitary gland. The thirst centers, by as yet unknown effector mechanisms, stimulate thirst.

When the effective circulating volume is reduced by more than 10 per cent, volume-dependent mechanisms stimulate ADH release. Activation of extrarenal baroreceptors by blood volume depletion produces afferent signals, carried by cranial nerves IX and X, which result in nonosmotic ADH release. Volume contraction also stimulates formation of angiotensin II, a potent stimulus to thirst.

The Antidiuretic Response. The cardinal characteristics of the antidiuretic response depend primarily on the integrated activity of two regions of the nephron: the medullary thick ascending limb of Henle, referred to as the diluting segment; and the collecting duct, which may be termed the concentrating segment.

The medullary thick ascending limb absorbs a large amount, possibly as much as 25 per cent, of the filtered load of sodium. Some of this reabsorbed sodium is trapped in the renal medullary interstitium, thus accounting in large part for the hyper-

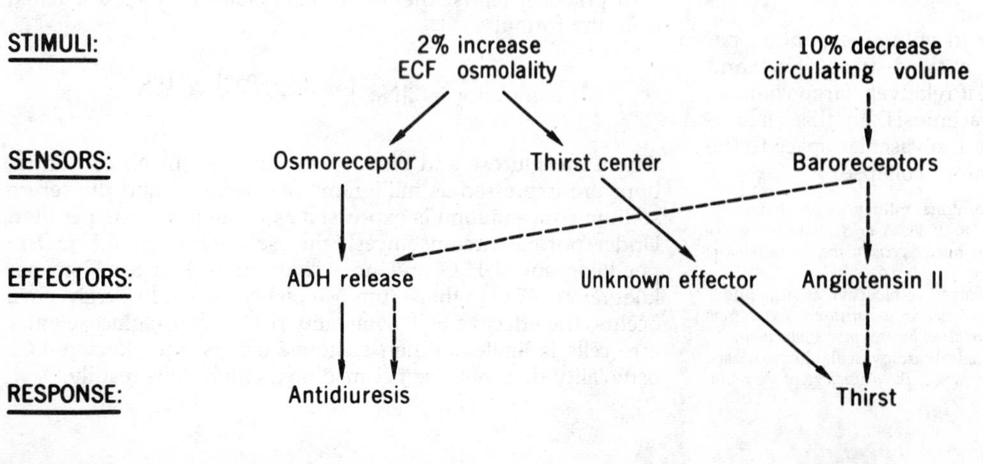

Figure 76–4. The water repletion reaction. The integrated operation of the sensor and effector mechanisms responsible for thirst and renal water conservation is shown. The response may be stimulated either by a 2 per cent decrease in ECF osmolality or a 10 per cent decrease in blood volume.

tonicity of the renal medullary interstitium. However, the medullary thick limb of Henle is also water impermeable. Consequently, salt abstraction from the thick limb of Henle accounts simultaneously for the development of medullary hypertonicity, thus permitting maximal antidiuresis in the presence of ADH and the appearance of maximally dilute urine in early distal convolutions. This permits in turn a maximal water diuresis when ADH is absent.

In normal individuals, approximately 18 liters daily of tubular fluid reaches the early distal tubule; the osmolality of this fluid is quite dilute, approximately 50 mOsm per kilogram of H_2O. Thus in the total absence of ADH and volume contraction, maximal rates of water diuresis include a urine volume of 18 liters daily having an osmolality of 50 mOsm per kilogram of H_2O. During antidiuresis, ADH increases the water permeability of collecting ducts (see Ch. 225). There is osmotic equilibration of tubular fluid with the hypertonic medullary interstitium, and consequently a reduction in urine volume, a concentration of urine, and a conservation of body water. When ADH is absent, the water permeability of collecting ducts is low and there is reduced absorption of tubular fluid, which escapes unchanged as hypotonic urine.

Reductions in the daily rate of salt absorption by the thick ascending limb reduce the ability to form a maximally dilute urine. When reduced volumes of glomerular filtrate reach the thick ascending limb, the volume of hypotonic tubular fluid formed by the diluting segment is correspondingly reduced. There may also be a reduction in the minimal urine osmolality reaching early distal convolutions.

Finally, since collecting ducts are partially permeable to water in the absence of ADH, a reduced volume of hypotonic fluid reaching collecting ducts equilibrates partially with the medullary interstitium, thereby limiting the ability to dilute urine maximally. In some experimental circumstances, sufficiently significant reductions in the rate of solute excretion result in formation of a hypertonic urine when ADH is absent.

To summarize, the disturbances in body fluid osmolality, both hypertonic and hypotonic, may be rationalized, to a large degree, by the interplay between the functions of the thick limb of Henle, serving as the diluting segment, and the ADH-sensitive collecting duct, which serves as the concentrating segment.

HYPOTONIC DISORDERS

DEFINITION. A hypotonic disorder is one in which the ratio of solutes to water in body fluids is reduced, and the serum osmolality and serum sodium are both reduced in parallel. True hypotonicity of body fluid must be distinguished from disorders in which the *measured* serum sodium is low while the *measured* serum osmolality is either normal or increased.

The distinction among these disorders is listed in Table 76–5. The measured serum sodium can be reduced either because of an increased concentration of small, nonsodium solutes restricted to the ECF or because of a laboratory artifact. In hyperglycemia or excessive mannitol administration, these solutes, which are restricted to the ECF, draw water from the cellular compartment. The serum sodium is therefore reduced even though the serum osmolality may be increased. When a small, nonsodium solute is distributed in total body water, as in ethanol intoxication or in azotemia, the serum osmolality rises but the serum sodium concentration remains normal. This observation, the so-called "osmolar gap," is particularly helpful in evaluating acutely ill, intoxicated patients.

In hyperlipemic or hyperproteinemic states, the volume of water in a given sample of serum sent for laboratory analysis is reduced. The flame photometer measures the total amount of sodium in a correspondingly reduced volume of water per unit volume of serum, and therefore reports a low serum sodium level. However, the measured serum osmolality, which is a colligative property of aqueous solutions, is measured as being normal, since the actual concentration of sodium per unit volume of water is normal.

ETIOLOGY AND PATHOGENESIS. Hyponatremia and simultaneous body water hypotonicity develop whenever water intake exceeds the sum of renal plus extrarenal water losses; in chronic hyponatremia, the net water intake and net water output may be equal. Thus hyponatremia and body fluid hypotonicity may occur when there is a primary increase in water ingestion, when the ability of the kidney to dilute urine maximally is limited, or when a combination of these factors is operative.

More specifically, we may consider two major classes of disorders resulting in dilutional hyponatremia. First, there may be an absolute increase in water intake that exceeds the ability of a normal kidney to excrete free water, as in *primary polydipsia*, often referred to as psychogenic polydipsia. Patients with this disorder ingest unusually large volumes of water, often in excess of 10 to 15 liters daily, and generally develop mild, clinically asymptomatic hyponatremia. Profound hyponatremia is rare in these patients because the ability of the kidney to excrete large volumes of maximally dilute urine is not impaired.

The second and most common reason for clinically significant hyponatremia is a disturbance in *water output* because of an inability of the kidney to excrete a maximally dilute urine. This inability to dilute urine maximally may occur (1) because of reductions in the rate of salt absorption by the diluting segment, that is, the thick ascending limb of Henle; (2) because of sustained nonosmotic release of the effector hormone ADH; and (3) because of a combination of these factors. Table 76–6 summarizes these disturbances in water output.

Reduced Sodium Delivery to Diluting Segments. The first group in Table 76–6 includes disorders in which a reduced sodium intake, without significant sodium depletion or ECF volume contraction, decreases the rate of sodium delivery to the diluting segment and consequently impairs either the maximal rate of dilute urine formation, the minimal urine osmolality, or both.

TABLE 76–5. DISTINCTION BETWEEN APPARENT AND REAL HYPOTONICITY

Condition	Measured Serum [Na]	Measured Serum Osmolality
True hypotonicity	↓	↓
Increased nonsodium ECF solutes		
Hyperglycemia	↓	↑
Mannitol administration	↓	↑
Increased nonsodium ECF and ICF solutes		
Ethanol	nl	↑
Ethylene glycol	nl	↑
Methanol	nl	↑
Isopropyl alcohol	nl	↑
Laboratory Artifact		
Hyperlipemia	↓	nl
Hyperproteinemia	↓	nl

TABLE 76–6. HYPONATREMIA REFERABLE TO IMPAIRED RENAL EXCRETION OF WATER

Reduced Sodium Delivery to the Diluting Segment
- Starvation
- Beer potomania
- ? Myxedema

Primary Excess of ADH
- SIADH
- Drug-induced ADH production
- Drug potentiation of ADH action
- Trauma
- Potassium depletion
- ? Myxedema
- ? Acute intermittent porphyria

Mixed Disorders
- Volume contraction (Addison's disease)
- Edema with deranged Starling forces (congestive heart failure, constrictive pericarditis, and cirrhosis)

Beer potomania, although an uncommon disorder, illustrates nicely this mechanism for hyponatremia. Patients with beer potomania derive a large part of their caloric intake from the ingestion of large volumes of beer, which contains little salt or protein. Because sodium and urea are the major urinary solutes, dietary restriction of these solutes, particularly sodium, increases the fractional rate of proximal sodium absorption, diminishes the rate of salt delivery to diluting segments, and in turn limits the daily rate of formation of dilute urine. For example, since the minimum urinary osmolality that can be achieved is approximately 50 mOsm per kilogram of H_2O, the excretion of 15 liters of highly dilute urine requires the excretion of 750 mOsm of solute. If the daily urinary solute excretion falls, the maximal daily rate of dilute urine formation is also reduced. Moreover, partial equilibration of reduced volumes of collecting duct fluid with the renal medullary interstitium impairs even further the daily excretion of dilute urine.

Hyponatremia due to reduced solute intake is not restricted to individuals with beer potomania but may occur during starvation, when intake may be dramatically reduced without parallel reductions in water intake. Hyponatremia due to starvation is now seen commonly in elderly nursing home patients who are inadequately supervised. In such patients, reduced dietary intake of sodium also reduces urinary diluting capacity by curtailing the rate of sodium delivery to the loop of Henle.

Patients with beer potomania or starvation are therefore to be distinguished from individuals in whom a reduced effective circulating volume accompanied by an increase in total body water or by a reduction in glomerular filtration rate reduces the rate of salt delivery to diluting segments and collecting ducts (see below). In short, beer potomania and starvation are classic examples in which a reduced rate of delivery to the diluting segment, in the absence of ADH release, blunts significantly urinary diluting power in the absence of profound gains or excesses in total body water.

Primary Effector ADH Excess. THE SYNDROME OF INAPPROPRIATE ADH PRODUCTION (SIADH). SIADH is a disorder in which hyponatremia occurs as a result of sustained endogenous production and release of ADH or ADH-like substances; the effective circulating volume is normal or increased and there are no other physiologic or pharmacologic stimuli to ADH release. The disorder occurs most commonly in association with pulmonary diseases, particularly bronchogenic carcinoma; in association with cranial disorders, including head trauma and infections of the central nervous system; and in association with a number of other neoplasms, notably pancreatic carcinoma. SIADH also seems to occur in acute intermittent porphyria. Finally, there is indirect evidence that a similar process may account in part for the hyponatremia seen in myxedema.

ADH, or a peptide having comparable biologic activity, is produced by tumors such as oat cell lung carcinoma, either by the primary tumor or by metastases, by adenocarcinoma of the pancreas, and by duodenal adenocarcinoma. Increased ADH levels, estimated either by bioassay or radioimmunoassay, have also been noted in patients with cranial disorders such as skull fractures, subdural hematomas, subarachnoid hemorrhage, and brain tumors, in acute intermittent porphyria, and possibly in myxedema. It is presumed that ADH release in cranial disorders occurs because of direct hypothalamic stimulation independent of osmotic stimuli. The causes for ADH production and release in nonmalignant pulmonary disorders, acute intermittent porphyria, and myxedema are unknown.

As a result of the sustained release of ADH or ADH-like substances, patients who develop SIADH retain ingested water, become hyponatremic and modestly volume expanded, and generally increase their body weight by 5 to 10 per cent. The volume expansion results in reduced rates of proximal tubular sodium absorption, and consequently a natriuresis, albeit at a net expansion of total body water. Since aldosterone secretion is stimulated by hyponatremia, it is possible that secretion of this mineralocorticoid may also contribute to reducing renal sodium losses in volume-expanded hyponatremic patients with SIADH. There are also increased urinary losses of substances like uric acid, whose excretion rates vary directly with effective circulating volume and with rates of sodium excretion. Consequently, hypouricemia is common in SIADH. The glomerular filtration rate is normal, as is adrenal and thyroid function.

The urine osmolality in patients with SIADH need not be hypertonic to plasma, but only inappropriately high for the level of serum osmolality. Patients with SIADH ordinarily have normal or increased rates of solute excretion and normal or increased effective circulating volumes. Hence the excretion of urine that is not maximally dilute in a setting of hyponatremia represents, in fact, inappropriate ADH-mediated antidiuresis.

OTHER CAUSES OF EXCESSIVE ADH PRODUCTION AND/OR RELEASE. Table 76–6 lists other circumstances in which an increased level of ADH is the primary factor responsible for hyponatremia. A number of commonly used drugs stimulate ADH release. These include vincristine, cyclophosphamide, carbamazepine, phenothiazines, morphine, barbiturates, chlorpropamide, amitriptyline, thiothixene, and clofibrate. Chlorpropamide also potentiates the effect of ADH on the water permeability of collecting ducts. The posterior pituitary peptide oxytocin (Pitocin) also has an antidiuretic action, although a much less potent one than does vasopressin. Thus the administration of intravenous hypotonic solutions containing oxytocin for the purpose of inducing labor may result in profound hyponatremia. Trauma or surgical stress also stimulates ADH release.

Ordinarily, diuretic-induced hyponatremia is related to volume contraction; this kind of body fluid dilution will be discussed below. However, chronic, severe potassium depletion induced by diuretics also can result in ADH release. A group of nonedematous patients has been described in whom increases in plasma antidiuretic activity occur in association with thiazide-induced hypokalemia and a reduced total body exchangeable potassium content. Hyponatremia, increased levels of antidiuretic activity in serum, and an inappropriately concentrated urine persist, so long as hypokalemia is present, even if extracellular fluid volume deficits are impaired. The mechanisms by which potassium depletion stimulates ADH release are unknown.

Mixed Disorders. Hyponatremia occurs commonly both in states of true volume contraction and in certain edematous states in which filling of the arterial tree is impaired. The former disorders include patients in whom both ECF and total body water are reduced; the latter group includes those patients with deranged Starling forces, notably local or systemic increases in venous pressure, which result in inadequate filling of the arterial tree. In both sets of disorders, two factors may contribute, individually or in unison, to the pathogenesis of hyponatremia: nonosmotic, volume-mediated ADH release and reductions in the rate of sodium delivery to the diluting segment.

Volume contraction is a potent nonosmotic stimulus to ADH release. Figure 76-5 shows the relations between osmotic and nonosmotic, volume-mediated stimuli and plasma ADH levels in experimental animals; entirely comparable responses occur in man. There is a linear relation between increases in plasma osmolality and increases in plasma ADH levels. However, the relation between blood volume depletion and plasma ADH levels is nonlinear. When more than 7 to 10 per cent blood volume depletion occurs, plasma ADH levels rise sharply and produce an antidiuretic effect even when the plasma osmolality is reduced below normal. In other words, volume-mediated, nonosmotic ADH release occurs primarily when circulatory dynamics are moderately to severely advanced; in that circumstance, volume-mediated stimuli override osmotically mediated ADH release, and hyponatremia ensues.

A second factor that accounts for hyponatremia in volume-contracted states is an inability to dilute urine maximally because the rate of sodium delivery to diluting segments in the thick ascending limb is reduced. This occurs because increased rates of proximal tubular sodium absorption are stimulated by

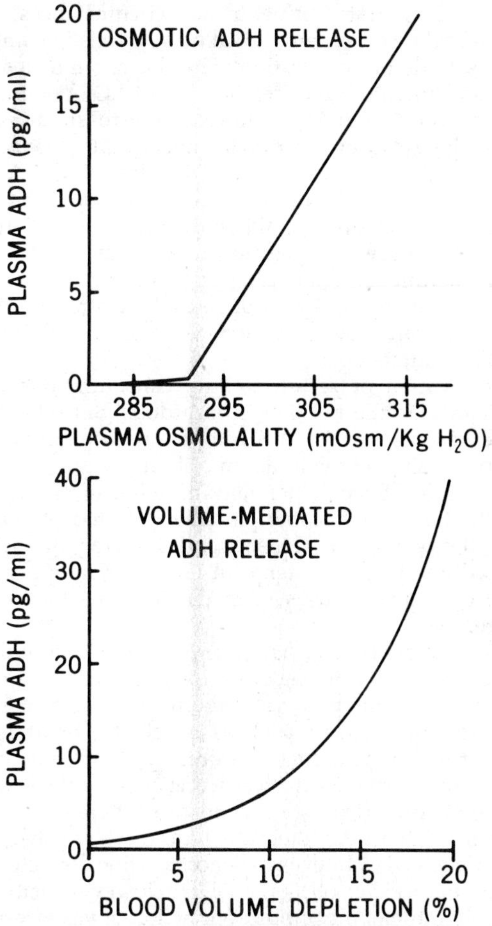

Figure 76–5. Relation between plasma ADH concentrations and either effective ECF osmolality (upper plot) or the percentage of blood volume depletion (lower plot). Note that the relation is linear with effective ECF osmolality but exponential with blood volume depletion. (Adapted from Dunn et al.: J Clin Invest 52:3212–3219, 1973.)

reduced sodium intake or by inadequate filling of the arterial tree in conditions with combined ECF volume expansion and reduced arterial tree filling. The significance of volume contraction as a pathogenic factor in this type of hyponatremia can be gauged by noting that hyponatremia occurs during volume contraction in experimental animals with pituitary diabetes insipidus.

Hyponatremia is a common feature of untreated Addison's disease and occurs because of a combination of circumstances. In mineralocorticoid deficiency, the combination of ECF volume contraction, glomerular filtration reduction, enhanced proximal tubular salt absorption, and volume-mediated, nonosmotic ADH release appears to be the major factor responsible for an inability to handle water loads. Glucocorticoid deficiency also impairs the ability to handle water loads, but there are conflicting views about the mechanisms responsible for this effect. One of the factors responsible for water retention is nonosmotic ADH release secondary to a reduction in effective circulating volume, which results from a glucocorticoid-mediated impairment in cardiac function.

Hyponatremia occurs commonly in advanced stages of disorders characterized by edema formation and a reduced effective circulating volume (Table 76–6), particularly in intractable heart failure and advanced hepatic cirrhosis with ascites. Reduced rates of salt delivery to diluting segments in these disorders clearly contribute to the impairment in water excretion. A limited number of radioimmunoassay measurements of plasma ADH levels in patients with heart failure or severe ascites also indicate that the plasma concentrations of this hormone are inappropriately high with respect to plasma osmolality. Nonosmotic ADH release may also contribute to the development of hyponatremia in these disorders. Furthermore, since nonosmotic ADH release occurs only with profound reductions in blood volume (Fig. 76–5), the occurrence of hyponatremia in congestive failure or cirrhosis probably indicates profound arterial underfilling. This observation correlates well with the ominous prognosis of hyponatremia in these disorders.

Other Hyponatremic States. Rarely, hyponatremia occurs in individuals in whom osmoreceptors appear to be "reset" downward. These individuals develop hyponatremia when the effective circulating volume is normal. However, in contrast to patients with SIADH, individuals with reset osmoreceptors develop a brisk water diuresis when the serum sodium is reduced sufficiently, suggesting that suppression of ADH release occurs at a lower plasma osmolality than normal.

Hyponatremia sometimes occurs in debilitated or severely ill patients without a gain in total body water and when the intracellular sodium concentration is increased. The disorder is referred to as the "sick cell syndrome." The activity of membrane-bound (Na^+ + K^+)-ATPase is also impaired in severely ill patients. Consequently, it is believed that the hyponatremia in the sick cell syndrome occurs because of redistribution of sodium from the ECF to the ICF.

CLINICAL MANIFESTATIONS. The clinical manifestations of hyponatremia are produced by the brain swelling that accompanies acute dilution of total body water and generally becomes manifest when the serum sodium concentration falls to 120 mEq per liter or less. The early symptoms include *lethargy, weakness,* and *somnolence,* which can proceed rapidly to *seizures, coma,* and *death.* Because untreated acute water intoxication is nearly uniformly fatal, it represents a medical emergency. In chronic hyponatremia, central nervous system manifestations are far less common, even when the serum sodium concentration is as low as 110 mEq per liter, because the loss of brain solutes, principally potassium chloride, minimize brain cell swelling for a given reduction in body water osmolality.

DIAGNOSIS. The diagnosis of hyponatremia is most commonly made from routine laboratory findings. Hyponatremia should also be considered whenever there is a sudden deterioration in central nervous system function, particularly in circumstances such as intractable heart failure, hepatic cirrhosis with ascites, or the administration of large volumes of intravenous fluids. When hyponatremia has been identified, the patient should be evaluated for the underlying condition that produced body fluid dilution. The evaluation should include a careful history and physical examination; measurement of the serum creatinine, BUN, and electrolytes; measurement of the urinary sodium concentration of the FE_{Na}; measurement of serum and urine osmolalities; and when appropriate, evaluation of thyroid and adrenal function.

The history and physical examination are generally adequate to recognize disorders such as beer potomania or compulsive water ingestion, or for noting the ingestion of drugs that stimulate ADH release or enhance ADH action. The presence of edema is characteristic of individuals in whom hyponatremia occurs because of a reduced effective circulating volume coupled with ECF volume expansion. In myxedema or Addison's disease, the typical clinical or laboratory findings of these disorders are generally present.

The most difficult differential diagnosis among hyponatremic disorders involves the distinction between patients who are modestly volume contracted and those who have SIADH. In both circumstances, the serum sodium and the serum osmolality are reduced, whereas the urine osmolality is inappropriately high with respect to the reduced serum osmolality. Nonosmotic water conservation in SIADH and in volume contraction is recognized by the presence of a urine osmolality greater than 120 to 150 mOsm per kilogram of H_2O in association with a reduced serum osmolality. The distinction between the two disorders therefore depends on a clinical and laboratory assessment of effective circulating volume.

Patients who are volume contracted may provide a history of volume losses or of diuretic ingestion and exhibit the signs of ECF volume contraction discussed previously in the section on Volume Depletion. When the volume losses are due to extrarenal causes, the urinary sodium concentration is less than 10 to 15 mEq per liter and the FE_{Na} is generally less than 1 per cent. The presence of hyperuricemia may also be a useful index to the possibility of ECF volume contraction. Prerenal azotemia may occur if the volume contraction is severe. Patients with SIADH are generally normovolemic or slightly volume expanded and therefore exhibit none of the signs of volume contraction. The serum BUN and creatinine are normal and the serum uric acid is generally reduced. The urinary sodium concentration usually exceeds 30 mEq per liter, and the FE_{Na} is greater than 1 per cent. Tests of adrenal function are normal.

The above studies usually discriminate between SIADH and extrarenal volume contraction. When ECF volume contraction is due to renal salt wasting, urinary sodium losses generally persist unless volume contraction is profound. Moreover, as noted previously (see Volume Depletion), the blood pressure and pulse may be normal in states of modest volume contraction. A useful diagnostic and therapeutic maneuver in this situation is to observe the results of water restriction. When water intake is restricted to 600 to 800 ml daily, patients with SIADH exhibit a highly characteristic response: A 2 to 3 kilogram weight loss is accompanied by correction of hyponatremia and cessation of salt wasting, usually over a period of two to three days. If weight loss fails to correct both hyponatremia and urinary sodium wasting simultaneously, the diagnosis of SIADH is doubtful. Rather, renal sodium wasting with ECF volume contraction, due to Addison's disease or one of the other renal salt losing disorders listed in Table 76–1, is the more probable diagnosis.

TREATMENT. The goal of treatment in hyponatremia is to correct body water osmolality and therefore restore cell volume to normal by raising the ratio of sodium to water in extracelluar fluid. The increase in ECF osmolality draws water from cells and therefore reduces their volume. The choice of therapeutic approach, and whether or not net sodium and water balance are adjusted to be positive or negative during therapy, depends on the serum sodium concentration, the rate at which hyponatremia has developed, the clinical status of the patient, and the underlying disorder.

Acute Hyponatremia. Acute hyponatremia associated with a serum sodium concentration below 120 to 125 mEq per liter and central nervous system manifestations requires immediate therapy. In volume-contracted states, the treatment of choice is to raise the serum sodium to 125 mEq per liter over a 6-hour interval by administering hypertonic 3 to 5 per cent saline. Since the desired effect is to correct body water osmolality, the amount of sodium administered must be sufficient to raise total body water osmolality to approximately 250 mOsm per kilogram of H_2O, that is, to approximately twice the desired serum sodium concentration. A convenient formula for calculating this sodium requirement is:

$$[125 - \text{measured serum } Na^+] \times 0.6 \text{ Body Weight} = \text{required mEq of } Na^+.$$

The serum sodium is in milliequivalents per liter, and the body weight is in kilograms. Since 60 per cent of body weight is water, the formula allows an estimate of the amount of sodium required to raise body water osmolality to 250 mOsm per kilogram of H_2O.

The administration of hypertonic saline solutions is hazardous in volume-expanded, salt-retaining states such as congestive heart failure. Furthermore, in SIADH associated with volume expansion and sodium wasting, the administration of hypertonic saline alone may be ineffective in correcting hyponatremia because the administered salt is excreted promptly in a relatively concentrated urine. In such circumstances, one may use normal saline or hypertonic saline solutions in combination with furosemide administration. The diuretic induces urinary salt loss and therefore reduces the risk of ECF volume expansion. Moreover, the diuresis induced by furosemide is characterized by the excretion of urine having a sodium concentration that is appreciably lower than that in plasma. Consequently, the combination of intravenously administered normal or hypertonic saline and a furosemide-induced diuresis of urine that is dilute with respect to plasma provides an effective way of raising the serum sodium in SIADH or other volume-expanded states. By adjusting the rates of salt administration to be less than urinary salt losses, reductions in ECF volume can be produced simultaneously.

Rapid elevation of serum sodium concentrations to levels greater than 125 mEq per liter is hazardous. Since loss of brain solute represents one of the compensatory mechanisms for preserving brain cell volume in dilutional states, a serum sodium of 140 mEq per liter may be relatively hypertonic to brain cells that have become partially depleted of solute as a result of hyponatremia. Consequently, raising the serum sodium rapidly to levels greater than 120 to 125 mEq per liter can result in central nervous system damage due to acute brain shrinkage.

Chronic Hyponatremia. Mild, asymptomatic chronic hyponatremia is generally managed by correction of the underlying disorder, when the hyponatremia occurs in volume contraction or in salt-retaining states such as congestive heart failure or hepatic cirrhosis with ascites. Chronic hyponatremia in SIADH may be easily corrected by restricting water intake to 800 to 1000 ml daily, provided that patients can adhere to the program of water restriction. An alternative approach involves the use of agents such as lithium or demeclocycline, which interfere with the renal tubular effects of ADH. However, neither agent consistently inhibits the antidiuretic action of vasopressin in all patients, and both agents have other adverse effects. As another alternative, some workers have recommended reducing renal ability for concentrating urine by administering large oral loads of urea, thereby producing a modest osmotic diuresis.

HYPERTONIC DISORDERS

DEFINITION. A hypertonic disorder is one in which the ratio of solutes to water in total body water is increased. All hypernatremic states are hypertonic. However, in some hypertonic disorders, the increase in effective ECF osmolality may be due to nonsodium solutes, for example, in uncontrolled hyperglycemia.

ETIOLOGY AND PATHOGENESIS. Hypernatremia develops whenever water intake is less than the sum of renal and extrarenal water losses; in chronic hypertonic states, net water balance may be zero. The most common causes for clinically significant hypernatremia occur as a consequence of three pathogenic mechanisms: (1) impaired thirst, (2) solute or osmotic diuresis, or (3) excessive losses of water, either via the kidneys or extrarenally. There may be combinations of these derangements. These disorders are grouped in Table 76–7 according to the primary pathogenic mechanism. There is also

TABLE 76–7. MAJOR CAUSES OF HYPERNATREMIA

Impaired Thirst
Coma
Essential hypernatremia
Solute Diuresis
Osmotic diuresis: diabetic ketoacidosis, nonketotic hyperosmolar coma, mannitol administration
Excessive Water Losses
Renal
Pituitary diabetes insipidus
Nephrogenic diabetes insipidus
Extrarenal
Sweating
Combined Disorders
Coma plus hypertonic nasogastric feeding

a group of miscellaneous disorders (such as hypokalemia, hypercalcemia, and interstitial renal disease) and chronic renal failure, which either impair partially renal urinary concentrating ability or blunt partially the responsiveness of collecting ducts to ADH. Such disorders rarely cause significant hypernatremia and will not be discussed further.

Inadequate Intake of Water. This problem occurs in patients who are comatose or otherwise unable to communicate thirst. Because of the exquisite sensitivity of thirst mechanisms to changes in effective body water osmolality, hypernatremia due to inadequate water intake is rare in conscious patients. Finally, in clinical terms, the hypertonic disorders that have particular relevance, because of their potentially lethal effects on the central nervous system, are those in which the osmolality increase is referable to increase in the concentrations of solutes largely restricted to the ECF, since these conditions lead to cellular shrinkage, particularly in the central nervous system.

Conscious patients with Cushing's syndrome or primary hyperaldosteronism commonly have slight elevations in the serum sodium. The reasons for hypernatremia in these disorders are not known.

"Essential hypernatremia" is another disorder in which an elevated serum sodium occurs in the conscious state. The defect in patients with essential hypernatremia appears to be an insensitivity of thirst centers and osmoreceptors to osmotic stimuli. However, both thirst and antidiuresis occur when these patients are volume contracted. Consequently, it has been inferred that volume-mediated stimuli to thirst and ADH release are intact in patients with essential hypernatremia. This disorder may be either congenital or acquired, sometimes in association with histiocytic infiltration of the central nervous system.

Osmotic Diuresis. This is another mechanism for producing renal water losses in excess of sodium losses and therefore hypertonicity. This occurs commonly in uncontrolled glycosuria and may occur during mannitol administration for increased intracranial pressure. Since these solutes are restricted to the ECF, the serum sodium is generally reduced in the early stages of osmotic diuresis, and the effective ECF osmolality is increased primarily by the impermeant nonsodium solute. In prolonged osmotic diuresis, net water losses may be sufficiently great that hypernatremia develops. In this circumstance, the effective ECF osmolality increase is due to the combined effects of hypernatremia and the nonsodium solute. Hypernatremia due to an osmotic urea diuresis can occur if large amounts of protein and amino acids are administered by nasogastric tube, or if tissue catabolism is great, as in burns. In this circumstance, hypernatremia is entirely responsible for the increased effective ECF osmolality.

Hypernatremia may also occur when large amounts of hypertonic sodium solutions are administered, particularly in patients whose renal function is compromised. Two common examples of this condition include the rapid intravenous administration of multiple ampules of sodium bicarbonate during cardiopulmonary resuscitation, and the administration of large amounts of sodium bicarbonate to patients with lactic acidosis.

Excessive Water Losses. Impairment of ADH production, release, or action, as in pituitary or nephrogenic diabetes insipidus, respectively, can lead to profound water deficits and to hypernatremia. In such circumstances, the urine volumes are large, the urine osmolality is low, and the net rate of solute excretion is low, in contrast to individuals undergoing osmotic diuresis, in whom rates of urinary solute excretion are elevated.

Striking water losses may also occur with excessive sweating, particularly during rigorous physical activity by untrained individuals exposed to a high humidity. This phenomenon plays a major role in the evolution of heat stroke.

Combined Disorders. Finally, hypertonic dehydration may occur as a combination of these events. A common example in modern clinical practice involves the injudicious administration of large amounts of carbohydrate or amino acids by nasogastric tube, coupled with limited amounts of water, in stroke patients unable to communicate thirst.

CLINICAL MANIFESTATIONS AND DIAGNOSIS. Since two thirds of body water is intracellular, primary water losses tend to have modest effects on circulating volume unless fluid losses are profound. Rather, the clinical manifestations are produced by brain shrinkage that results from increases in effective ECF osmolality. Thus the symptoms of hypertonicity produced either by hypernatremia or by impermeant nonsodium solutes such as glucose are referable to the central nervous system and range from somnolence and confusion to coma, respiratory paralysis, and death. The degree of symptomatology varies with the degree of hypertonicity and with the rate at which hypertonicity develops. In acute hypertonicity, symptoms generally appear when the effective ECF osmolality exceeds 320 to 330 mOsm per kilogram of H_2O, and coma and respiratory arrest may occur when the ECF osmolality exceeds 360 to 380 mOsm per kilogram of H_2O. Chronic hypertonicity generally produces fewer central nervous system manifestations, because brain cells accumulate idiogenic osmoles, which minimize the tendency to brain shrinkage.

TREATMENT. The treatment of acute hypernatremia requires the administration of dilute solutions, generally by an intravenous route. A hypotonic salt solution (half-normal saline) may be useful if significant volume contraction occurs in association with hypernatremia. Otherwise, a 5 per cent dextrose in water solution may be used. Three particular factors should be borne in mind when treating acute hypernatremia: (1) In the severely volume-contracted patient with severe hypernatremia, the administration of isotonic saline solutions has two advantages: it provides fluid resuscitation in impending cardiovascular collapse; and the isotonic salt solution, which is hypotonic with respect to the hypertonic patient, avoids unnecessary rapid falls in the serum sodium. (2) If 5 per cent dextrose in water solutions are administered at a rapid rate, hyperglycemia and osmotic diuresis may occur and hence aggravate the hypertonic state. In this circumstance, the use of a 2.5 per cent dextrose solution in one quarter normal saline is advisable. This solution has been particularly useful in treating hypernatremia associated with volume contraction in children with pituitary or nephrogenic diabetes insipidus. (3) Rapid correction of hypertonicity to a normal serum osmolality is hazardous. Since accumulation of idiogenic osmoles by brain cells is a compensatory mechanism for preserving brain volume in hypertonic disorders, a normal serum osmolality may be relatively hypotonic to brain cells that have accumulated idiogenic solutes. Hence if the serum osmolality is reduced rapidly, central nervous system damage due to brain swelling may occur. A useful guide to circumventing this difficulty is to reduce the serum sodium by no more than 1 mEq per liter during every 2 hours of the first two days of treatment.

Andreoli TE: The polyuric syndromes. *In* Andreoli TE, Hoffman JF, Fanestil DD (eds.): Physiology of Membrane Disorders. New York, Plenum Medical Book Company, 1978, pp 1063–1091. *A discussion of the physiology of the polyuric states, their differentiation one from another, and therapeutic approaches; extensively referenced.*

Arieff AI, Schmidt RW: Fluid and electrolyte disorders and the central nervous system. *In* Maxwell MH, Kleeman CR (eds.): Clinical Disorders of Fluid and Electrolyte Metabolism. New York, McGraw-Hill Book Company, 1980, pp 1409–1480. *This chapter is a superb review of the pathophysiology, manifestations, and treatment of the hyperosmolar syndrome; thoroughly referenced.*

Fichman MP, Vorherr H, Kleeman CR, Telfer N: Diuretic-induced hyponatremia. Ann Intern Med 75:853, 1971. *Description of hyponatremia in nonedematous patients taking diuretics who have hypokalemia and marked decreases in total body potassium, and whose hyponatremia is corrected by repletion of body potassium.*

Lifschitz MD, Stein JH: Hormonal regulation of renal salt excretion. Semin Nephrol 3:196, 1983. *A detailed analysis of the interplay between hormones and the kidney in regulating salt excretion.*

Miller M, Dalakos T, Moses AM, Fellerman H, Streeten DHP: Recognition of partial defects in antidiuretic hormone secretion. Ann Intern Med 73:721, 1970. *A concise guide to testing procedures for states of ADH insufficiency and a rational scheme for interpreting the test results.*

Narins RG, Jones ER, Stom MC, Rudnick MR, Bastl CP: Diagnostic strategies in disorders of fluid, electrolyte and acid-base homeostasis. Am J Med 72:496, 1982. *A useful clinical strategy for analyzing hypotonic and hypertonic disorders.*

Disturbances in Potassium Balance

PHYSIOLOGIC CONSIDERATIONS

The body contains approximately 3500 mEq of potassium, of which only 60 mEq, or about 2 per cent of the total, is extracellular. Under normal circumstances, external potassium balance depends on dietary potassium intake and renal potassium excretion; fecal potassium losses are only about 10 mEq per day unless diarrhea is present. Since 98 per cent of potassium is located intracellularly, primarily in skeletal muscle, regulation of the serum potassium concentration depends not only on external potassium balance, but also on potassium exchanges between the intracellular and extracellular compartments.

Transfer Between ICF and ECF

The intracellular compartment serves as a reservoir that protects the constancy of the ECF potassium concentration. In potassium-depleted states, a 1 mEq per liter fall in serum potassium requires the loss of about 100 to 200 mEq of potassium; hence the bulk of external potassium loss comes from the cellular compartment. Conversely, if large amounts of potassium are administered acutely, the rise in serum potassium is less than would be expected if the administered potassium were distributed solely in the ECF. In this situation, cellular uptake of potassium obviously occurs and prevents greater increases in the serum potassium concentration. This ability of cells to accumulate potassium can be enhanced strikingly by chronic administration of high potassium diets.

A number of *effector* mechanisms regulate the partition of potassium between the ICF and ECF. These include active and passive ionic transcellular transport processes.

ACTIVE TRANSPORT PROCESSES. The cardinal transport process regulating K^+ distribution between ICF and ECF is cell membrane bound (Na^+ + K^+)–ATPase, which actively transports potassium into cells and therefore counterbalances the passive leak of potassium from cells into interstitial fluid. Insulin is a second effector that promotes potassium transfer from ECF to ICF; this hormone promotes cellular uptake of potassium, independently of cellular glucose uptake, by increasing the activity of the (Na^+ + K^+)–ATPase. Furthermore, there is evidence that hyperkalemia may augment insulin release. Thus hyperkalemia may be the *sensor* that stimulates release of insulin, which then serves as an *effector* for potassium entry into cells. In addition, beta-adrenergic agents such as epinephrine and isoproterenol promote cellular uptake of potassium.

PASSIVE TRANSPORT PROCESSES. A number of passive effector mechanisms also regulate the partition of potassium between the ICF and ECF. First, alterations in ECF pH reproducibly shift potassium between the ICF and the ECF: Systemic acidosis, whether metabolic or respiratory, promotes potassium efflux from cells; while systemic alkalosis, either metabolic or respiratory, promotes cellular potassium uptake. As a general rule, a plasma reduction of 0.1 pH unit raises the serum potassium by 0.6 mEq per liter, while a plasma increase of 0.1 pH unit produces a similar reduction in serum potassium. The mechanisms for these pH-induced potassium shifts between ICF and ECF are not understood. It has also been suggested that increases in plasma bicarbonate concentrations may, by unknown mechanisms, promote potassium entry into cells independently of pH changes.

Second, cellular shrinkage produced by increases in effective ECF osmolality raises the intracellular potassium concentration and thereby increases the rate of passive potassium leakage from the ICF to the ECF. This potassium leakage may result in hyperkalemia when large glucose loads are administered to insulin-deficient diabetic patients who also have hyporeninemic hypoaldosteronism; the insulin lack limits cellular re-entry of potassium and the aldosterone deficiency limits renal potassium excretion. Increases in cell potassium concentrations produced by cellular shrinkage also contribute significantly to the hyperkalemia of diabetic ketoacidosis, because hyperglycemia raises cell potassium by cell shrinkage, and insulin lack prevents accelerated potassium re-entry into cells.

Finally, it was noted in the section on Osmolality Disturbances that brain cells lose potassium chloride when exposed to chronic ECF hypotonicity; a similar effect also occurs in renal tubular cells. However, muscle cells, which are the largest component of ICF potassium, do not appear to participate in this process. Consequently, hypotonic disorders, by themselves, have little effect on the serum potassium or on external potassium balance.

Renal Handling of Potassium

The renal handling of potassium differs strikingly from the way in which the kidneys process sodium. Sodium excretion involves filtration, partial tubular absorption, and appearance of nonabsorbed sodium as urinary sodium excretion. When dietary sodium intake is varied, there is a prompt adjustment in urinary sodium excretion, either in the upward direction when sodium intake is increased, or in the downward direction when sodium intake is curtailed.

In contrast, virtually all dietary potassium, ordinarily about 50 to 200 mEq per day, appears in the urine because of tubular secretion of potassium by terminal nephron segments. These regions of the nephron can increase rates of potassium secretion significantly if dietary potassium intake is augmented; and they carry out net absorption of potassium in kaliopenic states. In other words, these terminal nephron segments regulate external potassium balance by adjusting *renal output* to balance *intake*.

A convenient way of considering distal nephron handling of potassium, and the ways in which effector mechanisms modulate this process, are shown in Figure 76–6. The dashed lines indicate passive processes and the solid lines active transport processes. Basolateral membranes of all terminal nephron segments, including the thick limb of Henle, the distal tubule, and the collecting duct, all share two common characteristics: a passive leakage pathway for K^+ efflux and an active (Na^+ + K^+)–ATPase for cellular K^+ uptake. The apical membranes of these nephron segments also contain passive, potassium leakage pathways. In the thick ascending limb of Henle, apical membranes contain a furosemide-sensitive coupled entry step that involves electroneutral Na^+:K^+:$2Cl^-$ co-transport, driven by the electrochemical sodium gradient between lumen and cells. In distal tubular and collecting ducts, there is little evidence for the presence of such an apical membrane Na^+:K^+:$2Cl^-$ co-transport process. Rather, Na^+ entry into tubular cells appears to involve sodium-specific channels that are blocked by amiloride. Thus, in the ascending limb, coupled electroneutral sodium entry into cells does not result in luminal electronegativity (in fact, the lumen in the thick ascending limb is electropositive), whereas, in the distal tubule and collecting duct, amiloride-sensitive ionic sodium entry produces luminal electronegativity.

The majority of net K^+ secretion occurs in these latter two segments, driven indirectly by the rate of sodium entry into cells, which increases luminal electronegativity and increases the activity of basolateral (Na^+ + K^+)–ATPase, thus raising cell potassium concentrations. In the loop of Henle, little net potassium secretion occurs, because the lumen is electropositive and because coupled Na^+:K^+:$2Cl^-$ transport from lumen to cells recycles secreted potassium back into cells.

The major elements of the *effector systems* that regulate distal nephron potassium excretion include the rate of distal tubular sodium delivery, dietary potassium intake, plasma pH, aldosterone, impermeant anions, and tubular flow rates. When distal sodium delivery rates are increased, increased sodium entry into cells across apical membranes is accompanied by increased activity of pump (Na^+ + K^+)–ATPase, which tends to raise intracellular potassium concentrations. Either an increase in dietary potassium intake or an increase in plasma pH tends, as indicated above, to raise cellular potassium content.

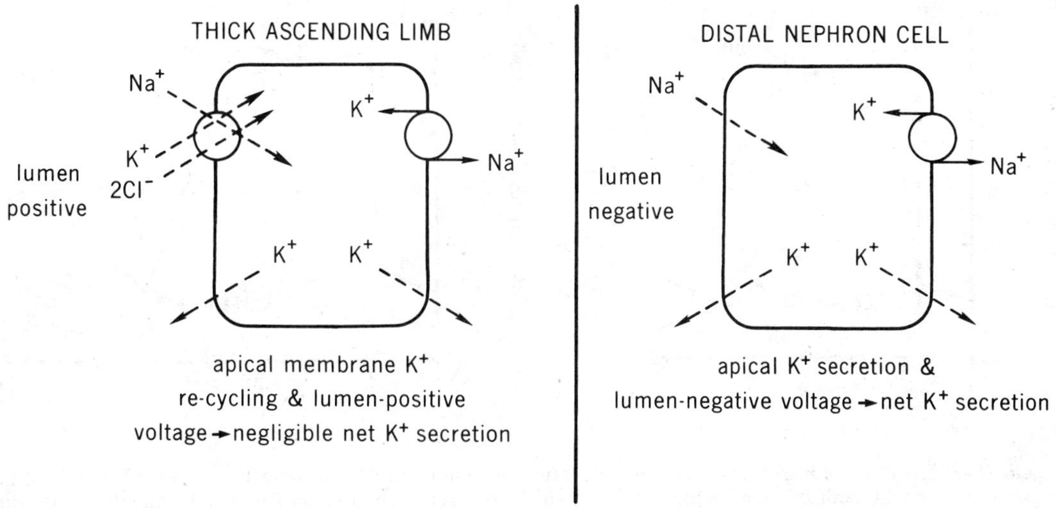

Figure 76–6. Handling of potassium in late nephron segments, including the thick ascending limb and the distal nephron. The dashed arrows represent passive transport processes and the solid arrows represent active transport processes. In the thick ascending limb, K^+ recycling into cells by Na^+:K^+:$2Cl^-$ co-transport, and the lumen-positive voltage, reduce the rate of net K^+ secretion. Most urinary K^+ comes from net K^+ secretion by terminal nephron segments.

Urinary excretion of impermeant anions such as sulfate, carbenicillin, and penicillin produces greater luminal electronegativity. Aldosterone and mineralocorticoids, whose kaliuretic effects may be dissociated from their sodium-sparing effects, increase the permeability of luminal membranes to potassium. These hormones may also augment distal tubular (NA^+ + K^+)–ATPase activity. While each of these factors has relevance, the rates of aldosterone secretion and distal salt delivery to terminal nephron segments are the cardinal variables.

In other words, each of the above factors modulates one or another portion of a generalized mechanism, namely, an electrochemical gradient favorable to the passive movement of potassium from tubular cells to urine and consequently to net potassium secretion. Conversely, reductions in sodium delivery, potassium restriction, reductions in plasma pH, and mineralocorticoid lack all reduce the magnitude of passive potassium movement from cells to tubular fluid and therefore tend to reduce net potassium secretion. Finally, increases in tubular flow rates, as in osmotic diuresis, also promote potassium secretion, while reductions in tubular flow rates reduce potassium secretion. The mechanism responsible for this effect is unknown.

The net rate of urinary potassium excretion in any given circumstance therefore depends on the interplay of these multiple factors in modulating the common effector mechanism for potassium secretion. For example, mineralocorticoid excess in primary aldosteronism commonly leads to severe potassium wasting. But this kaliuresis can be curtailed by dietary sodium restriction and accentuated by dietary sodium loading. Conversely, in hyporeninemic hypoaldosteronism, hyperkalemia may be prevented by insuring a liberal intake of sodium.

The renal adaptation to excess potassium loads occurs over a 24- to 36-hour period. Consequently, hyperkalemia from the large ingestion of oral potassium loads is uncommon in normal individuals. But the renal response to dietary potassium restriction is more sluggish and requires seven to ten days for full development. Even under the latter circumstances, urinary potassium losses are rarely less than 20 mEq daily.

Excitable Tissues and the ICF/ECF Potassium Ratio

The clinical consequences of hypokalemia and hyperkalemia are generally referable to changes in the excitable characteristics of heart, skeletal muscle, and smooth muscle. Excitable tissues, such as nerve, heart, and skeletal muscle, share certain common properties. At rest, excitable tissues are far more permeable to potassium than to sodium. The cell interior is electronegative with respect to extracellular fluid, and this voltage is largely determined by the logarithm of the ratio of intracellular (K_i) to extracellular (K_o) potassium concentrations. When excitable tissues are suddenly depolarized to their threshold voltage, there is a profound increase in membrane permeability to sodium and an accompanying increase in the sodium-to-potassium permeability ratio. This sodium entry into the cells of excitable tissues probably occurs through sodium-specific channels that have electronegative sites and are activated by sudden depolarization of excitable tissues to threshold. Thus during acute depolarization to threshold, the sodium channels are activated and sodium enters the cell passively and produces the initial spike of the action potential, during which time the cell interior becomes electropositive.

This voltage-dependent increase in sodium permeability during depolarization to threshold is the most fundamental characteristic of excitable tissues (except in those excitable tissues, such as the atrioventricular node, where Ca^{++} influx into cells is responsible for the action potential). However, if an excitable cell is partially depolarized in the resting state, the rate of rise of action potentials is reduced; the prolonged resting depolarization, by undefined mechanisms, reduces the increase in sodium permeability that accompanies the action potential. This effect of resting depolarization on reducing sodium permeability during action potentials is referred to as inactivation.

Repolarization of excitable cells occurs more slowly than depolarization. During repolarization, potassium permeability rises with respect to sodium permeability, and there is passive potassium efflux from the cell to the ECF. This potassium efflux restores the electronegativity of the cell interior. In nerve and skeletal muscle, potassium efflux occurs almost immediately after the initial spike of the action potential. In cardiac muscle, potassium efflux follows the absolute refractory period and coincides with the relative refractory period, or phase 3 of the cardiac action potential.

Hyperkalemia reduces the K_i/K_o ratio and consequently partially depolarizes electrical tissues at rest. Hyperkalemia also increases the potassium permeability of excitable cells. The results of these changes on cardiac excitation are illustrated in the left-hand panel of Figure 76–7. Because partial resting depolarization inactivates the rate of sodium entry into cells during excitation, the rate of phase zero depolarization is slower

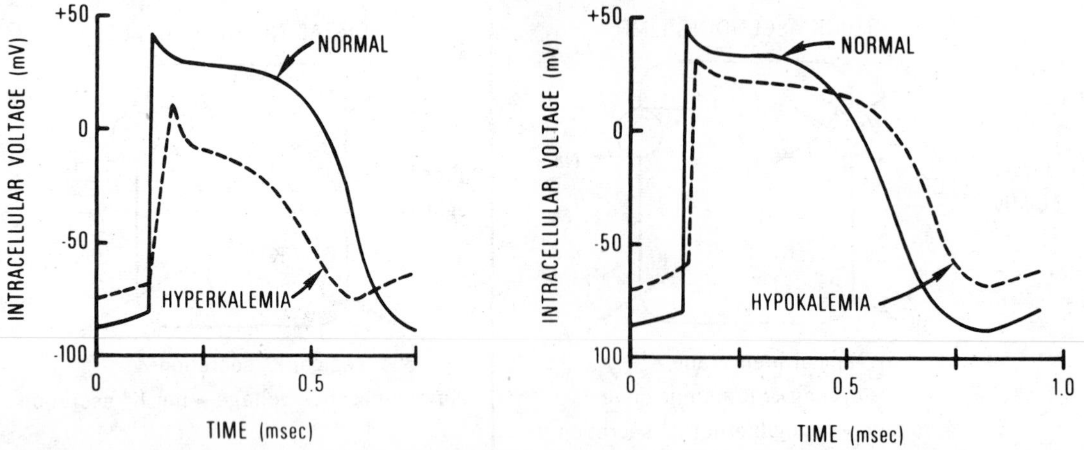

Figure 76–7. The effect of increases or decreases in serum potassium on the cardiac action potential. The solid lines represent the normal cardiac action potential; the dashed lines represent the cardiac action potential with either hyperkalemia (left panel) or hypokalemia (right panel).

and the peak of phase zero depolarization is markedly reduced. The increased potassium permeability accelerates repolarization and shortens the plateau phase. The net effect of progressive hyperkalemia is therefore to make the heart progressively refractory to excitation.

The effects of hypokalemia on excitable tissues are more complex. Because the K_i/K_o ratio rises in hypokalemia, one expects that excitable cells at rest would be hyperpolarized. While this occurs initially, resting depolarization eventually follows, because the high K_i/K_o ratio, by itself, reduces the potassium permeability of excitable cells. The effects of hypokalemia on cardiac muscle fibers are shown in the right-hand panel of Figure 76–7. At rest, the cell is partially depolarized because the reduced potassium permeability allows the high extracellular-to-intracellular sodium ratio to make the cell interior less negative. The initial spike of the action potential is less affected than in hyperkalemia because the reduced potassium permeability offsets the reduced sodium permeability during phase zero depolarization. Since potassium efflux determines the rate of repolarization, the reduced potassium permeability prolongs the relative refractory period. The net effect of these changes in cardiac tissue is to increase the likelihood of sinus bradycardia, and, because of a prolonged relative refractory period, the risk of arrhythmias. In skeletal muscle, the reduction in membrane permeability to potassium produced by hypokalemia leads, in severe hypokalemia, to generalized paralysis.

HYPOKALEMIA AND POTASSIUM DEPLETION

DEFINITION. Chronic hypokalemia generally reflects a reduction in total body potassium. As mentioned earlier, a 1 mEq reduction in serum potassium generally implies the net loss of 100 to 200 mEq of potassium from the body. In extreme body potassium depletion, the serum potassium may be as low as 1.5 to 2.0 mEq per liter. Acute reductions in serum potassium without parallel reduction in total body potassium occur when potassium is shifted from extracellular to intracellular compartments.

ETIOLOGY AND PATHOGENESIS. Hypokalemia and simultaneous potassium depletion occur whenever renal plus extrarenal potassium losses exceed potassium intake. In advanced body potassium depletion, intake and output of potassium may be equal. The four major causes for hypokalemia are given in Table 76–8.

Inadequate Intake. Reduced potassium intake may result in potassium depletion and hypokalemia because maximal renal conservation of potassium requires, as indicated above, seven to ten days. During this interval, the net renal potassium loss may be as much as 150 to 200 mEq.

Excessive Renal Losses. These disturbances of potassium balance are common. Many of the causes for renal potassium wasting can be analyzed in terms of factors that modulate the common effector system for potassium secretion. Mineralocorticoid excess accelerates distal tubular potassium secretion, as indicated in connection with Figure 76–6. Consequently, hypokalemia occurs regularly in primary hyperaldosteronism; in states of glucocorticoid excess such as Cushing's syndrome; and in secondary hyperaldosteronism, including accelerated hypertension, profound congestive heart failure, and the rarely occurring renin-producing tumors of the kidney. *Chronic licorice ingestion* can produce a syndrome that mimics primary hyperaldosteronism, because glycyrrhizinic acid, a component of licorice extract, has physiologic properties similar to aldosterone.

In *Bartter's syndrome,* sodium chloride wasting and secondary aldosteronism may contribute to potassium depletion. However, potassium depletion in Bartter's syndrome may also occur either when aldosterone secretion rates are normal or following bilateral adrenalectomy. Consequently, it is believed that a tubular defect in potassium handling also contributes to the hypokalemia of Bartter's syndrome (see also Ch. 83.5).

TABLE 76–8. MAJOR CAUSES OF HYPOKALEMIA

Inadequate Intake
Excess Renal Loss
Mineralocorticoid excess
Bartter's syndrome
Diuresis
Diuretics with a pre-late distal locus osmotic diuresis
Chronic metabolic alkalosis
Antibiotics
Carbenicillin
Gentamicin
Amphotericin B
Renal tubular acidosis
Distal, gradient-limited
Proximal
Liddle's syndrome
Acute leukemia
Ureterosigmoidostomy
Gastrointestinal Losses
Vomiting
Diarrhea, particularly secretory diarrheas
Villous adenoma
ECF → ICF Shifts
Acute alkalosis
Hypokalemic periodic paralysis
Barium ingestion
Insulin therapy
Vitamin B_{12} therapy

Virtually all diuretics having a locus of action prior to the late distal tubule (Table 76–4) increase urinary potassium losses. Enhanced sodium delivery to distal nephron segments is a major factor responsible for the kaliuresis produced by these diuretics, since sodium restriction or volume depletion tends to minimize diuretic-induced potassium losses. In the case of carbonic anhydrase inhibitors such as acetazolamide, inhibition of proximal bicarbonate absorption also accentuates potassium losses. Distal tubular segments are relatively impermeable to bicarbonate; consequently, increased delivery of bicarbonate to distal nephron regions has an impermeant anion effect that increases luminal electronegativity in these nephron regions.

Osmotic diuresis is commonly associated with increased renal potassium losses, because increased tubular flow rates enhance net potassium secretion. In diabetic ketoacidosis, renal potassium losses are therefore common. Yet patients with diabetic ketoacidosis and a reduced total body potassium commonly present with hyperkalemia, because metabolic acidosis tends to promote potassium shifts from the ICF to the ECF. Consequently, profound hypokalemia may develop if body potassium is not replenished concomitantly with insulin therapy and ECF volume expansion.

Potassium depletion is seen frequently in *chronic metabolic alkalosis.* When the alkalosis is associated with volume contraction, secondary hyperaldosteronism results in renal potassium losses. Potassium depletion in chronic metabolic alkalosis is also enhanced if bicarbonaturia is present, because of the impermeant anion effect produced by bicarbonate delivery to terminal nephron segments. In fact, the hypokalemia associated with upper gastrointestinal fluid losses, as in vomiting or nasogastric suction, is primarily the result of the renal potassium losses produced by secondary hyperaldosteronism and/or bicarbonaturia. The potassium losses from the upper gastrointestinal tract are small, since upper gastrointestinal tract fluid contains only about 10 mEq of potassium per liter.

Hypokalemia may develop during therapy with certain *antibiotics.* Carbenicillin or other penicillin-like antibiotics exist as sodium or potassium salts of impermeant anions and promote kaliuresis because they increase net sodium excretion and because of an impermeant anion effect. Amphotericin B increases the permeability of luminal membranes to potassium and therefore promotes potassium secretion. Gentamicin produces potassium losses by unknown mechanisms.

Hypokalemia and potassium depletion are common findings in *distal, gradient-limited renal tubular acidosis.* Increased distal sodium delivery and the impermeant anion effect produced by bicarbonate wasting account for most of the potassium losses seen in proximal renal tubular acidosis. Consequently, salt restriction, which enhances the rate of proximal sodium bicarbonate absorption in this disorder, also tends to correct potassium depletion. In gradient-limited distal renal tubular acidosis, hypokalemia may be accentuated by volume losses and secondary hyperaldosteronism. Other factors, not yet understood, also contribute to hypokalemia in this disorder. Hyperkalemia rather than hypokalemia commonly accompanies the hyperchloremic acidosis of interstitial disease (Type IV acidosis) (Ch. 83.2).

Liddle's syndrome is a rare tubular disorder characterized by hypokalemia, metabolic alkalosis, hypertension, and normal aldosterone secretion rates (Ch. 83.5). Therapy with triamterene, but not aldosterone antagonists such as spironolactone, ameliorates the disorder. These findings suggest that terminal nephron sodium avidity and potassium secretion independent of aldosterone are major factors in the pathogenesis of Liddle's syndrome. Thus in operational terms, Liddle's syndrome may be described as distal nephron hyperfunction, as regards Na^+ absorption and H^+ and K^+ secretion.

Gastrointestinal Losses. These provide the other major route for potassium depletion. As indicated above, potassium depletion associated with vomiting is referable primarily to renal potassium losses. However, diarrhea can produce significant potassium losses, since diarrheal fluid contains 30 mEq per liter of potassium. The most striking diarrheal potassium losses occur in secretory diarrheas, such as with non–beta islet cell tumors of the pancreas, which produce vasoactive intestinal polypeptide, and in laxative abuse. In both secretory diarrheas and chronic laxative abuse, hypokalemia appears referable to increased rates of K^+ secretion through apical membrane K^+ channels. Villous adenomas of the colon produce potassium depletion because of excessive colonic K^+ secretion from the adenoma. Hypokalemia is uncommonly seen in inflammatory bowel disease.

ECF-ICF Shifts. Acute hypokalemia with a normal total body potassium may occur because of potassium shifts from the ECF to the ICF. In *hypokalemic periodic paralysis,* acute shifts of potassium from the ECF to the ICF produce limb and trunk paralysis (Ch. 538). The periodic attacks are often precipitated by high carbohydrate meals. Patients with the disorder can often abort attacks by exercising affected muscles. The chronic use of acetazolamide can prevent attacks. A condition resembling hypokalemic periodic paralysis occurs with the ingestion of *barium salts* and is endemic in China, where the disorder is referred to as "Pa-Ping." Barium appears to produce hypokalemia by blocking K^+ channels in skeletal muscle and thus blocking efflux of potassium from ICF to ECF. *Insulin* therapy and *vitamin* B_{12} therapy also promote potassium shifts from the ECF to the ICF. This type of hypokalemia may also occur with thyrotoxicosis, especially in Oriental men.

CLINICAL MANIFESTATIONS. The clinical effects of potassium deficiency may be manifest in one or more organ systems, including skeletal muscle, heart, kidneys, and the gastrointestinal tract. The most serious disturbances are those affecting the neuromuscular system. At serum potassium concentrations in the range of 2 to 2.5 mEq per liter, *muscular weakness* is likely to occur; with more severe hypokalemia the patient may develop *areflexic paralysis,* in which case respiratory insufficiency is an immediate threat to survival. The severity of the neuromuscular disturbance tends to be proportional to the speed with which the potassium level has declined.

Losses of large amounts of potassium from skeletal muscle may be accompanied by *rhabdomyolysis* and *myoglobinuria.* Hence, rhabdomyolysis sometimes occurs in military recruits subject to severe exercise, sweating, and ECF volume contraction. The secondary hyperaldosteronism that follows excessive salt loss produces urinary potassium wasting and consequently potassium depletion. Potassium depletion secondary to malnutrition and vomiting is also one of the pathogenic mechanisms in alcoholic rhabdomyolysis.

The *electrocardiographic abnormalities* of potassium depletion affect primarily repolarization segments of the ECG, in keeping with effects of hypokalemia on the action potential. The common electrocardiograph manifestations of hypokalemia include sagging of the S-T segment, depression of the T wave, and elevation of the U wave. With marked hypokalemia, the T wave becomes progressively smaller and the U waves show increasing amplitude. In some cases, the merging of a flat or positive T wave with a positive U wave may be interpreted erroneously as a prolonged Q-T interval. Ordinarily, there are no serious clinical consequences from the abnormalities in cardiac excitation. In patients treated with digitalis, hypokalemia may precipitate serious *arrhythmias.*

Longstanding potassium depletion is apt to produce renal tubular damage, referred to as *hypokalemic nephropathy.* Potassium deficiency also affects smooth muscle of the gastrointestinal tract and can result in *paralytic ileus.*

TREATMENT. The treatment of hypokalemia involves replacement therapy with potassium salts and attempts to correct the underlying disorder. Since diuretic abuse is probably the most common cause for hypokalemia in routine clinical practice, every attempt should be made to identify diuretic ingestion.

Except in extreme circumstances, oral rather than parenteral potassium replacement is prudent. However, when gastrointestinal function is impaired, or when neuromuscular manifestations of hypokalemia are present, parenteral therapy with potassium may be advisable. Since potassium deficits involve both the ICF and the ECF, their correction requires the transfer of administered potassium from the ECF into the ICF. The major problem in parenteral therapy is to avoid intravenous administration of potassium at rates sufficiently great to produce hyperkalemia. A prudent protocol to follow is to add potassium chloride to intravenous solutions at a final concentration of 40 to 60 mEq per liter, and to administer no more than 10 to 20 mEq of potassium per hour. Except under unusual circumstances, the total amount of potassium administered daily should not exceed 200 mEq. The serum potassium should be monitored at appropriate intervals; the frequency of monitoring should be determined by the patient's clinical condition, by the initial serum potassium, by the rate at which the serum potassium changes in a given patient, and by the patient's renal function. Because the electrocardiographic manifestations of hypokalemia are subtle, the electrocardiogram should not be used as a guide to replacement therapy.

While potassium chloride is the salt of choice for intravenous potassium replacement, oral potassium chloride solutions are not well tolerated because of gastrointestinal irritation. Enteric coated potassium chloride tablets are to be avoided, because they produce small bowel ulcerations. A more convenient way to administer oral potassium is in the form of organic salts such as gluconate or citrate. This form of therapy is, however, not effective in hypokalemic metabolic alkalosis with hypochloremia. In this circumstance, chloride supplementation is required together with potassium replacement and is most easily achieved by administering sodium chloride supplementation.

HYPERKALEMIA AND POTASSIUM EXCESS

DEFINITION. Chronic hyperkalemia can occur with little or no increase in total body potassium. However, acute increases in serum potassium concentrations, produced by potassium shifts from the ICF to the ECF, can occur even when total body potassium is normal or reduced.

ETIOLOGY AND PATHOGENESIS. Hyperkalemia develops whenever the rate of potassium intake or the rate of potassium efflux from intracellular to extracellular fluids exceeds the sum of renal plus extrarenal potassium losses. The renal mechanisms for potassium excretion adapt efficiently to increases in the rate of potassium influx to extracellular fluid, particularly from dietary sources. Hence acute or chronic hyperkalemia due to exogenous potassium intake is uncommon, unless renal mechanisms for potassium excretion are compromised. In the latter setting, injudicious potassium administration may result in hyperkalemia. This occurs most commonly when intravenous potassium chloride is administered too rapidly; when potassium salts of antibiotics such as penicillin are administered; when transfusions are given with blood that has been stored for long periods of time; or when salt substitutes containing potassium are used. The occurrence of hyperkalemia in these settings usually requires that renal potassium excretion be impaired.

Acute or chronic hyperkalemia occurs most commonly either because of diminished renal excretion or because there is a sudden *transcellular shift* of potassium from the ICF to the ECF. The major causes of hyperkalemia are listed in Table 76–9 according to this format.

Diminished Renal Excretion. Hyperkalemia may occur in *acute oliguric renal failure* of any cause. In *chronic renal failure,* hyperkalemia generally does not occur until the glomerular filtration rate has reached markedly low levels. However, hyperkalemia may be precipitated in chronic renal failure either by the development of acidosis or, as indicated above, by the injudicious administration of potassium salts. Hyperkalemia also occurs with only modest reductions in the glomerular filtration rate, if there is impairment of potassium secretion by terminal

TABLE 76–9. MAJOR CAUSES OF HYPERKALEMIA

- **Diminished Renal Excretion**
  - Reduced GFR
    - Acute oliguric renal failure
    - Chronic renal failure
  - Reduced tubular secretion
    - Addison's disease
    - Hyporeninemic hypoaldosteronism
    - Potassium-sparing diuretics
- **Transcellular Shifts**
  - Acidosis
  - Cell destruction
    - Trauma, burns
    - Rhabdomyolysis
    - Hemolysis
    - Tumor lysis
  - Hyperkalemic periodic paralysis
  - Diabetic hyperglycemia
    - Insulin dependence plus aldosterone lack
  - Depolarizing muscle paralysis
    - Succinylcholine

nephron regions. This occurs in *Addison's disease, hyporeninemic hypoaldosteronism,* and with the injudicious administration of *potassium-sparing diuretics* such as triamterene or spironolactone. The tendency toward hyperkalemia in these circumstances can be aggravated by ECF volume contraction, which reduces sodium delivery to terminal nephron segments, or by acidosis, which promotes cellular potassium efflux.

Transcellular Shifts. The second class of disorders causing acute hyperkalemia includes situations in which there is an abrupt shift of potassium from the ICF to the ECF. This occurs in *acidosis* or in circumstances that result in *cell destruction;* the latter occurs commonly with tissue trauma, burns, rhabdomyolysis, or hemolysis, and with lysis of large masses of tumor cells. As indicated previously, hypokalemia predisposes to rhabdomyolysis. Thus the sudden occurrence of hyperkalemia in potassium-depleted patients is a diagnostic clue to the development of rhabdomyolysis.

Hyperkalemic periodic paralysis is an autosomal dominant disorder in which sudden increases in serum potassium result in muscle paralysis (Ch. 538). The hyperkalemia is often provoked by dietary potassium intake or by exercise. Myotonia occurs commonly in the disorder and appears either between attacks or immediately preceding attacks. The pathogenesis of the disorder is not understood. The acute paralytic attack can be treated by intravenous administration of calcium gluconate or glucose and insulin. Chronic treatment with diuretics such as acetazolamide minimizes the frequency of attacks.

Paradoxical hyperkalemia occurs when *sudden hyperglycemia* develops in insulin-dependent diabetics who also have interstitial renal disease and associated hyporeninemic hypoaldosteronism. The sudden increase in ECF osmolality draws water from cells, raises intracellular potassium concentrations, and therefore promotes passive potassium efflux from cells. The insulin lack minimizes cellular re-entry of potassium, and the aldosterone deficiency blunts renal potassium excretion. Insulin therapy promptly corrects the hyperkalemia. Finally, anesthetic agents or other drugs that cause a *depolarizing muscle paralysis,* such as succinylcholine, promote potassium efflux from muscle cells. The loss of cell electronegativity in this situation increases passive potassium efflux from muscle cells.

Pseudohyperkalemia may occur in thrombocytosis or leukocytosis, because clotting of blood promotes potassium release from these cells, and may be identified by noting that the *serum* potassium is elevated while the *plasma* potassium is normal. This kind of artifact occurs most commonly in patients with myeloproliferative disorders.

CLINICAL MANIFESTATIONS. The most important clinical manifestations of hyperkalemia relate to alterations in cardiac excitability. For this reason, the electrocardiogram is the single most important guide in appraising the threat posed by hyperkalemia and in determining how aggressive a therapeutic approach is necessary.

The electrocardiographic manifestations of hyperkalemia follow directly from the effects of hyperkalemia on cardiac action potentials (Fig. 76–7). The earliest manifestation of hyperkalemia, the development of peaked T waves, becomes manifest when the serum potassium exceeds 6.5 mEq per liter. This peaking of the T waves is a manifestation of the accelerated repolarization of the cardiac action potential produced by hyperkalemia. When the potassium concentration exceeds 7 to 8 mEq per liter, diminished cardiac excitability results in prolongation of the PR interval followed by a loss of P waves and widening of the QRS complex. These changes indicate progressive inexcitability of cardiac muscle, and are referable to hyperkalemia-induced inactivation of sodium permeability during the initial spike of the action potential. When the serum potassium exceeds 8 to 10 mEq per liter, the electrocardiogram may develop a sine wave pattern and cardiac standstill can occur.

The correlation between serum potassium concentrations and electrocardiographic abnormalities is approximate at best; in a given patient, progression from peaked T waves to a sine wave pattern may occur rapidly, particularly if the serum potassium concentration rises rapidly. Therefore, the development of peaked T waves in conjunction with hyperkalemia should be viewed as a serious disorder; more advanced electrocardiographic manifestations of hyperkalemia should be treated as life-threatening medical emergencies.

TREATMENT. Three kinds of maneuvers are used in the treatment of hyperkalemia: (1) agents such as glucose plus insulin or sodium bicarbonate, which promote the transfer of potassium from the ECF to the ICF; (2) maneuvers that enhance potassium elimination from the body, such as diuretics, exchange resins, and dialysis; and (3) the use of calcium, which does not alter serum potassium concentrations but counteracts the effects of hyperkalemia on cardiac excitability.

Both insulin and sodium bicarbonate promote potassium entry into cells. The administration of 25 grams of glucose, together with 10 units of regular insulin, is an effective way of reducing the serum potassium rapidly. The glucose may be administered over 30 minutes as a 20 per cent solution, or it may be given as a 50 per cent glucose solution. It is insulin that promotes potassium entry into cells; glucose is administered together with insulin to prevent hypoglycemia. In insulin-dependent diabetic patients in whom sudden hyperglycemia has precipitated the hyperkalemia, insulin administration alone suffices to reduce the serum potassium concentration.

The administration of 40 to 150 mEq of sodium bicarbonate intravenously over a 30- to 60-minute interval also promotes potassium entry into cells, particularly if acidosis is also present. This maneuver should be used with caution in patients with compromised renal function because of the risks of hypernatremia and of ECF volume overload.

None of the maneuvers described above removes potassium from the body. However, gastrointestinal potassium losses may be produced by the use of cation exchange resins in the sodium cycle, such as sodium polystyrene sulfonate (Kayexalate). Each gram of the resin contains approximately 1 mEq of sodium, and exchanges for about 1 mEq of potassium. This stoichiometry is, however, not precise, since the sodium form of the resin also exchanges for other cations in gastrointestinal secretions, including calcium. In chronic hyperkalemia, 20 grams of Kayexalate may be given three or four times a day in a 70 per cent solution of sorbitol. The sorbitol creates an osmotic diarrhea and enhances resin passage through the gastrointestinal tract. In acute circumstances, Kayexalate may also be administered by enema, generally as 100 grams of resin suspended in 200 ml of 20 per cent sorbitol. The use of chronic Kayexalate therapy in patients with chronic renal failure carries with it the risk of sodium overload.

In settings of extreme hyperkalemic cardiotoxicity, when P waves are absent and the QRS complexes are widened, the administration of calcium gluconate, 10 to 30 ml of a 10 per cent solution over a 10- to 20-minute interval, may be lifesaving. This approach should be undertaken with constant electrocardiographic monitoring and should be used with extreme caution in patients who have received digitalis. In the latter circumstance, calcium administration may unmask digitalis intoxication, especially if other agents are used simultaneously to reduce the serum potassium. Calcium salts should not be added to bottles of intravenous fluids containing bicarbonate, because water-insoluble calcium salts will form.

The effect of calcium salts in minimizing the cardiotoxic effects of hyperkalemia may be understood by noting, as described in the section on Physiologic Considerations, that depolarization of excitable tissues by elevating serum K^+ concentrations inactivates sodium channels and that the extracellular sides of these sodium channels are electronegative. Divalent cations such as calcium provide a remarkably effective way of screening these electronegative sites. Thus calcium salts raise the voltage gradient across sodium channels by screening electronegative surface charges of these channels on their extracellular fluid sides, and consequently restoring the voltage-dependent excitability of these channels.

Finally, acute hemodialysis or peritoneal dialysis provides another mechanism for potassium removal from the body. This approach is particularly advantageous in acute renal failure; when patients are volume-expanded and sodium administration may produce congestive heart failure; or when there is a continued efflux of large amounts of potassium from the ICF to the ECF, as in burns or rhabdomyolysis.

Armstrong CM: Some general properties of excitable tissues. *In* Andreoli TE, Hoffman JF, Fanestil DD (eds.): Physiology of Membrane Disorders. New York, Plenum Medical Book Company, 1978, pp 479. *A description of the ionic basis of the cardiac action potential.*

Cohen JJ: Disorders of potassium balance. Hosp Prac 14:119, 1979. *A brief discussion of the clinical manifestations and management of both hypokalemia and hyperkalemia.*

Cox M, Sterns RH, Singer I: The defense against hyperkalemia: The roles of insulin and aldosterone. N Engl J Med 299:525, 1978. *A concise review of the roles of insulin and aldosterone as effectors regulating both renal potassium excretion and the partition of potassium between the ICF and the ECF.*

Gennari FJ, Cohen JJ: Role of the kidney in potassium homeostasis: Lessons from acid-base disturbances. Kidney Int 8:1, 1975. *A discussion of renal potassium excretion in acute and chronic acid-base disturbances.*

Gordon AM, Luke IK: Disorders of muscle membranes: The periodic paralyses. *In* Andreoli TE, Hoffman JF, Fanestil DD (eds.): Physiology of Membrane Disorders. New York, Plenum Medical Book Company, 1978, pp 817. *A detailed description of pathophysiologic mechanisms involved in the periodic paralyses, together with an analysis of potassium-calcium interactions in modulating the excitability of sodium channels; extensively referenced.*

Harrington JT, Isner JM, Kassirer JP: Our national obsession with potassium. Am J Med 73:155, 1982. *An analysis of the risks of hypokalemia and strategies for potassium supplements in patients taking potassium-wasting diuretics.*

Nardone DA, McDonald WJ, Girard DE: Mechanisms in hypokalemia: Clinical correlation. Medicine 57:435, 1978. *An in-depth review of the basic mechanisms and pathophysiology of hypokalemia; extensively referenced.*

Disturbances in Acid-Base Balance

PHYSIOLOGIC CONSIDERATIONS

The pH of arterial blood and interstitial fluid normally ranges between 7.35 and 7.45, despite wide variations in dietary intake of acids or alkali. The arterial pH range over which cardiac function, metabolic activity, and central nervous system function can be maintained is narrow; the widest range of pH values compatible with life is from 6.8 to 7.8, or an interval of one pH unit. Lesser ECF pH changes, as small as 0.1 to 0.2 pH unit, can also significantly alter these body functions.

The major buffer system in extracellular fluid is the bicarbonate–carbonic acid pair. The relation between pH, bicarbonate, and carbonic acid concentrations in ECF may be expressed according to the familiar Henderson-Hasselbalch equation:

$$pH = pK + \log \frac{HCO_3^-}{H_2CO_3}$$

where pK is the carbonic acid dissociation constant, HCO_3^- is the plasma bicarbonate concentration, and H_2CO_3 is the plasma carbonic acid concentration. The H_2CO_3 concentration is given by $\alpha PaCO_2$ where α is the CO_2 solubility constant and has a value of 0.03, and $PaCO_2$ is the arterial carbon dioxide tension. Therefore with a $PaCO_2$ of 40 mm Hg, the Henderson-Hasselbalch equation becomes:

$$7.4 = 6.1 + \log \frac{24 \text{ mM/L}}{1.2 \text{ mM/L}}.$$

The arterial pH provides a qualitative but not quantitative index to total body water acid-base status because, at any given time, about two thirds of an acid or alkali load is buffered by proton shifts into or out of the ICF, respectively. For these reasons, some workers prefer to use the term "acidemia" for acidosis and "alkalemia" for alkalosis, to connote that plasma pH measurements provide quantitative information about the pH status of plasma and interstitial fluid, and only qualitative information about total body acid-base balance.

Proton shifts into the ICF, in acidosis, and out of the ICF, in alkalosis, provide an immediate buffering capacity that tends to minimize changes in ECF pH for any given acid or base load. Thus a convenient way to express the total body buffering capacity is as follows: Since bicarbonate is predominantly an extracellular anion, the total ECF bicarbonate content in a 70 kg man having 15 liters of ECF is (24 mEq per liter × 15 liters) or 360 mEq HCO_3^-. Since this represents only one third of total body buffering capacity, the latter is (360 mEq HCO_3^- × 3) or 1080 mEq. This quantity is often referred to as the "bicarbonate space," and may be calculated as:

$$(\text{arterial } HCO_3^- \times 0.6 \text{ body weight})$$

that is, using total body water as an index to total buffering capacity. The bicarbonate space is also an index to net acid excess or net base excess; if the arterial HCO_3^- concentration in a 70 kg man is reduced to 15 mEq per liter while the Pa_{CO_2} remains constant, the net acid excess (or net base deficit) is (24 − 15) mEq per liter × 42 liters = 378 mEq. Conversely, if the arterial HCO_3^- concentration rises to 33 mEq per liter while the Pa_{CO_2} remains constant, the net base excess (or acid deficit) is 378 mEq.

While proton shifts between the ECF and ICF help stabilize the plasma pH against acute fluctuations, the ultimate maintenance of pH balance requires that *input* of acid or base into the body be matched by *output* of acid or base, so that the HCO_3^-/H_2CO_3 ratio and the total bicarbonate content in the ECF remain constant. The cardinal systems involved in these external processes are the kidneys for bicarbonate balance and the lungs for carbon dioxide balance.

CO_2 Production and Elimination

VOLATILE ACID INPUT. The largest source of endogenous acid production is from combustion of glucose and fatty acids to carbon dioxide and water, or in other words, to a volatile acid. During aerobic glycolysis, that is, cellular respiration, glucose oxidation involves oxygen utilization and carbon dioxide production according to the reaction:

$$C_6H_{12}O_6 + 6O_2 \rightarrow 6CO_2 + 6H_2O.$$

Since red blood cells contain carbonic anhydrase (c.a.), carbon dioxide hydration in erythrocytes yields:

$$CO_2 + H_2O \overset{\text{c.a.}}{\rightleftarrows} H_2CO_3 \rightleftarrows H^+ + HCO_3^-.$$

The protons formed from carbonic acid dissociation are buffered by hemoglobin, while bicarbonate leaves red blood cells in exchange for chloride (the familiar chloride shift). In other words, carbon dioxide generation is equivalent to carbonic acid formation, and the bulk of hydrogen ion formed is buffered intracellularly.

A simple way of calculating the daily rate of volatile acid production is to note, from the above reactions, that the production of one mole of metabolic water and one mole of carbon dioxide represents, through dissociation of carbonic acid, the formation of one mole of hydrogen ions.

Since the molecular weight of water is 18, 1 liter of water contains about 55 moles of water. Consequently, the average rate of metabolic water production, about 400 ml daily, yields 22,000 millimoles of water and an equal number of carbon dioxide molecules. Thus, the rate of volatile acid production amounts to about 22,000 mEq of hydrogen ion daily. The cellular combustion of carbohydrates and fatty acids to carbon dioxide and water is remarkably efficient. Under normal circumstances, organic anions such as lactate and ketoacids, which derive from incomplete combustion of carbohydrates and fatty acids, have plasma concentrations of approximately 5 mEq per liter.

VOLATILE ACID OUTPUT. Pulmonary ventilation excretes the carbon dioxide formed by cellular respiration. During blood transit through the lungs, bicarbonate re-enters red blood cells and combines with protons to form carbonic acid, which dissociates to carbon dioxide and water. The carbon dioxide so formed diffuses freely through red blood cells and alveolar epithelium, so that the rate of carbon dioxide excretion is governed primarily by the rate of minute ventilation.

Under normal circumstances, the rate of cellular carbon dioxide production is relatively constant. When hyperpnea or hypoventilation develops, there is a transient loss or gain of carbon dioxide, respectively. However, in the steady state, the rate of carbon dioxide removal by the lung equals the rate of carbon dioxide production by cellular respiration whether there is normal ventilation, hyperpnea, or hypoventilation.

MODULATION OF RESPIRATION. The prime factors normally regulating alterations in the rate of minute ventilation are subtle changes in cerebrospinal fluid (CSF) pH or arterial pH. Sensor chemoreceptors in central medullary centers or in the carotid body are activated by small reductions in CSF pH or arterial pH, respectively; the pH reduction can result either from CO_2 accumulation or from nonvolatile acid accumulation, which reduces the plasma bicarbonate concentration. Under most circumstances, central medullary chemoreceptors provide the major impetus to altering ventilatory response, and the carotid body chemoreceptors serve as relatively minor stimuli to ventilation. The medullary respiratory centers therefore serve as the major *effector* mechanism for regulating carbon dioxide output by increasing ventilation rate.

The ventilatory response for carbon dioxide removal involves an increase in both tidal volume and respiratory rate. On an average, for every 1 mEq per liter reduction in plasma bicarbonate produced by metabolic acidosis, increased minute ventilation will produce a 1.2 mm Hg fall in the Pa_{CO_2}. Under most circumstances, the maximum reduction in Pa_{CO_2} produced by the hyperventilatory response to severe metabolic acidosis is to a Pa_{CO_2} of 12 to 15 mm Hg, and hyperventilation to Pa_{CO_2} values less than 10 mm Hg in metabolic acidosis almost never occurs. Conversely, an increase in arterial pH reduces the rate of minute ventilation and therefore results in CO_2 retention. For increases in plasma bicarbonate concentrations to 35 mEq per liter the Pa_{CO_2} usually remains 50 mm Hg. When profound metabolic alkalosis occurs, the Pa_{CO_2} may rise further, but virtually never exceeds 65 mm Hg.

Renal Bicarbonate Processing

In addition to volatile acid production due to carbon dioxide formation, cellular metabolism also results in the formation of a number of nonvolatile acids. The major source for nonvolatile acid production is the metabolism of sulfur-containing amino acids such as cysteine and methionine, which results in sulfuric acid formation. Consequently, the daily rate of nonvolatile acid production is closely related to dietary protein intake and to the rate of endogenous protein catabolism. Nonvolatile acids also derive from oxidation of phosphoproteins and phospholipids, which results in phosphoric acid formation; nucleoprotein degradation, which yields uric acid; and incomplete combustion of carbohydrates and fatty acids, which produces lactic acid and the ketoacids.

The daily rate of nonvolatile acid production under normal conditions is about 1 mEq per kilogram of body weight. Thus daily nonvolatile acid production would consume the total body fluid buffering capacity in about two weeks, were it not for the fact that the kidneys excrete nonvolatile acids, and in so doing, regenerate bicarbonate. Since the minimum urine pH ordinarily attainable is 5.0 and the amount of nonvolatile acid to be excreted is about 70 mEq daily, it is evident that renal hydrogen ion excretion, which is equivalent to renal bicarbonate regeneration, occurs mainly as protons trapped in an undissociated form by urinary buffers.

The kidneys also filter large quantities of bicarbonate daily: for a normal plasma bicarbonate concentration of 24 mEq per liter and a glomerular filtration rate of 180 liters daily, the net amount of bicarbonate filtered is approximately 4300 mEq daily, or about four times the total body buffering capacity. Thus, in addition to generating new bicarbonate, the renal tubules must also absorb filtered bicarbonate.

BICARBONATE REABSORPTION. Virtually all filtered bicarbonate is absorbed together with sodium by the proximal tubule. Consequently, the rate of proximal bicarbonate reabsorption is modulated by the same *effectors* that regulate proximal sodium absorption. Among these, the effective circulating volume exerts a central effect. Volume expansion, which resets glomerulotubular balance downward (see section on Volume Disorders), reduces the fractional rate of proximal bicarbonate reabsorption; the effect is sometimes termed "reducing the bicarbonate threshold." Conversely, volume contraction raises the bicarbonate threshold by increasing the fractional rate of proximal tubular sodium bicarbonate reabsorption.

Two other *effectors* regulate, in operational terms, the rate of bicarbonate reabsorption. One of these is the arterial Pa_{CO_2}: High Pa_{CO_2} values raise the apparent bicarbonate threshold, while low Pa_{CO_2} values reduce the rate of bicarbonate reabsorption. This factor accounts for the compensatory increase in plasma bicarbonate concentrations in respiratory acidosis. Second, hypokalemia also increases the rate of bicarbonate reabsorption, presumably by raising the intracellular hydrogen ion concentration. This factor accounts for the fact that, in hypokalemic, hypochloremic metabolic alkalosis associated with volume contraction, alkalosis can persist after volume deficits are restored. In this circumstance, correction of potassium deficits is required for correction of the alkalosis.

BICARBONATE REGENERATION. The excretion of nonvolatile acids and simultaneous renal regeneration of bicarbonate occur principally in distal nephron segments. Distal renal tubular cells hydrate carbon dioxide to carbonic acid, which dissociates to protons secreted into the urine, and bicarbonate anions, which are absorbed into blood. The secreted protons titrate urinary buffers, principally phosphate, while sodium is absorbed. Thus the overall reaction is:

$$\underset{(filtered)}{Na_2HPO_4} + H^+ + HCO_3^- \rightarrow \underset{(excreted)}{NaH_2PO_4} + \underset{(absorbed)}{NaHCO_3}$$

Titratable acid formation normally accounts for about one third of renal acid excretion. The remaining two thirds of acid excretion is accounted for by ammonia (NH_3) secretion by the sequence:

$$\underset{(filtered)}{NaR} + NH_3 + H^+ + HCO_3^- \rightarrow \underset{(reabsorbed)}{NaHCO_3} + \underset{(exorted)}{NH_4R}$$

where NaR is the filtered sodium salt of a nonvolatile acid, NH_3 is ammonia produced by renal tubular cells, and the protons and bicarbonate come from carbon dioxide hydration by tubular cells.

It is evident that distal acid excretion and bicarbonate absorption are accompanied by sodium absorption. Consequently, *effector* systems that enhance distal sodium absorption, such as aldosterone or increased rates of sodium delivery to terminal nephron segments, also promote terminal nephron hydrogen ion excretion. Three other *effector* mechanisms also increase the rate of hydrogen ion excretion. First, delivery of sodium to terminal nephron segments in association with impermeant anions such as sulfate favors proton movement from tubular cells to lumen. Second, hypokalemia enhances hydrogen ion excretion, particularly in sodium-acquisitive states, presumably because hypokalemia is accompanied by a fall in intracellular pH. Third, acidosis stimulates ammoniagenesis by renal tubular cells; consequently, in metabolic acidosis, increases in the rate of renal acid excretion are referable primarily to increased rates of ammonium excretion. In other words, these latter three effector systems enhance renal acid excretion by creating a favorable situation for proton transfer from tubular cells to urine. Conversely, aldosterone deficiency, alkalosis, or reduced rates of salt delivery to terminal nephron segments reduce renal capacity for acid excretion.

pH Disequilibria Between Plasma and CSF

Because central rather than arterial chemoreceptors are the prime sensors for pH-mediated changes in respiration, the ventilatory responses to pH changes mediated by respiratory processes or metabolic processes differ. The blood-brain barrier is freely permeable to carbon dioxide. Consequently, pH changes produced exclusively by hyperventilation or hypoventilation occur almost simultaneously in arterial plasma and in the CSF, and the respiratory response to primary increases or decreases in the Pa_{CO_2} occurs almost instantaneously. However, the blood-brain barrier imposes a lag in the rate at which arterial bicarbonate equilibrates with the CSF. Thus in metabolic acidosis, the arterial pH and bicarbonate concentration fall more rapidly than does the pH of the CSF; and in the metabolic alkalosis, the CSF pH and bicarbonate concentration rise more slowly than does the arterial plasma pH. Consequently, in the early stages of acute metabolic acidosis, there may be a 1- to 3-hour delay in the development of a maximal hyperventilatory response. Conversely, when metabolic acidosis is corrected rapidly, hyperventilation may persist for a few hours because of a delay in the rise of cerebrospinal fluid pH.

An unusual situation relating to this effect occurs in diabetic ketoacidosis and in certain other metabolic acidoses associated with impaired central nervous system function. In these situations, carotid body chemoreceptors rather than central medullary chemoreceptors can provide the major stimulus to respiration driven by a reduced arterial pH. The rapid correction of ECF acidosis by bicarbonate administration reduces the rate at which carotid body chemoreceptors drive ventilation. When this occurs, Pa_{CO_2} levels in plasma and in the CSF rise almost simultaneously; but because of a lag in the rate of bicarbonate entry into the CSF, the CSF bicarbonate/carbonic acid ratio tends to fall. In severe diabetic ketoacidosis, this situation can result in an actual fall in CSF pH simultaneously with a rise in arterial pH produced by intravenous bicarbonate administration.

DEFINITION OF ACID-BASE ABNORMALITIES

The arterial pH is determined by the ratio of the bicarbonate/carbonic acid buffer system, as expressed in the Henderson-Hasselbalch equation. These data also provide an index to total body acid-base balance, because the majority of body buffering occurs within cells. Acid-base disturbances can therefore occur either by altering the serum bicarbonate concentration, referred to as a "metabolic" disorder, or by altering arterial carbon dioxide tension, referred to as a "respiratory" disorder. A convenient way for considering these disturbances is illustrated in Figure 76–8, which illustrates pH isobars (for pH 7.0, 7.4, and 7.8) calculated according to the Henderson-Hasselbalch equation for the bicarbonate concentrations and Pa_{CO_2} values listed on the ordinate and abscissa, respectively.

TYPES OF ACID-BASE ABNORMALITIES. The left-hand panel in Figure 76–8 shows the directional changes in Pa_{CO_2} and bicarbonate concentrations that *initiate* the four basic types of acid-base abnormalities. *Respiratory acidosis* results from hypoventilation and reduces pH by raising the Pa_{CO_2}. *Respiratory alkalosis* results from hyperventilation and raises pH by reducing the Pa_{CO_2}. *Metabolic alkalosis* occurs when increases in the plasma bicarbonate concentration raise pH, and *metabolic acidosis* occurs when reductions in plasma bicarbonate reduce pH.

Any of these initial acid-base disturbances activates *compensatory responses,* illustrated in the right-hand panel of Figure 76–8, which tends to minimize the pH changes produced by the initial acid-base abnormality. By comparing the directional arrows in the left- and right-hand panels of Figure 76–8, it becomes evident that the initial disturbance in any of these four acid-base abnormalities tends to displace the arterial pH away from the pH 7.4 isobar and that the compensatory response partially restores arterial pH values toward the pH 7.4 isobar. The arterial pH, Pa_{CO_2}, and plasma bicarbonate concentrations illustrated in the right-hand panel of Figure 76–8 are the values usually observed clinically in the four primary acid-base disturbances.

We may now consider these primary acid-base abnormalities and the compensatory responses in more detail. In respiratory acidosis, increased rates of renal bicarbonate reabsorption raise plasma bicarbonate concentrations to offset increases in Pa_{CO_2} values. In chronic respiratory acidosis, renal bicarbonate absorption generally stabilizes the arterial pH close to the pH 7.4 isobar, if the arterial Pa_{CO_2} remains less than 55 mm Hg. However, in acute respiratory acidosis, the renal response to increases in arterial Pa_{CO_2} does not occur with sufficient rapidity to offset the pH derangement. Accordingly, for a given increase in Pa_{CO_2}, acidosis will be appreciably more severe in acute rather than chronic hyperventilation. In respiratory alkalosis, renal bicarbonate excretion minimizes the tendency to an increased arterial pH but generally is inadequate to prevent arterial pH increases, particularly in acute hyperventilatory states.

In metabolic acidosis, compensatory hyperventilation can reduce the arterial Pa_{CO_2} to 12 to 15 mm Hg, but in severe metabolic acidosis, it is never adequate to restore the arterial pH to normal. In metabolic alkalosis, plasma bicarbonate concentrations in excess of 35 mEq per liter result in a compensatory hypoventilation that can raise the Pa_{CO_2} to 50 mm Hg. In severe metabolic alkalosis, Pa_{CO_2} values as high as 60 to 65 mm Hg may occur, particularly in azotemic patients.

In addition to these four primary acid-base abnormalities, there may also occur *mixed disorders,* in which two primary acid-base abnormalities may exist simultaneously. In certain instances, a mixed acid-base disorder may result in pH, Pa_{CO_2}, and plasma bicarbonate concentrations that are entirely normal, even though two acid-base abnormalities are present simultaneously. Such a situation can arise, for example, in a patient with advanced chronic renal failure who develops metabolic alkalosis as a consequence of vomiting. The only clue to an acid-base abnormality in this circumstance might be increased plasma levels of phosphates and sulfates, that is, anions other than chloride or bicarbonate. Consequently, in addition to an estimate of the arterial pH, Pa_{CO_2}, and plasma bicarbonate concentrations, an evaluation of the *anion gap* is a virtual necessity in analyzing acid-base disturbances, particularly in the case of metabolic acidosis.

THE ANION GAP. Sodium is the principal cation in extracellular fluids. The sum of plasma chloride plus bicarbonate concentrations is less than the serum sodium concentration; the remaining anions required for electroneutrality, generally

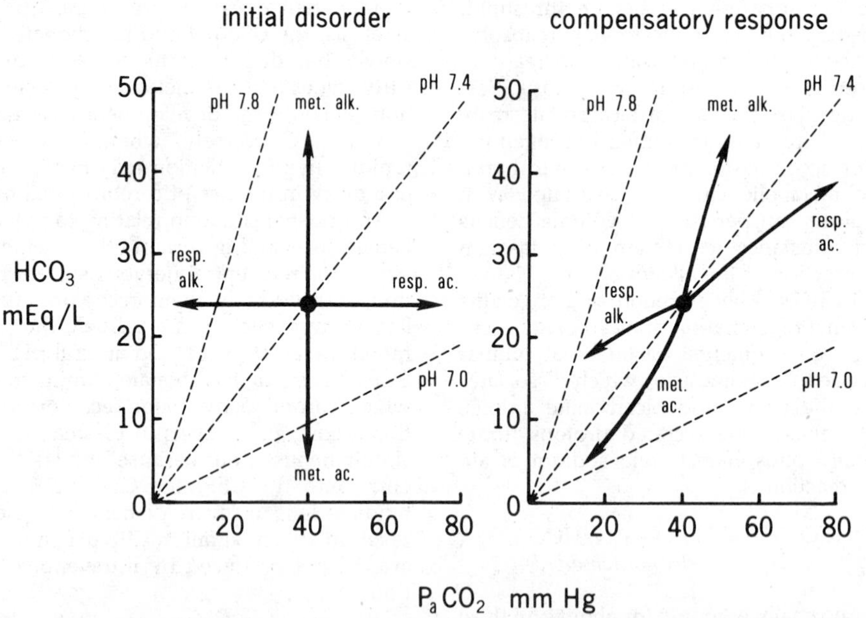

Figure 76–8. Schematic frame of reference for considering acid-base disturbances. The dotted lines are the pH isobars for pH values of 7.8, 7.4, and 7.0, computed from the Henderson-Hasselbalch equation for given combinations of arterial bicarbonate values (vertical axes) and arterial carbon dioxide tensions (horizontal axes). The graph on the left, labelled initial disorder, shows the initial derangement in HCO_3^- concentrations in metabolic acidosis and metabolic alkalosis and the initial Pa_{CO_2} derangement in respiratory acidosis and respiratory alkalosis. Note that each of the four changes in either HCO_3^- or Pa_{CO_2} tends to displace the arterial pH from the pH 7.4 isobar. The graph on the right, labelled compensatory response, indicates the general trend of pH, HCO_3^- and Pa_{CO_2} changes actually observed in the four primary acid-base disturbances: respiratory acidosis, respiratory alkalosis, metabolic acidosis, and metabolic alkalosis. Respiratory acidosis and alkalosis are accompanied by compensatory renal bicarbonate retention and loss, respectively. Metabolic acidosis and alkalosis are accompanied by compensatory hyperventilation and hypoventilation, respectively. Note that the compensatory response in each of the four acid-base disorders tends to restore arterial pH values toward the pH 7.4 isobar.

TABLE 76–10. MAJOR CAUSES OF METABOLIC ACIDOSIS

Normal Anion Gap	Increased Anion Gap
Bicarbonate Loss	**Reduced Excretion of Inorganic Acids**
Proximal renal tubular acidosis	Renal failure
Dilutional acidosis	**Accumulation of Organic Acids**
Carbonic anhydrase inhibitors	Lactic acidosis
Primary hyperparathyroidism	Ketoacidosis: alcoholic
Diarrheal states	diabetic
Small bowel drainage	starvation
Ureterosigmoidostomy	Ingestion: salicylates
Failure of Bicarbonate Regeneration	paraldehyde
Distal, gradient-limited renal tubular acidosis	methanol
Hyporeninemic hypoaldosteronism	ethylene glycol
Diuretics: triamterene, spironolactone	
Acidifying Salts	
Ammonium chloride	
Lysine hydrochloride	
Arginine hydrochloride	
Hyperalimentation	

not reported with routine serum electrolyte measurements, are referred to as unmeasured anions or as the anion gap. A convenient formula for calculating the anion gap is:

$$\text{Anion gap} = Na^+ - (Cl^- + HCO_3^-)$$

where Na^+, Cl^-, and HCO_3^- are the serum sodium, chloride, and bicarbonate concentrations, respectively. The anion gap includes primarily phosphates and sulfates derived from tissue metabolism, lactate and ketoacids arising from incomplete combustion of carbohydrates and fatty acids, and negatively charged protein molecules, principally albumin. The normal value for unmeasured anions, or the anion gap, is 10 to 12 mEq per liter; albumin and other proteins normally account for about half of the anion gap.

An *increased* anion gap generally indicates the presence of metabolic acidosis. Three kinds of disturbances, either alone or in combination, can produce metabolic acidosis with an increase in the anion gap. First, a reduction in glomerular filtration rate results in phosphate or sulfate retention. Second, lactic acid, beta-hydroxybutyric acid, and the ketoacids accumulate when there is either excessive production of these substances, incomplete combustion of glucose or fatty acids to carbon dioxide and water, or a combination of these two processes. Finally, exogenous ingestion of substances such as salicylates, methanol, or ethylene glycol lead to increased formation of organic acids and therefore increase the anion gap and produce metabolic acidosis.

A *reduced* anion gap provides an index to certain other disorders. The anion gap will be reduced if the sodium concentration falls while the chloride plus bicarbonate concentrations are unchanged; or in other words, when the concentration of another cation in serum is increased while the serum osmolality remains normal. This may occur in severe multiple myeloma of the IgG variety, since the myeloma proteins are cationic at pH 7.4. Hyperviscosity syndromes may also result in a reduced anion gap because of a laboratory artifact: when serum is excessively viscous, automatic pumps deliver decreased volumes of serum to a flame photometer, producing artifactual reductions in sodium concentrations. Lithium intoxication, hypermagnesemia, and hypercalcemia raise nonsodium cation concentrations sufficiently high to reduce the anion gap, but this circumstance occurs rarely.

The anion gap will also be decreased if the serum sodium concentration remains normal while the serum chloride plus bicarbonate concentrations are increased. This occurs most commonly in hypoalbuminemia. A low anion gap also occurs in bromide intoxication, since colorimetric techniques for serum chloride determinations give spuriously high values for chloride plus bromide when bromide is present in relatively high concentrations in serum.

METABOLIC ACIDOSIS

ETIOLOGY AND PATHOGENESIS. A convenient way to consider the metabolic acidoses is to divide them into two groups, those having a normal anion gap and those having an increased anion gap. Table 76–10 presents a classification of metabolic acidosis according to this format. The metabolic acidoses having a *normal anion gap* occur because the kidneys fail to reabsorb or regenerate bicarbonate, because there are extrarenal losses of bicarbonate, or because excessive amounts of substances yielding hydrochloric acid have been administered. The presence of a normal anion gap implies that the glomerular filtration rate is sufficient to excrete sulfates and phosphates, that there is no endogenous overproduction of organic acids, and that there has not been ingestion of substances that lead to organic acid accumulation.

NORMAL ANION GAP METABOLIC ACIDOSIS. ***Bicarbonate Losses.*** Bicarbonate losses occur either when the proximal tubule fails to absorb virtually all filtered bicarbonate, that is, when the apparent bicarbonate threshold is reduced, or when there are losses of bicarbonate from the gastrointestinal tract. Renal bicarbonate wasting occurs in *proximal renal tubular acidosis,* either alone or as part of the Fanconi syndrome. The apparent threshold for bicarbonate in this disorder is set below the normal value of 26 mEq of bicarbonate per 100 milliliters of glomerular filtrate, and may be as low as 15 to 20 mEq of bicarbonate per 100 milliliters of glomerular filtrate. Consequently, bicarbonate wasting occurs whenever the plasma bicarbonate is raised above the apparent renal threshold for bicarbonate (see Ch. 83.2).

For this reason, attempts to correct the acidosis by bicarbonate administration are generally unrewarding, because increases in the plasma bicarbonate produced by administering bicarbonate salts are accompanied by corresponding increases in bicarbonaturia. A promising new therapeutic approach to this disorder involves reducing the effective circulating volume by sodium restriction. This maneuver exploits the fact that ECF contraction resets glomerulotubular balance upward and consequently increases the fractional rate of sodium, and hence bicarbonate, reabsorption by the proximal tubule.

A converse of this situation is sometimes referred to as *dilutional acidosis.* Individuals who are volume expanded reduce the fractional rate of sodium bicarbonate absorption by the proximal tubule and consequently develop mild reductions in plasma bicarbonate concentrations. *Carbonic anhydrase inhibitors* such as acetazolamide inhibit proximal sodium bicarbonate absorption, resulting in metabolic acidosis. *Primary hyperparathyroidism* also reduces the apparent bicarbonate threshold in the proximal tubule; mild degrees of hyperchloremic acidosis are commonly noted in patients with this disorder.

Both pancreatic and small bowel secretions are rich in bicarbonate. Hence *diarrheal states* and *ileal drainage* can result in significant bicarbonate losses. *Ureterosigmoidostomy* results in metabolic acidosis because the colon can secrete bicarbonate in exchange for chloride. Thus in patients with this surgical procedure, urine reaching the colon is alkalinized by bicarbonate exchange for chloride, thereby producing a net bicarbonate loss.

Failure of Bicarbonate Regeneration. The second major group of disorders producing hyperchloremic acidosis includes those disorders in which the ability of the distal nephron to regenerate bicarbonate is impaired. *Distal, gradient-limited renal tubular acidosis* and chronic interstitial renal disease with *hyporeninemic hypoaldosteronism* are prototypes of this kind of metabolic acidosis. The nature of these two disorders is, however, different. In gradient-limited, distal renal tubular acidosis, proton secretion may be normal, but because the distal tubule is unable to maintain a steep urine-to-blood proton concentration gradient, secreted protons are recycled back to blood. The administration of large quantities of phosphate salts permits the excretion of large amounts of titratable acid in this disorder, because the pH of the phosphate buffer system is 6.8, that is, relatively high. Furthermore, potassium wasting and hypokalemia are common in distal, gradient-limited renal tubular acidosis, due at least in part to secondary hyperaldosteronism stimulated by sodium wasting.

In hyporeninemic hypoaldosteronism, which generally occurs in association with interstitial disease, the distal tubular derangements include diminished rates of sodium absorption and diminished rates of proton and potassium secretion. Consequently, sodium wasting with hyperkalemic, hyperchloremic acidosis are the hallmarks of this disorder. Finally, diuretics such as *triamterene, spironolactone,* and *amiloride,* which interfere with distal tubular sodium absorption, proton secretion, and potassium secretion, thus result in hyperkalemic, hyperchloremic metabolic acidosis (Table 76–4).

Acidifying Salts. The third major group of diseases producing hyperchloremic acidosis includes the administration of *acidifying salts* such as ammonium hydrochloride, lysine hydrochloride, or arginine hydrochloride; in each instance, metabolism of ammonium or the amino acids leads to hydrochloric acid formation. *Hyperalimentation* without the administration of adequate amounts of bicarbonate or bicarbonate-yielding solutes (such as lactate or acetate) can also produce hyperchloremic metabolic acidosis. The acidosis occurs because the synthetic amino acids used in hyperalimentation mixtures contain positively charged amino acids such as arginine, lysine, and histidine, which yield proton equivalents when metabolized.

INCREASED ANION GAP METABOLIC ACIDOSIS. Metabolic acidoses characterized by an increased anion gap occur either because the kidneys fail to excrete inorganic acids, such as phosphate or sulfate, or because there is net accumulation of organic acids.

Reduced Acid Excretion. Renal failure, either acute or chronic, results in metabolic acidosis with an increased anion gap due to retention of sulfates and phosphates. In chronic renal failure, metabolic acidosis occurs because the net amount of ammonium excreted daily falls as functional renal mass diminishes. The plasma bicarbonate concentration in most patients with chronic renal failure ranges between 16 and 20 mEq per liter. While this degree of acidosis appears relatively modest, the daily acid load is buffered by bone salts; this buffering may contribute to the osteopenia of chronic renal failure. In acute tubular necrosis, acidosis occurs because of generalized tubular dysfunction, including impaired net acid excretion. The plasma bicarbonate generally remains above 16 mEq per liter unless sepsis, profound hypoxia, or extensive tissue necrosis complicates the disorder.

Organic Acid Accumulation. Organic acid accumulation represents the second major cause for metabolic acidosis with an increased anion gap and is the most common cause for acute metabolic acidosis. Normally, the complete combustion of carbohydrates and fatty acids to carbon dioxide and water is highly efficient and results in the production of approximately 22,000 mEq of hydrogen ion per day. Thus it is evident that processes which impair cellular respiration, and therefore result in nonvolatile rather than volatile acid production, can lead to profound metabolic acidosis.

The syndrome of *lactic acidosis* results from impaired cellular respiration. Lactic acid is produced in muscle, red blood cells, and other tissues as a consequence of anaerobic glycolysis. Lactic acid oxidation involves reduction of nicotine adenine dinucleotide (NAD) by lactic acid dehydrogenase (*LDH*) according to the reaction:

$$\text{Lactate} + \text{NAD} \underset{}{\overset{LDH}{\rightleftarrows}} \text{pyruvate} + \text{NADH}$$

Cellular respiration involves mitochondrial oxidation of pyruvate and NADH to carbon dioxide and water. When lactic acidosis occurs because of impaired cellular respiration, the lactate-to-pyruvate (L/P) ratio rises, as does the NADH/NAD ratio. Thus glycolysis in a setting of impaired cellular respiration results in increased production of nonvolatile lactic acid. Lactic acidosis should not be confused with states in which serum lactate levels are elevated, with normal L/P and NADH/NAD ratios, in vigorous exercise, for example. Lactic acidosis is also characterized by negative serum nitroprusside (Acetest) reactions, since Acetest tablets react with acetoacetic acid and acetone, but not with beta-hydroxybutyric acid. In lactic acidosis, the beta-hydroxybutyric acid/acetoacetic acid ratio is elevated in parallel with the increased NADH/NAD ratio.

Lactic acidosis occurs most commonly in disorders characterized by inadequate oxygen delivery to tissues, such as shock, septicemia, and profound hypoxemia. Drug-induced lactic acidosis may occur with phenformin therapy and isoniazid toxicity; in both circumstances, oxygen utilization by tissues is thought to be impaired. Lactic acidosis also occurs in association with leukemia and diabetes mellitus. The presence of a negative Acetest reaction in patients with diabetic acidosis is a valuable clue to the coexistence of diabetic ketoacidosis and lactic acidosis. There is also a spontaneous, idiopathic form of lactic acidosis in debilitated patients, which is almost uniformly fatal.

A second group of disorders characterized by an anion gap metabolic acidosis includes those disorders in which cellular respiration may not be impaired, but accelerated rates of organic acid production, particularly from lipolysis, result in an increased anion gap. *Alcoholic ketoacidosis* occurs in patients with chronic alcoholism and a recent history of binge drinking, little or no food intake, and recurrent vomiting. Hypoglycemia may be present. The major pathogenic mechanism for alcoholic ketoacidosis seems to depend on accelerated rates of lipolysis, and hence on beta-hydroxybutyric acid production, because of reduced rates of insulin secretion referable to starvation. The Acetest reaction is variably positive and the beta-hydroxybutyrate/acetoacetate ratio is elevated. Lactate utilization is diminished in this disorder. Patients with alcoholic ketoacidosis have beta-hydroxybutyric acid, rather than lactic acid, as the principal nonvolatile acid. *Diabetic ketoacidosis* is the most common cause for metabolic acidosis with an increased anion gap, and occurs because of increased rates of ketogenesis due to insulin lack and inadequate carbohydrate combustion. *Starvation* produces metabolic acidosis by essentially the same mechanism: increased hepatic ketogenesis with reduced caloric intake.

Thus in a general sense, one may consider that alcoholic ketoacidosis, diabetic ketoacidosis, and starvation share at least one common feature: accelerated lipolytic ketogenesis due at least in part to insulin lack. Obviously, however, the approach to therapy varies in these disorders. In alcoholic ketoacidosis and starvation, caloric supplementation with carbohydrates, which stimulates insulin release, usually suffices. In diabetic ketoacidosis, insulin therapy simultaneously promotes carbohydrate combustion and diminishes lipolysis. Finally, in each of these disorders, volume expansion should accompany the above maneuvers.

Finally, a number of ingested substances can also result in severe metabolic acidosis with a large anion gap. *Salicylism* produces a complex set of acid-base abnormalities. Salicylates stimulate ventilation through central mechanisms; the reduction in Pa_{CO_2} can therefore result in reductions in plasma bicarbonate concentrations. Since salicylate is a relatively strong acid, the ingestion of large quantities of salicylate can, by itself, contribute to metabolic acidosis and an increased anion gap. Salicylates also interfere with mitochondrial function. As a consequence, a number of as yet unidentified organic acids accumulate in serum and are the major factors responsible for the anion gap acidosis of salicylism.

A number of other agents, including *paraldehyde, methanol,* and *ethylene glycol,* also produce severe metabolic acidosis with organic acid accumulation. In methanol poisoning, formic acid (an end product of methanol metabolism) accounts in large part for the reduction in serum bicarbonate concentration. In ethylene glycol intoxication, oxalic acid accumulation is not adequate to account entirely for the reduction in plasma bicarbonate; however, oxalate deposition in tissues is clearly a major factor in ethylene glycol toxicity. The organic acids responsible for an increased anion gap in paraldehyde intoxication have not been identified.

DIAGNOSIS AND TREATMENT. The diagnosis of metabolic acidosis requires analysis of serum electrolytes and, when indicated, measurement of arterial pH and Pa_{CO_2}. A cardinal clinical manifestation of metabolic acidosis is hyperventilation, which, when severe, is manifested as Kussmaul's respiration. However, in patients with chronic metabolic acidosis, hyperventilation may be difficult to detect clinically.

Severe metabolic acidosis exerts a negative inotropic effect on the heart, which depends, at least in part, on the fact that acidosis diminishes tissue responsiveness to catecholamines. Thus in lactic acidosis, negative inotropy sets the stage for a potentially lethal chain of events: poor tissue perfusion → lactic acidosis → decreased cardiac function → further reduction in tissue perfusion.

Acidosis also affects the delivery of oxygen to tissues. In acidosis, the Bohr effect shifts the oxyhemoglobin dissociation curve to the right. This compensatory mechanism permits the delivery of oxygen to inadequately perfused tissues. However, the protective characteristics of the Bohr effect may be offset by the effect of pH variation on red blood cell 2,3-diphosphoglycerate (2,3-DPG). Increases in red cell 2,3-DPG also shift the oxyhemoglobin dissociation curve to the right. However, acidosis tends to reduce red blood cell 2,3-DPG; this may offset partially the compensatory Bohr effect and therefore aggravate inadequate tissue oxygenation in acidosis.

Since metabolic acidosis is a manifestation of a variety of different diseases, the treatment of metabolic acidosis varies depending on the underlying process and on the acuteness and severity of the acidosis. However, certain general principles serve as useful guidelines for therapy: The principles can be formulated with respect to the classification of metabolic acidosis presented in Table 76–10. Those disorders characterized by *failure of bicarbonate regeneration* or *reduced excretion of inorganic acids* represent acidoses in which the kidneys fail to excrete a normal load of nonvolatile acid, or in other words, fail to regenerate approximately 70 mEq of bicarbonate daily. Thus the treatment of these metabolic acidoses requires removal of the offending agent, if patients are receiving triamterene or spironolactone, and the administration of relatively modest amounts of bicarbonate. In chronic renal failure, alkali therapy is generally not required unless the plasma bicarbonate falls below 16 to 18 mEq per liter. If the acidosis is more severe, bicarbonate supplementation in the form of Shohl's solution (see below) may be instituted. Caution should be exercised to avoid sodium overload or the appearance of tetany, if overalkalinization occurs.

In distal, gradient-limited renal tubular acidosis, the administration of 30 to 60 mEq of bicarbonate daily usually corrects the acidosis. This can be given conveniently in the form of Shohl's solution, which is a mixture of sodium citrate and citric acid; 1 ml of Shohl's solution yields the equivalent of 1 mmol of sodium bicarbonate. Potassium supplementation is also required in the disorder. In children with distal renal tubular acidosis, greater quantities of bicarbonate may be required to avoid growth retardation. Large-dose alkali therapy, in the range of 5 to 14 mEq alkali per kilogram daily, is required to prevent stunted growth in children with the disorder.

The therapy of patients with metabolic acidosis due to *external bicarbonate loss* varies with the nature of the disorder. As indicated above, sodium restriction and an attendant rise in the apparent bicarbonate threshold may be helpful in treating proximal renal tubular acidosis. In acute metabolic acidosis due to gastrointestinal losses, the net bicarbonate deficit may be roughly calculated, as indicated previously, from the reduction in "bicarbonate space," or total body buffering capacity, as:

$$(24 \text{ mEq per liter} - \text{measured plasma } HCO_3^-) \times 0.6 \text{ body weight (kg)}$$

Bicarbonate therapy should be instituted when the arterial pH falls below 7.1. It is prudent to administer sufficient sodium bicarbonate intravenously to raise the plasma bicarbonate concentration to 16 mEq per liter over a 12 to 24 hour interval, rather than to repair the entire bicarbonate deficit. Calculation of the bicarbonate deficit in this manner is valid only if there are no further bicarbonate losses. If the latter persist, as in cholera or other secretory diarrheas, the daily amount of bicarbonate given to maintain the plasma bicarbonate concentration in the range of 16 mEq per liter may actually exceed the calculated bicarbonate space.

The treatment of acidoses due to *accumulation of organic acids* varies with the disorder. In *lactic acidosis,* therapy should be directed toward improving tissue perfusion. Because the disorder results from a failure of conversion of lactic acid and other organic acids to carbon dioxide and water, large amounts of sodium bicarbonate, sometimes in excess of 1000 mEq per 24 hour period, may be required to avoid the development of lethal acidosis. The treatment is further complicated by the fact that the response to alkali therapy, in any given patient, is not predictable. The administration of large amounts of sodium bicarbonate (in the form of ampules containing 44.5 mmol of sodium bicarbonate per 50 milliliters) carries with it the risk of cellular shrinkage due to hypertonicity and circulatory overload due to ECF volume expansion. Hemodialysis or peritoneal dialysis to remove volume excess and to correct hypertonicity is therefore a valuable adjunct to the therapy of lactic acidosis when large amounts of alkali are required.

The treatment of *alcoholic ketoacidosis* generally requires only the administration of saline solutions and glucose. Alkali therapy should not be used unless the metabolic acidosis is in the lethal range. The same considerations apply to starvation ketosis. As indicated previously, the insulin release provoked by glucose administration suppresses lipolysis and consequently the overproduction of ketoacids.

In *diabetic ketoacidosis,* insulin therapy promotes glucose utilization and consequently complete oxidation of ketoacids; simultaneously, ketogenesis is reduced. Therefore alkali therapy is ordinarily not required in the disorder. Furthermore, because the hyperventilatory response to acidosis in some diabetic patients is governed by arterial rather than central medullary chemoreceptors, intravenous sodium bicarbonate administration may result in arterial alkalinization, a reduction in the rate of minute ventilation, and a potentially lethal fall in CSF pH. Sodium bicarbonate therapy in diabetic ketoacidosis should therefore be reserved for initial therapy of the disorder when the arterial pH is below 7.0 to 7.1 and cardiac contractility is impaired. Finally, because *salicylates, methanol,* and *ethylene glycol* are, by themselves, tissue toxins, appropriate therapy for these disorders may include not only alkalinization but also hemodialysis for removal of the offending agent.

METABOLIC ALKALOSIS

ETIOLOGY AND PATHOGENESIS. The maintenance of the plasma bicarbonate concentration depends on renal bicarbonate reabsorption and renal bicarbonate regeneration (that is, net acid excretion). Consequently, while metabolic alkalosis may be *initiated* by the loss of hydrogen ion from the body, for example during gastric drainage, the *maintenance* of a sustained metabolic alkalosis requires that the net rate of renal bicarbonate reabsorption and/or renal bicarbonate generation be greater than normal. In other words, a steady-state elevation of plasma bicarbonate concentration to levels greater than 24 mEq per liter requires increased activity of one or more of the effector mechanisms regulating bicarbonate handling by renal tubules. In normal individuals, it is therefore difficult to produce metabolic alkalosis by simple alkali loading.

Table 76–11 lists the major clinical causes of metabolic alkalosis. The table includes two disorders in which the apparent threshold for proximal bicarbonate reabsorption is increased, namely, volume contraction and potassium depletion; and disorders which increase net bicarbonate regeneration, including increased rates of distal salt delivery and mineralocorticoid excess, either primary or as a consequence of volume contraction. Table 76–11 also lists Liddle's syndrome, in which the pathogenesis of alkalosis is obscure.

Volume contraction can sustain metabolic alkalosis because of an increase in the apparent rate of bicarbonate reabsorption by the proximal tubule. The most common cause for initiating this kind of alkalosis is hydrochloric acid loss because of vomiting or gastric suction. In the early stages of gastric fluid losses, there is a modest sodium bicarbonate diuresis, but urinary sodium chloride excretion is reduced. As volume contraction becomes increasingly severe, sodium conservation occurs and potassium bicarbonate is excreted in an attempt to maintain pH homeostasis. Finally, when potassium depletion becomes severe, urinary sodium plus potassium excretion is sharply reduced and paradoxical aciduria occurs: the urine is acid while the plasma bicarbonate and pH are both elevated. *Contraction alkalosis* is a frequently misunderstood term; the designation should be reserved for those patients in whom metabolic alkalosis has developed and volume contraction maintains the alkalosis by increasing the apparent proximal tubular threshold for bicarbonate reabsorption. Thus contraction alkalosis is a mirror image of the dilutional acidosis listed in Table 76–10.

Potassium depletion from any cause, when sufficiently severe, can sustain metabolic alkalosis initiated by acid loss, for example, during gastric drainage. Presumably, potassium loss from cells is accompanied by increased hydrogen ion concentrations within cells, including renal tubular cells. Thus potassium depletion, when sufficiently severe, can raise the rate of renal tubular bicarbonate reabsorption and hence maintain a metabolic alkalosis. Consequently, when serum potassium concentrations are reduced to about 2 mEq per liter, metabolic alkalosis due to gastric fluid loss becomes resistant to saline but responsive to potassium chloride administration.

Situations in which there occurs *enhanced delivery of sodium chloride* to terminal nephron segments enhance renal acid excretion and therefore lead to metabolic alkalosis by increasing the rate of renal bicarbonate generation. This effect occurs with loop diuretics (Table 76–4), such as furosemide or ethacrynic acid, and with the proximal tubular diuretic metolazone. These diuretics also contribute to the maintenance of metabolic alkalosis by contracting ECF volume and by promoting potassium depletion. Salt wasting is common in *Bartter's syndrome*; metabolic alkalosis due to renal bicarbonate generation is therefore a common feature of the disorder. The administration of large amounts of *impermeant anions* such as carbenicillin also favors distal hydrogen ion secretion. Thus carbenicillin therapy is one of the few circumstances in which an increased anion gap and metabolic alkalosis can be produced simultaneously by the same agent.

TABLE 76–11. MAJOR MECHANISMS FOR METABOLIC ALKALOSIS

ECF volume contraction
Potassium depletion
Increased distal salt delivery
Mineralocorticoid excess
Liddle's syndrome
Bicarbonate loading (post-hypercapneic alkalosis)
Delayed conversion of administered organic acids

Mineralocorticoid excess, either primary or secondary, can also result in metabolic alkalosis because of renal bicarbonate generation. The disorder can occur in volume-expanded patients, for example, in primary hyperaldosteronism, in which the alkalosis is unresponsive to sodium chloride loading; and in patients with a reduced effective circulating volume and secondary hyperaldosteronism. The alkalosis of mineralocorticoid excess occurs primarily because of increased generation of bicarbonate by terminal nephron segments (or in other words, by increased renal acid excretion) and is clearly accentuated by potassium depletion. *Liddle's syndrome* is a disorder of unknown cause in which metabolic alkalosis, hypokalemia, and hypertension occur because of an increase in sodium avidity by terminal nephron segments, which can be blocked by triamterene therapy.

The disorders listed in Table 76–11, with the exception of post-hypercapneic alkalosis, result in metabolic alkalosis by two general kinds of mechanisms. First, metabolic alkalosis may be initiated by a loss of acid from nonrenal sources, for example, gastric fluid loss; and the kidney maintains the metabolic alkalosis by raising the rate of proximal tubular bicarbonate reabsorption. This is the primary mechanism responsible for the alkalosis associated with ECF volume contraction or potassium depletion. Second, the generation of metabolic alkalosis may occur intrarenally, because of increased rates of renal bicarbonate generation (or net acid excretion). This appears to be the major factor responsible for the alkalosis accompanying increased rates of salt delivery to the terminal nephron, mineralocorticoid excess, and Liddle's syndrome. Obviously, there may be considerable degrees of overlap. For example, loop diuretics increase rates of salt delivery to terminal nephron segments and therefore enhance bicarbonate generation. However, these agents also produce hypokalemia and ECF volume contraction, and as a consequence raise the apparent threshold for bicarbonate reabsorption. Likewise, in primary aldosteronism, increased distal nephron bicarbonate generation as a cause for alkalosis is accentuated by the effects of hypokalemia on bicarbonate reabsorption.

Under normal circumstances, it is nearly impossible to produce metabolic alkalosis by increasing dietary alkali intake. However in certain situations, *bicarbonate loading* can produce either a transient or a steady-state alkalosis. One such circumstance is *post-hypercapneic alkalosis.* Patients with chronic hypercapnia develop compensatory increases in plasma bicarbonate concentrations: On an average, chronic hypoventilation results in a 0.3 mEq per liter rise in serum bicarbonate for each 1.2 mm Hg increase in excess of a Pa_{CO_2} of 40 mm Hg. If ventilatory status is improved acutely, the Pa_{CO_2} will fall quickly but the plasma bicarbonate will remain elevated, particularly if the patient is salt-acquisitive because of congestive heart failure or ECF volume contraction. A common way for accentuating post-hypercapneic alkalosis is to maintain patients on ventilators having high positive end-expiratory pressures, which causes a central-tourniquet effect that reduces cardiac output.

Delayed conversion of *accumulated organic acids* is a second mechanism for producing transient metabolic alkalosis. This may occur after insulin therapy for diabetic ketoacidosis, during the recovery phase of lactic acidosis, and following high-efficiency hemodialysis. In the latter circumstance, acetate in the dialysis bath is taken up rapidly during dialysis. The accumulated acetate, which represents "potential bicarbonate," is then converted to bicarbonate after dialysis has been completed. Prolonged metabolic alkalosis because of alkali loading is a common feature of the *milk-alkali syndrome.* The alkalosis occurs because of prolonged ingestion of absorbable alkali in patients with impaired renal function due to hypercalcemic nephropathy. Frequent vomiting and attendant ECF volume contraction may also contribute to alkalosis in this disorder.

CLINICAL FEATURES AND DIAGNOSIS. There are no specific signs or symptoms of metabolic alkalosis. Relatively severe metabolic alkalosis can result in *cardiac arrhythmias.* Severe metabolic alkalosis can also result in severe *hypoventilation,* especially in patients with reduced renal function. *Tetany* and *increased neuromuscular irritability,* which are quite common in acute respiratory alkalosis, are very rare in chronic metabolic alkalosis. Rather, since hypokalemia generally accompanies metabolic alkalosis, *muscular weakness* and *hyporeflexia* are often seen in chronic metabolic alkalosis.

The diagnosis is inferred in most cases by routine measurements of serum electrolytes and can be confirmed by arterial blood gas analysis. Hypokalemia is generally present. The finding of an unexplained hypokalemic metabolic alkalosis is suggestive of the presence of Cushing's syndrome due to an extrarenal neoplasm.

The urinary chloride concentration is a useful index for distinguishing metabolic alkalosis due to volume contraction from that due to primary mineralocorticoid excess. In volume-contracted states, the urinary chloride concentration is generally less than 10 mEq per liter. However, volume-contracted patients with Bartter's syndrome and those taking diuretics generally have elevated urinary chloride concentrations. The combination of postural hypotension, hypokalemic metabolic alkalosis, and a urinary chloride concentration greater than 20 mEq per liter is therefore suggestive of diuretic abuse or Bartter's syndrome.

TREATMENT. In metabolic alkalosis associated with hypokalemia and volume contraction, appropriate therapy consists of volume expansion with saline solutions and potassium replacement (see section above on Disturbances in Potassium Balance). If the metabolic alkalosis is sufficiently severe that significant hypoventilation is present ($Pa_{CO_2} > 60$ mm Hg), the administration of dilute hydrochloric acid or other acidifying salts, such as lysine hydrochloride or arginine hydrochloride, may be required. The use of these amino acid salts carries with it the risk of hyperkalemia in excess of that expected simply from the change in arterial pH, presumably because these agents promote potassium efflux from cells. Neither ammonium chloride, lysine hydrochloride, nor arginine hydrochloride should be used in patients with liver disease.

If diuretic abuse can be identified, use of these agents should be discontinued. Indomethacin may correct partially the abnormalities of Bartter's syndrome, although potassium supplementation is almost invariably required. Triamterene is effective in preventing potassium wasting in Liddle's syndrome.

Hypokalemia and metabolic alkalosis due to primary hyperaldosteronism are best treated by potassium chloride supplementation, which tends to correct the metabolic alkalosis partially. Dietary sodium restriction in this disorder also tends to reduce renal potassium wasting. Of course, neither of these maneuvers provides definitive therapy for primary hyperaldosteronism.

RESPIRATORY ACIDOSIS

ETIOLOGY AND PATHOGENESIS. Respiratory acidosis occurs whenever there is impairment in the rate of alveolar ventilation. Carbon dioxide elimination involves the following sequence: Transfer of carbon dioxide from tissues to the lungs in the form of venous bicarbonate; formation of carbon dioxide within red blood cells by a reversal of the chloride shift, described previously in connection with tissue buffering mechanisms; perfusion of the lungs with systemic venous blood; diffusion of carbon dioxide from pulmonary capillaries to alveoli; and alveolar ventilation. Under normal circumstances, the rates of carbon dioxide hydration within red blood cells and of carbon dioxide diffusion from pulmonary capillaries into alveoli are sufficiently rapid that carbon dioxide accumulation is virtually synonymous with hypoventilation.

In chronic hypercapneic states, the rate of carbon dioxide elimination by the lungs equals the rate of carbon dioxide production by tissues, although the process occurs at a higher Pa_{CO_2}. Hence, a sudden increase in the Pa_{CO_2} tension in an individual with chronic hypercapnia indicates that an acute event, for example, pneumonia, has been superimposed on the chronic hypoventilatory disorder.

Acute respiratory acidosis may occur when there is a sudden depression of the medullary respiratory center, as in narcotic overdose or anesthesia; when there is paralysis of the respiratory muscles, as in profound hypokalemia, neuromuscular disorders (myasthenia gravis), or the administration of agents that impair neuromuscular transmission (aminoglycoside antibiotics); when there is airway obstruction, as in foreign body aspiration or profound bronchospasm; when trauma, such as flail chest, impedes ventilation; and when an acute insult is imposed on a chronic hypercapneic state.

Chronic respiratory acidosis generally occurs in individuals with chronic bronchitis, emphysema, and bullous lung disease; in patients with extreme kyphoscoliosis; and in individuals with extreme obesity (Pickwickian syndrome).

The arterial pH and plasma bicarbonate concentrations differ in acute and chronic respiratory acidosis. As indicated in the right-hand panel of Figure 76–8, the compensatory response to carbon dioxide retention is to increase the plasma bicarbonate concentration by raising the apparent threshold for bicarbonate reabsorption. In general, the plasma bicarbonate concentration rises by approximately 0.3 mEq per liter for every millimeter of mercury increase in the Pa_{CO_2} over 40 mm Hg, until the Pa_{CO_2} reaches 80 mm Hg. However, this compensatory increase in plasma bicarbonate concentration generally requires two to three days for complete expression. Consequently, in the early stages of acute respiratory acidosis, the plasma bicarbonate does not rise appreciably, and profound reductions in arterial pH are buffered largely by intracellular proton accumulation. Conversely, when chronic hypercapnia is relieved suddenly, there is a two- to three-day lag in renal bicarbonate excretion, which produces the post-hypercapneic alkalosis described in the preceding section.

These concepts are also useful in evaluating the possibility of mixed acid-base disorders occurring in association with respiratory acidosis. For example, since the rate of compensatory bicarbonate retention is delayed in acute respiratory acidosis, the presence of an elevated plasma bicarbonate concentration in a setting of acute carbon dioxide retention should be an index to the simultaneous occurrence of acute respiratory acidosis and metabolic alkalosis. Likewise, because renal bicarbonate reabsorption is an effective compensatory mechanism for chronic carbon dioxide retention, plasma bicarbonate concentrations below 28 to 30 mEq per liter in patients having chronic Pa_{CO_2} values in excess of 50 mm Hg should alert one to the possible coexistence of acute metabolic acidosis and chronic respiratory acidosis.

Since hypercapnia is synonymous with alveolar hypoventilation, patients with carbon dioxide retention are invariably hypoxemic. A compensatory polycythemia occurs commonly in chronic hypercapneic states.

CLINICAL MANIFESTATIONS. The clinical manifestations of respiratory acidosis vary depending on the severity of the disorder and on the rate at which carbon dioxide retention has occurred. Acute increases in Pa_{CO_2} values result in *somnolence, confusion,* and ultimately in *CO_2 narcosis. Asterixis* may also be present. Because carbon dioxide is a cerebral vasodilator, the blood vessels in the optic fundi are often dilated, engorged, and tortuous; in severe hypercapneic states, frank *papilledema* may occur.

TREATMENT. The only practical treatment for acute respiratory acidosis involves treatment of the underlying disorder and ventilatory support. The possibility of drug abuse should always be considered in otherwise healthy patients who suddenly develop acute respiratory depression; consequently, naloxone (Narcan) therapy should be considered in all comatose patients seen in the emergency room in whom no apparent cause for respiratory depression can be identified.

In patients with chronic hypercapnia who develop sudden increases in Pa_{CO_2} values, attention should be directed toward identifying factors such as pneumonia or pulmonary embolism that may have aggravated the underlying disorder. *Oxygen therapy in patients with chronic hypercapnia should be instituted with extreme caution, since hypoxemia may be the primary stimulus to respiration in this setting.* Consequently, in such patients, sudden increases in the arterial Pa_{O_2} produced by oxygen administration may result in cessation of respiration. The administration of alkalinizing salts has no place in the management of chronic respiratory acidosis.

RESPIRATORY ALKALOSIS

ETIOLOGY AND PATHOGENESIS. Respiratory alkalosis occurs when hyperventilation reduces the arterial Pa_{CO_2} and consequently increases arterial pH. Acute respiratory alkalosis is most commonly the result of severe anxiety, in which it is generally referred to as the hyperventilation syndrome. Acute hyperventilation may also occur because of damage to the respiratory centers; in acute salicylism; in fever and septic states; and in association with pneumonia, pulmonary emboli, or congestive heart failure. The disorder may also be produced iatrogenically by injudicious mechanical ventilatory support. Chronic hyperventilation occurs in the acclimation response to exposure to high altitudes (a low ambient oxygen tension), in advanced hepatic insufficiency, and in pregnancy.

During acute hyperventilation, plasma bicarbonate concentrations fall by approximately 3 mEq per liter when the Pa_{CO_2} falls to about 25 mm Hg. This fall in plasma bicarbonate is due largely to proton shifts from the ICF to the ECF and tends to minimize acute changes in arterial pH. In chronic hyperventilation, renal bicarbonate loss provides the compensatory response to the reduction in Pa_{CO_2}. In experimental studies with dogs, approximately two to four days are required for a maximum renal compensatory response, which involves approximately a 0.4 mEq per liter reduction in plasma bicarbonate concentrations for every millimeter of mercury fall in Pa_{CO_2}.

Hyperventilation and respiratory alkalosis may also occur, as mentioned previously, following the correction of metabolic acidosis, and particularly in diabetic ketoacidosis. In all likelihood, hyperventilation persists in this setting because of the lag in the rate at which plasma bicarbonate concentrations rise with respect to ECF bicarbonate concentrations during correction of metabolic acidosis.

CLINICAL MANIFESTATIONS AND TREATMENT. Chronic hyperventilation may be asymptomatic. The acute hyperventilation syndrome is characterized by *light-headedness, paresthesias, circumoral numbness,* and *tingling of the extremities. Tetany* occurs in severe cases. Both the acute metabolic alkalosis and the reduction in ionized calcium contribute to the increased neuromuscular excitability.

The treatment of acute respiratory alkalosis involves correction of the underlying disorder. When severe anxiety provokes the hyperventilation syndrome, air rebreathing with a paper bag generally terminates the acute attack. If this maneuver fails, sedation may also be required.

Adrogué HJ, Wilson H, Boyd AE, Suki WN, Eknoyan G: Plasma acid-base patterns in diabetic ketoacidosis. N Engl J Med 307:1603, 1982. *A systematic analysis of metabolic acidosis in diabetic patients.*

Emmett M, Narins RG: Clinical use of the anion gap. Medicine 56:38, 1977. *A review of concepts underlying the use of the anion gap in clinical practice.*

Gabow PA, Kaehny WD, Fennessey PV, Goodman SI, Gross PA, Schrier RW: Diagnostic importance of an increased serum anion gap. N Engl J Med 303:854, 1980. *A large prospective study in which the relation of an increased anion gap to the presence of organic acidosis is elevated.*

Garella S, Chang BS, Kahn SI: Dilution acidosis and contraction alkalosis: Review of a concept. Kidney Int 8:279, 1975. *An analysis of the concepts of dilution acidosis and contraction alkalosis.*

Garella S, Chazan JA, Cohen JJ: Saline-resistant metabolic alkalosis or "chloride-wasting nephropathy." Ann Intern Med 73:31, 1970. *A study of the pathogenesis of "saline-resistant" metabolic alkalosis in patients with severe potassium deficiency.*

Halperin ML, Hammeke M, Josse RG, Jungas RL: Metabolic acidosis in the alcoholic: A pathophysiologic approach. Metabolism 32:308, 1983. *The clinical spectrum of metabolic acidosis in alcoholic patients.*

Kreisberg RA: Lactate homeostasis and lactic acidosis. Ann Intern Med 92:227, 1980. *A good review of lactate metabolism and lactic acidosis; extensive bibliography.*

Levy LJ, Duga J, Girgis M, Gordon EE: Ketoacidosis associated with alcoholism in nondiabetic subjects. Ann Intern Med 78:213, 1973. *An examination of the factors which account for the ketoacidosis in nondiabetic, chronically alcoholic patients.*

Mitchell JH, Wildenthal K, Johnson RL: The effects of acid-base disturbances on cardiovascular and pulmonary function. Kidney Int 1:375, 1972. *The effects of acid-base disturbances on cardiac function, ventilation, oxygen-hemoglobin dissociation, and pulmonary circulation.*

Rector FC, Cogan MG: The renal acidoses. Hosp Pract 99-111, April, 1980. *An easy-to-read review of the mechanisms, diagnosis, and management of both proximal and distal renal tubular acidosis.*

Seldin DW, Rector FC: The generation and maintenance of metabolic alkalosis. Kidney Int 1:306, 1972. *An excellent and extensive review of the pathogenesis of chronic metabolic alkalosis.*

77. ACUTE RENAL FAILURE

Jared J. Grantham

DEFINITION

Acute renal failure is a syndrome characterized by a relatively rapid decline in renal function that leads to the accumulation of water, crystalloid solutes, and nitrogenous metabolites in the body. Clinically significant acute renal failure is usually associated with a daily increase in the serum creatinine and urea nitrogen levels (azotemia) greater than 0.5 and 10 mg per deciliter, respectively. *Oliguria,* a rate of urine flow less than 400 ml per day, is commonly observed, but in some cases the urine output may exceed this limit (*nonoliguric* acute renal failure). Complete cessation of urine flow, *anuria,* is relatively uncommon.

ETIOLOGY

Acute renal failure may be seen in a wide variety of clinical settings (Table 77–1). A systematic approach to the causes of acute renal failure facilitates diagnosis in the individual patient. It is important to remember that acute renal failure is a bilateral process, except in patients with only one functioning kidney.

Prerenal

Prerenal causes lead to renal failure by decreasing the effective perfusion of kidney parenchyma. An absolute decrease in blood volume (hypovolemia), the most common prerenal disorder, may be caused by skin, gastrointestinal, and renal losses of water and electrolytes, hemorrhage, and sequestration of fluids in body cavities. In some conditions the kidneys respond as though the blood volume were decreased, when in fact the measured volume is normal or even increased. These oliguric states include congestive heart failure (which may be precipitated by myocardial infarction or dysrhythmia), sepsis, anaphylaxis, and liver failure. Bilateral renal artery occlusion can occur spontaneously owing to emboli from the heart or from an atheromatous aorta. Embolism of atheroma occurs commonly in the course of difficult surgical procedures involving the abdominal aorta.

Postrenal

Although quite rare, *bilateral ureteral obstruction* may be due to calculi, shed papillae in analgesic nephropathy, thrombus,

TABLE 77–1. CAUSES OF ACUTE RENAL FAILURE SYNDROME

Location of Primary Disorder	Clinical Examples
Prerenal	
Absolute decrease in effective blood volume	Hemorrhage, skin losses (burns, sweating), GI losses (diarrhea, vomiting), renal losses (diuretics, glycosuria), fluid pooling (peritonitis, burns)
Relative decrease in blood volume (ineffective arterial volume)	Congestive heart failure, dysrhythmias, sepsis, anaphylaxis, liver failure
Arterial occlusion	Bilateral thromboembolism, thromboembolism of solitary kidney, aortic or renal artery aneurysm
Postrenal	
Ureteral obstruction	Bilateral or solitary kidney (calculi, neoplasm, clot, retroperitoneal fibrosis, iatrogenic)
Venous occlusion	Bilateral or solitary kidney (renal vein thrombosis, neoplasm, iatrogenic)
Intrarenal	
Vascular	Vasculitis, malignant hypertension, vasopressors, eclampsia, microangiopathy, hyperviscosity states, nonsteroidal anti-inflammatory drugs, hypercalcemia, iodinated radiocontrast agents
Glomerulus	Acute glomerulonephritis
Tubular injury	
Ischemia	Profound hypotension, postrenal transplant, vasopressors, microvascular constriction
Intratubular pigments	Hemoglobinuria, myoglobinuria
Intratubular proteins	Myeloma
Intratubular crystals	Uric acid, oxalate, sulfonamides, pyridium
Tubulointerstitial	Interstitial nephritis due to drugs, infection, radiation
Nephrotoxins	Antibiotics (gentamicin, kanamycin, neomycin, amikacin, tobramycin, streptomycin, cephaloridine, amphotericin B); metals (mercury, bismuth, uranium, arsenic, silver, cadmium, iron, antimony); solvents (carbon tetrachloride, glycol, tetrachlorethylene); iodinated contrast agents; streptozotocin, cisplatin

neoplasms, and iatrogenic causes. Commonly in bilateral obstruction one kidney is blocked for several days or weeks before obstruction of the contralateral kidney causes acute renal failure. Acute ureteral obstruction of a solitary kidney is seen occasionally. Acute renal failure can be caused by *urethral obstruction* due to prostatic hypertrophy, prostatitis, bladder and prostate tumors, bladder rupture, calculi, and iatrogenic causes. In hospitalized patients with indwelling urinary catheters, the patency and correct placement of the catheter should always be checked in the evaluation of acute renal failure.

Bilateral renal venous occlusion is rare but may be seen in hypercoagulable states, with intra-abdominal neoplasms, or secondary to surgical procedures.

Intrarenal

The renal arterial and arteriolar *blood vessels* may be involved in vasculitis, malignant hypertension, eclampsia, and microangiopathies. Pronounced vasospasm leading to acute renal failure may be seen in scleroderma, during systemic infusions of norepinephrine, secondary to the use of nonsteroidal anti-inflammatory compounds, iodinated radiocontrast agents, or diet pills, or in hypercalcemic states.

Glomerular inflammation (acute glomerulonephritis, Ch. 80) may cause acute renal failure by sharply reducing renal blood flow. *Renal tubules* are susceptible to a number of insults. *Ischemic* injury, sometimes progressing to frank necrosis, may be seen secondary to profound hypotension, especially in elderly persons. About one half of kidneys transplanted from cadaver sources undergo oliguric renal failure. The intravenous administration of powerful vasoconstrictors, such as norepinephrine, may cause acute ischemic tubular injury in certain susceptible patients. Renal tubules are susceptible to injury by high levels of urinary pigments (hemoglobinuria, myoglobinuria), especially in the setting of renal hypoperfusion and ischemia. Several serum proteins are potentially nephrotoxic, including kappa and lambda light chains, which may be abundantly excreted in patients with multiple myeloma. Renal tubules may be occluded by uric acid, oxalate, sulfonamide, or pyridium crystals, leading to acute renal failure.

A wide variety of chemicals are potential tubular toxins. Antibiotics of the aminoglycoside class (one of the most common iatrogenic nephrotoxins), streptomycin, cephaloridine, and amphotericin all injure renal tubules when given in excessive doses. These agents are apparently nephrotoxic even at low therapeutic doses in patients who are oliguric or hypotensive or who have underlying renal disorders. The combined effects of aminoglycosides and certain cephalothin drugs appear to be additive in causing acute renal failure. Heavy metal poisoning is seen rarely but may cause acute tubular necrosis and renal failure. Iodinated radiocontrast agents may directly injure renal tubules in patients with underlying disorders such as diabetes mellitus, systemic lupus erythematosus, and chronic renal insufficiency from nearly any cause. Chemotherapeutic agents such as streptozotocin and cisplatin almost routinely cause acute renal injury that may progress to acute renal failure. Phencyclidine, a psychotropic agent, has caused acute renal failure in a few patients.

INCIDENCE

Acute renal failure is a relatively common syndrome. The incidence in the general outpatient population is not known; in one study about 5 per cent of patients on medical and surgical units in a general hospital experienced an episode of acute renal failure. Approximately 60 per cent of cases are related to surgery or trauma; the remainder have medical or obstetric causes. Overall, about one half of cases of acute renal failure in hospitalized patients may be iatrogenic.

PATHOGENESIS

Ischemia and nephrotoxins are the most common causes of acute renal failure listed in Table 77–1. There are at least three important phases in the acute renal failure syndrome due to ischemia or nephrotoxins. In the first, or *initiation* phase, the kidneys are subjected to an insult that produces parenchymal injury (e.g., temporary cessation of renal blood flow; nephrotoxins or pigments; see Table 77–1 and Fig. 77–1). In some patients who are hypovolemic, the initiation phase can be overridden by plasma volume expansion and the acute renal failure syndrome aborted. More commonly, however, the initiation phase causes profound renal vasoconstriction and an initial decrease in renal blood flow. The initiation phase is followed by the *maintenance* phase, during which renal vasoconstriction may persist, thereby decreasing the formation of glomerular filtrate. The hydraulic permeability of the glomeruli is usually decreased, diminishing further the ability of glomeruli to form filtrate. In addition to factors operating within the glomeruli, injury to renal tubules causes the cells to slough from the basement membranes to form casts that can obstruct urine flow. Moreover, the damaged epithelium of the tubules allows the small amount of glomerular filtrate that is formed to leak back into the peritubular capillaries. These four factors, vasoconstriction, decreased glomerular permeability, intratubular obstruction, and tubular back leak of filtrate (Figs. 77–1 and 77–2), operate in concert to depress the effective glomerular filtration rate in the ischemic and nephrotoxic types of acute renal failure listed in Table 77–1.

In some cases the renal blood flow may return to relatively normal levels 24 to 48 hours after the initiation phase. Despite

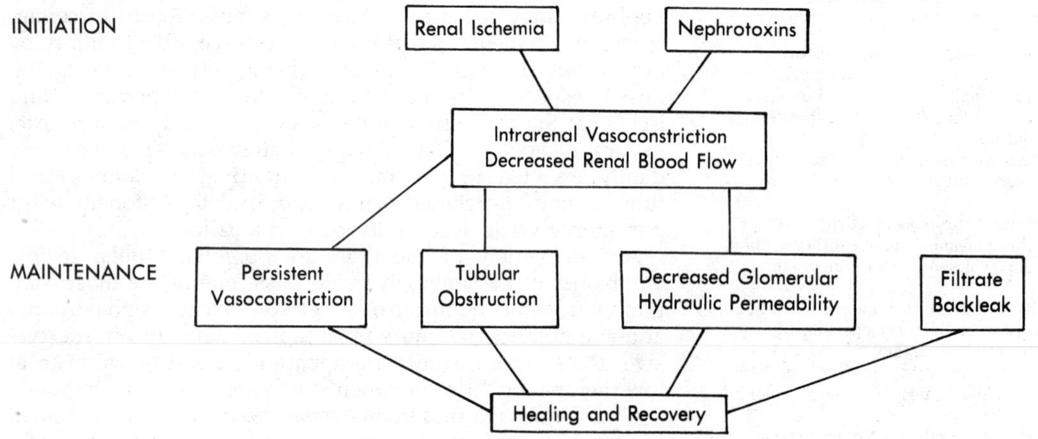

Figure 77–1. Pathogenesis of acute renal failure.

this, the glomerular filtration rate (GFR) remains very low owing to the decreased glomerular hydraulic permeability, tubular obstruction, or tubular back leak of filtrate.

The third stage in the pathogenetic sequence is the *recovery* phase. Provided that the initiating causes remit, healing of renal parenchyma and recovery of function may be expected in most types of acute renal failure.

CLINICAL MANIFESTATIONS

The onset of acute renal failure usually follows the initiating event by an interval varying from a few hours to as long as several days. Patients and physicians usually first notice a reduction in urine volume in the oliguric types of acute renal failure. Facial edema, tight fitting rings, and weight gain reflect the retention of water. Rarely pulmonary edema may be an initial manifestation. Renal pain is uncommon except in association with acute infection, urolithiasis, and tumors. Hematuria is seen in nephritic syndromes and vascular occlusive states but is uncommon in nephrotoxic and transient ischemic states.

The serum creatinine and urea levels rise steadily. In severely oliguric persons of average size the serum creatinine level rises about 1.5 to 2 mg per deciliter per day. When the measured increase in serum creatinine exceeds this range, one should consider hypercatabolic factors; when the measured increase is less, renal clearance of creatinine may be greater than the rate of urine volume flow would suggest. The serum urea nitrogen level usually rises in concert with the creatinine level. However,

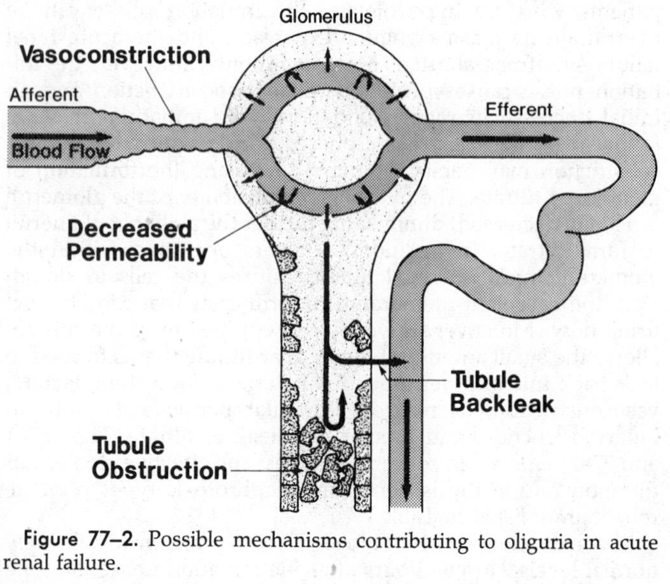

Figure 77–2. Possible mechanisms contributing to oliguria in acute renal failure.

urea production is altered by food intake, by tissue catabolism, and by blood within the intestines; consequently, the urea levels do not reflect the performance of the kidneys as well as do creatinine levels.

Hyperkalemia due to inadequate renal excretion of potassium may be life threatening early in the course of acute renal failure. Metabolic acidosis due to inadequate renal excretion of hydrogen ions is seen later on. Hyponatremia may be seen in patients who drink unlimited amounts of water or other fluids. Hypocalcemia, hyperphosphatemia, hyperuricemia, and anemia usually develop after several days unless there are mitigating factors such as rhabdomyolysis and hemolysis. Serum amylase levels may be twice normal in the absence of pancreatitis.

The uremic syndrome develops gradually, and in addition to the features mentioned above, is characterized by the progressive development of anorexia, nausea, vomiting, nervous irritability, hyperreflexia, asterixis, seizures, and coma. Hemorrhagic signs include ecchymoses, gastric and colonic hemorrhage, and pericarditis.

DIAGNOSIS

When renal failure is recognized it is important to determine the probable cause and remediable factors underlying kidney dysfunction. Table 77–2 lists several key components in the diagnostic approach to renal failure.

The initial objective is to determine if the renal failure is acute or chronic. The diagnostic evaluation starts at the patient's bedside. With conversant ambulatory patients the onset of renal dysfunction can usually be determined based on historical changes in urine output (oliguria, polyuria, nocturia), abnormal urine color, and changes in body weight. Chronic renal failure is further indicated by anemia, osteodystrophy, lipiduria, bilaterally small kidneys, neuropathy, and a modestly elevated serum level of uric acid.

TABLE 77–2. DIAGNOSTIC APPROACH TO RENAL FAILURE

1. Review of medical history, clinical setting, medications
2. Physical examination including evaluation of hemodynamic status
3. Urinalysis including careful sediment examination
4. Simultaneous chemical analysis of blood and urine. Osmolality, urea, creatinine, sodium, chloride, potassium, uric acid
5. Bladder catheterization if urethral obstruction suspected
6. Fluid-diuretic challenge
7. Radiologic studies
    - Plain abdominal roentgenogram
    - Ultrasonography
    - Radioisotope scans (pertechnetate ^{99m}Tc, ^{131}I-hippurate)
    - CT scan
    - Pyeloureterography
        - Intravenous pyelography
        - Retrograde pyelography
        - Antegrade (percutaneous) pyelography
8. Renal biopsy

In the differential diagnosis of acute renal failure it is important to distinguish among *prerenal, postrenal,* and *intrarenal* factors.

Prerenal Failure

Prerenal failure is suggested by a history of rapid weight loss, flu-like illness, lack of fluid ingestion, bleeding, nasogastric aspiration, diuretic therapy, or orthostatic dizziness. In prerenal failure due to *extracellular fluid volume contraction* the physical examination may reveal orthostatic hypotension and tachycardia, poor venous filling and a "thready" pulse, and peripheral vasoconstriction with cool extremities and dry mucous membranes. When prerenal failure occurs in *euvolemic or hypervolemic* patients, one usually finds signs of congestive heart failure or liver failure, including distended veins, a third heart sound, pulmonary rales and wheezes, ascites, jaundice, and peripheral edema.

Urinary indices (Table 77–3) show concentrated urine (relatively high specific gravity and osmolality), low fractional excretions of sodium and chloride, and a high urine to plasma creatinine ratio. Diuretics can diminish the diagnostic usefulness of urinary indices and should not be used prior to collecting urine for analysis. Urinalysis and urine sediment examination are usually unremarkable except for hyaline casts.

When the physical and chemical findings point to prerenal acute azotemic due to a *decrease in extracellular fluid volume,* a fluid challenge of 500 to 1000 ml of isotonic saline may stimulate urine formation in the average adult. In the author's opinion, mannitol and diuretics are contraindicated in volume-depleted patients with prerenal azotemia. In prerenal azotemia associated with an *expanded extracellular fluid volume,* diuretics may be indicated as part of the general plan to improve cardiac function.

Prerenal azotemia due to occlusion of renal arteries is revealed by radioisotope screening tests and arteriography. Urine output generally is scanty. Urinalysis may show hematuria and proteinuria, and urinary indices show an inability to concentrate urinary solutes (Table 77–3).

Postrenal Failure

Obstruction to the flow of urine may be acute or chronic (see Ch. 82). In most cases of acute obstruction of the *upper tract* the patient notices pain in the flank or lower abdominal regions and fluctuating urine output. *Urethral* obstruction usually causes urinary frequency, dribbling, and lower abdominal fullness. In urinary tract obstruction infected urine is commonly observed.

The onset of renal failure due to obstruction of the urinary drainage system can be difficult to determine. To cause renal failure the urinary drainage from both kidneys must be compromised; alternatively the patient may have only one kidney. Chronic progressive processes, such as retroperitoneal neoplasia, can obstruct the drainage of one ureter weeks or months before the contralateral ureter is obstructed. Obstructive uropathy should be suspected in patients with adenopathy, abdominal scars, palpable bladder, flank tenderness, prostatic enlargement, or pelvic masses with induration.

Urinary findings are nonspecific. The sediment contains leukocytes and erythrocytes in infected patients. The urinary indices are variable. In acute obstruction the indices are identical to those seen in prerenal failure; in obstructions more than two days in duration the indices are similar to those seen in intrarenal tubular injury (Tables 77–2 and 77–3).

When urethral obstruction is suspected bladder catheterization may be diagnostic. With upper tract obstruction ultrasonography in the hands of an experienced radiologist is the most useful diagnostic test. Rarely, acute obstruction of the urinary tract may occur without dilation of the renal pelvis and cannot be detected by sonography. The ^{131}I-hippurate scan is a noninvasive test that is useful for determining the potential for return of renal function in obstructive uropathy. Bilateral upper tract obstruction is usually nonsynchronous. In such cases the hippurate scan shows asymmetric accumulation of the isotope. The kidney showing the most intense uptake of hippurate is the best candidate for return of function after relief of obstruction. Intravenous pyelography is useful to localize the site of obstruction, but adequate renal function is needed to concentrate the contrast material in the urinary tract. Retrograde pyelography should be reserved for those cases in which the noninvasive methods are not available or those in which equivocal results have been obtained. In some cases the CT scan may provide anatomic confirmation of obstruction.

Occlusion of the renal veins is suggested by a history of a hypercoagulable state, pulmonary emboli, hematuria, or proteinuria. Urinary indices are not diagnostic. Radioisotope studies of renal perfusion may be suggestive, but definitive diagnosis depends on renal arteriography or venography.

TABLE 77–3. URINARY INDICES IN ACUTE RENAL FAILURE

Index	Prerenal	Acute Tubular Injury
Urine osmolality mOsm/kg H_2O	> 500	< 350
Urine sodium mEq/L	< 20	> 40
Urine/plasma creatinine	> 40	< 20
Fractional sodium excretion	< 1	> 1

Intrarenal Failure

Renal failure due to intrinsic dysfunction is suggested by a history of multisystem disease (e.g., SLE, vasculitis), fever, malaise, skin rash, hypertension, gross hematuria, hypotensive episode, or exposure to nephrotoxins.

The urinalysis is an invaluable guide in the diagnosis of intrarenal failure. Acute glomerulonephritis is characterized by hematuria, proteinuria, erythrocyte casts, and granular casts. Lipid bodies and broad waxy casts suggest a chronic process. Pus casts indicate acute or chronic interstitial inflammation. Urinary eosinophils are seen in allergic interstitial nephritis. Crystalluria is observed in urate and oxalate disorders. Physicians should be able to recognize these formed elements in the urine and should personally examine a freshly prepared urine sediment. Acute inflammation of the preglomerular arterioles may or may not be associated with alterations in glomerular capillaries. In the absence of glomerular capillary inflammation the urinalysis reflects ischemic tubular injury due to reduced renal blood flow. Acute tubular injury does not give specific urinary sediment findings, but celluluria, epithelial cell casts, and coarse granular casts should raise the index of suspicion.

Urinary indices (Table 77–3) are very helpful in differentiating between conditions that cause injury to preglomerular arterioles and glomeruli and those that cause acute tubular injury. In the former the indices show a prerenal pattern, whereas in acute tubular injury the fractional excretion of sodium is increased and the urinary osmolality approaches that of plasma. The conditions that may exhibit low or normal fractional sodium excretion at some point in the course of the acute renal failure syndrome are listed in Table 77–4.

TABLE 77–4. CONDITIONS ASSOCIATED WITH FRACTIONAL SODIUM EXCRETION (FE_{Na}) LESS THAN 1 PER CENT IN ACUTE RENAL FAILURE SYNDROME

Intense Intrarenal Vasoconstriction

1. Iodinated radiocontrast
2. Acute bilateral ureteral obstruction
3. Severe burns
4. Sepsis
5. Pigment excretion (myoglobin, hemoglobin)
6. Nonsteroidal anti-inflammatory drugs
7. Amphotericin B
8. Norepinephrine, dopamine
9. Liver disease
10. Cardiopulmonary bypass

Vascular Inflammation

1. Acute glomerulonephritis
2. Acute vasculitis
3. Renal transplant rejection

Radiologic tests are relatively nonspecific in the evaluation of intrarenal failure. The ^{131}I-hippurate scan shows accumulation of isotope in both kidneys if some renal perfusion is preserved and viable tubules remain. Renal arteriography may show microaneurysm formation in polyarteritis nodosa. Renal biopsy is usually indicated in the evaluation of glomerulonephritis, vasculitis, or interstitial nephritis but is not commonly used when pyelonephritis or acute tubular injury is suspected.

TREATMENT

There are at least four major objectives in the treatment of acute renal failure: (a) correct the reversible causes, (b) prevent additional injury, (c) convert oliguric to nonoliguric renal failure, and (d) provide general metabolic support during the maintenance and recovery phases of the syndrome.

Correct Reversible Causes

Prerenal and postrenal factors contributing to renal function should be corrected in so far as is possible. Drugs that interfere with renal perfusion or that are directly nephrotoxic should be stopped. In hypotensive patients the blood pressure should be restored by discontinuing antihypertensive drugs and administering isotonic volume-expanding solutions. In elderly patients with longstanding hypertension, a "normal" blood pressure of 110/70 may in fact be inadequate to generate glomerular filtrate. If there is doubt about the status of the plasma volume, an intravenous challenge of isotonic saline (500 to 1000 ml) is warranted. In the states listed in Table 77–4 associated with a low fractional sodium excretion due to intrarenal vasoconstriction, a volume challenge combined with 40 to 80 mg of intravenous furosemide may reverse the oliguric state, and in some cases prevent the maintenance phase of acute renal failure.

Prevention of Additional Injury

Radiocontrast agents are potentially harmful to patients in the maintenance phase of acute renal failure, and alternative diagnostic methods should be used whenever possible. CT scans are often done with contrast enhancement, and physicians are not always aware of this "hidden" source of iodinated radiocontrast material. Nonsteroidal anti-inflammatory drugs and nephrotoxic antibiotics should be avoided if possible. Drug dosages should be adjusted according to guidelines for renal failure, and plasma drug levels should be monitored when possible.

Convert Oliguria to Nonoliguria

Oliguria in and of itself is not harmful, and a normal urine flow rate does not accelerate the healing process in the acute renal failure syndrome. Nonetheless, experience shows that the management of patients with acute renal failure is simplified and the survival rate may be improved by converting oliguria to nonoliguria with diuretics and fluid administration. A trial of furosemide (2 to 10 mg per kilogram intravenous) is warranted. If urine output exceeding 40 ml per hour is achieved, additional doses of diuretic may be given periodically.

General Support

Conservative management without dialysis may be adequate in many cases. Indwelling urinary catheters should be avoided in uncomplicated cases. Intermittent catheterization using careful sterile technique is usually sufficient in oliguric obtunded patients. In all patients careful attention to fluid status is crucial to successful management. Daily weight measured by a competent assistant or physician is essential in the evaluation of changes in fluid balance. Catabolic patients may be expected to lose about 0.5 kg per day. As a rule of thumb, patients can be allowed to drink a volume of fluid (water, tea, coffee) equal to 500 ml plus the amount of the preceding 24-hour urine output. In febrile patients this fluid limit can be increased. In anorectic patients the fluids are given intravenously.

Sodium, potassium, and chloride are not given to patients in the maintenance phase of acute renal failure, except inadvertently in the food they eat. This may amount to about 1 mEq per kilogram of Na, K, and Cl daily. Protein intake is restricted to 0.7 to 1 gram per kilogram of body weight per day and is principally composed of foods high in essential amino acid content. Carbohydrates and fats are given to insure an adequate caloric intake. In patients who cannot eat, intravenous infusion of essential amino acids and glucose may be necessary, but this regimen contributes a considerable fluid load.

In addition to measurements of daily weight, fluid intake and fluid output, serial determinations of blood pressure (supine and upright), serum electrolytes, creatinine, urea nitrogen, and blood hematocrit are essential for patient management. Hyperkalemia exceeding 6 mEq per liter is a potentially serious complication that can be handled temporarily by ingestion of polystyrene sulfonate exchange resin (25 to 50 grams) in a solution containing sorbitol. Electrocardiographic changes showing widened QRS complexes or AV dissociation demand immediate treatment with intravenous sodium bicarbonate (88 mmol), glucose and insulin (25 units regular insulin per liter of 10 per cent glucose), and calcium gluconate (10 per cent solution, 10 to 30 ml). These measures will generally control the serum potassium level until dialysis can be initiated. (See Ch. 76 for a discussion of hyperkalemia.)

Dialysis may be necessary in certain patients in the maintenance phase of acute renal failure. The indications for dialysis include severe hyperkalemia (serum $K^+ > 6.5$ mEq per liter after treatment), severe metabolic acidosis (serum bicarbonate < 10 mEq per liter after bicarbonate therapy), pulmonary edema due to fluid overload, progressive azotemia (urea nitrogen $>$ 100, creatinine > 10 mg per deciliter), encephalopathy, seizures, bleeding diathesis, pericarditis, and uremic enteropathy.

In uncomplicated cases, peritoneal dialysis may be the most suitable method of treatment. This procedure avoids the wide shifts in blood volume and blood solute composition encountered in hemodialysis, and anticoagulants are not used. Peritoneal dialysis can be used for prolonged treatment if recovery of renal function is slow.

In many cases, one must remove solutes and water from the blood faster than can be achieved by peritoneal dialysis. Also, patients with acute renal failure frequently have pre-existing abdominal injuries. In such cases hemodialysis is the preferred dialytic method. One has rapid access to the circulation by percutaneous catheterization of femoral or subclavian veins. Alternatively, external plastic shunts can be placed in adjacent arteries and veins in the lower or upper extremities. In hemorrhagic states, systemic heparinization is not feasible, and regional anticoagulation with citrate or prostacyclin may be necessary.

PROGNOSIS

The prognosis for patient recovery must be viewed from at least two perspectives: (1) patient survival, and (2) recovery of renal function.

Patient Survival

With the advent of modern dialysis techniques few if any patients with the acute renal failure syndrome die of uremia. Death is usually a consequence of the underlying disease that caused the acute renal failure or secondary to trauma and/or sepsis. The mortality rate in traumatized septic patients with acute renal failure is disturbingly high (40 to 80 per cent).

Recovery of Renal Function

The prognosis for recovery of renal function depends on the nature of the underlying disorder that initiated the renal dysfunction. All acute renal failure due to prerenal causes is potentially reversible. In postrenal failure, renal function may be expected to stabilize or improve significantly if the obstruction is relieved.

Acute renal failure due to intrarenal causes has a variable outcome. Glomerulonephritis and vasculitis may respond to immunosuppressive therapy, with complete recovery of renal function. Acute renal failure due to renal tubular injury is usually reversible provided that the cause of ischemia is removed or nephrotoxins are avoided. Recovery of renal function to near normal levels is more likely in nonoliguric than in oliguric patients, and in subjects who have strong images by the ^{131}I-hippurate renal scan. The duration of the period of poor renal function is highly variable. Recovery of renal function takes longer in elderly patients than in young persons. Recovery is also prolonged in patients who develop acute renal failure in addition to a chronic renal disorder that compromises baseline function.

The major improvements in renal function usually appear in the first and second weeks after the beginning of the recovery phase. Some mild defects in renal function may persist for months or years after a bout of acute tubular injury.

PREVENTION

The opportunity for major prevention of acute renal failure is in the hands of physicians and surgeons. As noted, hospital-acquired acute renal failure was seen in nearly 5 per cent of all patients admitted to one general hospital; nearly one half of these cases were iatrogenic.

A few simple measures will diminish the incidence of acute renal failure acquired in the hospital: (1) Patients should be adequately hydrated before receiving iodinated radiocontrast material. (2) Adequate hydration is necessary before certain surgical procedures, specifically repair of abdominal aortic aneurysm and renal transplantation. (3) Adequate hydration is essential before and during chemotherapy using cisplatin and streptozotocin. (4) Pretreatment with allopurinol before chemotherapy of massive tumors will diminish uric acid excretion. (5) Nonsteroidal anti-inflammatory drugs should be avoided in patients with renal diseases. (6) Nephrotoxic antibiotics should be avoided or carefully monitored. (7) Antibiotic combinations that synergistically potentiate acute tubular injury should be avoided (gentamicin and cephalothin, for example).

Bennett WM, Muther RS, Parker RA, Feig P, Morrison G, Golper TA, Singer I: Drug therapy in renal failure: Dosing guidelines for adults. Ann Intern Med 93:62–89, 286–325, 1980. *A handy, well-referenced guide to drug dosages in acute renal failure.*

Brenner BM, Lazarus JM: Acute Renal Failure. Philadelphia, WB Saunders Co., 1983. *The pathogenesis and therapy of acute renal failure are discussed by several authorities in this well-referenced book.*

Harwood TH, Hiesterman DR, Robinson RG, Cross DE, Whittier FE, Diederich DA, Grantham JJ: Prognosis for recovery of function in acute renal failure. Arch Intern Med 136:916, 1976. *A simple noninvasive radioisotope test (^{131}I-hippurate) is shown to be useful in judging the prognosis for recovery of renal function.*

Hou SH, Bushinsky DA, Wish JB, Cohen JJ, Harrington JT: Hospital-acquired renal insufficiency: A prospective study. Am J Med 74:243, 1983. *A disturbing study that establishes in one hospital the risk for developing acute renal failure.*

Miller TR, Anderson RJ, Linas SL, Henrich WL, Berns AS, Gabow PA, Schrier RW: Urinary diagnostic indicies in acute renal failure. A prospective study. Ann Intern Med 89:47, 1978. *A well-designed study that documents the usefulness of urinary electrolyte measurements in determining the cause of acute renal failure.*

Porter GA: Nephrotoxic Mechanisms of Drugs and Environmental Toxins. New York, Plenum Press, 1982. *A comprehensive collection of essays by an excellent group of authorities who deal with topics of increasing clinical interest.*

78. CHRONIC RENAL FAILURE

Juha Kokko

INTRODUCTION

Chronic renal failure (CRF) is a functional diagnosis characterized by a progressive and generally irreversible decline in glomerular filtration rate (GFR). It is caused by a large number of diseases. Figure 78–1 summarizes the causes of chronic renal failure in North American patients on chronic maintenance

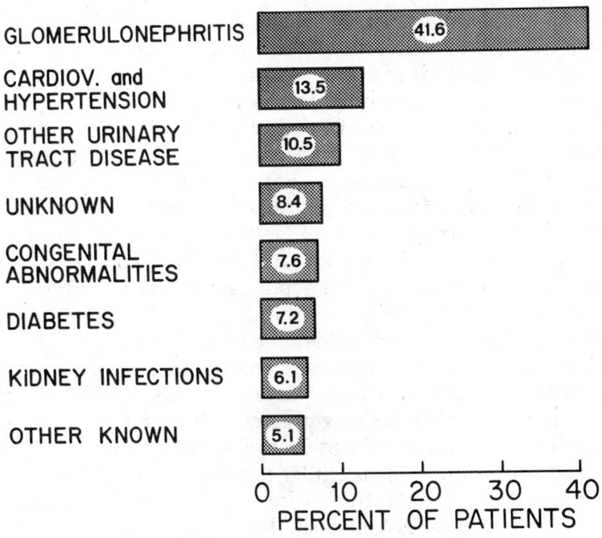

Figure 78–1. Histogram of primary renal diseases leading to dialysis. (Data based on National Registry data as represented by Wernman in Dialysis Transplantation 7:1034, 1978.)

dialysis according to 1978 figures from the National Dialysis Registry. In some geographic locations diabetes and hypertension are more common disease processes leading to dialysis than the National Dialysis Registry indicates for the entire country. In this classification "glomerulonephritis" is not a specific disease but reflects a heterogeneous group of glomerular disorders in which the common expression is renal failure. This chapter considers the pathophysiology and clinical manifestations of CRF, an approach to the patient with CRF, and principles of management.

PATHOPHYSIOLOGY AND CLINICAL MANIFESTATIONS

The clinical constellation of signs and symptoms of end-stage renal failure is known as the "uremic syndrome." In the initial phases of advancing renal failure most organ functions remain normal so that the patient often seeks medical attention only when his disease has progressed to the uremic stage. Normally the adult patient is unaware of advancing renal failure until the GFR has decreased to 20 ml per minute. At this phase adherence to strict therapeutic principles is of utmost importance to prevent the complications of CRF. When conservative medical management is no longer adequate, alternative approaches such as dialysis or transplantation (see Ch. 79) must be considered.

The uremic syndrome results from derangements of function of many systems of the body, although the prominence of specific symptoms may vary from patient to patient. No organ system is spared. The pathophysiology and clinical manifestations of uremia will be discussed by components even though this is arbitrary and not all of them may be present in the same patient. This clinical description will be followed by a short summary of the retained "toxins" that have been considered of importance in the development of the uremic syndrome.

Components of the Uremic Syndrome

WATER, ELECTROLYTE, AND ACID-BASE METABOLISM IN UREMIA. Renal and extrarenal compensatory mechanisms maintain electrolyte and water metabolism near normal until the late stages of renal failure. However, characteristic changes can occur at that time.

Potassium. The normal human dietary intake of potassium is 1 to 1.5 mEq per kilogram of body weight per day, more than 90 per cent of which is excreted by the kidneys. Essentially all the filtered potassium is normally reabsorbed so that only a small fraction is delivered to the early distal nephron. The potassium excreted in the urine has been largely secreted by nephron segments beyond the macula densa, chiefly by passive diffusion down an electrochemical gradient, and to a lesser extent by active transport processes. In each case intracellular concentration of potassium is important in net potassium secretion. The accumulation of potassium in the distal tubular cells is related to the activity of Na-K-ATPase in the basolateral region of the cell. The greater the activity of this pump, the higher the rise in intracellular potassium and the greater the secretory rate of potassium. The activity of Na-K-ATPase is controlled by diet and mineralocorticoid status (both high potassium diet and mineralocorticoids lead to high renal Na-K-ATPase). Both normal and uremic subjects adapt to high potassium diets by increasing potassium excretion per nephron. In addition, the gut increases its ability to secrete potassium in response to a rise in intracellular potassium concentration.

In spite of these adaptive processes, potassium homeostasis in CRF patients is not normal. In advanced CRF the serum potassium concentration tends to be higher than normal even though body stores of potassium are often reduced. Hyperkalemia can be accentuated by trauma, surgery, anesthesia, blood transfusion, increased acidosis, or sudden changes of dietary intake. It can produce the usual spectrum of cardiac abnormalities, but many patients are asymptomatic until cardiac arrest occurs. Occasional patients complain of muscle weakness or paresthesias. The major warning signs are those detected by electrocardiography.

Total body potassium content may be low in CRF: (1) Many patients with CRF have anorexia and reduced dietary intake of potassium. (2) There is greater than normal loss of intracellular potassium to extracellular compartments with subsequent loss from the body. Of special importance is the low intracellular content of potassium in muscle. The low intracellular potassium concentration may reflect a decrease in Na-K-ATPase activity, as well as displacement of intracellular potassium by hydrogen ion. Patients with chronic renal failure tolerate acute increases in serum potassium concentration with less cardiotoxicity than do patients without kidney disease. Vigorous dialysis can restore the intracellular concentration of potassium to normal, suggesting the removal of circulating inhibitor of potassium transport.

Sodium. The kidney has a remarkable capacity to maintain total body sodium content within normal limits until the very end stages of functional deterioration. To accomplish this the remaining nephrons of the CRF patient must excrete a proportionately greater quantity of dietary sodium to maintain total body sodium balance within normal limits. This observation has led to a search for a humoral factor(s) that might be responsible for the increased natriuresis per nephron of the failing kidney. Such a factor has been called a "natriuretic hormone," but to date the existence of this factor has not been convincingly demonstrated.

Sodium excretion can be varied only over a restricted range in renal failure, and this narrows as GFR declines. Nevertheless, most patients remain in sodium balance until their GFR is below 5 ml per minute. Rarely, patients exhibit inappropriate natriuresis; more commonly patients have a tendency toward sodium retention and volume expansion because their dietary intake exceeds the blunted ability of the diseased kidney to excrete the usual sodium load.

SODIUM WASTING. Those patients who have CRF and *salt-losing nephropathy* may lose sodium to the point of extracellular volume contraction and hypotension. These patients will require sufficient dietary salt to prevent their hypotensive symptoms. A wide variety of renal diseases may be associated with salt wasting, but the most common are pyelonephritis, medullary cystic disease, hydronephrosis, interstitial nephritis secondary to analgesic abuse, and milk-alkali syndrome. Presumably in these conditions the collecting ducts are incapable of reabsorbing sufficient quantities of delivered sodium.

SODIUM RETENTION. Some patients are unable to increase sodium excretion to appropriate levels with increases in sodium intake. Most of these patients come to a new steady state with total body weight a few pounds higher than their euvolemic weight. When these patients then receive an extra sodium load they usually excrete it promptly, thus maintaining their new state of volume expansion. They behave as if they have reset their feedback control system for sodium reabsorption. This situation is more common in patients with glomerular than with tubulointerstitial disease. These patients often have the physical findings of expanded extracellular fluid volume: hypertension, peripheral edema, pulmonary congestive state, enlarged heart, and functional flow murmur. The clinical picture is often interpreted as heart failure, and valvular heart disease is suspected erroneously. A small percentage of patients with normal cardiac output become relentless sodium retainers and require hemodialysis for volume control. These patients tend to be diabetic. Surreptitious intake of salt may play a role, but other unknown factors may also be of etiologic significance.

Acid-Base Balance. The kidney normally regulates blood pH within narrow limits by reabsorption (proximal tubule) and regeneration (distal tubule) of bicarbonate or by secretion of hydrogen (distal convoluted tubule and collecting duct segments) (Fig. 78–2). When diets high in alkali content are ingested, the kidney excretes less acid; whereas with acid ash diets and endogenous acid production, the kidney reabsorbs and regenerates bicarbonate and secretes hydrogen ion in amounts sufficient to maintain normal pH. A maximally acid urine in the human has a pH of 4.5 to 5.0. However, the total quantity of acid that can be excreted is a function of the amount of buffer that can be excreted. The excreted buffers may be filtered or generated. Quantitatively the most important filtered buffer is phosphate; the most important newly generated buffer is ammonium (Fig. 78–2).

In chronic renal disease with progressively fewer functioning nephrons there is progressively less ammonia produced for the titration of secreted acid. Thus in CRF the urine pH may be maximally acid, but the total amount of hydrogen ion is low. In disease processes that disproportionately affect the medulla, the ability to form maximally acid urine is lost early. Metabolic acidosis, which may be partially compensated by respiratory mechanisms, develops when exogenous intake and endogenous production of acid exceed renal excretory capacity. In metabolic acidosis there is recruitment of extrarenal buffering mechanisms. Either the excess hydrogen ions are buffered by bone salts and other extracellular mechanisms or they enter the cells to be buffered by intracellular mechanisms. These buffering mechanisms allow for maintenance of relatively stable, albeit lower than normal, blood bicarbonate concentrations when the urinary excretion rate cannot keep up with endogenous production of acid. Tissue stores of buffer are partly consumed over long periods of time. Loss of bone salts contributes to the development of osteomalacia and renal osteodystrophy. With recruitment of the various buffer mechanisms and with a decreased ability of the kidney to excrete various organic acids, there is a progressive rise in the "anion gap" $[N_2 - (Cl + HCO_3)]$, to around 20 to 24 mEq per liter, and a reciprocal decrease in plasma bicarbonate concentration. The serum bicarbonate concentration usually does not fall below 12 to 15 mEq per liter. Severe metabolic acidosis is uncommon in CRF. The blood pH normally does not drop below 7.25. If a patient with CRF is seen with an arterial blood pH below 7.25, a search should be made for causes of superimposed metabolic acidosis (e.g., diabetic ketoacidosis or lactic acidosis). This steady state metabolic acidosis with decreased bicarbonate is well tolerated by most patients with CRF, probably reflecting its slow development.

Another form of renal acidosis, distinct from the uremic acidosis described above, is type IV renal tubular acidosis (RTA) or hyporeninemic hypoaldosteronism with hyperkalemia and hyperchloremic acidosis. This set of chemical findings usually

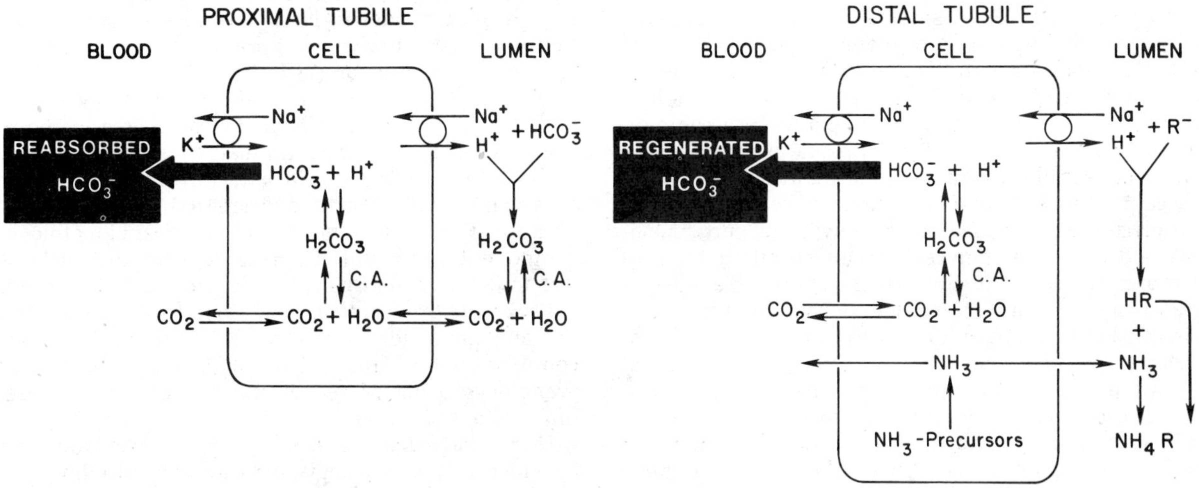

Figure 78–2. Schematic illustration of bicarbonate reclamation (reabsorption of filtered bicarbonate) by the proximal tubule and bicarbonate regeneration (formation of new bicarbonate by hydrogen secretion) by the distal tubule. C.A. in both panels signifies carbonic anhydrase. R represents nonabsorbable anion. Also indicated is the importance of NH_3 in the buffering of secreted hydrogen.

occurs in the early stages of CRF when GFR is moderately depressed to about 25 per cent of normal values. At this stage the kidney still has the capacity to excrete various organic acids, and therefore patients with type IV RTA, in contrast to those with uremic acidosis, have normal anion gaps. The exact incidence of this finding is not known, but it is not uncommon. type IV RTA is seen most frequently in diabetic patients with progressing renal failure or those with predominantly tubulo-interstitial disease. It is described further and compared with other types of RTA in Ch. 83.

Chloride. Patients with CRF are unable to regulate chloride excretion. For example, CRF patients excrete greater amounts of sodium when they are given an excess of sodium bicarbonate than following an equivalent amount of sodium chloride. With increased intake of NaCl there is retention of salt and fluid and weight gain. Many CRF patients are in a stable volume-expanded state. The preferential retention of chloride in CRF patients does not usually lead to a reciprocal decrease in bicarbonate concentration, and thus CRF patients tend to be proportionately hyperchloremic with respect to sodium concentration.

Calcium. The total serum calcium concentration in CRF patients is significantly lower than normal, although usually above 7.5 mg per deciliter. Great variability exists, and occasionally the calcium level is very low. CRF patients tolerate the hypocalcemia quite well, and rarely is a patient symptomatic from the decreased calcium concentration. Tetany is surprisingly uncommon. It is occasionally precipitated by the infusion of sodium bicarbonate, but the usual muscle twitching and cramping of CRF are unrelated to hypocalcemia.

CRF patients have decreased intestinal absorption of calcium, and in consequence fecal calcium loss exceeds that of normal subjects. Jejunal and ileal malabsorption of calcium in CRF can be corrected by oral administration of active vitamin D analogues with increases in serum calcium concentrations.

In addition, patients with either acute or chronic renal failure are resistant to the normal calcemic action of parathyroid hormone (PTH). The mechanism of resistance may be secondary to a decreased permissive effect of $1,25(OH)_2D_3$ on bone action of PTH. Renal osteodystrophy is discussed in Ch. 248.

A subgroup of CRF patients develops hypercalcemia after some months on hemodialysis. Most often the hypercalcemia is due to persistent secretion of PTH from glands that have previously undergone hyperplasia. Occasionally these patients become symptomatic with bone pain or exhibit signs of metastatic calcification. Parathyroidectomy may be indicated if other causes of hypercalcemia can be ruled out.

Magnesium. Patients with CRF tend to have modest elevations in serum magnesium concentration when GFR has fallen below 20 per cent of normal. Urinary excretion of magnesium is diminished, but intestinal magnesium absorption continues normally. Most CRF patients with hypermagnesemia have no associated symptoms or findings. Nevertheless, it is prudent to discontinue magnesium-containing antacids and cathartics in patients with GFR <20 ml per minute.

Phosphate. The most important determinant of serum phosphate level is the relationship between net reabsorption of phosphate from the gut and excretion of phosphate by the kidney. The serum phosphate concentration is significantly higher than normal in patients with GFR below 20 ml per minute.

The major reason for hyperphosphatemia is decreased excretion of phosphate with advancing renal disease. The retained phosphate is of major pathogenetic importance in the development of the secondary hyperparathyroidism of CRF. It is postulated that in the evolution of CRF there are periodic decreases in phosphate excretion as nephrons progressively drop out. The resultant increases in plasma phosphate concentration lead to reciprocal decreases in serum calcium concentration, increased secretion of PTH, and increased tubular rejection of phosphate. This adaptive mechanism will maintain a normal serum phosphate concentration until GFR has fallen to approximately 20 per cent of normal. However, if usual dietary phosphorus intake continues in patients with far advanced renal disease, these adaptive mechanisms cannot compensate fully and hyperphosphatemia ensues. If dietary phosphorus is decreased in proportion to the decrease in GFR, hyperphosphatemia can be prevented and the expected rise in serum parathyroid hormone blunted. In addition, intestinal absorption of phosphate can be reduced by use of compounds that bind phosphate in the gut in nonabsorbable form.

CARDIOVASCULAR ABNORMALITIES. Cardiovascular complications are common in patients with CRF and can be classified into three main categories: atherosclerosis and hyperlipidemia, hypertension, and pericarditis.

Atherosclerosis. Accelerated atherosclerosis is one of the major factors limiting the longevity of patients with chronic renal failure. Although the plasma lipid pattern may be normal in CRF, the most characteristic abnormality is elevated triglyceride concentrations with normal or slightly elevated plasma cholesterol levels (type IV). A smaller percentage of patients has type IIa or IIb hyperlipoproteinemia. The incidence of elevated triglyceride concentrations is increased in patients maintained on chronic hemodialysis as compared with nondialyzed patients. Cardiovascular death is particularly common after the fifth year of dialysis. There appears to be a positive relationship between the elevation of plasma triglycerides and the increased incidence of occlusive coronary disease. The cause of hypertriglyceridemia in CRF is unknown, but current evidence favors a defect in triglyceride removal rather than an increase in triglyceride production. The most probable cause of the decreased removal rate of very low density lipoproteins is a defect in hepatic lipoprotein lipase activity.

Hypertension. Hypertension is common in chronic renal disease, being present in the majority of patients at the onset of maintenance dialysis. At least two factors contribute to its high incidence in CRF: (1) The tendency toward sodium retention and volume expansion is perhaps the most important. Expansion of the extracellular volume is accompanied by an initial rise of cardiac output, which may persist, followed by a rise in peripheral resistance. Patients with volume-sensitive hypertension may have increasing problems with blood pressure control as they progress into renal failure. (2) Alterations of the renin-angiotensin axis are also important contributors to the pathogenesis of hypertension. Although the absolute plasma values for renin and angiotensin are variable in CRF, plasma renin activity is inappropriately high for the degree of sodium retention in most patients. This view is supported by the efficiency of angiotensin-coverting enzyme inhibitors in controlling hypertension, and by those few patients whose hypertension can be controlled only by bilateral nephrectomy.

Pericarditis. "Uremic pericarditis" is a term that refers to pericarditis of unknown etiology occurring in association with uremia. Conventionally pericarditis is not classified as "uremic" if an infectious etiology can be documented. Uremic pericarditis may occur before or after initiation of hemodialysis. It is most common in patients who are not dialyzed adequately. It is most likely caused by some unknown biochemical substance. Characteristically, the pericardial fluid is hemorrhagic. The onset of pericarditis is usually signaled by pain, often on the left side of the chest with respiratory accentuation. Pain is often severe and frequently associated with a friction rub. The friction rub can be loud, generalized, and even palpable. Tamponade can occur with signs of falling blood and pulse pressure, raised jugular venous pressure, and poorly perfused extremities. The hemorrhage is thought to originate from sheared pericardial capillaries that have developed in response to uremic inflammation of the pericardium.

HEMATOLOGIC ABNORMALITIES. Hematologic abnormalities are among the most consistent manifestations of uremia. These abnormalities include anemia, bleeding, and granulocyte and platelet dysfunction.

Anemia. Many patients with CRF have severely reduced hematocrits. Hematocrits in the 20 to 25 per cent range are not uncommon. The manifestations of anemia include pallor, tachycardia, a wide pulse pressure with accentuation by exercise, a systolic ejection murmur best heard over the pulmonary area, and the precipitation of angina pectoris in patients with underlying coronary artery disease.

The primary cause of anemia in CRF is a deficiency of erythropoietin, which is a glycoprotein normally produced in the kidney in response to anoxia. It is responsible for normal red blood cell differentiation from stem cells. The decreased erythropoietin may be the result of destruction of renal parenchyma, the presence of circulating inhibitors, or protein deprivation that in turn decreases erythropoietin production. The result is normochromic, normocytic anemia.

Other factors may contribute to anemia. Many patients on maintenance hemodialysis programs are iron deficient. Iron absorption from the gut may be decreased in CRF patients and restored to normal following hemodialysis. Furthermore, iron deficiency may develop in dialyzed patients because of frequent blood sampling, loss of blood in hemodialysis tubing and coils, and periodic accidental losses from hemodialysis access sites. Red blood cell survival is shortened in uremia, probably due to some extrinsic factor: (1) Red blood cells isolated from uremic patients and infused into nonuremic individuals have a normal life span. (2) Aggressive hemodialysis increases the red blood cell survival to or toward normal. In addition, many patients with CRF have added intrinsic erythrocytic factors contributing to anemia, which include decreased Na-K-ATPase activity, pentose phosphate dysfunction, microangiopathic hemolytic component as a result of hypersplenism, and folate deficiency due to its dialyzability in chronic hemodialysis patients.

Leukocyte Dysfunction. In addition to anemia, there are other hematologic abnormalities in CRF. Although the granulocyte count is usually normal, some patients have a tendency toward granulocytopenia. Moreover, the chemotactic response of granulocytes is subnormal.

Hemorrhagic Diathesis. A hemorrhagic tendency, manifested by epistaxis, menorrhagia, or excessive bleeding or bruising after trauma, is common in late renal failure but seldom life threatening. Whole blood clotting time and prothrombin time are usually normal. Bleeding time may be prolonged, perhaps related to the associated abnormalities of platelet function. Platelets are often decreased in number owing to increased peripheral destruction. In addition, there are functional defects such as decreased adhesiveness and aggregation. These abnormalities are often corrected by hemodialysis and may be secondary to a dialyzable uremic toxin. The hemorrhagic diathesis of uremia is discussed further in Ch. 166 and 167.

INFECTIONS. Most patients with CRF develop serious infections during the course of their disease. Theoretically, this assumed susceptibility to infection could be due to deranged or deficient humoral or cellular immunity, impaired inflammatory reaction, or increased exposure to pathogenic bacteria and viruses. Humoral immunity is, in general, intact. Although exceptions exist, most patients have a normal humoral response to vaccines. Cellular defense mechanisms are often deficient. Skin tests may show impairment of delayed hypersensitivity. Patients with CRF may have low lymphocyte counts, and their lymphocytes do not respond normally to mitogenic stimulation. Abnormal lymphocyte function may be due to some dialyzable factor, since it is nearly normal after vigorous dialysis or after suspension of lymphocytes harvested from uremic patients in nonuremic sera. The neutrophil count is usually normal in chronic renal failure, and it rises appropriately in response to infection. However, a transient decrease may occur following hemodialysis owing to sequestration of leukocytes in pulmonary capillaries. In addition, leukocytes of uremic subjects have a decreased ability to phagocytize bacteria. The chemotactic response of polymorphonuclear leukocytes is also depressed; this function improves with hemodialysis. Additionally, patients on hemodialysis are frequently exposed to bacterial and viral infections. Staphylococcal sepsis is not uncommon. The presumed portal of entry is cutaneous contamination through the arteriovenous hemodialysis access. Gram-negative sepsis also occurs with increased frequency. Often an infected urinary tract can be implicated as the cause. Superinfection with *Candida albicans* is very common, mainly affecting the buccal mucosa. There is a significant increase in frequency of hepatitis in dialysis patients owing to multiple transfusions and increased exposure, secondary to either hepatitis B virus or non-A non-B viruses. The disease is usually asymptomatic, but it can be severe. Approximately one third of CRF patients who contract hepatitis become chronic carriers.

GASTROINTESTINAL DISORDERS. Gastrointestinal symptoms are common in patients with uremia. Their symptoms have varying presentations and may be quite distressing. The most common early symptom is loss of appetite. Many uremic patients then progress to develop nausea and vomiting, sometimes severe enough to cause loss of salt and water leading to volume depletion and negative caloric balance causing weight loss. The specific cause of these symptoms has not been identified.

Gastrointestinal bleeding is also common in uremic patients. Often it is of minor magnitude detected by positive stool guaiacs, but it also can be severe. The gastrointestinal bleeding may be the result of scattered petechiae, ulceration, or other specific lesions. Undoubtedly the platelet defects contribute to the increased frequency of gastrointestinal bleeding characteristic of uremic patients.

OSTEODYSTROPHY. The term "renal osteodystrophy" is an all-inclusive term for the skeletal changes in uremia which include, in decreasing order of frequency, osteitis fibrosa, osteomalacia, osteoporosis, and osteosclerosis. Osteitis fibrosa is almost universal in terminal renal failure; it may be found in as many as 90 per cent of patients starting regular dialysis, the exceptions being those with rapidly progressive disease and a short experience of uremia. A substantial minority will exhibit abnormal radiographs, but very few will complain of bone tenderness or muscle weakness. Few patients survive more than a year or two on dialysis without evidence of bone disease. Osteomalacia is less common, and only a minority of patients will complain of bone pain. Retardation of growth occurs in children with renal insufficiency, often accompanied by musculoskeletal pain and muscle weakness. Clinical and radiologic features of rickets may be seen, but osteitis fibrosa is the most common lesion. Renal osteodystrophy is due in large part to increased parathyroid hormone (PTH) activity, deficiency in active vitamin D metabolites, and chronic acidosis. The pathogenesis and clinical features of renal osteodystrophy are discussed in greater detail in Ch. 248.

NEUROPATHY. Many patients with CRF have abnormalities in central and peripheral nervous system function. Tiredness, insomnia, and psychologic symptoms, including agitation, irritability, depression, regression, and rebellion, are common. Patients tend to have fewer such symptoms if they are eating a nutritious diet and are well dialyzed. Patients with secondary hyperparathyroidism caused by uremia have abnormal electroencephalograms (EEG) characterized by increased frequency of slow wave activity. Patients with secondary hyperparathyroidism caused by CRF may show improvement in their EEG and psychologic symptoms after parathyroidectomy. The mechanism by which PTH exerts these effects is not known, but in the uremic dog PTH increases brain calcium content and abnormal EEG changes of uremia require elevated levels of PTH. Brain calcium content is higher in patients with CRF than in patients who die without renal failure.

Peripheral neuropathy is also common in CRF. Clinical manifestations include painful paresthesias of extremities, twitchings, "restless leg syndrome," loss of deep tendon reflexes, muscular weakness, and occasional sensory deficits. Lower extremities are involved much more frequently than upper extremities. Diminished deep tendon reflexes and vibratory sense may be found, but the most reliable objective measurement of peripheral neuropathy in CRF is slowing of nerve conduction velocities. Peripheral neuropathy can be drug induced, but its pathophysiology in most patients is unknown. However, symptoms of neuropathy can be improved by prolonging the period of dialysis and by use of membrane dialyzers with larger membrane surface areas. Also, patients on chronic peritoneal dialysis have been said to have fewer symptoms than patients on extracorporeal hemodialysis. These findings suggest that the development of peripheral neuropathy is related to dialyzable uremic toxins of the "middle molecule" range.

MYOPATHY. Muscular weakness develops slowly, but it is common in patients with end-stage renal failure. Proximal muscles are affected more than distal muscles. It is not uncommon to see some wasting of the limb and cervical muscles. There are no distinct histologic features of uremic myopathy. The resting transmembrane potential difference of skeletal muscle cells is abnormally low, and the average mean duration of the action potential is significantly shortened in uremic individuals. In inadequately dialyzed uremic patients intracellular sodium and chloride contents are elevated, whereas potassium content is reduced. These findings are consistent with either increased permeability of the muscle membrane to these ions or a decrease in active efflux of sodium. However, it is doubtful that these are primary muscle membrane abnormalities, since all the abnormalities can be corrected by dialysis. Indeed, resting skeletal muscle membrane responses have been used as an index of adequacy of hemodialysis. Although a number of hormones and factors have been proposed as causal of uremic myopathy, the identity of such a factor(s) remains conjectural.

CARBOHYDRATE METABOLISM. Carbohydrate metabolism is often abnormal in patients with chronic renal failure. Glucose tolerance is reduced as shown by a rapid rise and delayed return to normal of the blood glucose concentration after an oral or intravenous glucose load. Fasting blood glucose values are normal or slightly elevated. This state of impaired glucose tolerance is often termed *uremic pseudodiabetes mellitus.* Severe hyperglycemia does not occur unless the patient receives a large load of glucose, e.g., during peritoneal dialysis with hypertonic glucose solutions. Nevertheless, the requirement for exogenous insulin decreases in insulin-dependent diabetics as renal failure progresses. At least two different mechanisms are responsible for the simultaneous coexistence of abnormal glucose tolerance and a decreased requirement for exogenous insulin: (1) enhanced peripheral resistance to insulin, and (2) a decreased renal clearance of insulin.

Increased peripheral resistance to insulin in uremia is manifested by a diminished forearm uptake of glucose in response to insulin, and elevated concentrations of circulating insulin as compared with normal subjects. A number of possibilities exist to explain the insulin resistance. First, some uremic substances may interfere with the action of insulin, since aggressive hemodialysis decreases exogenous requirements for insulin. Second, potassium deficiency may alter the nature of insulin released from the pancreas. Indeed, proinsulin to insulin ratios rise in nonuremic patients who are potassium deficient. Third, there is decreased binding of insulin to peripheral receptors in CRF. Fourth, low-protein diets may improve peripheral sensitivity to insulin. Whatever the reason(s), patients with CRF clearly have some degree of peripheral resistance to insulin.

Insulin is filtered and metabolized by the kidney. With progressing CRF the urinary clearance of insulin approaches GFR, presumably reflecting a decreased uptake of filtered insulin by the proximal convoluted tubule. Nevertheless, blood insulin concentrations rise owing to decreased extraction of insulin by renal tubular epithelial cells. These observations explain the decrease in insulin requirements of diabetics with progressing CRF, but it is also necessary to postulate a degree of peripheral resistance to insulin to explain the carbohydrate intolerance ("uremic pseudodiabetes") of nondiabetic subjects with CRF.

URIC ACID. Approximately two thirds of the total uric acid excretory load is normally removed each day by the kidney. With progression of CRF hyperuricemia is a consistent finding once GFR has decreased to 20 per cent of normal. However, the correlation between the rise of serum uric acid and the severity of chronic renal failure is poor. Only rarely does the serum uric acid concentration rise above 10 mg per deciliter unless dehydration is superimposed. Whether or not the elevated serum uric acid levels hasten the development of end-stage renal disease is not known.

PRURITUS. Generalized pruritus is a frequent symptom of CRF and is occasionally severe and intractable. Usually there are no dermatologic findings. To date no single causative factor has been identified. Implicated factors include some dialyzable product of uremia, high calcium-phosphorus product in extracellular fluid with deposition of calcium salts in the dermal structures, and abnormalities in nerve end plates. Symptomatic relief has been reported with more frequent dialysis, parathyroidectomy, dietary protein restriction, and exposure to sunburn spectrum of ultraviolet light.

Role of Retained Toxins

The kidney has a remarkable capacity to regulate the excretion of a variety of substances to maintain their blood concentrations at optimal levels. During the evolution of renal insufficiency until GFR is severely compromised this capacity is maintained by adaptive mechanisms whereby the remaining nephrons either metabolize or excrete greater than normal quantities of the substance in question. Adaptive mechanisms do not exist for substances that are freely filtered and neither reabsorbed nor secreted. Urea and creatinine are the classic examples of this group of compounds. Their clearance rates are close approximations of the glomerular filtration rate. However, most substances are not only filtered but also reabsorbed, secreted, or metabolized. In general, the blood concentrations of the latter group of substances do not rise until the later stages of renal disease. Many of the putative uremic toxins belong in this latter group.

The symptoms of uremia are, in part, caused by dialyzable substances that accumulate from failure of their renal excretion. Azotemic patients improve symptomatically after initiation of hemodialysis. No single substance has evolved as the cause of uremic symptoms. Multiple compounds no doubt contribute. The list of the suggested "uremic toxins" is long (e.g., guanidines, amines, phenols, indoles) and beyond the scope of this chapter. Urea and "middle molecules" (presumed polypeptides with molecular weights between 1000 and 1500) have received the most attention and will be discussed here.

UREA. Since blood urea nitrogen rises rapidly with decreasing GFR, and since intravenous injections of urea to animals produced neurologic symptoms, it was only natural to suspect that high urea concentrations produced uremic symptoms. However, this view is no longer held. For example, in studies in which patients were dialyzed for prolonged periods of time against a dialysate with a high concentration of urea, only minimal symptoms of headache, lethargy, emesis, or tremor were noted with postdialysis blood urea concentrations as high as 200 mg per deciliter. This is strong presumptive evidence that the clinical manifestations of chronic renal failure are not secondary to urea itself. In addition some patients have uremic symptoms at serum urea concentrations as low as 60 mg per deciliter. Therefore other factors in end-stage renal disease are of importance in producing uremic symptoms.

"MIDDLE MOLECULAR WEIGHT" TOXINS. The origin of the "middle molecular weight" toxin concept came from the clinical observation that patients who were peritoneally dialyzed had fewer uremic symptoms than patients who were hemodialyzed to the same blood urea concentration with small surface area dialyzers. It was argued that the peritoneum was more permeable to substances in the molecular weight range of 500 to 5000 than were the small pore hemodialyzers. Significant effort has been spent to identify specific compounds in this molecular range that might be toxic. Although a great number of compounds have been identified, there have been few correlative studies to establish "cause and effect" relationships. However, toxic effects of "middle molecules" isolated from uremic serum include inhibitions of hemoglobin synthesis, glucose utilization, lymphoblast transformation, leukocyte phagocytic activity, and nerve conductivity. Although the "middle molecular weight" toxin theory has not been established with certainty, clinical observations are consistent with the view that there are compounds in this molecular weight range that may play a role in the pathogenesis of the uremic syndrome.

APPROACH TO THE PATIENT WITH UREMIA

The principles of approach to the uremic patient are the same as toward any patient who comes to the attention of the physician. A detailed clinical history is imperative, with special emphasis on urinary tract symptoms such as nocturia, hematuria, dysuria, polydipsia, and polyuria. Also of special importance is a complete history of systemic diseases, of exposure to toxins and infections, and of renal diseases in the family. The medical history will often be of diagnostic significance. The physical examination should emphasize the blood pressure, retina, cardiovascular system, renal examination with auscultation for bruits and palpation of size, rectal examination for size of prostate in males, gynecologic examination for pelvic masses in females, extremity examination for edema and nail bed findings, and neuroskeletal examination for evidence of myopathy, neuropathy, and osteodystrophy. Laboratory tests should include a complete blood count and urinalysis.

Additional studies should be designed to elucidate whether a patient has acute reversible renal failure, acute worsening of CRF resulting from aggravating factors, or a chronic progressive disease. Again, the history is important. It is unlikely that a patient with acute renal disease is asymptomatic with elevations of serum creatinine and blood urea nitrogen above 10 and 100 mg per deciliter, respectively. On the other hand, patients, especially if young, with slowly progressing CRF are often asymptomatic with much higher elevations of serum creatinine and blood urea nitrogen. Thus, if in the absence of other diseases, a patient complains of nausea, vomiting, anorexia, and weakness and the creatinine and blood urea nitrogen are below 10 and 100 mg per deciliter, respectively, the chances are that the patient is suffering from an acute process. Unfortunately exceptions to this rule exist. Also, in chronic renal failure the hematocrit tends to be lower, phosphate concentration higher, uric acid concentration lower, and urine sediment more benign. However, none of these tests is specific enough to differentiate with certainty between acute and chronic renal failure.

X-ray determination of the kidney size can be helpful in determining the chronicity of renal disease. The x-rays can be in the form of plain abdominal films, tomograms, or intravenous urograms (if the blood urea nitrogen is less than 100 mg per deciliter). Of these the plain abdominal film is least expensive, free from complications, and often informative. Renal sonograms can be used to estimate renal size and identify hydronephrosis or cystic masses. If the kidneys are significantly reduced in size, this almost always indicates chronicity and irreversibility. Normal kidney size tends to favor an acute process, although exceptions exist. Chronic renal processes in which kidney size may be normal or larger than normal include polycystic renal disease, amyloidosis, scleroderma, and diabetes mellitus. Thus normal renal size does not rule out a chronic process.

It is also important to differentiate between renal versus extrarenal causes of azotemia. Extrarenal causes of progressive uremia may be either pre- or postrenal. Prerenal causes are those disease processes that decrease the blood flow to the kidneys. This may be due to true ECF volume depletion or to effective volume depletion as seen with cardiac and liver failure. Characteristic findings in prerenal azotemia are a disproportionate increase in the ratio of blood urea nitrogen to creatinine ($>10\times$) and low fractional urinary excretion (<1 per cent) of filtered sodium and chloride. Also, it is imperative to rule out postrenal causes of azotemia, namely lower or upper urinary tract obstruction. Lower urinary tract obstruction may be diagnosed by having the patient void completely and then measuring the residual urine volume in the bladder via catheterization. The presence of residual urine indicates lower urinary tract obstruction. Occasionally sufficient time has elapsed between voluntary voiding and insertion of the catheter so that "new" urine is formed. When the physician is unsure of the significance of 5 to 10 ml of residual urine he may elect to instill 20 to 40 ml of air into the bladder. If this air is passed (which the patient experiences as a "whistling" sound) during the next voiding, then the bladder can empty completely and lower urinary obstruction is ruled out. In males by far the most common cause is an enlarged prostate. Any time a uremic

TABLE 78–1. TREATABLE* TYPES OF PARENCHYMAL RENAL DISEASE

Acute hypertensive nephropathy
Analgesic nephropathy
Hemolytic-uremic syndrome
Hypercalcemic nephropathy
Lupus nephritis
Multiple myeloma
Oxalate nephropathy
Pyelonephritis
Renal vein thrombosis
Wegener's granulomatosis

*The mode of therapy and results in these disease processes are variable. All these processes may present with such severe end-stage renal disease that no form of conservative management is effective.

patient is seen with anuria, it is imperative that lower urinary tract obstruction be ruled out, especially if accompanied by symptoms such as hesitancy in initiating the urinary stream, slow urinary stream, and incontinence. Upper urinary tract obstruction can be established by ruling out residual urine in the bladder and demonstrating dilated renal calices, pelvis, and ureter(s) above the obstruction. This can be established by intravenous and retrograde pyelography or by renal sonograms. In addition to the dilated urinary tract systems, there characteristically exists delayed visualization and delayed clearance of the dye on intravenous urograms. The most common causes of upper urinary tract obstruction include renal stones, congenital obstruction, and bladder cancer.

Once it has been determined that uremia is secondary to renal parenchymal disease and not due to pre- or postrenal causes, the physician must determine if a treatable form of parenchymal disease is present. The most common forms of treatable renal disease are listed in Table 78–1. The following additional tests may be helpful and are often considered: renal arteriography and renal biopsy. In general, although renal arteriography produces excellent visualization of the kidney, it is of limited diagnostic value in patients with uremia. It may be helpful in patients suspected of having polyarteritis nodosa, tumors (although uremia is an uncommon association), and renal disease secondary to severe hypertension.

Renal biopsy may give a definitive histologic diagnosis provided it is performed before the disease has progressed to such a degree that the only possible morphologic interpretation is "end-stage kidney disease." Renal biopsy can be performed by a percutaneous route with local anesthesia or as an open biopsy under general anesthesia, but it should be carried out only by those who are trained in its use. The associated morbidity and mortality are low, but the possibility of complications nevertheless exists. For these reasons renal biopsy is probably indicated in only a small number of patients with uremia. While a consensus does not exist among nephrologists, biopsy should not be done unless the physician has strong feelings that the information to be gained will influence management. In our institution biopsies are not customarily performed in patients with chronic disease when the GFR is <20 ml per minute or the kidneys are small in size. Contraindications to renal biopsy include uncorrectable bleeding tendencies, severe hypertension, bacteriuria, suspicion of perinephric abscess, hydronephrosis, and extreme obesity. Biopsy is often useful in patients with normal sized kidneys and progressive renal disease if they have (or are suspected to have) nephrotic syndrome, collagen vascular disease (especially systemic lupus erythematosus), tubulointerstitial disease, or rapidly progressive glomerular disease.

MANAGEMENT

The management of CRF patients can be divided conveniently into three separate categories: treatment of aggravating factors, treatment of specific complications of uremia, and consideration of optimal diet and general principles in the long-term follow-up of patients with CRF. We will consider those principles of management that are common to all forms of CRF regardless of etiology.

Aggravating Factors

Patients with CRF are highly susceptible to factors that may cause a deterioration of renal function. These must be sought meticulously and treated immediately so that the underlying renal failure will not be worsened permanently. The most common of these factors are infection and volume depletion.

Infection. Infection of the urinary tract is especially common following instrumentation or catheterization of the bladder. Specific care should be directed toward evaluating the degree of proteinuria, pyuria, and bacteriuria and any changes from baseline abnormalities. Increased proteinuria and exaggerated pyuria suggest urinary tract infection, and call for a culture of clean-voided urine. If infection is documented, specific antibiotics are indicated. Care must be exercised to adjust the drug dosage for the degree of renal failure. A number of antibiotics are nephrotoxic, and the susceptibility to nephrotoxicity increases with advancing renal failure. Uremic patients are also more prone to other infections such as sepsis and pneumonia. These systemic infections in turn may compromise renal blood flow and result in worsening uremia.

Volume Depletion. Patients with CRF also are susceptible to volume depletion. Most often this is due to nausea, vomiting, diarrhea, or decreased intake of fluid. Thus physical signs of volume depletion should be sought. Urinary electrolyte measurements will often suggest volume depletion. Although CRF patients normally have an elevated fractional urinary excretion of sodium and chloride (the degree being dependent on the severity of the decrease in GFR), these patients are able to decrease their fractional excretion of sodium and chloride in response to volume depletion. A decrease in previously determined high fractional excretion of sodium and chloride of 2 per cent (or a decrease in fractional excretion to less than 1 per cent) is highly suggestive of either true or effective volume depletion. Patients with CRF may rapidly and irreversibly decrease their GFR with volume depletion, so it is imperative for treatment, either oral or intravenous fluid replacement, to be started as soon as feasible. Patients with CRF who are not on chronic dialysis should be hospitalized if there is any doubt that adequate volume repletion can be carried out on an outpatient basis.

Complications of Uremia

WATER AND ELECTROLYTE ABNORMALITIES. Treatment of altered states of calcium, phosphorus, and bicarbonate balance are discussed subsequently under Renal Osteodystrophy.

Hyperkalemia. The mean serum potassium is higher than normal, whereas the total body potassium content is lower than normal in CRF. Serum potassium concentrations up to 6 mEq per liter are well tolerated in CRF patients. However, patients with CRF have difficulty in excreting a sudden increase in potassium load. Therefore potassium concentrations above 6.0 mEq per liter should be treated. One should initially determine whether the hyperkalemia is a result of some aggravating factor such as volume depletion, tissue breakdown, transient worsening of acidosis, action of drugs such as spironolactone or triamterene, fever, or high intake of potassium; or whether hyperkalemia is a consequence of steady metabolic events. If hyperkalemia is of modest degree and due to some aggravating factor, the therapy should be directed toward correcting the source of hyperkalemia. However, if hyperkalemia is severe, paralysis of skeletal muscles and electrocardiographic changes may be present. This represents a medical emergency and requires immediate transfer of potassium intracellularly and rapid excretion of potassium from the body. There are two commonly accepted techniques for shifting potassium intracellularly. The first is the intravenous administration of 10 per cent glucose to which has been added 20 to 50 units of regular insulin per liter. The second is the intravenous administration of sodium bicarbonate at a rate of 2 to 3 ampules (88 to 132 mEq) in several minutes. A rapid shift of serum pH in an alkaline direction will allow potassium to enter cells in exchange for hydrogen. Also, if ECG changes of hyperkalemia exist, $CaCl_2$ or calcium gluconate may be given intravenously. Each ampule should be given slowly over a five-minute period and with extreme care if the patient is receiving digitalis. The intracellular shift of potassium often brings only temporary improvement, and measures to increase excretion of potassium should be instituted. If sufficient renal function exists, intravenous saline with furosemide will promote excretion of potassium. In addition, cation exchange renins such as sodium polystyrene sulfonate (Kayexalate) can be given orally in a dose of 20 to 30 grams three to four times a day or 50 grams rectally as a retention enema. When given orally it should be administered with 100 ml of 20 per cent sorbitol (many patients do not tolerate the commercially available 70 per cent sorbitol when given orally); or when given rectally, with 100 to 200 ml of 70 per cent sorbitol. Sorbitol will induce osmotic influx of fluid into the gut, which will cause diarrhea and excretion of potassium from the body. In addition, patients with little or no renal function should be dialyzed against potassium-free fluids until serum potassium starts to drop.

Abnormalities of Sodium Balance. Total body sodium content dictates total extracellular fluid volume. Although fractional excretion of sodium per nephron increases as renal disease progresses, patients with CRF are nevertheless susceptible to both volume contraction and volume expansion. Since even mild volume depletion may affect renal function adversely in CRF patients, it is prudent to maintain these patients in a somewhat expanded state (on the "wet side"). Volume sensitive hypertension and pulmonary edema will be limiting factors, but it is even more hazardous to keep a patient completely edema free. If a patient should develop orthostatic hypotensive symptoms, salt intake should be liberalized. Ideally, dietary salt intake should be decreased in proportion to the decrease in GFR. Some of the sodium should be given as sodium bicarbonate as described for renal osteodystrophy, below. If the patient is poorly compliant and becomes volume expanded, the use of diuretics such as furosemide or ethacrynic acid is indicated, assuming that underlying kidney function is sufficient to permit a satisfactory clinical response to these drugs. If volume expansion causes severe symptoms and does not respond to conventional techniques, acute peritoneal or hemodialysis is indicated. Hypo- and hypernatremia are treated with the same general principles of water restriction or free water administration as in any other patient. Neurologically symptomatic, life-threatening hyponatremia may require the administration of hypertonic sodium chloride, but this risks potential volume expansion. One should be prepared for the possibility of acute dialysis to remove extra volume.

CARDIOVASCULAR ABNORMALITIES. It is important to control the cardiovascular complications of CRF to realize the potential longevity of chronic hemodialysis. Hypertriglyceridemia and hypertension are the primary risk factors leading to accelerated atherosclerosis and high cardiovascular mortality. It is not clear whether the course of atherosclerotic vascular disease in CRF patients can be altered. Even patients who have undergone successful renal transplantation seem to have an increased incidence of cardiovascular deaths. Nevertheless, it seems advisable to adhere to the same dietary principles in patients with hypertriglyceridemia and CRF as in patients without CRF (see Ch. 48). If clofibrate is used, its dosage level should be decreased proportionately to the degree of renal failure to prevent its adverse side effects.

Hypertension is the result of numerous interrelated factors in CRF patients. It is most commonly volume dependent and volume sensitive. Thus one of the primary objectives is to decrease intravascular volume, an approach that will be sufficient to control hypertension in many patients. If the patient has an adequate urine volume, the judicious use of diuretics together with a decrease in the dietary intake of salt and water is indicated. Of the available diuretics, furosemide and ethacrynic acid are preferred because of their low renal toxicity. Volume can be removed in patients on dialysis by ultrafiltration during the procedure. If volume contraction is not sufficient, then the same general principles apply to the treatment of hypertension as in any other patient (see Ch. 47). Additional drugs such as methyldopa, hydralazine, and beta blockers such as propranolol and metoprolol may be required. Captopril, an oral inhibitor of angiotensin-converting enzyme, has been shown to be particularly useful in some patients. Minoxidil, a direct smooth muscle vasodilator, has also been advocated in a small group of patients with otherwise refractory hypertension. There still exists an extremely small number of patients with malignant hypertension that cannot be controlled by any medical regimen. These patients may respond to bilateral nephrectomy.

The diagnosis of uremic pericarditis requires hospitalization and treatment for fear of impending cardiac tamponade. The best initial therapy is daily dialysis for approximately a week. Indomethacin is not effective in uremic pericarditis. If pericarditis remains refractory to increased frequency of dialysis, intrapericardial injection of nonabsorbable steroids may prove therapeutic. Some patients will require partial pericardiectomy if they develop circulatory impairment that does not respond to medical management.

HEMATOLOGIC ABNORMALITIES. Anemia of CRF often improves with maintenance hemodialysis. The rise in hematocrit is not due to stimulation of erythropoietin production but rather to the removal of some circulating factor that inhibits the normal response to erythropoietin.

Besides achieving the best possible metabolic status of the patient with either hemodialysis or transplantation, there exist two general considerations for treatment of anemia: long-term medical treatment and transfusion. The general aim of medical treatment is to increase the hematocrit to values as high as possible without secondary side effects. Because patients with CRF, especially those on maintenance hemodialysis, are iron deficient, supplemental iron should be given. Iron can be given daily as a ferrous salt or on a periodic basis as intravenous iron dextran. Oral iron supplementation is inexpensive and is associated with very few side effects. Unfortunately, not all patients rebuild their iron stores to normal even if given 900 mg of ferrous sulfate per day. These patients probably do not absorb iron normally in spite of hemodialysis. They require periodic intravenous iron dextran. There is no consensus on frequency or dosage, and there is the potential of iron overload with hemosiderosis and occasional anaphylactoid reaction. While some patients have a gratifying hematologic response to periodic intramuscular injections of androgens, many patients do not respond at all (especially anephric patients) and many have untoward side effects to androgens. Most CRF patients do not have folate deficiency unless they are receiving maintenance dialysis treatment. Folic acid is dialyzable, and therefore it is standard practice to order small daily doses of folate (1 mg per day orally) in the hope of increasing erythropoiesis.

What are the indications for transfusion? Many CRF patients tolerate extraordinarily low hematocrits surprisingly well. This may be due to increased release of oxygen from hemoglobin during chronic anemia. Nevertheless, some patients do require periodic transfusions. If patients are unduly tired and unable to do routine tasks, packed red blood cell transfusions can be given in amounts sufficient to abate the symptoms. If such symptoms improve, this provides strong presumptive evidence that the weakness was due to anemia and not to uremia per se. It is rare that transfusions are necessary in CRF patients if the hematocrit is above 20 per cent. However, notable exceptions are provided by patients with angina pectoris. In these patients the physician may be forced to transfuse the patient even at hematocrit values in the low 30's. This situation may become more common as the mean age of dialysis patients becomes older.

INFECTIONS. Infections are more common in uremic than nonuremic patients. The general approach to the use of antibiotics should be the same in both groups of patients. Ideally the antibiotic dose should be adjusted by monitoring the serum concentration of the antibiotic. However, this often is not feasible and therefore after an initial normal loading dose, dosage levels must be adjusted for the degree of renal failure if the antibiotic is excreted by the kidney (Table 78–2). Some antibiotics are more nephrotoxic than others and nephrotoxicity is potentiated by CRF. If drug sensitivities allow a choice in treatment of a given infection, the physician should choose the least nephrotoxic antibiotic that is therapeutic.

RENAL OSTEODYSTROPHY (see also Ch. 248). Hyperparathyroidism, decreased amounts of active vitamin D metabolites, and chronic metabolic acidosis all contribute to the development of renal osteodystrophy as noted above. The goals of treatment are to normalize these abnormalities to the extent possible. If meticulous care is taken at the beginning of renal failure to keep serum phosphorus, calcium, and bicarbonate levels within the normal range by use of active vitamin D analogues, the development of renal osteodystrophy can be largely prevented. Since elevated phosphate concentrations contribute to the development of hypocalcemia and secondary hyperparathyroidism, it is prudent to decrease dietary phosphorus content. If patients are unable to comply with phosphate-deficient diets, antacids containing aluminum or magnesium salts can be used to decrease gut absorption of phosphate. The degree of phosphate absorption varies greatly from patient to patient, and the goal of dietary phosphate restriction and phosphate binders should be to maintain the serum phosphorus within the normal range. If the serum phosphorus concentration is normal, the serum calcium concentration should increase. However, if the calcium concentration remains low, oral calcium salts can be given. If vitamin D analogues are used for osteitis fibrosa, either 25-OHD (50 μg per day) or 1,25-$(OH)_2D$ (0.5 μg per day) may be effective. For "pure" osteomalacia neither metabolite may be effective, although 25-OHD has been shown to be useful in some instances. Care must be exercised that calcium does not rise to levels at which the calcium × phosphorus product is high enough to cause soft tissue calcification (i.e., >60). Hypercalcemia is the major hazard associated with the use of vitamin D analogues, especially with 1,25-$(OH)_2D$.

Chronic acidosis can lead to progressive bone resorption. Therefore patients with CRF and metabolic acidosis should be given oral alkali. One practical way to administer alkali is in the form of Shohl's solution (solution of citric acid and sodium citrate). Another inexpensive way is to prepare a solution of $NaHCO_3$ at home from baking soda and water to a final concentration of 1 mEq per milliliter. These solutions should be given in amounts sufficient to maintain serum HCO_3^- at 20 mEq per liter or greater. The dietary intake of sodium may have to be lowered to offset the increased sodium load that derives from oral alkali administration.

In an occasional patient all medical approaches are unsatisfactory either because of poor patient compliance or because they are initiated too late in the course of the osteodystrophy. In some patients bone pain and spontaneous fractures continue in spite of therapy. Parathyroidectomy should be reserved for patients with definite evidence of hypercalcemia who are considered treatment failures after an adequate trial of optimal medical management.

NEUROPATHY. No specific treatment exists for either central or peripheral neuropathy. However, both objective and subjective improvement may occur by prolonging the periods of dialysis and by use of larger surface area dialyzers. Also, gratifying improvement of peripheral neuropathy has been noted following successful renal transplantation.

MYOPATHY. No specific therapy exists for myopathy. Patients may improve dramatically with adequate dialysis. Some patients have shown improvement of myopathy following treatment with active vitamin D analogues.

CARBOHYDRATE METABOLISM. Abnormalities of carbohydrate metabolism in the nondiabetic patient are of no or minimal clinical significance. In the diabetic patient, insulin dosages must be adjusted to maintain serum glucose values at normal levels. Often smaller insulin doses will be adequate as CRF progresses.

URIC ACID. Although uric acid levels are consistently elevated in CRF, they are rarely much above 10 mg per deciliter. However, even if the uric acid levels are significantly higher there is little or no evidence to suggest that asymptomatic hyperuricemia should be treated. It is our practice to treat elevated uric acid levels in uremic patients only when there are tophaceous deposits or symptomatic gout. If treatment is elected, allopurinol is the drug of choice since patients with CRF do not respond to uricosuric agents. The allopurinol dose should be decreased to 100 mg per day in chronic uremic patients due to potential toxic side effects.

PRURITUS. No specific therapy has withstood the test of time in the treatment of pruritus. A few patients get relief following topical application of emulsified oils or the use of oral antihistamine agents. Some patients have benefited from lowering the serum phosphate concentration by phosphate binders. There are reports of beneficial effects of ultraviolet light. Parathyroidectomy has sometimes relieved intractable pruritus.

Diet

An appropriate diet can be critically important in the management of patients in chronic renal failure, for it may provide symptomatic improvement and also may slow the rate of loss

TABLE 78–2. ANTIBIOTIC DOSAGE IN CRF

Major Reduction in Dosage	Moderate Reduction in Dosage	Minor or No Reduction in Dosage	Agents That Should Not Be Used
Flucytosine	Ampicillin	Amphotericin B	Bacitracin
Gentamicin	Carbenicillin	Cefotaxime	Chlortetracycline
Kanamycin	Cefazolin	Cefoperazone	Nitrofurantoin
Oxytetracycline*	Cephaloridine	Chloramphenicol	
Streptomycin	Cephalothin	Clindamycin	
Tetracycline*	Cloxacillin	Doxycycline	
Tobramycin	Co-trimoxazole	Erythromycin	
Vancomycin	(trimethoprim-	Isoniazid	
	sulfamethoxazole)	Lincomycin	
	Methicillin	Nafcillin	
	Moxalactam		
	Oxacillin		
	Penicillin G		
	Ticarcillin		

*Although tetracyclines are not significantly nephrotoxic per se, their dosage should be reduced in CRF because of their hepatotoxicity with increased blood levels (especially with chlortetracycline) and because their antianabolic actions cause an increase in blood urea nitrogen disproportionate to the degree of renal failure. If tetracyclines are indicated in renal failure, doxycycline is the drug of choice because it is cleared by hepatic routes.

of residual renal function. Although nutritional and caloric intake should be individualized for obese and malnourished patients, some general principles are applicable to all patients. In general, the higher the amount of protein in the diet, the higher will be the serum urea concentration. This occurs because amino acids are metabolized to form urea in addition to all other nitrogenous waste products that have been implicated as factors causing the uremic syndrome. Reducing the amount of protein in the diet will lower the blood urea concentration and reduce symptoms. Moreover, the difficulties in controlling serum phosphorus and acidosis will be ameliorated, since a high-protein intake is always associated with a high intake of phosphates as well as other inorganic ions. However, if dietary protein is too low, protein malnutrition will occur with loss of strength, body weight, and muscle mass. This can be avoided if the protein requirements are met by providing 0.6 gram of protein per kilogram of body weight per day, of which at least 60 per cent contains proteins rich in essential amino acids, e.g., eggs, lean meat, and milk. Although a high calorie intake can improve nitrogen utilization at very low nitrogen intakes, it is not necessary to force large amounts of calories on these patients as long as minimum protein requirements are being met. Providing about 30 kilocalories per day generally suffices, although this may be lowered for obese patients or raised for patients weighing less than their ideal body weight. Accumulated waste products can be reduced even further by lowering the daily protein intake to approximately 20 grams of protein per day, but only if the diet is supplemented with essential amino acids or a mixture of essential amino acids and their alpha-ketoanalogues. Such a regimen will maintain adequate protein nutrition for prolonged periods of time in patients with advanced renal failure. Alpha-ketoanalogues of essential amino acids are aminated in the body to form essential amino acids and hence body protein. Nitrogen, which otherwise would have accumulated as waste products, is therefore used to build body proteins. Low-protein diets in which daily minimum requirements are met and the very low protein diet supplemented with mixtures of amino acids and alpha-ketoanalogues may slow the rate of loss of residual renal function and possibly postpone the time when therapy with chronic hemodialysis becomes necessary. Diets should be supplemented with the water-soluble B vitamins plus vitamin C and folic acid; there is no need to supply additional vitamin A or E. Vitamin D should be reserved for treatment of severe renal osteodystrophy. In general, there is no need to place a severe restriction on dietary sodium unless there is hypertension or edema. Most patients with chronic renal failure can readily excrete sodium until renal function is markedly impaired (creatinine clearances less than 10 ml per minute), but they cannot rapidly stop excreting salt when dietary sodium is markedly restricted. For most patients, the diet should contain at least 1.5 to 2 grams of sodium per day. As long as the amount of urine is greater than 1 liter per day, it is unusual to have to restrict potassium in the diet. Using these guidelines, uremic symptoms and the consequences of renal insufficiency can be controlled for most patients. Once chronic hemodialysis becomes necessary, the diet should be altered to meet the added requirements related to dialysis therapy.

General Principles of Follow-up

Patients with CRF should be seen at regular intervals to monitor the progress of their disease. The frequency of these visits will depend upon the presence of other diseases, e.g., hypertension and heart failure, and on how rapidly residual renal function is being lost. All patients should be seen at least every three months, at which time a medical history is taken

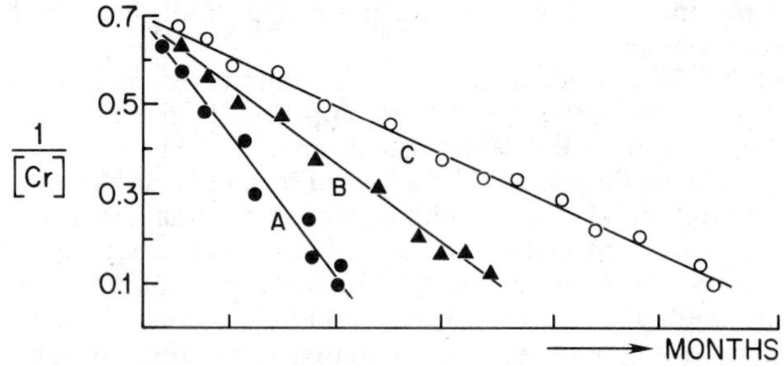

Figure 78–3. Plot of reciprocal of serum creatine concentration (vertical axis) against time (horizontal axis) in three hypothetical patients. This is a useful way to determine the rate of progression of CRF in a given patient, since each patient tends to have a predetermined slope reflecting the underlying cause of CRF. For example, patient A reflects rapidly progressing renal failure such as seen with diabetes mellitus, patient B might represent nephrosclerosis secondary to essential hypertension, and patient C might reflect the slower rate of progression of polycystic disease.

and a physical examination is performed. In addition, laboratory values including hematocrit, white count, serum urea nitrogen and creatinine concentrations, and electrolyte values should be obtained. Monitoring the progress of renal insufficiency is generally accomplished by measuring the serum creatinine concentration as an indirect index of GFR. Alternatively, 24-hour urine collections can be obtained to measure creatinine and urea clearances, since the average of these two values gives a close approximation of GFR. For most patients, the loss of residual renal function proceeds at a constant rate; this rate is different for each patient, although generally patients with polycystic renal disease have a slower rate of loss of renal function than those with diabetic nephropathy. To monitor the progress of the disease, the reciprocal of the serum creatinine concentration can be plotted against time for an individual patient, as shown in Figure 78–3. For most patients, this relationship is remarkably linear and can be used to estimate when a patient will become a candidate for maintenance hemodialysis. When the reciprocal of serum creatinine concentration reaches 0.1 or less (a creatinine concentration of 10 mg per deciliter), the patient is close to the time when dialysis becomes necessary. Moreover, a sudden change in the slope of this line can indicate that some other factor, such as obstruction, infection, or uncontrolled hypertension, is accelerating the rate of loss of residual renal function.

Bricker NS: Sodium homeostasis in chronic renal disease. Kidney Int 21:886, 1982. *This article is an examination of factors regulating sodium homeostasis in normal and chronic failure patients.*

Chan MK, Varghese Z, Moorhead JF: Lipid abnormalities in uremia, dialysis and transplantation. Kidney Int 19:625, 1981. *An excellent overview editorial that discusses clearly the complex lipid abnormalities in uremic and dialysis patients.*

DeLuca HF: The vitamin D hormonal system: Implications for bone diseases. Hosp Pract April 1980, pp 57–63. *Dr. DeLuca reviews clearly the factors important in the pathophysiology of renal osteodystrophy, with special emphasis on the central role of vitamin D.*

Fisher JW: Mechanism of the anemia of chronic renal failure. Nephron 25:106, 1980. *A nice editorial review which discusses the etiologic factors responsible for the anemia of chronic renal disease. This article puts forth evidence to suggest that erythropoietin deficiency has a central role in the development of anemia of end-stage renal disease.*

Knochel JP, Seldin DW: The pathophysiology of uremia: *In* Brenner BM, Rector FC (eds.): The Kidney. 2nd ed. Philadelphia, W. B. Saunders Company, 1981, pp 2137–2183. *A comprehensive synthesis of metabolic and endocrine abnormalities in uremia. This review chapter is especially good in discussing the pathogenesis of metabolic abnormalities of uremia. It has 251 well-chosen references.*

Mitch WE: Conservative management of chronic renal failure: *In* Brenner BM, Stein JH (eds.): Contemporary Issues in Nephrology, Chronic Renal Failure, Vol. 7. New York, Churchill Livingstone, 1981, pp 116–152. *A complete discussion of the principles and practice of dietary therapy of chronic renal failure.*

Wineman RJ: End-stage renal disease: 1978. Dialysis Transplantation 7:1034, 1978. *A review of demographic characteristics of end-stage renal disease as derived from the National Dialysis Registry.*

79. TREATMENT OF IRREVERSIBLE RENAL FAILURE

79.1. Dialysis

Robert G. Luke

Each year approximately 1 in 10,000 of the United States population develops end-stage renal disease (ESRD) and requires one of the various forms of renal replacement therapy: chronic hemodialysis in a center or at home, intermittent peritoneal dialysis—usually at home, continuous ambulatory peritoneal dialysis, or transplantation from a live-related or cadaveric donor. Most of the costs of such treatment are covered for almost all of the United States population by the Renal Medicare Program, and in 1983 approximately 80,000 patients participated in that program. The most common causes of end-stage renal disease are chronic glomerulonephritis, nephrosclerosis, chronic pyelonephritis (reflux nephropathy), diabetic glomerulosclerosis, and polycystic kidney disease. The overall incidence of end-stage renal disease is 4.5 times greater in blacks than in Caucasians; hypertensive nephrosclerosis accounts for 33 per cent of the cases in blacks but only 8 per cent in whites.

Choice of renal replacement therapy is dictated by the availability of a live-related donor (best results), the age of the patient (transplantation is less frequently performed over the age of 50 to 55 years), and the presence of important systemic extrarenal disease (which may preclude surgery or immunosuppression). Preliminary hemodialysis is usually necessary before transplantation. Home hemodialysis or intermittent peritoneal dialysis requires the support of a partner, an adequate home, self-motivation by the patient, and reasonably stable medical circumstances. Such patients have better rehabilitation and survival rates than those on in-center hemodialysis, but this may relate to patient selection factors. The cost of home dialysis is less than in-center dialysis. In general, patients are best served when all modalities of treatment for end-stage renal disease are readily available and well integrated.

TECHNICAL ASPECTS

As renal excretory function becomes progressively impaired, solutes accumulate in the body and eventually contribute to the uremic syndrome (see Ch. 78) and, ultimately, death. These solutes, especially those of low molecular weight such as urea, can be removed efficiently from the blood by the process of diffusion across a semipermeable membrane down a chemical concentration gradient (dialysis). Substances higher in concentration in the dialysate than in the plasma, such as bicarbonate, will diffuse into the plasma (Fig. 79–1). The membrane must be nontoxic and compatible with red blood cells, white blood cells, platelets, and plasma proteins. Either a synthetic membrane in the process of extracorporeal hemodialysis or, in peritoneal dialysis, the lining membrane of the peritoneal cavity is used.

Hemodialysis

Membranes of varying hydraulic conductivity and solute permeability can be used in dialyzers of varying surface area and extracorporeal blood volume (100 to 250 ml in adults) to accommodate patients of different sizes, including infants. To remove accumulated sodium chloride and water, ultrafiltration across artificial membranes is induced by a transmembrane hydrostatic pressure, either positive on the blood side or negative on the dialysate side (Fig. 79–1). The removal of over 1 liter of fluid per hour is feasible and predictable based on the ultrafiltration coefficient of the dialyzer.

The two most common types of dialyzer units in use today are the flat plate, in which blood flows through parallel plates of membrane alternating with dialysate flowing in the opposite direction, and the hollow-fiber "artificial kidney," in which blood flows through numerous hollow fibers of about 200 μ

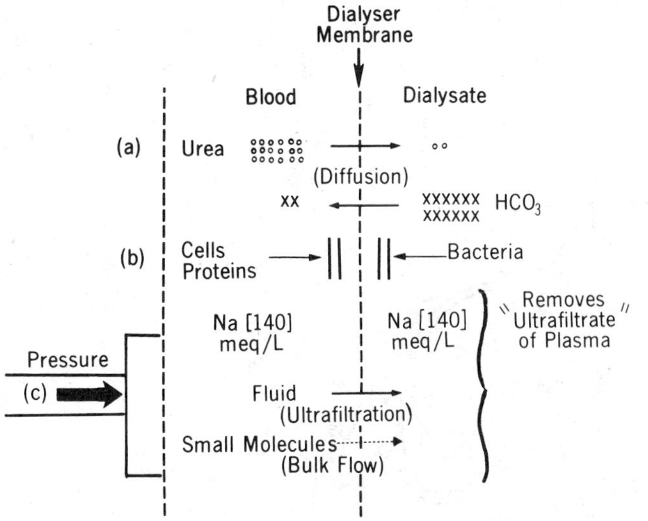

Figure 79–1. Mechanisms of removal of solute and fluid during dialysis. *(a)* Diffusion of urea from high concentration in blood into dialysate and of bicarbonate from higher concentration dialysate into lower concentration in the blood of patient with renal failure. *(b)* The dialysis membrane is impermeable to red blood cells and plasma proteins and to bacteria in the dialysate (but not to endotoxins). *(c)* The dialysate sodium is freely diffusible and determines the plasma sodium; fluid is removed by application of a transmembrane pressure (in peritoneal dialysis by increased glucose and hence osmotic pressure in the dialysate). The fluid is accompanied by small molecules such as sodium and chloride by convection (solvent drag).

internal diameter with dialysate flowing between the fibers, again in the opposite direction. The essential components of a dialysate delivery and monitoring system of an artificial kidney apparatus are shown in Figure 79–2. Blood flow rates of 200 to 300 ml per minute are usual. Heparin is given intermittently or infused continuously (1000 to 10,000 units in total) to prevent clotting of blood in the dialyzer during the usually 3- to 6-hour procedure; dosage is controlled by the whole blood or activated clotting time.

Dialysate is made up from concentrate and is either supplied (in large dialysis facilities) to each kidney via a central delivery system or made within each machine using concentrate and a proportioning system that dilutes the concentrate to provide physiologic dialysate. The latter contains normal serum levels of sodium and chloride, a variable potassium concentration (0 to 4 mEq per liter) depending on the patient's need for removal of potassium, and acetate (normally metabolized to bicarbonate) or bicarbonate (35 mEq per liter) to correct the renal failure patient's metabolic acidosis. Bicarbonate may be preferable to acetate as a source of base in some patients, either because acetate is not metabolized normally (in which case the normally transient increase in "anion gap" in the plasma will persist) or because it may contribute to hypotension during the hemodialysis procedure. A slight respiratory alkalosis is common during dialysis because of loss of CO_2 across the dialyzer and persists transiently at the end of the hemodialysis procedure because, although the extracellular base deficit has been corrected, the respiratory center continues to respond transiently to intracellular acidosis. Calcium levels in the dialysate—3.5 mEq per liter—are higher than ionized calcium levels in blood to allow a calcium influx from the dialysate, since most patients with chronic renal failure are in negative calcium balance. Dialysate flow rates are usually 500 ml per minute and thus the patient's blood "sees" 120 liters of fluid during a standard 4-hour dialysis. Various problems have occurred because of trace metals and other substances in the public water supply, but tap water is now routinely purified by reverse osmosis and/or deionization prior to its use in dialysate.

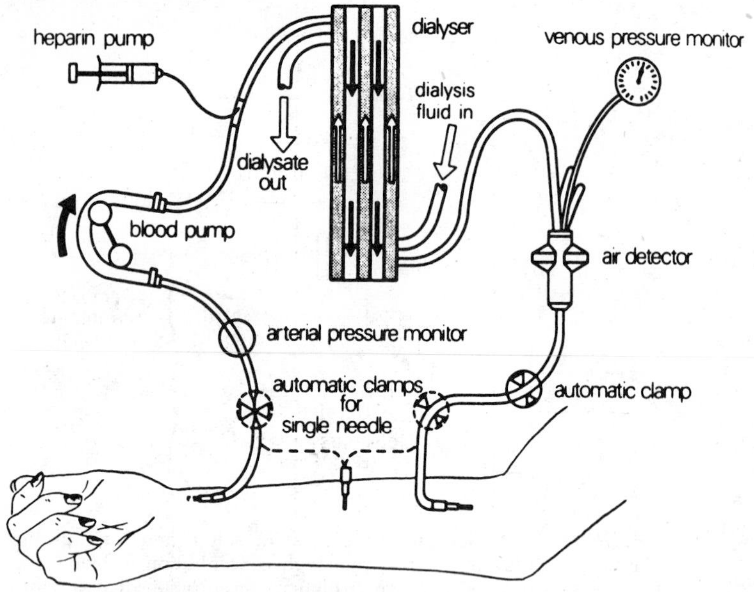

Figure 79–2. Essential components of a dialysis delivery system which, together with the dialyzer, makes up an "artificial kidney." In isolated ultrafiltration no dialysis fluid is used (bypass mode). Also shown is the apparatus for using a single needle for inflow and outflow of blood from the patient. (From Keshaviah PR, Shaldon S. *In* Drukker W, Parsons FM, Maher JF (eds.): Replacement of Renal Function by Dialysis. 2nd ed. Boston, Martinus Nijhoff Publishers, 1983, p. 224.)

Peritoneal Dialysis

In peritoneal dialysis clearances of low molecular weight substances are less than for hemodialysis (for example, a urea clearance of 20 to 25 ml per minute versus 150 ml per minute for hemodialysis), but clearance of some larger, perhaps also toxic, substances is greater because of the greater permeability of the peritoneal membrane to these larger molecules and the longer duration of treatment. When required, fluid removal is carried out by means of osmotic movement of water using high concentrations of glucose (1500 to 4500 mg per deciliter) in the dialysate. Exchange volumes during peritoneal dialysis are commonly 1 to 3 liters each hour. Acute dialysis can be carried out manually using bottles or plastic containers and a stylet catheter, which can be inserted at the bedside under local anesthesia. Several types of automated machines are available that make dialysate from concentrate, deliver set volumes of fluid into the abdomen, and then allow drainage after a set "dwell" time. The commonest type now in use is the cycler, which is relatively simple, uses commercially prepared dialysate in bottles, and automatically cycles up to a total of 16 liters of dialysate in and out of the abdomen for a period of 8 hours (often overnight). Because peritoneal dialysis is less efficient than hemodialysis, dialysis times are much longer (Table 79–1). Therefore chronic intermittent peritoneal dialysis is only practical for use at home.

CLINICAL USE

During hemodialysis, the major limiting factor for clearance of small molecular weight substances such as urea is the "unstirred layer" barrier to diffusion at the blood-membrane interface. Clearance does not increase significantly beyond blood flow rates of 250 ml and dialysate flow rates of 500 ml per minute; surface areas of 1.0 to 1.3 square meters are usually adequate to reduce blood urea by about 50 per cent during a 3- to 4-hour hemodialysis. In contrast, the limitation to clearance of a larger molecular weight substance such as inulin is the permeability of the membrane, and inulin clearance for most commonly used hemodialysis membranes is quite small (Table 79–1). The permeability of the peritoneal membrane (the effective surface area of which is estimated between 0.5 and 1 square meter in adults) for larger molecular weight substances is much greater than the artificial membranes, but dialysate flow rates in intermittent peritoneal dialysis are much less (35 ml per minute). Thus urea clearance for peritoneal dialysis is much less than for hemodialysis, and inulin clearance relatively greater (Table 79–1). Peritoneal blood flow has been estimated at 50 to 100 ml per minute and is clearly a factor that may critically limit clearance in states of markedly reduced cardiac output. Unfortunately the causes of toxicity in the uremic syndrome are poorly understood, so that the ideal dialysis regimen or membrane cannot be defined. Techniques that remove small molecular weight end products of protein metabolism, such as urea, are quite successful and compatible with prolonged survival and reasonable well-being, however.

TABLE 79–1. TIME-AVERAGED CLEARANCE (ml/min)*

Technique	Weekly Duration	Urea Clearance	B_{12} Clearance	Insulin Clearance
		(60)†	(1350)†	(5200)†
Hemodialysis	3 × 4 = 12 hrs	11 (160)‡	2.5 (30)	0.3 (4)
Intermittent PD	4 × 10 = 40 hrs	6 (25)	1.5 (7)	1.2 (5)
CAPD	Continuous	7	5	3
Normal kidney	Continuous	60	120	120

*Does not include residual renal function.
†Molecular weight (daltons).
‡Figures in parenthesis are actual clearances during procedure.
PD, peritoneal dialysis; CAPD, chronic ambulatory peritoneal dialysis.

Until the early 1960's hemodialysis was utilized exclusively for the treatment of acute renal failure, and each use required surgical cannulation of an artery and a vein. Development of the permanently inserted Scribner Teflon shunt between the radial artery and a forearm vein and containing a connector allowed repeated vascular access and made possible the management of irreversible renal failure by chronic intermittent hemodialysis. Today permanent vascular access is usually obtained by creation of an end-to-side arteriovenous fistula in the forearm or insertion of a prosthetic arteriovenous graft when the vessels themselves are inadequate.

Similarly, the use of the various forms of peritoneal dialysis for the chronic treatment of ESRD has depended on the development of a permanent indwelling peritoneal catheter. This is made of radiopaque Silastic 25 cm long and includes an intra-abdominal (located in the pelvis), subcutaneous (with a Dacron felt cuff barrier to bacteria at each end), and external segment. Most ESRD patients continue to be managed, however, by chronic in-center hemodialysis, and only about 20 per cent of all dialysis patients are on some form of home dialysis, including chronic ambulatory peritoneal dialysis.

Initiation of Dialysis

Before initiating chronic dialysis careful discussion with the patient and family should address the issue of whether such treatment is in the patient's best interest. For example, if there is extensive irremediable extrarenal disease, such as severe cerebrovascular disease or a painful malignancy, it may be wiser to continue conservative treatment only.

Initiation of dialysis should occur when conservative management of chronic renal failure is beginning to be inadequate but before the development of uremic symptoms. In general, dialysis becomes necessary at a creatinine clearance of 4 to 8 ml per minute or a serum creatinine of about 10 mg per deciliter. However the patient's general clinical state is more important than the level of blood urea nitrogen or creatinine. It is especially important to institute therapy before the onset of pericarditis, peripheral neuropathy, or an impaired nutritional state secondary to anorexia or other uremic gastrointestinal symptoms, as subsequent recovery is then quite prolonged and mortality rate increased. Vascular access should be placed, if feasible, a few months before dialysis so as to allow it to mature adequately. Of the permanent types of access, only the Scribner shunt is available for use immediately. If uremia develops abruptly, acute vascular access can be maintained for up to several weeks by an indwelling subclavian vein catheter or intermittently via the femoral vein.

In *diabetic nephropathy* renal failure may accelerate microangiopathic complications—especially retinopathy, gastropathy, and peripheral neuropathy—and many nephrologists therefore prefer to initiate replacement therapy earlier in such patients, perhaps when serum creatinine approximates 5 to 8 mg per deciliter. The progression of diabetic glomerulosclerosis to ESRD at that stage also tends to be quite rapid.

Hypertension is an important complication in most patients who reach end-stage renal disease. Antihypertensive medications can usually be tapered after initiation of dialysis, and blood pressure can be controlled by adjustment of plasma and extracellular fluid volume by ultrafiltration during dialysis and by dietary salt and water restriction. Sympatholytic drugs or drugs that cause postural hypotension are best avoided, since they interfere with the ability to remove fluid adequately by ultrafiltration. A reduction in urinary volume commonly accompanies the onset of dialysis because of lessening of solute osmotic diuresis. The concept of "dry weight" is a clinically important one in a chronic dialysis patient, regardless of modality of therapy. This is the postdialysis weight at which the patient has an acceptable blood pressure and a plasma volume adequate for avoiding symptoms of diminished cardiac output or of pulmonary congestion. Short-term changes in weight are always due to salt and water deficits or excesses, but careful supervision is required to detect changes in body mass in either direction over longer periods. Interdialytic weight gains should not exceed 2 to 3 kg but unfortunately often do so in patients who are not compliant with dietary salt and fluid restrictions.

Most dialysis patients thus have "volume-dependent" hypertension and require antihypertensive medications only if they are noncompliant with salt and water intake. In perhaps 10 per cent of patients, however, blood pressure is "renin dependent," and progressive ultrafiltration is accompanied by persistent rebound hypertension after hemodialysis due to rising circulating levels of angiotensin II. Previously bilateral nephrectomy was sometimes employed to control blood pressure in such patients, but the advent of such potent drugs as captopril and minoxidil has virtually eliminated the need for this procedure. Furthermore, it is especially important to avoid bilateral nephrectomy when some recovery of renal function may occur in time, as after an episode of primary or secondary malignant hypertension or after rapidly progressive glomerulonephritis. Indeed, anephric patients fare less well overall during chronic dialysis because of absence of erythropoietin production and, possibly, of 1,25-OH cholecalciferol, and because of loss of residual renal clearance of larger molecular weight substances.

Dialysis disequilibrium describes a syndrome in which confusion, headache, and focal neurologic signs develop owing to more rapid dialysis of solutes from the plasma than from the intracellular compartment, especially from the brain. Thus an osmotic gradient can be set up between brain cells and extracellular fluid and lead to cerebral edema. This complication usually occurs in patients with acute or chronic renal failure and uremic symptomatology and/or a very high blood urea nitrogen (BUN). Short dialysis with a low blood flow usually prevents this problem, which does not occur in maintained chronic dialysis patients and is extremely rare during initiation of any of the forms of peritoneal dialysis because of their lesser efficiency.

TABLE 79–2. RELATIVE INDICATIONS FOR PERITONEAL (PD) OR HEMODIALYSIS (HD) FOR MANAGEMENT OF ACUTE RENAL FAILURE

Clinical Circumstance	Comment
1. Recent cerebral surgery, vascular accident or trauma	PD preferred; risk of hemorrhage with heparin and of fluid shifts in brain during HD
2. Hypercatabolic states (e.g., multiple injuries)	HD preferred; PD may not provide adequate clearance of urea, etc.
3. Recent cardiac surgery or myocardial infarction	PD preferred; increased risks of hypotension and arrythmias with HD
4. Recent abdominal surgery	HD preferred; loss of fluid via incisions during PD; ileus requires surgical placement of PD catheter
5. Acute hemorrhage or severe coagulopathy	PD preferred; but in certain circumstances HD without heparin feasible
6. Complicating severe lung disease	HD preferred; PD may cause atelectasis and impair vital capacity by interfering with movement of diaphragm

Hepatitis B (Hb_sAg) is carried in the plasma of some patients with chronic renal failure, who therefore constitute a serious risk to dialysis staff and other patients, since there is repeated exposure to the patient's blood. Separate dialysis facilities and staff are needed for such patients if home dialysis or transplantation is not feasible. Routine monitoring for Hb_sA_g is now performed in negative patients, and active immunization is available and indicated for patients and staff. Non-A, non-B hepatitis also remains an epidemiologic problem.

Hemodialysis and acute intermittent peritoneal dialysis are also employed in the treatment of acute renal failure, the most frequent cause of which is acute tubular necrosis (see Ch. 77). These patients are often quite ill, and survival is aided by frequent "prophylactic" dialysis to maintain a BUN of less than 100 mg per deciliter. The relative merits of hemodialysis and peritoneal dialysis for acute renal failure are outlined in Table 79–2.

ROUTINE MANAGEMENT

Patients on chronic hemodialysis usually require a slightly reduced protein intake (0.8 to 1.0 gram per kilogram), but a more stringent control of salt and potassium intake, to maintain satisfactory levels of blood urea nitrogen, potassium, and blood pressure. Hyperkalemia remains a significant cause of death in chronic dialysis patients, usually due to dietary indiscretion. Monitoring of adequacy of dialysis requires a combination of assessment of clinical well-being, including nutritional state, and of BUN and serum electrolytes, including calcium and phosphorus. The BUN reflects urea production rates and is dependent on protein intake and endogenous protein catabolism as well as upon adequacy of urea removal by dialysis. Provided nutrition and protein intake are adequate, a BUN less than 90 to 100 mg per deciliter immediately prior to dialysis is usually acceptable. Plasma chemistries are checked monthly, or less often in stable home patients, in the absence of clinical problems. Adequate clearances can usually be achieved by a total of 12 (9 to 15) hours of hemodialysis per week on a thrice weekly schedule. In most patients supplemental oral base (sodium bicarbonate) is not required; serum HCO_3 should be kept above 20 mEq per liter in the predialysis blood. Dialysis is almost always inadequate to maintain serum phosphate in an acceptable range (3.5 to 5.0 mg per deciliter) and, as in the conservative management of renal failure, oral aluminum-containing phosphate binders are necessary. Constipation is a frequent result and needs treatment by, for example, the use of an osmotic cathartic such as 70 per cent sorbitol. Because of loss of water-soluble vitamins, including folic acid, from the blood during dialysis, routine administration of supplements of these substances is necessary. Oral iron is also given because there is a chronic small loss of blood that cannot be returned to the patient at the end of each dialysis. Anabolic steroids such as nandrolone decanoate can improve the red blood cell production in dialysis patients and hence are commonly administered.

COMPLICATIONS OF CHRONIC DIALYSIS (Table 79–3)

The major clinical complications experienced by patients on chronic dialysis are renal osteodystrophy, anemia, vascular access infections and thromboses, pericarditis, and ascites. The major cause of death remains cardiovascular disease, but the high incidence of coronary atherosclerosis probably reflects the risk factors of hypertension and hyperlipidemia (and perhaps of a high calcium-phosphate product) rather than any specific effects of chronic dialysis per se. Dialysis does cause some cardiovascular stress during the procedure owing to ultrafiltration and reduction of plasma volume and to a modest reduction in arterial oxygen levels (by 10 to 20 mm Hg). This latter is due either to hypocarbia secondary to loss of CO_2 across the dialyzer and/or to sequestration of blood leukocytes in alveolar capillaries after the activation of complement by the dialyzer membrane; a transient leukopenia is usual during the first hour of dialysis. Episodes of hypotension and hypoxia secondary to those dialysis effects frequently provoke angina in patients with coronary vascular disease.

Renal osteodystrophy is discussed elsewhere from the standpoint of both pathogenesis and treatment (see Ch. 248). Normal serum levels of calcium, phosphate, bicarbonate, and parathormone should be maintained. Calcium supplements, phosphate binders, and 1,25-OH cholecalciferol may be needed. Rarely soft tissue calcification, hypercalcemia, and progressive osteitis fibrosa cystica may necessitate subtotal parathyroidectomy. Osteomalacia usually responds to 1,25-OH cholecalciferol, but one resistant type, in which an excess of aluminum is found on bone biopsy, appears to respond only to diminishing bone aluminum by chelating agents such as desoxyferamine.

Anemia is a constant finding. The hematocrit in a well-dialyzed, well-nourished dialysis patient is usually in the range of 25 to 35 per cent. However, in anephric patients it is usually 12 to 20 per cent. Transfusion is not indicated unless anemia is contributing to symptoms, heart failure, or angina. The major cause of the anemia appears to be lack of erythropoietin together with depression of erythropoiesis by azotemia. Iron deficiency anemia is not uncommon and may be indicated by a lowered serum ferritin level. Eosinophilia is quite common in chronic dialysis patients and appears to be of little clinical importance.

TABLE 79–3. COMPLICATIONS IN PATIENTS ON CHRONIC DIALYSIS

Accelerated cardiovascular disease	During dialysis
Hypertension	Hypotension
Renal osteodystrophy	Cramps
Anemia	Bleeding
Serositis	Leukopenia with pulmonary sequestration of WBC's
Pericarditis	Hypoxia
"Dialysis ascites"	Electrolyte disturbances
Pleural effusion	Dialysis disequilibrium
Access infections and thrombosis	
Dialysis dementia	
Pseudogout, tenosynovitis	
Pruritus	
Poor nutrition	
Hepatitis B (Hb_sAg) carrier state	

Serositis as manifested by pleural effusion, ascites, or pericarditis may complicate chronic dialysis. The pathogenesis is not established, although onset often accompanies periods of infection, stress, or protein catabolism. The diagnosis in each case is dependent on elimination of other causes. In general the abnormal fluid has the characteristics of an exudate and, especially in the case of the pericardial sac, may be hemorrhagic. Patients with pericardial effusion may develop pericardial tamponade, especially during dialysis when intravascular volume and right heart pressure are being reduced. Atrial arrythmias are also common. If pericardial effusion occurs, dialysis should be carried out daily with very careful control of anticoagulation. If hemodynamic, radiologic, or ultrasonic assessment shows no improvement, surgical treatment by pericardial stripping or medical treatment by pericardiocentesis and insertion of a locally long-acting steroid such as triamcinolone is indicated. "Dialysis ascites" can be an intractable management problem. Poor nutrition and fluid overload often contribute, and insertion of a LeVeen shunt (one-way valve with bacterial filter between peritoneum and vena cava) may be necessary. Tuberculosis is an important differential cause of these complications, and diagnosis is dependent on histology and culture, since anergy is common. Pleural effusion is less common and less troublesome than pericarditis and ascites.

Access infections are commonly due to *Staphylococcus aureus* infection, may be associated with bacteremia or septicemia, or even bacterial endocarditis, and may require excision of the graft. Access problems are the most frequent cause of admission to hospital in the dialysis population. Steal syndromes may develop with pain in the hand during dialysis, especially in patients with diabetic vascular disease. Very high blood flows through fistulas may contribute to congestive heart failure, but this is quite unusual.

Dialysis dementia is a progressive fatal disease of the central nervous system associated with speech and motor defects, dementia, and seizures. It is now much less frequent, probably because of improved procedures for preparation of dialysate water and reduction in its aluminum content. Motor paralysis due to peripheral neuropathy is also now rare in well-dialyzed patients.

Pseudogout and *tenosynovitis* occur quite frequently in dialysis patients and respond well to drugs such as indomethacin. *Pruritus* is a troublesome symptom and is sometimes attributable to a high blood calcium-phosphate solubility product or to hyperparathyroidism. In some cases pruritus, despite correction of the above factors, remains resistant to treatment.

The dialysis procedure itself may be complicated by hypotension and muscle cramps; both are related to rates of ultrafiltration and usually respond to injections of small amounts of hypertonic fluids such as 0.3 M NaCl or 20 per cent mannitol. Contributory causes of hypotension are autonomic insufficiency, diminished cardiac function, and hypotensive drugs. In patients who are prone to ventricular ectopy it is important to avoid hypoxia by supplemental oxygen and rapid changes in serum potassium by modifying dialysate potassium concentration. This is especially true in patients on cardiac glycosides. Other complications of the dialysis procedure are air embolism, bleeding secondary to heparin, loss of blood due to clotting of the dialyzer, and electrolyte disturbances due to errors in the dialysate. Fortunately these are all now quite unusual. Indeed, death or serious morbidity due to complications of the hemodialysis procedure itself in properly trained or supervised patients is now exceedingly rare.

TABLE 79–4. CONTINUOUS AMBULATORY PERITONEAL DIALYSIS (CAPD)

Advantages	Disadvantages
Requires no machine	Peritonitis due to contamination during bag changes*
Maintains constant plasma solutes	Patient time: 4 exchanges at 30 to 40 minutes/7 days per week
Less restricted dietary intake	Loss of protein in dialysate (8 to 12 grams/day)—requires increased protein intake
Less expensive (?)	Hyperlipidemia and obesity (glucose in PD fluid)
No dependence on helpers or nurses	Long-term adequacy of peritoneal membrane as dialyzer (?)
Enhanced mobility	
Better control of blood pressure (?)	
Good control of blood glucose by intraperitoneal insulin in diabetic patients	
Less cardiovascular stress	

*Majority of cases can, however, be treated on an out-patient basis with intraperitoneal antibiotics.

CONTINUOUS AMBULATORY PERITONEAL DIALYSIS (CAPD)

Since its introduction in 1977 this technique has achieved widespread patient acceptance. It makes use of the fact that small molecular weight solutes reach complete equilibration with peritoneal fluid in 4 to 6 hours. Thus the patient exchanges 1.5 to 3.0 liters of sterile dialysate containing hypertonic glucose (1.5, 2.5, or 4.25 per cent) and physiologic electrolytes three to five times a day through a Tenckhoff peritoneal dialysis catheter and is able to maintain adequate removal of solutes and water. Table 79–4 lists the advantages and disadvantages of the technique. Since insulin-dependent diabetics have more complications of vascular access because of their vasculopathy and since regular insulin can be given in the dialysate with excellent control of the blood sugar, CAPD does offer advantages to patients with diabetic glomerulosclerosis. In infants and children the higher peritoneal surface area relative to body size also facilitates CAPD. In contrast to poorer dialysis of small molecular weight solutes as compared to hemodialysis, dialysis of larger molecules (>500 daltons) is increased (see Table 79–1). Larger "middle molecules" may accumulate in chronic hemodialysis patients and contribute to complications such as pericarditis. Many patients have been managed successfully by CAPD for several years, but long-term follow-up is not yet sufficient to be confident of the ultimate success of the procedure. Currently a significant number of patients change their mode of therapy in the first year.

LIMITATIONS OF DIALYSIS

For chronic dialysis, hemodialysis remains the "gold" standard, and many patients continue to do well after over 10 years on this form of treatment. The three-year survival rate for American patients aged 20 to 25 years is 85 per cent, for those 60 to 65 years, 60 per cent, and for those with diabetic renal disease, 40 per cent. This form of treatment is inherently limited, however, not only because of low clearances (see Table 79–1) but also because the endocrine and regulatory functions of the native kidney are not replaced by the "artificial kidney." Indeed, life saving as it is, the latter term is a misnomer; the patient with an endogenous creatinine clearance of even 15 ml per minute is usually better off than one on maintenance chronic dialysis or CAPD.

Drukker W, Parsons FM, Maher JF: Replacement of Renal Function by Dialysis. 2nd ed. Boston, Martinus Nijhoff Publishers, 1983. *This is a complete reference work for all technical and clinical aspects of dialysis.*

79.2. Renal Transplantation

William J. C. Amend, Jr.

HISTORICAL PERSPECTIVE. Clinical renal transplantation had its successful beginnings at the Peter Bent Brigham Hospital in 1954 with the successful implantation of a kidney from a healthy identical twin donor into a young patient with chronic renal failure. This predated by some years the technique of chronic, repetitive hemodialysis and offered hope to patients with chronic renal failure. Unfortunately, most patients do not have an identical twin donor. Success in extending this transplantation technique to patients who were genetically dissimilar to their organ donor (the donor being a relative, nonrelative, or cadaver, or even a subhuman primate) had to await the discovery and use of various immunosuppressant techniques. With chronic dialysis unavailable until 1963, however, these early attempts often resulted in loss, either through transplant rejection (with resultant fatal uremia) or through patient morbidity and death from the necessarily extensive and prolonged immunosuppressant treatments.

From 1960 until the present, advances have been made in organ preservation, knowledge of histocompatibility, tests in vitro involving pretransplant immunologic responses, immunosuppression, and aspects of patient management, so that there is a higher likelihood of transplant functional success coupled with reduced patient mortality. Over the past ten years, a greater utilization of both dialysis and transplantation has occurred from (1) technical and scientific improvements, (2) physician and patient awareness of treatment availability, and (3) economic support for its clinical applications (through legislative appropriation). These developments have permitted a close interdigitation and individualization of these two treatment methods for patients with chronic renal failure. At present, approximately 3500 patients per year receive a renal transplant, and approximately 70,000 patients per year receive some form of chronic dialytic support in the United States.

DONOR ASPECTS. Organ transplants can be generally divided into two types: (1) those from a living donor (related or nonrelated) and (2) those from a cadaver donor.

Living Donor. A prospective donor to a patient with chronic renal failure must meet certain criteria. The donor should have no significant medical history and be of an acceptable age (18 to 60 years). High motivation and normal emotional responses are necessary. Often a psychologic evaluation is recommended. Preliminary tissue-typing tests are performed, including ABO typing, HLA serotyping (human leukocyte antigen typing), and a direct lymphocyte crossmatch between donor lymphocytes and recipient sera. Biologic relatives are preferred, since there is probable tissue-typing compatibility. The post-transplant clinical response can be roughly predicted after this histocompatibility testing and with other immune tests performed in vitro (see Immunologic Aspects, below, and Ch. 436). Finally, the donor undergoes intensive medical testing, culminating in pyelography and renal arteriography. If these medical tests are completely normal, the person can serve as a low-risk donor with the probability of near normalization of renal function following a half-year period of compensatory renal hypertrophy in the remaining kidney. Recently, long-term studies of renal donors at many transplant centers have shown little functional deterioration, proteinuria, or hypertension for the subsequent 2 to 20 years.

Cadaver Donor. Cadaver donations come after death from brain trauma, subarachnoid bleeding, or some other sudden, terminal event that occurs in a previously healthy individual. After brain death has been determined, the next of kin is contacted for permission for organ donation. When permission is given, a transplant team or regional organ bank is contacted for organ procurement. The kidneys are removed and maintained at cold temperatures (4 to 6° C) with either a saline flush solution (cold preservation) or pulsatile perfusion (Belzer technique). The latter allows prolonged storage (up to 72 hours), but is occasionally accompanied by perfusion changes in the kidneys. While the kidneys are stored, the donor-recipient matching is performed at a histocompatibility laboratory, utilizing lymphocytes from donor lymph nodes obtained during the procurement procedure. These tests must be carried out rapidly (within 6 to 24 hours) in order to utilize the cadaver kidney before irreversible, storage-induced damage occurs. Computer-assisted analysis allows for the selection of recipients from a cadaver-transplant waiting list. This necessary speed of matching is in marked contrast to the methodical pretransplant immune testing (sometimes taking weeks) in live-related donor renal transplants.

RECIPIENT CHARACTERISTICS. The transplant recipient may have end-stage renal failure from a variety of causes. The most common are glomerulonephritis, diabetes mellitus, nephrosclerosis, and polycystic disease. Dialysis patients with severe chronic pulmonary disease, with known cancer within three years of surgery, or with known active infection are considered unsuitable transplant candidates.

Recurrent urinary tract infections, persistently high antiglomerular basement membrane antibody levels, or resistant forms of renin-dependent hypertension often indicate the need for pretransplant bilateral nephrectomy. Also, if ureteral reflux is demonstrated with or without positive urine cultures, preliminary bilateral nephrectomy is performed. Recipients with certain forms of renal disease must be carefully informed regarding the absolute and relative risks of recurrent disease possibilities.

IMMUNOLOGIC ASPECTS. ***Histocompatibility.*** Increasing degrees of genetic similarity between donor and recipient confer upon organ transplants increasing chances for successful transplant function. This is evident when the transplant experience using identical twins (isografts) and transplantation from different species (unmodified heterografts) are considered. In the former case, there is no genetic disparity and hence no likelihood of rejection. The transplant success in these instances relates to nonrejection factors such as technical problems or the possibility of recurrent disease. Heterografts are not currently performed, since unmodified, heterotopic antigens present a marked immune stimulus resulting in prompt rejection of this foreign tissue. More usually, organ transplants are performed between two genetically dissimilar members of the same species (allografts or homografts).

Histocompatibility is defined as the degree to which the tissues of two individuals are alike. Cell surface antigens (phenotypes appearing on white cells and endothelial cells) are determined by histocompatibility genes, known as the HLA system. Each genetic locus expresses its phenotypic information independently on human lymphocytes (T and/or B cells). A combination of five genetic loci within the sixth human chromosome is known as the major histocompatibility locus (MHL) and encompasses genotypes for both Class I and Class II antigens. There are probably other important histocompatibility loci, such as the MB and MT antigens, which are less well defined. In addition, there may be other histocompatibility gene sites on other chromosomes. The major histocompatibility complex of man is described more fully in Ch. 436.

The antigens of the serologically defined loci (such as A, B, C, and D_r) can be determined over six hours, whereas the antigens of the lymphocyte-defined loci (D) are determined by lymphocyte blastogenesis occurring in vitro over three to five days. A haplotype is that genetic information (from adjoining gene loci) that would be carried on any one chromosome. All individuals have leukocyte phenotypes that are made up of two haplotypes for the various HLA antigens.

Prior to a transplant, a patient with kidney failure undergoes tissue typing to assess his histocompatibility and to compare this to potential donors. By noting the various A, B, and D_r leukocyte phenotypes (and their distribution) in a family, such as in Figure 79–3, it is possible to construct haplotypes involving these three histocompatibility antigens. In the example shown, the patient is a two-haplotype match to one sister, one-haplotype match to two siblings and both parents, and a zero-haplotype match to one sister. The last sibling would be of the same match grade as a randomly obtained, live-related, or cadaver donor. In addition, ABO compatibility is currently felt to be necessary, so that donor selection includes both red-cell and white-cell tissue antigen systems. If there are no compatible relatives who might be a donor, the potential histocompatibility match from a nonrelative (living or cadaver donor) is shown in Figure 79–3.

As noted in Figure 79–4, functional survival of the transplant is excellent when two full haplotypes (HLA-identical) are shared and is less when only one haplotype is shared. Recently, many centers have employed pretransplant donor-specific blood transfusions, DST (see below under Immune Responses), for one-haplotype as well as zero-haplotype transplants (the latter being completely mismatched, such as a wife-husband match). Thus far, these are as successful as the pairs with the best HLA-match grades. Cadaver kidney transplant results are also depicted in Figure 79–4. HLA and A and B locus matching does not improve cadaver-donated graft success rates in most centers in the United States. On the other hand, pretransplant blood transfusions have an important beneficial effect on graft survival. Recently, matching for the D_r locus has improved cadaver graft success in some, but not all, regions of the United States.

Immune Responses. Organ transplants evoke a variety of responses in the recipient. If there has been previous sensitization (from blood transfusions, previous transplants, or pregnancy) a *hyperacute rejection* can immediately occur. This is based on a recipient antibody-donor endothelial cell reaction and resembles a Shwartzman phenomenon. Resultant cortical necrosis occurs with no treatment possible. This is avoided with carefully performed pretransplant donor-recipient lymphocyte crossmatching. This crossmatching must particularly involve a T-cell type crossmatch.

If a weaker degree of sensitization, perhaps to a minor histocompatibility locus, has occurred, a slightly delayed secondary humoral response can occur. This is termed an *acute accelerated rejection,* which is pathologically similar to the hyperacute rejection. This likewise is irreversible, but it occurs in a delayed manner two to six days post-transplant.

In the more usual circumstances, the allograft is initially invaded by recipient macrophage and monocyte cells. If antigenic differences to the allograft are noted, these cells will process the antigen with a T lymphocyte and activate this T cell in an antigen-specific manner. This cell then circulates back to the reticuloendothelial system (the so-called "afferent arc"). There these altered cells stimulate the central lymphoid system to elicit an immune response (through the "efferent arc"). The response in the central lymphoid system is usually a combination of cellular (T-cell mediated) and humoral (B-cell mediated) types. The former reaction appears to be the prime cause of the initial *acute transplant rejection,* occurring one to three weeks post-transplant. This acute rejection and its outcome depend in part on whether immunosuppressive treatment is effective and on whether certain forms of immune response cells predominate. The types of T cells that may be formed (with varying responses to immunosuppression) include suppressor cells, helper cells, or killer cells (cytotoxic T cells). Helper cell–augmented antibody formation might produce a pathologic picture similar to that seen in acute accelerated rejection. Such an acute rejection would be irreversible but occurring at a later date. Another poor transplant result is seen when circulating antibodies augment *cell-mediated cytotoxicity.* The immune response in a successfully treated rejection episode is often characterized by the host's development of suppressor cells and their dampening immunoregulatory effects. The allograft becomes less immunogenic or the host less responsive to this antigen-specific stimulus through a poorly understood adaptive response.

Later immune reactions against the allograft might occur through three mechanisms: (1) A continued slow antibody formation would first produce pathologic changes and finally clinically recognizable alterations associated with *chronic allograft rejection.* (2) Alterations in the allograft's antigenicity might occur following some sorts of infection, possibly including cytomegalovirus, Epstein-Barr, or other viral infection. This altered allograft antigenicity might then produce a *late immune response,* which might be similar in nature to an acute transplant rejection. (3) The recipient's own immune responses might be

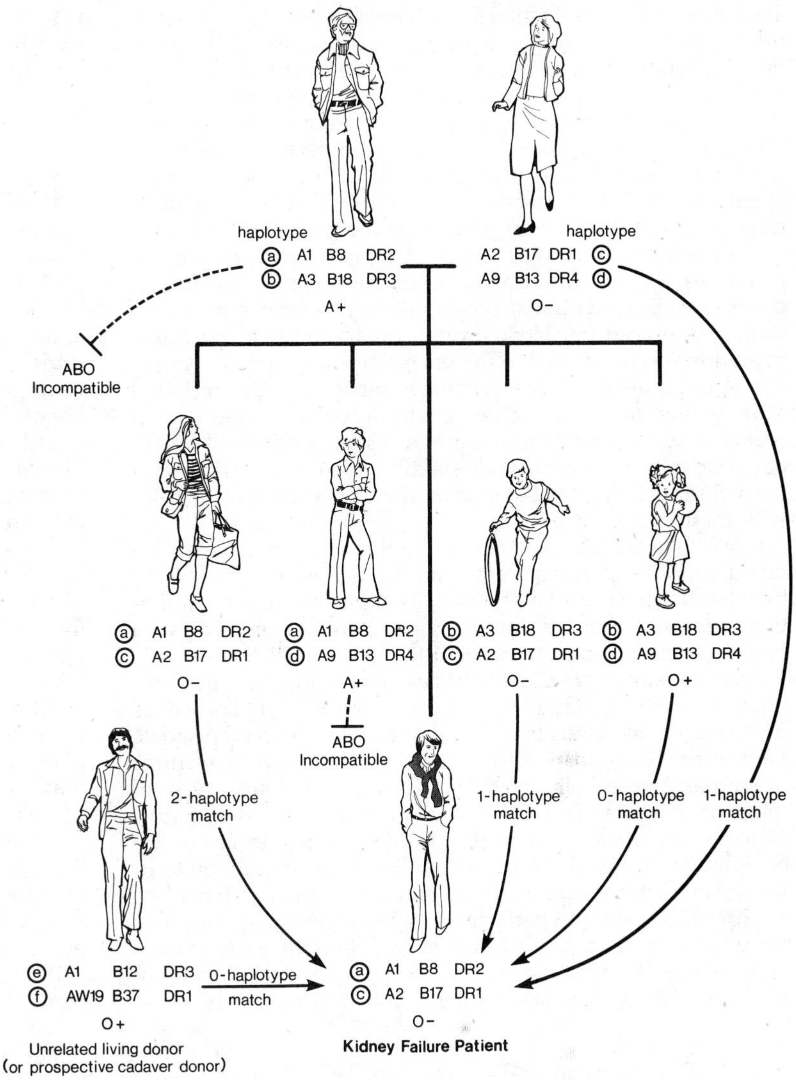

Figure 79–3. Family tree of HL-A genotypes and unrelated HL-A genotype.

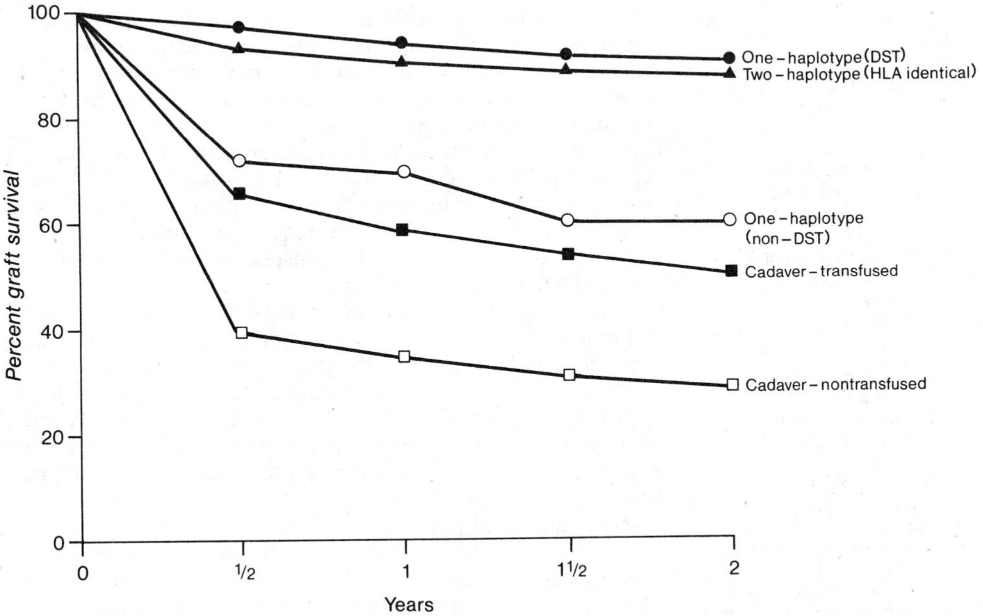

Figure 79–4. Actuarial allograft survivals of various types of renal homotransplants.

altered with a systemic infection and/or illness with a *change in the adaptive response* (e.g., reduction in suppressor cell formation). Alterations in immune responses are already noted in such systemic illnesses as sarcoidosis and viral hepatitis.

Transfusions have recently been shown to markedly improve transplant survivals of both cadaver and related-type transplants. The exact mechanism of this benefit is poorly understood, but may reflect both natural selection and recipient modification. The latter might include the possibility of inducing enhancing antibodies or of developing suppressor cell responses. Lately, interest has been renewed in the use of donor-specific blood transfusions prior to renal transplantation. With this procedure, blood from a prospective kidney transplant donor is transfused to the prospective renal failure patient before the transplant. This technique carries a risk of recipient sensitization, which must be serially tested by using careful lymphocyte crossmatch techniques. Less sensitization of potential recipients to these donor-specific blood transfusions has been observed if stored blood is used or if azathioprine is given with the transfusions.

CLINICAL ASPECTS. The clinical course following transplantation contains features which can be divided on a temporal basis, and which can be additionally separated into complications that are primarily immunologic, surgical, or medical in nature. These complications are listed in Table 79–5.

Early Immunologic Complications. As mentioned, the three types of early rejection seen post-transplant are known as hyperacute, acute-accelerated, and acute-rejection episodes. Pathologically, they are differentiated by characteristic features of humoral or cellular reaction. Clinically, the first type of rejection presents as frank intraoperative or early postoperative oligo-anuria, which must be quickly differentiated from surgical complications. Renal scan flow studies with pertechnetate or transplant arteriography show nonvisualization. Transplant nephrectomy must be performed. Acute-accelerated rejections occur several days post-transplant and present as fulminant rejections with fever, oliguria, tenderness, and enlargement of the graft. Often, thrombocytopenia and microangiopathic hemolytic anemia are found. Again, renal scans will reveal little or no allograft blood flow, consistent with cortical necrosis. The course is that of irreversible renal failure, which again results in the need for transplant nephrectomy. This form of rejection represents a secondary humoral or cell-mediated response.

TABLE 79–5. COMPLICATIONS FOLLOWING RENAL TRANSPLANTATION

	Early Complications (< 2 months)	Late Complications (> 2 months)
Immunologic	Hyperacute rejection Acute accelerated rejection Acute rejection	Acute rejection Chronic rejection
Surgical	Procurement/perfusion injury Urinary leak Obstruction	Lymphocele Reflux Obstruction-stone, cicatrization Renal artery stenosis
Medical	Renal failure—acute tubular necrosis, acute rejection	Progressive renal failure or nephrotic syndrome—chronic rejection, recurrent disease Transplant pyelonephritis Hypertension Atherosclerotic events Erythrocytosis
Immunosuppression-related	Impaired host defense—infections Moon facies, obesity Poor wound healing Gastrointestinal bleeding Leukopenia, thrombocytopenia Steroid psychosis	Impaired host defense—infections Moon facies, obesity Aseptic necrosis, osteoporosis Steroid myopathy Hypophosphatemia Cataracts Steroid hyperglycemia Neoplasia Hepatitis, pancreatitis

The most common type of rejection, acute rejection, occurs after the first week post-transplant. It is felt to be a primary, cell-mediated process against the foreign donor cells. It is characterized by allograft enlargement, fever, malaise, oliguria, hypertension, and reduced renal clearances. Renal scans will initially show a reduction in excretion with cortical retention, followed in several days by reductions in cortical uptake as well. If the rejection episode occurs during a period of acute tubular necrosis, its diagnosis may be delayed, being made either by serial scan assessment or by a transplant biopsy during a febrile episode. Elevated levels of urinary beta-2 microglobulins also help distinguish the rejection episode from coexisting acute tubular necrosis (ATN). Lymphocyturia is often found and may be helpful, along with a negative urine culture, in ruling out allograft pyelonephritis. Renal biopsies performed at this time reveal interstitial edema and foci of small lymphocytes in peritubular areas. Additional immunosuppressive therapy (with prednisone, antithymocyte globulin, allograft radiation) at this time usually has both anti-inflammatory and immunologic effects. The typical acute rejection episode lasts five to ten days, with some cases appearing to develop a postrejection ATN (with a prolonged recovery phase). Patients with multiple or severe early rejections have worse allograft functional outcomes (at one, two, and five years) than patients without. Acute rejection episodes occur more commonly (80 per cent versus 50 per cent) after cadaver renal transplantation than after live-donor transplantation. No rejection episodes occur after identical twin transplantation (isografts).

Early Surgical Complications. After cadaver transplantation, there may be initial ATN on the basis of donor-agonal changes, warm ischemia (in excess of 30 minutes), or excessive donor-sympathetic responses at or near the time of cadaver organ procurement. ATN per se does not affect the eventual transplant outcome. The patient will, however, require post-transplant dialysis. Rarely, storage or perfusion injury can occur. In either case, a technically poor result will occur with suboptimal renal function. Careful attention to the technical aspects of cadaver kidney procurement reduces these possibilities. These problems are usually not seen with live donor transplants, since there can be careful preoperative management of the donor's hydration status and a marked reduction in warm ischemic injury. Attentive surgical technique lowers the possibilities of vesicoureteral reflux, of urinary leak from the neocystostomy site, and of lymphocele formation.

Early Medical Complications. Medical problems initially noted post-transplant include continuing renal failure (from ATN or rejection), during which the patient requires dialysis. Hypophosphatemia can be seen after normal renal function is regained. Persisting secondary hyperparathyroidism causes exaggerated phosphaturia. This parathyroid hyperplasia usually regresses during the first half year following successful transplantation. Correction of the patient's anemia or an increase in a diabetic patient's daily insulin requirement gives a favorable transplant prognosis, since the transplanted kidney has already begun renal endocrine function.

Immunosuppression commonly used following renal transplantation may include one or a combination of glucocorticosteroids, azathioprine or cyclophosphamide, antithymocyte globulin, cyclosporin A, or some other lymphocyte depletion technique such as thoracic duct drainage or, more recently, total lymph node irradiation. All these therapies confer what is termed "nonspecific immunosuppression." Despite different mechanisms of action, generalized impairments of cell- or humoral-mediated immune responses are produced.

Hypercortisolism accounts for many of the undesired side effects and morbidity in renal transplant patients. In the early post-transplant period, poor wound healing, reduced host defenses, psychologic changes, and steroid-induced hyperglycemia are particularly common. The acquired moon facies is disturbing to most individuals. Growth may be retarded in children receiving daily glucocorticosteroids. In an attempt to reduce these problems, many transplant patients are shifted to once daily or alternate-day dose regimens (see Ch. 29). Other immunosuppressive agents also reduce host defenses in a nonspecific fashion. The patient becomes more susceptible to viral, protozoal, fungal, or bacterial infection. Infections, particularly pulmonary, must be aggressively diagnosed and specific treatment rapidly begun. The patient's immunosuppression should be reduced if infection is suspected, even at the potential risk of transplant rejection loss. Bone marrow suppression, liver abnormalities, or hemorrhagic cystitis can also occur from one or more of these antimetabolites. The type and dosage of the drugs must be adjusted with monitoring of these signs.

Late Immunologic Complications. Rarely does an acute rejection process occur more than two to three months after a transplant. This may occur either spontaneously or more frequently following an abrupt change in immunosuppressant therapy. Usually, rejection processes are more of a chronic, vascular type in the months to years following the transplant. Chronic rejections are clinically asymptomatic and are detected by renal functional abnormalities (progressive azotemia, proteinuria) and often have associated hypertension.

Late Surgical Complications. Late problems can be primarily of a urologic type. Vesicoureteral reflux is not seen if the reflux-correcting "tunnel" procedure is employed at the time of transplantation. Lymphoceles may not be detected until years after the transplant and can be associated with partial obstruction, infection, or hypertension. Since allografts are denervated, stone passage is painless and is usually associated only with (temporary) renal impairment, hematuria, or signs of an associated urinary tract infection.

Late Medical Complications. In the months and years following a renal transplant, several medical problems can affect patients. Atherosclerotic disease, already a noteworthy complication of dialysis, is frequently present. Predisposing risk factors include significant hypertension and lipid abnormalities seen during uremia and dialysis. Opportunistic infectious problems still occur. Careful evaluation for any post-transplant patient with a febrile illness is necessary. Fungal, protozoal, or viral infections are particularly serious and require rapid diagnosis and supportive therapy. Immunosuppression should be diminished if host resistance is compromised. Aseptic necrosis or osteonecrosis, particularly of weight-bearing joints, is an unfortunate complication seen in 15 per cent of these patients. It principally affects hip, knee, and shoulder joints and is related to pre-existing secondary hyperparathyroidism, in addition to the transplant corticosteroid therapy. Excellent rehabilitation therapy, however, can be provided with arthroplastic surgery. Hypertension frequently occurs after transplantation and may be related to rejection (either acute or chronic), residual kidney or renal pressor mechanisms (from the native kidneys), glucocorticoid or mineralocorticoid effects, urologic abnormalities (lymphoceles or obstruction), or transplant renal artery stenosis. Evaluation of severe hypertension necessitates a urologic and renovascular workup, with the frequent need for selective venous renin measurements from three kidney sites. Infusions of angiotensin-converting enzyme inhibitors might also be important in detecting renin-dependent, angiotensinogenic hypertension.

Certain forms of neoplasms are particularly noted in transplant patients. Cervical dysplasia and carcinoma may be related to herpes type 2 involvement. Excessive cases of so-called immunoblastic lymphoma, leukemia, and cutaneous malignancies have also been noted. However, a generalized increase of malignancies (solid tumors as well as other forms of lymphoproliferative disorders) has not been demonstrated. It is not known whether the immunosuppression lowers tumor surveillance in these patients, or whether the allograft alters the patient's own immune response (from a chronic antigen exposure). Rarely, a patient will develop post-transplant erythrocytosis. Such patients should be evaluated to establish the primary nature of this disorder. Often, recurrent phlebotomies are necessary for one to two years.

TABLE 79–6. RECURRENT DISEASES OF RENAL ALLOGRAFTS

Primary Disease	Comments
Membranous glomerulonephritis	Same immunologic pattern; appearance is similar to chronic rejection
Rapidly progressive glomerulonephritis	Fulminant course in isografts; "crescents" on pathology; graft failure
Anti-GBM glomerulonephritis	With and without preliminary bilateral nephrectomy; graft failure
Juxtamedullary focal glomerulosclerosis	With and without graft failure
IgA nephropathy	Immunofluorescence without disease
Membranoproliferative disease	
Type 1	With and without graft failure
Type 2 ("dense deposit")	Graft failure
Oxalosis	Deposits and graft failure
Cystinosis	Deposits without graft failure
Henoch-Schönlein syndrome	
Diabetes mellitus	Glomerular lesions nodular and diffuse; no graft failure (yet)

The transplant kidney may develop the nephrotic syndrome with or without clearance deterioration. Usually, particularly if the primary renal disease was nonimmunologic, this is secondary to chronic rejection. By pathologic examination, chronic rejection has elements of either a predominantly arteriolar lesion with an intimal reaction or of a glomerular lesion with generalized basement membrane thickening and mesangial proliferation. Clinically, progressive hypertension and proteinuria are hallmark features of early phases of chronic rejection, with the eventual development of intractable renal failure. On the other hand, patients with certain forms of renal disease (Table 79–6) may be predisposed to recurrence of the original disease in their allografts. This was first noted in a high frequency with identical twin transplants, but must be suspected in all patients with these primary renal diseases. Renal biopsy or immunologic tests must be performed for diagnosis. Treatment of such conditions in the allograft is the same as that of the primary disease. Transplant pyelonephritis is characterized by pain and swelling over the transplant, and usual accompanying renal functional deterioration. Potential urologic problems should be tested for in this circumstance.

Transplant patients often regain fertility, and contraceptive advice is indicated. Despite theoretical risks of genetic malformation and a higher incidence of miscarriage and spermatozoal malformation, no severe congenital malformations have been described, and many successful pregnancies and impregnations have occurred.

Psychologically, much anxiety and depression can occur with transplant- or immunosuppressive-related problems. The glucocorticoids directly affect the emotions of such patients, making the reactive nature of their emotional responses even more labile during such stresses. Despite an otherwise excellent physical status, some patients remain overly concerned that the transplant may "fail." Most patients with well-functioning renal transplants attain a degree of rehabilitation similar to their premorbid status.

Over a period of time, the patient seems to adapt immunologically to the transplant in a poorly understood manner. Even after an initial success of two years or more, there continues to be a relationship between the degree of histocompatibility and the long-range functional prognosis. There is a greater chance of late transplant failure in cadaver renal transplants than in forms of related renal transplants. Also, one-haplotype transplants do less well than fully matched sibling pairs. After an initial two years of transplant success, the T½ or half-life probabilities for two-haplotype transplants are 34 years, for one-haplotype transplants 10 years, and for cadaver transplants 7.5 years. This analysis is practically important when discussing the long-range prognosis with a transplant recipient. The prognosis of certain patient populations, those with diabetes, for instance, is lessened because of systemic complications in these groups.

When a patient rejects a first renal transplant within the first year, transplant nephrectomy is usually necessary. Rejected foreign tissue left in situ will produce a symptom constellation of fever, allograft tenderness, generalized malaise, cachexia, and weight loss. Transplants that undergo chronic rejection, if well tolerated, may be left in place.

Retransplantation (a second or third time) can be attempted if the first transplant fails. An effort is made to avoid similar histocompatibility antigens in subsequent transplants, or at least to assess whether specifically shared lymphocytotoxic antibodies have developed subsequent to the first transplant. A similar clinical course (regarding rejection probabilities) can be anticipated in later transplants, suggesting that the recipients' own immune regulation is an important factor in transplant success. Choosing a different immunosuppressive agent for a second transplant might be important to attain better transplant success.

This chapter on renal transplantation concludes with some comments on patient survival. Three to 5 per cent of patients receiving a cadaver renal transplant are at risk of dying each year. Recipients of related donor transplants have improved patient survival likelihoods. The risk of death in certain patient groups (transplant recipients with diabetes or other systemic disease) is higher. All are comparable to the chronic dialysis mortality experience if transplant units encourage close integration with dialysis. A successful transplant permits the best opportunity for complete rehabilitation of a patient with chronic renal failure.

Guttman RD: Renal transplantation. N Engl J Med 301:975, 1979. *Well-organized review of subject. Lengthy and complete reference list.*

Merrill JP: Dialysis versus transplantation in the treatment of end stage renal disease. Ann Rev Med 29:343, 1978. *Good review of the interrelationship between these two treatment methods.*

Strom TB: The improving utility of renal transplantation in the management of end-stage renal disease. Am J Med 73:105, 1982. *A thorough review of the subject, particularly good with the discussion of immunosuppression.*

80. GLOMERULAR DISORDERS

William G. Couser

About 60,000 patients in the United States require hemodialysis for chronic renal failure at an annual cost in excess of one billion dollars. Two thirds of these have some glomerular disease. First described in the writings of Richard Bright in the early nineteenth century, these diseases have subsequently intrigued many clinician-investigators who have attempted to separate and classify them solely on the basis of clinical manifestations and histopathology, the latter usually available only following autopsy. Inconsistent terminology and confusing classification systems proliferated, sufficient to befuddle generations of medical students. Until recently nephrologists usually concentrated on studying physiologic aspects of renal function about which more was known and upon which far more precise measurements could be made.

The past two decades have witnessed a marked improvement in this situation for several reasons: (1) Experimental models of glomerular diseases have been produced by immunizing animals with either renal antigens or various foreign proteins, thus confirming a long-held suspicion that most such diseases have an immunologic basis. (2) The histologic and functional abnormalities in these models were found to be associated with the development of immune deposits in glomeruli, demonstrated by immunofluorescence (IF) and electron microscopy (EM). (3) The factors that determine the quantity, size, and composition of these deposits have been studied systematically, and the mechanisms by which they lead to tissue injury have been defined. (4) The widespread application of percutaneous renal biopsy as a routine clinical diagnostic tool has allowed experimental observations to be applied to understanding the pathogenesis of glomerular lesions in man.

New concepts have emerged regarding how glomerular immune deposits form, the factors that determine glomerular permeability to protein in normal and diseased states, the immunogenetic basis for renal diseases, and the processes that lead from acute renal disease to progressive renal failure. Many of these advances are reviewed in Chapter 74. In this chapter, glomerular diseases are classified on a clinical basis into three groups: (1) primary renal diseases that usually present with the abrupt onset of hematuria, red cell casts, proteinuria, and decreased glomerular filtration rate (acute nephritic syndrome or glomerulonephritis [GN]); (2) primary renal diseases that usually present with the insidious onset of heavy proteinuria and relatively normal glomerular filtration rate (nephrotic syndrome); and (3) secondary glomerular diseases resulting from renal involvement by a variety of systemic illnesses, which may be either nephritic or nephrotic. This approach has the virtue of simplicity, but it is useful only if its limitations are fully appreciated. Separation between primary and secondary renal diseases is sometimes difficult and arbitrary. For example, IgG-IgA nephritis is recognized as a primary renal disease and Henoch-Schönlein purpura is classified as a secondary one, although they probably represent only differing clinical manifestations of the same process and often overlap. All of the diseases that present as acute GN may cause the nephrotic syndrome, although they do so uncommonly, and some nephrotic glomerular diseases may occasionally exhibit nephritic features.

IMMUNE MECHANISMS AND THE GLOMERULAR RESPONSE TO INJURY

Two immunologic mechanisms of glomerular disease are generally accepted (see Ch. 74 for details): (1) Rare patients develop glomerulonephritis due to deposition of antibody to glomerular basement membrane (GBM) antigens, which results in a typical uninterrupted linear staining pattern along all glomerular capillary walls by immunofluorescence microscopy (see Fig. 80–7). (2) Much more commonly glomerulonephritis is associated with discontinuous, or granular, deposits of immunoglobulin and complement (see Figs. 80–2*B*, 80–3*B*, and 80–8). These deposits may occur at three sites: (1) within the glomerular mesangium as in IgG-IgA nephropathy, Henoch-Schönlein purpura, and early lupus nephritis; (2) along the subendothelial surface of the capillary wall between endothelial cells and GBM, as seen in more severe forms of lupus nephritis and Type I membranoproliferative glomerulonephritis (MPGN); and (3) on the outer, subepithelial surface of the capillary wall, as in membranous nephropathy and the so-called subepithelial "humps" in post-streptococcal glomerulonephritis. Granular, or immune complex, deposits at mesangial and subendothelial sites can result either from the passive glomerular trapping of preformed immune complexes from the circulation, or they may form locally or in situ owing to initial glomerular localization of free antigens followed by antibody binding to them. Subepithelial immune complex deposits appear to form only on a local basis. Figure 80–1 illustrates schematically how immune deposits at each of these sites are related to normal glomerular structures and some of the morphologic lesions that result.

Several glomerular diseases that are believed to be immunologically mediated do not have immune deposit formation in glomeruli. For example, minimal change nephrotic syndrome (MCNS) exhibits a marked increase in capillary wall permeability without immune deposits or histologic changes; and idiopathic rapidly progressive glomerulonephritis (RPGN) is characterized by severe glomerular inflammatory changes with crescent formation without detectable immune deposits.

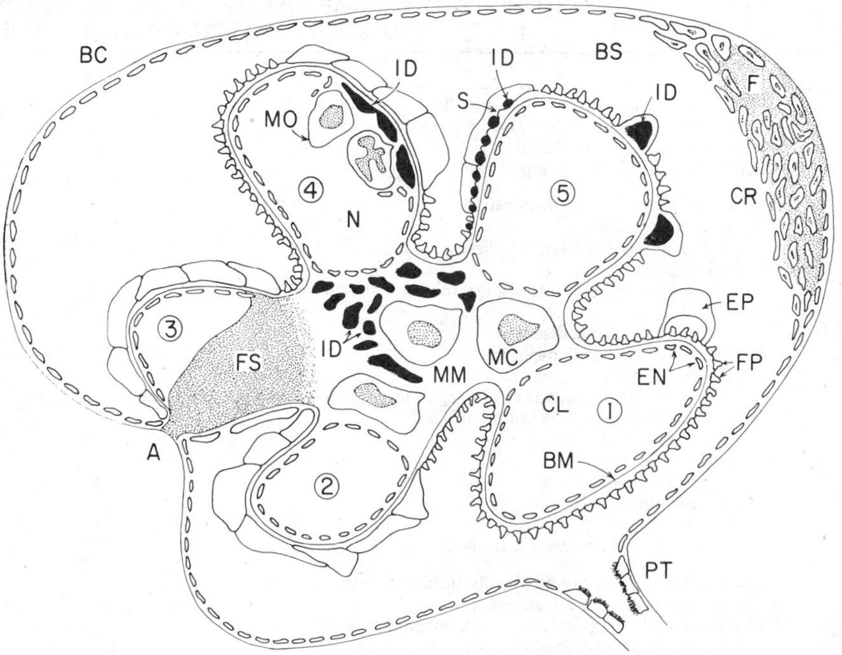

Figure 80–1. A highly schematized illustration of a cross-section of a single glomerulus showing normal glomerular architecture and some of the characteristic changes seen in glomerular diseases. One lobule with five capillary loops is illustrated within Bowman's capsule (BC). The capillary loops are supported by the intercapillary mesangium containing mesangial cells (MC) and mesangial matrix (MM). Note that the normal glomerular capillary wall (loop 1) is composed of three layers: Endothelial cells (EN), basement membrane (BM), and epithelial cells (EP) with epithelial cell foot processes (FP).

Loop 2 illustrates minimal change nephrotic syndrome with only diffuse effacement, or "fusion," of epithelial cell foot processes. Foot process effacement is also seen in other areas where increased capillary permeability with proteinuria would occur. In loop 3 a focal sclerotic lesion (FS) is seen with collapse of the capillary loop and adhesion (A) to Bowman's capsule. Immune complex deposits (ID) are shown in black at three sites: Within the mesangial matrix (loop 4); as subendothelial deposits between endothelial cells and basement membrane as seen in class IV SLE and type I MPGN (loop 4); and as the diffuse, finely granular subepithelial deposits of membranous nephropathy (left, loop 5) with intervening "spikes" (S) of basement membrane, or the larger, more widely spaced subepithelial humps (right, loop 5) seen in post-streptococcal glomerulonephritis. Mesangial and subendothelial deposits usually elicit an infiltrate of neutrophils (N) and monocytes (MO) that may displace endothelial cells and directly injure basement membrane, as shown in loop 4. With severe injury, fibrin (F) leakage into Bowman's space (BS) may induce formation of a cellular crescent (CR) composed of proliferating parietal epithelial cells and circulating mononuclear cells as shown from 1 to 3 o'clock. CL = Capillary lumen; PT = proximal tubule.

The type and severity of histologic and functional glomerular disease induced by immune deposits in glomeruli depend on many factors, including the quantity, composition, and site of the deposits. Most glomerular antibody deposits contain predominantly IgG, which activates complement via the classic complement pathway. When deposits are in mesangial and subendothelial sites they are accessible to circulating inflammatory cells. Chemotactic and immune adherence mechanisms recruit participation of neutrophils and macrophages, and these effector cells cause direct damage to glomeruli by release of proteolytic enzymes and toxic oxygen metabolites. An inflammatory glomerular lesion results, with clinical manifestations that include hematuria, proteinuria, and loss of renal function. IgA deposits activate complement less well and predominantly by the alternate complement pathway. When immune deposits form at a subepithelial site, as in membranous nephropathy, they are not accessible to circulating cells and the resulting lesion is a noninflammatory one, with the nephrotic syndrome apparently induced by a direct, probably membranolytic, effect of complement activation on capillary wall permeability. Thus, glomerular immune complex deposits may induce a spectrum of both clinical and histologic manifestations. The clinical consequences range from the acute nephritic syndrome with acute renal failure, as seen in some cases of post-streptococcal glomerulonephritis, to idiopathic nephrotic syndrome with normal renal function, as in membranous nephropathy. Table 80–1 lists the glomerular diseases, classified by the mechanisms that produce them and with their major clinical presentations noted.

ACUTE GLOMERULONEPHRITIS

Pathophysiology of the Acute Nephritic Syndrome

The terms *acute GN* and *acute nephritic syndrome,* which are synonymous, refer to the abrupt onset of hematuria and proteinuria, usually associated with some impairment in renal function and often with retention of salt and water, leading to hypertension and edema. Virtually all of these abnormalities are present in patients with post-streptococcal GN (PSGN) but are less frequently found in other causes of the acute nephritic syndrome. The most common primary renal diseases that produce the acute nephritic syndrome are summarized in Table 80–2, where their major distinguishing clinical and pathologic features are compared. The syndrome may also result from membranoproliferative glomerulonephritis (MPGN), which is discussed under diseases that cause the nephrotic syndrome, and from glomerular involvement in several of the systemic diseases to be discussed subsequently.

HEMATURIA. Hematuria is the hallmark of the acute nephritic syndrome. When hematuria is associated with proteinuria (> 500 mg per day) and red blood cell (RBC) casts, it usually reflects an acute glomerular inflammatory process that may have the potential for rapid loss of renal function. This contrasts with several less inflammatory lesions that present primarily with proteinuria and the nephrotic syndrome (see p. 578). RBC's probably reach the urine through breaks or "gaps" in the capillary wall and form casts as they become embedded in concentrated tubular fluid with an increased protein concentration. Hematuria and RBC casts may occasionally be seen in other diseases in which capillary wall disruption occurs, such as malignant hypertension and hereditary nephritis.

PROTEINURIA. In acute GN, proteinuria invariably accompanies hematuria but rarely exceeds 3.5 grams per day and is therefore in the "non-nephrotic" range. Proteinuria in acute GN reflects an increased urinary content of serum proteins due to some combination of three factors: (1) A generalized increase in the permeability characteristics of the glomerular capillary wall itself, (2) altered glomerular hemodynamics, and (3) mechanical disruptions in capillary wall structure. Thus proteinuria in acute GN is "nonselective" and contains serum globulins as well as albumin. The pathophysiology of glomerular protein excretion is discussed in more detail below under Nephrotic Syndrome.

IMPAIRED RENAL FUNCTION. When glomerular inflammation severe enough to cause hematuria and proteinuria is present, the glomerular filtration rate (GFR) is usually reduced. This may range from a minimal reduction in GFR with normal serum creatinine values to oliguria or anuria requiring dialysis. Multiple factors account for the reduced GFR, including the effects of acute immune injury on glomerular pathophysiology and

TABLE 80–1. GLOMERULAR DISEASES CLASSIFIED BY IMMUNOLOGIC MECHANISMS AND THEIR PRINCIPAL CLINICAL MANIFESTATIONS

	Nephritis	Nephrotic Syndrome
Anti-GBM Antibody Glomerulonephritis		
With pulmonary involvement (Goodpasture's syndrome)	Yes	Rare
Without pulmonary involvement	Yes	Rare
Complicating membranous nephropathy	Yes	Yes
Immune Complex Glomerulonephritis		
Primary renal diseases		
IgG-IgA nephropathy (Berger's disease)	Yes	Rare
Membranous nephropathy	No	Yes
Type I membranoproliferative glomerulonephritis (MPGN)	Yes	Yes
Idiopathic	Yes	Rare
Associated with systemic diseases		
Postinfectious glomerulonephritis		
Post-streptococcal	Yes	Rare
Following other bacterial, viral, fungal, mycoplasmal, protozoal, spirochetal infections	Yes	Variable
Subacute bacterial endocarditis (SBE)	Yes	Rare
"Shunt nephritis"	Yes	Yes
Visceral abscesses	Yes	No
Collagen-vascular diseases		
Systemic lupus erythematosus (SLE)	Yes	Yes
Henoch-Schönlein purpura (HSP)	Yes	Yes
Essential mixed cryoglobulinemia (EMC)	Yes	Yes
Diseases of Undefined but Probably Immune Pathogenesis		
Minimal change–focal sclerosis group	No	Yes
Idiopathic rapidly progressive glomerulonephritis (RPGN)	Yes	Rare
Type II MPGN (dense deposit disease)	Yes	Yes
Vasculitides: Polyarteritis nodosa (PAN)	Yes	Rare
Hypersensitivity vasculitis	Yes	No
Wegener's granulomatosis	Yes	Rare
Hemolytic-uremic syndrome (HUS) and thrombotic thrombocytopenic purpura (TTP)	Rare	No

the development of glomerular intracapillary thromboses, acute tubular necrosis secondary to glomerular ischemia, tubular obstruction by casts, and compression of the glomerular tuft by proliferating cells or epithelial cell crescent formation. The return of renal function to normal depends not only on cessation of the process that initiated the injury but also on the extent of irreversible structural changes that have occurred, such as necrosis, sclerosis, and fibrosis.

HYPERTENSION. Hypertension is a common manifestation of the acute nephritic syndrome in PSGN and may be a presenting sign in older patients. It is largely volume dependent, reflecting impaired renal excretion of sodium and water with reduced levels of plasma renin and aldosterone. Hypertension can generally be controlled by strict adherence to sodium restriction.

EDEMA. Edema in the acute nephritic syndrome, like hypertension, reflects extracellular fluid volume expansion due to renal retention of salt and water. The mechanisms of renal sodium retention in acute GN are poorly understood but include a reduced filtered sodium load as well as enhanced

TABLE 80–2. SUMMARY OF PRIMARY RENAL DISEASES THAT PRESENT AS ACUTE GLOMERULONEPHRITIS

Diseases	Post-Streptococcal Glomerulonephritis (PSGN)	IgG-IgA Nephritis	Goodpasture's Syndrome	Idiopathic Rapidly Progressive Glomerulonephritis (RPGN)
Clinical Manifestations				
Age and sex	All ages, mean 7, 2:1 male	15–35, 2:1 male	15–30, 6:1 male	mean 58, 2:1 male
Acute nephritic syndrome	90%	50%	90%	90%
Asymptomatic hematuria	Occasionally	50%	Rare	Rare
Nephrotic syndrome	10–20%	Rare	Rare	10–20%
Hypertension	70%	30–50%	Rare	25%
Acute renal failure	50% (transient)	Very rare	50%	60%
Other	1–3 week latent period	Follows viral syndromes	Pulmonary hemorrhage; iron-deficiency anemia	None
Laboratory Findings	↑ ASO titers (70%) Positive streptozyme (95%) ↓ C3-C9 Normal C1, C4	↑ Serum IgA (50%) IgA in dermal capillaries	Positive anti-GBM antibody	None
Immunogenetics	HLA B12, D "EN" (9)[1]	HLA Bw 35, DR4 (4)[1]	HLA DR2 (16)[1]	None established
Renal Pathology				
Light microscopy	Diffuse proliferation	Focal proliferation	Focal→diffuse proliferation with crescents	Crescentic GN
Immunofluorescence	Granular IgG, C3	Diffuse mesangial IgA	Linear IgG, C3	No immune deposits
Electron microscopy	Subepithelial humps	Mesangial deposits	No deposits	No deposits
Prognosis	95% resolve spontaneously 5% RPGN or slowly progressive	Slow progression in 25–50%	75% stabilize or improve if treated early	75% stabilize or improve if treated early
Treatment	Supportive	None established	Plasma exchange, steroids, cyclophosphamide	Steroid pulse therapy and/or plasma exchange

[1]Relative Risk

sodium reabsorption in either the distal nephron or deep juxtamedullary nephrons. Edema and fluid retention are seen in over 90 per cent of patients with acute PSGN but are less common in other diseases causing the acute nephritic syndrome. Unlike nephrotic edema, edema in the nephritic syndrome is often present in nondependent areas such as eyelids, face, and hands. The key to management is effective sodium restriction, since diuretics may not be effective in the acute stage of GN.

Glassock RJ, Cohen AH, Bennett CM, Martinez-Maldonado M: Primary glomerular diseases. *In* Brenner BM, Rector FC Jr. (eds.): The Kidney. 2nd ed. Philadelphia, W. B. Saunders Company, 1981, p 1351. *The introduction in this chapter contains a detailed analysis of the pathophysiology of the acute nephritic syndrome as defined by clinical and experimental studies.*

Isolated Hematuria

The presence of persistent abnormal hematuria (more than five RBC's per high power field in more than one fresh-voided urine specimen), without systemic disease, RBC casts, significant proteinuria, or impaired renal function, is a common medical problem that may or may not reflect renal parenchymal disease. It is more common in children and adolescents than in adults. A careful medical and urologic evaluation must be performed with appropriate laboratory, radiologic, and urologic procedures to exclude nonglomerular lesions of the urinary tract such as infection, prostatism, papillary necrosis, polycystic and medullary sponge kidney, renal or urinary tract tumors, arteriovenous malformations, renal stones, blood dyscrasias, and hemoglobinopathies. The "loin pain–hematuria syndrome" is a disorder usually seen in young women taking oral contraceptives who develop recurrent episodes of gross hematuria accompanied by loin pain and mild hypertension in the absence of proteinuria or reduced renal function. The condition appears to be benign and is reversible when oral contraceptives are discontinued.

If no cause of hematuria can be found and no evidence of systemic or renal disease is present, isolated hematuria appears to be a benign entity, and only careful follow-up is indicated. Renal biopsy would be performed in such patients only if evidence of progressive renal disease developed or if the patient required further evaluation for other purposes such as insurance or employment. When such patients do undergo renal biopsy, the results usually reveal a mild, nonprogressive form of glomerular disease, often focal GN with or without mesangial IgA deposits. Only about 20 per cent of such patients will have normal renal biopsies.

Burden RP, Dathan JR, Etherington MD, Guyer PB, MacIver AG: The loin-pain/hematuria syndrome. Lancet 1:897, 1979. *This paper reviews the clinical, pathologic, and angiographic findings in nine young women with this syndrome, which is an important one to recognize.*

Kupor LR, Mullins JO, McPhaul JJ: Immunopathologic findings of idiopathic renal hematuria. Arch Intern Med 135:1204, 1975. *A good review of biopsy findings in 80 patients with isolated hematuria that reveal a typical variety of mild glomerular lesions but a good long-term prognosis.*

Isolated Proteinuria

A more detailed discussion of proteinuria is given in Ch. 75. Like isolated hematuria, non-nephrotic range proteinuria *without* hematuria or decreased renal function may indicate a significant glomerular disease, but usually does not. When increased urinary protein excretion is suggested by qualitative analyses such as the dipstick, it must be confirmed by an accurate measurement of 24-hour protein excretion. Values in excess of 150 mg per day in adults, and 140 mg per square meter per day in children, are regarded as abnormal if an accurate 24-hour urine collection has been obtained. Abnormal protein excretion may be intermittent or persistent (fixed).

INTERMITTENT PROTEINURIA. The most common causes of intermittent proteinuria are *exercise*, assumption of the *upright position* (postural proteinuria), and *fever*. Up to 10 per cent of routine medical admissions may exhibit transient proteinuria. The basis for proteinuria in most of these conditions is probably hemodynamic (see above), although subtle alterations in glomerular architecture have not been excluded. Total protein excretion is usually less than 2.0 grams per day, renal function is normal, and 20-year follow-up studies have shown resolution of the proteinuria in a majority of cases with no evidence of progressive renal disease.

PERSISTENT PROTEINURIA. Persistent or fixed proteinuria can also occur without glomerular disease. *"Overflow" proteinuria* occurs when excess production of filterable, low molecular weight proteins exceeds the tubular reabsorptive capacity, as occurs with the production of lysozyme (molecular weight 14,000) in myelomonocytic leukemia or L-chains in plasma cell dyscrasias such as multiple myeloma. In some cases up to 5.0 grams of L-chains may be excreted daily. Another nonglomerular cause of proteinuria is renal tubular disease in which normal quantities of proteins such as lysozyme or beta$_2$ microglobulin are filtered but not reabsorbed. This can result in urinary excretion of up to 2.0 grams of such proteins daily in a variety of interstitial nephropathies and disorders of tubular function.

Isolated, fixed, non-nephrotic proteinuria of glomerular origin is associated with an increased incidence of hypertension and a somewhat decreased life expectancy in long-term follow-up studies, but progressive renal disease is rare. Renal biopsy in such patients usually reveals some glomerular abnormality. The spectrum of lesions in isolated proteinuria is wide and similar to that discussed above in isolated hematuria. In patients with fixed proteinuria of less than 2.0 grams per day without hematuria, systemic disease, or impaired renal function, renal biopsy is usually not performed unless a change in clinical status occurs or the patient requests a biopsy for other purposes.

Abuelo JG: Proteinuria: Diagnostic principles and procedures. Ann Intern Med 98:186, 1983. *A well-written summary of the different types of proteinuria, their causes and prognosis, with emphasis on the approach to evaluation of patients with mild proteinuria and normal renal function.*

SPECIFIC RENAL DISEASES THAT PRESENT AS ACUTE GLOMERULONEPHRITIS (GN) (see Table 80–2)

The prototype of acute postinfectious GN is post-streptococcal GN (PSGN), but glomerular disease may follow infection with a variety of other bacterial and nonbacterial agents: both gram-positive and gram-negative bacteria, viruses, mycoplasma, fungi, protozoa, helminths, and spirochetes. Many of these associations have been noted only in patients with endocarditis or infected ventriculoatrial shunts. It is important to distinguish between specific postinfectious glomerular diseases such as PSGN and the nonspecific role of many infections, particularly viral illnesses, in producing "exacerbations" of underlying glomerular disease. These exacerbations are usually evidenced by an increase in proteinuria and hematuria associated with the infection, usually without an intervening latent period.

Post-streptococcal Glomerulonephritis (PSGN)

Etiology, Incidence, and Epidemiology. GN occurs only following infection with a group A (beta hemolytic) streptococcus of nephritogenic M type, usually type 12 in the United States. Streptococcal pharyngitis is the most common antecedent event in the North, and PSGN occurs with a frequency of less than 5 per cent after a latent period of 6 to 20 days (average 10). The disease is often sporadic, occurs in the winter and spring, is more common in males, and is accompanied by serologic evidence of recent streptococcal infection in over 80 per cent of cases. In the South streptococcal pyoderma or impetigo is more common, the attack rate is higher (25 to 50 per cent), the latent period is longer (14 to 21 days, average 20), and the disease affects males and females equally, often occurring in epidemic form in more temperate climates in the summer and fall.

Pathogenesis. Granular immune complex deposits in glomeruli cause the clinical and histologic features of PSGN. The presence of these deposits, hypocomplementemia, and the latent period between infection and the onset of GN suggest that the disease is similar to experimental acute serum sickness, in which acute GN is mediated by formation of glomerular deposits containing antigen and antibody to it 8 to 10 days following a single injection of antigen (see Ch. 74). The deposits are thought to reflect glomerular trapping of circulating immune complexes, but they may also form on a local basis. Streptococcal antigens have been identified in glomerular deposits early in PSGN in some patients. The presence of C3 in the deposits and the prominent infiltrate of neutrophils and mononuclear cells in the acute stage suggest a lesion that is mediated by complement, neutrophils, and macrophages.

Pathology. Figure 80–2 illustrates the typical findings in acute PSGN by light microscopy, IF, and EM. The histologic lesion in PSGN is a diffuse (all glomeruli involved) proliferative GN with a marked hypercellularity involving glomerular endothelial and mesangial cells, as well as neutrophils and mononuclear cells with narrowing or occlusion of capillary loops (Fig. 80–2*A*). Proliferation of epithelial cells in Bowman's space results in formation of glomerular "crescents" in severe glomerular disease. Extensive crescent formation is seen in about 5 per cent of patients and correlates with a more severe initial disease and reduced likelihood of complete recovery. Coarsely granular deposits of IgG and C3 occur along the glomerular capillary walls and in the mesangium (Fig. 80–2*B*). By EM there are discrete electron-dense subepithelial nodules or "humps" (Fig. 80–2*C*) that persist for about eight weeks before resolution makes identification difficult. Subepithelial humps are a highly characteristic feature of PSGN, although they may occasionally be seen in other types of bacterial postinfectious GN and type I MPGN.

Clinical Findings. PSGN is the prototype of the acute nephritic syndrome and causes all of the findings discussed above under Pathophysiology of Acute Nephritic Syndromes. The disease is most common in children between 3 and 12 years of age, with a mean age of about 7, and is rare in infancy and in adults over 50. The typical presentation of PSGN is the abrupt onset of hematuria (90 per cent), which is usually evident as dark or *"smoky" urine*, accompanied by *malaise* and sometimes gastrointestinal symptoms such as abdominal pain, nausea, and vomiting. Central nervous system manifestations may include headaches and occasionally seizures. *Edema* is an early and frequent sign, often in a periorbital distribution most

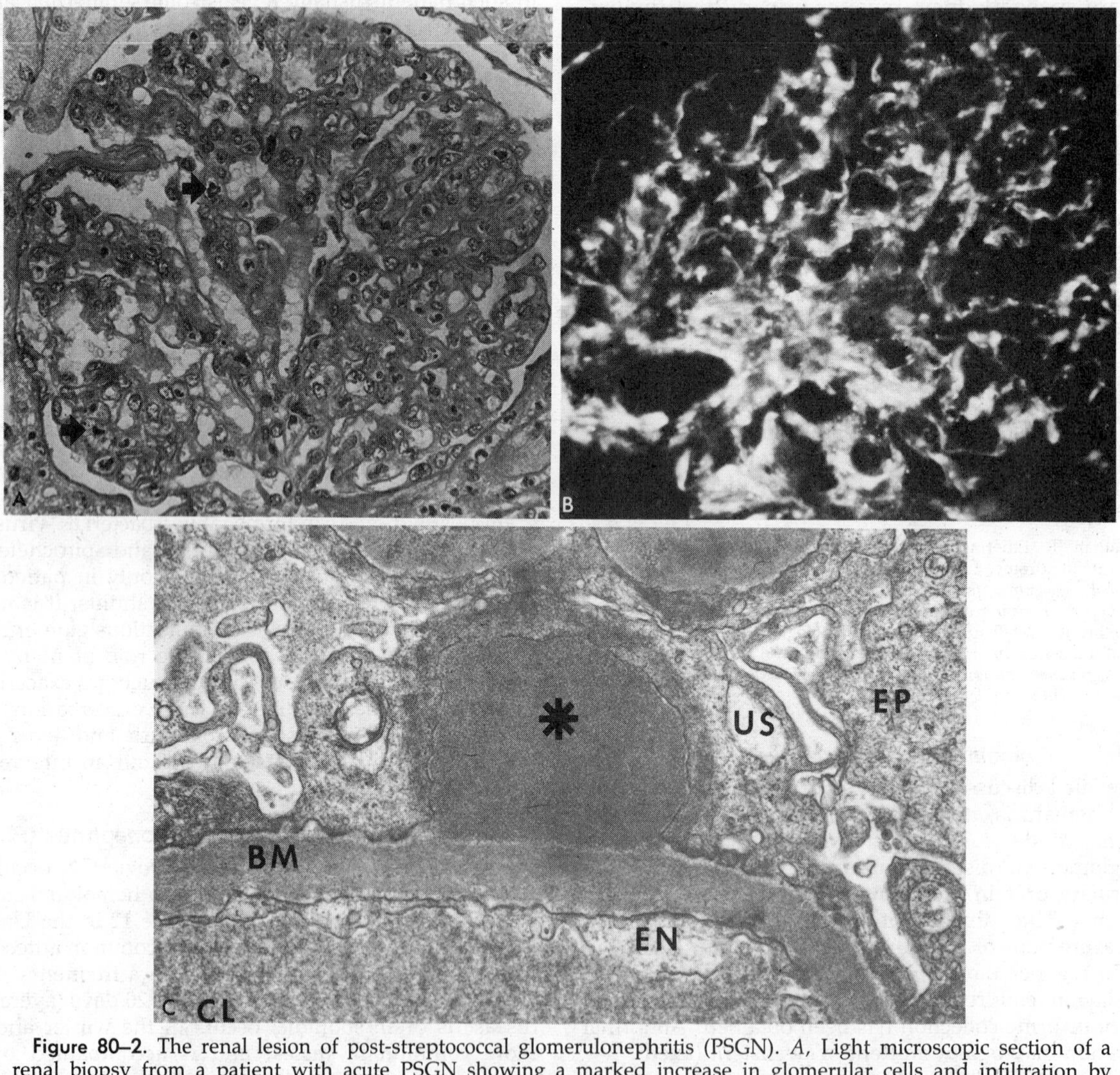

Figure 80–2. The renal lesion of post-streptococcal glomerulonephritis (PSGN). *A*, Light microscopic section of a renal biopsy from a patient with acute PSGN showing a marked increase in glomerular cells and infiltration by polymorphonuclear leukocytes (arrows) (periodic acid–Schiff stain; × 300). *B*, Immunofluorescent staining for IgG from the same biopsy reveals a coarse granular pattern of deposits on the capillary walls and in the mesangium (× 350). *C*, Electron microscopy in acute PSGN reveals a characteristic electron-dense "hump" on the subepithelial surface (*) with effacement of epithelial foot processes around the deposit. BM = basement membrane; CL = capillary lumen; EN = endothelial cell; EP = epithelial cell; US = urinary space (× 14,400). (Reproduced with permission from Couser WG, Salant DJ, Stilmant MM. *In* Flamenbaum W, Hamburger RJ (eds.): Nephrology. Philadelphia, JB Lippincott Company, 1982, pp 265–301.)

evident on arising and sometimes progressing to peripheral edema and anasarca. *Hypertension* is present in 60 to 70 per cent of patients and reflects renal retention of salt and water with volume overload. Proteinuria is usually present as well. About 20 per cent of hospitalized patients develop nephrotic range proteinuria (more than 3.5 grams per day), usually transiently and during the recovery phase. Renal function is impaired in about 50 per cent of patients.

Prognosis. Three clinical courses can be defined in PSGN: complete recovery, no recovery, or partial recovery with progressive disease. In over 90 per cent of cases complete recovery occurs with spontaneous diuresis in an average of four to seven days. Even patients who require dialysis during the acute phase usually recover spontaneously without specific therapy. However, abnormal hematuria and proteinuria may persist for up to two years. About 20 to 50 per cent of such patients have mild hypertension, slightly reduced inulin clearances, and increased urine protein excretion for many years as residua of the initial disease. Progressive renal disease is a very uncommon consequence of PSGN when renal function returns to normal and proteinuria is less than 500 mg per day.

Fewer than 5 per cent of patients with PSGN have oliguria lasting more than nine days; the prognosis in these patients is worse. Although spontaneous complete recovery has been reported in children with oliguria or anuria for up to 25 days, this is unusual. Patients who do recover after prolonged oliguria usually do not have extensive crescent formation on biopsy. Many patients with prolonged oliguria will have over 50 per cent of glomeruli involved with crescents. About half of these will still recover spontaneously. However, in the remainder, the disease behaves like rapidly progressive glomerulonephritis (RPGN) with no recovery at all or with only partial recovery of renal function, followed by persistent proteinuria and progressive renal disease leading to renal failure in months to years. Patients with PSGN who have oliguric renal failure lasting over one week, particularly adults, should undergo a renal biopsy. If extensive crescent formation is found they should be considered for therapy as outlined below under Treatment of RPGN.

Laboratory Features. Laboratory findings consist of an abnormal urinalysis, elevated antibodies against streptococcal exoenzymes, and reduced serum complement levels. The urinalysis usually reveals signs of glomerular inflammation with proteinuria, RBC's, WBC's, and casts. RBC casts are present in 60 to 85 per cent of cases when a freshly voided urine is examined. The urine is often concentrated and exhibits biochemical characteristics of prerenal azotemia, including a low urine sodium, indicating severe glomerular disease with good preservation of tubular function.

Beta-hemolytic streptococci are detected by culture in only 25 per cent of untreated patients, but serologic tests generally confirm recent streptococcal infection. The anti-streptolysin O (ASO) titer exceeds 200 Todd units within one to three weeks and may remain elevated for months. About 20 per cent of normal children may exhibit elevated ASO titers on random examinations. An increase in ASO titer may not be seen if penicillin therapy is initiated early or if the antecedent infection was in the skin. Antibodies to other streptococcal enzymes are usually elevated as well. The streptozyme test utilizes five of these antigens in a single assay and is quite sensitive and specific. Over 90 per cent of patients with PSGN have a reduced level of total hemolytic complement or C3 during the first two weeks of illness, with about 50 per cent returning to normal within three weeks and over 90 per cent within eight weeks. The pattern of complement component depression suggests alternate pathway activation, with levels of C1q and C4 usually normal.

Diagnosis. The differential diagnosis of acute GN with hypocomplementemia includes other forms of postinfectious GN such as SBE or shunt nephritis, SLE, and type I membranoproliferative glomerulonephritis (MPGN). Only MPGN is difficult to exclude by clinical and laboratory criteria. A similar pattern of alternate complement pathway activation is seen in MPGN, a disease that also may occasionally follow streptococcal infection (see p. 583), and MPGN must be considered when nephrotic range proteinuria and hypocomplementemia persist for longer than two months. The diagnosis of PSGN can usually be made by the presence of typical clinical features of the acute nephritic syndrome following a streptococcal infection by an appropriate latent period, and by hypocomplementemia and serologic evidence of recent streptococcal infection. Because patients with PSGN usually recover spontaneously and no specific therapy is indicated, the diagnosis is often made clinically without a renal biopsy. Biopsy is indicated, however, if atypical features are present, such as prolonged oliguria, anuria, persistent hypocomplementemia, the nephrotic syndrome, or clinical or serologic evidence of systemic disease.

Treatment. In most patients with PSGN there is no need for specific therapy, since spontaneous recovery can be anticipated. Antibiotics should be given if cultures are positive for group A streptococci, but penicillin therapy does not alter the incidence or severity of PSGN. Manifestations of sodium retention such as hypertension, edema, and congestive heart failure can usually be managed with careful sodium restriction, but diuretics and antihypertensive agents may be employed if necessary. Dialysis may be required temporarily in some patients, most of whom will still recover normal renal function spontaneously.

There are no data on which to base a recommendation for therapy in patients with prolonged oliguria and a crescentic glomerular lesion on biopsy. Although up to 50 per cent of such patients may recover spontaneously, the prognosis is sufficiently guarded to warrant considering therapy with pulse steroids or plasma exchange as outlined below under RPGN.

Nissenson AR, moderator: Post-streptococcal acute glomerulonephritis: Fact and controversy. Ann Intern Med 91:76, 1979. *An excellent overview of the microbiology, epidemiology, clinical manifestations, laboratory features, pathogenesis, and sequelae of PSGN, with 128 references.*

Nissenson AR, Mayon-White R, Potter EV, Mayon-White V, Abidh S, Poon-King T, Earle DP: Continued absence of clinical renal disease 7 to 12 years after poststreptococcal acute glomerulonephritis in Trinidad. Am J Med 67:255, 1979. *A thorough study of over 700 patients, with an excellent summary of the literature and review of the data on long-term prognosis in PSGN.*

Glomerulonephritis in Subacute Bacterial Endocarditis (SBE)

Glomerular disease in SBE ranges in severity from the proteinuria and hematuria seen in 70 per cent of patients, usually with normal renal function, to occasional cases of crescentic GN with acute renal failure. It is more common in chronic cases with right-sided cardiac involvement and negative blood cultures, as may occur in patients who abuse drugs. A wider variety of organisms have been implicated, most commonly *Staphylococcus aureus* and *Streptococcus viridans*. Serologic abnormalities are often present, including hypocomplementemia with activation of both the classic and alternate complement pathways, cryoglobulinemia, positive rheumatoid factor, and circulating immune complexes. Renal biopsy usually demonstrates a focal proliferative GN, often with necrosis and intracapillary thrombi. Granular deposits of IgG, IgM, and C3 occur in mesangial and subendothelial areas, implicating an immune complex rather than an embolic mechanism in the pathogenesis of the lesion. Renal function usually returns to normal following appropriate antibiotic therapy and eradication of the infection. However, recovery may be slow if the lesion is severe or crescents are present.

Gutman RA, Striker GE, Gilliland BC, Cutler RE: The immune complex glomerulonephritis of bacterial endocarditis. Medicine 51:1, 1972. *A good review of the clinical and pathologic features of nine cases of glomerulonephritis associated with SBE, emphasizing its immune complex origin.*

Perez GO, Rothfield N, Williams RC: Immune complex nephritis in bacterial endocarditis. Arch Intern Med 136:333, 1976. *This case illustrates the severity of renal involvement that may occur in SBE and its reversibility. Data linking the infecting organism to the glomerular immune deposits are also presented.*

Shunt Nephritis

Chronic intravascular infection may lead to GN in patients with ventriculoatrial shunts for hydrocephalus. Up to 20 per cent of such shunts become infected with *Staphylococcus albus* and a variety of other organisms. Patients develop chronic malaise, fever, weight loss, and anemia, much like the symptoms of SBE. However, the renal lesion, which resembles type I MPGN pathologically, is more frequently associated with heavy proteinuria and often the nephrotic syndrome. Laboratory findings resemble those in SBE, and cultures may be positive from the blood, cerebrospinal fluid, and shunt itself. The renal lesion resolves slowly in most patients following eradication of the infection, which requires shunt removal in many cases, as well as appropriate antibiotic therapy.

Groeneveld ABJ, Nommensen FE, Mullink H, Ooms ECM, Bode WA: Shunt nephritis associated with *Propionibacterium acnes* with demonstration of the antigen in glomeruli. Nephron 32:365, 1982. *This relatively typical case is well studied, and the discussion presents a thoroughly referenced review of the literature on this disease.*

Glomerulonephritis with Visceral Abscesses

This association, noted more commonly in Europe than in the United States, presents with an abrupt onset of acute renal failure associated with proteinuria, hematuria, and red cell casts in a patient with a pyogenic visceral abscess. Abscesses are most frequently located in the respiratory tract but have been reported at numerous other sites, including the abdomen, the uterus, and an infected aortofemoral graft. Endocarditis may be present but usually is not, and blood cultures are commonly negative. In contrast to PSGN, SBE, and shunt nephritis, serologic studies, including complement levels, are usually normal. A variety of bacteria have been implicated. The glomerular lesion is usually a proliferative GN with crescents present. IF and EM studies usually do not reveal immune deposits, so that the pathogenesis of this lesion is unclear. Recovery of renal function has occurred in about half of the patients reported with acute renal failure who were successfully treated to eradicate the infection, but the overall mortality is quite high.

Beaufils M: Glomerular disease complicating abdominal sepsis. Kidney Int 19:609, 1981. *A detailed review of nonstreptococcal postinfectious glomerulonephritis, including SBE as well as abscess related lesions. The frequency with which renal biopsies reveal glomerular disease as a cause of acute renal failure in patients with sepsis is striking, since most such patients would not be as extensively studied in the United States.*

IgG-IgA Nephritis (Berger's Disease)

Overview and Incidence. In 1968 Jean Berger reviewed 55 biopsies of children with so-called benign hematuria, idiopathic hematuria, or recurrent hematuria of childhood and noted a high frequency of mesangial IgA deposits and a variety of glomerular lesions, most commonly focal GN. IgG-IgA nephritis causes about 20 per cent of acute GN in the United States but is more common in France and Japan. It is the commonest cause of primary glomerular disease in Europe and Australia. The disease is now regarded as a monosymptomatic form of *Henoch-Schönlein purpura* (HSP), but clinical manifestations are milder than in HSP and are usually confined to the kidney. Because of its systemic manifestations, HSP is discussed on p. 587.

Pathogenesis. The pathogenesis of the renal lesion in IgG-IgA nephritis and HSP is not known. It appears to be a consequence of mesangial formation of immune deposits composed predominantly of IgA (see Fig. 80–3*B*). The IgA probably represents the antibody component of an immune complex containing a nonrenal antigen. In favor of this suggestion are studies showing that (1) serum levels of IgA immune complexes are elevated and correlate with clinical manifestations of the disease in some patients and (2) a similar glomerular lesion may develop in liver disease associated with elevated portal pressure and increased levels of IgA-containing immune complexes. The glomerular IgA deposits appear to be predominantly polymeric and of mucosal origin, which may reflect the association of disease activity with viral infections of the upper respiratory and gastrointestinal tracts.

Pathology. The typical lesion of IgG-IgA nephritis is seen by light microscopy to have a focal distribution, meaning that some glomeruli are involved while others are spared, and is also segmental, with lesions in some glomerular tufts but not others (Fig. 80–3*A*). Mesangial expansion and hypercellularity are common, but the characteristic lesion is a focal and segmental proliferative GN. When crescents are present they are usually small and rarely involve more than 30 per cent of glomeruli. Immune deposits are present diffusely in the mesangium of all glomeruli and contain IgA as the predominant immunoglobulin, accompanied by C3 in 60 per cent and IgG in 30 per cent of cases (Fig. 80–3*B*). C1q and C4 are usually absent, suggesting alternate complement pathway activation. Patients with deposits along the subendothelial aspect of the capillary wall or in the subepithelial space generally have more severe disease and more proteinuria.

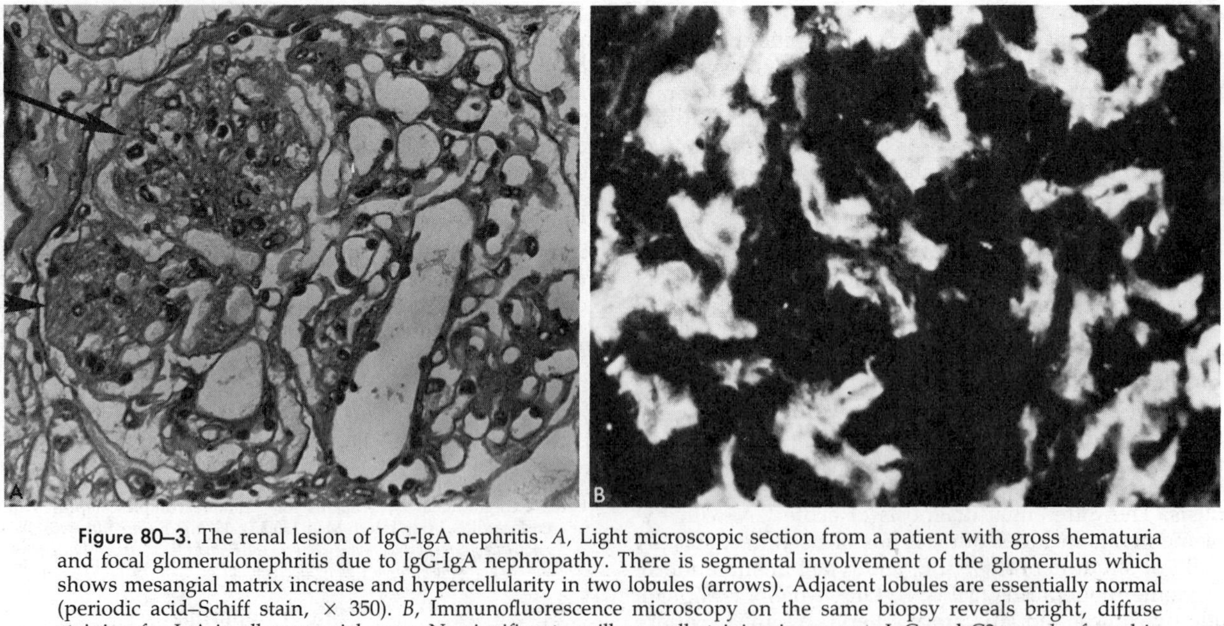

Figure 80–3. The renal lesion of IgG-IgA nephritis. *A,* Light microscopic section from a patient with gross hematuria and focal glomerulonephritis due to IgG-IgA nephropathy. There is segmental involvement of the glomerulus which shows mesangial matrix increase and hypercellularity in two lobules (arrows). Adjacent lobules are essentially normal (periodic acid–Schiff stain, × 350). *B,* Immunofluorescence microscopy on the same biopsy reveals bright, diffuse staining for IgA in all mesangial areas. No significant capillary wall staining is present. IgG and C3 may be found in a similar pattern but with less intensity (× 450). (Reproduced from Couser WG, Salant DJ, Stilmant MM. *In* Flamenbaum W, Hamburger RJ (eds.): Nephrology. Philadelphia, JB Lippincott Company, 1982, pp 265–301.)

Clinical and Laboratory Findings and Diagnosis. Berger's disease is two to three times more common in males than in females, and most cases present before the age of 35. The classic presentation is with *gross hematuria* that occurs coincident with, or immediately following (24 to 48 hours), a viral upper respiratory infection (50 per cent), flu-like illness (15 per cent), a gastrointestinal syndrome (10 per cent), or other infectious prodrome. Associated findings often include mild fever, malaise, myalgias, dysuria, and loin pain. The remainder of cases are identified during medical evaluation for persistent, asymptomatic hematuria or proteinuria. The absence of a latent period as well as normal levels of complement and anti-streptococcal antibodies, distinguishes this disease clinically from PSGN. Moreover, other features of the acute nephritic syndrome, including edema and hypertension, are seen in fewer than half of the patients. Only about 25 per cent of patients have impaired renal function during active disease, and the serum creatinine rarely exceeds 3 mg per deciliter. Proteinuria is usually less than 1 gram per day.

Gross hematuria usually lasts only two to six days, but microscopic hematuria often persists between attacks and may be what brings the patient to medical attention. Fifty per cent of patients will have only a single episode of gross hematuria. The remainder have recurring episodes for many years, usually "triggered" by viral infections.

There are no laboratory findings diagnostic of IgG-IgA nephritis. About half of all patients have elevated serum levels of IgA that do not correlate with disease activity. Circulating immune complexes containing IgA are present intermittently, and deposits of IgA, C3, and fibrin may be present in the dermal capillaries of normal skin. The incidence of this disease is greater in persons with HLA-Bw 35 and HLA-DR4 phenotypes.

Course and Prognosis. Progression to renal failure occurs in 15 to 20 per cent of patients within six months, and a 50 per cent death or dialysis rate is projected over 20 years. While there are no clinical or pathologic features that permit accurate prediction of progression, patients who tend to do worse are male, have a prolonged clinical course, develop hypertension or proteinuria exceeding 3 grams per day, or have extensive glomerular sclerosis present on biopsy.

Treatment. No specific form of therapy has been shown to alter the long-term clinical course of this disease. Rigorous control of hypertension is important. Mesangial deposits of IgA occur with a high frequency in renal allografts but rarely compromise graft function.

Nakamoto Y, Asano Y, Dohi K, Fujioka M, Iida H, Kida H, Kibe Y, Hattori H, Takeuchi J: Primary IgA glomerulonephritis and Schönlein-Henoch purpura nephritis. Clinicopathological and immunohistological characteristics. Q J Med 97:495, 1978. *This report details the clinical renal manifestations and renal pathology of 205 Japanese patients with IgG-IgA nephritis and 35 with HSP and concludes that the two diseases are manifestations of the same process.*

Southwest Pediatric Nephrology Study Group: A multicenter study of IgA nephropathy in children. Kidney Int 22:643, 1982. *A thorough description of the clinical and pathologic features of this disease in 62 children age 4 to 18 from the southwestern United States. The study emphasizes the difficulties in predicting course from initial pathologic features and presents a complete review of current data on progression and treatment.*

Rapidly Progressive Glomerulonephritis (RPGN)

Overview. The term RPGN is applied to any glomerular disease in which rapid loss of renal function occurs in association with extensive crescent formation in many glomeruli, usually over 50 per cent (Fig. 80–4). Volhard and Fahr first noted the association between crescents and a poor prognosis in 1914, and the term RPGN was first applied by Ellis in 1942 to a subset of patients who probably had PSGN with extensive crescents and an unfavorable outcome.

RPGN may occur in severe cases of a wide variety of glomerular diseases, which are listed in Table 80–3, or it may occur alone as a primary renal disease. The classification system used here is based on pathogenetic mechanisms. Accurate prognosis and selection of appropriate therapy require that the underlying mechanisms be defined. About 20 per cent of cases of RPGN are mediated by anti-GBM antibody deposition and

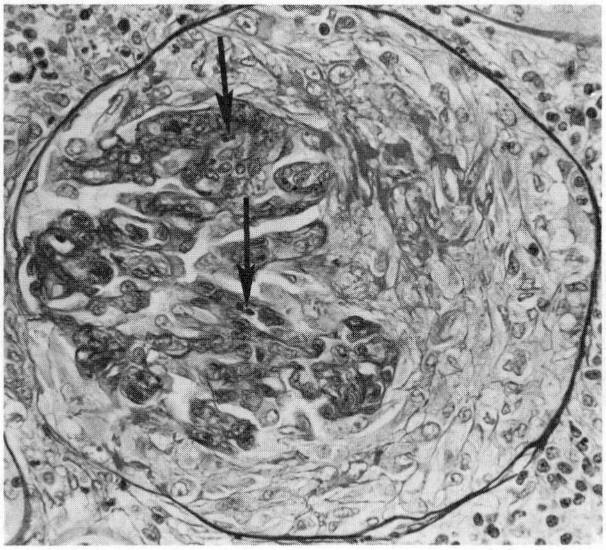

Figure 80–4. Light microscopy from a patient with idiopathic RPGN reveals the presence of a large cellular crescent in Bowman's space surrounding and compressing the glomerular capillary. A few polymorphonuclear leukocytes are seen in the glomerulus (arrows) (periodic acid–Schiff stain, × 275). (Reproduced from Couser WG, Salant DJ, Stilmant MM. *In* Flamenbaum W, Hamburger RJ (eds.): Nephrology. Philadelphia, JB Lippincott Company, 1982, pp 265–301.)

40 per cent by glomerular immune complex formation (usually in association with some systemic disease process such as PSGN or SLE), and 40 per cent are primary renal lesions with no significant glomerular immune deposits, which are classified here as idiopathic RPGN (Table 80–3).

RPGN DUE TO ANTI-GBM ANTIBODY. Although much is known of the mediation of immune glomerular injury from studies of experimental anti-GBM nephritis, this mechanism accounts for fewer than 5 per cent of cases of GN seen clinically. Anti-GBM GN is characterized by the abrupt onset of a proliferative GN, usually with crescents, and a characteristic linear deposition of IgG along the GBM by IF (Fig. 80–5). In about two thirds of cases, pulmonary hemorrhage accompanies GN,

TABLE 80–3. CLASSIFICATION OF RAPIDLY PROGRESSIVE (CRESCENTIC) GLOMERULONEPHRITIS

Type of RPGN	Frequency
Anti-GBM Antibody Mediated RPGN	20%
Goodpasture's syndrome	
Idiopathic anti-GBM nephritis	
Membranous nephropathy with crescents	
RPGN Associated with Granular Immune Deposits	40%
Postinfectious	
Post-streptococcal glomerulonephritis	
Bacterial endocarditis	
"Shunt" nephritis	
Visceral abscesses, other nonstreptococcal infections	
Noninfectious	
Systemic lupus erythematosus	
Henoch-Schönlein syndrome	
Mixed cryoglobulinemia	
Solid tumors	
Primary Renal Disease	
Membranoproliferative glomerulonephritis	
IgG-IgA nephropathy	
Idiopathic "immune complex" nephritis	
RPGN without Glomerular Immune Deposits	40%
Vasculitis	
Polyarteritis	
Wegener's granulomatosis	
Idiopathic RPGN	

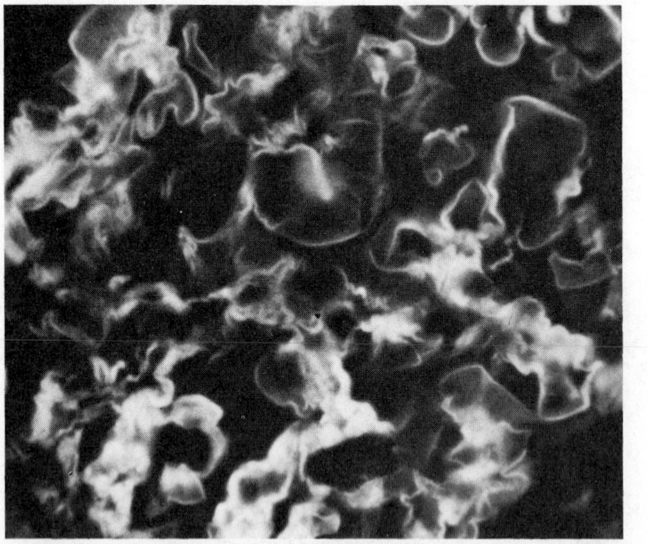

Figure 80–5. Immunofluorescence microscopy on a renal biopsy from a patient with Goodpasture's syndrome reveals continuous, uninterrupted, linear deposition of IgG along all capillary walls. This pattern is characteristic of anti-GBM disease (× 450). (Reproduced from Couser WG, Salant DJ, Stilmant MM. *In* Flamenbaum W, Hamburger RJ (eds.): Nephrology. Philadelphia, JB Lippincott Company, 1982, pp 265–301.)

and the disease is termed Goodpasture's syndrome. The remaining one third of patients have anti-GBM nephritis without pulmonary involvement.

Goodpasture's Syndrome. PATHOGENESIS. The events that initiate anti-GBM antibody production are not known. An initial pulmonary insult is suspected in many cases of Goodpasture's syndrome and may result in exposure of normally sequestered alveolar basement membrane antigens, resulting in production of anti-alveolar basement membrane antibody that cross-reacts with GBM. However, a similar antibody mediates the glomerular disease in anti-GBM nephritis without pulmonary hemorrhage, suggesting that other events also initiate antibody production. The development of lung hemorrhage appears to require the presence of prior lung damage to allow antibody deposition. Genetic factors are clearly important in this disease. There is a strong association with HLA-DRw2 (relative risk 15 to 34 times normal). Anti-GBM antibody production is a self-limited event lasting about two to four months. Exacerbations of disease associated with increased antibody levels may be triggered by infectious complications. Antibody binding to GBM mediates glomerular injury by mechanisms that involve complement activation and participation of both neutrophils and macrophages. Fibrin deposition in Bowman's space is believed to initiate glomerular crescent formation.

PATHOLOGY. The early histologic lesion in Goodpasture's syndrome is a focal proliferative and necrotizing GN that progresses to diffuse involvement with crescent formation. Extensive interstitial infiltrates may also be present, perhaps due to antibody deposition on tubular basement membranes. There is a characteristic, continuous, linear pattern of IgG deposition along the capillary wall, accompanied by C3 in about 70 per cent of cases (Fig. 80–5). Tubular basement membrane deposits may also occur. EM is not diagnostic.

CLINICAL FEATURES. Goodpasture's syndrome is a disease of young males (6:1 male-to-female ratio) characterized by a triad of *pulmonary hemorrhage, GN,* and *anti-GBM antibody production.* It usually begins with pulmonary hemorrhage manifest as hemoptysis, pulmonary alveolar infiltrates by x-ray, dyspnea, and iron deficiency anemia. The pulmonary symptoms are followed within days to weeks by development of hematuria, proteinuria, and rapid loss of renal function. Over half of patients with Goodpasture's syndrome are azotemic when first seen. Hypertension and fluid retention are uncommon. Preceding flu-like illness or exposure to other pulmonary toxins such as volatile hydrocarbon solvents and cigarettes is common. Until recently, 80 per cent of cases required treatment for end-stage renal disease within one year, although several patients with mild disease have recovered spontaneously. Up to 30 per cent of patients may die as a consequence of the pulmonary hemorrhage.

LABORATORY FINDINGS AND DIAGNOSIS. The only laboratory finding specific for anti-GBM nephritis is the demonstration of antibody to GBM in the serum or as linear deposits of IgG in glomeruli. The antibody can be detected quickly in serum by indirect IF using normal human kidney substrate in a test that is similar to the fluorescent antinuclear antibody test. The indirect IF assay is positive in 80 to 90 per cent of patients with Goodpasture's syndrome. A more sensitive radioimmunoassay is also commercially available and is positive in over 95 per cent of patients. There are rare false positives, usually in patients who have SLE. It is urgent to make a diagnosis and to initiate therapy early in RPGN of all types. An anti-GBM assay, as well as a renal biopsy, should therefore be obtained as soon as possible after the diagnosis of RPGN is suspected. The demonstration of anti-GBM antibody is critical, since a variety of other diseases may result in similar pulmonary and renal manifestations, including SLE, polyarteritis nodosa, Wegener's granulomatosis, and other forms of systemic necrotizing vasculitis.

TREATMENT. As in all forms of RPGN, the success of treatment is critically dependent upon how quickly it is initiated. The overall survival rate in Goodpasture's syndrome has risen from less than 10 per cent 15 years ago to over 50 per cent today owing to earlier diagnosis and detection of milder cases, better general medical care, and probably some improvements in specific therapy for the disease. There is little evidence that oral steroids or immunosuppressive agents alone significantly alter the course of the renal lesion. The pulmonary hemorrhage commonly responds to either high dose oral prednisone therapy or to intravenous "pulse" methylprednisolone (see treatment of RPGN below). However, steroid pulse therapy does not appear to benefit the renal lesion. Most centers now treat anti-GBM disease with vigorous plasma exchange therapy combined with prednisone, 1 mg per kilogram per day, and cyclophosphamide, 2 to 3 mg per kilogram per day. Plasma exchanges of up to 4 liters per day are performed on a daily or alternate-day basis until anti-GBM antibody is no longer detectable in the circulation and disease progression has halted. Therapy may require several weeks. Replacement is with albumin, or, when pulmonary hemorrhage is active, with fresh frozen plasma. Overall survival in anti-GBM nephritis appears to be improved by plasma exchange therapy. However, the response rate in patients who are oliguric on presentation or who have serum creatinines exceeding 6 mg per deciliter is very low, again emphasizing the need for early diagnosis. In patients with end-stage renal disease due to anti-GBM nephritis, renal transplantation appears to be safe if delayed until anti-GBM antibody is no longer detectable in the serum.

Anti-GBM Glomerulonephritis Without Pulmonary Hemorrhage. Some patients have the same anti-GBM antibody-mediated renal disease as seen in Goodpasture's syndrome, but antibody localization does not occur in lungs and pulmonary hemorrhage is therefore absent. The patients are generally older than those with Goodpasture's syndrome (mean age about 50), and males and females are equally affected. In all other respects, the clinical and pathologic findings, course, and treatment are the same as those discussed above for Goodpasture's syndrome. Because such patients present with an idiopathic form of acute RPGN without pulmonary hemorrhage, it is important that the possibility of anti-GBM nephritis be considered in all patients who present in this fashion, and that circulating anti-GBM antibody studies and renal biopsy be performed early.

Briggs WA, Johnson JP, Teichman S, Yeager HC, Wilson CB: Antiglomerular basement membrane antibody-mediated glomerulonephritis and Goodpasture's syndrome. Medicine 58:348, 1979. *An excellent description of the spectrum of clinical features, course and response to therapy in 11 patients with Goodpasture's syndrome and one patient with anti-GBM nephritis without pulmonary hemorrhage, accompanied by a complete literature review.*

Peters DK, Rees AJ, Lockwood CM, Pusy CD: Treatment and prognosis in antibasement membrane antibody-mediated nephritis. Transplant Proc 14:513, 1982. *These recent data on 41 patients are from the group that first popularized plasma exchange in the treatment of anti-GBM disease and emphasizes the lack of effect in patients with oliguria or creatinines exceeding 6 mg per deciliter and the importance of immunogenetic factors in determining prognosis. The paper contains data related to optimal frequency and duration of plasma exchange therapy.* (See also Hind et al., p. 578.)

RPGN DUE TO GLOMERULAR IMMUNE COMPLEX FORMATION. Patients with RPGN associated with granular deposits of immunoglobulin and complement in glomeruli account for about 40 per cent of all patients seen with crescentic GN. In most cases the glomerular disease is a manifestation of some well-defined systemic illness such as SLE, Henoch-Schönlein purpura, or other forms of vasculitis, or of another well-defined primary renal disease such as PSGN, MPGN, or rarely IgG-IgA nephropathy. In all of these disorders the correct diagnosis can usually be made from the associated clinical, laboratory, and pathologic findings. Prognosis depends considerably on the underlying disease. For example, about 50 per cent of patients with RPGN secondary to streptococcal infection will recover spontaneously without specific therapy, while in RPGN due to SLE spontaneous recovery virtually never occurs. Therapy for the glomerular disease per se is the same as that outlined below under treatment for idiopathic RPGN and includes the use of methylprednisolone pulse therapy and/or plasma exchange.

In about 10 to 20 per cent of this group, no definable systemic disease or other renal disease is present. The clinical features, course, and response to therapy are similar to those of patients with idiopathic RPGN without immune deposits (see below).

IDIOPATHIC RPGN. ***Overview and Incidence.*** RPGN as a primary renal disease, first described in 1968, is usually not associated with significant glomerular immune deposits. Although some patients were found to have anti-GBM nephritis without pulmonary hemorrhage, the majority of patients with idiopathic RPGN do not have the immunopathologic findings of either anti-GBM or immune complex nephritis.

Pathogenesis. The disease mechanism in idiopathic RPGN is undefined but probably is immune in nature. Whatever the mechanism leading to capillary wall damage, leakage of fibrin into Bowman's space apparently initiates epithelial cell proliferation and crescent formation. Some of the vague prodromal clinical manifestations, as well as the presence of crescentic GN without immune deposits, are quite similar to findings in several of the vasculitides. This disease may be a variant of vasculitis and may share a common pathogenetic mechanism, although inflammatory changes are confined primarily to the glomerular capillaries.

Pathology. There is extensive glomerular crescent formation with circumferential cellular crescents usually involving 50 to 100 per cent of glomeruli (see Fig. 80–4). Earlier cases may show fewer or smaller crescents and later ones reveal more fibrosis of crescents and glomerular obsolescence. There is a rough correlation between the percentage of glomeruli with crescents, the severity of clinical disease, and the prognosis. Changes in the glomerular tuft itself may be minimal. Prominent proliferative changes suggest a postinfectious etiology and a better prognosis. Interstitial changes are frequently prominent, and vasculitis is absent. Fibrinogen and fibrin polymers are present in the crescents. The glomeruli at most show only focal granular deposits of IgM and C3, which are generally regarded as nonspecific. EM may show "gaps" or rupture of the capillary wall but usually does not show immune deposits.

Clinical Manifestations and Diagnosis. Idiopathic RPGN is a disease of older patients (mean age 58). There is a slight male predominance. The disease tends to present in clusters. Many patients have a prodrome that resembles a viral illness with myalgias; arthralgias; loin, back, and abdominal pain; fever; and malaise. Minor hemoptysis is common, and fleeting pulmonary infiltrates may be seen by x-ray. No specific inciting events have been identified. RPGN presents as an acute nephritic syndrome, including *hematuria, proteinuria,* and *rapidly decreasing renal function,* often without hypertension or edema. As in anti-GBM nephritis, the progression of renal disease is usually very rapid, with up to 50 per cent of patients oliguric at the time of presentation and half of these sufficiently uremic to require immediate dialysis. The remaining patients may require dialysis within one to three weeks. At the time of presentation the disease is often relatively acute and potentially reversible.

The laboratory features of idiopathic RPGN are entirely nonspecific. ASO titers, antinuclear and anti-GBM antibodies, circulating immune complexes, and complement levels are normal or negative. The diagnosis is made by renal biopsy in a patient with deteriorating renal function, evidence of glomerular disease in the urine sediment, absence of anti-GBM antibody, and lack of clinical or serologic evidence of other systemic diseases such as SLE.

Treatment and Prognosis. The natural history of idiopathic RPGN is difficult to define, since virtually all patients receive some form of therapy. Review of all reported cases treated with oral steroids and/or cytotoxic agents reveals little apparent benefit and a death or dialysis rate of about 75 per cent in two years. Favorable prognostic factors include a young age at the time of onset, a history of a preceding infectious episode, absence of oliguria and hypertension, serum creatinine below 6 mg per deciliter at presentation, and fewer than 50 per cent crescents in the renal biopsy. Recently success rates approaching 75 per cent have been reported in small numbers of patients treated with either methylprednisolone pulse therapy or plasma exchange. In pulse therapy, methylprednisolone, 30 mg per kilogram to a maximum of 3 grams, is given intravenously over 20 minutes on a daily or alternate-day basis for three doses, followed by oral prednisone, 2 mg per kilogram, which is tapered over several months. About 75 per cent of patients, including some who were oliguric and on dialysis, have shown a dramatic response, with a return of renal function to normal or nearly normal levels. Responses have generally been evident within five to ten days and have continued over four to six weeks. However, long-term follow-up data in such patients are very limited, and some will progress to renal failure later despite an impressive initial response. Very similar results have been reported in patients treated with intensive plasma exchange (plus prednisone and cyclophosphamide). This treatment is extremely expensive and, compared to pulse therapy, probably has a higher incidence of complications, primarily bleeding and infection. Neither form of therapy has yet been shown in a prospective, controlled study to improve long-term patient or kidney survival over what might be achieved with more conservative measures. Until such data are available, the author's feeling is that both pulse therapy and plasma exchange probably do represent significant advances in the treatment of idiopathic RPGN. When high doses of steroids are to be used anyway, initiating this therapy with intravenous methylprednisolone has no major side effects, and there is evidence that it is more efficacious than oral prednisone in RPGN. If a response is not seen within days, plasma exchange should be considered following careful review of the patient's age, severity of disease, and other complicating medical factors, as well as the relative experience of individual centers with this form of therapy. A rational decision based on data cannot be made now regarding which of these forms of treatment is of greater benefit and whether any additional benefit accrues from employing both simultaneously.

The reported experience with renal transplantation in idiopathic RPGN is minimal, but the disease appears to recur rarely in allografted kidneys.

Couser WG: Idiopathic rapidly progressive glomerulonephritis. Am J Nephrol 2:57, 1982. *This recent review discusses the classification, clinical features, pathology, pathogenesis, and treatment of idiopathic RPGN in considerable detail, with 159 references.*

Hind CRK, Paraskevakou H, Lockwood CM, Evans DJ, Peters DK, Rees AJ: Prognosis after immunosuppression of patients with crescentic nephritis requiring dialysis. Lancet 1:263, 1983. *This paper reviews the experience with plasma exchange and immunosuppression in 48 patients with all forms of RPGN and acute renal failure requiring dialysis. No patients with acute anti-GBM disease responded, while about two thirds of patients with other forms of RPGN, including idiopathic, vasculitic, and Wegener's showed a sustained improvement in renal function. The urgency of early diagnosis is emphasized.*

Stilmant MM, Bolton WK, Sturgill BC, Schmitt GW, Couser WG: Crescentic glomerulonephritis without immune deposits. Clinico-pathologic features. Kidney Int 15:184, 1979. *This is the first paper to concentrate on the clinical features and pathology in 16 patients with what now appears to be the most common type of idiopathic RPGN.*

NEPHROTIC SYNDROME

The nephrotic syndrome is not a disease; it is a group of signs and symptoms commonly seen in patients with glomerular diseases that are characterized by a marked increase in capillary wall permeability to serum proteins rather than (or sometimes in addition to) glomerular inflammatory changes. The primary abnormality in nephrotic syndrome is the excretion of large amounts (greater than 3.5 grams per day) of protein in the urine. Other manifestations that may occur secondary to *proteinuria* include *hypoalbuminemia, edema, hyperlipidemia,* and *lipiduria*. In contrast to the acute nephritic syndrome, the onset of the nephrotic syndrome is usually insidious, gross hematuria and red cell casts are infrequent, and renal function is often normal at the time of presentation.

The list of diseases that may cause the nephrotic syndrome is extensive and includes virtually every disorder that may affect the glomerulus. About one third of adults and 10 per cent of children have the nephrotic syndrome as a manifestation of some systemic disease, usually diabetes, SLE, or amyloidosis. In two thirds of adults, and most children, the nephrotic syndrome is idiopathic and a manifestation of one of three types of primary glomerular disease: minimal change nephrotic syndrome (MCNS) or its variants, membranous nephropathy, or membranoproliferative glomerulonephritis (MPGN). The relative frequencies of these diseases and their identifying characteristics are presented for comparison in Table 80–4. It is important to note that the occurrence of the nephrotic syndrome in patients over 45 may be associated with occult malignancy. The association of Hodgkin's disease with MCNS and of solid tumors of the lung, breast, and GI tract with membranous nephropathy is discussed below. All of the diseases discussed in the section on acute GN can also cause the nephrotic syndrome, although they do not commonly do so.

Pathophysiology of the Nephrotic Syndrome

PROTEINURIA. Glomeruli are normally perfused with plasma containing over 60,000 grams of protein per day, but less than 150 mg of protein is excreted in the final urine. The filtration barrier, which includes the endothelial cells, basement membrane, epithelial cells, and slit diaphragms, restricts the transcapillary passage of proteins on the basis of their size, shape, and electrical charge. The size barrier is primarily at the level of the endothelial cells and GBM. It restricts filtration of molecules between about 18 and 42 Å and effectively prevents filtration of neutral molecules larger than 42 Å. Circulating proteins such as albumin (36 Å) are further restricted from crossing the capillary wall by an electrical charge barrier conferred by the polyanionic sialoprotein coating on endothelial and epithelial cells and heparan sulfate–containing glycosaminoglycans in the lamina rara externa and interna. Thus, molecules with a net negative charge (anionic) are less freely filtered, or encounter smaller "pores" in the capillary wall, than positively charged (cationic) molecules of the same size. Most serum proteins are anionic at physiologic pH and may be filtered in increased amounts if the charge barrier is reduced, as it is in some glomerular diseases.

Glomerular hemodynamic factors also alter protein filtration. Thus, in situations of reduced renal perfusion, renal blood flow (RBF) may be reduced while GFR is maintained by adaptive

TABLE 80–4. SUMMARY OF PRIMARY RENAL DISEASES THAT PRESENT AS IDIOPATHIC NEPHROTIC SYNDROME

	Minimal Change Nephrotic Syndrome[1] (MCNS)	Focal Glomerular Sclerosis[1] (FGS)	Membranous Nephropathy	Membranoproliferative Glomerulonephritis (MPGN) Type I	Type II
Frequency[1]					
Children	75%	10%	<5%	10%	
Adults	15%	15%	50%	10%	
Clinical Manifestations					
Age	2–6, some adults	2–6, some adults	40–50	5–15	
Sex	2:1 male	1.3:1 male	2:1 male	male-female	
Nephrotic syndrome	100%	90%	80%	60%	
Asymptomatic proteinuria	0	10%	20%	40%	
Hematuria	20%	60–80%	60%	80%	
Hypertension	10%	20% early	Infrequent	35%	
Rate of progression	Does not progress	10 years	50% in 10–20 years	10–20 years	5–15 years
Associated conditions	Allergy, Hodgkin's disease	None	Renal vein thrombosis, cancer, SLE	None	Partial lipodystrophy
Laboratory Findings	Manifestations of nephrotic syndrome	Manifestations of nephrotic syndrome	Manifestations of nephrotic syndrome	Low C1, C4, C3-C9	Normal C1, C4, low C3-C9 C3 nephritic factor
Immunogenetics	HLA B8, B12 (3.5)[2]	Not established	HLA-DRW3 (12–32)[2]	Not established	
Renal Pathology					
Light microscopy	Normal	Focal sclerotic lesions	Thickened GBM, spikes	Thickened GBM, proliferation, lobulation	
Immunofluorescence	Negative	IgM, C3 in lesions	Fine granular IgG, C3	Granular IgG, C3	C3 only
Electron microscopy	Foot process fusion	Foot process fusion	Subepithelial deposits	Mesangial and subendothelial deposits	Dense deposits
Response to Steroids	90%	15–20%	May slow progression	Not established	

[1]Approximate frequency as a cause of idiopathic nephrotic syndrome. About 10 per cent of adult nephrotic syndrome is due to various diseases that usually present with acute glomerulonephritis (Table 80–2).

[2]Relative risk.

changes in other determinants of GFR such as intracapillary hydraulic pressure. Under these circumstances the filtration fraction (GFR/RBF) is increased, resulting in a higher than normal protein concentration at the efferent end of the glomerular capillary. This may produce an increased diffusion of protein across the capillary wall, resulting in proteinuria in the absence of glomerular disease in situations such as congestive heart failure and other conditions of reduced renal perfusion (see isolated proteinuria below).

Proteinuria, the hallmark of the nephrotic syndrome, exceeds 3.0 to 3.5 grams per day in adults, or 40 mg per square meter per hour in children. Fixed nephrotic range proteinuria with the nephrotic syndrome generally occurs only in the presence of diffuse glomerular disease. The immune mechanisms that may cause an increase in the permselective properties of the glomerular capillary wall are reviewed in Ch. 74. These processes may induce a loss of net negative charge on the capillary wall, as appears to occur in MCNS, leading to a marked increase in urinary albumin excretion without significant change in the excretion of other serum proteins *(selective proteinuria).* Other diseases with extensive capillary wall immune deposits, such as membranous nephropathy, or disorders of basement membrane biochemistry or structure, such as those found in diabetes or hereditary nephritis, are associated with apparent structural defects and increased filtration of all serum proteins *(nonselective proteinuria).* Over 40 grams of protein may be excreted in the urine each day in some patients. It is this loss of protein that leads to the other clinical and biochemical manifestations of the nephrotic syndrome.

HYPOALBUMINEMIA. Serum albumin concentration decreases to less than 3.0 grams per deciliter when the rate of urinary protein loss and renal catabolism of filtered albumin (which may exceed 10 grams per day in the nephrotic syndrome) exceeds the rate of hepatic synthesis. Hepatic albumin synthesis is normally 12 to 14 grams per day in adults and may increase in the nephrotic syndrome but can be limited by various factors, including age, poor nutritional status, and liver disease. Thus, some patients may exhibit significant hypoalbuminemia with proteinuria of less than 10 grams per day, while others excreting larger amounts of protein are better able to maintain serum albumin levels.

EDEMA. Edema in the nephrotic syndrome results in part from a reduction in plasma oncotic pressure such that capillary hydraulic pressure exceeds oncotic pressure in peripheral capillaries and fluid leaves the capillaries. Although the reduction in effective circulating volume that occurs may result in increased renal retention of salt and water through normal compensatory mechanisms, over 50 per cent of patients with the nephrotic syndrome have normal or increased plasma volume and normal or low levels of plasma renin during sodium retention, suggesting a primary renal contribution to salt retention in the nephrotic syndrome through mechanisms that remain poorly defined.

HYPERLIPIDEMIA. Hyperlipidemia is common in the nephrotic syndrome and is inversely proportional to the serum albumin concentration. Hypercholesterolemia and elevated phospholipids are the most constant abnormalities observed, but increased levels of low and very low density lipoproteins, triglycerides, and chylomycrons are also seen. The primary mechanism appears to be increased hepatic synthesis of cholesterol, triglycerides, and lipoproteins, but reduced catabolism of these compounds has also been demonstrated.

LIPIDURIA. In a nephrotic urine sediment lipids are seen as free fat, oval fat bodies (degenerated renal tubular epithelial cells containing cholesterol esters), and fatty casts, all of which exhibit a Maltese cross pattern under polarizing light. Lipiduria parallels the level of urine protein excretion rather than the serum lipid levels.

Complications of the Nephrotic Syndrome

The most clinically important metabolic complications of the nephrotic syndrome are severe protein malnutrition, which may require appropriate nutritional supplementation, hypercoagulability with a tendency to form thrombi in both renal and peripheral veins leading to thromboembolic complications, and acute renal failure.

Hypercoagulability is thought to be a consequence of altered clotting factor levels in the nephrotic syndrome, including reduced levels of factors IX, XI, and XII; elevated levels of factors V and VIII, fibrinogen, and platelets; a reduction in levels of antithrombin III and antiplasmin; and increased susceptibility of platelets to aggregation. There is a high incidence (10 to 40 per cent) of thrombus formation in renal, pulmonary, and peripheral veins, and occasionally in arteries, with frequent thromboembolic phenomena. The incidence of renal vein thrombosis appears to be particularly high in patients with the nephrotic syndrome due to membranous nephropathy and MPGN. Routine anticoagulation is not indicated unless emboli occur.

Acute renal failure in the nephrotic syndrome very rarely occurs owing to rapid progression of the underlying renal disease, since most diseases that cause the nephrotic syndrome progress very slowly. However, acute renal failure does occur as a consequence of several potentially treatable disorders superimposed on nephrotic glomerular disease. These include (1) reduced renal perfusion due to low plasma volume, which can result in acute tubular necrosis, particularly following a surgical procedure or biopsy; (2) interstitial renal edema in patients with MCNS and significant peripheral edema, who may develop intrarenal swelling sufficient to produce increased intrarenal pressure, cessation of filtration, and acute renal failure (this may be reversible with diuretic therapy); (3) drug-induced allergic interstitial nephritis, particularly in patients receiving diuretic therapy; (4) bilateral acute renal vein thrombosis (which is rare); and (5) acute renal failure in patients receiving nonsteroidal anti-inflammatory drugs such as fenoprofen and naproxen. This may occur as a result of inhibition of prostaglandin-dependent glomerular plasma flow in states of volume contraction or from acute allergic interstitial nephritis, which may be accompanied by a reversible nephrotic syndrome with a glomerular lesion like that in MCNS.

Other complications that may also be associated with the nephrotic syndrome include reduced levels of IgG (which may dispose to bacterial infection), proximal tubular dysfunction with signs of Fanconi's syndrome, deficiencies of trace metals such as iron, copper, and zinc, and loss of vitamin D with development of osteomalacia and secondary hyperparathyroidism. Measurements of thyroid function such as T_4 radioimmunoassay and T_3 resin uptake may falsely suggest reduced function, but free T_4 and TSH levels are generally normal.

Bernard DB: Metabolic abnormalities in nephrotic syndrome. Pathophysiology and complications. *In* Brenner BM, Stein JH (eds.): Contemporary Issues in Nephrology. Vol 9. New York, Churchill Livingstone, 1982, p 85. *A review article that provides a current analysis of the pathogenesis and clinical significance of the numerous metabolic derangements reported in the nephrotic syndrome, including hypoalbuminemia, hyperlipidemia, coagulation abnormalities, endocrine abnormalities, and others.*

Coggins CH: Management of nephrotic syndrome. *In* Brenner BM, Stein JH (eds.): Contemporary Issues in Nephrology. Vol 9. New York, Churchill Livingstone, 1982, p 283. *A clear review of the approach to clinical management of each of the systemic manifestations of nephrotic syndrome independent of the glomerular disease that causes them.*

Reineck HJ: Mechanisms of edema formation in the nephrotic syndrome. *In* Brenner BM, Stein JH (eds.): Contemporary Issues in Nephrology. Vol 9. New York, Churchill Livingstone, 1982, p 31. *A clear and comprehensive analysis of this controversial topic, with suggestions on management.*

Primary Renal Diseases That Present as the Nephrotic Syndrome

Minimal Change Nephrotic Syndrome (MCNS)

As indicated in Table 80–4, MCNS accounts for about 75 per cent of cases of idiopathic nephrotic syndrome in children and up to 20 per cent in adults. Synonyms include minimal change disease, nephropathy or glomerulopathy, lipoid nephrosis, and nil disease.

Pathogenesis. The pathogenesis of MCNS is not known. The disease is characterized by a loss of net negative charge on the capillary wall and can recur promptly in the transplanted kidney, suggesting the presence of a circulating factor that neutralizes or destroys glomerular polyanion, resulting in loss of the charge barrier and a selective type of proteinuria. The association of MCNS with Hodgkin's disease, its responsiveness to steroids and alkylating agents, and the tendency for remission to follow some viral infections, particularly measles, have focused attention on the possibility of an abnormality in T lymphocytes, perhaps involving production of a lymphokine with properties that induce increased glomerular capillary permeability. However, attempts to demonstrate such a substance have not been successful thus far.

Pathology. By definition, the diagnosis of MCNS requires the absence of abnormalities by light microscopy and of immune deposits by IF. Diffuse epithelial cell foot process effacement, or "fusion," is the only abnormality usually seen by EM, but some morphologic abnormalities may occur in MCNS, including mild to moderate focal or diffuse proliferation of mesangial cells, mesangial deposits of IgM or C3 by IF, and the presence of focal glomerular sclerosis (FGS) by light microscopy. In the presence of FGS, response to steroids is poor, and progressive loss of renal function is commonly seen. This has led several authors to consider FGS as a separate disease (see below). However, in some patients the FGS lesion appears to develop late in the course of MCNS and may simply be a histologic marker of a more severe and less responsive form of MCNS mediated by a similar mechanism.

Mesangial proliferation and mesangial IgM deposits may occur together or separately and usually predict a poor (or delayed) response to steroids and an increased possibility of progression. As with FGS, there have been attempts to classify such patients into separate disease categories (mesangial-proliferative GN, IgM nephropathy). When progression occurs in patients with MCNS and mesangial proliferation and/or IgM deposits, glomeruli develop changes typical of FGS. Whether these morphologic or immunopathologic variants identify different disease mechanisms or simply reflect differences in severity or in host environment in patients with a similar underlying disease is not clear.

Clinical Features. The peak incidence of MCNS is in children two to six years of age, in whom it virtually always presents as a full-blown nephrotic syndrome. In childhood, males are affected twice as commonly as females. One third of patients will have a preceding upper respiratory tract infection or other identifiable antecedent event. In the absence of volume contraction, renal function and blood pressure are normal, but up to one third of patients may have a reduced GFR when first seen due to hypovolemia and reduced renal perfusion. Urine protein excretion may exceed 40 grams per day in severe cases, and serum albumin is less than 2.0 grams per deciliter in over 90 per cent of children. The complications of this disease are discussed above under complications of the nephrotic syndrome in general, with protein malnutrition, infections, thromboembolic phenomena, and acute renal failure as the problems of greatest clinical significance. In addition, there is an association between MCNS and Hodgkin's disease in which the nephrotic syndrome may be the presenting sign of an occult lymphoma.

Laboratory Findings. The laboratory findings in MCNS are those of the nephrotic syndrome of any etiology. Proteinuria is "selective" (greater than 90 per cent albumin) in about 85 per cent of cases. Complement levels are usually normal, but elevated levels of circulating immune complexes may be detected by non–complement-fixing assays. A consistent but poorly understood observation is a marked reduction in ASO titers (less than 100 Todd units).

Course and Treatment. Before steroids and modern antibiotics were available the spontaneous remission rate in MCNS was estimated at 25 to 40 per cent. During that era, the mortality rate in children exceeded 50 per cent in five years owing to infections or thromboembolic complications. The mortality rate now is about 7 to 12 per cent in nephrotic children and less than 2 per cent in those who respond to steroids. Some of this improvement reflects the development of effective antibiotics and better general medical care. Steroid therapy has never been shown in a controlled study to improve survival in patients with MCNS. However, the usual dramatic resolution of the nephrotic syndrome following steroid administration, as well as the fact that survival has improved since the presteroid era, has led to the widespread belief that such treatment is beneficial.

Conventional doses of oral prednisone are 60 mg per square meter per day in children and 2 mg per kilogram per day in adults, given daily for four weeks, followed by alternate-day therapy for four more weeks and then a tapering course over four to six months. Within four weeks, 90 per cent of children will have responded, and 90 per cent of adults will respond within about eight weeks. There is little value in continuing steroid therapy beyond eight weeks if abnormal levels of proteinuria persist. The 10 per cent of patients who fail to respond generally have FGS (see below).

Of the steroid responders, roughly 50 per cent will remain free of proteinuria or develop infrequent relapses that respond to steroids, eventually entering permanent remission. The remainder will either become "frequent relapsers" (more than twice a year) or steroid dependent, often with a high incidence of steroid side effects. Some can be managed conservatively with salt restriction, diuretics, and a high-protein diet. In children, the clinical manifestations of the nephrotic syndrome are usually more severe, and steroid toxicity may require the use of an additional drug. Either cyclophosphamide, 2 to 3 mg per kilogram per day (75 mg per square meter per day in children), or chlorambucil, 0.2 to 0.3 mg per kilogram per day, given for 8 to 12 weeks, has been shown to increase the frequency and duration of remission in steroid-sensitive MCNS. However, because of their gonadal toxicity and teratogenic potential, these agents should be used only when both the nephrotic syndrome and steroid side effects are severe. About half of such patients treated with a second drug are reported to be in remission four years later, suggesting that complete remission can be achieved with drug therapy in almost 90 per cent of patients with MCNS.

Donadio JV Jr: Primary glomerular diseases: To treat or not to treat. Contrib Nephrol 33:86, 1982. *An excellent, current, and objective review of the benefits of various forms of therapy in MCNS and other primary glomerular diseases.*

Grupe WE: Primary nephrotic syndrome in childhood. Adv Pediatr 26:163, 1979. *A good review of the clinical course, general management, and specific therapy of MCNS in children, including the use of cytotoxic drugs.*

Hoyer JR: Idiopathic nephrotic syndrome with minimal glomerular changes. *In* Brenner BM, Stein JH (eds.): Contemporary Issues in Nephrology. Vol 9. New York, Churchill Livingstone, 1982, p 145. *This is an excellent and current review of all aspects of MCNS, including the clinical features, pathogenesis, pathology, and treatment.*

Focal Glomerular Sclerosis (FGS)

Overview. FGS is a histologic lesion found in some patients with otherwise typical MCNS, and it correlates well with steroid resistance and progressive renal failure. Controversy exists regarding whether it should be classified as a separate glomerular disease or should be viewed as one end of a spectrum that ranges from pure steroid-responsive MCNS with no morphologic abnormalities to typical FGS. This spectrum includes patients who have either mesangial proliferation by light microscopy and/or mesangial IgM deposits with or without evidence of FGS. The author favors the view that mesangial proliferation, mesangial IgM deposits, and FGS are part of the MCNS spectrum. However, the clinical features of patients with idiopathic nephrotic syndrome and FGS in early biopsies are sufficiently different from those who do not have these lesions to warrant separate consideration.

Pathogenesis. The etiology and pathogenesis of the lesion of FGS are unknown. Presumably the basic mechanism underlying the generalized increase in capillary wall permeability may be the same as that in MCNS, and the structural lesion may be the consequence of either the greater severity of this process in such patients or the presence of some additional, as-yet-unidentified factor(s). Experimentally, a marked increase in mesangial trafficking and deposition of circulating macromolecules occurs in association with altered glomerular permeability. Mesangial dysfunction, with loss of contractile properties that are now thought to play a role in the regulation of local capillary loop hemodynamics, may precede the development of FGS. This could result in persistent glomerular vasodilatation, hypertension, and hyperfiltration, with consequent structural damage to the capillary wall by mechanisms similar to those described below under pathogenesis of chronic GN.

Pathology. The diagnosis of FGS is made by renal biopsy in which sclerotic lesions are seen only in some glomeruli (focal) and within an affected glomerulus are present only in some capillary loops (segmental). The presence of sclerosis involving occasional entire glomeruli (global sclerosis) is a common finding that increases with age in all patients and does not have prognostic significance. The FGS lesion itself is an expansion of the mesangial matrix with wrinkling and collapse of adjacent capillary loops, development of PAS-positive intracapillary hyaline deposits, adhesions to Bowman's capsule, and often foamy cells and focal epithelial cell proliferation (Fig. 80–6). Glomeruli that do not contain the lesion of FGS exhibit changes identical to those of MCNS, indicating that the increase in capillary permeability is a diffuse one not confined to the areas of sclerotic lesions. Interstitial infiltrates and tubular atrophy usually accompany lesions of FGS. IgM and C3 are frequently deposited nonspecifically in sclerotic lesions and may occasionally be seen more diffusely in the mesangium.

Clinical Features. FGS is present in 5 to 15 per cent of patients with idiopathic nephrotic syndrome and is associated with a higher frequency of hematuria (65 per cent), hypertension (10 per cent), and renal insufficiency unresponsive to volume expansion (10 per cent) than is seen in MCNS (Table 80–4). Sterile pyuria is also common. Proteinuria is nonselective, presumably reflecting the focal areas of structural damage to the capillary wall associated with lesions of FGS. While most patients have the nephrotic syndrome, a significant minority are detected with asymptomatic proteinuria, a finding that is rarely seen in MCNS. When all of these features accompany the finding of FGS in an early biopsy, only about 15 to 20 per cent of such patients will respond to steroid therapy and many of these do not remain steroid responsive. The presence of the nephrotic syndrome, hematuria, hypertension, decreased renal function, and mesangial hypercellularity on biopsy tend to indicate a poor prognosis.

A smaller group of patients appears to have clinically typical MCNS without hematuria or hypertension but shows early lesions of FGS on biopsy. Often such biopsies are obtained later in the course of the disease after several episodes of steroid-responsive nephrotic syndrome, and such patients may remain steroid responsive for many years and progress very slowly or not at all. When all patients with FGS on initial biopsy are studied, only about 40 per cent are in renal failure at the end of ten years.

Laboratory Features. There are no distinctive laboratory abnormalities, except for the increased incidence of hematuria and presence of nonselective proteinuria, that differentiate patients with FGS from those with pure MCNS.

Course and Treatment. Patients with FGS on initial biopsy, especially if hematuria, hypertension, and nephrotic syndrome are present, rarely respond to steroids and progress to renal failure in an average of about ten years. The level of proteinuria is clearly related to prognosis, and 80 per cent of all patients with non-nephrotic proteinuria retain normal renal function for over ten years. About 15 to 20 per cent of all patients with FGS and the nephrotic syndrome will show a response to steroids, sometimes months to years after therapy, a phenomenon that justifies a trial of steroid therapy as outlined above for MCNS in such patients. If steroid responsiveness is present, the prognosis is considerably better, and such patients may behave like those with MCNS. Alkylating agents such as cyclophosphamide and chlorambucil have been shown to increase the frequency and duration of steroid-induced remission in FGS as they have in MCNS. There is no evidence that immunosuppressive drugs are effective in steroid-resistant patients.

Patients with FGS who progress to renal failure have a high incidence of recurrent disease in renal transplants. Factors that have been correlated with recurrence include mesangial hypercellularity, a rapidly progressive course (less than three years), and receipt of a well-matched living-related donor transplant. In four antigen matches, the recurrence rate may be as high as 80 per cent, although it is less than 50 per cent for all patients with end-stage renal disease due to FGS. With recurrence, patients develop the nephrotic syndrome within a few hours to one week, accompanied by lesions of FGS in the transplant and usually a shortened graft survival. This phenomenon is important both in emphasizing the necessity for accurate diagnosis of renal disease in patients prior to transplantation and in selecting and counseling potential kidney donors.

Beaufils H, Alphonse JC, Guedon J, Legrain M: Focal glomerulosclerosis: Natural history and treatment. Nephron 21:75, 1978. *This study of 70 patients emphasizes the frequency of asymptomatic proteinuria in FGS, occasional responses to steroids, relationships of proteinuria to prognosis, and recurrence rate after transplantation.*

Tisher CC, Alexander RW: Focal glomerular sclerosis. *In* Brenner BM, Stein JH (eds.): Contemporary Issues in Nephrology. Vol 9. New York, Churchill Livingstone, 1982, p 175. *A comprehensive review article that discusses all aspects of this group of patients, including the relationship to MCNS, treatment, and prognosis.*

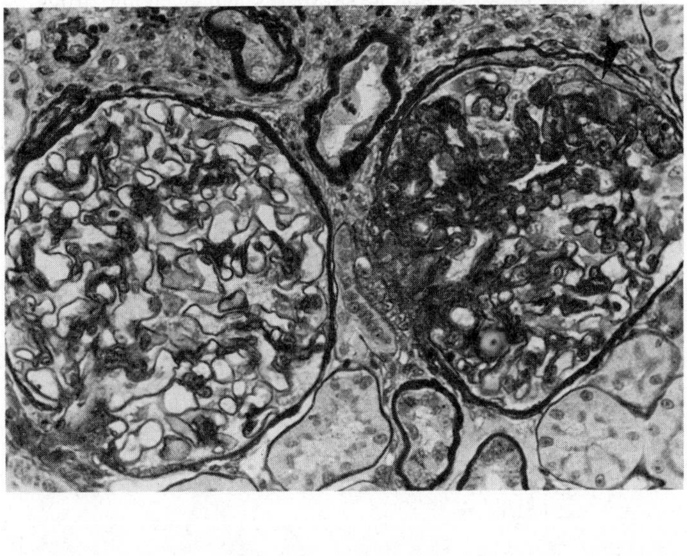

Figure 80–6. Renal biopsy from a patient with nephrotic syndrome, FGS, and decreased renal function. By light microscopy the glomerulus on the left appears almost normal with only slight mesangial matrix increase, while the glomerulus on the right is partially sclerotic with an adhesion to Bowman's capsule at one o'clock (arrowhead). Two atrophic tubules with thickened basement membranes in the upper part of the field are surrounded by fibrosis and mononuclear cells. (Periodic acid–Schiff stain, × 350.) (Reproduced from Couser WG, Salant DJ, Adler S, Bernard DB, Stilmant MM. *In* Brenner BM, Lazarus JM (eds.): Acute Renal Failure. Philadelphia, WB Saunders Company, 1983, p 403.)

HEROIN NEPHROPATHY. In some centers up to 25 per cent of new cases of FGS and 10 per cent of all cases of end-stage renal disease occur in young adults with a history of parenteral drug abuse, usually including heroin. Other renal lesions such as GN secondary to bacterial endocarditis, hepatitis B–associated membranous nephropathy, large vessel vasculitis, and interstitial nephritis related to embolized foreign material are also seen in addicts. However, the entity of nephrotic syndrome with FGS, hypertension, and rapidly progressive renal disease appears to be the most common drug-related lesion. Discontinuation of drug use has resulted in stabilization or improvement in renal function in some patients, but no other form of therapy has proven beneficial. The role of the injected drugs or other foreign substances in the pathogenesis of this lesion is not known.

Cunningham EE, Brentjens JR, Zielezny MA, Andres GA, Venuto RC: Heroin nephropathy. A clinicopathologic and epidemiologic study. Am J Med 68:47, 1980. *This paper reports 23 drug addicts with nephrotic syndrome, most of whom have FGS and progress to end-stage renal disease. It emphasizes the importance of this entity as a cause of chronic renal failure in some urban settings.*

Membranous Nephropathy

Overview. Membranous nephropathy is an uncommon disease in childhood but is the commonest cause of idiopathic nephrotic syndrome in adults, where it accounts for about 50 per cent of all cases (Table 80–4). As with all other causes of idiopathic nephrotic syndrome, the diagnosis can be made only by renal biopsy.

Pathogenesis. Although long considered a prototype of immune complex GN, circulating immune complexes are rarely present in idiopathic membranous nephropathy. Subepithelial immune deposits may result from antibody binding to a non-GBM glomerular antigen in a discontinuous subepithelial distribution or from exogenous antigens becoming localized at this site, usually on the basis of charge-charge interactions with glomerular anionic structures and then binding antibody in situ. It has not been established which of these mechanisms is the predominant one in man. The observations that patients with membranous nephropathy may have impaired immunoglobulin synthesis, low avidity antibodies, and monocyte suppressor cells suggest that the disease may be one of relative immune deficiency.

Subepithelial immune deposits appear to induce proteinuria by a complement-dependent mechanism that probably involves some activity of the terminal complement pathway to produce a lesion somewhere in the distal portion of the glomerular filtration barrier. The role played by inciting agents such as drugs (gold, *d*-penicillamine, captopril) or hepatitis virus in initiating this process is unknown. A strong association exists between idiopathic membranous nephropathy and HLA-DRw3 (relative risk about four), an association also noted in patients who develop membranous nephropathy while taking drugs. Although most cases are idiopathic, some develop in association with a variety of other conditions, including *drugs* (penicillamine, gold, captopril), infectious agents (hepatitis B, various parasitic infestations), *SLE,* and *malignancy,* particularly solid tumors of the lung, breast, and gastrointestinal tract. The nephrotic syndrome may be the presenting sign of an otherwise occult neoplasm, and older patients with idiopathic membranous nephropathy should be carefully evaluated for malignancy. An identical lesion occurs in about 15 per cent of patients with SLE and may be the presenting sign of this disease when other systemic and serologic manifestations are absent. Young females who present with what appears to be idiopathic membranous nephropathy must be carefully followed for later development of SLE. Other associations such as those with Sjögren's syndrome, mixed connective tissue disease, diabetes, thyroiditis, syphilis, sarcoidosis, and sickle cell disease are documented but rare.

Pathology. By light microscopy glomeruli may appear entirely normal early in membranous nephropathy, but as the disease progresses, a diffuse thickening of capillary walls occurs without any increase in glomerular cellularity (Fig. 80–7). A silver methenamine stain will usually demonstrate the spike-like extensions of basement membrane between areas of subepithelial deposits, and the subepithelial deposits themselves may be seen with a PAS stain. A diffuse, very finely granular pattern of immune deposits of IgG and usually C3 is found along the subepithelial surface of all capillary loops (Fig. 80–8). EM demonstrates electron-dense deposits in an exclusively subepithelial distribution with effacement of overlying foot processes (Fig. 80–9).

Clinical Manifestations. The mean age of onset of idiopathic

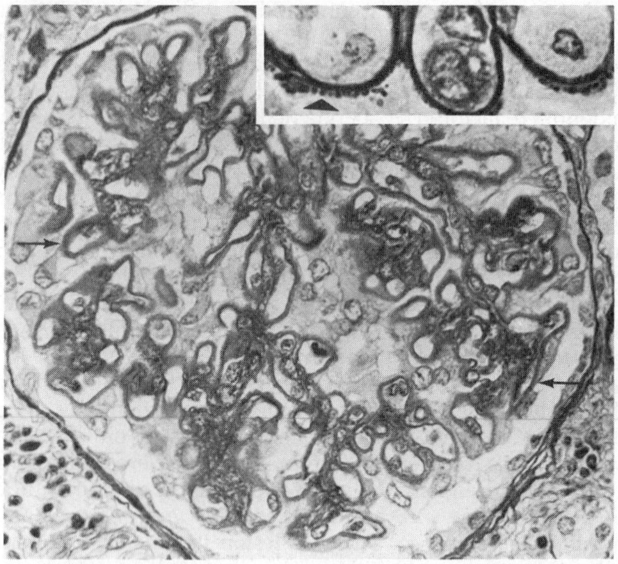

Figure 80–7. Light microscopy in early membranous nephropathy shows mininal thickening of the glomerular capillary walls (arrows) without any increase in cells or mesangial matrix. In the inset, three capillary loops stained with silver methenamine demonstrate the "spikes" of basement membrane between deposits (arrowhead) (periodic acid–Schiff stain, × 350; inset: silver methenamine stain, × 900). (Reproduced from Couser WG, Salant DJ, Stilmant MM. *In* Flamenbaum W, Hamburger RJ (eds.): Nephrology. Philadelphia, JB Lippincott Company, 1982, pp 265–301.)

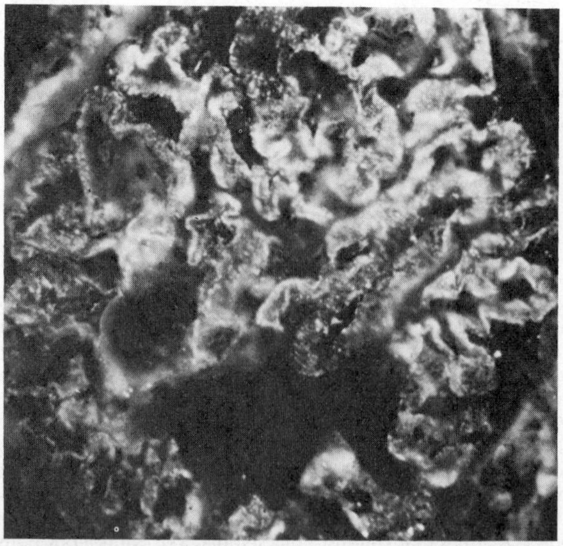

Figure 80–8. Immunofluorescence microscopy in membranous nephropathy demonstrates diffuse, finely granular staining for IgG (and C3) on all capillary walls, usually without mesangial deposits (× 400). (Reproduced from Couser WG, Salant DJ, Stilmant MM. *In* Flamenbaum W, Hamburger RJ (eds.): Nephrology. Philadelphia, JB Lippincott Company, 1982, pp 265–301.)

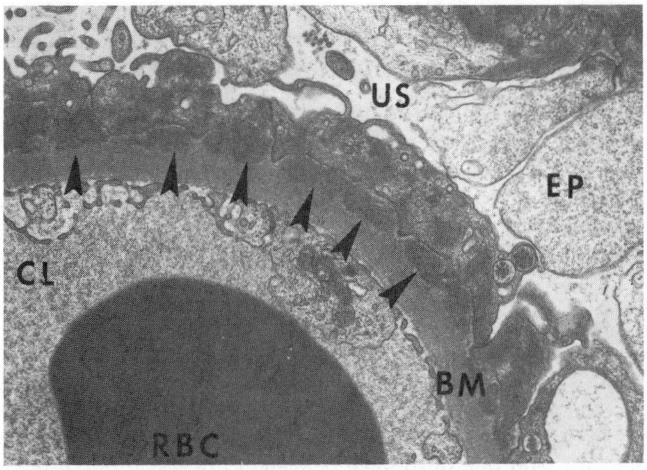

Figure 80–9. Electron micrograph of a glomerulus in membranous nephropathy showing many electron-dense subepithelial deposits (arrowheads) between the basement membrane and effaced epithelial cell foot processes. A red blood cell is present in the capillary lumen (× 15,000). BM = basement membrane; CL = capillary lumen; EP = epithelial cell; RBC = red blood cell. (Reproduced with permission from Couser WG, Salant DJ, Adler S, Bernard DB, Stilmant MM. *In* Brenner BM, Lazarus JM (eds.): Acute Renal Failure. Philadelphia, WB Saunders Company, 1983, p 406).

membranous nephropathy in the United States is 40 to 50, and males predominate about 2 to 1. However, the disease has been reported in patients as young as 2 and over 70. Over 80 per cent of patients present with the nephrotic syndrome, but 20 per cent may be seen first with asymptomatic proteinuria. Microscopic hematuria is present in about 60 per cent of cases in adults, but red cell casts are rare. Hypertension is uncommon and renal function is usually normal at the time of presentation. The association of membranous nephropathy with other disease processes has been discussed above under Pathogenesis.

Two complications of this disease are important: (1) Several patients have been reported to develop a *superimposed anti-GBM nephritis* with crescent formation and a clinical course similar to that of RPGN. This possibility must be considered in otherwise stable patients who experience a rapid deterioration in renal function accompanied by a nephritic urine sediment. (2) An incidence of *renal vein thrombosis* as high as 50 per cent has been reported in membranous nephropathy. Any patient in whom a thromboembolism is suspected should be studied for renal vein thrombosis and treated with long-term anticoagulation to reduce thromboembolic complications if a venous thrombosis is demonstrated.

Laboratory Studies. There are no laboratory abnormalities specific for idiopathic membranous nephropathy. Because of the frequency of various associated conditions, the laboratory workup should include determinations of antinuclear and anti-DNA antibody, serum complement levels, rheumatoid factor, cryoglobulins, hepatitis B antigen, VDRL, and tests to exclude diabetes. In older patients, a careful clinical and radiologic search for occult malignancy is justified. If the patient has unusual flank pain, hematuria, or a reason to suspect pulmonary emboli, the renal veins should be studied by venography.

Course and Treatment. The disease has a widely variable clinical course with substantial fluctuations in proteinuria and an uncertain prognosis. The spontaneous remission rate is about 25 per cent in adults. Another 25 per cent of patients will have persistent nephrotic range proteinuria for many years but will retain normal renal function. The remaining 50 per cent of adults, and 10 to 15 per cent of children, experience a slowly progressive deterioration of renal function that results in end-stage renal disease in an average of about 15 years, although more rapid progression may be seen. No clinical or pathologic criteria have been identified that will predict the future clinical course in an individual patient.

The variable clinical course in idiopathic membranous nephropathy makes any assessment of benefits from therapy difficult, since large numbers of patients must be followed in a prospective controlled fashion to obtain meaningful data. One such study in adults with idiopathic membranous nephropathy and normal renal function compared treatment with 100 to 150 mg of prednisone every other day for two months with a placebo and demonstrated a slower rate of deterioration in renal function in patients treated with prednisone. Several retrospective studies have reached similar conclusions. No effect of immunosuppressive agents has been clearly demonstrated. Until better data are available, alternate-day treatment with steroids for three to four months seems worthwhile and without significant morbidity.

Recurrent membranous nephropathy in transplants is rare but has been reported in several patients who have progressed to end-stage renal disease in a period of four years or less. Recurrence usually has not adversely affected graft survival. Significantly more cases of de novo membranous nephropathy have been reported in renal allografts than cases of recurrence, and the disease is a relatively common cause of the nephrotic syndrome in transplant patients.

Arnaout MA, Rennke HG, Cotran RS: Membranous glomerulonephritis. *In* Brenner BM, Stein JH (eds.): Contemporary Issues in Nephrology. Vol 9. New York, Churchill Livingstone, 1982, p 199. *A comprehensive review of the clinical, pathologic, pathogenetic, and therapeutic aspects of membranous nephropathy, with over 200 references.*

Cameron JS: Pathogenesis and treatment of membranous nephropathy (Nephrology Forum). Kidney Int 15:88, 1979. *A very complete and thoughtful discussion of membranous nephropathy by an experienced clinical investigator. It includes a review and discussion of the data on steroid treatment in this disease with Dr. Cecil Coggins.*

Collaborative Study of the Adult Idiopathic Nephrotic Syndrome. A controlled study of short-term prednisone treatment in adults with membranous nephropathy. N Engl J Med 301:1301, 1979. *A carefully controlled, prospective study of 72 patients with idiopathic membranous nephropathy, which concludes that a three-month course of alternate-day prednisone therapy slows the rate of deterioration in renal function.*

Membranoproliferative Glomerulonephritis (MPGN)

Overview. The term membranoproliferative glomerulonephritis (MPGN) refers to a clinicopathologic entity found primarily in young adults and characterized by idiopathic nephrotic syndrome, hypocomplementemia, and a histologic lesion having the lobular appearance of glomeruli with both thickening of the basement membrane and cellular proliferation. This entity has also been called lobular GN, chronic hypocomplementemic GN, and mesangiocapillary GN. These histologic and clinical features are probably common to at least two separate and perhaps unrelated diseases, which are now referred to as type I MPGN (that with subendothelial immune deposits) and type II MPGN (dense deposit disease). Type I MPGN is about twice as common as type II, and the two diseases cause about 10 per cent of cases of idiopathic nephrotic syndrome in both children and adults (Table 80–4). However, unlike the other glomerular diseases that cause idiopathic nephrotic syndrome, about 20 per cent of patients will present with an acute nephritic syndrome, and nephritic features are common in both of these diseases.

Pathogenesis. TYPE I MPGN. Several features of type I MPGN suggest that it is a chronic immune complex GN: (1) the granular deposits of IgG and C3 in a subendothelial and mesangial distribution, (2) the activation of the classic complement pathway, (3) the frequent presence of cryoglobulins and circulating immune complexes, (4) the presence of similar lesions in patients with some forms of postinfectious GN, including shunt nephritis and nephritis associated with chronic hepatitis B antigenemia, and (5) the production of similar lesions in animals immunized chronically with a foreign serum protein. However, the etiology of the disease, the nature of the antigen(s) involved, and the reasons for the chronicity of the process remain unknown.

TYPE II MPGN. This disease does not appear to be an immune

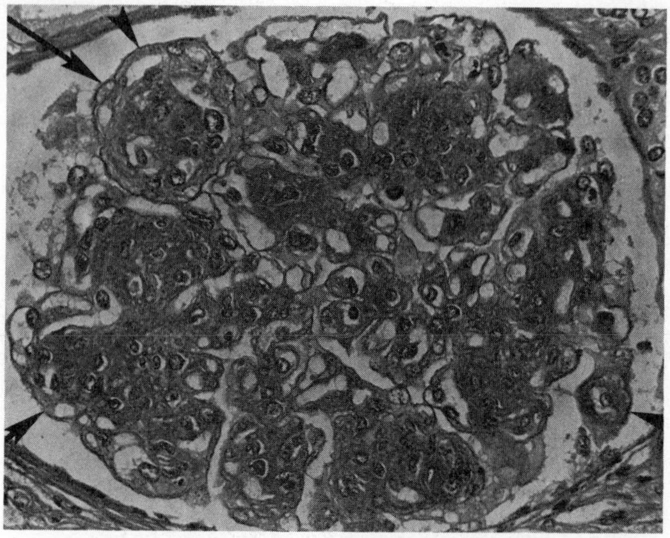

Figure 80–10. Light microscopy in membranoproliferative glomerulonephritis shows glomerular hypercellularity, segmental thickening of the basement membrane (arrowheads), and lobulation of glomerulus (arrows). (Periodic acid–Schiff, × 350.) (Reproduced from Couser WG, Salant DJ, Stilmant MM. *In* Flamenbaum W, Hamburger RJ (eds.): Nephrology. Philadelphia, JB Lippincott Company, 1982, pp 265–301.)

deposit disease, and the nature of the dense deposits remains unclear. Despite much study of the unique abnormalities in complement metabolism associated with this disease, and the identification of C3 nephritic factor in the serum, the role of the complement abnormalities, if any, in the pathogenesis of the disease remains undefined. There is no animal model of dense deposit disease, and similar lesions have not been described in other renal diseases.

Pathology. Type I MPGN. Light microscopy reveals a diffuse proliferative GN with thickening of the glomerular capillary walls, increase in mesangial cells and matrix, and a lobulated appearance of the glomerulus (Figure 80–10). The thickened capillary walls are due to subendothelial immune deposits and interposition of mesangial matrix between GBM and endothelium, resulting in a double contour, splitting, or "tram track" appearance of the capillary walls on silver stain. Crescents are present in less than 10 per cent of cases. Coarsely granular deposits of C3, and often of IgG, IgM, C4, properdin, and fibrin, occur in the mesangium and in peripheral capillary loops in a pattern much like that seen in diffuse proliferative, or class IV, SLE. By EM there are dense subendothelial and mesangial deposits present as well as mesangial matrix interposition with capillary wall thickening and narrowing of the capillary lumen.

Type II MPGN.The histologic findings in type II MPGN are very similar to those in type I disease except that crescents are present in up to 30 per cent of patients and correlate with a worse prognosis. The dense deposits may be seen as PAS-positive, ribbon-like deposits within the capillary wall as well as along Bowman's capsule and tubular basement membranes. C3 is present along the margins of these deposits, resulting in a double linear pattern on the capillary walls as well as surrounding deposits of similar material in the mesangium (mesangial rings). Granular immune deposits of IgG are much less common than in type I disease. EM reveals extensive replacement of the lamina densa with homogenous, dark-staining material that may also be seen in the mesangium, Bowman's capsule, and tubular basement membrane.

Clinical Features. There are only minor differences in the clinical manifestations of types I and II MPGN. What follows is a description of patients with the more common type I disease. The differences observed in type II disease are commented on below. MPGN is a disease of children and young adults, rarely seen before age five and relatively uncommon after age 30. Males and females are affected approximately equally. The nephrotic syndrome is the presenting sign in about 50 per cent of patients and develops during the course of the disease in over 80 per cent. Up to 20 per cent may present with an acute nephritic syndrome (which is more common in type II), and the remainder are detected with asymptomatic hematuria or proteinuria or both. Preceding upper respiratory tract infections have occurred in about half of patients with type I MPGN and may have been streptococcal. Hematuria is a common feature of the disease. Hypertension is present in one third, and 25 per cent have a reduced GRF on initial presentation.

The clinical course is quite variable. One third of patients develop end-stage renal disease within 6 to 10 years, one third have persistent nephrotic syndrome with relatively stable renal function, and one third have persistent non-nephrotic proteinuria or hematuria. Fewer than 5 per cent experience spontaneous remissions. In the long term at least 50 per cent of patients with type I will reach end-stage renal disease in 15 to 20 years, while type II progresses somewhat more rapidly (6 to 10 years). Poor prognostic signs in individual patients include a reduced GFR at onset, the presence of the nephrotic syndrome, early hypertension, gross hematuria, and the presence of either crescents or sclerosis on a renal biopsy.

Type I MPGN recurs in about 25 per cent of patients who receive renal transplants but rarely interferes with graft function.

The clinical features of type II disease which differ from type I include a higher frequency of both the nephrotic syndrome and acute nephritic episodes, a lower frequency of asymptomatic hematuria and proteinuria, more rapid progression to renal failure (probably due to the greater frequency of nephritic episodes), more frequent and persistent hypocomplementemia (see below), and a higher frequency of recurrence in transplants. Type II disease is also associated with partial lipodystrophy in some patients.

Laboratory Abnormalities. The laboratory abnormalities in type I MPGN include elevations in levels of circulating immune complexes in about 50 per cent of patients and fluctuating levels of complement with depression of both classic (C1q, C4) and alternate pathway components at some time in most patients. In type II disease, hypocomplementemia is more frequent and persistent, and only alternate pathway activation is usually seen with a reduction in C3 and other alternate pathway proteins such as properdin and factor B, while classic pathway components are usually normal. Most type II patients have a circulating IgG autoantibody (C3 nephritic factor, or C3 Nef) directed against the C3 convertase of the alternate complement pathway. The definitive diagnosis of either type I or type II MPGN can be made only by renal biopsy with complete IF and EM studies.

Treatment. Despite the fact that the pathogenesis of type I and type II MPGN is probably different, most therapeutic studies have not distinguished between the two, and results have been similar for both. Some authors have reported improvements or stabilization in renal function in patients treated with a "cocktail" of drugs, including steroids, cytotoxic agents, anticoagulants, and antiplatelet agents in various combinations, but this has usually resulted in a relatively high complication rate. Similar results have been obtained more recently using aspirin and other antiplatelet agents, and these studies need to be confirmed. Alternate-day steroid therapy appears to slow the clinical progression of these diseases and may preserve renal function, but often at the cost of relatively toxic reactions to steroids, primarily severe hypertension in children with type I MPGN. At the present time there is no generally accepted form of therapy that has been demonstrated to be of long-term benefit in this disease.

Cameron JS, Turner DR, Heaton J, Williams DG, Ogg CS, Chantler C, Haycock GB, Hicks J: Idiopathic mesangiocapillary glomerulonephritis. Comparison of types I and II in children and adults and long-term prognosis. Am J Med

74:175, 1983. *An excellent clinical review of 104 well-studied patients which discusses the clinical and laboratory findings in type I and II MPGN, the differences between children and adults, and the long-term prognosis and prognostic features.*

Kim Y, Michael AF, Fish AJ: Idiopathic membranoproliferative glomerulonephritis. *In* Brenner GM, Stein JH (eds.): *Contemporary Issues in Nephrology.* Vol. 9. New York, Churchill Livingstone, 1982, p 237. *A comprehensive review article that discusses all aspects of clinical manifestations, pathology, pathogenesis, and treatment of type I and type II MPGN with over 100 references.*

GLOMERULAR INVOLVEMENT IN SYSTEMIC DISEASES

The most common systemic diseases resulting in glomerular involvement are the various forms of vasculitis. With the group of diseases referred to as systemic necrotizing vasculitis, a distinction is made between necrotizing vasculitis involving medium-sized and larger vessels (the polyarteritis nodosa group including classic PAN, allergic granulomatosis, and "overlap" syndromes), and necrotizing vasculitis involving small vessels and capillaries (hypersensitivity vasculitis or microscopic PAN plus several well-defined clinical syndromes, including SLE, HSP, and mixed essential cryoglobulinemia). The only other common vasculitic syndrome with significant renal involvement is Wegener's granulomatosis.

Polyarteritis Nodosa (PAN)

Classic PAN, a disease of older adults sometimes associated with drug abuse (particularly amphetamines) and hepatitis B antigenemia, is described in detail in Ch. 451. Renal involvement, which occurs in 90 per cent of cases, is usually manifest first as hematuria with an active urine sediment and mild proteinuria. In 70 per cent of cases, the renal lesion is primarily an ischemic one caused by vasculitic involvement of arcuate and interlobular arteries. This is best demonstrated by abdominal angiography and is generally not seen on renal biopsy. Aneurysmal dilatation is present in renal, hepatic, and mesenteric vessels. In 30 per cent of patients, a focal necrotizing GN with crescents may be seen. Both types of glomerular involvement may sometimes occur in the same patient. Immune deposits are generally not found in the glomerulus, and the pathogenesis of the renal disease is uncertain. Renal failure is a major cause of death and may be either a slowly progressive process or develop acutely in association with accelerated hypertension. In patients with PAN who develop hypertension and acute renal failure, renal cortical necrosis is common, and there is little reversibility. More often, the disease is a slowly progressive one in which vigorous control of hypertension, use of oral steroids, and addition of cytotoxic agents such as cyclophosphamide have achieved five-year survivals of over 80 per cent of patients in uncontrolled studies.

Milder renal lesions may occur in the other two subgroups of this category. In allergic granulomatosis, allergic symptoms, asthma, pulmonary involvement, and eosinophilia are prominent features of the disease. In the overlap syndromes, both allergic manifestations and small vessel involvement may occur in the presence of the classic large vessel involvement seen in PAN.

Cupps TR, Fauci AS: The Vasculitides. Philadelphia, WB Saunders Company, 1981. *This monograph outlines the most commonly utilized classification system for vasculitis, as well as the clinical features, pathogenetic aspects, and therapeutic recommendations for the major vasculitic syndromes.*

Wegener's Granulomatosis

Wegener's granulomatosis is a granulomatous rather than a necrotizing vasculitis but also involves large vessels, usually of the upper and lower respiratory tract and kidney (see Ch. 452). The disease presents most frequently in the fourth or fifth decade of life and affects more males than females. Presenting signs usually are respiratory and include purulent rhinorrhea, painful sinusitis, otitis, keratoconjunctivitis, oral ulcerations, and multiple bilateral nodular pulmonary infiltrates. Renal involvement eventually develops in over 80 per cent of patients and untreated may result in the death of up to 30 per cent. Early renal involvement is manifest by hematuria, proteinuria, and mild renal impairment with a focal and necrotizing proliferative GN, usually without immune deposits. However, severe diffuse necrotizing and crescentic GN may develop rapidly. Necrotizing granulomatous vasculitis may be seen in biopsies of the respiratory tract but is often not evident in renal biopsies. The presence of granulomas may be the only pathologic finding that distinguishes Wegener's granulomatosis from PAN. Spontaneous improvements in renal disease have not been reported. There are no characteristic laboratory abnormalities in Wegener's granulomatosis. Although the diagnosis can usually be made on clinical grounds, a renal biopsy is generally performed early in the disease to identify potentially severe renal involvement that may be clinically silent and to distinguish Wegener's granulomatosis from other diseases with pulmonary and renal manifestations, such as Goodpasture's syndrome, which would be treated differently. Prognosis and therapy are discussed in Ch. 452.

Fauci AS, Haynes BF, Katz P, Wolff SM: Wegener's granulomatosis: Prospective clinical and therapeutic experience with 85 patients for 21 years. Ann Intern Med 98:76, 1982. *This paper from the NIH describes in detail the clinical manifestations of 85 patients with Wegener's granulomatosis and the treatment protocol now used to induce remissions in over 90 per cent of patients.*

Hypersensitivity Vasculitis (Microscopic PAN, Allergic Vasculitis, Leukocytoclastic Angiitis)

This disease is a form of systemic necrotizing vasculitis of small vessels in which the clinical manifestations do not fall into a well-recognized syndrome such as SLE, HSP, or essential mixed cryoglobulinemia (see Ch. 450). The disease is believed to be a manifestation of immune complex formation in small vessels and frequently follows exposure to some offending antigen such as an infectious agent, drug, or foreign protein by about a seven- to ten-day latent period. However, about half of patients will not have an identifiable antecedent event. The skin is most commonly involved, with palpable purpura. Other frequent manifestations include microangiopathic hemolytic anemia and pulmonary infiltrates with hemoptysis.

Clinical renal involvement is present in about 50 per cent of cases and is usually manifest initially as asymptomatic proteinuria associated with a focal necrotizing GN on biopsy. Impairment in renal function is present in 20 to 40 per cent of cases, and up to 10 per cent may develop acute oliguric renal failure. On biopsy, these patients generally have extensive necrotizing glomerular lesions with abundant crescent formation and negative IF studies. Treatment considerations are similar to those outlined above for idiopathic RPGN, including high-dose steroid pulse therapy and possibly plasma exchange. There is more evidence to support the use of additional cytotoxic agents, such as cyclophosphamide, in the treatment of RPGN due to vasculitis than is present in idiopathic RPGN.

Systemic Lupus Erythematosus (SLE)

The current diagnostic criteria and clinical manifestations of SLE are considered in more detail in Ch. 447. This section will discuss only the renal involvement in this systemic necrotizing vasculitis. About 70 per cent of patients will have clinical manifestations of renal disease ranging from microscopic hematuria and proteinuria to an acute nephritic syndrome with acute renal failure and typical nephrotic syndrome. Renal biopsies reveal some abnormalities in most patients.

CLASSIFICATION. The most common classification system used for renal involvement in SLE is the World Health Organization (WHO) classification based on histopathologic criteria (Table 80–5).

Normal Kidneys (Class I). Only very rarely do patients with diagnostic criteria for SLE have entirely normal kidneys by light microscopy, IF, and EM, and they do not have clinical manifestations of glomerular disease.

Minimal or Mesangial Lupus Nephritis (Class II). This is the earliest and mildest form of renal involvement in SLE and is

TABLE 80–5. HISTOLOGIC CLASS, CLINICAL PRESENTATION, AND PROGNOSIS IN SLE NEPHRITIS

Histologic Type	WHO Class	Frequency (%)*	Proteinuria (%)	Nephrotic Syndrome† (%)	Azotemia‡ (%)	Death (%)	Uremic Death (%)
Normal	I	<5					
Mesangial	II	15	68	0	12	18	0
Focal proliferative	III	20	100	15	18	30	11
Diffuse proliferative	IV	50	100	87	75	58	36
Membranous	V	15	100	88	20	38	6

*Per cent of patients biopsied with SLE who show this lesion.
†Proteinuria exceeding 3.0 grams per 24 hours.
‡Serum creatinine exceeding 1.2 mg per deciliter or BUN exceeding 25 mg per deciliter.

characterized by mesangial deposits of immunoglobulin and C3 with (Class IIB) or without (Class IIA) focal proliferative changes by light microscopy. Clinical manifestations of proteinuria and hematuria are present in most patients, but the nephrotic syndrome and renal insufficiency are very uncommon and do not develop unless progression to a more severe lesion occurs, as happens in about 20 per cent of patients. Complement levels are often normal. Five-year survival is over 90 per cent, and no specific therapy is indicated for the renal lesion.

Class III (Focal Proliferative Lupus Nephritis). This is a stage in a continuum between mesangial lesions alone and diffuse proliferative lupus nephritis. Focal proliferative changes are present in fewer than 50 per cent of glomeruli, but all glomeruli contain immune deposits of IgG, IgA, C3, and usually IgM and fibrin-related antigens. Deposits are predominantly mesangial, but occasional subendothelial deposits may be seen. All patients have proteinuria, but the nephrotic syndrome and renal insufficiency occur in fewer than 20 per cent and may remit following steroid therapy. Serologic abnormalities including hypocomplementemia are more severe than in Class II disease. Long-term prognosis with this lesion is also good (90 per cent five-year survival). However, there is a relatively high incidence of transformation to Class IV disease, resulting in a reduction in five-year survival to about 70 per cent, with almost half of the deaths occurring from renal failure. The most reliable predictor of progression is probably the presence of subendothelial deposits by EM.

Class IV (Diffuse Proliferative Lupus Nephritis). This is the severest of the proliferative glomerular lesions in lupus, with proliferation seen in over 50 per cent of glomeruli, frequently with crescent formation and necrosis. Extensive mesangial and subendothelial deposits contain all immunoglobulins, C3, and fibrin. Mesangial and subendothelial deposits are present by EM, often with subepithelial deposits as well. Proteinuria is seen in all patients, and nephrotic range proteinuria is present in 50 per cent at onset and 90 per cent some time during the course of the disease. Renal function is decreased in 75 per cent at the time of presentation, and serologic evidence of disease activity, including hypocomplementemia, elevated levels of anti-DNA antibody, and circulating immune complexes, is present in most patients. The long-term prognosis for this lesion has improved considerably over the years, with most centers now achieving survival rates of about 75 per cent at five years. The best prognosis is in those patients in whom a remission of the nephrotic syndrome and normalization of serologic parameters are achieved within one year of starting therapy.

Class V (Membranous Lupus Nephritis). About 15 per cent of patients with SLE will develop a glomerular lesion that may be indistinguishable from idiopathic membranous nephropathy with extensive subepithelial deposits of all immunoglobulins and C3. The nephrotic syndrome and a slowly progressive renal disease are common (see Table 80–4). The level and avidity of anti-DNA antibody are often low in such patients, who may have undetectable levels of antinuclear antibody at the time of presentation. The incidence of systemic manifestations of SLE and serologic abnormalities in general is also lower in patients with a membranous lesion. Some transformation can occur from Class V to Class IV, and vice versa, but the long-term prognosis for patients with this lesion does not differ significantly from those with Class II disease. As in idiopathic membranous nephropathy, there appears to be an increased incidence of renal vein thrombosis. No treatment is indicated for the renal lesion per se, although steroid therapy as discussed under idiopathic membranous nephropathy should be given serious consideration.

SEROLOGIC MONITORING. The serologic tests that have been correlated with renal disease activity in SLE include measurements of antibody to double-stranded DNA (particularly if the *Crithidia luciliae* assay is used and only complement-fixing antibodies are measured); levels of C3, C4, and CH 50, with C4 probably the most sensitive; immune complexes measured by solid phase C1q assay; and cryoglobulin levels. While there are reports of a general correlation between abnormalities in each of these laboratory parameters and disease activity in large numbers of patients, there is considerable disagreement about the utility of such measurements in predicting renal disease activity and adjusting therapy in individual patients. The best parameters for following the activity of renal disease remain the serum creatinine level, urine protein excretion, and careful examination of the urine sediment.

TREATMENT OF LUPUS NEPHRITIS. The introduction in the 1950's of high-dose steroid therapy for patients with severe renal disease resulted in an increase in two-year survival from close to zero to about 25 per cent, and there is little disagreement that steroids do have a beneficial effect in lupus nephritis. Usually high-dose steroid therapy is given for a period of four to six weeks and subsequently tapered and adjusted according to responses in renal function, serologic parameters, and extrarenal disease. In the two decades since the introduction of steroid therapy, there has been a steady increase in survival rates to over 80 per cent five-year survival in Class IV disease and 90 per cent in other patients. However, most large prospective studies have shown no long-term beneficial effects on renal function from the addition of immunosuppressive drugs such as azathioprine or cyclophosphamide to a conservative steroid regimen. These agents have no established role in the long-term treatment of lupus nephritis.

In acute disease with rapid deterioration of renal function, initiation of steroid therapy with pulse methylprednisolone (see treatment of RPGN above) may result in a more rapid return to maximal levels of renal function but has no apparent long-term beneficial effect compared to high-dose oral steroids. The role of plasma exchange therapy in the management of patients with lupus nephritis and rapidly deteriorating renal function is currently undergoing controlled study. Early anecdotal results have been favorable. This form of therapy should be considered in patients with severe disease and deteriorating renal function who are refractory to high-dose steroids. With the development of renal failure, disease activity in SLE usually subsides. Renal transplantation has been carried out in a large number of patients without significant problems.

Baldwin DS: Clinical usefulness of the morphological classification of lupus nephritis. Am J Kidney Dis 2 (Suppl. 1):142, 1982. *This is an excellent and updated overview of the relationship between the various histologic classes of lupus nephritis, clinical manifestations of renal disease, transitions, and long-term course. The paper references several older but more detailed analyses of the same type. This journal contains the entire proceedings of a 1981 conference on lupus nephritis, including excellent reviews of the pathology, pathogenesis, and treatment.*

Coggins CH: Overview of treatment of lupus nephropathy. Am J Kidney Dis 2 (Suppl. 1):197, 1982. *A short, concise, and thoughtful summary of a large and very confusing literature. It reviews the evidence for a beneficial effect of steroids in lupus nephritis and the lack of evidence for a beneficial effect of cytotoxic drugs and discusses the role of renal biopsy in evaluating this disease.*

Glassock RJ (ed.): Glomerulonephritis in systemic lupus erythematosus. Am J Nephrol 1:53, 1981. *The discussion of this case by a pathologist, rheumatologist, and nephrologist deals with most of the issues of major clinical concern in managing patients with lupus nephritis and includes 91 references. Like most discussions of therapy, the approach advocated here is arbitrary and would be regarded as too aggressive by some.*

Henoch-Schönlein Purpura (HSP)

This disease, also referred to as Henoch-Schönlein syndrome or anaphylactoid purpura, is another systemic necrotizing vasculitis of small vessels in which systemic manifestations include palpable purpura (100 per cent) on the lower extremities and buttocks due to a leukocytoclastic vasculitis of dermal vessels, arthralgias of large joints, usually the knees and ankles (70 per cent), gastrointestinal involvement with colic and bleeding (25 per cent), and renal involvement (see Ch. 167). About 30 per cent of patients have clinical evidence of renal disease in the form of hematuria or acute nephritic syndrome. Except for the systemic manifestations, the disease is very similar in its morphologic and clinical characteristics to IgG-IgA nephropathy but is of somewhat greater severity. Typically the disease presents with an acute nephritic syndrome, usually without edema or hypertension, developing within three months of the onset of other systemic manifestations of HSP. Many patients have an infectious episode prior to the onset of renal disease. In contrast to IgG-IgA nephritis, in adults the renal lesion may be quite severe. Up to 25 per cent of adults may develop a severe crescentic lesion with RPGN. The nephrotic syndrome has been reported to develop in over 50 per cent, and progressive renal failure occurs in at least 25 per cent of patients. The renal involvement is must less severe in children. Predictors of progressive disease include presentation with an acute nephritic syndrome, nephrotic syndrome, crescents, and subepithelial deposits or subendothelial "lead-shot" lesions by EM. Most patients have self-limited episodes of renal involvement, usually lasting one week or less. However, recurrences are common.

Laboratory features are not distinctive and do not differ from those described for IgG-IgA nephritis. Renal biopsy may reveal a spectrum of lesions ranging from focal mesangial proliferation to diffuse crescentic GN, but the most characteristic lesion is a focal necrotizing GN in which necrosis and fibrin deposition are more common than in IgG-IgA nephritis. IF and EM findings do not differ from those in IgG-IgA nephritis with diffuse mesangial deposits of IgA and lesser amounts of IgG and complement. IgA deposits are also present in dermal capillaries of involved or uninvolved skin.

The pathogenesis of HSP is unknown but is presumed to be immunologic. The various possibilities are outlined above in the discussion of IgG-IgA nephropathy. Reports of patients with typical IgG-IgA nephritis who later develop the systemic manifestations of HSP, IgG-IgA nephritis and HSP in identical twins, and similar immunogenetic associations in the two diseases, as well as the clinical, histologic, and immunopathologic similarities, strongly suggest that a common underlying disease mechanism is involved.

No treatment has been shown to be of benefit in patients with recurrent episodes of acute nephritis or patients with slowly progressive loss of renal function. Short courses of steroids may be useful in controlling systemic manifestations but do not appear to benefit the renal lesion. Patients who develop crescents and a clinical picture of RPGN should be considered for treatment as outlined above under idiopathic RPGN.

Meadow AR, Glasgow EF, White RHR, Moncrieff MW, Cameron JS, Ogg CS: Schönlein-Henoch nephritis. Q J Med 41:241, 1972. *This older article provides an excellent review of the clinical features in a large series of adult patients with HSP.*

Vashikawa N, White RHR, Cameron AH: Prognostic significance of the glomerular changes in Henoch-Schönlein nephritis. Clin Nephrol 16:223, 1981. *This study describes 83 children followed for a mean of six years and provides considerable data on the long-term course of the disease while identifying several clinical and pathologic parameters that predict a poor outcome.*

Essential Mixed Cryoglobulinemia (EMC)

Low concentrations of mixed cryoglobulins, usually Type III with polyclonal IgG and IgM with rheumatoid factor activity, are seen in a variety of immune glomerular disorders, autoimmune diseases, vasculitides, and neoplastic syndromes where they rarely produce symptoms (Ch. 450). Type II mixed cryoglobulins, composed of monoclonal IgM rheumatoid factor and polyclonal IgG, are characteristic of a disorder called essential mixed cryoglobulinemia (EMC), in which dependent vascular purpura, Raynaud's phenomenon, arthralgias, weakness, and GN are the principal clinical manifestations. Cryoprecipitates from these patients often contain hepatitis B antigen. The disease is one of middle age and affects females somewhat more often than males.

Renal involvement is present in about 40 per cent of cases and is usually preceded by purpura and arthralgias. The severity of renal disease ranges from microscopic hematuria and proteinuria to an acute nephritic syndrome with acute renal failure. In contrast to most of the other vasculitic syndromes, the nephrotic syndrome is a rather frequent occurrence, and severe hypertension is common. Laboratory abnormalities include a markedly elevated sedimentation rate, cryoglobulins, rheumatoid factor activity, and an artifactual decrease in levels of early complement components, with C3 and later components often normal. The glomerular lesion is a diffuse proliferative and exudative GN, sometimes accompanied by vasculitis, with large PAS-positive proteinaceous deposits present in many capillaries. The subendothelial capillary deposits are composed predominantly of IgG and IgM, with lesser amounts of C3 and fibrin. In patients with acute nephritic syndrome and renal failure the prognosis is poor. However, in all patients with renal disease, over 50 per cent may recover with or without therapy, and the survival rate at ten years is about 75 per cent. Although steroids and cytotoxic agents alone have not been shown to be of consistent benefit in the renal lesion, recent reports suggest that plasma exchange therapy may improve the prognosis in patients with severe renal disease.

Tarantino A, DeVecchi A, Montagnino G, Imbasciati E, Mihatsch MJ, Zollinger HU, Barbiano Di Belgiojoso G, Busnach G, Ponticelli C: Renal diseases in essential mixed cryoglobulinaemia. Q J Med 197:1, 1981. *A detailed review of the renal manifestations, biopsy findings, and long-term course in 44 patients with EMC and renal disease, emphasizing the spectrum of disease and prognosis.*

Thrombotic Microangiopathy (Hemolytic Uremic Syndrome and Thrombotic Thrombocytopenic Purpura)

Hemolytic uremic syndrome (HUS) and thrombotic thrombocytopenic purpura (TTP) are referred to collectively by some authors as thrombotic microangiopathy. The two disorders can be clinically indistinguishable, probably have a common, although poorly understood, pathogenesis, and respond to similar therapy.

HEMOLYTIC UREMIC SYNDROME (HUS). HUS is a syndrome of microangiopathic hemolytic anemia, thrombocytopenia, and renal impairment which usually occurs abruptly in children about three to ten days following episodes of gastroenteritis or viral upper respiratory tract infections. A similar syndrome occurs less commonly in adults, often associated with complications of pregnancy or during the postpartum period (postpartum acute renal failure) or associated with the use of oral contraceptives. Acute renal failure develops in up to 60 per cent of children but usually resolves spontaneously within about two weeks with only supportive therapy. Chronic renal failure occurs in only 10 per cent of patients, usually those who suffer loss of renal function in a gradual, progressive manner, who have oliguria lasting longer than two weeks, or who have total anuria. Laboratory features of the disease include microangiopathic hemolytic anemia, thrombocytopenia, increased numbers of reticulocytes, elevated bilirubin levels, reduced haptoglobin levels, and elevated levels of fibrin split products, usually with only minimal laboratory evidence of disseminated intravascular coagulation. In TTP (see below) levels of fibrin split products are less commonly elevated. The glomerular lesion is one of intimal hyperplasia of arterioles and intracapillary fibrin thrombi, sometimes with areas of focal necrosis. The anemia and thrombocytopenia are presumably due to trapping of platelets and destruction of red cells in the areas of capillary thrombosis. The pathogenesis of the syndrome is unknown but probably involves glomerular endothelial cell injury by some as-yet-unidentified circulating factor, with subsequent fibrin deposition and thrombosis. Decreased endothelial cell production of prostacyclin, a vasodilator and inhibitor of platelet aggregation, has been reported but may be a secondary event.

Only supportive therapy, including early dialysis, is required in typical HUS in children, since the rate of spontaneous recovery is very high. In adults, the prognosis is considerably worse because renal involvement is more severe and development of bilateral cortical necrosis more common. This is particularly true in cases associated with pregnancy and oral contraceptives. No form of therapy has been determined to be effective in HUS, although aspirin, antiplatelet agents, heparin, fresh frozen plasma infusions, and plasma exchange have all been advocated by some authors. In adults with severe disease, treatment with plasma exchange as described below for TTP, in addition to steroids, antiplatelet agents, and aspirin, is probably indicated.

THROMBOTIC THROMBOCYTOPENIC PURPURA (TTP). TTP is clinically and pathologically very similar to HUS (see Ch. 167). The differences that distinguish this end of the spectrum of thrombotic microangiopathy are (1) a more common occurrence in young adults, (2) fever as a frequent manifestation of the disease, (3) neurologic abnormalities that tend to predominate and cause death, and (4) a lesser degree of renal involvement with acute renal failure in only about 10 per cent of cases. Hematuria is the most common manifestation of renal disease. Proteinuria, generally less than 5 grams per day, and a serum creatinine in excess of 2 mg per deciliter occur in about 50 per cent of cases. Histologically the renal lesion is the same as that in HUS. TTP has a considerably worse prognosis than HUS, with about a 75 per cent mortality within three months, and spontaneous recovery is rare.

A wide variety of therapeutic regimens have been employed in TTP, including all of those listed above for HUS as well as intravenous infusion of prostacyclin and vigorous plasma exchange. The most promising results have been obtained with plasma exchange, often in combination with fresh plasma, antiplatelet agents, and steroids, a regimen that has produced rather dramatic clinical remissions in several patients with apparently severe and advanced disease. In refractory cases, splenectomy may confer an additional benefit.

Ponticelli C, Rivolta E, Imbasciati E, Rossi E, Mannucci PM: Hemolytic uremic syndrome in adults. Arch Intern Med 140:353, 1980. *This paper emphasizes the severity of renal involvement and worse prognosis in this syndrome in adults compared to children.*

Ridolfi R, Bell WR: Thrombotic thrombocytopenic purpura. Report of 25 cases and review of the literature. Medicine 60:413, 1981. *This is a comprehensive review article covering clinical features, renal involvement, pathology, and pathogenesis of TTP, with a detailed and current approach to therapy and over 200 references.*

CHRONIC GLOMERULONEPHRITIS

Chronic GN is not a separate disease. It represents the progressive stage of any of the primary or secondary glomerular diseases discussed in this chapter prior to development of end-stage renal disease. Thus, PSGN, IgG-IgA nephritis, RPGN, focal glomerular sclerosis, membranoproliferative glomerulonephritis, membranous nephropathy, and SLE, as well as diseases such as hereditary nephritis, may result in chronic GN with progressive loss of renal function, proteinuria, abnormal urine sediments, and diminishing renal size. About 60 to 70 per cent of all cases of end-stage renal disease result from some form of chronic GN. In the early stages these lesions can be accurately diagnosed by renal biopsy and sometimes successfully treated. It is difficult to define a level of renal function below which attempts to make an accurate diagnosis are no longer useful. However, in patients with chronic disease, small kidneys, and creatinine clearances below 15 ml per minute, the changes on renal biopsy are rarely diagnostic, and there is little reversible component to the renal damage.

The clinical features of chronic GN are noteworthy only for the frequency with which progressive renal disease is asymptomatic. About 50 per cent of patients will present with advanced renal insufficiency without a clear past history of renal disease. In most patients with chronic renal failure and creatinine clearances below 25 ml per minute, progression to renal failure is inexorable. The rate of progression can be quite accurately predicted from plots of the reciprocal of serum creatinine concentration versus time and is quite consistent for individual patients although not for specific diseases. The clinical manifestations of chronic renal failure are discussed in more detail in Ch. 78.

In end-stage glomerular disease the renal cortex is thin, and glomeruli are acellular, sclerotic, and often surrounded by collagenous material. Tubular atrophy, interstitial fibrosis, and cellular infiltrates are widespread. The mechanisms by which acute renal injury leads to progressive loss of renal function have not been well defined. In some acute inflammatory diseases such as RPGN, immune injury may be so severe that glomeruli are irreversibly destroyed by ischemia, necrosis, and thrombosis, resulting in acute renal failure and end-stage renal disease without a chronic or progressive phase. However, in most diseases progression is a much slower process that appears to continue long after the initial disease process has resolved. Attempts to document secondary immune mechanisms, such as antibodies to altered glomerular components or cell-mediated immunity to renal antigens, have not produced convincing evidence for such processes.

Recent studies suggest that the primary mechanisms of progression in glomerular disease may be hemodynamic. Loss of functioning nephron mass from an acute injury results in an adaptive increase in glomerular capillary plasma flow rates and transcapillary hydraulic pressure gradients (*glomerular hyperfiltration)* to maximize the GFR. Hyperfiltration appears to result in increased capillary permeability to protein and structural glomerular damage when sustained above a certain level over time. The histologic manifestation of this form of glomerular injury is focal glomerular sclerosis—a process that characterizes virtually all progressive renal diseases and results in gradual loss of filtering surface area. The process by which glomerular hyperfiltration leads to sclerosis is unclear but may involve mesangial cell as well as capillary wall injury, leading to abnormal production of matrix constituents that form the sclerotic lesion. Glomerular hyperfiltration induced experimentally can be substantially modified by restricting dietary protein intake. This raises the possibility that changes in dietary protein may be beneficial in slowing or halting progression in a variety of chronic renal diseases. The role of nutritional therapy in chronic renal disease has not yet been defined but is the subject of intensive ongoing investigation.

Brenner BM, Meyers TW, Hostetter TH: Dietary protein intake and the progressive nature of kidney disease: The role of hemodynamically mediated glomerular injury in the pathogenesis of progressive glomerular sclerosis in aging, renal ablation and intrinsic renal disease. N Engl J Med 307:652, 1982.

This is an elegant example of how recent basic physiologic studies can be correlated with older clinical and experimental observations to support a new hypothesis that attributes progressive glomerular sclerosis to adaptive changes in glomerular hemodynamics (hyperfiltration). If correct, this insight could have profound implications for the treatment of chronic renal disease.

Glassock RJ, Cohen AH, Bennett CM, Martinez-Maldonado M: Primary Glomerular Diseases. *In* Brenner BM, Rector FC Jr (eds.): The Kidney. Philadelphia, W. B. Saunders Company, 1981, p 1394. *This chapter presents a detailed discussion of the clinical and pathologic features, course, and therapy of chronic GN and is extensively referenced.*

Maschio G, Oldrizzi L, Tessitore N, D'Angelo A, Valvo E, Lupo A, Loschiavo C, Fabris A, Gammaro L, Rugiu C, Panzetta G: Effects of dietary protein and phosphorus restriction on the progression of early renal failure. Kidney Int 22:371, 1982. *These are the first published clinical data in man suggesting that moderate dietary restriction of protein (0.6 grams per kilogram) may significantly slow progression of chronic renal disease of several etiologies.*

81. TUBULOINTERSTITIAL DISEASES

81.1 Introduction to Interstitial Nephritis and Interstitial Nephropathy

Martin Goldberg

DEFINITION AND ETIOLOGIES. Bacterial infection of the kidneys was once thought to be a major cause of chronic nonglomerular renal disease; hence the term chronic pyelonephritis. This entity was characterized by chronic inflammation and fibrosis involving primarily the renal interstitium and the structures passing through it, including the renal tubules and the renal vasculature. Many noninfectious conditions (see below) can produce identical histopathologic alterations without evidence of concomitant infection. It is now known that most cases of chronic interstitial renal disease in the adult (whether or not they are associated with inflammation) are *not* primarily caused by bacterial infections: (1) only a minority of patients with interstitial disease have a clear previous history of acute renal infection; (2) there is little evidence that chronic bacteriuria per se (a risk factor for acute pyelonephritis) leads to chronic progressive renal disease with renal failure; and (3) bacterial infection, when present, is usually preceded by another primary cause of chronic interstitial nephritis.

Chronic interstitial nephropathy is a clinicopathologic syndrome in which the primary process involves the renal interstitium and related structures and with time is associated with a number of characteristic functional abnormalities. When associated with interstitial inflammation, this condition is best termed *chronic interstitial nephritis.* Frequently the pathologic process may involve only atrophy, sclerosis, or even neoplastic infiltration such that *interstitial nephropathy* (or tubulointerstitial disease) is a more appropriate term. Table 81–1 provides an etiologic classification of the chronic interstitial nephropathies, including the common causes of chronic interstitial nephritis. Most of the causes of interstitial nephropathy are amenable to medical or surgical therapy. Approximately 90 per cent of the cases of chronic interstitial nephritis are due to potentially remediable causes. This contrasts strikingly with chronic glomerulonephritis in the adult, in which commonly the precise etiology is unknown and specific therapy is lacking. The acute forms of interstitial nephritis are discussed in Ch. 74 and 85, and many of the chronic forms are discussed individually in the chapters that follow. Some additional mechanisms will be commented on here.

Obstructive Nephropathy. Obstruction in the urinary tract distal to the renal papillae is the primary cause of more than half the interstitial nephritides. Obstruction may be due to a variety of congenital and acquired lesions that may occur from the ureteropelvic junction to the urethral meatus. Regardless of the cause, the mechanism of the structural renal damage and associated functional disorders is related to the increased pressure within the urinary tract transmitted to the nephrons within the kidney. When unilateral, the characteristic damage occurs to one kidney, but renal failure does not develop (except in cases of a solitary kidney); in bilateral obstruction renal failure is characteristic. Obstruction may be complete or partial, each of which produces different clinical syndromes. The primary event, obstruction to the flow of urine in the presence of continued urine formation by the kidney and ureteropelvic peristalsis proximal to the obstruction, is followed shortly by a rise in intraluminal hydrostatic pressure within the proximal

TABLE 81–1. THE ETIOLOGIC SPECTRUM OF CHRONIC INTERSTITIAL NEPHROPATHY

1. Obstructive nephropathy (see Ch. 82)
   a. Congenital
   b. Acquired
2. Toxic nephropathies (see Ch. 81.3)
   a. Drugs
      (1) Analgesics
      (2) Antibiotics (aminoglycosides, cephalosporins)
      (3) Mithramycin
      (4) Amphotericin
   b. Heavy metals
      (1) Lead
      (2) Cadmium
      (3) Bismuth
      (4) Beryllium
      (5) Lithium carbonate (may cause severe tubular dysfunction; severe renal failure is rare)
3. Metabolic nephropathies
   a. Intrarenal crystal nephropathy
      (1) Urate (gout, urate overproduction states)
      (2) Calcium salts (nephrocalcinosis)
         (a) Hypercalcemic states
         (b) Hyperoxaluria
         (c) Renal tubular acidosis (distal types)
      (3) Cystinosis
   b. Hypokalemic (kaliopenic) nephropathy (causes tubular dysfunction; questionable cause of renal failure)
4. Immunologic interstitial nephropathies
   a. Systemic lupus erythematosus (see Ch. 447)
   b. Renal transplant rejection (see Ch. 79.2)
   c. Drug-induced allergic interstitial nephritis (incomplete recovery from the acute episode)
      (1) Most commonly associated with methicillin, penicillin, ampicillin, rifampin, sulfonamides, phenindione, phenytoin
      (2) Less commonly associated with oxacillin, nafcillin, cephalosporins, thiazide diuretics, furosemide, nonsteroidal anti-inflammatory drugs, allopurinol, cimetidine
   d. Sjögren's syndrome (mechanism not proven)
   e. Interstitial nephritis associated with primary glomerulonephritis (see Ch. 80)
      (1) Focal glomerulosclerosis
      (2) Membranoproliferative glomerulonephritis
      (3) Membranous glomerulonephritis
      (4) Hereditary nephritis (Alport's)
      (5) Goodpasture's disease
      (6) IgA nephropathy
5. Infiltrative processes involving the interstitium
   a. Amyloidosis
   b. Lymphomas
   c. Leukemias
   d. Plasma cell myeloma
   e. Waldenström's macroglobulinemia ("plymphocyte" infiltration)
6. Infectious interstitial nephritis
   a. Chronic (nonobstructive) pyelonephritis (pyogenic bacterial infection is rarely a primary cause of renal failure in the adult)
   b. Tuberculous nephritis
   c. Mycotic nephritis (rare except in the immunocompromised host)
7. Noninfectious granulomatous nephritis
   a. Sarcoidosis
   b. Idiopathic
8. Physical and environmental factors
   a. Balkan nephropathy
   b. Radiation nephritis (see Ch. 81.3; also has a vascular injury component)
9. Cystic diseases of the kidney (see Ch. 90)
   a. Congenital polycystic disease
   b. Medullary cystic disease
10. Vascular nephropathy
   a. Benign nephrosclerosis (longstanding)
   b. Chronic renal artery obstruction
      (1) Atherosclerosis
      (2) Fibromuscular hyperplasia
      (3) Polyarteritis
   c. Sickle hemoglobinopathies
11. Idiopathic interstitial nephropathy

ureters and pelvis. This is transmitted to the nephrons within the kidney, leading ultimately to a reduction in GFR. The magnitude of the fall in GFR depends on the completeness of obstruction and the magnitude of the pressure rise.

Obstruction in the urinary tract is the single most important cause of chronic renal bacterial infection, such that the pathogenesis and rate of progression of the renal disease are often due to a combination of pressure nephropathy and bacterial pyelonephritis. Frequently the infection is initiated by some form of diagnostic or therapeutic instrumentation of the urinary tract. The topic of obstructive nephropathy is discussed more extensively in Ch. 81.2.

Chronic (Nonobstructive) Pyelonephritis. Chronic progressive pyelonephritis resulting from bacterial infection of the kidney is a rare cause of chronic renal failure in the absence of obstruction or other primary causes of renal disease. It is true that acute pyelonephritis heals with some scarring, and it is possible that the scar tissue may be excessive and lead to significant deformity of the renal architecture. Multiple acute episodes followed by extensive scarring could theoretically lead to renal failure. Well-documented descriptions of this process in the adult are few in number. The growing kidney is more likely to develop deforming scars following acute infection than is the mature kidney. Reports of postinfectious renal sclerosis and atrophy are more common in the pediatric literature, and it is likely that previous childhood infection is responsible for the unilateral contracted kidney sometimes seen on urography in the adult.

Immunologic Interstitial Nephropathies. Immunologic injury to the interstitium and the various nonglomerular structures associated with it may be an important factor contributing to certain chronic renal diseases. Our present understanding of these phenomena is rudimentary. In the table are listed several conditions in which immunologic insults are known to occur, such as systemic lupus erythematosus (SLE) and renal transplant rejection, which are discussed in Ch. 447 and 79.2, respectively. Although renal disease in SLE is characteristically due to primary glomerulonephritis, immune complexes have been observed in the tubular interstitial region. Furthermore, occasionally lupus nephritis and other immunologically mediated glomerulonephropathies may be manifest primarily as a chronic interstitial nephropathy. The same is true for chronic renal transplant rejection, although the immunologic mechanisms are different.

Acute allergic interstitial nephritis is probably an immunologically mediated disease related to drug hypersensitivity. Some studies have suggested the involvement of immune complexes, whereas others have implicated antitubular basement membrane antibodies. The typical clinical syndrome associated with this entity (which may be caused by a variety of drugs; see Table 81–1) is acute renal failure, with a tendency toward recovery within several weeks or less (see Ch. 81.3). In a few instances, however, recovery may be incomplete and the disease may progress into a clinical syndrome typical for a chronic interstitial nephropathy. It is possible that many cases of chronic idiopathic interstitial nephropathy may have been of immunologic origin.

Balkan Nephropathy. This is a chronic progressive interstitial disease of insidious onset and unknown cause, restricted to a rural area of 120 by 30 miles around the Danubian Gates tributaries and occurring mainly in farmers living in the flat river bottom land of Yugoslavia, Rumania, and Bulgaria. It is due to an acquired toxic or infectious factor that produces a severely contracted, atrophic kidney and advanced renal failure, typically at ages 30 to 40 years.

Idiopathic Interstitial Nephritis. In approximately 10 per cent of patients with the clinicopathologic syndrome of interstitial nephritis, a cause cannot be discovered. There is nothing about the clinical manifestations, course, and prognosis in these patients that specifically differentiates them from other interstitial nephritides with known causes. It is likely that this percentage will decrease as our knowledge about exogenous (environmental) or endogenous (metabolic) nephrotoxins increases.

PATHOLOGY. Despite the varied causes, the pathology of the interstitial nephritis is generally nonspecific except in certain instances associated with obstruction or with infiltration by neoplastic cells or deposition of certain proteins (e.g., amyloid) or certain crystals (e.g., urate, oxalate, or calcium salts). Grossly, in the advanced stages, the kidneys are smaller than normal and usually irregular in outline, a manifestation of multiple scars. Dilatation of one or more calices associated with overlying cortical scars is thought by some to be pathognomonic of bacterial infection, but this concept remains controversial.

Microscopically, there is typically a chronic inflammatory process of the interstitium involving mainly lymphocytes, plasma cells, and fibroblasts. These are associated with a heavy deposition of collagen and ground substance containing substantial quantities of mucopolysaccharide. The tubular cells are atrophic and flat, and the tubular configuration is distorted by surrounding fibrous tissue. These latter changes are often associated with dilated tubular lumens filled with eosinophilic casts. The tubular basement membranes are characteristically thickened. The glomeruli appear to be involved secondarily late in the disease process. Characteristically they are surrounded by a cuff of fibrous tissue, and the glomerular tuft undergoes fibrosis and hyalinization in the advanced stages. Involvement of the vasculature is variable, but in those patients with hypertension (approximately 50 per cent of patients with interstitial nephritis) arteriolar nephrosclerosis may be seen. Since most of the renal interstitium resides in the medulla, this structure and its papillae are heavily involved in a sclerosing and deforming process. Occasionally frank papillary necrosis may occur, particularly in the nephropathy associated with overuse of analgesic drugs.

COMMON CLINICAL AND PATHOPHYSIOLOGIC MANIFESTATIONS. Despite the multiple causes of chronic interstitial renal disease, each of which may be associated with one or more specific clinical manifestations (e.g., hydronephrosis in obstructive uropathy, clinical gout in urate nephropathy, urinary stones in certain metabolic diseases), the clinical and laboratory features of the interstitial renal disease per se are remarkably similar. Episodes of acute infection are not common unless associated with another predisposing factor such as urinary tract obstruction. If a remediable or reversible factor can be removed or treated at any stage of the disease prior to the terminal phases, the condition has a remarkable propensity to stabilize, and progression may be arrested or retarded. Characteristically there are few symptoms and signs before the *insidious onset of renal failure* with its concomitant uremic syndrome. At this late stage anorexia, nausea, vomiting, fatigue, weight loss, and anemia appear, along with the other classic manifestations of end-stage renal disease (see Ch. 78). Prior to these late stages, the major manifestations of interstitial nephritis occur in certain laboratory tests (see below).

Hypertension is frequently present in advanced chronic interstitial nephritis, but it occurs less commonly than with chronic glomerulonephritis (approximately 50 per cent of cases in the former, compared to >80 per cent in the latter), and the severity of the hypertension appears to be less in primary interstitial disease than in glomerulonephritis. Occasionally chronic interstitial nephritis may be associated with episodes of acute hypotension caused by sodium depletion and hypovolemia as a consequence of impaired renal conservation of sodium.

LABORATORY: URINALYSIS. The urine sediment usually contains no pathognomonic abnormalities. It may be entirely normal, but frequently it contains moderate numbers of red blood cells, white blood cells, and tubular epithelial cells. White blood cell casts may be present during active infection. Heavy proteinuria is not a characteristic feature. Dipstick examination usually reveals trace to 1+ proteinuria; 24-hour protein excretion is characteristically less than 2.5 grams and usually less than 1.5 grams. When present, the increased urinary protein contains a lesser fraction of albumin than in glomerulonephritis and a higher fraction of so-called tubular proteins such as lysozyme or beta-2 microglobulin, which are sometimes used as markers of tubular proteinuria.

RENAL FUNCTIONAL ABNORMALITIES AND THEIR PATHOPHYSIOLOGY. Although not diagnostic, certain changes in renal tubular function occur in chronic interstitial nephritis which are more characteristic and occur earlier than with chronic glomerulonephritis. Since a large portion of the involved interstitium is in the renal medulla, the structures in this region (the loop of Henle, vasa recta, interstitial cells, and collecting ducts) exhibit functional abnormalities relatively early in the course of the disease. Frequently evidence of dysfunction of the distal nephron or of the renal medulla is present with only moderate degrees of azotemia. The most important tubulointerstitial functional abnormalities in chronic interstitial nephritis are (1) impaired concentrating ability, (2) impaired renal conservation of sodium, (3) renal acidosis, often associated with hyperchloremia, (4) impaired renal excretion of potassium and hyperkalemia even when oliguria or severe acidosis is absent, and (5) certain endocrine deficiencies.

Impaired Renal Concentrating Capacity. The normal concentrating mechanism requires not only the intactness of the specific structures involved, thin and thick limbs of the loop of Henle, cortical and medullary collecting tubules and ducts, and the vasa recta, but also a normal anatomic configuration of these structures in relation to each other and the medullary interstitium. Since the interstitial nephropathies primarily distort or displace the medullary architecture, the complex system responsible for generating the medullary concentration gradient is disorganized. This disorganization may occur with only minimal reduction in glomerular filtration rate (GFR). Hence, marked impairment in urine concentration (maximum urine osmolality [U_{max}] less than 500 to 600 mOsm per kilogram) after 12 to 16 hours of fluid deprivation is a common finding before severe azotemia occurs; when GFR reduction becomes moderate to severe (serum creatinine >6.0 to 7.0 mg per deciliter), the U_{max} is isotonic to plasma and may even be less than plasma despite the administration of vasopressin.

Impaired Renal Conservation of Sodium. Fine regulation of sodium excretion (under the influence of hormonal and other controlling factors) occurs in the terminal segments of the nephron, including the collecting system of tubules and ducts. Hence, it is not surprising that patients with chronic interstitial nephropathy exhibit "salt-wasting" relatively early in their disease. This usually means an inability to eliminate sodium from the urine or sharply reduce its excretion when dietary changes or pathophysiologic events require this homeostatic adaptation to prevent severe contraction of the extracellular fluid volume or hypovolemia. Hence, abrupt dietary sodium restriction is rarely indicated in these patients, since they characteristically cannot reduce sodium excretion below 50 to 75 mEq per day without experiencing the consequences of hypovolemia. Furthermore, such patients must be observed closely during bouts of intercurrent gastroenteritis in order to provide early replacement of fluid and electrolyte deficits which would tend to produce further deterioration of renal function.

Renal Acidosis. The distal nephron is important in the renal excretion of acid (hydrogen ions). In these segments hydrogen ions are secreted to react with the urinary buffers, ammonia, and monohydrogen phosphate. Also, the terminal nephron is a site for the addition of ammonia buffer into the tubular fluid. These processes are necessary to regenerate the bicarbonate buffer in body fluids which is consumed by the daily production of 60 to 80 mEq of hydrogen ions from the catabolism of proteins and the incomplete combustion of carbohydrates. The major defect in acid excretion in patients with chronic interstitial nephritis is a reduction in ammonium excretion. This reduces the capacity of the kidney to eliminate "metabolic" hydrogen ions, leading to a decreased bicarbonate concentration in body fluids. As the acidosis develops, the renal tubules reabsorb a greater proportion of the filtered sodium as sodium chloride. Hence, hyperchloremic acidosis is typically observed; when azotemia is moderate (serum creatinine <4.0 mg per deciliter), the anion gap (the difference between the serum sodium concentration and the sum of the bicarbonate and chloride concentrations) may be normal, rising only in the advanced stages of the disease. This "tubular" acidosis of chronic interstitial nephritis is different, however, from classic renal tubular acidosis in that there is no major problem in secreting hydrogen ion against a gradient in the former condition. Hence, minimal urine pH is usually normal (<5.5).

Impaired Renal Excretion of Potassium. Hyperkalemia is not uncommonly found in patients with chronic interstitial nephritis. This not only is seen in the oliguric end-stages of the disorder (typical of all end-stage renal disease), but also may occur without oliguria. There are several mechanisms contributing to this abnormality which are secondary to impaired ability of the kidney to eliminate potassium. First, acute metabolic acidosis increases the rate of movement of potassium ions from cellular to extracellular fluid while concomitantly reducing the renal tubular secretion of potassium in the distal nephron. Since patients with interstitial nephropathy have a propensity for acidosis (see above), hyperkalemia is a frequent associated finding and may be rapidly corrected by the administration of alkali. Second, hyperkalemia may occur in these patients in the absence of both acidosis and oliguria. Two pathophysiologic mechanisms have been observed in some of these patients, the relative frequency and importance of which remain to be determined: (1) In some patients, hyperkalemia has been associated with *hyporeninemia and hypoaldosteronemia* (both unresponsive to sodium depletion). Hence mineralocorticoid deficiency resulting from either a primary abnormality in renal renin secretion or an abnormality in the adrenal response to changes in serum potassium appears to account for the hyperkalemia in this group. Interestingly, most subjects with interstitial nephritis in this category have had diabetes mellitus. (2) In another group of patients, the hyperkalemia has been associated with an apparent intrinsic tubular defect in potassium secretion, unresponsive to endogenous and exogenous mineralocorticoid.

Renal Endocrine Deficiencies. An additional consequence of interstitial damage is abnormal renal hormonal activity. Renin, erythropoietin, and 1,25-dihydroxy vitamin D_3 appear to be made in the interstitium. A decrease in renin production occurs in the syndrome of *hyporeninemic hypoaldosteronism,* which is characterized by hyperkalemia and which is not specifically related to the level of azotemia. This syndrome appears to occur mainly in patients who have chronic interstitial nephropathy. *Decreased erythropoietin* production is the major cause of the anemia of chronic renal failure. It might appear reasonable to assume that the production of erythropoietin would be decreased to a greater degree (relative to the level of renal failure) in chronic interstitial nephropathy than in glomerular disease. It is the impression of many nephrologists that chronic interstitial nephropathy is complicated by more severe anemia than is chronic glomerular disease. The *1-hydroxylation of 25-hydroxy vitamin D* also occurs in the renal interstitium. It appears that a higher proportion of patients with chronic interstitial nephropathy have significant renal osteodystrophy than do patients with the same degree of renal impairment from primary glomerular disease. It is not known, however, whether the renal osteodystrophy is worse because 1-hydroxylation is disordered at an earlier stage or because the same level of abnormality in 1-hydroxylation is present for a longer period of time as a consequence of the slower progression of the renal failure.

RENAL IMAGING (UROGRAPHY, ULTRASONOGRAPHY, AND CT SCAN). The radiologic picture of the urinary tract is generally nonspecific. The specificity relates to some of the causes of the interstitial nephritis: e.g., hydronephrosis and hydroureter in obstructive uropathy, the occurrence of papillary necrosis in analgesic-associated nephropathy and sickle cell disease. Early in the course, the renal size and outlines may be normal, but bilaterally small kidneys are generally characteristic. The renal outlines are typically irregular due to cortical scar formation, and the calices are frequently distorted and often dilated and blunted. Occasionally the urogram may be normal. In recent years renal ultrasound and the CT scan have supplemented or even replaced urography in helping to delineate the causes and stages of various interstitial nephropathies. Thus, ultrasound is rapidly becoming the initial (and often the ultimate) diagnostic procedure in obstructive nephropathy and cystic diseases of the kidney. Both ultrasound and the CT scan may be extremely useful in defining the site and extent of intrarenal stones.

RENAL BIOPSY. As already stated, the histopathology of chronic interstitial nephritis is nonspecific with regard to etiology. Early in the course, the typical cortical biopsy specimen may show no abnormalities despite the presence of severe disease in the juxtamedullary and medullary areas. The most valuable use of renal biopsy is to exclude glomerulonephritis when this is a differential diagnostic problem (which is *not* commonly the case).

COURSE. The time course of chronic interstitial nephropathy is quite variable. If the primary cause can be treated *early* in the disease, progression is often retarded, and occasionally some improvement in renal function may occur. This is most dramatic in the relief of urinary tract obstruction. If the cause cannot be eliminated or the disease has progressed to an advanced stage, the subsequent rate of progression toward end-stage is often slower than occurs in chronic glomerulonephritis at comparable levels of renal dysfunction. Episodes of apparent acute deterioration of renal function can often be reversed by appropriate administration of fluids and electrolytes to treat hypovolemia, acidosis, or hyperkalemia.

TREATMENT. Specific therapy should be directed toward the primary causative factors (see below). In the presence of urinary infection, antimicrobial therapy is generally indicated as described in Ch. 85. An initial attempt should be made to eradicate the offending organisms. Often this is impossible, and a maintenance program designed to reduce the number of urinary pathogens may be in order. Management of hypertension and chronic renal failure (including dialysis and transplantation) is similar to that in other chronic renal diseases (see Ch. 47 and 78).

Andres G, Brentjens J, Kohli R, Anthone R, Anthone S, Ballah T, Montes M, Mookerjee BS, Premzyna A, Sepulveda M, Venulo R, Elwood C: Histology of human tubulo-interstitial nephritis associated with antibodies to renal basement membranes. Kidney Int 13:480, 1978. *A carefully conducted collaborative immunopathologic study of patients with interstitial nephritis in whom reasonable evidence of an immunologic mechanism (i.e., antibody formation against tubular basement membranes) is strongly implicated as a major pathogenetic factor. The prevalence of this phenomenon as a major factor in human interstitial nephritis is still unknown.*

Cotran RS: Tubulointerstitial diseases. *In* Brenner B, Rector FC Jr (eds.): The Kidney 3rd ed. Philadelphia, W. B. Saunders Company, 1981. *A comprehensive review of modern concepts of interstitial nephropathy by a distinguished experimental nephropathologist. Emphasis is on etiology, pathogenesis, and histopathology.*

DeFronzo RA: Hyperkalemia and hyporeninemic hypoaldosteronism. Kidney Int 17:118, 1980. *A well-written review of the important hormonal and renal physiologic factors contributing to hyperkalemia, mainly in patients with various types of interstitial nephropathies. An excellent discussion of pathophysiology.*

Freedman LH: Interstitial renal inflammation, including pyelonephritis and urinary tract infection. *In* Earley LE, Gottschalk CW (eds.): Strauss and Welt's Diseases of the Kidney. Boston, Little, Brown & Company, 1979, p 817. *A comprehensive modern review of pathogenesis, diagnosis, and management of interstitial nephritis and renal and urinary infection.*

Heptinstall RH: Pathology of the Kidney. 3rd ed. Boston, Little, Brown & Company, 1983, p 1172. *This section in one of the standard textbooks of renal pathology contains excellent photographs of the histopathology of Balkan nephropathy.*

McCluskey RT: Cell mediated mechanisms in renal diseases. Kidney Int 21 (Suppl 11):S6, 1982. *This is a scholarly and critical current review of cellular mechanisms involved in immunologic renal diseases with an excellent discussion of such processes involved in tubulointerstitial disease, including drug-induced interstitial nephritis and the rule of anti-tubular basement membrane antibodies.*

Murray T, Goldberg M: Chronic interstitial nephritis: Etiological factors. Ann Intern Med 82:453, 1975. *This clinical study represents the most recent observations in a group of adult patients with interstitial nephropathies, indicating that infection per se is not a significant cause of renal failure without accompanying obstruction or other predisposing mechanical, toxic, or metabolic factors. Further, this study suggests that 90 per cent of patients with interstitial nephropathy have a potentially remediable cause.*

81.2. Analgesic-Associated Nephropathy

Martin Goldberg

In the past three decades increasing numbers of patients with chronic interstitial nephritis associated with the ingestion of large quantities of analgesic drugs have been reported from various parts of the world. Until the past decade, the importance of analgesic-associated nephropathy (AAN) as a cause of chronic renal disease in the United States was thought to be minor, but recent observations strongly suggest that this is not the case. In fact it is likely that AAN accounts for at least 6 per cent of all patients with chronic renal failure and at least 20 per cent of patients with interstitial nephropathies in the United States.

Proof of the causal relationship between analgesics and renal disease is lacking, but circumstantial epidemiologic evidence as well as experimental studies in animals has convinced most observers that AAN is a specific entity with potentially important implications from the standpoint of public health and preventive medicine.

ETIOLOGY. In the earlier reports of AAN, phenacetin was implicated as the most important single nephrotoxic agent. Further clinical and experimental observations have strongly suggested, however, that nephrotoxicity and chronic renal disease are more likely to occur from ingestion of mixtures of aspirin and phenacetin (or related drugs such as acetaminophen) than from ingestion of either drug alone. The quantity of drugs required to produce renal damage is not known. Nevertheless the risk of developing renal disease appears to be higher following consumption of a cumulative dose of more than 1 kg of either aspirin or phenacetin (when taken in combination). This corresponds to ingestion of 6 or more tablets per day of most of the commonly available analgesic combinations for a period of three years or more. Actually, most patients with AAN have taken considerably more than this amount for longer periods of time when the disorder is first diagnosed.

PATHOGENESIS AND PATHOLOGY. Experiments in animals indicate that the major metabolic products of both aspirin and phenacetin are concentrated in the kidney. Further, acetaminophen (into which almost all phenacetin is converted within one hour of administration) accumulates in the renal medulla paralleling the normal medullary gradient for urea which is most concentrated at the papillary tip. Hypotheses have been proposed (but not yet proved) that suggest a synergistic toxic action of the metabolites of the two drugs. In this formulation, the phenacetin metabolites may produce oxidative damage to the medullary tissues, whereas salicylates simultaneously inhibit the major tissue defenses against oxidative damage (i.e., glucose-6-phosphate dehydrogenase).

The earliest morphologic changes occur in the inner medulla of the kidney and appear to be interstitial sclerosis (with minimal inflammation) and tubular degeneration and atrophy. With time focal areas of papillary and medullary necrosis develop, and occasionally the papillary tip may necrose entirely into the renal pelvis. Subsequently, the entire medulla undergoes a sclerosing and degenerative process, and at this stage there develops an infiltration with mononuclear inflammatory cells. The renal tubules undergo marked atrophy associated with thickening of their basement membranes. Finally the fibrotic and inflammatory process extends to the cortical interstitium. Secondarily marked degeneration and atrophy of the cortical structures develop, including ultimately periglomerular fibrosis, glomerular sclerosis, and arteriolar nephrosclerosis. At this late stage the kidney is grossly contracted and deformed with medullary and cortical scars.

Renal functional changes occur concomitantly with the pathologic alterations. Prior to the development of azotemia, the classic pathophysiologic changes of chronic interstitial nephritis may be manifest—especially fixed isosthenuria and a tendency toward a metabolic acidosis with a normal anion gap. The acidosis worsens with increasing renal insufficiency, and ultimately impaired renal sodium conservation may be an important feature.

CLINICAL MANIFESTATIONS. Analgesic-associated nephropathy characteristically occurs over the age of 30, and two thirds to three fourths of the patients have been women. Most patients attribute their ingestion of analgesics to headaches or backaches, and many feel that the drugs provide them with a significant "mood elevation." In fact, psychoneurotic problems are characteristic of this group of patients, particularly anxiety, depression, and hypochondriasis. Although a majority of the patients obtain these drugs directly as proprietary preparations, many receive them through prescriptions by physicians who are unaware that they are perpetuating the continued toxic exposure to the kidneys.

In most patients, the clinical manifestations are subtle or minimal until advanced renal failure develops. The patient with AAN may be seen by the physician for several reasons: for complaints concerning the original cause of the overuse of analgesics (e.g., headache, backache); acute urinary tract symptoms (e.g., colic, secondary infection, frequency, dysuria, hematuria); manifestations of chronic interstitial nephritis (e.g., nocturia, metabolic acidosis, salt wasting); manifestations of chronic renal failure (e.g., anemia, fatigue, uremia, hypertension); or manifestations of extrarenal effects of the continued analgesic overuse (e.g., gastrointestinal complaints, anemia).

The gastrointestinal disturbances (present in half the patients) include upper gastrointestinal bleeding secondary to gastritis or peptic ulcer, symptoms of peptic ulcer aggravated by the drugs, and nonspecific dyspepsia. A number of these patients have undergone gastrointestinal surgery.

Anemia is present in most patients with AAN and is not necessarily related to the degree of renal failure. It appears to be due to a combination of the toxic effects of phenacetin and similar drugs on the red blood cell to produce methemoglobinemia, the effects of chronic gastrointestinal blood loss, and the effects of uremia.

Hypertension, present in approximately half the patients, is typically mild and benign in character. It is usually discovered after the initial diagnosis of the renal disease.

A dramatic event which occurs at some time in a minority of patients with AAN is ureteral colic associated with passage of fragments of necrotic papillae. This is frequently associated with hematuria (gross or microscopic) and manifestations of acute pyelonephritis secondary to obstruction. Occasionally the patient may experience the passage of tissue which is a fragment of a necrosed renal papilla.

A troublesome and common characteristic of analgesic overusers is their reluctance to admit to the use of analgesics or to report the true amount of analgesic consumption. Such patient denial often occurs despite specific interrogation by the physician.

In addition to chronic renal failure, there is increasing evidence that patients taking large doses of analgesic mixtures might be predisposed to certain malignancies. Recent epidemiologic studies from Switzerland, Scandinavia, and North Carolina strongly suggest that patients with AAN have an increased risk of developing transitional cell carcinomas of the urinary tract, particularly of the renal pelvis.

LABORATORY FINDINGS. Laboratory findings typically include evidence of azotemia and anemia. The latter may be normochromic, normocytic, or hypochromic microcytic with evidence of iron deficiency. Urinalysis is nonspecific and exhibits the characteristics of interstitial nephritis, as already discussed. Pyuria and hematuria are often unassociated with positive urine cultures. White blood cell casts in the sediment may be seen during a bout of acute pyelonephritis. Positive urine bacterial culture results are found in only approximately half of the patients at some point of their course. A substantial number of patients develop renal failure without any evidence of past infection despite multiple cultures of the urine.

DIAGNOSIS. The two most important elements in the diagnosis are the documentation of a history of ingestion of sufficient amounts of analgesics and the presence of a chronic interstitial nephritis unexplained by any other known preexisting cause such as obstruction, stone disease, or gout.

As discussed, the history is frequently difficult to obtain because of denial characteristics of many of these patients. It is essential to speak with members of the family living in the same household or with the patient's pharmacist if the diagnosis of AAN is a possibility.

Evidence for papillary necrosis clinically or radiologically should significantly raise the suspicion of diagnosis of AAN. Other causes such as diabetes mellitus, obstructive uropathy, and sickle cell disease rarely are associated with passage of sloughed papillae.

Intravenous urography has been abnormal in as many as 90 per cent of these patients. Often it is nonspecific and shows calyceal distortion and clubbing associated with small kidneys. A common finding is the appearance of the radiopaque medium in tracts extending from the calices; less often (20 to 40 per cent of patients) the classic radiologic findings of papillary necrosis (such as a "ring sign") may be seen.

PROGNOSIS AND TREATMENT. The natural history may be significantly influenced by the cessation of analgesic ingestion. Patients with renal disease who continue their drug consumption invariably develop progressive renal failure leading to end-stage disease over a period of five to ten years after initial diagnosis. On the other hand, cessation of heavy analgesic use can result in prolonged periods of apparent stabilization of renal function in many patients with AAN (usually in those with a serum creatinine less than 5.0 mg per deciliter). In a few patients, actual improvement in GFR with a fall in serum creatinine level may occur even with apparent end-stage disease. This knowledge emphasizes the importance of early diagnosis of AAN and insistence that the patient discontinue the chronic ingestion of analgesic combinations.

PREVENTION. Increased awareness of and reduction of excessive use or abuse of analgesic mixtures should lead to a decreased incidence. Furthermore, elimination of the specific offending agent, if known, would be the ideal preventive approach. Unfortunately we do not have this precise information. On the other hand, reports from Canada, Scandinavia, and Scotland, which have banned phenacetin from over-the-counter analgesic mixtures, indicate a decreased incidence of analgesic nephropathy since removal of the drug.

Clive DM, Stoff JS: Renal syndromes associated with nonsteroidal antiinflammatory drugs. N Engl J Med 310:563, 1984. *A recent and comprehensive review of this important topic, with 157 references. A good starting point for further reading.*

Cove-Smith JR, Knapp MS: Analgesic nephropathy: An important cause of chronic renal failure. Q J Med 47:49, 1978. *An excellent descriptive analysis of experience with 55 patients with analgesic nephropathy followed, in some cases, up to 84 months by the same observers.*

Dubach UC, Rosner B, Pfister E: Epidemiologic study of abuse of analgesics containing phenacetin. N Engl J Med 308:357, 1983. *This is the best and most carefully conducted controlled epidemiologic study available on analgesic nephropathy, performed on 623 subjects from Switzerland who were observed over a decade. It clearly documents that heavy users of analgesics have a higher incidence of both abnormal kidney function and kidney-related mortality than causal users or nonusers.*

Gonwa TA, Corbett WT, Schey HM,. Buckalew VM Jr: Analgesic associated nephropathy and transitional cell carcinoma of the urinary tract. Ann Intern Med 93:249, 1980. *This is a carefully conducted epidemiologic study representing the first such report from North America which strongly incriminates analgesic abuse or overuse as a risk factor for transitional cell carcinoma of the renal pelvis.*

Murry T, Goldberg M: Analgesic associated nephropathy in the USA: Epidemiological, clinical and pathogenetic features. Kidney Int 13:64, 1978. *A summary of the problem in the USA, where it has only recently been recognized as an important cause of chronic renal disease throughout the country.*

Wilson DR, Gault MH: Declining incidence of analgesic nephropathy in Canada. Can Med Assoc J 127:500, 1982. *This is an important report of a survey of Canadian nephrologists in 1980, seven years after federal legislation banned the sale of phenacetin in combination with salicylates. It found that the incidence of AAN had decreased by 50 per cent, confirming the findings of similar surveys in Scandinavia and Scotland.*

81.3. Toxic Nephropathy

Bryan T. Emmerson

DEFINITION

Originally, the term toxic nephropathy was used to refer to acute renal damage from an exogenous poison. A cause and effect relationship between the toxin and the renal disease was usually obvious, the degree of renal damage was related to the dose of the toxin, and the damage was often reversible when the toxin ceased to act. The meaning was then extended to cover both acute and chronic processes. However, the establishment of an etiologic association between the toxic agent and the renal disease was often more difficult in the latter case, and required prolonged study of chronically exposed individuals. More recently, it has become clear that chemicals other than direct nephrotoxins may produce renal disease, so that *the concept of a toxic nephropathy now includes any adverse alteration in renal function or structure caused by an exogenous chemical or abnormal body constituent.* Thus renal damage caused by immunologically mediated reactions to foreign substances is classified with the toxic nephropathies. In such cases, the relationship between the causative agent and the renal disease is less clear and the development of the renal damage is less predictable because of the wide variations in the immune responsiveness of individuals. Moreover, remission is less likely to occur on removal of the initiating agent. The concept of toxic nephropathy also includes damage to the kidney by abnormal concentrations of normal body constituents, such as hypercalcemia, hyperuricemia, hypokalemia, and hypomagnesemia. These topics are dealt with elsewhere, and will not be considered further here. Renal damage from excessive analgesic consumption is such an important variety of toxic nephropathy that it is dealt with separately in Ch. 81.2. The renal manifestations of drug-induced lupus erythematosus and the renal damage from drug-induced hemolysis, methemoglobinuria, or thrombotic thrombocytopenic purpura have also been excluded from detailed consideration in this chapter.

INCIDENCE

Incidence varies greatly in different parts of the world, depending in part on the number and variety of nephrotoxic agents in the environment. However, reported frequencies are rarely a reliable indication of true incidence. The diagnosis of a toxic nephropathy depends, first, upon awareness and, second, upon recognition of the causative agent; both may present major difficulties. Thus the early detection of renal damage by a putative nephrotoxin may be difficult because of the large functional reserve of the kidney and the lack of simple tests to demonstrate minor degrees of functional impairment. Once the nephrotoxic potential of a particular agent has become widely appreciated, further cases of nephrotoxicity relating to its use tend no longer to be reported. In different geographical areas, toxic nephropathy accounts for between 5 and 25 per cent of cases of acute renal insufficiency and failure. This incidence will change as new agents come into use, as their nephrotoxicity is recognized, and as their use subsequently declines, or as their intrinsic nephrotoxicity is modified, a pattern observed with the aminoglycoside antimicrobials. Moreover, many of the renal diseases of still unknown etiology may prove to have a toxic cause.

SUSCEPTIBILITY OF THE KIDNEY TO TOXINS

Many factors contribute to the special susceptibility of the kidney to damage by chemicals, the major ones being its concentrating and excretory functions. The toxic effect of most substances depends upon the *concentration achieved at the effector site,* and high concentrations of toxic substances may occur during their excretion within tubular fluid and tubular epithelial cells. In the case of medullary damage, the countercurrent mechanism may also contribute. The volume of glomerular filtrate is large, and tubular epithelial cells have a high metabolic rate, transporting large amounts and a wide variety of substances (both endogenous and exogenous) during secretory and excretory processes. The flow rate and pH of the tubular fluid, as well as the presence of renal disease, may also affect the concentration of toxin to which tubular epithelial cells are exposed. These cells are particularly prone to damage during the period of neonatal development. The kidney is also liable to involvement in a broad spectrum of immunologically mediated disease, the fine structure of the glomerulus being important in determining the specific localization of immune complexes. When one considers the wide variety of substances absorbed from an increasingly complex environment and needing to be excreted (even large amounts of Worcestershire sauce are said to cause renal damage), it is perhaps surprising that the kidney is able to handle so many without developing lesions.

PATHOGENETIC MECHANISMS

Renal dysfunction caused by exogenous agents can result from dose-related cytotoxicity, an immunologically mediated nephropathy, and prerenal or postrenal mechanisms (Table 81–2).

CONCENTRATION-DEPENDENT CYTOTOXICITY. The usual and most important variety of toxic nephropathy is related to the cytotoxic effect of various exogenous protoplasmic poisons. The damage to the kidney is usually related to the degree of exposure and depends upon the concentration of the toxin to which the cell is exposed, both directly and during the concentration and transport processes involved in excretion. At the molecular level, the precise mechanism of cytotoxicity is complex and not well understood. When the concentration of toxin is low, only altered function of the involved cells may be apparent—in the proximal tubule by the *Fanconi syndrome,* and in the distal tubule by *failure of concentrating capacity and acid excretion.* If the concentration of toxin is high, on the other hand, necrosis of tubular cells may occur—in the proximal tubule leading to the *syndrome of acute renal failure,* and in the distal tubule leading to either *nephrogenic diabetes insipidus* or *renal tubular acidosis.* Disseminated intravascular coagulation may be superimposed on any of these acute processes as an additional pathogenetic mechanism. The concentration of some toxins may also be increased by the medullary countercurrent mechanism, which appears to be a factor in analgesic-induced papillary necrosis (see Ch. 81.2).

IMMUNE-MEDIATED NEPHROPATHY. Immune mechanisms also are involved in some varieties of renal damage from exogenous substances. With some agents, information is insufficient to determine whether the renal damage is due to cytotoxic or to immune mechanisms, or whether both may be acting. In *immune-mediated nephropathy* the extent of the renal damage is unrelated to the dose of the toxic agent and its development is less predictable. It is often associated with systemic manifestations of hypersensitivity and is likely to recur on a second

TABLE 81–2. PATHOGENETIC MECHANISMS OF TOXIC RENAL DAMAGE

1. Concentration-dependent cytotoxicity, dose-related; superimposed acute renal failure and intravascular coagulation—e.g., metal-induced acute tubular necrosis or chronic nephropathy
2. Immune-mediated nephropathy
   a. With systemic hypersensitivity—e.g., methicillin-induced acute interstitial nephritis
   b. Without systemic manifestations—e.g., gold-induced glomerulonephritis or nephrotic syndrome
   c. Hypersensitivity angiitis—e.g., sulfonamide sensitivity
3. Prerenal: reduced renal blood flow or glomerular filtration rate—e.g., dehydration, anaphylactic reaction, hypotension
4. Postrenal: tubular or ureteric obstruction—e.g., crystal nephropathy, retroperitoneal fibrosis

exposure to the causative agent. Circulating antibodies to the causative agent may sometimes be demonstrable, and cell-mediated immune mechanisms may also play a pathogenetic role.

Hypersensitivity angiitis, sometimes with Henoch-Schönlein purpura, occurring as a reaction to an exogenous agent such as sulfonamide, may result in renal disease. Glomeruli may be involved when various processes leading to a glomerulonephritis are invoked as a response to an exogenous agent. Immune complexes, such as those occurring during gold therapy, may be deposited beneath, and induce a response on the part of, the epithelial cells of the glomerular capillary. It has been suggested that petroleum products may be involved in the genesis of Goodpasture's syndrome, in which circulating antibodies against glomerular basement membrane have been found. In drug-induced systemic lupus erythematosus, circulating immune complexes may cause damage to tubules as well as glomeruli. Damage to tubules may also be found in the presence of antibodies to tubular basement membrane. These have been said to develop following primary cytotoxic damage to tubular cells.

An immunologically mediated *acute interstitial nephritis* is also an important variety of toxic nephropathy. The best example is the reaction to methicillin, in which hematuria and deterioration of renal function occur. Kidney size is usually increased in acute cases. The characteristic histologic lesion consists of edema and infiltration of interstitial tissues, chiefly by T lymphocytes and plasma cells, but also by eosinophils and occasional polymorphonuclear leukocytes, in the absence of interstitial fibrosis. Dilatation of tubules may be seen, occasionally with casts; there may also be degeneration and necrosis of tubular epithelial cells in the most severely affected areas with atrophy of tubules. Characteristically, the glomeruli and vessels are normal, whereas antibody to tubular basement membrane has been noted on immunofluorescence. Those agents, such as rifampin and phenindione, that can lead to prolonged anuria and impairment of renal function may cause tubular atrophy and interstitial fibrosis as well as focal aggregations of lymphocytes and plasma cells.

PRERENAL AND POSTRENAL MECHANISMS. Disordered fluid and electrolyte balance or an anaphylactic reaction to a therapeutic agent may cause a reduction in renal blood flow and a corresponding fall in the glomerular filtration rate. Treatment with drugs that inhibit protein synthesis, such as the tetracyclines, can also contribute to nitrogen retention. Postrenal causes are relatively uncommon, the most important being tubular obstruction by sulfonamide or uric acid crystals, or ureteral obstruction from retroperitoneal fibrosis resulting from treatment with methysergide or practolol.*

The various pathogenetic mechanisms mentioned are not mutually exclusive, and various combinations may occur, as illustrated subsequently.

ASSOCIATED CLINICAL SYNDROMES

With such a wide variety of pathogenetic mechanisms, the clinical presentation may be extremely varied. The traditional toxic nephropathy following exposure to a poison is most likely to present with either tubular dysfunction or the syndrome of acute renal failure. If exposure has been prolonged, chronic renal failure may develop. The clinical manifestations of the immunologically mediated forms of renal disease include the nephritic syndrome, the nephrotic syndrome, and the acute or chronic renal failure of interstitial nephritis. Combinations of several of these syndromes may occur simultaneously or sequentially at different phases of exposure to a toxic agent. The recognition of any of the syndromes is greatly facilitated by information concerning renal function prior to contact with any potential nephrotoxin. The syndromes are included here to facilitate the subsequent consideration of particular nephrotoxic agents.

*Investigational drug.

RENAL TUBULAR DYSFUNCTION. Although the clinical manifestations may vary widely, three syndromes are seen with toxic renal damage severe enough only to impair tubular function. (1) The *Fanconi syndrome,* a term used broadly to imply renal impairment in which tubular dysfunction is more severe than glomerular dysfunction (Ch. 83.5). Its manifestations include glycosuria, aminoaciduria and phosphaturia, and sometimes hypokalemia. It is seen in several metal nephropathies, and in that caused by degraded tetracycline. (2) Impairment of urine concentrating capacity leading to *nephrogenic diabetes insipidus* with polyuria and polydipsia, as seen in nephrotoxicity caused by lithium, fluoride, and demeclocycline (Ch. 226). (3) Impairment of acid excretion leading to *renal tubular acidosis,* as develops in the nephrotoxicity caused by amphotericin B (Ch. 83.2).

ACUTE RENAL FAILURE. This may occur in varying degrees of severity, and may be detected only if one is alert to the possibility. In its milder form, slight proteinuria with an increased excretion of cells and casts in the urine may be found, with a fall in urine volume and the appearance of azotemia. An example of this may be seen in nephrotoxicity caused by the aminoglycoside antimicrobials. In its most acute form, such as that occurring after the ingestion of inorganic salts of mercury, the clinical pattern will be that of acute tubular necrosis with the early development of oliguria or anuria and a dramatic cessation of renal function (see Ch. 77). This is potentially reversible after removal of the causative agent.

The syndrome of acute renal failure caused by *acute interstitial nephritis* usually presents with deterioration of renal function, often associated with oliguria, developing some days or weeks after exposure to the causative agent. Hematuria, either microscopic or macroscopic, and proteinuria are commonly seen, together with systemic manifestations such as fever, rash, arthralgia, eosinophilia, and sometimes disordered liver function. Mostly, the renal insufficiency is of moderate degree and is associated either with oliguria or with polyuria if the urine-concentrating mechanism is impaired. Remission usually occurs after withdrawal of the causative agent; however, if it is continued, the associated acute renal insufficiency may become chronic, leading to permanent renal impairment. Steroid therapy after withdrawal of the causative agent has appeared to hasten remission in some cases.

CHRONIC RENAL INSUFFICIENCY AND FAILURE. When caused by renal damage by toxic agents, the syndrome of chronic renal insufficiency will usually be indistinguishable clinically from that following renal damage of any other cause. The typical syndrome is described in Ch. 78. In some of these situations, there may be slowly progressive deterioration of renal function, even in the absence of continuing toxic concentrations of the initiating agent. In such cases, hypertension with consequent vascular sclerosis may be important in producing the progressive damage. Chronic lead nephropathy represents a typical example of this variety of toxic nephropathy.

THE GLOMERULONEPHRITIC SYNDROME. Glomerular involvement in an immune-mediated response to an exogenous toxin may present with the clinical features of a glomerulonephritis, with insidious proteinuria, hematuria, and nitrogen retention. When proteinuria becomes sufficient to induce hypoalbuminemia and edema, the nephrotic syndrome (see Ch. 80) may result. Typical examples occur with a wide variety of therapeutic agents, such as penicillamine, trimethadione, and gold, and with certain exogenous noxious agents such as snake venom, poison ivy, bee sting, or pollens.

Linton AL, Clark WF, Driedger AA, Turnbull I, Lindsay RM: Acute interstitial nephritis due to drugs. Ann Intern Med 93:735, 1980. *Report of nine cases, with literature review.*

Muehrcke RC, Volini FI, Morris AM, Moles JB, Lawrence AG: Acute toxic nephropathies: Clinical pathologic correlations. Ann Clin Lab Sci 6:477, 1976. *A review of acute renal failure of toxic origin, including the authors' extensive clinical experience in this area. Extensively referenced.*

Porter GA (ed.): Nephrotoxic mechanisms of drugs and environmental toxins.

TABLE 81–3. SOME COMMON OR IMPORTANT NEPHROTOXINS

Antimicrobial and chemotherapeutic agents: Aminoglycosides (streptomycin, neomycin, gentamicin); cephalosporins (cephaloridine, cephalothin); penicillins (methicillin and ampicillin); sulfonamides; tetracycline, demeclocycline; rifampin, ethambutol; amphotericin B
Metallic salts: lead, cadmium, mercury, gold, lithium, uranium, copper, bismuth, thallium, arsenic and arsine, platinum, silicon
Therapeutic agents: phenindione, D-penicillamine, phenytoin, trimethadione, paramethadione, furosemide, streptozotocin, nonsteroidal anti-inflammatory drugs, sulfinpyrazone, allopurinol, analgesics (salicylates and aspirin-phenacetin combinations), paracetamol, cimetidine
Anesthetic agents: methoxyflurane, enflurane
Radiographic contrast media, especially those used in high concentration for angiography and cholecystography
Hydrocarbons and organic solvents: carbon tetrachloride, tetrachloroethylene, ethylene glycol
Osmotic agents: low molecular weight dextrans
Physical agents: radiation, heat stroke, electroshock
Miscellaneous: potassium bromate, carbon monoxide, snake and spider venom, mushroom poisoning

This list is not comprehensive and the omission of a substance does not imply the absence of nephrotoxicity.

New York, Plenum Medical Book Company, 1982. *Multiauthor book concerning mechanisms of action of a wide range of nephrotoxins. Partly experimental but some excellent clinical chapters.*

Roxe DM: Toxic nephropathy from diagnostic and therapeutic agents. Am J Med 69:759, 1980. *Review and commentary with 140 references.*

Singer I, Forrest JN: Drug-induced states of nephrogenic diabetes insipidus. Kidney Int 10:82, 1976. *An extensive review of normal and disordered mechanisms of water excretion with special consideration of lithium, demeclocycline, and methoxyflurane.*

SOME IMPORTANT NEPHROTOXINS (Table 81–3)

Antimicrobial and Chemotherapeutic Agents

Dose-related nephrotoxicity is generally greater if (1) *even apparently minor renal insufficiency* (such as occurs with increasing years, and which may not produce nitrogen retention) *is present prior to therapy,* (2) *two potentially nephrotoxic agents are used together,* or (3) *exposure is prolonged.* In the presence of pre-existing renal disease, it may be possible to avoid nephrotoxicity by modifications of dosage which prevent the development of toxic serum concentrations.

Appel GB, Neu HC: The nephrotoxicity of antimicrobial agents. N Engl J Med 296:663, 722, 784, 1977. *Comprehensive three-part review of all antimicrobial agents; 272 references.*

Bennett WM, Singer I, Golper T, Feig P, Coggins CJ: Guidelines for drug therapy in renal failure. Ann Intern Med 86:754, 1977. *Ten pages of tables listing pharmacokinetic variables, adjustments in renal failure and toxic effects; 615 references.*

Whelton A: Antibacterial chemotherapy in renal insufficiency. A review. Antibiot Chemother 18:1, 1974. *Extensive clinical, pharmacologic, and toxicologic review; 234 references.*

AMINOGLYCOSIDES. These agents bind to renal tissue, and a large proportion of a given dose is rapidly excreted by the kidney. All are potential dose-related nephrotoxins which affect primarily the proximal tubule and present chiefly as acute renal insufficiency, sometimes with oliguria. Since nephrotoxicity is related to the serum concentration and the duration of therapy, the initial dosage regimen should be determined from a consideration of lean body weight and renal function and subsequently adjusted according to the measured serum concentrations of the aminoglycoside. Renal function should be monitored during therapy.

Streptomycin exhibits low nephrotoxicity, but renal function must be monitored in order to prevent accumulation of the drug and resulting ototoxicity. Neomycin, the most toxic aminoglycoside, is too toxic for parenteral use and is restricted to topical application or irrigation and to bowel sterilization by oral administration. Some neomycin is absorbed systemically from both these routes, however, and toxic serum concentrations, with nephrotoxicity and ototoxicity, may occur if renal excretory function is impaired.

Gentamicin accumulates in proximal tubular cells, whence it is only slowly eliminated. Clinically significant nephrotoxicity with nitrogen retention is not infrequent, and dosage should be calculated with care, with monitoring of serum gentamicin and creatinine and urea concentrations. The risk of renal damage may be increased by associated therapy with cephalosporins or diuretics or by potassium depletion. When acute tubular necrosis develops, hemodialysis may be needed, and, although the lesion is potentially reversible, recovery may be slow and incomplete.

Tobramycin has less nephrotoxic potential than gentamicin, but the relative risk for amikacin remains to be established. Careful calculation of dose and monitoring of serum levels are important. Both are effectively removed by hemodialysis.

Cronin RE: Aminoglycoside nephrotoxicity: Pathogenesis and prevention. Clin Nephrol 11:251, 1979. *Reviews mechanism of, and factors predisposing to, nephrotoxicity, and how nephrotoxicity in the clinical setting may be minimized.*

VANCOMYCIN. Although there is little recent evidence for serious nephrotoxicity, this drug, which is now largely used for resistant staphylococcal infections, is ototoxic and should be used as a potential nephrotoxin. Dosage should be guided by serum concentrations.

CEPHALOSPORINS. The original cephalosporin, cephaloridine, demonstrated dose-related nephrotoxicity and should no longer be used. Cephalothin, although certainly less nephrotoxic, may

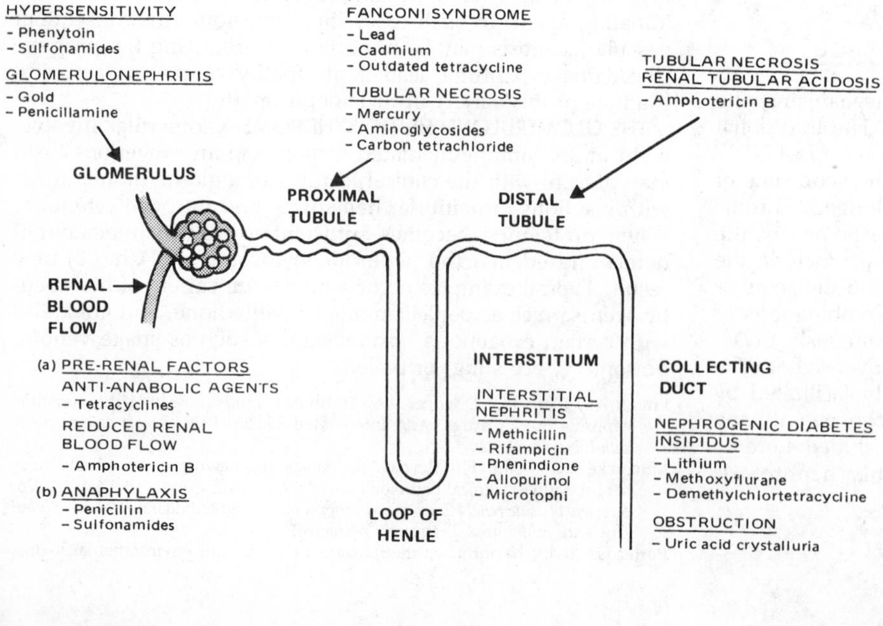

Figure 81–1. Pattern of nephron dysfunction attributable to particular nephrotoxins.

still on rare occasions induce renal damage in man, although this appears to be significantly less than that of even the newer aminoglycosides. The new cephalosporins, cefuroxime and cefamandole, and the cephamycin, cefoxitin, seem to have minimal nephrotoxic potential.

Cephalosporins are rapidly excreted by tubular excretory mechanisms probably within the proximal convoluted tubule, and high concentrations are achieved within the tubular epithelial cells. Nephrotoxicity seems to be a particular risk if high dosage is used in patients with pre-existing renal disease. Although some reports have suggested that the lesion is an acute interstitial nephritis, immunofluorescence has been negative and there has been no clear evidence of antibody production. Other factors promoting nephrotoxicity include concurrent diuretic therapy, dehydration or plasma volume depletion, and the simultaneous administration of aminoglycoside antibiotics.

There are many reports of nephrotoxicity during combined therapy with cephalosporins and aminoglycosides. It presents clinically as dose-related reversible acute renal failure. It is particularly likely in very ill patients with possible pre-existing renal disease exposed to high serum antibiotic concentrations for more than five days. Such concurrent administration follows the general rule of increased nephrotoxicity when two potential nephrotoxins are administered simultaneously.

Annotation: Cephalosporin nephrotoxicity. Lancet 1:962, 1979. *Helpful review; 8 recent references.*

PENICILLIN DERIVATIVES. Penicillin preparations do not exhibit direct or dose-related nephrotoxicity. Renal damage may develop during an anaphylactic reaction to penicillin, particularly if hypotension occurs. There is also some evidence of a hypersensitivity type of angiitis developing after penicillin therapy which may affect the kidney, producing lesions in the glomerular tufts. However, the main renal lesion, associated in particular with the semisynthetic penicillins, is an acute interstitial nephritis of allergic origin. Although it is chiefly seen after methicillin therapy (one in five patients) and occasionally after ampicillin therapy, it can probably be a rare complication of therapy with any of the penicillin derivatives. Methicillin nephropathy usually presents, some days after the beginning of treatment, with fever, a rash and eosinophilia; with hematuria, which may be macroscopic; and with steadily progressive renal insufficiency. Eosinophils can usually be found in the patient's urine. Histologically, the glomeruli are normal and the tubules show only patchy changes, but there is interstitial edema with infiltration by lymphocytes, monocytes, plasma cells, and eosinophils. In some such cases, serum antibodies to the penicilloyl antigen have been detected, and immunofluorescence has been noted along both the tubular and the glomerular basement membrane. The postulated mechanism has been the development of an immune response to an antigen-protein complex resulting from the coupling of the penicilloyl hapten to a renal structural protein producing a cell-mediated type of immune response. Subsequent exposure to the same or a different penicillin has usually resulted in an exacerbation of the renal disease.

The management of penicillin-induced acute interstitial nephritis includes both withdrawal of the cause and careful management of any associated acute renal insufficiency. The limited evidence available suggests that prednisone significantly speeds resolution of the renal lesion, and should be used, particularly in the more severe cases. Heparin may be added if there is evidence of intravascular fibrin deposition.

Galpin JE, Shinaberger JH, Stanley TM, et al.: Acute interstitial nephritis due to methicillin. Am J Med 65:756, 1978. *Description of 14 patients, eight of whom received prednisone therapy.*

SULFONAMIDES. Nephrotoxic reactions to the sulfonamides, relatively frequent during their early years of use, are now quite uncommon. There is probably no dose-related nephrotoxic effect. The main problem was related to crystallization of the sulfonamide within the renal tubules, leading to hematuria and an obstructive uropathy with oliguria and progressive renal failure. The tendency to crystallization of sulfonamides depended upon the sulfonamide concentration, the solubility of the particular compound, and the pH of the tubular fluid or urine. It is preventable by maintenance of a dilute alkaline urine. The newer sulfonamides are appreciably more soluble, and the risk of sulfonamide crystalluria is low.

An allergic reaction to the sulfonamides is relatively common, unrelated to the dose used. Some of the manifestations resemble an acute interstitial nephritis; an immune complex glomerulonephritis and a necrotizing angiitis have also been reported. Such reactions were particularly associated with the use of the long-acting sulfonamides. Although the sulfonamide component of co-trimoxazole (trimethoprim-sulfamethoxazole) can cause any of these reactions, serious renal toxicity has been rare in patients with normal renal function; it is more common in renal insufficiency, in which the dose of co-trimoxazole should be reduced.

TETRACYCLINE. The tetracyclines inhibit the utilization of amino acids for protein synthesis and increase urea production. This is a particular problem in patients with stable chronic renal failure in whom the excretion of the tetracycline is also delayed and its metabolic effect intensified. The tetracyclines also promote an increase in salt and water excretion which, in patients with chronic renal failure, leads to weight loss, acidosis, and a fall in the creatinine clearance. This can result in a marked deterioration of renal function and even death in subjects with pre-existing renal disease. *Doxycycline* elimination is unchanged in chronic renal failure. Hence, although it has a slight antianabolic effect, it does not cause an exacerbation of renal failure in patients with renal disease and is the tetracycline of choice in this situation.

The consumption of outdated and deteriorated tetracyclines has caused a reversible Fanconi syndrome. This has been associated with glycosuria (sufficient at times to cause polyuria and weight loss), phosphaturia, and aminoaciduria, together with proteinuria which has varied from mild to considerable. There is often associated evidence of renal tubular acidosis, and the patients have usually shown hypokalemia, hypouricemia, and hypophosphatemia. Some have also had polyuria. These features have usually resolved within a month.

Demethylchlortetracycline (demeclocycline) can cause impairment of renal concentrating power in normal subjects and can induce a reversible nephrogenic diabetes insipidus with polyuria and polydipsia. The effect is dose related and reversible, and demethylchlortetracycline is used in the treatment of the chronic syndrome of inappropriate secretion of antidiuretic hormone. It is thought to act by inhibiting the generation of cyclic AMP and its action in promoting osmotic water flow through membranes. Its use has been associated with the development of nonoliguric renal failure in patients with cirrhosis.

Montoliu J, Carrera M, Darnell A, Revert L: Lactic acidosis and Fanconi's syndrome due to degraded tetracycline. Br Med J 283:1576, 1981. *Detailed case report.*

Oster JR, Epstein M, Ulano HB: Deterioration of renal function with demeclocycline administration. Curr Ther Res 20:794, 1976. *Describes acute renal insufficiency in a patient with hepatic cirrhosis and ascites; elevated plasma demeclocycline concentration.*

ANTITUBERCULOUS AGENTS. Patients receiving therapy with *rifampin (rifampicin)* may develop influenza-like symptoms of chills, malaise, vomiting, and fever, which are followed by oliguria, leading to acute renal failure. This often remits after rifampin is withdrawn. Most patients affected in this way have received a prior course of rifampin for between one and twelve months, and the syndrome has developed on starting a second course of the drug. Although the initial evidence suggested that the acute renal failure was related to an acute tubular necrosis produced by vasomotor mechanisms, the lesions have recently been regarded as fitting more an acute interstitial nephritis, and occasionally immunoglobulin deposits have been seen around the tubules. Some of these patients have also had positive Coombs' test results, and others a positive macrophage migration inhibition reaction. Anti-rifampin antibodies have been found in the serum of many affected patients, but have been absent in a few. However, these antibodies have also been demonstrated in serum from patients receiving regular daily therapy with rifampin in the absence of any complications. It is likely therefore that the renal lesions develop as a response to a critical level of antigen-antibody complex which occurs when rifampin therapy is intermittent. Clinical manifestations may vary from mild renal insufficiency to severe renal failure requiring dialysis.

The use of *ethambutol* has also been occasionally associated with an episode of acute renal failure which has remitted after withdrawal of the drug, only to leave persistent impairment of renal function in some cases. The pathologic changes suggested an interstitial nephritis, and, although this appears to be a rare development, observation of renal function during administration of ethambutol seems to be warranted. Ethambutol also causes hyperuricemia by lowering urate clearance, but this mechanism does not appear to be involved in the causation of the acute renal failure. Acute interstitial nephritis with allergic skin manifestations has, on rare occasions, been attributed to para-aminosalicylate.

Nessi R, Bonoldi GL, Redaelli B, DiFilippo G: Acute renal failure after rifampicin. A case report and survey of the literature. Nephron 16:148, 1976. *Reviews 36 cases and suggests an immunologic basis for the renal disease.*

AMPHOTERICIN B. This drug, used only in systemic fungal infections, causes nephrotoxicity in most patients. It is strongly protein bound, is not dialysable, and is slowly excreted from the body, largely by nonrenal routes. One of its earliest actions is to alter the permeability of cellular membranes. This effect on the luminal membrane of the renal tubular epithelium leads to a failure of hydrogen ion excretion and an increased urinary loss of potassium ions. Thus one of its earliest manifestations is the development of a distal type of renal tubular acidosis, with hypokalemia. A rise in the pH of the morning urine may be observed with the impairment of hydrogen ion excretion, and this will usually precede any fall in glomerular filtration rate. There is also a tendency to both uricosuria and phosphaturia, probably indicating proximal tubular damage, and there may be impairment of renal concentrating power similar to a nephrogenic diabetes insipidus. Of major importance, however, is the steady decrease in glomerular filtration rate, which is in proportion to the dose of amphotericin B administered and which has been attributed to renal vasoconstriction. This may progress to the syndrome of acute tubular necrosis. The associated renal insufficiency is potentially reversible at low dosage, and a slow recovery of function usually occurs. However, irreversible renal failure may develop with a sufficiently high dose. The histologic findings are primarily those of necrosis of both the proximal and distal tubules, together with a characteristic nephrocalcinosis in which calcium deposits are present within both tubules and the renal interstitium. Vacuolization of the smooth muscle cells in the media of arteries and arterioles has also been observed.

Because it is used chiefly in life-threatening situations, treatment may have to be continued despite developing nephrotoxicity. This may sometimes be mitigated by a reduction in the dose or in its frequency. In each case, the risk of nephrotoxicity must be weighed against the risk of the underlying disease. The varied sequelae of nephrotoxicity which have been described must be diagnosed and any dehydration and sodium or potassium depletion corrected early. Although a good urine volume should be maintained, there is no convincing evidence that the concurrent administration of mannitol reduces nephrotoxicity.

Burgess JL, Birchall R: Nephrotoxicity of amphotericin B, with emphasis on changes in tubular function. Am J Med 53:77, 1972. *Describes features of progressive tubular and glomerular damage in patients treated with amphotericin B.*

Metal Nephropathies

The pathogenesis of renal damage resulting from metals may be either by a direct, dose-dependent, and reversible toxicity or mediated by immune mechanisms. The spectrum of clinical manifestations will depend particularly on the acuteness and severity of exposure and its duration, and on the responses, particularly the immunologic responses, of the host. In general, their nephrotoxicity may be attributed to their reactivity with sulfhydryl groups. Any of the associated clinical syndromes may occur, although an acute interstitial nephritis is rare. Establishing an etiologic association between a metal and the renal lesion may be difficult enough in the acute nephropathies and may require extensive epidemiologic studies in the chronic nephropathies. The manifestations of the renal responses to the more important metals are shown below (Table 81–4).

LEAD. Acute lead poisoning is probably the most common metal intoxication, especially in children (see Ch. 565). Lead paint is one of the most common sources, and lead can be absorbed either by children sucking fingers contaminated with lead paint and ingesting paint flakes or industrially during demolition of old buildings. Contaminated water, food, or utensils may cause sporadic lead poisoning. Contamination of "moonshine" produced in illicit lead-containing stills in the southern United States is a common source.

Acute lead poisoning is seen most frequently in the summer, possibly because of the enhancement of lead absorption by vitamin D. Acute lead intoxication may cause symptoms which at times are vague, but which may include intestinal colic, anemia, peripheral neuritis, or an encephalopathy with optic neuritis. The kidney is frequently involved, but symptoms may be few and specific search is often needed to demonstrate the acute nephropathy. Histologically, proximal tubular degeneration is seen, together with the presence of eosinophilic (acid-fast) intranuclear inclusion bodies. Swelling of the mitochondria is found with an impairment of their oxidative and phosphorylative functions. These intranuclear inclusions contain sulfhydryl groups and consist of a lead-protein complex. Such cells, still containing eosinophilic intranuclear inclusion bodies, may sometimes be detected in the urine during an acute lead nephropathy. Mild proteinuria is often found, with an increased excretion of casts. Glycosuria and aminoaciduria, manifestations of the Fanconi syndrome, are frequent. Nitrogen retention may be seen in more severe cases. The lesion, however, is usually reversible, and regeneration of the proximal tubular epithelial cells occurs.

TABLE 81–4. MANIFESTATIONS OF METAL NEPHROTOXICITY

	Acute Nephropathy			
Metal	*Tubular Necrosis*	*The Fanconi Syndrome*	**Chronic Nephropathy**	**Nephrotic Syndrome**
Lead	+	+	+	0
Cadmium	+	+	+	0
Mercury	+	0	?	+
Gold	+	0	+	+
Uranium	+	+	+	0
Copper	+	+	+	0
Bismuth	+	+	+	0
Thallium	+	0	0	+

Long-continued low-grade exposure to lead may cause chronic lead nephropathy. Such exposure was seen particularly in Queensland, Australia, where acute lead poisoning was common in children until 1930, owing to the ingestion of powdered and flaking lead paint from weathered verandah railings. Careful epidemiologic follow-up subsequently established a greatly increased incidence of chronic renal disease in those children who had suffered from acute lead poisoning, and a positive correlation of the renal disease with increased lead stores in bone has incriminated lead etiologically. The prolonged ingestion of lead-contaminated water in Scotland has also been associated with raised blood lead concentrations, renal insufficiency, and hyperuricemia. A similar syndrome to that seen in Queensland has been detected among "moonshine" drinkers in the southern United States, where the "moonshine" has been prepared in stills with lead condensers. Increased and prolonged industrial exposure to lead has also been associated with chronic renal insufficiency with hypertension and gout. However, even when features of excessive lead absorption and storage can be shown, it may be difficult to establish lead as the cause of any associated chronic renal disease in the individual.

In Queensland, criteria for establishing a diagnosis of *chronic lead nephropathy* include (1) the presence of uniform and equal contraction of both kidneys, (2) the presence of longstanding chronic renal disease with slow progression, (3) exclusion of an alternative cause for the renal disease, and (4) definite evidence of excessive past lead absorption. As continuing manifestations of lead intoxication were absent, evidence for the last-named aspect could be obtained either by demonstrating an increased content of lead in bone (usually skull bone) or by the presence of an increased excretion of lead in urine after a standardized dose (1 gram) of calcium EDTA. Those who developed their acute lead intoxication during childhood often had impairment of mental functions as well. Another associated feature in chronic lead nephropathy is the presence of disproportionate hyperuricemia and gouty arthritis; gout is usually regarded as being rare in patients with chronic renal failure, whereas gout is seen in half the patients with chronic lead nephropathy. The disproportionate hyperuricemia in this condition is due to reduced renal excretion of urate. Pathologically, the kidneys show uniform granular contraction and fibrosis. The likely sequence of events includes severe renal damage with destruction of nephrons during the acute lead intoxication, followed by the disappearance of the damaged tissue during childhood and adolescence, the onset of hypertension in early adult life, and the gradual onset and progression of chronic renal failure with the development of the granular contracted kidneys.

The management of chronic lead nephropathy is essentially that of the conservative management of chronic renal failure. However, a much slower rate of progression may be expected than in glomerulonephritis, and the normalization of the plasma levels of urate, phosphate, and bicarbonate is desirable to minimize complications. Unless there are signs of acute lead intoxication, the administration of calcium disodium EDTA does not benefit the renal lesion. If it is to be given because signs of acute lead intoxication are present, the dose of calcium EDTA should be reduced in proportion to the reduced glomerular function.

Emmerson BT: Chronic lead nephropathy. Kidney Int 4:1, 1973. *An historical review with special emphasis on the diagnosis and pathology in Queensland; 60 references.*

CADMIUM. Cadmium can produce both an acute nephropathy with proximal tubular lesions and a chronic nephropathy. It has a high affinity for sulfhydryl groups, thereby damaging disulfide bonds and also leading to a disturbance of energy production at the cellular level, which may lead to cellular necrosis. Cadmium is used in the metal plating industry and can be leached by acid from cadmium-plated containers or volatilized by heating, leading to acute respiratory symptoms (see Ch. 565). Severe and acute exposure, which often occurs via the respiratory tract, may lead to renal tubular and cortical necrosis. Chronic cadmium poisoning occurs both in cadmium workers and in the nearby population following industrial contamination of the countryside. During this less severe exposure, a "tubular" proteinuria comprising low molecular weight proteins (between 15,000 and 40,000) is found. This urinary protein consists largely of β_2 microglobulins, immunoglobulin light chains, and lysozyme. Many persons from areas chronically polluted with cadmium are found to show this "tubular" type of proteinuria and also, in the early stages, aminoaciduria and glycosuria. Impaired concentrating ability and features of renal tubular acidosis may also occur. Some of these features may increase the tendency to form renal calculi, and persistent hypercalciuria may lead to a painful osteomalacia which, in Japan, is referred to as "itai-itai byo" or "ouch-ouch" disease. With continuing exposure, and often even without further exposure, progressive renal damage occurs. At this stage, the pathologic findings are similar to those in chronic lead nephropathy, but the presence of hypercalciuria and the absence of urate retention permit chronic cadmium nephropathy to be distinguished clinically from that caused by lead.

On diagnosis of cadmium intoxication, removal from exposure and reduction of cadmium intake are desirable when possible. The renal tubular acidosis and any other defects of tubular function may have to be compensated by specific supplements. There is concern for added nephrotoxicity from chelating agents in this condition, so that calcium EDTA should be used with great care, if at all.

Adams RG, Harrison JF, Scott P: The development of cadmium-induced proteinuria, impaired renal function, and osteomalacia in alkaline battery workers. Q J Med 38:425, 1969. *Classic paper recording the sequelae of 12 years of industrial exposure.*

MERCURY. Mercury, probably the most nephrotoxic metal, causes cellular damage by combining with sulfhydryl groups of the mitochondrial membrane and by inhibiting sulfhydryl-containing enzyme systems. Mercurial compounds are used extensively in many industrial processes, and there have been areas of environmental contamination by mercurial waste (see Ch. 565). Mercurials were used in medicine as organic mercurial diuretics, as mercury-containing ointments and skin lotions, and as calomel; none is extensively used any longer. Absorption may occur from the skin or mucous surfaces or by inhalation, the last-named route being possible with metallic mercury.

Significant absorption of mercurial compounds may lead to systemic symptoms with circulatory collapse and oliguria. Acute ingestion of mercurial salts should be treated urgently by gastric lavage with a fluid containing milk and egg albumin, intended to combine with mercury, and charcoal may be added to adsorb any uncombined compound. Absorbed mercury is rapidly bound to renal tissue and is only slowly excreted. Oliguria develops early, at which time the urine is likely to show proteinuria with cellular casts and increased numbers of red and white cells. Occasionally glycosuria and aminoaciduria are seen, but the toxicity is such that these are only transient. Calcification of the necrotic proximal tubules occurs more commonly when this is due to mercury than to other metals. Regeneration of the tubules may occur, provided that the damage is not too great.

Because of its considerable toxicity, measures to prevent mercury intoxication are of great importance. Absorbed mercury is rapidly bound to protein, so that early treatment with dimercaprol (BAL) in full dosage is usually indicated. This may have to be combined with early and frequent dialysis to remove dimercaprol-mercury complexes which may not otherwise be eliminated if there is associated oliguria or anuria.

Mercurials have also been implicated in the nephrotic syndrome. This occurred particularly when organic mercurial diuretics were given to patients with pre-existing renal disease. The proteinuria is glomerular in type, and symptoms of hypersensitivity may sometimes be detected. Light microscopy is frequently normal, but electron microscopy provides evidence of an immune-complex type of glomerulonephritis with epimembranous electron dense deposits, extension of the basement membrane between the deposits, and fusion of the epithelial foot processes. Removal from the mercury exposure will often produce a fall in the mercury excretion and a remission in the proteinuria.

Mercury has also been said to induce a chronic renal lesion, but the evidence is not strong that this can develop other than as a residual damage after an acute toxic nephropathy. Proteinuria has been recorded in workers with chronic exposure to mercury, and this has been observed to subside after removal from exposure. There are few pathologic or epidemiologic studies in such patients, and the lack of any relationship between exposure and response suggests that this might be a mild variety of immune complex glomerulonephritis such as has been considered above for the mercury-induced nephrotic syndrome. However, residents of Minamata Bay in Japan have suffered chronic organic mercurial exposure. Although this primarily caused neurologic disorders, affected persons showed tubular proteinuria. The demonstration of this type of proteinuria may therefore provide an early indication of renal damage from organic mercurials.

Chugh KS, Singal PC, Uberoi HS: Rhabdomyolysis and renal failure in acute mercuric chloride poisoning. Med J Aust 2:125, 1978.

Iesato K, Wakashin M, Wakashin Y, Tojo S: Renal tubular dysfunction in Minamata disease. Ann Intern Med 86:731, 1977. *Demonstrates tubular proteinuria with renal tubular epithelial antigen and beta-2-microglobulinuria in patients with organic mercury poisoning.*

Tubbs RR, Gephardt GN, McMahon JT, Pohl MC, Vidt DG, Barenberg SA, Valenzuela R: Membranous glomerulonephritis associated with industrial mercury exposure. Am J Clin Pathol 77:409, 1982. *A study of pathogenetic mechanisms.*

GOLD. Gold salts are used in the treatment of rheumatoid arthritis. Parenteral gold is initially bound to plasma proteins, but with an increase in tissue binding the amount of gold in the circulation steadily falls. Gold tends to accumulate particularly in the kidneys, where, in the first few days, it is seen chiefly in the proximal tubular epithelial cells. It is later present in the distal tubules and within interstitial macrophages, where it may persist for up to 30 years after its last administration.

Toxic reactions to gold result chiefly in dermatitis, bone marrow depression, or nephrotoxicity. The kidneys are involved in only a small proportion of such reactions, and renal damage usually manifests first either as microscopic hematuria or proteinuria. Mild proteinuria may remit despite continuation of therapy. Nephrotoxicity in the form of acute tubular necrosis with anuria may rarely be seen. The more common type of reaction, however, consists of the development of an immune complex glomerulonephritis, with proteinuria varying in degree from mild to sufficiently heavy to cause the nephrotic syndrome. Its development is not dose related. Intracytoplasmic gold inclusions are seen in proximal tubule cells, together with subepithelial deposits of electron dense material (presumably immune complexes) within the glomeruli with fusion of epithelial cell foot processes. However, gold is absent from the glomerular lesions. Subsequently, by a process of synthesis of basement membrane by the glomerular epithelial cells, the subepithelial deposits are displaced toward the endothelial side. Ultimately, these deposits may be eliminated and the basement membrane restored. Repair is usually incomplete, however, and the appearance is that of a chronic membranous glomerulonephritis. Resolution may take up to a year and may be incomplete in a third of patients.

Viol GW, Minielly JA, Bistricki T: Gold nephropathy. Arch Pathol Lab Med 101:635, 1977. *Study of three patients by light and electron microscopy, immunofluorescence, and x-ray fluorescence spectroscopy; discusses pathogenetic mechanisms.*

LITHIUM. Lithium is eliminated from the body almost exclusively by the kidney. Although renal toxicity has long been recognized, its importance has become apparent only since the more widespread use of lithium carbonate in serious affective disorders, such as the manic-depressive psychoses. Long-term therapy, even in doses yielding plasma lithium concentrations within the accepted safety range, can lead, in about 25 per cent of patients, to failure of renal concentrating capacity with polyuria and polydipsia. This is unresponsive to vasopressin and represents an acquired nephrogenic diabetes insipidus. A mild distal acidification defect can also be demonstrated. Maintenance of a dilute urine and the administration of lithium in divided doses may be preventive. The effect appears to be largely dose dependent and to be potentially reversible. Renal concentrating ability should be checked regularly during therapy. Patients who develop polyuria should not be allowed to become salt depleted, because this results in increased proximal tubular reabsorption of both salt and lithium, thereby leading to a higher serum lithium concentration with associated features of systemic, particularly neurologic, toxicity. Withdrawal of phenothiazine therapy or the institution of indomethacin or diuretic therapy in patients stabilized on lithium is also likely to increase the serum lithium concentration. Acute renal failure and the nephrotic syndrome are seen infrequently. Hemodialysis is the most effective means of removing lithium during intoxication. Reversible histologic changes have been found in the distal convoluted tubules, but lithium has not been definitely implicated in the etiology of the chronic interstitial fibrosis that is commonly seen in psychiatric patients. Nor is there evidence that appropriate lithium treatment leads to chronic renal damage.

Hansen HE: Renal toxicity of lithium. Drugs 22:461, 1981. *An extensive review and bibliography.*

Walker RG, Bennett WM, Davies BM, Kincaid-Smith P: Structural and functional effects of long-term lithium therapy. Kidney Int 21:513, 1982. *A comparison of renal function and structure in pre- and post-lithium treated patients.*

URANIUM. Uranium is less nephrotoxic than either mercury or lead. Its chemical toxicity overshadows any associated radiation hazard. Accidental or industrial toxicity is rare in man because of the great care exercised with its use. After parenteral administration, it accumulates in the renal cortex and is excreted via the kidney. Acute or intense exposures may cause nephrotoxic tubular lesions, which may present either with acute renal failure or as specific abnormalities of tubular function. Workers exposed to uranium have shown aminoaciduria and glycosuria, but catalasuria is the most sensitive index of toxic tubular damage. Impairment of renal concentrating ability and acid excretion has been noted. There are few reports of chronic exposure in man, but prolonged high dosage in animals has led to granular contracted kidneys with cortical narrowing.

COPPER. Acute poisoning with copper salts occurs during attempted suicide in some countries. Tubular degeneration and necrosis with acute renal failure are seen in the more severe cases, but it is difficult to tell whether this is a direct nephrotoxic lesion from copper or is secondary to the associated hemolysis, hemoglobinuria, and shock. Copper is nondialyzable, and hemodialysis is of no value in its elimination; peritoneal dialysis may be of benefit.

Hepatolenticular degeneration (Wilson's disease), caused by a genetically determined reduction in ceruloplasmin, the copper-binding serum protein, is associated with deposition of copper in both the liver and the kidney. In the kidney, this results in areas of focal tubular necrosis corresponding with the site of maximal copper deposition. The functional defects of the Fanconi syndrome are seen with tubular proteinuria, generalized aminoaciduria, phosphaturia, uricosuria, and distinctive hypercalciuria. Defective urinary acidification may also be present. Glomerular filtration rate steadily falls, although the fall rarely causes clinical symptoms. The chronic copper overload and the resultant functional tubular lesions are reversible by penicillamine therapy.

BISMUTH. Soluble bismuth compounds may be taken either accidentally or with suicidal intent and have been administered in the treatment of warts. The kidney, which is the main excretory route for bismuth, retains bismuth tenaciously for long periods. Acute bismuth nephrotoxicity can lead to acute renal failure with tubular necrosis. Although potentially reversible, there is a high mortality. Less intense exposure may lead to the Fanconi syndrome with proteinuria, glycosuria, aminoaciduria, phosphaturia, uricosuria, and a salt-losing state. Refractile yellowish-brown inclusion bodies, usually intranuclear, may be found in the kidney for up to 30 years after exposure. Although dimercaprol (BAL) has been used in acute intoxications, experience with this use is limited and there is only limited evidence of a beneficial effect.

Urizar R, Vernier RL: Bismuth nephropathy. JAMA 198:187, 1966. *Describes renal manifestations of bismuth toxicity and reviews 30 case reports.*

THALLIUM. Thallium is used chiefly as a rat poison or for denaturing alcohol. Although it is largely excreted by the kidneys and is concentrated in them, renal lesions are a relatively unimportant part of the syndrome of thallitoxicosis (see Ch. 565). Proteinuria is seen, and the urine also contains erythrocytes and granular casts. In more severe lesions, nitrogen retention with either oliguria or polyuria may develop. In such cases, toxic changes occur in the proximal convoluted tubules. One case of the nephrotic syndrome has been reported.

Renal elimination of thallium is promoted by an active diuresis. Although the amount eliminated is not large in comparison with that by other routes, hemodialysis is also effective and should be used at an early stage, particularly if there is any associated renal failure.

Pedersen RS, Olesen AS, Freund LG, Solgaard P, Larsen E: Thallium intoxication treated with long term haemodialysis, forced diuresis and Prussian blue. Acta Med Scand 204:429, 1978. *Measures progressive concentrations of thallium in urine, dialysis bath fluid, and the arterial and venous lines of the dialyzer.*

ARSENIC. The dramatic gastrointestinal manifestations of arsenical intoxication overshadow the associated toxic nephropathy. In its mildest form, the urine may contain protein, casts, erythrocytes, and leukocytes. Oliguria, nitrogen retention, and acute renal failure may develop, but it is difficult to differentiate the direct metal nephrotoxicity from that of any associated shock. In the presence of normal renal function, therapy with dimercaprol (BAL) is indicated. Arsenic is effectively removed by hemodialysis, and this should be used, either with or without dimercaprol, if the patient is oliguric or anuric. Arsine poisoning (AsH_3) is accompanied by impaired renal function, but this is due more to the associated hemolysis than to any direct nephrotoxic effect.

Giberson A, Vaziri ND, Mirahamadi K, Rosen SM: Haemodialysis of acute arsenic intoxication with transient renal failure. Arch Intern Med 136:1303, 1976. *Measures arsenic in serum and urine and calculates removal during dialysis.*

PLATINUM. Platinum compounds are potentially nephrotoxic because they are concentrated within and eliminated by the renal tubules. The coordinate metal complex, cis-platin, which is a useful antineoplastic agent, results in dose-dependent injury to the proximal and distal tubules, leading to both acute and chronic renal insufficiency. Renal wasting of potassium and magnesium (with hypocalcemia) is not infrequent and appropriate replacement is indicated. The maintenance of a good urine flow rate reduces the risk of nephrotoxicity.

Blachley JD, Hill JB: Renal and electrolyte disturbances associated with cis platin. Ann Intern Med 95:628, 1981. *Well referenced review.*

SILICON. Inhalation of silica can occasionally lead to the development of a multisystem disorder with proteinuria and a rapidly progressive variety of glomerulonephritis. The renal lesion appears to be in part immunologically mediated and in part directly nephrotoxic.

Bolton WK, Suratt PM, Sturgill BC: Rapidly progressive silicon nephropathy. Am J Med 71:823, 1981. *Describes four patients with silica exposure who develop a connective tissue disorder with heavy proteinuria and a glomerulonephritic picture.*

Therapeutic Agents

Renal damage from therapeutic agents, although a rare occurrence, may develop unpredictably, usually as part of an abnormal immune response to a foreign substance. Features of an adverse drug reaction involving other organs, particularly the skin and liver, are often present. Any of the associated clinical syndromes listed may occur, although those resulting from cytotoxic mechanisms occur least frequently. Many of the agents to be considered cause renal damage so rarely that monitoring of renal function is not indicated during their routine use.

PHENINDIONE. On rare occasions, patients treated with phenindione may develop an acute interstitial nephritis with acute renal failure. In such cases, dermatitis and hepatitis are often present, and the macrophage migration inhibition test may be positive. Some may present with the nephrotic syndrome. The severity of the renal failure varies greatly, but it may be prolonged and at times irreversible. When renal complications are recognized, the drug should be withdrawn and, if the renal lesion is severe, steroid therapy used.

McMenamin RA, Davies LM, Craswell PW: Drug induced interstitial nephritis, hepatitis and exfoliative dermatitis. Aust NZ J Med 6:583, 1976. *Describes four cases of interstitial nephritis, two attributable to phenindione and two with multiple drug exposure.*

D-PENICILLAMINE. D-Penicillamine, originally used in the treatment of hepatolenticular degeneration and in some metal intoxications, is now being used more frequently for rheumatoid arthritis. Mild proteinuria occurs commonly, and this sometimes settles with lowering of the dose. However, the proteinuria may become heavy, and up to 30 per cent of patients develop the nephrotic syndrome. This, too, is potentially reversible on cessation of the drug, although remission may be delayed and incomplete in some patients. Renal complications force cessation of therapy in up to 20 per cent of patients.

The mechanism responsible appears to be an immunologic one, and examination of renal biopsies has shown electron-dense deposits, presumably of immune complexes, present on the epithelial surface of the glomerular basement membrane, together with fusion of the foot processes of the epithelial cells. IgG and complement have been identified in relation to these deposits. A rare complication of therapy has been the development of the syndrome of lung hemorrhage with nephritis. In such cases, the clinical picture has been of a rapidly progressive glomerulonephritis and the pathologic findings those of a focal proliferative glomerulonephritis, with prominent epithelial crescent formation. However, the linear immunofluorescence characteristic of Goodpasture's syndrome has not been present.

Annotation. Penicillamine nephropathy. Br Med J 282:761, 1981. *Reviews management of patients who develop proteinuria during penicillamine treatment.*

ANTICONVULSANTS. A hypersensitivity reaction to *phenytoin* (diphenylhydantoin) may involve the kidney, causing the syndrome of acute renal failure. Associated features have included skin lesions, varying from a rash to exfoliative dermatitis, and signs of hepatitis or myositis, which were sometimes accompanied by fever and lymphadenopathy. Some of the features have suggested an arteritis. The lesion is usually reversible on withdrawal of the drug, although sometimes steroid treatment has been needed.

Oxazolidinediones. Proteinuria, which may become heavy enough to induce the nephrotic syndrome, may occur in patients receiving trimethadione or paramethadione, sometimes after years of treatment. The proteinuria usually responds to withdrawal of the drug, but there is a wide variation in the rate of recovery, from a prompt fall to a gradual remission over six to twelve months. Some have remitted with continuing treatment at a lower dose. On light microscopy, the kidney has usually appeared normal, although occasional minor glomerular abnormalities have been found. Infiltration of the glomeruli with eosinophils has also been reported, suggesting an allergic reaction. In this case, immunofluorescence was negative for immunoglobulin and electron microscopy showed an irregular thickening and splitting of the glomerular basement membrane, which contained a variety of deposits different from those of membranous glomerulonephritis. Some patients with persistent disease have been treated successfully with steroids and immunosuppressive drugs, but in view of the recovery which occurs following simple withdrawal of the drug—albeit at a variable rate—it is difficult to obtain clear evidence that such therapy changed the natural history of the disease. However, remission following withdrawal and steroid therapy has not been invariable, and renal failure and death have occurred.

Bar-Khayim Y, Teplitz C, Garella S, Chazan JA: Trimethadione-induced nephrotic syndrome. A report of a case with unique ultrastructural renal pathology. Am J Med 54:272, 1973. *Describes infiltration of glomerular capillary loops by eosinophils.*

DIURETICS. The thiazide diuretics, as well as furosemide and acetazolamide, have all on rare occasions been implicated in the etiology of allergic interstitial nephritis with acute renal failure. Sometimes there have been features of a hypersensitivity angiitis. However, the case for an etiologic association is not absolute, as many of the patients had also received other drugs; augmentation of nephrotoxicity may be involved.

NONSTEROIDAL ANTI-INFLAMMATORY DRUGS. Renal lesions attributed to phenylbutazone have been seen after as little as 2 grams administered over a six-day period, and are due to a sensitivity mechanism. Although rare, they have presented either as acute renal failure (with or without oliguria), as acute interstitial nephritis, as membranous glomerulonephritis, or as an allergic angiitis, sometimes with manifestations of thrombotic thrombocytopenic purpura.

Acute renal failure may develop during therapy with a wide range of these drugs and is usually due to one of two mechanisms. Rarely, an acute interstitial nephritis may develop, with unusually heavy proteinuria. More frequently, the renal failure is due to alterations in renal blood flow secondary to inhibition of prostaglandin synthesis. This is more likely to develop in patients with volume contraction (such as with diuretic therapy) or in the presence of even minor degrees of renal insufficiency. Hyperkalemia is often severe. See Ch. 81.2 for a more extensive discussion of this important topic.

Clive DM, Stoff JS: Renal syndromes associated with nonsteroidal antiinflammatory drugs. N Engl J Med 310:563, 1984. *A recent, comprehensive review; well referenced.*

DRUGS ALTERING URATE CONCENTRATIONS. The potent uricosuric, *sulfinpyrazone*, has been reported to cause a typical acute interstitial nephritis which resolved on cessation of therapy. A second challenge with the drug caused a mild recurrence of the syndrome. Acute tubular necrosis has also been reported. Therapy with *allopurinol* has also been associated with the development of an acute interstitial nephritis, probably as a cell-mediated hypersensitivity response. In these cases there is often evidence of angiitis with skin lesions, fever, and eosinophilia, and the histologic findings are characteristic of acute interstitial nephritis. Glomerulonephritic lesions have been seen in some. Reactions to allopurinol have occurred in patients with previously normal renal function, but are more likely to occur in patients with pre-existing renal disease. The risk is probably less if a lower dose is used. Because of the severe associated nonrenal complications of fever, angiitis, and skin reaction, prednisone has usually been administered and has appeared to produce a more rapid improvement in renal function. However, therapy has often been needed for months, and earlier withdrawal has been followed by a relapse of fever and renal insufficiency. On occasion, despite steroid therapy, the renal insufficiency has been severe and prolonged and at times fatal.

ANTI-CANCER AGENTS. The nephrotoxic potential and manifestations of anti-cancer drugs vary with the particular agent. Renal function should be assessed prior to therapy and a good urine flow rate initiated and maintained. *Methotrexate* and its metabolite tend to precipitate in the renal tubule following active secretion by tubular cells. Nephrotoxicity during high dose therapy can be minimized by an alkaline diuresis.

The *nitrosoureas* streptozocin and semustine frequently cause nephrotoxicity. Proteinuria is early, often with manifestations of the Fanconi syndrome, such as glycosuria, phosphaturia, and uricosuria, with proximal (Type II) renal tubular acidosis. Nitrogen retention, which may progress despite cessation of treatment, is frequent. In some patients, an insidiously progressive interstitial fibrosis may develop months after cessation of treatment.

Flurane Anesthetics

Many anesthetic agents lead to a transient reduction in renal blood flow and glomerular filtration rate, but are not specifically nephrotoxic. The use of methoxyflurane and, to a lesser extent, enthrane as anesthetic agents has been associated with renal dysfunction in the immediate postoperative period. When this occurs, it presents as a vasopressin-resistant polyuric renal failure, which is usually transient and remits within 10 to 20 days. The loss of renal concentrating power with a persistently negative fluid balance leading to dehydration suggests damage to the distal nephron. However, the initial polyuric phase may pass into a later oliguric phase with typical features of acute renal failure, which either may remit after weeks or months or may persist as chronic renal insufficiency for years. These developments are largely a reflection of the concentration and duration of administration of the anesthetic agent. The associated renal insufficiency varies greatly in severity, clinical presentation, and persistence.

Methoxyflurane is metabolized to fluoride and oxalate. Fluoride inhibits enzyme systems involved in sodium transport in the ascending limb of the loop of Henle and the early distal tubule. The threshold for nephrotoxicity is a plasma fluoride concentration of 40 or 50 μmole per liter, although lower concentrations have been associated with nephrotoxicity in patients with pre-existing renal disease. After methoxyflurane anesthesia, calcium oxalate crystals are frequently noted in the urine and, when toxicity occurs, intratubular and interstitial calcium oxalate crystals have been noted within the kidney. This oxalate deposition is thought to be relatively less important than the fluoride in the induction of renal damage. Histologic changes vary greatly, depending upon the stage and degree of toxicity. In the early stages, degeneration and necrosis of tubular epithelial cells and tubular dilatation are seen, whereas in those patients with persisting renal insufficiency increasing interstitial fibrosis is found.

Fluoride is rapidly excreted while the urine flow rate is good, so that a diuresis is important in prophylaxis. However, toxic levels may persist if oliguria occurs early. The finding of a high serum fluoride concentration in an oliguric patient therefore would support the early use of hemodialysis. Management otherwise is that appropriate for the stage of acute or chronic renal failure, with electrolyte and fluid supplements during the period of nephrogenic diabetes insipidus. The condition can be prevented by limiting the concentration and duration of methoxyflurane which is administered, particularly in subjects with even mild pre-existing renal disease, and by avoiding the simultaneous use of other potentially nephrotoxic drugs.

Gottlieb LS, Trey C: The effects of fluorinated anesthetics on the liver and kidneys. Ann Rev Med 25:411, 1974. *Detailed description of the clinical syndrome and histopathology of methoxyflurane-induced renal disease; 40 references.*

Radiographic Contrast Media

The major urographic and angiographic media in use are triiodinated benzoic acid derivatives—diatrizoate, iothalamate, and metrizoate. The methylglucamine salts have less endothelial toxicity than sodium salts and are preferable for coronary and cerebral angiography, whereas sodium salts are preferred for excretion urography. Occasional patients, particularly those with a history of allergy or asthma, may demonstrate idiosyncratic reactions to radiographic contrast media with widely varying manifestations, sometimes appearing as an anaphylactoid reaction and sometimes as acute renal failure. Their development is usually not dose dependent.

Although increasing amounts of contrast media are being used to provide better definition of the kidneys and urinary tract, the incidence of nephrotoxic reactions to these agents remains very low. The various contrast agents are excreted by glomerular filtration and are concentrated in the renal tubular fluid without active tubular secretion; the concentration in the urine may be up to 100 times that in the plasma. Toxicity is basically dependent upon the concentration of medium achieved at the cellular level. High dose excretion urography is only rarely associated with direct tubular toxicity, the risk of nephrotoxicity being related to *(1) the state of hydration, (2) the presence of pre-existing renal disease, and (3) the dose of contrast medium administered*. Thus it is chiefly a risk in patients with diabetes or myeloma, in the presence of dehydration, stasis, or obstruction to urine flow, or when larger doses or repeated exposures occur to media with a high iodine content. Although dehydration seems to be the dominant factor in renal failure after urography in multiple myeloma, contrast media are better avoided in such patients if possible. Urography is particularly dangerous in juvenile-onset diabetics with moderate to severe grades of renal failure. In all situations, the risk is greatly reduced by the avoidance of dehydration.

Nephrotoxicity is somewhat more of a hazard with selective renal angiography, and even after nonrenal angiography. However, the renal vascular bed tends to react to high concentrations of contrast media by vasoconstriction (whereas in other vascular beds vasodilatation may occur), and this may lead to varying degrees of acute renal failure. A similar renal reaction may occur after cardiac angiography, especially in the presence of diabetic renal disease. The initial clinical manifestation is usually oliguria occurring within 24 hours of the procedure and lasting up to five days, associated with nitrogen retention. Although it is usually completely reversible, prolonged impairment of renal function has occurred in occasional cases. This nephrotoxicity has been attributed variously to altered renal hemodynamics and erythrocyte crenation and agglutination from the viscous hypertonic medium, tubular obstruction caused by dye-protein interactions, and direct toxicity to tubular epithelial cells. However, it may also develop when increased concentrations of contrast medium occur because of faulty placement of the intra-arterial catheter, reduced blood flow to a small kidney, injection of a branch artery, or wedging of a catheter tip in a narrowed renal artery, causing both delayed transit time of the dye and local renal ischemia. Many radiographic contrast agents are also uricosuric, and an acute uric acid nephropathy has been invoked. However, acute renal failure has occurred with these agents despite the maintenance of a vigorous diuresis and the prevention of a high urinary urate concentration, so that uric acid does not seem to have an etiologic role in any associated renal damage.

CHOLECYSTOGRAPHY. Contrast media, such as iopanoic acid and ipodate, which are used for oral cholecystography, or iodipamide and ioglycamate, which are used for intravenous cholangiography, have all on occasion been associated with acute tubular necrosis, but the risk is much less with the newer agents. Dehydration is unnecessary in cholecystography and, because of the associated hazard, should be prevented, if necessary by prior water ingestion. The risk of nephrotoxicity is otherwise increased if multiple or repeated doses of contrast medium are given, if there has been a recent intravenous cholangiogram, if there is significant renal disease, or in the presence of hepatic disease with reduced hepatic excretion of contrast medium. The Dubin-Johnson syndrome is a contraindication to cholangiography.

Thus renal complications from radiographic contrast media may be minimized by using the lowest necessary dose of medium (especially if the normal route of elimination is impaired), together with the maintenance of a good urine flow rate. Should acute renal failure supervene, the management is that of this condition from whatever cause, and dialysis may be required.

Ansari Z, Baldwin DS: Acute renal failure due to radiocontrast agents. Nephron 17:28, 1976. *Describes 25 patients, of whom 20 had impaired renal function prior to the procedure.*

Byrd L, Sherman RL: Radiocontrast-induced acute renal failure. Medicine 58:270, 1979. *Reviews incidence (0.15 per cent), risk factors, pathogenesis, and clinical presentations; 85 references.*

Knapp MS: Renal failure after contrast radiography. Br Med J 287:3, 1983. *Recent editorial review.*

Organic Solvents and Hydrocarbons

CARBON TETRACHLORIDE. Carbon tetrachloride is widely used as a solvent and dry cleaning fluid, occasionally in fire extinguishers, and rarely as a vermifuge. Absorption is usually by inhalation (this is aggravated by exposure in confined spaces) or following ingestion. Its toxicity is enhanced by alcohol, probably because of the increased activity of drug-metabolizing enzymes, leading to an increase in its conversion to ethylchlorformate. Being lipid-soluble, it is concentrated in tissue fat stores, the brain, and bone marrow. Either carbon tetrachloride itself or its metabolites have a direct toxic effect on the liver and kidney parenchyma, leading to centrilobular necrosis in the liver and degeneration of the proximal and, to a lesser extent, the distal tubular epithelium of the kidney.

The early clinical manifestations of intoxication involve the gastrointestinal and central nervous systems. Nausea, vomiting, and abdominal pain are common, and headache, confusion, convulsions, and coma may occur. A toxic hepatitis with jaundice is a later development. This is considered in further detail in Ch. 121. Renal complications may be delayed for up to a week and range from proteinuria, with microscopic hematuria and casts, to oliguria, passing into the full syndrome of acute renal failure. However, because of the associated hepatic disease, the rise in blood urea nitrogen is disproportionately low and the serum creatinine concentration should be used as the index of renal function. Bleeding tendencies may occur, caused by hypoprothrombinemia, disseminated intravascular coagulation, and hypofibrinogenemia. Carbon tetrachloride may be demonstrated in expired air or blood by infrared spectrophotometry. Trichloroethylene and tetrachloroethylene, although less toxic, may lead to similar renal complications.

Carbon tetrachloride is not dialyzable. If exposure has been acute, removal to an area with adequate ventilation is essential. Management is like that of acute renal failure from other causes, including dialysis as indicated. The nephrotoxic lesion is potentially reversible following a single exposure, and the mortality in well managed cases is less than 20 per cent.

Nielsen VK, Larsen J: Acute renal failure due to carbon tetrachloride poisoning. Acta Med Scand 178:363, 1965. *Describes five cases, commenting on diagnostic difficulties, and reviews 128 cases collected from the literature.*

ETHYLENE GLYCOL. Ethylene glycol and its congeners are aliphatic alcohols used as freezing point depressants. They are potently nephrotoxic following ingestion, which usually occurs by error or in the search for an ethanol substitute. Initial symptoms are often encephalitic, with confusion, convulsions, and coma. A severe acidosis is often present at this stage. Features of myocarditis and myositis may become apparent and, prior to the development of oliguria, crystals of calcium oxalate may be seen in the urine, together with microscopic hematuria. When oliguria and anuria supervene, the clinical pattern is that of acute renal failure, which may remit or, if the damage has been severe enough, may pass into a chronic uremia. The pathologic findings result from the metabolism of ethylene glycol to oxalate and other toxic intermediates; the brilliant birefringent crystals of calcium oxalate are found in a wide variety of tissues. In the kidney, they are seen within the lumens of the proximal tubules, many of which also demonstrate tubular necrosis.

Ethylene glycol is dialyzable so that early dialysis is indicated. As it is metabolized by alcohol dehydrogenase, its metabolism can be delayed by the simultaneous administration of ethanol

(10 grams per hour). The most important aspect of management is the maintenance of a vigorous diuresis, using both mannitol and intravenous furosemide or ethacrynic acid. Acidosis should also be corrected. Institution of these measures soon after diagnosis or soon after the detection of hematuria with calcium oxalate crystalluria may prevent the development of acute renal failure, and this treatment may be needed for several days until all the ingested ethylene glycol has been metabolized. Should acute renal failure develop, therapy is essentially that of this condition with frequent dialysis. Ultimate prevention depends upon the widespread appreciation of its toxicity and the hazard of storage in improper containers.

Vale JA, Prior JG, O'Hare JP, Flanagan RJ, Feehally J: Treatment of ethylene glycol poisoning with peritoneal dialysis. Br Med J 284:557, 1982. *Reports three cases and comments on management.*

HYDROCARBONS. Most toxins exert their primary effect upon renal tubules, and tubular necrosis has been described after exposure to diesel oil, and a reversible Fanconi syndrome, renal tubular acidosis, and acute renal failure after *glue sniffing*. However, it has also been suggested that some hydrocarbon solvents may induce glomerular injury. Initially, Goodpasture's syndrome was linked with exposure to petroleum products, and more recently an increased incidence of exposure to inhaled hydrocarbon solvents has been reported in patients with proliferative glomerulonephritis and some other renal diseases with nonspecific types of glomerular disease. The proposed mechanism involves immune complex formation. Although the association remains of interest, causality has not yet been established.

Osmotic Nephropathy and Low Molecular Weight Dextrans

Swelling and vacuolation of proximal tubular epithelial cells may be seen histologically in the severe glycosuria of diabetes, following the use of mannitol as a diuretic, or after the use of hypertonic sucrose to relieve cerebral edema. However, such lesions have no functional significance. On the other hand, the use of dextrans with a molecular weight of less than 60,000, with the aim of improving vascular flow, has not infrequently been associated with the development of oliguria and acute renal failure. Some of these patients have had acute allergic or anaphylactic reactions, and others have developed an acute hypersensitivity glomerulonephritis. Most of the persons who developed acute renal failure following the use of these low molecular weight dextrans, however, have had severe generalized vascular disease. Animal experiments have shown that anuria is likely to develop after their use when reduced perfusion of the kidney leading to reduced filtration pressure is present. These dextrans are readily filterable, and the concentration of the dextran which occurs in the tubules may promote plugging when there is slowing of flow. Thus in clinical practice, it is wise to limit dextran administration to 1 liter per day and to cease its administration if the urine flow rate is less than 1500 ml per 24 hours, or if the blood urea is more than 60 mg per 100 ml (10 mmol per liter). When renal complications are developing, the decline in urine flow rate is usually gradual and can be treated, and probably prevented, by a mannitol- or drug-induced diuresis. These are thought to act by preventing the development of high intratubular concentrations of dextran.

Feest TG: Low molecular weight dextran: A continuing cause of acute renal failure. Br Med J 2:1300, 1976. *Brief report of seven case histories.*

Radiation

The development of *radiation nephritis* is now uncommon, being largely prevented by shielding the kidney during irradiation and controlling the dose reaching the kidney during radiotherapy of malignancies near the kidney. Pathologically, the main lesion appears to affect the capillary endothelium of the glomeruli, possibly by interfering with its ability to produce the ground substance of the basement membrane. Subsequent death of these cells within two to three months is thought to cause local activation of the coagulation system and secondary vascular damage, leading to a response by mesangial cells and variable thickening and splitting of the glomerular basement membrane. Thus some glomeruli appear to be hyalinized, whereas some show fibrinoid necrosis and focal scarring. In addition, the epithelium and basement membranes of tubules are damaged, resulting in degeneration and collapse of tubules and diffuse interstitial changes which, in the acute phase, may consist of edema and, in the chronic stages, progressive fibrosis. Immunofluorescent studies are usually negative. Vascular lesions of the medium and small arterioles may also occur with intimal proliferation, degeneration of smooth muscle, fibrinoid necrosis, and thrombosis. The renal plasma flow falls steadily with doses of radiotherapy exceeding 400 rads, and there is also impairment of tubular function. At cumulative therapeutic doses of between 2000 and 2500 rads, a progressive decrease in glomerular filtration rate is found, and clinical manifestations are seen. These are usually not apparent until six to eight months or more after the irradiation has occurred. The clinical pattern is variable, depending upon the severity of the lesion, and may range from a relatively acute renal dysfunction to the development of chronic renal damage. Hypertension, which may be either benign or, more frequently, severe, is a common development. In acute radiation nephritis, malignant hypertension is a major problem and there is a high mortality. The more chronic varieties show a moderate degree of proteinuria with impaired concentrating power and usually a steady decline in renal function unless malignant hypertension supervenes. Vigorous treatment of any associated hypertension is vital, but the management of the associated acute or chronic renal insufficiency does not differ from that of other causes. If only one kidney is involved and control of hypertension is difficult, nephrectomy may result in remission of the hypertension. A more general discussion of radiation injury is found in Ch. 562.

Keane WF, Crosson JT, Staley NA, Anderson WR, Shapiro FL: Radiation-induced renal disease. A clinicopathologic study. Am J Med 60:127, 1976. *Light, electron microscopic, and immunofluorescent studies were performed on renal tissue from two patients whose renal insufficiency developed within 12 months of abdominal irradiation.*

82. OBSTRUCTIVE NEPHROPATHY

Floyd C. Rector, Jr.

Obstruction of the urinary tract may produce profound structural and functional changes in the kidneys and, if uncorrected, may result in complete, irreversible loss of renal function. Early diagnosis and appropriate correction, therefore, are essential for preserving or restoring renal function and preventing the progression to end-stage renal failure. The obstructing lesions may occur at any site in the urinary tract from the renal tubules to the terminal urethra. The clinical presentation is variable, depending on the site of obstruction and whether the obstruction is acute or chronic, complete or partial, unilateral or bilateral, or complicated by urinary tract infection.

INCIDENCE AND ETIOLOGY. In a large series of autopsies the prevalence of hydronephrosis varied from 3.5 to 3.8 per cent. Clinically significant urinary tract obstruction occurs less frequently than noted at postmortem examination; nevertheless it is a rather common disease in all age groups. Hydronephrosis is a contributing factor to destruction of renal function in 15 to 25 per cent of uremic patients.

Obstructive uropathy can result from three general types of obstruction (Table 82–1): (1) mechanical obstruction of the lumen of the urinary tract; (2) functional or anatomic abnormalities of the ureter, bladder, or urethra; or (3) compression from masses or processes extrinsic to the urinary tract. The prevalence of the various causes of obstruction varies with age and sex. The most common causes are congenital abnormalities of the urinary tract (e.g., urethral valves, vesicoureteral reflux, cystocele) in children, pregnancy and pelvic malignancy in women, renal stones in young men, and prostatic hypertrophy in elderly men. Acute ureteral obstruction from calculi results

TABLE 82–1. CAUSES OF OBSTRUCTIVE UROPATHY

- Intraluminal
  - Stone
  - Bladder tumor
  - Papillary necrosis
  - Clot
  - Ureteral tumor
  - Bence Jones proteinuria
  - Acute urate nephropathy
- Intramural
  - Congenital
    - Ureteropelvic dysfunction (10 per cent bilateral)
    - Ureterovesical stricture (simple or ureterocele)
    - Bladder neck obstruction
    - Pinpoint meatus
  - Acquired
    - Urethral stricture
    - Ureteral stricture (tuberculosis, etc.)
    - Neurogenic bladder dysfunction
- Extramural
  - Prostatic obstruction
  - Ureteropelvic juncture—vessels, bands, etc.
  - Aortic aneurysm
  - Periureteral fibrosis
  - Retroperitoneal tumor or nodes
    - Extraurinary growth (carcinoma of colon, diverticulitis)
  - Pelvic tumor
  - Inadvertent ligature

in the hospitalization of 1 out of 1000 Americans each year. Benign prostatic enlargement occurs in 80 per cent of men over 60 years, and 10 per cent of these require surgery for the correction of obstruction. Vesicoureteral reflux is most common in young girls, but also occurs to some extent in approximately 5 per cent of adults. Neurogenic bladder dysfunction is a serious medical problem frequently complicated by incontinence, recurrent urinary tract infection, bladder stones, and hydronephrosis; this disorder can occur secondary to traumatic injuries of the spinal cord or to metabolic and neurologic diseases (diabetes mellitus, multiple sclerosis, myelodysplasia, senile dementia, and vascular disease).

PATHOLOGY AND PATHOPHYSIOLOGY. Obstruction of the lower urinary tract produces profound structural and functional changes in the kidney and, if complete, can irreversibly destroy renal function within four to six weeks. This is the consequence of combined mechanical and hormonal factors (Table 82–2). Superimposition of urinary tract infection or renal immunologic injury (antibody formation secondary to the release of renal antigens into the circulation) will accelerate and intensify this destruction of renal function.

Immediately following obstruction of one ureter, pressures in the pelvis and tubules increase, causing the pelvis and tubules to dilate and the renal papillae to become flattened. Secondary to the increased tubular pressure and dilatation there is a marked decrease in glomerular filtration rate, disruption of the junctional complexes between tubular cells permitting backleak of solutes from tubule lumen to blood, and inhibition of sodium reabsorption and potassium and hydrogen secretion in the distal nephron.

Concomitant with these mechanical changes there is stimulation of prostaglandin production within the kidney. Increased levels of PGI_2 (prostacyclin) stimulate the release of renin (sufficient to cause acute hypertension) and produce vasodilation of the renal cortex. Increased levels of PGE_2 produce vasodilation of the renal medulla, block the action of vasopressin, and further inhibit salt transport in the loop of Henle and distal nephron. As a consequence of these hormonal changes there is an initial rise in renal blood flow, lasting four to six hours. Thereafter, renal blood flow progressively falls to levels of 10 to 15 per cent of normal despite continued increased production of PGI_2 and PGE_2. This fall in blood flow is the result of intense renal vasoconstriction produced by increased levels of the prostaglandin derivative thromboxane A_2, one of the most potent vasoconstrictors known. Associated with these mechanical and hormonal changes the kidney becomes severely ischemic, with many nephrons ceasing to function. The residual nephrons have reduced filtration rates and impaired ability to conserve sodium, secrete potassium, and acidify and concentrate the urine. The tubules progressively atrophy, the medulla is destroyed, and by four to six weeks the cortex consists of only a thin shell of connective tissue with few remaining glomeruli.

If the obstruction is corrected prior to this stage of irreversible renal damage, there may be significant recovery of renal function. Experimental studies in dogs have shown 45 to 50 per cent recovery after two weeks of complete obstruction, 15 to 30 per cent recovery after three to four weeks of obstruction, but no recovery after six weeks of complete obstruction.

In contrast to the changes observed with complete obstruction, with partial obstruction, particularly if bilateral, the renal pelvis may become tremendously dilated, holding 2 to 3 liters of urine, and yet structure and function of the renal cortex may be relatively well preserved. Functionally, filtration rate and blood flow may be only slightly (or moderately) reduced, and the major abnormality may be the inability to concentrate the urine and/or secrete potassium and hydrogen ions.

TABLE 82–2. EFFECTS OF OBSTRUCTION ON RENAL FUNCTION

- I. Mechanical
  - A. Increased tubular pressure
    1. Disruption of junctional complexes—increased tubule permeability
    2. Decreased collecting duct Na transport; decreased H^+ and K^+ secretion
    3. Decreased GRF
  - B. Increased renal interstitial pressure
    1. Altered proximal reabsorption
    2. Impaired countercurrent function
- II. Hormonal
  - A. Increased PGI_2 synthesis
    1. Stimulated renin release
    2. Cortical vasodilatation
  - B. Increased PGE_2 synthesis
    1. Medullary vasodilatation
    2. Inhibition of vasopressin action
    3. Inhibition of aldosterone action
    4. Inhibition of Cl^- transport in thick ascending limb
  - C. Increased thromboxane A_2 synthesis
    1. Cortical vasoconstriction
    2. Decreased number of functioning nephrons
  - D. Retained natriuretic factors in blood
- III. Other
  - A. Decreased glomerular permeability
  - B. Decreased mesangial clearance of immune complexes

CLINICAL MANIFESTATIONS OF URINARY TRACT OBSTRUCTION. The clinical manifestations of urinary tract obstruction depend on the site of obstruction and on whether it is acute or chronic. Patients with obstruction below the bladder (prostate, urethra) may have decreased force and caliber of the urinary stream, intermittency, postvoid dribbling, hesitancy, and nocturia. Neurogenic dysfunction of the bladder with incomplete emptying may cause urgency, frequent urination, and urinary incontinence (overflow incontinence). These symptoms, however, do not occur with obstruction at higher levels in the urinary tract. Urinary tract obstruction may also present as asymptomatic hydronephrosis, as renal colic, as either acute or chronic renal failure, or occasionally as a specific renal tubular disorder (Table 82–3).

Pain. The pain associated with urinary tract obstruction is produced by distention of the renal capsule, and the intensity of the pain is related to the rate of distention. With chronic, low grade obstruction the renal collecting system can be tremendously dilated without producing pain. This form of obstruction will be discovered either accidentally or during the workup for urinary tract infection, renal failure, or renal tubular abnormalities. Occasionally, in patients with chronic asymptomatic hydronephrosis the urinary tract may become acutely and painfully distended during a diuresis induced by large fluid intake (e.g., water, beer). Therefore, intermittent flank pain induced by fluid intake should suggest the presence of

TABLE 82–3. CLINICAL MANIFESTATIONS OF URINARY TRACT OBSTRUCTION

1. Lower tract symptoms: urgency, hesitancy, incontinence, nocturia
2. Chronic hydronephrosis
   a. Asymptomatic
   b. Intermittent pain
3. Renal colic
4. Renal failure
   a. Acute
      (1) Intratubular
      (2) Lower tract
   b. Chronic
      (1) Hydronephrosis
      (2) Infection ± lithiasis
      (3) Interstitial nephritis
      (4) Reflux nephropathy
      (5) Papillary necrosis
5. Recurrent urinary tract infection
6. Renal tubule dysfunction
   a. Concentration defect
      (1) Nocturia, polyuria
      (2) Nephrogenic diabetes insipidus
   b. Distal renal tubular acidosis
   c. Potassium secretory defect
7. Hypertension
   a. Acute—renin dependent
   b. Chronic—volume dependent
8. Polycythemia
9. Postobstructive diuresis

urinary tract obstruction. Pain induced by urination should suggest vesicoureteral reflux. Acute obstruction of a ureter with a stone may produce one of the most severe forms of pain encountered in clinical medicine. Usually the pain is located in the lower abdomen or flank, radiating into the groin on the obstructed side.

Renal Failure. Chronic obstruction of one kidney will result in unilateral hydronephrosis if the obstruction is partial, and in a nonfunctioning kidney if the obstruction is complete. Unilateral obstruction will not produce renal failure if the opposite kidney is functional. However, obstruction of a single functioning kidney or bilateral obstruction can give rise to either acute or chronic renal failure.

Acute renal failure secondary to obstruction is usually associated with severe oliguria or anuria, although it may occasionally present as "high output" acute renal failure. Variable output from day to day should suggest the presence of lower urinary tract obstruction. Acute renal failure can arise from sudden occlusion of the lower urinary tract or from widespread intratubular obstruction secondary to precipitation of Bence Jones protein in patients with multiple myeloma or of uric acid in patients with myeloproliferative disorders treated with chemotherapy.

Urinary tract obstruction is an important pathogenetic factor in 15 to 25 per cent of patients with end-stage renal failure and uremia. This progression to chronic renal failure can occur as a consequence of progressive hydronephrosis or by the destructive effects of recurrent urinary tract infections. In fact, it is unusual for chronic, recurrent pyelonephritis to occur in the absence of mechanical problems in the lower urinary tract. Urinary tract obstruction may also produce chronic interstitial nephritis unrelated to infection. Recently, several patients with chronic vesicoureteral reflux have been found to have severe chronic glomerulonephritis. The mechanism is not known, but it has been postulated to be an immune complex type of nephritis triggered by antibody production against renal antigens released from the damaged kidneys.

Infection. Recurrent urinary tract infection may be superimposed on urinary tract obstruction and present with the typical symptoms of fever, flank tenderness, and dysuria. The incidence of urinary tract infection ranges from 8 to 15 per cent in patients with urinary tract obstruction who have not been previously instrumented. Instrumentation (bladder catheters, cystoscopy), neurogenic bladder dysfunction, and bladder stones all increase the incidence of chronic infection. Once infection is established in the obstructed urinary tract, it is extremely difficult to eradicate and may contribute significantly to morbidity and the rate of destruction of renal function.

Tubular Dysfunction. A small percentage of patients may present with renal tubular abnormalities as the principal manifestation of their urinary tract obstruction. The most frequent of these abnormalities is inability to concentrate the urine. Usually, this is characterized by isosthenuria, nocturia, and modest polyuria, but occasionally may express itself as vasopressin-resistant nephrogenic diabetes insipidus with the excretion of large volumes (greater than 4000 ml per day) of dilute urine. The factors contributing to the defect in concentrating ability are destruction of the renal medulla and the antagonistic effects of PGE_2 against the renal action of vasopressin. Occasionally, patients with obstruction may present with renal tubular acidosis of the distal type, characterized by hyperchloremic acidosis with an inability to lower urine pH below 6.0 in response to acid loading. Less commonly, patients with obstruction may present with hyperkalemia secondary to a renal tubular defect in potassium secretion. When hyperkalemia occurs it is invariably associated with hyperchloremic acidosis.

Hypertension. Hypertension occurs in approximately 30 per cent of patients with acute unilateral obstruction. The hypertension tends to be mild and transient (rarely lasting longer than one week) and is caused by increased renin secretion. In general, hypertension is not a feature of chronic unilateral obstruction, although there have been a few cases of high renin hypertension reported, which were corrected by removal of the obstructed kidney. In contrast, a high percentage of patients with chronic bilateral hydronephrosis have hypertension. These patients do not have elevated renin levels, and the hypertension appears to be the consequence of retained salt and water.

Polycythemia. A rare manifestation of obstructive nephropathy is polycythemia. In the small number of patients in which this disorder has been observed, the erythrocytosis rapidly resolves following nephrectomy and is thought to be due to abnormal production of erythropoietin by the obstructed kidney.

Postobstructive Diuresis. Following the surgical correction of lower urinary tract obstruction the patient may undergo a marked diuresis ("postobstructive diuresis"). Both clinically and experimentally, postobstructive diuresis is associated with bilateral, but not with unilateral, obstruction. In most instances the diuresis is transient and does not result in significant contraction of extracellular volume. In these cases the diuresis is the consequence of the excretion of salt, urea, other solutes, and water retained during the period of obstruction, and continues until the volume and composition of the extracellular fluid return to normal. In a few instances, however, the diuresis represents a true salt and water wastage, with depletion of extracellular volume and its associated findings (e.g., postural hypotension, tachycardia). Recent experimental studies suggest that a natriuretic factor, normally excreted into the urine, is retained during periods of bilateral obstruction and causes salt wasting when the obstruction is released. There also appears to be a vasopressin-resistant component to the diuresis, possibly caused by high levels of renal prostaglandins.

DIAGNOSIS AND EVALUATION. Urinary tract obstruction should be suspected in patients who have lower urinary tract symptoms (diminished stream, urgency, hesitancy, incontinence); recurrent urinary tract infections; pain in the flank, groin, or lower abdomen; abdominal masses; or unexplained uremia or oliguric acute renal failure. The patient's history should be evaluated for previous stone disease, drug ingestion, diabetes mellitus, or neurologic disorders. The physical examination should evaluate the abdomen and flanks for pain or masses, the external genitalia, the prostate in men, and the pelvic structures in women. In selected circumstances, postvoiding urine volume measured by bladder catheterization may provide the key to diagnosis. This test, however, must be performed with great care to avoid inducing infection.

In patients presenting with acute oliguric renal failure, other causes of oliguria-anuria must be excluded. These include (1) extracellular volume depletion, (2) renal arterial or venous occlusion, (3) acute glomerular disease or vasculitis, (4) cortical necrosis, (5) acute tubular necrosis, and (6) urinary tract obstruction. Workup of these patients should include history of drug exposure (antibiotics, radiopaque dyes, analgesics, chemotherapy), evidence for multiple myeloma or uric acid nephropathy, and status of extracellular fluid volume. The urine should be carefully examined for red cell casts, renal tubular cell casts (renal failure casts), urate crystals, and red cells. Urine sodium concentration is helpful in that it should be low (less than 10 mEq per liter) in prerenal azotemia, acute glomerular disease, or renal vasculitis, but will be relatively high in acute tubular necrosis and urinary tract obstruction.

The key to the diagnosis of urinary tract obstruction is the demonstration of a dilated urinary collecting system. One of the most useful techniques for identifying dilatation of the renal pelvis, particularly in acutely oliguric patients, is B-mode ultrasonography. This technique is rapid and noninvasive and avoids the potential hazards of radiocontrast dyes. The intravenous urogram with nephrotomography is also a useful procedure in patients in whom radiocontrast agents are not contraindicated. In the presence of renal failure it is necessary to use a higher dose of dye. In most patients, even those with severe reduction of GFR, there should be adequate visualization to determine kidney size, whether there are one or two kidneys, and whether the renal pelvis is dilated. If the obstruction is acute, the nephrogram will be delayed but quite dense, whereas if the obstruction is more chronic, the nephrogram will be faint. Delayed films, 24 to 36 hours after dye injection, may be necessary to visualize the renal pelvis and collecting system sufficiently to identify the site of obstruction. In performing these tests it must be remembered that the renal pelvis may not be dilated at the time of study if the obstruction is partial and/or intermittent, or if the patient is severely volume depleted. In evaluating patients with intermittent flank pain, it is important, therefore, to perform the study at a time when the patient is having pain or after induction of osmotic or water diuresis. In severely ill patients, it is important to correct any deficits of extracellular volume prior to the test.

Once the presence of urinary tract obstruction is established, more complex urologic procedures such as retrograde pyelography, percutaneous antegrade pyelography, cystoscopy, and voiding cystograms may be needed to identify the site of vesicoureteral reflux and the functional status of the bladder. Renal scans are helpful in determining the relative function of the two kidneys, and are particularly useful in determining the residual function of a unilaterally obstructed kidney.

TREATMENT. The general aims of therapy are (1) relief from the symptoms of obstruction, (2) prevention or eradication of infection, and (3) preservation of renal function. Obstruction complicated by infection and sepsis is a potentially lethal disease requiring relief of obstruction as soon as possible. Complete obstruction, uncomplicated by infection, is not a medical emergency, but should be evaluated and corrected promptly for optimal preservation of renal function. In this situation uremia, if present, should first be treated by dialysis before proceeding with surgical correction of the obstruction. Elective repair of urinary tract obstruction is indicated in patients with recurrent urinary infections, persistent pain, urinary retention, recurrent bleeding, or progressive renal damage. Simple uncomplicated postvoid residual urine, vesicoureteral reflux, and dilation of the collecting system are not indications for surgery.

The specific method used for relief of obstruction depends on the general status of the patient, whether the situation requires an emergency or elective procedure, the location of the obstruction, whether the obstructing lesion is benign or malignant, whether the obstruction is mechanical or neurogenic, and the functional status of the obstructed kidney.

In the septic patient requiring an emergency procedure, the obstruction can be relieved either by urethral or ureteral catheters or by percutaneous placement of a nephrostomy tube into the dilated renal pelvis. These bypass procedures can also be used electively in the presence of complete obstruction to gain time for diagnostic studies and the evaluation of residual renal function. Occasionally, one may elect to leave these diversion tubes in place permanently. Despite the inevitable urinary infection associated with the presence of these tubes, the patients may survive for years with little or no further loss of renal function. However, whenever possible, the tubes should be removed and a more definitive procedure performed. If the obstructed kidney is nonfunctional and has no chance of recovering function (chronic obstruction or complete acute obstruction for more than three to four months), then nephrectomy may be the most judicious procedure. A discussion of surgical procedures is beyond the scope of this chapter.

Acute obstruction of a ureter with a renal stone is usually transient and will correct spontaneously in 85 to 90 per cent of the cases. If the stone is greater than 5 mm, it may become impacted in the ureter and require surgical removal within a few days. If a stone lodged in the ureter does not produce complete obstruction, one can delay for two to four weeks to see if spontaneous passage will occur. If the stone is not passed, it should then be surgically removed. Manipulation or removal of ureteral stones by a basket catheter is sometimes successful, but this procedure runs the risk of ureteral injury with subsequent stricture.

Functional obstruction secondary to neurogenic bladder is a complicated and difficult management problem. Helpful maneuvers are frequent voiding, double voiding, suprapubic pressure on the bladder during voiding, and the use of cholinergic drugs. Intermittent catheterization may also be used, with the addition of anticholinergic or sympathomimetic drugs to prevent incontinence between catheterizations. More severe cases may require a permanent indwelling catheter or, preferably, surgical reimplantation of the ureters into an ileal conduit.

Beck LH, Stein JH, Earley LE: Obstructive uropathy. *In* Earley LE, Gottschalk CW (eds.): Strauss and Welt's Diseases of the Kidney. 3rd ed. Boston, Little, Brown & Company, 1979. *An extensive review of the pathophysiology of obstructive uropathy written for nephrologists.*

Klahr S (Guest Editor): Obstructive uropathy. *In* Kurtzman N (ed.): Seminars in Nephrology, Vol II, No 1, March, 1982. *A superb multiauthored review of the physiologic, biochemical, and hormonal changes in the obstructed kidney.*

Muldowney FP, Duffy GT, Kelly DG, Duff FA, Harrington C, Freaney R: Sodium diuresis after relief of obstructive uropathy. N Engl J Med 274:1294, 1966. *This study demonstrated that in most patients the natriuresis and diuresis following relief of obstructive uropathy are the consequence of the excretion of salt and water retained during the period of obstruction. The process continues until the patients achieve a normal body fluid and sodium content. Evidence of true salt wasting, causing clinically significant salt depletion, is very unusual.*

Needleman P, Wyche A, Bronson SD, Holmberg S, Morrison AR: Specific regulation of peptide-induced renal prostaglandin synthesis. J Biol Chem 254:9772, 1979. *Complete ureteral obstruction activates the biochemical pathways for the synthesis of prostaglandins and thromboxanes in the kidney.*

Okegawa T, Jonas PE, DeSchryver K, Kawasaki A, Needleman P: Metabolic and cellular alterations underlying the exaggerated renal prostaglandin and thromboxane synthesis in ureter obstruction in rabbits. J Clin Invest 71:81, 1983. *Acute unilateral ureteral obstruction produces an inflammatory reaction in the obstructed kidney with an interstitial infiltrate of monocytes and fibroblasts. These inflammatory cells account for the increased cyclooxygenase activity and the exaggerated production of PGE_2 and thromboxane A_2.*

Wright FS, Howards SS: Obstructive injury. *In* Brenner BM, Rector FC Jr (eds.): The Kidney. 2nd ed. Philadelphia, W. B. Saunders Company, 1981. *A very comprehensive review of the physiology of the lower urinary tract and the pathogenesis of obstructive unopathy. This chapter provides a good overview of the various surgical procedures available for the different causes of lower urinary tract obstruction.*

Yarger WE, Schocken DD, Harris RH: Obstructive nephropathy in the rat: Possible roles for the renin-angiotensin system, prostaglandins, and thromboxanes in postobstructive renal function. J Clin Invest 65:400, 1980. *Following the relief of complete unilateral obstruction in the rat, the kidney remains vasoconstricted with low blood flow and filtration rate. This is the consequence of excessive thromboxane production. Inhibition of thromboxane synthesis prevents the vasoconstriction.*

83. SPECIFIC RENAL TUBULAR DISORDERS

83.1. Introduction

Martin G. Cogan

The diverse reabsorptive functions of the kidney are generally segregated such that specific nephron segments are responsible for specific transport functions. As described in Ch. 73, the proximal nephron is responsible for the reabsorption of most of the filtered bicarbonate, glucose, amino acids, uric acid, phosphate, and low molecular weight proteins. The loop of Henle reabsorbs over half the filtered sodium chloride as well as divalent cations. The distal nephron (including the cortical and medullary collecting ducts), under the influence of aldosterone, reabsorbs the final quantity of sodium, secretes hydrogen ions to lower the pH of the urine and titrate buffers, and secretes potassium ions. The terminal collecting ducts can be induced by antidiuretic hormone to permit water reabsorption and thereby cause urinary concentration.

Genetic and acquired conditions exist that can affect one or more of the reabsorptive or secretory transport processes within each of these nephron segments, as illustrated in Table 83–1. Depending on the transport sites affected, these diseases therefore lead to abnormal wastage or retention of specific solutes. For instance, within a given nephron segment, there may be a selective transport defect for a single solute (e.g., bicarbonate in proximal renal tubular acidosis or glucose in renal glycosuria) or for a class of solutes (e.g., dibasic amino acids in cystinuria). Alternatively, those solutes modulated by a specific hormone may be affected by a hormone-deficient or -resistant state (e.g., in hypoaldosteronism or diabetes insipidus). Finally, there are diseases that affect all solutes normally transported by a given nephron segment (e.g., all proximally transported solutes in Fanconi's syndrome). Luminal, cellular, or peritubular components of the overall transport process can be responsible for each of these situations. The following sections describe some of the more common transport defects of the individual nephron segments.

83.2. Renal Tubular Acidosis (RTA)

Martin G. Cogan

The renal tubular acidoses are a group of hyperchloremic metabolic acidoses characterized by impaired renal acidification. Proton secretion by the kidney is incapable of maintaining the plasma bicarbonate concentration at a normal level even though endogenous acid production (from diet, metabolism, and gastrointestinal base loss) is not elevated. As summarized in Table 83–2, defective renal hydrogen ion secretion may be manifested as an inability to reabsorb bicarbonate by the proximal nephron (proximal, or Type II RTA) or an inability to excrete sufficient urinary net acid by the distal nephron. Such failure to excrete net acid may in turn be due to an isolated defect in lowering the urinary pH (classic distal, or Type I RTA), a total failure of the hydrogen ion and potassium secretory function of the distal nephron (generalized distal, or Type IV RTA), or the inability to produce or excrete sufficient ammonium (RTA of glomerular insufficiency). Type III is an outdated designation that is no longer used. Figure 83–1 summarizes the sites of defective renal acidification in RTA.

TABLE 83–1. CLINICAL SYNDROMES DUE TO NEPHRON TRANSPORT DEFECTS

Proximal Nephron
Nonselective: Fanconi's syndrome
Selective
Amino acidurias
Glycosurias
Proximal RTA
Uric acid disorders
Calcium/phosphate disorders
Loop of Henle
? Bartter's syndrome
Distal Nephron (Distal Tubule and Collecting Ducts)
Classic distal RTA
Hypoaldosteronism and generalized distal RTA
Hyperaldosteronism
Other potassium secretory disorders
Renal salt wasting
Loop and Medullary Collecting Ducts
Diabetes insipidus
SIADH
Other concentrating/diluting disorders

PROXIMAL (TYPE II) RTA

PATHOPHYSIOLOGY. The proximal nephron reabsorbs 85 to 90 per cent of the filtered bicarbonate, predominantly by Na^+/H^+ exchange and the enzymatic degradation of H_2CO_3 to CO_2 and H_2O by carbonic anhydrase. Interference with the normal operation of Na^+/H^+ exchange or of carbonic anhydrase activity will therefore result in excess delivery of bicarbonate to the distal nephron and, because of the limited distal bicarbonate reabsorption capacity, into the urine. Thus, the urinary wastage of $\geq$ 15 per cent of the filtered bicarbonate load at a normal blood bicarbonate concentration is pathognomonic of proximal RTA. The excess delivery of the relatively impermeant bicarbonate to the distal nephron also results in accelerated potassium secretion and hypokalemia. As the plasma bicarbonate concentration and filtered load fall owing to defective proximal bicarbonate reabsorption and subsequent urinary bicarbonate wastage, absolute bicarbonate delivery to the distal nephron progressively decreases. At a certain point, usually when the plasma bicarbonate concentration is 15 to 18 mM, the distal nephron can cope with the delivery out of the proximal tubule. At this stage, bicarbonaturia disappears, urinary pH can be lowered normally, and net acid excretion equivalent to endogenous acid production resumes. Acid-base homeostasis is reestablished at the expense of metabolic acidosis.

Defective proximal acidification can be the result of drugs or disorders that affect the physical integrity of the proximal nephron cells, inhibit carbonic anhydrase, or allow dissipation of the sodium gradient from lumen to cell, the energy source for driving proton extrusion. If the lumen-to-cell sodium gradient is disrupted either from disturbances of metabolism or from increased cell sodium permeability, other sodium cotransported solutes (such as glucose, amino acids, phosphate, urate) also may be affected, creating the full-blown Fanconi syndrome (see Ch. 83.5).

SYMPTOMS AND ETIOLOGIES. Manifestations of the proximal RTA are attributable to acidemia (growth retardation, anorexia and malnutrition, volume depletion), potassium depletion (muscular weakness, polyuria, nocturia, polydipsia), and disordered calcium/phosphate/parathormone/vitamin D metabolism (osteomalacia and other bone disease). Proximal RTA is a rare disorder, ascribable to multiple myeloma, genetic defects (cystinosis, Wilson's disease, fructose intolerance), heavy metals (lead, mercury, cadmium), drugs that inhibit carbonic anhydrase (acetazolamide), and vitamin D–deficient/secondary hyperparathyroid states.

DIAGNOSIS AND TREATMENT. Laboratory findings of proximal RTA are those of a hyperchloremic, hypokalemic metabolic acidosis. When the patient is acidemic, the urine is acidic and net acid excretion equals endogenous acid load (Table 83–2). When bicarbonate is infused to normalize the plasma bicarbonate concentration, massive bicarbonaturia results ($\geq$ 15 per cent of the filtered load). Proximal RTA is usually not isolated but rather associated with the full Fanconi syndrome.

Therapy of the underlying disease should be undertaken if possible (e.g., multiple myeloma) or offending drugs or toxins discontinued (e.g., heavy metals). When this is not possible,

TABLE 83–2. RENAL TUBULAR ACIDOSES

Type	Renal Defect	Plasma [K$^+$]	Proximal Acidification: HCO_3^- Reabsorption (During HCO_3^- Loading)	Distal Acidification: $U_{pH_{min}}$ (During Acidosis)	Distal Acidification: $(U_{NH_4^+}\cdot V) + (U_{TA}\cdot V)$ (During Acidosis)
Proximal (Type II)	↓ Proximal acidification	↓	↓	< 5.5	N
Classic distal (Type I)	↓ Distal pH gradient	↓	N	> 5.5	↓
Generalized distal (Type IV)	↓ Aldosterone action	↑	N	< 5.5	↓
Glomerular insufficiency	↓ NH_3 production	N	N	< 5.5	↓

Abbreviations: $U_{pH_{min}}$ = minimal urinary pH; $(U_{NH_4^+}\cdot V) + (U_{TA}\cdot V)$ = urinary ammonium plus titratable acid excretion; N = normal.

proximal RTA is treated with large amounts of sodium and potassium bicarbonate. As the plasma bicarbonate concentration rises with treatment, distal bicarbonate delivery increases, causing more potassium wasting and the need for further potassium supplementation. Because of the inability to fully correct the disorder with bicarbonate alone, volume contraction utilizing diuretics is also used to stimulate fractional proximal bicarbonate reabsorption. Therapy with vitamin D is indicated when signs of vitamin D deficiency exist.

CLASSIC DISTAL (TYPE I) RTA

PATHOPHYSIOLOGY. The distal nephron (especially the cortical and medullary collecting ducts) is normally capable of lowering the urine pH fully 2 to 3 pH units below that of blood to titrate filtered buffers (principally phosphate) to form titratable acids and endogenously produced ammonia to form ammonium. If the distal nephron is incapable of lowering the luminal pH below 5.5 when challenged by metabolic acidosis, a classic distal RTA is present. Because of the inappropriately high urine pH, net acid excretion (titratable acid plus ammonium minus bicarbonate) is subnormal, less than acid production by the body. Accelerated potassium secretion occurs, presumably because there is reduced competition by proton secretion for the electrochemical driving forces in the distal nephron. The acidification defect may result from an insufficient number of proton-secreting pumps in the distal nephron. Alternatively, there may be backleak of acid across the luminal membrane, so that establishment of a pH gradient is prevented even when proton secretion is normal (Fig. 83–1).

SYMPTOMS AND ETIOLOGIES. Distal RTA is found both in infants and children and in adults. Symptoms may be of acidosis or hypokalemia, as described above. Nephrocalcinosis and nephrolithiasis are common, either as a cause or as a result of classic distal RTA. However, bone disease is not as frequent as in proximal RTA. Classic distal RTA may also be genetic (most frequently autosomal dominant), or due to autoimmune diseases (Sjögren's syndrome, systemic lupus erythematosus, chronic active hepatitis, primary biliary cirrhosis, and other hypergammaglobulinemic states), drugs and toxins (amphotericin, toluene), and various tubulo-interstitial diseases.

DIAGNOSIS AND TREATMENT. The findings of hyperchloremic, hypokalemic metabolic acidosis with an inappropriately high urine pH (> 5.5) and diminished net acid excretion confirm the diagnosis (Table 83–2). In individuals with a normal plasma bicarbonate concentration, the failure to lower urine pH to < 5.5 following an acute acid challenge with NH_4Cl defines the syndrome of incomplete classic distal RTA (see Ch. 76 for details of the NH_4Cl test). Proximal bicarbonate reabsorption as tested by bicarbonate loading is normal. Treatment with alkali is generally very effective. The daily dose of alkali in adults is 1 to 3 mEq per kilogram, to compensate for the normal acid production by the body plus a small amount of urinary bicarbonate wastage. In contrast to proximal RTA, urinary potassium wasting is ameliorated with alkali therapy. Children require more alkali, about 5 to 14 mEq per kilogram per day.

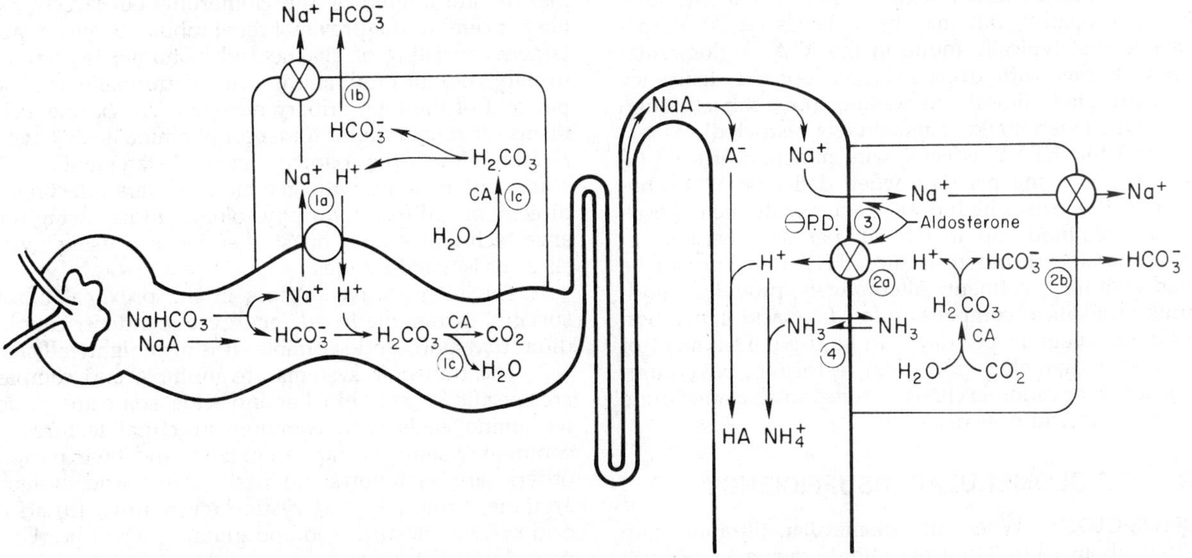

Figure 83–1. Sites of impaired renal acidification. In the left side of the figure are shown the possible sites of disordered proximal hydrogen ion secretion in a model of a proximal tubule cell. Proximal RTA may be a consequence of an impaired Na^+/H^+ antiporter or lumen-to-cell sodium gradient (1a); disturbed HCO_3^- exit (1b); or inhibition of carbonic anhydrase, CA (1c). The possible sites of disordered acidification in a model of a distal tubule cell are shown in the right side of the figure. Classic distal RTA is a consequence of a qualitative or quantitative problem of the proton pump or proton back leak (2a) or of impaired bicarbonate exit (2b). Generalized distal RTA results from a disturbance of aldosterone-dependent sodium reabsorption as well as potassium and proton secretion (3). The RTA of glomerular insufficiency results from diminished ammonia availability (4).

Prognosis with respect to stabilization of glomerular filtration rate in adults or growth in children is excellent with provision of adequate alkali therapy.

GENERALIZED DISTAL (TYPE IV) RTA

PATHOPHYSIOLOGY. When sodium is reabsorbed in the distal nephron under the influence of aldosterone, a lumen-negative potential difference is generated, favoring secretion of potassium and hydrogen ions. Disruption of potassium and hydrogen secretion may therefore be ascribable to a defect in the integrity of the distal nephron cell, deficient aldosterone production or action, diminished sodium reabsorption, or shunting of the lumen-negative potential by enhanced chloride reabsorption. Any of these processes will lead to diminished total hydrogen ion and potassium excretion and therefore metabolic acidosis with hyperkalemia. The hyperkalemia will also serve to independently depress renal ammoniagenesis, which exacerbates the defect in renal acidification. The ability to reabsorb bicarbonate (a proximal nephron function) and to lower the urinary pH normally (a qualitative distal nephron function at low buffer strength) remains intact (Table 83–2).

SYMPTOMS AND ETIOLOGIES. The symptoms of generalized distal RTA in children or adults usually relate to the acidosis itself or occasionally to the neuromuscular consequences of hyperkalemia. The most common forms of generalized distal RTA are due to reduction in aldosterone level or prevention of its action. The adrenal synthesis of aldosterone may be directly impaired, as in Addison's disease or in inherited enzymatic defects, such as 18- or 21-hydroxylase deficiencies. More commonly, primary hyporeninemia due to diabetic nephropathy, hypertensive nephrosclerosis, or tubulo-interstitial diseases can also reduce aldosterone levels. Finally, end-organ unresponsiveness to mineralocorticoid with high circulating levels of aldosterone can be found in various tubulo-interstitial diseases, especially those that have a predilection for the medulla and papilla of the kidney (e.g., analgesic abuse, sickle cell disease, and obstructive nephropathies).

DIAGNOSIS AND TREATMENT. Generalized distal RTA is unique among the hyperchloremic metabolic acidoses in being a hyperkalemic disorder. Glomerular filtration rate is invariably reduced in the forms associated with hyporeninemia or tubulo-interstitial nephropathy, but may be at levels ($\geq$ 30 ml per minute) above that typically found in the RTA of glomerular insufficiency. Forms with overt mineralocorticoid deficiency may have associated clinical salt wasting (i.e., salt excretion exceeding intake when intake is moderately restricted).

Treatment of this RTA is effected with mineralocorticoid (9-α-fludrocortisone 0.1 mg per day) when deficient. When hyporeninemia is the cause, high doses of the synthetic mineralocorticoid are required (up to 0.5 mg per day) because of associated mineralocorticoid resistance. Hypertension can be precipitated with this treatment. Alternatively, providing modest amounts of alkali to compensate for daily acid generation (1 to 3 mEq per kilogram per day) can be used. Treatment of the hyperkalemia by dietary potassium restriction, potassium-wasting diuretics, or cation-exchange resins can also ameliorate or even correct the acid-base disorder.

RTA OF GLOMERULAR INSUFFICIENCY

PATHOPHYSIOLOGY. When the glomerular filtration rate (GFR) falls to about 20 to 30 ml per minute owing to intrinsic glomerular or tubulo-interstitial disease, a normokalemic metabolic acidosis is frequently found. The cause of this acidosis is thought to be either deficient ammonia production or impairment in the urinary trapping of ammonia as ammonium. In either case, proximal bicarbonate reclamation and the ability to lower the urine pH to $<$ 5.5 are intact, but the failure to generate sufficient acid excretion to equal intake results in systemic acidosis.

SYMPTOMS AND ETIOLOGY. The degree of metabolic acidosis is generally mild, and plasma bicarbonate concentration is usually $>$ 15 mEq per liter. The acidemia has been suggested by some investigators to exacerbate the osteodystrophy of progressive renal disease. Although tubulo-interstitial diseases are thought to produce this form of RTA more commonly than glomerular diseases, this distinction has been difficult to verify. This hyperchloremic metabolic acidosis should be distinguished from the high anion gap (normochloremic) metabolic acidosis due to retained organic acids that usually occurs when glomerular insufficiency is more severe (GFR $<$ 20 ml per minute). The two acidoses may coexist.

DIAGNOSIS AND TREATMENT. A hyperchloremic, normokalemic metabolic acidosis that occurs when GFR falls to about 20 to 30 ml per minute is typical of the RTA of glomerular insufficiency. Although net acid, specifically ammonium, excretion is subnormal, the urine pH is appropriately acidic (Table 83–2). Mineralocorticoid levels are not diminished. An elevated anion gap (uremic acidosis) is generally seen only when GFR is $<$ 20 ml per minute. Treatment consists of 1 to 3 mEq per kilogram per day of alkali therapy to compensate for daily acid ingestion and production.

Arruda JAL, Kurtzman NA: Mechanisms and classification of deranged distal urinary acidification. Am J Physiol 239:F515, 1980. *This paper provides a critical and insightful examination of the causes of classic and generalized distal RTA.*

Cogan MG, Rector FC Jr, Seldin DW: Acid-base disorders. *In* Brenner BM, Rector FC Jr (eds.): The Kidney. 2nd ed. Philadelphia, WB Saunders Company, 1981, pp 841–907. *This chapter is a comprehensive review of acid-base homeostasis, including the RTA's.*

Harrington JT, Cohen JJ: Metabolic acidosis. *In* Cohen JJ, Kassirer JP (eds.): Acid-Base. Boston, Little, Brown & Company, 1982, pp 121–226. *This chapter describes the pathophysiology and clinical manifestations of metabolic acidoses.*

Rector FC Jr, Cogan MG: The renal acidoses. Hosp Pract 15:99, 1980. *This article provides an introduction to the diagnosis and pathophysiology of the hyperchloremic metabolic acidoses.*

Schambelan M, Sebastian A, Biglieri EG: Prevalence, pathogenesis and functional significance of aldosterone deficiency in hyperkalemic patients with chronic renal insufficiency. Kidney Int 17:89, 1980. *This paper provides one of the most comprehensive reviews of the heterogeneous causes of generalized distal (Type IV) RTA.*

83.3. Renal Hyperaminoacidurias

Lloyd H. Smith, Jr.

L-Amino acids, of which approximately 20 are present in plasma, are filtered by the glomerulus but largely reabsorbed (95 per cent) in the proximal renal tubule. Some aminoaciduria, largely consisting of glycine and histidine, is normal, but the urinary content of all amino acids is normally less than 2 to 3 per cent of the total urinary nitrogen. The biochemical mechanisms for renal tubular transport of amino acids have not been clearly defined; the following general statements are based on studies of patients with genetic disorders affecting transport directly or indirectly, on physiologic studies using renal clearance techniques, and on studies in vitro using renal cortical slices or isolated tubules:

1. The reabsorptive process in the proximal tubule is site specific, carrier mediated, energy dependent, coupled to sodium transport, and saturable. It is also highly efficient.

2. The transport systems are multiple and complex. Some are specific for individual amino acids; some are group specific for amino acids with common structural features. The five common systems so far recognized, and their prototypic disorders, are as follows: (a) basic amino acid system: lysine, arginine, ornithine, and cystine (cystinuria); (b) acidic amino acid system: aspartic acid and glutamic acid (dicarboxylic aminoaciduria); (c) neutral amino acid system I: proline, hydroxyproline, and glycine (renal iminoglycinuria); (d) neutral amino acid system II: the remaining neutral α-amino acids not listed above (Hartnup disease); and (e) β-amino acid system: β-alanine, β-aminoisobutyric acid, taurine (hyper-β-alaninemia).

3. The renal tubular transport systems for amino acids are often shared by the epithelial cells of the gut mucosa, but seem

not to be phenotypically expressed in other cells. For example, certain genetic disorders (cystinuria, Hartnup disease) may affect both the renal tubule and gut mucosa, but no defects have as yet been demonstrated in other tissues.

PATHOGENETIC MECHANISMS. Based on these considerations, it is convenient to classify hyperaminoaciduria as being due to one of three pathogenetic mechanisms:

1. *Saturation of the transport mechanisms.* The filtered load of the amino acid is abnormally increased, generally owing to a block in its further metabolism. This is sometimes called "overflow" aminoaciduria. As a subset of this category, the overflow of one amino acid may compete with another amino acid for a common transport system, producing a combined "overflow-renal" aminoaciduria.

2. *Specific abnormality of the transport mechanism.* There is an inherited abnormality of the reactive site which reduces the ability of the renal tubule to transport a specific amino acid or group of amino acids. The filtered load of the amino acid is normal, or may be reduced because of renal wastage, and other functions of the renal tubule, including the transport of other amino acids, are unimpaired. This category is called selective renal aminoaciduria.

3. *General abnormality of the transport mechanism.* There is an inherited or acquired abnormality which interferes with the structural or functional integrity of the proximal renal tubule, especially with the utilization of metabolic energy for active transport. The impairment of amino acid transport is not selective and results in generalized renal aminoaciduria.

The overflow aminoacidurias are not, strictly speaking, renal diseases, and they will be discussed in Ch. 187–194. Table 83–3 presents a classification of the renal hyperaminoacidurias. The generalized renal aminoacidurias are usually associated with derangement of other tubular functions, often in a pattern termed Fanconi's syndrome (see Ch. 83.5). Cystinuria and its variants hypercystinuria and hyperdibasic aminoaciduria are discussed in Ch. 83.4. The other specific renal aminoacidurias are all very rare and will be summarized briefly.

HARTNUP DISEASE. Named for the propositus family, Hartnup disease is a rare (1 in 16,000 births) inherited disorder of the renal tubule and the gut mucosa characterized by impaired transport of a specific group of neutral α-amino acids (alanine, serine, threonine, valine, leucine, isoleucine, phenylalanine, tyrosine, tryptophan, and histidine). These amino acids, together with glutamine and asparagine, are excreted in the urine in amounts approximately five to ten times greater than normal, as readily demonstrable by chromatographic studies. Amino acids in other specific groups (basic, acidic, β-amino acids, glycine, and imino acids) are transported normally and are not increased in urine. Hartnup urine also contains increased amounts of indoles and indican, derived from bacterial metabolism of tryptophan which fails to be normally absorbed in the gut.

The clinical manifestations are those of pellagra (see Ch. 217)—intermittent skin rash especially in sun-exposed areas, cerebellar ataxia, and psychiatric disturbances. L-Tryptophan is metabolized in part via the kynurenine pathway to nicotinamide, normally supplying as much as 50 per cent of that cofactor. In Hartnup disease there is secondary tryptophan deficiency owing to its diminished absorption, and therefore a marginal supply of nicotinamide. Symptoms and signs of pellagra tend to occur when nutrition is inadequate, adding diminished dietary intake of nicotinamide to impaired synthesis from its endogenous precursor, L-tryptophan. No other adverse effects of the transport defects in the gut and kidney have been demonstrated, although it has been speculated that products of the bacterial metabolism of other poorly absorbed amino acids might contribute to the pathogenesis of the clinical findings. The diagnosis should be considered in patients with the clinical findings of pellagra in the absence of dietary deficiency and can be readily established by the chromatographic demonstration of the characteristic pattern of aminoaciduria. Hartnup disease is transmitted as an autosomal recessive trait, not expressed phenotypically in heterozygotes, so that sibs of newly discovered cases should be investigated. The treatment of Hartnup disease is that of a balanced diet supplemented by nicotinamide (40 to 250 mg per day), which suffices to prevent pellagra.

TABLE 83–3. RENAL HYPERAMINOACIDURIAS

Selective renal aminoacidurias
Cystinuria (cystine, lysine, arginine, ornithine)
Hypercystinuria (cystine)
Hyperdibasic aminoaciduria (lysine, arginine, ornithine)
Hartnup disease (neutral amino acids, excluding glycine and imino acids)
Iminoglycinuria (proline, hydroxyproline, glycine)
Dicarboxylic aminoaciduria (glutamic acid, aspartic acid)
Histidinuria (histidine)
Lysinuria (lysine)
Generalized renal aminoacidurias
Inherited
Idiopathic Fanconi's syndrome, Wilson's disease
Cystinosis, Lowe's syndrome, galactosemia
Hereditary fructose intolerance, congenital renal tubular acidosis
Acquired
Heavy metal poisoning (lead, mercury, cadmium)
Outdated tetracycline, multiple myeloma
Hyperparathyroidism, acute tubular necrosis
Nutritional disturbances (potassium depletion, vitamin D deficiency, kwashiorkor)

IMINOGLYCINURIA. This rare (1 in 16,000 to 20,000 births) autosomal recessive trait is characterized by selective impairment of the renal tubular reabsorption of proline, hydroxyproline, and glycine. In some homozygotes gut mucosal transport of these amino acids may be similarly defective. No clinical abnormalities have been ascribed to iminoglycinuria, which is usually discovered by chance during survey of urinary amino acids. Genetic heterogeneity has been demonstrated in the linkage of the renal and gut defects, in the severity of the transport defect, and in the presence or absence of isolated hyperglycinuria as a marker of the heterozygous state. No treatment for this benign variation is indicated.

DICARBOXYLIC AMINOACIDURIA. This selective defect in the renal tubular transport of aspartic acid and glutamic acid has been described in only two unrelated patients. Clearance of these dicarboxylic acids exceeded the glomerular filtration rate, indicating net tubular secretion. In one patient but not the other an analogous gut mucosal defect appeared to be present. No clinical findings can as yet be attributed to the transport defect of these two nonessential amino acids.

HISTIDINURIA AND LYSINURIA. A selective aminoaciduria for histidine has been described in two sibs with mental retardation. *Lysinuria,* without impairment of cystine, ornithine, and arginine, has been discovered in one child with mental retardation, seizures, and poor growth and development. In histidinuria and lysinuria the respective transport defects were present in both the renal tubule and the gut mucosa.

Jepson JB: Hartnup disease. *In* Stanbury JB, Wyngaarden JB, Fredrickson DS (eds.): The Metabolic Basis of Inherited Disease. 4th ed. New York, McGraw-Hill Book Company, 1978, p 1563. *This is the most complete review of the clinical syndrome of Hartnup disease and its interesting pathogenesis whereby a defect in the absorption of an essential amino acid, tryptophan, results in a secondary vitamin deficiency syndrome, pellagra.*

Rosenberg, LE, Scriver CR: Disorders of amino acid metabolism. *In* Bondy PK, Rosenberg LE (eds.): Metabolic Control and Disease. 8th ed. Philadelphia, W. B. Saunders Company, 1980, p 583. *This chapter contains an authoritative review of the biochemical, physiologic, and clinical aspects of the known disorders of amino acid transport and metabolism.*

Scriver CR: Familial Iminoglycinuria. *In* Stanbury JB, Wyngaarden JB, Fredrickson DS, Goldstein JL, Brown MS (eds.): The Metabolic Basis of Inherited Disease. 5th ed. New York, McGraw-Hill Book Company, 1983, p 1792. *This chapter gives an extensive discussion of this rare, benign disorder of transport with emphasis on pathogenetic mechanisms. 87 references.*

83.4. Cystinuria

Samuel O. Thier

DEFINITION. Cystinuria is a disorder of amino acid transport affecting the brush border of the epithelial cells of the renal tubules and the gastrointestinal tract. The clinical disease is inherited as a complex autosomal recessive trait characterized by the precipitation of cystine in the urine. Cystine, the least soluble naturally occurring amino acid, precipitates as crystals that form urinary tract calculi, which may cause colic, obstruction, infection, and ultimately renal insufficiency.

PREVALENCE. The overall prevalence of the disease as determined by newborn screening is about 1 in 7,000, which makes cystinuria one of the more common inherited disorders. The prevalence ranges from 1 in 2,000 in England to 1 in 15,000 in the United States.

ETIOLOGY AND PATHOGENESIS. Cystinuria results from an absent or defective transport mechanism for cystine and the dibasic amino acids in the brush border of the proximal renal tubule and the small intestine. This results in an aminoaciduria that is renal in origin and highly selective. Excessive quantities of cystine and the dibasic amino acids lysine, arginine, and ornithine are excreted despite a normal or reduced filtered load of these amino acids. The mixed disulfide of homocysteine-cysteine is also excreted in excess quantities and appears to be a normal plasma constituent that shares the defective renal transport mechanism. A comparable transport defect has been demonstrated in the intestine. Reports of an increased prevalence of cystinuria among patients with neurologic defects do not appear to be explicable on the basis of transport abnormalities; cystine does not share transport mechanisms with the dibasic amino acids in the brain. Furthermore, studies of a large group of homozygous cystinuric patients did not reveal an increased prevalence of mental deficiency.

Patients homozygous for cystinuria excrete from 250 to more than 1000 mg of cystine per gram of creatinine per day. At least three phenotypes of homozygous cystinuria are defined on the basis of intestinal amino acid transport studies in vitro and in vivo in the homozygote and urinary amino acid excretion in the heterozygote. In Type I homozygotes intestinal transport of all involved amino acids in vitro is abnormal and the intestinal absorption of cystine in vivo is markedly reduced. Heterozygotes have normal urinary amino acid excretion. Type II homozygotes have defective transport of dibasic amino acids, but not of cystine in vitro; absorption of cystine in vivo is reduced. Heterozygotes have elevated urinary cystine and lysine excretion (incompletely recessive). Type III homozygotes have normal gut transport in vitro and in vivo. Heterozygotes have an incompletely recessive pattern of urinary amino acid excretion. Complex heterozygotes, that is, individuals who resemble the homozygotes but who have inherited two different mutations on the same allele, have been described (for example, Type I-III, I-II, or II-III).

CLINICAL MANIFESTATIONS AND DIAGNOSIS. The disease occurs equally in both sexes. Males are more severely affected and have a higher mortality rate, perhaps related to urinary tract anatomy, with a greater likelihood of urethral obstruction. Although the peak of clinical expression is in the second and third decades, the disease may appear at any time from the first year of life to as late as the ninth decade. Renal colic is the most common presenting symptom. Recurrent calculi may be associated with obstruction, subsequent infection, and eventual loss of renal function. Infection, hypertension, or renal failure may be the initial clinical presentations.

The disulfide bond of cystine renders stones radiopaque, although less dense than calcium stones. The stones may be single, multiple, or present as staghorn calculi. The presence on roentgenogram of a smooth staghorn calculus with multiple smooth satellite stones is highly suggestive of cystinuria. Infection may produce mixed cystine-calcium stones or cystine-free stones. Cystine may also act as a nidus for calcium oxalate stone formation, much as uric acid does.

Cystinuria should be considered in every patient with urinary calculi or recurrent urinary tract colic. The solubility of cystine in acid urine is between 300 and 400 mg per liter and increases in alkaline urine. Therefore, the first morning specimen or other concentrated urine, particularly when acidified, is most likely to show the typical hexagonal plate cystine crystals. The cyanide-nitroprusside test is a useful screening procedure. Since a positive nitroprusside test may also be seen in patients excreting homocystine, beta-mercaptolactate disulfide, and acetone, the diagnosis of cystinuria should be pursued by thin layer chromatography or high voltage electrophoresis, which will disclose increased quantities of cystine, lysine, arginine, and ornithine. Amino acid excretion can then be quantitated by ion exchange chromatography, or cystine excretion alone may be quantitated following its electrolytic reduction to the thiol, which can be colorimetrically measured.

Cystinuria has been associated with hyperuricemia, hemophilia, retinitis pigmentosa, muscular dystrophy, muscular hypotonia, mongolism, and hereditary pancreatitis; it also occurs as an isolated aminoaciduria with hypocalcemic tetany. The original observation that cystinuric patients are shorter than the general population, perhaps because of the malabsorption of essential amino acids, has not been substantiated.

TREATMENT. The goals of medical treatment of cystinuria are to reduce the excretion and increase the solubility of cystine. Surgical therapy has been directed at (1) attempts to dissolve cystine calculi by alkaline irrigation, (2) removal of cystine stones by lithotomy, and (3) the transplantation of a noncystinuric kidney to replace one destroyed by cystinuria.

Cystine is the metabolic product of the essential amino acid methionine. The results of nutritionally adequate diets low in methionine have been variable. Avoidance of excess methionine intake is reasonable, but discomforting diets are not indicated.

The solubility of cystine may be enhanced by maintaining a urine volume sufficient to keep the urine cystine concentration below 300 mg per liter. In a patient excreting 1 gram of cystine per day, this will require more than 4 liters of fluid intake. Fluid must not simply be ingested at random but must be distributed to maintain a high flow of dilute urine over all 24 hours. Thus, the intake of water at bedtime and again at 2 or 3 A.M. will reduce the important problem of supersaturation of the urine at night when the urine flow and the pH are low. Hydration therapy is successful in preventing stone formation in approximately two thirds of patients who adhere to it. Cystine solubility can also be enhanced by an alkaline pH but does not increase significantly until the pH is above 7.5. The administration of bicarbonate, citrate, and carbonic anhydrase inhibitors has been advocated and seems theoretically reasonable.

For those patients who continue to form stones on a low methionine diet, high fluid intake, and alkalinization, the use of D-penicillamine is recommended. This drug, through a disulfide exchange reaction, forms a mixed disulfide of penicillamine-cysteine that is significantly more soluble than cystine. On adequate penicillamine therapy, usually 1 to 2 grams per 24 hours, cystine excretion may be kept below 200 mg per gram of creatinine, the level at which stone formation is minimal. The undesirable side effects of penicillamine dictate that it be restricted to patients in whom more conservative therapy has failed or who have lost one kidney from cystine stone disease. As many as 50 per cent of patients receiving the drug will develop allergic reactions, usually fever and rash; rarely, arthralgias occur. More severe reactions include nephrotic syndrome and pancytopenia, both of which may be reversible when the drug is discontinued. Epidermolysis, thrombocytopenia, loss of taste, and a fatal Goodpasture-like syndrome have also been reported. Therapy should be initiated with close supervision to monitor hypersensitivity reactions. In patients developing such reactions, adequate results have been obtained by readministering the medication at low doses and gradually increasing the dosage over one to two months. Since penicillamine may react with pyridoxine, supplemental pyridoxine phosphate is recommended. Thus far, no interference with growth has been noted in children taking penicillamine, and although great caution is indicated, pregnancies have been successfully completed in women receiving the drug. N-acetyl-

D-penicillamine, a related compound, has been reported to be as effective and to have fewer side effects. Mercaptopropionylglycine, which also forms a mixed disulfide with cysteine, has been reported to be as effective as penicillamine in preventing stones, and to be free of serious side effects. Initial studies in the United States, however, indicate that in patients previously sensitive to penicillamine there is a high incidence of serious side effects to mercaptopropionylglycine. In addition to fever and rash, heavy proteinuria and pemphigus foliaceus have been reported.

Chlordiazepoxide has been found to reduce cystine crystalluria by as-yet-undefined mechanisms. Finally, there are conflicting reports as to whether glutamine can reduce cystine excretion.

Cystine stones can be dissolved by irrigating the urinary tract with alkaline solutions of N-acetyl-penicillamine, D-penicillamine, and trimethamine. Since the defect in cystinuria resides in the transport epithelium of the genetically affected person, a kidney from a noncystinuric donor would be expected to remain disease free when transplanted into a cystinuric subject. This has, in fact, been the case. Chronic dialysis remains an appropriate therapy for end-stage renal failure.

Halperin EC, Thier SO, Rosenberg LE: The use of D-penicillamine in cystinuria: Efficacy and untoward reactions. Yale J Biol Med 54:439, 1981. *A review of penicillamine and comparison to fluid and alkalinization therapy.*

Segal S, Thier SO: Cystinuria. *In* Stanbury J, Wyngaarden J, Fredrickson D, Goldstein J, Brown M (eds.): The Metabolic Basis of Inherited Disease. 5th ed. New York, McGraw-Hill Book Company, 1983, pp 1774–1791. *A thorough chapter dealing with clinical, genetic, and physiologic aspects of cystinuria.*

83.5. Other Renal Tubular Disorders

Robert W. Schrier

BARTTER'S SYNDROME

Bartter's syndrome was originally diagnosed in a five-year-old boy, and the majority of subsequent reports have been in children. Recently, an autosomal recessive pattern of genetic inheritance has been suggested in childhood cases. The pathogenesis of Bartter's syndrome, however, remains unknown. Bilateral adrenalectomy has failed to correct the abnormalities, and the defect appears to be one of primary renal potassium or chloride wasting. Adults have been diagnosed as having Bartter's syndrome. In many of the adult patients, however, specific causes of chronic volume depletion have been present which could lead to a condition mimicking Bartter's syndrome. These patients have been designated with the diagnosis of pseudo-Bartter's syndrome.

PRESENTING COMPLAINTS. The musculoskeletal, gastrointestinal, and genitourinary tracts primarily account for the presenting signs and symptoms in patients with Bartter's and pseudo-Bartter's syndrome. The majority of these presenting problems result from the *hypokalemia* that consistently accompanies these syndromes. The patients frequently present with polyuria, polydipsia, and enuresis, and may have evidence of renal failure. These hypokalemic syndromes are also associated with muscle weakness and muscle cramps. Patients may have carpopedal spasm with positive Trousseau and Chvostek signs. Growth retardation is a frequent accompaniment of Bartter's syndrome in children. Some patients present with vomiting, anorexia, constipation, and abdominal pain. A flat plate of the abdomen may provide evidence of ileus.

DIAGNOSTIC FEATURES. The diagnostic features of Bartter's syndrome include (1) hypokalemia secondary to renal potassium wasting (urine potassium >20 mEq per liter), (2) metabolic alkalosis with serum bicarbonate >30 mEq per liter with arterial pH >7.45, (3) elevated plasma levels of renin and aldosterone with resistance to the pressor effect of exogenous angiotensin II, (4) hyperplasia of the renal juxtaglomerular apparatus, (5) normal blood pressure and absence of edema, (6) urinary chloride >20 mEq per liter, and (7) additional findings, including hyperuricemia, hypomagnesemia, nephrogenic (vasopressin-resistant) diabetes insipidus, and increase in urinary excretion of prostaglandins.

DIFFERENTIAL DIAGNOSIS. Many of the features of Bartter's syndrome can be mimicked by other disorders. *Surreptitious diuretic abuse* for cosmetic or other reasons may present with hypokalemic alkalosis associated with hyperreninemia and hyperaldosteronism. These patients also are normotensive without edema, exhibit excessive excretion of urinary prostaglandins, and have urinary chloride concentration >20 mEq per liter. Urinary or plasma diuretic levels may be necessary to confirm the diagnosis of pseudo-Bartter's syndrome in these patients. *Surreptitious vomiting* or prolonged nasogastric suction also mimics most of the features of Bartter's syndrome except that urinary chloride is <20 mEq per liter; however, severe potassium depletion from any cause may lead to renal chloride wasting (urine chloride >20 mEq per liter). *Excessive exposure to adrenocortical hormones,* including Cushing's syndrome, primary hyperaldosteronism, ectopic ACTH-producing tumors, and licorice ingestion, presents with hypokalemic metabolic alkalosis but is associated with an elevation of blood pressure. Lower gastrointestinal losses of potassium can be distinguished from Bartter's syndrome because fecal bicarbonate losses cause metabolic acidosis rather than alkalosis. Moreover, unless severe potassium depletion leads to a chloride-losing nephropathy, the urinary chloride concentration is <20 mEq per liter. Some gastrointestinal disorders with *diarrhea,* however, may be associated with relatively more chloride than bicarbonate loss, e.g., occasionally with a villous adenoma, and therefore present with a hypokalemic metabolic alkalosis. Surreptitious cathartic abuse, malabsorption, and infectious causes of diarrhea are examples of circumstances that must be excluded prior to establishing the diagnosis of Bartter's syndrome. With surreptitious cathartic abuse, melanosis coli may be observed on colonoscopy. A pink or red color of a stool homogenate or other extract of urine suggests cathartic abuse secondary to phenolphthalein; loss of haustral markings with a "garden hose" appearance of nonshortened colon by radiographic studies also suggests cathartic abuse. *Chronic renal sodium and potassium wasting* may occasionally cause a pseudo-Bartter's syndrome in association with medullary cystic disease, renal tubular acidosis, partial urinary tract obstruction, or vesicoureteral reflux. Recently, a new hypokalemic entity has been described in children. It is associated with hypokalemia, normal blood pressure, and hyperreninemia, but in contrast to patients with Bartter's syndrome these patients have been found to have hypo- rather than hyperaldosteronism. The pathogenesis of this new disorder is unknown.

TREATMENT. The treatment of pseudo-Bartter's syndrome is aimed at the primary causative disorder. Pseudo-Bartter's syndrome secondary to surreptitious vomiting, or to diuretic or cathartic abuse, is difficult to treat because of the patient's psychologic dependence on the vomiting, diuretics, or cathartics. Many treatments for Bartter's syndrome have been tried, particularly in an effort to correct the renal potassium wasting. Blockade of mineralocorticoid receptors with spironolactone, suppression of renin release with beta-adrenergic blockers such as propranolol, and magnesium replacement have met with only minimal success. Because of the findings of increased urinary prostaglandin excretion, inhibition of prostaglandin synthetase (cyclooxygenase) with drugs such as indomethacin has been used to treat patients with Bartter's syndrome. These agents have led to sodium retention, suppression of plasma renin and aldosterone, diminished urinary prostaglandin excretion, less renal potassium wasting, and at least partial correction of the hypokalemia; however, some of these patients eventually escape from the beneficial effects of these agents. Captopril, an angiotensin-converting enzyme inhibitor, has been recently administered to patients with Bartter's syndrome with some improvement in the hypokalemia and the vascular resistance to angiotensin. However, until the specific cause of Bartter's syndrome is better delineated, a more rational therapeutic approach may not be possible.

Anderson RJ, Schrier RW: Potassium metabolism in Bartter's and pseudo-Bartter's syndrome. Ciba Monograph, 1980. *This paper reviews the clinical features of Bartter's syndrome as well as the other clinical causes of conditions that may mimic Bartter's syndrome (pseudo-Bartter's syndrome).*

Bergstein JM, Weinberger MH: Hypokalemia, normal blood pressure, and hyperreninemia with hypoaldosteronism. J Pediatr 99:561, 1981.

Dunn MJ: Prostaglandins and Bartter's syndrome. Kidney Int 19:86, 1981. *This editorial reviews the potential pathogenetic role of prostaglandins in Bartter's syndrome.*

Gill JR, Bartter FC: Evidence for a prostaglandin-independent defect in chloride reabsorption in the loop of Henle as a primary cause of Bartter's syndrome. Am J Med 65:766, 1978. *This paper suggests that a defect in chloride reabsorption in the ascending limb of Henle's loop is the initiating cause of Bartter's syndrome.*

LIDDLE'S SYNDROME

The presence of hypokalemic metabolic alkalosis and hypertension suggests excessive mineralocorticoid activity such as occurs with primary hyperaldosteronism (Ch. 230). Because of the mineralocorticoid-mediated retention of sodium and extracellular fluid volume expansion, these patients have suppressed plasma renin activity independent of whether the source of the aldosterone excess is an adrenal adenoma, adrenal carcinoma, or adrenal hyperplasia. Patients with Liddle's syndrome have hypertension, hypokalemic metabolic alkalosis, low plasma renin activity, but *low* rather than high aldosterone activity. These findings and the observed increase in distal tubular sodium reabsorption in this familial disorder suggest the excess of a yet-to-be-identified mineralocorticoid hormone. In addition to Liddle's syndrome, the differential diagnosis in patients with hypokalemic alkalosis, hypertension, low plasma renin, and low or normal plasma aldosterone includes (1) glucocorticoid excess—Cushing's syndrome, ectopic ACTH from tumors, or exogenous glucocorticoid administration; (2) excess desoxycorticosterone (DOC) in adrenogenital syndrome—17-α-hydroxylase deficiency with absence of adrenal androgens and estrogens leading to failure of secondary sexual development, or 11-hydroxylase deficiency with androgen excess and virilism; (3) adrenal carcinomas that excrete excess DOC; and (4) excess ingestion of licorice containing glycyrrhizinic acid, which has mineralocorticoid activity.

Liddle GW, Bledsoe T, Coppage WS: A familial renal disorder simulating primary aldosteronism but with negligible aldosterone secretion. Tr Assoc Am Physicians 76:199, 1963. *This is the original description of a familial entity that mimics primary hyperaldosteronism but in which aldosterone activity is suppressed.*

RENAL GLYCOSURIA

Renal glycosuria is defined as the excretion of excessive amounts of glucose in the urine in the presence of normal filtered loads of glucose. Implicit in this definition is an abnormality in tubular glucose transport. Such an abnormality can occur in association with generalized proximal tubular dysfunction; these abnormalities will be discussed below under Fanconi's syndrome. *Familial renal glycosuria* is an isolated defect in renal glucose transport in which intestinal glucose transport is normal. The renal tubular defect in glucose transport can occur secondary to a decrease in maximal tubular reabsorption (TmG) of glucose (Type A) or an increase in splay of the titration curve of glucose reabsorption, giving a reduced threshold for glycosuria (Type B). These two entities are shown in Figure 83–2. Renal glycosuria is inherited as an autosomal recessive trait. Mild and severe Type A glycosuria and Type B glycosuria can exist in the same pedigree. Obligate heterozygotes may have modest defects and mild, often intermittent glycosuria; homozygote children have severe defects in glucose transport with profound glycosuria. The diagnosis of familial renal glycosuria includes (1) exclusion of other causes of melituria (pentosuria, fructosuria, sucrosuria, maltosuria, galactosuria, lactosuria); (2) glucosuria in the presence of a normal filtered load of glucose and a normal (or slightly flat) glucose tolerance test; (3) exclusion of other tubular defects such as excessive uricaciduria, phosphaturia, and aminoaciduria; (4) family history of glucosuria (inconstant), usually mild in the parents if present; and (5) absence of the progression to diabetes mellitus. Familial glycosuria is a benign disease that has an excellent prognosis and requires no treatment. Insulin administration, when a diagnosis of diabetes mellitus is mistakenly made, may lead to hypoglycemic episodes. So can prolonged starvation in the presence of substantial urinary losses of glucose, e.g., in Type A homozygote patients. Glucosuria without hyperglycemia also may be observed in either pregnant women or patients with renal disease and glomerular filtration rates less than 15 ml per minute.

Krane SM: Renal glycosuria. *In* Stanbury JB, Wyngaarden JB, Fredrickson DS (eds.): The Metabolic Basis of Inherited Disease. 4th ed. New York, McGraw-Hill Book Company, 1978, pp 1607–1617. *This chapter presents a thorough discussion of renal and metabolic studies in the various types of renal glycosuria.*

RENAL PHOSPHATE WASTING

Renal phosphaturia occurs with primary and secondary *hyperparathyroidism* and also as an integral part of generalized dysfunction of proximal tubule transport (Fanconi's syndrome;

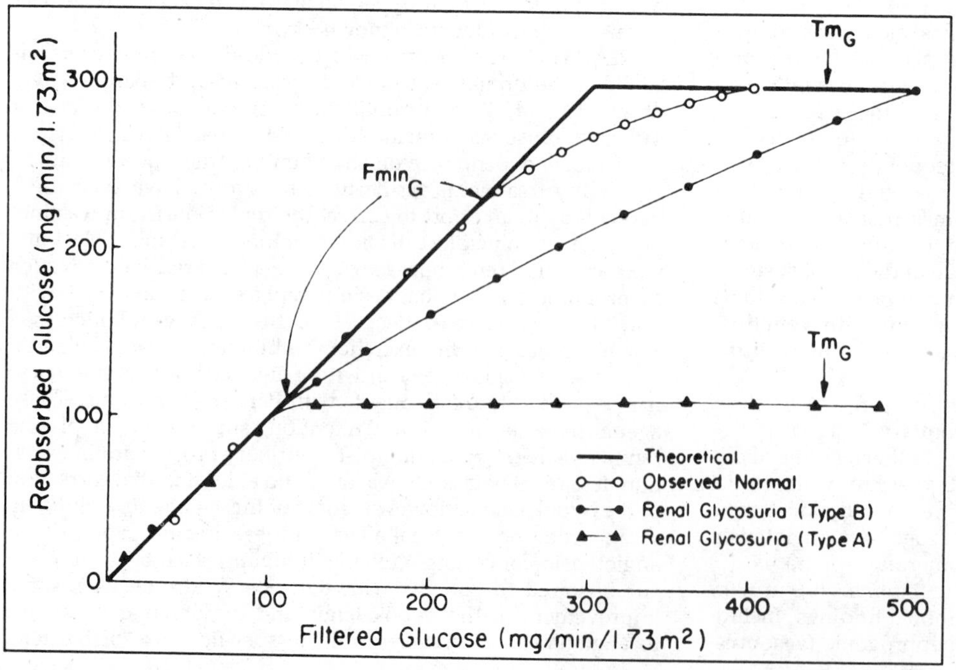

Figure 83–2. Glucose titration curves in man illustrating normal renal tubular reabsorption of glucose in contrast to the two forms of renal glycosuria (Types A and B). (From Elsas LJ, Rosenberg LE: Renal glycosuria. *In* Earley LE, Gottschalk CW (eds.): Strauss and Welt's Diseases of the Kidney. 3rd ed. Boston, Little, Brown & Company, 1979.)

see below). *Pseudo-vitamin D deficiency rickets* or vitamin D-dependent rickets is inherited as an autosomal recessive trait and is due to a defective or absent hydroxylation of 25-OH vitamin D_3 to $1,25(OH)_2$ vitamin D_3. The resultant decrease in gastrointestinal calcium absorption causes hypocalcemia, which increases parathyroid hormone release; the high circulating levels of parathyroid hormone account for the diminished renal phosphate reabsorption, phosphaturia, and hypophosphatemia. All defects, including the rickets and hypophosphatemia, are corrected by physiologic doses (1 μg per day) of $1,25(OH)_2$ vitamin D_3.

Vitamin D-resistant rickets (also called familial hypophosphatemic rickets) is inherited by an X-linked dominant gene and is not responsive to treatment with vitamin D or known vitamin D analogues alone. Rickets (children) and osteomalacia (adults) are hallmarks of the disease; although serum $1,25(OH)_2$ vitamin D levels in these patients are low, vitamin D supplementation alone does not correct the bone disease, phosphaturia, or hypophosphatemia. A defect in both renal and intestinal phosphate transport has been found. A combination of phosphate supplementation and vitamin D is necessary to treat effectively the bone disease and hypophosphatemia. Renal phosphate wasting, *hypophosphatemic osteomalacia,* and impaired conversion of 25-OH vitamin D_3 to its $1,25(OH)_2$ derivative have also been described with giant cell tumors of bone. Removal of the tumor corrects these abnormalities, but the cause of the defect is unknown. A similar clinical syndrome may occur in connection with reparative granulomas and soft tissue hemangiomas. Certain diuretics (e.g., furosemide), the Syndrome of Inappropriate Antidiuretic Hormone Secretion (SIADH), primary hyperaldosteronism, and saline infusion can also result in increased urinary excretion of phosphate. Also see Ch. 207 for a discussion of hypophosphatemia.

Fukomoto Y, Tarii S, Tsukiyama K, et al.: Tumor-induced vitamin D–resistant hypophosphatemic osteomalacia associated with proximal renal tubular dysfunction and 1,25-dihydroxyvitamin D deficiency. J Clin Endocrinol Metab 94:873, 1979. *This report from Japan summarizes the international experience with this intriguing syndrome and presents further evidence that there is an associated block in the synthesis of 1,25-dihydroxycholecalciferol as the cause of osteomalacia.*

Rasmussen H, Anast C: Familial hypophosphatemic rickets and vitamin D–dependent rickets. *In* Stanbury JB, Wyngaarden JB, Fredrickson DS, Goldstein JL, Brown MS (eds.): The Metabolic Basis of Inherited Disease. 5th ed. New York, McGraw-Hill Book Company, 1983, p 1743. *This is an authoritative discussion of these rare genetic disorders which emphasizes current knowledge of the pathogenesis. There are 238 references and an excellent discussion of vitamin D metabolism as well.*

FANCONI'S SYNDROME

CLINICAL FEATURES. Fanconi's syndrome is characterized by a constellation of disturbances of proximal tubular dysfunction, including aminoaciduria, glycosuria, phosphaturia, bicarbonaturia, kaliuresis, and uricaciduria. As a result of these defects, hypophosphatemic rickets (children) or osteomalacia (adults), renal tubular acidosis, hypokalemia, and hypouricemia may be the presenting conditions. The hypokalemia may be associated with a nephrogenic diabetes insipidus and resultant polyuria. Growth retardation in children with Fanconi's syndrome may result from chronic acidosis, renal potassium and phosphate wasting, and possibly amino acid wasting. The renal phosphate wasting and hypophosphatemia may decrease 1,25 dihydroxyvitamin D_3 in both adults and children, thus contributing to the osteomalacia and rickets. A distinct type of proteinuria may also be present, including urinary losses of serum hormones, light chains, and small protein molecules.

ETIOLOGY. The inborn and acquired causes of Fanconi's syndrome are included in Table 83–4. Fanconi's syndrome may be acquired or associated with a hereditary enzymatic disorder. In addition, a primary hereditary disorder (idiopathic Fanconi's syndrome) has been identified and is unassociated with any known disease. Of the acquired causes of Fanconi's syndrome, *multiple myeloma* is the most common. Many of these patients do not have a monoclonal serum spike, and Fanconi's syndrome frequently precedes the development of the myeloma. Thus, adults with Fanconi's syndrome should have immunoelectrophoresis performed on concentrated urine; Bence Jones proteinuria is consistently found in these patients. *Amyloidosis* with or without multiple myeloma is another acquired cause of Fanconi's syndrome. Both *Sjögren's syndrome* and *renal transplantation* may cause proximal tubular dysfunction and Fanconi's syndrome in addition to distal tubular dysfunction. Various *heavy metals* have been incriminated as causes of Fanconi's syndrome, including mercury, lead, cadmium, uranium, and strontium. Maleic acid administration provides an excellent experimental model of Fanconi's syndrome. Several *drugs* have also been found to cause Fanconi's syndrome, including 6-mercaptopurine, streptozotocin, and outdated tetracycline; the latter is probably no longer a cause of Fanconi's syndrome, since citric acid has been removed as a preservative. Aminoglycosides and *chronic renal failure* may be associated with evidence of proximal tubular dysfunction, perhaps because of direct nephrotoxicity in the former instance and secondary hyperparathyroidism in the latter.

TABLE 83–4. ETIOLOGIES OF FANCONI'S SYNDROME

Inborn	Acquired
Cystinosis	Multiple myeloma
Wilson's disease	Amyloidosis
Galactosemia	Sjögren's syndrome
Heredity fructose intolerance	Nephrotic syndrome
Tyrosinemia	Renal transplantation
Lowe's syndrome	Vitamin D deficiency
Glycogenosis	Heavy metals
Vitamin D–resistant rickets	Lead, mercury, cadmium, uranium, strontium
	Drugs
	Outdated tetracycline, maleic acid, 6-mercaptopurine, streptozocin, aminoglycosides

PATHOGENESIS. It has been suggested that many of these acquired renal disorders may be associated with a defect in the conversion of 25-hydroxycholecalciferol to 1,25-dihydroxycholecalciferol in the renal cortex. The deficiency of the latter hormone (rather than, or in addition to, renal phosphate wasting) may account for both the bone disease and some of the tubular transport defects associated with Fanconi's syndrome. It has also been shown that light chains will inhibit Na^+-K^+ ATPase activity, maleic acid will decrease ATP stores, and cadmium will diminish both. Either defect will lead to a generalized defect of proximal transport function and thus cause Fanconi's syndrome.

Cystinosis, an autosomal recessive disorder, is the most common cause of Fanconi's syndrome in children. Cystine crystals are found in the cornea, conjunctiva, bone marrow, liver, reticuloendothelial cells, and kidney. The infant (nephropathic) form leads to rickets, Fanconi's syndrome, and renal impairment. The adult form (Cogan's syndrome) is generally diagnosed incidentally during a slit-lamp examination; this form has a benign course without evidence of renal impairment, but cystine crystals are present in the conjunctiva, cornea, and bone marrow. With end-stage renal failure renal transplantation may be undertaken successfully without evidence of recurrence in the grafted kidney. Cysteamine has been reported to be an effective therapeutic agent.

Other hereditary causes of Fanconi's syndrome include *Wilson's disease,* which appears to occur secondary to copper accumulation in the renal cortex. Penicillamine may chelate the copper and at least partially reverse the functional renal impairment. *Hereditary fructose intolerance* is a genetic disorder characterized by a deficiency of fructose-1-phosphate aldolase in kidney and liver so that fructose-1-phosphate accumulates in these tissues. With avoidance of fructose intake this disorder is benign. *Lowe's syndrome* (oculocerebrorenal syndrome) is a hereditary cause of Fanconi's syndrome in males, characterized by growth retardation, mental retardation, hypotonia, bilateral congenital cataracts, and glaucoma. *Tyrosinemia* and *galactosemia* are other rare disorders resulting from enzyme defects which may be accompanied by proximal tubular dysfunction and Fanconi's syndrome.

Roth KS, Foreman JW, Segal S: The Fanconi syndrome and mechanisms of tubular transport dysfunction. Kidney Int 20:705, 1981.
Schneider JA, Schulman JD: Cystinosis. *In* Stanbury JB, Wyngaarden JB, Fredrickson DS, Goldstein JL, Brown MS (eds.): The Metabolic Basis of Inherited Disease. 5th ed. New York, McGraw-Hill Book Company, 1983, p 1844. *An extensive review of the clinical and metabolic features of cystinosis with an emphasis on pathogenesis. 272 references.*

84. DIABETES AND THE KIDNEY

Bryan D. Myers

INCIDENCE AND PREVALENCE

Among the 15,000 patients entering chronic dialysis and kidney transplantation programs in the United States each year, the development of end-stage renal failure can be attributed to diabetes mellitus in approximately 25 per cent. Diabetic glomerulopathy, a complex disorder associated with a diffuse expansion of collagenous components of the glomerulus, is the predominant cause of the renal failure. The diabetic patient is also prone to other renal diseases such as pyelonephritis, papillary necrosis, and obstructive nephropathy that occasionally cause or exacerbate renal failure (Ch. 82 and 85). Diabetic patients are particularly likely to get hyporeninemic hypoaldosteronism and exhibit the syndrome of generalized distal (Type IV) RTA (Ch. 83.2). Diabetic patients with severe glomerulopathy are most susceptible to these associated renal disorders as well. Most victims of end-stage diabetic renal disease will have longstanding Type I diabetes, defined here as juvenile-onset and insulin-dependent diabetes (see Ch. 230). Patients with Type II diabetes, characterized by a more advanced age of onset and not requiring insulin for control of hyperglycemia, are not spared from diabetic glomerulopathy and compose a substantial minority among diabetic patients in end-stage renal failure programs.

CLINICAL AND LABORATORY FEATURES OF DIABETIC GLOMERULOPATHY

The natural history of diabetic glomerulopathy has been best documented in Type I patients who have been subjected to prolonged serial observations. Early abnormalities of glomerular function and structure appear to be invariable in all Type I diabetics, but only 30 to 50 per cent will develop a progressive, proteinuric form of diabetic glomerulopathy. The evolution of the glomerulopathy in this subset of Type I diabetics may be thought of as a continuum of glomerular injury. As illustrated in Figure 84–1, the continuum may be divided into three stages. The first stage of occult glomerulopathy cannot be diagnosed by conventional laboratory techniques and lasts for approximately ten years. It is followed by two clinically evident stages of increasingly severe glomerular injury. Both are identified by the presence of proteinuria, while the milder, intermediate second stage merges with the advanced third stage with the development of azotemia. In considering the clinical and laboratory features of this prolonged and progressive glomerular disease, it is useful to review each stage separately.

Stage 1—Occult Diabetic Glomerulopathy

During this stage, the Type I diabetic patient is devoid of clinical symptoms and signs of glomerulopathy. The most striking laboratory finding is a 20 to 40 per cent *elevation of the glomerular filtration rate* (GFR) above that found in age-matched normal controls. Although ultrastructural alterations can be demonstrated in the glomerular capillary wall and mesangium in the early stages of the disease, they do not appear to account for the observed glomerular hyperfiltration. Striking elevations of GFR in poorly controlled diabetic patients can be lowered within a matter of hours following restoration of normoglycemia. A parallel *increase in renal plasma flow,* measured by the clearance of *p*-aminohippurate, and also reversible by lowering blood glucose levels, points to a hemodynamic basis for the hyperfiltration. Notwithstanding the responsiveness of vasomotor regulation in the kidney to alterations in the metabolic milieu, GFR tends to remain elevated even with good metabolic control of the diabetic state. Not until proteinuria ushers in the intermediate second stage of the glomerulopathy does the GFR tend to fall into the normal range.

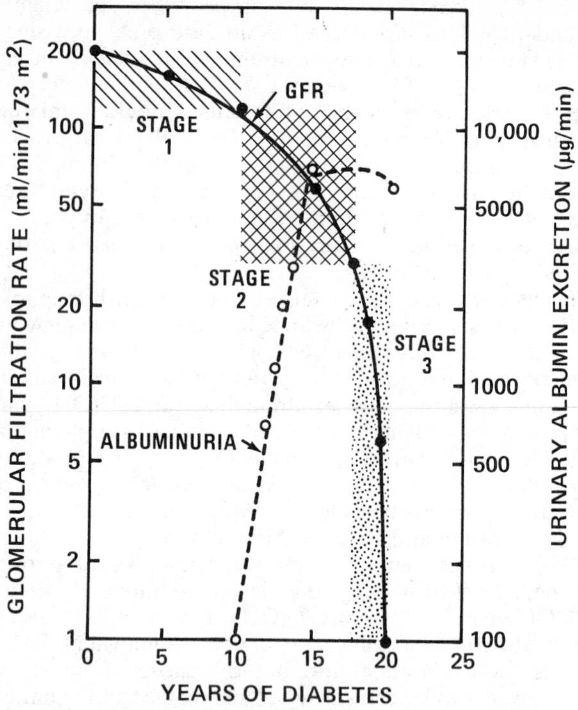

Figure 84–1. The glomerular filtration rate (●—●) and albumin excretion rate (○--○) have been plotted against time to chart a hypothetical course typical of diabetic glomerulopathy. The course of the disease has been divided into three stages, which are described in the text.

The stage 1 glomerular hyperfiltration is accompanied by a subtle increase in the urinary albumin excretion rate that is not measurable by conventional techniques. Healthy adolescents and young adults excrete albumin in their urine at rates of up to 15 µg per minute. Many patients with Type I diabetes of short duration excrete albumin at rates in excess of 15 µg per minute but less than the 100 µg per minute, which is roughly the threshold detectable by conventional techniques. This "*microalbuminuria*" is inferred to represent an increase in the transglomerular filtration of albumin rather than a decrease in tubular reabsorption of a normal, filtered albumin load. Microalbuminuria tends to be associated with the most striking degrees of hyperfiltration observed among Type I diabetics, suggesting that it may also have a hemodynamic basis. It is exaggerated by exercise, which causes an increase in the intraluminal hydraulic pressure of the glomerular capillaries, and is blunted, although not abolished, by restoration of normoglycemia.

Early in the course of Type I diabetes there is a consistent *increase in kidney size.* Hyperfiltration, renal hyperemia and enlargement, and microalbuminuria are all characteristic of this early occult stage, but hypertension, an important complication of diabetic glomerulopathy, is not prevalent. The incidence of hypertension in large diabetic populations without proteinuria is no different from that in nondiabetic populations.

Stage 2—Intermediate Diabetic Glomerulopathy

This stage is heralded by the development of persistent, easily measurable proteinuria. Once proteinuria has become manifest its magnitude tends to reflect the rate of deterioration of glomerular capillary wall function that typifies the second stage of diabetic glomerulopathy. As indicated in Figure 84–1, proteinuria tends to increase exponentially with time and to be related inversely to GFR.

After several years of proteinuria, urinary losses reach nephrotic proportions (> 3.5 grams per 24 hours) and the patient will frequently become edematous. The proteinuria is also paralleled by an increasing prevalence of hypertension. Thus stage 2, intermediate diabetic glomerulopathy, is characterized by *increasing proteinuria, declining GFR,* and the development of *hypertension* and *edema.*

The proteinuria of stage 2 diabetic glomerulopathy has no pathognomonic characteristics, but several features distinguish it from other glomerular diseases: (1) From the onset of the second stage, immunoglobulins and other large plasma proteins are excreted in the urine in large quantities along with albumin, i.e., there is no size selectivity. (2) Persistent and massive urinary losses of plasma proteins in stage 2 diabetic glomerulopathy are rarely accompanied by hypoproteinemia. Inasmuch as the conventional definition of the nephrotic syndrome requires hypoproteinemia in addition to massive proteinuria and edema, stage 2 diabetic glomerulopathy does not truly exemplify the nephrotic syndrome. An important role in edema formation is ascribed to reduction of plasma oncotic pressure in patients with the nephrotic syndrome as classically defined; the absence of these phenomena in stage 2 diabetic glomerulopathy implicates alternate mechanisms of edema formation. (3) The renin-angiotensin-aldosterone system tends to be depressed in stage 2 glomerulopathy. In fact this entity probably constitutes the most common example of hyporeninemic hypertension. Despite the tendency of diabetics with stage 2 glomerulopathy to become edematous, plasma aldosterone concentration and the urinary excretion rate of aldosterone are frequently depressed. Thus both the mechanism by which edema is formed and the basis for the widespread prevalence of hypertension in stage 2 diabetic glomerulopathy remain obscure.

Stage 3—Advanced Diabetic Glomerulopathy

The third, advanced stage represents the terminal 2 or 3 years of what is typically a 20- to 25-year process. Its onset is delineated by the development of *azotemia.* Retention of urea, creatinine, and other nitrogenous compounds will generally become apparent once the GFR has declined to less than one third of normal levels. As with the intermediate stage that precedes it, GFR in the third and terminal stage of diabetic glomerulopathy has been observed to decline at rates approaching 1 ml per minute per month. Thus in the prototypical case illustrated in Figure 84–1, GFR is predicted to decline from a normal value approximating 120 ml per minute at the onset of stage 2 to zero at the end of stage 3 over a period of 10 years. Not only does GFR decline irrevocably, resulting in progressive azotemia, but *edema* and *hypertension* tend to worsen in the third and final stage of the disease. Similarly, *proteinuria* continues to be massive and *hypoproteinemia* finally results. Although reduced plasma protein concentration and the lowered GFR serve to lower the filtered protein load, urinary protein excretion rate is maintained at massive levels, reflecting increasing leakiness of the glomerular capillary wall to large plasma proteins.

By the time the third, advanced stage of diabetic glomerulopathy is reached, *widespread microangiopathy* involving the retinae and peripheral nerves is invariable. Although its extent varies among patients, retinopathy is frequently associated with visual impairment sufficient to result in functional blindness. The effects of peripheral and more particularly of autonomic neuropathy may be equally devastating. This is particularly true when autonomic neuropathy results in partial paresis of the bladder. Progressive urinary retention may exacerbate renal insufficiency in stage 3 glomerulopathy by resulting in a superimposed obstructive nephropathy. Obstructive nephropathy in turn may predispose the already vulnerable patient to ascending pyelonephritis and/or ischemic papillary necrosis, thereby compromising renal function even further. (For more detailed discussion of obstructive nephropathy, see Ch. 82.)

Given the prolonged duration of diabetes mellitus, by the time stage 3 glomerulopathy is reached many patients will be 40 years of age or more, an age group in which atherosclerosis, accelerated in part by the presence of longstanding hypertension, will adversely affect several organ systems. Coronary artery disease, cerebrovascular disease and stroke, and peripheral vascular disease are all common in the third stage of diabetic glomerulopathy, and account collectively for the majority of fatalities. The eventual need for substitution therapy in end-stage renal failure programs occurs in a setting, therefore, in which serious extrarenal complications are prevalent and impair the effectiveness of rehabilitation generally achieved by such therapy.

DIAGNOSIS

Proteinuria due to diabetic glomerulopathy is accompanied by typical changes of glomerular histopathology. These include a striking accumulation of matrix components of the mesangium and a widening of the glomerular capillary wall due to a thickened glomerular basement membrane. The former change results in an acellular expansion of the mesangium, which is most commonly diffuse in nature and hence termed diffuse intercapillary glomerulosclerosis. Not infrequently mesangial matrix accumulation occurs in a segmental fashion, resulting in the formation of acellular spherical nodules at the center of single or multiple peripheral glomerular lobules (Fig. 84–2), referred to as nodular glomerulosclerosis. A nodular accumulation of mesangial matrix material, indistinguishable from that observed in diabetic subjects, has been associated with dysproteinemia, notably that associated with a monoclonal proliferation of B lymphocytes or plasma cells. Provided that the latter entity is excluded, however, the finding of diffuse or nodular glomerulosclerosis in a proteinuric diabetic subject is diagnostic of diabetic glomerulopathy.

A diagnosis of diabetic glomerulopathy can be made with a high degree of certainty in a proteinuric diabetic patient, without resort to biopsy, which carries a finite risk for the patient. Background and proliferative retinopathy, for example, are correlated strongly with the presence of diffuse or nodular glomerulosclerosis in a proteinuric diabetic. The diagnostic probability can be further strengthened by using noninvasive imaging techniques, such as ultrasonography or nephrotomography, to demonstrate kidney enlargement. Nephrotoxic acute renal failure caused by contrast agents occurs more commonly in patients with diabetic glomerulopathy than in any other patient category. For this reason nephrotomography (or other radiologic procedures) should be performed without the use of contrast agents whenever possible. The coexistence of retinopathy and nephromegaly in diabetic patients with proteinuria is so constant that the performance of a diagnostic renal biopsy need be considered only when these factors are absent, particularly when the duration of diabetes is less than 10 years. Under these circumstances, a renal biopsy has frequently revealed other primary glomerulopathies such as minimal change nephropathy, membranous glomerulopathy, and proliferative glomerulonephritis (Ch. 80).

PATHOGENESIS AND PATHOPHYSIOLOGY

The diabetic state per se is the presumed forerunner of glomerulopathy. Glomerular basement membrane (GBM) wid-

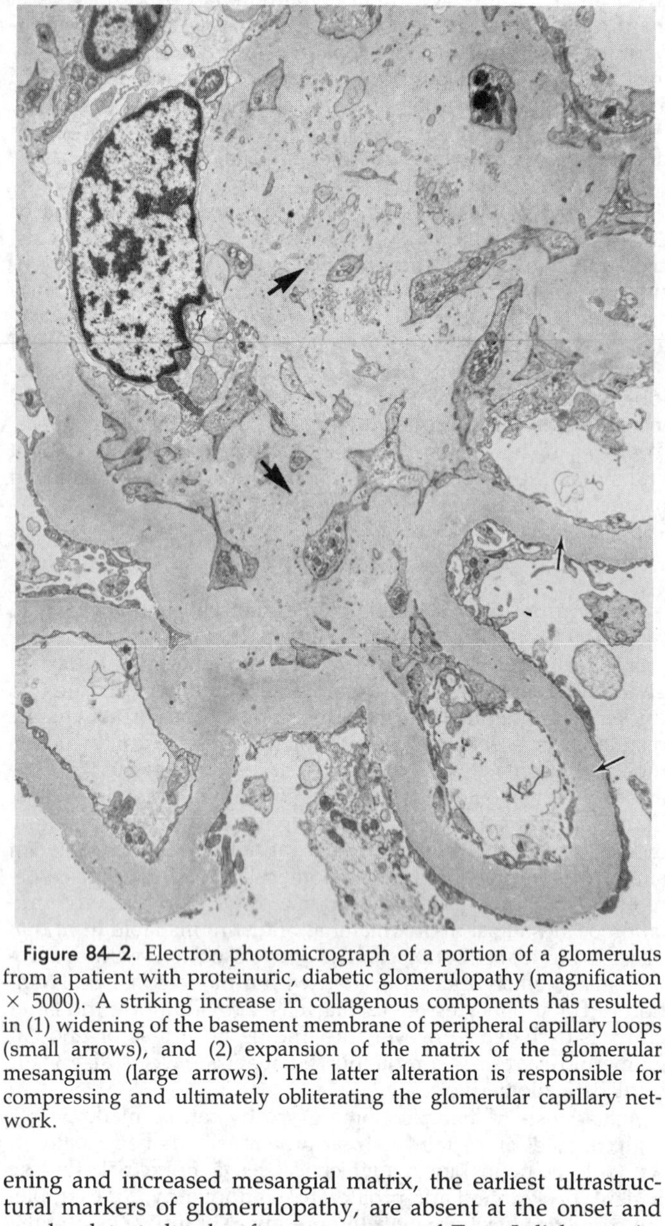

Figure 84–2. Electron photomicrograph of a portion of a glomerulus from a patient with proteinuric, diabetic glomerulopathy (magnification × 5000). A striking increase in collagenous components has resulted in (1) widening of the basement membrane of peripheral capillary loops (small arrows), and (2) expansion of the matrix of the glomerular mesangium (large arrows). The latter alteration is responsible for compressing and ultimately obliterating the glomerular capillary network.

ening and increased mesangial matrix, the earliest ultrastructural markers of glomerulopathy, are absent at the onset and can be detected only after some years of Type I diabetes. An identical sequence has been observed in experimental diabetes induced in a variety of mammalian species with the use of pancreatic beta cell toxins or pancreatectomy.

As in humans, GFR is substantially elevated in the rat with experimental diabetes of short duration. Micropuncture techniques have demonstrated that the early hyperfiltration is a consequence of altered vasomotion in the major resistance vessels of the renal cortex. Dilatation of the efferent and especially the afferent glomerular arterioles results in an elevation of glomerular capillary perfusion rate and pressure. By contrast, those determinants of GFR that are intrinsic to the glomerular capillary wall, namely hydraulic conductivity and the surface area available for filtration, are unaltered. Thus hyperfiltration early in the course of diabetes appears to have a purely hemodynamic basis. It remains to be determined which factor(s) associated with the diabetic state are responsible for the deranged renal vasoregulation. Although hyperglycemia per se has been implicated, augmented levels of glucagon and growth hormone are usual accompaniments of diabetic hyperglycemia, and each of these hormones is capable of inducing a rise in GFR. The renal hemodynamic alterations associated with onset of diabetes precede the development of histopathologic changes in glomeruli. It has been suggested that they serve as a stimulus for the ensuing accumulation of mesangial matrix components and hence the subsequent glomerulosclerosis. The application of a unilateral renal artery clip (the so-called two kidney Goldblatt hypertension model) in the diabetic rat is associated with *less* severe glomerulosclerosis in the clipped kidney, which is protected from the transmission of elevated arterial pressure into the glomerular capillaries.

Whether or not glomerular capillary hypertension and hyperperfusion are the proximate causes of an accumulation of mesangial matrix components, there seems little doubt that this lesion is responsible for the progressive reduction of GFR that typifies the second and third stages of clinical diabetic glomerulopathy. As shown in Figure 84–2, expansion of the mesangial matrix occurs at the expense of the surrounding glomerular capillary loops, with progressive reduction of the surface area available for filtration. By the time the end of the third stage of diabetic glomerulopathy has been reached, the mesangium will have encroached upon most glomerular capillary loops to the point that they have become almost totally obliterated.

The process by which the glomerular basement membrane becomes widened has also been presumed to be responsible for the alteration in the glomerular capillary wall, causing it to be permeable to large plasma proteins. Surprisingly, however, there is no correlation whatsoever between glomerular basement membrane width and proteinuria. While the structural basis of proteinuria remains obscure, the functional nature of the disturbance in glomerular permselectivity has been elucidated by the use of in vivo physiologic techniques in which the clearance of probe filtration markers of graded size has been used to define the size-selective properties of the glomerular filter. One such study has revealed that proteinuria in diabetic glomerulopathy can be accounted for by the development within the glomerular capillary wall of a subpopulation of enlarged, protein-permeable pores. In contradistinction to the diffuse widening of the basement membrane seen by electron microscopy (Fig. 84–2), the enlarged pores can be estimated to be few in number and to behave as isolated defects in the glomerular capillary wall.

PROGNOSIS AND TREATMENT

The profound loss of filtering surface area and the disruption of glomerular membrane pores that underlie the progressive glomerular hypofiltration and increasing proteinuria of stage 2 and 3 glomerulopathy in diabetics are unlikely to be reversible. Attempts to maintain blood glucose in such patients in a normal range have failed to prevent or attenuate the progression of renal insufficiency. Meticulous control of hypertension, however, may slow the rate of decline of GFR. Together with antihypertensive therapy, attention to and correction of coexistent cardiac failure, obstructive nephropathy, pyelonephritis, and other events that may lower GFR independently of the glomerulopathy represent the mainstay of therapy of proteinuric glomerulopathy.

Based on our current understanding of the pathophysiology and pathogenesis of diabetic glomerulopathy, a major effort should be made to prevent the disease from entering the progressive downhill course that follows the advent of the second stage of the glomerulopathy. Initial data from several longitudinal, prospective studies indicate that if blood glucose can be maintained permanently in a normal range, progression from the early occult stage of the injury may be averted. Presumably, prevailing pressures and flows in the glomerular capillary network will be lowered along with the blood glucose level and an important potential stimulus for progressive glomerulosclerosis removed. Thus, no effort should be spared to identify the 30 to 50 per cent of diabetic patients at special risk of developing progressive glomerulopathy. Such patients should be referred to specialized facilities where their insulin requirement can be carefully evaluated and its replacement facilitated by custom-tailored regimens that employ constant infusion devices or multiple daily insulin injections. Among the patients who should be thus targeted are those with trace proteinuria (<500 mg per 24 hours) and those with retinopathy in the absence of proteinuria.

Once end-stage renal failure has supervened the diabetic patient should be referred for treatment to a dialysis and/or transplantation center (Ch. 78 and 79). Many diabetic patients respond favorably to and enjoy a good quality of life with these modalities of treatment. With special attention to the unique problems of the diabetic patient with renal failure, the survival rates achieved with chronic hemodialysis or with chronic ambulatory peritoneal dialysis, or following renal transplantation, are today approaching those achieved for nondiabetic patients.

Bryer-Ash M, Ammon RA, Luetscher JA: Increased inactive renin in diabetes mellitus without evidence of nephropathy. J Clin Endocrinol Metab 56:557, 1983. *The abnormalities in the renin-angiotensin system in diabetic glomerulopathy are clearly delineated.*

Hostetter TH, Troy JL, Brenner BM: Glomerular hemodynamics in experimental diabetes mellitus. Kidney Int 19:410, 1981. *An elegant micropuncture study demonstrating the hemodynamic basis for glomerular hyperfiltration in early experimental rat diabetes.*

Hostetter TH, Rennke HG, Brenner BM: The case for intrarenal hypertension in the initiation and progression of diabetic and other glomerulopathies. Am J Med 72:375, 1982. *A lucid review of the pathophysiology of diabetic glomerulopathy citing virtually every important reference to this subject.*

Kimmelstiel P, Wilson C: Intercapillary lesions in glomeruli of kidney. Am J Pathol 12:83, 1936. *A landmark paper written 15 years after the introduction of insulin. It contains a classic description of nodular diabetic glomerulosclerosis, often referred to after the authors as the Kimmelstiel-Wilson kidney.*

Mauer SM, Steffes MW, Azar S, Sandberg SK, Brown DM: The effects of Goldblatt hypertension on development of the glomerular lesions of diabetes mellitus in the rat. Diabetes 27:733, 1978. *A landmark study establishing the etiologic importance of the metabolic milieu and hemodynamic factors in diabetic glomerulopathy.*

Mogensen CE: Progression of nephropathy in long-term diabetics with proteinuria and effect of initial anti-hypertensive treatment. Scand J Clin Lab Invest 36:383, 1976. *The best prospective study of progressive glomerular dysfunction in longstanding human diabetes.*

Myers BD, Winetz JA, Chui F, Michaels AS: Mechanisms of proteinuria in diabetic nephropathy: A study of glomerular barrier function. Kidney Int 21:96, 1982. *Modern physiologic techniques and mathematical modeling are used to describe the glomerular capillary wall as an ultrafiltration membrane; the defect in the glomerular filter of proteinuric diabetics is elucidated.*

Osterby R, Gundersen HJG, Hørlyck A, Koustrup JP, Nyberg G, Westberg G: Diabetic glomerulopathy: Structural characteristics of the early and advanced stages. Diabetes 32:79, 1983. *A review of the authors' use of electron microscopy and elegant morphometric techniques to chart the evolution and progression of diabetic glomerulopathy.*

Viberti GC, Pickup JC, Jarret JC, Keen H: Effect of control of blood glucose on urinary excretion of albumin and β_2 microglobulin in insulin-dependent diabetes. N Engl J Med 300:638, 1979. *The relationship between microalbuminuria and control of early diabetes is well illustrated.*

Viberti GC, Bilous RW, Mackintosh D, Keen H: Monitoring glomerular function in diabetic nephropathy. Am J Med 74:256, 1983. *A careful prospective study of the effects of metabolic control on proteinuric glomerulopathy. Its message is pessimistic.*

85. URINARY TRACT INFECTIONS AND PYELONEPHRITIS

Vincent T. Andriole

DEFINITION

Urinary tract infection is a phrase used to describe both microbial colonization of the urine and tissue invasion of any structure of the urinary tract. Bacteria are most commonly responsible, although yeast, fungi, and viruses may, on occasion, produce urinary tract infection. Urinary tract infections may be relatively mild, such as the "honeymoon cystitis" syndrome, or catastrophic, such as a perinephric abscess in a diabetic. Urinary tract infections are often categorized according to the site of infection. While this separation is convenient for the purpose of discussion, it is often not possible to make the distinction between the various types of infections on clinical grounds alone.

Significant bacteriuria refers to the presence of bacteria in the urine in sufficient numbers to denote active infection rather than contamination. A bacteria count over 100,000 organisms per milliliter in a fresh "clean catch" specimen is a reliable indicator of active infection of the urinary tract but does not indicate whether the infection is cystitis or pyelonephritis.

Asymptomatic bacteriuria refers to the multiplication of large numbers of bacteria in the urine without producing symptoms. Dysuria and frequency in the absence of significant bacteriuria are common problems among young women. This entity has been called the *acute urethral syndrome* and is often caused by *Chlamydia trachomatis*.

Cystitis and *acute pyelonephritis* are symptomatic infections of the bladder and kidney, respectively. *Perinephric and renal abscesses*, uncommon complications of urinary tract infections, usually occur (1) in urinary tract obstruction, (2) in bacteremia, in particular with staphylococcal or candidal bacteremia, and (3) in immunocompromised individuals, particularly diabetics.

Complicated infections refer to the presence of bacteriuria in association with structural or neurologic defects in the voiding mechanism (vesicoureteral reflux, neurogenic bladder), foreign bodies (stones or indwelling catheter), or intrinsic renal disease (diabetic nephropathy or polycystic renal disease).

Chronic pyelonephritis refers to the pathologic and radiologic findings of chronic cortical scarring, tubulointerstitial damage, and deformity of the underlying calyx. Chronic bacterial pyelonephritis can be *active* or *inactive*. The *active* form occurs in patients with persistent *complicated* infection, whereas the *inactive* form consists of focal sterile scars of a past infection. Recurrent infection can result in multiple scars combined with active foci of infection. In the absence of obstruction, reflux, foreign bodies, or an immunocompromised host (notably the diabetic patient), urinary tract infections rarely cause the shrunken, scarred kidneys of end-stage chronic pyelonephritis.

A variety of other disease states can produce renal lesions that mimic "chronic pyelonephritis." Characteristics identical to bacterial pyelonephritis can be observed, in the absence of infection, in patients who suffered from severe vesicoureteral reflux in childhood. This entity, *reflux nephropathy*, refers to the radiographic triad of intrarenal reflux and vesicoureteral reflux, scarring, and loss of parenchymal mass in the absence of other obstructive lesions and can ultimately lead to end-stage renal failure with scarred, shrunken kidneys. Recent evidence suggests that "reflux nephropathy" may result from "autoimmune" renal damage rather than bacterial infection of the kidney. Nevertheless, the combination of recurrent infection and reflux nephropathy can also result in chronic pyelonephritis. *Analgesic nephropathy* may produce papillary necrosis and may also mimic bacterial pyelonephritis on x-ray.

PATHOGENESIS

The normal urinary tract is free of bacteria except for some organisms normally present near the external meatus and some staphylococci and diphtheroids normally found in the distal urethra. Urine, as a culture medium, generally supports bacteria multiplication. However, high concentrations of urea and hyperosmolality (which are present in the renal medulla), an acid pH, and urinary organic acid are generally unfavorable to bacterial growth. In addition, the dynamics of the urinary flow (washout) and antibacterial properties of the lining membrane of the urinary tract and of the vaginal and periurethral epithelial cells appear to be important defense mechanisms.

Urinary tract infections result most commonly from ascending transurethral invasion of the bladder by pathogenic gram-negative aerobic bacilli normally present in the large bowel and in the perineum, particularly of women. In the sequence of infection, bacteria migrate from the anus to the periurethral area and along the urethra into the bladder, where infections occur if the organisms become established within this organ. This pathogenic mechanism helps explain the higher rate of urinary tract infection in women, whose urethras are shorter than those of men, and the marked frequency of the urinary infection associated with instrumentation of the urethra and the bladder.

Other possible pathways from the lumen of the intestine to

the urinary passages and the kidney include the hematogenous and lymphatic routes. The hematogenous route is a less common mechanism for renal infection, and generally, but not always, requires antecedent structural damage to the kidney. Staphylococcal bacteremia can produce multiple microabscesses in the kidney *(renal carbuncle).* Disseminated *Candida albicans* infections in the immunocompromised host can involve the kidney. Finally, septic emboli, particularly in the setting of bacterial endocarditis, represent a classic mode for hematogenously disseminated infection of the kidney.

The renal medulla, because of its unique hypertonicity, is much more susceptible to infection than the cortex. In experimental pyelonephritis, as few as 10 to 100 *Escherichia coli* may produce infection in the medulla, whereas 100,000 are required to infect the cortex. The increased susceptibility of the medulla is thought to be due to impaired leukocyte mobilization and phagocytosis in the hypertonic environment.

Microbial virulence factors are also important in the pathogenesis of symptomatic urinary infections. *E. coli* strains isolated from patients with pyelonephritis are more likely to (1) possess large amounts of K (capsular) antigen, (2) adhere in larger numbers to human urinary epithelial cells, and (3) possess surface pili, than are strains found in asymptomatic bacteriuria. The virulence of *Proteus* species may be related to their urease content and ammonia production.

CLINICAL MANIFESTATIONS

The symptoms of the acute urinary tract infections are varied and include frequency, dysuria, burning pain on urination, suprapubic discomfort, passage of cloudy and occasionally blood-tinged urine, fever, costovertebral angle tenderness or flank pain, and rigors. Urinary tract symptoms, particularly dysuria, occur in 20 per cent of women each year, although only half of these women seek medical attention. Approximately one third of these women will have the acute urethral syndrome (urethritis), one third will have bladder bacteriuria (cystitis), and one third will have renal infection.

In general, clinical grounds form an uncertain basis for separating patients with the acute urethral syndrome from those with either bladder or renal bacteriuria because of the high degree of overlap among these three groups of disorders. Thus, frequency, burning, and suprapubic pain are found approximately equally in all three groups of patients. Costovertebral angle tenderness and fever may be present as frequently in patients with the acute urethral syndrome as in those with renal bacteriuria. Rigors occur almost equally (15 per cent) in patients with the acute urethral syndrome and those with cystitis. Similarly, tenderness in the region of one or both kidneys occurs not infrequently in lower urinary tract infections. However, a sudden rise in body temperature to 38.9° to 40.6°C, shaking chills, aching costovertebral or flank pain, and symptoms of sepsis are more characteristic of acute pyelonephritis than of cystitis or urethritis.

Laboratory tests show a polymorphonuclear leukocytosis and an abnormal urinary sediment in both cystitis and pyelonephritis. In both disorders, the urine may be laden with leukocytes, but white blood cell casts are more typical of pyelonephritis. Stain of the sediment reveals numerous bacteria, usually gram-negative bacilli, and urine cultures confirm the presence of significant bacteriuria. Cultures of blood may also be positive in some cases of pyelonephritis. A simple but convenient way of identifying infection of the urinary tract is by examining the unspun urine: the microscopic presence of bacteria from an unspun urine specimen generally indicates more than 100,000 colonies per milliliter of urine.

Impaired renal function or acute hypertension is rarely seen in acute pyelonephritis, but renal concentrating ability may be impaired. There must also be subclinical forms of acute pyelonephritis because tests that differentiate "upper" (kidney) from "lower" (bladder) infection often indicate the presence of renal infection in the absence of flank pain or fever. Procedures such as ureteral catheterization and bladder washout are considered to be research maneuvers. Search for antibody-coated bacteria in the urine as a marker of renal bacteriuria may be performed, but the sensitivity and specificity of this test are not optimal. Pyelonephritis at times presents with symptoms that do not point to the urinary tract. Some patients may have only backache without demonstrable renal tenderness. Others have upper or lower abdominal pain together with symptoms of disturbed gastrointestinal function. Some complain only of general fatigue.

In the absence of obstructive lesions of the urinary tract or host immunocompromise, as in diabetics, upper or lower urinary tract infections are generally self-limited, lasting 10 to 14 days. When obstruction or host immunocompromise is present, pyelonephritis may be complicated by papillary necrosis, perinephric abscess, or renal carbuncle. These complications should be suspected when persistent flank pain, fever, and leukocytosis are unresponsive to otherwise adequate chemotherapy (see below).

Acute urinary tract infection complicated by pyelonephritis may occur in patients subjected to urethral instrumentation, particularly long-term indwelling catheters. Sepsis from pyelonephritis is a major cause of death in individuals having neurologic disorders requiring long-term indwelling catheters.

DIAGNOSIS

Significant Bacteriuria

The concept of "significant bacteriuria" was introduced to distinguish between those bacteria that actually multiply in the urine and bacteria that are contaminants. This distinction can be made by knowledge of the site and manner in which the urine is collected from the patient, and by enumeration of the number of organisms present in the sample. The criterion of 100,000 or more organisms per milliliter of urine for the diagnosis of significant bacteriuria is an excellent operational definition when the clear-voided method is used to collect specimens, since contaminants will usually be present in numbers ranging from 1,000 to 10,000 colonies per milliliter. In contrast, organisms found in urinary tract infection grow well in urine and usually achieve concentrations of greater than 100,000 colonies per milliliter.

The clean-voided method, in both males and females, provides reliable results if the urine is collected with proper cleansing and processed promptly. Because the reliability of the method can vary with experience and care, overdiagnosis can be avoided by obtaining multiple specimens, particularly in the asymptomatic patient. Finally, as indicated above, the unspun urinary sediment can be examined for bacteria.

Bacterial counts lower than 100,000 colonies per milliliter may occur in patients with true bacteriuria, but can be established as valid indices of infection only when the same species of bacteria can be isolated repeatedly. Isolation of multiple species from the urine usually indicates contamination, especially in the asymptomatic person.

Urine collected by suprapubic aspiration or bladder catheterization is less likely to be contaminated. In this instance, bacterial counts of less than 100,000 organisms per milliliter are likely to be significant.

Bacteriologic Findings

The species of bacteria most likely to be recovered from individuals with bacteriuria depends upon prior history of infection, prior antimicrobial therapy, hospitalization, and instrumentation of the urinary tract. The bacterial flora found in individuals with symptomatic bacteriuria is no different from that in cases of cystitis or pyelonephritis. Enterobacteriaceae are the most common organisms identified. *E. coli* acccounts for more than 80 per cent of all species recovered in uncomplicated cases, whereas *Proteus, Klebsiella, Enterobacter, Pseudomonas,* enterococci, and staphylococci are more often found in patients who have had previous infection or instrumentation. Occasionally, *Serratia marcescens, Acinetobacter, Candida albicans,* and *Cryptococcus neoformans* may produce infection of the urinary tract in diabetics and in immunosuppressed or corticosteroid-treated patients. Coliforms are also the most common organisms (40 per cent) responsible for the acute urethral syndrome, although *Staphylococcus saprophyticus* (5 per cent) and *Chlamydia trachomatis* (25 per cent) are responsible for some cases. Patients with the acute urethral syndrome caused by *Chlamydia trachomatis* have pyuria but sterile bladder urine when cultured with standard bacteriologic media.

Anaerobes are commonly present in the distal urethra and the vagina and are abundant in the gut, but they rarely produce urinary tract infection. Suprapubic aspiration of urine or examination of tissues is needed to prove anaerobic infections. When responsible, anaerobes are usually associated with complicated, longstanding infections.

Microscopic Methods

Rapid diagnostic methods are available either by preparation of a Gram's stain of unsedimented urine and examination with an oil immersion lens, or by study of the centrifuged urinary sediment for bacteria, employing the high-dry objective under reduced light, with or without methylene blue stain. The Gram's stain correlates about 80 to 90 per cent with quantitative culture. Examination of the unstained sediment is also very helpful and can be done during routine examination for formed elements. A useful criterion for a positive sediment is the presence of many (preferably more than 20) obvious bacteria. Pyuria is arbitrarily defined as 10 or more leukocytes per high power field in the centrifuged specimen. Some erythrocytes may be seen in the urine, and gross hematuria may occur when inflammation in the bladder is intense. Proteinuria is not common in urinary tract infections. There is, however, one exception to the latter statement: specifically, in acute fulminant pyelonephritis, as in other severe acute interstitial nephritides, rather significant degrees of proteinuria may occur transiently.

Radiology

Radiographic evaluation of the urinary tract is undertaken to detect correctable lesions that may contribute to the severity or recurrence of urinary tract infections. Evaluation is indicated in men with any type of urinary tract infection or in instances of documented bacteremia. In women, urography is indicated after three or four recurrences of lower or upper tract infection, and in instances where a seven- to ten-day course of antibiotics fails to eradicate the infection.

EPIDEMIOLOGY AND NATURAL HISTORY

Bacteriuria in the newborn population has been difficult to study because of problems inherent in urine collection. Cultures of urine obtained by bladder puncture suggest a prevalence of 1 to 2 per cent. Infection of the urinary tract in this age group may be part of a generalized, life-threatening gram-negative sepsis and is more common in boys than girls. Symptomatic urinary infections are more prevalent among girls in preschool years and are often associated with obstructive or neurogenic lesions. Urologic investigation is valuable in this age group. *Urologic evaluation is mandatory in males of any age because of the high frequency of structural abnormalities found* (valves, malformation, and obstructive and neurogenic lesions).

The prevalence of bacteriuria among school girls is 1 to 2 per cent; it is only 0.03 per cent in boys of the same age. The prevalence of bacteriuria in females rises about 1 per cent per decade.

Urinary infection is common after marriage. The pathogenesis of the "honeymoon cystitis" syndrome remains unclear. Physical factors associated with sexual activity in previously sexually nonactive women may play a prominent role. Many patients with "honeymoon cystitis" (up to 50 per cent) will have dysuria due to local irritation rather than infection, and this should be clearly differentiated by culture.

Bacteriuria of pregnancy varies from 2 to 6 per cent, depending upon age, parity, and socioeconomic group. Acute symptomatic pyelonephritis will develop later in pregnancy in approximately 20 per cent of these women. However, there is no evidence that isolated episodes of pyelonephritis in pregnant women lead to chronic urinary tract infections after these women cease child-bearing activities. Early detection and treatment of bacteriuria in pregnancy will prevent the emergence of symptomatic infection.

Elderly women may have frequencies of bacteriuria as high as 10 per cent; this rate may increase in hospitalized patients, particularly diabetics. Bacteriuria in the male begins to appear in "prostate years" and is often initiated by instrumentation.

Role of Instrumentation

Bacteriuria persists in 1 to 2 per cent of relatively healthy individuals following a single catheterization; the risk is higher in the debilitated patient and in males with prostatic obstruction. With open indwelling catheter drainage, bacterial colonization exceeds 90 per cent within three to four days. This may lead to life-threatening pyelonephritis and gram-negative sepsis. Fortunately, it is largely preventable by (1) careful criteria for catheterization and (2) use of aseptic closed drainage. The catheter should be removed as soon as it is no longer needed.

Intermittent self-catheterization coupled with abdominal pressure may be of benefit in patients with neurogenic bladders and may result in minimal urinary tract infections.

TREATMENT

The goal of treatment is to eradicate bacteria from the urinary tract in order to relieve symptoms, prevent renal damage, and diminish the likelihood of spread of infections to other sites. Prophylaxis is used to prevent recurrent symptomatic infection. Suppression, although rarely effective, is used to diminish the number of bacteria in the urine or tissues. Indications for therapy depend on the potential of infection to give rise to symptoms or damage to the urinary tract and the likelihood that treatment will be effective.

Asymptomatic Bacteriuria

There is considerable debate as to whether to treat *asymptomatic bacteriuria* in females. In the absence of underlying structural or neurologic lesions the likelihood is slight that renal damage will occur. Furthermore, short courses of therapy, when effective, are commonly followed by reinfection. In contrast, asymptomatic bacteriuria occurring during pregnancy should definitely be treated to prevent symptomatic illness in the third trimester.

It also seems reasonable to treat infection in asymptomatic individuals who are known to be at high risk for recurrent symptomatic infection or who may have major predisposing factors to renal disease, such as diabetes or polycystic kidneys, or who have anatomic or neurologic abnormalities. If the treatment fails to eradicate asymptomatic infections in such individuals, further treatment should be reserved for acute symptomatic episodes. Bacteriuria in the elderly is frequent, usually uncomplicated, and highly recurrent. It should not be treated overzealously if simple measures fail, because the toxicity and expense of therapy may outweigh the risk of disease.

Symptomatic Urinary Tract Infection

Acute uncomplicated episodes of symptomatic bacteriuria localized to the lower urinary tract (bladder or urethra) can be treated effectively with oral single-dose therapy, either amoxicillin, 3 grams, or co-trimoxazole (trimethoprim, 0.32 grams, plus sulfamethoxazole, 1.6 grams), two double-strength tablets. Single-dose therapy will usually fail to eradicate either renal bacteriuria or complicated infections. Symptomatic urethritis caused by *Chlamydia trachomatis* should respond to oral doxycycline (100 mg twice daily for seven days).

Pyelonephritis requires a 7- to 14-day or longer course of therapy. Complicated infections in which obstruction or a foreign body is not removed may not respond to such a course. Hematogenous pyelonephritis requires specific therapy directed at the invading organism.

The choice of an oral or parenteral agent depends upon the severity of the infection and the patient's ability to take the oral agent. Drugs are selected on the basis of cost, side effects, and antibacterial spectrum. Antimicrobial susceptibility tests should be used to guide therapy of recurrent episodes. Effective oral agents include sulfonamides, tetracyclines, ampicillin, amoxicillin, cinoxacin, cephalosporins, co-trimoxazole, trimethoprim, or nitrofurantoin. The last three drugs are useful in recurrent infections, because emergence of resistant strains occurs infrequently.

The initial attack of urinary tract infection is usually due to *E. coli,* which is sensitive to most antimicrobial agents and therefore may be treated "blindly" with the agents described above with equal success. However, the widespread use of these agents for other infections has decreased their previous reliability. For example, approximately 40 per cent of *E. coli,* including those that are community-acquired, are now resistant to ampicillin.

When therapy is successful, bacteriuria should disappear within 24 hours even if pyuria and symptoms continue. A repeat urine culture should be obtained after 72 hours of treatment. A positive culture at this time denotes treatment failure. It is important to recognize bacteriologic failure early and to change to another drug. Parenteral agents, such as ampicillin, a cephalosporin, or an aminoglycoside, may be required in some instances or when the patient is too ill to receive an oral agent. A follow-up culture one week after the completion of antimicrobial therapy is recommended to document a cure.

Some authors recommend routine follow-up cultures several times over the ensuing year to detect recurrent bacteriuria, but this practice is prohibitively expensive and difficult to justify on medical grounds in asymptomatic patients.

Recurrent Infections

Recurrence of infection in the few weeks after treatment is usually due to persistence of the same focus, whereas later recurrence, particularly in females, is more often a result of reinfection. Frequent recurrent infections may be managed by either close follow-up and treatment of each episode or by prophylaxis with nitrofurantoin, trimethoprim, or co-trimoxazole as a single bedtime dose.

Urinary antiseptics such as methenamine mandelate or hippurate require an acid urine, preferably at pH 5.5, and are of little value unless their use is accompanied by agents that consistently lower urinary pH, such as high-dose ascorbic acid (1000 mg daily). Methenamine, however, is an effective "suppressant" agent and is best used after infection is eradicated by a more effective drug.

Prophylaxis when given for three to six months is effective for recurrent infections of the reinfection type in women. Cessation of prophylaxis, however, results in a significant incidence of recurrence in individuals having structural abnormalities of the urinary tract or intrinsic renal structural defects. In those circumstances prophylaxis should be reinstituted. Generally, the therapeutic agent should be changed if bacteriuria persists during treatment. This latter circumstance usually means an organism resistant to the agent is now colonizing the urine. Prophylaxis is ineffective in patients with indwelling catheters and will only lead to emergence of resistant bacteria.

The patient should be instructed to drink fluids generously and void frequently. Double voiding in patients with vesicoureteral reflux is recommended. Voiding after sexual intercourse is felt by some to decrease the chance of recurrent infection, but postcoital use of prophylactic agents is probably more effective.

Complicated Infections

Complex urinary infections, i.e., those in the presence of obstructive uropathy, neurogenic bladders, or catheters, are exceedingly difficult to eradicate. They are often best left untreated except for management of acute episodes. Suppressive therapy should be considered ineffective if bacterial populations in the urine are not reduced to less than 1000 per milliliter. The key to management is relief of obstruction or the removal of foreign bodies. Intermittent catheterization has benefited some patients with neurogenic bladders.

COMPLICATIONS

While most urinary tract infections, including pyelonephritis, are self-limited and easily treated, there are three severe complications of pyelonephritis with which the clinician must be familiar: *renal papillary necrosis, renal abscess* (renal carbuncle), and *perinephric abscess.* In general, these complications are uncommon and occur most often in the setting of underlying structural renal abnormalities or host immunocompromise (particularly diabetes).

Renal Papillary Necrosis

Renal papillary necrosis, an ischemic necrosis of the renal papilla and adjacent portions of the renal medulla, may be seen in association with severe pyelonephritis, diabetes mellitus, sickle cell anemia, obstructive uropathy, and analgesic abuse. Although infection appears to be the most important factor in the pathogenesis of this lesion, the peculiarities of blood supply of the medulla must also be a factor. This helps explain the frequent occurrence of the lesion in patients with diabetes and generalized vascular disease, as well as the role of obstruction, which must impair blood supply to this area. The zone of necrosis may occur from the extreme tip of the pyramid as far proximal as the corticomedullary junction. Eventually this may slough, with migration of chunks of necrotic tissue down the urinary passages.

The clinical manifestations of renal papillary necrosis are intensification of symptoms of pre-existing pyelonephritis. There may be pain in the lumbar region, colicky pain along the ureteral radiation, hematuria, and high fever. Manifestations of gram-negative bacteremia may supervene. This lesion should be considered in elderly patients with diabetes who show rapid deterioration in clinical status with signs of active pyelonephritis and increasing renal decompensation.

The diagnosis can sometimes be made by finding pieces of renal medullary tissue in the urinary sediment. Pyelography may demonstrate the scarring and asymmetry of chronic pyelonephritis, plus cavities and sinuses in the region of the papilli. The classic ring-shadow pattern results from detachment of a papilla and its outline within the contrast-filled cavity.

Therapy should be directed toward control of infection and measures employed to improve the status of patients who have diabetes mellitus or who are habitual abusers of analgesic agents.

Renal Abscess

Renal abscesses usually occur as a result of extension of a pyelonephritic process. Up to one third of the cases, however, arise from hematogenous spread from a distant focus. In the latter instance, virulent organisms such as *S. aureus* are likely to be involved.

A renal abscess may be identified by intravenous pyelography, ultrasonography, or computed tomography. It should be suspected whenever a urinary tract infection fails to respond to an adequate (two-week) course of appropriate antibiotics. Blood and urine cultures may be negative, so antibiotic regimens may need to be established empirically to cover gram-negative rods and staphylococci. Surgical drainage is usually required in addition to parenteral antibiotics, although early diagnosis may eliminate the need for surgery in some patients.

Perinephric Abscess

Perinephric abscesses are notoriously difficult to diagnose. They have an insidious onset, with symptoms usually present for over two weeks at the time of presentation. Fever and unilateral flank pain are common presenting symptoms. The diagnosis should be considered in the evaluation of any patient with a fever of unknown origin. A recent history of urinary tract infection should alert one to the possibility of a perinephric abscess, although this piece of history is often absent. Over two thirds of patients with perinephric abscesses have either diabetes or kidney stone disease.

Perinephric abscesses occur almost exclusively from the rupture of an intrarenal abscess. Diagnosis can be established by ultrasonography, computed tomography, or fluoroscopy that shows restricted motion of the involved kidney on respiration. Surgical drainage is mandatory.

Andriole VT: Current concepts of urinary tract infections. *In* Weinstein L, Fields BN (eds.): Seminars in Infectious Disease, Vol III. New York, Thieme-Stratton, Inc, 1980, pp 89–130. *The author's review of practical diagnostic methods, microbiologic concepts, host defenses, clinical syndromes, and treatment of urinary tract infections.*

Bailey RR (ed.): Single Dose Therapy of Urinary Tract Infection. Balgowlah, ADIS Health Science Press, 1983. *A multiauthor text on single-dose therapy in adults and children.*

Bailey RR: The relationship of vesicoureteral reflux to urinary tract infection and chronic pyelonephritis-reflux nephropathy. Clin Nephrol 1:132, 1973. *An excellent review of the subject of reflux nephropathy.*

Kunin CM: Detection, Prevention and Treatment of Urinary Tract Infections. 3rd ed. Philadelphia, Lea & Febiger, 1979. *An excellent text that describes the pathogenesis, management, and prevention of urinary infections.*

Mayrer AR, Miniter P, Andriole VT: Immunopathogenesis of chronic pyelonephritis. Am J Med 75 (Suppl 1B):59, 1983. *Recent studies describing immunologic mechanisms of renal injury and scarring, which produce an histopathologic picture of chronic pyelonephritis.*

Stamm WE, Koutsky LA, Benedetti JK, Jourden JL, Brunham RC, Holmes KK: Chlamydia trachomatis urethral infections in men. Ann Intern Med 100:47, 1984. *An excellent study and review of this underdiagnosed type of infection.*

Stamm WE, Wagner KF, Amsel R, Alexander ER, Turck M, Counts GW, Holmes KK: Causes of the acute urethral syndrome in women. N Engl J Med 303:409, 1980. *A detailed description of the various etiologies of the acute urethral syndrome in women.*

86. VASCULAR DISORDERS OF THE KIDNEY

J. Caulie Gunnells, Jr.

RENAL INFARCTION FROM ARTERIAL THROMBI AND EMBOLI

Vascular occlusions involving major or minor renal arteries or veins may result in systemic hypertension or loss of functioning renal mass, or both. Hypertension and renal failure occur more commonly following occlusive disease of the renal arterial than of the venous circulation. This chapter will be devoted primarily to acute renal arterial occlusive disease. The clinical features of renovascular hypertension are reviewed in detail in Ch. 47 and will not be covered here. In addition, since the end results of primary renal infarction from renal artery thrombi are essentially the same as those from renal emboli, these conditions will be considered together.

Not covered in this chapter are two forms of "functional" or "relative" renal ischemia usually occurring without demonstrable intrinsic occlusive renal arterial lesions: acute tubular necrosis and acute renal cortical necrosis. They are discussed in Ch. 77.

Renal infarction may be segmental or may involve the entire kidney. The extent of ischemic injury reflects (1) the size and number of the renal artery or arteries involved, (2) the nature of vascular insult, (3) the extent of coexistent vascular or parenchymal renal disease, and (4) the presence of capsular and collateral vessels. Fortunately, approximately 30 per cent of individuals have multiple main renal arteries, a well developed capsular circulation arising from vessels other than the main renal arteries, and a complex bifurcation of secondary and tertiary renal artery vessels. Therefore segmental rather than total renal infarction is a more common clinical event.

Renal arterial obstruction with infarction may occur as a result of *thrombosis* (superimposed on arteriosclerosis or fibrous dysplasia, aneurysm of the renal artery, aortic dissection, periarteritis nodosa, vasculitis, sickle cell disease, scleroderma, profound hypotension, and polycythemia) or *embolism* (mural thrombi or vegetations, cholesterol crystals or plaques, intravascular tumors [atrial myxoma], or foreign bodies). In addition, renal infarction may occur as a complication of *severe trauma*, with total interruption of the vascular supply to one or both kidneys. Therefore after extensive trauma, even in the absence of hematuria, it may be advisable to obtain early some diagnostic assessment of the integrity of the blood supply to the kidney.

CLINICAL PICTURE. Total or segmental renal infarction is suggested by a history of flank pain, fever, leukocytosis, and transient gross and/or microhematuria, together with an elevated lactic acid dehydrogenase value and rapidly progressive renal failure without evidence of renal stone or obstructive uropathy. The coexistence of heart disease (murmur, myocardial infarction, arrhythmia) suggests a major renal artery embolism, whereas the presence of severe abdominal aortic and/or peripheral vascular disease with hypertension suggests either a major renal artery thrombus or progressive microembolic disease. In addition, the onset of severe hypertension or the acceleration of prior hypertension may occur with renal ischemia.

Intravenous urography with nephrotomography and renal scintiscans are equally effective in demonstrating the absence of function in one or both kidneys. The renal scintiscan may provide important initial baseline data for follow-up study without exposure to the potential toxicity of contrast media. Abdominal angiography should be reserved for patients who are candidates for surgical or mechanical intervention.

TREATMENT. Long-term anticoagulation is efficacious in the treatment of renal artery embolism. Surgery should be considered only for patients with bilateral embolization or with an embolus to a single functional kidney. In the patient with a major renal artery thrombosis, surgery offers a hope of restoring some degree of renal function together with improvement in blood pressure. Successful revascularization of the kidney following oliguria and renal failure of up to 38 days' duration has been reported. The success of these surgical procedures depends upon the nature of the coexistent cardiovascular disease, the presence of collateral flow, and the combined skill and experience of the surgeon and radiologist. Increasing interest and demonstrated effectiveness of transluminal balloon angioplasty in the treatment of these patients are encouraging. In addition, the use of intra-arterial streptokinase in renal artery embolism appears promising.

Selected patients will benefit from transient dialysis while awaiting re-establishment of effective renal blood flow.

PROGNOSIS. The nature, extent, and severity of the underlying cardiac disease most often predicts the outcome of patients with renal artery embolus. The extent and type of abdominal aortic vascular disease is more important in renal artery thrombosis.

Edwards BS, Stanson AW, Holley KE, Sheps SG: Isolated renal artery dissection. Presentation, evaluation, management, and pathology. Mayo Clin Proc 57:564, 1982. *An excellent review of 35 cases.*

Fischer CP, Konnak JW, Cho KJ, Eckhauser FE, Stanley JC: Renal artery embolism: Therapy with intra-arterial streptokinase infusion. J Urol 125:402, 1981. *Authors' experience together with review of literature.*

Lessman RK, Johnson SF, Coburn JW, Kaufman JM: Renal artery embolism: Clinical features and long-term follow-up of 17 cases. Ann Intern Med 89:477, 1978. *An excellent detailed review and follow-up of one of the larger series of patients with renal artery embolism; emphasizes the nonoperative management.*

Sniderman KW, Sos TA: Percutaneous transluminal recanalization and dilatation of totally occluded renal arteries. Radiology 142:607, 1982. *A report of seven patients treated by this technique.*

Wasser WG, Krakoff LR, Haimov M, Glabman S, Mitty HA: Restoration of renal function after bilateral renal artery occlusion. Arch Intern Med 141:1647, 1981. *An up-to-date review of the medical and surgical management with good bibliography.*

RENAL VEIN THROMBOSIS

Renal vein thrombosis may occur as a primary or secondary event, and as an acute or chronic process. It may be unilateral or bilateral and may involve the major renal vein, smaller renal venous radicles, or both. Renal vein thrombosis in the adult population is usually of the chronic secondary variety and associated with heavy proteinuria and other features of the nephrotic syndrome, regardless of the extent or location of anatomic involvement. The acute primary variety almost always occurs in children, usually under the age of two years, in a clinical setting of an acute illness characterized by volume contraction, dehydration, gastroenteritis, and a fulminant, rapidly progressive, and often fatal clinical course with bilateral hemorrhagic renal infarction. The remainder of this discussion will be directed to the more common adult form of chronic renal venous thrombosis and its associated clinical features.

Renal vein thrombosis is reported to occur in approximately 20 to 25 per cent of patients with the nephrotic syndrome. This figure is not precise, since diagnostic renal venography has not been performed in all reported series. Renal vein thrombosis occurs most frequently in patients with membranous glomerulopathy; less commonly in association with membranoproliferative glomerulonephritis and renal amyloidosis; and infrequently or rarely in patients with focal sclerosing glomerulopathy, nil or minimal change disease, diabetic nephropathy, and collagen vascular disease. Renal vein thrombosis is rarely a primary event in the adult population. In addition to its occurrence with primary parenchymal renal disease, renal vein thrombosis has been described in patients with inferior vena caval thrombosis, congestive heart failure, pregnancy, constrictive pericarditis, trauma, and morbid obesity.

A relatively high incidence of thromboembolic events occurs in patients with nephrotic syndrome, suggesting a hypercoagulable state that perhaps accounts for the frequently associated renal vein thrombosis. Several abnormalities of the coagulation sequence have been described in nephrotic patients that could produce intravascular thrombosis, but the pathogenesis of the proposed hypercoagulable state remains unsettled.

CLINICAL SETTING. Clinical features of renal vein thrombosis are, for the most part, those of nephrotic syndrome—namely, massive edema and proteinuria. On rare occasions, flank pain in association with gross or microhematuria may occur. Systemic hypertension is not uncommon. Rarely the patient may present with thromboembolism (pulmonary emboli) as the initial manifestation of renal vein thrombosis.

LABORATORY FEATURES. The urinalysis exhibits heavy qualitative proteinuria with quantitative protein excretion in the nephrotic range (see Ch. 80 for other biochemical features of the nephrotic syndrome). Attention has been directed toward two features of renal vein thrombosis; protein excretion is usually markedly increased, and there may be a high incidence of initially decreased renal function, with an ensuing progressive decline in glomerular filtration rate.

Intravenous urography may demonstrate enlarged renal outlines with stretching of the calyces secondary to interstitial edema. The subsequent development of venous collaterals produces scalloping of the upper portion of the ureter. Conclusive anatomic diagnosis of renal vein thrombosis is best established by phlebography of the inferior vena cava and both renal veins. β-scan ultrasonography and computed tomography may also be useful in the diagnosis of vena caval and renal vein thrombosis.

HISTOPATHOLOGY. The major histologic features of renal vein thrombosis reflect the associated underlying renal disease. Indeed, in unilateral renal vein thrombosis the contralateral kidney demonstrates similar or identical findings as in the ipsilateral kidney, indicating the pathogenetic importance of the underlying primary renal disease. Renal vein thrombosis may result in (1) relatively more interstitial edema and fibrosis as compared to glomerular alterations; (2) a peculiar glomerular margination and stasis of leukocytes; and (3) fibrin deposition in some renal venous channels.

PROGNOSIS. Patients with renal vein thrombosis and underlying primary parenchymal renal disease have a poorer prognosis than patients with similar forms of renal disease without renal vein thrombosis. More rapid deterioration in renal function and greater degrees of proteinuria result. In the absence of renal functional loss, the other most important factor in an unfavorable prognosis is the demonstration of existent or potential extrarenal thromboembolic episodes. Careful assessment for evidence of pulmonary embolization is of particular importance. It has been recommended that baseline noninvasive radioactive pulmonary scans be obtained in patients with renal vein thrombosis as an aid in establishing prognosis and making clinical decisions relative to therapy.

TREATMENT. Anticoagulation remains the mainstay of therapy, primarily because of the ever-present threat of recurrent extrarenal thromboembolism. Unfortunately, treatment must be extended for long periods of time and is not without additional problems in patients with renal disease.

To date the role of surgery in the treatment of chronic renal vein thrombosis has not been established.

Adrenocortical steroids and cytotoxic drugs may be indicated for the underlying primary renal disease. However, in view of a possible thrombotic tendency in steroid-treated patients, their use in patients with renal vein thrombosis needs careful monitoring.

Harrington JT, Kassirer JP: Renal vein thrombosis. Ann Rev Med 33:255, 1982. *An excellent clinical review with practical information.*

Llach F, Papper S, Massry SG: The clinical spectrum of renal vein thrombosis: Acute and chronic. Am J Med 69:819, 1980. *Updated observation of a group with long interest and experience with renal vein thrombosis.*

Massry SG, Vaziri ND: Renal vein thrombosis and the nephrotic syndrome. *In* Massry SG, Glassock RJ (eds.): Textbook of Nephrology, Vol 2. Baltimore, Williams & Wilkins, 1983, p. 6.62. *Contains extensive information on clotting abnormalities in the nephrotic syndrome.*

Trew PA, Biava CG, Jacobs RP, et al.: Renal vein thrombosis in membranous glomerulopathy. Medicine 57:69, 1978. *An updated and extensive review of the association of renal vein thrombosis with membranous glomerulopathy.*

Wagoner RD, Stanson AW, Holley KE, Winter CS: Renal vein thrombosis in idiopathic membranous glomerulopathy and nephrotic syndrome: Incidence and significance. Kidney Int 23:368, 1983. *An excellent study of 27 patients with membranous glomerulopathy.*

87. RENAL DISEASE IN PREGNANCY

John P. Hayslett

The detection and clinical management of renal disease in the gravid female is complicated by concern for fetal development and survival, as well as for the health of the patient. In addition, clinical evaluation must account for physiological changes in volume status and renal function that accompany pregnancy.

RENAL FUNCTION IN PREGNANCY. Pregnancy is characterized by a gradual, cumulative retention of 500 to 900 mEq of sodium and 6 to 8 liters of water, which are distributed between maternal extracellular fluid and the fetus. Despite an expansion in plasma volume of 30 to 45 per cent, mean blood pressure falls approximately 15 per cent due to a reduction in peripheral vascular resistance. The glomerular filtration rate increases by 30 to 50 per cent by the twelfth week of gestation; the elevation is sustained until term and is position dependent (Fig. 87–1). An evaluation of glomerular filtration rate should take into account expected levels during gestation and should not compare measured values to reported normal values obtained in the nonpregnant individual. Because of the marked position dependence, a convenient way of measuring filtration rate in

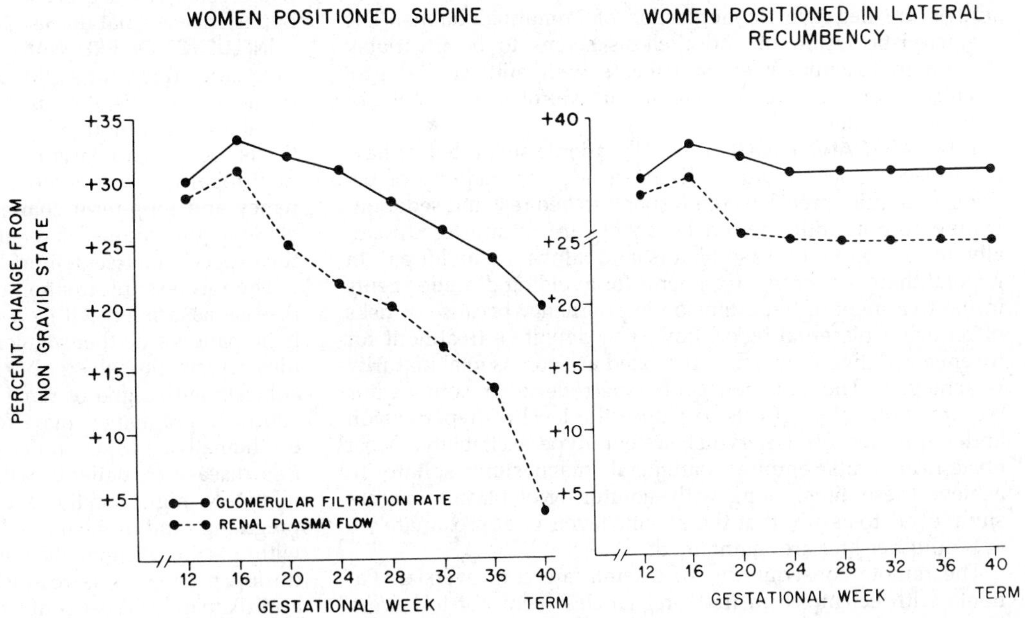

Figure 87–1. The early increment of glomerular filtration rate and effective renal plasma flow is position dependent and is sustained if subjects are studied in lateral recumbency. (Adapted from Pippig L: Clinical aspects of renal disease during pregnancy. Med Hyg 27:181, 1969. *In* Lindheimer MD, Katz AI: Kidney Function and Disease in Pregnancy. Philadelphia, Lea and Febiger, 1977.)

later pregnancy is with a timed (e.g., four hours) water-loaded creatinine clearance with the woman positioned in the lateral recumbent position.

Owing to the increase in glomerular filtration rate and expanded plasma volume, the levels of creatinine and blood urea nitrogen fall to approximately 0.5 mg per deciliter and 9 mg per deciliter, respectively. Plasma concentrations above 0.8 mg per deciliter of creatinine and 13 mg per deciliter of urea nitrogen should alert the physician to the possibility of renal insufficiency. Plasma osmolality falls from approximately 280 mOsm · Kg H_2O^{-1} to 270 owing to a resetting of the osmostat; plasma uric acid falls to 3 to 4 mg per deciliter and plasma bicarbonate to approximately 20 mEq per liter (owing to mild respiratory alkalosis). Glucosuria and aminoaciduria may occur during pregnancy as a result of a transient reduction in the renal threshold of absorption. The ureters dilate during pregnancy and for as long as 12 weeks post partum with no implication of outflow obstruction.

TOXEMIA OF PREGNANCY

DEFINITION. Toxemia, unique to human pregnancy, is characterized by hypertension, edema, and proteinuria. Clinically the syndrome is divided into the stages of preeclampsia and eclampsia, the latter when convulsions have occurred. Onset is usually insidious after the thirty-second week of pregnancy, but it may occur as early as the twenty-fourth week. In women with a hydatidiform mole, toxemia has been reported to occur in the first trimester. The usual sequence is edema and hypertension, followed by proteinuria, although proteinuria may occasionally precede hypertension. Signs of toxemia spontaneously subside after delivery. Clinical criteria for diagnosis vary depending on changes of blood pressure considered to be abnormal in pregnancy. In general, hypertension in the third trimester is defined by a blood pressure measurement of 140/85 mm Hg or greater if sustained for four to six hours, or an increase of 30 mm Hg or more in systolic blood pressure and 15 mm Hg or more in diastolic pressure above values measured during the early stages of pregnancy. The major differential diagnosis involves a distinction between toxemia, essential hypertension, and primary renal disease, although toxemia can be superimposed on the other two clinical entities.

INCIDENCE. Toxemia of pregnancy occurs worldwide with an incidence that varies between 2 per cent and 25 per cent in different populations. In the United States the quoted incidence is 6 to 7 per cent. Individuals with a poor socioeconomic status are at higher risk for developing the syndrome; the incidence is reduced after introduction of adequate prenatal care with special attention to weight gain and monitoring of blood pressure. The syndrome occurs predominantly in primigravidas and in multiparous women over 35 years of age.

CLINICAL MANIFESTATIONS. Clinical symptoms may include headache, visual disturbances, and apprehension. While diastolic hypertension may be prominent, systolic blood pressure seldom exceeds 160 mm Hg except when associated with underlying hypertension. Funduscopic examination may reveal segmental arteriolar narrowing and a generalized glistening fundus indicative of retinal edema. The ocular changes reflect vasoconstriction. Signs of central nervous system hyperexcitability are regarded as ominous, since they often precede convulsions with a high maternal and fetal death rate. Laboratory findings include a rate of protein excretion usually less than 2 grams per day, but higher levels in the range seen in the nephrotic syndrome may occur. There is a reduction in glomerular filtration rate and renal plasma flow to about 60 per cent of that in pregnancy control subjects. Owing to elevated levels of glomerular filtration rate in normal pregnancy, however, blood urea and serum creatinine levels may not appear to be elevated in toxemic patients, especially if compared to nonpregnant control values. Plasma uric acid levels rise in toxemia to about 5.0 mg per deciliter in mild toxemia and to over 7.0 mg per deciliter in severe states, owing to a fall in its renal clearance. It is suggested that uric acid levels provide a guide for estimating severity of toxemia.

PATHOGENESIS AND PATHOLOGY. The cause of toxemia is not understood. Plasma levels of aldosterone and renin are lower in toxemic women than in normal pregnant individuals but still may be inappropriately high in relation to salt intake and volume status. Many primigravidas who eventually develop toxemia exhibit increased sensitivity to the pressure effects of infused angiotensin many weeks before they become hypertensive. In addition, although a reduction in placental blood flow is found in toxemia, it is not known whether this is a primary change or is secondary to systemic hypertension.

The histopathologic renal changes in toxemia, primarily confined to the glomerulus, are termed *glomerular capillary endotheliosis*. The glomeruli are large and swollen, with encroachment on capillary lumina by swollen and vacuolated endothelial and mesangial cells. Occasionally, small subendothelial deposits and fibrin deposits may be seen, but immunofluorescence studies are negative for deposition of immunoglobulins. The characteristic lesion of endotheliosis seems to be invariably present in toxemia, even in patients with mild clinical preeclampsia, but resolves during an interval of a few weeks or months after delivery.

TREATMENT AND PROGNOSIS. All patients suspected of having preeclampsia should be hospitalized. The majority of patients with mild preeclampsia respond to bed rest and sedation. If they do not, antihypertensive agents are administered, usually in the form of vasodilators and alpha methyldopa. In general there are strong arguments for avoiding diuretic agents in the treatment of hypertension in pregnancy because of risks of reducing placental blood flow. The definitive treatment for toxemia is delivery, which is indicated as soon as fetal maturity is achieved. The occurrence of hyperreflexia or convulsions requires immediate efforts to reduce the level of hypertension and depress central nervous system hyperexcitability. Most obstetrical units employ parenteral magnesium sulfate to achieve these aims, along with monitoring of plasma magnesium levels to assure that therapeutic levels of approximately 6 to 8 mEq per liter are maintained.

The remote consequences of toxemia are controversial. Patients with eclampsia in first pregnancies seem not to have a higher incidence of subsequent hypertension than does the general population. The prevalence of late hypertension has been found to be increased in multiparous patients with eclampsia.

RENAL PARENCHYMAL DISEASES

Pregnancy may occur in women with pre-existing renal disease; during pregnancy women may acquire the same kinds of disease that exist in the nongravid state. Three important clinical questions concerning these patients warrant further discussion: (1) What are the criteria that help to distinguish preeclampsia from other causes of renal dysfunction? (2) Does pregnancy adversely influence the course of the underlying renal or systemic disease? (3) Does the presence of renal insufficiency or nephrotic syndrome significantly reduce the likelihood for a successful fetal outcome?

DIFFERENTIAL DIAGNOSIS OF RENAL DISEASE IN PREGNANCY. Since the clinical hallmarks of preeclampsia, e.g., hypertension, proteinuria, and edema, are also manifested by most other types of renal parenchymal disease, a diagnostic evaluation cannot be based on these clinical features alone. Preeclampsia does not occur before the twenty-fourth week of gestation, except in hydatidiform mole or multiple gestation pregnancies. The differential diagnosis is therefore simplified if clinical signs of renal disease are known to exist prior to conception or in the early stages of pregnancy. In patients who are not observed until the last trimester of pregnancy, however, identification of the cause of renal dysfunction is often difficult. The renal biopsy finding of the pathognomonic changes of preeclampsia provides the only absolute method of confirming the diagnosis of toxemia. When it is necessary to establish the diagnosis, renal biopsy should be performed during the week immediately following delivery. During pregnancy, therefore, management in most cases must rely on a presumed clinical diagnosis. Since the clinical manifestations of preeclampsia usually resolve spontaneously within four to six weeks post partum, persistence of hypertension, proteinuria, or renal insufficiency strongly suggests a primary renal disease.

Information on the relative incidence of the various causes of hypertension and proteinuria during gestation has been reported in a large series of patients in whom the diagnosis was confirmed by renal biopsy performed within six days of delivery. In most of these patients a presumed diagnosis of preeclampsia was made during pregnancy. Among primigravidas the incidence of preeclampsia, primary renal disease, and hypertensive glomerulosclerosis was 83 per cent, 12 per cent, and 5 per cent, respectively. In multiparous patients, in contrast, preeclampsia occurred in only 38 per cent of patients, while renal disease accounted for 26 per cent of cases, and hypertensive renal disease for 24 per cent.

INFLUENCE OF PREGNANCY ON UNDERLYING RENAL DISEASE. Pregnancy does not significantly alter the course of preexisting primary renal disease due to either glomerular or tubulointerstitial injury. Although increased proteinuria, often to nephrotic levels, occurs in nearly one half of patients with a glomerulonephropathy, there is no constant relationship between pregnancy and long-term changes in glomerular filtration rate. In general, the course of renal disease in these patients follows the expected course defined by the underlying pattern of injury.

There is less information on the effect of pregnancy on renal disease associated with systemic disorders. Pregnancy in diabetic patients neither accelerates the onset of diabetic glomerulosclerosis nor alters the natural cause of renal disease in subjects with signs of renal dysfunction before conception. In contrast, pregnancy may adversely influence systemic lupus erythematosus (SLE), reflected in relapse and exacerbations of this disease in patients with an established diagnosis and a relatively high incidence of de novo onset of SLE during pregnancy and in the immediate postpartum period. In patients with no clinical signs of active SLE before pregnancy the course during pregnancy is relatively mild and the live birth rate is approximately 90 per cent. In contrast, about half of all patients with clinical evidence of active SLE at the time of conception have subsequent exacerbations, which are often severe and associated with increased fetal loss.

An increase in urinary protein excretion in subjects with glomerulonephropathies is common during pregnancy and frequently results in the clinical manifestations of nephrotic syndrome. Sodium retention usually tends to become more severe in the last trimester. In most cases the level of proteinuria spontaneously returns to pregestational levels after delivery. Low birth weight has been reported by some to correlate directly with low serum albumin levels, but this finding has not been found in all patient series. An increase in the rate of edema formation should be anticipated during the later stages of pregnancy in patients with moderate or severe proteinuria and can be blunted by the introduction of a diet with low sodium content. The use of diuretics in pregnancy is controversial because of the possible induction of reduced placental blood flow. Conservative measures including dietary measures and bed rest are preferred. The judicious use of natriuretic agents may be useful in patients who fail to respond to conservative measures and has not been shown to increase fetal death.

INFLUENCE OF RENAL DISEASE ON FETAL OUTCOME. In the absence of hypertension and severe renal insufficiency, e.g., serum creatinine greater than 2.0 mg per deciliter, the live birth rate is greater than 90 per cent in most patients with primary renal disease. Pregnancies associated with mild to moderate renal insufficiency, however, result in an increased rate of preterm delivery and small-for-gestational-age births. Severe renal insufficiency reduces the incidence of live births to 20 to 50 per cent. Since there is no evidence that pregnancy alters the natural course of primary renal diseases or most types of renal disease due to systemic disease, early termination of pregnancy is not indicated on medical grounds. Clinical management should include control of hypertension and careful monitoring of fetal growth to maximize the likelihood of fetal maturity at birth.

ACUTE RENAL FAILURE IN PREGNANCY

Acute renal failure during pregnancy results from severe injury to tubular epithelial cells due to renal ischemia or to the action of nephrotoxic agents (Ch. 74). The cell injury may be reversible, with an eventual complete restoration of renal function; it may be irreversible and lead to renal cortical necrosis. Renal cortical necrosis is characterized by the development of fibrosis within the cortex in a diffuse or patchy pattern, with relative sparing of the medullary portions of the kidney. Although cortical necrosis is uncommon in nonpregnant individuals, it is a frequent complication of obstetric conditions, especially in subjects beyond the age of 30 years and in association with abruptio placentae. It has been suggested that increased reactivity of the renal vasculature to vasoactive amines in pregnancy and local activation of coagulation may play an important role in the induction of tissue injury leading to cell death.

In addition to the usual causes of acute renal failure, some types of renal insults are unique to pregnancy. Septic abortion and hyperemesis gravidarum may cause renal failure in early pregnancy, while severe preeclampsia, placenta previa, and abruptio placentae are causative factors in the later stages of pregnancy. Clinical management of acute renal failure in pregnancy is comparable to that in nonpregnant patients (Ch. 77). Because of the reported high rate of fetal death, delivery should be performed as soon as the maternal condition has been stabilized and fetal maturity is ascertained. There is inadequate experience with dialysis treatment in gravid patients with acute renal failure to assess its possible usefulness.

Katz AI, Davison JM, Hayslett JP, Singson E, Lindheimer MD: Pregnancy in woman with kidney disease. Kidney Int 18:192, 1980. *An analysis of a large series of pregnancies associated with primary renal disease. An excellent source for references.*

Pritchard JA: Management of preeclampsia and eclampsia. Kidney Int 18:259, 1980. *A clear and concise description of the regimen used to treat toxemic women in obstetrical units.*

88. HEREDITARY CHRONIC NEPHROPATHIES

Wadi N. Suki

Several genetically transmitted renal disorders of unknown pathogenesis may fall under this heading. This chapter will discuss two of these disorders, Alport's syndrome and the nail-patella syndrome. Some hereditary disorders of renal tubular function are described in Chapter 83. Other genetic disorders that may be associated with renal disease are listed in Table 88–1.

ALPORT'S SYNDROME

DEFINITION. Also known as "chronic hereditary nephritis," this syndrome is characterized by the familial occurrence in successive generations of a progressive nephritis, more severe in males, manifested invariably by hematuria and frequently associated with a sensorineural hearing deficit.

GENETICS. The mode of transmission in most kindreds is consistent with autosomal dominant inheritance with discrepant penetrance in the two sexes, males being affected earlier and more severely than females. Male and female offspring of an affected female are at equal risk (1 in 2) for inheriting this disorder, whereas male offspring of an affected male are at a greatly reduced risk (1 in 8) compared to the female (1 in 2). Autosomal recessive and sex-linked dominant inheritance also have been described in certain kindreds, suggesting that this disorder may be genetically heterogeneous.

INCIDENCE AND PREVALENCE. Several hundred kindreds of all races and geographic origins have been described. While its exact incidence is unknown, Alport's syndrome accounts for nearly 5 per cent of patients with end-stage renal disease.

PATHOLOGY AND PATHOGENESIS. Early in the disease the kidneys may be normal or large in size, but they shrink with progression of the disease. Under light microscopy the glomeruli may be normal or show some hypertrophy of epithelial cells and increase in mesangial matrix. Later changes will consist of mesangial cell proliferation, thickening and splitting of capillary walls, thickening of Bowman's capsule, tubular cell atrophy, thickening and splitting of the tubular basement membrane, interstitial fibrosis, and the presence of foam cells. Electron microscopy characteristically reveals both thinning and irregular thickening of the glomerular and tubular basement membranes, with splitting of the lamina densa into several lamellae separated by lucent zones containing electron-dense round granulations.

The etiology and pathogenesis of Alport's syndrome are unknown. It has been speculated that an inherited abnormality of the noncollagenous glycopeptides of the glomerular basement membrane may be responsible for thinning and rupture followed by repair and focal thickening.

CLINICAL MANIFESTATIONS. By the age of six years the disease would have been discovered in 70 per cent of patients, the rest being discovered at any age thereafter up to and well into adulthood. Persistent or intermittent microscopic hematuria is universally present. Gross hematuria may occur in 60 per cent of patients, especially after exercise or respiratory infections. Proteinuria is present in 70 per cent of patients. It is usually mild but reaches the nephrotic range in 25 per cent of patients. Sensorineural hearing loss in the high frequency (4000 to 8000 Hz) range is observed in 40 to 60 per cent of patients, predominantly males. Its presence may require audiometric testing, but it may progress to clinical deafness. Ocular disorders, especially anterior and posterior lenticonus and spherophakia, are seen in 15 per cent of patients. The renal disease may be mild and nonprogressive, especially in women, or may progress with the development of azotemia and hypertension culminating in chronic renal failure and uremia. Progression occurs

TABLE 88–1. INHERITED RENAL DISEASES

- Disorders of Tubular Function
  - Proximal tubule
    - Cerebro-oculorenal syndrome of Lowe
    - Cystinosis (Fanconi's syndrome)
    - Cystinuria
    - Galactosemia
    - Glycogen storage (von Gierke's) disease
    - Glycinuria
    - Hartnup disease
    - Hepatolenticular degeneration (Wilson's disease)
    - Hereditary fructose intolerance
    - Hypophosphatemic vitamin D–resistant rickets
    - Iminoaciduria
    - Proximal renal tubular acidosis
    - Pseudohypoparathyroidism
    - Renal glucosuria
  - Distal/collecting tubule
    - Distal renal tubular acidosis
    - Nephrogenic diabetes insipidus
- Disorders of Renal Structure
  - Agenesis
  - Cystic disorders
    - Hepatocerebrorenal syndrome of Zellweger
    - Medullary sponge kidney
    - Medullary cystic disease
    - Polycystic kidney disease, adult type
    - Polycystic kidney disease, infantile type
    - Renal retinal dysplasia
  - Duplication
  - Renal malformations with extrarenal anomalies
- Biochemical Disorders
  - Alkaptonuria
  - Cystinosis
  - Diabetes
  - Glycosphingolipidosis (Fabry's disease)
  - Hepatolenticular degeneration (Wilson's disease)
  - Hyperuricemia
  - Oxalosis
  - Xanthine oxidase deficiency
- Systemic Disorders
  - Amyloidosis
  - Asphyxiating thoracic dystrophy (Jeune's disease)
  - Charcot-Marie-Tooth disease
  - Laurence-Moon-Biedl syndrome
  - Osteo-onychodysplasia (nail-patella syndrome)
- Hereditary Chronic Nephropathies
  - Benign recurrent hematuria
  - Hereditary chronic nephritis
  - Hereditary chronic nephritis with hyperprolinemia
  - Hereditary chronic nephritis with thrombocytopathy
  - Hereditary immune nephritis
  - Infantile nephrosis

predominantly in males, with a predilection to those with massive proteinuria, deafness, and lenticonus. Renal failure may occur in childhood or in adulthood, and in affected males usually before age 40 years. Affected females may experience decline of renal function during pregnancy.

In several kindreds patients with classic Alport's syndrome have been reported to have thrombocytopenia with giant platelets manifested clinically by bruising, epistaxis, and gastrointestinal bleeding, and in the laboratory by prolonged bleeding time. A few cases have also been associated with hyperprolinemia (Ch. 191).

DIAGNOSIS. The presence of progressive renal disease in one family member younger than age 50, other than the proband, and the presence of neural hearing loss in the patient or a relative, is the basis for the diagnosis of Alport's syndrome in a patient with hematuria with or without proteinuria, azotemia, or hypertension. Differential diagnosis includes benign familial hematuria, a nonprogressive disorder characterized by a uniformly thin glomerular capillary basement membrane; and IgA nephropathy (Berger's disease), a glomerulonephritis with distinctive findings on light, electron, and especially immunofluorescent microscopic examination of the renal glomerulus. The audiometric findings, ocular manifestations, and family history, coupled with the changes in the glomerular and tubular basement membrane, usually should distinguish Alport's syndrome from other renal disorders.

TREATMENT. There is no specific treatment for Alport's syndrome, and no therapy is known to alter its course. Only conventional management of progressive renal disease is available. Peritoneal dialysis or hemodialysis and related or cadaveric donor kidney transplantation have been utilized with degrees of success at least matching those in other renal disorders. In fact, improvement of hearing deficit has been reported after renal transplantation.

NAIL-PATELLA SYNDROME

An autosomal dominant trait also known as osteo-onychodysplasia, this disorder of mesenchymal tissue is characterized by atrophic or absent fingernails, hypoplasia or aplasia of the patella, accessory conical iliac horns, thickening of the scapula, and subluxation of the radial heads at the elbow. In 40 per cent of patients the kidneys may be involved, as manifested by mild proteinuria and rarely hematuria. Occasionally the nephrotic syndrome and progression to renal failure (27 per cent) may be observed. Light microscopy shows glomerular cellular proliferation, mesangial sclerosis, and basement membrane thickening. Electronmicroscopy reveals areas of rarefaction in the lamina densa of the glomerular basement membrane filled with bundles of curvilinear fibrils having the typical periodicity of collagen. No specific therapy exists for this disorder. Renal transplantation has been carried out without evidence of recurrence of the disease in the transplanted organ.

Bennett WM, Musgrave ME, Campbell RA, Elliott D, Cox R, Lovrien EW, Beals RK, Porter GA: The nephropathy of the nail-patella syndrome. Am J Med 54:304, 1973. *A good description of the renal disorder in the nail-patella syndrome.*

Guhler C, Levy M, Broyer M, Naizot C, Gonzales G, Perrin D, Habib R: Alport's syndrome. A report of 58 cases and a review of the literature. Am J Med 70:493, 1981. *An excellent review of the clinical and histologic features of Alport's syndrome in children.*

89. RENAL CALCULI

Charles Y. C. Pak

DEFINITION. Renal calculi (kidney stones, nephrolithiasis) are abnormal concretions occurring in the kidneys, consisting of crystalline components and an organic matrix. They are typically located within the calyces or pelvis and may become lodged in the ureter or bladder as they are passed. Nephrolithiasis should be differentiated from nephrocalcinosis, calcification of renal parenchyma. Stones originating in the bladder (bladder stones) are rare in industrialized countries, although they were common in antiquity and are still frequent in certain countries in Southeast Asia.

Nephrolithiasis affects 0.1 to 1 per cent of the population, with a recurrence rate in afflicted individuals of 50 to 80 per cent. Calcareous (calcium-containing) renal stones account for 80 to 95 per cent of stones and are principally composed of calcium oxalate and calcium phosphate, usually occurring as mixtures. The remaining stones are composed of uric acid, cystine, magnesium ammonium phosphate (struvite), and rarely xanthine (Table 89–1).

ETIOLOGY AND PATHOGENESIS. Renal stones form by an initial crystallization of a nidus (termed nucleation) from a supersaturated urine with subsequent crystal growth and aggregation of the nidus into a macroscopic stone. Kidney stones are not simply masses of crystals. They usually have an organic matrix that gives form, cohesiveness, and sometimes a remarkably regular structure to the stone (Fig. 89–1). At the present time abnormalities in the amount or composition of stone matrix have not been demonstrated to be important in stone pathogenesis. It is impossible to dissolve the amounts of calcium, oxalate, and phosphate present in normal urine in 1 or 2 liters of distilled water. Obviously, therefore, there are substances present in normal urine that impede crystallization and sustain supersaturation. These normal inhibitors are not fully characterized but seem to include pyrophosphate, magnesium, citrate, and certain organic macromolecules (such as glycosaminoglycans).

All patients with stones are presumed to have some physiologic derangement that makes them susceptible to stone formation, although no cause can be demonstrated by current techniques in 5 per cent of patients. These derangements alter urinary concentration of stone-forming constitutents and of inhibitors to cause supersaturation and facilitated nucleation, crystal growth, and aggregation (Table 89–2). Supersaturation of crystalloids can result from (1) too little urine output (a concentrated urine) or (2) an absolute increase in the amount of a stone constituent excreted over a period of time. Most attention has been directed toward metabolic abnormalities that increase the amount of stone constituents in urine.

There are other factors that may be important in stone pathogenesis beyond the concentration of the stone crystalloid in the urine: (1) *Urine pH.* The formation of a stone may be acutely dependent on pH (uric acid, magnesium ammonium phosphate), moderately so (calcium phosphate, cystine), or essentially independent (calcium oxalate). (2) *Stasis.* Most embryonic stones are probably harmlessly washed out in the urine. Stasis allows time for the nascent stone to grow. (3) *Reduction in the concentration of inhibitors of crystallization in the urine.* This may be of great importance, and indirect methods have been described to define an increased tendency toward crystallization at given concentrations of calcium, oxalate, and phosphate in the urine of stone formers. Hypocitruria has now been directly measured as a contributing cause of stones. (4) *Heterogeneous nucleation.* Crystallization may begin in a supersaturated solution that is seeded with a crystal of a different (heterogeneous) composition but one that has an analogous

TABLE 89–1. COMPOSITION OF RENAL STONES

Type	Percentages
Calcium oxalate	70
Calcium phosphate	10
Hydroxyapatite	
Brushite	
Tricalcium phosphate	
Carbonate apatite	
Magnesium ammonium phosphate	5–10
Uric acid	<5
Cystine	1
Xanthine	<1

Some stones occur as mixtures. Percentages are calculated for the predominant stone types.

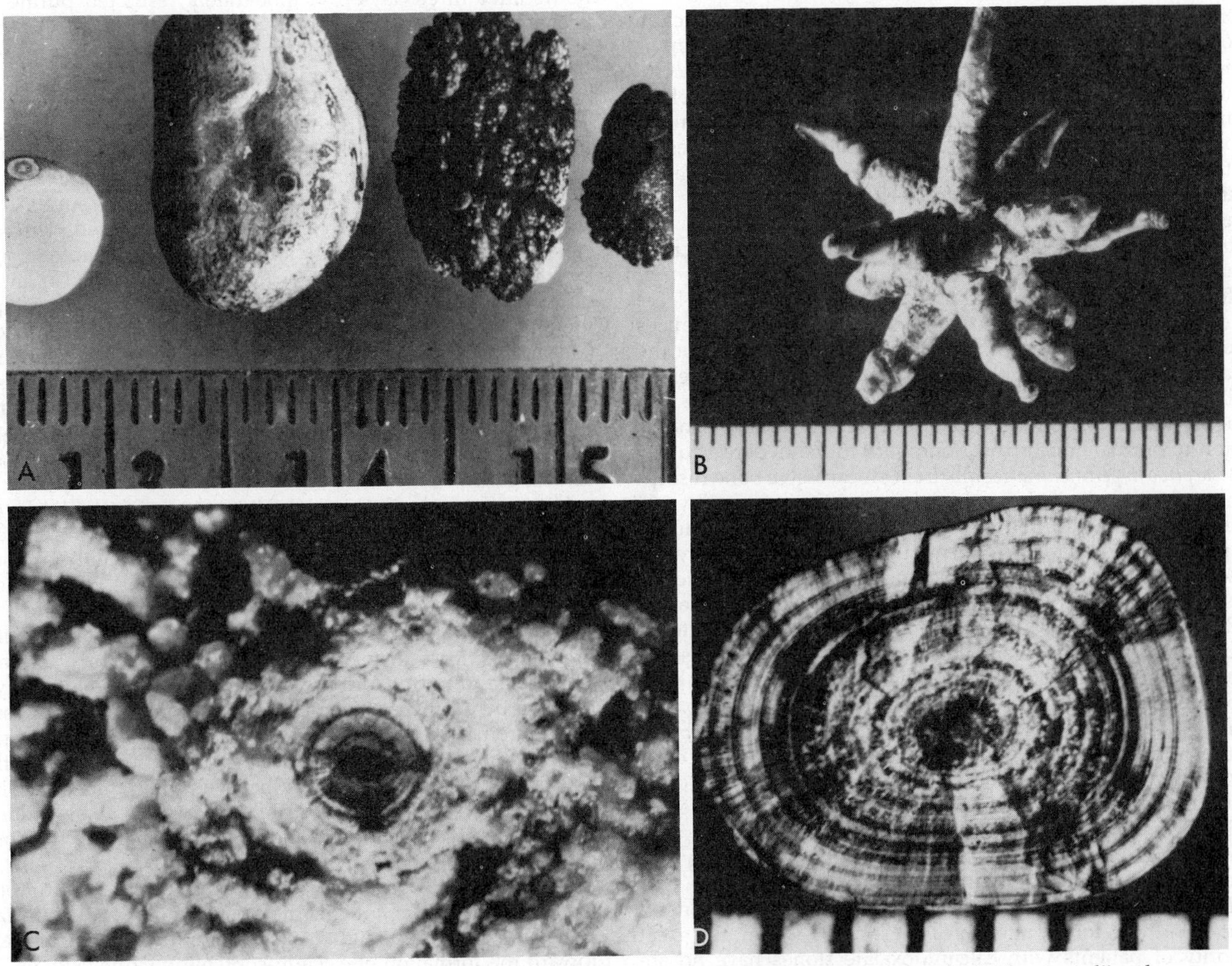

Figure 89–1. Gross appearance of selected kidney stones. *A,* Calcium oxalate monohydrate calculi ("hempseed" and "mulberry"). *B,* Calcium oxalate monohydrate "jackstone." *C,* Central nucleus of calcium oxalate monohydrate, intermediate zone of calcium oxalate monohydrate and apatite, and outer coarse crystals of magnesium ammonium phosphate. *D,* Alternating light and dark laminations and central nucleus of a pure urine acid stone. (From Prien EL, Prien EL Jr: Composition and structure of urinary stone. Am J Med 45:654, 1968, with permission.)

surface topography. This process of one crystal growing on the surface of another is known as epitaxy. Many stones are mixed in composition and perhaps represent epitaxial growth. Of greatest practical importance, however, calcium oxalate crystals can be nucleated by uric acid or sodium hydrogen urate crystals. This is the presumed cause of the calcium oxalate stone diathesis associated with hyperuricosuria (see below).

TABLE 89–2. PATHOGENESIS OF NEPHROLITHIASIS

Cause	Percentage of Patients with Stones	Sex Predominance
Idiopathic hypercalciuria		
Absorptive hypercalciuria	40–60	Male
Renal hypercalciuria	5–15	Equivalent
Primary hyperparathyroidism	4–10	Female
Hyperoxaluria		
Primary	Rare	Equivalent
Enteric	2	Equivalent
Hyperuricosuric calcium oxalate nephrolithiasis	10–40	Male
Hypocitraturia	15–40	Male
Renal tubular acidosis	1	Equivalent
Uric acid lithiasis	<5	Male
Cystinuria	1	Equivalent
Infection (struvite stones)	<10	Female
No metabolic cause found	5	Male

Hypercalciuria. As noted, calcium is a constituent of 80 to 95 per cent of kidney stones. Hypercalciuria is the single most frequent abnormality found in patients with stone diathesis. Hypercalciuria is often statistically defined and varies with body size and diet. In general the normal upper limit for urinary calcium is 300 mg per day on a diet containing 1000 mg of calcium per day (some use a figure of 4 mg per kilogram per day), and 200 mg per day on a diet with a daily composition of 400 mg of calcium and 100 mEq of sodium (urinary calcium tends to parallel urinary sodium so that dietary sodium should ideally be controlled). Hypercalciuria can result from (1) enhanced absorption from dietary sources, (2) primary renal wastage with secondary enhanced absorption, or (3) excessive resorption from storage in bone. These different forms will be discussed briefly.

Absorptive hypercalciuria, the most common abnormality, is encountered in 40 to 60 per cent of patients with kidney stones. Increased absorption of dietary calcium may rarely occur from excessive ingestion of milk and other dairy products, from vitamin D excess (Ch. 244), or from the altered vitamin D metabolism associated with sarcoid (Ch. 67). Absorptive hypercalciuria usually refers, however, to a primary idiopathic increase in intestinal absorption of calcium. The disorder (or disorders) tends to be familial. The consequent rise in serum calcium concentration tends to suppress parathyroid function. Hypercalciuria ensues from the increased renal filtered load of calcium and the reduced renal tubular reabsorption of calcium associated with parathyroid suppression. Serum calcium is typically maintained within the normal range because of compensatory hypercalciuria. Some patients may show hypophosphatemia and high serum 1,25-dihydroxyvitamin D (hypophosphatemic absorptive hypercalciuria). It has been suggested that the enhanced renal synthesis of 1,25-dihydroxyvitamin D resulting from renal phosphate "leak" accounts for the enhanced intestinal absorption of calcium.

Renal hypercalciuria, as a form of "idiopathic hypercalciuria," occurs less commonly than absorptive hypercalciuria and originates from an impaired renal tubular reabsorption (renal leak) of calcium. The ensuing decline in serum calcium causes secondary hyperparathyroidism, which in turn stimulates the renal synthesis of 1,25-dihydroxyvitamin D. Thus, the skeletal mobilization and intestinal absorption of calcium may be secondarily increased, effects that restore serum calcium concentration to normal and further contribute to the hypercalciuria.

Resorptive hypercalciuria results from an excessive bone resorption, most commonly from the hypersecretion of parathyroid hormone. Four to 10 per cent of all kidney stones are caused by primary hyperparathyroidism (Table 89–2); conversely, 10 to 40 per cent of patients with primary hyperparathyroidism present with renal stones. The hypercalcemia of hyperparathyroidism causes hypercalciuria by augmenting the renal filtered load of calcium. The intestinal calcium absorption may also be increased secondarily, consequent to parathyroid hormone–dependent stimulation of the synthesis of 1,25-dihydroxyvitamin D; this increased calcium absorption further contributes to the hypercalciuria. Hypercalciuria secondary to net bone resorption is also seen in thyrotoxicosis, multiple myeloma, pseudohyperparathyroidism of malignancy, metastatic diseases of bone, and immobilization (acute osteoporosis) and with spontaneous or iatrogenic Cushing's syndrome. In only the latter two syndromes are kidney stones common.

Hyperoxaluria. Oxalate is the second most common constituent of kidney stones, after calcium (Table 89–1), but the great majority of patients with calcium oxalate stones have no abnormality of oxalate metabolism. Sustained hyperoxaluria, which may be defined as the excretion of greater than 60 mg of oxalate per 1.73 M^2 per 24 hours, occurs only (1) in primary hyperoxaluria, two rare genetic disorders described in Ch. 182, (2) in pyridoxine deficiency, (3) rarely with excessive ingestion of ascorbic acid, and (4) from enhanced absorption of dietary oxalate, termed enteric hyperoxaluria.

Enteric hyperoxaluria, which is encountered in approximately 2 per cent of patients with stones, occurs typically in patients with ileal disease (ileal resection, jejunoileal bypass surgery, inflammatory disease of the small bowel). In ileal disease in which there is malabsorption of fat, intraluminal content of divalent cations, particularly calcium, may be reduced by being bound to unabsorbed fatty acids. Thus, calcium is not normally available to bind and limit oxalate absorption. The resulting enlarged free intestinal oxalate pool increases absorption and renal excretion of oxalate. Oxalate absorption may be stimulated primarily as well, especially in the colon, since patients with ileostomies do not have hyperoxaluria. Low urine volume (from an excessive intestinal loss of fluid) and defective urinary inhibitor activity (from an impaired renal excretion of citrate and magnesium) probably contribute to calcium stone formation in ileal disease.

In hypercalciuria associated with increased calcium absorption (e.g., absorptive hypercalciuria), a mild increase in oxalate excretion to the higher ranges of normal may be found (up to 50 mg per day). The total amount of oxalate absorbed from the gut may be high because more calcium is absorbed and less calcium is available intraluminally to bind oxalate.

Uric Acid Stones. Approximately two thirds to three fourths of the uric acid synthesized in the body is excreted in the urine. The rest is excreted in the intestine and largely destroyed by bacterial degradation. Uric acid excretion varies widely with diet. Urinary values greater than 600 mg per 1.73 M^2 per 24 hours after three days of a moderately restricted purine diet probably represent endogenous overproduction. In the study of patients with kidney stones it is more important to measure uric acid excretion on the patient's usual diet. Here an excretion of >750 mg for women and >800 mg for men would be considered abnormally high.

Uric acid stones usually form in urines with a pH of less than the dissociation constant for uric acid (5.5), especially when there are absolute increases in uric acid (hyperuricosuria). Thus, the amount of urinary free uric acid is increased. Uric acid stones often occur in primary gout, which may be accompanied by low urinary pH and hyperuricosuria (Ch. 195), or in secondary causes of purine overproduction, such as myeloproliferative states, glycogen storage disease, and malignancy. Chronic diarrheal syndromes (ulcerative colitis, regional enteritis, jejunoileal bypass surgery) may cause uric acid stones by inducing net alkali deficit and lowering urine volume (thereby reducing urinary pH and augmenting urinary concentration of uric acid). Most patients with uric acid stones do not have clinical gout.

Hyperuricosuric Calcium Oxalate Stone Diathesis. Hyperuricosuria may be the only discernible biochemical abnormality associated with calcium oxalate stones (10 per cent), although it often coexists with hypercalciuria (30 per cent). Most patients with hyperuricosuric calcium oxalate nephrolithiasis do not suffer from clinical gout. The hyperuricosuria is usually dietary in origin, since a history of high purine intake may often be disclosed and normal urinary uric acid excretion values may be restored by purine restriction. Less commonly, hyperuricosuria results from a primary overproduction of uric acid. The urinary pH typically exceeds 5.5, so that dissociated urate rather than uric acid predominates. It is believed that urates facilitate crystallization of calcium oxalate, either directly by inducing heterogeneous nucleation or indirectly by removing macromolecular inhibitors through adsorption.

Hypocitruria. Citrate, alone or as a complex with other urinary components, inhibits the crystallization of calcium salts. Thus, hypocitruria would be expected to increase the tendency toward the formation of calcium-containing kidney stones. The normal range of urinary excretion of citrate is 300 to 1100 mg per day. Hypocitruria is encountered in renal tubular acidosis and enteric hyperoxaluria owing to reduced renal synthesis or increased tubular reabsorption of citrate and in infection from bacterial degradation of citrate. It is also often found with other causes of calcium nephrolithiasis (10 to 45 per cent) and may occur as the sole abnormality (5 per cent). The cause for hypocitruria often remains unknown.

Renal Tubular Acidosis. Although more commonly associated with nephrocalcinosis, distal (Type I) renal tubular acidosis may present with nephrolithiasis. The cause for stone formation is multifactorial and probably includes hypercalciuria (from induced renal leak of calcium by acidosis), enhanced dissociation of phosphate, an increased saturation of calcium phosphate (from high urinary pH), and an impaired inhibitor activity (from defective excretion of citrates). Renal tubular acidosis is described in greater detail in Ch. 83.2.

Cystinuria. A cystine kidney stone forms only in a patient with the genetic disorder cystinuria (Ch. 83.3). Other forms of amino aciduria are not associated with the excretion of enough cystine to form stones. Cystinuria is characterized by a disturbance in renal and intestinal handling of lysine, arginine, ornithine, and cystine. Stone formation, occurring in a minority of patients with cystinuria, is the result of an excessive renal excretion of cystine and its low solubility in urine. Cystine solubility is pH dependent; at pH 5, 300 mg of cystine may be dissolved in each liter of urine, whereas at pH 7.5, 500 mg of cystine may go into the solution. Many patients with cystinuria excrete substantially more than 300 mg of cystine per day.

Infection. Urinary tract infections with urea-splitting organisms may be associated with renal stones of struvite (magnesium ammonium phosphate) and varying amounts of calcium phosphate. Ammonia formed by enzymatic degradation of urea by bacterial urease undergoes hydration to form ammonium and hydroxyl ions. The resulting alkalinity of urine augments dissociation of phosphate to form more triphosphate ions and reduces the solubility of struvite. Thus, the urinary environment becomes supersaturated with respect to struvite. Although struvite stones may form de novo from infection alone, they may sometimes occur as a complication of other causes of renal calculi, such as hypercalciuria. The presence of a struvite stone is presumptive evidence for concurrent or previous urinary tract infection.

Idiopathic Stone Diathesis. In approximately 5 per cent of patients, *no metabolic cause* may be discerned. In some patients, low urine volume because of disdain for drinking fluids may contribute to stone formation. Nephrolithiasis may also be found in association with *renal structural abnormalities,* such as ectopic kidney, polycystic kidney, and horseshoe kidney. In this situation it is generally believed that stones, usually composed of struvite or calcium phosphate, form secondarily to urinary tract infection. Medullary sponge disease is often associated with calcareous renal calculi. There is no convincing evidence that the structural abnormality causes stone formation, since metabolic abnormalities (such as the three forms of hypercalciuria) are usually disclosed in medullary sponge disease, in similar distribution to that of patients without this disease.

CLINICAL MANIFESTATIONS. Patients with renal stones may be asymptomatic; may pass small, sandlike concretions with relatively little pain; or may experience severe symptoms from ureteral obstruction, localized trauma, or infection. Renal colic is the manifestation of ureteral spasm produced by the irritation of a stone and accompanying obstruction. Microscopic hematuria is almost invariably present; gross hematuria, even clots, may sometimes accompany renal colic. Pain may begin in the costovertebral angle or the flank and may migrate toward the groin; sometimes pain moves into and may be most severe in the testis or penis in the male. Pain may subside after the stone or clot has passed, but the process may take several hours, even days, if the stone is impacted or if ureteral swelling impedes migration. Women frequently report that the pain of renal colic is more severe than that of labor. Infection arising from stones may lead to fever, flank tenderness, dysuria, and frequency of urination.

DIAGNOSIS. ***Initial Screen.*** The first step in the diagnosis of the cause of a kidney stone is to secure the stone for analysis, if at all possible. The analysis should preferably be carried out by a crystallographic technique, which can sometimes reveal the sequence of stone formation from the central nidus to the periphery.

All patients with renal stones should have a careful history, abdominal roentgenographic examination, urinalysis and culture, and a routine blood screen.

A positive family history of renal calculi suggests absorptive hypercalciuria or, more rarely, cystinuria, primary hyperoxaluria, or Type I renal tubular acidosis. Absorptive hypercalciuria should be suspected in middle-aged white men who have a history of recurrent calcium-containing stones and a family history of renal stones. Renal hypercalciuria may be present in patients with a history of recurrent urinary tract infection, especially if the infection preceded the onset of the stone disease. A high calcium diet may aggravate the stone disease in those with an intestinal hyperabsorption of calcium. Patients with gout may form stones of either uric acid or calcium oxalate. A history of chronic diarrhea, ileal disease, or intestinal surgery should arouse the suspicion of uric acid or calcium oxalate stones (enteric hyperoxaluria). A high purine intake may cause hyperuricosuria and contribute to stone formation in hyperuricosuric calcium oxalate nephrolithiasis. Acetazolamide may impair renal acidification and cause formation of calcium phosphate stones. Excessive ingestion of vitamin D and of oxalate-rich foods (such as spinach and brewed tea) may increase oxalate excretion.

Calcium-containing stones, struvite stones, and cystine stones are radiopaque. Uric acid stones and the rarely encountered xanthine and 2,8-dihydroxyadenine stones are radiolucent (see Ch. 196). A staghorn calculus suggests a cystine or struvite stone. Positive urine culture for *Proteus, Pseudomonas, Klebsiella,* or *Staphylococcus* in association with an alkaline urine indicates that the stone is probably struvite. On a routine blood screen, primary hyperparathyroidism is suggested by hypercalcemia and hypophosphatemia (Ch. 246); hypophosphatemic absorptive hypercalciuria by normocalcemia and hypophosphatemia; and defective acidification by the electrolyte picture of hyperchloremic metabolic acidosis.

In-Depth Evaluation. The objective of in-depth evaluation, applicable particularly to those with recurrent calculi, is to discern the specific metabolic cause for the nephrolithiasis. Ideally, it should include a measure of parathyroid function (serum immunoreactive parathyroid hormone); 24-hour urinary calcium (on defined diets with respect to calcium and sodium intake); 24-hour urinary calcium, oxalate, uric acid, citrate, total volume, and pH (on random diets); and a measure of renal tubular reabsorption and intestinal absorption of calcium (from urinary calcium during fasting and following excessive oral ingestion of calcium). Hypercalciuria should be defined with respect to the particular diet during which urinary calcium is determined as noted above. If the stone is not known to be calcium containing, a qualitative test for urine cystine is indicated.

The nature of parathyroid function distinguishes the three forms of *hypercalciuria.* Primary hyperparathyroidism is suggested by parathyroid stimulation in the setting of hypercalcemia, absorptive hypercalciuria by normal or suppressed parathyroid function with normocalcemia and hypercalciuria, and renal hypercalciuria by parathyroid stimulation with normocalcemia and hypercalciuria. Fasting urinary calcium is invariably increased in renal hypercalciuria and is frequently elevated in primary hyperparathyroidism, whereas it is typically normal in absorptive hypercalciuria. Intestinal calcium absorption is always increased in absorptive hypercalciuria and is often high in renal and resorptive hypercalciurias.

In *enteric hyperoxaluria,* urinary calcium is typically low (<100 mg per day) and urinary oxalate high (often >100 mg per day). Serum calcium and magnesium may be low, parathyroid function may be stimulated, metabolic acidosis may be present, and urinary citrate is low (<100 mg per day).

Urinary uric acid consistently exceeds 600 mg per day and pH is greater than 5.5 in *hyperuricosuric calcium oxalate nephrolithiasis.* Urinary pH is usually low (<5.5) *in uric acid lithiasis* and high (>7) in *struvite* lithiasis. Urine pH is inappropriately high (>6) in Type I *renal tubular acidosis.*

TREATMENT. Kidney stones are heterogeneous in pathogenesis and not infrequently are manifestations of a generalized multisystem disorder. By and large kidney stones cannot be treated medically in the sense of causing their dissolution. The goal of treatment is to stop growth or new formation of stones by correcting the specific underlying physicochemical and physiologic derangements. Stone prophylaxis often entails a prolonged program. It is particularly important, therefore, to ensure patient compliance, few complications, and reasonable costs.

General Treatment. The initial treatment program, applicable to all patients with renal calculi, consists of a high fluid intake to assure a minimum urine volume of 2 liters per day. At least 3 liters of fluids should be drunk each day, distributed throughout the day. In general, any fluid (with the exception of milk and oxalate-rich tea in certain disorders to be enumerated) may be consumed. In patients with intestinal hyperabsorption of calcium, dairy products and certain calcium-rich foods should be avoided. Oxalate intake should be restricted in patients with enteric hyperoxaluria. An excessive dietary intake of sodium should be discouraged, since this may enhance calcium excretion. Urinary tract infection should be vigorously treated.

Activity of Stone Diathesis. As noted, as many as 1 per cent of the population may have a kidney stone at some time. Some patients, usually men, have a single calcium oxalate stone in middle life and are not subsequently affected. Clearly it would not be wise to begin a lifetime program of pharmacologic intervention without some knowledge of the prognosis of the stone diathesis in the individual patient. In the absence of remediable disorders, such as primary hyperparathyroidism, it is often wise following a first stone episode to institute the general measures noted above and then to follow patients carefully with sequential radiographs to document whether new stones are forming or old stones enlarging before more vigorous measures are instituted.

Specific Medical Treatment. Specific programs may be required when the aforementioned conservative measures are ineffective in controlling stone formation and there is continued activity of stone diathesis.

Treatment of Hypercalciuria. The surgical removal of abnormal parathyroid tissue is clearly the treatment of choice for kidney stones secondary to the hypercalciuria of primary hyperparathyroidism. Following parathyroidectomy, serum 1,25-dihydroxyvitamin D, intestinal calcium absorption , and urinary calcium decline toward normal. Parathyroidectomy may also ameliorate the extrarenal manifestations of primary hyperparathyroidism, such as bone disease and peptic ulcer disease (Ch. 99). Similarly, the hypercalciuria of vitamin D excess, sarcoid, thyrotoxicosis, multiple myeloma, and malignancies and the acute osteoporosis of immobilization may respond to specific therapies directed to those systemic entities. Most frequently, however, the problem remains as to how to reduce urine calcium in the group of disorders known collectively as idiopathic hypercalciuria. Several agents that have proved to be useful will be individually discussed.

Thiazides (and related compounds such as chlorthalidone) are unique among diuretics in their ability to augment the renal tubular reabsorption of calcium and therefore to reduce urinary calcium. At a dosage of hydrochlorothiazide of 50 mg twice a day, or an equivalent amount of related drugs, thiazides represent the treatment of choice for renal hypercalciuria. Thiazides correct the renal leak of calcium and thereby reverse the sequence of parathyroid hyperactivity, increased synthesis of 1,25-dihydroxyvitamin D, and enhanced absorption of intestinal calcium. The urinary saturations of calcium oxalate and calcium phosphate are reduced. The efficacy of thiazides is shown in Figure 89–2. Thiazides are equally effective in the control of absorptive hypercalciuria. Although the reduction in urinary calcium has not been shown to be followed by an appropriate fall in intestinal calcium absorption, there is no substantive evidence for osteosclerosis or soft tissue calcification. However, thiazides should not be used in resorptive hypercalciuria, because they may provoke hypercalcemia. Hypokalemia secondary to thiazides should be treated, because it may cause hypocitraturia and lower urinary inhibitor activity. There is recent evidence that amiloride, a potassium-sparing diuretic, may share the hypocalciuric action of thiazide.

Sodium cellulose phosphate should be used only in patients with normophosphatemic absorptive hypercalciuria in whom hypercalciuria cannot be controlled by dietary calcium restriction. When given orally, it forms a nonabsorbable complex with calcium that is then excreted in the feces. About 2.5 to 5 grams of this resin with each meal is sufficient to limit the amount of luminal calcium available for absorption and to restore normal urinary calcium. This reduces urinary saturation of calcium salts, particularly that of calcium phosphate, without overly stimulating parathyroid function or causing bone disease. Urinary oxalate may increase, because less calcium may be available intraluminally to complex oxalate, so that a moderate dietary restriction of oxalate is recommended. Oral magnesium supplementation should be provided, since this drug also binds magnesium. Sodium cellulose phosphate is contraindicated in primary hyperparathyroidism, in renal hypercalciuria, and in states of normal intestinal calcium absorption because of stimulating parathyroid function and producing or aggravating bone disease.

Orthophosphates, as neutral or alkaline soluble salts of sodium and/or potassium, are potentially absorbable from the intestinal tract, unlike sodium cellulose phosphate. When given orally (at a dosage of 1.5 to 2.0 grams of phosphorus per day), they decrease urinary calcium and increase urinary phosphate. They reduce urinary saturation of calcium oxalate, although they may increase that of calcium phosphate. Moreover, urinary inhibitor activity may be increased, probably consequent to the increased renal excretion of inhibitors, such as pyrophosphate and citrate. Orthophosphates are optimally indicated in the management of hypophosphatemic absorptive hypercalciuria, because of the possibility that they may compensate for the renal leak of phosphate and restore normal serum 1,25-dihy-

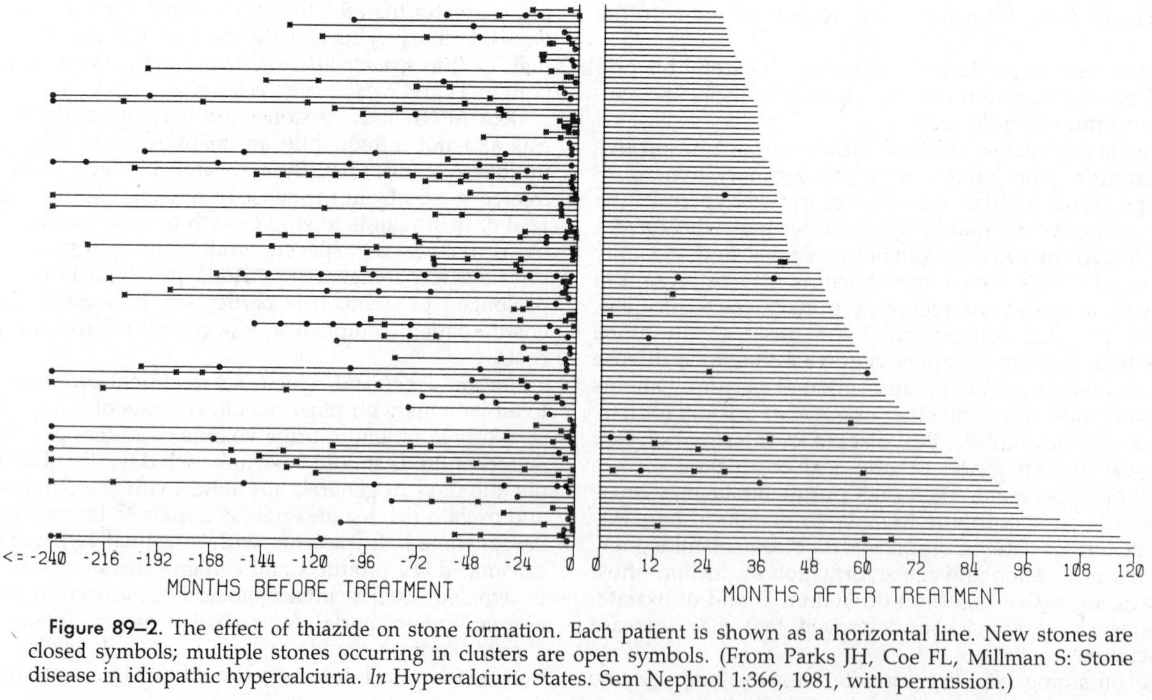

Figure 89–2. The effect of thiazide on stone formation. Each patient is shown as a horizontal line. New stones are closed symbols; multiple stones occurring in clusters are open symbols. (From Parks JH, Coe FL, Millman S: Stone disease in idiopathic hypercalciuria. *In* Hypercalciuric States. Sem Nephrol 1:366, 1981, with permission.)

droxyvitamin D and calcium absorption. They may also be useful in the management of normocalciuric patients who suffer from calcium-containing stones because of a presumed deficiency of urinary inhibitors. Orthophosphates are contraindicated in moderate or severe hypercalcemia and in renal failure because of the danger of metastatic calcification and in urinary tract infection because of the danger of struvite or calcium phosphate (hydroxyapatite or brushite) stone formation.

Treatment of Enteric Hyperoxaluria. Oral administration of large amounts of calcium or magnesium has been recommended for the control of nephrolithiasis of enteric hyperoxaluria. Although urinary oxalate may decrease, the concurrent rise in urinary calcium may obviate the beneficial effect of this therapy in some patients. Cholestyramine does not generally cause a sustained reduction in oxalate excretion. A limitation of dietary oxalate intake and alkali therapy may be helpful in lowering oxalate and increasing citrate in urine.

Treatment of Hyperuricosuric Calcium Oxalate Stone Diathesis. This form of hyperuricosuria usually results from a diet high in purine precursors of uric acid. It should therefore be subject to effective dietary therapy. Unfortunately many patients cannot or do not chose to maintain this dietary restraint. Allopurinol, 300 mg per day orally, will produce normal or subnormal levels of urinary uric acid and thereby may inhibit urate-induced crystallization of calcium oxalate.

Treatment of Renal Tubular Acidosis. In renal tubular acidosis, citrate or bicarbonate salt of sodium or potassium (60 to 120 mEq per day in divided doses) sufficient to correct the acidosis may reduce urinary calcium and augment citrate excretion, even though urinary pH remains elevated (see Ch. 83.2 for details).

Treatment of Uric Acid Stones. In uric acid stone diathesis, administration of bicarbonate or citrate may increase urinary pH and create an environment in which uric acid (as its sodium salt) is more soluble. Moderate amounts of alkali (40 to 60 mEq of bicarbonate per day in divided doses), sufficient to raise urinary pH to a range of 6 to 6.5, are recommended. Alkali therapy may be complicated by the formation of calcium stones, especially at high dosages. The potassium salt rather than sodium salt of bicarbonate or citrate may be preferable in preventing this complication. If hydration and alkali therapy are ineffective, allopurinol should be used to decrease uric acid stone formation. See the discussion in Ch. 195 on Gout for more details.

Treatment of Cystinuria (see Ch. 83.4). If a high fluid intake and alkali therapy are ineffective in reducing cystine concentration below saturation in cystinuria, *D-penicillamine* (2 grams per day in divided doses) may be required. This compound reduces urinary cystine content by forming a more soluble mixed disulfide with cysteine. Unfortunately, penicillamine treatment may be complicated by serious side effects, including nephrotic syndrome, dermatitis, and pancytopenia. An investigational drug, alpha-mercaptopropionylglycine, may exert similar action on cystine excretion, with apparent reduced toxicity.

Treatment of Struvite (Magnesium Ammonium Phosphate) Stones. If a longstanding effective control of infection with urea-splitting organisms can be achieved, there is some evidence that new struvite stone formation can be averted, or some dissolution of existing stones may be achieved. Unfortunately, such a control is difficult to obtain with antibiotic therapy alone. It is difficult to clear the infection completely from an existing struvite stone because the stone often harbors the organisms within its interstices. Even if sterilization of urine is achieved by antibiotic therapy, reinfection often occurs from harbored organisms. Addition of acetohydroxamic acid, a urease inhibitor, at a dosage of 250 mg three times per day, may be more effective in controlling struvite stone formation. If not, surgical removal of stones should be considered.

Treatment of Hypocitraturia. *Potassium citrate* (40 to 80 mEq per day in divided doses) may increase urinary citrate and inhibit crystallization of calcium salts in hypocitraturic calcium nephrolithiasis (occurring in the absence of obvious acidosis or infection).

SURGICAL TREATMENT. Surgical removal of stones may become mandatory when nephrolithiasis is complicated by obstruction or infection. When the obstructing stone is too large to pass, ureterolithotomy or pyelolithotomy may be required. Small stones in the ureter may be removed by a flexible "basket" passed retrograde. When the stone is the source of intractable infection, particularly by urea-splitting organisms, nephrolithotomy is generally recommended. Recently, less invasive surgical techniques have been introduced, including stone removal via percutaneous nephroscope, and extracorporeal shock wave lithotripsy.

Broadus AE, Insogna KL, Lang R, et al.: Evidence for disordered control of 1,25-dihydroxyvitamin D production in absorptive hypercalciuria. N Engl J Med 311:73, 1984. *New evidence about the pathogenesis of this most common cause of stone diathesis.*

Coe FL: Nephrolithiasis: Pathogenesis and Treatment. Chicago, Year Book Medical Publishers, 1978. *A detailed review of current concepts of cause and treatment of calcareous as well as noncalcareous stones.*

Coe FL: Prevention of kidney stones. Am J Med 71:514, 1981. *A succinct, thoughtful essay that explores the general approaches available to prevent stone formation.*

Millman S, Strauss AL, Parks JH, et al.: Pathogenesis and clinical course of mixed calcium oxalate and uric acid nephrolithiasis. Kidney Int 22:366, 1982. *A useful review of the intriguing and important interactions of uric acid and oxalate in stone pathogenesis.*

Pak CYC: Medical management of nephrolithiasis. J Urol 128:1157, 1982. *A description of selective treatment for different forms of calcium nephrolithiasis.*

Pak CYC, Britton F, Peterson R, Ward D, Northcutt C, Breslau NA, McGuire J, Sakhaee K, Bush S, Nicar M, Norman DA, Peters P: Ambulatory evaluation of nephrolithiasis. Classification, clinical presentation and diagnostic criteria. Am J Med 69:19, 1980. *A detailed description of the outpatient protocol that provides diagnostic criteria for different causes of nephrolithiasis.*

Pak CYC, Galosy RA: Propensity for spontaneous nucleation of calcium oxalate. Quantitative assessment for urinary FPR-APR discriminant score. Am J Med 69:681, 1980. *A detailed description of physiologic and physicochemical actions of various drugs available for control of stone formation.*

Sherrard DJ: Metabolic causes of nephrolithiasis. West J Med 138:541, 1983. *A useful general overview.*

90. CYSTIC DISEASES OF THE KIDNEY

Kenneth D. Gardner, Jr.

GENERAL CONSIDERATIONS

The renal cystic diseases are a group of heterogeneous disorders that share a single characteristic: cystic deformity of the kidney. They account for 10 per cent of all end-stage renal disease. They affect infants, children, adults, and the elderly. They do not always cause symptoms or signs. When a cause of morbidity, however, they usually present with one or more of the symptoms and signs listed in Table 90–1.

Their definitive diagnosis depends heavily on radiographic and sonographic techniques. Cysts as small as 0.3 to 0.5 cm, depending on location in the kidney, may be detected by modern sonographic and computer-assisted tomographic techniques (Fig. 90–1).

Biopsy, open or percutaneous, sometimes is used, but when cysts are sparse or deep within the kidney, it may yield cyst-free tissue. Neither negative radiographic studies nor negative renal biopsy results rule out renal cystic disease with 100 per cent reliability.

TABLE 90–1. FREQUENTLY ENCOUNTERED SYMPTOMS AND SIGNS AMONG THE RENAL CYSTIC DISEASES

Abdominal pain
Abdominal swelling
Palpable intra-abdominal mass(es)
Recurrent urinary tract infections
Hematuria (gross or microscopic)
Progressive renal failure
Anuria (rare)
Proteinuria<1 to 3 grams per day

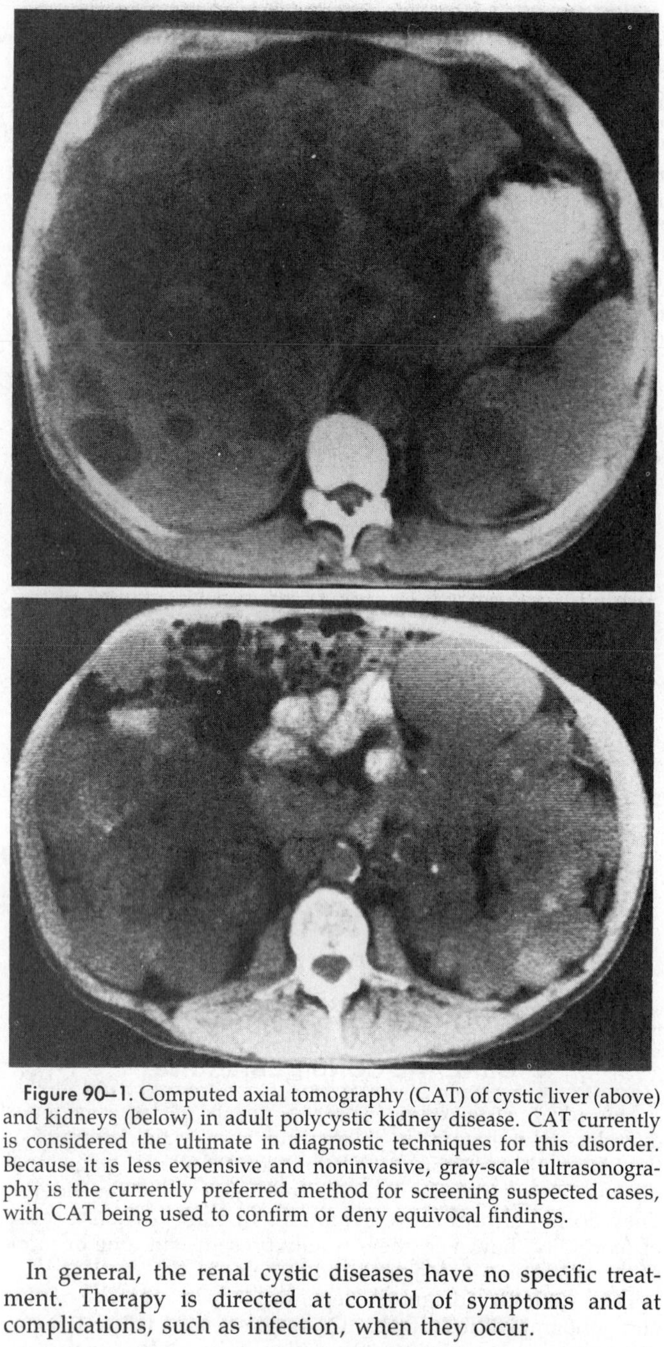

Figure 90–1. Computed axial tomography (CAT) of cystic liver (above) and kidneys (below) in adult polycystic kidney disease. CAT currently is considered the ultimate in diagnostic techniques for this disorder. Because it is less expensive and noninvasive, gray-scale ultrasonography is the currently preferred method for screening suspected cases, with CAT being used to confirm or deny equivocal findings.

In general, the renal cystic diseases have no specific treatment. Therapy is directed at control of symptoms and at complications, such as infection, when they occur.

CLASSIFICATION

A classification of renal cystic disease in seven major categories appears in Table 90–2. These categories include heritable, congenital, and acquired conditions. Seven renal cystic disorders are relatively common and will be considered here in some detail: infantile and adult polycystic kidney disease, the simple cyst, acquired renal cystic disease, medullary cystic disease, medullary sponge kidney, and multicystic dysplasia.

Bernstein J: A classification of renal cysts. *In* Gardner KD Jr (ed.): Cystic Diseases of the Kidney. New York, John Wiley & Sons, 1976, pp 7–30. *Genetic, anatomic, and clinical criteria are combined to form a scheme that has a place for virtually every form of cystic lesion in the human kidney.*

TABLE 90–2. CLASSIFICATION OF THE RENAL CYSTIC DISEASES*

I.	Polycystic disease (includes *recessive* and *dominantly inherited* forms)
II.	Renal cysts in hereditary syndromes
III.	*Simple cysts, solitary and multiple*
IV.	Segmental and unilateral cystic disease
V.	*Acquired cystic disease*
VI.	Renal medullary cysts (includes the *nephronophthisis–medullary cystic disease complex* and *medullary sponge kidney*)
VII.	Renal dysplasia (includes *congenital multicystic kidney*)

*After Bernstein J, Gardner KD Jr: *In* Harrison JH et al. (eds.): Campbell's Urology. 5th ed. Philadelphia, W. B. Saunders Company, in press.

POLYCYSTIC KIDNEY DISEASE

In polycystic disease, the kidneys are characterized by massive enlargement and diffuse cyst formation. When ages at onset are analyzed, two peaks are found. In the minority of cases, diagnosis is made at birth or during the first decade of life. In the majority of cases, illness appears between the fourth and sixth decades. These two forms of polycystic kidney disease are designated as *childhood* and *adult.* They are distinguished by genetic, morphologic, and clinical criteria.

Childhood Polycystic Disease

The incidence of childhood polycystic kidney disease (CPKD) is not known. Among live births, estimates of its occurrence range between 1 in 6000 and 1 in 14,000. It has appeared in from 1 in 225 to 1 in 450 autopsies.

CPKD is inherited as a recessive trait. The number of cases reported is relatively small.

Based on kindreds in which a specific constellation of clinical signs seems to breed true, four varieties of CPKD have been described: *perinatal, neonatal, infantile,* and *juvenile.* The four variants are distinguished from one another by the extent to which kidneys and liver are affected, by differences in the evolution of clinical symptoms and signs, and by the ages at which death occurs.

Renal cystic disease predominates in the *perinatal* form; death occurs in the first few weeks of life. Hepatic fibrosis and signs of portal hypertension predominate in the *juvenile* form; death may not occur until young adulthood. The *neonatal* and *infantile* variants are intermediate to these extremes.

These subtypes are not universally accepted. Some believe that there is but one condition in which the less serious the renal lesion, the more apt the individuals are to live until hepatic fibrosis becomes clinically significant. At present data are insufficient to settle this difference in opinion.

Microscopically the kidneys in CPKD show greatly dilated collecting tubules interspersed between wedges of normal renal parenchyma. In kidneys from patients who have survived several years, the dilated tubules assume a more rounded, typically cystic appearance.

CPKD should be distinguished from adult-onset polycystic kidney disease (APKD) and congenital multicystic kidney (CMK). Grossly the kidney in CPKD has a smooth, rather than bosselated, surface. When the organ is cut, one sees fusiform, radially oriented rather than round cysts on the cut surface. Kidneys with the appearance typical of APKD are found infrequently in children and infants, so age alone is not a valid discriminant. CMK is almost never familial, is often segmental or unilateral, and is a form of renal dysplasia.

Renal cysts may accompany congenital hepatic fibrosis. The cystic lesion is found in only half the cases, and is mild. The hepatic lesion is one of periportal fibrosis and bile duct proliferation. Again, because of a relative lack of experience, there is continuing disagreement as to whether these cases can or cannot be distinguished from CPKD.

Blyth H, Ockenden BG: Polycystic disease of kidneys presenting in childhood. J Med Genet 8:257, 1971. *A classic discussion, helpful to the understanding of this relatively uncommon lesion.*

Lieberman E, Salinas-Madrigal L, Gwinn JL, Brennan LP, Fine RN, Landing BH: Infantile polycystic disease of the kidneys and liver: Clinical, pathological and radiological correlations and comparison with congenital hepatic fibrosis. Medicine 50:277, 1971. *Arguments toward the concept that childhood polycystic disease is a single spectrum of clinical illness.*

Adult Polycystic Kidney Disease

DEFINITION AND INCIDENCE. Adult polycystic kidney disease (APKD) is the most common form of renal cystic kidney disease in adults, aside from the simple renal cyst. It appears once in every 500 autopsies and affects an estimated 300,000 people in the United States. It is responsible for renal failure in 10 per cent of patients coming to transplantation or dialysis. It is heritable, occurring as a mendelian dominant trait. Typically, renal function is normal during the first few decades of life. Renal failure is attributed to progressive cyst formation and appears during the fifth decade of life, with terminal renal failure ensuing over the next ten years.

EPIDEMIOLOGY. The pathologic lesion characteristic of APKD has been recognized for a century. Credit for recognizing its hereditary nature is extended to Cairns, a British urologist. Dalgaard has reported the largest number of families, 284, and his monograph remains the classic on APKD. Gene penetrance is 100 per cent by 80 years of age, meaning that if a genetically predisposed individual survives to that age, there is 100 per cent probability that polycystic kidneys will be present. In any affected family, renal failure tends to appear at about the same age. Heritable factors influence not only the morphologic characteristics of APKD but also the timing of its clinical evolution.

PATHOGENESIS AND PATHOLOGY. The pathogenesis of APKD is unknown. One early suggestion was that tubules in these kidneys were obstructed, either by "salts" of uric acid or by a failure of the two segments of nephrons to join properly during development of the kidney. Later studies demonstrated that most cystic nephrons in APKD are in communication with glomeruli and final urinary space, making obstruction a far less attractive pathogenetic possibility. More recently, partial, not total, tubular obstruction and altered compliance of tubular basement membrane have been suggested. Whatever the pathogenetic mechanism, it has its effect over time in genetically preconditioned kidneys that initially are grossly normal in structure and function.

The kidney from end-stage APKD is variably enlarged, sometimes to the size of an American football. Its surface is covered with countless cysts that are filled with yellow, white, brown, or black fluid. Microscopically, cysts appear to compress adjacent, otherwise normal renal tissue.

Analyses demonstrate that cystic contents have a composition that is characteristic of either proximal tubular or distal tubular fluid, suggesting that cyst walls continue to function.

CLINICAL MANIFESTATIONS. The classic clinical findings in APKD are a *positive family history, bilateral flank masses, elevated blood pressure,* and *uremia.* Flank pain is the earliest symptom. It begins months to years before detectable renal enlargement. Renal failure follows nephromegaly. This sequence of events—discomfort, then deformity, then dysfunction—and the impression one gets on microscopic evaluation that cysts are compressing normal renal tissue have given rise to the concept that cyst expansion is responsible for renal failure in APKD.

Patients come to the attention of physicians because of pain, bleeding, urinary tract infection, nephrolithiasis, or obstructive uropathy. Rarely an affected individual may present with anuria caused by expansion of strategically located cysts to the point that urinary outflow from otherwise functioning kidneys is obstructed.

Liver disease also occurs in APKD. However, it differs dramatically from the hepatic lesion of CPKD. Cyst formation, not hepatic fibrosis, can be demonstrated in up to 30 per cent of APKD cases. Rarely or never is there evidence of hepatic dysfunction. *Liver cysts* are demonstrated only because they are looked for by ultrasonography or radioisotopic scanning in known cases of APKD. Cysts in other organs also can be found, although their frequency is far less. In approximately 10 per cent of cases, *berry aneurysms* in the cerebral circulation are present. In a small percentage of cases cerebral vascular accidents occur.

DIAGNOSIS. Diagnosis of APKD rests on the clinical manifestations already discussed. The family history is positive for renal disease in 75 per cent of reported cases. Inattentiveness to history-taking, inadequate autopsy data, and new mutations are considered to account for failure to ascertain a positive family history in 100 per cent of cases. Depending on the stage of the disease, any degree of abnormality may be found on urinalysis or in the level of azotemia. Massive proteinuria (>3 grams per 24 hours) is rare and should raise the possibility of complicating disease or an alternative diagnosis. In many cases, anemia is not marked, possibly because the polycystic kidney retains significant erythropoietic capability. Renal sodium wasting and nephrolithiasis occur, but not with the severity or frequency seen in medullary cystic disease or sponge kidney.

APKD must be differentiated from hydronephrosis, pyelonephritis, renal neoplasm, and medullary sponge kidney. Sonographic and radiographic techniques will disclose bilateral massive cyst formation and enlarged kidneys in APKD. Because polycystic kidneys may be unusually susceptible to infection, retrograde pyelography is best avoided in making a diagnosis.

TREATMENT AND PROGNOSIS. Treatment is nonspecific and symptomatic. Renal transplantation and dialysis will prolong life once end-stage renal failure occurs. Genetic counseling is important. Because renal failure typically appears after the childbearing years, transmission of the condition from generation to generation is assured. All children of an affected individual are threatened by the specter of renal failure later in life, even though only one in every two on the average will actually be involved. Management of families with APKD requires participation of the physician, geneticist, social worker, surgeon, and often psychiatrist.

Dalgaard OZ: Bilateral polycystic disease of the kidneys: A followup study of 284 patients and their faimilies. Acta Med Scand 158 (Suppl 328), 1957. *An impressive clinical study, done by a young physician, and still the single most important piece of writing on the subject.*

Evan AP, Gardner KD Jr, Bernstein J: Polypoid and papillary epithelial hyperplasia: A potential cause of ductal obstruction in adult polycystic disease. Kidney Int 16:743, 1979. *Visual evidence supporting one hypothesis of the pathogenesis of this form of renal cystic disease.*

Grantham JJ: Polycystic kidney disease: A predominance of giant nephrons. Am J Physiol 244 (Renal Fluid Electrolyte Physiol 13):F3-F10, 1983. *An update on APKD from the viewpoint of the renal physiologist.*

Hartnett M, Bennett W: Extrarenal manifestations of cystic kidney disease. *In* Gardner KD Jr (ed.): Cystic Diseases of the Kidney. New York, John Wiley & Sons, 1976, pp 201–219. *An excellent review of the nonrenal complications.*

SIMPLE CYSTS

The renal cortex may be the site of single or multiple simple cysts. These are thin-walled structures that usually bulge from the surface of the kidney and contain a sterile, clear ultrafiltrate of plasma. Evidently, they arise as a degenerative process; they are common in the elderly and rare in the infant. They can reach prodigious size, but most frequently they are small, asymptomatic, and discovered incidentally during the course of urography or autopsy.

Simple renal cysts are of importance for at least two reasons. First, when multiple they may cause diagnostic confusion with the polycystic or multicystic kidney. Second, they may be the site of neoplasia.

Radiographically visible calcification in the wall of a simple renal cyst ("eggshell" calcification) is not reliable as evidence of a benign cystic lesion. Transcutaneous aspiration of a simple renal cyst, especially if its locaiton is near the lower pole, is a relatively easy, safe procedure and can help distinguish between simple cyst and cystic neoplasm. It should be performed only when pyelography or sonography has established the presence of a definitely cystic renal mass. It is especially useful in the elderly or the severely ill patient, for whom the risks of arteriography or surgery may be increased.

Characteristically, fluid from the simple cyst contains nonmalignant cells on cytologic examination, is straw colored, and has low concentrations of lactic dehydrogenase (LDH), protein, and fat. Necrotic or cystic neoplasms, in contrast, contain fluid in which malignant cells and blood may be evident and whose concentrations of fat and protein are high. When cyst fluid is bloody, the odds are roughly one in three that carcinoma is present. LDH concentrations are low in cystic malignancies but are high in the presence of inflammation.

After fluid removal, contrast medium may be injected into the cystic space. Simple cysts usually have a smooth wall and fill completely. Neoplastic cysts, in contrast, usually exhibit multiloculation, incomplete filling, and a shaggy or irregular lining.

Jackman RJ, Stevens GM: Benign hemorrhagic renal cysts. Radiology 110:7, 1974. *How the benign renal cyst differs from cystic renal malignancy.*

Lang EK, Johnson B, Chance HL, Enright JR, Fontenot R, Trichel BE, Wood M, Brown M, St. Martin EC: Assessment of avascular renal mass lesions: The use of nephrotomography, arteriography, cyst puncture, double contrast study and histochemical and histopathologic examination of the aspirate. South Med J 65:1, 1972. *The clinical approach to simple renal cysts and masses.*

Spence HM, Singleton R: Cysts and cystic disorders of the kidney: Types, diagnosis, treatment. Urol Survey 22:131, 1972. *Urologic view of renal cysts.*

Thornbury JR: Needle aspiration of avascular renal lesions. Correlation of contrast medium injection with cytologic and arteriographic diagnosis. Radiology 105:299, 1972. *More on cyst aspiraton and its interpretation.*

ACQUIRED RENAL CYSTIC DISEASE

In recent years a growing number of reports document the appearance of cysts in the previously noncystic kidneys of patients on long-term hemodialysis. A curiosity at first, acquired renal cystic disease now is emerging as a clinically significant, perhaps common, disorder. Prospective and retrospective studies from several countries describe its appearance in 30 to 50 per cent of patients maintained for three or more years on hemodialysis.

Clinically acquired cystic disease is not benign. Cysts may rupture or bleed spontaneously. More disturbing is the frequency with which neoplasia and malignant disease accompany the disorder. Ishikawa et al. examined kidneys from four individuals on dialysis for five or more years. All had cysts; three had adenocarcinoma, and multiple adenomas were found in the fourth. The index report of Dunnill and associates describes cysts in kidneys of 14 of 30 patients. Six of the 14 had tumors, multiple in five.

The signs of malignant change in the setting of acquired cystic disease are not specific: hematuria, pain, and asymmetric renal enlargement. The appearance of one more of these signs in the chronic dialysis patient should spur an aggressive search for renal malignancy by ultrasonography or CT scan.

Dunnill MS, Millard PR, Oliver D: Acquired cystic disease of the kidneys: A hazard of long-term intermittent maintenance haemodialysis. J Clin Pathol 30:868, 1977. *The cornerstone paper on this unsuspected complication of hemodialysis.*

Ishikawa I, Saito Y, Onouchi Z, et al.: Development of acquired cystic disease and adenocarcinoma of the kidney in glomerulonephritis chronic hemodialysis patients. Clin Nephrol 14(1):1–6, 1980. *Cyst formation and neoplasia occur at alarming rates among 94 Japanese dialysis subjects.*

NEPHRONOPHTHISIS–CYSTIC RENAL MEDULLA COMPLEX

DEFINITION. A characteristic appearance of the kidney in this disorder gives the complex its name. There is bilateral involvement. The kidneys are shrunken and scarred, and contain a variable number of small intramedullary and corticomedullary cysts. Microscopically, interstitial nephritis is present in varying degrees of severity. Signs and symptoms of the complex include a positive family history of anemia, renal salt-wasting, failure to thrive in children, and progressive renal failure.

INCIDENCE AND PREVALENCE. More than 300 examples of the complex have been reported. Not all are typical. Renal cysts are not described in some 15 per cent of cases. The family history is negative for renal disease in about 15 per cent. Renal salt-wasting has been documented in fewer than 25 patients, although it has not universally been sought. The anemia is not disproportionate to the degree of renal failure.

EPIDEMIOLOGY. Four variants of the complex are distinguished by genetic criteria: isolated cases, recessively inherited cases with or without retinal pathology, and dominantly transmitted disease. Sporadic cases may reflect the occurrence of the complex in an only child or a new mutation in the general population; or medullary cysts might occur as an acquired rather than a heritable trait in rare instances.

In approximately 50 per cent of reported patients the recessive mode of transmission appears most likely. There has been consanguineous mating in several families. Both sexes are equally involved. Self-selection among involved families may account for a ratio of greater than one affected to three unaffected siblings. This variant is called *familial juvenile nephronophthisis*.

Retinal pathology, typically retinitis pigmentosa, and recessive inheritance characterize an additional 17 per cent of reported cases. This variant of the complex is designated *renal-retinal dysplasia*.

In about 18 per cent of published cases, a dominant pattern of inheritance is documented. Consanguinity and retinal pathology have never been observed among these individuals. This variant is designated *adult-onset medullary cystic disease*.

Affected individuals with dominantly transmitted disease are significantly older at the times of onset of renal failure and death. Thus, as is the case in polycystic kidney disease, differing modes of inheritance are distinguished by differing ages at onset and death.

A defect in urinary concentrating ability has been reported among the parents or siblings of an affected individual on ten occasions. This evidence, tenuous as it is, raises the possibility that a heterozygous state of the complex exists.

PATHOGENESIS. Nothing is known of the pathogenesis of the complex. The disease has not recurred in transplanted kidneys, making it impossible to implicate a genetically determined, circulating, cystogenic nephrotoxin as its cause. Under light microscopy tubular atrophy, round cell infiltration, periglomerular fibrosis, and small noncortical cysts characterize the renal lesion. Involvement is always bilateral and symmetrical, even at the microscopic level. Microdissection reveals cyst formation along collecting tubules and loops of Henle but nowhere else along the nephron.

CLINICAL MANIFESTATIONS. Affected patients come to medical attention because of uremia or because the diagnosis has been made or is under consideration in a relative. Eighty per cent of patients describe nocturia, polyuria, polydipsia, or enuresis. Weakness, pallor, and disordered bone growth (in children) follow in descending order of frequency.

Hypertension is relatively infrequent, occurring in roughly one third of azotemic subjects. This low incidence may be due to subclinical salt-wasting, but such a phenomenon has not been established among these patients as a group. In some patients, renal salt-wasting may reach tremendous proportions, exceeding 250 mEq of sodium per day. Renal function may transiently improve in such individuals when salt and water deficits are replaced.

The earliest clinical sign of involvement may be diminution of maximal urinary concentrating ability. It has been described in six instances in which other evidence of the complex ultimately evolved. More experience is necessary before the value of this test as a diagnostic tool can be established. Hair color has been touted as a helpful sign in diagnosing affected cases. In one series, affected individuals had red or blond hair. Because most other case reports do not indicate hair color, the validity of this sign also remains in doubt.

Instances of the complex have been reported in patients with a horseshoe kidney, congenital hepatic fibrosis, and the Laurence-Moon-Biedl syndrome.

There are several negative features that distinguish the complex from other renal cystic disorders. Nephromegaly does not occur. Cyst formation is restricted to the kidneys; cysts (and aneurysms) are not found in other organs. Nephrocalcinosis and urolithiasis, with one exception, have not been reported. The urinalysis is remarkable for its lack of pathology, even in late uremia. Significant hematuria, proteinuria, cylindruria, and bacteriuria are unusual, so much so that when markedly abnormal urines are demonstrated repeatedly, alternative diagnoses should be considered.

DIAGNOSIS. Instances of the complex must be differentiated from all those conditions in which there is progressive azotemia and diminishing renal size. A family history that is positive for renal disease is helpful, more so if postmortem specimens of renal tissue from relatives disclose the typical lesion. Renal arteriography with tomography has been helpful in making antemortem diagnoses, although small cysts can be missed. Similarly, renal biopsy, open or closed, is diagnostic when interstitial nephritis and cysts are found. Because cysts lie deep in the kidney substance, however, it is the more common experience to remove renal tissue without cysts. One is left, then, with the lesion of interstitial nephritis and all the diagnostic possibilities that it intimates.

TREATMENT AND PROGNOSIS. Genetic counseling, hemodialysis, and renal transplantation offer hope for prevention and for prolongation of life among affected individuals. As with adult polycystic kidney disease, individuals affected because of dominantly inherited disease often have procreated before becoming ill. No reliable means currently exists to differentiate affected from nonaffected children in these kindreds.

Renal salt-wasting should be treated with salt and water in amounts sufficient to maintain adequate blood volume and optimal renal function. Appropriate antibiotics should be used to treat recurrent urinary tract infection, but there is no evidence that they slow progression of the disease.

Gardner KD Jr: Juvenile nephronophthisis and renal medullary cystic disease. *In* Gardner KD Jr (ed.): Cystic Diseases of the Kidney. New York, John Wiley & Sons, 1976, pp 173–185. *A summation of published experience with these lesions.*

Mena E, Bookstein JJ, McDonald FD, et al.: Angiographic findings in renal medullary cystic disease. Radiology 110:277, 1974. *Excellent portrayals of medullary cystic disease and the importance of arteriography to its accurate diagnosis.*

Schimke, RN: Hereditary renal-retinal dysplasia. Ann Intern Med 70:736, 1969. *The first of a growing number of reports on this variant. Well-written.*

Strauss MB: Clinical and pathological aspects of cystic disease of renal medulla. Ann Intern Med 57:373, 1962. *The modern classic. The author's child is reported.*

MEDULLARY SPONGE KIDNEY

Medullary sponge kidney (MSK) is a relatively common, roentgenographically diagnosed disorder of the intrapyramidal or intrapapillary segments of the renal collecting tubules, characterized by ectasia sometimes to the point of actual cyst formation. Estimates of its frequency in the general population range between 1 in 5000 and 1 in 20,000. It is found in approximately 1 in 200 individuals with urologic disease.

Infection, tubular obstruction, and heritable factors have been considered in the pathogenesis of MSK. Although evidence of chronic papillary infection is found in many patients, most authorities consider infection to be a secondary feature. The lesion is rare in infants and children, most cases having been reported in adults. Intraluminal deposits of uric acid are commonplace in children, but MSK is not. Therefore in utero obstruction of the distal nephron by "salts" is considered a remote possibility to account for the lesion. A role for heritable factors in the transmission of MSK is suggested by the facts that nine families are described in which MSK has affected two or more individuals (in one family, three consecutive generations were affected), and that instances of MSK are reported in association with other heritable diseases (e.g., the Ehlers-Danlos syndrome). Most authorities, however, consider MSK to be a congenital, not heritable, lesion.

The kidney in MSK is usually normal in size, but may be slightly enlarged (in 30 per cent of cases) when cystic changes are marked. The cut surface exhibits intrapyramidal cysts which contain calcareous deposits in approximately 50 per cent of cases. The cysts are, in fact, dilated collecting tubules. Any number from one to all renal pyramids in either or both kidneys may be affected. Microscopically, the most constant feature is a variably severe infiltration of the interstitium with inflammatory cells, usually most pronounced nearest the pelvis of the kidney.

Diagnosis of MSK is based on radiographic or clinical grounds. Many cases are identified incidentally, during the workup for hematuria, stones, recurrent urinary tract infection, or other conditions in which intravenous pyelography is indicated. During intravenous pyelography, contrast medium concentrates in the ectatic or cystic tubules. Calculi are located in the same regions. When one is careful to take films after the nephrographic phase and before pelvocalyceal filling is complete, contrast medium can be seen to fill the ectatic intrapyramidal tubules. As calices empty, contrast medium persists in the ectatic intrapyramidal tubules. At present, there is not general acceptance that milder forms of MSK exist. For example, the *pyramidal blush,* which is seen frequently during routine pyelography, is considered by some to be an early stage of the MSK lesion; most radiourologists consider it an unrelated and perhaps even normal finding. The issue is unsettled.

When uncomplicated by stone formation or infection, MSK may go undetected. On the other hand, when complications intervene, debilitating disease and even renal failure may occur. Over two thirds of affected individuals with clinically overt disease have impairment in maximal urinary concentrating ability. Five instances of distal tubular renal acidosis have been reported, although in most patients with MSK the urinary acidifying ability is normal. Hypercalciuria occurs in 40 per cent of patients. Its mechanism has not been established. Renal salt-wasting in mild proportions also may be seen but does not reach the degree of severity noted in the nephronophthisis–cystic renal medulla complex.

In one large series, renal colic was the most frequent presenting complaint in complicated cases of MSK. Hematuria, either microscopic or macroscopic, and acute urinary tract infection together constituted the second most frequent set of presenting complaints. Renal failure and elevated blood pressure are unusual.

MSK has been reported in patients ranging in age from 3 weeks to 71 years of age. It is more frequent in women. In one series, approximately 50 per cent of the patients had proteinuria and hyperuricemia.

Uncomplicated MSK follows a benign clinical course. Radiographic evidence of progression has been documented in fewer than 15 per cent of patients. It consists only of slight changes in the size or distribution of dilated collecting tubules. Among symptomatic patients, the disease runs a variable course. One may enjoy long symptom-free periods, while another will require repeated hospitalizations for lithiasis or recurrent urinary tract infection.

One patient in ten is regarded as having a poor prognosis. Partial or total nephrectomy, when the disease is unilateral, has been curable. However, the disease does progress asynchronously in the two kidneys in some instances. Therefore care must be exercised not to perform nephrectomy in an individual with asymmetric but bilateral involvement.

The differential diagnostic possibilities for MSK include all those conditions in which nephrocalcinosis and nephrolithiasis occur: hyperparathyroidism, milk-alkali syndrome, multiple myeloma, sarcoidosis, tuberculosis, vitamin D intoxication, and so on. Among these possibilities, Ekström et al. consider hyperparathyroidism the most common. Renal papillary necrosis may mimic the appearance of MSK on excretory urography. Papillary necrosis, however, is usually acute and occurs most frequently in patients with diabetes mellitus, sickle cell anemia, obstruction, analgesic abuse, and recurrent urinary tract infection. On pyelography, MSK can be confused with childhood polycystic kidney disease; differentiation can be made on clinical grounds. The experienced radiologist will have no difficulty distinguishing MSK from calyceal diverticula and calyceal cysts.

MSK has been reported to accompany a variety of other clinical diseases, including the Ehlers-Danlos syndrome, horseshoe kidney, ectopic kidney, and mongolism. MSK has accompanied congenital total hemihypertrophy in 17 instances; the lesion of MSK sometimes is on the same side as the hemihypertrophy and sometimes on the opposite.

The efficacy of stone-preventive measures in MSK has not been established; but on the grounds of "nothing ventured, nothing gained," it would appear worthwhile to institute them in patients with frequent episodes of urolithiasis.

Ekström T, Engfeldt B, Lagergren C, et al.: Medullary Sponge Kidney. Stockholm, Almqvist and Wiksell, 1959. *Still the comprehensive work on the subject.*

Kuiper JJ: Medullary sponge kidney. *In* Gardner KD Jr (ed.): Cystic Diseases of the Kidney. New York, John Wiley & Sons, 1976, pp 151–171. *An updated review.*

Parks JH, Coe FL, Strauss AL: Calcium nephrolithiasis and medullary sponge kidney in women. N Engl J Med 306:1088, 1982. *A comprehensive study of stone formation and MSK—one of the first.*

Yendt ER: Medullary sponge kidney and nephrolithiasis. N Engl J Med 306:1106, 1982. *Editorial comment on the preceding article.*

CONGENITAL MULTICYSTIC KIDNEY (CMK)

CMK or multicystic renal dysplasia may be encountered at any age. It is perhaps the most common cause of an abdominal mass in infancy.

DEFINITION. *Renal dysplasia* is "a disturbance in nephrogenesis that results in a conversion of all, a segment, or multiple microscopic foci of one or both kidneys to structures which do not recapitulate any stage in normal nephrogenesis." In CMK, one finds nests of normal renal tissue that are scattered among cysts, variably differentiated mesenchyme, weirdly branching tubules lined by atypical epithelium, and foci of fatty, cartilaginous, and hematopoietic tissue.

ETIOLOGY. The majority of dysplastic (multicystic) kidneys occur in association with obstruction. When the entire kidney is involved, ipsilateral ureteral atresia or stenosis is found in 90 per cent of cases. When a segment of kidney is affected, drainage from the affected segment likewise is abnormal. This association therefore implicates obstruction during development as the causative mechanism of CMK.

CLINICAL MANIFESTATIONS. Bilateral diffuse involvement, because of the absence of functioning renal tissue, is incompatible with life. Unilateral or segmental involvement is not, however, and such cases may go undiscovered unless an abdominal mass is present or infection, trauma, hemorrhage, or hypertension supervenes and leads to the diagnosis. Urinalyses and tests of renal function are within normal limits in the affected adult. The roentgenographic picture is characteristic: a nonfunctioning segment or mass of renal tissue to which an arterial supply can be identified with difficulty if at all, and from which no continuity of ureteral drainage can be demonstrated. Rim-like calcifications in cyst walls strengthen the diagnosis.

INCIDENCE. Because of its frequently silent nature, the true incidence of CMK is not known. Among reported cases, each sex and each kidney are affected with equal frequency. A positive family history generally is absent, although scattered reports of involvement in twins, siblings, and relatives have appeared.

DIAGNOSIS. In adulthood, the discovery of CMK usually is incidental to the workup of an abdominal mass, intra-abdominal calcification, hypertension, recurrent urinary tract infection, or abdominal pain or discomfort. Infants or children suffering from a variety of teratologic syndromes may have renal dysplasia as one abnormality. Usually involvement outside the kidney dominates the clinical picture in these cases, however, and the finding of renal dysplasia is of importance only to the geneticist and pathologist.

The segmental or unilateral forms of CMK occur only rarely among several members of a given family. On these grounds it is distinguished from PKD, which is always bilateral and familial. Congenital unilateral hydronephrosis is a frequent cause of an abdominal mass in children and is distinguished from CMK by the usual persistence of residual renal function, a ureter that is of normal caliber distal to the obstructed site and a massively dilated pelvocalyceal system, and a patent renal artery on the involved side. Among adults, differentiation may be difficult between CMK and renal agenesis. Renal function is absent in both. In renal agenesis, retrograde pyelography shows only a small stump of ureter or is unsuccessful because no ureteral orifice can be found; no flank mass, renal artery, or eggshell calcifications can be demonstrated. Ultimately surgical exploration may be required to make the distinction.

PROGNOSIS AND TREATMENT. The prognosis of CMK among adults is excellent. Malignant change has not been reported. Should the involved kidney become infected or be traumatized, nephrectomy may be required.

Bernstein J: The morphogenesis of renal parenchymal maldevelopment (renal dysplasia). Pediatr Clin North Am 18:395, 1971. *A lucid explanation of exactly what is meant by renal dysplasia.*

Gur A, Siegel NJ, Davis CA, Kashgarian M, Hayslett JP: Clinical aspects of bilateral renal dysplasia in children. Nephron 15:50, 1975. *The clinical approach. Practical.*

Spence HM: Congenital unilateral multicystic kidney: An entity to be distinguished from polycystic kidney disease and other cystic disorders. J Urol 74:693, 1955. *Differential diagnosis. Practical and informative. A must-read.*

91. ANOMALIES OF THE URINARY TRACT

Richard D. Williams

Congenital aberrations of the urinary tract occur in over 10 per cent of the population. They vary in severity from lesions incompatible with life to those that are insignificant and detected only incidentally during studies prompted by unrelated causes. Often the anomalies, although not intrinsically detrimental, predispose to infection, lithiasis, and chronic renal failure, which lead to their recognition.

KIDNEY

ANOMALIES OF NUMBER. *Bilateral renal agenesis* is rare (1 in 4800 births), more frequent in males (3 to 1 ratio), and typically accompanied by oligohydramnios, Potter's facies, and pulmonary hypoplasia; this complex results in death within a few days of birth. *Unilateral renal agenesis* is more common (1 in 1100 births), generally involves the left kidney, and is seen more often in males (ratio 1.8 to 1). Renal absence is considered secondary to lack of a ureteral bud. Occasionally, a presumptive diagnosis of unilateral renal absence may be made in males when an ipsilateral vas deferens is absent on palpation. In only 10 per cent of renal agenesis cases is the adrenal absent. Extrarenal tissue or *supernumerary kidneys* are extremely rare (only 60 cases have been described); they are distinct from ureteral and calyceal duplication to be described later.

ANOMALIES OF POSITION (ECTOPIA). These are due to abnormal renal ascent: They include lumbar and pelvic and the less common thoracic or crossed ectopic varieties. As a group they occur in 1 in 900 cases and reach clinical significance only when they are mistaken for tumor during exploratory surgery or because of associated genital anomalies. Anomalies of fusion fall into this same category, since the abnormality leads to lack of ascent; *fused pelvic kidneys* or *horseshoe kidneys* (typically fused at their lower poles) are prevented from normal ascent by the inferior mesenteric artery. These latter two anomalies are associated with recurrent infection and calculi in 10 to 20 per cent of patients, and to a high incidence of ureteropelvic junction obstruction. *Nephroptosis* is the descent toward the pelvis of a normally ascended kidney when the upright posture is assumed; it is seen in adults and is perhaps due to poor renal fixation in the retroperitoneum. This condition, which is not an anomaly per se, is usually asymptomatic and rarely, if ever, needs surgical correction. Anomalies of rotation, commonly termed *malrotation*, are due to incomplete ventromedial rotation during ascent and are rarely related to any functional abnormality.

ANOMALIES OF THE RENAL PARENCHYMA. There is a heterogenous group of cystic and dysplastic lesions of the kidney. The most important group of disorders are those that produce cystic abnormalities, described in detail in Ch. 90. *Renal dysplasia* occurs in several forms: (1) *Multicystic kidneys* are malformed, nonfunctioning, generally unilateral, and invariably associated with ipsilateral ureteral atresia. When both kidneys are involved the manifestations and prognosis are similar to those in patients with bilateral renal agenesis. (2) *Segmental dysplasia* or *hypoplasia* is rare; it is not usually associated with significant renal complications, except in the bilateral and generalized form. (3) *Total renal dysplasia* is associated with lower urinary tract obstruction such as *posterior urethral valves* or functional bladder outlet obstruction, as in the *"prune-belly" syndrome.*

RENAL VASCULATURE

Multiple renal arteries occur in 15 to 20 per cent of the population. They are of little significance, except when they are inadvertently injured during an operation or (rarely) when they cause calyceal infundibular obstruction or (more often) *ureteropelvic junction obstruction. Congenital renal artery aneurysms* are infrequent; they are differentiated from acquired lesions by their location at the bifurcation of the main renal artery or at a distal branch point. The lesions require surgical treatment only if resulting hypertension is uncontrolled or if they are calcified or have a diameter of more than 2.5 cm. *Congenital arteriovenous fistulas* are rare but may result in hematuria, hypertension, and/or cardiac failure (if large), necessitating surgical intervention.

COLLECTING STRUCTURES AND URETER

Calyceal anomalies include *diverticuli, hydrocalycosis, megacalycosis,* and *infundibular stenosis.* They are clinically important only when urinary stasis results in recurrent infection and/or stone formation. *Ureteropelvic junction obstruction* is one of the more frequent causes of hydronephrosis in childhood. Bilaterality is not unusual and the condition is often asymptomatic; however, flank pain (particularly following diuresis), urinary infection, and gross hematuria (following minor trauma) are frequent findings on presentation. Relief of symptoms as a rule follows surgical repair (pyeloplasty), although normalization of the radiologic abnormality is infrequent.

Ureteral duplication is the most common ureteral anomaly; it may be incomplete, with the duplicated ureters combining to form only one entrance per side into the bladder, or complete, with two or more ureters coursing toward the bladder on one or both sides. Most often all completely duplicated ureters enter the bladder. The ureter from the lower pole often obtains poor implantation within the bladder, which may result in vesicoureteral reflux and possibly recurrent infection and hydroureteronephrosis. Ureteral ectopia can also occur in the absence of duplication but results in similar sequelae.

Ureteral reflux may be unrelated to duplication but due to an abnormal implantation of the ureter into the bladder with a resulting poorly developed trigone and deficient lower ureteral muscle. This condition can cause recurrent urinary infection in children; however, surgical reimplantation is necessary only in severe cases. Other ureteral anomalies include *ureterocele,* a congenital distal ureteral meatal stenosis; *megaloureter,* an abnormality of the ureteral musculature allowing massive ureteral dilatation, often without calyceal distortion; *ureteral valves; ureteral diverticuli;* and *retrocaval ureter,* an anomaly of the formation of the vena cava causing the ureter to course behind the cava.

BLADDER

Anomalies of the bladder are very infrequent and include (1) *complete absence* (agenesis), which results in a persistent cloaca; (2) *duplication,* which may be complete with separate ureteral openings drained by separate urethras, or incomplete with a septum or hour-glass deformity; (3) *urachal* anomalies, which may appear as a patent connection to the umbilicus, a *diverticulum* at the dome of the bladder, or a *urachal cyst* along the course of the partially obliterated urachus; and (4) *exstrophy,* which is the most common severe anomaly of the bladder.

Exstrophy represents a midline defect in closure of the bladder wall, lower abdominal muscles, pubic bones, and anterior urethra *(epispadias).* The *"prune-belly" syndrome* is a complex anomaly in which absence of the abdominal muscles is associated with bilateral cryptorchidism, ureteral dilatation and reflux, and an irregular capacious bladder with a dilated proximal urethra.

URETHRA

Hypospadias is the most common urethral anomaly in males (1 in 300 live births). The lesion results from failure of ventral fusion of the urogenital folds. It may present as a ventrally displaced meatus on the distal penile shaft or, in more severe forms, with the meatus opening more proximal on the shaft or in the perineum. These latter forms are often associated with a ventral penile chordee. Isolated *epispadias* (failure of dorsal closure of the urethra) occurs in males or females and is usually associated with incontinence. Congenital *urethral strictures* are infrequent. Although *meatal stenosis* is common, it is thought to be acquired, inasmuch as it generally is seen only in circumcised boys. Congenital *urethral diverticuli* are not rare, yet they generally are small and of no consequence. Finally, *megalourethra,* a markedly dilated anterior urethra, often associated with poor development of the erectile corpora, is rarely seen.

Arey LB: Developmental Anatomy. 7th ed. Philadelphia, W.B. Saunders Company, 1974. *The most complete text describing the derivation of congenital anomalies.*

Perlmutter AD, Retik AA, Bauer SB: Anomalies of the upper urinary tract. *In* Harrison et al.: Campbell's Urology. 4th ed. Philadelphia, W.B. Saunders Company, 1979, p 1309. *A complete and well-referenced treatise of the subject.*

92. TUMORS OF THE KIDNEY, URETER, AND BLADDER

Richard D. Williams

Benign and malignant renal tumors are either primary in the kidney and its surrounding connective tissue or collecting structures, or secondary (involving the kidney from adjacent organs or distant sites of origin). By definition, any mass within the kidney is a "renal tumor," but only solid masses are considered in this chapter. Cystic lesions of the kidney are discussed in Ch. 90. A classification of renal tumors is presented in Table 92–1.

APPROACH TO THE PATIENT WITH A RENAL MASS

In the past, most renal masses were detected on excretory urograms (IVP) during an evaluation prompted by signs or symptoms of disease (Table 92–2). Surgical exploration was often necessary for definitive diagnosis and treatment. Today,

TABLE 92–1. CLASSIFICATION OF RENAL TUMORS

Benign Tumors
Adenoma
Oncocytoma
Mesoblastic nephroma
Hamartoma-angiomyolipoma
Leiomyoma
Hemangioma
Primary Malignant Tumors
Renal cell carcinoma (adenocarcinoma)
Nephroblastoma (Wilms' tumor)
Urothelial carcinoma (renal collecting system and pelvis)
Sarcoma
Secondary Malignant Tumors (Direct Extension or Metastatic)
Adrenal carcinoma
Retroperitoneal sarcoma, pancreas, colon
Lung, stomach, breast
Reticuloendothelial—lymphoma and Hodgkin's disease, and hematologic—leukemia and multiple myeloma

TABLE 92–2. PRESENTING SYMPTOMS OR LABORATORY ABNORMALITIES IN 309 PATIENTS WITH RENAL CELL CARCINOMA

Initial Symptom or Abnormality	Per Cent of Total
"Classic triad" (gross hematuria, pain, abdominal mass)	9
Hematuria	59
Abdominal mass	45
Pain	41
Weight loss	28
Anemia	21
Tumor calcification on x-ray	13
Symptoms from metastases	10
Fever	7
Incidental finding	7
Hypercalcemia	3
Erythrocytosis	3
Acute varicocele	2

Adapted from Skinner DG, Colvin RB, Vermillion CD, Pfister RC, Leadbetter WF: Diagnosis and management of renal cell carcinoma. Cancer 28:1165, 1971.

there are multiple new modalities for the accurate diagnostic study of renal masses, and because of their sensitivity an increasing number of incidental renal masses are being identified in asymptomatic patients. A systematic algorithmic approach should result in less than 10 per cent of renal masses being indeterminate prior to surgery (Fig. 92–1). Its use can also often obviate the requirement for surgical definition.

The IVP with nephrotomography is still the study of first choice and can accurately define 75 per cent of renal masses. A demonstrated renal mass will require renal ultrasonography (US) to determine more accurately whether the mass is cystic or solid. If the mass fulfills all US criteria for a simple cyst (65 per cent of renal masses), there is little need for further workup, inasmuch as US is over 95 per cent accurate (Ch. 90). In the symptomatic patient, however, further workup, including cyst puncture or computed tomographic (CT) scan or both, may be appropriate. When a mass is suspected on IVP but not confirmed on US (15 per cent of cases), either an isotopic scan of the renal cortex or renal CT is required, particularly in symptomatic patients.

If the mass on US is solid or complex (20 per cent of cases), a renal CT scan (both with and without intravenous injection of iodine contrast) has replaced renal arteriography as the next diagnostic step. CT is as accurate as, and obviates the potential morbidity of, angiography in defining renal masses. Contrast enhancement of the usually highly vascular renal cancer on a CT study leaves little doubt as to the nature of a solid mass. In addition CT can give sufficient local staging information to allow definitive surgical management. When contrast enhancement is coupled with areas of a negative CT number (relative tissue density in Hounsfield units) typical of fat, a diagnosis of angiomyolipoma is appropriate and no further workup or immediate treatment will be required. In indeterminate cases, arteriography or needle aspiration or both may be needed to define the diagnosis further; however, in these unusual cases, final definition will likely require surgery.

In general, the nature of primary renal parenchymal masses in adults will be readily defined via this algorithm. Another advance that might further shape the algorithm suggested above is magnetic resonance imaging (MRI). Early studies suggest that MRI is currently equal to CT in diagnosing renal masses but possibly better in local tumor staging, determining intravascular tumor extension, and defining hemorrhage within renal lesions. With the advent of paramagnetic agents capable of contrast-like enhancement, MRI may permit differentiation between tumor types.

Clayman RV, Williams RD, Fraley EE: Current concepts in cancer: Pursuit of the renal mass. N Engl J Med 300:72, 1979. *This paper presents a proper perspective on the role of surgical exploration in the evaluation of renal masses.*

Hricak H, Williams RD, London PL, Kaufman L: NMR imaging of the human kidneys—Part II: Renal masses. Radiology 147:765, 1983. *An initial report emphasizing the potential of MRI in defining renal masses.*

Richie JP, Garnick MD, Seltzer D, Bettmann MA: CT scan for diagnosis and staging of renal cell cancer. J Urol 129:1114, 1983. *A substantial series of patients studied by CT with surgical correlation of results.*

Weyman PJ, et al.: Comparison of computed tomography and angiography in the evaluation of renal cancer. Radiology 137:417, 1980. *Establishes computed tomography as a modality equal to angiography in the diagnosis of renal malignancies.*

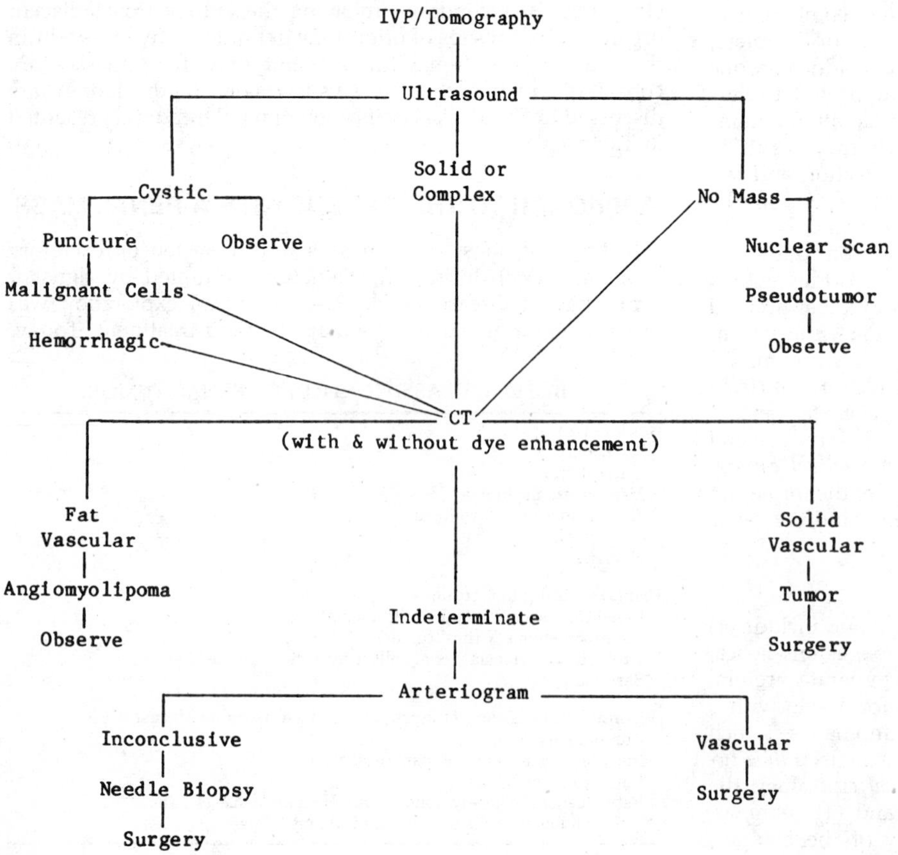

Figure 92–1. Algorithm for the definition of renal masses.

BENIGN RENAL TUMORS

Renal adenoma is the most common benign solid parenchymal lesion. Those under 3 cm in size have been designated as "benign," yet they tend to occur in circumstances similar to lesions larger than 3 cm (which are considered cancerous), i.e., in patients above 40 years of age, with a male to female ratio of 2 or 3 to 1. Small "renal adenomas" (< 3 cm) are virtually indistinguishable histologically from renal adenocarcinomas and a few have in fact metastasized. Since the biology of these small tumors cannot be predicted preoperatively, most urologic oncologists consider them to be malignant and recommend radical nephrectomy. Trials of a subtotal nephrectomy in highly selected lesions are appropriate, however, since there are surprisingly good survival rates following partial nephrectomy for renal cancer in solitary kidneys and after subtotal nephrectomy in bilateral disease, and since the diagnosis of small asymptomatic renal tumors is increasing because of the liberal use of CT scanning.

Renal oncocytoma is a recently recognized subtype of adenoma that has a characteristic pale brown gross appearance and contains cells with an acidophilic cytoplasm. These tumors, although sometimes several centimeters in size, are generally asymptomatic. The typical spoke-wheel pattern on angiography is not sufficiently specific to exclude a malignant lesion preoperatively, and therefore treatment continues to be radical nephrectomy.

Mesoblastic nephroma, a benign congenital renal tumor of early childhood, must be distinguished from the highly malignant nephroblastoma or Wilms' tumor. Unlike the latter, however, the mesoblastic nephroma is commonly diagnosed at birth or within the first few months of life. The prognosis is excellent; complete surgical resection is curative, and neither chemotherapy nor radiotherapy is required.

Hamartoma-angiomyolipoma is seen most often in adult patients with tuberous sclerosis (adenoma sebaceum, epilepsy, and mental retardation) and is often detected as a result of retroperitoneal hemorrhage. The tumors may be quite large and commonly multiple and bilateral. As their name implies, they contain vascular, adipose, and smooth muscle elements. The diagnosis can be difficult to establish for patients without the stigmata of tuberous sclerosis. Computed tomography, however, can define these tumors by exhibiting a negative CT number in areas of fat within the mass and can in addition delineate multiple and bilateral tumors with more clarity. The asymptomatic patient with typical CT findings of fat within the tumor does not require surgery, however, as the prognosis is excellent without treatment.

A variety of *other benign renal tumors* include *fibroma,* a renal parenchymal, capsular, or perinephric fibrous mass; *lipoma,* adipose deposition within or around the kidney, often perihilar or within the renal sinus; *leiomyoma,* a not uncommon retroperitoneal tumor that may arise from the renal capsule or renal vascular walls; and *hemangioma,* occasionally accounting for hematuria with an elusive cause. Because these and other less common benign tumors are not frequently seen, it is often quite difficult to establish a diagnosis. When these tumors are accompanied by symptoms or produce a renal mass with calyceal distortion, the final diagnosis is generally made by the pathologist after the kidney is removed.

Lieber MM, Tomera KM, Farrow GM: Renal oncocytoma. J Urol 125:481, 1982. *An excellent discussion of the diagnosis, pathology, and treatment of this recently recognized entity.*

Pitts WR, Kazam E, Gray G, Vaughan ED: Ultrasonography, computed tomography, and pathology of angiomyolipoma of the kidney: Solution to a diagnostic dilemma. J Urol 124:907, 1980. *Description of the use of CT to define angiomyolipoma, forming the basis for conservative management.*

PRIMARY MALIGNANT TUMORS

RENAL CELL CARCINOMA. Renal cell carcinoma is the most common renal malignancy in adults, accounting for just under 10 per cent of all malignancies and approximately 7500 deaths per year in the United States. The tumor is also called renal adenocarcinoma, Grawitz' tumor, hypernephroma, and nephrocarcinoma, although renal cell carcinoma (RCC) has become a universally accepted designation. RCC appears to arise from cells of the proximal convoluted tubule. Risk factors include cigarette smoking and maleness (ratio of 2 or 3 to 1). Persons with HLA antigen types BW44 and DR8 may be more prone to develop renal cancer. RCC is occasionally familial and is more common in patients with von Hippel–Lindau disease, horseshoe kidneys, and adult polycystic kidney disease. Histologically, RCC is of three varieties: the classic "clear cell" type characterized by uniformly large, cholesterol-laden cells with small nuclei and rare mitoses; a granular cell type exhibiting a darker staining cytoplasm containing numerous mitochondria, and more numerous mitoses; and an uncommon spindle cell variety that has fusiform cells and variability in cell size.

Clinical Manifestations. The classic presenting triad of *hematuria, flank pain,* and a *palpable abdominal mass* is seen in less than 20 per cent of patients and among those only with far advanced local tumors (Table 92–2). Gross or microscopic hematuria alone, however, is present in approximately 60 per cent of patients with RCC. The detection of renal tumors in asymptomatic patients has increased, but nearly 50 per cent of patients continue to have local extension or metastatic disease at the time of diagnosis. Because of its protean manifestations and propensity for curious metastatic sites, RCC has been dubbed the "internist's tumor" (Table 92–3). Indeed, paraneoplastic syndromes are common in patients with RCC: *pyrexia* (fever as a presenting symptom occurs in approximately 20 per cent of cases), *hypertension* (10 to 15 per cent), *erythrocytosis* (3 to 8 per cent), *hypercalcemia* (3 to 5 per cent), *anemia* (10 to 20 per cent), and *hepatic dysfunction* (1 to 3 per cent). The paraneoplastic syndromes may raise suspicion of RCC but they do not suggest metastases; neither are they prognostic, since removal of the primary tumor when there is no demonstrated metastasis will usually eliminate the associated syndrome. Hepatic dysfunction (Stauffer's syndrome), characterized by elevated levels of alkaline phosphatase and alpha$_2$ globulin, prolonged prothrombin time, and a low serum level of albumin, all in the absence of hepatic metastases, is an exception to this rule, since in such cases there is an unexplained high recurrence rate after definitive treatment of localized disease.

Diagnosis. There is no specific diagnostic laboratory test for RCC. The physician must often suspect RCC in patients with unexplained constitutional symptoms. The diagnostic evaluation relies on the algorithm previously described for investigation of a renal mass (Fig. 92–1). A mass suspected on IVP with tomograms should be confirmed by ultrasonography. If it is solid on US, an abdominal CT scan will, in approximately 80

TABLE 92–3. SOME UNUSUAL OR SYSTEMIC MANIFESTATIONS OF RENAL CELL CARCINOMA

Fever
Weight loss, inanition
Anemia
Erythrocytosis
Leukemoid reaction, eosinophilia
Thrombocytosis
Hypercalcemia (PTH, prostaglandins)
Hypertension (with or without renin ↑)
Cushing's syndrome (ACTH)
Stauffer's syndrome (hepatopathy)
Galactorrhea (prolactin)
Amyloidosis
Congestive heart failure (A/V fistula)
Thrombophlebitis
Inferior vena cava obstruction
Left varicocele
Budd-Chiari syndrome
von Hippel-Lindau disease

Adapted from Cronin RE, et al.: Renal cell carcinoma: Unusual systemic manifestations. Medicine 55:191, 1976.

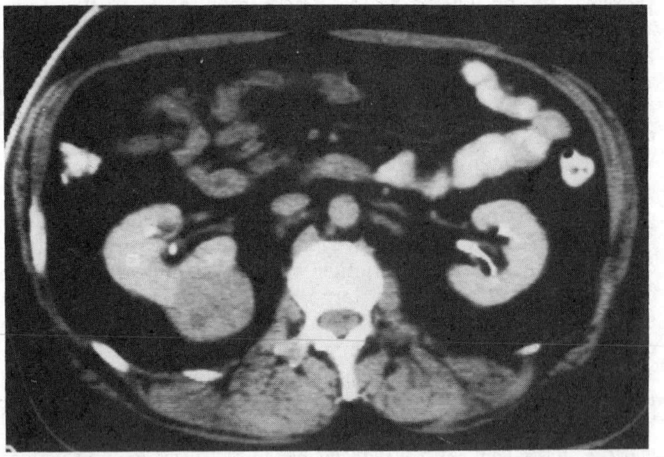

Figure 92–2. Contrast-enhanced abdominal CT scan showing renal cell cancer in the right kidney.

per cent of cases, be sufficient to establish the diagnosis (Fig. 92–2). A renal vein or caval thrombus is common and may change the surgical approach to treatment, so the presence of a thrombus should be determined by ultrasonography or CT scanning. In equivocal cases a venacavogram may be necessary for definition and/or determination of the cephalad extent of the thrombus before operation. The CT scan may be capable of determining local extension and/or local lymph node involvement, although it has not been found to be specific enough in most cases to obviate exploratory surgery for confirmation.

Staging and Treatment. It is important to determine the presence of metastases before determining therapy. No benefit has been ascribed to removal of the primary tumor in patients with known metastases unless the patient is symptomatic, the metastasis is solitary and amenable to resection, or a promising medical therapeutic protocol is planned (see below). Spontaneous regression of metastases following surgical removal of the primary tumor is calculated at 0.5 per cent, whereas the surgical mortality is nearly 1 per cent. The primary metastatic sites beyond the ipsilateral adrenal and local lymph nodes are lung and long bones. A chest roentgenogram and CT and a radionuclide bone scan are routine staging modalities. Lymphangiography has not been helpful in staging RCC patients.

Therapy of RCC depends entirely on the staging system summarized in Table 92–4. In patients with Stages I, II, and III B, treatment consists of a radical nephrectomy, which includes removal of the kidney and ipsilateral adrenal intact within its surrounding fascia, as well as removal of a possible intracaval thrombus. The local hilar lymph nodes will be included, but a formal para-aortic node dissection is not warranted. The prognosis for patients so treated approximates a 60 to 70 per cent five-year survival. Patients with lymph node involvement (Stage III A, C) have a 25 to 35 per cent five-year survival, and those with distant metastases (Stage IV) generally have less than a 10 per cent five-year survival.

Treatment of metastatic disease has included radiotherapy, chemotherapy, and immunotherapy, with none of these modalities emerging as clearly beneficial in effecting long-term survival. Hormonal therapy with medroxyprogesterone has less than a 10 per cent response rate. A variety of other hormonal agents including testosterone, tamoxifen, nafoxidine, and estramustine have similarly shown few responses. Approximately 20 per cent of patients with metastatic RCC were reported to respond to vinblastine, but this has not been subsequently confirmed. The combination of vinblastine and CCNU is currently the standard treatment, but short-term responses are obtained in only up to 20 per cent of patients. Immunotherapy with BCG, *Corynebacterium parvum,* and xenogeneic immune RNA has been tried with limited success. Current trials of human leukocyte interferon are reported to show up to a 30 per cent response rate with an occasional complete remission, but these studies, which are in progress, will require confirmation. Although radiation therapy is not important in primary treatment, it can provide short-term control of symptomatic bone metastases.

TABLE 92–4. STAGING SYSTEM FOR RENAL CARCINOMA

Stage I	Tumor confined to the renal parenchyma
Stage II	Tumor involving the perinephric fat or adrenal but confined within Gerota's fascia
Stage III A	Tumor involving regional nodes
B	Tumor thrombus in renal vein or vena cava
C	Tumor involving lymph nodes and renal vein or vena cava
Stage IV	Tumor extending into adjacent organs (liver, colon, pancreas, duodenum) or distant metastases

Cronin RE, Kaehny WD, Miller PD, et al.: Renal cell carcinoma: Unusual systemic manifestations. Medicine 55:291, 1976. *This article presents eight cases with unusual aspects of RCC and contains a comprehensive review of the literature.*

DeKernion JB: Treatment of advanced renal cell cancer—traditional methods and innovative approaches. J Urol 130:2, 1983. *A superb and inclusive review of the current treatment of disseminated RCC.*

Holland JM: Cancer of the kidney—natural history and staging. Cancer 32:1030, 1973. *The classic article on RCC containing a complete description of the staging system.*

Quesada JR, Swanson D, Trinidade A, Gutterman JU: Renal cell cancer: Antitumor effects of leukocyte interferon. Cancer Res 43:940, 1983. *The initial paper describing improved results with human leukocyte interferon in the treatment of metastatic RCC.*

Richie JP, Garnick MD: Primary renal and ureteral cancer. *In* Rieselbach RE, Garnick MB (eds.): Cancer and the Kidney. Philadelphia, Lea & Febiger, 1982, pp 662–706. *An excellent general review in a book devoted to the interrelationships of neoplastic diseases and renal disease. 185 references.*

Richie JP, Skinner DG: Renal neoplasia. *In* Brenner BM, Rector FC Jr (eds.): The Kidney. 2nd ed. Philadelphia, W. B. Saunders Company, 1981, pp 2109–2134. *An inclusive discussion of the protean clinical findings and therapy of RCC patients with 140 references.*

NEPHROBLASTOMA. Nephroblastoma (Wilms' tumor) is the second most common solid tumor of childhood (exceeded in incidence only by neuroblastoma). It is diagnosed in one third of cases when the child is under the age of 2 and in two thirds of cases when the child is under the age of 4.

Clinical Manifestations and Diagnosis. The tumor is palpable in as many as 80 per cent of cases and is often noted by a parent. Pain is initially present in 50 per cent of cases, hematuria (usually microscopic) in 10 to 20 per cent, and hypertension in approximately 60 per cent. The diagnosis is established first by IVP, which commonly shows calyceal distortion. Calcification within the mass occurs in 10 to 15 per cent of cases. Abdominal CT scans are useful to determine tumor extension and the possibility of bilaterality (this occurs in approximately 7 per cent of patients). Arteriography is not currently utilized.

If there still is doubt about the differential diagnosis (after the studies just described are done), measurement of urine vanillylmandelic acid should help rule out neuroblastoma. The metastatic workup should be directed to the lungs, liver, and opposite kidney. A chest roentgenograph and CT and an abdominal CT are sufficient. Nephroblastoma, as is the case with RCC, often produces a tumor thrombus in the inferior vena cava which may have to be delineated by venacavography. Abdominal ultrasound is also a reasonable alternative to establish this possibility.

Treatment. The development of successful treatment of nephroblastoma (Wilms' tumor) is rightfully heralded as one of the most significant advances in cancer therapy of the past few years. The prognosis has improved from a 25 per cent survival in the 1960's to a current rate of over 85 per cent disease-free survival, if there is no distant dissemination or unfavorable histology.

The initial treatment of nephroblastoma is complete surgical removal of the primary tumor and kidney, even when there are metastases. A transabdominal approach will allow the safest access and the necessary visibility of the liver, para-aortic nodes, and contralateral kidney for complete staging. Occasionally radiotherapy or chemotherapy may be required preoperatively to decrease the bulk of massive tumors. Combined therapy is indicated postoperatively in all patients but is dependent upon accurate staging, completeness of surgical extirpation, and tumor histology. A tumor confined to the kidney in children under 2 years of age requires only postoperative administration of actinomycin D and vincristine, whereas for all others the best results are obtained with radiation therapy to the tumor bed plus administration of actinomycin D and vincristine. Doxorubicin has also been shown to be an active agent in the treatment of this disease. Additional areas of current investigation are (1) radiation therapy and the addition of doxorubicin to vincristine and actinomycin D for patients with extensive local disease and favorable histology, and (2) radiation therapy with triple drug versus quadruple drug (addition of cyclophosphamide) for cases with unfavorable histology (anaplasia or sarcomatous elements). Wilms' tumor may occasionally be seen in adults; similarly, RCC occurs but rarely in children.

D'Angio GJ, et al.: The treatment of Wilms' tumor—results of the second National Wilms' Tumor Study. Cancer 47:2302, 1981. *A follow-up of the first NWTS report establishing improved results with complete staging and chemotherapy only in younger patients.*

Leape LL: Diagnosis and management of Wilms' tumor and neuroblastoma. *In* Skinner DG, Dekernion JB (eds.): Genitourinary Cancer. Philadelphia, W. B. Saunders Company, 1978, pp 179–199. *A complete and erudite discussion of all aspects of the diagnosis and management of the two most common solid malignancies of childhood.*

UROTHELIAL TUMORS. Malignant tumors of the urothelial lining of the urinary tract include those involving the collecting structures of the kidney (renal pelvis and calyces), ureter, and bladder. These tumors are transitional cell cancers (TCC) in over 90 per cent of cases, with an occasional squamous cell carcinoma (often in association with chronic inflammation due to stone formation in the upper tracts, and with *Schistosoma haematobium* infestation in the bladder), and rarely adenocarcinoma (commonly associated with embryologic hindgut remnants such as a persistent urachus in the dome of the bladder). TCC tends to be multifocal, occurring bilaterally in the upper tracts in a few cases but with an increasing frequency of simultaneous occurrence or recurrences in the ureter and particularly in the bladder. In each location there is a strong association of TCC with cigarette smoking, exposure to certain industrial chemicals (particularly aromatic amines), and chronic abuse of phenacetin-containing analgesics.

TCC of the Renal Pelvis and Calices. CLINICAL MANIFESTATIONS AND DIAGNOSIS. The presenting finding is gross or microscopic hematuria in more than 80 per cent of cases. In contrast to RCC, constitutional symptoms and paraneoplastic syndromes are few. Generally the diagnosis is made by the finding of a filling defect in a calix, infundibulum, or renal pelvis on IVP. Ultrasonography can be utilized to eliminate the possibility of a nonopaque calculus. Examination of the urine by an experienced cytologist can be diagnostic of TCC, although the site will be undetermined. A repeat IVP with compression and/or cystoscopy with retrograde pyelography, including ureteral wash or brush cytology, may be required to establish the diagnosis. CT scanning may be useful in determining local extent of tumor but is usually unnecessary. Arteriography is generally not diagnostically useful. The tumors tend to metastasize to lung and bone, and therefore a chest roentgenogram and CT and a bone scan are often indicated. Since these tumors tend to be multifocal, careful preoperative scrutiny of the opposite side of the urinary tract (on IVP) and of the bladder and urethra by direct cystourethroscopy is recommended.

TREATMENT AND PROGNOSIS. Treatment of renal urothelial cancer is radical nephroureterectomy, with removal of the entire ureter. Because 40 to 50 per cent of patients will have or develop similar tumors within the bladder, direct cystourethroscopy is a necessary postoperative routine, usually done quarterly the first year, twice the second year, and then annually.

Most of these tumors are low grade and noninvasive, and the five-year tumor-free survival rate after complete removal of the ipsilateral upper tract is more than 90 per cent. Patients with high grade and/or invasive lesions, however, have a poor prognosis (< 15 per cent five-year survival). Chemotherapeutic combinations, which have begun to show activity in TCC of the bladder, may also be efficacious in metastatic TCC of the upper tracts (see below).

TCC of the Ureter. CLINICAL MANIFESTATIONS AND DIAGNOSIS. These tumors are most often detected secondary to gross or microscopic hematuria, but occasionally present with renal colic due to obstructing blood clots. Diagnosis is commonly made by the finding of a ureteral filling defect on IVP. If the ureter is totally obstructed with a resultant lack of contrast excretion, cystoscopy and retrograde ureterography are required to demonstrate the lesion. As in renal pelvis TCC, ureteral urine or brush cytology can be diagnostic. Abdominal CT scans can aid in local staging, as can chest roentgenograms, and CT and bone scanning assist in detecting distant metastases.

TREATMENT AND PROGNOSIS. Prognosis is determined by the histologic grade of the lesion and the depth of invasion. Selected low grade lesions may be successfully treated by segmental resection, particularly in patients with renal insufficiency or a solitary kidney, but the definitive approach remains nephroureterectomy, as in renal pelvis TCC. Prognosis of low grade noninvasive lesions is greater than 85 per cent five-year survival, but for the higher grade, usually invasive lesions the prognosis is dismal. Treatment of metastatic disease is rarely successful; however, as with TCC of the renal pelvis, the newer combinations of chemotherapy are promising (see below).

TCC of the Bladder. Bladder cancer affects over 20,000 people and accounts for nearly 10,000 deaths annually in the United States. Men are affected at least twice as often as women.

CLINICAL MANIFESTATIONS AND DIAGNOSIS. Hematuria occurs at presentation in 68 per cent of patients and classically is total (throughout the stream) whether microscopic (as tested by a three-glass test) or gross. The degree of hematuria does not parallel the size of the lesion. Bladder irritability (frequency and dysuria) in the absence of infection is also a common (25 per cent) presenting complaint, particularly in males.

Intravenous pyelography is not sufficiently sensitive to detect small bladder tumors, but it is helpful in detecting upper tract TCC in the 10 per cent of patients with simultaneous lesions and in predicting bladder wall invasion in patients with concomitant unilateral ureteral obstruction. Urine cytology may establish the diagnosis of TCC but not the site. Definitive diagnosis requires cystoscopy and transurethral bladder biopsy under anesthesia, at which time a bimanual examination can predict whether the tumor has extended beyond the bladder wall. Metastases are local into adjacent pelvic structures and lymph nodes and distant to lungs and bones, and therefore staging of deeply invasive tumors is by chest roentgenograms, CT of the chest and abdomen, and bone scanning.

TREATMENT AND PROGNOSIS. Nearly 80 per cent of bladder TCC's are low grade and noninvasive (stage 0) or invade only into the lamina propria (stage A). Patients with such lesions have an 85 per cent five-year survival rate when treated by complete transurethral resection of the tumor(s). The lesions tend toward multiple recurrences in more than 50 per cent of patients and therefore cystoscopic surveillance is a mandatory postoperative routine. Intravesical chemotherapy with thiotepa, doxorubicin, mitomycin C, or more recently BCG has been used successfully for prophylaxis in patients with multiple or recurrent superficial low grade tumors, resulting in an approximate 50 per cent reduction in recurrences. Importantly, only about 20 per cent of patients presenting with superficial bladder TCC will subsequently develop high grade and/or invasive disease.

Unfortunately 80 per cent of patients with invasive bladder TCC are found so at initial presentation. In patients with deeply invasive disease, stage B_1 refers to superficial muscle invasion, stage B_2 to deep muscle invasion, and stage C to full-thickness bladder wall invasion. In the absence of metastases current best efforts at cure of invasive disease require preoperative radiation therapy (2000 R) to the bladder and pelvis, followed by pelvic lymphadenectomy and radical cystectomy (complete removal of the bladder and prostate in males and the bladder, urethra, and uterus in females). This approach affords a 50 to 60 per cent five-year survival rate in patients with stage B_1, B_2, or C disease. Patients with pelvic lymph node (stage D_1) or distant metastases (stage D_2) have less than a 15 per cent five-year survival rate.

Metastatic disease is difficult to treat, but recent combination chemotherapy with vinblastine, methotrexate, and cisplatinum is showing a durable 30 per cent complete remission rate. This significant advance, if consistent, may alter the surgical approach to bladder TCC in the future.

SARCOMAS. Renal sarcomas are rare; they include rhabdomyosarcoma, liposarcoma, fibrosarcoma, osteogenic sarcoma, and, most commonly, leiomyosarcoma. In general, sarcomas are quite malignant and usually detected at a late stage, and thus have a poor prognosis. The diagnostic approach is similar to that for RCC. Treatment is surgical with wide local excision; however, local recurrence and subsequent distant metastases are the rule.

Cummings KB: Nephroureterectomy: Rationale in the management of transitional cell carcinoma of the upper urinary tract. Urol Clin North Am 7:769, 1980. *A complete discussion of the important elements in determining the need for radical surgery in TCC of the upper urinary tract.*

Gittes RF: Tumors of the bladder. *In* Harrison et al.: Campbell's Urology. 4th ed. Philadelphia, W. B. Saunders Company, 1978, pp 1033–1070. *A detailed discussion of the epidemiology, diagnosis and staging, and treatment of bladder TCC.*

SECONDARY MALIGNANT TUMORS

Tumors of the lung, stomach, and breast most commonly metastasize to the kidney, but the metastases are usually clinically silent except for occasional microscopic hematuria. More than 50 per cent of patients with primary lung cancer have renal metastases at autopsy. Routine use of staging abdominal CT in a variety of primary malignancies is expected to increase the premorbid diagnosis of secondary renal tumors. Adjacent tumors of the adrenal, colon, and pancreas, and sarcomas may spread contiguously into the kidney. Reticuloendothelial tumors, such as lymphoma and Hodgkin's disease, and hematologic malignancies, such as leukemia and multiple myeloma, may infiltrate the kidney, but this type of renal involvement is almost never primary or symptomatic. Other forms of renal involvement in multiple myeloma are described in Ch. 163.

Part XI
GASTROINTESTINAL DISEASES

93. INTRODUCTION

Marvin H. Sleisenger

Digestive diseases in the United States account for a large part of the economic burden of illness, of total days of illness among adults, of all admissions to general hospitals, and of all major surgical operations. The prompt recognition of digestive disease and its treatment are thus plainly important. In order best to discharge this responsibility, knowledge of the pathophysiologic basis for signs and symptoms of gastrointestinal disease is most helpful. This introduction to the chapters on gastrointestinal diseases will be concerned with this broad subject.

APPROACH TO THE PATIENT WITH GASTROINTESTINAL DISEASE. In the approach to a patient with gastrointestinal disease the physician must obtain an accurate history of illness, correctly interpret the principal symptoms of digestive disease, conduct a thorough physical examination in which findings often characteristic of specific gastrointestinal diseases and syndromes are assiduously sought, and make intelligent use of laboratory tests and other diagnostic aids. An accurate history of digestive disease requires attention to details which mark the duration of the disability, establishing relationships between the waxing and waning of symptoms and external factors such as stress, eating, or fasting. Understanding the pathophysiologic basis of symptoms and signs helps greatly to establish the location, nature, and urgency of the problem.

The majority of patients with digestive disease have had their illness for years. The common diseases are chronic: acid-peptic disease affecting the esophagus, stomach, or duodenum; alcoholic disease of the liver and pancreas; calculous biliary tract disease; inflammatory bowel disease; postprandial dyspepsia; and irritable bowel. To be sure, some gastrointestinal diseases may be acute and even catastrophic; the acute abdomen is a general phrase of importance in both medical and surgical practice.

This introduction sets the stage for the study of specific diseases and disorders of the digestive system. It reviews the importance of a thorough history and physical examination. The common symptoms and signs of gastrointestinal disease are also reviewed in the context of their pathophysiologic basis.

THE VALUE OF A THOROUGH HISTORY. The duration of symptoms in patients with digestive diseases ranges from moments to decades. In an emergency room a physician may be called to see a previously healthy person suffering the symptoms and displaying the signs of an acute intra-abdominal disorder requiring a rapid decision about whether surgery is indicated. The next patient seeking his care may be an elderly person with a problem of four or more decades' duration. This patient is also ill but does not appear to be. Differences exist in the incidences of digestive problems in patients' families, in their reactions to stress, in their dietary habits, in the degree of involvement of other organ systems, and in the degree to which their illnesses affect general health and activity.

The natural history of many gastrointestinal diseases is marked by characteristic patterns of symptoms. Complaints often have a particular intensity, a periodicity (time of day, month, or season), and a relationship to fatigue, stress, eating, or drinking alcohol. For example, patients with irritable bowel tend to have low grade, nagging, cramp-like lower abdominal distress for decades. The distress may be aggravated by certain foods, and may wax and wane with the appearance and disappearance of stress. While the discomfort may be intense at times, its intensity contrasts with the acute, sudden, and excruciating pain of the patient with an acutely obstructed ureter or common bile duct, a perforated duodenal ulcer, or an acutely ischemic small intestine. Pain of gastrointestinal disease may be intermediate between acute and chronic, and between severe and mild, e.g., the epigastric distress of duodenal ulcer. It rarely incapacitates and is usually relieved quickly with appropriate therapy. However, a change in these characteristics, i.e., increased duration and less relief with antacids, may signal a possible penetration and deserves special attention. Complications are common in the natural history of many other gastrointestinal diseases. The patient with longstanding irritable bowel may also have diverticulosis and suddenly rupture a diverticulum. Knowledge of the natural history of digestive diseases is essential to understanding changes in patterns of symptoms, particularly pain.

The *locus* and *timing* of the distress are important in determining which organ of the digestive tract is affected. Upper abdominal discomfort related to meals usually means that the stomach, duodenum, gallbladder, or pancreas is the site of the problem. Periumbilical pain one half hour or so postprandially may indicate that the small intestine is involved. When the discomfort is in the lower abdomen and is associated with abnormal bowel habit or relieved by bowel movement or flatus, the colon is likely to be at fault. The *nature* of the pain is also important. Aching pain is characteristic of ulcer disease, boring pain of pancreatic disease, and cramping pain of both small and large intestine.

The presence of associated symptoms is important in evaluating gastrointestinal disease. Fever, arthritis, conjunctivitis, uveitis, and erythema nodosum may all be associated with the diarrhea of chronic inflammatory bowel disease. Continuing weight loss and evidence of malnutrition with vitamin deficiencies usually reflect a serious organic disease (however, such malnutrition may result from anorexia or satiety related to serious neuropsychiatric problems). Type and location of pain, presence of diarrhea, a relationship of symptoms to diet and alcohol, and history of prior surgery all help the clinician better to define the disease underlying the malnutrition and possible malabsorption. The historical facts associated with *weight loss* due to digestive disease are crucial for correct diagnosis. Is anorexia due to depression or physical illness? If the appetite is normal, is decreased intake due to *dysphagia, nausea, early satiety*, or *fear* of postprandial symptoms? Some individuals lose weight, despite good appetite and adequate food intake, because of *malabsorption* or *occult intra-abdominal malignancy*. The chronic alcoholic may get enough calories from ethanol to supply energy needs and may not lose weight; however, his diet lacks important ingredients such as essential amino acids and fatty acids, vitamins, minerals, and electrolytes.

EMOTION AND STRESS. *Emotion* and *stress* play a large role in many gastrointestinal disorders. Patients who are massively obese or who have anorexia nervosa are emotionally disturbed, and their eating habits are expressions of that disturbance extended over prolonged periods of time. These aberrant eating habits may represent bizarre but unconscious attempts at resolution of family conflicts, for example. No clear association among personality, stress, and the pathogenesis of duodenal ulcer has been established. Nevertheless, it is clear that recurrence of symptoms can often be correlated with emotional tension.

It has long been held that emotion plays a role in the pathogenesis of ulcerative colitis, but patients with this disease have not been shown to have an abnormal prevalence of psychiatric illness or an abnormal number of "critical life incidents." There is a higher incidence of both psychoneurotic behavior and critical life incidents in patients with irritable bowel than in those with ulcerative colitis.

By definition a personality disorder underlies the habitual abuse of alcohol, which occurs in many patients with diseases of the digestive system. No amount of effort in treating the esophagus (reflux esophagitis), stomach (erosive gastritis), pancreas (acute and chronic pancreatitis), or liver (acute alcoholic hepatitis, cirrhosis) will favorably affect the clinical course of these patients without attention to the basic problem.

THE PHYSICAL EXAMINATION: COMMON SIGNS OF GASTROINTESTINAL DISEASE. Certain signs of serious illness must be sought on physical examination of patients with complaints of digestive disease. The abdominal findings in patients with acute abdominal problems that require immediate surgery are discussed in Ch. 114.

Evidences of Malnutrition. Malnutrition is common in serious gastrointestinal diseases. It is characterized principally by signs of weight loss, mainly disappearance of fat depots and decreased muscle mass. Malnutrition is often associated with signs of *vitamin* and *mineral deficiencies.* Erythroderma, glossitis, cheilosis, muscle tenderness, angular stomatitis, bronzing of exposed skin, nasolabial seborrhea, dementia and peripheral neuropathy all reflect deficiency of B soluble vitamins. Glossitis, peripheral neuropathy, and lemon-tinted pallor may reflect vitamin B_{12} deficiency. Rough skin may be due to hyperkeratosis follicularis (vitamin A deficit?) or perifolliculitis of vitamin C deficiency. Petechiae, ecchymoses, or other evidences of easy bruising may reflect vitamin K deficiency. Pallor and glossitis may be due to folate deficiency while pallor, lingual atrophy, koilonychia, and splenomegaly point to iron deficiency. Petechiae and ecchymoses may reflect vitamin K deficiency; failure to grow, kyphosis, and skeletal deformities are evidences of vitamin D lack. Xerophthalmia results from insufficient vitamin A. Deficiencies of trace metals may be suspected on physical examination. Copper and zinc deficiencies are associated with loss of taste acuity, and zinc deficiency with severe dermatitis, hyperpigmentation, as well as alopecia and evidence of dementia. Central nervous system damage, due principally to deficiency of vitamin B_1 and ranging from recent ophthalmoplegia and confusion to dementia and cerebellar ataxia, may be noted, particularly in alcoholics.

Patients with *protein deficiency* not only lose subcutaneous fat and muscle mass but also they may have edema, decreased turgor and dyspigmentation of skin and dryness, brittleness, and lightening of hair, hepatomegaly, and mental dullness. Inadequate protein slows growth of children and impairs bone integrity in adults. Protein malnutrition caused by gastrointestinal disease is usually not selective, being coupled with subnormal caloric intake, and this is called *protein-calorie malnutrition.* Lack of essential fatty acids leads to skin eczema.

Other Important Signs. Physical signs pointing to disease in a particular organ system are also important. Thus, jaundice, hepatomegaly, splenomegaly, ascites, and spider angiomas all indicate chronic and severe liver disease. Palpable abdominal masses may be found in malignancies of the gastrointestinal tract, Crohn's disease, intraperitoneal abscesses, or lymphoma. Abdominal distention with evidence of gas-filled loops of bowel is often noted in patients with malabsorption resulting from diffuse proximal small bowel disease or from conditions associated with bacterial overgrowth.

Fever may be present during periods of inflammatory activity in patients with acute and chronic inflammatory disease of the gut, pancreatitis, cholecystitis, cholangitis, lymphoma, abscesses (intra-abdominal, hepatic, retroperitoneal, and perirectal), and acute progressive infarction of the bowel. The duration of fever varies and reflects the nature of the underlying disease. For example, fever is present for hours in acute suppurative cholangitis or acute small bowel infarction, and for days or even weeks in alcoholic hepatitis, Crohn's disease, pancreatitis with extensive necrosis or sepsis, abscesses (including liver), or lymphoma.

PATHOPHYSIOLOGIC BASIS FOR COMMON SYMPTOMS OF GASTROINTESTINAL DISEASE. An understanding of the pathophysiologic basis of the important symptoms of digestive disease will help in their correct interpretation and thus in arriving at an effective plan for diagnosis and treatment.

Anorexia. Disturbances of appetite, such as *anorexia* and *early satiety*, are common in digestive disease. *Anorexia* is the absence of hunger; i.e., despite the clear need for nutrient, the sensations of hunger are not felt. *Satiety* is the loss of the desire to eat after ingesting food. The control of both appetite and satiety resides in the hypothalamus. Bilateral *satiety centers* in the ventral medial portion of the hypothalamus regulate food intake by controlling more lateral hypothalamic *feeding centers.* The satiety center is thought to be activated after feeding by a high arteriovenous difference of glucose with suppression of the feeding center. Free fatty acids also stimulate the satiety center with disappearance of hunger after feeding. The release of gut hormones with feeding, particularly cholecystokinin (CCK), glucagon, bombesin, and somatostatin, may lead to satiety. These peptides, which delay gastric emptying when given exogenously, may endogenously delay gastric emptying after meals in man.

The precise roles of gastric distention and rate of gastric emptying on inhibition of feeding are not yet defined. It is likely that hormones, mainly CCK, by delaying gastric emptying and thus maintaining distention, cause satiety. In turn, hormonal action depends upon intact vagal afferent innervation of the stomach. On the other hand, the low interprandial A-V difference of glucose is thought not only to suppress the satiety center (thus activating the feeding center) but also thereby to initiate the unpleasant symptom complex called *hunger.* It is accompanied by so-called "hunger contractions" of the stomach; however, hunger is still experienced in the absence of such contractions. Appetite is the desire for food after hunger ceases. It is controlled on a more conscious level.

The causes of anorexia are both physical and psychologic. Anorexia nervosa is a psychologic disorder in which appetite virtually does not exist and hunger is markedly reduced. Anorexia is a nonspecific symptom in that it is associated with many organic diseases, intestinal and extraintestinal. The depression of appetite in some gastrointestinal diseases, such as carcinoma of the pancreas or stomach, is not well understood. In many patients anorexia is clearly associated with continuing intra-abdominal pain or fever; in others, with chronic or recurrent nausea.

Hyperphagia. The complex factors underlying excessive feeding include (1) inability to regulate energy intake according to nutritive value for the food, (2) cultural influences, (3) possible failure of normal response to feeding; i.e., failure of release of peptides that delay gastric emptying or defective receptor mechanism for them, and (4) a hypothalamic lesion, although this has not as yet been demonstrated in humans. Another group, usually young females, will alternate cramming of food ("bulimia") and vomiting with periods of anorexia.

Abdominal Pain. The most frequent symptom that brings a patient with digestive disease to the physician is pain, most commonly abdominal, but not infrequently located in the chest or back. Pain warns the patient of possible imminent tissue damage and is usually caused by anoxia, inflammation, or stretching of smooth muscle or organ capsules. Pain from the viscera and peritoneum is mediated by the sympathetic nervous system. The afferent endings are located in the smooth muscle of hollow organs, in the peritoneum, and in organ capsules. These afferents are identified with dermatomes which correspond with segments of the spinal cord. They travel with afferents from the periphery. This association is the basis of *referred pain* to extra-abdominal structures.

Pain originating from hollow viscera is called *visceral;* it is midline, dull, and often associated with nausea. The location depends upon the organ involved. Pain from the esophagus is usually felt over the site but occasionally in the suprasternal notch. Pain from the stomach and duodenum is epigastric or to the right of the midline in the epigastrium. Jejunal and ileal pain is often periumbilical, although distal ileal pain may be perceived in the right lower quadrant. Colonic pain is lower abdominal in location, often poorly localized. Pain from the gallbladder and common bile duct is in the right upper quadrant or epigastrium; when severe, it is often also felt in the midline of the upper back. Pancreatic pain is midline or to the left of the epigastrium and often radiates through to the midline of the upper back.

Pain may be felt at a site distant from the organ involved, either by referral or by involvement of neighboring structures. Thus, an abscess in the right lower quadrant over the psoas may refer its pain to the hip or groin; spasm of the esophagus may lead to pain felt down the inner aspect of the left upper arm, as in the pain of myocardial ischemia. The pain in the trapezius ridge areas of the shoulders may be associated with irritation of the diaphragmatic pleura by an inflammatory process such as a subdiaphragmatic abscess. The physician must be familiar with the common areas of pain reference and with the influence on pain patterns of involvement by contiguity.

Intra-abdominal pain is often due to *inflammation* or *ischemia*. Edema and spasm narrow the involved segment; smooth muscle proximal to the narrowed gut stretches, causing pain. In addition, ischemia and inflammation lower the pain threshold by releasing local bradykinin, serotonin, histamine, prostaglandins, and lactic acid. Pain is due in part also to the stretching of smooth muscle in blood vessels. Sensory nerve fibers may be directly involved by a tumor (e.g., paraspinal sensory nerve roots may be entrapped by cancer of the pancreas, other retroperitoneal malignancies, or abscesses).

Initially visceral pain is felt in the midline and is dull in character regardless of the organ involved. As inflammation or ischemia progresses, the pain will shift gradually to the site of the organ affected. Thus, in a matter of hours the pain of acute appendicitis shifts from the midline to the right lower quadrant, and that of cholecystitis from the midline to the right upper quadrant.

Varying degrees of urgency characterize different pains in the abdomen. Intelligent diagnosis and management depend upon correct interpretation of the quality, intensity, duration, and location of pain. This assessment, taken together with the findings on physical examination, is the basis for the differential diagnosis, further studies, and management.

The patient's behavior during the pain is also important in correct interpretation. Pain caused by stretching of smooth muscle of the gut, ureter, or common bile duct is colicky. The patient tends to be restless, and the pain is not aggravated by movement. The patient with peritoneal irritation, on the other hand, prefers to lie quietly, since jarring or movement exacerbates the pain.

FACTORS AFFECTING INTENSITY AND PERCEPTION OF PAIN. The patient's description of pain is influenced by neural, psychologic, and cultural factors. Perception is reduced by environmental stress, as in battle. Likewise, depression blunts perception. The neural influences reside within the spinal cord, particularly the dorsal horns, which integrate central and peripheral impulses with those of pain, altering them before they reach the brain. Perception is also affected by cultural influences, ranging from demonstrativeness to stoicism. Finally, age affects pain perception. Patients in the 8th decade and beyond often have a significant rise of pain threshold. Degree of discomfort is often disproportionately low even with sepsis, perforation, and infarction in this group.

Vomiting. Vomiting is the rapid evacuation of gastric contents in retrograde fashion from stomach through mouth. It must be distinguished from *rumination,* the asymptomatic regurgitation of food, rechewing, and reswallowing. It is immediately due to a forceful contraction of the abdominal muscle with the cardia and mouth open. It is the final stage of a three-part act. The first is *nausea,* a most unpleasant feeling, difficult to define but universally recognizable. Gastric motor activity is diminished, and duodenal pressure increases with reflux of duodenal contents into the stomach. Nausea is followed by *retching,* which comprises spasmodic respiratory movements opposed by expiratory contractions of the abdominal muscles and raises the cardia of the stomach, an important preparatory maneuver. Paraphenomena of vomiting include hypersalivation, some reverse peristalsis of the small intestine, evidences of abnormal vagal stimulation (principally bradycardia), and the urge to defecate. Vomiting is controlled by bilateral vomiting centers in the dorsal portions of the lateral reticular formation of the medulla, activated by so-called chemoreceptor trigger zones (CTZ).

Drugs cause nausea and vomiting by stimulating the chemoreceptor trigger zones; this pathway also mediates the nausea and vomiting of motion sickness, uremia, diabetic ketoacidosis, and general anesthetics. Vagal afferents may also stimulate the vomiting centers, bypassing the chemoreceptor trigger zones. Examples include distention of the smooth muscle of the gut, particularly when sudden; substances noxious to the mucosa of the stomach such as copper sulfate or mustard; and irritation and inflammation of the peritoneum. Thus, a large number of diseases and disorders that affect the intestine, bile ducts, ureters, and peritoneum are associated with nausea and vomiting. The symptom complex is often nonspecific and not helpful in differential diagnosis of intra-abdominal disorders. Additional pathways to the vomiting center are stimulated by noxious smells and tastes, but the location of the involved supramedullary receptors is not known.

TYPES OF VOMITING. Important features of vomiting that may characterize a particular category of underlying disease are its amount, duration, content, and relationship to meals.

When a patient vomits during or immediately after a meal, it is most likely to be psychogenic, although such vomiting, particularly after a heavy meal, may be due to edema and spasm of the pylorus associated with a pyloric canal ulcer. (However, in these latter cases, the patient often has pain that is relieved by emesis, in contrast to failure of pain relief by vomiting in patients with cancer of the pancreas or biliary tract disease, for example.) Vomiting an hour or more after a meal is more compatible with gastric outlet obstruction, acute pancreatitis, or motility disorder of the stomach (diabetic neuropathy, postvagotomy). Vomiting of material eaten many hours previously also fits in the category of organic obstruction. Often patients with chronic outlet obstruction will have large, dilated stomachs and on examination will be noted to have a succussion splash. This sign is important in distinguishing psychogenic from organic obstruction in chronic vomiting. Alcoholics, pregnant women, and uremics have nausea and vomiting early in the morning on arising. Some patients with increased intracranial pressure may have vomiting unassociated with meals or nausea; classically, it has been described as projectile or forceful, although this is by no means always the case.

Large amounts of vomitus, food and secretions, usually indicate nearly complete or complete obstruction. This may also result, however, from severe gastric atony and dilatation, or, in rare instances, from hypersecretion of gastric juice in the Zollinger-Ellison syndrome without outlet obstruction.

QUALITY OF VOMITUS. *Content* of the vomitus is important in the determination of the underlying disorder. Undigested food indicates a gastric outlet obstruction. If there is blood in the vomitus, an inflammatory or malignant disease of the stomach should be suspected. Vomitus without bile indicates that the problem is prepyloric, whereas consistent appearance of bile suggests that the problem is postpyloric. The presence of bile may signify only that the increase in pressure in the duodenum was sufficiently great that, with a relaxed pylorus, duodenal contents entered the stomach preceding evacuation. Large volume vomitus of high acidity (pH 1.5 or less) suggests gastrinoma, although outlet obstruction with an active duodenal ulcer may have a similar output.

Odor may also be helpful. A fecal smell to vomitus suggests low intestinal obstruction, a fistula between the stomach and colon or between the upper small intestine and colon, or bacterial overgrowth of the stomach or small intestine (longstanding obstruction).

Nausea and vomiting that follow the recent onset of a persisting abdominal pain provide a clue to a likely important event within the abdomen, an event that often requires hospitalization and, in some cases, surgery.

CLASSIFICATION OF DISEASES AND DISORDERS ASSOCIATED WITH VOMITING. The major categories of disorders associated with vomiting are summarized in Table 93–1.

Psychogenic vomiting, a chronic and complex disturbance, takes place immediately after eating or during the meal. It is often self-induced and, although chronic, is compatible with good health over many years. It is frequently associated with anorexia nervosa or follows the binge eating of bulimia.

The clinical entities associated with nausea and vomiting which command immediate attention are *intra-abdominal, intracranial,* and *metabolic diseases.* In the abdomen they include gastric outlet obstruction; intestinal obstruction; gastrointestinal inflammation; perforation of a viscus; peritonitis; pancreatitis; abscess; acute distention of smooth muscle in bile ducts, the ureter, and the small intestine; and acute ischemia. In general, nausea and vomiting often follow severe pain, extra-abdominal as well as intra-abdominal. In addition, ileus of the intestine and stomach, and acute gastric dilatation with atony, no matter what the cause, are often associated with nausea and vomiting. In these instances, organic outlet obstruction or intestinal obstruction cannot be demonstrated.

Intracranial disease causing increased intracranial pressure (tumor, hematoma), many *toxic* and *metabolic encephalopathies* (including infection), migraine headache, and *gastric neuropathies* are examples of neurologic diseases associated with vomiting.

In medical practice nausea and vomiting are most commonly *drug induced.* The list of offending drugs is lengthy; most drugs are capable of causing nausea and vomiting in susceptible individuals. Whether the afferent stimuli originate from the action of drugs on the gastrointestinal tract or from the direct effect of drugs on the chemoreceptor zone is not clear in most instances. Anticholinergic agents, however, may cause vomiting by inhibiting motor activity in patients with partial outlet obstruction. The most common causes of gastric outlet obstruction are chronic ulcer disease of the pylorus or duodenum and antral carcinoma.

COMPLICATIONS OF VOMITING (Fig. 93–1). The major consequences of prolonged vomiting include *dehydration, hypokalemia,* and *alkalosis.* Dehydration is due to fluid loss. Hypokalemia results from exchange of sodium for potassium in the renal tubule in an effort to conserve sodium lost in vomitus, from diminished potassium intake, and from loss of potassium in the vomitus. Alkalosis follows loss of hydrogen ions in the vomitus and is exacerbated by a contraction of extracellular fluid, with noncommensurate loss of bicarbonate and shift of hydrogen into cells resulting from potassium deficiency. Sodium depletion results from loss of sodium in the vomitus and, in some instances, renal loss of sodium. Urine is concentrated; a variable amount of bicarbonate is lost, depending upon whether or not the renal transport maximum (Tm) for bicarbonate is exceeded. The urinary excretion of sodium, potassium, and chloride is low if the Tm for bicarbonate is not exceeded. On the other hand, if the Tm for bicarbonate is

TABLE 93–1. COMMON DISEASES AND DISORDERS ASSOCIATED WITH NAUSEA AND VOMITING

Psychogenic
Drug-induced
Intra-abdominal problem:
Colic, sepsis, perforated viscus
Inflammation: ischemia
Toxins and poisons (ingested, inhaled, injected)
Metabolic disorders and diseases
Gastric outlet obstruction
Duodenal and high small bowel destruction
Intracranial diseases
Viral gastroenteritis
Cyclic vomiting, childhood
Pregnancy
Due to pain, intra-abdominal or extra-abdominal

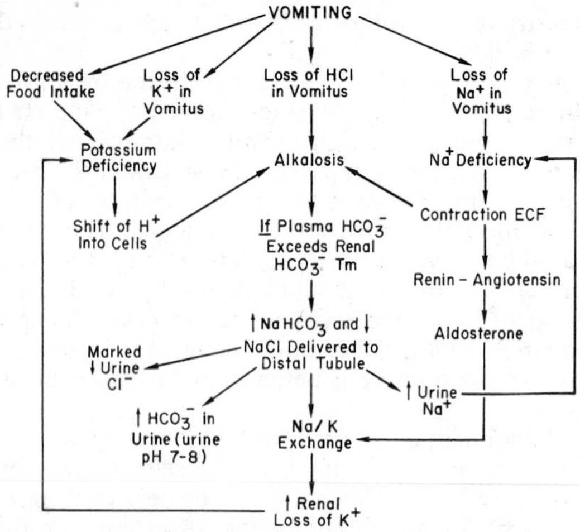

Figure 93–1. Metabolic consequences of vomiting. (From Feldman M: In Sleisenger MH, Fordtran JS [eds.]: Gastrointestinal Diseases. 3rd ed. Philadelphia, W. B. Saunders Company, 1983.)

exceeded, sodium, potassium, and bicarbonate will be high in the urine, and urine chloride will be low.

Signs and symptoms that result from the metabolic consequences of vomiting include muscle weakness, polydipsia, impaired urinary concentration, and abdominal distention (caused by hypokalemia); muscle cramps, weakness, somnolence, and even stupor (caused by hyponatremia and marked dehydration); and hypotension and low urinary output (caused by dehydration and intravascular volume contraction).

Change in Bowel Habit: Constipation and Diarrhea. Normal bowel habit ranges from one bowel movement per three to four days to three to four stools per day. Generally patients readily discern significant changes in their own pattern. Some persons may have only one stool per week or longer for many years. Severe constipation may be lifelong, as in congenital aganglionosis of the colon (Hirschsprung's disease). The definition of diarrhea is also difficult. It is not based entirely on numbers of bowel movements, although patients with diarrhea most frequently have more than three bowel movements per day. The definition most often used is based on volume—a daily stool bulk that exceeds 150 ml. A patient may have three or more small bowel movements a day but not be considered to have diarrhea. The physician who is consulted for longstanding constipation or diarrhea is obliged to investigate the complaint. Hitherto undiagnosed chronic treatable disease may be found.

Change in bowel habit must always be taken seriously even if it has occurred gradually over many months or even years. The recent onset of constipation or diarrhea may represent a reaction to stress, a change in diet, an enteric infection, malignancy of the colon, or a result of a metabolic disease. The majority of patients with nonorganic causes of constipation (bowel movement frequency of less than two per week) will increase the number of movements to three or more if placed on a high fiber diet. A few patients will complain of lifelong inability to have bowel movements without vigorous catharsis or enemas. Such patients may also have megacolon and require investigation of the innervation of the distal colon. Increasing constipation may be a chronic manifestation of a systemic disease such as myxedema or of the effects of drugs such as phenothiazines or anticholinergics. A decreasing caliber of stool, on the other hand, may connote organic obstruction and may be due to a constricting malignancy of the distal colon.

The onset of diarrhea of more than a few weeks' duration necessitates investigation (see Ch. 102). Its significance depends in part on its accompanying features. Thus, if associated with bleeding and fever in a recent traveler, an enteric infection (shigellosis or amebiasis) is suggested. At the other extreme is the individual with diarrhea for many years and a bowel habit characterized by several loose, nonbloody movements after breakfast each day and occasionally after the evening meal.

This individual appears healthy, is active, has no systemic symptoms, and most likely has irritable bowel syndrome (IBS). In between these extremes are many diseases associated with diarrhea.

Chronic diarrhea may or may not be associated with weight loss. If the patient is losing weight, the question of *malabsorption syndrome* must be addressed (see Ch. 103). Patients with this syndrome have abnormal stools—bulky, light in color, foul smelling, greasy in appearance and character. Weight loss might be due to associated anorexia or fear of eating because of discomfort following meals, both symptoms resulting possibly from an inflammatory or malignant disease of the intestine, liver, or pancreas. Does the diarrhea persist despite the patient's abstaining from eating? If so, a secretory tumor of the pancreas, thyroid, or enterochromaffin tissue may be responsible. On the other hand, if the diarrhea is ameliorated by restricting food and fluid and if the stool water prior to such restriction has contained lower than normal concentrations of sodium and potassium, a disorder causing so-called osmotic diarrhea must be suspected. It results from the intraluminal generation of osmotically active material from unabsorbed disaccharides, hexoses, fatty acids, and amino acids. The bacterial metabolites of these substances are osmotically active, drawing fluid into the lumen of the intestine. The amount and rate of transit are such that the colon cannot reabsorb most of the water and electrolyte presented to it. A more extensive discussion of the pathophysiology of diarrhea and its differential diagnosis is presented in Ch. 102.

Gastrointestinal Bleeding. Gastrointestinal bleeding may be gross or occult. Gross bleeding may be caused by a variety of disorders, including erosions of the stomach, tears and varices of the lower esophagus, ulcers of the duodenum, vascular tumors of stomach and small intestine (particularly leiomyomas), vascular dysplasias of the right colon, sudden severe ischemia of the small and large intestine, diverticula of the colon, or rupture of arterial aneurysms or of bypass aortic grafts into the gut lumen. The bleeding may be dramatic clinically, particularly if bright red blood has been vomited or passed in large quantities from the rectum. Many patients, however, note only black, tarry stools. Regardless of the character of the bleeding, the patient's condition is determined by the amount and rapidity of loss. Most often such persons require hospitalization, emergent study, and appropriate treatment, including emergency surgery. Gastrointestinal bleeding is discussed in Ch. 113.

Cardiovascular Responses to Acute Gastrointestinal Hemorrhage. Tachycardia is the earliest response to loss of blood volume in otherwise healthy persons, and it is accentuated by change in position from lying to standing. With continuing hemorrhage diastolic hypotension appears. At first it is evident only when the patient assumes an upright or standing posture; later it is present without change in position. A fall in diastolic blood pressure is not ordinarily noted until the patient has lost in excess of 20 to 25 per cent of intravascular volume within a few hours. Systolic hypotension is noted with continuing hemorrhage and also will not be appreciated early unless the patient assumes an upright posture.

The decreased cardiac output of significant acute gastrointestinal hemorrhage is manifested in the skin as coolness and a clammy moisture, occasionally with peripheral cyanosis. Decreasing cardiac output and cerebral ischemia cause confusion, agitation, or obtundation. With the upright posture, patients may note symptoms of blurred vision, roaring in the ears, vertigo, or a dizzy sensation; in severe cases or in later life, patients may suffer syncope. The aging brain is very sensitive to hypoperfusion and, hence, anoxia. In the elderly and those with compromised cerebral circulation, hypoperfusion may initiate cerebral thromboses. Even in those who are still alert, changes in the electroencephalogram may be noted.

Fall in cardiac output is often accompanied by changes in cardiac function. Thus, patients with significant arteriosclerotic disease of the coronary arteries may develop angina pectoris, and even without pain ischemic changes on the electrocardiogram such as S-T segment depression or T wave inversion are common. On occasion the patient suffers an acute myocardial infarction. Oliguria is a common manifestation in patients with severe blood loss from the gastrointestinal tract. At onset of bleeding, urinary osmolality and specific gravity are increased and sodium concentrations are usually less than 20 mEq per liter. With severe shock and marked renal hypoperfusion, acute cortical or tubular necrosis may supervene. The gastrointestinal tract itself is not immune from the manifestations of a severe decrease in cardiac output brought about by hypovolemia. The liver is not severely injured unless hypotension is severe and prolonged. However, the tubular gastrointestinal tract, particularly the small bowel beyond the ligament of Treitz, cecum, transverse colon, and descending colon, may suffer the effects of ischemia (see Ch. 105). Nonocclusive ischemia of these areas of the tubular gastrointestinal tract can be associated with a rapid deterioration of the patient.

With occult bleeding, patients may or may not have other symptoms indicative of disturbance in a particular part of the gastrointestinal tract. Many elderly persons complain of the effects of a progressive anemia. Unexplained iron deficiency with stools containing occult blood in such patients often reflects carcinoma of the cecum and right colon. Between these extremes are patients who intermittently pass small amounts of blood by rectum. These are patients who must be suspected of having malignancy, ischemia, or inflammatory disease of the distal colon. Chronic occult bleeding in elderly persons, particularly those with aortic valve disease, may be due to angiodysplastic lesions of the gut, particularly of the cecum and right colon.

Intestinal Gas. Patients are frequently bothered by symptoms caused by intestinal gas. These are *eructation*, the distress of *bloating* with borborygmi, and *excessive flatus*.

The major intraluminal gases are nitrogen (N_2), carbon dioxide (CO_2), and methane (CH_4); all these gases but N_2 are produced in the bowel lumen. About 600 ml of gas is passed per rectum per day, of which over 400 ml is produced enterically. The amount of hydrogen and CO_2 depends to a significant degree upon the diet. Unabsorbed carbohydrate and protein, particularly greens and vegetables, are broken down by colonic bacteria to yield hydrogen and carbon dioxide. CH_4 is produced by only about one third of the adult population.

Although complaints referable to intestinal gas have classically been attributed to excessive air swallowing, it is clear that this habit is not responsible for a major contribution either to the amount of intestinal gas or to the symptoms. Normally, swallowed air is quickly expelled. It may cause distress in only a very limited number of persons who do not normally expel it.

Eructation (Belching). Air that is expelled by belching is usually that recently swallowed into the esophagus. Repeated belching may on occasion be associated with serious organic disease, particularly with gastric outlet obstruction or gastric dilatation. The vast majority of patients who belch frequently in order to relieve distress are overanxious (constantly swallowing air, thus the word "aerophagia").

Abdominal Distress of Distention (Bloating). Bloating and "gas pains" have classically and erroneously been thought to be due to excessive gas. In fact, abnormal intestinal motor activity usually accounts for these symptoms. Usually, the intestinal contents move along in an orderly fashion, stimulated particularly by eating. Disorders of motility both in the small bowel and in the colon may move gas faster than normal. However, there may be areas of resistance to rapid passage owing to organic disease or, more commonly, to motor dysfunction associated with spasm, noted particularly in the irritable bowel syndrome. Bowel proximal to a narrowed area dilates, whether narrowing is a stricture or spasm, stretching the smooth muscle and eliciting pain of a cramping nature. Organic causes of disturbed motility may also underlie these symptoms, e.g., progressive intestinal obstruction caused by a stricture or tumor. Recent onset of these complaints always warrants thorough investigation.

The *irritable bowel syndrome* is associated with a motor disturbance and often with abdominal bloating. The discomfort of these patients may indeed be due to gas, albeit in normal amounts. It may be alleviated by dietary exclusion of gas-forming foods, including lactose, thus relieving complaints of many years to decades.

EXCESSIVE FLATUS (GAS PER RECTUM). Excessive flatus results from ingesting foods notorious as substrates for gas formation, from an overgrowth of gas-producing bacteria in the gastrointestinal tract, or from malabsorption of carbohydrates (e.g., lactase deficiency). Patients have excessive gas resulting from bacterial action on unabsorbed carbohydrate in the colon (or in the small gut if there is bacterial overgrowth), with release of hydrogen as the most important gas but also of CO_2. Only about one third of normal individuals produce intestinal methane, but a larger number (80 per cent) of patients with cancer of the colon do so. Methane production presumably reflects a special bacterial colonization of the colon. Some patients have normal amounts of flatus per day but complain of increased frequency of flatus following a meal. This complaint is most likely due to a hyperactive gastrocolic reflex, which characterizes many patients with irritable bowel syndrome.

Patients who pass more than a normal amount of gas may complain of bloating and pain. Analysis of flatus demonstrates unusually high percentages of hydrogen and carbon dioxide. Whether it is due to a particular disease of the small intestine, pancreatic insufficiency, bacterial overgrowth of the small intestine, or lactase deficiency requires definition. Excessive colonic production of gas also may be caused by the ingestion of abnormal amounts of fruit and vegetables which contain nonabsorbable carbohydrates, and may respond to dietary restriction of lactose, legumes, and wheat.

Jaundice. Jaundice is due to elevated levels of either conjugated or unconjugated bilirubin in plasma and extracellular fluid. It is a common and important sign of disease of the liver or biliary tract, or of hemolysis. Hyperbilirubinemia may result from excessive production of bilirubin (hemolysis), reduced excretion of bilirubin into the bile (liver disease), or obstruction of the flow of bile into the intestine (biliary tract disease). Rarely jaundice is caused by hereditary diseases producing defects in the hepatic uptake of bilirubin or its glucuronidation. Impaired capacity to secrete conjugated bilirubin into the bile may also be due to inherited metabolic defects. The pathophysiology of bilirubin metabolism is discussed in greater detail in Ch. 117.

Jaundice is not usually detectable in natural light below plasma bilirubin levels of 2 to 2.5 mg per deciliter. Jaundice caused by conjugated bilirubin is associated with dark urine, since conjugated bilirubin is water soluble and therefore excreted in the urine. On the other hand, nonconjugated bilirubin is lipid soluble and protein bound so that it is not excreted in the urine.

The most common cause of jaundice is injury to the hepatocyte by virus, toxin, or drug. The clinical significance of jaundice in a patient therefore depends to a large extent on its duration, intensity, and relationship to possible infection or drug use, and on the presence or absence of factors that may cause obstruction (cholelithiasis). On the other hand, gradually progressive jaundice in an elderly person not taking hepatotoxic drugs and with no evidence of viral infection most frequently indicates a periampullary malignancy obstructing the extrahepatic ductal system. Pruritus is common in many patients with jaundice; it may be due to severe intrahepatic cholestasis, extrahepatic obstruction, recurrent jaundice of pregnancy, or primary biliary cirrhosis.

The clinical evaluation of jaundice requires careful note of the possibility of viral hepatitis, particularly B virus and non-A, non-B viruses in the non-Western world. In the Western world alcohol is by far the most common liver toxin. Careful search on physical examination for evidences of liver disease is crucial in evaluating patients with jaundice. The presence of masses, particularly of a palpable gallbladder, is a most important finding. In many instances, the routine laboratory examinations, including liver function tests, are of great help but must be interpreted with caution. The differential diagnosis of jaundice may require use of the specialized diagnostic techniques discussed in Ch. 94 and 95.

Most patients with gastrointestinal disease complain of one (or more) of the symptoms and demonstrate some of the signs that have been discussed. The significance attached to these signs and symptoms determines which road to diagnosis and treatment will be taken. This approach to patients ensures intelligent reference to detailed descriptions of the clinical possibilities and leads to wise choices of tests and procedures. In the chapters that follow, symptoms and signs will be more fully described in terms of specific diseases of the various organs constituting the digestive system, and a wide range of diagnostic tests and procedures will be included. In this way the science of medicine and gastroenterology is brought to bear on good patient care.

Sleisenger MH, Fordtran JS: Gastrointestinal Disease, Part 1, Pathophysiology. 3rd ed. Philadelphia, W. B. Saunders Company, 1983.

Smith LH Jr, Thier SD (eds.): Pathophysiology: The Biological Principles of Disease. 2nd ed. International Textbook of Medicine, Vol. 1. Philadelphia, W. B. Saunders Company, 1985.

94. DIAGNOSTIC IMAGING PROCEDURES IN GASTROENTEROLOGY

Robert N. Berk

In the past decade several innovative techniques have been introduced in radiology for the detection of diseases of the gastrointestinal tract, liver, pancreas, spleen, and retroperitoneum. These remarkable new procedures have extended the diagnostic capability of radiologists far beyond that which was previously possible with conventional plain abdominal radiography and barium studies. These techniques include abdominal ultrasonography, computed tomography, radionuclide scanning, visceral angiography, endoscopic retrograde cholangiopancreatography, and percutaneous transhepatic cholangiography. Nuclear magnetic resonance, the latest of these innovations, is not yet generally available in clinical practice.

ABDOMINAL ULTRASONOGRAPHY

Ultrasonography or echography employs sound waves in the range above human hearing which are generated by a piezoelectric crystal. The sound waves are reflected from tissue interfaces depending on differences in acoustical impedance. These echoes are recorded by the same crystal that generates the waves and are displayed as a cross-sectional image in longitudinal, transverse, or oblique planes. The early instruments were capable of producing images only in black and white, whereas the new gray-scale scanners display the image in multiple shades of gray, which permits more accurate characterization of the ultrasonic properties of tissues and better resolution of anatomic structures. Real-time scanning devices, similar to a fluoroscope except that ultrasound is used rather than x-rays, are now available. With these instruments motion, such as vascular pulsations, can be identified and studied.

Greater skill and effort are required to produce a sonographic image with maximal diagnostic information than are necessary for conventional radiography. The operator must have exact knowledge of the diagnostic problem involved and must individualize each examination. However, sonography has the

Acknowledgment: I wish to express my appreciation to Robert J. Stanley, M.D., and Stuart S. Sagel, M.D., Washington University School of Medicine, St. Louis, for providing the illustrations of computed tomography.

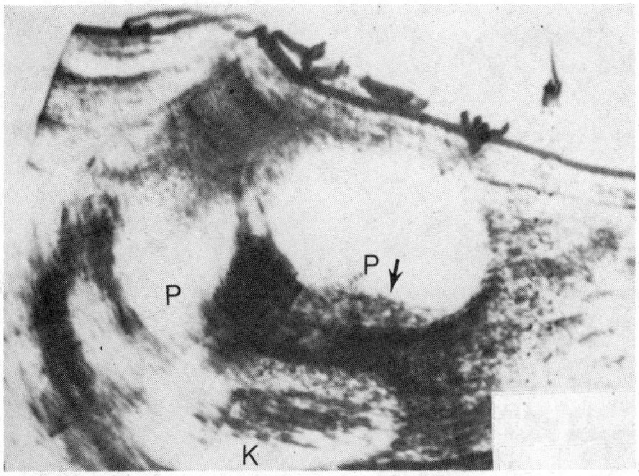

Figure 94–1. Ultrasound scan showing a bilobulated pancreatic pseudocyst (P). Longitudinal section made to the left of the midline and viewed with the patient's head on the observer's left. K, Kidney. Note the inflammatory debris in the dependent portion of the cyst (arrow).

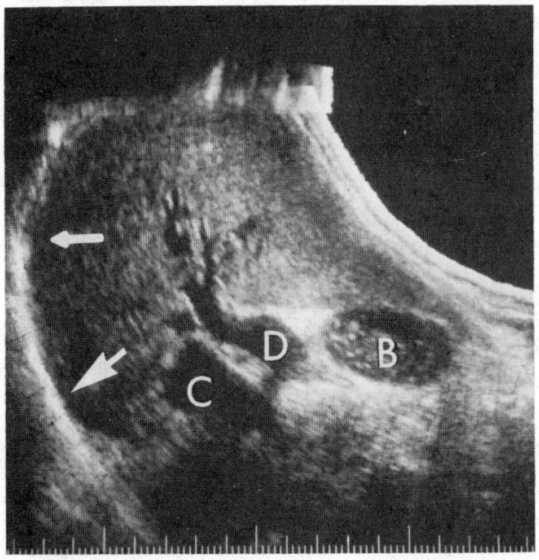

Figure 94–2. Ultrasound scan showing dilated bile ducts (D) in a patient with obstructive jaundice due to carcinoma of the head of the pancreas. Longitudinal scan made to the right of the midline and viewed with the patient's head to the observer's left. The dilated common bile duct (D) lies in front of the inferior vena cava (C). Dilated intrahepatic bile ducts, the gallbladder (B), and the diaphragm (arrows) are visible. The carcinoma cannot be identified in this plane.

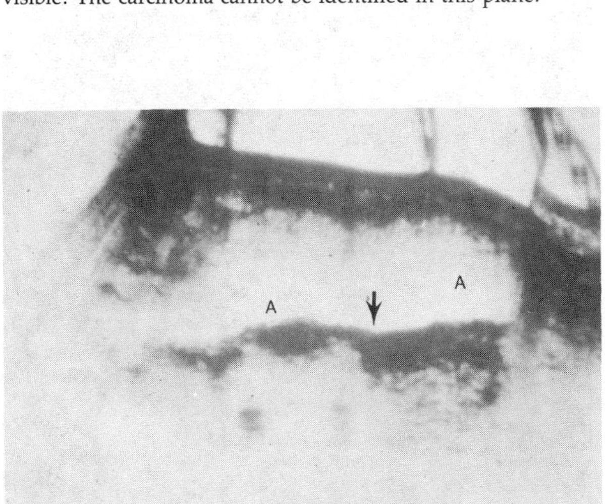

Figure 94–3. Ultrasound scan showing a large aneurysm (A) of the abdominal aorta. Longitudinal scan made through the midline and viewed with the patient's head to the observer's left. The absence of internal echoes in the aneurysm and the good definition of the posterior border (arrow) indicate that it is fluid filled.

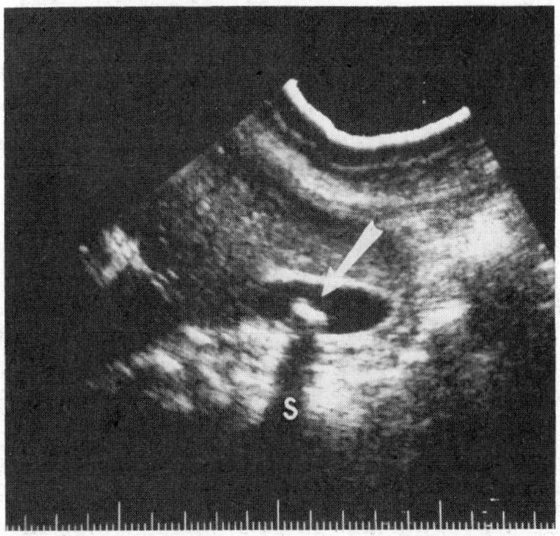

Figure 94–4. Ultrasound scan showing a single gallstone in the gallbladder (arrow). Longitudinal section to the right of the midline and viewed with the patient's head to the observer's left. The gallstone casts an acoustical shadow (S) because it does not transmit the ultrasound. The scale at the bottom indicates intervals of 1 cm.

major advantage of being entirely noninvasive, and the ultrasound waves have no known harmful effects. Consequently, there are no risks involved in the examination. This offers the additional advantage that serial studies can safely be performed to follow the course of an illness and the results of treatment.

Since ultrasound is transmitted poorly through air, gas in the intestinal lumen interferes with an adequate examination. This may be an insurmountable problem in patients with paralytic ileus. However, since sonography is not dependent on the presence of fat to identify the abdominal viscera as are procedures that use x-rays, diagnostic examinations can still be achieved in cachectic patients in whom there is paucity of intra-abdominal fat.

Ultrasonography of the abdomen produces an image of a cross-section of the liver, gallbladder, pancreas, spleen, and kidneys. The examination is useful in the detection of intra-abdominal masses, which may be as small as 2 cm in diameter. Furthermore, it is usually possible to distinguish between cysts and tumors. Fluid-filled structures such as cysts transmit ultrasound readily, so that there are few internal echoes and the posterior boundary of the mass is easily identified. Solid tumors transmit ultrasound poorly, internal echoes are evident, and the posterior margin of the lesion is not well defined. Consequently, ultrasonography is ideally suited for the identification of pancreatic pseudocysts, intra-abdominal abscess, and cysts of the liver and spleen (Fig. 94–1). Dilated bile ducts in the liver in cases of obstructive jaundice, splenic and hepatic hematomas in patients with trauma, and aneurysms of the abdominal aorta can be visualized (Figs. 94–2 and 94–3). The gallbladder and gallstones can be recognized in patients in whom opacification of the gallbladder with cholangiography and cholecystography is impossible (Fig. 94–4). Solid masses such as carcinoma of the pancreas, hepatic metastases, and hepatomas can be detected. The diagnosis of pancreatitis can often be made by detecting diffuse enlargement of the pancreas. Finally, the presence of ascites can be readily established, even when only small amounts of fluid are present.

Berk RN, Ferrucci JT, Fordtran JS, et al.: The radiological diagnosis of gallbladder disease, an imaging symposium. Radiology 141:49, 1982. *A good review of the role of all of the imaging modalities in the diagnosis of gallbladder disease.*

Berk RN, Leopold GR, Fordtran JS: Imaging of the gallbladder. Adv Intern Med 28:387, 1983. *A succinct analysis of gallbladder sonography.*

Ferrucci JT: Body ultrasonography. N Engl J Med 300:538, and 590, 1979. *A classic overview of the entire subject.*

Whalen JP: Radiology of the abdomen: Impact of the new imaging methods. Am J Roentgenol 133:585, 1979. *Valuable analysis of the most efficacious use of ultrasound, CT, and other diagnostic techniques in a variety of clinical circumstances. A must for anyone wanting further information.*

COMPUTED TOMOGRAPHY

Computed tomography (CT) is a technique of radiography in which minor differences in x-ray absorption, not evident by conventional radiograph techniques, are made visible by computer processing of x-rays transmitted through the body. In 1969, Hounsfield originated the concept that the use of a computer would permit recovery of a large amount of information concerning soft tissues which had previously been lost because of superimposition of data and insensitivity of traditional methods of recording the radiographic image. He devised a method in which a cathode x-ray tube display of the processed information gives a gray scale image of a transverse section of the body (Fig. 94–5).

Anatomic definition is more precise with CT than with ultrasonography, but the equipment necessary for CT is extremely expensive, and the radiation dose is not inconsequential. Although intestinal gas does not interfere with CT scanning, absence of fat in malnourished patients impairs the quality of the CT image.

Like ultrasonography, CT is useful in the detection of hepatic metastases, cysts, and abscesses. Tumors and cysts of the kidney and retroperitoneal lymphadenopathy and other masses can be identified. Pancreatitis produces diffuse enlargement of the pancreas, which is visible on the CT scan. Carcinoma of the pancreas has the same density as the normal pancreatic parenchyma, but the tumor can be recognized by detecting focal enlargement of the pancreas and obliteration of adjacent fat planes (Fig. 94–6). At this time CT has only limited applicability in parenchymatous disease of the liver. However, nodularity in advanced cirrhosis and radiolucency in fatty infiltration of the liver can be identified (Fig. 94–7). CT plays a valuable role in differentiating jaundice caused by biliary obstruction from cholestasis caused by parenchymal disease. In the former, dilated bile ducts can be identified in the liver and in the porta hepatis (Fig. 94–6). Finally, the gallbladder can be seen on CT because of the difference in x-ray absorption between the hepatic parenchyma and bile (Fig. 94–5). Consequently, enlargement of the gallbladder and cholelithiasis can be identified.

In many cases, CT and ultrasonography are complementary diagnostic examinations. This is particularly true in diseases involving the liver, spleen, pancreas, and kidneys. However, the retroperitoneum is better evaluated with CT than with ultrasonography, whereas ultrasonography has advantages in the diagnosis of gallbladder disease and aneurysms of the abdominal aorta.

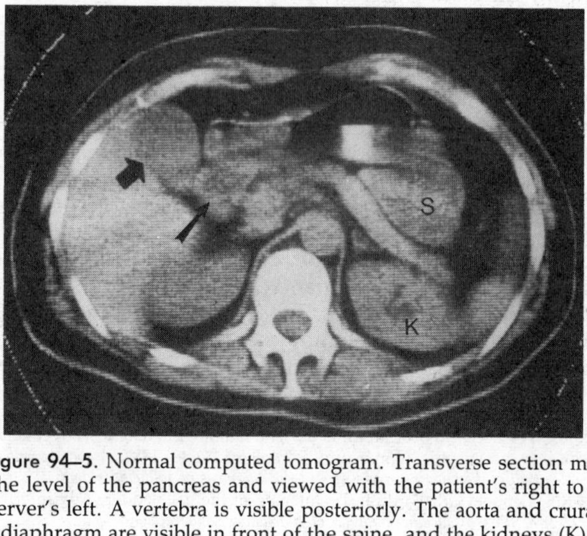

Figure 94–5. Normal computed tomogram. Transverse section made at the level of the pancreas and viewed with the patient's right to the observer's left. A vertebra is visible posteriorly. The aorta and crura of the diaphragm are visible in front of the spine, and the kidneys (K) are evident laterally. The body and tail of the pancreas lie between the fluid-filled stomach (S) in front and the kidney posteriorly. The bile-filled gallbladder (thick arrow) lies in front of the liver. The second portion of the duodenum (thin arrow) is adjacent to the head of the pancreas.

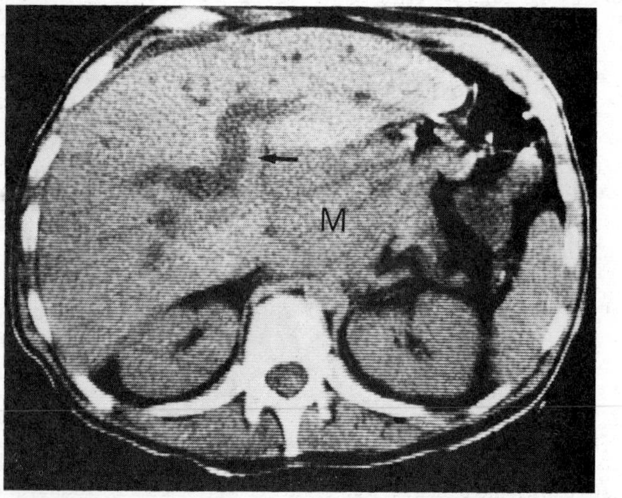

Figure 94–6. Computed tomogram in a patient with obstructive jaundice due to carcinoma of the pancreas. Transverse section made at the level of the pancreas and viewed with the patient's right to the observer's left. The spine and kidneys are evident posteriorly. The tubular structures are dilated (arrow), bile-filled bile ducts within the liver. There is a large mass (M) in the head of the pancreas.

Freeney PC, Lawson TL: Radiology of the pancreas. New York, Springer-Verlag, 1983. *Succinct text with magnificent illustrations.*

Moss AA, Schrumpf JD, Schnyder P, Korobkin M, Shimshak RR: Computed tomography of focal hepatic lesions. Radiology 131:427, 1979. *A profusely illustrated analysis.*

Siegelman SS, Copeland BE, Saba GP, et al.: Computed tomography of fluid collections associated with pancreatitis. Am J Roentgenol 134:1121, 1980. *A classic article.*

Snow JH, Goldstein HM, Wallace S: Comparison scintigraphy, sonography and computed tomography in the evaluation of hepatic neoplasms. Am J Roentgenol 132:915, 1979. *Excellent discussion of the relative value of these modalities.*

Wittenberg J: Computed tomography of the body. N Engl J Med 309:1160, 1983.

RADIONUCLIDE IMAGING

Progressive improvements in radiopharmaceuticals and imaging devices in the past decade have resulted in increased

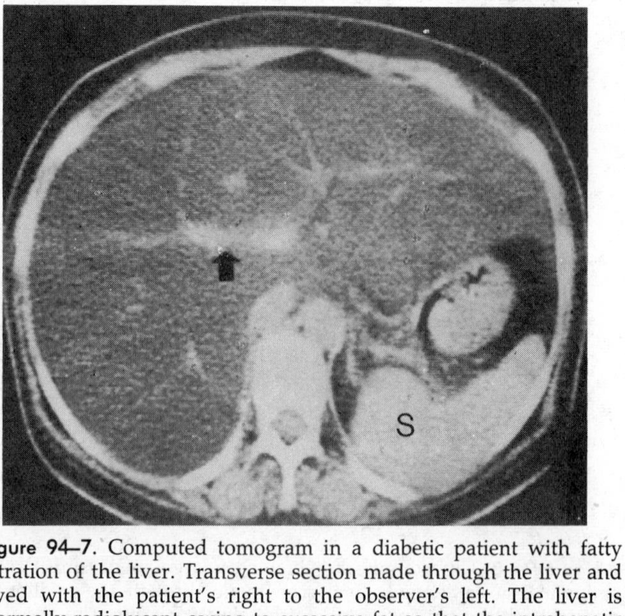

Figure 94–7. Computed tomogram in a diabetic patient with fatty infiltration of the liver. Transverse section made through the liver and viewed with the patient's right to the observer's left. The liver is abnormally radiolucent owing to excessive fat so that the intrahepatic vascular tree is visible (arrow). The normal density of the liver is the same as that of the spleen (S).

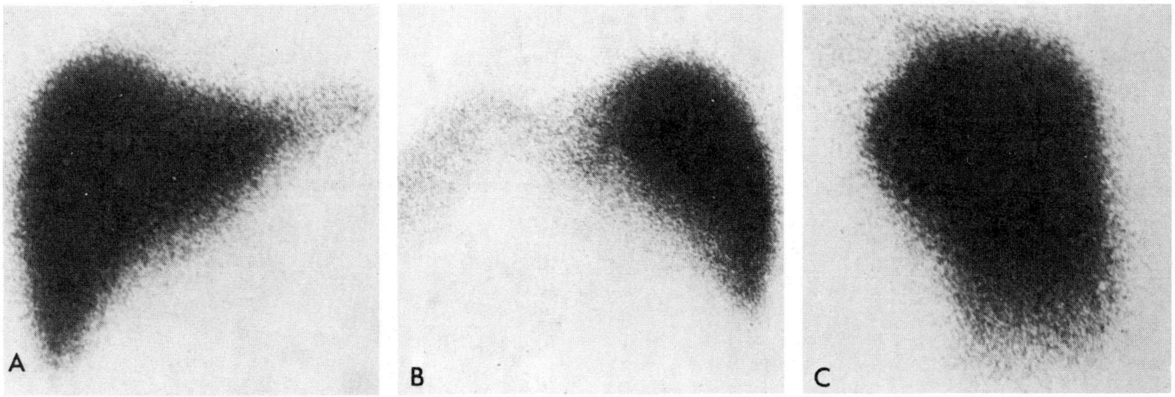

Figure 94–8. Normal technetium-99m–labeled sulfur colloid radionuclide image. The normal liver is well seen. *A,* Anterior projection. *B,* Posterior projection. *C,* Right lateral projection.

accuracy of radionuclide imaging in the diagnosis of intra-abdominal disease. The degree of resolution of anatomic details of the nuclear medicine techniques is less than that of other radiographic procedures, but this disadvantage is offset by the lack of morbidity or mortality and the versatility of the radionuclide techniques.

Radiopharmaceuticals used for the evaluation of the liver include colloidal suspensions that undergo phagocytosis by the Kupffer cells (technetium-99m–labeled sulfur colloid) and substances that are excreted by the polygonal cells (iodine-131–labeled rose bengal and technetium-99m iminodiacetic acid [HIDA]). In addition, gallium-67 and indium-111-bleomycin are useful agents because of their tendency to concentrate in hepatic tumors and abscesses.

Liver scanning is useful to (1) evaluate the size, shape, and position of the liver; (2) diagnose hepatic masses such as tumors, abscesses, and hematomas; (3) estimate the extent of hepatocellular disease in such conditions as cirrhosis; and (4) determine the cause of jaundice (Figs. 94–8 to 94–11).

A major limitation in liver imaging with radionuclides is the difficulty inherent in detecting a small lesion of decreased uptake (cold spot) in a background of diffuse radioactivity in the normal tissue (Fig. 94–9). It is possible that in the future radiopharmaceuticals will be developed to label the abnormal tissue rather than the normal parenchyma, thereby increasing the resolution of the test. At present, lesions that are located at the periphery of the liver and those in the left lobe are more easily seen. The minimal resolution of the technique is approximately 1 cm in the left lobe and 2 cm in the right lobe. Even with the newer techniques, the overall accuracy for detecting liver metastases is approximately 80 per cent. At present, combining radionuclide imaging with biochemical tests such as alkaline phosphatase, serum albumin, and serum glutamic oxaloacetic transaminase provides the best screening test for the detection of liver metastases.

Subphrenic abscesses are relatively easy to identify by combining liver and lung imaging in which the abscess produces a separation between the two visualized organs (Fig. 94–9). Gallium-67 scanning is a convenient supplement to the procedure and is particularly useful when a pleural effusion is a possible cause of the separation.

Iodine-131 rose bengal and technetium-99m HIDA are useful to distinguish jaundice caused by hepatic parenchymal disease from that caused by obstruction of the biliary tract. In patients with high grade obstructive disease of the biliary tract, there is increased concentration in the biliary tree and lack of excretion into the small bowel. The test is not reliable in the presence of low grade obstruction. In these cases measurement of the urinary and fecal excretion of the radioisotope is a more accurate indication of biliary obstruction than the radionuclide image. Patients with parenchymal disease have generalized decreased concentration of the radiopharmaceutical in the liver.

Exquisite visualization of the gallbladder and bile ducts is provided by 99m-Tc HIDA scintigraphy even in the presence of hyperbilirubinemia (Fig. 94–11). Nonvisualization of the gallbladder with opacification of the common bile duct in patients who have not had a cholecystectomy is accurate evidence for the diagnosis of acute cholecystitis. Because the procedure is quick, safe, and reliable even in jaundiced patients with serum bilirubin up to 6 mg per deciliter, it is preferred over intravenous cholangiography and is used to replace or supplement sonography of the gallbladder.

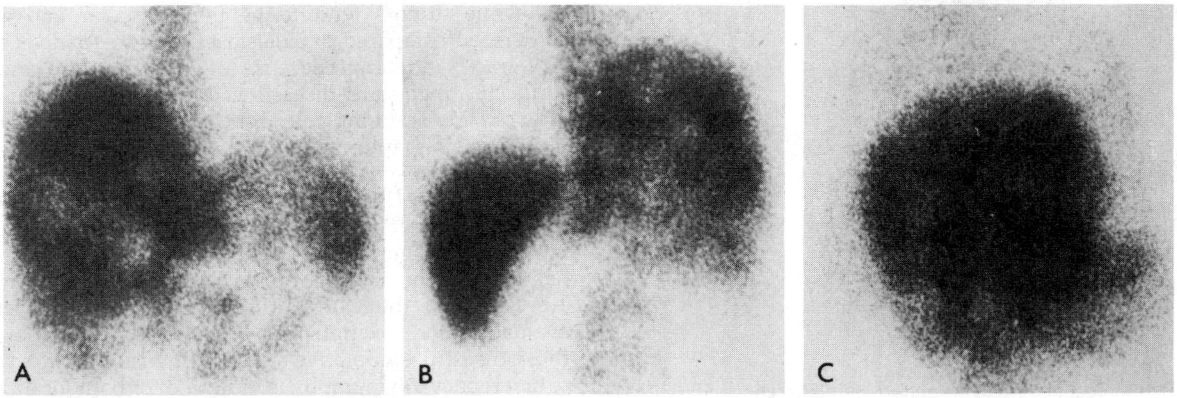

Figure 94–9. Technetium-99m–labeled sulfur colloid radionuclide image showing multiple metastases in the liver from carcinoma of the lung. Multiple "cold" areas are visible in the liver. Note also increased uptake in the bone marrow. *A,* Anterior projection. *B,* Posterior projection. *C,* Right lateral projection.

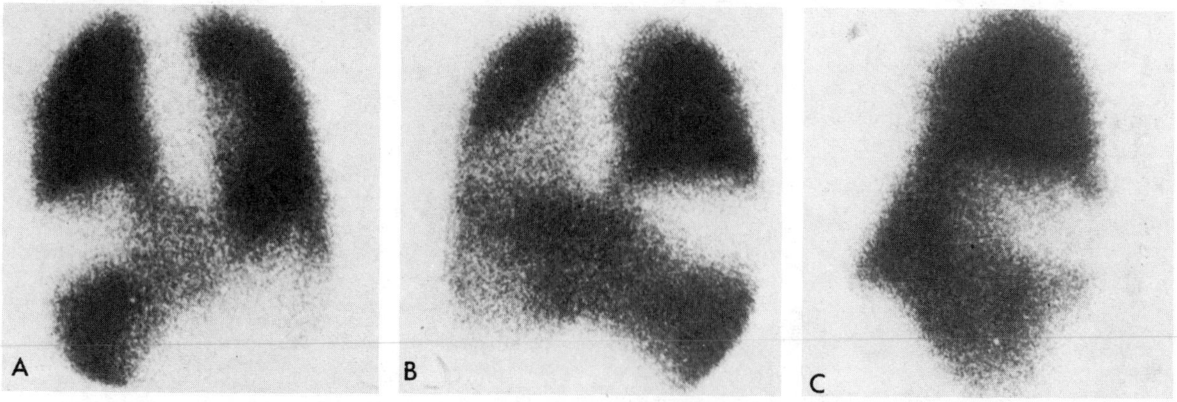

Figure 94–10. Combined liver-lung scan showing a subphrenic abscess. The examination was done with technetium-99m–labeled sulfur colloid and technetium-99m–labeled macroaggregated albumin. Note the separation between the right lung and the liver due to the abscess. *A*, Anterior projection. *B*, Posterior projection. *C*, Right lateral projection.

Phagocytosis of technetium-99m–sulfur colloid by the spleen provides a valuable method for evaluating the spleen. This technique can be used to (1) determine the presence of splenomegaly, (2) detect accessory spleens, (3) diagnose a subcapsular hematoma, and (4) identify space-occupying lesions such as a cyst or tumor.

The affinity of technetium-99m–pertechnetate for gastric mucosa makes this radiopharmaceutical useful for the detection of Meckel's diverticula and ectopic gastric mucosa in the esophagus (Barrett's epithelium). Eighty-five per cent of symptomatic Meckel's diverticula contain functioning gastric mucosa, so the technique is useful in a high percentage of patients.

Freeman LM, Blaufor MD: Gastrointestinal diseases—update. Semin Nucl Med 12:1, 104, 1982. *A comprehensive review.*

Lunia S, Parthasarathy K, Bakshi S, Bender MA: Evaluation of 99mTc–sulfur colloid liver scintiscans and their usefulness in metastatic workup; review of 1424 studies. J Nucl Med 16:62, 1975. *A concise analysis.*

Petasnick JP, Ram P, Turner DA, Fordham EW: Comparison of hepatic imaging by various modalities. Semin Nucl Med 9:8, 1979. *Excellent summary of relative roles of the new imaging modalities.*

Weismann HS: Cholescintigraphy. *In* Berk RN, Ferrucci JT, Leopold GR (eds.): Radiology of the Gallbladder and Bile Ducts. Philadelphia, W. B. Saunders Company, 1983, pp 261–314. *A thorough review.*

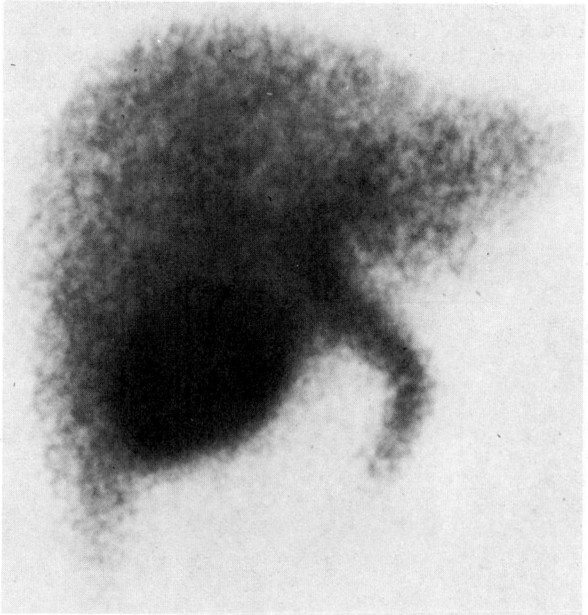

Figure 94–11. Technetium-99m–labeled iminodiacetic acid (HIDA) radionuclide image showing a normal gallbladder and bile duct. In cases of acute cholecystitis with cystic duct obstruction, the gallbladder fails to visualize.

VISCERAL ANGIOGRAPHY

Techniques for vascular catheterization, contrast materials, and radiographic equipment for visceral angiography have improved remarkably since the introduction of the Seldinger technique for the percutaneous insertion of a catheter into an artery or vein in 1953. The ability to perform subselective catheterization of intra-abdominal vessels and new methods to magnify the radiographic image have improved definition of vascular abnormalities. Procedures for interventional angiography have been devised in which selective occlusion of vessels can be accomplished through the arterial catheter for the control of gastrointestinal bleeding, preoperative devascularization of tumors, and treatment of arteriovenous malformations. Progress in visceral angiography has led to pharmacoangiography, in which drugs are injected through the arterial catheter to enhance opacification, differentiate between normal and tumor vessels, control gastrointestinal bleeding, and treat hepatic metastases.

The introduction of ultrasonography and computed tomography has made it necessary to re-evaluate the role of visceral angiography in the diagnosis of tumors of the pancreas and liver. Arteriography is an invasive procedure associated with small but significant morbidity. Furthermore, the ability of angiography to detect pancreatic carcinoma in a curable stage and to differentiate it from pancreatitis has been disappointing (Fig. 94–12). Contrarily, angiography is obviously still a valuable tool for the diagnosis of vascular tumors of the liver such as angiomas, hemangioendotheliomas, benign hepatic adenomas, and most primary hepatomas (Fig. 94–13). The accuracy of angiography in the diagnosis of hepatic metastases depends on the vascularity of the metastases relative to the normal hepatic parenchyma. Metastases from hypernephromas and endocrine tumors tend to be hypervascular and are easily recognized compared to metastases from the pancreas, alimentary tract, and lung. Because of greater safety and relative simplicity, metastatic disease of the liver is best diagnosed by radionuclide scanning, ultrasonography, or computed tomography. Angiography should be reserved for special situations in which the results of other procedures are not conclusive.

Angiography is accurate in the diagnosis of splenic and hepatic rupture (Fig. 94–14). However, the introduction of peritoneal lavage for the detection of intraperitoneal bleeding has reduced the need for more complex diagnostic procedures. Nevertheless, the extent of liver injury can sometimes be evaluated more accurately by angiography than at surgery. In these cases, postoperative angiography is often indicated.

Emergency angiography is indicated for both localization and therapy in the management of patients with acute gastrointestinal bleeding (Fig. 94–15). Not only may bleeding sites be demonstrated by contrast medium extravasation, but also the

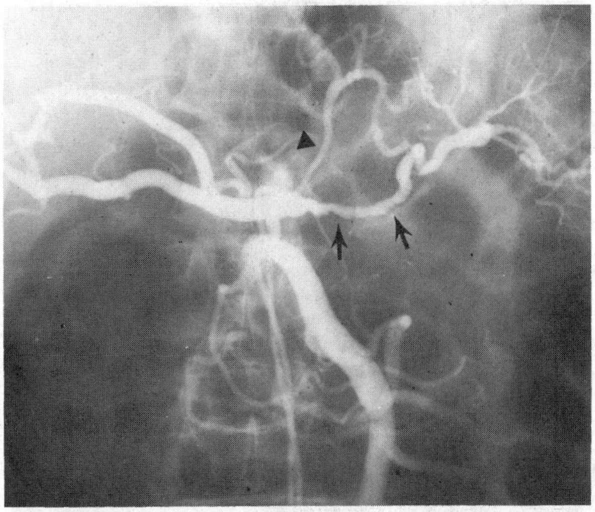

Figure 94–12. Early arterial phase from a combined celiac and superior mesenteric artery angiogram in a patient with carcinoma of the pancreas. There is irregular encasement of the splenic (arrows) and left gastric (triangle) arteries indicative of invasion by carcinoma of the pancreas.

hemorrhage may be stopped with infusions of vasoconstricting agents or by means of transcatheter vessel occlusion with blood clots and other materials. The intra-arterial infusion of vasopressin is effective in controlling bleeding in 80 per cent of patients with gastric mucosal bleeding and in 60 per cent of those with bleeding duodenal ulcers. On the basis of present evidence it appears that intra-arterial infusion of vasopressin has no benefit over continuous low dose intravenous infusion of the drug in the control of bleeding from esophageal varices.

The majority of patients with massive rectal bleeding have hemorrhage from colonic diverticula or vascular ectasias, usually on the right side of the colon (Fig. 94–15). Following identification of the bleeding site by angiography, selective

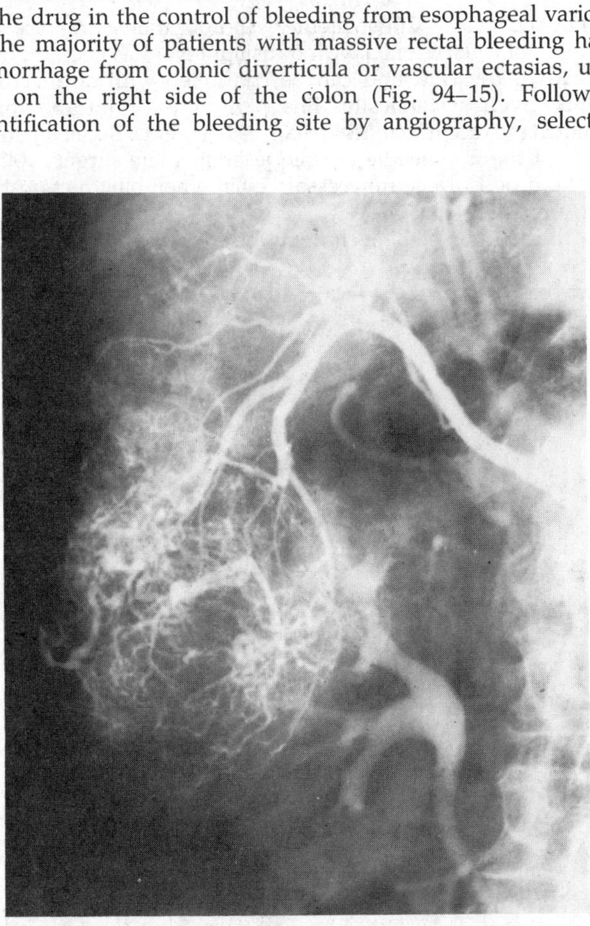

Figure 94–13. Late arterial phase from a subselective hepatic artery angiogram showing a highly vascular hepatoma of the right lobe of the liver. A large mass is apparent with abnormal vessels and pooling of contrast material. Contrast material also is visible in the pyelocaliceal structures of the right kidney.

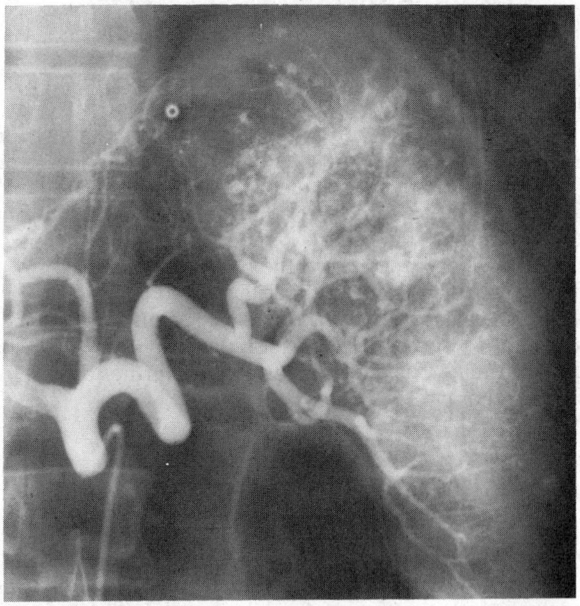

Figure 94–14. Late arterial phase from a celiac artery angiogram showing a ruptured spleen. Irregular pooling of contrast material in the spleen is apparent in the upper pole with loss of the uniform sinusoidal opacification in the lacerated area.

vasopressin infusion through the catheter acutely controls the hemorrhage in 90 to 95 per cent of patients.

Baum S, Rosch J, Dotter CT, et al.: Selective mesenteric arterial infusions in the management of massive diverticular bleeding. N Engl J Med 288:1269, 1973. *Succinct description of this therapeutic innovation by authorities on the subject.*

Bookstein JJ, Greenway GD: Gastrointestinal hemorrhage: Angiography and transcatheter therapy. *In* Teplick JG, Haskin ME (eds.): Surgical Radiology. Vol 1, Philadelphia, W. B. Saunders Company, 1981, pp 789. *A fine summary of both diagnosis and treatment of gastrointestinal bleeding.*

Reuter SR, Redman HC: Gastrointestinal Angiography. Philadelphia, W. B. Saunders Company, 1977. *Excellent monograph covering every aspect of the subject.*

Witkins RA, Viamonte M: Interventional Radiology. Oxford, Blackwell Scientific Publications, 1982. *A detailed description of therapeutic maneuvers using the angiographic catheter.*

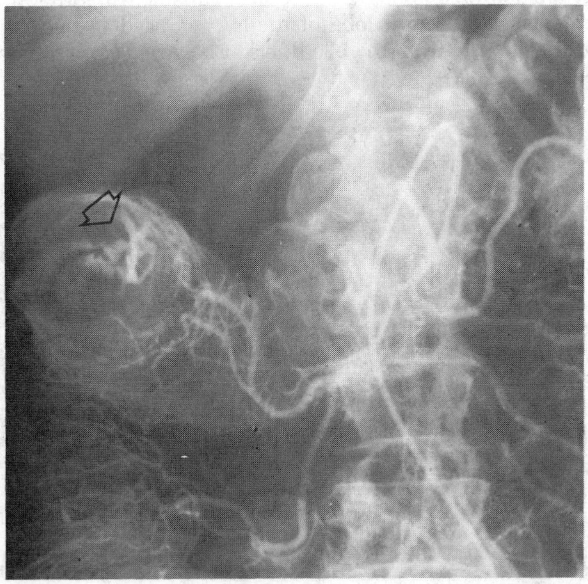

Figure 94–15. Late arterial phase from a superior mesenteric artery angiogram showing pooling of contrast material in the lumen of the hepatic flexure due to hemorrhage from colonic diverticulum (arrow). Opacification of the wall of the colon is evident, and there is faint visualization of the portal vein.

ENDOSCOPIC RETROGRADE CHOLANGIOPANCREATOGRAPHY

Endoscopic retrograde cholangiopancreatography (ERCP) is a diagnostic modality that has been made possible by the development of the fiberoptic endoscope. With this instrument it is possible to insert a small catheter into either the common bile duct or the pancreatic duct through the papilla of Vater under direct vision. Radiographic contrast material can then be injected through the catheter under fluoroscopic control to opacify the biliary tree and/or the pancreatic duct (Fig. 94–16). Consequently, radiographic opacification of the biliary tree is possible when impaired liver function or common duct obstruction precludes successful opacification with oral cholecystography or intravenous cholangiography. A further discussion of ERCP is contained in Ch. 95.

PERCUTANEOUS TRANSHEPATIC CHOLANGIOGRAPHY

The introduction of the fine needle technique for percutaneous transhepatic cholangiography has made it possible to opacify the biliary tree safely in a high percentage of patients regardless of obstruction of the bile ducts. Consequently, the procedure is an important tool for the evaluation of patients with jaundice.

A flexible, 23-gauge needle with an outer diameter of 0.7 mm, 15 cm in length, is inserted into the liver percutaneously from the right midaxillary line. The tip of the needle is positioned in the hepatic parenchyma to the right of the twelfth thoracic vertebra under fluoroscopic guidance. Radiographic contrast material is injected slowly as the needle is withdrawn. Recognition of the site of contrast material deposition is readily made fluoroscopically. Contrast material in the hepatic parenchyma persists; contrast material in hepatic or portal venous radicles flows away rapidly; whereas contrast material in the bile ducts persists and moves slowly toward the porta hepatis. Insertion of the needle can safely be repeated several times if the bile ducts are not visualized on the initial trial. When the bile ducts are identified, contrast material is injected in sufficient quantities to fill the biliary tree and multiple radiographs are made.

Because the needle has an external diameter of only 0.7 mm, only a small hole is made in the liver capsule. In addition, the substance of the right lobe of the liver is used to tamponade any bile leakage from the bile ducts or bleeding from the portal or hepatic veins. Consequently, complications are rare and usually mild. Bacteremia with transient fever has been reported in 7 to 10 per cent and can be controlled with antimicrobial agents given systemically. Bile peritonitis or intraperitoneal hemorrhage occurs in less than 2 per cent. Because of the safety of the fine needle technique, immediate surgery following the procedure is unnecessary even when bile duct obstruction is present.

With the fine needle technique the success rate of opacifying

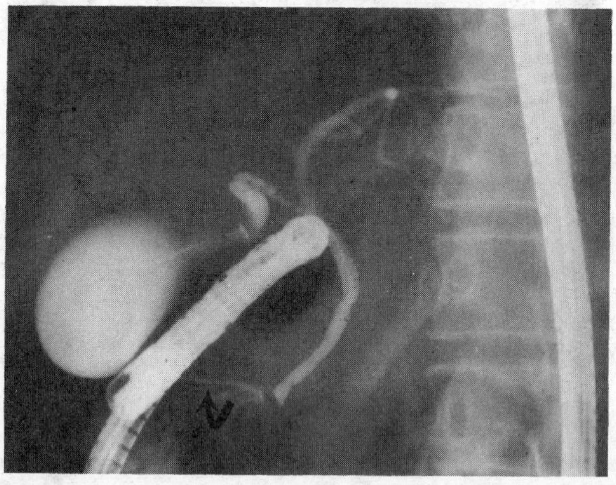

Figure 94–16. Normal endoscopic retrograde cholangiogram. The gallbladder, cystic duct, common hepatic duct, and common bile duct are visible. Note the endoscope with the tip positioned opposite the papilla of Vater. A catheter (arrow) has been inserted into the papilla of Vater under direct vision.

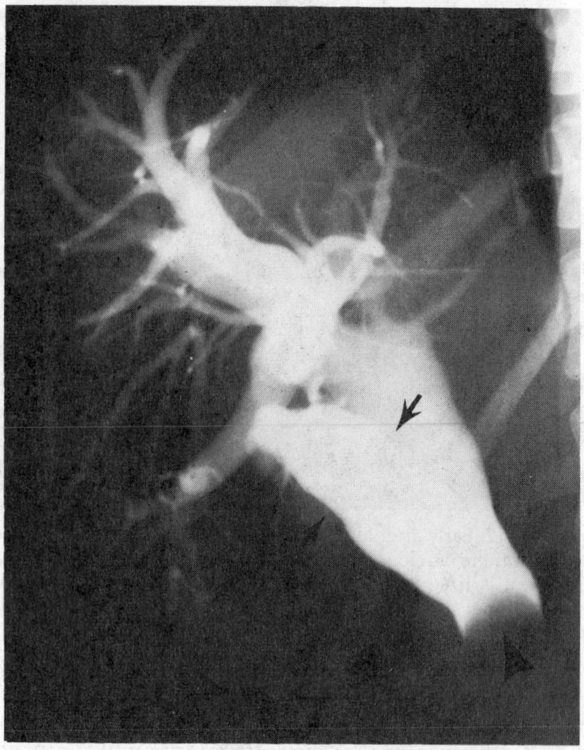

Figure 94–17. Fine needle percutaneous transhepatic cholangiogram in a jaundiced patient showing marked dilatation of the biliary tree due to an obstructing gallstone in the common bile duct (arrowhead). The cystic duct (arrows) and intrahepatic ducts are dilated. The gallbladder is not filled.

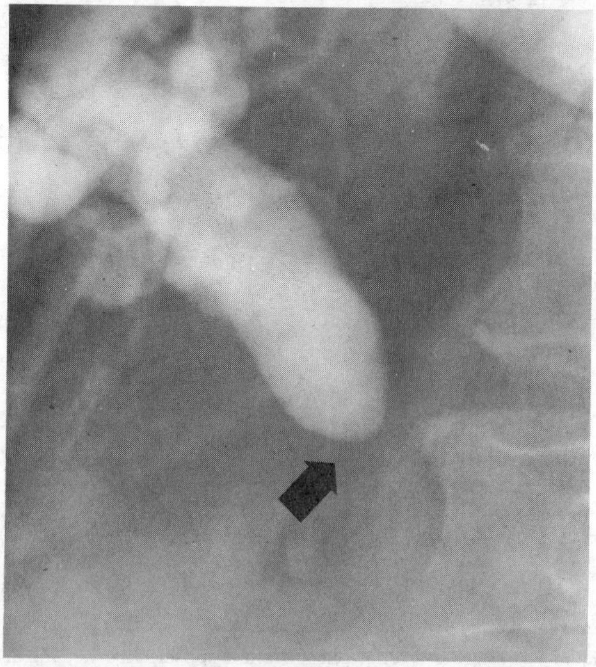

Figure 94–18. Fine needle transhepatic percutaneous cholangiogram in a jaundiced patient showing obstruction of the common bile duct due to carcinoma of the pancreas. Note the marked dilatation of the bile duct with the abrupt tapering at the point of obstruction (arrow).

the biliary tree is 100 per cent in patients with bile duct dilatation and between 60 and 80 per cent when the bile ducts are normal. The skill required of the operator is modest compared to that necessary to perform retrograde endoscopic cholangiography. The time and the cost required to perform percutaneous cholangiography are considerably less.

Percutaneous cholangiography permits the differentiation of jaundice caused by obstruction of the bile duct from that caused by parenchymal disease and provides valuable information for the surgeon concerning the cause, location, and extent of the biliary obstruction prior to surgery (Figs. 94–17 and 94–18). The procedure can be followed by an interventional technique such as transhepatic biliary drainage or dilation of a bile duct stricture performed via a catheter inserted percutaneously.

Berk RN, Ferrucci JT, Leopold GR: Radiology of the Gallbladder and Bile Ducts: Diagnosis and Intervention. Philadelphia, W. B. Saunders Company, 1983. *A complete and lucid review.*

Mueller PR, Harbin WP, Ferrucci JT, et al.: Fine needle transhepatic cholangiography; reflections after 450 cases. Am J Roentgenol 136:85, 1981. *A lucid discussion by experts on the subject.*

NUCLEAR MAGNETIC RESONANCE

Cross-sectional images of the body can be obtained without x-ray by the use of nuclear magnetic resonance (NMR) (Figs. 94–19 and 94–20). This phenomenon involves the combined effect of a magnetic field and radiofrequency radiation on protons (hydrogen nuclei). Summarized briefly, protons spin and act as magnetic compasses. When placed in a strong magnetic field they tend to become aligned with the field, producing a net magnetic vector in the sample. A radiofrequency pulse of a specific frequency is used to alter the energy state of the protons. This displaces the net magnetic vector by an amount determined by the strength and duration of the pulse. After the pulse is removed, the protons emit energy in the form of a radiofrequency signal as they return to their original orientation. When a gradient is introduced in the magnetic field, the frequency emitted by the radiated protons varies with their position in the gradient. The signal can then be used to form a proton map or two-dimensional image of the portion of the body being studied. NMR is discussed further in Ch. 21.

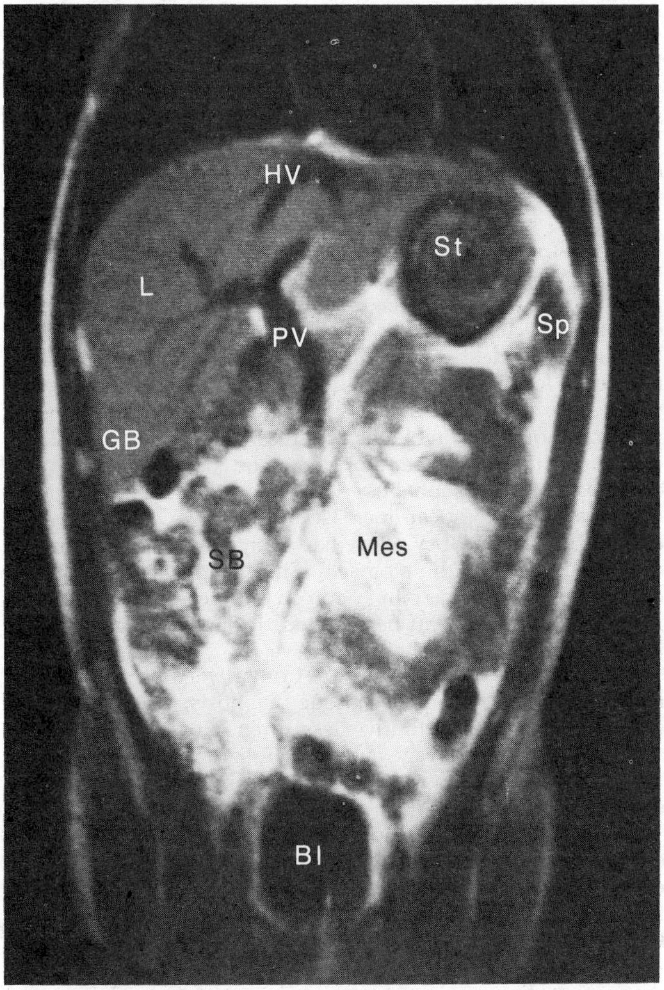

Figure 94–19. Normal nuclear magnetic resonance image. Anterior coronal section. General Electric Company, Milwaukee, Wisconsin. (L = liver, Sp = spleen, St = stomach, GB = gallbladder, HV = hepatic veins, PV = portal vein, SB = small bowel, Mes = mesentery, Bl = bladder.)

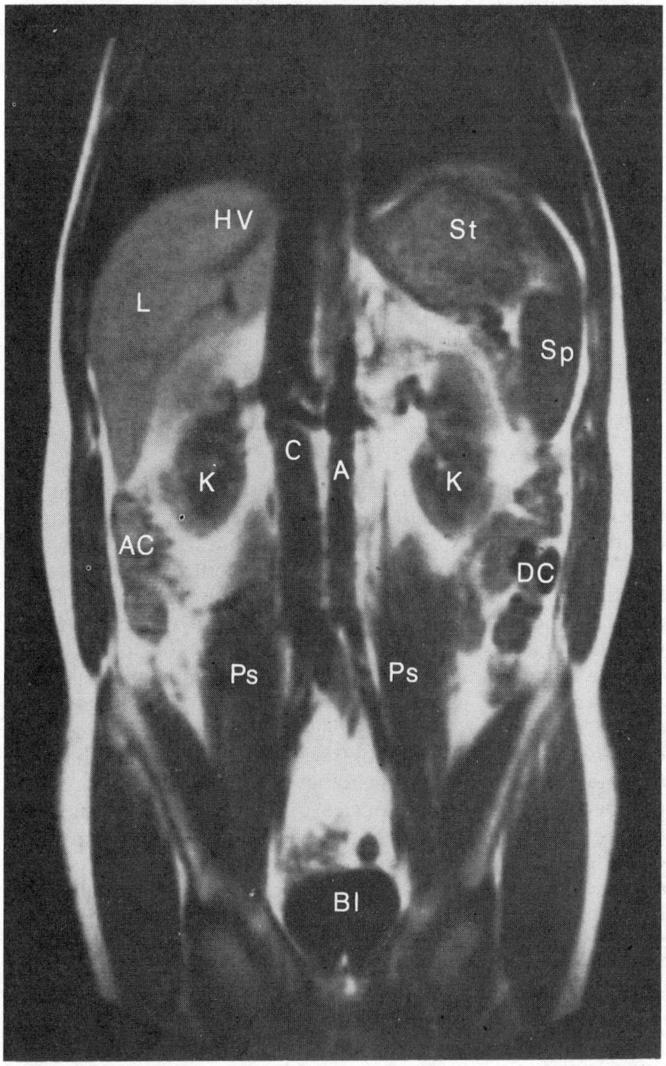

Figure 94–20. Normal nuclear magnetic resonance image. Posterior coronal section. General Electric Company, Milwaukee, Wisconsin. (L = liver, Sp = spleen, St = stomach, C = inferior vena cava, A = aorta, K = kidney, AC = ascending colon, DC = descending colon, Ps = psoas muscle, Bl = bladder, HV = hepatic veins.)

The advantage of NMR compared with computed tomography is that there is better contrast resolution between normal tissues with NMR. NMR images allow discrimination between normal and abnormal tissues, because of the differences in relaxation times. For instance, the signal from a tumor differs from that of adjacent normal tissue. NMR does not involve ionizing radiation and has no known harmful effects; images can be obtained in any plane. Flow prevents blood from emitting a signal, so the lumen of normal arteries and veins appears as black tubes (Fig. 94–20).

The disadvantages of the new technique include the high cost of the machine, difficulties associated with having a powerful magnetic field in a hospital environment, and concern over the effect of the magnetic field on cardiac pacemakers, surgical clips, and metallic prostheses. Calcium is not detected by NMR, and the lungs are inaccessible.

Kressel HY, Axel L, Thickman D, et al.: NMR imaging of the abdomen. Am J Roentgenol 141:1179, 1983. *Early results in 45 patients.*

Pykett IL: NMR imaging in medicine. Sci Am 246:78, 1982. *An excellent, understandable review of the physical principles of NMR.*

Young IR, Bailes DR, Burl M: Initial clinical evaluation of whole body NMR tomography. J Comput Assist Tomogr 6:1, 1982. *First insights into the clinical potential of NMR imaging.*

95. GASTROINTESTINAL ENDOSCOPY

Paul Sherlock

Remarkable progress in fiberoptic endoscopy during the last two decades has affected the management of many gastrointestinal disorders. Major technical advances include forward-viewing endoscopes with complete tip control and sufficient length to permit direct visualization of mucosal lesions as far distal as the descending duodenum, and of the entire colon with the colonoscope. Newer instruments allow a 45-degree oblique angle for wider viewing in narrow tubular areas such as the esophagus, gastric antrum, duodenum, and parts of the colon. The forward-viewing panendoscope and the oblique instrument are highly versatile, with single or double channels to obtain specimens for histology and cytology. Snares for polypectomy and large biopsies can be inserted through the biopsy channel of both the upper panendoscope and the colonoscope. Electrocautery and laser probes can be inserted, and their usefulness in the treatment of gastrointestinal bleeding is currently being investigated. The side-viewing instruments are used primarily for visualizing the ampulla of Vater and for cannulation of the common bile duct and pancreatic duct. All these instruments allow multiple observers during a procedure, and 35-mm still photographs and 8- or 16-mm movies and videotape recordings can be taken.

The diagnostic accuracy of endoscopy is dependent upon the skill and experience of the endoscopist. Endoscopic findings should be documented by photographs or videotape whenever possible. Individuals with minimal training should be discouraged from performing endoscopy, as this may lead to diagnostic error and/or complications—cogent reasons for comprehensive endoscopic training programs, preferably as part of residency programs in gastroenterology or surgery. Teaching endoscopy as an isolated technical procedure may lead to improper application, excessive use and cost, faulty interpretation of findings, and inappropriate decisions for patient care.

There are multiple indications for diagnostic and therapeutic endoscopy. Substantiation by controlled studies for some of these indications is lacking, as is consensus as to the proper sequencing of radiologic, nuclear, ultrasonic, and endoscopic studies. New endoscopic techniques must be tested for effectiveness, risk, cost and suitability for specific problems. Controlled studies are needed to compare endoscopy with other diagnostic and therapeutic procedures. We need clinical algorithms to decide logically which procedure should be done and when.

Endoscopy is contraindicated in patients with severe acute cardiac or pulmonary disease and should not be done if perforation of the gastrointestinal tract is suspected or if the patient is uncooperative.

Premedication may be important in individual patients. Parenteral diazepam and meperidine reduce the rate of unsatisfactory patient cooperation to less than 1 per cent. Emptying the stomach prior to upper gastrointestinal endoscopy may be necessary to improve visualization and prevent aspiration pneumonia if pyloric obstruction is suspected or after recent food intake. This is not necessary in the usual patient undergoing endoscopy, since retained secretions can be aspirated through the suction channel. Topical anesthesia with gargle or spray to the posterior pharynx is usually necessary for upper endoscopy.

ESOPHAGOGASTRODUODENOSCOPY (Panendoscopy)

Endoscopy of the esophagus, stomach, and duodenum is generally done with a single forward-viewing panendoscope with cytology and biopsy capability. The side-viewing instrument is occasionally used for more thorough evaluation of areas of the stomach and duodenum not adequately visualized by the forward-viewing instrument. It has been helpful in examining the ampullary region of the second portion of the duodenum for tumors and clarifying the nature of duodenal abnormalities, especially in the presence of a deformed bulb. Given the capability of the forward-viewing instrument, the stomach and duodenum should be examined even when symptoms suggest only esophageal disease because of the frequency of associated pathology.

Histologic and cytologic diagnosis can be made with a high degree of accuracy, using a biopsy and cytology brush inserted through the open channel in the endoscope. The brush or lavage cytology method, utilizing the Papanicolaou staining technique, has increased the diagnostic yield of upper gastrointestinal tumors.

Complications from upper panendoscopy include perforation. This is extremely rare with the newer fiberoptic instruments, and occurs more often in the cricopharyngeus area of the upper esophagus. Perforations have occurred through Zenker's diverticula and through areas of tumor during or following endoscopic manipulation in both the esophagus and stomach. Extreme bleeding from the biopsy site, aspiration pneumonia, sepsis, thrombophlebitis from intravenous medication, and cardiovascular complications from the procedure or the premedication—although rare—must be anticipated.

CANCER. Endoscopy has increased the diagnostic yield of upper gastrointestinal cancer and has been found to be accurate in 85 to 92 per cent of cases. When endoscopy is combined with brush and/or lavage cytology as well as biopsy, the diagnostic accuracy can be in the range of 95 to 99 per cent. For a high diagnostic yield four to six biopsies must be obtained from each lesion. Perhaps even more important is the selection of areas to be biopsied. Areas covered by normal-appearing mucosa should be avoided, whereas areas of nodularity or discoloration should be biopsied. The best results can be obtained in the esophagus, where a combination of tissue biopsy and cytology can increase the positive yield to as high as 100 per cent. Biopsy alone has been less productive in the esophagus than in the stomach, since esophageal tumors are often stenotic and the biopsy forceps do not reach the tumor. The cytology brush can be inserted through the stenotic area to brush the center of the tumor.

Tumors of the stomach that are primarily exophytic or mass-like usually yield a positive tissue diagnosis, whereas tumors that are primarily infiltrative less often provide a diagnostic specimen. Pulsatile lavage cytology, utilizing a dental irrigating unit, can be added to the brushing and biopsy to increase the diagnostic yield.

Using endoscopy, biopsy, and cytology, gastric lymphoma, either primary or secondary, can be diagnosed in 70 to 88 per cent of cases. When suspected lymphoma is confirmed by tissue diagnosis, the management of the patient will be significantly influenced.

Malignant gastric ulcers usually provide a positive tissue diagnosis when six or more biopsies are obtained from the inner edge of the ulcer margin and from the four quadrants rather than from the outer edge. The base of the ulcer should not be biopsied, since one may obtain only necrotic nondiagnostic material. The highly accurate assessment of the nature of a gastric ulcer that is obtained by endoscopy has virtually eliminated the debate regarding the benign versus malignant character of a gastric ulcer seen on x-rays (see Fig. 99–6). The role of endoscopy in patients with ulcerating gastric lesions will depend upon both the radiographic appearance and the clinical situation. In considering the need for endoscopy, etiologic factors should be considered, such as ingestion of ulcerogenic drugs or a coexistent active duodenal ulcer. Follow-up endoscopy should be considered (1) when complete healing is not demonstrated in 6 to 12 weeks; (2) when symptoms persist even though the x-ray indicates complete healing; (3) if initial endoscopic appearance and/or histology were not clearly benign; and (4) if the ulcer was initially found only on endoscopy.

Gastric polyps are rare lesions in standard-risk patients. The incidence of malignancy in the polyp varies with its size, with those over 2 cm having a significant risk. Small hyperplastic polyps do not have to be removed, but large ones may require removal by snare-cautery technique similar to that used for colonic polyps. Gastric ulcer at the site of polyp removal is a frequent complication. Gastric bleeding or perforation is unusual.

UPPER GASTROINTESTINAL BLEEDING. Upper gastrointestinal panendoscopy is a very accurate means of determining the presence and site of upper gastrointestinal bleeding. Bleeding lesions are precisely identified more frequently by endoscopy than by barium meal radiography. However, the beneficial effects of precise diagnosis on patient outcome are presently unclear. Endoscopy should locate and identify the bleeding source even with multiple lesions, determine whether or not bleeding is continuous and from an arterial source, and determine whether a vessel is visible in an ulcer base. Therapeutic choices are often influenced by these observations, but current studies suggest that endoscopy in acute gastrointestinal bleeding may not alter outcome. If controlled trials of endoscopic methods for controlling bleeding, such as laser probes, use of solutions for sclerosing of esophageal varices, or electrocautery, prove to be safe and effective, more accurate endoscopic diagnosis may affect the outcome in a very favorable manner. A more extensive discussion of the approach to the patient with upper gastrointestinal bleeding is found in Ch. 112.

MISCELLANEOUS INDICATIONS. Upper endoscopy may have a role for patients with symptoms of dysphagia, odynophagia, unexplained heartburn, unresponsive abdominal pain, duodenal ulcer pain, or gastric outlet obstruction. Unexplained radiologic lesions, gastrointestinal hemorrhage, surveillance of patients at high risk for stomach cancer, symptoms and signs after gastric surgery, chemotherapy, or radiation therapy all may require endoscopic evaluation. Endoscopy is also useful in the removal of foreign bodies, dilatation of esophageal strictures, and the placement of tubes in patients with unresectable esophageal cancer.

ENDOSCOPIC RETROGRADE CHOLANGIOPANCREATOGRAPHY

Endoscopic retrograde cholangiopancreatography (ERCP) utilizes the side-viewing flexible endoscope. An experienced, skilled endoscopist with a cooperative, appropriately sedated patient can pass the instrument, enter the duodenum, and identify and cannulate the papilla in as little as 10 to 20 minutes in 75 to 80 per cent of attempts (see Fig. 94–16). It is often easier to cannulate the main pancreatic duct than the common bile duct. Reasons for failure include compression of the duodenal wall by tumor, carcinoma involving the papilla itself, location of the papilla within a duodenal diverticulum, previous surgery in the area, duodenal stricture or stenosis, and Billroth II gastric resection.

The indications for ERCP are (1) confirmation of an abnormal or equivocal CT scan in pancreatic cancer; (2) confirmation of the diagnosis of sclerosing cholangitis; (3) obstructive jaundice, especially in the patient with abnormal coagulation factors for whom percutaneous transhepatic cholangiography might be dangerous; (4) placement of nasobiliary and internal biliary stents for palliation of malignant bile duct obstruction; and (5) performing endoscopic sphincterotomy for removal of common bile duct stones or for papillary stenosis.

Complications from ERCP include injection pancreatitis, cholangitis, and drug reactions. Pancreatitis most often occurs within 24 hours of the procedure and is usually mild and well tolerated. Fluoroscopic monitoring to prevent overdilatation of the pancreatic ducts may not be sufficient to prevent its occurrence. Cholangitis, which occurs in about 1 per cent of patients, can lead to severe sepsis and death. Cholangitis does not generally occur in the setting of a normal biliary tree. Prompt antibiotic therapy and surgery should be considered when retrograde cholangiography demonstrates an obstructed biliary tree.

RETROGRADE PANCREATOGRAPHY. After the papilla is cannulated for pancreatography, Renografin-60 is injected under fluoroscopic control into the pancreatic duct and x-ray films are taken. The radiographic interpretation, particularly of minor pancreatic duct abnormalities, may be a source of controversy, since there are normal variations in ductal architecture. Occasionally pancreatography is complicated by duct anomalies, the most common of which is incomplete fusion of the dorsal and ventral portions of the gland, causing only the small ventral portion to visualize. This may result in an incorrect diagnosis of pancreatic cancer.

The most common dilemma is differentiating between carcinoma of the pancreas and chronic pancreatitis (Fig. 95–1). The two may coexist. One often sees chronic pancreatitis distal to a cancer involving the proximal duct. Carcinoma may develop in the setting of pre-existing pancreatitis. Cutoff or stenosis of the pancreatic duct with tapering at the point of occlusion is the most striking finding of carcinoma. Stricture of the duct may suggest neoplastic origin when the secondary branches in the area of the stricture are absent. When the common bile duct is involved with carcinoma of the head of the pancreas, the narrowing or cutoff of both the pancreatic and bile ducts strongly suggests pancreatic cancer. Although some confusion exists in interpreting pancreatograms, endoscopic pancreatography plays an important role in the evaluation of patients with possible pancreatic cancer. Unfortunately, symptomatic pancreatic cancer diagnosed by ERCP in most patients is inoperable (see Ch. 108).

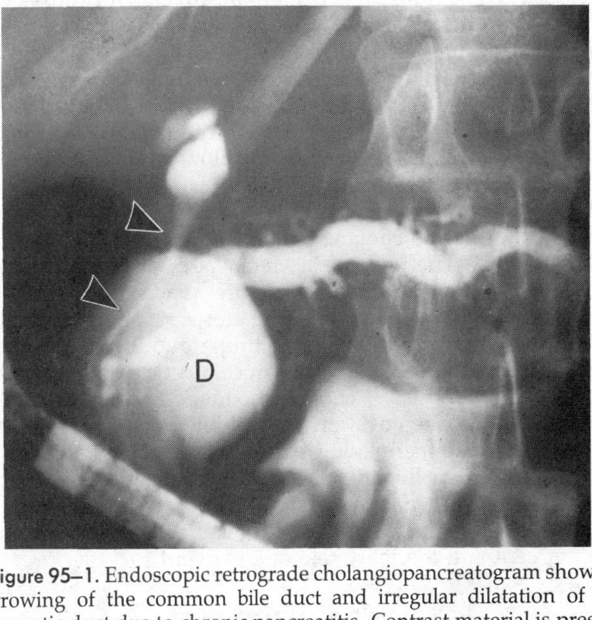

Figure 95–1. Endoscopic retrograde cholangiopancreatogram showing narrowing of the common bile duct and irregular dilatation of the pancreatic duct due to chronic pancreatitis. Contrast material is present in a duodenal diverticulum (D) and in the fourth portion of the duodenum. Note saccular dilatation of the branches of the pancreatic duct and the smooth tapered appearance of the common bile duct (arrows).

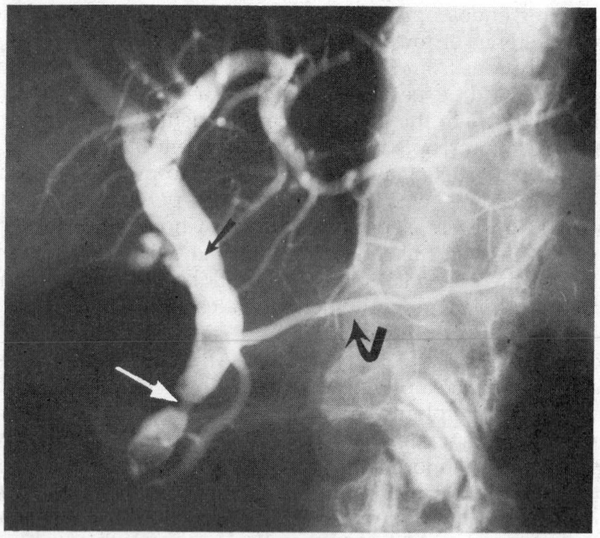

Figure 95–2. Endoscopic retrograde cholangiopancreatogram showing gallstones and a stricture (white arrow) of the common bile duct. The patient had a previous cholecystectomy. Note the cystic duct remnant (black arrow), mild dilatation of the common bile duct, and the normal pancreatic duct (curved arrow). The endoscope had been removed prior to the radiograph.

Lavage cytology, lavage carcinoembryonic antigen (CEA) from the pancreatic duct via the endoscope, brushing devices, and a special biopsy forceps passed into the ampulla have had limited use, and the success has not been striking in increasing the diagnostic yield. Direct visualization of both the biliary and pancreatic ductular systems through a thin cholangiopancreatoscope passed through the instrument channel of an enlarged master scope has also had limited use and success. Both stones and cancer can be visualized with this technique, but further investigation is needed.

RETROGRADE CHOLANGIOGRAPHY. Cholangiography via the endoscope (Fig. 95–2) has been useful in the evaluation of the jaundiced patient with a success rate of approximately 75 per cent. Retrograde cholangiography can delineate common bile duct obstruction from both benign and malignant causes and can identify normal or abnormal hepatic ducts. Cytology can be obtained from the bile duct in a similar manner as from the pancreatic duct. Thin needle percutaneous transhepatic cholangiography is usually recommended before ERCP as the procedure to be used in evaluating the jaundiced patient, particularly if the hepatic ducts are shown by ultrasound or computed tomography (CT) scan to be dilated. However, one cannot evaluate the duodenum and papilla or obtain pancreatography during a thin needle cholangiogram.

OTHER USES. The endoscopic removal of retained common duct stones by an electrosurgical wire attached to the ERCP catheter or by cutting the papilla (endoscopic sphincterotomy) has been extensively utilized in Europe and is being investigated in the United States. The procedure is also being used for papillary stenosis. A choledochoduodenostomy is created that facilitates the removal of retained bile duct stones and the placement of semipermanent endoprosthesis for palliation in this setting of malignant bile duct obstruction. Experience suggests that the danger of endoscopic sphincterotomy is considerably less than that from surgery, with a morbidity rate of 8 per cent and mortality rate of 1 per cent.

LAPAROSCOPY

Laparoscopy (peritoneoscopy) involves the creation of a pneumoperitoneum and the endoscopic inspection of the anterior abdominal space. The laparoscope is introduced through a puncture in the abdominal wall. Preferably the procedure is carried out with local anesthesia and light sedation. The technique has been very helpful in determining the etiology of hepatomegaly and ascites; diagnosing metastatic cancer of the liver and peritoneum; determining operability and curability in patients with cancer; and guiding needles for biopsy of solid organs, masses, or the peritoneum. The accuracy of laparoscopic diagnosis has been above 90 per cent in experienced hands. Findings established at laparoscopy can change a clinical impression and alter treatment plans in as many as 40 per cent of patients.

The greatest application of this technique is in diagnosing focal liver disorders such as metastatic carcinoma. This is especially true at an early stage when tumor nodules are small and widely scattered, decreasing the probability of a positive hit by a blind percutaneous biopsy. More than two thirds of the liver can be examined at laparoscopy. It is estimated that 70 to 80 per cent of the liver surface can be seen if a tilt table is used and a probe is utilized to lift the liver.

At laparoscopy biopsy can be visually guided with an accuracy of over 90 per cent. Even with two biopsies and aspiration cytology, blind percutaneous biopsy or biopsy aimed at scan defects does not reach the accuracy of laparoscope-guided biopsy. Laparoscopy is also useful when liver malignancy is suspected and blind biopsy is negative and when a scan shows only a left lobe defect.

Laparoscopy with local anesthesia is reasonably safe as an invasive test. Mild complications such as subcutaneous gas dissections occur in about 1 in 100 procedures. More serious complications such as bleeding or bowel perforation occur in about 1 to 2 per 1000 procedures. Mortality is less than 1 per 1000. In general, morbidity and mortality are slightly greater than percutaneous liver biopsy and considerably less than laparotomy.

Adhesions around the liver, usually from prior surgery obscuring areas of interest and restricting hepatic mobility, are one of the main problems in the laparoscopic diagnosis of liver neoplasms. Omentum may also adhere to the liver, limiting the view of the hepatic surface; ascites may obscure an abnormal area. Neoplasms may be localized to areas such as the posterior and very superior surfaces not routinely seen at laparoscopy. Intrahepatic subsurface lesions, which occur as a unique type of involvement in about 10 per cent of liver metastases, may be missed, but they can be suspected by a bulge or contour change on the liver surface.

In jaundiced patients the laparoscopic assessment of the liver and gallbladder may differentiate intrahepatic from extrahepatic cholestasis as well as various types of cirrhosis. If there is blockage of the common bile duct below the cystic duct, the gallbladder will be tense and distended. The advantage of laparoscopy in the jaundiced patient is the ability to make a tissue diagnosis when the biliary obstruction is caused by cancer and if metastases are present in the liver or peritoneum. The diagnosis of unsuspected ascites can also be made. Tissue may be obtained safely and reliably from the liver surface with a cytology brush to avoid the risk of bile leakage when there is extrahepatic biliary obstruction.

The ability of laparoscopy to detect small early metastases to the liver has been applied to staging various malignancies before treatment, particularly in carcinoma of the lung. In primary hepatocellular carcinoma, laparoscopy may be very helpful in staging for possible surgical cure. The peritoneum and diaphragm can be evaluated for evidence of metastatic spread. It can be determined if both lobes of the liver are involved by multifocal tumor and whether diffuse cirrhosis is present, which would preclude a major hepatic resection.

Laparoscopy appears to be highly accurate for staging Hodgkin's disease, and the assessment of liver involvement has a diagnostic yield approaching the laparotomy standard. Laparoscopy is not quite as accurate as laparotomy with non-Hodgkin's lymphoma, but because of its lower morbidity laparoscopy still offers an important means of achieving a pathologic diagnosis of liver involvement.

FIBEROPTIC SIGMOIDOSCOPY AND COLONOSCOPY

Fiberoptic sigmoidoscopy and colonoscopy have enabled direct visualization of the entire colon. The completely movable tip in an arc of 360 degrees with four-way tip deflection allows negotiation of the rectosigmoid and the flexures. In addition there is capability for biopsy, brush cytology, lavage cytology, and photographic documentation of observed lesions. Polyps can be removed by the cautery-snare technique. Fibercolonoscopy frequently provides information that can influence the diagnosis and treatment of both benign and malignant diseases of the colon. Integration of these techniques with the double contrast barium enema, fecal occult blood testing, tumor markers, biopsy, and cytology has provided impressive diagnostic and therapeutic capability.

The 60-cm flexible sigmoidoscope allows for more thorough examination of the rectosigmoid area and may result in better patient acceptance than the 25-cm rigid sigmoidoscope. The changing pattern of distribution of cancer in the colon and rectum toward more proximal involvement is an important consideration for the future application of sigmoidoscopy in asymptomatic patients. The time required for flexible sigmoidoscopy is about twice that required for rigid sigmoidoscopy. As would be expected, the yield from flexible sigmoidoscopy is higher than that from rigid sigmoidoscopy owing to the more extensive area of examination. The disadvantages of flexible sigmoidoscopy are the greater time and expertise required, the more costly equipment, and higher maintenance cost. A 30- to 35-cm flexible sigmoidoscope is now available that is less expensive than the 60-cm scope and requires less training in its use.

Fiberoptic colonoscopy has revolutionized our diagnostic and therapeutic capabilities when dealing with disease of the colon. It has extended the routine endoscopic observation of the colon from 25 cm to the entire colon. Polyps and cancers not visualized on barium enema are frequently detected at colonoscopy.

CANCER OF THE COLON (see Ch. 106). Patients should be considered for colonoscopy if they present with symptoms suggesting neoplastic disease or unexplained colonic disease, or with gross or occult blood in the stool. Colonoscopy is useful to confirm or clarify the results of barium enema or to search for additional synchronous lesions, both adenomas and cancer. Colonoscopy has also been useful in patients who have had partial colonic resection not only for examination of the remaining colon but also for examination of the anastomotic site that may be beyond reach of the sigmoidoscope. Biopsy and brushing of the anastomotic site are critical for postoperative surveillance of patients who have had recent colorectal cancer.

INFLAMMATORY BOWEL DISEASE (see Ch. 104). Most patients with inflammatory bowel disease do not require colonoscopy. However, when adequate data are not available from clinical, sigmoidoscopic, or radiologic studies, colonoscopy may prove an important aid in the diagnosis and management of patients with ulcerative colitis and Crohn's disease. When it is clinically necessary to differentiate between ulcerative and granulomatous colitis, colonoscopy with multiple biopsies may be helpful. Colonoscopy can determine the anatomic extent of the inflammatory process. It is occasionally useful preoperatively in patients with Crohn's colitis in whom radiologic examination has not yielded sufficient information for planning optimal surgical resection. When there is strong clinical suspicion of inflammatory bowel disease despite negative sigmoidoscopy and barium enema, colonoscopy with biopsy may determine the presence or absence of colitis.

Proctosigmoidoscopy with biopsy of suspicious lesions and barium enema are still important diagnostic techniques for following patients with ulcerative colitis. However, because of the more uniform distribution of cancers superimposed on ulcerative colitis and the frequent inability of the examiner to reach the 25-cm level, the 25-cm sigmoidoscope does not detect the majority of cancers.

Diagnostic colonoscopy in ulcerative colitis has usually been performed to investigate an abnormality seen on previous barium enema. The two most common problems requiring endoscopic resolution are strictures and mass lesions. Although most strictures are benign, some may be malignant and carcinoma may spread submucosally, narrowing the lumen circumferentially. Multiple biopsies may fail to reveal the presence of carcinoma within such a stricture. During colonoscopy pseudopolyps need not be biopsied, since they have no malignant or premalignant potential. When multiple polypoid lesions are present throughout the colon, it may not be possible for the endoscopist to differentiate visually among a pseudopolyp, a neoplastic polyp, and carcinoma. These polyps should be biopsied when they are larger than 1 cm, have surface friability, are of a color different from the adjacent pseudopolyps, or have an irregular surface configuration.

Utilizing biopsy and brush and lavage cytology via the colonoscope, it is now possible to clarify suspicious areas, particularly structures beyond the reach of the standard rigid sigmoidoscope. Exfoliative cytology is an underutilized technique that may be helpful in detecting in situ an early carcinoma of the colon in patients with ulcerative colitis, as it has with cervical cancer.

Colonoscopy provides the ability to obtain multiple biopsies throughout the colon for evaluation of dysplasia which, if severe, is considered a neoplastic alteration of the mucosa comparable to anaplastic epithelium found in colonic adenomas. When moderate to severe dysplasia is a consistent finding, colectomy is recommended. Since dysplastic changes may be patchy in distribution, the colonoscope affords the ability to visualize mucosal abnormality for biopsy as well as to take multiple random biopsies throughout the colon in search of dysplastic change. A regular program of colonoscopy surveillance for dysplasia may be needed when a patient has had total colitis for more than seven to ten years.

In patients with inflammatory bowel disease colonoscopy is contraindicated in the presence of fulminant colitis, toxic megacolon, suspected perforation, or peritonitis.

LOWER GASTROINTESTINAL BLEEDING (see Ch. 113). Colonoscopy has very little role in patients with acute hemorrhage from the lower gastrointestinal tract. The blood may obstruct vision and make detection of lesions difficult. Angiographic procedures may be preferable. However, chronic blood loss requires investigation by colonoscopy. The presence of diverticulosis on barium enema in patients with blood in the stool does not always explain the reason for the blood. An occult carcinoma and significant-sized polyps have been found in several series when colonoscopy has been done. Other lesions such as angiodysplasia, particularly of the proximal colon, may be the cause. These lesions can often be seen on colonoscopy and are well seen on angiography.

POLYPOSIS (see Ch. 106). Diagnostic colonoscopy is appropriate in certain patients in whom the risk for the development of carcinoma of the colon is increased. These include persons with a family history of familial polyposis or cancer syndromes or a personal history of neoplastic colorectal polyp or cancer. Endoscopic surveillance of these persons is important. In patients with the familial polyposis syndrome when the colon has not yet been resected, endoscopy with biopsy and cytology is necessary to detect early developing cancer. Preoperative colonoscopy may discover synchronous colon lesions when barium enema shows carcinoma. The type of follow-up after removal of a solitary polyp or carcinoma is controversial. Studies are underway utilizing colonoscopy and/or barium enema with air contrast to answer this question.

Most polyps can be completely removed by cautery-snare technique during colonoscopy (Fig. 95–3). The safety of this procedure has been substantiated by the low incidence of complications in numerous series. This technique avoids the need for many laparotomies that previously would have been done when the polyp found on barium enema was beyond reach of the sigmoidoscope. The morbidity, mortality, and cost

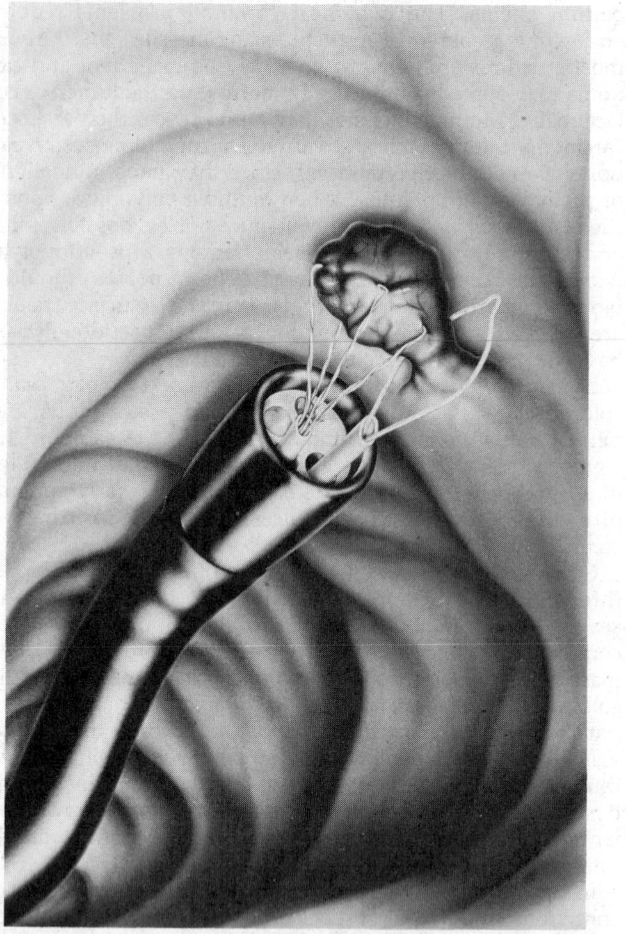

Figure 95–3. Schematic drawing of removal of pedunculated polyp via double channel fiberoptic colonoscope. The multiprong forceps has the head of the polyp, while the snare, which is attached to an electrocautery apparatus, is looped around the base of the polyp. Polyps can easily be removed through the single channel colonoscope without the aid of forceps. (Courtesy of Mr. Ingram Chodorow.)

of colonoscopic polypectomy are significantly less than polypectomy by laparotomy. The latter is justified only when an endoscopist is unable to safely remove the entire lesion or when infiltrating cancer is present in the polyp. It must be determined by controlled studies whether removal of polyps will lessen the incidence of colonic cancer. This concept is based on the opinion that most cancers arise in pre-existing polyps and is suggested in a study in which the sigmoidoscopic removal of all polyps reduced the anticipated incidence and invasiveness of subsequent development of cancer of the rectosigmoid.

FUTURE OF ENDOSCOPY

Future prospects in endoscopy include even smaller diameter instruments to allow more thorough examination of the upper gastrointestinal tract and improved diagnostic techniques, including lavage with dyes and chemicals and assays of tumor-associated antigens and enzymes. Longer endoscopes may also place the small bowel under direct scrutiny. The dramatic progress in therapeutic endoscopy such as polypectomy and the removal of common duct stones may subsequently include the control of gastrointestinal bleeding, utilizing electrodes, tissue glues, and laser beams inserted through the endoscope. Needles to instill sclerosing solutions for esophageal varices are also being investigated.

The fiberoptic endoscope has added an enormous dimension to our diagnostic and therapeutic capabilities. The future promises continued advances. This remarkable technology should result in cost-effective care for the management of patients with gastrointestinal disease.

Boyce HW Jr: Laparoscopy. *In* Schiff L (ed.): Diseases of the Liver. 5th ed. Philadelphia, J. B. Lippincott Company, 1982, pp 333–348. *An excellent description of laparoscopic indications, contraindications, technique, and pathology.*

Cotton PB: Progress Report: ERCP. Gut 18:316, 1977. *A superb review of the technical aspects, methods, success rates, complications, radiologic aspects, and clinical relevance of diagnostic ERCP.*

Decker W, Tytgat GN: Diagnostic accuracy of fiberendoscopy in detection of upper intestinal malignancy: A follow-up analysis. Gastroenterology 73:710, 1977. *Review of fiberendoscopic studies in 1005 patients revealed an overall correct endoscopic interpretation in 92.7 per cent of 135 patients with gastric malignancy. Diagnosis was correct in 98.8 per cent, owing largely to the number of biopsies (GTR>10) in gastric ulcer patients.*

Eastwood GL: Does early endoscopy benefit the patient with active upper gastrointestinal bleeding? Gastroenterology 72:737, 1977. *Immediate fiberoptic endoscopy has been used extensively in upper gastrointestinal bleeding with expectation that early diagnosis would lead to reduced morbidity and mortality. However, this has not been borne out in prospective studies to date.*

Kurtz RC, Lightdale CJ, Winawer SJ, Sherlock P: Endoscopy and gastrointestinal neoplasia: Diagnosis and management. *In* Hickey RC (ed.): Current Problems in Cancer. Chicago, Year Book Medical Publishers, 1980. *Extensive review of upper panendoscopy, fiberoptic colonoscopy, sigmoidoscopy, ERCP, and laparoscopy for diagnosis and management of neoplasia and management of complications of neoplastic disease.*

Proceedings of the NIH Consensus Workshop on Upper Gastrointestinal Bleeding. Dig Dis Sci (suppl):1, 1981. *Papers on the value of endoscopy in upper gastrointestinal bleeding that were used as background for the consensus workshop outlining the role of endoscopy in this condition.*

Rogers BHG, Silvis SE, Nebel OT, Sugawa C, Mandelstam P: Complications of flexible fiberoptic colonoscopy and polypectomy. Gastrointest Endosc 22:73, 1975. *In 25,298 diagnostic colonoscopies there was a morbidity of 0.32 per cent and a mortality of 0.008 per cent. The most common complication from diagnostic colonoscopy was perforation (0.22 per cent). In 6214 colonoscopic polypectomies a morbidity of 2,3 per cent was reported with no mortality. The most common complication was hemorrhage (1.9 per cent).*

Rubin CE, Silverstein FE, McDonald G: Indications for fiberoptic endoscopy. Viewpoints Dig Dis 10: No 5, Nov 1978. *Excellent brochure by American Gastroenterological Association which outlines approach to 20 common problems indicating when endoscopy is useful and when superfluous or possibly harmful.*

Safrany L: Duodenoscopic sphincterotomy and gallstone removal. Gastroenterology 72:338, 1977. *"Clinical Trends and Topics" paper on excellent results with sphincterotomy for choledocholithiasis and papillary stenosis, with overall mortality of 1.2 per cent and emergency laparotomy as a result of the procedure of 2.5 per cent. Complication and mortality rates appear lower than with equivalent conventional surgical techniques.*

Silvis SE, Rohrmann CA, Vennes JA: Diagnostic accuracy of endoscopic retrograde cholangiopancreatography in hepatic, biliary and pancreatic malignancy. Ann Intern Med 84:438, 1976. *Report of 73 successful studies in which diagnosis of tumor was made in 67 patients for diagnostic yield of 92 per cent. Hallmark of malignancy was obstruction and stenosis. Study indicates that malignant disease of pancreas and biliary tract is adequately assessed by this method.*

Simeone JF, Wittenberg J, Ferrucci JT: Modern concepts of imaging of the pancreas. Invest Radiol 15:6, 1980. *Review of progress in imaging techniques of the pancreas comparing ultrasound, computed tomography, and endoscopic retrograde cholangiopancreatography.*

Sivak MV Jr, Levin B (eds.): ERCP: Diagnostic and therapeutic aspects—An international symposium. Gastrointest Endosc 28:197, 1982. *Selected papers from the Cleveland Clinic course indicating the role of ERCP in modern gastroenterology.*

Williams CB, Waye JD: Colonoscopy in inflammatory bowel disease. Clin Gastroenterol 7:701, 1978. *Authoritative discussion of usefulness, indications, and contraindications of colonoscopy in all forms of inflammatory bowel disease, including differential diagnosis between ulcerative colitis and Crohn's disease and the cancer risk in ulcerative colitis.*

Winawer SJ, Leidner SD, Boyle C, Kurtz RC: Comparison of flexible sigmoidoscopy with other diagnostic techniques in the diagnosis of rectocolonic neoplasia. Dig Dis Sci 24:277, 1979. *Comparison of flexible and rigid sigmoidoscopy in 108 patients, indicating greater yield of both adenomas and cancers using flexible instrument inserted to greater distance with improved patient tolerance.*

96. ORAL MEDICINE

Sol Silverman, Jr.

Many oral diseases representing local and systemic conditions must be recognized by the physician for appropriate treatment or referral. Signs and symptoms of many of these diseases, as well as effective management, can be quite variable. Fortunately, most oral diseases are benign and noncontagious. Many of the conditions are progressive, making correct diagnosis and early treatment important factors in minimizing morbidity. Precancerous lesions and malignancies occur frequently enough to be of constant concern in the differential diagnosis. Some of the most common and clinically important oral diseases will be reviewed briefly in this chapter.

DENTAL CARIES

Caries (tooth decay) is possibly the most widespread human disease and the greatest cause of loss of teeth prior to the age of 35.

ETIOLOGY. Bacteria, substrate, and a susceptible tooth are required for the carious lesion. Although a variety of microorganisms can be responsible for dental decay, the most important appear to be certain streptococcal strains. Substrate for bacterial growth is a critical factor; primarily carbohydrates in the form of sucrose have been shown to be most harmful in promoting dental plaque, bacterial growth, and the carious lesion. Most natural teeth are susceptible to decay unless preventive measures are instituted.

SIGNS AND SYMPTOMS. Early decay can be detected by careful clinical examination and x-ray evaluation. When the lesion becomes moderately advanced, missing tooth structure, surface softness, discoloration, and sensitivity become apparent.

MANAGEMENT. Treatment requires removal of the carious material by instrumentation and replacement by a suitable dental material. Prevention entails the following points:

1. Proper hygiene to reduce dental plaque (polysaccharide matrix adherent to tooth surface promoting bacterial proliferation). This can be accomplished by brushing, preferably with a fluoride dentifrice, vigorous mouth rinsing, and flossing.

2. Diet (reducing carbohydrates, preferably sucrose-source foods) to minimize a major component of plaque and the most effective bacterial substrate.

3. Fluoride, to produce a more acid-resistant tooth structure, to enhance tooth remineralization, and to interfere with bacterial growth. A fluoride supplement of approximately 1 mg daily during tooth development has been shown to be an effective means of reducing dental decay. The amount of fluoride depends upon that occurring in the communal water supply and the amount of water consumed daily. Daily fluoride mouth rinses and topical applications by the dentist also are very effective supplements for children, as well as for adults who continue to have caries problems. This is particularly true in adults with reduced saliva (i.e., Sjögren's syndrome, irradiation effects, drug-induced xerostomia). Reliable epidemiologic studies indicate that fluoride ingestion does not increase the risk for development of cancer.

Leverett DH: Fluorides and the changing prevalence of dental caries. Science 217:26, 1982. *Studies reviewed documenting the reduction of dental caries through fluoride in community water supplies, individual usage (dentifrices, mouth rinses, and supplements) and incorporation in food processing.*

Newbrun E: Sugar and dental caries: A review of human studies. Science 217:418, 1982. *Studies reviewed indicating that frequent or high intake of sugary foods predisposes to dental decay.*

DENTAL ABSCESS

If the carious process (bacterial infection with tooth decalcification) progresses to the dental pulp, pulpitis (inflammation of the dental pulp) ensues. Spontaneous sensitivity and reactions to temperature changes are often the first signs. The pulpitis may be reversible if the carious process is removed; however, if it continues, abscess formation takes place. The abscessed tooth is manifested by pain that may be spontaneous, in response to temperature changes or to pressure. Dental abscesses can sometimes be caused by deep fillings or trauma, which initiates the pulpal inflammatory process.

DIAGNOSIS. The abscessed tooth is classically diagnosed by its tenderness to slight percussion, reactivity to heat, and a periapical radiolucency visualized in dental x-rays. Progression of the abscess can lead to severe pain, swelling, lymphadenopathy, and fever. The discomfort may be continuous or intermittent, and cannot always be localized to the offending tooth.

Occasionally abscess formation is not accompanied by symptoms and is detected by routine x-ray examination. In these cases the dental abscess or granuloma often converts into a cyst or may develop a fistular tract, establishing chronic low grade drainage ("gumboil" or parulis).

Ludwig's angina can be a rare complication if appropriate drainage, removal of the infectious source, or effective antibiotics are not instituted.

MANAGEMENT. Emergency care involves drainage, antibiotics (preferably penicillin, with erythromycin being used in penicillin-sensitive individuals), and analgesic drugs. Definitive treatment is by endodontic therapy (root canal filling) or extraction.

PERIODONTAL DISEASE

This condition is the most common cause for the loss of teeth beyond the age of 35. Periodontal disease is manifested by the loss of dental bone support (alveolar process of mandible and maxilla), which creates dental pockets (gingival and bony crevices around the teeth). This further promotes accumulation of bacteria, debris and calculus formation, worsening of the inflammatory process, further acceleration of bone loss, and loosening of the teeth. This process may be accompanied by gingivitis, purulent exudates, swelling, and pain.

ETIOLOGY. Although the most common cause of periodontal disease is poor hygiene (formation of plaque and calculus), in some individuals causative factors remain unknown. Bacterial toxins and inflammation are the common denominators, and immunologic mechanisms have been implicated. Inheritance does not play an important role. In addition to staining tooth structure, tobacco usage has been shown to increase the risk for gingivitis, periodontal disease, and earlier loss of teeth. Diabetes also encourages periodontal disease by suppressing local cell systems that control bacterial proliferation and inflammation. Associations between periodontal disease and other metabolic diseases, gastroenteropathies, and nutritional deficiencies have not been established. The loss of bone through the aging process is a common denominator, and periodontal disease in younger persons is extremely rare, even with poor hygiene.

DIAGNOSIS. Early periodontal disease may go unrecognized, since it is often asymptomatic and without clinically obvious signs. As periodontal disease continues, however, it usually can be detected by gingival erythema and swelling, tooth mobility, and a gingival exudate associated with discomfort or pain. Periodontal disease is confirmed by examination for dental pockets and more accurately assessed by loss of bone seen in x-rays. Certain conditions, such as histiocytosis, hypophosphatasia, and the Papillon-Lefèvre syndrome, can simulate precocious periodontal disease when the jaw bones are affected and teeth are lost prematurely.

PREVENTION AND TREATMENT. Optimal home care (brushing, rinsing, and flossing) and periodic dental office prophylaxes (curettage and polishing) are extremely important factors in removing the causative dental plaque (similar but not identical to plaque causing dental caries). For advanced periodontal disease, surgical alterations of gingiva and alveolar bone, as well as splinting teeth together, may be helpful in slowing or preventing further deterioration. In acute flares, hydrogen peroxide mouth rinses (3 per cent H_2O_2 with equal parts warm water) and antibiotics (preferably penicillin) are usually effective. Although a nutritious diet is important, this will not prevent periodontal disease. Effective human vaccines are not yet available.

Murphy NC, Newman MG: Update and commentary on periodontics; Applying recent discoveries to your practice. J Calif Dent Assoc 9:41, 1981. *Critical assessment of causative factors, pathogenesis, and control of periodontal disease.*

ACUTE GINGIVITIS

This condition, often referred to as acute necrotizing ulcerative gingivitis (ANUG) and Vincent's infection, does not follow any epidemiologic patterns, and there is no evidence that it is contagious. With proper microbiologic testing methods, it does seem to be often associated with fusiform and spirochete

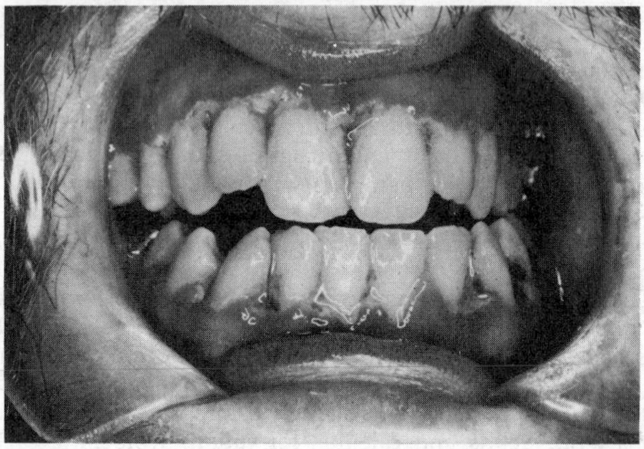

Figure 96–1. Acute necrotizing ulcerative gingivitis. Note typical necrosis of marginal gingiva. These signs, associated with pain and fetid odor, were present for one week.

organisms. Poor oral hygiene and suboptimal nutrition are frequently found. ANUG can mimic gingival changes occasionally seen in individuals with blood dyscrasias or viral infections.

DIAGNOSIS. The condition is usually characterized by its acute nature associated with pain, fetid oral odor, and gingival ulcerations (Fig. 96–1). There may be associated tendency toward bleeding. Most often there is no associated fever or lymphadenopathy, but malaise may be present.

The diagnosis is established by ruling out other, more serious systemic disease and by response to treatment. This condition differs from chronic gingivitis, which may be asymptomatic and due to poor home care, irritating fillings, or pocket formation (incipient periodontal disease).

TREATMENT. The most conservative approach is by improving oral hygiene, hydrogen peroxide mouth rinses (3 per cent H_2O_2 mixed with equal parts warm water), and dental prophylaxis. Adequate nutrition is important, and antibiotics are useful in case of fever, lymphadenopathy, or severe oral signs and symptoms. Penicillin is the drug of choice (1000 to 1500 mg daily), with erythromycin in similar dosages an alternative. If good home care is continued, recurrence is unlikely.

When ANUG does not respond to treatment, other diseases must be considered, requiring more extensive laboratory tests. Diseases such as erythema multiforme, lichen planus, pemphigoid, and pemphigus may mimic a chronic or subacute gingivitis. In these instances a biopsy will assist the diagnosis and corticosteroids will control signs and symptoms.

APHTHOUS ULCERS

Aphthous ulcers (canker sore, ulcerative stomatitis) occur in up to 40 per cent of the population. There appears to be a genetic tendency, since offspring of parents with aphthous ulcers have a greater risk for developing them. Aphthae usually appear by age 20 and without sex preference. There is a tendency to have fewer and less severe attacks as time progresses. Viral, bacterial, or other causative agents have never been proved; immunologic factors are being implicated. Certain foods, fever, and stress may bring on attacks in predisposed persons.

DIAGNOSIS. The diagnosis of aphthae is made by clinical appearance and history. Most commonly they appear as shallow, pseudomembrane-covered ulcerations with a surrounding erythematous halo. They are often tender and heal spontaneously in one or two weeks. Aphthae may occur as multiple small ulcers, or sometimes they appear as single large ulcerations (major aphthae), which usually incur more pain and a longer healing period (Fig. 96–2). This implies a difference in the host and not the disease. Some patients will never be free of ulcers; as one ulcer heals, others occur.

Blood examinations or smears are not helpful. Biopsies show nonspecific inflammation and ulceration; the initial inflammatory cell is the lymphocyte. The larger lesions can mimic more serious diseases, since the inflammatory process involves underlying musculature, causing more induration and pain.

Aphthous ulcers may be associated with inflammatory bowel disease and Behçet's syndrome. In the differential diagnosis care must be taken not to confuse aphthae with the oral manifestations of erythema multiforme, erosive lichen planus, primary herpetic stomatitis, pemphigoid, pemphigus, drug reactions, and mucosal manifestations of blood dyscrasias.

TREATMENT. Frequently, special treatment is unnecessary. Empirical approaches, using bland mouth rinses, topical preparations, vitamins, and mild sedatives and analgesics, may be helpful in some persons. The most effective management is by administering short courses of corticosteroids systemically. Frequently less than 40 mg prednisone daily for two to three days will give adequate control of signs and symptoms (this also confirms the inflammatory nature of aphthae). The dosage and duration of corticoid treatment may vary with individual patients and their characteristic patterns of disease. Vaccines and antibiotics have not proved beneficial.

Olson JA, Greenspan JS, Silverman S: Recurrent aphthous ulcerations. J Calif Dent Assoc 10:53, 1982. *Comprehensive review of clinical features, pathogenesis, and management.*

ORAL HERPETIC INFECTIONS

Herpes simplex virus (HSV) infects the mouth in a variety of ways. Diagnostic techniques are usually impractical, and treatment is supportive. Evidence for a contagious nature is lacking. A history of these lesions has not been associated with an increased risk for cancer.

COLD SORE (HERPES LABIALIS). The most common bothersome lesion is the cold sore. In the prone individual the latent virus is activated by an external irritant (cold, fever, trauma) and yields the characteristic vesicle or vesicles that subsequently scab and usually take one to three weeks to heal. The lesion is not associated with any rise in HSV antibody titer, and no effective preventive or therapeutic agents (vaccines, vitamins, ointments, and antivirals) are available. Therefore, an empirical approach with which any patient gets the best result is still indicated (see Ch. 555).

RECURRENT INTRAORAL HSV. Intraoral recurrent herpetic lesions should not be confused with recurrent aphthous ulcers. Recurrent herpetic infections are rare and only occur on the gingiva or hard palate. They are usually characterized by shallow, small, irregular erosive lesions on an erythematous mucosa. Pain is usually no more than moderate, and the lesions are usually self-limiting in seven to ten days.

PRIMARY HERPETIC GINGIVOSTOMATITIS. Primary herpetic gingivostomatitis is the most acute form of oral herpetic infec-

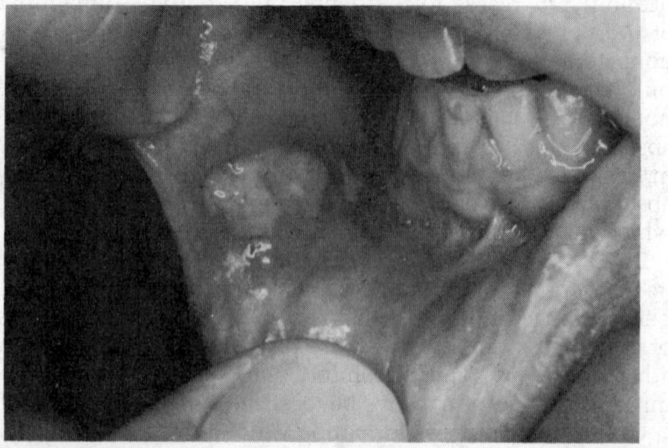

Figure 96–2. Aphthous ulcers. These idiopathic ulcerations usually do not exceed 5 to 6 mm in size and heal in 10 to 14 days. This large (major) aphthous ulcer had been present for one month and did not heal for two months.

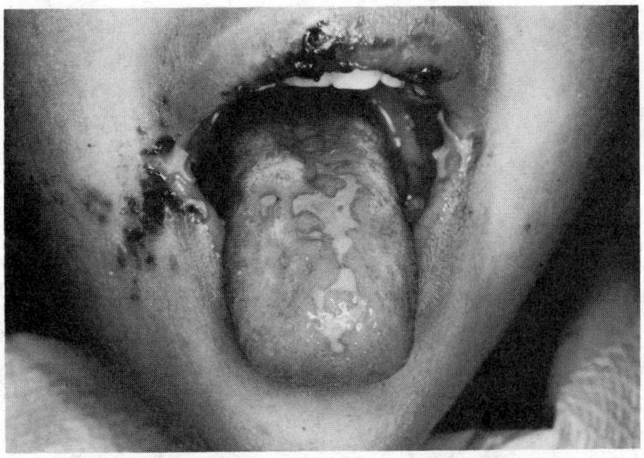

Figure 96–3. Primary herpetic gingivostomatitis in a five-year-old youngster. These acute attacks render lifelong immunity.

tion. Usually 90 per cent of the population are infected before puberty, but most persons do not develop noticeable lesions or complaints. Signs and symptoms can include ulcerations on an erythematous and edematous mucosa (Fig. 96–3). This is often accompanied by lymphadenopathy, fever, and malaise, which can be confused with more serious illnesses. The condition is self-limiting; signs and symptoms usually become progressively severe for one week and disappear by the end of the second week. Treatment is supportive with antipyretic-analgesic agents, rest, and nutritional supplements.

During the course of disease, HSV antibody titer rises at least four-fold and confers lifelong immunity. Blood tests usually show only a slight lymphocytosis. Cytologic smears show pseudogiant cells (squamous) typical of the herpetic infection.

Approximately 10 per cent of adults, as shown by seroepidemiologic study, either did not become infected in childhood or have not developed adequate antibodies. Therefore, this infection is not limited to children. Adult infections of primary herpetic gingivostomatitis are usually more severe than the childhood form. Both forms can be mistaken for more severe diseases such as erythema multiforme, infectious mononucleosis, blood dyscrasias, and pemphigus. Persons who are immunosuppressed, e.g., cancer and kidney transplant patients, have an increased risk for developing a primary herpetic stomatitis. Systemic antiviral agents have not proved effective in controlling these conditions.

Shillitoe EJ, Silverman S Jr: Oral cancer and herpes simplex virus—a review. Oral Surg 48:216, 1979. *Reviews the biology of HSV and describes its pathogenesis in oral diseases.*

CANDIDIASIS (Moniliasis, Thrush)

Candida albicans (see Ch. 372) is a normal oral flora resident in about 30 to 40 per cent of the population. For reasons always not clearly understood, the fungi can become overpopulated and produce clinical signs and symptoms. Most frequently oral candidal infections are associated with antibiotic use (suppressing oral bacterial flora and making more carbohydrate substrate available), diabetes mellitus, xerostomia, immunosuppression, and the wearing of dentures (poor hygiene).

DIAGNOSIS. Oral candidiasis is often recognized by complaints of generalized mouth discomfort. It may be acute or chronic. While examination frequently reveals the typical surface creamy white fungal colonies, often the manifestation is that of irregular or widespread erythema (Fig. 96–4). Occasionally there will be erosive changes. Angular cheilitis is a common finding.

Since the clinical appearance is often only suggestive, smears or cultures (to observe pseudomycelia and spores) may be required to confirm the diagnosis. If biopsies are obtained, special staining with the periodic acid–Schiff (PAS) method may show the fungus, which grows in the most superficial epithelial stratum.

TREATMENT. The first step in treatment is to rule out underlying factors, such as hyperglycemia, xerostomia, and anemia. Hydrogen peroxide–saline mouth rinses (3 per cent H_2O_2 diluted with equal parts warm saline) are helpful. Specific treatment includes orally dissolving nystatin vaginal troches (100,000 units three or four times daily). Nystatin suspension is not as effective, since the contact time with the oral mucosa is much less. Clotrimazole tablets (10 mg dissolved orally five times daily) appear to be equally or more effective than the nystatin. Recent trials with ketoconazole taken systemically appear to offer an alternative to oral dissolution, which some individuals find objectionable. The angular cheilitis is most effectively treated with Mycolog cream (nystatin-neomycin-gramicidin-triamcinolone). Oral candidiasis does not appear to be contagious or related to infections at other sites. Unless the underlying cause is identified and corrected, oral infections can recur.

Mackowiak PA: The normal microbial flora. N Engl J Med 307:83, 1982. *Reviews microbial florae and their interrelationships in health and disease.*

Renner RP, et al.: The role of *C. albicans* in denture stomatitis. Oral Surg 47:323, 1979. *Reviews biology of oral* Candida, *techniques for measurement and differential diagnosis of clinical appearance. In a control study, increased fungal infections in denture wearers were shown.*

GLOSSITIS

Inflammatory conditions of the tongue are moderately common and quite variable. The asymptomatic glossitis may be due to the aging process (atrophy of the filiform papillae) or due to such idiopathic conditions as geographic tongue (glossitis migrans) and median rhomboid glossitis (central papillary atrophy). Occasionally glossitis may reflect a blood dyscrasia or a variety of debilitating diseases involving malnutrition. By careful clinical examination, history, and ruling out other dis-

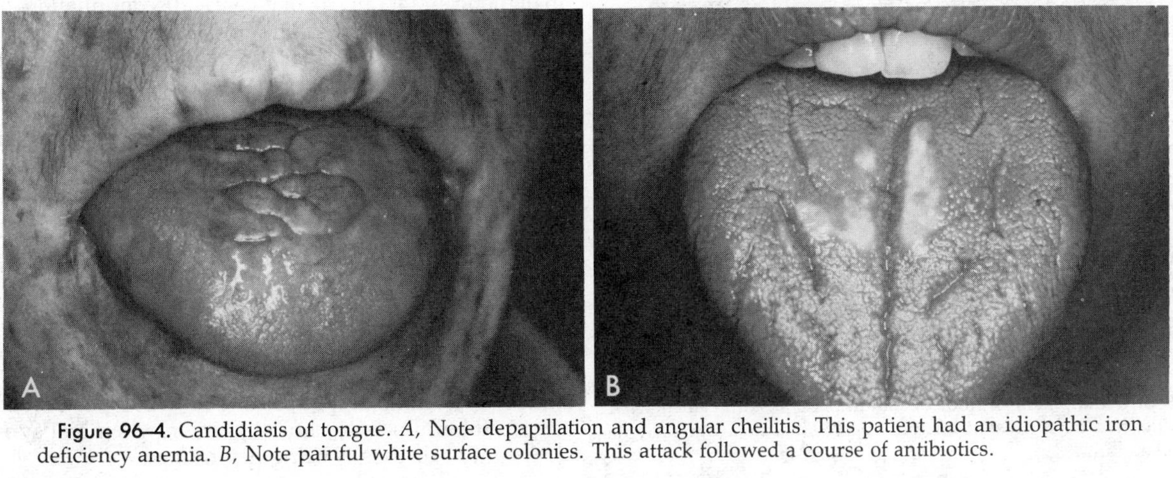

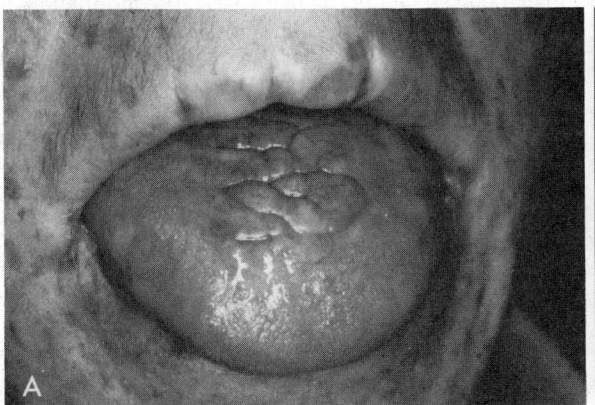

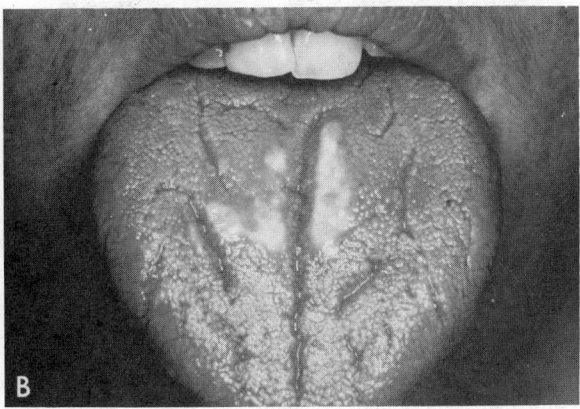

Figure 96–4. Candidiasis of tongue. *A,* Note depapillation and angular cheilitis. This patient had an idiopathic iron deficiency anemia. *B,* Note painful white surface colonies. This attack followed a course of antibiotics.

eases, the asymptomatic atrophic tongue can usually be classified.

The complex clinical problems are associated with patients having symptomatic glossitis (glossopyrosis, glossodynia). Frequently examination of the tongue will not reveal any specific lesions or depapillation. The symptoms are often a manifestation of anxiety or depression. Occasionally the glossitis may be due to a drug reaction. Xerostomia or dehydration may be causative factors, and candidiasis must be ruled out. Rarely, anemia or hyperglycemia may induce these changes. Glossitis is not caused by poor oral hygiene, dentures, or other tooth-related problems. Tobacco use may contribute to the discomfort, as may certain foods. In many cases the etiology remains unknown, and by default they are classified as psychogenic.

MANAGEMENT. Approach to the patient with a symptomatic tongue usually involves a careful history and consideration of discontinuing or altering drugs. Tobacco must be discontinued, at least temporarily. Blood dyscrasias and hyperglycemia should be ruled out with the appropriate tests. Inspection for any obvious dental or oral pathology is in order, and these should be corrected even though it is unlikely that they may play a role. Occasionally a malignancy of the tongue may create these symptoms; therefore, a careful examination must be performed. Reassuring a patient that there is no sign of malignancy is sometimes an important part of management. Candidiasis should be eliminated by appropriate cultures or smears, or by instituting a short trial of topical antifungal agents.

A systematic pharmacologic approach, including placebos, vitamins, tranquilizers, and antidepressant agents, may be utilized after the other diagnostic approaches are exhausted. Occasionally sialogogues (pilocarpine) or anti-inflammatory agents (corticoids) are helpful. If all these approaches fail and a diagnosis cannot be established, then any acceptable supportive therapy may be attempted, i.e., hypnosis, biofeedback, or even periodic recall visits for reassurance.

LEUKOPLAKIA-ERYTHROPLAKIA

These terms designate white and red patches that may occur on any oral mucosal surface (Figs. 96–5 and 96–6). There may be associated discomfort, and an etiologic factor is not always apparent.

MANAGEMENT AND DIAGNOSIS. The first practical approach is to remove all irritants, such as tobacco use, ill-fitting dentures, poor hygiene, spicy or hot foods, and any other potentially injurious habits, in order to see if the lesions are reversible. If not, representative biopsies should be obtained. Most often leukoplakia will be a manifestation of benign hyperkeratosis and erythroplakia a reflection of epithelial atrophy and

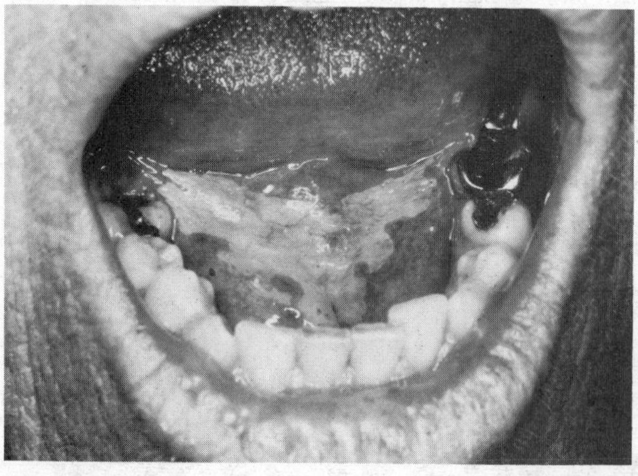

Figure 96–5. Leukoplakia of floor of mouth. This lesion, which was asymptomatic, had been present for four years. The cause was related to cigarette smoking.

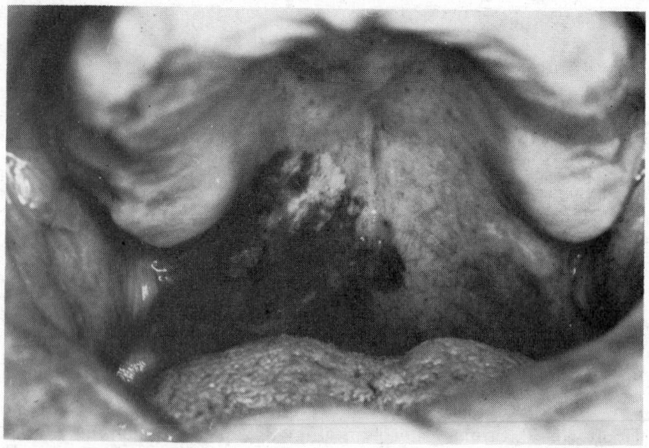

Figure 96–6. Erythroplakia of oropharynx. The lesion was slightly painful and had been noticed for four months. Risk for malignant transformation is high.

inflammation. If a lesion cannot be classified as any specific disease entity, then at the very least it should be followed closely because of the risk for malignant transformation (thus the term precancerous lesion). If the biopsy indicates dysplasia, then a more aggressive attempt should be made to remove these lesions surgically. Resection does not guarantee permanent control or cancer prevention.

DIFFERENTIAL DIAGNOSIS. Occasionally a white- and/or red-appearing oral lesion may already be a squamous carcinoma. Alternatively, it may represent a classifiable benign lesion such as lichen planus, erythema multiforme, or pemphigoid. In these latter conditions, topical or systemic corticosteroids will help confirm the diagnosis by at least partial control of the lesion. For leukoplakia and erythroplakia, corticosteroids, keratinolytic agents, vitamin A, and other approaches have not been uniformly effective.

Silverman S Jr, Gorsky M, Lozada F: Oral leukoplakia and malignant transformation. A follow-up study of 257 patients. Cancer 53:563, 1984. *Describes profiles and establishes risk factors in patients with precancerous oral lesions.*

ORAL CANCER

Cancer of the mouth accounts for about 4 per cent of all cancers. The tongue is the most common site, although it may occur in any mouth site. More than 90 per cent are squamous carcinomas, commencing in the oral epithelial lining. The average age of onset approximates 60 years, and there is a 2 to 1 male to female prevalence. Oral cancer occurs in all ethnic groups.

ETIOLOGY. The increased risk and cause-effect relationship among tobacco use, alcohol consumption, and mouth cancer have been well documented. Abstinence is significant in preventive measures. Since patients with one oral cancer have an extremely high risk for developing second head and neck malignancies (about 20 per cent), discontinuation of tobacco and alcohol is critical. Although various forms of oral irritation, food carcinogens, and herpesvirus have been implicated, studies have not confirmed an associated risk factor. Familial tendencies have not been demonstrated.

DIAGNOSIS. There are no reliable signs or symptoms associated with mouth cancer (Fig. 96–7). This causes patient delay in seeking professional advice, and conversely the varied features often delay diagnostic procedures. The most common finding is that of a painful ulceration associated with induration. Early malignant changes often can appear as essentially asymptomatic white and/or red surface patches. Patients often describe these changes as lumps or irritations.

Biopsy is the only acceptable method of diagnosis. Exfoliative cytology and vital staining with toluidine blue (1 per cent aqueous toluidine blue, decolorized with 1 per cent acetic acid) are useful adjuncts to clinical opinion when biopsy is delayed or extent of disease is being determined.

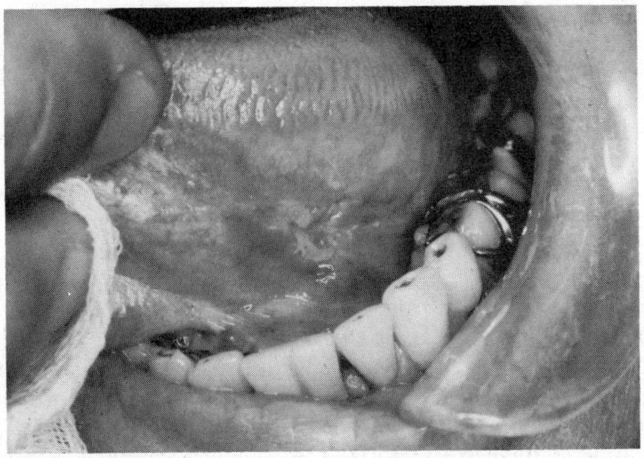

Figure 96–7. Oral squamous carcinoma. This early cancer at the junction of the tongue and mouth floor had been noticed for three weeks. It was at first mistaken for a traumatic ulcer.

TREATMENT. The survival rate for oral cancer is relatively poor, in most studies averaging less than 50 per cent. This is usually due to late detection, promoting lesions that are locally extensive with diffuse margins, large tumor volume, and spread to the neck (cervical lymphadenopathy). While spread to neck nodes is rather common, approximating 50 per cent, involvement of other organ systems occurs in less than 15 per cent of advanced cases.

Curative therapy utilizes radiation and surgery. Often these modalities are used in combination, which seems to increase cure rates slightly, although also increasing morbidity. In advanced cases chemotherapy is also used (most effective drugs include methotrexate, bleomycin, and cisplatinum); the sequences, dosages, and combinations vary.

REHABILITATION. Rehabilitation is essential, since treatment often compromises appearance, function, and attitude. For surgical defects maxillofacial prosthetic appliances are very effective. Paraprofessionals are useful in improving speech and swallowing defects. Radiation, which is frequently used, alters saliva and taste, interfering with oral comfort and nutrition. Dietary consultation can often assist food acceptance. Xerostomia usually can be improved by the administration of pilocarpine, 5 mg four times a day, if more conservative methods (sugarless gum or candy drops) are unsuccessful. Supplements of elemental zinc (up to 100 mg daily) have improved taste perception in some patients. Jaw bone and mucosal necrosis is also increased with radiation, and special care must be taken regarding dental procedures, extractions, and other forms of dental trauma. The risk is proportional to the radiation dosage, becoming most critical above 6500 rads. Antibiotics and time will often control the necrosis; however, surgery is sometimes required.

Silverman S Jr, Gorsky M, Greenspan D: Current trends in the occurrence of oral cancer. Early detection of oral carcinoma. J Dermatol Allergy 6:26, 1983. *Comprehensive review of epidemiology, etiology, diagnosis, staging and survival; many tables and photos; selected references.*

97. DISEASES OF THE ESOPHAGUS

Charles E. Pope II

CLINICAL SYMPTOMATOLOGY

The esophagus would seem to be a relatively simple portion of the gastrointestinal tract. Its duty, the transport of solid, liquid, and gas, usually is performed unobtrusively. The structure of the esophagus is not complex. Yet malfunction can lead to such trivial complaints as heartburn or overwhelming clinical problems such as aspiration, obstruction, and hemorrhage. A good clinical history will often be the most valuable diagnostic test. The laboratory diagnosis of esophageal malfunction often leads our therapeutic capabilities.

Esophageal disorders can be expressed by a group of symptoms that are unique to this organ. The esophagus also shares other symptoms with the rest of the gastrointestinal tract. The clinician should concentrate on the unique symptoms, as further investigations will usually uncover an esophageal cause.

DYSPHAGIA. Consciousness of bolus arrest during swallowing, even if transient, is a symptom indicating esophageal dysfunction. The patient will usually use the term "sticks," "hesitates," "pauses," or "hangs up," and will often indicate the site of dysphagia with a finger.

Bolus arrest closely associated with the act of swallowing is dysphagia. The sensation of a substernal lump present one half hour after eating is not dysphagia. Most patients consider mild dysphagia a normal phenomenon "I just swallowed something that was too big." Thus, often they will not spontaneously mention the presence of dysphagia unless questioned closely.

Dysphagia may result from inability to propel the bolus from the pharynx into the esophagus, so-called "transfer dysphagia." It is most commonly associated with diseases of the muscle or neural control of the pharynx and is perceived in the neck. Dysphagia usually is felt in the suprasternal notch, or substernally. The exact location of the sensation is of little use in pinpointing the site of bolus arrest. Dysphagia for a liquid bolus usually indicates an esophageal motor disorder; dysphagia for solids can be seen either with an organic obstruction (stricture or cancer) or secondary to esophageal motor disorders.

The patient's response to dysphagia can also provide useful information about the cause of the dysphagia. If the bolus must be regurgitated, and if an attempt to force the bolus down with water is met by a sudden return of the fluid, then an organic obstruction should be suspected. If the patient is able to force the bolus down by posturing, by performing a Valsalva maneuver, by repeated swallowing, or by ingesting fluid, then a motor disorder is more likely. Inexorable progression of dysphagia over months usually signals the presence of organic narrowing, either a lumen-obliterating carcinoma or a stricture caused by active peptic esophagitis.

Dysphagia is never an expression of a pure psychiatric disorder; it is not a manifestation of hysteria. Some patients with well-established esophageal disease such as achalasia, will report that their dysphagia is often worse at a time of severe emotional tension. Such observations have led many patients (and unfortunately some physicians) to believe that dysphagia is a matter for the psychiatrist rather than the gastroenterologist. Such an opinion can lead to subsequent embarrassment or tragedy, especially if an esophageal carcinoma is overlooked.

ODYNOPHAGIA. Pain upon swallowing, odynophagia, is another cardinal symptom of esophageal disease. Bolus arrest producing dysphagia can sometimes progress to a sensation of pain as esophageal obstruction continues. However, odynophagia usually occurs during the transit of the bolus and disappears once the swallowed material has left the esophagus. It may be mild in intensity so that the patient is merely aware of the location of the swallowed bolus. This is most commonly seen in patients with reflux disease. It can be of such intensity that the patient will refuse to swallow any solids or liquids and will expectorate saliva. Odynophagia can be seen after involvement of the mucosa by *reflux,* by *radiation,* or by *viral infections.* Odynophagia can be an uncommon manifestation of carcinoma, or of a localized ulcer caused by a lodged tablet. Odynophagia thus localizes a process to the esophagus, but gives us no clue as to pathogenesis.

HEARTBURN (PYROSIS). Heartburn or pyrosis is the most common manifestation of esophageal disease, so much so that it is difficult to recruit "normal" subjects, if strict histories are taken to eliminate any who have ever had heartburn. The term "burning" rather than "pain" is usually used, although heartburn can increase in intensity until it is perceived as pain. Patients commonly illustrate heartburn with a movement of the open hand up and down the sternum. This is in contrast to the stationary tightly clenched fist of angina pectoris. Heartburn is usually relieved, even if only temporarily, by taking antacids. A constant burning, unrelieved by antacids, may well be of esophageal origin, but it does not represent heartburn. Heartburn is often worse after recumbency or lifting; and may follow overeating or alcoholic indiscretion.

REGURGITATION. Regurgitation of fluid contents into the mouth often accompanies heartburn. Sometimes such regurgitation is associated with eructation; often it accompanies bending over, lifting, or lying down at night. The bitter regurgitated fluid is often described as yellow-brown or green. Regurgitation at night may lead to stridor or to wheezing, a hoarse voice, and other respiratory symptoms from unrecognized reflux. Less commonly, regurgitated fluid is not from the stomach or duodenum, but from fluid retained in an *achalasic esophagus* or in a large *pharyngeal diverticulum.* An uncommon but fascinating process that can be confused with regurgitation is *rumination.* In this condition, recently eaten food is propelled back into the mouth from the stomach by a strong contraction of the abdominal wall musculature. It commonly is rechewed, reswallowed, and again returned to the mouth.

ESOPHAGEAL COLIC. In addition to the discomfort from severe reflux which can advance from heartburn into pain, abnormal motor activity of the esophageal muscle can cause severe pain clinically indistinguishable from angina pectoris in terms of intensity, radiation, relationship to exercise, and even response to nitroglycerin. Chest pain of esophageal origin can radiate directly through to the back, and is often found in patients who also notice dysphagia. Esophageal colic can last from five to ten seconds to hours.

HEMATEMESIS. Although vomiting blood is less specific for esophageal disease than are many of the symptoms listed above, hematemesis can signal the presence of esophageal varices, of mucosal ulceration resulting from esophageal reflux, of a rent of the mucosa of the lower esophagus, or, uncommonly, of an ulcerating carcinoma or leiomyoma of the esophagus. Although bleeding from the esophagus may be life threatening, more often it is a slow ooze, usually caused by esophageal reflux disease, which presents clinically as an iron deficiency anemia.

Pope CE II: Chapters on the esophagus. *In* Sleisenger MH, Fordtran JS (eds.): Gastrointestinal Disease. 3rd ed. Philadelphia, W. B. Saunders Company, 1983, pp 145–155, 407–504. *Reference textbook on esophageal disease. Good source for recent references.*

Vantrappen G, Hellemans J: Disease of the Esophagus. Berlin, Springer-Verlag, 1974. *An exhaustive reference book on the esophagus. Strong on the European experience.*

GASTROESOPHAGEAL REFLUX DISEASE

DEFINITION. Gastroesophageal reflux disease (GERD) refers to the varied clinical manifestations of reflux of stomach and duodenal contents into the esophagus. It is preferable to the term "reflux esophagitis" because the latter expression tends to mean different things to the clinician, the endoscopist, and the pathologist. Although it may be associated with a sliding hiatus hernia, "symptomatic hiatus hernia" is a term that tends to put the emphasis on the wrong anatomic entity and pathophysiology. Gastroesophageal reflux disease can be characterized by any combination of symptoms and radiologic, endoscopic, or pathologic changes. In its milder manifestations, it is a common disease; its most florid state is uncommon but may be life threatening.

PATHOGENESIS. Several factors must work in concert to produce clinical effects of esophageal reflux. All persons will demonstrate short bursts of reflux if monitored with an intraesophageal pH probe over 24 hours. This reflux is seen postprandially and usually in the upright position. Those in whom reflux has produced symptoms or pathologic changes will demonstrate more prolonged episodes of reflux, which tend to occur at night. The factor or factors that cause this difference are not known. However, important differences between persons with and without reflux might help explain these findings.

The *lower esophageal sphincter* (LES) is a specialized bundle of circular muscle at the lower end of the esophagus with different physical and pharmacologic characteristics when compared to the circular muscle above and below it. There is a tendency for mean LES pressure to be significantly lower in subjects with GERD as compared with normals, but LES pressures are not very useful in predicting whether reflux is present in an individual patient unless the pressure is very low. The most common event associated with reflux appears to be an *inappropriate relaxation of the lower esophageal sphincter,* i.e., LES relaxation unassociated with either swallowing or the distention of the esophageal body by refluxed fluid. Thus, two abnormalities of LES may be associated with reflux: a sphincter with very low tone as measured by lower esophageal sphincter pressure, or inappropriate relaxation of a normally competent sphincter.

Several factors are important in removing refluxed material. The upright position facilitates esophageal emptying by gravity. Peristaltic waves initiated by swallowing or by esophageal distention help remove the refluxed material. Acid placed within the esophagus is cleared less well by patients with GERD than by normal subjects, even though the manometric tracings seen in both groups seem identical.

The composition and perhaps the quantity of the refluxed material also play a role in the production of GERD. Gastric acid and pepsin seem clearly important in the pathogenesis of GERD. Bile salts and possibly pancreatic enzymes may be responsible in those patients in whom acid is absent. The combination of bile salts plus acid is more injurious to the esophageal than either agent alone. Other less well studied pathogenetic factors such as altered or abnormal esophageal mucus, swallowed saliva of high bicarbonate content, and diminished resistance of the esophageal mucosa to digestion may be important in the inflammation of the esophagus in GERD.

Esophageal squamous epithelium reacts to reflux by an increase in the basal cell or germinative layer. The dermal pegs are increased in height and may become more vascular. If the process becomes more severe, the epithelial layer is destroyed, with the appearance of microulcers and classic signs of inflammation in the lamina propria such as infiltration with polymorphonuclear leukocytes and edema. Even deeper lesions cause first submucosal, then muscular inflammation and fibrosis, resulting in an esophageal stricture. Why reflux is so common, yet inflammation and stricture formation so relatively uncommon, is not known.

Other conditions can be associated with the pathogenesis of reflux. Reflux during pregnancy, once thought to be due to the increased abdominal pressure from the fetus, may be due mainly to diminished LES pressure caused by extra estrogen and progesterone. Weight gain also tends to aggravate reflux through an unknown mechanism. As expected, resection of the lower esophageal area for cancer or myotomy for achalasia can lead to severe postoperative reflux (see below).

ROLE OF HIATUS HERNIA. The presence of a hiatus hernia is now considered to be much less of a factor in GERD than previously thought. Some radiologists find hiatus hernias in a large percentage of patients, no matter what the reason for the examination. Others rarely demonstrate a hiatus hernia. Since it is no longer necessary to demonstrate a hiatus hernia in order to understand, diagnose, or treat GERD, it seems appropriate not to spend a great deal of time trying to define whether a hiatus hernia is present or absent in dealing with most patients with GERD. The important entity to investigate is reflux, not hiatus hernia.

SYMPTOMS OF GASTROESOPHAGEAL REFLUX DISEASE. *Heartburn* is the most common manifestation of GERD. It can vary from an occasional mild burning after overeating to an ever present, severe discomfort that severely limits a patient's life style. It may be accompanied by *regurgitation* of gastric contents either into the mouth or into the respiratory tree. This latter group of patients may complain of nocturnal wheezing, hoarseness, a need to clear the throat repeatedly, and a sensation of deep pressure at the base of the neck. This group of symptoms may be the primary clinical presentation and more prominent than the classic symptoms of GERD.

Dysphagia is often present in those with significant GERD. Although dysphagia may be severe and even mark the onset of stricture formation, it usually is mild and must be carefully sought. Dysphagia of GERD is for solids, and the dysphagia is usually overcome by swallowing repeatedly or by washing down the bolus with some water. Dysphagia without anatomic strictures has been noted in about three fourths of patients scheduled for antireflux surgery. Many patients with GERD will not complain of bolus arrest, but rather of being aware of the location of each solid morsel as it travels down the esophagus.

Blood loss may result from esophageal erosion and shallow ulcers. Rarely producing life-threatening hemorrhage, the erosions are much more likely to weep quietly over a prolonged period of time, producing iron deficiency anemia. Some of these patients have very few other clinical manifestations of GERD, and the condition is discovered by endoscopy during an evaluation of occult gastrointestinal bleeding. Patients who vigorously and repeatedly abuse alcohol seem prone to develop severe erosive esophagitis with bleeding; this lesion heals with abstinence from alcohol without other major antireflux therapy.

DIAGNOSIS. The history and clinical manifestations of GERD are the most important diagnostic aids in the establishment of the diagnosis; objective testing is used to quantify the extent and severity of the process. In the evaluation of an individual, questions to be answered dictate the appropriate test.

Does reflux exist and if so, to what degree? This question might arise either if another condition such as pulmonary disease is present and a causal relationship is being sought, or if some idea of the frequency and extent of reflux is important. Reflux during a barium swallow in adults is uncommon unless vigorous provocative maneuvers are employed. When spontaneous reflux of barium is seen, it usually denotes free reflux. Children reflux barium more easily than do adults. The pH probe can be used either for short-term studies of 15 to 30 minutes or for more prolonged periods (24 hours). If repeated bursts of reflux are demonstrated during a 15-minute period, then severe reflux is present. At the same time, the ability of the esophagus to clear itself of refluxed acid can be evaluated. Usually a manometric catheter is attached to the pH probe in order to locate it in the esophagus; this catheter can also estimate the LES pressure. Only very low values of LES pressure such as 1 to 2 mm Hg (normal, about 20 mm Hg) are of prognostic value.

Reflux can be measured noninvasively by scanning of the esophageal area with a gamma camera after placing a solution of ^{99m}Tc sulfur colloid in the stomach. An abdominal binder is used to stress the gastroesophageal junction if free reflux is not seen. This technique seems to be of most value in infants and children, who tolerate esophageal tubes very poorly.

Could reflux be responsible for the patient's symptoms? This question might be asked if pain is the predominant symptom rather than more classic heartburn. This question can be answered with the same catheter assembly used to measure LES pressure and acid reflux. After a five-minute period of dripping normal saline through one of the pressure catheters whose opening has been localized to the upper esophagus, this infusion is changed to 0.1 N hydrochloric acid without the patient's knowledge. Reproduction of the symptoms within 30 minutes of acid infusion (usually four to five minutes into the infusion) and rapid disappearance of the symptom with a switch back to saline infusion suggests an esophageal cause of the discomfort.

As another approach, the patient is asked to signal the time of discomfort during prolonged pH monitoring of the esophagus. If the patient signals discomfort at the same time that reflux is demonstrated by the pH probe, then a causal relationship is made more likely. Prolonged pH monitoring is not used widely clinically because of the expense of hospitalization. The development of portable pH monitors may make this approach more feasible.

What has reflux done to the esophageal mucosa? A barium swallow will detect gross changes such as stricture formation or a deep esophageal ulcer, but will miss the much more common shallow ulcerations and erosions. These will be detected by direct inspection with the endoscope. Only discrete lesions such as erosions and ulcerations should be taken as proof of esophageal damage; such endoscopic findings as erythema, edema, or friability are subject to wide interobserver variation. If the mucosa appears absolutely normal, as it is in approximately one third of patients with moderate to severe symptoms of GERD, then suction biopsy can demonstrate the changes of reflux (Fig. 97–1).

A logic tree of how these tests might be used is shown in Table 97–1. A patient whose symptoms are severe enough to seek medical attention might be screened with a barium swallow. Uncommonly, reflux will be demonstrated, a stricture found, or a deep ulcer seen. This might lead to immediate endoscopy for more complete evaluation. If a patient presents with hematemesis and reflux symptoms, then endoscopy might appropriately be used as the first step (since a barium swallow is not likely to show reflux, a stricture, or an ulcer). After first evaluation, it is appropriate to begin therapy (see Treatment, below). Only if there is a poor response to therapy should an acid perfusion test be used to confirm the diagnosis. At the same time, the presence of reflux can be checked, an estimate of LES pressure and acid clearance obtained, and the presence or absence of peristaltic waves evaluated.

More intensive therapy should be instituted at this point. If it fails and the patient is still symptomatic, endoscopy can be employed to see if gross disease is still present in the face of maximal therapy. If the appearance of the mucosa is normal grossly in the presence of overwhelming symptoms, then suction biopsies can be obtained to search for objective evidence of reflux damage. This scheme will restrict extensive testing to those who have failed medical therapy and who are presumably candidates for surgical treatment. This algorithm can be modified if the patient has blood loss or severe dysphagia. Endoscopy should follow a screening barium x-ray examination.

COMPLICATIONS OF GASTROESOPHAGEAL REFLUX DISEASE. ***Esophageal Stricture.*** Of the many who complain of symptoms of GERD, only a few will develop esophageal strictures. Usually beginning at the lower end of the esophagus, strictures may migrate over years to the mid-esophagus or higher. Columnar epithelium will be found below the stricture. Presumably those who develop strictures have had deep circumferential ulceration of the esophageal mucosa owing to reflux damage. Instead of having healing with only minimal submucosal and muscular fibrosis, these patients develop esophageal obstruction with a narrowed esophageal lumen. If reflux can be controlled, these strictures will disappear.

Dysphagia is the clinical hallmark of esophageal stricture formation. Unlike the relatively mild dysphagia seen in uncomplicated GERD, the dysphagia in patients with strictures tends to be constant and slowly progressive, causing the patient to alter the type of food taken. If a bolus becomes arrested in the stricture, it is usually necessary for the bolus to be regurgitated back into the mouth before further intake of food or fluids is possible.

Strictures are most easily evaluated by barium swallow. Sometimes the extent of the strictured area is overestimated unless the esophagus below the stricture can be fully distended by barium. For mild strictures, the ingestion of a bread or marshmallow bolus can draw attention to slight luminal narrowing when the bolus impacts there. Once demonstrated, endoscopy with biopsy and/or brush cytology is in order to make certain of the benign nature of the stricture.

Esophageal Ulcer. In addition to the more common shallow

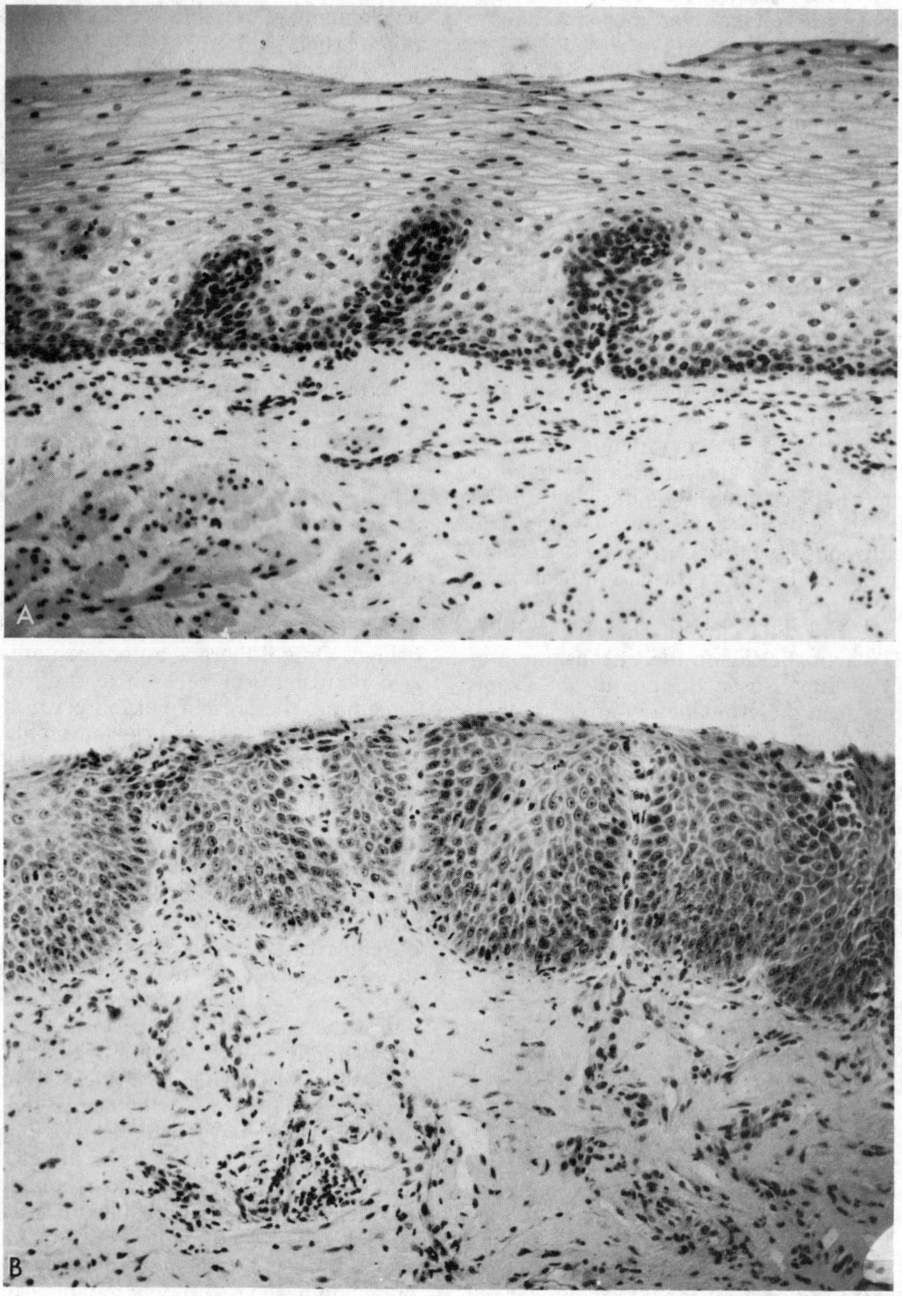

Figure 97–1. *A,* Normal esophageal histology. This suction biopsy is taken from an asymptomatic individual without reflux. Note that the basal cell layer is relatively thin and that the dermal pegs extend less than halfway to the free surface of the biopsy. *B,* Histology seen in GERD. This suction biopsy is taken from a patient with symptomatic and pH-probe proven reflux. The basal layer is quite thick and the pegs extend to the free surface.

ulcerations, deep esophageal ulcers may complicate severe GERD. These ulcers, which retain barium and usually project outside the wall of the esophagus, characteristically produce severe and unrelenting pain, often with radiation of the pain through to the back. Brisk hemorrhage is another manifestation, either from erosion through to an esophageal artery or, more catastrophically, into the nearby aorta. The presence of an ulcer can be suspected on a barium swallow and confirmed endoscopically. The ulcer is usually found to reside in columnar (Barrett's) epithelium.

Columnar Epithelium. In some patients who have suffered severe esophageal ulceration as a result of GERD, the healing epithelium is replaced not with squamous epithelium but with a specialized columnar epithelium. This occurs in at least three distinct histologic types. The most common type appears villiform, and the epithelium contains goblet cells. Less commonly, the mucosa resembles the junctional-type epithelium found between the normal esophageal mucosa and the gastric fundic mucosa. It contains cardiac-type mucosa glands and no parietal or chief cells. Least common is gastric fundus–type epithelium containing parietal and chief cells. This epithelium can sometimes, but not always, be recognized endoscopically by its brighter red color and patchy distribution. Serial studies in patients with prolonged severe reflux show that the junctional zone between squamous and columnar epithelium can progress orad over years. Columnar epithelium is found at and below mid-esophageal strictures and around deep esophageal ulcers, although it can be found on routine biopsy of patients with severe GERD. Its major clinical importance is not only as a marker of severe reflux but also as a precursor for adenocarcinoma of the esophagus (see under Esophageal Tumors.).

Pulmonary Aspiration. If refluxed material breaches the up-

TABLE 97–1.

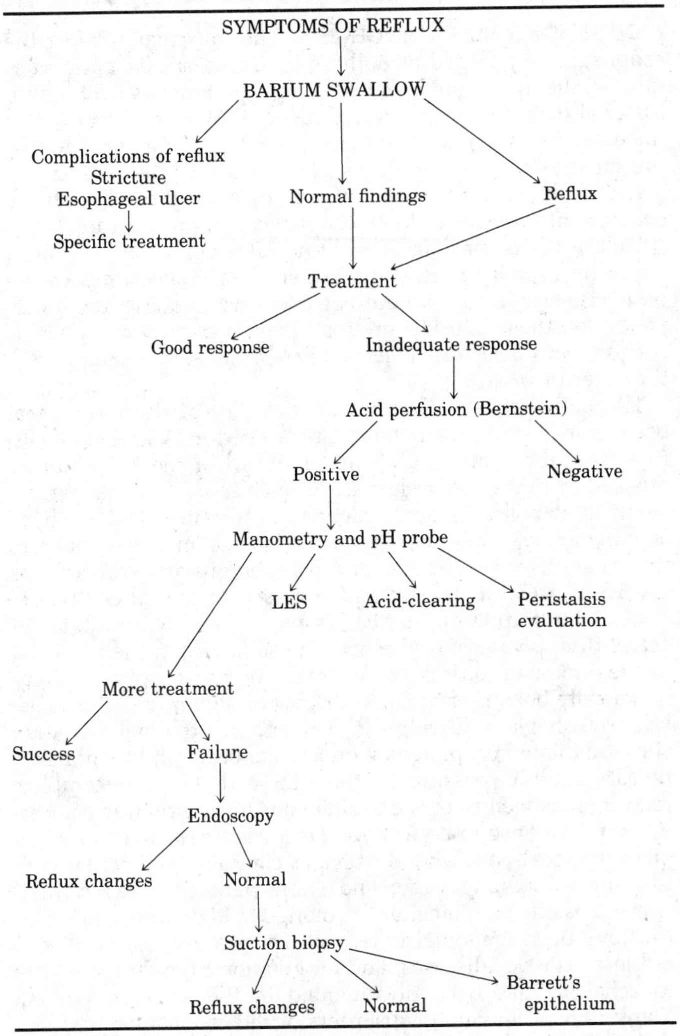

per esophageal sphincter, it may easily spill into the larynx and tracheobronchial tree. Some patients react to such a spill with intense respiratory stridor. Others seem to tolerate the presence of refluxed contents in the larynx and tracheobronchial tree with milder laryngeal or respiratory symptoms. It is even possible that the gastric contents do not have to reach the larynx; instillation of acid in the esophagus of susceptible individuals while they are in the upright posture can be shown to cause closing of small bronchial airways, presumably by a vagal reflex.

None of the clinical features of pulmonary aspiration (Table 97–2) is pathognomonic. Taken together they point toward reflux and aspiration as a possible etiology. Diagnostic proof of the relationship is difficult with current techniques. Radioisotopes placed in the stomach have been demonstrated the next morning to be in the lungs by gamma camera scanning, but this cannot be demonstrated in the majority of patients. Only correction of reflux with subsequent disappearance of pulmonary symptoms can prove the relationship.

TREATMENT OF GASTROESOPHAGEAL REFLUX DISEASE AND ITS COMPLICATIONS. *Medical Management.* Most mildly symptomatic patients with reflux and some moderately afflicted

TABLE 97–2. CLINICAL FEATURES OF PULMONARY ASPIRATION

1. Onset of "asthma" in patients over 30 years without a family history of asthma or industrial exposure
2. Nocturnal or early morning cough
3. Nocturnal wheezing
4. Hoarseness, especially on arising
5. The need to clear the throat repeatedly
6. A feeling of constant pressure deep in the neck

TABLE 97–3. TREATMENT OF GASTROESOPHAGEAL REFLUX DISEASE

Simple Measures

1. Elevation of head of the bed
2. Avoidance of food and fluid intake before bedtime
3. Liquid antacid (aluminum hydroxide-magnesium hydroxide) one and three hours after meals and at bedtime
4. Avoidance of cigarettes, alcohol
5. Weight loss

Measures for Resistant Cases

1. Alginic acid–antacid (Gaviscon), 15 ml four times a day
2. Bethanechol (Urecholine),* 10 or 25 mg four times a day
3. Cimetidine,* 300 mg four times a day

*This use is not listed in the manufacturer's directive.

individuals can be helped by manipulations designed to alter the frequency or type of esophageal reflux. Many patients respond to the simple measures outlined in Table 97–3. Elevation of the head of the bed by 6 to 8 inches is the simplest and most effective form of therapy. Twenty-four–hour pH monitoring has shown that this simple measure decreases the frequency and length of reflux episodes. The use of pillows to elevate the thorax does not work well, as patients tend to roll off the pillows during the night. A plywood wedge under the mattress can be used if the bed frame cannot be moved. Avoiding food and fluid for at least three hours before retiring decreases the amount of material available for reflux at night. Avoidance of food that the patient finds distressing, such as fatty foods, chocolate, and onions, makes sense but has never been subjected to clinical trial.

Neutralization of acid is approached by taking 30 ml of aluminum hydroxide–magnesium hydroxide antacid one and three hours after meals and at bedtime. In recalcitrant cases, hourly antacids may be tried, with substitution of pure aluminum hydoxide gel to control diarrhea produced by the magnesium ion. Most patients will not tolerate such a regimen for long.

An attempt should be made to have the patient stop smoking, drinking alcohol, and overeating. Most patients, however, apparently prefer to suffer with reflux symptoms than to give up these mainstays of life.

If these simple measures are not effective, then more vigorous treatment is indicated. Alginic acid–antacid, 15 ml after each meal and at bedtime, has been shown to be more effective than placebo and as effective as antacids. It is worth trying, but often will not control symptoms of severe reflux. Bethanechol* is a parasympathomimetic agent that can be used in doses of 10 or 25 mg four times a day. Cimetidine,* 300 mg four times a day, although not approved for therapy of heartburn, improves symptoms significantly when compared with placebo. Its effect on objective signs of reflux such as esophageal erosions is less well established.

Surgical Management. In a patient in whom adequate trial of medical management as outlined above has not brought good results in a six-month period, and in whom there is good objective evidence of reflux, surgical correction of reflux should be considered. Surgical therapy was originally aimed at ablation of hiatus hernias; often the hernia was repaired but reflux and symptoms continued unabated. Current surgical therapy, regardless of exact techniques, attempts to restore sphincter competence by surrounding the lower end of the esophagus with a cuff of gastric fundal muscle. This is done either completely, as in the Nissen fundoplication, or partially (Hill repair, Belsey repair).

It is difficult to choose one operation or method over another, as most published surgical reports do not carefully define the exact indications for the operation, the length and type of preoperative medical management, or the use of objective tests pre- and postoperatively. Follow-up tends to be short and incomplete; the postoperative assessments are usually made by those responsible for choosing or operating upon the patients.

*This use is not listed in the manufacturer's directive.

Therefore, no firm statement can be made about the true efficacy of surgery in the correction of reflux.

A surgeon experienced in the techniques of antireflux surgery is necessary for good postoperative results. Most antireflux surgery is performed deep in the abdomen with poor visability; technique is all important. Although some individual surgeons have enviable postoperative results, antireflux surgery has a relatively poor reputation in many medical communities. Currently, a conservative approach toward antireflux surgery seems indicated.

Treatment of Complications. *Esophageal strictures,* if mild, can be handled by careful attention to dietary intake, improvement of dentition, and institution of medical therapy. If this approach is unavailing, then mechanical bougienage of the stricture is indicated. Either weighted rubber dilators (Hurst; Maloney) or steel olives passed with a wand (Eder-Puestow) can be used by someone familiar with these techniques. With the latter instrument, even very tight long strictures can be dilated, preferably under radiologic control. Once the lumen is restored to a diameter of 13 to 15 mm, most patients swallow without difficulty. If the stricture is stable and requires dilation only every four to six months, nothing else is necessary.

Some patients will not tolerate dilation or require vigorous dilation every three to four weeks. This is an indication for definitive antireflux operation, following which the stricture will regress. Unfortunately, many strictures persist after attempts at antireflux surgery. Esophageal replacement by colon, jejunum, or stomach is a surgical maneuver of last resort; such procedures have relatively high morbidity and mortality. Those afflicted by strictures often have significant lung and cardiovascular disease that makes them unsuitable operative candidates.

If a patient has a peptic stricture that does not respond to dilation and if surgery is deemed too risky because of the patient's age or condition, irradiation of the stomach may be tried. Fifteen hundred rads to the stomach is usually well tolerated and produces anacidity for weeks to months after therapy is completed. Acid production usually returns at a later date, but often at a lower level. This procedure sometimes facilitates dilation of the stricture.

Esophageal ulcers also represent a major therapeutic problem. Although cimetidine therapy may heal an ulcer, antireflux surgery, if tolerated, is a more reliable mode of treatment. If not, gastric radiation can be employed as in esophageal stricture.

Columnar epithelium may be premalignant. There is no way short of esophageal resection to make certain that the epithelium can be removed. Adequate antireflux therapy will cause regression of columnar epithelium in a rare patient, but further study is necessary before antireflux surgery can be recommended as a treatment for columnar epithelium. The effect of long-term cimetidine therapy on either recurrence of esophagitis or on the columnar epithelium is not known.

Treatment of the pulmonary complications of reflux depends on the age of the patient. Infants who present with recurrent bronchitis can be treated by postural methods and by thickening the formula. In adults, attention to posture at night is most important (see above). Since diagnostic methods that establish a direct causal relationship between reflux and lung disease are lacking, caution is advised in offering surgery to those who present with primary pulmonary problems and in whom reflux is demonstrated.

DeMeester TR, Johnson LF, Kent AH: Evaluation of current operations for the prevention of gastroesophageal reflux. Ann Surg 180:511, 1974. *The only randomized surgical trial of different antireflux operations.*

Dodds WF, Hogan WJ, Helm JF, Dent J: Pathogenesis of reflux esophagitis. Gastroenterology 81:376, 1981. *Exhaustive discussion of causes of reflux disease.*

Richter JE, Castell DO: Gastroesophageal reflux. Ann Intern Med 97:93, 1982. *Good coverage of diagnosis and therapy.*

MOTOR DISORDERS OF THE ESOPHAGUS

DEFINITION AND PATHOGENESIS. The muscular tube of the esophagus is guarded at both ends by specialized bundles of muscle, the upper and lower esophageal sphincters (UES, LES). Material from the oropharynx is injected at a high velocity (in the case of liquids), and precise coordination is required to link the muscles of the oropharynx, UES, body of the esophagus, and LES into a functional unit. Failure of any or all of these components will result in an esophageal motor disorder.

Failure of the oropharyngeal and UES units can be caused either by primary muscle disease such as *myotonia dystrophica* or *dermatomyositis* or by neurologic lesions involving the innervation of these muscle groups. *Brain stem infarcts, multiple sclerosis,* and *amyotrophic lateral sclerosis* serve as examples for the latter process.

The pathogenesis of motor abnormality of the esophageal body is less well understood. The striated muscle that constitutes the upper one quarter to one third of the body can be affected by primary muscle disease, such as *myotonia dystrophica,* or by metabolic disease affecting muscle function, such as *hypothyroidism.* The smooth muscle seems more resistant to muscular disease, but the intrinsic nervous network can be involved in *Chagas' disease* and *achalasia.* In the latter disease, there is infiltration of Auerbach's plexus with lymphocytes or actual disappearance of the neuron cell bodies in the plexus.

The motor disorders of the body of the esophagus have historically been classified as *achalasia* or *diffuse spasm.* In achalasia dysphagia and esophageal retention predominate; x-ray shows a dilated esophagus with a distal beak, and manometry reveals a high pressure in the LES with no or incomplete relaxation as well as only simultaneous low amplitude contractions in response to a swallow. *Diffuse spasm* is a combination of esophageal colic and dysphagia clinically; segmental contractions shown by x-ray; and some peristaltic waves interspersed with simultaneous, prolonged, high-amplitude contractions on a manometric record. There are many variations of these "classic" diseases, and progression from diffuse spasm to achalasia has been documented in the same individual. Many nonspecific motor disorders of the esophagus exist that do not fit these two syndromes. The pathophysiology of these nonspecific disorders has not been described. It seems best at the present state of knowledge to be descriptive of the features of a motor disorder without being too precise about an actual name of the disorder.

SYMPTOMS. The type of symptom produced is a function of the level and extent of the problem. *Weakness of the oropharyngeal musculature* may cause *transfer dysphagia*—the inability to propel a solid or liquid bolus from the pharynx to the esophagus. Patients are aware usually that they cannot begin the act of deglutition. Solids are usually more trouble than liquids. Palatal weakness may lead to *nasal regurgitation* of fluids or to *laryngeal aspiration* because of muscular failure to seal off the larynx. Such weakness may be signaled by a nasal quality of the voice.

Incoordination of UES relaxation has been suggested as a cause of transfer dysphagia and for the production of Zenker's diverticulum, but current high-fidelity methods fail to show such incoordination. Transfer dysphagia accompanied by a prominent cricopharyngeal impression on a barium swallow ("cricopharyngeal achalasia") similarly shows no defect in relaxing or in timing when studied by modern manometric methods.

Motor disorders in the body of the esophagus produce either *dysphagia* or *pain,* or both. The dysphagia may be intermittent or continuous. It may be manifest both for solids and for liquids. It is rare for the arrested material to be regurgitated; often posturing (throwing the shoulders back and extending the neck) or a Valsalva maneuver will help the material pass into the stomach.

Pain or esophageal colic is the other major clinical presentation of motor disorders. The pain is usually substernal, described as a feeling of pressure or aching, radiating to the back as well as to the neck, jaw, and arms. It can range in intensity from a transient discomfort to an overwhelming, agonizing pain similar to that of a major myocardial infarction or dissecting aortic aneurysm. The pain may last for only five to ten seconds or may be present for hours. The differentiation between angina pectoris and esophageal colic may be impossible on clinical grounds; both may be related to exercise, have the same intensity and distribution, and respond to sublingual nitroglycerin.

Failure of the lower esophageal sphincter may present with two separate symptom complexes. If the sphincter fails to relax on deglutition (as occurs in achalasia), there will be dysphagia and retention of contents in the body of the esophagus. This failure coupled with loss of peristalsis (achalasia) leads to marked esophageal retention, regurgitation, and overflow of esophageal contents into the tracheobronchial tree. If there is primary muscle failure of the sphincter as occurs in *scleroderma,* then massive reflux and the consequences of GERD will follow.

DIAGNOSIS. A careful history is essential in choosing the correct diagnostic tools for evaluating esophageal motor disorders. If the difficulty is thought to be in the oropharynx and upper esophageal sphincter, a cineradiograph would offer the most information. The cine film allows for frame-by-frame analysis of this rapidly moving portion of the gastrointestinal tract. Incoordination of tongue and palate, unilateral pharyngeal weakness, and aspiration of small amounts of barium into the trachea on swallowing can be shown. Air double contrast examinations of the pharynx can elucidate an unsuspected hypopharyngeal carcinoma. A diverticulum or prominence of the cricopharyngeal muscle can also be seen. Manometric examination of the hypopharynx and upper esophageal sphincter has been disappointing.

Radiology offers the best chance of diagnosis when the motor disorders have relatively static changes. In achalasia the body of the esophagus commonly dilates with retention of food, secretions, and barium (Fig. 97–2). Special attention can be paid to the terminal end of the esophagus. In achalasia, there is a smooth tapering beak. Any irregularity of this beak should lead to a vigorous search for an infiltrating neoplasm of the cardia, which can exactly mimic achalasia clinically and radiologically.

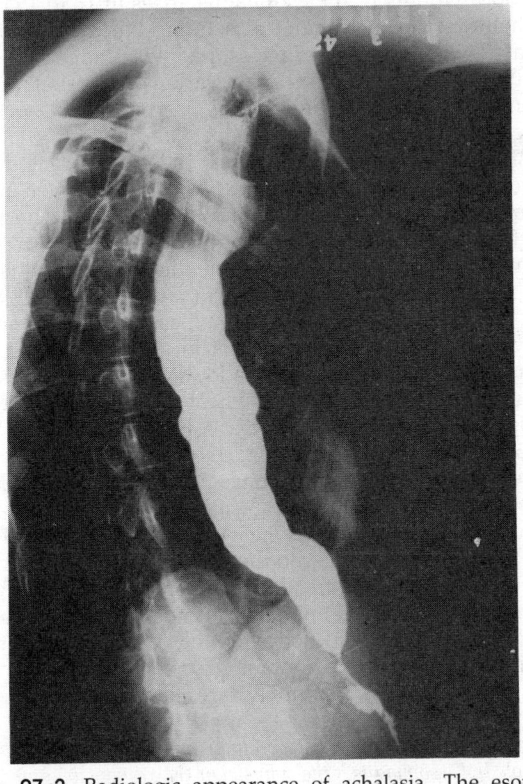

Figure 97–2. Radiologic appearance of achalasia. The esophageal body is dilated and terminates in a narrowed segment. (Courtesy of Dr. FE Templeton. From Pope CE II: *In* Sleisenger MH, Fordtran JS [eds.]: Gastrointestinal Disease. 3rd ed. Philadelphia, W. B. Saunders Company, 1983.)

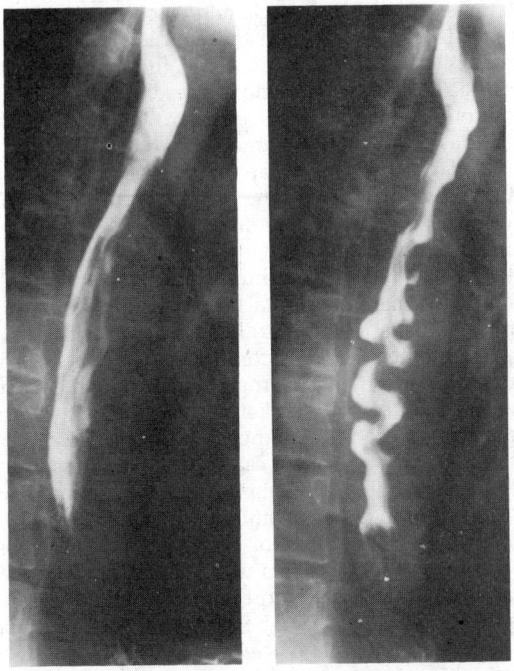

Figure 97–3. Radiologic appearance of diffuse spasm. Two spot films were taken within ten seconds of each other. A fairly normal appearance on the left changes rapidly to an appearance of numerous contractions. (Courtesy of Dr. CA Rohrmann. From Pope CE II: *In* Sleisenger MH, Fordtran JS [eds.]: Gastrointestinal Disease. 3rd ed. Philadelphia, W. B. Saunders Company, 1983.)

If the esophageal muscle is atonic, as is seen in far advanced scleroderma, barium and even air will be retained for long periods of time in the supine position. Assumption of the upright position will rapidly clear the barium from the esophagus and leave a double contrast view of a dilated esophagus.

The radiologist has more difficulty when the motor abnormality is more intermittent, as shown in Figure 97–3. Such a radiologic appearance is not always evidence for a clinically important motor disorder; elderly patients will often show similar radiologic findings and yet be totally asymptomatic.

Manometric examination allows more prolonged evaluation of esophageal motor function and is the only method that allows lower esophageal sphincter function to be directly determined. Normally, a swallow causes a peristaltic wave to be detected sequentially by pressure detectors spaced along the esophagus. Aperistalsis (no response to a swallow), simultaneous single or multiple contractions, prolonged contractions of high amplitude and low velocity, and spontaneous activity not related to swallowing can be recorded. Some of the "classic" patterns associated with diseases are listed in Table 97–4. Many

TABLE 97–4. CLASSIC MANOMETRIC FINDINGS

Disease	LES	Body
Achalasia	High resting pressure; no relaxation or incomplete on deglutition	Low amplitude simultaneous contractions on deglutition; some peristalsis in top 1 to 2 cm of esophagus
Diffuse spasm	Normal or high resting pressure; occasionally premature closure	Some peristaltic waves; other swallows followed by baseline elevation with superimposed simultaneous contractions
Scleroderma	Normal or low resting pressure; occasionally no sphincter pressure detectable	Low amplitude peristaltic waves or total aperistalsis except in upper 2 to 4 cm of esophagus

subjects present with dysphagia and/or chest pain in different patterns. It is best to describe the radiologic and manometric findings in the individual patient and then try to relate them to the classic syndrome most closely resembled. Also, progression from one syndrome (diffuse spasm) to another (achalasia) over time has often been documented.

Manometric examination can be of special benefit in the evaluation of chest pain if the patient happens to have an attack of chest pain during the examination. If the chest pain is accompanied by motor activity that allows the manometrist to predict onset, intensity, and disappearance of the chest pain by watching the manometric tracing, the diagnosis of an esophageal origin of chest pain is firmly established. Similarly, if pH is being simultaneously monitored and the episodes of chest pain correlate closely with drops in intraesophageal pH, an esophageal origin of pain is likely. Conversely, if typical chest pain occurs but there is no change in motor activity or pH over control values, an esophageal cause of pain is unlikely. Unfortunately, such definitive statements can only be made in about 20 per cent of the patients examined.

Pharmacologic stimulation of the esophagus has been employed for diagnostic purposes using such agents as mecholyl, pentagastrin, bethanechol, and ergonovine, but no universally successful stimulus has yet been found. The possibility of serious coronary ischemia or cardiac arrhythmia with ergonovine limits the usefulness of this agent.

Endoscopy has little usefulness in the evaluation of most motor disorders except for inspection of the cardia with a retroflexed view from the stomach to rule out an infiltrating carcinoma. Possibly transport of radionuclides as measured by a gamma camera will aid in the detection and evaluation of motor disorders.

TREATMENT. Of the various motor disorders of the esophagus, only *achalasia* seems amenable to relief. Since the problem in achalasia is one of obstruction of the lower end of the esophagus by a sphincter that will not relax, all forms of therapy are directed at relief of this obstruction. Short-term improvement in clinical symptoms and in scintigraphic esophageal emptying has been reported, both with isosorbide dinitrate, a long-acting nitrate, and nifedipine, a calcium channel blocker. The place of long-term pharmacologic management of achalasia has not been established. Dilation with a large Hurst bougie may give temporary relief; a few patients have been maintained for long periods of time with weekly self-dilations. Much more effective is brusk dilation with a pneumatic bag under x-ray control. This should be performed by an expert, since the rate of perforation even in good hands is about 5 to 15 per cent. Bag dilation is preferable initially on all patients.

Surgery is reserved for those in whom bag dilation fails or those who do not wish to be exposed to the risk of perforation. Direct section of the lower esophageal sphincter muscle (myotomy) is carried out, sparing some gastric muscle fibers to prevent postoperative reflux (Heller procedure). Amazingly, after both bag dilation and myotomy, manometry reveals return of normal peristalsis in 20 per cent of those with achalasia. This observation is difficult to explain in view of the degeneration of Auerbach's plexus in the intramural nervous network, thought to explain the pathogenesis of this disease.

Treatment of most other motor disorders is much more difficult. Patients with diffuse spasm can be given nitroglycerin or anticholinergics, but the results are disappointing. Balloon dilation has also been suggested to be of benefit in diffuse spasm, but it is difficult to understand how stretching of the lower esophageal sphincter segment would benefit a process that involves the entire esophageal body. Division of all the circular muscle with a long myotomy has been tried, but the long-term results of this procedure are not always favorable.

Treatment of other nonspecific motor disorders associated with chest pain can be equally frustrating. Prescribing sublingual nitroglycerin is justifiable. If it is ineffective, long-acting nitrate therapy will probably not work. Anticholinergic drugs will benefit only a few. Preliminary uncontrolled reports on the use of calcium channel blocking drugs are promising. Only meperidine (Demerol) has been uniformly useful. Obviously this medication is not a good long-term solution to the problem. Long myotomies have been tried in selected patients; occasional good long-term results have been obtained. It would seem wise not to subject any patient to myotomy until that patient had been observed manometrically during an attack, and an esophageal origin of pain firmly established.

The treatment of *scleroderma* and other conditions marked by aperistalsis revolves mostly around the associated reflux. If there is no obstruction at the lower end of the esophagus, either by a malfunctioning sphincter or by an organic narrowing, aperistalsis is amazingly well tolerated, usually with only mild dysphagia for solids. Caution should be employed in offering antireflux surgery to patients with scleroderma, as a tight fundoplication without any peristalsis in the body of the esophagus will lead to severe dysphagia.

Castell DO: Achalasia and diffuse esophageal spasm. Arch Intern Med 136:571, 1976. *Review article on both syndromes.*

Vantrappen G, Janssens J, Hellemans J, Coremans G: Achalasia, diffuse esophageal spasm and related motility disorders. Gastroenterology 76:450, 1979. *This article details variations and interrelationships between various motor disorders, and also shows return of peristalsis in some patients with achalasia after bag dilation.*

ESOPHAGEAL TUMORS

ETIOLOGY AND PATHOGENESIS. Carcinoma of the esophageal epithelium, both squamous cell and adenocarcinoma, is by far the most common and important tumor of the esophagus. Benign neoplasms (leiomyoma, papilloma, and fibrovascular polyps) are rarer by far. Squamous cell cancer has an incidence of 4 per 100,000 in males (United States), rising to 130 per 100,000 in North China. It is associated with both alcohol intake and tobacco smoking in countries where these substances are used. Esophageal cancer occurs more commonly in those who have developed squamous cancers of the head and neck, in those with lye strictures, and in patients with untreated or inadequately treated achalasia.

Adenocarcinoma of the esophagus arises in 10 to 15 per cent of patients with columnar epithelium (Barrett's epithelium) associated with chronic reflux esophagitis. Indeed, transition of columnar epithelium through various stages of atypia to adenoma and carcinoma in situ has been described within the same esophagus in those with Barrett's epithelium.

SYMPTOMS. In Western countries, the most common clinical symptom of carcinoma is *progressive dysphagia* over a six- to eight-month period until only liquids can be taken. The obstruction reflects circumferential involvement of the esophageal wall by tumor and does not occur until the cancer is biologically rather far advanced. The dysphagia may be accompanied by a *steady, boring pain,* which signals mediastinal involvement and inoperability. In the Orient but not in the United States, pain is often a relatively early sign of a localized and thus resectable tumor. Unexplained persistent chest pain should always be investigated by a careful double contrast x-ray view of the esophagus or by endoscopy (Fig. 97–4).

More advanced lesions manifest themselves with *halitosis, weight loss,* and *coughing after drinking fluid.* The last-named symptom is caused either by near-complete esophageal lumen obstruction with overspill into the larynx or by the development of a tracheoesophageal fistula. Hoarseness from involvement of the recurrent laryngeal nerve by tumor and hematemesis are unusual symptoms. Nail bed clubbing can be seen with both benign and malignant tumors. Hypercalcemia and excess ACTH production are extremely rare manifestations of esophageal carcinoma.

Since dysphagia is the most common presenting symptom of neoplasm of the esophagus, the physician is responsible for making absolutely certain that cancer is not the cause of dysphagia. Early diagnosis affords the only chance for cure. Early diagnosis allows the patient, family, and physician to plan better all aspects of the patient's future.

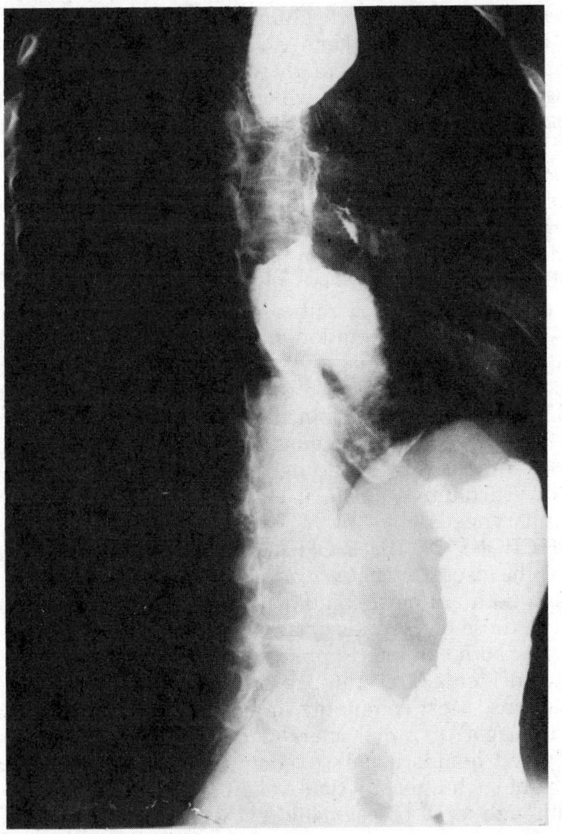

Figure 97–4. Obstructing carcinoma of the esophagus. Note an extraluminal collection of barium demonstrating a localized perforation in the tumor mass.

DIAGNOSIS. The clinical suspicion of a cancer of the esophagus should lead immediately to an esophagogram, possibly with double contrast techniques. Any irregularity, especially if it narrows the lumen, mandates further evaluation. If dysphagia is present, the radiologist should give a bolus of barium-soaked bread or a large marshmallow to discover any possible sites of arrest.

In the presence of symptoms but a normal barium swallow, endoscopy with biopsy and brushing of any suspicious lesion for examination of tissue and of exfoliated cells is indicated. The endoscopist should always obtain a good retroflexed view of the cardia from below to make certain that an adenocarcinoma of the gastroesophageal junction has not been overlooked.

If narrowing has been seen by barium swallow, then endoscopy with biopsy and cytologic brushings of the involved area must be done. With the fiberoptic endoscope, numerous blind biopsies from as deep in the lesion as possible will be most helpful. Biopsy of visible tissue will often reveal only inflammatory tissue. Sometimes as many as eight or nine biopsies must be obtained before tumor is recovered.

Exfoliative cytology will sometimes give a higher degree of positive results than will biopsy if the cells are collected properly and evaluated by a highly competent laboratory. The collecting tube must pass through the lesion and obtain gastric contents to ensure an adequate specimen for study. Diagnostic accuracy of exfoliative cytology depends on meticulous technique. In most hospitals biopsy must be relied upon.

Once a tumor is identified, certain procedures in addition to chest films are essential for staging before a therapeutic decision is reached. A careful physical examination for nodal metastases, bronchoscopy for evidence of tracheal involvement, liver function tests plus ultrasound or nuclear medicine scan for metastases, and probably CT scanning for mediastinal nodal involvement are necessary before the final therapeutic plan is decided upon. A chest roentgenogram is mandatory.

TREATMENT. The ideal form of treating cancer of the esophagus, either for cure or for palliation, has not yet been developed. No series exists in which patients were carefully staged with the best noninvasive methods available and then randomized to different treatment modalities. Treatment choices still reflect local custom and personal prejudices of physicians, surgeons, and radiotherapists interested in this disease.

Surgical resection of lower one third squamous carcinoma and adenocarcinoma is preferred in most centers if the patient does not have widespread metastases. Surgery offers the benefit of rapidly restoring esophagogastric continuity. Perhaps only one quarter of all patients presenting to a medical-surgical center will have a resectable tumor; of these patients 20 per cent will not survive the operative period, and five-year survival will be only 5 to 10 per cent, even with extensive resections. Long-term survival cannot be predicted in the individual case by the operative findings. There is growing enthusiasm for palliative resection with restoration of gastrointestinal continuity with stomach or colon. Surgical results in China and Japan are better than those quoted for the United States, with hospital deaths of 5 per cent and five-year survivals of 20 to 30 per cent. Whether this represents better technical skill, a different type of patient, or earlier diagnosis is not certain.

Radiotherapy is employed in upper one third lesions and often in middle third tumors as well. This form of therapy has little hospital mortality, although it carries some short-term and long-term morbidity. With ideal home situations, radiotherapy can be carried out on an outpatient basis. Approximately 40 per cent of tumors cannot be destroyed with conventional 6000 rad therapy. Combination of pre- and postoperative radiation with resective therapy has been employed, but there is no good evidence that such combined therapy is better. Adenocarcinomas occasionally respond to radiotherapy but are not as radiosensitive as squamous cell carcinomas.

When obvious extraesophageal spread is present, palliation with bougienage to restore and maintain an adequate esophageal lumen may be done. If performed with a wire guide under fluoroscopic guidance, such therapy is not hazardous in skilled hands. If dilation does not offer lasting relief, then a Silastic tube can be placed perorally for relief of esophageal obstruction. Such tubes are also of great benefit in the treatment of a malignant tracheoesophageal fistula.

Choice of therapy will depend on the location and size of the lesion, presence or absence of spread, cell type, and the skills of the medical community. Until an adequate randomized trial after adequate staging is carried out, choice of treatment modality will continue to be a matter of preference.

Earlam R, Cunha-Melo JR: Oesophageal squamous cell carcinoma. Br J Surg 67:381, 457, 1980. *Two articles present exhaustive literature reviews of surgical and radiotherapy of esophageal carcinoma.*

George FW: Radiation management in esophageal cancer. Am J Surg 139:795, 1980. *A review of radiotherapy of cancer of the esophagus, with some suggestions for future directions of investigation.*

Parker EF, Moertel CG: Carcinoma of the esophagus: Is there a role for surgery? Am J Dig Dis 23:730, 1978. *A discussion of the advantages and disadvantages of surgical therapy of cancer of the esophagus.*

OTHER CONDITIONS

RINGS AND WEBS. During early development, the lumen of the esophagus becomes completely obliterated and then is recanalized to form the adult hollow viscus. It is not too surprising that a failure of this process leads to atresia or a residual web. Such webs usually occur in the upper esophagus, often with eccentric openings; occasionally they are multiple. A much more common web or ring is located in the terminal esophagus, has a symmetrical opening, and is usually at the junction between squamous and the normal transitional or columnar epithelium of the stomach (Fig. 97–5). This latter ring (Schatzki's ring) can be demonstrated in many individuals if cine studies of the lower esophageal zone are used. It produces symptoms infrequently but in a characteristic manner. An

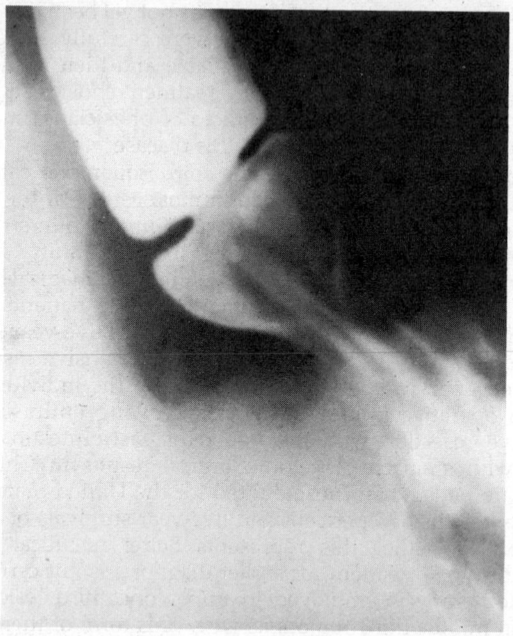

Figure 97–5. Lower esophageal ring (Schatzki's ring). This ring consists of a symmetrical thin web located in the terminal esophagus. (From Pope CE II: *In* Sleisenger MH, Fordtran JS [eds.]: Gastrointestinal Disease. 3rd ed. Philadelphia, W. B. Saunders Company, 1983.)

acquired web located in the postcricoid area is sometimes associated with iron deficiency anemia.

All these types of webs or rings cause dysphagia for solids, and the impacted bolus usually has to be regurgitated. The lower esophageal ring (Schatzki's ring) has a characteristic clinical presentation that allows the diagnosis to be made by history. Every three to four months, after a bolus of meat or bread, the patient will complain of dysphagia and total inability to swallow solids or liquids. The bolus will be regurgitated, and then the patient can continue to eat normally. If the patient comes to the emergency room with an impacted bolus of meat, nothing will be seen after the impacted bolus is removed with the operating endoscope, and the disorder will be labeled as "hysterical dysphagia." The lower esophageal ring is not well seen with the rigid endoscope, as the lower portion of the esophagus cannot be distended enough to force the ring into prominence.

Treatment of all webs involves mechanical disruption either with a dilator or with the endoscope. Treatment of the iron deficiency anemia is said to cause the postcricoid webs to disappear. Only very rarely will a surgical approach to a web or ring be necessary.

DIVERTICULA OF THE ESOPHAGUS. Zenker's diverticulum of the pharynx is not anatomically an esophageal diverticulum, as its neck is above the upper esophageal sphincter muscle, but custom has dictated its inclusion in description of esophageal diverticula. An epiphrenic diverticulum usually occurs on the right side of the esophagus just above the lower esophageal sphincter. Other diverticula are at the level of the carina, and are known as traction diverticula, although traction by scar tissue is rarely demonstrated. Scleroderma is occasionally associated with numerous wide-mouthed diverticula scattered along the length of the esophagus. Large amplitude motor waves have been associated with mid-body diverticula, and either achalasia or motor incoordination with epiphrenic diverticula.

Symptoms vary widely; many diverticula are found by accident during barium examination of the esophagus. If a patient with dysphagia is found to have a diverticulum, it is difficult to tell whether the diverticulum or the associated motor disorder is the cause. Zenker's diverticulum often has a classic symptom complex, particularly when it becomes large. It retains saliva and food particles, which may either be aspirated or cause repeated postprandial throat clearing with production of liquid and food particles. Patients with this type of diverticulum can often press on the neck and empty the diverticulum. The pouch can become so large that it can compress the esophagus anteriorly and obstruct it. In the presence of diverticula great caution must be exercised in passing tubes into the esophagus or stomach. Zenker's diverticulum is a special problem, since tubes naturally enter it rather than the esophageal opening, and the risk of perforation into the mediastinum is great. Traction and epiphrenic diverticula do not require treatment. Zenker's diverticulum, if large, may require diverticulectomy or diverticulopexy with coincident section of the cricopharyngeus muscle. Most techniques for diverticulectomy automatically accomplish cricopharyngeal section at the same time. If the diverticulum is small, it may regress after section of the cricopharyngeus.

INFECTIONS OF THE ESOPHAGUS. Two major infections involve the esophagus: *Candida* and *herpesvirus* infections. Although both are most common in immunocompromised hosts such as those on steroids or undergoing cancer chemotherapy, either or both can infect apparently healthy hosts. Both can be found incidentally at autopsy or during endoscopy for other indications. Most commonly, infection of the mucosa leads to odynophagia of rather marked degree. Dysphagia for both solids and liquids usually accompanies the odynophagia and can be of such intensity that weight loss is rapid.

Although x-ray occasionally reveals a shaggy mucosa in the case of monilial involvement, and occasionally even a stricture, endoscopy is the best method of detecting and confirming infectious involvement. *Candida* can present as isolated white plaques, which can be confused with glycogenic acanthosis, or progress to form confluent ulcerations with an overlying membrane. Herpesvirus tends to produce isolated ulcers, but extensive involvement can produce confluent ulcerations. Biopsy of the ulcerated area usually shows either invasive hyphae of *Candida* or characteristic nuclear changes of the squamous cells when herpesvirus is present. Cytologic washings occasionally demonstrate the same change.

Treatment is dependent on correct identification of the etiologic agent. For *Candida* infection, an assessment of the degree of severity is needed. For mild disease, topical therapy with 250,000 units of nystatin (Mycostatin) every two hours will suffice. For more serious infections, low-dose intravenous amphotericin therapy has been successful, the dose being individualized on the basis of weight and renal status. Treatment with miconazole and ketoconazole appears promising. For severe esophageal infections, ketoconazole should be given in doses of 200 mg to 400 mg per day for eight to ten days. Herpesvirus infection is treated symptomatically with viscous lidocaine.

ESOPHAGEAL INJURIES. ***Caustic Ingestion.*** Caustic burns of the esophagus occur in children by accident; adults usually suffer such burns because of suicide attempts. Lye crystals, and especially liquid lye preparations for drain cleaning, are the most common cause. The speed of lye injury is so great that attempts to neutralize the caustic are futile. Detergents and Clorox also find their way into the esophageal lumen of both children and adults. The history is all important, but the degree of esophageal injury still must be assessed endoscopically as an emergency. Significant esophageal damage has been seen even without oral burns; conversely, oral burns do not necessarily mean that the material has reached the esophagus. If there is no esophageal reaction after apparent caustic ingestion, further care directed toward the esophagus will not be necessary.

The accepted therapy of a definite lye or caustic burn remains unsupported by clinical trials. For burns with solid lye or other solid agents, steroids have been recommended, at an initial dose of 80 mg per day, tapering to 20 mg per day until esophageal healing. Most clinicians also use broad-spectrum antibiotics such as ampicillin, 500 mg four times a day. If liquid lye has been the damaging agent, serious consideration of emergency esophagogastrectomy is in order, as lesser measures have been met with unacceptably high mortality.

Damage by Medication. A new form of iatrogenic illness of the esophagus has recently become evident. Ingested pills tend to lodge in the esophagus and damage the mucosa in a localized area. Tetracycline, doxycycline, ascorbic acid, and quinidine have all been indicted, and the list will undoubtedly grow. Normal individuals can retain small capsules in the esophagus, even when swallowing in the upright position. The clinical syndrome consists of steady burning or chest pain, accompanied by local odynophagia, all occurring four to six hours after ingestion of one of the offending capsules or tablets. Endoscopy (not clinically necessary) usually shows a localized mucosal ulcer, which heals without a scar within a week. Symptomatic therapy is adequate, but prophylaxis seems to be a more practical idea. Pills of the offending class should be taken in the upright position with several swallows of water.

Esophageal Trauma. The esophagus is well protected by the thoracic cage, but can be involved either by blunt trauma (automobile accidents) or by penetrating missiles (gunshots, knives). Often the surgeon's attention is directed toward more life-threatening damage to heart, lungs, or major blood vessels, and it is understandable that a rent in the esophagus may thus be overlooked. This unfortunate oversight, however, will be followed by mediastinitis, which may worsen an already grave situation. Iatrogenic perforation with endoscope, dilator, or, very rarely, nasogastric tube leads to a similar complication.

Vomiting itself can cause esophageal injury, either mucosal (*Mallory-Weiss*) or through-and-through rupture (*Boerhaave's syndrome*). The mucosal lesion first described by Mallory and Weiss has been recognized much more frequently since the advent of rapid emergency endoscopy with fiberoptic endoscopes. Classically, the patient has repeated attacks of retching, productive at first of gastric contents, and later of bright red blood. One quarter of patients shown to have a Mallory-Weiss tear have no prior history of vomiting. The tear is usually in the gastric mucosa just below the gastroesophageal junction, although it can extend through the junction and up into the esophageal mucosa. Diagnosis of this condition is almost always made at endoscopy; the rent is usually seen as the endoscope is being withdrawn from the stomach into the esophagus. The majority of such lesions heal with conservative therapy. Angiographic or surgical therapy is necessary in less than 5 per cent.

Vomiting can also cause a complete tear in the esophageal wall. Unlike the Mallory-Weiss lesion, the tear in Boerhaave's syndrome is located above the gastroesophageal junction on the left side. It usually follows vomiting, but other marked increases in intra-abdominal pressure such as lifting a heavy weight or straining at stool have been associated with a tear. The clinical diagnosis can be extremely difficult; often patients with esophageal rupture are thought to have a myocardial infarct, pneumothorax, a perforated viscus, or pancreatitis. Air in the mediastinum or the rapid appearance of a hydrothorax on the left usually leads to the correct diagnosis.

The diagnosis of esophageal perforation can usually be established by a cautious radiographic examination with water-soluble material. Barium may be used only if a rent is not demonstrated by the water-soluble agent. Immediate surgical repair is the accepted method of treatment of esophageal perforation. In those too ill for surgery, treatment consists of nasogastric suction, antibiotics, and subsequent mediastinal drainage if necessary.

Pope CE II: Rings and webs; Diverticula; Involvement of the esophagus by infections, systemic illnesses, and physical agents. *In* Sleisenger MH, Fordtran JS (eds.): Gastrointestinal Disease. 3rd ed. Philadelphia, W. B. Saunders Company, 1983, pp 476–479, 491–504. *Textbook review of these various conditions.*

98. GASTRITIS

Charles T. Richardson

DEFINITION. Inflammation of the stomach mucosa may be diffuse and involve all parts of the stomach or localized to the fundus and body or antrum. Even within a specific area (e.g., the antrum), inflammation may be diffuse or localized. Gastritis is classified as acute or chronic primarily on the basis of histologic and/or endoscopic findings and long-term clinical follow-up. Acute gastritis is believed to be a self-limited disease, whereas chronic gastritis by definition persists for long periods of time.

ACUTE GASTRITIS

ETIOLOGY. Drugs (such as aspirin and ethanol), bile salts, and pancreatic enzymes damage the gastric mucosa and are believed to cause both acute and chronic gastritis (see Chronic Gastritis, below). How these chemical agents cause gastritis is not known. They are thought to disrupt the so-called "gastric mucosal barrier" (the ability of gastric mucosa to restrict movement of hydrogen ions from lumen to mucosa), thereby allowing back-diffusion of acid and pepsin, and in this manner to contribute to the development of gastritis. Inhibition of prostaglandin synthesis by these drugs also may be a factor.

Acute gastritis also occurs in the setting of severe medical or surgical illnesses such as respiratory failure, sepsis, renal failure, hypotension, or trauma. This form of acute gastritis is called "stress" ulceration and may produce "stress" bleeding. Although the exact pathogenesis of "stress"-related gastritis is not known, mucosal ischemia is believed to be an important factor. Gastric acid is also likely to be involved, since in experimental models mucosal damage does not occur in the absence of acid. Bile and pancreatic juice may also be contributing factors.

An epidemic form of acute gastritis of unknown etiology has been reported associated with decreased gastric acid secretion (hypochlorhydria). Since gastritis occurred in a number of different persons who were in contact with each other over a relatively brief period of time, an infectious etiology was suspected; however, an organism has not been identified.

Additional causes of acute gastritis include roentgen irradiation, ingestion of corrosive substances, ingestion of staphylococcal exotoxin, and bacterial infections. Gastritis caused by bacterial infection is called acute phlegmonous gastritis. This is a rare but fulminant and often fatal form of acute gastritis. Streptococci are most commonly the cause, although staphylococci, *Escherichia coli,* and *Proteus* have been cultured from stomachs of patients with acute phlegmonous gastritis.

CLINICAL MANIFESTATIONS. Patients with acute gastritis secondary to aspirin or "stress" often have hematemesis and/or melena and may have pain, nausea, and vomiting. This form of acute gastritis is called acute hemorrhagic or erosive gastritis. At times, bleeding can be so severe that patients develop hypotension or shock.

Finding acute gastritis on biopsy does not necessarily mean that a patient has clinically important disease, since as many as 30 per cent of otherwise healthy, asymptomatic persons can have acute gastritis on biopsy. Also, some forms of acute gastritis with known cause, such as acute irradiation gastritis, are not associated with symptoms. However, patients with other causes of gastritis may have symptoms. For example, some patients with epidemic gastritis with hypochlorhydria have epigastric pain, nausea, and vomiting.

The physical examination in patients with acute gastritis is usually normal unless bleeding or other illnesses such as liver disease or arthritis are present. If bleeding occurs, the patient may have a reduced hematocrit, increased blood urea nitrogen, and a positive nasogastric aspirate or stool guaiac test for blood.

TABLE 98–1. TYPES OF GASTRITIS, METHOD OF DIAGNOSIS, AND ENDOSCOPIC, BARIUM X-RAY, AND/OR HISTOLOGIC FINDINGS

Types of Gastritis	Method of Diagnosis	Endoscopic, Barium X-Ray, and/or Histologic Findings
Acute		
Drug-induced (salicylates or other nonsteroidal anti-inflammatory drugs or alcohol)	Endoscopy	Congested mucosa with petechial hemorrhages and erosions.
	Histology	Neutrophils and mononuclear cells infiltrate the lamina propria; edema and hemorrhage distort the glands; inflammatory cells fill the pits and glands forming small abscesses.
Stress-induced (secondary to severe medical or surgical diseases or trauma)	Endoscopy	Erythema, petechial hemorrhages and erosions cover most of the mucosa.
	Histology	Inflammatory cells (primarily neutrophils) infiltrate the lamina propria; edema and hemorrhage distort the glands; pit and gland abscesses and focal sloughing of surface cells can be seen.
Chronic		
Superficial	Histology	Inflammatory cells (neutrophils, lymphocytes, plasma cells, and a few eosinophils) are limited to the gastric pits and upper lamina propria.
Atrophic	Histology	Inflammatory cells are located superficially but also invade deeper into the lamina propria; thinning of the mucosa with loss of glandular elements and intestinal metaplasia may occur.
Gastric atrophy	Histology	More severe form of atrophic gastritis; a marked reduction in mucosal thickness with loss of parietal and chief cells occurs; only a few inflammatory cells are present.
Special Types		
Giant Hypertrophic	Endoscopy or barium x-ray	Large folds are usually confined to the fundus and body but may involve the antrum.
	Histology	Hyperplasia of mucus, parietal, and chief cells; large cystic spaces containing mucus are often seen.
Eosinophilic	Endoscopy or barium x-ray	Rigid, nondistensible antrum and/or thickened mucosal folds are usually seen.
	Histology	Eosinophils infiltrate the lamina propria, submucosa, and muscular layers.
Granulomatous	Endoscopy or barium x-ray	Involved portions of the stomach are narrowed and rigid.
	Histology	Granulomas are found in the mucosa and submucosa and occasionally can be found in the muscular layer and serosa.

Unless there are concomitant diseases, other laboratory studies are usually normal (see Ch. 113).

DIAGNOSIS. Most clinically significant forms of acute gastritis are diagnosed by endoscopy (Table 98–1). For example, in acute gastritis secondary to aspirin or "stress," the gastric mucosa often appears congested and petechial hemorrhages, erosions, and superficial ulcerations cover the mucosal surface. These changes may be diffuse, although the fundus and body are most severely affected.

On biopsy, inflammatory cells (usually neutrophils and mononuclear cells) infiltrate the lamina propria, whereas the glandular areas are distorted by edema and hemorrhage. Exudate often fills the gastric pits and/or glands (pit and/or gland abscesses). In severe forms of gastritis (e.g., aspirin- or "stress"-induced), focal sloughing of surface epithelial cells can occur, producing superficial erosions and ulcerations.

NATURAL HISTORY. The major feature differentiating acute from chronic gastritis is the tendency for mucosal changes in acute gastritis to revert to normal. The time over which this occurs depends on the type of acute gastritis and on the method used to detect the endpoint. For example, in acute hemorrhagic gastritis the endoscopic appearance of the gastric mucosa may revert to normal within 24 to 48 hours after bleeding has stopped. Histologic reversion to normal may require a longer period of time.

Some patients with epidemic gastritis with hypochlorhydria have had moderate to severe gastritis on biopsy from two to five months after initial diagnosis, and moderate gastritis even up to 12 months. Acute gastritis is a reversible lesion, but histologic abnormalities may persist for months in some forms of acute gastritis. Whether acute gastritis progresses to chronic gastritis in some patients is not known.

TREATMENT. Most patients with acute gastritis do not require treatment. For example, acute gastritis found on biopsy in asymptomatic, healthy persons need not be treated. Treatment with antacids may be warranted in symptomatic patients who have a histologic diagnosis of acute gastritis and in whom other causes of symptoms have been excluded. Since there have been no controlled clinical trials evaluating antacids in the treatment of acute gastritis, the effectiveness and dosage are not known.

Patients with acute hemorrhagic gastritis present special therapeutic problems. Many of these patients experience severe upper gastrointestinal bleeding that requires treatment, including fluid and blood replacement and nasogastric lavage. Since acid and pepsin probably play a role in the pathogenesis, it seems reasonable to reduce gastric acidity and concomitantly peptic activity with antacids and/or cimetidine or ranitidine. Surgical therapy is to be avoided if at all possible because of its inordinately high morbidity and mortality.

Initially, an antacid (usually 30 ml of a liquid Al-Mg preparation) is prescribed every hour during the day and night; higher doses or more frequent administration may be needed in some patients. A combination of antacid plus cimetidine or ranitidine has been recommended by some physicians. Measurement of intragastric pH every hour and administration of medications in doses to keep intragastric pH above 3.5 have been suggested. Such a regimen prevents "stress"-induced ulcerations and bleeding in a large percentage of critically ill patients; however, there is no evidence that maintaining pH above 3.5 controls bleeding or assists in healing acute hemorrhagic gastritis once it occurs.

CHRONIC GASTRITIS

CLASSIFICATION. Chronic gastritis is usually classified on the basis of mucosal histology and/or the anatomic portion of the stomach involved. Although endoscopic and radiologic criteria for classifying chronic gastritis have been reported, gastric mucosal biopsy is the most reliable means of diagnosis. Biopsies should be obtained from several different areas, since chronic gastritis may be a localized disease.

HISTOLOGY. Chronic gastritis is divided into superficial gastritis, atrophic gastritis, and gastric atrophy (Table 98–1). When inflammatory cells are limited to the gastric pits and upper lamina propria, gastritis is classified as superficial. In atrophic gastritis inflammatory cells invade deeper into the lamina propria and glandular epithelium. Lymphoid follicles may also be seen. As the disease progresses, thinning of the mucosa occurs with loss of glandular elements. In some patients intestinal metaplasia develops with loss of parietal and chief cells and development of goblet cells, absorptive cells, and intestinal villi. Finally, in patients with gastric atrophy, parietal and chief cells are absent, mucosal thickness is reduced markedly, and only a small number of inflammatory cells are present.

LOCATION. Chronic atrophic gastritis has been divided into Type A and Type B, based primarily on the anatomic portion of the stomach involved and the presence or absence of parietal cell antibodies. In Type A gastritis the fundus and body of the stomach are involved, whereas the antrum is relatively normal. Parietal cell antibodies are found in a large percentage of patients, and pernicious anemia may develop. On the other hand, in Type B gastritis the antrum is involved primarily, although inflammation is found frequently in the fundus and body. Parietal cell antibodies do not occur. Immunologic, functional, and clinical differences between these two types of gastritis will be discussed below.

ETIOLOGY. The causes of chronic gastritis are unknown, although a number of mechanisms have been postulated. For example, radiation injury, nutritional deficiencies, endocrine disorders, and infectious diseases have been postulated but not proved to cause chronic gastritis. Repeated insults to the gastric mucosa by mechanical, thermal, or chemical agents have also been thought to cause chronic mucosal changes. Long-term alcohol or aspirin ingestion may lead to chronic gastritis, although this has not been clearly established.

Reflux of duodenal juice into the stomach is believed to irritate gastric mucosa and perhaps lead to chronic gastritis. Lysolecithin, which is formed when phospholipase A from pancreatic juice reacts with lecithin from bile, appears to be the most damaging constituent of refluxed duodenal juice. Lysolecithin, bile, and pancreatic juice are postulated to initiate the process leading to gastritis by removing the mucus layer from the epithelial surface. This leads to damage of the "mucosal barrier," allowing diffusion of gastric acid and pepsin into the mucosa. This, in turn, leads to further mucosal damage.

Immunologic injury may play a role in the pathogenesis of chronic gastritis in some patients. Patients with atrophic gastritis of the fundus and body (Type A gastritis) usually have antibodies against parietal cells, and some, but not all, of these patients develop pernicious anemia. Approximately 90 per cent of patients with pernicious anemia have parietal cell antibodies. Many also have antibodies to intrinsic factor, which may be of two types: (1) a blocking antibody which reacts with the vitamin B_{12}–intrinsic factor binding site and blocks the binding of vitamin B_{12} and intrinsic factor; or (2) a binding antibody which can react either with intrinsic factor alone or with intrinsic factor–vitamin B_{12} complex.

Antibody to gastrin-producing cells has been found recently in a few but not all patients with gastritis primarily involving the antrum (Type B gastritis). This finding adds further support for the role of immunologic abnormalities in the development of chronic gastritis. These patients do not have parietal cell or intrinsic factor antibodies and do not develop pernicious anemia.

Whether parietal cell and other cellular antibodies lead to mucosal destruction or whether they are markers of mucosal damage caused by other mechanisms is not known. Repeated injection of cellular antibodies can lead to gastric atrophy and decreased acid secretion in laboratory animals, suggesting that development of antibodies may be the initiating event. Serum of some patients with pernicious anemia has been found to contain an autoantibody that is cytotoxic to canine gastric mucosal cells. On the other hand, patients with adult-onset hypogammaglobulinemia can develop gastric atrophy and pernicious anemia even though they do not have antibodies to parietal cells or intrinsic factor.

Genetic influences also have been implicated in the development of chronic gastritis. Family members of patients with pernicious anemia have a higher incidence of atrophic gastritis, achlorhydria, vitamin B_{12} malabsorption, and parietal cell and intrinsic factor antibodies than does the general population. The role of genetics in patients with chronic gastritis who do not have pernicious anemia has not been adequately explored.

Theoretically, gastric atrophy could also develop from the absence of a mucosal trophic factor such as gastrin, urogastrone, or epidermal growth factor, or from end-organ resistance to one of these factors. So far, there are no studies evaluating these possibilities.

CLINICAL MANIFESTATIONS. As with acute gastritis, many patients with chronic gastritis and no other underlying disease are asymptomatic and have a normal physical examination. For example, it is rare for patients with pernicious anemia to have symptoms related to gastritis or gastric atrophy. Symptoms such as nausea, vomiting, and epigastric pain can occur in patients with chronic gastritis; however, studies have shown a poor correlation between presence or absence of symptoms and histologic evidence of gastritis. Thus, a biopsy diagnosis of chronic gastritis should not be used as the sole explanation for upper gastrointestinal symptoms, and other causes such as peptic ulcer disease, gastric cancer, or cholelithiasis should be excluded.

Other clinical findings in patients with chronic gastritis relate to abnormalities in laboratory studies. Gastric acid secretion usually is lower than normal and is especially low or absent in patients with atrophic gastritis or gastric atrophy. Decreased secretion of pepsin also occurs. Patients with gastritis involving the fundus and body but sparing the antrum (Type A gastritis) usually are hypo- or achlorhydric and have elevated serum gastrin concentrations presumably secondary to an alkaline antral pH (sometimes as high as in patients with Zollinger-Ellison syndrome). When gastritis involves the antrum primarily (Type B gastritis), acid secretion is usually diminished but serum gastrin concentration is in the normal range.

In patients with pernicious anemia, the vitamin B_{12} absorption test (Schilling test) is abnormal when performed in the absence of exogenous intrinsic factor, and in untreated patients signs and symptoms of vitamin B_{12} deficiency may develop. Some patients with pernicious anemia have clinical and laboratory evidence of other diseases such as Hashimoto's thyroiditis, hypothyroidism, hyperthyroidism, insulin-dependent diabetes mellitus, or vitiligo.

NATURAL HISTORY. Chronic gastritis is a longstanding disease that increases in frequency with advancing age. The individual patient is thought to progress over time from superficial gastritis to chronic atrophic gastritis to gastric atrophy, but this has not been established. It is also not known whether all patients who later in life are found to have gastric atrophy initially had superficial gastritis. In one study, patients with chronic superficial gastritis were followed for 10 to 20 years. Superficial gastritis persisted, relatively unchanged, in half of the patients, whereas progression to atrophic gastritis occurred in most of the remainder. Reversion to normal was also noted in a few patients.

Associations have been reported between chronic gastritis and gastric polyps, benign gastric ulcer, and gastric cancer. Although benign gastric ulcers usually occur in an area of chronic superficial or atrophic gastritis, it is not known whether gastritis precedes and perhaps leads to gastric ulcer formation or whether gastritis develops in response to ulceration. Gastric cancer may occur more frequently in patients with both Types A and B gastritis; however, numerically the incidence is higher in Type B.

TREATMENT. Most patients with chronic gastritis do not require treatment for the following reasons: (1) the pathogenesis of chronic gastritis is poorly understood; thus, it is difficult to design rational therapy; (2) most patients with chronic gastritis are asymptomatic; and (3) there is no evidence that therapy prevents sequelae such as gastric atrophy, pernicious anemia, or cancer.

Although pernicious anemia cannot be prevented, it seems reasonable to follow patients with known gastric atrophy for development of either signs or symptoms of pernicious anemia or low serum B_{12} levels. Glucocorticoid therapy can partially reverse the gastric mucosal changes in patients with pernicious anemia, but chronic therapy with steroids is impractical and dangerous.

Patients with pernicious anemia should be evaluated for other diseases such as thyroid disease or diabetes mellitus, and their relatives should be screened for pernicious anemia. Whether or not patients with pernicious anemia and/or gastric atrophy should be screened periodically for gastric cancer is controversial.

SPECIAL TYPES OF GASTRITIS

GIANT HYPERTROPHIC GASTRITIS. Several relatively uncommon clinical syndromes are characterized by gastric mucosal hypertrophy. These syndromes are usually included under the heading of giant hypertrophic gastritis, although inflammatory cells are not always present. The most commonly recognized syndrome is *Menetrier's disease,* which is characterized by gastric mucosal hypertrophy, hyposecretion of gastric acid, increased loss of protein from the stomach, edema, weight loss, and occasionally pain, nausea, and vomiting. Another syndrome, *hypertrophic hypersecretory gastropathy,* is similar but is associated with hypersecretion of acid. These syndromes are more commonly found in men than in women and usually occur between the ages of 30 and 50, although a childhood variety has been described. Gastric atrophy and parietal cell antibodies have been reported as late developments in a few patients.

Diagnosis is based on clinical findings, appearance of large mucosal folds on upper gastrointestinal x-ray series or endoscopy, and histologic appearance of mucosal biopsies (Table 98–1). Large mucosal folds are usually limited to the fundus and body of the stomach, although the antrum may be involved. Mucosal biopsy reveals hyperplasia of all three glandular elements—parietal, chief, and mucus-secreting cells. Because of the enlarged folds, other diseases such as Zollinger-Ellison syndrome, infiltrating carcinoma, lymphoma, or amyloid must be excluded.

In some patients medical therapy with anticholinergic drugs has led to reduced gastric secretion, decreased protein loss, and clinical improvement. Cimetidine also has been reported to decrease protein loss, although the mechanism is unknown. One or both of these therapies should be tried prior to surgical intervention. Some patients have been treated successfully with vagotomy and pyloroplasty. In a few patients, persistent, severe protein loss or recurrent gastrointestinal hemorrhage may necessitate total gastrectomy.

EOSINOPHILIC GASTRITIS (GASTROENTERITIS). Eosinophilic infiltration of the gastrointestinal tract can involve the stomach and/or small intestine. Peripheral eosinophilia also commonly occurs. The pathogenesis is poorly understood, although allergic or immunologic factors are thought to be involved. Both IgE-mediated and IgE-independent mechanisms have been implicated.

Gastric involvement is usually limited to the antrum. On biopsy eosinophils infiltrate the mucosa and the muscular layer (Table 98–1). This leads to antral rigidity and thickening of mucosal folds. Delayed gastric emptying and/or gastric outlet obstruction may occur. On x-ray it is often difficult to differentiate eosinophilic gastritis from granulomatous disease or neoplasm. Clinically, patients usually present with pain, nausea, and vomiting. Occasionally, eosinophils may invade the serosa, leading to ascites.

Eosinophilic gastritis is often a self-limited disease, but in some patients symptoms persist or recur. Corticosteroid therapy has been useful in alleviating obstructive signs and symptoms as well as ascites.

GRANULOMATOUS GASTRITIS. Granulomas can be found in the stomach as part of generalized diseases such as tuberculosis, histoplasmosis, sarcoidosis, syphilis, or Crohn's disease, or may be limited to the stomach and unassociated with other diseases. Two examples of the latter are eosinophilic granuloma (a separate disease from eosinophilic gastritis) and isolated (idiopathic) granulomatous gastritis.

On upper gastrointestinal x-ray the involved portions of the stomach appear rigid and narrowed and the x-ray appearance is often similar to that of malignancy (Table 98–1). The antrum is most often involved, although granulomas can be found also in the mucosa of the body and fundus. Mucosal biopsies reveal granulomas in the mucosa and submucosa, and in surgical specimens granulomas have been found in the muscular layer and serosa. Ulcerations may also occur. Because of the malignant appearance on x-ray, cancer must be ruled out in all patients by multiple biopsies and/or cytology.

Because of problems with differentiating granulomatous gastritis from malignancy, the condition in most patients is diagnosed at the time of surgery. If the diagnosis of granulomatous gastritis is made preoperatively, a search should be made for a primary disease and therapy should be tailored to the specific disease (e.g., tuberculosis). If an etiology cannot be found and malignancy has been excluded, the patient should be observed for several weeks since spontaneous resolution of isolated granulomatous gastritis has been reported. If resolution does not occur, surgical therapy is indicated.

GASTRITIS FOLLOWING GASTRIC SURGERY. Gastritis is a common histologic and endoscopic finding after either a subtotal gastrectomy or antrectomy has been performed for peptic ulcer disease. This form of gastritis is often referred to as bile reflux or alkaline gastritis, reflecting the theory that it is caused by the reflux of bile or pancreatic juice or both into the gastric remnant. Features believed to be compatible with the diagnosis include (1) epigastric pain, heartburn, nausea, and vomiting (often vomiting of bile-containing material) and/or weight loss; (2) presence of bile in the gastric remnant; (3) endoscopic evidence of gastritis; and (4) histologic evidence of gastritis. None of these features, however, are specific for the diagnosis. For example, such symptoms frequently occur following ulcer surgery with or without histologic or endoscopic evidence of gastritis. Furthermore, histologic or endoscopic changes can occur in postoperative patients who are asymptomatic. The presence of bile in the gastric remnant also does not mean necessarily that patients have bile-induced gastritis, because it is very easy for bile and other duodenal contents to reflux into the gastric remnant. Thus, caution should be exercised in making the diagnosis of bile reflux gastritis.

Cholestyramine or aluminum hydroxide antacids, as bile acid–binding agents, have been given to patients with postgastrectomy gastritis, but usually do not alleviate symptoms or reverse the histologic appearance of gastritis. As noted, bile acids alone may not be responsible for symptoms associated with "bile reflux gastritis;" other substances such as pancreatic secretions may be needed. Corrective surgery has consisted of procedures designed to divert duodenal contents away from the gastric remnant. The most commonly used operation is called a Roux-en-Y diversion. Some but not all studies have shown this procedure to be successful in relieving symptoms. Thus, surgery should be reserved for patients with incapacitating symptoms.

Hastings PR, Skillman JJ, Bushnell LS, Silen W: Antacid titration in the prevention of acute gastrointestinal bleeding: A controlled, randomized trial in 100 critically ill patients. N Engl J Med 298:1041, 1978. *This study demonstrates that the incidence of stress-related upper gastrointestinal bleeding in critically ill patients can be reduced by maintaining intragastric pH above 3.5 with antacid.*

Meyer JH: Reflections on reflux gastritis. (Editorial.) Gastroenterology 77:1143, 1979.

Moody FG, Cheung LY, Simons MA, Zalewsky C: Stress and the acute gastric mucosal lesion. Am J Dig Dis 21:148, 1976. *Evaluates the relationship between mucosal ischemia and the development of acute mucosal lesions.*

Ramsey EJ, Carey KV, Peterson WL, Jackson JJ, Murphy FK, Read NW, Taylor KB, Trier JS, Fordtran JS: Epidemic gastritis with hypochlorhydria. Gastroenterology 76:1449, 1979. *Histologic, functional, and clinical characteristics of an epidemic of acute gastritis are detailed.*

Ritchie WP Jr: Acute gastric mucosal damage induced by bile salts, acid and ischemia. Gastroenterology 68:699, 1975. *Concludes that a combination of mucosal ischemia and topically applied acid and bile salts is necessary for development of acute hemorrhagic gastritis.*

Siurala M, Salmi HG: Long-term follow-up of subjects with superficial gastritis or a normal gastric mucosa. Scand J Gastroenterol 6:459, 1971. *This biopsy study reports results of a 16- to 20-year follow-up of subjects with an initially normal gastric mucosa or superficial gastritis.*

Weinstein WM: Gastritis. *In* Sleisenger MH, Fordtran JS (eds.): Gastrointestinal Disease. 3rd ed. Philadelphia, W. B. Saunders Company, 1983, pp 559–578.

99. PEPTIC ULCER

99.1. Pathogenesis

Charles T. Richardson

DEFINITION

Ulcers are defects in the gastrointestinal mucosa that penetrate the muscularis mucosa. This distinguishes them from superficial erosions that do not extend through the muscularis mucosa. Peptic ulcers usually occur in the stomach, pylorus, or duodenal bulb but also can develop in the eosphagus and the postbulbar duodenum. In patients with markedly increased acid secretion (as in Zollinger-Ellison syndrome) ulcers sometimes develop in the distal duodenum and jejunum. Peptic ulcers occasionally occur in the ileum in or near Meckel's diverticula.

Originally, all ulcers in the upper gastrointestinal tract were believed to be caused by the aggressive action of hydrochloric acid and pepsin on the mucosa. Thus they became known as "peptic ulcers." Although acid and pepsin are secreted by most patients with benign ulcers, they are not the only causes of ulcers. Ulcers probably result from a number of different pathogenetic mechanisms in which luminal aggressive factors overcome mucosal defenses against them. Mechanisms believed important in the pathogenesis of ulcer disease are discussed in greater detail below.

NORMAL PHYSIOLOGY

STRUCTURE. The stomach is divided into four anatomic regions: the cardia, fundus, body, and antrum (Fig. 99–1). *Parietal cells,* which secrete acid, and *chief cells,* which secrete pepsinogen, are located primarily in the fundus and body, although a few are found in the antrum. *Gastrin (G) cells* are located in the antrum.

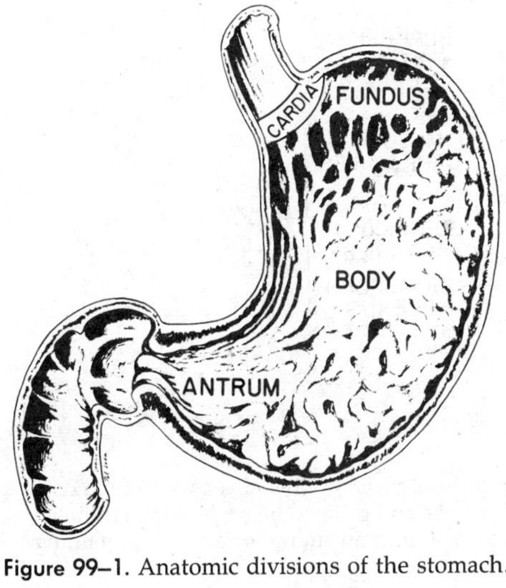

Figure 99–1. Anatomic divisions of the stomach.

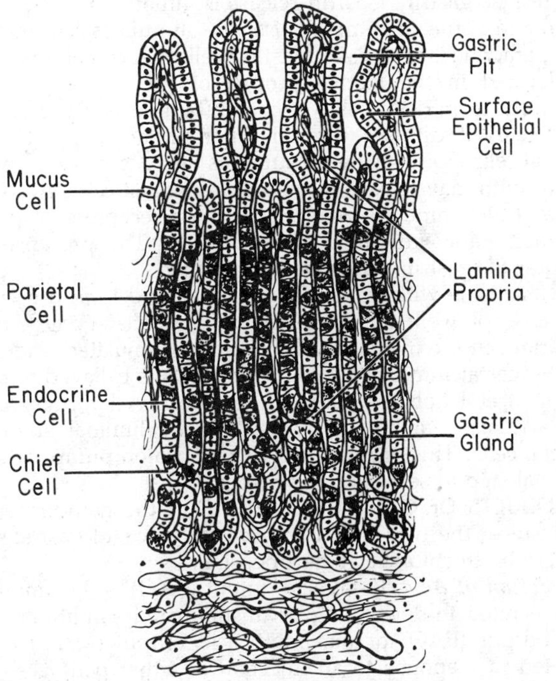

Figure 99–2. Diagram demonstrating the cell types lining the pits and glands of the gastric mucosa.

Gastric mucosa is made up of a series of pits and glands (Fig. 99–2). The pits contain surface epithelial cells while the glands contain mucus, parietal, endocrine, and chief cells. Normal gastric juice is a mixture of parietal secretion (acid) and nonparietal secretions (mucus, bicarbonate, sodium, and pepsin).

CONTROL OF GASTRIC SECRETION. Three endogenous chemicals (acetylcholine, gastrin, and histamine) stimulate acid secretion (Fig. 99–3): (1) *Acetylcholine* is believed to be a neural transmitter and is released by vagal efferent neurons. Vagal stimulation of acid secretion occurs when humans see, smell, taste, chew, or think about appetizing food. Local neurons within the wall of the stomach also release acetylcholine and are activated when the stomach is distended. (2) *Gastrin* is a hormone responsible for acid secretion. Protein in food is the most potent stimulant of gastrin release, but calcium, other cations such as magnesium, and alkalinization of the antrum

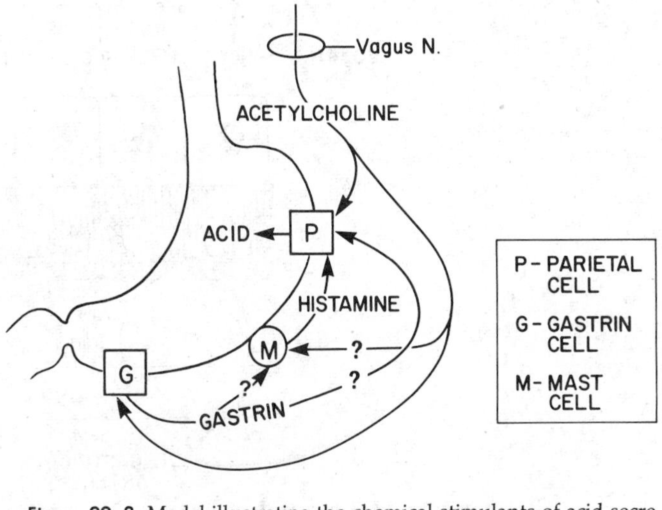

Figure 99–3. Model illustrating the chemical stimulants of acid secretion. Acetylcholine originates in the vagus nerves; gastrin is released from gastrin cells (G) in the antrum; and histamine is liberated from mast cells in the lamina propria of the gastric mucosa.

also release gastrin. Gastrin release is inhibited by acid within the lumen of the antrum. (3) *Histamine* stimulates acid secretion via a paracrine mechanism. Mastlike cells that contain histamine are located in the lamina propria of the stomach in close proximity to parietal cells. When histamine is liberated from mast cells, it diffuses through intercellular spaces to reach parietal cells. Some evidence suggests that gastrin or acetylcholine or both may release histamine from mast cells. Acetylcholine and histamine are believed to act on receptors on parietal cell membranes to cause acid secretion. The presence of a receptor for gastrin is less well established.

Mechanisms within parietal cells that lead to acid secretion also are not well defined. It is believed that cyclic AMP is important in the mediation of histamine-stimulated acid secretion while calcium entry into parietal cells is believed to play a role in acetylcholine-stimulated secretion. A hydrogen/potassium ATPase enzyme is located on the luminal surface of parietal cells. This enzyme serves as a proton pump, which is the final step in secretion of hydrogen ions.

PRODUCTS OF GASTRIC SECRETION. In the pathogenesis of peptic ulcer the two most important products of gastric secretion are hydrochloric acid and pepsin.

Secretion of Acid. Basal acid output (BAO) is the amount of acid secreted under fasting or unstimulated conditions. Peak acid output (PAO) or maximum acid output (MAO) is acid secreted in response to an injection of either pentagastrin or histamine, the maximal amount of acid that a normal subject or patient with ulcer disease can secrete. MAO reflects the number of parietal cells in an individual and the ratio of BAO to MAO represents the fraction of parietal cell mass functional under basal conditions. Thus, if a patient has an increased amount of gastrin, acetylcholine, or histamine near parietal cells or if there is increased sensitivity of parietal cells to normal amounts of these stimulants, BAO will be increased as will the BAO/MAO ratio. Such a patient is said to have a basal hypersecretory state (see below).

Upper and lower limits of normal acid secretion are shown in Table 99–1. Men secrete more acid than women. This can be explained, in part, by differences in body size, but men secrete more acid than women even when corrections are made for weight and lean body mass.

TABLE 99–1. UPPER (ULN) AND LOWER (LLN) LIMITS OF NORMAL ACID SECRETION IN HEALTHY MEN AND WOMEN

	Acid Output (mmol/hr)*			Basal/ Maximum
	Basal	*Peak*	*Maximum*	
Men (N = 116)				
ULN	10.5	60.6	46.3	0.31
LLN	0	11.6	8.0	0
Women (N = 62)				
ULN	5.6	40.1	30.2	0.29
LLN	0	8.0	5.0	0

*Acid output (volume of gastric juice times concentration of acid) is measured in 15-minute intervals and is expressed in mmol/hr. Basal acid output is the sum of acid secreted during four 15-minute periods. Peak acid output is the sum of the highest two 15-minute periods after pentagastrin or histamine stimulation multiplied by two. Maximum acid output is the sum of four 15-minute intervals after pentagastrin or histamine stimulation.

Secretion of Pepsin. Pepsin is secreted into the lumen as an inactive precursor, pepsinogen. Pepsinogen secretion usually accompanies acid secretion. Although mechanisms controlling pepsinogen secretion are less well understood, cholinergic stimulation is believed to be a major mediator. Once pepsinogen is secreted into the gastric lumen, it is converted by acid to pepsin, the active enzyme. The optimal pH for conversion of pepsinogen to pepsin ranges between 1.8 and 3.5.

MAINTENANCE OF NORMAL MUCOSAL INTEGRITY. Several mechanisms are believed important in protecting gastric and duodenal mucosa from damage by acid, pepsin, bile, pancreatic enzymes, and other possible aggressive factors. These defensive mechanisms include mucus, bicarbonate, mucosal blood flow, cell renewal, and possibly endogenous prostaglandins. Most of the information available presently regarding these mechanisms has been obtained from in vitro experiments or studies in animals. Methods are being developed currently to evaluate these mechanisms in humans.

Mucus. This secretory product is a gel that forms a thin, protective coat over superficial mucosal cells (Fig. 99–4). Mucus has several functions: (1) to protect underlying cells from mechanical forces of digestion; (2) to lubricate the mucosa, assisting movement of food over mucosal surfaces; (3) to retain water within the mucus gel and thereby provide an aqueous environment for underlying cells; and (4) to form an unstirred layer impeding, but not blocking, diffusion of hydrogen ions

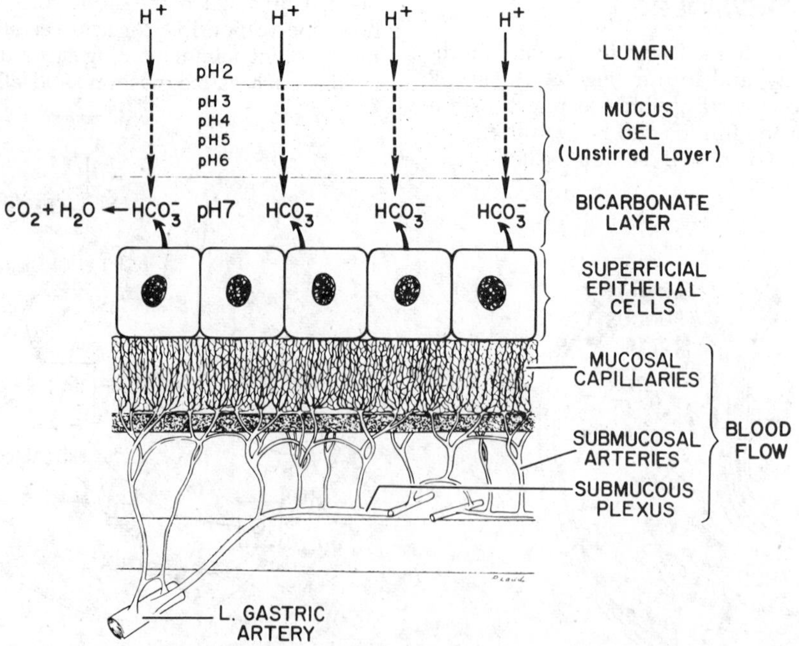

Figure 99–4. Model illustrating mechanisms maintaining mucosal integrity. Superficial epithelial cells secrete mucus and bicarbonate that aid in maintaining a pH gradient between lumen and mucosa and protect the underlying epithelial cells from damage by acid and pepsin. Mucosal blood flow is also believed to be a mechanism important in maintaining mucosal integrity.

from the lumen to the apical membrane of epithelial cells. Under normal conditions, mucus is constantly being produced but also is being removed continuously by mechanical forces during mixing and grinding of food and by pepsin, which degrades mucus into soluble glycoprotein subunits. However, secretion and degradation of mucus remain in equilibrium.

Bicarbonate. A bicarbonate-rich fluid is secreted by surface epithelial cells in the stomach and duodenum and also by Brunner's glands in the duodenum. Although some bicarbonate reaches the lumen, much of the secreted bicarbonate remains below or within the mucus layer (Fig. 99–4). Thus, the mucosal surface is in contact with fluid that contains a high pH relative to the lumen of the stomach. Under normal conditions, hydrogen ions are neutralized by bicarbonate (producing carbon dioxide and water) as they diffuse through the mucus gel layer. A pH gradient is thus established between the lumen and surface epithelial cells.

Mucosal Blood Flow. The rich blood supply of the stomach and duodenum is important in maintaining normal mucosal integrity. Gastric and duodenal mucosae are supplied by arborizing mucosal capillaries that traverse the glandular area of the stomach and duodenum. Beneath the muscularis mucosa, an extensive system of submucosal arteries and a submucous plexus of arteries and veins regulate the blood supply to surface epithelial cells (Fig. 99–4).

Cell Renewal. Normal cell renewal is also an important factor in maintaining mucosal integrity. Cells are constantly dying and are being replaced by new cells. In order for this system to function normally, there must be a balance between cell loss and cell renewal. Disruption of this steady state may lead to mucosal damage.

Endogenous Prostaglandins. Prostaglandins (PG) may play a role in maintaining mucosal integrity. Exogenous prostaglandins, primarily PGE_2, stimulate mucus and bicarbonate secretion, increase mucosal blood flow, and enhance protein synthesis that may be important in cell renewal. The mucosal protective ability of prostaglandins has been labeled "cytoprotection." Whether endogenous prostaglandins activate mucosal protective mechanisms in a manner similar to exogenous prostaglandins has not been established.

ABNORMALITIES IN PATIENTS WITH DUODENAL OR GASTRIC ULCERS

GENETIC PREDISPOSITION. Heredity has been postulated to play a role in the pathogenesis of ulcer disease in some patients, and several families with a high incidence of ulcers have been described. The mechanism(s) whereby genetic factors contribute to ulceration in these families is unclear. Originally, it was believed that familial aggregations of ulcer disease represented polygenic inheritance because the genetics of peptic ulcer could not be explained by a single autosomal, sex-linked, dominant, or recessive defect. Polygenic or multifactorial disorders are believed to be caused by the interaction of several genes with environmental factors. Thus, the hereditary component in ulcer disease was believed to reflect the combined contribution of many different genes in an individual patient. More recently, polygenic inheritance has seemed less likely than genetic heterogeneity. In this form of inheritance a number of genetically determined abnormalities share a common clinical manifestation—in this case, the ulcer crater. A number of rare genetic syndromes are associated with peptic ulcer disease. Multiple endocrine neoplasia I syndrome is the most common example (Ch. 240). Additionally, several pathophysiologic abnormalities believed to be associated with increased acid and pepsin secretion or increased gastric emptying have been discovered and several of these have been found in "ulcer families." For example, several families have been described in whom an increased level of serum pepsinogen I was inherited as an autosomal dominant trait. Since serum pepsinogen I concentrations reflect chief cell mass and correlate with maximum acid output, members of these families may have developed ulcers because of either increased pepsin or acid secretion or increased secretion of both. Other abnormalities, such as those leading to diminished mucosal defense, may be inherited also. The true importance of hereditary factors in the pathogenesis of peptic ulcer disease has not been established.

ABNORMALITIES IN SECRETION OF ACID AND PEPSIN. Approximately 40 per cent of patients with duodenal ulcer disease have acid secretion rates above the upper limits of normal shown in Table 99–1. The remainder have values within the normal range. Since pepsinogen secretion usually accompanies acid secretion, approximately the same percentage of ulcer patients will have increased or normal pepsinogen secretion.

Most patients with gastric ulcers have either normal or lower than normal acid secretion rates. Only a minority of patients with gastric ulcer disease (for example, a few patients with Zollinger-Ellison syndrome) have secretion rates above the normal range. The fact that most gastric ulcer patients have normal or lower than normal acid secretory rates does not exclude acid and pepsin as the cause of gastric ulcer disease in an individual patient but suggests that other factors may be involved (see below). This same concept applies to patients with duodenal ulcers who have normal rates of acid secretion.

There are three known mechanisms for increased basal acid secretion: (1) increased stimulation by *gastrin* (Zollinger-Ellison syndrome, retained antrum syndrome, and antral gastrin (G) cell hyperplasia or hyperfunction); (2) increased stimulation by *acetylcholine* (vagal hyperfunction); and (3) increased *histamine* stimulation (systemic mastocytosis or basophilic leukemia). Other causes of basal hypersecretion may exist, but so far they have not been described. Ulcers presumably occur in patients with these disorders because of increased levels of acid and pepsin. All of the currently recognized syndromes causing increased basal acid secretion are rare. Of the group Zollinger-Ellison syndrome is the most common and will be discussed separately (see Ch. 99.6).

REFLUX OF BILE AND PANCREATIC JUICE. Bile acids, lysolecithin, and pancreatic enzymes are believed to be aggressive factors that lead to ulceration in some patients, especially some of those with gastric ulcers. It has been postulated that duodenal contents reflux into the stomach causing gastritis that, in turn, predisposes to gastric ulceration. Some patients with gastric ulcers may have an incompetent pyloric sphincter that allows reflux of bile or pancreatic enzymes or both into the stomach.

Two mechanisms have been proposed whereby bile and pancreatic juice may damage gastric mucosa: first, alteration of mucus overlying surface epithelial cells reducing its protective effect, and second, damage to the so-called gastric mucosal barrier (the ability of the stomach to maintain electrical and hydrogen ion concentration gradients between lumen and blood). When these protective mechanisms are disrupted, the mucosa becomes more permeable to the damaging effects of acid and pepsin. Although bile and pancreatic juice have been postulated as the cause of ulcers in some patients, a cause and effect relationship has not been clearly established.

ABNORMALITIES OF MUCOSAL DEFENSE. Little is known at the present time about how disruptions in mucosal integrity may lead to ulceration, although there are several theoretical ways in which this might occur. For example, some patients may secrete *reduced amounts of mucus* or *structurally abnormal mucus*. Both could lead to a weaker mucus gel layer.

Diminished blood flow also may lead to cell injury and ulceration in some patients. Gastric mucosal ischemia is believed to be a factor in the pathogenesis of acute mucosal injury, as occurs in patients with severe medical or surgical illnesses (stress ulceration). Whether similar reductions in blood flow contribute to the development of chronic gastric or duodenal ulcers is not known. There are fewer collateral blood vessels on the lesser curvature of the stomach compared to the greater curvature. Whether this anatomic difference in blood supply leads to reduced blood flow to the lesser curvature with subsequent ulceration in some patients is not known, but most gastric ulcers do occur on the lesser curvature.

Decreased bicarbonate secretion is a theoretical possibility as a cause for diminished mucosal defense. Reduced pancreatic bicarbonate secretion into the lumen of the duodenum could lead to increased acidity in the duodenal bulb with subsequent duodenal ulceration. There is no evidence, however, that patients with pancreatic insufficiency have a higher incidence of duodenal ulcers. Possible *abnormalities in cell renewal* in the pathogenesis of peptic ulcer is entirely speculative at the present time.

EMOTIONAL STRESS. The mechanism(s) by which emotional stress might contribute to ulcer disease in some patients is unclear. Certain emotions such as hostility, resentment, guilt, and frustration are associated with increased gastric acidity. Furthermore, basal acid secretion has been reported to increase during stressful interviews and prior to surgery in ulcer patients or before difficult school examinations in healthy subjects. Two patients have been described recently who developed acid hypersecretion and gastric ulcer disease during periods of severe emotional stress. With alleviation of stress, acid secretion diminished and symptoms and ulcerations disappeared. Thus, it appears that certain emotions can cause increased acid secretion that in turn may lead to ulceration in certain patients. Emotional stress may alter factors that maintain mucosal integrity and thereby result in ulcers because of decreased mucosal defense. Although emotional stress is likely to be a factor in the pathogenesis of ulcer disease in some patients, its exact role is uncertain.

DELAYED GASTRIC EMPTYING. For a number of years delayed gastric emptying was believed to be a major factor in the pathogenesis of gastric ulcer disease. It was postulated that delayed gastric emptying caused retention of food in the stomach; in turn, this retention led to increased gastrin release, higher rates of acid secretion, and gastric ulceration. Prolonged gastric emptying, perhaps due to antral hypomotility, was also believed to cause stasis and delayed clearing of duodenal contents (bile and pancreatic enzymes) that had refluxed into the stomach. This in turn could damage gastric mucosa, cause gastritis, and lead to ulceration. Neither of these proposed pathogenetic mechanisms was ever established. Currently delayed emptying is believed to be related to ulceration in only a minority of patients.

EXOGENOUS FACTORS. The most important exogenous factors that have been associated with peptic ulcer disease are cigarette smoking and the use of nonsteroidal anti-inflammatory drugs. The possible association with adrenocorticosteroid therapy, infectious agents, or with alcohol or caffeine is much more tenuous.

Cigarette Smoking. Whether cigarette smoking is related to the pathogenesis of ulcer disease is unclear, although epidemiologic data suggest an association between the two: (1) Smoking is more common among patients with ulcers than among control subjects. (2) There is a positive correlation between the quantity of cigarettes smoked and the prevalence of ulcer disease. (3) Death due to peptic ulcer disease is more likely among patients who smoke than among those who do not. (4) Duodenal ulcers are less likely to heal in cigarette smokers than in nonsmokers. Whether this applies also to patients with gastric ulcers is not known.

Two mechanisms have been postulated whereby smoking may lead to ulceration: reduction of pyloric sphincter pressure and decreased pancreatic bicarbonate secretion. Smoking has been shown to reduce pyloric sphincter pressure in some patients with gastric ulcers. This, in turn, may lead to increased duodenogastric reflux of bile and pancreatic enzymes into the stomach with subsequent damage to the gastric mucosa. Nicotine reduces pancreatic bicarbonate secretion and may thereby lead to duodenal ulcers by impairing neutralization of acid by bicarbonate in the duodenal bulb. There is no proof, however, that either of these mechanisms actually causes ulceration.

Nonsteroidal Anti-inflammatory Drugs. These medications inhibit prostaglandin synthesis and cause decreased mucus and bicarbonate secretion, diminished mucosal blood flow, and perhaps reduced cell renewal. Aspirin and other nonsteroidal anti-inflammatory drugs cause superficial mucosal erosions in the stomach, presumably by reducing the factors believed important in maintaining mucosal integrity. It is unclear, however, whether these drugs also cause chronic gastric or duodenal ulcers. Several epidemiologic studies indicate that chronic gastric ulcers occur more frequently in patients taking large doses of aspirin than in control populations. In spite of these results, a definite relationship between the intake of aspirin and other nonsteroidal anti-inflammatory drugs and the development of chronic ulcers has never been established. These drugs may play a role in the pathogenesis of chronic gastric ulcers in some patients. Their role in the development of duodenal ulcers seems less likely.

Adrenocorticosteroid Therapy. Several epidemiologic studies suggest an association between treatment with adrenocorticosteroid therapy and peptic ulcer disease, especially in patients who have been treated with large doses of prednisone. Results from other studies have arrived at different conclusions; the relationship between steroid therapy and ulcer disease remains controversial.

Infectious Agents. Cytomegalovirus (CMV) has been isolated from gastric ulcers in a few patients receiving immunosuppressive drugs and in patients with post-transfusion CMV mononucleosis. *Candida albicans* also has been found in gastric ulcers in several patients. Whether these organisms caused the ulcers or whether the organisms were there secondarily is not known. Herpesviruses have never been isolated from gastric or duodenal ulcers, but one study indicated that antibodies to *Herpesvirus* type I occurred more frequently and in higher titers in patients with duodenal ulcers than in control subjects.

Alcohol or Caffeine-Containing Beverages. Even though both of these substances stimulate acid secretion, there is no evidence that either causes gastric or duodenal ulcers.

Allen A: Structure and function of gastrointestinal mucus. *In* Johnson LR (ed.): Physiology of the Gastrointestinal Tract. New York, Raven Press, 1981, pp 617-639. *This is an excellent review of the role of mucus in upper gastrointestinal physiology.*

Feldman M, Richardson CT: Gastric acid secretion in humans. *In* Johnson LR (ed.): Physiology of the Gastrointestinal Tract. New York, Raven Press, 1981, pp 693-707. *This chapter reviews the physiology of acid secretion and gastrin release in humans.*

Grossman MI (ed.): Peptic Ulcer. A Guide for the Practicing Physician. Chicago, Year Book Medical Publishers, Inc., 1981. *This book is an objective review of recent information relative to the pathogenesis of peptic ulcer disease including the role of environmental and hereditary factors.*

Richardson CT: Gastric Ulcer. *In* Sleisenger MH, Fordtran JS (eds.): Gastrointestinal Disease. 3rd ed. Philadelphia, W. B. Saunders Company, 1983, pp 672-693. *The factors involved in the pathogenesis of gastric ulcer are discussed.*

Soll AH, Isenberg JI: Duodenal ulcer diseases. *In* Sleisenger MH, Fordtran JS (eds.): Gastrointestinal Disease. 3rd ed. Philadelphia, W. B. Saunders Company, 1983, pp 625–672. *The pathophysiologic abnormalities found in various groups of duodenal ulcer patients are discussed.*

99.2. Epidemiology, Clinical Manifestations, and Diagnosis

Lawrence R. Schiller

EPIDEMIOLOGY

Peptic ulcer disease is a common disorder affecting approximately a quarter of all men and a sixth of all women in the United States, as judged by the presence of scars in the stomach and duodenum at autopsy. However, only 5 to 10 per cent of all individuals develop *symptomatic* peptic ulcer in their lifetime. Although ulcer disease is a common cause of morbidity, it is a relatively rare cause of death. The yearly incidence of symptomatic peptic ulcer disease in the United States is approximately

18 per 10,000 adults, but the current mortality rate is only 2.5 per 100,000.

Ulcer incidence varies by site, sex, and age. Symptomatic duodenal ulcer is more common than symptomatic gastric ulcer in both men (5.5 to 1) and women (2.8 to 1). Men are twice as likely as women to develop a duodenal ulcer but equally as likely to develop a gastric ulcer. Duodenal ulcer usually first produces symptoms between the ages of 25 to 55 years (peak occurrence at age 40) and gastric ulcer most commonly between 40 and 70 years of age (peak occurrence at age 50).

Some investigators report a recent decline in hospitalization and mortality rates for peptic ulcer disease, suggesting that the prevalence of peptic ulcer may be declining in the United States. It is unclear whether this reflects an actual change in the prevalence of peptic ulcers, a change in the criteria for hospitalization, or a change in the way mortality data are recorded. Studies from other countries suggest that morbidity and mortality from ulcer disease vary widely with geography and may not be declining with time. Before 1900 duodenal ulcer was a rarity and gastric ulcer was a disorder diagnosed mainly in young women. The reasons for reported changes in prevalence and sex incidence with time and for geographic differences are not known.

SYMPTOMS

DYSPEPSIA. Peptic ulcer usually presents as a painful upper abdominal disorder with the constellation of symptoms known as *dyspepsia*. Dyspepsia is poorly defined by both patients and physicians and often includes such symptoms as nausea, vomiting, anorexia, and fullness and bloating in addition to pain or discomfort. Most patients thought to have ulcers because of "typical dyspepsia" are not found to have peptic ulcer by x-ray or endoscopy but instead have other diseases or are classified as having "non-ulcer" (functional) dyspepsia.

A list of clinical features and their frequency in gastric ulcer, duodenal ulcer, and "non-ulcer" dyspepsia is provided in Table 99–2. It is impossible to differentiate these conditions from each other or from other diseases producing upper abdominal symptoms, such as cholelithiasis, by any one clinical feature. In practice physicians make the correct diagnosis on the basis of history in patients with dyspepsia less than 50 per cent of the time. In contrast, recent attempts to use structured questionnaires and computer-generated multivariate analysis of clinical findings have been remarkably successful in predicting diagnoses in patients with upper abdominal symptoms (80 to 90 per cent correct). This suggests that information leading to a correct diagnosis is contained within the history, but that physicians may be obtaining or analyzing the data incorrectly.

TABLE 99–2. CLINICAL FEATURES OF GASTRIC ULCER, DUODENAL ULCER, AND "NON-ULCER" DYSPEPSIA*

Clinical Feature	Gastric Ulcer (%)	Duodenal Ulcer (%)	"Non-Ulcer" Dyspepsia (%)
Features of pain:			
Primary pain location			
Epigastric	67	61–86	52–73
Right hypochondrium	6	7–17	4
Left hypochondrium	6	3–5	5
Radiation to back	34	20–31	24–28
Frequently severe	68	53	37
Gnawing pain	13	16	6
Clusters (episodic)	16	56	35
Occurs at night	32–43	50–88	24–32
Within 30 min of food	20	5	32
Increased by food	24	10–40	45
Food relief	2–48	20–63	4–32
Not related to food or variable	22–53	21–49	22–65
Relief by alkali	36–87	39–86	26–75
Anorexia	46–57	25–36	26–36
Weight loss	24–61	19–45	18–32
Nausea	54–70	49–59	43–60
Vomiting	38–73	25–57	26–34
Heartburn	19	27–59	28
Fatty food intolerance	—	14–72	53
Bloating	55	49	52
Belching	48	59	60

*From Soll AH, Isenberg JI: Duodenal ulcer disease. *In* Sleisenger MH, Fordtran JS (eds.): Gastrointestinal Diseases, 3rd ed. Philadelphia, W.B. Saunders Company, 1983, pp 625–672.

PAIN. The clinical diagnosis of ulcer disease has usually been based on the location of pain, its character, and the factors aggravating or alleviating it. For example, ulcer pain is classically described as being located in the epigastrium and as burning or gnawing in character. Pain in this location also occurs in a majority of patients with "non-ulcer" dyspepsia, however, and pain of this character actually occurs in a minority of patients with either gastric or duodenal ulcer (Table 99–2). Some patients describe ulcer pain as a cramping sensation not unlike hunger pangs, but descriptions of the character of pain are often hard to obtain in an unbiased way and are difficult to assess. Typical ulcer pain is said to be relieved by ingestion of food or antacids, but this is also quite variable. A better predictor of the presence of peptic ulcer (especially duodenal ulcer) is an episodic pattern of pain. Individual episodes of pain usually are short-lived, lasting for minutes rather than hours. Episodes of pain usually occur in clusters lasting from days to weeks, interspersed with long symptom-free periods. Some patients with ulcer report annual recurrences of pain during particular seasons such as spring or fall. Patients with a history of peptic ulcer who present with a recurrence of their typical symptoms can usually be assumed to have a recurrence and can be managed accordingly.

The cause of ulcer pain remains unknown. Ulcer pain is usually attributed to increased acidity at the ulcer site and the relief of pain to a decrease in luminal acidity. This theory is consistent with the typical onset of pain several hours after a meal, when gastric empyting has reduced the buffering capacity of gastric contents and intraluminal acidity rises. Attempts to induce pain by perfusing the ulcer site with acid have not uniformly produced pain, however. In several studies ingestion of placebo with no buffering capacity was as effective as ingestion of active antacid in relieving ulcer pain. In addition, ingestion of food sometimes worsens pain. Alternative mechanisms for the production of ulcer pain have been proposed, such as abnormal gastric or duodenal motor function, but are similarly unproved.

COMPLICATIONS. Peptic ulcers frequently fail to produce dyspepsia or pain and therefore may present de novo as a complication, such as bleeding, obstruction, or perforation. These are discussed in Chapter 99.5.

PHYSICAL EXAMINATION

The physical examination is usually not helpful in uncomplicated peptic ulcer disease. Epigastric tenderness is an insensitive and nonspecific finding and correlates poorly with the presence of an active ulcer crater. When ulcer disease is complicated by obstruction, perforation, penetration, or bleeding, important physical findings may be present (see Ch. 99.5).

Rarely, peptic ulcer is associated with multisystem syndromes that may produce physical findings. For instance, systemic mastocytosis, stiff skin syndrome, pachydermoperiostosis, and multiple lentigenes-ulcer syndrome may have cutaneous findings. Ulcer-tremor-nystagmus syndrome and amyloidosis may produce both peptic ulcer and neurologic findings.

DIAGNOSTIC VISUALIZATION

The diagnosis of ulcer depends on visualizing the ulcer crater by radiography or endoscopy. Radiography is well tolerated even in patients in fragile condition, readily available, and comparatively inexpensive, making it an excellent screening test. However, radiography may miss as many as 20 per cent of peptic ulcers. Endoscopy is more accurate and allows directed biopsy and cytology of suspicious lesions but cannot always be done safely in uncooperative patients or those whose condition is unstable. In the United States, where endoscopy currently costs from three to five times as much as radiography, upper gastrointestinal radiographs, preferably with both single contrast and double contrast techniques, are often the initial diagnostic test. In symptomatic patients with no abnormalities on x-ray and in patients with ulcer in whom symptoms do not subside on therapy, endoscopy can establish or exclude the diagnosis of ulcer disease or can show that symptoms are related to an unhealed ulcer. In situations in which there is little difference in cost between endoscopy and x-ray, endoscopy is preferable in the investigation of patients with dyspepsia because of its greater sensitivity in diagnosis.

DUODENAL ULCER. If a duodenal ulcer is demonstrated by x-ray (Fig. 99–5) no further diagnostic evaluation is necessary and treatment can be started. Since duodenal ulcers are rarely malignant, endoscopic biopsy is not necessary. Follow-up examinations to assess healing of a duodenal ulcer need not be done routinely. Patients with duodenal ulcer are usually treated for a fixed length of time if symptoms subside (see Ch. 99.3).

GASTRIC ULCER. If a gastric ulcer is found on x-ray (Fig. 99–6), malignancy should be rigorously excluded, particularly if there is any possibility that the ulcer may be malignant. Gastric ulcers are especially suspected of malignancy if (1) the ulcer is located completely within the gastric wall or in an intraluminal mass, (2) there is nodularity of the ulcer base or of adjacent gastric mucosa, or (3) there are no folds radiating to ulcer margin, (4) the ulcer is large, and (5) there is histamine- or pentagastrin-fast achlorhydria. Malignancy can best be excluded by direct endoscopic visualization of the gastric ulcer to obtain brush cytologic specimens and to obtain a minimum of six to eight pinch biopsy specimens for careful pathologic examination. This approach will lead to an accurate diagnosis in more than 95 per cent of cases. Some investigators recommend that patients with benign appearing gastric ulcers not have endoscopy initially but that malignancy be excluded by

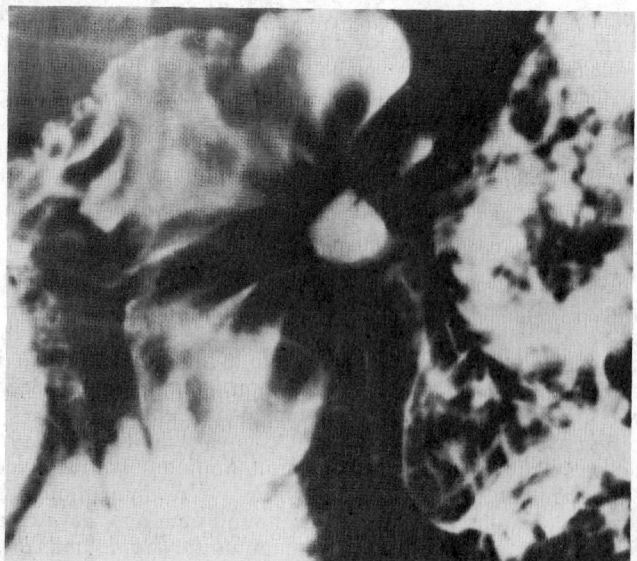

Figure 99–5. Duodenal ulcers are recognized when barium is retained within an ulcer niche. In this example barium has collected in an ulcer at the base of the duodenal bulb along the posterior wall. Folds radiate to the margin of this ulcer. (From Goldberg HI: *In* Sleisenger MH, Fordtran JS [eds.]: Gastrointestinal Disease. 2nd ed. Philadelphia, W. B. Saunders Company, 1978).

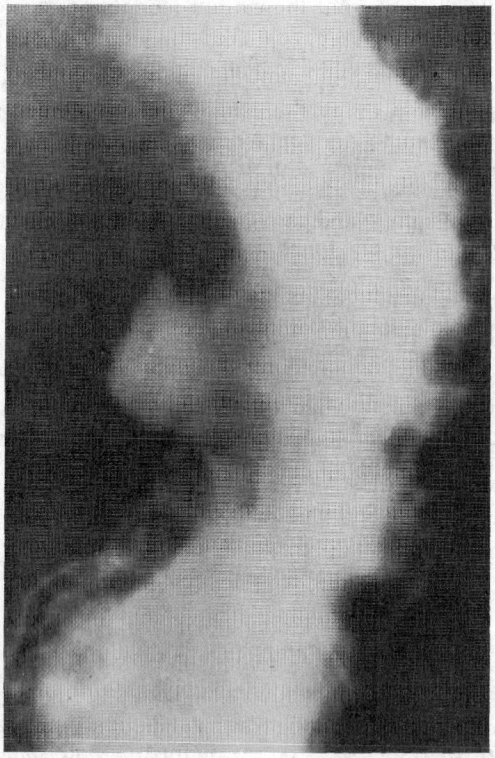

Figure 99–6. This ulcer of the lesser curve of the stomach demonstrates several features typical of benign gastric ulcers: The ulcer crater projects beyond the contour of the gastric wall, the margin of the ulcer crater is sharply defined and smooth, the ulcer is surrounded by a broad lucent band—an ulcer collar—resulting from edema at the ulcer orifice, and mucosal folds radiate from the ulcer collar. (From Goldberg HI: *In* Sleisenger MH, Fordtran JS [eds.]: Gastrointestinal Disease. 2nd ed. Philadelphia, W. B. Saunders Company, 1978.)

repeating an x-ray study or by endoscopy after a period of therapy to prove that the ulcer has healed. Whether initially endoscoped and found benign or not, all gastric ulcers should be followed to healing. This can be done by repeating the x-ray examination or by endoscopy after treatment for 8 to 12 weeks to allow healing to occur. Endoscopic examination and biopsy are clearly indicated in patients in whom gastric ulcers do not heal within this time.

LABORATORY STUDIES

SERUM GASTRIN LEVELS. Radioimmunoassay of gastrin is useful in screening patients with known ulcer disease for Zollinger-Ellison syndrome and other rare hypersecretory states. The reasons for identifying these patients are (1) they may have a more severe course marked by excessive complications such as bleeding, obstruction, or perforation; (2) therapy is different, particularly surgical therapy (see Ch. 99.4); (3) associated but undiagnosed diseases of other organs, such as multiple endocrine neoplasia type I, may cause morbidity; and (4) gastrinomas associated with Zollinger-Ellison syndrome may be malignant and cause death from metastasis. Early recognition of Zollinger-Ellison syndrome makes possible effective control of symptoms and sometimes allows resection of tumor and cure of the disease (Ch. 99.6).

Measurement of serum gastrin concentrations in all patients with peptic ulcer disease is not cost effective because the incidence of Zollinger-Ellison syndrome is low (less than 1 per cent of patients with peptic ulcer disease). Table 99–3 lists the selective clinical situations in which obtaining a fasting serum gastrin level may be useful, although even with this selectivity the likelihood of identifying a patient as having Zollinger-Ellison syndrome is low.

If fasting serum gastrin concentrations are elevated ($>$ 200 pg per milliliter), gastric acid secretion should be measured in

TABLE 99–3. CLINICAL SITUATIONS IN WHICH MEASUREMENT OF SERUM GASTRIN LEVELS IS INDICATED

Family history of peptic ulcer
Ulcer associated with hypercalcemia or other manifestations of multiple endocrine neoplasia type I
Multifocal peptic ulcer
Peptic ulceration of postbulbar duodenum or jejunum
Peptic ulceration associated with diarrhea*
Chronic unexplained diarrhea*
Enlarged gastric folds on upper GI x-ray
Before surgery for "intractable" ulcer
Recurrent ulcer after ulcer surgery

*Not due to antacid ingestion.

order to prove that gastrin levels are not elevated in response to hypochlorhydria or achlorhydria, such as that due to pernicious anemia, atrophic gastritis, gastric cancer, or vagotomy. A finding of high serum gastrin levels and increased basal acid output limits the differential diagnosis to only a few entities (Table 99–4). If both fasting gastrin levels and basal acid secretion are very high (> 1000 pg per milliliter and > 15 mmol per hour, respectively), a diagnosis of Zollinger-Ellison syndrome is likely.

When fasting gastrin levels or basal acid outputs or both are less markedly elevated and the diagnosis of Zollinger-Ellison syndrome is unclear, the response of serum gastrin concentration to an intravenous injection of secretin may be helpful. In individuals with Zollinger-Ellison syndrome, intravenous injection of pure Secretin-Kabi 2 U per kilogram of body weight results in a prompt and pathognomonic rise of gastrin of > 200 pg per milliliter within 2 to 10 minutes. Patients with other hypergastrinemic conditions (Table 99–4) and normal individuals do not show this elevation. Gastrin secretion rises with calcium infusion also, but this rise is less reliable diagnostically than that following injection of secretin.

Differentiation of other rare hypergastrinemic syndromes (Table 99–4) can be made on the basis of (1) history of ulcer surgery (retained antrum syndrome, discussed in Ch. 99.4) or small bowel resection, (2) demonstration of gastric outlet obstruction by x-ray or endoscopy, (3) laboratory evidence of renal failure, or (4) response of serum gastrin levels to a meal. Patients with antral G cell hyperplasia or hyperfunction more than double their already elevated fasting gastrin levels after ingestion of a protein meal. Patients with Zollinger-Ellison syndrome do not usually have this exuberant response to a meal.

ACID SECRETORY TESTING. Gastric acid secretion is measured by placing a vented nasogastric tube in the gastric antrum under fluoroscopic guidance and aspirating gastric juice with a suction pump. By measuring the volume and acid concentration (determined either by titration to pH 7.0 or indirectly from pH measurements), the quantity of acid secreted by the stomach can be calculated. Basal acid output (BAO) is defined as the amount of acid produced during four consecutive 15-minute periods. V_{max} for acid secretion is estimated by injecting a maximally effective dose of a gastric secretagogue. Pentagastrin (6 μg per kilogram), the biologically active carboxyl-terminal fragment of gastrin, is preferred for this purpose. Histamine or betazole (Histalog) can also be used. Stimulated secretion is expressed as peak acid output (PAO, the sum of the two highest consecutive 15-minute periods after injection multiplied by 2) or as maximal acid output (MAO, the sum of four consecutive 15-minute periods after injection). Values for acid secretion in healthy subjects and ulcer patients are shown in Table 99–1. In the absence of hypergastrinemia, measurement of gastric acid secretion is usually unnecessary in patients with peptic ulcer. Basal and peak acid output are increased in duodenal ulcer patients as a group (see Ch. 99.1), but knowledge of the level of acid secretion has no therapeutic implications for the individual patient at present. Measurement of acid secretion rates is sometimes useful preoperatively so that postoperative values can be compared and the effect of the operation on acid secretion can be assessed (see Ch. 99.4).

TABLE 99–4. CAUSES OF INCREASED FASTING SERUM GASTRIN CONCENTRATIONS AND INCREASED BASAL ACID OUTPUT

Zollinger-Ellison syndrome
Retained antrum syndrome
Massive small bowel resection (?)
Chronic gastric outlet obstruction (?)
Renal failure
Antral G cell hyperplasia or hyperfunction

DIFFERENTIAL DIAGNOSIS

Peptic ulcer can usually be distinguished from painful intestinal disorders that customarily produce discomfort in the periumbilical or lower quadrants of the abdomen (e.g., appendicitis or diverticulitis). Disorders affecting the viscera of the upper abdomen or chest are more difficult to differentiate from peptic ulcer disease (Table 99–5). Differentiation of these disorders can often be made by considering the acuteness of pain, lack of response to eating or antacids, changes of pain with changes in position, radiation of pain, and the presence of physical findings such as rebound tenderness, all of which are atypical in uncomplicated peptic ulcer disease. Because ulcer disease is common and ulcer symptoms are often variable, however, peptic ulcer must be considered as a possible cause of abdominal symptoms even in patients with atypical symptoms.

ZOLLINGER-ELLISON SYNDROME. Patients with Zollinger-Ellison syndrome (gastrinoma) most characteristically have exceptionally aggressive peptic ulcer disease with frequent symptomatic relapses complicated by bleeding or perforation. Some, however, have no active ulcer disease but seek medical aid instead with symptoms of reflux esophagitis or chronic diarrhea, or because of either local or metastatic tumor. The presence of the Zollinger-Ellison syndrome is suggested by (1) a strong family history of ulcer, (2) endocrine disturbances consistent with multiple endocrine neoplasia syndrome type I (MEN I) (see later discussion), (3) chronic diarrhea, (4) rapid symptomatic recurrence, (5) multiple ulcers, or (6) recurrent postoperative peptic ulcers. The diagnostic tests required to establish this diagnosis have been noted earlier. Gastrinomas are further discussed in Ch. 99.6.

FUNCTIONAL DYSPEPSIA. *Functional dyspepsia* is diagnosed when a symptomatic individual is not found to have an ulcer or other structural disease, such as cholelithiasis. It has been estimated that 20 to 30 per cent of patients with this diagnosis eventually develop peptic ulcer; therefore, some of these patients may really have evanescent ulcers that evade diagnosis. Women in their twenties are especially likely to have this condition. Some of these patients have a disruption of normal gastric motor function. Gastrokinetic agents such as metroclopramide or domperidone or alpha-adrenergic agonists such as ephedrine or lidamidine have been found to reverse both symptoms and motor dysfunction in some of these patients. Longer clinical trials are needed before such therapy can be generally recommended for patients with functional dyspepsia.

GASTRIC CANCER. Many patients with gastric cancer present with dyspepsia (Ch. 100). This diagnosis should be considered

TABLE 99–5. COMMON DISEASES THAT MAY PRODUCE EPIGASTRIC PAIN SIMULATING PEPTIC ULCER

Myocardial infarction
Pleurisy
Pericarditis
Esophagitis
Cholecystitis
Pancreatitis
Irritable bowel syndrome

in particular when dyspepsia is associated with weight loss or evidence of occult gastrointestinal blood loss in an elderly individual or when x-ray or endoscopic appearances of gastric ulcer are suspicious for malignancy. However, a diagnosis of cancer should also be considered in any individual with a benign-appearing gastric ulcer, since roughly 2 to 5 per cent of such ulcers contain foci of gastric carcinoma.

MISCELLANEOUS DISORDERS. A variety of other diseases can produce dyspepsia that may mimic that of peptic ulcer. These conditions include *infiltrative diseases* of the stomach such as hypertrophic gastritis, tuberculosis, syphilis, Crohn's disease and other granulomatous gastritides (see Ch. 98); *duodenal obstruction* by polyps, webs, or an annular pancreas; and *intestinal parasitosis* by giardia or strongyloides. More common diseases causing dyspeptic symptoms include *biliary tract disease* and *pancreatitis*. These can often be differentiated from ulcer disease by history, but tests such as sonography, cholecystography, and serum amylase determinations are usually necessary to confirm their diagnosis.

de Dombal FT: Analysis of foregut symptoms. *In* Baron JH, Moody FG (eds.): Butterworth's International Medical Reviews, Gastroenterology 1, Foregut. London, Butterworth & Co Ltd, 1981, pp 49-66. *Excellent review of new approaches to foregut symptoms, including multivariate analysis.*

Jensen RT, Gardner JD, Raufman J-P, Pandol SJ, Doppman JL, Collen MJ: Zollinger-Ellison syndrome: Current concepts and management. Ann Intern Med 98:59, 1983. *Recent review of diagnosis and management of Zollinger-Ellison syndrome.*

Richardson CT: Gastric ulcer. *In* Sleisenger MH, Fordtran JS (eds.): Gastrointestinal Disease. 3rd ed. Philadelphia, W. B. Saunders Company, 1983, pp 672-693. *Clinical features of gastric ulcers are reviewed in depth.*

Soll AH, Isenberg JI: Duodenal ulcer diseases. *In* Sleisenger MH, Fordtran JS (eds.): Gastrointestinal Disease. 3rd ed. Philadelphia, W. B. Saunders Company, 1983, pp 625-672. *Detailed review of current concepts of duodenal ulcer disease.*

Thompson WM, Kelvin FM, Gedgaudas RK, Rice RP: Radiologic investigation of peptic ulcer disease. Radiol Clin North Am 20:701, 1982. *Review of state of the art for radiology of peptic ulcer with many excellent examples.*

99.3. Medical Therapy

Walter L. Peterson

In the healthy human stomach and duodenum there is an effective balance between the potential of gastric acid and pepsin to damage mucosal cells and the ability of these cells to protect themselves from injury. Disruption of this balance leads to peptic ulcers. In some patients the imbalance occurs primarily because of acid (and pepsin) hypersecretion, in others primarily because of some abnormality in mucosal defense, and in still others because of both mechanisms. However, once an ulcer has formed, healing may be promoted by manipulating either factor, regardless of which was primarily responsible for the ulcer. For example, although aspirin is believed to produce a gastric ulcer by disrupting mucosal defense in some way, the ulcer may be treated by a drug that reduces gastric acidity, such as cimetidine.

Therapeutic agents for peptic ulcer disease can be classified as those that act primarily by reducing levels of acid and pepsin in the gastric lumen and those that act primarily by enhancing mucosal defense. Since pepsin's activity is pH dependent, reduction of acidity reduces peptic activity simultaneously.

DRUGS THAT REDUCE GASTRIC ACIDITY

Gastric acidity may be reduced either by inhibiting secretion of acid from parietal cells or by neutralizing acid that has been secreted.

INHIBITION OF ACID SECRETION. Secretion may be reduced either by blocking the interaction of histamine or acetylcholine with their receptors on parietal cells (histamine *H_2-receptor antagonists* or *antimuscarinic drugs*) or by interfering with the intracellular machinery of the parietal cell (*prostaglandins* or *substituted benzimidazoles*) (Fig. 99–7).

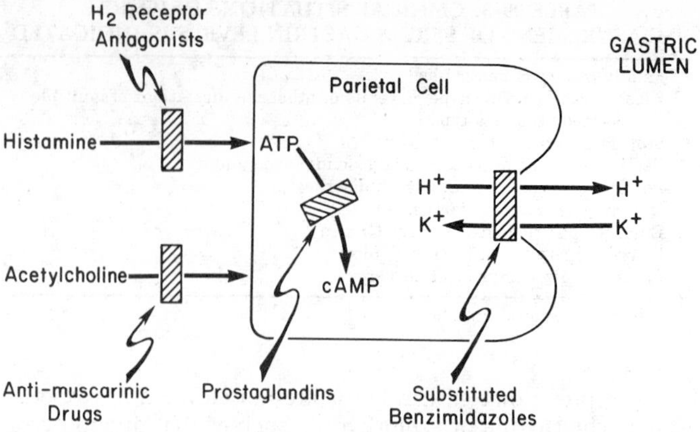

Figure 99–7. Sites of action of four drugs employed to inhibit acid secretion.

H_2-RECEPTOR ANTAGONISTS. The effects of histamine are mediated through H_1 and H_2 receptors. H_1 receptors are located in the smooth muscle of the bronchus and small bowel and H_2 receptors are located on parietal cells and the uterus. H_1 receptors are blocked by classic antihistamines such as diphenhydramine (Benadryl), while H_2 receptors are blocked by specific H_2-receptor antagonists.

The first commercially available H_2-receptor antagonist was *cimetidine* (Tagamet), whose structure, like histamine, contains an imidazole ring. Cimetidine reduces fast- and food-stimulated gastric acid secretion by about 95 per cent and 75 per cent, respectively, in its customary dose of 300 mg, but the drug has a relatively short (six hours) duration of effect. Side effects with cimetidine, which are uncommon and almost always reversible, include mental confusion (especially in elderly patients with hepatic or renal insufficiency), gynecomastia, impotence, and interaction with other commonly prescribed drugs. Cimetidine competitively antagonizes the metabolism (via the cytochrome P-450 system) of warfarin, theophylline, propranolol, phenytoin, chlordiazepoxide, and diazepam. Although blood levels of these drugs rise when given concomitantly with cimetidine, the clinical importance of such rises is unsettled. *Ranitidine* (Zantac), which possesses a furan ring, is the second H_2-receptor antagonist to gain widespread human use. Its putative advantages over cimetidine include a five- to ten-fold increase in potency (and hence a twice daily administration), and to date fewer reported side effects. It does not cross the blood-brain barrier well and therefore may not cause mental confusion. Although it has less of an effect on the cytochrome P-450 system, it may also interfere with the metabolism of drugs.

ANTIMUSCARINIC DRUGS. The classic antimuscarinic drugs reduce fast- and food-stimulated acid secretion by about 50 per cent and 30 per cent, respectively. However, these drugs also block other muscarinic receptors and produce unwanted side effects such as drowsiness, blurred vision, and urinary hesitancy. The centrally active tricyclic antidepressant drugs trimipramine and doxepin also possess antimuscarinic properties. Pirenzipine is a tricyclic antimuscarinic compound that does not cross the blood-brain barrier and therefore has no antidepressant activity or central nervous system side effects. Pirenzipine (not available in the United States) is believed to block certain types of muscarinic receptors (e.g., those controlling acid secretion) at doses that do not block other muscarinic receptors (e.g., those controlling heart rate and smooth muscle contraction). Thus, acid secretion can be controlled by doses of drug too small to produce side effects such as tachycardia and bladder atony.

PROSTAGLANDINS. Several methylated analogues of prostaglandin E_2 have been shown to reduce gastric acid secretion, probably by interfering with generation of cyclic AMP in the parietal cell. However, doses of drug needed to accomplish this often result in diarrhea. Therefore, prostaglandins in doses that reduce acid secretion may have limited use as ulcer therapy.

SUBSTITUTED BENZIMIDAZOLES. This class of drugs, the prototype of which is omeprazole, is an extremely potent inhibitor of gastric acid secretion. These drugs inhibit H^+/K^+ ATP-ase, an enzyme found at the acid secretory surface of parietal cells that mediates final transport of hydrogen ions (via exchange with potassium ions) into the gastric lumen (Fig. 99–7). There is a prolonged duration of action, even when blood levels of drug are undetectable. Studies are underway to determine pharmacologic and safety profiles of these drugs.

NEUTRALIZATION OF GASTRIC ACID. Antacids react with hydrochloric acid to form a salt and water, thereby reducing gastric acidity. Sodium bicarbonate, a classic antacid, is not recommended for long-term use because of its short duration of action and its propensity to produce alkalosis and sodium retention. Neither is calcium carbonate suggested for therapy of peptic ulcer because it may cause acid rebound (sustained hypersecretion of gastric acid after antacid has emptied from the stomach) and may cause the milk-alkali syndrome. Antacids most widely recommended are those containing varying proportions of magnesium and aluminum hydroxide. Serious side effects with these two compounds are uncommon. However, antacids containing proportionately larger amounts of magnesium hydroxide often produce diarrhea, whereas those with large amounts of aluminum hydroxide may produce constipation. All antacids can result in "taste fatigue" for individual patients. Most antacids used today are relatively low in sodium content.

Beyond individual preferences for antacid flavors, patients with ulcer may choose any of the commercially available magnesium and aluminum hydroxide antacids as long as neutralizing capacity is considered. Most clinical studies with antacids specify doses in terms of in vitro neutralizing capacity (for example, 140 mmol seven times per day), and antacids vary in potency. Table 99–6 lists several commonly prescribed antacids with the volume required to neutralize 70 or 140 mmol of hydrochloric acid in vitro.

DRUGS THAT ENHANCE MUCOSAL DEFENSE

Mucosal protection is more of a conceptual term than one with a firm definition because it is not known exactly what constitutes "mucosal defense." Mucus, bicarbonate secretion, and blood flow may all play roles, and some of the drugs that "enhance mucosal defense" may indeed affect these variables. However, a more general description of these drugs is that they exert a beneficial effect on an ulcer *without affecting luminal gastric acidity*. Since they do not belong in the first group, they fall by default into the second group.

SUCRALFATE. Sucralfate (Carafate) is the aluminum hydroxide salt of a sulfated disaccharide, sucrose octasulfate. It is virtually unabsorbed and without important side effects. In an acidic environment, some of the aluminum hydroxide radicals dissociate, leaving sucrose with one to seven ionized sulfate groups. These negatively charged ions are insoluble, viscous, and adherent to positively charged necrotic tissue proteins in the bases of ulcers. The exact mechanisms of action are not understood. It has been suggested that sucralfate forms a shield over an ulcer crater, preventing acid from reaching regenerating ulcer tissue. It has also been suggested that the drug adsorbs bile acids or pepsin or both in the lumen. Finally, recent evidence suggests that sucralfate may stimulate the generation of local prostaglandins. The drug should not be taken at the same time as food, antacids, or other medications. Binding with food or antacids may limit the effectiveness of the drug and binding of the drug by other medications may limit their absorption.

TABLE 99–6. VOLUMES (IN ML) OF SEVERAL COMMONLY PRESCRIBED LIQUID ANTACIDS REQUIRED TO NEUTRALIZE 70 OR 140 MMOL OF HYDROCHLORIC ACID

	70 mmol	140 mmol
Maalox Therapeutic Concentrate Mylanta II	15	30
Gelusil II	20	40
Maalox Mylanta Gelusil Riopan Alternagel*	30	60
Amphojel*	50	100

*Aluminum hydroxide antacids.

PROSTAGLANDINS. Prostaglandins play a poorly defined role in mucosal integrity, but their absence may permit development of ulcers of the stomach and duodenum. When given exogenously in small doses that do not affect acid secretion, both naturally occurring prostaglandins and their methylated analogues may heal peptic ulcers. The mechanisms of this effect are unclear, but probably include stimulation of mucus (which could shield the mucosa much like sucralfate) and stimulation of gastric bicarbonate (a nonparietal secretion that could act as an endogenous antacid). Side effects in such small doses are negligible. These drugs are not yet available in the United States.

BISMUTH. Tripotassium dicitrato-bismuthate (DeNol), a complex bismuth salt, chelates with protein (e.g., necrotic ulcer tissue) at acidic pH levels. Its mechanism of action is probably much like sucralfate's and, like sucralfate, the drug is poorly absorbed. Thus side effects are minor. The drug in liquid form has an unpleasant odor and, like all bismuth compounds, it will darken stools. DeNol is unavailable in the United States.

LICORICE EXTRACTS. Carbenoxolone is a synthetic derivative of glycyrrhetic acid, a substance found in licorice. It appears to promote ulcer healing by several mechanisms. The drug produces thick mucus, inhibits peptic activity (independent of pH), and may actually increase the longevity of mucosal cells. Because carbenoxolone possesses licorice's aldosterone-like side effects (salt retention, hypertension, hypokalemia), it is not the preferred drug for peptic ulcer therapy; it is unavailable in the United States.

TREATMENT OF PATIENTS WITH PEPTIC ULCER

At this writing, four drugs are available in the United States as first line therapy for patients with peptic ulcers: cimetidine, ranitidine, antacids, and sucralfate. Because of their side effects, currently available antimuscarinic drugs should be used as adjunctive therapy only. While selecting one of the first line drugs, a physician should also be aware of several factors that at one time or another have been considered important in ulcer therapy.

COMPLEMENTARY FACTORS IN PEPTIC ULCER THERAPY. Factors to consider in this category include diet, smoking, alcohol or analgesic use, sedatives, and the need for hospitalization.

Diet. Diet therapy was once the standard in the treatment of peptic ulcer disease. Now, it is clear that no specific diet is of proven benefit in ulcer therapy. Patients should avoid whatever foods cause them discomfort but otherwise eat whatever they like. Because food, especially milk, stimulates acid secretion, between meal or bedtime snacks should be taken in moderation.

Smoking. There are many important reasons (other than the presence of a peptic ulcer) to encourage patients to stop smoking. However, the data are very persuasive that patients who do not smoke experience ulcer healing more often and more rapidly than those who smoke. The mechanism of this adverse effect on peptic ulcers is not known.

Alcohol. There is no evidence that alcohol ingestion retards ulcer healing. Nevertheless, because alcohol damages gastric mucosa, patients with ulcers who choose to drink should be advised to drink in moderation.

Analgesics. Drugs that inhibit prostaglandin synthesis (aspirin, nonsteroidal anti-inflammatory drugs) can produce gastric ulcers and therefore patients with this disorder should stop the drugs if possible. Although the evidence that these drugs cause duodenal ulcer is unconvincing, patients with refractory or bleeding duodenal ulcer should be advised not to take them.

Sedatives. Although emotional stress may play a role in the pathogenesis of peptic ulcers in some patients, routine use of sedative drugs is of no proven benefit in ulcer therapy.

Hospitalization. Hospitalization should be reserved for patients with complications of ulcer disease (bleeding, perforation, penetration, obstruction) (see Ch. 99.5) or patients with ulcer pain refractory to routine medical management. In other situations, hospitalization is not warranted and has not been shown to lead to more rapid healing.

TREATMENT OF PATIENTS WITH UNCOMPLICATED DUODENAL ULCER. In selecting a drug with which to treat a patient with duodenal ulcer (or gastric ulcer, see below), four factors must be considered: effectiveness, safety, convenience, and cost (Table 99–7).

Effectiveness. All four drugs are equally effective in hastening healing of duodenal ulcer when compared with placebo. Cimetidine (in doses of 300 mg with meals and at bedtime or 400 mg twice daily), ranitidine (150 mg twice daily), antacids taken seven times daily, or sucralfate (1 gram four times daily) produce ulcer healing in 70 per cent of patients by four weeks of therapy and in almost 90 per cent of patients by six weeks. Each also promptly relieves ulcer pain, although often not significantly better than placebo.

Safety. Although side effects do occur with these drugs, they are uncommon and usually not serious. As examples, one can anticipate diarrhea occurring with large doses of magnesium hydroxide antacid or one may need to monitor serum levels of some drugs (e.g., theophylline or phenytoin) when taken in conjunction with cimetidine.

Convenience. Antacids have been proven effective only when taken seven times daily, an inconvenience for many patients. Sucralfate is taken one hour *before meals,* a time period not always readily anticipated by patients. Ranitidine's twice daily dosage may be more convenient than cimetidine's four times daily regimen. However, recent studies suggest that cimetidine may also be taken in twice-daily dosage (Table 99–7).

Cost. Cost varies according to the regimen and the locale where the drug is purchased. As shown in Table 99–7, antacid in large doses is the most expensive regimen in Dallas, followed by ranitidine, sucralfate, and cimetidine.

Recommendation. Patients should initially be treated with adequate doses of a single drug. Cimetidine or ranitidine are the first line drugs of choice, primarily because of convenience, with cimetidine perhaps having the advantage of lower cost. Sucralfate and antacids are just as effective as H_2-receptor antagonists but are somewhat less convenient. Treatment should continue for four to six weeks, and if the patient is symptom free, the medication is stopped. Documentation of ulcer healing by x-ray or endoscopy is unnecessary in the patient with routine duodenal ulcer.

APPROACH TO PATIENTS WITH DUODENAL ULCER IN WHOM FIRST LINE THERAPY FAILS. Failure of first line therapy for duodenal ulcer is defined as the development of a complication (bleeding, perforation, penetration) while the patient is on therapy or persistence of ulcer symptoms after several weeks of therapy. For patients who do not require surgery, there are several alternatives for continued medical therapy. Changing to a different drug and/or increasing drug dosage and/or combining two drugs are options. There are no data to support any of these particular approaches.

If symptoms persist after one or more changes in medical therapy, surgery should be considered (see Ch. 99.4). However, before it is performed, the patient should undergo endoscopy to verify the existence of an unhealed ulcer, compliance with the medication regimen should be established, and the Zollinger-Ellison syndrome should be excluded. A period of medical therapy in a hospital may benefit some patients with peptic ulcer disease of this severity.

TREATMENT OF PATIENTS WITH GASTRIC ULCER. Cimetidine in a dose of 300 mg four times daily will lead to complete healing in 85 per cent of benign gastric ulcers by eight weeks. Early reports suggest that results with ranitidine will be comparable. Liquid antacids in doses of 70 mmol (15 to 50 ml) (Table 99–7) seven times daily produce results comparable to those with cimetidine, although once again the inconvenience of such a regimen may be a disadvantage. Results of sucralfate therapy are currently being evaluated.

Because the specter of malignancy exists with gastric ulceration (not a problem with duodenal ulcer), special efforts are taken to make sure that the ulcer is benign and that it heals completely. Assuming that endoscopic biopsies were taken at the time of initial diagnosis and showed no evidence of malignancy, proof of healing can be obtained either by x-ray or endoscopy. Unless the ulcer was very large initially, it will usually heal in eight weeks. If the ulcer is unhealed at this time, repeat endoscopic biopsies should be taken to confirm the benignity of the ulcer and if no evidence of tumor is found, medical therapy should be continued for another four to eight weeks. Since very few of these ulcers that have not healed after eight weeks of cimetidine therapy will ultimately heal if the same dose of cimetidine is continued, the dose of drug should either be increased or antacids added. A specific duration for continued therapy should be specified (e.g., another four or eight weeks), after which the patient should be operated upon if the ulcer has not healed.

LONG-TERM MAINTENANCE THERAPY. Once an ulcer has healed with full-course therapy, long-term treatment with cimetidine (400 mg at bedtime for duodenal ulcer; 400 mg twice daily for gastric ulcer) or ranitidine (150 mg at bedtime) will significantly reduce the high incidence of recurrent ulcer (as high as 70 to 80 per cent in one year). However, not every patient requires such therapy. Patients who have bled from an ulcer should receive maintenance therapy in the hope that rebleeding will not occur and that surgery will not be necessary. Maintenance therapy is also given to those patients with frequent or especially severe recurrences for whom surgery must otherwise be considered. Unless a patient is a poor operative candidate, surgery is recommended if the ulcer recurs during maintenance therapy.

TABLE 99–7. COMPARISON OF DRUGS TO TREAT DUODENAL (DU) AND GASTRIC (GU) ULCERS

Drug	Dose	Regimen	Effective For: DU	Effective For: GU	Cost to Patient for 30 Day Course‡
1. Cimetidine	300 mg	qid	Yes	Yes	$37–39
	400 mg	bid	Yes	Not Tested	$34–37
2. Ranitidine	150 mg	bid	Yes	Yes*†	$48–52
3. Antacids (see Table 99–6)	70 mmol	1&3h pc and hs	Yes†	Yes	$34–42§
	140 mmol	1&3h pc and hs	Yes	Not Tested	$68–84
4. Sucralfate	1 gram	qid	Yes	Yes*†	$36–39

*Not approved by U.S. FDA at time of writing.
†Not studied in U.S.
‡Range of four drug stores in Dallas, Texas (Sept., 1983).
§Maalox therapeutic concentrate (Rorer, Inc.).

TREATMENT OF PATIENTS WITH ZOLLINGER-ELLISON SYNDROME. Patients with Zollinger-Ellison syndrome (ZES) pose a special problem. Because of constant gastrin-induced hypersecretion of acid, they are always at risk of ulceration and ulcer complications. The treatment is discussed under the heading Zollinger-Ellison syndrome.

Collen MJ, Howard JM, McArthur KE, et al.: Comparison of ranitidine and cimetidine in the treatment of gastric hypersecretion. Ann Intern Med 100:52, 1984. *It was concluded that ranitidine was threefold more potent than cimetidine and did not have the antiandrogen side effects.*

Freston JW: Cimetidine-I. Development, pharmacology, and efficacy. II. Adverse reactions and patterns of use. Ann Intern Med 97:573, 728, 1982. *A scholarly, in-depth review of cimetidine.*

Isenberg, JI, Peterson, WL, Elashoff JD, et al.: Healing of benign gastric ulcer with low-dose antacid or cimetidine. A double-blind, randomized, placebo-controlled trial. N Engl J Med 308:1319, 1983. *A well-done study demonstrating clearly the efficacy of cimetidine for treatment of gastric ulcer.*

Peterson WL, Richardson CT: Pharmacology and side effects of drugs used to treat peptic ulcer. *In* Sleisenger MH, Fordtran, JS (eds.): Gastrointestinal Disease. 3rd ed. Philadelphia, W. B. Saunders Company, 1983, pp 708–725. *A more comprehensive review of ulcer therapeutic agents.*

Richardson, CT: Gastric ulcer. *In* Sleisinger MH, Fordtran JS (eds.): Gastrointestinal Disease. 3rd ed. Philadelphia, W. B. Saunders Company, 1983, pp 672–693. *Includes a detailed discussion of clinical results with therapeutic agents for gastric ulcer.*

Soll AH, Isenberg JI: Duodenal ulcer diseases. *In* Sleisenger MH, Fordtrans JS (eds.): Gastrointestinal Disease. 3rd ed. Philadelphia, W. B. Saunders Company, 1983, pp 625–674. *Presents for duodenal ulcer what the preceding reference does for gastric ulcer.*

Walt RP, Trotman IF, Frost R, et al.: Comparison of twice-daily ranitidine with standard cimetidine treatment of duodenal ulcer. Gut 22:319, 1981. *One of the larger studies demonstrating comparability of ranitidine and cimetidine in treatment of duodenal ulcer.*

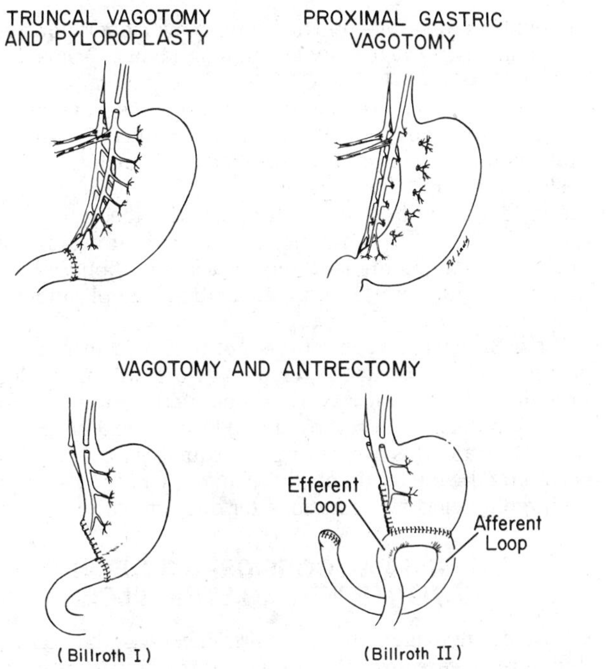

Figure 99–8. Model illustrating surgical procedures for peptic ulcer disease.

99.4. Surgical Therapy

Richard C. Thirlby

INDICATIONS

Peptic ulcers can be managed medically in most patients. However, surgery may be required to treat patients with complications of ulcers (hemorrhage, perforation, or obstruction) or patients with intractable ulcer disease. The decision to operate for intractability is difficult and is made primarily on subjective criteria. The physician and the patient must decide when pain and multiple ulcer recurrences become tolerable or intractable. Usually, patients should be considered for surgery when they have failed medical management. Failure of medical therapy occurs when an ulcer does not heal on medication, when ulcers recur during maintenance medical treatment, or after multiple ulcer recurrences. Pain, interruption of livelihood or lifestyle, and history of major complications all influence the decision to refer patients for surgery. Pain per se is not an indication. Endoscopy should be performed before surgery to document the presence of an active ulcer in a patient with intractable pain, because the pain may arise from another cause.

SURGICAL PROCEDURES

SUBTOTAL GASTRECTOMY. Subtotal gastrectomy (65 to 75 per cent gastrectomy) was the standard operation for duodenal ulcer disease for many years. This procedure was effective in preventing ulcer recurrence in 90 to 95 per cent of cases, but the incidence of long-term postoperative complications was excessive (Table 99–8). This procedure is no longer recommended for treating patients with duodenal ulcers but is occasionally used in treating patients with gastric ulcers (see below).

TRUNCAL VAGOTOMY AND PYLOROPLASTY. Vagotomy eliminates cephalic (vagal) stimulation of acid secretion and reduces basal acid output by 80 to 90 per cent and maximal (peak) acid output by 50 to 60 per cent. Truncal vagotomy also denervates the antral pump mechanism, leading to delayed gastric emptying. This can be overcome by adding a drainage (gastric emptying) procedure to vagotomy either as a pyloroplasty (Fig. 99–8) or a gastrojejunostomy.

Operative mortality with vagotomy and pyloroplasty is less than 1 per cent (Table 99–8). Even when this procedure is performed as an emergency, operative mortality is relatively low in contrast to an operative mortality of 9 to 15 per cent after emergency vagotomy and antrectomy (see below). Vagotomy and pyloroplasty usually constitute the surgical treatment of choice for bleeding ulcers and are also used by some surgeons to treat patients with intractable ulcer disease.

TRUNCAL VAGOTOMY AND ANTRECTOMY. Resection of the gastric antrum, or antrectomy, removes gastrin-containing mucosa and diminishes the gastric phase of food-stimulated acid secretion. Antrectomy alone reduces acid secretion, but the combination of an antrectomy with a vagotomy leads to an even greater reduction in acid output.

The combination of truncal vagotomy and antrectomy (Fig. 99–8) is frequently considered the standard elective operation for duodenal ulcer disease because ulcers recur rarely after this procedure. However, operative mortality is approximately 1 per cent, and long-term postoperative complications occur

TABLE 99–8. SURGICAL PROCEDURES FOR TREATMENT OF PEPTIC ULCER DISEASE

	Operative Mortality		Late Postoperative Complications					Incidence of Recurrent Ulcers
			Dumping		Diarrhea			
	Elective	Emergent	Mild*	Severe	Mild*	Severe	Weight Loss	
Subtotal gastrectomy	1%	10%	60%	5%	15%	0%	50%	5–10%
Truncal vagotomy and pyloroplasty	<1%	<7%	20%	2%	20%	2%	5–39%	7–10%
Truncal vagotomy and antrectomy	1%	9–15%	30%	2–5%	20–30%	2%	10–42%	1%
Proximal gastric vagotomy	0.1%	1%	0.5%	0%	1–2%	0%	0–5%	10%

*Nearly all patients have some change in bowel habits. Numbers are averages of many series and reflect clinically important symptoms.

frequently (Table 99–8). Therefore, newer operations such as proximal gastric vagotomy are gaining favor in some centers.

PROXIMAL GASTRIC VAGOTOMY. The parietal cell mass can be selectively denervated (proximal gastric vagotomy) (Fig. 99–8) while antral innervation and motor function remain intact. This operation reduces acid secretion while maintaining normal gastric emptying. Since many of the late sequelae of other acid-reducing procedures (e.g., dumping, diarrhea) are secondary to abnormal gastric emptying, the theoretic advantage of proximal gastric vagotomy is to reduce acid secretion with minimal mortality and long-term postoperative complications (Table 99–8).

Proximal gastric vagotomy is not indicated in patients with gastric outlet obstruction, active pyloric channel ulcers, or prepyloric ulcers. However, complicated peptic ulcer disease (history of bleeding or perforation) or high acid outputs do not contraindicate this procedure. Proximal gastric vagotomy is becoming the operation of choice in many hospitals for patients undergoing elective operations for duodenal ulcers.

SPECIAL CONSIDERATIONS IN PATIENTS WITH GASTRIC ULCERS

Surgical management of gastric ulcers is the same as for duodenal ulcers except that gastric cancer is a concern in patients with nonhealing gastric ulcers. If endoscopy with multiple biopsies and brush cytology specimens indicates that a gastric ulcer is benign, cancer is excluded with 95 to 98 per cent certainty (see Ch. 100). However, if an ulcer has not healed after 12 weeks of medical management (15 weeks in patients with initial ulcers >2.5 cm in diameter), surgery is usually indicated to exclude the possibility of cancer.

While proximal gastric vagotomy is currently the procedure of choice for most patients with duodenal ulcers, antrectomy alone is indicated in most patients with gastric ulcers (Fig. 99–8). Sometimes a subtotal gastrectomy is performed to remove more of the gastric ulcer–prone epithelium. Vagotomy is usually not necessary, because many patients with gastric ulcers have normal or low acid secretion rates. A few patients, on the other hand, also have duodenal ulcers and may require vagotomy in addition to an antrectomy.

LATE POSTOPERATIVE COMPLICATIONS

POSTPRANDIAL DUMPING. This can occur whenever the pyloric mechanism is disrupted, either by pyloroplasty, gastroduodenostomy (Billroth I) (Fig. 99–8), or gastrojejunostomy (Billroth II). The dumping syndrome occurs most often after truncal vagotomy and antrectomy and rarely develops after proximal gastric vagotomy (Table 99–8). The syndrome is transient in most patients and can be managed by dietary manipulations (see below).

Postprandial dumping syndrome is divided into early and late symptoms. *Early* symptoms occur immediately after a meal and are both intestinal (nausea, vomiting, epigastric pain, diarrhea, and dyspepsia) and vasomotor (flushing, dizziness, tachycardia, and diaphoresis). The initiating event is believed to be rapid gastric emptying, and symptoms may be caused by several pathophysiologic events: (1) duodenal or jejunal distention produced by the food bolus, (2) contraction of circulating blood volume due to displacement of fluid into the hyperosmolar solution in the gut (especially after consumption of carbohydrates) and (3) release of vasoactive hormones (serotonin, bradykinin, vasoactive intestinal peptide).

Late postprandial dumping symptoms occur one to three hours after a meal and are believed to result from hypoglycemia. The mechanism is presumed to be a rapid rise in blood glucose after ingestion of a large carbohydrate meal. This leads to an exaggerated insulin response followed by reactive hypoglycemia.

Treatment of the dumping syndrome is largely dietary (Table 99–9). Medications such as serotonin antagonists or antimuscarinic drugs are ineffective in most patients. Reconstructive surgery aimed at slowing the transit of food through the small intestine (using reversed intestinal segments) may be indicated in the 2 to 5 per cent of patients who are severely disabled.

POSTVAGOTOMY DIARRHEA. Diarrhea is common following gastric surgery, especially when vagotomy is included. In some patients (20 to 30 per cent), diarrhea is clinically important and in 2 per cent it is incapacitating (Table 99–8). The pathogenesis is unclear, and diagnosis of postvagotomy diarrhea should not be made with excluding *inflammatory bowel disease, lactose deficiency, celiac sprue,* or other causes of diarrhea, because gastric surgery may unmask previously silent diseases.

Treatment of postvagotomy diarrhea is largely dietary (Table 99–9). Medications (antidiarrheal agents, opiates, cholestyramine, and aluminum hydroxide–containing antacids) may be helpful in some patients. Approximately 2 per cent of patients will require reoperation (using reversed intestinal segments) to control disabling diarrhea.

WEIGHT LOSS. Weight loss occurs frequently after antrectomy (Table 99–8). In general, it develops in proportion to the extent of gastric resection and occurs most commonly after a Billroth II gastrojejunostomy (Fig. 99–8). Weight loss after gastric surgery most commonly results from inadequate caloric intake. Early satiety resulting from a small gastric remnant, especially after a generous antrectomy, may cause patients to limit meal size. Fear of eating because of postprandial symptoms or diarrhea may also prevent patients from consuming adequate caloric intake. Other causes of weight loss include bacterial overgrowth that can occur in the afferent limb (blind loop) of a Billroth II anastomosis (Fig. 99–8), relative pancreatic insufficiency, and in rare cases celiac sprue. Bacterial overgrowth leads to hydrolysis of conjugated bile salts and also damage to small intestinal absorptive cells. In turn, this causes malabsorption of fat, fat-soluble vitamins, and other nutrients. Bacteria also utilize vitamin B_{12}; this may lead to B_{12} deficiency. Relative pancreatic insufficiency and malabsorption may occur after a Billroth II anastomosis because of dilution of enzymes by rapid gastric emptying and, to a lesser extent, because of poor mixing of food in the efferent loop with pancreatic enzymes and bile (Fig. 99–8).

Antibiotics or surgical conversion of a Billroth II to a Billroth I anastomosis will reduce bacterial overgrowth and may restore vitamin B_{12}, fat, and fat-soluble vitamin absorption toward normal. Converting a Billroth II to a Billroth I anastomosis also may increase absorption by better mixing of food with pancreatic secretions, which further reduces malabsorption. Weight loss and malabsorption may be helped also by dietary manipulations (Table 99–9), antidiarrheal drugs, pancreatic enzymes, or a gluten-free diet in patients with celiac sprue.

ANEMIA. Anemia after surgery for ulcer disease can be caused by deficiency of iron, vitamin B_{12}, or folate. Iron deficiency is frequent after gastric resection. Malabsorption of iron and bleeding from recurrent ulcers or peristomal gastritis contribute to iron deficiency, although the exact mechanism(s) is unclear. Vitamin B_{12} deficiency may occur either because of atrophic gastritis (loss of parietal cells that secrete intrinsic factor) or because of bacterial overgrowth in the afferent loop of a Billroth II anastomosis (Fig. 99–8). Folate deficiency is uncommon and presumably is caused by malabsorption of folate from food and by decreased ingestion of dietary folate.

TABLE 99–9. DIETARY TREATMENT OF DUMPING SYNDROMES AND POSTVAGOTOMY DIARRHEA

1. Follow low carbohydrate, high protein, high fat diet.
2. Avoid refined carbohydrates and concentrated carbohydrates such as sugar, jelly, cake, pie, pudding, candy; substitute complex carbohydrates such as starch.
3. Eat six small meals a day.
4. Drink fluids between meals rather than immediately before or during meals.
5. Eat slowly.

Evaluation of anemic patients after surgery for peptic ulcer requires measurements of serum iron, B_{12}, and folate and assessment of stool for blood. Parenteral administration of vitamin B_{12} (1000 μg per month intramuscularly) and oral or intravenous iron (Imferon) may be required if deficiencies are documented. If bacterial overgrowth is suspected in patients with a Billroth II anastomosis, antibiotics (e.g., tetracycline, 250 mg four times daily) may be helpful.

ALKALINE REFLUX GASTRITIS AND ESOPHAGITIS. Reflux of duodenal contents, particularly bile, into the gastric remnant is believed to cause gastritis and esophagitis (see Ch. 98). Symptoms include continuous, burning abdominal pain, frequently exacerbated by eating, nausea, and vomiting of bile-containing material. Establishing reflux and inflammation as the cause of symptoms is difficult, since many asymptomatic postgastrectomy patients have similar endoscopic or histologic findings. Furthermore, no test definitively confirms that this gastritis is caused by reflux.

Results of medical treatment with drugs that bind bile salts (cholestyramine or aluminum hydroxide–containing antacids) are poor. Roux-en-Y jejunal interposition prevents reflux of duodenal contents into the gastric remnant and esophagus and may relieve symptoms in some patients. However, it is difficult to select patients who may benefit from this operation, because the diagnosis is often in doubt.

AFFERENT LOOP SYNDROME. This can occur in patients who have a Billroth II type gastroenterostomy (Fig. 99–8). Symptoms occur when pancreatic and biliary secretions collect in a partially obstructed afferent loop, causing distention and pain. Eventually, the fluid bypasses the partial obstruction, rushes into the stomach, and provokes vomiting. Thus, the symptom complex is characterized by postprandial cramping epigastric pain followed by projectile vomiting. Pain usually is relieved after vomiting. The vomitus is voluminous, contains bile, and does not contain food because food has left the stomach and passed through the efferent loop. Management of severe symptoms requires operative revision of the gastrojejunal anastomosis.

POSTOPERATIVE RECURRENT PEPTIC ULCER

Postoperative ulcers can develop in the stomach, the duodenum, or the jejunum in patients with a Billroth II gastrojejunostomy (marginal ulcer) (Fig. 99–8). The incidence varies for the different operations (Table 99–8). The clinical presentation is usually characterized by pain. However, complications such as bleeding, obstruction, or perforation may occur. Diagnosis of postoperative recurrent ulcer is best made by endoscopy because upper gastrointestinal barium studies are poor at identifying postoperative ulcers, particularly after a Billroth II gastrojejunostomy.

Incomplete vagotomy is responsible for postoperative recurrent ulcers in the majority of patients. Other uncommon causes include *Zollinger-Ellison syndrome, retained antrum syndrome, ulcerogenic drugs* (aspirin or other nonsteroidal anti-inflammatory drugs), *silk surgical sutures* at the anastomosis, or *antral G cell hyperplasia.* Serum gastrin concentrations should be measured in all patients with recurrent ulcers to rule out Zollinger-Ellison syndrome (see Ch. 99.6).

Sham feeding is the best test for diagnosis of incomplete vagotomy. This test makes use of the fact that the thought, sight, smell, and taste of food stimulates acid secretion via vagal pathways to the stomach (see Ch. 99.1). An appetizing meal is presented to a patient, and the meal is chewed but not swallowed. Acid output is measured during the test by aspirating gastric secretions through a nasogastric tube. Acid output induced by sham feeding that is greater than 10 per cent of pentagastrin-stimulated peak acid output implies incomplete vagotomy. The insulin test, or Hollander test, of vagal function is no longer recommended because it is dangerous; hypoglycemic seizures, myocardial infarction, and deaths have been reported. It is also less reliable and less specific than the sham feeding test.

Until recently, the treatment of postoperative recurrent ulcers caused by incomplete vagotomy was surgical. The advent of histamine H_2-receptor antagonists has made medical management the first choice. Postoperative recurrent ulcers will heal with histamine H_2-receptor antagonists in 60 to 90 per cent of patients, and reoperation may not be necessary. Long-term maintenance therapy (cimetidine 400 to 800 mg at bedtime) is required in most patients to prevent further recurrence. The indications for reoperation in patients with recurrent ulcer secondary to incomplete vagotomy are (1) failure to heal with cimetidine or ranitidine, (2) recurrence on maintenance therapy with H_2-receptor antagonists, (3) a complication (bleeding, obstruction, or perforation) associated with recurrent ulcer or (4) noncompliance with long-term medical therapy. The choice of reoperation should be individualized. If sham feeding confirms incomplete vagotomy, transthoracic revagotomy usually should be performed if the patient has had an emptying procedure such as pyloroplasty or a type of gastroenterostomy such as Billroth I or II at the initial operation. Antrectomy may be indicated in some patients who have had only a vagotomy as their initial procedure.

Bushkin FL, Woodward ER (eds.): Postgastrectomy syndromes. Major Problems in Clinical Surgery, Vol 20. Philadelphia, W. B. Saunders Company, 1976, pp 1–167. *Concise monograph emphasizing the pathophysiology and surgical treatment of postgastrectomy syndromes.*

Feldman M: Postoperative recurrent ulcer. *In* Sleisenger MH, Fordtran JS (eds.): Gastrointestinal Disease. 3rd ed. Philadelphia, W. B. Saunders Company, 1983, pp 749–756. *Excellent review of pathogenesis and evaluation of postoperative recurrent ulcer.*

Jordan PH, Jr: Operations for peptic ulcer disease and their early postoperative complications. *In* Sleisenger MH, Fordtran JS (eds.): Gastrointestinal Disease. 3rd ed. Philadelphia, W. B. Saunders Company, 1983, pp 739–748. *A general review of the surgical treatment of peptic ulcer disease including indications for surgery and a description of the operations.*

Knight CD, VanHeerden JA, Kelly KA: Proximal gastric vagotomy: Update. Ann Surg 197:22, 1983. *Seven-year experience with proximal gastric vagotomy in 298 patients evaluated and treated at the Mayo Clinic.*

99.5. Complications

Mark Feldman

Approximately one of three patients with peptic ulcer disease experiences a complication such as *bleeding, perforation,* or *obstruction* at some point. A complication may be the first manifestation or it may occur later in the course of ulcer disease. Patients with a peptic ulcer in the pyloric channel or postbulbar duodenum, patients with combined duodenal and gastric ulcer, and patients with Zollinger-Ellison syndrome are especially likely to experience ulcer complications. There has been a recent 30 per cent decline in hospitalizations for duodenal ulcer complications in the United States. This decline preceded introduction of histamine H_2-receptor antagonists for peptic ulcer therapy. During the same time period, hospitalizations for gastric ulcer complications increased slightly. The reason(s) for these trends in hospitalizations for ulcer complications are uncertain.

The clinical presentation, methods of diagnosis, and therapy of the major ulcer complications differ. For this reason, each complication will be discussed separately, although a patient simultaneously may have more than one complication.

BLEEDING

Bleeding is the most common complication of peptic ulcer disease, occurring in 15 to 20 per cent of patients with duodenal ulcer and 10 to 15 per cent of patients with gastric ulcer at some time during their course. The risk of bleeding is unrelated to duration of ulcer disease; one out of four patients will have no history of ulcer disease when they present with bleeding. The mortality rate for a single bleeding episode of approximately 7 per cent has not changed in the past several decades.

Hemorrhage results from erosion of the ulcer into a blood vessel (Ch. 113). The most common sign of acute bleeding is melena, with or without hematemesis. Although these symptoms usually indicate major blood loss (> 1000 ml), melena may occur with loss of as little as 50 to 75 ml of blood. In some patients with major hemorrhage, gastrointestinal transit of blood may be so rapid that the stool is bright red or maroon. Moreover, a nasogastric aspirate may not always contain blood if active bleeding from a duodenal ulcer does not reflux into the stomach. Thus, the combination of hematochezia and a bloodless, nasogastric aspirate does not always indicate a lower (colonic) source of bleeding. The hemoglobin and hematocrit on admission may not reflect the severity of bleeding if sufficient time has not elapsed to allow for compensatory hemodilution. Therefore, the severity of acute bleeding is better assessed by the blood pressure and pulse rate measured in the supine and the upright positions. A supine systolic blood pressure <100 mm Hg and a supine pulse rate >100 beats per minute suggest major blood loss, as do a fall in blood pressure >10 mm Hg and an increase in pulse >20 beats per minute after the patient assumes an upright position.

Although peptic ulcer is the commonest source of acute upper GI bleeding (accounting for 40 to 50 per cent of cases), the differential diagnosis includes esophagogastric varices, erosive and hemorrhagic gastritis, and Mallory-Weiss laceration. Less common causes include benign and malignant gastric neoplasm, esophagitis, duodenitis, vascular lesion (e.g., angiodysplasia, arteriovenous malformation), and aortoenteric fistula in patients with an aortic graft. Peptic ulcers may also cause chronic or intermittent bleeding resulting in iron deficiency anemia. In such instances, it may be necessary to exclude other causes of chronic blood loss such as colonic cancer before attributing the bleeding to a peptic ulcer.

There are certain factors that, if present, adversely affect clinical outcome in patients with bleeding peptic ulcers. These include (1) severe, continuing hemorrhage (arbitrarily defined as the need for three or more units of blood in the first 24 hours or six or more units in the first 48 hours after pre-existing losses have been replaced; (2) early rebleeding usually occurring within three to five days of initial stabilization; (3) age greater than 60 years; (4) underlying associated diseases, especially involving the cardiovascular system, lungs, and liver (particularly active alcoholic liver disease); (5) presence of gastric ulcer as opposed to duodenal ulcer; and (6) endoscopic visualization of a blood vessel or clot in the base of an ulcer. If a visible vessel is present, there is at least a 50 per cent likelihood of ulcer rebleeding while the patient is in the hospital.

If continuous bleeding occurs or if major rebleeding occurs in the hospital, it is customary to proceed to surgery. Urgent surgery is required in approximately 15 per cent of patients with bleeding peptic ulcers. Mortality rates after emergency ulcer surgery are two- to three-fold higher than after elective surgery. Emergency surgical therapy for bleeding duodenal ulcer consists of suture ligation of the bleeding vessel along with either (1) truncal vagotomy and pyloroplasty or (2) truncal vagotomy and antrectomy. Emergency vagotomy and pyloroplasty has a higher in-hospital rebleeding rate than truncal vagotomy and antrectomy but a lower mortality rate. There is insufficient information at present regarding proximal gastric vagotomy without drainage (also known as parietal cell vagotomy, highly selective vagotomy, selective proximal vagotomy, and superselective vagotomy). For bleeding gastric ulcer, distal gastrectomy that includes the ulcer in the resected specimen is usually carried out. If the ulcer is quite proximal in the stomach, the ulcer is usually biopsied and ligated, followed by distal gastrectomy. Although emergency surgery stops bleeding in 90 to 95 per cent of cases, there is little evidence that subsequent rebleeding is prevented by these operations.

If urgent surgery is unnecessary because bleeding ceases spontaneously (as is usually the case), the patient is observed for several days in the hospital. Various measures have been employed in these patients, including nasogastric suction, antacid therapy, and inhibition of gastric acid-pepsin secretion with either cimetidine or anticholinergics. None of these measures, alone or in combination, has been proved to prevent rebleeding in the hospital, although a recent study has suggested that ranitidine may prevent early rebleeding from duodenal ulcer. Other antisecretory agents such as somatostatin and secretin and also tranexamic acid, an antifibrinolytic compound, have shown some promise in early clinical studies, but more data are needed.

Once a patient bleeds from a peptic ulcer, he has a 30 to 50 per cent chance of bleeding again from an ulcer, a two-fold or greater risk than the overall ulcer population. This 30 to 50 per cent risk remains approximately the same after a second or third bleeding episode. No relationship exists between the severity of the initial bleeding event and the severity of subsequent bleeding. There is no evidence as yet that chronic medical therapy or conventional surgical therapy reduces this 30 to 50 per cent risk of rebleeding. It is thus debatable whether, after initial stabilization and ulcer healing, a patient with one, two, or more bleeding episodes should (1) be given no treatment, (2) be placed on chronic "ulcer prophylaxis" with low doses of cimetidine or ranitidine, or (3) undergo elective ulcer surgery.

PERFORATION

An ulcer that extends through the entire wall of the duodenum or stomach may have either of three outcomes: (1) rupture into the peritoneal cavity with spillage of duodenal or gastric contents *(free perforation)*; (2) erosion into and confinement by a solid organ such as pancreas, liver, or spleen *(penetration)*; or (3) perforation into a hollow viscus such as the common bile duct, gallbladder, or intestine *(fistula formation)*.

Free perforation occurs in 6 to 11 per cent of patients with duodenal ulcer and in 2 to 5 per cent of patients with gastric ulcer. Perforation may occur as an initial manifestation of ulcer disease but more often occurs during the course of known disease. Free perforation occurs more commonly in men than in women. Duodenal ulcers that perforate are usually anterior, while bleeding duodenal ulcers are more often posterior. A duodenal ulcer may occasionally perforate posteriorly into the lesser sac and cause back pain rather than signs of generalized peritonitis. Most perforated gastric ulcers arise from the lesser curvature. In approximately 10 per cent of cases, peptic ulcer perforation is complicated by significant bleeding.

The characteristic clinical feature of free perforation is the sudden onset of severe, constant abdominal pain that reaches maximal intensity rapidly. The pain is initially present in the upper abdomen but quickly becomes generalized. Movement exacerbates the pain so that the patient prefers to lie on his back without moving. Marked abdominal tenderness to palpation is present and there is diffuse boardlike rigidity of the abdominal wall musculature. Hypotension and tachycardia are usually present because of intraperitoneal fluid losses. Hemoconcentration and leukocytosis are usually present, whereas fever often is absent. The serum amylase is mildly elevated in one out of six patients. Upright abdominal radiographs will show free air (pneumoperitoneum) in approximately 75 per cent of cases. If pneumoperitoneum is not evident and there is strong clinical suspicion of perforation, it may be necessary to administer a water-soluble contrast agent orally to demonstrate extravasation. However, a definite diagnosis of perforated peptic ulcer often is not established until surgery is performed. The differential diagnosis of perforated ulcer is discussed in Ch. 99.2.

Certain atypical presentations or perforation may occur: (1) In some individuals, a perforation will rapidly close with only minimal contamination of the peritoneal cavity and with rapid, spontaneous clinical improvement. (2) Abdominal pain and physical findings may be less impressive in elderly patients and also in patients with neurologic and/or psychiatric problems. Such patients may present with unexplained shock. (3) Fluid may leak into the peritoneal cavity slowly and collect in the right paracolic gutter, resulting in a clinical presentation simulating acute appendicitis.

Treatment of free perforation can be surgical or medical. In most cases surgery is carried out to establish the diagnosis and to patch the perforation with a piece of omentum (Graham closure). There is controversy as to whether definitive ulcer surgery also should be carried out at the time of perforation. Some physicians will perform either vagotomy and pyloroplasty or truncal vagotomy and antrectomy for duodenal ulcer (or distal gastrectomy for gastric ulcer) if there has been a long history of ulcer disease or previous ulcer complications. Recently, proximal gastric vagotomy along with closure has been used successfully in patients with perforated duodenal ulcers. If perforation occurred more than 8 to 12 hours earlier, definitive surgery is usually not performed because of extensive peritoneal soiling. Some physicians close the perforation and defer definitive ulcer surgery until another indication is present (intractable pain, pyloric stenosis). In one recent study, half of patients treated by simple closure of the perforation were asymptomatic up to six years after surgery. However, 8 per cent of patients in that study had a second perforation, usually within one year. If the patient has a perforated gastric ulcer and resection of the stomach is not carried out, the ulcer should be biopsied because 10 per cent of perforated gastric ulcers are malignant. Medical therapy of free perforation that is diagnosed early is usually reserved for elderly or high-risk patients who may not tolerate surgery. This treatment consists of nasogastric suction, intravenous fluids, and systemic broad-spectrum antibiotics. Some patients whose perforation appears to have become sealed off and are improving rapidly may also be treated medically.

Mortality from free perforation is approximately 5 to 15 per cent for duodenal ulcer and somewhat higher for gastric ulcer, especially if the gastric ulcer is near the cardia. The most important factors associated with a poor outcome in perforated duodenal ulcer are longstanding (>48 hrs) perforation prior to surgery; preoperative shock; serious concurrent illnesses; and possibly older age.

Penetration into solid organs such as the pancreas occurs with an uncertain frequency because penetration can be diagnosed with certainty only at surgery or autopsy. These patients almost always have a long history of ulcer disease and usually present with intractable ulcer pain.

Fistula is an uncommon form of perforation. When this complication occurs, duodenal ulcers usually perforate into the common bile duct, whereas gastric ulcers usually perforate into the colon or duodenum. Patients with duodenocholedochal fistula may be asymptomatic but have air in the biliary tree, or they may present with cholangitis and abnormal liver function tests. The fistula is usually demonstrated by upper GI series, in which case barium refluxes from the duodenal bulb into the biliary tree. The fistula may close during medical treatment, although surgery may be required in some cases. Gastrocolic fistula caused by perforated gastric ulcer is often associated with aspirin ingestion. These patients may have diarrhea and malabsorption. The usual treatment is surgical. A gastric ulcer in the antrum may also perforate into the duodenal bulb, resulting in two channels from the stomach to duodenum ("double pylorus").

OBSTRUCTION

Gastric outlet obstruction occurs in approximately 5 per cent of patients with duodenal ulcer or gastric ulcer and is especially common if the ulcer is located in the pyloric channel. Obstruction is caused by edema, smooth muscle spasm, fibrosis, or a combination of these processes. Although obstruction usually occurs in patients who have had ulcer disease for many years, a patient occasionally may present with obstruction as the initial manifestation of ulcer disease. Mortality rates from obstruction in peptic ulcer disease are 7 to 26 per cent depending on the age of the patient and the presence or absence of associated diseases.

Characteristically, symptoms of delayed gastric emptying—nausea, vomiting, epigastric fullness or bloating, anorexia, and early satiety—are present. Anorexia, early satiety, vomiting, and a fear of eating (sitophobia) may contribute to significant weight loss. Epigastric pain is commonly present and may be relieved temporarily by vomiting. Symptoms usually have been present for weeks or months upon presentation. Vomiting may be delayed an hour or more after eating, is often copious in amount, and may contain stale, undigested food or blood but no bile. Physical examination may reveal volume depletion (hypotension, tachycardia, and dry skin and mucous membranes), visible peristalsis in the epigastrium, or a succussion splash over the stomach.

A clinical suspicion of gastric retention is enhanced if any of the following objective measurements are present: (1) aspiration of >300 ml gastric fluid four or more hours after a meal (a large bore tube may be necessary for this); (2) aspiration of >200 ml gastric fluid the morning after an overnight fast; or (3) removal of >400 ml gastric fluid 30 minutes after instilling 750 ml isotonic saline into the empty stomach *(saline load test)*. Gastric retention may be appreciated on a plain abdominal film (large, dilated stomach containing solid debris) and documented by upper GI series or radionuclide scintigraphy. Gastric retention is not always caused by gastric outlet obstruction. Gastric retention can be secondary to gastric atony, as in diabetic gastroparesis, following vagotomy, or as a side effect of medications. The presence of gastric outlet obstruction usually can be established by endoscopy or upper GI series. Gastric outlet obstruction is caused by peptic ulcer disease in 80 to 90 per cent of cases. The other common cause is carcinoma of the antrum. Less common causes include gastric lymphoma, pancreatic carcinoma, pancreatitis, adult hypertrophic pyloric stenosis, eosinophilic gastritis, Crohn's disease, antral caustic stricture, antral polyp, and annular pancreas.

Laboratory studies usually reflect intravascular volume depletion (hemoconcentration, prerenal azotemia) and a hypokalemic, hypochloremic metabolic alkalosis due to vomiting. If extensive weight loss has occurred, hypoalbuminemia, cutaneous anergy, and a low serum transferrin concentration may be present. The urine is usually concentrated and contains little chloride (<10 mEq per liter), but the urinary sodium concentration and pH are variable depending on the renal threshold for bicarbonate.

Therapy of gastric outlet obstruction has three goals: gastric decompression and resolution of obstruction, replacement of fluids and electrolytes, and nutritional support. Gastric decompression is accomplished by continuous nasogastric suction for at least 72 hours. With prolonged obstruction, gradual gastric dilatation occurs and this interferes with the contractile function of gastric smooth muscle. Electrolyte disturbances such as hypokalemia can also contribute to gastric motor dysfunction. A saline load test, performed serially, may have prognostic value. For example, a return of >300 ml after 24 hours of nasogastric suction suggests that obstruction will not resolve and that surgery will probably be required. After 72 hours, a return of <200 ml is a favorable sign and usually indicates that the tube can be removed and the patient fed. Intravenous fluids and electrolytes are given to replace pre-existing and current losses. Isotonic saline containing 10 to 20 mEq of potassium chloride per liter is satisfactory in most cases. Losses of gastric acid from continuous aspiration can be curtailed by administering cimetidine in a dose of 300 mg intravenously every four to six hours. If suction is carried out for only a few days, it may suffice to provide calories with 5 per cent dextrose solution intravenously, along with soluble vitamins. However, if it appears that prolonged suction will be necessary and that surgery is imminent, parenteral intravenous hyperalimentation should be instituted. This is especially valuable if the patient has lost significant lean body mass.

The percentage of patients with obstruction who respond to

medical management varies considerably from series to series, but an average figure is 50 per cent. The ultimate response to medical therapy is related to relative degrees of edema and spasm and fibrosis, because edema and spasm may resolve. An uncertain percentage of patients who respond to medical therapy and are discharged have obstruction again within the next several years and may undergo surgery at that time. However, obstruction may resolve on medical therapy and may not recur for many years. Thus, it is prudent to attempt medical management rather than to proceed directly to surgery. Such an approach may have benefits even if surgery is performed because it allows time for the obstructed stomach to decompress and regain tone, for electrolyte disturbances to be corrected, and for nutritional status to be improved.

If obstruction does not resolve in three to seven days, surgery is usually necessary. There is controversy as to which operation is best: subtotal gastrectomy with gastrojejunostomy, vagotomy and antrectomy, vagotomy and pyloroplasty, or vagotomy and gastrojejunostomy. Some surgeons are reluctant to perform any type of vagotomy in an obstructed stomach for fear of postoperative gastric atony, although this complication is uncommon. Gastrojejunostomy without resection or vagotomy is associated with a high ulcer recurrence rate (30 to 40 per cent). Recently, proximal gastric vagotomy combined with intraoperative dilation of the stenotic pylorus has been introduced, although there is not yet sufficient experience to evaluate this technique.

Boey J, Wong J, Ong GB: A prospective study of operative risk factors in perforated duodenal ulcers. Ann Surg 195:265, 1982. *In this study it was found that concurrent medical illness, preoperative shock, and perforation of more than 48 hours were associated with increased mortality.*

Dawson J, Cockel R: Ranitidine in acute upper gastrointestinal haemorrhage. Br Med J 285:476, 1982. *Only three of 27 patients who bled from duodenal ulcer rebled while taking oral ranitidine compared with 11 of 26 patients taking placebo.*

Drury JK, McKay AJ, Hutchison JSF, Joffe SN: Natural history of perforated duodenal ulcers treated by suture closure. Lancet 2:749, 1978. *These authors favor simple oversewing and a "wait and see" policy toward perforated duodenal ulcer.*

Elashoff JD, Grossman MI: Trends in hospital admissions and death rates for peptic ulcer in the United States from 1970 to 1978. Gastroenterology 79:750, 1980. *Careful epidemiologic study that analyzes duodenal and gastric ulcer separately.*

Jordan PH: Proximal gastric vagotomy without drainage for treatment of perforated duodenal ulcer. Gastroenterology 83:179, 1982. *This author advocates proximal gastric vagotomy at the time of perforation.*

Storey DW, Bown SG, Swain CP, Salmon PR, Kirkham JS, Northfield TC: Endoscopic prediction of recurrent bleeding in peptic ulcers. N Engl J Med 305:915, 1981. *Patients with vessels visible in the ulcer crater at endoscopy had a 56 per cent chance of rebleeding in the hospital.*

Walker C: Complications of peptic ulcer disease and indications for surgery. *In* Sleisenger MH, Fordtran JS (eds.): Gastrointestinal Disease. 3rd ed. Philadelphia, W. B. Saunders Company, 1983, pp 725–738. *Comprehensive review with extensive references.*

99.6. Zollinger-Ellison Syndrome

Charles T. Richardson

DEFINITION

The Zollinger-Ellison syndrome, when first described in 1955, consisted of the triad of a non-beta islet cell tumor of the pancreas, hypersecretion of gastric acid, and severe peptic ulcer disease. A humoral substance postulated to be produced by the tumor was later demonstrated to be gastrin. With further experience the Zollinger-Ellison syndrome has now been defined as: (1) an increased serum gastrin concentration, (2) an increased basal acid output plus an increased ratio of basal to peak (pentagastrin-stimulated) acid output, and (3) peptic ulcer disease and/or diarrhea. Not all patients with an elevated serum gastrin concentration and hypersecretion of acid have tumors that can be identified at surgery. Presumably, their tumors are too small to be found at laparotomy or there is hyperplasia of the islets of Langerhans, a condition known as *microadenomatosis*.

CLINICAL MANIFESTATIONS

Zollinger-Ellison syndrome occurs most frequently between ages 35 and 65 years and is more common in men than in women.

Abdominal pain resulting from an ulcer is the most common clinical finding in patients with this syndrome. Such ulcers usually occur in the duodenal bulb but also may develop in the postbulbar duodenum, the jejunum, stomach, or esophagus. Complications of ulcer disease such as bleeding or perforation occur in 40 to 50 per cent of patients at some time during their course and may be the presenting manifestation. *Diarrhea* is a frequent complaint and may precede ulceration in some patients or occur without ulcers in others (5 to 10 per cent). *Fat malabsorption* (steatorrhea) is occasionally noted.

About 20 to 30 per cent of patients with Zollinger-Ellison syndrome have multiple endocrine neoplasia (MEN I) syndrome and thus have a hereditary form of peptic ulcer disease. These patients may have parathyroid or pituitary tumors and clinical findings such as hypercalcemia, renal stones, or increased prolactin levels. It is unlikely that peptic ulcer disease occurs in increased frequency in association with parathyroid adenomas except in patients who also have MEN I syndrome.

PATHOPHYSIOLOGY

Peptic ulcers in patients with Zollinger-Ellison syndrome presumably result from increased secretion of acid and pepsin driven by excessive amounts of circulating gastrin. Gastrin also has a trophic effect on parietal (acid secreting) cells that leads to an increased parietal cell mass. Since parietal cell mass correlates with maximum acid output, some patients with Zollinger-Ellison syndrome also have increased maximum (peak) acid outputs.

Diarrhea results almost exclusively from the large volumes of fluid secreted by the stomach and is relieved in most patients by aspirating gastric juice via a nasogastric tube or more conveniently by treating patients with H_2-receptor antagonists (see below). Independent of stimulating acid secretion, gastrin may also play a role in the development of diarrhea by reducing intestinal absorption of water and electrolytes.

Steatorrhea may occur for several reasons. First, acid damages small bowel epithelial cells. This, in turn, causes a mucosal defect that limits transport of fat and perhaps other nutrients across the mucosa. Second, pancreatic lipase is inactivated by acid. This leads to decreased breakdown of triglycerides and contributes to fat malabsorption. Third, acid may decrease the amount of conjugated bile acids in the duodenum and upper jejunum. This results in inadequate formation of micelles; this, in turn, may lead to fat malabsorption.

DIAGNOSIS

Zollinger-Ellison syndrome should be suspected in patients who have: (1) ulcers in unusual locations such as the postbulbar duodenum or jejunum, (2) ulcers that persist despite medical treatment, (3) ulcers and diarrhea, (4) abnormally large gastric folds or thickened duodenal and/or jejunal folds, (5) ulcers and manifestations of other endocrine tumors such as renal stones, (6) a family history of ulcer disease, and (7) recurrent ulcers after ulcer surgery.

These criteria call for measurement of the serum gastrin concentration (Table 99–3). If the level is abnormally high, a gastric analysis should be performed. Zollinger-Ellison syndrome is a likely diagnosis if the serum gastrin level is elevated, basal acid output is increased (>10.6 mmol per hour in men and 5.6 mmol per hour in women), and the ratio of basal to peak acid output (pentagastrin stimulated) is greater than 0.40. The diagnosis can be confirmed by performing a secretin stimulation test (see Ch. 99.2). This test is especially helpful in patients with serum gastrin concentrations or basal acid outputs that are only slightly increased. A positive secretin test along with an increased serum gastrin concentration and basal acid output establishes the diagnosis of Zollinger-Ellison syndrome in over 95 per cent of patients.

Tumors are found at surgery in 40 to 70 per cent of patients with Zollinger-Ellison syndrome and are usually located in the pancreas. Tumors have also been found in the duodenum, stomach, greater omentum, transverse mesocolon, and other areas of the peritoneal cavity. Angiography or sonography is usually not helpful in localizing gastrinomas. Computerized axial tomography, on the other hand, is occasionally useful in determining the location of tumors and should be obtained prior to laparotomy. Since some gastrinomas have been found in the stomach or duodenum, upper endoscopy also should be performed to look for tumors. Techniques such as intraoperative sonography or transhepatic venous sampling to measure gastrin from tributaries draining the pancreas or duodenum have been helpful in some centers in localizing tumors, but these tests are not available in most hospitals.

THERAPY

For many years total gastrectomy was the treatment of choice for patients with the Zollinger-Ellison syndrome. All of the acid-secreting mucosa as well as the antrum was removed with subsequent cure of peptic ulcers and diarrhea. However, many of the late postoperative complications that occur in patients with ordinary peptic ulcer disease developed with even greater frequency and severity after total gastrectomy. Furthermore, mortality was higher with total gastrectomy than with other surgical procedures for ulcer disease.

With the advent of H_2-receptor antagonists it has become possible to treat patients medically. Antagonism of the H_2-receptor with either cimetidine or ranitidine effectively reduces acid secretion in most patients and decreases symptoms related to the disease. However, larger than normally prescribed doses as well as more frequent administration are often required. For example, 600 mg cimetidine every four hours* or 300 mg ranitidine every eight hours may be necessary to reduce acid secretion adequately. A few patients have required as much as 5 to 10 grams of cimetidine daily. The dose of cimetidine or ranitidine may be reduced by treating patients concomitantly with an antimuscarinic drug such as glycopyrrolate or isopropamide (see Fig. 99–7), since antimuscarinic drugs have been shown to enhance the inhibitory effect on acid secretion of H_2-receptor antagonists.

Medical treatment with H_2-receptor antagonists is not ideal for two reasons: First, complications of ulcer disease have occurred in some patients, and second, medical therapy does not provide an opportunity to search for resectable tumors, more than half of which are believed to be malignant. Because of this, a reasonable approach to treating patients with Zollinger-Ellison syndrome is laparotomy to search for resectable tumors present in about 20 to 30 per cent of patients, followed by medical therapy with H_2-receptor antagonists if all functioning tumor has not been removed at surgery.

In an effort to reduce failures of medical therapy, vagotomy may be combined with H_2-receptor antagonists in some patients to reduce acid secretion and add to the inhibitory effect of cimetidine or ranitidine. Even though treatment with H_2-receptor antagonists is still necessary in most patients, the dose of medication can be reduced in many patients treated with this approach. This form of therapy remains experimental, but preliminary results are promising.

McGuigan JE: The Zollinger-Ellison Syndrome. *In* Sleisenger MH, Fordtran JS (eds.): Gastrointestinal Disease. 3rd ed. Philadelphia, W. B. Saunders Company, 1983, pp 693–705. *A review of the pathophysiology, diagnosis, and treatment of Zollinger-Ellison syndrome.*

Jensen RT, Gardner JD, Raufman J-P, Pandol SJ, Doppman JL, Collen MJ: Zollinger-Ellison syndrome: Current concepts and management. Ann Intern Med 98:59, 1983. *A review of the literature relative to current diagnosis and treatment of Zollinger-Ellison syndrome including the experience with patients treated at the National Institutes of Health.*

---

*May exceed maximum recommended daily dose.

100. NEOPLASMS OF THE STOMACH

Paul Sherlock

The majority of gastric neoplasms are malignant, in contrast to the colon where the reverse is true. Although gastric carcinoma is steadily decreasing in the United States, it still represents a major public health problem throughout the world. In some countries it is the most frequent cancer and the leading cause of death from cancer. In the United States gastric carcinoma is responsible for 90 to 95 per cent of malignant disease of the stomach. It is difficult to estimate the percentage of primary lymphomas, since many of these involve the stomach secondarily. A reasonable estimate is that 5 per cent of all primary gastric malignancy is Hodgkin's disease (HD) and non-Hodgkin's lymphoma, particularly the latter since HD rarely involves the stomach as a primary site. The sarcomas, including leiomyosarcoma, liposarcoma, neurogenic sarcoma, and fibrosarcoma, are all relatively rare malignant tumors that may involve the stomach. Leiomyosarcoma of the stomach represents about 1 per cent of gastric cancers.

CARCINOMA OF THE STOMACH

EPIDEMIOLOGY. The incidence of gastric cancer varies markedly in different areas of the world. It is extremely common in Japan, Latin America west of the Andes, some parts of the Caribbean, and Eastern Europe; moderately common in Finland, Austria, and Czechoslovakia; and uncommon in the United States, Australia, New Zealand, and other Anglo-Saxon countries. Fluctuations may occur within smaller geographic areas, such as an extremely high incidence of gastric cancer in northern Wales and a considerably lower incidence in the rest of the British Isles. Colorectal cancer tends to be rare where gastric cancer is common and vice versa. The low incidence in the United States is a recent development, since gastric cancer was the most common known cancer in the United States 40 to 50 years ago. Other countries that previously had a high incidence have also begun to show a decrease. The reasons for this are unknown. Environmental factors are considered important in the etiology of gastric cancer as evidenced by populations migrating to areas of either low or high risk and taking on the risk of the area of migration. Japanese moving to Hawaii have a decreased incidence of gastric cancer in subsequent generations, and there is a further reduction with migration to the mainland. The incidence of colonic cancer increases with this migration.

ETIOLOGY. *Dietary influences* are thought to be important, but exhaustive epidemiologic research has not clarified the factors involved. Consumption of barbecued meats, smoked or pickled fish and sauces, and alcohol, and deficiencies of magnesium and vitamin A have all been postulated but unproved as causes of gastric cancer.

Nitrosamines are powerful carcinogens for animals. They can be formed easily from common, secondary, tertiary, and quaternary amines by combining these with nitrite (the nitrosation reaction). This reaction can take place under varying conditions of pH and temperature, so that nitrosamines may be formed in the soil, under conditions of food storage, during food preparation such as frying bacon, or in the body. Bacteria may play a role by catalyzing the amine nitrite union or by reducing nitrate to nitrite. Thus the achlorhydric stomach is considered a favorable site for nitrosamine synthesis. The necessary amines can be found in many foods and medications, whereas nitrate and nitrites are found naturally in food and water and are present in food preservatives. Ascorbic acid (vitamin C) blocks the nitrosation reaction in the test tube. The increased intake of vitamin C and refrigeration have been postulated to be responsible for the decrease in gastric cancer in this country over the last few decades. Although the hypothesis concerning nitrites and gastric cancer is attractive, much more work is needed to substantiate this theory.

Blood group A is associated with a 20 per cent higher incidence of gastric cancer even in areas of the world where gastric cancer is rare. This fact and the aggregation of gastric cancer in certain families have raised the possibility of a genetic component. Demonstrating familial occurrence is not enough to prove that hereditary factors are important in the etiology of gastric cancer, since familial concentrations may be due either to genetic factors or to common environmental influences.

Pernicious anemia has a less firm association with cancer of the stomach than previously thought and the linkage is probably through gastritis. When pernicious anemia becomes clinically manifest, the gastric mucosal abnormality has been present for at least several years. Gastric cancer probably develops slowly; cytologic abnormalities suggesting in situ carcinoma have been observed for as long as 20 years in some patients.

Atrophic gastritis is usually present with gastric cancer, characterized by cellular infiltration, loss of normal parietal and chief cells, and intestinalization. Achlorhydria is associated with this type of gastritis. Carcinoma of the stomach may also develop from the intestinal tissue present in the intestinalized atrophic stomach. Chronic gastritis may therefore be a premalignant state.

Adenomatous polyps of the stomach, especially those larger than 2 cm, may occasionally give rise to carcinoma. Most stomach polyps are hyperplastic and do not become malignant. Such adenomatous polyps can be associated with anacidity, pernicious anemia, or infiltrating carcinoma developing elsewhere in the stomach. The stomach with a polyp requires vigilance.

Subtotal resection for benign peptic ulcer disease results in a two- to three-fold increase in gastric stump carcinoma when compared with the normal population. The interval between resection and development of stump carcinoma is usually between 15 and 30 years, although shorter intervals have been noted. The development of chronic atrophic gastritis, which may commence several years following resection, appears to be a major pathogenic factor for increased risk. Biliary, pancreatic, and intestinal reflux into the stomach remnant may contribute to the development of cancer. *Immunologic deficiencies,* particularly the common variable type, may lead to a greater predisposition to gastric cancer.

It is doubtful that a benign gastric ulcer degenerates into a malignant lesion. Since chronic atrophic gastritis is common with both benign and malignant gastric ulcers, the underlying predisposing factor may be atrophic gastritis.

INCIDENCE AND PREVALENCE. It is estimated that there were 23,000 new cases of gastric cancer and 14,000 deaths from gastric cancer in the United States in 1980. Although this is a substantial number, a dramatic decline in the incidence of stomach cancer has occurred here and in many other countries. The magnitude of the decline varies. In the United States the age-adjusted mortality rate for males dropped from 28 per 100,000 in 1930 to 9.7 per 100,000 in 1967. The rate of decline has been the steepest among U.S. whites and in the older age group of all race-sex categories. Carcinoma of the stomach occurs most frequently between the ages of 50 and 70 years and is rare in patients younger than 30 years. The incidence and mortality rise steeply with age. Rates are higher in males than females by 2 to 1. The ratio approaches unity in patients younger than 30 and older than 80. The incidence of gastric cancer is higher for U.S. blacks than whites, but the marked difference noted earlier in the century is diminishing. Risk of gastric cancer is greatest among those of low socioeconomic status.

PATHOLOGY. Carcinoma of the stomach is adenocarcinoma that usually is manifested pathologically in one of four ways: (1) Most often it appears as a bulky mass with deep central ulceration projecting into the lumen and invading the wall. (2) The tumor may infiltrate and narrow a portion of the lumen, most often in the antrum. Less commonly the infiltration extends throughout the entire stomach, resulting in *linitis plastica*—a fixed, nondistensible stomach with absence of normal folds and a narrowed lumen. (3) Polypoid or exophytic carcinoma with or without a stalk may occur and be difficult to distinguish from a benign polyp on x-ray. (4) More rarely, carcinoma of the stomach may occur as a superficially spreading tumor involving only the mucosal surface and producing a granular appearance. This is unlike linitis plastica, which extends through the entire thickness of the wall.

Gastric carcinomas may be well differentiated adenocarcinomas or may be so anaplastic as to resemble diffuse histiocytic lymphoma or sarcoma. A true carcinoma in situ is rarely found and is confined entirely to the glands. This is more commonly seen at the surface of large adenomatous polyps of the stomach.

In about 75 per cent of patients with carcinoma of the stomach the tumors are found in the distal third. The lymphatic flow from such tumors is in the direction of the subpyloric nodes and porta hepatis and along both curvatures. The tumor very rarely spreads to the pancreaticolineal nodes, in contrast to proximal and midstomach lesions. Celiac and pancreatic nodal involvement occurs from lesions in all areas. In addition to invasion of lymph nodes, gastric carcinoma invades local structures: the lower end of the esophagus by submucosal spread, the pancreas, the transverse colon, the peritoneum, and, rarely, the duodenum. Hematogenous spread results in pulmonary, pleural, liver, brain, and bone metastases.

CLINICAL MANIFESTATIONS (Table 100–1). Early carcinoma of the stomach is frequently asymptomatic. *Anorexia* and *weight loss* are nonspecific symptoms and not well correlated with the size of the tumor. *Early satiety,* particularly with linitis plastica; *bloating; dysphagia; epigastric distress;* or more severe epigastric boring pain may be later symptoms. *Vomiting* is commonly a later symptom that may be caused by pyloric obstruction but may occur with other levels of obstruction. Vomiting also occurs without obstruction and may be secondary to the motility disturbance that a fixed mass in the wall produces. The pain is similar to that of peptic ulcer in about one fourth of patients, particularly when the tumor has ulcerated. In most patients, however, the pain usually occurs after eating and is not relieved by food or antacids. Boring pain radiating to the back may indicate penetration of the tumor into the pancreas.

Dysphagia may occur with more proximal lesions, particularly when they have invaded the area around the cardioesophageal junction or spread submucosally to the esophagus, which is common in fundal lesions. Weakness and fatigue from *anemia* caused by chronic occult blood loss is common, although massive bleeding and hematemesis are unusual. Angina pectoris, congestive heart failure, and cerebral ischemia may occur because of the anemia. Perforation occurs in a small percentage of patients and can simulate peptic ulcer. When the tumor metastasizes, symptoms will depend upon organ involvement and may include jaundice, diarrhea, bone pain, cough, fever, hiccups, central nervous system disturbances, and abdominal bloating from ascites.

TABLE 100–1. ADENOCARCINOMA OF THE STOMACH

Associated With	Clinical Manifestations
Environment—geographical differences	Anorexia, early satiety, weight loss
Diet—? nitrosamines	Dysphagia, vomiting, weakness
Blood group A	Epigastric distress to severe, boring pain
Atrophic gastritis (pernicious anemia)	Anemia, occult blood in stools
Adenomatous polyps (> 2 cm)	Epigastric mass, signs of metastases
Subtotal resection for benign ulcer disease	Rare—Virchow's node, Blumer's shelf, Trousseau's syndrome, acanthosis nigricans

Physical examination during the early stages of gastric carcinoma may be completely unremarkable. Later there may be signs of weight loss and anemia. When the tumor has disseminated, hepatomegaly from metastases, jaundice, or ascites from peritoneal implants may be present. Splenomegaly may occur if the portal or splenic vein is invaded. A palpable *epigastric mass* is present in less than one half of patients and usually, but not always, indicates extensive involvement. Left supraclavicular adenopathy (Virchow's node), a nodular perirectal wall (Blumer's shelf), or umbilical nodules give evidence of metastatic spread.

Several extragastric signs may precede the detection of an underlying malignancy. These include recurrent thrombophlebitis (Trousseau's syndrome), acanthosis nigricans, a verrucous hyperpigmented elevated skin lesion involving primarily the flexor spaces of the body; neuromyopathy characterized by localized sensory and/or motor disturbances; or profound central nervous system involvement with abrupt onset of confusion, memory defects, hostility, or ataxia. More detailed descriptions of the paraneoplastic syndromes are contained in specific chapters in Part XIV.

Laboratory studies usually disclose iron deficiency or megaloblastic anemia if the tumor is associated with untreated pernicious anemia. *Occult blood in the stool,* even with a single determination, is present in about one half of the patients. Most patients have gastric acid present but in reduced amounts. A few have achlorhydria after maximal stimulation with pentagastrin. A few have hypersecretion, especially with antral tumors. Therefore the presence of acid does not ensure that carcinoma is not present. An ulcerating lesion with achlorhydria on maximal stimulation almost certainly indicates a malignant tumor; elevated carcinoembryonic antigen almost invariably means disseminated disease. Abnormalities in liver function, particularly a markedly elevated alkaline phosphatase and 5′nucleotidase, suggest liver metastases. Microangiopathic hemolytic anemia has been reported in several patients with gastric cancer. Rarely, protein-losing enteropathy occurs with ulcerated carcinomas of the stomach.

DIAGNOSIS. ***Roentgenologic Diagnosis.*** Most gastric cancers will be suspected on roentgenologic examination (Fig. 100–1). The standard upper gastrointestinal series has been refined to include barium contrast studies capable of detecting very small lesions. With the gastric mucosa covered by a thin layer of barium and distended with air or gas, multiple projections are taken, which outline almost the entire stomach surface. Refinement of technique can be accomplished by using high density barium, CO_2, simethicone for gas dispersion, and glucagon to induce gastroparesis. With such methods films showing fine detail may be produced and small mucosal lesions visualized.

The radiologist is usually able to define the characteristics of a benign versus malignant lesion and is on occasion even able to suggest a histologic diagnosis. For example, lymphoma of the stomach may be suspected by the extensive involvement, multiple shallow ulcerations, and giant rugal hypertrophy caused by infiltrative disease, and by the fact that the duodenum may be involved in the neoplastic process. A gastric ulcer often gives difficulty, but radiologic accuracy is in the range of 80 per cent. Characteristic radiographic signs that suggest a malignant lesion are the presence of an ulcer in a mass, irregular folds stopping short of the ulcer crater, and an irregular ulcer base. It is essential to determine the nature of the ulcer by endoscopy with biopsy and cytology when any doubt exists. Generally the location of an ulcer is not too important in determining malignancy. However, if the ulcer is in the fundus of the stomach, there is a higher index of suspicion; if it is within 1 cm of the pylorus it is almost always benign. Ulcers on the greater and lesser curvatures have about equal frequency of malignancy. Rigidity, loss of distensibility, unchanging contour, and irregular peristalsis are characteristic of a malignant lesion; when extensive infiltration from linitis plastica is present, a "leather bottle" appearance may result.

Endoscopy with Biopsy and Cytology. Fiberoptic endoscopy has increased the diagnostic yield over radiology alone and has been found to be accurate in 85 to 92 per cent of cases. When combined with biopsy and brush cytology, the diagnostic accuracy is in the range of 95 to 99 per cent in various series. About one half of early gastric cancers present as small ulcerations; some have slight elevation or depression of the adjacent mucosa. The next most common type is a small polyp. Appearance at endoscopy may be misleading. Directed tissue sampling techniques, such as forceps biopsy or brush or directed lavage cytology, should be used on any suspicious area whether it is raised, depressed, discolored, or ulcerated. With more advanced carcinoma a specific tissue diagnosis can also be achieved with high accuracy by directed forceps biopsy and cytology techniques. The use of endoscopy to diagnose malignancies of the stomach is described in greater detail in Ch. 95.

Other Techniques. Maximal gastrin-stimulated gastric acid determination defines achlorhydria. This is helpful in differentiating benign from malignant ulceration of the stomach but is less important now with fiberoptic endoscopy, biopsy, and cytology.

Immunologic tests for the detection of gastric malignancy have been described. Elevation of carcinoembryonic antigen (CEA) is a late finding in gastric carcinoma but can define

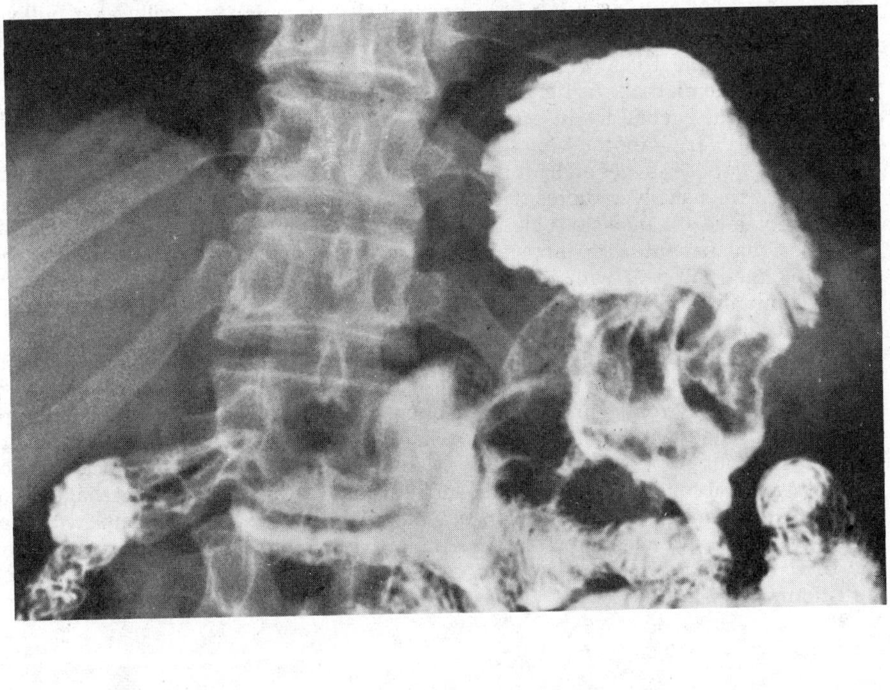

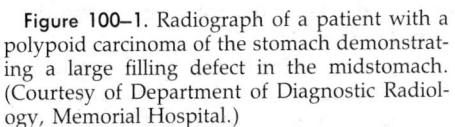

Figure 100–1. Radiograph of a patient with a polypoid carcinoma of the stomach demonstrating a large filling defect in the midstomach. (Courtesy of Department of Diagnostic Radiology, Memorial Hospital.)

metastatic disease before it is clinically evident. The immunologic detection of fetal sulfoglycoprotein antigen (FSA) in the gastric juice of patients with cancer has been noted. The sulfoglycoprotein of carcinomatous gastric juice often has blood group A glycoprotein, which has been associated with gastric cancer.

TREATMENT. At present *surgery* provides the only satisfactory curative treatment for gastric cancer. The high frequency of regional node metastases plays a major role in the choice of the surgical procedure and the results of various therapeutic efforts. When the tumor is localized in the distal portion of the stomach, the omentum as well as nodes in the region of the porta hepatis and the pancreatic head are dissected, and a generous subtotal gastrectomy is performed. For tumors in the pars media and the proximal stomach, total gastrectomy may be indicated to obtain an adequate margin and for dissection of the predictable lymphatic spread in all directions. Distal pancreatectomy and splenectomy are usually necessary. There is little doubt that operative mortality is greater after total gastrectomy than after subtotal resection, and the procedure should be avoided whenever possible.

With extensive bleeding or obstruction, a palliative limited subtotal gastric resection can be done even in the presence of residual cancer. Palliative total gastrectomy should almost never be done. Resection of recurrent cancer in the gastric remnant may be of considerable palliative value even when a cure is not obtained. Occasionally a long-term survival follows resection of recurrent disease.

Chemotherapy is often suggested for unresectable gastric adenocarcinoma in an effort to decrease symptoms and prolong survival. The most widely used drug has been 5-fluorouracil (5FU), with an overall partial response rate of 15 to 20 per cent. Other agents such as mitomycin C, doxorubicin (Adriamycin), and the various nitrosoureas have also been used as single agents with varying response.

Combinations of chemotherapeutic agents have shown some increased activity in obtaining responses in gastric cancer. Combinations currently under active investigation are methyl-1,3-cis-(2-chlorethyl)-1-nitrosourea (methyl-CCNU), vincristine (Oncovin), and 5FU; and mitomycin-C, 5FU, and cytosine arabinoside (Ara-C). The combination utilizing mitomycin-C, 5FU, and doxorubicin has shown significant activity with increased response rates to about 40 per cent and increased survival and is currently the treatment of choice.

Adjuvant chemotherapy following apparently curative surgery is an attractive concept for gastric carcinoma because of its high recurrence rate. Micrometastases are undoubtedly frequently present after surgery, and it has been postulated that chemotherapy might be most effective against such minimal disease. However, multiple trials with single agents have not been successful. Several trials using adjuvant chemotherapy with combinations of agents are in progress and may provide an answer to this very important question.

Radiation therapy is generally unsatisfactory, since gastric carcinomas are usually radioresistant. Occasionally palliation may be obtained for persistent bleeding, obstruction, or pain. An occasional patient with inoperable gastric carcinoma has had prolonged survival with radiation therapy. A controlled study combining 5FU with radiation therapy for inoperable metastatic disease resulted in a synergistic effect in both response rate and survival. Further studies are needed utilizing this combination modality.

Patients with gastrointestinal cancer frequently have complications associated with their disease or its treatment which require vigorous supportive treatment. Many aspects of the patients' general condition require consideration and treatment, including the management of infection; anemia; gastrointestinal bleeding; fluid and electrolyte loss secondary to vomiting, diarrhea, or fistula formation; disabling ascites; pain; and poor nutrition.

Total parenteral nutrition is being utilized more frequently to supply the daily caloric requirement of patients with gastric cancer. Preoperative and postoperative use of this modality enables patients to withstand the rigors of surgery and to tolerate more effectively the postoperative period, including the use of chemotherapy.

PROGNOSIS. The five-year survival rate depends upon whether or not adjacent lymph nodes contain cancer. The presence of perigastric lymph node metastases indicates a less than 15 per cent chance for survival. Early diagnosis plays a role in prognosis because a long period of time between the onset of cancer and its diagnosis favors lymphatic spread. In the Japanese studies, resection of gastric cancer limited to the mucosa and submucosa had almost a 70 per cent cure rate; when disease was limited to the mucosa, cure rate was 90 to 95 per cent. Linitis plastica and infiltrating lesions have a very poor prognosis as compared with polypoid or exophytic disease. Gastric cancer presenting as peptic ulcer has a five-year survival rate of 25 or 35 per cent, which is better than most other varieties except for the superficially spreading type.

PREVENTION. Until we learn more of the etiologic factors in gastric carcinoma we cannot practice primary prevention. We can only practice a limited degree of secondary prevention i.e., detect the disease at a very early stage to prevent its devastating consequences. The mass survey approach utilized in Japan is not practical in the United States because of the relatively low incidence of gastric cancer. Patients in high risk groups—those with achlorhydria, chronic atrophic gastritis, adenomatous polyps of the stomach, pernicious anemia, subtotal gastric resection, immunologic deficiencies, occult blood in the stool, or other symptoms—should be put under surveillance.

LYMPHOMA OF THE STOMACH

Primary lymphoma represents about 5 per cent of all primary malignant tumors of the stomach, and non-Hodgkin's lymphoma accounts for most of these. It is extremely rare for Hodgkin's disease (HD) to involve the stomach as a primary lesion. Patients with lymphoma are generally about a decade younger than those with carcinoma of the stomach, and males are affected more frequently. Pain is the most frequent symptom, and mild anemia is common owing to gastrointestinal bleeding (which on occasion can be massive). A palpable mass is the most common presenting physical finding. Studies of maximal stimulation of gastric acid secretion have not been done in a large group of patients, but achlorhydria seems to be unusual. Secondary lymphoma involving the stomach is common in the course of disseminated lymphoma but is difficult to diagnose.

Lymphoma of the stomach frequently presents radiographically as a bulky mass and less frequently as a diffusely infiltrating tumor—the most common form of secondary lymphoma—giving the appearance of large folds on upper gastrointestinal series, frequently associated with multiple nodular defects and ulcerations (Fig. 100–2). Lymphoma of the stomach often resembles superficially spreading carcinoma, linitis plastica, or solitary adenocarcinoma. Gastroscopy with directed biopsy and brush cytology gives a higher yield than was previously appreciated. Exophytic lesions provide a diagnosis in about 88 per cent of cases; the infiltrative type does not yield as high an accuracy.

Pseudolymphoma is a gastric lesion that may be confusing. This diffuse or discrete lesion is an atypical inflammatory response in the region of benign gastric ulcers. It is frequently difficult for the pathologist to differentiate pseudolymphoma from a true lymphoma.

In patients with lymphoma of the stomach there is a significant incidence of nontumorous lesions such as stress ulcer, hemorrhagic gastritis, and monilial gastritis. Therefore in such patients with upper gastrointestinal bleeding or other symptoms referable to the stomach, it is important that a careful diagnostic approach be undertaken to determine the possible nontumor cause of the sign or symptom.

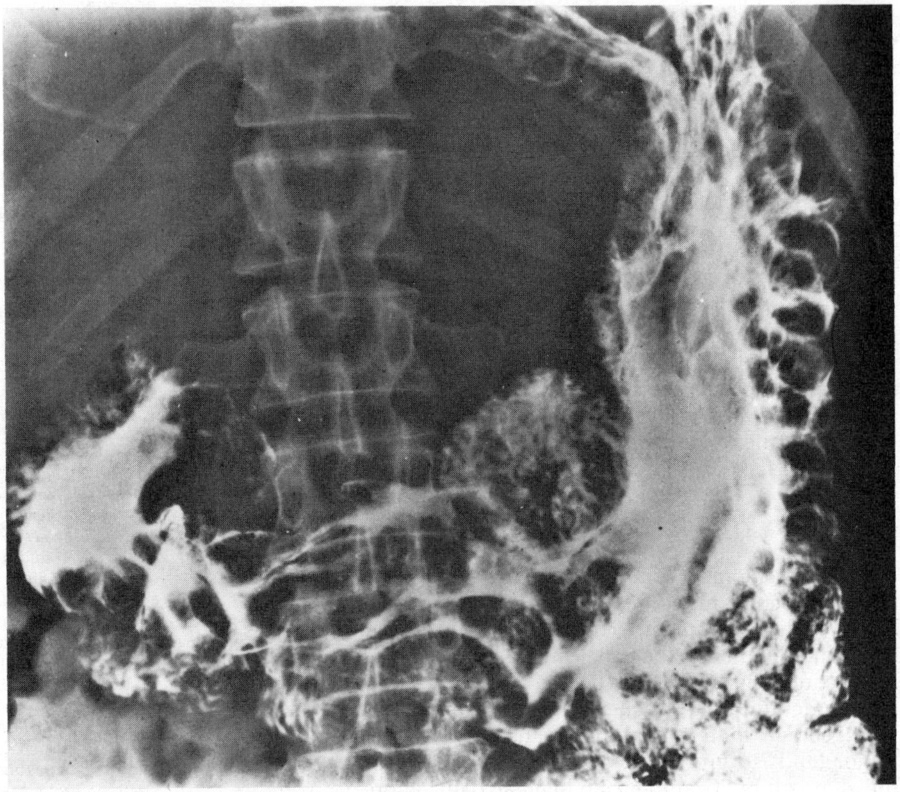

Figure 100–2. Radiograph of a patient with lymphoma of the stomach demonstrating the very large polypoid-appearing folds throughout the stomach. (Courtesy of Department of Diagnostic Radiology, Memorial Hospital.)

Treatment of primary lymphoma of the stomach is usually surgical resection followed by 3600 to 4000 rads of radiotherapy, particularly if lymph nodes are involved. Some have advocated radiotherapy alone because of the marked sensitivity of lymphoma to radiation. If lymphoma involves the stomach secondarily, radiotherapy or chemotherapy or both are indicated. The five-year survival following surgery for primary lymphoma of the stomach is in the range of 50 per cent for non-Hodgkin's lymphoma and less for HD, suggesting that HD is already disseminated when initially found in the stomach. The best prognosis for primary tumors occurs with small lesions confined to the stomach, differentiated into tumor follicles without lymph node involvement and with only superficial infiltration of the wall.

OTHER MALIGNANT TUMORS OF THE STOMACH

Leiomyosarcoma of the stomach represents about 1 per cent of gastric cancers and may present with a large intramural mass with central ulceration. Systemic symptoms are minimal, but massive bleeding or a palpable mass of which the patient is aware may be the presenting complaints. The tumor may be slow growing; five-year survival following resection is in the range of 50 per cent. Metastases to the liver and nodes are common, but these patients have a better prognosis than those with other metastatic tumors. Liposarcoma, fibrosarcoma, myxosarcoma, and neurogenic sarcoma are extremely rare and present with symptoms similar to those of leiomyosarcoma. Neurogenic sarcoma can be associated with von Recklinghausen's disease.

Metastatic disease to the stomach from other sites is not common but may simulate primary gastric cancer. Malignant melanoma and breast and lung carcinomas are the most frequent offenders. In breast cancer the metastatic lesions may be ulcerative, of linitis plastica type, or polypoid.

LEIOMYOMAS AND BENIGN TUMORS

Leiomyomas are commonly found at postmortem examination but are rarely of clinical significance. They occur equally in men and women, and are usually found in the midportion and antrum of the stomach. They may grow toward the mucosa, encroach on the lumen, and cause mucosal effacement and secondary ulceration. They may grow in the direction of the serosa, producing a mass that is predominantly extrinsic. Simultaneous inward and outward growth results in a dumbbell shape. These are also characteristic of leiomyosarcomas, and differentiation on x-ray or gastroscopy is difficult. Bleeding is common and epigastric pain may simulate peptic ulcer disease. On roentgen examination the findings are usually an intramural filling defect with or without secondary ulceration. Gastroscopic examination reveals effaced but normal mucosa overlying the mass. Central ulceration may be seen.

Asymptomatic leiomyomas need not be removed while symptomatic lesions are excised locally.

Neurofibroma occasionally associated with von Recklinghausen's disease, neuroma, lymphangioma, ganglioneuroma, lipoma, carcinoid, and hamartoma associated with Peutz-Jeghers syndrome all may involve the stomach. About 10 per cent of hamartomas of the stomach and duodenum in Peutz-Jeghers syndrome become malignant.

ADENOMAS

Adenomas of the stomach are relatively rare lesions. They occur in 1 to 2 per cent of patients with achlorhydria but may be single or multiple in as high as 20 per cent of patients with pernicious anemia. They are more common in the body and antrum. Most polyps of the stomach are hyperplastic, not neoplastic, and do not become malignant. Villous adenomas are rare. Adenomatous polyps are the usual neoplastic type of polyp. These tumors are more frequent in men than in women and are generally seen in patients over 50. Well over 90 per cent of patients with adenoma of the stomach are achlorhydric. The lesion may be sessile or pedunculated with a well defined stalk composed of a thin strand of connective tissue covered by an epithelial layer.

Bleeding, dyspepsia, and nausea are the most common symptoms of gastric polyposis, but most patients are asymptomatic. The diagnosis may be strongly suspected when a rounded smooth defect in the stomach on upper gastrointestinal series or a mass covered by mucosa with or without a stalk is detected by x-ray or endoscopy.

The size of polyps strongly influences management. It is rare for a polyp under 2 cm to show malignant change. In view of their potential for malignancy (present and future) sessile lesions larger than 2 cm or polyps of any size causing significant symptoms should be removed. Pedunculated polyps can now be safely removed by cautery-snare technique via the fiberoptic endoscope. For sessile polyps of more than 2 cm diameter, a segmental gastric resection may be necessary to rule out carcinoma. If carcinoma is diagnosed histologically at the time of surgery, subtotal gastric resection should be done. Diffuse or multiple polyposis involving a large segment of stomach may mask frank carcinoma. Subtotal gastrectomy may be done, although patients with multiple gastric polyps have been followed for as long as 20 years without developing difficulties.

TUMORS OF THE DUODENUM

Adenocarcinoma of the duodenum is very rare but is more common than lymphoma, which, in turn, arises more commonly in the jejunum and ileum. The second and third portions of the duodenum are the usual sites of adenocarcinoma. Cancer in the duodenal bulb is exceedingly rare. Adenocarcinoma of the duodenum more frequently affects men and develops at a younger age than carcinoma of the stomach or colon. The tumor tends to grow into the lumen or to invade the wall of the duodenum. Cramping abdominal pain, anorexia, weight loss, vomiting, and melena are common. Jaundice or fever may result from obstruction of the ampulla of Vater or the common bile duct when the carcinoma involves the second portion of the duodenum. The tumor may simulate benign postbulbar ulceration. The diagnosis is usually made by radiologic examination and confirmed by endoscopy. Pancreaticoduodenectomy is necessary. Five-year survival ranges between 4 and 15 per cent.

Lymphoma, leiomyosarcoma, carcinoid, metastatic cancer, and benign tumors may involve the duodenum, and these are discussed in more detail in Ch. 106. In general, these lesions are manifested as an intramural and submucosal mass with the exception of lymphoma and metastatic cancer, which frequently are exophytic and ulcerate. Any tumor, benign or malignant, may occur in a diverticulum at the descending portion of the duodenum. Aberrant pancreatic tissue may produce a submucosal filling defect in the duodenum, which may resemble a neoplastic lesion. Also, hyperplasia or adenoma of Brunner's glands may produce multiple polypoid defects in the duodenal bulb and is frequently associated with hypersecretion, duodenal ulcer and, rarely, Zollinger-Ellison syndrome. A prominent ampulla of Vater may resemble a neoplastic lesion radiographically. Endoscopy may be necessary to clarify the situation.

Brooks JJ, Enterline HT: Primary gastric lymphomas. A clinicopathologic study of 58 cases with long-term follow-up and literature review. Cancer 51: 701, 1983. *A large series of primary gastric lymphomas with long-term follow-up (average 12.8 years). Five- and ten-year survival rates were 57 and 46 per cent, respectively. Statistically significant prognostic variables were smaller tumor size, superficial mural invasion (submucosal only), and pathologic stage I disease.*

Correa P: Epidemiology of gastric cancer and its precursor lesions. *In* Decosse JJ, Sherlock P (eds.): Gastrointestinal Cancer I. The Hague, Martinus Nijhoff, 1981, pp 119–130. *A very thorough review of the epidemiologic aspects of gastric cancer and its precursors. The role of diet and nitrate intake is evaluated.*

Correa P: Chronic gastritis as a precursor of cancer. *In* Sherlock P, Morson BC, Barbara L, Veronesi U (eds.): Precancerous Lesions of the Gastrointestinal Tract. New York, Raven Press, 1983, pp 145–153. *This fine review discusses evidence from clinical and epidemiologic studies indicating that before gastric cancer develops, most patients go through a lengthy and complex series of mucosal changes, which constitute the precursor status. These histologic changes are reviewed.*

Dahm K: Cancer of the gastric stump. *In* Sherlock P, Morson BC, Barbara L, Veronesi U (eds.): Precancerous Lesions of the Gastrointestinal Tract. New York, Raven Press, 1983, pp 165–186. *Cancer is a late complication in the gastric stump in patients undergoing subtotal gastric resection for benign ulcer. This review discusses etiology, pathology, diagnosis and surveillance recommendations. Experimental observations suggest that duodenal or jejunal gastric reflux contributes to the carcinogenic sequence.*

Decker W, Tytgat GN: Diagnostic accuracy of fiberendoscopy in detection of upper intestinal malignancy. A follow-up analysis. Gastroenterology 73:710, 1977. *Review of fiberoptic endoscopy studies in 1005 patients revealed overall correct endoscopic interpretation in 92.7 per cent. Of 135 patients with gastric malignancy the diagnosis was correct in 98.8 per cent largely because of the number of biopsies (>10) obtained in gastric ulcer patients.*

Diehl JJ, Hermann RE, Cooperman AM, Hoerr SO: Gastric carcinoma. A ten-year review. Ann Surg 198:9, 1983. *This presents data on 164 patients with gastric adenocarcinoma during the period 1970–1980. Despite the routine use of fiberoptic endoscopy the majority of gastric cancers were advanced at diagnosis; their prognosis of these cancers remains discouraging.*

Dupont JB, Lee JR, Burton GR, Cohn I: Adenocarcinoma of the stomach: Review of 1,497 cases. Cancer 41:941, 1978. *A 25-year series demonstrated resectability rate of 48 per cent. Five-year survival was 7.4 per cent overall and varied from 2.0 per cent after esophagogastrectomy to 22.1 per cent after radical subtotal gastrectomy and 30.3 per cent for localized disease.*

Macdonald JS, Schein PS, Wooley PV, et al.: 5-Fluorouracil, Adriamycin and mitomycin-C (FAM) combination chemotherapy for advanced gastric cancer. Ann Intern Med 93:533, 1980. *This combination showed 42 per cent response rate in 62 patients.*

Ming SC: Gastric carcinoma. A pathological classification. Cancer 39:2475, 1977. *The classification described provides a simple basis for evaluation of various aspects of gastric cancer.*

Nelson RS, Lanza FL: The endoscopic diagnosis of gastric lymphoma. Gastrointest Endosc 21:123, 1975. *Describes characteristic endoscopic picture of malignant lymphoma of stomach with its multicentric masses and central volcano ulcer.*

Phillips JC, Lindsay JW, Kendall JA: Gastric leiomyosarcoma: Roentgenologic and clinical findings. Am J Dig Dis 15:239, 1970. *The typical clinical and roentgenologic findings are reviewed in 11 patients. The tumors were predominantly exogastric lesions. Ulcerations were present in five cases. Hemorrhage, fever, abdominal pain and a palpable abdominal mass are helpful clinical points.*

Sakita T, Oguro Y, Takasu S, Fukutomi H, Miwa T, Yoshimori M: Observations on the healing of ulcerations in early gastric cancer. Gastroenterology 60:835, 1971. *Significant healing was observed in 71 per cent of malignant gastric ulcers found in a group of 122 cases of early gastric cancer. A plea for careful endoscopic follow-up of gastric ulcer is made.*

Winawer SJ, Posner G, Lightdale CJ, Sherlock P, Melamed M, Fortner JG: Endoscopic diagnosis of advanced gastric cancer. Factors influencing yield. Gastroenterology 69:1183, 1975. *Study in 50 patients using forward viewing panendoscopy. Diagnostic yield was higher for exophytic lesions than for infiltrative tumor, and directed brush cytology alone was more productive than directed biopsy alone. Combination of infiltrative character and location in antrum or cardia often resulted in nondiagnostic biopsy and cytology specimens.*

101. DISORDERS OF GASTROINTESTINAL MOTILITY

Sidney Phillips

Normal Motility of Stomach, Small Intestine, and Colon

MOTILITY AND OTHER FUNCTIONS OF THE BOWEL. Motility is a general term that embraces all movements of the gastrointestinal tract and its contents. As such, the subject encompasses contractions of smooth muscle, the intraluminal pressures thereby developed, and the transit of contents that results from gradients of pressure. Movements of chyme along the bowel are modified by the actions of specialized segments of intestine, the sphincters, and the whole is integrated by neural and humoral levels of control. Motility is best understood teleologically, i.e., as a process that facilitates the other, more fundamental functions of the gut.

After solid food is chewed and moistened by saliva, it moves rapidly, in small boluses, into the stomach. Acting as a simple conduit, the esophagus is well served by strong bands of smooth muscle, integrated toward propulsive peristaltic motility, that push solid food to the stomach, even against the forces of gravity. Moreover, the lower and upper esophageal sphincters prevent acid-peptic reflux from corroding the esophageal mucosa and entering the bronchial tree. (Ch. 97 covers esophageal function and disease in detail.)

The stomach has three major functions: (1) accommodating meals of variable volumes, (2) grinding of solid food into small particles, and (3) the finely tuned process of gastric emptying. This last function is an important control of the load of chyme presented to the small bowel for digestion and absorption. Thus, the gastric fundus exhibits "receptive relaxation," a decrease in basal tone that is mediated by vagal reflexes and that reduces pressure in the body and fundus during a meal. Receptive relaxation provides accommodation for that meal, and food remains in the stomach for acid-peptic digestion to proceed. Later in the postcibal period basal tone returns; this increase in intraluminal pressure facilitates emptying of the liquid phase of mixed meals. Meanwhile, the antrum has developed strong, rhythmic peristaltic contractions that propel food to the prepyloric antrum. However, in the digestive phase, the pylorus allows little emptying of solids; rather, solids are ground against the terminal antrum, triturated, and retropelled to the proximal antrum for another cycle of grinding. Only later does the antrum allow small solids (<1 mm) to pass through. By a combination of these forces and the integrated action of duodenal musculature, pressure gradients are developed whereby gastric emptying is controlled very precisely. Sensitive receptors in the duodenal mucosa respond to intraluminal fat and hydrogen ions or hypertonicity of the contents, setting in motion a feedback mechanism that further brakes emptying. In this way, contents entering the duodenum are prepared for their subsequent contact with pancreaticobiliary secretions. These controls are disturbed most dramatically when the pylorus is destroyed surgically; dumping syndromes or gastric stasis may be unfortunate, and all too common, sequelae.

Transit through the small bowel is steady but slow, a series of gentle to and fro movements of chyme, well suited to the mixing of food with digestive enzymes. Further, exposure of digestive products to the absorptive cells is maximized. Moreover, a normal pattern of motility is important in maintaining relative sterility of the small bowel. Disordered motility leads to bacterial overgrowth ("blind loop syndrome") and a malabsorption syndrome (see Ch. 103).

The colon can be thought of as two functional entities. The proximal half dehydrates its contents, removing salt and water very effectively. In addition, it stores feces, which undergo bacterial biotransformation by the fecal flora. Some components of dietary fiber can be digested only in this way. The motor activity of this segment subserves these functions of storing and mixing via its back and forth movements and mixing waves (haustra). The distal colon and rectum store formed stools until evacuation is convenient. The necessary propulsion and excretion are achieved by coordination of peristaltic contractions and voluntary elevations of intra-abdominal pressure. The anal sphincters relax in concert with these propulsive forces.

GASTROINTESTINAL SPHINCTERS. In physiologic terms, a sphincter is an area of high intraluminal pressure within the bowel. Sphincters separate areas of lower pressure and thus are able to modify the flow of intestinal contents. Sphincters respond to appropriate stimuli, distention or changes of pressure within the adjacent bowel, by either tightening or relaxing. Sphincters may be recognized anatomically by the presence of specialized bands of muscle (upper esophageal sphincter) or may be associated with no clearly defined or unique tissue (lower esophageal sphincter) (see Ch. 97). The pylorus has a concentrated bundle of circular muscle characteristic of a sphincter, but it contracts and relaxes in concert with adjacent bowel. Functionally, the pylorus is not clearly distinct from the antrum or duodenum and can be considered as having only certain characteristics of a "sphincter." The ileocecal junction has the appearance of a valve but behaves more like a true sphincter. One of its important roles is to prevent reflux of fecal flora into the small intestine. The anal sphincters are well developed anatomically and function as true sphincters.

ELECTRICAL AND MECHANICAL CORRELATES OF MOTILITY. Contractions of smooth muscle cells are determined by the state of polarization-depolarization of the cell membranes, contraction occurring only when action potentials ("spikes") are superimposed on an appropriate background level of depolarization. Throughout the stomach and intestines a baseline fluctuation of basal electrical activity is present in the muscularis, as measured by extracellular electrodes embedded in the muscle layers. This omnipresent "basic electrical rhythm" (BER, slow wave or pacesetter potential) originates at specific sites ("pacemakers") located in the proximal stomach, proximal duodenum, and mid-colon. The potentials so generated, at 3 per minute in stomach, 12 per minute in duodenum, and 6 per minute in the colon, spread distally along muscle bundles, thus establishing a maximal frequency at which the smooth muscle can contract. In other words, antral pacesetters of 3 per minute establish this as the maximal rate of antral contractions, and the corresponding rate in the proximal duodenum is 12 per minute. In the small bowel this rate slows progressively, in a caudad direction along the bowel, so that the terminal ileal rate is 8 to 9 per minute. When spike discharges are present on any slow wave complex, adjacent smooth muscle contracts and a pressure-sensitive probe will record an increase of intraluminal pressure. Circumstances in the colon are more complex. The major rate for the BER is 6 per minute, but another, slower pattern (3 per minute) can be seen. The colonic pacemaker is located in the transverse colon, and pacesetter potentials spread distally and proximally. Such a system may well provide the basis for to and fro movement in the colon, allowing storage, desiccation, and fermentation in the cecum. The local frequency of pacesetter potentials establishes the maximal rate at which the bowel can contract at that locus. However, not all pacesetter potentials have action potentials; in other words, the smooth muscle may contract at its maximal rate, not contract at all, or exhibit any intermediate level of activity. The state of fasting or feeding is a major determinant of the degree of muscular activity that actually occurs.

FASTING AND POSTCIBAL MOTILITY. The fasting bowel is not quiescent but exhibits cycles of contractility which are interrupted by food. With a periodicity of approximately two hours, an intense burst of motor activity begins in the stomach, in which every pacesetter potential has an action potential associated with it. Thus, the antrum contracts at its maximal rate of 3 per minute, and contractions are uniformly powerful. This wave of activity passes caudally through duodenum, jejunum, and ileum. The velocity of this "front" is such that on reaching the terminal ileum another "front" (or migrating motor complex) originates in the stomach. At any single locus, a cycle of activity lasts approximately two hours during fasting, each intense burst of motility lasting 5 to 15 minutes. The remainder of the two-hour cycle is taken up with quiescence (lasting about one hour—"phase I"), intermittent contractile activity (about 45 minutes—"phase II"), and then the migrating complex ("phase III"). The migrating complex has been described by Code as the "interdigestive housekeeper." The function proposed is one of sweeping secretions, desquamated cells, and food residue distally in preparation for another meal. Food interrupts the cycle, replacing it with the "fed pattern" of intermittent contractions (similar to phase II) that last for four to ten hours. Whereas transit is rapid in phase III of fasting, it is slower after a meal.

CONTROL OF GASTROINTESTINAL MOTILITY. The cholinergic system has important control of the proximal gut. Vagal denervation impairs receptive relaxation of the stomach and, by reducing gastric accommodation to large volumes, speeds the emptying of liquids. Vagal denervation also diminishes the important duodenal "brake" on gastric emptying. On the other hand, antral contractions are also weakened by vagotomy, and hence the grinding and emptying of solids are reduced. The sympathetic nervous system becomes more important in the distal bowel, particularly in the coordination of rectal contractions and relaxation of the anal sphincters. A third autonomic system ("noncholinergic-nonadrenergic") also exists, although the exact neurotransmitters responsible for it are as yet unclear. Among the candidates are ATP ("purinergic"), dopamine-like compounds, and the gastrointestinal hormones (neuropeptides such as vasoactive intestinal polypeptide, neurotensin, substance P, enkephalins). The coordination between neural and humoral control of motility is still under study. Some gastrointestinal hormones or neuropeptides may act locally on adjacent epithelial cells or nervous tissue, exhibiting a so-called "paracrine" function.

A number of gastrointestinal hormones can alter gastrointestinal motility, but whether they have physiologic roles is unclear. Cholecystokinin-pancreozymin contracts the gallbladder and intestinal smooth muscle. Other stimulating hormones include gastrin and motilin, and inhibitory hormones include secretin, glucagon, vasoactive intestinal polypeptide, and gastric inhibitory polypeptide.

CLINICAL ASSESSMENT OF GASTROINTESTINAL MOTILITY. Measuring the rate of movement of barium suspensions is the traditional index of motility, but not a very satisfactory one. Barium suspensions are dense, behave as liquids, and hence are inappropriate for determining the transit of water or solids. Moreover, barium, unlike food, lacks the effect of nutrients. As a result, the study of barium transit is helpful only when gross abnormalities are present. Similar criticism pertains to the gastric emptying of a saline "meal" (saline load test). Some have evaluated the transit of barium mixed with food ("barium hamburger"). This technique is difficult to quantify and has not been widely used. Gastric emptying of solids and liquids can be measured by external gamma camera techniques, using suitably labeled markers of the liquid and solid phases of "meals." These approaches are likely to gain more clinical acceptance in the future. The measurement of intraluminal pressures by transducers or water-filled catheters is used in research studies but has gained little clinical acceptance except in the esophagus.

Christensen J: Motility of the colon. *In* Johnson LR (ed.): Physiology of the Gastrointestinal Tract. New York, Raven Press, 1981. *Complete review with 185 references of the basic mechanisms; includes some material on pathophysiology of disease.*

Kelly KA: Motility of the stomach and gastroduodenal junction. *In* Johnson LR (ed.): Physiology of the Gastrointestinal Tract. New York, Raven Press, 1981. *Comprehensive review of the physiology of the region; contains all major references to basic mechanisms.*

Wingate DL: Backwards and forwards with the migrating complex. Dig Dis Sci 26:641, 1981. *Complete historical and scientific review of small intestinal motility with emphasis on the normal physiology. Referenced extensively.*

Disorders of Gastroduodenal Motility

PATHOPHYSIOLOGY OF VOMITING

Vomiting is the major manifestation of abnormal gastroduodenal motility; it is the forceful expulsion from the mouth of material from the upper gastrointestinal tract. When projectile, the symptom suggests mechanical obstruction, but less disturbed progression of chyme may produce effortless regurgitation. Vomiting has both central causes, which are discussed in Ch. 93, and peripheral causes, e.g., intra-abdominal stimulation of the vomiting reflex (e.g., peritonitis) or mechanical obstruction of the upper gut (e.g., pyloric stenosis).

Vomiting depletes the body of fluids, electrolytes, and hydrochloric acid and leads to dehydration, alkalosis, and secondary hypokalemia. The composition of gastric juice varies from hypochlorhydria (e.g., obstructing carcinomas) to hyperchlorhydria (e.g., Zollinger-Ellison syndrome), and the metabolic disturbances of vomiting vary accordingly. In its severest form, alkalosis secondary to vomiting causes a progressive rise of blood pH and plasma bicarbonate and severe hypochloremia. In an attempt to compensate for losses of hydrogen ion, the kidneys excrete bicarbonate and the pH of urine rises. Urinary loss of water and sodium, along with bicarbonate, exaggerates the dehydration of gastric losses and the concomitant decreased oral intake. If the kidney excreted enough $NaHCO_3$ to balance losses of HCl, acid-base balance would be maintained, but at a perilous cost—severe depletion of extracellular fluid (ECF) volume. The renal tubules exchange sodium for potassium and, when potassium is depleted, for hydrogen ions. Treatment for gastric alkalosis requires replacement of lost chloride and sodium, with proportionately more chloride than sodium in reference to their normal ratios in ECF. Replacing potassium loss may require up to 100 to 200 mEq of KCl intravenously per day if urine output is adequate. Intravenous KCl should generally not be given at a rate exceeding 10 mEq per hour for this type of parenteral replacement.

When loss is less severe, replacement therapy is achieved orally, allowing the kidneys to correct acid-base and electrolyte imbalance. Antiemetic drugs such as prochlorperazine (Compazine) or chlorpromazine (Thorazine) are useful, but extrapyramidal side effects should be monitored if the dose exceeds 30 to 50 mg daily. Dimenhydrinate (Dramamine) and trimethobenzamide (Tigan) suppress the vomiting chemoreceptors and are less toxic but also probably less effective as antiemetics. Delta-9-tetrahydrocannabinal (THC) has been shown to be effective in reducing the nausea and vomiting that accompany cancer chemotherapy. Metoclopramide (Reglan) speeds gastric emptying and has gained wide acceptance as an antiemetic. The drug, though correcting impaired gastric emptying, does not augment normal emptying.

Kassirer JP, Schwartz WB: The response of normal man to selective depletion of hydrochloric acid: Factors in the genesis of persistent gastric alkalosis. Am J Med 40:10, 1966. *This classic study, in which gastric acid was removed from healthy volunteers by gastric aspiration, observes the development of alkalosis and the effects of treatment. It still forms the basis of our understanding of this metabolic disorder.*

PYLORIC STENOSIS: GASTRIC OUTLET OBSTRUCTION

ETIOLOGY AND PATHOGENESIS. A transient syndrome occurs when acute peptic ulcers involve the pyloric canal. A chronic, cicatricial condition often complicates recurrent ulceration in the pyloroduodenal region, and vomiting may be severe. Carcinoma is also a cause of gastric outlet obstruction. In infants, hypertrophy of pyloric muscle may occur, leading to severe degrees of obstruction. Hypertrophic pyloric stenosis occurs rarely in adults, although in later life it is difficult to distinguish a specific "hypertrophic syndrome" from the multiple, variable manifestations of chronic peptic ulcer disease.

Congenital Hypertrophic Pyloric Stenosis

INCIDENCE. This lesion occurs in 2 to 4 infants per 1000 live births, is more common in firstborn children, and four to five times more frequent in males. A familial incidence is reported, as is an increased incidence in twins. Some degree of muscle spasm is present, since partial relaxation may occur during anesthesia or with the use of anticholinergic drugs.

CLINICAL MANIFESTATIONS. The infant usually seems normal at birth, but regurgitation is noted at one to three weeks post partum and rapidly progresses to projectile vomiting, dehydration, and weight loss but without anorexia. The vomitus contains no bile. Gastric peristalsis may be visible, and the hypertrophied pylorus may be palpable in the epigastrum.

DIAGNOSIS. The radiologic appearances are characteristic: an elongated, narrow, pylorus surrounded by the hypertrophied muscle, which may be seen as a soft tissue shadow. In adults, the pyloric region may protrude proximally into the antrum, resembling a uterine cervix at endoscopy.

TREATMENT. After correction of acid-base and electrolyte imbalance, a trial of anticholinergics and small feedings is justified in milder examples, but surgical correction will usually be necessary. Pyloromyotomy in the fashion of Ramstedt is performed; a simple longitudinal incision of the circular muscle suffices, with an excellent prognosis. In adults, resection of the pylorus and distal antrum with vagotomy is usually advisable.

POSTOPERATIVE DISORDERS

Surgical therapies for peptic ulcer disease often result in profound alterations of the finely tuned process of gastric emptying (see also Ch. 99). The most radical surgical procedures for peptic ulceration resect the antrum and pylorus, thus removing the physical effect of the distal stomach in the grinding of solid food, as well as removing the pyloric sieve. The lesser procedure of total gastric vagotomy is usually combined with pyloroplasty or gastroenterostomy ("drainage"), since reduced antral grinding in the vagotomized stomach leads to retention of solids. If the "drainage" maneuver is less than adequate, stagnation of solids may occur, although, at the same time, gastric emptying of liquids may be excessively rapid. This "dumping" of liquids is readily explicable by impairment of vagally innervated receptive relaxation of the proximal stomach, a process that permits storage of volume without undue elevation of intragastric pressure. Thus, after gastric surgery many disorders of gastric emptying are encountered, including rapid emptying of liquids (dumping syndrome), reduced emptying of solids (gastroparesis), or a combination of both. Certain mechanical complications of gastroenterostomy are also recognized, including obstruction of afferent jejunal loops and intussusception of jejunal limbs into the gastric remnant. The least traumatic surgical procedure, proximal gastric vagotomy, reduces gastric hypersecretion by denervation of the parietal cells alone. Innervation of the antrum and pylorus being preserved, gastric emptying is minimally affected.

Diagnostic steps for the patient with postoperative problems include a careful history, which must determine the exact temporal relationship of symptoms to meals, degree of nausea, nature of vomitus, and ability to handle liquid or solid diet. Barium meal examination is often unhelpful, testing as it does only the emptying of a dense liquid without nutrient content. However, failure to empty some barium by 30 minutes or retention of most barium at six hours signals a severe abnormality. Endoscopy may reveal fasting retention of foods or solid masses (bezoars) in the stomach, and is useful to exclude mechanical obstruction. This common and confusing syndrome may be better evaluated in the future by the use of γ-labeled mixed meals monitored by external gamma cameras, thus allowing selective evaluation of emptying patterns for labeled liquids and solids.

Dumping Syndrome

DEFINITION, CLINICAL FEATURES, AND INCIDENCE. This symptom complex of sweating, weakness with orthostatic features, tachycardia, and sometimes diarrhea following meals, occurs transiently in one third or more of patients after gastric surgery. Although most common and severe after gastric resection and gastroenterostomy (Billroth II), it may complicate any operation for peptic ulceration. Symptoms appear as soon after surgery as patients begin a regular diet. Although usually subsiding by 3 to 12 months after surgery, symptoms may persist and be debilitating. Liquid meals, especially those containing large amounts of carbohydrate, are most likely to evoke symptoms. Patients learn that recumbency minimizes symptoms and often discover that avoidance of sugars and desserts helps.

ETIOLOGY AND PATHOGENESIS. No other syndrome in gastroenterology has received more scrutiny and yet yielded so little uniform information as to its cause and rational treatment. Hypovolemia caused by pooling of interstitial fluid in the gut (as a result of uncontrolled entry of hyperosmolar fluids into the small bowel), hypoglycemia, and hormonal imbalance have received most attention. Among the humoral agents incriminated are the gastrointestinal hormones serotonin and neurotensin. The symptoms can be mimicked in some patients by depletion of extracellular volumes (and corrected by volume expansion), by hypoglycemia, and by distention of a balloon in the small intestine.

DIAGNOSIS. The diagnosis is established by the characteristic history and the exclusion of other diseases likely to produce similar symptoms. Radiology and endoscopy of the upper gastrointestinal tract are required to rule out organic or mechanical problems.

TREATMENT. Reassurance that the symptoms will subside with time will often be sufficient treatment. Patients should be advised to eat small meals, separating fluids from the more solid components of major meals. Lying down after large meals may help, as will avoidance of sweetened drinks and desserts. The prognosis is good with regard to major incapacitation, although minor symptoms may continue indefinitely if certain combinations of diet and activity are pursued.

Gastroparesis and Bezoars

DEFINITION AND PATHOPHYSIOLOGY. Many patients demonstrate mild degrees of gastric retention of solids after gastric surgery, although few (<10 per cent) have major problems. Motility studies reveal diminished phase III activity ("motor fronts") in the stomach but normal cyclic activity in the small bowel. However, the degree to which motility is impaired is not correlated closely with clinical manifestations, and individual susceptibility of patients is still unexplained.

CLINICAL MANIFESTATIONS. Postprandial fullness, nausea, and vomiting are the major features. Occasionally, solid material may completely obstruct the stoma or the esophagus. The most important consequence, however, is superficial ulceration of the stomach, which often bleeds.

DIAGNOSIS. Bezoars are detected by barium meal examination or endoscopy. The latter procedure has additional therapeutic potential, since boluses can be broken up mechanically and washed into the small intestine or removed by gastric lavage. Barium studies reveal intraluminal filling defects, often of massive dimensions.

TREATMENT. Physical disruption of bezoars by endoscopy, repeated gastric lavage, or both will be helpful. Chemical disruption by papain or cellulase has been successful also. Patients should then be advised to chew their food well and avoid large amounts of raw fruit and vegetables. Metoclopramide can accelerate the delayed emptying of solids after gastric surgery, although most studies report only short-term benefits. Metoclopramide (10 mg) or bethanechol (5 mg) has been shown experimentally to stimulate gastric contractions and to speed emptying of solids.

PROGNOSIS. In general, dietary measures and gradual recovery of gastric contractile function can be expected to alleviate symptoms. In some patients, however, a permanent change in eating patterns is required.

Intussusception

Jejunal intussusception into the stomach may occur after Billroth II gastric resection or, less often, after gastroenterostomy. Although it is sometimes asymptomatic, pain and gastric outlet obstruction may result. The radiologic picture of a "coiled spring" filling defect and the endoscopic appearances are characteristic. When intussusception is severe, surgical correction is required.

Malagelada JR: Physiological basis and clinical significance of gastric emptying disorders. Dig Dis Sci 24:657, 1979. *Review of gastroparesis, postsurgical and diabetic, including pathophysiology, diagnosis, and treatment.*

Meyer JH: Chronic morbidity after ulcer surgery. *In* Sleisenger MH, Fordtran JS (eds.): Gastrointestinal Disease. 3rd ed. Philadelphia, W. B. Saunders Company, 1983, p 757. *Comprehensive review of all major problems seen after all types of gastric surgery. Includes pathophysiology, clinical features, and treatment; contains 117 references.*

GASTROPARESIS DIABETICORUM

DEFINITION AND INCIDENCE. Severely impaired gastric emptying without evidence of mechanical obstruction is a well recognized complication of diabetes mellitus. It is unknown whether lesser degrees of gastric stasis are responsible for milder symptoms and the variable control of blood sugar so common in diabetics with longstanding disease.

PATHOGENESIS AND CLINICAL FEATURES. The cause is unknown, but autonomic denervation of the proximal gut seems likely. Patients may be of any age and either sex, and are usually "juvenile-onset" diabetics whose disease is of more than ten years' duration. Retinopathy, nephropathy, and other complications are common. The pathophysiologic features are an absence of phase III activity "fronts" in the distal stomach, with the motor pattern of the small bowel being normal. Nausea, vomiting, poor and variable control of blood sugar levels, and weight loss are the major presenting symptoms. Esophageal reflux, esophagitis, and even repeated episodes of Mallory-Weiss syndrome from vigorous vomiting may be seen.

DIAGNOSIS. The clinical picture is characteristic, but mechanical obstruction must be excluded by radiology and upper gastrointestinal endoscopy. Fluoroscopy may suggest reduced antral contractions or display retained food and secretions.

TREATMENT AND PROGNOSIS. Dietary management with soft foods well cooked and chewed should be instituted, since pharmacologic maneuvers provide little long-term benefit. Metoclopramide is certainly the best agent available at this time (Fig. 101–1). Unfortunately, drug resistance is common and long-term benefit is less common. Cholinergic agents (bethanechol 5 to 10 mg) are worthy of trial, but are not often effective. Surgical treatment (e.g., gastroenterostomy) may be attempted, but only temporary benefit should be anticipated.

Malagelada JR, Rees WDW, Mazzotta LJ, Go VLW: Gastric motor abnormalities in diabetic and postvagotomy gastroparesis: Effect of metoclopramide and bethanechol. Gastroenterology 78:286, 1980. *Experimental study of diabetics and postgastrectomy patients, some with and some without evidence of gastroparesis. The abnormality in symptomatic subjects, a loss of gastric phase III activity, was partly corrected by drug treatment.*

MISCELLANEOUS CONDITIONS

Gastric diverticula are uncommon, single, and asymptomatic. True diverticula are always located in the upper quarter of the stomach, usually on the posterior wall. Their only significance is in their diagnostic confusion with peptic ulcers or ulcerating neoplasms. Endoscopy may be required for this differentiation. Pseudodiverticula are scarred areas of dilatation, usually in the prepyloric antrum, in association with peptic ulcer disease.

Gastric volvulus is torsion of the stomach along its long axis, the esophagogastric junction and pylorus remaining fixed. Large hiatal hernias or diaphragmatic defects may be predisposing factors. An acute volvulus is often an abdominal emergency, particularly if the gastric blood supply is compromised. The chronic form is more common; bloating, regurgitation, dysphagia, and pain may occur and the diagnosis is made radiologically. Surgical treatment is required for acute volvulus and for severe symptomatic chronic volvulus.

Acute dilatation of the stomach is best considered as a localized form of paralytic ileus (see below); it is seen after abdominal operations or immobilization in body casts, during diabetic ketoacidosis, or as an acute side effect of anticholinergics. Compulsive air swallowers are most prone to this disorder, and any of the aforementioned causes may be aggravated by apprehension, which increases the tendency for aerophagia. Distention of the stomach may become massive if nasogastric suction is not instituted, and mucosal bleeding may lead to "coffee-ground" emesis.

Aerophagia is a normal accompaniment of swallowing, but may be exaggerated in anxious persons, leading to epigastric bloating. Bloating often induces patients to attempt repeated belches. Each of these perpetuates the swallowing of gas and its trapping in the stomach. Organic disease must be excluded, and the chewing of gum and ingestion of carbonated beverages should be avoided. The most effective therapy is a simple explanation of symptoms.

Disorders of Small Bowel Motility

INTRODUCTION

Normally progression of food through the small intestine is slow and steady, and an extensive spreading out of chyme allows its maximal contact with the digestive-absorptive surface. Although the "head" of a barium meal may reach the terminal ileum in one to two hours, mean transit time (for 50 per cent of a meal) is slower and the "tail" is even more delayed. This pattern of transit through the small bowel has led to the unsubstantiated proposal that "intestinal hurry" is a cause of malabsorption and diarrhea. Although appealing, the concept has received little experimental scrutiny. The only documented examples of intestinal hurry are those examples of "short bowel syndrome," seen after extensive resection of the small bowel, and the malabsorption that accompanies jejunoileal bypass. In these conditions, the major defect is inadequate contact between chyme and the digestive-absorptive surface (see Ch. 103).

The chronic stasis of delayed transit through the small intestine, from any cause, is often accompanied by an overgrowth of intestinal flora, since normal motility helps maintain the relative sterility of the small bowel. The *"blind loop syndrome"* can be produced experimentally by ganglionic blocking drugs (nonobstructive or adynamic ileus) and by partial mechanical obstruction. The blind loop syndrome occurs clinically (1) in conditions causing stasis (chronic obstruction, giant jejunal diverticula, and surgical blind pouches), (2) when a fistula is present between the colon and the upper bowel, and (3) with disturbances of the interdigestive motor complex (see Ch. 103).

ILEUS: ADYNAMIC AND MECHANICAL

DEFINITION AND ETIOLOGY. Ileus signifies impairment of caudad transit of intestinal contents. It can be subdivided into two broad categories: (1) adynamic or paralytic and (2) mechanical. The difference between these categories is important clinically: mechanical causes are usually treated surgically, whereas adynamic ileus requires medical management. Adynamic ileus occurs in association with abdominal surgery or

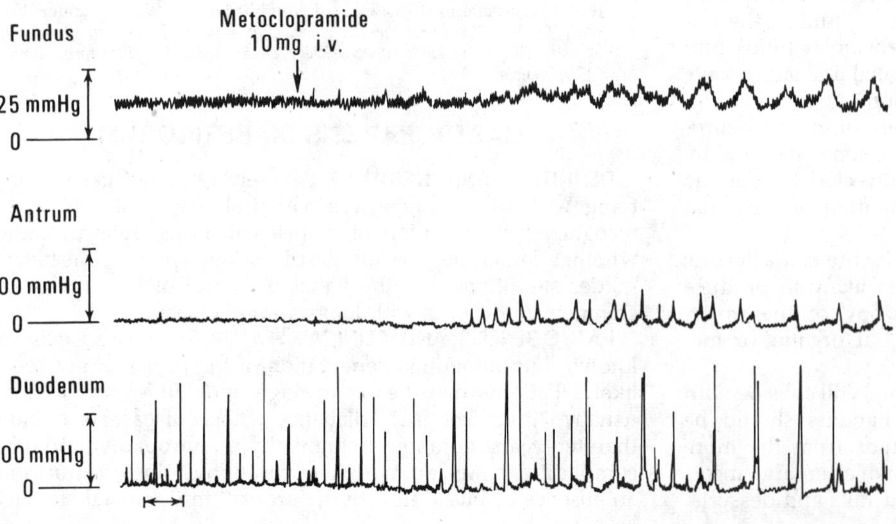

Figure 101–1. Effect of intravenous metoclopramide on fundic, antral, and duodenal motility in a patient with diabetic gastroparesis. Note the absence of pressure changes in the stomach before treatment, although duodenal activity is normal. Metoclopramide causes pressure waves to develop in the fundus and antrum. (From Malagelada JR, et al.: Gastroenterology 78:286, 1980. Reproduced with permission of the authors and publishers.)

external trauma, when the peritoneum is exposed to irritants (bacterial toxins, bile, blood, pancreatic enzymes, or intestinal contents), in severe electrolyte imbalance, and after intra-abdominal vascular accidents. The etiopathogenesis is unknown, although disordered sympathetic tone is presumed. Ileus can also be induced by ganglionic blocking drugs.

Mechanical obstruction may occur at any level of the small bowel or colon; it can be separated pathogenetically into lesions lying outside the bowel (e.g., adhesive bands, obstructed hernias), those within the wall (e.g., intramural tumors, hematomas, strictures), and those within the lumen (e.g., epithelial tumors, foreign bodies, intussusception).

PATHOPHYSIOLOGIC CONSEQUENCES. In both forms of obstruction, distal progression of air, saliva, food, and secretions ceases. The proximal bowel distends and its function becomes compromised, further reducing absorption and propulsion. In experimental obstruction of the canine small intestine, absorption from distended bowel segments diminishes after 6 to 12 hours and is replaced by secretion of sodium and water. Increased intraluminal pressure, elevation of portal venous and lymphatic pressures, ischemia, and the toxic effects of rapid bacterial multiplication in the involved segment are among the mechanisms proposed to account for these changes.

Once obstruction is established, edema, petechial hemorrhages, and finally necrosis and gangrene develop in the bowel wall. These changes are most pronounced when occlusion or strangulation of the vasculature occurs, as in closed-loop obstruction, which produces exceedingly high intraluminal pressure. Excessive permeability of the damaged intestinal mucosa allows proteins to leak from blood into the intestinal lumen; conversely, bacteria and their toxins enter the damaged and permeable mucosa. Peritonitis, therefore, frequently complicates untreated obstruction. Additional injury to ischemic mucosa may be caused by compounds in the intestinal lumen, including pancreatic enzymes, bile acids, and bacterial enterotoxins. The sequence whereby untreated obstruction leads to irreversible shock and death is uncertain. Extracellular fluid volume depletion, free perforation of the bowel, bacterial toxins, gram-negative septicemia, and splanchnic vasoconstriction all have been implicated. The general role of bacteria is well established experimentally, since mortality from obstruction is reduced in newborn or germ-free animals, or when broad-spectrum antibiotics have been given previously.

Hypovolemia, hyponatremia, and hypochloremia are the major abnormalities observed. During the course of ileus, several liters of extracellular fluid may become sequestered in the intestine. Experimental obstruction of the distal small bowel results in leakage of as much as 50 per cent of the plasma volume into this "third space." Additional fluid may accumulate in the peritoneal cavity. The total fluid loss varies with the site, duration, and degree of obstruction. Plasma concentrations of electrolytes are initially normal, since the fluid lost is isotonic, but the patient usually becomes thirsty and drinks sodium-poor fluid, so that hyponatremia develops. Severe vomiting depletes chloride, and alkalosis may be prominent in obstruction of the upper intestine. Impairment of renal function secondary to hypovolemia and starvation, with consequent ketosis, may combine to produce mild acidosis.

CLINICAL MANIFESTATIONS. The symptoms and signs depend on the level of obstruction, its duration, and whether the cause is obstructive or adynamic. Paralytic ileus may cause little pain and be manifested only by abdominal distention and vomiting. When present, pain is less severe and rhythmic than in mechanical obstruction. Increased volumes of aspirate obtained from nasogastric suction and oliguria may be early manifestations of paralytic ileus in the patient already under close observation, e.g., postoperatively. The symptoms of mechanical obstruction are vomiting, cramping abdominal pain, distention, and obstipation. When obstruction is episodic, relief may be heralded by watery, voluminous stools. When proximal, obstruction produces earlier vomiting, epigastric or mid-abdominal pain, and minimal distention. Distal obstructive lesions are associated with less vomiting, lower abdominal pain, and more prominent abdominal distention with obstipation. Physical signs are those of the metabolic disorder, particularly extracellular dehydration and hypovolemia, abdominal distention with variable tenderness, and a mass that might indicate the underlying lesion. Bowel sounds are high pitched, frequent, and rushing in mechanical obstruction. Adynamic ileus has lesser physical signs; distention is prominent, but tenderness is less pronounced unless the ileus is associated with peritonitis. Bowel sounds are infrequent to absent early in ileus in contrast to mechanical obstruction. Bowel sounds may disappear later in the course of mechanical obstruction.

DIAGNOSIS. Plain abdominal x-ray films are vital for diagnosis, to determine the level of obstruction, and to distinguish mechanical from adynamic ileus. Air-fluid levels in obstructed bowel will be seen in upright or lateral decubitus films. Mechanical obstruction often also demonstrates a sharp demarcation between dilated bowel above and collapsed bowel below the point of obstruction. Such a transition is not seen in ileus, in which dilatation is uniform throughout small and large intestines.

Colonic gas shadows are recognized by the presence of haustra, which are asymmetrical and do not extend across the entire diameter of the bowel. Valvulae conniventes of the small bowel are regular, symmetrical shadows across the entire diameter. Contrast material will pool above an obstruction and should not be given by mouth. Proctosigmoidoscopy and a barium enema, without preparation, can be performed cautiously when the obstruction is thought to be in the colon. Other diagnostic measures to determine a cause of ileus should then be considered. Overall metabolic evaluation will include measurements of serum electrolytes and the status of acid-base balance, blood urea, hematocrit, and serum protein levels, as well as careful monitoring of urine volume.

TREATMENT. The primary goals of therapy for ileus or obstruction are (1) intestinal decompression, (2) restoration or maintenance of fluid and electrolyte balance, and (3) treatment of the cause. Most instances of adynamic ileus are transient, and a medical approach can achieve all three goals. However, when the obstruction is mechanical, initial decompression is achieved by intubation but definitive decompression and removal of the obstruction usually requires surgery.

Nasogastric aspiration is usually sufficient for decompression, because this removes air before it reaches the intestine. Fluid replacement is aimed at replacing the lost water, sodium, chloride, and potassium. This is achieved by intravenous infusions of isotonic sodium chloride, alternating with 5 per cent glucose and potassium (up to 40 mEq per hour), provided that urine flow is adequate (over 50 ml per hour). Central venous pressure should be monitored to assure adequate replacement as well as to avoid fluid overload, particularly in patients with compromised cardiovascular reserve. Repeated observations are made of serum electrolytes as well as blood pressure, urinary output, and hematocrit. Alkalosis or acidosis should be corrected. When fever, leukocytosis, or signs of peritonitis suggest perforation or strangulation, appropriate antimicrobials are administered to suppress growth of intestinal bacteria. Strangulation with impending gangrene demands surgery within six hours.

Jones RS: Intestinal obstruction, pseudo-obstruction, and ileus. *In* Sleisenger MH, Fordtran JS (eds.): Gastrointestinal Disease, 3rd ed. Philadelphia, W. B. Saunders Company, 1983, p 308. *A more detailed description of the causative lesions, clinical features and practical management of obstruction of the small and large intestine.*

INTESTINAL PSEUDO-OBSTRUCTION

DEFINITION. Pseudo-obstruction implies a syndrome with clinical features akin to mechanical obstruction but for which there is no obstructive lesion. When the episode is single and transient, pseudo-obstruction is more appropriately included among examples of adynamic ileus. Thus, the term should be applied to chronic or recurrent episodes of obstruction. The underlying causes are either unknown or untreatable diseases, and pseudo-obstruction has a poor prognosis.

ETIOLOGY. So-called "primary idiopathic pseudo-obstruction" has no known cause. It affects families, and the defect appears to be transmitted as an autosomal dominant trait. Relatives of patients with the syndrome may have only radiologic and manometric evidence of abnormal intestinal motility or the full-blown disease. Primary pseudo-obstruction can be subdivided into (1) hollow visceral myopathy and (2) autonomic neuropathies. Pseudo-obstruction also occurs as a manifestation of other diseases (Table 101–1), termed secondary intestinal pseudo-obstruction.

PATHOGENESIS. The pathophysiology of both primary or secondary forms is unknown, but the mechanisms are probably diverse. Category 1 of Table 101–1 includes diseases in which the smooth muscle itself is directly replaced by infiltrates, fibrous tissue, or other noncontractile elements. Category 2 lists diseases in which intramural nervous tissue is involved, either destroyed (Chagas' disease) or histologically intact but functionally disturbed ("ganglioneuromatosis"). Category 2 also includes diseases with extensive denervation, as when there is other evidence of autonomic dysfunction with involvement of the urinary bladder (diabetes mellitus and other neuropathies). Disturbances of hormonal regulation of intestinal function may also be of importance. Certain drugs as listed in Table 101–1 may occasionally be associated with pseudo-obstruction.

CLINICAL MANIFESTATIONS. Patients with pseudo-obstruction may be of any age but, as anticipated from the nature of the underlying causes, are more often middle aged or older. The clinical presentation may vary from one of persistent symptoms of moderate severity to more acute episodes of distention and vomiting, closely mimicking the more common circumstance of mechanical obstruction. The symptoms and signs are those of retarded transit and stagnation of intestinal contents, a variable spectrum of dysphagia, regurgitation, vomiting, distention, obstipation, diarrhea, and malabsorption. Abdominal pain is quite variable also and, when prominent, makes differentiation from mechanical obstruction quite difficult. Manifestation of neuromuscular incoordination of other systems, notably the urinary bladder, may be present, as may the features of any underlying disease. Severe and chronic pseudo-obstruction may produce malnutrition and inanition.

TABLE 101–1. CAUSES OF SECONDARY INTESTINAL PSEUDO-OBSTRUCTION*

1. *Diseases involving intestinal smooth muscle ("intestinal myopathies")*
   - Collagen vascular diseases
     - Scleroderma
     - Dermatomyositis
     - Polymyositis
     - Systemic lupus erythematosus
   - Amyloidosis
   - Primary muscular diseases
     - Myotonic dystrophy
     - Progressive muscular dystrophy
2. *Neurologic diseases ("Intestinal neuropathies")*
   - Chagas' disease
   - Hirschsprung's disease
   - Familial autonomic dysfunction
   - Parkinson's disease
3. *Endocrine diseases*
   - Hypothyroidism
   - Diabetes mellitus
   - Hypoparathyroidism
   - Pheochromocytoma
4. *Drug effects*
   - Phenothiazines, tricyclic antidepressants, antiparkinsonian drugs, ganglion blockers, clonidine
5. *Miscellaneous associations*
   - Ceroid deposits in bowel
   - Nontropical sprue
   - Jejunal diverticulosis

*Modified, with permission of the authors, from Faulk DL, Anuras S, Christensen J: Gastroenterology 74:922, 1978.

DIAGNOSIS. The diagnosis of pseudo-obstruction requires the painstaking exclusion of mechanical obstruction. Free flow of contrast must be demonstrated after a barium meal with small bowel follow-through and with a barium enema. Failure to recognize a correctable mechanical obstruction may have grave consequences. The differentiation of pseudo-obstruction from slowly progressive distal obstruction (as, for example, with carcinoid tumors, radiation enteritis, and other fibrosing lesions) can also be quite difficult. Adjunctive evidence of a generalized disorder of muscle function can be obtained from motility studies of the esophagus, from cystometric studies, and from clinical evidence of underlying disease. When malabsorption is present, other causes of steatorrhea must be excluded. In some instances, exploratory laparotomy cannot be avoided and full thickness biopsy of involved intestine can be helpful.

TREATMENT. Pharmacologic treatment of pseudo-obstruction, although rational, has generally been unrewarding. Cholinergic agents and metoclopramide have the most appeal but are usually ineffective; hormones such as cholecystokinin-pancreozymin and a related peptide, cerulein, have also been tried with poor results. Corticosteroids have not augmented motility or reduced steatorrhea. Elevated serum levels of prostaglandins have been reported, as has partial relief with indomethacin. However, in an uncommon disease with an unpredictable natural history, any therapeutic information is largely anecdotal. Acute episodes require nasogastric suction and parenteral fluids, sometimes leading to parenteral alimentation. When a "blind loop syndrome" is present, antibiotics can be helpful. Surgical resection of more severely affected segments can help very occasionally but should not be entertained lightly; each laparotomy merely increases the likelihood of adhesive obstruction, further confusing an already complex problem. The prognosis is poor, and some patients have required total (home) parenteral nutrition.

Carney JA, Go VLW, Sizemore GW, Hayles AB: Alimentary tract ganglioneuromatoses. N Engl J Med 295:1287, 1976. *Description of patients with a syndrome of megacolon and/or other features of pseudo-obstruction. The histologic feature of ganglioneuromatosis was present, and patients had features of multiple endocrine adenomatosis, Type 2B.*

Snape WJ Jr: Pseudo-obstruction and other obstructive disorders. Clin Gastroenterol 11:3, 1982. *Succinct review of pathophysiology and clinical features of the syndrome. Contains all major original references.*

DIVERTICULA OF THE SMALL INTESTINE

Duodenal diverticula are common and only rarely of any significance. Although a few examples of ulceration and bleeding have been documented, duodenal diverticula are of little diagnostic significance in upper gastrointestinal hemorrhage. Diverticula are equally common in patients with hemorrhage as in those having barium studies for other reasons. Jejunal diverticula are important when stasis and bacterial overgrowth occur, resulting in the "blind loop syndrome" (see Ch. 103).

Meckel's diverticulum is the most common congenital abnormality of the gut, occurring in 2 per cent of the population. Meckel's diverticula are situated 30 to 90 cm proximal to the ileocecal sphincter on the antimesenteric wall of the ileum. Although usually 5 to 7 cm in length, they can be much longer. Gastric mucosa is present within the lumen in about one third of these diverticula. They are usually asymptomatic, but occasionally bleed, perforate, become inflamed, or obstruct the ileum. The presence of gastric mucosa and the capacity of this tissue to take up selectively radioisotopes of technetium form the basis of a diagnostic test using external gamma-camera scintillography. The diverticulum "lights up" and can be occasionally identified in this way.

Disorders of Colonic Motility

INTRODUCTION

The colon's multiple functions—desiccation of feces, bacterial metabolism of unabsorbed materials, storage of stools, and voluntary defecation—are served by a complex pattern of motility. The walls of the cecum and ascending and transverse colons show radiologic indentations ("haustra") that correspond to low pressure mixing waves, as recorded by intraluminal pressure transducers. These waves are thought to provide a "back and forth" mixing that facilitates reabsorption of salt and water. This motor pattern probably also increases the digestive potential for bacterial enzymes on dietary fiber. Transit through the descending colon is more rapid, although feces are stored in the sigmoid region. Entry of stools into the rectum triggers a coordinated sequence of rectal events, voluntary elevations of intra-abdominal pressure, and relaxation of the anal sphincters whereby controlled and voluntary defecation is possible (Fig. 101–2).

Dietary fiber may modify colonic motor function. It was initially defined imprecisely as "crude dietary fiber," but modern analytical techniques have now identified the important components of fruits, vegetables, and the outer shells of cereals that constitute fiber. The major components of fiber are celluloses (large, unbranched polymers of glucose), hemicelluloses (highly branched polymers of five-carbon sugars), pectins (gel-forming carbohydrates), and lignins (noncarbohydrate polymers of phenylpropanes). The differing chemical compositions within each of these classes and wide variations among the natural sources of fiber in foods contribute to the variable clinical effects of different fibers. In most instances, fiber decreases transit time through the colon and increases fecal bulk while undergoing some degree of digestion by the fecal flora. Fiber is resistant to digestion by mammalian enzymes. Gases (hydrogen, carbon dioxide, and, in one third of adults, methane) and organic anions (butyrate, proprionate, acetate) are generated. Undigested components of fiber have physical effects on feces by entrapping ions and water within their complex matrices. Fiber deficiency has been incriminated in several colonic diseases, including simple constipation, diverticulosis, hemorrhoids, and carcinoma of the colon.

Vahovny GV, Kritchevsky D: Dietary Fiber in Health and Disease. New York, Plenum Press, 1982. *A simple but comprehensive monograph that contains much that will be useful for clinicians wishing to know more about modern views on fiber. Excellent chapters on "what is fiber," physical properties of fiber in the bowel, and effects of fiber on colonic function.*

SIMPLE CONSTIPATION: LAXATIVES AND THEIR ABUSE

DEFINITION. Most normal adults experience brief episodes of constipation when their living habits change abruptly, and yet a precise definition of constipation is difficult and subjective. Normal frequency of stools is approximately three or more per week; moreover, defecation should be painless, not require undue straining, and be satisfyingly complete. Patients may complain of constipation if any of these criteria is not fulfilled. In order to determine whether a patient has constipation, stool frequency and fecal weight should be measured over a period of two weeks during which the intake of fiber in the diet is adequate and no constipating drugs are being taken. On such a schedule a stool should be passed with ease at least every other day. Only then can a decision be made that constipation is deserving of complete evaluation.

ETIOLOGY. Constipation is a symptom and not a disease. The major causes are listed in Table 101–2. In many instances a combination of factors will be present, e.g., diets that contain little fiber, complicated by drugs that constipate, being ingested by an individual who is debilitated, with poor muscular tone, and who has a poor habit for defecation. Clearly, the list of underlying causes in Table 101–2 dictates that constipation that continues despite the program outlined above must be evaluated carefully.

PATHOGENESIS. The major abnormality is slow transit of feces through the colon, an abnormality that can be documented best by observing the time required for small radiopaque pellets to be excreted. There is no evidence that fluid absorption by the colon is excessive, except to the degree that augmented absorption can be explained by slower transit. In most instances of secondary constipation a pathogenic mechanism cannot be specified.

CLINICAL MANIFESTATIONS AND DIAGNOSIS. Many symptoms are falsely attributed to constipation; these include halitosis, distention, belching, rectal gas, abdominal discomfort, headache, and even temper tantrums. However, severe fecal impaction can cause intestinal obstruction with spurious ("overflow") diarrhea, stercoral ulceration with bleeding, and even acute abdominal crises. Features of underlying disease may be present by history or on physical examination. Other physical findings may include tenderness of the colon to abdominal palpation and sigmoidoscopic visualization of melanosis coli, a superficial, brown pigmentation of the rectal mucosa that is seen in persons who use anthraquinone laxatives habitually. Abuse of laxatives can have other serious sequelae (see below).

TREATMENT. When treatable diseases are excluded, it is im-

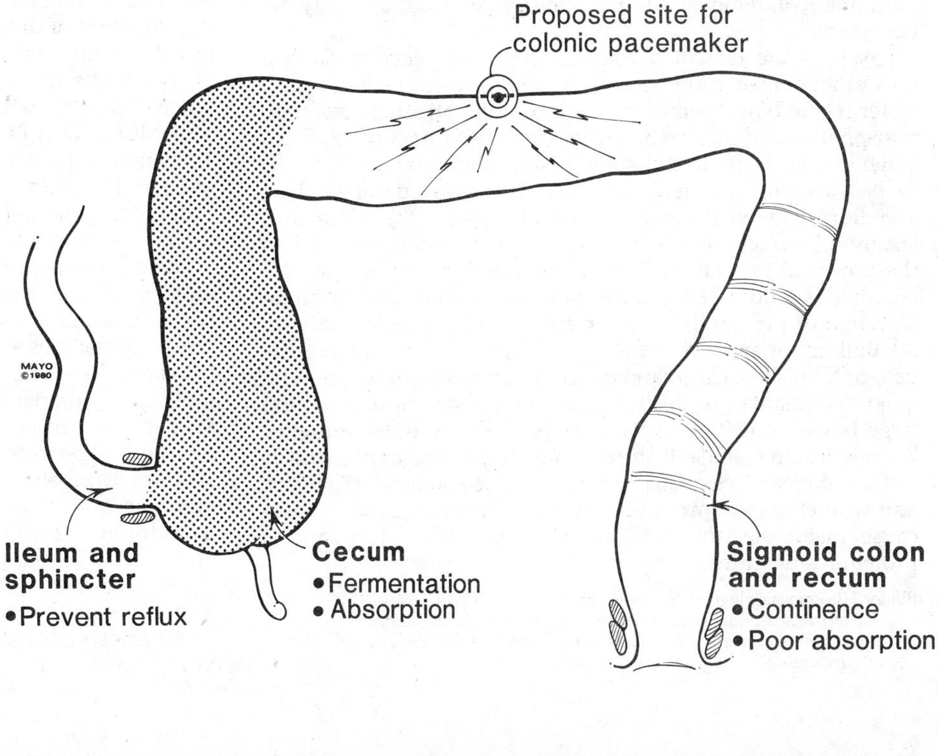

Figure 101–2. Conceptual framework for considering regional localization of colonic motor function. The proximal portions are concerned more with absorption and fermentation, the distal colon and rectum with continence and defecation.

TABLE 101–2. MAJOR CAUSES OF CONSTIPATION

1. *"Functional causes"*
   Fiber-deficient diets
   Inadequate evacuatory habits
   Variants of "irritable bowel syndrome"
   Psychoses and mental deficiency
   Debilitation and extreme old age
2. *Colonic diseases*
   Chronic obstructive lesions (e.g., tumors, strictures)
   Ulcerative proctitis
   Collagen vascular diseases with muscular abnormalities
3. *Rectal diseases*
   Stricture (e.g., ulcerative colitis, postsurgical)
   Painful conditions (fissure, abscess)
   Prolapsed rectal mucosa
   Rectocele
4. *Neurologic diseases*
   Hirschsprung's disease
   Ganglioneuromatosis
   Chagas' disease
   Intestinal pseudo-obstruction
   Spinal cord injuries and disease
   Parkinson's disease
   Cerebral tumors and cerebrovascular disease
5. *Metabolic diseases*
   Porphyria
   Hypothyroidism
   Hypercalcemia
   Pheochromocytoma
   Uremia
6. *Drugs*
   Analgesics, antacids (calcium and aluminum compounds), anticholinergics, anticonvulsants, antidepressives, bismuth salts, ganglion blockers, heavy metal poisonings, drugs for parkinsonism and psychotherapy

portant to educate the patient as to the colon's functions, so that the patient can develop better habits. Establishment of a daily ritual, aided by an increase in dietary fiber through use of fruit and vegetables or the addition of psyllium hydrophilic colloids (Metamucil), should be the major approach. Patients need to be told that such agents are not cathartics and that a prompt evacuation will not follow their use. The patient should gradually increase a regular (three times daily) dosage of psyllium hydrophilic colloids until an effect is achieved, and then continue that dosage. One teaspoonful (7 grams) of powder three times a day may suffice, as an example. Chronic use of more potent laxatives should be avoided. In fecal impaction, enemas may soften and dislodge hard feces; suppositories and "wetting agents" may also help. When all else fails, manual removal, under appropriate sedation, may be necessary.

Laxatives are classified conventionally into several classes: (1) Osmotic agents are poorly absorbed molecules that retain water in the bowel lumen through osmotic pressure. Sulfates, phosphates, and magnesium salts are in this category. (2) Stool softeners, such as dioctyl sodium sulfosuccinate, are thought to be "wetting agents," although they also stimulate fluid secretion in a way similar to the next class. (3) "Stimulant laxatives," which vary in potency from the relatively mild to the powerful purgatives, include phenolphthalein, senna, the biguanides, and castor oil. All these drugs stimulate intestinal secretion of fluid and also augment propulsive motor activity. (4) Bulking agents are derivatives of plant fiber. For regular use, only this last class can be considered totally harmless. The major stimulants can destroy intramural nerve plexuses in the large bowel, causing "cathartic colon." This serious sequel of lifelong laxative abuse features a radiologic appearance similar to that of ulcerative colitis, a "pipestem" colon lacking haustra and with abnormal propulsive activity. Laxative abuse can also cause major electrolyte imbalance, mild steatorrhea, and a protein-losing enteropathy.

Binder HJ: Pharmacology of laxatives. Ann Rev Pharmacol Toxicol 17:355, 1977. *Succinct review of newer classification of laxatives, including sections on influence of laxative on fluid absorption and secretion, intestinal motility, and side effects of laxative abuse.*

DeVroede GV: Constipation: mechanisms and management. *In* Sleisenger MH, Fordtran JS (eds.): Gastrointestinal Disease. 3rd ed. Philadelphia, W. B. Saunders Company, 1983, p 288. *This is the most complete scientific evaluation of constipation. By focusing on the important underlying diseases, the author develops a strong approach that will not always be needed for simpler examples. But valuable understanding of this common and variable symptom will arise from careful review, and the clinician wishing to understand this common symptom will gain much from such review.*

IRRITABLE BOWEL SYNDROME

DEFINITION AND INCIDENCE. The key features of the irritable bowel syndrome are abdominal discomfort, alterations of bowel habit, and no demonstrable organic cause. It is the most common gastrointestinal disorder in Western societies, constituting up to 50 per cent of all referrals for subspecialty opinion. It is more common in women than men, and occurs in the middle years of life. Numerous terms are applied to the syndrome, but several are inappropriate and even harmful. The entity is not an inflammation, and thus "mucous" or "spastic" *colitis* is incorrect. A far worse consequence, though, is that patients with irritable bowel might have their problems compounded by false associations with another major disease, chronic ulcerative colitis. Functional diarrhea is sometimes considered as a separate entity, although irritable bowel syndrome may be characterized by episodes of diarrhea, often alternating with constipation.

ETIOLOGY AND PATHOGENESIS. Although causative mechanisms are unknown, it is likely that the syndrome includes a number of entities for which specific causes will eventually be uncovered. For example, the definition of lactase deficiency has allowed some patients who earlier would have been designated as having irritable bowel to receive a specific diagnosis and therapy. Further, examples are seen in which the initial manifestations of specific disease entities, such as nontropical sprue or pancreatic insufficiency, are beyond the sensitivity of current diagnostic approaches. The underlying disease declares itself only later. Psychologic and social stresses are often present in patients with irritable bowel syndrome, and may be related in a temporal sense to exacerbations of symptoms. They are thought to be at least aggravating factors, but may be causative.

Investigations of the pathophysiology have centered on motility studies of the colon. The colonic neuromusculature is abnormally sensitive to stress in the irritable bowel syndrome. Thus, although basal contractions are not very different from normal, meals, emotional stresses, mechanical distention, and pharmacologic stimuli elicit greater numbers of more powerful contractions. In the sigmoid colon, higher intraluminal pressures have been incriminated as a mechanism for pain and the development of diverticula and muscular hypertrophy. Studies of colonic myoelectrical activity reveal an increased incidence of waves at a rate of 3 per minute and fewer at 6 per minute, when compared with control subjects.

CLINICAL FEATURES. Particular traits of personality have been attributed to patients with irritable bowel syndrome. They are often rigid, methodical persons who are conscientious, with obsessive-compulsive tendencies. Depression and hysteria are the most common psychiatric illnesses.

Abdominal pain is the most common complaint. This pain may be of any type or severity, but characteristically is not severe enough to interfere with sleep. Pain is often related to meals, sometimes suggesting peptic ulcer disease, and possibly triggered in the colon by the "gastrocolic reflex." Colonic motility is augmented regularly by food, although an intact stomach and an intact nervous system are not required. Thus, the term "gastrocolic reflex" is a misnomer. Pain may be relieved by passing flatus, which is often thought by the patient to be excessive in amount. Variants of irritable bowel syndrome include the "splenic flexure syndrome," in which colonic gas appears to be localized to that region. In fact, volumes of intestinal gas are not increased in the irritable bowel syndrome; rather, the patient is overly sensitive to normal volumes of gas, or to intestinal distention by balloons. Some disturbance of bowel habit is always present as diarrhea, constipation, or a variable pattern. Stools are described as marbles, pellets, and "rabbity"; mucus and undigested food are described but are of no significance. Bleeding is not a feature unless hemorrhoids are also present, and weight loss does not occur unless depression is a major feature. Associated features—emotional lability, lethargy, headaches, and benign cardiovascular symptoms—are likely psychosomatic manifestations. The program of investigation, which includes stool analysis, clinical laboratory surveys, proctosigmoidoscopy, and barium enema, is designated to eliminate underlying organic disease.

TREATMENT AND PROGNOSIS. Sympathetic explanation of the nature of the disorder and a careful exclusion of other diseases of the colon with subsequent reassurance are keys to successful management of these patients. A positive approach can be taken; irritable bowel syndrome is *not* a "wastebasket" but a disorder of colonic function with an as yet unknown pathogenesis. Drug therapy should be avoided if at all possible. Psychoneuroses may require treatment, and severe pain may require a non-narcotic analgesic. Anticholinergic spasmolytics may also be helpful, and episodes of diarrhea may require treatment with antimotility agents. Constipation should be explained and treated with hydrophilic colloids and diet (see above). Patients should eliminate foods from the diet *only* when a specific food predictably increases symptoms and when exclusion of that food has been shown to help. The rigid use of a "low residue" diet has no place, and may well aggravate many features of the syndrome. The disorder is chronic, and it is unlikely to be modified greatly by any single measure. The aim should be to reduce symptoms to a tolerable level that interferes minimally with the patient's normal activities.

Connell AM: Motility and its disturbances. Clin Gastroenterol 11:3, 1982. *Excellent monograph with chapters covering irritable bowel syndrome, emotions and the gastrointestinal tract, and diverticular disease.*

DIVERTICULOSIS COLI

DEFINITION AND INCIDENCE. Colonic diverticula are outpouchings of mucosa through the muscular layers and therefore contain no smooth muscle in their walls. They occur in close proximity to the teniae coli, where the muscular coats of the colon are perforated by an arteriole. The prevalence of colonic diverticula increases with age above 30 to 40 years, and they are present in over 50 per cent of octagenarians in the United States. Since most patients remain asymptomatic, simple diverticulosis is more an anatomic abnormality than it is a disease. However, the term "diverticular disease" is often applied to a spectrum that extends from uncomplicated diverticula, which are thought by some to be variants of the irritable bowel syndrome, to the serious complications of diverticula: bleeding, perforation, and diverticulitis (see Ch. 114).

PATHOGENESIS. Diverticula with muscle hypertrophy seem to be related to spasm of colonic muscle with raised luminal pressures and muscular hypertrophy in the sigmoid colon. "Simple" diverticula have no associated hypertrophy of muscle or evidence for high intraluminal pressures. The former or "spastic" type has been related both to irritable bowel syndrome and to a deficiency of fiber in the Western diet. Fiber is thought to protect by increasing fecal bulk, which, in turn, increases the diameter of the colon. By Laplace's law, the smaller the radius of a cylinder, the greater the pressure generated at a given tension. It is proposed that heightened pressure herniates mucosa and submucosa through the wall of the colon at points of intrinsic weakness. The fiber theory rests to a large extent on the increased incidence of spastic diverticulosis in Western society when compared to societies in which more fiber is ingested. This theory is supported by the increased incidence of diverticulosis in the past century, associated with increasing refinement of the Western diet. The pathogenesis of "simple" diverticula is unknown.

CLINICAL FEATURES. Most patients with diverticula are asymptomatic. When diverticula are present in patients with irritable bowel syndrome, it is virtually impossible to determine their role in the cramping left lower quadrant pain, constipation, or alternating constipation and diarrhea of which these individuals complain. Episodes of more severe distress, lasting for hours or a few days, are classified clinically as *acute diverticulitis.* Although tenderness and a sausage-shaped mass may be noted in the left lower quadrant, fever and leukocytosis characteristic of diverticulitis are absent in bouts of "diverticular disease." On occasions, however, there will be clinical overlap between the symptoms of "diverticular disease" and those of diverticulitis. Bleeding of two types can be seen with diverticula, those with or without diverticulitis. Minimal or occult bleeding may complicate either form of the disease. Significant gross bleeding is seen most often in asymptomatic patients, and is less common in those with diverticulitis. Such bleeding from diverticula at any level of the colon, often requiring transfusions of blood, is a common cause of severe rectal bleeding in older patients. It is the most serious symptom of "diverticular disease."

DIAGNOSIS. The diagnosis of diverticula in the colon is by barium enema examination. The diverticula are seen as outpouchings, particularly in the sigmoid colon. Muscular spasm and hypertrophy may be present, giving a "sawtooth," asymmetrical pattern to the barium column. In appropriate cases evidence of diverticulitis should be sought—i.e., extraintestinal flow of barium, indicating chronic perforation of the bowel. The differential diagnosis from carcinoma can be difficult, or impossible in some instances. Proctosigmoidoscopy may be painful but may reveal diverticula, luminal spasm, and fixed angulation of the sigmoid from prior disease.

TREATMENT. The only plausable program for treating diverticula of the colon is designed to increase stool bulk; the aim is to prevent constipation and the development of high pressures within the lumen of the colon. Bran, hydrophilic colloids, and dietary supplements of vegetables and fruits should be used. However, the clinical success of these programs is still uncertain. Spasmolytic anticholinergics and nonopiate analgesics may be needed. Narcotics increase intraluminal pressure and should be avoided. During follow-up visits an assessment must be made as to whether the episodes of pain represent diverticulitis, since this diagnosis raises the question of surgical treatment if recurrences are frequent. (For a discussion of treatment of diverticulitis see Ch. 97.)

Almy TP, Howell DA: Diverticular disease of the colon. N Engl J Med 302:324, 1980. *This medical progress article gives an excellent summary of current knowledge concerning the pathogenesis, clinical picture, and treatment of colonic diverticula. It also supplies 119 pertinent references.*

MEGACOLON: CONGENITAL (HIRSCHSPRUNG'S DISEASE) AND ACQUIRED

DEFINITION. Hirschsprung's disease is colonic dilatation resulting from a functional obstruction of the rectum, where there is a congenital absence of intramural neural plexuses ("aganglionosis") and a "narrow segment." Acquired megacolon may be secondary to any of the causes of constipation discussed under that heading and may be assumed if colonic dilatation was not present at an earlier examination.

INCIDENCE. Congenital aganglionosis occurs in 1 of each 5000 live births, is five to ten times more common in boys, is more common in sibs of probands, and is more common in children with Down's syndrome or other congenital abnormalities. Acquired megacolon occurs in the young, the very old, and the infirm.

PATHOGENESIS. Aganglionosis is due to arrest of the caudad migration of cells from the neural crest cells that are destined to develop as intramural plexuses; thus, the aganglionic segment always extends from the internal anal sphincter a variable distance proximally. In most instances, the aganglionic segment is within the rectum and sigmoid colon; involvement of very short segments, only the region of the anal sphincters, has also been described. The aganglionic segment is permanently contracted, causing dilatation proximal to it. Pressure studies of the anorectal segment demonstrate an absence of normal relaxation of the internal sphincter in response to rectal distention. This abnormality is absent in acquired megacolon, which has no specific pathogenesis but is merely the extreme end-result of severe constipation of many possible causes.

CLINICAL MANIFESTATIONS AND DIFFERENTIAL DIAGNOSIS. Children with congenital megacolon have obstipation, intestinal obstruction, and meconium ileus in the first days of life. Later in life the presentation is less dramatic. It does not then mimic acute intestinal obstruction, but is characterized by severe constipation and recurrent fecal impactions. Although most children have difficulty before the second month of life, very short segment aganglionosis may not cause severe symptoms until after infancy.

Congenital megacolon must be differentiated from other causes of neonatal intestinal obstruction, particularly intestinal atresia and imperforate anus. The differential diagnosis from acquired megacolon is also important. Fecal incontinence is common in acquired megacolon but does not occur in Hirschsprung's disease. Other underlying causes of severe constipation (Table 101–2) should also be sought. Digital examination of the rectum shows the rectum to be empty in congenital megacolon; barium enema (Fig. 101–3) usually confirms the absence of stool from the rectal ampulla and will demonstrate the narrowed distal segment in three fourths of patients. In acquired megacolon, dilatation of the bowel extends as far distal as the anal sphincter. Definitive diagnosis of Hirschsprung's disease is made by the absence of ganglion cells from Meissner's and Auerbach's plexuses, as seen in a full thickness biopsy of the rectum. Hirschsprung's disease can be excluded when ganglion cells are seen within Meissner's submucosal plexus in more superficial biopsies; however, failure to see ganglion cells may be due to faulty technique, and their absence from punch or suction biopsies is not diagnostic of congenital megacolon.

TREATMENT. When a diagnosis of congenital megacolon is established, the treatment of choice is definitive surgery, although preliminary decompression by a colostomy may be necessary to relieve acute obstruction. In other instances, decompression can be achieved by a regular program of enemas. A number of surgical approaches are well established, and the procedure of choice should be left to the surgeon.

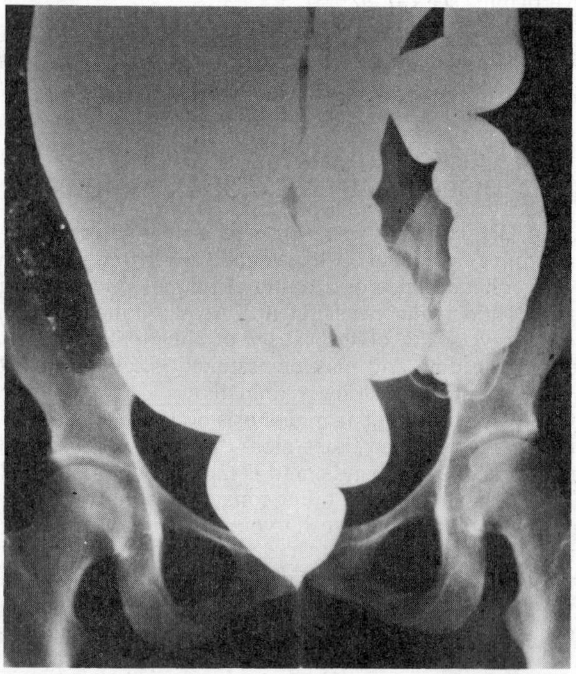

Figure 101–3. Radiologic appearances of the colon in an adult with chronic constipation. The colon is dilated (megacolon) with a smooth tapering down to a narrowed segment of rectosigmoid and rectum. These appearances are typical of Hirschsprung's disease (congenital megacolon). The patient had aganglionosis from the mid-sigmoid colon distally.

Treatment of acquired megacolon is medical. It involves disimpaction of feces by laxatives and enemas, a retraining of bowel habits, and behavioral modifications.

Phillips SF: Megacolon: Congenital and acquired. *In* Sleisenger MH, Fordtran JS (eds.): Gastrointestinal Disease. 3rd ed. Philadelphia, W. B. Saunders Company, 1983, p 112. *A description of congenital and acquired megacolon in children, including clinical features, diagnosis, and treatment.*

MOTOR DYSFUNCTION IN SPINAL CORD TRANSECTION

DEFINITION. Whether due to trauma or intrinsic neurologic disease, cord transection causes a predictable disturbance of gastrointestinal motility, the recognition and management of which is key to adequate acute and long-term management of these patients.

PATHOGENESIS. The exact level of denervation and the rapidity of onset, instantaneous in many traumatic transections but slower with some intrinsic diseases, will modify the clinical picture. However, three clinical stages can be generally recognized.

CLINICAL FEATURES AND TREATMENT. In the acute stage of spinal shock, motility, transit, and evacuation are markedly depressed. Although most emphasis has been placed upon the symptoms of obstipation and abdominal distension, acute gastric dilatation and paralysis of the small intestine can also be serious complications. This phase, which lasts usually only a few days, may require nasogastric suction, rectal decompression, and the use of stimulants (e.g., neostigmine [Prostigmin] 0.3 to 0.5 mg). During a second stage, automatic reflex activity of the bowel is established. By this time, the functions of the upper gut are usually near normal but emptying of the colon may require suppositories or digital removal to reinforce reflex defecation. In the chronic stage of "reconditioning," bulking agents, stool softeners, and a program featuring planned attempts at stooling will be required. Postprandial timing and a sitting posture will be helpful at this point. The anal sphincteric reflexes are retained in most paraplegics.

Guttmann L: Spinal Cord Injuries: Comprehensive Management and Research. 2nd ed. Oxford, Blackwell Scientific, 1976. *The most comprehensive discussion of pathophysiology, clinical features and practical therapy of this problem; written by the pioneer of systematic care for spinal injuries.*

102. DIARRHEA

John S. Fordtran

DEFINITION AND INTRODUCTION

Diarrhea is best defined as an abnormal increase in stool liquidity and in daily stool weight (>180 grams). It is usually associated with increased stool frequency and is often accompanied by urgency, perianal discomfort, incontinence, or a combination of all three. It must be recognized that some patients have increased frequency and liquidity of stools even when their stool weight is less than 180 grams. Therefore, the definition is not perfect.

Since diarrhea results from disturbances in the normal flow and transport of gut fluids, the normal physiology of the human digestive tract with respect to water and electrolyte absorption and secretion will first be considered.

NORMAL PHYSIOLOGY

DELIVERY, FLOW, AND ABSORPTION RATES. In fasting people, the intestine contains very little fluid. However, when people eat three normal meals per day, about 9 liters of fluid is delivered to the proximal duodenum. Approximately 2 liters of this fluid is from ingested food and liquids, the rest being digestive secretions.

The volume of chyme that passes through different segments of the small bowel depends on the type of food that has been eaten. For example, meals containing high concentrations of sugar are hypertonic, and when such meals are ingested, the volume of material passing through the jejunum is even greater than the volume that enters the proximal duodenum. On the other hand, after isotonic or hypotonic meals (such as a meal of steak, potatoes, and tea), the volume of fluid traversing the jejunum is much less than that which was delivered to the duodenum. (These considerations are especially important in patients who have had gastric surgery or intestinal resection.) In either case, the osmolality of chyme is adjusted toward that of plasma as fluid travels through the duodenum and upper jejunum, and by the time chyme reaches the ileum, most of the dietary sugars, amino acids, and fats have been absorbed. Therefore, fluid arriving at the ileum is mainly an isotonic salt solution, similar in its ionic makeup to plasma. The ileum absorbs much, but not all, of this salt solution. About 1 liter per day of unabsorbed ileal fluid is emptied into the colon. This fluid is isotonic and resembles plasma with regard to its sodium and potassium concentrations, but the concentrations of chloride and bicarbonate are approximately 70 and 60 mEq per liter, respectively.

The colon can absorb 2 to 4 liters of isotonic salt solution per day (even more in patients with secondary hyperaldosteronism associated with salt depletion). Theoretically the colon could absorb all of the 1 liter of fluid presented to it each day. However, the presence of nonabsorbable and osmotically active solutes from the diet and from bacterial action, a relatively slow rate of absorption from the rectosigmoid, and timely bowel movements prevent complete fluid absorption and desiccation of the fecal mass. About 100 ml of fluid is excreted in the feces; its sodium and chloride concentrations are about 50 mEq per liter, while the potassium concentration is about 90 mEq per liter. This fluid also contains a high concentration of volatile fatty acids (from bacterial action on nondigestible carbohydrates), which dissipate most of the unabsorbed or secreted bicarbonate ions and which often cause stool fluid to be hypertonic to plasma. Since the gastrointestinal tract does not have a diluting mechanism, the osmolality of fecal fluid is never less than the osmolality of plasma.

To summarize, daily volumes of fluid traversing the duodenum are 9 liters, traversing the ileocecal valve area are 1 liter, and traversing the anal sphincter are 0.1 liter. Stated in another way, the small bowel absorbs 8 liters of fluid per day and empties 1 liter into the colon, and the colon absorbs 0.9 liter. Theoretically 2 to 4 liters of fluid would have to be delivered to the colon per day before diarrhea would ensue, provided that delivery rates were steady, the fluid contained no abnormal solutes, and colon function was normal. Unfortunately, the latter qualifications do not apply in many gastrointestinal diseases.

TRANSPORT PHYSIOLOGY. The mechanisms responsible for fluid absorption differ in different regions of the gut and in different species. According to the model for the ileum shown in Figure 102–1, the brush border membrane contains a carrier that facilitates the simultaneous entry of Na^+ and glucose into the cells; Na^+ cannot enter without glucose. A separate pair of exchange carriers works together to facilitate the simultaneous and electrically neutral entry of Na^+ and Cl^-. Na^+ enters in exchange for H^+, and Cl^- enters in exchange for HCO_3^-. If these two exchange carriers operate at the same rate, Na^+ and Cl^- are absorbed in equal amounts, and H^+ and HCO_3^- are secreted in equal amounts and react in the lumen to form CO_2 and water. However, the anion carrier usually operates more rapidly than the cation carrier, and there is a net secretion of HCO_3^-. (This accounts for the high concentration of HCO_3^- and the low concentration of Cl^- in fluid which the ileum delivers to the colon.) Once inside the cell (via either the Na^+/H^+ exchange or the Na^+-glucose carrier), Na^+ is pumped out of the cell across the basolateral membrane by a pump that is probably an Na^+-K^+ ATPase. Chloride and glucose exit the basolateral membrane by facilitated or passive diffusion.

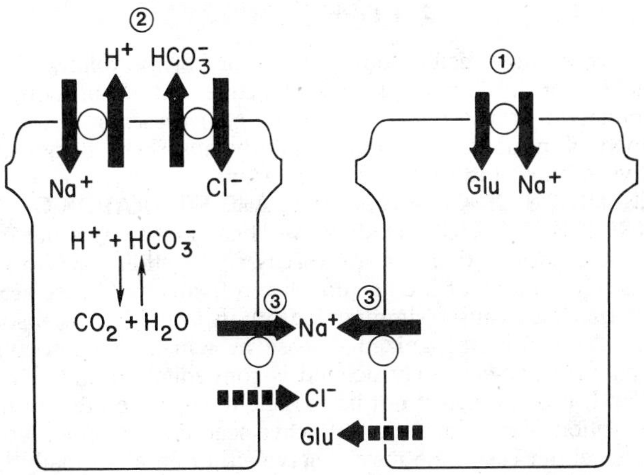

Figure 102–1. Active transport mechanisms in the human ileum. *1,* Brush border glucose-sodium carrier. *2,* Double exchange carriers for neutral NaCl entry. *3,* Basolateral membrane sodium pump.

Sodium pumping at the basolateral membrane causes a potential difference (PD) across the mucosa (serosal side positive). However, the tight junctions between small bowel mucosal cells (the "shunt pathway") are "leaky," and passive diffusion of anions (in the absorptive direction from lumen to plasma) or cations (in the secretory direction) readily dissipates the PD. Therefore, the residual PD across small bowel mucosa is only 2 to 4 mV.

Colonic cells and colonic transport are somewhat different. The brush border membrane apparently has a carrier for Na^+ which is not influenced by glucose or other actively absorbed nonelectrolytes (glucose is not absorbed in the colon). There is no convincing evidence for Na^+-H^+ exchange, but the brush border membrane appears to have an anion exchange carrier that facilitates chloride absorption and bicarbonate secretion. The tight junctions are "tight," so the electrical gradient generated by the basolateral membrane pump is sustained. The PD is, therefore, about 30 mV (serosal side positive).

Potassium movement in all regions of the gut is passive, in response to electrochemical gradients. Thus, passive potassium absorption in the colon is retarded (owing to the high lumen negative PD), and the potassium concentration in fecal fluid is much higher than in plasma (up to 100 mEq per liter). Water movement throughout the gut is passive, secondary to osmotic pressure gradients generated by active solute transport.

NORMAL SMALL BOWEL SECRETION. Small intestinal cells normally secrete as well as absorb electrolytes and water, with the secretion rate normally being of less magnitude than the absorption rate, so that the net effect of small bowel transport processes is absorption of fluid. (Although it is possible that the same cell might both absorb and secrete, the putative small bowel secretion probably originates in crypt cells, whereas absorption takes place from villous cells.) This is an extremely important concept, because it means that a hormone or toxin might reduce net absorption rate in either of two ways: (1) by stimulating secretion, and (2) by inhibiting absorption. In either case, the observed effect is reduced absorption. Similarly, a hormone or a toxin might cause small bowel secretion by stimulating active secretion, so that it overwhelms the normal absorptive process; or a hormone or a toxin could cause secretion by inhibiting absorption, so that the normal small bowel secretion is unmasked. In fact, many toxins and hormones appear capable of both stimulating secretion and inhibiting normal absorption (see below). In patients with diarrhea caused by toxins or hormones, it is difficult to ascertain which of these factors is predominant.

In the colon, absorption takes place from the surface epithelial cells. There is no evidence for or against a normal colonic secretion.

PATHOPHYSIOLOGY

Diarrhea may result from one or more of the following: (1) deletion or inhibition of normal active ion absorption; (2) stimulation of intestinal ion secretion; (3) presence in the gut lumen of unusual amounts of poorly absorbed, osmotically active solutes; and (4) deranged intestinal motility.

INHIBITION OF ION ABSORPTION AND STIMULATION OF ION SECRETION (SECRETORY DIARRHEA). These first two pathophysiologic causes of diarrhea are discussed together for two reasons. First, many of the hormones and toxins that cause active secretion also cause (simultaneously) an inhibition of absorption. (The only recognized disease in which the absorptive mechanism is selectively deleted is congenital chloridorrhea.) Second, it is difficult if not impossible to separate inhibition of absorption from stimulation of active secretion in clinical studies. In either case, one may observe either an abnormally low absorption rate or intestinal secretion. (See Normal Small Bowel Secretion, above.)

Figure 102–2 illustrates the current concepts about what happens when the cyclic AMP concentration of mucosal cells is elevated by any one of several diseases (see below). First, the neutral mechanism for NaCl entry into the cell is inhibited, resulting in an inhibition of absorption through this pathway. Second, an anion secretory process is stimulated. In contrast to carrier-mediated neutral NaCl entry, the Na^+-glucose entry mechanism and the basolateral sodium pump are not affected by high intracellular concentration of cAMP, and sodium and glucose entering the cell via this carrier can be transported across the basolateral membrane at a normal rate. The normality of this glucose-sodium absorptive process makes oral glucose-saline solution therapy effective in the correction of salt and water depletion in patients with cholera and related diseases.

Although the biochemical mechanisms are not defined, there appear to be other causes of inhibition of ion absorption and/or stimulation of ion secretion which are not related to a high concentration of mucosal cell cyclic AMP. These abnormalities in ion transport may be mediated by changes in intracellular calcium concentration, or by cyclic nucleotides other than cAMP. Some clinically important causes of inhibition of ion absorption and/or stimulation of ion secretion are listed in Table 102–1.

Clinically, diseases that cause diarrhea by virtue of inhibition of ion absorption or stimulation of ion secretion are called

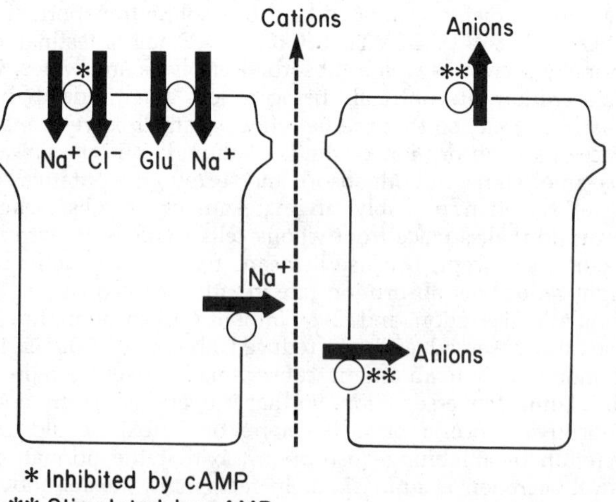

Figure 102–2. Model of cyclic AMP–mediated change in intestinal transport. Active anion secretion is stimulated (**), and there is inhibition of neutral NaCl entry across the brush border membrane (*). The glucose-sodium entry carrier and the basolateral membrane sodium pump are intact. Cations are secreted passively via the tight junction pathway. See Field et al. for a more detailed discussion.

TABLE 102–1. SOME CAUSES OF SECRETORY DIARRHEA*

I. Agents that activate the adenylate cyclase-cAMP system
 A. Cholera toxin
 B. Heat labile toxin of *E. coli*
 C. *Salmonella* enterotoxin
 D. Vasoactive intestinal polypeptide (VIP)
 E. Prostaglandins
 F. ? Dihydroxy bile acids, long-chain fatty acids
II. Agents that probably do not activate the adenylate cyclase-cAMP system
 A. Heat stable toxin of *E. coli*
 B. Enterotoxins of *Clostridium perfringens, Pseudomonas aeruginosa,* and *Klebsiella pneumoniae*
 C. Calcitonin
 D. Serotonin
 E. Castor oil, phenolphthalein
III. Chronic secretory diarrhea
 A. Pancreatic cholera syndrome (VIP, calcitonin)
 B. Medullary carcinoma of thyroid (calcitonin, prostaglandins)
 C. Ganglioneuroma and ganglioneuroblastoma
 D. Malignant carcinoid syndrome (serotonin)
 E. Villous adenoma of the rectum
 F. Surreptitious laxative abuse
 G. Fatty acid and bile acid malabsorption

*Agents or diseases that produce diarrhea by virtue of inhibition of ion absorption and/or stimulation of ion secretion.

"secretory diarrhea." Secretory diarrhea can usually be recognized by the following features: First, the diarrhea persists during a two-day fast. This is due to net intestinal secretion and/or failure to reabsorb fasting digestive secretions. Second, there is no (or only a small) fecal solute gap.* This means that the osmolality of fecal fluid can be accounted for entirely or almost entirely by electrolytes. These two criteria hold in most instances, but not in fatty acid–induced secretory diarrhea, in which a fast will cause the diarrhea to subside, and not completely in some malabsorption syndromes, in which multiple pathophysiologic events occur simultaneously.

OSMOTIC DIARRHEA. Osmotic diarrhea is caused by accumulation of poorly absorbable solutes in the gut lumen. There are three main subtypes: (1) ingestion of poorly absorbable solutes, such as some laxatives; (2) maldigestion of ingested food; and (3) failure to transport an osmotically active dietary nonelectrolyte (glucose, for example), which is normally absorbed by a special mechanism. Being osmotically active, these poorly absorbed solutes cause water and salts to be retained within the intestinal lumen, resulting in diarrhea. (The osmolality of small bowel fluid is the same as that of plasma, but the effective osmotic pressure of the luminal fluid is higher than that of plasma owing to the presence of the nonabsorbable solute.)

Osmotic diarrhea stops when the patient fasts (or stops ingesting the poorly absorbable solute). Furthermore, the fecal fluid has a large solute gap, i.e., normal electrolytes do not account for much of fecal fluid osmolality. In osmotic diarrhea resulting from carbohydrate malabsorption, the concentration in stool of volatile fatty acids is high and the pH is low because of fermentation. In some instances it is necessary to measure magnesium and other specific ions in the stool to identify the cause of osmotic diarrhea, especially in surreptitious laxative abuse.

Normal fecal fluid, which can be isolated from stool by dialysis methods, often has a modest solute gap (mainly because of unabsorbed carbohydrates and their bacterial products). Therefore, the presence of a solute gap is suggestive of osmotic diarrhea only if stool volume losses are substantially higher than normal. For example, a modest osmotic gap with a stool volume of only 200 ml per 24 hours would not by itself be highly suggestive of osmotic diarrhea.

DERANGED INTESTINAL MOTILITY. On a priori grounds, three major derangements might cause diarrhea. First, abnormally reduced peristalsis may allow bacterial overgrowth in the small bowel (see Ch. 103). Second, "intestinal hurry" may reduce contact time between the small bowel mucosa and its contents,

*Fecal solute gap = (osmolality) − 2 ([Na] + [K]). The factor of 2 is to account for anions in stool.

and thus result in delivery of abnormally large and qualitatively abnormal fluid loads to the colon. This occurs in spite of the fact that absorption in the small bowel is normal per unit of time. Third, premature emptying of the colon caused by an abnormality of its contents, or by intrinsic colonic "irritability" or inflammation, results in a reduced contact between luminal contents and colonic mucosa, and therefore increased volume and liquidity of the stools. Some diarrheal diseases apparently caused mainly or in part by deranged motility are irritable bowel syndrome, malignant carcinoid syndrome, postvagotomy diarrhea, diarrhea resulting from diabetic neuropathy, diarrhea resulting from thyrotoxicosis, and the diarrhea associated with postgastrectomy dumping syndrome. Abnormal motility may also contribute to acute diarrhea caused by infections.

DIAGNOSIS

Although the cause of diarrhea is obvious in many clinical situations, in many others it is not. Here we are concerned with a diagnostic approach to the patient with diarrhea in whom the cause is unknown.

HISTORY AND PHYSICAL EXAMINATION. When the stools are consistently large, the underlying cause of diarrhea is likely to be located in the small bowel or in the proximal colon. By contrast, in small volume diarrhea, in which the patient has frequent urges to defecate but passes only small amounts of feces or mucus, the disorder is usually in the left colon and rectum. Passage of blood mixed in with the diarrheal stool usually indicates inflammation of the mucosa, less often a neoplasm. Passage of nonbloody mucus suggests irritable bowel syndrome, as does a history of small volume diarrhea alternating with constipation. Frothy stools and excessive flatus suggest fermentation of unabsorbed carbohydrates. Excessively foul stools suggest putrefaction of unabsorbed amino acids. Visible oil or fat indicates severe steatorrhea. Fecal soiling (incontinence) suggests an anal sphincter defect. Diarrhea in a patient with features of anorexia nervosa suggests laxative abuse.

The drugs the patient is taking should be carefully noted. The following are especially likely to cause diarrhea: antibiotics, antacids, antihypertensive agents, thyroxine, digitalis, propranolol, quinidine, colchicine, potassium supplements, lactulose, and ethanol. The possibility of laxative intake should always be considered.

There are, of course, many other pertinent facts obtainable from the history, including previous surgery, symptoms of systemic illness, travel location, and related illnesses in family members. In chronic and recurrent diarrhea, an association of exacerbation of diarrhea with emotional stress should be sought, although in many patients whose pattern of diarrhea and clinical course fit with what is called irritable bowel syndrome, no such association can be established. The patient's sexual history should be taken, since male homosexuals have a high incidence of shigellosis, giardiasis, and other intestinal infections, as well as the usually recognized venereal diseases.

The physical examination may reveal clues to the cause of diarrhea. Some physical findings, as well as other clinical associations, that may assist in the diagnosis of diarrhea are listed in Table 102–2.

CLINICAL CLASSIFICATION. If the cause of diarrhea is not apparent after the history and physical examination, it is helpful to place the patient in one of the following categories, on the basis of information obtained from the history: (1) acute diarrhea (duration less than two weeks); (2) traveler's diarrhea; (3) chronic and recurrent diarrhea; (4) diarrhea of unknown origin (when previous more or less complete diagnostic workups did not reveal the diagnosis); and (5) incontinence (when the patient may complain of "diarrhea," but the major disability is caused by fecal incontinence). Some of the most likely diagnostic possibilities in each of these categories are listed in Table 102–3. Traveler's diarrhea, diarrhea of unknown origin, and incontinence are discussed later in this chapter.

TABLE 102–2. CLUES TO DIAGNOSIS OF DIARRHEA FROM OTHER SYMPTOMS, SIGNS, AND LABORATORY TESTS

Symptom or Sign Associated with Diarrhea	Diagnoses To Be Considered
Arthritis	Ulcerative colitis, Crohn's disease, Whipple's disease
Liver disease	Ulcerative colitis, Crohn's disease, bowel malignancy with metastasis to liver
Fever	Ulcerative colitis, Crohn's disease, amebiasis, lymphoma, tuberculosis
Marked weight loss	Malabsorption, inflammatory bowel disease, cancer, thyrotoxicosis
Eosinophilia	Eosinophilic gastroenteritis, parasitic disease
Lymphadenopathy	Lymphoma, Whipple's disease
Neuropathy	Diabetic diarrhea, amyloidosis
Postural hypotension	Diabetic diarrhea, Addison's disease, idiopathic orthostatic hypotension
Flushing, large liver	Malignant carcinoid syndrome
Proteinuria	Amyloidosis
Perianal disease or right lower quadrant abdominal mass	Crohn's disease
Purpura	Celiac disease
Peptic ulcer	Zollinger-Ellison syndrome, antacid therapy, gastrocolic fistula
Following cholecystectomy	? Bile acid malabsorption
Frequent infections	Immunoglobulin deficiency
Immunodeficiency	Giardiasis, nodular lymphoid hyperplasia, celiac sprue
Hyperpigmentation	Whipple's disease, celiac disease, Addison's disease
Good response to corticosteroids	Ulcerative colitis, Crohn's disease, Whipple's disease, Addison's disease, pancreatic cholera, eosinophilic enteritis
Good response to antibiotics	Bacterial overgrowth in small intestine, tropical sprue, Whipple's disease, celiac disease

DIAGNOSTIC TESTS. ***Routine Examination of Stool.*** Unless the diagnosis is readily apparent from the history and physical examination, certain relatively simple studies on the stool should routinely be carried out. Regardless of the clinical classification, the information obtained will usually narrow the diagnostic possibilities.

STAIN FOR PUS. The presence or absence of intestinal inflammation can often be ascertained by examination of a stained stool specimen. Wright's or methylene blue stains are satisfactory. The presence of large numbers of white blood cells is diagnostic of inflammation. The presence of rare scattered white cells is within normal limits.

In patients with acute or traveler's diarrhea, pus in the stool suggests invasion of the mucosa by *Shigella, E. coli, E. histolytica, Salmonella*, gonococci, *Campylobacter*, or other invasive organisms. In general, shigellosis and invasive *E. coli* infections cause more pus than *Salmonella* and *E. histolytica*. Antibiotic-associated colitis may or may not be associated with pus. Diarrhea caused by noninvasive organisms that produce enterotoxins (toxigenic *E. coli*, for example), viruses, and *Giardia* are not associated with pus in the stool.

In patients with chronic and recurrent diarrhea or in diarrhea of unknown etiology, pus suggests colitis of some type, be it idiopathic ulcerative colitis, Crohn's colitis, antibiotic-associated colitis, amebic colitis, ischemic colitis, or tuberculous colitis. Pus is especially abundant in idiopathic ulcerative colitis, and tends to be less so in amebic colitis. Absence of pus on a single examination does not, of course, absolutely rule out any of these entities. Radiation-induced disease of the large or small bowel and Crohn's disease limited to the small intestine may or may not be associated with pus in the stool. Pus is not present in the stools of patients with irritable bowel syndrome, most causes of malabsorption syndrome, laxative abuse, or giardiasis, and sometimes pus is not present in patients with amebic colitis.

OCCULT BLOOD. Occult (or gross) blood in association with diarrhea usually indicates inflammation, and therefore usually has the same significance as pus in the stools (see above). When blood is present in diarrheal stools that do not contain pus, one should think of amebiasis, neoplasms of the colon, heavy metal poisoning, and acute ischemic damage to the gut.

SUDAN STAIN FOR FAT. If excess fat is present on Sudan stain, steatorrhea is probably present, and the various causes of malabsorption syndromes should be considered (see Ch. 103). Most such patients will have chronic and recurrent diarrhea; steatorrhea in a patient with acute or traveler's diarrhea suggests giardiasis.

ALKALINIZATION. A pink color following alkalinization indicates phenolphthalein ingestion as the cause of diarrhea. The test is so easily and quickly done, and the significance of a positive result so great, that it should be carried out routinely in patients with chronic diarrhea.

Other Tests. Patients with chronic diarrhea in whom the diagnosis is not evident should have a hemogram, chemical profile, and urinalysis. Evidence of systemic illness will have obvious implications on the etiology of diarrhea, and some of these associations are listed in Table 102–2.

The more direct studies most likely to help establish the diagnosis should be evident from the likely causes of diarrhea that are listed in Table 102–3. The order in which tests are carried out, assuming that further tests are necessary, will vary according to the physician's intuition in a particular patient. Certain of the diagnostic tests deserve brief discussion here.

SEARCH FOR INFECTIOUS AND PARASITIC ORGANISMS. It is important to complete the examination for parasites and to have adequate bacterial cultures in progress prior to examination of the patient with radiologic contrast media, because barium interferes with successful demonstration of pathogens. Failure to find *Giardia* in stool samples is not strong evidence against giardiasis; sometimes it is necessary to examine duodenal fluid in order to demonstrate this organism. Special culture methods are required if the presence of gonococcal, *Campylobacter*, and *Yersinia* infections are to be established. Serologic tests for amebae and lymphogranuloma venereum may assist in the diagnosis in some patients. Finally, tests for clostridial toxin will help in the specific diagnosis of antibiotic-associated colitis.

TABLE 102–3. SOME CAUSES OF DIARRHEA IN FIVE DIFFERENT CLINICAL CATEGORIES

A. Acute diarrhea
  1. Viral, bacterial, and parasitic infections
  2. Food poisoning
  3. Drugs (acute or chronic)
  4. Fecal impaction
  5. Heavy metal poisoning (acute or chronic)
B. Traveler's diarrhea
  1. Bacterial infections
    a. Mediated by enterotoxins, e.g., heat labile and/or heat stable producing *E. coli*
    b. Mediated mainly by invasion of mucosa and inflammation, e.g., invasive *E. coli, Shigella, Campylobacter*
    c. Mediated by combination of invasion and enterotoxins, e.g., *Salmonella*
  2. Viral and parasitic infections
C. Chronic and recurrent diarrhea
  1. Irritable bowel syndrome
  2. Inflammatory bowel disease
  3. Parasitic infections
  4. Malabsorption syndromes, lactase deficiency
  5. Drugs (acute or chronic)
  6. Heavy metal poisoning (acute or chronic)
D. Chronic diarrhea of unknown origin (previous workup failed to reveal diagnosis)
  1. Surreptitious laxative abuse
  2. Irritable bowel syndrome
  3. Unrecognized inflammatory bowel disease
  4. Bile acid malabsorption
  5. Other cause of chronic diarrhea that was previously overlooked
E. Incontinence
  1. Cause of sphincter dysfunction
    a. Anal surgery for fissures, fistulas, or ? hemorrhoids
    b. Episiotomy or tear during childbirth
    c. Anal Crohn's disease
    d. ? Diabetic neuropathy
    e. Idiopathic
  2. Cause of diarrhea—same as under C and D

PROCTOSIGMOIDOSCOPY. Provided that stool specimens are accurately examined (see above), proctosigmoidoscopy is usually of little help in patients with acute and traveler's diarrhea. (An exception to this statement is in antibiotic-associated diarrhea, in which proctoscopy may reveal pseudomembranes.) On the other hand, proctosigmoidoscopy is often essential in patients with chronic and recurrent diarrhea and in patients with diarrhea of unknown etiology. It is especially apt to be abnormal in those whose stools contain pus and/or blood; it is usually normal in patients with diarrhea caused by the various malabsorption syndromes.

Proctosigmoidoscopy because of diarrhea should be done without enemas, laxatives, or suppositories. Such preparations may wash away exudate, distort the mucosa, induce trauma, and by these means obscure evidence of disease or create the false impression of disease. In almost all instances fecal matter can easily be aspirated or pushed aside, and since most abnormalities are diffuse, fecal matter does not interfere greatly with a satisfactory examination. The presence of solid stool in the rectum of a patient who supposedly has diarrhea is also revealing, suggesting an acute diarrhea that is subsiding, that the patient may have irritable bowel syndrome, or that the diarrhea is secondary to fecal impaction.

Since proctitis may not be evident grossly, even to the experienced eye, mucosal smears should always be obtained and stained for pus. In my opinion, irritable bowel syndrome should not be diagnosed until after a stained mucosal smear has shown that pus is not present. Stained smears are preferable to biopsy in most patients because they never cause bleeding, because they can be interpreted within minutes after they are obtained, and because they are less expensive.

The mucosa should be carefully examined for melanosis coli, although melanosis may be present microscopically even if it is not present grossly.

RECTAL BIOPSY. Provided that smears are done (see above), biopsy is not specifically helpful in the workup of most patients with diarrhea. The main disorders that might be detected by biopsy but not by smears and stool examination are amyloidosis, Whipple's disease, granulomatous inflammation, melanosis coli, and schistosomiasis. Biopsy is indicated in patients with diarrhea of unknown origin, especially in a search for melanosis coli and unsuspected colitis that may not have been evident grossly.

Rectal biopsy is best done with small forceps, rather than with the large type that comes with most proctoscopy sets. The biopsy should be taken from the posterior wall of the rectum on a valve. Although the risk is uncertain, some clinicians believe that a rectal biopsy with large forceps predisposes to a colonic perforation if a barium enema is done within ten days of the biopsy.

QUANTITATIVE FECAL FAT. Quantitatively collected stools (usually for 72 hours) should be analyzed for fat content: (1) when malabsorption is suggested by the history and physical examination, (2) when the qualitative test for fecal fat is positive, or (3) routinely in patients with diarrhea of unknown origin. If steatorrhea is present, the differential diagnosis of malabsorption syndrome can be pursued (see Ch. 103). Of course, the results of this test must be interpreted with knowledge of the approximate intake of dietary fat. Stool weight in grams (which is equivalent to stool volume in milliliters) should also be noted and recorded (see below).

TWENTY-FOUR–HOUR STOOL VOLUME. For reasons indicated under History and Physical Examination, above, knowledge of stool volume helps localize the region of the intestine that is most likely responsible for diarrrhea, and in several instances specific information on stool volume is of great diagnostic help. For example, stool volumes greater than 500 ml per day are rarely seen in patients with irritable bowel syndrome, and stool volumes of less than 1000 ml per day provide evidence against pancreatic cholera syndrome. Also, very large measured stool volumes will alert the physician to the need for vigorous fluid replacement therapy.

Collection of 24-hour stool specimens is easy to do in the initial phases of diarrhea workup, prior to barium x-rays, enemas, or other preparations. With a little effort, it can be accurately done on an outpatient basis. If a record of stool frequency is kept, the average volume of each stool can be calculated and the results may give useful insight.

In special instances, e.g., in diarrhea of unknown origin, it is useful to measure stool electrolytes and osmolality and to determine whether or not the diarrhea persists during a 48-hour fast (while the patient is given glucose and salt solutions intravenously). These results will help establish whether the diarrhea is secretory or osmotic in type (see Pathophysiology, above). Except in congenital chloridorrhea, the sum of the sodium and potassium concentrations always exceeds the chloride concentration in fecal fluid.

Vasoactive Intestinal Polypeptide (VIP) and Related Hormones. If diarrhea of unknown origin has lasted longer than four weeks, is secretory in type, and is severe (>1 liter per day and/or associated with hypokalemia and salt and water depletion), and if surreptitious laxative abuse and organic disease of the gastrointestinal tract have been excluded, such patients may have pancreatic cholera syndrome. It is only in this rare subgroup of patients that serum assay for VIP, prostaglandins, calcitonin, and other gastrointestinal hormones is likely to be helpful. Because these assays are imperfect, and because pancreatic cholera syndrome is a very rare disorder, high values should be interpreted with caution.

Therapeutic Trials. In some instances, therapeutic trials are indicated as diagnostic tests. (Obviously, in most instances, the results must be considered suggestive rather than conclusive.) These may include pancreatic enzymes, antibiotics (also as part of Schilling test), metronidazole or quinacrine (for giardiasis), cholestyramine (for bile acid malabsorption), indomethacin (for prostaglandin synthetase inhibition), and various diets (lactose-free, carbohydrate-free, low fat, and avoidance of any specific food to evaluate the unlikely possibility of food allergy).

SPECIAL CONSIDERATIONS

IRRITABLE BOWEL SYNDROME (FUNCTIONAL DIARRHEA). In most patients this diagnosis is readily evident from the history of intermittent diarrhea and constipation associated with abdominal pain, and from the lack of signs or symptoms of systemic illness. A minimum of diagnostic studies is needed in such patients (see Ch. 101).

However, persistent or recurrent diarrhea in the face of a negative workup raises the possibility that the diarrhea is "functional" or "psychogenic" in origin, even though initially this may have seemed unlikely. At this point, it is well to review the characteristics of diarrhea in patients with irritable bowel syndrome. First, it is usually intermittent and associated with pain, but it may be constant and painless. Second, the stools are usually small in volume by history, and measured stool volumes larger than 500 ml per day weigh heavily against this diagnosis. Third, the diarrhea does not usually wake the patient from sleep. In addition to these considerations, there should be no evidence of organic disease. The degree to which organic causes of diarrhea should be specifically ruled out (in patients whose pattern of diarrhea is consistent with irritable bowel syndrome) varies, depending on the age of the patient and severity of the clinical problem. In particularly troublesome, persistent, and refractory diarrhea, a thorough evaluation may be indicated, and therapeutic trials may be appropriate.

If these criteria are met, it is reasonable to make a diagnosis of irritable bowel syndrome, although it should be recognized that doing so does not imply that the pathogenesis or etiology of the diarrhea has necessarily been explained. It is likely that there are several causes of what we now call irritable bowel syndrome, including emotional stress, postdysentery malfunction, food intolerances, subclinical malabsorption, bile acid malabsorption, and others waiting to be discovered.

TRAVELER'S DIARRHEA. This term is usually applied to patients who get diarrhea within two weeks of traveling to a tropical location and in whom the diarrhea runs a self-limited course lasting one to ten days. It is caused by a variety of infectious organisms that somehow overcome natural defense mechanisms, such as gastric acidity, propulsive small bowel motility, and local immunologic reactions. The most common cause of traveler's diarrhea is enterotoxin-producing forms of *E. coli*. Certain *E. coli* liberate either a heat labile (LT) or a heat stable (ST) enterotoxin, both of which are under genetic control of bacterial plasmids. The initial pathogenetic event is colonization of the small bowel by such an organism, a phenomenon facilitated by epithelial receptors for filamentous bacterial appendages called pili. The resulting adherence to the small bowel mucosa allows toxins to accumulate in the lumen of the small intestine. The toxins cause an increase in either cAMP (LT) or cGMP (ST) or both, and intestinal secretion results from mechanisms similar to that illustrated in Figure 102–2. These toxins apparently have no effect in the colon.

Some other causes of traveler's diarrhea are listed in Table 102–3. Shigellosis and invasive *E. coli* cause diarrhea mainly by virtue of mucosal invasion, whereas in salmonellosis mucosal invasion and an enterotoxin are both involved in the pathogenesis of diarrhea. In some instances traveler's diarrhea is probably caused by viral infection, and in a few instances it is caused by infection with *E. histolytica*, *Giardia*, or strongyloidosis. In the latter parasitic infections, the diarrhea often lasts longer than ten days and may become chronic. In some instances giardiasis contracted during travel causes the delayed onset of diarrhea several weeks after the traveler has returned home. Even in studies in which elaborate diagnostic studies are available, the cause of traveler's diarrhea cannot be established in about one third of cases.

There are thus many causes of traveler's diarrhea. The presence of chills, fever, tenesmus, cramping, pus, or blood suggests mucosal invasion by a bacterial organism, whereas the absence of these findings is suggestive of enterotoxin-mediated diarrhea. Stool volumes are usually low, but occasionally they may be as voluminous as in cholera. Large volume secretory diarrhea acquired during travel is most likely caused by enterotoxin-producing organisms or by *Salmonella*. Occasionally such diarrhea can be caused by *Giardia*. Large volume diarrhea associated with pus in the stools is probably due to a *Salmonella* infection.

The incidence of traveler's diarrhea can be reduced, but not eliminated, by good hygiene and by a wide variety of prophylactic antibiotics. However, antibiotic prophylaxis is not generally recommended by experts, because the risks outweigh the benefits. The risks include toxic reaction to the antibiotic, promotion of resistant strains, rebound diarrhea when the antibiotic is stopped, and possible encouragement of the proliferation of more serious infections such as salmonellosis or typhoid fever. The incidence of traveler's diarrhea can also be reduced by ingestion of bismuth subsalicylate (Pepto-Bismol), 60 ml four times a day. This compound apparently inhibits colonization by enterotoxin-producing organisms. Whether or not smaller doses would be effective has not been established.

In about 20 per cent of cases, traveler's diarrhea lasts longer than 14 days. Giardiasis, amebiasis, and antibiotic-associated diarrhea or colitis (if the patient was treated with an antibiotic) should be suspected in such patients. If the diarrhea becomes chronic, tropical sprue, postdysentery irritable bowel syndrome, and postdysentery lactase deficiency should be suspected.

Treatment is usually supportive and symptomatic, and antibiotics are usually not advisable (see Therapy, below).

CHRONIC DIARRHEA OF UNKNOWN ORIGIN. This category

refers to patients in whom a more or less complete diagnostic evaluation in the recent past has failed to reveal the cause of chronic diarrhea. As was indicated in Table 102–3, the most likely causes of diarrhea in these patients, if indeed a specific diagnosis can be established, are *surreptitious laxative ingestion* and *irritable bowel syndrome.* If the patient has had episodes of salt and water depletion requiring intravenous therapy, hypokalemia, or a preoccupation with weight control, the likelihood of laxative abuse is increased. A rare patient in this category will turn out to have pancreatic cholera syndrome or one of its variants. Of course, almost any cause of diarrhea could have been missed during a previous "complete" evaluation, and all reasonably likely possibilities should be considered, earlier x-rays reviewed, and so forth. Some unusual and easily overlooked causes of chronic diarrhea are listed in the tables.

Assuming that the routine evaluation discussed above does not yield the likely diagnosis, the following studies are suggested: (1) Determination of stool volume, osmolality, and electrolytes in an attempt to classify the diarrhea as osmotic or secretory in type and to determine whether one is dealing with a large volume or small volume diarrhea. (2) Check of stool and urine for phenolphthalein and for other laxatives if possible. (3) Search of the patient's room and belongings for laxatives. (Some clinicians think it is unethical to search a patient's room. I think it is unethical not to do so in this group of patients, since if the diagnosis of surreptitious laxative abuse is missed, the patient will be subjected to many needless and to some potentially hazardous tests and therapies.) (4) Test for bile acid malabsorption, if this test is available. (5) Rectal biopsy.

If the patient is not taking laxatives or other drugs that can cause diarrhea or hypokalemia, further workup will be determined by what is found when stool volume and electrolytes are measured. If stool volumes are less than 500 ml per day, it is likely that the patient will ultimately be classified as having irritable bowel syndrome, although the tables should be used in an effort to make certain that other likely diseases have been excluded. If stool volumes are greater than 1 liter per day and the diarrhea is secretory in type, the causes of chronic secretory diarrhea listed in Table 102–1 should be considered. If the diarrhea is osmotic in type, the cause of the solute gap should be determined; carbohydrate malabsorption, a saline type laxative such as magnesium sulfate, ingestion of bran, and use of sorbitol (as a sugar substitute) are most likely.

INCONTINENCE. Most patients whose major disability is due to fecal incontinence present to their physician with "diarrhea." Either they are embarrassed to mention the incontinence or they interpret it as a manifestation of severe diarrhea. If patients do mention incontinence, the physician also usually attributes it to voluminous diarrhea. However, in most such instances these patients are suffering primarily from a defect in the continence mechanisms, rather than severe diarrhea. As a matter of fact, quantitative stool collections usually reveal rather small fecal volumes, even though stools are soft to liquid in consistency. In any case, the major problem in most such patients is in the anal continence mechanisms. Some causes of such defects are listed in Table 102–3.

Anal sphincter training may improve sphincter function and reduce the frequency of incontinent episodes. It is also important to establish the cause of diarrhea if possible, since effective therapy of the diarrhea will usually prevent further incontinence. Symptomatic therapy with opiate drugs is helpful in some patients. There is recent interest in surgical treatment for incontinence, but no good prospective studies have been done. No therapy for incontinence in diarrhea patients, whether involving drugs, biofeedback, or surgery, has included objective data that convincingly establish its benefit.

THERAPY

The most satisfactory therapy is to cure the underlying disease. When this is not possible, certain drugs may ameliorate the disease and thus reduce the severity of diarrhea (prednisone for inflammatory bowel disease is an example). In a few instances, the disease cannot be ameliorated but there is fairly specific therapy for the diarrhea, such as cholestyramine for bile acid malabsorption. It is hoped that a specific and potent inhibitor of intestinal secretion will soon be developed. Phenothiazine drugs inhibit intestinal secretion caused by cholera toxin and *E. coli* enterotoxins, but fear of side effects has limited their clinical application. An alternative hope is to discover a drug that will enhance the normal rate of absorption, and thus overcome the effect of a secretagogue. So far, no practical and useful drug in this category has been developed.

At present, unfortunately, in many patients the disease process responsible for diarrhea cannot be satisfactorily suppressed and specific therapy is lacking. Supportive and symptomatic therapy is required in such instances.

FLUID REPLACEMENT. The most important aspect of therapy in acute and traveler's diarrhea, and in some patients with chronic diarrhea, is prevention or correction of salt and water depletion. This can be done by oral ingestion of liquids and salty foods, oral glucose-saline solutions, or intravenous fluid therapy, as dictated by the clinical situation. Two points deserve emphasis. First, soft drinks, tea, and citrus juices contain little if any sodium chloride (even Gatorade contains only 23 mEq per liter sodium chloride). Second, oral glucose-saline solutions or liquids plus salty foods will actually worsen the diarrhea (in terms of stool volume) as they help correct fluid depletion.

AVOIDANCE OR TREATMENT OF PERIANAL DISCOMFORT. Apparently helpful therapy consists of (1) avoidance of soap, toilet paper, washcloths and towels; (2) gentle washing with warm water on absorbent cotton after each bowel movement, followed by gentle, thorough drying with absorbent cotton; (3) if seepage is present, absorbent cotton retained next to the anal orifice and held in place by snug underwear; (4) sitz baths for 10 minutes two or three times a day; and (5) hydrocortisone creams (1 per cent). In addition to these measures, patients may obtain relief by additional gentle cleaning with soft pads containing witch hazel (Tucks). Locally applied anesthetic ointments may be transiently helpful, but ointments restrict perspiration and anesthetics may irritate the perianal skin, so these agents should be used only for short periods of time. It is important to recognize specific treatable conditions, such as perianal moniliasis.

OPIATES. Codeine, diphenoxylate with atropine (Lomotil), and loperamide reduce urgency, bowel movement frequency, and stool volume in a wide variety of acute or chronic diarrheal illnesses. This is not to say that they have a beneficial effect in every patient; but they do in most, so that when groups of patients are studied, both stool frequency and stool volume are reduced to a statistically significant extent. Of the three drugs, loperamide and codeine are usually somewhat superior to diphenoxylate; loperamide may have less tendency than codeine to cause addiction. Codeine, however, is much less expensive. In chronic diarrhea, the drugs may be given once a day in a maximal tolerated dose, or several times daily in smaller doses.

Opiate drugs are generally thought to reduce diarrhea through reducing the propulsive activity of the gut and thereby reducing stool frequency. This mechanism might also enhance contact time between intestinal mucosal and luminal contents. Assuming that at least part of the gut mucosa is in an absorbing and not a secretory state, this would allow greater absorption of fluid and thereby reduce stool volume. Opiates have also been reported to stimulate active chloride absorption, and to have antisecretory action against several secretagogues. It has been suggested that these effects account for a major part of the antidiarrheal activity of opiate drugs. This concept has not been convincingly established in clinical situations using therapeutic doses of opiate drugs.

Opiate drugs should not be used in patients with severe ulcerative colitis with impending toxic megacolon, and there is suggestive evidence that they may prolong the duration of diarrhea in patients with shigellosis, and perhaps in diarrheal diseases caused by other invasive bacteria and in antibiotic-associated diarrhea. Opiates are hazardous in patients with liver disease, and they should not be used in young children. These reservations notwithstanding, opiates are often of benefit in the symptomatic relief of diarrhea in adult patients, including those with less severe ulcerative colitis and with many acute infectious diarrheal illnesses. Obviously, they should be prescribed only when diarrhea is causing significant disability.

There are rare case reports suggesting that opiate drugs can be a cause of paradoxical diarrhea.

BISMUTH SUBSALICYLATE. As already noted, bismuth subsalicylate apparently prevents infection with enterotoxin-producing *E. coli* organisms. In addition, this agent will bring mild symptomatic relief in patients with acute infectious diarrhea, whether bacterial or viral in origin. The mechanism of the effect is unknown. The dose is 30 to 60 ml every 30 minutes for eight doses. Patients should be warned that this medication may turn their stools black. If the patient is on other medications, possible drug interaction should be considered.

ANTIBIOTICS IN ACUTE AND TRAVELER'S DIARRHEA. For at least two reasons, antibiotics should not usually be used. First, in most patients they will not shorten the duration of illness. Second, their use risks the development of antibiotic-associated diarrhea or colitis, superimposed on whatever was causing the diarrhea in the first place. This greatly confuses the problem if the diarrhea becomes chronic.

In mild disease (small volume diarrhea, no chills or fever, no blood or pus in the stool), antibiotics should not be prescribed unless a specific indication emerges from the bacteriology and parasitology laboratory. In patients who are severely ill, especially if they have blood or pus in the stool, antibiotic therapy aimed at shigellosis is reasonable, pending the result of stool culture.

Binder HJ (ed.): Mechanisms of Intestinal Secretion. New York, Alan R. Liss, Inc., Kroc Foundation Series, Vol. 12, 1979. *A detailed examination of the mechanisms of intestinal secretion. Twenty-two chapters by different experts, with an emphasis on basic research.*

Field M, Fordtran JS, Schultz SG (eds.): Secretory Diarrhea. Bethesda, Maryland, American Physiological Society, 1980. *Sixteen chapters by different experts on various aspects of the pathophysiology of secretory diarrhea. The emphasis is on basic research, although there is a highly original chapter on the pharmacology of antidiarrheal drugs by DW Powell and M Field.*

Krejs GJ, Fordtran JS: Diarrhea. *In* Sleisenger MH, Fordtran JS (eds.): Gastrointestinal Disease. 3rd ed. Philadelphia, W. B. Saunders Company, 1983, pp 257–279. *A detailed description of the physiology of the human intestinal tract with regard to water and electrolyte movement and the pathophysiology of chronic diarrhea.*

Lambert HP (ed.): Infections of the GI Tract. Clin Gastroenterol 8:No 3, 1979. *Twelve excellent chapters by different experts dealing with pathophysiology of diarrhea, viral infections, pathogenic mechanisms in bacterial diarrhea,* E. coli, Shigella, *food poisoning, typhoid and paratyphoid fever,* Campylobacter *enteritis, traveler's diarrhea, antibiotic-associated colitis, antibiotic resistance, and antimicrobial agents. The book contains much practical and clinically useful information.*

Read NW, Harford WV, Schmulen AC, Read MG, Santa Ana CA, Fordtran JS: A clinical study of patients with fecal incontinence and diarrhea. Gastroenterology 76:747, 1979. *This article emphasizes the importance of fecal incontinence in patients with chronic diarrhea. Mechanisms of normal continence are discussed and diagnostic tests are proposed.*

Read, NW, Krejs GJ, Read MG, Santa Ana CA, Morawski SG, Fordtran JS: Chronic diarrhea of unknown origin. Gastroenterology 78:264, 1980. *A detailed account of the clinical problems encountered in patients with intractable and difficult-to-diagnose chronic diarrhea.*

103. MALABSORPTION

103.1. Pathophysiology and Diagnosis

Robert M. Glickman

The malabsorption syndrome is a constellation of symptoms and signs that are the direct result of altered intestinal absorption of fat, protein, carbohydrate, minerals, and vitamins. Occasionally, diseases may selectively impair the absorption of a given nutrient or vitamin, with a correspondingly more restricted deficiency state because certain absorptive processes are restricted to limited portions of the gastrointestinal tract. In order to treat malabsorption, the physician should clearly define the absorptive defects, relate them to the abnormal function of a portion of the gastrointestinal tract, and uncover the disease entity or entities responsible.

MECHANISMS OF NORMAL ABSORPTION

Normal absorption refers to the processes by which the end products of digestion leave the intestinal lumen, traverse the intestinal epithelial cells, and gain entrance to the general circulation by way of either the portal vein or the lymphatics. The products of digestion (amino acids, fatty acids, sugars) must make intimate contact with the microvillus membrane of the intestinal epithelial cell to allow efficient cellular uptake. Both intestinal peristalsis and contraction of individual microvilli assist molecules to penetrate an "unstirred layer" adjacent to microvilli. Decreased intestinal peristalsis (i.e., visceral neuropathy, scleroderma) increase the barrier effect of this unstirred layer. Nutrients cross the cell membrane by one or both of two processes, *active transport* or *passive transport*.

Active transport moves substances across the cell membrane against a chemical or electrical gradient at the cost of metabolic work with the expenditure of energy. Active transport is "saturable," since the rate of transport levels off as luminal electrochemical activity of the ion increases.

Passive transport, requiring no energy, is the passage of a molecule across a membrane barrier according to chemical concentration and electrical gradients. Examples are the absorption of fatty acids, water, and bile salts in the jejunum. Some ions are simply carried across by water moving into the cell, "solvent drag."

FAT ABSORPTION. Fat absorption is a multi-step process involving the coordinated participation of several organs and is carried out very efficiently. Under normal conditions less than 5 per cent of ingested fat (about 100 grams daily) is recovered in the stool. As shown in Figure 103–1, the overall process of fat absorption can be conveniently considered as being composed of several processes within three phases: (1) luminal phase, (2) mucosal phase, and (3) secretory phase (lymphatic or portal venous transport).

Intraluminal Digestion. Most dietary fat is ingested in the

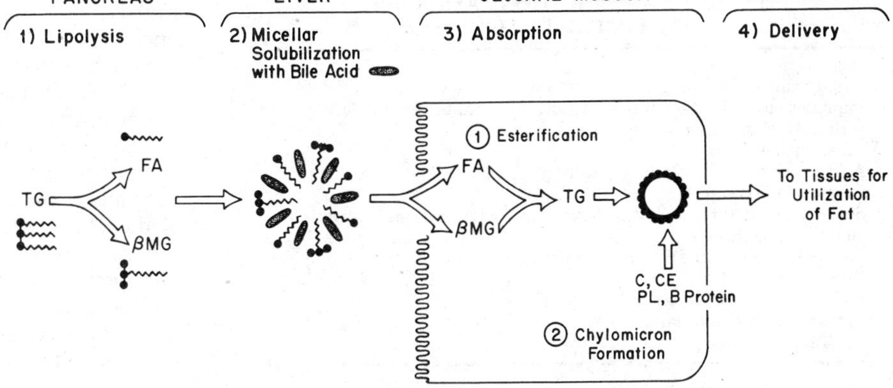

Figure 103–1. Schematic of intestinal absorption, showing the participation of pancreas, liver, and intestinal mucosal cell in fat absorption. (From Wilson FA, Dietschy JM: Gastroenterology 61:911, 1971. Copyright 1971, The Williams & Wilkins Company, Baltimore.)

form of triglycerides containing three long chain fatty acids on a glycerol backbone. Triglyceride undergoes some hydrolysis in the stomach through the action of lingual and gastric lipases. The major role of the stomach, however, is in emulsification of lipid for slow release into the duodenum. Most lipolysis of triglyceride occurs in the duodenum catalyzed by pancreatic lipase, which hydrolyzes triglyceride to yield free fatty acids and one molecule of β-monoglyceride. In addition to lipase, the pancreas must also secrete an additional pancreatic factor, colipase, which facilitates the interaction between lipase and triglyceride, permitting efficient hydrolysis. The presence of bile salts and a pH greater than 4 are also required for optimal lipase activity. The release of cholecystokinin-pancreozymin (CCK-PZ) from duodenal epithelial cells stimulates pancreatic secretion and contraction of the gallbladder, providing pancreatic enzymes and bile salts. *Secretin,* released from duodenal mucosa by gastric acid, stimulates the secretion of bicarbonate-rich pancreatic fluid and thereby raises duodenal pH to permit effective lipolysis.

The pathogenesis of impaired lipolysis can be classified with respect to abnormalities of these physiologic variables (Table 103–1). Lipolysis releases monoglyceride and fatty acids that are more water soluble than the parent triglyceride. Efficient absorption depends on *micelle* formation in which these lipid moieties interact with conjugated bile salts in mixed aggregates or micelles. A "critical micellar concentration" is maintained by efficient mechanisms that conserve the total bile salt pool, which is only 2 to 4 grams, by an enterohepatic circulation whereby about 95 per cent of bile salts are actively absorbed in the terminal ileum and returned to the liver by the portal venous system. This bile acid pool is recycled several times during the course of a meal, totaling up to 30 grams per day. Thus, at most, 600 mg of bile salts needs to be synthesized by the liver each day, an amount equal to that lost in the stool.

Significant amounts of fat may be absorbed in the absence of bile salts. Conditions of impaired micelle formation and decreased lipid absorption are shown in Table 103–2.

Mucosal Phase. Lipids that have been incorporated into luminal micelles diffuse more readily to the microvillus membrane where they are thought to be taken up passively because of their solubility in the lipid rich surface membrane. A low molecular weight, cytosolic protein, fatty acid binding protein, avidly binds fatty acids and appears to function as an intracellular transport protein for long chain fatty acids. These fatty acids are transported to the smooth endoplasmic reticulum, where they are re-esterified with monoglyceride to form triglyceride. Absorbed cholesterol is also largely esterified with fatty acids yielding cholesterol esters, the major transport form for cholesterol. After re-esterification of lipids, the intestine must synthesize phospholipids and specific proteins (apoproteins) in order to incorporate these nonpolar lipids into lipoproteins, the major transport vehicles for lipid transport in lymph and plasma. These polar components are added to the surface of the lipid droplet, producing lipoproteins called *chylomicrons.* The synthesis of apoprotein B, a chylomicron apoprotein, is of particular importance for triglyceride transport, since it is obligatory for chylomicron formation and secretion. Abetalipoproteinemia (discussed below) represents a genetic defect of apoprotein B synthesis with consequent impairment of chylomicron formation.

Secretory Phase. Once the intracellular phase of chylomicron formation is complete, the particles are concentrated in the Golgi apparatus and then are discharged through the lateral basal portion of the cell to the interstitium and mesenteric lymph to be delivered via the thoracic duct to the vena cava.

Most triglyceride absorption takes place in the upper jejunum, although the ileum is capable of chylomicron formation and secretion. It does so when jejunal function is impaired (i.e., jejunal resection). C6 to C10 fatty acids and triglycerides containing these fatty acids are transported by alternative mechanisms. In general, these triglycerides are better absorbed than long chain triglycerides, since (1) they are more completely hydrolyzed by pancreatic lipase; (2) they are less dependent on micellar solubilization; (3) approximately 30 per cent of unsplit medium chain triglycerides can be directly taken up into the intestinal epithelial cell and subsequently hydrolyzed by a mucosal lipase to fatty acids; and (4) unlike long chain fatty acids, medium chain fatty acids do not require resynthesis to triglyceride and can pass directly into the portal venous system. These represent major therapeutic advantages for lipid absorption in patients with a variety of malabsorption syndromes. Medium chain triglycerides exist in low concentrations in normal diets but are available for therapeutic use (see below).

Fat-soluble vitamins (A, D, E, K) are absorbed after micellar solubilization and are transported into lymph with chylomicrons. In the case of vitamin A, the free vitamin is esterified in the intestinal epithelial cell with a molecule of fatty acid, and vitamin A ester is then incorporated into chylomicrons.

PROTEIN AND AMINO ACID ABSORPTION. Dietary protein, as well as endogenous protein from intestinal secretions and desquamated cells, cannot be absorbed intact in nutritionally significant amounts and so must first be digested. Although gastric proteases or pepsins may initiate protein digestion, the role of gastric digestion is not a major one. In contrast, the proteolytic enzymes in pancreatic secretions have a major role in protein digestion. Secreted as inactive enzymes or zymogens, pancreatic proteases must be activated by a small intestinal mucosal enzyme, enterokinase, which is liberated by the presence of food in the duodenum. Trypsin, liberated from trypsinogen by enterokinase, is thought to activate the other pancreatic proteases from their zymogens. Endopeptidases (trypsin, chymotrypsin, elastase) cleave internal peptide bonds, whereas exopeptidases cleave peptide bonds at the carboxy terminus. The resultant products are a mixture of peptides of variable length (two to six amino acids) as well as single amino acids. Oligopeptides are quantitatively the major product (70 per cent) of pancreatic proteases; further hydrolysis of these oligopeptides to free amino acids is accomplished by peptidases located either on the microvillus membrane or in the cytosol of the enterocyte. The composition and chain length of an individual peptide appear to influence the subcellular site of peptide

TABLE 103–1. CONDITIONS ASSOCIATED WITH IMPAIRED LIPOLYSIS

Postgastrectomy
Rapid transit ("dumping")
Improper emulsification of triglyceride, bicarbonate, and lipase, e.g., Billroth II anastomosis
Altered duodenal pH
Acid hypersecretion—Zollinger-Ellison syndrome
Decreased CCK-PZ release
Severe intestinal mucosal destruction, e.g., sprue, regional enteritis
Pancreatic insufficiency
Loss of lipase and bicarbonate secretion
Chronic pancreatitis
Pancreatic duct obstruction
Decreased luminal bile salts
See Table 103–2

TABLE 103–2. CONDITIONS ASSOCIATED WITH IMPAIRED MICELLE FORMATION

Decreased hepatic synthesis of bile salts
Severe parenchymal liver disease
Decreased delivery of bile salts to the intestinal lumen
Biliary obstruction (stone, tumor, primary biliary cirrhosis)
Cholestatic liver disease
Decreased effective concentration of conjugated bile acids
Increased acidity (Zollinger-Ellison syndrome)—decreased ionization of bile salts with increased proximal absorption
Drugs affecting micelle formation—neomycin, cholestyramine
Stasis syndromes with secondary bacterial overgrowth and bile salt deconjugation
Increased intestinal loss of bile salts
Ileal disease or resection

hydrolysis. The final products of peptide hydrolysis are amino acids that are directly absorbed into the portal vein.

Distinct active transport systems have been described in the intestinal mucosal cell for neutral and basic amino acids. These systems transport the L form of the amino acid, require energy, and depend on luminal sodium for activity. In addition to specific amino acid transport systems, transport of di- and tripeptides across the microvillus membrane into the cell has been described. Certain peptides are preferentially transported into the enterocyte without brush border hydrolysis. This mechanism may explain why severe nutritional disturbances are uncommon in diseases such as Hartnup disease despite a severe defect in the transport of neutral amino acids. Presumably, small peptides can enter the enterocyte through independent transport systems; there they undergo cytoplasmic hydrolysis, with subsequent absorption of amino acids.

From the aforementioned considerations protein malabsorption would be expected in diseases causing pancreatic insufficiency, those which impair enterocyte function, or those which decrease the absorbing surface.

CARBOHYDRATE ABSORPTION. Carbohydrate, in the form of starches, sucrose, and lactose, is a major component of diets throughout the world. All carbohydrate must be digested to a final monosaccharide product before it can be transported from the intestinal epithelial cell into the portal vein. Carbohydrate digestion is accomplished by initial pancreatic hydrolysis, with the resultant oligosaccharides split into their component monosaccharides by specific hydrolytic enzymes located in the microvillus membranes of the enterocyte. Pancreatic amylase, an α-amylase, hydrolyzes interior α1,4 linkages of starch, but not α1,6 linkages. Therefore the principal products of amylase action are maltose and maltotriose. Amylase action is extremely efficient, with most starch hydrolysis occurring in the duodenum. These oligosaccharides, as well as dietary sucrose and lactose, require further hydrolysis by specific microvillus membrane disaccharidases for absorption. Sucrase, lactase, and α-dextrinase (isomaltase) each participate in specific hydrolysis of sucrose, lactose, maltose, and maltotriose, as well as α-limit dextrins, liberating glucose and fructose (from sucrose), glucose and galactose (from lactose), and glucose (from maltose and α-dextrins). These monosaccharides traverse the brush border and gain entry into the cell by specific transport processes which are stereospecific and require sodium. Galactose and glucose share the same transport system, whereas fructose is transported by facilitated diffusion. Xylose is actively transported via the glucose-galactose transport system. Glucose is transported into the cell probably bound (with sodium) to a protein carrier. Monosaccharides are transported out of the cell by active sodium extrusion across the basolateral aspect of the enterocyte via a sodium pump and then moved into the portal vein.

From the aforementioned considerations, one could predict malabsorption of dietary carbohydrates in the following circumstances: (1) severe pancreatic insufficiency; (2) selective deficiency of brush border disaccharidases, i.e., sucrase or lactase deficiency; (3) generalized impairment of brush border and enterocyte function, i.e., sprue, extensive regional enteritis; and (4) loss of mucosal surface, i.e., short bowel syndromes.

VITAMIN B_{12} ABSORPTION. Vitamin B_{12} (cobalamin), synthesized by microorganisms, is found almost exclusively in foods containing animal protein, from which it must be liberated and absorbed via a specific intestinal transport system. Vitamin B_{12} is liberated from food by cooking and by the action of acid and pepsin in the stomach. In order to be absorbed, the vitamin must combine with *intrinsic factor,* a glycoprotein synthesized and secreted by the gastric parietal cell. The B_{12}–intrinsic factor complex is the only form in which the vitamin can be absorbed by a specific transport system in the ileum. Vitamin B_{12} also avidly binds to other glycoproteins present in saliva, gastric juice, bile, and intestinal juice called R binders, but these complexes cannot be absorbed by the ileum. In fact, pancreatic proteases degrade the R binders in the duodenum and permit vitamin B_{12} to associate with intrinsic factor. The B_{12}–intrinsic factor complex is bound to specific receptors on the microvillus membrane of the entire ileum, with maximal activity in the terminal ileum. After a lag period of several hours, cobalamin appears in the ileal cell and is absorbed into the portal circulation bound to a transport protein, transcobalamin II. Intrinsic factor is not absorbed. From these considerations it is possible to predict that impaired B_{12} absorption would result from intrinsic factor deficiency (pernicious anemia), failure to degrade R binders (pancreatic insufficiency), diseased or absent ileum (regional enteritis, ileal resection, sprue). In addition, bacterial overgrowth may be associated with a decreased absorption of vitamin B_{12} (discussed below).

FOLIC ACID ABSORPTION. Dietary folic acid is present in foods in the form of polyglutamates; these are hydrolyzed to monoglutamates, probably via an enzyme found on the microvillus membrane. The absorption of monoglutamates is thought to be an active process at low concentrations of folate, but folate may be passively transported at higher concentrations. Folic acid is recycled to some degree by an enterohepatic circulation. Although most cases of folic acid deficiency are dietary in origin (in contrast to vitamin B_{12} deficiency), extensive duodenal and jejunal involvement with disease (i.e., celiac disease) may result in folate deficiency.

WATER AND ELECTROLYTE ABSORPTION. Water and electrolyte absorption takes place largely in the small intestine. Water moves across the membrane passively, i.e., secondary to osmotic gradients. The rate of water absorption in the small gut is five to ten times that in the stomach. To some extent water follows the active transport of glucose and electrolytes, moving with them to maintain isotonicity of intraluminal contents. The small intestine usually absorbs over 7 liters of water per day, representing ingested water and reabsorption of gastrointestinal secretions.

Sodium transport is in part an active process that is linked to an exchange with H^+ in both jejunum and ileum. A similar exchange mechanism for Cl^- and HCO_3^- exists only in the ileum. In vitro studies indicate that a Na^+ pump mechanism may be operative. In humans, Na^+ transport is enhanced by absorption of glucose in the jejunum, either via this mechanism or by being "dragged" into the cell by the water in which glucose is carried. Some Na^+ also moves passively, i.e., down a gradient across the mucosa. Potassium movement seems to be passive, diffusing from the lumen proximally and into the lumen distally.

The amount of water and sodium absorbed represents the difference between influx from lumen to blood and efflux in the reverse direction. This net flux is diminished by hypertonicity of the intraluminal solution and is increased by hypotonicity. Changes in concentration of sodium in the lumen depend on relative rates of exchange of both sodium and water between blood and lumen.

During diarrhea, sodium concentration increases with increasing stool volume, and beyond 3 liters approaches values close to that of plasma. Conversely, potassium concentration progressively decreases.

CALCIUM AND IRON ABSORPTION. *Calcium* is absorbed mainly in the duodenum by an active process that is principally regulated by vitamin D. While vitamin D is absorbed from the diet as a fat-soluble vitamin that is transported from the intestine via chylomicrons, the dietary form of the vitamin (vitamin D_3) must be metabolized initially by the liver (25-hydroxylation) and then by the kidney (1-hydroxylation) to form the major active form of the vitamin 1,25-dihydroxycholecalciferol ($1,25(OH)_2D_3$) (Ch. 244). This conversion is responsive to parathyroid hormone levels, which in turn are regulated by the calcium requirement. $1,25(OH)_2D_3$ stimulates intestinal calcium absorption through mechanisms that have been elucidated only in part. The activated vitamin, now more properly considered a hormone, localizes in the nucleus of the enterocyte, leading to synthesis of calcium-binding protein, alkaline phosphatase, and a calcium-activated ATPase, all of which may participate in active calcium transport. Calcium absorption is also influenced by luminal pH and the presence of excessive amounts of insoluble or poorly soluble anions (fatty acids), which can bind calcium in the lumen, making it unavailable for absorption.

Iron is absorbed actively in an amount sufficient to balance normal losses through cell desquamation and minor bleeding. This requires about 0.5 to 1.0 mg in the adult man and postmenopausal woman and about 1.2 to 1.8 mg for women during the years of normal menstruation. The rate of iron absorption can be increased five to eight times during iron deficiency. Absorption, which occurs principally in the duodenum, is a two-step process of uptake and transfer. Uptake is dependent upon oxidative metabolism. The transfer of Fe through the serosa to the circulation is probably the rate-limiting step. In plasma iron is bound to a specific globulin, *transferrin*, which transports it to tissues for storage, particularly to the liver. Iron absorption is diminished in chronic infection and by prior administration of large amounts of iron, and is increased in iron deficiency and during active erythropoiesis. Animal hemoglobin is an important source of iron in the human, and in fact is that form of iron most rapidly absorbed, followed by Fe^{++} and then Fe^{+++}. Heme is readily absorbed as the intact molecule from which iron is split within the cell by heme oxygenase. Some iron is released from heme intraluminally and is taken up directly by the cells.

Absorption of inorganic iron depends upon its release from dietary compounds to which it is originally bound. Absorption of both Fe^{+++} and Fe^{++} is enhanced by chelation with ascorbic acid, carbohydrates, and amino acids at the pH of normal gastric juice. These complexes remain soluble at the alkaline pH of the duodenum where iron is absorbed. Diminished iron absorption is associated with achlorhydria, because an acid pH is needed to solubilize ferric iron for chelation with ascorbic acid and other substances, in which form it is absorbed. However, ferrous iron may also be chelated at an alkaline pH. Overall, iron absorption is regulated by the state of repletion, content of iron in absorbing cells, and factors affecting erythropoiesis. The influence of gastric and pancreatic juice proteins which bind iron is still uncertain. Iron absorption is also discussed in Ch. 131 and 206.

TABLE 103–3. CLASSIFICATION OF MALABSORPTION SYNDROME

I. Category 1: Defective intraluminal hydrolysis or solubilization
- A. Primary pancreatic insufficiency
- B. Secondary pancreatic insufficiency
- C. Deficiency of conjugated bile acids
- D. Bacterial overgrowth (bile acid deconjugation)
  - 1. Blind loops
  - 2. Multiple strictures and jejunal diverticula
  - 3. Fistulas
  - 4. Postgastrectomy
  - 5. Scleroderma and pseudo-obstruction

II. Category 2: Mucosal cell abnormality and inadequate surface
- A. Primary mucosal cell disorders
  - 1. Disaccharidase deficiency and monosaccharide malabsorption
  - 2. Abetalipoproteinemia
  - 3. Vitamin B_{12} malabsorption
  - 4. Cystinuria and Hartnup disease
- B. Small bowel disease
  - 1. Celiac disease
  - 2. Whipple's disease
  - 3. Nongranulomatous ileojejunitis
  - 4. Allergic and eosinophilic gastroenteritis
  - 5. Amyloidosis
  - 6. Small bowel ischemia
  - 7. Crohn's disease (granulomatous enteritis)
- C. Inadequate surface

III. Category 3: Lymphatic obstruction
- A. Lymphoma
- B. Tuberculosis and tuberculous lymphadenitis
- C. Lymphangiectasia

IV. Category 4: Infection
- A. Tropical sprue
- B. Acute infectious enteritis
- C. Parasitoses

V. Category 5: Multiple defects
- A. Subtotal gastrectomy
- B. Distal ileal resection, disease, or bypass
- C. Radiation enteritis

VI. Category 6: Unexplained
- A. Hypogammaglobulinemia
- B. Carcinoid syndrome
- C. Hypothyroidism
- D. Diabetes mellitus
- E. Mastocytosis
- F. Hyperthyroidism and hypoadrenocorticism

VII. Category 7: Drug-induced malabsorption
- A. Cholestyramine
- B. Colchicine
- C. Irritant laxatives
- D. Neomycin
- E. p-Aminosalicylic acid
- F. Phenindione

CAUSES OF THE MALABSORPTION SYNDROME

The principal diseases and disorders that may give rise to the malabsorption syndrome are listed in Table 103–3. These conditions are discussed in detail in a subsequent portion of this chapter and are presented only in brief outline at this point. They can be divided conveniently into seven categories, based upon pathologic and pathophysiologic considerations.

CLINICAL MANIFESTATIONS

The signs and symptoms of the malabsorption syndrome include weight loss, anorexia, abdominal distention, borborygmi, muscle wasting, and passage of abnormal stools that are characteristically light yellow to gray, greasy, and soft. In many instances frequent movements are noted, but occasionally there is only one very bulky stool per day. The patient may describe the stools as sticky or malodorous. There may be difficulty in flushing the stool down the toilet because of excess stickiness. The traditional description of steatorrhea as "floating" stools because of their fat content is incorrect; they float because of their gas. In addition, edema, ascites, skeletal disorders, peripheral and circumoral paresthesias, tetany, and, rarely, convulsions may be observed.

The clinical features and the pathophysiological basis of the signs and symptoms of the malabsorption syndrome are detailed in Table 103–4. The symptoms may be intermittent or low grade, so that medical attention is not sought for a very long time—more than 35 years in some instances of adult celiac disease. They may complain only of fatigue and depression, and may lose weight only during the early months of illness.

In more severe malabsorption secondary manifestations such as bleeding or skeletal pain may predominate. In some patients borborygmi and abdominal distention are the complaints, while others seek help for weakness or dyspnea secondary to anemia.

Persistent or severe cramping periumbilical or right lower quadrant pain not relieved by movements is frequently seen in patients with *Crohn's disease* and, with stricturing and obstruction, may become chronic and associated with distention and emesis. Diffuse periumbilical pain is often suffered by patients with *nongranulomatous ileojejunitis, lymphoma, eosinophilic gastroenteritis, radiation enteritis, amyloidosis,* and, occasionally, *adult celiac disease.* Patients with *chronic pancreatitis* usually suffer recurrent deep epigastric pain that radiates to the midback; in patients with *lymphoma* of the small intestine and mesentery, the pain may be cramping (obstruction) or steady and intense (local invasion or spread).

Patients with malabsorption owing to *ischemia* of the small gut have periumbilical or midabdominal cramping pains 30 minutes after meals and may fear to eat. Those with *hypogammaglobulinemia* may have other historical evidences of immunoglobulin deficiency (repeated infections, or even symptoms suggesting malignancy). *Eosinophilic gastroenteritis* may be highlighted by a specific "food allergy" or by a history of skin,

TABLE 103–4. CORRELATION OF LABORATORY DATA WITH ABSORPTIVE DEFECTS AND SIGNS AND SYMPTOMS OF THE MALABSORPTION SYNDROME

Clinical Features	Laboratory Evidence	Pathophysiology
Muscle wasting; small stature; edema	↓ Serum albumin	*Impaired protein metabolism* ↓ Absorption ↓ Intake
Skeletal deformity; pain fractures	X-ray: demineralization; collapsed vertebrae	↑ Enteric loss ↓ Synthesis
Weight loss; pale, bulky stools	↑ Fecal fat ↓ Serum cholesterol, carotene	*Impaired absorption and excess loss of:* Fat
Paresthesias; tetany; + Chvostek; Trousseau; bone pain; fractures	↓ Serum Ca^{++}; ↓ or normal $PO_4^{\equiv}$; ↑ alkaline phosphatase; x-ray: Looser's lines, Milkman's fractures; ↑ osteoid seams; ↓ serum Mg^{++}	Fat-soluble vitamins and calcium Vitamin D, calcium, magnesium
Bleeding: ecchymoses, hematuria	↑ Prothrombin time with response to vitamin K	Vitamin K
Hyperkeratosis follicularis	↓ Serum carotene, vitamin A tolerance	Vitamin A
G Paresthesias; neuropathy A L N O	Macrocytic anemia; megaloblastosis; ↓ serum B_{12} and ↓ absorption B_{12}	Vitamin B_{12}
E S M S I I	Macrocytic anemia; megaloblastosis; ↓ serum folic acid	Folic acid
A T Koilonychia I S	Microcytosis, hypochromia; ↓ serum iron and ↓ saturation iron binding protein; ↓ iron in marrow	Iron
Dehydration; nocturia	↓ Plasma volume	Water
Muscle cramps, weakness	↓ Serum Na^{+}	Sodium
Muscle flaccidity, weakness; ↓ tendon reflexes, arrhythmias	↓ Serum K^{+}; EKG abnormalities	Potassium
Cheilosis; neuritis; dermatitis, glossitis; muscle weakness	↑ Urinary 5-HIAA, indican; ↓ serum B_{12}, folic acid	Vitamin B complex; folic acid, vitamin B_{12}
Abdominal distention, flatulence; diarrhea	Low to flat oral glucose tolerance curve; ↓ absorption d-xylose; ↓ oral lactose tolerance; ↓ or absent rise of blood glucose after oral sucrose; ↓ or absent rise of blood reducing substances after oral galactose; fluid levels on x-ray; stools: acid pH, + Clinitest	Impaired hydrolysis of disaccharides, particularly lactose and sucrose, or ↓ absorption of monosaccharides and amino acids

nasopharyngeal, bronchial, or other allergy. Virulent peptic ulcer disease *(Zollinger-Ellison syndrome)* will usually highlight the history of malabsorption caused by gastric hypersecretion. Diarrhea associated with carbohydrate will be noted from childhood in those with *disaccharidase deficiency* or *monosaccharide malabsorption*. Surgical scars and associated histories will characterize cases of *massive resection, gastrectomy* and *ileal resection, bypass procedures,* and *blind loops*. Those with *enteroenteric* or *enterocolic fistulas* as well have a long history of inflammatory disease, usually Crohn's disease, or malignancy. Hepatobiliary tract disorders will have features of chronic obstruction of the common bile duct or of chronic intrahepatic disease.

Physical examination early in the course may be unimpressive, with perhaps only some smoothness of the edges of the tongue or minimal abdominal distention. Later it will reveal one or more evidences of malnutrition and multiple vitamin deficiencies: pallor, diffuse brownish pigmentation of the skin but not of the mucous membranes, hyperkeratosis, petechiae or ecchymoses, muscle wasting, edema, abdominal distention, skeletal deformity (particularly kyphosis), positive Chvostek and/or Trousseau signs, glossitis, cheilosis, impaired vibration sense, deep muscle pain, and clubbing of the fingers. In addition, signs of various underlying diseases listed in Table 103–3 may be noted.

The malabsorption syndrome may be fatal, owing to the nature of the underlying disease (lymphoma, pancreatic carcinoma, progressive scleroderma, or granulomatous enteritis) or to the complications of malabsorption, which include superimposed infection, hypokalemia, or progressive inanition.

PATHOPHYSIOLOGIC BASIS FOR CLINICAL MANIFESTATIONS

Table 103–4 correlates the various absorptive defects and vitamin deficiencies, the clinical signs and symptoms, and the abnormalities of the routine laboratory tests in the malabsorption syndrome. Rarely does a patient manifest all the findings listed in Table 103–4, but many patients will exhibit many of them.

IMPAIRED PROTEIN METABOLISM: WEIGHT LOSS, EDEMA. Impairment of protein metabolism is reflected by decreased muscle mass and lowered serum protein levels. It may result from several factors. Synthesis may be below normal owing to defective protein absorption, diminished intake, or associated liver disease. Catabolism or breakdown is accelerated because of inadequate intake and absorption of carbohydrate. Decreased serum albumin may result also from abnormal loss of protein into the lumen of the gut, so-called *protein-losing enteropathy* (see below). *Hypogammaglobulinemia,* both congenital and acquired, has also been associated with steatorrhea, but the defective fat absorption cannot be related directly to low plasma globulins.

The emaciation and weakness may be extreme and may erroneously suggest far advanced malignancy.

CLINICAL EFFECTS OF STEATORRHEA. Excess loss of fat in the stool deprives the body of substantial numbers of calories and contributes greatly to weight loss and malnutrition. The irritative effect of unabsorbed hydroxylated long-chain (C18) fatty acids may contribute to the diarrhea with its severe losses of water, electrolytes, and other nutrients. In addition, fatty acids bind calcium and reduce its absorption. Intraluminal calcium normally inhibits the absorption of dietary oxalate by precipitating it as calcium oxalate in the gut. When unabsorbed fatty acids bind calcium, oxalate absorption is abnormally enhanced, resulting in calcium oxalate kidney stones, particularly in patients with massive small bowel resections. Flatulence, fluid in loops of small intestine, and abdominal distention may be related to both diminished fat absorption and excessive carbohydrate fermentation. Failure to absorb fat-soluble vitamins A, D, and K also results in a variety of serious symptoms, as recorded in Table 103–4.

VITAMIN D DEFICIENCY: HYPOCALCEMIA AND SKELETAL DISEASE IN MALABSORPTION SYNDROME; HYPOMAGNESEMIA. Low serum calcium results from failure of normal absorption owing both to vitamin D deficiency and to binding of calcium by unabsorbed fatty acids. Symptoms and signs caused by depression of ionized plasma calcium are listed in Table 103–4 and are described in detail in Ch. 243.

Low levels of serum calcium stimulate parathyroid activity. Increased secretion of parathormone raises the level of blood calcium both by direct effect upon bone and by a renal mechanism. These processes lead to osteitis fibrosa. In addition, the low product of calcium and phosphorus in extracellular fluid impairs the mineralization of osteoid, resulting in osteomalacia. Osteomalacia principally affects the spine, rib cage, and long bones, with or without fractures (Milkman's fractures), and may cause extreme pain, particularly of the spine, pelvis, and legs (see Ch. 244).

In patients with poor protein nutrition, in part caused by malabsorption or protein-losing enteropathy (see below), particularly in postmenopausal women and elderly men, *osteoporosis* is an additional cause of osteopenia.

Hypomagnesemia may also be noted in the malabsorption syndrome, causing symptoms that are identical with those of hypocalcemia. Differentiation is accomplished by the finding of lowered serum magnesium and by disappearance of symptoms only after administration of magnesium chloride or sulfate. Hypomagnesemia may also dramatically reduce the responsiveness of the parathyroids to hypocalcemia. Indeed, correction of magnesium deficiency may be essential to restoration of normal calcium by action of the parathyroid glands (see Ch. 208).

VITAMIN K DEFICIENCY: BLEEDING DIATHESIS IN MALABSORPTION SYNDROME. As noted, *bleeding*, particularly subcutaneous, nasal, urinary, vaginal, and occasionally gastrointestinal, is not uncommon in the malabsorption syndrome and may be the principal symptom. Defects in coagulation result from deficiency of factors II, VII, IX, and X owing to impaired absorption of fat-soluble vitamin K. In addition, severe folate deficiency may be accompanied by thrombocytopenia, which may also contribute to the bleeding diathesis.

VITAMIN A DEFICIENCY. In the malabsorption syndrome *hyperkeratosis follicularis* may be noted, but *nyctalopia* is very rare.

VITAMIN E DEFICIENCY. Vitamin E levels are often depressed in the malabsorption syndrome, reflecting fat-soluble vitamin malabsorption. While there was previously uncertainty whether vitamin E deficiency resulted in specific signs or symptoms, there is increasing evidence that deficiency of the vitamin may lead to progressive neurologic disease. Demyelinating disorders of the central nervous system have been reported in severe, prolonged vitamin E deficiency associated with abetalipoproteinemia (see below) as well as severe fat malabsorption secondary to biliary atresia. Thus neurologic disease associated with fat malabsorption should suggest vitamin E deficiency as a potential cause.

MANIFESTATIONS OF ABNORMAL CARBOHYDRATE ABSORPTION. The abnormal carbohydrate absorption results in diminished glycogen stores in liver and muscle. Also, intraluminal fermentation of sugars contributes greatly to abdominal distention and flatulence. Failure to hydrolyze disaccharides, particularly lactose *(disaccharidase deficiency)*, results in watery diarrhea as well as these local abdominal complaints (see below). Bacterial conversion of unabsorbed carbohydrate yields volatile fatty acids which may cause diarrhea by inhibiting water and sodium absorption by the colon.

VITAMIN B_{12} DEFICIENCY (see also Ch. 135). Deficiency of vitamin B_{12} or folic acid may cause a macrocytic anemia with a megaloblastic bone marrow, whereas iron deficiency will cause a microcytic hypochromic anemia. With deficiency of vitamin B_{12}, folic acid, and iron, anemia with mixed features will be present. The major diseases and disorders of B_{12} deficiency are listed in Table 103–5. Pernicious anemia is the only one among them that has B_{12} absorption significantly corrected by giving intrinsic factor with it. The various B_{12} absorption tests are found in Table 103–5. Impaired vitamin B_{12} absorption and megaloblastosis may also be noted occasionally in patients with *adult celiac disease* usually reflecting severe disease involving the ileum.

FOLIC ACID DEFICIENCY (see also Ch. 135). Folic acid deficiency may also underlie *megaloblastosis* and *anemia*. As there is often an associated deficiency of vitamin B_{12}, diagnosis may be established only by the finding of low serum folic acid levels (less than 5.0 ng per milliliter), or of a reticulocytic response to administration of minimal daily effective dosage (0.05 to 0.5 mg parenterally). Usually, however, folic acid deficiency is corrected by adequate diet or oral supplementation.

GLOSSITIS AND PERIPHERAL NEUROPATHY. *Glossitis* and *peripheral neuropathy* can in part be attributed to deficiency of vitamin B_{12}. Since combined system disease may be induced or exacerbated by administration of folic acid, *vitamin B_{12} stores in tissues must be replenished before administration of folic acid alone for megaloblastic anemia.*

IMPAIRED IRON ABSORPTION (see also Ch. 131). Iron absorption may be subnormal except when the malabsorption syndrome is due to uncomplicated pancreatic insufficiency. Most often the iron deficiency is caused by poor absorption owing either to mucosal disease or to inability to release inorganic iron from organic compounds. However, occult blood loss may contribute to the anemia. Iron deficiency anemia is very common in *adult celiac disease* and may be noted also in the later stages of *tropical sprue.* When associated with deficiencies of folic acid and vitamin B_{12}, iron deficiency may not become apparent until these substances are repleted. Incorporation of iron into young marrow red blood cells requires both folic acid and vitamin B_{12}.

DIMINISHED ABSORPTION OF WATER AND ELECTROLYTES. *Dehydration, weakness,* and *hypotension* occur commonly in the malabsorption syndrome. Large amounts of water and electrolytes are lost if diarrhea is severe or if stools are very loose or bulky. Absorption of water in adult celiac disease is slower than normal; the small intestine, in fact, secretes water and sodium. Diuresis after a water load is delayed, and as a consequence patients with steatorrhea often have nocturia.

TABLE 103–5. ABSORPTION OF ^{60}Co-VITAMIN B_{12} IN MEGALOBLASTIC ANEMIA ASSOCIATED WITH SELECTED DISORDERS

Result After:	Pernicious Anemia and Total Gastrectomy	Adult Celiac Disease*	Blind Loop Syndrome	Primary Malabsorption of Vitamin B_{12} or Ileal Resection	Tropical Sprue	Pancreatic Insufficiency*
Vitamin B_{12}	Low	Low-normal or low	Low	Low	Normal or low	Normal-low†
Vitamin B_{12} + intrinsic factor	Normal	No change	No change	No change	No change	No change
Vitamin B_{12} after antimicrobial therapy	Low	No change	Normal	No change	Normal or low	No change
Vitamin B_{12} after gluten-free diet	No change	Normal	No change	No change	No change	No change
Vitamin B_{12} + bicarbonate	No change	No change	No change	No change	No change	Normal‡
Vitamin B_{12} + pancreatic extract	No change	No change	No change	No change	No change	Normal

*Rare in adult celiac disease: very rare in pancreatic insufficiency.
†Rare to be low.
‡Return to normal more likely with pancreatic extract than with bicarbonate.

Hyponatremia not caused by renal loss responds readily to administration of sodium, and symptoms of sodium depletion—weakness, lethargy, nausea, cramps—rapidly disappear. *Hypokalemia*, if severe, causes muscle flaccidity, weakness, and cardiac arrhythmias.

VITAMIN B COMPLEX DEFICIENCY: DERMATITIS, NEURITIS, AND CHEILOSIS. Although *glossitis, neuritis* (peripheral neuropathy), and *dermatitis* in the malabsorption syndrome have been attributed to deficiency of B vitamins, proof of impaired absorption of these substances (vitamins B_1, B_2, and B_6) is not at hand. Perhaps deficiency results from metabolic action of abnormal bacterial flora that ordinarily do not inhabit the small bowel. However, conclusive demonstration of this mechanism also is lacking, particularly in *adult celiac disease*. Moreover, administration of vitamin B complex ($B_{1, 2, 6, 12}$) does not always cure the glossitis, which may be partially due to iron deficiency.

DIAGNOSIS

A high index of suspicion of the diagnosis is essential for those with minimal complaints and seemingly normal-appearing stools. The clues to diagnosis of the malabsorption syndrome are the history, symptoms, signs, and laboratory abnormalities listed in Tables 103–3 to 103–5 that relate to malabsorption of fat and other substances, particularly fat-soluble vitamins, protein, iron, and vitamin B_{12}. The average patient will complain of rather bulky, light-colored stools, often with increased frequency (but not necessarily so), abdominal distention, and variable weight loss and, occasionally, of a bleeding tendency, paresthesias, bone pain, or symptoms of anemia.

Laboratory Diagnosis

The pathophysiologic basis for the abnormal findings of the laboratory tests has been described and is presented in Table 103–4. The particular values of the individual tests in arriving at a diagnosis are considered in Table 103–6. The essential diagnostic tests, excluding routine blood studies (complete blood count, determination of Ca^{++}, K^{+}, and prothrombin time), include measurement of 72-hour stool fat, serum carotene, d-xylose absorption, tests of pancreatic function, tests for bacterial overgrowth, roentgenographic study of small bowel, tests for vitamin B_{12} absorption, and biopsy of the small intestine.

MEASUREMENT OF STOOL FAT: SERUM CAROTENE. The most important feature in the diagnosis of the malabsorption syndrome is steatorrhea; accurate measurement of fecal fat is therefore extremely important. The only reliable method is the chemical analysis of a 72-hour stool collection while the patient is ingesting 80 to 100 grams of fat per day. Normal excretion of fecal fat in these circumstances is 6.0 grams or less per 24 hours or 6 to 9 per cent of ingested fat (Table 103–6). Often a qualitative Sudan stain for fat globules on a suspension of stool will give an indication of significant steatorrhea. The test is simple, relatively sensitive, and is effective for screening. However, it cannot substitute for a quantitative fecal fat determination for the definitive diagnosis of steatorrhea. Eosin staining of a stool suspension may also reveal striated muscle fibers that suggest maldigestion, most often the result of pancreatic insufficiency.

This test is essential for diagnosis, because only in the so-called primary mucosal cell abnormalities (except for abetalipoproteinemia) is fat absorption normal (Table 103–3). Steatorrhea, however, does not indicate into which category of malabsorptive disorders the patient falls. If fecal fat is elevated, a roentgenographic study of the small intestine as well as a d-xylose test must be performed. Increasingly, small bowel biopsy is being done routinely if pancreatic disease is unlikely. Finally, determinations that reflect bacterial overgrowth (intestinal stasis) are required either when the roentgenographic studies display a *blind loop, jejunal diverticula, strictures, enteroenteric* or *enterocolic fistula*, or the marked intestinal stasis of *scleroderma* or when the biopsy is normal.

Depressed levels of serum carotene will usually be found in patients with steatorrhea. This test is useful in "screening" those in whom the malabsorption syndrome is suspected, but it cannot substitute for a fat determination.

D-XYLOSE ABSORPTION (Table 103–6). The absorption of the pentose d-xylose is a useful index for the absorption of carbohydrates in the study of malabsorption. Twenty-five grams is given orally; if the patient does not vomit, has no delay in gastric emptying, is well hydrated, and has normal kidney function, 4.5 grams or more will be excreted in a five-hour collection of urine. It is absorbed actively like glucose, but its metabolism is not as rapid as that of glucose, and its renal excretion does not depend upon a threshold. As a measure of carbohydrate absorption, the use of d-xylose is more reliable than an oral glucose tolerance test. In patients over 60, renal excretion diminishes; in such individuals, as well as in patients with delayed gastric emptying, liver disease with ascites, or renal disease, blood levels are measured and should reach at least 20 mg per deciliter in two hours.

The absorption and therefore the excretion of d-xylose is significantly diminished (less than 4.5 grams in five hours) in patients with intestinal *disease* affecting particularly the *jejunum*, after *massive resection*, and in marked *bacterial overgrowth*, presumably owing to bacterial action or mucosal damage. Note that d-xylose does not require intraluminal digestion and therefore is independent of pancreatic function. The procedure thus serves to separate patients with intestinal mucosal disease or deficiency from those with pancreatic insufficiency and from normal subjects. Xylose absorption may also be tested by measuring blood levels after administration of ^{14}C xylose.

Normal d-xylose absorption is strong evidence against the diagnosis of *adult celiac disease*. An abnormal result, however, casts strong doubt upon the diagnosis of *pancreatic insufficiency*. The test is also valuable in gauging the effect of therapy when pretreatment values have been low.

TESTS FOR UNABSORBED CARBOHYDRATE. Disaccharidase deficiency may result from isolated deficiency of a single disaccharidase (i.e., lactase, sucrase), from generalized mucosal damage (i.e., sprue), from inadequate surface (massive small bowel resection), or from bacterial overgrowth in the small intestine. In each instance, unabsorbed carbohydrate is broken down by colonic bacteria to yield hydrogen and short chain fatty acids. This results in an acid pH of the stool, which can easily be tested with pH paper. In addition, short chain fatty acids are osmotically active and result in an osmotic gap in the stool. If diarrheal fluid has an osmolarity much higher than twice the sum of the sodium and potassium concentrations, other substances must account for a significant fraction of the osmolarity (see Ch. 102). In the case of carbohydrate malabsorption, fermentation products of carbohydrates are responsible. Traditional diagnosis of specific disaccharidase malabsorption has been made by measuring blood monosaccharide values after oral administration of the suspected carbohydrate in question. These tests are outlined in Table 103–6. In addition, the increase in breath hydrogen after administration of the offending carbohydrate can be measured in expired air (breath hydrogen test). This test is reliable and noninvasive and is becoming increasingly used in helping to establish the diagnosis of bacterial overgrowth syndrome, as well.

PANCREATIC FUNCTION. Evaluation of pancreatic function by measurement of volume and bicarbonate concentration of duodenal aspirates after appropriate stimulation or concentration of enzymes after a test meal is in order if the d-xylose test is normal and roentgenographic study of the small intestine is normal or equivocally so in patients with demonstrated steatorrhea. It is clearly indicated if biopsy is normal and there is no other apparent disease or disorder. Subnormal response strongly indicates pancreatic insufficiency or pancreatic ductal obstruction, although normal values do not exclude these possibilities.

TABLE 103–6. LABORATORY TESTS COMMONLY EMPLOYED TO STUDY MALABSORPTION

	Normal Values	Malabsorption Syndrome*
Serum:		
Albumin	4.0 to 5.2 grams/dl	Diminished
Carotene	0.06 to 0.4 mg/dl	Diminished, particularly in small bowel disease
Calcium	9.0 to 10.5 mg/dl	Diminished, particularly in small bowel disease
Cholesterol	150 to 250 mg/dl	Diminished
Potassium	3.5 to 4.7 mEq/L	Diminished
Magnesium	1.7 to 2.0 mEq/L	Diminished
Vitamin B_{12}	100 to 700 $\mu\mu$g/ml	Diminished, particularly in tropical sprue and bacterial overgrowth
Folic acid	5 to 21 ng/ml	Diminished, particularly in small bowel disease
Plasma:		
Prothrombin time	Control value	Elevated
Tolerance tests:		
d-Xylose (25 grams orally)	Urinary excretion of 4.5 grams or greater per 5 hours	Diminished in diseases of the mucosa, particularly celiac disease, and in intestinal stasis (normal in pancreatic insufficiency)
Glucose (100 grams orally)	35 mg/dl over fasting plasma level	"Flat curve" in celiac disease and diseases of intestinal wall and in monosaccharide malabsorption
Lactose (50 to 100 grams orally) (2.0 grams/kg in children)	Rise in blood glucose of 20 mg/dl	Low to flat curve in primary lactose deficiency, celiac disease, and diseases of the intestinal wall
Sucrose (100 grams orally)	Rise in blood glucose of 20 mg/dl	Low to flat in celiac disease and disease of intestinal wall
Vitamin B_{12} (μc ^{60}Co B_{12})	>7% urine excretion/24 hours	Decreased with intestinal stasis, ileal dysfunction, or resection
Stool fat:		
Chemical determination (80 to 100 grams fat daily)	<6 grams/24 hours or 6–9% of ingested fat	Increased
Miscellaneous:		
Indican (urinary excretion)	Less than 100 mg/24 hours	More than 200 mg in bacterial overgrowth
5-HIAA (urinary excretion)	1.7 to 8.0 mg/24 hours	20 to 600 mg in malignant carcinoid syndrome
Breath tests:		
^{14}C Glycine-cholate orally	Minute amounts $^{14}CO_2$/4 to 8 hours	Elevated in bacterial overgrowth, ileal dysfunction or bypass
^{14}C xylose orally	Minute amounts $^{14}CO_2$/4 to 8 hours	Elevated in bacterial overgrowth
Glucose (50 grams orally)	Minute amounts H_2/4 to 8 hours	Elevated in bacterial overgrowth
Lactulose (10 grams orally)	Minute amounts H_2/4 to 8 hours	Elevated in bacterial overgrowth
Lactose (50 grams orally)	Minute amounts H_2/4 to 8 hours	Elevated in lactase deficiency

*Usual findings. Some values for serum tests may be normal in some patients, e.g., carotene, calcium, and vitamin B_{12} in pancreatic insufficiency and calcium in tropical sprue.

TESTS FOR BACTERIAL OVERGROWTH. Bacterial overgrowth as a cause for malabsorption syndrome may be present in a large number of diseases in which there is either small bowel stasis or contamination by lower gut organisms. Bacterial overgrowth in the small intestine may be detected by so-called "breath tests," culture of jejunal aspirates, and assessment of vitamin B_{12} absorption (Table 103–5).

Breath Tests. These include oral administration of ^{14}C glycine-cholate or ^{14}C xylose with measurement over four to six hours of expired $^{14}CO_2$. In diseases of bacterial overgrowth in the small intestine and of the terminal ileum, bacteria (small intestinal in the former situation and colonic in the latter) will deconjugate a significant amount of orally administered ^{14}C glycine-cholate before it is absorbed; likewise, bacteria in the upper small intestine will attack xylose, releasing $^{14}CO_2$. In both instances $^{14}CO_2$ quickly diffuses into the circulation and can be measured in expired air. Normally, only a minute quantity of $^{14}CO_2$ is detectable in four to six hours; however, when bacteria are present in the small gut, $^{14}CO_2$ excretion in breath is elevated many fold after ingestion of ^{14}C glycine-cholate or ^{14}C xylose. Expired $^{14}CO_2$ will be elevated after ^{14}C glycine-cholate is ingested in patients with disease, resection, or bypass of the terminal ileum, as well. Breath hydrogen is markedly increased with bacterial overgrowth after either glucose or lactulose is ingested; it is also greatly elevated in patients with lactose deficiency after ingestion of oral lactose (Table 103–6).

Tryptophan Metabolites. Urinary levels of indoxylsulfate (indican) over 100 mg per 24 hours reflects bacterial overgrowth. High levels of urinary 5-hydroxyindoleacetic acid (5-HIAA) are present in malignant carcinoid syndrome associated with malabsorption (Ch. 242).

Culture of Jejunal Aspirates. Techniques for culture of jejunal aspirates for fastidious anaerobic bacteria (clostridia, fusiforms, bacteroides) while difficult are increasingly available for diagnosis of bacterial overgrowth. Usually, the upper small intestine appears bacteria free in about one third of normal subjects; in the remainder, gram-positive or facultative anaerobes are present (lactobacilli and enterococci) in concentrations of 10^1 to 10^3 organisms per gram of content. Coliforms may be transiently present but rarely exceed 10^3. Normally, the terminal ileum has concentrations of organisms approaching 10^5 to 10^8 per gram, and these include gram-negative coliforms and bacteroides. In the colon enormous concentrations of anaerobes—bacteroides, lactobacilli, and clostridia—are usually present. When these organisms, particularly bacteroides and lactobacilli (but also clostridia and coliforms), luxuriate in the small intestine, the so-called bacterial overgrowth syndrome results (see Bacterial Overgrowth, Ch. 103.2).

Cultures of aspirates may now be obtained via sterile polyethylene tubes. Precise microbiologic technique for anaerobic organisms must, however, be practiced or the exercise will be futile. If such culture techniques are available, the finding of greater than 10^4 organisms per milliliter of jejunal aspirate would be considered abnormal.

ROENTGENOGRAPHIC STUDIES. Diagnosis of the malabsorption syndrome may be facilitated by recognition of changes in the roentgenograms of the small bowel which point to bacterial overgrowth and include *strictures* or *fistulas, blind loops* usually from previous surgery (Fig. 103–2), or marked *stasis,* as in scleroderma. Dilatation of the proximal jejunum with "flocculation" and "scattering" of barium, slight coarsening of valvulae conniventes, and rather oddly shaped collections called "moulage," point strongly to *adult celiac disease* (Fig. 103–3). Such changes, but particularly disordered transit and markedly thickened folds, may be noted in *Whipple's disease, amyloidosis, radiation enteritis, hypoproteinemia, Zollinger-Ellison syndrome,* and

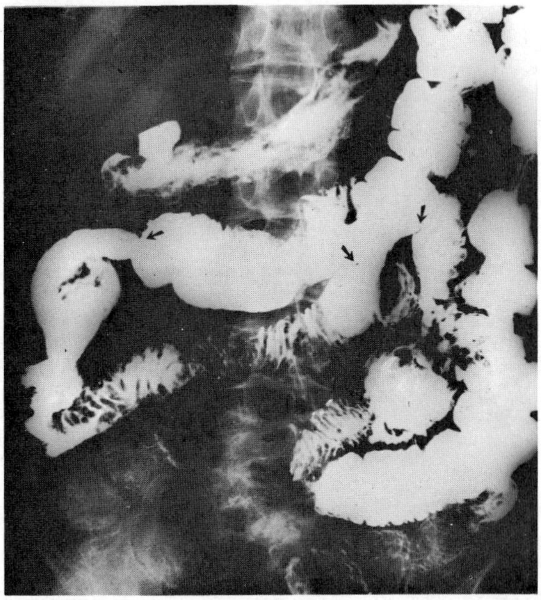

Figure 103–2. Small bowel series showing postoperative terminal ileum (arrow on left) and ileotransverse colostomy stoma (between arrows on right). Note the blind loop.

eosinophilic enteritis. Small mucosal nodules may be noted in so-called *lymphoid nodular hyperplasia* associated with hypogammaglobulinemia and giardiasis.

VITAMIN B_{12} ABSORPTION. Vitamin B_{12} absorption is tested by oral administration of radioactive vitamin B_{12} and measuring its excretion in the urine over a 24-hour period. The absorbed radioactive B_{12} is "flushed out" by the intramuscular administration of 1000 μg of nonlabeled B_{12}. Greater than 7 per cent of the administered dose should be excreted. The absolute values depend upon the dose of labeled B_{12}.

The conditions that cause malabsorption of vitamin B_{12} are listed in Table 103–5, where details of differential diagnosis by variations of the labeled B_{12} absorption test (Schilling test) are also given.

JEJUNAL HISTOLOGY. Histologic study of jejunal mucosa obtained by suction biopsy technique has further aided differential diagnosis of the malabsorption syndrome. The procedure is easily performed with one of several available tubes (Rubin tube or Crosby capsule). Prothrombin time must be normal. Characteristic findings have been associated with *celiac disease* in both children and adults and in *tropical sprue, Whipple's disease, amyloidosis,* and *eosinophilic gastroenteritis.* In some instances alterations may be noted in diffuse nongranulomatous *ileojejunitis,* in *lymphoma,* after *gastrectomy,* in *hypogammaglobulinemia* with steatorrhea, in patients with intestinal *lymphangiectasia* associated with protein-losing enteropathy who have dilated lacteals, and in individuals with *radiation enteritis, mastocytosis,* or severe *drug reactions.* Fat-laden epithelial cells are found in *abetalipoproteinemia.* Certain parasites, namely, *Giardia lamblia, Coccidioides immitis,* and *Cryptosporidia* have also been found on biopsy.

A section of normal jejunal mucosa is shown in Figure 103–5. The villi are long, delicate, and frond-like; the lining columnar epithelium is regular with basal orientation of nuclei. The crypts are normal, and cellular infiltration of the lamina propria is minimal. In well-oriented sections villus height is normally three to four times the height of crypts. Proper interpretation of jejunal histology depends upon correct (perpendicular) sectioning of the specimen, which, in turn, requires correct mounting before fixing.

The jejunal histology in *adult celiac disease and tropical sprue* is strikingly abnormal. In evaluation of small bowel biopsies from such patients, particular attention must be directed to configuration of the villi, morphology of the epithelial cells with their brush border, and the degree of the chronic inflammatory cell infiltration. The severity of changes may be graded from mild to moderate to severe. In the *severe* group (total villous atrophy) the changes consist of complete flattening of the mucosal

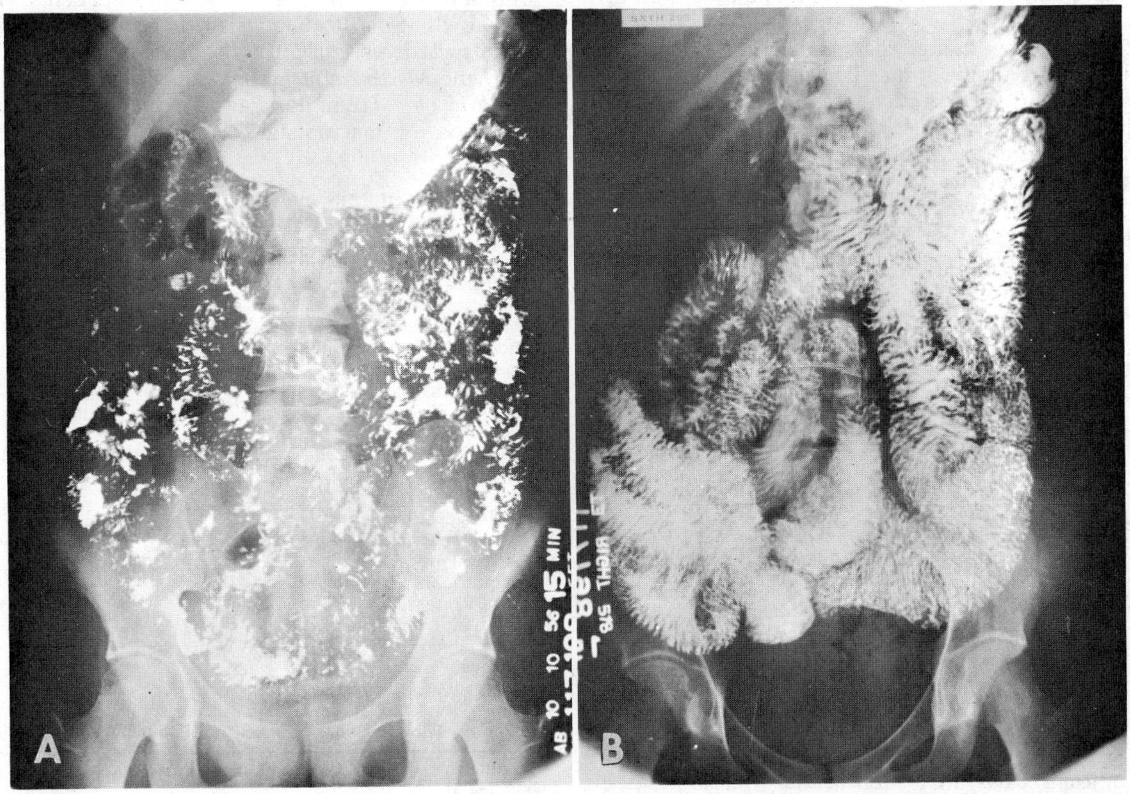

Figure 103–3. Small bowel roentgenographic series in patient (M.S.) with adult celiac disease. *A,* Before treatment. *B,* Six weeks after elimination of gluten from the diet. Note that the severely disordered pattern has improved.

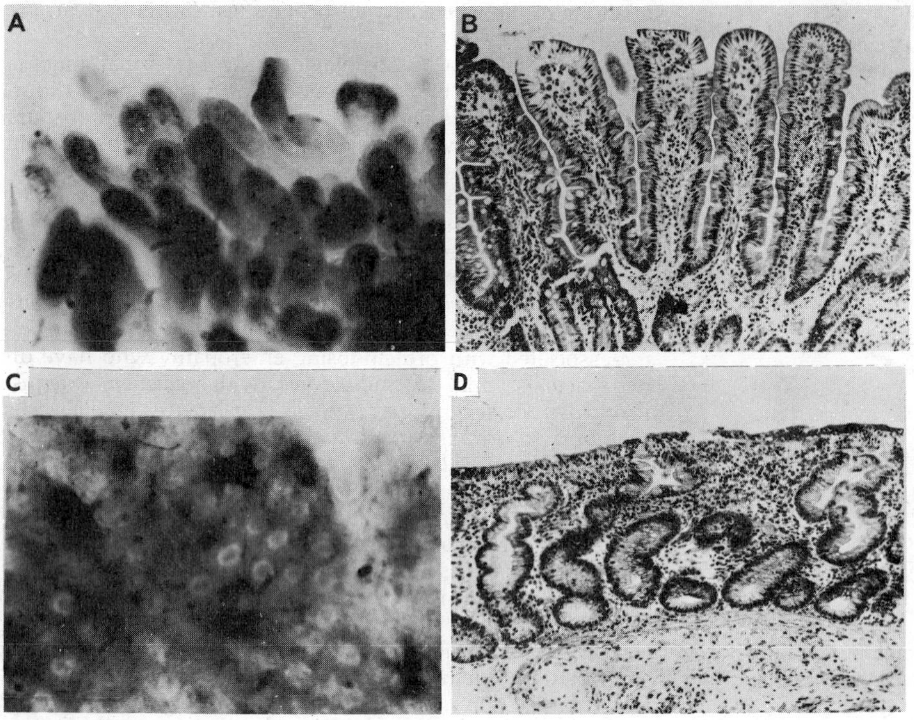

Figure 103–4. Comparison of dissecting microscopy and light microscopy of jejunal biopsy specimens from a normal person (*A, B*) and a patient with adult celiac disease (*C, D*). *A*, Finger-like villi vs. *B*, normal villous pattern. *C*, "Mosaics" vs. *D*, total villous atrophy.

surface without detectable villi or, at best, only very short and broad villi. Generally, there is a dense infiltration of chronic inflammatory cells and disorganization of the epithelial cells with a sparse brush border (Fig. 103–4). In the *mild* group (partial villous atrophy), the villi are formed but still are shorter and broader than normal. In some areas the villi approach normal in all respects. The epithelial cells with brush border generally may be nearly normal and the cellular infiltration is mild. In the *moderate* subdivision (subtotal villous atrophy), changes ranging between those of the mild and severe groups are noted.

Total villous atrophy, although characteristic of celiac disease, is not specific. Occasionally, it may be noted in *tropical sprue*, and, in patchy fashion, in *bacterial overgrowth syndrome, infectious gastroenteritis, kwashiorkor, giardiasis, lymphoma*, or *Whipple's disease*; it has also been reported in *diffuse nongranulomatous ileojejunitis* (often "ulcerative"), as well as in patients with *congenital hypogammaglobulinemia* in whom plasma cells are absent in the lamina propria. Some of the last-named will respond to a gluten-free diet and thus have adult celiac disease as well. The classic findings are also present in so-called *collagenous sprue*, in which there is also a broad band of collagen between surface cells and lamina propria.

Varying degrees of villous atrophy have also been noted (but not responsive to gluten elimination) in patients with *eosinophilic gastroenteritis*, in some *parasitoses*, and in *intestinal ischemia, dermatitis herpetiformis, soy bean sensitivity, radiation enteritis, tuberculosis, viral enteritis*, and conditions caused by *colchicine* and *neomycin*. Mild inflammatory cell infiltration of the lamina propria has been noted in biopsies from patients with bacterial overgrowth. Specific diagnosis may also be made histologically of *strongyloidiasis, capillariasis, coccidiosis*, including *cryptosporidium*, and *Mycobacterium avian intracellulare*.

In *Whipple's disease* the diagnosis may be made by the demonstration of macrophages laden with periodic acid–Schiff

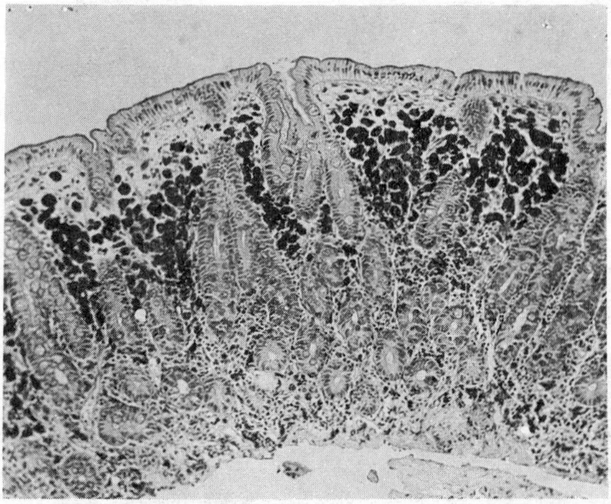

Figure 103–5. Jejunal biopsy from a patient with Whipple's disease. Periodic acid–Schiff stain. Note macrophages laden with stained material in the lamina propria.

TABLE 103–7. SMALL INTESTINAL BIOPSY IN THE DIAGNOSIS OF MALABSORPTION

*Diagnostic small bowel biopsy**
- Whipple's disease
- Abetalipoproteinemia
- Immunodeficiency syndromes
- Intestinal lymphoma
- Eosinophilic gastroenteritis
- Systemic mastocytosis
- Parasitic diseases (giardiasis, coccidiosis, strongyloidiasis, capillariasis, cryptosporidiosis)

Abnormal but not diagnostic small bowel biopsy†
- Celiac sprue
- Tropical sprue
- Unclassified sprue
- Infectious gastroenteritis
- Bacterial overgrowth
- Malnutrition
- Crohn's disease
- Intestinal lymphangiectasia

Usually normal small bowel biopsy
- Pancreatic disease
- Postgastrectomy malabsorption
- Primary (isolated) disaccharidase deficiency
- Bile salt deficiency syndromes (see Table 103–2)

*Although certain of the lesions may be patchy, the changes are diagnostic when found.

†Although many of the observed changes will be characteristic, they are not diagnostic of a single disease entity.

staining material in lymph nodes or in the lamina propria of the intestinal wall. In addition, total villous atrophy may be noted (Fig. 103–5). Electron microscopic studies during the active phase of the disease have revealed membranous structures, which may represent an infectious agent outside the macrophages. Deposits of amyloid have been found in the submucosa of the jejunum in patients with *amyloidosis*, particularly within the walls of arterioles.

Examination of fresh biopsy specimens under the dissecting microscope may yield information about a number of diseases of the small intestine associated with malabsorption. The normal patterns of *finger-like villi* are seen in Figure 103–5. A most extreme change is noted with total villous atrophy, with *"mosaics"* or *"brain patterns"* as the picture under the dissecting microscope. Examples of this classification are presented in Figure 103–4. Table 103–7 lists the utility of small bowel biopsy in various conditions which may be associated with the malabsorption syndrome.

103.2. Management

Marvin H. Sleisenger

DIFFERENTIAL FEATURES AND TREATMENT OF INDIVIDUAL FORMS OF THE MALABSORPTION SYNDROME

The presenting clinical picture of the malabsorption syndrome includes a wide range of symptoms—bulky stools, flatulence, distention, anorexia, weight loss, weakness, glossitis, paresthesias, bleeding, bone pain. A careful history is of extreme importance in differential diagnosis. Particular attention must be paid to bowel habits in childhood, family history, previous illnesses and surgical operations, and dietary habits (including consumption of alcohol). A history of symptoms commonly associated with diseases that might underlie the malabsorption must be sought. Valuable clues may also be derived from a careful physical examination. In this way diagnosis of *tropical sprue, adult celiac disease, Whipple's disease, hypothyroidism, hyperthyroidism, hypoparathyroidism, scleroderma, lymphoma,* and other disorders which may underlie malabsorption is facilitated.

The malabsorption syndrome must be differentiated from a wide variety of conditions characterized by a bleeding diathesis, by skeletal pain with or without fracture, by evidence of vitamin B deficiency and extreme malnutrition, or by chronic diarrhea. Diagnosis of the malabsorption syndrome as a cause for these symptoms and signs must first, however, be based upon demonstration of abnormal fat absorption.

As the patient with the malabsorption syndrome may have extreme weight loss, weakness, hypotension, and diffuse pigmentation, differentiation from *Addison's disease* must be made. Abnormalities of serum calcium, carotene, or plasma prothrombin and impaired absorption of fat and xylose indicate the presence of the malabsorption syndrome (Table 103–6).

The principal distinctive features of the individual forms of the malabsorption syndrome are discussed according to the seven categories of Table 103–3.

There are numerous conditions that can produce the malabsorption syndrome. Its treatment must be individualized for optimal effectiveness. In contrast to the often gratifying response to dietotherapy shown by patients with *adult celiac disease,* or to antimicrobials by patients with *Whipple's disease, bacterial overgrowth,* and *tropical sprue,* successful management of malabsorption resulting from various other diseases or alterations of the gastrointestinal tract is often difficult. Dosage schedules for agents used in the treatment of malabsorption syndrome are listed in Table 103–8.

Category 1: Defective Intraluminal Hydrolysis or Solubilization

PRIMARY PANCREATIC INSUFFICIENCY. Pancreatic insufficiency results from *chronic relapsing pancreatitis, carcinoma of the pancreas,* or *cystic fibrosis,* or occurs *after extensive resection* of the gland. In the first three instances, it is due to extensive parenchymal destruction and/or obstruction of the major ductal system. In chronic pancreatitis with malabsorption (see Ch. 107), the patient is frequently diabetic, the gland is often calcified, and frequently, but not always, there is a history of recurrent attacks of inflammation. Occasionally the dominant symptoms of *carcinoma of the pancreas* are those of malabsorption rather than pain, anorexia, or jaundice. *Cystic fibrosis* is most often clinically apparent in early childhood; however, the diagnosis is often made in young adults.

Whatever the cause of pancreatic insufficiency, failure of lipolysis results in moderate to severe steatorrhea, depending to some degree on the amount of gland remaining. Patients with this disease may show evidence of deficiency of either vitamin B_{12} or fat-soluble vitamins. In contrast to adult celiac disease, d-xylose absorption is normal in pancreatic insufficiency. The diagnosis of pancreatic insufficiency is documented by analysis of duodenal fluid after stimulation of the pancreas.

SECONDARY PANCREATIC INSUFFICIENCY. Since pancreatic lipase is inactivated at an acid pH, conditions characterized by excessive gastric acid secretion, such as non-β islet cell tumor of the pancreas (Zollinger-Ellison syndrome) or massive small bowel resection, are associated with significant steatorrhea. A low pH in the upper small gut also precipitates bile salts and causes mild histologic abnormalities. Dilution of pancreatic hydrolytic enzymes because of rapid gastric emptying is responsible for an apparent pancreatic insufficiency after subtotal gastrectomy and pyloroplasty with vagotomy.

DEFICIENCY OF CONJUGATED BILE ACIDS. An insufficient concentration of conjugated bile acids in the upper intestine may be caused by severe liver disease, prolonged extrahepatic biliary tract obstruction, diminished bile acid pool, or a significant reduction of conjugated bile acids resulting from bacterial overgrowth (see below). The result is diminished hydrolysis of triglycerides and steatorrhea because of insufficient conjugated bile acids for normal micelle formation.

Distal *ileectomy,* severely *diseased terminal ileum,* or *ileal bypass* (surgical or via cholecystocolonic fistula), by disrupting the enterohepatic circulation of conjugated bile acids, also diminishes the bile acid pool and causes steatorrhea, of a degree roughly proportional to the length of the resected, diseased, or bypassed segment. Further, since bile acid absorption is subnormal, these substances make contact with colonic mucosa, inhibiting water and salt absorption, particularly in the ascending colon. Diarrhea results, the so-called *choleretic enteropathy,* with three to six loose to soft movements per day. When less than 100 cm of terminal ileum is involved, both the steatorrhea and diarrhea are mild. Patients with more than 100 cm of ileum resected generally lose from 15 to 30 grams of fat in stools per day. This large degree of steatorrhea may be due in small part to loss of absorptive function of the ileum, although it is likely that the diminished bile acid pool is mainly responsible.

A decreased conjugated bile acid pool with steatorrhea is also notable in primary or *secondary biliary cirrhosis* in which cholestasis is a prominent feature. It is surprising, however, that the steatorrhea of complete biliary tract obstruction is moderate, indicating other mechanisms for absorption in addition to proximal uptake of micellar lipid. Malabsorption of fat in *postnecrotic* (macronodular) or *portal* (micronodular) *cirrhosis* is usually mild unless *chronic pancreatitis* (usually caused by alcohol) is also present.

BACTERIAL OVERGROWTH (INCREASED BILE ACID DECONJUGATION). Steatorrhea and vitamin B_{12} deficiency anemia may result from alterations in the anatomy of the small intestine, particularly surgically created *"blind" loops; enteroenteric, enterocolic,* or *gastrojejunocolic fistulas; afferent loop stasis* after subtotal gastrectomy and gastrojejunostomy; or *chronic obstruction* caused by adhesions or strictures, *jejunal diverticula,* or diseases with *motor abnormalities* such as scleroderma and pseudo-ob-

TABLE 103–8. REPRESENTATIVE DOSAGES FOR AGENTS USED IN MANAGEMENT OF PATIENTS WITH THE MALABSORPTION SYNDROME

1. CALCIUM
   Oral: Calcium gluconate (91 mg Ca^{++}/gram), 5 to 10 grams three times daily, or calcium carbonate (500 mg Ca^{++}/tablet), 1 to 2 grams daily in divided doses
   Intravenous: Calcium gluconate injection; U.S.P. 10 per cent solution (9.1 mg Ca^{++}/ml), 10 to 30 ml administered slowly intravenously, depending upon response
2. MAGNESIUM
   Oral: Magnesium gluconate, 500 mg tablets (29 mg Mg^{++} per tablet), 1 to 4 grams daily in divided doses
   Intramuscular: (20% sol.) 10 ml two or three times daily
   Intravenous: Magnesium sulfate, 0.5 per cent solution, up to 1000 ml at a rate not faster than 1.0 mEq/minute
3. IRON
   Oral: Ferrous sulfate, 325 mg three times daily
   Intramuscular: (Imferon); must be calculated according to severity of anemia; detailed instructions accompany preparation
4. FAT-SOLUBLE VITAMINS
   a. VITAMIN A
      Oleovitamin A capsules, U.S.P. (25,000 units per capsule), 100,000 to 200,000 units daily in severe deficiencies; maintenance, 25,000 to 50,000 units daily
   b. VITAMIN D
      Synthetic oleovitamin D, U.S.P. (10,000 U.S.P. units vitamin D/gram), 30,000 units daily; increase dosage as necessary to raise serum calcium to normal; dosage varies considerably, depending on response as determined by level of serum calcium and urinary calcium
   c. COMBINATION A AND D VITAMINS
      Concentrated oleovitamins A and D U.S.P. (50,000 to 65,000 U.S.P. A units and 10,000 to 13,000 U.S.P. D units/gram) may be used rather than separate preparations
   d. VITAMIN K
      Oral: Menadione, U.S.P., 4 to 12 mg daily; vitamin K_1 tablets (Mephyton), 5 to 10 mg daily
      Intravenous: (bleeding episodes—acute situations): vitamin K_1 (Mephyton), 50 mg ampule; administer 50 mg slowly over ten-minute period; repeat in eight to twelve hours if prothrombin time has not returned to normal
5. FOLIC ACID, U.S.P. (5 mg tablets)
   Dose: Initial, 5 mg daily for one month; maintenance, 1 mg daily
6. VITAMIN B_{12} INJECTION, U.S.P. (15 μg/ml)
   Dose: Initial, 100 μg daily for two weeks; maintenance, 100 μg monthly; if combined system disease is present, a more intensive program is indicated
7. VITAMIN B COMPLEX
   Any multivitamin preparation that contains daily requirements (thiamine 1.6 mg, riboflavin 1.8 mg, and niacin 20 mg); use two tablets daily; intramuscular preparations are available for severe deficiencies
8. PANCREATIC SUPPLEMENTS, ORAL
   Recently these agents have been shown to be more effective when given with 300 mg cimetidine at mealtimes and snacks.

8. PANCREATIC SUPPLEMENTS, ORAL *(Continued)*
   a. Pancrease (enteric coated microspheres), 2 or 3 during meals and snacks
   b. Viokase (0.3 gram tablet), 6 tablets with each meal and snacks
   c. Cotazym (0.3 gram capsule), 5 capsules with meals and snacks
9. BROAD-SPECTRUM ANTIMICROBIALS FOR BACTERIAL OVERGROWTH
   Oral: Tetracycline (0.25 gram), 1.0 gram per day in divided doses for 10 to 14 days; ampicillin (0.25 gram), 1.0 to 2.0 grams per day in divided doses; sulfisoxazole (0.5 gram), 1.0 to 2.0 grams daily in divided doses; gentamicin, 3.0 mg/kg per day in divided doses; repeated courses often necessary or administration for three to four days each week indefinitely
10. HUMAN ALBUMIN, SALT POOR (0.25 gram/ml)
    Intravenous administration of 50 to 100 grams each day for three to seven days to elevate a severely depressed serum albumin level
11. GLOBULIN, IMMUNE SERUM (0.165 gram/ml)
    Intramuscular injection of 0.05 ml/kg each three to four weeks in patients with hypogammaglobulinemia and recurrent infection
12. ADRENOCORTICOSTEROIDS
    Prednisolone or prednisone, 30 to 60 mg orally for 10 to 14 days; 5.0 to 15.0 mg maintenance dose daily
13. ANTIDIARRHEAL AGENTS
    Oral: Diphenoxylate hydrochloride (2.5 mg), 5.0 mg twice or three times daily; deodorized tincture opium, 10 drops twice to three times per day; imodium (2 mg capsules), 4 mg followed by 2 mg for each unformed stool, not more than 16 mg per day; loperamide 2 mg once or twice daily
14. CHOLESTYRAMINE, ORAL RESIN
    4.0 gram dose, three times daily, before feedings
15. CALORIC SUPPLEMENTATION
    Oral: (a) Medium-chain triglyceride (MCT) "Home or Hospital Mix" (MCT: 45 per cent calories; caseinate, 15 per cent; dextrose, 40 per cent): ingredients homogenized with H_2O to 1 liter (MCT: 75 mg; caseinate, 60 grams; dextrose, 160 grams); keep at 20° C for one year; defrost day's formula each morning; give three ounces at meals; gradually increase between-meal feedings to six ounces; Portagen (MCT: 45.0 grams fat/quart; 30 cal/oz; 10 per cent carbohydrate): formula mix; prepare according to instructions; give 16 oz every day
    (b) Hydrolyzed protein, amino acids, lactose free, low residue: Vivonex or Flexical, 1 kcal/ml; feed 24 ml daily in divided portions, orally or by tube
    (c) Intact protein, lactose free, low residue: Ensure or Isocal, 1 kcal/ml; feed 2400 ml daily in divided portions
    Peripheral intravenous: 500 ml 10% fat emulsion plus 3 liters of 10% dextrose per 3.5% amino acid solution per 24 hours yields 1500 calories; add electrolytes, vitamins, and trace minerals
16. DRUGS FOR PARASITES
    Oral: Thiabendazole (25 mg/kg/day): strongyloidiasis, two to three days; *Capillaria philippinensis,* 30 days; *A. duodenale, N. americanus,* 25 mg/kg/day twice daily for two days
    Oral: Metronidazole* (0.25 gram), 0.25 gram three times daily for seven days, or quinacrine, three times daily for seven days for *Giardia lamblia*

*This use is not listed in the manufacturer's directive.

struction. The common denominator in all these conditions is bacterial overgrowth, which results from stasis in a segment of small bowel caused by anatomic factors, motor abnormalities, or contamination of small bowel by large bowel content. In general, a total bacterial count of greater than 10^6 organisms per gram or 10^4 bacteroides per gram is significant and may be considered responsible for impairment of intraluminal solubilization of hydrolyzed lipid. Bacteria play a role in the malabsorption of *tropical sprue,* and after *subtotal gastrectomy* and Billroth II gastrojejunostomy. Overgrowth rarely is responsible for malabsorption in the diarrhea of *diabetic neuropathy.* Patients with the bacterial overgrowth syndrome may also have severe diarrhea as well as steatorrhea, possibly owing to impairment of Na^+ and water absorption by hydroxy fatty acids that result from bacterial action on unabsorbed fatty acids. Also, volatile fatty acids, products of fermentation of sugars and amino acids, may cause diarrhea by inhibiting water and salt absorption by the colon (see Ch. 102).

The mechanism of the malabsorption of vitamin B_{12} and fat caused by bacterial overgrowth is clear. Vitamin B_{12} is utilized by multiplying anaerobic organisms. Fat absorption is impaired by deconjugation of bile acids by bacterial enzymes. The decline in concentration of conjugated bile acids below a critical level impairs micelle formation, reducing uptake of lipid by the mucosa. Concentration of free bile acids is increased intraluminally; their absorption from the proximal small gut by passive diffusion is rapid; and their serum levels are elevated. High levels of free fatty acids may also inhibit cellular resynthesis of triglycerides. In patients with bacterial overgrowth less than 20 per cent of intraluminal fat may be in a micellar phase 45 minutes after ingestion of a lipid meal (normal: more than 50 per cent). Since hydrolysis of fat is not impaired, steatorrhea is principally the result of impaired micelle formation.

Although the jejunal villi are not entirely normal in jejunal biopsy specimens of patients with bacterial overgrowth, demonstrating some infiltration of the lamina propria with lymphocytes, plasma cells, and occasionally polymorphonuclear cells, along with mild blunting, the appearance is usually quite different from the picture in adult celiac disease.

"Blind" Loops. A loop of intestine is "blind" either when it is disconnected from the main stream (rare) or when intestinal contents may gain access to it but not readily egress from it.

An example would be a partly defunctionalized terminal ileal loop that has been partially excluded by either side-to-side or end-to-side ileotransverse colostomy (Fig. 103–2). Stasis and overgrowth of bacteria take place with subsequent invasion of the upper small intestine.

Multiple Strictures and Jejunal Diverticula. Strictures result from diffuse *granulomatous ileojejunitis, tuberculosis,* or *x-radiation* therapy. Frequently these patients have crampy abdominal pain, bloating, and other symptoms of progressive luminal narrowing, as well as other evidences of their underlying diseases. Most multiple jejunal diverticula are probably acquired. Stasis of intestinal content in these pockets of bowel leads to bacterial overgrowth. It is interesting that many of these patients are achlorhydric.

Fistulas. Fistulas may complicate gastric or intestinal neoplasm or granulomatous enteritis, involving stomach, small gut, and colon (gastrocolic), small gut and colon (enterocolic), or loops of small gut (enteroenteric). Malabsorption may also, of course, result from exclusion of significant lengths of absorbing surface from the main stream by large fistulas (gastroileostomy).

The diagnosis is greatly aided by a history of previous chronic enteric disease or of surgical procedure. Roentgenographic examination will often establish the diagnosis by the demonstration of one of these diseases or alterations. Frequently, however, the cause may not be demonstrated.

The megaloblastic anemia commonly associated with the "blind loop" syndrome will, unlike pernicious anemia, respond to the administration of broad-spectrum antimicrobial drugs. After 10 to 14 days of such therapy (ampicillin or tetracycline, 1.0 gram daily in divided dose), absorption of vitamin B_{12} is usually, but not always, restored to normal (Table 103–5). In contrast to those with pernicious anemia and many with *jejunal diverticula,* these patients usually secrete hydrochloric acid.

Postgastrectomy. Afferent loop stasis after gastrectomy and gastrojejunostomy (Billroth II) is a cause for steatorrhea and malabsorption and may be due in part to bacterial contamination of the afferent loop (see Category 5).

Scleroderma and Pseudo-Obstruction (see also Ch. 448). Severe involvement of the small bowel by *scleroderma* may cause malabsorption. Muscle atrophy and fibrosis impair mobility, causing stasis and often serious ileus. Jejunal biopsy reveals normal villi, but there may be an increased number of inflammatory cells in the lamina propria.

Bacterial overgrowth is the principal factor in the steatorrhea and malabsorption of most patients with scleroderma involving the small intestine.

Pseudo-obstruction of the small and large intestine is a rare condition, reflecting an abnormality of gut smooth muscle function, and characterized by periodic episodes of prolonged ileus. It may be secondary to degeneration of gut smooth muscle or autonomic innervation of unclear etiology. *Amyloidosis* of the gastrointestinal tract is an example of acquired pseudo-obstruction and results in malabsorption secondary to bacterial overgrowth.

Treatment of Defective Intraluminal Hydrolysis

PRIMARY PANCREATIC INSUFFICIENCY. Replacement of digestive enzymes is important in the treatment of patients with *primary pancreatic exocrine insufficiency.* Among the available sources of enzymes are a commercial pancreatic extract, pancreatin, U.S.P.; a preparation containing whole raw pancreas, Viokase; one containing hog pancreas extract, Cotazym; and a porcine pancreatic enzyme concentrate, Pancrease. Doses of these preparations are listed in Table 103–8; occasionally, it may be necessary to increase the recommended amounts. Replacement therapy is most effective when it is given in divided doses with four to six meals daily. Potency may in some cases be increased if cimetidine, 300 mg, is given orally one hour before the extracts. Some patients with primary pancreatic insufficiency do not absorb vitamin B_{12} normally, although this is rarely responsible for megaloblastic anemia. This defect may not be corrected by giving bicarbonate alone. Pancreatic extracts, however, will increase absorption to normal.

SECONDARY PANCREATIC INSUFFICIENCY. Hypersecretion of acid caused by *non-β islet cell tumor* (Zollinger-Ellison syndrome) is best treated by large doses of H_2 blockers, occasionally with potent anticholinergic agents (see Ch. 99.6). After *massive small bowel resection,* gastric hypersecretion may appear and be relieved by vagotomy and pyloroplasty. This condition also, however, may be successfully treated with adequate doses of an H_2 blocker, either cimetidine or ranitidine. Fortunately, hypersecretion is transient in most patients after massive small bowel resection. Relative pancreatic insufficiency after surgery for peptic ulcer disease (subtotal gastrectomy, pyloroplasty and vagotomy) also should be treated with pancreatic extract (Table 103–8).

DEFICIENCY OF CONJUGATED BILE ACIDS. Patients in whom insufficient bile reaches the intestine pose a difficult problem in treatment unless their lesions are surgically correctable. The keystone of medical management is a balanced diet without restriction of fat. In some patients additional calories can be provided by medium-chain triglycerides that do not require bile salts for absorption. For patients with chronic *cholestatic liver disease* it is important to provide calcium and fat-soluble vitamins A, K, and D in adequate amounts (Table 103–8). The demineralization of bone in patients with prolonged biliary obstruction results from osteoporosis and osteomalacia. Adequate supplements of vitamin D and calcium not only may prevent further osteomalacia but also may increase calcium deposition. More recently, a synthetic compound, 1α-OH-D_3, has been effectively used in patients with vitamin D deficiency and demineralization. Because inactivity contributes to the skeletal demineralization, maximal ambulation must be encouraged.

BACTERIAL OVERGROWTH (BILE ACID DECONJUGATION). The surgical correction of the strictures, diverticula, fistulas, or blind loops associated with bacterial overgrowth may effect a permanent cure and is, when feasible, the therapy of choice.

In some patients with malabsorption syndrome associated with either *subtotal* (Billroth II) or *total gastrectomy* or *scleroderma,* long-term antimicrobial therapy should be undertaken. Ampicillin or tetracycline, 1.0 gram per day, should be given for 10 to 14 days, and intermittently every other day for three days each week thereafter (Table 103–8). Many of these patients, similar to those with bacterial overgrowth from other disorders, require continuous treatment. Rotation of antimicrobial drugs may be advisable in an effort to avoid the emergence of drug-resistant microbial populations. Aspiration of jejunal contents for cultures or serial breath tests may be necessary for therapeutic guidance (Table 103–6). If organisms are not susceptible to the more usually employed drugs, courses of gentamicin, 3 mg per kilogram daily, may be given. All these drugs should be used in a rotational scheme. Occasionally, some patients with recurrent *Crohn's disease* and strictures or fistulas, in whom the surgical approach is not feasible, will have to be managed in a similar fashion.

In addition to the assessment of clinical response, efficiency of antimicrobial therapy may be judged by the return of the bile salt breath test and urinary indican to normal or nearly normal levels.

USE OF MEDIUM-CHAIN TRIGLYCERIDES (Table 103–8). Feeding preparations of medium-chain triglycerides, composed of fatty acids with six to ten carbons, appears to be valuable in a number of diseases that cause malabsorption, including those associated with defective intraluminal hydrolysis or solubilization of fat (see above).

Medium-chain triglycerides are most effective in those with pancreatic insufficiency who are also being given supplements of pancreatic enzymes (see above) and in patients with deficiency of conjugated bile salts (particularly biliary tract obstruction or bile fistulas).

Category 2: Mucosal Cell Abnormality and Inadequate Surface

Primary Mucosal Cell Disorders

DISACCHARIDASE DEFICIENCY AND MONOSACCHARIDE MALABSORPTION. Inability to split disaccharides because of disaccharidase deficiency (lactase or sucrase and isomaltase) may be primary or secondary to damage of the mucosa. Primary lactase deficiency may be congenital (rare) or, more commonly, acquired as an isolated defect that develops later in life. Symptoms may appear during infancy, childhood, or adulthood. Bacterial fermentation of unsplit lactose produces lactic and other organic acids which increase osmotic load with water entering the lumen. Diarrhea, cramping abdominal pain, borborygmi, and flatulence result from ingestion of milk and milk products. Weight loss and steatorrhea are usually mild and appetite is good, although infants and children may not thrive well. This pathophysiologic concept applies equally to *sucrase deficiency* when sucrose is ingested.

Lactase deficiency is by far the most common, particularly in blacks, and is more common in the yellow races than in whites. Dietary deficiency of lactose is not the cause. Adults diagnosed as having irritable colon syndrome (see Ch. 101) may coincidentally be deficient in jejunal lactase. The reason for the clinical appearance of the disorder in adulthood is not clear. It is also occasionally unmasked after subtotal gastrectomy or by increased milk ingestion as therapy for a peptic ulcer. Since no disease of the mucosal cells is evident histologically, the deficiency is thought to be primary, but its clinical development is somehow acquired. Adequate mucosal lactase levels are present in infancy but progressively decrease in adulthood in those affected.

Diagnosis of lactase deficiency may be made by the measurement of blood glucose after the oral administration of lactose (Table 103–6). A rise of less than 20 mg per deciliter is abnormal, and if the patient's blood glucose rises normally after he ingests a mixture of glucose-galactose of equal amount, lactase deficiency is extremely likely. Diagnosis may be confirmed only by the finding of low lactase activity in a jejunal biopsy specimen, although the diagnosis is usually established less invasively. Occasionally, these patients have lactosuria after administration of 50 grams of lactose during the lactose tolerance test.

The hydrogen breath test is becoming increasingly used in the diagnosis of carbohydrate malabsorption, including lactose deficiency. Excess breath hydrogen is generated by colonic bacteria from unabsorbed lactose given orally (Table 103–6).

Treatment of primary lactase deficiency is by elimination of milk and milk products from the diet, which often dramatically relieves all symptoms. It may also be beneficial to patients with the secondary variety of deficiency until the primary disease responds to appropriate treatment. Lactase-deficient patients may vary in their ability to tolerate dietary lactose and may tolerate some dietary lactose. This is often determined by the patient.

Depression of lactase activity is also secondary to certain diseases affecting the brush borders of jejunal mucosal cells, such as *celiac disease;* but it is also found after *massive* small bowel *resection* and in *nonbacterial jejunitis, infectious diarrhea of childhood, Giardia lamblia infection, Whipple's disease, cystic fibrosis,* and *Crohn's disease.*

Deficiency of *sucrase* is rare; it is associated with deficiency of isomaltase. It is a homozygotic deficiency affecting perhaps as many as 2 in 1000 individuals in the population. Symptoms include watery diarrhea and borborygmi, after ingesting sucrose.

Diagnosis of sucrase deficiency may be made by failure of blood glucose to rise at least 20 mg per deciliter after ingestion of 100 grams of sucrose or by excessive breath hydrogen after ingesting sucrose (Table 103–6). Treatment may be either elimination or marked reduction of sucrose, dextrins, and starches from the diet.

Congenital *glucose-galactose malabsorption* is present from birth and is exacerbated by all sugars broken down to these hexoses. Diagnosis is made by failure of these children to absorb either of these substances. Treatment consists of feeding fructose or fructose precursor–containing foods.

ABETALIPOPROTEINEMIA (ACANTHOCYTOSIS). Abetalipoproteinemia is a disease characterized by a morphologic defect of erythrocytes, "spiny red cells," absent serum beta-lipoproteins, very low serum cholesterol, and a very low plasma triglyceride that fails to rise after triglyceride ingestion. The intestinal mucosal biopsy is characteristic with epithelial cells engorged with triglyceride droplets even after an overnight fast. These findings are compatible with a defect in chylomicron formation. In abetalipoproteinemia the intestinal cells do not contain apoprotein B, which is obligatory for normal fat absorption. Steatorrhea may be severe in infants but characteristically is mild in adults. Concomitant neurologic disease (ataxia, nystagmus, motor incoordination, retinitis pigmentosa) develops in the second or third decade and often is disabling. Its pathogenesis is unknown; however, the severe vitamin E deficiency that invariably is found has been implicated. Substitution of medium-chain triglycerides for ordinary triglycerides has led to weight gain, since chylomicron formation and lymphatic absorption are not required. Supplementation with vitamins A and E may also be required. Aggressive therapy with large doses of vitamin E may be required to raise plasma levels and is thought to slow the progression of the disease.

VITAMIN B_{12} MALABSORPTION. Very rarely, primary malabsorption of the vitamin B_{12}–intrinsic factor complex is noted, perhaps owing to absence of a specific but unidentified "receptor" in the ileal mucosa (Imerslund's syndrome). These patients have been shown to have adequate intrinsic factor, normal ileal histology and calcium concentration, and alkaline pH. Treatment is monthly injections of vitamin B_{12} intramuscularly (Table 103–8).

CYSTINURIA AND HARTNUP DISEASE. Rarely, patients may have genetic disorders of intestinal transport of amino acids. In *cystinuria* dibasic amino acids are involved—cystine, arginine, lysine, and ornithine (see Ch. 83.4); in *Hartnup disease,* neutral amino acids—e.g., phenylalanine and leucine. Tryptophan deficiency leads to nicotinamide deficiencies with rash, dementia, and ataxia. These patients are cured with adequate oral nicotinamide or adequate oral protein, because they absorb small peptides normally (see Ch. 83.3).

Small Bowel Disease

These diseases include *adult celiac disease, Whipple's disease, nongranulomatous ileojejunitis, eosinophilic gastroenteritis, amyloidosis, small bowel ischemia,* and *Crohn's disease.*

ADULT CELIAC DISEASE (SPRUE). Adult celiac disease (gluten-sensitive enteropathy, celiac sprue, nontropical sprue) is an important cause of chronic malabsorption in temperate climates.

Etiology and Pathogenesis. The disease is caused by damage to differentiated villus epithelial cells in response to the ingestion of dietary gluten. The majority of these patients have an abnormal reaction of the small intestinal mucosa to a fraction of gluten; however, the exact component causing the damage is unknown. In celiac disease mucosal cell turnover is increased, with a marked proliferation of essentially normal crypt cells thought to represent a compensation to villus cell damage. These changes result in the characteristic histologic picture of villous atrophy, crypt hypertrophy, and columnar to cuboid change of villus cells with damage to the microvillus membrane (see Fig. 103–4). Malabsorption is primarily due to decreased uptake and transport of nutrients secondary to the marked loss of absorptive surface area and severe damage to the remaining villus cells. In addition, the jejunum of most untreated patients has been shown to be in a net secretory state for water and salt, further contributing to the diarrhea.

Although the pathogenesis of celiac disease remains unknown, increasing evidence suggests that genetic factors are of importance. Ten to 15 per cent of first degree relatives of patients with the disorder have abnormal intestinal biopsies although they are asymptomatic. The intestinal cell damage seems to be mediated by immunologic mechanisms. Histologically the intestine is infiltrated with lymphocytes and plasma cells. A gluten challenge in patients in remission results in a rapid accumulation of plasma cells and lymphocytes in the mucosa before histologic damage is evident. These cells have been shown to produce antigluten antibodies. Genetic factors may be important in explaining this presumed immunologic sensitivity to gluten. Celiac disease, for example, shows a strong association with two histocompatibility antigens, HLA-B8 and HLA-DW3, which are present in 60 to 90 per cent of patients (antigen frequency 20 to 30 per cent in the general population). An additional antigen has been described on the surface of B lymphocytes from patients with sprue (70 to 80 per cent of patients versus 15 per cent of normals) and is present in 100 per cent of parents of patients. Although the precise relationship of these genetic factors in the pathogenesis of the disease is uncertain, it is possible that these genes in combination code for a receptor on the surface of intestinal epithelial cells which binds gluten.

Clinical Manifestations and Diagnosis of Celiac Disease. The manifestations of celiac disease typically begin in infancy after weaning and the introduction of cereals. Commonly, the symptoms of celiac disease disappear in later childhood and in adolescence, despite continued malabsorption. Although the clinical remission is sometimes permanent, the classic features of adult celiac disease may appear during the third to sixth decades. The patients then may present with a spectrum of disability, ranging from mild discomfort and diarrhea with perhaps some anemia to severe illness with an extreme degree of malabsorption, foul-smelling diarrheal stools, skeletal disorders, bleeding phenomena, and symptoms of hypocalcemia. At times the disease may be characterized by one manifestation that may dominate the clinical picture. Thus iron deficiency anemia, folate deficiency, or osteopenic bone disease may be present without obvious diarrhea or steatorrhea, thus delaying the correct diagnosis. There are no pathognomonic physical signs in this disease. There may be any degree of malnutrition, as evidenced by muscle wasting and edema. Hypotension and abdominal bloating are very common. Occasionally, there is clubbing of the fingers and pigmentation similar to that of Addison's disease. The disease may appear clinically after gastric resection for peptic ulcer. Signs and symptoms of celiac disease and their pathophysiologic bases are noted in Table 103–4.

Roentgenography of the small bowel gives findings that are characteristic but not specific. Frequently the only change is an altered pattern with some dilatation of proximal loops of small bowel and minimal coarsening of the jejunal folds. More severe impairment is manifested by marked dilatation of small bowel segments and clumping of the barium meal, with a waxy cast appearance of bowel segments (the "moulage" sign) (Fig. 103–3). Modern colloidal suspensions of barium do not result in flocculation, and x-ray abnormalities may be minimal. As mentioned previously, the routine laboratory studies used in establishing the presence of the malabsorption syndrome are not specific. In general, abnormal studies will point to mucosal cell dysfunction. d-Xylose absorption is almost always abnormal, reflecting jejunal damage. The extent of the lesion may be roughly correlated with clinical severity. Vitamin B_{12} absorption is often normal but may be depressed if disease is extensive and involves the ileum. The diagnosis of celiac disease requires an intestinal biopsy showing total or subtotal villus atrophy. This histologic picture is not specific for celiac disease, but the diagnosis is untenable in its absence. Because the disease results from toxicity induced by a dietary component, the proximal bowel is always involved. Since the biopsy appearance is only *compatible* with celiac disease, a firm diagnosis can only be made when withdrawal of gluten from the diet (see below) results in a clinical remission. The vast majority of patients with adult celiac disease respond favorably to an adequate gluten-free diet; no other condition will respond so dramatically or so completely. Nevertheless, an empiric trial of a gluten-free diet in the absence of an intestinal biopsy compatible with sprue is to be discouraged. The diet is difficult to follow and failure to respond may have alternative interpretations. Since a gluten-free diet must be followed for life, there should be no shortcuts in making a definitive diagnosis.

Treatment of Celiac Disease. The basis for the use of the gluten-free diet in adult celiac disease lay in observations of its beneficial effects in the celiac syndrome of children. These patients cannot tolerate cereals with high gluten content. Thus when wheat, rye, oats, and barley are eliminated from the diet, diarrhea and steatorrhea cease, appetite improves, and rapid weight gain ensues.

The gluten-free diet excludes all cereal grains except rice and corn. To follow this diet, all labels must be carefully scrutinized to eliminate completely products that contain wheat, rye, barley, and oats as "fillers" (e.g., ice cream, salad dressings, canned foods, condiments, candy). As substitutes for the usual grains, rice, corn, and soy flours may be used. A wheat starch flour (Cellu Products Company) is available. Beer and ale must be avoided, because they contain cereal residues; however, whiskies can be used, because the offending agent is not contained in the distillate. All other foods, except milk and milk products if they cause symptoms owing to lactase deficiency, are permitted, including fats. In general, the diet should be well balanced and high in protein. The complete diet is available in standard nutrition texts.

A substantial majority of the patients with adult celiac disease have responded to this diet, showing symptomatic improvement within a few days or a week (Fig. 103–6). Most clinical remissions will occur within two months, although a rare patient may require as long as 12 months. Weight gain has been so striking that patients have voluntarily restricted their caloric intake. Absorption of d-xylose returns to normal within a few weeks of elimination of gluten. Steatorrhea diminishes remarkably in all instances, but fat absorption returns completely to normal only in those patients who carefully eliminate all gluten. A rare patient will not respond (see below). Follow-up biopsies demonstrate return to normal of mucosal histology in 50 per cent of patients who maintain that they adhere strictly to their diet, and marked improvement in most others. It is difficult to ascertain whether those who do not respond are ingesting some gluten. The physician should, however, also suspect other diseases that are associated with nongluten-sensitive villous atrophy (*hypogammaglobulinemia*, particularly with *Giardia lamblia*; *lymphoma*; *collagenous sprue*; *Whipple's disease*; and *diffuse nongranulomatous ileojejunitis*). In these conditions villous atrophy is patchy.

Corticosteroids produce significant improvement in adult celiac disease without entirely correcting the steatorrhea or biochemical abnormalities. These agents should be used for long-term therapy only in patients whose condition is refractory to the gluten-free diet, because impaired protein metabolism and osteoporosis are troublesome features in this chronic condition.

Occasionally, a patient with adult celiac disease is critically ill, with severe diarrhea, wasting and anorexia, and serious protein and electrolyte depletion. There may also be bleeding, tetany, and edema. This situation demands a rigorous therapeutic regimen, employing intravenous vitamin K and calcium as well as infusions of salt-poor albumin (Table 103–8). In such cases corticosteroids may be lifesaving by greatly stimulating

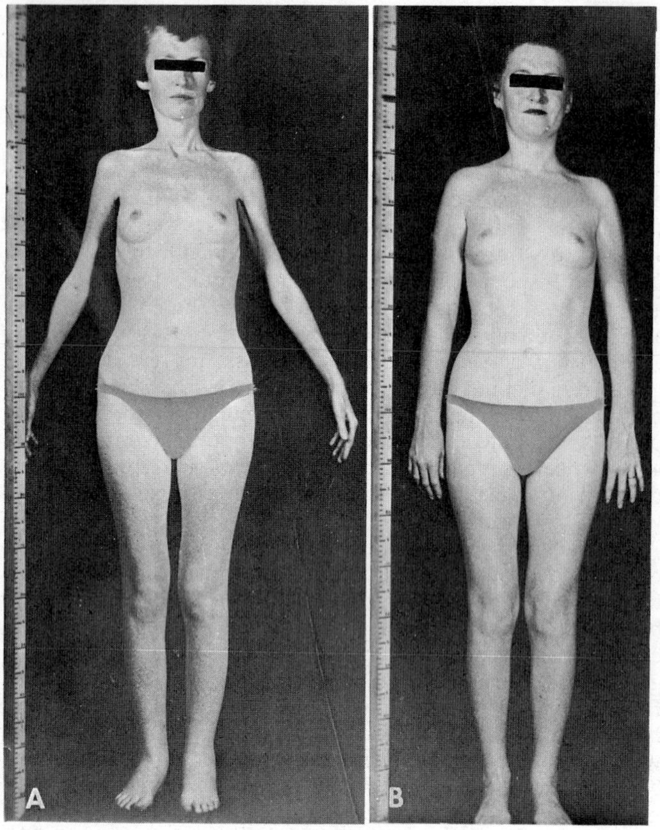

Figure 103–6. Appearance of patient (M.S.) with adult celiac disease. *A,* Before treatment. Note wasting and edema. *B,* Six weeks after elimination of gluten from the diet.

the appetite and perhaps by increasing absorption. Initially, either corticotropin, 30 units, or prednisone, 60 mg, should be given intravenously over an eight-hour period daily. Often a clinical response will be noted in 10 to 14 days, when oral prednisone in gradually decreasing doses can be instituted. Simultaneously, a gluten-free diet should be offered, and, as the patient's condition improves, drug therapy should be discontinued by gradual reduction in dosage over three to four weeks. These patients should remain on such dietotherapy permanently. Supplements (vitamins D and K, calcium, iron, folic acid, B-soluble vitamins, and vitamin B_{12}) are gradually withdrawn as clinical and chemical improvement proceeds; the program is set by results of reported essential laboratory determinations and personal observations.

Special Considerations and Complications of Adult Celiac Disease. Lymphoma and Carcinoma. The incidence of primary small bowel lymphoma and carcinoma in patients with adult celiac disease is high, about 13 per cent in a large collected series, with lymphoma contributing 10 per cent. Abdominal pain, weight loss, bleeding, obstruction, and perforation are the cardinal clinical features of this fatal complication. It is believed that lymphoma is more common in those not treated with a gluten-free diet, although this is not firmly established. Relapse in those who have responded, associated with suggestive symptoms, should alert the physician to the possibility.

Small Bowel Ulceration. Nonmalignant ulcers of the jejunum and ileum may complicate celiac disease, and are manifested by exacerbation of severe diarrhea, abdominal pain, fever, and severe hypoproteinemia secondary to protein-losing enteropathy (see below). Perforation, bleeding, and/or obstruction are late manifestations. While a variety of treatments have been tried (corticosteroids, immunosuppressive agents), they are usually ineffective (see Ch. 114).

Neurologic Complications. A syndrome similar to subacute combined degeneration of the spinal cord is noted early in celiac disease, despite remission with a gluten-free diet and in the absence of vitamin B_{12} deficiency (see Ch. 482).

Celiac Disease and the Skin. Dermatitis herpetiformis, a pruritic skin disorder characterized by vesicles and papules, is associated in the majority of patients with an abnormality of the jejunal mucosa identical with that of celiac disease. There is a similar increased frequency of HLA antigens as seen in sprue. The lesion tends to be patchy in its distribution, and most patients have no overt malabsorption. The small bowel lesion returns to normal after a gluten-free diet, and although the skin disorder may require additional therapy, it may also respond to gluten restriction. Partial and total villous atrophy have also been noted in psoriasis.

A rare patient with adult celiac disease who does not respond entirely to the diet may also have relative *pancreatic insufficiency,* i.e., the release of secretin and CCK is diminished. These patients require oral pancreatic extract (Table 103–8).

Collagenous Sprue. This disease resembles adult celiac disease in that it has the identical histologic picture, but it is not responsive to gluten elimination. By definition, therefore, these patients do not have celiac disease but rather a form of refractory sprue. Later, collagen is extensively deposited in the lamina propria beneath the epithelium. Early in the course some patients may respond to corticosteroids, but frequently no treatment is effective and the prognosis is poor.

Hyposplenism. An occasional patient with the adult celiac syndrome will have splenic atrophy with hyposplenism and diminished immunologic response to antigens.

WHIPPLE'S DISEASE. In Whipple's disease, or lipophagic intestinal granulomatosis (intestinal "lipodystrophy"), there is a heavy infiltration of the intestinal wall and lymphatics by macrophages filled with glycoprotein. It is a generalized disease with steatorrhea as its principal feature, and it occurs predominantly in males in the fourth to seventh decades.

It may be difficult to differentiate this entity from other serious to fatal causes of malabsorption, particularly *lymphoma* and *tuberculosis.* Several manifestations such as polyserositis and postprandial pain are seen in all three diseases. However, nondeforming arthritis is most characteristic of Whipple's disease and is frequently the initial complaint. Also, there may be symptoms of central nervous system involvement in Whipple's disease. When gastrointestinal symptoms occur, the disease usually progresses rapidly with marked diarrhea, weight loss, weakness, and symptoms of anemia and deficiencies of fat- and water-soluble vitamins. Physical findings that suggest this disorder include lymphadenopathy, found in 40 per cent of the patients, and the various manifestations of polyserositis. Fever may be noted in about one third of the patients. Indefinite plastic or doughy abdominal masses have been described in approximately one quarter of the patients. The most consistent findings in the routine laboratory studies are anemia and an increased sedimentation rate; eosinophilia is occasionally present. Classically, steatorrhea is severe, with d-xylose absorption depressed. The roentgenographic findings in the small bowel are nonspecific, usually showing a sprue-like pattern. Often there is a marked thickening of small bowel mucosal folds, suggesting an infiltrative process. Occasionally, severe protein-losing enteropathy may be seen, presumably secondary to infiltration of abdominal lymph nodes and lymphatic obstruction.

The diagnosis of Whipple's disease depends on the finding of periodic acid–Schiff (PAS) positive macrophages infiltrating the involved tissues. The diagnostic procedure of choice is peroral intestinal biopsy. The proximal intestine is invariably involved even early in the course of the disease. The pathognomonic finding is the identification of macrophages containing PAS-positive material in the lamina propria of the small intestine (Fig. 103–5). There may be patchy villous atrophy and evidence of lymphatic obstruction (lymphangiectasia) from infiltrated abdominal lymph nodes. Electron microscopic studies clearly show numerous small bacilli in patients with active disease; however, the responsible agent has not been cultured or identified to date. These characteristic pathologic changes can also be seen in peripheral or abdominal lymph nodes. In cases with central nervous system involvement (uncommon), PAS-positive cells have also been seen in cerebrospinal fluid.

Treatment of Whipple's Disease. Antimicrobial drugs by mouth are effective in treating Whipple's disease. Continuous treatment with penicillin G, 0.25 gram four times daily, or broad-spectrum antimicrobials, tetracycline or ampicillin, always brings about remission. The dose of tetracycline or ampicillin is 1.0 gram daily. The duration of therapy with antimicrobials is determined by the clinical response. Such treatment should probably be maintained indefinitely; otherwise, symptoms may return. Histologic as well as clinical improvement is noted after a period of weeks to months, with loss of diarrhea, reappearance of appetite, and tremendous gain of weight. The PAS-positive material slowly disappears from the mucosa, and the bacilliform bodies are no longer visible on electron microscopy. When remission has been sustained for nine months to one year, antimicrobial agents may be given intermittently, i.e., every other day or for three consecutive days each week (Table 103–8).

The symptoms of Whipple's disease may respond to corticosteroid therapy, as do those of other diseases characterized by arthritis and polyserositis, but the overall result of such treatment is not satisfactory. The desperately ill patient should be given both glucocorticoids intravenously *and* parenteral antimicrobial agents until the improvement of the patient permits withdrawal of the former agent.

NONGRANULOMATOUS ILEOJEJUNITIS. Steatorrhea and malabsorption may result not only from the complications of Crohn's disease *(strictures, fistulas,* or *massive resections)* (see Ch. 104) but also from nongranulomatous inflammation of a large segment of the small intestine, particularly the jejunum. The small intestine is diffusely inflamed; mesenteric nodes are slightly enlarged, and serosal lymphatics are dilated.

The onset of this latter illness is abrupt, with fever (39 to 40.5° C), pain, and diarrhea; signs and symptoms of malabsorption may predominate in a matter of one to two weeks. Splenomegaly, occurring in 20 per cent of these patients with fever, may suggest an initial diagnosis of abdominal lymphoma. Diffuse inflammatory changes in roentgenograms of the small bowel may be indistinguishable from that of a wide variety of conditions associated with the malabsorption syndrome. The leukocyte count is elevated, and serum albumin falls rapidly to 1.5 to 2.5 grams per deciliter. Diagnosis is usually made either by the response to treatment or by surgical exploration (see Ch. 114).

Treatment of Nongranulomatous Ileojejunitis. In diffuse nongranulomatous ileojejunitis, corticosteroids may have a dramatic effect upon the clinical symptoms, including those that are due to malabsorption. The protein-losing enteropathy remits as the inflammation subsides. Fever and diarrhea disappear; appetite and strength return as serum albumin rises.

Such patients, often acutely ill with fever and diarrhea, usually respond to intravenous corticotropin, 40 units daily, given over an eight-hour period for 10 to 14 days, or to prednisolone, 40 to 60 mg daily. With recovery, the dosage is tapered. Unfortunately, some of these patients have a relentless, refractory course and die of bowel perforation or intercurrent sepsis in two to three months, and the long-range outlook for permanent remission of this disease in those who initially respond is likewise not good (Ch. 114).

ALLERGIC AND EOSINOPHILIC GASTROENTERITIS. This syndrome is characterized by malabsorption, varying degrees of gastrointestinal bleeding, protein-losing enteropathy, and infiltration of the small intestinal mucosa by eosinophils in the absence of vasculitis. In a minority of instances in adults, the disease appears to be a response to an allergen such as milk protein, meat, or fish. Even in the absence of an offending agent, these patients have histories of hay fever, eczema, and asthma, particularly in childhood, or other food idiosyncrasies.

The symptoms—cramping pain, diarrhea, weight loss, nausea, fever, and a degree of malabsorption—are related to the location and extent of the disease in the small bowel. Fat loss in stool is about 15 to 20 grams per day. If the stomach is also involved, epigastric pain, vomiting, and bleeding are common. Marked eosinophilia is a constant finding and is greater than 20 per cent and Charcot Leyden crystals can be found in the stool. The disease tends to be chronic with recurrent symptoms. Roentgenographic examination often reveals a nonspecific "malabsorption pattern" with coarsened folds of jejunum. Hypoproteinemia caused by protein-losing enteropathy may be severe and may be associated with marked edema and ascites. Iron deficiency anemia resulting from occult gastrointestinal bleeding is common in children.

Another form of this disease is so-called *eosinophilic granuloma,* in which the process consists of localized nodular or pedunculated infiltrative eosinophilic lesions (involving the submucosa and muscle layer) without allergy or peripheral eosinophilia. *Eosinophilic gastroenteritis* may also involve the serosa of the bowel as well as peritoneum, with ascites the predominant manifestation.

Treatment of Eosinophilic Gastroenteritis. Effective therapy consists of withdrawal of offending foods, particularly milk for children and fish or a particular meat in some adults. In sicker patients, prednisone, 20 to 40 mg daily orally with gradual tapering to a low maintenance dose, will bring remission of major symptoms and decrease of eosinophilia. With remission, edema and infiltrate of the jejunal mucosa also disappear in patients with no involvement of deeper layers. Biopsy differentiates this disease from granulomatous enteritis and tuberculosis. The clinical picture, typical history, eosinophilia, obvious allergies, characteristic biopsy findings, and response to treatment are sufficient to establish the diagnosis.

Often the diagnosis can be made by gastroscopic biopsy of the antrum if involved.

AMYLOIDOSIS. Either the primary or the secondary form of the disorder may affect the gastrointestinal tract and cause malabsorption. Diffuse crampy pain and ileus are the most frequent abdominal symptoms. Roentgenographically, amyloidosis of the bowel is characterized by dilated loops of bowel, occasionally with thickening of the jejunoileum and slow passage of the barium meal through the intestines. The diagnosis is made by tissue study.

Treatment is supportive, because the disease is too extensive for resection. If it is secondary to chronic infection or granulomatous disease, successful management of the underlying disorder may rarely be helpful. In view of the altered intestinal motility that may accompany intestinal amyloidosis, bacterial overgrowth may be present and may represent a treatable element of malabsorption.

SMALL BOWEL ISCHEMIA. Chronic ischemia of the small bowel, caused by atherosclerosis of the celiac, superior, and inferior mesenteric arteries, may occasionally cause malabsorption, presumably because of impairment of mucosal cell function. No histologic damage, however, has been demonstrated in such instances (see Ch. 105).

The blood supply to the small intestine is occasionally severely compromised in patients with so-called collagen vascular disease, particularly *periarteritis nodosa* and *systemic lupus erythematosus.* It is also affected in *Behçét's disease, Degos' disease,* and *Henoch-Schönlein purpura.* Degos' disease is characterized by necrotic skin lesions and, like Behçét's, may terminate in infarction of the gut due to necrotizing vasculitis.

CROHN'S DISEASE. This important disease of the small bowel may cause malabsorption in a number of ways: by extensive damage to the mucosa; by multiple strictures (bacterial overgrowth); by fistulas between small bowel and colon (bacterial overgrowth); or by necessitating ileectomy (defective solubilization and loss of absorptive surface) or massive resection (inadequate surface and defective solubilization). Bacterial overgrowth and defective solubilization are discussed in Category 1 above; inadequate surface, a portion of Category 2, is discussed below. The clinical picture of diffuse Crohn's disease of the small intestine is discussed in Ch. 104.

Inadequate Surface

Most absorption takes place in the duodenum and first 90 cm of the jejunum. Patient survival is now reasonably certain with 90 to 120 cm of remaining normal small bowel following surgical resections, and survival is possible with shorter segments provided that caloric intake is adequate. This length of jejunum is sufficient for normal carbohydrate absorption and, in most instances, for maintenance of positive nitrogen balance. The postoperative course is influenced by the site of resection—jejunum or ileum. Thus vitamin B_{12} absorption will be subnormal if a large length of ileum has been removed; conversely, sacrifice of a corresponding amount of jejunum will more seriously impair absorption of fat, calcium, and folic acid.

During the past decade, *jejunoileal bypass* has been performed on morbidly obese patients to achieve weight loss. The common procedure is the so-called "14 and 4," in which 14 inches of proximal jejunum is anastomosed to 4 inches of terminal ileum. The proximal end of excluded bowel is closed, and the distal end is anastomosed to colon. The effect of this procedure is a marked malabsorption identical to that which follows massive resection of small bowel (see below). Although enormous losses of pounds ensue in most patients—usually 25 to 45 per cent of preoperative weight in one to two years—some undesirable sequelae, not related to intestinal deficiency, are observed. These include severe hepatic dysfunction, arthritis, motor disturbances (colonic pseudo-obstruction) of the gut, and oxalate kidney stones. Care must always be taken to replete inevitable losses of water, electrolytes, calcium, magnesium, and vitamins caused by the diarrhea that follows the operation (Table 103–8).

The three common causes for extensive resection of large segments of the small intestine are (1) *recurrent regional enteritis,* (2) *mesenteric vascular disease,* particularly thrombosis of the superior mesenteric artery, and (3) *malignant processes* involving the blood supply of the small bowel.

TREATMENT. Inadvertent surgical *jejunocolostomies* or *gastroileostomies,* which sidetrack large segments of small intestine, and unsuccessful jejunoileal bypass must be corrected surgically as soon as possible.

The patient who has had an *extensive resection of the small intestine,* nearly always right colon, ileum, and part of distal jejunum, requires continuous and meticulous medical care. For weeks or even for one or two months, nutrition may be adequately maintained by intravenous hyperalimentation using fluids containing calories, protein, minerals, and vitamins. Usually, 3 liters daily of standard solutions may satisfy nutritional requirements for an adult. The physician must learn the local and systemic complications of such therapy (Ch. 220).

Oral feedings should be initiated as soon as possible, preferably containing substances that require minimal hydrolysis and are easily absorbed. Such refined preparations as Ensure have been useful, because they contain simple sugars and amino acids; however, as with all hypertonic preparations, diarrhea may be aggravated.

For periods of up to 12 months postoperatively, the remaining segment of intestine will show progressive improvement in absorptive capacity, associated with elongation and dilatation. Since the amount of fat absorbed is proportional to the amount presented to the absorbing surface, the maximal intake of fat that does not cause symptoms is desirable. Regardless of which segment or its part—ileum or jejunum—remains, the diet should be high in protein. Frequent feeding (six times daily) should be recommended and may consist in part of protein and amino acids (Table 103–8). Vitamins A, D, and K and the B-complex vitamins as well as calcium, iron, and magnesium may be given orally. In general, a high protein intake will adequately maintain the serum albumin; however, occasionally, infusions of salt-poor albumin must be given.

Supplementation of the diet by medium-chain triglycerides (see above; Table 103–8) has been of distinct benefit to patients with massive small bowel resection, diminishing diarrhea and helping to stabilize weight by improving fat absorption; however, weight gain attributable principally to medium-chain triglycerides in these patients is slight. Drugs that decrease intestinal motility, such as diphenoxylate hydrochloride (5.0 mg twice or three times daily), anticholinergics (propantheline, 15 to 30 mg twice to three times daily), loperamide (2 mg once or twice daily) and/or small doses of tincture of opium (10 drops twice to three times daily), or codeine (30 to 60 mg twice to three times daily) may help reduce diarrhea (Table 103–8).

In certain patients, usually after massive resection of the small bowel, insufficient bowel remains to support nourishment by the oral route. Recent technologic advances in intravenous hyperalimentation have enabled this procedure to be carried out chronically at home. Although not generally available, this has permitted survival in cases that would otherwise have been fatal.

Category 3: Lymphatic Obstruction

LYMPHOMA. The malabsorption syndrome secondary to lymphoma of the small bowel and mesentery may be clinically and roentgenographically identical to the classic picture of adult celiac disease. Several features, however, suggest the correct diagnosis. The symptoms of this disease are likely to be of much shorter duration and to include crampy abdominal pain and fever. Lymphadenopathy and hepatosplenomegaly do not appear until late in the course. Although intramural small bowel masses may be present in some cases, the roentgenographic study of the intestine generally does not reveal them. Abdominal ultrasound or CT scan may reveal enlarged retroperitoneal lymph nodes or a retroperitoneal mass. Unexpectedly, the usual therapeutic measures, such as diet, fat-soluble vitamins, and vitamin B_{12}, may lead to a temporary clinical and laboratory remission. The incidence of malabsorption syndrome caused by small bowel lymphoma is difficult to ascertain. It appears that as many as 10 per cent of patients with adult celiac disease may develop lymphoma. Although lymphatic obstruction is important in the pathophysiology of steatorrhea in lymphoma, widespread disease of the intestine will also contribute significantly to the malabsorption.

The diagnosis is usually established by laparotomy necessitated by some complication of the underlying disease, such as bleeding, perforation, or obstruction. In some patients, the diagnosis may be made from jejunal tissue obtained by peroral biopsy. The average duration of this illness after onset of symptoms is 13 months, despite resection and roentgen therapy.

Primary intestinal lymphoma, with malabsorption, may be a chronic condition in certain parts of the world, particularly in the Middle East in young Arabs and Sephardic Jews. The clinical picture strongly resembles adult celiac disease in terms of chronicity and jejunal villous atrophy; however, most of these patients do not respond to elimination of gluten, and peroral biopsies will show evidence of lymphoma in the majority. These young Middle Easterners may survive for as long as ten years. Lymphoma also complicates *α-chain disease* in which heavy chains of IgA are produced excessively.

Treatment. Treatment of lymphoma of the small bowel and mesentery includes local resections as well as radiotherapy, and possibly therapy with chlorambucil and steroids or cyclophosphamide when the disease is disseminated (see Ch. 106 and 158). Despite this program, the course is frequently progressive, the average duration of life after onset of symptoms being one to two years.

INTESTINAL TUBERCULOSIS AND TUBERCULOUS LYMPHADENITIS. Tuberculosis may result in a malabsorption syndrome through involvement of the mesenteric lymph nodes, although in some cases there may be associated disease of the intestinal wall, and in others, bacterial overgrowth. It is rare in the United States, and it occurs almost always in persons with a history of severe pulmonary or lymph node tuberculosis.

Fever, palpable abdominal masses, a positive tuberculin skin test, evidence of old or recent disease on chest roentgenography, and calcification of mesenteric and pelvic lymph nodes on flat film all suggest the diagnosis, which may be confirmed by culture of sputum or gastric juice. Rarely, stool culture may be useful, but only if the other secretions are demonstrably free of tubercle bacilli. Roentgenographic studies, both barium enema and small bowel series, are particularly helpful when there is also deformity of the ileocecal segment resulting from hyperplastic lesions. Often exploratory laparotomy with node or bowel biopsy is necessary for diagnosis. The treatment of tuberculosis is discussed in Ch. 298.

LYMPHANGIECTASIA. In addition to the diseases just discussed, several other conditions may rarely cause the malabsorption syndrome by lymphatic blockade. These include *primary lymphangiectasia,* a genetically determined disease characterized by mild to moderate diarrhea, mild steatorrhea, and protein-losing enteropathy (see below), certain *protozoan diseases* (see Category 4), *the reticuloendothelioses, metastatic tumor* to the mesenteric nodes, and *neoplastic invasion of the main lymphatic channels* in the retroperitoneal tissues. *Retractile mesenteritis* and *retroperitoneal fibrosis* are diseases of unknown etiology characterized by inflammatory fibrosis in the retroperitoneum that may cause lymphatic obstruction. In general these disorders of lymphatic obstruction may result in a characteristic intestinal biopsy showing dilated lacteals. Chylous ascites may be present reflecting lymphatic obstruction, and peripheral lymphopenia is often also seen. Diarrhea, mild steatorrhea, and hypoalbuminemia of primary lymphangiectasia due to protein-losing enteropathy (see below) may be alleviated by a low fat diet with added medium-chain triglycerides.

Category 4: Infection

TROPICAL SPRUE. Tropical sprue can be differentiated from adult celiac disease. The disease occurs primarily in persons residing in certain areas of the Far East, India, and the Caribbean or in Westerners who visit tropical countries. Both nutritional deficiencies and bacterial contamination of the small gut appear to play causative roles. This disease responds to administration of broad-spectrum antimicrobial drugs, suggesting, but not proving, that infection is responsible. Although a single causative organism has not been isolated, jejunal bacterial overgrowth with a variety of enteric organisms has been frequently found. Some of these bacteria may produce enterotoxins, which may damage the intestine and contribute to the symptoms. Histologic changes suggestive of tropical sprue may be noted in persons newly arrived in the tropics; such changes may often be associated with an acute enteritis and a variable degree of malabsorption. Although the remarkable clinical improvement that follows folic acid therapy strongly suggests a vitamin deficiency, tropical sprue is not seen in some areas of the world where the population has a marginal or even inadequate diet. Conversely, it has been noted in people with adequately "balanced" diets.

Clinically, the patient complains of fatigue, asthenia, weight loss, glossitis, stomatitis, cheilosis, and hyperkeratosis. Bleeding caused by hypoprothrombinemia and clinical evidence of calcium depletion are rare. Later, edema and anemia (megaloblastic) appear.

Laboratory investigation reveals mainly steatorrhea and megaloblastic anemia. Small bowel roentgenographic findings and histologic changes of the jejunum are the same as those in adult celiac disease except that *total villous atrophy* is not as commonly encountered in tropical sprue. In many tropical areas, however, asymptomatic persons often have histologic abnormalities suggestive of tropical sprue, making tissue diagnosis very difficult. Other routine laboratory studies, including d-xylose absorption, are also comparable in the two diseases.

Treatment for Tropical Sprue. The therapy for this disease with antimicrobial drugs is very effective. A low fat, high protein diet, and migration to a temperate climate, are also helpful. Administration of a broad-spectrum antimicrobial (tetracycline, 1.0 gram daily by mouth) along with 10 mg of folic acid daily is the best treatment and frequently brings remission, with disappearance of diarrhea and glossitis and gain in appetite and weight. However, response may be slow in some patients, and normal absorption and jejunal histology may not be noted for six months or longer. Parenteral vitamin B_{12} should be given for two months (Table 103–8). For those not responding completely within six months of treatment with antimicrobials and folic acid, therapy should be continued for as long as absorption continues to improve.

When remission has been achieved, 5.0 mg of folic acid daily is the maintenance therapy. In the presence of achlorhydria, addition of vitamin B_{12} to the regimen should be considered unless absorption of ^{60}Co B_{12} is normal (Table 103–8). If absorption of vitamin B_{12} remains subnormal after remission, monthly injections should be given.

ACUTE INFECTIOUS ENTERITIS. Bacterial and viral infections may cause transient but severe malabsorption with steatorrhea, diminished calcium absorption, and reduced levels of serum calcium and proteins and plasma prothrombin. With recovery, absorption returns to normal. Agents responsible, often in epidemics, include shigellae, enteropathic *E. coli, V. cholerae, V. parahaemolyticus,* some salmonellae, *C. perfringens,* staphylococci, *Yersinia,* and enteroviruses. (Details of diagnosis and treatment of these disorders are discussed in the appropriate chapters of Part XIX.)

Treatment. These patients may recover without specific antimicrobial therapy, provided that fluids and electrolytes have been rapidly and adequately replaced. Such infections are apt to attack patients who travel to tropical countries or are debilitated, or who have had abdominal surgery, particularly those also given broad-spectrum antimicrobials.

PROTOZOAN AND HELMINTHIC DISEASES. Protozoan or helminthic diseases are a common cause of malabsorption in many tropical areas and are particularly associated with malnutrition. Because tropical sprue is also endemic in many of these countries, it is often difficult to assign a cause of malabsorption, especially in view of the histologic changes (blunting of villi, cellular infiltration of the lamina propria) which are present in many asymptomatic individuals who are malnourished with or without parasites. Some of these patients with mild to moderate steatorrhea (10 to 15 grams per 24 hours), however, have malabsorption syndrome caused by *hookworm, strongyloidiasis, Capillaria philippinensis, coccidiosis, giardiasis,* and *tapeworm infestations.* Parasites must be isolated and identified, and response to therapy, clinically, biochemically, and histologically, must be forthcoming before definite etiologic attribution of the malabsorption and malnutrition to parasitic infection can be made. (For details of diagnosis and treatment of parasitoses, see the relevant chapters of Part XX.)

Patients with *Giardia lamblia* infection of the small bowel may suffer from malabsorption, particularly individuals with *subtotal gastrectomy; hypogammaglobulinemia; selective IgA deficiency;* or *severe malnutrition.* The role played by the parasite is not completely clear despite demonstration of its invasion of the mucosa and report of improvement in absorption after treatment with metronidazole* (0.75 gram orally daily for seven days) or quinacrine (0.1 gram three times daily for one week). Villous atrophy that may be associated with the giardiasis of hypogammaglobulinemia may be reversed with effective therapy for the parasite (see below, Category 6). In all doubtful cases it is wise to treat the patient (Table 103–8).

Category 5: Multiple Defects

SUBTOTAL GASTRECTOMY. Steatorrhea and malabsorption after subtotal gastrectomy and gastrojejunostomy (Billroth II) or total gastrectomy are attributable to (1) loss of reservoir

*This use is not listed in the manufacturer's directive.

function with rapid emptying and dispersion of food through the small intestine, thereby diluting the normal output of pancreatic enzymes; or (2) stasis with bacterial contamination of the afferent loop of a Billroth II gastrojejunostomy. Deficiency of vitamin B_{12} will inevitably follow total gastrectomy, the lag period being determined by the liver store of the vitamin. Absorption of calcium and iron may also be impaired after gastric resective surgery and when severe will result in an elevated serum alkaline phosphatase, metabolic bone disease, and microcytic hypochromic anemia.

Treatment. As yet no preparation of pure conjugated bile acids is available for treatment. Pancreatic extracts may be tried in selected cases, although when given alone they have not produced consistent improvement. However, when pancreatic extract is combined with broad-spectrum antimicrobials (ampicillin or tetracycline, 1.0 gram per day in divided dosage) in the treatment of patients after Billroth II operations, fat absorption may improve. In some patients bacterial contamination—probably originating in the afferent loop—plays an important etiologic role in the malabsorption syndrome that follows this procedure. Conversion of Billroth II to Billroth I has been reported to reduce steatorrhea in some patients.

Patients who have undergone Billroth II procedures should receive a high-calorie diet rich in protein, with frequent feedings containing as much fat as can be tolerated, in order to maintain good nutrition. After a total gastrectomy, 30 to 100 μg of vitamin B_{12} intramuscularly must be given monthly. Calcium, iron, and the fat-soluble vitamins may be added to this regimen as needed or when diarrhea or steatorrhea is so severe that deficient absorption of these substances may be anticipated (Table 103–8).

DISTAL ILEAL RESECTION, DISEASE, OR BYPASS. As noted, resection, often required for *Crohn's disease* or *vascular insufficiency, ileal bypass* for *obesity*, or extensive ileal disease causes deficiencies of vitamin B_{12} and bile salts. Malabsorption is also in part due to loss of the reserve capacity of the ileum for absorbing fat, a function that is carried on because proximal fat absorption is impaired by deficiency of bile salts.

Vitamin B_{12} should be replaced parenterally, as in pernicious anemia. If the megaloblastic anemia that appears does not respond entirely to vitamin B_{12}, folic acid should be added to the regimen (Table 103–8).

Treatment with cholestyramine, a bile salt–binding resin, is indicated and will often ameliorate the diarrhea caused by the effect of unabsorbed bile acids upon the colon. It is often most effective in ileal resections of less than 100 cm when steatorrhea is usually mild. With resections of greater than 100 cm, however, it may increase steatorrhea by further diminishing the bile acid pool. No replacement therapy for the bile acid deficiency is currently available clinically. Steatorrhea will be reduced, however, by feeding medium-chain triglycerides in place of dietary lipid (Table 103–8). *Hyperoxaluria* with renal stones may also be present and results from increased oxalate absorption secondary to steatorrhea and bile salt effects on the colonic mucosa. Therapy consists of a low oxalate diet, reduction of steatorrhea by substituting medium-chain triglycerides for dietary fat, and use of cholestyramine and oral calcium supplements to precipitate oxalate in the bowel lumen.

RADIATION ENTERITIS. A few patients who receive high dosage x-ray therapy to the abdomen will develop a malabsorption syndrome on the basis of radiation injury to the bowel. Since the reaction to injury is slow, symptoms do not appear for weeks to months after exposure. Large doses cause ulceration of the mucosa and endarteritis of submucosal vessels with transmural necrosis, followed by scarring with strictures and permanent loss of function of the small intestine. In some instances stasis caused by obstruction *(bacterial overgrowth)* and *lymphatic obstruction* contribute. Jejunal biopsy may reveal patchy villous atrophy. Unlike celiac disease, there is no crypt hypertrophy and mitoses are decreased. Treatment consists of correction of stenosed loops causing obstruction, replacement therapy for those with irreversible damage or inadequate surface, and broad-spectrum antimicrobials for those with bacterial overgrowth resulting from multiple strictures (see above).

Category 6: Unexplained

HYPOGAMMAGLOBULINEMIA. The role of intraluminal immunoglobulins, particularly IgA, in maintaining the structure and function of the intestinal tract is not known, because their antibacterial activity as antibodies is minimal. Patients with hypogammaglobulinemia may, however, have steatorrhea and diminished d-xylose absorption. Evidence at hand indicates that most (if not all) of these patients have a deficiency of both plasma IgA and IgG and of intestinal IgA. Some patients have only plasma IgA ("selective") deficiency. IgM may be increased in serum and intestine in patients with selective IgA deficiency. The intestinal histology in diffuse hypogammaglobulinemia reveals normal histology or patchy villous atrophy, but *plasma cells are absent* and lymphocytes are reduced in all cases. Occasionally, it shows so-called "nodular lymphoid hyperplasia," and rarely it causes a granulomatous lesion. A high percentage of these patients with malabsorption have *Giardia lamblia* infestation of their intestinal fluid, and in some the organism invades the mucosa. A rare patient will have *celiac disease*.

Treatment. Of those with villous atrophy, a rare patient will have a good to excellent response to the gluten-free diet. Antimicrobial drugs and injections of gamma globulin appear to be ineffective. The key to successful management appears to be eradication of giardiasis with quinacrine or metronidazole* (Table 103–8). Symptoms remit, absorption improves (including d-xylose), and villi regenerate.

METASTATIC MALIGNANT CARCINOID SYNDROME. The presenting symptoms of this disease may be those of malabsorption. Steatorrhea may be caused in part by an increased production of 5-hydroxytryptamine (serotonin), which markedly increases gastrointestinal motility, lymphatic obstruction of the mesentery of the small bowel, and ileal dysfunction. Treatment is that used for carcinoid syndrome in general. Methysergide (8.0 to 12.0 mg per day, orally) and cyproheptadine (12 to 16 mg per day in divided doses) have been reported to decrease diarrhea in this disease. Small doses of tincture of opium or diphenoxylate or loperamide may alleviate diarrhea. Parachlorphenylalanine, which inhibits synthesis of 5-HTP, may control diarrhea but has undesirable side effects on the central nervous system. After ileal resection cholestyramine may be helpful.

HYPOPARATHYROIDISM AND PSEUDOHYPOPARATHYROIDISM. Steatorrhea and deficient parathyroid function are associated. The mechanism by which parathormone is involved in fat absorption or transport is unknown. With vitamin D_2 therapy, diarrhea decreases, steatorrhea disappears, serum carotene and albumin levels rise, vitamin B_{12} absorption increases, and the roentgenographic appearance of the small bowel becomes normal. Diagnosis of hypoparathyroidism as a basis for malabsorption may be established by measuring parathormone levels (see Ch. 246). Mild malabsorption (fecal fat about 10 grams per 24 hours) has been reported in pseudohypoparathyroidism because in this disease parathormone does not facilitate the effect of vitamin D upon calcium absorption. The effect of hypocalcemia per se upon intestinal absorption is not known. As noted above, magnesium deficiency secondary to malabsorption may diminish both parathormone secretion and its effectiveness on target tissues (see also Ch. 208). Magnesium deficiency must therefore be carefully ruled out in all patients who present with malabsorption and the clinical and laboratory findings of hypoparathyroidism.

Treatment. Administration of vitamin D and calcium will correct hypocalcemia and improve fat absorption as well as other manifestations of disease.

DIABETES MELLITUS. Patients with longstanding diabetes mellitus may have severe diarrhea (see Ch. 101). Some with diarrhea will also have steatorrhea and malabsorption, and the condition in these patients is usually not well controlled by

*This use is not listed in the manufacturer's directive.

dietary means or insulin, or both. A high percentage of such patients also have some evidence of neuropathy. In these patients, the intestinal difficulty may be due to involvement of the autonomic innervation of the small bowel, because they also have orthostatic hypotension, inability to perspire, and impotence. Changes in the microbial flora or mesenteric vascular insufficiency may also contribute to the malabsorptive state. A rare response to broad-spectrum antimicrobials supports the former hypothesis; however, careful bacteriologic studies of intestinal contents in patients with diabetic neuropathy and diarrhea reveal that bacterial overgrowth is a rare cause for the steatorrhea. Although exocrine function is usually normal in diabetes, some patients have *pancreatic insufficiency*, for which replacement therapy should also be given (Table 103–8) (see Ch. 107). An increased incidence of *adult celiac disease* has also been reported in diabetics.

MASTOCYTOSIS. Patients with overproduction of mast cells suffer not only from urticaria pigmentosa but also from gastrointestinal symptoms. Perhaps the latter result from overproduction of histamine and of serotonin. Malabsorption is rare in these individuals. The lamina propria of the jejunal mucosa may or may not be infiltrated with mast cells; villi may be absent or stunted. Whether fat absorption is also impaired because of gastric hypersecretion or increased intestinal transit has not been determined. (See Ch. 438.)

HYPERTHYROIDISM AND HYPOADRENOCORTICISM. Some patients with hyperthyroidism have steatorrhea. The pathogenesis is not understood. Steatorrhea is due in part to excessive intake of fat in the diet (more than 120 grams per day). Successful therapy returns fat absorption to normal. Likewise, steatorrhea has been found in patients with Addison's disease in whom replacement therapy has corrected it.

Category 7: Drug-Induced Malabsorption

Some commonly used drugs may cause malabsorption. *Cholestyramine*, in doses of 12.0 or more grams per day, by binding bile salts renders them inactive in the process of fat solubilization and causes mild steatorrhea (7.0 to 15.0 grams of fat per day). *Colchicine* ingestion leads to mild malabsorption of fat (about 9.0 grams of fecal fat per day), protein, and d-xylose by affecting epithelial cell replication and function. Certain *irritant laxatives*, presumably by markedly increasing transit, likewise may cause mild steatorrhea. *Neomycin*, frequently administered to patients with severe hepatic disease, causes steatorrhea, increased fecal loss of nitrogen, and impaired d-xylose absorption. The degree of malabsorption is dose related and may be noted with as little as 4.0 grams per day. It causes some blunting of villi and of their absorptive cells, reduces hydrolysis of fat, and precipitates bile salts. *Bacitracin, polymyxin,* and *kanamycin* may also cause malabsorption. Large doses (twice normal) of *p-aminosalicylic acid* lead to mild steatorrhea and decrease in absorption of d-xylose. *Phenindione*, an anticoagulant, may also cause steatorrhea. Anticonvulsants such as *phenytoin* in some way cause folic acid deficiency, as do *oral contraceptive* agents. Aluminum hydroxide–containing antacids inhibit the absorption of dietary phosphate owing to binding in the intestinal lumen. Prolonged use can lead to a phosphorus depletion syndrome with hypophosphatemia, hypercalciuria, nephrolithiasis, osteomalacia, muscle weakness, anorexia, and mild hemolysis.

MALABSORPTION SYNDROME AND ENTERIC LOSS OF PROTEIN (Protein-Losing Enteropathy)

Hypoalbuminemia in the absence of liver disease, inadequate protein intake, or albuminuria manifested by edema or ascites may be due to excessive loss of serum protein into the intestine—so-called *protein-losing enteropathy*. This loss has been noted in patients with mucosal ulceration of the stomach, small bowel, or colon; with mucosal disease without ulceration; or in lymphatic obstruction (Table 103–9). Intestinal lymphatic dilatation without obvious cause is also associated with abnormal enteric protein loss (Fig. 103–7).

TABLE 103–9. CLASSIFICATION AND THERAPY OF DISEASES ASSOCIATED WITH ENTERIC LOSS OF PLASMA PROTEIN

Disease	Therapy
A. Mucosal ulceration:	
Gastric carcinoma	
Gastric lymphoma	Surgical resection
Multiple gastric ulcers	
Colonic cancer	
Granulomatous enteritis	
Diffuse nongranulomatous ileojejunitis	Corticosteroids
B. Mucosal disease without ulceration:	
Rugal hypertrophy (Ménétrier's, etc.)	Resection, if local
Celiac disease	Gluten elimination
Tropical sprue	Antimicrobials; folic acid
Whipple's disease	Antimicrobials
Allergic gastroenteropathy	Elimination diet; steroids
Bacterial or parasitic enteritis	Antimicrobial drugs
Gastrocolic fistula	Resection
C. Lymphatic abnormalities:	
Capillaria philippinensis	Thiabendazole
Primary lymphangiectasias	Low-fat diet or medium-chain triglycerides
Lymphenteric fistula	Resection
Lymphoma	Chemotherapy
Constrictive pericarditis	Pericardiectomy
Tricuspid valvular disease	Rx of heart failure

Allergy to milk protein and, in rare cases, to cereals or even meat may underlie *protein-losing enteropathy* by affecting the small intestine. Biopsy is normal or shows mild infiltration of the lamina propria with eosinophils; the disorder usually begins in childhood; it is characterized by hypoproteinemia and edema; an iron deficiency anemia is common, as is diarrhea; eosinophilia is a prominent feature. This condition may well be a milder form of *eosinophilic gastroenteritis* in which both protein-losing enteropathy and malabsorption may be more serious (see above).

CLINICAL PICTURE. As noted, the clinical picture may be dominated by signs and symptoms of hypoproteinemia. In most instances, the patient complains of some abdominal symptoms related to the underlying disease.

DIAGNOSIS. The diagnosis of protein-losing enteropathy should be suspected in any patient with low serum albumin without liver disease or proteinuria. Since globulins may be lost as well, the characteristic hyperglobulinemia found in the hypoalbuminemia of cirrhosis is absent. An absolute lympho-

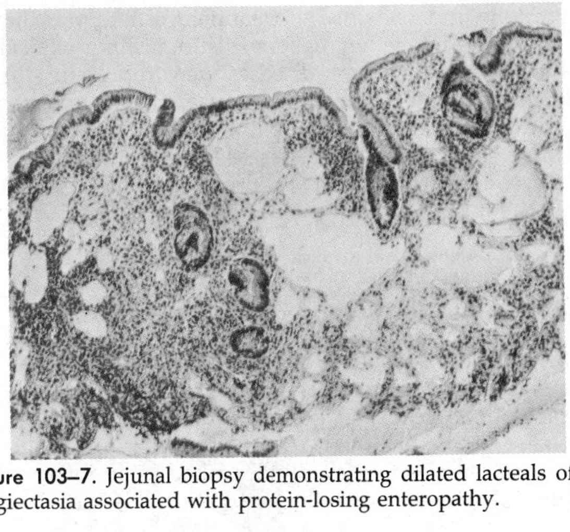

Figure 103–7. Jejunal biopsy demonstrating dilated lacteals of lymphangiectasia associated with protein-losing enteropathy.

cytopenia may also be found. The abnormal loss may be confirmed by abnormal fecal excretion of ^{51}Cr after intravenous injection of ^{51}Cr albumin or by a rapid decay curve after intravenous ^{51}Cr chloride or ^{131}I-albumin.

TREATMENT. The treatment of protein-losing enteropathy is based upon the pathogenesis of the disorder and is outlined in Table 103–9.

PROGNOSIS OF MALABSORPTION SYNDROME

The outlook for the patient with malabsorption syndrome depends upon both the nature of the underlying disease and the institution of appropriate therapy. Proper treatment, of course, implies correct diagnosis. The prognosis may be highly favorable (properly treated adult celiac disease) or highly unfavorable (systemic sclerosis involving the bowel), as discussed under the specific entities.

Bayless TM, et al.: Lactose and milk intolerance: Clinical implications. N Engl J Med 292:1156, 1975. *A brief but useful report of a study of the prevalence and clinical importance of lactose and milk intolerance in 166 male patients of different ethnic backgrounds.*

Klipstein FA: Tropical sprue in travellers and expatriates living abroad. Gastroenterology 80:590, 1981. *An excellent discussion of the differential diagnosis and treatment of tropical sprue, in which the problem is usually chronic contamination of the small bowel by enteric pathogens.*

Sleisenger MH (ed.): Malabsorption and nutritional support. Clin Gastroenterol 12:No. 2, 1983. Chapters 1–13; 16, 17. *An up-to-date symposium that covers the general topic of malabsorption in excellent detail. This is a good starting point for an in-depth study of this topic.*

Sleisenger MH, Fordtran JS (eds.): Gastrointestinal Disease. 3rd ed. Philadelphia, W. B. Saunders Company, 1983. Chapters 15–17; 49–51; 53; 57–66; 73, 74. *Chapters dealing with physiology and nutrient absorption and diseases causing malabsorption in a leading gastroenterological text. Excellent bibliographies.*

Trier JS, et al.: Celiac sprue and refractory sprue. Gastroenterology 75:307, 1978. *A clinical conference that presents a well-balanced overview of the pathogenesis, pathophysiology, clinical features, treatment, and complications of sprue (59 references).*

104. INFLAMMATORY BOWEL DISEASE

104.1. Introduction

Irwin H. Rosenberg

Inflammatory bowel disease is a generic term that refers to idiopathic chronic inflammatory diseases of the intestine, principally *ulcerative colitis* and *Crohn's disease*. Ulcerative colitis, as the name implies, is an inflammatory, ulcerating process of the colon; Crohn's disease is a transmural granulomatous enteritis that may involve any part of the intestine, but primarily the distal small intestine and colon. These two conditions of unknown etiology share a number of clinical, epidemiologic, immunologic, and genetic features, including extraintestinal complications and response to treatment. Therefore, they are often considered together despite distinguishing clinical and pathologic features. These diseases may represent different pathologic responses to a common cause, or they may turn out to be unrelated in etiology and pathogenesis. These two major forms of inflammatory bowel disease will be discussed separately for convenience, but it will prove useful to compare and contrast them throughout.

104.2. Crohn's Disease

Irwin H. Rosenberg

DEFINITION. *Crohn's disease* is a subacute and chronic inflammatory process of unknown cause that may involve any part of the intestinal tract, especially the distal ileum, colon, and anorectal region. Although earlier reports are suggestive, Crohn's disease was first clearly described as an inflammatory condition of the terminal ileum by Burrill Crohn and his colleagues in 1932 and called *regional ileitis*. Shortly thereafter reports of similar transmural granulomatous inflammation of portions of the small and large bowel made the term "regional enteritis" more appropriate. A similar granulomatous inflammation of the colon, distinguishable from ulcerative colitis, was subsequently described and termed "Crohn's disease of the large intestine." The pattern in over 50 per cent of patients with Crohn's disease is *ileocolitis*, involvement of the distal small bowel with variable, segmental involvement of the colon. *Ileitis* is a common designation for Crohn's disease confined to the ileum. *Crohn's colitis* refers to predominant involvement of the colon.

EPIDEMIOLOGY. Like ulcerative colitis, Crohn's disease is more common in northern Europe and the United States, less frequent in central Europe and the Middle East, and infrequent in Asia and Africa. Crohn's disease has a prevalence roughly half that of ulcerative colitis. However, the incidence and prevalence of Crohn's disease has, until recently, been rising while that of ulcerative colitis is remaining stable. In the United States this disease affects 50,000 to 100,000 patients at any time, with 5,000 to 10,000 new cases diagnosed each year. The incidence of Crohn's disease is approximately equal in males and females. The age of onset profile of Crohn's disease is shown in Figure 104–1. Crohn's disease is uncommon before age ten; the peak incidence occurs in the next two decades and declines thereafter. A later peak of incidence has been reported at 55 to 60 years but whether this represents a true secondary peak or the effect of hospitalization for other disorders (e.g., ischemic bowel) remains uncertain.

American blacks and American Indians are at less than one fifth the risk of the white population for inflammatory bowel disease. There is growing evidence that the incidence of inflammatory bowel disease in blacks is rising. In Japan the incidence of inflammatory bowel disease has been relatively low, but now is rising steadily. The prevalence of Crohn's disease is six times higher for Jewish men and three times higher for Jewish women. The incidence of inflammatory bowel disease among Jews in Israel is lower than that of Jews in the United States or in northern Europe. Israeli Jews of European (Ashkenazic) ancestry are at considerably greater risk than are Jews of Mediterranean or Middle Eastern (Sephardic) ancestry. Inflammatory bowel disease occurs with equal frequency in urban and rural populations. Some of these demographic features are summarized in Table 104–1.

FAMILIAL-GENETIC PATTERN. There are definite familial clusters of patients with both ulcerative colitis and Crohn's disease.

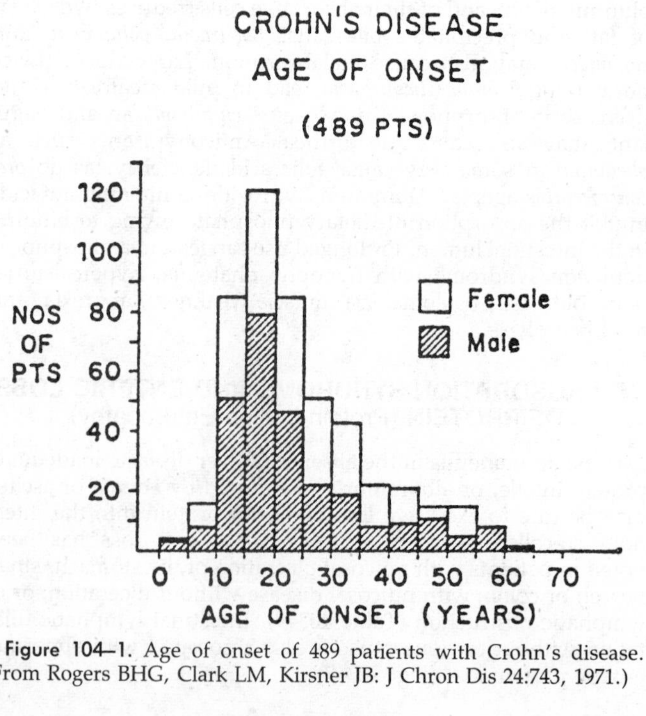

Figure 104–1. Age of onset of 489 patients with Crohn's disease. (From Rogers BHG, Clark LM, Kirsner JB: J Chron Dis 24:743, 1971.)

TABLE 104–1. DEMOGRAPHIC FEATURES OF CROHN'S DISEASE

Worldwide distribution
More common in whites than nonwhites
Increased frequency among European stock
More common among Jews (especially Ashkenazi) than non-Jews (3 to 8 times)
Most frequent age of onset: 15 to 30 years
Aggregation in families
Increasing incidence over past 20 years (1.4 to 4 times)

Modified from Donaldson RM, Jr: *In* Sleisenger MH, Fordtran JS (eds.): Gastrointestinal Disease. 3rd ed. Philadelphia, W. B. Saunders Company, 1983.

In one large series, 17.5 per cent of patients had a positive family history for a similar disorder. As many as five members in a single family with inflammatory bowel disease have been reported. Three fourths of family clusters involve either ulcerative colitis or Crohn's disease, but in one fourth of such families both ulcerative colitis and Crohn's disease are found in the same pedigree. Disease concordance has occurred in some but not all monozygotic twins.

ETIOLOGY AND PATHOGENESIS. Both Crohn's disease and ulcerative colitis are diseases of unknown etiology. The patterns of prevalence described above suggest both host and environmental factors. Individual susceptibility factors are suggested by the specific ethnic patterns of occurrence and the phenomenon of family clustering. Familial occurrence might also represent exposure of the patient and family members to common environmental factors. Parallel trends in disease incidence with increasing technologic development in Asia as well as Europe and the United States also suggest environmental factors. Some of the many and disparate theories of the etiology of Crohn's disease will be reviewed briefly.

Psychogenic Factors. Significant emotional events have often seemed to be temporally related to the onset or exacerbation of inflammatory bowel disease, leading to the hypothesis that psychogenic factors are important in its etiology or pathogenesis. The nervous system may profoundly influence the motor, secretory, vascular, and metabolic functions of the digestive system, but it is difficult to conceive how these variables would lead to the type of segmental involvement of transmural inflammation often seen in Crohn's disease. Psychogenic factors are probably important only in their contribution to symptomatic exacerbations.

Infectious Origin. Both the clinical and the pathologic manifestations of Crohn's disease and ulcerative colitis suggest the possibility that intestinal bacteria are involved in the etiology of the inflammation or as secondary invaders: (1) Intestinal bacterial counts are increased. (2) The fever and toxemia often present are suggestive of the absorption of bacteria or bacterial toxic products, and bacteria have been cultured from portal vein blood at the time of surgery. (3) The use of antibiotics or the substitution of parenteral for oral nutrition (which sharply decreases the quantity of intestinal bacteria) may lead to significant clinical improvement in both forms of inflammatory bowel disease. Several bacterial agents including cell wall-deficient bacteria and variant strains of normal gut flora have been proposed, but evidence for a direct etiologic role is lacking. *Yersinia enterocolitica* infection can produce an acute ileitis and *Campylobacter* and *Clostridium difficile* have been reported in association with exacerbations of Crohn's disease, but these agents are not implicated in the etiology.

Tissues from patients with Crohn's disease or with ulcerative colitis have been reported repeatedly to produce inflammatory lesions when injected either into the footpad or the ileal wall of mice or rabbits. Multicenter reappraisal of the animal model and "viral isolation" studies, using standardized methods and laboratory exchange of tissue homogenates, has failed to confirm the original observations. Nevertheless the search for microbiologic agents represents one current approach to understanding the etiology of the inflammatory bowel diseases.

Immunologic Factors. Whether or not microorganisms are directly implicated in the etiology of these diseases, they may be involved in their pathogenesis in concert with altered immune mechanisms. Some of the extraintestinal manifestations of inflammatory bowel disease suggest the presence of antigen-antibody complexes in these sites. Circulating lymphocytes from patients with inflammatory bowel disease may be cytotoxic to cultures of human fetal or adult colonic epithelial cells. Responses of circulating lymphocytes to nonspecific mitogens are generally intact, especially in patients with ulcerative colitis. Some abnormalities of proportions or numbers of circulating B and T lymphocytes, particularly T-suppressor cells, have been reported. Serum concentrations of the major immunoglobulin classes follow no predictable pattern among patients with ulcerative colitis or Crohn's disease and fail to show a consistent relationship to the state of activity or severity of the diseases. None of these immunologic changes have been clearly shown to be implicated in the etiology or pathogenesis of inflammatory bowel disease. A recent focus on the function of lymphocytes and macrophages isolated from the intestinal tissue itself may provide more direct insights relevant to local immune phenomena.

MEDIATORS OF INFLAMMATION. Prostaglandins, together with leukotrienes and kinins, are potential mediators of some of the inflammatory responses. Through their ability to stimulate adenylate cyclase and ion secretion in the bowel, prostaglandins may contribute to diarrhea as well. Increased amounts of prostaglandin metabolites have been observed in rectal mucosa of patients with active colitis but not during remission.

PATHOLOGY. Crohn's disease may involve any segment of the alimentary canal or any combination of segments. There are, however, pathologic changes that characterize the inflammatory process in any segment of involved bowel. The involved portion of the bowel, usually the distal ileum and adjacent right colon, is thickened and hyperemic with some serosal fibrin deposition and adhesions between adjacent loops of bowel (Fig. 104–2). The adjacent mesentery is commonly thickened with migration or "creeping" of mesenteric fat onto the serosal surface of the bowel. Mesenteric lymphatics are engorged, and mesenteric lymph nodes are commonly enlarged and matted.

Diseased segments of bowel wall are thickened. The mucosa may be nearly normal or only mildly hyperemic, or there may be elongated linear ulcerations, usually in the long axis of the bowel. In more advanced cases the mucosal architecture is destroyed by multiple ulcerations, with only small islands of mucosa remaining. Numerous aphthoid ulcers may be present in the mucosa (Fig. 104–3). Deep ulcers or clefts may extend into the thickened and edematous submucosa and sometimes through to the serosal surface.

Fistulas form readily in this setting of a transmural inflammation when deep ulceration and fissures combine with obstruction and stenosis to form a penetrating, pressure-relieving pathway to adjacent and adherent loops of bowel or other viscera, and sometimes to the abdominal wall. Ileoileal, ileosigmoid, and ileocecal communications are most common, but communication with other parts of the gastrointestinal tract, including the stomach, duodenum, and gallbladder, has been reported. Fistulas may also occur from the intestine to the urinary bladder, the renal collecting system, and the female genital tract, most often, the vagina.

The inflammatory process involves all layers of the bowel and consists of infiltration of lymphocytes, histiocytes, and plasma cells with characteristic aggregation to form noncaseating granulomas. Focal granulomas are found in about half of the cases; in the remainder, well-defined lymphoid aggregates are found.

These pathologic changes and their progression correlate with many of the important clinical manifestations of Crohn's disease. Abdominal pain and cramps reflect the narrowed lumen and partial obstruction that result from thickening of the bowel wall. Diarrhea may represent disordered mucosal

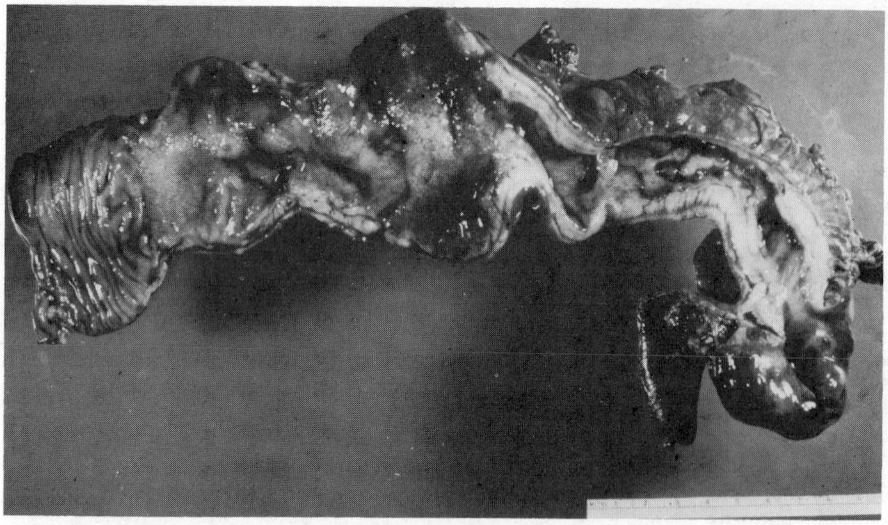

Figure 104–2. Resected specimen of ileum showing thickening of the wall, loss of normal mucosa, scarring, and stricture in Crohn's disease. "Creeping fat" is visible on the serosal surface.

absorptive–secretory function or abnormal motility of either small or large bowel. The transmural inflammation increases adherence of loops of bowel, producing signs of peritoneal irritation and the formation of abdominal masses.

CLINICAL PRESENTATION. When Crohn's disease affects primarily the distal small intestine (*Crohn's ileitis* or *regional enteritis*), the most characteristic clinical pattern emerges. A young person, usually in the second or third decade, will present with a period of episodic abdominal pain, largely postprandial and often periumbilical, occasionally with low grade fever and mild diarrhea. Such episodes often remit spontaneously but recur with increasing frequency and severity, with pain eventually localizing to the right lower quadrant.

The *abdominal pain* often has the characteristics of partial intestinal obstruction, made worse by eating and improved by rest, local heat, and fasting. The effect of early ileitis on bowel habits may be variable. *Diarrhea* is rarely more severe than four or five stools daily, and rectal bleeding is uncommon. *Weight loss* is frequent. In children growth retardation and delayed sexual maturation may be the presenting clinical feature in Crohn's disease. The patient may be aware of *tenderness in the right lower quadrant* and even of a palpable mass in that region. A history of *aphthous ulcerations of the mouth* may be obtained. The similarity of this presentation to that of acute appendicitis commonly results in an abdominal exploration, and diagnosis is then made surgically. When the involvement of the small intestine is more diffuse in the syndrome of jejunoileitis, the presentation may include more diffuse abdominal pain and more prominent weight loss, growth retardation, and sometimes peripheral edema.

In Crohn's colitis or ileocolitis the presentation is characterized by lower abdominal, crampy pain worsened by eating, by diarrhea, and by fever. Crohn's colitis tends to be more subtle in onset than ulcerative colitis and thus may not be diagnosed until anemia or other systemic complications predominate.

One third of all patients with Crohn's disease and one half with Crohn's colitis develop perirectal or perianal fistulas with pain, mass, purulent drainage, and often fever. Perianal complications may represent communication of a fistulous tract from the small bowel along the presacral gutter to the perirectal area, but more commonly are a complication of deep, penetrating ulceration in Crohn's colitis of the lower colon. When drainage is impaired, local abscess formation occurs.

Extraintestinal manifestations such as arthritis, ankylosing

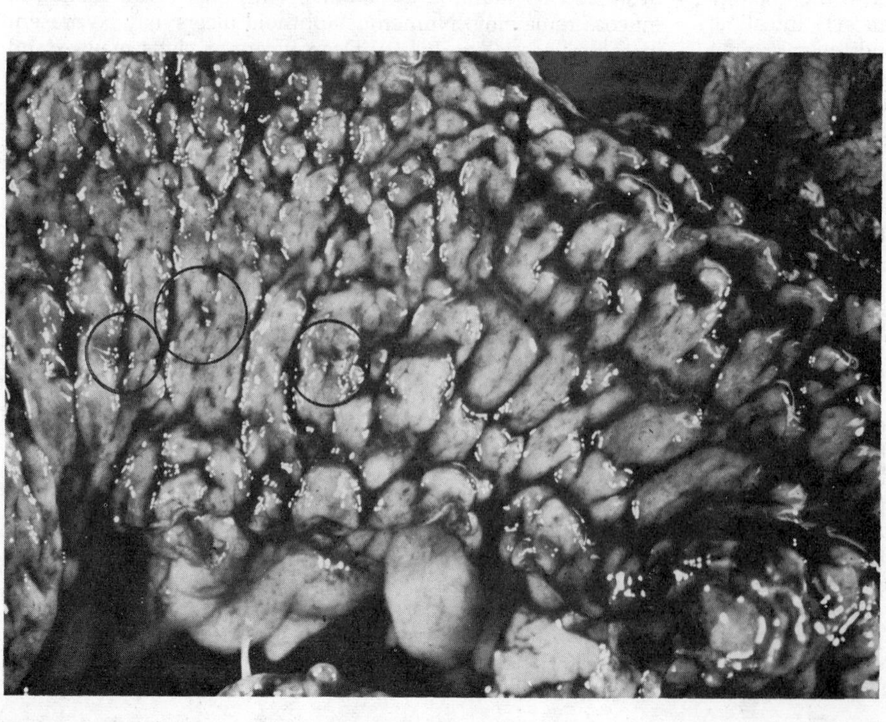

Figure 104–3. Close-up photograph of "cobblestone" appearance of colonic mucosa in Crohn's colitis formed by linear and transverse ulcerations and intervening mucosa. Aphthoid ulcers are identified by circles.

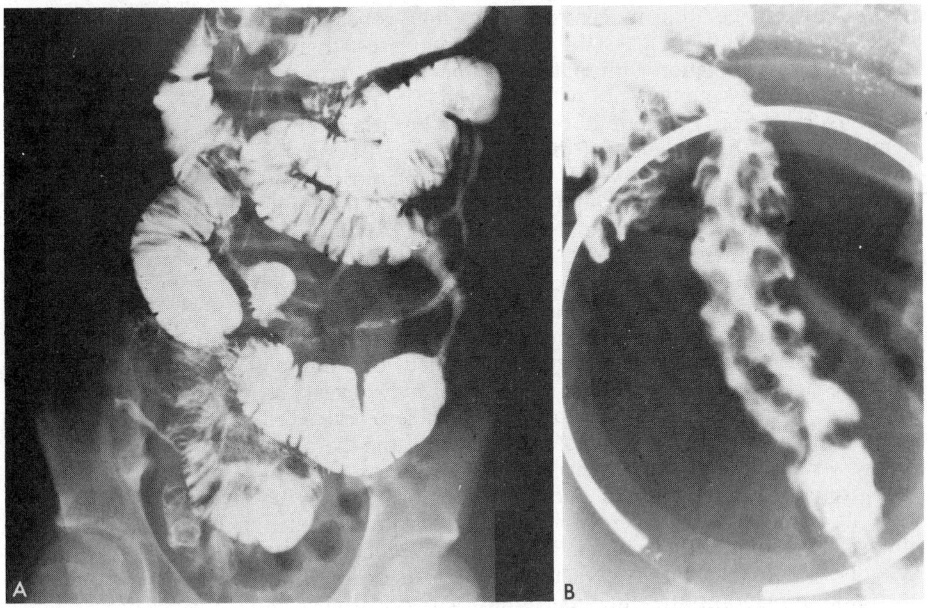

Figure 104–4. *A*, Small bowel radiograph in Crohn's disease demonstrating extensive jejunoileitis with areas of narrowing and mucosal damage alternating with "skip areas" of more normal bowel. *B*, Cobblestone appearance of the terminal ileum in Crohn's disease.

spondylitis, and erythema nodosum may precede or strongly influence the presenting syndrome. These extraintestinal manifestations of Crohn's disease will be discussed subsequently.

DIAGNOSIS. The diagnosis of Crohn's disease may be delayed for months or even years in patients whose symptoms are subtle and insidious and in those in whom extraintestinal manifestations focus attention away from the bowel. Crohn's disease should be suspected in patients of any age, but particularly in those in the younger age groups, when there is a history of recurrent episodes of abdominal pain worsened by eating, and a change in bowel habits with intermittent or persisting diarrhea. The presence of pain, tenderness, and a mass in the right lower quadrant should strongly heighten the suspicion of this diagnosis. A history of weight loss is common. In addition, unexplained arthritis, perianal disease, recurrent fevers, or, in children, cessation of normal growth should raise the question of Crohn's disease even if gastrointestinal symptoms are minimal.

Physical Examination. A moderately ill patient may be pale, underweight, and febrile (temperature seldom greater than 38° C). An abdominal examination often demonstrates tenderness or a mass in the right lower abdominal quadrant. The bowel sounds may be hyperactive. Examination of the extremities may reveal signs of large joint arthritis or, rarely, clubbing. Uveitis, iritis, and skin manifestations (see below) may occasionally be present. Peripheral edema may reflect protein depletion. Examination of the rectum and perianal area may identify perianal fistulas, fissures, or an abscess. A purulent vaginal discharge in a woman with Crohn's disease is strongly suggestive of enterovaginal fistula.

Radiographic Examination. The diagnosis of Crohn's disease depends in considerable measure on the presence of characteristic radiographic findings in the bowel. The abdominal plain film may demonstrate dilated loops of small bowel in the presence of partial obstruction. The diagnosis depends, however, upon upper and lower intestinal barium contrast studies (Figs. 104–4 and 104–5). Characteristic changes on the small bowel roentgenogram include segmental narrowing, obliteration of the normal mucosal pattern with or without evidence of ulceration, enteroenteric fistula formation, or the classic "string sign" of the contrast medium shown on segmental films of the terminal ileum, particularly when changes are localized to the most distal small bowel and the adjacent right colon (Fig. 104–4).

Most radiologists prefer air contrast radiography of the colon to delineate the presence or extent of disease in the large bowel (Fig. 104–5). In 85 per cent of patients with Crohn's disease of the large bowel there will also be involvement of the distal small bowel, which is best demonstrated by antegrade barium studies as described above. It is important to distinguish between "backwash ileitis" associated with ulcerative colitis and true mucosal involvement of ileal Crohn's disease. In Crohn's colitis there is a characteristic asymmetrical and segmental pattern with areas of disease separated by areas of apparently normal colonic tissue.

The most subtle changes in the small bowel are thickening and edema of the valvulae conniventes. Earliest changes in the large bowel are the appearance of small aphthous ulcers on air contrast examinations. Loss of haustral markings may be a subtle early finding. Mucosal ulcers are likely to be longitudinal. When severe ulcerative disease is present, the alternation of

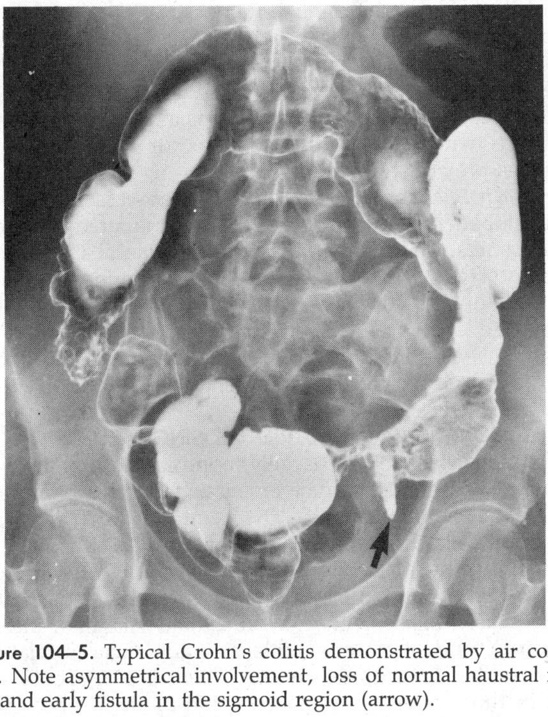

Figure 104–5. Typical Crohn's colitis demonstrated by air contrast exam. Note asymmetrical involvement, loss of normal haustral markings, and early fistula in the sigmoid region (arrow).

ulcers with regenerating mucosa produces the "cobblestone" appearance (Fig. 104–4*B*). As the disease progresses, there is increasing scar formation with total loss of mucosal pattern and narrowing of the segments of involved bowel. The presence of fistulous tracts from one loop of bowel to another can often be demonstrated. The presence of distinctly narrowed segments of bowel need not be taken as clear evidence of cicatricial and irreversible obstruction. These findings are often manifestations of severe edema and thickening of the bowel and may improve substantially following treatment. The newer technique of enteroclysis—installation of barium directly into the small bowel by tube—may add precision to small intestinal studies.

Laboratory Diagnosis. No laboratory test is diagnostic for Crohn's disease. Anemia may result from blood loss, or iron or folate deficiency. Examination of the stool may reveal the presence of occult blood and increased fat. Fecal leukocytes call attention to inflammatory processes as a basis for the diarrhea. A low serum albumin reflects malnutrition and increased enteric protein loss. Low serum calcium or magnesium may be seen in patients with severe diarrhea and steatorrhea. An abnormal Schilling test of vitamin B_{12} absorption reflects extensive disease or resection of the ileum. Other tests of intestinal absorption, including the quantitative fecal fat, xylose absorption test, and lactose absorption test, are helpful in assessing the extent and severity of disease. Analyses of the circulating levels of iron, folate, vitamin B_{12}, 25-hydroxy vitamin D, and plasma zinc may demonstrate evidence of micronutrient depletion.

Proctosigmoidoscopy. In contrast to ulcerative colitis the rectum is uninvolved in more than half of the patients with Crohn's disease. Proctosigmoidoscopy may simply show mild erythema associated nonspecifically with diarrhea. Rarely, a biopsy of the normal-appearing rectum will reveal inflammatory changes and even granuloma, but such biopsies are not a regular part of the diagnostic evaluation.

Colonoscopy. Colonoscopy may be valuable in determining the extent and severity of colonic involvement and in evaluating strictures or polypoid masses. Colonoscopic biopsies are helpful for verification of the diagnosis in difficult cases, but should be avoided in patients with acutely symptomatic colitis.

LOCAL COMPLICATIONS. Chronic, transmural inflammation of the bowel with progressive scarring leads to a number of local complications. Hemorrhage is uncommon, but *chronic blood loss* leading to iron deficiency often occurs. Local scarring and narrowing of the bowel lead to *intestinal obstruction* of varying severity. Free *intestinal perforation* occurs rarely; more often there is fistulous communication between loops of bowel or into matted mesentery, which presents as a tender, inflammatory mass with fever. Fistulas can occur in any abdominal viscus, as previously noted.

Perianal fistulas and related fissures and abscesses affect nearly half of all patients with Crohn's disease. Indurated, nonhealing rectal fissures, draining perianal fistulas, or local abscesses may cause local pain, fever, and progressive perineal distortion. Abscesses must be drained, with special attention to the integrity of the anal sphincter muscles and the threat of fecal incontinence. A judicious and persistent combination of bowel rest, dietary, drug, and surgical therapy is required (see Treatment).

MALABSORPTION AND NUTRIENT-LOSING ENTEROPATHY. Predictably, malabsorption is largely found in those patients with extensive inflammatory involvement or following partial resection of the small intestine. The ileum is the major site of absorption of both vitamin B_{12} and bile salts. Ileitis may therefore result in malabsorption of this vitamin as well as steatorrhea on the basis of the interrupted enterohepatic circulation of bile salts. Malabsorption of fat-soluble vitamins, including vitamin D, and of water-soluble vitamins such as folate, has been reported in Crohn's disease. There is a tendency, especially in those who have had resection of the ileocecal valve, to develop bacterial overgrowth, which further contributes to malabsorption. Enteric protein loss through the damaged epithelium may be an important contributor to protein and associated trace metal depletion. The reader is referred to Ch. 103 for a more extensive discussion of malabsorption.

TABLE 104–2. EXTRAINTESTINAL MANIFESTATIONS OF THE INFLAMMATORY BOWEL DISEASES

Nutritional and metabolic abnormalities
Weight loss
Hypoalbuminemia—nutritional, protein-losing enteropathy
Growth retardation in children
Vitamin deficiencies
Deficiencies of calcium, magnesium, or zinc
Hematologic abnormalities
Anemia—bleeding, Fe deficiency, folate deficiency
Leukocytosis, thrombocytosis
Skin and mucous membrane
Pyoderma gangrenosum
Erythema nodosum
Stomatitis with multiple aphthous ulcers
Arthritis
Ankylosing spondylitis, sacroiliitis (HLA-B27 associated)
Peripheral arthritis of large joints
Hepatic and biliary manifestations
Fatty liver
Pericholangitis
Sclerosing cholangitis
Cirrhosis
Gallstones
Carcinoma of the bile ducts
Renal complications
Kidney stones—uric acid, calcium oxalate
Obstructive uropathy
Fistulas to urinary tract
Amyloidosis (rare)
Eye complications
Conjunctivitis, episcleritis
Iritis

SYSTEMIC AND EXTRAINTESTINAL COMPLICATIONS (see Table 104–2.) ***Nutritional Complications.*** Nutritional complications are common in inflammatory bowel disease. The majority of patients admitted to the hospital will exhibit some degree of nutritional depletion. Assessment of the nutritional status should be part of the initial evaluation of the patient in order to recognize and treat nutritional complications early. Deficiency of protein, calories, minerals, vitamins, and trace metals are well documented in both Crohn's disease and ulcerative colitis. These deficiencies may result from inadequate dietary intake, malabsorption, or intestinal loss of protein, as noted above. In addition, increased nutritional requirement relating to the chronic inflammatory response and faster cell turnover in the diseased gut is probable but less well documented.

Growth Retardation. Retarded skeletal growth, often with a delay in sexual maturation, is frequently observed in children whose onset of Crohn's disease occurs before puberty. In some patients a slowing or arrest of linear growth occurs years before the diagnosis of Crohn's disease is made and may be the condition that brings the patient to medical attention. The pathogenesis of growth retardation is complex. No hormonal deficiencies have been demonstrated in these patients. Corticosteroids administered daily in high doses for colitis or Crohn's disease may suppress growth in some patients. Lower doses or alternate-day steroid therapy may allow restoration of normal growth by suppressing the activity of the disease. Abnormalities of intestinal absorption have not been prominent in those patients carefully studied. Caloric insufficiency may result from a dietary intake that is limited by the young patient in response to abdominal pain and diarrhea. Protein, vitamin, and mineral deficiencies are less regular.

Hepatobiliary Complications. Hepatobiliary complications of Crohn's disease (and of ulcerative colitis) include a spectrum from clinically inapparent histologic abnormalities through progressive and sometimes life-threatening liver disease. The possibility that chronic or intermittent portal bacteremia or the return from the gut to the liver of toxic metabolic products, such as lithocholic acid, may be responsible for hepatic injury has been suggested but not proved. Neither viral hepatitis after blood transfusion nor drug toxicity can account for a significant proportion of liver disease in these patients. *Fatty infiltration* of the liver is found in virtually all biopsy or autopsy specimens of patients with inflammatory bowel disease. Abnormalities other than fatty infiltration are found in the majority of liver specimens obtained by needle biopsies in patients with inflammatory bowel disease: *pericholangitis* (50 to 70 per cent), *chronic active hepatitis, cirrhosis,* extrahepatic obstruction associated with *primary sclerosing cholangitis,* and, most rarely, *carcinoma of the bile ducts.* Fewer than 25 per cent of such patients will have increased alkaline phosphatase activity; jaundice is even less common. However, when serious or progressive liver disease is present histologically, liver function tests are usually abnormal.

Pericholangitis refers to a lymphocytic inflammatory response in the entire portal triad, not only periductal as the name implies. Most patients with pericholangitis demonstrated by biopsy are asymptomatic, and the majority have normal liver function tests. Some may have recurring episodes of cholestasis, jaundice, and pruritus with increased serum alkaline phosphatase. In a few patients the full picture of ascending cholangitis, shaking chills, fever, and jaundice will occur. Recurrent right upper quadrant pain may cause diagnostic confusion with gallstone disease, which is also more common in patients with Crohn's disease. Occasionally, pericholangitis will progress to cirrhosis. Those patients with pericholangitis found incidentally on liver biopsy at the time of surgery without a history of cholangitis or hepatic function abnormalities are likely to have a benign course without progressive hepatic deterioration.

Sclerosing cholangitis is an uncommon inflammatory and sclerosing lesion of extra- and intrahepatic bile ducts causing biliary obstruction and recurrent cholangitis. Its relationship to pericholangitis is uncertain. In some patients inflammation extends from the portal triads to the intra- and extrahepatic ducts. The extent of anatomic abnormality is best determined by endoscopic retrograde cholangiography. Corticosteroids are often used to suppress inflammation, and antibiotics are used to treat episodes of cholangitis. In some patients adequate bile drainage may have to be established surgically. Carcinoma of the bile ducts, although extremely rare in Crohn's disease, is sometimes seen in the setting of sclerosing cholangitis.

Gallstones develop with increased frequency in patients with Crohn's disease whether or not bile duct abnormalities exist. This tendency is often attributed to bile salt malabsorption in the diseased ileum, leading to a diminished bile salt pool and a relative increase in the ratio of cholesterol to bile salts in bile.

Renal Complications. Renal complications in Crohn's disease include *obstructive uropathy, nephrolithiasis, fistulas* to the renal collecting system, and, rarely, *amyloidosis.* Fistulas from the bowel to the renal excretory system may present as the passage of gas or fecal material in the urine. The diagnostic changes may be more subtle and simply involve recurrent episodes of pyuria or infection. Right-sided hydronephrosis resulting from cicatricial and inflammatory obstruction of the right ureter may be asymptomatic, and some advocate the regular use of intravenous pyelography in the full evaluation of the patient with Crohn's disease. Corrective surgery by unsheathing of the right ureter may prevent progressive destruction of the right kidney.

The most common renal complication is *nephrolithiasis.* There is an increased incidence of uric acid stones in both Crohn's disease and ulcerative colitis, probably related to increased cell turnover and the excretion of a concentrated urine of increased acidity. The most frequent type of kidney stone in patients with Crohn's disease, however, is composed of calcium oxalate as its main crystalloid. Patients with extensive disease of the distal small intestine, particularly those who have had resections of the distal small bowel, have excessive absorption of dietary oxalate and low urinary excretion of citrate and are therefore at increased risk for the formation of calcium oxalate stones (see Ch. 89 for more details).

Miscellaneous Complications. Both *peripheral arthritis* and *spondylitis* occur in Crohn's disease as in ulcerative colitis, affecting approximately 10 to 20 per cent of patients. *Erythema nodosum* is seen in approximately 9 per cent of patients with Crohn's disease, but *pyoderma gangrenosum* and *erythema multiforme* are rare. Ocular complications include *episcleritis* and *iritis* in 3 to 4 per cent of the patients.

DIFFERENTIAL DIAGNOSIS. The classic presentation of Crohn's disease with a characteristic history, a palpable right lower abdominal mass, and typical radiographs offers little diagnostic challenge. The presentation, however, may be highly variable. With an acute onset, Crohn's disease may be mistaken for appendicitis, particularly in a young person with right lower quadrant rebound tenderness and leukocytosis. Diarrhea, however, is uncommon in appendicitis. If progression of symptoms and signs is rapid and the opportunity to diagnose Crohn's disease by the typical x-ray findings is not feasible, exploration may be necessary. An *appendiceal abscess* is particularly difficult to distinguish from a mass associated with Crohn's disease by x-ray.

Infection by *Yersinia enterocolitica* causes an acute or subacute mesenteric adenitis and may produce diarrhea, abdominal pain, and fever. Infection by *Campylobacter fetus* may resemble acute or subacute colitis. Successful diagnosis requires attention to the specific requirements for culturing these organisms. Distinction of Crohn's disease from *ileocecal tuberculosis* or from fungal infections involving the bowel is usually possible on epidemiologic grounds. Intestinal tuberculosis is rare in the United States and western Europe and is usually seen in native-born Americans only in the presence of extensive pulmonary tuberculosis. Persons raised in areas where milk-borne tuberculosis is common often have ileocecal tuberculosis without pulmonary disease.

Benign lymphoid hyperplasia of Peyer's patches in the ileum is seen on barium x-ray in children and young adults in a setting of infection or fever. This benign condition is distinguishable from Crohn's disease on radiographic grounds, since no mucosal abnormality or luminal narrowing occurs.

Patients with a more chronic course present a more extensive differential diagnosis. *Nongranulomatous ulcerative jejunoileitis,* another inflammatory condition of the small bowel of unknown etiology, has more prominent malabsorption, protein-losing enteropathy, and nonspecific shallow small bowel ulcers on intestinal biopsy. This distinction in rare cases, however, requires exploration and surgical biopsies.

Lymphoma or *lymphosarcoma* of the small bowel may produce a picture similar to that of Crohn's disease. Once initiated, the symptoms of this malignant process are usually more persistent and more rapidly progressive than those of Crohn's disease. Palpable abdominal masses tend to be firmer. A diffuse nodularity of the bowel without segmental narrowing characteristic of Crohn's disease on small bowel series suggests abdominal lymphoma. Occasionally *carcinoid* of the ileum or other malignancies will be extensive and invasive enough to be mistaken for Crohn's disease by radiography.

Radiation enteritis involving the distal ileum and colon after pelvic irradiation for carcinoma is distinguished from Crohn's disease mainly by history.

Eosinophilic gastroenteritis may present with diarrhea, malabsorption, and protein-losing enteropathy, but the pattern of the intestinal involvement demonstrated by radiographic or endoscopic techniques, peripheral blood eosinophilia, and intestinal biopsy are distinguishing features.

When Crohn's disease involves the duodenum or stomach, it may be mistaken for duodenal ulcer disease, or even the Zollinger-Ellison syndrome when there are multiple ulcerating lesions. The pain pattern tends to be different in these conditions. Crohn's disease causes more persistent or postprandial abdominal pain and symptoms of obstruction. Endoscopy and biopsy in addition to x-ray findings may be helpful in distinguishing these conditions from Crohn's disease.

For distinction between Crohn's ileitis and backwash ileitis

TABLE 104–3. A COMPARISON OF THE CLINICAL AND PATHOLOGIC FEATURES OF CROHN'S COLITIS AND ULCERATIVE COLITIS

Feature	Crohn's Colitis	Ulcerative Colitis
Intestinal		
Malaise, fever	Common	Uncommon
Rectal bleeding	Sometimes	Common
Abdominal tenderness	Common	May be present
Abdominal mass	Very common (especially with ileocolitis)	Not present
Abdominal pain	Very common	Unusual
Fistulas	Very common	Very uncommon
Endoscopic		
Rectal disease	Occasionally	Very common
Diffuse, continuous symmetrical involvement	Uncommon	Very common
Aphthous or linear ulcers	Common	Very unusual
Cobblestoning	Common	Very unusual
Friability	Unusual	Very common
Radiologic		
Continuous disease	Uncommon	Very common
Ileal involvement	Very common	"Backwash ileitis"
Asymmetry	Very common	Uncommon
Strictures	Common	Uncommon
Fistulas	Very common	Uncommon
Pathologic		
Discontinuity	Common	Uncommon
Rectal involvement	Uncommon	Common
Intense vascularity	Uncommon	Common
Ileal involvement	Common	Nonexistent
Aphthous ulcers	Common	Very uncommon
Transmural involvement	Common	Very uncommon
Lymphoid aggregates	Common	Uncommon
Crypt abscesses	Uncommon	Very common
Granulomas	Common	Uncommon
Linear clefts	Common	Uncommon

associated with ulcerative colitis and for the differentiation of Crohn's colitis and ulcerative colitis, the reader is referred to Table 104–3.

TREATMENT. There is no known cure for Crohn's disease. Treatment is empirical and is directed at alleviating the symptoms and manifestations of the disease. Symptomatic remissions may occur during therapy, or even in its absence, but the disease is lifelong, and surveillance by the physician must be a continuing process. In addition to medical and sometimes surgical management, general support is very important, including attention to the psychologic stresses imposed by the disease on the patient and the family. In addition, the physician must anticipate, identify, and, when possible, prevent the common nutritional and metabolic complications described above.

Medical Management. Medical management of Crohn's disease requires a comprehensive assessment of the clinical status of the patient. It is particularly important to determine the extent and severity of the disease, largely by radiologic and proctoscopic methods, and to assess the presence or absence of the complications. Only on the basis of this complete information, and a knowledge of the patient as an individual, can a full program of nutritional, drug, and supportive therapy be rationally planned.

Nutritional Treatment. Nutritional assessment is based on a careful diet history to determine the extent of calorie insufficiency, to document weight loss, and to analyze nutritional status on the basis of body measurements and laboratory tests. In prepubertal patients assessment of growth pattern is a critical part of the evaluation.

For ambulatory patients dietary goals should be set which are adequate for the nutritional needs of the patient but which minimize stress on the inflamed and often narrowed segments of bowel. Evidence of lactose intolerance should be sought by history and when possible confirmed by *blood* or *breath test analysis* (see Ch. 103). Removal of lactose-rich foods, such as milk and ice cream, in the lactase-deficient patient may have a prompt symptomatic benefit. In many patients with cramping and diarrhea, decreasing the intake of fiber-containing foods may be beneficial, and in those with steatorrhea a decrease of fat intake to 70 to 80 grams per day may substantially improve diarrhea. Attention to restoration of an adequate diet must always accompany these deletions.

The hospitalized patient presents a different management problem. More than half of such patients suffer from deficiencies of calories, protein, certain vitamins, and minerals. Most such patients take an inadequate diet limited by the worsening of intestinal symptoms after eating. One approach in such patients is to put the inflamed and narrowed bowel "at rest" by removing the stimulus of food intake on intestinal secretion and motility. Many patients derive symptomatic benefit from partial rather than total bowel rest with the delivery of nutrients enterally in the form of low residue–defined formula diets. Rarely can adequate nutritional maintenance be achieved by the oral intake of these formula diets owing to limitations of palatability. The use of small caliber nasogastric tubes for continuous or intermittent drip provides a well tolerated alternative means of delivery that is often associated with a marked decrease in bacterial flora, stool frequency, and symptoms. In more severely ill patients, and in those who cannot tolerate enteral feeding or who lack adequate intestine for absorption, total parenteral nutritional support is used increasingly.

For the severely malnourished patient, total parenteral nutrition can be used to achieve nutritional repletion during the diagnostic investigation, to prepare the nutritionally depleted patient for surgery, and, when required, to maintain the patient through the postoperative period. For the patient with a short bowel disability following major intestinal resections, total parenteral nutrition can be used in the immediate postoperative period or even for prolonged nutritional support at home until the adaptive responses permit oral nutritional maintenance. In patients with fistulas total parenteral nutrition and bowel rest may lead to closure of the fistulas with sustained remission in 20 to 50 per cent of patients. The combination of nutritional support therapy and corticosteroids appears more effective than either modality alone.

Specific attention to vitamin and mineral depletion will help in the management of anemia and bone disease and should aid the healing process and the overall sense of well-being. Calcium and magnesium losses may be particularly high in the presence of poor intake, severe diarrhea, and steatorrhea. Vitamin D deficiency may lead to metabolic bone disease in Crohn's disease patients, particularly after intestinal resection. This deficiency can usually be corrected with adequate amounts of oral vitamin D, approximately 4000 IU daily. Vitamins can usually be replaced by a therapeutic multivitamin preparation containing three to five times the normal daily requirement. Zinc deficiency should be considered, especially in patients with prolonged and severe diarrhea who may require replacement therapy. In patients on parenteral nutrition, addition of trace metals to parenteral fluids is mandatory.

Therapy in Growth-Retarded Patients. The young patient whose growth is retarded presents a special challenge. In some patients the institution of a medical regimen, including sulfasalazine or corticosteroids, preferably on an alternate-day regimen, will suppress symptoms and disease activity sufficiently to improve dietary intake and restore growth. Restoring normal nutrition is crucial to success of medical therapy. Nutrition may be restored, by total parenteral nutrition, including episodic administration at home, or by administering a defined, minimal residue formula diet by enteral tube. Surgery, timed to permit a maximal growth spurt during puberty, is recommended by some for intractable disease in ulcerative colitis or Crohn's ileocolitis unresponsive to medical management. In such instances the possibility of a period of relative freedom from symptoms and potential growth restitution must be balanced against the strong likelihood of recurrence of Crohn's disease and the need for repeated resections later.

Sulfasalazine. Containing both a sulfonamide, sulfapyridine, and a salicylate in azo linkage, sulfasalazine is the most commonly used drug in inflammatory bowel disease. Sulfasalazine in the usual dose of 3 grams a day orally has been established by means of a national cooperative study as effective treatment for the management of exacerbations of Crohn's disease, particularly of Crohn's disease of the colon. Sulfasalazine in combination with prednisone was not better than prednisone alone in treatment of an acute exacerbation of Crohn's disease. The effectiveness of sulfasalazine in Crohn's disease limited to the small intestine remains in question. No drug regimen has been proved to reduce recurrences of Crohn's disease after clinical remission, whether spontaneous, induced by drugs, or after resective surgery. Still in many centers sulfasalazine therapy, once instituted, is maintained. Side effects of sulfasalazine treatment are discussed in Ch. 104.3.

Antimicrobial Therapy. Despite the fact that no specific microbiologic agent has been implicated in the etiology or pathogenesis of Crohn's disease (see above), antibiotics are often used empirically in this inflammatory disorder. Parenteral antibiotics are commonly used in the acutely ill patient with fever and signs of peritoneal irritation and sometimes as an adjunct in programs for bowel rest or with corticosteroid therapy. The use of antibiotics including tetracycline and trimethoprim in ambulatory patients with Crohn's disease has yielded some promising results, but these observations require confirmation in controlled trials.

Metronidazole has a broad spectrum of activity against anaerobic bacteria that predominate in the gastrointestinal tract and are present in markedly increased numbers in inflammatory bowel diseases. Metronidazole has been used as an adjunct in the management of perianal fistula in Crohn's disease with reported success. A recent controlled trial has demonstrated the efficacy of metronidazole, 10 mg per kilogram per day in divided doses, in the management of acute exacerbations of Crohn's disease.

Corticosteroid Therapy. Corticosteroids are used to suppress inflammation in the bowel and the coincident systemic manifestations of inflammation. The decision to use corticosteroids in Crohn's disease is one that should be taken with care. Prednisone in doses of 0.25 to 0.75 mg per kilogram for four months is usually effective in the treatment of an exacerbation of Crohn's disease, but prolonged corticosteroid use does not seem to prevent exacerbations of the disease. Therefore, the usual practice is to treat the acute exacerbation with 40 to 60 mg of prednisone per day for two to four weeks followed by tapering doses as symptoms permit. Some patients, unable to be tapered off prednisone, may continue to take low doses for protracted periods. In prepubertal patients it is particularly important to give corticosteroids on an alternate-day regimen if at all possible to reduce growth retardation. Such an alternate-day regimen should be used when possible even in adult patients.

Immunosuppressive Therapy. Azathioprine* has been used with reported encouraging results in the general management of patients with Crohn's disease, but these studies have been largely uncontrolled. In Crohn's disease, as well as in ulcerative colitis, the use of daily doses of 1.0 to 1.5 mg per kilogram has permitted the lowering of corticosteroid doses without symptomatic exacerbation in controlled trials. As a single agent, however, azathioprine demonstrated no superiority over a placebo in a four-month trial. When 6-mercaptopurine is used for longer periods, it may be effective in the management of some patients with Crohn's disease if sufficient time is allowed for the immunosuppressive effects to be accomplished. Toxic side effects may limit the use of these agents (see Ch. 176).

Antidiarrheal Drugs. Patients may be symptomatically improved by drugs given to diminish intestinal motility and diarrhea. Loperamide, diphenoxylate, tincture of opium, or paregoric can be used to reduce diarrhea in Crohn's disease. Anticholinergic drugs are helpful in some patients in diminishing stool frequency. All these antimotility drugs should be used carefully, with special attention to narcotic dependence in the case of codeine, paregoric, and opium. Symptoms of obstruction may be exacerbated with all of these drugs.

Surgery for Ileitis or Ileocolitis. Surgical resection of bowel involved in Crohn's disease is occasionally required, but is undertaken with reluctance because of the high rate of recurrence of the disease. In one study recurrence after resection of the involved distal small bowel or ileum and adjacent colon was 50 per cent in five years, 75 per cent in ten, and 91 per cent in fifteen. Still there is a prominent place for surgery in the management of many patients with Crohn's disease. Surgery is clearly indicated for high grade intestinal *obstruction* unresponsive to medical therapy, for *perforation*, and for *fistulas* to other abdominal organs such as the bladder. Patients lacking these clear indications may undergo resective surgery for *intractable disease* with the knowledge that recurrence is likely but still seeking temporary symptomatic relief. Surgery in the adolescent with growth retardation has been discussed earlier. The most common operation is resection of the involved portions of the terminal ileum with an ileocolonic anastomosis. Such an anastomosis should retain as much of the right colon as possible, since the right colon may be critical in determining the extent of debility from postiliectomy diarrhea.

Surgery for Crohn's Colitis. Indications for surgery in Crohn's colitis are similar to those for ulcerative colitis (see Ch. 104.3). Uncontrolled bleeding, perforation, and toxic dilatation are rarer than in ulcerative colitis but may occasionally demand acute surgical intervention. Most commonly surgery is performed for clinical intractability of the disease despite full medical management. Intractability usually means inability to work or function socially despite therapy, inadequate growth and development in children, unresolved perianal complications, or unremitting systemic complications such as iritis or liver disease. The surgical approach may be that of total proctocolectomy and resection of involved terminal ileum with ileostomy, or a total colectomy with ileosigmoid, ileorectal, or ileoanal anastomosis. For any resection with internal anastomosis, recurrence rate is in excess of 75 per cent in ten years. In many patients a period of several years of relative freedom from symptoms without ileostomy makes ileorectal or ileosigmoid anastomosis the surgical approach of choice. For patients with extensive involvement of colon, including the rectum, total proctocolectomy with ileostomy is usually performed. The need for surgical revision of the ileostomy, usually caused by complications resulting from recurrent inflammatory disease, may be as high as 40 per cent in five years. The actual rate of recurrence of Crohn's disease after ileostomy is uncertain but is probably less than 15 per cent in five years. Thus Crohn's colitis, in contrast to ulcerative colitis, is not cured by total proctocolectomy.

PROGNOSIS. Crohn's disease exacts a very substantial cost in altered patient life style and in regular, often intensive medical care. A pattern of remissions and exacerbations is usual. Although disease-free intervals may extend for years and rarely for decades, the most characteristic and discouraging feature of Crohn's disease is its almost relentless tendency to recur despite intensive medical treatment or after surgery. The benefits of some years free of symptoms after surgical resection are substantial in many patients. About 50 per cent of patients require surgical treatment eventually. Surgery is rarely if ever curative, however, so every effort should be made to manage all aspects of the patient's illness. Overall mortality attributed to Crohn's disease or its complications ranges from 5 to 18 per cent in various reports. It is lower in patients with disease limited to the small intestine.

The outlook for patients with Crohn's disease has improved steadily with advances in general and supportive treatment. Further progress may be expected as our understanding of the etiology of Crohn's disease increases.

*This use is not listed in the manufacturer's directive.

Donaldson RM Jr: Crohn's disease. *In* Sleisenger MH, Fordtran JS (eds.): Gastrointestinal Disease. 3rd ed. Philadelphia, W. B. Saunders Company, 1983, p 1088. *Excellent, balanced review of all phases of Crohn's disease, supplemented by illustrative radiographs and 129 references.*
Greenstein AJ, Janowitz HD, Sachar DB: The extraintestinal complications of Crohn's disease and ulcerative colitis: A study of 700 patients. Medicine 55:401, 1976.
Kirsner JB, Shorter RG: Recent developments in "nonspecific" inflammatory bowel disease. N Engl J Med 306:775, 837, 1982. *A current and authoritative review with emphasis on concepts of etiopathogenesis.*
Mendeloff AI: The epidemiology of inflammatory bowel disease. Clin Gastroenterol 9:259, 1980. *A comprehensive review and critique comparing the behavior of Crohn's disease and ulcerative colitis in a volume devoted to inflammatory bowel disease.*
The National Cooperative Crohn's Disease Study. Gastroenterology 77:825, 1980. *Twelve articles summarizing the results of a cooperative study, clinical characteristics, drug therapy, diagnostic studies, complications, and adverse reactions.*

104.3. Ulcerative Colitis

Bernard Levin

DEFINITIONS. Ulcerative colitis is a chronic disease of unknown etiology characterized by inflammation of the mucosa and submucosa of the large intestine. The inflammation usually involves the rectum down to the anal margin and extends proximally in the colon for a variable distance. Terms in common usage refer to the anatomic extent of the disease: *pancolitis* for involvement of the entire colon; *ulcerative proctitis* or *proctosigmoiditis* for diseases limited to the rectum or rectosigmoid; and *left-sided colitis* for disease of the descending colon.

Ulcerative colitis has an estimated incidence of 2 to 7 cases per 100,000 and a prevalence of 40 to 100 cases per 100,000 population in the United States. For ulcerative proctitis both the incidence and prevalence are roughly comparable to those for colitis. Although both Crohn's disease and ulcerative colitis are being increasingly recognized, there is no evidence that the incidence of ulcerative colitis is actually increasing. In the United States between 200,000 and 400,000 persons suffer from inflammatory bowel diseases, with about 30,000 new cases diagnosed each year. Ulcerative colitis affects women more frequently than men and exhibits a bimodal age distribution, with a first peak of incidence between the ages of 15 and 20 years and a secondary small peak at ages 55 to 60 (Fig. 104–6). The incidence of ulcerative colitis in blacks may be as low as one third that in whites, and its incidence among Jews is about three to five times greater than among non-Jews.

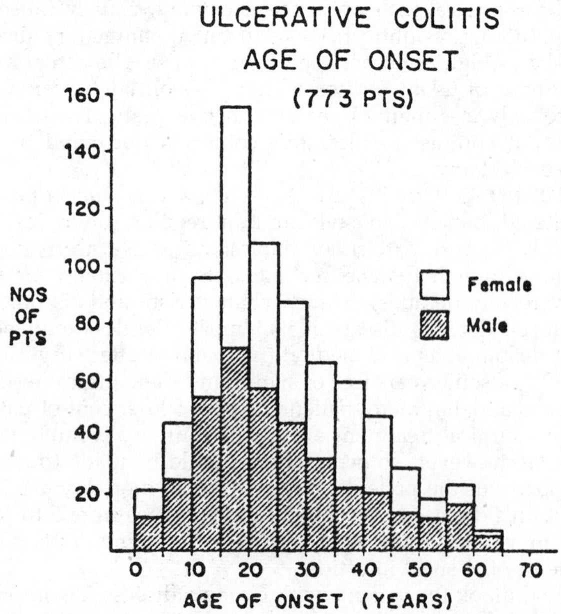

Figure 104–6. Age of onset in 773 patients with ulcerative colitis. (From Rogers BHG, Clark LM, Kirsner JB: J Chron Dis 24:743, 1971.)

FAMILIAL AND GENETIC FEATURES. There is an increased familial incidence of inflammatory bowel disease, both for ulcerative colitis and Crohn's disease, but without a clear-cut pattern of inheritance. In one study about 4 per cent of a control population had a family history of inflammatory bowel disease, whereas 11 per cent of those with chronic inflammatory bowel disease had a family history of these disorders. The onset of disease in patients from affected families occurred at a lower age than in those without family histories.

Patients with inflammatory bowel disease and ankylosing spondylitis have a likelihood of 50 to 90 per cent of possessing the histocompatibility antigen HLA-B27, whereas the antigen is found in 6 to 9 per cent of the control population. The antigen is present in even higher prevalence in patients with spondylitis without inflammatory bowel disease (see Ch. 445). An increased incidence of ankylosing spondylitis has been reported in relatives of patients with ulcerative colitis or Crohn's disease. These findings continue to arouse interest in genetic factors in the pathogenesis of chronic inflammatory bowel disease.

ETIOLOGY AND PATHOGENESIS. The etiology of chronic ulcerative colitis is unknown. Furthermore, no satisfactory animal model of the human disorder has been discovered.

Considerable debate has occurred about the role of psychosomatic factors in the initiation and further development of ulcerative colitis. Once the illness has become manifest, it is often impossible to distinguish its influences on behavior from the patient's premorbid personality. Any illness characterized by severe diarrhea, rectal bleeding, and a variety of constitutional symptoms, especially when occurring in a young, previously healthy person, constitutes a stressful situation and can destroy a patient's self-confidence. Regressive behavior may result. Hospitalized children with colitis are often compulsively neat, demanding, and immature for their age. Adults may exhibit exaggeration of dependency needs during periods of active disease. Conflicting data exist about the occurrence of significant life-stress crises at the time of onset of the disease.

Ulcerative colitis is characterized by an inflammatory reaction in the bowel resembling that caused by known microbiologic pathogens such as *Shigella*. However, no organism has been reproducibly demonstrated to be responsible for the condition. Nevertheless, microbial infection remains a possible cause because of the recent recognition of "new" bacterial causes of enteritis and colitis (*Yersinia enterocolitica* and *Campylobacter fetus* ssp. *jejuni*). The possible role of viral agents in the etiology of inflammatory bowel disease is discussed in more detail in relation to Crohn's disease (see Ch. 104.2).

An immunologically mediated pathogenetic mechanism is suggested by the frequent presence of personal and family histories of atopic diseases in patients with ulcerative colitis and the concomitant presence of conditions such as erythema nodosum, arthritis, uveitis, and vasculitis. Circulating anticolon antibodies have been described in ulcerative colitis, but these remain of unknown significance. The beneficial effects of corticosteroid therapy for ulcerative colitis are consistent with its immunosuppressive as well as its anti-inflammatory effects.

Some of the extraintestinal manifestations of ulcerative colitis such as skin rashes, arthritis, and vasculitis suggest immune complex deposition. Activation of the alternative complement pathway in ulcerative colitis is suggested by the observations of normal or elevated levels of C3PA and markedly reduced levels of properdin convertase in sera from patients with extraintestinal complications of the disease.

Antilymphocyte antibodies have been found in up to 40 per cent of patients with ulcerative colitis, and in up to 50 per cent of family members and unrelated household contacts of patients with inflammatory bowel disease. In contrast these antibodies were found in only 4 per cent of control family members. Lymphocytotoxic antibodies have been found in sera from patients with inflammatory bowel disease and from their unaffected spouses more frequently than sera from age-matched controls and their spouses. Such data suggest exposure to a common environmental agent, but genetic factors must also be implicated since there is an increased prevalence of lymphocytotoxic antibody in sera from consanguineous relatives without household contact as well.

Lymphocytes from many patients with either ulcerative colitis or Crohn's disease will kill colonic epithelial cells in tissue culture. The sera from such patients contain a factor that allows normal peripheral blood cells also to kill colonic epithelial cells. The pathogenetic role of these alterations in cellular immunity is not established.

Observations of immunologic events at the intestinal mucosal level have suggested decreased spontaneous antibody secretion in intestinal mononuclear cells compared with peripheral blood mononuclear cells, which showed increased synthesis and secretion of IgG, IgM, and IgA. This suggests the possibility that a primary mucosal immunodeficiency in the bowel of patients with inflammatory bowel disease weakens the mucosal barrier, thereby facilitating both a local inflammation and a heightened systemic immune response.

PATHOLOGY. Pathologic changes in the colon in ulcerative colitis readily predict the clinical features of the disease. In 75 per cent of patients disease involves only the left side of the colon. In the remainder, the entire colon is involved (pancolitis). Extensive vascular engorgement and mucosal ulceration result in bleeding. The damaged mucosa is less able to absorb sodium and water, and watery diarrhea results. Iron deficiency anemia results from blood loss, and hypoalbuminemia may reflect transmucosal loss of protein. The histologic changes in ulcerative colitis are nonspecific, but the chronicity and distribution pattern are characteristic.

Ulcerative colitis involves primarily the mucosa of the colon. Unlike the segmental lesions of Crohn's disease, the mucosa is inflamed continuously, occasionally terminating at some point in the colon where the abnormality gradually changes to a normal appearance over a distance of a few centimeters. The involved mucosa is red and granular and bleeds diffusely. The macroscopic lesions may progress from small, petechial ulcerations to deeper, linear ulcers separated by islands of inflamed but intact mucosa. In severe cases, large areas of the colon may be denuded (Fig. 104–7).

The inflammatory process begins with increased numbers of inflammatory cells in the lamina propria: plasma cells, lymphocytes, monocytes, eosinophils, and polymorphonuclear leukocytes. Capillary dilatation causes hyperemia and vascular engorgement. Polymorphonuclear cells accumulate near the tips of the crypts of Lieberkühn. The crypt epithelium shows degenerative changes or even frank necrosis, with extension of the inflammatory process into the surrounding tissue causing characteristic microabscesses (Fig. 104–8). These crypt abscesses may coalesce by lateral enlargement to produce shallow ulcerations of the mucosa extending down to the lamina propria. Alternatively, the mucosa may be undermined on three sides, leaving an area of ulceration adjacent to an attached fragment of the mucosa. Such resulting mucosal excrescences may be seen as pseudopolyps on radiologic or endoscopic examination.

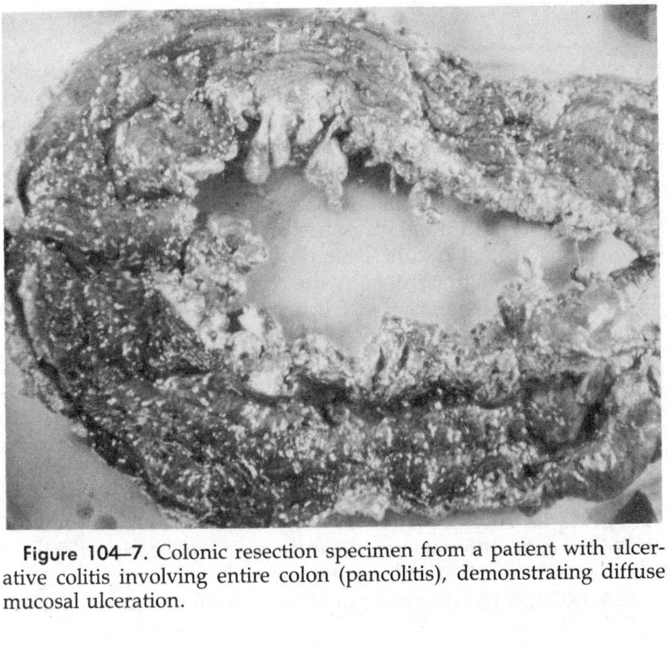

Figure 104–7. Colonic resection specimen from a patient with ulcerative colitis involving entire colon (pancolitis), demonstrating diffuse mucosal ulceration.

Some of the features of ulcerative colitis result from the attempts of the inflamed colon to regenerate or repair the destroyed crypts. Regenerating crypts become distorted, branching, and diminished in number and contain goblet cells. Highly vascular granulation tissue may develop in denuded areas. Collagen may be deposited in the lamina propria, and the muscularis mucosae may hypertrophy.

The alternating processes of superficial ulceration and granulation followed by re-epithelialization can lead to the development of polypoid excrescences. These are inflammatory polyps (pseudopolyps) that are not neoplastic. Longstanding disease gives rise to hyperplasia of the muscularis mucosae, and this change, accompanied by postinflammatory fibrosis, causes shortening of the colon. The haustrations are lost, and the large bowel has the appearance of a smooth tube. Strictures may be caused by the localized fibromuscular hyperplasia; a distinction must be made between these and malignant strictures.

In the most severe cases, the inflammation can involve the submucosa and even the serosa and lead to perforation. In toxic dilatation of the colon, a particularly severe and acute form of this disease, the diameter of the lumen of the colon is greatly increased and the bowel wall is thinned, with a serious risk of spontaneous perforation.

CLINICAL MANIFESTATIONS AND COURSE. The five most common symptoms of ulcerative colitis are *rectal bleeding, diarrhea, abdominal pain, weight loss,* and *fever.* The patient is usually in the second, third, or fourth decade of life at the onset of symptoms. Ulcerative colitis may begin in a subtle manner or with catastrophic suddenness. Patients may relate the acute onset of symptoms to a recent emotional upset, to an upper respiratory infection, or occasionally to oral antibiotic therapy.

When signs and symptoms of colonic inflammation (including malaise, lower abdominal discomfort, and an increased number of bowel movements with rectal bleeding) are not marked, the designation *mild ulcerative colitis* is often used. This form of the disease, which accounts for roughly half of all patients with ulcerative colitis, is less likely to be recognized and may not be diagnosed for months or even years. The mortality is negligible, and the long-term prognosis for these patients does not differ from that of a control population. The development of colonic cancer in mild ulcerative colitis is about one seventh of that occurring in the more severe forms of the disease.

Moderate ulcerative colitis describes a more abrupt onset of the disorder, typically associated with four to five loose and bloody bowel movements per day. In this form of the disease, which accounts for about 30 per cent of ulcerative colitis, abdominal cramps may be severe and may awaken the patient at night. Low grade fever, fatigue, and malaise may be prominent symptoms, as may some of the extracolonic manifestations (see below). The patient may have anorexia and weight loss. Some patients with moderate colitis may become progressively worse, with increasingly severe diarrhea, bleeding, and fever. The immediate mortality in patients with moderate colitis is low because of the efficacy of corticosteroid therapy, but the long-term prognosis for avoiding colectomy is guarded. Exacerbations of the disease often occur and may require intensive medical management over extended periods. The risk of developing cancer of the colon is increased and probably affects this group most significantly.

Severe or fulminant ulcerative colitis presents usually in a dramatic fashion with *profuse diarrhea, rectal bleeding,* and *fever,* which may be as high as 39° C. This form of the disease occurs

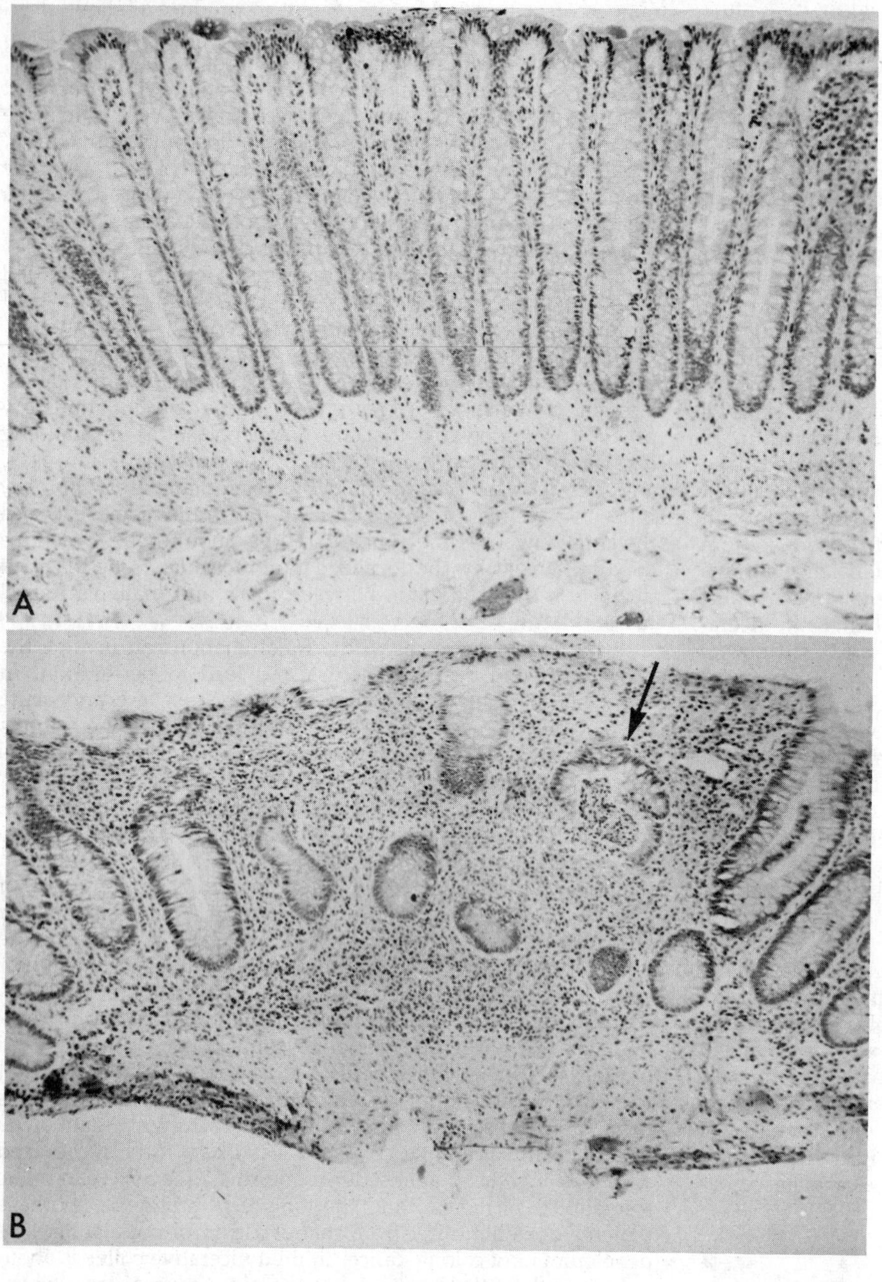

Figure 104–8. Rectal biopsies from *(A)* a normal patient and *(B)* a patient with ulcerative colitis. In *B*, note mucosal atrophy, branching of a gland, cellular infiltration, and crypt abscess *(arrow)*. × 100. (From Cello JP: In Sleisenger MH, Fordtran JS [eds.]: Gastrointestinal Disease. 3rd ed. Philadelphia, W. B. Saunders Company, 1983.)

in about 15 per cent of patients with ulcerative colitis. Abdominal cramps, rectal urgency, and profound weakness are common presenting symptoms. Intermittent nausea, anorexia, and weight loss are also present. Occasionally patients with initially less severe disease may worsen and present a picture of fulminant colitis. Physical examination reveals an acutely ill, pale, weak, and febrile patient. Tachycardia, hypotension, and even shock may be present. Examination of the abdomen reveals generalized tenderness; localized tenderness, especially with "rebound," signals the onset of peritoneal irritation. This suggests that the inflammatory process has extended beyond the mucosa. Absence of bowel sounds should suggest the diagnosis of toxic dilatation, and this serious complication must be carefully excluded.

TOXIC DILATATION OF THE COLON (TOXIC MEGACOLON). In severe ulcerative colitis, the patient may become gravely ill with signs and symptoms of a general toxic state associated with abdominal pain, distention, rebound tenderness, and dilatation of the diameter of the colon on plain abdominal roentgenograms to 6 cm or greater (Fig. 104–9). In a patient with severe active colitis, toxic megacolon may be precipitated by a barium enema examination (and its antecedent preparation), potassium depletion, or anticholinergic or narcotic medication. The complication may also develop spontaneously. Medications that may decrease colonic motility should be avoided in these patients. Severe inflammation disrupts the neural and muscular elements that maintain normal tone. This allows the intraluminal pressure to expand the colon well beyond its normal width. Bacteria overgrow and are thought to produce toxins that intensify the complication and contribute to the hazard of peritonitis. Diffusion of these toxic products into the systemic circulation contributes to the toxic state.

Clinical signs include fever, tachycardia, dehydration, and abdominal tenderness and distention. The loss of bowel sounds is a significant finding. The colon is found to be dilated with severe mucosal disease demonstrated by a plain film of the abdomen (Fig. 104–9). Marked leukocytosis, hypokalemia, anemia, and hypoalbuminemia are frequently present. The mortality rate in toxic dilatation of the colon may be as high as 20 to 30 per cent. Intensive medical therapy with early colectomy can decrease mortality (see Treatment).

DIAGNOSIS. The diagnosis of ulcerative colitis is usually made

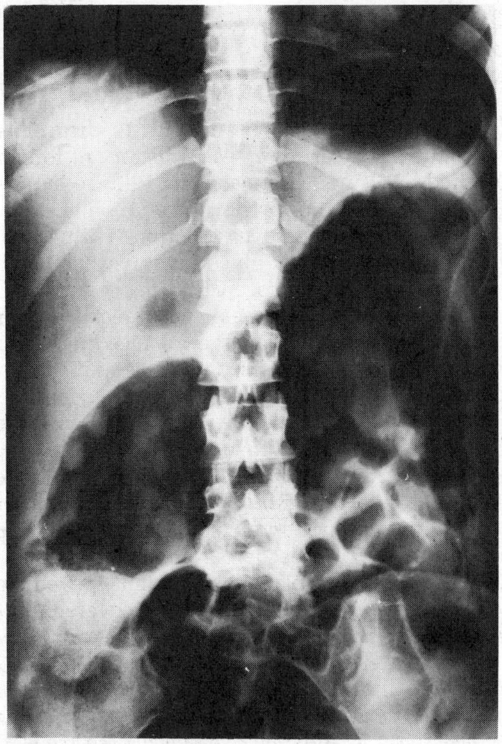

Figure 104–9. Plain film of the abdomen from a patient with ulcerative colitis and toxic megacolon. Note that the air in the colon silouettes an irregular colonic mucosa. (From Cello JP: In Sleisenger MH, Fordtran JS [eds.]: Gastrointestinal Disease. 3rd ed. Philadelphia, W. B. Saunders Company, 1983.)

on the basis of its clinical features, the demonstration of inflammation of the rectal and sigmoidal mucosa on proctosigmoidoscopy, and the exclusion of specific infections by appropriate stool culture and examination for parasites. The diagnosis may be supported by radiologic examination, fiberoptic colonoscopy, and rectal biopsy.

Proctosigmoidoscopy. This is the most reliable diagnostic study in ulcerative colitis because the observer may inspect the mucosa directly. This examination is indicated in every patient with rectal bleeding. At the same time, fresh stool samples may be obtained for culture and microscopy to determine the presence of fecal leukocytes or trophozoites. The mucopurulent exudate should be aspirated, mixed with a drop of warm saline, and examined microscopically for motile, hematophagous trophozoites of *E. histolytica.* It is important to exclude the diagnosis of amebiasis before beginning corticosteroid therapy.

The gross appearance of the rectal mucosa is nonspecific in acute colitis. Specific causes such as shigellosis and *Campylobacter* infections should be excluded by cultures obtained at the time of proctosigmoidoscopy. Particularly, but not exclusively, in patients with prior antibiotic therapy acute colitis may be caused by the enterotoxin of *Clostridium difficile.* Such patients may have endoscopic features of pseudomembranous colitis (see Ch. 278). It is preferable to avoid enemas prior to proctosigmoidoscopy in a patient suspected of having ulcerative colitis because they may confuse by irritating normal rectal mucosa and by aggravating mild abnormalities. Despite its name, in the early phases ulcerative colitis does not produce visible ulcers, but rather the red, diffusely bleeding, granular mucosa looks as though it has been gently sandpapered. Edema and erythema produce a markedly reddened, swollen mucosa with a diminished vascular pattern, the changes of hyperemia, petechiae, and fragility.

In moderate colitis, purulent exudate and discrete small ulcers appear. Gross pus and spontaneous diffuse bleeding mark severe colitis, and there may be large areas of ulceration. After appropriate therapy in mild cases, the appearance of the rectum may return to normal or near normal; however, repeated attacks with attempts at healing may cause loss of the normal vascular pattern, fine or coarse granularity of the mucosa, blunting of the normally sharply angulated rectal valves, and inflammatory polyps composed of tags of damaged mucosa and heaped-up granulation tissue. After many cycles of inflammation and healing, the bowel may scar and become stenosed.

Rectal Biopsy. A biopsy usually is not necessary to make the diagnosis of ulcerative colitis if the clinical and sigmoidoscopic features are typical. However, there may be certain instances in which biopsy is helpful: (1) to exclude other forms of colitis such as Crohn's disease of the colon, pseudomembranous colitis, or amebic colitis; (2) to search for mucosal dysplasia in cancer surveillance in patients with longstanding colitis; or (3) to confirm equivocal sigmoidoscopic findings in a patient with a history suggestive of ulcerative colitis.

Radiography. The patient who is ill with moderate or severe colitis should not be subjected to barium enema examination. In such patients radiologic examination is unnecessary for diagnosing ulcerative colitis and may be dangerous. Preparation of the patient by use of cathartics and enemas will worsen the condition significantly.

In the acutely ill patient the plain abdominal film should be employed in the initial evaluation. The extent of disease can be predicted by observing the patterns of fecal residue in the colon as well as the mucosal outline and haustral patterns. Failure to recognize early a grave complication such as toxic megacolon increases the risk of morbidity and mortality. The diagnosis of toxic dilatation is made on both clinical and radiographic grounds. Patients suspected of having toxic megacolon (fever, abdominal tenderness and distention, decreased or absent bowel sounds) may be seen on plain film to have dilatation of the mid-transverse colon to a diameter of 6 cm or more (Fig. 104–9).

Barium enema examination may provide the following important information: (1) When sigmoidoscopy confirms the diagnosis of colitis, and after specific infectious causes have been excluded, it helps to determine the extent and severity of the mucosal lesions. If the sigmoidoscopy is negative in a patient with rectal bleeding and diarrhea, barium examination will be helpful in making the diagnosis of another cause such as neoplasm, Crohn's disease of the colon, or ischemic colitis. (2) In patients with equivocal findings at sigmoidoscopy or on a rectal biopsy, it may demonstrate features of ulcerative colitis more proximally. (3) The barium enema may detect complications such as colonic cancer in patients with longstanding colitis.

The postevacuation film of a single contrast barium enema also provides information about mucosal detail. Unless the double contrast (barium and air) technique is used, however, fine mucosal abnormalities may be overlooked and the extent of the involvement underestimated.

In the acute stage of ulcerative colitis, fine granularity reflects mucosal edema and hyperemia. As the disease progresses, superficial erosions develop and adherent barium produces a stippled appearance. Tiny ulcerations may be seen as these enlarge, and "collar-button"–like projections appear that involve the colon circumferentially. As the disease progresses, the normal colonic mucosal surface is lost; however, it may regenerate with healing. Inflammatory polyps may appear as rare or numerous intraluminal filling defects (Fig. 104–10). The inflammatory process also may affect the muscular layers of the colon, producing a smooth, foreshortened colon without haustra. After recovery from a first attack, haustral markings may reappear. After longstanding mucosal and submucosal thickening in some patients with ulcerative proctitis or colitis, the presacral space may enlarge. This is seen best on a lateral view of the barium-filled rectum.

A small bowel follow-through radiographic study should be performed after acute symptoms are controlled to help exclude

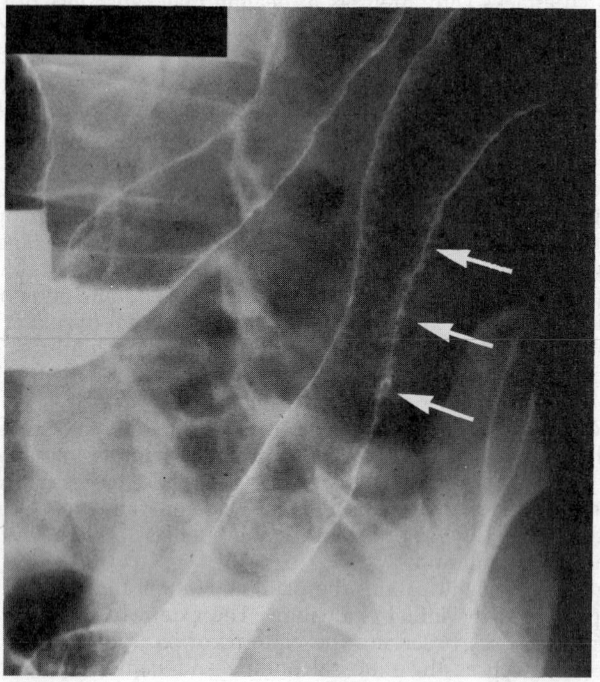

Figure 104–10. Double contrast enema in patient with active ulcerative colitis with discrete collar button ulcers (arrow) in an anhaustral and diffusely granular colon.

the diagnosis of Crohn's disease. In ulcerative colitis involving the entire colon, the ileocecal valve may be dilated and incompetent. The terminal ileum may be dilated, but discrete ulceration is seen only when Crohn's disease is present.

Colonoscopy. Colonoscopy has little place in the diagnosis of acute ulcerative colitis and may be hazardous because of the risks of perforation and hemorrhage. Since the entire colon may be examined by colonoscopy, it is extremely useful in the patient who does not have acute and severe symptoms when the diagnosis and extent of inflammatory bowel disease are uncertain. Colonoscopy is most commonly used in obtaining multiple biopsies in patients with longstanding colitis in a search for neoplastic changes.

DIFFERENTIAL DIAGNOSIS. Numerous other causes of diarrhea must be considered in the differential diagnosis of ulcerative colitis, but the clinical presentation, sigmoidoscopic findings, and radiologic features are used to make a definite diagnosis. The differential diagnosis of rectal bleeding includes hemorrhoids, colonic adenomas and carcinomas, angiodysplastic lesions, bleeding disorders, and diverticular disease. The differential diagnosis of gastrointestinal bleeding is discussed in greater detail in Ch. 113.

Viral infections, bacillary dysentery, and toxigenic strains of *E. coli* may cause acute colitis and occasionally simulate ulcerative colitis. Diarrhea is a prominent symptom of these diseases, but rectal bleeding is uncommon except in *shigellosis,* which rarely lasts more than a few days. *Campylobacter* infections may closely mimic nonspecific ulcerative colitis. Its diagnosis is particularly important, since this infection responds well to appropriate antibiotic therapy. *Salmonella* infections may present as an acute or subacute diarrheal disorder. *Yersinia enterocolitica* produces an acute bacterial ileitis and mesenteric adenitis, which more closely resemble an acute attack of Crohn's disease.

Ischemic colitis is more common in elderly individuals and often causes a segmental form of colitis. Typically, roentgenographic features of "thumbprinting" caused by intramural hemorrhage are observed. Infarction of the colon, affecting primarily the right side of the colon, may be seen in young women taking oral contraceptives. This clinical picture of acute lower abdominal pain, fever, and rectal bleeding may resemble acute ulcerative colitis, but the course will help distinguish this entity.

Amebiasis may occasionally be difficult to distinguish from ulcerative colitis in its early phases. A history of foreign travel may be elicited but is not essential. Mild, diffuse hyperemia on sigmoidoscopic examination is not uncommon. Later, distinctive features include discrete large ulcers with overhanging edges. Fresh preparations of mucopus must be examined for the presence of trophozoites (see Ch. 385).

Gonococcal proctitis may present with rectal burning and diarrhea, a mucopurulent discharge, or bleeding. On sigmoidoscopic examination, generalized redness and edema of the rectal mucosa may be indistinguishable from ulcerative proctitis. The rectal discharge should be cultured for gonococci.

Pseudomembranous colitis is usually associated with a pre-existing history of antibiotic use. This condition is generally related to the growth of *Clostridium difficile,* which produces a toxin that can be identified in stools. In patients with pseudomembranous colitis, proctoscopic examination reveals raised, initially small, yellowish plaques on intensely red and later ulcerated mucosa. The plaques may be covered by mucus, which must be swabbed off before the plaque can be seen. The mucosa bleeds when the membrane is stripped.

The following diseases also may cause rectal inflammation: *histoplasmosis, leukemic* and *lymphomatous infiltration, solitary ulcer syndrome, malakoplakia,* and *lymphogranuloma venereum.* The last-named disorder presents with the passage of blood, mucus, and pus from the rectum, but patients also may have perianal fistulas and inguinal adenopathy. Patients with *radiation proctitis* will have a history of radiation therapy for cancer of the cervix, prostate, or testis, but the proctoscopic appearance is indistinguishable from that of nonspecific ulcerative colitis.

The most difficult differential diagnosis is that between ulcerative colitis and Crohn's disease of the colon. *Crohn's colitis* presents with diarrhea but usually not with rectal bleeding. Crohn's colitis also is frequently associated with perianal lesions. Characteristic features of these two diseases are compared in Table 104–3. Clinical data, endoscopic examinations, and barium enemas can differentiate Crohn's disease of the colon from ulcerative colitis in 80 to 85 per cent of patients with inflammatory bowel disease. In approximately 15 to 20 per cent of patients differentiation is not possible, and the type of colitis remains undetermined. The differentiation is useful in that it affects the approach to treatment and the assessment of prognosis.

LOCAL COMPLICATIONS. Local complications include hemorrhoids, anal fissures, perianal or ischiorectal suppuration, rectovaginal fistulas, and rectal prolapse. These complications appear most frequently when diarrhea is severe. Anal fissures improve with control of the colitis. Perirectal abscesses and rectal fistulas heal with incision and drainage of abscesses and unroofing of fistulous tracts.

More significant complications include massive hemorrhage, colonic strictures, inflammatory polyps, adenomatous polyps, adenocarcinoma, and toxic dilatation. *Massive hemorrhage* occurs in about 5 per cent of patients. Prompt replacement of circulating blood volume, correction of hypoprothrombinemia, and early colectomy if bleeding is uncontrollable are the principles of management of this condition.

Colonic strictures are seen in some patients on barium examination or during colonoscopy. Occasionally these apparent strictures may be due to spasm and will disappear after the intravenous administration of glucagon. It is essential to ensure that strictures are benign by colonoscopic biopsy and brushing cytology. Nevertheless it is not always possible to exclude a deeply infiltrating carcinoma by these means, and colectomy should be considered if any doubt exists about the diagnosis. *Inflammatory polyps* do not require removal except in cases in which it is impossible to distinguish them grossly from true adenomas. *Adenomatous polyps,* when identified, should be removed at the time of colonoscopy. Their association with

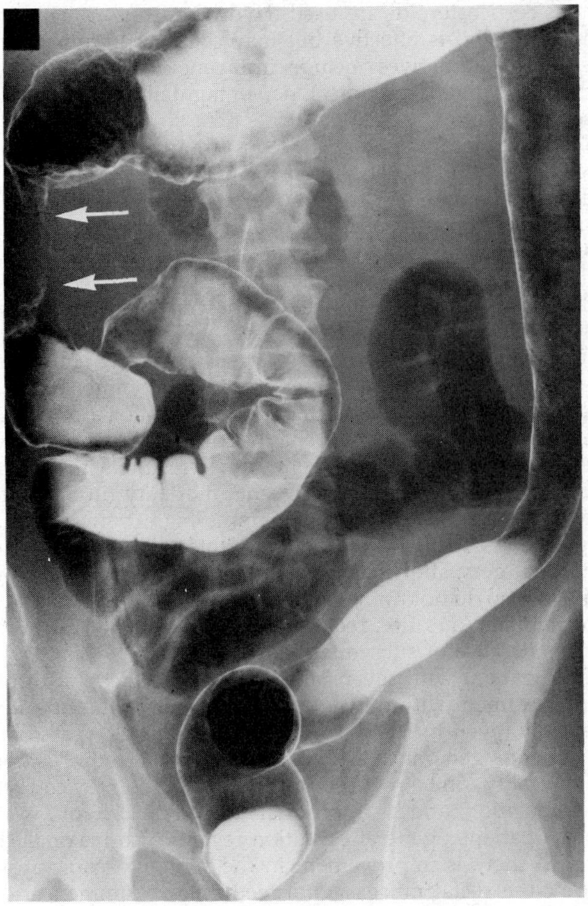

Figure 104–11. Double contrast enema in patient with chronic ulcerative colitis illustrating anhaustral colon, diffuse mucosal granularity, and carcinoma in the ascending colon (arrows).

carcinoma of the colon is of particular significance in the patient with longstanding colitis, and the patient's colon warrants careful evaluation for the presence of other adenomas or carcinoma (see Ch. 106).

Carcinoma of the large bowel occurring as a complication of ulcerative colitis is correlated with the extent of disease and its duration (Fig. 104–11). The overall prevalence of cancer in all patients with ulcerative colitis is between 3 and 5 per cent. For those with pancolitis and a duration of disease greater than ten years, the risk is 10 to 20 times greater than that of the general population (see Fig. 106–5). In children ulcerative colitis usually involves the entire colon; more adults have disease limited to the distal colon. The risk of developing cancer is similar in both children and adults with universal disease, viz. 13 per cent after 15 years, 23 per cent after 20 years, and 42 per cent after 25 years of the disease.

The patients who develop colonic cancer are often in a quiescent stage of their illness, and diagnosis often is delayed because the symptoms of bleeding or diarrhea may be attributed initially to a recurrence of the colitis. The tumors in colitis may be flat and small and not detectable even by expert colonoscopic and radiologic techniques. The prognosis of carcinoma of the colon in ulcerative colitis tends to be worse than that developing in the absence of colitis, because the diagnosis is often made late and the lesions are often multifocal and display a high grade of malignancy.

Some physicians advocate elective proctocolectomy after 10 to 12 years of the active ulcerative colitis to avoid progression to colonic cancer. The patient, however, may be very reluctant to undergo this procedure, particularly if the colitis or the side effects of medication are minimal. In biopsies obtained at proctoscopy or colonoscopy, the presence of epithelial dysplasia (neoplastic change) in the mucosa may provide an early indication of increased vulnerability to colonic cancer. Multiple biopsies are required and interpretation by an experienced pathologist is essential. These issues are discussed in detail in Ch. 87.

EXTRAINTESTINAL COMPLICATIONS (see Table 104–2). Two characteristic skin lesions occur in ulcerative colitis: *pyoderma gangrenosum* and *erythema nodosum*. *Erythema nodosum* is characterized by the appearance of dull, red, raised, painful nodules usually on the skin of the legs. This lesion, which is more common in women than in men, is roughly correlated with the activity of the mucosal disease and is likely to develop when arthritis also accompanies the attack of colitis. It is seen in both ulcerative colitis and Crohn's disease. *Pyoderma gangrenosum* is seen in 5 per cent of patients with ulcerative colitis and is characteristic of that disease. The lesion starts with the appearance of a furuncle on the skin and later appears as a painful, indurated area surrounded by violaceous, undermined skin. Topical and systemic corticosteroids have been used to suppress the colonic inflammation with parallel improvement of the lesions of pyoderma gangrenosum. Favorable responses to dapsone (Avlosulfon) therapy also have been reported.

There are two separate types of *joint involvement* in ulcerative colitis and Crohn's disease: (1) sacroiliitis with or without ankylosing spondylitis, and (2) a specific form of peripheral arthritis. The prevalence of *ankylosing spondylitis* in chronic ulcerative colitis and Crohn's disease varies from 1.6 to 12.6 per cent, at least 30 times more common than in the general population. The symptoms of ankylosing spondylitis are pain and stiffness in the spine with loss of normal lumbar lordosis. *Sacroiliitis* may be symptomatic or associated only with mild pain in the region of the sacroiliac joints. On routine radiologic examination, changes compatible with sacroiliitis were identified in approximately 20 per cent of patients with ulcerative colitis and Crohn's disease. When spondylitis occurs unassociated with ulcerative colitis, the histocompatibility antigen HLA-B27 is found in roughly 90 per cent of patients. Seventy-five per cent of patients with ankylosing spondylitis who have simultaneous inflammatory bowel disease have this antigen. The *peripheral arthritis* associated with both Crohn's disease and ulcerative colitis occurs in about 10 to 12 per cent of patients with both conditions. The arthritis is a transient, acute, painful swelling that usually affects one or more large joints and is accompanied by a sterile serous joint effusion. The knees are commonly affected, but any joint may be involved. Arthritis rarely precedes the onset of the inflammatory bowel disease but may begin at any time during its course. It is more common in patients with extensive bowel involvement and at times of a flare-up of intestinal symptoms. Peripheral arthritis is more common in patients with perianal disease.

There appears to be a *hypercoagulable state* in ulcerative colitis, with reported increases in the platelet count and in the plasma levels of factor V, factor VIII, and fibrinogen. This may account for the enhanced susceptibility to thromboembolic phenomena exhibited by these patients.

Conjunctivitis, iritis, and/or episcleritis occur as complications in 3 to 10 per cent of patients with ulcerative colitis or Crohn's colitis (and a smaller percentage of those with regional enteritis). Iritis is the most important because of its threat to vision. There is a high incidence of iritis in patients with both spondylitis and colitis. Iritis presents as a red, painful eye with discomfort increased in the dark owing to pupillary dilatation. *Stomatitis* with multiple aphthous ulcers may occasionally be severe.

The incidence of *kidney stones*, particularly urate stones, in patients with ulcerative colitis is approximately twice that in the normal population. Following colectomy and ileostomy, the incidence of urate stones may be as high as 20 times normal. Prevention is best achieved by ensuring adequate hydration and reducing urine acidity, but may on occasion require the use of allopurinol (see Ch. 89).

Hepatobiliary complications of both ulcerative colitis and

Crohn's disease range from asymptomatic *pericholangitis* to *sclerosing cholangitis, chronic active hepatitis* and *cirrhosis,* and *bile duct carcinoma.* The *nutritional abnormalities* commonly seen in patients with ulcerative colitis are usually not as severe as those seen with Crohn's disease, but growth retardation is not unusual (see Ch. 104.2).

TREATMENT. Management of the patient with ulcerative colitis requires a comprehensive review of the patient's medical, nutritional, and psychologic needs. Ulcerative colitis tends to follow an acute relapsing course with quiescent intervals in some patients, during which the rectal mucosa may appear normal. No method other than colectomy is known to cure ulcerative colitis. During remission treatment is designed to prevent relapse. In patients with chronic active inflammation, therapy is intended to suppress inflammation.

General Therapy. Dietary and nutritional decisions are important in the management of ulcerative colitis and of Crohn's disease (see Nutritional Treatment in Ch. 104.2). The fiber content of the diet should be reduced during periods of diarrhea. In lactose intolerant patients restriction of lactose intake (avoidance of dairy products) may ameliorate the diarrhea. Alternatively, bacterial lactase is commercially available and may be used to reduce the lactose content of milk to well tolerated levels. Nutritionally balanced, minimal residue liquid nutritional formulas are available and are acceptable as supplements to most patients. In the severely ill, catabolic patient, parenteral alimentation may be employed to put the bowel at rest, largely to prepare patients for colectomy or for the postoperative recovery period.

The causes of anemia may be multiple and may include the anemia of chronic illness (see Ch. 134), blood loss with resulting iron deficiency, or folate deficiency. Oral iron may be poorly tolerated, necessitating the use of parenteral iron. Folate deficiency is associated with sulfasalazine therapy as well as with inadequate dietary intake owing to reduction in folate-containing foods such as fresh fruits and leafy vegetables.

In the patient with mild or moderate colitis, agents to reduce diarrhea may be useful. These include diphenoxylate with atropine (2.5 to 5 mg), codeine (15 to 30 mg), deodorized tincture of opium (6 to 10 drops), paregoric (4 to 8 ml), or loperamide (2 to 4 mg) before meals and at bedtime. Tincture of belladonna (10 drops) four times a day and other anticholinergics may be used to decrease abdominal cramps. Extreme care must be exercised in the use of these medications in the moderately ill patient because of the risk of precipitating toxic dilatation.

Nonspecific measures include attention to psychologic stresses in the patient's life, often involving interactions with close relatives. Patients should be encouraged to have adequate amounts of rest and sleep. As with any other chronic illness, patient education is important in enabling the patient and family to understand the nature of the disease and its effects on the individual. Formal psychiatric counseling is reserved for a minority of patients, although most benefit from a sympathetic, supportive relationship with their physicians, which may involve modest amounts of psychotherapy.

Therapy for Severe Acute Colitis. Early diagnosis and recognition of this condition are important in reducing mortality. An early decision between intensive medical treatment and immediate surgery may be necessary, particularly if there is evidence of perforation or of peritonitis, or if there is uncontrollable hemorrhage. Toxic dilatation is perhaps the most threatening type of acute severe ulcerative colitis. Failure of toxic dilatation to respond to medical management within 24 to 36 hours is ominous, since the mortality of such patients is very high unless colectomy is performed. Adequate replacement of circulating plasma volume with crystalloid, plasma, and blood is essential. Broad-spectrum antibiotics (usually chloramphenicol plus an aminoglycoside or ampicillin plus an aminoglycoside in combination with metronidazole) and intravenous corticosteroids are used. Hydrocortisone, 300 mg intravenously daily, is effective but may cause sodium and water retention. Alternatives include intravenous prednisolone, 60 mg daily, or methylprednisolone, 48 mg daily, in four divided doses.

Successful treatment depends on prompt recognition, early surgical consultation, and intensive resuscitative, antibacterial, and anti-inflammatory therapy. Important measures include intravenous fluids, plasma, blood, nasogastric suction, antibiotics, and intravenous corticosteroids. It is essential that the patient be re-evaluated every four to six hours by the physician and surgeon, and that plain abdominal films be obtained twice daily. Failure to respond to maximal therapy within 24 to 36 hours makes prompt surgical intervention essential. Usually the surgeon will choose to perform an abdominal colectomy with ileostomy, leaving the rectum in place for a subsequent operation when the patient has recovered from this severe episode. Early surgical intervention has resulted in decreased mortality in the acute phase. Overall mortality (in both medically and surgically treated patients) is high, between 12 and 30 per cent. About one fifth of patients with toxic dilatation require surgery after failure to respond to medical treatment. Patients who do not undergo surgical therapy during the attack of toxic dilatation often require elective surgery within 6 to 12 months because of subsequent failure of medical therapy.

If the patient with severe ulcerative colitis does not respond to full treatment within five to ten days, many clinicians advise colectomy (even in the absence of toxic megacolon) as soon as the patient's general condition has been stabilized. Postoperative mortality can be reduced by earlier operation, by correction of malnutrition, and by appropriate antibiotic therapy.

If the patient's general condition responds to maximal therapy and there is improvement in the sigmoidoscopic appearance of the rectal mucosa, oral feeding can commence along with the use of oral corticosteroids. If liquids are tolerated well, solid foods are added gradually as tolerated. Sulfasalazine, 2 to 4 grams orally daily, is usually then added. The oral corticosteroid dose should initially be about 40 mg of prednisone a day. If the clinical response continues to be satisfactory, this dose can be reduced by 5 mg daily every week to a dose of 20 mg of prednisone daily. This dose should be administered for a period of six to eight weeks before it is slowly tapered. Slow reductions in dosage sometimes help individual patients to withdraw eventually from this medication. Repeated brief courses of steroids for treatment of recurrences do not cause as many disabling side effects as does continuous use. Alternate-day dosage is associated with fewer side effects, but this regimen may have diminished symptomatic benefit in some patients. An alternate-day regimen may be of particular value in prepubertal children to avoid the growth suppression of large daily doses of corticosteroids.

Moderate to Mild Acute Colitis. For mild or moderate attacks of colitis, hospitalization is usually not required. In addition to the general measures already described, sulfasalazine is used with or without corticosteroids, depending on the severity of diarrhea and systemic symptoms. For mildly symptomatic colitis with predominantly left-sided disease, oral sulfasalazine and topical corticosteroid therapy are often satisfactory.

Corticosteroid can be applied locally to the rectal and colonic mucosa as hydrocortisone (100 mg) administered in 100 ml of saline either by enema or by slow rectal infusion. This volume of fluid always reaches the sigmoid colon, but the proximal spread is variable. Approximately one third is absorbed systemically. Suppositories and foam can be used for disease confined to the rectum. Newer nonabsorbed topical corticosteroid preparations diminish systemic side effects.

Sulfasalazine is largely unabsorbed and is metabolized by colonic bacteria to sulfapyridine and 5-aminosalicylic acid. The 5-aminosalicylic acid may exert a therapeutic effect by interfering with prostaglandin synthesis, a mediator of inflammation. Synthesis of prostaglandin E_2 by cultured rectal mucosa from patients with colitis and prostaglandin synthetase activity of the rectal mucosa are increased in active colitis. Adverse reactions to sulfasalazine, including headaches, arthralgias, nausea, skin rashes, and mild hemolysis, occur in up to 15 to 20 per cent of patients. More severe blood dyscrasias, high fever, leukopenia, and agranulocytosis are rare. A reversible loss of fertility may occur in some patients. Many of these side effects occur in patients taking 4 grams or more of sulfasalazine per day; reduction to a dose of 2 to 3 grams is often effective. Sulfapyridine is acetylated in the liver after absorption before being excreted in the urine. Many of the patients with adverse effects are genetic slow acetylators. Sulfasalazine is effective in treating moderate colitis, and continued treatment lessens the frequency of recurrent attacks. Newer compounds, such as sustained release 5-aminosalicylic acid, have been devised to transport this compound into the colon without sulfapyridine.

Active Chronic Colitis. For patients with chronic symptoms resulting from persistent inflammation, topical corticosteroids in addition to sulfasalazine and antidiarrheal preparations are used. Azathioprine* may be of benefit in the rare patient who is dependent on corticosteroids and for whom surgical management is inappropriate. In general, there is a reluctance to use azathioprine in children or in adults who have not completed their families in view of the mutagenic potential of the drug. The aim in quiescent colitis is to prolong remission. Sulfasalazine (2 to 3 grams per day orally) has been demonstrated to be effective.

Surgical Therapy. Proctocolectomy with construction of an ileostomy cures ulcerative colitis and leads to a remission or improvement in many of the peripheral manifestations. Absolute indications for subtotal or total colectomy are (1) *perforation,* with or without abscess formation; (2) *colonic carcinoma,* for which total proctocolectomy and lymph node dissection are required; and (3) *massive hemorrhage.* Relative indications are as follows: (1) Severe acute colitis with or without toxic dilatation of the colon (toxic megacolon), with failure to respond to maximal therapy. The current trend is toward earlier surgical intervention in this group of patients after restoration of plasma volume, administration of antibiotics, corticosteroids, and total parenteral nutrition for as long as possible preoperatively. In the absence of toxic dilatation many clinicians are willing to wait for seven to ten days before advising surgery. It is indefensible to extend medical therapy in a patient who continues to bleed and who has high fever, tachycardia, severe diarrhea, depleted intravascular and extravascular volumes, hypoalbuminemia, and electrolyte depletion. (2) Failure of medical management. The patient with chronic symptoms or frequent relapses over a period of five years or longer, particularly in the face of corticosteroid-induced complications, has the promise of improved quality of life after proctocolectomy and ileostomy. Although this decision is particularly difficult in children, it should not be delayed, since the risk of growth retardation in children is great (see Growth Retardation, Ch. 104.2). (3) Suspicion of cancer. In a patient with extensive colitis of long duration the presence of dysplastic changes or a mass lesion with overlying dysplasia may be used as a basis for recommending proctocolectomy. Other considerations may include chronic symptoms or the presence of a highly suspicious persisting stricture even after endoscopic biopsy and cytology have failed to reveal malignancy.

The internist, surgeon, and stoma therapist all play an important role in the pre- and postoperative education and management of the patient with proctocolectomy and ileostomy. The mortality of elective proctocolectomy is approximately 1 to 3 per cent. Over two thirds of patients have no postoperative complications such as hemorrhage, intra-abdominal sepsis, or intestinal obstruction. Between 10 and 15 per cent of patients with a standard ileostomy (Brooke) following proctocolectomy will require some form of surgical revision of the stoma. The reoperation rate for the continent ileostomy (Kock) is as high as 20 to 30 per cent in some series and postoperative complications and dysfunction not requiring operation are common. The continent ileostomy is contraindicated in Crohn's disease, in fulminating ulcerative colitis, in cases of diagnostic uncertainty, in emotionally unstable patients, and when experienced surgeons are unavailable. Other, rare complications include impotence (less than 2 per cent, in contrast to a universal incidence after an abdominoperineal resection for carcinoma of the rectum) and damage to the ureters. Healing of the perineal wound may be delayed for up to six months. Patients who are about to undergo or have undergone proctocolectomy with ileostomy will benefit from referral to groups such as the Ileostomy Association or Ileoptomists. Ingenious procedures are under investigation with the goal of preserving rectal muscle and anal sphincter function. These include ileoanal anastomosis after construction of an ileal reservoir in the pelvis.

ULCERATIVE COLITIS AND PREGNANCY. About one third of patients with inactive ulcerative colitis have exacerbation and about two thirds with active disease have worsening of their condition either during pregnancy or in the early postpartum period. For those with continuing active colitis the worsening is likely to occur in the first trimester. When the first attack of ulcerative colitis occurs during pregnancy or the postpartum period, symptoms are often severe. About 10 per cent of pregnancies in women with ulcerative colitis will terminate in spontaneous abortions.

The general diagnostic and therapeutic measures previously described apply to pregnant patients. Radiographic studies should be minimized and proctoscopy performed only when necessary, especially during the first trimester. The usual indications for corticosteroid therapy apply. Sulfasalazine therapy during pregnancy has not been reported to have adverse effects on the fetus. Azathioprine is not used during pregnancy, although no adverse effects upon the fetus have been reported. Therapeutic abortion has little place in the management of pregnant patients with ulcerative colitis except for the rare instances of women in the first trimester who are desperately ill and are likely to lose the child. Women with quiescent ulcerative colitis should not be discouraged from pregnancy. In the presence of active colitis, pregnancy should be postponed until control of the colitis has been achieved for at least one year.

ULCERATIVE PROCTITIS. Ulcerative proctitis probably represents ulcerative colitis limited to the rectum. Typically the patient presents with mild or moderate rectal bleeding, rectal tenesmus, and an increased number of bowel movements. Symptomatic episodes recur periodically several times a year.

The macroscopic and microscopic features are similar to those described previously for ulcerative colitis, although only the distal 3 to 10 cm of the rectum may be involved. On sigmoidoscopy there is usually a sharp line of demarcation between the distal inflammatory process and normal proximal rectal or lower sigmoid mucosa.

Therapy includes the general measures described for ulcerative colitis, with the use of sulfasalazine, 2 to 4 grams per day by mouth, and topical corticosteroids. Commonly used preparations include enemas containing 100 mg of hydrocortisone or 40 mg of methylprednisone, administered once daily. Steroid suppositories (25 mg of hydrocortisone) or steroid foam (90 mg of hydrocortisone per dose) may be inserted into the rectum once or twice daily. Newer forms of therapy under investigation include topical 5-aminosalicylic acid and nonabsorbable corticosteroids. Response to treatment is usually very satisfactory, although occasional patients may remain symptomatic despite intensive therapy.

PROGNOSIS OF ULCERATIVE COLITIS. The outlook for recovery from a first attack of ulcerative colitis is very good. Mortality, which is about 5 per cent, occurs almost exclusively in those who have a severe form of the disease involving the entire colon. The mortality is higher in patients over 60 years, approximately 17 per cent, compared to 2 per cent in patients between ages 20 and 59. Toxic megacolon has a mortality rate of about 20 per cent. Death generally results from the complications of massive hemorrhage, systemic infections, pulmonary

*This use is not listed in the manufacturer's directive.

embolism, or associated cardiac disorders. Better medical therapy and earlier colectomy for patients who do not respond to medical therapy have improved the overall acute prognosis.

After the first attack about 10 per cent of patients will have a remission lasting up to 15 years or more. An additional 10 per cent will experience continuously active colitis. The remainder (75 per cent) experience remissions and exacerbations of their disease over the ensuing years irrespective of the severity of the initial attack. About one fifth of patients with ulcerative colitis require proctocolectomy at some stage in their illness. After the first postoperative year, the long-term prognosis for patients with colectomy for ulcerative colitis is similar to that of the general population. With continuous improvements in medical and surgical management, long-term prognosis for both survival and quality of life continues to improve.

Hodgson HJF: Assessment of drug therapy in inflammatory bowel disease. Br J Clin Pharm 14:159, 1982. *A detailed discussion of the methods of evaluation of the effectiveness of medical treatment.*

Kelly KA, Phillips SF, Beahrs OF: The continent ileostomy. *In* Kirsner JB, Shorter RG (eds.): Inflammatory Bowel Disease. 2nd ed. Philadelphia, Lea and Febiger, 1980. *The authors review their experience with the Kock ileostomy emphasizing careful preoperative selection, meticulous intraoperative technique, and conscientious postoperative care.*

Kirsner JB, Shorter RG (eds.): Inflammatory Bowel Disease. Philadelphia, Lea and Febiger, 1980. *An in-depth monograph with chapters by leading authorities on incidence trends, pathology, etiology, and medical and surgical therapy.*

Kirsner JB, Shorter RG: Recent developments in "nonspecific" inflammatory bowel disease. N Engl J Med 306:775, 837, 1982. *A current review of various aspects of new investigations in ulcerative colitis and Crohn's disease.*

Riddell RH, Goldman H, Ransohoff DF, et al.: Dysplasia in inflammatory bowel disease: Standardized classification with provisional clinical applications. Hum Pathol 14:931, 1983. *A definitive description of colonic dysplasia including an illustrative atlas.*

105. VASCULAR DISEASES OF THE INTESTINE

James H. Grendell

ANATOMY, PHYSIOLOGY, AND PATHOPHYSIOLOGY OF THE MESENTERIC CIRCULATION

The intra-abdominal portions of the digestive tract receive their blood supply almost entirely from three relatively large arteries arising from the aorta. The anatomy of these vessels, including their anastomotic interrelationships and potential for collateral formation, determines the consequences of acute or chronic vascular occlusion.

The celiac axis, the most cephalad of the three major arteries, usually originates at a level between the twelfth thoracic and the first lumbar vertebrae, passing next to the median arcuate ligament of the diaphragm (Fig. 105–1). Its branches supply the liver and biliary structures (hepatic artery), spleen (splenic artery), and the stomach (left gastric and gastroepiploic, short gastrics, and branches of the gastroduodenal, including the right gastroepiploic). The gastroduodenal artery gives rise to the superior pancreaticoduodenal arteries, which not only provide part of the blood supply to the pancreas and duodenum but also form anastomoses with the inferior pancreaticoduodenal arteries, which are derived from the superior mesenteric artery. These interconnections, the pancreaticoduodenal arcades, are an important potential route for collateral blood flow between the celiac and the superior mesenteric arteries.

The superior mesenteric artery originates behind the pancreas at the level of the first lumbar vertebra, just caudal to the celiac axis (Fig. 105–2). In addition to the inferior pancreaticoduodenal arteries, the superior mesenteric artery gives rise to branches supplying the small and large intestines from the distal duodenum to the distal transverse colon. These intestinal branches form a series of three or four arcades before entering the wall of the intestine as arteriae rectae. Although there is considerable potential for collateral flow within the primary and secondary arcades, the arteriae rectae appear to represent end arteries, and few, if any, important anastomotic connections are present within the bowel wall itself. Accordingly, selective occlusion of these more distal vessels, as may occur in vasculitis, may lead to segmental infarction.

The inferior mesenteric artery, the smallest of the three major arteries, supplies the distal transverse colon, the descending and sigmoid colon, and the proximal portions of the rectum. Its branches form a series of arcades ending in arteriae rectae similar to what is found in the superior mesenteric artery's distribution. Branches of the inferior mesenteric artery connect with those of the superior mesenteric artery via the arch of Riolan ("meandering mesenteric artery") and the marginal artery (Fig. 105–2), and with the inferior and middle rectal branches of the hypogastric (internal iliac) arteries.

In general, veins parallel arteries in the smaller branches and for portions of the main mesenteric trunks. However, rather than entering the vena cava directly, the superior mesenteric and splenic veins join to form the portal vein, which enters the liver after receiving additional blood from the gastric circulation via the coronary vein. The inferior mesenteric vein usually drains into the splenic vein.

The blood supply to the intra-abdominal portion of the gastrointestinal tract is richly endowed with anastomotic interconnections that help protect against the consequences of occlusive vascular disease. If the occlusive process is chronically

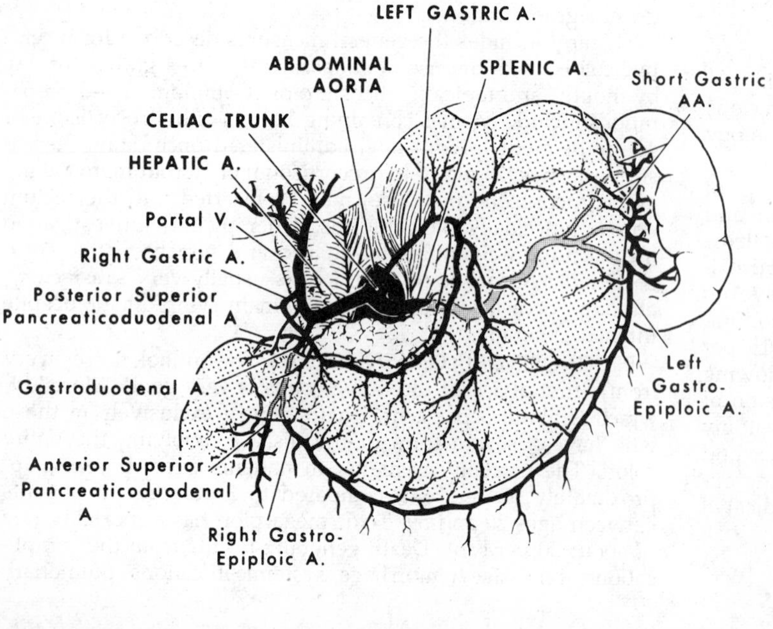

Figure 105–1. Arterial supply to the stomach and duodenum, showing major branches of the celiac axis and the superior portion of the pancreaticoduodenal arcades. (From Grendell JH, Ockner RK: *In* Sleisenger MH, Fordtran JS [eds.]: Gastrointestinal Disease. 3rd ed. Philadelphia, W. B. Saunders Company, 1983.)

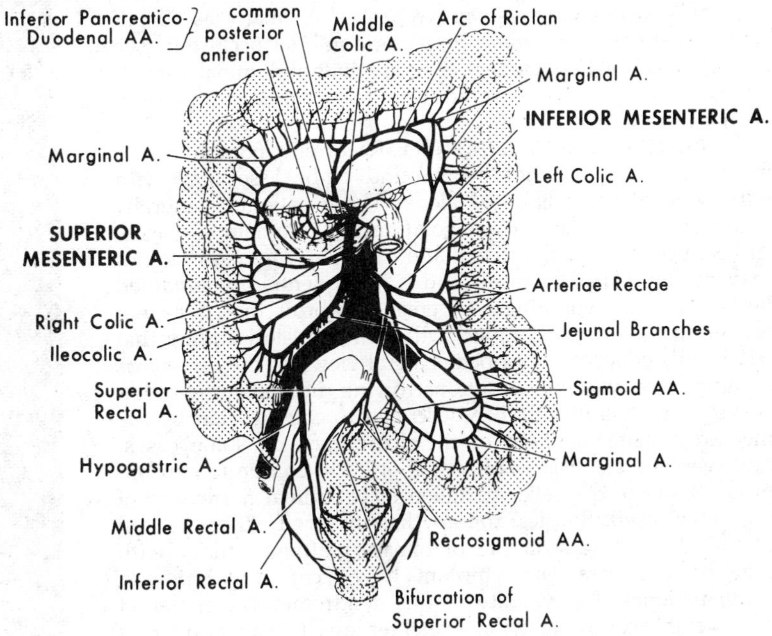

Figure 105–2. Arterial supply to the small and large intestines, showing the inferior portion of the pancreaticoduodenal arcades and the anastomoses between superior and inferior mesenteric arteries (arc of Riolan or "meandering mesenteric," and the marginal artery). (From Grendell JH, Ockner, RK: *In* Sleisenger MH, Fordtran JS [eds.]: Gastrointestinal Disease. 3rd ed. Philadelphia, W. B. Saunders Company, 1983.)

progressive, these interconnections usually permit sufficient collateral flow to maintain intestinal viability. In fact it is possible for *all* of the intra-abdominal digestive tract to be adequately supplied by only one of its three primary arterial sources. Conversely, the collateral supply may be only marginally adequate or nonexistent in certain areas, such as the arteriae rectae and intramural arteries. Also potentially vulnerable are the "watershed" areas in the distal transverse colon and splenic flexure and at the junction of the superior and middle portions of the rectum, where branches of the inferior mesenteric artery anastomose with branches of the superior mesenteric and hypogastric arteries, respectively. This may, in part, explain why segmental infarction of the colon occurs most commonly in the region of the splenic flexure and rectosigmoid.

The mesenteric circulation is regulated by three different means: (1) *Intrinsic regulation* or local modulation of blood flow occurs in response to changes in arteriolar transmural pressure or to alterations in tissue oxygenation in order to maintain adequate blood flow and oxygen delivery. Examples of this include the vasodilatation observed after brief periods of arterial occlusion (reactive hyperemia) and during digestion of a meal (functional hyperemia). Functional hyperemia may also, in part, be due to the effects of regulatory gastrointestinal peptides. (2) *Extrinsic neurologic regulation* of intestinal blood flow is mediated by sympathetic postganglionic fibers originating from the splanchnic nerves, which cause constriction of arteries and arterioles and a reduction in intestinal blood flow. Continued stimulation of these nerves, however, leads to a partial or in some cases complete recovery of flow (autoregulatory escape). (3) *Circulating endogenous and exogenous agents* may affect mesenteric blood flow. Increased arteriolar resistance is caused by α-adrenergic agonists, vasopressin, angiotensin II, prostaglandin F_2, and digitalis glycosides. Vasodilatation and increased blood flow result from the actions of β-adrenergic agonists, prostaglandin E_1, and the gut hormones cholecystokinin, gastrin, and glucagon.

The microcirculation of the intra-abdominal digestive organs is controlled by (1) the arteriole that, as the major site of resistance, is the most important local determinant of overall mesenteric blood flow, and (2) the precapillary sphincter, which determines capillary perfusion.

Several factors are important in determining the extent, severity, or possible reversibility of ischemic processes or events. The first of these is the abruptness of a vascular occlusion; more gradually occlusive processes may permit development of collaterals. A second factor is size and configuration of a vessel; emboli most commonly enter the large, obliquely situated superior mesenteric artery. A third factor is the level of involvement of a localized occlusive process. Vasculitis involving arteriae rectae or intramural arteries does not allow for development of collateral blood flow and may result in ischemia of a limited segment of intestine.

Intestinal ischemia may occur in hypoxic or low cardiac output states in the absence of an anatomic obstruction to blood flow (nonocclusive intestinal infarction). It is postulated that this may result from (1) the formation of toxic superoxide anions, (2) loss of the protective function of small intestinal brush border glycoproteins against the deleterious effects of luminal pancreatic proteases and bacterial toxins, or (3) shunting of oxygen from the villus tip caused by a countercurrent exhange resulting from the arrangement of blood vessels in the villus.

CHRONIC INTESTINAL ISCHEMIC SYNDROMES

ABDOMINAL ANGINA. This uncommon syndrome is due to severe atherosclerosis involving at least two of the three major arterial supplies to the intestine. There is usually a history of intermittent dull or cramping midabdominal pain characteristically beginning 15 to 30 minutes after eating and lasting for one to two hours. This is the period of increased intestinal blood flow and oxygen consumption required for digestion and absorption. Patients may also have lost a substantial amount of weight due mainly to a decrease in food consumption resulting from fear of the pain associated with eating. Mild to moderate malabsorption may also be present. Physical examination usually uncovers evidence of atherosclerotic disease involving other vessels. The presence or absence of an abdominal bruit is not of diagnostic value. A presumptive diagnosis may be made on the basis of a strongly suggestive history and the angiographic demonstration of significant ($>$ 50 per cent) narrowing of at least two of the three major arteries. Often there is evidence of collateral flow. Many patients who are asymptomatic may show similar angiographic findings. Surgical treatment has included bypass, endarterectomy, and reimplantation procedures with significant relief of symptoms in most patients. Percutaneous transluminal angioplasty has also been employed successfully and offers the possibility that nonoperative approaches may also prove useful. As many as 50 per cent of patients with acute mesenteric arterial occlusion (see below) give a history suggestive of previous abdominal angina. Successful treatment of chronic intestinal ischemia may prevent such a catastrophic outcome.

CELIAC COMPRESSION SYNDROME. Recurrent abdominal pain in some individuals has been found to be associated with narrowing of the celiac axis alone. These patients, generally younger women in otherwise good health, complain of epigastric pain of variable frequency and duration. The pain may or may not be related to meals and is infrequently accompanied by nausea and vomiting. An epigastric bruit that does not radiate to the lower abdomen is the only physical finding that has been frequently described. Lateral views of the celiac axis at angiography demonstrate narrowing near its origin. At surgery this has usually been ascribed to compression by the median arcuate ligament of the diaphragm. In some cases, however, the stenosis has been reported to be due to neurofibrous tissue of the celiac ganglion or to intimal narrowing of the vessel itself. Surgical therapy has involved either division of the obstructing structure or bypass grafting, usually with relief of symptoms. The symptoms have recurred with time in some patients. The validity of this syndrome is a matter of considerable controversy for several reasons: (1) similar degrees of celiac axis narrowing have been found incidentally at angiography or autopsy in a substantial number of patients without symptoms of this syndrome, and (2) stenosis of the celiac axis alone would not be expected to result in symptomatic intestinal ischemia because of mesenteric collateral vessels. Some investigators believe that the pain is not truly ischemic but may arise in the celiac ganglion, which is removed or disrupted by most surgical treatments for this syndrome. Resolution of this controversy will require more precise clinical and pathophysiologic definition of the syndrome, including detailed follow-up studies. Surgery should be reserved for those patients with preoperative angiographic evidence of celiac stenosis who would otherwise undergo exploratory laparotomy for disabling and unexplained abdominal pain. At operation a thorough search for other disorders should precede treatment for presumed celiac compression syndrome.

ACUTE INTESTINAL ISCHEMIC SYNDROMES

ACUTE BOWEL INFARCTION: MESENTERIC ARTERIAL OCCLUSION. Gradual occlusion of one or sometimes even two of the three major mesenteric arteries may be asymptomatic because of the development of adequate collateral circulation. However, when intestinal blood flow falls below a critical level, ischemic necrosis of the supplied areas will result. Most commonly this is due to advanced *atherosclerotic disease* affecting at least two of the major visceral branches of the aorta. Generally the most proximal segments of these arteries are most severely involved. In addition to *embolism,* which is discussed below, other causes of mesenteric arterial occlusion include dissecting *aortic aneurysm, fibromuscular hyperplasia,* and *systemic vasculitides,* which may involve the mesenteric arteries at any level from the major arterial trunks to the intramural arteries. An association has also been reported with the use of *oral contraceptives.*

DIAGNOSIS. The early diagnosis of acute intestinal infarction is often difficult. The history usually is not very helpful, but evidence of "abdominal angina" (see above) or other conditions predisposing to thrombosis may aid in the evaluation. Patients frequently have *severe abdominal pain* that initially may be colicky in nature and periumbilical in location. Bowel sounds not only may be present but may even be hyperactive. At this stage the patient's complaint of pain often appears out of proportion to physical findings or laboratory studies. As ischemia progresses, pain becomes constant and poorly localized. Systemic manifestations become prominent and severe, including *tachycardia, hypotension, fever, leukocytosis, acidosis,* and the presence of *blood* in nasogastric aspirate, vomitus, or stool. It has been suggested, on the basis of small numbers of patients and experimental animal studies, that elevations in serum and peritoneal fluid phosphate concentration may be sensitive indicators of intestinal infarction. Abdominal x-rays usually show evidence of an *ileus* with distended, thick-walled loops of bowel and air-fluid levels (Fig. 105–3). Gas in the intestinal wall or portal vein is a late finding. Ultimately, when ischemic necrosis becomes transmural, signs of *peritonitis,* including bloody peritoneal fluid, appear. At this point, the prognosis (with or without surgery) is extremely poor.

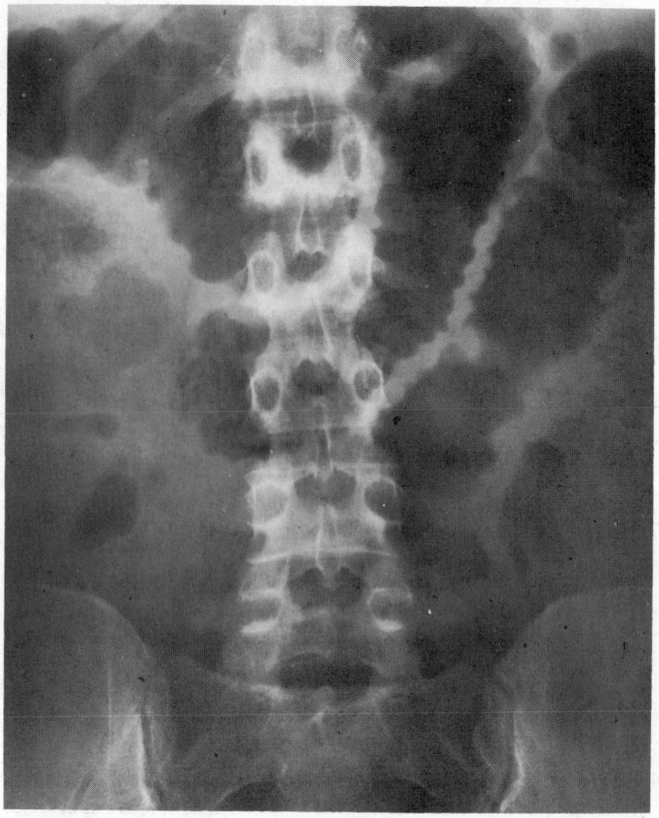

Figure 105–3. A supine abdominal x-ray in a patient with acute infarction of the small intestine showing dilated loops of small bowel with irregular thickening of the bowel wall.

The early diagnosis of bowel infarction depends upon a high index of suspicion and exclusion of other conditions likely to present as an acute abdomen. A decision regarding extensive radiographic studies, especially angiography, in patients with suspected bowel infarction must be individualized. For the patient in whom signs of peritonitis are present, suggesting that perforation may have already occurred, the information to be obtained from further studies may not justify the necessary delay in surgical management. However, earlier in the course, angiography may help define the nature and extent of the occlusive process or, in the absence of major vessel occlusion, suggest the diagnosis of nonocclusive infarction. Interpretation, however, is often difficult and clinical judgment is based only in part on surgical findings. Computed tomography shows promise of becoming a rapid, noninvasive means of confirming the diagnosis of acute bowel infarction by identifying characteristic changes in the appearance of the bowel wall and mesentery.

TREATMENT. Initial supportive therapy, aimed at stabilization of the patient's condition prior to surgery, includes nasogastric suction, replacement of fluid and electrolyte deficits, administration of broad-spectrum antibiotics after blood cultures have been obtained, and cardiopulmonary support, if needed. As soon as the patient's condition is adequately stabilized and the diagnosis strongly suspected, prompt surgical exploration should be performed. At surgery, resection of necrotic bowel is the primary objective. An attempt may be made to revascularize the remaining viable intestine by bypass graft or endarterectomy if the patient's condition is sufficiently stable to perform the additional surgery.

At the time of operation it is important but sometimes difficult to define the limits of viable bowel in order to resect completely irreversibly diseased intestine while at the same time avoiding unnecessary development of the short bowel syndrome. It is often necessary to perform a "second-look" operation 12 to 36 hours after the initial exploration to identify and resect any additional bowel that in the interim proves to be nonviable. Infarction of large segments of intestine carries essentially a 100 per cent mortality rate without surgery. Even with surgery the mortality rate is > 50 per cent in most series because of delay in diagnosis or because of other complicating factors such as advanced age or atherosclerotic disease involving other vital organs.

Mesenteric vasculitis (e.g., as may occur in lupus erythematosus, polyarteritis nodosa, dermatomyositis, rheumatoid vasculitis, and Henoch-Schönlein purpura) may cause segmental intestinal infarction not conforming to the distribution of the major arteries. Vascular occlusion may not be demonstrable angiographically if only intramural arteries and arterioles are involved. Although some patients may require emergency surgery for intestinal necrosis and perforation, these complications are less common than with occlusions of the major arteries or their principal branches. In some cases the acute episode may resolve spontaneously, which may leave the patient with a segmental stricture demonstrable by barium contrast studies.

MESENTERIC ARTERY EMBOLISM. Emboli to the mesenteric circulation most commonly involve the superior mesenteric artery because of its size and the oblique angle of its origin from the aorta. These emboli usually arise from mural thrombi in the heart in patients with atherosclerotic or valvular heart disease, but may also arise from vegetations of bacterial endocarditis, atrial myxomas, valvular prostheses, or from atherosclerotic plaques in the thoracic or upper abdominal aorta, either spontaneously or during angiography. Patients may have a history of previous embolic episodes or exhibit evidence of simultaneous peripheral embolization (e.g., to the brain or extremities). Typically patients describe the *abrupt onset of severe midabdominal cramping pain,* accompanied by vomiting or diarrhea. Although patients may feel and appear severely ill, early in the course objective physical findings are sparse. If the diagnosis is not made promptly and appropriate treatment undertaken, a mesenteric embolus will lead to bowel infarction. Angiography may demonstrate mesenteric artery occlusion in the absense of collateral circulation, indicating the acute nature of the process. Computed tomography may also strongly suggest the diagnosis early in the course of the disease in a patient with acute onset of abdominal pain of unknown source (Fig. 105–4). Following supportive measures as needed to stabilize the patient's condition, immediate exploration with embolectomy and resection of any infarcted bowel is indicated. A "second look" procedure will sometimes be necessary. The characteristic setting in which mesenteric embolism occurs, as well as its abrupt onset, offers a greater opportunity for early diagnosis and treatment. For this reason, and because the patients generally are younger, the prognosis is more favorable than for most nonembolic causes of bowel infarction. Some patients who are successfully treated by embolectomy without need for bowel resection may develop a transient malabsorption syndrome persisting for several months.

NONOCCLUSIVE INTESTINAL INFARCTION. In some patients clinical findings suggestive of mesenteric arterial occlusive disease or embolism occur without a demonstrable obstruction to arterial flow. This syndrome, now recognized with increasing frequency, usually occurs in the setting of severe congestive heart failure, shock, hypoxia, or a recent myocardial infarction. The clinical course often evolves more slowly than is seen with occlusive processes. Occasionally a precipitating event is not identifiable. The use of α-adrenergic vasoconstrictors (and possibly digitalis glycosides) may also contribute to the development of this process. Because of its high degree of metabolic activity, the mucosa has the greatest requirement for intestinal blood flow of the various layers of the bowel wall. Thus it will show the earliest evidence of ischemic injury. At times, it may be the only portion to undergo hemorrhagic infarction. However, infarction may ultimately become transmural and occur in a patchy and irregular distribution, not conforming to the area supplied by a major vessel. Early angiography is useful to exclude a major vessel occlusion, which would usually require vascular surgery. In at least 50 per cent of such patients angiography reveals irregular narrowing of the major arterial branches and arcades (due to spasm) and impaired filling of the intramural vessels. Therapy consists of supportive measures and surgical exploration to resect infarcted bowel if the patient's situation suggests the need for this. Selective infusion of vasodilators into the mesenteric circulation has been suggested but its therapeutic efficacy remains to be established. This syndrome generally carries a very poor prognosis, primarily because it is usually associated with shock or severe cardiopulmonary disease.

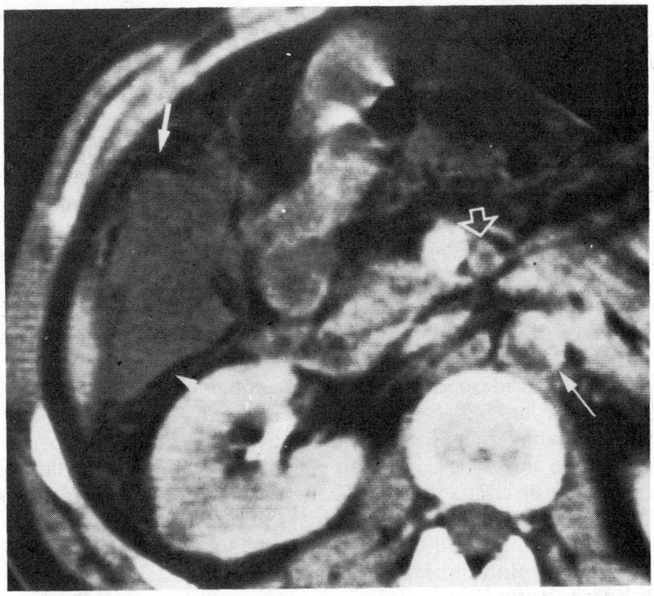

Figure 105–4. An abdominal CT scan following contrast administration in a patient with infarction of the distal ileum and ascending colon due to an embolus from a cardiac mural thrombus which occluded the superior mesenteric artery. The clear arrow shows the occluded superior mesenteric artery which fails to be opacified by the contrast agent, unlike the superior mesenteric vein seen adjacent to it on the left. The thick white arrows show gas within the wall of the ascending colon. The thin white arrow points to the abdominal aorta which contains atherosclerotic plaque or thrombus. (Courtesy of Michael P. Federle, M.D.)

ISCHEMIC COLITIS. Ischemic injury to the colon may be caused by advanced atherosclerosis or interruption of the colonic blood supply during surgery (e.g., abdominal aortic aneurysmectomy, aortoiliac reconstruction, abdominoperineal resection), or may occur in association with "hypercoagulable" states, amyloidosis, vasculitis, ruptured aortic aneurysm, colorectal cancer, or the use of oral contraceptive agents. In addition, nonocclusive colonic ischemia may occur in states of low cardiac output or hypoxia. The syndrome of ischemic colitis may be quite variable in its extent, severity, and prognosis. However, extensive infarction and perforation appear to be infrequent. Localized or segmental ischemia is more common, particularly affecting those areas of the colon that lie on the "watershed" between two adjacent arterial supplies; i.e., the splenic flexure (superior and inferior mesenteric arteries) and the rectosigmoid (inferior mesenteric and internal iliac arteries). Characteristically patients over the age of 50 are most often affected with *abrupt onset of lower abdominal cramping pain, rectal bleeding* and, to variable degrees, *vomiting* and *fever*. Some patients give a history of similar symptoms occurring intermittently for weeks to months before presentation. Left-sided abdominal tenderness and peritoneal signs may be present, as well as evidence of generalized atherosclerotic disease. Sigmoidoscopy may be normal, may show evidence of mild nonspecific proctitis, or may reveal a spectrum of findings including multiple discrete ulcers, blue-black hemorrhagic submucosal blebs, or an adherent pseudomembrane. Angiography generally has not proved useful in the diagnosis of patients in this setting. The differentiation of ischemic colitis from infections of the colon, diverticulitis, and idiopathic inflammatory bowel disease (ulcerative colitis, Crohn's disease of the colon) may be very difficult. Initial management consists of general supportive measures including antibiotics. In those patients in whom perforation or infarction of viscus appears likely, early surgical exploration is indicated; however, many patients will improve without surgery. Subsequent barium enema will often show a characteristic picture of intramural hemorrhage and edema including "thumbprinting," tubular narrowing, and "sawtooth" irregularity (Fig. 105–5). Some patients will proceed to complete resolution of the clinical process and x-ray abnormalities. Others will develop a residual stricture that eventually may require surgical resection.

MESENTERIC VENOUS THROMBOSIS. This condition, which accounts for about 5 to 15 per cent of patients with intestinal ischemia, almost always involves the superior mesenteric vein. It is associated with a variety of conditions: stasis in the mesenteric venous bed (portal hypertension, congestive heart failure), abdominal neoplasms, intra-abdominal inflammation (peritonitis, abscess, inflammatory bowel disease), abdominal surgery and trauma, a variety of presumed hypercoagulable states (antithrombin III deficiency, polycythemia vera), and use of oral contraceptives. Occasionally a predisposing condition is absent. Patients may have abrupt onset of a clinical picture indicative of acute bowel infarction; however, many others have a more gradual course with development of progressive abdominal discomfort over a period of weeks. Physical findings are nonspecific. The presence of a small amount of bloody peritoneal fluid is typical and may be an important clue to the diagnosis in patients with a subacute clinical course. Selective superior mesenteric angiography shows intense spasm of the arteries to the involved segment of bowel and absence of venous drainage.

Following initial supportive care to stabilize the patient's condition, an operation should be performed to resect infarcted or severely ischemic bowel. Reconstructive venous surgery is not generally possible. Because there is about a 25 per cent rate of recurrent thrombosis within the first several weeks postoperatively, anticoagulation is recommended except in patients who have underlying disease processes that would make this too hazardous. A "second look" operation to search for recurrent thrombosis may also be required if there is unexplained clinical deterioration following initial surgery. In general the prognosis is more favorable than for patients with mesenteric arterial disease, with reported mortality as low as 20 per cent.

MISCELLANEOUS DISORDERS

INTRAMURAL INTESTINAL HEMORRHAGE. This may follow abdominal trauma or in the setting of ischemic bowel injury, vasculitis, or bleeding diatheses. Some patients have a picture suggesting a perforated viscus (severe abdominal pain, tenderness, leukocytosis), but most have cramping abdominal pain and vomiting suggestive of partial or complete bowel obstruction. Hematemesis or melena and fever may be present. Occasionally a palpable abdominal mass caused by the presence of a hematoma may be noted. Barium studies of the small intestine typically show a "stacked coins" or "thumbprint" appearance. Usually intramural intestinal hemorrhage can be managed conservatively with nasogastric suction, intravenous hydration and electrolytes, and correction of an underlying coagulopathy, when possible. In those patients with high grade or unremitting intestinal obstruction, or in whom signs of peritonitis develop (suggesting perforation), surgery is necessary.

PARAPROSTHETIC-ENTERIC AND AORTOENTERIC FISTULAS. Following aortic aneurysmectomy and other procedures in which vascular prostheses are placed in the abdomen or retroperitoneum, fistulas may form between the graft and adjacent bowel. This may occur as early as several weeks postoperatively but in most cases is delayed by at least two years. This complication usually results from local infection or damage to the intestine or its blood supply at surgery, with subsequent erosion of the bowel wall by the graft. Patients may present with massive upper or lower gastrointestinal bleeding or both that may be rapidly fatal without emergency surgery. In a number of patients, however, bleeding may be initially intermittent, resembling that from a number of more common lesions. In these patients, early consideration of this diagnosis with urgent

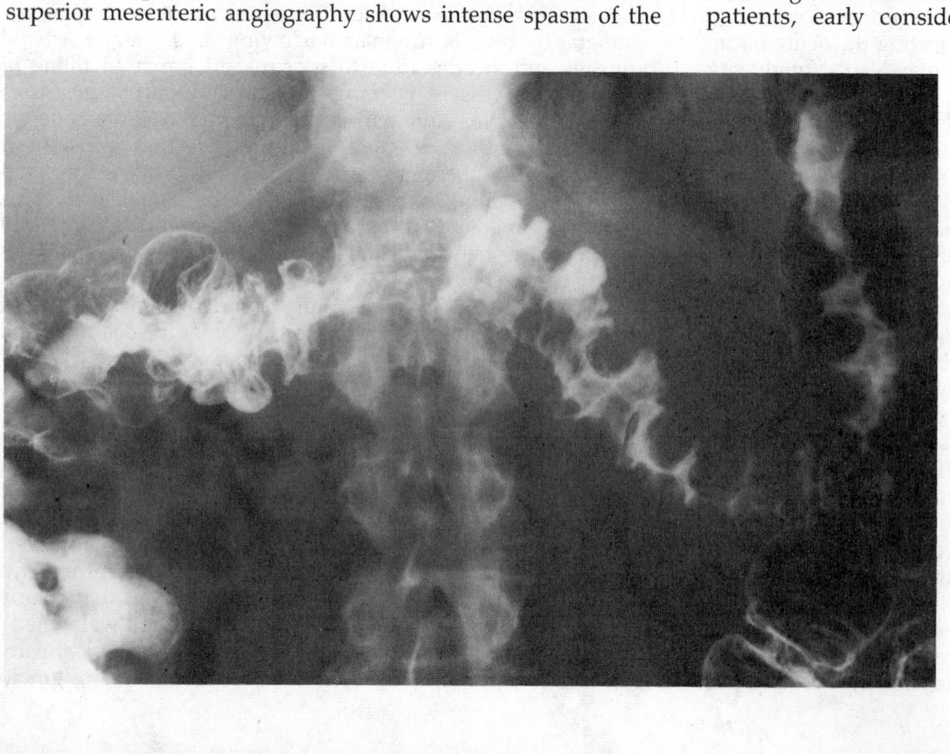

Figure 105–5. A barium enema in a patient with ischemic colitis showing narrowing and "thumbprinting" (nodular indentations of the bowel wall) in the distal transverse colon. This is one of the "watershed" areas of the colon between two adjacent arterial supplies (superior and inferior mesenteric arteries) where ischemia is more likely to develop.

evaluation by upper endoscopy, radiolabeled red blood cell studies, computed tomography, and/or angiography may be required to establish the diagnosis and need for surgical intervention.

Unoperated abdominal aortic aneurysms and aneurysmal dilatations of other major abdominal arteries may erode into the gastrointestinal tract, causing upper or lower gastrointestinal bleeding or both of various degrees of severity.

SUPERIOR MESENTERIC ARTERY SYNDROME. This uncommon syndrome of postprandial epigastric pain, distention, and vomiting has been attributed to compression of the third portion of the duodenum between the superior mesenteric artery anteriorly and the fixed retroperitoneal structures posteriorly. This has been described as occurring most commonly in individuals who have lost a substantial amount of weight or are of "asthenic habitus," and in children with rapid growth in the absence of corresponding weight gain or who have been fixed in a position of hyperextension by a cast following spinal injury or surgery. Barium contrast studies show distention of the proximal duodenum, and lateral aortograms have shown a narrowing of the angle between the aorta and the superior mesenteric artery. The differental diagnosis includes generalized disorders of gastrointestinal motility such as scleroderma, and anorexia nervosa. Recommended treatment has included the use of small feedings and elemental diets with the patient lying prone or on the left side in the knee-chest position after eating. In refractory cases duodenal mobilization or duodenal-jejunal bypass has reportedly been effective in relieving symptoms. Since apparent compression of the duodenum by the superior mesenteric artery does not prove clinically significant obstruction, the diagnosis of this syndrome must be made only after other possible causes of duodenal stasis have been excluded.

VASCULAR MALFORMATIONS INCLUDING ANGIODYSPLASIA. Hemangiomas of the small intestine are very uncommon vascular tumors found throughout the bowel, particularly the jejunum. They represent one of the causes of gastrointestinal bleeding that may be very difficult to locate. These lesions are most reliably diagnosed by abdominal angiography.

Vascular malformations can occur in the gastrointestinal tract in association with diseases involving the skin such as the *hereditary hemorrhagic telangiectasia (Osler-Weber-Rendu) syndrome, blue rubber bleb nevus syndrome,* and the *CREST syndrome* (calcinosis, Reynaud's phenomenon, esophageal hypomotility, sclerodactyly, and telangiectasia). In addition, vascular malformations may occur as a primary process *(angiodysplasia)* chiefly involving the colon but also occurring in the stomach or small intestine. This latter process is being increasingly recognized as a frequent cause of lower intestinal bleeding, especially in patients over the age of 60. An association of angiodysplasia with aortic stenosis has also been reported but not fully established.

Angiodysplastic lesions consist of ectatic, tortuous submucosal veins and groups of ectatic mucosal vessels lying just under the colonic epithelium or at times on the luminal surface unprotected by any intestinal epithelium. The etiology of these lesions remains uncertain. One theory suggests that they develop as a result of chronic low grade obstruction of the submucosal veins as they penetrate the muscularis propria; another theory proposes that these lesions develop because of chronic mucosal ischemia.

Larger vascular malformations including primary angiodysplastic lesions may be visualized by selective mesenteric arteriography. Many of these lesions are small and are best demonstrated by endoscopy. Such lesions are present in a large number of older individuals without apparent gastrointestinal blood loss. For those patients who have chronic or recurrent gastrointestinal blood loss without other apparent cause, surgery has been recommended if vascular malformations could be identified and localized (e.g., right colectomy for lesions in the cecum). This approach is often unsatisfactory and bleeding may recur either because some lesions in other parts of the gastrointestinal tract may not have been appreciated at the initial evaluation or because new lesions may subsequently

develop. For these reasons, nonoperative endoscopic approaches are being evaluated to obliterate vascular malformations by such techniques as electrocoagulation or laser photocoagulation.

Boley SJ, Brandt LJ, Veith FJ: Ischemic disorders of the intestines. Curr Probl Surg 15(4):1, 1978. *A comprehensive and extensively referenced review of this area. The authors espouse an aggressive approach to the management of nonocclusive ischemia that is not universally accepted.*

Bynum TE, Jacobson ED: Nonocclusive intestinal ischemia. Arch Intern Med 139:281, 1979. *A concise editorial summary of the issues involved in the pathophysiology and management of this disorder. Most of the points considered are still valid today.*

Croft RJ, Menon GP, Marston A: Does "intestinal angina" exist? A critical study of obstructed visceral arteries. Br J Surg 68:316, 1981. *A provocative report demonstrating the difficulty in relating gastrointestinal symptoms to angiographic findings.*

Federle MP, Chun G, Jeffrey RB, Rayor R: Computed tomographic findings in bowel infarction. Am J Roentgenol 142:91, 1984. *This article demonstrates the potential value of computed tomography in the diagnosis of vascular diseases of the intestine.*

Grendell JH, Ockner RK: Vascular diseases of the bowel. *In* Sleisenger MH, Fordtran JS (eds.): Gastrointestinal Disease. 3rd ed. Philadelphia, W. B. Saunders Company, 1983, p 1543. *A comprehensive survey including pathophysiology, diagnosis, and management.*

Kiernan PD, Pairolero PC, Hubert JP Jr, Mucha P Jr, Wallace RB: Aortic graft-enteric fistula. Mayo Clin Proc 55:731, 1980. *A detailed review of the clinical features, management, and prognosis of this entity.*

Rogers DM, Thompson JE, Garrett WV, Talkington CM, Patman RD: Mesenteric vascular problems. A 26-year experience. Ann Surg 195:554, 1982. *This article describes an extensive surgical experience with a variety of vascular diseases of the intestine.*

Weaver GA, Alpern HD, Davis JS, Ramsey WH, Reichelderfer M: Gastrointestinal angiodysplasia associated with aortic valve disease: Part of a spectrum of angiodysplasia of the gut. Gastroenterology 77:1, 1979. *An extensive review with excellent endoscopic photographs of representative lesions.*

106. NEOPLASMS OF THE LARGE AND SMALL INTESTINE

Sidney J. Winawer

NEOPLASMS OF THE LARGE INTESTINE

Adenocarcinoma of the large intestine is a worldwide health problem of major importance, especially in western countries. The incidence of this cancer in the United States is more than 120,000 per year; more than half of those affected will die of their disease within five years of the time of diagnosis. With the exception of skin cancer, cancer of the colon, along with lung cancer and breast cancer, is one of the three leading malignancies in this country in terms of annual new cases. New concepts and new technologies for diagnosis and treatment of this cancer have evolved over the past few years, providing opportunities for earlier detection and improved survival.

The colon is the site of a variety of other malignant tumors. Its second most common primary malignant tumor is the epidermoid or squamous cell carcinoma of the anal canal and rectum. Other primary malignant tumors that can involve the colon include lymphomas, leiomyosarcomas, and malignant carcinoid tumors as well as direct invasion by tumors from adjacent sites such as stomach, uterus, ovary, and prostate. Rarely tumors from such sites as breast and lung metastasize to the colon.

The most frequent tumors that involve the large intestine are adenomas, which may be found in as many as 5 to 10 per cent of asymptomatic patients over the age of 40 on routine proctosigmoidoscopy. A variety of other benign tumors, including lipomas, leiomyomas, and benign carcinoid tumors, occur in the colon. Of these all are rare except for lipomas of the ileocecal valve. Adenomas of the large intestine will be discussed first because of their frequency and their association with cancer of the colon.

Polyps of the Colon

A polyp in a generic sense is any lesion that arises from the surface of the gastrointestinal tract and protrudes into the lumen (Fig. 106–1). Polyps are usually defined pathologically as overgrowths of epithelial tissue that may be either hyperplastic or neoplastic, benign or malignant, and of various histopathologic subtypes. They are noted clinically in the large bowel as negative shadows in the lumen demonstrated by barium enema or by direct visualization during proctosigmoidoscopy or colonoscopy. They may be single or multiple, pedunculated (on a stalk) or sessile (flat and without a stalk), and sporadic in occurrence or part of a dominantly transmitted familial polyposis syndrome. Their importance lies in their frequency, their occasional production of symptoms (bleeding), and most of all their potential for malignant transformation. They are to be distinguished from pseudopolyps, which have an inflammatory mass in association with normal epithelium.

PATHOLOGY. In addition to carcinoma of the large intestine, which may present as a polypoid mass, four distinct types of benign polyps arise from colonic epithelium: (1) hyperplastic (metaplastic), (2) tubular adenomas, (3) villous adenomas, and (4) mixed type. *Hyperplastic polyps,* which account for about 25 per cent of all polyps and for most of the polyps of the rectum, tend to be small and asymptomatic, and are not considered to be neoplastic, based on the histologic criteria of normal cellular differentiation and a sharp line of demarcation between the polyp and the normal mucosa. *Neoplastic polyps* or adenomas have the same distribution in the colon as do cancers of the colon and account for most of the polyps above the area of the rectum. They are usually less than 1 cm in diameter (75 per cent), may be sessile or pedunculated, and represent localized neoplastic tumors of colonic epithelium. Histologically they have abnormal cellular differentiation and exhibit predominantly tubular structure. *Villous adenomas* typically are spongy, exophytic, and larger than adenomatous polyps (60 per cent > 2 cm). They exhibit a predominantly glandular pattern representing overgrowth of poorly differentiated cells from the base of the crypts of Lieberkühn. They have a high association with malignant transformation. *Mixed type adenomas* contain both tubular and villous components, and the villous component tends to increase with the size of the polyp.

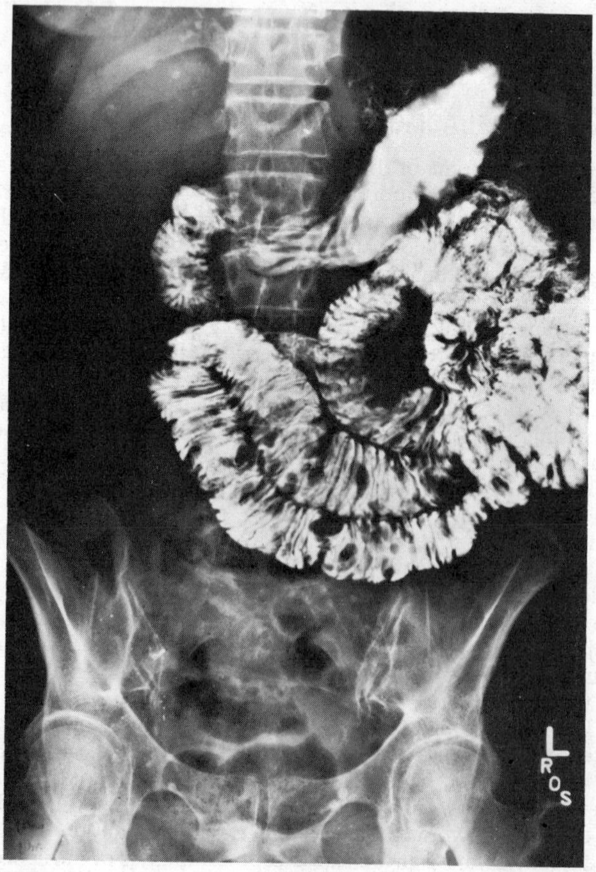

Figure 106–1. Barium study of the upper gastrointestinal tract showing multiple polyps of the small bowel in a patient with Peutz-Jeghers syndrome.

RELATIONSHIP OF COLONIC ADENOMAS TO CANCER. The evidence that links benign adenomas (the neoplastic polyps classified as adenomas, mixed, or villous) to adenocarcinoma of the colon is compelling: (1) the epidemiology of adenocarcinomas and adenomas of the colon is similar wherever studied in the world; (2) adenocarcinomas of the colon occur in the same anatomic distribution as adenomas of the colon; (3) the risk for colorectal cancer is high in patients with a prior history of adenomas, but is lower if adenomas are removed; (4) as adenomas grow in size, the frequency of finding cancer in the adenoma increases; (5) residual adenomatous tissue can sometimes be found in colorectal cancers on pathologic examination; and (6) the association of cancer and adenomas is particularly strong in the inherited colorectal cancer syndromes, with adenocarcinomas having been documented to have arisen from the underlying adenomas. In brief, there is now very little doubt that colorectal cancer arises from an antecedent premalignant tumor of the colon, the benign adenoma.

The premalignant nature of adenomas is related to size and histology. The frequency of cancer in adenomas is 1 per cent in adenomas less than 1 cm in size; 10 per cent in adenomas between 1 and 2 cm in size; and as high as 50 per cent in some reports in adenomas greater than 2 cm in size. The relationship of cancer to adenomas is much greater in adenomas with villous components than in adenomas without villous components. Cancer in adenomas is usually well differentiated and occurs most commonly in the tip of the adenoma without invasion of the muscularis mucosae. These are called in situ or focal cancers and are not immediately dangerous. Less commonly, cancers in adenomas invade the muscularis mucosae, and therefore have the potential to grow down the stalk, invade lymphatics, involve adjacent lymph nodes, and metastasize.

The occurrence of adenomas signifies an important transformation of the colonic mucosa to a premalignant state. Thus, it is understandable that additional adenomas often concurrently exist (synchronous adenomas) and others will appear subsequently (metachronous adenomas). The synchronous rate for adenomas is 50 per cent, and the metachronous rate is 30 to 40 per cent. Synchronous and metachronous rates for colorectal cancers are 1.5 to 5 per cent and 5 to 10 per cent, respectively. Multiple adenomas appear to be associated with a higher frequency of metachronous adenomas and metachronous cancers.

CLINICAL MANIFESTATIONS. Most polyps are asymptomatic. When symptoms do occur, they most frequently result from *bleeding* (hematochezia or iron deficiency anemia, depending on the location of the polyp and the rate of blood loss). When polyps are very large they may rarely cause *abdominal pain* from partial intestinal obstruction or from induced intussusception. Villous adenomas may rarely result in *watery diarrhea* with severe potassium depletion or in excessive secretion of mucus with loss of sufficient protein to produce hypoalbuminemia (an unusual form of "protein-losing enteropathy").

TREATMENT AND FOLLOW-UP. Because of the association of polyps with cancer of the colon, it is recommended that they be removed when identified.

Colonoscopic Polypectomy. Pedunculated polyps of any size can be removed by cautery snare through the colonoscope (see Fig. 95–3). Sessile polyps smaller than 2 cm can generally also be removed by cautery snare through the colonoscope. Controversy exists as to whether polyps larger than 2 cm should be removed by colonoscopy or by surgery. Although large sessile polyps can be excised segmentally via the colonoscope, this approach is challenged because many of them already are cancerous, the risk of complications during removal is significantly increased, and the completeness of removal is uncertain. Since there is also risk involved in surgery, each case must be individualized. Suspicion that a polyp may be a polypoid adenocarcinoma warrants a biopsy and brushing for cytology. If the diagnosis of carcinoma is confirmed, surgery is indicated. Benign-appearing polyps are totally excised, not biopsied, and the entire polyp is submitted for pathologic examination. Polyps up to 7 or 8 mm in size can be removed by a combination of biopsy and fulguration. This is a particularly rapid and effective means for treating these small lesions.

After endoscopic polypectomy the patient must be followed periodically. Usually a repeat colonoscopy is performed one year later to search for missed synchronous lesions, and then approximately every three years thereafter to search for metachronous lesions. If the patient has multiple adenomas, colonoscopy is often done annually for several years.

Focal cancer in an adenoma demands special consideration. If the cancer is in the tip of the polyp and has not penetrated the muscularis mucosae, no further surgery need be done. If the cancer has penetrated the muscularis mucosae and lymphatic invasion has been demonstrated, if the cancer is poorly differentiated, or if it has extended down to the line of cautery, then follow-up laparotomy and segmental resection are indicated. In such circumstances there will be approximately a 5 per cent frequency of regional lymph node metastases.

Inherited Polyposis Syndromes of the Large and Small Intestines

There are a number of heritable syndromes characterized by polyposis of the intestine with or without additional extraintestinal manifestations. Some of these syndromes have a greatly increased frequency of cancer, and some have a slightly increased frequency of cancer.

Familial polyposis of the colon, an autosomal dominant trait, is characterized by multiple adenomas of the large intestine and rarely of the ileum as well (Fig. 106–2). In this disorder, which occurs approximately once each 8000 births, hundreds and sometimes thousands of polyps develop throughout the entire colon, beginning in childhood. Virtually all patients with familial polyposis develop carcinoma of the colon by age 40, so subtotal colectomy should be carried out early in adult life in affected persons. An intensive survey of other family members must be conducted because of the inheritance pattern; some cases occur without a family history and probably represent spontaneous mutations.

Gardner's syndrome is a dominantly transmitted disorder characterized by the triad of adenomas of the colon, bone tumors

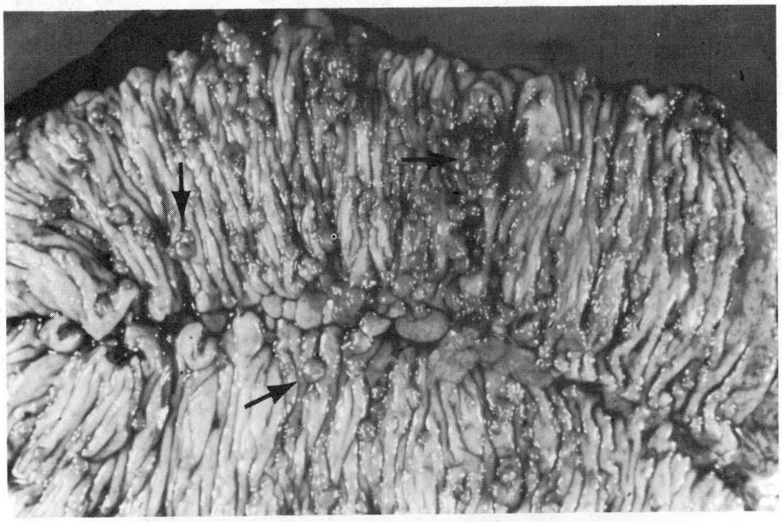

A

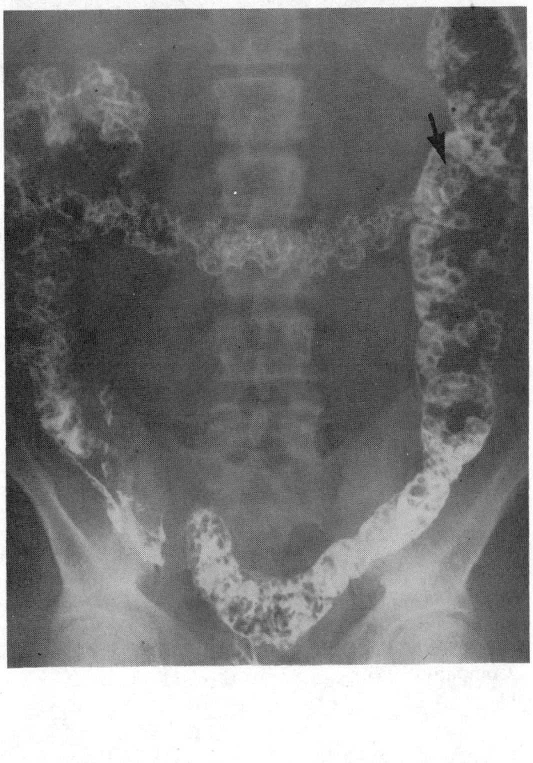

B

Figure 106–2. *A,* Patients with familial polyposis have multiple adenomatous polyps carpeting the colon, as demonstrated in this gross specimen. Note that the colon is diffusely studded with sessile and occasional pedunculated adenomatous polyps (arrows). Many of the larger polyps contain villous elements, and occasionally villous adenomas are found. Although no carcinoma was seen in this patient, nearly all patients will eventually develop colorectal carcinoma if surgery is not performed. *B,* This barium enema examination of a patient with familial polyposis represents diffuse studding of the large bowel with adenomatous polyps. Note the marked variation in size of these polyps. Although this patient did not have osteomas or soft tissue tumors, the barium enema is similar to that seen in Gardner's syndrome. (From Boland CR, Kim YS: *In* Sleisenger MH, Fordtran JS [eds.]: Gastrointestinal Disease. 3rd ed. Philadelphia, W. B. Saunders Company, 1983.)

(osteomas), and soft tissue tumors (lipomas, sebaceous cysts, fibromas, fibrosarcomas) (Fig. 106–3*A*). Other associated features include retroperitoneal fibrosis, supernumerary teeth, and a tendency toward the development of carcinomas of the thyroid, adrenal, and duodenum in the region of the ampulla of Vater. There may be osteosclerosis of the skull in addition to the osteomas of the mandible and maxillary regions. The colonic polyps resemble those of familial polyposis and have the same potential for malignancy. The treatment is therefore subtotal colectomy and a careful survey for other affected members of the family.

Turcot's syndrome represents the rare association of adenomas of the colon with a variety of tumors of the central nervous system. The polyps have a high frequency of malignant transformation. The central nervous system lesions have included medulloblastoma, ependymoma, and glioblastoma. The mode of transmission is thought to be autosomal recessive, although this is unclear.

Peutz-Jeghers syndrome is a rare familial disorder, with autosomal dominant transmission, characterized by multiple intestinal polyposis and mucocutaneous pigmentation (Fig. 106–3*B*). The polyps, which occur in the small intestine, large intestine, and stomach, are mostly hamartomas rather than true adenomas and as such have a low potential for malignant transformation. It is estimated that 2 to 3 per cent of patients with this syndrome develop adenocarcinoma of the intestinal tract, with the small intestine being more frequently involved than the colon. Pigmentation is particularly marked in the buccal mucosa, in the hard and soft palate, on the lips, on the soles of the feet, on the dorsum of the hands, and around the mouth and nostrils. More rarely exostoses, ovarian tumors, and polyps of the bladder and nose have been described. Surgical removal of gastric and small bowel polyps is reserved only for complications such as bleeding or intestinal obstruction. True adenomas can occur in the colon in this disorder. These can usually be removed endoscopically.

Generalized juvenile polyposis refers to a familial syndrome with autosomal dominant transmission characterized by hamartomatous polyps in the colon and rectum and to a lesser extent in the small intestine and stomach. Symptoms usually begin in the first decade of life with bleeding, diarrhea, and abdominal pain. There are no extraintestinal manifestations. There seems to be an increased incidence of carcinoma of the intestine in families with generalized juvenile polyposis, probably from true adenomas that occur with higher frequency in these families.

Cronkhite-Canada syndrome refers to the rare association of generalized intestinal polyposis, dystrophy of the fingernails, alopecia, and cutaneous hyperpigmentation. The polyps are hamartomas; no familial association has been clearly established.

Adenocarcinoma of the Colon

EPIDEMIOLOGY. Colorectal cancer is more prevalent in the developed countries, suggesting a relationship to economic development. Its incidence is high in North America, New Zealand, and Europe and low in South America, Africa, and Asia. The United States has one of the highest rates of colorectal cancer in the world. Migrants to a particular geographic area assume the colonic cancer risk of that area. This is well illustrated by the higher incidence of the disease among blacks in America as compared to those in Africa, in Puerto Ricans who have migrated to the mainland as compared to those in Puerto Rico, and in first and second generation Japanese immigrants to Hawaii and the mainland United States as compared to Japanese in Japan. In the United States the incidence of colorectal cancer is higher in the north than in the south, in urban areas as compared to rural areas, and in whites as compared to blacks. There is a slightly increased risk among certain occupations such as asbestos workers and factory woodworkers.

ETIOLOGY. Migrant studies strongly suggest that *environmental factors,* particularly *diet,* are important in the etiology of colorectal cancer. There is a low incidence of appendicitis, adenomas, diverticulosis, ulcerative colitis, and colorectal cancer in the South African Bantu and other African populations in which diets contain more fiber and less animal fat than is the case with diets in more developed areas. High fiber diets produce rapid intestinal transit so that any potential carcinogen is in contact with the mucosa for a shorter period of time. The various components of fiber may bind carcinogens or cocarcin-

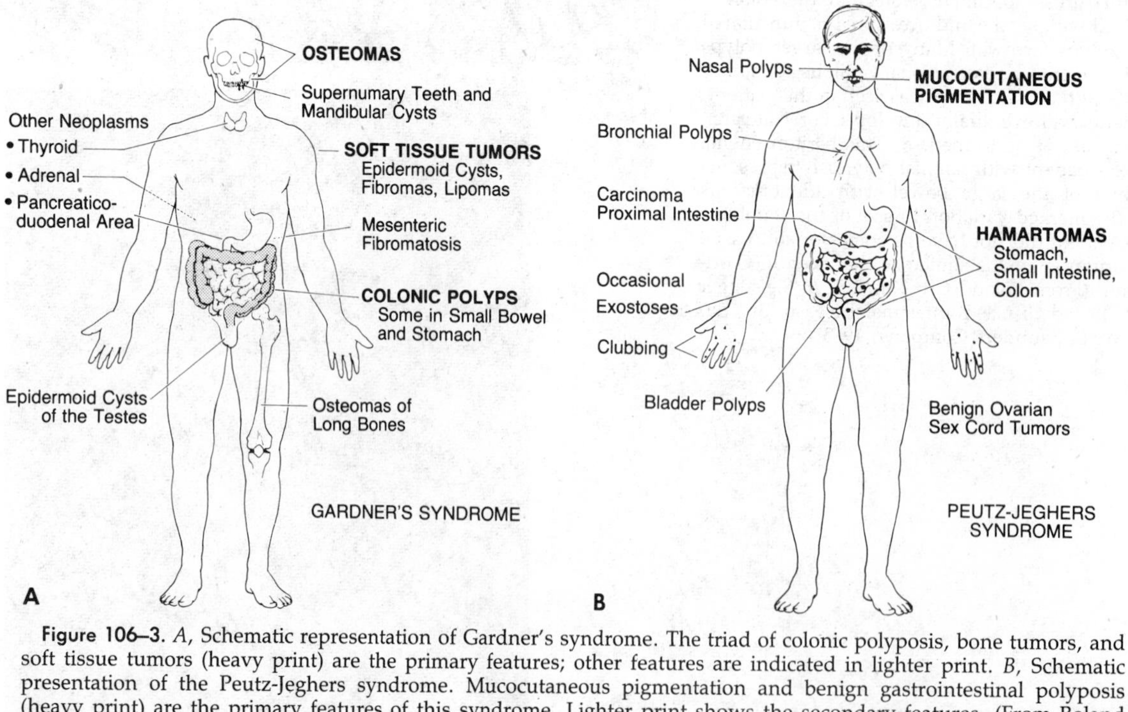

Figure 106–3. *A,* Schematic representation of Gardner's syndrome. The triad of colonic polyposis, bone tumors, and soft tissue tumors (heavy print) are the primary features; other features are indicated in lighter print. *B,* Schematic presentation of the Peutz-Jeghers syndrome. Mucocutaneous pigmentation and benign gastrointestinal polyposis (heavy print) are the primary features of this syndrome. Lighter print shows the secondary features. (From Boland CR, Kim YS: *In* Sleisenger MH, Fordtran JS [eds.]: Gastrointestinal Disease. 3rd ed. Philadelphia, W. B. Saunders Company, 1983.)

ogens or increase intraluminal bulk and thereby dilute carcinogens. A direct association between *increased fat and animal protein* intake (particularly beef) in the western diet and the rising incidence of colonic cancer has been suggested. In Japan, the intake of fat (mostly unsaturated) provides only 12 per cent of the total caloric intake; in the United States fat intake represents 40 to 44 per cent of the total caloric intake. It has been postulated that the western diet with its high beef and fat content favors the establishment of bacterial flora capable of producing enzymes such as beta glucuronidase and azoreductase, resulting in increased metabolism of acid and neutral sterols to carcinogens and cocarcinogens. Studies are in progress concerning putative mutagens in feces, including nitrosamide, which has been demonstrated in the feces of persons on high beef diets. Reduction in mutagenicity and in levels of nitrosamide in the stool has been noted in patients on high doses of ascorbic acid and alpha tocopherol. Obviously much remains to be learned about the proposed relationship of diet to colorectal cancer, concerning both the validity of the association and the chemical link between diet and the induction of neoplastic transformation.

SUSCEPTIBILITY. In addition to general risk factors that influence susceptibility on a broad basis (Table 106–1), there are a number of specific factors that affect risk in the individual (see accompanying table). One of these factors is age. The risk for colorectal cancer begins to increase slightly at age 40 and more sharply at age 50, doubling with each decade and reaching a maximum at age 75 (Fig. 106–4). Additional risk factors include a prior history of colorectal cancer or adenoma, a prior history of female genital cancer, underlying ulcerative colitis of long standing, and a family history of one of the inherited colon cancer syndromes (see below).

Prior Colonic Cancer or Adenoma. Patients who have had one colorectal cancer are at increased risk for a subsequent colorectal cancer (metachronous lesion) occurring at a future time from the initial or index lesion. A prior adenoma of the colon also increases risk for subsequent colorectal cancer. The association of adenomas and cancer of the colon has been previously discussed in detail.

Ulcerative Colitis. One third of deaths related to chronic ulcerative colitis (CUC) are due to colorectal cancer, which occurs in an overall incidence 7 to 11 times greater in patients with CUC than in the general population. The risk of cancer in ulcerative colitis can be related to two recognized variables: (1) the duration of active colitis, and (2) the anatomic extent of colonic involvement by the pathologic process.

The relationship between duration of ulcerative colitis and the cumulative risk of colorectal cancer for both adults and

TABLE 106–1. COLORECTAL CANCER RISK FACTORS*

Standard Risk:	Age over 40, men and women
High Risk:	Inflammatory bowel disease
	History of female genital or breast cancer
	History of colonic cancer or adenoma
	Peutz-Jeghers syndrome
	Familial polyposis syndromes
	Family cancer syndromes
	Hereditary site-specific colonic cancer
	History of juvenile polyps
	Immunodeficiency disease

*From Stearns MW Jr (ed.): Neoplasms of the Colon, Rectum, and Anus. New York, John Wiley & Sons, 1980, pp 9–22. Reprinted with the kind permission of the publisher.

children is shown in Figure 106–5. In adults the risk begins to rise after seven years, and 20 per cent of patients with cancer and CUC develop their malignancies between seven and ten years from the onset of colitis. Extent of colonic involvement by CUC also affects risk for cancer. Pancolitis carries a greater risk than colitis confined to the left side of the colon, where risk appears later, approximately 15 years after onset. Colitis confined to the rectosigmoid carries minimal risk, and ulcerative proctitis appears to have no increased risk for cancer. The high risk for cancer in ulcerative colitis has been considered by some investigators to be an overestimate resulting from referral of many patients with ulcerative colitis and cancer to centers that have reported the association.

In recent years a small subgroup (10 to 15 per cent) of patients with longstanding CUC has been identified by biopsy as having dysplasia of the colonic mucosa as an indicator for risk of cancer. When severe (high grade) dysplasia is found, approximately 50 per cent of patients will be found to have simultaneous cancer; with moderate (low grade) dysplasia, approximately one third of patients have cancer. Approximately 80 per cent of patients with CUC and colorectal cancer have dysplasia on biopsy. Although there are difficulties in histologic interpretations and dysplastic changes may be patchy, nevertheless the general concept is an important one; the demonstration of dysplasia has potential value in identifying those patients with CUC who are at greatest risk for colorectal cancer.

Patients with granulomatous colitis are also at higher risk for colorectal cancer than the general population, but considerably less so than patients with CUC. Once again, risk is related to the duration of disease.

Heredity and Colonic Cancer. Inherited predisposition to

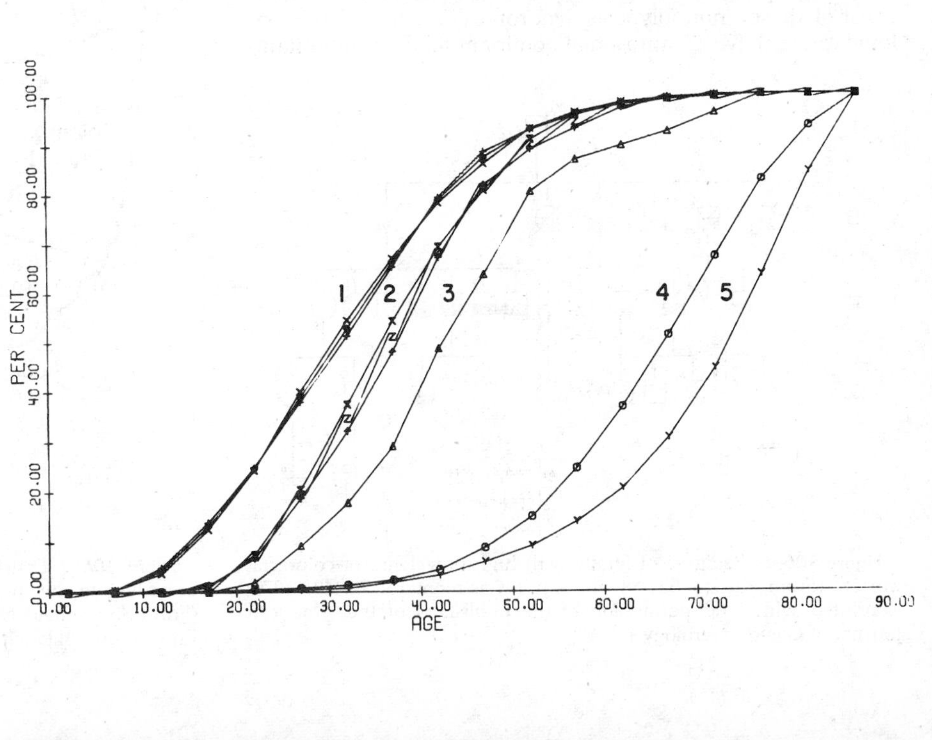

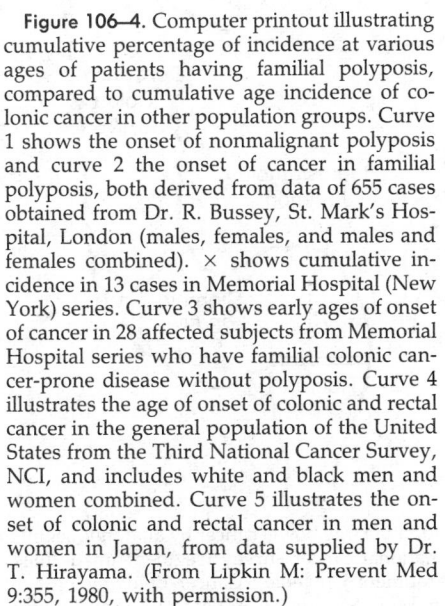

Figure 106–4. Computer printout illustrating cumulative percentage of incidence at various ages of patients having familial polyposis, compared to cumulative age incidence of colonic cancer in other population groups. Curve 1 shows the onset of nonmalignant polyposis and curve 2 the onset of cancer in familial polyposis, both derived from data of 655 cases obtained from Dr. R. Bussey, St. Mark's Hospital, London (males, females, and males and females combined). × shows cumulative incidence in 13 cases in Memorial Hospital (New York) series. Curve 3 shows early ages of onset of cancer in 28 affected subjects from Memorial Hospital series who have familial colonic cancer-prone disease without polyposis. Curve 4 illustrates the age of onset of colonic and rectal cancer in the general population of the United States from the Third National Cancer Survey, NCI, and includes white and black men and women combined. Curve 5 illustrates the onset of colonic and rectal cancer in men and women in Japan, from data supplied by Dr. T. Hirayama. (From Lipkin M: Prevent Med 9:355, 1980, with permission.)

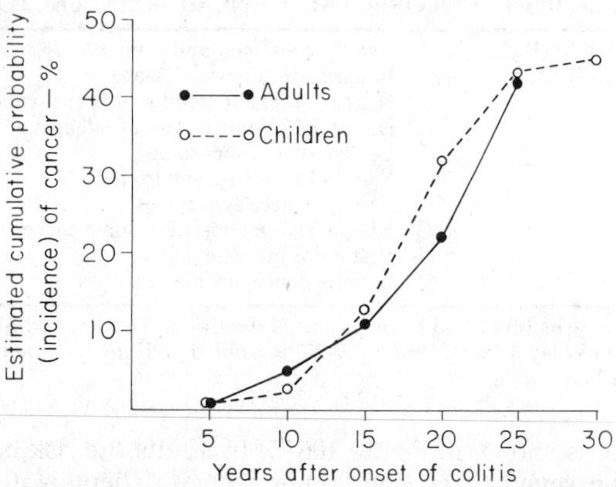

Figure 106–5. Graphs illustrating estimated cumulative incidence with time of cancer complicating ulcerative colitis in adults and children with panproctocolitis. (From Stauffer JQ: *In* Sleisenger MH, Fordtran JS [eds.]: Gastrointestinal Disease. 2nd ed. Philadelphia, W. B. Saunders Company, 1978.)

colonic cancer can be divided into two major categories: the polyposis type (familial polyposis, Gardner's syndrome, juvenile polyposis, Peutz-Jeghers syndrome, and Turcot's syndrome) and the nonpolyposis types (site-specific colonic cancer, the familial cancer syndromes, and Muir's [Torre's] syndrome). The familial polyposis syndromes have been discussed previously.

When it is stated that certain patients with a heritable predisposition to colonic cancer belong to a "nonpolyposis group," it is meant only that the colon is not carpeted by a myriad of small polyps. There is increasing evidence, however, that even in this group colorectal cancer develops from adenomas as in the familial polyposis syndromes. These adenomas are either single or multiple but if multiple are only in small numbers. Three major patterns are seen in this group: (1) Cancer confined to the colon and rectum (site-specific). In site-specific colonic cancer the transmission from generation to generation is only for colorectal cancer. (2) Multifocal cancer involving other sites in the gastrointestinal tract or the female sex organs (ovary, uterus, and breast) as well as the colon and rectum. This is sometimes called the "family cancer syndrome." (3) Muir's (Torre's) syndrome, a rare disorder resulting in multiple adenocarcinomas and epidermoid carcinomas in many organs in association with a large number of sebaceous cysts.

All of these "nonpolyposis syndromes" associated with colonic cancer have an autosomal dominant mode of inheritance

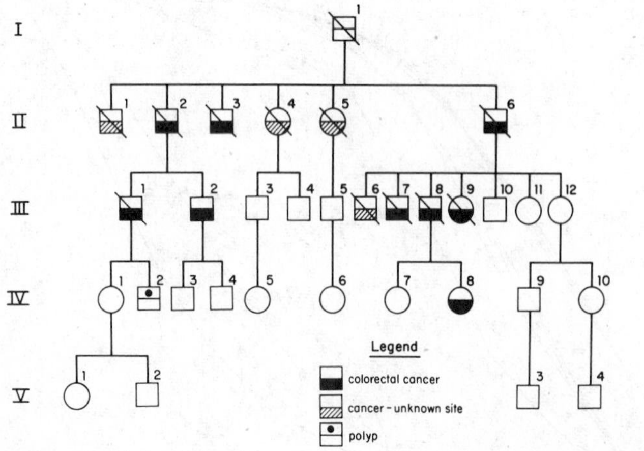

Figure 106–6. Pedigree of family with high prevalence of colorectal cancer. (From Kussin SZ, et al.: Am J Gastroenterol 72:448, 1979. Reprinted with kind permission of the publishers of the American Journal of Gastroenterology.)

with a high degree of penetrance. Multiple cancers within the colon often occur at a young age (under 40), with risk beginning as young as age 20. The majority of cancers in this group are on the right side of the colon, in contrast to those occurring in the usual patient or in patients with familial polyposis or Gardner's syndrome.

Beyond the clear-cut dominant transmission of predisposition to colonic cancer described above or that seen in the familial polyposis syndromes, there are other ill-defined, probably polygenic influences on the development of these malignant lesions (Fig. 106–6). The first-degree relatives (parents, siblings, children) of patients who have had a single colorectal cancer have a three-fold greater frequency of colorectal cancers than is expected in the average population. Families with autosomal dominant patterns of inheritance are easy to identify by family history. The significance of one affected first-degree relative is difficult to determine. The likelihood of genetic factors being present with two or more first-degree relatives with colorectal cancer is much greater. The pattern of the cancer can provide clues to the presence of an inherited predisposition, i.e., such factors as colorectal cancer in a first-degree relative under the age of 40, particularly on the right side of the colon, or bilateral premenopausal breast cancer in the family. Better indicators are obviously needed to identify the presence or absence of genetic factors in the predisposition of individuals or families to develop colorectal cancer.

PATHOLOGY. Approximately 50 per cent of adenocarcinomas of the colon occur in the distal 25 cm of large bowel (Fig. 106–7). This percentage was higher in the past, but there has been a "proximal migration" of neoplasia in the colon in recent years. The distal descending colon and upper sigmoid represents another frequent site of colorectal cancer, as do the cecum and ascending colon. Cancer is much less frequent in the transverse colon. On the left side of the colon, cancers are commonly annular and tend to obstruct; on the right side of the colon, they are primarily polypoid. In fact, either of these gross patterns can occur anywhere in the colon, and all colonic cancers commonly ulcerate and bleed. Metastatic spread from carcinoma of the colon occurs by direct invasion of surrounding structures, by way of regional lymphatics, or less commonly by multiple peritoneal implants. Of distant organs the liver is most frequently involved, but metastases may also occur to lung, and to bone and brain, rarely.

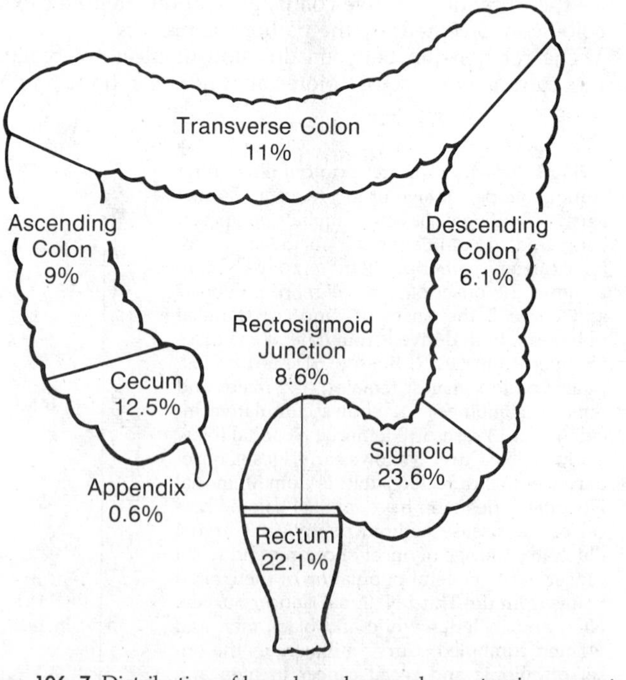

Figure 106–7. Distribution of large bowel cancer by anatomic segment according to the third national cancer survey (segment unspecified). (From Shottenfeld D, Fraumeni J Jr [eds.]: Cancer Epidemiology and Prevention. Philadelphia, W. B. Saunders Company, 1982, pp 703–727.)

CLINICAL MANIFESTATIONS. Adenocarcinomas of the colon, especially those on the right side, are often clinically silent for a long period of time. The most common symptoms relate to *bleeding* (anemia with its many manifestations or hematochezia) and *obstruction* (change in bowel habits, sometimes pain). When the lesion is in the right colon, the bleeding is often occult since the blood tends to be well mixed with stool and therefore escapes notice. Tumors of the cecum and ascending colon rarely obstruct, at least early in their course, so that a change in bowel habits or pain is less useful as an early symptom. Polypoid lesions of the left side of the colon may be associated with frequent and sometimes loose stools. With obstructing left-sided lesions, changes in bowel habits are usually those of gradual but progressive constipation, tenesmus, or a reduction in stool caliber, and hematochezia is much more frequent. Because of the frequency of tumor ulceration and bleeding, testing chemically for occult blood is an excellent survey technique and leads to an earlier diagnosis with a greater chance for cure. The general symptoms of malignancy—weakness, malaise, anorexia, weight loss—are frequent but nonspecific. Adenocarcinoma of the colon may present with a localized perforation, which becomes sealed off, or signs of peritonitis (fever, generalized discomfort, rebound tenderness) when the perforation enters freely into the abdominal cavity. An abdominal mass or the signs and symptoms of metastasis to the liver may rarely be the earliest complaints.

Cancers at the mucocutaneous junction or in the anal canal or rectum may present with rectal bleeding, change in bowel habits, mass, or perineal pain. These can also present with symptoms referable to invasion of adjacent organs, including hematuria, urinary frequency, or vaginal fistulas.

DIAGNOSIS. ***Differential Diagnosis.*** The diagnosis of colorectal cancer must be considered when patients present with a change in bowel habits, a recent decrease in caliber of the stool, rectal bleeding, unexplained abdominal pain, or iron deficiency anemia. Overall the most common causes for bright red rectal bleeding are non-neoplastic, but the frequency of neoplastic lesions as the cause for bleeding increases progressively over age 40 and is especially high in those with a family history of colonic cancer. Bright red rectal bleeding can also be caused by angiodysplasia of the colon, diverticulosis, and a variety of other benign and malignant tumors of the colon (see Ch. 113).

A change of bowel habits can be produced by many other neoplastic lesions as well as by several benign disorders. Change in the caliber of the stool to a pellet type with more difficulty in passage is as common in progressive diverticular disease and muscle hypertrophy of the colon as in colonic malignancy (see Ch. 101). Diarrhea and incontinence can be a manifestation of many colonic and small intestinal diseases in addition to colorectal cancer. A recent change in bowel habits in one who has always had regular bowel habits, particularly if the person is at risk for colorectal cancer, clearly raises the possibility of a colonic neoplasm. The character of rectal bleeding cannot distinguish benign from neoplastic disorders. Blood appearing only on the toilet paper is indeed most commonly from hemorrhoids or a fissure, but it can also be from rectal cancer. Although a profuse bleeding episode is more likely to be the result of angiodysplasia, diverticulosis, ulcerative colitis, or ischemic colitis, it may be due to a large ulcerating neoplasm of the right colon.

Metastatic Colonic Cancer. Metastases of colon cancer may be present before resection or may occur after it, producing different patterns of symptoms. Metastases to liver with progressive hepatomegaly may produce pain from distention of the liver capsule. Spread within the pelvis can result in pressure on the urinary bladder, obstruction of the rectosigmoid, sciatic nerve pain, and sometimes small bowel obstruction. Metastases to lung and bone are usually silent until very advanced. Intra-abdominal metastases may produce multiple areas of small and large bowel obstruction. Implants on the peritoneum sometimes cause ascites. Metastatic lesions can also occur in the skin, within the subcutaneous tissues, in suture lines, and within the bowel lumen. Intraluminal recurrences of colorectal cancer are unusual and follow surgery performed under adverse circumstances such as obstruction, or a low anterior resection for rectal cancer that leaves only a very narrow distal margin free of tumor. When tumor recurs within the colon, it more commonly is an intra-abdominal growth from the serosa into the lumen.

Diagnostic Approach. The history, physical examination, and common laboratory tests are essential for early diagnosis of colonic cancer. The history should combine the patient's symptoms with important clues such as the prior removal of an adenoma or even of a colorectal cancer, a history suggesting ulcerative colitis, or a family history suggesting one of the inherited colonic cancer syndromes. Physical examination may reveal evidence for Peutz-Jeghers syndrome, soft tissue tumors suggesting Gardner's syndrome, or the possibility of Muir's syndrome, and will provide clues as to any possible spread of the tumor to the liver, peripheral nodes, or skin. The digital rectal examination is important to determine the presence of a low lying tumor or of perianal or pelvic disease. Laboratory testing might reveal iron deficiency anemia, occult blood in the stool, or an abnormality of liver function. Evaluation of the patient would also include a chest roentgenogram to search for pulmonary metastases.

When patients have symptoms or signs of colorectal cancer, the digital rectal examination should be followed by proctoscopy and barium enema and, in most cases, colonoscopy. Proctoscopy may be performed with a rigid instrument, but this has had poor patient acceptance and physician application. Flexible sigmoidoscopes are more comfortable for the patient and have produced a much higher diagnostic yield because of the more complete insertion (see Ch. 95). The combination of proctoscopy and barium enema is the first step in the investigation of patients in whom colorectal neoplasm is suspected. A double contrast barium enema is more revealing of mucosal lesions than the single column study. In a well-prepared patient the vast majority of colorectal cancers can be detected by the combination of these two techniques. A barium enema should not be ordered without a prior proctoscopy, since there may be a distal lesion that could be obstructive and result in a perforation during the examination if the radiologist is not alerted to its presence. In addition, the patient may not have a neoplastic lesion but may have another disease, such as ulcerative colitis, which can readily be diagnosed by proctoscopy. If this disease is very active, a barium enema may in fact be undesirable.

Colonoscopy should be done in patients in whom proctoscopy and barium enema have not revealed the basis for their symptoms. Colonoscopy will be successful in uncovering many lesions not detected by the barium enema, especially polyps but also cancers. Colonoscopy is also desirable in patients who have had an abnormality detected by barium enema. If the lesion detected radiologically appears to be cancer, it should be located endoscopically and confirmed by biopsy. In addition, a search for synchronous lesions and polyps should be carried out. If the lesion seen on x-ray is clearly an obstructing cancer of the left side, then colonoscopy is not necessary and may actually be hazardous. When the barium enema has uncovered only a polyp, colonoscopy can be utilized to remove the polyp, to search for other polyps, and to rule out an associated malignancy.

During colonoscopy, tissue sampling would include not only biopsies but also brushings for cytology, which increases the sensitivity of tissue diagnosis. Saline lavage through the colonoscope allows for aspiration of cells freshly exfoliated for cytologic study (see Ch. 95). Lavage is usually done only in special circumstances such as longstanding, quiescent ulcerative colitis. Lavage can be helpful to determine whether a mass lesion in a patient with diverticulosis is a diverticular abscess or neoplastic mass. In longstanding ulcerative colitis, biopsies are useful to look for dysplasia as an indication of premalignancy. These are usually obtained from the cecum to the rectum at 10-cm intervals.

TREATMENT. ***Surgery.*** The goal of treatment for primary malignant neoplasms of the colon is to remove them as completely as possible. The best hope for cure is surgical removal of the segment of colon harboring the neoplasm, including omentum with lymph nodes. Cancers of the right and left colons are treated by hemicolectomies; cancer of the sigmoid and upper rectum above 5 cm from the anal verge is resected anteriorly with removal of a wide margin of normal colon above and below the tumor. In low anterior resections, the surgeon wishes to leave 2 to 3 cm of tumor-free margin distal to the tumor. Lesions within 4 to 5 cm of the anal verge are usually treated by a combined abdominal-perineal resection (APR). It is desirable to do a lower anterior resection rather than an APR if at all possible, since APR is not associated with increased survival and leaves the patient with a permanent colostomy. The recent availability of staplers allows the surgeon to do a low anterior resection of tumors closer to the anal verge than previously possible.

Epidermoid cancers in the anal canal may be treated by local excision if superficial. If deeper, an APR is required. A period of preoperative radiation and chemotherapy in these cases will usually shrink the tumor and improve the likelihood of successful resection.

Patients may require surgery for palliation as well as for cure. Obstruction usually requires a colostomy, followed at a later time by closure of the colostomy. In most patients with obstruction, however, a primary resection and colostomy can usually be accomplished in one stage. Carcinoma which has perforated also is usually treated by primary resection and colostomy with later closure of the colostomy. Patients with obvious metastatic disease may require surgery for their tumor if it bleeds or obstructs significantly. Palliative treatment with radiation and/or chemotherapy of the metastases may then proceed.

Radiation Therapy. Radiation may be used preoperatively and in patients who have evidence of recurrent disease, especially in the pelvis, or localized recurrences intra-abdominally. Adjuvant use of radiation and chemotherapy in rectal cancer has been associated with a longer tumor-free interval after surgery. Radiation has occasionally been used for extensive liver metastases in patients who have not responded to chemotherapy and have considerable pain from distention of the liver capsule, but at the hazard of producing radiation hepatitis and hepatic coma.

Chemotherapy. Chemotherapy of colorectal cancer is used for metastatic disease and as adjuvant therapy in patients at high risk for recurrence but who have no known residual disease. Unfortunately chemotherapeutic agents are usually unsuccessful in the treatment of adenocarcinoma of the colon. 5-Fluorouracil (5-FU) has been disappointing because of its poor efficacy. Methyl-CCNU in combination with 5-FU, or with 5-FU and streptozotocin, is being investigated. Most combination agent trials have not been very encouraging. For epidermoid cancers of the anal canal, the combination of mitomycin C and 5-FU in sequence with radiation has been effective in producing tumor regression preoperatively. Chemotherapy is most effective for liver metastases, and is not as effective as radiation for pelvic recurrence or an isolated single mass. Current trials suggest that there may be some benefit for adjuvant chemotherapy in patients with rectal cancer judged histologically to be at high risk of recurrence, but as yet no benefit has been demonstrated for patients with colonic cancer. There has also been interest in direct infusion of the liver with floxuridine (FUDR) and other agents through a surgically placed catheter connected to a pump implanted subcutaneously. The efficacy of this method compared to systemic chemotherapy is being studied in patients with liver metastases.

Most other primary malignancies of the colon are treated by resection. Metastatic disease to the colon may require surgery for obstruction or bleeding. Disseminated cancers involving the colon, such as lymphoma, melanoma, or breast cancer, usually require systemic treatment for the primary tumor.

PROGNOSIS AND FOLLOW-UP. The overall ten-year survival for patients after surgery for colorectal cancer is approximately 42 per cent. The survival correlates directly with the stage of the disease: cancer confined to the mucosa, 80 to 90 per cent ten-year survival; cancer extending through all areas of the bowel wall, 60 to 80 per cent; and cancer involving the regional lymph nodes, 50 to 60 per cent. Rectal cancers with node involvement, especially when they are low lying, have a lower ten-year survival than colonic cancers with node involvement.

Patients with regional node involvement may be entered into a program of adjuvant chemotherapy. Synchronous cancers and polyps that have not been removed either preoperatively or at the time of surgery should be removed within a few months postoperatively. At that time the anastomosis is usually brushed for cytologic study for any possible seeding that may have occurred at surgery. Colonoscopy can be repeated a year later and every three years thereafter, since new polyps require two to three years to grow large enough to have a premalignant potential. After surgery, patients without known metastases and not treated with adjuvant chemotherapy should be seen for history, physical examination, and laboratory tests (hematocrit, stool for occult blood, and liver function tests) at intervals of approximately every three months the first two years, then every six months through the fifth year, and annually thereafter.

CEA AND ESTABLISHED COLONIC CANCER. Measurement of circulating carcinoembryonic antigens (CEA) is not a reliable screening test for the early diagnosis of colonic cancer. There is some indication, however, that CEA levels may rise before any other clinical or laboratory abnormalities appear in patients with recurrent colonic cancer after surgery. The common cause for such an increase in the CEA is widespread metastatic disease, particularly involving the liver. In a few patients, however, rising CEA may reflect a small localized, potentially resectable intra-abdominal metastasis. Although still investigational, it has been suggested that the CEA be performed monthly during the first year postoperatively and perhaps every three months in the second and third years. If a significant rise in the CEA is detected, the patient should undergo an intensive investigation, including liver function tests, liver scan, colonoscopy, and chest x-ray; if all are negative, a "second look" exploration should be considered to search for a localized, potentially resectable intra-abdominal metastasis. In patients who have a rising CEA with negative workup, there is an 80 per cent chance of finding recurrent tumors, most of which are resectable. However, it is possible that this approach to recurrent disease not only would not help the patient but also would detract from the quality of life.

PREVENTION OF COLORECTAL CANCER. Prevention may be defined as (1) primary, the identification and eradication of agents in the environment that produce colorectal cancer, and attempted control of genetic factors; and (2) secondary, the identification and eradication of premalignant lesions, and the detection and resection of cancer while it is still curable. No effective primary preventive measures are now available. Despite the previously cited evidence that diet may be related in some way to the evolution of colorectal cancer, there is no current proof that proscription of any diet in favor of a low fat and high fiber regimen would be effective.

Secondary prevention as defined above has been more rewarding with the introduction of better methods of screening for early cancer or premalignant adenomas. Effective screening requires the application of relatively simple and inexpensive tests to a large number of people in order to identify those who are likely to have disease. There are several critical questions to consider in any screening program: (1) What are the expected benefits in terms of survival of those patients whose disease is discovered by screening tests and treated, and in terms of the possible mortality reduction from colorectal cancer in the entire screened population? (2) Can high-risk subgroups be identified?

(3) Are effective screening tests available? (4) Are community health resources adequate for the diagnostic workup and treatment of persons with positive screening tests? (5) What are the costs, patient compliance, and risks of screening?

It is justifiable to consider screening for colorectal cancer in the United States, since it is a high-risk country by worldwide epidemiologic standards. It is assumed that earlier diagnosis would lead to longer survival. In general, screening programs that have been in progress for colorectal cancer have demonstrated earlier staging and better survival of patients with cancer detected through screening but have not had sufficient time to prove that the screened group has a lower mortality from colorectal cancer. Screening for rectosigmoid cancer with periodic sigmoidoscopy may lead to earlier detection and improved long-term survival and even to a less than expected incidence of cancer at this anatomic site, probably because of identification and eradication of polyps. Screening for colorectal cancer can be classified in two ways: general screening of patients at average risk, and screening of patients in high-risk subgroups.

Average-Risk Patients. In average-risk groups (all of those not in one of the defined high-risk groups), suggested screening includes testing stool specimens for occult blood annually with impregnated guaiac slides (Hemoccult, SmithKline Diagnostics, Sunnyvale, California) and by sigmoidoscopy every three to five years (Fig. 106–8). Guaiac solutions, Hematest, and benzidine have been discarded because of too many false-negative and false-positive results. Testing with six slides over a period of three days, with the patient making smears from two different parts of the same stool each day while on a high fiber, meat-free diet, has resulted in detection of early colorectal cancer. Current trials using this approach have been promising but need further time for long-term results. This test is useful only in totally asymptomatic patients and should not be used as a substitute for clinical judgment in patients who have symptoms of neoplastic disease or who have already reported a history of rectal bleeding. The effective utilization of this test requires follow-up studies of patients who have positive tests, positive being defined as one or more positive slides. Diagnostic workup must include not only a double contrast barium enema but also colonoscopy to search for lesions that are missed by the barium enema and an UGI series if no colonic neoplasm is detected. Approximately 50 per cent of patients with positive tests will have neoplastic lesions, mostly adenomas but also colorectal cancers. More specific fecal occult blood tests using immunologic methods are being evaluated. The fecal occult blood test is not very sensitive for rectosigmoid tumors and therefore is complemented by sigmoidoscopy. Rigid sigmoidoscopes have been used; however, flexible scopes of 35 to 60 cm in length have been tested and appear to increase the yield of polyps and cancers and provide a more comfortable examination.

High-Risk Groups. GENETIC. Familial polyposis requires early surgery. Patients with a family history of polyposis or Gardner's syndrome should have sigmoidoscopy at least annually, beginning at puberty. Female patients with a history of genital or breast cancer should have periodic fecal occult blood testing and sigmoidoscopy, beginning as soon as they are identified. Patients with site-specific colonic cancer or the family cancer syndrome must be examined with barium enema and/or colonoscopy beginning at age 20, since one cannot comfortably rely only on fecal occult blood testing in these very high-risk patients. A reasonable screening approach would be a fecal occult blood test annually and colonoscopy every three to five years. The search would be primarily for adenomas, for which the colonoscope is much more sensitive than x-ray. The number of patients with nonpolyposis inherited colon cancer syndromes is not known, but probably is greater than currently appreciated.

PRIOR ADENOMA OR COLONIC CANCER. Patients with a prior history of adenoma or colonic cancer should be examined periodically by colonoscopy. Once the colon has been cleared of all synchronous lesions, screening every three to five years is sufficient, since excisable metachronous lesions usually do not develop sooner and often require years to evolve.

SCREENING FOR COLORECTAL CANCER

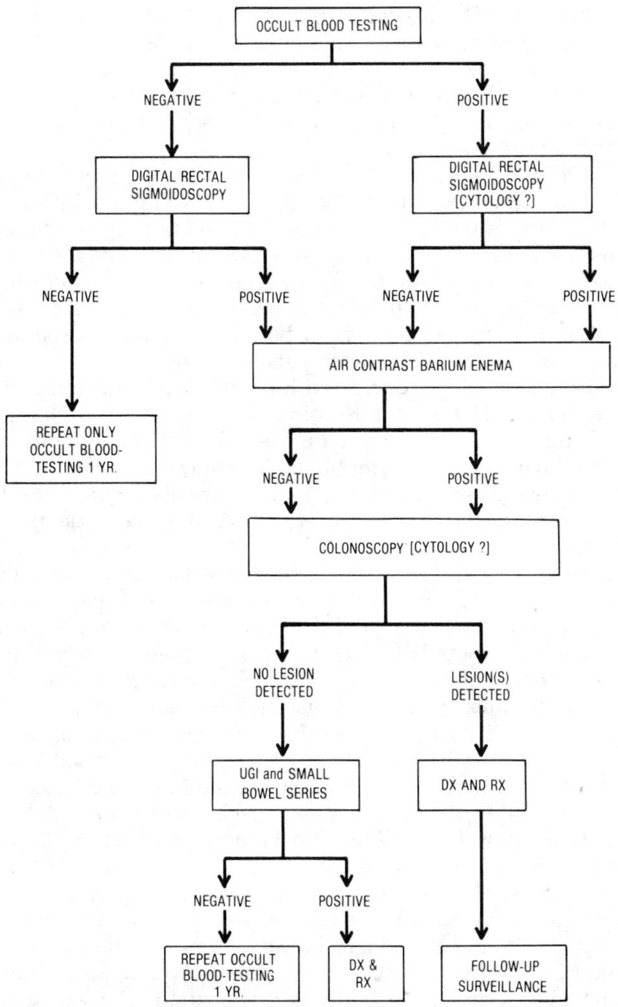

Figure 106–8. This screening approach is currently in process and under evaluation at Memorial Hospital, New York, N.Y., and is suggested for asymptomatic people 40 years of age and over without any other associated risk factors. It can also be considered for people at increased risk because of past history or family history, but should be instituted at a younger age. The initial testing of stools for occult blood is of no value in the presence of known associated colonic disease. Cytologic lavage is incorporated in the above schema where it is currently being done in this program, but its role in the asymptomatic patient is yet to be determined. Colonoscopy is suggested even in the presence of positive findings, to search for synchronous lesions and/or clarify the nature of demonstrated abnormalities. (From Winawer SJ, et al.: Gastroenterology 70:783, 1976. Reprinted with the kind permission of the publishers.)

ULCERATIVE COLITIS. No well established data exist on the optimal detection of cancer early in ulcerative colitis or granulomatous colitis, or at what intervals screening should be conducted. One suggestion is that multiple biopsies be obtained by colonoscopy once a year or once every other year after the patient has had universal colitis for seven years or left-sided colitis for 15 years. If moderate or severe dysplasia is seen on these biopsies and confirmed in several specimens at several examinations, total colectomy should be considered. Patients with granulomatous colitis should be evaluated endoscopically if they have a change in their symptoms or develop a stricture (which may harbor a tumor).

NEOPLASMS OF THE SMALL INTESTINE

EPIDEMIOLOGY. Cancer is rare in the small intestine; only about 2000 cases occur in the United States each year. Small bowel cancer, like cancer of the large intestine, is more common in developed Western countries than in underdeveloped countries. With rare exceptions, the incidence for males is higher than that for females.

ETIOLOGY AND RISK FACTORS. Some cancers originating in the small intestine are related to pre-existing premalignant states, such as Crohn's disease of the small intestine or gluten-sensitive enteropathy. Small intestinal cancer may rarely develop from polyps of the Peutz-Jeghers syndrome or from polyps in patients with familial polyposis or Gardner's syndrome. The incidence of small bowel malignancy, especially lymphoma, is also increased in patients with various hereditary syndromes involving decreased humoral or cellular immunity. Lymphoma is by far the most common malignancy complicating celiac disease. A particular type of small intestinal lymphoma, called Mediterranean lymphoma, is endemic in the Middle East, affecting Sephardic Jews, Arabs, Armenians, and Iranians; environmental factors in the area have not been adequately studied.

Several hypotheses have been suggested to explain this striking rarity of small intestinal malignancies, especially adenocarcinomas, as compared to adenocarcinomas of the colon. The bacterial population of the colon, quantitatively much greater than that of the small intestine, may convert bile acids or other products to carcinogens. Ingested carcinogens may be diluted in the small intestine by the large volume of liquid present there. Also, the transit time through the small bowel is much faster than through the colon, limiting the exposure of the small intestinal epithelium to carcinogens. The rapid cell proliferation of the small intestinal mucosa may also be important in preventing malignancy.

PATHOLOGY. Four types of neoplasms, adenocarcinomas, carcinoids, lymphomas, and leiomyosarcomas, account for over 95 per cent of malignant small bowel tumors. The most common tumor of the small intestine is asymptomatic benign carcinoid, most often found at postmortem examination. The most common tumor detected clinically in the small intestine is metastatic malignancy (lymphoma, melanoma, and carcinoma of the breast, kidney, ovary, and testicle). Adenocarcinomas are most common in the proximal small intestine, and carcinoids and lymphomas are most common in the distal small intestine.

CLINICAL MANIFESTATIONS. Small carcinoid tumors are asymptomatic, but larger carcinoid tumors can obstruct or bleed. The vast majority of symptomatic carcinoid tumors produce features of the carcinoid syndrome; the primary tumor of the small intestine is asymptomatic (see Ch. 242). Leiomyosarcomas often cause bleeding, and lymphomas present with a spectrum of clinical manifestations, including intestinal obstruction, bleeding, fever, or malabsorption. Adenocarcinomas have characteristic clinical presentations, depending on their location: in the postbulbar area they may simulate peptic ulcer disease; in the periampullary area they can obstruct the common bile duct causing jaundice; and beyond the periampullary area they can obstruct the bowel. Adenocarcinomas of the distal small bowel usually develop as a complication of Crohn's disease and are most often found at surgery in patients operated on for longstanding Crohn's disease and obstruction. The clinical manifestation of benign polyps of the small intestine is usually bleeding. Most, however, are silent.

DIFFERENTIAL DIAGNOSIS. Tumors of the small intestine that present with bleeding or obstruction of the small bowel must be differentiated from many other causes of these symptoms. Bleeding can be secondary to Meckel's diverticulum, vascular anomaly, or duodenal ulcer, among other diagnoses. Obstruction can be due to adhesions, internal hernias, volvulus, or strictures. Obstructive jaundice can be due to tumors in the area of the ampulla as well as to carcinoma of the pancreas, bile duct cancer, impacted common duct stone, acute pancreatitis, and many other causes. Investigation of a patient with suspected small bowel tumor depends on the location and the clinical presentation. Patients presenting with atypical duodenal ulcer disease usually require upper gastrointestinal x-rays. Patients presenting with obstructive jaundice usually require sonography and either percutaneous transhepatic cholangiography or ERCP. Those with small intestinal obstruction require a period of decompression followed by radiologic study of the small bowel. Where tumors are accessible to direct visualization, such as the terminal ileum by colonoscopy and ileoscopy, or the upper duodenal area by upper gastrointestinal endoscopy, the procedures should be performed to confirm the presence of tumor and to obtain a tissue diagnosis.

THERAPY. Treatment is primarily surgical for adenocarcinomas, leiomyosarcomas, and malignant carcinoids. Primary lymphoma of the small intestine is usually treated surgically, although in poor-risk patients radiation therapy may provide the same benefit. Radiation therapy may be used postoperatively if there is evidence of spread beyond the bowel wall. If the lymphoma of the small intestine is part of a disseminated process, then chemotherapy is usually the treatment of choice (see Ch. 158).

PROGNOSIS AND PREVENTION. The prognosis of small intestinal adenocarcinomas is generally poor, with survival extremely low for the majority of patients. The prognosis for leiomyosarcoma and primary lymphomas of the small bowel is good if the lesion can be entirely removed by surgical resection, but this is rarely possible. Patients with malignant carcinoid tumors may survive for long periods, even after extensive metastases (see Ch. 242).

So little is known of the etiology of carcinoid tumors and leiomyosarcomas of the small bowel that no speculation regarding their prevention can be made. Primary small intestinal lymphomas could possibly be decreased in the Middle East by public health measures that decrease the high incidence of chronic bowel inflammation and parasitic infestation in this area. Diagnosis and treatment of celiac disease may reduce the frequency of superimposed malignancies. Surgical resection, rather than bypass, for Crohn's disease may decrease the incidence of adenocarcinoma in this high-risk group. In Peutz-Jeghers and multiple polyposis syndromes, adenomas in the duodenum could be monitored and potentially removed endoscopically.

General Review

Winawer SJ, Sherlock P: Malignant neoplasms of the small and large intestine. *In* Sleisenger MH, Fordtran JS (eds.): Gastrointestinal Disease. 3rd ed. Philadelphia, W. B. Saunders Company, 1983, pp 1220–1249.

Epidemiology

Schottenfeld D, Winawer SJ: Large intestine. *In* Schottenfeld D, Fraumeni J Jr (eds.): Cancer Epidemiology and Prevention. Philadelphia, W. B. Saunders Company, 1982, pp 703–727. *A critical overview of the present concepts in the worldwide epidemiology of large bowel cancer.*

Etiology

Weisburger JH, Reddy BS, Spingarn NE, Wynder EJ: Current views on the mechanism involved in the etiology of colorectal cancer. Burkitt DP: Fibre in the aetiology of colorectal cancer. Goldin B: The role of diet and the intestinal flora in the etiology of large bowel cancer. *In* Winawer SJ, Schottenfeld D, Sherlock P (eds.): Colorectal Cancer: Prevention, Epidemiology, and Screening. Progress in Cancer Research, Vol 13. New York, Raven Press, 1980, pp 19–41. *This series of papers reviews the evidence for the three major factors (fat, fiber, and bacterial flora) currently felt to be important in the etiology of colorectal cancer.*

Screening and Risk

Devroede G: Risk of cancer in inflammatory bowel disease. *In* Winawer SJ, Schottenfeld D, Sherlock P (eds.): Colorectal Cancer: Prevention, Epidemiology, and Screening. Progress in Cancer Research. Vol. 13, New York, Raven Press, 1980, pp 325–334. *This paper carefully examines the relative risk among the subgroups of patients with inflammatory bowel disease.*

Gilbertsen VA, Nelms JM: The prevention of invasive cancer of the rectum. Cancer 41:1137, 1978. *Unique long-term study demonstrating the impact of proctosigmoidoscopy on the natural history of rectosigmoid cancer.*

Kussin SZ, Lipkin M, Winawer SJ: Inherited colon cancer: Clinical implications. Am J Gastroenterol (State of the Art) 72:448, 1979. *A review of the literature of inherited colonic cancer with a focus on the possible link of genetic factors to sporadic cancer.*

Winawer SJ, Sherlock P, Schottenfeld D, Miller DG: Screening for colon cancer. Gastroenterology 70:783, 1976. *Presentation of a rational approach to the consideration of risk factors as a basis for screening. A resource.*

Diagnosis

Hunt RH, Waye JD: Colonoscopy: Techniques. Clinical Practices and Colour Atlas. London, Chapman and Hall, 1981. *An extremely informative book on all aspects of colonoscopy.*

Winawer SJ, Leidner SD, Hajdu SI, Sherlock P: Colonoscopic biopsy and cytology in the diagnosis of colon cancer. Cancer 42:2849, 1978. *This paper presents data on the usefulness of tissue sampling techniques and discusses their clinical application.*

Treatment

Stearns MW Jr: Neoplasms of the Colon, Rectum, and Anus. New York, John Wiley & Sons, 1980. *Many aspects of treatment of colorectal cancer are presented in depth in this monograph, which is written by Memorial Sloan-Kettering Cancer Center physicians, including surgery, chemotherapy, and radiation.*

Carcinoembryonic Antigen (CEA)

Zamcheck N: Current status of CEA. *In* Winawer SJ, Schottenfeld D, Sherlock P (eds.): Colorectal Cancer: Prevention, Epidemiology, and Screening. Progress in Cancer Research. Vol. 13. New York, Raven Press, 1980, pp 219–234. *The current status of CEA in the follow-up of patients after surgery is discussed in detail in this paper by one of the senior investigators in the field.*

Prevention

Lennard-Jones JW, Morson BC, Ritchie JK, Shove DC, Williams CB: Cancer in colitis: Assessment of the individual risk by clinical and histological criteria. Gastroenterology 73:1280, 1977. *Evidence for dysplasia as an important tool in patients with ulcerative colitis is presented by the group that first called attention to the concept.*

Sherlock P, Lipkin M, Winawer SJ: The prevention of colon cancer. A combined clinical and basic science seminar. Am J Med 68:917, 1980. *Screening is examined from the viewpoint of the spectrum of risk, with heavy emphasis on markers being investigated in high-risk groups.*

Winawer SJ: Screening for colorectal cancer: An overview. Cancer 45:1093, 1980. *An overview of the issues that are involved in considerations of screening.*

Winawer SJ, Fleisher M, Baldwin M, Sherlock P: Current status of fecal occult blood testing in screening for colorectal cancer. Ca 32:100, 1982. *A comprehensive review of the background and status of fecal occult blood testing.*

Small Intestine

Lightdale CJ, Koepsell TD, Sherlock P: Small intestine. *In* Schottenfeld D, Fraumeni JF Jr (eds.): Cancer, Epidemiology and Prevention. Philadelphia, W. B. Saunders Company, 1982, pp 692–702. *An excellent review of various epidemiologic and etiologic aspects of small intestinal tumors.*

107. PANCREATITIS

Michael D. Levitt

The pathogenesis of pancreatitis remains obscure and treatment is therefore supportive rather than specific. Only in the area of diagnostic procedures have there been major recent advances. The physician can now diagnose acute and chronic pancreatitis accurately, but the ability to influence the course of the disease has progressed little during the past 10 years.

NORMAL ANATOMY AND PHYSIOLOGY OF EXOCRINE PANCREAS. The exocrine pancreas consists of acinar cells that synthesize digestive enzymes. These enzymes reside in zymogen granules within the cells and are deposited into the central ductule of the acinus. The ductules coalesce to form larger ducts, finally draining into the main pancreatic duct (Wirsung), which empties into the duodenum at the ampulla of Vater. Pancreatic secretion is stimulated by two hormones produced in the duodenum: (1) secretin, which is released in response to acid in the duodenum, stimulates a pancreatic juice high in volume and [HCO_3^-]; (2) cholecystokinin-pancreozymin (CCK-PZ), which is released in response to fatty acids and amino acids in the duodenum and results in a secretion rich in enzymes.

The enzymes secreted by the pancreas are grouped into those that digest starch (amylase), fat (lipases), and protein (trypsin and other proteolytic enzymes). The proteolytic enzymes are secreted in an inactive form, thus preventing autodigestion of the pancreas. Trypsinogen is activated to trypsin in the duodenal lumen, and trypsin then activates the other proteolytic enzymes. Protease inhibitors in the pancreas and pancreatic juice provide additional protection against autodigestion.

CLASSIFICATION OF PANCREATITIS. Pancreatitis is classified as acute or chronic by clinical or pathologic criteria. Clinically, an attack of pancreatitis is defined as *acute* if the patient becomes asymptomatic following recovery, whereas in *chronic* pancreatitis the patient has persistent pain or insufficient exocrine or endocrine pancreatic secretion. The term *relapsing* denotes recurrent attacks that may occur in either acute or chronic pancreatitis. The pathologic findings in acute pancreatitis range from mild interstitial edema (which may not warrant the designation of pancreatitis), to acute inflammatory infiltrate, to necrosis and hemorrhage with virtually complete destruction of the gland. Since laparotomy is contraindicated in acute pancreatitis, pancreatic pathology is seldom documented by examination of tissue. Chronic pancreatitis is characterized by the disappearance of acinar tissue and the presence of fibrosis, calcification, and cyst formation. Frequency data for pancreatitis are limited. Pancreatitis will occur in roughly 0.5 per cent of the population and accounts for about one death annually per 100,000 population.

Acute Pancreatitis

PATHOGENESIS. The final common pathway of acute pancreatitis is thought to be autodigestion by activated enzymes. Although the exact mechanism that provokes this process of autodigestion remains speculative there is an association between pancreatitis and the clinical conditions listed in Table 107–1. Familiarity with these conditions is useful clinically, since the diagnosis of pancreatitis is often suggested by the coexistence of one of these states, and the prevention of recurrent pancreatitis usually hinges on the elimination of the predisposing condition. No cause of acute pancreatitis is uncovered in about 15 per cent of cases.

In the United States, the majority of patients with acute pancreatitis have alcoholism or gallstones as an etiologic factor. Alcoholic pancreatitis develops in susceptible persons after heavy ethanol ingestion for many years. Chronic alcoholism may produce proteinaceous plugs in the small pancreatic ducts, causing atrophy of the acini drained by the obstructed duct. These chronic, irreversible pathologic changes antedate the first attack of acute pancreatitis, and 10 per cent of alcoholics develop pancreatic insufficiency without a recognized acute attack. The factors triggering the superimposition of an acute attack on this chronic process are not understood.

Patients with gallstone pancreatitis virtually always have gallstones in their feces, whereas a much lower frequency of fecal stones is found in patients with gallstones who do not have pancreatitis. Thus, passage of a gallstone through the ampulla of Vater creates conditions favorable to the development of pancreatitis. This condition is not simply obstruction, since ligation of the ampulla does not cause pancreatitis. Rather, some factor such as reflux of biliary or duodenal contents or stimulation of pancreatic secretion appears necessary to produce pancreatitis. This "large duct" form of pancreatitis differs from the "small duct" type observed in alcoholics in that the

TABLE 107–1. ETIOLOGIC FACTORS IN PANCREATITIS

- Alcoholism
- Biliary tract disease
- Trauma—postoperative, abdominal injuries, post-ERCP
- Infections—mumps, coxsackievirus and echovirus, mycoplasma, parasitosis
- Metabolic—hyperlipidemia, hyperparathyroidism, pregnancy, uremia, post-renal transplant
- Drugs
  - Multiple reports
    - Immunosuppressive—corticosteroids, azathioprine, L-asparaginase
    - Diuretics—thiazides, furosemide, ethacrynic acid
    - Miscellaneous—phenformin, oral contraceptives, tetracycline
  - Rare or questionable reports
    - Acetaminophen, isoniazid, rifampin, propoxyphene
- Vascular—shock. lupus erythematosus, periarteritis, atheromatous embolism
- Mechanical—pancreas divisum, and ampullary stenosis, ampulla of Vater tumor, duodenal diverticula, duodenal Crohn's disease, duodenal surgery
- Penetrating duodenal ulcer
- Familial

former seldom leads to chronic pancreatitis or pancreatic calcifications and is cured by cholecystectomy.

Postoperative pancreatitis is the third most commonly identified cause of acute pancreatitis. Although pancreatitis may follow any type of abdominal surgery, biliary tract procedures and retroperitoneal node dissections have the highest incidence of this complication.

Hypertriglyceridemia, often with lactescent serum, occurs in about 15 per cent of patients with acute pancreatitis. Many of these patients are alcoholics who have an underlying abnormality of lipid metabolism, which is particularly pronounced during the acute attack. The apparent decrease in frequency of attacks of pancreatitis following dietary therapy for hypertriglyceridemia suggests that hyperlipidemia is a cause of pancreatitis.

Vascular insufficiency of the pancreas is a more common cause of pancreatitis than is generally recognized. Pancreatitis (usually asymptomatic) was observed in postmortem examination of 10 per cent of patients who died with hemorrhagic shock. Pancreatitis is a well-recognized complication of ischemia resulting from vasculitis or cholesterol emboli.

Pancreas divisum is a common (5 per cent) anatomic variant in which the portion of the pancreas (tail, body, and part of head) derived from the embryological dorsal pancreas is drained through the duct of Santorini and the minor papilla rather than via the duct of Wirsung and the ampulla of Vater. Pancreas divisum occurs in 20 to 25 per cent of patients with otherwise unexplained pancreatitis. Presumably, this variant drainage is sometimes inadequate, although sphincterotomy of the minor ampulla has yielded only equivocal benefit in the prevention of pancreatitis.

A number of drugs have been linked to the development of pancreatitis (Table 107–1). This linkage is generally rather weak with the exception of antimetabolites such as L-asparginase, which is associated with a 10 per cent frequency of pancreatitis. Frequently it is difficult to exclude the possibility that pancreatitis is a complication of the disease for which the drug was prescribed. For example, the high frequency of pancreatitis reported in patients taking diuretics may reflect the increased incidence of pancreatitis in patients with various forms of vascular disease.

Pancreatitis may be inherited as an autosomal dominant trait, which often begins in childhood. This type of pancreatitis has an increased incidence of late-developing pancreatic carcinoma.

CLINICAL PRESENTATION. The hallmark of acute pancreatitis is *abdominal pain.* This diagnosis should be considered in every patient presenting with abdominal discomfort. The time from onset to peak intensity of the pain ranges from seconds to hours. The pain, which tends to be steady rather than colicky, varies in intensity from minor to agonizing. At the onset of the attack, the pain is often localized to the epigastrium and left upper quadrant, but as the attack progresses, it becomes diffuse and radiates to the back. The back pain results from retroperitoneal irritation and is partially relieved by flexing the trunk. Acute pancreatitis may be relatively painless, and massive hemorrhagic necrosis of the gland, frequently in postoperative patients, may be an unexpected postmortem finding. *Vomiting* occurs in 70 to 90 per cent of the cases, but often brings about only minimal relief of the abdominal discomfort. The past medical history is important, since pancreatitis is usually associated with one of the underlying conditions listed in Table 107–1, and there frequently is *a previous history* of similar attacks of pain.

Nonspecific physical findings include fever, tachycardia, and hypotension. *Abdominal tenderness* is virtually always present; however, abdominal guarding and rigidity may be surprisingly slight, given the apparent distress of the patient. Although rarely palpable on initial examination, an abdominal mass subsequently develops in 10 to 20 per cent of patients. Occasionally, in hemorrhagic pancreatitis, retroperitoneal blood dissects into the flanks or around the umbilicus, producing Grey Turner's or Cullen's sign, respectively.

History and physical examination are seldom diagnostic of acute pancreatitis, and the differential diagnosis includes all causes of abdominal pain. Features favoring the existence of pancreatitis include a left upper quadrant component of the pain (as opposed to the right-sided nature of gallbladder pain), steady pain (as opposed to the colic of bowel disease), vomiting that does not relieve pain (the discomfort of gastritis and bowel obstruction are transiently relieved by vomiting), and abdominal rigidity less than that expected for pain (perforated peptic ulcer has marked rigidity). The absence of a condition associated with pancreatitis (Table 107–1) reduces the possibility of pancreatitis, whereas a previous history of documented pancreatitis is the single most reliable indicator that the present attack is also due to pancreatitis.

LABORATORY TEST. ***Amylase.*** In few disease states does the diagnosis rely so heavily on a single laboratory determination as is the case with acute pancreatitis and the measurement of serum amylase. The patient with abdominal pain and an elevated serum or urine amylase level is usually considered to have pancreatitis, whereas a patient with identical symptoms and physical findings but normal amylase levels seldom is diagnosed as having pancreatitis. The sensitivity and specificity of the amylase measurements cannot be evaluated, since the actual presence or absence of pancreatitis is seldom verified by some independent, more reliable technique.

Amylase is produced in large quantity by the pancreas, salivary glands, and certain malignant tumors, and in lesser quantity by the fallopian tubes and lungs. Normally, most of the amylase secreted by the pancreas and salivary glands enters and is confined to the gut. A small fraction enters the plasma accounting for the normal serum amylase activity, of which about two thirds is salivary isoamylase and one third pancreatic isoamylase.

In pancreatitis, increased quantities of pancreatic amylase escape into the lymph and blood flow of the pancreas. An increase in pressure in the pancreatic duct owing to obstruction or injection of contrast material during endoscopic retrograde cholangiopancreatography (ERCP) causes amylase to regurgitate into the plasma usually with little or no accompanying inflammation.

Amylase is cleared from the plasma with a half-life of about two hours, about 20 per cent being excreted in the urine. Two thirds of the amylase filtered by the glomerulus is normally reabsorbed or catabolized by the renal tubule.

A variety of conditions other than pancreatitis may cause an elevated serum amylase level. Inflammation or trauma to the salivary glands causes excessive release of salivary amylase into the serum. Chronic, unexplained elevations of serum amylase activity are almost always due to increases in salivary-type isoamylase, although there is usually no clinical evidence of salivary gland disease. In mesenteric infarction and perforated peptic ulcer, amylase from the intestinal lumen may leak into the circulation. These conditions must always be differentiated from pancreatitis in patients with abdominal pain and hyperamylasemia. Ruptured ectopic pregnancy, ovarian cysts, and various forms of pulmonary disease have also been reported to be associated with elevations of serum amylase. A chronic, very high serum amylase level may result from the production of amylase by metastatic tumors originating in the lung, reproductive tract, or pancreas. Serum amylase levels may also be elevated because of slow clearance from the blood. Uncomplicated renal failure is commonly associated with serum amylase values up to two times normal; higher levels suggest associated pancreatitis. Macroamylasemia is an asymptomatic state in which amylase is bound to serum proteins, thus forming a complex that is slowly cleared from the serum. Confusion results when the macroamylasemic patient has associated abdominal pain.

The rate of excretion of amylase in the urine is increased out of proportion to the serum amylase level in pancreatitis and may be elevated when the serum amylase is normal. This disproportionate elevation apparently results from the inhibition of tubular reabsorption of amylase in acute pancreatitis; thus, a greater portion of the filtered amylase appears in the urine. Although a more sensitive indicator of pancreatitis than is the serum level, the urinary amylase may be falsely normal when renal failure complicates pancreatitis. Spuriously elevated values occur in virtually all the nonpancreatitic conditions that cause hyperamylasemia (except macroamylasemia and renal disease) and in a variety of conditions with proximal renal tubular malfunction, including thermal burns, diabetic acidosis, and postoperative states.

Measurement of the ratio of the renal clearance of amylase and of creatinine (C_{Am}:C_{Cr})* has been used as an indicator of the efficiency with which the kidney excretes amylase relative to creatinine. C_{Am}:C_{Cr} (normal values: 1 to 4 per cent) is elevated in most patients with acute pancreatitis, reduced in macroamylasemia, and normal to low in patients with salivary hyperamylasemia.

Serum amylase originates from a variety of organs in addition to the pancreas, but serum lipase, trypsin, or pancreatic isoamylase are derived almost entirely from the pancreas. These enzymes, although technically more difficult to measure than amylase, may therefore provide in the future a more specific and sensitive indicator of pancreatitis.

The appropriate interpretation of amylase measurements may be summarized as follows. The patient with an acute attack of abdominal pain and an elevated serum amylase activity in all likelihood has acute pancreatitis, provided that perforated ulcer and bowel infarction are excluded. An elevated urinary amylase with a normal serum amylase is suggestive, but less diagnostic, of pancreatitis. The height of the amylase elevation does not correlate with the severity of the pancreatitis. For example, extremely high values, which return to normal over one to two days, are often associated with the passage of common duct stone and minimal, if any, inflammation of the pancreas. Elevation of amylase activity beyond seven days is usually associated with relatively severe pancreatitis, and a protracted clinical course and elevation for more than 14 days suggests the possibility of a pseudocyst or pancreatic ascites. Chronic elevations of serum amylase activity associated with mild or no abdominal symptoms are seldom due to pancreatic disease but rather to renal failure, macroamylasemia, salivary hyperamylasemia, or tumor hyperamylasemia. The use of C_{Am}:C_{Cr} should be restricted largely to patients with hyperamylasemia of unknown origin. A high ratio suggests pancreatitis; a normal ratio, salivary hyperamylasemia; and a very low value, macroamylasemia. Serum isoamylase assay can readily distinguish pancreatic from salivary hyperamylasemia. Serum lipase levels can also be used to distinguish pancreatic from salivary hyperamylasemia, since lipase is not produced by the salivary gland.

Other Laboratory Tests. A variety of other laboratory values may be abnormal in pancreatitis. The leukocyte count is usually elevated. Early in the course of acute pancreatitis, the hematocrit often rises to supranormal levels owing to *hemoconcentration* resulting from the massive loss of serum into the peritoneal and retroperitoneal spaces. *Hyperglycemia* often occurs, possibly resulting from increased glucagon and/or decreased insulin release. The serum in pancreatitis is frequently lactescent, and for unknown reasons the serum amylase level is frequently normal in this situation. *Hypocalcemia* is indicative of severe pancreatitis and is postulated to result from sequestration of calcium in soaps in areas of fat necrosis. In addition, there is a probable failure of the usual mechanisms that regulate calcium homeostasis. The presence of any of these nonspecific findings—elevated hematocrit, hyperglycemia, hypocalcemia, or hyperlipemia—in a patient with abdominal pain should always arouse suspicion of acute pancreatitis. Methemalbuminemia results from the extravascular destruction of hemoglobin and is the only laboratory finding that directly indicates that the pancreatitis is hemorrhagic. Evidence of cholestasis (elevated serum bilirubin and alkaline phosphatase) occurs in as many as 25 per cent of patients with acute pancreatitis, owing to compression of the common bile duct as it passes through the edematous pancreas. The cholestasis usually clears spontaneously in seven to ten days.

Roentgenograms. Roentgenograms of the abdomen should be obtained to rule out the presence of free air, signifying a perforation. In pancreatitis nonspecific ileus is usually observed. Somewhat more specific for pancreatitis, but not diagnostic, are localized gas collections in loops of bowel overlying the pancreas.

Imaging Techniques. Until recently, the pancreas could be only indirectly visualized radiographically via its impression on other viscera. The development of techniques to visualize the pancreas directly by means of ultrasound, computed tomography (CT), and ERCP has marked a great advance. The role of ultrasound and CT scanning in the diagnosis of acute pancreatitis has not been fully established. Both techniques show a diffusely enlarged pancreas in 70 to 90 per cent of patients during an acute attack of pancreatitis (Figs. 107–1 and 107–2). It is not clear if such visualization appreciably enhances the diagnostic accuracy of the cheaper and quicker amylase assay. ERCP exacerbates acute pancreatitis and is contraindicated during an acute attack.

TREATMENT. About 50 per cent of patients with acute pancreatitis have relatively mild and self-limited disease and probably would recover without benefit of medical therapy; 40 per cent are quite ill but survive their attack; and 10 per cent succumb despite the best of therapy. Virtually all deaths occur during the first or second attack of acute pancreatitis, recurrent attacks having a very low mortality rate. It is frequently difficult

A
 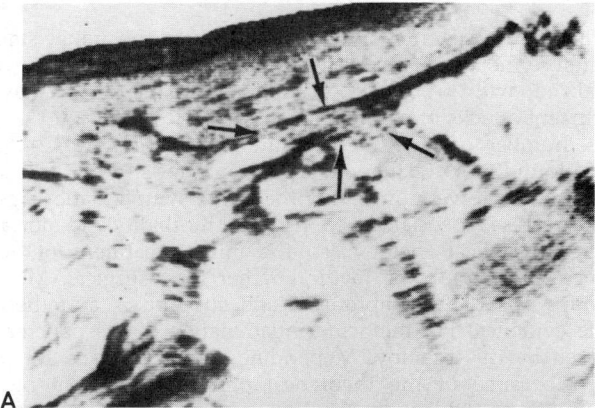
B
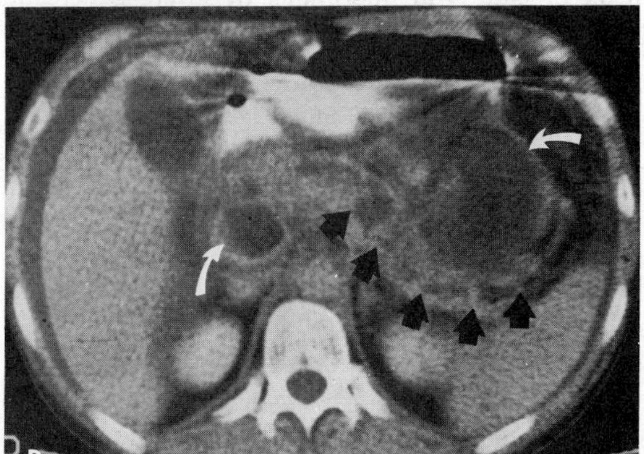

Figure 107–1. Normal pancreas demonstrated by ultrasound (above) and computed tomography (below). (Courtesy of Dr. Eugene P. DiMagno, Mayo Medical School, Rochester, Minnesota.)

---

*Calculated as follows: $C_{Am}:C_{Cr} = \frac{[Am]\ urine}{[Am]\ serum} \times \frac{[Cr]\ serum}{[Cr]\ urine}$

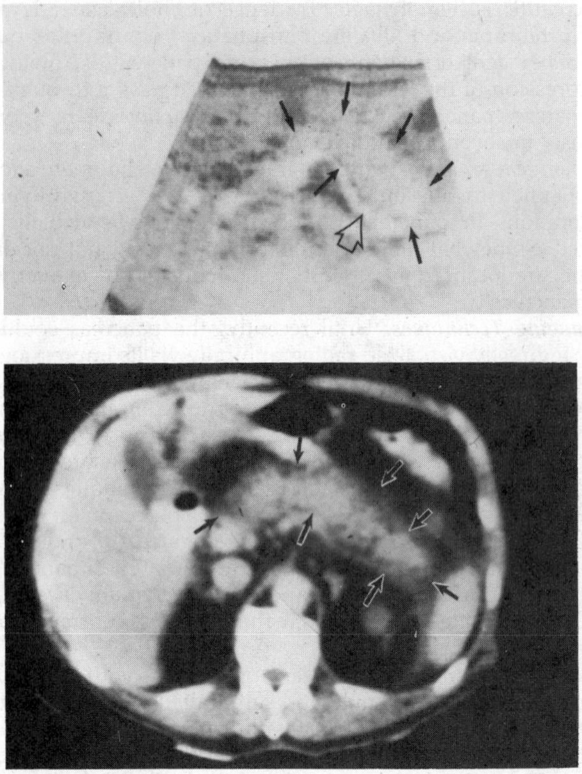

Figure 107–2. Diffusely enlarged pancreas of acute pancreatitis demonstrated by ultrasound (above) and computed tomography (below). The large arrow on the sonogram points to the splenic vein. (Courtesy of Dr. Henry I. Goldberg, Department of Radiology, University of California at San Francisco.)

to judge the severity of the attack during the initial stages; therefore most patients with acute pancreatitis should be hospitalized, with a possible exception being the patient having recurrent attacks of chronic pancreatitis.

A number of objective measurements (Table 107–2) have been found to correlate with a poor prognosis.

Surgical intervention during the acute, symptomatic stage of pancreatitis is associated with a greater morbidity and mortality than is medical therapy, so the initial treatment of acute pancreatitis should be medical rather than surgical. Medical therapy is largely symptomatic and supportive, and there is little evidence that the acute inflammation of the pancreas is altered by this therapy. Meperidine should be used for pain relief because of the theoretical problem of spasm of the sphincter of Oddi with morphine. In severe pancreatitis, as much as 6 to 10 liters of plasma and blood may be sequestered in the retroperitoneal and peritoneal spaces. Prompt replacement of these losses with colloid or whole blood is probably the single most important aspect of the initial medical therapy. Such volume replacement probably accounts for recent sharp declines in the frequency with which acute renal failure complicates pancreatitis. In addition, this therapy helps maintain perfusion of the pancreas, a factor that seems to diminish the severity of experimental pancreatitis. Cautious insulin therapy is indicated for marked hyperglycemia, and intravenous calcium may be required for hypocalcemia.

For years, the major objective of therapy for acute pancreatitis was to "put the pancreas at rest" by reducing the humoral stimuli to pancreatic secretion. To this end, the patient received no oral alimentation and gastric suction was carried out to prevent gastric HCl from entering the duodenum, thus minimizing secretin release. This therapy was based on limited evidence of benefit in experimental pancreastitis and on the clinical observation that the abdominal pain of pancreatitis appeared to subside more rapidly following the initiation of nasogastric suction. Two recent controlled studies in mild to moderately severe pancreatitis failed to demonstrate any significant benefit from nasogastric suction and in such patients this form of therapy is optional. The value of suction in severe hemorrhagic pancreatitis has not been confirmed; however, the associated ileus that invariably complicates severe pancreatitis provides a strong indication for nasogastric suction. The use of peritoneal dialysis to remove toxins in the peritoneal cavity should be considered when the patient's condition deteriorates despite standard medical therapy. A randomized trial of peritoneal dialysis showed striking short-term benefit in severe pancreatitis; however, late deaths due to sepsis resulted in similar overall mortalities for the dialyzed and control groups.

A number of therapies have been shown to be ineffective in controlled studies: proteolytic enzyme inhibitors such as aprotinin (Trasylol), glucagon to reduce pancreatic secretion, anticholinergics to reduce gastric and pancreatic secretion, and prophylactic antibiotics to prevent infection in the pancreatic bed.

COMPLICATIONS. The most important complications associated with acute pancreatitis are listed in Table 107–3. In the absence of these complications, recovery usually occurs in one to two weeks. A frequent cause of death during the first few weeks of the illness is the development of the *adult respiratory distress syndrome* (ARDS) secondary to increased alveolar capillary permeability. Prompt recognition and treatment with O_2 and positive end-expiratory pressure (PEEP) breathing appear to be lifesaving in some of these patients. Necrosis, edema, and hemorrhage in the pancreatic bed and surrounding tissues may lead to formation of two types of mass lesions, which can be differentiated by sonography. A *phlegmon* is a solid, inflamed mass of pancreatic tissue that usually subsides spontaneously. A *pseudocyst* is a cystic collection of fluid and necrotic debris whose walls are variously formed by the pancreas and other surrounding organs (Fig. 107–3). Pseudocysts often communicate with a pancreatic duct and are, therefore, rich in pancreatic enzymes. A serious complication of either phlegmons or pseudocysts is the development of an *abscess*, which is usually heralded by increasing pain, hectic fever, and leukocytosis. Immediate surgical drainage of the lesion is indicated, since nonoperative therapy carries a mortality of nearly 100 per cent.

TABLE 107–2. ADVERSE PROGNOSTIC SIGNS IN ACUTE PANCREATITIS*

On admission:
- Age over 55
- Leukocyte count over 16,000/mm^3
- Blood glucose over 200 mg/dl
- Serum LDH over 350 IU/L
- Serum GOT over 250 sigma Frankel U/dl

During initial 48 hours:
- Hematocrit decrease over 10%
- BUN rise over 5 mg/dl
- Serum calcium below 8 mg/dl
- Arterial P_{O_2} below 60 mm Hg
- Base deficit over 4 mEq/L
- Estimated fluid sequestration over 6 L

*If fewer than three of these signs are present, mortality is negligible (<1 per cent) and few are seriously ill. If more than four signs are present, mortality may be 25 per cent and an additional 50 per cent of patients are seriously ill.

TABLE 107–3. COMPLICATIONS OF ACUTE PANCREATITIS

Pancreatic—phlegmon, pseudocyst, abscess, ascites, hemorrhage
Contiguous organs—portal venous thrombosis, bowel necrosis, intraperitoneal bleeding, obstruction of common duct
Systemic
- Cardiovascular—hypotension, nonspecific ST-T changes, pericardial effusion
- Pulmonary—pleural effusion, shock lung, atelectasis
- Renal—acute renal failure
- Gastrointestinal—gastritis
- Hematologic—disseminated intravascular coagulation
- Metabolic—hypocalcemia, hyperglycemia, hypertriglyceridemia
- Fat necrosis—subcutaneous, bone
- Central nervous system—psychosis

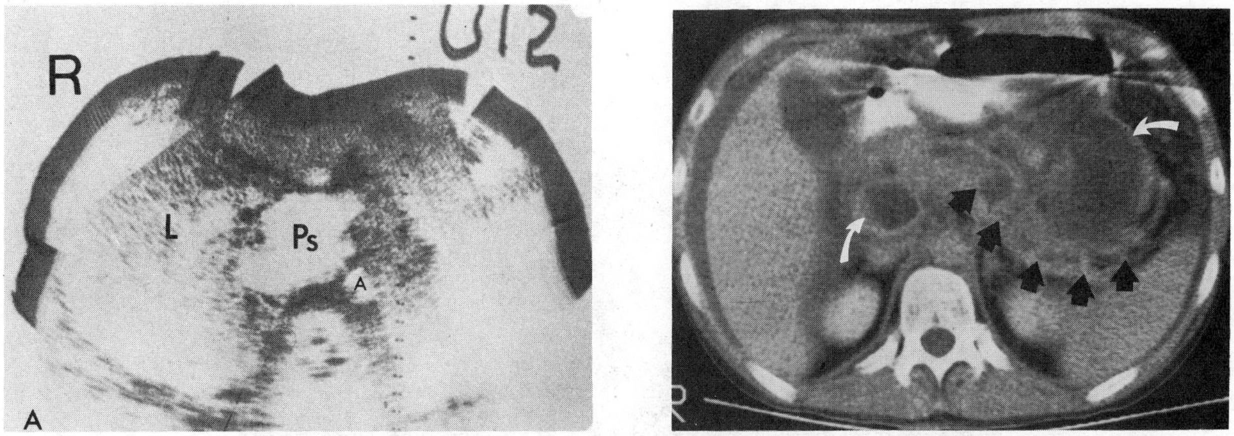

Figure 107–3. *A,* A pseudocyst demonstrated by ultrasound. Ps = pseudocyst; A = aorta; L = liver; R = right of patient. (Courtesy of Dr. Dennis A. Sarti, Dept. of Radiological Sciences, University of California at Los Angeles, and Radiology 125:789, 1977.) *B,* A CT scan through the region of the tail, body, and head of the pancreas demonstrates the presence of two pancreatic pseudocysts (curved white arrows). The larger of the two extends from the tail of the pancreas anteriorly to compress a portion of the greater curvature of the stomach, here denoted by contrast material in the dependent portion and an air/fluid level. The smaller of the two is well circumscribed and located in the head of the pancreas. Both pseudocysts are of low CT density and well-described margins. In addition, the pancreatic duct (black arrows) is dilated and irregular in contour, a finding typical of a chronic pancreatitis. (Courtesy of Dr. Henry Goldberg, University of California at San Francisco.)

Although large pseudocysts are usually palpable, smaller cysts are detected only by sonography or CT scanning. Many pseudocysts (particularly the smaller ones) are relatively asymptomatic and resolve spontaneously; some pseudocysts (usually the larger ones) cause marked discomfort and have the potentially lethal complications of hemorrhage or perforation. It is usually safe to follow smaller, asymptomatic pseudocysts or larger, uncomplicated cysts that are diminishing in size. The cyst that is expanding or causing appreciable discomfort should be drained, either surgically via anastomosis of the cyst to the gut or percutaneously via a needle. The indications for the traditional surgical as opposed to the newer percutaneous procedures remain to be determined. Complications of abscess, hemorrhage, or rupture require immediate surgical intervention.

It is very important to prevent the recurrence of acute pancreatitis by the treatment of conditions listed in Table 107–1. Abstinence from ethanol frequently does not prevent the progression of alcoholic pancreatitis but may reduce the frequency and severity of attacks. Studies to rule out the presence of gallstones are mandatory, since cholecystectomy in such patients nearly always prevents subsequent attacks. Cholecystectomy usually should be carried out after the subsidence of symptoms but during the initial hospitalization. Treatment of hypertriglyceridemia with a low calorie, low fat diet, as well as abstinence from alcohol, seems to prevent some subsequent attacks of hyperlipemic pancreatitis. Hypercalcemia as the cause of pancreatitis may be obscured during the acute attack and should be excluded by a serum calcium determination following recovery. ERCP should be performed in patients who have had more than one attack of otherwise unexplained pancreatitis. Lesions, potentially correctable by surgery, which may be detected by ERCP include small gallstones missed by sonography, an isolated stricture in the main pancreatic duct, an undetected pseudocyst, pancreas divisum, or ampullary stenosis.

Chronic Pancreatitis

ETIOLOGY. Chronic pancreatitis may be associated with most of the conditions listed in Table 107–1, with the exception of gallstone disease, which only produces recurrent acute attacks. Alcoholism is by far the most common cause of chronic pancreatitis in the United States; in some parts of the world, protein-calorie malnutrition is the major cause.

PATHOPHYSIOLOGY. In chronic alcoholism (with or without superimposed acute pancreatitis), proteinaceous plugs in the pancreatic ducts apparently lead to atrophy of the acinar tissue, fibrous tissue replacement, and dilatation of the ductular system. Calcification of these ductular plugs accounts for the diffuse stippled calcification of the pancreas observed in about 30 per cent of patients. Pseudocysts are also a frequent finding. The normal secretion of pancreatic enzymes far exceeds that required for digestion, and malabsorption occurs only when enzyme secretion falls to less than 10 per cent of normal. Clinically significant malabsorption of fat-soluble vitamins is relatively rare in pancreatic insufficiency (as compared with small bowel mucosal disease), since normal lipolysis is relatively unimportant for the absorption of the fat-soluble vitamins. The pathophysiology of pancreatic malabsorption is discussed in detail in Ch. 103. Impaired glucose tolerance is common, but diabetic ketosis and coma are rare. The vascular, neurologic, and renal complications of diabetes mellitus are seldom seen in the hyperglycemia of chronic pancreatitis. Vitamin B_{12} malabsorption occurs in about 50 per cent of patients with chronic alcoholic pancreatitis, because of failure to digest B_{12} binding proteins, but pernicious anemia is relatively uncommon.

CLINICAL MANIFESTATIONS. *Pain* is the predominant symptom in about 90 per cent of patients. It may take the form of recurrent acute attacks often superimposed on a background of low grade abdominal pain or relatively constant pain usually aggravated by food ingestion. The discomfort is most often epigastric and in the left upper quadrant with radiation to the back, and is characteristically relieved by forward flexion of the trunk. Physical examination of the abdomen usually reveals less abdominal tenderness than expected in view of the often disabling pain of which the patient complains.

As the disease progresses, insufficient pancreatic secretion results in *malabsorption* manifested by the passage of bulky, foul-smelling stools. The failure to digest triglycerides may result in the passage of fat droplets that float as a visible scum on the toilet water, a finding which indicates that the steatorrhea is due to pancreatic insufficiency rather than small bowel mucosal disease. The combination of malabsorption and poor oral intake often leads to appreciable weight loss. Malabsorption is described more extensively in Ch. 103.

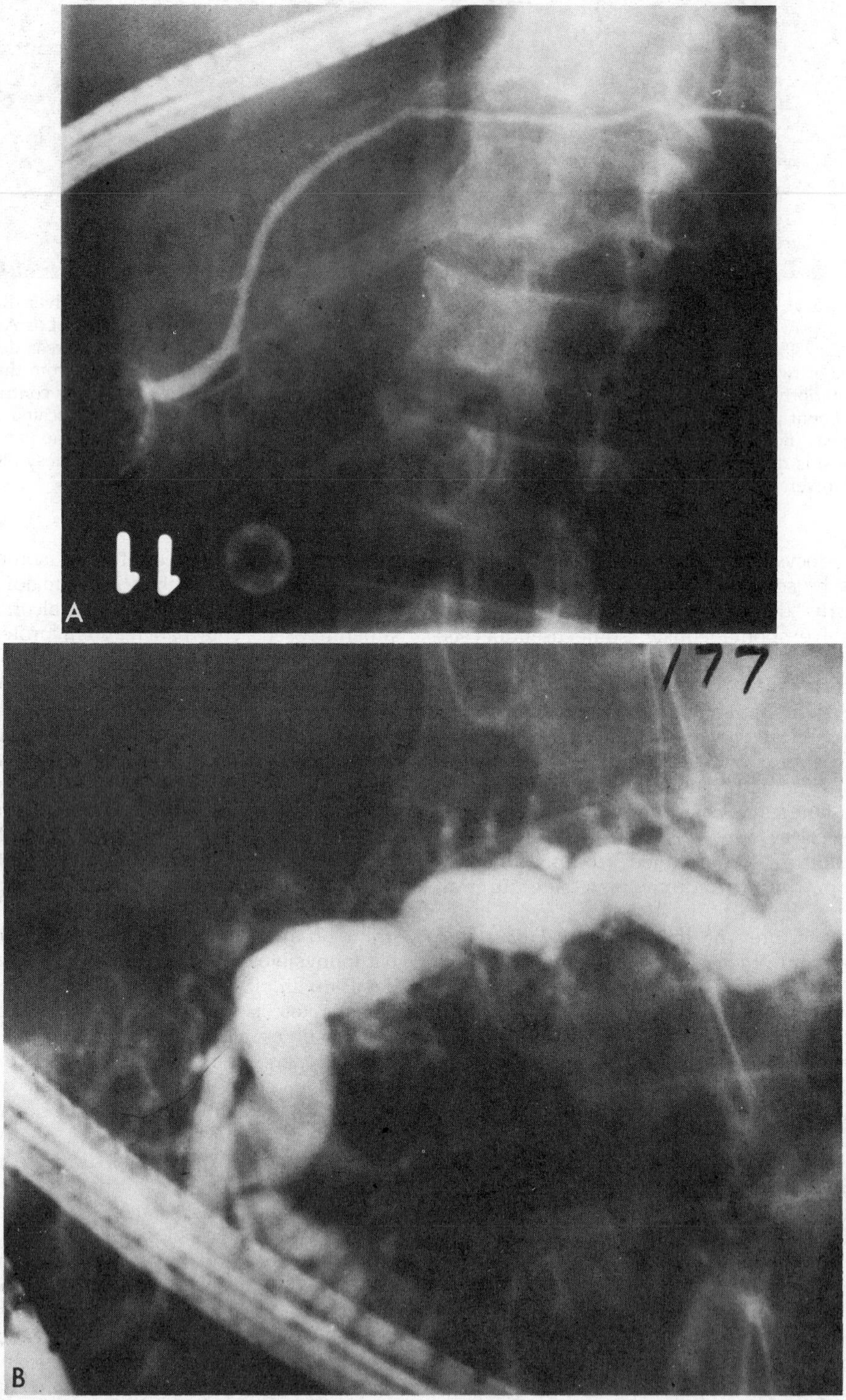

Figure 107–4. Normal pancreatic ductogram as demonstrated by ERCP *(A)*, contrasted with dilatation of ductal system in chronic pancreatitis *(B)*. (Courtesy of Dr. Stephen E. Silvis, Chief, Specialized Diagnostic and Treatment Unit, Medical Service, Veterans Adminstration Medical Center, Minneapolis, Minnesota.)

Less common clinical manifestations of chronic pancreatitis include cholestasis caused by compression of the common duct as it passes through the head of the pancreas; subcutaneous fat necrosis presenting as erythematous, tender nodules, usually on the lower extremities; and intramedullary fat necrosis, causing bone pain.

DIAGNOSIS. The diagnosis of chronic pancreatitis usually requires no additional laboratory confirmation in the alcoholic patient with a past history of acute pancreatitis who subsequently develops chronic abdominal pain and steatorrhea. When the patient presents with chronic abdominal pain and steatorrhea without previous history of acute pancreatitis, the usual diagnostic problem is to distinguish chronic pancreatitis from carcinoma of the pancreas. Diffuse, stippled pancreatic calcification is observed radiographically in about 30 per cent of patients with chronic pancreatitis and is virtually diagnostic. Sonography or CT scanning should be the next step to rule out the presence of a solid, localized pancreatic mass suggesting carcinoma, and to demonstrate calcifications not seen with a survey abdominal film. If the existence of chronic pancreatitis remains in doubt, it may be useful to measure pancreatic secretory function by collecting duodenal aspirate during secretin stimulation. Pancreatic secretion in chronic pancreatitis usually has decreased [HCO_3^-] and low output of enzymes; however, similar results may be observed in carcinoma of the pancreas. ERCP is almost always diagnostic in chronic pancreatitis. The main pancreatic duct is found to be irregularly strictured and dilated ("chain of lakes"), and the major branches have a "beaded" appearance owing to dilatation (Fig. 107–4). In pancreatic carcinoma a localized stricture of the main duct is observed, with dilatation distal to the stricture.

TREATMENT. Chronic symptomatic pancreatitis denotes irreversible pathologic damage to the pancreas. Although the course of the disease may not be modified, the conditions that predispose to pancreatitis (particularly alcoholism) should be eliminated if possible.

Pain. Pain is the predominant problem of most patients with chronic pancreatitis. In fact, there are few benign diseases associated with such persistent, disabling pain for which current medical or surgical therapy is so unsatisfactory. The cause of the pain is unclear, although its frequent relation to food ingestion suggests that pancreatic secretion plays a role. Large doses of pancreatic supplements appear to reduce the pain of some patients, presumably via a negative feedback on pancreatic secretion. Efforts should be made to treat with nonaddicting analgesics, such as salicylates or acetaminophen. Unfortunately, most patients with chronic pancreatitis sooner or later become addicted to narcotics and the withdrawal of the narcotics is difficult to achieve. Dietary regimens or other forms of medical manipulation are rarely useful in the management of the pain. Fortunately, as the pancreatitis "burns out" the pain often gradually disappears, leaving exocrine and endocrine deficiency as the major clinical problems.

Because of the inadequacy of medical therapy, a variety of surgical procedures have been employed for the treatment of the pain of chronic pancreatitis. If the patient has a localized stricture of the main pancreatic duct or a pseudocyst, resection of the pancreas distal to the stricture or drainage of the cyst may produce remarkable improvement. However, most patients do not have such surgically treatable lesions. Although widely employed in the past, sphincterotomy and various procedures designed to interrupt the pain fibers from the pancreas appear to be of limited value. The Puestow procedure is designed to allow free drainage of the entire pancreatic duct into the small bowel. The main pancreatic duct is "filleted" along its entire linear extent, and a loop of jejunum is then anastomosed longitudinally over the opened duct. There is disagreement as to the benefit derived from the Puestow procedure. At best, not more than two thirds of patients obtain some pain relief, and most studies have not taken into account the decreasing pain that is part of the natural history of chronic pancreatitis.

Exocrine Deficiency. A second problem associated with chronic pancreatitis is malabsorption and diarrhea caused by deficient secretion of pancreatic enzymes. This problem can be controlled, although absorption is frequently not normalized, by the administration of 4 to 8 capsules of a pancreatic enzyme preparation with each meal. A low pH in the stomach irreversibly denatures the pancreatic enzyme. Therefore if malabsorption does not respond to pancreatic supplements, the additional administration of antacids or cimetidine to raise the pH of the stomach will enhance delivery of active enzyme into the duodenum and improve absorption. The treatment of pancreatic exocrine deficiency is described in greater detail as part of the general approach to patients with malabsorption (see Ch. 103).

PROGNOSIS. Few patients die of chronic pancreatitis per se. The incidence of carcinoma of the pancreas is, at most, only slightly increased above normal, except in the familial form of pancreatitis. Thus, the prognosis is largely a function of the associated alcoholism or of other diseases that may be associated with chronic pancreatitis.

Arvanitakis C, Cooke AR: Diagnostic tests of exocrine pancreatic function and disease. Gastroenterology 74:932, 1978. *Extensive review and bibliography of exocrine pancreatic function tests.*

Ettien JT, Webster PD III: The management of acute pancreatitis. Adv Intern Med 25:169, 1980. *Excellent review and bibliography of treatment of acute pancreatitis.*

Field BE, Hepner GW, Shabot MM, Schwartz AA, State D, Worthen N, Wilson R: Nasogastric suction in alcoholic pancreatitis. Dig Dis Sci 24:339, 1979. *Controlled study showing no benefit from nasogastric suction in acute pancreatitis.*

Husband JC, Meire HG, Kreel L: Comparison of ultrasound and computer-assisted tomography in pancreatic diagnosis. Br J Radiol 50:855, 1977. *Compares the images of the ultrasound and computed tomography in acute and chronic pancreatitis.*

Isaksson G, Ihse I: Pain reduction by an oral pancreatic enzyme preparation in chronic pancreatitis. Dig Dis Sci 28(2):97, 1983. *Provides data on controlled trial of pancreatic supplements for control of pain of chronic pancreatitis.*

Ranson JH: The surgical treatment of acute pancreatitis. NY Acad Med Bull 58:601, 1982. *Review of surgical intervention in acute pancreatitis.*

Ranson JHC, Rifkind KM, Turner JW: Prognostic signs and nonoperative peritoneal lavage in acute pancreatitis. Surg Gynecol Obstet 143:209, 1976. *Evaluates the prognostic significance of various clinical and laboratory findings in acute pancreatitis.*

Sarles H: Chronic calcifying pancreatitis—chronic alcoholic pancreatitis. Gastroenterology 66:604, 1974. *Review of pathogenesis of chronic, alcoholic pancreatitis.*

Sleisenger MR, Fordtran JS (eds.): Gastrointestinal Diseases. 3rd ed. Philadelphia, W. B. Saunders Company, 1983. *Excellent review of acute and chronic pancreatitis.*

Winship D, et al.: Pancreatitis: Pancreatic pseudocysts and their complications. Gastroenterology 73:593, 1977. *Review of etiology, diagnosis, course, and treatment of pseudocysts.*

108. CARCINOMA OF THE PANCREAS

John P. Cello

DEFINITION. Carcinoma of the pancreas is an insidiously developing, relentlessly progressive, and nearly universally fatal malignancy arising in the epigastric retroperitoneum. Over 90 per cent of carcinomas of the pancreas are adenocarcinomas, derived from the simple cuboidal epithelium of the pancreatic duct. Five per cent of adenocarcinomas of the pancreas are of islet cell origin, often manifested early by the secretion of hormones. These islet cell malignancies are discussed in Ch. 232. Even rarer forms of pancreatic malignancy include acinar cell, epidermoid, adenocanthomas, sarcomas, and cystadenocarcinomas.

INCIDENCE AND EPIDEMIOLOGY. Carcinoma of the pancreas is responsible for over 24,000 new cases of cancer and 20,000 cancer-related deaths annually in the United States. This accounts for 5 per cent of all cancer-related deaths among both men and women. It is the second most common tumor of the digestive system (after colonic cancer) and the fourth most common cause of cancer deaths. Men are more frequently afflicted than women (2:1 in most clinical studies). Although carcinoma of the pancreas may be seen in patients at any age, the mean age of onset is the seventh and eighth decades of life.

Over the past half century a gradual increase in the age-adjusted mortality rate from carcinoma of the pancreas has been noted in Western society. During this period, carcinoma of the stomach (which had been the most common cause of cancer-related deaths in men) has decreased in incidence, and has been surpassed as a cause of cancer-related deaths by carcinoma of the pancreas. The reasons for this dramatic decrease in age-adjusted mortality rates for carcinoma of the stomach and the corresponding surge in deaths from carcinoma of the pancreas are unknown. In addition to advancing age and possibly diabetes mellitus, carcinoma of the pancreas is increased in incidence among heavy smokers. Chronic hereditary pancreatitis but not alcoholic pancreatitis may likewise be a risk factor for pancreatic cancer. A strong association between coffee consumption and pancreatic cancer was identified in one study of 369 patients with pancreatic malignancy. After adjustment for cigarette smoking, the relative risks for no coffee, one to two cups per day, three to four cups, and five or more cups were 1.0, 2.1, 2.8, and 3.2, respectively.

PATHOPHYSIOLOGY AND CLINICAL MANIFESTATIONS (see Table 108–1). Ductal adenocarcinoma of the pancreas is characterized by a dense fibrotic scirrhous or desmoplastic reaction producing a compact hard mass of tissue in the retroperitoneum. The pancreas lacks a mesentery. It lies adjacent to the bile duct and other vital porta hepatis structures, and is surrounded by duodenum, stomach, and colon; the most common clinical manifestations of pancreatic cancer are those related to the encroachment on these adjacent structures. There are few characteristic signs or symptoms that immediately point to a diagnosis of pancreatic cancer. At the time of diagnosis more than half of the patients complain of vague, dull *epigastric abdominal pain* occasionally going to the back. This usually implies invasion of adjacent retroperitoneal organs or splanchnic nerves. *Insidious weight loss* with anorexia and occasionally with a curious aversion for meats, accompanied by a metallic taste in the mouth, diarrhea, weakness, and vomiting, may also be seen. The *vomiting* may signal gastric or duodenal invasion or extensive peritoneal metastases. *Hematemesis* and *melena* may likewise be noted by patients with duodenal or gastric involvement as the tumor erodes into these richly vascularized adjacent structures. *Jaundice* is noted in over 50 per cent of patients, the vast majority of whom unfortunately have large tumor masses arising from the head of the pancreas and encasing the distal common bile duct. On occasion, however, a small focal mass in the head of the pancreas will obstruct the distal common bile duct and produce early jaundice. About one quarter of the patients with pancreatic malignancy have a large, hard palpable abdominal mass noted at the time of presentation. Occasionally, the jaundice and weight loss may be accompanied by a palpable, distended gallbladder *(Courvoisier's sign)*, which is suggestive of the obstructing periampullary lesion. Patients with carcinoma of the pancreas may also have *thrombophlebitis*, *psychiatric disturbances*, or *diabetes mellitus*.

DIAGNOSIS. The insidious development of pancreatic malignancy without characteristic signs or symptoms and its low five-year survival rate have given rise to the search for newer, more sensitive and specific diagnostic tests. Most patients with pancreatic cancer will have *anemia* resulting from nutritional deficiency, indolent blood loss into the bowel, or the anemia of "chronic disease." An *elevated erythrocyte sedimentation rate* is common, as is the presence of blood in the stools on chemical testing. On occasion, the obstructive jaundice together with blood loss into the duodenum may produce a characteristic *silver-colored stool*.

TABLE 108–1. SYMPTOMS AND ROUTINE LABORATORY TESTS IN CARCINOMA OF THE PANCREAS

Symptom*	Percentage	Laboratory Test†	Percentage Abnormal
Abdominal pain	74	Alkaline phosphatase	82
Jaundice	65	5′-Nucleotidase	71
Weight loss	60	LDH	69
Diarrhea	27	SGOT	64
Weakness	21	Albumin	60
Constipation	8	CEA (>5.0 ng/ml)	57
		Bilirubin	55
Hematemesis/melena	7	Amylase	17
Vomiting	6	α-Fetoprotein	6
Abdominal mass	1		

*Modified from Anderson A, Bergdahl L: Am Surg 42:173, 1976.
†Modified from Fitzgerald PJ, Fortner JG, Watson RC, et al.: Cancer 41:868, 1978.

Serologic biochemical tests cannot definitively make or exclude the diagnosis of pancreatic malignancy (see Tables 108–1 and 108–2). On occasion, patients with pancreatic malignancy will have *elevated serum amylase* due to associated pancreatitis. *Elevation of serum alkaline phosphatase* occurs commonly in patients with pancreatic malignancy and is due either to distal common bile duct obstruction or to multiple hepatic metastases. In patients with bile duct obstruction, relentlessly progressive *hyperbilirubinemia* is noted, with the direct-reacting fraction predominant. *Elevated carcinoembryonic antigen* (CEA) has been noted in over 70 per cent of patients with pancreatic malignancy. CEA elevation is not specific for either pancreatic cancer or gastrointestinal tract malignancies in general (see Ch. 172). Elevated CEA levels are noted in patients with cirrhosis, chronic pancreatitis, renal failure, and other nongastrointestinal malignancies. Other serologic markers such as *α-fetoprotein* (AFP), *human chorionic gonadotropin* (HCG), ferritin, RNA-ase, and oncofetal antigen have been reportedly elevated in small numbers of patients with pancreatic malignancies.

Galactosyltransferase isoenzyme II (GT-II) has recently been reported as more sensitive and specific than other "tumor" markers for pancreatic malignancy. Sixty-seven per cent of patients with pancreatic cancer had detectable serum levels of GT-II compared with only 1.7 per cent of patients with benign disease. However, GT-II was likewise noted in 55 per cent of patients with other malignancies (Table 108–2). Neither these nor other serologic or biochemical tests should be used to make or exclude the diagnosis of pancreatic malignancy.

The *upper gastrointestinal tract series* may demonstrate widening of the "C-loop" of the duodenum and mass indentation along the medial aspect of the descending duodenum in patients with cancer of the pancreatic head. Anterior displacement of the stomach and/or displacement of the ligament of Treitz from the greater curvature of the stomach may be noted in patients with carcinoma of the pancreatic body or tail. Occasionally, *hypotonic duodenography* may demonstrate a clearer mass indentation of the second portion of the duodenum. The upper gastrointestinal series is, however, a poor screening test in making the early diagnosis of pancreatic malignancy, especially in patients with carcinoma of the body and tail of the pancreas.

TABLE 108–2. EVALUATION OF SENSITIVITY AND SPECIFICITY OF TESTS FOR PANCREATIC CANCER

	Ultrasound Positive in*	CT Positive in	ERCP Positive in	CEA Positive in	GT-II Positive in
Pancreatic cancer	64%	79%	93%	34%	67%
Other malignancies	13%	7%	0	26%	55%
Benign diseases	1%	4%	0	2%	2%

*"Positive in" refers to an imaging result suggestive of pancreatic cancer or an abnormally high serum level of CEA or GT-II (galactosyltransferase II). (Modified from Podolsky DK, McPhee MS, Alpert E, et al.: N Engl J Med 304:1313, 1981.)

The abdominal imaging techniques of ultrasonography and computed tomography (CT) (see Ch. 94) have markedly enhanced our ability to visualize the pancreas. Pancreatic malignancy is characteristically seen on either *ultrasound* or *CT scanning* as either an asymmetrically or uniformly enlarged and nonhomogeneous pancreas (see Fig. 94–6). In addition to the mass enlargement of the pancreas, marked dilation of the extrahepatic and intrahepatic bile ducts will be readily apparent in patients with bile duct obstruction (see Fig. 94–2). Metastases to the liver and peripancreatic lymph nodes may also be detected by either ultrasound or CT scanning. The sensitivity and specificity of both ultrasound and CT scanning in pancreatic cancer exceed 80 per cent. The larger mass lesions will almost certainly be demonstrated by both ultrasound and CT. However, the lower limits of resolution in both techniques are in the range of 1 to 2 cm; thus small foci of malignancy in the pancreas, especially those not altering the contour of the gland, may be overlooked. Nonetheless, these two tests are the most helpful in identifying patients with pancreatic disease.

Many invasive diagnostic procedures are available for investigating tumors of the pancreas (see Ch. 94). *Angiography* will usually demonstrate displacement of the pancreatic arcades or tumor encasement of celiac, splenic, gastroduodenal, or superior mesenteric arteries (see Fig. 94–12). Moreover, the venous phase of the angiogram may demonstrate occlusion of the splenic vein and portal vein. With *secretin or cholecystokinin (CCK) stimulation of the pancreas,* the volume of pancreatic juice that can be collected via a duodenal sump (Dreiling) tube is characteristically decreased but the bicarbonate and trypsin concentrations remain normal. *Transhepatic cholangiography* (THC) in patients with pancreatic malignancy obstructing the common bile duct will usually demonstrate a long irregular tapered segment of the common bile duct as it passes through the pancreatic malignancy (see Fig. 94–18). Difficulty may be encountered, however, in differentiating malignant stricturing of the distal common bile duct caused by pancreatic malignancy from that produced by scarring in a patient with chronic pancreatitis.

Endoscopic retrograde pancreatography provides the only means of visualizing the pancreatic duct (see Ch. 95). Since most pancreatic cancer is ductal adenocarcinoma, even small mass lesions can be demonstrated to occlude branches of the main pancreatic duct. The characteristic finding of an abrupt cutoff of the pancreatic duct or the stricturing of both pancreatic and common bile duct (so-called "double duct sign") is virtually diagnostic of pancreatic carcinoma (Fig. 108–1).

Histologic demonstration of malignancy by *intraoperative transduodenal biopsy* was previously the only means of obtaining tissue for diagnosis. *Fluid cytology* collected by duodenal aspiration at the time of secretin stimulation or collected during endoscopic retrograde pancreatography (ERCP) may demonstrate malignant cells in an appreciable number of patients. *Guided fine needle aspiration cytology* of the pancreas is now possible using either ultrasonographic or computed tomographic guidance. In most series, 80 to 90 per cent sensitivity and 100 per cent specificity in the presence of pancreatic cancer have been demonstrated.

LOGICAL USE OF DIAGNOSTIC METHODS. A schematic approach to the diagnosis of pancreatic cancer is summarized in Figure 108–2. In the patient with the suspicion of pancreatic malignancy, ultrasonography should be performed first. If the ultrasound scan is inadequate in visualizing the pancreas, a computed tomographic study should then be done. In those patients with an accessible pancreatic mass, a guided aspiration biopsy or cytologic examination of the mass lesion should be performed, using either ultrasound or CT guidance. In those patients with histologic or cytologic confirmation of malignancy, appropriate therapy may be initiated. In patients with ultrasonographic or CT demonstration of a markedly dilated common bile duct, a transhepatic cholangiogram (THC) should demonstrate changes compatible with pancreatic malignancy. In patients with small focal enlargement or pancreatic calcification, ERCP should be performed to differentiate focal pancreatic disease such as malignancy from either chronic pancreatitis or a normal gland. A normal ultrasound scan and/or CT with a normal ERCP (all of which can and should be done on an outpatient basis) virtually excludes pancreatic cancer.

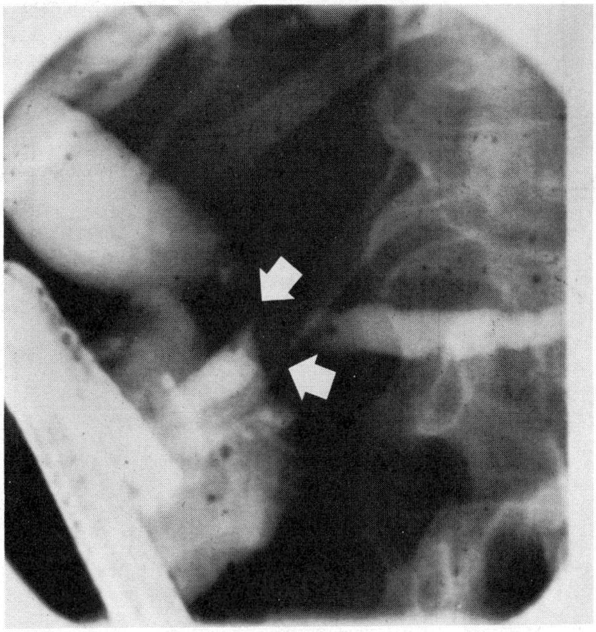

Figure 108–1. Endoscopic retrograde cholangiopancreatography (ERCP) in carcinoma of the head of the pancreas. A classic "double duct sign" is seen with stricturing of both the distal common bile duct and pancreatic duct (arrows). A markedly enlarged proximal common bile duct is filled with contrast material. A 2-cm pancreatic adenocarcinoma was successfully removed by Whipple's resection. However, death occurred within six months of recurrent disease.

DIFFERENTIAL DIAGNOSIS. There are no characteristic signs or symptoms of carcinoma of the pancreas, especially for a cancer arising in body or tail of the gland. In patients *without* jaundice, the vague abdominal pains, anorexia, weight loss, and malaise are all nonspecific and may be difficult to distinguish from those in patients with gastric ulcer, gastric cancer, other intra-abdominal malignancies, chronic pancreatitis, and even severe depression. In a reliable elderly patient, however, these complaints should lead to a suspicion of pancreatic or other malignancy. Epigastric abdominal masses from pancreatic cancer should be distinguished from an enlarged left hepatic lobe, gastric or colonic masses, large omental metastases, and pancreatic pseudocyst or chronic pancreatitis.

Most patients with carcinoma of the pancreatic head have obstructive jaundice. Other periampullary malignancies such as ampullary, duodenal, and cholangiocarcinomas and porta hepatis node metastases should be differentiated from pancreatic cancer, since many periampullary malignancies tend to have better prognoses than pancreatic cancer following radical surgery. Benign conditions causing obstructive jaundice, such as common bile duct gallstones, chronic pancreatitis, or bile duct strictures, must always be clearly differentiated from malignant obstruction of the bile duct. Intrahepatic cholestasis from drugs, toxins, hepatitis, abscess, cirrhosis, and even alcoholic hepatitis must be distinguished from extrahepatic cholestasis, usually by employing biochemical tests and noninvasive imaging techniques.

THERAPY. The main forms of therapy for carcinoma of the pancreas are surgery, chemotherapy, and radiation therapy. Whipple's resection (pancreaticoduodenotomy) or subtotal or total pancreatectomy should be reserved for patients with small focal mass lesions without any evidence of involvement of adjacent vascular structures or distal metastases. The operative

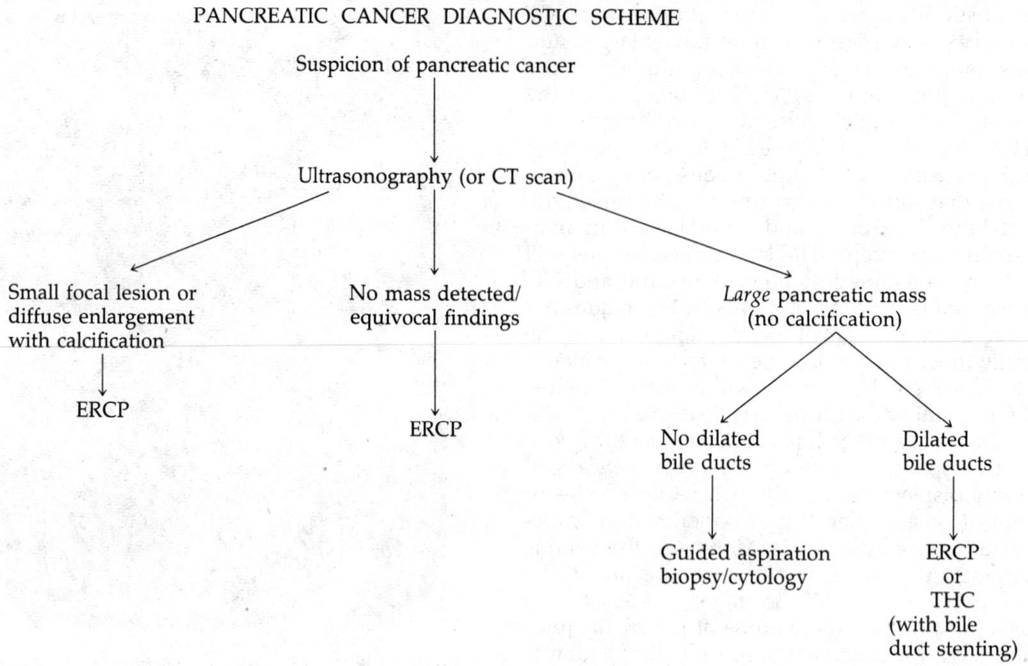

Figure 108–2. Pancreatic cancer diagnosis.

mortality of Whipple's procedure is 20 per cent, with a mean five-year survival of only 5 per cent. Mean survival in an unselected series of patients undergoing Whipple's resection is not significantly better than with the palliative biliary bypass alone. Total pancreatectomy, combining the en bloc resection of pancreas and spleen, has been shown to improve mean survival when compared to palliative bypass and Whipple's resection. Marked improvements in mean survival with total pancreatectomy occur only in patients with disease confined exclusively to the pancreatic bed. In patients with large bulky tumor masses obstructing the common bile duct, palliative surgical bypass with a choledochojejunostomy may be considered. Percutaneous transhepatic stenting of the common bile duct may likewise palliatively decompress the dilated biliary tree. Percutaneous transhepatic external drainage may also be employed to relieve the obstructive jaundice and its attendant pruritus. These latter two techniques, in experienced hands, should be employed rather than laparotomy palliative duct decompression in poor-risk surgical patients with large bulky tumors.

Chemotherapy may offer palliation in patients with nonresectable pancreatic malignancy. However, studies using 5-fluorouracil (5FU), carmustine (BCNU), and other chemotherapeutic agents have not demonstrated substantial improvements in mean survival time. Larger studies with controlled groups are necessary before recommending the routine use of chemotherapy.

Radiation therapy with standard supravoltage techniques provides palliation in 70 per cent of patients with nonresectable pancreatic malignancy, and can result in improved mean survival when compared to historic controls. In preliminary studies, heavy particle beam radiation employing a cyclotron guided by computed tomography has resulted in impressive palliation in patients with nonresectable pancreatic malignancy.

Cello JP: Carcinoma of the pancreas. *In* Sleisenger MH, Fordtran JS (eds.): Gastrointestinal Disease. 3rd ed. Philadelphia, W. B. Saunders Company, 1983, pp 1514–1527. *This recent review covers the general topic of carcinoma of the pancreas and contains an extensive and up-to-date list of 54 references.*

Fitzgerald PJ, Fortner JG, Watson RC, Schwartz MK, Sherlock P, Benua RS, Cibilla AL, Schottenfeld D, Miller D, Winawer SJ, Lightdale CJ, Leidner SD, Nisselbaum JS, Menendez-Botet DJ, Poleski MH: The value of diagnostic aids in detecting pancreas cancer. Cancer 41:868, 1978. *Thorough analysis is made of the diagnostic accuracy of invasive and noninvasive tests in 184 patients suspected of having pancreatic cancer. CT scanning, celiac angiography, alkaline phosphatase, and* ^{75}*Se-selenomethionine, in that order, had the highest percentage of correct diagnoses.*

Itoh K, Yamanaka T, Kasahara K, Koike M, Nakamura A, Hayaski A, Kimura K, Morioka Y, Kawai T: Definitive diagnosis of pancreatic carcinoma with percutaneous fine needle aspiration biopsy under ultrasonic guidance. Am J Gastroenterol 71:469, 1979. *This work describes the "skinny needle" aspiration biopsy technique for pancreatic cancer. Ultrasound is used in this study, but CT scanning will most likely prove the superior visualization technique to assist in guided biopsy.*

MacMahon B, Yen S, Trichopoulos D, Warren K, Nardi G: Coffee and cancer of the pancreas. N Engl J Med 304:630, 1981. *The authors analyzed use of tobacco, alcohol, tea, and coffee in 369 patients and 644 controls. A weak positive association was noted between pancreatic cancer and cigarette smoking, but no association with use of cigars, pipe tobacco, alcohol, or tea. Three or more cups of coffee were associated with a relative risk of pancreatic cancer of 2.7.*

Podolsky D, McPhee MS, Alpert E, Warshaw AL, Isselbacher KJ: Galactosyltransferase isoenzyme II in the detection of pancreatic cancer: comparison with radiologic, endoscopic and serologic tests. N Engl J Med 304:1313, 1981. *GT-II was the most sensitive (67 per cent) and specific (98 per cent) for discriminating between benign and malignant pancreatic disease. As a single test, only ERCP was more sensitive than GT-II. When GT-II was combined with ultrasound or with CT, sensitivities of 92 and 88 per cent, respectively, were noted.*

109. FOOD POISONING

David F. Altman

Food poisoning, which may be defined as clinical syndromes arising from the ingestion of food that either is contaminated or is itself toxic, may cause illness in three distinct ways: (1) by its contamination with microorganisms or their products (most common); (2) by its contamination with poisonous chemicals; or (3) by ingestion of poisonous plants or animals.

As the gastrointestinal tract is the mode of entry for these various contaminants, most illnesses associated with food poisoning involve some form of gastroenteritis, with either upper or lower gastrointestinal manifestations predominating. Other syndromes are often identifiable by extraintestinal (particularly neurologic) signs and symptoms. It is difficult to identify single cases of foodborne disease unless the incubation period is very short or the clinical syndrome distinctive because of the frequency of minor gastrointestinal illnesses. Foodborne disease is usually recognized only when an outbreak occurs and several persons experience a similar illness after ingesting a common food.

Overall, fewer than half of the known outbreaks of foodborne disease are attributed to a specific etiologic agent. Nevertheless it is important to attempt to define the etiology of such an outbreak. Prophylaxis against secondary spread of an infection may be important (e.g., in shigellosis). A more accurate prognosis for the victim may become available, as some illnesses are self-limited and short-lived, whereas others may have a chronic residual effect. Perhaps most important, faulty food handling or storage techniques may be identified and further outbreaks prevented.

To facilitate identification of possible agents in foodborne illness, such syndromes can be classified by their incubation period and the type of clinical symptoms (see Table 109–1). With the possibilities thus limited, specific sampling of food or bacteriologic cultures of blood or stool may quickly lead to the correct diagnosis.

BACTERIAL FOOD POISONING

As an aid to diagnosis and therapy, bacterial food poisoning can be conveniently classified as (1) that due to the ingestion of living microorganisms, (2) that due to the ingestion of a toxin produced by microorganisms in food prior to its ingestion, or (3) that due to enterotoxins produced in the gut by pathogens only after their ingestion.

The most important "infectious" types of food poisoning, requiring ingestion of living organisms, are *Salmonella* gastroenteritis and *Shigella* dysentery, which are dealt with in Ch. 283 and 285, respectively. Other organisms responsible in this way include *Campylobacter jejuni, Escherichia coli, Vibrio cholerae, Vibrio parahaemolyticus, Bacillus cereus,* and *Clostridium perfringens.* In addition, an epidemic of listeriosis transmitted by food and a foodborne outbreak of streptococcal pharyngitis have both been reported.

The "toxin" type of food poisoning most often identified is due to *Staphylococcus aureus.* The syndrome of botulism caused by ingestion of the toxin produced by *Clostridium botulinum* is discussed in Ch. 279.

Staphylococcal Food Poisoning

ETIOLOGY. This form of food poisoning is caused by an enterotoxin produced by multiplying staphylococci before the contaminated food is ingested. Nearly all strains known to elaborate enterotoxins are coagulase-positive *Staphylococcus aureus;* however, some coagulase-negative strains have also been incriminated. The two major sources of contamination are human carriers (usually nasal or skin) and cows with mastitis, the former accounting for nearly 90 per cent of outbreaks. Staphylococcal food poisoning requires not only contamination of food with the microorganisms but also a period of some hours during which they may multiply, as may occur during slow cooling after cooking or if food is held at ambient temperature. Subsequent reheating may destroy the organism but not the remarkably heat-resistant toxin, and it is the latter that causes the clinical illness.

PATHOGENESIS, CLINICAL MANIFESTATIONS, AND TREATMENT. Little is known about the mode of action of the enterotoxins. In experimental animals they cause destruction of gastrointestinal mucosal cells and evoke an inflammatory response. Effects on other organ systems, including the emetic centers in the brain, also have been postulated. Symptoms usually begin two to four hours after ingestion of the toxin, heralded by salivation and followed rapidly by nausea, vomiting, abdominal cramping, and diarrhea. The illness usually is short, rarely lasting 24 hours, and often is subsiding by the time medical attention is sought. It may occasionally be life threatening, especially in the elderly or in persons with other serious illness. Therapy is supportive and symptomatic, the primary goal being to restore extracellular fluid volume with parenteral fluids as necessary. Antibiotic therapy may worsen the course of the illness.

PREVENTION. Proper food handling is essential for the prevention of staphylococcal food poisoning. Sanitary measures and personal hygiene can prevent contamination of the food to some degree. More importantly, food handlers must recognize that enterotoxin is not produced at ordinary domestic refrigerator temperatures. Foods should not be left to cool slowly, especially in large containers, and should be taken from the refrigerator (and reheated, if required) immediately before serving.

Clostridial Food Poisoning

ETIOLOGY. *Clostridium perfringens* Type A has been the third most common bacterial cause of food poisoning in the United States for the last several years. Clostridial poisoning typically occurs in fairly large outbreaks. The organism is ubiquitous, being found in most samples of raw meat, human and animal feces, flies, soil, and dirt from kitchens. Both heat-sensitive and heat-resistant strains have been known to cause outbreaks. The conditions necessary for an outbreak generally include the cooking of meat, poultry, or beans at a temperature (usually less than 100° C) high enough to kill vegetative forms but insufficient to destroy heat-resistant spores. Oxygen is driven out of the food, thereby lowering the oxidation-reduction potential of the medium. During slow cooling the spores germinate, encouraged by the relatively anaerobic environment and the rich supply of amino acids and other growth factors. If the food is not reheated to a temperature high enough to inactivate the recently multiplied organism, ingestion may result in illness.

PATHOGENESIS AND CLINICAL MANIFESTATIONS. Ingestion of living organisms is necessary for the production of clostridial food poisoning, but the pathogenesis of the clinical manifestations remains to be defined. Several toxins have been suggested, but none is clearly responsible for human disease. The incubation period is usually 8 to 12 hours after ingestion, but may be as long as 24 hours. The usual symptoms are abdominal cramps and diarrhea; vomiting is rare, as are headache, chills, and fever. The illness is self-limited, rarely lasting more than 24 hours. Treatment rarely is necessary and should always be

TABLE 109–1. CLINICAL INDICATORS OF THE ETIOLOGY OF FOODBORNE ILLNESS

Predominant Symptomatology	Mean Incubation Period			
	< 2 Hours	2–7 Hours	8–14 Hours	> 14 Hours
Upper intestinal	Heavy metals	*S. aureus* *B. cereus*		
Lower intestinal			*C. perfringens* *B. cereus*	*V. cholera* Enterotoxic or invasive *E. coli* *Shigella* spp. *V. parahaemolyticus*
Both upper and lower gastrointesinal				*Salmonella* *V. parahaemolyticus*
Extragastrointestinal, i.e., some gastrointestinal plus others, usually paresthesias or other abnormal sensory complaint	Scombrotoxin Shellfish toxin Mushroom toxin (early)	Ciguatoxin	Mushroom toxin (delayed)	*C. botulinum*

confined to efforts at symptomatic relief. The few deaths recorded have been in elderly or debilitated patients.

PREVENTION. Food is best served immediately after cooking. If it is to be kept, it should be cooled rapidly. Cooked meat should always be kept either cold, below 5° C, or hot, over 60° C. This is especially true of food prepared in large batches.

Vibrio Parahaemolyticus Food Poisoning

V. parahaemolyticus is a gram-negative facultative anaerobe found in marine water and fauna throughout the world. It lives in sediment of coastal and estuarian waters during cold winter months. As the temperature rises in spring and summer, the organism leaves the sediment and colonizes animal life, especially shellfish and crustaceans. Not all strains are pathogenic.

The pathogenesis of the illness is not clearly defined, and different serotypes may produce disease by different mechanisms. The presence of fecal leukocytes and occasionally bloody diarrhea implies bacterial invasion and damage of the gut mucosa.

Virtually all outbreaks of *V. parahaemolyticus* food poisoning have occurred during warm months of the year and have been associated with the ingestion of raw or improperly refrigerated seafood. Although originally described in Japan, cases have occurred in other parts of Asia and on the Atlantic, Gulf, and Pacific coasts of the United States. The incubation period is usually between 12 and 24 hours, but has been as long as 96 hours. Explosive watery diarrhea is present in more than 90 per cent of cases, with nausea, vomiting, and abdominal cramps as common accompaniments. Fever, headache, and chills occur less often. The diagnosis is suspected when a typical illness occurs after eating seafood, and is confirmed by recovery of the organism from stool. Treatment is rarely necessary, as the illness infrequently lasts more than two days. However, in protracted cases, antibiotic treatment with tetracycline or ampicillin may shorten the illness.

Prevention depends on the recognition both of the potential for contamination of seafood with *V. parahaemolyticus* during warm months and of the predisposition of organisms to multiply under conditions of inadequate refrigeration. Cooked seafood may also become cross-contaminated when stored under proper conditions with a raw source.

Bacillus Cereus Food Poisoning

Bacillus cereus is an aerobic, motile, spore-forming, gram-positive rod that has been increasingly recognized as a cause of foodborne disease. There appear to be two separate clinical forms of the disease. An emetic form, clinically identical to staphylococcal food poisoning, is associated with contaminated fried rice. A diarrheal form has a longer incubation period and predominantly lower gastrointestinal symptoms, reminiscent of *Clostridium perfringens* food poisoning. Cell-free filtrates derived from *B. cereus* strains responsible for this latter form of illness stimulate the adenylate cyclase–cyclic AMP system in intestinal epithelial cells, and their activity is destroyed by heat, thus resembling cholera enterotoxin. The illnesses are usually mild and self-limited, and antibiotics are not indicated. No fatalities have been reported. As the organism commonly occurs in soil and in many dried or processed foods, careful food handling is most important in prevention of the disease. *B. cereus* may be found in uncooked rice, for example, and heat-resistant spores may survive boiling. If the rice is left unrefrigerated, the spores may then germinate and produce toxin. Flash frying or rewarming before serving is often not sufficient to destroy the preformed, heat-stable toxin. The disease thus can be prevented by prompt refrigeration of boiled rice.

Barker WH Jr, Gangarosa EJ: Food poisoning due to *Vibrio parahaemolyticus*. Ann Rev Med 25:75, 1974. *A comprehensive review of the bacteriology and pathogenesis of this illness.*

Centers for Disease Control: Foodborne Disease Outbreaks Annual Summary 1980, issued February 1983. *An annual compendium of reports of foodborne diseases in the USA, with analysis of vehicles of transmission and contributing factors to contamination for each type of infection identified.*

Horowitz MA: Specific diagnosis of foodborne disease. Gastroenterology 73:375, 1977. *A clinician's guide to the clinical and epidemiologic differential diagnosis of foodborne diseases.*

Loewenstein MS: Epidemiology of *Clostridium perfringens* food poisoning. N Engl J Med 286:1026, 1972. *A brief review of the sources and nature of this illness, with particular attention to food handling mistakes most often incriminated.*

Minor TE, Marth EH: Staphylococci and Their Significance in Food. New York, Elsevier Scientific Publishing Company, 1976. *A comprehensive monograph on staphylococcal food contamination, the roles of various foodstuffs in outbreaks, and methods of prevention.*

Schlech WF III, Lavigne PM, Bortolussi RA, et al.: Epidemic listeriosis—Evidence for transmission by food. N Engl J Med 308:203, 1983. *This is a thorough account of a heretofore suspected but unproved type of food-related illness.*

Terranova W, Blake PA: *Bacillus cereus* food poisoning. N Engl J Med 298:143, 1978. *A brief but comprehensive review of the various forms of this illness.*

CHEMICAL FOOD POISONING

Food poisoning caused by chemicals may be related either to the accidental contamination of food prior to its preparation or during storage or to a food additive or preservative. Thus, various forms of metallic poisoning, discussed in Ch. 565, can occur when food, particularly acid liquids, comes in contact with certain metals, especially cadmium, copper, tin, or zinc.

The so-called Chinese restaurant syndrome, in which individuals develop sensations of burning skin, facial pressure, chest pressure, and headaches 10 to 20 minutes after eating certain Chinese foods (especially won ton soup), has been attributed to the use of monosodium L-glutamate (MSG). The symptoms appear to be a pharmacologic effect of MSG, obeying a dose-effect relationship, but with a widely variable threshold for an oral dose.

Sodium nitrite, widely used as a preservative in smoked meats, has been blamed for the "hot dog headache" seen in some persons. In addition, because of its metabolism to nitrosamines it is suspected to be a potential carcinogen, although evidence for this is inconclusive.

Schaumburg HH, Byck R, Gerstil R, Mashman JH: Monosodium L-glutamate: Its pharmacology and role in the Chinese restaurant syndrome. Science 163:826, 1969. *A careful analysis of MSG pharmacology and its dose-effect relationships.*

POISONOUS ANIMALS AND PLANTS

Fish and Shellfish Poisoning

Vertebrate fish may contain various toxins capable of causing human illness. Most commonly this is due to toxin contained in musculature (ichthyosarcotoxins), of which nine types have been described. The most common fish poisonings worldwide—ciguatera, scombroid, and puffer fish poisoning—are attributable to ichthyosarcotoxins.

Two forms of shellfish poisoning, paralytic and neurotoxic, have been described. These are caused by toxins derived from dinoflagellates contaminating the shellfish.

CIGUATERA FISH POISONING. Ciguatera fish poisoning is caused by ciguatoxin, a lipid-soluble, heat-stable substance for which chemical structure has not been determined. More than 400 fish species have been implicated, generally bottom-dwelling shore fish found in temperate and tropical zones.

The onset of the illness usually occurs one to six hours after, but may be as soon as a few minutes or as long as 30 hours after, ingestion of toxic fish. Gastrointestinal symptoms, including abdominal cramps, nausea, vomiting, and diarrhea, predominate at the outset, along with numbness and paresthesias of the lips, tongue, and throat. Paresthesias may later involve the extremities, and in severe cases there may be abnormal temperature sensations, cranial nerve palsies, hypotension, bradycardia, and even respiratory paralysis. Acute symptoms usually subside within a few days, and require only symptomatic, supportive therapy. However, weakness and sensory disturbances may persist for months or years.

SCOMBROID FISH POISONING. Scombroid fish poisoning is the only form of ichthyosarcotoxism in which toxins are formed by the action of bacteria, in this case particularly *Proteus morgani*, on fish flesh. The chemical nature of the scombrotoxin is unknown, but it is thought to consist of histamine and related substances. Most fish that have caused outbreaks are members of the suborder *Scombroidea*, most commonly mahi-mahi, tuna, mackerel, and bonito. Symptoms begin within a few minutes of ingestion and resemble those of a histamine reaction: flushing, headache, dizziness, abdominal cramps, nausea, vomiting and diarrhea, and occasionally urticaria and generalized pruritus. The illness has a median duration of four hours in the reported outbreaks. Antihistamines have provided symptomatic relief. Production of the toxin is inhibited by proper refrigeration, perhaps reflecting the temperature optimum of 20 to 30° C for the enzymatic conversion of histidine to histamine. Improper refrigeration of fresh-caught fish has been observed in most outbreaks of this illness.

PUFFER FISH POISONING (TETRODON POISONING). Many puffer fish found in the Pacific, Atlantic, and Indian Oceans are inherently toxic. The tetrodotoxin found in their viscera is a neurotoxin, and its effects are nearly identical to the saxitoxin that produces paralytic shellfish poisoning (see below).

PARALYTIC SHELLFISH POISONING. Paralytic shellfish poisoning is caused by the ingestion of bivalve mollusks contaminated with the neurotoxin of the dinoflagellates *Gonyaulax catanella* or *Go. tamarensis.* Although a "red tide," related to "blooming" of the dinoflagellates, has been associated with paralytic shellfish poisoning, not all red tides are toxic, and some outbreaks have occurred in the absence of a red tide. The structure of the toxin of *Go. catanella,* saxitoxin, has been characterized, and it appears to act by blocking the propagation of nerve and muscle action potentials.

The illness begins within 30 minutes of ingestion of a toxic mollusk and is characterized by paresthesias of the mouth, lips, face, and extremities and by nausea, vomiting, and diarrhea. In more severe cases, muscle weakness or paralysis and respiratory embarrassment may occur. Deaths, though rare, have occurred within the first 12 hours. Treatment consists of a cathartic or enema in severe cases to remove unabsorbed toxin. Gastric lavage may be used if vomiting has not occurred. Mechanical ventilatory assistance may be required.

NEUROTOXIC SHELLFISH POISONING. *Gymnodinium breve* is a toxic dinoflagellate that causes a red tide off both the Gulf and Atlantic coasts of Florida. Within three hours of the consumption of shellfish contaminated with this toxin, patients experience paresthesias, abnormal temperature sensations, ataxia, nausea, vomiting, and diarrhea. The disease is self-limited and milder than paralytic shellfish poisoning. No deaths have been reported.

MUSHROOM POISONING

Of the more than 2000 identified species of mushrooms, fewer than 50 are poisonous. However, even expert mycologists may have difficulty identifying poisonous species. Moreover, with the increased interest in "organic" foods and in the hallucinogenic substances found in certain species, poisoning from the ingestion of wild mushrooms has been increasing in frequency.

The principal toxin is amanitine, which contains cyclic octapeptides. Phalloidin, another putative toxin, appears to have some hepatocellular toxicity, but mushrooms with phalloidin but without amanitine have been consumed without ill effect. Amanitine selectively inhibits nuclear RNA polymerase II. Mushrooms containing these toxins belong to the genera *Amanita* and *Galerina. Amanita verna* (the "destroying angel"), *A. virosa,* and *A. phalloides* (the "death cap") are the species most often associated with mushroom poisoning in the United States, and *A. phalloides* accounts for more than 90 per cent of such deaths in Europe.

Symptoms of *A. phalloides*–type mushroom poisoning characteristically occur in three stages. The first is characterized by the abrupt onset of abdominal pain, nausea, vomiting, and diarrhea 6 to 24 hours after ingestion. This may be accompanied by severe fluid and electrolyte disturbances and fever. The second stage, occurring during the next 24 to 48 hours, involves worsening of hepatic and renal function despite resolution of the initial symptoms. Finally, during the third and fourth days after ingestion, hepatic and renal function deteriorate, accompanied occasionally by cardiomyopathy and coagulopathy, convulsions, coma, and death. The mortality rate is between 40 and 90 per cent.

The diagnosis of mushroom poisoning may be difficult. The delayed onset of symptoms may cause patients not to associate the illness with the ingestion of wild mushrooms. The mushroom toxins can be detected in gastric aspirate, vomitus, or stool by thin layer chromatography in some laboratories. Treatment remains exclusively supportive, including renal dialysis when indicated. Thioctic acid has been used experimentally since 1968 as an antidote for *A. phalloides*–type mushroom poisoning, but this treatment now appears to be ineffective.

Plant Alkaloids, Mycotoxins, and Other Poisonings

These various forms of food poisoning remind us of historic knowledge of the pharmacologic effect of plant alkaloids and other toxicants found naturally in foods. Although formerly used with therapeutic intent, plant alkaloids are now more often ingested accidentally and often in large doses. Reports now appear of digitalis intoxication from home-brewed teas made with foxglove or oleander; diarrhea from senna tea, which contains the stimulant cathartic anthraquinone; and liver failure from *Senecio longilobus,* which contains highly hepatotoxic pyrrolizidine alkaloids. Other highly toxic plants include *Atropa belladonna* (deadly nightshade) and *Datura stramonium* (thorn apple, jimson weed), whose berries and seeds can cause an atropine effect; *Conium maculatum* (hemlock), which contains several alkaloids with severe central nervous system depressant effects; and *Phytolacca americana* (pokeweed), whose leaves and berries have strong emetic properties.

Lathyrism, a slowly progressive spastic paraplegia, is associated with the ingestion of sweet peas of the species *Lathyrus sativus.* Large amounts of this may be ingested during famines in Africa and Asia. The toxic principle appears to be beta-aminoproprionitrile. Interestingly, this substance when given to poultry and other experimental animals, causes degeneration of the aortic media, with resulting dissecting aortic aneurysms or aortic rupture. This effect is not seen in man.

Mycotoxins may contaminate some moldy foods. Ergotism is the most familiar syndrome caused by this ingestion (see Ch. 411). Other mycotoxins, including aflatoxin, have been identified. This product of *Aspergillus flavus* contaminates grains stored in warm, damp areas, and has been associated with the development of hepatocellular carcinoma. Small amounts of aflatoxin have been found in commercial peanut butter in the United States.

Hughes JM, Merson MH: Fish and shellfish poisoning. N Engl J Med 295:1117, 1976. *A thorough review of the pathophysiology and clinical manifestations of this group of illnesses.*

Olson KR, Pond SM, Seward J, et al.: *Amanita phalloides*–type mushroom poisoning. West J Med 137:282, 1982. *This is a comprehensive review of the clinical manifestations of mushroom poisoning, the various species involved and a brief guide to their identification. Therapeutic options are presented.*

Poisoning associated with herbal teas. Morb Mort Wkly Rep 26:257, 1977. *Case reports and discussions of several types of herbal poisonings.*

Wogan GN: Mycotoxins. Ann Rev Pharmacol 15:437, 1975. *A review of the current understanding of the pharmacology and health impact of mycotoxins.*

110. DISEASES OF THE RECTUM AND ANUS

David F. Altman

DISEASES OF THE RECTUM

INTRODUCTION. The rectum primarily serves a storage function by allowing convenient disposition of fecal waste. Most diseases of the rectum involve some inflammatory change that alters neuromuscular control over defecation and results in symptoms of constipation or diarrhea, tenesmus, and urgency.

The sigmoidoscope and forceps biopsy instruments are most useful to examine the rectum. In contrast, the barium enema gives poor resolution in the rectum and therefore is unreliable as a primary diagnostic tool. Sigmoidoscopy using flexible fiberoptic instruments permits more of the rectum and sigmoid to be examined with decreased patient discomfort.

PROCTITIS. Inflammatory disease of the rectum may be caused by radiation injury, trauma from a foreign body, ischemia or infection, or other processes. Chronic inflammatory disease of unknown etiology, perhaps related to more generalized inflammatory bowel diseases, is a frequent occurrence.

INFECTIOUS PROCTITIS. Inflammatory disease in the rectum may be caused by several infectious agents. The syndromes of bacillary dysentery and amebiasis are discussed in Ch. 285 and 385, respectively. Venereally transmitted diseases, especially gonorrhea, syphilis, and lymphogranuloma venereum, may involve the rectum primarily (see Ch. 302, 303, and 306). These diseases have their greatest impact in the male homosexual population; e.g., asymptomatic rectal carriage of gonorrhea may be detected in up to two thirds of tested subjects, and frequent sexual contact permits rapid spread of the infection.

Diagnosis of anorectal gonorrhea is best made by obtaining culture material with a sterile cotton swab inserted approximately 2.5 cm into the anal canal, swept around a peripheral arc for 10 seconds, and then inoculated immediately on selective growth medium. Rarely, disseminated gonococcal infection with bacteremia has been reported after anorectal gonorrhea. Treatment is the same as for other localized gonococcal infections (see Ch. 302).

Herpes simplex virus is known to cause an acute proctitis in homosexual men. Anorectal pain and discharge are the most common presenting complaints, and these are often accompanied by constipation, tenesmus, and hematochezia. Neurologic involvement, with urinary bladder dysfunction, paresthesias, erectile difficulties, and gluteal or thigh pain, is also seen. Proctoscopy will often show an acute distal proctitis with ulcerations. Rectal biopsy shows acute inflammation, and intranuclear inclusions, if seen, confirm the diagnosis. Treatment is supportive and symptoms resolve spontaneously, although there may be periodic recurrences.

NONSPECIFIC ULCERATIVE PROCTITIS. Nonspecific ulcerative proctitis most commonly produces symptoms of rectal bleeding, tenesmus, and often a mucosanguineous anal discharge. The bleeding seldom is severe, and patients with diarrhea often describe no increase in stool volume but rather frequent passage of small amounts of mucus or blood. Systemic symptoms, such as fever and weight loss, rarely occur. Indeed, the patient usually feels remarkably well in spite of the primary complaints noted above. Extraintestinal manifestations of inflammatory bowel disease, especially arthritis, uveitis, and dermatitis, also are rare. The diagnosis is made when (1) sigmoidoscopy reveals inflammation of the rectal musoca with a clearly demarcated upper border above which the mucosa is normal, (2) the remainder of the colon and small intestine is found to be normal by barium x-ray and/or colonoscopy, and (3) a rectal biopsy demonstrates changes indistinguishable from those of chronic ulcerative colitis.

Differential diagnosis includes Crohn's ileocolitis, radiation proctitis, and infectious disease of the rectum, especially bacillary dysentery, amebiasis, lymphogranuloma venereum, and gonorrheal proctitis. A detailed history and physical examination, appropriate cultures of stool and rectal mucus, biopsy, and serologic studies for chlamydiae should suffice to distinguish among these possibilities.

Treatment is primarily that of more generalized inflammatory bowel disease, with the exception that systemic corticosteroids are rarely or never used. Topical corticosteroids, administered once or twice daily either as suppositories or as enemas, often provide a satisfactory response. Sulfasalazine or other poorly absorbed sulfa preparations may also be used either orally or rectally. With treatment the disease usually runs a course with periodic exacerbations. Rectal strictures may occur, but carcinoma of the rectum seems to be only a small risk. However, biannual sigmoidoscopy is warranted to follow the course of the illness. Fewer than 15 per cent of patients with ulcerative proctitis develop diffuse ulcerative colitis.

FECAL IMPACTION AND STERCORAL ULCER. Incomplete evacuation of feces over an extended period of time may result in the formation of an obstructing mass of firm stool in the distal colon or rectum. *Fecal impaction* occurs most often in children with undiagnosed congenital megacolon or psychiatric disorders, in patients with painful anal diseases, and in elderly, debilitated, or sedentary persons. Patients may complain only of a sensation of fullness in the lower abdomen, anorexia, and malaise. Liquid stool above the fecal mass may distend the proximal colon and then pass around the obstruction. This may be misinterpreted as diarrhea, and inappropriate treatment may be instituted. The diagnosis is most easily made on digital rectal examination, but when the impaction is located more proximally in the sigmoid colon, only an abdominal mass may be felt.

A large fecal impaction usually requires both administration of enemas and mechanical disimpaction digitally. Treatment consisting of saline enemas and oral mineral oil is usually successful once the fecal mass has been broken up. More extraordinary enema solutions have included milk and molasses in equal volumes and water-soluble x-ray contrast material. Warm oil or soapsuds enemas rarely are necessary; in fact, they may be injurious to the rectal mucosa.

Fecal impactions may be associated with the development of intestinal obstruction, volvulus, megacolon, or rectal prolapse. Colonic perforation can occur spontaneously, usually during the attempted passage of the fecal mass. More often, perforation is iatrogenic and is signaled by the onset of fever, abdominal pain and distention, or shock shortly after disimpaction. Surgical treatment is required, and without early diagnosis mortality is high.

Stercoral ulcers in the rectum and colon probably result from pressure necrosis produced by the fecal mass. The ulcer is irregular and has a dark gray or purple outline. Biopsies reveal little inflammation. The ulcer heals rapidly after the mass is removed, but complications of bleeding or perforation have been reported.

Prevention of recurrent impaction is essential. In patients with illnesses predisposing to the development of impaction, prophylaxis may consist of the use of stool-wetting or bulk-forming agents. Mild laxatives may also be used when necessary.

SOLITARY RECTAL ULCER. Discrete, usually single ulcerations of unknown cause may develop in the rectum as well as in other areas of the colon. Solitary ulcer of the rectum is commonly a chronic condition in which the patient complains of painless passage of blood and/or mucus with stool and, less frequently, of dull rectal pain. In contrast, ulcers in the proximal colon usually cause acute abdominal pain. Although this condition has been called solitary ulcer, sigmoidoscopy reveals multiple lesions in 30 per cent of patients. Usually located 7 to 10 cm from the anal verge, the ulcers are shallow and occasionally have heaped-up or nodular borders. The ulcers may be round, linear, or irregular in outline and average 2 cm in diameter. They are chronic, lasting many years, and no treatment has been uniformly successful. Fortunately, complications are rare. The cause of solitary rectal ulcers has not been established. Trauma does not appear to be a major factor. Possibly the ulcer is related to the unusual entity *colitis cystica profunda*, with the ulcer resulting from rupture of cystic degeneration of heterotopic colonic mucosa. Solitary rectal ulcer must be distinguished from other diagnostic possibilities requiring more specific therapy, particularly carcinoma, Crohn's disease, and lymphogranuloma venereum. Biopsy of the rim of the ulcer is most helpful in diagnosis.

PROCTALGIA FUGAX. Proctalgia fugax is episodic severe rectal pain, probably related to spasm of the coccygeus and levator ani muscles. Anorectal infection, fracture of the coccyx, or chronic prostatitis may cause symptoms that mimic those of proctalgia fugax. Chronic trauma from poor sitting posture is said to be causative, but psychologic factors often are prominent. The pain is severe, lasting up to 45 minutes, and even may awaken the patient from sleep. The physical examination is generally normal except for muscle tenderness detected on digital rectal examination. Warm baths, muscle massage, and improvement of posture often constitute successful therapy. In most patients, the symptoms resolve spontaneously over a period of months to years.

Trauma to the coccyx can result in severe pain, termed *coccygodynia*. This may also be related to muscle spasm secondary to the trauma. The diagnosis is made by eliciting pain during movement of the coccyx, and treatment consists of administration of warm sitz baths, massage of the spastic muscles, tranquilizers such as diazepam, and local anesthetic injections.

Chronic ischemia of the rectum may also cause severe anorectal pain accompanied by fecal incontinence and rectal bleeding. This is most often seen in patients over age 50 and may follow anal surgery. Arteriography may show inferior mesenteric artery occlusion or a vascular steal.

Devroede G, Vobecky S, Masse S, et al.: Ischemic fecal incontinence and rectal angina. Gastroenterology 83:970, 1982. *A brief but comprehensive description of this entity, including histology, radiography and rectal manometry.*

Folley JH: Ulcerative proctitis. N Engl J Med 282:1362, 1970. *This remains the most comprehensive review of the clinical features of this illness.*

Goldberg M, Hoffman GC, Wombolt DG: Massive hemorrhage from rectal ulcers in chronic renal failure. Ann Intern Med 100:397, 1984. *Reports of the occurrence of solitary rectal ulcers in patients with chronic renal failure.*

Goodell SE, Quinn TC, Mkrtichian PA-C, et al.: Herpes simplex virus proctitis in homosexual men: Clinical, sigmoidoscopic and histopathological features. N Engl J Med 308:868, 1983. *This series of articles provides an overview of the etiology, diagnosis, and management of anorectal infections seen in homosexual men.*

McMillan A, Lee FD: Sigmoidoscopic and microscopic appearance of the rectal mucosa in homosexual men. Gut 22:1035, 1981. *In a study of 100 men who practiced anal intercourse, the authors demonstrated the presence of proctitis on both gross and histologic inspection, without microorganisms identified.*

Quinn TC, Corey L, Chaffee RG, et al.: The etiology of anorectal infections in homosexual men. Am J Med 71:395, 1981.

Quinn TC, Goodell SE, Mkrtichian PA-C, et al.: *Chlamydia trachomatis* proctitis. N Engl J Med 305:195, 1981.

DISEASES OF THE ANUS

By virtue of its strategic location and function, diseases of the anus occasion many complaints. Most patients with common anal disorders can be well cared for without surgery or referral to a proctologist.

HEMORRHOIDS. Hemorrhoids are dilated veins of the hemorrhoidal plexuses in the anal canal and lower rectum. By age 50, fully 50 per cent of people have hemorrhoids. *Internal hemorrhoids* arise from the superior (internal) hemorrhoidal venous plexus and are covered by rectal mucosa. *External hemorrhoids* are dilatations of the inferior (external) hemorrhoidal plexus and are covered with pain-sensitive anoderm and perianal skin. The pathogenesis of hemorrhoids remains controversial. In the traditional view they are varicosities caused by increased intra-abdominal pressure (often owing to pregnancy or to the straining involved in passage of scybalous stool). On the other hand, hemorrhoids develop early in pregnancy prior to significant uterine enlargement, and furthermore bleeding from hemorrhoids is not of dark but rather of bright (arterial) blood. Thus alternative views suggest the possibility of a rich arteriovenous network at the anus that might be under some degree of hormonal influence. Manometric studies of the anal sphincters in patients with internal hemorrhoids often show elevated resting pressures and abnormal low frequency pressure waves undulating at less than two cycles per minute. These changes are found in 40 per cent of patients with hemorrhoids but in only 5 per cent of people without hemorrhoids. It has been postulated that these pressure changes contribute to the development of the hemorrhoids.

The diagnosis is usually made when bleeding, thrombosis, or prolapse ensues. Chronic bleeding is associated with internal hemorrhoids and may be severe enough to cause iron deficiency anemia. Thrombosis of external hemorrhoids may be painful, and the examiner sees a small, very tender, tense bluish lump in the anal canal. Prolapse of an internal hemorrhoid usually is mild, but eventually the hemorrhoid may become irreducible, leading to thrombosis. The differential diagnosis is not difficult; however, rectal bleeding should not be attributed to hemorrhoids until completion of anorectal examination including sigmoidoscopy.

Conservative therapy, consisting of warm sitz baths, and stool softeners, usually suffices for hemorrhoids that cause only scant bleeding or minimal discomfort. Internal hemorrhoids that bleed persistently or prolapse are most successfully treated with band ligation, in which a rubber band is placed over the base of the hemorrhoid with a special apparatus, the band causing necrosis and sloughing of the hemorrhoid in about seven days. Alternatively, fusiform internal hemorrhoids can be sclerosed by the submucosal injection of a sclerosing agent (e.g., 5 per cent phenol in oil) into the tissue at the upper pole of the hemorrhoid (not into the hemorrhoid itself). These measures are not appropriate for the pain-sensitive external hemorrhoids. When these thrombose, the clot can be excised under local anesthesia. If pain is subsiding when the patient comes for treatment, simple therapy with analgesics, sitz baths, and stool softeners will usually suffice. Ointments and suppositories widely advertised for therapy of hemorrhoids have at best limited value.

ANORECTAL ABSCESS AND FISTULA. *Anorectal abscesses* are infections of the tissue spaces in and adjacent to the anorectum. Clinical features, dependent on the size and location of an abscess, usually include a throbbing, constant pain either in the perianal area or higher in the rectum. A large abscess may produce fever. The abscess is palpated externally near the anus or internally by digital rectal examination. These abscesses are classified according to their location in the anatomic spaces. The perianal abscess, just beneath the anal skin, is the most common. Other sites include the ischiorectal fossa, the intermuscular plane between the internal and external sphincters, the pelvirectal space above the levator ani and below the pelvic peritoneum, and the retrorectal space. Infection usually arises in an anal crypt. Patients with Crohn's disease, hematologic disorders, and other immune-deficient states are particularly susceptible to the development of anorectal abscesses. Prompt surgical drainage of the abscess is the treatment of choice.

Anorectal fistulas, hollow fibrous tracts lined by granulation tissue and connecting the anal canal or rectum with the perianal skin, may result from the rupture or surgical drainage of an anorectal abscess. Such fistulas may also develop from tuberculosis, Crohn's disease, carcinoma, radiation therapy, lymphogranuloma venereum, and anal fissures. Patients complain of the constant and irritating drainage of pus, blood, mucus, and occasionally stool. Treatment requires both control of the underlying disease and surgical fistulotomy.

ANAL FISSURE. An anal fissure is a longitudinal elliptical or rounded defect which occurs in the anoderm (usually in the posterior midline) and which extends into the anal canal as far as the pectinate line. The cause is most often anal trauma, usually the passage of a large firm stool. The patient complains of severe tearing or burning anal pain and occasionally of the passage of a few drops of blood. A swelling at the lower end of the fissure, the "sentinel pile," may be perceived as an anal mass. Chronic spasm and inflammation can lead to anal stenosis. Observation of fissures out of the midline or of multiple fissures should raise the question of inflammatory bowel disease, carcinoma, tuberculosis, syphilis, or other venereal disease. Most fissures heal spontaneously, and local anesthetics, sitz baths, and stool softeners give good results in most cases. Chronic fissures may require surgical excision or sphincterotomy.

PRURITUS ANI. Itching of the perianal skin is a symptom, not a diagnosis. The causes are many and varied. Principal categories of etiologies include anorectal diseases (e.g., fistulas, fissures, neoplasms); dermatologic diseases (psoriasis, eczema, seborrheic dermatitis); contact dermatitis (including reaction to agents commonly used to treat the pruritus); infections and parasites (especially pinworms, scabies, and pediculosis); poor hygiene; and systemic diseases, especially diabetes mellitus and chronic liver disease. Also, many patients are thought to have pruritus on the basis of irritant stools. Normal feces are weakly acid, and diarrheal stools tend to be alkaline, which may be irritating to perianal skin. Specific therapy of one of the aforementioned conditions is the preferred approach; however, most patients require a general regimen, including avoidance of topical agents, laxatives, and tight underclothing, and careful hygiene after defecation with use of nonmedicated talcum powder if necessary. Occasionally, patients benefit from the sparing application of 1 per cent hydrocortisone to the skin, especially at night when the symptoms seem to be worst. Anecdotal reports suggest benefit from the use of *Lactobacillus acidophilus* preparations or malt soup extract (Maltsupex) to produce a more acid colonic flora.

ANAL MALIGNANCY. Epidermoid carcinomas of the anus of various histologic types (e.g., squamous cell, basal cell, cloacogenic) constitute about 2 per cent of cancers of the large bowel. The lesions tend to spread widely both directly into the perianal structures and via lymphatic and hematogenous metastases. Bleeding, pain, and a mass are the usual presenting symptoms. Pruritus, mucoid drainage, and change in bowel habits may also occur. Surgical excision is necessary except in the anoderm well below the pectinate line where small lesions may respond to irradiation. Overall five-year survival rates of 60 per cent have been reported for surgically treated patients.

Other malignancies more rarely seen in the anus include malignant melanoma, mucinous adenocarcinoma, and extramammary Paget's disease. Each of these may produce trivial symptoms and may have widely metastasized by the time of discovery. Wide surgical excisional biopsy must be performed for a suspected lesion. Abdominoperineal resection is still the treatment of choice, but its impact on survival in melanoma is unclear.

Kaposi's sarcoma of the perianal skin, anus, and rectum may occur, particularly as a manifestation of the acquired immune deficiency syndrome (AIDS). In fact this may be the earliest manifestation of the syndrome. Symptoms are rare, as is clinically significant bleeding. Local therapy of isolated lesions with radiation has been successful in selected cases, but this does not address the problem of the underlying immune defect.

FECAL INCONTINENCE. Anal sphincter dysfunction can be a most devastating result of perianal disease, anal surgery, or certain neurologic diseases. Various surgical reconstructive techniques have been employed with some success. Operant conditioning, using biofeedback techniques, has been highly successful in some individuals, and the long-term result has been good.

Engel BT, Nikoomanesh P, Schuster MM: Operant conditioning of rectosphincteric responses in the treatment of fecal incontinence. N Engl J Med 290:646, 1974. *A report on the successful biofeedback techniques used in incontinent patients.*

Schrock TR: Diseases of the anorectum. *In* Sleisinger MH, Fordtran JS (eds): Gastrointestinal Disease. 3rd ed. Philadelphia, W. B. Saunders Company, 1983, p 1280. *An excellent review of diagnosis and treatment of common anorectal disorders.*

Thomson H: Piles: Their nature and management. Lancet 2:494, 1975. *A concise review of the controversies of pathogenesis and management of hemorrhoids.*

111. DISEASES OF THE PERITONEUM

Michael D. Bender

ANATOMY AND PHYSIOLOGY. The peritoneum is a continuous mesothelial membrane that lines the abdominal cavity and its contained viscera. The peritoneal cavity is subdivided by peritoneal reflections and mesenteric attachments into several compartments or recesses, which are clinically important because they determine the location and spread of pathologic processes such as abscesses and metastases. The omentum, a double layer of fused peritoneum, plays an important role in peritoneal defense mechanisms by closing perforations, containing infection, and providing blood supply. The microvascular anatomy of the peritoneum consists of long straight vessels arranged in two layers at right angles to each other, which helps account for the efficiency of the peritoneal membrane as an exchange interface.

The visceral peritoneum does not contain pain receptors; afferent stimuli are transmitted via the visceral autonomics. In contrast, the parietal peritoneum is supplied by spinal nerves that also innervate the abdominal wall. As a result, irritation of the parietal peritoneum produces well localized somatic pain, whereas irritation of the visceral peritoneum produces a less well defined discomfort that is poorly localized. The diaphragmatic portion of the peritoneum is supplied by the phrenic nerve centrally and by intercostal nerves peripherally. As a result, pain caused by diaphragmatic irritation may be referred either to the shoulder or to the thoracic and abdominal wall.

The peritoneal surface, a semipermeable membrane, allows for the passive diffusion of water and solutes between the abdominal cavity and the subperitoneal vascular (blood and lymphatic) channels. In general, water and solutes of molecular weight less than 2000 are absorbed from the peritoneal cavity via the blood vascular system; larger molecules and particulate substances enter the lymphatics. Movement of particles from the peritoneal cavity into the subdiaphragmatic lymphatics is facilitated by discontinuities that exist between the peritoneal mesothelial cells and the lymphatic endothelial cells. Basement membranes are scanty or absent so that particles of substantial size may move freely from the abdominal cavity into the subdiaphragmatic lymphatics, a process that may be facilitated by respiratory motion of the diaphragm itself. Water and electrolytes equilibrate rapidly (within 2 hours) between the blood vascular compartment and the free peritoneal cavity. *Net* fluid movement from the abdominal cavity into the plasma occurs at a maximal rate of approximately 30 to 35 ml per hour in both normal persons and in patients with portal hypertension and ascites. This rate cannot be exceeded despite vigorous diuresis; rather such diuresis only serves to remove fluid from other body compartments, and may cause hypovolemia. The importance of transperitoneal fluid exchange is also illustrated in peritonitis, in which fluid movement into the peritoneal cavity caused by increased vascular permeability can be rapid and massive and may lead to hypotension and shock.

The peritoneum heals readily after damage. Peritoneal injuries normally heal without the formation of adhesions, but in the presence of infection, ischemia, or foreign bodies, adhesions may result. In these situations, fibrinogen released into the peritoneal cavity is converted to fibrin, and then to fibrous adhesions.

DIAGNOSIS. The cardinal symptoms of peritoneal disease are *abdominal pain* and *ascites*. More variable in their occurrence are fever, distention, nausea and vomiting, and altered bowel habits. Direct tenderness, rebound tenderness, and involuntary spasm of the abdominal musculature are the major signs of peritoneal irritation. These signs and symptoms may be minimal or absent in the elderly or debilitated patient and will vary, depending on the location, cause, and acuteness of the underlying process. Because of this, peritoneal disease should be considered in any patient whose abdominal pain is difficult to diagnose.

Radiographically, ascites may be manifested by abdominal haziness, separation of bowel loops, or widening of the flank stripe on plain abdominal films. Otherwise, peritoneal disease reflects itself indirectly on barium contrast studies. Angulation, separation, or rigidity of bowel loops may indicate visceral peritoneal involvement. *Ultrasonography* and *computed tomography* may be useful in demonstrating relatively small amounts of peritoneal fluid, and especially in distinguishing free fluid from cystic masses. Computed tomography also has occasionally been successful in the demonstration of peritoneal implants and in the examination of the retroperitoneum.

If ascites is present, *abdominal paracentesis* is essential to establish its cause (see below). *Peritoneal biopsy,* particularly with the Cope needle, is a relatively simple and safe bedside technique that may yield a positive diagnosis of neoplastic or infectious causes in 50 to 60 per cent of cases. *Peritoneoscopy,* performed under the proper circumstances by a physician experienced in this technique, can be accomplished with little morbidity or mortality. A successful examination may obviate the need for exploratory surgery and may permit biopsy under direct vision of involved portions of the peritoneum or liver. If a diagnosis cannot be made in a patient with obvious peritoneal disease by means of the aforementioned procedures, *exploratory laparotomy* may be necessary.

ASCITES

CLINICAL FEATURES. The accumulation of fluid within the peritoneal cavity is a common clinical finding with a wide range of causes. Its pathophysiology varies with the cause and includes abnormalities in portal venous hydrostatic and colloid osmotic pressure, hepatic lymph formation, splanchnic lymphatic drainage, renal sodium and water excretion, and subperitoneal capillary permeability. In addition, leakage from disrupted abdominal structures may accumulate in the peritoneal cavity. The pathophysiology of ascites associated with portal hypertension is considered in Chapter 126.

Small amounts of ascites may be asymptomatic, but as it increases the patient becomes aware of abdominal distention and a sense of fullness and discomfort. Larger amounts of ascites, especially if the abdomen is tensely distended, may cause respiratory distress, anorexia, nausea, early satiety, pyrosis, or frank pain. Body weight may vary, depending on the state of nutrition and the underlying disease process. On physical examination the flanks bulge, and a fluid wave may be demonstrable. Shifting dullness is somewhat more sensitive but may be nonspecific. Although it is difficult to detect less than 1.5 to 2 liters of fluid, placing the patient on his hands and knees and percussing flatness over the dependent abdomen (puddle sign) may demonstrate smaller amounts. Indirect evidence such as penile or scrotal edema, umbilical herniation, or pleural effusion may suggest the presence of ascites.

As mentioned previously, diagnosis of the presence of ascites may be facilitated by plain abdominal films, ultrasound, or computed tomography.

EVALUATION OF ASCITES FLUID. Once the diagnosis of ascites is made by examination, imaging techniques, or paracentesis, laboratory analysis of the fluid removed is essential to determine its cause. Evaluation of ascites fluid includes inspection, with laboratory determination of protein, cell count and differential, culture, amylase, lactic dehydrogenase, cytology, and lipid concentration.

Fluids with protein concentrations *exceeding 3 grams per 100 ml* are designated exudates, and below these values, transudates. Diseases usually but not invariably associated with transudative ascites include congestive heart failure, inferior vena cava obstruction, Budd-Chiari syndrome, hypoalbuminemia, cirrhosis, Meigs' syndrome, and vasculitis. Exudates are common in neoplasms, tuberculosis, myxedema, and pancreatic ascites. Although this classification is useful, exceptions in both directions occur not infrequently. For this reason, ascitic protein concentrations must be interpreted only in the context of all other clinical and laboratory findings.

A large number of red cells suggests the diagnosis of neoplasm, especially hepatocellular or ovarian carcinoma. An ascitic fluid leukocyte count of more than 500 per cubic millimeter is strongly suggestive of a peritoneal inflammatory process, such as infection or tumor infiltration. A predominance of polymorphonuclear leukocytes suggests acute bacterial infection, whereas lymphocytes and monocytes characterize chronic inflammatory disease, especially tuberculosis, but there are exceptions. Cytologic examination is essential if malignancy is suspected and may be expected to yield accurate results in more than half of cases. Other chemical determinations may be helpful in diagnosis. LDH is often increased in neoplastic ascites. Peritoneal fluid amylase is greatly increased in pancreatic ascites; triglyceride concentrations exceed those of plasma in chylous ascites. Samples of fluid should be cultured for bacteria, acid-fast bacilli, or fungi in the appropriate clinical setting, such as fever, undiagnosed pain, or deterioration in a patient with cirrhosis.

TREATMENT: GENERAL CONSIDERATIONS. Although small or moderate amounts of ascites are often only esthetically displeasing, ascites frequently has a detrimental effect on the overall sense of well-being of the patient. Massive ascites may require urgent removal for severe abdominal discomfort, respiratory distress, cardiac dysfunction, or ulceration or impending rupture of an umbilical hernia. Paracentesis is the method of choice for rapid removal of fluid, as it rapidly reduces intra-abdominal pressure and improves cardiac performance. Concern has been expressed that removal of large volumes of fluid incurs the risk of hypovolemia and hypotension, especially in the vasodilated cirrhotic. Generally speaking, however, one should not hesitate to remove ascites in sufficient volume to treat complications, as the removal of small or moderate amounts is usually well tolerated.

In patients with intractable disabling massive ascites that does not respond to repeated paracentesis or diuretic therapy, peritoneovenous shunting has been successful. Because of numerous complications, careful consideration must be given before recommending peritoneovenous shunting (see Ch. 126). Details of nutritional and diuretic management of ascites is discussed in Chapter 126.

DIFFERENTIAL DIAGNOSIS OF ASCITES. Although a wide variety of disease processes may be associated with the presence of ascites, more than 90 per cent of patients with this complication are found to have *cirrhosis, neoplasm, congestive heart failure,* or *tuberculosis.* For purposes of classification, causes of ascites may be divided into diseases not involving the peritoneum on the one hand (Table 111–1) and diseases of the peritoneum on the other (Table 111–2). Of those cases not associated with peritoneal disease, cirrhosis is by far the most common; it is considered in Chapter 125. Portal hypertension caused by diseases of the heart and great veins account for a substantial number of patients with ascites of obscure origin. Included in this group are patients with congestive heart failure, constrictive pericarditis, and inferior vena cava and hepatic vein obstruction (Budd-Chiari syndrome). Clinically, patients with these conditions may not be readily distinguishable from those with hepatic cirrhosis; a high index of suspicion is necessary, and special procedures may be required in order to establish or exclude the diagnosis.

Hypoalbuminemia of any cause, including nephrotic syndrome and protein-losing enteropathy, may be associated with a classically transudative ascites.

Various endocrine conditions may be associated with ascites. These include *myxedema,* in which the fluid is typically protein-rich, and diseases of the ovary, among them *Meigs' syndrome,* in which transudative ascites is associated with ovarian fibroma or cystadenoma, struma ovarii, and "ovarian overstimulation syndrome."

TABLE 111–1. CAUSES OF ASCITES NOT ASSOCIATED WITH PERITONEAL DISEASE*

I. Portal hypertension
  A. Cirrhosis
  B. Hepatic congestion
    1. Congestive heart failure
    2. Constrictive pericarditis
    3. Inferior vena cava obstruction
    4. Hepatic vein obstruction (Budd-Chiari syndrome)
  C. Portal vein occlusion
II. Hypoalbuminemia
  A. Nephrotic syndrome
  B. Protein-losing enteropathy
  C. Malnutrition
III. Miscellaneous
  A. Myxedema
  B. Ovarian disease
    1. Meigs' syndrome
    2. Struma ovarii
    3. Ovarian overstimulation syndrome
  C. Pancreatic ascites
  D. Bile ascites
  E. Chylous ascites
  F. Urine ascites and nephrogenic ascites

*From Bender MD, Ockner RK: *In* Sleisenger MH, Fordtran JS (eds.): Gastrointestinal Disease. 3rd ed. Philadelphia, W. B. Saunders Company, 1983.

Pancreatic ascites usually occurs in the presence of chronic pancreatitis or pseudocyst. The most common etiologic factors are alcohol and trauma. The ascites fluid amylase concentration is elevated, often to extremely high levels. Diagnosis of ductal disruption and pseudocyst leakage is usually possible with endoscopic retrograde pancreatography. Drainage of the pseudocyst and repair of duct injury often have been effective in managing this complication, particularly in traumatic cases. In the chronic alcoholic with pancreatic ascites, a trial of conservative management is indicated before surgery is undertaken. Leakage of bile may be associated with the development of *bile ascites,* a condition for which surgical repair of the biliary tract is usually necessary. This situation is not necessarily associated with the fulminant clinical picture of fever, leukocytosis, and peritonitis, i.e., bile peritonitis, which appears to result from superimposed infection.

TABLE 111–2. DISEASES OF THE PERITONEUM*

I. Infections
  A. Bacterial peritonitis
  B. Tuberculous peritonitis
  C. Fungal diseases
    1. Candidiasis
    2. Histoplasmosis
    3. Coccidioidomycosis
    4. Cryptococcosis
  D. Parasitic diseases
    1. Schistosomiasis
    2. Enterobiasis
    3. Ascariasis
    4. Strongyloidiasis
    5. Amebiasis
II. Neoplasms
  A. Secondary malignancy
  B. Primary mesothelioma
  C. Pseudomyxoma peritonei
III. Granulomatous peritonitis
  A. Exogenous
  B. Endogenous
  C. Iatrogenic
IV. Miscellaneous
  A. Vasculitis
  B. Familial paroxysmal peritonitis (familial Mediterranean fever)
  C. Eosinophilic gastroenteritis
  D. Whipple's disease
  E. Gynecologic disease
    1. Endometriosis
    2. Deciduosis
    3. Gliomatosis
    4. Leiomyomatosis
    5. Dermoid cyst
    6. Melanosis
  F. Splenosis
  G. Sclerosing peritonitis
  H. Peritoneal lymphangiectasia
  I. Peritoneal loose bodies and cysts
  J. Peritoneal encapsulation

*Modified from Bender MD, Ockner RK: *In* Sleisenger MH, Fordtran JS (eds.): Gastrointestinal Disease. 3rd ed. Philadelphia, W. B. Saunders Company, 1983.

Chylous ascites is due to the presence of lipoproteins and chylomicrons in the peritoneal cavity. These lipid-rich particles impart a turbidity to the fluid that facilitates its diagnosis. However, not all turbid abdominal fluids are "chylous." Establishment of the diagnosis requires direct evidence that the turbidity is indeed the result of neutral lipid, a determination best made by analysis of the fluid for triglyceride concentration. Other turbid abdominal fluids may be due to cellular debris and are designated *pseudochylous ascites,* a condition occasionally associated with abdominal neoplasm or infection. The differential diagnosis of true chylous ascites depends upon its chronicity and the age of the patient. *Chronic chylous ascites* in adults is caused in over 80 per cent of cases by abdominal neoplasm, usually lymphoma, with associated obstruction and disruption of the abdominal lymphatics resulting from extensive lymph node involvement. *Acute chylous ascites* ("chylous peritonitis") is associated with abrupt onset of abdominal pain. In some cases, this syndrome is due to trauma, intestinal obstruction, or rupture of a chylous cyst, but identifying a specific cause may not be possible even at laparotomy. In children, congenital malformations of the lymphatics, including intestinal lymphangiectasia, account for a higher proportion of the cases of chylous ascites.

Urine ascites may result from trauma to the urinary tract, high grade obstruction caused by posterior urethral valves in the neonate, or renal transplantation. Ascites also may occur in a few patients maintained on chronic hemodialysis. The cause of this is not defined, but it appears to reflect a number of factors, including prior peritoneal dialysis or infection, fluid overload, hypertension, poor nutrition, or hypoalbuminemia. Management may be difficult, but if aggressive dialysis does not help, renal transplantation seems to offer the best chance of relieving chronic ascites.

INFECTIONS OF THE PERITONEUM

ACUTE BACTERIAL PERITONITIS. Bacterial peritonitis most commonly results from perforation of an abdominal viscus caused by trauma, obstruction, infarction, neoplasm, foreign bodies, or primary inflammatory disease. The details of differential diagnosis are discussed in Chapter 52. The peritoneum has several defense mechanisms in response to bacterial contamination. First, bacteria may be cleared from the peritoneum via the diaphragmatic lymphatics. Second, opsonins, polymorphonuclear leukocytes, and macrophages enter the peritoneal cavity where phagocytosis of bacteria can occur. Finally, the peritoneum and omentum can contain localized infections and enclose small visceral perforations, in part by exudation of fibrin-containing fluid.

Regardless of etiology, abdominal pain, nausea, vomiting, tachycardia, and fever are usually present. The severity of these symptoms is related to the extent of contamination; in generalized peritonitis, shock is often present and may be profound, whereas signs and symptoms may be minimal if infection is localized. In severe cases, there may be exquisite diffuse direct and rebound tenderness and rigidity of the abdomen; bowel sounds are usually diminished or absent, and distention may be present. Despite its dramatic presentation, recognition of acute peritonitis may be difficult in those patients in whom the clinical manifestations are masked or suppressed, such as the elderly patient or those receiving corticosteroids. In these patients, a high index of suspicion is necessary, since minor or isolated signs such as tachycardia or unexplained hypotension may herald peritonitis.

Laboratory findings are nonspecific and may include leukocytosis, hemoconcentration (from fluid loss into the peritoneum), and subdiaphragmatic air or distended intestinal loops on plain abdominal films.

The principal systemic complications of peritonitis are septicemia, shock, ileus, and widespread organ failure including respiratory, renal, hepatic, and cardiac failure. Local complications include wound infection, abscess, anastomotic breakdown, and fistula formation.

The initial management of peritonitis includes restoration of fluid and electrolyte balance, institution of nasogastric suction to reduce distention and improve pulmonary function, oxygen, analgesics to control pain, and early antibiotic therapy. In advanced peritonitis, polymicrobial aerobic and anaerobic organisms are usually found, requiring broad-spectrum coverage. This may include aminoglycosides for aerobes, clindamycin or metronidazole for anaerobes, and possibly ampicillin to cover enterococci. Cephalosporins have also been popular for their broad-spectrum coverage. Total parenteral nutrition may be necessary in severe peritonitis with major catabolic losses.

The decision to operate must be individualized, but in those patients who are seen early after a recognized perforation of a viscus and who are good operative candidates, surgery usually should be undertaken as soon as it is feasible. However, in a few patients who are very poor operative risks, it may be desirable to attempt to control the process nonoperatively and to encourage its localization by antibiotic drugs and other conservative measures. Localized abscesses so formed may be drained later when circumstances are more favorable.

Despite the use of antibiotics, modern anesthesia, and intensive support systems, the mortality of generalized peritonitis remains at 50 per cent.

ABDOMINAL ABSCESSES. Intra-abdominal abscesses form from a collection of necrotic tissue, bacteria, and white blood cells contained in one of the spaces of the peritoneal cavity and walled off from the rest of the peritoneal cavity by inflammatory adhesions. The origin of abscesses is diverse, but the contamination is almost invariably derived from endogenous gut flora that escapes as a result of inflammatory perforation, ischemia, traumatic injury, or a surgical procedure. Abscesses within the abdomen localize in three distinct areas: the subphrenic spaces, the intermesenteric area (including the paracolic gutters and interloop areas), and the pelvis. The subphrenic and pelvic localizations reflect the dependent position of these spaces in the recumbent patient, and the effect of diaphragmatic movement in drawing fluid up into the subphrenic spaces.

Accurate diagnosis of intra-abdominal abscesses is often a difficult challenge, particularly in immunologically depressed patients with malignancy or malnutrition or patients receiving perioperative antibiotics; all of these may mask clinical signs of sepsis. Fever is the most reliable finding. Other signs and symptoms include malaise, pain, nausea, vomiting, anorexia, tachycardia, abdominal tenderness, and abdominal distention. Leukocytosis with a left shift in the differential count, the usual finding, may be absent. Elevated bilirubin or hepatic enzymes may be a clue to the presence of intra-abdominal sepsis. A subphrenic localization is suggested by thoracic symptoms and signs including dyspnea, chest pain, decreased breath sounds, dullness, and radiologic evidence of impaired diaphragmatic motion, pleural effusion, or atelectasis. Pelvic localization is suggested by urinary or rectal symptoms and careful vaginal or rectal examination.

Diagnosis is facilitated by imaging procedures. Plain films may reveal nonmovable gas bubbles, often with air fluid levels, and barium contrast studies may suggest a mass by displacement of normal structures. Technetium liver-lung scanning may localize subphrenic abscesses. Ultrasonography, computerized tomography, and gallium citrate-76 or indium-111 leukocyte labeling are newer modalities that may help diagnose abscesses not visualized by other means. Occasionally the diagnosis is made only at the time of abdominal exploration.

Antimicrobial therapy usually suppresses the process and helps to contain it but may also obscure its recognition. Surgical drainage remains the definitive therapy, although recently percutaneous catheter drainage has been shown to be efficacious for certain abscesses.

PRIMARY (SPONTANEOUS) BACTERIAL PERITONITIS. Bacterial peritonitis may occur in the absence of an acute intra-abdominal precipitating factor. In this circumstance, the offending organism may not be enteric, and the syndrome is more likely to occur in patients who have pre-existing ascites, impaired immunologic defenses, or a cause for bacteremia such as localized infection elsewhere in the body or indwelling catheters. A widely recognized example of this circumstance is the child with nephrotic syndrome and ascites who develops primary peritonitis, but urinary tract infection may now be a more common predisposing factor in children. The mortality rate associated with this entity has diminished considerably during recent decades because of the availability of antimicrobial drugs.

More common is spontaneous bacterial peritonitis in patients with advanced, decompensated cirrhosis and ascites. This syndrome is discussed in Chapter 126.

OTHER INFECTIONS. *Tuberculous peritonitis* is discussed in detail in Chapter 298. It should be emphasized that this disorder may present in a variety of ways, ranging from an acute abdomen to an insidiously developing, otherwise unexplained ascites resembling (or associated with) cirrhosis. Accordingly, its presence should be suspected in all patients with ascites, with or without an apparently adequate cause. Fewer than half of the patients have active disease elsewhere in the body, and tuberculosis skin testing and appropriate cultures of ascites fluid for tubercule bacilli should be regarded as routine in the evaluation of ascites. The diagnosis is strongly suggested by a high percentage of lymphocytes in the abdominal fluid and may be confirmed by means of a positive culture, peritoneal biopsy, laparoscopy, or if necessary exploratory laparotomy. The very satisfactory response of this condition to appropriate chemotherapy adds to the importance of early diagnosis.

Fungal and parasitic diseases may be associated with peritoneal involvement and occasionally with ascites. The most common fungal peritonitis is due to *candidiasis*, which may occur after contamination of the peritoneal cavity caused by perforated ulcer, trauma, surgery, or peritoneal dialysis. Other disorders, including histoplasmosis, coccidioidomycosis, cryptococcosis, ascariasis, amebiasis, and schistosomiasis, are quite uncommon, but deserve consideration in otherwise unexplained cases of peritoneal disease with or without ascites.

TUMORS OF THE PERITONEUM

SECONDARY CARCINOMATOSIS. Secondary malignancy is the most common form of neoplastic involvement of the peritoneum. More than 75 per cent of such tumors are classified as adenocarcinoma, but peritoneal involvement by sarcoma, lymphoma, leukemia, carcinoid, and multiple myeloma has been described. Ascites formation in these patients appears to result from the combination of increased capillary permeability and obstruction of channels that drain the peritoneal cavity by way of the subdiaphragmatic lymphatics. The clinical picture is usually that associated with advancing malignancy, including weakness and weight loss, and variable complaints referable to the abdomen such as pain, distention, nausea, or vomiting. Radiographic findings may include angulation, fixation, or displacement of intestinal loops, or submucosal edema reflecting lymphatic obstruction. Ultrasonography or computed tomography may help confirm the presence of ascites and associated mass lesions. On abdominal paracentesis, the fluid obtained usually has a high LDH and protein content (more than 3.0 grams per deciliter); cellular composition is variable, and occasionally the fluid is grossly bloody. The diagnosis is reliably made in most patients by means of cytology or peritoneoscopy, but surgical exploration occasionally may be necessary.

Treatment of this condition involves the intraperitoneal administration of antitumor agents, including alkylators, antimetabolites, or radioactive isotopes. Unfortunately, the prognosis of patients in this advanced stage of malignancy is poor. Intra-abdominal quinicrine or other sclerosing agents have occasionally been successful in producing a fibrous serositis, thereby obliterating the free peritoneal space and reducing further fluid exudation, but the usefulness of this approach is limited by the frequent occurrence of fever, nausea, vomiting, and abdominal pain.

Salt restriction and diuretics may be tried but are often unsuccessful. Paracentesis is useful, and removal of large volumes may be well tolerated; although it may reduce body protein stores, it is often indispensible for patient comfort. In selected patients, peritoneovenous shunting affords palliation in 75 per cent of cases.

PRIMARY MESOTHELIOMA. Primary mesotheliomas are tumors arising from the epithelial and mesenchymal elements of the mesothelium. Approximately 25 per cent involve the peritoneum, often in association with the more frequent pleural localization. Exposure to asbestos is the most established etiologic factor (see Ch. 559), although it is unclear if asbestos fibers produce peritoneal disease by passage from the intestinal lumen, penetration of the diaphragm, or via retrograde lymphatic transport.

Mesothelioma is most common in males over the age of 50 and is associated with the gradual onset of abdominal pain and distention, anorexia, nausea, vomiting, weight loss, and ascites. Blood counts and chemistries are rarely helpful, and barium contrast films reveal nonspecific findings. Ultrasonography and computed tomography demonstrate ascites in sheetlike masses that may suggest the diagnosis. Paracentesis yields an exudate that may be hemorrhagic, and high fluid hyaluronic acid concentrations suggest the diagnosis. Peritoneoscopy reveals extensive studding of peritoneal surfaces with nodules and plaques. However, laparotomy is often necessary to provide adequate biopsies and rule out a primary neoplasm. Even with biopsy or cytologic specimens, the variable histologic characteristics of epithelial and mesenchymal elements may make it difficult to differentiate from other malignancies.

The prognosis of peritoneal mesothelioma is exceedingly poor, with a median survival of about one year after diagnosis. Death usually results from cachexia or obstruction rather than metastatic disease. Tumor response and increased survival have been reported after chemotherapy (especially doxorubicin) and/or radiotherapy, but treatment is undergoing continued evaluation.

PSEUDOMYXOMA PERITONEI. Pseudomyxoma peritonei is a rare condition in which the peritoneal cavity becomes distended with a mucinous semisolid translucent material. The two major causes of this "mucinous ascites" are mucinous cystadenomas and cystadenocarcinomas of the ovary and appendix, although other tumors of the genitourinary and gastrointestinal tract have been associated with the process. Extensive pseudomyxoma is invariably associated with cystadenocarcinomas, although they may be low grade.

The condition usually presents as an increase in abdominal girth with little in the way of other clinical signs of disease. At surgery, the abdominal cavity is found to contain gelatinous material existing in a variety of states, including cystic masses, lying freely without apparent attachment, or anchored to the peritoneal surface. If the tumor is indeed malignant, it appears to be low grade and rarely metastasizes. As a result, the course of the disease is prolonged and is characterized by recurrent episodes of intestinal obstruction and fistula formation. The most promising therapeutic approach at present appears to be one that combines surgical removal of the ovary, appendix, and as much mucin as possible with intraperitoneal installation of an alkylating agent.

GRANULOMATOUS PERITONITIS. The peritoneum responds to a wide variety of stimuli with a granulomatous inflammatory reaction. *Exogenous* causes include mycobacteria, parasites, fungi, or organic material; *endogenous* causes are rare and include keratin in squamous tumors, meconium, sarcoidosis, and Crohn's disease. The most common etiology is *iatrogenic*, due to contamination at the time of surgery from starch, talc, cotton, or wood fibers used in surgical gloves, gowns, or drapes. *Starch granulomatous peritonitis* presents two to nine weeks postoperatively with pain, tenderness, fever, distention, nausea, and vomiting, and may suggest adhesions or abscesses. If it is considered, the diagnosis can be made by demonstrating starch granules in peritoneal fluid. Short-term indomethacin or corticosteroids often speeds recovery.

MISCELLANEOUS DISEASES OF THE PERITONEUM. The peritoneal membrane may be affected by a wide variety of systemic diseases, including systemic lupus erythematosus (see Ch. 447) and other collagen vascular diseases, Whipple's disease (see Ch. 104), familial Mediterranean fever (see Ch. 209), and eosinophilic gastroenteritis (see Ch. 162). Rarely, unusual tissues deposit on the peritoneum, which may cause low grade peritoneal symptoms or be mistaken for metastatic carcinoma. Examples include endometrial, decidual, glial, and splenic tissue. Several other unusual conditions affecting the peritoneum have been described (Table 111–2) including sclerosing peritonitis, mesothelial hyperplasia and metaplasia, peritoneal lymphangiectasis, and peritoneal loose bodies, cyst, and encapsulation.

Antman KH: Malignant mesothelioma. N Engl J Med 303:200, 1980. *A concise update of epidemiologic, pathologic and clinical aspects, including current approaches to treatment.*

Bender MD, Ockner RK: Ascites. *In* Sleisenger MH and Fordtran JS (eds.): Gastrointestinal Disease. 3rd ed. Philadelphia, W. B. Saunders Company, 1983, p 335.

Bender MD, Ockner RK: Diseases of the peritoneum, mesentery and diaphragm. *In* Sleisenger MH, Fordtran JS (eds.): Gastrointestinal Disease. 3rd ed. Philadelphia, W. B. Saunders Company, 1983, p 1569. *A broad review, extensively referenced.*

Sones PJ: Percutaneous drainage of abdominal abscesses. Am J Roentgenol 142:35, 1984. *A current review describing the indications, technique, and results of percutaneous abscess drainage.*

Wilson SE, Finegold SM, Williams RA: Intra-abdominal Infection. McGraw-Hill Book Company, New York, 1982. *A comprehensive monograph on all aspects of this subject, with excellent chapters on the pathophysiologic and clinical aspects of peritonitis and abdominal abscesses.*

112. DISEASES OF THE MESENTERY AND OMENTUM

Michael D. Bender

GENERAL CLINICAL FEATURES. Patients with mesenteric disease usually have nonspecific symptoms such as abdominal pain, distention, or intestinal obstruction. The most frequent physical finding is a mass, which may be mobile. There are no specific laboratory findings, but mesenteric disease may be suspected if calcifications, displacement of bowel loops, or pressure deformities are observed radiographically. Ultrasonography and computed tomography are useful in identifying mesenteric and omental masses. However, definitive diagnosis usually depends on direct inspection and biopsy, either surgically or by peritoneoscopy.

MESENTERIC INFLAMMATORY DISEASE. This syndrome includes a spectrum of conditions ranging from acute inflammation to a chronic fibrosing process associated with intestinal obstruction, ascites, and steatorrhea. Included are such conditions as "mesenteric panniculitis" and "retractile mesenteritis." The cause of this syndrome is not known, but it is believed to represent the sequel to some inciting event such as trauma, infection, or ischemia in the mesentery. Fat necrosis occurs, evoking an inflammatory reaction with subsequent scarring and granuloma formation.

The condition is most commonly seen in males and in late adulthood. The acute syndrome ("mesenteric panniculitis"), which constitutes the presentation of 60 per cent of cases, is characterized by recurring abdominal pain, weight loss, nausea, vomiting, and fever. In most patients, a tender abdominal mass is palpable; leukocytosis may or may not be present. The remaining 40 per cent of cases are identified by the discovery of a mass on examination or at surgery. Radiographic examination is nonspecific, showing the effects of an abdominal mass and variable scarring that includes displacement and separation of intestinal loops with angulation, stenosis, and extrinsic compression. In some patients the condition evolves into a more chronic process ("retractile mesenteritis"), characterized by continuing pain, fever, weight loss, and various signs of intestinal obstruction, ascites, and steatorrhea. At surgery, the small bowel mesentery is found to be the principal site of involvement; it is thickened and fibrotic, particularly at the root. Resection of the mass is often not possible, and generally should not be attempted. Microscopically in mesenteric panniculitis there is infiltration of adipose tissue by foamy macrophages and lymphocytes, with fat necrosis, fibrosis, and calcification. In retractile mesenteritis, the thickening and fibrosis are more pronounced, and there is less evidence of acute necrosis and inflammation. Infrequently, the mesocolon or parietal peritoneum may be involved, or the process may occur in association with retroperitoneal fibrosis.

Although long-term experience with this syndrome is limited, most patients seem to have prolonged survival; most become asymptomatic after a period of months to years, whereas a minority exhibits the more chronic symptoms noted earlier. The role of corticosteroids is uncertain; although they may be effective in the management of those patients in whom acute symptoms predominate, there is no evidence that they affect the long-term prognosis or progression of the disease. In 15 per cent of patients, malignant lymphomas develop; the basis for this apparent association is not known.

MESENTERIC AND OMENTAL CYSTS AND TUMORS. Mesenteric cysts usually develop as the result of anomalies in the mesenteric lymphatic system but may also consist of enteric or urogenital epithelium or coelomic mesothelium. They may spontaneously wax and wane in size; usually they do not cause symptoms in patients less than 10 years of age. Symptoms are related to the size and position of the cyst, which on physical examination is nontender, round, and mobile. Spontaneous rupture, hemorrhage, or infection may occur, but these complications are unusual. Treatment consists of surgical excision.

Mesenteric tumors are rare and usually arise from the cellular elements normally present in the mesentery. They include fibromas, myxomas, lipomas, and other less common neoplasms of mesenchymal or neural origin. Most are well differentiated, low grade fibrosarcomas that produce symptoms such as pain, weight loss, abdominal mass, and compression of adjacent organs. They may be treated successfully by surgical excision. Others are more highly malignant and may metastasize distantly. *Mesenteric lymphoid tumors* also occur, and certain of these have been associated with unexplained abnormalities in iron metabolism with hypochromic microcytic anemia. *Metastatic tumors* of the mesentery are more common than primary tumors and are usually due to enlarged lymphomatous or carcinomatous lymph nodes.

Tumors of the omentum, unlike those of the mesentery, are chiefly muscular in origin (leiomyomas, leiomyosarcomas). About 40 per cent of these are malignant and cause symptoms by virtue of local invasion and development of an abdominal mass; distant metastasis is unusual.

MISCELLANEOUS DISEASES. *Torsion of the omentum* is an acute surgical condition that mimics acute appendicitis or cholecystitis. It usually occurs in patients over age 30 and causes right-sided abdominal pain with nausea, vomiting, fever, leukocytosis, and occasionally a mass. Omentectomy is indicated. *Idiopathic primary omental infarction* presents a similar clinical picture, and is invariably diagnosed only at laparotomy. *Mesenteric fibromatosis* is a benign noninflammatory fibrous proliferation of the mesentery, which occurs mainly in patients with familial polyposis of the colon or Gardner's syndrome.

Bender MD, Ockner RK: Diseases of the peritoneum, mesentery and diaphragm. *In* Sleisenger MH, Fordtran JS (eds.): Gastrointestinal Disease. 3rd ed. Philadelphia, W. B. Saunders Company, 1983. *A broad review, extensively referenced.*

Kipfer R, Moertel C, Dahlin D: Mesenteric lipodystrophy. Ann Intern Med 80:582, 1974. *A well-documented, extensive series with good data on the natural history of mesenteric inflammatory disease.*

113. GASTROINTESTINAL HEMORRHAGE

Walter L. Peterson

Gastrointestinal (GI) hemorrhage is a common clinical problem. Despite increased availability of intensive care units and improved methods of diagnosis, mortality from upper gastrointestinal hemorrhage is still approximately 10 per cent, which represents almost no decline over the past 30 years. The most likely reason for this observation is that the efficacy of available therapy is little better today than 30 years ago. This is especially true for the group of patients who account for the largest share of overall mortality, i.e., those with bleeding esophageal varices. This chapter describes general considerations in the management of the patient with gastrointestinal hemorrhage. The most important goals in this regard are (1) hemodynamic stabilization of the patient, (2) cessation of bleeding by the least invasive technique possible, and (3) prevention of recurrent hemorrhage. The overall approach to the patient with GI hemorrhage is shown in Figure 113–1.

RECOGNITION OF GASTROINTESTINAL HEMORRHAGE

PRESENTING SIGNS AND SYMPTOMS. Patients with GI hemorrhage have either obvious efflux of blood from the GI tract or no external manifestation (i.e., occult bleeding). Efflux of blood is manifested as (1) *hematemesis,* in which bright red or "coffee-ground" material is vomited; (2) *melena,* which is black, tarry, sticky, odoriferous stool;* and (3) *hematochezia,* the passage of bright red or maroon stool. Occult bleeding may occur with (1) signs and symptoms of *hypovolemia;* (2) *anemia,* either symptomatic or detected only by routine laboratory screening; or (3) chemical evidence of *occult blood* in the stool.

OBJECTIVE CONFIRMATION. Objective evidence that blood has entered the GI tract may be obtained by examining the stool or gastric aspirate for blood. If blood is not grossly evident, a chemical test for occult blood—for example, Hemoccult—can be performed. False positive results occur in 1 to 2 per cent of stool specimens, more often if the patient is taking oral iron

*Melena must not be confused with dark stools produced by iron, licorice, or bismuth compounds.

Recognition of hemorrhage
and
assessment of severity
↓
Resuscitation
↓
Differentiation of upper
from lower GI hemorrhage
↓
Empiric therapy for
upper GI hemorrhage
↓
Diagnosis
↓
Treatment

Figure 113–1.

preparations. Vitamin C may produce false negative tests. The hematocrit should always be measured to substantiate blood loss from any source or site, although the hematocrit may be normal immediately after an acute bleeding episode (see below).

RAPIDITY AND MAGNITUDE OF HEMORRHAGE. After confirming that a patient is bleeding (or recently has bled), the physician must determine whether it is continuing, determine its rapidity and magnitude, and begin resuscitation. These are important steps that must precede any concern for the site of gastrointestinal hemorrhage, whether upper or lower.

The rapidity of hemorrhage is gauged initially by the manner in which bleeding is manifested. Hematochezia or repeated episodes of copious hematemesis suggest brisk hemorrhage, as does inability to clear the nasogastric aspirate of bright red blood with gastric lavage. The ultimate measure of rapidity of hemorrhage remains the amount and rapidity of blood transfusions required to restore and maintain the vascular volume.

The magnitude of hemorrhage can be estimated by the clinical presentation. Melena can be produced experimentally by as little as 100 to 200 ml of blood, although in clinical practice the presence of melena almost always indicates at least 500 ml of blood loss. Upper gastrointestinal (UGI) bleeding manifested by hematochezia suggests losses of 1000 ml or more. By contrast, as little as 25 ml blood loss will produce a guaiac-positive stool.

Acute blood losses greater than 1000 ml are more accurately estimated by evidence of hypovolemia manifested by tachycardia, hypotension, or a fall in blood pressure upon change of position (orthostatic hypotension). These signs must be evaluated with knowledge of the physiologic compensatory responses following an acute GI hemorrhage (see below). To interpret these signs too literally may lead to underestimation of the severity of the hemorrhage, a cardinal danger in the management of such patients.

PATHOPHYSIOLOGY OF ACUTE BLEEDING. The hematocrit and blood pressure measured initially in a bleeding patient reflect three basic factors: (1) the volume of blood lost, (2) the rate at which it is lost, and (3) the extent of endogenous volume replacement. Following loss of 20 per cent of the circulating blood volume (1000 ml), there is an immediate fall in blood pressure, a rise in heart rate, and peripheral vasoconstriction. The hematocrit initially remains unchanged. Only as fluid enters the vascular space from extravascular compartments does the hematocrit fall and blood pressure rise. The heart rate may soon return to normal or actually fall below normal, and may therefore be an unreliable sign of the severity of a hemorrhage. As noted, the level of the hematocrit depends on the rapidity and completeness of dilution of the remaining blood as well as the severity of the hemorrhage. An isolated hematocrit reading, unless low, is of little help.

The blood pressure is the most important sign of the state of blood volume and most accurately mirrors the severity of the situation. However, it is also affected by the patient's age, preexisting blood pressure, and ability to mobilize fluid. For example, a dehydrated patient who bleeds acutely may be unable to restore volume. The resulting blood pressure will be low and the hematocrit may remain normal or high. A low hematocrit, low blood pressure, or rapid heart rate usually indicates a severe hemorrhage. A normal hematocrit, normal blood pressure, or normal heart rate must be interpreted with caution.

INITIAL THERAPY

RESUSCITATION. Initial therapy (resuscitation) is independent of the source of bleeding. Rather, it is dependent on the rapidity and magnitude of hemorrhage. Generally, patients should be placed in an intensive care unit unless it is clear that the bleeding is mild or chronic and the patient does not require resuscitation. It is also prudent to obtain surgical consultation to follow the patient through resuscitation, diagnosis, and therapy, so that rapid surgical assistance is available if needed. Resuscitation is directed toward supporting the vascular volume and providing adequate tissue oxygenation. Large intravenous catheters should be inserted, at times into a large central vein, and fluids begun. The physician must remember that the dilutional effect of exogenous fluids will lower the hematocrit. Nasal oxygen (2.0 to 3.0 liters per minute) may be necessary, particularly for elderly persons or those with cardiac or pulmonary disease. Urine output and systemic blood pressure should be closely monitored and, if necessary, central venous or pulmonary wedge pressures as well. Blood is sent for typing and crossmatching as well as for other laboratory data (especially determinations of clotting factors). An electrocardiogram and chest x-ray should be obtained and, to record the patient's progress, a flow sheet for fluids, vital signs, and other values is initiated.

The blood products administered depend upon the rapidity of hemorrhage and the resources of individual blood banks. Patients with active bleeding should receive whole blood if possible; but if packed red blood cells must be used to treat active bleeding, fresh frozen plasma should be given with every 4 to 6 units.

In patients whose plasma volume has been restored from extravascular compartments, packed red blood cells are sufficient. Packed cells are indicated especially in elderly patients with chronic bleeding who are in shock and in whom whole blood may produce vascular volume overload. Fresh frozen plasma should be given to patients whose bleeding has ceased only if there are demonstrated needs. For example, patients with cirrhosis may have special needs for clotting factors present in fresh frozen plasma.

When and how much blood is transfused varies from patient to patient and is dependent upon several factors. These include the volume of blood lost, the presence or absence of continuing hemorrhage, the chronicity of blood loss, and the patient's clinical response to blood loss. For example, a young patient may tolerate without transfusion a hematocrit of 25 per cent or less quite well, especially if bleeding has been chronic; on the other hand, an older patient, at the same hematocrit, may have postural hypotension, confusion, or angina pectoris and require transfusion. Patients with continuing hemorrhage usually require blood regardless of the absolute hematocrit level. A hematocrit of 30 per cent has proved to be a satisfactory level to achieve with transfusions. Nevertheless, the requirements for numbers of units of blood must often be determined individually, based on the patient's clinical status.

DISTINGUISHING BETWEEN UPPER AND LOWER GASTROINTESTINAL HEMORRHAGE

As restorative therapy is begun, thought should be given to whether the source of bleeding is from the upper or lower gastrointestinal tract. Hematemesis connotes a source of bleeding above the ligament of Treitz. Melena results from the breakdown of blood during its transit through the intestinal tract. The longer blood remains in the GI tract, the more likely melena will occur. Therefore, melena occurs most often from upper GI bleeding lesions and only occasionally from bleeding sites as distal as the right colon. Hematochezia represents either a very rapid, massive (1000 ml) UGI hemorrhage or, more likely, a lower intestinal source. Hypovolemia, anemia, or occult stool blood may be manifestations of either upper or lower GI hemorrhage. To confirm or detect a UGI source, a nasogastric tube is placed. A bloody aspirate is diagnostic of UGI hemorrhage; a clear aspirate effectively rules out active bleeding from the esophagus and stomach. When the gastric aspirate is negative for blood, the source of bleeding is usually lower GI, but an actively bleeding postpyloric lesion (such as duodenal ulcer) may still be present. Obviously the nasogastric aspirate may be negative if bleeding has ceased.

Other findings in UGI bleeding include hyperactive bowel sounds, leukocytosis, low grade fever, and elevation of the

BUN. Elevation of the BUN in acute UGI bleeding probably represents a combination of (1) absorption of a high protein load (approximately 15 grams of globin plus plasma proteins per 100 ml of blood) with resulting increased synthesis of urea and (2) hypovolemia with reduced renal perfusion.

EMPIRIC THERAPY FOR UPPER GASTROINTESTINAL HEMORRHAGE

If the patient is suspected of having UGI hemorrhage, a nasogastric tube is placed to document that its source is esophageal, gastric, or (in many cases) immediately postpyloric and to gauge the rapidity of bleeding. If the aspirate is a flow of fresh blood, this tube is withdrawn and is replaced with a large bore orogastric tube for gastric lavage. Large volumes (500 to 1000 ml) of iced saline or tap water are lavaged through the orogastric tube, although room temperature fluids may function as well. The fluid is removed from the stomach by gravity drainage, avoiding excess suction, which can damage the gastric mucosa. Gastric lavage serves several purposes: the rate of bleeding is gauged, blood clots are evacuated, and hemostasis may be promoted. Although cause and effect have not been proved, gastric lavage is associated with cessation of such bleeding in 85 to 90 per cent of patients. No therapeutic intervention, including cimetidine, has been shown to improve upon the results obtained with lavage alone. The amount of lavage fluid required varies from patient to patient. Gastric contents will clear in some with 1 to 2 liters of fluid, whereas in others 10 or more liters may be required.

If bleeding does not subside during lavage, levarterenol (Levophed, 8 mg in 100 ml of normal saline) may be instilled into the stomach through the nasogastric tube. Such local vasoconstrictor therapy may be effective as a stopgap measure, although no controlled evidence is available to prove its effectiveness.

If hemorrhage ceases during lavage, empiric therapy should be begun for the most common cause of UGI hemorrhage in the nonalcoholic—i.e., peptic ulcer. One such approach is to maintain gastric pH as close to neutrality as possible during the initial 24 to 72 hours when recurrent hemorrhage is most likely. This may be accomplished by blocking acid secretion with an H_2-receptor blocking agent and monitoring gastric pH hourly. Hourly doses of supplemental antacids (beginning with 30-ml aliquots of an aluminum-magnesium preparation) are then instilled through the nasogastric tube to maintain the pH near 7. When a particular dose of antacid is found that will reliably maintain the pH near 7, the nasogastric tube can be withdrawn and antacids given orally. After three days, therapy is continued with standard doses of ulcer medication (see Ch. 99).

DIAGNOSTIC APPROACH TO DETERMINE THE SPECIFIC CAUSE OF HEMORRHAGE

To this point in a patient's course, attention has been directed toward establishing that GI hemorrhage has occurred, determining its rapidity and magnitude, localizing the source as upper or lower GI, and initiating resuscitation. During this time, it is important to obtain a careful history and perform a thorough physical examination. Although the information obtained often provides only valuable clues, it may at times be diagnostic. The subsequent approach to treatment depends on whether or not bleeding continues or ceases with initial therapy.

UPPER GASTROINTESTINAL HEMORRHAGE. Helpful historic information includes prior episodes of bleeding, associated illnesses (e.g., cirrhosis), medications taken (especially analgesics and anticoagulants), or prior abdominal surgery (for peptic ulcer or for placement of aortic vascular prostheses). Has the patient experienced epistaxis or hemoptysis? Does the patient tell of dyspepsia, heartburn, or retching prior to hematemesis, which may indicate peptic ulcer, reflux esophagitis, or a Mallory-Weiss mucosal tear, respectively? On physical examination, the physican should look for cutaneous manifestations of underlying diseases such as Osler-Weber-Rendu syndrome, Ehlers-Danlos syndrome, pseudoxanthoma elasticum, and the blue rubber bleb nevus syndrome. Is there adenopathy to suggest malignancy? Or jaundice, palmar erythema, spider angiomas, or hepatosplenomegaly to suggest cirrhosis?

If Hemorrhage Continues Despite Initial Therapy. If bleeding continues even after vigorous gastric lavage, further therapy may be invasive and will differ depending upon the actual source of bleeding. Therefore, rapid, accurate diagnosis is required and is best achieved with panendoscopy. In the occasional situation in which bleeding is so brisk as to preclude visualization by endoscopy, and if time will allow, arteriography will often delineate an actively bleeding arterial site. If none is found, venous bleeding from varices is inferred. Radioisotopic techniques (see below) might also visualize the site of bleeding. Arteriography, however, offers the potential advantage of permitting infusion of vasoconstrictor drugs into the offending vessel as a means of treatment. Barium studies of the UGI tract are not appropriate in this setting, because only potential bleeding sites can be seen and because the contrast material may hinder further diagnostic procedures such as endoscopy or arteriography.

Rapid bleeding from fistulization of an aortofemoral bypass graft into the duodenum is a special situation. The nasogastric aspirate is often clear, but melena or marked hematochezia suggests a UGI site. In a patient with an aortofemoral graft, endoscopy of the esophagus, stomach, and proximal duodenum should be done immediately to exclude a bleeding site other than a graft-enteric fistula. The fistula itself, if present, is rarely seen at endoscopy. Arteriography may not reveal the bleeding from the graft and should not be done. Immediate surgery is indicated in patients with grafts if no other site of hemorrhage is visualized.

If Hemorrhage Ceases with Initial Therapy. In most patients, (85 per cent or more), hemorrhage ceases with initial therapy or is not active at the time of admission and urgent diagnosis is not required. Most patients should undergo either a barium UGI series or panendoscopy for diagnostic evaluation. The UGI series is a safe, inexpensive procedure that will detect most UGI malignancies and many peptic ulcers. This is especially true if a double-contrast x-ray examination is performed. Panendoscopy is more specific and sensitive, and hence a more accurate diagnostic tool (especially for superficial bleeding lesions). However, making a diagnosis may not have an impact on patient outcome, since therapy is often the same regardless of the bleeding lesion.

Angiography is rarely indicated in patients who cease bleeding, for it will detect only abnormal vascular patterns that are rare and may or may not be the actual source of bleeding. Nevertheless, in selected cases of UGI bleeding in which UGI x-rays and endoscopy are unrevealing, arteriography may be helpful (see The Diagnostic Dilemma, below).

LOWER GASTROINTESTINAL HEMORRHAGE. Remote and recent historical points that are important in assessing lower gastrointestinal hemorrhage include a prior history of rectal bleeding (hemorrhoids, diverticulosis, or polyps), a recent change in stool caliber (colonic cancer), acute abdominal pain with bleeding (ischemic colitis), or recurrent or bloody diarrhea (inflammatory bowel disease). A history of familial colonic polyposis or of an aortofemoral bypass graft would also be very important. On physical examination, one should palpate for abdominal masses, look for external hemorrhoids, and note any masses present on digital rectal examination. Inflammatory bowel disease or familial polyposis may have extracolonic manifestations involving skin, bones, or joints (see Ch. 104 and 106).

If Hemorrhage Continues Despite Initial Therapy. Anoscopy and proctosigmoidoscopy can detect lesions involving the lower 20 to 25 cm of the colon such as hemorrhoids, polyps, inflammatory bowel diseases, ischemic colitis, or rectosigmoid cancer. On many occasions, however, all that can be seen is blood coming from somewhere above the level reached by the instruments. While an angiography team is being assembled, it is reasonable to perform a quick upper endoscopy to exclude a postpyloric bleeding site in the UGI tract. If endoscopy is negative, and if bleeding persists, angiography will sometimes localize the site of lower intestinal bleeding, although perhaps not the specific lesion (see above for the approach to possible bleeding from aortofemoral grafts). This is especially helpful in patients bleeding from diverticula or vascular anomalies. Intra-arterial infusions of vasopressin may even stop the bleeding before surgical intervention is required. Barium enema examination should not be performed, as it will preclude subsequent angiography. Colonoscopy is difficult in the face of continuing hemorrhage, but may be performed if bleeding slows to an ooze.

Detection of intestinal extravasation of a radioisotope such as technetium-99m (^{99}Tc)–labeled sulfur colloid is a noninvasive means to localize active bleeding. ^{99}Tc sulfur colloid is rapidly cleared from the blood by the liver and spleen, which means that bleeding may be detected only a short time. Attachment of ^{99}Tc to the patient's own red blood cells avoids this problem. While important therapeutic decisions should probably not be based solely on the results of radionuclide scanning until more experience has been gained, this technique may at the least be a helpful screening test prior to arteriography.

If Hemorrhage Ceases with Initial Therapy. Patients whose bleeding ceases spontaneously during resuscitation should in most instances undergo proctoscopy and then be observed for 48 hours before further diagnostic evaluation. A barium enema is not performed before this time for fear of being unable to utilize arteriography (because of residual barium) should hemorrhage recur. After 48 hours a barium enema is usually obtained. In some patients, the results of the barium enema, when coupled with the clinical findings, may complete the evaluation. In others, the barium enema is considered a complementary prelude to colonoscopy. Colonoscopy may be performed (after cleansing the colon) to confirm or biopsy lesions detected by barium enema, to exclude other sources of bleeding in the large number of patients who may have diverticulosis as an incidental finding, and to detect mucosal lesions or small polyps missed by barium enema. Patients who experience recurrent hemorrhage during the 48-hour waiting period may require angiography or, if bleeding again ceases, early colonoscopy without a preliminary barium enema. If evaluation of the patient with presumed lower GI bleeding is unrewarding, UGI sources should be excluded with an UGI series and possibly endoscopy; lesions below the ligament of Treitz but above the terminal ileum may be sought with a small bowel series (see The Diagnostic Dilemma, below).

SPECIFIC CAUSES OF HEMORRHAGE AND THEIR TREATMENT

The causes of GI bleeding are shown in Table 113–1. The ligament of Treitz is generally considered the dividing point for upper and lower GI lesions. However, because jejunal and ileal lesions are so rarely the cause of GI bleeding, lower GI bleeding almost always comes from the colon.

UPPER GASTROINTESTINAL HEMORRHAGE. The three most common causes of serious upper gastrointestinal bleeding are peptic ulcer, acute mucosal lesions, and esophageal varices.

Peptic ulcer (gastric, duodenal, or postsurgical anastomotic ulcers) will in most cases require urgent surgery if bleeding does not cease. Although nonoperative techniques using endoscopic electrocoagulation or laser photocoagulation are becoming increasingly available, their role has been far from clarified and they should still be considered experimental modalities. If bleeding ceases, therapy after the first three days (see above) is the same as for nonbleeding ulcers, i.e., antacids, sucralfate, or histamine H_2-receptor antagonists (see Ch. 99). *Acute mucosal lesions* (esophagitis, gastritis, or Mallory-Weiss tears) that continue bleeding often respond to intra-arterial infusions of vasoconstrictor drugs such as vasopressin, thereby precluding the need for surgery. Such treatment, of course, necessitates catheterization of visceral arteries, usually the celiac. In some centers embolic therapy with blood clot or Gelfoam is also used. If bleeding ceases, acute mucosal lesions are treated with measures to reduce gastric acidity, although Mallory-Weiss lesions usually require no specific therapy. If aspirin is believed to be the cause of acute gastritis, other analgesics should be substituted. This should be done cautiously, since most other analgesics (with the exception of enteric coated aspirin) also may cause gastritis. "Stress" gastritis can be prevented in patients predisposed to this lesion by the prophylactic administration of frequent, large doses of a potent antacid.

Continuing hemorrhage from *esophageal or gastric varices* is a condition for which no therapy has been convincingly shown to be satisfactory. A low-dose, constant intravenous infusion of vasopressin* (0.1 to 0.4 unit per minute) is often recommended. However, recent evidence suggests that this therapy may be no better than placebo at stopping variceal bleeding. Balloon tamponade will often stop the bleeding but at a substantial risk of esophageal perforation or pulmonary aspiration. Because emergent or even urgent surgery for variceal hemorrhage carries with it an extremely high mortality in patients with cirrhosis of the liver, new techniques such as transhepatic obliteration of varices or endoscopic sclerotherapy have been developed. Because the transhepatic angiographic technique requires puncture of a diseased, easily bleeding liver, and because there are more endoscopists available than angiographers, endoscopic sclerotherapy has more or less been given pre-eminence. If hemorrhage has ceased, and depending upon the individual circumstances, consideration may be given to means of preventing future episodes of hemorrhage. These consist of portal vein decompressive surgery, repeated endoscopic injections of varices with a sclerosing solution, or perhaps propranolol, a beta-blocking agent that lowers portal pressure.

Malignant lesions producing UGI hemorrhage are usually treated surgically while rare *vascular lesions* such as Osler-Weber-Rendu syndrome or angiodysplasia may respond either to experimental thermal obliteration with endoscopic electro- or laser coagulation or, if localized, to segmental surgical resection.

LOWER GASTROINTESTINAL HEMORRHAGE. *Hemorrhoids* are treated medically with sitz baths and lubricating suppositories, by banding, or surgically, depending on the severity and frequency of bleeding episodes (see Ch. 110). *Ischemic colitis, inflammatory bowel disease,* and *cancer* only rarely produce bleeding severe enough to necessitate immediate surgery and are managed as they would be if hemorrhage had not been the presenting symptom. Hemorrhage from *diverticulosis* that continues after initial therapy may respond to intra-arterial vasopressin therapy. If not, diagnostic arteriography may localize the bleeding site to permit segmental colonic resection rather than subtotal colectomy. *Vascular malformations* located by arteriography may also respond to intra-arterial vasopressin. Indication for elective surgical resection of diverticula or vascular malformations that cease bleeding either spontaneously or with vasopressin depend upon the severity and frequency of bleeding episodes.

THE DIAGNOSTIC DILEMMA

The diagnostic approach to patients with gastrointestinal hemorrhage just described will not lead to diagnosis in many patients. Fortunately such failure is not detrimental to most, particularly during a period of observation. Nevertheless, failure to locate and define the source of bleeding jeopardizes patients with multiple episodes of hemorrhage that require

*This use is not listed in the manufacturer's directive.

TABLE 113–1. CAUSES OF GI BLEEDING

Upper GI	Upper or Lower GI	Lower GI
Duodenal ulcer	Neoplasms	Hemorrhoids
Gastric ulcer	Carcinoma	Anal fissure
Anastomotic ulcer	Leiomyoma	Diverticulosis
Esophagitis	Sarcoma	Meckel's diverticulum
Gastritis	Hemangioma	Ischemic bowel disease
Mallory-Weiss tear	Lymphoma	Inflammatory bowel disease
Esophageal varices	Melanoma	Solitary colonic ulcer
Hematobilia	Polyps	Intussusception
Menetrier's disease	Arterial-enteric fistulas	
	Vascular anomalies	
	Osler-Weber-Rendu	
	Blue rubber bleb nevus	
	CREST syndrome	
	Arteriovenous malformations	
	Angiodysplasia (vascular ectasia)	
	Hematologic diseases	
	Elastic tissue disorders	
	Pseudoxanthoma elasticum	
	Ehlers-Danlos	
	Vasculitis syndromes	
	Amyloidosis	

repeated hospitalizations and blood transfusions, particularly high-risk elderly patients with a potentially curable lesion.

There are at least three reasons that a diagnosis of the bleeding lesion fails. First, it may be in a location that is relatively inaccessible to standard x-ray procedures and endoscopy. The best example is a lesion of the small bowel, i.e., a middle GI lesion. Second, there may be single or multiple lesions that are potential bleeding sites, and documentation of the one responsible may be virtually impossible. Third, the lesion responsible for the hemorrhage may be overlooked because of its subtle manifestation or because diagnosticians are unfamiliar with the lesion.

Lesions of the small bowel include tumors, vascular malformations, or Meckel's diverticula. An infusion small bowel series, in which a tube is positioned in the third portion of the duodenum to allow a controlled, steady infusion of barium, permits the radiologist to follow the column of barium more closely than with the standard small bowel series. Tumors of the small bowel may be detected with this technique. If this procedure is unrewarding, visceral angiography may detect abnormal vascular patterns of tumors or vascular malformations, although contrast material will not enter the lumen unless bleeding is active (at least 0.5 ml of blood loss per minute). Meckel's diverticula are sources of bleeding primarily in young patients and may at times be localized by using a technetium isotopic scan. This test is often difficult to interpret.

Confirmation that a lesion is actually the site of hemorrhage requires either endoscopy or arteriography performed while the patient is bleeding. In the UGI tract this may be of particular importance in patients with esophageal varices, whereas in the lower GI tract it is important in the patient with suspected bleeding from diverticulosis or angiodysplasia. For example, a patient may present with a lower GI hemorrhage that ceases spontaneously. Barium enema discloses diverticula, and colonoscopy reveals no other lesions. If the patient at a later time has another hemorrhage, arteriography may demonstrate that a diverticulum is bleeding in a particular area of the colon, or it may disclose a lesion such as angiodysplasia which was overlooked on colonoscopy. The role of radionuclide scanning in patients whose conditions present a diagnostic dilemma remains to be settled.

Vascular malformations are subtle lesions with which many physicians may be unfamiliar. These range from the hereditary telangiectasias of Osler-Weber-Rendu to angiodysplasia, which may account for an important proportion of GI hemorrhage in elderly patients. This lesion is believed to be an acquired one that develops as part of the aging process. In theory, many years of low grade obstructions of submucosal veins ultimately lead to small arteriovenous communications in the mucosa and submucosa. This lesion was originally recognized by arteriography as a cause of bleeding in the cecum and may be responsible for a substantial proportion of bleeding episodes previously ascribed to right-sided diverticula. Because many of these malformations are submucosal, they cannot always be seen by colonoscopy or at surgery.

More recently, angiodysplasias arising in the mucosa have been described endoscopically. These vascular lesions have been found both in the cecum and in the UGI tract. They are described as bright red, flat, and fern-like. As more endoscopists become familiar with this lesion, it will likely become a more frequently listed cause of both upper and lower gastrointestinal hemorrhage in the elderly.

Treatment of angiodysplasia localized to the cecum and ascending colon may be treated with right hemicolectomy. In fact, some investigators suggest resection after the first episode of hemorrhage. An alternative form of therapy, as yet experimental, is thermal coagulation, using electrocoagulation or laser. This technique would appear expecially useful when there are multiple, widely scattered lesions or when they are present in the UGI tract and surgical resection would result in undesirable postoperative complications.

Athanasoulis CA, Waltman AC, Novelline RA, Krudy AG, Sniderman KW: Angiography, its contribution to the emergency management of gastrointestinal hemorrhage. Radiol Clin North Am 14:265, 1976. *A detailed review of diagnostic and therapeutic angiography by one of its pioneers.*

Boley SJ, DiBiase A, Brandt LJ, Sammartano RJ: Lower intestinal bleeding in the elderly. Am J Surg 137:57, 1979. *Emphasizes the increasing awareness of angiodysplasia as a cause of lower intestinal hemorrhage in the elderly.*

Dronfield MW, Langman MJS, Atkinson M, Balfour TW, Bell GD, Vellacott KD, Amar SS, Knapp DR: Outcome of endoscopy and barium radiography for acute upper gastrointestinal bleeding: Controlled trial in 1037 patients. Br Med J 284:545, 1982. *A very large trial evaluating the benefit of early endoscopy in acute upper gastrointestinal bleeding.*

Fleischer D: Etiology and prevalence of severe persistent upper gastrointestinal bleeding. Gastroenterology 84:538, 1983. *A nice evaluation of severe upper gastrointestinal bleeding.*

Gilbert DA, Silverstein FE, Auth DC, Rubin CE: Nonsurgical management of acute nonvariceal upper gastrointestinal bleeding. *In* Spaet TH (ed.): Progress in Hemostasis and Thrombosis, Vol IV. New York, Grune & Stratton, 1978, pp 349–395. *The definitive work concerning nonsurgical therapy; especially good with new endoscopic techniques.*

Graham DY, Davis RE: Acute upper gastrointestinal hemorrhage. New observations on an old problem. Digest Dis 23:76, 1978. *A concise work dealing with diagnosis of upper gastrointestinal hemorrhage.*

Graham DY, Smith JL: The course of patients after variceal hemorrhage. Gastroenterology 80:800, 1981. *Demonstrates the dismal prognosis for variceal bleeders.*

Peterson WL: Gastrointestinal bleeding. *In* Sleisenger MH, Fordtran JS (eds.): Gastrointestinal Disease. 3rd ed. Philadelphia, W. B. Saunders Company,

1983, pp 177–207. *A much expanded, fully referenced review of gastrointestinal bleeding.*
Schiller KFR, Cotton PB: Acute upper gastrointestinal hemorrhage. Clin Gastroenterol 7:595, 1978. *Excellent overview of upper gastrointestinal hemorrhage, with extensive bibliography.*
Zinner MJ, Zuidema GD, Smith PL, Mignosa M: The prevention of upper gastrointestinal tract bleeding in patients in an intensive care unit. Surg Gynecol Obstet 153:214, 1981. *The best study of prophylactic prevention of "stress" bleeding.*

114. MISCELLANEOUS INFLAMMATORY DISEASES OF THE INTESTINE

Marvin H. Sleisenger

Acute Appendicitis (Including the Acute Abdomen)

DEFINITION. Appendicitis is acute inflammation of the vermiform appendix. It is rare before the age of two and reaches a peak incidence in the second and third decades. The vast majority of patients are between the ages of 5 and 30. Although incidence of the disease declines after the age of 40, the annual incidence is about 1.5 per thousand for males and 1.9 per thousand for females between the ages of 17 and 64. The disease is important because it is common and curable; it therefore constitutes the most important entity in the differential diagnosis of the acute abdomen.

PATHOLOGY. Usually, the appendix is swollen, hyperemic, warm, and covered with exudate. However, in the early stages it may appear only slightly discolored and, in the late stages, gangrenous with perforation. Microscopically, the picture ranges from some acute inflammatory cells in the lumen and mucosa to acute inflammatory changes transmurally with superficial mucosal ulcerations; in advanced stages, one or more perforations may be noted, particularly in patients over the age of 60.

ETIOLOGY AND PATHOGENESIS. The initiating event in acute appendicitis appears to be obstruction, followed by increased intraluminal pressure, reduced venous drainage, thrombosis, hemorrhage, edema, and bacterial invasion of the wall. The appendiceal artery (an end artery) becomes occluded and perforation results.

Calculi are thought to be the most common cause of the initial obstruction. A small percentage of inflamed appendices contain a radiologically demonstrable calculus, as compared with 2.7 per cent of normal ones. Gangrene and perforation are more common in appendices with calculi. The calculi are composed of inspissated fecal material, calcium phosphate–rich mucus, and inorganic salts. Although fecaliths are more common in populations eating a low fiber diet, the incidence of appendicitis is decreasing in the West, and 70 per cent of patients with acute appendicitis do not have calculi. Alternative pathogenetic mechanisms include obstruction by parasites, lymphoid hyperplasia associated with viral infections, and twisting of the appendix by adhesions. An additional theory is malfunction of a valve system at the entrance of the appendix.

CLINICAL PICTURE AND DIAGNOSIS. The duration of appendicitis is usually 12 to 48 hours from onset to hospitalization. Over 95 per cent complain of *pain* at onset, classically referred to the epigastric or periumbilical areas and later localizing in the right lower quadrant. This sequence, however, is not found in all patients and is notably absent in *retrocecal appendicitis.* Further, a significant number will not localize clearly to the right lower quadrant, the pain being either diffuse or in the lower abdomen. In *pelvic appendicitis* the pain may be in the left lower quadrant. When retrocecal, the pain may be referred to the thigh or right testicle. Dysuria is present frequently in both types of appendicitis.

Pain referred to the mid-epigastrium is due to stretching of the organ during early inflammation. Initially it is vague and mild, but it gradually increases over about four hours and may be colicky. It tends to subside, and when the process has reached the serosa and the peritoneum, it localizes over the site of disease. In some patients distress appears to be alleviated at the time of perforation; after perforation, localization of pain will depend on whether or not the process is quickly walled off locally. Thus if the spreading infection is not contained, generalized abdominal discomfort of variable severity will result. *Anorexia* and *nausea* (with or without vomiting) are the second and third most frequent symptoms. In almost all instances, pain precedes the appearance of these other complaints, and its principal feature is *persistence.* About 10 per cent of patients will have constipation; diarrhea is uncommon. Temperature usually ranges between 38 and 38.6°C; higher levels usually indicate perforation.

PHYSICAL EXAMINATION. The findings on physical examination depend not only upon the stage of the inflammation but also upon the age of the patient. Tenderness to palpation is the most common (99 per cent), important, and reliable sign; indeed without it, diagnosis is unlikely. It is usually confined to McBurney's point (one finger) in the right lower quadrant, corresponding to the usual location of the organ. However, although rectal tenderness is present in about one third of patients, it may be so severe as to indicate pelvic peritonitis and thus probable *pelvic appendicitis.* On initial examination in a minority of patients, a mass may be felt in the right lower quadrant or in the pelvis or transrectally. Localized rebound pain is found in 75 per cent. Generalized rebound tenderness indicates diffuse peritonitis. Bowel sounds may be present or absent; absence associated with distention and generalized rebound tenderness is consistent with perforation and diffuse peritonitis. The patient with acute appendicitis often does not seem ill. The physician must not be deceived; the diagnosis rests upon persisting pain and localized tenderness.

On occasion, tenderness may be elicited in the case of retrocecal appendicitis by stretching the psoas by hip extension. Very rarely, because of the odd location of the appendix, tenderness may be in the right upper quadrant or even the left lower quadrant.

LABORATORY FINDINGS. Laboratory studies consistently show a leukocytosis with an increase in polymorphonuclear cells—over 10,000 per cubic millimeter and greater than 75 per cent, respectively. Urinalysis is usually normal; however, about 15 per cent of patients have either a slight amount of protein or mild pyuria or hematuria. Presence of a calcified fecalith in the right lower quadrant on flat film of the abdomen is helpful, but it is present in only a small percentage of patients. Other findings on flat film include possible obliteration of the right psoas shadow, right lower quadrant sentinel loop ileus, and a right lower quadrant soft tissue mass with or without gas bubbles. With perforation and generalized peritonitis, fluid in the peritoneal cavity and obliteration of the peritoneal lines may be noted.

DIFFERENTIAL DIAGNOSIS OF APPENDICITIS AND OF THE ACUTE ABDOMEN. Appendicitis is first on the list of conditions causing acute abdominal pain that require surgery or immediate consultation with a surgeon. Here a few principles regarding the acute surgical abdomen in the setting of the differential diagnosis of acute appendicitis will be reviewed.

Pain Characteristics. Conditions associated with pain of sudden onset include *perforated viscus* or *acute ischemia* (although acute ischemia does not always cause acute or severe pain in the elderly); occasionally, the onset of pain in *acute small bowel obstruction, choledocholithiasis, ureteral obstruction,* and *dissection of an abdominal aortic aneurysm* may also be abrupt. The more gradual onset of pain usually indicates an inflammatory lesion, including appendicitis. However, the pain of diffuse *inflammatory bowel disease* is not localized as it is in appendicitis, except as a consequence of perforation or fistulization in Crohn's disease. The pain of pelvic inflammatory disease is usually associated with menstruation and has been present for 24 or more hours, whereas appendicitis pain is more often intermenstrual and rarely is suffered so long except with perforation.

The type and radiation of the pain also help in differential diagnosis. For example, evidence of irritation of the diaphragm may be found on the right in *acute cholecystitis* and on the left in *acute pancreatitis;* sudden severe pain referred to the tips of the shoulders, associated with diffuse intra-abdominal pain and, later, distention, is more typical of perforated viscus, particularly *peptic ulcer. Ureteral obstruction* causes pain which is frequently referred to the genitalia or groin. Steady continuous pain is more characteristic of inflammation, as in appendicitis; on the other hand, intermittent or crampy pain is more characteristic of *obstruction of a hollow viscus* such as the gallbladder or small bowel.

Pain precedes nausea and vomiting in *appendicitis;* on the other hand, vomiting may be an early symptom of *acute cholecystitis or acute pancreatitis.* Bile-stained vomitus associated with acute cramping upper abdominal pain suggests *small bowel obstruction;* blood in the vomitus points toward a mucosal lesion proximal to the third portion of the duodenum. Relief of pain by vomiting suggests *gastric outlet obstruction.* Vomiting, of course, may accompany any intra-abdominal conditions, particularly if the patient is in great pain and has ileus or generalized peritonitis.

Physical Findings. Physical examination of the patient with an acute abdomen is of great importance, and the range of findings expected in acute appendicitis has been discussed. Localized tenderness and temperature elevation associated with continuing pain over a period of hours reflect either *localized peritonitis,* with or without perforation, or *vascular necrosis* of an ischemic organ. In such instances, the temperature is approximately 38.5 to 39.5°C. Higher temperatures are more often associated with urinary tract infections or bacterial pneumonias. A continuing rising pulse rate likewise indicates the possibility of gangrene or perforation of a viscus.

Diffuse peritonitis is reflected by resistance of movement and change in position because of accentuation of pain; on the other hand, colic caused by *obstruction* of bile ducts, ureter, or small bowel early in its course is associated with restless movement. Later, in biliary tract and small bowel obstruction, infection and compromise of the blood supply may ensue and will cause the appearance of signs of localized tissue necrosis and peritonitis. The abdomen should be carefully examined for scars of previous surgery that may now underlie an *intestinal obstruction* caused by adhesions; hernias must be sought. A succussion splash indicates marked *gastric outlet obstruction.*

In examining the patient with an acute abdomen, the physician should palpate in that quadrant which is farthest removed from the site of distress. The important findings that indicate a surgical condition include persistent localized tenderness with unequivocal rebound, indicating localized peritonitis, and guarding. Guarding must be interpreted circumspectly, because it may be voluntary or involuntary. If it is the latter, underlying peritoneal irritation is likely. Generalized involuntary guarding is a classic finding for a perforated intra-abdominal viscus. The presence of an abdominal mass not previously noted, particularly when associated with other findings of inflammation, gangrene, or perforation, is very strong evidence for a surgical condition. Likewise, free air in the abdominal cavity, as evidenced by distention, absence of bowel sounds, and absence of liver dullness in the setting of acute abdominal pain, reflects a perforated viscus. Bowel sounds may be more active and high pitched in early obstruction or continuously active in diffuse acute inflammation (nonsurgical) of the small bowel. With increasing distention of small bowel loops, the sounds become less frequent and more high pitched. Bruits are an important finding, because they may reflect the presence of *arterial aneurysms,* the dissections of which may be the cause for the abdominal pain.

Rectal examination is crucial in differential diagnosis. Unequivocal tenderness indicates pelvic inflammation, and a mass usually reflects the presence of an abscess. As noted above, this examination often reveals positive findings in acute appendicitis. A glove specimen of stool must always be examined for occult blood. In females with acute abdominal pain, pelvic examination is essential to complement a careful gynecologic history.

Laboratory Aids in Diagnosis. The laboratory examination, consisting of urinalysis, complete blood count, serum electrolytes, BUN and creatinine, x-ray examination of the abdomen and chest, and sonography of the abdomen is essential in differential diagnosis of the acute abdomen.

A *polymorphonuclear leukocytosis* strongly substantiates an acute intra-abdominal process with inflammation or necrosis; a low hematocrit reflects a disorder that is also capable of producing bleeding—*mucosal ulcerations, intestinal carcinoma, ischemia,* or *dissecting aneurysms.* An elevated hematocrit and BUN suggest dehydration, usually caused by vomiting and deficient fluid intake.

Urinalysis is vital in differential diagnosis, because the presence of pyuria, particularly white cell casts and bacteria on the smear of urinary sediment, is strong evidence for urinary tract infection and interdicts surgical exploration. Microscopic hematuria (numerous red cells) suggests stone or tumor of the genitourinary tract; red cell casts, on the other hand, suggest glomerulitis. A few scattered white and red cells may be seen in the sediment of about 20 per cent of patients with acute appendicitis. Examination of a *stool specimen* for blood and white blood cells is indicated in patients with right lower quadrant pain, fever, and *diarrhea. Salmonella* enterocolitis (and other bacterial infections) may be confused with acute appendicitis.

Important blood chemistries are *serum amylase,* elevation of which usually reflects acute pancreatitis; however, it may not be elevated in chronic relapsing pancreatitis, and it is elevated in other conditions such as *perforated peptic ulcer, strangulated obstruction* of the small bowel with perforation, *acute cholecystitis, cholangitis, acute renal failure,* and *ruptured tubal pregnancy.*

Roentgenographic Studies in the Acute Abdomen. Roentgenologic examinations of importance include chest films, flat film of the abdomen, intravenous pyelogram, and CT scans. The flat and upright films of the abdomen may show free air in the peritoneal cavity, reflecting a perforation of a hollow viscus (80 per cent of cases are due to perforated ulcer, followed by perforated diverticulum and appendicitis). They also support the diagnosis of acute small bowel obstruction, indicate the likelihood of calculus disease of either gallbladder or urogenital tract, outline a large obstructed stomach, and reveal a variety of soft tissue masses that may reflect cysts or abscesses. Collections of extraintestinal gas often point to abscesses; occasionally, the biliary tree may be outlined by air, thus revealing a fistula to bowel. Diffuse calcification of the region of the pancreas indicates chronic pancreatitis. As noted, calculi in the right lower quadrant may rarely help in the diagnosis of acute appendicitis. Flat film of the abdomen also may yield findings characteristic of acute pancreatitis, including "sentinel" loops and a "cut-off" of the colon. A cross-table lateral view will outline an abdominal aortic aneurysm. A routine chest x-ray is essential in order to reveal free intraperitoneal air under the diaphragm, to demonstrate pneumonia, or to show an elevated diaphragm on the left with or without pleural effusion and partial atelectasis as noted in acute pancreatitis, or on the right, reflecting subphrenic abscess. A barium enema showing a patent appendix is evidence against acute appendicitis.

Sonography may demonstrate gallstones, dilated common bile duct and intrahepatic ducts, collections of fluid including abscesses, defects in the liver, obstruction of the urinary tract, enlargement ("phlegmon") of the pancreas in acute pancreatitis or by an inflammatory pseudocyst, or an enlarged abdominal aorta or lymph nodes. Ultrasound may also indicate *colonic diverticulitis, Crohn's disease, intramural hemorrhage,* or *intussusception* by revealing a thickened bowel wall. It may also help in diagnosing *"closed loop" obstruction.* Radionuclides given intravenously may help by visualizing the gallbladder (technetium-99m, "IDA" compounds), or by localizing an intra-abdominal abscess (gallium citrate-67). Visualization of the gallbladder by technetium-99m scan renders the diagnosis of acute cholecystitis highly unlikely. CT scans may help in the occasional patient suspected of having *acute pancreatitis* or its complications, particularly when sonography has been technically poor, in localizing abscesses, and in detecting *traumatic injuries*, particularly lacerations and subcapsular hematomas of liver, spleen, and kidneys. An intravenous pyelogram may establish the patency of the urinary tract or, conversely, establish ureteral obstruction or hydronephrosis unilaterally. Examination of the upper gastrointestinal tract with nonbarium-containing radiopaque substances (Gastrografin) may help in the diagnosis of perforated ulcer.

Nonsurgical conditions that cause acute abdominal pain are important in the differential diagnosis of acute appendicitis. Chief among these are *pyelonephritis, pneumonia, pulmonary infarction, acute myocardial infarction*, and *pericarditis*, all of which may cause acute upper abdominal pain. Acute distention of the liver and its capsule resulting from *acute right heart failure* may simulate *acute cholecystitis; acute hepatitis*, viral or toxic (including alcohol), may closely simulate acute biliary tract disease. In these instances, however, an enlarged tender liver will be felt. Further, SGOT determinations will be markedly elevated. (However, acute obstruction of the common duct with cholangitis may transiently raise SGOT to levels of 1000 units or more for 24 to 48 hours.)

Systemic diseases, such as *sickle cell disease, acute intermittent porphyria, tabes dorsalis, heavy metal poisoning*, and *diabetic neuropathy*, all may present pictures simulating an acute surgical abdomen.

Acute pancreatitis, still considered a nonsurgical condition unless caused by common bile duct obstruction, usually is characterized by pain of many hours' to days' duration, associated with a history suggestive of biliary tract disease or indicative of acute and chronic alcoholism, and in its early stages abdominal tenderness is usually localized to the epigastrium. Markedly elevated plasma amylase (within 48 hours of onset) or elevated urinary amylase-creatinine clearance (>3.5 per cent) will help establish the diagnosis.

SPECIAL CONSIDERATIONS IN DIFFERENTIAL DIAGNOSIS OF ACUTE APPENDICITIS. Great care must be extended to establish the diagnosis of this condition in the very young and very old. Children with diffuse abdominal pain that is preceded by anorexia, nausea, and vomiting and often associated with diarrhea are more likely to have *acute infectious gastroenteritis*, in some cases due to *Yersinia enterocolitica* or *pseudotuberculosis*. Acute enteric infection with *Salmonella* must always be suspected, particularly in young adults with right lower quadrant pain, fever, and diarrhea. *Acute mesenteric adenitis*, presumably caused by viral illnesses and often associated with diffuse abdominal pain, is frequently confused with acute appendicitis in children. The difficulty is in those patients in whom there is some right lower quadrant tenderness and slight elevation of the white count. In such instances a diagnosis must be established at operation, because it is far safer to undertake a negative exploration than to neglect removal of an acutely inflamed appendix. Clinical differentiation of acute appendicitis from *Meckel's diverticulitis* is impossible. The acute onset of *Crohn's disease* involving terminal ileum may be very difficult to distinguish from acute appendicitis, although such patients usually have cramping abdominal pain and diarrhea.

In young women diagnosis is confused by problems in the reproductive system, such as *ruptured graafian follicles, twisted ovarian cysts, ectopic pregnancy, dysmenorrhea, ruptured endometrioma*, and *acute pelvic inflammatory disease. Ruptured ectopic pregnancy* is usually of dramatic suddenness and is often associated with shock and massive blood loss; these findings in a pregnant woman make the diagnosis virtually certain. The *ruptured graafian follicle* is noted in midcycle; fever and leukocytosis are uncommon. Tenderness on moving of cervix on vaginal examination points toward a *twisted ovarian cyst*, the pain of which is out of proportion to the general well-being of the patient. The pain of *gonococcal salpingitis* is more diffuse and tenderness is not so well localized as in appendicitis. Localized pain and tenderness in a pregnant woman whose pregnancy remains normal and who is not bleeding indicate probable appendicitis.

The differential diagnosis of appendicitis in the elderly may also be difficult. The classic picture is seldom noted, the history may be inadequate or misleading because of infirmity or the effects of medication, and the appendix perforates early. Findings on physical examination are usually not as dramatic, and, despite complications, fever may only be slightly elevated. Accuracy in diagnosis of patients over 60 years of age is below 70 per cent, and the incidence of perforation without a localized or generalized peritonitis at surgery is nearly 70 per cent—more than twice as high as all other age groups combined.

In elderly patients the principal problems in differential diagnosis are *cholecystitis, diverticulitis, mesenteric thrombosis, intestinal obstruction, incarcerated hernia*, and *perforated ulcer*.

Right-sided acute diverticulitis may simulate acute appendicitis in every respect. In a few instances, *left-sided diverticulitis* may localize tenderness to the right lower quadrant, because the sigmoid is often more redundant in the elderly. The patient also may have an episode of diarrhea associated with cramping or steady lower abdominal pain, slight temperature elevation, and, later, evidence of moderate to complete large bowel obstruction. When differential diagnosis is difficult, a cautious barium enema may help greatly in excluding acute diverticulitis as the cause of the problem.

Conversely, elderly patients must not be subjected to the risk of exploration falsely. Accordingly, all efforts should be extended to make certain that *acute myocardial* or *pulmonary infarction, pneumonia*, or other systemic disease or toxin is not responsible for acute abdominal pain simulating appendicitis.

TREATMENT. Unless strongly contraindicated, the only therapy for acute appendicitis is surgical removal of the appendix. Since mortality correlates with perforation and, except in elderly patients, perforation correlates with duration of symptoms, early diagnosis and appendectomy are essential for the lowest acceptable morbidity and mortality for the disease. To avoid the catastrophe of unoperated-upon acute appendicitis, normal appendices may have to be removed in 20 to 25 per cent of patients.

In patients in whom complications (*perforation, peritonitis*, and *abscess*) have already occurred or are suspected, dehydration must be corrected, continuous nasogastric suction started, and gentamicin, 1.0 to 1.5 mg per kilogram, and clindamycin, 1.6 to 2.5 grams per day, parenterally, should be initiated prior to surgery.

Patients with obvious acute appendicitis for whom no surgeon is available may be treated with head-up position of the bed; intravenous fluids; gentamicin, 1.0 to 1.5 mg per kilogram, clindamycin, 1.6 to 2.4 grams and ampicillin, 2.0 grams intravenously in divided doses daily; and nasogastric suction. The chance for recovery in otherwise healthy individuals with this program is surprisingly good. However, these patients must be scheduled for appendectomy six weeks later, or appendicitis is likely to recur.

MORBIDITY AND MORTALITY OF SURGERY. Overall, about 15 per cent of patients with acute appendicitis develop complications postoperatively; this figure is about 35 per cent in those with perforation and localized peritonitis at the time of surgery and is 70 per cent in those with perforation and generalized peritonitis. The complications include *wound infection, intra-abdominal abscess*, mechanical *small bowel obstruction, fecal fistula*, and, much more rarely, *intraperitoneal hemorrhage. Pylephlebitis* is extremely rare (1 in 1000).

The overall mortality of acute appendicitis ranges from 0.18 to 1.6 per cent and is due principally to the interrelated factors of age and perforation. Indeed, mortality over the age of 60 ranges from 6.4 to 14 per cent. The cause of death in this group may be attributed equally to septic and nonseptic complications.

Jess P, Bjerregaard B, Brynitz S, Holst-Christensen J, Kalaja E, Lund-Kristensen J: Acute appendicitis. Prospective trial concerning diagnostic accuracy and complications. Am J Surg 141:232, 1981.

Lewis FR, Holcraft JW, Boey J, Dunphy JE: Appendicitis. A critical review of diagnoses and treatment in 1000 cases. Arch Surg 110:677, 1975. *An excellent discussion of differential diagnosis in which the authors point out the features of conditions for which appendicitis is mistaken.*

Schrock TR: Acute appendicitis. *In* Sleisenger MH, Fordtran JS (eds.): Gastrointestinal Disease. 3rd ed. Philadelphia, W. B. Saunders Company, 1983, p 1268. *A concise yet comprehensive article on every aspect of the subject. A handy reference.*

Talbert JL, Zuidema GD: Appendicitis. A reappraisal of an old problem. Surg Clin North Am 46:1101, 1966. *A comprehensive review of this disease with appropriate emphasis upon pitfalls of diagnosis.*

Yusuf MF, Dunn E: Appendicitis in the elderly: Learn to discern the untypical picture. Geriatrics 34:73, 1979.

Way LW: Abdominal pain and the acute abdomen. *In* Sleisenger MH, Fordtran JS (eds.): Gastrointestinal Disease. 3rd ed. Philadelphia, W. B. Saunders Company, 1983, p 217. *An excellent chapter containing all important information on diagnosis of the acute abdomen, identifying the cause and the accepted approaches to management.*

Diverticulitis of the Colon

DEFINITION. Diverticulitis of the colon is a focal inflammation in the wall of the apex of a diverticulum, most commonly of the sigmoid, caused by inspissated feces. It is more common in those with multiple diverticula that have appeared at an early age. Peridiverticulitis results from necrosis with micro- or macroperforation. An abscess then forms, its size depending on the size of the rupture; small ones may subside with scarring while larger abscesses involve pericolonic tissue and may even dissect along, or within, the bowel wall. Occasionally they rupture into contiguous organs (bladder, ureter, vagina, and small bowel).

CLINICAL PICTURE. The predominant clinical symptoms of diverticulitis are *pain* and *fever*. The pain is usually prominent and is frequently constant. Most commonly, it is localized in the left lower quadrant, because the sigmoid and descending colon are the sites of the largest number of diverticula. The patient may have a few loose stools or become constipated, and only rarely is rectal bleeding noted. Bleeding from diverticula is not associated with inflammation and perforation. It is usually bright red and may be copious. Bleeding colonic diverticula must be differentiated from ischemic colitis, acute amebic and *Shigella* dysenteries, ulcerative colitis, and tumors of the colon (see Ch. 113). When the perforation and sepsis are of sufficient magnitude, the patient may also have chills with fever as high as 39 to 39.5°C. Usually, however, the fever is low grade, between 38 and 39°C.

Although the pain may be somewhat intermittent and even colicky at onset, it usually becomes steady and is of the same quality as noted in acute appendicitis. Indeed, acute diverticulitis has often been referred to as "left-sided appendicitis." The patient may seek medical help after only a few hours or, when the situation is not so severe, after a few days of lingering but nagging lower quadrant pain and low-grade fever. Rarely, a *diverticulum* of the *right colon* will perforate, causing right lower quadrant pain with fever, closely simulating appendicitis. Diagnosis is usually made at laparotomy.

Physical examination is extremely important in establishing the diagnosis. Since the process usually quickly involves the serosal surface and peritoneal cover, marked, localized tenderness will be found, both direct and rebound. Frequently, a tender mass may be discerned. When present for more than a few days, this mass may be astonishingly firm, even hard, and the distinction grossly from carcinoma is almost impossible. The abdomen is often slightly distended. Rectal examination also will be painful, because inflamed bowel is often within reach of the finger; also, a mass may be palpable if a sizable abscess has formed.

In some instances the patient will have complications of diverticulitis: *dysuria, pyuria, pneumaturia,* or *passing gas or feces through the vagina*. These symptoms are due to perforation of bladder or vagina by the diverticulitis (colovesical and colovaginal fistulas). The vast majority of these patients, usually elderly, do not relate these symptoms to a prior attack of severe pain. The presenting symptom may be septic fever, caused by pericolic, pelvic, or subdiaphragmatic abscess. The inflammatory process may penetrate other pelvic organs, but such fistulization is often clinically undramatic. Rarely, the diverticulum perforates freely. In this instance the signs of free perforation are evident; that is, distention of the abdomen, generalized rebound tenderness, and absent bowel sounds. It is unusual also for diverticulitis to cause persistent colonic obstruction (see below).

DIAGNOSIS. Diverticulitis should be suspected particularly in patients with known diverticula who develop fever, leukocytosis, and signs of pericolic and peritoneal inflammation in the left lower quadrant. The diagnosis is even more likely if a mass is palpable. Fever between 38.5 and 39° C is also compatible with the diagnosis; when the process is more extensive and with formation of a *pericolic abscess* and its complications, the temperature is usually over 39° C, and the white count is proportionately higher. Urinalysis will reflect varying degrees of involvement of the urinary tract by this septic process; that is, with mild ureteral irritation a few red and white cells may be seen in the urinary sediment, but with direct involvement of the ureter or invasion of the ureter or the bladder, the urine may be frankly septic and contain large numbers of red cells.

Some patients suffer much left flank pain owing to *hydronephrosis* resulting from obstruction of the ureter by a *pericolic abscess*. An intravenous pyelogram shows no function or an obstructed kidney on the left.

The use of x-rays is of crucial importance in the diagnosis, especially a flat film of the abdomen. Evidence of pericolic perforation and abscess formation may be suspected from collections of air and fluid in the left lower quadrant. Free air may be seen under the diaphragm in instances of free perforation. Occasionally, the proximal colon may be slightly dilated, indicating partial colonic obstruction. Rarely is obstruction complete. Sonography may reveal a localized thickening of the wall of the involved colon. Later, sonography and scintigraphy (gallium citrate-67) may localize an abscess.

Sigmoidoscopy should be carefully performed with minimal preparation. Air insufflation should not be used, and the importance of the examination is to exclude other conditions (see below). Usually with diverticulitis the instrument cannot be passed beyond the rectosigmoid junction, which is occluded by fixation, angulation, and spasm.

Clinicians debate the advisability of using a barium enema in the diagnosis of diverticulitis, particularly in its acute phase. The concern is that the increased intraluminal pressure may cause perforation. The history, physical examination, and laboratory information are sufficient to make the clinical diagnosis in the vast majority of instances, and barium enema should await some subsidence of the acute phase of the illness. The exceptions to this dictum are those instances in which the *acute ischemic colitis* of the left colon and perforation of a left colonic carcinoma cannot otherwise be excluded.

The roentgenographic features characteristic of diverticulitis are the presence of barium outside a diverticulum, the delineation of a pericolic mass (Fig. 114–1), or the demonstration of a fistula originating in the colon. In some instances the distinction between diverticulitis and carcinoma or Crohn's disease may be difficult (see below). The presence of irregularity, thickening, or even a sawtooth appearance of the bowel is not sufficient to make the diagnosis of diverticulitis, because these are typical for diverticula without perforation.

After diagnosis of diverticulitis has been established, intravenous pyelography should be done to ascertain whether or not obstructive involvement of the urinary tract is present, particularly on the left side. In some instances, as noted above, urinary symptoms may be the predominant feature, and radio-

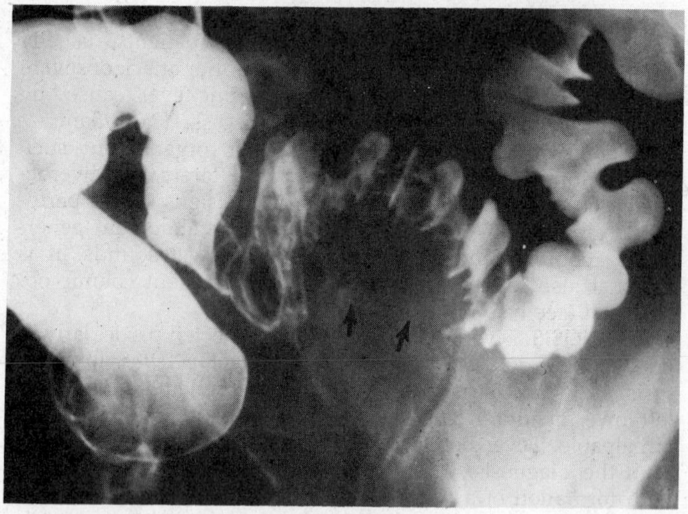

Figure 114–1. A paracolic mass that deforms and displaces the sigmoid lumen is delineated in a patient with diverticulitis and a palpable left lower quadrant mass (From Almy TP, Naitove A: *In* Sleisenger MH, Fordtran JS [eds.]: Gastrointestinal Disease. 3rd ed. Philadelphia, W. B. Saunders Company, 1983.)

graphic examination of the urinary tract may have to be performed early.

DIFFERENTIAL DIAGNOSIS. For many years symptoms of *diverticulosis* have been attributed incorrectly to diverticulitis. *Diverticulosis* may periodically be associated with marked local tenderness, a palpable sigmoid loop, and some degree of large bowel obstruction, and thus the picture suggests diverticulitis. However, such patients do not have fever, the localized tenderness gradually recedes, the white count is not elevated, and there is no evidence of involvement of contiguous organs. Barium enema will reveal an irregular luminal contour with a narrowed sigmoid, possibly even a so-called "sawtooth" appearance of the mucosa. Barium must be noted outside the diverticulum, a fistula seen, or evidences of a pericolic or intramural mass detected before the diagnosis of diverticulitis is definitely made.

Carcinoma of the colon must be distinguished from diverticulitis because of similarity of age during which both diverticulitis and cancer of the colon appear. The differential diagnosis is especially difficult, because in about 25 per cent of patients with diverticulitis the lumen is narrowed, suggesting carcinoma. Differentiation from cancer is more difficult if diverticulitis has appeared insidiously. Chronic obstruction, more persistent rectal bleeding, and weight loss are more characteristic of *cancer*. However, the tumor may be obscured on barium enema in 50 per cent of patients with diverticula. Localized tenderness with rebound, leukocytosis, and fever support the diagnosis of diverticulitis. In some cases, however, it may be impossible to distinguish the two conditions, especially when the barium enema has features common to both; i.e., a mass, luminal irregularities, and partial obstruction. In such patients colonoscopy may be very helpful in excluding cancer. Rapid disappearance of the obstruction strongly suggests diverticulitis. In some patients correct diagnosis can be made only at surgery, and, in a few, only from surgical biopsy or by the disappearance of the occlusion following colostomy.

Crohn's disease of the colon may be difficult to exclude in the face of marked luminal narrowing or multiloculated channels parallel to the bowel wall on x-ray. Clinically, although both may produce pain, partial obstruction and lower abdominal mass, some rectal bleeding, fever, and leukocytosis, the past history differs. The patient with Crohn's colitis usually will have had previous episodes of lower abdominal pain, fever, and diarrhea. Sigmoidoscopy may reveal the rectum to be involved with granulomatous disease. Also, evidence elsewhere in the bowel of granulomatous disease, such as cobblestoning, long intramucosal sinus tracts, and skip areas, will help in the differential diagnosis (see Ch. 104).

Ischemic colitis of the left colon in elderly patients may produce signs and symptoms of bowel necrosis and localized peritonitis that are difficult to distinguish from diverticulitis. In these instances, gross rectal bleeding is prominent, and a barium enema is of crucial importance, because so-called "thumb printing" will be found in ischemic colitis, especially in the area of the splenic flexure and descending colon (see Ch. 105).

TREATMENT OF DIVERTICULITIS. Patients with low grade fever and no evidence of mass, fistula, or obstruction may be treated with clear liquids by mouth and ampicillin (2.0 grams) or a cephalosporin (4.0 to 6.0 grams) per day in divided dosage intravenously. If the patient has fever of 39° C or more or has a tender mass or other evidence of greater extent of infection, gentamicin, 1.0 to 1.5 mg per kilogram, and clindamycin, 1.6 to 2.4 grams, are given parenterally in divided doses daily. In such patients nasogastric suction and intravenous fluids are given to maintain intramuscular volume, urinary output, and electrolyte balance. About 50 per cent of complicated cases will require surgery. Surgical consultation must be obtained early in all cases in which a mass is palpable or when there is suspicion of peritonitis or involvement of a contiguous organ.

Most patients respond well to this type of therapy with abatement of the fever, tenderness, and evidence of partial obstruction. Long-term therapy becomes identical with that for diverticulosis (see Ch. 101).

COMPLICATIONS AND INDICATIONS FOR SURGERY. Surgical intervention is necessary for the complications of diverticulitis such as an *enlarging mass* despite therapy, *generalized peritonitis, persisting intestinal obstruction*, or the development of a *fistula*. Elective surgery is indicated for recurrent attacks of diverticulitis and for the inability to exclude a carcinoma as the cause for persisting deformity after recovery from the acute phase.

Almy TP, Howell DA: Diverticular disease of the colon. N Engl J Med 302:324, 1980. *A marvelously lucid update of every aspect of the subject.*

Almy TP, Naitove A: Diverticula of the colon. *In* Sleisenger MH, Fordtran JS (eds.): Gastrointestinal Disease. 3rd ed. Philadelphia, W. B. Saunders Company, 1983. pp 896–910. *A complete description of etiology, pathogenesis and clinical pictures and complications of colonic diverticula, including diverticulitis.*

Hughes LE: Complications of diverticular disease: Inflammation, obstruction and bleeding. Clin Gastroenterol 4:147, 1975. *Excellent review of the principal complications of diverticulitis with much information on management of them.*

Larson DM, Masters SS, Spiro HM: Medical and surgical therapy in diverticular disease—a comparative study. Gastroenterology 71:734, 1976.

Welch CE, Malt RA: Abdominal surgery. N Engl J Med 300:648, 705, 765, 1979. *A clear summary of the recent advances in diagnosis and management of diverticulitis.*

Radiation Enterocolitis

Damage to the small intestine and colon may result from radiation therapy for abdominal and pelvic malignancy.

INCIDENCE. Incidence of severe radiation injury varies between 2.5 and 25 per cent of patients treated with radiotherapy for pelvic and intra-abdominal malignancy. Minor degrees of damage are common, as evidenced by impaired ileal absorption of conjugated bile acids in many women who are irradiated for pelvic cancer. It is noted most commonly after the total dosage exceeds 5000 rads. Transient histologic inflammatory change may, however, be found in the rectal mucosa of nearly 75 per cent of individuals receiving such therapeutic irradiation. The small intestine is more frequently affected than the rectum.

PATHOGENESIS AND PATHOLOGY. Damage results from interference with replication of radiosensitive epithelial cells, particularly of the crypt, leading to varying degrees of damage to the mucosal surface. Often it is reversible if dosage is not too great or treatment is not prolonged. Such damage may follow dosage of less than 5000 rads. Damage to the mesothelial cells of the small submucosal arterioles results in varying degrees of occlusion and mucosal transmural necrosis. Accordingly, hyperemia and ulceration of the mucosa are frequent. With extreme damage, diffuse edema is followed by extensive fibrosis with multiple strictures and irreversible damage. Such serious damage is more common in diabetics, in those with previous abdominal surgery, and in patients with serious vascular disease.

The pathologic changes range from diminution of crypt cell mitosis and shortening of villi of the small intestine to varying degrees of hyperemia, edema, and inflammatory cell infiltration of the mucosa. Mucosal thickness decreases. Progress of damage is marked by crypt abscesses, sloughing of epithelial cells, and, later, mucosal ulcerations, diffuse or localized, are found. Two to 12 months after radiotherapy, the damage to the blood vessels becomes prominent. In these instances, repair of acute damage does not ensue. The mucosa and submucosa become progressively ischemic and fibrotic. *Abscesses* and *fistulas* may form with sinus tracts between loops of intestine and between intestine and neighboring organs. A more general discussion of radiation injury is found in Ch. 562.

CLINICAL PICTURE. Symptoms may appear early, that is, during the first or second week of therapy, or late, that is, six months or more after completion of therapy. Early, diarrhea and mild rectal bleeding may appear, resembling ulcerative colitis. Sigmoidoscopy reveals an edematous mucosa which may be friable; in more extreme instances, the acute changes also reveal a patchy or diffusely necrotic mucosa.

Later, symptoms of radiation include gross rectal bleeding, decrease in stool caliber, and progressive difficulty in defecation with marked constipation, all indicating severe rectal involvement. Small intestinal symptoms result from either fibrosis and obstruction or fistulization and abscess formation. If the damage is especially diffuse, malabsorption may be noted, as described in Ch. 103.

DIAGNOSIS. Diagnosis of radiation enteritis is suspected with any of the aforementioned symptoms in patients who have received significant radiation. Sigmoidoscopy shows a picture which ranges from variable degrees of edema to a markedly inflamed and necrotic mucosa. Multiple telangiectases are common, as is rectal stricture. Since most cases are fairly clear cut, biopsy is usually not indicated.

Barium studies of the intestine are not specific and range from changes of diffuse edema and spasm to diffuse fibrosis with strictures, fistulas, and ulceration in more severe cases. Thus the picture may resemble localized malignancy in the colon or diffuse granulomatous disease in the small intestine. Long strictured areas may also be noted, however, in the colon.

Differential diagnostic usefulness of small vessel angiography of the intestine in radiation enteritis remains to be confirmed.

TREATMENT. Improving methods for monitoring radiotherapy and delivering rads in small increments will probably reduce the incidence of this complication; however, the increasing incidence of malignancy and of the efficacy of radiotherapy will probably increase the total number of such patients.

Symptoms caused by early reaction consist of mild diarrhea and perhaps some minimal bleeding that can be managed by reduction of dose by 10 per cent, with the judicious use of tranquilizers, anticholinergic drugs, local analgesics, agents that increase stool bulk, and warm sitz baths for those with rectal involvement. An elemental diet free of gluten, milk protein, and lactose may benefit patients with early radiation reaction. If watery diarrhea is a problem, treatment with cholestyramine (4 to 12 grams per day) to bind bile salts may help greatly. If rectal bleeding is prominent, treatment with steroid retention enemas should be initiated as in ulcerative colitis (see Ch. 104). If the bleeding is more significant, transfusions may be required and even, possibly, surgery. Rectal strictures may be dilated, provided that it is early in their course and they are not extensive. Lubricants and stool softeners are often helpful; however, the progress to symptomatic occlusion of the lumen may necessitate proximal colostomy. Fistulas should be resected and abscesses drained. Resection of bowel and anastomoses are hazardous in view of the impaired blood supply.

In patients with malabsorption, treatment is as outlined in Ch. 103.

PROGNOSIS. Prognosis depends on the extent and degree of damage, the age of the patient, the course of the underlying malignancy, and whether or not the patient has systemic vascular disease. Unfortunately, extensive disease of the colon usually means significant disease in the small intestine. The prognosis is guarded in those with ulceration, fibrosis, or fistulas in whom repeated resections or other major surgical procedures must be carried out. In such cases, age and cardiovascular status are also crucial determining factors.

DeCosse JJ, Rhodes RS, Wentz WB, Reagan JW, Dwarken HJ, Holden WD: The natural history and management of radiation-induced injury of the gastrointestinal tract. Ann Surg 170:369, 1969. *One of the better accounts of the evolution of radiation enteritis available. Still current despite its age.*

Earnest DH, Trier JS: Radiation enterocolitis. *In* Sleisenger MH, Fordtran JS (eds.): Gastrointestinal Disease. 3rd ed. Philadelphia, W. B. Saunders Company, 1983, pp 1259–1267. *A comprehensive discussion of the radiation damage to small and large gut.*

Goldstein F, Khory J, Thornton JJ: Treatment of chronic radiation enteritis and colitis with salicylazosulfapyridine and systemic corticosteroids. Am J Gastroenterol 65:201, 1976.

Small Intestinal Ulceration: Isolated and Diffuse

ISOLATED NONSPECIFIC ULCERS

This inflammatory disease of unknown etiology is rare. About 75 per cent are ileal and 25 per cent jejunal. Often they are multiple. Formerly these ulcers were often attributable to ingestion of enteric-coated potassium chloride. Such ulceration may also be associated with *vascular disease, hematologic disorders, granulomatous diseases, trauma, infections,* and *neoplasia.*

The clinical picture consists of periumbilical colicky pain and perhaps nausea and vomiting. Frequently, however, the patient presents with small bowel obstruction, bleeding, or perforation. Duration of illness is usually weeks to months but may be years. Accordingly, examination may show signs of obstructions, or peritonitis may be present.

Laboratory investigation is normal unless the patient has been bleeding or has had protracted vomiting; plain films of the abdomen are of great value if small bowel is obstructed or has perforated. Barium contrast studies in the uncomplicated cases are most often unrevealing, although in rare instances ulceration and narrowing may be noted. Upper endoscopy may reveal the ulcer or ulcers if located in the high jejunum.

Treatment for the disease is conservative if no complications have occurred. If the involved segment is bleeding, perforated, or stenotic, it should be resected.

Brandborg LL: Other infections, inflammatory and miscellaneous diseases of the small intestine. *In* Sleisenger MH, Fordtran JS (eds.): Gastrointestinal Disease. 2nd ed. Philadelphia, W. B. Saunders Company, 1978, p 1076. *An excellent account of acute inflammatory and ulcerative diseases of the small intestine.*

Lawrason FD, Alpert E, Mohr FL, et al.: Ulcerative-obstructive lesions of the small intestine. JAMA 191:641, 1965. *A comprehensive, worldwide survey of this disease, indicating a large number of associated diseases.*

DIFFUSE ULCERATION OF JEJUNUM AND ILEUM

Diffuse ulceration of the small bowel may be found in *adult celiac disease (celiac sprue), lymphoma,* and idiopathic *chronic ulcerative enteritis* (also known as *chronic ulcerative nongranulomatous jejunoileitis*). Patients with *gluten-sensitive enteropathy (celiac sprue)* may develop diffuse ulceration of jejunum and ileum, usually signaling a rapid decline in their clinical course despite elimination of gluten from the diet, with increased diarrhea, malabsorption, and in some patients perforation or hemorrhage. In instances of mild degrees of ulceration, steroids may induce remission; however, the majority are refractory to medical therapy and require appropriate resection of involved gut. Mortality in this group is high. The condition in patients with lymphoma and diffuse ulceration also is often refractory to resection and radiotherapy.

Chronic ulcerative enteritis and *eosinophilic gastroenteritis* affect the small intestine, usually in patients under 50. They are characterized by diarrhea, weight loss, variable degrees of malabsorption, and protein-losing enteropathy. *Chronic ulcera-*

tive enteritis is a much graver illness, often with fever, ascites and edema, a rapidly progressive course unresponsive to steroids, and a high mortality. The etiology is unknown. Biopsy, peroral or at laparotomy, reveals nonspecific diffuse inflammation and mucosal ulcers. Prednisolone, 60 to 100 mg intravenously daily over two to three weeks, may be associated with remission in about one half of these patients. Infection, intraperitoneal or systemic, is the common cause of death.

Eosinophilic gastroenteritis may be localized to stomach, small intestine, or colon—so-called *eosinophilic granuloma*. It consists of infiltration by sheets of eosinophils into the submucosal and muscle layers. It is associated with systemic illnesses or peripheral eosinophilia and appears in the fourth to sixth decades. Steroids are often effective, but surgery may be indicated. *Universal eosinophilic gastroenteritis*, on the other hand, is a disease of younger persons, is often associated with allergies, always has a peripheral eosinophilia (greater than 20 per cent), affects stomach and small intestine diffusely, and is associated with diarrhea, crampy pain, weight loss, hypoalbuminemia, and often occult bleeding. Rarely, it responds to elimination of certain foods, particularly fish or meat. Most patients, however, require treatment with steroids, usually short-term (ten days to two weeks), but some may require long-term administration of 10 mg of prednisolone daily.

Bayless TR: Small intestinal ulceration: Isolated and diffuse. *In* Sleisenger MH, Fordtran JS (eds.): Gastrointestinal Disease. 3rd ed. Philadelphia, W. B. Saunders Company, 1983. *Excellent clarification and description of isolated and diffuse ulceration of the small gut.*

Greenberger N: Allergic disorders of the intestine and eosinophilic gastroenteritis. *In* Sleisenger MH, Fordtran JS (eds.): Gastrointestinal Disease. 3rd ed. Philadelphia, W. B. Saunders Company, 1983. *A concise review of eosinophilic disease of the gut.*

Part XII
DISEASES OF THE LIVER, GALLBLADDER, AND BILE DUCTS

115. CLINICAL APPROACH TO LIVER DISEASE

Robert K. Ockner

The liver plays a central and varied role in many essential physiologic processes. It is the sole source of albumin and many other plasma proteins, and of blood glucose in the postabsorptive state; it is the major site of lipid synthesis and source of plasma lipoproteins; and it is the principal organ in which a wide variety of endogenous and exogenous substances such as ammonia, steroid hormones, drugs, and toxins undergo biotransformation. To the extent that biotransformation "detoxifies" or inactivates a substance, the liver may be viewed as serving a regulatory or protective function for the whole organism; to the extent that such biotransformation results in the formation of toxic products, as in the case of certain drugs, the liver may bear the brunt of their adverse effects.

The clinical manifestations of liver diseases are also varied. Moreover, the clues by which the clinician may be first alerted to the existence of liver disease, even when advanced, may be subtle, consisting of seemingly trivial information gleaned during a careful history (e.g., increased fatigue, or the reversal of sleep pattern or personality change of early hepatic encephalopathy), physical examination (e.g., prominence of breast tissue and small testes in a man with cirrhosis, or excoriation reflecting pruritus), or routine laboratory screening tests (e.g., mild decreases in one or more of the formed elements of the blood because of portal hypertension–associated hypersplenism). Careful assessment is equally important in the patient with obvious liver disease, to address more complex questions. For example, does what seems to be acute hepatitis in fact represent relapse of previously subclinical chronic hepatitis, or δ-agent infection in a hepatitis B carrier? (See Ch. 120.) Or does the deteriorating course of a patient with known cirrhosis represent the natural progression of the disease, or a superimposed common bile duct stone, adverse drug reaction, or hepatocellular carcinoma?

HISTORY. Some very *nonspecific symptoms* may be important evidence of liver disease, including fatigue, malaise, fever, change in sleep pattern or behavior, diminished libido, anorexia, weight loss, nausea, and vomiting. *Pruritus* is an important symptom of *cholestasis* (impaired bile secretion), and may be present in the absence of jaundice. *Jaundice* is often first noted by family members or friends, and, especially in dark-skinned individuals, may appear first as a yellow discoloration of the conjunctivae *("scleral icterus")*. Since jaundice in most forms of liver and biliary disease reflects cholestasis (see below), such patients will often observe that stool color lightens while urine gets darker as the excretion of "bile pigments" is diverted from bile to urine. Right upper quadrant *abdominal discomfort* or *pain* may reflect a rapidly enlarging liver with distention of Glisson's capsule because of acute hepatic inflammation or congestion, an acutely inflamed gallbladder, common bile duct obstruction by an impacted gallstone, or abscess or tumor in the liver or adjacent areas.

The history may provide important clues to the presence of *complications of liver disease*, especially those reflecting *portal hypertension* and *portal-systemic shunting*. Early hepatic *encephalopathy* may cause subtle changes in affect or sleep pattern. More overt symptoms include episodic somnolence, confusion, combativeness, ataxia, incoordination, or obtundation. A history of *abdominal swelling* suggests ascites, and may be most easily recalled by the patient as a change in the fit of clothing, possibly associated with *edema*. Ascites may also occur in many other conditions, including hepatic vein or inferior vena cava occlusion, congestive cardiac failure and constrictive pericarditis, and a wide variety of neoplastic and inflammatory processes (see Ch. 111). A history of *gastrointestinal bleeding* in a patient with liver disease may suggest esophageal varices, but can also reflect other lesions such as *gastritis*, *Mallory-Weiss syndrome*, and *peptic ulcer*.

The history is of major importance in the identification of potentially significant *etiologic* or *predisposing factors*. Viral hepatitis is suggested by a history of contact with jaundiced persons, exposure to persons known to have hepatitis or to a common source of hepatitis, ingestion of uncooked or steamed clams, prior blood transfusion, work with subhuman primates, employment in certain health professions (especially in dialysis or transplantation units), accidental inoculation, sexual promiscuity (especially in the homosexual community), sharing of needles, travel to geographic areas with inadequate public health programs, and consumption of water or uncooked vegetables in such areas. Foreign travel may also suggest parasitic disease such as amebic liver abscess. Q fever hepatitis may occur in individuals in proximity to livestock. Exposure to drugs, ethanol, and other potential dietary, occupational, or environmental toxins must be reviewed in detail. The information obtained may require supplementation or corroboration by family members or other close associates, especially in regard to ethanol consumption. It is often possible to document previous liver function through recourse to *medical records*, and this is particularly useful in evaluating the chronicity of liver disease. A *family history* of jaundice, liver disease, or neonatal jaundice may suggest an inherited disorder such as Wilson's disease, α_1-antitrypsin deficiency, or hemochromatosis.

PHYSICAL EXAMINATION. Scleral *icterus* may be detected at a serum bilirubin concentration as low as 2.0 to 2.5 mg per deciliter. Although *spider telangiectasias*, most prominent around the shoulders and upper trunk, and *palmar erythema* are nonspecific and may be present to a limited extent in normal subjects (especially women in pregnancy), they are potentially important signs of liver disease, and usually imply chronicity. Excoriations reflect pruritus and suggest significant cholestasis, not necessarily accompanied by jaundice. *Xanthomas* and *xanthelasmas* are not specific for hepatobiliary disease, but may be a sign of prolonged cholestatic hypercholesterolemia. Changes in hair pattern, gynecomastia, and small or soft testes may reflect the *hormonal changes* that accompany cirrhosis in men. Prominence of cutaneous veins in the epigastrium or around the umbilicus may indicate a *portal-systemic collateral circulation* and, therefore, portal hypertension.

Examination of the heart and lungs may provide evidence of congestive cardiac failure, constrictive pericarditis, or diseases of the lungs or pleura that may be associated with liver dysfunction, cause pain referred to the abdomen, or reflect processes involving the subdiaphragmatic regions such as tumor or abscess.

Examination of the *liver* should include documentation of its *size*, and is best recorded both as the distance to which the lower edge extends below the costal margin, and its overall vertical span as determined by percussion. These dimensions should be related to a reproducible landmark such as the midclavicular line. The *form* and *consistency* of the liver should be noted: e.g., smooth, with a sharp edge; nodular and rock-hard; firm with a rounded and irregular edge. A rapidly decreasing liver size during the course of severe acute hepatitis may be a sign of massive hepatic necrosis. An abdominal mass, tenderness, or muscular spasm may suggest secondary involvement of the liver or biliary passages by a neoplastic or inflammatory process. *Ascites*, most readily detected as dullness or bulging in the flanks, fluid wave, or shifting dullness, may be caused by advanced liver disease, or superimposed infectious or neoplastic processes.

A diffusely tender and enlarged liver suggests hepatitis or congestion, whereas tenderness in a relatively limited area at or below the lower margin in the region of the interlobar fissure may reflect acute cholecystitis. A visible or palpable gallbladder is abnormal and may be an important sign of primary gallbladder pathology, or of cystic or common bile duct obstruction, the latter usually neoplastic (Courvoisier's sign). Splenomegaly may be the first evidence of portal hypertension of any cause, or may reflect primary splenic pathology such as neoplasm or infection.

Neurologic evaluation is of particular importance with respect to signs of hepatic encephalopathy. These are discussed in detail in Ch. 127, but, as noted, these may be very subtle, consisting initially of a personality change, a mild confusional state, or lethargy. A *flapping tremor* ("asterixis"), characteristic of metabolic encephalopathy of any cause, is usually present in more obvious cases. In advanced hepatic encephalopathy almost any form of neurologic abnormality may be present, including seizures, lateralizing signs, and abnormal posturing. Despite this, it is essential in patients with liver disease to consider other causes of central nervous system pathology such as the effects of ethanol, sedatives or other toxins, hypoglycemia, trauma, hemorrhage, infection, and primary or secondary neoplasms.

Schiff L, Schiff E (eds.): Diseases of the Liver. Philadelphia, J. B. Lippincott Company, 1982.

Sherlock S: Diseases of the Liver and Biliary System. Oxford, Blackwell Scientific Publications, Ltd., 1981.

Wright R, Alberti KGMM, Karran S, Millward Sadler GH (eds.): Liver and Biliary Disease. London, W. B. Saunders Company, 1979.

Zakim D, Boyer T (eds.): Hepatology: A Textbook of Liver Disease. Philadelphia, W. B. Saunders Company, 1982.

Four current and comprehensive textbooks that serve to introduce the topic and provide literature references dealing with the broad field of hepatobiliary structure, function, and disease.

116. HEPATIC METABOLISM IN LIVER DISEASE

Robert K. Ockner

Intermediary metabolism may be profoundly disturbed in liver disease. The resulting changes may be integral components of the disease process, but in some instances their clinical significance and prominence overshadow those of the liver disease itself.

CARBOHYDRATE METABOLISM. Except during the absorption of dietary carbohydrate, maintenance of blood glucose levels depends entirely on the liver. Two distinct mechanisms are involved: *glycogenolysis* and *gluconeogenesis.* In glycogenolysis, glucose is released from hepatic glycogen by the enzyme phosphorylase, the activity of which is stimulated by a series of events triggered by the interaction of glucagon or epinephrine with specific liver cell surface receptors. Insulin, conversely, stimulates the incorporation of glucose into hepatic glycogen. Normal hepatic glycogen stores are sufficient to sustain blood glucose concentrations in the absence of exogenous carbohydrate for only about 24 hours; beyond that, maintenance of blood glucose in the fasting state depends entirely on hepatic gluconeogenesis. Gluconeogenesis, i.e., the de novo synthesis of glucose, largely from lactate, pyruvate, and amino acid precursors, is stimulated by glucagon and epinephrine and inhibited by insulin.

Thus, the normally functioning liver is responsive to a continually changing nutritional and hormonal milieu. During the fed state (relative glucose and insulin excess), glucose production (gluconeogenesis and glycogenolysis) is minimal; instead, dietary glucose either is stored as glycogen or is converted to fatty acids *(lipogenesis)*, largely to be secreted from the liver in the form of triglyceride-rich lipoproteins and destined for storage in adipose tissue. In the fasting state, the process is reversed, and relative glucagon excess with respect to insulin favors energy consumption rather than energy storage. Thus, liver glycogen is mobilized, and gluconeogenesis is increased; glucose is no longer diverted to lipogenesis, but is exported into plasma. The decrease in fatty acid synthesis is associated with increased fatty acid oxidation, which becomes the principal energy source for the liver.

In liver disease, disturbances in glucose homeostasis usually produce *hypoglycemia* or *glucose intolerance.* Mild hypoglycemia (blood glucose concentrations between 45 and 60 mg per deciliter) occurs in about 50 per cent of patients with uncomplicated acute viral hepatitis. As a rule, these patients are not hyperinsulinemic; rather, hypoglycemia may reflect several hepatic abnormalities, including diminished glycogen stores, diminished glycogenolytic response to glucagon, diminished gluconeogenesis, and impaired repletion of hepatic glycogen during the fed state. In most cases, the hypoglycemia is not clinically significant, but in very severe acute liver injury of any cause, such as virus- or drug-induced massive hepatic necrosis or Reye's syndrome, hypoglycemia may be an important component of the syndrome of acute liver failure. Hepatic hypoglycemia may also occur in the absence of overt liver damage. For example, *alcoholic hypoglycemia* classically occurs in persons whose only important source of calories over a period of days is ethanol; hypoglycemia in this setting reflects both a depletion of hepatic glycogen stores and inhibition of gluconeogenesis by ethanol. Hypoglycemia should be considered in the differential diagnosis of altered mental status in any patient with significant acute liver disease or exposure to ethanol or other toxins.

Glucose intolerance, on the other hand, is more typically associated with chronic liver disease and cirrhosis. Plasma insulin concentrations tend to be high, suggesting a state of *insulin resistance.* Both insulin receptor number and binding affinity have been found to be diminished in peripheral blood monocytes, suggesting a more generalized receptor defect. In addition, insulin resistance may in part reflect increased plasma glucagon concentrations and in part a diminished insulin effect on the liver because the hormone is diverted to the peripheral circulation via portal-systemic shunts. Regardless of the mechanism, the glucose intolerance associated with chronic liver disease, per se, is rarely of clinical significance. Such patients may also have disorders such as *hemochromatosis* and *chronic pancreatitis,* in which *diabetes mellitus* may also contribute to glucose intolerance.

LIPID METABOLISM. The liver plays a central role in the metabolism of fatty acids and other lipids and lipoproteins. Of the total daily turnover of plasma *free fatty acids* (FFA), about one third enter the liver, where they are esterified to triglycerides or other esters, or undergo oxidation, largely in the mitochondria. The balance between esterification and oxidation is closely regulated, as is the rate of de novo fatty acid synthesis. In the fasting state, fatty acid synthesis is inhibited, whereas fatty acid oxidation is increased at the expense of the esterification pathways. In the fed state, de novo fatty acid synthesis and esterification are favored, whereas oxidation is diminished. Exclusive of dietary sources and de novo synthesis, a total of approximately 60 to 70 grams of plasma FFA (>200 mmol) is taken up by the liver each day in the average adult, and in the fasting state fatty acids are the major energy source for the liver. Interference with hepatic fatty acid metabolism may either cause or be caused by clinically significant abnormalities of hepatic structure and function.

Fatty liver usually reflects excess accumulation of triglyceride, which may be deposited as large vacuoles displacing the nucleus, or as small droplets, in which the nucleus remains central. It may be viewed as an imbalance between the rate of triglyceride biosynthesis on the one hand, and the rate of triglyceride disposition (primarily secretion into plasma in the form of very low density lipoproteins) on the other. This imbalance may result from many factors which can affect either or both sides of the equation. Conditions associated with large vacuolar fatty liver include obesity, protein-calorie malnutrition (e.g., kwashiorkor, jejunoileal bypass), diabetes mellitus, corticosteroid therapy, and ethanol ingestion (see Ch. 125). Small droplet fat accumulation (see below) is characteristic of obstetric fatty liver (acute fatty liver of pregnancy), Reye's syndrome, Jamaican vomiting sickness, and tetracycline and valproic acid hepatotoxicity and, occasionally, is ethanol-related. Accumulation of triglyceride in the liver cell is usually associated with hepatomegaly and reflects abnormal liver function, but does not *by itself* appear to cause severe, progressive, or lasting liver damage.

Conversely, interference with fatty acid oxidation at any of several stages may have profound consequences. For example, *alcoholic ketosis* is attributed to an ethanol- or acetaldehyde-mediated impairment of the tricarboxylic acid cycle, resulting in incomplete oxidation of the two-carbon fragments derived from β-oxidation of fatty acids. A far more profound derangement of hepatic function is caused by hypoglycin, a low molecular weight compound present in the unripened fruit of the ackee tree and the cause of *Jamaican vomiting sickness.* In this disorder, hypoglycin metabolites are converted to coenzyme A thioesters and to carnitine derivatives. Since these cannot be metabolized further, they effectively sequester the cellular carnitine pool. Fatty acid oxidation is inhibited, and there is a corresponding decrease in ATP production and gluconeogenesis. Continuing fatty acid esterification under these conditions leads to a form of fatty liver characterized by *small droplet fat* deposition, associated in severe cases with liver failure and hypoglycemia. Despite the histopathologic and clinical similarities between this entity and *Reye's syndrome, obstetric fatty liver,* and *tetracycline* and *valproic acid hepatotoxicity,* in none of these latter conditions has the pathogenesis been fully elucidated.

Another clinically important aspect of hepatic lipid metabolism concerns the synthesis of *cholesterol* and *bile acids* and the excretion of biliary lipids. The liver is the major source of endogenously synthesized cholesterol (approximately 0.5 grams per day). Together with cholesterol of dietary origin, this newly synthesized cholesterol enters a "metabolically active" hepatic cholesterol pool, from which is derived the cholesterol destined for secretion into bile or into plasma (in lipoproteins), for synthesis of liver cell membranes, and for conversion to bile acids. Bile acid synthesis accounts for the disposition of approximately half of the total daily turnover of cholesterol and, as such, is an important determinant of body cholesterol stores. Relative rates of secretion of bile acids, cholesterol, and phosphatidyl choline (lecithin) into bile are important factors in the pathogenesis of cholesterol gallstones, but the mechanism(s) by which the secretion of these substances is effected and controlled is poorly understood.

AMINO ACID AND PROTEIN METABOLISM. Except for the immunoglobulins, most plasma proteins, including albumin, clotting factors, transferrin, α_1-antitrypsin, and the nonalimentary lipoproteins, are synthesized in the liver. The synthesis of each is controlled by specific regulatory mechanisms. In all cases, however, synthesis and secretion are dependent on the integrity of many aspects of cell function, including the transcriptional mechanisms in the nucleus, the translational mechanisms in the rough endoplasmic reticulum, and the secretory mechanisms in the Golgi apparatus. Despite these common features, individual proteins are affected differently in liver disease. This nonuniformity may result from several factors such as the availability of an essential *nutritional* component (e.g., the vitamin K–dependent clotting factors), *hormonal* influences (e.g., very low density lipoproteins), *genetic* determinants (e.g., ceruloplasmin or α_1-antitrypsin), the effects of drugs or toxins (e.g., the warfarin-like anticoagulants or ethanol) or the response of selected proteins such as fibrinogen (and other "acute phase reactants," including C-reactive proteins, caeruloplasmin, haptoglobin, and transferrin) to inflammatory processes. In addition, the *kinetics* of synthesis and turnover of a particular protein are major determinants of response of its plasma concentration to acute liver injury. In general, plasma concentrations of proteins of which the turnover is rapid (e.g., clotting factors, plasma half-time of hours to days) are more likely to be depressed by severe acute liver injury than are those of proteins that turn over more slowly (e.g., albumin, plasma half-time of 2½ to 3 weeks). Finally, *catabolism* of certain plasma proteins may be accelerated (e.g., clotting factors in *disseminated intravascular coagulation,* or albumin in *protein-losing enteropathy*). For these reasons, although liver disease generally tends to depress the plasma concentration of proteins of hepatic origin, plasma concentrations of such proteins may not accurately reflect the severity of the liver disease in a given patient. Interpretation of the prothrombin time, partial thromboplastin time, and serum albumin concentrations in the evaluation of liver disease is discussed in Ch. 118.

Amino acids, in addition to their obvious importance in protein synthesis, also participate in other reactions in the liver. Of special significance is the role of certain amino acids as precursors for gluconeogenesis, as discussed above. Amino acids may undergo *transamination,* in which the α-amino group is transferred to an α-keto acid, as in the alanine transaminase (ALT)–mediated deamination of alanine to pyruvate; the resulting transfer of the amino group to α-ketoglutarate converts this acceptor to glutamate. Alternatively, amino acids may undergo *oxidative deamination;* in this case, an α-keto acid is formed as the amino group is converted to ammonium ion and, ultimately, to urea (see below).

BIOTRANSFORMATION AND DETOXIFICATION. The liver is the major site of chemical modification of a wide variety of exogenous drugs and toxins, as well as endogenous substances such as hormones. The reactions potentially involved are numerous and, in many instances, involve the cytochrome P-450–dependent microsomal mixed function oxidase system. The basic principles of drug disposition are discussed in Ch. 22, but several aspects warrant special emphasis in the context of liver function and disease. First, while biotransformation of an endogenous or exogenous substance may *inactivate* it or render it more suitable for urinary or biliary excretion, there are many examples of compounds upon which activity or toxicity is conferred by this process. A number of clinically significant hepatotoxins are *activated* in this way, and there is reason to suspect that some "idiosyncratic" hepatic drug reactions may reflect individual differences in drug metabolism rather than an immunologic response (see Ch. 121). Second, diseases of the liver may seriously impair the biotransformation of exogenous substances, thereby resulting in an *increased sensitivity* to certain drugs (e.g., sedatives and opiates), or may enhance the biologic effect of endogenous hormones (e.g., contributing to the feminizing effects of chronic liver disease) or toxins (e.g., diminished hepatic conversion of ammonia to urea in hepatic encephalopathy). Finally, one substance may significantly influence the hepatic biotransformation of another. Examples of this particular form of *drug-drug interaction* include the well recognized induction of the microsomal drug-metabolizing system by prior administration of phenobarbital and its inhibition by various toxins.

A particularly important hepatic detoxification pathway converts *ammonium ion* to urea via the Krebs-Henseleit *urea cycle,* in which ornithine, citrulline, argininosuccinate, and arginine are intermediates, and that involves both mitochondrial and cytosolic components (see Fig. 192–1). Glutamate, formed from NH_4^+ and α-ketoglutarate, is the principal NH_2 donor. Ammonium ion is produced in abundance in the intestinal tract, especially the colon, by the bacterial degradation of luminal proteins and amino acids, and of endogenous urea, 25 per cent of the daily production of which diffuses into the intestinal lumen. The NH_4^+ so formed diffuses into the portal circulation and is transported to the liver, where it is converted to urea by the mechanism described above. As discussed in Ch. 127, *hepatic encephalopathy* in part reflects the failure of this important detoxification process (or of analogous pathways for other *enterogenous toxins*) because of extensive acute liver cell necrosis or direct entry of portal blood into the peripheral circulation via spontaneous or surgically created portal-systemic shunts.

Arias IM, Popper H, Schachter D, Shafritz D: The Liver: Biology and Pathology. New York, Raven Press, 1982. *An in-depth and well-documented presentation of many more basic aspects of normal and abnormal hepatic structure and function.*
Zakim D, Boyer T (eds.): Hepatology: A Textbook of Liver Disease. Philadelphia, W. B. Saunders Company, 1982.

117. BILIRUBIN METABOLISM AND HYPERBILIRUBINEMIA

Bruce F. Scharschmidt

BILIRUBIN METABOLISM (see Fig. 117–1)

BILIRUBIN CHEMISTRY. Bilirubin consists of four pyrrole rings linked by three carbon bridges. Unconjugated bilirubin is virtually water insoluble at physiologic pH because its –COOH and –NH groups are involved in strong intramolecular hydrogen bonds and are therefore unable to interact with water. These intramolecular hydrogen bonds are disrupted by conjugation of the –COOH groups with glucuronic acid as occurs in the liver cell, thus greatly enhancing the aqueous solubility of the molecule and altering its biologic properties. In contrast to the more polar water-soluble conjugates, relatively nonpolar unconjugated bilirubin diffuses across most biologic membranes such as the blood-brain barrier, placenta, and intestinal and gallbladder epithelium. It is excreted in bile in only trace amounts. Thus, hepatic conjugation confers upon bilirubin the properties that permit its elimination from the body and thereby prevents damage to the central nervous system. Exposure of bilirubin to light appears reversibly to convert unconjugated bilirubin to one of several isomers that are also unable to form intramolecular hydrogen bonds, and hence have increased water solubility. These photoisomers are excreted by the liver without conjugation; this may be the primary mechanism by which phototherapy lowers serum bilirubin concentration in the neonate with impaired conjugation.

BILIRUBIN FORMATION. Bilirubin is formed by selective cleavage of the heme ring at the α-methene bridge. Daily bilirubin production in adults averages about 4 mg per kilogram, of which about 70 per cent results from degradation of the heme moiety of hemoglobin in senescent erythrocytes. Most of the remainder results from the breakdown of nonhemoglobin hemoproteins in the liver, principally the cytochromes P-450. A minor fraction of bilirubin production results from premature destruction of newly formed erythrocytes in the bone marrow or circulation. In certain clinical disorders (e.g., megaloblastic anemia) destruction of young or developing erythroid cells is increased and may account for a substantial proportion of total bilirubin production. The most common cause of increased bilirubin production in humans is increased breakdown of hemoglobin heme resulting from hemolysis.

Senescent erythrocytes are normally sequestered and degraded in the mononuclear phagocytic cells of the spleen, liver, or bone marrow. In contrast, the heme moiety of methemalbumin, methemoglobin, free hemoglobin, and haptoglobin-bound hemoglobin is taken up and catabolized by hepatic parenchymal cells. Microsomal heme oxygenase, the heme-cleaving enzyme, is most abundant in the liver, spleen, and bone marrow, and exhibits substrate-mediated induction by heme or hemoglobin. The conversion of heme to biliverdin, which is rate limiting for bilirubin formation, is followed by reduction of biliverdin to bilirubin by cytosolic biliverdin reductase. The reason why mammals convert nontoxic, water-soluble biliverdin to water-insoluble bilirubin is unclear. Recent studies suggest, however, that bilirubin, unlike biliverdin, is able to cross the placenta.

BILIRUBIN BINDING TO PLASMA PROTEINS. Unconjugated bilirubin is bound reversibly to albumin at a primary high affinity site ($3 \times 10^7 M^{-1}$). At plasma concentrations exceeding its molar equivalence with albumin (about 35 mg per deciliter), bilirubin binds to at least two low-affinity sites from which it can be displaced by other organic anions or a reduction in pH. A variety of compounds, including certain sulfonamides, penicillin derivatives, furosemide, and radiographic contrast media, may displace bilirubin from its albumin binding sites and increase the risk of kernicterus in neonates. Presumably because of its tight albumin binding and low water solubility, unconjugated bilirubin is not excreted in urine. Conjugated bilirubin is somewhat less tightly bound to albumin than is bilirubin. It is filtered to a greater extent at the glomerulus, is incompletely reabsorbed by the renal tubules, and therefore does appear in the urine in small amounts in patients with conjugated hyperbilirubinemia.

In addition to the reversible binding to albumin just described, a bilirubin fraction has recently been identified that binds very tightly, perhaps covalently, to albumin. It has been detected only in patients with hepatobiliary disease, in whom it may constitute a substantial proportion of direct-reacting fraction as measured by conventional assays (see below). While its clinical significance remains unclear, its presence helps explain the different results obtained with various techniques for measurement of bilirubin in serum. It also may help explain the occasionally extremely slow resolution of hyperbilirubinemia in patients convalescing from hepatitis or in whom biliary obstruction has been relieved, as well as the disappearance of bilirubinuria in these patients prior to the resolution of jaundice.

HEPATIC BILIRUBIN TRANSPORT. Hepatic uptake of bilirubin and other organic anions such as sulfobromophthalein across the sinusoidal membrane displays several features characteristic of carrier-mediated transport, including saturability and competition. Uptake of bilirubin and other substances tightly bound to protein is facilitated by large fenestrations in the cells of the sinusoidal lining that permit plasma proteins to enter the space of Disse and directly contact the hepatocyte plasma membrane.

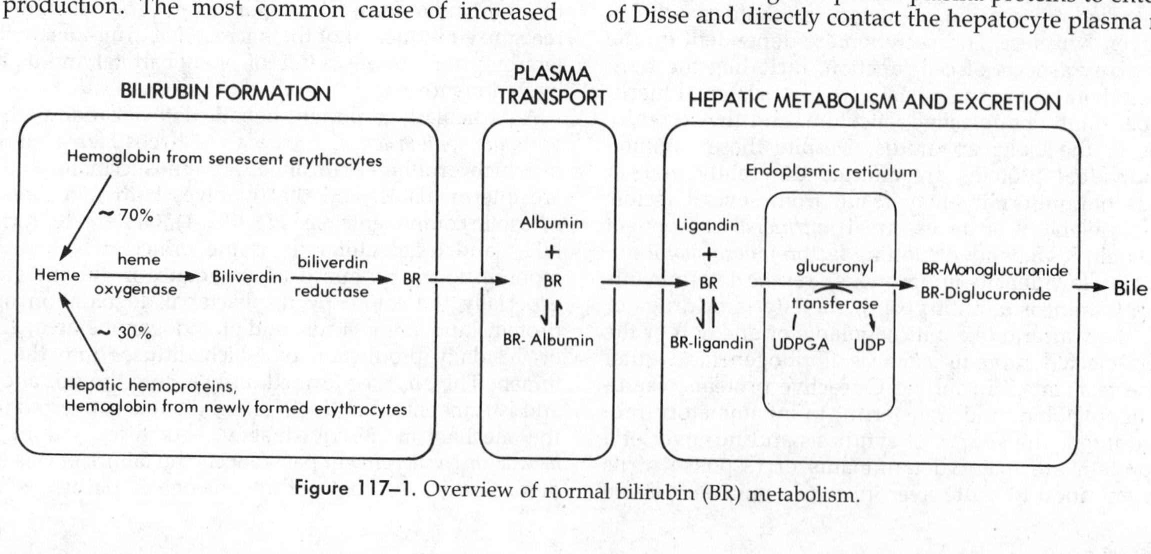

Figure 117–1. Overview of normal bilirubin (BR) metabolism.

Uptake of albumin-bound bilirubin by the putative membrane carriers may indeed be facilitated by transient binding of the albumin-bilirubin complex to the cell surface. Once inside the liver cell, bilirubin and other organic anions appear to bind to cytoplasmic proteins such as ligandin. Ligandin, which constitutes 5 per cent of cytoplasmic protein in rat liver, may alter net uptake by reducing bilirubin efflux back into plasma. In addition to transport through the cytoplasm, bilirubin may be directly transferred from the plasma membrane to the membranes of the endoplasmic reticulum, where conjugation occurs.

In the process of conjugation, the carboxyl groups of one or both propionic acid side chains of bilirubin are esterified, usually with glucuronic acid. Glucose and xylose conjugates are formed in trace amounts only. Formation of bilirubin mono- and diglucuronide is catalyzed by microsomal UDP-glucuronyltransferase. Transport of conjugated bilirubin from the hepatocyte into bile, like the uptake step, seems to show saturability and competition and therefore is presumably carrier mediated. Excretion and/or conjugation, but not uptake, appear to be rate limiting for overall bilirubin transport from blood to bile. It is at present uncertain whether the excretory process is active, i.e., intrinsically concentrative and energy requiring, or equilibrative. Bilirubin diglucuronide predominates in human bile, with the isomeric monoglucuronides present in small amounts.

ENTEROHEPATIC CIRCULATION. Absorption of conjugated bilirubin from the gallbladder and small intestine is negligible. In the terminal ileum and colon, bilirubin is converted by bacterial enzymes to a complex series of colorless tetrapyrroles collectively termed the urobilinogens. There is a generally poor correlation between bilirubin production and urobilinogen excretion, so that measurement of fecal urobilinogen is of limited diagnostic value. Up to 20 per cent of urobilinogen is reabsorbed, and 90 per cent of this is promptly re-excreted by the liver, with much of the remainder appearing in urine. Although it is frequently assumed that the clay-colored (acholic) stool present with biliary obstruction results from diminished excretion of bilirubin and urobilinogen, the normal brown color of stool may actually be due to other nonbilirubin pigments, perhaps of plant origin, which are also excreted in bile and undergo enterohepatic circulation.

CONCENTRATION IN PLASMA. The use of newer assay techniques indicates that virtually all circulating bilirubin in healthy adults is unconjugated. In contrast, circulating bilirubin in patients with hepatocellular or biliary tract disease consists predominantly of mono- and diconjugates. By comparison with newer techniques, the conventional diazo-assay, which is employed in most clinical laboratories, tends to overestimate total plasma bilirubin concentration in patients with hepatobiliary disease, perhaps because of the detection of pigment covalently bound to albumin. Moreover, determination of conjugated bilirubin based on measurement of the direct-reacting fraction is frequently in error. Nonetheless, for practical clinical application, conventional laboratory techniques are generally adequate. Plasma bilirubin concentration, which ranges normally between 0.3 and 1.0 mg per deciliter, varies directly with bilirubin production and inversely with hepatic bilirubin clearance. Thus, it is possible to interpret all forms of hyperbilirubinemia in terms of increased production and/or decreased clearance.

INHERITED DISORDERS OF BILIRUBIN METABOLISM

The hereditary disorders of hepatic bilirubin metabolism constitute a heterogeneous group of disorders characterized by an impaired ability of the liver to transport or conjugate bilirubin (Table 117–1). The common and benign entity of *Gilbert's syndrome* and the exceedingly rare and almost uni-

TABLE 117–1. THE HEREDITARY DISORDERS OF HEPATIC BILIRUBIN METABOLISM

	Gilbert's Syndrome	Type I Crigler-Najjar Syndrome	Type II Crigler-Najjar Syndrome	Dubin-Johnson Syndrome	Rotor's Syndrome
Incidence	Up to 7% of population	Very rare	Uncommon	Uncommon	Rare
Inheritance	? Autosomal dominant	Autosomal recessive	? Autosomal dominant	Autosomal recessive	Autosomal recessive
Defect(s) in bilirubin metabolism	Decreased hepatic UDP-glucuronyl-transferase activity, (?) slow hepatic bilirubin uptake, associated mild hemolysis in up to 50% of patients	Absent hepatic UDP-glucuronyl-transferase activity	Markedly decreased or undetectable UDP-glucuronyltransferase activity	Impaired biliary excretion of conjugated bilirubin	Impaired biliary excretion of conjugated bilirubin
Plasma bilirubin concentration (mg/dl)	≤3 in absence of fasting or hemolysis, predominantly unconjugated	17–50, usually >20, all unconjugated	6–45, usually <20, all unconjugated	1–25, usually <7, about 60% conjugated	1–20, usually <7, about 60% conjugated
Clinical sequelae	None	Death in infancy of kernicterus in almost all cases	Usually none, rarely kernicterus	Probably none	Probably none
Plasma sulfobromophthalein disappearance rate	Mildly abnormal in some patients (45-minute retention <15%)	Usually normal	Usually normal	Slow initial disappearance with frequent secondary rise (45-minute retention <20%)	Markedly slowed, no secondary rise (45-minute retention 30–50%)
Oral cholecystography	Normal	Normal	Normal	Faint or non-visualization	Usually normal
Hepatic histology (light microscopy)	Normal, occasionally increased lipofusion	Normal	Normal	Coarse pigment in centrolobular cells	Normal
Reduction of plasma bilirubin concentration by phenobarbital	Yes	No	Yes	Minimal	Unknown
Diagnosis	Clinical and laboratory findings, response to fasting occasionally helpful, liver biopsy not usually necessary	Clinical and laboratory findings, lack of response to phenobarbital	Clinical and laboratory findings, response to phenobarbital	Clinical and laboratory findings, sulfo-bromophthalein disappearance, urinary coproporphyrin excretion	Clinical and laboratory findings, sulfobromophthalein disappearance
Treatment	None necessary	None uniformly effective	Phenobarbital if bilirubin concentration markedly elevated	None available, avoid estrogens (may worsen jaundice)	None available

formly lethal Type I *Crigler-Najjar syndrome* represent opposite ends of this spectrum. Routine tests of liver function are generally normal in all these disorders, but a variety of abnormalities in the hepatic handling of bilirubin and other cholephilic anions such as sulfobromophthalein have been described. Many of these disorders, including Gilbert's syndrome, the *Dubin-Johnson syndrome,* and *Rotor's syndrome,* may mimic acquired hepatobiliary disease. They are all of interest because of the insight they provide into hepatic bilirubin transport and conjugation.

GILBERT'S SYNDROME. Because of its frequency (up to 7 per cent of the population), Gilbert's syndrome is the disorder most likely to be encountered by the clinician. Mild unconjugated hyperbilirubinemia is recognized most commonly during the second and third decades of life because of the presence of scleral icterus, often first noted with fasting, or as an incidental laboratory finding. Although a variety of nonspecific symptoms have been described, these may well be due to anxiety, and it is unlikely that any significant symptoms are attributable to Gilbert's syndrome itself. Gilbert's syndrome results from a decrease in the hepatic clearance of unconjugated bilirubin, but the precise reason for this decrease remains unclear. Evidence supporting both impaired conjugation and impaired hepatic bilirubin uptake exists. The diagnosis of Gilbert's syndrome used to require the absence of hemolysis. However, more recent studies in which the syndrome has been diagnosed by the characteristic decrease in clearance of radiobilirubin from plasma indicate that up to one half of patients have a very slight decrease in red cell survival detectable by ^{51}Cr-labeling; Gilbert's syndrome may also occasionally be found in patients with overt hemolysis (e.g., congenital spherocytosis). The principal clinical importance of this disorder is that it can be confused with more serious acquired hepatobiliary disease. From a practical standpoint, the diagnosis of Gilbert's syndrome is made by demonstrating low grade unconjugated hyperbilirubinemia in a patient with a normal physical examination and otherwise repeatedly normal laboratory tests of liver function. Normal fasting and postprandial concentrations of bile acids in serum are also helpful in excluding liver disease. Liver biopsy demonstrating normal histology is rarely necessary. An exaggerated hyperbilirubinemic response to fasting, lipid withdrawal, or nicotinic acid administration has been found to be helpful by some investigators but these tests are neither sensitive nor specific enough to warrant routine use. In patients with overt hemolysis, direct measurement of hepatic bilirubin clearance may be necessary to establish the diagnosis. Gilbert's syndrome and the other inherited disorders of hepatic bilirubin metabolism are outlined in the accompanying table.

BENIGN RECURRENT CHOLESTASIS. In contrast to the inherited disorders, in which hepatic bilirubin metabolism or excretion is selectively impaired, this entity is characterized by recurrent attacks of cholestasis manifested by pruritus, conjugated hyperbilirubinemia, and elevated serum levels of alkaline phosphatase and bile salts. Individual attacks may persist from weeks to months, do not result from biliary obstruction, and typically remit spontaneously. Attacks frequently begin in childhood, recur at highly variable intervals, and do not generally lead to cirrhosis or decreased longevity. The etiology of this disorder is unknown, but an inherited basis is postulated because of its early age of onset and familial nature.

There are also inherited forms of hemolytic anemia (e.g., hereditary spherocytosis), which may produce modest unconjugated hyperbilirubinemia owing to increased bilirubin production. These disorders are discussed in detail in Ch. 137.

ACQUIRED HYPERBILIRUBINEMIA

HEMOLYSIS. Hemolysis increases bilirubin production and generally produces low grade unconjugated, indirect-reacting hyperbilirubinemia. Because of the enormous reserve of the hepatic bilirubin transport mechanism, hepatic bilirubin clearance remains constant, and plasma bilirubin concentration increases linearly with bilirubin production rate in most individuals. Since the bone marrow cannot increase erythrocyte production more than about eight-fold, ongoing *steady-state hemolysis* by itself cannot account for a sustained increase in plasma unconjugated bilirubin concentration above 4 to 5 mg per deciliter. Concentrations consistently exceeding this indicate hepatic dysfunction irrespective of the presence of hemolysis. In contrast, *acute hemolysis,* even in patients with normal hepatic function, may produce elevations in total plasma bilirubin concentration that greatly exceed 5 mg per deciliter, as well as an increase in the conjugated fraction. The increase in conjugated pigment indicates that the maximal hepatic excretory capacity for bilirubin has temporarily been exceeded.

INEFFECTIVE ERYTHROPOIESIS. Bilirubin production is increased and hence the plasma concentration of unconjugated, indirect-reacting bilirubin may be elevated in a variety of disorders associated with ineffective erythropoiesis. Markedly increased ineffective erythropoiesis is the basis of the rare disorder known as *shunt hyperbilirubinemia* or *idiopathic dyserythropoietic jaundice.*

FASTING HYPERBILIRUBINEMIA. Fasting causes an increase in the plasma concentration of unconjugated, indirect-reacting bilirubin owing primarily to a decrease in hepatic bilirubin clearance. This effect may be particularly marked in patients with Gilbert's syndrome and the Type II Crigler-Najjar syndrome. Both dietary composition and total caloric intake are important, since a normocaloric but lipid-free diet produces a response similar to that observed with complete fasting, and the effect of complete fasting is reversed by feeding small amounts of lipid. The mechanism of the decrease in hepatic bilirubin clearance with fasting is unclear. A slight increase in bilirubin production contributes to fasting hyperbilirubinemia.

POSTOPERATIVE HYPERBILIRUBINEMIA. Postoperative hyperbilirubinemia (also called postoperative intrahepatic cholestasis or postoperative jaundice) usually occurs in patients who have undergone major surgery. The incidence of postoperative hyperbilirubinemia (>2 mg per deciliter) is about 15 per cent following open heart surgery compared with about 1 per cent after elective abdominal surgery, and may be increased in patients with pre-existing liver disease. Hyperbilirubinemia, usually predominantly conjugated, occurs from one to ten days after surgery, can become quite marked, and is typically accompanied by a two- to four-fold elevation of the alkaline phosphatase and 5′-nucleotidase with minimally abnormal transaminase levels and prothrombin time. The etiology of the hyperbilirubinemia is probably multifactorial, with both increased bilirubin production (from breakdown of transfused erythrocytes and resorption of hematomas) and impaired hepatic excretory function (from hypotension, hypoxemia, or bacteremia) being potentially important contributing factors. Postoperative hyperbilirubinemia is usually benign and resolves as the overall condition of the patient improves. It is important to distinguish it from postoperative jaundice caused by biliary obstruction or hepatocellular necrosis resulting from shock, anesthetic injury, or post-transfusion hepatitis. Hepatocellular necrosis resulting from shock, anesthetic injury, or hepatitis is typically accompanied by markedly abnormal transaminase levels and prothrombin time.

DIFFUSE HEPATOCELLULAR INJURY. Hyperbilirubinemia associated with disorders such as viral hepatitis reflects one aspect of a global insult to hepatocellular function. The hyperbilirubinemia is of importance primarily as an index of the severity of hepatocellular injury. In unusual cases in which hyperbilirubinemia seems disproportionate to the hepatic injury, as reflected by serum transaminase levels and prothrombin time, a search for causes of increased bilirubin production (e.g., hemolysis) or decreased hepatic bilirubin clearance (e.g., infection) is worthwhile.

MISCELLANEOUS. Mild unconjugated hyperbilirubinemia is occasionally found in a variety of unrelated conditions. *Cyclic premenstrual unconjugated hyperbilirubinemia* appears related to serum progesterone levels. Administration of *chenodeoxycholic acid* and certain drugs such as *propranolol, rifampin,* and *probenecid* has been associated with mild, reversible unconjugated hyperbilirubinemia in the absence of overt hepatic jaundice.

Gollan JL, Schmid R: Bilirubin update: Formation, transport, and metabolism. *In* Popper H, Schaffner F (eds.): Progress in Liver Diseases. Vol VII. New York, Grune and Stratton, 1982, pp 261–283. *A comprehensive review of recent developments in bilirubin metabolism.*

Weiss JS, Gautam A, Lauff JJ, Sundberg MW, Jatlow P, Boyer JL, Seligson D: The clinical importance of a protein-bound fraction of serum bilirubin in patients with hyperbilirubinemia. N Engl J Med 309:147, 1983. *A concise description of the protein-bound fraction—in whom it occurs and what it means.*

Wolkoff AW: Bilirubin metabolism and hyperbilirubinemia. *In* Berk PD (ed.): Seminars in Liver Diseases. New York, Thieme-Stratton, Inc., 1983, pp 1–82. *A series of short and authoritative reviews generally focusing on issues of clinical relevance.*

118. LABORATORY TESTS IN LIVER DISEASE

Robert K. Ockner

Unlike tests employed in the clinical evaluation of other organ systems (e.g., arterial blood gases, creatinine clearance, plasma hormone assays), "liver function" tests for the most part are highly empirical, and often do not indicate either the integrity of liver function or the severity of a disease process. Despite this, and provided that their limitations are recognized, they may be useful in screening for hepatobiliary diseases, diagnostic evaluation, and following the course of the disease. In this chapter, the generally available laboratory tests for the diagnosis of hepatobiliary disease are discussed with regard to physiology, pathophysiology, and clinical usefulness.

BILIRUBIN. The metabolism of bilirubin and its measurement are discussed in detail in Ch. 117.

TRANSAMINASES. *Transaminases (aminotransferases)* catalyze the transfer of amino groups from aspartate or alanine to α-ketoglutarate. The enzymes are named either by the products of the reaction (glutamic and oxalacetic, or glutamic and pyruvic transaminases, SGOT or SGPT, respectively) or, as is currently preferred, by the amino-group donor (aspartate or alanine transaminases, AST or ALT, respectively). Specific isozymes of AST are present in liver cell mitochondria and cytoplasm, whereas ALT is confined to the cytoplasm. Increased serum transaminase activity in liver disease is assumed to reflect leaking from injured cells. Transaminases are not present in appreciable concentrations in urine. Although present in bile, activity there does not reflect that in serum, and clearance of these enzymes from plasma does not depend on secretion into bile or urine. Since the mechanisms and determinants of transaminase clearance are not understood, interpretation of serum activity is necessarily empirical. Generally, the height of the transaminase activity reflects the severity of hepatic necrosis, but there are important exceptions. In even the most severe forms of acute *alcoholic hepatitis,* for example, levels seldom exceed 200 to 300 IU per liter. In contrast, serum transaminase activities of 1000 IU or more are often present in mild uncomplicated acute *viral hepatitis* or sudden high grade *biliary obstruction,* as may occur during passage of a gallstone. Conversely, initially elevated serum transaminase activities may fall as the clinical course of massive hepatic necrosis deteriorates, suggesting that the liver is so severely damaged that little enzyme activity remains.

Despite these caveats, the serum transaminase activities may be helpful in certain circumstances: First, they are useful as *screening tests* for liver disease. Although AST levels may be increased in diseases of other organs (e.g., myocardium and skeletal muscle), values more than ten times the upper limit of the normal range usually reflect hepatic or biliary pathology. Moreover, the ALT is relatively specific for hepatobiliary disease. In the context of other clinical and laboratory findings, identification of the source of increased serum transaminase activity is not usually difficult. Second, it is distinctly uncommon for the AST to exceed 15 times the upper limit of normal in bile duct obstruction, except when it occurs suddenly, or is associated with cholangitis. Third, in contrast to most other forms of parenchymal liver disease, in which the ALT activity usually equals or exceeds the AST, in *alcoholic hepatitis* this relationship is reversed, and this may be useful diagnostically. Finally, transaminase values are often useful in monitoring the course of acute or chronic parenchymal liver disease, although, as noted, they are potentially misleading in certain circumstances.

ALKALINE PHOSPHATASE. This group of enzymes is present in many tissues, including liver, bile ducts, intestine, bone, kidney, placenta, and leukocytes; hepatic alkaline phosphatase itself appears heterogeneous. The phosphatases catalyze the release of inorganic phosphate from a phosphate ester substrate, at alkaline pH. Their biologic function is unknown, except for an apparent relationship to bone deposition. Normally, serum alkaline phosphatase activity reflects mainly the liver and bone isozymes. In some persons, especially those of blood types O or A who are secretors of the ABO red cell antigens and are positive for the Lewis antigen, intestinal alkaline phosphatase may account for 20 to 60 per cent of total serum activity. In the later stages of pregnancy, the placental contribution may be substantial. More recently a number of less common sources of alkaline phosphatase have been identified. These include a variant associated with hepatoma, and the so-called *Regan isozyme.* The latter is apparently identical to the placental enzyme, but originates in a variety of tumors, especially lung; it also may be detected rarely in the serum of normal subjects.

Serum alkaline phosphatase activity may be increased in many conditions not associated with hepatobiliary disease, including bone disorders, pregnancy, normal growth, and occasionally the presence of malignancy not involving either bone or liver (e.g., the Regan isozyme), and for this reason the organ or tissue of origin must be identified. In some cases, this is obvious because of other clinical and laboratory findings. When the source is less apparent, several methods are available to differentiate hepatobiliary from other isozymes, such as heat stability or electrophoretic separation of isozymes. Most practical and available is the measurement of the serum *5′-nucleotidase, leucine aminopeptidase,* or *γ-glutamyl transpeptidase* activities, which tend to parallel that of alkaline phosphatase in hepatobiliary disease, but do not usually increase in bone disease. However, the first two of these may increase during pregnancy (see below).

Serum hepatobiliary alkaline phosphatase activity is usually increased in bile duct obstruction, parenchymal disease, or infiltrative or mass lesions of the liver. This increased serum activity reflects increased enzyme synthesis rather than decreased biliary excretion or leakage from damaged cells. Although the highest levels usually occur with bile duct obstruction, very high values may also be associated with intrahepatic cholestasis or infiltrative or mass lesions. On the other hand, it is most unusual for the serum alkaline phosphatase activity to remain relatively normal in the presence of significant bile duct obstruction, especially in association with jaundice. Conversely, elevated alkaline phosphatase may be the only clinically apparent abnormality in bile duct stricture or in lesions that produce obstruction of a single hepatic lobe or segment. As many as one third of patients with isolated elevations of serum hepatobiliary alkaline phosphatase activity may have no demonstrable underlying liver or biliary disease.

LEUCINE AMINOPEPTIDASE, 5′-NUCLEOTIDASE, AND γ-GLUTAMYLTRANSPEPTIDASE. Leucine aminopeptidase (LAP) is an ubiquitous cellular peptidase whereas 5′-nucleotidase (5′-NT) is a plasma membrane enzyme that cleaves the inorganic phosphate from adenosine- or inosine-5′-phosphate. The serum activity of both enzymes usually increases in cholestasis, and their major clinical value is that they may be of help in identifying the source of an elevated serum alkaline phosphatase activity.

Since these enzymes may be elevated in late pregnancy, they are most useful in the nonpregnant patient. Although an elevated serum activity of either of these enzymes suggests an hepatobiliary origin of an increased alkaline phosphatase, the converse is not true, and liver alkaline phosphatase occasionally may be increased while the others remain normal.

Gamma-glutamyl transpeptidase (GGTP) is present in many tissues. It increases in serum not only in hepatobiliary disease but also after myocardial infarction, in neuromuscular diseases, in pancreatic disease in the absence of biliary obstruction, and during the ingestion of ethanol and other inducers of hepatic microsomal enzymes. The GGTP has been proposed as a sensitive screening test for hepatobiliary disease, and for the monitoring of abstinence from ethanol. This test may be used to identify the source of an alkaline phosphatase elevation, but it offers no clear advantage over the other available tests.

ALBUMIN AND GLOBULIN. *Albumin* is synthesized exclusively in the liver at a rate of 100 to 200 mg per kilogram of body weight per day. The synthetic rate is influenced by systemic or liver disease and by nutritional state, thyroid hormone, glucocorticoids, plasma colloid osmotic pressure, and toxins such as ethanol and carbon tetrachloride. The mechanism of albumin degradation in health is not known; the rate is increased in exfoliative dermatitis, severe burns, nephrotic syndrome, and protein-losing enteropathy. Thus, albumin concentration, which reflects the balance between synthesis and degradation or loss, may be importantly influenced by factors other than the functional state of the liver, and therefore this test is not specific. On the other hand, if other factors can be excluded, hypoalbuminemia may be an important sign of liver disease, and serum albumin concentration may be a useful indicator of changing hepatic function. Although hypoalbuminemia reflects diminished synthesis in some patients with cirrhosis and ascites, in others synthesis is normal and hypoalbuminemia is caused by a redistribution among the extracellular fluid compartments, including the peritoneal cavity.

Serum globulins are of limited diagnostic utility in hepatobiliary diseases. As a group, they are heterogeneous with respect to site and regulation of production, physical properties, and physiologic function. Their concentration, as measured by serum protein electrophoresis or salt fractionation, may be influenced by a wide variety of hepatic and extrahepatic factors and disease states. The mechanism for their increased serum concentration in liver disease is not fully understood, but probably is multifactorial, and may include stimulus to increased antibody production resulting from increased entry of bacterial antigens into the systemic circulation, or release of antigenic material from injured liver cells. An important exception to this generalization is the finding of a diminished concentration of the α_1-globulin fraction as demonstrated by serum protein electrophoresis. Since approximately 85 per cent of this fraction is accounted for by α_1-antitrypsin, a decrease in its concentration may be an important sign of an α_1-antitrypsin deficiency, an inherited disorder associated with neonatal hepatitis, cirrhosis, and pulmonary emphysema (see Ch. 124). Elevated IgM concentrations are common in primary biliary cirrhosis, but other clinical, laboratory, and imaging procedures are of greater diagnostic value. Diffuse increases in globulin concentrations are commonly seen in cirrhosis, and may be especially pronounced in HBsAg-negative chronic active hepatitis (see Ch. 122).

PROTHROMBIN TIME. This test, usually performed by the one-stage (Quick) method, measures the rate at which prothrombin in citrated plasma is converted to thrombin in the presence of added calcium, tissue thromboplastin, and activated clotting factors. It depends on the plasma concentration not only of prothrombin but also of other clotting factors synthesized in the liver, including V, VII, X, and fibrinogen. Prothrombin time (or, expressed as a percentage of a standardized control sample, prothrombin content) may be abnormal if plasma concentrations of prothrombin itself or of the other important factors are reduced below a critical level. This may reflect an increased rate of degradation, as in disseminated intravascular coagulation, a decreased rate of synthesis, or both.

Synthesis of fibrinogen, prothrombin and of factors V, VII, IX, X, XI, XII, and XIII occurs in the liver. Synthesis of prothrombin and factors VII, IX, and X depends on an adequate supply of *vitamin K,* which activates preformed polypeptides in the liver by stimulating the synthesis of the calcium-binding residue, γ-carboxyglutamic acid. Thus, an abnormal prothrombin time that reflects decreased production of these factors may be caused rarely by *inherited abnormalities,* and much more commonly by *vitamin K deficiency, liver disease,* or both. Vitamin K is abundant in many foods, and a portion of the vitamin that is produced by intestinal bacteria may also be available to the host. Thus, deficiency of the vitamin is most often caused by one of the *malabsorption syndromes,* including biliary obstruction and other causes of cholestasis. Rarely, it may reflect antimicrobial suppression of intestinal bacteria. Any acute or chronic liver disease may cause an abnormal prothrombin time if the synthesis of essential clotting factors is impaired. In acute liver disease, hypoprothrombinemia often indicates an unfavorable prognosis.

An abnormal prothrombin time may be of diagnostic value in the evaluation of the jaundiced patient. In general, when it is prolonged on the basis of vitamin K deficiency alone, e.g., because of cholestasis-induced malabsorption, it will return to near normal levels within hours after parenteral administration of vitamin K. In contrast, when clotting factor synthesis is diminished because of parenchymal liver disease, response to vitamin K may be slight or absent. Unfortunately, for several reasons this simple and attractive diagnostic approach does not always reliably differentiate obstructive from parenchymal liver disease. First, hypoprothrombinemia may reflect more than one factor, e.g., biliary obstruction associated with parenchymal liver disease or disseminated intravascular coagulation. Second, vitamin K malabsorption and a prolonged but correctable prothrombin time may result from cholestasis of any cause, including parenchymal disease such as primary biliary cirrhosis, cholestatic hepatitis, and drug-induced cholestasis. Finally, a partial response to vitamin K administration may be misleading. Because of these shortcomings, the response of an abnormal prothrombin time to parenteral vitamin K administration must be interpreted in the context of other available information.

The *partial thromboplastin time* is used to assess the "intrinsic" clotting mechanism, and reflects the activity of all clotting factors except for platelet factor 3, factor XIII, and factor VII. For this reason, the test is complementary to the prothrombin time and may indicate deficiencies of other clotting factors or the presence of a circulating anticoagulant.

SERUM LIPIDS AND LIPOPROTEINS. Parenchymal liver disease and bile duct obstruction may be associated with significant abnormalities in serum lipids and lipoproteins. In acute parenchymal liver disease, there may be loss of the α_1-lipoprotein band normally present on serum lipoprotein electrophoresis, reflecting abnormal composition and physical properties of the high density lipoproteins. There may also be a transient hypertriglyceridemia, reflecting the presence in serum of abnormal low density lipoproteins rich in triglycerides. These changes appear attributable in part to deficient activity of plasma lecithin: cholesterol acyltransferase (LCAT), an enzyme of hepatic origin that esterifies plasma cholesterol. The changes are transient, and with resolution of the acute liver injury, plasma lipids and lipoproteins return to their previous state.

In cholestasis the serum concentrations of unesterified cholesterol and phospholipids are increased, and the development of xanthomas and xanthelasma is related to the severity and duration of this abnormality. Of the increased plasma unesterified cholesterol, a major fraction is accounted for by the presence of an abnormal low density lipoprotein, designated *LPX.* LPX consists mainly of unesterified cholesterol and phosphatidyl choline (lecithin), in a 1:1 molar ratio, with a small amount of protein, largely a mixture of albumin and the C apolipoproteins. In negative-staining electron microscopy, LPX assumes the shape of a disc that may form rouleaux. The similarity of the lipid composition LPX to that of bile (primarily free cholesterol and lecithin), together with other evidence, suggests that it represents the entry into plasma either of biliary lipid or of lipid from the hepatocyte normally destined for secretion into bile. LPX is not currently of value in the differential diagnosis of jaundice. Its concentrations are correlated with the far simpler determination of plasma free cholesterol concentration, but not with other tests of liver function.

MITOCHONDRIAL ANTIBODY. In approximately 90 per cent of patients with primary biliary cirrhosis, serum contains antibodies directed against a lipoprotein component of the inner mitochondrial membrane. The antibodies are neither organ nor species specific, and are demonstrated by immunofluorescent techniques employing rat kidney, liver, and stomach and human thyroid, stomach, and kidney. They include the three main immunoglobulin classes and are complement fixing. In patients with primary biliary cirrhosis, the titer is not related to the increased level of serum IgM or the stage or severity of the disease.

Mitochondrial antibodies are also present in up to 25 per cent of patients with chronic active hepatitis and postnecrotic cirrhosis and in 7 to 8 per cent of asymptomatic relatives of patients with primary biliary cirrhosis. They are rarely present in extrahepatic biliary obstruction. A small percentage of patients with nonhepatic diseases may also exhibit positive tests; these include the collagen-vascular disorders, thyroiditis, myasthenia gravis, Addison's disease, autoimmune hemolytic anemia, and chronic biologic false-positive reactions for syphilis. Five types of mitochondrial antibodies have thus far been identified; the first (M_1) is the type usually found in primary biliary cirrhosis. Mitochondrial antibodies are demonstrable in only 0.4 to 0.7 per cent of the general population.

In the differential diagnosis of jaundice the mitochondrial test is useful in two respects. First, a negative result renders the diagnosis of primary biliary cirrhosis unlikely but does not exclude it. Second, because of its rarity in extrahepatic biliary obstruction, a positive result tends to suggest parenchymal liver disease, but it does not exclude bile duct obstruction. Since the incidence of gallstones in patients with primary biliary cirrhosis is approximately 40 per cent, and is also increased in other forms of cirrhosis, the mitochondrial antibody test cannot be regarded as a reliable basis for distinguishing "medical" from "surgical" jaundice.

ANTINUCLEAR AND SMOOTH MUSCLE ANTIBODIES. Either or both of these tests may be positive in a variable percentage of patients with chronic active hepatitis, usually among those cases not associated with hepatitis B infection. They have also been demonstrated in a minority of patients with primary biliary cirrhosis. As is true of the mitochondrial antibody, these factors are neither organ nor species specific. They probably do not play a role in pathogenesis. The presence of these antibodies in serum may suggest but does not differentiate among chronic hepatitis, postnecrotic cirrhosis, or primary biliary cirrhosis, and clearly does not exclude a bile duct lesion.

TESTS FOR HEPATITIS VIRUS INFECTION. These tests and their clinical significance are discussed in Ch. 120.

URINE AND STOOL EXAMINATIONS. The presence of bilirubin in urine indicates that a significant fraction of plasma bilirubin is conjugated, and is strong evidence of hepatobiliary disease. Jaundice in the absence of bilirubinuria indicates an exclusively unconjugated hyperbilirubinemia, i.e., reflecting hemolysis, ineffective erythropoiesis, or an inherited disorder of bilirubin conjugation. For several reasons, urine and fecal *urobilinogen* determinations usually do not provide useful information in the evaluation of hepatobiliary disease (see Ch. 124). Testing of stool for occult blood is essential, and may provide the first evidence of an alimentary tract lesion related or unrelated to hepatobiliary disease, a bleeding diathesis, or an explanation for the appearance of hepatic encephalopathy. In selected cases, depending on the clinical circumstances, stool culture or examination for ova and parasites may provide information of importance in the diagnosis of liver disease.

HEMATOLOGIC TESTS IN LIVER DISEASE. Diseases of the liver may be associated with a wide variety of hematologic abnormalities, including qualitative and quantitative changes in the formed elements, and in clotting function. The abnormalities depend not only on the etiology of the liver disorder but also on whether it is acute or chronic, or associated with complications such as liver failure or portal hypertension.

In acute liver disease not associated with liver failure, major changes in the formed elements are uncommon and consist primarily of mild anemia, reflecting either low grade hemolysis or marrow depression. Macrocytosis may be present. Slight leukopenia is not uncommon, and often is associated with atypical lymphocytes.

Rarely, a severe aplastic anemia may complicate acute viral hepatitis. The pathogenesis is unknown, the prognosis is very poor, and treatment is largely ineffective. In other forms of acute liver disease, hematologic abnormalities, e.g., marrow suppression, may be caused by toxins such as ethanol or drugs. Zieve's syndrome also occurs in the alcoholic. It consists of hemolytic anemia and hypertriglyceridemia; the basis for this association is not understood. Coagulopathy may complicate massive hepatic necrosis, reflecting depressed hepatic synthesis of clotting factors or disseminated intravascular coagulation.

In chronic liver disease, a number of abnormalities of the erythrocytes may be present. Target cells, often associated with cholestasis, result from an expansion of the cell membrane, with relative preservation of the cholesterol to phospholipid ratio. Spur cells (acanthocytes) are most often found in advanced cirrhosis, usually alcoholic, and reflect a more profound relative and absolute increase in membrane free cholesterol.

Red cells, white cells, and platelets may be decreased in patients with portal hypertension, primarily because of hypersplenism. A number of other abnormalities may be present, but to a large extent these are caused by associated nutritional, pathologic, or pharmacologic influences. Examples include iron deficiency, megaloblastic, and sideroblastic anemias.

LIVER BIOPSY. Performed by a blind technique or under direct vision during laparoscopy, this procedure is of value in the diagnosis of diffuse or localized parenchymal diseases (e.g., cirrhosis, chronic hepatitis, hemochromatosis) and hepatomegaly. Because bile duct obstruction is often associated with nonspecific parenchymal changes, biopsy is not ordinarily a preferred initial diagnostic procedure in the evaluation of the patient with cholestatic jaundice. Rather, imaging and cholangiographic methods are more rewarding in this setting. Liver biopsy requires the cooperation of the patient, except in infants, and normal clotting function. Relative or absolute contraindications include the presence of biliary sepsis, right pleural disease, ascites, coagulopathy, and high grade bile duct obstruction.

IMAGING TECHNIQUES AND CHOLANGIOGRAPHY. These techniques are discussed in detail in Ch. 94. In the following chapter, their utility is considered briefly in the context of the diagnosis of jaundice.

Arias IM, Popper H, Schachter D, Shafritz D: The Liver: Biology and Pathobiology. New York, Raven Press, 1982. *An in-depth and well-documented presentation of many more basic aspects of normal and abnormal hepatic structure and function.*

Popper H, Schaffner F (eds.): Progress in Liver Diseases. Vol VI. New York, Grune & Stratton, 1979. *A collection of 38 authoritative reviews of the "state of the art" in diverse aspects of liver structure, function, and disease. Very useful as a primary source of information and of pertinent references.*

Zakim D, Boyer T (eds.): Hepatology: A Textbook of Liver Disease. Philadelphia, W. B. Saunders Company, 1982.

119. APPROACHES TO THE DIAGNOSIS OF JAUNDICE

Robert K. Ockner

As discussed in Ch. 117, jaundice may be caused by a wide range of disorders. Excluding hemolysis, ineffective erythropoiesis, and congenital errors of bilirubin metabolism (any of which may be present *in addition to other causes*), jaundice can be broadly classified as *intrahepatic* or *extrahepatic*. Included among the intrahepatic causes are (1) hepatocellular diseases such as viral or drug-induced acute or chronic liver disease, (2) various metabolic and infiltrative disorders such as anoxia, Wilson's disease, and metastatic tumor, and (3) disorders of the intrahepatic biliary system such as primary biliary cirrhosis, intrahepatic sclerosing cholangitis, and congenital disorders associated with cystic dilatation of the smaller bile ducts. Extrahepatic causes of jaundice, i.e., large bile duct obstruction, include choledocholithiasis, bile duct strictures, chronic pancreatitis with bile duct compression, and tumors affecting the bile duct itself or critically situated contiguous structures such as lymph nodes in the porta hepatis, the ampulla of Vater, or the head of the pancreas.

In view of the magnitude and diversity of the differential diagnosis, the clinical approach must be equally broad. A careful history and physical examination are of paramount importance, emphasizing a search for clues that might suggest a cause such as exposure to a jaundiced person or a potentially toxic drug (viral or drug-induced hepatitis), an antecedent history of pruritus and xanthelasma (chronic cholestasis such as primary biliary cirrhosis), recurrent abdominal pain and nausea (gallstone disease), chronic ulcerative colitis (sclerosing cholangitis), or epigastric pain, weight loss, and distended gallbladder (cancer of the head of the pancreas). Routinely available laboratory studies are also helpful (see Ch. 118). In general, serum aminotransferase activities do not exceed 10 to 15 times the upper limit of normal in patients with bile duct obstruction, unless there is superimposed bacterial cholangitis or the obstruction occurs suddenly, and is high grade. In the latter instance, usually associated with impaction of a gallstone in the common bile duct, the aminotransferase level, which may exceed 1000 IU, usually also falls quite rapidly (over a few days) toward normal. Alkaline phosphatase activities usually exceed two to three times normal, but very high values may be seen in both intrahepatic and extrahepatic processes. Elevation of serum cholesterol tends to suggest chronic cholestasis but is of little help in differential diagnosis. Amylase activity may be elevated because of pancreatitis induced by passage of a gallstone that also causes bile duct obstruction, or may reflect pancreatitis of some other cause that secondarily causes compression of the intrapancreatic portion of the distal common bile duct. Hepatitis serologies may help in diagnosis, but obstructive biliary disease may be superimposed on chronic parenchymal liver disease such as chronic hepatitis B or cirrhosis.

Despite the seemingly limitless number of diagnostic possibilities and of permutations and combinations of clinical and laboratory findings, the clinical evaluation (that based on history, physical examination, and routine laboratory tests) is quite accurate and serves to identify correctly the cause of jaundice in 80 to 85 per cent of cases. It is for confirmation of these clinical diagnoses (when needed) and for the elucidation of the clinically more obscure processes that other diagnostic procedures are available. The availability and accuracy of these procedures has increased dramatically in recent years, and the decision regarding their proper use has become a critically important part of the judgmental process involved in the management of these problems.

The diagnostic approach to the jaundiced patient does not lend itself readily to generalizations or inflexible algorithms. Rather, a host of highly individual factors must be taken into account. These include the evolving clinical course and current status of the patient; the differential diagnosis; the availability, reliability, and safety of the available diagnostic tests in a given institution; and the experience and judgment of a consulting surgeon. Despite these reservations, some general guidelines are valid in many instances and may serve, with appropriate modification, as the basis for an approach to diagnosis.

First, as noted above, the diagnosis in most patients will be obvious or strongly suggested by routine clinical and laboratory findings. For example, if the patient appears to have viral or drug-induced acute hepatitis, if this presumptive diagnosis is supported by appropriate laboratory studies, and if the patient is doing well, more elaborate or invasive studies are usually unnecessary as continuing observation and follow-up studies will suffice.

Second, if more information is needed in a patient with unexplained cholestatic jaundice, *liver biopsy* is often not helpful, since in many cases of parenchymal cholestasis the histopathology is nonspecific. Moreover, parenchymal liver disease not only does not exclude biliary tract disease but may in fact predispose to it (e.g., the increased incidence of gallstones in cirrhosis). Thus, although biopsy can be performed with reasonable safety in the presence of bile duct obstruction, in most cases it will not be the initial diagnostic procedure of choice.

Of the available radiographic and imaging procedures, *ultrasound* and *CT scanning* are attractive because they are noninvasive and provide accurate information concerning caliber of the bile ducts. Because of its lesser cost, the absence of radiation exposure, and its ability to detect stones in the gallbladder accurately, ultrasound may be preferred. However, these two tests suffer from a finite, albeit small error rate (both false positives and false negatives) in the diagnosis of bile duct obstruction. This is not unexpected in view of the fact that these techniques provide information as to the *caliber* of the bile duct; the presence or absence of biliary obstruction can only be *inferred*. Clearly, the syndrome of biliary tract obstruction is so varied that the relationship between completeness and duration of the obstructive process on the one hand and the caliber of the ducts on the other must also vary. For these reasons, the noninvasive tests, although useful in initial assessment, may not be definitive.

Direct cholangiography is currently the most reliable approach to the nonoperative diagnosis of cholestatic jaundice. It may be accomplished either percutaneously, with the Chiba ("skinny") needle, or endoscopically. In most centers, the probability of duct visualization with the percutaneous transhepatic technique approaches 100 per cent in the presence of bile duct obstruction. The success rate with parenchymal jaundice is variable but generally lower. The procedure is rapid and simple, is readily performed in most institutions, and involves minimal cost and technical experience. For these reasons, percutaneous transhepatic cholangiography represents the best combination of accuracy, speed, low risk, and low cost, and therefore is suggested as the single most valuable of the currently available invasive techniques (see also Ch. 94).

Endoscopic retrograde cholangiography, although more demanding of patient and physician, more expensive, and more time consuming, nonetheless has a definite place. It can be safely performed in the patient with abnormal clotting function, whereas the percutaneous study cannot. It may demonstrate duct pathology when the percutaneous approach has failed, and may be especially suitable in those patients in whom the intrahepatic bile ducts are not dilated, or in whom there may be associated pancreatic disease. Finally, it may permit a direct therapeutic approach in certain cases, e.g., endoscopic sphincteroplasty and stone extraction for patients with retained impacted common bile duct stones or gallstone-associated pancreatitis. Each of these procedures carries with it certain risks, which are discussed in Ch. 95.

Scharschmidt BF, Goldberg HI, Schmid R: Approach to the patient with cholestatic jaundice. N Engl J Med 308:1515, 1983. *A concise summary, useful approach, and comprehensive bibliography.*

Vennes JA, Bond JH: Approach to the jaundiced patient. Gastroenterology 84:1615, 1983. *A balanced editorial addressing the clinical problem in general and two accompanying articles in particular.*

120. ACUTE VIRAL HEPATITIS

Robert K. Ockner

DEFINITION. Acute viral hepatitis is caused by any of several agents and presents as a spectrum of syndromes ranging from entirely subclinical and inapparent to rapidly progressive and fatal. In most cases, it is self-limited and uncomplicated, but, depending on the viral agent involved, there is a variable incidence of clinically significant extrahepatic manifestations or of progression to chronic liver disease. These diseases represent an infection by a viral agent with relative or absolute predilection for the hepatocyte. After a variable incubation period, viral replication in the liver cell approaches a maximum, followed by the appearance of viral components in body fluids and/or excreta, liver cell necrosis with an associated inflammatory response, changes in laboratory tests of liver function, and symptoms and signs of liver damage. The immunologic response of the host appears to play an important but not fully defined role in pathogenesis.

ETIOLOGY. Viral hepatitis is caused by three major agents and several minor ones. The vast majority of cases are accounted for by hepatitis viruses A and B, and the so-called "non-A non-B" agents, of which there appear to be at least two. Selected characteristics of each are summarized in Table 120–1, and each is considered in greater detail below. Other viral agents that cause an acute hepatitis syndrome include the Epstein-Barr virus (infectious mononucleosis), cytomegalovirus, herpes simplex, yellow fever, and rubella; the clinical disorders caused by these agents are considered in greater detail elsewhere in the text. More recently recognized is the delta (δ) agent, which may cause an acute or chronic hepatitis syndrome limited to those individuals with simultaneous or pre-existing hepatitis B virus infection (see below).

PATHOLOGY. The lesion of ordinary acute hepatitis A, B, and non-A non-B consists of focal necrosis of individual hepatocytes associated with a mononuclear inflammatory response, and expanded portal areas that are infiltrated predominantly by lymphocytes and in which bile ducts may be especially prominent (bile duct "proliferation"). There is often a variable, but usually minor, degree of necrosis of hepatocytes bordering the portal areas (so-called periportal hepatitis or "piecemeal necrosis"). Necrosis of an individual liver cell, whether periportal or within the lobule, is usually reflected in its replacement by a cluster of mononuclear cells, or may be represented by balloon degeneration or by a shrunken cell with homogeneously eosinophilic cytoplasm and a condensed pyknotic nucleus ("acidophil body"). The regular pattern of the cords of hepatocytes is disrupted, mitotic figures and cholestasis are common, and Kupffer cells are prominent. Although these features are characteristic of typical acute viral hepatitis, they are not specific, individually or collectively. Thus, the same overall pattern of injury is seen in certain forms of drug-induced liver disease, and its individual components are seen in many processes of diverse etiology and duration. Mononuclear cell portal infiltrates, periportal hepatitis, and bridging or confluent necrosis may be especially prominent in chronic forms of hepatitis.

More severe variants of the acute necrotic process include "bridging" necrosis, "confluent" or "submassive" necrosis, and massive necrosis. In these, the necrotic process simultaneously involves contiguous groups of cells rather than single cells in isolation. As a result, there may be variable collapse or condensation of stroma. "Bridging" necrosis, so named because the contiguous zones of necrosis may extend between (i.e., "bridge") adjacent portal and/or central areas, may be a necessary, if not sufficient, antecedent to evolution to a subacute form of hepatitis with progressive deterioration of liver function leading over several months to death in liver failure, or to chronic hepatitis or to cirrhosis, but such a predisposition is not conclusively established. Thus, bridging necrosis is compatible with complete clinical and histologic recovery and therefore does not per se constitute evidence of chronic or progressive liver disease.

Submassive and massive hepatic necrosis are reflected in a more severe clinical course and a less favorable prognosis. Massive necrosis, in which broad areas of hepatocytes are destroyed, with condensation of stromal elements and portal structures (bile ducts and vessels), is usually manifested clinically as fulminant hepatic failure (see Ch. 127). This syndrome is characterized by severely deranged liver function, hepatic encephalopathy, and a high case fatality rate. In survivors, however, despite the severity of the acute process, a chronic course is unusual and liver histology typically returns nearly to normal.

In the recovery phase there is regeneration of hepatocytes and a largely complete restoration of normal lobular architecture. It is distinctly uncommon for the healing that follows a circumscribed acute hepatitis to be accompanied by fibrous scar formation or by nodular regeneration; in the latter, hepatocytes cluster in an abnormal configuration lacking a central vein and other components of the normal lobular architecture. These two manifestations of an *abnormal* healing process (fibrosis and nodular regeneration) are the essential components of cirrhosis, a form of chronic liver disease that almost always reflects ongoing injury and repair rather than a single acute event.

CLINICAL AND LABORATORY MANIFESTATIONS. The earliest symptoms of acute viral hepatitis typically are nonspecific, predominantly constitutional and gastrointestinal. They may include malaise, fatigue, anorexia, nausea, vomiting, and arthralgias, and may suggest a "flu" or upper respiratory syndrome to both patient and physician. Classically, the patient may describe a loss of taste for coffee or cigarettes. Fever, if present, is usually mild. Abdominal discomfort may reflect an enlarged tender liver. Arthritis occurs in 10 to 15 per cent of cases; in hepatitis B it appears to represent immune complex deposition, but it also occurs with similar frequency in hepatitis

TABLE 120–1. CHARACTERISTICS OF COMMON CAUSATIVE AGENTS OF ACUTE VIRAL HEPATITIS

	Hepatitis A	Hepatitis B	Hepatitis Non-A Non-B (Two or More Agents)
Causative agent	27 nm RNA virus	42 nm DNA virus; core and surface components	Apparent similarities to hepatitis B virus
Transmission	Fecal-oral; H_2O-, foodborne	Parenteral inoculation, or equivalent; direct contact	Same as for B; also, common-source outbreaks
Incubation period	2–6 weeks	4 weeks–6 months	2–20 weeks
Period of infectivity	2–3 weeks in late incubation and early clinical phases	During HBsAg-positivity (occasionally only with anti-HBc positivity)	Unknown
Massive hepatic necrosis	Rare	Uncommon	Uncommon
Carrier state	No	Yes	Yes
Chronic hepatitis	No	Yes	Yes
Prophylaxis (see text)	Hygiene; immune serum globulin	Hygiene; hepatitis B immune globulin; vaccine	Hygiene; ? immune serum globulin; avoid commercial blood

A, in which immune complexes have not been demonstrated. Urticaria may occur occasionally.

After a period of several days to a week or more, the prodromal phase may lead to an icteric phase. The earliest clinical manifestation of a rising serum concentration of direct-reacting bilirubin is bilirubinuria, followed by a lightening of stool color, scleral icterus, and, in light-skinned individuals, frank jaundice. Constitutional symptoms often abate during the icteric phase, especially in children, in whom the disease is characteristically less severe. In adults, the gastrointestinal components of the prodrome may persist or even increase for a time. If cholestasis worsens, pruritus may cause increasing discomfort.

Physical findings are variable and depend on the stage of the illness. The only objective finding during the prodrome, apart from mild fever, may be an enlarged and tender liver, associated in perhaps 20 per cent with splenomegaly. Jaundice may or may not appear; indeed, it is likely that the vast majority of cases remain anicteric. Excoriations reflect the intensity of pruritus. Spider nevi occasionally develop during an acute hepatitis, but since their appearance is unusual, it should suggest the possibility of a more chronic process.

Laboratory studies are highly variable, but almost by definition the clinical onset is accompanied by rising activities of serum transaminases; usually the ALT (SGPT) exceeds the AST (SGOT). An elevated serum bilirubin is predominantly direct reacting; very high concentrations, e.g., greater than 15 to 20 mg per deciliter, indicate a severe lesion, or may reflect associated hemolysis. The alkaline phosphatase is usually moderately increased, whereas serum albumin concentration may decrease slightly. A diffuse hyperglobulinemia is common. Prothrombin time is prolonged in more severe cases, and a persisting or increasing prolongation is an unfavorable prognostic sign. Mild and clinically insignificant hypoglycemia occurs in perhaps 50 per cent of cases; more profound hypoglycemia may complicate fulminant hepatic failure. Hematologic tests are also quite variable. Usually, the total leukocyte count is normal or slightly decreased and atypical lymphocytes may be present. In more severe cases, total leukocytes may be increased, with relative or absolute neutrophilia. Hemoglobin and hematocrit are usually relatively normal, but occasionally there may be a coincidental hemolytic process, and rarely the course is complicated by aplastic anemia. Urinalysis is usually nonspecific except for the presence of bilirubin.

An important aspect of the laboratory approach to acute viral hepatitis is the etiologic serodiagnosis, made possible by recent advances in the virology of this group of diseases. Although establishing a specific etiologic diagnosis will not usually influence management, it may have a bearing on prognosis, and is particularly useful epidemiologically and for the immunization of contacts. These tests are discussed below, under Hepatitis A, Hepatitis B, and Prevention.

After an icteric phase lasting usually from several days to several weeks, the patient enters a convalescent phase in which there is gradual improvement in symptoms and laboratory tests. The healing process may require several weeks, during which time residual weakness and malaise are common. Normalization of laboratory tests is usually complete within four months. Persistence of abnormalities beyond six months suggests that the process may have become chronic; in this circumstance, liver biopsy may be indicated if there is no evidence of continuing improvement.

COMPLICATIONS AND EXTRAHEPATIC MANIFESTATIONS. The two most important complications of acute viral hepatitis are massive hepatic necrosis (fulminant hepatitis) and progression to chronic hepatitis. Fortunately, these are uncommon, especially in hepatitis A, in which chronicity does not occur and massive necrosis is less common than in hepatitis B and non-A non-B.

Massive hepatic necrosis with fulminant hepatic failure occurs in fewer than 1 per cent of cases of acute viral hepatitis and is usually signaled by deepening jaundice, increasing prothrombin time, and hepatic encephalopathy, which, in its earliest stages, may appear only as a subtle personality change. Serum transaminases may remain high but in many cases will fall, often in association with a decrease in liver size. These changes are assumed to reflect extensive loss of parenchymal mass and, in the presence of other evidence of a deteriorating course, are unfavorable prognostic signs. The diagnosis and management of acute hepatic failure and encephalopathy are considered in greater detail in Ch. 127.

Evolution to chronic hepatitis is a more common complication of acute hepatitis B and non-A non-B. It is suggested by persistence of abnormal serum transaminases, with or without other laboratory abnormalities and clinical symptoms, beyond an arbitrarily selected end-point. Authorities differ as to where that end-point belongs; guidelines range from four to twelve months, but most would accept six months as reasonable. Clearly, however, judgments must be individualized as to when an acute process becomes chronic (or, more pragmatically, when investigations such as liver biopsy should be performed). For example, as long as the patient continues to show evidence of clinical and laboratory improvement, there is little to be gained from a more vigorous diagnostic or therapeutic approach. Conversely, evidence suggestive of chronic liver disease (e.g., signs of portal hypertension or progressive deterioration of laboratory tests) appearing before six months may justify earlier diagnostic intervention. Since many of the histopathologic features associated with chronic hepatitis also may be components of an acute process, however, liver biopsies obtained too early in the course may be difficult to interpret and potentially misleading. Chronic hepatitis is also considered under Hepatitis B and Hepatitis Non-A Non-B, below, and in greater detail in Ch. 122.

The *cholestatic hepatitis syndrome* occurs occasionally as a complication of acute viral hepatitis. Patients may exhibit a relatively prolonged course dominated by cholestatic features, including pruritus, dark urine, light stools, direct-reacting hyperbilirubinemia, and alkaline phosphatase elevation. Little is known of the specific viral etiology or pathophysiologic basis for this syndrome. Almost without exception, however, the prognosis is favorable. The major problem in management posed by this variant is its occasionally difficult differentiation from biliary obstruction and the possible need to exclude disorders such as gallstones, stricture, and tumors by means of appropriate imaging and cholangiographic techniques.

Aplastic anemia may very rarely complicate the icteric or convalescent phase of acute viral hepatitis. Its pathogenesis is unknown, and its prognosis poor. Among the relatively few survivors, there is no clear evidence of a beneficial effect of glucocorticoids or anabolic steroid treatment. Other formed elements may also be depressed, and pancytopenia, agranulocytosis, and thrombocytopenia have been reported.

Extrahepatic manifestations of acute viral hepatitis also include *arthralgias* and *arthritis*, and *urticaria*. These are usually most prominent during the prodromal phase and, in hepatitis B, appear to reflect deposition of immune complexes. They also may occur in non-B hepatitis. Other manifestations of hepatitis B infection, such as *glomerulonephritis* and *vasculitis*, are also associated with immune complex deposition and are discussed in Ch. 80 and 62, respectively. A tentative association of *essential mixed cryoglobulinemia* with hepatitis B infection also has been reported. *Pancreatitis* is found in 12 to 40 per cent of cases of fatal acute viral hepatitis, and serum amylase activity may be elevated in up to 30 per cent of nonfatal cases; the true overall incidence and mechanism of pancreatitis in viral hepatitis are not known. Myocarditis, pneumonitis, and other extrahepatic manifestations are rare, and in their presence other systemic disorders should be considered.

SPECIFIC ETIOLOGIC CATEGORIES OF VIRAL HEPATITIS

HEPATITIS A. This form of hepatitis is also referred to as "infectious hepatitis," "short-incubation hepatitis," or "MS-I hepatitis." The causative agent (hepatitis A virus) is a 27 nm diameter RNA virus that is readily and almost exclusively transmitted via the fecal-oral route. In this important respect it differs significantly from hepatitis B and most cases of non-A non-B. Accordingly, when the etiology of water-borne, point-source, food-handler–related, and institutional hepatitis outbreaks has been defined, hepatitis A almost invariably has been implicated. A form of non-A non-B hepatitis may also be spread by contaminated water supplies. In addition, hepatitis A occurs sporadically and is spread by direct person-to-person contact; there appears to be an increased incidence among promiscuous homosexuals. Spread of hepatitis A in day care centers may involve not only children but also the staff and the families of affected children. Although parenteral transmission is theoretically possible, it must occur rarely. The incidence of the disease appears to correlate in a general way with personal hygiene and the efficacy of public health measures, as suggested by the apparent influence of socioeconomic status on the incidence of hepatitis A antibodies (anti-HAV), which averaged 45 per cent in one study of an urban population in the United States and approximated 90 per cent in residents of Costa Rica. Since there is no evidence for the existence of a chronic form of hepatitis A or a carrier state, the "reservoir" for the virus appears to consist of the large number of clinically inapparent acute cases, as well as those persons in the late incubation period of overt hepatitis A who shed virus prior to the clinical onset.

Hepatitis A infection typically has an incubation period of two to six weeks. Fecal shedding of virus occurs during the final week of the incubation period and the prodromal phase, and declines as serum transaminases reach maximal levels (Fig. 120–1 and Table 120–1). Although there is a transient viremia during this interval, parenteral transmission of the disease is very rare. Viral shedding in stool declines as antibody (anti-HAV) appears in serum. Initially, antibody is predominantly of the IgM class, but an IgG antibody soon appears, and after several weeks to a few months the IgM antibody disappears. The IgG antibody persists in serum for many years; its exclusive presence indicates prior experience with, and immunity to, the hepatitis A virus. The presence of the IgM antibody, on the other hand, indicates current or very recent infection (Table 120–2). Shedding of virus is limited to a two- to three-week period; there is no evidence for a carrier state or chronic hepatitis A. An IgA antibody to HAV appears in the feces of patients at about the time fecal shedding of virus ceases and persists for several weeks.

TABLE 120–2. SEROLOGIC TESTS IN VIRAL HEPATITIS

Agent	Terminology	Definition	Significance
Hepatitis A (HAV)	Anti-HA	Antibody to HAV	
	IgM type		Current infection or convalescence
	IgG type		Current or previous infection; indicates immunity
Hepatitis B (HBV)	HBsAg	HBV surface antigen	Positive in most cases of acute or chronic infection
	HBeAg	"e" antigen; HBV core component	Transiently positive in acute hepatitis, and in some chronic cases; reflects Dane particle concentration and infectivity
	Anti-Hbc (IgM or IgG)	Antibody to HBV core antigen	Positive in all acute and chronic cases and in carriers; thus, marker of HBV infection; not protective
	Anti-HBe	Antibody to "e" antigen	Transiently positive during convalescence and in some chronic cases and carriers; not protective; reflects low infectivity and possible integration of HBV DNA into host genome
	Anti-HBs	Antibody to surface antigen	Becomes positive late in convalescence in most acute cases; protective

The acute illness itself is quite diverse in its clinical manifestations and course. The majority of cases probably are clinically inapparent, especially in children, or are perceived as a nonspecific "flu" syndrome. Jaundice, when it occurs, is usually mild. Symptoms usually subside and serum transaminases return to normal within three to four months. Rarely, hepatitis A causes massive hepatic necrosis and fulminant hepatic failure, but this complication is much less common than in hepatitis B and non-A non-B.

The ease with which hepatitis A is transmitted among contacts and via water and food, as well as the demonstrated efficacy of immune serum globulin in prevention or amelioration of the disease, underscores the value of individual and public health measures to control the spread of the infection. The application of these to the management of the individual patient and his contacts is discussed below.

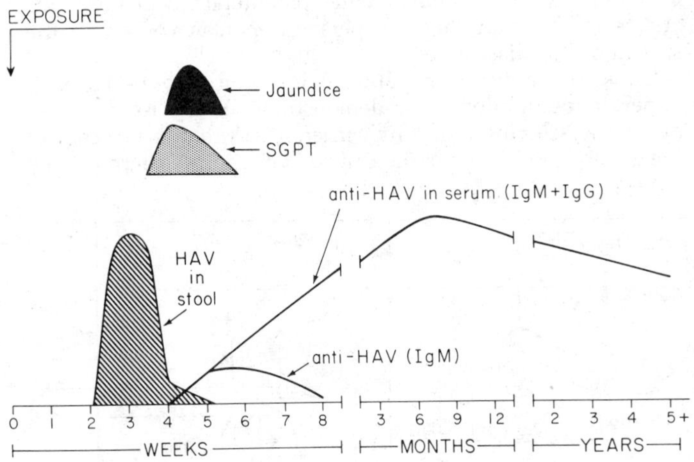

Figure 120–1. Sequence of clinical and laboratory findings in a patient with hepatitis A. Fecal shedding of virus is brief in duration, and ends with the appearance of anti-HAV in serum. (From Krugman S, Gocke DJ: Viral Hepatitis. Philadelphia, W. B. Saunders Company, 1978.)

HEPATITIS B. In marked contrast to hepatitis A, hepatitis B virus infection may cause a wide variety of acute or chronic hepatic and extrahepatic diseases, as well as a chronic carrier state. Its presentation as an acute hepatitis is typical of those cases that previously were designated "serum hepatitis," "homologous serum jaundice," "long-incubation hepatitis," or "MS-II hepatitis," although it is now apparent that many of these cases may also represent non-A non-B hepatitis (see below). The hepatitis B virus (HBV) differs in almost every respect from hepatitis A (Tables 120–1 and 120–2; Fig. 120–2). The complete infective virion, or *"Dane" (HBV) particle,* is a DNA virus of 42 nm diameter, consisting of antigenically distinct surface and core components. The *surface coat* is largely lipid and protein, and may exist in serum or other body fluids either as a component of the Dane particle or as separate 20 nm diameter spheres or cylinders. Its major antigenic determinant (hepatitis B surface antigen, HBsAg) includes several subtypes (d, y; w, r), and can be detected by sensitive radioimmunoassay techniques in the serum of at least 75 per cent of infected persons during the acute disease (Fig. 120–2). The hepatitis B virus *core* consists of circular DNA, DNA polymerase, and other determinants, which include the hepatitis B core antigen (HBcAg) and two or three related "e" antigens (HBeAg). The biologic significance of HBcAg and HBeAg is not fully understood, but each elicits a humoral antibody response (anti-HBc and anti-HBe, respectively) during the course of the hepatitis B infection, and these may be of diagnostic or prognostic significance. Recently it has become possible to detect HBV-DNA in serum by molecular hybridization. This appears to be a very sensitive test for the presence of infective virus and may become generally available in the foreseeable future.

In contrast to hepatitis A, *transmission* of hepatitis B by the fecal-oral route is relatively unimportant; infection may follow oral ingestion, but large doses appear necessary. Instead, the virus is present in virtually all body fluids and excreta, and transmission of this disease occurs primarily via parenteral routes. Therefore, it usually requires either overt inoculation (e.g., transfusion, or injection via a contaminated needle) or intimate personal contact (e.g., between sexual partners, patients and health professionals, and mother to newborn infant). The disease occurs with an increased frequency among sexual partners of acutely infected individuals, as well as among chronically exposed persons, including health professionals and patients exposed to blood and blood products (e.g., workers and patients in clinical laboratories, dialysis and oncology units), the sexually promiscuous (especially male homosexuals), drug users who share needles, and handlers of primates (which are susceptible to infection). In urban centers, hepatitis B may account for up to 50 per cent of sporadic cases of acute hepatitis, even in the absence of documented parenteral inoculation. This attests to the importance of person-to-person contact in the spread of this disease.

Unlike hepatitis A, hepatitis B infection may be chronic, either in association with demonstrable liver disease or in otherwise seemingly healthy carriers. Less than 1 per cent of the general population of the United States and Western Europe is HBsAg-positive. This low incidence contrasts with incidence of anti-HBs of about 10 per cent in the same population, providing additional evidence that in most patients with acute hepatitis B the infection is self-limited and followed by immunity, and only infrequently leads to chronic liver disease or a carrier state. The incidence of HBsAg-positivity is much higher in less developed areas (up to 15 per cent) and among certain subpopulations with increased exposure and/or impaired immunity, such as patients with Down's syndrome, leprosy, or lymphoproliferative disorders, addicts, and patients undergoing dialysis. In addition to acute cases, therefore, these chronically infected individuals constitute the "reservoir" that serves to perpetuate the virus. Historically, it is likely that transmission of the disease has occurred not so often via overt parenteral inoculation but rather via sexual contact, or from mother to newborn. In the latter instance (*"vertical transmission"*), i.e., in infants born to mothers with acute or chronic infection, there is a high probability that the neonate will acquire the disease. This is especially likely when the mother develops acute hepatitis B in late pregnancy or early postpartum, or has chronic hepatitis. Transmission appears to correlate with the presence of HBeAg in maternal serum, reflecting the concentration of Dane particles. Characteristically, these infants remain chronically infected for many years, either as "carriers" or with a persisting low grade and chronic hepatitis. They are probably at increased risk of developing hepatocellular carcinoma (see Ch. 128). Vertical transmission may be an important mechanism by which the reservoir of the virus is sustained from generation to generation.

The *incubation period* of acute hepatitis B, as defined by the appearance of clinical symptoms, varies between four weeks and six months, with an average of about 50 days (if the incubation period is defined instead in terms of the interval between exposure and the first *serologic* evidence of viremia, it may be as brief as two weeks, especially after exposure to large parenteral doses). Two weeks to two months prior to the clinical onset, HBsAg becomes detectable in serum (see Fig. 120–3 and Table 120–2). At about the time of the clinical onset and the rise in serum transaminase activities anti-HBc becomes detectable. Initially, an IgM anti-HBc is present in high titer and persists for several months to one year; thereafter IgG anti-HBc predominates; as of the time of this writing, tests for the detection of IgM anti-HBc are not generally available. IgG anti-HBc persists for up to several years after acute hepatitis, and is present in all chronic carriers. It appears to play no role in host defenses; rather, it serves as a reliable marker of hepatitis B infection currently or within the preceding few years. The Dane particle markers (HBeAg and DNA polymerase) usually become detectable in serum prior to the rise in transaminase. The duration of HBsAg positivity is highly variable, and may persist for a few days to two to three months; persistence beyond this time may indicate a chronic course. Characteristically, HBsAg becomes undetectable prior to the appearance of anti-HBs. This antibody can be demonstrated in 80 to 90 per cent of patients, usually late in convalescence, and indicates relative or absolute immunity. Its appearance generally suggests a successful response to the infection, but there are exceptions to this in certain patients with chronic hepatitis (see Ch. 122).

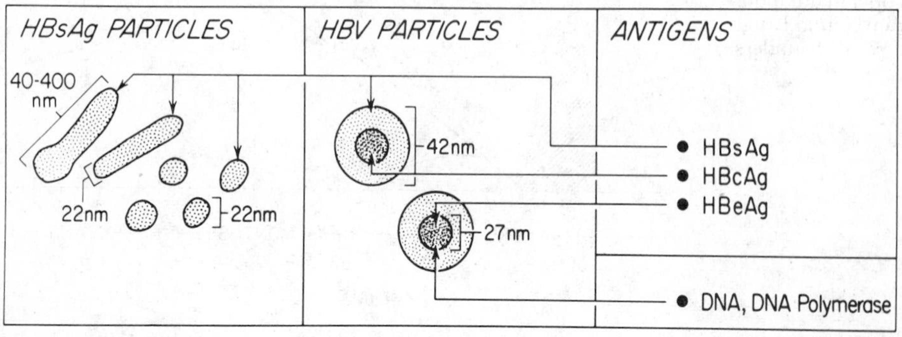

Figure 120–2. Forms of HBV in plasma, showing location of the various components and antigenic determinants. (From Koff RS: *In* Sanford JP, Luby JP (eds.): The Science and Clinical Practice of Medicine. Infectious Diseases. Vol. 8. New York, Grune & Stratton, 1981, by permission.)

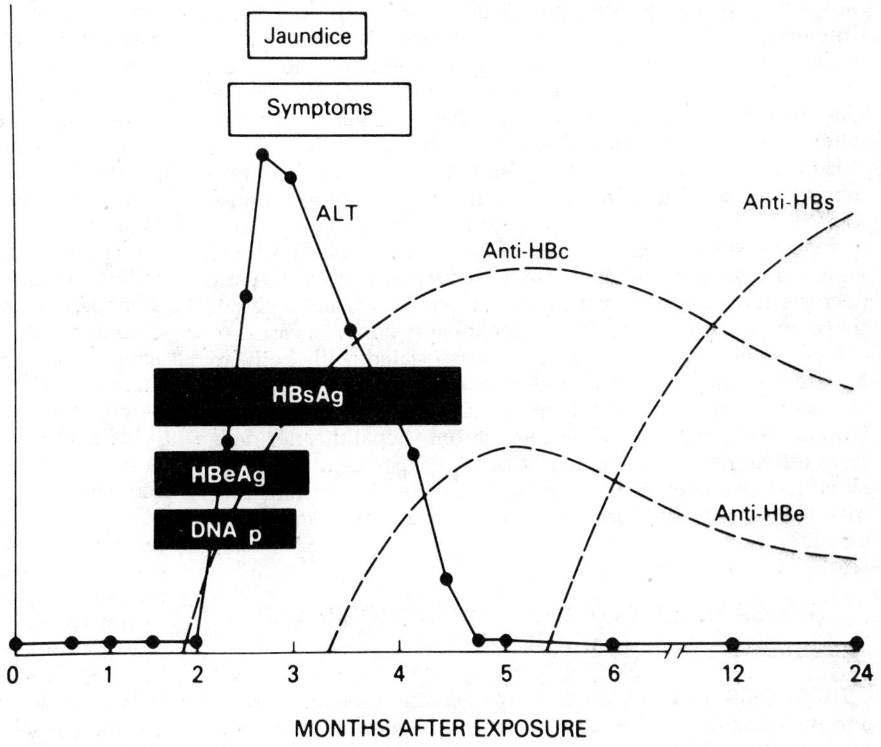

Figure 120–3. Sequence of clinical and laboratory findings in a patient with acute hepatitis B, followed by recovery. HBsAg-emia is the initial manifestation. "Dane particle markers" (HBeAg and DNA polymerase) precede the ALT rise and are transient. Anti-HBc appears during the acute illness; after the disappearance of HBsAg and before the appearance of anti-HBs, anti-HBc may be the only marker of hepatitis B infection. (From Schafer DF, Hoofnagle JH: Serological diagnosis of viral hepatitis. Viewpoints Dig Dis 14(2):6, 1982.)

Several important qualifications should be noted in interpreting the results of hepatitis B serologic tests. First, in a significant number of patients with acute hepatitis B the serum is negative for HBsAg, presumably because the antigen is very low in titer or evanescent. For this reason, a single negative HBsAg test does not exclude the diagnosis. Anti-HBc is more sensitive in this regard and may be the only serologic indication of hepatitis B infection. A negative test for anti-HBc effectively excludes the diagnosis. On the other hand, a positive test for anti-HBc in an HBsAg-negative serum could merely reflect a prior episode of hepatitis B. These HBsAg-negative, anti-HBc positive patients may be classifiable on the basis of the anti-HBs: if this test is positive early in the course of an acute hepatitis, it is evidence against the diagnosis of acute hepatitis B. When testing for IgM anti-HBc becomes generally available, the detection of this marker would suggest recent acute rather than pre-existing chronic HBV infection, as noted above. In those IgM-anti-HBc negative subjects in whom HBV infection appears to have antedated the acute illness, the possibility of superimposed infection by the δ agent or a non-A non-B virus must be considered.

The *clinical course* of acute hepatitis B is more variable and usually more prolonged than that of hepatitis A. It is also more often associated with extrahepatic manifestations, including urticaria and other rashes, arthritis, and, much less commonly, glomerulonephritis and vasculitis. The immune complexes that appear to cause these extrahepatic manifestations consist of HBsAg, anti-HBs, and complement components. Glomerulonephritis and vasculitis are also associated with chronic hepatitis B infection, and are not necessarily accompanied by apparent liver disease. Indeed, up to one third of all cases of polyarteritis nodosa may be caused by or associated with hepatitis B virus infection.

Approximately 90 per cent of patients with acute hepatitis B recover completely and become HBsAg negative. Fewer than 1 per cent develop massive hepatic necrosis, but this complication is more common than in hepatitis A. Of the 10 per cent of patients who remain HBsAg-positive beyond three or four months, a significant number will clear the antigen over a period of six months to a year or more without developing evidence of chronic hepatitis. Many of those with prolonged HBsAg positivity, however, appear destined either to become chronic carriers or to develop chronic persistent or chronic active hepatitis (see Ch. 122).

Delta (δ)-agent infection is a more recently recognized complication of hepatitis B. The δ agent is an incomplete RNA virus that requires antecedent or simultaneous HBV infection in order to infect the host cell. The agent exists in plasma in a coat of HBsAg and is present in the nuclei of infected hepatocytes. δ-Agent infection is reflected by the presence of anti-δ antibody in serum (IgM acutely; IgG chronically); almost invariably the serum is positive for HBsAg and anti-HBc and, in most, anti-HBe. It is most commonly found among intravenous drug addicts and recipients of multiple transfusions. In subjects who are acutely and simultaneously infected with HBV and δ there is no apparent increase in the probability that chronic hepatitis will ensue. In individuals chronically infected with HBV, however, superimposed acute δ infection usually also becomes chronic and is associated with the histopathologic findings of chronic active hepatitis. Acute δ infection may cause fulminant hepatic failure. At this time, tests for δ-agent infection are not generally available.

HEPATITIS NON-A NON-B. A large number of cases of acute viral hepatitis are caused by at least two other agents. Progress is being made in the identification of these agents, but it still is not possible to document the infection on a routine basis. Consequently, the designation "non-A non-B" remains appropriate, since these forms of hepatitis are essentially diagnoses of exclusion.

Non-A non-B hepatitis is the major cause of *post-transfusion hepatitis.* It occurs in approximately 5 to 10 cases per 1000 transfusions, and can be transmitted in whole blood, packed cells, platelets, plasma, and especially clotting factor concentrates. The incidence of post-transfusion hepatitis B has been greatly reduced by screening of donors for HBsAg. Non-A non-B also is a common cause of hepatitis in needle users and accounts for 20 per cent or more of sporadic cases, i.e., those not associated with obvious contact or parenteral inoculation. A significant number of those cases of hepatitis previously referred to as "serum hepatitis" or "homologous serum jaundice" actually represented non-A non-B hepatitis infections. Conversely, it is also now clear that some cases of "non-A non-B" hepatitis actually represent δ-agent infection. Moreover, recent evidence suggests that certain monoclonal antibodies may detect HBsAg in subjects otherwise negative for this determinant and therefore classified as non-A non-B.

Hepatitis B and non-A non-B also have many similar clinical manifestations. Thus, the incubation period of non-A non-B hepatitis is longer than that of hepatitis A, ranging from two to twenty weeks, with an average of eight weeks. The acute illness is also quite variable. The incidence of massive hepatic necrosis appears comparable to that of hepatitis B, and together these two categories account for the great majority of cases.

Finally, non-A non-B hepatitis is associated with both an apparent carrier state (inferred from the fact that it may be transmitted by blood from apparently healthy donors) and chronic hepatitis. The incidence of chronic hepatitis after non-A non-B transfusion hepatitis exceeds 25 per cent, but in a significant number of such patients the disease is mild and may spontaneously subside or remit after a year or more (see Ch. 122).

GENERAL APPROACHES TO DIAGNOSIS AND MANAGEMENT

DIAGNOSIS. In its classic presentation, the presumptive diagnosis of acute viral hepatitis is readily suggested by a compatible history and physical examination, in association with laboratory evidence of hepatocellular injury, i.e., significantly increased serum transaminases. Because all of these features are nonspecific, however, it is essential that other possible etiologic factors be considered, such as use of medications or illicit drugs, alcohol, exposure to environmental or industrial toxins, and the possible acquisition of unusual infections as suggested by travel or residence in rural or less well developed areas. Exposure to viral hepatitis itself is suggested by contact with jaundiced persons or persons known to have developed hepatitis, sexual promiscuity (especially among male homosexuals), transfusion of blood or blood products, or the sharing of needles by drug users. Among health professionals, workers in dialysis and oncology units, surgeons, dentists, and clinical laboratory technicians are at increased risk, as is anyone in direct contact with blood, blood products, or other body fluids. Despite the importance of a careful inquiry into these possible risk factors, many patients with acute viral hepatitis will report no significant exposures.

A careful and complete physical examination will help establish the diagnosis (tender hepatomegaly is the most common finding) and help exclude other processes that occasionally mimic acute viral hepatitis, such as acute hepatic congestion, disseminated sepsis or liver abscess, or biliary tract disease with or without cholangitis.

Serodiagnosis of viral hepatitis is now possible, within certain limitations (see Hepatitis A and Hepatitis B, above). A positive test for the IgM class of anti-HAV, or a rising titer of total anti-HAV is strong evidence for acute hepatitis A. Conversely, if the test for anti-HAV is negative well into the convalescent phase, the diagnosis is excluded. A single positive test for anti-HAV is of little diagnostic value, since this could reflect a previous infection.

Although an acute hepatitis syndrome associated with HBsAg-positivity has been taken as presumptive evidence for acute hepatitis B, none of the tests generally available at this time permit early and unequivocal diagnosis or exclusion of this entity. An important exception is that the presence of anti-HBs or the absence of anti-HBc early in the course of an acute hepatitis tends to exclude acute HBV infection. Since the classic pattern in which both HBsAg and anti-HBc are positive acutely may not be present in all cases (although anti-HBc itself is virtually always positive), a single negative test for HBsAg does not definitively exclude acute hepatitis B. Medical records, if available, may be of help by providing information about prior liver function tests, hepatitis serologies, or blood donation. Since donated blood has been screened routinely for HBsAg since 1972, such information may be quite helpful in the evaluation of hepatitis B serologies. It seems likely that, as tests for IgM anti-HBc, anti-δ, and the non-A non-B agents become available, accurate serodiagnosis of hepatitis syndromes will be greatly facilitated.

If a *liver biopsy* is performed, it may demonstrate the pathologic features of acute viral hepatitis. However, these are nonspecific, and in the vast majority of cases biopsy is not indicated. Its use should be reserved for patients in whom the diagnosis is uncertain or in whom there is concern regarding chronicity or a deteriorating course, or any circumstance in which documentation of the histopathology may influence management. In the most severely ill patients biopsy may not be possible because of abnormalities of clotting function.

DIFFERENTIAL DIAGNOSIS. Acute viral hepatitis A, B, and non-A non-B may be mimicked by a large number of other acute infections and noninfectious processes. Infections include other viruses such as cytomegalovirus, Epstein-Barr virus (infectious mononucleosis), and yellow fever; and nonviral processes such as Q fever, secondary syphilis, leptospirosis, salmonellosis, pyogenic and amebic liver abscess, malaria, and toxoplasmosis. A wide variety of drugs and toxins may injure the liver and cause a clinical syndrome that can resemble viral hepatitis (see Ch. 121). Inborn errors of metabolism such as Wilson's disease may also lead to acute hepatic necrosis. Acute hepatic congestion secondary to cardiac failure or venous occlusion, cholecystitis, and acute biliary obstruction should also be excluded. Finally, the possibility that what appears to be acute hepatitis may in fact represent the exacerbation of chronic hepatitis should be considered.

MANAGEMENT. There is no specific treatment for acute viral hepatitis. Major emphasis is placed on symptomatic and supportive care and on the prevention of transmission. Prevention is considered in detail below.

Most patients with acute viral hepatitis do not require hospitalization and are appropriately managed at home. Rest is advisable, but strict confinement to bed is not necessary beyond what is dictated by the patient's own sense of fatigue and malaise. No specific dietary measures are indicated, but most patients find a low-fat, high-carbohydrate diet more palatable. During the most severe phases of the illness, anorexia and nausea may be so extreme that oral intake of any kind is minimal. In such instances, attention to fluid balance is important, and it may be necessary to advise the intake of small amounts of clear fluids at frequent intervals. Although there is an appropriate reluctance to administer medication to the patient with liver disease, judicious use of small doses of antinausea agents such as hydroxyzine, trimethobenzamide, and even prochlorperazine is occasionally necessary and usually well tolerated. As the patient's symptoms decrease and appetite improves, intake can be liberalized, usually according to taste. Alcoholic beverages should be avoided throughout the course of the acute illness. Ambulation and activity may be increased as symptoms and laboratory tests improve; the most useful advice is that such activity should be limited so as to avoid causing fatigue. The decision to return to employment or school must take into consideration the patient's symptoms, the strenuousness of the work, and the potential for transmission of the disease; this, in turn, is a function of the viral etiology and the closeness of contact with others. In general, transmission is quite unlikely after two to three weeks in hepatitis A, whereas spread of hepatitis B or non-A non-B ordinarily requires direct person-to-person contact.

Hospitalization is indicated for those patients in whom severe nausea and vomiting prevent maintenance of adequate fluid balance, in whom there is evidence of progressive deterioration, especially with encephalopathy or prolongation of prothrombin time, or in whom invasive diagnostic studies are indicated.

There is no convincing evidence to justify the use of corticosteroids in acute hepatitis, regardless of its severity. The management of fulminant hepatitis poses special problems in patient monitoring and support, and is discussed in detail in Ch. 127.

PREVENTION. The entire area of hepatitis prophylaxis has been dramatically changed by the availability of an effective vaccine for hepatitis B. In this vaccine, the immunizing antigen is HBsAg, prepared from donor sera; an appropriate immune response is reflected by the appearance of anti-HBs. Similarly, the hepatitis A virus has been propagated in tissue culture, offering the hope that for this disease also a vaccine will be available in the foreseeable future. Finally, continuing progress in the identification, isolation, and characterization of non-A non-B viral hepatitis agents suggests the possibility of active immunization, although not for some time. Pending the advent of generally available and effective vaccines for all of the viral causes of acute hepatitis, prevention must depend mainly on personal hygiene and public health measures directed at minimizing the exposure of potentially susceptible individuals, and on the appropriate use of passive immunization.

The use of public health and hygienic measures rests on the premise that body fluids and excreta of infected individuals are potentially infective. Clearly there are certain exceptions, depending on the specific virus involved, the clinical stage of the infection, the amount of potentially infective material involved, and the nature of the exposure. For example, because of the ease with which hepatitis A is spread via the fecal-oral route, contact of such patients with others should be minimized, and their excreta and essentially all materials handled by them during their brief period of infectivity should be carefully disposed of. In contrast, hepatitis B is not commonly spread via the fecal-oral route. Although excreta are to be regarded as infective in these patients, the more important concern is transmission via puncture by contaminated needles (or equivalent exposure to infective material) or intimate personal (sexual) contact, especially during the period of HB_sAg positivity. Non-A non-B hepatitis more closely resembles hepatitis B in its transmissibility, but common-source outbreaks analogous to those caused by hepatitis A virus have recently been documented. Because of these differences among the agents and differences in the approach to passive immunization, serologic diagnosis of the acute viral hepatitis case is useful, even though most patients with these disorders may be expected to do well regardless of etiology. In practice, however, rapid serodiagnosis is not always possible, and for this reason certain generalizations regarding the early management of the patient and his contacts are appropriate and are discussed below, along with measures for specific agents.

Hepatitis A. Since the infection is spread primarily via the fecal-oral route, including transmission by handling food, in drinking water, and potentially by fomites, strict attention to hygiene on the part of the patient and his attendants, whether in home or hospital, is of utmost importance during the period of viral shedding (Fig. 120–1). Direct body contact should be limited to that necessary for care; attendants should wear gloves, and careful handwashing is appropriate. Food, utensils, clothing, linen, needles, and excreta should be handled separately and carefully, also by gloved attendants. The virus is readily inactivated by boiling or by exposure to formalin, chlorine, or ultraviolet irradiation. In the hospital setting, strict isolation is not usually required for cooperative and informed patients with hepatitis A. In the home, similar measures should be implemented to the extent possible.

Close contacts of patients with hepatitis A should receive passive immunization with immune serum globulin as soon as possible, preferably within the first few days. The official recommended dose is 0.02 ml per kilogram up to a maximum of 2 ml, although up to 5 ml has been advocated. This would apply to immediate family members, sexual contacts, or others with whom the patient has been in close contact during the presumed period of infectivity. Casual contacts in the workplace or school probably do not require passive immunization unless there is reason to suspect mutual handling of food, beverages, or contaminated items. On the other hand, it is important to inquire about other possible cases among work or classroom associates. If there is reason to suspect a possible point-source outbreak, then all similarly exposed persons should receive immune serum globulin, and appropriate epidemiologic information obtained.

The mode of transmission of hepatitis A also renders its prevention a matter of concern for those who intend to travel in areas where public health and sanitation measures may be suboptimal. In such circumstances, drinking water, fresh fruits and vegetables, and shellfish may be contaminated and should be avoided if possible. For these persons, administration of a standard dose (0.02 ml per kilogram) of immune serum globulin may be expected to afford protection for up to three months; for longer periods, a dose of 0.05 ml per kilogram is recommended and should be repeated at four- to six-month intervals.

Hepatitis B. Although this agent is less readily transmitted via the fecal-oral route, due consideration should be given to the general hygienic measures outlined for hepatitis A, in both home and hospital. Transmission ordinarily requires direct contact with the patient or the equivalent of a parenteral inoculation of infective material. Thus, in the home, children are far less likely than the spouse to acquire hepatitis B from an acutely infected adult. In the hospital, strict isolation may not be necessary if excreta, needles and other medical supplies, and personal utensils are identified, carefully handled, and discarded.

Passive immunization with immune serum globulin enriched in anti-HBs (Hepatitis B Immune Globulin, or HBIG) is protective against hepatitis B infection in certain circumstances, and when used in accordance with established guidelines. Because this material is expensive (approximately $250 to $300 for the prescibed two doses of 0.05 to 0.07 ml per kilogram each, four weeks apart), it should not be used indiscriminately. At present, its use is officially recommended in the following specific situations:

1. Inoculation of material known to be contaminated with the hepatitis B virus, e.g., inadvertent puncture of a health professional by a needle from an HBsAg-positive patient, or accidental transfusion of HBsAg-positive blood or blood products.
2. Splash of HBsAg-positive material into the eye or on an open skin wound or eruption, as may occur in a laboratory accident or during a surgical or diagnostic procedure.
3. Ingestion of HBsAg-positive material, as may occur during a laboratory pipetting accident.

Less well established and more controversial indications for the use of HBIG include (1) sexual partners of patients with *acute* hepatitis B (partners of patients with chronic hepatitis B presumably have been previously exposed); and (2) infants born to HBsAg-positive mothers, especially those who have had acute hepatitis B during the final trimester of pregnancy or first two months post partum, or who are positive for both HBsAg and HBeAg at the time of delivery.

In any case, the rational use of HBIG depends on two essential components. First, it must be documented that the material to which the person has been exposed contains HBsAg, and this requires identification of the source and appropriate serologic confirmation. For example, accidental puncture of the skin by one of several used needles in a disposal container effectively precludes meeting this requirement and, therefore, the use of HBIG. Second, the exposed person must actually be at risk. If, at the time of exposure, he is already positive for HBsAg (i.e., infected) or anti-HBs (i.e., immune), nothing will be gained from the administration of anti-HBs (HBIG). Ideally, therefore, the serologic status of both "donor" and "recipient" should be documented before the decision to administer HBIG is made. In practice, however, this is not usually possible within the few days' interval after exposure in which HBIG appears to be most effective. As a practical alternative to this dilemma, one possible approach is to immediately obtain serum from both the "donor" and the person at risk. Pending results of the HBsAg assays, the latter may be given 5 ml of ordinary immune serum globulin. HBIG may be administered later, if indicated by the test results. This approach represents a compromise between the need to institute early passive immunization on the one hand and to avoid indiscriminate use of HBIG on the other, and at a cost which is small relative to that of the HBIG itself. Other approaches are possible. In the family situation, the value of administering HBIG to the spouse remains controversial, but it is generally accepted that its use is not required for children since they are at low risk.

Hepatitis B Vaccine. As noted, a safe and effective vaccine has been developed for the prevention of hepatitis B. It became generally available in the summer of 1982, after extensive field trials in the homosexual population, in which there is a high incidence of hepatitis B and a high and predictable rate of acquisition of the infection owing to frequent and promiscuous sexual contacts in certain segments of this population. The vaccine consists of highly purified and triple-inactivated HBsAg obtained from the serum of chronic carriers. It is administered in three 20 μg doses initially, and one and six months later, and regularly elicits production of anti-HBs in the recipient. (Smaller doses are used for children, and larger doses for dialysis and immunocompromised patients.) The vaccine appears safe, but is not recommended by the manufacturer for use in pregnant women or infants under the age of three months. Among subjects who have completed the three-dose immunization, protection against hepatitis B infection approaches 100 per cent. Although the duration of this protection remains unclear, it probably is of the order of five years.

The vaccine is recommended for use in high-risk groups and individuals. These include, but are not limited to, health professionals (especially those with high exposure risk such as surgeons, dentists, and dialysis workers), susceptible dialysis patients and those subject to multiple transfusions (e.g., hemophiliacs), certain residents and staff of custodial care institutions, and sexually active and promiscuous male homosexuals. Preliminary evidence suggests that it is also effective, when the first vaccine dose is combined with HBIG, in the passive-active immunization of health professionals after accidental needle stick, and (beginning at three months) in infants born to HBsAg-positive mothers. The cost effectiveness of screening of potential vaccine recipients (e.g., anti-HBs determination) varies with the circumstance. In general, in those groups in which prevalence of hepatitis B is relatively low, screening is not cost effective, whereas it is useful in groups with a high prevalence (e.g., the homosexual community). For most health professionals, screening is marginally cost effective and depends on the prevalence of hepatitis B infection in the particular subgroup. In any case, it is established that administration of the vaccine to individuals already infected or immune is without harmful sequelae.

Hepatitis non-A non-B. There is at present no generally available means of documenting exposure to, or infection by, this group of agents, but it appears to be transmitted in a manner that more closely resembles that of hepatitis B than hepatitis A. Thus close personal contact and parenteral inoculation appear necessary, suggesting that prophylactic measures suitable for hepatitis B are appropriate.

A problem largely confined to non-A non-B hepatitis at present is that of post-transfusion hepatitis. The single most effective means of reducing the incidence of this disorder is the exclusion of blood obtained from commercial (paid donor) sources. A variety of screening methods have been studied. While there is a correlation between aminotransferase activity in donor unit plasma and the probability of post-transfusion hepatitis in a recipient, the cost-benefit factors remain unclear and at present such screening is not routinely used. The possible role of pre-exposure (i.e., pretransfusion) immune serum globulin in the prevention of the disorder remains unclear, and at present immune serum globulin is not officially recommended for its prevention.

Alter HJ (ed.): Hepatitis B. Sem Liver Dis 1:1, 1981. *A minisymposium in which clinically relevant aspects of acute and chronic hepatitis B infection are discussed by a group of recognized experts.*

Dienstag JL: Hepatitis A virus: Identification, characterization and epidemiologic investigations. *In* Popper H, Schaffner F (eds.): Progress in Liver Diseases. New York, Grune & Stratton, 1979, pp 343–370. *A comprehensive review of basic and clinical aspects of hepatitis A.*

Dienstag JL: Non-A, non-B hepatitis. Gastroenterology 85:439, 743, 1983. *A thorough consideration of putative agents and a current summary of clinical, epidemiologic, and prophylactic aspects.*

Favero MS, Maynard JE, Leger RT, Graham DR, Dixon RE: Guidelines for the care of patients hospitalized with viral hepatitis. Ann Intern Med 91:872, 1979. *Specific recommendations based on current concepts of epidemiology. A useful guide.*

Gregory P: Steroid therapy in severe viral hepatitis. N Engl J Med 294:681, 1976. *Convincing evidence that corticosteroids are not helpful, and potentially harmful, in severe acute viral hepatitis.*

Immunization Practices Advisory Committee. Immune globulins for protection against viral hepatitis. MMWR 30:423, 1981. *CDC recommendations concerning passive immunoprophylaxis.*

Immunization Practices Advisory Committee. Inactivated hepatitis B virus vaccine. Ann Intern Med 97:379, 1982. *Official recommendations regarding the use of hepatitis B vaccine.*

Jacobson IM, Dienstag JL: The delta hepatitis agent: Viral hepatitis, type D. Gastroenterology, 86:1614, 1984. *Excellent and well-referenced editorial that summarizes current concepts and recent progress toward the understanding of basic and clinical aspects of this newer facet of hepatitis B infection.*

Szmuness W, Alter JH, Maynard JE: Viral Hepatitis. 1981 International Symposium, Philadelphia, Franklin Institute Press, 1982. *Proceedings of a March 1981 International Symposium. New progress and current concepts in virtually all aspects of the field are presented, discussed, and referenced.*

Tong MJ, Thursby M, Rakela J, McPeak C, Edwards VM, Mosley JW: Studies on the maternal-infant transmission of the viruses that cause acute hepatitis. Gastroenterology 80:999, 1981. *The report of a large study of vertical transmission of hepatitis viruses.*

121. TOXIC AND DRUG-INDUCED LIVER DISEASE

Robert K. Ockner

DEFINITION AND GENERAL PRINCIPLES OF DIAGNOSIS AND MANAGEMENT

Pharmacologic and chemical agents may produce a wide variety of acute or chronic liver diseases. At the one extreme they may take the form of asymptomatic and seemingly inconsequential abnormalities in liver function, whereas at the other they may include fatal acute massive hepatic necrosis or progressive chronic hepatitis, cirrhosis, and liver failure. This spectrum of histopathologic changes, clinical and laboratory features, and prognosis therefore is as broad as that of all other forms of liver disease. Several characteristics of these disorders create special problems for the clinician. First, the mere *association* of a given drug with disturbed liver function does not necessarily imply causality, either in an individual case or in general, and this problem accounts for much of the uncertainty in the field. Second, in a specific instance it may be unclear whether liver dysfunction is caused by a drug, by the underlying disorder for which the implicated drug is being used, by some other concurrent treatment, or by an independent process. Furthermore, in most forms of drug-induced liver injury, there exist important yet poorly understood differences in individual susceptibility. Although some of these differences may be immunologically mediated, this has not been established, and other factors such as differences in drug metabolism are probably of greater significance. Finally, not only may the histopathologic changes seen in drug-induced liver injury be very similar to those of other common entities such as viral hepatitis or biliary obstruction, but some drugs may produce more than one kind of lesion.

Since most forms of drug-induced liver injury are not associated with a specific histopathology, diagnosis must depend chiefly on the history of exposure, consistent clinical, laboratory, and (when appropriate) biopsy findings, and improvement subsequent to removal of the presumed toxin. For those agents that produce small droplet lipid deposition, such as tetracycline or valproic acid, or those that produce prominent centrilobular necrosis, such as acetaminophen (especially when associated with significant blood levels of the drug), the diagnosis can be made with reasonable certainty on the basis of laboratory and biopsy findings. In most instances, however, unequivocal diagnosis cannot be made without demonstration of recurrent liver damage in response to rechallenge with the implicated drug. With rare exceptions, however, this maneuver is not justified; moreover, for those agents that cause a viral hepatitis–like reaction (e.g., halothane or isoniazid), there is the distinct possibility of a severe or even fatal outcome. Although assumption of such risks may be necessary on rare occasions, in most instances some degree of diagnostic uncertainty is acceptable as long as the patient is improving and alternative drugs are available.

The appropriate management of drug-induced liver disease consists of discontinuation of the implicated drug(s) and supportive care for acute hepatitis or liver failure as needed. Only in acetaminophen hepatoxicity is there convincing evidence that specific pharmacologic intervention is beneficial (see below). There is no clear evidence that corticosteroids are of value in the treatment of drug-induced liver disease, although they may suppress systemic manifestations, especially when there is an associated serum sickness–like syndrome. Complications of hepatic adenomas, whether or not estrogen-associated, may require a surgical approach.

HISTOPATHOLOGIC CLASSIFICATION OF DRUG-INDUCED LIVER DISEASE

The classification shown in Table 121–1, although useful conceptually, should not obscure the fact that a given agent may cause more than one form of liver injury. For example, isoniazid may produce a nonspecific focal hepatitis, an acute viral hepatitis–like lesion, or chronic active hepatitis, whereas oral contraceptives may cause hepatocellular cholestasis or liver cell adenoma, and have been implicated in hepatic vein thrombosis.

Zonal necrosis is most commonly produced by hepatotoxins that cause a predictable and dose-related injury that also can be produced in laboratory animals. Examples include the centrilobular necrosis associated with *carbon tetrachloride* and *acetaminophen* toxicity. For these and some other agents, toxicity depends on their conversion in the liver cell to a toxic derivative. Despite the predictability and dose dependency that characterize this class of agents, there are significant differences in individual susceptibility, in part reflecting differences in rates of conversion to toxic products. The acute lesion either is fatal or is followed by essentially complete recovery. A similar lesion may result from chronic exposure, but it is not certain that this leads to progressive liver disease and cirrhosis.

TABLE 121–1. CLASSIFICATION OF DRUG-INDUCED LIVER DISEASE

Category	Examples
Predictable hepatotoxins with zonal necrosis	Acetaminophen, carbon tetrachloride
Nonspecific hepatitis	Aspirin, oxacillin
Viral hepatitis-like reactions	Halothane, isoniazid, phenytoin
Cholestasis	
Noninflammatory	Estrogens, 17-α-substituted steroids
Inflammatory	Chlorpromazine, antithyroid agents
Fatty liver	
Large droplet	Ethanol, corticosteroids
Small droplet	Tetracycline, valproic acid
Granulomas	Phenylbutazone, allopurinol
Chronic hepatitis	Methyldopa, nitrofurantoin
Tumors	Estrogens, vinyl chloride
Vascular lesions	6-Thioguanine, anabolic steroids

Nonspecific hepatitis consists of isolated foci of liver cell necrosis and inflammation, without the characteristic features of viral hepatitis. It also appears to exhibit a variable dose dependency. Neither the mechanism of the injury nor the basis for individual differences in susceptibility is known. Examples include *aspirin* and *oxacillin*.

Viral hepatitis–like reactions may mimic the broad spectrum of clinical, histopathologic, and prognostic variants of viral hepatitis, from an acute uncomplicated process, to bridging or submassive necrosis, to fatal massive necrosis. Examples include *halothane, isoniazid, methyldopa, sulfonamides,* and *phenytoin*. There are marked differences in individual susceptibility to this form of injury, accounting for its sporadic occurrence and for the common belief that it represents a form of drug allergy. Although there appears to be a specific antibody to hepatocyte surface membranes in the serum of patients with severe halothane hepatitis, it is not certain whether this is important in pathogenesis or represents a secondary immune response to membrane antigens exposed during the halothane-induced injury. Furthermore, in the hepatitis associated with isoniazid and phenytoin, there is increasing evidence that cell injury is mediated by a toxic drug metabolite. Thus, differences in individual susceptibility need not imply an immunologic mechanism but may reflect the influence of genetic, dietary, environmental, or pharmacologic factors on drug metabolism.

Cholestasis is a very common manifestation of drug-induced liver injury, and takes two distinct forms. In the first, caused principally by *natural and synthetic estrogens* and by *17α-substituted androgenic and anabolic steroids*, there is usually little or no evidence of hepatocellular necrosis or a substantial inflammatory response. The injury is most simply viewed as the impaired secretion of bile by the liver cell, probably reflecting a direct steroid effect on the physical properties of cellular membranes or the activities of enzymes involved in this process. Although large doses may minimally impair bile secretion in most subjects, certain persons seem especially sensitive. These differences in individual susceptibility clearly are not allergic, and appear at least in part genetically determined. The lesion is completely and rapidly reversible.

In the second form of cholestatic injury, there is significant hepatocellular necrosis and portal and lobular inflammation; acidophil bodies and eosinophils are variably present. Systemic features, including fever, rash, and arthralgias, are not uncommon. This form of injury is produced by a broad group of agents, including the *phenothiazines, oral hypoglycemic* and *antithyroid* agents, and the *macrolide antibiotics* (e.g., erythromycin estolate). Its prognosis is generally favorable and complete recovery may be expected, except in very few individuals in whom chlorpromazine leads to a prolonged but ultimately resolving cholestatic course; rarely, the reaction may prove fatal. Marked differences in individual susceptibility associated with systemic features have suggested drug allergy as the basis for this form of injury. Chlorpromazine, however, is converted to a number of variably toxic metabolic products; this may account not only for the frequently abnormal liver function observed in patients receiving large doses for prolonged periods but also for the smaller number who develop the overt inflammatory and necrosing cholestatic lesion.

Fatty liver usually represents the accumulation of triglyceride within the hepatocyte, and also may occur in two forms. In the most common, associated with *ethanol, corticosteroids, protein-calorie malnutrition, obesity, uncontrolled diabetes mellitus,* and after *jejunoileal bypass*, the fat accumulates in large droplets that displace the liver cell nucleus and confer upon it an adipocyte-like appearance. Despite this distortion, liver function may be well preserved.

A much less common pattern is seen in association with *tetracycline* or *valproic acid* hepatotoxicity, and occasionally with alcoholic liver disease, and superficially resembles that seen in *Reye's syndrome, obstetric fatty liver,* and *Jamaican vomiting sick-*

ness. It consists of fat deposited in smaller droplets throughout the liver cell, the nucleus remaining central. This pattern is usually associated with significant, occasionally fatal, disturbances in liver function.

Granulomas are found in the liver in certain forms of drug-induced liver injury, and may be associated with extrahepatic granulomas and prominent systemic features. Included among the agents responsible are *phenylbutazone, quinidine, allopurinol, phenytoin, halothane,* and *hydralazine*.

Chronic hepatitis has been associated with an increasing number of drugs, including *methyldopa, isoniazid, sulfonamides, nitrofurantoin, dantrolene, acetaminophen,* and *aspirin*. Although these agents more often cause acute liver injury, prolonged use may occasionally result in a chronic progressive process leading in some instances to cirrhosis. In many cases, the lesion is largely or completely reversible, but in severe cases this may require many months after the drug is discontinued. Rarely, progressive liver failure and death may ensue despite cessation of the drug. *Ethanol* abuse occasionally is associated with a lesion similar to that of chronic active hepatitis.

Tumors caused by drugs and other chemical agents may be of several types, including *hepatic adenoma (and possibly hepatocellular carcinoma)* associated with *oral contraceptive* use, and *angiosarcoma* caused by prolonged exposure to *vinyl chloride* monomer or Thorotrast. The mechanism by which these tumors are produced is not known, but their clinical and laboratory features generally resemble those of similar tumors occurring "spontaneously." A possible exception is the apparently greater size, vascularity, and tendency to sudden hemorrhage of hepatic adenomas associated with oral contraceptive use (see Ch. 128).

Vascular lesions of several kinds occasionally are caused by drugs. Oral contraceptives have been implicated as a cause of hepatic vein thrombosis. Hepatic *veno-occlusive disease*, a process that affects the smaller tributaries of the hepatic vein, has been associated with the use of *antitumor agents*, including *6-thioguanine* and *cytarabine* as well as with ingestion of *pyrrolidizine alkaloids*, e.g., from plants of *Senecio* and *Crotelaria* species ("bush tea poisoning"). *Oral contraceptives* and *anabolic steroids* have been identified as causes of *peliosis hepatis*, a condition in which the liver lobule contains extrasinusoidal blood-filled spaces; this lesion is also seen in certain chronic wasting neoplastic and inflammatory diseases.

SELECTED EXAMPLES OF DRUG-INDUCED LIVER DISEASE

ACETAMINOPHEN. Hepatotoxicity caused by acetaminophen is a classic example of a predictable, dose-dependent form of zonal necrosis. This readily available agent has been used with increasing frequency in suicide attempts. It causes death in acute liver failure, often associated with renal failure, and usually with doses in excess of 10 to 15 grams. Within several hours patients develop nausea, vomiting, and hypotension. This initial phase may then subside and the patient may exhibit few symptoms, but over the next 24 to 48 hours there appears clinical and laboratory evidence of progressive deterioration of liver function.

The injury apparently is caused by toxic products of acetaminophen biotransformation; above threshold levels these toxic products overwhelm the capacity of detoxification mechanisms (e.g., conjugation with glutathione or other acceptors) and appear to react directly with critical cell constituents. The rate of formation of these toxic products reflects not only drug dose but also the activity of the cytochrome P-450–dependent microsomal drug metabolizing system. When the activity of this pathway has been stimulated by inducers such as phenobarbital or ethanol, increased amounts of toxic product are formed. The activity of this pathway and the availability of endogenous acceptors such as glutathione are probably important determinants of individual differences in susceptibility to acetaminophen toxicity. In addition, glutathione is important in many and diverse aspects of cell function; thus, depletion of this critically important substance may have major adverse effects apart from its unavailability to combine with toxic drug metabolites.

Although acute toxicity usually requires a dose in excess of 10 to 15 grams, the clinical history is quite unreliable as the basis for assessing prognosis in a given case. Far more useful is the acetaminophen plasma level: when it exceeds 200 mg per liter at four hours, 100 mg per liter at eight hours, or 50 mg per liter at 12 hours after ingestion, severe liver damage may occur. Subsidence of the early gastrointestinal symptoms is not necessarily a favorable prognostic sign, and measurement of the plasma concentration is important both for prognosis and for treatment. Treatment of the higher risk patients with N-acetylcysteine* within the first ten hours after ingestion may significantly improve chances for survival. N-acetylcysteine has been thought to act by providing additional cysteine for glutathione synthesis, but other possible mechanisms are not excluded. The recommended dose of N-acetylcysteine (Mucomyst) is 140 mg per kilogram orally initially, followed by maintenance doses of 70 mg per kilogram every four hours for a total of 72 hours. (In Britain, an intravenous preparation is available, and is administered as follows: 150 mg per kilogram initially over 15 minutes, 50 mg per kilogram over the next four hours and 100 mg per kilogram over the next 16 hours.) In all cases, supportive care is also indicated, and early gastric aspiration may permit recovery of a substantial portion of the ingested dose. In survivors, recovery is virtually complete; there is no evidence of chronic progressive liver disease, but in some cases serum bile acid concentrations may be increased, and there may be residual hepatic fibrosis.

In addition to the acute effects of a massive overdose, acetaminophen may also cause liver injury when taken chronically at doses within the therapeutic range (3 to 8 grams per day). On liver biopsy, either centrilobular necrosis or a picture suggestive of chronic hepatitis may be found. This injury is fully reversible after the drug is discontinued.

ASPIRIN. Usually in doses in excess of 3.0 grams per day, aspirin may cause abnormalities in serum transaminases and other liver function tests, associated with a biopsy picture of either a nonspecific or chronic hepatitis. Not unexpectedly, these effects are seen most often in patients with diseases such as juvenile and adult rheumatoid arthritis and systemic lupus erythematosus, in which chronic high dose salicylate therapy is commonly employed. The mechanism of the injury is not known, but its clear-cut dose dependency suggests a toxic effect of either aspirin or a product of its biotransformation.

The diagnosis of aspirin hepatotoxicity should be suspected in any subject on high-dose salicylate therapy with abnormal liver function. Serum salicylate concentrations will usually be found to exceed 20 mg per deciliter. The injury is rapidly and completely reversible when salicylates are discontinued. A potential source of confusion may arise when liver functions are abnormal in a patient with features of "autoimmune" disease and a liver biopsy suggestive of chronic active hepatitis. If the patient is taking salicylates and the serum salicylate concentration is compatible, this constellation of findings should suggest salicylate hepatotoxicity and should be managed accordingly, before giving consideration to corticosteroid treatment for chronic active hepatitis.

There has been recent concern regarding aspirin treatment of viral syndromes in children and its possible etiologic or contributory role in the development of Reye's syndrome. While conclusive evidence for a causal relationship is lacking, caution is advised in the use of aspirin in such circumstances.

CHLORPROMAZINE. This agent characteristically produces a cholestatic reaction, associated with variable local and systemic symptoms, including fever, anorexia, nausea, abdominal discomfort, and, occasionally, rash. On biopsy, hepatocellular and canalicular cholestasis is found, together with a significant but variable lobular and portal inflammatory infiltrate and liver cell

*This use is not listed in the manufacturer's directive.

necrosis. The sporadic occurrence of this reaction, and its systemic features and frequently associated eosinophilia, suggested "drug allergy." However, recent evidence suggests that chlorpromazine causes a form of toxic liver injury. Thus, among those using this drug in high doses or for prolonged periods, there is a high incidence of abnormal liver function. Furthermore, in acute animal experiments, chlorpromazine at doses approximating those used clinically causes an acute dose-related impairment of bile secretion. Finally, certain chlorpromazine metabolites have been shown to affect adversely several factors necessary for the formation of bile. Individual differences in susceptibility to chlorpromazine cholestasis may reflect corresponding differences in the rate of formation of the more toxic metabolites.

The prognosis of chlorpromazine cholestasis is generally favorable. Rarely, patients may exhibit a prolonged course resembling primary biliary cirrhosis despite discontinuation of the agent, but in these cases eventual recovery, even after three to four years, also is the rule. Fatal hepatic necrosis is also rare. Therapeutic intervention, other than discontinuation of the drug and symptomatic support (e.g., cholestyramine or colestipol for pruritus), is not indicated; if cholestasis is prolonged, replacement of fat-soluble vitamins may be necessary.

ERYTHROMYCIN ESTOLATE. The lauryl sulfate salt of propionyl erythromycin may cause a cholestatic reaction with components of inflammation and necrosis of liver cells. A similar reaction occasionally has been associated with erythromycin ethylsuccinate and erythromycin propionate. Erythromycin estolate hepatotoxicity often presents as an acute syndrome of a right upper quadrant pain, fever, and variable cholestasis, and there are several well-documented cases in which such patients were subjected to major surgery for presumed cholecystitis or cholangitis. The prognosis for the hepatic lesion is uniformly excellent, but the reaction may be expected to recur if the drug is readministered. The mechanism of the injury is unknown.

HALOTHANE. This anesthetic agent is now generally accepted as a rare cause of a viral hepatitis-like reaction and, even more rarely, of fatal massive hepatic necrosis. The mechanism of the injury is unknown, but an immunologic basis is suggested by the fact that most clinically apparent cases occur in persons with a history of prior exposure to halothane or a related agent, and by the presence of antibodies to hepatocyte surface membranes in patients' serum (see above). On the other hand, halothane is predictably hepatotoxic in animals when circumstances favor its metabolism via reductive pathways. Halothane hepatitis usually becomes evident approximately seven to ten days after anesthesia, but with repeated exposures the interval between administration and the clinical onset decreases. The course is indistinguishable from that of viral hepatitis and may terminate fatally within days, progress to rapid and complete recovery, or exhibit a more prolonged course with eventual recovery. Despite earlier evidence to the contrary, single exposure halothane hepatitis does not appear to lead to chronic hepatitis.

ISONIAZID (INH). The overall incidence of clinical hepatitis among persons taking *isoniazid* (INH) for single drug chemoprophylaxis against tuberculosis approximates 1 per cent, with a case fatality rate of about 10 per cent. Clinically and histologically, the disease resembles the wide spectrum of viral hepatitis, and may appear as a relatively mild acute process, a subacute or chronic hepatitis, or fatal massive necrosis. There is an important age effect on incidence, which may exceed 2 per cent among persons over the age of 50. Most cases become manifested within two to three months after the start of the drug, but the onset may be delayed for up to 12 months. Despite earlier reports to the contrary, there seems to be no apparent relationship between acetylator status (rapid as opposed to slow acetylators) and risk of hepatotoxicity.

In addition to the 1 per cent overall incidence of overt hepatitis, there is approximately a 10 to 20 per cent incidence of subclinical liver injury, manifested by mild to moderate increases in serum transaminase activity reflecting a focal nonspecific hepatitis. The laboratory abnormalities associated with this lesion appear nonprogressive and will subside in most patients despite continued administration of the drug.

The mechanism of neither of these two forms of expression of isoniazid hepatotoxicity is fully understood. However, there is evidence that a toxic metabolite may be involved. There is no evidence to suggest "drug allergy"; indeed, patients with isoniazid hepatitis usually lack clinical manifestations, such as skin rash and arthralgias, which might suggest drug allergy.

The clinical presentation of isoniazid hepatitis may be nonspecific, consisting initially of a "flu" syndrome or low grade fever. For this reason, any patient receiving isoniazid should be followed at regular intervals and advised to report intercurrent symptoms. If these are found to be associated with clinical or laboratory evidence of disturbed liver function, the drug should be discontinued, pending further evaluation. A more difficult question concerns the appropriate management of the patient with an asymptomatic transaminase elevation early in the course of isoniazid treatment. Since there is at least a 90 per cent probability (especially in younger patients) that this finding reflects a transient and self-limited event rather than significant hepatitis, it is not generally recommended that liver function tests be routinely monitored in patients taking isoniazid. However, a several-fold elevation in transaminase levels in a patient over 35 years of age, even in the absence of symptoms, must be regarded as potentially serious and may be sufficient to justify discontinuation of the drug. As a general rule, the risk-benefit ratio for isoniazid chemoprophylaxis rises rapidly after age 35, and in this group it is often best to err on the side of caution by stopping the drug when in doubt.

The management of suspected isoniazid hepatitis, apart from discontinuing the drug, is supportive. Fulminant hepatic failure should be treated as described in Ch. 127. There is no evidence that corticosteroids are of value in either acute or chronic forms of the disease.

RIFAMPIN. This antituberculous agent may cause liver injury. This agent reversibly impairs the hepatic uptake of bilirubin and sulfobromophthalein from plasma; it is also an inducer of the microsomal cytochrome P-450–dependent drug-metabolizing system. This latter effect has been cited as the mechanism by which rifampin may cause an unusually precipitous and severe form of isoniazid hepatitis when the two agents are administered together, but this possible drug interaction is not conclusively established. Rifampin itself has been implicated as a cause of acute hepatitis, but in most reported cases isoniazid was also being used; thus, the true incidence of rifampin hepatitis is unknown.

METHYLDOPA. This drug appears to be the only important antihypertensive agent with a significant incidence of hepatotoxicity. It is similar to isoniazid in that minor and apparently inconsequential abnormalities in liver function occur in perhaps 5 per cent of subjects, whereas overt acute or chronic hepatitis is much less common. There is a high incidence of serologic indicators of altered immunity in users of this drug, but hepatic injury does not correlate with Coombs test positivity and may be mediated by a toxic drug metabolite. Most reported cases have resembled acute viral hepatitis, but this agent is also important among the growing list of drugs implicated as causes of chronic active hepatitis.

ORAL CONTRACEPTIVES. These hormonal agents have been associated with several adverse effects on the hepatobiliary system: (1) hepatocellular cholestasis, (2) hepatic vein thrombosis, (3) liver cell neoplasia, and (4) increased predisposition to cholesterol gallstone formation.

The *cholestatic effects* of oral contraceptives are largely attributable to the estrogenic component. Among oral contraceptive users, the majority exhibit subtle disturbances in bile secretory function (e.g., as demonstrated by measurement of the transport maximum for sulfobromophthalein), whereas only a few develop clinical cholestasis, with associated pruritus and jaundice. Histologically, there is usually little or no inflammation or hepatocellular necrosis. The syndrome is completely reversible, usually within two to three months, when the pill is discontinued. An entirely analogous situation may occur during the later stages of pregnancy, in which subclinical or mild cholestasis is common (decreased BSP T_{max} or mild pruritus), whereas clinically overt cholestasis ("recurrent intrahepatic cholestasis of pregnancy") is unusual and resolves rapidly after parturition. Cholestasis of pregnancy can be reproduced by subsequent administration of estrogens; it may be caused by a direct physical effect of the natural or synthetic estrogen on membrane components important in the bile secretory process. The obvious marked individual differences in susceptibility to this effect, although clearly not related to "drug allergy," are not well understood. The possible importance of genetic factors is suggested by the higher incidence of this problem among women with the Dubin-Johnson syndrome, the substantial differences in its incidence among descendants of certain Indian tribes in Chile, apparently unrelated to current location, diet, or other environmental factors, and the recent documentation of the familial occurrence of recurrent cholestasis of pregnancy.

Treatment of oral contraceptive–induced cholestasis consists of discontinuation of the drug, and symptomatic support (e.g., bile acid sequestrants for pruritus) as needed. Resolution should be rapid and complete; persistence of abnormalities beyond two or three months, or worsening at any time after the pill is discontinued, suggests the possibility that the agent may have simply unmasked some pre-existing clinically inapparent condition, and additional diagnostic evaluation may be indicated.

Kopanoff DE, Snider DE Jr, Caras GJ: Isoniazid-related hepatitis. Am Rev Respir Dis 117:991, 1978. *A detailed review of available clinical data to date, with recommendations concerning follow-up and monitoring. A USPHS Cooperative Surveillance Survey from the Center for Disease Control.*

McMaster KR, Hennigas GR: Drug-induced granulomatous hepatitis. Lab Invest 44:61, 1981. *A current summary of implicated agents, with histopathologic documentation.*

Mitchell JR, Jollow DJ: Metabolic activation of drugs to toxic substances. Gastroenterology 68:392, 1975. *A good discussion of the basic concepts of the hepatotoxicity of drug metabolites.*

Ockner RK: Drug-induced liver disease. *In* Zakim D, Boyer T (eds.): Hepatology. Philadelphia, W. B. Saunders Company, 1982, pp 691–722. *A classification and summary of pharmacologic agents that may cause liver injury, including consideration of mechanisms and clinical aspects.*

Prescott LF, Illingworth RN, Critchley JAJH, Stewart MJ, Adam RD, Proudfoot AT: Intravenous N-acetylcysteine: The treatment of choice for paracetamol poisoning. Br Med J 2:1097, 1979. *Convincing recent support for an aggressive approach to treatment. A case is made for the superiority of the intravenous route, although studies in the United States currently are based on oral administration.*

Zimmerman HJ (ed.): Drug-induced liver disease. Semin Liver Dis 1:89, 1981. *A useful, multiauthored summary of recent advances and perspectives.*

Zimmerman HJ: Hepatotoxicity. The Adverse Effects of Drugs and Other Chemicals on the Liver. New York, Appleton-Century-Crofts, 1980. *Currently the most comprehensive and authoritative single source on the subject. Well-organized, readable, and thoroughly referenced.*

122. CHRONIC HEPATITIS

Robert K. Ockner

GENERAL CONSIDERATIONS

DEFINITION. Chronic hepatitis is a sustained inflammatory process in the liver lasting more than six months to one year. It encompasses a wide spectrum of syndromes of diverse etiology, pathogenesis, histopathology, and clinical manifestations. In most, there is a variable element of hepatocellular necrosis. In its more severe forms, this inflammatory and necrotic process may lead to collapse of stromal elements, distortion of the lobular architecture, and a reparative process consisting of fibrosis and nodular regeneration (i.e., cirrhosis). The cell necrosis is associated with an inflammatory response that may be predominantly portal, periportal, or lobular in its distribution.

ETIOLOGY. Chronic hepatitis (Table 122–1) can be caused by *hepatitis B* (with or without δ agent superinfection) and *non-A non-B* virus infection, *drugs* and *toxins* (see below and Ch. 121), and *inborn errors of metabolism* such as *Wilson's disease* and *α_1-antitrypsin deficiency*. In addition, there are one or more poorly understood types of *unknown etiology* in which clinical and laboratory features suggest but do not prove an immunologically mediated process.

TABLE 122–1. CAUSES OF CHRONIC HEPATITIS

Chronic viral infections
Hepatitis B
Hepatitis B with superimposed δ-agent
Hepatitis non-A non-B
Drugs and toxins
Acetaminophen
Aspirin
Dantrolene
Ethanol
Isoniazid
Methyldopa
Nitrofurantoin
Oxyphenisatin
Sulfonamides
Wilson's disease
α_1-Antitrypsin deficiency
Idiopathic (? "autoimmune")

CLINICAL AND LABORATORY MANIFESTATIONS AND DIAGNOSIS. Patients with chronic hepatitis may be entirely asymptomatic and exhibit only minimal abnormalities in routine laboratory tests, or may be incapacitated by progressive liver failure and the complications of portal hypertension. At any given time, the clinical and laboratory features may not correlate well with histopathology or long-term prognosis. For this reason, and because concepts of the natural history and response to treatment are changing for some of these disorders, decisions regarding diagnosis, management, and prognosis are often difficult and uncertain. These aspects of the various chronic hepatitis syndromes are considered in greater detail in the balance of this chapter.

PATHOLOGY. In most forms of chronic hepatitis there is a prominent portal inflammatory reaction, consisting mainly of mononuclear cells, especially small lymphocytes and plasma cells. There is also variable necrosis and inflammation involving hepatocytes immediately adjacent to the portal area. In this *periportal hepatitis* (or *"piecemeal necrosis"*) the inflammatory process invades the peripheral portions of the hepatic lobule, so that individual liver cells or nests of cells are isolated within the inflammatory zone. Periportal hepatitis (piecemeal necrosis) is not specific for chronic hepatitis, and often is present in uncomplicated acute hepatitis and several other processes. For this reason it does not necessarily reflect a chronic or progressive process, and its significance can only be judged in the context of associated pathologic and clinical findings.

The lobular architecture may be substantially disrupted, as indicated by extension of the portal inflammatory and necrotic process into the lobule to a depth sufficient to span adjacent portal and/or central areas, i.e., *"bridging necrosis."* Although bridging necrosis can occur as part of an otherwise uncomplicated and self-limited acute hepatitis, it reflects a more severe injury that has a greater propensity to lead to progressive deterioration over a period of weeks to months (*"subacute hepatic necrosis"*) or to chronic active hepatitis and cirrhosis. Thus, its presence, or the presence of submassive necrosis or significant fibrosis in a patient with liver disease lasting more than six months, suggests a chronic and progressive process. Paradoxically, among survivors of the most extreme forms of acute liver injury, i.e., massive hepatic necrosis, chronic progressive liver disease is uncommon. Although the classification of chronic hepatitis that follows is based on histopathology, overlap is common, and differentiation of one from the other may be difficult.

CHRONIC PERSISTENT HEPATITIS

DEFINITION AND PATHOLOGY. Chronic persistent hepatitis is a nonprogressive inflammatory process largely confined to the portal areas. There is little or no periportal or lobular hepatitis; significant fibrosis and cirrhosis are absent. Of the small number of patients with acute hepatitis B whose illness becomes chronic, most will be found to have this lesion, and it is the most common form of chronic hepatitis. By definition, the diagnosis of persistent hepatitis is not appropriate if there is significant stromal collapse, fibrosis, or nodular regeneration.

CLINICAL AND LABORATORY MANIFESTATIONS. Chronic persistent hepatitis may be entirely asymptomatic or associated with nonspecific symptoms, including fatigue, anorexia, abdominal discomfort, or right upper quadrant pain. Extrahepatic manifestations such as arthritis, glomerulonephritis, and vasculitis are rare. Jaundice, if present, is usually very mild. Physical findings are usually limited to palmar erythema, a few spider telangiectasias, and mildly tender hepatomegaly; the spleen occasionally is slightly enlarged. By definition, complications of advanced liver disease and portal hypertension, such as evidence of a collateral circulation, ascites, and encephalopathy, are absent.

Laboratory abnormalities are also mild, and include moderate increases in serum transaminases, bilirubin, and globulins. Albumin concentration and prothrombin time are usually normal. The serum is positive for HBsAg in perhaps 20 to 30 per cent of patients; other serologic tests such as mitochondrial, smooth muscle, and antinuclear antibodies are usually negative.

DIAGNOSIS, PROGNOSIS, AND MANAGEMENT. In any patient with persisting abnormalities of liver function, ethanol or other potential hepatotoxins should be discontinued, at least temporarily, to determine their possible significance. Because its clinical and laboratory features are totally nonspecific, the diagnosis of persistent hepatitis cannot be made without liver biopsy, but even biopsy does not always make it possible to distinguish this syndrome with certainty from chronic active hepatitis. The outlook is favorable, in that progression to cirrhosis or liver failure does not occur. However, the syndrome may last for ten years or more, and may cause continuing or intermittent discomfort or disability. Because of the difficulties inherent in the biopsy diagnosis of this group of disorders, continuing observation is important. Evidence of significant clinical deterioration may indicate the presence of a more serious process such as chronic active hepatitis, cirrhosis, or hepatocellular carcinoma and would be reason to consider repeating the liver biopsy. No specific treatment is indicated or available for chronic persistent hepatitis. Symptomatic and nutritional support are appropriate, and exposure to potential hepatotoxins should be avoided. For patients in whom alcohol has been excluded etiologically, small amounts of alcoholic beverages are permissible if they do not cause worsening of symptoms or laboratory tests. A form of chronic persistent hepatitis may be found in those patients in whom corticosteroid treatment has induced a remission in pre-existing chronic active hepatitis. The prognosis of this variant is less favorable, since about 50 per cent of such patients may have relapse after steroid therapy is discontinued.

CHRONIC LOBULAR HEPATITIS

This is a less well defined variant of chronic hepatitis in which the predominant lesion is a scattered single-cell necrosis in the lobule, with a relatively minor portal inflammatory component. It is, in effect, a form of unresolved acute hepatitis. As in the case of chronic persistent hepatitis, it does not appear to progress to cirrhosis or liver failure. Aside from those few patients in whom HB_sAg is positive and presumed causative, a specific etiology is not identifiable.

CHRONIC ACTIVE HEPATITIS

DEFINITION. This is the most serious form of chronic hepatitis because of its potential for progression to cirrhosis and liver failure. It has been designated by a number of other essentially synonymous terms, such as *lupoid hepatitis, autoimmune hepatitis, plasma cell hepatitis, chronic aggressive hepatitis,* and *chronic active liver disease.*

ETIOLOGY. Approximately 20 per cent of cases are associated with, and presumably caused by, *chronic hepatitis B infection,* with or without superimposed δ-agent infection (see Ch. 120). Chronic active hepatitis may also follow non-A non-B hepatitis. Drugs that can cause the syndrome include *dantrolene, isoniazid, methyldopa, nitrofurantoin, oxyphenisatin,* and *sulfonamides.* Chronic use of *acetaminophen, aspirin,* and *ethanol* occasionally may cause similar changes, as may *Wilson's disease* and *α_1-antitrypsin deficiency.* In a large number of cases the etiology is unknown, although many of this group exhibit clinical features and serologic abnormalities suggestive of autoimmunity. Despite such suggestive evidence, however, a truly "autoimmune" basis for chronic hepatitis has not been conclusively established, and in many instances phenomena that might be considered to reflect such a mechanism are also found in that form of the disease associated with hepatitis B virus infection. With time, specific etiologies may be identified for additional subsets of chronic active hepatitis.

PATHOLOGY. The syndrome is characterized by expansion of portal areas, which are infiltrated by lymphocytes and plasma cells, by periportal hepatitis, and by a variable degree of bridging necrosis, collapse, and fibrosis. In one third or more of patients, macronodular cirrhosis is present at the time of diagnosis. Except for the characteristic features of α_1-antitrypsin deficiency, which can be demonstrated by histochemistry, the various causes of chronic active hepatitis cannot be differentiated from one another on the basis of pathology.

CLINICAL MANIFESTATIONS. The course of chronic active hepatitis may be highly variable. The onset is usually insidious, but in perhaps one third of cases may resemble an acute hepatitis. It may affect all age groups and both sexes. However, HBsAg-negative cases occur mainly in young adult females, often associated with a more severe course and "autoimmune" features, whereas HBsAg-positive cases are more common in older males, and are often minimally symptomatic. Patients may be asymptomatic, or may exhibit a wide range of local or constitutional symptoms typical of liver disease, such as fatigue, malaise, fever, anorexia, jaundice, or ascites.

Extrahepatic manifestations are often quite prominent and at times may dominate the clinical picture, especially in young females. These include amenorrhea, various skin rashes, glomerulonephritis, polyserositis, thyroiditis, vasculitis, Sjögren's syndrome, pneumonitis, depression of the formed elements of the blood, and an apparently increased incidence of ulcerative colitis.

Physical findings may also be quite variable. Patients may exhibit only a few spider telangiectasias, possibly with mild enlargement of liver and/or spleen, and may or may not be jaundiced. In advanced cases with cirrhosis, patients may have ascites, evidence of collateral circulation, or encephalopathy. In young women, acne and hirsutism may reflect the hormonal effects of chronic liver disease. Evidence of other extrahepatic manifestations may also be prominent, as noted above.

LABORATORY FINDINGS. Transaminases are usually elevated over a range from minimally abnormal to in excess of 1000 IU. Globulins usually are diffusely increased, and albumin often is low. The alkaline phosphatase is usually only slightly to moderately increased; major increases should suggest the possibility of biliary tract disease or infiltrative or mass lesions. Prothrombin time generally reflects the severity of the disease but may also be influenced by vitamin K deficiency. Because of their variability, the laboratory tests often poorly reflect the pathologic process; for this reason they do not always provide a reliable basis for the assessment of natural history or response to treatment.

Chronic active hepatitis is often characterized by the presence of a number of unusual but nonspecific immunoglobulins in serum, especially in patients who are negative for HBsAg.

These include smooth muscle antibodies (positive in about two thirds), antinuclear antibodies (about one half), and antimitochondrial antibodies (about one third). Antibodies to a liver plasma membrane protein also have been demonstrated; their significance is unknown.

DIAGNOSIS. Diagnosis of chronic active hepatitis requires liver biopsy. In addition to the pathology, it is essential to establish a specific etiology, if possible, e.g., chronic hepatitis B infection, drugs, ethanol, Wilson's disease, or α_1-antitrypsin deficiency. Exposure to drugs and toxins usually can be identified by means of a careful history, including, when appropriate, questioning of family members or friends. A positive test for HBsAg suggests that hepatitis B virus infection is causative, but even in these persons drugs and toxins also should be considered. Conversely, some cases of chronic active hepatitis may be caused by hepatitis B virus despite HBsAg-negative serum (in these patients serum has been positive for anti-HBc and occasionally anti-HBs as well, and recently it has been possible to demonstrate HBV DNA in serum by molecular hybridization). Wilson's disease should be excluded in any patient with chronic hepatitis who is under the age of 40. Appropriate tests for this purpose include slit-lamp examination for Kayser-Fleischer rings, and measurement of serum ceruloplasmin and urinary copper excretion. If all tests are negative, additional studies are not necessary; when the suspicion persists, measurement of liver copper concentration or incorporation of radioactive copper into serum ceruloplasmin may be necessary (see Ch. 205). α_1-Antitrypsin deficiency can be excluded by protease-inhibitor phenotyping of serum and, in liver biopsy specimens, by the absence of PAS-positive material in hepatocytes after diastase treatment of the tissue section.

The *differential diagnosis* includes *chronic persistent hepatitis, postnecrotic cirrhosis,* and some cases of *primary biliary cirrhosis* in which clinical and pathologic features may resemble those of chronic active hepatitis.

TREATMENT. Treatment of chronic active hepatitis not attributable to drugs, Wilson's disease, or α_1-antitrypsin deficiency has been studied in several large clinical trials. The great majority of patients included for study were symptomatic and had clinically obvious liver disease, and most were negative for HBsAg; however, criteria for inclusion, treatment programs, controls, and duration of follow-up differed substantially among the studies.

Generally, *corticosteroids,* with or without low-dose azathioprine, improve laboratory test results, reduce symptoms, suppress the inflammatory response seen on biopsy, and decrease short-term and long-term morbidity and mortality. Thus, in the Mayo Clinic study, a favorable clinical, biochemical, and histologic response was seen initially in 56 per cent of patients, whereas spontaneous improvement occurred in only 20 per cent of placebo-treated controls; early mortality and progression to cirrhosis were also decreased. Similarly favorable results were observed in studies conducted at other institutions.

Despite this seemingly beneficial overall response, several factors that importantly influence the natural history and response to treatment must be considered in making the decision to institute a chronic treatment program with potentially significant adverse effects. First, chronic hepatitis does not usually progress to cirrhosis or liver failure in the absence of bridging necrosis on liver biopsy; the absence of such changes would tend to weigh against the use of corticosteroids. Second, there is no information regarding natural history, or evidence that corticosteroids are of benefit in asymptomatic chronic active hepatitis. Third, HBsAg-positive patients respond less well (or not at all) to corticosteroids than do those who are HBsAg-negative. Fourth, a substantial percentage of patients with non-A non-B post-transfusion chronic active hepatitis may improve spontaneously after a year or longer. Finally, since many patients with chronic active hepatitis would fail to meet the criteria for inclusion in some of the published series, any decision regarding their treatment is necessarily an extrapolation from a limited study population.

In view of this substantial uncertainty concerning the value of corticosteroids in certain subsets of chronic active hepatitis, it is very difficult to make broadly applicable recommendations as to their use. In general, however, an initially favorable response would most likely be expected in a young, HBsAg-negative female with progressive disease characterized by prominent symptoms and "autoimmune" features, and no recent transfusion or other exposure to non-A non-B hepatitis. (In more recent follow-up analysis of the Mayo series, however, it was found that the presence or absence of "autoimmune" features did not substantially affect the response to treatment among non-B chronic hepatitis patients.) HBsAg-positive patients with relatively mild symptoms will benefit little or not at all from corticosteroid treatment. Since there appear to be exceptions, such decisions must be individualized.

In the Mayo Clinic study, an initial daily dose of 60 mg of prednisone or of 30 mg of prednisone combined with 50 mg of azathioprine, tapering gradually over several weeks to months to a daily maintenance dose of 20 mg of prednisone or 10 mg of prednisone plus 50 mg of azathioprine, was found to be most effective. The azathioprine was of no value when given alone, but permitted use of the lower prednisone dose, thereby reducing the incidence of significant steroid-related complications, which otherwise approximated 60 per cent. Alternate-day treatment was less effective. If a favorable response is not observed within two to three months, treatment should be discontinued.

Patients being treated for chronic active hepatitis should be examined and have their liver function determined periodically. The possible side effects of drug treatment should be monitored and liver biopsies should be repeated at intervals of six months to one year, depending on the circumstances. Return of liver enzymes to a level less than twice the upper limit of normal, together with a liver biopsy showing subsidence of the inflammatory and necrotic process to a picture similar to that of persistent hepatitis, is considered a successful response and warrants an attempt gradually to discontinue treatment. In about 50 per cent of patients, this attempt will succeed and additional corticosteroid treatment will not be needed. In the remainder, evidence of relapse may suggest the need for reinstitution of therapy.

In some patients with chronic hepatitis B, a relapse—either spontaneous or following immunosuppressive therapy—may be followed by an apparent remission associated with seroconversion from HBe-positive to anti-HBe-positive and loss of other "Dane particle markers" from serum. This seroconversion is considered to represent a change from a replicative to an integrated state of the HBV-DNA. However, patients in this latter phase of the disease are still subject to reactivation of their disease, either spontaneous or associated with immune suppression.

Unfortunately the disease may eventually progress to cirrhosis despite an apparently favorable clinical response, especially in those patients in whom repeated recurrences of activity require treatment over a period of three years or longer. Over these longer intervals the advisability of continued corticosteroid therapy must be judged not only on the basis of symptoms and laboratory and biopsy findings but also in recognition of the possibility of diminishing returns in the face of increasing risks. The possible effectiveness of other experimental approaches to the treatment of chronic active hepatitis, including the use of interferon and adenine arabinoside, remains to be determined.

SPECIAL CLINICAL PROBLEMS

Two circumstances are encountered in clinical practice with sufficient frequency that they deserve particular comment with reference to diagnostic approach and management.

UNEXPECTED ELEVATION OF SERUM TRANSAMINASES. The advent and common use of multiphasic laboratory screening techniques have led to the identification of individuals in whom transaminase activities are abnormal but who lack clinical evidence of liver disease. If the abnormal finding is confirmed, and if it does not reflect muscle or other extrahepatic disease, it may have either of two possible implications: (1) it may reflect a subclinical acute process (e.g., acute viral hepatitis), or (2) it may reflect a chronic process (e.g., chronic toxic or viral hepatitis). If the patient is asymptomatic or nearly so, a period of observation is appropriate, and follow-up studies and hepatitis serologies should be obtained. Alcohol and potentially hepatotoxic drugs and toxins should be avoided. Improvement would presumably reflect resolution of a self-limited process or the response to removal of a toxin, e.g., ethanol. Worsening of the results may herald the clinical onset of a more overt syndrome, the proper evaluation of which would depend on the circumstances. Persistence of the abnormality beyond six to twelve months may reflect a chronic hepatitis and may justify liver biopsy.

HEPATITIS B SURFACE ANTIGEN POSITIVITY. Approximately 0.1 to 0.2 per cent of the population of the United States is positive for HBsAg. At any given time, most of these persons exhibit no overt evidence of liver disease, and are designated "carriers." The meaning of the term "carrier" varies, however, and has been used to include all chronically positive individuals, or only those who have no apparent liver disease.

The practical question of significance concerns the management of the patient with a positive test. If the result is confirmed, it could indicate (1) a subclinical acute hepatitis B, (2) chronic hepatitis (persistent or active) or cirrhosis, or (3) a "healthy" carrier state. Although differentiation of these conditions may require liver biopsy, HBsAg-positive persons who have no clinical or laboratory evidence of liver disease usually have normal or nonspecific biopsy findings. For the few among this group of *asymptomatic persons with normal liver function tests* who may have chronic active hepatitis on biopsy, there is no evidence that corticosteroid treatment is indicated. Therefore, these individuals can be followed at intervals without first obtaining a liver biopsy. Those HBsAg-positive persons who do have clinical and/or laboratory signs of liver disease should be managed in accordance with the severity and duration of the process; persistence of the abnormalities beyond six months may suggest a chronic hepatitis and the need for liver biopsy.

Becker MD, Scheuer PJ, Baptista A, Sherlock S: Prognosis of chronic persistent hepatitis. Lancet 1:53, 1970. *An important early and well-documented clinical and pathologic description, including long-term follow-up.*

Berman M, Alter HJ, Ishak KG, Purcell RH, Jones EA: The chronic sequelae of non-A non-B hepatitis. Ann Intern Med 91:1, 1979. *Documentation of the frequency and prognosis of chronic hepatitis in a group of multiply transfused patients.*

Boyer JL: Chronic hepatitis—a perspective on classification and determinants of prognosis. Gastroenterology 70:1161, 1976. *A useful framework for understanding histologic classification.*

Czaja AJ, Ammon HV, Summerskill WHJ: Clinical features and prognosis of severe chronic active liver disease after corticosteroid-induced remission. Gastroenterology 78:518, 1980. *Long-term follow-up of the Mayo Clinic study.*

Czaja AJ, Davis GL, Ludwig J, Baggenstoss AH, Taswell HF: Autoimmune features as determinants of prognosis in steroid-treated chronic active hepatitis of uncertain etiology. Gastroenterology 85:713, 1983. *Follow-up data in chronic non-B disease, indicating little difference between patients with and without "autoimmune" features.*

Czaja AJ, Ludwig J, Baggenstoss AH, Wolf A: Corticosteroid-treated chronic active hepatitis in remission. Uncertain prognosis of chronic persistent hepatitis. N Engl J Med 304:1, 1981.

Davis GL, Hoofnagle JH, Waggoner JG: Spontaneous reactivation of chronic hepatitis B virus infection. Gastroenterology 86:230, 1984. *A series of cases in which clinically significant reactivation was not preceded by immunosuppressive therapy.*

Hoofnagle JH, Dusheiko GM, Seeff LB, Jones EA, Waggoner JG, Bales ZB: Seroconversion from hepatitis B e antigen to antibody in chronic type B hepatitis. Ann Intern Med 94:744, 1981. *Information on natural history and possible implications of spontaneous changes in the e-anti-e system with time.*

Kirk AP, Jain S, Pocock S, Thomas HC, Sherlock S: Late results of the Royal Free Hospital prospective controlled trial of prednisone therapy in hepatitis B surface antigen negative chronic active hepatitis. Gut 21:78, 1980.

Liaw Y-F, Chu C-M, Chen T-J, Lin D-Y, Chang-Chien C-S, Wu C-S: Chronic lobular hepatitis: A clinicopathological and prognostic study. Hepatology 2:258, 1982. *A generally benign disorder warranting no specific treatment.*

Schalm SW, Summerskill WHJ, Gitnick GL, Elveback IR: Contrasting features and responses to treatment of severe chronic active liver disease with and

without hepatitis B_s antigen. Gut 17:781, 1976. *Important evidence that HBsAg-positive patients respond less well, or not at all, to corticosteroid treatment.*

Scott J, Gollan JL, Samourian S, Sherlock S: Wilson's disease presenting as chronic active hepatitis. Gastroenterology 74:645, 1978. *A thorough clinical and pathologic description of 17 patients presenting with features of chronic active hepatitis. Emphasis is placed on the often difficult problem of differential diagnosis.*

Scullard GH, Smith CI, Merigan TC, Robinson WAS, Gregory PB: Effects of immunosuppressive therapy on viral markers in chronic active hepatitis B. Gastroenterology 81:987, 1981. *Evidence that viral replication may be potentiated.*

Shafritz DA, Shouval D, Sherman HI, Hadziyannis SJ, Kew MC: Integration of hepatitis B virus DNA into the genome of liver cells in chronic liver disease and hepatocellular carcinoma. N Engl J Med 305:1067, 1981. *Evidence for the possible basis for the link between HBV infection and liver cancer.*

Wright EC, Seeff LB, Berk PD, Jones A, Plotz PH: Treatment of chronic active hepatitis. An analysis of three controlled trials. Gastroenterology 73:1422, 1977. *A very thorough review and critique of three major trials, the results of which have formed the basis for many of the current concepts in this area.*

123. PARASITIC, BACTERIAL, FUNGAL, AND GRANULOMATOUS LIVER DISEASE

Bruce F. Scharschmidt

PARASITIC DISEASE OF THE LIVER AND BILIARY TRACT

The parasitic disorders of humans are discussed in detail in Part XX. Those parasitic disorders that commonly involve the liver and biliary tract are outlined in Table 123–1, and certain points will be re-emphasized here. With respect to diagnosis, the most important first step is a carefully obtained history of travel or residence in an endemic area and potential exposure to the parasite. For example, prior travel or residence in Central Africa or the Middle East in a patient with hepatomegaly and portal hypertension suggests the diagnosis of *schistosomiasis*, particularly if a history of swimming in fresh water followed by pruritus or fever is obtained. In East Asia, prior ingestion of raw or undercooked freshwater fish in a patient with biliary disease should raise the possibility of *clonorchiasis* or *opisthorchiasis*. A history of cattle or sheep raising in a patient being investigated for an hepatic mass should suggest *echinococcosis* and interdict the use of needle biopsy until the possibility of a cystic lesion has been excluded. Ingestion of uncooked freshwater plants (e.g., watercress) from cattle- or sheep-raising areas may be an important clue to the presence of *fascioliasis*, and a history of contact with pet cats and dogs, particularly puppies, is typically obtained from patients with *toxocariasis*.

Tender hepatomegaly and eosinophilia are commonly present during the invasive phase of many helminthic disorders, including *ascariasis, toxocariasis, strongyloidiasis, schistosomiasis*, and *fascioliasis*, yet the diagnosis may not be suspected until weeks, months, or even years later when complications resulting from the presence of eggs or the adult parasite appear. At this time, eosinophilia may no longer be present. With the exception of echinococcosis, serologic and skin tests are of limited value in the helminthic disorders, and the diagnosis generally requires demonstration of larvae or ova in feces or tissue.

Protozoan disorders also frequently involve the liver, and *malaria* is among the most common causes of hepatomegaly worldwide. However, hepatic involvement in malaria and in most protozoan infections represents a relatively minor component of the overall clinical disorder. The outstanding exception is *amebiasis*, of which hepatic amebic abscess is the most life-threatening manifestation (see Liver Abscess, below). In comparison to the helminthic disorders, protozoan infections are less frequently accompanied by eosinophilia and can more often be diagnosed by serologic tests.

Treatment of the helminthic disorders is discussed in Ch. 387 to 423. In addition to eradication of the parasite, biliary tract surgery may be necessary in patients with ascariasis, clonorchiasis, opisthorchiasis, or fascioliasis who develop com-

TABLE 123–1. COMMON PARASITIC DISEASES OF THE LIVER AND BILIARY TRACT

Disorder (Organism)	Principal Endemic Areas	Nature of Hepatic Involvement		
		Pathophysiology	*Manifestations*	*Diagnosis*
Helminthic disorders				
Ascariasis *(Ascaris lumbricoides)*	Worldwide; most common in underdeveloped areas of Asia, Africa, and tropics	Initially larvae carried to liver by portal blood; later, adult worms may enter the biliary tree from the intestine and deposit eggs	Occasional hepatomegaly and fever during larval migration; later, granuloma formation, biliary obstruction, biliary colic, cholangitis, and stone formation	Identification of ova in feces
Toxocariasis *(Toxocara canis, T. cati)*	North and South America, Europe, India	Larval migration in hepatic parenchyma (visceral larva migrans)	Hepatomegaly, granuloma formation	Identification of larvae in tissue, serologic testing
Strongyloidiasis *(Strongyloides stercoralis)*	Tropics	Larval invasion of liver with hyperinfective syndrome (rare)	Granuloma formation	Identification of larvae in stool or duodenal juice, filarial complement fixation test
Echinococcosis *(Echinococcus granulosus, E. multilocularis)*	Worldwide	Growth of larval form (hydatid cyst) in liver	Signs and symptoms of an hepatic mass, cyst rupture, secondary infection, rarely portal hypertension with *E. multilocularis*	Serologic tests, including hemagglutination and complement fixation
Schistosomiasis *(Schistosoma mansoni, S. japonicum)*	East Asia, Central Africa, Middle East, and South America	Adult worms live in portal venous system, eggs carried to liver by portal blood	Granuloma formation, hepatomegaly, portal hypertension and its complications	Identification of eggs in feces or tissue (e.g., rectal mucosa, liver)
Clonorchiasis *(Clonorchis sinensis)*	East Asia	Worms grow and deposit eggs in bile ducts	Granuloma formation, biliary obstruction and infection, stone formation, cholangiocarcinoma	Identification of ova in stool
Opisthorchiasis *(Opisthorchis felineus, O. viverrini)*	Europe, Asia, and Thailand	Worms grow and deposit eggs in bile ducts	Similar to clonorchiasis	Identification of ova in stool
Fascioliasis *(Fasciola hepatica)*	Worldwide	Larvae migrate through hepatic parenchyma to the bile ducts	Hepatomegaly and fever during invasive phase; later, biliary obstruction and infection	Identification of ova in stool
Protozoan disorders				
Amebiasis *(Entamoeba histolytica)*	Worldwide	Invasion of hepatic parenchyma	Signs and symptoms of hepatic abscess, extension and rupture into adjacent structures	Serologic tests, including gel diffusion precipitin and indirect hemagglutination, for tissue invasion; sigmoidoscopy and stool examination for intestinal infection
Malaria *(Plasmodium falciparum, P. vivax, P. ovale, P. malariae)*	Africa, Asia, Central and South America	Pre-erythrocytic (all types) and exoerythrocytic stages (except *P. falciparum*) present in liver	Centrolobular necrosis with acute *P. falciparum* infection hepatosplenomegaly with chronic malaria	Identification of plasmodia in blood smear
Visceral leishmaniasis *(Leishmania donovani)*	Mediterranean basin, Asia, Africa, South America	Infection of mononuclear phagocytic cells of liver and other organs	Hepatosplenomegaly, fever	Identification of parasite in tissue, serologic testing
Toxoplasmosis *(Toxoplasma gondii)*	Worldwide	Parasite multiplication in liver	Hepatosplenomegaly	Serologic tests, including indirect fluorescent antibody test and Sabin-Feldman dye test; isolation of organism from tissue or body fluid
Trypanosomiasis *(Trypanosoma brucei, T. gambiense, T. rhodesiense)* *(T. cruzi)*	Tropical Africa South and Central America	Hepatic involvement during acute systemic phase	Hepatosplenomegaly, hepatocellular necrosis and jaundice occasionally with *T. rhodesiense* infections	Identification of parasite in blood, tissue, or cerebrospinal fluid; serologic testing

plications such as biliary obstruction, infection, or stone formation. Patients with schistosomiasis and recurrent life-threatening hemorrhage caused by esophageal varices may be candidates for portacaval anastomosis. However, all adult worms should be eradicated prior to such surgery to prevent systemic dissemination of ova. The treatment of amebic liver abscess is discussed later in this chapter. Treatment of other protozoan disorders involving the liver is discussed in Ch. 378 to 386.

MYCOTIC LIVER DISEASE

Hepatic involvement is frequently absent or constitutes a minor component of mycotic disease in man, but virtually all fungal infections, when disseminated, can involve the liver. These include histoplasmosis, cryptococcosis, mucormycosis, aspergillosis, coccidioidomycosis, North and South American blastomycosis, candidiasis, sporotrichosis, and actinomycosis. Hepatic pathologic changes may include granulomas, hepatocellular necrosis, and abscesses. The manifestations, diagnosis, and treatment of mycotic disease are discussed in detail in Ch. 365 to 376.

HEPATIC MANIFESTATIONS OF SYSTEMIC BACTERIAL INFECTION

Many systemic infections can be accompanied by minor abnormalities of standard liver function tests and, less commonly, jaundice. Since these changes typically occur in the absence of demonstrable invasion of the hepatic parenchyma by the infecting organism(s), they are generally attributed to the hepatic effects of various toxins. For example, bacterial endotoxin may impair hepatocellular function, and has been implicated in the cholestasis occasionally associated with gram-negative bacterial infections. Staphylococcal exotoxin(s) appears responsible for the cholestasis that sometimes accompanies the toxic shock syndrome. Fever and hypoxemia also adversely affect liver cell function. Infection by gram-positive cocci (particularly pneumococcus), gram-negative cocci (e.g., gonococcus), and gram-negative bacilli (particularly *E. coli* infections in infants) may all be accompanied by jaundice. The jaundice and/or abnormal liver function tests in these patients resolve with successful treatment of the infection, and the importance of these abnormalities lies primarily in the fact that they may be mistaken for other disorders such as viral hepatitis or biliary tract obstruction.

In addition, certain organisms can affect the liver directly. Hepatic invasion by streptococci or salmonellae is a rare cause of liver dysfunction and a hepatitis-like illness. Gonococcal perihepatitis (*Fitz-Hugh–Curtis syndrome*) typically occurs in women with concomitant or recent pelvic inflammatory disease and causes an acute inflammatory reaction in the hepatic capsule accompanied by right upper quadrant pain and fever. "Violin-string" adhesions between the anterior abdominal wall and liver surface may result. *Treponema pallidum* may also invade the liver, and secondary syphilis is accompanied by an hepatitis-like illness in up to 10 per cent of cases. Hepatitis associated with secondary syphilis differs from most other forms of acute hepatic injury in that it is typically associated with a markedly elevated alkaline phosphatase activity in serum.

LIVER ABSCESS

Pyogenic Liver Abscess

DEFINITION. A pyogenic liver abscess is a macroscopic collection of pus within the hepatic parenchyma that results from bacterial infection.

ETIOLOGY. Enteric flora (particularly *E. coli* and *Klebsiella*) and pyogenic gram-positive cocci (particularly *S. aureus*) are common causes of pyogenic liver abscess. With appropriate culture techniques, anaerobic bacteria have been isolated from one half or more of pyogenic abscesses, and multiple bacterial species are present in about two thirds of all cases. Mycotic and mycobacterial infections are unusual causes of macroscopic hepatic abscess. Failure to isolate any organism from a presumed pyogenic abscess occurs relatively frequently and may reflect inappropriate sample handling or culture technique or misdiagnosis of an amebic abscess.

INCIDENCE. Liver abscess is an uncommon disorder, accounting for less than 1 per cent of most necropsy series. This relative infrequency is somewhat surprising when one considers the large blood flow to the liver and its strategic position between the portal and systemic circulations.

PATHOGENESIS. The most common predisposing cause for pyogenic hepatic abscess is currently biliary tract disease, including acute cholecystitis as well as disorders leading to obstruction of the ductal system. Infection in areas drained by the portal venous system (e.g., appendicitis, diverticulitis) may also result in pylephlebitis and pyogenic hepatic abscess, but this occurs less frequently now than in the preantibiotic era. Other important predisposing causes include direct extension from adjacent structures other than the biliary tree (subphrenic or perinephric abscess), penetrating or blunt abdominal trauma, septicemia, and infection arising in necrotic primary or secondary tumor deposits. In many cases, no predisposing cause is apparent. Pyogenic liver abscesses may be single or multiple. Multiple small abscesses occur particularly frequently in association with pylephlebitis, biliary tract obstruction with cholangitis, and septicemia. Pyogenic abscesses related to intra-abdominal infection occur most commonly in the right hepatic lobe, possibly as a result of preferential flow to this area from the superior mesenteric vein.

CLINICAL MANIFESTATIONS. The symptoms of hepatic abscess are usually those of a systemic febrile illness lasting from several days to weeks, although multiple small abscesses related to cholangitis or septicemia tend to appear dramatically and suddenly. No characteristics of the fever pattern reliably distinguish hepatic abscess from abscesses elsewhere in the body. In addition to fever and symptoms of chronic illness, such as weight loss and anorexia, patients may complain of abdominal pain or distention. Jaundice is present in up to 20 per cent of cases and often indicates concomitant biliary tract disease with cholangitis. Extension or rupture into the pleural, pericardial, or peritoneal space occurs less commonly with pyogenic than with amebic abscesses.

The most common physical findings are hepatomegaly and right upper quadrant tenderness. However, unlike the liver in acute hepatitis, a point of maximal tenderness may be demonstrable by palpation or percussion. Even without extension into the pleural space, basilar rales or an elevated or fixed right hemidiaphragm may be present.

DIAGNOSIS. Routine laboratory studies are not particularly helpful. As with any abscess of comparable duration and severity, leukocytosis and anemia are frequently present. Alkaline phosphatase is elevated in most cases, and other liver function tests may be normal to mildly abnormal. Marked hyperbilirubinemia is uncommon.

Radiologic studies are frequently useful. Roentgenograms of the chest reveal abnormalities such as elevation of the right hemidiaphragm, basilar atelectasis, or pleural effusion in about half of cases. Radionuclide scanning is positive in 80 to 90 per cent of reported cases, but may fail to detect small abscesses. Ultrasound is often of value in distinguishing an abscess from a solid tumor or simple cyst, and computed tomography may be very useful when radionuclide scanning and/or ultrasound examination are inconclusive.

Blood cultures have been positive in up to 40 per cent or more of reported cases and should be obtained routinely when an hepatic abscess is suspected. On the basis of clinical findings and chest roentgenograms, pyogenic liver abscesses are most commonly mistaken for pneumonia, hepatitis, cholecystitis, or cholangitis.

TREATMENT. When an hepatic abscess is strongly suspected on the basis of clinical, laboratory, and radiologic findings, blood cultures should be drawn and antibiotic therapy begun. Antibiotics should be chosen to include coverage for gram-negative enteric bacteria and anaerobic organisms as well as possibly for *S. aureus*. If amebic abscess is a possibility, empiric therapy for this disorder (e.g., metronidazole) should be included.

Although surgical drainage of large solitary abscesses has long been the accepted approach to therapy and is still strongly recommended by many authorities, there are now several reported series of patients treated successfully without surgery. If such a nonoperative approach is chosen, accessible lesion(s) should be aspirated both to confirm the diagnosis and obtain material for Gram's stain and culture. Aspiration is best performed under sonographic or computed tomographic guidance and should be performed after beginning antibiotic therapy and instituting appropriate supportive measures (Fig. 123–1). The therapeutic value of percutaneous drainage is not established; however, it is probably appropriate to drain as much of the abscess content as possible at the time of the diagnostic aspiration, and consideration should be given to leaving in a drainage catheter. Antibiotic therapy should be modified as necessary on the basis of the results of cultures of blood or abscess content. Antibiotics are generally administered parenterally for the first 10 to 14 days and continued for a total of four to six weeks. Even in patients successfully treated by this approach, abnormalities on radionuclide scanning may persist for months.

Surgical consultation is appropriate for all patients in whom

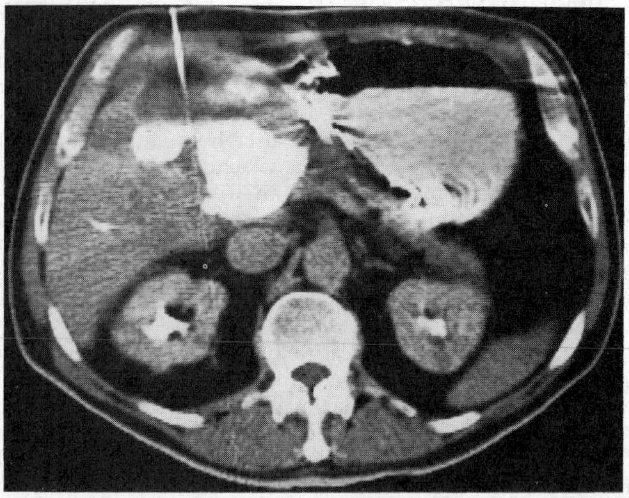

Figure 123–1. Computed tomogram showing CT-directed needle aspiration of a liver abscess. The needle is seen as the thin dense linear object entering the liver from the anterior abdominal wall. Contrast material has been introduced into the abscess cavity through the needle in order to outline the extent of the abscess.

hepatic abscess is strongly suspected, even if the nonoperative approach just outlined is elected, because emergency surgery may be necessary in patients who fail to respond to this treatment or in patients who suffer complications from percutaneous aspiration or drainage. For patients with multiple small abscesses not amenable to surgical drainage, antibiotic administration with attempted aspiration of the largest, most accessible lesions is the only therapy possible, and antibiotics must frequently be administered for several months in such cases. Conversely, surgical intervention is generally necessary for patients in whom the abscess(es) is due to a predisposing surgical disorder such as intra-abdominal sepsis or biliary tract obstruction. Percutaneous drainage of the biliary system may also be at least temporarily useful in the latter group (see Ch. 129).

PROGNOSIS. The prognosis for patients with pyogenic hepatic abscesses has improved considerably since antibiotics have become available, but this remains a serious illness with reported mortality rates ranging from 10 to 60 per cent. The prognosis is adversely affected by the presence of multiple abscesses that cannot be surgically drained, advanced age, underlying malignancy, or extension or rupture into the pleural, pulmonary, or pericardial cavities.

Amebic Liver Abscess

INCIDENCE. In developed countries, such as the United States, liver abscess is most commonly of bacterial origin. In contrast, amebic liver abscess predominates in areas of the world in which sanitation is poor and is a relatively common disorder in some countries. For example, over 2000 cases of amebic liver abscess were treated during a 20-year period at a single medical unit in South Africa. The factor(s) that predispose to liver abscess in a patient with intestinal amebiasis are unknown. A more general discussion of amebiasis is found in Ch. 385.

CLINICAL MANIFESTATIONS. The clinical and laboratory features of amebic liver abscess are very similar to those of a pyogenic liver abscess. Approximately 10 per cent of patients have symptoms of more than two weeks' duration, and occasionally symptoms have been present for months. While fever and leukocytosis are typical features of an amebic abscess, very high fever and a leukocyte count in excess of 20,000 per cubic millimeter may represent clues to secondary bacterial infection. Less than one half of patients have a history of recent diarrhea suggestive of intestinal amebiasis, and *E. histolytica* are identified in the stool of only one third of patients with an abscess. Extension of the abscess into the pleural space commonly causes cough, dyspnea, pleurisy, or even symptoms of a bronchohepatic fistula. Overall, extension or rupture into the pleural, pericardial, or peritoneal cavity occurs in up to 10 per cent of patients. Rupture into the pericardial or peritoneal cavities is particularly frequent with abscesses in the left lobe.

DIAGNOSIS. Routine laboratory studies, chest roentgenogram, radionuclide scan, ultrasound examination, and computed tomography reveal abnormalities very similar to those of pyogenic abscess. Although amebic abscesses are most commonly solitary and located in the right lobe, they may be multiple and can occur in other locations.

Serologic testing is extremely valuable in the diagnosis of amebic liver abscess. Indirect hemagglutination, the standard test performed by the Parasitology Division of the Centers for Disease Control in Atlanta, is positive in more than 90 per cent of patients with amebic liver abscess, and antibody titers remain elevated for many years. The gel diffusion precipitin test, which is available in most state laboratories and many local hospitals, is similarly positive in more than 90 per cent of cases, but reverts to negative in most patients within one year after successful treatment. This fact can be an advantage in distinguishing active disease from past infection. Recent reports suggest that immunoassay for *E. histolytica* antigens in serum may prove valuable in the diagnosis of acute infection, but these reports will require confirmation.

TREATMENT. For patients with an amebic abscess, medical therapy alone is usually sufficient. Metronidazole (750 mg three times daily for ten days) is the drug of choice, and some authorities recommend that an intestinal amebicide such as diiodohydroxyquin (650 mg three times daily for 20 days) be given in addition. Chloroquine (500 mg daily for 10 weeks) is reportedly equally effective, but the long duration of treatment and lack of efficacy against intestinal amebae render it less desirable. A variety of alternative regimens also exist (see Ch. 385). Most patients report rapid symptomatic improvement after both forms of therapy and are afebrile by the end of the first week. However, since metronidazole is also effective against anaerobic bacteria present in pyogenic liver abscesses, a favorable therapeutic response to this agent cannot, by itself, be considered proof of an amebic versus a pyogenic abscess. Rare treatment failures have been reported, and it is particularly important in such cases to make sure that any concomitant intestinal infection has been eradicated. The role of needle aspiration in the treatment of amebic abscess is controversial. Some advocate it routinely and report excellent results; however, there are no controlled studies to support the therapeutic value of aspiration, and most patients recover with medical therapy alone. Aspiration should be undertaken only by skilled personnel, after appropriate medical therapy has been begun, and is probably most appropriate for patients with impending rupture as evidenced by increasing pleural or pericardial reaction or progressive hepatic enlargement, particularly with abscesses in the left lobe. Surgery is rarely necessary.

PROGNOSIS. The prognosis in uncomplicated amebic abscess is excellent with appropriate medical therapy, the mortality being as low as 1 per cent in some series. With extension or rupture into the pleural, pericardial, or peritoneal space, the mortality increases sharply. Even after successful treatment, resolution of the radionuclide scan defect caused by an amebic abscess may require many months.

GRANULOMATOUS DISEASE OF THE LIVER

ETIOLOGY. The liver is one of the most frequent sites in the body for granuloma formation. By virtue of its large number of mononuclear phagocytic cells and strategic location, the liver clears the circulation of many substances, including microorganisms, antigens, and immune complexes. In addition, the liver is the major site of metabolism of many drugs and toxins. These factors help account for the 2 to 10 per cent incidence of granulomas found in liver biopsies.

Hepatic granulomas have been reported in association with a wide variety of infectious and other systemic illnesses, hepatobiliary disorders, and drugs or exogenous agents (Table 123–2). Since granulomas are not a rare finding in liver biopsy material, it is possible that many of the reported associations, including some of those listed in Table 123–2, are spurious. For example, granulomas have been reported in association with viral hepatitis, fatty liver, and alcoholic cirrhosis. However, granulomas are distinctly unusual in these disorders, and a second unrecognized process was likely to have been present in reported cases. These disorders have therefore been excluded from Table 123–2.

PATHOLOGY. Granulomas in the liver, as elsewhere, consist of a compact collection of mature mononuclear phagocytes. In well developed granulomas, these phagocytic cells take the form of epithelioid cells. Giant cells and necrosis are frequent additional features, but their presence is not necessary for the pathologic diagnosis of granuloma. Although the morphologic features of the granuloma itself are seldom characteristic enough to permit a determination of etiology, this is occasionally possible (e.g., acid-fast bacilli in tuberculosis, ova in schistosomiasis, larvae in toxocariasis, fibrinoid ring plus central clear space in Q fever, birefringent granules in starch granuloma or in foreign substance injection as with parenteral drug abuse). The location of the granuloma or the presence of coexisting parenchymal liver disease may also be helpful, as in granulomatous arteritis and primary biliary cirrhosis.

CLINICAL MANIFESTATIONS. The predominant clinical manifestations are generally those of the underlying disorder. In many of the entities listed in Table 123–2, hepatic dysfunction either is not detectable or constitutes a minor component of the illness. Hepatomegaly is present in more than one half of all patients, whereas splenomegaly is less frequent. In the absence of a primary hepatobiliary disorder, peripheral stigmata (vascular spiders, palmar erythema) and complications (portal hypertension, ascites, encephalopathy) of chronic liver disease are uncommon. Overall, serum alkaline phosphatase and transaminase are mildly to moderately elevated in up to two thirds of patients, and hyperbilirubinemia occurs in approximately one quarter of the cases. However, these generalizations do not apply to many individual cases. For example, portal hypertension is a frequent complication of schistosomiasis, and certain patients with sarcoidosis have striking cholestasis and jaundice.

TABLE 123–2. HEPATIC GRANULOMAS (REPORTED ASSOCIATIONS)

Infections	*Hepatobiliary disorders*
Bacterial, mycobacterial, spirochetal	Primary biliary cirrhosis
Tuberculosis	Chronic active hepatitis
Atypical mycobacteria	Granulomatous hepatitis
Tularemia	Jejunoileal bypass
Brucellosis	*Systemic disorders*
Leprosy	Sarcoidosis
Typhoid fever	Wegener's granulomatosis
Granuloma inguinale	Vineyard sprayer's lung
Syphilis	Inflammatory bowel disease
Whipple's disease	Chronic granulomatous disease
Listeriosis	Allergic granulomatosis
Melioidosis	Granulomatous arteritis-polymyalgia rheumatica
BCG immunotherapy	Melanoma
Viral	Hodgkin's disease
Infectious mononucleosis	Lymphoma
Cytomegalovirus	*Exogenous agents*
Chickenpox	Phenylbutazone
Influenza B	Alpha-methyldopa
Lymphogranuloma venereum	Sulfonamides
Rickettsial	Carbamazepine
Q fever	Hydralazine
Fungal	Procainamide
Coccidioidomycosis	Quinidine
Histoplasmosis	Allopurinol
Cryptococcosis	Phenytoin
Actinomycosis	Halothane
Blastomycosis	Penicillin
Aspergillosis	Nitrofurantoin
Nocardiosis	Chlorpromazine
Torulopsosis	Chlorpropamide
Candidiasis	Clofibrate
Parasitic	Oral contraceptives
Amebiasis	Beryllium
Giardiasis	Copper sulfate
Schistosomiasis	Parenteral foreign material (starch, talc, silicon, etc.)
Clonorchiasis	
Fasciolasis	
Toxocariasis	
Ascariasis	
Toxoplasmosis	
Strongyloidiasis	
Ancyclostomiasis	
Tongue worm (pentastomida)	

DIAGNOSIS. Because hepatic granulomas are associated with a variety of disorders, many of which are infrequently encountered in clinical practice, the differential diagnosis of granulomatous disease of the liver is one of the most challenging problems in medicine. The histopathologic features and location of the granuloma(s) seldom indicate the etiology, and cultures of the biopsy specimen are usually negative. For example, acid-fast bacilli are demonstrable by appropriate stains in about 10 per cent of biopsies from patients with tuberculosis, and culture is also infrequently positive. In most cases, the finding of hepatic granulomas serves mainly to direct attention to the broad class of diseases known to cause a granulomatous response in the liver, and the specific diagnosis depends on cultures and/or biopsies from other sites, serologic tests, or skin tests.

The workup should begin with a careful interview, probing previous illnesses, travel, occupational and environmental exposures, and drug use or abuse. Physical examination should include careful inspection of the skin and palpation of lymph nodes. A chest roentgenogram is valuable in detecting sarcoidosis and tuberculosis as well as certain fungal diseases. Serial thin sections of the biopsy material with special stains should be obtained to increase the likelihood of detecting acid-fast bacilli, fungi, ova, or foreign material. Bacterial, mycobacterial, and fungal cultures of the biopsy material as well as blood and possibly bone marrow should be obtained when the biopsy is performed as part of an investigation of fever. The appropriateness of additional tests, cultures, and biopsies depends upon the individual clinical circumstances. Despite a thorough search, a satisfactory cause for the granuloma(s) is not discovered in 20 per cent or more of cases. Such patients in whom no satisfactory explanation for the hepatic granulomas can be found and who have fever of unknown origin have been designated as having *granulomatous hepatitis.* The existence of granulomatous hepatitis as an entity distinct from sarcoidosis has been disputed.

TREATMENT AND PROGNOSIS. The treatment is that of the underlying disorder. When the underlying disorder can be successfully treated or an offending drug or exposure terminated, clinical and biochemical evidence of liver dysfunction typically disappears. The granulomas themselves, however, may persist for a variable length of time, depending on the rapidity with which the inciting agent is mobilized. Patients with granulomatous hepatitis have generally responded favorably to administration of corticosteroids. However, this approach should not be undertaken unless a thorough search has failed to reveal a cause for the granulomas and generally unless a trial of antituberculous therapy has failed.

Berger LA, Osborne DR: Treatment of pyogenic liver abscesses by percutaneous needle aspiration. Lancet 1:132, 1982. Herbert DA, Rothman J, Simmons F, Fogel DA, Wilson S, Ruskin J: Pyogenic liver abscesses: Successful nonsurgical therapy. Lancet 1:134, 1982. *These two articles summarize the results in 25 patients treated nonoperatively.*

Drugs for parasitic infections. Med Letter 24:5, 1982. *A recent, concise summary of this topic.*

Harrington PI, Gutierrez JJ, Ramirez-Ronda CH, Quinones-Soto R, Bermudez RH, Chaffey J: Granulomatous hepatitis. Rev Infect Dis 4:638, 1982. *An exhaustively referenced and thorough review of the disorders associated with hepatic granulomas.*

Patterson M, Healy GR, Shabot JM: Serologic testing for amoebiasis. Gastroenterology 78:136, 1980. *A practical guide to the use of serologic tests in the diagnosis of intestinal and hepatic amebic infection.*

Peters RS, Gitlin N, Libke RD: Amebic liver abscess. Ann Rev Med 32:161, 1981. *A concise review of amebic liver abscess, with a practical clinical orientation.*

124. INHERITED, INFILTRATIVE, AND METABOLIC DISORDERS INVOLVING THE LIVER

Bruce F. Scharschmidt

The liver is involved in a variety of inherited, infiltrative, and metabolic disorders. Most of the disorders included in this chapter, e.g., Wilson's disease, hemochromatosis, the glycogen and lipid storage diseases, and amyloidosis, are discussed here only with respect to their hepatic involvement. A more comprehensive treatment of these entities can be found elsewhere in this textbook.

ALPHA$_1$-ANTITRYPSIN DEFICIENCY

Alpha$_1$-antitrypsin (A_1AT) deficiency is an inherited disorder associated with a decreased concentration of A_1AT in serum (see Ch. 60). This glycoprotein, which is found in other body fluids as well as in serum, inhibits a variety of proteolytic enzymes, including pancreatic trypsin, chymotrypsin, and elastase, as well as certain proteases produced by leukocytes and macrophages. It is normally present in a concentration of about 200 mg per deciliter in serum, where it accounts for 90 per cent of total antitrypsin activity and a major portion of the alpha-1-globulin fraction. A_1AT production is controlled by codominant alleles, and more than 25 different alleles have been identified by starch gel electrophoresis of serum. The most common allele at the P_i (protease inhibitor) locus is termed M (allele frequency 0.94 to 0.95 in the United States). The most important variant is Z, since P_iZZ accounts for virtually all patients with severe A_1AT deficiency. The liver plays a critical role in the pathophysiology of the disorder, as evidenced by the observation that A_1AT levels return to normal after liver transplantation and the P_i phenotype converts to that of the donor.

Severe A_1AT deficiency is associated with early-onset emphysema in some individuals, liver disease in others, and occasionally both liver and lung disease. The pathogenesis of the disorder is unclear, because only about 10 per cent of individuals with P_iZZ phenotype develop overt liver disease in childhood. The deficiency state, by itself, is not sufficient to produce disease. Liver disease related to A_1AT deficiency typically presents with signs and symptoms of cholestasis in the first few days to weeks of life. In a minority of infants, cholestasis persists or worsens and is associated with liver failure and death in a few years. Cholestasis typically remits by six months in the remaining patients, about half of whom nevertheless develop cirrhosis. The long-term prognosis for these children is uncertain. An as yet undefined proportion of infants with P_iZZ phenotype who do not develop neonatal cholestasis have also been shown to have elevated transaminase levels in serum and fibrosis or cirrhosis on liver biopsy. The importance of A_1AT deficiency as a cause of liver disease in adults is less clear. Severe deficiency, P_iZZ phenotype, is probably associated with an increased incidence of cirrhosis in adults, and several studies suggest that heterozygous A_1AT deficiency phenotypes MZ and SZ may account for some cases of chronic active hepatitis or cryptogenic cirrhosis. A_1AT deficiency may also predispose to the development of hepatocellular carcinoma.

The diagnosis of A_1AT deficiency can be suspected from serum protein electrophoresis and confirmed by measurement of A_1AT in serum either as trypsin inhibitory activity or by immunoassay. However, definitive diagnosis requires determination of protease inhibitor phenotype by electrophoresis. This is particularly true of individuals with heterozygous A_1AT deficiency who may have serum levels of A_1AT in the low normal range. Patients with the Z allele also exhibit characteristic rounded eosinophilic cytoplasmic inclusions in periportal hepatocytes. These inclusion bodies are immunologically related to A_1AT but differ in certain amino acids as well as in their content of sialic acid and other sugars. Importantly, such eosinophilic inclusions have been recently described as an apparently acquired defect in patients with alcoholic liver disease and are thus not diagnostic of inherited A_1AT deficiency. There is currently no specific therapy for this disorder; however, a number of patients have successfully undergone transplantation.

WILSON'S DISEASE

Wilson's disease is an autosomal recessive disorder with a prevalence worldwide of about 1 in 30,000 (see Ch. 205). Its clinical and pathologic manifestations result from excessive accumulation of copper in many tissues, including the brain, liver, cornea, and kidneys. Although the primary genetic defect remains undetermined, impaired biliary copper excretion rather than enhanced absorption is the cause of the copper accumulation. Unfortunately, the diagnosis of this treatable disorder is often missed or delayed because of its rarity and diverse presentations. Hepatic disease is a common initial clinical manifestation in childhood and adolescence and may take the form of a self-limited illness resembling viral hepatitis, fulminant hepatic failure, or chronic active hepatitis. A majority of patients with fulminant hepatic failure die despite initiation of D-penicillamine therapy. Rarely, Wilson's disease may present as an hepatic disorder in later life. More commonly, however, adults with Wilson's disease have prominent neurologic dysfunction, and hepatic disease, although invariably present on biopsy, does not dominate the clinical picture. The diagnosis and treatment of Wilson's disease are discussed in detail in Ch. 205; however, certain points merit special emphasis here. First, while the combination of an abnormally low ceruloplasmin level in serum and Kayser-Fleischer rings establishes the diagnosis, about 15 per cent of patients having Wilson's disease presenting with hepatic manifestations have serum ceruloplasmin concentrations in the low normal range and about one half of patients who seek medical help with chronic active hepatitis or fulminant hepatic failure have not yet developed Kayser-Fleischer rings. If the diagnosis of Wilson's disease is uncertain, a biopsy should be performed for quantitative copper determination. If coagulation abnormalities preclude a biopsy, measurement of incorporation of orally administered radiolabeled copper into ceruloplasmin or measurement of serum copper or urinary copper excretion may be useful.

HEMOCHROMATOSIS

Hemochromatosis is among the more common genetic disorders, with a calculated homozygous frequency of about 1 in 300 to 1 in 400 in certain high prevalence areas. Although the molecular basis of the underlying defect responsible for enhanced intestinal iron absorption remains undetermined, recent genetic studies have clarified the phenotypic expression of this disease. Persons homozygous for the hemochromatosis allele, which is in close linkage with HLA-A3 on chromosome 6, show progressive accumulation of hepatic iron and usually develop clinical evidence of disease in the fourth, fifth, or sixth decades of life. Heterozygotes may also show abnormal accumulation of hepatic iron, but the absolute amounts present are much less than in homozygotes and clinical evidence of iron overload rarely develops.

Hepatic iron overload is most commonly manifested as moderate to marked hepatomegaly with initially well preserved liver function. Esophageal varices, ascites, and impaired hepatic synthetic function are present in more advanced cases. Other important clinical features include abnormal skin pigmentation, glucose intolerance, cardiac involvement, hypogonadism, and arthropathy. Hepatocellular carcinoma develops in up to one third of patients. With appropriate phlebotomy therapy hepatic function frequently improves, and there are case reports that suggest regression of apparent cirrhosis.

Screening for hemochromatosis is probably best accomplished by measurement of transferrin saturation and serum ferritin. A saturation exceeding 50 per cent is present in nearly all homozygotes over 20 years of age, and a value less than 50 per cent largely precludes the diagnosis. However, the positive predictive value of a transferrin saturation exceeding 50 per cent is relatively low. In contrast, a transferrin saturation exceeding 80 per cent is a much more reliable indicator of hemochromatosis. Serum levels of ferritin are a generally accurate reflection of tissue iron stores and exceed 1000 ng per ml in most patients. However, occasional families with hemochromatosis and normal serum ferritin levels have been described and, conversely, serum ferritin is typically elevated out of proportion to tissue iron stores in patients with hepatocellular necrosis. If either of these tests suggests iron overload, liver biopsy with quantitative iron determination and histochemical stains for iron should be performed. A variety of noninvasive methods for measurement of hepatic iron have been proposed for use in patients who cannot undergo a liver biopsy, including dual-energy computed tomographic scanning, nuclear magnetic resonance, and magnetic susceptibility measurement. Clinical experience with these techniques is as yet limited. Hemochromatosis is discussed in detail in Ch. 206.

STORAGE DISEASES

The glycogen storage diseases may present as disorders of the liver as well as of the heart and musculoskeletal system. Hepatomegaly is a prominent feature of most of these disorders, whereas splenomegaly is found primarily in Type IV and less commonly in Type III. Patients with Types I and III glycogen storage disease frequently survive childhood and may be encountered by the physician treating adults. Portacaval anastomosis may improve growth and reverse certain metabolic abnormalities in selected Type I patients, although the mechanism for these beneficial effects is uncertain. The glycogen storage diseases are discussed in detail in Ch. 179. In addition to glycogen, the liver abnormally stores fatty acids, cholesterol, or complex lipids in the lipid storage disorders as well as various mucopolysaccharides and mucolipids. Although hepatomegaly is common to most of these disorders, the clinical consequences are attributable largely to involvement of the nervous and musculoskeletal systems.

PROTOPORPHYRIA

Protoporphyria is a disorder characterized by increased protoporphyrin content in erythrocytes, plasma, feces, and liver. It is inherited as an autosomal dominant and results from a deficiency of heme synthase (ferrochelatase), the enzyme that catalyzes the formation of heme from protoporphyrin and iron. It is most conveniently diagnosed by demonstrating an elevated level of erythrocyte protoporphyrin. Protoporphyria is usually a mild disorder manifested by photosensitivity and, rarely, hemolysis. Hepatobiliary complications include pigment gallstones and infrequent hepatic failure. To date, about 18 cases of hepatic failure associated with protoporphyria have been reported. The hepatic failure, typically heralded by cholestasis, is associated with and presumably results from massive hepatic accumulation of birefringent crystals of protoporphyrin. Interruption of the enterohepatic circulation of protoporphyrin with cholestyramine or activated charcoal was reported to deplete hepatic protoporphyrin deposits and restore liver function to normal in three patients with mild disease, but it is unlikely that such treatment would be helpful in patients with severe cholestasis and established hepatic failure. At present, there is no way of identifying the small proportion of patients with protoporphyria who will develop significant hepatic disease.

CYSTIC FIBROSIS

In infants with cystic fibrosis, amorphous-eosinophilic material in bile ducts and ductules, presumably representing inspissated secretions, may produce cholestasis (see Ch. 64). Later manifestations include cholangitis, fibrosis, and obstructive biliary cirrhosis. Up to 20 per cent of patients who survive to adolescence have cirrhosis with portal hypertension, and bleeding from esophageal varices represents a significant cause of morbidity in this older age group. The mortality of shunt surgery in these patients is high, but long-term survivors are reported. Since liver disease with portal hypertension has even been reported as a first manifestation of cystic fibrosis, the diagnosis should be considered in a young patient with otherwise unexplained liver disease.

AMYLOIDOSIS

Amyloid deposition in the liver is common in amyloidosis of all types (see Ch. 163). Hepatomegaly is present in approximately one half of patients with systemic amyloidosis, splenomegaly is present in about 10 per cent of patients, and mild elevation of the serum alkaline phosphatase is the most common biochemical abnormality. Cutaneous stigmata of chronic liver disease (e.g., spider angiomas, palmar erythema) and portal hypertension are unusual. Intrahepatic cholestasis with marked elevation of the serum bilirubin and alkaline phosphatase concentrations occurs in about 5 per cent of patients. Although early case reports suggested that percutaneous liver biopsy was particularly hazardous in patients with amyloidosis, subsequent experience with current biopsy techniques has failed to demonstrate excessive risk. However, the diagnosis of amyloidosis can usually be established without resorting to liver biopsy.

SARCOIDOSIS

Hepatic involvement in sarcoidosis represents a continuum from the presence of asymptomatic granulomas to cases in which hepatic involvement represents a prominent part of the overall clinical picture (see Ch. 67). Approximately two thirds to three quarters of patients with sarcoidosis have demonstrable hepatic granuloma, making the liver one of the most commonly involved organs in this disease. These figures, however, may be artificially high, since they are derived in part from autopsy studies of patients with extensive disease and from patient series in which the diagnosis was established by liver biopsy. Nonetheless, liver biopsy is often of value in establishing the diagnosis of sarcoidosis.

About 20 per cent of patients with sarcoidosis have hepatomegaly, and up to 40 per cent have abnormal liver function tests, most commonly a mild elevation of the alkaline phosphatase. Overt hepatic involvement is present in fewer than 20 per cent of patients. This may take several forms, including (1) hepatomegaly, generally with splenomegaly, and multiple abnormal liver function tests; (2) chronic cholestasis, which may closely mimic primary biliary cirrhosis; and (3) portal hypertension and its manifestations. The characteristic histologic feature of hepatic sarcoidosis is the presence of granulomas, frequently located in portal tracts. Chronic portal tract inflammation, hepatocyte poikilocytosis and anisocytosis, fibrosis, and even cirrhosis may be accompanying findings. Little information is available regarding the response of these hepatic lesions to corticosteroids, but a therapeutic trial can be justified if significant symptoms are present and tuberculosis and other disorders producing hepatic granuloma have been excluded.

ENTERIC BYPASS

Hepatic disease related to enteric bypass surgery has typically been reported in patients who have had extensive bypass procedures for treatment of marked obesity. Jejunocolic bypass, an early operation, has now largely been abandoned because of a high incidence of complications, including cirrhosis and hepatic failure. The jejunoileal bypass procedure is less frequently associated with life-threatening liver disease. Hepatic abnormalities are nevertheless common following even jejunoileal bypass and may take several forms. The most common is simple fatty change. Fatty change is present in up to two thirds of markedly obese patients prior to bypass surgery, and hepatic lipid content increases during the period of weight loss. Fatty change in some patients is accompanied by fibrosis. Cirrhosis ensues in up to 5 per cent of patients, and death from liver failure accounts for a substantial proportion of the early postoperative mortality of 2 to 4 per cent. Liver disease may occur more frequently among older patients undergoing intestinal bypass and among patients who exhibit the greatest degree of weight loss. Histologic features are similar to those of alcoholic liver disease, including the presence of alcoholic hyaline. Longer term follow-up studies suggest that hepatic abnormalities may not appear until several years after surgery in some patients.

The pathogenesis of these hepatic changes is unclear. Weight loss itself does not account for the progressive postoperative fat accumulation, since this does not occur in nonoperated obese patients who lose weight through dietary measures. However, hepatic disease resembling alcoholic hepatitis and even cirrhosis have been described in abstinent patients with obesity who have not undergone bypass surgery. Protein depletion, leading to a kwashiorkor-like state, may contribute to the fatty change. Increased production in the gut of potentially toxic substances may also play a role. For example, increased delivery of chenodeoxycholate to the colon results in increased production of the potentially hepatotoxic bile salt lithocholate. The bypassed segment may also serve as a site for bacterial overgrowth and production of potentially toxic bacterial products.

Laboratory studies of hepatic function are frequently abnormal in the first few postoperative months following bypass surgery even in the absence of serious liver disease. Conversely, the absence of abnormal hepatic function tests or clinical evidence of liver disease during the first postoperative year does not preclude the possible later development of significant liver disease. Deterioration of synthetic or excretory function as evidenced by an abnormal prothrombin time that does not respond to vitamin K administration, hypoalbuminemia, or hyperbilirubinemia is an ominous sign. Biopsy is the only reliable way of assessing the severity of hepatic disease, and some advocate follow-up biopsies in all patients. Certain patients seem to respond favorably to oral or parenteral administration of amino acid solutions. Serious and persistent hepatic disease is an indication for re-establishing normal bowel continuity. Gastroplasty may be preferred in many obese patients as a way of achieving weight loss. It is technically demanding but is only rarely associated with the many metabolic complications, including liver disease, that follow jejunoileal bypass.

INFLAMMATORY BOWEL DISEASE

Liver function tests may be transiently abnormal in up to one half of patients with chronic ulcerative colitis and Crohn's disease, but clinically significant liver disease is much less common. A variety of histologic abnormalities have been described in patients with inflammatory bowel disease, but accurate estimates of their prevalence are not available. *Pericholangitis,* defined as portal tract inflammation with or without periductular fibrosis, has been found in 5 to 30 per cent of biopsies. It is often asymptomatic and follows a benign course but has been associated with jaundice in some instances. Direct cholangiography has revealed sclerosing cholangitis in a substantial proportion of patients with pericholangitis, suggesting that these two disorders may be part of the same disease spectrum (see Ch. 104). Other histologic findings have included fatty change, chronic hepatitis, cirrhosis (1 to 5 per cent of cases), amyloidosis, and the presence of granulomas. Portal bacteremia or other toxins in portal blood have been implicated in the pathogenesis of pericholangitis. However, the precise relationship of pericholangitis and other lesions to the underlying bowel disease is unclear. The differential diagnosis of jaundice in the setting of inflammatory bowel disease also includes gallstones, bile duct carcinoma, sclerosing cholangitis, and/or pericholangitis.

No specific therapy is available for these hepatic abnormalities. Treatment should be directed at the underlying bowel disease, although this does not reliably produce improvement in the hepatic disorder. Progression of serious liver disease in ulcerative colitis has been reported to be halted by colectomy in some patients; however, progression of hepatic disease has been observed in other patients following colectomy, so this approach cannot be generally recommended.

TOTAL PARENTERAL NUTRITION

Total parenteral nutrition has been associated with hepatomegaly, mild to moderate elevation of alkaline phosphatase, generally minimal transaminase elevation, and occasionally jaundice. Liver biopsy in these patients has frequently revealed fatty change, cholestasis, and mild periportal inflammation. Some of these abnormalities have been due to the underlying disease or complicating infection, but total parenteral nutrition, by itself, can produce elevated serum bile salt levels and occasionally hyperbilirubinemia in both infants and adults. The degree of abnormality appears related to the duration and amount of parenteral alimentation. Hepatic function generally returns to normal when total parenteral nutrition is discontinued, although elevation of the alkaline phosphatase may persist for several weeks. Modifying the infusate by lowering the calorie-to-nitrogen ratio or decreasing the total caloric intake has also been reported to reverse the hepatic abnormalities. Total parenteral nutrition also appears to predispose patients to the development of gallstones and cholecystitis, and these possibilities should be kept in mind when evaluating a patient receiving parenteral nutrition for hepatobiliary disease.

PREGNANCY

Liver size, liver function tests, and liver histology remain normal during uncomplicated pregnancy. The increased concentrations of alkaline phosphatase that typically occur in the second and third trimesters are usually of placental origin. *Hyperemesis gravidarum* of sufficient severity to require hospitalization may be accompanied by minor abnormalities in standard liver function tests. Focal hepatic necrosis, hemorrhage, and occasionally liver rupture are findings in women dying from *eclampsia. Acute fatty liver of pregnancy* can be defined as a syndrome of acute hepatic dysfunction that develops in late pregnancy, is associated with microvesicular fat accumulation in hepatocytes, and resolves with delivery. It typically becomes apparent after the 30th week of gestation and is manifested initially by constitutional symptoms, often with abdominal pain, followed in many instances by overt evidence of hepatic failure including encephalopathy and jaundice. In the past, intravenous tetracycline therapy was incriminated in some cases, but this is rarely true at present. The only known treatment is termination of the pregnancy. Earlier reports suggested that the disorder was associated with a very high mortality rate, but more recent reports suggest that there is a spectrum of disease severity and that milder cases without frank hepatic failure occur and have a favorable prognosis. It also appears that acute fatty liver may, at least in some instances, fall within the spectrum of hepatic dysfunction associated with pre-eclampsia or eclampsia, as these two disorders occasionally share certain features including onset in late pregnancy, increased incidence in young primiparas, the presence of coagulopathy, hypertension, and proteinuria, and resolution upon delivery. *Cholestasis of pregnancy* generally occurs in the last four months of gestation (range 7 to 39 weeks). It is characterized by pruritus sometimes followed by jaundice. It typically resolves within two weeks of delivery, and frequently recurs in subsequent pregnancies or with administration of oral contraceptives. Serum alkaline phosphatase and bile salts are increased, and hyperbilirubinemia may be present. Serum transaminase is also frequently mildly elevated. Although generally considered a benign condition, cholestasis of pregnancy has been associated with an increased incidence of premature labor and postpartum hemorrhage.

CIRCULATORY DISTURBANCE

Hepatic function and histology are commonly altered in patients with cardiovascular disease. Disorders associated with an elevation of systemic venous pressure typically produce hepatic venous congestion manifested by hepatomegaly, minor abnormalities of liver function tests, and centrolobular congestion without necrosis; occasionally it can also cause marked hepatic tenderness, cholestasis, and/or hepatocellular necrosis with striking transaminase elevation. Longstanding hepatic congestion may lead to cardiac cirrhosis with fibrous bands joining centrilobular areas (see Ch. 125). When hypotension is superimposed, even transiently, on hepatic congestion, severe centrilobular necrosis, transaminase levels exceeding 1000 units, marked hyperbilirubinemia, and hypoprothrombinemia may result. Associated clinical features closely mimic those of viral hepatitis. Differentiating this disorder from viral hepatitis may be particularly difficult, since hepatic dysfunction often does not become obvious until several days after the resolution of the circulatory failure. Unlike viral hepatitis, however, serum transaminase levels frequently fall very rapidly and may approach normal within days. If the circulatory insult is brief, patients usually recover from their hepatic injury uneventfully. Fatal fulminant hepatic failure has been reported, however. A similar form of acute hepatic injury is occasionally seen in persons without pre-existing cardiovascular disease who suffer severe or prolonged hypotension, or in patients with severe isolated left heart failure.

Alagille D: α-1-Antitrypsin deficiency. Hepatology, 4:11S, Jan-Feb Suppl. 1984. *A concise review of the clinical course of 45 children with neonatal cholestasis and A_1AT deficiency.*

Gollan JL: Diagnosis of hemochromatosis. Gastroenterology 84:418, 1983. *A concise and well-referenced summary of diagnostic tests for hemochromatosis.*

Hocking MP, Duerson MC, O'Leary P, Woodward ER: Jejunoileal bypass for morbid obesity. Late follow-up in 100 cases. N Engl J Med 308:995, 1983. *A summary of complications in patients with intact bypasses followed for more than five years.*

McCullough AJ, Fleming CR, Thistle JL, Balebus WP, Ludwig JT, Dickson ER: Diagnosis of Wilson's disease presenting as fulminant hepatic failure. Gastroenterology 84:161, 1983. *This article summarizes the clinical features of this presentation of Wilson's disease and the value of various tests other than liver biopsy in making the diagnosis.*

Steven MM: Pregnancy and liver disease. Gut 22:592, 1981. *A thoroughly referenced review of this topic.*

Zakim D, Boyer TD: Hepatology. Philadelphia, W. B. Saunders Company, 1982. *Consult chapters 12, 33, 42, 43, 44, and 48 for current, authoritative, and well-referenced reviews of the disorders discussed briefly in this chapter.*

125. CIRRHOSIS OF THE LIVER

Thomas D. Boyer

GENERAL CONSIDERATIONS. Cirrhosis is an irreversible alteration of the liver architecture, consisting of hepatic fibrosis and areas of nodular regeneration. When the nodules are small (less than 3 mm), uniform, and encompass one lobule, the term micronodular or unilobular cirrhosis is applied. In macronodular or multilobular cirrhosis the nodules exceed 3 mm, vary in size, and encompass more than one lobule. Frequently, features of both micro- and macronodular cirrhosis are present in the same liver. Etiologic diagnosis may be impossible from the gross and microscopic appearance of the cirrhotic liver and must therefore be based on history, physical examination, biochemical and serologic tests, and histochemical stains. The causes of cirrhosis are listed in Table 125–1.

Patients with cirrhosis may have one of two general types of manifestations: (1) signs or symptoms related to hepatocellular necrosis, which are similar to those of acute hepatitis and include jaundice, nausea and vomiting, and tender hepatomegaly; or (2) signs or symptoms of the complications of cirrhosis, which are largely due to the rise in intrahepatic vascular resistance that leads to portal hypertension and its complications (ascites, formation of portal-systemic collaterals, encephalopathy, splenomegaly, and bleeding esophageal and gastric varices). Other, less specific manifestations of cirrhosis include gynecomastia, spider angiomas, parotid hypertrophy, and testicular atrophy. Patients frequently present a mixed picture with features of both hepatocellular necrosis and portal hypertension.

Since agents that cause cirrhosis may have systemic effects as well, extrahepatic features may dominate the clinical picture with little or no evidence of liver disease. For example, patients with alcoholic liver disease frequently have complaints referable to the central nervous system, peripheral nerves, heart, muscles, and gastrointestinal tract. Patients with diseases such as primary biliary cirrhosis may have prominent eye and skin disorders. Patients with hemochromatosis may present with diabetes mellitus or arthritis, and patients with Wilson's disease, with central nervous system dysfunction, before liver disease becomes apparent. Thus, cirrhosis is frequently a subclinical illness, and a high index of suspicion may be necessary to establish a correct diagnosis.

ALCOHOLIC LIVER DISEASE

DEFINITION AND INCIDENCE. Alcoholic liver disease is a serious sequela of the chronic abuse of ethanol. There are three histopathologic lesions associated with ethanol abuse: *fatty liver, alcoholic hepatitis,* and *cirrhosis.* Alcohol is the most common

TABLE 125–1. CAUSES OF CIRRHOSIS

Drugs and toxins
Alcohol
Methyldopa
Methotrexate
Isoniazid
Perhexiline maleate
Oxyphenisatin
Infections
Hepatitis B and non-A non-B
Syphilis (tertiary)
Biliary obstruction
Carcinoma (pancreatic or bile duct)
Chronic pancreatitis
Common duct stones
Strictures
Cystic fibrosis
Biliary atresia
Metabolic
Wilson's disease
Hemochromatosis
Pediatric—α_1-antitrypsin deficiency, galactosemia, hereditary fructose intolerance, glycogen storage disease Type IV, tyrosinosis
Cardiovascular
Chronic right heart failure
Budd-Chiari syndrome
Veno-occlusive disease
Miscellaneous
Chronic active hepatitis
Primary biliary cirrhosis
Sarcoidosis
Indian childhood cirrhosis
Jejunoileal bypass
Neonatal hepatitis
Cryptogenic

cause of liver disease in the Western world, and alcoholic cirrhosis is discovered at from 1.6 to 9.9 per cent of all necropsies in the United States. The peak incidence is in patients 40 to 55 years of age; however, patients in their twenties may be seen with advanced alcoholic liver disease. The male to female ratio is 2:1.

ETIOLOGY AND PATHOGENESIS. *The relationship between alcohol abuse and cirrhosis* is well established. Epidemiologic studies have shown that the incidence of cirrhosis and the per capita consumption of alcohol are directly related, and that countries with the greatest alcohol consumption also have the highest incidence of cirrhosis. Neither the pattern of drinking (spree versus daily) nor the type of alcoholic beverage consumed appears to be important in the genesis of liver disease. The single most important factor is the average daily consumption of ethanol. Levels of daily ethanol consumption exceeding 40 to 80 grams for 10 to 15 years are associated with an increase in the incidence of cirrhosis. Women may be more susceptible to the toxic effects of ethanol than men, and a lower daily consumption of ethanol by women may lead to cirrhosis. As the daily level of alcohol consumed rises, the time required for the development of cirrhosis is reduced.

Ethanol is an hepatotoxin. Administration of alcohol to humans or animals leads to the development of fatty liver (hepatic steatosis). The mitochondria and endoplasmic reticulum of hepatocytes are altered morphologically and functionally. Ethanol also causes lactic acidemia, hyperuricemia, and hypoglycemia. Many of the effects of ethanol reflect its metabolism, which is catalyzed primarily by the cytosolic enzyme alcohol dehydrogenase as shown:

$$\underset{\text{Ethanol}}{CH_3CH_2OH} \xrightarrow[\text{NAD}^+ \longrightarrow \text{NADH + H}^+]{\text{Alcohol dehydrogenase}} \underset{\text{Acetaldehyde}}{CH_3CHO}$$

(Other metabolic pathways via a microsomal ethanol oxidizing system or a catalase system appear to be of minor importance, except perhaps at high ethanol concentrations.) The acetaldehyde formed from ethanol is then oxidized to acetate by acetaldehyde dehydrogenase with NAD^+ as a cofactor. The limiting step in the rate of metabolism of ethanol is the availability of the cofactor NAD^+, which is converted to NADH during the aforementioned two reactions. This increased reducing potential in the cell favors the conversion of pyruvate to lactate. When blood levels of ethanol are high (more than 200 mg per deciliter), the resulting lactic acidemia decreases the clearance of urate by the kidneys and hyperuricemia develops. Recent studies suggest that at lower levels of ethanol ingestion (blood level $\leq$ 150 mg per deciliter) increased production of urate is the cause of hyperuricemia. Inhibition of gluconeogenesis and fasting hypoglycemia may also follow ethanol abuse. This is discussed further in Ch. 116. Fatty acid oxidation is impaired and the esterification of fatty acids to triglycerides is increased. These effects, together with a relative defect in lipoprotein secretion, lead to the development of a fatty liver. The metabolism of ethanol may lead to increased levels of acetaldehyde in the blood and probably within the hepatocyte. Acetaldehyde is a reactive molecule and may interact with proteins and membrane lipids, causing alterations in their structure and function, which may lead to cell injury and death.

Although the metabolic effects of ethanol are relatively well understood, the mechanism by which it causes chronic liver disease is not. There is evidence for impaired protein synthesis and secretion, mitochondrial injury, lipid peroxidation, cellular hypoxia, and cell-mediated and antibody-mediated cytotoxicity, but the relative importance of each of these in producing sustained cell injury is unknown.

Ethanol fed to animals (baboons may be an exception) receiving an otherwise balanced diet has not been shown to cause alcoholic hepatitis or cirrhosis. In addition, only 10 to 20 per cent of alcoholics and one third of baboons develop cirrhosis despite similar levels of ethanol ingestion. Thus, *genetic, nutritional,* or *environmental* factors may act in concert with ethanol to cause liver disease.

Malnutrition is a common finding in alcoholics who have both poor diet and reduced intestinal absorption of dietary nutrients. Administration of ethanol to patients with active alcoholic liver disease does not appear to impair recovery if the patients also receive a balanced, high-calorie diet. Lesions identical to those of alcoholic hepatitis may develop following jejunoileal bypass for obesity, a condition in which protein malnutrition is common. Thus, malnutrition appears to potentiate the adverse effects of alcohol. Other factors, such as simultaneous exposure to other hepatotoxins, may also be important in the genesis of liver injury; however, further investigation is required to define their role. Alcoholism and alcoholic liver disease are more common in certain populations and within families, but there is no evidence of a genetically determined abnormality in the metabolism of ethanol that renders them more susceptible to liver injury.

DIAGNOSIS. The diagnosis of alcoholic liver disease should be considered in any patient who consumes more than 40 grams of ethanol daily. Tender hepatomegaly, fever, and jaundice are suggestive of alcoholic hepatitis whereas ascites and venous collaterals suggest cirrhosis. Many patients, however, will lack any distinctive clinical features such that a firm diagnosis cannot be established without liver biopsy. In addition, up to 20 per cent of patients with clinical features of alcohol liver disease are found on liver biopsy to have another type of hepatic disorder.

PATHOLOGY, CLINICAL PRESENTATION, AND THERAPY. Alcohol causes three major pathologic lesions and clinical illnesses: *fatty liver, alcoholic hepatitis, and cirrhosis.* Each of these may occur as an isolated event, or they may be present in any combination in a single patient. Therefore, although the three lesions will be described as single entities, many patients have all three and will have a mixed clinical picture. The histologic pattern is not specific for alcohol alone but may also be found in patients with Indian childhood cirrhosis, in the livers of patients who have undergone jejunoileal bypass for obesity, or as an unusual accompaniment of obesity or diabetes mellitus. Patients treated with the vasodilator perhexiline maleate also may develop a lesion identical to alcoholic liver disease.

Fatty Liver. *Fatty liver* is the most common biopsy finding in alcoholics. The fat, either centrilobular or diffuse in location, is present in large droplets, which occupy most of the volume of the hepatocyte. Occasionally, the fat is present in small droplets, resembling the lesion of Reye's syndrome or fatty liver of pregnancy. Patients with fatty liver are usually asymptomatic, but on occasion they may have abdominal pain, icterus, or vague gastrointestinal complaints. The liver is enlarged and may be tender, but is of normal consistency. Ascites, venous collaterals, and the stigmata of chronic liver disease, if present, are not attributable to the fatty liver per se, but reflect more serious lesions. The laboratory tests are only mildly abnormal in fatty liver. Jaundice, when present, is usually mild (bilirubin below 5 mg per deciliter), although intense cholestasis occasionally develops in patients with fatty liver. The AST, if elevated, is only modestly so (less than five times normal). The serum albumin and globulin are abnormal in about 25 per cent of patients. Patients with alcoholic fatty liver alone have an excellent prognosis. Withdrawal of the alcohol leads to a rapid resolution of the clinical illness and histologic lesion (fat disappears within three to six weeks). On rare occasion, these patients die suddenly from multiple fat emboli to the lungs.

Alcoholic Hepatitis. *Alcoholic hepatitis* (acute sclerosing hyaline necrosis) is a serious sequela of alcoholism because it may lead to hepatic failure or to cirrhosis. The pathologic lesion is most severe in central areas, and consists of hepatocellular necrosis and the triad of (1) *alcoholic hyalin,* (2) *infiltration by polymorphonuclear leukocytes,* and (3) *increased intralobular connective tissue* with or without occlusion of the hepatic venules and sclerosis of terminal hepatic (central) veins. Alcoholic hyalin

(Mallory body) is an eosinophilic intracellular aggregate of proteinaceous material that is characteristically perinuclear in location. The origin of alcoholic hyalin is uncertain although it may be formed by intermediate filaments. It is present in only 30 per cent of liver biopsies in which the diagnosis of alcoholic hepatitis can be made on clinical and other histologic criteria. Alcoholic hyalin is not specific for alcoholic liver disease, since it has also been found in the livers of patients with Wilson's disease, primary biliary cirrhosis, hepatocellular carcinoma, and diabetes mellitus, as well as following jejunoileal bypass. It can also be induced in animals by feeding griseofulvin. The infiltration of polymorphonuclear leukocytes frequently is associated with foci of cell injury or is near cells that contain Mallory bodies. Central vein sclerosis may be severe enough to cause a severe outflow block and portal hypertension in the absence of cirrhosis.

The clinical features of alcoholic hepatitis encompass a broad spectrum of patients, ranging from those who are asymptomatic to those with hepatic failure. Patients commonly complain of anorexia, nausea, vomiting, abdominal pain, and weight loss. Tender hepatomegaly is present in at least 80 per cent of patients. Ascites, jaundice, fever (37.2 to 39.4° C), splenomegaly, and encephalopathy are common but not invariable. Although fever is common, bacterial infection should be excluded since such patients are at an increased risk for developing pneumonia, urinary tract infections, sepsis, and bacterial peritonitis. The AST is frequently elevated; however, the degree of elevation is modest (less than 10 times normal) and is lower than expected for the amount of hepatocellular necrosis present. The ALT may be normal and is almost always less than the AST. The AST/ALT ratio frequently exceeds two. This is in contrast to viral hepatitis, in which the AST frequently exceeds 15 to 25 times normal and the ALT is equal to or greater than the AST. Hyperbilirubinemia is common (60 to 90 per cent) in alcoholic hepatitis, and it may be marked (20 to 30 mg per deciliter). The alkaline phosphatase is usually elevated to less than three times normal, but an occasional patient has a cholestatic picture in which the alkaline phosphatase is unusually high. Prolongation of the prothrombin time, hypoalbuminemia, and hyperglobulinemia may be present. The white blood cell count frequently is elevated (>10,000) and may exceed 30,000 to 40,000 per cubic millimeter. Patients with alcoholic hepatitis may develop the hepatorenal syndrome, and a rising BUN and creatinine are poor prognostic signs.

Treatment for alcoholic hepatitis is nonspecific. Patients with alcoholic hepatitis should receive a well-balanced diet, high in calories (2500 to 3000 kcal). Protein should be included in the diets unless encephalopathy is present. Anorexia is frequent, and tube or intravenous alimentation may be necessary. There is evidence for an immunologic-mediated injury in alcoholic hepatitis; therefore, corticosteroids have been used in the treatment of these patients. The administration of prednisone has not been shown to decrease the morbidity or mortality of patients with mild to moderate disease. Use of steroids to treat patients with severe alcoholic hepatitis is controversial and cannot be recommended on the basis of available evidence. Agents such as propylthiouracil, penicillamine, and colchicine have also been used in the treatment of alcoholic hepatitis, but current information regarding the efficacy of these newer forms of therapy is insufficient to warrant usage.

The *prognosis* for patients with alcoholic hepatitis is much worse than for those with fatty liver. Some patients who stop drinking may have complete resolution of the lesion. In most patients, however, alcoholic hepatitis persists (with clinical improvement), progresses to cirrhosis, or leads to hepatic failure and death. The hospital mortality for patients with severe disease (who cannot have biopsy or who have encephalopathy) exceeds 40 per cent, whereas for those with milder disease the expected death rate is 10 per cent or less.

Alcoholic Cirrhosis. *Alcoholic cirrhosis,* although usually micronodular, can be macronodular or of a mixed type. Micronodular cirrhosis is not specific for alcoholic liver disease, as it has also been seen in other conditions. Histologically, there are dense bands of connective tissue joining portal and central areas. Scarring is most severe in the central regions, and there may be collagen deposits in the space of Disse. Nodules are usually regular in size. In addition, alcoholic hepatitis frequently coexists, as well as varying amounts of cholestasis, iron, and fat.

Clinically, cirrhosis is an asymptomatic disease in 10 to 20 per cent of patients. It is also commonly present in association with alcoholic hepatitis, and signs of acute liver injury may dominate the clinical picture. Patients may also have ascites, gastrointestinal bleeding, or encephalopathy. The liver may be large or small and usually has a firm consistency. Spider angiomas, palmar erythema, parotid enlargement, testicular atrophy and gynecomastia (men), menstrual irregularities (women), and muscle wasting are frequently found; however, these findings are not specific for alcoholic cirrhosis. Upper abdominal pain associated with bloody ascitic fluid, right upper quadrant bruit, or a friction rub over the liver suggests hepatocellular carcinoma.

The *laboratory abnormalities* present in patients with cirrhosis may be similar to those of alcoholic hepatitis. The AST is normal to mildly elevated, and bilirubin is only slightly increased unless the picture is complicated by alcoholic hepatitis, hemolysis, sepsis, hepatic failure, or carcinoma. Anemia is a common finding. The cause of the anemia is multifactorial, including blood loss, folate and pyridoxine deficiency, hemolysis, and the toxic effect of ethanol on the bone marrow. Hypersplenism or bone marrow suppression by ethanol may lead to thrombocytopenia or leukopenia. The serum sodium and potassium may be low in patients with ascites. Hypomagnesemia and hypophosphatemia are common, as is a mild respiratory alkalosis. The BUN and creatinine are increased in patients who have been treated with excessive diuretics or who are developing hepatorenal failure.

The *treatment* of alcoholic cirrhosis is also nonspecific. Deficiencies of vitamins (folate, thiamin, pyridoxine, vitamin K) and minerals (magnesium, phosphate) should be corrected. The sodium content of the diet need not be reduced unless there is sodium retention by the kidneys. Protein restriction is necessary only when there is clinical evidence of hepatic encephalopathy.

The *prognosis* for patients with alcoholic cirrhosis is dependent upon two features: presence of complications and continued abuse of alcohol. Patients without ascites, jaundice, or gastrointestinal bleeding have a better prognosis than those with these complications. Continued alcohol abuse reduces the expected five-year survival to only 40 per cent, whereas it is 60 per cent or greater in those who abstain.

Galambos J: Cirrhosis. Philadelphia, W. B. Saunders Company, 1979. *An excellent monograph that reviews cirrhosis and its complications.*

Orrego H, Israel Y, Blendis LM: Alcoholic liver disease: Information in search of knowledge. Hepatology 1:267, 1981. *A review of the possible causes of ethanol-mediated hepatic injury.*

Zakim D, Boyer TD, Montgomery C, Kanas N: Alcoholic liver disease. *In* Zakim D, Boyer TD (eds.): Hepatology: A Textbook of Liver Disease. Philadelphia, W. B. Saunders Company, 1982, p 739. *A complete review of the pathogenesis, pathology, clinical presentation, and treatment of alcoholic liver disease.*

PRIMARY BILIARY CIRRHOSIS

DEFINITION AND ETIOLOGY. Primary biliary cirrhosis is a cholestatic disorder that develops because of progressive destruction of small and intermediate-sized intrahepatic bile ducts. The extrahepatic biliary tree and larger intrahepatic bile ducts are patent. The cause of primary biliary cirrhosis is unknown. The injury to the bile ducts is thought to be on an immunologic basis, as there is a high frequency of serum autoantibodies, elevated levels of immunoglobulins (especially IgM), circulating immune complexes, and a reduced cell-mediated immune response in patients with this disease. In addition, the injured bile ducts are surrounded by lymphocytes and, on occasion, by granulomas. These findings, however, are nonspecific and do not establish the etiologic agent or agents responsible for the disease. Genetic factors may also be important, as the disease has been described in a mother and daughter, in siblings, and in twins. In addition, the incidence of positive tests for antimitochondrial antibodies in relatives of patients with primary biliary cirrhosis is increased. The high female preponderance suggests that estrogens or progesterone may be important in the pathogenesis of this disease.

PATHOLOGY. Primary biliary cirrhosis is best described pathologically as progressive, nonsuppurative, destructive cholangitis. This disorder can be separated into four histopathologic stages: *ductal, ductular, scarring,* and *cirrhotic*. The lesions in the first two stages are distributed unevenly and may therefore be absent in needle biopsies of the liver. The characteristic lesion (ductal or Stage 1) consists of damaged interlobular and septal bile ducts surrounded by a dense infiltrate of lymphocytes and plasma cells. Well-formed granulomas are frequently seen near the injured bile ducts. In Stage 2 (ductular) of the disease, there is proliferation of bile ductules and reduction in the number of bile ducts. Portal fibrosis may be present or absent and granulomata are found less often than in Stage 1. Later, as the inflammation subsides, there is an increase in scarring most marked in portal areas with fibrous septa extending into the lobule (Stage 3). When cirrhotic (Stage 4), the liver may lose all of the characteristic lesions. Bile ducts are few in number in both Stages 3 and 4 and this paucity of bile ducts may be the only clue to the diagnosis of primary biliary cirrhosis. In one quarter of the cases, alcoholic hyalin is identifiable in the biopsy. Histologic features of chronic active hepatitis may also be present, leading to difficulties in diagnosis.

CLINICAL MANIFESTATIONS (Table 125–2). Ninety per cent of patients with primary biliary cirrhosis are female. The disease has been found in patients as young as 23 and as old as 72; however, the majority of patients are of ages 40 to 60. The onset is usually marked by *pruritus,* although the condition in an increasing number of patients is being diagnosed at an asymptomatic stage. The diagnosis is made in these latter patients when hepatomegaly is found or an elevated alkaline phosphatase is noted on an automated screening panel. The itching may start during pregnancy or with the use of birth control pills. Following delivery or withdrawal of the medication, the itching usually continues; this is in contrast to *cholestasis of pregnancy,* in which pruritus resolves following parturition. Itching leads to excoriative dermatitis and thickening and darkening of the skin. Hepatomegaly and less frequently splenomegaly may be found at the time of diagnosis. *Jaundice* rarely precedes the onset of pruritus, and may follow it by several years. *Portal hypertension* and *hepatic failure* are usually late events, and ascites or bleeding esophageal varices are uncommon presenting features. *Hypercholesterolemia,* secondary to the decreased biliary excretion of cholesterol, may be severe enough to produce xanthomas. *Osteomalacia* or more commonly *osteoporosis* may develop in these patients. The cause of the bone disease is incompletely understood; however, malabsorption of vitamin D and calcium are important pathogenic factors.

TABLE 125–2. CLINICAL FEATURES OF PRIMARY BILIARY CIRRHOSIS

Signs and Symptoms	Laboratory
Female preponderance (> 90%)	Antimitochondrial antibodies (> 90%)
Pruritus	Elevated alkaline phosphatase, cholesterol, IgM, serum bile acids, and bilirubin
Jaundice	**Associated Diseases**
Skin hyperpigmentation	Sjögren's syndrome
Hepatosplenomegaly	Scleroderma/CREST syndrome
Xanthelasma/xanthoma	Arthritis
Bleeding diathesis (vitamin K deficiency)	Autoimmune thyroiditis
Bone pain (osteoporosis/osteomalacia)	Renal tubular acidosis
Ascites/variceal hemorrhage (late)	

Copper accumulates in the livers of patients with primary biliary cirrhosis because it cannot be efficiently secreted into the bile. The levels of hepatic copper may reach levels equal to those found in Wilson's disease, and rarely *Kayser-Fleischer rings* have been described.

ASSOCIATED DISEASES. Primary biliary cirrhosis is associated with a variety of disorders. *Sjögren's syndrome* with dryness of the eyes and mouth is present in at least 70 per cent of patients when specific tests (Schirmer test, buccal biopsy, and others) are used (Ch. 449). *Scleroderma* and the *CREST syndrome* (calcinosis, Reynaud's phenomenon, esophageal hypomotility, sclerodactyly, telangiectasia) are both increased in frequency in patients with primary biliary cirrhosis. The prevalence of *arthritis,* both seropositive and seronegative, is increased in these patients. *Thyroid autoantibodies* are found in about 25 per cent of patients, and in the antibody-positive patients thyroid dysfunction (primarily hypothyroidism) is common. *Renal tubular acidosis* also is present in patients with primary biliary cirrhosis. The pathogenesis of the renal tubular acidosis is unknown but it may be secondary to deposition of copper in renal tubules.

LABORATORY FINDINGS. The *alkaline phosphatase* is elevated in almost all patients with primary biliary cirrhosis, although it may be normal in asymptomatic patients. The elevation is usually two to six times normal, but can be more than ten times normal. The serum bilirubin is usually normal or mildly elevated until the later stages of the disease are reached. Serum bile acids and cholesterol are increased frequently. Serum *immunoglobulin M* levels are increased in 75 per cent of patients with primary biliary cirrhosis. The finding, however, is not specific. Hypoprothrombinemia and hypocalcemia may be present and reflect deficiencies of vitamins K and D. The serum transaminases are normal to mildly elevated. Eighty-four to 98 per cent of patients with primary biliary cirrhosis have *circulating antimitochondrial antibodies.* This antibody is directed toward an antigen in the inner mitochondrial membrane. The antibody is neither species nor organ specific. Antimitochondrial antibodies may be present in patients with HBsAg-negative chronic active hepatitis, cryptogenic cirrhosis, and collagen vascular diseases; however, the test is negative in patients with extrahepatic obstruction unless they also have primary biliary cirrhosis or chronic active hepatitis. A small percentage of patients (5 to 30 per cent) with primary biliary cirrhosis have antinuclear antibodies in their serum.

DIAGNOSIS. The diagnosis of primary biliary cirrhosis is established by finding a positive antimitochondrial antibody test and the characteristic pathology (Stage 1 or 2) on liver biopsy. It may be necessary to exclude extrahepatic obstruction in some patients in whom the diagnosis of primary biliary cirrhosis cannot be made with certainty, as *extrahepatic biliary obstruction* can clinically mimic primary biliary cirrhosis. Also, patients with primary biliary cirrhosis have an increased incidence of gallstones, which may cause biliary obstruction. Biliary tract disease may be excluded by either transhepatic or endoscopic retrograde cholangiography.

THERAPY AND PROGNOSIS. No specific therapy for primary biliary cirrhosis is available. Corticosteroids are not known to be effective in this disease and will aggravate the bone disease. Azathioprine has been found to be an ineffective form of therapy for patients with primary biliary cirrhosis. D-Penicillamine has been shown to reduce hepatic copper and to improve some hepatic biochemical tests. Improvement in survival has not been shown convincingly and there is a high incidence of side effects from penicillamine. Further experience is required in the use of D-penicillamine before it can be recommended.

The treatment of primary biliary cirrhosis is directed toward its complications and includes correction of specific deficiency states and reduction in the pruritus. Dietary fat may be reduced to 40 grams daily to decrease steatorrhea and improve calcium absorption. Medium-chain triglycerides are absorbed directly into the portal vein without the presence of intraluminal bile salts, and these may be given as a dietary supplement. If the prothrombin time is prolonged, vitamin K (10 mg) is given intramuscularly every four weeks. Although studies performed to date are inconclusive, the osteomalacia may be preventable. General measures included exposure to sunlight (10 to 20 minutes daily) and dietary supplementation with vitamin D and calcium. The serum 25(OH)D level should be measured and, if low, it should be increased to the normal range with oral vitamin D. If the serum 25(OH)D levels fail to increase with vitamin D therapy, then oral 25(OH)D, 100 to 200 μg daily, may be given. Hepatic osteomalacia may be effectively treated with either oral 25(OH)D or 1,25-$(OH)_2D$. Hepatic osteoporosis does not appear to respond to treatment with metabolites of vitamin D. During the administration of vitamin D or its metabolites, the serum and urine calcium must be monitored closely to prevent development of hypercalcemia. See Ch. 245 and 249 for further discussions of osteomalacia and osteoporosis, respectively.

The cause of the pruritus is unknown, but it may be secondary to increased tissue levels of bile salts. Cholestyramine and colestipol are anion exchange resins that bind bile salts in the intestines, preventing their reabsorption in the terminal ileum. Eight to 12 grams of cholestyramine is given daily preceding meals in divided doses. Fat-soluble vitamins should not be given at the same time as the resin. The hypercholesterolemia may also respond to cholestyramine therapy. Clofibrate should not be used in these patients, as there may be a paradoxical increase in the serum cholesterol.

Patients with primary biliary cirrhosis who are asymptomatic have a good prognosis, with a ten-year survival similar to age-matched controls. Patients who present with symptoms have, in contrast, an average life expectancy of 5.5 to 11 years. The development of jaundice, ascites, or cirrhosis is associated with a poor prognosis.

Arnaud S: 25-Hydroxyvitamin D_3 treatment of bone disease in primary biliary cirrhosis. Gastroenterology 83:137, 1982. *Reviews the problem of osteoporosis in patients with liver disease, especially primary biliary cirrhosis.*

Christensen E, Crowe J, Doniach D, Popper H, Ranek L, Rodes J, Tygstrup N, Williams R: Clinical pattern and course of disease in primary biliary cirrhosis based on an analysis of 236 patients. Gastroenterology 78:236, 1980. *Describes the presenting features and clinical course of a large number of patients.*

Long R, Scheuer PJ, Sherlock S: Presentation and course of asymptomatic primary biliary cirrhosis. Gastroenterology 72:1204, 1977. *Patients presenting without hepatic symptoms but who were found fortuitously, frequently because of an increased alkaline phosphatase. An important study because prognosis is quite different when compared to symptomatic patients.*

Matloff DS, Alpert E, Resnick RH, Kaplan MN: A prospective trial of D-penicillamine in primary biliary cirrhosis. N Engl J Med 306:319, 1982. *This study failed to show a positive effect of penicillamine on symptoms or survival.*

Roll J, Boyer J, Barry D, Klatskin G: The prognostic importance of clinical and histologic features in asymptomatic and symptomatic primary biliary cirrhosis. N Engl J Med 308:1, 1983. *Defines the clinical and pathologic features that predict survival.*

SECONDARY BILIARY CIRRHOSIS

DEFINITION, ETIOLOGY, AND PATHOLOGY. Secondary biliary cirrhosis is an uncommon sequela of longstanding obstruction of the biliary tree. Obstruction is usually present for more than one year (mean of about six years) before cirrhosis develops; however, intervals as short as four months from the onset of obstruction (jaundice) to the diagnosis of cirrhosis have been reported. Cirrhosis or fibrosis may also develop in the absence of jaundice in patients with prolonged partial biliary tract obstruction as may be seen in chronic pancreatitis. In adults, obstruction is due to gallstones, strictures, carcinoma, chronic pancreatitis, or sclerosing cholangitis. In children, biliary atresia and cystic fibrosis are common causes of secondary biliary cirrhosis.

The liver is usually enlarged and dark green in color. The surface is granular or occasionally nodular. The lobular pattern is usually preserved until the cirrhosis is advanced. The portal tracts are widened owing to fibrosis and proliferation of bile ducts. The hepatic parenchyma may contain bile plugs, infarcts, or lakes. There is focal hepatocellular necrosis. As the cirrhosis progresses, the fibrous septa extend into the hepatic parenchyma, forming pseudolobules. In advanced cirrhosis, there is nodular regeneration.

CLINICAL MANIFESTATIONS. *Jaundice* is common but not invariable and the level of jaundice may fluctuate. Patients with strictures or stones may have suffered recurrent bouts of cholangitis or biliary colic. *Pruritus* is also a common complaint and may precede the onset of icterus. If the pruritus is severe, itching may lead to thickening and darkening of the skin. Xanthelasma and xanthomas may appear. *Steatorrhea* with diarrhea may be a major complaint, and *bone disease* may develop owing, in part, to malabsorption of vitamin D and calcium. Splenomegaly is common. Ascites and gastrointestinal bleeding develop later in the course of the disease and are uncommon presenting complaints.

LABORATORY TESTS. The serum bilirubin is usually moderately increased (3 to 15 mg per deciliter). The alkaline phosphatase is also almost always increased; however, in 25 to 30 per cent, the elevation is less than twice normal. The AST is usually elevated, but the elevations are moderate. The prothrombin time may be prolonged and may improve with vitamin K administration. Hypoalbuminemia and hyperglobulinemia may also be present. Serum cholesterol and bile acids may be increased. *Lipoprotein X*, an abnormal lipoprotein, is found commonly in patients with extrahepatic obstruction (see Ch. 118). Lipoprotein X is also present in other forms of liver disease, and its absence does not exclude extrahepatic obstruction. Elevations of the white blood cell count in patients with extrahepatic obstruction suggest the presence of cholangitis or an hepatic abscess.

THERAPY AND PROGNOSIS. Relief of the biliary obstruction is the only specific form of treatment. In patients in whom the obstruction cannot be relieved, the correction of vitamin deficiencies and the use of cholestyramine to relieve itching, as outlined for the treatment of primary biliary cirrhosis is warranted. In addition, there may be recurrent episodes of cholangitis requiring antibiotic treatment.

The prognosis for patients with carcinoma is poor, with most dying because of the malignancy and not because of the liver disease. The mortality for patients with benign obstructions (stone or stricture) depends on whether or not the obstruction can be relieved. When the obstruction cannot be relieved, mortality is high; however, survival may be prolonged (years) before the patient dies from hepatic failure or bleeding esophageal varices. Surgical relief of the biliary obstruction improves survival, although ascites and esophageal varices may develop later. The development of these complications, usually many years after apparently successful surgery, may be due to subclinical recurrence of partial biliary obstruction.

Littenberg G, Afroudakis A, Kaplowitz N: Common bile duct stenosis from chronic pancreatitis: A clinical and pathologic spectrum. Medicine 58:385, 1979. *Reviews the effects on the liver of biliary obstruction secondary to chronic pancreatitis.*

Scobie BA, Summerskill W: Hepatic cirrhosis secondary to obstruction of the biliary system. Am J Dig Dis 10:135, 1965. *Although an old reference, it is one of the few that describe a large number of patients with secondary biliary cirrhosis.*

CRYPTOGENIC CIRRHOSIS

DEFINITION AND ETIOLOGY. Cryptogenic (macronodular or postnecrotic) cirrhosis is any cirrhosis for which the etiology is unknown. The liver contains little or no necrosis or inflammation and has no diagnostic pathologic lesions (for example, alcoholic hepatitis); it lacks any specific lesions demonstrable by histochemical stains, e.g., α_1-antitrypsin or iron; and specific serologic tests, e.g., HBsAg, anti-HBc, AMA, and ceruloplasmin, are negative. It is assumed that most cases represent the end-stage of a previously active, chronic, or recurrent hepatitis, but alcoholic and other chronic liver diseases give rise to a very similar form of coarsely nodular cirrhosis. Cases previously called cryptogenic cirrhosis have been reported to be due to type B hepatitis despite the absence of detectable levels of HBsAg in the plasma. In these cases, HBV antigens were demonstrable in the liver cells and the serum was positive for anti-HBc. Cryptogenic cirrhosis should become a less frequent diagnosis as our understanding of the causes of liver disease increases and we develop tests for agents such as non-A, non-B hepatitis.

PATHOLOGY. The liver is usually small and its surface distorted by large regenerative nodules (macronodular), which may be several centimeters in diameter. The liver between the nodules appears to be collapsed and fibrotic. The microscopic appearance of the liver is one of regenerative nodules separated by connective tissue. The portal areas may be infiltrated by mononuclear cells, but the liver cells are well preserved, and active hepatocellular necrosis or hepatic steatosis is minimal or absent.

CLINICAL MANIFESTATIONS. Cryptogenic cirrhosis may remain clinically silent for many years and frequently is discovered unexpectedly, often during the evaluation of an unrelated condition. When the disease becomes "clinically manifest," its signs and symptoms are usually related to portal hypertension and include ascites, splenomegaly, hypersplenism, bleeding esophageal varices, or hepatic encephalopathy. The liver may be of normal size or small. Splenomegaly is common; spider angiomas, ascites, and abdominal wall venous collaterals may also be present. Serum transaminases and bilirubin are usually normal to slightly increased. Hyperglobulinemia is common and may be the only laboratory abnormality.

DIAGNOSIS. Cryptogenic cirrhosis is a diagnosis of exclusion and is based on histologic and clinical evidence of cirrhosis in the absence of a definable etiology (see Table 125–1). Wilson's disease and hemochromatosis, although uncommon, are specifically treatable and should therefore be carefully excluded (see Ch. 205 and 206). A small number of patients with cryptogenic cirrhosis have chronic hepatitis B infection despite the absence in the serum of detectable levels of HBsAg. Measurement of anti-HBc may be helpful in identifying these patients. Testing for antimitochondrial antibodies, ANA, and an LE preparation will help exclude primary biliary cirrhosis and chronic active hepatitis. α_1-Antitrypsin deficiency may be excluded by appropriate histochemical stains and serologic tests (see Ch. 124). Findings of hepatic congestion on biopsy may be indicative of occult cardiac disease or hepatic vein occlusion. A previous history of alcoholism may be the only evidence for alcohol as the cause of the cirrhosis.

TREATMENT AND PROGNOSIS. Specific therapy for this type of cirrhosis is lacking. Complications such as ascites, encephalopathy, and gastrointestinal bleeding should be managed as discussed in Ch. 113, 126, and 127. Patients who have asymptomatic cirrhosis may do quite well with a good five-year prognosis; however, the onset of ascites or bleeding esophageal varices is a poor prognostic sign.

CARDIAC CIRRHOSIS

ETIOLOGY. Cardiac cirrhosis is an uncommon complication of severe, prolonged, recurrent right heart failure of any etiology, although it is usually caused by rheumatic heart disease (mitral or aortic stenosis with tricuspid regurgitation), cardiomyopathy, or constrictive pericarditis.

PATHOLOGY. The gross appearance of the liver in acute hepatic failure is one of alternating red and pale areas (nutmeg liver). The red areas are congested central areas of the hepatic lobule, whereas the pale areas are the preserved hepatocytes. With recurrent bouts of heart failure, the centrilobular hepatocytes atrophy and fibrosis develops. The fibrosis is most marked in the central areas, and with time fibrous septa extend out into the rest of the lobule. Regenerative nodules develop later and they arise from the periphery of the hepatic lobule.

CLINICAL MANIFESTATIONS, DIAGNOSIS, AND THERAPY. The clinical picture is usually dominated by the cardiac disease. Differentiation of patients with acute hepatic congestion from those with cardiac cirrhosis is difficult, as the clinical features are similar (see Ch. 124). The liver may be small or enlarged and firm. When tricuspid regurgitation is present, the absence of hepatic pulsation suggests cirrhosis. Ascites and splenomegaly are common. The bilirubin is usually only mildly increased, and either the unconjugated or conjugated pigment may predominate. The AST is often moderately elevated but may be normal if the heart failure is controlled. The prothrombin time may be prolonged, and in the presence of significant liver disease Coumadin and related anticoagulants should be used with caution. The diagnosis of cardiac cirrhosis is established by performing a liver biopsy. However, in most situations, this is not warranted.

Reduction in the incidence of rheumatic fever and tuberculosis as well as advances in cardiovascular surgery in the Western world have made cardiac cirrhosis an uncommon disease. Its prognosis depends largely upon the course of the cardiac disease. If the latter can be successfully treated, hepatic function improves and liver disease stabilizes.

Dunn GD, Hayes P, Breen K, Schenker S: The liver in congestive heart failure: A review. Am J Med Sci 265:174, 1973. *Reviews both acute and chronic heart failure and their effects on the liver.*

126. MAJOR SEQUELAE OF CIRRHOSIS

Thomas D. Boyer

PORTAL HYPERTENSION

ANATOMY AND PHYSIOLOGY OF PORTAL VENOUS SYSTEM. The portal venous system begins in the capillaries of the intestines and terminates in the hepatic sinusoids. The portal vein is formed by the confluence of the superior and inferior mesenteric veins and splenic vein.

The liver receives about 1500 ml of blood each minute, two thirds of which is provided by the portal vein. The hepatic artery provides 40 to 60 per cent of the oxygen supply to the liver. The liver offers little resistance to the flow of blood, and the pressure within the sinusoids is low (less than 5 mm Hg above the pressure in the inferior vena cava). Since the veins in the portal system lack valves, increased resistance to flow at any point between the splanchnic venules and the heart will increase pressure in all vessels on the intestinal side of the obstruction.

DEFINITION AND PATHOGENESIS. Portal hypertension represents an increase in the hydrostatic pressure within the portal vein or its tributaries. This is manifested clinically by the development of portal-systemic collaterals, splenomegaly, and/or ascites. Since portal hypertension may be present in the absence of clinical findings, it may be detectable only by measurement of pressures in the portal system. Pressures within the hepatic sinusoids may be measured by catheterizing the hepatic veins (wedged hepatic vein pressure). Alternatively, the portal vein pressure may be measured directly by transhepatic or umbilical vein catheterization or at surgery. Portal hypertension is present when the wedged hepatic vein pressure is more than 5 mm Hg higher than the inferior vena cava pressure or when the portal vein pressure recorded at surgery exceeds 18 to 22 mm Hg (25 to 30 cm of water). Portal hypertension is generally considered to be a progressive disorder. The portal pressure, however, may decrease as the liver disease improves, i.e., alcoholic hepatitis. Portal hypertension also can be an acute and transient phenomenon, as may occur with acute right heart failure. Since the pressure in any vascular system is directly proportional not only to resistance but also to flow, portal hypertension may result from either increased blood flow in the portal vein or increased resistance to flow within the portal venous system.

Increased portal venous blood flow is an unusual cause of portal hypertension for two reasons. First, the flow in the hepatic artery is responsive to the flow and pressure within the portal vein. Increases in portal vein flow cause a reflex decrease in hepatic artery blood flow, thereby tending to maintain a rela-

TABLE 126–1. CAUSES OF PORTAL HYPERTENSION

Increased hepatic blood flow
Splenomegaly not due to liver disease
Arteriovenous fistula
Diseases of cardiovascular system
Portal vein occlusion
Splenic vein occlusion
Hepatic vein occlusion
Veno-occlusive disease
Web lesion or thrombosis of inferior vena cava
Congestive heart failure–constrictive pericarditis
Liver diseases
Cirrhosis—all causes
Congenital hepatic fibrosis
Schistosomiasis
Idiopathic portal hypertension
Sarcoidosis
Alcoholic hepatitis
Partial nodular transformation

tively normal sinusoidal pressure. Second and most important, the outflow resistance from the liver is very low. Increases in portal vein flow must therefore be large to cause a significant increase in portal venous pressure.

Increased resistance to venous flow is the most common mechanism for the development of portal hypertension. Liver disease accounts for the majority of cases; however, occlusion of the portal or hepatic veins and cardiac disease also cause increased resistance to flow and increases in portal pressure. The diseases causing portal hypertension are listed in Table 126–1 and discussed below.

CLINICAL MANIFESTATIONS. The clinical presentation of portal hypertension depends to a certain extent upon its cause. Essentially all forms may present with either *bleeding esophageal varices* or *splenomegaly* with or without *hypersplenism*. In portal vein thrombosis, as the liver is normal, ascites and jaundice are unusual. *Ascites* and other signs of hepatic disease (jaundice, spiders, encephalopathy) are common clinical features of cirrhosis. Occlusion of the hepatic veins almost always leads to development of ascites and varying degrees of hepatic dysfunction. Thus, the clinical findings may be important clues to the cause of the portal hypertension.

The development of portal-systemic collaterals is the major complication of portal hypertension. There are several vessels that may form collaterals. The veins that lie in the mucosa of the gastric fundus and esophagus are of greatest clinical interest because, when dilated, they form gastric and esophageal varices (Fig. 126–1). The remnant of the umbilical vein may also dilate. If flow through this vessel becomes great enough, a loud venous hum may be audible over the path of the umbilical vein (Cruveilhier-Baumgarten syndrome). The umbilical vein enters the left portal vein, and therefore, if a venous hum is present, the cause of the portal hypertension must be intrahepatic or in the hepatic veins or inferior vena cava. Large collaterals also may form between the splenic and renal (chiefly left) veins. Dilated abdominal wall veins are common in patients with portal hypertension and are especially prominent when the patient stands. The hemorrhoidal veins may also act as collaterals. However, the dilatation of these vessels is so common in normal individuals that their presence is of little diagnostic use. Varices may also form in unusual locations within the intestines (e.g., ileostomies, upper small bowel, and ascending, descending, and sigmoid colons), and these may bleed.

DISEASES CAUSING PORTAL HYPERTENSION (see Table 126–1). *Arteriovenous fistulas* may form between an artery and the portal vein or one of its tributaries as a consequence of abdominal trauma, liver biopsy, carcinoma (either intra- or extrahepatic), or rupture of an arterial aneurysm (e.g., splenic). An upper abdominal bruit or a palpable thrill at surgery suggests this diagnosis in any patient with portal hypertension. The fistula can be localized by celiac angiography and is usually surgically correctable.

Splenomegaly resulting from hematologic diseases such as polycythemia rubra vera and myelofibrosis or an infiltrative process such as Gaucher's disease may, in rare instances, lead to portal hypertension. The enlarged spleen receives high blood flows from the splenic artery, leading to high flows within the splenic vein which are thought to cause the rise in portal pressure. These diseases also frequently involve the liver, and the infiltrative process may increase intrahepatic resistance. However, the principal event in the genesis of the portal hypertension appears to be the high portal vein blood flow, since splenectomy usually cures the portal hypertension.

Splenic vein thrombosis may be caused by pancreatitis, abdominal trauma, or a locally invasive tumor. Pressure is increased only in areas drained by the splenic vein, whereas pressure in the portal vein is normal. The diagnosis should be suspected in a patient with gastric or esophageal varices but a normal liver biopsy, and is established by celiac angiography. Splenectomy is curative.

Portal vein thrombosis may develop following abdominal trauma or intra-abdominal sepsis, or in association with cirrhosis or hepatocellular carcinoma. However, in the majority of cases the cause is unknown. This is primarily a disease of children, although adults may also develop portal vein thrombosis. The diagnosis is again suggested by the presence of portal hypertension in a patient with a normal liver biopsy. The diagnosis is established by angiography. Thrombi also may be identified using ultrasound or by CT scan. The surgical management of these patients may be difficult because of the absence of a patent vein to use for making a portal-systemic shunt.

Thrombosis of the hepatic veins (Budd-Chiari syndrome) may follow abdominal trauma or the use of birth control pills, or may occur in patients with diseases such as polycythemia rubra vera and paroxysmal nocturnal hemoglobinuria, which have an associated hypercoagulable state. Patients with hepatic vein

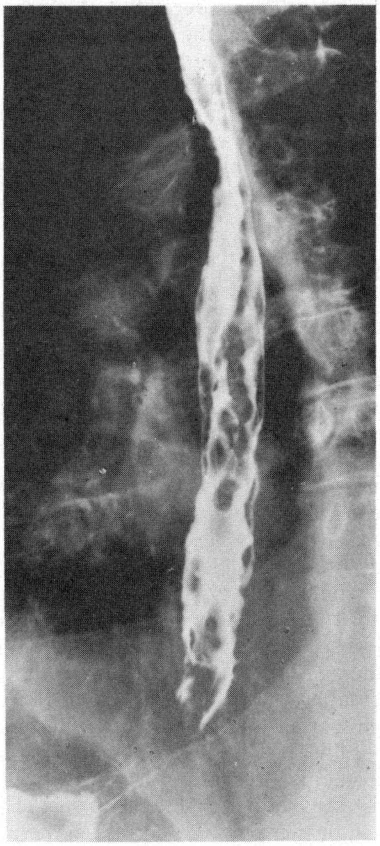

Figure 126–1. Barium esophagogram, demonstrating large varices involving the lower two thirds of the esophagus. Courtesy of T. Munyer. (From Zakim D, Boyer TD [eds.]: Hepatology: A Textbook of Liver Diseases. Philadelphia, W. B. Saunders Company, 1983.)

thrombosis may develop an acute, subacute, or chronic illness in which abdominal pain and ascites are the major features. The liver is usually enlarged and tender. Elevations of the serum transaminases and bilirubin are usually mild, although they can be increased significantly in patients who have an acute illness. The initial clinical diagnosis is usually cirrhosis, and the correct diagnosis is not suspected until centrilobular congestion is seen on liver biopsy. Catheterization of the inferior vena cava and hepatic veins is a useful test in the evaluation of these patients. The presence of thrombi in the inferior vena cava can be established. The diagnosis of hepatic vein thrombosis is made by finding the characteristic pathology on liver biopsy, excluding cardiac disease that causes a similar histologic lesion, and inability to catheterize the hepatic veins. The outlook for patients with hepatic vein thrombosis is poor, with mortality rates of 50 to 90 per cent. Recently, the use of side-to-side portacaval shunts in these patients has been thought to prolong survival. Further experience is required before the proper role of this procedure can be evaluated. The use of anticoagulants has not been shown to affect survival.

Veno-occlusive disease (nonthrombotic occlusion of hepatic venules) also causes a Budd-Chiari–like syndrome. Veno-occlusive disease develops in patients who have ingested plants containing pyrrolidizine alkaloids, who have been treated for malignancy with certain chemotherapeutic agents, or following bone marrow transplantation. It also is a common finding in patients with alcoholic hepatitis and cirrhosis. The disease is thought to be due to a toxic injury to the endothelium of the affected vessels. The occluded venules may be present in a liver biopsy, and an abnormal vascular pattern is found when contrast is injected into the hepatic veins.

Thrombi, tumor, or a membrane in the inferior vena cava may obstruct the hepatic veins and give a clinical picture similar to that of hepatic vein thrombosis, with the additional features of peripheral edema and stasis dermatitis. Membranous obstruction near the terminus of the inferior vena cava has been described in all areas of the world but is most frequently observed in South Africa and the orient. These patients also have a high incidence of hepatocellular carcinoma. The reasons for this latter association are unclear. Catheterization of the inferior vena cava will identify the obstructing lesion. Removal of the membrane surgically is sometimes possible and leads to resolution of the portal hypertension. Thrombectomy is usually not helpful.

Cirrhosis causes portal hypertension by increasing the intrahepatic vascular resistance. The increased resistance is thought to occur because of compression of vessels by regenerative nodules and narrowing of portal vessels within the fibrous tissue. In alcoholic liver disease, serious portal hypertension may develop without cirrhosis. In some patients with acute alcoholic hepatitis, there is progressive obliteration of the central veins with resultant centrilobular fibrosis. These patients develop a severe outflow block, which leads to the formation of ascites or esophageal varices.

Portal hypertension due to noncirrhotic portal fibrosis may occur in four conditions. In *schistosomiasis*, the adult worm resides in the intestinal venules. The eggs are shed into these vessels and are swept into the portal vein and into the liver, where they lodge in and obstruct the portal venules. The host's immune response to the eggs leads to destruction of the portal venules and, in combination with the occlusion of the vessels by the eggs, portal hypertension develops. (Schistosomiasis is discussed more fully in Ch. 396.) *Idiopathic portal hypertension* (Banti's syndrome) is a disease in which there is portal hypertension, no cirrhosis, and a patent portal vein. The liver biopsy may be normal, or there may be fibrosis in the periportal areas and in the space of Disse. The disease process is progressive, with the liver eventually becoming small and fibrotic. A similar clinical picture may be seen in patients exposed to arsenic, vinyl chloride, and copper salts. *Congenital hepatic fibrosis* is also a disease that causes portal hypertension without cirrhosis. In the portal areas, there is marked hyperplasia of the bile ducts and stellate fibrosis. This condition may be present in association with cystic liver disease and Caroli's disease (intrahepatic ductal ectasia). There is also an associated polycystic renal lesion in many patients. The development of portal hypertension is the major consequence of this form of liver disease, as hepatic function is well maintained. Hepatic *sarcoidosis* may rarely lead to hepatic fibrosis and portal hypertension.

DIAGNOSTIC APPROACH TO PORTAL HYPERTENSION. The existence of portal hypertension should be suspected in any patient with ascites or splenomegaly. The presence of portal hypertension is established when portal-systemic collaterals are found. One may find collaterals on physical examination (dilated abdominal wall or umbilical veins), or they may be identified in the esophagus or stomach by a gastrointestinal series or by endoscopy. In addition to establishing the presence of portal hypertension, its etiology must also be identified, since some causes (splenic vein thrombosis) may be curable. A liver biopsy will provide useful information as to the presence of liver disease; central venous congestion suggests hepatic vein thrombosis or cardiac disease. If the biopsy is not diagnostic, then catheterization of the hepatic veins may be performed. Recording of an elevated pressure will establish the presence of liver disease. Also, inferior vena cava or hepatic vein thrombosis may be found during catheterization of the hepatic veins. If the wedge pressure is normal, then the cause of the portal hypertension is (1) occlusion of the portal vein or its tributaries, (2) liver disease that involves the periportal areas and portal venules (schistosomiasis or idiopathic portal hypertension) and therefore does not increase the wedge pressure, or (3) increased flow in the portal vein. Celiac angiography will usually differentiate among this group of patients. Ultrasonography or computed tomographic scans may also be used to identify thrombi in the portal vein.

BLEEDING ESOPHAGEAL AND GASTRIC VARICES

PATHOGENESIS. Hemorrhage from esophageal varices is a major complication of portal hypertension. The mortality in adult patients with cirrhosis varies from 30 to 60 per cent for each bleeding episode. The varices form because of increased pressure in the portal vein. Bleeding from varices may occur when the portal pressure exceeds 11 to 12 mm Hg above inferior vena cava pressure. However, not all patients with pressures above these levels have bleeding varices. Why some varices bleed is unknown, although large varices are more likely to bleed than smaller ones; reflux esophagitis and ascites do not appear to be important in the genesis of bleeding.

CLINICAL MANIFESTATIONS. The most common presentation is hematemesis. The bleeding may be massive with the rapid development of shock, or the bleeding may stop spontaneously only to recur later. On occasion, the patient may only complain of hematochezia or melena without an antecedent history of hematemesis. Features suggesting underlying liver disease such as hepatomegaly, ascites, or jaundice may be present or absent, depending on the etiology of the portal hypertension and the activity of the underlying hepatic disease.

DIAGNOSIS AND TREATMENT. The care of the patient with gastrointestinal bleeding is discussed in detail in Ch. 113, and here we will emphasize only a few points. The restoration of the patient's blood volume takes precedence over all other therapies and diagnostic tests. The blood volume should be corrected rapidly but not excessively, since overexpansion may lead to the development of ascites or renewed bleeding. Proof that esophageal or gastric varices are the source of hemorrhage depends on endoscopy, since, even in those with known varices, 30 to 50 per cent will be bleeding from other lesions (especially gastritis).

The bleeding from varices in many patients stops without any specific therapy. The *medical management* of patients who continue to bleed includes *vasopressin, endoscopic sclerosis of varices*, and *balloon tamponade*. Chronic therapy with *propranolol* has recently been reported to lower the wedged hepatic vein pressure and prevent recurrent hemorrhage from esophageal varices. The effect of propranolol on portal pressure is incompletely understood and the efficacy of this form of therapy is unproved. The use of propranolol for the prevention of variceal hemorrhage cannot currently be recommended.

Vasopressin is a potent vasoconstrictor and it is believed to act by constricting the splanchnic arterioles, which results in a fall in portal flow and thus a drop in portal pressure. This drug should be given only to patients who can be carefully monitored, preferably in an intensive care unit. Pitressin is infused into a peripheral vein at a rate of 0.2 to 0.4 unit per minute. This therapy will provide temporary control in about 60 per cent of patients. Unfortunately, about half of those initially controlled will have rebleeding, and the use of vasopressin has little effect on morbidity or mortality. The gastric and esophageal varices lie in the mucosa of the gastric fundus and esophagus and are therefore susceptible to *balloon tamponade.* Tamponade is best accomplished by inserting a tube that has a gastric and an esophageal balloon (Sengstaken-Blakemore tube). Once placed in the stomach, the gastric balloon is inflated and pulled into the cardia of the stomach, tamponading the varices. If bleeding does not stop, then the esophageal balloon is inflated. This therapy is effective in controlling hemorrhage in 70 to 90 per cent of patients. There is a significant risk of aspiration during balloon tamponade, and 50 to 60 per cent of the patients will hemorrhage again. During endoscopy, the *direct injection of esophageal varices* with sclerosing agents has been described as a method for the acute control of bleeding and for the long-term management of these patients. Also, *transhepatic cannulation and thrombosis of varices* has been reported to be an effective form of therapy. Both of these new methods are associated with serious side effects and require further clinical experience before their role in the management of bleeding varices is established.

Surgical therapy for portal hypertension involves the anastomosis of the high pressure portal system to the low pressure systemic venous system. This is accomplished by creating a *portal-systemic shunt.* There are two basic types of shunts. One is *nonselective,* in that the entire portal-venous system is decompressed. The end-to-side and side-to-side portacaval and mesocaval shunts are nonselective. *Selective* shunts decompress only the varices. The pressure remains high in the portal vein, and portal flow into the liver is preserved. Thus, the varices are decompressed with a minimal disruption of the normal hepatic circulation. The distal splenorenal shunt is of this type. The selective shunt may cause less encephalopathy than the nonselective types of shunts without improving survival.

There are four clinical situations in which portal-systemic shunts have been used. (1) *Hypersplenism* is not an indication for a portal-systemic shunt, because the reduction in formed elements in the blood is usually not of clinical significance. (2) The *prophylactic shunt* is made in patients with cirrhosis and varices but who have never bled. Prophylactic shunts shorten survival compared to unoperated controls, with death from hepatic encephalopathy and liver failure. Thus prophylactic shunts should not be performed. (3) *Emergency shunts* may be used to control hemorrhage in actively bleeding patients. However, the operative mortality may exceed 50 per cent, so that emergency shunts should be used rarely and in a select group of patients. The indications for this operation are still controversial. (4) *Therapeutic portal-systemic shunts* are used in patients who have bled at least once from varices. Operations in these patients have been shown to stop further bleeding from varices effectively. Unfortunately, the patient's survival is not improved significantly because of an increased incidence of hepatic encephalopathy and liver failure when compared to unoperated controls. Possibly these results could be improved upon by better selection of patients for the operations. As might be expected, the majority of patients with poor hepatocellular function, i.e., those who are jaundiced with hypoalbuminemia, ascites, encephalopathy, and poor nutrition, tolerate a portal-systemic shunt less well than do patients without these complications of liver disease. Patients with more severe liver disease may well be better managed by sclerosis of their varices than by shunt operations. The morbidity and mortality from bleeding esophageal varices will remain high until current therapies are refined and new ones developed.

Boyer TD: Portal hypertension and its complications. *In* Zakim D, Boyer TD (eds.): Hepatology: A Textbook of Liver Disease. Philadelphia, W. B. Saunders Company, 1982, pp 464–499. *A current review of portal hypertension and its causes.*

Conn HO: Propranolol in the treatment of portal hypertension: A caution. Hepatology 2:741, 1982. *An editorial that counsels caution in the use of propranolol and reviews critically previously published reports.*

Mitchell MC, Boitnott JK, Kaufman S, Cameron JL, Maddrey WC: Budd-Chiari syndrome: Etiology, diagnosis and management. Medicine 61:199, 1982. *An excellent review of hepatic vein thrombosis.*

Reynolds TB, Donovan AJ, Mikkelsen WP, Redeker AG, Turrill FL, Weiner JM: Results of a 12-year randomized trial of portacaval shunt in patients with alcoholic liver disease and bleeding varices. Gastroenterology 80:1005, 1981. *Excellent controlled trial of therapeutic portacaval shunts. Reviews previous studies.*

Smith JL, Graham D: Variceal hemorrhage: A critical evaluation of survival analysis. Gastroenterology 82:968, 1983. *A careful evaluation of survival following an episode of hemorrhage from varices.*

ASCITES

DEFINITION. Ascites is the presence of excess fluid in the peritoneal cavity. It is most frequently due to cirrhosis, but there are numerous other causes (see Ch. 111), and it cannot be assumed that the appearance of ascites is indicative of cirrhosis. For this reason, patients with a recent onset of ascites must be thoroughly evaluated to establish its cause.

PATHOGENESIS (Table 126–2). Ascites forms in patients with portal hypertension because of changes in the formation and reabsorption of hepatic and splanchnic lymph and because of alterations in the metabolism of salt and water by the kidneys.

Splanchnic Lymph Formation. Increases in portal venous pressure cause a rise in the pressure within the splanchnic capillaries, resulting in loss of fluid into the interstitial space. The capillaries of the intestine restrict the loss of protein to the interstitial space, and an oncotic gradient develops between the capillary and the extravascular space. This oncotic gradient returns the majority of the fluid to the capillary, and any fluid loss is usually removed by the intestinal lymphatics. For this reason, diseases that elevate the pressure only in the splanchnic bed, e.g., portal vein thrombosis, cause ascites uncommonly. The contribution of splanchnic lymph to the formation of cirrhotic ascites is uncertain.

Hepatic Lymph Formation. The endothelial lining of the hepatic sinusoids is discontinuous and does not effectively restrict plasma protein loss with even slight increases in sinusoidal pressure. Thus, in contrast to the intestines, the oncotic gradient between the sinusoids and extravascular space is small, and much of the fluid entering the interstitial space is not returned to the vascular space. For these reasons the concentration of plasma proteins is not a major factor in the pathogenesis of ascites associated with liver disease. These large amounts of fluid lost into the interstitial space must be returned to the vascular space via hepatic lymphatics. When the rate of formation of lymph exceeds the rate of removal, then fluid "weeps" out of the lymphatics and into the peritoneal cavity. Diseases that cause marked elevations of the sinusoidal

TABLE 126–2. FACTORS IN THE PATHOGENESIS OF CIRRHOTIC ASCITES

1. Increased hydrostatic pressure in hepatic sinusoids and splanchnic capillaries.
2. Overproduction of hepatic and splanchnic lymph secondary to (1), leading to a transudation of lymph into peritoneal space.
3. Limited or reduced reabsorption of water and protein by peritoneal lymphatics.
4. Sodium retention by the kidney secondary to hyperaldosteronism, increased sympathetic activity, alterations in metabolism of prostaglandins and kinins, and altered renal hemodynamics.
5. Impaired renal water excretion, in part caused by increased levels of ADH.

pressure, e.g., cirrhosis and hepatic vein thrombosis, therefore commonly cause ascites.

Peritoneal Reabsorption. The peritoneum plays an active role in the reabsorption of the ascitic fluid. Water and protein are reabsorbed by the lymphatics in the peritoneal membrane. The intra-abdominal pressure and character of the peritoneum are important factors in determining the rate of removal. The amount of fluid removed by the peritoneal lymphatics is variable but usually does not exceed 800 to 1000 ml every 24 hours.

Renal Function. An important factor in the genesis of ascites is the *retention of sodium* by the kidney. During the formation of ascites there is a positive sodium balance despite a total body sodium that is greater than normal. The pathogenesis of the sodium retention by the kidney is understood poorly; however, there is increased reabsorption of sodium by both proximal and distal tubules. The increased reabsorption of sodium may be mediated, in part, by increased plasma levels of aldosterone, increased sympathetic activity, and alterations in the renal production of prostaglandins and kinins. Reduced renal blood flow resulting from vasoconstriction also leads to enhanced sodium reabsorption.

CLINICAL MANIFESTATIONS AND DIAGNOSIS. Patients with ascites complain of increasing abdominal girth. The presence of ascites on physical examination is suggested by the findings of shifting dullness, a ballotable liver, or a fluid wave. Small amounts of ascites may be identified with an abdominal ultrasound. Once the presence of ascites is suspected, a diagnostic paracentesis should be performed. The character of the ascitic fluid in cirrhosis is variable; however, 80 to 90 per cent of patients have an ascitic fluid protein concentration of less than 3 grams per deciliter. The low protein content of the ascitic fluid may reflect a change in the permeability characteristics of the sinusoids of the cirrhotic liver (i.e., capillarization of the sinusoids) and the contribution of low protein splanchnic lymph. The ascitic fluid lactic dehydrogenase concentration is also low. The ascitic fluid white blood cell count is less than 500 per cubic millimeter in 90 per cent of patients with cirrhosis, and mononuclear cells predominate (>75 per cent).

MANAGEMENT. Resolution of the acute hepatic injury, following withdrawal of ethanol or a specific course of therapy, may reduce portal hypertension, and ascites may resolve spontaneously. In many patients, however, ascites is chronic and specific therapy is warranted. Accumulation of ascitic fluid occurs only in patients who are in positive sodium balance; therefore, *restricting sodium intake* will diminish or stop the accumulation of ascitic fluid. Diets containing 250 to 500 mg of sodium (10 to 20 mEq) are adequate to achieve sodium balance in most patients. With improvement in liver function, sodium retention may diminish and the patients will begin to lose their ascites. The kidney is also unable to excrete a water load normally in some patients with ascites, and *fluid restriction* (1000 to 1500 ml daily) is sometimes necessary to prevent hyponatremia. Recent studies have shown high blood levels of antidiuretic hormone in cirrhotic patients with hyponatremia. Many patients do not lose their ascites or edema with sodium restriction, and the use of *diuretics* becomes necessary. Spironolactone and triamterene act on the distal tubule and cause a natriuresis with sparing of potassium. Spironolactone, 150 to 400 mg daily, causes a diuresis in patients with mild to moderate sodium retention. Furosemide, thiazides, and ethacrynic acid are more potent diuretics and cause both a natriuresis and potassium wasting. Furosemide, 40 to 80 mg daily, in combination with spironolactone or triamterene, causes a diuresis in most patients with ascites. All diuretics cause a loss of fluid from the plasma. This fluid is then replaced by the reabsorption of ascitic or edema fluid. The rate of fluid lost should therefore not exceed the rate at which the ascites and edema may be reabsorbed. The maximal rate of reabsorption of ascitic fluid varies widely; however, fluid losses of 1 kg daily in patients with edema and ascites and 0.5 kg daily in those with only ascites are well tolerated. The BUN and electrolytes must be monitored for the development of azotemia and hypokalemia. The use of diets very low in sodium (250 to 500 mg) is possible in the hospital; however, this is rarely possible in an outpatient setting. Therefore, preceding discharge from the hospital, the patient's sodium intake should be increased (1 to 2 grams daily) and diuretics adjusted so that he is still in negative sodium balance.

A few patients with cirrhosis will not respond to diuretic therapy. Treatment in the hospital with increasing doses of diuretics leads to azotemia or hepatic encephalopathy. Other patients are controlled in the hospital but, upon discharge, rapidly reaccumulate their ascitic fluid. If these patients are incapacitated by the ascites, they may be candidates for other therapies. The *peritoneovenous (LeVeen) shunt* consists of a tube placed subcutaneously between the peritoneal cavity and the superior vena cava. There is a pressure-activated one-way valve that allows peritoneal fluid to enter the vascular space but prevents the backflow of blood into the tube. This shunt may be effective in controlling ascites; however, its use is associated with episodes of disseminated intravascular coagulation, sepsis, and frequent shunt thrombosis, thus limiting its application only to patients who have severe and incapacitating ascites. Even in this latter group of patients, its use is controversial. The shunt should not be used in patients whose condition can be managed by other therapies. Repeated *abdominal paracentesis* of 1 to 2 liters of ascitic fluid is a poor form of long-term therapy for resistant ascites. Patients presenting with massive ascites and difficulty in breathing, however, may be improved dramatically by the removal of 1 to 2 liters of fluid. Attempts to increase the venous oncotic pressure by infusions of albumin or plasma are not likely to cause sustained diuresis and is an expensive form of therapy.

SPONTANEOUS BACTERIAL PERITONITIS. Patients with cirrhosis and ascites may develop spontaneous bacterial peritonitis. There is no obvious cause for the peritonitis, i.e., perforation of the bowel, and it appears to occur because of bacterial seeding of the ascitic fluid via the lymph or blood or by bacteria traversing the bowel wall. The frequency of this complication in patients with ascites may be increasing, and its early recognition is essential (mortality exceeds 60 to 90 per cent even if treated). The clues to the diagnosis are the presence of fever, abdominal pain or tenderness, or decreased bowel sounds in a patient with ascites. The diagnosis should also be suspected in patients with the sudden onset of hepatic encephalopathy or hypotension. Patients may be asymptomatic and the diagnosis suggested only by finding an elevated ascitic fluid white blood cell count, or by a positive ascitic fluid culture. The diagnosis is established by an abdominal paracentesis, which should be performed in patients with onset of new ascites or in those with a change in their clinical course. The ascitic fluid white blood cell count is usually above 500 per cubic millimeter (93 per cent of cases), and more than 50 per cent of the cells are polymorphonuclear leukocytes. The ascitic fluid pH also is lower than the blood pH. Bacteria may be identified on Gram's stain. The ascitic fluid and blood should be cultured and treatment instituted before the results of culture are known, as delays in therapy may increase mortality. The organisms most frequently cultured are Enterobacteriaceae (mainly *E. coli*) and Group D streptococci, *Streptococcus pneumoniae*, and *Streptococcus viridans*. Other bacteria are cultured less frequently, and anaerobic bacteria are uncommon isolates. Initial antibiotic therapy should therefore include both an aminoglycoside or newer cephalosporin antibiotic and ampicillin. The response to therapy is monitored by the fever pattern and by changes in the ascitic fluid white blood cell count. If therapy is effective, the ascitic fluid white blood cell count falls and the predominant cell again becomes mononuclear. Antibiotic therapy is continued for 10 to 14 days.

HEPATORENAL SYNDROME

DEFINITION AND PATHOGENESIS. The hepatorenal syndrome (functional renal failure) is a decrease in renal function that develops in a patient with serious liver disease in whom all other causes of renal dysfunction are excluded. The kidneys lack serious pathologic lesions. If the liver disease improves, normal renal function returns. The pathogenesis of the hepatorenal syndrome is unknown. There is intense intrarenal vasoconstriction and redistribution of blood flow. In addition, the plasma levels of renin and aldosterone are increased. These changes may be due to a reduced "effective" plasma volume in some patients.

CLINICAL MANIFESTATIONS. Patients developing the hepatorenal syndrome frequently have severe hepatic disease and therefore are jaundiced and have other signs and symptoms of liver disease. Almost all of the patients with this syndrome have ascites. The illness is marked by oliguria. The urine is usually free of protein, and the urine sediment is normal. The urine sodium is low (<10 mEq per liter), the urine-to-plasma creatinine ratio is high (>30:1), and the urine-to-plasma osmolality ratio is greater than 1.0. These urine findings are different from those of acute tubular necrosis, in which the urine sodium is high (>30 mEq per liter), the urine-to-plasma creatinine ratio is low (<20:1), and the urine is isosmotic to plasma. The progression of the renal failure is variable, with some patients having a complete loss of renal function over several days, whereas in others the serum creatinine slowly increases over several weeks as the liver function gradually worsens.

DIFFERENTIAL DIAGNOSIS. Patients with liver disease may develop renal failure for a variety of reasons. These patients commonly receive diuretics and may develop prerenal azotemia. Renal function will improve with withdrawal of the medication. Acute tubular necrosis may occur following an episode of hypotension (bleeding or sepsis) or during fulminant hepatitis and can be distinguished from hepatorenal failure by the urine findings. Drugs (antibiotics, especially aminoglycosides, and nonsteroidal anti-inflammatory medications) may cause worsening of renal function in patients with cirrhosis. Acute pyelonephritis, with or without papillary necrosis, may also cause renal failure in patients with liver disease.

THERAPY AND PROGNOSIS. Specific causes of renal failure should be looked for and excluded. Any medications that are potential nephrotoxins should be withdrawn. A brief trial of plasma expansion with monitoring of urine output and serum creatinine may be attempted, in order to exclude hypovolemia as a cause of the renal failure. The volume of fluid infused should be limited (1000 ml), as overexpansion of the plasma volume may precipitate variceal hemorrhage. Infusions of vasodilators may transiently improve renal function; however, this does not improve survival. Uremia may be treated by dialysis; however, overall survival is again not improved. The use of peritoneovenous shunts in these patients is being investigated, but their efficacy is as yet unproven. The prognosis for patients with the hepatorenal syndrome is poor, with over 90 per cent dying during hospitalization, usually from liver failure or complications of portal hypertension. Definitive therapies must await a better understanding of the pathogenesis of this syndrome.

Alpern RJ: Renal sodium retention in liver disease. West J Med 138:852, 1983. *A review that provides new ideas about an old problem.*

Epstein M: Peritoneovenous shunt in the management of ascites and the hepatorenal syndrome. Gastroenterology 82:790, 1982. *An authoritative review of the good and bad effects of the peritoneovenous shunt.*

Epstein M (ed.): The Kidney in Liver Disease. 2nd ed. New York, Elsevier Biomedical, 1982. *A complete review of the renal functional alterations in liver disease. Multiple authors contributed to this work.*

Hoefs JC, Canawati HN, Sapico FL, Hopkins RR, Weiner J, Montogomerie JZ: Spontaneous bacterial peritonitis. Hepatology 2:399, 1982. *Describes the clinical features and hospital course of patients with spontaneous peritonitis.*

Perez-Ayuso RM, Arroyo V, Planas R, Gaya J, Bory F, Rimola A, Rivera F, Rodes J: Randomized comparative study of efficacy of furosemide versus spironolactone in nonazotemic cirrhosis with ascites. Relationship between the diuretic response and the activity of the renin-aldosterone system. Gastroenterology 84:961, 1983. *Spironolactone was shown to be a more effective diuretic than furosemide in this group of patients.*

Witte C, Witte M, Dumont A: Lymph imbalance in the genesis and perpetuation of the ascites syndrome in hepatic cirrhosis. Gastroenterology 78:1059, 1980. *Attempts to define the factors responsible for the formation of ascites. The authors introduce new theories and discuss old ones. Requires careful reading.*

127. ACUTE AND CHRONIC HEPATIC FAILURE WITH ENCEPHALOPATHY

Bruce F. Scharschmidt

The syndrome of hepatic encephalopathy, including current concepts of pathogenesis, its accompanying clinical manifestations, and diagnosis and treatment, is discussed in the first part of this chapter. Special considerations apply depending upon the underlying liver disease, and are discussed separately for fulminant hepatic failure and chronic liver disease. Finally, the possible role of hepatic transplantation in patients with end-stage liver disease is briefly reviewed.

THE SYNDROME OF HEPATIC ENCEPHALOPATHY

DEFINITION AND SIGNIFICANCE. Hepatic encephalopathy (also called hepatic coma or portal-systemic encephalopathy) represents a constellation of neurologic signs and symptoms accompanying advanced, decompensated liver disease of all types and/or extensive portal-systemic shunting. For the clinician, recognition of these signs and symptoms often represents an important clue to the presence of deteriorating liver function or superimposed complications. In addition, repeated neurologic evaluation of the encephalopathic patient provides valuable information regarding the patient's course and prognosis.

PATHOGENESIS. The pathogenesis of hepatic encephalopathy remains unclear. A variety of clinical observations indicate that the encephalopathy is at least partially attributable to toxic materials that are derived from the metabolism of nitrogenous substrate in the gut and that bypass the liver through anatomic or functional shunts. This is the origin of the term *portal-systemic encephalopathy*, often used interchangeably with hepatic encephalopathy. Several putative gut-derived toxins have been identified on the basis of their presence in increased amounts in the blood or cerebrospinal fluid of some encephalopathic patients. *Ammonia* and *mercaptans* result from the degradation of urea or protein and sulfur-containing compounds, respectively, and both can produce coma when administered in large doses to animals. The presence of mercaptans in the breath of some encephalopathic patients probably accounts for the characteristic sweetish musty odor termed *fetor hepaticus*. Ammonia-induced changes in central nervous system metabolism include depletion of glutamic and aspartic acids and ATP. While often present in increased amounts in the blood or cerebrospinal fluid or both, the absolute concentration of ammonia, ammonia metabolites including glutamine, and mercaptans correlates only roughly with the presence or severity of encephalopathy. *Gamma-aminobutyric acid* is also produced in the gut and is present in increased amounts in the blood of patients and animals with hepatic failure. It is the principal inhibitory neurotransmitter in the mammalian brain, and the sedative-hypnotic effects of benzodiazepines and barbiturates are believed to be mediated via the γ-aminobutyric neurotransmitter system. A role for γ-aminobutyric acid in hepatic encephalopathy is supported by the observation that visual evoked potentials in animals with hepatic failure mimic those of benzodiazepine-induced or barbiturate-induced coma but differ from those of comatose states caused by administration of ether, ammonia, or mercaptans. Abnormal neurotransmission is also the cornerstone of a separate hypothesis, which holds that accelerated entry of *aromatic amino acids* into the central nervous system results in decreased synthesis of normal neurotransmitters such as norepinephrine and enhanced synthesis of *false neurotransmitters* such as octopamine. Other compounds such as *fatty acids* are also present in blood in increased amounts and have been proposed as potentially toxic. Finally, several studies have demonstrated impaired integrity of the *blood-brain barrier* in animals with acute hepatic failure, and it is possible that hepatic

TABLE 127–1. STAGES OF HEPATIC ENCEPHALOPATHY

Stage I	Varied manifestations, including apathy, lack of awareness, euphoria, anxiety, restlessness, shortened attention span
Stage II	Lethargy, drowsiness, disorientation
Stage III	Deep somnolence (but patient can at least transiently be aroused)
Stage IV	Coma (absent verbal response)

encephalopathy may represent the combined effects of a number of toxins acting on an unusually susceptible nervous system.

NEUROLOGIC MANIFESTATIONS. The personality and mental changes of hepatic encephalopathy are frequently divided into stages as outlined in Table 127–1. Although this staging of encephalopathy is generally useful, marked individual variations occur, and many patients do not show an orderly progression of symptoms. Moreover, the clinical grading scale is relatively insensitive. Standardized testing has revealed psychomotor abnormalities in a high proportion of patients with cirrhosis in whom conventional neurologic examination is normal. Such *subclinical encephalopathy* is potentially important inasmuch as it may be associated with impaired functional capacity, including job performance and ability to drive an automobile. Patients with hepatic encephalopathy also display a characteristic spectrum of abnormal neurologic signs. Early signs may include asterixis, myoclonus, hyperactive muscle stretch reflexes, facial grimacing, and blinking, as well as primitive reflexes such as suck, snout, and grasp. As encephalopathy progresses, extensor toe responses, clonus, and decerebrate or decorticate posturing may be observed. Generalized flaccidity with absent reflexes occurs preterminally.

In addition to the acute, reversible signs and symptoms already mentioned, some patients with longstanding liver disease and portal-systemic shunting develop *irreversible neurologic dysfunction.* This infrequent form of hepatic encephalopathy may be characterized by prominent and persistent motor abnormalities, which include tremor, rigidity, slurred speech, oral-facial dyskinesia, choreoathetosis, and ataxic gait. Spastic paraparesis is another unusual manifestation of advanced chronic liver disease and portal-systemic shunting.

As with other types of metabolic encephalopathy, asymmetrical neurologic findings can occur but are unusual, and brainstem reflexes such as the pupillary light response, oculovestibular response, and oculocephalic response are typically preserved until very late. Thus, asymmetric neurologic signs or abnormal brainstem reflexes may suggest a structural lesion of the central nervous system such as a subdural hematoma. Seizures, like asymmetrical findings, are uncommon in the absence of alcohol withdrawal and should alert the clinician to the possibility of a structural lesion or hypoglycemia. In addition to its value in differential diagnosis, the neurologic examination may be helpful in assessing prognosis in the comatose patient. For example, the disappearance of pupillary reactivity, of the oculocephalic or oculovestibular response, or of deep tendon reflexes is associated with a very poor prognosis in all types of metabolic encephalopathy, including hepatic encephalopathy (but excluding drug overdose). Electroencephalographic changes are sensitive indicators of hepatic encephalopathy but are not specific for this disorder. They include symmetrical slowing observed initially over the frontal areas with later spreading laterally and posteriorly.

DIAGNOSIS. There is no single laboratory test or clinical finding that can unequivocally establish the diagnosis of hepatic encephalopathy. Rather, the diagnosis is based upon the presence of compatible neurologic signs and symptoms in a patient with advanced liver disease and exclusion of other possible causes of the neurologic abnormalities. Routine laboratory studies including electrolytes, calcium, blood urea nitrogen, creatinine, glucose, and standard liver function tests are of help primarily in excluding other causes of metabolic encephalopathy and evaluating the presence and severity of hepatic disease. Toxicologic screening is also appropriate when ingestion of sedatives or toxins capable of altering neurologic function is suspected. Determinations of blood ammonia and cerebrospinal fluid levels of glutamine are helpful when markedly elevated. However, levels correlate only roughly with mental status. These tests are therefore of limited value in most circumstances. Structural lesions such as a subdural hematoma are often a consideration and may require special radiologic studies. Other causes of encephalopathy such as the Wernicke-Korsakoff syndrome, sepsis, or meningitis must also be excluded, depending on the clinical circumstances.

TREATMENT. ***Supportive Care.*** There is no clinically established way of initiating hepatic regeneration or improving hepatic function; the management of patients with hepatic encephalopathy is therefore largely supportive. A thorough search should be made to detect and correct factors that may precipitate or aggravate encephalopathy (Table 127–2). All nonessential drugs should be stopped—particularly sedatives and potentially hepatotoxic agents. For the occasional patient who demonstrates manic disorientation as an early manifestation of encephalopathy, soft restraints are preferable to sedative hypnotic agents. Therapy should also be directed at decreasing the production of ammonia and other substances that result from enteric bacterial metabolism of nitrogenous substrates. Blood urea nitrogen should be lowered if possible since urea diffuses into the gut and is a substrate for ammonia production. Gut cleansing should be accomplished by enema and by oral administration of cathartics such as magnesium citrate. It is also generally appropriate to restrict dietary protein to about 40 grams per day in mildly encephalopathic patients and eliminate it in patients with more advanced or progressive encephalopathy. Several additional points regarding protein merit consideration. First, *vegetable protein* appears somewhat less likely to induce encephalopathy than animal protein and may be useful in the long-term management of patients with chronic or recurrent encephalopathy. Second, preliminary studies suggest that protein administration may be beneficial in patients with acute alcoholic hepatitis. Since protein-calorie malnutrition may play a role in the pathogenesis of this disorder, judicious administration of 40 to 80 grams of protein, with careful observation, may be appropriate for patients with alcoholic hepatitis and even moderate encephalopathy. Finally, several investigators believe that oral or parenteral administration of *branched chain amino acids* is beneficial in the treatment of hepatic encephalopathy, by virtue of their ability to compete with aromatic amino acids for entry into the central nervous system and normalize neurotransmitter metabolism (see above). To date, such recommendations are based largely on uncontrolled clinical observations.

In addition to these measures aimed at decreasing nitrogenous substrate, ammonia production should be further inhibited by oral administration of a poorly absorbable antibiotic, such as neomycin in a dose of 1 to 2 grams every six hours, or by administration of lactulose. Lactulose (β-1,4-galactoside-fructose) is neither metabolized nor absorbed in the upper small bowel and is metabolized by ileal and colonic bacteria to organic acids. It is as effective as neomycin in lowering blood ammonia and reversing encephalopathy in patients with chronic liver

TABLE 127–2. HEPATIC ENCEPHALOPATHY—COMMON PRECIPITATING FACTORS

Deterioration in hepatic function
Drugs (sedative or potentially hepatotoxic agents)
Gastrointestinal hemorrhage
Increased dietary protein
Azotemia
Hypokalemia
Infection
Constipation
Anesthesia and surgery
Hypoxia
Diuretics (hypokalemia, alkalosis, and hypovolemia)

disease. The mechanisms of action of lactulose may include increased bacterial assimilation of ammonia, decreased ammonia production, and possibly trapping of ammonia as NH_4^+ or ammonia precursors in the bowel lumen made more acidic by its metabolism. Lactulose therapy is commonly initiated by administering 50 ml of the syrup orally every two hours until diarrhea ensues. Thereafter, the dose is decreased to that amount necessary to produce two to four soft stools per day. Lactulose can also be given by retention enema. Although it has been assumed that the administration of neomycin with lactulose might impair the effectiveness of lactulose by inhibiting the bacteria responsible for its metabolism, recent studies suggest that concomitant administration of the two agents may be useful in selected patients.

FULMINANT HEPATIC FAILURE

ETIOLOGY. Fulminant hepatic failure is defined as hepatic failure with Stage III or IV encephalopathy developing in less than eight weeks in a patient without pre-existing liver disease. It develops most commonly as a complication of viral hepatitis (usually B or non-A non-B), but may also result from exposure to a potentially hepatotoxic drug (e.g., acetaminophen) or anesthetic (halothane), exposure to a frank hepatotoxin (e.g., carbon tetrachloride or yellow phosphorus), or from certain less common hepatic disorders (e.g., acute hepatic vein occlusion, acute fatty liver of pregnancy) and infections (herpes simplex virus). Reye's syndrome may present a similar clinical picture; however, it differs from most forms of fulminant hepatic failure in its presumed pathogenesis, its rarity beyond the second decade of life, and by the accumulation of microvesicular fat in hepatocytes.

DIAGNOSIS. The diagnosis of fulminant hepatic failure requires the presence of Stage III or IV encephalopathy in a patient with severe, acute liver disease. Synthetic function of the liver as reflected by the prothrombin time is nearly always markedly abnormal. Serum bilirubin concentration is less helpful, since some patients may become very ill rapidly and progress to coma before the serum bilirubin is markedly elevated. Serum transaminase levels are usually elevated early in the illness but do not reliably distinguish between fulminant hepatic failure and acute hepatitis without encephalopathy.

TREATMENT. A thorough search should be made to detect and correct factors that may precipitate or aggravate encephalopathy (Table 127–2); however, encephalopathy in fulminant hepatic failure primarily reflects the severe nature of the underlying liver injury, and correcting potential precipitating factors is less likely to produce objective benefit than it is in patients with encephalopathy complicating chronic liver disease. In addition to the aforementioned general measures, special attention must be directed to those complications that frequently occur in patients with fulminant hepatic failure. *Hypoglycemia* is common and results from impaired glycogenolysis and gluconeogenesis. Frequent monitoring of blood glucose is necessary, and administration of 2 to 3 liters per day of a 10 per cent dextrose solution is often advisable. *Hyponatremia,* which is typically due to a combination of impaired renal clearance of free water and administration of excessive free water in the form of dextrose solutions, may require water restriction. *Hypokalemia,* which increases renal ammonia production, should be corrected. *Azotemia* frequently occurs and may result from hypovolemia, hepatorenal syndrome, or acute tubular necrosis. Hypovolemia should be corrected when present. Survival in patients with fulminant hepatic failure and either the hepatorenal syndrome or acute tubular necrosis does not appear to be improved by dialysis. In the patient with severe hypoprothrombinemia and serious *bleeding,* administration of fresh frozen plasma is appropriate in addition to measures directed more specifically at the source of hemorrhage. The risk of gastrointestinal bleeding in patients with fulminant hepatic failure has been shown to be reduced by prophylactic administration of the H_2-receptor antagonist cimetidine. However, on the basis of studies in other critically ill patient groups, prophylactic administration of antacids is probably more effective and generally advisable. There is no evidence that heparin improves survival in patients with *disseminated intravascular coagulation* with hepatic failure. The risk of pulmonary, genitourinary, and other *infections* should be minimized by proper positioning of the patient to prevent aspiration and by judicious use of genitourinary and intravenous catheters. *Bacteremia* is a frequent complication of fulminant hepatic failure, with streptococci, *Staphylococcus aureus,* and *E. coli* being the most commonly isolated organisms. *Hypoxemia* is commonly present even in the absence of obvious pulmonary pathology; it may result from both functional right-to-left shunting and ventilation perfusion imbalance and should be corrected by administration of oxygen. *Pulmonary edema* may occur in the absence of left heart failure and may require mechanical ventilation with positive end-expiratory pressure. *Hypotension* is common even in the absence of sepsis or bleeding and results from reduced systemic vascular resistance. However, pressors are often ineffective or only transiently effective. *Respiratory alkalosis* is a common early finding and requires no treatment. *Metabolic acidosis,* which occurs rarely and may be due to lactic acid accumulation, should be treated with bicarbonate. *Cerebral edema* is present in over half of patients dying of fulminant hepatic failure and may result in intracranial herniation. Moreover, in conjunction with systemic hypotension, it reduces cerebral perfusion and may cause brain death. Corticosteroids do not appear to be of benefit, but a single controlled study suggests that direct monitoring of intracranial pressure and treatment of intracranial hypertension with mannitol significantly improves survival. Treatment of clinically evident intracranial hypertension, manifested by unequal or abnormally reactive pupils, myoclonus, and/or decerebrate posturing, is certainly appropriate. Unfortunately, clinical signs may be an insensitive way of detecting intracranial hypertension. The decision regarding invasive intracranial pressure monitoring must thus be carefully individualized.

Experimental Measures. Because the mortality of fulminant hepatic failure is high even with optimal supportive care, a variety of other forms of therapy have been tried. Some of these, *corticosteroid administration, exchange transfusion,* and administration of *L-dopa* or *hepatitis B hyperimmune globulin* (for hepatitis B), have been shown to be ineffective by controlled prospective clinical trials. Similar controlled observations for the remaining measures, which include *amino acid infusion, plasmapheresis, hemodialysis, total body washout, cross circulation* with a human volunteer or baboon, or *extracorporeal perfusion* through a human cadaver liver, pig liver, or baboon liver are not available. However, the reported uncontrolled observations strongly suggest that these experimental forms of therapy offer *no advantage* over conventional supportive care. Several reports suggest that *charcoal hemoperfusion* may improve survival, but the efficacy of this treatment needs to be established by controlled trials.

PROGNOSIS. The short-term prognosis for patients with fulminant hepatic failure who progress to coma is poor, the average reported survival being about 20 per cent. In contrast, the outlook for those patients who do survive an episode of fulminant hepatic failure with coma is quite good. Virtually all patients have returned to their previous state of health within two to three months, and follow-up liver biopsies have usually demonstrated no or minimal abnormalities. Patients with persistent biochemical or histologic abnormalities have frequently been found to have had pre-existing liver disease or to have continuing exposure to toxic or infectious agents, as for example through parenteral drug abuse.

CHRONIC LIVER DISEASE WITH ENCEPHALOPATHY

ETIOLOGY. Hepatic encephalopathy may also occur in patients with chronic liver disease, usually cirrhosis with portal-systemic shunting. Some patients with cirrhosis may be chronically encephalopathic. In most, however, encephalopathy tends to occur acutely and intermittently. In this latter group, the occurrence of encephalopathy reflects a worsening of hepatic function and/or the presence of one or more precipitating factors (Table 127–2).

DIAGNOSIS. As with fulminant hepatic failure, diagnosis requires the presence of signs and symptoms compatible with hepatic encephalopathy in a patient with underlying chronic liver disease. Routine tests of liver function are typically abnormal but are of little value in differential diagnosis. Unlike fulminant hepatic failure, encephalopathy in patients with chronic liver disease may be accompanied by only minimally abnormal liver function tests. A markedly elevated or rising prothrombin time in an encephalopathic patient with known chronic liver disease suggests superimposed acute hepatocellular necrosis. It is extremely important in patients with chronic alcoholic liver disease to exclude other causes of metabolic encephalopathy (e.g., hypoglycemia, alcohol intoxication, Wernicke-Korsakoff syndrome), meningitis, or structural lesions such as subdural hematoma.

TREATMENT. Unlike fulminant hepatic failure, encephalopathy in the patient with chronic liver disease is frequently not due to acute hepatocellular necrosis, but rather results from one or more potentially reversible precipitating factors. The essential first step in the management of these patients is to identify and, when possible, correct such factors as are outlined in Table 127–2. Additional general measures as outlined earlier for the treatment of hepatic encephalopathy should be undertaken. A small number of patients with chronic hepatic encephalopathy fail to respond to standard measures, and preliminary clinical studies suggest that administration of ornithine salts of branched-chain keto acids or bromocriptine may be helpful in this selected patient group.

The complications and additional supportive care required for these patients are similar to those described for fulminant hepatic failure. Overall, however, the severity and frequency of complications (e.g., hypoglycemia) are less than with fulminant hepatic failure. The various forms of experimental therapy that have been tried in fulminant hepatic failure also have no established role in the management of patients with chronic liver disease with encephalopathy.

PROGNOSIS. Because encephalopathy in patients with chronic liver disease is frequently precipitated by potentially reversible factors, the short-term prognosis is better than in fulminant hepatic failure. Most patients survive the acute episode, particularly if the encephalopathy is not attributable to a sudden deterioration of hepatic function. However, because the underlying chronic liver disease is commonly irreversible and slowly progressive, the long-term prognosis is guarded.

HEPATIC TRANSPLANTATION

The first orthotopic liver transplantation in a human was performed in 1963. Since then, more than 600 transplants have been performed worldwide and the frequency of transplant procedures continues to increase; indeed, well over half of all transplants have been performed since January 1, 1980. As a result of newer immunosuppressive therapy, better supportive care, and improved surgical techniques, the survival of patients having transplantation for nonmalignant conditions has also steadily improved. The most frequent indication for hepatic transplantation has been end-stage nonalcoholic cirrhosis, and the three-year survival of patients in this group having transplants since 1980 is about 41 per cent. A relatively small number of patients with alcoholic cirrhosis has received liver transplants and the three-year survival among these patients has been only 20 per cent. The other major disease categories for which hepatic transplantation has been performed, listed in order of frequency, and the corresponding three-year survivals for patients undergoing transplantation since 1980, are as follows: biliary atresia (60 per cent); hepatocellular carcinoma (20 per cent); cholangiocarcinoma (less than 10 per cent); metabolic disorders, predominantly α_1-antitrypsin deficiency (60 per cent); sclerosing cholangitis (25 per cent); Budd-Chiari syndrome (47 per cent); and other miscellaneous disorders.

Given the lack of satisfactory therapeutic alternatives for most patients with end-stage liver disease and the anticipation of continued improvement in survival among transplant recipients, it is likely that transplantation will be used with increasing frequency for a variety of chronic hepatic disorders. As of yet, liver transplantation has had little application to patients with fulminant hepatic failure. This is largely a result of the difficulties inherent in procuring a donor liver within a short period of time and in transporting a critically ill and unstable prospective recipient to a transplant center for major surgery. With an increasing number of centers performing transplants, increasingly efficient donor organ procurement, and possibly development of auxiliary liver transplantation in which the recipient's own liver is left in place, transplantation may become a realistic possibility for selected patients with fulminant hepatic failure.

Canalese J, Gimson AE, Davis C, Davis M, Mellon PJ, Williams R: Controlled trial of dexamethasone and mannitol for the cerebral oedema of fulminant hepatic failure. Gut 23:625, 1982. *A controlled study reporting improved survival with aggressive monitoring of intracranial pressure and treatment with mannitol.*

Conn HO, Leevy CM, Vlahcevic ZR, Rodgers JB, Maddrey WC, Seef L, Levy LL: Comparison of lactulose and neomycin in the treatment of chronic portal-systemic encephalopathy. A double-blind controlled trial. Gastroenterology 72:573, 1977. *A skillfully designed prospective study in patients with cirrhosis and chronic portal-systemic encephalopathy. Provides useful information regarding clinical assessment of encephalopathy as well as administration of lactulose and neomycin.*

Flute PT: Clotting abnormalities in liver disease. *In* Popper H, Schaffner F (eds.): Progress in Liver Diseases. New York, Grune & Stratton, 1979, pp 301–322. *A concise review of the role of the liver in blood clotting with emphasis on practical applications.*

Gazzard BG, Portmann B, Murray-Lyon JM, Williams R: Causes of death in fulminant hepatic failure and relationship to quantitative histologic assessment of parenchymal damage. Quart J Med 44:615, 1975. *An analysis of 132 patients with fulminant hepatic failure, one of the largest series ever compiled.*

Gimson AE, Mellon PJ, Branch S, Canalese J, Williams R: Earlier charcoal hemoperfusion in fulminant hepatic failure. Lancet 2:681, 1982. *An uncontrolled study reporting apparently improved survival with this treatment.*

Hoyumpa AM Jr, Desmond PV, Avant GR, Roberts RK, Schenker S: Hepatic encephalopathy. Gastroenterology 76:184, 1979. *A concise review with illustrative case material emphasizing the clinical features and treatment of hepatic encephalopathy.*

Karvountzis GC, Redeker AG, Peters RL: Long-term follow-up studies of patients surviving fulminant viral hepatitis. Gastroenterology 67:879, 1974. *Clinical, biochemical, and histologic findings in 22 patients surviving acute hepatitis with encephalopathy.*

Plum F, Hindfelt B: The neurological complications of liver disease. *In* Vinken PJ, Bruyn GW (eds.): Handbook of Clinical Neurology. Amsterdam, North Holland Publishing Company, 1976, pp 349–377. *The clinical description of neurologic abnormalities is a particularly valuable part of this comprehensive review.*

Schafer DF, Jones EA: Potential neural mechanisms in the pathogenesis of hepatic encephalopathy. *In* Popper H, Schaffner F (eds.): Progress in Liver Diseases. New York, Grune & Stratton, 1982, pp 615–627. *A concise review with emphasis on the possible role of gamma-aminobutyric acid in hepatic encephalopathy.*

Scharschmidt BF: Human liver transplantation: Analysis of data on 540 patients from four centers. Hepatology, 4:95S Jan-Feb Suppl, 1984. *A recent summary of the results of liver transplantation in humans.*

Uribe M, Marquez MA, Ramos GG, et al.: Treatment of portal-systemic encephalopathy with vegetable and animal protein diets: A control crossover study. Dig Dis Sci 27:1109, 1982. *A controlled study of different protein sources with important practical details regarding diet.*

Van Dyke RW, Scharschmidt BF: Hepatic encephalopathy and hepatic failure. *In* Watts D (ed.): Gastrointestinal Disease. Los Altos, CA, Lange Medical Publications, 1984 (In press). *A recent comprehensive review of the topic.*

Zieve L: Hepatic encephalopathy: Summary of present knowledge with an elaboration on recent developments. *In* Popper H, Schaffner F (eds.): Progress in Liver Diseases. New York, Grune & Stratton, 1979, pp 327–342. *A concise summary of recent investigations regarding the pathogenesis of hepatic encephalopathy.*

128. HEPATIC TUMORS

Bruce F. Scharschmidt

A variety of tumors occur in the liver. Each has certain distinctive features with respect to pathology, pathogenesis, clinical presentation, treatment, and/or prognosis, and these are discussed here under the headings Benign and Malignant Hepatic Tumors. The diagnostic approach to a patient with a suspected hepatic neoplasm is discussed at the end of this chapter.

BENIGN HEPATIC TUMORS

Hepatocellular Adenoma

Hepatocellular adenomas occur almost exclusively in women. These tumors are most frequently detected during the child-bearing years, particularly the third and fourth decades of life, but are occasionally found in postmenopausal women as well. Adenomas most commonly occur in the right lobe of the liver, are solitary in about one third of the cases, and are often quite large, with up to one half being 10 cm or more in diameter. Hepatocellular adenomas are usually well circumscribed, may be surrounded by a pseudocapsule, and often show areas of bile stasis, hemorrhage, and necrosis. Microscopically, these tumors consist of a monotonous array of normal to slightly atypical hepatocytes without portal tracts or bile ducts. Kupffer cells are markedly reduced in number or absent, and a few arteries and thin-walled veins are present.

The preponderance of this tumor in women suggests a hormonal role in its pathogenesis, and there is strong circumstantial evidence implicating oral contraceptives. The number of reported cases of this tumor has increased dramatically since oral contraceptives were introduced in 1960. A literature review in 1974 cited only 67 cases, yet it is estimated that about 300 hepatocellular adenomas are now diagnosed annually in the United States, and nearly 90 per cent of these are associated with oral contraceptive use. Moreover, some adenomas have clearly regressed in a period of months to years after oral contraceptives were discontinued. The risk of developing this tumor appears to increase steadily with increasing duration of oral contraceptive use, and the annual incidence is estimated to be 3 to 4 per 100,000 in women who have taken oral contraceptives continuously for several years. Although not generally regarded as a premalignant lesion, there are rare instances in which hepatocellular carcinoma appears to have arisen in an hepatocellular adenoma.

Most patients with hepatocellular adenoma present with signs and symptoms of an abdominal mass, tumor infarction, or intratumor hemorrhage (pain, fever, leukocytosis), or tumor rupture (pain, hemoperitoneum, circulatory collapse). Because the true incidence of these tumors is unknown, the actual proportion that ruptures cannot be determined. However, about one third of patients with hepatocellular adenoma develop intra-abdominal hemorrhage, and the mortality in this group is approximately 20 per cent.

Because Kupffer cells are infrequent or absent, hepatocellular adenomas usually appear as a defect ("cold spot") on ^{99m}technetium–sulfur colloid scans. They show a range of angiographic appearances from hypovascular to hypervascular. The management of hepatocellular adenomas is a matter of some debate. Complete surgical excision is commonly undertaken because of the high incidence and mortality of tumor rupture. In patients taking oral contraceptives that can be discontinued, a trial period of observation with repeated radionuclide scans is also justifiable, particularly if the location, size, or number of tumors would make resection hazardous.

Focal Nodular Hyperplasia

Focal nodular hyperplasia, which shows a female to male predominance of 2:1 to 7:1, has also been referred to as pseudotumor, focal cirrhosis, and hepatic hamartoma. Despite distinctive pathologic features, focal nodular hyperplasia and hepatocellular adenoma have often been confused in the medical literature. Unlike hepatocellular adenoma, a firm link between focal nodular hyperplasia and oral contraceptives has not been established. Focal nodular hyperplasia generally is a solitary tumor in the right lobe. It has a characteristic grossly lobulated appearance on cut section, which is produced by a central fibrous core with septa radiating in a stellate pattern. Hemorrhage and necrosis are rare. Microscopically, these fibrous septa contain bile ductules and inflammatory cells and are surrounded by normal or slightly atypical hepatocytes as well as Kupffer cells.

Unlike hepatocellular adenomas, focal nodular hyperplasia does not usually produce symptoms and is generally found incidentally at surgery or necropsy. In up to 20 per cent of the cases, it presents as an upper abdominal mass. Portal hypertension has been reported in association with multiple lesions, and rupture is rare. Because these tumors contain Kupffer cells, they frequently take up ^{99m}technetium–sulfur colloid normally and may appear as voids, hot spots, or some combination of these on scan. Occasionally they exhibit uniform uptake of isotope equivalent to that of normal liver and are not visualized by ^{99m}technetium–sulfur colloid scan. They are characteristically hypervascular on angiography with a visible capillary blush. Since focal nodular hyperplasia has no known malignant potential, asymptomatic lesions can be followed nonoperatively if resection would be difficult or hazardous. If encountered unexpectedly at surgery, simple wedge biopsy is appropriate if complete excision would be difficult.

Hemangioma

Cavernous hemangioma is probably the most common benign hepatic tumor, with a 0.4 to 7.3 per cent incidence in necropsy series and a predominance in females. The great majority of hemangiomas are found incidentally at surgery or necroscopy. These lesions can, however, present with signs and symptoms of an abdominal mass, infarction, rupture, or thrombocytopenia and hypofibrinogenemia.

Despite their vascular nature, hemangiomas may appear as a cold spot on radionuclide scanning, even with rapid sequence imaging. Their presence can occasionally be suspected on plain roentgenogram of the abdomen by the presence of calcified spicules radiating from the center of the lesion. The angiographic appearance of dense and persistent tumor staining is virtually diagnostic. Computed tomographic studies with rapid sequential imaging following the bolus injection of intravenous contrast material may also provide diagnostically useful information in many cases. The definitive treatment of symptomatic hepatic hemangiomas is surgical resection. There are also case reports of regression following radiotherapy or hepatic artery ligation.

Other Benign Tumors

A variety of less common benign liver tumors may also occur in adults. They usually produce no symptoms unless very large. Included in this group are *bile duct adenomas, bile duct cystadenomas, fibromas, lipomas, leiomyomas, mesotheliomas, teratomas,* and *myxomas. Nodular regenerative hyperplasia* is a condition characterized by multiple nodules of varying size arising in a noncirrhotic liver. The nodules are composed of liver plates that are two cells thick. An association with rheumatoid arthritis, Felty's syndrome, CREST syndrome, oral contraceptives, and a variety of drugs is reported. The most common manifestation of nodular regenerative hyperplasia is portal hypertension.

MALIGNANT HEPATIC TUMORS

Hepatocellular Carcinoma

EPIDEMIOLOGY. In the United States and Western Europe, hepatocellular carcinoma (hepatoma) is increasing in incidence but remains relatively uncommon, accounting for less than 1 per cent of all causes of death at autopsy and 2.5 per cent or less of all malignancies. In certain other areas of the world, including parts of sub-Saharan Africa, Southeast Asia, Japan, Oceania, and Greece, hepatocellular carcinoma is the most frequent or one of the most frequent malignancies and an important cause of overall mortality. Hepatocellular carcinoma is predominantly a disease of males and usually arises in a cirrhotic liver. The risk appears to be greatest in cirrhosis associated with hemochromatosis and hepatitis B virus infection, low in primary biliary cirrhosis and Wilson's disease, and intermediate in alcoholic and cryptogenic cirrhosis. Compelling evidence indicates that chronic hepatitis B virus infection may predispose to hepatocellular carcinoma: (1) The aforementioned areas of the world in which hepatocellular carcinoma is most prevalent are the same areas in which hepatitis B virus infection is most common. (2) Serologic evidence of hepatitis B virus infection is much more common in patients with hepatocellular carcinoma than in controls, an observation that has been made in all parts of the world including the United States. (3) Prospective studies have indicated that the incidence of hepatocellular carcinoma is several hundred-fold higher in individuals with hepatitis B virus infection than in noninfected controls. (4) Analysis of tumor tissue in patients with serologic evidence of hepatitis B virus infection has indicated the presence of hepatitis B virus integrated into the host genome. (5) Woodchucks infected with a virus that appears to be a close relative of the hepatitis B virus that infects humans are predisposed to the development of hepatocellular carcinoma.

In most cases, hepatocellular carcinoma develops in a cirrhotic liver. However, in about one quarter of all hepatitis B virus–associated cases, no hepatic fibrosis is present. Epidemiologic evidence has also suggested a link between hepatocellular carcinoma and ingestion of aflatoxins, mycotoxins produced by *Aspergillus flavus*, a mold that can grow in warm moist areas and contaminate peanuts and stored grains. Case reports have also suggested a link between hepatocellular carcinoma and α_1-antitrypsin deficiency and administration of androgenic steroids, Thorotrast, and possibly estrogenic steroids in the form of oral contraceptives (Table 128–1).

CLINICAL FEATURES. The most common presenting symptoms of hepatocellular carcinoma are *abdominal pain*, the presence of an *abdominal mass*, and *weight loss*. Hepatocellular carcinoma may also present with rupture and hemoperitoneum, obstructive jaundice, unexplained deterioration in a patient with cirrhosis, or a variety of unusual manifestations, including erythrocytosis, hypercalcemia, and hypoglycemia. Hepatomegaly is present in about two thirds of patients. Other suggestive physical findings include the presence of a bruit, hepatic friction rub, or bloody ascites. Hepatocellular carcinoma may invade and obstruct the portal and hepatic veins and metastasizes most often to regional lymph nodes and the lungs. Alpha-fetoprotein levels in serum greater than 1000 ng per ml or progressively rising levels are highly suggestive of hepatocellular carcinoma. Unfortunately, only a minority of patients with hepatocellular carcinoma in most parts of the world, including the United States, have elevations of this magnitude, and low level elevations up to about 200 ng per ml are relatively nonspecific. For this reason, α-fetoprotein has proved disappointing in the screening of high risk populations in Japan, where only about 50 per cent of patients with tumors less than 5 cm in size had elevations greater than 200 ng per ml, and less than 20 per cent had levels exceeding 1000 μg per ml. Hepatocellular carcinomas typically fail to take up ^{99m}technetium–sulfur colloid but accumulate ^{67}gallium normally on radionuclide scan, and they generally appear as an irregular hypervascular mass with tumor "staining" and arterial displacement and/or encasement on angiography.

TREATMENT AND PROGNOSIS. The results of current treatment for hepatocellular carcinoma are discouraging. In the United States, median survival from the time of diagnosis is about six months, and survival appears to be even shorter in African patients. Because of the advanced stage of the disease at the time of diagnosis and the frequent coexistence of severe liver disease, only a small fraction of patients are candidates for hepatic resection. Adriamycin alone or in combination with

TABLE 128–1. HEPATOCELLULAR CARCINOMA

Incidence From 1–7 per 100,000 to > 100 per 100,000 in high-risk areas **Sex** 4:1 to 8:1 male predominance, except fibrolamellar carcinoma **Associations** Cirrhosis Hepatitis B virus infection (usually with cirrhosis) Hemochromatosis (with cirrhosis) Aflatoxin ingestion Thorotrast α_1-antitrypsin deficiency **Common Clinical Presentations** Abdominal pain Abdominal mass Weight loss Deterioration of liver function	**Unusual Manifestations** Bloody ascites Tumor emboli to lung Obstructive jaundice Obstruction of hepatic or portal veins Bloody ascites Metabolic (erythrocytosis, hypercalcemia, hypercholesterolemia, carcinoid syndrome, sexual changes, hypoglycemia, acquired porphyria) **Suggestive Clinical or Laboratory Findings** Hepatic bruit or friction rub α-fetoprotein ↑ (> 400 ng/ml)

other agents has produced objective tumor response in up to 50 per cent of patients, but has minimally affected survival. Radiation therapy has also yielded disappointing results. Hormonal therapy has been tried, but experience with this approach is too limited to judge its value. As discussed in Ch. 127, transplantation has been performed in over 100 patients with unresectable hepatocellular carcinoma, and the three-year survival among such patients has been about 15 per cent.

Recently a variant of typical hepatocellular carcinoma termed fibrolamellar carcinoma has been described. This tumor differs from the typical form of the disease in that it usually occurs in young adults without underlying cirrhosis, lacks the usual male predominance, is associated with a longer survival when untreated, and has been cured surgically in between 10 and 30 per cent of cases.

Other Primary Hepatic Malignancies

Cholangiocarcinoma occurs much less frequently than hepatocellular carcinoma, and shows an association with clonorchiasis in the Far East. It may present with obstructive jaundice when it involves major ducts in the area of the hepatic hilum. Truly mixed hepatocellular cholangiocarcinomas are rare. Angiosarcoma, an unusual tumor associated with vinyl chloride exposure as well as arsenic and Thorotrast administration, frequently causes thrombocytopenia and has a propensity to rupture, causing hemoperitoneum and circulatory collapse. Other unusual primary hepatic malignancies of adults include cholangiocellular carcinoma, cystadenocarcinoma, squamous carcinoma, and hepatoblastoma.

As with hepatocellular carcinoma, treatment of these hepatic malignancies has been unsatisfactory. Resection is seldom possible. About 40 patients with cholangiocarcinoma have undergone liver transplantation, and the three-year survival in this group has been about 7 per cent.

Tumors Metastatic to Liver

The liver and lung are the most frequent sites of metastatic malignancy, and metastases constitute the largest group of hepatic tumors in adults. Necropsy studies have demonstrated hepatic metastases in more than half of patients with primary malignancies having portal venous drainage (e.g., stomach, colon, and pancreas). Other solid tumors that frequently metastasize to the liver include melanoma and tumors of the lung, oropharynx, and bladder. Next to the spleen, the liver is also the most common extranodal site of involvement by Hodgkin's disease, the non-Hodgkin's lymphomas, and malignant histiocytosis (histiocytic medullary reticulosis).

DIAGNOSTIC APPROACH TO THE PATIENT WITH A SUSPECTED HEPATIC NEOPLASM

Most hepatic neoplasms present as a right upper quadrant or epigastric mass. Additional clinical features that may provide clues regarding the specific type of tumor have been noted above and include pre-existing cirrhosis (hepatocellular carcinoma), portal or hepatic vein thrombosis (hepatocellular carcinoma), oral contraceptive use (hepatocellular adenoma), abdominal pain with hemoperitoneum and hypotension (hepatocellular adenoma; less commonly angiosarcoma, hepatocellular carcinoma, hemangioma), and unusual systemic manifestations (hepatocellular carcinoma). Cholangiocarcinoma and hepatocellular carcinoma can cause biliary obstruction, but this may potentially result from strategically located tumors of all types.

Physical examination most commonly reveals hepatomegaly or a discrete mass. The presence of a bruit or friction rub may suggest hepatocellular carcinoma but is not specific. Alkaline phosphatase and transaminase elevations are the most common biochemical abnormalities. In general, however, liver function tests are neither specific nor particularly helpful in the diagnosis of hepatic tumors and may be entirely normal in some patients. Uncommon biochemical abnormalities in patients with hepatocellular carcinoma include the presence of a variant alkaline phosphatase, erythrocytosis, or hypercholesterolemia. A markedly elevated and/or progressively rising α-fetoprotein level is strongly suggestive of hepatocellular carcinoma.

Examination of tissue is ultimately required for the unequivocal diagnosis of hepatic tumors. In a patient with a known extrahepatic malignancy and clinical or biochemical evidence of hepatic metastases, radionuclide scanning is a reasonable first step in the workup and can be expected to reliably detect solid metastases greater than 2 to 3 cm in diameter. The finding of single or multiple defects on radionuclide scan is consistent with metastatic disease, and a percutaneous biopsy can be expected to recover tumor in 50 to 75 per cent of such cases. Two biopsies performed through the same skin site and cytologic examination of the tissue core and aspirated fluid appear to enhance the yield. The biopsy should be directed at a palpable nodule or radionuclide scan defect when possible. In patients with lymphoreticular malignancies, percutaneous biopsy is less sensitive in demonstrating hepatic involvement than wedge biopsy obtained at laparotomy, and histologic evidence of hepatic involvement may be found even in the absence of clinical, biochemical, or radionuclide scan abnormalities.

The workup of a patient with a suspected primary hepatic tumor must be individualized on the basis of the relative risks and benefits of establishing a diagnosis. Radionuclide scanning is again often helpful, but abnormalities can be very difficult to interpret in patients with diffuse hepatocellular disease or cirrhosis. Radionuclide scans may detect 50 per cent or less of hepatocellular carcinomas less than 5 cm in diameter. Ultrasound examination or computed tomography, particularly following intravenous injection of iodinated contrast media, appears to be more sensitive than radionuclide scanning in the detection of small tumors and may be useful also in excluding a cyst. Angiography may occasionally permit a definite diagnosis, as with an hemangioma, and is helpful in assessing resectability. In the patient with a solitary, apparently resectable lesion, preoperative biopsy is frequently unnecessary. Two additional factors must be taken into account when assessing the appropriateness of a preoperative biopsy. First, needle biopsy of primary lesions such as hemangioma, angiosarcoma, and possibly hepatocellular adenoma is potentially dangerous owing to their propensity to hemorrhage, and biopsy of a possible echinococcal cyst is contraindicated. Second, definitive diagnosis of hepatocellular adenoma and focal nodular hyperplasia, which consist predominantly of normal or minimally abnormal hepatocytes, may be difficult from examination of a needle biopsy alone. In the patient who is not a candidate for surgery or in whom information regarding tumor type will importantly influence decisions regarding further evaluation and therapy, a diagnosis can often be established by needle biopsy. Compared with percutaneous biopsy, a laparoscopic approach facilitates directed biopsy of visible tumor deposits and may permit control of bleeding. Inspection of the liver at laparoscopy for evidence of cirrhosis or tumor deposits not evident from radiologic studies may also aid in determining the resectability of a lesion. A percutaneous aspiration biopsy directed by computed tomography should also be considered in patients with small or deep-seated lesion. Non-neoplastic lesions that may mimic hepatic tumors include regenerative nodules, anomalous hepatic lobulation, cysts, and abscesses.

Conn H: Rational use of liver biopsy in the diagnosis of hepatic cancer (editorial). Gastroenterology 62:142, 1972. *A concise summary of the diagnostic yield of liver biopsy for metastatic cancer.*

Isahk KG, Rabin L: Benign tumors of the liver. Med Clin North Am 59:995, 1975. *A concise yet comprehensive review based on the uniquely rich experience at the Armed Forces Institute of Pathology.*

Kerlin P, Davis GL, McGill DB, Weiland LH, Adson MA, Sheedy PF II: Hepatic adenoma and focal nodular hyperplasia: Clinical, pathologic, and radiologic features. Gastroenterology 84:994, 1983. *A concise review comparing and contrasting these two common benign hepatic neoplasms.*

Kew MC, Geddes EW: Hepatocellular carcinoma in rural Southern African blacks. Medicine 61:98, 1982. *A review of 585 cases of hepatocellular carcinoma.*

Locker GY, Doroshow JH, Zwelling LA, Chabner BA: The clinical features of hepatic angiosarcoma: A report of four cases and a review of the English literature. Medicine 58:48, 1979. *A review of current information about this unusual tumor.*

Shinagawa T, Ohto M, Kimura K, et al.: Diagnosis and clinical features of small hepatocellular carcinoma with emphasis on the utility of real-time ultrasonography: A study in 51 patients. Gastroenterology 86:495, 1984. *A review of the clinical features, biochemical abnormalities, and utility of conventional imaging techniques in the diagnosis of hepatocellular carcinomas less than 5 cm in diameter.*

129. DISEASES OF THE GALLBLADDER AND BILE DUCTS

Biliary tract disorders result from a variety of congenital, inflammatory, metabolic, infectious, neoplastic, and parasitic conditions. These conditions often present in subtle ways and can pose challenging diagnostic problems. Ongoing improvements in diagnostic and therapeutic techniques have allowed the clinician to diagnose patients with biliary tract disease more quickly and to treat them more effectively.

129.1. Normal Physiology of Bile Formation

Peter F. Malet

Bile is an isotonic mixture of the secretion of hepatocytes and ductular epithelial cells. The volume of bile ranges from 500 to 1500 ml per day, depending on the amount and kind of food ingested. The canalicular fraction of bile, produced by the hepatocytes, is the largest and is bile salt dependent. A smaller component of canalicular bile may be related to active transport of electrolytes by the hepatocytes.

A second alkaline fraction of bile flow, the ductular secretion, is generated by an active transport of Na^+ and HCO_3^-, stimulated by secretin, cholecystokinin, and gastrin.

Under basal (fasting) conditions, tonic contraction of the sphincter of Oddi diverts about half of hepatic bile from the common duct and duodenum into the gallbladder, where it is concentrated by active reabsorption of Na^+, Cl^-, and HCO_3^- and passive resorption of H_2O. The gallbladder reabsorptive mechanism is capable of concentrating gallbladder bile ten-fold and can halve its volume in one hour.

Cholecystokinin, released from the intestinal mucosa after meals by fat, amino acids, and H^+, simultaneously stimulates the gallbladder to contract and the sphincter of Oddi to relax, emptying bile into the duodenum.

Bile salts are synthesized by hepatocytes from cholesterol by a multi-step process, the rate-limiting step of which is catalyzed by 7α-hydroxylase. The two primary bile salts (synthesized in the liver) are cholate and chenodeoxycholate; these are conjugated before secretion with either glycine or taurine to improve solubility. Secretion of bile salts involves active transport across the biliary canalicular membrane. After entering the gut, bile salts aid in fat absorption and then are largely reabsorbed in the ileum; those that reach the colon are partially deconjugated and converted by bacterial 7α-dehydroxylation to the secondary bile salts: these are deoxycholate and lithocholate. Deoxycholate is absorbed from the colon, reconjugated in the liver, and excreted in bile. Lithocholate is poorly reabsorbed and is sulfated as well as reconjugated during hepatic transfer. Sulfation reduces reabsorption during cycling. Deoxycholate continues to recycle within the enterohepatic circulation. The average bile salt composition of bile is 35 per cent chenodeoxycholate, 35 per cent cholate, 25 per cent deoxycholate, 2 per cent ursodeoxycholate, and 2 per cent lithocholate; each is conjugated with glycine or taurine in a ratio of 3:1. Bile salts are secreted in the form of micelles containing phospholipids (mainly lecithin), and cholesterol. These lipids account for 90 per cent of biliary solids.

Intestinal reabsorption of bile salts, which is about 95 per cent for a single passage, occurs by passive diffusion throughout the gut and by active transport within the terminal ileum. The reabsorbed bile salts are largely bound to albumin in portal blood, and are then almost completely removed by the hepatocytes in a single passage through the liver. The bile salt pool, normally 1.8 to 3.0 grams, passes through the liver and gut more than twice during each meal, producing six to eight cycles daily (i.e., each day about 20 to 30 grams of bile salts enters the duodenum). During an average day involving three meals, bile salts are in continuous motion with peaks of secretion following meals. At night, when the majority of the secreted hepatic bile enters the gallbladder, the intestinal concentration of bile salts is much lower. Conservation of bile salts in this enterohepatic circulation is so efficient that only 15 to 25 per cent (500 to 800 mg) of the bile salt pool must be replaced by hepatic synthesis of new bile salts daily. If the efficiency of enterohepatic conservation is impaired by conditions such as biliary fistula, Crohn's disease, or ileal resection, hepatic synthesis of bile salts increases. The maximal synthetic rate (5 grams per day) will be insufficient to restore intraluminal concentrations to normal if external losses exceed this amount.

Besides electrolytes, other solids of bile are bilirubin that has been conjugated in the liver with glucuronic acid (Ch. 117), proteins, low concentrations of the end-products of drug and hormone metabolism and metals such as calcium, iron, copper, and zinc.

Bile salts are amphophiles, possessing water-soluble and fat-soluble sides. In an aqueous medium they are distributed randomly until a critical concentration (about 2mM) is reached, at which point spontaneous aggregation forms multimolecular structures called micelles. In micelles, the bile salt molecules line up with their hydrophilic portions facing the solvent (water) and their hydrophobic portions facing each other (see Fig. 103–1). The hydrocarbon center of the micelle can incorporate biliary lecithin and cholesterol, and the entire aggregate remains water soluble. The addition of lecithin, a water-insoluble compound, enhances the ability of bile salt micelles to incorporate other lipids. The ultimate cholesterol-carrying capacity of bile depends on the relative amounts of bile salt and lecithin (Fig. 129–1) as well as the total lipid concentration.

129.2. Pathophysiology of Gallstone Disease

Peter F. Malet

In Western cultures about 75 per cent of gallstones are composed principally of cholesterol (cholesterol gallstones) and 25 per cent of calcium bilirubinate and other calcium salts (pigment gallstones). Overall, about 15 per cent of gallstones

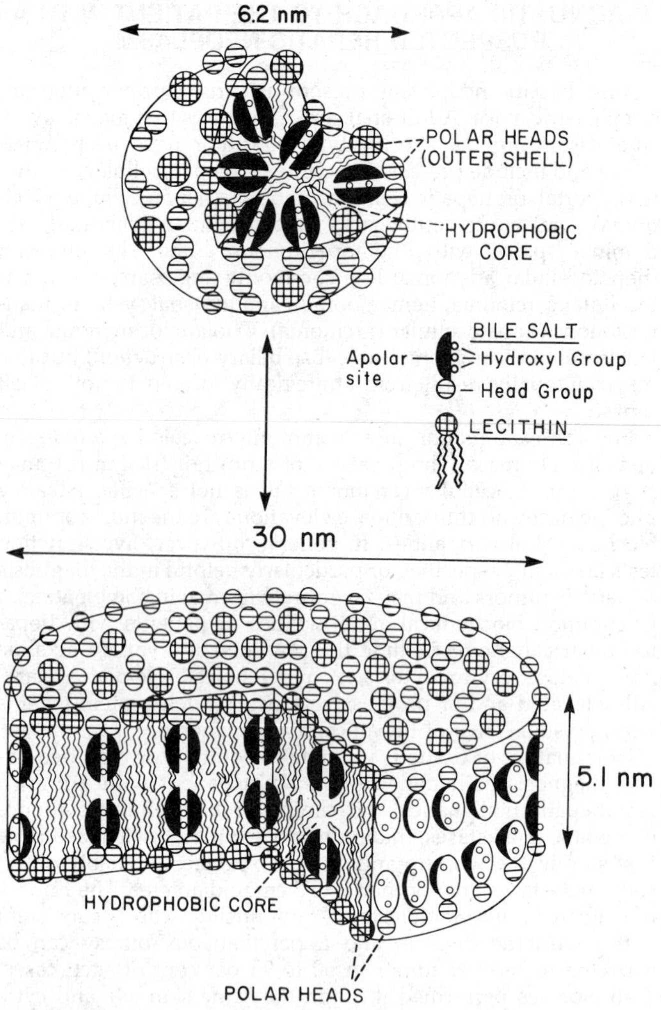

Figure 129–1. Dimorphic structure of biliary mixed lipid micelle which has recently been shown to exhibit a sphere → disc transition, depending upon whether the solution is bile salt-rich (sphere) or lecithin-rich (disc). The lecithin-rich micelle is larger and capable of dissolving and transporting a much larger amount of cholesterol. The transition depends upon the bile salt-lecithin molar ratio present in the micelle but may also be influenced by other constituents present in native bile. Bile salt molecules in both micellar forms are thought to form pairs (dimers) to avoid contact of the hydroxyl groups (solid circles) with the apolar environment of the micellar core. (Adapted with permission from Muller K: Biochemistry 20:404, 1981. Copyright 1981 American Chemical Society.)

are radiopaque, about two thirds of which are pigment and one third are cholesterol stones. The symptoms caused by gallstones are the same regardless of the chemical composition and to a large extent are independent of size. Stones less than 3 to 4 mm in diameter can cause pain and jaundice by passage through the cystic and common bile ducts while larger stones can cause pain by intermittently becoming impacted in the neck of the gallbladder.

CHOLESTEROL GALLSTONES. Cholesterol stones are usually yellow-green to tan and are round or faceted. They may be single or multiple; most range in size from 1 mm to 3 to 4 cm. Cholesterol accounts for from 50 to 100 per cent of stone weight, the remainder consisting of mucin glycoproteins and less than 10 per cent calcium bilirubinate and/or other calcium salts. These stones affect three times as many women as men, the difference beginning at puberty and declining after menopause. The incidence is higher with multiparity and with the use of birth control pills, which suggests an influence of female sex hormones. The incidence in blacks, whites, and American Indians increases in that order. About 75 per cent of American Indian women over age 25 and 90 per cent of those over age 60 are affected. In the United States, 20 per cent of 75-year-old men and 35 per cent of 75-year-old women have stones at autopsy. Environmental and dietary influences are important, since the incidence in blacks in Africa is much lower than blacks in the United States.

Cholesterol, which is insoluble in water, is normally carried in bile within bile salt–lecithin micelles. A prerequisite to cholesterol gallstone formation is an excess of cholesterol in relation to micellar carrying capacity, a circumstance that may result from decreased bile salt or increased cholesterol concentration in bile.

Figure 129–1 is a phase diagram on which any aqueous mixture of bile salt, lecithin, and cholesterol can be represented by a point indicating the molar percentage each contributes to total lipids. The cholesterol of mixtures that fall in the lower left area exists in stable micellar (completely clear) solution. Outside this area, in patients with gallstones, cholesterol forms either a metastable solution, which is clear initially but forms crystals after standing, or a supersaturated solution containing either liquid or solid crystals of cholesterol.

Bile of patients with gallstones has relatively more cholesterol than that of normal persons. In patients with gallstones, bile is supersaturated with cholesterol as it emerges from the liver, implicating the hepatocytes rather than the gallbladder as the cause of the abnormality. Most patients with gallstones have a decreased total bile salt pool size and their hepatocytes have decreased amounts of the enzyme 7α-hydroxylase. These observations suggest that diminished bile salt secretion is a factor in the genesis of lithogenic bile in many patients. Another factor, particularly associated with obesity, is increased cholesterol secretion into hepatic bile.

The relationship between cholesterol and bile salt output is such that when bile salt secretion drops, the cholesterol to bile salt ratio climbs and the bile becomes more lithogenic. During fasting, bile salts are sequestered in the gallbladder, hepatic secretion drops, the rate of cholesterol secretion persists, and the bile becomes more lithogenic. Supersaturation of bile is therefore common in humans without stones after overnight or prolonged fasting.

Cholesterol saturation of bile appears to be a necessary but not a sufficient condition for cholesterol gallstone formation. Supersaturated bile from patients without gallstones does not form cholesterol crystals, even on prolonged incubation, while bile of identical lipid composition from patients with stones usually contains or forms such crystals. The gallbladder is considered to be important in gallstone formation, possibly by supplying a nidus for crystallization such as mucin glycoproteins secreted by the epithelium or by providing an area of stasis to facilitate precipitation. For example, stone formation occurs predominantly in the gallbladder and cholesterol gallstones rarely recur after cholecystectomy.

PIGMENT GALLSTONES. Pigment stones are subdivided into two categories, black and brown stones, on the basis of differing compositional and clinical characteristics. *Black pigment stones* are usually under 1 cm, irregular in shape, and glassy on cross section. They form in the gallbladder and are composed of calcium bilirubinate, bilirubin polymers, calcium phosphate and carbonate, and mucin glycoproteins. There is no relationship between black stones and obesity, parity, saturation of bile with cholesterol, or bile salt pool size. Rather, old age and less than ideal weight are associated with black stone formation in the general population. There is no sexual predisposition; American Indians are rarely, and Scandinavians infrequently, affected. The concentration of unconjugated bilirubin is increased in the bile of many patients with these stones; however, cirrhosis and hemolytic diseases, which predispose to the development of these stones, are not present in most patients.

Brown pigment stones (calcium bilirubinate) have alternate layers of calcium bilirubinate or calcium salts of fatty acids. Bilirubin often precipitates with calcium because β-glucuronidase of bacterial, biliary epithelial, or hepatic origin deconjugates bilirubin diglucuronide to less soluble bilirubin. The fatty acids of biliary lecithin may be similarly precipitated as calcium salts because of hydrolysis by phospholipases. These stones are much more common in the Orient; the incidence decreases with the westernization of the culture and diet. They can form either in the gallbladder and/or in intra- or extrahepatic biliary ducts. In Western nations, they form primarily in the common bile duct after cholecystectomy for cholesterol stones. Unlike in the West, in the Orient stones frequently recur after removal and are associated with massive dilatation of the biliary tract and an accompanying cholangiohepatitis (recurrent pyogenic cholangitis), often resulting in secondary biliary cirrhosis and hepatic failure.

DISSOLUTION OF GALLSTONES. Attempts have been made to dissolve gallstones by reversing some of the pathogenetic mechanisms just described. Chenodeoxycholate (CDC), 12 to 15 mg per kilogram per day orally, will dissolve a substantial proportion of radiolucent cholesterol gallbladder stones within two years. CDC causes the bile to become unsaturated by mechanisms that are still unclear. Ursodeoxycholate (UDCA), the 7β-hydroxyl epimer of CDC, has a similar effect, and apparently is less hepatotoxic (slight to moderate rises of AST and ALT levels) and diarrheogenic. These compounds are ineffective for dissolution of pigment stones, of radiopaque stones, of stones in nonfilling gallbladders, and of stones in obese patients. Candidates for dissolution treatment are significantly symptomatic patients who are bad risks for surgery because of other illnesses or who are elderly. Stones will usually dissolve in one or two years in 30 to 40 per cent of patients who receive CDC in a dose of 12 to 15 mg per kilogram daily. Relative contraindications to therapy include chronic liver diseases, chronic diarrhea, and peptic ulcer disease. Women who may become pregnant should not be treated because of the potential for harmful effects of CDC on the fetus. When treatment is discontinued after initial dissolution, gallstones return in up to 50 per cent of patients within five years.

PATHOPHYSIOLOGY OF BILIARY OBSTRUCTION. Obstruction caused by a stone is the primary cause of all manifestations of gallstone disease. Obstruction of the cystic duct by gallbladder stones distends the gallbladder, producing biliary pain. If the obstruction persists, acute cholecystitis may ensue. The intermediary steps from obstruction to acute inflammation are discussed later. Whether complications such as empyema or perforation develop depends on whether secondary infection occurs. Cholecystectomy cures cholecystitis, but cholecystostomy, which only relieves the obstruction, will eliminate all the clinical manifestations of the disease.

Obstruction of the common duct may produce pain, jaundice, pruritus, infection, and biliary cirrhosis, and, as with gallbladder disease, surgical procedures that decompress the duct upstream from the stone eliminate these manifestations. The situation in the ductal system differs from that in the gallbladder, however, because when ductal pressure exceeds about 25 cm per H_2O, bile is refluxed into blood. Pressures in this range and even higher commonly accompany mechanical obstruction and are probably aggravated by infection. Regurgitation of ductal bacteria into the systemic circulation may explain why cholangitis is often accompanied by systemic bacteremia, chills, and high fever. Fortunately, obstruction of the common duct by stones is rarely complete. With unrelieved ductal obstruction, biliary cirrhosis gradually develops. Three months is the shortest time in which cirrhosis occurs and the earliest cases follow neoplastic (high-grade) obstruction.

OBSTRUCTIVE JAUNDICE. Patients with biliary obstruction often present with jaundice. The approach to the clinical evaluation of jaundice is described in detail in Ch. 119.

129.3. Roentgenologic and Other Imaging Tests

Peter F. Malet

Biliary disease usually results from obstructive lesions; radiologic techniques, if successful in outlining the system, are often diagnostic. The choice and timing of these direct and indirect

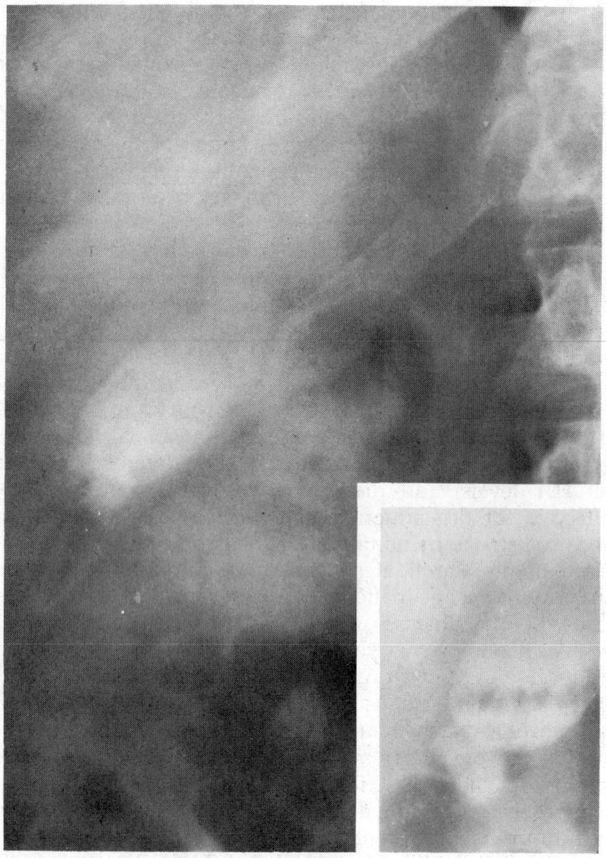

Figure 129–2. Oral cholecystogram, showing gallstones. In this case the stones are considerably less distinct on the supine than on the upright film (inset), where they float as a layer.

procedures depend upon the diagnostic strategy of the clinician. They are discussed in greater detail in Ch. 115.

Plain roentgenograms can demonstrate the 10 to 15 per cent of gallstones that contain enough calcium to be radiopaque, but the relationship of the stones to the gallbladder or bile ducts is not always obvious. Emphysematous cholecystitis, air in the bile ducts, and calcium in the wall of the gallbladder also have diagnostic appearances on plain films.

Oral cholecystography requires that the patient swallow tablets of iopanoic or tyropanoic acid, which are then absorbed from the gut, excreted in bile, and concentrated in the gallbladder. If the gallbladder is opacified, stones in the lumen are shown as radiolucent defects (Fig. 129–2). The gallbladder may not be opacified for several reasons: if the drug is not taken; if the patient has been fasting for several days immediately before taking the tablets; if absorption by the gut or excretion by the liver is faulty; if the cystic duct is blocked; or if the diseased gallbladder mucosa cannot concentrate the bile. If hepatic and intestinal function are normal, nonopacification is 95 per cent reliable in indicating gallbladder disease.

Ultrasonography of the biliary tree may demonstrate gallstones or dilatation of the intrahepatic or extrahepatic ductal system (Fig. 129–3). Real-time ultrasonography is very reliable in detecting gallbladder stones (false positives are uncommon); gallbladder stones will be missed, however, in a small percentage of cases. Unfortunately less than one third of common duct stones are identified. Ductal dilatation is detected in about 90 per cent of cases of proven obstruction.

Percutaneous transhepatic cholangiography (PTC) involves direct percutaneous puncture of an intrahepatic duct by a needle inserted through the eighth or ninth right intercostal space into the center of the liver. An abnormal clotting mechanism, ascites, and severe cholangitis are contraindications. PTC has proved particularly valuable in diagnosing gallstones within the biliary tract, biliary strictures, and neoplastic obstruction of the bile ducts (Fig. 129–4). A technically successful study can be obtained in nearly all patients with dilated ducts and in 70 per cent of patients with normal-sized ducts.

Endoscopic retrograde cholangiopancreatography (ERCP) involves cannulation of the common bile duct and pancreatic duct through the ampulla of Vater via the duodenoscope (Fig. 129–5). With experience, a successful study of one or both ducts is possible in 80 to 90 per cent of attempts. ERCP is particularly useful in patients with normal-sized bile ducts or in whom pancreatic disease as a cause of bile duct obstruction is strongly suspected.

Both PTC and ERCP are usually contraindicated in active cholangitis, because as ductal pressure increases during injection of the contrast material, severe uncontrollable sepsis may

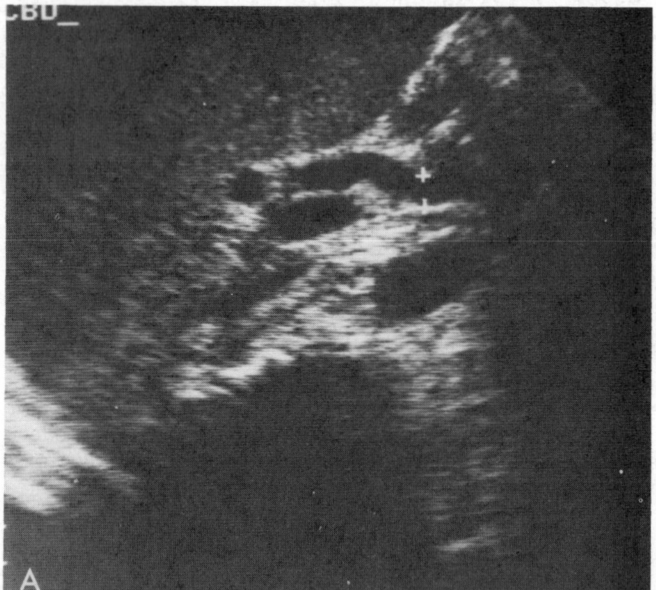

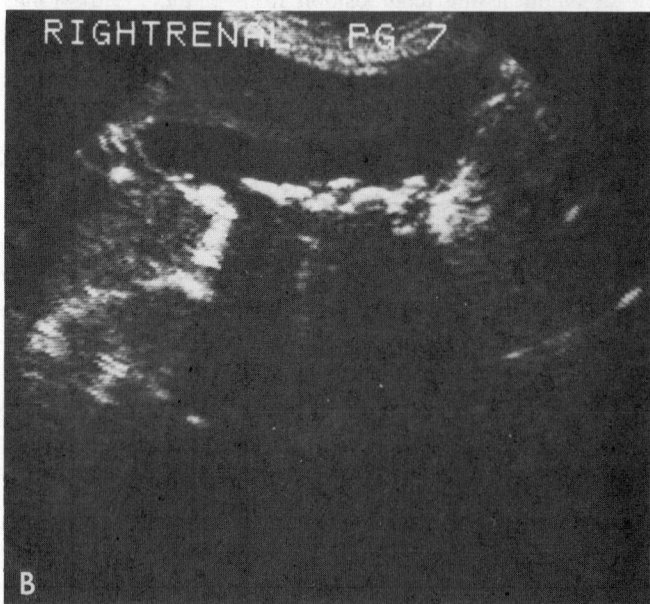

Figure 129–3. *A*, Ultrasonography of extrahepatic biliary tract showing a dilated common bile duct (the width of the duct measured between the two white markers is 8.3 mm); the portal vein is seen as the anechoic area directly beneath the common bile duct. *B*, Ultrasonography of a gallbladder containing gallstones that appear as numerous echogenic foci within the gallbladder lumen with distal acoustic shadowing, that is, paucity of echoes distal to the stones. These stones were an incidental finding during ultrasonography of the kidneys. (Courtesy of Dr. Peter Arger.)

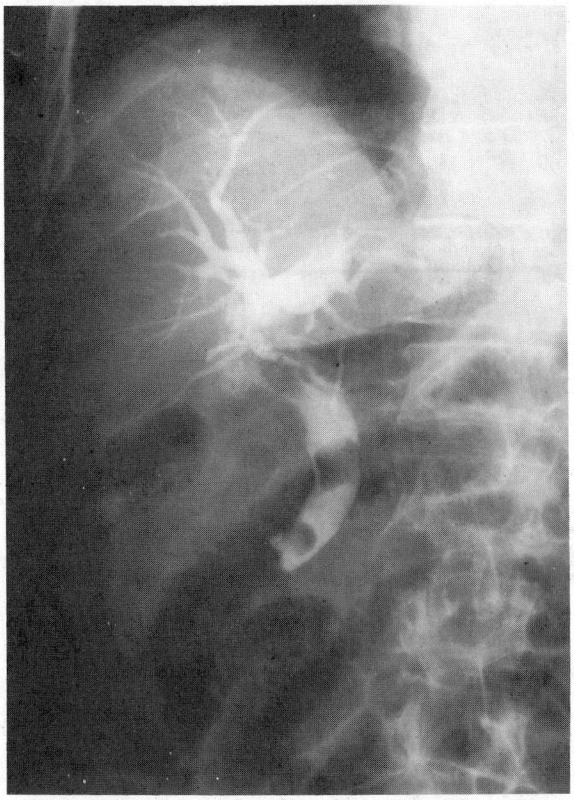

Figure 129–4. Percutaneous transhepatic cholangiogram demonstrating a dilated common bile duct and intrahepatic bile ducts secondary to obstruction by a gallstone in the distal common bile duct. This patient had a prior cholecystectomy. (Courtesy of Dr. Gordon McLean.)

be produced. Patients undergoing either of these procedures should usually be premedicated with antimicrobial agents regardless of whether there is a history of cholangitis. Ductal dilatation usually indicates distal obstruction by neoplasm, stricture, or stone. The correlation between dilatation and obstruction is inexact because (1) the ducts may be dilated from previous disease or surgery although currently unobstructed, (2) cirrhosis or cholangitis may stiffen the ducts enough to prevent dilatation, and (3) lesions characterized by intermittent obstruction (e.g., common duct stones, stricture) may produce dilation followed by spontaneous decompression; ducts may appear undilated if the patient is examined after the duct has spontaneously decompressed.

Radionuclide imaging of the biliary tree may be accomplished by intravenous injection of a ^{99m}Tc-labeled derivative of iminodiacetic acid (e.g., HIDA, PIPIDA, or DESIDA). Normally a high quality image of the biliary tree appears within 30 minutes after administration of the radionuclide agent. This test is becoming the procedure of choice in verifying the diagnosis of acute cholecystitis. Filling of the ducts but not of the gallbladder supports the diagnosis of cholecystitis due to obstruction of the cystic duct by a stone. A false-negative study is rare; however, false-positive (nonfilling) studies are seen in patients with severe illnesses such as pancreatitis and cholestatic liver disease, and in those receiving intravenous hyperalimentation. Ultrasonography and CT scanning are more useful in detecting common bile duct obstruction.

There is very little role for intravenous cholangiography (IVC) because of its limited diagnostic accuracy and the availability of more sensitive and specific tests such as PTC and ERCP, which provide much more contrast within the biliary tree.

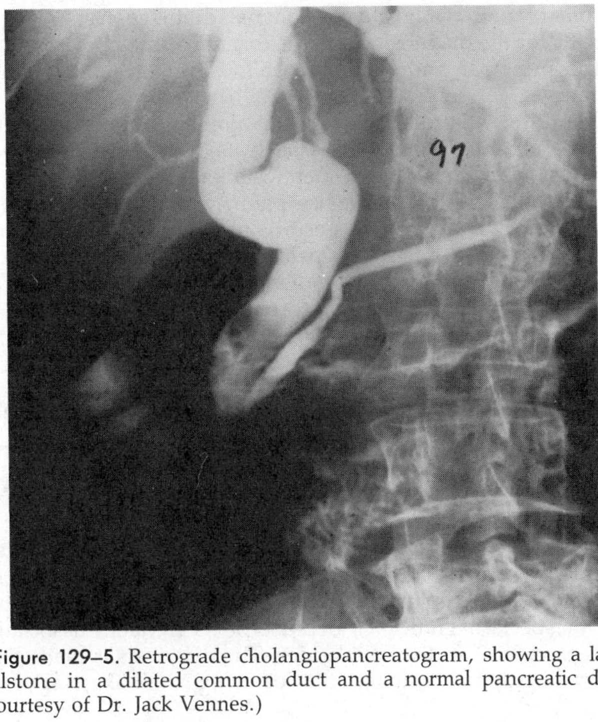

Figure 129–5. Retrograde cholangiopancreatogram, showing a large gallstone in a dilated common duct and a normal pancreatic duct. (Courtesy of Dr. Jack Vennes.)

129.4. Clinical Categories of Gallbladder and Biliary Tract Disease

ASYMPTOMATIC GALLSTONES

Roger D. Soloway

It has been estimated that 30 to 50 per cent of patients in the United States with gallstones are asymptomatic (Fig. 129–6), and that about 1.5 per cent of patients with gallstones undergo cholecystectomy each year. Mortality from gallstone disease is reasonably low under a conservative plan of management of treating only those who present with symptoms. Asymptomatic patients may therefore be followed expectantly with prophylactic cholecystectomy reserved for the following two exceptions: (1) diabetics, because their mortality from acute cholecystitis is 10 to 15 per cent, and (2) patients with calcified gallbladders, often associated with carcinoma of the gallbladder. Symptomatic cholelithiasis carries a 33 per cent risk of producing a complication requiring surgery within five years. Asymptomatic patients with gallstones have an 18 per cent chance of developing biliary pain in 20 years and only 3 per cent will require a cholecystectomy.

CHRONIC CHOLECYSTITIS

Peter F. Malet

Chronic cholecystitis is the most common symptomatic nonacute manifestation of cholecystolithiasis. Often, however, the pathologic findings in the gallbladder wall and the clinical manifestations of gallstone disease correlate poorly.

In some patients the gallbladder is severely affected, often the result of previous attacks of acute cholecystitis, with shrinking, scarring and thickening of the wall, adhesions to adjacent viscera, and patchy replacement of the mucosa by granulation tissue or collagen. Nonopacification following oral cholecystography is frequent in such patients. At the other extreme the gallbladder is grossly normal with only slight thinning of the mucosa, mild patchy scarring and inflammation, and a normal oral cholecystogram.

Cholesterolosis, resulting from submucosal cholesterol-laden macrophages, is present in about 5 per cent of cases and gives the mucosal surface the appearance of a strawberry. Cholesterolosis may occur without gallstones and may be asymptomatic or associated with pain.

CLINICAL MANIFESTATIONS. Chronic cholecystitis commonly produces a steady *pain* located in the epigastrium or right upper

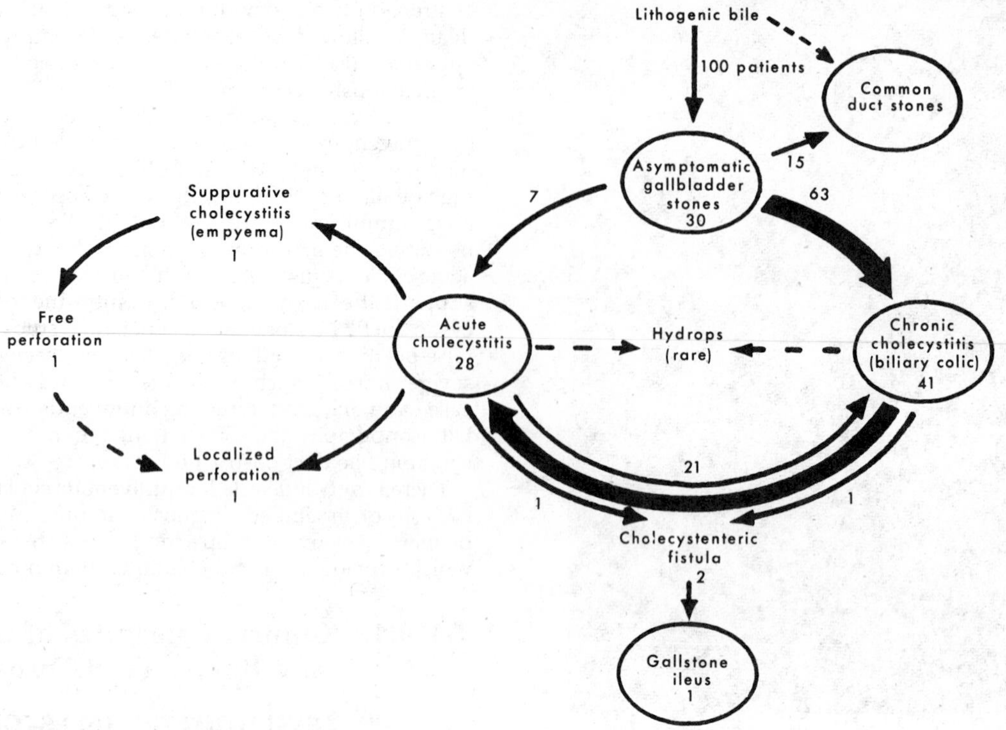

Figure 129–6. Natural history of cholecystolithiasis. The major clinical syndromes are contained in the ovals, and the numbers represent the approximate percentage of patients with gallstone disease who present in that way.

quadrant, thought to be caused by gallbladder distention arising from transient obstruction of the cystic duct by a gallstone. The onset of pain takes only a few minutes; it quickly reaches a plateau in intensity that may range from moderate to excruciating and after 30 minutes to several hours it subsides gradually. The pain usually does not wax and wane like intestinal colic. Nausea and vomiting may accompany the attack and only a vague residual ache or soreness may remain after the acute pain has dissipated. Tenderness, muscular guarding, a palpable mass, fever, and leukocytosis are absent, distinguishing this condition from acute cholecystitis. Many patients have simultaneous pain referred to the back near the scapula or to the right shoulder area. Some attacks may be related to ingestion of an especially large or fatty meal. Attacks may occur daily or as seldom as once every few years. Dyspepsia, fatty food intolerance, flatulence, heartburn, and belching may occur but are not helpful diagnostically because they often occur in persons with normal gallbladders.

Hydrops of the gallbladder refers to its distention with mucus and gallstones; it may develop from cystic duct obstruction in chronic cholecystitis. Hydrops produces constant discomfort in the right upper quadrant and a palpable mass without the clinical findings of acute cholecystitis.

DIAGNOSIS. An oral cholecystogram will demonstrate the gallstones in about two thirds of patients, but in the others the gallbladder does not opacify. In the latter case, a second dose of the cholecystographic agent should be given and the x-rays repeated. If nonopacification persists and liver function and intestinal absorption are normal, gallbladder disease can be inferred with a high degree of certainty.

About 2 to 3 per cent of patients with gallstones will have adequate opacification of the gallbladder during an oral cholecystogram and do not demonstrate calculi, either because the stones are too small to be seen or because they are of the same radiographic density as the contrast medium. Real-time ultrasonography should be used in such patients, because it is 95 to 99 per cent sensitive in detecting gallbladder stones. It also has the advantage of allowing examination of the common bile duct, pancreas, and adjacent liver at the same time without radiation exposure.

In a few patients with typical biliary pain in the absence of demonstrable gallstones by cholecystography or ultrasonography, examination of bile for crystals may prove helpful. A sample of bile is obtained from an orally placed duodenal tube and is examined microscopically for the presence of cholesterol or calcium bilirubinate crystals. In addition, the bile can be incubated at 37° C for 48 hours to look for formation of microcrystals of cholesterol. In the presence of what seems to be biliary pain, a positive duodenal drainage test is highly specific for the diagnosis. On gross examination, cholesterolosis is the principal finding in the gallbladder of some of these patients.

The differential diagnosis includes other common causes of chronic abdominal symptoms such as peptic ulcer and pancreatitis, which may have manifestations similar to those of chronic cholecystitis. Radicular pain from spinal lesions may mimic biliary pain. Angina pectoris may cause pain thought to be abdominal, just as biliary pain may be felt in the precordial region. Postprandial pain or discomfort may result from the irritable bowel syndrome or intestinal tumors.

COMPLICATIONS. *Choledocholithiasis* is the most common complication, affecting about 15 per cent of patients with cholecystolithiasis. The incidence of common duct stones increases with advancing age. Patients with symptomatic chronic cholecystitis often eventually develop an attack of acute cholecystitis. About two thirds of patients with acute cholecystitis have previously had symptomatic chronic cholecystitis. *Mirizzi's syndrome* results from extrinsic compression of the common hepatic or common bile duct by a large stone passing through the cystic duct. Obstructive jaundice may develop. Calcification of the gallbladder (*"porcelain gallbladder"*) is an uncommon condition but of special significance because of its frequent association with carcinoma of the gallbladder. The diagnosis is made from the radiographic demonstration of an eggshell-like rim of calcium in the gallbladder wall. Adenocarcinoma of the gallbladder is found mainly in elderly patients with cholelithiasis, most of whom have had biliary symptoms for many years.

TREATMENT. Dietary changes, anticholinergics, and antacids have no effect on the course of the disease, but they sometimes provide temporary symptomatic relief. Analgesics should be used for relief of pain. Cholecystectomy is the treatment of choice. At operation the common bile duct is inspected, operative cholangiograms are obtained, and the common duct is explored if there is evidence of choledocholithiasis.

Cholecystectomy relieves symptoms from chronic cholecystitis. Loss of the gallbladder does not impair gastrointestinal function. The mortality of elective cholecystectomy is under 0.5 per cent. In patients over 70, however, mortality rises to 2 to 3 per cent; most of the postoperative deaths are a result of preexisting cardiopulmonary diseases.

ACUTE CHOLECYSTITIS

Roger D. Soloway

Acute cholecystitis usually produces acute right subcostal pain and tenderness. However, acute inflammation of the gallbladder is revealed at less than 20 per cent of cholecystectomies.

PATHOGENESIS. Filling the gallbladder of a dog with concentrated bile and obstructing the cystic duct produces acute inflammation. If the gallbladder is empty or distended with physiologic saline solution instead of bile, cystic duct obstruction is tolerated without inflammation. Obstruction is associated with the release of phospholipase from the gallbladder epithelium that can hydrolyze lecithin, releasing lysolecithin, an epithelial toxin. Simultaneously the epithelial barrier coating of mucin glycoproteins may be acutely disrupted, making the epithelium susceptible to injury by the detergent action of the concentrated bile salts.

Bacterial infection is secondary to biliary obstruction rather than primary. Bacteria are not present in the gallbladders of patients with chronic cholecystitis and cholesterol or black pigment gallstones. Early in acute cholecystitis, the gallbladder bile is positive for bacteria by culture in 50 per cent of cases, but within a week after onset the figure reaches 90 per cent. Although infection is secondary, it may be ultimately responsible for the most serious sequelae of acute cholecystitis, empyema and perforation.

Acalculous cholecystitis, accounting for 5 per cent of cases, is more common in men and in patients with unrelated sepsis. Some cases have been associated with prolonged fasting after major trauma, e.g., war injuries or surgical operations, some with *Salmonella typhosa,* and some with polyarteritis nodosa or ischemia of other causes. At operation the bile is viscous and full of sludge. Perforation is more frequent, and the outcome is generally worse than in acute calculous cholecystitis.

PATHOLOGY. Early inflammation with subserosal edema, mucosal ulcerations, and submucosal hemorrhages progresses slowly to cellular infiltration of the wall after three to four days, which reaches its greatest intensity at the end of the first week. During the second week, patchy mural gangrene, small intramural abscesses, and collagen deposition all appear. Resolution of the acute changes takes another week or more.

The term *empyema* describes the rare entity of a pus-filled gallbladder characterized clinically by a septic form of acute cholecystitis. No documented case has occurred in the last 2500 operations at our hospital. Gangrene and perforation are most common in the fundus where the blood supply is meager or in the neck where stones become impacted. With perforation, gallbladder contents may spill into the free abdominal cavity (bile peritonitis) or, more often, are confined by adhesions (pericholecystic abscess). Sometimes an adherent viscus is penetrated, making a cholecystenteric fistula through which the gallstones and pus may be discharged. Fistulization is most frequent with the duodenum, but jejunal and colonic fistulas have been described. A large gallstone passing through to the small gut may obstruct it to produce *gallstone ileus.*

Chronic obstruction of the cystic duct causes *hydrops* (mucocele), a condition in which the gallbladder is distended with uninfected mucus *(white bile).* Hydrops may result either from resolved acute cholecystitis or from cystic duct obstruction without inflammation.

CLINICAL MANIFESTATIONS. An attack of acute cholecystitis begins with *abdominal pain* that increases gradually in severity. The pain is usually located in the right subcostal region from the start, but it sometimes begins in the epigastrium or left upper quadrant and then shifts to the region of the gallbladder as inflammation progresses. Two thirds or more of patients have had previous attacks of biliary colic. Early in the attack the patient may expect the symptoms to subside spontaneously as had happened before with similar pains, and medical aid is often not sought until 48 hours or more. Referred pain may be experienced in the back at the scapular level. Patients in their 70's or 80's may have few or no localizing symptoms.

Anorexia, nausea, and *vomiting* are often present but vomiting is rarely severe enough to be confused with bowel obstruction and is generally less than in acute pancreatitis. In the absence of complications, chills are rare and the temperature is about 38° C. Chills and high fever suggest suppurative cholecystitis or associated cholangitis.

The right subcostal region is tender to palpation, and involuntary muscle spasm generally limits the examination. If the patient takes a deep breath while the subhepatic area is being palpated, heightened tenderness arrests inspiration *(Murphy's sign).*

In somewhat more than a third of the patients, a distended, tender gallbladder can be distinctly felt, an important finding that confirms the suspected diagnosis. The gallbladder cannot be felt in the rest of the patients because of obesity, rigidity of the abdominal wall, or a deep subhepatic location, or because it is small and shrunken from previous inflammation. Other related conditions characterized by a tender mass in the same area are pericholecystic abscess, acute cholecystitis complicating carcinoma of the gallbladder, torsion of the gallbladder, or the rare case of gallbladder distention in obstructive cholangitis (e.g., suppurative cholangitis and Oriental cholangiohepatitis).

About 20 per cent of patients with acute cholecystitis have mild *jaundice* caused by edema of the nearby common duct or more likely by common duct stones. Rarely a tumor of the bile ducts is the underlying cause.

With treatment, improvement is usually noticeable within the first 12 to 24 hours, and the signs and symptoms gradually subside over three to seven days. Persistent severe pain, a rise in temperature or leukocyte count (> 10,000 per cubic millimeter), appearance of shaking chills, or of more severe local or generalized abdominal tenderness all indicate progression of the disease and suggest the need for surgery.

Empyema (suppurative cholecystitis) can produce systemic toxicity and mild rises in bilirubin, alkaline phosphatase, and the transaminases, and may herald perforation. If this severe infection is controlled with antimicrobial drugs, a large tender gallbladder may remain palpable for several weeks, and return of well-being is similarly prolonged.

DIAGNOSIS. The diagnosis is strongly suggested by the clinical manifestations just described. Roentgenograms of the abdomen may show calcified gallstones or an enlarged gallbladder. Ultrasonography is probably the simplest and most reliable method of detecting gallbladder stones in these patients. Oral cholecystograms are diagnostically unreliable because of unpredictable absorption and excretion of the contrast agent and should not be scheduled until four to six weeks after the attack.

Radionuclide scanning following intravenous administration of ^{99m}Tc DESIDA or related compounds is the procedure of choice to verify a clinical impression of acute cholecystitis. If the gallbladder fills, the diagnosis of acute cholecystitis is quite unlikely. If the bile duct fills but the gallbladder does not, the diagnosis is strongly supported.

In the differential diagnosis, acute pancreatitis, acute appendicitis, and perforated peptic ulcer are the conditions that most often cause major problems. Furthermore, acute cholecystitis and acute pancreatitis may coexist.

In women, *gonococcal perihepatitis* (Fitz-Hugh–Curtis syndrome), caused by intra-abdominal spread of the infection to the right upper quadrant, may be mistaken for acute cholecystitis, but adnexal tenderness is usually present on pelvic examination. A cervical smear usually reveals gonococci, and the patients are younger, often have higher fever, and are in less distress than would be expected with cholecystitis. Shoulder pain and a friction rub over the liver, common in the Fitz-Hugh–Curtis syndrome, are not found in uncomplicated acute cholecystitis.

Acute hepatitis, either viral or alcoholic, sometimes produces marked right upper quadrant pain and tenderness. A history of recent binge drinking, high transaminase levels, and liver biopsy aid differentiation. Pneumonitis, pyelonephritis, and acute cardiac disease (particularly right-sided failure) all on occasion may cause acute pain suggestive of cholecystitis. The use of ^{99m}Tc DESIDA will distinguish between the unusual location of pain in these disorders and acute cholecystitis.

TREATMENT. Most patients with acute cholecystitis will improve with either expectant treatment or cholecystectomy performed during the acute attack. In general, the decision regarding the kind of treatment should include the following considerations (Fig. 129–7): (1) Whether the diagnosis is secure; (2) whether biliary complications have occurred or appear imminent; and (3) the overall condition of the patient (operative risk).

Upon the patient's admission to the hospital, nasogastric suction should be started and fluids given intravenously to correct dehydration. In many elderly patients, the acute biliary condition may aggravate pre-existing cardiac, pulmonary, or renal disease, and produce a more ominous prognosis if surgery is delayed or if adequate treatment is not given.

Antimicrobials are of principal value to treat suppurative complications. If the patient is seen shortly after symptoms begin, and if local signs and symptoms are mild, antimicrobial therapy need not be given. Ampicillin (2 grams) or a cephalosporin (4 to 6 grams) in divided doses parenterally is adequate, except in patients with empyema or perforation in whom an aminoglycoside (i.e., gentamicin 1.0 to 1.5 mg per kilogram) plus clindamycin (600 mg), given parenterally every eight hours, would be preferable.

Cholecystectomy is generally considered the optimal therapy for acute cholecystitis, but only after the diagnosis is confirmed and the patient adequately prepared for operation. Many physicians still prefer to reserve surgery during the acute attack for those patients who develop complications and for those who become worse or fail to improve. For patients who respond to nonoperative management, interval cholecystectomy is generally recommended four to eight weeks later. Although nonoperative therapy is still common practice, about 25 per cent of patients managed in this way require urgent operation for worsening disease.

About 30 per cent of patients are good surgical risks; in these patients, the diagnosis is obvious within 12 to 24 hours, and cholecystectomy can be scheduled promptly. Another 30 per cent are good surgical candidates, but the gallbladder cannot be felt. In this situation the diagnosis should be regarded as tentative, and a ^{99m}Tc DESIDA scan should be performed preoperatively to verify the clinical impression.

Another 30 per cent of patients will have serious coexistent cardiac, respiratory, or other disease whose treatment takes precedence. The cholecystitis should be treated expectantly while the other problems are being corrected. Progression of

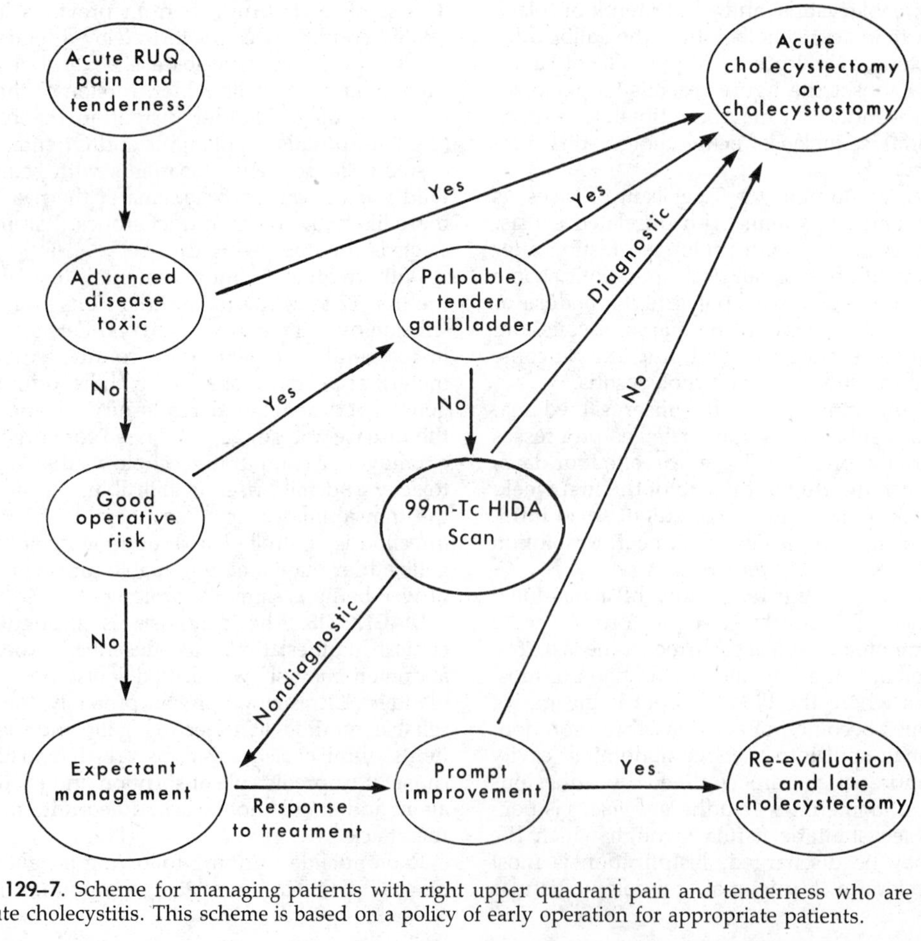

Figure 129–7. Scheme for managing patients with right upper quadrant pain and tenderness who are thought to have acute cholecystitis. This scheme is based on a policy of early operation for appropriate patients.

local abdominal findings requires continued re-evaluation, balancing the risks of operation with the risks of continued delay.

About 10 per cent of patients require emergency surgery for complications present on admission or that appear later during observation and medical management. When emergency operation becomes necessary, cholecystostomy may sometimes be preferable to cholecystectomy in the seriously ill patient. In this procedure, the fundus is incised, stones and pus are removed from the lumen, and the organ is decompressed by catheter drainage, allowing the acute infection to resolve. Patients who recover should undergo cholecystectomy six to eight weeks later. Those who continue to be poor surgical risks may be followed expectantly if postoperative cholecystography shows that the gallbladder and common duct contain no residual stones. If stones are present, interventional radiologic techniques can be used to remove gallbladder stones through the cholecystectomy tract after four to six weeks of tract maturation and ERCP can be utilized to remove ductal stones. In seriously ill patients, the cholecystostomy tube can be left in place indefinitely.

After the cholecystostomy tube is removed from a patient whose biliary system contains no calculi, within the first year about 50 per cent of patients develop new stones and additional symptoms. Eventually, 90 per cent of patients will again develop stones.

COMPLICATIONS. In *emphysematous cholecystitis,* a rare variant of acute cholecystitis, gas of bacterial origin can be seen in the gallbladder lumen and adjacent tissues. Clinically, emphysematous cholecystitis causes the same signs and symptoms as acute cholecystitis. Men are affected twice as frequently as women, about 30 per cent of patients have diabetes mellitus, and the gallbladder is acalculous in about half the cases. Gas does not develop until 24 to 48 hours after the attack begins, at which time a radiolucent halo outlines the lumen and an air-fluid level may be seen on upright films. Subserosal and then pericholecystic emphysema appear with time. Differential diagnosis of the x-ray findings includes cholecystenteric fistula, appendiceal or subhepatic abscess, and, rarely, lipomatosis of the gallbladder. In about half the cases the gas-forming organisms are clostridia, and the rest are *E. coli,* streptococci, and other bacteria of intestinal origin. Treatment is the same as for acute cholecystitis, but the somewhat more aggressive nature of emphysematous cholecystitis and the association with diabetes mellitus indicate that prompt surgery is usually required.

Perforation is usually manifested by greater sepsis and more marked abdominal signs. Perforation may take any of three forms: (1) free perforation into the abdominal cavity, (2) localized (contained) perforation with pericholecystic abscess, and (3) perforation into another viscus with fistula formation.

Free perforation, which has a 25 per cent mortality, is fortunately the least common type. It usually occurs early in the attack, often within the first three days, suggesting that when gangrene develops this quickly it cannot be walled off by adjacent viscera or the omentum. Clinically, free perforation classically causes toxicity with high temperatures (greater than 39° C), leukocytosis over 15,000 per cubic millimeter, and diffuse abdominal tenderness and rigidity. In more than half the cases, the correct diagnosis is unsuspected until laparotomy or autopsy, because a clear-cut history of preliminary right upper quadrant pain is often lacking. The incidence of missed diagnosis should decrease with the increased use of ultrasonography and CT scans. Treatment consists of intravenous antimicrobial therapy and emergency laparotomy with cholecystectomy.

Localized perforation most often appears in the second week of the attack at the peak of the inflammatory reaction. The diagnosis should be suspected with increasing local signs, especially when a mass suddenly appears. In most cases cholecystectomy can be performed, but in a severely ill patient, cholecystostomy and drainage of the abscess may be wiser.

Fistula formation usually involves the nearby second portion of the duodenum or, less commonly, the colon, jejunum, stomach, or common bile duct. Rare fistulas have entered the renal pelvis or bronchus, or extended through the abdominal wall (empyema necessitatis). After intestinal fistulization the contents of the gallbladder are discharged into the gut, often aborting the acute attack. Clinically, the fistula itself may not be suspected because it produces no unique findings; many are discovered incidentally during a later cholecystectomy. In the absence of biliary obstruction a cholecystenteric fistula is not necessarily of pathophysiologic significance. Cholecystocolonic fistulas may cause malabsorption from diversion of bile or from heavy bacterial contamination of the upper gut. If a particularly large gallstone enters through the fistula, it may obstruct the intestine, a condition called *gallstone ileus.*

PROGNOSIS. The mortality of acute cholecystitis of 5 to 10 per cent is almost confined to patients over 60 years of age with serious associated disease. Suppurative complications are more common in the elderly, who can tolerate them least. In most instances, localized perforation can be managed satisfactorily at operation. Free perforation is considerably more ominous (25 per cent mortality) but is rare.

In patients who are treated expectantly, recurrent biliary symptoms are so common that an elective cholecystectomy should be planned in most cases. Another acute attack is not nusual during the month or two of waiting.

GALLSTONE ILEUS

Roger D. Soloway

Gallstone ileus is an intestinal obstruction usually seen in elderly women and is caused by a gallstone lodged in the gut lumen. The stone, passing through a cholecystenteric fistula, most often enters the gut in the duodenum, less commonly the jejunum, ileum, colon, or stomach. It is often assumed that the initial event responsible for fistula formation is an attack of acute cholecystitis, but only 30 per cent of patients with gallstone ileus give a history of recent right upper quadrant pain. After entering the gut, the gallstone moves downstream until it becomes too large for the intestinal lumen to accommodate. Gallstones, usually over 2.5 cm in diameter, most frequently obstruct the terminal ileum; they will block the colon only if its lumen has been narrowed by intrinsic disease.

On physical examination the findings are those of small bowel obstruction. Sometimes the large stone can be felt as a mass on abdominal, vaginal, or rectal examination, but it is rarely correctly identified. Roentgenograms usually show air in the biliary tree if the films are carefully examined, and in some cases a radiopaque gallstone can be identified at the leading edge of the obstruction. Treatment consists of removing the obstructing gallstone through a small enterotomy. It is generally wise to leave the biliary disease undisturbed initially, because elderly patients tolerate long procedures poorly, and nothing much is gained by repairing the fistula primarily. Postoperatively, many patients become asymptomatic and the fistula closes spontaneously; for them, expectant management is best. About 50 per cent will require cholecystectomy.

The mortality rate is 15 to 20 per cent because of delay in diagnosis and cardiopulmonary complications.

CHOLEDOCHOLITHIASIS AND CHOLANGITIS

Roger D. Soloway

In Western countries choledocholithiasis is usually the result of passage of gallstones formed in the gallbladder into the common duct. About 15 per cent of patients with cholelithiasis are thought to develop choledocholithiasis. Once in the common duct, the stones may pass into the duodenum, but the frequency of this event is not known and is clinically greatly underestimated. Less commonly, stones form in a dilated duct behind a longstanding obstruction by stones, stricture, or ampullary stenosis. About 5 per cent of patients with choledocholithiasis have no gallbladder stones; in such cases it is assumed that all the gallbladder stones escaped into the duct or more rarely that the stones formed primarily in the common duct. Stone type helps to determine site of origin: cholesterol or black stones more likely form in the gallbladder while almost all brown stones in patients in Western countries form in the bile ducts.

CLINICAL MANIFESTATIONS. The natural history of choledocholithiasis is incompletely known. About 30 to 40 per cent of patients are asymptomatic at the time of diagnosis, implying a relatively benign course in many cases. Obstruction by stones of the biliary or pancreatic ducts may produce any of the following syndromes: biliary colic, jaundice (without pain), cholangitis, pancreatitis, or a combination of these (Fig. 129–8). Secondary hepatic effects of persistent obstruction include biliary cirrhosis or hepatic abscesses.

Intermittent cholangitis, consisting of biliary colic, jaundice, and fever and chills *(Charcot's triad)*, is the most common presenting symptom complex. In the absence of previous biliary surgery it is almost diagnostic of choledocholithiasis in Western countries. Intermittency of symptoms is quite characteristic, a manifestation of intermittent partial obstruction. Whenever pain, chills with fever, and jaundice fluctuate together over a span of a few days or a week, cholangitis from biliary obstruction is almost certainly the cause. In a typical attack chills may precede the other symptoms, and bilirubinuria may follow. Epigastric or right upper quadrant pain, indistinguishable from biliary pain caused by gallbladder stones, is steady and very severe. Pain may be referred to the right infrascapular area, the upper back, the right shoulder, or even the precordium, suggesting coronary artery or esophageal disease.

The severity of fever and chills varies widely from the usual mild transient illness to overwhelming sepsis with shock (see *Suppurative Cholangitis*, below). In the average case, the temperature rises to 38.5 to 40° C, preceded by chills and positive

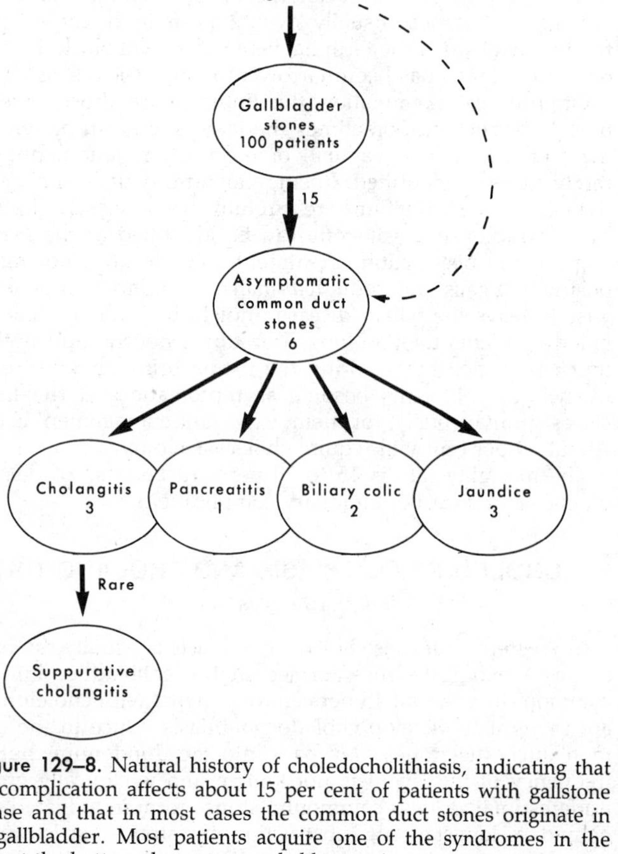

Figure 129–8. Natural history of choledocholithiasis, indicating that this complication affects about 15 per cent of patients with gallstone disease and that in most cases the common duct stones originate in the gallbladder. Most patients acquire one of the syndromes in the ovals at the bottom, but many probably remain asymptomatic.

blood cultures. Localized tenderness in the subcostal region may be associated with extreme guarding and rigidity, but more often the local findings are minimal or intermittent and are usually less severe than in acute cholecystitis.

In most cases of common duct obstruction caused by stones, the gallbladder does not become distended because it is scarred and inelastic, and the obstruction is recent, partial, and transient, the obverse of Courvoisier's law: i.e., a distended nontender gallbladder in a jaundiced patient signifies neoplastic obstruction of the bile duct.

DIAGNOSIS. In cholangitis the leukocyte count averages 15,000 per cubic millimeter but may go much higher in severe cases. Bilirubin values are usually in the range of 2 to 4 mg per deciliter and are uncommonly higher than 10 mg per deciliter. Elevated serum alkaline phosphatase and 5′-nucleotidase levels indicate extrahepatic obstruction. The AST generally remains below 200 units; however, transiently it may exceed 1000 units. In these instances the prompt drop within 48 hours allows differentiation from viral hepatitis and suggests the diagnosis of obstruction.

The same conditions considered for the patient with chronic cholecystitis must be excluded for biliary pain caused by ductal calculi. In patients who have had a cholecystectomy, differentiation between choledocholithiasis and biliary stricture as the cause of cholangitis usually depends on radiologic demonstration of the ducts. When the presenting syndrome is painless cholestatic jaundice, other causes, especially periampullary and biliary neoplasms, must be considered. With neoplastic obstruction the bilirubin averages about 18 mg per deciliter and rarely fluctuates. Although jaundice from stones may be as intense, the level of bilirubin is characteristically less than 10 mg per deciliter and it may rise and fall episodically. The diagnosis of intrahepatic cholestasis from causes such as drugs, viral hepatitis, or pregnancy should usually be reached by exclusion only after opacification of normal bile ducts by percutaneous transhepatic cholangiography or endoscopic retrograde cholangiopancreatography. Gallstone disease is common in cirrhosis, so choledocholithiasis and alcoholic liver disease may coexist.

Common duct stones may cause acute pancreatitis indistinguishable clinically from that resulting from alcohol or other causes and unaccompanied by specific signs of biliary disease. Pancreatitis caused by biliary calculi, despite numerous attacks, rarely progresses to pancreatic calcification, chronic pain, and pancreatic insufficiency, as so often occurs in the alcoholic variety. The pancreatitis is much more severe, more protracted, and more frequently hemorrhagic. Gallstone disease should be ruled out in every patient with acute pancreatitis, because further damage during such an episode and future attacks can be avoided if the gallstones are removed by cholecystectomy.

TREATMENT. The potential seriousness of cholangitis warrants hospitalization for diagnosis and treatment in most cases. After blood cultures are drawn, antimicrobial drugs effective against enteric organisms are given by the parenteral route. At present a regimen of a cephalosporin or ampicillin for mild attacks or an aminoglycoside plus clindamycin in severe infection is likely to control the infection. Failure to obtain a rapid response may mean that the organisms were not susceptible to the initial drugs, justifying the addition of another drug or a shift from the initial regimen on the basis of the result of cultures and drug susceptibility tests. The margin between mild and severe illness is small; antimicrobial therapy should be expected to control the acute attack within 48 to 72 hours, and if there is no improvement or worsening after this period, emergency surgery must be considered seriously.

More than 90 per cent of patients respond satisfactorily to treatment, with an orderly attempt at diagnosis allowed. If oral cholecystography or ultrasonography has previously demonstrated gallbladder stones, laparotomy is indicated, and additional studies aimed at demonstrating the ductal pathology are usually not necessary. In patients with jaundice, acute pancreatitis, or upper abdominal pain who have had a cholecystectomy in the past, ultrasonography should be performed; direct opacification of the ducts can be attempted by percutaneous transhepatic or, preferably, retrograde endoscopic cholangiopancreatography. Both kinds of direct cholangiography are potentially hazardous in active cholangitis and should be postponed if possible until infection is well controlled, proceeding then only under the protection of antimicrobial therapy. However, decompression of the bile duct using a nasobiliary catheter or a sphincterotomy may provide the control needed when there is evidence of duct obstruction.

Deciding between endoscopic and surgical approaches to the management of choledocholithiasis can be done only on a case by case basis until further guidelines, based on comparative studies, are available. If the gallbladder is present, cholecystectomy should be done, and the common duct is opened and emptied of stones. A T tube is usually left in the duct to decompress biliary pressure in the postoperative period and to provide a route for subsequent cholangiograms. With accurate diagnosis and treatment, choledocholithiasis is cured by cholecystectomy and choledocholithotomy. Recurrent ductal stone formation occurs infrequently except when the duct has become markedly dilated.

In patients with advanced disease, the common duct may be so packed with hundreds of stones that it is dilated to 3 cm or more in diameter. Rarely, the intrahepatic ducts become markedly dilated and contain innumerable brown stones, making complete extraction technically impossible. In either of these situations recurrent or persistent choledocholithiasis is almost certain unless a choledochoduodenostomy, sphincteroplasty, or Roux-en-Y choledochojejunostomy is performed to create a wide conduit between the duct and intestine through which residual and recurrent stones can pass. A hepaticojejunostomy with or without a hepatic segmental resection of the affected area of the intrahepatic ductal system may be necessary.

Selected patients with choledocholithiasis who previously have had a cholecystectomy may be satisfactorily treated by endoscopic sphincterotomy. Using the side viewing duodenoscope, a wire is passed into the bile duct and the sphincter divided by electrocautery. Common duct stones 1 cm or smaller will usually pass into the duodenum. This technique may be unsuccessful with large stones or when the common duct is greatly dilated. Bleeding and pancreatitis are the principal complications but are infrequent. The mortality of the procedure is less than 1 per cent in experienced hands.

RETAINED COMMON DUCT STONES. The methods for detecting duct stones at operation are about 95 per cent reliable, which means, unfortunately, that a few are overlooked only to be discovered on postoperative T tube cholangiograms. There are two approaches to eliminate residual stones without another laparotomy. Neither method should be tried until four to six weeks postoperatively. One technique depends on the ability of mono-octanoin (glyceryl-1-mono-octanoate) to dissolve cholesterol gallstones. Mono-octanoin is infused into the duct at 5 ml per hour; care must be exercised to avoid producing pressures in the duct greater than 30 cm H_2O during infusion. The retained stones disappear in about two thirds of patients within a four to eight day treatment period. There is no solvent known to be effective against black pigment stones. A combination of mono-octanoin and chenodeoxycholate has been successful against brown stones.

Instrumental extraction is somewhat simpler, faster, and the treatment of choice. Under image intensification fluoroscopy the T tube is pulled out, a Dormia ureteral basket is passed into the duct, and the stone is grasped and withdrawn. The best plan usually is to try instrumental extraction first and dissolution if it fails. If neither mechanical extraction nor chemical dissolution is successful, transendoscopic sphincterotomy may allow the stone to pass into the duodenum. If that technique is unsuccessful, reoperation is necessary.

SUPPURATIVE CHOLANGITIS. The severest form of cholangitis, suppurative cholangitis, involves the same causative factors as the "nonsuppurative" form but differs in that obstruction is complete, ductal contents become purulent, and clinically the manifestations of sepsis overshadow those of cholestasis. Hypotension and mental changes such as lethargy or confusion appear in addition to right upper quadrant pain, chills, fever, and jaundice. Some elderly patients may be hypothermic and have minimal clinical signs. Because infection in the face of the high-grade obstruction progresses so rapidly, the serum bilirubin does not reach very high levels before the patient becomes moribund from sepsis. Costly delays in diagnosis are frequent, a consequence of failure to recognize the significance of mild icterus and abdominal pain in a patient with sepsis. All but a few cases involve complications of choledocholithiasis, the others occurring with biliary stricture or neoplastic obstruction, usually from bile duct carcinoma with or without sclerosing cholangitis.

Laboratory tests reveal evidence of cholestasis with bilirubin values between 2 and 5 mg per deciliter and elevated serum levels of alkaline phosphatase, 5′-nucleotidase, and transaminases. The leukocyte count varies from subnormal to 40,000 per cubic millimeter.

Tenderness is present to palpation in the right upper quadrant, but rigidity is rare. In some cases secondary cholecystitis develops, and an enlarged tender gallbladder may be found on abdominal examination. Ultrasonography may show dilated bile ducts. Percutaneous transhepatic cholangiography would be extremely hazardous. Diagnosis rests on recognizing the evidence of biliary obstruction and its relationship to the sepsis, and on verifying the initial impression by an ultrasound scan. After initial resuscitation—consisting of intravenous infusions, antimicrobial drugs (gentamicin or tobramycin plus clindamycin parenterally) and measures to restore cardiac, pulmonary, or renal function—decompression of the duct by emergency laparotomy or transendoscopic sphincterotomy offers the only hope of saving the patient. Biliary stents have been placed endoscopically to reduce obstruction and systemic sepsis. Hypoglycemia has been found in some patients whose depressed cerebral function seemed to improve with infusion of hypertonic glucose solutions.

At surgery when choledochotomy is performed, pus often squirts from the duct owing to the high pressure. If the patient's condition permits, thorough exploration can be performed to correct the obstruction by removing stones, repairing a stricture, or bypassing a tumor. Insertion of a T tube proximal to the obstruction is sufficient in patients who are unable to tolerate a longer operation, but sometime later it will be necessary to perform a second more definitive procedure before the T tube can be removed. The mortality rate is about 50 per cent, resulting from septic shock, renal failure, acute hepatic insufficiency, or a combination of these complications.

BILIARY STRICTURE

Peter F. Malet

Biliary stricture almost always results from surgical injury to the duct and usually follows cholecystectomy rather than procedures on the duct itself such as deliberate choledochotomy for common duct exploration. The first sign of trouble postoperatively might be excessive flow of bile through drains or the appearance of jaundice or cholangitis. Biliary stricture may also result from external trauma or scarring produced by choledocholithiasis.

Injury to the duct that is identified early can sometimes be successfully repaired. Partial biliary obstruction and intermittent cholangitis weeks or months after cholecystectomy constitute a serious and challenging clinical problem. The symptoms resemble those of cholangitis with choledocholithiasis. Laboratory evidence consists of leukocytosis and elevated serum levels of bilirubin, alkaline phosphatase and transaminases. The jaundice and cholangitis are generally mild and transient, and infection generally responds promptly to antimicrobial therapy. Diagnosis can be made with visualization of the biliary tract by either PTC or ERCP. With persistent obstruction over several years, secondary biliary cirrhosis with portal hypertension or multiple intrahepatic abscesses may develop.

Differential diagnosis includes all the various causes of obstructive jaundice and cholangitis, but in most cases the major consideration is choledocholithiasis. A useful differential feature is that the initial symptoms of stricture usually begin within two years after cholecystectomy, whereas a symptom-free interval longer than this is common with residual or recurrent common duct stones.

In all but a few cases an attempt should be made to repair the stricture surgically by creating a new unobstructed conduit between normal duct on the hepatic side of the lesion and the proximal intestine rather than attempting direct end-to-end anastomosis of the duct after excision of the lesion. The overall success rate of these operations is about 75 per cent with an operative mortality of 10 per cent.

Balloon catheter dilatation of a short stricture at the time of either PTC or ERCP may be useful in some patients, particularly those who are poor operative risks. This involves the insertion into the bile duct of a balloon-tipped catheter; inflation of the balloon stretches the narrowed area and allows greater bile flow.

OTHER CAUSES OF BILE DUCT OBSTRUCTION

Peter F. Malet

Duodenal and pancreatic tumors are common causes of obstruction in the middle-aged or elderly. These important diseases are discussed in Ch. 106 and 108. Common bile duct obstruction may also be caused by a variety of uncommon disorders. Jaundice, biliary colic, and episodes of cholangitis may be caused by sclerosing cholangitis in patients with ulcerative colitis or by Oriental cholangiohepatitis in a recent immigrant from Southeast Asia. Rare causes are compression by neoplastic or inflammatory paraductal lymph nodes or by duodenal Crohn's disease.

SCLEROSING CHOLANGITIS. *Sclerosing cholangitis,* a condition of unknown cause, consists of benign nonbacterial chronic inflammatory narrowing of the bile ducts. The entire ductal system is involved in over half the cases; less commonly, the process may be confined to the extrahepatic or intrahepatic portion. The ratio of males to females is 3:2, and the peak incidence occurs in the third and fourth decades. About one half of the cases are associated with *ulcerative colitis* (Ch. 104). The severity of sclerosing cholangitis does not parallel the activity of the colitis and colectomy does not improve the cholangitis. Other much less commonly associated diseases are *retroperitoneal fibrosis, regional enteritis,* and *Riedel's thyroiditis.*

The initial complaint may be jaundice or pruritus, although both eventually appear in most cases. There may be mild upper abdominal pain and sometimes fever, but a clinical picture resembling bacterial cholangitis is uncommon in the absence of previous surgical exploration or instrumentation of the ducts. Hepatomegaly may be present in some cases; when secondary cirrhosis develops, ascites or splenomegaly are found.

Jaundice may be constant or fluctuating, and bilirubin values are usually in the range of 2 to 10 mg per deciliter. The alkaline phosphatase is quite high and remains elevated despite variations in clinical manifestations. Antimitochondrial antibodies are absent. Other liver function tests are normal until late in the illness when hepatic failure develops.

Percutaneous transhepatic cholangiography or preferably endoscopic retrograde cholangiopancreatography is required to establish the diagnosis. The x-rays show diffuse irregular ductal narrowing with attenuation of the peripheral intrahepatic ducts. One third of patients develop gallstones behind the strictured bile ducts; these are usually brown pigment gallstones. When considering a differential diagnosis, a single short stenosis (1 to 2 cm) of the duct more likely represents a neoplasm or traumatic stricture than sclerosing cholangitis. More diffuse stenosis may be difficult to distinguish from diffuse ductal carcinoma.

Treatment with corticosteroids or immunosuppressants has not been proved to be generally effective, but a few patients do respond. A trial of treatment is advocated by some experts. Cholestyramine is useful for pruritus. Antimicrobials are necessary if bacterial cholangitis develops.

In symptomatic patients, the aim of therapy is to relieve biliary obstruction. If a segmental stricture is present, balloon dilatation can be attempted either percutaneously or endoscopically if the lesion is in the common bile duct. Balloon dilatation may have to be repeated intermittently to provide sustained relief of obstruction; there is the risk of inducing bacterial cholangitis, particularly with the endoscopic approach. Percutaneous catheter drainage is another option but often does not provide adequate drainage of all obstructed areas in diffuse disease. Surgical therapy is warranted in some cases in order to stent diffuse disease or to bypass severe distal common bile duct disease. Significant palliation follows surgery in most cases but is not usually permanent. Most patients have episodic remissions and exacerbations, during which secondary biliary cirrhosis develops. Death may follow uncontrollable biliary sepsis with hepatic abscesses, liver failure, or bleeding from esophageal varices.

STRUCTURAL ABNORMALITIES. *Choledochal cysts* occasionally produce their initial clinical manifestations in young adults, presenting with jaundice, pain, or cholangitis. Diagnosis requires transhepatic or retrograde cholangiography; CT scan or ultrasonography can provide information about surrounding structures. The most definitive surgical procedure is excision of the cyst, followed by Roux-en-Y choledochojejunostomy.

Caroli's disease consists of saccular intrahepatic bile duct dilatations that most often becomes symptomatic in patients between the ages of 20 and 50, because of intrahepatic stone formation and cholangitis. Two forms are recognized: (1) disease of the ducts only and (2) ductal disease associated with hepatic fibrosis and medullary sponge kidney (most common). The latter patients often have complications of portal hypertension before cholangitis or obstructive jaundice appears. Antimicrobial therapy may control attacks of cholangitis, and surgical procedures to facilitate ductal emptying or to extract stones may help in some cases, but the intrahepatic anomaly cannot be definitively corrected unless lobectomy is possible for single lobe involvement.

Duodenal diverticula usually arise within 1 to 2 cm of the hepatobiliary ampulla. They may obstruct the common duct by anatomic distortion of its duodenal entry, by diverticulitis, or by an enterolith (of bile acids) in the sac. Even in jaundiced patients, however, most duodenal diverticula are only incidental findings; but when definite proof implicates them in ductal obstruction, either choledochoduodenostomy or Roux-en-Y choledochojejunostomy is the treatment of choice.

PANCREATITIS. *Pancreatitis* can produce transient jaundice by obstruction of the distal common duct where it is encased by pancreatic tissue. Prolonged obstruction can result from pressure by an adjacent pseudocyst or entrapment of the distal common bile duct in severe pancreatic scarring from chronic pancreatitis. Diagnosis may be delayed in alcoholic patients in whom elevated bilirubin values are usually attributed to hepatocellular disease. Persistent elevation of alkaline phosphatase in an alcoholic should raise suspicion of the possibility of biliary obstruction, particularly if pancreatic calcification is present on plain abdominal x-rays. Jaundice resulting from chronic pancreatitis requires choledochoduodenostomy or Roux-en-Y anastomosis of jejunum to the gallbladder or common bile duct.

HEMOBILIA. *Hemobilia* classically presents with biliary colic, obstructive jaundice, and occult or gross intestinal bleeding. There is a delay in diagnosis in many cases because the presentation is not typical or the condition is not considered in the differential diagnosis of upper gastrointestinal bleeding. Most cases are caused by hepatic injury from external or operative trauma with secondary bleeding into the ductal system. Other causes include biliary or hepatic neoplasms, ductal rupture of an hepatic artery aneurysm, hepatic abscess, gallstones or following percutaneous needle biopsy of the liver or cholangiography. Hemobilia in the Orient accompanies both biliary parasitism with *Ascaris lumbricoides* or cholangiohepatitis. Hemobilia following trauma is best treated by hepatic artery ligation, which is well tolerated except when there is advanced parenchymal disease; otherwise, direct management of the causative lesion is necessary.

PARASITIC DISEASE. An *echinococcal hepatic cyst* can rupture into the ducts and can give rise to biliary colic, jaundice, and cholangitis (Ch. 393). Treatment involves surgical removal of the obstructing hydatid debris and daughter cysts from the ducts and excision of the parent cyst from the liver after attempts are made to sterilize its contents with absolute alcohol or hypertonic saline (30 per cent) solution. *Ascariasis* may produce biliary colic, jaundice, and cholangitis by worm invasion into the bile ducts from the duodenum (Ch. 406). Treatment entails antimicrobial drugs for the cholangitis and then piperazine after the acute symptoms are controlled. If progressive cholangitis occurs despite medical therapy, common duct exploration and extraction of the worms may be necessary.

ORIENTAL CHOLANGIOHEPATITIS. *Oriental cholangiohepatitis*, or recurrent pyogenic cholangitis, is a common form of recurrent cholangitis in the Orient associated with brown pigment gallstone formation throughout the biliary tract. The cause is unclear but possibilities include parasites in the ducts (although *Clonorchus sinensis* is found in only 20 per cent of cases) and a low protein diet. Most patients present with acute cholangitis; those with recurrent cholangitis may develop liver abscesses, biliary enteric fistulas, or sepsis. In advanced cases, one (usually the left) or both lobar ducts may become honeycombed with scars or abscesses, producing atrophy of the hepatic parenchyma. Direct cholangiography is necessary for a definitive diagnosis. Sphincteroplasty or choledochojejunostomy is usually performed to remove stones and sludge and provide adequate biliary drainage. Cholecystectomy or partial hepatic resection is required when the gallbladder or localized hepatic segments are involved.

CARCINOMA OF THE GALLBLADDER

Roger D. Soloway

In the United States in 1978, there were approximately 2500 deaths from carcinoma of the gallbladder, a number equal to the mortality from benign disease of the biliary tract. Gallbladder cancer accounts for 1 per cent of all cancer deaths and 3 per cent of gastrointestinal malignancies. Women affected outnumber men by 3 to 1, and the average age is 70. Because 85 per cent of cases occur in patients with gallstones, cholelithiasis is thought to be etiologically important; gallbladder cancer develops in fewer than 1 per cent of patients with cholelithiasis. The disease is 5 to 10 times more frequent in American Indian populations, in which group it is the most common gastrointestinal tumor in women.

Most gallbladder carcinomas are adenocarcinomas, the remainder being squamous cell carcinomas. The earliest spread is usually by metastasis to the hilar lymph nodes and adjacent hepatic parenchyma followed by direct extension to the liver and hilar structures. Distant metastases appear relatively late.

The patients have one of the following clinical pictures: (1) unremitting deep jaundice from common duct and hepatic involvement; (2) acute cholecystitis, usually with a palpable mass; (3) chronic cholecystitis with intermittent right upper quadrant pain; and (4) advanced disseminated carcinoma. The diagnosis is not often considered preoperatively, but in some instances clinical clues are present. In about two thirds of patients a mass can be felt and in one third there is local tenderness. In all but a few cases the oral cholecystogram does not opacify, and even when it does, the tumor can rarely be demonstrated. The diagnosis can be suspected on ultrasound if an intraluminal gallbladder mass is identified that does not change with position. Pathologic studies indicate that all apparent tumor would be removed in 25 per cent of cases by cholecystectomy, resection of a rim of adjacent liver, and dissection of the common duct lymph node chain. Even in this favorable group the five-year survival rate is 5 per cent. Most patients live for only a few months after the diagnosis.

BENIGN TUMORS AND PSEUDOTUMORS OF THE GALLBLADDER

Peter F. Malet

Adenomyomatous hyperplasia, also called adenomyomatosis, is the most common of these lesions; there is hyperplasia of the mucosa with formation of intramural diverticulae. Typically, neoplastic or inflammatory changes are absent. Adenomyomatosis is usually diagnosed by oral cholecystography as a sessile filling defect with a central umbilication and small peripheral opaque areas representing diverticula. A few cases are associated with episodic pain that can be cured by cholecystectomy, but most often adenomyomatosis is asymptomatic.

Cholesterol polyps are a focal form of cholesterolosis consisting of submucosal macrophages filled with cholesterol and located at a villous tip. Generally, multiple polyps are present. The polyp is attached to the mucosa by a fragile stalk that can easily be broken. Cholecystectomy is indicated if the patient has abdominal pain for which there is no other apparent cause.

Papillary and nonpapillary *adenomas* are the only true benign neoplasms of the gallbladder. Most adenomas are pedunculated; about two thirds are multiple. They appear as filling defects on oral cholecystography. It is doubtful that many gallbladder carcinomas arise from adenomas, because adenomas are much less common than carcinomas of the gallbladder.

TUMORS OF THE BILE DUCT

Roger D. Soloway

The main cause of early morbidity from tumors of the bile duct is biliary obstruction with gradual hepatocellular damage or secondary hepatobiliary infection. Tumors of the bile ducts are rarely benign. Papilloma, the most frequent, is often multifocal and therefore difficult to cure. Adenomas and granular cell tumors are localized but are often difficult to treat surgically without radical excision. This section will be directed primarily to discussion of malignant tumors, but many of the same principles of pathophysiology and diagnosis will apply to the rare benign tumors.

Except for a rare squamous cell tumor, bile duct malignancies are adenocarcinomas with either a scirrhous or a papillary pattern. Grossly, three types of pathologic presentations occur: focal stricture, diffuse thickening, and nodular mass. The first two varieties can easily be mistaken for a benign process such as post-traumatic stricture or sclerosing cholangitis. In many cases, spread is confined to local lymph node metastases or hepatic invasion for months or years before there is more widespread abdominal or systemic involvement. The common hepatic duct or common bile duct is the site of origin in about two thirds of the cases. The eponym *Klatskin tumor* is often used to refer to adenocarcinoma at the bifurcation of the common hepatic duct. By contrast with carcinoma of the gallbladder, cholelithiasis is found in only one third of patients, and men slightly outnumber women. The average age at diagnosis is 70 years. A number of cases have been reported in younger patients with ulcerative colitis. Since some of these patients had previously undergone colectomy, it is thought that elimination of the diseased colon is not protective. Sclerosing cholangitis is a recognized complication in these same patients and may have identical clinical features, especially when it primarily affects the extrahepatic bile ducts. In the Orient, infestation with *Clonorchis sinensis* probably contributes to the higher incidence of intrahepatic cholangiocarcinoma.

CLINICAL MANIFESTATIONS. The typical patient presents with unremitting severe jaundice, mild deep-seated upper abdominal pain, and weight loss. Pruritus is reported by many, usually but not always, after the onset of jaundice. Pain, present in over half the patients, is not colicky and tends to be steady; fever and chills are absent. Hepatomegaly without splenomegaly is found on abdominal examination. Tumors of the common duct sparing the cystic duct often produce in addition to jaundice a distended nontender palpable gallbladder *(Courvoisier's law).* Most patients have occult blood in the stool.

The serum bilirubin exceeds 10 mg per deciliter in most cases, with a mean value of around 18 mg per deciliter. The complete obstruction of the ductal system results in a bilirubin of 30 mg per deciliter or higher. The alkaline phosphatase is raised and AST may be slightly elevated, although rarely higher than 200. Obstruction of the right or left hepatic system alone causes 10 to 30-fold increase in alkaline phosphatase with normal levels of bilirubin. Serum proteins are most often normal. The prothrombin time may be prolonged but responds to parenteral vitamin K. Serum cholesterol is usually elevated and averages about 400 mg per deciliter.

DIAGNOSIS. Ultrasonography or CT scan shows dilatation of the intrahepatic bile ducts. Transhepatic or retrograde cholangiography demonstrates marked ductal dilatation and the site of the block. Only a benign stricture of the duct is likely to create a similar radiographic picture, but if the patient has had no previous biliary surgery, benign stricture is extremely unlikely.

The differential diagnosis includes primary biliary cirrhosis and drug-induced cholestatic jaundice. In neither of these conditions does the bilirubin generally reach levels over 12 to 15 mg per deciliter. Xanthelasma, found often with primary biliary cirrhosis, are only rarely seen with neoplastic obstruction. Antimitochondrial antibodies can be demonstrated in the serum of most patients with primary biliary cirrhosis. Sclerosing cholangitis, usually associated with chronic inflammatory bowel disease, is characterized by intermittent attacks of pain, jaundice, and fever. It also shows a characteristic pattern on transhepatic cholangiography or ERCP.

Choledocholithiasis and biliary stricture are less likely to present with deepening jaundice and weight loss. The jaundice fluctuates, is milder, and is usually associated with fever. Transhepatic cholangiogram or ERCP will help to exclude these diseases.

TREATMENT. Unfortunately, complete excision of the tumor is often impossible, because unexpendable anatomic structures are involved early. Nevertheless, a few cures can be expected when radical surgery is judiciously employed, and palliation is often lengthy and of excellent quality.

With proximal lesions, the findings at surgery consist of a collapsed gallbladder and a small common duct. Distal lesions require radical pancreaticoduodenectomy (Whipple's procedure) for complete removal. Because this operation has a 15 per cent mortality, it should be performed only if no gross tumor would be left behind. Tumors of the supraduodenal duct are sometimes amenable to complete resection. Localized tumors of the bifurcation of the hepatic duct are best treated by excision, even though microscopic deposits of tumor usually remain in the bed of the dissection. Reconstruction involves use of a Roux-en-Y hepaticojejunostomy.

For tumors with local or distant spread the goal is palliation. If duodenal obstruction is unlikely, the treatment of choice is percutaneous or endoscopic stenting of the biliary tract with catheters having multiple portholes above and below the point of bile duct obstruction. Either tube can be changed periodically to prevent plugging. Distal tumors can be bypassed by cholecystojejunostomy or other types of biliary-enteric anastomoses. For unresectable tumors at the junction of the hepatic ducts (Klatskin tumors) a tube may be placed in the duct to maintain bile flow by spanning the tumor; the hepatic end is brought out directly through the liver substance, and the duodenal end is brought out through a choledochotomy (the U tube technique). Holes in the intraductal and intraintestinal portions of the tube allow bile to reach the gut from the liver. When debris begins to plug the lumen, as usually happens within 6 to 12 months, the tube can easily be replaced without reoperation. Radiotherapy is usually recommended after excision; chemotherapy has not been effective.

PROGNOSIS. Cure is achieved in 5 to 10 per cent, and many patients survive in good condition for several years or more following palliative excision. If biliary drainage can be maintained with a tube, patients with unresectable lesions occasionally do well for a year or two. Death eventually results from hepatic replacement with tumor or intrahepatic sepsis from recurrent ductal obstruction.

POSTCHOLECYSTECTOMY SYNDROME

Roger D. Soloway

After cholecystectomy, 10 per cent of patients continue to have significant abdominal symptoms. In most patients, the explanation for continued postoperative symptoms is that the gallstone disease was not the cause of their preoperative complaints. Patients with typical biliary pain are more often relieved by cholecystectomy than those with the vague symptoms of fatty food intolerance, dyspepsia, or flatulence. Success of cholecystectomy also correlates with the extent of pathologic change in the gallbladder wall; patients with persistent symptoms more often had minimal scarring and a functioning gallbladder.

In others, postcholecystectomy complaints can be attributed to overlooked disease, especially choledocholithiasis, pancreatitis, peptic ulcer, or irritable bowel syndrome. These possibilities must be investigated by appropriate studies.

Stenosis of the sphincter of Oddi (ampullary stenosis), biliary dyskinesia, neuroma of the cystic duct stump, and other cystic duct remnant lesions are conditions that have returned to clinical favor as causes of the postcholecystectomy syndrome along with objective tests for detection such as ERCP with manometry and ^{99m}Tc DESIDA scanning.

Renewed interest in ampullary stenosis and biliary dyskinesia has followed the development of methods to perform endoscopic sphincterotomy. Early results suggest that a minority of patients with episodic biliary colic in the absence of stones have hypertension, dysmotility, and/or stenosis of the sphincter of Oddi. The appearance of a narrowed sphincter alone is insufficient to document either stenosis or dyskinesia. A provocative test has been used that involves injection of morphine (10 mg) and neostigmine methylsulfate (1 mg) intramuscularly. Pain and a rise in serum amylase levels are indications of ampullary stenosis. The results of this test, however, do not correlate with sphincter of Oddi pressures, and the test is sometimes positive in normal subjects. Clinicians should remain skeptical about a diagnosis of ampullary stenosis when the principal finding is abdominal pain. The diagnosis is more secure in patients with recurrent pancreatitis, cholangitis, choledocholithiasis, and/or dilated bile duct, whose sphincter appears tight on x-ray and will accept only a small probe. Treatment consists of division of the sphincter at operation or transendoscopically. Patients with recurrent pancreatitis should have an operative pancreatic septectomy in addition—division of that portion of the pancreas separating the distal common bile duct and pancreatic duct, thereby dividing that portion of the sphincter that extended onto the pancreatic duct.

Convincing evidence has been submitted to document the importance of each of the aforementioned conditions in specific cases. Dyskinesia of the common duct and sphincter without stenosis is very difficult to establish as a cause of the syndrome. Perhaps further data from manometric studies will elucidate a relationship between motor abnormalities and postoperative pain. In the management of such patients with chronic abdominal pain in the absence of objective findings, exploratory laparotomy has a low rate of success for diagnosis and surgical correction of minor variations in the gut anatomy usually fails to cure.

Boey JH, Way LW: Acute cholangitis. Ann Surg 191:264, 1980. *This article describes the spectrum of severity of acute cholangitis and how severity relates to the underlying cause, and makes recommendations for therapy.*

Boyer JL: New concepts of mechanisms of hepatocyte bile formation. Physiol Rev 60:303, 1980. *A comprehensive review of this subject.*

Brandt-Rauf PW, Pincus M, Adelson S: Cancer of the gallbladder: A review of 43 cases. Hum Pathol 13:48, 1982. *A review of the clinicopathological findings, epidemiology, and natural history of this virtually incurable disease.*

Chitwood WR Jr, Meyers WC, Heaston DK, Herskovic AM, Mc Leod ME, Jones RS: Diagnosis and treatment of primary extrahepatic bile duct tumors. Am J Surg 143:99, 1982. *Covers the subject in detail.*

Dolgin SM, Schwartz JS, Kressel HY, Soloway RD, Miller WT, Trotman BW, Soloway AS, Good LI: Identification of patients with cholesterol or pigment gallstones using discriminant analysis of radiographic features. N Engl J Med 304:808, 1981. *Clinically useful method of identifying many black pigment stones.*

Gracie WA, Ransohoff DF: The natural history of silent gallstones: The innocent gallstone is not a myth. N Engl J Med 307:798, 1982. *The only article describing a group of patients with truly asymptomatic gallstones.*

Grundy SM: Mechanism of cholesterol gallstones formation. Sem Liver Dis 3:97, 1983. *A comprehensive up-to-date review of the biochemistry leading to cholesterol supersaturation of bile.*

Jarvinen HJ, Hastbacka J: Early cholecystectomy for acute cholecystitis. A prospective randomized study. Ann Surg 191:501, 1980. *This controlled trial demonstrates the advantages of early surgery over expectant management for acute cholecystitis.*

Kern F Jr: Epidemiology and natural history of gallstones. Sem Liver Dis 3:87, 1983. *Most recent review on currently implicated factors in gallstone formation.*

Maton PN, Iser JH, Reuben A, Saxton HM, Murphy GM, Dowling RH: Outcome of chenodeoxycholic acid (CDCA) treatment in 125 patients with radiolucent gallstones. Medicine 61:86, 1982. *Factors influencing efficacy, withdrawal, symptoms and side effects, and postdissolution recurrence.*

Mauro MA, McCartney WH, Melmed JR: Hepatobiliary scanning with 99mTc-PIPIDA in acute cholecystitis. Radiology 142:193, 1982. *Assessment of sensitivity of this technique in diagnosis.*

Scharschmidt BF, Goldberg HI, Schmid R: Current concepts in diagnosis: Approach to the patient with cholestatic jaundice. N Engl J Med 308: 1515, 1983. *Excellent review on the most efficient approach to distinguishing intrahepatic from extrahepatic cholestasis.*

Schoenfield LJ, Lachin JM: Chenodiol (chenodeoxycholic acid) for dissolution of gallstones: The National Cooperative Gallstone Study. A controlled trial of efficacy and safety. Ann Intern Med 92:257, 1981. *Definitive paper on chenodiol safety and efficacy in a dose of 750 mg daily (8–10 mg/kg).*

Trotman BW, Soloway RD: Pigment gallstone disease: Summary of the National Institutes of Health—International Workshop. Hepatology 2:879, 1982. *Up to date summary—60 references.*

Way LW, Dunphy JE: Biliary stricture. Am J Surg 124:287, 1972. *Description of the diagnosis and results of surgical therapy for biliary stricture.*

Wenckert A, Robertson B: The natural course of gallstone disease. Gastroenterology 50:376, 1966. *This is one of the more commonly quoted series on the natural history of gallstone disease; the study involved a group containing both symptomatic and asymptomatic patients.*

Wiesner RH, LaRusso NF: Clinicopathologic features of the syndrome of primary sclerosing cholangitis. Gastroenterology 79:200, 1980. *A review of 50 patients with sclerosing cholangitis.*

Part XIII
HEMATOLOGIC DISEASES

130. INTRODUCTION

David G. Nathan

This introduction is primarily intended to provide a general background to diagnostic hematology and marrow function. The remaining chapters in Part XIII emphasize fundamental physiologic principles and provide descriptions of relatively common hematologic disorders with the hope that the entire Part will influence the reader to consider such diseases broadly and systematically.

The nonmalignant disorders of erythrocytes, phagocytes, and platelets, including their precursors and progenitors, are initially discussed. Then follows a description of the acute and chronic proliferative disorders that involve the cells of the marrow and lymphoid systems, a series of chapters that ends with a discussion of bone marrow transplantation. The final chapters of Part XIII are devoted to a review of the disorders of the fluid phase of blood coagulation and the vascular purpuras.

DIAGNOSTIC HEMATOLOGY. The circulating blood cells are the products of the terminal differentiation of recognizable precursors. In fetal life hematopoiesis occurs throughout the reticuloendothelial system. In the normal adult, the process of terminal differentiation of the recognizable precursors of erythrocytes, granulocytes, and platelets occurs exclusively in the marrow cavities of the axial skeleton with some extension into the proximal femora and humeri, but the space is highly expandable when the demand for blood cell production is accelerated (Fig. 130–1).

Observations of differentiated blood cells by enumeration and relatively simple morphologic studies of properly prepared blood films provide the essential cornerstone of diagnostic hematology. Automated blood counts and cell sizing now provide both reproducibility and enhanced diagnostic capacity. For example, early red cell production failure may be heralded by unexpected macrocytosis. Peripheral blood cell morphology offers insight into the rate of effective hematopoiesis; the state of marrow nutrition with respect to vitamin B_{12}, folic acid, and iron; the presence of acquired and congenital disorders of the membrane; the energy metabolism or the hemoglobin of erythrocytes that leads to their accelerated destruction; the differential diagnosis of infections; the presence of allergic reactions; the acquired or congenital abnormalities of intracellular organelles; and the invasion of the marrow by malignant cells or infectious agents. The contributions of morphologic techniques to hematologic diagnosis depend entirely upon the adequacy of specimen preparation and the skill of the observer. Egregious errors are made when diagnostic pronouncements are based on inadequate material. The slavish enumeration of individual cells is rarely of aid without careful overall inspection and positive searches for diagnostic clues that are relevant to the case at hand. Morphology can be particularly misleading if the observer does not understand that many kinds of disorders induce similar changes in shape, particularly in the red cells.

Although circulating lymphocytes appear to be terminally differentiated cells, they are instead capable of rapid proliferative responses to appropriate stimuli during which they resume the appearance of relatively undifferentiated precursors. At this stage they are often called "atypical," even though this blastic transformation is entirely appropriate. The functional subsets of lymphoid cells are not readily demonstrable by inspection, although recent experience has shown that "killer" lymphocyte function may be associated with larger cells that contain granules. Obtaining that important information requires studies of lymphocyte function and studies with specially prepared antibodies reactive with lymphocytes.

Well-prepared marrow films and biopsy specimens also contribute important information such as total marrow cellularity, the presence of invading malignant cells or infectious granulomas, the adequacy of the numbers of megakaryocytes, the ratio of myeloid to erythroid precursors, the state of marrow cell nutrition, the presence of abnormal storage cells, and even the deposition of abnormal crystals. In brief, the blood lends itself to biopsy and to structural, chemical, and functional studies far more readily than does any other human organ. Its cellular elements are diverse, bearing in common only a joint ancestral cell, origin in the marrow, and the property of being transported through vessels suspended in plasma.

PRECURSORS OF CIRCULATING BLOOD CELLS. ***Erythrocytes.*** Much of the progress of differentiation of erythroid precursors can be appreciated morphologically, particularly the onset of hemoglobin synthesis and the maturation and extrusion of the nucleus. The salient features of the morphologic changes that occur during erythroid precursor development are related to biochemical alterations summarized in Figure 130–2. During this process each proerythroblast may give rise to approximately eight erythrocytes. The transit time from proerythroblast to emergence of reticulocytes is approximately five days. The transit time may decrease during anemic stress to as little as two days by means of skipped divisions. The red cells that emerge under conditions of stress are macrocytic and may contain as much as 25 per cent fetal hemoglobin (F cells). They may also bear additional fetal characteristics, particularly the presence of i antigen on their surfaces. More quantitative analyses of the transit of erythroid precursors during the process of maturation may be appreciated from the use of radioactive iron that, when injected intravenously, accumulates preferentially in the newly synthesized ferritin of proerythroblasts and ultimately emerges in peripheral blood incorporated into reticulocyte hemoglobin. The use of surface scanning following infusion of ^{59}Fe-labeled transferrin reveals the site as well as the rate of intramedullary erythropoiesis. This is largely an investigative and not a clinical tool except for cases in which the anatomic site of erythropoiesis needs to be determined, such as in myeloid metaplasia. A qualitative assessment of erythroid precursor activity throughout the body may be gained from injection of ^{111}Indium chloride and marrow scintigraphy. ^{111}Indium binds to transferrin and is incorporated into immature marrow erythroid precursors. Body scanning then reveals the distribution of marrow (Fig. 130–3).

Granulocytes. The process of intramedullary granulocyte maturation involves changes in nuclear configuration and the accumulation of specific intracytoplasmic granules. A model that describes the production and kinetics of neutrophils is shown in Figure 130–4 (see also Ch. 147 and 148). It is highly compartmentalized. The relatively small peripheral blood pool is divided into two compartments in equilibrium, the circulating and the marginating pools. These pools provide entrance into the tissues. The level of peripheral cells is buffered by an immense marrow reserve of identifiable precursors, some of which are in the mitotic compartment and some in the maturing and storage compartment. The kinetics of proliferation of these recognizable precursors have been studied using labeled precursors of DNA. These so-called labeling indices, from which estimates of cell cycle times can be derived, have served as important approaches to the study of pharmacology and toxicity of chemotherapeutic agents.

Platelets. The differentiation of committed megakaryocytes, the precursors of platelets, involves a nuclear endoreduplication phenomenon which produces 16N and 32N megakaryoblasts. The endoreduplication ceases at the stage of the mature megakaryocyte. Platelet shedding from megakaryocytes is accomplished by the formation of multiple demarcation membranes within the cytoplasm of the cell, usually visible only by electron microscopy. Although the platelet appears at first to be a simple tissue fragment (Fig. 130–5), its functions are diverse and

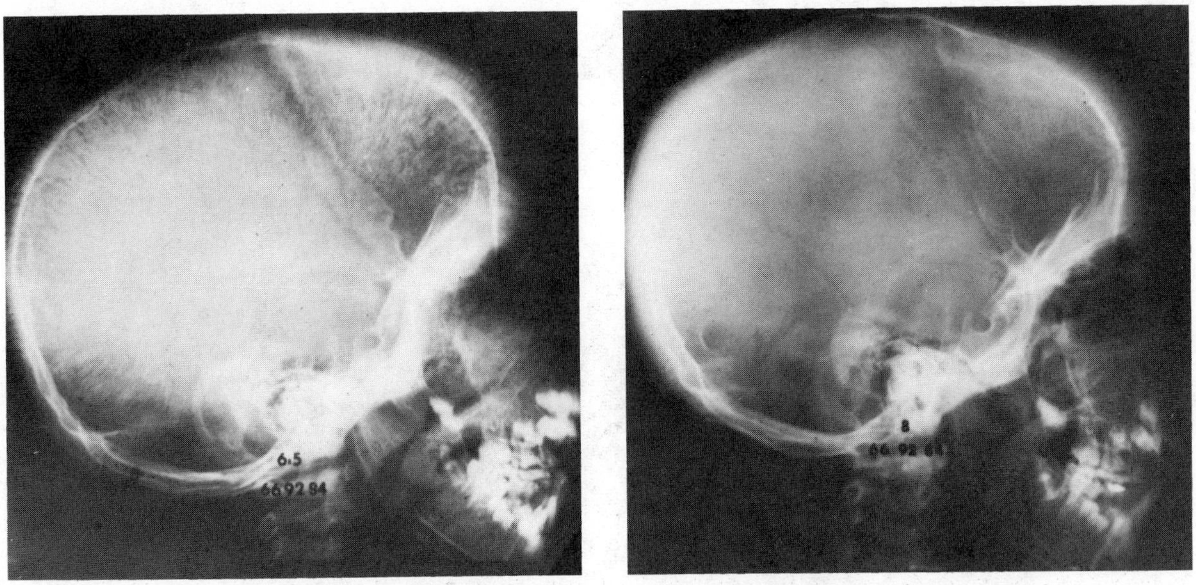

Figure 130–1. Roentgenograms of the skull of a patient with homozygous beta thalassemia at the age of 6½ years *(left),* before splenectomy and transfusion therapy, and at the age of eight years *(right),* after splenectomy and transfusion therapy to control anemia. Note the marked "hair-on-end" appearance in the left-hand radiograph, signifying expansion of the marrow space. (From Nathan DG: N Engl J Med 286:586, 1972.)

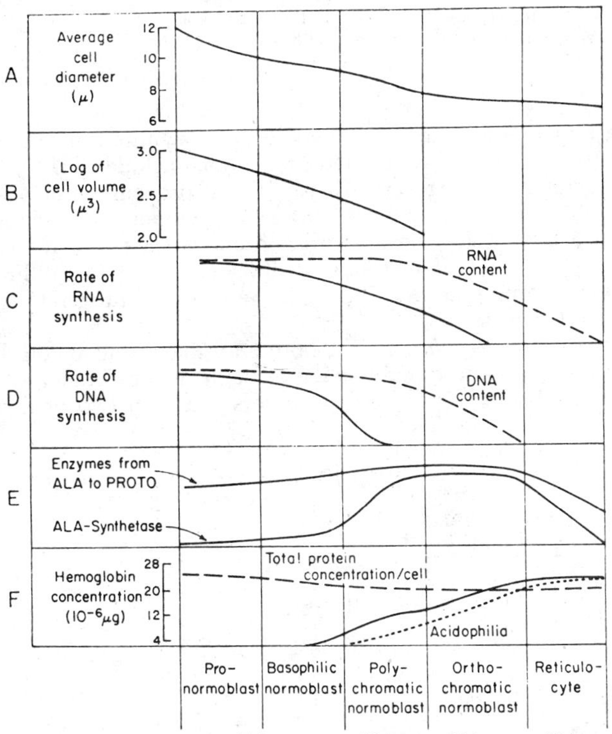

Figure 130–2. Erythroid maturation: alterations in cell size, rates of DNA and RNA synthesis, enzymes involved in heme synthesis, and hemoglobin concentration. Substances listed in the left-hand column are represented by corresponding solid black lines. Unless specified, graphs represent relative values. ALA refers to δ-aminolevulinic acid; PROTO refers to protoporphyrin. It will be noted that considerable protein synthesis takes place during the earliest phase. Following this the nucleolus disappears but mitochondria remain. As the content of DNA decreases and the concentration of RNA starts to fall, hemoglobin begins to appear, increasing rapidly in amount. (From Granick S, Levere RD: In Moore CV, Brown EB [eds.]: Progress in Hematology, Vol IV. New York, Grune & Stratton, 1964. Reprinted by permission of Grune & Stratton.)

hemostatically versatile. It must selectively adhere to abnormal surfaces and then sequentially secrete, aggregate, fuse, and retract in order to ensure a firm platelet-fibrin plug. In the process it assists in the coagulation cascade, synthesizes prostaglandins, and releases ADP and a variety of other substances of known and unknown function.

Lymphocytes. The geography of lymphocyte precursor maturation and differentiation is considerably more complex than that of the other hematopoietic cells. Primitive lymphoid precursors of B cell origin arise in the marrow, spleen, and lymph nodes where they continue their maturation and differentiation. Primitive T cell precursors arise in the marrow, travel to the thymus where they undergo further differentiation, and are finally exported to the spleen, lymph nodes, and marrow where they establish their final residence and perform many of their functions. Both T and B cells enter the peripheral blood circulation that delivers them to tissue sites at which their functions may be required or their unbridled activity may cause disease (see Ch. 427). Circulating lymphocytes represent only a tiny fraction of the total lymphocyte pool. Analysis of these circulating cells may not reflect the nature of the total pool.

HEMATOPOIETIC PROGENITORS. The recognizable marrow precursors of the differentiated peripheral blood cells tend to occupy the attention of hematologists, but they are rarely primary causes of the hematopoietic cytopenias. It is true that various toxins or nutritional deficiencies can so seriously damage the orderly progression of precursor differentiation that effective production of fully differentiated blood cells is embarrassed. In general, however, deficient or excessive production of blood cells is due to abnormalities of *undifferentiated progenitor cells.* They must themselves undergo vital processes of maturation and amplification to give rise to the recognizable precursors of circulating differentiated blood cells.

Progenitor Maturation. Pluripotent stem cells are few in number, but the initial stages of their development lead to committed progenitors of the lymphoid and myeloid systems (Fig. 130–5). These committed progenitors are destined to produce the differentiated, recognizable precursors of the specific types of blood cells. Pluripotent stem cells are capable of slow but indefinite self-renewal, whereas the committed progenitor cells are not capable of indefinite self-renewal. They "die by differentiation," and their numbers depend on influx

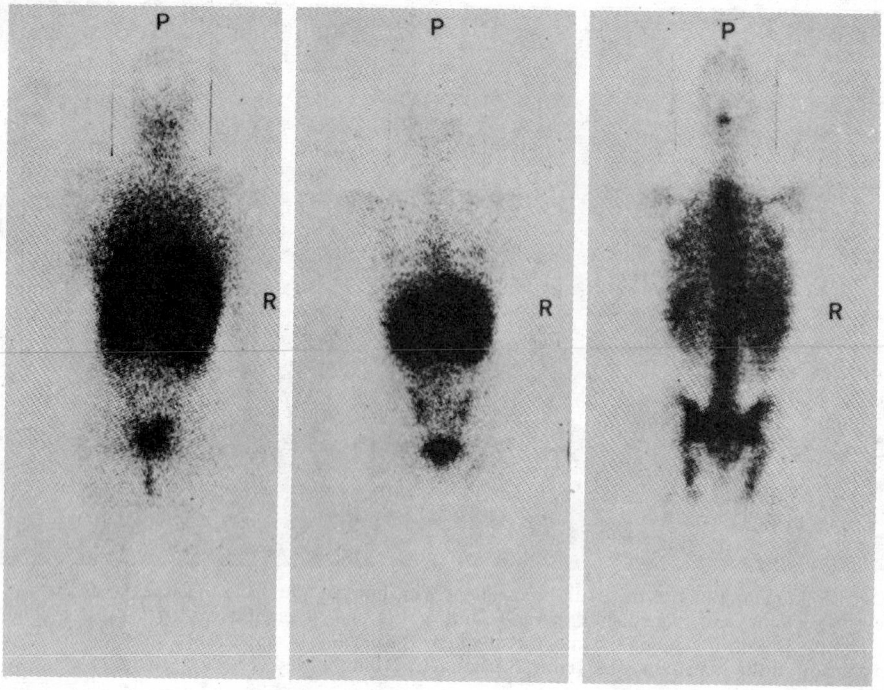

Figure 130–3. Spectrum of $^{111}InCl$ scintigraphic patterns in patients with idiopathic aplastic anemia. On the *left* is the scintigram of a patient prior to marrow transplantation. There is no marrow activity. In the *middle* is the scintigram of a patient with borderline uptake within the marrow. On the *right* is a normal scintigram of a patient after transplantation. Liver activity is seen in all three patients, and splenic activity is seen in one. (From McNeil BJ, Rappeport JM, Nathan DG: Br J Haematol 34:599, 1976.)

from the pluripotent stem cell pool. The committed erythrocyte, phagocyte, and platelet progenitors and the precursors to which they give rise emerge as the result of the maturation of a tripotential progenitor usually called CFU-S for the spleen colony–forming unit described by Till and McCulloch in mice. They observed hematopoietic colonies in the spleens of lethally irradiated mice rescued with bone marrow cells of histoidentical donors. The spleen colonies contained megakaryocyte, granulocyte, and erythroid precursors. A small fraction of CFU-S is found to be replicating or in the act of DNA synthesis at any one time. As more committed progenitors are formed, the fraction of these cells undergoing DNA synthesis increases. These increasingly committed progenitors include CFU-M, the progenitors of megakaryoblasts; CFU-C, progenitors of phagocytic precursors; and BFU-E, the erythroid burst–forming units which ultimately give rise to erythroid precursors. This last-named process of maturation ultimately leads to erythroid colony–forming units, CFU-E, the immediate progenitors of proerythroblasts.

Progenitor Regulation. The hormones that regulate both the amplification and differentiation of the hematopoietic progenitors are beginning to become understood, and two of them,

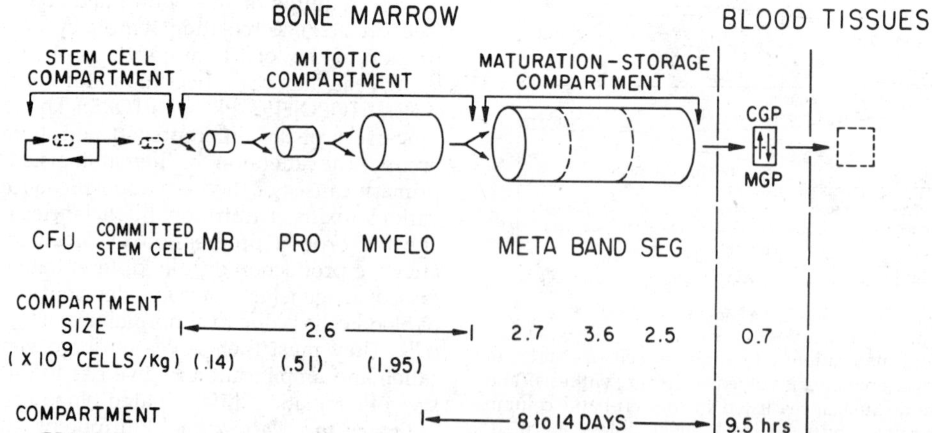

Figure 130–4. Model of the production and kinetics of neutrophils in man. The marrow and blood compartments have been drawn to show their relative sizes. The compartment transit times as derived from labeling studies with $DF^{32}P$ and tritiated thymidine are shown on the next to last line and the last line. The less obvious symbols in the figure include CGP, the circulating granulocyte pool; MGP, the marginating granulocyte pool; CFU, the tripotential stem cell; MB, myeloblast; and PRO, promyelocyte. (From Wintrobe MM, Lee RG, et al.: Clinical Hematology. 7th ed. Philadelphia, Lea & Febiger, 1974, p 244.)

THE PROGENITOR BASIS OF HEMATOPOIESIS

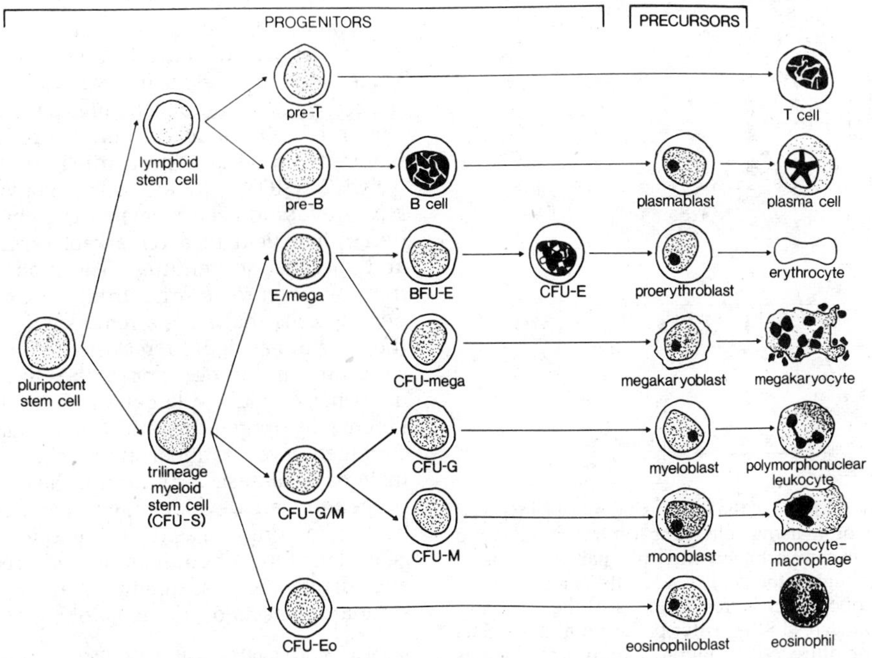

Figure 130–5. A schematic outline of the progenitor basis of hematopoiesis. Note the progressive restriction in the potential for terminal differentiation of the progenitors as they mature from left to right in the drawing. They finally form the recognizable marrow precursors from which the circulating blood cells, shown on the far right, are derived. Not shown in this outline is the process of self-renewal of fractions of the progenitor cell populations, particularly the immature progenitors. Also not shown is the progressive amplification of progenitors and precursors as they mature and differentiate. The bipotential erythroid-megakaryocyte progenitor shown in this drawing and referred to in the text has been demonstrated in the mouse, but not definitely in man.

erythropoietin and colony-stimulating activity, have been purified. Thrombopoietin is the least characterized, but it is now possible to grow colonies of megakaryocytes in the presence of impure preparations of the hormone. Colony-stimulating activity (CSA), a product of macrophages and T lymphocytes, exists in several molecular forms. It is required for the formation of in vitro colonies of granulocytes and macrophages. Its role in vivo is not as well defined. Both CSA and erythropoietin are glycoproteins. Erythropoietin is largely produced in the kidney in the adult in response to hypoxia and/or anemia and can also be produced in the liver, particularly in fetuses. Its deficiency in renal disease contributes to the anemia observed in uremia. Very rare patients with autoantibodies to erythropoietin have red cell aplasia. There is increasing evidence that primitive BFU-E do not differentiate to form red cells in response to erythropoietin without the assistance of inducer hormones that can be derived from T lymphocytes, adherent cells, or a class of nonadherent, non-T cells yet to be clearly defined.

The process of maturation of the erythroid progenitor cells is accompanied by increasing size and an increased sensitivity to erythropoietin. In fact, it is in the later stages of erythroid progenitor maturation that marked amplification of the numbers of progenitors occurs in response to erythropoietin.

Progenitors and Marrow Failure. The hematopoietic progenitors can be detected in the null cell fraction of peripheral blood and in the mononuclear Ia+ cell fraction of marrow. Interactions of progenitor cells and the various factors produced by neighboring inducer cells are presently subjects of intensive scrutiny because it is now apparent that the major disorders of bone marrow failure are due largely to progenitor cell loss or dysfunction. For example, the various aplastic anemias, paroxysmal nocturnal hemoglobinuria, the leukemias, and polycythemia vera are the results of various types of progenitor cell dysfunction or failure. Whether some of these represent primary diseases of progenitor cells and some diseases of inducer cells is yet to be determined. In rare cases antibodies with activity against progenitors have been detected. In certain other cases abnormal lymphocytes appear to suppress progenitor cell function.

Progenitor Cell Therapy. The fact that progenitor cells are relatively resistant to isolation, storage, and freezing has led to the expanding utilization of bone marrow transplantation as an important form of therapy of many hematologic disorders. In this treatment the host is rendered completely deficient both immunologically and hematologically, and the progenitor cells from a compatible donor are transfused. In other approaches now under consideration, the marrows of leukemic individuals may be rendered free of leukemic cells by a variety of techniques and reinfused after storage into the same donors. During the storage period the donors receive intensive ablative therapy. The frozen marrow cells are then infused to reconstitute hematopoietic function.

MARROW ANATOMY. Although most cases of bone marrow failure and malignancy are due to disorders of progenitors, the total microenvironment in which progenitors, inducer cells, and precursors interact to form mature differentiated peripheral blood cells is complex and subject to severe dysfunction. This is an obvious problem in myelofibrosis, or in infectious granulomatosis of the marrow. But certain other forms of bone marrow failure, such as aplastic anemia itself, may also be due to more subtle forms of microenvironmental failure. The marrow cavity is a vast network of vascular channels or sinusoids that separate groups of hematopoietic cells, including fat cells. The hematopoietic cells are found in the intrasinusoidal spaces. Clumps of megakaryocytes are found adjacent to marrow sinuses. They shed platelets, the fragments of their cytoplasm, directly into the lumen. This reduces the requirement for movement of bulky megakaryocytes, a mobility characteristic

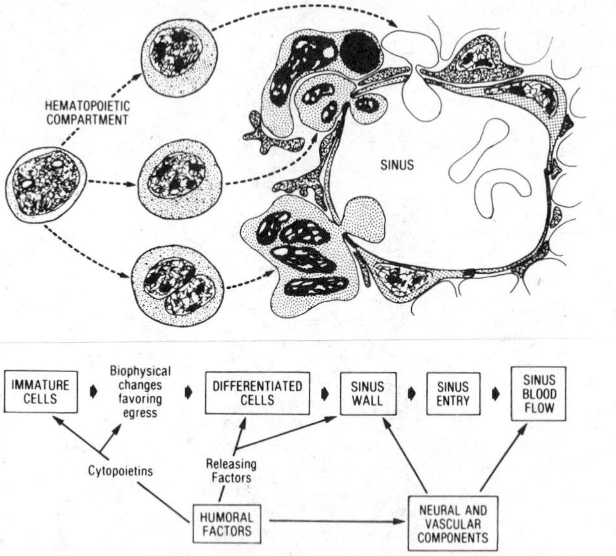

Figure 130–6. A schematic diagram of the factors that may be involved in controlling the release of marrow cells. The central relationship between the hematopoietic compartment and the marrow sinus is depicted. The drawing highlights the similarity of the egress process for the three major hematopoietic cells: reticulocytes in the top pathway, granulocytes and monocytes in the center pathway, and platelets in the lower pathway. Immature cells undergo biophysical changes under the influence of cytopoietins that favor egress. In the case of reticulocytes, enucleation precedes egress. This is shown by the solid black inclusion in the perisinal macrophage representing nucleophagocytosis antecedent to digestion of the erythroblast nucleus. The cytoplasmic protrusion of the megakaryocyte presumably detaches itself from the cell and will further fragment into platelets in the circulation. (From Lichtman MA, Chamberlain JK, Santillo PA: *In* Silber R, LoBue J, Gordon AS [eds.]: The Year in Hematology, 1978. New York, Plenum Medical Book Company, 1978, p 274.)

of the granuloid and erythroid differentiated precursors as they approach the point at which they egress from the marrow. The vascular and hematopoietic compartments are lined by reticular cells that form the adventitial surfaces of the vascular sinuses and extend cytoplasmic processes to create a lattice for the mesh of endothelial cells and fibronectin on which blood cells are found. The lattice is illustrated by reticulin stains of marrow sections and scanning electron photomicrographs. A schema of the egress of cells from marrow is shown in Figure 130–6.

KINETICS OF HEMATOPOIESIS. The marrow microenvironment supporting the progenitors and precursors must provide for the normal steady state rates of renewal of the cellular elements of blood. Under homeostatic conditions, the production rates precisely equal destruction rates. The average life span of a human red cell is approximately 120 days. This means that approximately 5×10^4 red cells must be produced per day per microliter of blood in an adult. The average life span of platelets is seven to ten days for a daily production rate of 2×10^4 platelets per microliter of blood. The white blood cell compartment exhibits more complex kinetics. Granulocytes are rapidly turned over with an approximate intravascular life span of 6 to 12 hours in humans. To maintain a level of circulating granulocytes of 5×10^3 per microliter requires a daily production that is roughly comparable to that of red cell and platelet production, approximately 2×10^4 cells per microliter of blood. At the opposite extreme in terms of life span is the lymphocyte, which can exhibit lifetimes measured in months, or even years. This long life span of lymphocytes suggests that the daily renewal of certain lymphocyte progenitors occurs at a rate substantially lower than that of the progenitors of the other formed elements of blood. The various symptoms of complete marrow failure are closely related to the life span and the turnover of the peripheral cells of the blood. Thus, patients with complete marrow failure initially lose granulocytes and therefore usually present with enhanced susceptibility to infection. Petechial bleeding caused by platelet deficiency rapidly follows, and finally pallor and symptoms of anemia occur. Loss of circulating lymphocytes and cellular immune function is an unusual event in such circumstances.

The turnover of red cells and platelets can be measured for diagnostic purposes, using $Na_2{}^{51}CrO_4$ as a labeling agent. Both the red cell and the platelet life spans can be estimated and the site of the red cell destruction determined. This can be a useful maneuver in decisions regarding splenectomy.

CONCLUSION. Modern cell biology and molecular genetics have revolutionized hematology, changing it from a largely descriptive field to a remarkable amalgamation of diagnostic and therapeutic ventures. The realization that differentiated marrow precursors arise from a population of lymphoid-appearing cells that have a remarkable developmental biology of their own has led to reclassification of the marrow failure syndrome and to new approaches to therapy, particularly with bone marrow transplantation. In addition, inquiries into the kinetics of progenitors and differentiated precursors have encouraged more rational approaches to the chemotherapy of malignant diseases. As approaches to the actual isolation of progenitors are developed, enumeration of these cells will soon be as commonplace as the evaluation of precursors and mature cells. This kind of enumeration will require specific antibodies and diagnostic instruments that are taking their places as standard aspects of the hematology of the 1980's.

Burakoff SJ, Lipton JM, Nathan DG: Recapitulation of the immune response and hematopoietic system in bone marrow transplantation. *In* Nathan DG (ed.): Bone marrow transplantation. Clin Haematol 12:695, 1983. *A brief up-to-date review of regulation of hematopoiesis in two volumes devoted to basic and clinical aspects of marrow transplantation.*

Graber S, Krantz S: Erythropoietin and the control of red cell production. Ann Rev Med 29:51, 1978. *An excellent review of the details of erythropoietin function and clinical applications.*

Lichtman MA, Chamberlain JK, Santillo PA: The factors thought to contribute to the regulation of egress of cells from marrow. *In* Silber R, LoBue J, Gordon AS (eds.): The Year in Hematology, 1978. New York, Plenum Medical Book Company, 1978. *An excellent review of marrow anatomy and function.*

Metcalf D, Moore MAS: Hematopoietic cells. *In* Neuberger A, Tatum EG (eds.): Frontiers of Biology, Vol 24. Amsterdam, North Holland Publishing Company, 1971. *This is the "bible" of hematopoiesis, particularly with respect to techniques and the history of the development of cell biology in this field.*

Nathan DG, Housman DE, Clarke BJ: The pathophysiology of hematopoiesis. *In* Nathan DG, Oski F (eds.): Hematology in Infancy and Childhood. 2nd ed. Philadelphia, W. B. Saunders Company, 1980. *A general review of the physiology of hematopoiesis emphasizing physiology and clinical correlations.*

Quesenberry P: Hematopoietic stem cells. N Engl J Med 301:755, 1979. *A brief review of progenitor cell function.*

Thomas ED (ed.): Aplastic anaemia. Clin Hematol 7:No. 3, 1978. *A compendium of articles in which hematopoietic dysfunction is assessed at the progenitor cell level.*

Weiss RE, Reddi AH: Appearance of fibronectin during the differentiation of cartilage, bone and bone marrow. J Cell Biol 88:630, 1981. *Contains an excellent array of photomicrographs of developing marrow cells within a fibronectin framework.*

131. INTRODUCTION TO THE ANEMIAS

Alan S. Keitt

Humans live in tenuous equilibrium with their life blood. Elaborate mechanisms have evolved to extract the nutrients for blood formation from available food stores and to conserve them by efficient recycling. The transition from hunter-gatherer to agricultural societies resulted in the replacement of most readily absorbable heme iron in the human diet by poorly absorbable iron in grains, thus rendering this balance precarious for a large part of the world's population. Other evolutionary strategies have concentrated genes for various red cell abnormalities that enhance survival in malarial areas but at the cost of producing anemia within a large minority of the population of these regions. Parasitic infestations and frequent pregnancies produce stress on iron balance in the same underdeveloped and populous areas. As a result of these combined nutritional, genetic, and parasitic factors, the global hematocrit is by no

TABLE 131–1. PATHOPHYSIOLOGIC CLASSIFICATION OF ANEMIAS

I. Hypoproliferative anemias
  A. Marrow aplasias (Ch. 132)
  B. Myelophthisic anemia (Ch. 132)
  C. Anemia of chronic disease (Ch. 134)
  D. Anemia with organ failure
    1. Renal failure
    2. Hepatic failure
    3. Hypothyroidism
    4. Hypopituitarism
  E. Anemia with blood dyscrasias
II. Maturation defects
  A. Cytoplasmic
    1. Hypochromic anemias (Ch. 134)
  B. Nuclear
    1. Megaloblastic anemias (Ch. 135)
  C. Combined
    1. Myelodysplastic syndromes (Ch. 523)
III. Hemolytic anemias (Ch. 136)
  A. Immune hemolysis (Ch. 138)
  B. Primary membrane defects (Ch. 137)
  C. Hemoglobinopathies (Ch. 142)
  D. Enzymopathies (Ch. 137)
  E. Toxic hemolysis—physical/chemical (Ch. 132 and 138)
  F. Traumatic hemolysis (Ch. 138)
  G. Hypersplenism (Ch. 138)
IV. Dilutional anemias
  A. Pregnancy
  B. Splenomegaly
  C. Waldenström's macroglobulinemia

means optimal; anemia is perhaps the most frequent and significant worldwide health problem. Anemia does not have the same impact on the population of western societies, but it remains a cardinal indicator of disease and requires careful consideration and treatment.

Although defined by numbers, anemia is in reality a *process* that evolves within a clinical context. For the experienced hematologist, this clinical context is analogous to habitat for the ornithologist. A brief glance through the binoculars is often sufficient to identify the microspherocytes of autoimmune hemolytic anemia in a patient known to have systemic lupus erythematosus just as one instantly recognizes a wood duck in the woods because that is where it belongs. In the same vein, an unfamiliar stray may be noticed by the alert observer when it occurs outside of its usual clinical context. The importance of habitat in hematologic diagnosis cannot be overemphasized and is often neglected in the current proliferation of sequential algorithms for the diagnosis of anemia. Such constructions, which are based primarily on laboratory data, may fail to take into account changes occurring over time and often provide only a single point of entry to the process of anemia.

The great majority of anemias are diagnosed and treated by nonhematologists. Except for the primary blood dyscrasias, the diagnostic classification of the anemias is relatively simple and logical. One such classification is presented in Table 131–1, but readers are encouraged to construct their own set of anemia algorithms using the following discussion as a guide.

DEFINITION OF ANEMIA

Anemia is defined as a reduction in either the volume of red blood cells (termed the hematocrit or packed cell volume [PCV]) or the concentration of hemoglobin in a sample of peripheral venous blood when compared with similar values obtained from a reference population. Normal values for red blood cell measurements are given in Table 131–2. By convention the normal range is defined to include 95 per cent of a reference population that is assumed to have a normal (Gaussian) distribution. In this definition 2.5 per cent of "normal individuals" will fall below this arbitrary statistical limit and be classified as anemic. Some of these individuals in the general population will be truly anemic while others are statistical outliers. Unfortunately this statistical definition of anemia may fail to detect truly anemic patients whose hematocrits have decreased significantly without leaving the defined normal range. Here, the only valid reference figure is a previous hematocrit in that individual.

RED CELL MASS. Anemia can be more rigorously defined as a reduction in red cell mass (a misnomer for the total volume of circulating erythroid cells in the body). Red cell mass can be accurately measured by isotope dilution using ^{51}Cr-labeled red cells, a procedure usually employed to establish increased red cell mass, i.e., erythrocytosis, rather than anemia. This measurement is occasionally useful for assessing anemia in patients with marked splenomegaly in whom the peripheral hematocrit underestimates the true red cell mass (see below).

ALTERATIONS IN PLASMA VOLUME. Fluctuations in plasma volume from either technical or physiologic factors may cause variations in the hematocrit of normal individuals. Prolonged stasis associated with venipuncture (> 1 minute) causes leakage of plasma from occluded capillaries with a consequent rise in hematocrit. A marked shift in plasma volume may occur upon ambulation after a period of recumbency with a consequent fall in hematocrit of up to 10 per cent. A large increase in plasma volume in the third trimester of pregnancy causes a lowering of peripheral venous hematocrit despite a modest increase in red cell mass.

EFFECTS OF AGE, SEX, AND ALTITUDE. Adult levels of hematocrit are reached by late childhood in females. The higher hematocrit of males as compared with females begins at puberty as a result of stimulation of hematopoiesis by androgenic hormones.

Whether the hematocrit normally declines with aging is controversial. With age the cellularity of the bone marrow is progressively replaced by fat and in men over 60 the incidence of anemia increases progressively as well. Some studies show similar trends in women. Iron deficiency and chronic diseases are common in this age group but seem not to account entirely for the increased incidence of anemia. Mild anemia in the elderly, therefore, must still be considered as an indicator of potential ill health, but investigation of these patients frequently fails to indicate a precise etiology.

The hematocrit is increased in individuals living at high altitudes as an appropriate response to diminished oxygen content of the atmosphere and blood. This effect can be noticed above 4000 feet where significant desaturation of hemoglobin begins. The definition of anemia therefore requires adjustment to the altitude at which the individual lives.

COMPENSATION FOR ANEMIA

INCREASED PLASMA VOLUME. Initial symptoms of patients with anemia are related to efforts by the body to compensate for the diminished oxygen supply. Later symptoms of progressive anemia reflect failure of these compensatory mechanisms. The symptoms and signs differ markedly depending on the

TABLE 131–2. SELECTED HEMATOLOGIC VALUES IN NORMAL INDIVIDUALS OF VARIOUS AGES*

Age	Hemoglobin (gm/dl) mean (−2SD)	Hematocrit (%) mean (−2SD)	MCV cu microns mean (−2SD)
1–3 days	18.5 (14.5)	56 (45)	108 (95)
0.5–2 yrs	12 (10.5)	36 (33)	78 (70)
12–18 yrs			
Male	14.5 (13)	43 (37)	88 (78)
Female	14.0 (12)	41 (36)	90 (78)
18–49 yrs			
Male	15.5 (13.5)	47 (41)	90 (80)
Female	14 (12.0)	41 (36)	90 (80)

*Values selected from Dallman PR: *In* Rudolph A (ed.): Pediatrics, 16th ed. New York, Appleton-Century-Crofts, Inc., 1977, p 1111. The values were derived by Coulter Counter. Values in parentheses represent two standard deviations below the mean, or the lower limit of normal assuming a normal distribution.

acuteness of onset of the anemia. The abrupt loss of 30 per cent of the circulating blood volume in a patient with gastrointestinal hemorrhage will result in marked postural hypotension, a fall in cardiac output, shunting of blood from skin to central organs, thirst, and air hunger (Ch. 113). In contrast, the gradual loss of 30 per cent of the circulating red cell mass in a patient with pernicious anemia may occur without any symptoms at all. The major difference lies in the blood volume, which is maintained by a proportionate increase in plasma volume as a compensatory response in most chronic anemias but is compromised in acute hemorrhage. Because the central blood volume is maintained until very late in the course of a progressive chronic anemia, such patients are susceptible to volume overload by transfusions. The injudicious administration of whole blood and even packed red cells may precipitate acute congestive heart failure in a previously well compensated individual.

INCREASED CARDIAC OUTPUT. In chronic anemias cardiac output increases to circulate fewer red cells through the tissues more frequently. This process is abetted by the diminished viscosity of blood at low hematocrits but is ultimately limited by the capacity of the heart to respond to the increased work. An early sign of failing compensation in gradual onset anemias is postural hypotension associated with symptoms of dizziness, throbbing headaches, and dyspnea on exertion.

REDUCED AFFINITY OF HEMOGLOBIN FOR OXYGEN. In anemia the oxyhemoglobin dissociation curve usually shifts in a manner to increase the quantity of oxygen released in tissues without appreciably altering the quantity of oxygen bound in the lungs (see Fig. 139–4). Red cell 2,3 diphosphoglycerate (2,3 DPG) regularly increases in anemic patients to mediate this effect. Maximum elevation of RBC 2,3 DPG increases oxygen delivery only about 30 per cent, but this is a highly efficient form of compensation requiring no significant expenditure of energy.

Level of Anemia at Which Symptoms Are Produced

The level of anemia at which symptoms occur is highly variable among individuals as would be expected from the widely differing degrees of physical activity, physical conditioning, circulatory adequacy, and sensitivity or stoicism of the population. In otherwise healthy individuals symptoms are usually present when the hemoglobin falls below 7 or 8 grams per deciliter.

Exceptions to this general rule are not infrequent. An occasional patient with a gradual onset anemia may deny all symptoms despite a hemoglobin of 5 grams per deciliter. Conversely, and more commonly, patients with mild anemia of 9 or 10 grams of hemoglobin per deciliter may complain bitterly of fatigue and lassitude. A careful search for underlying systemic disease or depression is warranted in these patients. Finally, because oxygen transport is much more compromised by impaired circulation than by diminished oxygen carrying capacity per se, patients with vascular or cardiac disease may become symptomatic with milder degrees of anemia. For example, angina, claudication, transient ischemic attacks, and cardiac failure can occur or be exacerbated with relatively mild anemia. In essence, each organ within each patient sets its own functional definition of anemia.

EVALUATION OF THE ANEMIC PATIENT

The remainder of this chapter outlines in considerable detail a general approach to the anemic patient. This involves the construction and interpretation of an initial data base that will guide subsequent diagnostic strategy. The confirmatory diagnostic procedures for specific types of anemia are detailed in the other chapters of this section and will be mentioned only briefly here. Good practice dictates that this initial data base be collected and analyzed prior to the random ordering of procedures or consultations, since it will provide definitive diagnoses in a surprisingly large number of patients and point toward efficient diagnostic approaches in most of the others.

Assessing the Clinical Context

The answers to six basic questions provide the essential information with which to include or exclude the great majority of anemias.

1. Is the patient truly anemic?

The answer to this seemingly trivial but in fact crucial question requires an awareness of all of the aforementioned factors that can affect the normal hematocrit as well as appreciation of the insidious nature of mistakes in sampling and measurement of blood. An unexpected and isolated low hematocrit in an otherwise completely normal clinical context bears repeating before an intensive investigation is undertaken.

Does the decreased hematocrit reflect a true decrease in red cell mass? Congestive heart failure and iatrogenic fluid overload commonly cause dilutional anemia that disappears once a diuresis is obtained. In patients with giant splenomegaly, red cells may be concentrated in the enlarged spleen and diluted in an increased plasma volume that is in general proportional to their degree of splenomegaly. Both maldistribution and dilution contribute to the frequently observed reduction in peripheral venous hematocrit in such individuals who may have a normal red cell mass. This phenomenon should be distinguished from hypersplenism in which the red cells (or other elements) are destroyed by the spleen. In contrast, dehydrated or severely burned patients may have significant anemia that is masked by diminished plasma volume.

2. Is the anemia inherited or acquired?

Heritable forms of anemia are almost always intrinsic to the red cell or marrow while acquired anemias more often result from extrinsic factors. This distinction, often of fundamental aid in diagnosis, is by no means always simple because of the episodic nature and variable severity of many genetic disorders, particularly those involving red cells. An inherited susceptibility to hemolysis, for example, may require exposure to an oxidant drug or severe infection in order for anemia to occur (e.g., G-6-PD deficiency in blacks). Patients may be unaware of mild to moderate lifelong anemias until they have a routine blood test or develop symptoms during pregnancy or after a severe febrile infection.

A positive family history suggests an inherited red cell disorder. Because of the concentration of genes for certain hemoglobinopathies and enzyme defects in various African, Mediterranean, and oriental populations, detailed information concerning racial background is pertinent. Clustering of involvement on one side of the family may give clues to autosomal dominant or sex-linked modes of transmission, while a history of consanguinity may accompany autosomal recessively transmitted diseases. The absence of family history by no means excludes a genetic mechanism of transmission, even in dominantly inherited disorders such as hereditary spherocytosis, which may arise by spontaneous mutation in a significant number of cases. The absence of congenital anemia can be implied in regular blood donors who will have been screened by the blood bank prior to each donation.

3. Is there evidence for blood loss?

Iron deficiency anemia is the most common anemia in the general population; it almost always results from blood loss in the developed western societies. Because of the frequency of iron deficiency a careful search for blood loss is mandatory in the initial evaluation of an anemic patient. Women of reproductive age are at particular risk because of the combined iron losses of menstruation (estimated at 20 to 30 mg per month) and pregnancy (estimated at 500 mg). Estimation of menstrual loss is difficult and requires specific questioning concerning the frequency of periods, the duration of heavy flow, the frequency of changing pads or tampons, and the appearance of clots.

Gastrointestinal bleeding caused by ulcers, cancers, anomalous vessels, and parasites is a frequent source of blood loss.

The gastrointestinal route is virtually the only significant occult source of bleeding. Thus iron deficiency is a frequent presenting manifestation of otherwise unsuspected gastrointestinal pathology, which must be carefully sought once bleeding has been documented.

A number of causes of blood loss that are frequently forgotten are listed below:

1. Diagnostic phlebotomy. Hospitalized patients, especially children and patients receiving intensive care, may undergo extensive phlebotomy. Individuals with low iron stores (most menstruating females) are at risk for developing iron deficiency as a result, while patients with other marrow impairments will be slow to make up the loss.
2. Regular blood donation.
3. Soft tissue bleeding after trauma or surgery. Fractured hips in the elderly are notorious for copious tissue bleeding. Iron is not readily salvaged from such hematomas.
4. Urinary loss of hemosiderin in chronic intravascular hemolysis.
5. Pulmonary bleeding in idiopathic pulmonary hemosiderosis.
6. Bleeding in patients with hemostatic defects including hemophilias and hereditary hemorrhagic telangiectasia.

A useful ancillary question that may uncover the presence of iron deficiency relates to the frequent ingestion of starch, clay, or ice. Craving for non-nutritive material, or *pica*, is common in patients with iron deficiency. In black cultures, clay has been a favorite substance since antiquity, and starch seems to be a modern equivalent. Another favorite material is ice, crushed or in cubes, which is also used by whites. Not all individuals who use these materials are iron deficient: there is a cultural as well as a physiologic component. Curiously, the craving for such substances often disappears within 24 hours of treatment with medicinal iron. Iron metabolism is more extensively discussed in Ch. 133 and 206.

4. Is there evidence for hemolysis?

Hemolytic anemias are considerably less common than are the anemias of iron deficiency or chronic disease and may be more difficult to recognize. Inherited disorders of the red cell show a very wide spectrum of severity for reasons that are not entirely clear. The more severe cases, which are encountered in hospitals and hematology clinics, are easily recognized. In milder cases, however, the patient may be unaware of the disease.

The answers to several questions are important for the initial data base. First, the patient should be asked if he has ever had jaundice, or yellowing of skin or eyeballs, and if he has ever had hepatitis. The key to suspecting inherited hemolytic anemias is the presence of constant or episodic jaundice. While the hepatic conjugating mechanism can handle a considerable increase in bilirubin production consequent to the breakdown of hemoglobin, the exacerbation of hemolysis occurring during severe febrile infections often causes visible jaundice. This combination frequently leads to the misdiagnosis of recurrent hepatitis. However, not all patients with intrinsic red cell defects give this history—some are able to handle the bilirubin load without visible jaundice.

Second, the patient should be asked if he has ever noticed darkening of the urine resembling tea or cola. Bile is characteristically absent from the urine in patients with hemolysis because the predominant form of bilirubin in the plasma is unconjugated and is tightly bound to albumin (Ch. 117). However, during periods of increased hemolysis, alternate products of bilirubin degradation called *dipyrroles* sometimes appear in the urine, causing considerable darkening in its color. For most patients, dark urine means concentrated urine so that specific questioning concerning the color is essential in order to exclude simple dehydration. Other causes of dark urine include hemoglobinuria in patients with moderate to severe intravascular hemolysis and biliuria in patients with liver or biliary tract disease. A careful search for symptoms of gallbladder disease in the patient or the family is warranted because of the frequency with which patients with chronic hemolytic disorders develop pigment stones.

As *exceptions,* megaloblastic anemias and severe dyserythropoietic states, which show marked ineffective erythropoiesis (also termed intramedullary hemolysis) can also cause jaundice. Similarly, resorption of large tissue hematomas may suggest hemolysis because of the resulting anemia and jaundice.

5. Has the patient been exposed to medication or toxins that can result in anemia?

The frequency with which individuals ingest or inhale medications and recreational drugs and the ubiquitous nature of chemical toxins require that a careful search be made for such exposures in an anemic patient. Drug-induced anemias (lumping together both medications and chemical toxins) may be associated with marrow aplasia, maturational defects, and hemolysis by both direct or immune mediated mechanisms. While it is frequently difficult to establish cause and effect between a given chemical and anemia, certain drugs are notoriously involved and a history of their use should always be sought. Alcohol is probably the most common toxin associated with anemia. The various categories and some specific agents are listed in Table 131–3.

6. Is there a systemic illness or any nonhematologic organ dysfunction?

Assessment of the habitat within which an anemia arises requires a careful search for systemic illness or organ dysfunction.

THE ANEMIA OF CHRONIC DISEASE (ACD). Most patients with active inflammatory disease or advanced malignancy show a characteristic mild to moderate anemia. The severity of the anemia is in general related to the intensity of the inflammation or the extent of malignant spread, although occasionally relatively localized tumors may present with prominent systemic symptoms and anemia. Weight loss, fever, and night sweats may indicate underlying systemic inflammation. Chronic infections such as subacute bacterial endocarditis and active inflammatory processes such as rheumatoid arthritis and inflammatory bowel disease are almost always associated with ACD. The diagnosis of ACD and its differentiation from iron deficiency are discussed in Ch. 133.

NONHEMATOLOGIC ORGAN DYSFUNCTION. Patients with diminished renal, hepatic, or endocrine function are often anemic. The pathogenesis of these anemias is multifactorial, and

TABLE 131–3. DRUGS THAT MAY CAUSE ANEMIA

Agents associated with marrow aplasia*
Antineoplastic drugs—antimetabolites, alkylating agents
Antibiotics—chloramphenicol
Anticonvulsants—phenylhydantoin
Insecticides
Solvents—benzene
Anti-inflammatory drugs—phenylbutazone
Agents associated with hemolytic anemia
Oxidant drugs†
Antibiotics—sulfonamides, sulfones
Antimalarials—primaquine
Analgesics—acetanilid
Miscellaneous compounds—methylene blue, naphthalene, phenylhydrazine, fava beans
Immune mediated
Penicillin, stibophen, alpha methyldopa, quinine, etc.
Agents causing maturation defects
Alcohol
Folate antagonists—trimethoprim, triamterene, methotrexate
Heme synthesis antagonists—INH, lead
Agents causing GI blood loss
Aspirin, nonsteroidal anti-inflammatory agents

*See Ch. 132 for a more complete listing.
†Hemolytic primarily in G-6-Pd deficient individuals.

there are relatively few constant distinguishing features. In each case, a significant degree of organ failure must be present to result in anemia. Therefore they are relatively easily excluded by simple measurement of renal, hepatic, thyroid, or pituitary function. The association of specific anemias with diseases of various organ systems is listed in Table 131–4.

The organ system most intimately involved with the hematopoietic system is the GI tract, the function of which is crucial for the absorption of nutrients and vitamins essential for blood formation. These rather tenuous absorption mechanisms are vulnerable to disturbance by a variety of gastrointestinal disorders. Some, such as previous surgical removal of the stomach or terminal ileum—organs that combine in the process of vitamin B_{12} absorption—are easily detected whereas others such as the autoimmune gastritis of pernicious anemia or the malabsorption of celiac disease may be more subtle and require a high index of suspicion. Fortunately, deficiency of iron, vitamin B_{12}, or folic acid can usually be suspected as a result of rather simple laboratory procedures that may lead to subsequent recognition of the underlying GI dysfunction.

ANEMIA ASSOCIATED WITH IMMUNE DYSCRASIAS. Immune dysfunction, due either to dysregulation or neoplasms or both, are commonly complicated by anemias. Autoimmune hemolytic anemia is classically associated with systemic lupus erythematosus or with B cell neoplasms, particularly chronic lymphocytic leukemia (CLL) or diffuse large cell (histiocytic) lymphomas. The hallmark of this combination is a positive Coombs' test (Ch. 136). Another B cell neoplasm, multiple myeloma, commonly presents with anemia due to marrow invasion or suppression or both. Thus the triad of skeletal symptoms (usually low back pain), renal dysfunction, and anemia should always prompt a search for myeloma.

TABLE 131–4. DISEASE-RELATED ANEMIAS

Organ/System	Disease	Associated Anemia
Immune	B cell neoplasms: lymphomas, CLL, myeloma	Autoimmune hemolysis, marrow replacement, ? marrow suppression
	Collagen-vascular disease	Autoimmune hemolysis, ACD, myelofibrosis
	Thymoma	Pure red cell aplasia
Gastrointestinal	Immune gastritis	Pernicious anemia
	Gastrectomy	B_{12}, iron deficiency
	Celiac disease	Folate deficiency
	Crohn's disease	ACD, folate, B_{12} deficiency
Liver	Laennec's cirrhosis	Folate deficiency, "spur cell" anemia
	Wilson's disease	Hemolysis
	"Pigment" gallstones	Chronic hemolysis
Kidney	Renal failure	Hypoproliferative
	Hematuria	Sickle cell disease or trait, iron deficiency
	Hemolytic-uremic syndrome	Microangiopathic hemolysis
Endocrine	Hypothyroidism	Hypoproliferative, pernicious anemia
	Hypogonadism	Hypoproliferative (males)
	Hypopituitarism	Hypoproliferative
Pregnancy		Unmasking a congenital anemia, iron, folate deficiency, dilutional anemia
Heart	Valvular stenosis or prosthesis	Traumatic hemolysis, iron deficiency
	Endocarditis	ACD
Pulmonary	Pulmonary hemosiderosis	Iron deficiency
Musculoskeletal	Rheumatoid arthritis	ACD
	Congenital deformities	Fanconi's, Diamond-Blackfan anemia
	Myopathies	Red cell enzyme deficiencies
Neurologic	Combined systems disease	B_{12} deficiency
	Neuropathy, encephalopathy	Lead and arsenic poisoning

TABLE 131–5. PHYSICAL FINDINGS IN VARIOUS ANEMIAS

Physical Finding	Associated Anemia
Skin	
Jaundice	Hemolysis, liver disease
Petechiae	Blood dyscrasia, autoimmune hemolysis with ITP
Telangiectasia	Iron deficiency
Spider angiomata	Liver disease
Facies	
Frontal bossing, maxillary prominence, hypertelorism	Severe congenital hemolysis
Eyes	
Scleral icterus	Hemolysis, liver disease
Retinal hemorrhages	Severe anemia of any cause
Mucous Membranes	
Glossitis	B_{12}, folate, or iron deficiency
Angular cheilosis	Iron deficiency
Lymph Nodes	
Generalized adenopathy	Malignant lymphoma, blood dyscrasias
Cardiac	
Valvular murmurs	Traumatic hemolysis, bacterial endocarditis
Abdominal	
Splenomegaly	Hypersplenism, chronic leukemias, hemolysis, etc.
Hepatomegaly	Liver disease
Pelvic and Rectal	
Hemorrhoids, masses	Blood loss
Extremities	
Symmetrical joint deformity	Rheumatoid arthritis, ACD, and iron deficiency
Congenital anomalies	Constitutional marrow aplasias
Leg ulcers	Chronic hemolysis, esp. sickle cell disease
Myopathy	Rare red cell enzymopathies
Neurologic	
Diminished vibration, position sense, dementia	Vitamin B_{12} deficiency
Neuropathy	Lead poisoning
Mental retardation, spastic paresis	Rare red cell enzymopathies

The Physical Examination

As in the evaluation of any systemic disorder, a complete physical examination is essential in the patient who presents with anemia. However, particular attention should be paid to the presence of certain key findings that are of help in classifying the anemia (Table 131–5).

The Initial Laboratory Data Base

An essential minimum laboratory data base, most of which is obtained on every hospitalized patient, includes a complete blood count (or hemogram), an examination of the peripheral blood smear (usually performed as part of the leukocyte differential), examination of at least one stool for occult blood, and a reticulocyte count. These readily available procedures provide powerful and sometimes definitive diagnostic information.

THE HEMOGRAM. Modern automated cell counters provide a great deal of information to the physician for remarkably little effort by the laboratory. These instruments are designed to detect the passage of individual blood cells through either an electrically charged aperture or a laser beam. The resulting change in impedance or in light scatter as the cell passes is counted and quantitated. The size of the impedance change is proportional to the size of the cell causing it. Thus both the number and size distribution of cells are measured, which allows for derivation of the total volume of red cells (the hematocrit), as well as separation between cells of different sizes (red cells and platelets).

Red Cell Indices. The mean corpuscular volume (MCV) is the most useful of the red blood cell indices. Most hematologists consider the range of MCV's between 80 and 100 cubic microns as normal, although the actual range defined by statistical criteria is somewhat narrower.

The MCV provides a convenient basis for separating anemias into groups that are microcytic (less than 80 cubic microns), normocytic (80 to 100 cubic microns), and macrocytic (greater than 100 cubic microns). This classification is useful but limited by the fact that the great majority of anemic patients fall within the normocytic group and must be distinguished by other means.

MICROCYTOSIS. The MCV has been particularly useful in detecting the presence of iron deficiency and the various forms of thalassemia. Carriers of beta thalassemia trait have MCV's that are almost always less than 80 and usually less than 70 cubic microns (Ch. 141). The alpha thalassemia traits are somewhat milder, with MCV's in the 70's. Moderate to severe iron deficiency is also associated with a decreased MCV. In general the hematocrit is much lower in iron deficiency than in thalassemia trait at a similar MCV. Severe inflammatory disease can induce iron deficient erythropoiesis in the anemia of chronic disease (ACD). While usually normocytic, occasionally such patients are quite microcytic despite normal or increased iron stores. Other causes of reduced MCV include defects in heme synthesis such as lead poisoning or inherited sideroblastic anemia (Table 131–6).

MACROCYTOSIS. Macrocytosis, often 130 cubic microns or more, is characteristic of severe megaloblastic anemias caused by either folate or B_{12} deficiency (Ch. 135).

An *exception* is the rather common occurrence of alpha thalassemia in blacks that can mask the macrocytosis seen in pernicious anemia. Similarly, combined nutritional deficiency of iron and B_{12} or folic acid, such as often occurs during pregnancy or in alcoholics, can result in severe anemia with a normal MCV. Here the key to the diagnosis may rest in the accompanying leukocyte abnormalities of hypersegmentation.

Primary marrow diseases, especially aplastic anemias and refractory anemias associated with myelodysplastic syndromes, commonly have a moderately elevated MCV. Many moderate or severe hemolytic disorders are also macrocytic because of the presence of large prematurely released reticulocytes.

The mean corpuscular hemoglobin (MCH) and mean corpuscular hemoglobin concentration (MCHC), which are derived indices, provide ancillary information concerning cell size and hemoglobin content but are rarely as helpful as the MCV. The Coulter apparatus is relatively insensitive to elevation of the MCHC that is known to occur in spherocytic disorders.

The Leukocyte and Platelet Count. Anemia should always be assessed in relation to total marrow function. Anemia with a diminished leukocyte and platelet count—pancytopenia—suggests either primary marrow disease, megaloblastic anemia, or hypersplenism. A bone marrow study is frequently needed to establish the diagnosis of pancytopenia.

TABLE 131–6. MICROCYTIC AND MACROCYTIC ANEMIAS

Microcytosis (MCV < 80μ³)	Macrocytosis (MCV > 100μ³)
Iron deficiency	Megaloblastic anemias
Thalassemias	Chemotherapy
Anemia of chronic disease (usually normocytic)	Reticulocytosis
	Aplastic anemias
Sideroblastic anemias Hereditary Lead poisoning	Hypothyroidism
	Sideroblastic anemias Acquired
Severe red cell fragmentation Burns Hereditary pyropoikilocytosis	Myelodysplasias Chromosome (5q−) deletion

THE RETICULOCYTE COUNT. The reticulocyte is a young cell newly released from the bone marrow. Normal circulating reticulocytes in a nonanemic individual are morphologically indistinguishable from more mature red cells and must be counted after staining with new methylene blue. The percentage of cells showing bluish clumps or strands of RNA in 500 or 1000 total cells is referred to as the reticulocyte count. The normal reticulocyte circulates for approximately 24 hours before maturing and may spend a brief portion of that time in the spleen. Because normal red cells survive for an average of 120 days, the normal reticulocyte count is approximately 1 per cent (range 0.5 to 1.8 per cent). Anemia of any cause, by decreasing the denominator of the fraction by which the reticulocyte is derived, will increase the count. For this reason the count is customarily corrected to a "normal" hematocrit of 45 per cent:

$$\text{Corrected retic count} = \text{retic count} \times \text{patient Hct}/45$$

Additional corrections of the reticulocyte count have been proposed that take into consideration the increased time of maturation of the "stress" reticulocytes released prematurely from the marrow in severe anemia. These may circulate for considerably longer than 24 hours but are also subject to a variable period of sequestration in the spleen. The uncertainty associated with estimating true reticulocyte maturation time in the circulation makes the interpretation of an elevated count a semiquantitative exercise. While reticulocytosis is a hallmark of hemolytic anemia, it gives no information about longevity of red cells; rather it reflects entirely the ability of the marrow to respond.

Reticulocytosis is most readily interpreted by several measurements over a significant time span. This allows one to assess whether the hematocrit is rising and the reticulocytosis is sustained. Persistent reticulocytosis of 5 per cent or greater (corrected) with a stable hematocrit over several weeks is highly suggestive of a continuing hemolytic process.

An *exception* occurs when the corrected reticulocyte count may not always be elevated in chronic hemolytic states and occasionally may fall precipitously to near zero. This so-called *aplastic crisis* is often associated with viral infection in children and occasionally with folic acid deficiency, especially during pregnancy in females with chronic hemolysis.

Reticulocytosis with a rising hematocrit suggests either a transient hemolytic episode, such as might occur in G-6-PD deficiency with an exposure to an oxidant drug, or recovery from blood loss. Recovery of marrow function after reversible suppression, such as correction of B_{12} or folic acid deficiency, will also cause marked transient reticulocytosis with a rising hematocrit.

A markedly decreased corrected reticulocyte count of less than 0.5 per cent implies a primary suppression of the marrow rather than just inadequate response to anemic stress. The causes of marrow failure are discussed in Ch. 132. Severe reticulocytopenia (0.1 per cent or less) implies aplasia of the marrow, either aplastic anemia or its variant pure red cell aplasia. Reticulocyte counts are sometimes expressed as an absolute number, rather than as a percentage. A normal value represents 1 per cent of five million red cells or approximately 50,000 reticulocytes per cubic millimeter. Levels below 20,000 reticulocytes per cubic millimeter represent severe reduction in marrow output.

In the great majority of anemias that represent varying combinations of marrow inadequacy and peripheral loss or destruction of red cells, reticulocytes fall in an indeterminate range within the extreme values given above.

STOOLS FOR OCCULT BLOOD. Testing at least one and preferably three stools for the presence of blood is a mandatory procedure in all anemic patients for reasons outlined previously. Bleeding may be intermittent and can be missed unless several tests are performed.

TABLE 131–7. USEFUL FINDINGS FROM PERIPHERAL BLOOD MORPHOLOGY

Abnormalities in Red Cell Morphology	Associated Anemias
Target cells	
Predominant	HbCC disease or trait, obstructive liver disease
Occasional	Iron deficiency, thalassemias, postsplenectomy
Howell-Jolly bodies	Hyposplenism
Oval macrocytes with hypersegmented neutrophils (more than 5% PMN's with 5 or more lobes)	B_{12} or folic acid deficiency
Sickle forms	Sickle cell disease or variants
Schistocytes	Traumatic or microangiopathic hemolysis
Prominent basophilic stippling	Lead poisoning, pyrimidine 5′ nucleotidase deficiency
Nucleated red cells	Severe hypoxic stress, invasion of marrow by tumor, fibrosis, granulomata
"Bite" cells—Heinz bodies (special stain)	Oxidant hemolysis
Microspherocytes (smooth)	Hereditary spherocytosis, autoimmune hemolytic anemia
Microspherocytes (rough = echinocytes)	Glycolytic enzyme defects (esp. postsplenectomy)
Extreme microspherocytes with budding and debris	Burns, hereditary pyropoikilocytosis
Elliptocytes	
Predominant	Hereditary elliptocytosis
Occasional	Iron deficiency, hypochromic anemias

EXAMINATION OF THE PERIPHERAL BLOOD SMEAR. Careful examination of a well-prepared peripheral smear completes the initial assessment of the anemic patient. The diagnostic information to be gained from an educated appraisal of the blood morphology exceeds that of any other simple laboratory test. In addition to abnormalities in red cells, abnormal leukocytes or platelets can also contribute valuable diagnostic information. It would be misleading to claim that most anemias can be diagnosed from the peripheral smear alone. However, the large number of anemic processes that can be excluded by the smear as well as the frequency of definitive abnormalities make it highly useful.

Several points deserve emphasis when looking at a peripheral blood smear from a patient with anemia: (1) It is crucial to be aware of the treacherous effects of artifact on red blood cell morphology. Routine differential counts and platelet estimations are frequently performed on blood smears that are totally inadequate for evaluation of red cells. (2) One must seek not only the particular abnormal red cell that may give a clue to diagnosis, but also must evaluate the background morphology in which it arises. The frequency of poikilocytosis in anemia is such that one can find almost any cell one wishes by looking long enough. Thus several schistocytes found in association with numerous other abnormal shapes are insufficient evidence that traumatic hemolysis is a major cause of the anemia. Marked poikilocytosis usually represents either the effects of dyspoiesis due to nutritional or dysplastic disorders of the marrow or fragmenting accidents to red cells that occur in the circulation.

TABLE 131–8. INDICATIONS FOR BONE MARROW EXAMINATION IN ANEMIA

Presence of nucleated red cells
Pancytopenias
Absence of reticulocytes
Presence of immature leukocytes
Monoclonal gammopathies
Definitive estimation of iron stores
Suspicion of sideroblastic anemia
Moderate to severe anemia of unknown cause
Combined nutritional deficiencies

TABLE 131–9. SOME USEFUL ANCILLARY TESTS WHEN THE DATA BASE IS UNREVEALING

Coombs' test
Sedimentation rate
Creatinine
Liver function tests
Thyroid profile
Serum protein electrophoresis
Serum iron and transferrin

The distinction between these alternatives is often difficult and may depend on ancillary data including marrow examination. In contrast, a particular abnormality such as spherocytosis when it occurs as a significant minority finding in an otherwise relatively normal cell population assumes more significance. (3) It should be noted that splenectomy greatly enhances the range of morphologic diversity in almost any anemia.

A list of relatively specific aberrations in red cell morphology and their associated anemias is given in Table 131–7.

EXAMINATION OF THE BONE MARROW IN EVALUATION OF ANEMIAS

The most common anemias—those associated with blood loss, chronic disease, hemolysis, or nutritional deficiency—do not normally require an examination of the marrow for definitive diagnosis. The available tests for assessing the sufficiency of iron, vitamin B_{12}, and folic acid in serum, when coupled with assessment of response to a therapeutic trial, are generally quite sufficient for simple deficiencies. Difficulties arise, however, in the complex case in which combined deficiencies or chronic disease is present. Since nutritional anemias, particularly in patients with alcoholism, are often multiple, marrow examination may be the only means to establish the adequacy of iron stores in the setting. Similar problems arise in iron deficiency when combined with chronic inflammatory disease such as active rheumatoid arthritis.

Virtually all of the other indications for marrow examination involve the suspicion of a primary blood dyscrasia or the invasion of the marrow space by an extrinsic tumor or infection. Examination of aspirated smears in general gives superior cytologic information while the core biopsy provides crucial information concerning the overall cellularity, as well as the presence of fibrosis, tumor, or granulomas. Both procedures are complementary and are best performed together when the diagnosis is in doubt.

Firm indications for marrow examination in anemia are listed in Table 131–8.

Careful assessment of the initial data base will almost always reveal diagnostic clues to follow. The definitive diagnostic approaches to the various disorders are described in the accompanying chapters. A list of useful ancillary procedures when no hints can be extracted from the data base are given in Table 131–9.

The approach to the patient with anemia. *In* Wintrobe MM: Clinical Hematology. Philadelphia, Lea and Febiger, 7th ed. 1974, pp 529–565. *A more leisurely approach to the subject with the usual comprehensive perspective and extensive historical references that have characterized this work throughout its many editions.*

Blood volume. *In* Mollison PL: Blood Transfusion in Clinical Medicine. Oxford, Blackwell Scientific Publications, 7th ed. 1983, pp 65–92. *A gold mine of information concerning the many factors influencing blood volume in health and disease. Much of this material is not generally referenced in hematology texts.*

132. ANEMIA DUE TO FAILURE OF PROGENITOR CELLS

Alan S. Keitt

The hematopoietic system consists of primitive migratory pluripotential stem cells, their progeny, and certain habitats to which these cells are attracted to undergo differentiation. The organization of these habitats is determined not by the derivatives of the stem cells but rather by specialized supporting

TABLE 132–1. CLASSIFICATION OF THE ETIOLOGY OF APLASTIC ANEMIA AND RELATED DISORDERS

- I. Aplastic Anemias
  - Acquired
    - Idiopathic
    - Autoimmune
    - Drugs
      - Cytotoxic
      - Dose-related
      - Idiosyncratic
    - Toxic chemicals
    - Radiation
    - Infections–hepatitis
    - Pregnancy
    - Paroxysmal nocturnal hemoglobinuria
  - Constitutional
    - Familial or congenital
    - Fanconi's anemia
    - Dyskeratosis congenita
- II. Unicellular Aplasias
  - Pure red cell aplasia
    - Acquired
      - Thymoma
      - Idiopathic
      - Autoimmune
      - Drugs and toxins
      - Transient erythroblastopenia of childhood
    - Constitutional
      - Diamond-Blackfan anemia
  - Agranulocytosis
    - Acquired
      - Idiopathic
      - Drugs and toxins
      - Felty's syndrome
      - Thymoma
    - Constitutional
      - Congenital
      - Familial–benign, severe, cyclic
      - Reticular dysgenesis
  - Thrombocytopenia
    - Acquired
      - Idiopathic
      - Autoimmune–systemic lupus erythematosus
      - Drugs and toxins
      - Neonatal–rubella or cytomegalovirus infections
    - Constitutional
      - Amegakaryocytic thrombocytopenia (associated with congenital anomalies)
      - Autosomal recessive thrombocytopenia

cells that provide a framework in which the hematopoietic and lymphoid cells may operate. These organs are components of the reticuloendothelial system, named for the fibroblastic and endothelial cells that make up their supporting matrix. They share certain homologies in their vascular architecture, namely a system of cords and sinuses, which are lined by the supporting cells. In subprimates and during fetal life, all of the reticuloendothelial organs may harbor active hematopoietic tissue. In mature primates, however, the liver, spleen, and lymph nodes assume other specialized functions, and only the bone marrow continues to support effective hematopoiesis.

Marrow failure may arise by two basically distinct mechanisms: the aplastic and myelophthisic anemias. The *aplastic anemias* represent failure of the stem cell to undergo differentiation, either because of intrinsic damage, inhibition, or interruption of its interactions with its particular microenvironment. The *myelophthisic anemias* result from loss of essential habitat for hematopoiesis due to destruction of the macroenvironment of the bone marrow by neoplastic or inflammatory tissue. This latter group will be considered briefly in a separate section at the end of this chapter.

THE APLASTIC ANEMIAS

Definition

APLASTIC ANEMIA. This refers to a diverse group of potentially severe marrow disorders characterized by peripheral pancytopenia and a marrow that is largely devoid of hematopoietic cells but that retains the basic marrow architecture or stroma with replacement of hematopoietic cells by large amounts of fat. Aplastic anemia has been classified as "severe" when at least two of the following three criteria are present: (1) anemia with a corrected reticulocyte count <1 per cent, (2) neutrophils <500 per cubic millimeter, (3) platelets < 20,000 per cubic millimeter. In addition, marrow hypocellularity must be present (estimated as < 25 per cent of marrow space). Mild to moderate cases that do not fulfill the aforementioned necessary criteria may become severe and vice versa.

UNICELLULAR APLASIAS. Isolated deficiencies of each of the main hematopoietic cell lines, i.e., pure red cell aplasia (PRCA), occur somewhat less commonly than typical aplastic anemia. In some instances the unicellular aplasias may progress to frank aplastic anemia with pancytopenia, but a significant number of other cases will remain "pure." The unicellular aplasias exhibit relatively normal cellularity of the bone marrow with selective dropout of one set of precursors. These disorders presumably arise from failure of a "committed" rather than a pluripotential stem cell. There is no clear means at the present time of separating these disorders from those in which primitive but recognizable precursors of a given cell line occur in the marrow but show a "maturation arrest."

CONSTITUTIONAL APLASIAS. Inherited forms of the disease, both pancellular and unicellular, have been designated as constitutional aplasias. These frequently arise in combination with various congenital anomalies and probably involve fundamental intrinsic abnormalities of stem cells.

Etiology

The multiple causes and diverse nature of the various bone marrow failure syndromes are classified in Table 132–1. Approximately 50 per cent of cases arise de novo and are thus considered idiopathic. The remaining cases are associated with exposure to an extremely diverse array of chemicals or ionizing radiation or occur in the context of a neoplastic, autoimmune, or infectious disease. There is little apparent clinical difference between the idiopathic and secondary forms of the disease.

DRUG-RELATED APLASIAS. ***Dose-Dependent Aplasias.*** Chemotherapeutic agents used in the treatment of various neoplasms are virtually uniform in their cytotoxicity for hematopoietic stem cells. The resulting aplasia is usually reversible and its severity depends on the amount of drug exposure. Agents that are cycle specific such as cytosine arabinoside and methotrexate act preferentially on the more mature stem cells, which are known to have a higher mitotic rate than the more primitive pluripotential stem cells. As a result, patients manifest pancytopenia prior to the depletion of the pluripotent stem cells on which ultimate marrow regeneration depends. Other agents such as busulfan attack both cycling and noncycling stem cells and therefore can lead to prolonged or irreversible aplasia unless used with great caution. Certain other drugs that are not used for chemotherapy show reversible, dose-related marrow suppression as an adverse side effect. These include phenytoin, phenothiazines, thiouracil, methicillin, and chloramphenicol.

Idiosyncratic Aplasias. Another large group of seemingly unrelated drugs, which may or may not show dose-related marrow suppression, is associated with the rare occurrence of disastrous aplasia in a small fraction of exposed individuals. The prototype of this group is chloramphenicol, for many years the leading cause of idiosyncratic drug-related aplastic anemia. Chloramphenicol has restricted usage in developed countries, but it is still widely available and heavily used in Third World countries, where accurate assessment of fatalities is unavailable.

In contrast to the dose-dependent aplasias, idiosyncratic reactions may occur weeks or months after exposure to small amounts of chloramphenicol. The frequency of this reaction is estimated between 1:24,000 to 1:40,000 of the exposed population. In one large series, recognition of aplasia occurred within 38 days of exposure in 50 per cent of affected individuals but not until more than 130 days from exposure in another 10 per

TABLE 132–2. CHEMICAL AND PHYSICAL AGENTS ASSOCIATED WITH THE DEVELOPMENT OF PANCYTOPENIA AND A HYPOPLASTIC MARROW*

ANTINEOPLASTIC AGENTS: alkylating agents, antimetabolites, antimitotic agents, antibiotics, radiation

ANTIMICROBIAL AGENTS: *chloramphenicol, organic arsenicals, quinacrine,* streptomycin, penicillin, methicillin, oxytetracycline, chlortetracycline, sulfonamides, sulfisoxazole (Gantrisin), sulfamethoxypyridazine (Kynex), amphotericin B

ANTICONVULSANTS: mephenytoin (Mesantoin), *trimethadione (Tridione),* phenacemide (Phenurone), phenytoin, ethosuximide (Zarontin)

ANTITHYROID DRUGS: carbethoxythiomethylglyoxaline (Carbimazole), methylmercaptoimidazole (Tapazole) potassium perchlorate, propylthiouracil

ANTIDIABETIC AGENTS: tolbutamide, chlorpropamide, carbutamide

ANTIHISTAMINES: tripelennamine (Pyribenzamine)

ANALGESICS: *phenylbutazone,* acetylsalicylic acid, indomethacin, carbamazepine (Tegretol)

SEDATIVES AND TRANQUILIZERS: meprobamate, chlorpromazine, promazine, chlordiazepoxide (Librium), mepazine

MISCELLANEOUS: *gold compounds,* acetazolamide (Diamox)

TOXIC CHEMICALS: solvents (*benzene,* glue, toluene, carbon tetrachloride), insecticides (chlorophenothane [DDT], parathion, chlordane, pentachlorophenol), bismuth, mercury, arsenic, colloidal silver

*Adapted from Wintrobe MM: Clinical Hematology. Philadelphia, Lea & Febiger, 1974. Drugs associated with 20 or more reported cases are in italics.

cent. A latent period does not always occur; the rapid development of severe aplasia during therapy is not uncommon.

Chloramphenicol also manifests reversible dose-related marrow suppression primarily affecting erythroid precursors probably as a result of its inhibition of mitochondrial protein and heme synthesis. This effect of chloramphenicol is associated with prominent vacuolization and sideroblastic changes in developing erythroblasts.

There is evidence from studies of identical twin concordance that some patients who develop severe idiosyncratic aplasia from chloramphenicol have an underlying genetic susceptibility. The nature and frequency of this putative sensitivity is unknown. The management and prognosis of chloramphenicol-related aplasia does not differ from that of other idiosyncratic drug reactions or of the idiopathic form of the disease and will be discussed subsequently. Drugs that have been associated with the development of marrow aplasias are listed in Table 132–2.

ENVIRONMENTAL TOXINS. Solvents and insecticides comprise the major group of toxins that have been linked to aplastic anemia. Of these, benzene is the most important and has received the most experimental attention. Benzene appears to have an unpredictable and heterogeneous effect on marrow function and may induce various combinations of aplasia, myelofibrosis, or frank leukemia. The abnormalities in marrow function may arise during or years after exposure to benzene. Most recognized cases have resulted from rather heavy and prolonged industrial exposures. Aplastic anemia after glue sniffing has been well documented and probably relates to the presence of benzene derivatives in glues.

INFECTIONS. ***Hepatitis.*** Severe aplastic anemia may follow an episode of apparent viral hepatitis. The nature of the preceding hepatitis has not usually been established, but a recent study failed to find serologic evidence of prior infection with either hepatitis A or B in 14 of 16 cases. Aplasia after hepatitis is twice as common in males as in females and usually occurs in patients under 20 years of age. The hepatitis is not unusually severe, whereas the subsequent aplasia is often quite severe and has a high mortality.

Epstein-Barr Virus. Aplasia has also been reported to follow Epstein-Barr (EB) virus infections, although some of these individuals may have received antibiotics so that attribution of cause and effect is not as well established as is the case in hepatitis. In boys with the X-linked immunodeficiency syndrome, in which severe and often fatal EB virus infections are common, a significant incidence of aplastic anemia has been noted. The onset of aplasia is precipitous and highly lethal, with death occurring within one week.

Parvovirus. Selective transient loss of erythroid precursors in the marrow with reticulocytopenia is a well-recognized occurrence in patients with congenital hemolytic anemias and has been termed *aplastic crisis.* Although the suppression of erythropoiesis is self limited, the rapid fall of hematocrit that is a result of the short life span of the remaining red cells may induce severe life-threatening anemia. The clinical history of such patients suggests that a viral syndrome usually precedes these episodes. Recently, human parvovirus infection has been linked to aplastic crisis in hereditary spherocytosis and sickle cell anemia, and the virus has been shown to selectively inhibit erythroid progenitors in cell cultures.

A similar, sudden cessation of erythropoiesis has also been noted in previously normal children and has been termed *transient erythroblastopenia of childhood* (TEC). Many of these children also have an apparent viral illness from two weeks to two months prior to the onset of reticulocytopenia. The possible relationship of TEC to parvovirus infection remains to be established. An autoimmune basis for TEC has been suggested by the finding of an IgG serum inhibitor of erythroid colony formation in some patients.

PRELEUKEMIA. Most forms of marrow aplasia, both acquired and congenital, have been associated with the occasional development of acute leukemia. One characteristic sequence of events occurs in children who present with typical aplastic anemia but respond rapidly to corticosteroid therapy. These patients ultimately relapse with typical acute lymphocytic leukemia of childhood. Acute myeloid leukemias may arise after years of mild or moderate marrow aplasia, particularly in patients with exposure to benzene or radiation.

Pathogenesis

The diversity of genetic, environmental, and clinical associations with the aplastic anemias makes the idea extremely unlikely that a single pathogenetic mechanism can explain the disease in all cases. Two general processes seem to account for the majority of occurrences of marrow aplasia: (1) an intrinsic inherited or acquired defect in a primitive stem cell that renders it unable to differentiate, (2) an immunologically mediated disturbance that damages the normal stem cell or prevents it from finding the appropriate cellular or microenvironmental milieu in which it can mature. The complex cellular and humoral interactions that are required for normal hematopoiesis are discussed in Ch. 130.

Elucidation of the pathogenesis of aplastic anemia has been aided by recent clinical observations involving bone marrow transplantation and the use of various immunosuppressing agents in the treatment of patients with this disease:

1. Approximately half of patients with aplastic anemia who have received marrow infusions from an identical twin demonstrate engraftment with rapid, complete, and prolonged recovery of marrow function. The original cases have now been followed for more than ten years without relapse. This relatively pure therapeutic experiment strongly suggests that the patient lacks functional stem cells that are present in the donated marrow. It further suggests that the marrow microenvironment is able to accept and sustain normal stem cell differentiation and that inhibitory factors, either cellular or humoral, are unlikely to be involved in this subgroup of patients.

2. In the other half of the attempted transplants between identical twins the donated marrow is rejected by the aplastic recipient. Most of these patients can subsequently be engrafted after a course of cyclophosphamide and show long-term complete recovery of marrow function similar to the previously mentioned group. The action of cyclophosphamide in these

patients is unclear. It may serve to interrupt permanently an immune process that prevents normal stem cell differentiation. Colony formation in marrow cell cultures from a healthy twin has been shown to be suppressed by mononuclear cells from the aplastic recipient, most likely by suppressor T cells. Successful culture of both erythroid and granulocytic colonies from marrows of some patients with aplastic anemia has been described to occur only after removal of their T cells.

An alternative explanation for the effect of cyclophosphamide suggests that the cytotoxic drug may be eliminating defective stem cells that occupy a limited number of architectural niches. As a result of this cellular debridement the drug would allow access of the transplanted stem cells to the particular microenvironmental site that is required for induction of differentiation. Insufficient data exist with which to distinguish these alternative possibilities.

3. Additional evidence that immune mechanisms may be operative in the pathogenesis of some forms of aplastic anemia lies in the improvement noted in from 30 to 65 per cent of patients with severe aplasia treated with antilymphocyte or antithymocyte globulin preparations. The responses to antithymocyte globulin differ markedly from those obtained with marrow transplantation. Improvement may take several months to occur and is usually incomplete, with persistence of moderate or even severe cytopenias. However, transfusion requirements often disappear and granulocytes and platelet counts may rise above critical levels for infection or bleeding. While this mode of therapy goes under the rubric of immunosuppression, these are complex heterologous antisera that may have many targets in addition to the immune cells against which they are raised.

4. The pathogenetic role of autoimmunity has a firmer basis in some of the unicellular aplasias, particularly in pure red cell aplasia, which often arises in patients with other manifestations of immune dysfunction. Thymoma, hypogammaglobulinemia, monoclonal gammopathy, antinuclear antibodies, and Coombs-positive hemolysis have all been reported in association with PRCA. Serum inhibitors of erythropoiesis have been described using marrow culture techniques. Immunoglobulin fractions derived from affected patients have shown specific staining of erythroblast nuclei by immunofluorescence as well as complement-dependent cytolysis of erythroblasts. These patients also frequently respond to combinations of prednisone or cyclophosphamide; reduction in the post-treatment level of serum inhibitor has been demonstrated in some instances.

Marrow aplasia syndromes are associated with agents that are known to be both cytotoxic and leukemogenic (e.g., alkylating agents, benzene, and ionizing radiation) as well as with consitutional disorders that may terminate in acute leukemia (e.g., Fanconi's anemia). This implies that intrinsic genetic damage to stem cells may prevent normal differentiation programs. The degree to which the proliferative potential of these damaged stem cells is preserved may then determine whether aplasia or leukemia ensues. Marrow failure in other cases seems to be associated with inhibition of normal stem cell differentiation, perhaps as a result of cellular or humoral autoimmunity. It is premature to invoke immune marrow suppression in most patients with aplastic anemia. Further investigation with refined marrow culture techniques, particularly in the identical twin transplants, is urgently needed.

Clinical Description

ONSET. Aplastic anemia affects individuals of all ages, although there is a sharp increase in incidence over the age of 65. The overall incidence of the disease was approximately 25 new cases per million persons per year in a large, carefully monitored Swedish population. The five-fold increase in patients over 65 may be attributable to their much greater exposure to medications. The clinical features of the disease relate almost entirely to the effects of inadequate numbers of functional peripheral blood cells. The onset is usually insidious but may be dramatic depending on the severity and rapidity with which the aplasia progresses. Bleeding manifestations may be the first indication of severe disease. These include gingival bleeding, epistaxis, and petechial hemorrhages, all of which are characteristic of severe thrombocytopenia. Fatigue and pallor are usually noted at presentation. Infections frequently begin with bacterial invasion of vulnerable areas of the GI tract, namely the oropharynx or the rectum. Opportunistic infections are unusual at presentation but may occur in patients with very low lymphocyte counts and after immunosuppressive therapy. Systemic symptoms are not prominent unless there is extensive infection, and weight loss is unusual.

PHYSICAL EXAMINATION. Pallor is frequent; its absence in a patient with the acute onset of petechial hemorrhages is much more likely to be associated with immune thrombocytopenic purpura. Retinal hemorrhages are not uncommon and correlate with the severity of anemia rather than thrombocytopenia. The spleen is not enlarged; splenomegaly strongly suggests an underlying blood dyscrasia or hypersplenism rather than marrow aplasia. The constitutional forms of marrow aplasia (Fanconi's anemia, dyskeratosis congenita, Diamond-Blackfan anemia, and others) are frequently associated with congenital anomalies that should be carefully noted. The onset of marrow disease in some of the constitutional disorders may occur in the second or third decade so they must be considered in the differential diagnosis of aplasia in the young adult or adolescent.

Diagnosis

The diagnosis of aplastic anemia is usually straightforward. It is based on the combination of peripheral cytopenias with the characteristic empty marrow replaced with fat.

PERIPHERAL BLOOD FINDINGS. The basic structural framework of the marrow remains relatively intact, so the peripheral red cells do not show marked abnormalities except for a tendency toward macrocytosis. The degree of macrocytosis depends on the extent to which primitive stem cells are recruited under the conditions of extreme anemic stress. The direct progeny of these earliest stem cells show the characteristics of fetal red cells, i.e., an increased amount of fetal hemoglobin, expression of the little i antigen, and macrocytosis. Nucleated red cells occur rarely in simple aplasia; their presence raises the possibility of a myeloproliferative or myelophthisic process instead. The total lymphocyte count may be normal but is often very low in severe cases and after therapy with steroids or other immunosuppressive agents.

BONE MARROW FINDINGS. The fatty marrow with empty stroma is the key diagnostic feature. Residual foci of mainly erythropoietic tissue are often found, however, that can alter the impression of aspirated material. A large needle biopsy (> 1 cm) is an essential adjunct in evaluating the degree of aplasia. It is important to obtain marrow outside of areas that have been irradiated previously for any reason. If a single biopsy and aspirate are equivocal, repeating is warranted.

Assessment of marrow cellularity is at best semiquantitative, and the degree of hypocellularity has not been shown to correlate well with prognosis. This probably results from unavoidable heterogeneity of sampling this large organ. Benign lymphoid nodules may be found; this finding must not be confused with involvement by malignant lymphoma. The unicellular aplasias arise in the setting of normal marrow cellularity with absence of a single cell line. In some cases of PRCA, as well as in agranulocytosis, immature precursors may be found in the absence of any mature forms.

ANCILLARY STUDIES. Because of the frequent association of paroxysmal nocturnal hemoglobinuria (PNH), the *Ham's test* or *sucrose hemolysis test* is frequently performed in patients with marrow aplasia, especially if there is any degree of reticulocytosis (Ch. 138). Occasional patients have had hypogammaglobulinemia; therefore, measurement of serum immunoglobulins is warranted. A search for thymoma should be performed by CT scan in patients with pure red cell aplasia. When there is a

TABLE 132–3. CAUSES OF PANCYTOPENIA

A.	Aplastic anemias (Table 132–1)
B.	Myelophthisic anemias (Table 132–4)
C.	Hypersplenism
D.	Megaloblastic anemias
E.	Myelodysplastic syndromes
F.	Overwhelming sepsis

question of a constitutional aplasia, skeletal and renal x-rays are indicated to assess the presence of congenital anomalies.

Marrow culture studies show impaired colony formation in virtually all cases. In the future it is likely that refined culture techniques capable of demonstrating cellular or humoral inhibition of hematopoiesis will assume increasing importance in guiding therapy.

DIFFERENTIAL DIAGNOSIS. A list of causes of peripheral pancytopenia is presented in Table 132–3. The most important distinction to be made in assessing aplastic anemia is to exclude the presence of leukemia, which may occasionally be characterized by marked marrow hypocellularity and pancytopenia. Splenomegaly, circulating immature cells, and increased marrow reticulin all suggest a primary blood dyscrasia or myelofibrosis rather than simple aplasia.

Management

INITIAL ASSESSMENT OF SUITABILITY FOR MARROW TRANSPLANTATION. The initial assessment of the patient with aplastic anemia is a crucial period requiring mature clinical judgment. On the one hand, patients with severe disease who present with bleeding and marked anemia will often require transfusion support; however, the chance for successful bone marrow engraftment is compromised in patients who have received prior transfusions. *The current treatment of choice for patients with severe disease who have an HLA compatible donor is bone marrow transplantation.* The initial task of the physician is to assess the likelihood that marrow transplantation will be needed and to obtain rapid referral to an appropriate facility in which this form of therapy is regularly performed. This admonition should not exclude the use of stabilizing transfusions under life-threatening circumstances; rather, it should encourage haste in obtaining referral and in performing HLA typing of potential donors. Criteria for severe disease have been previously defined. Most transplant centers require that the peripheral blood and marrow values persist for at least three weeks before drastic therapies are undertaken. It is of course crucial to discontinue any potentially toxic medications and to remove the patient from any unusual environmental source of toxins during this period. The details of the procedure and the results of bone marrow transplantation in aplastic anemia are covered in Ch. 165. Because of the unavailability of suitable donors and the poor results of transplantation in older patients, most patients with this disease must be treated by other means.

SUPPORTIVE CARE. Supportive care has assumed an increasingly important role in survival of aplastic anemia patients both before and after various therapeutic interventions. The care of such patients is complex and should be carried out, whenever possible, in a setting with adequate technical resources and experienced personnel.

Transfusions. Transplant candidates should have transfusion only when absolutely necessary because of the risk of sensitization and subsequent graft rejection. The number of donors should be restricted, and family members must be avoided until the question of transplantation is decided. Complete phenotyping of major and minor red cell antigens should be performed prior to transfusion. This will aid in the detection of red cell alloantibodies should they develop after repeated transfusions. The use of frozen red cells diminishes the development of leukocyte alloantibodies, but washed, leukocyte-poor packed cells are a more widely available and usually satisfactory substitute. Additional aspects of chronic transfusion therapy including the use of iron chelators to reduce iron overload are discussed in Ch. 141.

Granulocyte transfusions have no prophylactic benefit and may actually increase mortality because of the transmission of cytomegalovirus. Their current role in the aplastic patient is controversial; they may occasionally be of benefit in a patient with established septicemia who has failed to respond to appropriate antibiotics (Ch. 150).

Platelet transfusions are of undoubted value to the bleeding patient, but their continued use is limited by the development of alloantibodies that render the patient refractory to random donor platelets. Such patients may benefit from platelets obtained by pheresis of an HLA compatible donor. The onset of such refractoriness is highly variable, and a significant minority of patients seem to tolerate random donor platelet support for long periods.

Aplastic patients frequently tolerate very low platelet counts with only cutaneous bleeding in the form of petechiae and traumatic ecchymoses. While conventional teaching has held that a count below 20,000 is the threshold value for a high risk of bleeding, it may in fact be much lower (Fig. 132–1). Platelets should be reserved for actual bleeding episodes or the suspicion of cerebral hemorrhage. Patients with demonstrable increments after transfusions may reasonably be given prophylaxis as the count falls below 5000 or 10,000 per cubic millimeter.

Many hematologists believe that small doses of prednisone (15 mg daily) reduce capillary bleeding in severely thrombocytopenic patients. The data in Figure 132–1 indicate an apparent enhancement of GI bleeding in patients taking somewhat larger doses of prednisone. Thus the rationale for low-dose therapy remains in some doubt. The side effects of 15 mg of prednisone are sufficiently low that a trial is reasonable in patients with troublesome bleeding.

General Measures. Suppression of menstruation by appropriate hormonal manipulation is indicated for females with excessive blood loss. Aspirin and all antiplatelet medications should be avoided. Scrupulous attention to aseptic technique in administering intravenous infusions, avoidance of intramuscular injections, careful attention to handwashing by personnel, and isolation from obviously infected visitors are important. Rigid adherence to "reverse isolation" impedes proper nursing care without a corresponding benefit in reducing infections,

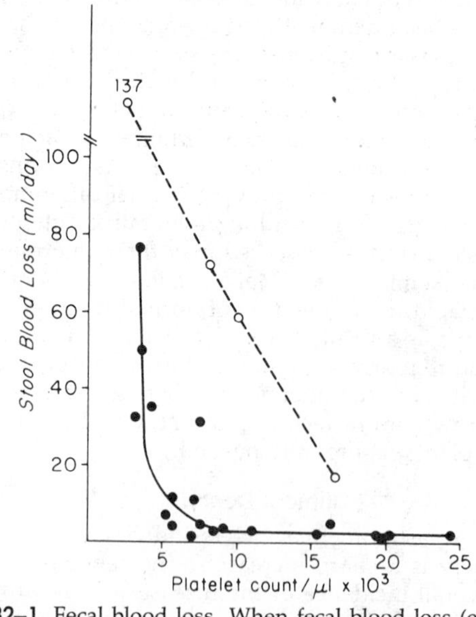

Figure 132–1. Fecal blood loss. When fecal blood loss (expressed as ml of blood/day) was determined in 20 aplastic thrombocytopenic patients (●), blood loss was less than 5 ml/day at platelet counts greater than 10,000/μl. At platelet counts between 5,000 and 10,000/μl blood loss averaged 9 ml ± 7/day. At levels less than 5,000/μl blood loss was markedly elevated at 50 ml ± 20/day. Prednisone in dosages of 20 to 60 mg/day markedly increased bleeding at any given platelet level (○). (From Slichter SJ, Harker LA: Thrombocytopenia. Clin Hematol 7:523, 1978.)

which are largely acquired from endogenous or ubiquitous flora. Management of these infections in the compromised host is discussed in Ch. 257.

THERAPY DIRECTED AT REVERSAL OF APLASIA. ***Immunosuppression.*** One of the most urgent issues in the management of patients with aplastic anemia involves the use of immunosuppressing agents. Reports from several centers in both Europe and the United States attest to the potential benefit of antilymphocyte globulin preparations in some patients. Various antisera, some derived against human thymocytes and others against lymphocytes, have been employed. The differences in reactivity of these products against lymphoid cells probably contributes to the apparent diversity of results that have been reported. However, there is clear evidence of efficacy, which is most notable in the randomized controlled study performed by Champlin and co-workers.

The efficacy of antithymocyte globulin therapy is being further tested in a multicenter trial in the United States. If the preliminary results are confirmed it can offer an important adjunctive form of therapy in the many patients for whom marrow transplantation is not feasible.

High doses of prednisone have been used for immunosuppression in patients with aplastic anemia. While most reported studies have failed to show benefit, one recent study described a number of complete remissions. The hazards of very high doses of corticosteroids, i.e., overwhelming fungal or other opportunistic infections, when combined with marrow aplasia, necessitate that this mode of therapy be considered experimental until its role can be more properly assessed.

Immunosuppression has a more clearly defined role in the treatment of unicellular aplasias, especially in pure red cell aplasia. Combinations of cyclophosphamide and other cytotoxic agents and prednisone have induced excellent remissions in PRCA, but the disease eventually recurs in most individuals. About one third of patients with PRCA and thymoma have had remissions after thymectomy.

Androgens. Because androgenic compounds stimulate erythropoiesis, testosterone as well as various other orally active derivatives have been employed in aplastic anemia. In general, early reports of remission induction by androgens in severe aplastic anemia have not been confirmed as occurring more frequently than spontaneous regressions. However, patients with less severe aplasia, who presumably have a higher number of committed erythroid progenitors for stimulation by androgens, frequently show improved hematocrit and lessened transfusion requirements. Occasional patients are androgen dependent and have relapsed repeatedly when androgens are discontinued. Granulocyte and platelet responses are much less common than is a rise in hematocrit. Both the injectable forms of testosterone enanthate (5 to 8 mg per kilogram once weekly) and synthetic oral agents, e.g., oxymethalone (2 to 4 mg per kilogram daily) have shown responses. Toxicity is significant; both groups of drugs cause masculinization with hirsutism, acne, fluid retention, and clitoral enlargement. The oral agents are associated with additional hepatic toxicity, including cholestatic jaundice and hepatocellular carcinoma.

Prognosis

Patients with aplastic anemia appear to fall into two major subgroups: (1) a severely affected group as previously defined with a high mortality (perhaps as high as 96 per cent with no treatment) by six months, and (2) a mildly to moderately affected group with a considerably better outlook. Before the era of bone marrow transplantation and intensive supportive care the overall mortality in all patients was from 55 to 75 per cent. The long-term fate of the survivors is unclear. Some enter an apparently complete remission while others manifest continued mild cytopenia. In addition to the standard criteria for severe disease, the following factors have adverse prognostic significance: male sex, absence of macrocytosis, acuteness of onset, persistence of severe cytopenias after the first month, and presence of more than 70 per cent lymphocytes in the marrow. Early improvement in cell counts confers a correspondingly improved prognosis while deterioration in mild to moderate cases places these patients in the high-mortality group. Unfortunately there is little with which to predict these transitions. The etiology of the aplasia seems to have little prognostic significance, with the possible exception of those occurring after hepatitis. Acute leukemia in patients who have been carefully studied at the onset and found to lack excess blasts in the marrow probably occurs in less than 1 per cent of cases.

Marrow transplantation in the severely aplastic patient has dramatically improved survival to more than 80 per cent of previously untransfused patients. Graft-versus-host disease continues to be a major problem in 20 to 50 per cent of survivors but does not appear to change the long-term survival figures (Ch. 165).

Myelophthisic Anemias

Myelophthisis is an archaic term for any pathologic process that obliterates the normal marrow architecture. The microcirculatory anatomy of the marrow normally serves to retain developing hematopoietic cells within extravascular spaces, called *cords,* until they are sufficiently mature to gain access to the general circulation by crossing the cordal-sinusoidal boundary. If this delicate network is disrupted, abortive attempts at hematopoiesis occur, which result in the release of immature blood cells into the peripheral blood. The presence of circulating nucleated red blood cells, myelocytes, or blasts and giant platelets is termed *leukoerythroblastosis.* This is a frequent although not invariable accompaniment of myelophthisis (Fig. 132–2). Transient leukoerythroblastosis may occur without myelophthisis under conditions of extreme erythropoietin-mediated marrow stress such as acute hemorrhage, abrupt hypoxemia, or severe chronic hemolysis.

The pathologic processes that cause myelophthisis can be usefully divided into four general categories (Table 132–4). Metastatic carcinoma has replaced tuberculosis as the most commonly associated condition. Many of these neoplastic marrow processes incite an intense fibrotic reaction that may obscure the malignant cells. The hematopoietic disorders that are most likely to cause myelofibrosis, idiopathic myelofibrosis, and chronic myelogenous leukemia are associated with marked megakaryocytic hyperplasia. Acute leukemias and well-differentiated lymphoid neoplasms, although they may totally replace the normal marrow, only rarely elicit a leukoerythroblastic response, for reasons that are not entirely clear.

The diagnosis of myelophthisis is frequently suggested by the presence of nucleated red blood cells or other immature forms on the peripheral smear. The total leukocyte and platelet count may be decreased if marrow replacement is extensive; however, there may be marked leukocytosis in idiopathic myelofibrosis or when a leukemoid reaction occurs. Teardrop-shaped red cells are commonly present along with other poikilocytes (Fig. 132–2). Occasionally the diagnosis is suggested by abnormal bone films showing focal lytic or blastic lesions, or a more widespread increase in bone density as in idiopathic myelofibrosis.

Definitive diagnosis of myelophthisis depends on adequate examination of the bone marrow (Fig. 132–2). Because the aspirate is characteristically "dry," a needle or surgical biopsy is essential. The marrow involvement is often patchy and residual areas of normal or hyperplastic marrow may be found. Demonstration of increased reticulin fibers in the marrow biopsy with silver stains is a useful adjunct in myelofibrotic conditions. A careful search for malignant cells embedded within the fibrotic tissue should always be performed.

The therapy of myelophthisic anemias is entirely dependent on the recognition and appropriate treatment of the underlying pathologic process. Successful treatment of breast or prostatic carcinomas, either by cytotoxic or hormonal agents, can lead

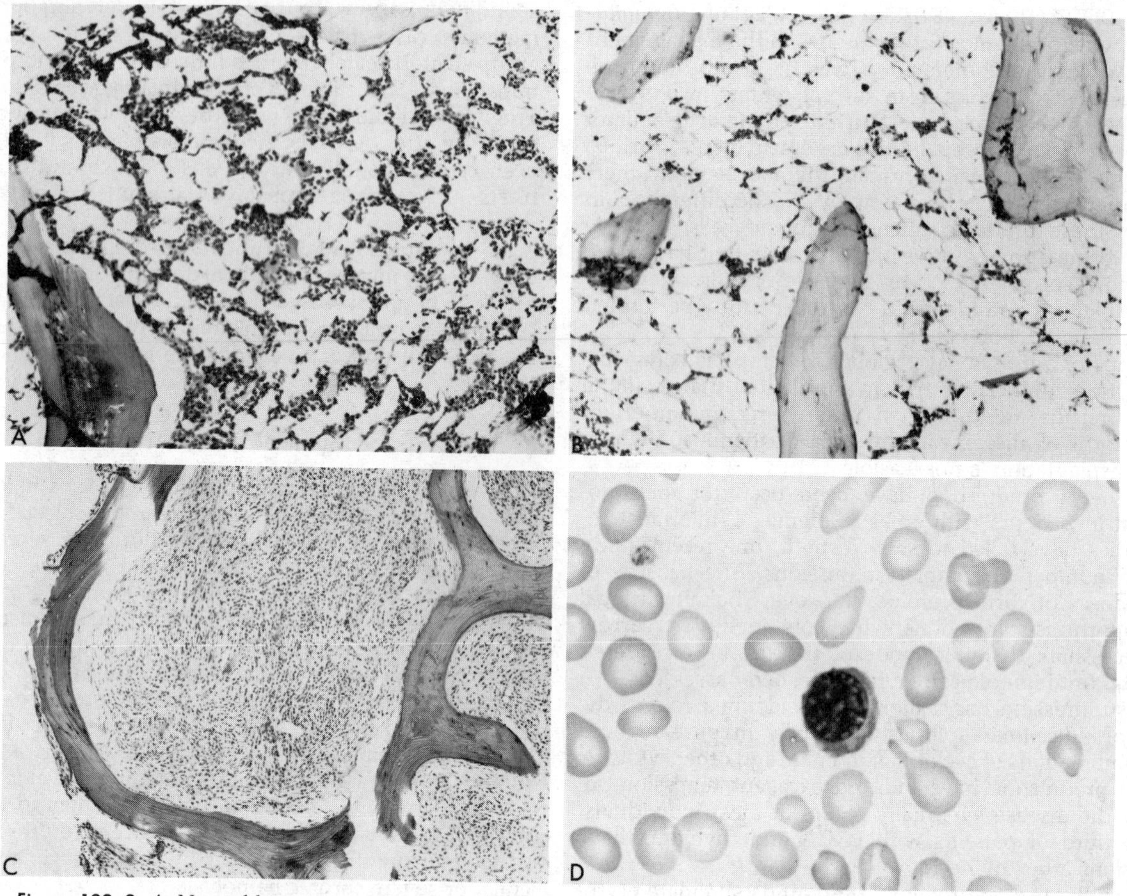

Figure 132–2. *A,* Normal bone marrow biopsy. Note even mixture of hematopoietic tissue and fat. *B,* Bone marrow biopsy from a patient with aplastic anemia. Note the increase in fat at the expense of normal hematopoietic tissue. *C,* Bone marrow biopsy from a woman with metastatic breast carcinoma. Note the dense fibrosis. *D,* Peripheral smear from a patient with idiopathic myelofibrosis. Note frequent teardrop forms and the nucleated red cell.

to complete resolution of the myelophthisis and recovery of normal marrow function. A dramatic example of the reversibility of the myelophthisic process has been demonstrated in the childhood disease osteopetrosis. This condition has recently been linked to an inherited defect in the mononuclear phagocytic system that is manifested by decreased osteoclast function. The resulting overgrowth of bony trabeculae that obliterates the marrow space can be completely reversed by bone marrow transplantation with restoration of normal hematopoiesis.

TABLE 132–4. CAUSES OF MYELOPHTHISIS

A. Neoplastic Infiltration of the Marrow
1. Hematologic malignancies
   Leukemias—acute and chronic
   Lymphomas–Hodgkins and non-Hodgkins
   Plasma cell myeloma
   Hairy cell leukemia
2. Nonhematologic malignancies
   Carcinomas–esp. breast, prostate, lung, stomach
   Neuroblastoma

B. Myelofibrosis
1. Primary (idiopathic)
2. Secondary–chronic myeloid leukemia, cancers, vasculitis (lupus, rheumatoid arthritis)

C. Granulomatous infections
1. Tuberculosis
2. Fungi

D. Metabolic Abnormalities
1. Lipid storage diseases–Gaucher's, etc.
2. Osteopetrosis

Alter BP, Rappeport JM, Parkman R: The bone marrow failure syndromes. *In* Nathan DG, Oski FA (eds.): Hematology of Infancy and Childhood. 2nd ed. Philadelphia, W. B. Saunders Company, 1981, pp 168–249. *An inclusive review with over 700 references currently in revision for a new edition. It is particularly useful for the inherited forms of marrow failure.*

Champlin R, Ho W, Gale RP: Antithymocyte globulin treatment in patients with aplastic anemia. A prospective randomized trial. N Engl J Med 308:113, 1983. *A report of the first controlled trial of antithymocyte globulin in aplastic anemia from a single institution.*

Rappeport JM, Nathan DG: Acquired aplastic anemias: Pathophysiology and treatment. Adv Intern Med 27:547, 1982. *The most readable of the many current reviews of the subject. A balanced presentation of alternative concepts of pathogenesis.*

Storb R, Thomas ED, Buckner CD, et al: Marrow transplantation for aplastic anemia. Sem Hemat 21:27–35, 1984. *A concise updating of the worldwide experience with marrow transplants for aplastic anemia including their toxicities.*

133. NORMOCHROMIC NORMOCYTIC ANEMIAS

James P. Kushner

The normocytic normochromic anemias are those in which the average cell size (MCV) and the average cell hemoglobin concentration (MCHC) are normal. These anemias occur in association with a large number of diseases, and the mechanisms responsible for the anemia are quite diverse. Frequently, the anemia is only a minor manifestation of a systemic disease of much more serious consequence. The anemia, however, may be the first detected evidence of disease and the finding of anemia may lead to studies resulting in correct diagnosis of an underlying disorder.

TABLE 133–1. CLASSIFICATION OF THE NORMOCYTIC NORMOCHROMIC ANEMIAS

I. Anemia with appropriate marrow response
  A. Acute posthemorrhagic anemia
  B. Hemolytic anemia (may be macrocytic when there is pronounced reticulocytosis) (Ch. 136–138)
II. Anemia with impaired marrow response
  A. Marrow hypoplasia
    1. Aplastic anemia (Ch. 132)
    2. Pure red cell aplasia (Ch. 132)
  B. Marrow infiltration
    1. Infiltration by malignant cells
    2. Myelofibrosis (Ch. 154)
    3. Inherited storage diseases
  C. Decreased erythropoietin production
    1. Kidney disease
    2. Liver disease
    3. Endocrine deficiencies
    4. Malnutrition
    5. Anemia of chronic disease (Ch. 134)

In spite of their highly variable causes, it is possible to approach normocytic normochromic anemias with a classification scheme that can direct the diagnostic investigation (Table 133–1). Central to this classification is the determination of whether the bone marrow is responding appropriately to a given degree of anemia. A normally functioning bone marrow can accelerate the rate of erythropoiesis up to eight-fold. Accelerated eyrthropoiesis by a normal bone marrow is reflected by an increase in the reticulocyte count. Reticulocytosis can be detected on routinely stained smears by the finding of a population of large polychromatophilic red cells. When reticulocytosis is pronounced the MCV may be moderately elevated because of the contribution of the large young erythrocytes to the measurement of the average cell size. Reticulocytosis is a manifestation of an appropriate marrow response to hemolytic anemia (see Ch. 136) and to acute posthemorrhagic anemia. These two conditions can generally be differentiated on clinical grounds.

When evidence of accelerated erythropoiesis in response to anemia is *not* found, it is likely that the underlying disorder is directly or indirectly affecting the bone marrow. Intrinsic marrow disease should be strongly suspected when leukopenia and thrombocytopenia are also found, or when morphologic abnormalities are found on the blood smear. These morphologic abnormalities include nucleated red cells, teardrop-shaped poikilocytes, immature granulocytes, and large platelets or megakaryocyte fragments (dwarf megakaryocytes). Marrow aspiration and biopsy are nearly always indicated in the face of these findings.

When anemia is found in association with an impaired marrow response and no signs of intrinsic marrow disease are detected, it is likely that an underlying disease is producing an indirect effect on red cell production. Renal disease, liver disease, and a variety of endocrine disorders indirectly affect erythropoiesis in association with a reduction in erythropoietin production. The pathogenesis of the anemia of chronic disease may also involve this mechanism, in addition to the defect in the mobilization of reticuloendothelial iron stores (Ch. 134).

Acute Posthemorrhagic Anemia

DEFINITION. The anemia caused by loss of a large volume of blood may occur as a result of trauma or because of an underlying disease that affects blood vessels or the coagulation mechanism. Bleeding may be obvious when profuse hemorrhage occurs from a body orifice or from an external wound. If bleeding occurs within a body cavity, tissue space, or the gastrointestinal tract, the nature of the problem may not be immediately appreciated (Ch. 113). The manifestation of hemorrhage depends on the rate and magnitude of the bleeding and the time elapsed between the acute hemorrhage and the first clinical observations.

CLINICAL MANIFESTATIONS AND DIAGNOSIS. The characteristic sequence of events following a single acute hemorrhage can be divided into two phases. The first, lasting up to three days, reflects the volume of blood loss and is dominated by the manifestations of hypovolemia. Anemia may not be detected by measurement of the volume of packed red cells (VPRC) or hemoglobin. The second phase occurs after the body has restored the blood volume to normal or near normal, and is characterized by the findings of anemia and reticulocytosis.

As outlined in Table 133–2, a normal individual can rapidly lose up to 20 per cent of the blood volume without any signs or symptoms. Limited signs of cardiovascular distress appear with losses up to 30 per cent of the blood volume, but shock gradually appears only when the blood loss exceeds 30 to 40 per cent of the blood volume. As the plasma volume and red cell mass are reduced in proportional amounts, the VPRC and hemoglobin fail to reflect the magnitude of blood lost. Clinical signs and symptoms must be used initially to estimate the degree of blood volume depletion and in planning emergency treatment. When blood loss is more gradual the plasma volume may be restored by endogenous mechanisms, and very large volumes of blood can be lost without clinical manifestations of shock.

Anemia is first detected following expansion of the plasma volume. In recumbent patients most of the plasma volume expansion has occurred by 24 hours; this expansion mainly is caused by movement of water and electrolytes into the intravascular space. In ambulatory patients plasma volume expansion occurs more slowly, mainly through the mobilization of albumin from extravascular sites. The VPRC may not reach the minimum value until three or four days after the hemorrhagic episode. Erythropoietin secretion is stimulated shortly after the appearance of the anemia, and hyperplasia of marrow erythroid elements then begins.

A reticulocytosis is usually detected three to five days after the hemorrhagic episode, and maximum reticulocyte counts are reached at six to eleven days. The degree of reticulocytosis is related to the magnitude of hemorrhage but rarely exceeds 14 per cent. During the period of maximum reticulocytosis, polychromatophilia and macrocytosis can be detected on the peripheral blood smear, and the MCV may become transiently increased. If the initial evaluation is done during this state, the findings may be mistaken for those of hemolytic anemia. Differentiation from hemolytic anemia may be difficult if bleeding has occurred into a body cavity or tissue space, because resorption of blood from these areas often results in an increased production of unconjugated bilirubin and even mild jaundice. In contrast to the reticulocyte response both the platelet count and the leukocyte count may rise dramatically within hours of an hemorrhage. Platelet counts as great as 1000

TABLE 133–2. CLINICAL MANIFESTATIONS OF ACUTE BLOOD LOSS IN OTHERWISE HEALTHY INDIVIDUALS

Percentage of Blood Volume Lost	Amount Lost (ml)	Clinical Manifestations
10–20	500–1000	Usually none; vasovagal syncope may occur in 5%; tachycardia in response to exercise; mild postural hypotension may be noted
20–30	1000–1500	Few changes supine; light-headedness and hypotension commonly occur when upright; marked tachycardia in response to exertion
30–40	1500–2000	Blood pressure, cardiac output, central venous pressure, urine volume reduced even when supine; thirst, shortness of breath, clammy skin, sweating, clouding of consciousness and rapid, thready pulse may be noted
40–50	2000–2500	Severe shock, often resulting in death

$\times 10^9$ per liter may be detected within one to two hours and leukocyte counts of 20 to 35 $\times 10^9$ per liter may be reached by two to five hours. Elevated platelet and leukocyte counts generally return to normal within three to five days.

TREATMENT. During the hypovolemic phase therapy should be directed at stopping the hemorrhage, combating shock, and restoring the blood volume. Restoration of the blood volume may be achieved by intravenous infusion of electrolyte solutions; colloid solutions of plasma protein, albumin, or dextran; or fresh whole blood. Complete reliance on fresh whole blood in the emergency situation is unwise for several reasons. First, large amounts of type O Rh-negative whole blood are required. If typing and cross-matching are done prior to transfusion, there may be a dangerous delay in therapy. Second, allergic transfusion reactions may restrict volume expansion or even produce plasma volume contraction. For the emergency situation, electrolyte solutions, albumin, or dextran are preferred.

Rapid infusion of Ringer's lactated or normal saline solution is the most widely used fluid therapy for hemorrhagic shock. An initial infusion of two to three times the volume of the estimated blood loss is administered. Because these solutions are rapidly distributed throughout the intravascular and extravascular compartments, they must be supplemented with colloid solutions. When large volumes of electrolyte solutions are infused most patients develop peripheral edema and elderly patients may develop pulmonary edema.

The colloidal preparations in wide use include a 6 per cent solution of high molecular weight dextran (dextran 70), a 10 per cent solution of low molecular weight dextran (dextran 40), and a 5 per cent solution of albumin in normal saline. Infusions of dextran 70 produce an initial volume effect slightly greater than the amount infused. Dextran 70 is slowly cleared over one to two days, allowing time for normal physiologic mechanisms to replace the volume lost. Dextran 40 has the advantage of an initial volume effect of nearly twice the amount infused. The lower molecular weight material is more rapidly cleared, however, and the volume-expanding effect is dissipated by 24 hours, before normal volume replacement mechanisms are maximal. Acute renal failure has occurred in a few patients receiving dextran 40. With either dextran solution, volumes in excess of one liter may interfere with platelet adhesiveness and the normal coagulation cascade. A solution of 5 per cent albumin in normal saline has the advantage of producing a known volume effect in the hypovolemic patient, but this preparation is relatively costly and time is required for preparation. A hypertonic albumin preparation containing 120 mEq of sodium lactate, 120 mEq of sodium chloride, and 12.5 grams of albumin per liter provides a predictable volume effect and minimizes interstitial fluid leakage. Use of hypertonic solutions requires careful monitoring of arterial and central venous pressures to avoid fluid overload.

Once the emergency has been dealt with, the bleeding lesion identified, and the bleeding stopped, attention can be directed to the anemia. The anemia itself rarely requires specific therapy and provision of a high protein diet and oral iron supplementation will suffice in most cases. Blood transfusions may be reserved for those situations in which rapid correction of the anemia is required, as in preparation of the patient for surgery.

Adamson J, Hillman RS: Blood volume and plasma protein replacement following acute blood loss in normal man. JAMA 205:609, 1968. *A classic study of acute blood loss and its treatment.*

Holcroft JW: Shock. *In* Way LW (ed.): Current Surgical Diagnosis and Treatment. 6th ed. Los Altos, Lange Medical Publications, 1983, p 192. *The management of acute blood loss and other aspects of shock from the surgeon's viewpoint.*

Mollison PL: Blood Transfusion in Clinical Medicine. 7th ed. Oxford, Blackwell Scientific Publications, 1983. *The "bible" for detailed analysis of the measurement of blood volume and its restoration by transfusions.*

Moss GS, et al.: Colloid or crystalloid in resuscitation of hemorrhagic shock: A controlled clinical trial. Surgery 89:434, 1981. *A prospective randomized study showing that, in most cases, volume expansion with simple electrolyte solutions is appropriate therapy.*

Shine KI, et al.: Aspects of the management of shock. Ann Intern Med 93:723, 1980. *An up-to-date review of the advantages and disadvantages of the available volume expanders.*

Other Normocytic Normochromic Anemias

ANEMIA OF CHRONIC RENAL INSUFFICIENCY. In contrast to the anemia found in association with most chronic diseases, the anemia associated with renal failure may be quite severe. Many factors may contribute to the anemia. Folate may be lost into the dialysate in patients receiving chronic dialysis therapy. Iron deficiency may develop because of blood loss from the genitourinary or gastrointestinal tracts or into the hemodialysis coil. Microangiopathic hemolytic anemia may occur in patients with renal failure because of malignant hypertension, or in the hemolytic-uremic syndrome. In the absence of any of these mechanisms the degree of anemia correlates roughly with the elevation of the blood urea nitrogen and creatinine. Although red cell survival may be moderately shortened, the mechanism underlying the anemia is mainly reduced red cell production. Failure of the erythropoietin-secreting function of the kidney appears to be responsible for the impaired marrow response to the anemia.

Blood transfusions are infrequently required. The VPRC rarely drops below 15 per cent, and most patients tolerate this degree of anemia remarkably well. Chronic dialysis therapy may result in a modest reduction in the degree of anemia, provided that folate or iron deficiency does not develop as a complicating factor. Androgens may be useful for patients who do not tolerate anemia well and require repeated transfusions. Weekly intramuscular injections of nandrolone decanoate (100 mg) or the oral administration of fluoxymesterone (10 to 30 mg per day) have proved effective in reducing transfusion requirements. Following a successful renal homograft, normal and even supranormal VPRC values may be achieved.

ANEMIA IN CIRRHOSIS AND OTHER LIVER DISEASE. Anemia is a frequent manifestation of liver disease; the pathogenetic mechanisms responsible may be more varied than those underlying the anemia of chronic disease. The anemia is generally normocytic and normochromic but occasionally it may be mildly macrocytic. It is unusual for the MCV to exceed 115 fl in the absence of advanced folate deficiency with frank megaloblastic changes in the marrow. Etiologic factors implicated in the pathogenesis of the anemia associated with liver disease include chronic alcoholism and its effect on erythropoiesis; iron deficiency due to blood loss from gastritis, peptic ulcer, varices, and deficient coagulation factors; sequestration of erythrocytes and other formed elements of the blood by the enlarged spleen resulting from portal hypertension; exaggeration of the degree of anemia because of the increased plasma volume associated with cirrhosis; and alterations in the lipid composition of erythrocyte membranes.

ANEMIAS ASSOCIATED WITH ENDOCRINE DISORDERS. Anemia frequently accompanies disorders of the pituitary gland, the thyroid gland, the adrenal glands, and the gonads. In general the anemia is mild and by itself produces few symptoms. Reduced tissue oxygen requirements as a result of the endocrine disturbance may result in diminished renal production of erythropoietin. Loss of the stimulating effect of androgens on erythrocyte production may be a factor in some cases. Endocrine disorders tend to begin insidiously; the early symptoms are generally no more specific than fatigue and lassitude. When initial laboratory testing reveals anemia, the diagnostic studies may be directed to the hematopoietic system. Unless endocrine disease is included in the differential diagnosis of a normocytic normochromic anemia, the primary diagnosis may be overlooked.

Anagnostou A, Fried W, Kurtzman NA: Hematological consequences of renal failure. *In* Brenner BM, Rector FC (eds.): The Kidney. 2nd ed. Philadelphia, W.B. Saunders Company, 1981. *A comprehensive treatise on the subject, with over 400 references.*

Eichner ER: The hematologic disorders of alcoholism. Am J Med 54:621, 1973. *A*

review of the hematologic effects of the pathogenetic agent responsible for most cases of advanced liver disease.
Williams WJ, Beutler E, Erslev AJ, Lichtman MA (eds.): Hematology. 3rd ed. New York, McGraw-Hill Book Company, 1983. *Extensive references to the anemias associated with renal and endocrine disorders.*

134. HYPOCHROMIC ANEMIAS

James P. Kushner

Anemias associated with a subnormal average cell hemoglobin concentration (MCHC) are classified as hypochromic. When the average cell size (MCV) is also reduced the anemia is classified as hypochromic, microcytic. Hypochromia and microcytosis can be detected either by examination of the stained blood smear or by calculation of the erythrocyte indices (Table 134–1). The widespread use of electronic cell counting equipment makes available the erythrocyte indices at the same time that anemia is usually detected by the finding of subnormal values for the hemoglobin concentration and the volume of packed red cells (VPRC).

The developing erythrocyte requires iron, protoporphyrin, and globin for the biosynthesis of hemoglobin. Hypochromic anemias, characterized by deficient hemoglobin synthesis, can be divided into three groups depending on which of the three components required for hemoglobin biosynthesis is deficient (Table 134–2).

IRON DEFICIENCY ANEMIA

DEFINITIONS. Iron deficiency anemia occurs when body iron stores become inadequate for the needs of normal erythropoiesis. Body iron stores must be exhausted before red cell production is restricted; therefore, anemia occurs at a late stage of iron deficiency. In its fully developed form iron-deficient erythropoiesis is characterized by hypochromia and microcytosis of the circulating erythrocytes, low plasma iron and ferritin concentrations, and a transferrin saturation of about 15 per cent or less. Iron deficiency anemia is a sign of disease and is not in itself a complete diagnosis.

PREVALENCE. Iron deficiency is the most common cause of anemia throughout the world, although it is difficult to define precisely its prevalence. Published studies vary in the reported incidence of iron deficiency because of differences in the criteria used to identify iron deficiency as well as in the nature of the population sampled in terms of age, sex, economic status, and local environmental factors. In parts of Africa and India, where marginal dietary intake and excessive iron loss due to intestinal parasites are present together, over half the population may suffer from iron deficiency anemia.

In most developed countries about 3 per cent of men, 20 per cent of women, and over 50 per cent of pregnant women are deficient in iron as judged by plasma iron levels. As judged by serum ferritin levels, iron stores are greatly reduced in about 25 per cent of children, 30 per cent of adolescents, 30 per cent of menstruating women, 60 per cent of pregnant women, and 3 per cent of men.

IRON METABOLISM. The total iron content of a healthy human subject remains within relatively narrow limits. Loss of iron from the body is precisely matched by absorption of iron from food. Iron loss is not due to "excretion" in the usual sense but rather to loss of intact cells containing iron. Epithelial cells from the gastrointestinal and urinary tracts, and from the skin, account for the normal daily iron loss in men of about 1 mg. In women, menstrual flow, childbearing, and lactation are additional routes of iron loss.

The body iron content in normal adult men is about 50 to 55 mg per kilogram of body weight and in women is about 35 to 40 mg per kilogram. This difference reflects the high incidence of iron deficiency in women and does not indicate any fundamental differences in iron metabolism between the sexes. Most of the body iron is found in hemoglobin, with smaller amounts in myoglobin and iron storage compounds (Table 134–3). Only a minute portion is found in plasma, where it is bound to transferrin.

The metabolism of iron is dominated by its role in hemoglobin synthesis. Iron incorporated into hemoglobin is utilized over and over again through an internal cycle, the *iron cycle* (Fig. 134–1). The plasma iron compartment, in which iron is bound to the transport protein transferrin, is central to this cycle. Iron moves from the plasma to erythroid precursor cells in the marrow. These cells synthesize hemoglobin and, with maturation, are released into the circulation. At the end of their 120-day life span the red cells are ingested by macrophages, principally in the splenic sinusoids, and the iron is extracted from the hemoglobin by the enzyme heme oxygenase. A small portion of this iron is stored in macrophages as ferritin or hemosiderin, but most is returned to the plasma where it becomes bound to transferrin, completing the cycle. In the normal adult male about 30 mg of iron completes the iron cycle daily. One to 2 mg of iron leaves the plasma daily and enters the liver and other tissues where it is utilized for the synthesis of other hemoproteins such as cytochromes and myoglobin.

ABSORPTION. The average intake of iron in the meat-containing diet in the United States is about 10 to 30 mg per day, but much greater variations occur in different parts of the world. Only 5 to 10 per cent of dietary iron (about 1 mg) is absorbed daily in order to balance precisely the amount lost. The amount of iron absorbed can increase up to five-fold if body iron stores are depleted or if erythropoiesis is accelerated. The amount absorbed decreases in states of iron overload or if there is

TABLE 134–1. RED CELL INDICES* IN HYPOCHROMIC AND MICROCYTIC ANEMIAS

	MCV (fl)	MCHC (g/dl)	MCH (pg)
Normal	83–96	32–36	28–34
Hypochromic	83–100	28–31	23–31
Microcytic	70–82	32–36	22–27
Hypochromic-microcytic	50–79	24–31	11–29

*Variations in the methods for measuring the red blood cell count, the volume of packed red cells, and the hemoglobin concentration could change the values slightly.

TABLE 134–2. CLASSIFICATION OF ANEMIAS CHARACTERIZED BY DEFICIENT HEMOGLOBIN SYNTHESIS AND THE PRESENCE OF HYPOCHROMIC ERYTHROCYTES

I. Disorders of iron metabolism
  A. Iron deficiency anemia
  B. Anemia of chronic disease
  C. Hereditary atransferrinemia
  D. Congenital hypochromic microcytic anemia with iron overload (Shahidi-Nathan-Diamond syndrome)
II. Disorders of porphyrin and heme synthesis: sideroblastic anemias
  A. Acquired sideroblastic anemias
    1. Idiopathic refractory sideroblastic anemia
    2. Complicating other diseases
    3. Associated with drugs or toxins—ethanol, INH, lead
  B. Hereditary sideroblastic anemias
    1. X chromosome–linked
    2. Autosomal recessive
III. Disorders of globin synthesis
  A. The thalassemias (Ch. 141)
  B. Hemoglobinopathies characterized by unstable hemoglobins (Ch. 143)

TABLE 134–3. DISTRIBUTION OF IRON IN THE BODY

	Iron Content (mg)		% of Total Body Iron	
Compound	*Men (70 kg)*	*Women (50 kg)*	*Men*	*Women*
Hemoglobin	2670	1500	69.6	73.1
Myoglobin	350	220	9.1	10.7
Heme enzymes	8	7	0.2	0.3
Transferrin	6	5	0.2	0.2
Ferritin-hemosiderin	800	320	20.9	15.7
Total	3834	2052	100.0	100.0

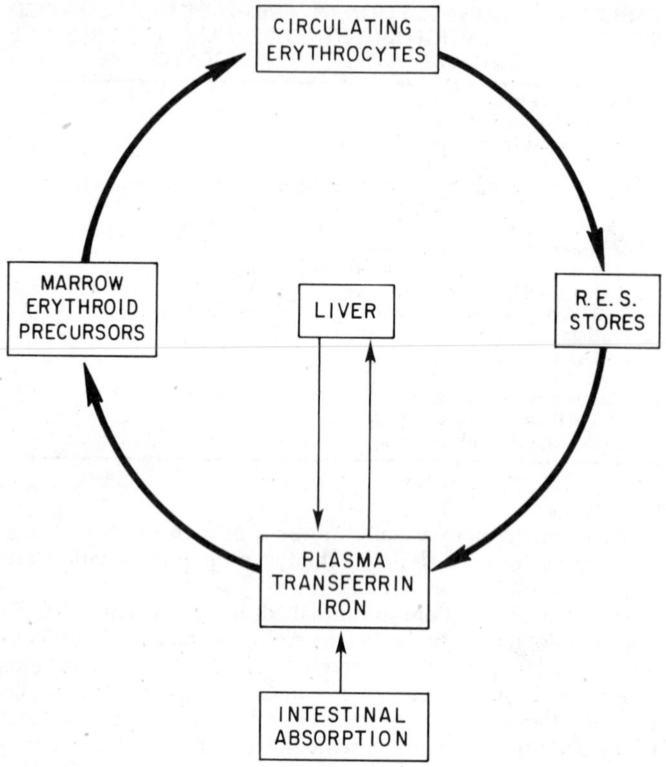

Figure 134–1. The internal iron cycle. In the plasma, iron (Fe) bound to transferrin is transported to the marrow where it is transferred to developing red blood cells and incorporated into hemoglobin. The mature red blood cells are released into the circulation and after 120 days are ingested by macrophages in the reticuloendothelial system (RES). Here the iron is extracted from hemoglobin and returned to plasma, completing the cycle.

erythroid hypoplasia. Total body iron balance is thus regulated at the absorptive step; the precise mechanism by which this control is accomplished has not been defined. Iron is absorbed chiefly in portions of the intestine proximal to the mid-jejunum and very little is absorbed in more caudal intestinal segments.

Iron is absorbed by two distinct pathways in humans, one for iron in heme and the other for iron in ferrous and ferric iron salts. Heme iron is derived from the hemoglobin, myoglobin, and other heme proteins in foods of animal origin. Exposure to the acid and proteases of gastric juice liberates the heme from its apoprotein. Heme is rapidly taken up by gastrointestinal epithelial cells and the iron is made available by enzymatic degradation of the porphyrin macrocycle. The absorption of heme iron is influenced very little by other dietary components.

The "bioavailability" of nonheme dietary iron, however, varies greatly. Availability is dependent on the oxidation state and solubility of the iron and the presence of chelating substances in the diet. Factors modifying the form in which iron is presented to the intestinal mucosal cell play an important role in the amount of iron that can be absorbed. At the acidic pH normally found in the stomach, both ferrous and ferric iron are soluble. Patients who have undergone gastrectomy, or who are achlorhydric for other reasons, demonstrate impaired absorption of iron. Cimetidine, a potent inhibitor of gastric acid secretion, may also impair the absorption of dietary iron. In the duodenum, as the pH rises, ferric iron is readily converted to insoluble ferric hydroxides. Agents such as ascorbic acid may promote iron absorption by reducing some ferric iron to ferrous iron, which remains soluble at neutral pH. Dietary constituents such as citrate may enhance the solubility of inorganic iron and hence enhance absorption. Phytates, neutral detergent fibers, and other substances present in cereals, grain, and corn impair iron absorption by binding iron as relatively insoluble complexes.

The clinical significance of the various luminal factors that influence iron absorption may be minimal in United States society, where the diet provides relatively large amounts of heme iron. In developing countries, however, diets are generally characterized by low meat content and high content of grains and vegetables. Such diets, with low heme iron content and high content of substances that impair nonheme iron absorption, may not meet the iron demands of many individuals. The manipulation of dietary iron content by large scale iron supplementation programs has been instituted in both developed and underdeveloped countries. The incidence of iron deficiency in the population is decreased by such programs, but the risks to individuals predisposed to iron loading remain to be determined (Ch. 206).

Entry of iron into the mucosal cell at the brush border has generally been considered a passive phenomenon, but recent studies with samples of normal human duodenal mucosa demonstrated that inhibitors of oxidative phosphorylation and glycolysis inhibit iron uptake. In addition, the uptake of iron from the intestinal lumen appears to be regulated. The uptake of ^{59}Fe by duodenal mucosal cells in iron-deficient individuals exceeds that in normal subjects by two- or three-fold. Although correction of the anemia in iron-deficient subjects by red cell transfusion does not decrease iron uptake, repletion of body iron stores restores the kinetics of iron uptake to normal. Once iron enters the mucosal cell it must be transported to the serosal surface of the intestine, where iron enters the plasma. Iron

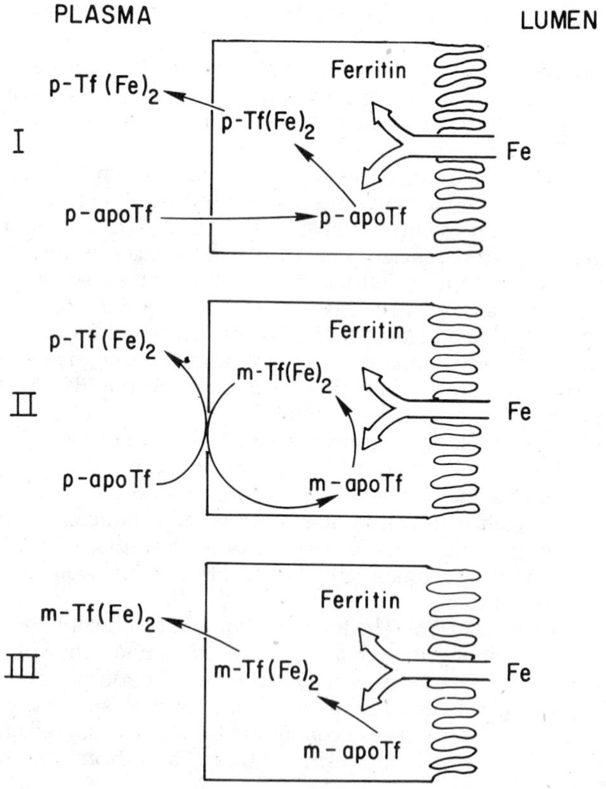

Figure 134–2. Three models for iron transport from the intestinal lumen into the plasma. (I) Plasma apotransferrin (P-apoTf) enters the mucosal cell on the serosal side, binds ferric iron, and then returns to the plasma as diferric transferrin (P-Tf$(Fe)_2$). (II) Ferric iron is bound by a specific mucosal apotransferrin (m-apoTf), becoming mucosal diferric transferrin (m-Tf$(Fe)_2$). The ferric iron is transferred to P-apoTf at the cell membrane. (III) Ferric iron is bound by m-apoTf. M-Tf$(Fe)_2$ then exits the mucosal cell on the serosal side and is subsequently used for iron transport throughout the body. In all three models, iron absorbed from the intestinal lumen may be diverted to ferritin. (From Ward JH et al: *In* Fairbanks VF [ed.]: Current Hematology and Oncology. Vol. 3. New York, John Wiley & Sons, 1984, p 5.)

within the mucosal cell can have two fates. One is to be incorporated into ferritin within the cytosol of the mucosal cell. Most ferritin iron does not ultimately reach the plasma but is lost from the body when the intestinal mucosal cell is sloughed after its three- to four-day life span. Iron not incorporated into mucosal cell ferritin is transported across the cell and ultimately appears in plasma as ferric iron bound to transferrin. A transferrin has been identified within the cytosol of mucosal cells and may serve as a "shuttle protein" transporting iron within the cell. The process of intracellular transport has not been precisely defined, but various models have been suggested that are compatible with available experimental evidence (Fig. 134–2). In all models, iron, once within the cell and oxidized to the ferric state, is directed to either transferrin or ferritin. The transferrin is either synthesized by the mucosal cell or transferred into the mucosal cell from the plasma. Iron then leaves the cell bound to transferrin. Although transferrin appears to play a central role in iron absorption, other mechanisms must also be available, because the rare patients with congenital atransferrinemia show no evidence of deficient absorption.

TRANSPORT. Transferrin, the iron transport protein in plasma, is a glycoprotein with an approximate molecular weight of 80,000. The liver is the major source of transferrin synthesis and the protein is equally distributed in the intravascular and extravascular spaces. Transferrin is capable of binding two iron atoms in the ferric state. In normal subjects the plasma concentration of transferrin is about 2.5 to 3.0 grams per liter. Plasma transferrin is usually quantified in terms of the amount of iron it will bind, a measure called the *total iron-binding capacity* (TIBC). In normal subjects only about one third of the available transferrin binding sites are occupied (TIBC = 33 per cent). Although there is a diurnal variation in plasma iron concentration, with the highest values in the morning and the lowest in the evening, no diurnal variation occurs in the TIBC. Although a number of genetically determined electrophoretic variants of transferrin have been demonstrated, all subtypes appear to function normally as iron transport proteins.

Transferrin has no known function other than as a transport protein and is reused for many cycles of iron transport. With the exception of very small amounts of iron in ferritin, all the iron in plasma is carried by transferrin. The affinity of transferrin for iron is sufficiently high that, theoretically, less than one free iron atom might be present in a liter of blood.

Significant physiochemical differences exist between the two iron-binding sites of transferrin when iron uptake and release are studied in vitro. In spite of these differences the two iron-binding sites function equivalently in the delivery of iron to cells in vivo. The two iron-binding sites are located on separate "halves" of the molecule but about 40 per cent of the amino acid sequence in the two halves is identical. This homology lends credence to the theory that transferrin arose from a duplication of a gene for an antecedent iron transport protein with a single iron-binding site. The evolutionary advantage of the doubled structure may be the reduction of losses in the glomerular filtrate.

CELLULAR UPTAKE. The initial event in the transfer of iron to cells is binding of diferric transferrin to specific, high affinity receptors on the cell surface. When receptors are lost because of cell maturation (as occurs in developing erythrocytes in vivo) or artificial manipulations in vitro, the ability of the cell to take up iron from transferrin is lost. The transferrin receptor, in most cells studied, exists as a dimer with a subunit molecular weight of about 90,000. As cellular iron uptake is directly proportional to the number of transferrin cell surface receptors, it follows that cells with a high iron demand should have large numbers of receptors. The biosynthesis of hemoglobin by erythroid cells has a high iron requirement, and the human reticulocyte may have as many as 300,000 receptors per cell. Developing erythroid cells in the bone marrow may have even more.

In the process of iron uptake by cells the transferrin recep-

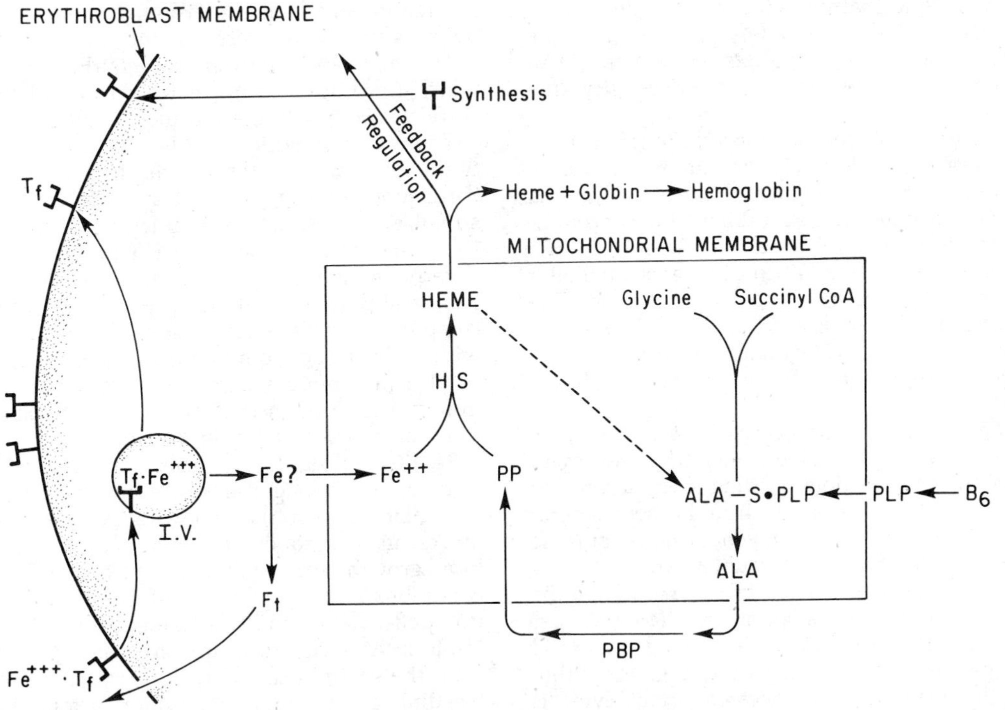

Figure 134–3. Diagrammatic representation of heme biosynthesis within the erythroblast. The relationships between the iron pathway, the porphyrin biosynthetic pathway, the vitamin B_6 pathway, and the synthesis of transferrin receptors are illustrated. The biosynthesis of porphyrins is dependent upon the availability of pyridoxal phosphate as a cofactor at the rate limiting Δ-aminolevulinic acid synthase step. The biosynthesis of heme requires both protoporphyrin and iron. Iron uptake is dependent upon the interaction of diferric transferrin with high affinity cell surface receptors. Receptor synthesis is regulated by heme; when heme synthesis is impaired, more receptors are synthesized and the cell takes up more iron. T_f represents transferrin, ⊤ receptors for diferric T_f, I.V. the acidic, nonlysosomal intermediate vesicle, Fe^{+++} ferrous iron, PP protoporphyrin, PBP porphyrin biosynthetic pathway, ALA Δ-aminolevulinic acid, ALA-s Δ-aminolevulinic acid synthase, PLP pyridoxal-5′ -phosphate, and B_6 vitamin B_6.

tor–diferric transferrin complex is internalized into an acidic, nonlysosomal vesicle (Fig. 134–3). At the acidic pH of the vesicle, iron is readily dissociated from diferric transferrin but the resulting apotransferrin remains bound to the receptor. The transferrin receptor–apotransferrin complex is transported back to the cell surface where, at neutral pH, the apotransferrin is liberated and becomes available for another cycle of iron binding and release.

Once iron enters the cell, two events occur. One is the delivery of iron to the mitochondria, where it is enzymatically incorporated into protoporphyrin to form heme. The other is the incorporation of iron into ferritin, a compound that may function as an intermediate or as an iron storage compound.

STORAGE. Iron-free apoferritin is a spherical protein made up of 24 subunits that surround a central cavity. The central cavity of each apoferritin molecule can potentially store more than 4000 molecules of iron. When iron is present in the central cavity, the protein is termed ferritin. The importance of ferritin as an iron storage compound is emphasized by the wide distribution of structurally similar ferritins in both plant and animal tissues.

A number of isoferritins with differing isoelectric points have been demonstrated. Two different ferritin subunits exist, termed H (the major subunit of heart ferritin) and L (the major subunit of liver ferritin). These may be present in differing quantities within a given ferritin molecule leading to heterogeneity. It appears that the H and L subunits are derived from different genetic loci.

Ferritin meets the requirement of cells for an efficient form of iron storage. It has a large capacity to store iron, maintains a reserve storage capacity (few ferritin molecules are iron-replete), and can quickly both take up and release iron. Thus, within the cell, ferritin may function as a stable iron reservoir or a short-term intermediate in intracellular iron transport. Ferritin aggregates are visible by light microscopy in developing erythroid cells when bone marrow smears are stained with Prussian blue. These "siderotic granules" are found in the cytosol of normal developing erythroblasts and are absent in erythroblasts obtained from subjects with iron deficiency anemia.

Small amounts of iron-poor ferritin (mostly apoferritin) circulate in plasma and can be accurately measured by a widely available radioimmunoassay. The origin and function of plasma ferritin is unknown, but under most conditions the concentration of ferritin in the plasma correlates directly with body iron stores. Normal values range from 12 to 325 ng per milliliter with a mean of about 125 for men and 55 for women. The concentration of ferritin in iron-deficient individuals is less than 10 ng per milliliter, whereas in individuals with iron overload the concentration is proportional to the increase in tissue storage iron.

Hemosiderin is an insoluble iron aggregate with a ratio of iron to protein that is high. It is derived from ferritin; however, the precise nature of the reactions leading from ferritin to hemosiderin have not been resolved. Iron in hemosiderin disappears from tissues after repeated venesections, but the mechanism by which iron is mobilized is unknown.

THE MACROPHAGE. While net iron uptake occurs through the intestinal mucosa, most transferrin-bound iron (over 95 per cent) reflects iron recycled from damaged or aged red blood cells by macrophages in the spleen and other organs. Within the macrophage the membrane of ingested erythrocytes is disrupted and the iron in hemoglobin is oxidized to the trivalent state, forming methemoglobin. The heme and globin are dissociated and the iron liberated from hemin (ferric-protoporphyrin) by the microsomal enzyme heme oxygenase, yielding iron and biliverdin. In order to meet a variable demand for iron, macrophages maintain a storage pool in ferritin and hemosiderin. Under normal conditions the amount of iron entering the macrophage approximates that leaving and there is little interchange between iron newly liberated from hemin and iron in the storage pool. Iron from recently destroyed erythrocytes passes quickly through the macrophage and appears in the plasma bound to transferrin.

When the red cell mass is expanding and erythrocytes are being produced more rapidly than they are being destroyed (e.g., following an acute hemorrhage), iron is mobilized from macrophages. The amount of iron leaving the macrophage under these conditions exceeds that entering. When red cell destruction exceeds production (e.g., in aplastic anemia), the amount of iron entering the macrophage exceeds that leaving and iron is deposited in stores. The control mechanism coupling the rate at which iron leaves the macrophage to the rate of erythrocyte production is unknown. Mobilization of iron from the storage pool is interfered with by infection, inflammation, and malignancy; such interference may be responsible for the anemia associated with chronic disease.

FERROKINETICS. Ferrokinetic studies, based on tracking ^{59}Fe as it moves from the plasma transferrin to the bone marrow and into circulating erythrocytes, make it possible to assess rates of both effective erythropoiesis and ineffective erythropoiesis. The term *ineffective erythropoiesis* refers to the production of defective erythrocytes that are destroyed before they leave the marrow (or very shortly thereafter). A small proportion of erythropoiesis is ineffective even in normal subjects, but in conditions such as megaloblastic anemia, thalassemia, and sideroblastic anemias, ineffective erythropoieses becomes greatly exaggerated. The plasma ^{59}Fe disappearance, expressed as the half-life ($t\frac{1}{2}$), is normally between 60 and 120 minutes. More rapid disappearance (a shorter $t\frac{1}{2}$) is found in iron deficiency and conditions with accelerated erythropoieses (such as polycythemia and hemolytic anemias). A long $t\frac{1}{2}$ indicates erythroid hypoplasia. The *plasma iron transport rate* (PIT) is a measure of the rate at which iron leaves the plasma. The PIT is a good index of total erythropoiesis, whether effective or ineffective. The PIT correlates well with the total nucleated red cell mass and the rate of red cell production. However, when erythropoiesis is reduced, or when the degree of transferrin saturation is high, the interpretation of the PIT is complicated by transfer of iron to tissues other than marrow.

The *erythrocyte iron turnover rate* (EIT) measures the rate at which iron moves from marrow to circulating red cells, and correlates well with the reticulocyte index.

The *marrow transit time* (MTT) evaluates the responsiveness of the marrow to erythropoietin. In general there is an inverse correlation between the MTT and the degree of erythropoietic stimulation. In situations characterized by an appropriate marrow response to anemia the MTT may be less than 24 hours.

Ferrokinetic measurements are useful for clinical and investigational purposes but are only approximations. Sophisticated computer analysis of plasma iron disappearance curves coupled with body surface counting over the liver, spleen, and sacrum may yield a more accurate assessment of the rates at which iron moves through the iron cycle, but such analyses are not routinely employed for clinical purposes.

PATHOGENESIS. Iron deficiency comes about as a late manifestation of prolonged negative iron balance caused by one or a combination of the following factors: inadequate dietary intake, malabsorption, blood loss, repeated pregnancies, and rapid growth during childhood. As daily iron loss under normal conditions is very small (about 1 mg), assigning the cause of iron deficiency in adults to inadequate intake or malabsorption implies chronicity measured in years. Iron losses that occur from the gastrointestinal tract or through excessive menstrual bleeding are far more important factors. Factors leading to negative iron balance can be divided into two broad categories: decreased iron uptake and increased iron loss (Table 134–4).

Decreased Iron Uptake. The daily dietary iron requirement for healthy adult men is about 5 to 10 mg. For premenopausal women the daily dietary requirement is higher, roughly 7 to 20 mg daily. In the United States the average diet contains about 6 mg per 1000 calories. The average man therefore consumes more iron than needed but many women subsist on

TABLE 134–4. FACTORS PRODUCING NEGATIVE IRON BALANCE AND IRON DEFICIENCY

I. Decreased iron uptake
  A. Inadequate diet
  B. Impaired absorption
    1. Achlorhydria
    2. Gastric surgery
    3. Celiac disease
    4. Pica
II. Increased iron loss
  A. Gastrointestinal bleeding (Ch. 113)
    1. Neoplasm
    2. Duodenal and gastric ulcers
    3. Hiatal hernia
    4. Gastritis from salicylates, other drugs, or toxins
    5. Diverticulosis
    6. Ulcerative colitis and regional enteritis
    7. Hookworm
    8. Meckel's diverticulum
    9. Hemorrhoids
    10. Arteriovenous malformations
  B. Menometrorrhagia
  C. Repeated blood donations
  D. Repeated pregnancies
  E. Hemoglobinuria due to chronic intravascular hemolysis
  F. Hereditary hemorrhagic telangiectasia
  G. Idiopathic pulmonary hemosiderosis
  H. Disorders of hemostasis

a marginal iron uptake. Because of the adequacy of their diets and their larger iron stores, males in the United States rarely develop iron deficiency solely on the basis of an inadequate dietary intake of iron. Even in women some factor in addition to poor diet is usually necessary before overt anemia develops.

Gastric acid facilitates the absorption of ferric iron in the diet (although it has little effect on heme iron or ferrous iron), and iron deficiency is a frequent complication following gastric operations. Additional factors that impair iron absorption after gastrectomy include rapid intestinal transit and bypass of the most active sites of iron absorption in the duodenum (as occurs in the Billroth II or Polya procedures). Malabsorption of iron may also occur in patients with adult celiac disease, and rarely iron deficiency anemia may be the dominant manifestation of celiac disease.

Impaired absorption of iron because of interactions with food substances such as phytates and vegetable fibers has been discussed. The ingestion of unusual substances, a practice known as *pica,* may also impair iron absorption. Although pica may be a manifestation of iron deficiency, in certain cultural groups the compulsive ingestion of substances such as clay (geophagia) or starch (amylophagia) may lead to iron deficiency. In the United States the practice appears to be most common in black women in the southern states. Clay interferes with iron absorption by acting in the gut as an ion exchange resin. Laundry starch is a carbohydrate with a very low iron content. When it is consumed in large quantities to the exclusion of other foods, a dietary deficiency of iron results.

Increased Iron Loss. Gastrointestinal bleeding is by far the most common cause of iron deficiency in men and is second only to menstrual loss as a cause in women. Repeated pregnancies without iron supplementation are a less common cause of iron deficiency in women.

Although any hemorrhagic lesion of the gastrointestinal tract may cause iron deficiency (Table 134–4), those most likely to do so are associated with chronic occult bleeding and the steady loss of small amounts of blood. In order to estimate the effect of blood loss on iron balance it is convenient to consider that 1.0 ml of blood contains about 0.4 mg iron. A steady blood loss of as little as 4 to 5 ml per day (1.6 to 2.0 mg iron) can result in negative iron balance and depletion of iron stores over several years. *Iron deficiency in men and in postmenopausal women must be considered to result from blood loss unless some other cause can be proven.* This is a critical dictum because iron deficiency anemia may be the first sign of a cancer of the gastrointestinal tract and the anemia may lead to the diagnosis when the tumor is in an operable stage. Carcinoma of the cecum, for example, is often clinically silent until the symptoms of anemia appear.

Blood loss from erosive gastritis due to aspirin ingestion is becoming an increasingly frequent cause of iron deficiency. Chronic ingestion of as few as two aspirin tablets daily may lead to blood loss of up to 4.5 ml per day.

CLINICAL MANIFESTATIONS. Iron deficiency anemia is not a disease; it is a sign of disease. In some patients, iron deficiency anemia is discovered incidentally when the presenting signs and symptoms are those of the disease that led to the deficiency. In some patients signs and symptoms of both the underlying disease and the iron deficiency are found together. In others only the symptoms of iron deficiency are present and the disease leading to the deficiency is occult.

The onset of iron deficiency anemia is insidious and the progression of symptoms is gradual. Patients are often able to accommodate quite well to the anemia and may continue to perform strenuous work with few symptoms. Fatigue, irritability, palpitations, dizziness, breathlessness, and headache are all common complaints of symptomatic individuals with anemia of any type and do not in themselves suggest iron deficiency as the cause of the anemia. However, some clinical findings do specifically suggest the presence of iron deficiency.

Chlorosis, a peculiar greenish pallor of iron-deficient adolescent girls, was frequently described in the decades between 1890 and 1910, although now is rarely noted. Oral lesions associated with iron deficiency include angular stomatitis (ulcerations or fissures at the corners of the mouth), atrophy of the lingual papillae, and varying degrees of glossitis. *Ozena* (chronic atrophy of the nasal mucosa associated with a foul-smelling discharge) occurs in some patients with iron deficiency anemia, particularly in southeastern Europe. Thinning and flattening of nails and finally the development of spoon-shaped nails (koilonychia) have been described in patients with advanced iron deficiency.

The association of dysphagia, angular stomatitis, and lingual abnormalities with iron deficiency anemia (Plummer-Vinson or Paterson-Kelly syndrome) is rarely noted in the United States but is quite common in Great Britain and Scandinavia. The dysphagia is due to the development of a mucosal web at the juncture of the hypopharynx and esophagus. Multiple webs may develop, usually extending from the anterior wall of the esophagus into the lumen. Occasionally they may encircle the lumen, forming a cufflike structure. In other patients a stricture with or without a web may be found, drastically constricting the opening into the esophagus at the level of the cricoid cartilage. Relief of the dysphagia requires rupturing of the webs or dilatation of the stenosis, because repletion of the iron stores alone is not effective. Other gastrointestinal complaints such as anorexia, pyrosis, flatulence, nausea, belching, and constipation are common in association with advanced iron deficiency anemia.

Pica, as already mentioned, can be a cause of iron deficiency but it also may be a striking manifestation of iron deficiency. The ingestion of ice (pagophagia) is particularly common. Many patients compulsively eat one or other food items; oddly, the object of the unnatural dietary craving usually contains very little iron.

The spleen is slightly enlarged in about 10 per cent of patients with iron deficiency anemia. There are no specific pathologic changes in the organ and the splenomegaly recedes with correction of the iron deficiency. Neuralgic pains, numbness, and tingling without objective neurologic abnormalities are reported by 15 to 30 per cent of patients and rarely iron deficiency anemia may lead to increased intracranial pressure, papilledema, and the clinical picture of pseudotumor cerebri.

LABORATORY FINDINGS. The degree of anemia is variable and depends upon the duration of iron-limited erythropoiesis. Because of the hypochromia the hemoglobin concentration is usually reduced to a greater degree than the VPRC. The mean corpuscular volume (MCV), mean corpuscular hemoglobin

(MCH), and mean corpuscular hemoglobin concentration (MCHC) are all usually reduced. The degree of change in the red cell indices is related to both the duration and the severity of the anemia. Average values for patients with hemoglobin concentrations of 8 to 9 grams per deciliter are MCV of 74 fl, MCHC 28 grams per deciliter, and MCH of 20 pg.

A well-stained blood smear reveals an increase in the area of central pallor in the individual red corpuscles (hypochromia), microcytes, and marked variations in cell size (anisocytosis) and shape (poikilocytosis) (Fig. 134–4 and color plates 2 and 3). The plasma iron concentration is generally less than 50 μg per deciliter and the total plasma iron-binding capacity (the transferrin concentration) is greater than 350 μg per deciliter. As a result the transferrin saturation is less than 15 per cent. The plasma ferritin concentration is generally less than 10 ng per milliliter. The last enzymatic reaction leading to the biosynthesis of heme (the ferrochelatase or heme synthase reaction) requires both iron and protoporphyrin as substrates. In iron deficiency excess protoporphyrin accumulates in the developing erythrocyte and is retained by the circulating erythrocytes. As a result the free erythrocyte protoporphyrin (FEP) is elevated, generally about five times normal (normal range, 30 to 80 μg per deciliter of red cells). Automated fluorimeters are making the FEP determination available in many routine clinical laboratories.

Both the percentage and the absolute number of reticulocytes are usually normal. The osmotic fragility of the erythrocytes may be normal, but more often there is increased resistance to hemolysis in hypotonic salt solutions. Although the leukocyte count is usually normal, in very chronic iron deficiency a slight decrease in the absolute number of granulocytes may be seen. The platelet count is usually elevated to levels of about two to three times normal and returns to normal after therapy. Rarely, in severe, longstanding iron deficiency anemia, mild thrombocytopenia may be noted.

Examination of the bone marrow is generally not required to establish a diagnosis of iron deficiency anemia. An exception is the clinical situation when suspected iron deficiency coexists with a chronic disease. Although anemias associated with chronic disease may mimic iron deficiency (see below), they can be distinguished by examination of the marrow. In iron deficiency the marrow is usually normocellular and there is mild erythroid hyperplasia. Macrophage iron is absent or severely reduced. Fewer than 10 per cent of the marrow normoblasts contain siderotic granules visible with Prussian blue staining. In the anemia of chronic disease macrophage iron stores are normal or increased; however, as in iron deficiency, very few normoblasts contain siderotic granules.

The sequence of laboratory changes in slowly developing iron deficiency is fairly predictable. Initially, as iron stores are depleted, the serum ferritin concentration falls. At the earliest stage of iron deficiency the transferrin concentration rises, the plasma iron concentration falls, and the FEP increases. When anemia first appears the morphology of the circulating erythrocytes and the erythrocyte indices are generally normal. As the anemia progresses the morphology becomes clearly hypochromic and microcytic and the indices reflect this.

TREATMENT. *Every effort must be made to recognize and if possible correct the underlying cause.* This should be possible in most patients. A simpler goal is correcting the anemia and replenishing body iron stores.

Iron is highly effective in treating iron deficiency but has no other legitimate therapeutic use. Iron exerts no beneficial effect on any of the anemias not caused by iron deficiency. A large number of preparations containing iron have been promoted for the oral treatment of iron deficiency, but none have any advantage over simple ferrous salts (ferrous sulfate, ferrous gluconate, and ferrous fumarate). Ferrous sulfate is the standard preparation for oral use. A daily dose of about 200 mg of elemental iron produces an optimal response. This dose is achieved with three ferrous sulfate tablets (each tablet contains 60 mg of elemental iron) given in divided doses with or just after a meal. Iron is best absorbed when the stomach is empty, but gastric irritation is extremely common when iron is taken this way. In spite of some reduction in absorption when iron is taken with meals, the gain in patient compliance is worth this slight disadvantage. Enteric-coated preparations, designed to reduce gastric irritation by retarding dissolution of the iron, cannot be recommended because with them the most actively absorbing regions of the intestine are bypassed and absorption is markedly reduced. Although large doses of ascorbic or succinic acid will increase iron absorption as much as 20 to 30 per cent, they add greatly to the expense of therapy. Most of the preparations containing iron and ascorbate include very small amounts of ascorbate, and iron–succinic acid preparations are not widely available.

Some patients given oral iron therapy complain of gastrointestinal symptoms (nausea, epigastric pain, cramps, diarrhea); however, it is rare that these symptoms are severe enough to require discontinuation of therapy. Gastric symptoms appear to be dose related and patients intolerant of full therapeutic doses may be able to take a dose of 120 mg per day. Gastric symptoms may be minimized by gradually increasing the dose during the first week of therapy. Regardless of the form of oral therapy used, it is important to continue treatment for 6 to 12 months after the anemia has been corrected. The prolonged therapy allows for repletion of iron stores.

When adequate doses of iron are given, there is often a rapid subjective improvement with a reduction of fatigue, lassitude,

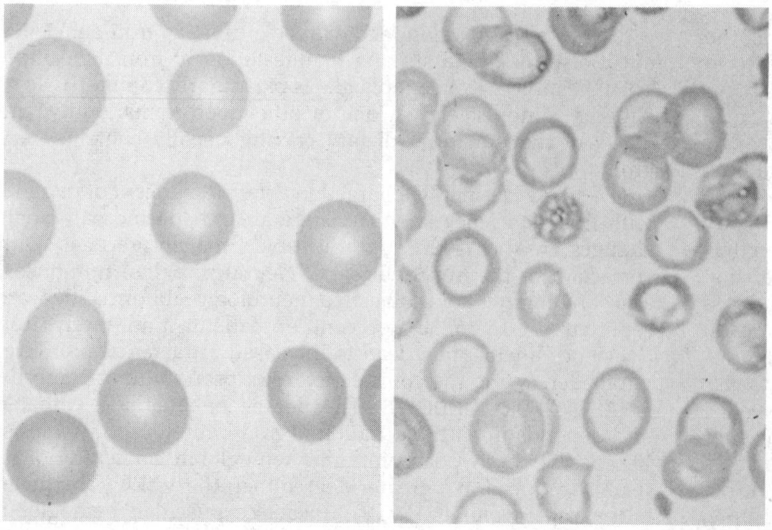

Figure 134–4. Blood smear from a patient with advanced iron deficiency anemia (*right*) and from a normal subject (*left*). The red cells from the iron deficient subject are poorly hemoglobinized (hypochromic), smaller than normal (microcytic), and vary in size and shape (anisocytosis and poikilocytosis). (Wright's stain, × 1000.)

and other nonspecific symptoms. This response may occur within two or three days, before any evidence of a hematologic response can be detected. An increase in the number of reticulocytes is the first sign of hematologic response, and a maximum value of 5 to 10 per cent is usually achieved after about ten days of therapy. The height of the reticulocyte peak and the rate of hemoglobin regeneration are proportional to the severity of the anemia. With only slight to moderate degrees of anemia a pronounced reticulocyte response cannot be expected. Although the hemoglobin concentration increases more rapidly at low levels than at high, it takes about two months to reach normal values regardless of the starting level.

It is not rare to encounter patients said to have iron deficiency anemia unresponsive to oral iron therapy. The following possible explanations for failure to respond to iron should be considered: (1) The diagnosis is incorrect and the anemia is not due to iron deficiency; (2) a complicating illness is present that dampens the expected response to iron therapy; (3) the patient failed to take the iron preparation as prescribed; (4) an ineffective iron preparation was prescribed; (5) the patient is continuing to lose iron in excess of intake; and rarely (6) there is malabsorption of iron.

Parenteral iron therapy should be reserved for patients who (1) are unable to tolerate iron compounds given orally, (2) repeatedly fail to heed instructions or are incapable of following them, (3) are losing blood at a rate too rapid to be compensated by oral iron intake, (4) have a disorder such as ulcerative colitis or regional enteritis in which symptoms may be aggravated by oral iron therapy, or (5) are unable to absorb iron from the gastrointestinal tract.

Iron-dextran complex (Imferon) containing 50 mg of iron per ml is the preparation of choice for parenteral administration. The total dose required to correct the anemia and to replenish stores can be calculated by the following formula:

$$\text{Iron to be injected (mg)} = [15\text{-patient's Hb(g/dl)}] \times \text{body weight (kg)} \times 3.$$

Iron-dextran can be given intramuscularly or intravenously. Intravenous administration does not appear to have a higher incidence of adverse effects than the intramuscular route. Anaphylactic reactions are rare (0.1–0.6 per cent), but fever, arthralgia, myalgia, and regional adenopathy occur in about 5 per cent of patients. Intramuscular injections should be made into the upper outer quadrant of the buttock, and the skin displaced laterally prior to injection to prevent staining of the skin by reflux of the dark-brown iron solution along the injection path. A test dose of 0.5 ml should be given initially to test for hypersensitivity. Generally 2.5 ml are injected into each buttock (total 5 ml or 250 mg of iron) daily. Intravenous administration permits larger doses to be given in a single injection; thus the discomfort and inconvenience of repeated intramuscular injections can be avoided. After testing for hypersensitivity, 10 ml (500 mg of iron) of undiluted iron-dextran may be administered over about a five-minute period. In Great Britain and Europe it is usual to administer the entire dose calculated by the formula in a single intravenous infusion. A 1:20 dilution of iron-dextran in saline is prepared and administered at an initial flow rate of 20 drops per minute. After five minutes, if no side effects are observed, the rate is increased to 40 to 60 drops per minute. Dextrose solutions should not be used as a diluent because the incidence of superficial phlebitis may be as high as 25 per cent with this vehicle.

PROGNOSIS. The prognosis in iron deficiency relates only to the underlying disorder causing the anemia. Patients rarely if ever die of iron deficiency anemia itself, but may die of the underlying cause. Recurrence of iron deficiency anemia after treatment is common, emphasizing the importance of identifying and effectively treating the cause of the iron deficiency.

HYPOCHROMIC ANEMIAS NOT CAUSED BY IRON DEFICIENCY

Once iron deficiency has been excluded as the cause of a hypochromic anemia, a limited number of diagnostic possibilities remain. A presumptive diagnosis is generally possible after analysis of the history and physical examination and the basic hematologic parameters. If the diagnosis remains obscure, a useful approach is to segregate the diagnostic possibilities on the basis of an accurate determination of the serum iron. When the serum iron is reduced to levels at which the transferrin saturation is less than about 15 per cent, only iron deficiency and the anemia of chronic disease need be considered.

Hypochromic anemias due to defects in globin biosynthesis (the thalassemias and hemoglobinopathies characterized by unstable hemoglobins) are discussed in Ch. 141 and 143.

THE ANEMIA OF CHRONIC DISEASE

The anemia of chronic disease is not always hypochromic; however, because of its association with hypoferremia, it is best discussed under the heading of hypochromic anemias. Although the anemia of chronic disease is usually normocytic and normochromic, hypochromia and even microcytosis may be the dominant morphologic abormalities. When microcytosis is present it is usually not as marked as in iron deficiency. The MCV rarely falls below 72 fl.

DEFINITION. A mild to moderate anemia frequently accompanies chronic infections, inflammatory diseases such as rheumatoid arthritis, and cancers. Since these are so common, the anemia of chronic disease is frequently encountered and may be second only to iron deficiency anemia in overall incidence. The anemia of chronic disease is defined by the presence of a chronic disease, anemia, and hypoferremia despite abundant quantities of iron in macrophage stores.

ETIOLOGY AND PATHOGENESIS. Three factors seem to interact in the pathogenesis of the anemia: (1) impaired flow of iron from macrophages to plasma, (2) decreased erythrocyte life span, and (3) inadequate marrow response to the mild hemolysis.

Characteristically, the serum iron is decreased, total iron binding capacity is reduced (a point often useful in differentiating the anemia from iron deficiency anemia), and transferrin saturation is subnormal. Injection of ^{59}Fe-labeled red cells (or labeled hemoglobin) reveals rapid clearance by reticuloendothelial cells but defective reutilization of the iron for new hemoglobin synthesis. In bone marrow aspirates stained for iron there is an increase in hemosiderin and ferritin in the macrophages; however, the number of red cell precursors containing siderotic granules is reduced. A decrease in the amount of iron available for heme biosynthesis results in the production of hypochromic erythrocytes and, as in iron deficiency, an increase in free erythrocyte protoporphyrin (FEP) to levels of three to five times normal. In contrast to iron deficiency anemia the FEP increases slowly and does not become clearly abnormal until significant anemia has developed. A humoral factor has been implicated in the pathogenesis of the abnormal iron metabolism. This factor, termed *leukocyte endogenous mediator* (LEM), is released from neutrophils and macrophages during phagocytosis or after stimulation by bacterial toxins. LEM is a low molecular weight protein that, when injected into experimental animals, produces the abnormalities of iron metabolism that characterize the anemia of chronic disease.

The erythrocyte life span is about 80 days rather than the normal 120 days. When red cells from a patient with the anemia of chronic disease are transfused into normal subjects they survive normally. Conversely, normal red cells have a shortened survival when transfused into patients with anemia. This suggests that an extracorpuscular factor is involved in the pathogenesis of the hemolysis. However, no such factor has yet been identified. Normally the bone marrow should be able to compensate for such a modest reduction in erythrocyte survival. Failure of the marrow to do so implies that impaired production capacity is important in the pathogenesis of the anemia. The marrow response to anemia is under the control of erythropoietin. In patients with the anemia of chronic disorders erythropoietin levels are usually lower than expected for the degree of anemia. The marrow, however, is capable of responding appropriately to erythropoietin when the hormone is injected or when erythropoietin production is stimulated by hypoxia or cobalt administration. The precise mechanism causing failure of erythropoietin release in response to the slowly developing anemia is unknown.

The three basic abnormalities are inter-related in the pathogenesis of the anemia. For example, the response to erythropoietin suggests that the hormone directly or indirectly affects the block in iron metabolism. It appears that balance is eventually reached between the three factors and thus the anemia is only mild to moderate and does not generally progress to the point at which transfusion therapy is required.

CLINICAL MANIFESTATIONS. Because this type of anemia occurs in association with so many diseases, the clinical manifestations vary widely. Although the signs and symptoms of the underlying disorder usually overshadow those of the anemia, in occasional patients the anemia is the first sign of the underlying disease.

DIAGNOSIS. The anemia develops during the first few months of the underlying illness and rarely progresses thereafter. The VPRC generally remains constant in a range between 25 and 40 per cent. The red cell morphology is usually normal as is the reticulocyte count. The characteristic iron determinations are a transferrin saturation less than 15 per cent with a normal serum ferritin. In the marrow there is a decrease in the number of erythroid precursors containing cytoplasmic iron granules (sideroblasts), but reticuloendothelial cells contain normal or increased iron stores. Despite the hemolysis, the usual manifestations of increased blood destruction are absent. The serum bilirubin and the excretion of urobilinogen are generally normal.

TREATMENT. Correction of the anemia depends upon successful treatment of the underlying disease. Blood transfusions are not usually necessary because the anemia is generally mild to moderate and is not progressive. Therapy with cobalt, androgenic steroids, and corticosteroids offers more potential for harm than good. The block to iron flow cannot be bypassed and the administration of oral or parenteral iron is of no benefit. When bleeding causes superimposed iron deficiency, the administration of iron will restore hemoglobin levels to those of the underlying chronic disorder but not back to normal.

SIDEROBLASTIC ANEMIA

DEFINITION. When hypochromic anemia is associated with hyperferremia and an increased transferrin saturation, a diagnosis of sideroblastic anemia is suggested. The sideroblastic anemias are a heterogeneous group of disorders associated with various defects in the porphyrin biosynthetic pathway. Porphyrin biosynthetic defects lead to diminished synthesis of heme, which in turn may be associated with an increase in cellular iron uptake (Fig. 134–3). The sideroblastic anemias are characterized by the association of anemia with the presence of an abnormal erythroid precursor in the marrow. The abnormal precursor, the ringed sideroblast, is a normoblast containing excessive deposits of iron within mitochondria. These iron laden mitochondria, because of their perinuclear distribution, account for the Prussian blue–positive granules forming a full or partial ring around the nucleus of the ringed sideroblast (Fig. 134–5). Normal sideroblasts contain one to four Prussian blue–positive ferritin aggregates in the cytoplasm and no visible iron in mitochondria.

PATHOGENESIS AND CLASSIFICATION. Mitochondrial iron excess appears to be a consequence of defective heme synthesis. A population of hypochromic erythrocytes, common to all the sideroblastic anemias, is morphologic evidence of the synthetic defect. Other common characteristics include abnormalities in

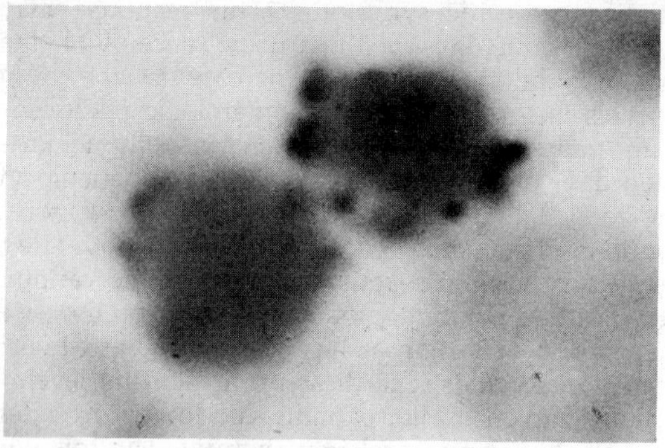

Figure 134–5. Ringed sideroblasts in an iron stain of bone marrow from a patient with idiopathic refractory sideroblastic anemia. The dark granules arranged around the nucleus of the normoblasts represent iron-laden mitochondria. (Prussian blue stain, × 1000.)

porphyrin biosynthesis; an increase in total body iron stores; an increase in the serum iron concentration, often to the point of complete saturation of transferrin; and kinetic evidence of ineffective erythropoiesis. It is customary to divide the sideroblastic anemias into two groups depending on whether the disorder appears to be acquired or inherited (Table 134–2).

Acquired Sideroblastic Anemias

IDIOPATHIC REFRACTORY SIDEROBLASTIC ANEMIA. This acquired disease of older adults has an unknown pathogenesis. The anemia develops insidiously and is often discovered during a routine examination. The anemia is usually slightly macrocytic. Examination of the peripheral blood smear reveals two populations of erythrocytes. One is entirely normal and the other is macrocytic and quite hypochromic with prominent basophilic stippling. Leukocyte and platelet counts are usually normal but leukopenia is occasionally noted and either moderate thrombocytopenia or thrombocytosis has been reported. Free erythrocyte protoporphyrin (FEP) is increased but the precise enzymatic defect(s) in porphyrin biosynthesis has not been defined. About 30 to 40 per cent of patients have a palpable spleen. Therapy with pyridoxine or folic acid is not successful and only rare patients respond to androgens. The median survival for patients with idiopathic refractory sideroblastic anemia is about ten years; most patients require no therapy. Transfusion therapy should be kept to a minimum because the chronic administration of erythrocytes has led to transfusional hemochromatosis. Therapy with daily subcutaneous infusions of deferoxamine may be of value to selected patients who require repeated transfusion. The condition in about 10 per cent of patients eventually shows evidence of transformation to acute leukemia.

SIDEROBLASTIC ANEMIA COMPLICATING OTHER DISEASES. Acquired sideroblastic anemia associated with other diseases and with drugs or toxins is quite common; however, the anemia is usually only mild. Inflammatory diseases such as rheumatoid arthritis, neoplasms, and a variety of primary hematologic disorders have all been associated with a secondary sideroblastic anemia. The treatment, course, and prognosis are all related to the nature of the associated disease.

SIDEROBLASTIC ANEMIA ASSOCIATED WITH DRUGS OR TOXINS. Sideroblastic anemia is a common complication in hospitalized alcoholics. Withdrawal of alcohol results in a reticulocytosis and disappearance of the ringed sideroblasts within five to ten days. *Alcohol* may cause sideroblastic anemia by interfering with pyridoxine metabolism and thus indirectly affecting the activity of Δ-aminolevulinic acid synthetase, the rate-limiting enzyme in the porphyrin biosynthetic pathway. This mechanism likely also underlies the sideroblastic anemia occasionally seen in association with the administration of the antituberculous agent *isonicotinic acid hydrazide* (INH). The sideroblastic anemia that occurs in *lead poisoning* is caused by the inhibition by lead of the enzyme that converts Δ-aminolevulinic acid to porphobilinogen (Δ-aminolevulinic dehydratase) and the enzyme heme synthetase (ferrochelatase). As a result of these two enzymatic defects it is possible to screen for lead poisoning by detecting either increased urinary excretion of Δ-aminolevulinic acid or a markedly increased FEP.

Hereditary Sideroblastic Anemias

Hereditary sideroblastic anemia is almost always a disease of males and is most likely inherited as an X-linked recessive trait. Although the anemia is usually detected in the late teenage years, in rare cases the anemia is found first in either infancy or adult life. The anemia is severe (average blood hemoglobin 6.5 grams per deciliter) and the red cell indices indicate marked microcytosis and hypochromia. The inherited defect in some way involves the interaction between Δ-aminolevulinic acid synthetase and its cofactor pyridoxal phosphate. Individuals with hereditary sideroblastic anemia are not pyridoxine deficient; however, large amounts of vitamin B_6 produce partial correction of the anemia.

Beutler E, Fairbanks VF: The effects of iron deficiency. *In* Jacobs A, Worwood M (eds.): Iron in Biochemistry and Medicine II. New York, Academic Press, 1980, pp 394–428. *An extensive review of both the hematologic and nonhematologic manifestations of iron deficiency.*

Jacobs A (ed.): Disorders of iron metabolism. Clin Hematol 11:1, 1982. *A collection of review articles covering basic physiology, clinical diagnosis, and patient management of iron deficiency, sideroblastic anemias, and iron overload.*

Kushner J, Cartwright GE: The sideroblastic anemias. *In* Advances in Internal Medicine. Vol 22. Chicago, Year Book Medical Publishers, 1976, pp 229–250. *A review of both clinical and experimental studies.*

Miescher PA, Jaffe ER, Finch CA (eds.): Semin Hematol 19:1, 1984. *An issue of a respected review journal devoted to the clinical aspects of iron deficiency and excess.*

Ward JH, Kushner JP, Kaplan J: Iron: Metabolism and Clinical Disorders. *In* Fairbanks VF (ed.): Current Hematology and Oncology. Vol 3. New York, John Wiley & Sons, 1984, pp 1–50. *An up-to-date review of basic iron metabolism with an extensive list of recent references.*

Williams WJ, Beutler E, Erslev AJ, Lichtman MA (eds.): Hematology. 3rd ed. New York, McGraw-Hill Book Company, 1983. *A comprehensive textbook of hematology with an excellent presentation of basic iron metabolism and its application to clinical medicine.*

Wintrobe MM, Lee GR, Boggs DR, et al. (eds.): Clinical Hematology. 8th ed. Philadelphia, Lea & Febiger, 1981. *The oldest standard textbook of hematology with an exhaustive description of the clinical manifestations of iron deficiency anemia.*

135. MEGALOBLASTIC ANEMIAS

William S. Beck

DEFINITION. Megaloblastic anemia (often a pancytopenia) is due to impaired DNA synthesis and is manifested by a readily recognized pattern of morphologic changes in bone marrow and blood cells that include giantism of these cells—and indeed of all proliferating cells in most cases—and various evidences of retarded cell division. The anemia is ordinarily macrocytic—i.e., the mean corpuscular volume (MCV) exceeds 100 cu μm—although not all macrocytic anemias are megaloblastic.

ETIOLOGY. Megaloblastic anemia is easily diagnosed in most cases. However, the differential diagnosis of the underlying disorder may be more difficult because defective DNA synthesis can have many causes. It is convenient to divide the megaloblastic anemias into three major etiologic categories: (1) those that are associated with vitamin B_{12} (cobalamin) deficiency and respond to vitamin B_{12} therapy, (2) those that are associated with folate deficiency and respond to folic acid (pteroylmonoglutamate) therapy, and (3) those unresponsive to vitamin B_{12} or folic acid therapy. Deficiencies of vitamin B_{12} and folate may themselves have a great many specific causes. Pernicious anemia, for example, is but one cause of vitamin B_{12} deficiency. Accurate differential diagnosis is important because it guides the choice of therapy and usually discloses a significant underlying disorder.

The major etiologic categories and their underlying causes are summarized in Table 135–1. Vitamin B_{12} deficiency and folate deficiency are by far the most common categories. Together with iron deficiency anemia they constitute the bulk of the so-called nutritional anemias, which are among the most common of human ills. Both vitamin deficiencies lead to tissue coenzyme deficiencies that are usually corrected easily by repletion of the lacking vitamin. Hematopoiesis then reverts from megaloblastic to normoblastic. Other mechanisms obviously account for the megaloblastic anemias that are unresponsive to therapy with vitamin B_{12} and folic acid.

The approach to a patient suspected of megaloblastic anemia should proceed through several orderly steps. First, it is determined from the reticulocyte count and other tests whether a macrocytic anemia is due to bone marrow failure or erythrocyte loss or destruction. If marrow failure, the presence of megalo-

TABLE 135–1. ETIOLOGIC CLASSIFICATION OF THE MEGALOBLASTIC ANEMIAS

Category	Etiologic Mechanisms
I. *Vitamin B_{12}* deficiency	
A. Decreased ingestion	Poor diet, lack of animal products, strict vegetarianism
B. Impaired absorption	1. Intrinsic factor deficiency Pernicious anemia Gastrectomy (total and partial) Destruction of gastric mucosa by caustics Anti-IF antibody in gastric juice Abnormal intrinsic factor molecule 2. Intrinsic intestinal disease Familial selective malabsorption (Imerslund's syndrome) Ileal resection, ileitis Sprue, celiac disease Infiltrative intestinal disease (e.g., lymphoma, scleroderma) Drug-induced malabsorption 3. Competitive parasites Fish tapeworm infestations (*Diphyllobothrium latum)* Bacteria in diverticula of bowel, blind loops 4. Chronic pancreatic disease
C. Increased requirement	Pregnancy Neoplastic disease Hyperthyroidism
D. Impaired utilization	Enzyme deficiencies Abnormal serum vitamin B_{12} binding protein Lack of transcobalamin II Nitrous oxide administration
II. *Folate deficiency*	
A. Decreased ingestion	Poor diet, lack of vegetables Alcoholism Infancy
B. Impaired absorption	Intestinal short circuits Steatorrhea Sprue, celiac disease Intrinsic intestinal disease Anticonvulsants, oral contraceptives, other drugs
C. Increased requirement	Pregnancy, infancy Hyperthyroidism Hyperactive hematopoiesis Neoplastic disease, exfoliative skin disease
D. Impaired utilization	Folic acid antagonists: methotrexate, triamterene, trimethoprim Enzyme deficiencies
E. Increased loss	Hemodialysis
III. *Unresponsive to vitamin B_{12} or folate therapy*	1. Metabolic inhibitors Purine synthesis: 6-mercaptopurine, 6-thioguanine, azathioprine Pyrimidine synthesis: 6-azauridine Thymidylate synthesis: 5-fluorouracil Deoxyribonucleotide synthesis: hydroxyurea, cytosine arabinoside, severe iron deficiency 2. Inborn errors Lesch-Nyhan syndrome Hereditary orotic aciduria Deficiency of formininotransferase, methyltransferase, etc. 3. Unexplained disorders Pyridoxine-responsive megaloblastic anemia Thiamine-responsive megaloblastic anemia Erythremic myelosis (Di Guglielmo's syndrome)

blastosis is established by demonstrating in blood and bone marrow the characteristic morphologic features to be described below. The broad etiologic category is then elucidated with serum vitamin assays and other procedures to be discussed. One then seeks a specific causal mechanism, administers specific treatment, and observes the response to treatment.

PATHOGENESIS AND PATHOLOGY OF MEGALOBLASTIC ANEMIA. The following discussion deals with the general features of megaloblastic anemia per se, irrespective of cause. The features of vitamin B_{12} and folate deficiency, irrespective of cause, and the major disorders responsible for these deficiencies will then be discussed.

Mechanism of Megaloblastosis. Megaloblasts contain a substantially increased amount of RNA and a normal or slightly increased amount of DNA per cell, the former presumably accounting for the cytoplasmic basophilia (blue color) in Wright's-stained smears. Tritiated thymidine is readily incorporated into the DNA of megaloblasts. Hence, DNA synthesis can occur. There is, however, impairment of a critical step in the pathway of DNA synthesis—the synthesis of thymidylate (dTMP). In addition, there is a sharp increase in intracellular dUMP and dUTP levels and thus of the dUTP/dTTP ratio. As a result there is significant misincorporation of uracil into DNA. Much of this uracil is removed by an "editorial" enzyme system, but lack of available dTTP blocks final DNA repair. Hence, DNA is fragmented and DNA replication and cell division are blocked, while synthesis of RNA and protein proceed normally. Prolongation of this state results in permanent loss of the capacity for cell division and eventual cell death. In megaloblastic bone marrow the degree of impairment of DNA synthesis varies from cell to cell and from cell series to cell series. Usually, it is more severe among erythrocyte precursors than granulocyte percursors.

Morphology of Megaloblastic Cells. (Color plate 2*F*.) The features characteristic of the megaloblastic state are seen most vividly in the Wright's-stained smear of aspirated bone marrow. Among *erythrocyte precursors* megaloblastic changes occur at all stages of development. They are larger than corresponding cells of the normoblastic series and often have a higher than normal ratio of cytoplasmic area to nuclear area. Promegaloblasts, the most immature of the series and the most easily recognized, display brilliantly colored, deeply basophilic (blue), granule-free cytoplasm and lavender-tinted chromatin with a distinctive open and fine-grained texture that contrasts with strand-like pronormoblast chromatin. As the cell matures, the chromatin retains its odd texture and is slow to form coarse deeply basophilic clumps. Development of a dense pyknotic nucleus like that of an orthochromatic normoblast either fails to occur or is delayed. With the appearance of hemoglobin, the apparent maturity of the cytoplasm contrasts sharply with the apparent immaturity of the nucleus—a feature termed *nuclear-cytoplasmic asynchronism* or *dissociation*. All of these changes are less well developed in mild or incipient megaloblastic anemias, or in megaloblastic anemias associated with iron deficiency.

Granulocyte precursors may also display nuclear-cytoplasmic asynchronism and enlargement, most strikingly at the metamyelocyte stage. A "giant metamyelocyte" has ragged chromatin and a relatively large nucleus, sometimes of bizarre shape, that takes stain poorly and may be pinched off in several places, in anticipation perhaps of later hypersegmentation.

The *bone marrow* is extremely cellular, especially when anemia is severe. Megaloblastic changes may be seen in all cell lines, although major changes may be limited to the erythroid cells. Many mitotic figures (i.e., cells in metaphase) are found among them. The myeloid to erythroid ratio typically falls from 3 to about 1. Megaloblastic granulopoiesis is more evident in infection, in which increased granulocyte production has been stimulated. Unless iron deficiency is present, iron in reticulum cells is increased.

In the *blood*, erythrocytes display striking variations in size and shape and are normochromic (unless iron deficiency coexists) and macrocytic, with MCVs ranging from 100 to more than 140 cu μm. Macro-ovalocytes, large oval-shaped erythrocytes up to 14 μm in diameter, are usually present (Color plate 2*E*). The reticulocyte count is often lower than normal, both in absolute and relative (percentage) terms. Erythrocyte changes become more severe as the anemia worsens. When the hematocrit is low (<20 per cent), nucleated red cells may appear in the blood.

Many neutrophils have more than four segments; occasionally some have up to 16 segments. Hypersegmented neutrophils, or macropolycytes, may be quite large. This is a significant finding, because it is not masked by coexisting iron deficiency and in folate deficiency tends to occur before bone marrow cells are overtly megaloblastic. Hypersegmentation is probably due to abnormalities of nuclear division and chromatin.

Megaloblastosis actually occurs in all proliferating body cells, which share the underlying defect in DNA synthesis. Thus epithelial cells of buccal mucosa, stomach, and vagina all display typical morphologic and biochemical abnormalities. These changes in many patients with vitamin B_{12} and folate deficiency account for such phenomena as glossitis (and mouth soreness), secondary gastric atrophy (and dyspepsia), and secondary malabsorption.

Pathophysiologic Features of the Megaloblastic State. Whatever its cause, megaloblastic anemia is associated with two pathophysiologic abnormalities: ineffective erythropoiesis and moderate hemolysis.

Ineffective erythropoiesis is indicated by (1) the marked increase in marrow erythroid precursors and the high ratio of erythroid precursors to released erythrocytes; (2) increase in plasma iron turnover to three to five times the normal level, despite the fact that iron uptake by individual erythroid precursors is normal; (3) decreased rate of reappearance of labeled plasma iron in blood erythrocytes; and (4) various signs of intramedullary destruction of megaloblasts. These include increased production of "early-labeled peak" bilirubin and endogenous carbon monoxide, phagocytosis of megaloblastic erythroid precursors by marrow reticulum cells, and high serum levels of lactic dehydrogenase (isozymes 1 and 2, which come from erythroid percursors) and muramidase (from leukocyte precursors). Other findings are slight to moderate increases in serum bilirubin, iron, and iron saturation, and decreases in haptoglobin (owing to ongoing hemolysis) and, in some patients, serum uric acid (owing to decreased DNA synthesis). Even when serum uric acid is not depressed, it usually rises sharply soon after the start of specific therapy.

Ineffective erythropoiesis causes intramedullary *hemolysis*. A substantial degree of extramedullary hemolysis also occurs. Erythrocyte life span is moderately decreased (to one half to one third normal) when patient erythrocytes are infused into normal subjects. This, of course, is classic evidence of an intracorpuscular defect. Decreased survival of normal erythrocytes infused into untreated patients suggests the presence of an extracorpuscular defect as well.

Inadequate production of myeloid cells accounts for the neutropenia of megaloblastic anemia. Elevated serum muramidase levels reflect the increased rate of intramedullary myeloid cell destruction. Thus, the mechanism of leukopenia is ineffective granulopoiesis. Ineffective thrombopoiesis also occurs; its pathophysiology parallels that of ineffective erythropoiesis and granulopoiesis. A decreased rate of platelet production (despite the presence of megakaryocytes) accounts for the mild to moderate thrombocytopenia observed in many patients with megaloblastic anemia.

Unless iron deficiency is present, ineffective erythropoiesis is inevitably associated with features suggesting iron overload: elevated plasma iron and iron saturation, increased plasma iron turnover, decreased incorporation of plasma iron into circulating hemoglobin, accumulation of iron in marrow retic-

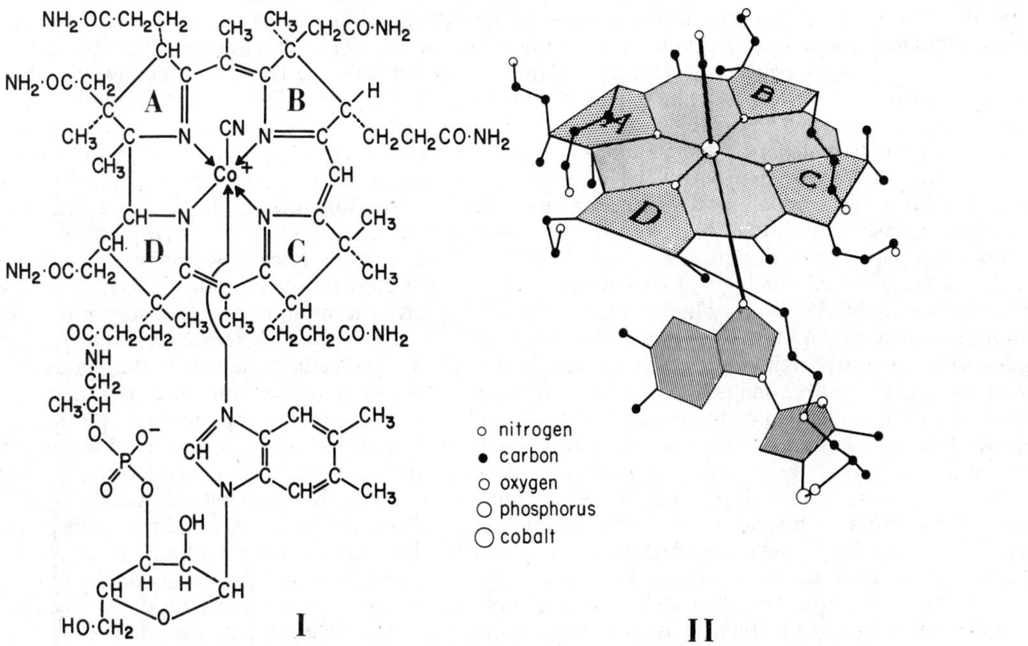

Figure 135–1. Chemical structure of vitamin B_{12}. *Formula I,* Molecular structure of cyanocobalamin. *Formula II,* Semidiagrammatic representation of three-dimensional structure showing relations of planar and nucleotide moieties. Hydrogen atoms and a number of oxygen atoms are omitted. (From Beck WS: N Engl J Med *266*:708, 1962.)

ulum cells, and increased iron stores in the liver (hepatic siderosis) and other tissues.

MEGALOBLASTIC ANEMIA OF VITAMIN B_{12} DEFICIENCY. Classic studies of pernicious anemia led directly or indirectly to much of our early knowledge of vitamin B_{12}. Until the demonstration by Minot and Murphy in 1926 of the successful treatment of pernicious anemia by liver feeding, the disease was almost invariably fatal. Potent liver extracts soon replaced liver feeding, but difficulties plagued investigators attempting to purify the anti–pernicious anemia principle of liver. Vitamin B_{12} was finally discovered in 1948 when proportionality was found between the nutrient activity of liver extracts in cultures of *Lactobacillus lactis* Dorner and their therapeutic activity in pernicious anemia. The resulting microbiologic assay rapidly facilitated purification and identification of the vitamin.

Metabolic and Nutritional Aspects of Vitamin B_{12}. Vitamin B_{12} is synthesized only by certain microorganisms. Wherever it is found in nature, it can be traced to microorganisms growing in soil, sewage, intestine, or rumen. Animals thus depend ultimately upon microbial synthesis for their vitamin B_{12} supply. Foods in the human diet that contain vitamin B_{12} are essentially those of animal origin: meat, liver, fish, eggs, and milk. The average daily diet in Western countries contains 5 to 30 μg of vitamin B_{12}, of which only 1 to 5 μg (the minimal daily requirement) is absorbed. Total body content is 2 to 5 mg in an adult man; approximately 1 mg is in the liver. Hence, a deficiency state will not develop for several years after cessation of vitamin B_{12} absorption.

The vitamin B_{12} molecule (Fig. 135–1) includes a porphyrin-like moiety (termed *corrin*) and a central cobalt atom. The four cobalamins of importance in animal cell metabolism are *cyanocobalamin* (CN-Cbl) and its analogue *hydroxocobalamin* (OH-Cbl), and two coenzyme forms—*adenosylcobalamin* (AdoCbl) and *methylcobalamin* (MeCbl). In adenosylcobalamin, a 5′-deoxyadenosyl moiety is the ligand of cobalt. This compound, the main storage form of vitamin B_{12} in liver, is the coenzyme of *methylmalonyl CoA mutase,* an enzyme catalyzing the final step in the pathway of propionic acid metabolism, in which methylmalonyl CoA is converted to succinyl CoA. This is the major AdoCbl-dependent reaction in animal tissues. Methylcobalamin, which occurs in small amounts in liver but is the major cobalamin in serum, is the coenzyme for the conversion of homocysteine to methionine (Fig. 135–2). This methyltransferase enzyme serves primarily as a means for converting N^5-methyltetrahydrofolate (N^5-methyl FH_4) to tetrahydrofolate (FH_4).

Impairment of DNA synthesis in vitamin B_{12} deficiency has been attributed to slowing of the cobalamin-dependent pathway of methionine synthesis. This sequesters folate as N^5-methyl FH_4, a form that is unavailable to the critical thymidylate synthetase reaction. This theory, the so-called "methylfolate trap" theory, is supported by the occurrence in vitamin B_{12} deficiency of elevated serum folate (N^5-methyl FH_4) levels. Folate coenzymes in tissues are in the form of polyglutamates. The enzyme converting folate (folylmonoglutamate) to folylpolyglutamate is most active with FH_4 as substrate and is relatively inactive with N^5-methyl FH_4. When the latter form

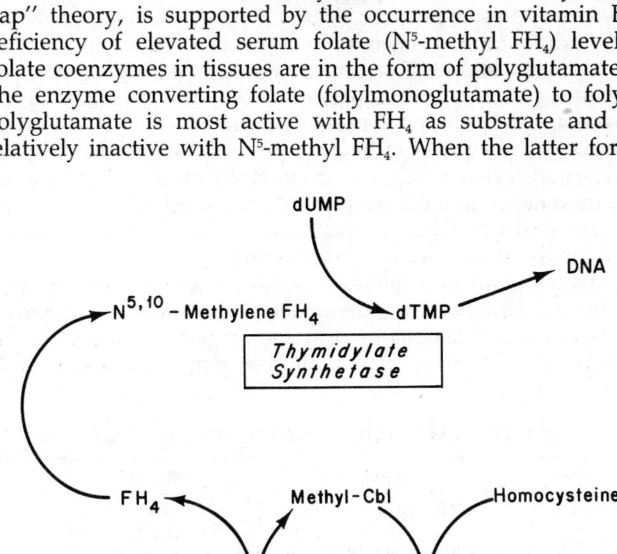

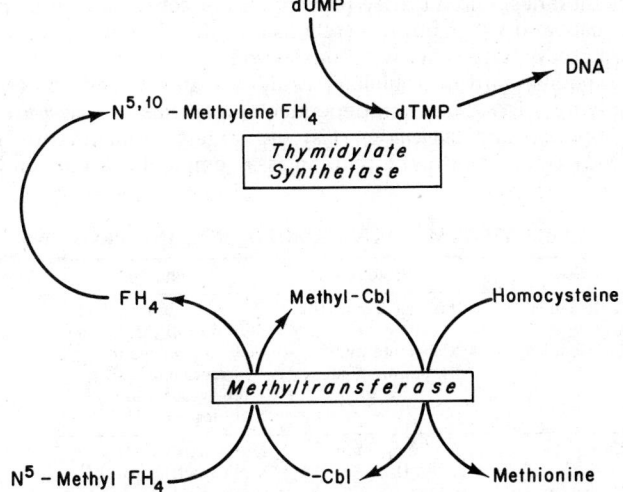

Figure 135–2. Diagram of relationship between N^5-methyl FH_4: homocysteine methyltransferase and thymidylate synthetase. In vitamin B_{12} deficiency, folate is sequestered as N^5-methyl FH_4. This ultimately deprives thymidylate synthetase of its folate coenzyme ($N^{5,10}$-methylene FH_4) and thereby impairs DNA synthesis.

accumulates in vitamin B_{12} deficiency, it is unavailable for conversion to folylpolyglutamate, and thymidylate synthetase is further deprived of its essential cofactor. This situation accounts for depressed levels of folylpolyglutamates in vitamin B_{12}–deficient tissues.

Vitamin B_{12} in food is liberated by peptic enzymes and acid in gastric juice. The vitamin is then bound by one or more proteins in gastric juice. Electrophoresis reveals two binders or classes of binders in gastric juice, one with slow and one with rapid mobility, that have been designated *S-proteins* and *R-proteins,* respectively. This terminology has been retained in the general classification of vitamin B_{12}–binding proteins (Table 135–2), although "cobalophilin" and "haptocorrin" have been recommended in place of R-protein. Of the several vitamin B_{12}–binding proteins in gastric juice, one is intrinsic factor (IF), an S-protein that, like HCl, is secreted by the parietal cells in man. Gastric R-protein may be largely of salivary origin. R-B_{12} complexes may be converted to IF-B_{12} with the participation of pancreatic proteases. The stable IF-B_{12} complex encounters specific mucosal receptors in the microvilli of the ileum that bind to a specific site on the IF molecule. Attachment requires neutral pH, Ca^{++}, or other divalent cations, but no energy. Vitamin B_{12} is transferred into the ileal cell and ultimately transferred to portal vein blood. Thus, IF is essential for the intestinal absorption of ingested vitamin B_{12}.

Secretion of IF parallels HCl secretion and is a glycoprotein of molecular weight 44,000 that binds a molecule of cobalamin with high affinity. Two types of anti-IF antibodies occur. "Blocking" antibodies prevent binding of vitamin B_{12} by IF and show little species specificity. "Binding" antibodies combine with IF-B_{12} and with free IF without impairing its ability to bind vitamin B_{12}. Both types of antibodies occur in sera of some patients with pernicious anemia.

R-proteins, which occur in serum, leukocytes, saliva, gastric juice, milk, and virtually all body cells, promote uptake of vitamin B_{12} by mitochondria and other organelles within cells. R-proteins have a relatively low level of binding specificity. This property may give them a role in binding biologically inert corrin and cobalamin analogues.

Normal plasma contains 175 to 725 pg per milliliter of vitamin B_{12} (normal range varying with method and laboratory). All of it is protein bound. The three major vitamin B_{12}–binding proteins of plasma are designated *transcobalamin I* (TC I), *transcobalamin II* (TC II), and *transcobalamin III* (TC III). TC I and TC III are R-proteins; TC II is an S-protein. They have only two known functions: TC II transports cobalamins through cell membranes, and all three prevent loss of cobalamins in urine, sweat, and other body secretions. As noted above, they undoubtedly have other functions as well.

The standard microbiologic assay of serum vitamin B_{12} (employing such cobalamin-dependent organisms as *Lactobacillus leichmannii* and *Euglena gracilis*) was largely supplanted in the 1960's by a radioisotope dilution assay employing a vitamin B_{12} binder. The higher results obtained with the isotopic assay were recently explained by the discovery in serum (and tissues) of a class of vitamin B_{12} analogues that are not assayed as vitamin B_{12} by microorganisms. They are assayed as vitamin B_{12} by isotopic procedures when the binder is an R-protein, but not when it is IF. In other words, the relatively low binding specificity of R-proteins produced a falsely high value in early isotopic serum vitamin B_{12} assays. Recently developed isotopic methods using IF as binder yield results in agreement with those of microbiologic assays. In addition, it raised many interesting questions. What is the source and fate of these analogues? Do they have pathophysiologic significance? Is it one of the roles of R-proteins, especially those of gastric juice, to bind these compounds (which may be of dietary origin) in order to minimize their absorption in the intestine?

TABLE 135–2. MAJOR VITAMIN B_{12}-BINDING PROTEINS

Source	Protein(s)	Function	Class*
Gastric juice	Intrinsic factor (IF)	Promotes absorption of vitamin B_{12} in ileum	S
Gastric juice	"Cobalophilin(s)" "Haptocorrin(s)"	May be involved in formation of IF-B_{12}; binds cobalamin analogues	R
Plasma	Transcobalamin I (TC I)	May participate in plasma transport of vitamin B_{12}	R
Plasma	Transcobalamin II (TC II)	Promotes entry of vitamin B_{12} into cells	S
Plasma (and granulocytes)	Transcobalamin III (TC III)	Unknown	R

*Based on electrophoretic mobility. R = rapid; S = slow.

Vitamin B_{12} Deficiency. The clinical picture of human vitamin B_{12} deficiency includes the nonspecific manifestations of megaloblastic anemia and its sequelae—e.g., megaloblastosis, slowly progressing anemia, glossitis, elevated serum lactic dehydrogenase—that occur as well in folic acid deficiency (and are described above), *plus* certain specific features that make possible the diagnosis of vitamin B_{12} deficiency, irrespective of the underlying cause. These include neurologic abnormalities, decreased serum vitamin B_{12} level, methylmalonic aciduria, and a characteristic response to vitamin B_{12} therapy and lack of response to therapy with physiologic doses of folic acid.

Neurologic symptoms occur late in some but not all patients. Curiously, they can occur in the absence of megaloblastic anemia. The neurologic syndrome, typical of vitamin B_{12} deficiency and not seen in folate deficiency, classically consists of symmetrical paresthesias (tingling and numbness) in feet and fingers, with associated disturbances of vibratory sense and proprioception, progressing to spastic ataxia with "*subacute combined system disease*" of the spinal cord, i.e., degenerative changes of the dorsal and lateral columns. In fact, the picture is more often chronic than subacute and more varied and complex. The ankle jerks are usually absent, and there is often a severe loss of postural sense. There are extensor plantar reflexes. Clinical signs include cerebral abnormalities, irritability, somnolence, "megaloblastic madness," and perversion of taste, smell, and vision with central scotomas and occasional optic atrophy. Tobacco amblyopia, a curious visual disorder in vitamin B_{12}–deficient smokers, has been attributed to the tendency of cyanide in tobacco smoke to convert a diminished supply of vitamin B_{12} coenzymes to metabolically inert cyanocobalamin. Neurologic involvement is associated with a defect in myelin synthesis. Its mechanism is still unknown. Several theories have been proposed, among them chronic cyanide intoxication, and the synthesis and incorporation into myelin of abnormal fatty acids produced as a result of competition between acetyl CoA and accumulated methylmalonyl CoA in the biosynthetic pathway of fatty acids. In its early stages the neurologic syndrome can be reversed by vitamin B_{12} therapy. In time, however, such chronic manifestations as spinal cord disease become irreversible.

A decreased serum vitamin B_{12} level is decisive diagnostic evidence. Clinical signs generally appear when the serum level is below 80 to 100 pg per milliliter. Serum folate is elevated when serum vitamin B_{12} is depressed unless there is coexisting folate deficiency. Methylmalonic aciduria is also a sensitive index of vitamin B_{12} deficiency except in rare cases in which it is due to an inborn error of metabolism. It does not occur in folate deficiency. Normal subjects excrete only traces of methylmalonate, i.e., 0 to 3.5 mg per 24 hours. Levels are variably elevated in vitamin B_{12} deficiency, sometimes to >300 mg per 24 hours. In practice, assay of urinary methylmalonate is rarely necessary.

Vitamin B_{12} therapy of vitamin B_{12} deficiency produces within hours an improved sense of well-being. An abrupt reticulocyte crisis begins several days after the start of therapy (Fig. 135–3). Reversal of clinical abnormalities then ensues. A partial response follows large (i.e., pharmacologic) doses of folic acid (5 mg per day), although the hematocrit is not fully restored

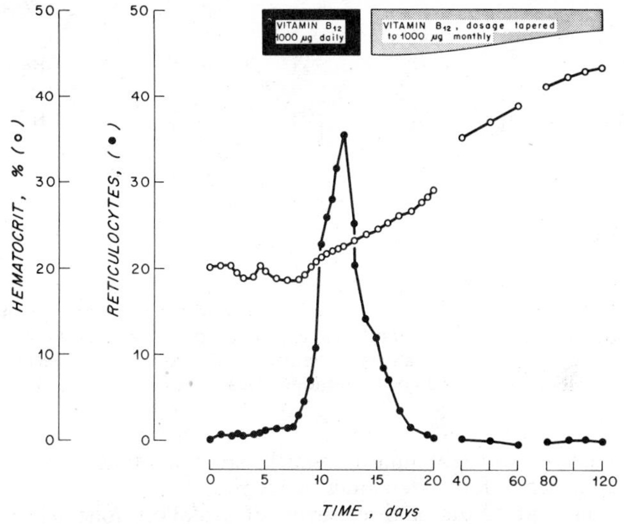

Figure 135–3. Time course of reticulocyte count and hematocrit level during treatment of pernicious anemia with vitamin B_{12}. (From Beck WS, Goulian M: *In* DiPalma J [ed.]: Drill's Pharmacology in Medical Practice. 4th ed. New York, McGraw-Hill Book Company, 1971.)

to normal, and patients previously without neurologic symptoms may suffer an acute onset of such symptoms. However, small (i.e., physiologic) doses of folic acid (200 to 400 μg per day) produce no response in vitamin B_{12} deficiency, whereas they produce good responses in folic acid deficiency.

Specific Deficiency Syndromes. Deficiency of vitamin B_{12}, as of all vitamins, may result from inadequate intake, abnormally increased requirements, or impaired utilization in the tissues (see Table 135–1). Deficiency of vitamin B_{12} results from poor diet only rarely. Reported instances have occurred mainly in vegetarians who also avoid dairy products and eggs. Most often deficiency is the result of diminished intestinal absorption of various etiologies. The most common cause is pernicious anemia, discussed below, in which a gastric mucosal defect decreases IF synthesis. Other and less common causes include total (occasionally subtotal) gastrectomy; pancreatic disease, in which lack of proteases in the duodenum appears to interfere with formation of IF-B_{12}; overgrowth of intestinal bacteria in the "blind loop" syndrome, strictures, anastomoses, diverticula, and other conditions producing intestinal stasis; infestation with the vitamin B_{12}–utilizing fish tapeworm *Diphyllobothrium latum* (once a common condition in Scandinavian countries); and organic disease of the ileum that interferes with vitamin B_{12} absorption despite the presence of adequate IF. Vitamin B_{12} deficiency resulting from increased requirements occurs mainly in pregnancy, presumably arising from the superimposition of fetal demands upon a background of poor nutrition. Impaired utilization of vitamin B_{12} occurs in various genetic defects, involving deletions or defects of methylmalonyl CoA mutase, TC II, and enzymes in the pathway of cobalamin adenosylation.

PERNICIOUS ANEMIA. Once a fatal disease and now the physician's favorite for its rich history, scientific importance, and cheerful prognosis, pernicious anemia is an atrophic gastropathy that leads to deficient IF secretion and eventual vitamin B_{12} deficiency. Because pernicious anemia was first described by Thomas Addison of Guy's Hospital, the term "addisonian pernicious anemia" is sometimes used to distinguish true pernicious anemia from the regrettably named "nonaddisonian pernicious anemia" (i.e., vitamin B_{12} deficiency arising from such other causes as ileitis or acquired gastric atrophy following inflammatory gastritis).

The incidence of pernicious anemia is age related, most cases occurring after the age of 40. Typically, it affects older north Europeans of fair complexion. An exception is its apparent predilection for young black women. A genetic basis for pernicious anemia is suggested by its high incidence in Scandinavians, a relatively inbred population, and by the occurrence of the disease or related abnormalities (e.g., achlorhydria) in patients' families. An underlying autoimmune process is suggested by the fact that many patients have serum binding or blocking anti-IF antibodies. Although such antibodies can block IF function if they enter the intestine, they are not responsible for cessation of IF synthesis. Anti-IF antibodies also occur in the absence of pernicious anemia in the serum of patients with diabetes mellitus, thyroid disease, and other diseases. Serum from pernicious anemia may also contain antibodies against gastric parietal cell cytoplasm and thyroid acinar cell cytoplasm. Pernicious anemia occurs frequently in patients with thyrotoxicosis, Hashimoto's thyroiditis, and several other diseases (hypogammaglobulinemia, vitiligo, rheumatoid arthritis, and gastric carcinoma).

Clinically, there is a slow onset of megaloblastic anemia and laboratory signs of vitamin B_{12} deficiency. If untreated, the patient may eventually develop neurologic symptoms. Diagnostic features are achlorhydria after histamine stimulation and decreased levels of IF in gastric juice as revealed by direct assay in vitro (which is performed routinely in Europe but infrequently in the USA) or by decreased vitamin B_{12} absorption in an in vivo test of vitamin B_{12} absorption. In the absorption test known as the *Schilling test*, a fasting patient ingests 0.5 microcurie (0.5 to 2.0 μg) [^{57}Co]cyanocobalamin at time zero. A dose (1 mg) of unlabeled cyanocobalamin is injected at two hours, and radioactivity is measured in a 24-hour urine collection. If excretion of radioactivity is low, the test is repeated (in no less than five days) by the same procedure, except that 60 mg of hog IF is given orally with the radioactive vitamin B_{12}. If poor excretion and therefore presumably poor absorption was due to IF deficiency, the result with the addition of exogenous IF should be normal. If excretion is still low, ileal disease may be suspected. Renal disease with impaired glomerular filtration may delay excretion of radioactivity in the Schilling test. Since the Schilling test includes an injection of vitamin B_{12}, it is a therapeutic commitment if therapy has not already been initiated.

Juvenile pernicious anemia includes four entities: (1) true pernicious anemia, which occurs infrequently between ages 2 and 14; (2) congential IF lack, with no other abnormality of gastric secretion and no anti-IF antibody; (3) production of a biologically inert IF (one case reported); and (4) familial selective malabsorption of vitamin B_{12} (Imerslund's syndrome) with normal absorption of other nutrients and normal gastric secretion of IF and HCl. The Schilling test reveals decreased vitamin B_{12} uncorrected by IF. Presumably, there is a defect of specific mucosal receptors for IF–B_{12}.

Therapy. Therapy consists in the parenteral administration of vitamin B_{12} (hydroxocobalamin or cyanocobalamin) in amounts that are ultimately sufficient to provide the 2 to 5 μg needed for the daily requirement and to replete liver stores and other reservoirs, which normally contain 2 to 5 mg of vitamin B_{12}. Because of its low cost and lack of toxicity, doses in excess of need are generally given. Parenterally administered vitamin B_{12} is bound to plasma proteins and cellular binding sites. If much more than 100 μg is given parenterally in a single dose, delay in encountering vacant binding sites promptly leads to renal excretion of unbound vitamin. Since hydroxocobalamin is bound more tightly by binding proteins than cyanocobalamin, it is less rapidly excreted by the kidney and more effective in achieving high serum vitamin B_{12} levels. Hypokalemia sometimes develops early in the course of treatment, especially in severely deficient patients, as a result of a sudden increase in the need for potassium in young red cells abruptly returning to normal hematopoiesis. The following treatment schedule is used in the author's clinic: (1) 500 to 1000 μg intramuscularly daily for two weeks; (2) the same dose twice weekly for an additional four weeks or until the hematocrit is normal; and (3) the same dose once monthly for the lifetime of the patient. A dosage schedule of 500 to 1000 μg every two weeks for six months is recommended for patients with neurologic manifestations. Neurologic symptoms persisting beyond 12 to 18 months are usually irreversible.

Oral vitamin B_{12}–IF preparations are not recommended, since the condition often becomes refractory to therapy. Oral therapy with vitamin B_{12} alone (500 to 1000 μg daily) should be reserved for the occasional patient who for some reason cannot receive parenteral therapy. This mode of therapy depends on intestinal absorption by passive diffusion, a process that is often unpredictable. Patients receiving oral medication who feel well may stop their medication. The patient with pernicious anemia should understand that he must be treated for life.

Since the response to vitamin B_{12} occurs within 48 to 72 hours, it is seldom necessary to subject the patient to the risks, discomfort, and expense of blood transfusion.

There is no need for iron therapy in pernicious anemia unless there is evidence of associated iron deficiency or reason to expect that tissue iron reserves are deficient—as, for example, in women of early middle age who may have had heavy menstrual losses or several pregnancies. In such cases, hemoglobin and erythrocyte regeneration is delayed until iron is given. There is no need to administer folic acid or ascorbic acid in addition to the vitamin B_{12}, provided that the patient takes an adequate diet. As long as vitamin B_{12} is given, folic acid therapy causes no harm. It is commonly elected to administer both vitamin B_{12} and folic acid to distressed patients with severe megaloblastic anemia without awaiting the diagnostic workup. In this situation, as in all cases of megaloblastic anemia, it is mandatory to obtain serum samples for vitamin assays before therapy starts.

With the exception of hereditary methylmalonic aciduria, vitamin B_{12} deficiency of whatever cause is the only valid indication for vitamin B_{12} therapy. It has been recommended, nevertheless, for many disorders in which there is no evidence of deficiency, especially for various types of neuropathy, liver disease, dermatologic disorders, and allergies, and as a "tonic" or appetite stimulant. The usefulness of vitamin B_{12} in these circumstances has not been proved, and its use for such purposes is not recommended. The administration of vitamin B_{12} to stimulate growth in underdeveloped children is also of dubious value.

MEGALOBLASTIC ANEMIA OF FOLATE DEFICIENCY. Converging lines of nutritional research led to the discovery of folic acid in the mid-1940's. In 1948 crystalline folic acid was obtained from liver and its structure confirmed by organic synthesis. Although experimental folic acid deficiency was known to produce megaloblastic anemia, it was not immediately recognized that folic acid is not the anti–pernicious anemia principle of liver, which was identified a year later. Confusion arose when folic acid therapy produced notable reticulocyte responses in pernicious anemia. Hemoglobin regeneration was incomplete, however, and relapses and neurologic complications occurred during treatment. Liver extracts active in pernicious anemia were then found by direct assay to contain little or no folic acid. Thus, it was recognized that vitamin B_{12} deficiency is the basis of the megaloblastic anemia of pernicious anemia and that folate deficiency is a distinctive cause of megaloblastic anemia.

Metabolic and Nutritional Aspects of Folic Acid. Folic acid is the trivial name for *pteroylmonoglutamic acid* (Fig. 135–4), parent compound of the large family of compounds known collectively as "folate" or "folates." The molecule contains three moieties: a pteridine derivative, a *p*-aminobenzoic acid residue, and an L-glutamic acid residue. The first two combined constitute pteroic acid; hence folates are pteroylglutamates. Folic acid occurs in nature largely in the form of folylpolyglutamates, in which multiple glutamic acid residues are attached by peptide linkages to the γ-carboxyl group of the preceding glutamic acid residue. The synthetic folic acid used therapeutically is folylmonoglutamate. However, folylmonoglutamates are converted

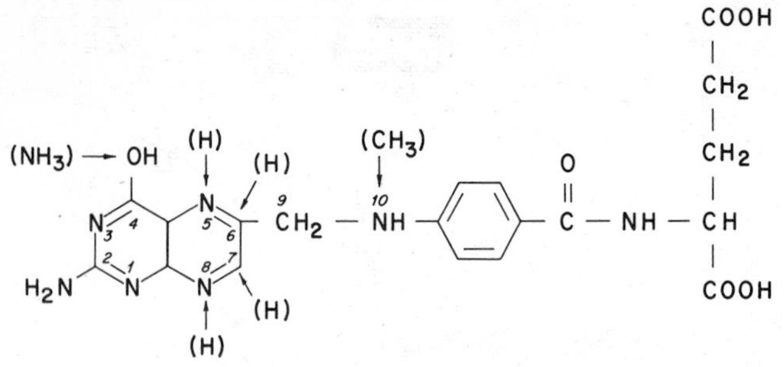

Figure 135–4. Chemical structure of folic acid (pteroylmonoglutamic acid). Substituents in parentheses are attached at the sites shown in the several folate derivatives described in the text. (From Beck WS [ed.]: Hematology. 3rd ed. Cambridge, Mass., MIT Press, 1981.)

in cells to polyglutamates, which are apparently the true coenzymes of folate-dependent enzymes.

Folic acid occurs at three levels of oxidation: folic acid (F); 7,8-dihydrofolic acid (FH_2); and 5,6,7,8-tetrahydrofolic acid (FH_4). Reduction of F to FH_4 is a necessary prerequisite to the participation of folic acid in enzyme reactions. In this reduction, F is reduced to FH_2, which is then reduced to FH_4. In animal cells both reactions are catalyzed by a single NADPH-linked enzyme, *dihydrofolate reductase,* which is notably sensitive to inhibition by folate analogues containing a 4-amino group (Fig. 135–4) such as aminopterin and amethopterin, later renamed methotrexate (MTX).

The folate family consists largely of FH_4 derivatives bearing one of several "one-carbon" substituents on N^5 or N^{10} (or both). Specific enzymes interconvert many of these compounds. Folate derivatives differ in their ability to support various microorganisms. The major form of folate in human serum is N^5-methyl FH_4 (a monoglutamate), which is assayed with *Lactobacillus casei.* Satisfactory isotope dilution assay procedures are now available for the assay of serum folate.

In metabolism, FH_4 is a catalytic self-regenerating acceptor-donor of one-carbon units in anabolic and catabolic reactions involving one-carbon transfers. A number of metabolic systems in animal tissues are known to require folate coenzymes. Thymidylate synthesis is the key reaction impairment that in folate deficiency produces major clinical manifestations (see Fig. 135–2). Methylation of deoxyuridylate to thymidylate, catalyzed by the enzyme thymidylate synthetase, is an essential step in the biosynthesis of DNA. Impairment of thymidylate synthesis in folate deficiency slows DNA synthesis with resulting megaloblastic transformation. Folate also participates in the breakdown of histidine and its catabolic product, formiminoglutamic acid (abbreviated FIGlu). Interference with this system in folate deficiency has no morbid effects, but it provides the basis for a diagnostic test for folate deficiency. When insufficient FH_4 is present to accept the formimino group, FIGlu accumulates in the urine, where it is easily detected.

Green leaves are rich sources of folate, the richest being asparagus, broccoli, spinach, and lettuce, each of which contains >1 mg of folate per 100 grams dry weight. Folates are also found in liver, kidney, yeast, and mushrooms. An average daily American diet, prepared without special precautions, contains approximately 200 μg of folate by *S. faecalis* assay and an additional 400 to 500 μg of folate that is active only with *L. casei.* Excessive cooking, particularly with large amounts of water, can remove or destroy a high percentage of the folate in foods. The minimal daily adult requirement for folic acid, or its derivatives, is 50 to 200 μg. Body reserves of folic acid are relatively much smaller than those of vitamin B_{12}. When a subject receiving a normal ration is switched to a daily intake of 5 μg per day, megaloblastic anemia develops in about four months. Folic acid requirements are increased during growth, in pregnancy, and in various diseases.

Folate Deficiency. The clinical picture of human folate deficiency includes nonspecific manifestations of megaloblastic anemia which are similar to those observed in vitamin B_{12}

deficiency—megaloblastosis, glossitis, elevated serum lactic dehydrogenase—*plus* certain specific features that make possible the diagnosis of folate deficiency, irrespective of the underlying cause. These include decreased serum folate levels (normal, 6 to 15 ng per milliliter), decreased red cell folate levels (normal, 150 to 600 ng per milliliter cells), and full clinical response to therapy with physiologic doses of folic acid. Features suggestive but not diagnostic of folate deficiency in a patient with megaloblastic anemia are lack of neurologic changes of the type seen in vitamin B_{12} deficiency, normal serum vitamin B_{12} and urine methylmalonic acid levels, and a history of circumstances almost certain to lead to folic acid deficiency, e.g., poor diet, malabsorption, or alcoholism.

Specific Deficiency Syndromes. As shown in Table 135–1, the major categories of folate deficiency are those due to decreased intake, increased requirements, and impaired utilization. Decreased intake is by far the most common. Because body folate reserves are small, deficiency develops rapidly in persons on an inadequate diet. As noted, excessive cooking may also promote deficiency, especially among peoples who live on finely divided foods such as rice. Megaloblastic anemia occurring in chronic liver disease is usually due to folate deficiency resulting from poor diet and impaired hepatic storage of folate. The macrocytic anemia accompanying liver disease is often normoblastic and unresponsive to folic acid therapy. Nutritional folate deficiency is often associated with multiple vitamin deficiencies. In such patients, a history of gross dietary inadequacy is usually easy to obtain. Folate is normally absorbed in the upper third of the small intestine and commonly malabsorbed in nontropical sprue (celiac disease) as described in Ch. 103. Tropical sprue is a malabsorptive disorder of unknown etiology that occurs frequently and endemically in the tropics—notably the West Indies, the Indian subcontinent, and Southeast Asia. It can be acquired by residents of temperate climates who go to the tropics, sometimes persisting long after return from the tropics. It may be due in part to deficiency of dietary folate, the malabsorption resulting from secondary gastrointestinal changes. Treatment with folic acid alone usually reverses all abnormalities, including defective folate absorption. Other causes of malabsorption are noted in Table 135–1. Low serum folate levels in patients receiving phenytoin (Dilantin) have been attributed to a reversible drug-induced malabsorption of folylpolyglutamate. Oral contraceptives have recently been shown to block deconjugation of folylpolyglutamate in certain women.

Pregnancy increases requirements for folate. Although true anemias of pregnancy are commonly due to iron deficiency or multiple nutritional deficiencies, two thirds of anemic pregnant women are folate deficient. Its frequency is attributable both to meager folate reserves and to the fact that pregnancy increases daily requirements for folate five- to ten-fold, especially in the last trimester. The presence of multiple fetuses, poor diet (a frequent result of anorexia or nausea), infection, and lactation may further increase requirements. The capacity of the fetus to take up folic acid (and other nutrients) at the expense of the mother, even when the available supply is markedly reduced, is both remarkable and unexplained. Folic acid supplementation is desirable during pregnancy not only because requirements are increased but also because there is a suspected association between severe folate deficiency and such complications of pregnancy as abruptio placentae, embryopathology, spontaneous abortion, and bleeding. The folate requirement also rises sharply in hemolytic anemias associated with acute or chronic overactivity of the bone marrow and in most neoplastic diseases, especially metastatic cancer and the leukemias. The deficiency presumably reflects competitive utilization of the vitamin by tumor cells, a phenomenon that resembles the preemption of maternal nutrients by a fetus.

Impaired utilization of folate is caused by administration of 4-aminopteroylglutamates, aminopterin and methotrexate, powerful inhibitors of dihydrofolate reductase that can deplete folate coenzymes in tissues within hours. Citrovorum factor (leucovorin, folinic acid, N^5-formyl FH_4) effectively counteracts the actions of MTX by bypassing the inhibited reductase and is useful in the treatment of toxicity.

Therapy. Folic acid is usually administered orally in 1 mg tablets. Oral therapy is satisfactory for most needs. Even in the presence of intestinal malabsorption, the relatively large doses used ordinarily permit sufficient absorption to achieve repletion. The usual dose is 1 to 2 mg daily, although doses in excess of 1 mg are seldom necessary. Folic acid in these doses also partially corrects the hematopoietic and gastrointestinal manifestations of vitamin B_{12} deficiency. Neurologic abnormalities, however, may progress with disastrous results. This is the principal danger in the uncritical use of folic acid. Therapy for four to five weeks is usually adequate to replenish stores and correct anemia. Therapy is continued until diet or underlying problems are corrected. In some patients (e.g., with malabsorption, chronic hemolysis, chronic exfoliative skin disease, or renal failure requiring hemodialysis), it must continue indefinitely.

A parenteral preparation containing 5 mg per milliliter of the sodium salt may be used in severely ill patients, in certain cases of malabsorption, or in patients incapable of taking oral medication. Citrovorum factor is available as a parenteral therapeutic preparation. Its main clinical indication is severe intoxication by folic acid antagonists that block folate reduction. In the absence of such inhibition, little is accomplished by treating folate deficiency with this compound instead of folic acid.

MEGALOBLASTIC ANEMIA UNRESPONSIVE TO VITAMIN B_{12} OR FOLIC ACID. Megaloblastic anemia is occasionally unaccompanied by vitamin B_{12} or folic acid deficiency and fails to respond to therapy with either vitamin. In some cases, folate or vitamin B_{12} deficiency coexists with megaloblastic anemia but is not responsible for it. Most of these occurrences arise in three situations (see Table 135–1): therapy with an antimetabolite drug that interferes with DNA synthesis (common), inborn error of metabolism (rare), and refractory megaloblastic anemia of undetermined etiology, which is probably due to somatic mutation leading to loss of an enzyme in the pathway of DNA synthesis. Except for various dysplastic features, megaloblasts in the bone marrows of these patients generally resemble those in vitamin-deficiency megaloblastic anemia. It can be assumed therefore that the defect in all is an impaired capacity to duplicate DNA at a normal rate. Drug-induced megaloblastosis is potentially reversible. However, those cases caused by genetic error or acquired refractory megaloblastosis are irreversible and unfortunately difficult to treat with any but supportive measures.

Babior BM (ed.): Cobalamin: Biochemistry and Pathophysiology. New York, John Wiley & Sons, 1975. *A standard work that includes essays on all aspects of vitamin B_{12}. Although somewhat outdated in certain particulars, some of these articles are classics.*

Beck WS: Metabolic aspects of vitamin B_{12} and folic acid. Erythrocyte disorders—anemias related to disturbance of DNA synthesis (megaloblastic anemias). *In* Williams WJ, Beutler E, Erslev AJ, Lichtman MA (eds.): Hematology. 3rd ed. New York, McGraw-Hill Book Company, 1983, pp 311–331, 434–465. *Sections of a standard hematology text that covers the megaloblastic anemias in detail. Extensive bibliographies.*

Blair JA (ed.) Chemistry and Biology of Pteridines: Pteridines and Folic Acid Derivatives. Proceedings of The Seventh International Symposium on the Chemistry and Biology of Pteridines and Folic Acid Derivatives, St. Andrews, Scotland, September 21–24, 1982. New York, Elsevier–North Holland, 1983. *Proceedings of an important meeting giving an up-to-date profile of current activities in the folic acid field.*

Castle WB: The conquest of pernicious anemia. *In* Wintrobe MM (ed.): Blood, Pure and Eloquent. A Story of Discovery, of People, and of Ideas. New York, McGraw-Hill Book Company, 1980, pp 283–318. *An engrossing historical essay by the one who in 1929 discovered intrinsic factor.*

Kolhouse JF, Kondo H, Allen NC, Podell E, Allen RH: Cobalamin analogues are present in human plasma and can mask cobalamin deficiency because current radioisotope dilution assays are not specific for true cobalamin. N Engl J Med 299:785, 1978. *By exploring the long recognized differences between results from isotopic and microbiologic assays, these authors discovered cobalamin analogues in plasma and established new guidelines for the assay of serum vitamin B_{12}.*

Lindenbaum J: Status of laboratory testing in the diagnosis of megaloblastic anemia. Blood 61:624, 1983. *A brief current guide to available methods. The author agrees with everything in it except the remarks on the deoxyuridine suppression test (see following paper by Pelliniemi and Beck).*

Pelliniemi TT, Beck WS: Biochemical mechanisms in the Killmann experiment: Critique of the deoxyuridine suppression test. J Clin Invest 65:449, 1980. *Although the widely recommended procedure known as the deoxyuridine suppression test is said to measure thymidylate synthesis reliably, this paper shows that considerable "suppression" still occurs in cells in which thymidylate synthesis has been deliberately obliterated and thus casts doubt on the test's reliability.*

Rosenberg LE: Disorders of propionate and methylmalonate metabolism. *In* Stanbury JB, Wyngaarden JB, Frederickson DS, Goldstein JL, Brown MS (eds.): The Metabolic Basis of Inherited Disease. 5th ed. New York, McGraw-Hill Book Company, 1983, p 474. *A thorough review of a group of inborn errors that may cause laboratory findings that could confuse an observer who is not alert to the possibilities. 191 references.*

Zagalak B, Friedrich W (eds.): Vitamin B_{12}: Proceedings of the Third European Symposium on Vitamin B_{12} and Intrinsic Factor. University of Zürich, March 5–8, 1979, Zürich, Switzerland. New York, Walter de Gruyter, 1979. *A survey of activities of the world's investigators in the fields of cobalamin chemistry, physiology, and pathophysiology. A fitting record of an important meeting that gives an astonishing reminder of the field's scientific depth.*

136. HEMOLYTIC DISORDERS: INTRODUCTION

Manuel E. Kaplan

PATHOPHYSIOLOGY OF HEMOLYSIS. Human red blood cells normally survive for approximately 120 days after they are released from the bone marrow as reticulocytes, being destroyed only after they have become senescent. With advancing cell age the activities of various red cell enzymes decline, and the cells become denser and less deformable. Phagocytic cells of the spleen and liver are believed to recognize and destroy effete red cells, although splenectomy does not extend the red cell life span beyond 120 days.

A hemolytic disorder is defined as premature destruction of red cells, which may occur either because inherently defective red cells are produced or because noxious factors are present in the intravascular environment. Intrinsic abnormalities that predispose to hemolysis may occur in the red cell membrane, or in its contained hemoglobin or enzymes. These are, for the most part, genetically determined. In contrast, the environmental abnormalities that prejudice red cell survival are almost all acquired. A classification of the causes of hemolytic anemia is given in Table 136–1.

To measure red cell survival, anticoagulated venous blood is incubated with radioactive chromium (^{51}Cr) to label intracellular hemoglobin and is then reinfused. Normally 50 per cent of the injected ^{51}Cr activity disappears from the blood (t½) in 29 ± 3 days rather than at 60 days, because ^{51}Cr is an imperfect label and slowly elutes from the red cells. Nevertheless, the results of such studies are clinically informative because rates of hemolysis are reliably quantified and the sites of red cell destruction can be identified by external scanning utilizing a collimated gamma scintillation counter.

TABLE 136–1. CLASSIFICATION OF THE CAUSES OF HEMOLYTIC ANEMIA

I. Congenital hemolytic disorders (see Ch. 137)
  A. Membrane defects
  B. Enzyme defects
    1. Embden-Meyerhof pathway defects
    2. Hexose monophosphate shunt defects
  C. Hemoglobin defects
    1. Structural (hemoglobinopathies) (see Ch. 142)
    2. Synthetic (thalassemias) (see Ch. 141)
  D. Other
II. Acquired hemolytic disorders (see Ch. 138):
  A. Sequestrational hemolysis (hypersplenism)
  B. Immune hemolytic disorders
    1. Alloimmune
    2. Autoimmune
    3. Drug-induced
  C. Paroxysmal nocturnal hemoglobinuria
  D. Due to toxins and metabolic abnormalities
  E. Due to red cell parasites
  F. Due to red cell trauma

CONSEQUENCES OF HEMOLYSIS. Accelerated destruction of red cells may occur intravascularly or, more commonly, after the cells have been culled from the circulation (sequestered).

Intravascular Hemolysis. Following intravascular hemolysis, hemoglobin is released into the plasma and is bound by haptoglobin, an alpha globulin synthesized by the liver. The haptoglobin concentration of blood, normally about 100 mg per 100 ml, reflects the rate of haptoglobin synthesis and catabolism. Haptoglobin synthesis is usually diminished in patients with parenchymal liver disease and may be increased in various inflammatory disorders, in which it acts as an acute phase protein. Free (uncomplexed) haptoglobin has a half-life of approximately four days. In contrast, hemoglobin-haptoglobin complexes are removed from the plasma within minutes, primarily by hepatic reticuloendothelial cells that catabolize both components of the complex. Haptoglobin catabolism usually exceeds haptoglobin synthesis in patients with significant intravascular hemolysis, and plasma haptoglobin levels fall, frequently to undetectable levels. If the quantity of hemoglobin entering the plasma exceeds the binding capacity of haptoglobin, hemoglobin appears in the glomerular filtrate, primarily as a 32,000 dalton alpha-beta dimer. The dimers are readily absorbed by cells of the proximal tubules that convert heme iron into ferritin and hemosiderin. After the tubular cells are sloughed, hemosiderin can be detected in the urinary sediment with a Prussian blue stain. Hemoglobinuria, which occurs only when the filtered load of alpha-beta dimer exceeds the absorptive capacity of the tubular cells, connotes rapid intravascular hemolysis. Persistent urinary loss of hemosiderin or hemoglobin or both may result in iron deficiency.

Hemoglobin in the plasma is unstable. Its heme prosthetic groups tend to dissociate and bind either to hemopexin, a beta globulin, or to albumin forming methemalbumin. Neither of these heme-protein complexes appears in the urine unless significant proteinuria is present. Because heme-hemopexin complexes are cleared rapidly from the blood, serum levels of hemopexin, like haptoglobin, are typically reduced or absent in the presence of significant intravascular hemolysis.

Erythrocytes contain high concentrations of the enzyme lactic dehydrogenase (LDH). Consequently, very high LDH levels are found in patients with intravascular hemolysis.

Extravascular Destruction. In most hemolytic disorders red cell destruction occurs extravascularly rather than intravascularly. Red cells are sequestered primarily within the spleen or liver or both and are phagocytized in situ. Although only a small fraction of the hemoglobin they contain escapes into the plasma, plasma haptoglobin levels characteristically fall, particularly when hemolysis is longstanding. However, plasma hemoglobin levels do not rise significantly, and no hemoglobinuria or hemosiderinuria occurs. Serum LDH levels are usually elevated, but not to the degree seen in intravascular hemolysis.

Hemoglobin derived from hemolyzed red cells is normally catabolized by reticuloendothelial cells to unconjugated, indirect-reacting bilirubin. As each heme tetrapyrrol ring is opened, one molecule of carbon monoxide is elaborated. The rate of formation of endogenously produced carbon monoxide has been used to quantify red cell destruction in vivo. However, this may not accurately reflect the rapidity of hemolysis since ineffective erythropoiesis (destruction of immature red cells in the bone marrow) also contributes to carbon monoxide formation. Unconjugated bilirubin produced by phagocytic cells is bound by albumin. The concentration of unconjugated bilirubin in the serum of a patient reflects the quantity of heme catabolized and the rate at which the liver is able to convert it into the direct-reacting, water-soluble product (Ch. 129). Serum levels of conjugated bilirubin are typically normal in patients with uncomplicated hemolytic disorders. Bilirubinuria does not occur unless the patient has concomitant hepatocellular or biliary disease.

Bone Marrow Response. The loss of circulating red cells results in an erythropoietic stimulus to the bone marrow proportional to the decline in the oxygen-carrying capacity of the blood. The normal bone marrow responds by increasing commensurately its erythropoietic activity. When examined morphologically, bone marrows of hemolyzing patients characteristically exhibit erythroid hyperplasia. Consequently, unless an underlying neoplastic disorder such as leukemia or lymphoma is suspected, diagnostic bone marrow studies are usually not indicated. The intensity of the marrow's erythropoietic response to hemolysis, which may reach a maximum of approximately eight times normal, is reflected by a retriculocytosis in the peripheral blood. The reticulocyte percentage alone does not adequately reflect the degree of marrow compensation. This may be more reliably gauged by calculating the reticulocyte index (patient hematocrit times percentage reticulocytes/normal hematocrit). In some patients a sustained reticulocytosis may compensate fully for the increased red cell destruction, and there is no anemia. More commonly, bone marrow compensation is incomplete so that anemia, of greater or lesser severity, supervenes. If bone marrow function is compromised by such factors as infection or folate deficiency the reticulocyte count will fall and the anemia will rapidly worsen because of the ongoing hemolytic process.

DIFFERENTIAL DIAGNOSIS OF HEMOLYTIC DISORDERS. ***The Diagnosis of Hemolysis.*** The presence of hemolysis as the cause of anemia is generally not difficult to establish. The clinical diagnosis is usually based on the presence of a sustained reticulocytosis in a patient exhibiting no evidence of blood loss or of increasing hemoglobin concentration. Some, or rarely in severe cases all, of the following findings may occur:

1. *Evidence of enhanced marrow response:* polychromatophilia, reticulocytosis, marrow erythroid hyperplasia.
2. *Evidence for excessive release of red cell components:* (a) plasma—unconjugated bilirubin ↑, LDH ↑, haptoglobin ↓, hemopexin ↓, methemalbumin +, free hemoglobin ↑; (b) urine—hemosiderin +, hemoglobin +.
3. *Measurement of red cell survival:* ^{51}Cr chromate tagging.

The problem remains to determine the cause of the hemolytic process (see Table 134–1). Hemolysis is caused either by an abnormality of the red cell or an abnormality in its environment, the circulatory system in which the red cell resides. Red cell abnormalities associated with hemolysis may be congenital (genetically determined) or acquired. Congenital red cell defects resulting in hemolysis may involve the cell membrane, erythrocyte enzymes, or the contained hemoglobin. Acquired red cell defects that predispose to hemolysis may occur (1) under conditions of grossly abnormal (dysplastic) red cell maturation (such as marked deficiencies of iron, B_{12}, or folate) with bone marrow production and elaboration into the circulation of severely misshapen erythrocytes, and (2) in paroxysmal nocturnal hemoglobinuria (Ch. 138). More commonly, acquired hemolytic disorders are due to the presence in the circulation of such noxious factors as red cell antibodies, activated complement components, chemical or metabolic "toxins," and parasites.

Clinical Findings. A patient with hemolysis may present with diverse complaints and physical findings that reflect the rapidity, underlying etiology, and pathophysiologic mechanism of red cell destruction. Patients with congenital hemolytic disorders are frequently anemic and intermittently jaundiced early in life. Usually a suggestive family history of anemia, jaundice, cholelithiasis, splenomegaly, and/or therapeutic splenectomy can be elicited. A significant proportion of patients with acquired hemolysis have an identifiable underlying disease such as systemic lupus erythematosus (SLE) or chronic lymphocytic leukemia (CLL). Patients with rapidly falling hemoglobin resulting from hemolysis of any cause commonly complain of fatigue, palpitations, breathlessness, postural dizziness, and worsening of pre-existing angina. Physical examination typically discloses pallor, mild jaundice, and frequently splenomegaly. Other signs and symptoms referable to specific underlying disease may also be present: joint discomfort in SLE, painful acrocyanosis in cold agglutinin disease, lymphadenopathy in CLL.

Laboratory Findings. Patients with significant hemolysis typically exhibit reticulocytosis with polychromasia on peripheral smear, unconjugated hyperbilirubinemia, decreased to absent serum haptoglobin levels, erythroid hyperplasia of the bone marrow, and elevated serum LDH levels. In fact, as noted earlier, these findings form the basis of diagnosing an anemia as being hemolytic. Hemoglobinemia, hemoglobinuria, and hemosiderinuria occur only when rapid intravascular hemolysis is present. Significant intravascular red cell destruction occurs in relatively few situations, e.g., G-6-PD deficiency, certain infections (*C. welchii,* falciparum malaria), paroxysmal nocturnal hemoglobinuria, paroxysmal cold hemoglobinuria, incompatible transfusions, and as a result of traumatic disruption of red cell membranes by excessive heat or mechanical stress.

The morphologic appearance of red cells is frequently abnormal in hemolyzing patients. Occasionally the abnormalities are so typical that they indicate the correct diagnosis (Table 136–2).

Further Studies. The overall clinical picture with which a hemolyzing patient seeks medical help is usually sufficiently informative to suggest a rational diagnostic approach. These approaches for a presumed congenital process include osmotic fragility test, glucose-6-phosphate dehydrogenase and pyruvate kinase screening tests, and hemoglobin electrophoresis; for a presumed acquired process they include direct antiglobulin (Coombs') test and Ham's test for PNH.

TREATMENT OF HEMOLYTIC ANEMIA. Only general supportive measures will be discussed here since effective therapy usually requires definition of the cause and pathophysiologic mechanisms underlying the specific disease processes, as described in the subsequent two chapters.

Severely anemic patients should be placed at temporary bed rest to reduce cardiac output. Nasal oxygen may afford symptomatic relief. Transfusions with packed red cells should be utilized to correct hemodynamic abnormalities rather than to treat low hemoglobin or hematocrit values. To avoid iatrogenically induced hypervolemia, transfusions should be administered slowly. The physician must consider the potential dangers of transfusions, particularly in patients with autoimmune hemolytic disorders (see Ch. 138).

To maintain accelerated erythropoiesis, chronically hemolyzing patients require extra quantities of folic acid. Therefore, daily oral supplementation with folic acid, 1 to 2 mg per day, is recommended. If concomitant vitamin B_{12} deficiency is suspected, the serum B_{12} concentration should be measured. If low, parenteral vitamin B_{12} should also be administered.

SPECIFIC HEMOLYTIC DISORDERS. The purpose of this brief introduction is merely to provide a background of the common pathophysiology of the hemolytic anemias as well as a general classification (Table 136–1). The anemias are discussed more

TABLE 136–2. MORPHOLOGIC ABNORMALITIES OF RED CELLS IN VARIOUS HEMOLYTIC DISORDERS

	Hemolytic Disorder	
Abnormality	*Congenital*	*Acquired*
Permanently sickled cells	Sickle cell anemia	—
Fragmented cells (schistocytes)	Unstable hemoglobins (Heinz body anemias)	Microangiopathic processes Prosthetic heart valves
Spur cells (acanthocytes)	Abetalipoproteinemia	Severe liver disease
Spherocytes	Hereditary spherocytosis	Immune, warm antibody type
Target cells	Thalassemia Hemoglobinopathies (Hgb C)	Liver disease
Agglutinated cells	—	Immune, cold agglutinin disease

extensively in Ch. 134 and 135. Specific hemolytic diseases resulting from intracorpuscular abnormalities (usually caused by genetic abnormalities of the red cell membrane, of red cell enzymes, or of hemoglobin) are presented in the following chapter. Chapter 138 summarizes the acquired hemolytic disorders.

137. HEMOLYSIS DUE TO INTRACORPUSCULAR ABNORMALITIES

Harry S. Jacob

Introduction

In acquired hemolytic anemias environmental stresses cause shortened red cell survival; in congenital hemolytic anemias red cells are usually intrinsically defective. The ultimate proof of intrinsic abnormality requires cross-transfusion studies in which the suspect cells, labeled with an appropriate radioactive material, are infused into a normal recipient. An excessively rapid disappearance of circulating radioactivity (red cells) is noted. Careful history-taking frequently provides ample support for suspicion that congenital hemolytic anemia involving an intrinsic red cell abnormality is present: (1) A history of similar disorders in several members of the patient's family is often elicitable. (2) These disorders are usually present from birth, so that childhood episodes of jaundice and anemia are frequently noted. (3) Since such patients suffer lifelong overproduction of bilirubin, signs and symptoms of cholelithiasis often occur at a uniquely early age.

Congenital hemolytic anemia may be due to an inherited abnormality of the erythrocyte membrane or of its cytoplasm. The erythrocyte membrane must serve both as a semipermeable barrier to cations (with sodium, potassium, and calcium being the most important in considerations of normal red cell viability) and as a flexible envelope that must provide the cell sufficient deforming capacity to allow for its journeys through small capillaries—many with smaller diameters than those of the erythrocytes themselves. A unique filtering apparatus exists in the spleen in which the vascular wall separating cords from sinusoids is fenestrated. The erythrocytes must pass through this "filter," the apertures of which are smaller by half than its diameter, to escape splenic sequestration and destruction. Deformability is an important determinant of red cell survival, and much interest has recently centered on elucidation of intrinsic (and acquired) abnormalities in membrane flexibility as they may relate to hemolytic processes.

The cytoplasm of erythrocytes contains hemoglobin and enzymes required for cellular production of energy (mainly in the form of adenosine triphosphate [ATP]) and of reducing capacity (mainly stored as NADPH). Genetic deficiencies of single enzymes frequently lead to shortened red cell survival and congenital hemolytic anemia, whereas mutations in the molecular structure of hemoglobin can also produce diminished survival, particularly when the mutant hemoglobin manifests abnormal solubility. Thus hemoglobins that tend to gel (hemoglobin S or sickle hemoglobin), to precipitate (as in certain unstable hemoglobinopathies), or to crystallize (hemoglobin C) cause premature red cell destruction, probably by diminishing cellular deformability. The abnormal hemoglobins are discussed in Ch. 142 and 143. This chapter will discuss abnormalities of the erythrocytic membrane and of the enzymes of the glycolytic pathway that are associated with hemolysis.

Although the nature of the intrinsic defects in congenital hemolytic anemia may differ widely, cellular destruction in these disorders generally occurs in reticuloendothelial organs, such as the spleen and liver, rather than intravascularly.

Membrane Abnormalities

HEREDITARY SPHEROCYTOSIS (HS)

DEFINITION. This condition is inherited as an autosomal dominant disorder and is found throughout the world; however, its incidence seems highest in northern Europeans, in whom rates of 1 in 5000 have been reported. The disorder is characterized by the presence in peripheral blood smears of numerous abnormally shaped red cells that are generally spheroidal, lacking the usual central pallor of normal biconcave discocytes. Blood smears obtained after splenectomy, which produces virtually complete remission of hemolysis, may contain large numbers of spiculated (acanthocytic) cells as well.

CLINICAL MANIFESTATIONS. (See Table 137–1.) The key clinical manifestations of HS are *anemia, splenomegaly,* and *jaundice.* Three different modes of presentation are commonly encountered. Generally children are only minimally anemic most of the time, because increased marrow production of erythrocytes matches the increased destruction rates, so that the hemolytic process is well compensated. However, without warning, or frequently during intercurrent, particularly viral, infections, bone marrow function diminishes and the young patient becomes rapidly and severely anemic to levels that on occasion produce congestive heart failure. These so-called *"aplastic crises"* are observed usually during the first six years of life. Often, however, the compensatory increase in bone marrow function is well enough maintained so that the condition goes undiscovered until adulthood. With time, splenic enlargement, which is detectable in the great majority of patients, tends to worsen progressively with attendant increase in hemolytic rate and less efficient compensation. Although episodic worsening of unconjugated hyperbilirubinemia (secondary to increased hemoglobin catabolism) occurs at all ages, adults frequently present with sudden onset of more severe jaundice—now caused by conjugated hyperbilirubinemia. The explanation is that *bilirubinate gallstones*, a manifestation of many chronic hemolytic processes, are commonly encountered in young adult HS patients. Since such stones are usually small, they tend to enter and occlude the common bile duct. Finally, the condition in some patients escapes detection until old age, when bone marrow function normally becomes sluggish; previous compensation of hemolysis now wanes, and anemia becomes obvious and frequently dangerous. This normal senescent process is exacerbated in many elderly patients by concomitant folic acid deficiency because of the increased folate requirements attendant on chronic increased marrow turnover; this combination may produce severe anemia with congestive heart failure.

In addition to these more common manifestations, *chronic ulceration of ankle skin* occurs in 10 to 15 per cent of adult patients. Rarer but potentially interesting syndromes that coexist with HS have also been described. Since the erythrocyte membrane is abnormal in this disorder (see below), the occurrence of abnormality in nonhematologic tissues invites speculation that defects in membrane composition might be more

TABLE 137–1. HEREDITARY SPHEROCYTOSIS

Clinical Manifestations	Laboratory Abnormalities
Anemia	Spherocytosis (Fig. 137–1)
Splenomegaly	Elevated MCHC
Jaundice	Osmotic fragility ↑
from hemolysis	Autohemolysis during 48-hour incubation
from bilirubinate gallstones	Abnormalities in family
Aplastic crisis (usually before age 6)	
Chronic leg ulcers (10–15% of adults)	
Rare	
Coincident spinal cord dysfunction	
Familial myocardiopathy	

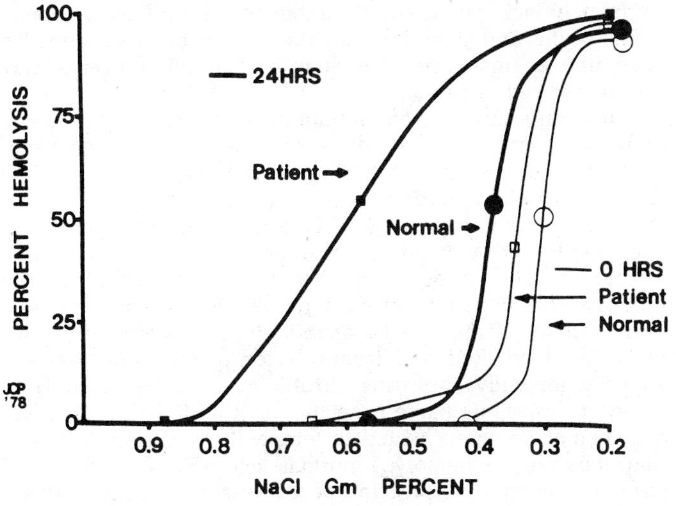

Figure 137–1. The osmotic fragility of red cells in hereditary spherocytosis. The figure shows the effect of 24-hour incubation.

generalized. The coincident syndromes include (1) unconjugated hyperbilirubinemia that continues despite correction of hemolysis by splenectomy, suggesting the diagnosis of Gilbert's syndrome; (2) spinal cord dysfunction, producing a multiple sclerosis–like illness; and (3) an unusual coincidence of familial myocardiopathy with HS in several recently examined families. With regard to the latter two syndromes, it is tantalizing that spectrin, a critical cytoskeletal protein of erythrocytes, has been identified in the central nervous system and in cardiac myocytes.

DIAGNOSIS. *Spherocytosis* is usually evident in peripheral blood smears, strongly suggesting the diagnosis of HS, particularly in patients with childhood hemolytic anemia and history of similar abnormalities in other family members (Color plate 2*K*). The red cells are somewhat dehydrated and thereby have *elevated MCHC levels.* In fact, an observed MCHC above 36 is itself strong evidence of HS, although it should be noted that patients may acquire spherocytosis with similarly elevated MCHC during episodes of particularly severe immune hemolytic anemia.* The most useful confirmatory test for HS is assay of *osmotic fragility.* This test measures the amount of hemolysis suffered by red cells placed in a gradient series of hypotonic solutions. It is rendered even more specific for HS if suspect whole blood is incubated for 24 hours at 37° C before the fragility assay; hereditary spherocytes markedly increase in osmotic fragility when so stressed, compared with the minimal increase manifested by normal cells (Fig. 137–1). By increasing incubation time to 48 hours, one notes excessive spontaneous hemolysis of hereditary spherocytes in their own plasma—the so-called *"autohemolysis test."* Characteristically, this excessive autohemolysis is markedly lessened by addition of large amounts of glucose to the incubated cells.

When the diagnosis of HS is established, close relatives should be investigated for unsuspected disease. These same tests are frequently useful in uncovering mildly affected new patients. Gene penetrance is low in this disease, and both parents of established HS patients are completely normal in 5 to 20 per cent of families. Nonetheless, other close relatives may be affected when the parents seemingly are not.

PATHOGENESIS. Spherocytes are less deformable than normal biconcave discocytes. This single characteristic is probably the most critical to the hemolytic process and makes the spleen the specific organ of entrapment and destruction. The spleen—in fact, a filter—contains a unique microvasculature in which 1 to 3 μ diameter holes perforate the membrane that separates splenic cords from splenic sinusoids. Hereditary spherocytes cannot change their shape sufficiently for 7 μ erythrocytes to traverse these constraining apertures, and thus they become sequestered and ultimately destroyed by splenic cord macrophages. This intrinsic red cell abnormality is exacerbated by the acidotic environment of the splenic red pulp—an environment that suppresses erythrocyte glycolytic metabolism and thus reduces ATP production. Since ATP is somehow required for maintenance of normal membrane flexibility, its deficiency worsens the already existing stiffness of spherocytes and renders them even less likely to escape from the splenic cords. The underlying cause of the decreased flexibility of hereditary spherocytes is not completely understood, but evidence is accumulating that different defects in structural proteins of the erythrocyte membrane may cause HS in different kindreds. Most attention in this regard has been given to two filamentous proteins, *spectrin* (a myosin-like protein) and a topographically related one, *actin.* Evidence of mutation in spectrin in unrelated families has recently been provided, and a spherocytic hemolytic anemia has been described in inbred mice in which erythrocytes lack spectrin.

In addition to its stiffness, the hereditary spherocyte membrane is hyperpermeable to sodium ions, which serves to promote intracellular sodium accumulation, particularly when metabolic energy production (ATP) flags. Water is accumulated concomitantly with sodium, resulting in cellular swelling, which, in turn, further jeopardizes the escape of stressed spherocytes through the apertures of the splenic microvasculature.

TREATMENT. Many hematologists advise that *splenectomy* be performed in virtually all patients, with surgery delayed until the age of six if possible. Conversely, some physicians choose to postpone splenectomy in mild cases because compensation seems excellent. Such conservative decisions should be infrequent in view of the increased likelihood of cholelithiasis and the progressive splenomegaly with increasing hemolysis, which occurs later in life at a time when bone marrow compensation is diminishing. In the pediatric age group an excellent growth spurt and feeling of well-being are commonly noted following splenectomy. Nevertheless, children seem to be particularly at risk to develop pyogenic infections (particularly with pneumococci and *H. influenzae*) following splenectomy for any cause. Thus the use of *prophylactic antimicrobial agents* (generally penicillin, 250 mg twice daily) in all nonhypersensitive, splenectomized patients is strongly urged; this prophylaxis should be continued for at least two years following the surgery and perhaps for longer periods in small children. The need for lifelong prophylaxis following splenectomy is uncertain. Polyvalent *pneumococcal polysaccharide vaccine* should also be given prior to elective splenectomy.

An interesting complication of splenectomy, albeit rare, provides insight into spleen physiology. On occasion a small spleen remnant is inadvertently left in the abdomen at the time of splenectomy. By a process evidently akin to work hypertrophy, this remnant may grow after several years into a full-sized spleen, and hemolysis, which has been in complete remission, may recur. Regeneration is documented by splenic scan, and re-splenectomy becomes necessary. Such regrowth is particularly likely if the spleen is lacerated by the surgeon or by blunt abdominal trauma.

Transfusions are rarely required, except in the aplastic crises seen in some children. Until splenectomy can be accomplished, *folic acid therapy* (1 mg three times a day) is suggested in order to prevent deficiency of this vitamin, which is excessively utilized in HS (and other chronic hemolytic syndromes); such supplementation helps sustain increased bone marrow proliferative activity. Finally, no patient should be diagnosed and treated for HS without also making a careful *search for the disorder in close family members.* It is particularly tragic when

*Spherocytosis on blood smears can also be seen (along with fragmented erythrocytes) in microangiopathic hemolytic anemias, in severely burned patients, and in those with overwhelming clostridial bacteremia. In the last-named case this is due to the detergent action on red cell membranes of phospholipases released by clostridial organisms.

severe anemia of HS occurs in elderly, poor-operative-risk patients whose condition might have been discovered earlier by such epidemiologic concern.

HEREDITARY ELLIPTOCYTOSIS

Hereditary elliptocytosis is closely allied to hereditary spherocytosis in most respects and has a similar prevalence (1 per 5000). However, red cells tend to be oval or elliptical rather than spheroidal, and only about 10 per cent of affected patients manifest significant shortening of red cell survival. It is only in this small proportion that osmotic fragility abnormalities, similar to those of HS, can be detected. Diagnosis is made by blood smear examination, and the defect appears to be inherited as a dominant trait. The close association with HS is particularly noted in some families in which some members have blood smears typical of hereditary spherocytosis, whereas other members appear to have elliptocytosis. Furthermore, the hereditary elliptocyte membrane also may possess abnormal spectrin or actin or other structural proteins—an implication made previously for hereditary spherocytes. In those patients who manifest hemolysis, the spleen is the specific site of sequestration and destruction, and splenectomy induces long-term remission. Splenectomy is rarely required in this very mild syndrome.

HEREDITARY STOMATOCYTOSIS AND OTHER RARE MEMBRANE ABNORMALITIES

Stomatocytosis is characterized by red cells with a linear, slit-like area of central pallor as seen on stained films and of bowl-shaped erythrocytes when perceived in wet preparations. Several different membrane abnormalities probably underlie stomatocytic shape, and most of these produce very mild or no hemolysis. Moderate increases in red blood cell membrane permeability to cations (particularly sodium and potassium) have been discerned in many affected persons. Recent data suggest that an abnormality in protein-protein interactions in the red cell membrane may underlie the disorder, at least in some patients. There is also other evidence that abnormal membrane structure is involved: (1) rare erythrocytes that completely lack membrane Rh antigens (Rh null cells) appear stomatocytic, and (2) typical stomatocytes can be experimentally generated by intercalating various amphiphilic reagents into normal red cell membranes.

Other rare intrinsic abnormalities that presumably affect erythrocyte membranes produce red cells with aberrant water content. Thus swollen, water-logged red cells (*"hydrocytosis"*) and, conversely, dehydrated, shrunken red cells (*"desiccocytosis"*) occur rarely in patients with severe congenital hemolytic anemias. In both situations, it is inferred that abnormalities in membrane cation and, secondarily, water permeability reflect inborn errors in structural elements of the erythrocyte membrane. Finally, families with *"hereditary pyropoikilocytosis"* have been described. Red cells from affected patients are bizarrely shaped, generally appearing shrunken and dehydrated. The disorder derives its name from the fact that the abnormal red cells hemolyze when heated to temperatures 2 to 3° C below that required to hemolyze normal cells (50° C). Since the structural membrane protein spectrin melts at exactly 50° C, this protein may be mutant (and thus denatures at lower than normal temperatures) in hereditary pyropoikilocytes; evidence of this has recently emerged. The hemolytic anemia associated with this intriguing abnormality may be severe and only moderately improved by splenectomy.

Enzyme Deficiencies

The mature human erythrocyte depends upon the glycolytic pathway for normal energy metabolism (Fig. 137–2). Most of the enzymes in this pathway have been found to be selectively deficient in activity in various families with congenital hemolytic states. In many cases the exact mechanism by which enzyme deficiency produces hemolysis is only partially understood. Normally, red cells metabolize about 90 per cent of incorporated glucose anaerobically through the Embden-Meyerhof pathway—the major products of which are adenosine triphosphate (ATP) and 2,3-diphosphoglycerate (2,3-DPG). ATP acts to preserve membrane flexibility and thus is critical in providing necessary deformability for erythrocytes to flow through the microvasculature. It is not surprising that deficiencies of Embden-Meyerhof pathway enzymes frequently engender premature sequestration and destruction of erythrocytes in reticuloendothelial organs, such as the spleen and liver. The

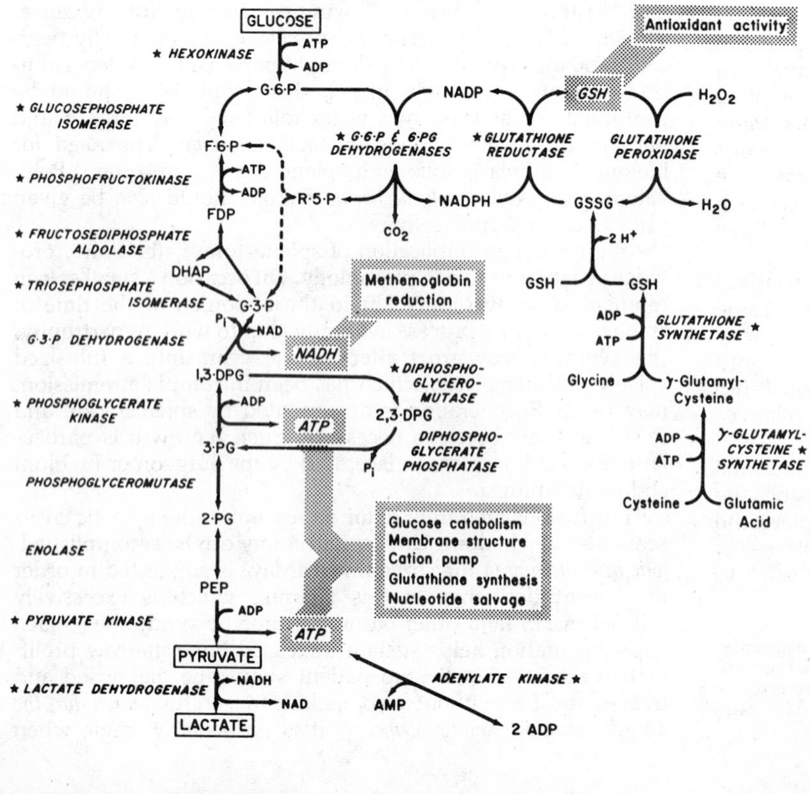

Figure 137–2. Glycolytic pathways and glutathione metabolism in the human erythrocyte. Stars indicate erythrocyte enzymes for which severe deficiency has been established. (From Valentine WN: Hemolytic anemia and inborn errors of metabolism. Blood 54:549, 1979. By permission.)

other product of glycolysis, 2,3-DPG, influences the binding of oxygen to hemoglobin, so that abnormalities in the Embden-Meyerhof pathway may alter oxygen delivery to tissues quite apart from inducing shortened red cell survival. About 10 per cent of glucose is metabolized by erythrocytes through the hexose monophosphate shunt, the sole producer of the reducing substance NADPH. Thus deficiencies of enzymes in this pathway produce red cells with a propensity to be damaged by various oxidative stresses—particularly those imposed by certain pharmacologic agents.

DEFECTS IN EMBDEN-MEYERHOF PATHWAY GLYCOLYTIC ENZYMES

PYRUVATE KINASE DEFICIENCY. Pyruvate kinase (PK) deficiency accounts for about 95 per cent of patients with enzyme deficiencies in the anaerobic pathway of erythrocytic glycolysis productive of congenital hemolytic anemia. The pattern of inheritance is recessive in most of the glycolytic enzyme–deficient hemolytic anemias, and the deficiency may be manifest in nonhematologic tissues; coincident abnormalities such as neurologic dysfunction may thereby result.

In PK deficiency, heterozygous parents are hematologically normal but can be detected by erythrocyte enzyme assay. Affected homozygotes usually have unimpressive blood smears, although crenated spheres are sometimes seen. As with most of the other glycolytic enzyme deficiencies, moderate to marked *hemolytic anemia* occurs, which is readily apparent in most patients during childhood. A strong *family history*, the occurrence of *premature gallstones*, and *splenomegaly* all mimic the manifestations of hereditary spherocytosis (HS); however, splenomegaly is generally not as marked as in HS. Several mutant PK enzymes that can produce hemolytic anemia have now been described. The osmotic fragility test is not particularly helpful, although *autohemolysis* (hemolysis after 48 hours of sterile incubation) is generally abnormally increased; but unlike the situation in hereditary spherocytosis, such hemolysis is not thwarted by glucose supplementation. This simple screening test (and the lack of spherocytes on blood smears) helps differentiate PK deficiency from HS, the other common congenital hemolytic anemia of childhood. The definitive test for PK deficiency is assay of enzyme activity in red cell hemolysates. This assay should be done in evaluating all childhood hemolytic anemias, especially when blood smears are relatively normal and when family (particularly sibling) histories are positive for other cases of possible hemolytic anemia. The PK enzymatic step is beyond the 2,3-DPG synthetic one so that 2,3-DPG tends to accumulate in erythrocytes of patients with PK deficiency. Since this important glycolytic intermediate may increase oxygen delivery from hemoglobin to tissues, anemic PK-deficient patients may be less handicapped than expected from consideration of hemoglobin levels alone. Relatively simple assay methods for the PK enzyme and for 2,3-DPG are now available in many clinical laboratories.

Hemolysis in PK deficiency is generally attributed to impaired glycolysis with concomitant deficient ATP generation. It seems likely that the small population of crenated spherocytes that are generally seen in PK-deficient blood smears are destined for rapid destruction in reticuloendothelial tissues. ATP is constantly required to pump intracellular calcium outward; its sluggish production in PK deficiency may produce the stiffened, dehydrated echinocytes (spiculated cells) characteristic of this disorder. Reticulocytes, but not mature red cells, still contain viable mitochrondria, which are efficient organelles for producing ATP by oxidative phosphorylation. This additional synthetic mechanism should presumably protect these young cells from lysis in this disorder. However, entrapment of PK-deficient cells—even reticulocytes—in the acidotic and anaerobic splenic environment probably further diminishes their ATP production. This may explain why reticulocyte levels often strikingly increase in PK deficiency following splenectomy, despite the partial amelioration of the hemolytic rate produced by the operative procedure. That is, in the absence of the spleen, mitochondrial ATP production in reticulocytes permits their relative metabolic advantage to be expressed as increased survival time. Splenectomy in PK deficiency is much less effective than in hereditary spherocytosis, and should be recommended, after infancy, only for severely affected patients, generally those requiring transfusions. All patients harboring PK-deficient red cells should be given folic acid supplementation (1 mg three times a day), and family members should be screened for heterozygosity and genetically counseled.

OTHER GLYCOLYTIC ENZYME DEFICIENCIES. Numerous other red cell glycolytic enzyme deficiencies that lead to sporadic congenital hemolytic anemia in families have also been described, but are rare occurrences (Valentine). Some are associated with neurologic dysfunction. Any patient with a congenital hemolytic process should have assays performed of all the glycolytic enzymes—assays that are currently available in only a few research laboratories throughout the world. After PK deficiency the next most commonly encountered of the red cell glycolytic abnormalities is *hexokinase deficiency*, a particularly instructive pathophysiologic error. Hexokinase is the first enzyme in red cell glycolysis, so that its deficiency decreases several glycolytic intermediates. Indeed, 2,3-DPG levels are low (in contrast to high levels with PK deficiency), and thus oxygen delivery to tissues is probably particularly inefficient. Patients with hexokinase deficiency have poorer exercise tolerance than those with PK deficiency despite similar levels of anemia, perhaps reflecting secondary 2,3-DPG deficiency.

DEFICIENCY IN ENZYME ACTIVITY RELATED TO THE HEXOSE MONOPHOSPHATE (HMP) SHUNT PATHWAY

Glucose-6-Phosphate Dehydrogenase (G-6-PD) Deficiency

The enzyme G-6-PD initiates the HMP shunt pathway, which normally consumes about 10 per cent of the glucose metabolized by the red cell (Fig. 137–2). This pathway generates NADPH, the major reducing compound synthesized by the red cell. Thus cells deficient in G-6-PD (or, more rarely, any of the other enzymes of the HMP shunt pathway) are hypersusceptible to damage by various oxidative stresses.

PATHOGENESIS OF HEMOLYSIS. A sequence of damage to erythrocyte constituents results when undefended oxidation occurs of: (1) ferrohemoglobin to ferrihemoglobin (methemoglobin); (2) reduced glutathione, which is present in large amounts in intact red cells, to its oxidized form; (3) sulfhydryl groups of the globin chains of hemoglobin. The globin chains denature and precipitate to form *Heinz bodies*. Such precipitates frequently attach to the inner surface of the red cell membrane; there, presumably by limiting deformability, they cause premature cell destruction. Any red cell—even those with normal HMP shunt metabolism—can be oxidatively damaged if stress is great enough. For example, certain oxidant drugs such as phenylhydrazine cause hemolytic anemia even in normal persons. In contrast, patients harboring red cells with a deficiency in one or another HMP shunt enzyme hemolyze when exposed to normally innocuous doses of oxidant compounds.

During the Korean War approximately 15 per cent of black American soldiers given the prophylactic antimalarial drug primaquine developed explosive hemolytic anemia. Intensive study of this extraordinary circumstance eventually showed that 10 to 15 per cent of black American males harbor red cells deficient in G-6-PD. Deficiency is inherited as a sex-linked trait, the gene coding for G-6-PD being located on the X chromosome. Thus the defect is fully expressed in male hemizygotes and female homozygotes, but is generally only minimally manifest in female heterozygotes. In such heterozygotes, two populations of red cells have been demonstrated by histochemical methods—normal and G-6-PD–deficient cells in varying proportions. This "mosaicism" constituted the first proof that one of the two X chromosomes (with its constituent genes) is randomly inactivated in somatic cells of females—the *Lyon hypothesis*.

Several different qualitative mutations in the G-6-PD enzyme that lead to quantitative deficiency (probably through accelerated in vivo enzyme inactivation) have been discovered in nearly all ethnic groups. Highest incidences of deficiency occur in malaria endemic areas. As with sickle cell anemia, this suggests that erythrocytic G-6-PD deficiency somehow protects against fatal varieties of malaria. Presumably a selective advantage is provided the host with this defect in parts of the world where malaria is or has been an important cause of morbidity. Protection might accrue from the fact that the malaria parasite itself imposes an oxidative stress on the red cells it invades. G-6-PD–deficient red cells, being unable to withstand this oxidative stress, prematurely hemolyze, foreshortening the required intraerythrocytic period for parasite maturation and propagation.

There are two common red cell G-6-PD isozymes, which are demonstrated by starch gel electrophoresis: Type A is found in about 30 per cent of American blacks, including most of those who are enzyme deficient; Type B is found in about 70 per cent of blacks and in nearly all whites.

MANIFESTATIONS IN BLACKS. The most common type of G-6-PD deficiency is found in blacks; about 10 per cent of American blacks, 8 to 20 per cent in West Africa, but only 2 per cent of South African Bantus harbor deficient red cells. Enzyme activity is reduced to about 15 per cent of normal in affected males, whereas in heterozygous females levels range from normal to those nearly as deficient as in affected males. In the latter females, random inactivation of the X chromosomes carrying normal G-6-PD genes has by chance evidently been excessive. Red cell survival is virtually normal in G-6-PD–deficient blacks unless the patients are subjected to oxidative stress, usually imposed by derivatives of several commonly utilized drugs. In addition, certain infections (pyogenic and infectious hepatitis) as well as diabetic ketoacidosis can also trigger hemolytic episodes in these patients. More than 40 drugs have been found to produce hemolysis in G-6-PD–deficient persons. These include the antimalarial drugs primaquine and quinine (the latter, it should be noted, is also used in popular beverages), antipyretics and analgesics such as phenacetin (commonly) and aspirin (only in large doses), the nitrofurans (such as Furadantin), sulfones, many sulfonamides, para-aminosalicylic acid, probenecid, quinidine, and water-soluble analogues of vitamin K, to name but a few. In addition, mothballs, which contain naphthalene, are not infrequently ingested by children who may develop explosive hemolysis if G-6-PD deficient. In fact, severe acute hemolytic episodes have been reported in black infants simply exposed to diapers stored in mothballs.

Hemolytic episodes induced by oxidant drugs in G-6-PD–deficient patients may be exacerbated or, in fact, triggered de novo by unrelated medical conditions. Thus bacterial infections can lead to hemolysis, perhaps because oxidant compounds, including hydrogen peroxide, are generated by phagocytizing white cells; such substances, by impinging on neighboring G-6-PD–deficient red cells, may bring about their destruction. In addition, an acquired inefficiency in red cell HMP shunt metabolism may occur in some patients who become uremic. Excessive hemolysis may thus occur in G-6-PD–deficient blacks for reasons unrelated to oxidant drug exposure.

Regardless of the triggering event, the kinetics of hemolysis are similar in G-6-PD–deficient blacks given oxidant drugs. Following a lag period of approximately two to three days, explosive destruction of red cells occurs. Elevated methemoglobin levels and the occurrence of Heinz bodies are frequently, but not always, perceptible indicators of oxidative damage, often having disappeared by the time hemolysis is obvious. Frequently, circulating red cells appear on blood smears with apparent pieces missing from their perimeters. Presumably these missing portions originally contained Heinz bodies which were pitted in the constraining filtration apertures of the spleen; thus, such morphology suggests that oxidative hemolysis is occurring. Hemoglobinemia and hemoglobinuria are usually of moderate degree during the explosive episode, but typically hemolysis is limited in duration, since only relatively old cells are vulnerable. That is, the more nearly normal G-6-PD activity found in younger red cells, which become more abundant in the circulation in response to hemolysis, protects them from excessive oxidative damage. Consequently, the red cell count may return to normal even though administration of the offending drug is continued, and diagnosis of the deficiency by assay of red cell enzyme activity may be difficult during this equilibrium phase when reticulocytosis is marked. Confirmation of the clinical diagnosis often must await the return to normal of the red cell age distribution.

MANIFESTATIONS IN OTHER POPULATIONS. G-6-PD deficiency in populations other than blacks is usually more severe, with red cell enzyme activity in most cases in the range of 0 to 5 per cent of normal. In addition, reduced G-6-PD activity is frequently observed in leukocytes and platelets, as well as red cells, in these patients. At least 100 different forms of G-6-PD have been demonstrated among white and Oriental populations by precise biochemical characterization of the enzymes. Greeks, Sardinians, Chinese, and Thais are populations with particularly frequent (1 to 10 per cent) incidences of G-6-PD deficiency. Deficient patients may manifest moderate chronic hemolytic anemia in the absence of drugs that can become dangerously severe with extrinsic oxidative challenge. In addition, hemolysis may worsen during episodes of acidosis, uremia, and infection. Generally, the spleen is not enlarged and osmotic fragility studies are normal. As might be expected, splenectomy is not useful in this disorder. *Favism* is a special type of G-6-PD–deficient hemolysis, and is observed almost solely in Mediterranean patients with the deficiency. This acute hemolytic disorder occurs after ingestion of Italian broad (fava) beans or, on occasion, after inhalation of pollen from the plant *Vicia faba* by patients with Mediterranean variety G-6-PD–deficient red cells. The hemolytic episode may be severe enough to cause death and occurs even in female heterozygotes. It has been speculated that two genes are necessary for favism to occur—one coding for G-6-PD deficiency, and the other for a unique type of metabolic degradation of a fava bean constituent that renders it especially oxidant. During the acute episode Heinz bodies are frequently seen in blood smears, as is methemoglobinemia.

G-6-PD–deficient white infants, particularly when premature, seem particularly prone to develop neonatal jaundice caused by excessive hemolysis. In addition, marked potentiation of hemolysis with dangerous hyperbilirubinemia may occur if the deficient newborn is inadvertently given water-soluble synthetic vitamin K preparations (even if these drugs are administered to the mother before delivery). In Hong Kong, for example, G-6-PD deficiency is the most common cause of severe neonatal jaundice leading to kernicterus. The propensity to develop marked neonatal jaundice in G-6-PD deficiency may reflect the fact that other red cell enzymes utilized in the defense against oxidative stresses, such as glutathione peroxidase, are also somewhat diminished even in normal infant red cells.

PREVENTION OF G-6-PD DEFICIENCY HEMOLYSIS. At least 100 million persons in the world have red cell G-6-PD deficiency, so that efforts to screen populations at high risk, using one of many simple screening tests for this deficiency, should be encouraged. Screening performed when the patient is well can serve to forewarn both patient and physician of hypersusceptibility to oxidant drugs. Ironically, for reasons described above, many deficient patients reside in areas where prophylactic antimalarials are commonly employed. Fortunately, some of these (e.g., chloroquine) are less liable to cause hemolysis than others (e.g., primaquine).

Other Deficiencies Related to the HMP Shunt Pathway

Deficiency of *6-phosphogluconate dehydrogenase* has been described, although its relationship to hemolysis is not yet clear. *Glutathione reductase* deficiency has also been described in several patients, although it now seems clear that this deficiency is rarely or never inherited, but instead is commonly caused by dietary riboflavin lack. This vitamin is a constituent of the coenzyme FAD, required for glutathione reductase activity, and its therapeutic administration ameliorates the red cell defect in virtually all patients. Absent red cell glutathione with an associated chronic hemolytic state has been reported to be due to genetic deficiency in either of the two enzymes involved in the synthesis of this important thiol compound—i.e., with *γ-glutamylcysteine synthetase* or *glutathione synthetase* deficiencies. With deficiency of the latter enzyme chronic neurologic disease may occur, but the causal relationship between the degenerative neurologic abnormality and the enzyme deficiency has not yet been established. Although a relatively mild hemolytic state has been reported to be due to *glutathione peroxidase* deficiency, the fact that most normal newborns harbor red cells with diminished levels of this enzyme makes it uncertain whether true genetic deficiency occurs.

ACQUIRED HYPERSUSCEPTIBILITY OF NORMAL RED CELLS TO OXIDATIVE STRESS. Patients with certain diseases of the gastrointestinal tract, particularly those leading to intestinal stasis, often harbor red cells that are hypersusceptible to oxidative stress. Overgrowth of bacteria in the small intestine may in some way be etiologic, as such patients frequently lose their oxidant hypersusceptibility when treated with nonabsorbable antimicrobials. The not uncommon hemolytic episodes noted when patients with ulcerative colitis are treated with sulfonamides, such as Azulfidine, may reflect this bacterial-induced reduction in red cell oxidant defense mechanisms. The nature of the putative bacterial toxins remains to be elucidated. An analogous, and frequently overlooked, hemolytic anemia occurs in patients with dermatitis herpetiformis who are given sulfones, such as dapsone. Since patients with this dermatologic condition frequently suffer from coexistent small intestine disease, hemolysis probably reflects oxidant hypersensitivity—a suggestion supported by the finding of scalloped (Heinz body–pitted?) red cells under these circumstances. Patients need not suffer intestinal disease or inherited erythrocyte enzyme deficiency to develop oxidant drug–induced hemolysis; excessive drug levels will shorten red cell survival in otherwise perfectly healthy people. Finally, 10 to 25 per cent of uremic patients acquire a defect in red cell HMP shunt activity. As with bacterial toxins, the nature of the uremic toxin is currently unknown. Affected patients are prone to hemolyze during hemodialysis, particularly if exposed to various oxidants, such as chloramine, commonly used to purify urban water supplies. In addition, the use of sulfonamides in the treatment of genitourinary infections in patients with chronic renal failure should be considered a potential exacerbator of the anemia suffered by such patients.

Other Intracorpuscular Abnormalities

The hemoglobinopathies and thalassemias, many of which are associated with hemolytic anemia, are considered in Ch. 141 to 144. Individual patients have been described with congenital hemolytic anemias caused by various other intrinsic red cell abnormalities. Thus a family manifesting increased membrane lecithin is an example of an intrinsic defect in red cell lipid homeostasis. A family with chronic hemolytic anemia in which red cells contain *excessive* adenosine deaminase attests to the importance of ATP in red cell integrity. In affected patients the excessive deamination of adenosine evidently lowers the availability of this purine for synthesis of ATP, which, in turn, is relatively deficient; red cell survival concomitantly diminishes. A congenital hemolytic anemia associated with pyrimidine nucleotidase deficiency is easily suspected in that basophilic stippling of red cells is striking in peripheral blood smears. In this condition pyrimidines accumulate intracellularly because of the deficiency of pyrimidine nucleotide catabolic enzyme. The accumulated material or the ribosomes containing it evidently precipitates into basophilic-staining particles. Similar stippling and hemolysis occurs in patients intoxicated with lead, which potently inhibits pyrimidine nucleotidase.

Finally, a large proportion of patients with erythropoietic porphyria have hemolytic anemia that may be partially relieved by splenectomy. It is presumed that the excessive porphyrins of this disease act as free radical generators that produce oxidative damage to red cells not unlike that noted with oxidant drug ingestion in G-6-PD–deficient patients.

Beutler E: Abnormalities of the hexose monophosphate shunt. Semin Hematol 8:311, 1971. *Review of biochemical and clinical abnormalities in the oxidant hemolytic anemias.*

Blood cell membranes. Semin Hematol 16:Nos. 1 and 2, 1979. *Review of normal and abnormal biochemistry of human red cell membranes and their relevance to red cell survival.*

Blood cell cytoskeleton. I. Red cell membrane skeleton. Semin Hematol 20:No. 3, 1983. *Review of membrane components involved in shape and deformability of red cells and their abnormalities in some hereditary hemolytic anemias.*

Oski FA, Marshall BE, Cohen PJ, Sugerman HJ, Miller LD: Exercise with anemia: The role of the left-shifted or right-shifted oxygen-hemoglobin equilibrium curve. Ann Intern Med 74:44, 1971. *Description of 2,3-DPG in ameliorating or potentiating clinical symptoms in two enzyme-deficient hemolytic anemias.*

Valentine WN: Hemolytic anemia and inborn errors of metabolism. Blood 54:549, 1979. *Review of biochemical and clinical abnormalities in hemolytic anemias associated with glycolytic enzyme deficiencies.*

138. ACQUIRED HEMOLYTIC DISORDERS

Manuel E. Kaplan

Hemolysis resulting from congenital, intrinsic defects of the red cell has been discussed in Ch. 137. Hemolysis can also result from a variety of acquired abnormalities of the erythrocyte and of the circulatory system in which it functions (see Table 136–1). In these disorders red cells are usually formed normally but are destroyed prematurely as a result of immunologic, physical, or chemical injury. The general manifestations of the acquired hemolytic anemias do not differ from those resulting from inherited intracorpuscular defects (Ch. 137).

SEQUESTRATIONAL HEMOLYSIS (HYPERSPLENISM)

By virtue of its unique vascular architecture, the normal spleen carefully sieves circulating red cells (Ch. 164). Arterial blood enters the spleen via arterioles in the white pulp. In the red pulp these arterioles communicate with either endothelial-lined sinuses or with closed, nonendothelialized cords that contain numerous fixed macrophages. To re-enter the venous circulation, red cells in the splenic cords must squeeze through narrow (3 μ) fenestrations between epithelial cells that line the splenic sinuses. Poorly deformable red cells are unable to meet this challenge and are destroyed by splenic cord macrophages. The splenic filtration barrier does not significantly jeopardize the survival of normal nonsenescent red cells. However, when the spleen becomes enlarged, it may randomly entrap and destroy normal red cells. This pathologic process is called *hypersplenism*. The differential diagnosis of splenomegaly is discussed in Ch. 164. In patients with hypersplenism the rapidity of hemolysis is poorly correlated with overall spleen size. Indeed, patients with marked splenomegaly may show little or no reduction in red cell survival.

Hypersplenism is best treated by effectively managing the underlying disease process. Splenectomy is rarely indicated; the procedure should be limited to patients who are transfusion-dependent and are reasonable operative risks and whose condition is refractory to medical therapy. Splenectomized individuals, particularly the young (under age ten), are statistically more likely to develop fulminant bacteremias and are less able to mount an effective primary (IgM) immune response to certain antigens. Consequently, the indications for splenectomy and its inherent risks should be carefully weighed before it is recommended.

IMMUNE HEMOLYTIC ANEMIAS

MECHANISMS OF IMMUNE HEMOLYSIS. In patients with immune hemolysis red cell destruction results from the binding of antibodies or complement components or both to the erythrocyte membrane. This may occur as a result of autoimmunization, of alloimmunization, or of exposure to certain drugs.

TYPES OF ANTIBODIES. Antibodies hemolyze red cells in vivo through various mechanisms on the basis of their structure, concentration, immunologic properties (complement fixing activity), the optimal temperature at which they are active, and the density and topographic distribution of the membrane antigens with which they combine. IgM red cell antibodies are generally agglutinating, complement-fixing, and active at colder temperatures. In contrast, most IgG red cell antibodies are fully active at 37° C, have little or no agglutinating activity, and vary in their ability to fix complement. IgA red cell antibodies usually occur in conjunction with IgG and/or IgM red cell antibodies, have no complement-fixing activity, and destroy red cells poorly.

ROLE OF COMPLEMENT. Most IgM and some IgG red cell antibodies activate the classical complement pathway after combining with membrane antigens. C1 binds to the Fc region of immunoglobulin heavy chains, develops esterase activity, and splits C4 into two fragments, C4a and C4b (Ch. 428). C4b attaches to the red cell membrane and binds C2, which in turn dissociates into C2a and C2b. C4b-2a complexes cleave C3 into C3a and C3b. C3b also binds directly to the membrane and is capable of activating both the alternative complement pathway (through factors B and D) and the membrane "attack" complex (C5-9) of the complement cascade. Insertion of activated C5-9 into the red cell membrane results in loss of membrane integrity. If complement activation continued unimpeded, life-threatening intravascular hemolysis would invariably ensue. However, the process is restrained by inhibitors normally present in plasma (factor I) and within the red cell membrane itself, which serve to block effective generation of the membrane attack components. However, red cells bearing fragments of activated complement components, i.e., C4b, C3b, C3bi (inactive C3b), and C3dg, are removed from the circulation and prematurely destroyed, primarily by hepatic macrophages that have receptors for these complement cleavage products.

HEMOLYSIS WITHOUT COMPLEMENT ACTIVATION. Red cells sensitized with IgG antibodies that fail to fix complement are sequestered and destroyed primarily within the splenic cords. Here they come into prolonged and intimate contact with macrophages bearing membrane receptors for the Fc component of the IgG molecule. The sensitized cells may be totally engulfed or undergo partial phagocytosis. Partially phagocytized red cells may reseal their membranes and, having lost proportionately more membrane than cytoplasm, assume a microspherocytic configuration. If the cells survive and re-enter the circulation, their abnormal shape testifies to their previous encounter with splenic macrophages. These spherocytic cells are particularly vulnerable since their deformability has been impaired and they retain significant membrane antibody.

DETECTION OF ANTIBODIES. The presence of red cell antibodies may be suspected from the appearance of freshly collected venous blood. IgM antibodies induce prompt red cell agglutination at room temperature. IgG antibodies are usually nonagglutinating but may so markedly reduce the negative charge (zeta potential) normally present on red cell surface that the cells are strongly aggregated by fibrinogen and other plasma macromolecules.

The *direct antiglobulin (Coombs') test* is most frequently used to detect immunoproteins present on the red cell membrane. This test measures the ability of a polyspecific antiserum that contains antibodies specific for human immunoglobulins and complement components to agglutinate a washed, dilute suspension of the patient's red cells. More precise identification of the membrane-bound immunoproteins may help to delineate the etiology and pathophysiologic mechanisms underlying a patient's hemolytic disorder. Consequently, when a positive direct antiglobulin test is obtained using a polyspecific reagent, the patient's red cells should be tested with various monospecific antisera that detect individual immunoglobulin classes or complement components. Almost all patients with immune hemolytic disorders exhibit a positive direct antiglobulin reaction. In the small percentage of patients (< 5 per cent) in whom this test is negative, more sensitive immunologic techniques may disclose increased concentrations of red cell–associated immunoproteins.

The *indirect antiglobulin test* detects serum antibodies capable of attaching to normal red cells. The serum is first incubated with a panel of serologically defined normal red cells. After the cells are washed, membrane-associated immunoprotein is sought by the antiglobulin reaction. Although in clinical situations the direct and the indirect Coombs' tests are frequently ordered together, only the former provides unequivocal evidence of an immune hemolytic process.

HEMOLYSIS DUE TO ALLOANTIBODIES. Alloantibodies capable of destroying transfused but not autologous red cells are products of immunologic responses to (1) bacteria that normally colonize the large intestine (giving rise to so-called "natural antibodies" that cross-react with allogeneic erythrocyte antigens), (2) transfused, imperfectly matched red cells, or (3) antigens of fetal red cells that entered the maternal circulation during pregnancy or at delivery.

Alloimmune red cell antibodies present in a patient's serum may be detected by agglutination of normal cells or by the indirect antiglobulin reaction. Since these antibodies have specificity for nonself antigens, they are harmless unless the patient is transfused with allogeneic red cells bearing the immunizing antigen. Consequently, it is crucial that these antibodies be detected in patients requiring transfusions and in pregnant women. In the latter, IgG red cell alloantibodies that gain access to the fetal circulation may induce erythroblastosis fetalis.

AUTOIMMUNE HEMOLYTIC ANEMIAS. Autoimmune hemolytic disorders are characterized by antibodies with specificity for autologous red cell antigens. The pathophysiologic mechanisms that result in autoantibody production are not fully understood. B lymphocyte clones capable of producing autoantibodies to red cells probably exist in everyone. They do not normally synthesize detectable quantities of autoantibody because their activities are suppressed by immunoregulatory T lymphocytes. If this suppressor mechanism is deranged, red cell autoantibodies may be produced in quantities sufficient to trigger red cell destruction. Certain diseases—infections, neoplasias, or collagen-vascular disorders—appear to stimulate the development of autoimmune hemolysis. The hemolytic disorders that result are therefore categorized as "secondary." In primary or idiopathic autoimmune hemolytic disorders no underlying or predisposing diseases can be detected.

AUTOIMMUNE HEMOLYTIC DISEASE DUE TO IgG, WARM-REACTING ANTIBODIES

CLINICAL MANIFESTATIONS. *Disease Associations.* In approximately 40 per cent of patients IgG-mediated autoimmune hemolytic anemia occurs secondary to an underlying disease, usually neoplastic or collagen-vascular in origin. Chronic lymphocytic leukemia and, less frequently, other lymphoproliferative disorders are the most commonly associated malignancies. There is a well-documented relationship between ovarian teratoma and warm immunohemolytic anemia. Systemic lupus erythematosus is the most frequently associated collagen-vascular disorder; less common are systemic sclerosis and rheumatoid arthritis. Occasional patients with ulcerative colitis present with warm autoimmune hemolysis.

Symptoms and Signs. Since the rate of red cell destruction, degree of anemia, and presence of underlying disease differ from patient to patient, a highly variable clinical picture can result. If hemolysis occurs suddenly, the patient usually presents with symptoms and signs related to severe anemia, i.e., pallor, fatigue, exertional dyspnea, dizziness, and palpitations. When hemolysis is more gradual, the anemia is usually less severe, and the patient may be relatively asymptomatic. On physical examination mild jaundice and splenomegaly are commonly present.

Laboratory Findings. The degree of anemia is variable and there are usually normal numbers of white cells and platelets. In occasional patients immune thrombocytopenia occurs in conjunction with immune hemolysis *(Evans' syndrome).* The mean corpuscular volume (MCV) may be increased, sometimes strikingly so (> 115 fl). When spherocytosis is prominent, the mean corpuscular hemoglobin concentration (MCHC) is usually elevated. The peripheral blood film typically discloses rouleaux formation, significant anisocytosis and poikilocytosis with numerous microspherocytes, and increased numbers of large polychromatophilic reticulocytes. Nucleated red cells may be present, particularly when hemolysis is rapid. The reticulocyte count is almost always elevated. Other typical laboratory findings include hyperbilirubinemia of the unconjugated type, diminished to absent serum haptoglobin, normal or slightly elevated plasma hemoglobin levels, and no urine hemosiderin. The direct antiglobulin test discloses only IgG or IgG and complement (C3dg). The indirect antiglobulin test may be positive or negative, a positive result implying that the red cell autoantibody has been produced in excess. Antibody eluted from the patient's red cells may exhibit specificity for well-defined red cell antigens, particularly in the Rh system. More commonly the eluted antibody is found to be a "panagglutinin," reacting with all normal red cells tested.

DIFFERENTIAL DIAGNOSIS. Since underlying diseases are present in almost half the patients with warm autoimmune hemolytic anemia, appropriate diagnostic studies to define them should be undertaken. The possibility of a lymphoproliferative disorder, a collagen-vascular disease, or drug-induced immune hemolysis must be considered. If the hemolytic disorder appears to be acquired but the direct antiglobulin test is negative, paroxysmal nocturnal hemoglobinuria (PNH) and various nonimmunologic causes of hemolysis (hypersplenism, a microangiopathic process) must be sought. If there is no evidence for these, the patient may have an immune hemolytic process that can be demonstrated only by immunologic studies more sensitive than the antiglobulin test. Alternatively, this may be inferred from a patient's objective clinical response to an empiric therapeutic trial of steroids.

TREATMENT. If an underlying disease process is identified, it should be treated. This frequently results in marked improvement of the accompanying hemolysis. Mild hemolysis may require no therapy.

Glucocorticoids. Patients with more rapid hemolysis should be treated with oral steroids equivalent to 1 to 2 mg of prednisone per kilogram per day, in single daily or divided (thrice daily) doses. If the patient is very symptomatic because of severe anemia, initial treatment with intravenous hydrocortisone, 400 to 800 mg per day, may be preferred followed by daily oral prednisone in divided doses. Improvement will usually occur within five to ten days, evidenced by increasing hemoglobin and hematocrit levels and decreasing reticulocytosis. At this time steroid therapy can be given as a single daily dose. Over the succeeding three to four weeks, the daily steroid dosage can usually be tapered, at five- to seven-day intervals, to a daily dose of approximately 20 mg of prednisone. During this time blood counts and reticulocyte counts should be checked periodically. Thereafter, the dose of steroids should be decreased more slowly, every two to three weeks by 5 mg per day, as long as the reticulocyte count does not rise significantly and the hemoglobin level remains stable. In occasional patients it may be possible to discontinue steroids entirely without exacerbating the hemolysis. More commonly, significant hemolysis persists and patients require daily maintenance steroid therapy, 5 to 10 mg of prednisone daily, or 10 to 30 mg on alternate days, which results in fewer undesirable side effects (Ch. 29).

The mechanism of the corticosteroid effect in warm autoimmune hemolytic disorders is not fully understood. Steroids appear to diminish the number, and possibly the binding strength, of monocyte and macrophage Fc receptors, thereby decreasing the ability of these cells to bind and destroy IgG-sensitized red cells. Prolonged therapy with steroids may suppress antibody synthesis; however, this effect certainly does not explain the prompt, frequently dramatic clinical improvement seen in most patients.

If the response to corticosteroid therapy is unsatisfactory, i.e., (1) hemolysis and anemia are not significantly improved within two weeks after initiating high-dose steroid therapy or (2) unacceptably large daily doses of steroids (> 15 to 20 mg of prednisone) are required to maintain hematologic improvement, other therapeutic approaches must be considered.

Splenectomy. ^{51}Cr red cell survival and sequestration studies should be performed, if possible, before splenectomy is undertaken. Typically they will disclose significantly reduced RBC survival (t½ = 5 to 15 days), and the spleen will be the major, if not exclusive, site of red cell destruction. In such a patient splenectomy is advisable and should result in marked hematologic improvement. Occasionally significant hemolysis persists after splenectomy. This usually results from intense red cell sensitization with IgG autoantibody, and characteristically responds to small maintenance doses of steroids. In patients in whom ^{51}Cr sequestration studies reveal the liver to be a major site of red cell destruction, the direct antiglobulin test usually discloses complement (C3dg) as well as IgG. Splenectomy results in less effective control of hemolysis in such patients, favorable responses being achieved in only 30 per cent. Consequently, a trial of immunosuppressive therapy may be preferred prior to splenectomy.

Immunosuppressive Drugs. At present either oral azathioprine* (Imuran), 50 to 200 mg per day, or cyclophosphamide* (Cytoxan), 50 to 150 mg per day, is the immunosuppressive agent most frequently employed in patients with warm immune hemolytic anemia. Responses are variable and usually not very dramatic. However, their use in patients whose conditions are refractory to steroids may permit reduction in the excessive steroid dosages required for maintenance.

Transfusion. Before hemolysis is adequately controlled by steroid therapy, severely anemic patients may require red cell transfusions. Transfusion is particularly hazardous when the patient has a positive indirect antiglobulin test because donor-patient compatibility cannot be ensured by cross-matching techniques. The serum of such a patient frequently contains a panagglutinating autoantibody reactive with red cells from all prospective donors. More importantly, the autoantibody may mask the presence of a red cell alloantibody that may be capable of provoking intravascular hemolysis of transfused red cells. To distinguish these antibodies, patient red cells from which autoantibody has been eluted are used to absorb totally autoantibody from the patient's serum. The absorbed serum is then tested for alloantibody activity with potential donor cells. In addition, blood banks usually attempt to identify possible blood group specificity of antibody eluted from a patient's red cells and of the serum antibody. Following these studies, donor red cells "most compatible" with the patient are selected for transfusion. Usually patients with autoimmune hemolysis can be safely transfused when these precautionary steps are taken. Donor cells should be administered slowly, with the patient being closely observed for symptoms and signs suggestive of a possible hemolytic transfusion reaction, the diagnosis and treatment of which are described in Ch. 146).

COURSE AND PROGNOSIS. In patients with secondary autoimmune hemolytic disorders the clinical course and ultimate

*This use is not listed in the manufacturer's directive.

prognosis are generally determined by the underlying disease process. Autoimmune hemolysis due to warm IgG antibodies is usually well controlled by corticosteroid therapy or splenectomy or both. Uncontrollable hemolysis resulting in death rarely occurs. All evidence of the disease may disappear in some patients. More commonly a positive direct antiglobulin test persists, and the patient experiences recurrent episodes of hemolysis that may require steroid therapy. The condition in splenectomized patients is generally more stable hematologically than that in patients managed by medical therapy alone. Major causes of death include thromboembolic disease and complications of chronically impaired host defense mechanisms caused by corticosteroids, splenectomy, or immunosuppressive drugs.

AUTOIMMUNE HEMOLYTIC DISEASE DUE TO COLD-REACTING ANTIBODIES

Cold-reacting red cell antibodies combine most avidly with erythrocyte membrane antigens at grossly subphysiologic temperatures (0 to 4° C). They exhibit characteristic "thermal amplitudes," i.e., maximum temperatures beyond which they are unable to combine effectively with their antigens. Pathologic cold antibodies produce clinical hemolysis because they retain significant immunologic reactivity at temperatures that are achievable in vivo (30 to 32° C). Thus, if the thermal amplitude of a red cell antibody does not extend to 30° C, the antibody will have no relevance pathophysiologically. IgM cold-reacting antibodies occur most commonly. Because they strongly agglutinate red cells in the cold, they are designated as *cold agglutinins.* Rare IgA cold agglutinins have been described; however, these antibodies do not produce hemolysis in vivo because they lack complement-fixing activity. Cold-reacting IgG red cell autoantibodies are occasionally encountered. They are intensely complement fixing and are responsible for producing the disease picture of paroxysmal cold hemoglobinuria.

COLD AGGLUTININ DISEASE. ***Pathophysiology.*** IgM cold agglutinins are normally present in human serum but have no known function and may represent by-products of polyclonal immunologic responses to viruses and other microorganisms. Cold agglutinins in serum are detected and quantified in serum by the cold agglutinin titer, i.e., the maximal serum dilution, at 4° C, that retains red cell agglutinating activity. Normal cold agglutinins are harmless because they are present in low concentrations in serum (titers ≤ 1:32) and exhibit low thermal amplitudes. Usually, but not always, the higher the patient's cold agglutinin titer, the broader the thermal amplitude of the cold antibody, and the greater the probability that the patient will experience hemolysis.

The synthesis of cold agglutinins may increase in response to certain infections, especially mycoplasma, viral (EB, cytomegalovirus), and protozoal (trypanosomiasis, malaria) infections. Titers of these polyclonal agglutinins usually peak within two to three weeks of onset, but rarely do antibody concentrations rise sufficiently to provoke clinically apparent hemolysis.

Cold agglutinin disease occasionally appears in patients with lymphoproliferative disorders, particularly histiocytic lymphoma. Indeed, hemolytic anemia may be the initial manifestation of the lymphoma. In these patients, the cold agglutinins are predictably monoclonal, containing either kappa or lambda light chains. Occasionally the antibody may be present in such a high concentration that it is detectable as a spike on serum protein electrophoresis.

Idiopathic cold agglutinin disease occurs most frequently in elderly patients in whom, by definition, no underlying infectious or neoplastic process can be identified. The cold agglutinin is almost always monoclonal kappa IgM.

Cold agglutinins react with polysaccharide components of red cell membrane glycolipids and glycoproteins immunochemically related to human ABO blood group antigens. Some of these polysaccharide antigens are better expressed on adult erythrocytes (designated I), and others on fetal red cells (i). Cold agglutinins that react significantly more strongly with adult red cells are said to exhibit anti-I specificity, whereas those that combine better with fetal (cord) erythrocytes show anti-i specificity. I and i are not alleles and both antigens are usually expressed on adult, as well as on fetal, red cells. However, the red cells of rare, otherwise normal individuals express only one or the other. Very infrequently patients with cold agglutinin disease have antibodies that exhibit exclusive anti-I or anti-i reactivity. Some cold antibodies that react equally well with adult and cord cells fail to agglutinate red cells pretreated with proteolytic enzymes and are said to show anti-PR specificity. Identification of the major reactivity of a cold agglutinin (anti-I, -i, or -PR) and its clonality may be clinically informative, since cold agglutinins produced in various diseases show different characteristic patterns of reactivity (Table 138–1).

Mechanisms of Hemolysis. High thermal amplitude cold agglutinins bind to red cells in the cooler portions of the circulation and initiate agglutination and complement activation via the classical pathway. Complement-mediated intravascular hemolysis may ensue. However, this occurs minimally or not at all in most patients because propagation of the complement cascade is effectively aborted before membrane damage occurs. Activation of the earlier components of the classical pathway (C1, 4, 2, and 3), as previously described, results in the binding of C3b (EC3b) to the red cell membrane. EC3b is so rapidly cleaved by the plasma C3 inactivator (factor I) that it is unable to trigger effective activation of the membrane attack components of complement (C5-9). Factor I activity is significantly enhanced by cofactors in the plasma (factor H) and in the red cell membrane itself. EC3b is progressively cleaved into EC3bi (inactive, membrane-bound C3b) and EC3dg, which are not able to propagate complement activation, and appear, to some degree, to inhibit binding of additional cold agglutinin to the red cell membrane. Although significant intravascular hemolysis is prevented, red cells bearing complement fragments are prematurely removed from the circulation and destroyed, primarily by hepatic macrophages.

Clinical Manifestations. In patients with postinfectious cold agglutinin disease, hemolysis is usually self-limited and mild. In contrast, idiopathic and lymphoma-associated cold agglutinin syndromes are accompanied by persistent hemolysis that is usually worse in winter. After exposure to cold, the patient may experience a picture of painful acrocyanosis, similar to Raynaud's phenomenon, induced by intense red cell autoagglutination. Unlike Raynaud's, there is usually no antecedent blanching or reactive hyperemia, and local gangrene does not occur. Severe chilling may accelerate hemolysis to such a degree that hemoglobinuria results.

Diagnosis. On physical examination the patient may be mildly jaundiced. As the patient's blood is drawn, the red cells may clump so rapidly that the blood appears to clot even in the presence of an anticoagulant. Warming of the anticoagulated blood to 37° C rapidly restores its normal appearance. Electronically measured blood counts are frequently inaccurate because of the intense autoagglutination at room temperature. The red count and MCV measurement are particularly affected, leading to distortion of the calculated hematocrit. This situation

TABLE 138–1. RELATIONSHIP BETWEEN COLD AGGLUTININ STRUCTURE AND SPECIFICITY IN VARIOUS DISEASES

	Specificity		
Structure	*Anti-I*	*Anti-i*	*Anti-PR*
Polyclonal/oligoclonal (κ + λ)	*Mycoplasma pneumoniae*	Infectious mononucleosis	
Monoclonal			
κ	Idiopathic cold agglutinin disease	Lymphoma	Idiopathic cold agglutinin disease
λ		Lymphoma	

should be recognized by alert laboratory personnel. The reticulocyte count is not uncommonly only mildly increased; this suggests suboptimal bone marrow compensation. The cold agglutinin titer is invariably elevated, and the direct antiglobulin test discloses C3dg. Typically, serum haptoglobin levels are decreased and LDH concentrations increased.

Treatment. When an underlying disease process is identified, it should be treated appropriately. Patients should be told to avoid exposure to the cold and to dress warmly. Treatment with daily chlorambucil,* 2 to 4 mg orally, improves the condition in some patients with idiopathic cold agglutinin syndrome, probably by reducing the synthesis of cold agglutinin. Glucocorticoids and splenectomy are generally of no benefit. If rapid hemolysis persists despite treatment, it may be advisable for the patient to move to a warmer climate.

PAROXYSMAL COLD HEMOGLOBINURIA. Paroxysmal cold hemoglobinuria (PCH) is an exceedingly rare autoimmune hemolytic disorder caused by IgG cold-reacting antibodies directed against the ubiquitous P blood group antigen. PCH was first described in patients with tertiary syphilis, but now more commonly accompanies certain viral infections. It may occur as an idiopathic process. The cold antibody is nonagglutinating but activates complement so efficiently that intravascular hemolysis results. Following exposure to cold, patients typically experience chills, fever, headache, and diffuse pain in the abdomen, back, and legs accompanied by hemoglobinuria. The direct Coombs' test is usually weakly positive for IgG and complement. PCH is diagnosed by demonstrating the presence, in the patient's serum, of the *Donath-Landsteiner antibody.* Normal red cells are mixed with the patient's serum and a source of complement and chilled (0 to 4° C). Thereafter, the cell suspension is incubated at 37° C for 45 to 60 minutes. The appearance of hemolysis is presumptive evidence of the Donath-Landsteiner antibody. When PCH accompanies a viral infection, hemolysis is usually self-limited, requiring only supportive therapy and protection of the patient from cold. In some patients hemolysis may periodically recur or become chronic. It may respond to treatment with glucocorticoids or to immunosuppressive drugs such as cyclophosphamide.

IMMUNE HEMOLYSIS DUE TO DRUGS. A number of drugs may cause immune hemolytic anemia. Three distinct mechanisms have been described:

1. *Drug binding to red cells.* When administered intravenously, certain immunogenic drugs, exemplified by penicillin, bind tightly to erythrocyte membranes. If drug-specific antibodies are produced, they attach to red cells at membrane sites occupied by the drug. In the case of penicillin-induced immune hemolysis, the offending antibody is characteristically IgG and is noncomplement fixing. In vivo, it binds to penicillin-modified red cells and induces their destruction by a mechanism essentially identical to that seen in warm autoimmune hemolytic anemia, i.e., IgG-sensitized red cells are sequestered primarily within the spleen and destroyed by Fc receptor-bearing macrophages. The direct antiglobulin test discloses only IgG. The antipenicillin specificity of the red cell antibody can be demonstrated by indirect antiglobulin testing. IgG eluted from the patient's red cells, as well as antibody that may be present in the patient's serum, fails to combine with normal erythrocytes unless the cells have been pretreated with penicillin. Since hemolysis promptly ceases soon after penicillin is discontinued, corticosteroid therapy is usually unnecessary.

2. *Innocent bystander hemolysis.* Most drugs that induce immune hemolytic anemia in humans (sulfonamides, phenothiazines, quinine, stibophen) bind primarily to plasma proteins rather than to red cells. They are weakly immunogenic but may, in some patients, stimulate the synthesis of drug-specific complement-fixing antibodies. Consequently, the patient's erythrocytes are bathed in plasma containing activated complement components generated by drug-antibody complexes. C3b binds directly to the red cell membrane complement receptor (CR1). By mechanisms previously described, CR1-bound C3b may activate the membrane attack complex of complement (C5-9) with sufficient rapidity to provoke intravascular hemolysis; or may be so promptly cleaved by factor I, the plasma C3b inactivator, that intravascular hemolysis is precluded. Intact red cells that bear complement fragments may be sequestered and prematurely destroyed, primarily by hepatic macrophages. The direct antiglobulin test reveals only membrane-associated complement cleavage products, primarily C3dg. Efforts to elute immunoprotein from the patient's red cells are unusually unsuccessful. The indirect antiglobulin test is characteristically negative; however, if the offending drug is added to normal erythrocytes suspended in the patient's serum with a source of complement, hemolysis may occur, and indirect Coombs' testing of the nonhemolyzed cells may disclose membrane-associated complement fragments. After the drug is discontinued, hemolysis generally subsides very promptly, and patients usually require no additional therapy.

3. *Drug-induced autoimmune hemolytic anemia.* A pure IgG direct antiglobulin test appears in approximately 15 per cent of patients chronically treated with methyldopa (Aldomet). However, only 10 per cent of the Coombs'-positive patients develop clinically apparent hemolysis. Antibodies eluted from the patients' red cells combine readily with normal erythrocytes in the absence of methyldopa, thereby displaying true autoimmune reactivity. Patients treated with levodopa or mefenamic acid (Ponstel), a nonsteroidal anti-inflammatory drug, may develop similar erythrocyte autoantibodies. By unknown mechanisms these agents probably interfere with immunoregulatory processes that suppress the synthesis of red cell autoantibodies. Moreover, it is not clear why hemolysis occurs in only a small percentage of Coombs'-positive methyldopa-treated patients. The mechanism of cell destruction appears identifical to that seen in warm autoimmune hemolytic anemia, i.e., splenic sequestration and red cell destruction by Fc receptor-positive macrophages. Hemolysis usually subsides within one to three weeks after methyldopa is discontinued, but a positive direct antiglobulin test may persist for many months. Although the hemolysis responds to steroid therapy, this therapy is rarely required. If methyldopa is readministered to a patient who has fully recovered from methyldopa-induced hemolysis, no anamnestic autoimmune response usually occurs. Hemolysis may recur, but only after a prolonged treatment period.

PAROXYSMAL NOCTURNAL HEMOGLOBINURIA

Paroxysmal nocturnal hemoglobinuria (PNH) is an acquired hemolytic disorder resulting from the proliferation of an abnormal clone of stem cells whose progeny are uniquely susceptible to complement-mediated membrane damage. Its etiology is not known. Since patients with PNH are unusually prone to develop aplastic anemia or acute leukemia, it may represent a "preneoplastic" transformation of hematopoietic stem cells. The disease is quite rare; however, it is probably underdiagnosed because its manifestations are frequently protean. It occurs with greatest frequency in early adulthood, but has been described in young children and in the very elderly.

PATHOPHYSIOLOGY. PNH red cells, granulocytes, and platelets are inordinately sensitive to the lytic effects of complement. The patient's peripheral blood frequently contains two or three subpopulations of red cells differing in their sensitivity to complement (I = normally sensitive cells, II = cells of intermediate sensitivity, and III = very sensitive cells). When PNH red cells are exposed to complement activated in vitro by either the classical or the alternative pathway, PNH II and III cells bind much greater quantities of C3b than do normal red cells. The rate of red cell destruction in vivo correlates well with the proportions of circulating red cells that are PNH II and III.

Spontaneous, limited in vivo activation of the alternative complement pathway appears to occur normally. This may result in binding of C3b to the red cell membrane complement receptor (CR1), resulting in EC3b. EC3b exerts positive feedback

*This use is not listed in the manufacturer's directive.

on the alternative pathway through factors B and D to generate additional C3b that may bind to unoccupied red cell CR1. EC3b may potentially trigger activation of C5–9, resulting in intravascular hemolysis. Normal human red cell membranes express activity (designated factor H–like) that facilitates rapid inactivation of membrane-bound C3b by factor I, the plasma C3b inactivator. PNH red cells are functionally deficient in factor H–like activity, which may account for their marked susceptibility to complement-mediated hemolysis.

Platelets and granulocytes from PNH patients are also abnormally sensitive to activated complement in vitro. Although the in vivo survival of PNH platelets has been reported to be normal, their enhanced susceptibility to complement activation may underlie the thrombotic diathesis commonly seen in these patients. Functional abnormalities of the PNH granulocyte have also been described.

CLINICAL MANIFESTATIONS. The diagnosis of PNH must be considered in all patients with chronic hemolysis, particularly when associated with hemoglobinuria, pancytopenia, or unusual venocclusive events. During episodes of rapid hemolysis, patients commonly experience diffuse abdominal and back pain that has been attributed to ischemia resulting from microcirculatory thrombi. Not infrequently major thromboses occur involving the hepatic, splenic, portal, or cerebral veins. On physical examination pallor and scleral icterus are common. The degree of anemia is highly variable, ranging from mild to severe. The reticulocyte count may be inappropriately low given the severity of the anemia. The MCV may be normal, slightly increased, or diminished, depending upon the degree of reticulocytosis and the presence of accompanying iron deficiency. Mild thrombocytopenia and granulocytopenia occur commonly. The peripheral blood smear reveals no autoagglutination, spherocytosis, or red cell fragmentation. The direct antiglobulin test is usually negative. Bone marrow cellularity varies from markedly hypoplastic to profoundly hyperplastic, and iron stores are usually reduced or absent. Erythroid elements predominate and cell maturation is typically normoblastic.

Because red cell destruction occurs intravascularly, the serum LDH is elevated, serum haptoglobin levels are reduced or absent, and hemosiderinuria is present. Frank hemoglobinuria usually occurs only intermittently and is most apparent after periods of sleep, when the urine is concentrated.

DIAGNOSIS. The diagnosis of PNH requires that the patient's red cells show excessive susceptibility to complement-mediated hemolysis in vitro. This is most frequently demonstrated by mixing the red cells with freshly collected normal human serum that has been mildly acidified *(Ham's test).* Hemolysis, which results from activation of the alternative pathway, is highly specific but unfortunately the Ham's test is too insensitive to detect all patients with PNH. The simpler *sucrose hemolysis test,* which results in complement activation via the classical pathway, is much more sensitive than the Ham's test but is less specific, with positive results occurring in some patients with myeloproliferative disorders. Low levels of neutrophil alkaline phosphatase and red blood cell acetyl cholinesterase occur commonly in PNH patients, but are nonspecific. Occasionally these measurements are used to confirm the diagnosis.

Other causes of intravascular hemolysis and hemoglobinuria that should be considered in the differential diagnosis include (1) hemolytic transfusion reactions, (2) paroxysmal cold hemoglobinuria, (3) red cell hemolysins such as those present in snake venoms and *C. welchii* exotoxin, (4) traumatic intravascular hemolysis as occurs in thrombotic thrombocytopenic purpura or march hemoglobinuria, and (5) G-6-PD deficiency (Ch. 137).

TREATMENT. Erythropoiesis may be enhanced with folic acid, iron, and androgen therapy. In some patients iron administration may provoke increased hemolysis and hemoglobinuria. This may be prevented by prior transfusion and probably results from the increased destruction of newly produced, complement-sensitive reticulocytes. Androgen administration may significantly improve the anemia. A six- to eight-week trial of oral fluoxymesterone or oxymesterone (5 to 50 mg per day), or of intramuscular nandralone decanoate (25 to 200 mg once weekly), is usually sufficient to identify androgen-responsive patients.

By unknown mechanisms steroid therapy (equivalent to 0.25 to 1 mg of prednisone per kilogram per day) significantly slows acute hemolytic episodes in some patients, and chronically administered low-dose steroids may reduce ongoing hemolysis. Daily steroids should not be administered except in life-threatening situations because of their unacceptable side effects and the increased danger of overwhelming bacterial or fungal sepsis. Alternate-day prednisone therapy, in dosages ranging from 15 to 40 mg, has been reported to improve more than 50 per cent of patients so treated.

Most patients with PNH eventually require blood transfusions. Initially donor red cells survive normally and suppress the production of the patient's abnormal red cells resulting in marked clinical improvement. Following repetitive transfusions, however, patients are prone to develop hemosiderosis and to produce alloantibodies to red cell, neutrophil, platelet, and even to plasma protein antigens. Once alloimmunization has occurred, further transfusion therapy is difficult, since it may be followed by rapid destruction of recipient (as well as of donor) red cells. Even compatible transfusions may trigger increased hemolysis of patient red cells and hemoglobinuria, probably because the donor packs contain small quantities of activated complement. If evidence of increased hemolysis follows transfusion of packed donor red cells, only washed red cells or frozen and reconstituted red cells should be administered.

PNH patients may require anticoagulation because they are susceptible to major thromboembolic events. Since heparin therapy has been reported to exacerbate hemolysis in some patients, it must be used with caution. Vitamin K antagonists can usually be employed without difficulty, but it is not yet clear whether continuous prophylactic anticoagulation with coumadin derivatives is clinically beneficial.

Although bone marrow transplantation has been reported to have successfully eradicated the PNH clone in selected patients, this approach must be regarded as experimental at this time.

PROGNOSIS. The course of PNH is exceedingly variable. Most patients survive fewer than ten years from the time of diagnosis. In a small percentage of patients all disease manifestations spontaneously subside, possibly reflecting disappearance of the aberrant clone. More commonly, patients experience waxing and waning hemolysis, which may be exacerbated by immunologic stress such as infection, transfusion, and immunization. Thrombotic events, primarily venous, account for much of the morbidity and mortality. With time, marrow function progressively deteriorates, and a clinical picture more closely resembling aplastic anemia may gradually ensue. In approximately 5 per cent of patients the disease evolves into acute myeloblastic leukemia.

HEMOLYSIS CAUSED BY CHEMICALS

A number of chemicals may directly interact with and injure red cells, resulting in hemolysis. These toxins range in complexity from inorganic cations (arsenic and copper) and simple organic compounds such as chloramine to complex biologic substances produced by microorganisms, plants, and lower animals. Arsenic and copper injure red cells probably by binding to membrane sulfhydryl groups. Copper-induced hemolysis has been observed in hemodialyzed patients, and may be responsible for the transient hemolytic episodes observed in patients with Wilson's disease.

Purification of urban water supplies with alum and chlorine results in the generation of chloramine, a potent oxidant. If chloramine is not efficiently removed from tap water that is used for hemodialysis, it may swiftly induce methemoglobin and Heinz body formation, resulting in rapid hemolysis.

Amphotericin is a lipophilic fungal product that binds avidly in vitro to red cell membrane lipids. In occasional patients it may provoke hemolysis, presumably by altering red cell membrane stability.

C. welchii, spiders, and snakes produce potent lipolytic toxins capable of damaging red cell membrane integrity, thereby provoking intravascular hemolysis. Marked spherocytosis of circulating red cells is commonly seen. Less rapid hemolysis of uncertain etiology may accompany severe infection with other bacteria *(D. pneumoniae, E. coli, S. aureus)*. Castor beans and certain species of mushrooms contain hemolysis-inducing toxins.

HEMOLYSIS CAUSED BY METABOLIC ABNORMALITIES

SPUR CELL HEMOLYTIC ANEMIA. Patients with a significant hepatocellular disease are frequently anemic. Blood loss, folate deficiency, alcohol-induced marrow dysfunction, and hypersplenism may contribute to the etiology of the anemia. However, in a small percentage of patients with end-stage cirrhosis, a clinical picture of rapid hemolysis develops with the appearance of numerous acanthocytes (spiculated, occasionally spur-shaped red cells).

Pathophysiology. Red cell membrane cholesterol and phospholipids exist in dynamic equilibrium with plasma lipids. In many patients with severe parenchymal liver disease, abnormal plasma lipoproteins appear to unload cholesterol and phospholipids onto the erythrocyte membrane. As a result the membranes spread and the cells thin out to become "target cells." The molar ratio of cholesterol to phospholipids in target cells is normal, and these cells usually survive normally. In patients with spur cell hemolytic anemia, excess cholesterol accumulates in the red cell membrane unaccompanied by parallel increases in phospholipids. This may be caused by an abnormal circulating low-density lipoprotein containing an increased ratio of free cholesterol:phospholipids. Red cell deformability is markedly reduced, and the cells are prematurely destroyed within the congested, hypertrophied spleen.

Clinical Manifestations. Patients with spur cell hemolytic anemia characteristically exhibit marked splenomegaly and signs of advanced cirrhosis including jaundice, ascites, varices, and neurologic manifestations of hepatic encephalopathy. The anemia is usually severe, perhaps in part because of concomitant gastrointestinal blood loss. The peripheral smear contains numerous acanthocytes and polychromatophilic reticulocytes. The direct antiglobulin test is negative. Red cells are sequestered by the spleen and have shortened survival.

Diagnosis. The presence of a significantly elevated reticulocyte count and numerous spur cells on peripheral smear in a patient with end-stage cirrhosis is diagnostic of this syndrome. When normal compatible red cells are incubated with the patient's plasma in vitro, they become acanthocytic.

Prognosis and Treatment. Spur cell hemolytic anemia carries an exceedingly poor prognosis, almost all patients dying within months because of the associated liver disease. The beneficial effects of transfusion are limited since normal cells survive no better than autologous cells in these patients. Splenectomy may slow the rate of hemolysis in selected patients but is exceedingly hazardous because of the severity of the liver disease.

HYPOPHOSPHATEMIA. Hemolysis may occur in patients with profoundly depressed serum phosphorus levels (< 1 mg per 100 ml) (Ch. 207). Hypophosphatemia of this degree occurs primarily in severely malnourished patients, particularly when they consume excessive quantities of phosphate-binding antacids. Erythrocyte ATP levels fall, the cells become poorly deformable, and hemolysis occurs primarily within the spleen.

HEMOLYSIS CAUSED BY RED CELL PARASITES

MALARIA. *Malarial infections*, particularly with *Plasmodium falciparum*, are probably the most common cause of hemolytic anemia worldwide (Ch. 378). Merozoites parasitize red cells and utilize for their own purposes hemoglobin, enzymes, and substrates, thereby metabolically depriving infected erythrocytes. As a result, the osmotic fragility and cation permeability of parasitized red cells are altered. Infected red cells may display new membrane antigens; this may help to explain the positive direct antiglobulin tests reported in some patients with falciparum malaria. Red cell destruction appears to occur primarily in the spleen, and splenomegaly is almost universally present in patients with chronic malarial infection. Rarely, rapid intravascular hemolysis with hemoglobinuria (blackwater fever) occurs soon after antimalarial therapy is initiated. It is not clear whether the infection or the drug plays the more important role in this phenomenon.

BABESIOSIS. *Babesia* are protozoans that parasitize red cells of many animal species (Ch. 384). Several cases of babesia-induced hemolytic anemia have been reported in humans. Although wood ticks are the usual vector, the disease may be transmitted by transfusion of infected red cells. The disease has been reported most frequently in the northeastern United States (Martha's Vineyard and Nantucket). Intraerythrocytic parasites can usually be seen in Giemsa-stained peripheral blood films.

BARTONELLOSIS. *Bartonella bacilliformis*, a bacterial species endemic to South America, grows on the surface of red cells rather than within them (Ch. 296). The disease is transmitted by the bite of the sand fly. Hemolysis is acute in onset and rapid, the red cells being sequestered by both liver and spleen. The peripheral blood smear typically discloses rod-shaped organisms on the erythrocyte surface and large numbers of normoblasts and reticulocytes. The infection responds well to treatment with penicillin, tetracyclines, streptomycin, or chloramphenicol.

HEMOLYSIS RESULTING FROM TRAUMA TO RED CELLS

When subjected to excessive mechanical stress, circulating red cells may hemolyze. The forces responsible may be generated extracorporeally or intravascularly. For example, fragmentational hemolysis may result from excessive intravascular shear stress originating in critically narrowed heart valves, pathologic shunts (arterial or arteriovenous), cardiac valve prostheses, poorly endothelialized vascular surfaces, or microvascular thrombi. In these situations hemolysis is characteristically accompanied by morphologic evidence of red cell fragmentation. Similarly red cell membranes may be injured by heat with resulting hemolysis. Temperatures higher than 49° C destabilize the normal human red cell membrane. Red cells, when heated in vitro, are observed to undergo membrane budding and fragmentation. Patients who have suffered extensive burns may show evidence of profound red cell membrane damage with prominent spherocytosis on peripheral smear. In some cases, hemoglobinemia and hemoglobinuria occur. The major syndromes of traumatic hemolysis will be summarized briefly.

MARCH HEMOGLOBINURIA. As red cells circulate through narrow vessels overlying the bones of the hands and feet, they may be traumatized by repetitive, relatively uncushioned forces generated by prolonged marching, running, karate blows, and a variety of other activities. Intravascular hemolysis accompanied by hemoglobinemia and hemoglobinuria may result. Interestingly, no red cell morphologic abnormalities are apparent in the peripheral blood film during, or immediately following, the physical activity that precipitated the hemolytic episode.

FRAGMENTATIONAL HEMOLYSIS DUE TO CARDIAC PATHOLOGY OR ABNORMALITIES OF LARGE VESSELS. Cardiac abnormalities involving primarily the left side of the heart, where pressures are high, may predispose to hemolysis. These include aortic stenosis (acquired and congenital), severe aortic regurgitation, and ruptured sinus of Valsalva. Significant red cell fragmentation may also occur as a result of traumatic arteriovenous fistulas, or therapeutic aortofemoral bypass procedures. In patients with these abnormalities hemolysis is usually mild.

More rapid hemolysis occurs, not uncommonly, in patients who have received prosthetic heart valves. Hemolysis is more likely to occur with aortic rather than mitral prostheses, artificial valves rather than those of biologic (porcine) origin, metallic valves rather than Silastic, cloth-covered valves, and with defective or poorly functioning valves that exhibit ball variance or paravalvular leaks.

Clinical Manifestations. Rapid intravascular hemolysis accompanied by hemoglobinemia and hemoglobinuria occurs in occasional patients. More commonly, patients present with increasing anemia, reticulocytosis, and numerous fragmented red cells (schistocytes) on peripheral blood film. Findings typical of significant intravascular hemolysis are usually present, i.e., low to absent haptoglobin levels, increased serum LDH concentrations, and hemosiderinuria. Chronic urinary iron loss may result in iron deficiency. Although usually negative, a positive direct Coombs' test has been found in a few patients with prosthetic heart valves for reasons that are not understood.

Treatment. Patients should be advised to limit their physical activities in an effort to reduce cardiac output and thereby to slow the rate of hemolysis. Oral iron, 300 mg of ferrous sulfate three times a day, should be given to correct iron deficiency, or rarely parenteral iron (iron-dextran) or transfusions may be required. If the rate of hemolysis necessitates chronic transfusion, it may be preferable to replace the prosthesis.

FRAGMENTATIONAL HEMOLYSIS DUE TO ABNORMALITIES WITHIN THE MICROCIRCULATION (MICROANGIOPATHIC HEMOLYTIC DISORDERS). ***Pathophysiology.*** Red cells may be fragmented when they are forced to flow through small vessels that have been partially occluded by microthrombi. Excessive shear forces are generated as the cells encounter and become tethered to fibrin strands, which may bisect and fragment the erythrocytes. The microthrombi may be formed as a result of (1) an underlying coagulopathy, i.e., disseminated intravascular coagulation (DIC), (2) an injury to the vascular endothelium, or (3) an unknown mechanism. Pathophysiologic processes that trigger DIC commonly induce endothelial injury as well; however, the reverse is frequently not true. Diseases associated with diffuse microvascular pathology may involve none of the characteristic findings of DIC. Consequently, in most patients with microangiopathic hemolytic disorders, the predominant etiologic factor (i.e., coagulation or vascular injury) can be discerned.

Disseminated intravascular coagulation (DIC) results when procoagulant is introduced into the systemic circulation (Ch. 167). Coagulation factors are consumed, thrombus formation occurs, and fibrinolytic mechanisms are secondarily activated. Patients with significant DIC characteristically have thrombocytopenia, abnormally prolonged plasma coagulation studies (prothrombin time, activated partial thromboplastin time) reflecting decreased concentrations of certain clotting factors (particularly V, VIII, and fibrinogen), and increased plasma concentrations of fibrin degradation products (FDP), which may prolong the thrombin time. DIC may be triggered by infections, particularly with gram-negative organisms; amniotic fluid embolism; and disseminated neoplasms that synthesize the elaborate potent procoagulants. Although patients with severe DIC may be critically ill, hemolysis is usually mild.

Diffuse or localized vascular lesions may induce red cell fragmentation, e.g., cavernous hemangiomas (Kassabach-Merritt syndrome), renal allografts undergoing rejection, malignant hypertension, eclampsia, vasculitic processes (rickettsial infections, periarteritis nodosa, Wegener's granulomatosis), and disseminated neoplasms. The severity of hemolysis ranges from mild to severe. Coagulation abnormalities mimicking those of DIC are usually absent.

Thrombotic thrombocytopenic purpura (TPP) (Ch. 166), the hemolytic uremic syndrome of children, and mitomycin C–induced hemolytic uremic syndrome of adult cancer patients are highly fatal disorders of unknown etiology that closely resemble one another clinically. Patients with these disorders develop rapid fragmentational hemolysis, thrombocytopenia, and renal failure with little or no laboratory evidence of DIC despite the presence of diffuse microvascular thrombi. TTP is characterized by microangiopathic hemolytic anemia, thrombocytopenia, and fluctuating, frequently bizarre neurologic abnormalities. Fever and renal involvement occur in more than 90 per cent of patients. The disease is seen in all age groups but occurs most commonly in young and middle-aged females. Possible precipitating factors include pregnancy, a variety of infections, various drugs (oral contraceptives, sulfonamides, penicillamine), and systemic lupus erythematosus. Hyaline microthrombi are diffusely present in arterioles and capillaries. Thrombi occur most frequently in the brain, heart, pancreas, adrenals, kidneys, and lymph nodes. They are composed primarily of agglutinated, disrupted platelets and fibrin-like material.

Pathophysiology. A variety of pathophysiologic mechanisms have been invoked to explain the pathogenesis of this disorder. The plasma of some patients contains a platelet aggregating substance that, according to some investigators, is not a clotting factor or an immunoglobulin. Its activity is inhibited by normal plasma. Others suggest that the platelet aggregating substance is a multimer of the normal factor VIII:von Willebrand factor (vWF) complex, possibly identical to that produced by cultured human endothelial cells. VIII:vWF multimers aggregate platelets in the presence of polycations. These findings suggest that some patients with TTP are unable to depolymerize VIII:vWF multimers, normally produced by endothelial cells, into normal factor VIII:vWF complexes.

Plasma from some TTP patients, unlike normal plasma, fails to stimulate normal endothelium to synthesize prostacyclin (PGI_2), a potent inhibitor of platelet aggregation. The infusion of normal plasma into such patients has been reported to increase in vivo synthesis of PGI_2. Serum from some patients with TTP has been found to contain IgG antibodies cytotoxic for endothelium. Endothelial damage in vivo may expose subendothelial collagen that induces platelet aggregation. The clinical management and treatment of TTP are discussed in Ch. 166.

TABLE 138–2. TYPICAL FINDINGS IN MICROANGIOPATHIC SYNDROMES OF VARIOUS ETIOLOGIES

		Coagulation Abnormalities (on a scale of 0 to 3)		
Etiology	*Rate of Hemolysis*	*Thrombocytopenia*	*Decreased Clotting Factors*	*Increased FDP**
DIC*				
Infection or malignancy	Slow	2–3	1–3	2–3
Endothelial damage				
Cavernous hemangioma	Slow to moderate	2–3	0–Tr	0–Tr
Malignant hypertension	Slow to moderate	0–Tr	0	0
Vasculitis	Mild	0–Tr	0	0
Malignancy	Moderate to rapid	0–Tr	0–Tr	0–Tr
Unknown				
TTP,* hemolytic-uremic syndrome	Rapid	3	0	0–Tr

*FDP = fibrin degradation products; DIC = disseminated intravascular coagulation; TTP = thrombotic thrombocytopenic purpura.

Clinical Manifestations. Table 138–2 summarizes the typical features of various syndromes associated with a microangiopathic blood picture.

Diagnosis. The diagnosis of a microangiopathic hemolytic disorder is based on the demonstration of schistocytes, grossly misshapen, sharply angulated erythrocytes that occasionally appear helmet-shaped (Color plate 2J), usually in association with reticulocytosis, diminished to absent serum haptoglobin levels, increased serum LDH concentrations, and hemosiderinuria. Hemoglobinemia and hemoglobinuria occur infrequently.

Immune Hemolytic Anemia

Fearon DT, Wong WW: Complement ligand-receptor interactions that mediate biological responses. Ann Rev Immunol 1:243, 1983. *A recent, lucid review of a complex topic, i.e., mechanisms of complement activation and of the pathologic implications of the binding of activated complement components to cell membranes.*

Frank MM, Schreiber AD, Atkinson JP, Jaffee CJ: Pathophysiology of immune hemolytic anemia. Ann Intern Med 87:210, 1977. *An easily comprehended review of the mechanisms of immune red cell destruction.*

Packman CH, Leddy JP: Drug-related immunologic injury of erythrocytes. *In* Williams WJ, Beutler E, Erslev E, Lichtman MA (eds.): Hematology. 3rd ed. New York, McGraw Hill Book Company, 1983, pp 647–652. *A concise, penetrating summary of drug-mediated immune hemolytic anemia in a standard textbook of hematology.*

Rosse WF: Cold agglutinins and hemolytic anemia: Clinical correlations. *In* Franklin EC (ed.): Clinical Immunology Update. New York, Elsevier/North Holland, 1979, pp 211–226. *A comprehensive review for aficionados of cold agglutinins.*

Wolach B, Heddle N, Barr RD, Zipursky A, Pai KRM, Blajchman MA: Transient Donath-Landsteiner haemolytic anaemia. Br J Haematol 48:425, 1981. *A new look at an old disease. PCH in children is rarely paroxysmal and is seldom precipitated by cold.*

Paroxysmal Nocturnal Hemoglobinuria

Pangburn MK, Schreiber, RD, Müller-Eberhard HJ: Deficiency of an erythrocyte membrane protein with complement regulatory activity in paroxysmal nocturnal hemoglobinuria. Proc Natl Acad Sci USA 80:5430, 1983. *An exciting new finding that may clarify the membrane abnormality in PNH.*

Rosse WF: Paroxysmal nocturnal hemoglobinuria. West J Med 132:219, 1980. *A review of the pathophysiology of PNH and its relationship to stem cell abnormalities.*

Rosse WF: Treatment of paroxysmal nocturnal hemoglobinuria. Blood 60:20, 1982. *A brief review of the treatment of PNH by a physician who has had vast clinical experience with this disease.*

Other

Abdalla S, Weatherall DJ, Wickramasinghe SN, Hughes M: The anaemia of *P. falciparum* malaria. Br J Haematol 46:171, 1980. *An interesting but far from definitive clinical study on possible mechanisms of hemolysis in children with malaria.*

Bowdler AJ: Splenomegaly and hypersplenism. Clin Haematol 12:467, 1983. *A thoughtful, comprehensive review of a topic that has generated controversy for many years.*

Cooper RA: Influence of increased membrane cholesterol on membrane fluidity and cell function in human blood cells. J Supramol Struct 8:413, 1978. *An excellent review of the pathophysiologic mechanisms of red cell membrane changes in liver disease.*

Crexells C, Aericide N, Bonny Y, Lepage C, Campau L: Factors influencing hemolysis in valve prostheses. Am Heart J 84:161, 1972. *A comprehensive summary of fragmentational hemolysis induced by cardiac valve prostheses.*

Lorhmann HP, Adam W, Heymer B, Kubanek B: Microangiopathic hemolytic anemia in metastatic carcinoma. Ann Int Med 79:368, 1973. *Prospective identification of fragmentational hemolysis in patients with malignancy with a discussion of possible mechanisms.*

Ridolfi RL, Bell WR: Thrombotic thrombocytopenic purpura. Medicine 60:413, 1981. *A thorough review of the clinical features of TTP with an extensive bibliography.*

139. HEMOGLOBIN STRUCTURE AND FUNCTION

Alan N. Schechter

The interior of the normal erythrocyte contains a 5 mM solution of hemoglobin, corresponding to about 280 million hemoglobin molecules per cell. Each molecule is a tetramer composed of two pairs of polypeptide chains to which four heme moieties are bound. The ability of the hemoglobin molecule to bind oxygen reversibly allows the erythrocyte to transport oxygen from the lungs to the tissues. The complex structure of the hemoglobin molecule allows it to bind, transport, and release oxygen with extraordinary efficiency. As a result of advances in molecular biology during the last several decades, the relationship between the structure and function of hemoglobin is very well understood. It is now possible to explain the pathophysiology of diseases related to hemoglobin at the molecular, and even atomic, level.

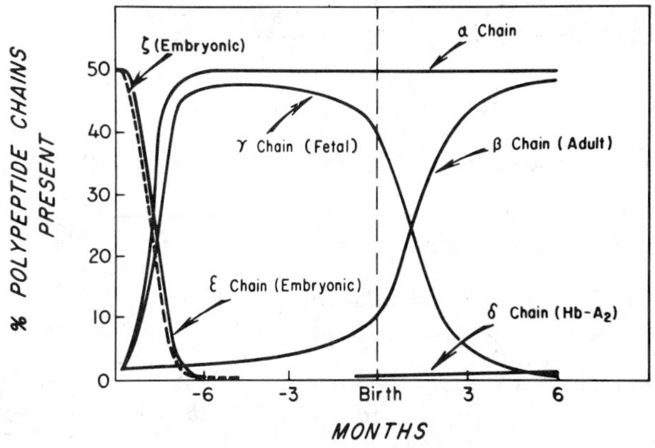

Figure 139–1. A diagram of the relative abundance of various human globin chains during development. The data upon which the diagram is based are incomplete because of the difficulty of obtaining fetal material. (From Bunn HF, Forget BG: Hemoglobin: Molecular, Genetic, and Clinical Aspects. Philadelphia, W. B. Saunders Company, 1985.)

STRUCTURE. The normal hemoglobins of the adult are hemoglobins A (about 97 per cent of the total), A_2 (about 2 per cent), and F (about 1 per cent). The protein, or globin, of each of these is composed of two α polypeptide chains and in addition two β (in hemoglobin A), two δ (in hemoglobin A_2), or two γ (in hemoglobin F) polypeptide chains. In the last decade an additional α-like globin, the ζ chain, and an additional β-like globin, the ϵ chain, have been discovered. These chains, with the α and γ chains, form hemoglobins which are detected in the early embryo: hemoglobin Gower 1 ($\zeta_2\epsilon_2$), hemoglobin Portland ($\zeta_2\gamma_2$), and hemoglobin Gower 2 ($\alpha_2\epsilon_2$). The α and α-like globins each have 141 amino acid residues; the β and β-like globins each have 146 residues.

The sequence of appearance, and sometimes disappearance, of the six polypeptide chains known to be synthesized by human beings is illustrated in Figure 139–1. The factors that control the sequential appearance of these polypeptides are poorly understood. The "switching" process from one hemoglobin to another is mainly related to the age of the fetus or infant and has not been clearly shown to be determined by the site of erythropoiesis, humoral factors, or the appearance of different clones of cells. Understanding of the molecular and cellular mechanism of this process is a major goal of contemporary research.

The chromosomal arrangement of the genes for these six polypeptide chains has been elucidated by somatic cell fusion, nucleic acid hybridization, and restriction endonuclease mapping techniques. Figure 139–2 shows that the human α-like genes are arranged on chromosome 16 and the β-like genes are on chromosome 11. The genes for the α chains appear in two functional copies that code for identical polypeptides. Of the two ζ genes, only the one on the 5′ (left) of the gene cluster appears to be functional. Chromosome 11 seems to have but one copy of the β, δ, and ϵ genes but two copies of the γ gene. The two γ genes differ at only one nucleotide in the regions coding for protein.

The exact sequence of nucleotides in the regions of DNA corresponding to these genes and in many of the regions separating them has been determined. The nucleotide sequences of the genes that specify amino acids in each of the polypeptides are interrupted by stretches of DNA, or intervening sequences, that do not code for amino acids in the hemoglobin molecule. The details of these sequences and other noncoding sequences are described in Ch. 140. Little is known of their significance. The elucidation of the anatomy of the human hemoglobin genetic region at this level of detail is

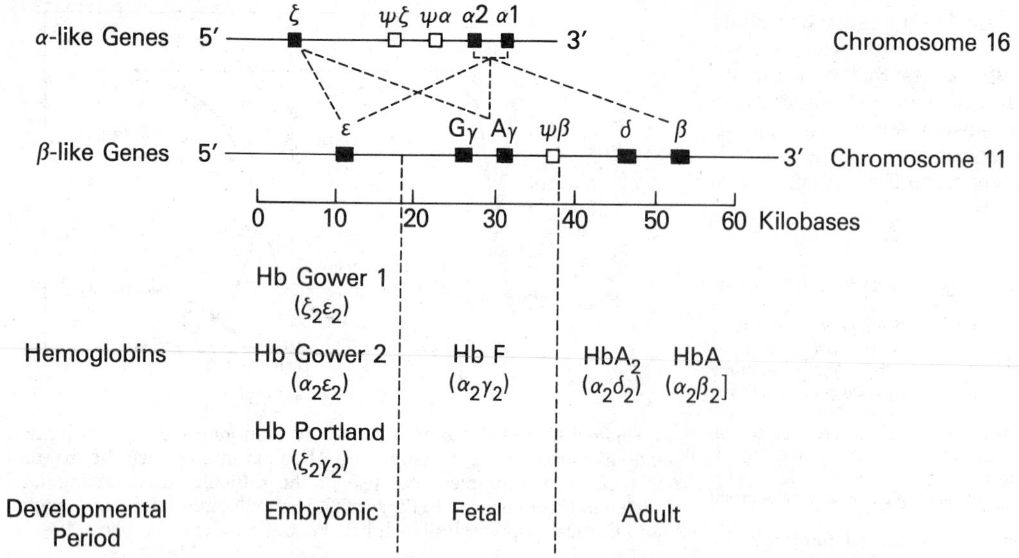

Figure 139–2. A diagram of the arrangement of the clusters of human α-like and β-like globin genes on chromosomes 16 and 11 and the embryonic, fetal, and adult hemoglobins that result from the combinations of the various globin chains encoded by these genes. The ψ genes are similar to globin genes but do not code for protein. Distances along the chromosome are expressed in terms of 1000 nucleotide pairs (a kilobase).

providing information about regulatory genetic functions as well as structural genetic elements, as described in Ch. 141.

While globin messenger RNA synthesis reaches a maximum in the early erythroblast series, globin polypeptide synthesis reaches a peak at about the level of the polychromatophilic erythroblast and continues into the reticulocyte stage. There appears to be little enzymatic processing of the globin polypeptides, except for removal of the amino-terminal methionine residue. The molecular details of the combination of the polypeptides with heme and with each other to form the hemoglobin tetramer are not fully understood, except that the importance of electrostatic interaction between chains has recently been recognized. Each cell contains three or more types of polypeptide chains, and they combine roughly in proportion to their concentrations. As long as synthesis of α (and α-like) chains and β (and β-like) chains is balanced, as it is in the normal person, the hemoglobin in the red cell is formed of two pairs of chains and is largely stable for the life span of the erythrocyte. If chain synthesis or degradation is unbalanced as in certain diseases, discussed in Ch. 141, then surplus chains will accumulate. Excess α chains remain monomeric, whereas the excess β chains form tetramers (β_4, hemoglobin H), as do the excess γ chains (γ_4, hemoglobin Barts). All of these surplus chains are unstable compared to normal hemoglobin and precipitate within the erythrocyte, shortening its life span and thus causing hemolytic anemias.

Each of the polypeptide chains of the hemoglobin molecule is folded into a compact subunit of dimensions 44 × 44 × 25

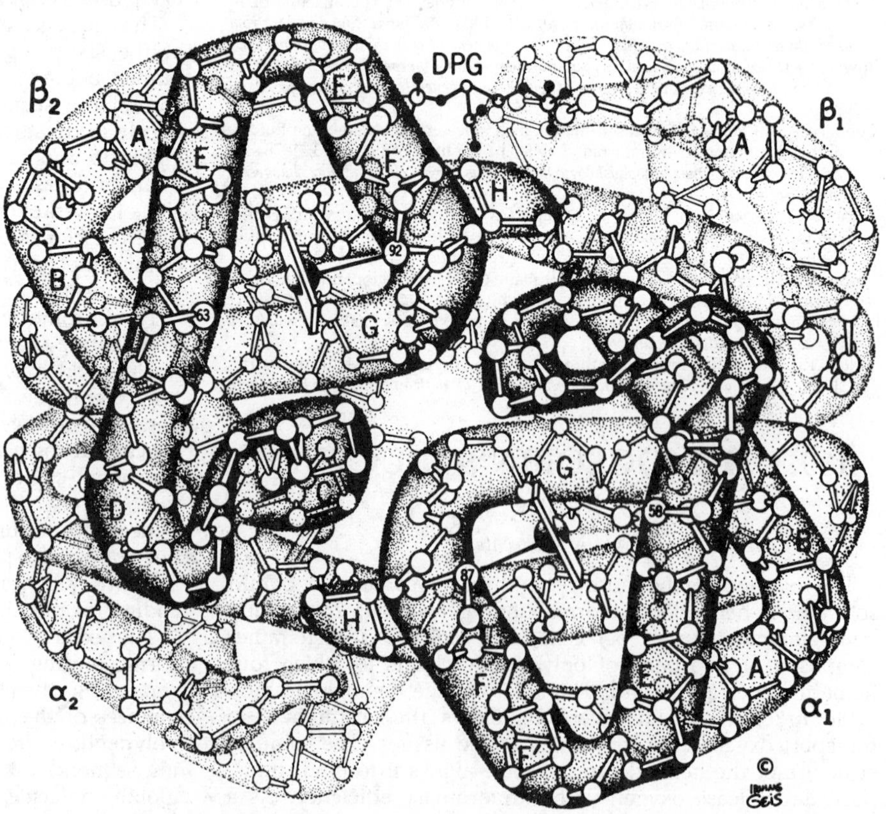

Figure 139–3. An artist's representation of the atomic model of human deoxyhemoglobin based on high-resolution x-ray crystallography analyses. This view is at right angles to the true symmetry axis that relates the two αβ dimers, arbitrarily designated $\alpha_1\beta_1$ and $\alpha_2\beta_2$. The backbone of the polypeptide chain of each subunit and the arrangements of the helices (A to H) and of the heme groups are shown. The bonding of the iron to the "proximal" histidine (residue 87 in the α chain and 92 in the β chain) is denoted as a solid line. The distal histidine residues are 58 in the α chain and 63 in the β chain. The position of the DPG molecule is slightly shifted for clarity. (Copyright 1981 by Irving Geis, 4700 Broadway, New York, New York, 10040.)

horizontal human Deoxyhemoglobin "Front View"

Å, with seven or eight stretches of α helix, designated A to H (Fig. 139–3). The heme group is at right angles to the surface of the protein. The folding patterns of the different hemoglobin polypeptide chains are quite similar to each other, even more so than the homologies in their amino acid sequences would suggest. The α (and α-like) subunits and the β (and β-like) subunits pair to form asymmetric dimers, denoted arbitrarily $\alpha_1\beta_1$ and $\alpha_2\beta_2$ (see Fig. 139–3). These dimers of unlike chains are the fundamental structural units of the hemoglobin tetramer. In the cell the hemoglobin molecules continually dissociate into dimers and reassociate into tetramers. Hybrid tetramers of dissimilar dimers can form. Thus, in a cell that contains significant amounts of hemoglobins A and F, the following species will be present: $\alpha_2\beta_2$ ($[\alpha\beta]_2$), $\alpha_2\gamma_2$ ($[\alpha\gamma]_2$), and $\alpha_2\beta\gamma$ ($[\alpha\beta\alpha\gamma]$).

The heme prosthetic groups are in four largely hydrophobic pockets, one being formed in each globin polypeptide chain by the amino acid side chains of the E and F helices on either side of the heme and of the G and H helices at the interior. The iron atoms are at the center of the porphyrin molecules, bound in a square array to the four nitrogen atoms of each pyrrole ring. In addition, the iron is tightly bound to the nitrogen atom of the imidazole side chain of the histidine residue at position 8 of the F helix (the "proximal" histidine). Oxygen or other small molecules such as carbon monoxide bind on the opposite or "distal" side of the heme in a very compact pocket formed by a number of amino acid side chains.

The nonaqueous environment around the iron atom allows it to remain in the ferrous state even in the presence of oxygen molecules, and imparts to the iron-oxygen bond a coordination character that makes its strength intermediate between a non-covalent and a covalent bond. This property is important in allowing the reversibility of oxygen binding. Despite this, some oxidation to the ferric form occurs naturally. A methemoglobin-reduction system exists in the erythrocyte, utilizing reduced nicotinamide adenine dinucleotide and the enzyme methemoglobin reductase, to keep the iron atoms in the ferrous form. This system, and other related enzymatic pathways, will be discussed in more detail in Ch. 145.

FUNCTION. In the range from normal arterial Po_2 values (100 mm Hg) to normal tissue Po_2 values (thought to be around 40 mm Hg), hemoglobin oxygen saturation decreases from about 100 per cent to about 75 per cent (see Fig. 139–4). Much more oxygen can be released if a further fall in tissue Po_2 values

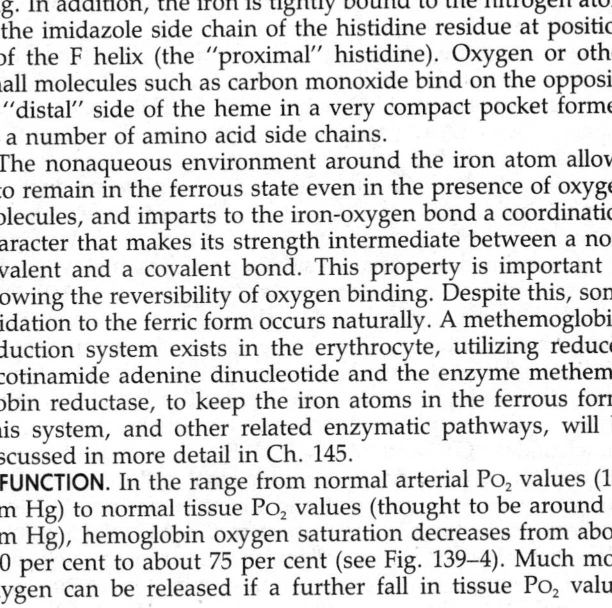

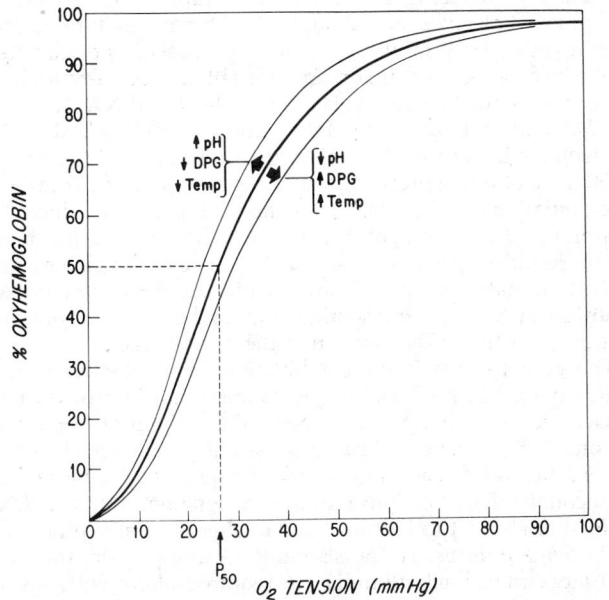

Figure 139–4. The oxygen binding curve for human hemoglobin A under physiologic conditions (dark curve). The affinity will be shifted by changes in pH, DPG concentration, and temperature as indicated. P_{50} represents the oxygen tension at half saturation. (From Bunn HF, Forget BG: Hemoglobin: Molecular, Genetic, and Clinical Aspects. Philadelphia, W. B. Saunders Co., 1984.)

occurs. The great physiologic benefit of hemoglobin results from both the sigmoidal shape of the oxygen binding curve and the fact that the hemoglobin tetramer has a relatively reduced oxygen affinity (or "shift to the right") as compared to its own subunits or to myoglobin. This allows efficient discharge of oxygen in peripheral tissues.

The normal, relatively low oxygen affinity of hemoglobin is due to the interactions of the subunits with each other, and to the binding of protons (the Bohr effect) and the molecule 2,3-diphosphoglyceric acid (DPG) to the hemoglobin tetramer. For reasons that are not completely understood, tetramers of hemoglobin composed of pairs of unlike chains have reduced oxygen affinity as compared to the subunits alone. In the pH region from 7.4 to 7.0, the binding of protons—which increases as pH is lowered—further decreases the oxygen affinity of hemoglobin, i.e., it shifts the oxygen equilibrium curve further to the right (Fig. 139–4). This results in more oxygen being released at a given Po_2, which is very useful since the pH is reduced in the tissues as compared to the capillaries of the lung. Thus the Bohr effect promotes oxygen delivery.

The discovery of the effect of DPG on reducing the oxygen affinity of hemoglobin tetramers has clarified many aspects of the physiology of oxygen transport. DPG, which is normally roughly equimolar with hemoglobin in the erythrocyte, binds reversibly to the region of the hemoglobin tetramer formed by the amino-terminal ends of each of the β chains (Fig. 139–3). One molecule of DPG binds to each hemoglobin tetramer. The binding affinity of DPG for deoxygenated hemoglobin is much greater than for oxygenated hemoglobin. DPG thus stabilizes the deoxygenated form of hemoglobin, increases its concentration relative to the oxygenated form, and so decreases the overall oxygen affinity, i.e., it causes a shift to the right of the oxygen equilibrium curve (Fig. 139–4). DPG binding to deoxygenated hemoglobin is proportional to its concentration in the erythrocyte, and thus oxygen affinity is inversely related to DPG levels. Variation in intracellular DPG, by mechanisms only poorly understood, appears to be a major physiologic mechanism for adjusting oxygen transport in the human being.

The binding of carbon dioxide to hemoglobin as carbamino complexes also lowers oxygen affinity. This process, however, is a relatively minor one in the red cell, and it is estimated that only 10 per cent of metabolically produced carbon dioxide is transported in this manner.

The sigmoidal nature of the oxygen equilibrium curve itself contributes greatly to the efficiency of hemoglobin by causing a release of much oxygen over a narrow range of tissue Po_2 values. (Roughly 250 million molecules of oxygen per red cell are released to the tissues in each cycle.) The shape of the binding curve is due to interactions or cooperativity within and between the dimers of the hemoglobin tetramer. The basis for these interactions at the level of individual atomic groups is still the subject of much debate, but the overall picture seems clear. Deoxygenated hemoglobin exists in a well defined arrangement of each polypeptide chain with respect to the heme group (tertiary structure) and with respect to each other (quaternary structure), called the T or tense form. Oxygenated hemoglobin has a significantly changed tertiary and quaternary structure, called the R or relaxed form. As oxygenation of each hemoglobin tetramer proceeds, the change in structure occurs in a relatively all-or-none manner, rather than being a gradual structural transition. This property leads to the cooperative or sigmoidal oxygen equilibrium curve.

The trigger for this structural transition is the binding of oxygen to the iron atoms and the resulting changes in the sizes and positions of these iron atoms and the orientations of the heme groups themselves within the polypeptide chains. The most direct result of these changes in the iron atoms and the heme groups is to lead to movements of the proximal histidine residues and the F helices. These movements, in turn, cause further changes in the arrangement of the globin polypeptides and interactions among amino acid side chains, within and between subunits. The final result is that the stable quaternary structure of the oxygenated hemoglobin is significantly different from that of the deoxygenated form. The deoxygenated and the oxygenated forms of human hemoglobin have been studied in detail by x-ray crystallography. As described in Ch. 144, this information has been extremely useful in understanding the molecular basis for altered function in certain hemoglobins. In addition, the molecular basis of the polymerization of deoxygenated sickle hemoglobin is explicable with this information, as described in Ch. 142.

Bunn HF, Forget BG: Hemoglobin: Molecular, Genetic, and Clinical Aspects. Philadelphia, W. B. Saunders Company, 1984. *The best single reference to all aspects of the study of hemoglobin.*

Dickerson RE, Geis I: Hemoglobin: Structure, Function, Evolution, and Pathology. Menlo Park, Benjamin/Cummings Publishing Company Inc., 1983. *A sophisticated and magnificently illustrated introduction to hemoglobin structure and function.*

Fermi G, Perutz MF: Haemoglobin and Myoglobin: Atlas of Molecular Structures in Biology. Vol 2. New York, Oxford University Press, 1981. *An introduction to information and conclusions from the structure.*

Ho C, et al. (eds.): Hemoglobin and Oxygen Binding. New York, Elsevier-North Holland, 1982. *A summary of biophysical studies of structure and function relationships in hemoglobin.*

Stamatoyannopoulos G, Nienhuis AW (eds.): Globin Gene Expression and Hematopoietic Differentiation. New York, Alan R. Liss, Inc., 1983. *An excellent introduction to the molecular genetics of hemoglobin.*

140. HEMOGLOBIN SYNTHESIS

Arthur W. Nienhuis

The red cell is one of the most uniquely specialized cells in the body. Lacking a nucleus and therefore devoid of any proliferative potential or even the ability to renew its own protein constituents, the red cell is totally adapted to carrying oxygen and carbon dioxide for its brief life span of approximately 120 days. The red cell's unique membrane constituents give it flexibility, allowing passage through even the narrowest capillaries and egress from the red pulp into the sinusoids of the spleen. The oxygen and carbon dioxide transport properties of the red cell depend on its content of hemoglobin. Hemoglobin amounts to more than 95 per cent of the cytoplasmic protein of the red cell; each cell contains 30 pg (approximately 280 million molecules) of this protein. In this chapter we will consider briefly the mechanism of hemoglobin synthesis, beginning with an outline of the flow of genetic information from gene to protein. Also germane are the mechanisms by which red cells come to contain hemoglobin to the virtual exclusion of most other proteins.

FLOW OF INFORMATION FROM GENE TO PROTEIN. ***Chromatin Structure.*** The nuclei of human cells contain chromatin, a complex of histone core particles called nucleosomes around which the DNA double helix is coiled. Nonhistone chromosomal proteins are thought to play a role in establishing higher order structures of chromatin so that the relatively vast amount of DNA may be packed into a cell's small nucleus. Furthermore, nonhistone proteins are thought to include regulatory factors which establish the structure of a restricted number of genes in a specialized cell to allow their exclusive expression. For example, the globin genes in erythroid cells have been shown to be in an active conformation, whereas in brain cells the globin genes are included among those genes whose conformation in chromatin render them inaccessible for transcription. The nature of these regulatory factors and the manner in which they interact with specific genes to promote their expression have only recently become accessible to experimental study.

Gene Structure. The DNA sequences that encode for a specific protein are not co-linear with the messenger RNA (mRNA) for that protein. Rather the coding portions of the gene, now called exons, are interrupted by a variable number of introns or intervening sequences of DNA. All functional globin genes studied to date have two introns and therefore three exons, as is diagrammatically shown for the human β globin gene in Figure 140–1. Considering the structure of the gene from left to right (5′ to 3′), the first exon encodes for the first 30 amino acids of β globin, the second encodes for the next 74 amino acids, and the last encodes for the remaining 42 amino acids. The smaller intron in the human β globin gene is 130 base pairs in length, whereas the larger is 850 base pairs in length. In general, the α globin genes have a similar structure, although the larger intron is only 150 base pairs long.

Globin mRNA Metabolism. Transcription of the β globin gene to produce its RNA copy probably begins at a point in the DNA that encodes for the 5′ end of mature mRNA. The major transcriptional control signals are in the promoter region. Conserved sequences required for accurate and efficient initiation of transcription by RNA polymerase include the "ATA" and "CAT" boxes at 31 and 76 nucleotides before the start site of transcription, respectively, and a duplicated "CACA" box just upstream from "CAT" (Fig. 140–1). Single nucleotide substitutions in these conserved regions have been identified in thalassemia globin genes (Ch. 141); these mutations cause decreased globin gene expression leading to deficient hemoglobin synthesis.

The entire gene, including its two introns, is copied into a co-linear RNA molecule. Transcription continues beyond those sequences represented in globin mRNA. The nucleotide sequence, "AATAAA," serves as a signal for cleavage of the transcription product and addition of a series of adenines to form the poly A track. The primary transcription product, the β globin mRNA precursor, is a 1600–1700 nucleotide molecule. During transcription, it is also modified at the 5′ end by addition of a guanosine diphosphate residue and several methyl groups in a series of reactions referred to as "capping" (Fig. 140–1).

The DNA sequences found at the exon-intron boundaries, when transcribed into RNA, serve as signals for precise and efficient splicing of the RNA transcript. Comparison of more than 100 exon-intron boundaries has lead to the identification of the consensus splice sequences shown in Figure 140–1. The dinucleotides "GT" and "AG" at the 5′ and 3′ ends of introns, respectively, are obligatory for functional splicing. The other nucleotides are not invariant and therefore are referred to as *consensus* nucleotides. As discussed in Ch. 141, single nucleotide substitutions in either obligatory or consensus nucleotides at the exon-intron boundaries of thalassemia globin genes cause abnormal RNA splicing, and therefore globin mRNA deficiency. Normally, processing is efficient and rapid; 95 per cent of precursor molecules are thought to become mature mRNA within only a few minutes of their synthesis. Approximately 100 molecules of precursor are present in each erythroblast compared with 20,000 to 50,000 molecules of mRNA.

Globin mRNA Structure. The mature mRNA is 600 to 650 nucleotides in length. Beginning from the cap site, the first 40 to 50 nucleotides represent an untranslated part of the mRNA. The initiation codon (AUG) signals the point at which the beginning of protein synthesis occurs. The next 423 (α) or 438 (β) nucleotides specify the protein sequence of the globin. Next is the terminator or stop codon, UAA in α and β globin mRNA, followed by 80 to 100 nucleotides that make up the 3′ untranslated part of the mRNA and then the poly-A track.

The genetic code is the combination of all possible codons that may specify the 20 amino acids that occur in protein. Four nucleotides can be put together in 64 different triplets or codons. The genetic code is degenerate in the sense that all codons are used; each amino acid is specified by more than one codon. Each codon requires a separate transfer RNA (tRNA) to allow it to be translated during protein synthesis.

Protein Synthesis. To translate mRNA into protein, the small and large ribosomal subunits are required along with several protein initiation, elongation, and termination factors and a complement of tRNA molecules. The initiator tRNA carries the amino acid methionine. Protein synthesis begins when this tRNA binds to an initiation factor and then subsequently is bound to the ribosome as specified by its anticodon, TAC, which interacts with the initiator codon. The codon next in line

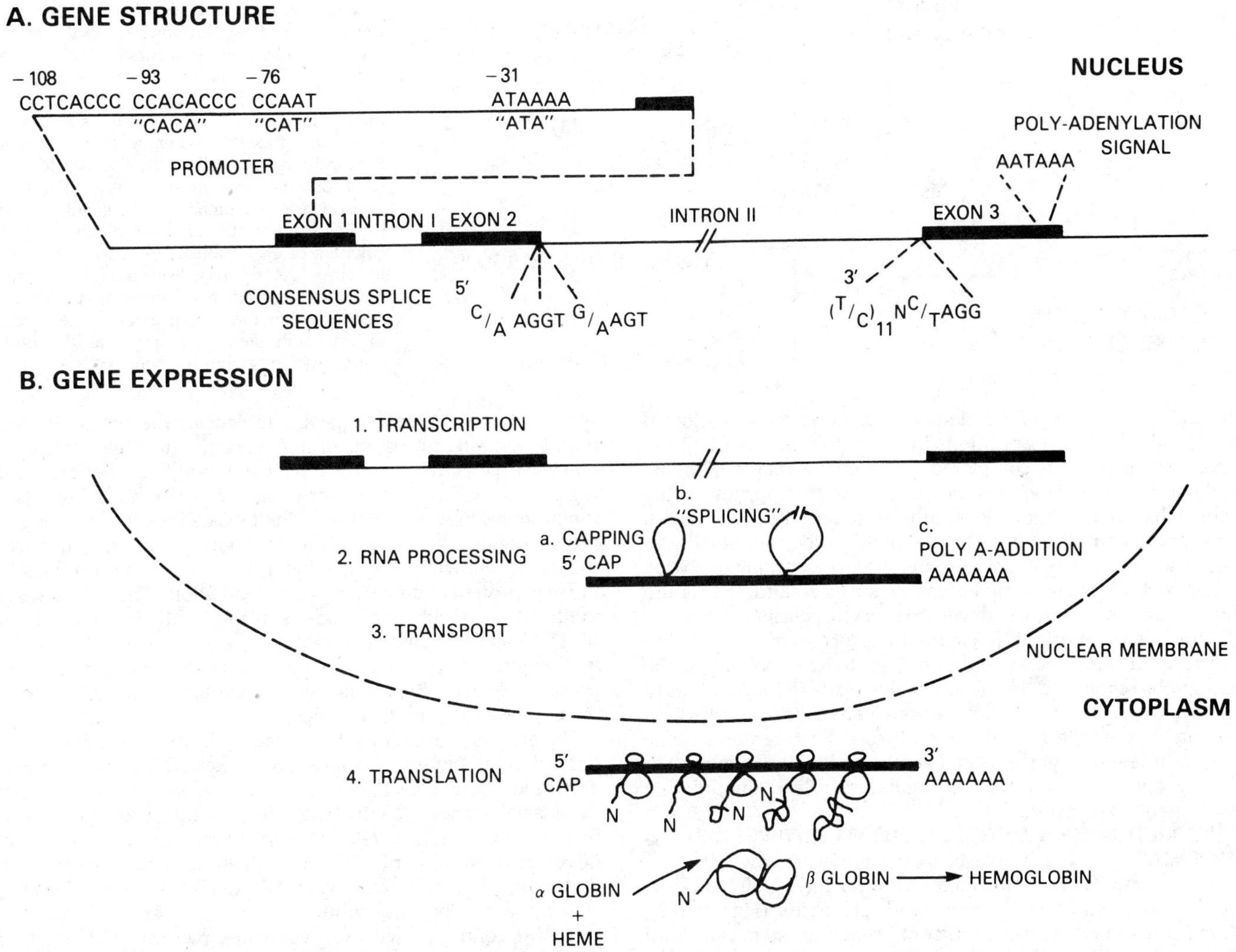

Figure 140–1. Structure and expression of the normal human β globin gene. The three exons encode for β globin; these coding sequences are interrupted by two introns or intervening sequences. Certain segments of the promotor region ("boxes") are conserved in many globin genes. The actual sequence of these "boxes" in the β globin gene promoter is shown. The splice sequences shown represent the consensus of those found at many exon-intron boundaries. Those actually found in the β globin gene resemble the consensus sequence but are not identical. C = cytosine, T = thymine, A = adenine, and G = guanine. The processes involved in gene expression include transcription of the gene, processing of the primary RNA transcript, transport of the mRNA from nucleus to cytoplasm, and translation of the mRNA into β globin.

in both human and α and β globin mRNA is GUG, which specifies valine. A tRNA for valine is bound to the ribosome as its anticodon, CAC, recognizes the valine codon in mRNA. A peptide bond is then formed between methionine and valine. The mRNA is then translocated on the ribosome, and the next codon is ready to be read. This series of reactions continues until the terminator codon is encountered, at which point the ribosomal subunits and a completed globin molecule are released from the mRNA by the action of a termination factor. Each mRNA molecule may serve simultaneously as a template for the synthesis of several globin molecules. The protein synthesis mechanism appears to be quite general; no specific factors are required to translate a particular mRNA.

The globins undergo a number of postsynthetic modifications. Removal of the methionine residue, donated by the initiator tRNA, occurs on the polyribosome before synthesis of the globin polypeptide is complete. After assembly into hemoglobin, nonenzymatic glycosylation reactions give rise to a variety of minor electrophoretic variants. The extent of these reactions is proportional to the life span of the erythrocyte and to mean blood glucose levels. The major glycosylated form is designated hemoglobin A_{1C}. It has a glucose molecule linked by means of Schiff base to the amino-terminus of the β chain. Since glycosylation varies directly with blood sugar level, measurements of such modified hemoglobins can be used to evaluate control of diabetes mellitus. Perhaps even more important, these modifications of hemoglobin may be the prototype of many other nonenzymatic glycosylation reactions, which could be the pathophysiologic mechanism for damage to various intracellular and extracellular proteins leading to the complications of diabetes mellitus.

IRON ACCUMULATION AND HEMOGLOBIN SYNTHESIS. To obtain the considerable amount of iron required for hemoglobin synthesis, the red cell utilizes membrane receptors specific for the iron transport protein transferrin. The transferrin receptor complex is transiently internalized into the red cell within an endocytic vesicle. The pH within the vesicle is lowered by active ion transport, thereby releasing iron from transferrin. The receptor-apotransferrin complex is then returned to the cell surface, where apotransferrin is released. Ferritin appears to act as an intermediary in the movement of iron through the cytoplasm to its ultimate destination in the mitochondrium, where it is combined with protoporphyrin to form heme by action of the enzyme heme synthetase. Synthesis of protopor-

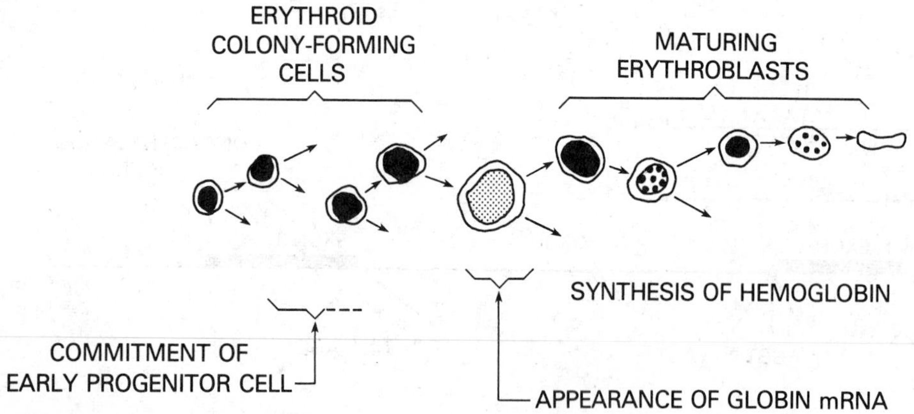

Figure 140–2. Regulation of hemoglobin synthesis during erythropoiesis. Two general classes of cells are the precursors of circulating red cells. Erythroblasts at various stages of maturation may be recognized within the bone marrow; these cells and circulating reticulocytes are engaged in hemoglobin synthesis. Erythroid stem cells, the progenitors of erythroblasts, are present within the bone marrow in very small numbers but may be detected by virtue of their ability to form colonies of erythroblasts in semi-solid media in vitro. As discussed in the text, current evidence suggests that commitment to expression of either the γ or β globin genes occurs in erythroid stem cells prior to the initial appearance of globin messenger RNA.

phyrin is by a series of reactions catalyzed by enzymes found in relatively high concentrations in erythroblasts (see Ch. 203).

Nascent or partially completed globin chains may bind heme while still on the polyribosome as soon as that portion of the globin that binds heme is synthesized and folded into an appropriate conformation. The assembly of the individual globins into the hemoglobin tetramer occurs spontaneously by virtue of both their complementary surfaces and their high concentrations within the developing erythroblasts.

Heme has important roles in the process of hemoglobin synthesis in addition to being an essential component of the hemoglobin molecule. Heme deficiency leads to inactivation of a critically required initiation factor, leading to a marked reduction in the rate of protein synthesis. Furthermore, heme may stimulate the synthesis and accumulation of globin mRNA directly and thus may have a regulatory role in modulating globin gene expression.

PRODUCTION OF HEMOGLOBIN DURING ERYTHROBLAST DEVELOPMENT. The erythroblasts in the bone marrow exhibit a series of amplification divisions during which globin mRNA accumulation and hemoglobin synthesis occur (Fig. 140–2). Thus from a very limited number of progenitor stem cells with high proliferative potential are produced a large number of highly specialized but terminally differentiated red cells.

Only 0.1 to 0.5 per cent of the total RNA synthesized in the earliest erythroblasts is globin mRNA, yet the globin mRNA species ultimately represents 95 per cent of the total mRNA present in reticulocytes. This remarkable accumulation of globin mRNA to the exclusion of other mRNA molecules appears to be the result primarily of two factors. First, globin mRNA is remarkably stable during erythroid differentiation. Indeed, there seems to be no degradation of globin mRNA following its synthesis until the reticulocyte stage of maturation. In contrast other mRNA species decay with a half-life of approximately 20 hours and are destabilized to decay even faster toward the end of erythroblast maturation. Also, during the later phases of erythroid maturation, synthesis of other mRNAs declines precipitously, whereas that of globin mRNA appears to continue until just prior to nuclear exclusion. Thus the remarkable stability and the continued synthesis of globin mRNA during all phases of erythroid maturation appear to account for its accumulation to the exclusion of other mRNA species.

MECHANISM OF PRODUCTION OF SPECIFIC HEMOGLOBINS. Fetal red cells contain predominantly Hb F, whereas adult red cells contain Hb A (see Ch. 139). Selective expression of the γ and β genes appears to be modulated at the level of transcription. The precursor to β globin mRNA is present in a lower concentration in fetal erythroblasts than is the precursor to γ mRNA, whereas in adult erythroblasts the β globin mRNA precursor is present in considerably higher concentration than that for γ mRNA. Thus, the pattern of hemoglobin synthesis accurately reflects the relative accumulation of the two mRNA species. Several clues suggest a molecular mechanism(s) that might regulate the transcription of individual globin genes. Nuclease sensitivity studies have shown that the promoter regions of expressed genes are "open" in chromatin, allowing for protein-DNA interactions. The DNA sequences of the promoter region of the individual globin genes are distinctly different, allowing for specific interaction with nonhistone nuclear proteins involved in gene regulation. The frequency of methylation of cytosine residues, a postsynthetic modification of DNA, varies inversely with gene expression and could further alter the interaction of promoter regions with regulatory proteins. Much effort is currently directed at identification of these putative regulatory molecules.

Factors that influence the relative level of expression of individual globin genes appear to be exerted on very primitive erythroid stem cells. Experimental analysis of colonies of erythroblasts formed in vitro indicate that those which develop from the stem cells in fetal liver make Hb F, whereas colonies developing from stem cells in adult bone marrow make predominantly, but not exclusively, Hb A. Thus the primitive stem cells appear to become committed at some very early stage in their differentiation with respect to the pattern of hemoglobin synthesis in their progeny erythroblasts.

Nienhuis A, Propper R: The thalassemias: Disorders of hemoglobin synthesis. *In* Nathan D, Oski F (eds.): Hematology of Infancy and Childhood. 2nd ed. Philadelphia, W. B. Saunders Company, 1981, pp 726-799. *A detailed account of the thalassemic disorders, with a more extensive discussion of gene expression and hemoglobin synthesis than that included here.*

Stamatoyannopoulos G, Nienhuis AW (eds.): Globin Gene Expression and Hematopoietic Differentiation. New York, Alan R. Liss, Inc., 1983. *This volume represents the proceedings of a symposium on hemoglobin switching held in September of 1982. As such it is an authoritative account by workers in the field of our current understanding of the globin genes and their expression.*

Stamatoyannopoulos G, Papayannopoulou T, Brice M, Kurachi S, Nakamoto B, Lim G, Farquhar M: Cell biology of hemoglobin switching I. The switch from fetal to adult hemoglobin formation during ontogeny. *In* Stamatoyannopoulos G, Nienhuis AW (eds.): Hemoglobins in Development and Differentiation. New York, Alan R. Liss, Inc., 1981. Papayannopoulou T, Nakamoto B, Kurachi S, Kurnit D, Stamatoyannopoulos G: Cell biology of hemoglobin switching II. Studies on the regulation of fetal hemoglobin synthesis in human adults. *In* Stamatoyannopoulos G, Nienhuis AW (eds.): Hemoglobins in Development and Differentiation. New York, Alan R. Liss, Inc., 1981. *These detailed reviews by major contributors to the problem of hemoglobin switching and erythroid stem cell differentiaiton should be consulted by those with a serious interest in this topic.*

141. THE THALASSEMIAS

Arthur W. Nienhuis

The thalassemias are hereditary anemias that occur because of mutations that affect the synthesis of hemoglobin. In β thalassemia there is deficient synthesis of β globin, whereas in α thalassemia there is deficient synthesis of α globin. Reduced synthesis of one of the two globin polypeptides leads to deficient hemoglobin accumulation, resulting in hypochromic and microcytic red cells. These red cell abnormalities are the

TABLE 141–1. CLINICAL CLASSIFICATION OF THE THALASSEMIAS

I. Severe beta thalassemia (Cooley's anemia)	Severe anemia, growth retardation, hepatosplenomegaly, bone marrow expansion, and bone deformities
A. Thalassemia major	Transfusion-dependent
B. Thalassemia intermedia	No regular transfusion requirement
II. Thalassemia trait (α or β)	Mild anemia with microcytosis and hypochromia
III. Hb H disease (α-thal)	Moderately severe hemolytic anemia, icterus, and splenomegaly
IV. Hydrops fetalis (α-thal)	Death in utero caused by severe anemia
V. Silent carrier (α or β)	Hematologically normal

most constant and characteristic features of this group of disorders. Table 141–1 contains a clinical classification of the thalassemias presented in the order in which they will be discussed in this chapter.

The incidence and prevalence of these conditions is highly variable. Most common is thalassemia trait, a mild, clinically insignificant anemia that apparently protects individuals from malaria (see below), and therefore through natural selection it has become extremely common in certain parts of the world. Thalassemia trait generally represents the heterozygous form of either α or β thalassemia. Hence where thalassemia trait is common, homozygous, more severely affected patients will be found frequently. In the United States, the incidence of β thalassemia is highest among ethnic groups originating from the Mediterranean area, parts of Africa, and Asia, whereas the incidence of α thalassemia is highest among those from Asia. Generally the incidence of thalassemia trait in these ethnic groups is 3 to 5 per cent. Approximately 1000 patients with more severe forms of thalassemia are known in the United States.

SEVERE β THALASSEMIA (Cooley's Anemia)

Severe β thalassemia occurs in patients who are homozygous for mutations that lead to a decrease in β globin synthesis. Because both β globin genes are affected, there is marked deficiency in β globin synthesis but α globin synthesis continues at an approximately normal rate. Accumulation of a large excess of α chains for which there are no β chains with which to combine has several serious deleterious effects. α Globin is highly insoluble and forms large intracellular inclusions. These interfere with the cell cycle in the bone marrow, retard the passage of red cells from the bone marrow, and reduce the survival of red cells in the circulation by virtue of membrane damage and splenic trapping. Marked ineffective erythropoiesis is the hallmark of this disorder because α inclusions interfere with erythroblast maturation, leading to intramedullary death of many red cell precursors. Severe anemia stimulates erythropoietin production, leading to erythroid stem cell and erythroblast proliferation. The vastly expanded erythroid cell mass results in osteoporosis with a potential for pathologic fractures. Extramedullary hematopoiesis is also often seen, and compression of vital structures, particularly the spinal cord, may occur as a consequence. Because of marrow expansion and bony deformities of the skull and facial bones, patients with severe β thalassemia often have a mongoloid appearance with prominent epicanthal folds referred to as a "chipmunk facies."

Patients with severe β thalassemia may be divided into two groups on the basis of their requirement for blood transfusion. Those with thalassemia major have an absolute requirement for blood without which severe anemia leads to death in infancy or early childhood. In contrast, patients with thalassemia intermedia are able to maintain their hemoglobin at 6 to 7 grams per deciliter without transfusion. This level is compatible with fairly normal growth and development, and many of these patients survive into adulthood.

Thalassemia Major

CLINICAL FEATURES. At birth patients with thalassemia major are nearly normal hematologically, since γ globin synthesis is normal and Hb F production is therefore adequate. However, as the switch from Hb F to Hb A is completed during the first year of life, the deficiency in β globin production becomes evident. By six to nine months of age, severe anemia reflected by pallor, poor growth, or inadequate food intake leads the anxious parents to bring the infant to the physician, at which time examination reveals the presence of marked hepatosplenomegaly. The hemoglobin may be 3 to 6 grams per deciliter, and the red cells exhibit the characteristic severe microcytosis, hypochromia, and red cell fragmentation. Demonstration of thalassemia trait (see below) in both parents is usually sufficient to establish the diagnosis. Study of the infant's blood shows low or absent Hb A, a large amount of Hb F, and an increase in the amount of Hb A_2 to 4 to 10 per cent of the total (normal <2.5 per cent). Biosynthetic studies, a tool of the research laboratory, may be employed to show the deficiency of β globin production.

CLINICAL COURSE. Prior to the use of regular blood transfusions, these children were grossly deformed because of expansion of the marrow spaces of the skull (see Fig. 130–1). Severe osteoporosis led to pathologic fractures, and anemia caused weakness and inanition. Death by two to three years of age was common. Blood transfusions were initially given infrequently for palliation, but gradually physicians interested in this condition came to recognize that regular transfusion to nearly normal hemoglobin levels could be used to suppress all disease manifestations. Growth and bone development of such hypertransfused children are normal, and in fact they are virtually indistinguishable from other children if the hypertransfusion regimen is started at a very early age. If transfusions are given less frequently, the patient may exhibit some stigmata of the untreated disorder—bony deformities, growth retardation, and hepatosplenomegaly.

THE PROBLEM OF IRON OVERLOAD. Because humans have a very limited ability to excrete iron, regular blood transfusions inevitably lead to a vast accumulation. Each unit of packed red cells contains approximately 200 mg of iron, so that by the age of 12 the average thalassemic, having received 125 to 150 units of packed cells, will have accumulated 25 to 30 grams of excess iron. This amount compares to the normal 3 to 4 grams found in adults, 75 per cent of which is present in red cells as hemoglobin. Excess iron deposition occurs in virtually all organs. Most cells have a considerable ability to cope with this extra iron by making ferritin and its partial degradation product hemosiderin. Nonetheless, cell damage occurs by virtue of iron-catalyzed peroxidation of membrane lipids and release of the enzymes from lysosomes rendered labile by their content of hemosiderin granules. Thus tissue hemosiderosis (excess iron) leads ultimately to the clinical condition secondary hemochromatosis. The liver, endocrine glands, and particularly the heart are the primary target organs (see Ch. 206).

Liver dysfunction is mild in the thalassemic patient with secondary hemochromatosis. Typically the liver is enlarged several centimeters below the right costal margin, and the transaminases are two to four times above the normal limits. Despite a 20- to 30-fold increase in iron concentration over normal, liver biosynthetic function as reflected by the concentration of serum albumin and various clotting factors is preserved. Fibrosis, invariably present on liver biopsy, may progress to frank cirrhosis anatomically, but clinical evidence of cirrhosis is rare.

As noted above, the course of adequately transfused thalassemic patients is essentially normal until the age of 10 to 12. Then growth failure is a frequent and distressing complication for both the child and parents. The mechanism for this growth failure is not known; growth hormone levels are generally normal, but the serum somatomedin concentration may be low. Failure of growth is accompanied by lack of pubescence. Primary hypogonadism is exceedingly common. The mechanism is usually a failure of the pituitary to produce adequate amounts of FSH and LH. Diabetes mellitus, hypothyroidism, and, rarely, hypoparathyroidism with tetany are additional complications that may occur particularly in patients who are in their late teenage years or early 20's.

Cardiac disease in the patients with severe β thalassemia may take three forms: pericarditis, congestive heart failure, and cardiac arrhythmias. Recurrent attacks of acute pericarditis are manifested by chest pain, often pleuritic and affected by a change of position, accompanied by fever and occasionally a pericardial friction rub. These attacks are usually self-limited, lasting four to seven days. Treatment consists of bed rest, aspirin, and other anti-inflammatory agents such as indomethacin in appropriate doses. Rarely constrictive pericarditis may require a pericardectomy.

Congestive heart failure is to be expected ultimately in patients with secondary hemochromatosis unless death occurs early by virtue of cardiac arrhythmias. Careful echocardiographic studies have suggested that iron deposition begins by the age of five to six years. By ten or twelve years, when the patient has received more than 100 units of blood, left ventricular dysfunction may be demonstrated by radionuclide cineangiography during the physiologic stress of exercise. Clinical congestive heart failure is usually a late complication; most patients die within twelve months of the onset of definite evidence of heart failure. Treatment with digoxin in doses adequate to achieve therapeutic blood levels may be quite helpful. Appropriate use of diuretics and vasodilator therapy may be extremely useful in providing palliation and extending the life span of these patients.

Atrial and ventricular ectopy is present in 24-hour electrocardiographic recordings in virtually all patients who have received more than 150 units of packed red cells. High grade ventricular ectopy with couplets, short runs of ventricular tachycardia, and multiple ventricular foci are of ominous prognostic significance. Ectopy may be extremely distressful to the patient, particularly at night when it is often most severe. Tachyrhythmias such as ventricular tachycardia and/or ventricular fibrillation occur despite therapy and are frequent causes of death in patients with severe thalassemia on regular transfusions. The pharmacologic treatment of cardiac arrhythmias is described in Ch. 50.

The prognosis of patients with thalassemia major is determined by the cardiac disease. The average age of death is 17 years, although a few patients may survive to their mid-20's. Because of this grim prognosis, a considerable effort has been focused on attempts to reduce the iron burden in these patients.

THE ROLE OF SPLENECTOMY. Splenic enlargement is frequent and often causes functional hypersplenism as manifested by an increasing transfusion requirement. Careful documentation of the patient's needs will often alert the physician to the development of hypersplenism as the need for blood rises. An average patient on a hypertransfusion regimen designed to maintain the hemoglobin at a level greater than 10 grams per deciliter will require 250 ml of packed cells per kilogram per year. If substantially more blood is required, the spleen should be removed. Leukopenia and thrombocytopenia, if present, are indicators of the presence of hypersplenism and should lead to prompt splenectomy.

The complication of splenectomy in this patient population is a risk of sudden overwhelming sepsis by encapsulated organisms. For this reason delay of splenectomy until after the age of four is highly desirable. Splenectomized patients should receive Pneumovax and may be placed on daily penicillin prophylaxis. More important, each patient should be given a small supply of a broad-spectrum antibiotic such as ampicillin to be taken orally in appropriate doses if high fever develops and immediate medical attention cannot be obtained.

CHELATION THERAPY. The only drug available for use in removal of iron is deferoxamine (Desferal). This drug has an extremely high affinity for trivalent iron, and despite extensive clinical use it appears to be relatively free of serious toxicity. Its disadvantages are that it must be given parenterally and that it has a very short serum half-life. Thus most drug, given as a single intramuscular injection, is rapidly excreted without binding any iron. To maximize the efficacy of the drug, a technique has been devised to administer it subcutaneously by using a small mechanical infusion pump. A needle is inserted into the subcutaneous tissue of the abdomen, and the drug is infused very slowly over a period of eight to twelve hours. With 1.5 grams of Desferal, two to three times more iron may be removed than by a single daily intramuscular injection. Often daily excretion of 30 to 40 mg of iron may be achieved in older patients and may lead to overall negative iron balance despite continued transfusion therapy provided that the drug is used at least five times per week. Current data indicate that this regimen will retard the rate of iron accumulation in the liver and reduce liver fibrosis. As yet not enough time has elapsed since the introduction of the subcutaneous regimen to determine whether it will slow the progression or prevent the onset of cardiac disease. The greatest probability of successfully preventing iron damage is in patients in whom treatment is begun early, preferably by the age of five years. Vitamin C in small doses (150 to 250 mg per day) given orally may increase the amount of iron excretion in response to deferoxamine infusions, although some evidence suggests that this agent may enhance tissue iron toxicity particularly to the heart, and therefore it should be used with caution in older patients.

Thalassemia Intermedia

Those patients with severe β thalassemia who maintain their hemoglobin levels above 6.0 to 7.0 grams per deciliter have a generally better prognosis. Individual patients with thalassemia intermedia generally have large amounts of Hb F, significant amounts of Hb A_2, and variable amounts of Hb A in their red cells. Iron accumulation may occur because of increased gastrointestinal absorption and ultimately may lead to secondary hemochromatosis with endocrine and cardiac dysfunction, but most patients with thalassemia intermedia survive into adulthood and many have children. Splenectomy may become necessary if evidence of hypersplenism is present. Osteoporosis may be severe, as these patients' erythroid mass is not suppressed. A disabling form of arthritis has been described. Large masses of erythroid tissue in extramedullary sites may cause organ dysfunction. Particularly distressing is spinal cord compression with paraplegia, although usually local radiation will reverse this condition. Any or all of these complications may ultimately lead to the use of a regular transfusion regimen in patients with thalassemia intermedia despite their marginally adequate hemoglobin levels. Such treatment has the added benefit of preventing the disfiguring facial abnormalities.

Genetically this condition is heterogeneous. Often the red cells of both parents exhibit stigmata of thalassemia trait, although frequently one parent may be a silent carrier of the thalassemia gene (see below). In such persons the impairment of β globin synthesis is so mild that the red cells are normal, but when the abnormal β gene is paired with another affected by a more severe β thalassemia mutation, thalassemia intermedia results. Elucidation of many thalassemia mutations at the molecular level has revealed marked quantitative variability ranging from 50 to 100 per cent reduction in β globin mRNA production (see below). Many patients are doubly heterozygous for two different mutations. The clinical heterogeneity of the β thalassemias reflects the many combinations of mutations that may be present in individual patients. Other genetic modifiers of the β thalassemia phenotype include α thalassemia mutations and genetic variants characterized by increased Hb F production. Coinheritance of an α thalassemia gene decreases α globin production leading to partial correction of the highly deleterious imbalance in α and β biosynthesis. Increased γ globin synthesis resulting in increased Hb F production compensates directly for deficient β globin production.

THALASSEMIA TRAIT

CLINICAL CHARACTERISTICS. Common to both α and β thalassemia is a condition referred to as thalassemia minor or trait. This condition generally occurs in individuals who are heterozygous for a mutation affecting α or β globin synthesis (see below). Characteristically the red blood cells are small and contain less hemoglobin than normal; the mean corpuscular volume averages 65 cubic microns (range 56 to 74), whereas the mean corpuscular hemoglobin averages 21 pg (range 20 to 23). Normal values for these parameters are 88 ± 5 and 30 ± 2, respectively. The total red cell count is often increased to 10 to 20 per cent above the normal range, so that anemia, if present, is mild. Rarely the packed cell volume may be as low as 30 per cent; values of 32 to 38 per cent are more typical. Splenomegaly is said to occur but is distinctly unusual, and other causes should be sought if this physical finding is present. No clinical symptoms may be attributed to the presence of thalassemia trait.

DIFFERENTIAL DIAGNOSIS. A characteristic feature of β thalassemia trait is an elevation of Hb A_2. This minor hemoglobin accounts for only 2 or 3 per cent of the total in normal red cells, but in thalassemia trait it may be elevated in the range of 4 to 8 per cent in more than 90 per cent of persons with this condition. Similarly, Hb F is often elevated to 1.5 to 2.5 per cent, although in rare types of thalassemia trait it may be as high as 10 to 15 per cent. In normal red cells, Hb F accounts for less than 1 per cent of the total. The minor hemoglobins, Hb A_2 and Hb F, are either normal or slightly decreased in patients with α thalassemia.

The differential diagnosis of thalassemia trait includes a consideration of iron deficiency. This diagnosis can be excluded only by measurement of the serum iron, total iron binding capacity, and serum ferritin. If these values are normal in patients whose red cells are severely microcytic, but in whom anemia, if present, is mild, the diagnosis of thalassemia trait can be considered established. The distinction between α and β thalassemia depends on the measurement of the minor hemoglobins. If these are normal, the diagnosis of α thalassemia is most likely, although rare subjects with β thalassemia also have normal levels of Hb A_2 and Hb F.

GENE FREQUENCY. Thalassemia trait is thought to protect persons from malaria, particularly during the early years of life when immunity is not yet established and fatal cerebral malaria caused by *Plasmodium falciparum* may occur. This selective advantage accounts for the high frequency of thalassemia genes in regions where malaria has been endemic for the past two millennia. These include the Mediterranean basin particularly, but also large parts of Asia and Africa. The gene frequency may be as high as 20 per cent in certain populations.

HEMOGLOBIN H DISEASE

PATHOPHYSIOLOGY. An anemia of moderate severity characterized by hypochromia, microcytosis, striking red cell fragmentation, and the presence of a fast migrating hemoglobin on electrophoresis occurs in patients who have a moderately severe deficiency in α globin production. The genetics of this condition will be considered later in this chapter. The fast migrating "hemoglobin" has the globin subunit composition $β_4$. It may account for up to 30 per cent of the total hemoglobin in these patients. Because the $β_4$ tetramer exhibits no cooperativity and has an extremely high oxygen affinity, it is functionally useless in oxygen transport. Thus patients with a significant amount of Hb H functionally have a more severe anemia than measurement of the hemoglobin concentration might suggest.

Hb H is an unstable tetramer. Thus as the red cell ages and loses its ability to withstand oxidative stress, Hb H may precipitate, forming inclusions that cause hemolysis. Oxidant drugs such as the sulfonamides may exacerbate hemolysis. Because the $β_4$ tetramer is soluble during the early phases of the red cell's life span, erythropoiesis in the bone marrow is effective and the anemia is generally not as severe as that seen in patients with β thalassemia who have an equivalent impairment in β globin production.

CLINICAL FEATURES. The average patient with Hb H disease maintains gainful employment, marries, and reproduces. Usually the anemia is moderate with a hemoglobin concentration of 7 to 10 grams per deciliter, although occasional patients may have more severe anemia. Moderate splenomegaly is often present. Splenectomy may be considered, but the occurrence of severe postoperative thrombocytosis with a propensity for recurrent pulmonary emboli makes this procedure inadvisable except in patients with unequivocal clinical evidence of hypersplenism as manifested by leukopenia, thrombocytopenia, and a worsening anemia or a transfusion requirement in a previously stable patient. Other therapeutic measures include prescription of folic acid, avoidance of oxidant drugs and iron salts, prompt treatment of infection, and judicious use of transfusions. Acquired Hb H disease has been described as a complication in patients with various forms of myeloproliferative and myelodysplastic disorders. In such patients, treatment and prognosis are related to the primary disorder.

HYDROPS FETALIS

The birth of stillborn infants from parents who both have α thalassemia trait reflects the severest form of α thalassemia. These infants are grossly edematous or hydropic because of congestive heart failure that occurs as a result of severe anemia. Their failure to produce any α globin results in the production of only Hb Barts ($γ_4$) and Hb H ($β_4$) during the later parts of gestation. Both these hemoglobins are nonfunctional in oxygen transport, so that once the embryonic hemoglobins disappear from the circulation early in fetal development, life is no longer possible. A high incidence of toxemia of pregnancy has been noted in mothers of hydropic infants. Prenatal diagnosis of this condition is possible (see below) and should be followed by prompt termination of the pregnancy.

SILENT CARRIER

The silent carrier state was first recognized among the α thalassemia syndromes. One parent of a patient with Hb H disease usually has all the features of α thalassemia trait, whereas the other has normal-appearing red cells with no anemia. Similarly, progeny of persons with Hb H disease fall into two groups: those having α thalassemia trait, and those with apparently normal hemoglobin production. In the silent carrier, the defect in α globin synthesis is so mild that no impairment in hemoglobin synthesis is evident, although when the mutation is paired genetically with a more severe impairment of globin synthesis, e.g., α thalassemia trait, Hb H disease occurs. A similar silent carrier state has also been described among the β thalassemia syndromes. Thalassemia intermedia occurs in those who inherit one thalassemia gene from a silent carrier and a second from a person with thalassemia trait.

THE GENETICS OF THE α THALASSEMIA SYNDROMES

As described in Ch. 139, the α globin genes in humans are duplicated. Thus two genes are found on each chromosome 16, making a total of four in each diploid cell. Four clinical states are seen in α thalassemia: silent carrier, thalassemia trait, Hb H disease, and hydrops fetalis. These conditions occur in persons who have one, two, three, or four α globin genes affected by mutations that reduce α globin synthesis.

The most frequent mutation that leads to α thalassemia is gene deletion. In the silent carrier one of the two genes on one chromosome 16 is missing, whereas the other two genes on the other chromosome 16 are normal. α Thalassemia trait can occur by two mechanisms. Persons who have two chromosomes with only one α gene will exhibit α thalassemia trait. This form is most common in the black population. Hb H disease is distinctly uncommon in this population, since offspring of two persons each of whom is homozygous for the one α gene chromosome can only have α thalassemia trait and not Hb H disease. In the Oriental population, α thalassemia trait occurs most commonly in those who lack both α genes on one chromosome and have the normal two on the other. Mating of such a person with a silent carrier who has one chromosome having only one α gene can lead to children with Hb H disease. Hydrops fetalis occurs among offspring of parents both of whom are heterozygous for chromosomes lacking both normal α globin genes.

In addition to the deletion mutations, many nondeletional types of α thalassemia have been described. Molecular characterization of several has revealed a diversity of defects involving either RNA splicing, polyadenylation, mRNA translation, or α globin stability. These mutations are similar to those in β thalassemia globin genes; their effects on RNA metabolism will be discussed in more detail in the next section.

THE MOLECULAR GENETICS OF THALASSEMIA

The β thalassemia mutations may be separated into two classes: β^{+} thalassemia, in which there is synthesis of a small amount of normal β globin, and β^{0} thalassemia, which in the homozygote is manifested by no β globin production at all. Similarly, nondeletional types of α thalassemia may abolish (α^{0}) or decrease (α^{+}) alpha globin production. Many mutations having specific effects on gene expression have been characterized by molecular cloning, DNA sequencing, and functional characterization. Each of the several steps in RNA metabolism—transcription, processing, transport, or mRNA translation—has been found to be affected by one or more individual mutations. The variable quantitative effect of the individual mutations on globin production has been clarified by these molecular studies.

PROMOTER MUTATIONS. Four globin genes, each of which has a single nucleotide substitution in the promoter region, have been isolated from different individuals with β thalassemia. Three of the mutant genes have substitutions in the "ATA" box (see Fig. 140–1). These mutations reduce promoter function to 20 to 25 per cent of normal, but some β globin mRNA is produced from these genes; hence they cause β^{+} thalassemia. The other promoter mutant characterized to date has a G substituted for C at the position 87 nucleotides from the start site for transcription in the first of the conserved "CACA" boxes. This mutation reduces promoter function to 10 per cent of normal and hence is a more "severe" thalassemia gene than those with the "ATA" box substitution.

SPLICING MUTATIONS. These are among the most common of mutations that cause thalassemia; 14 such mutant genes have already been described. Figure 141–1 contains a few illustrative examples classified by the manner in which they affect splicing of the globin mRNA precursor. Mutations that occur within the splice junction sequence decrease or abolish normal splicing at that site and often are accompanied by splicing at other sites that are not normally used. A substitution in the invariant GT, as shown in the example (Fig. 141–1*A*), abolishes splicing, making this a β^{0} gene, whereas substitutions in consensus nucleotides at the splice junction have a quantitative effect on splicing and hence are β^{+} mutations.

An interesting class of mutations are those that create an alternate site for splicing. These may occur within introns or, as shown in the examples in Figure 141–1*B*, within coding sequence (exons). These substitutions occur within regions of the precursor RNA molecule that resemble the consensus splice

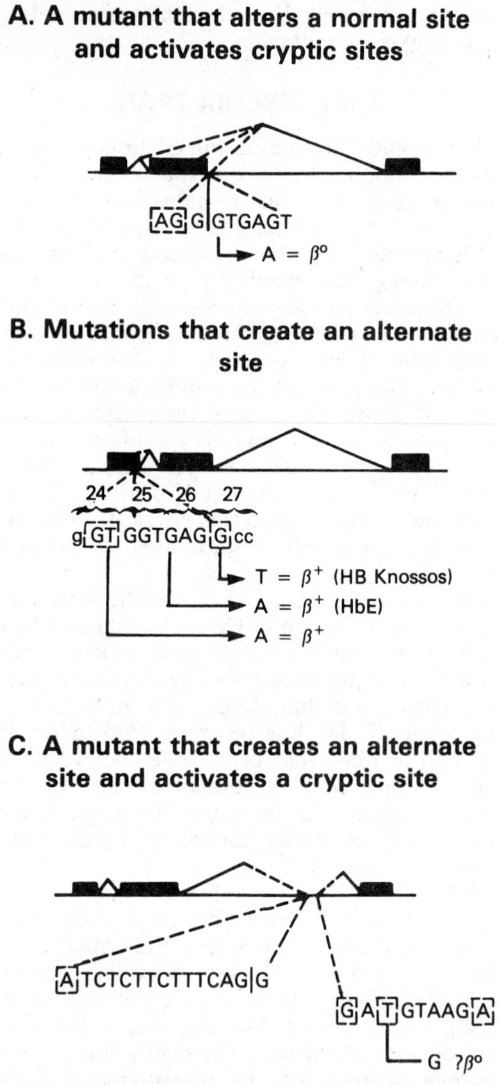

Figure 141–1. Thalassemia mutations that alter the splicing of the β globin gene transcript. *A*, The nucleotides, guanine (G) and thymine (T), are obligatory for normal splicing. Replacement of the G with adenine (A) abolishes normal splicing and leads to abnormal splicing at otherwise cryptic sites. *B*, Several different mutations at this position in the transcript create an alternate site that leads to abnormal splicing. This segment of the normal transcript includes the obligatory dinucleotide, GT, and matches the consensus sequence in all but the nucleotides in the boxes. Single nucleotide substitutions activate this otherwise inactive site. *C*, A substitution toward the end of intron II creates an alternate splice site. A normally cryptic site further upstream in the intron is also involved in a splicing reaction with exon 2–intron II splice junction, resulting in formation of a processed globin RNA that retains a portion of the sequence transcribed from intron II. Therefore, it cannot be translated into β globin.

junction sequence (see Fig. 140–1) but lack some critical element necessary for splicing. Nucleotide substitutions that add that element to the potential splice junction sequence lead to its activation, causing abnormal splicing and hence a thalassemic effect. Substitution of A for T in codon 24 of the β globin gene does not alter the amino acid sequence (GGT and GGA both encode for glycine) but creates an alternative splicing site. The other two mutations illustrated in Figure 141–1*B* (Hb E and Hb Knossos) alter both protein structure and the splicing pattern. Such structural mutants that are also characterized by decreased synthesis are referred to as *thalassemic hemoglobinopathies*.

A class of mutations that has interesting implications for control of splicing are those that create an alternate site and also activate cryptic splice sites remote from the mutation. There is a potential or cryptic splice site in the β globin gene transcript that matches the consensus splice junction sequence nearly perfectly and yet this site is used rarely if ever during normal splicing. Use of an alternative site, created by a thalassemia mutation, apparently alters the secondary structure of the precursor RNA molecule, leading to splicing at the otherwise cryptic site (Fig. 141–1C).

A POLYADENYLATION MUTATION. The sequence "AATAAA" is one of the signals that leads to cleavage of the globin gene transcript and addition of the poly A track (see Fig. 141–1). An α thalassemia gene isolated from an individual with Hb H disease has G substituted for A, altering the polyadenylation signal to "AATAGA." Most of the RNA transcript is not processed correctly and is prematurely degraded, although a small amount of normal α globin mRNA is produced by this mutant gene. Thus it is an α^+ thalassemia gene.

MUTATIONS THAT AFFECT mRNA TRANSLATION. Among the more common mutations in thalassemia genes are those that lead to premature termination of mRNA translation. Single nucleotide substitutions or small deletions that alter the mRNA reading frame introduce codons that signal the termination of protein synthesis on the abnormal mRNA. For example, substitution of thymine for cytosine in codon 39 introduces the stop codon UAG at that position. This abnormal β globin mRNA can be read only through codon 38, yielding a small, nonfunctional remnant of β globin. Premature termination mutations cause β^0 (or α^0) thalassemia.

Common mutations that cause α thalassemia are chain termination mutations. As described in Ch. 140, the completed globin molecule is released from the polyribosome when the protein synthetic apparatus encounters the normal terminator codon UAA. A single nucleotide change in this terminator codon will convert it to a codon that is functional for the insertion of any one of several amino acids, depending on the exact nucleotide that is substituted. In this case protein synthesis continues into the part of the mRNA that is usually untranslated, leading to the synthesis of a protein that may be as many as 30 amino acids longer than normal. Such an elongated α globin is found in Hb Constant Spring. This protein accounts for only 1 to 2 per cent of the total α globin in the cells of patients with Hb Constant Spring and their red cells exhibit the stigmata of thalassemia trait.

MUTATIONS THAT AFFECT GLOBIN STABILITY. Certain mutations may alter globin sequence and lead to instability and thus have a thalassemic effect despite a normal rate of synthesis of the mutant globin. Among the more dramatic of this class of mutations is one that leads to substitution of leucine for proline at position 125 of the α globin found in Hb Quong Sze. This mutation was discovered upon sequencing of the abnormal α gene and evidence of $\alpha^{\text{Quong Sze}}$ instability was subsequently obtained in vitro. Because of its marked instability, $\alpha^{\text{Quong Sze}}$ could not be detected in the red cells of the affected individual. Hb Quong Sze, like Hb E, is another of the thalassemic hemoglobinopathies characterized by both deficient net globin production and a structural abnormality.

DELETION MUTATIONS. Deletions causing α thalassemia have been described earlier. Small deletions that leave one of the two α globin genes intact on a chromosome are classified as α^+ mutations, while large deletions that remove both α genes are considered α^0 mutations. In contrast to α thalassemia, in which gene deletion is the most common mutation, gene deletion is rarely the mechanism for β thalassemia. A few patients of Indian ancestry have been found to have a deletion that has removed the 3′ half of the β globin gene and a small amount of flanking DNA. A special kind of deletion has resulted in the δβ fusion gene present in a few Italian patients who produce Hb Lepore. An unequal crossover during meiosis has led to the fusion gene that encodes for a globin that has the N-terminal sequence of δ globin and the C-terminal sequence of β globin. This globin is produced in very small amounts; hence this gene leads to thalassemia trait or thalassemia major in heterozygotes or homozygotes, respectively.

Several large deletions that have removed two or more genes from the β cluster have been characterized. The β thalassemia mutations have resulted in loss of the δ and β genes; the $^{A}\gamma\delta\beta$ thalassemia deletions include the $^{A}\gamma$ gene in addition. One interesting form of γδβ thalassemia has resulted in loss of all but the β gene and yet this β gene does not function. These observations suggest that the DNA sequences remote from a gene can nonetheless influence its expression. Two deletions have resulted in loss of the entire β-like gene cluster.

MUTATIONS THAT INCREASE Hb F PRODUCTION

About 1 per cent of the hemoglobin in adult blood is Hb F. This fetal hemoglobin is found in 2 to 10 per cent of red cells; these cells—called F cells—contain roughly 4 to 8 pg of Hb F and 24 to 28 pg of adult hemoglobin. As discussed in Chapter 140, these F cells originate during the differentiation of erythroid progenitor cells. F cell number and therefore Hb F levels are genetically determined in man.

Increased Hb F in individuals who are homozygous for β thalassemia mainly reflects amplification of the F cell population. In the bone marrow, those erythroblasts producing small amounts of γ globin have less of an excess in α globin synthesis and therefore are more likely to survive and leave the bone marrow. By this mechanism, the 1 per cent of γ synthesis in the bone marrow cell population may be amplified 10- to 40-fold in the peripheral blood. Of more interest from the aspect of gene control are those mutations that alter Hb F production by genetic mechanisms.

There are two general classes of deletion mutations that increase Hb F production in adults. The δβ thalassemia mutations are characterized by production of 5 to 12 per cent of Hb F in heterozygotes, while *hereditary persistence of fetal hemoglobin* (HPFH) deletion mutations are characterized by production of 25 to 30 per cent. Most of the red cells in heterozygous individuals with HPFH contain Hb F, whereas heterozygotes with δβ thalassemia mutations have Hb F in only 25 to 30 per cent of their red cells. These mutations have been carefully characterized structurally in an attempt to define the basis at the DNA level for these differing phenotypes. Figure 141–2 illustrates one of the more interesting differences. Just in front of the δ globin gene are found two members of a family of moderately repetitive DNA sequences called the *Alu family*. Each of the three deletions that produce the δβ thalassemia phenotype leave one or both of these Alu elements intact, whereas both HPFH deletions remove all or most of both. The manner by which Alu elements might influence expression of nearby genes forms the basis of many ongoing studies.

Another category of mutations that cause HPFH leave the β-like gene cluster intact and therefore are referred to as *nondele-*

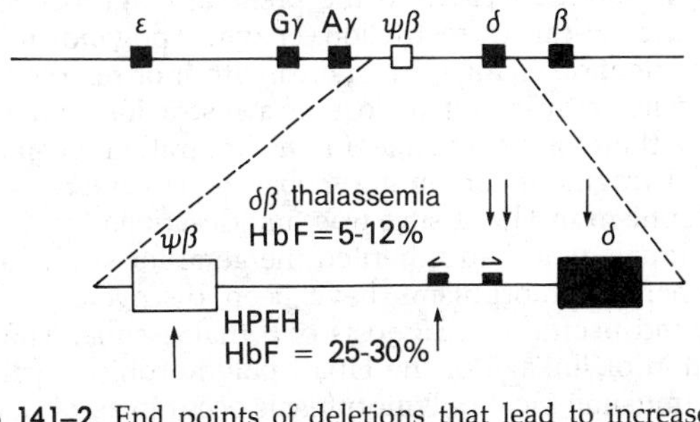

Figure 141–2. End points of deletions that lead to increased Hb F production in adults. The small black boxes (with overlying arrows) indicate the position of members of the Alu family of moderately repetitive DNA sequences. Each member is approximately 300 base pairs long and there are more than 500,000 members in the human genome. The two members in this position are oriented in opposite directions. The three δβ thalassemia mutations, the end points of which are indicated by the vertical arrows above the line, leave one or both of the repetitive sequences intact. In contrast, the HPFH mutations, the end points of which are indicated by the vertical arrows below the line, remove all or most of both Alu members. The deletions extend downstream (to the right) to remove the β globin gene and variable amounts of additional DNA.

tion mutations. Nondeletion HPFH mutations are characterized by a heterogenous distribution of Hb F in red cells (heterocellular) in contrast to the pancellular distribution of Hb F in heterozygotes with the deletion type of HPFH. There may be many different heterocellular HPFH mutations; genetic studies indicate that at least some are not linked to the β-like gene cluster. These mutations are therefore of particular interest because they may affect the function of protein molecules that influence the level of γ gene expression.

PRENATAL DIAGNOSIS

Because of the serious consequences of severe β thalassemia (Cooley's anemia), prenatal diagnosis of this condition with subsequent therapeutic abortion is thought by many to be highly desirable. Two general strategies have made this a feasible undertaking. The first approach is based on the fact that small amounts of β globin synthesis may be detected in the early mid-trimester fetus (see Ch. 139). In fetuses who have inherited two genes for β thalassemia, no β globin or very small amounts are produced at a time when normal fetuses are producing approximately 10 per cent β globin. By using sophisticated obstetric techniques, blood may be obtained from the umbilical vein and used for biosynthetic measurements of the globin synthetic pattern. Low or absent β globin synthesis occurs in homozygous fetuses, whereas intermediate levels are found in heterozygotes. This strategy has been widely applied in parts of Greece and Italy and has led to a significant reduction in the incidence of the severe form of β thalassemia in certain populations.

A second strategy for prenatal diagnosis relies on the study of DNA prepared from amniotic fluid cells of potentially affected persons. The globin genes in such DNA samples may be characterized by the techniques referred to as restriction endonuclease mapping. The DNA is digested with an enzyme that cuts at a specific nucleotide sequence. Among the million or so fragments generated from human DNA are those few that include the globin genes. The DNA is resolved electrophoretically, transferred to a nitrocellulose paper, and annealed to a radioactive probe specific for globin gene sequences. Depending on the enzyme used, a characteristic set of fragments containing globin gene sequences is generated. In persons who have inherited a mutation reflected by deletion of all or part of a globin gene, a change in a position of a particular fragment will serve to indicate the presence of such a mutation. Many cases of α thalassemia and rare cases of β thalassemia may be diagnosed in this way.

More widely applicable to the prenatal diagnosis of thalassemias are so-called restriction enzyme polymorphisms. A single nucleotide change, in an area within or remote from the globin gene, may result in loss of a restriction endonuclease site and therefore a change in the migration position of a particular fragment containing globin gene sequences. Such a polymorphism in Hpa I site, was first described by Kan (1978) in individuals who had inherited the gene for sickle hemoglobin. Other polymorphisms have been discovered and have been found useful for diagnosis of β thalassemia. The unique association or linkage of the Hpa I polymorphism with the β^S gene is unusual; most polymorphisms occur in association with both normal and abnormal β globin genes. Hence a different method of analysis is required rather than simple characterization of a single restriction endonuclease site.

Several restriction endonuclease sites—each of which is polymorphic, either present (+) or absent (−)—may be used to define the haplotype of the β globin gene region on a specific chromosome. Eighty to 90 per cent of the time a single mutation is associated or linked to a single set of restriction endonuclease polymorphisms, a single haplotype. Once the haplotype associated with a particular mutation in an ethnic group is known, haplotype analysis may be used to define the frequency of that mutation in that group. The normal β globin gene is found linked to all haplotypes. Hence, simple haplotype analysis cannot be used for prenatal diagnosis directly. Extensive family studies or study of DNA from an affected or completely normal child is necessary before haplotype analysis can be applied for prenatal diagnosis in that family.

An alternative approach utilizing DNA analysis for prenatal diagnosis is now feasible because several frequent mutations have been defined by DNA sequencing. Synthetic oligonucleotide probes, one specific for the normal gene and one specific for a particular abnormal gene, can be used to discriminate between the normal and abnormal genes in amniotic fluid DNA. This method is simple and direct but requires that several probes be available for each of the mutations that occur frequently in the population for whom prenatal diagnosis is offered. Technical innovations to increase sensitivity and specificity and the ready synthesis of specific probes will undoubtedly make this the method of choice for prenatal diagnosis in the future.

Of course the application of prenatal diagnosis requires appropriate screening and identification of persons at risk. Thalassemia trait can usually readily be identified by virtue of the morphologic changes in the red cells. Confirmation of the diagnosis depends on measurement of hemoglobin A_2 and Hb F.

EXPERIMENTAL THERAPY

Knowledge of globin gene structure and regulation has suggested a means to activate the structurally normal but inactive γ globin genes in individuals with severe β thalassemia. Increased γ globin synthesis is desirable because it partially compensates for the deficiency of β globin production and decreases the relative excess of α globin. DNA is modified after synthesis by methylation of cytosine residues. Expressed genes are relatively undermethylated compared to unexpressed DNA sequences. For example, the γ globin genes are undermethylated in fetal erythroid cells, but after the switch to adult hemoglobin synthesis the γ globin genes are fully methylated in adult erythroid cells. 5-Azacytidine inhibits DNA methylation and has been shown to activate genes in tissue culture cells and in experimental animals. Administration of 5-azacytidine to patients with severe β thalassemia under defined experimental protocols has resulted in increased γ globin synthesis and improvement in red cell production and survival. The effect is transient, lasting only two to three weeks. Reluctance to administer a potentially carcinogenic and toxic drug for longer periods has limited the use of 5-azacytidine to experimental studies of a few severely affected patients. Nonetheless these encouraging results have prompted a search for other effective and less toxic drugs that may make pharmacologic stimulation of the γ globin genes a useful approach for treatment of severe β thalassemia.

Cure of severe β thalassemia can be achieved by bone marrow transplantation from an HLA identical, unaffected sibling. A few patients have already been cured by this method. This procedure carries a 10 to 40 per cent risk of death or significant graft-versus-host disease (GVHD). Transplantation in infancy, preferably before transfusions are given, increases the probability of successful engraftment and reduces the risk of this disease. However, adequate transfusion therapy and effective chelation may provide 20 or more years of good-quality life for newborns. Thus, the availability of bone marrow transplantation raises a significant ethical dilemma for parents and physicians. In the future, refinements in the treatment of GVHD and transplantation techniques may permit wider application of bone marrow transplantation as treatment for patients with severe β thalassemia.

Alter BP: Prenatal diagnosis in hemoglobinopathies and other hematological diseases. J Pediatr 95:501, 1979. Orkin SH: Prenatal diagnosis of hemoglobin disorders by DNA analysis. Blood 63:249, 1984. *These reviews summarize the successful efforts made to develop techniques for prenatal diagnosis of the hemoglobinopathies.*

Ley TJ, Griffith P, Nienhuis AW: Transfusion hemosiderosis and chelation therapy. Clin Haematol 11:437, 1982. *This detailed review describes the pathogenesis of transfusional hemochromatosis and summarizes evidence related to the beneficial effects achieved with chelation therapy.*

Ley TJ, DeSimone J, Anagnou NP, Keller GH, Humphries RK, Turner PH, Young NS, Heller P, Nienhuis AW: 5-Azacytidine selectively increases γ globin synthesis in a patient with β^+ thalassemia. N Engl J Med 307:1469, 1982. *This paper reports the first use of 5-azacytidine to stimulate γ globin synthesis. The molecular effects and the proposed mechanism of action are described.*

Nienhuis AW, Anagnou NP, Ley TJ: Advances in thalassemia research. Blood, in press, 1984. *This review describes the molecular mechanisms of thalassemia and summarizes therapeutic approaches, both conventional and experimental.*

Orkin SH, Kazazian HH Jr, Antonarakis SE, Goff SC, Boehn CD, Sexton JP, Waber PG, Giardina PJV: Linkage of β thalassemia mutations and β globin gene polymorphisms with DNA polymorphisms in human β globin gene cluster. Nature 296:627, 1983. Trisman R, Orkin SH, Maniatis T: Specific transcription and RNA splicing defects in five cloned β thalassemia genes. Nature 302:591, 1983. *These are two classic papers that describe strategies used to identify mutations, determine their frequencies in populations in which thalassemia genes are common, and to characterize these mutations as to their functional consequences.*

Weatherall DJ, Clegg JB: The Thalassemia Syndromes. 3rd ed. Oxford, Blackwell Scientific Publications, Ltd., 1981. *This superb monograph describes the clinical aspects, genetics, and interactions of the various thalassemia syndromes. It should be consulted by anyone with a serious interest in thalassemia.*

142. SICKLE CELL ANEMIA AND ASSOCIATED HEMOGLOBINOPATHIES

Bernard G. Forget

DEFINITION. The sickle cell syndromes are due to the inheritance of a gene for a structurally abnormal β globin chain subunit of adult hemoglobin, the β^S chain of Hb S ($\alpha_2\beta^S_2$). The structural abnormality of the β^S globin chain consists of a single amino acid substitution or replacement: valine instead of the normal glutamic acid at position number 6 of the β polypeptide chain. Hb S can be found in the heterozygous state (Hb SA or sickle cell trait), in the homozygous state (Hb SS, sickle cell anemia, or sickle cell disease), in association with other structural hemoglobin variants (i.e., Hb SC and SD disease), in association with β thalassemia (Hb S–β thalassemia or sickle–β thalassemia syndromes), or in association with the thalassemia-like disorder termed hereditary persistence of fetal hemoglobin (Hb SF or Hb S-HPFH). The structural abnormality of Hb C, a nonsickling hemoglobin, also consists of a single amino acid substitution at residue number 6 of the β globin chain: in the β^C chain lysine replaces glutamic acid. Clinical syndromes associated with the inheritance of Hb C include Hb SC disease and homozygous Hb C disease.

PREVALENCE AND GENETICS. The sickle cell syndromes are particularly prevalent in black persons of African or Afro-American ancestry. However, the gene is also found at a lower frequency in persons of Mediterranean ancestry (southern Italians, Sicilians, and Greeks), in Saudi Arabia, and in India. The highest gene frequencies occur in equatorial Africa, in the so-called "malaria belt." The heterozygous state for Hb S (sickle cell trait) probably confers a biologic advantage against infection with falciparum malaria, and for this reason the gene frequency for Hb S has achieved high levels through natural selection in geographical areas of endemic malaria. In the United States the prevalence of the sickle cell trait in blacks is 8 to 10 per cent and the number of homozygous persons approaches 50,000, or 1 in 400 births. In certain areas of western Africa (Ghana and Nigeria), the prevalence of Hb SA can reach 25 to 30 per cent. The prevalence of Hb CA in black Americans is approximately 3 per cent. Gene mapping studies using restriction endonuclease analysis of cellular DNA to identify polymorphisms of nucleotide sequence in the DNA around the β^S globin gene have disclosed an unexpected heterogeneity of polymorphisms linked to the sickle β-globin genes in different individuals, suggesting multiple independent origins of the sickle gene.

PATHOPHYSIOLOGY. The sickling phenomenon resulting from aggregation or polymerization of Hb S molecules causes two major phenomena in affected persons: (1) a chronic compensated hemolytic anemia and (2) vaso-occlusive crises resulting in pain and tissue damage caused by infarction. These two phenomena are directly related to the physicochemical properties of the Hb S molecule and result from alterations of red cell metabolism and red cell rheology as a consequence of the sickling phenomenon.

The sickling phenomenon occurs only when the Hb S molecule is in the deoxy conformation (see Ch. 139). When Hb S is in the oxy conformation it has essentially normal physicochemical properties. In the deoxy conformation, Hb S molecules can aggregate with one another into long polymers and are aligned to form a gel of liquid crystals that are also called tactoids. The sickling process goes through a number of stages, as illustrated diagrammatically in Figure 142–1. In the process of nucleation, Hb S molecules form small aggregates, which then grow by addition of successive Hb S molecules. The larger aggregates then align themselves to form linearly arranged fibers that constitute a paracrystalline gel. These fibers can be detected as helical electron dense tube-like structures by electron microscopy (Fig. 142–1). The end result of the polymerization process is the transformation of the intracellular contents of the red cell from a fluid liquid to a viscous gel. The amount of Hb S polymer within red cells increases progressively as the percentage of oxygen saturation of the hemoglobin decreases. When the amount of polymer is sufficiently high, the red cells may assume the typical sickle or holly leaf shape associated with sickled erythrocytes (Fig. 142–2). The shape change of the erythrocyte is a passive phenomenon in which the red cell membrane conforms to the shape that is assumed by the intracellular gel of polymerized hemoglobin. The sickling phenomenon is reversible: with reoxygenation of the Hb S molecules the aggregated molecules disassociate, the gel becomes liquid, and the erythrocyte, if it has sickled, can return to its normal shape, as long as the red cell membrane has not become altered to form an irreversibly sickled cell (see below).

A number of factors can influence the rate and degree of Hb S aggregation in red cells. One of the most important determinants is the concentration of Hb S and of total hemoglobin within the red cell. In general the higher the percentage of Hb S, the more severe the sickle syndrome. Factors such as cellular dehydration that increase the mean corpuscular hemoglobin concentration (MCHC) will greatly facilitate sickling by increasing the opportunity and frequency of contact between Hb S molecules. The importance of hemoglobin concentration on sickling is underscored by the clinical observation that the co-inheritance of α thalassemia together with sickle cell anemia is generally (but not universally) associated with less severe hemolysis. The milder clinical course of Hb S–β thalassemia is also thought to be due in part to the associated hypochromia. The length of time during which Hb S remains deoxygenated is also very important: the chances of Hb S polymerization will be enhanced with any increase in the transit time of the red cell through the microcirculation. The presence of other hemoglobins within the red cell can also influence sickling. In general, at a constant MCHC, any other non-S hemoglobin molecules in the red cell, by a simple dilution effect, will decrease the opportunity of contact between Hb S molecules. In addition, the type of non-S hemoglobin present can differentially affect sickling: fetal hemoglobin (Hb F) participates much less readily than normal Hb A in polymer formation, whereas certain mutant hemoglobins such as Hb C and Hb D, although nonsickling per se, will participate in gelation more readily than Hb A. Finally, acidosis can enhance sickling by decreasing oxygen affinity (see Ch. 139) and thereby increasing the amount of deoxy Hb S in the red cell.

The sickling phenomenon results in two major red cell disturbances. The first is damage to the red cell membrane, as a result of repeated episodes of sickling and unsickling. Sickle red cells are "leaky": they tend to lose K^+ and water and eventually become dehydrated, the resulting increase in MCHC probably enhancing further sickling. The red cell membrane

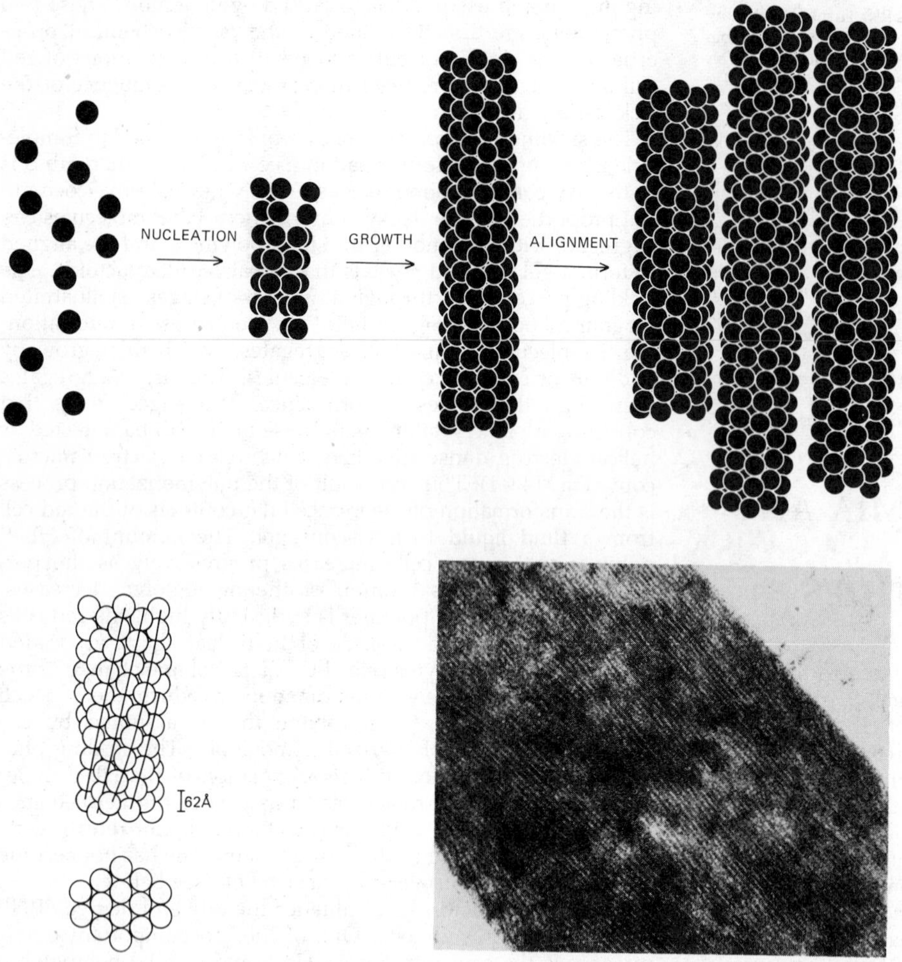

Figure 142–1. *Top,* Schematic representation of mechanism of deoxyhemoglobin S polymerization (sickling). Each circle represents a deoxyhemoglobin S tetramer: $\alpha_2\beta_2^S$. *Lower left,* Molecular model, based on electron microscopy, of the helical arrangement of deoxyhemoglobin S tetramers in a fiber of polymerized Hb S molecules; side view (above) and cross section or end-on view (below). *Lower right,* Electron micrograph (longitudinal section) of deoxyhemoglobin S gel in a sickled erythrocyte.

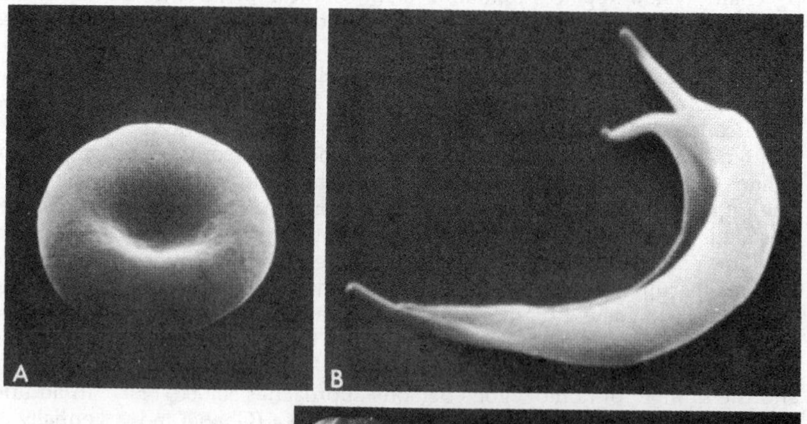

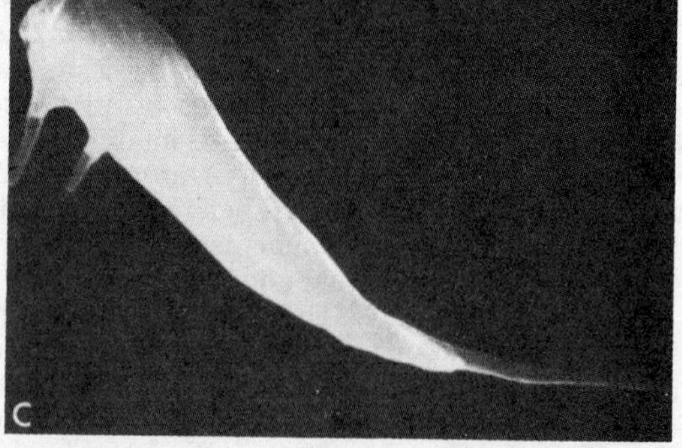

Figure 142–2. Scanning electron micrographs of oxygenated (A) and deoxygenated (B and C) SS erythrocytes. (Courtesy of Dr. James White.)

tends to accumulate calcium and becomes altered in other ways such that it may assume a rigid conformation in the sickle shape, thus forming an irreversibly sickled cell (or ISC), a cell that has the sickle shape even though the hemoglobin within it may not be in the aggregated state. As a result of these phenomena the red cells become rigid and relatively nondeformable, and are sequestered and prematurely destroyed within the reticuloendothelial system. This series of events constitutes the basis for the shortened red cell survival and hemolytic anemia that invariably accompany sickle cell anemia.

The second major disturbance relates to the flow properties of red cells containing substantial amounts of polymerized Hb S. Such cells are much less deformable than normal red cells and their flow through the microcirculation is greatly retarded. Stasis of blood flow promotes further polymerization of Hb S in other erythrocytes—the so-called "vicious viscous sickle cycle." Occlusion of the microvasculature by the viscous mass of erythrocytes leads to ischemia and eventual infarction of the tissue downstream from the obstruction, and results in a painful crisis and/or tissue damage.

The pathogenesis of some of the other clinical manifestations associated with sickle syndromes cannot be as easily attributed directly to the sickling phenomenon. The increased susceptibility of these patients to various types of infections is probably related to a number of different factors, including absence of spleen function owing to autoinfarction and, in certain patients, defective opsonization of bacteria by the alternative pathway (properdin system). The retardation of growth and development cannot be solely explained by endocrine dysfunction caused by organ damage from sickling but may be related to more ill-defined factors such as the anemia and general debility of these patients.

CLINICAL MANIFESTATIONS. ***Sickle Cell Trait.*** Persons who are heterozygous for Hb S are essentially asymptomatic. They should not have any anemia attributable to the hemoglobinopathy. Any anemia in such persons should be investigated for other secondary causes. Symptoms resulting from vaso-occlusion occur only in extreme circumstances of severe hypoxia such as flying in unpressurized aircraft. However, a universal finding in sickle cell trait is microinfarction of the renal medulla presumably owing to the ambient hyperosmolarity that is thought to lead to dehydration of the red cells, an increased MCHC, and sickling; as a result, in affected persons the urine is unconcentrated and isosthenuria is manifested. Painless hematuria can also occasionally be attributed to microinfarction of the renal medulla, although the other usual causes should be ruled out before painless hematuria in persons with sickle cell trait is attributed to the sickling phenomenon.

Sickle Cell Disease. THE ANEMIA. Patients homozygous for Hb S invariably have a chronic compensated hemolytic anemia of variable severity. In general the hematocrit ranges between 20 and 30 per cent and the hemoglobin between 6.5 and 10 grams per deciliter. The hemolysis is compensated by increased erythropoiesis manifested as an elevated reticulocyte count in the range of 10 to 25 per cent. Mild jaundice and indirect hyperbilirubinemia are also present as a reflection of the hemolysis. The degree of the anemia is usually stable in a given patient, although occasional hypoplastic or aplastic crises can occur owing to suppression of erythropoiesis at the time of infectious episodes and result in a rapid decrease in the reticulocyte count and a precipitous drop in the hemoglobin and hematocrit levels. Infection with a particular parvovirus has been implicated in the pathogenesis of aplastic crises. Another cause of rapid worsening of the anemia is the acute splenic sequestration crisis (a sudden pooling of large volumes of blood in the spleen) that can occur in younger patients with sickle cell anemia before autoinfarction of the spleen or in older patients with Hb SC disease and Hb S–β thalassemia in whom the spleen is not infarcted and may in fact be enlarged. There is some controversy as to whether or not a hyperhemolytic state can be associated with sickle cell anemia. From what is known of the basis for the hemolysis in this condition, there is no pathophysiologic mechanism for variable or accelerated hemolysis resulting from sickling alone. In general, the anemia and hemolysis in sickle cell disease do not increase or worsen during vaso-occlusive painful crises. If hemolysis suddenly worsens, one should look to other secondary causes that may be responsible, such as an associated glucose-6-phosphate dehydrogenase deficiency and exposure to an oxidant stress from drugs or an acute infection. Finally, in patients with marginal nutritional status and increased requirements, such as during pregnancy, folic acid deficiency can develop and aggravate the anemia—the so-called megaloblastic crisis of sickle cell disease.

VASO-OCCLUSIVE CRISES. The major disability suffered by patients with sickle cell anemia is related to painful vaso-occlusive crises and secondary end-organ damage as a direct consequence of the sickling phenomenon and occlusion of the microvasculature of one or another organ, most commonly the bones of the trunk and extremities. The episodes are characterized by sudden onset of excruciating pain in the back, chest, or extremities. There is frequently no identifiable precipitating event, although infections may be associated with the onset of the episode. Other predisposing factors include dehydration, acidosis, or increased hypoxia such as during a pulmonary infection. A low grade fever may be associated with the painful attacks, although not necessarily. In general, the onset of fever will occur one or two days after the onset of pain and will parallel the degree of tissue necrosis resulting from the ischemic infarction. The painful attacks last for variable periods of time, ranging from a few hours to a few days depending on the extent of the vaso-occlusive phenomenon and the rapidity with which treatment is initiated and is successful in reversing the occlusive episode. In general there are no external signs such as heat, swelling, or tenderness of the soft tissues over the affected bones. However, if the bone infarction occurs in proximity to a joint, an effusion can develop. Bone infarction may be difficult to differentiate from osteomyelitis, and definitive diagnosis of the latter must ultimately rely on positive bacterial cultures from aspirated material.

When the vaso-occlusive process occurs in the vasculature of organs other than bones, the clinical manifestations are primarily related to damage of the affected organ. Common acute vaso-occlusive clinical syndromes include cerebrovascular accidents (i.e., hemiplegia and seizures) caused by involvement of the cerebral vasculature; the acute chest syndrome associated with occlusion of the pulmonary vessels, which can be difficult to differentiate from acute pulmonary infarction caused by emboli or from acute pulmonary infections; hepatic crisis, with marked hyperbilirubinemia and other abnormal liver function tests, which can be difficult to differentiate from acute hepatitis or choledocholithiasis; priapism resulting from vaso-occlusion within the corpus cavernosum; and acute renal papillary infarction with hematuria and/or obstruction of the urinary collecting system.

More chronic complications include refractory skin ulcers of the leg, usually in the vicinity of the medial malleolus, an area that has poor collateral circulation; and variable degrees of renal insufficiency resulting from the combination of repeated infarctions and infectious episodes. All patients manifest the inability to concentrate the urine and have isosthenuria. Microinfarction in the peripheral retina is initially asymptomatic, but may lead to the formation of new blood vessels that are fragile and can hemorrhage, causing retinal detachment and blindness. For this reason periodic eye examinations are important to recognize and treat the early asymptomatic lesion before it progresses to the point of causing visual disturbances. Finally, repeated bone infarcts in the vicinity of joints can lead to secondary degenerative arthritis, and gradual infarction of the head of the femur results in aseptic necrosis of the hip.

OTHER CLINICAL MANIFESTATIONS. Clinical manifestations of sickle cell anemia not directly related to the sickling phenomenon include increased susceptibility to infections, cholelithiasis, and abnormal growth and development. The increased susceptibility to infections is probably related at least in part to absent spleen function and in some cases to an abnormality of the properdin opsonization pathway. In early childhood, septicemia and meningitis caused by encapsulated organisms such as *Diplococcus pneumoniae* and *Hemophilus influenzae* are common. In later life common infectious episodes include recurrent pneumonias, urinary tract infections, and osteomyelitis. The predisposition to osteomyelitis is probably related to the repeated bone infarcts that can form a nidus for infection. Although osteomyelitis caused by *Salmonella* occurs almost exclusively in patients with sickle cell anemia or one of the other sickle cell syndromes, *Staphylococcus aureus* is still the most common causative organism of osteomyelitis in these syndromes.

Cholelithiasis is very common, and can be manifested at a young age; it is caused by the chronic hemolysis that results in increased bilirubin production. Episodes of cholecystitis and choledocholithiasis can easily be confused with abdominal and hepatic sickle cell crises. The causes of delayed growth and development are poorly understood. Delayed puberty can result in late closure of the epiphyses and an asthenic habitus.

Other Sickle Cell Syndromes. The anemia and the hemolysis are less severe in the other sickle syndromes, such as Hb SC disease and sickle–β thalassemia, in which there is somewhat less propensity for sickling than in homozygous Hb SS disease. In these conditions the anemia frequently ranges between hemoglobin levels of 10 and 12 grams per deciliter, and the reticulocyte counts are usually less than 10 per cent, frequently in the range of 5 per cent.

In general the vaso-occlusive manifestations resulting from sickling are also less frequent and less severe in Hb SC disease and in sickle–β thalassemia than in sickle cell anemia, although all of the complications previously described for sickle cell anemia can also occur in these conditions. However, in contrast to sickle cell anemia, splenomegaly in adults is usually present in these syndromes and splenic infarcts and acute splenic sequestration crises can occur. The ocular complications of sickling also tend to occur more frequently in Hb SC disease than in sickle cell anemia and can in fact be the presenting symptoms. Complications associated with pregnancy also tend to occur more frequently in Hb SC disease than in sickle cell anemia. Sickle–β^0 thalassemia, in which Hb A is totally absent, is generally more severe than sickle–β^+ thalassemia and can be as clinically severe as sickle cell anemia.

DIAGNOSIS. The diagnosis of the various sickle syndromes relies on two types of tests: (1) screening tests to detect the presence of Hb S on the basis of its physicochemical properties, and (2) more definitive tests for the precise diagnosis of the particular genetic syndrome involved.

Two types of screening tests for the detection of Hb S are in current use. Both tests simply detect the presence of some Hb S in erythroid cells but do not differentiate sickle cell trait from the other sickle syndromes. The standard "sickle cell preparation" consists of mixing blood with a solution of sodium metabisulfite, which totally deoxygenates the blood and thus induces sickling that can be observed under the microscope. A second screening test is a solubility test which consists of mixing blood with a solution of high ionic strength and observing the mixtures for turbidity; normal hemoglobin will give a clear solution, whereas any Hb S in the solution will precipitate to give a turbid solution through which one cannot see the lines of an indicator card. Both tests, if properly done, are highly specific and accurate. The solubility test has the advantages that a microscope is not needed and that the test solution is relatively stable.

Once Hb S is detected by screening tests, hemoglobin electrophoresis should be carried out for precise diagnosis of the sickle syndrome. Table 142–1 summarizes the results obtained by hemoglobin electrophoresis in the various sickle cell syndromes as well as other associated clinical and laboratory findings that are useful in the differential diagnosis. In general, routine hemoglobin electrophoresis at pH 8.6 will suffice to establish the diagnosis. However, a few exceptions to this rule require additional tests to confirm or establish the suspected diagnosis. Because other hemoglobin variants can have the same electrophoretic mobility as Hb S at pH 8.6, electrophoresis in citrate agar at pH 6.1 should be performed to confirm the diagnosis (see Table 142–1). The distinction between Hb SS disease and Hb S–β^0 thalassemia can be very difficult to establish, since electrophoretic findings are similar in both cases. The Hb A_2 level should be elevated in Hb S–β thalassemia, but precise quantitation of Hb A_2 in the presence of Hb S is sometimes unreliable. Findings that should establish the diagnosis of Hb S–β^0 thalassemia rather than Hb SS disease include (1) the presence of hypochromia and microcytosis indicated by low MCV and MCH; (2) family study showing that one parent or an offspring has β thalassemia trait rather than sickle cell trait; (3) experimental studies of globin chain synthesis using labeled amino acid precursors (see Ch. 141), demonstrating decreased synthesis of β^S chains relative to α chains (β^S/α = 0.5 to 0.6); and (4) the finding of splenomegaly and the absence of ISCs on peripheral blood smear. The rare but interesting syndrome of Hb S–HPFH will also give hemoglobin electrophoretic findings similar to those of Hb SS disease but with an unusually high level of Hb F in the range of 30 per cent. Such patients, however, are not anemic and should be asymptomatic. The diagnosis can be confirmed by family study showing the absence of sickle cell trait and presence of heterozygosity for HPFH in a parent or offspring. Study of the distribution of Hb F within individual red cells, using the acid elution test of Betke and Kleihauer, will show uniform distribution of Hb F in Hb S–HPFH but heterogeneous distribution of Hb F in Hb

TABLE 142–1. DIFFERENTIAL DIAGNOSIS OF SICKLE CELL SYNDROMES

Genotype	Clinical Condition	Hemoglobin Electrophoresis Findings					Other Associated Findings
		Hb A	*Hb S*	*Hb A_2*	*Hb F*	*Hb C*	
SA	Sickle cell trait	55–60%	40–45%*	2–3%	~1%	—	Asymptomatic; no anemia
SS†	Sickle cell anemia	0	85–95%	2–3%	5–15%	—	Usually clinically severe; Hb F distributed heterogeneously among red blood cells
S–β^0 thal	Sickle cell–β thalassemia	0	70–80%	3–5%	10–20%	—	Moderate severity; splenomegaly in over half of the cases; Hb F distributed heterogeneously among red blood cells; hypochromia and microcytosis
S–β^+ thal	Sickle cell–β thalassemia	10–20%	60–75%	3–5%	10–20%	—	
SC‡	Hb SC disease	0	45–50%	2–3%	~1%	45–50%	Moderate severity; splenomegaly; many target cells on blood smear
SF (S-HPFH)	Sickle-hereditary persistence of fetal hemoglobin	0	70–80%	1.5–2%	20–30%	—	Uniform distribution of Hb F among all red cells; asymptomatic; no anemia

*Persons with associated α thalassemia trait have lower levels of Hb S, usually in the range of 26 per cent. The finding of a (nonsickling) hemoglobin with the mobility of Hb S but in much lower amounts (5 to 15 per cent) is suggestive of the Hb Lepore trait (see Ch. 141). Hypochromia and microcytosis are usually associated with these conditions.

†Hb SD disease gives similar electrophoretic findings at pH 8.6, but can be distinguished from Hb SS disease by hemoglobin electrophoresis in citrate agar at pH 6.1.

‡Hb S–O Arab and Hb SE diseases give similar electrophoretic findings at pH 8.6, but can be distinguished from Hb SC disease by hemoglobin electrophoresis in citrate agar at pH 6.1. Hb A_2 co-migrates with Hb C at pH 8.6 and can only be quantitated by column chromotography.

SS disease. Inheritance of Hb D (another relatively common β chain hemoglobinopathy in blacks) along with Hb S can also mimic homozygosity for Hb S, since Hb D comigrates with Hb S on electrophoresis at pH 8.6. Hb SD disease is not as clinically severe as sickle cell disease, and the diagnosis can be established by performing hemoglobin electrophoresis at neutral or acid pH, which separates the two hemoglobins. Similarly, Hb SC disease can be confused with the inheritance of Hb S along with a second hemoglobin variant that has a similar electrophoretic mobility to Hb C at pH 8.6, such as Hb O Arab or Hb E. These syndromes can be distinguished from Hb SC disease by electrophoresis in citrate agar at pH 6 to 7.

The peripheral blood smear in individuals with Hb SS disease (Color plate 2*I*) usually shows variable numbers of irreversibly sickled cells (ISCs) ranging between 5 and more than 50 per cent. In general the number of ISCs is relatively stable for a given patient, and there is a rough correlation between the number of ISCs and the severity of the hemolytic anemia. There is no correlation between the number of ISCs and the frequency or presence of vaso-occlusive crises. The peripheral blood smear, in addition to ISCs, will usually show variable numbers of target cells and occasional Howell-Jolly bodies owing to absent spleen function. Other hematologic findings related to functional asplenia include the presence of target cells and somewhat elevated leukocyte counts and platelet counts. Examination of the peripheral blood smear can also be helpful in differential diagnosis of the sickle syndromes. In general significant numbers of ISCs will be found essentially only in homozygous SS disease and not in the other sickle syndromes. Large numbers of target cells are characteristic of the inheritance of Hb C in either the heterozygous or the homozygous state.

TREATMENT. Despite extensive knowledge of the molecular basis and physical chemistry of the sickling phenomenon, there is still no specific molecular therapy available for the treatment or prevention of sickling. A number of compounds have been tested, and new compounds continue to be sought, that might interfere with sickling in vivo and be useful clinically. Unfortunately no such compound is currently available. Another potential molecular approach to the prevention of sickling would be to reactivate or increase fetal hemoglobin synthesis in the majority of the erythroid cells of affected patients to render them similar to the red cells of patients with Hb S–HPFH, a clinically mild syndrome. The first successful enhancement of Hb F levels in patients with sickle cell anemia and homozygous β thalassemia (see Ch. 141) has recently been accomplished by the administration of the chemotherapeutic agent 5-azacytidine* to a small number of patients. The rationale for this therapy resided in the findings that the drug causes demethylation of DNA and that active genes are usually hypomethylated whereas the inactive fetal γ globin genes of adults are hypermethylated; administration of the drug to baboons had previously resulted in increasing circulating Hb F levels. However, this therapy should be considered highly investigational at this time and restricted in its general applicability until the long term toxicity of the drug, including carcinogenicity, is established.

The cornerstones of therapy in sickle cell anemia have therefore not changed in recent years and continue to consist in the administration of the following supportive measures: oxygen, large volumes of intravenous fluids (preferably hypotonic and alkaline), analgesics to control the pain, and, when indicated, antibiotics to treat any associated bacterial infection. When administering fluids to patients with sickle cell anemia, it should be remembered that these patients have a fixed renal water loss owing to inability to concentrate urine, and that they are frequently dehydrated on presentation because of associated infection and fever. The amounts of administered intravenous fluids should therefore be increased to two to three times of what would be considered a normal maintenance volume. Patients with sickle cell disease are frequently marginally hypoxic because of chronic pulmonary disease. Even though they do not appear to be cyanotic, monitoring of arterial P_{O_2} is important, especially if there is an associated chest syndrome, and vigorous administration of oxygen should not be overlooked during the treatment of an acute sickle cell crisis. The role of alkali is controversial, and certainly if the patient is mildly acidotic, this acidosis should be corrected since it can potentiate the propensity of deoxy Hb S molecules to aggregate.

The role of blood transfusions and partial exchange transfusions is controversial in the treatment of acute vaso-occlusive crises of sickle cell disease. In general there is very little rationale for performing partial exchange transfusions simply for a painful vaso-occlusive crisis in a nonvital organ. Nevertheless such treatment may be occasionally indicated to interrupt an unusually prolonged painful crisis or when a patient is virtually continually disabled by frequent recurrent crises. In cases of life-threatening vaso-occlusive episodes or when there is a threat of severe organ damage such as in acute cerebrovascular accidents and priapism, partial exchange transfusions should be promptly carried out because no other effective form of therapy is available. It is also generally agreed that patients who have suffered one cerebrovascular accident are likely to have recurrent life-threatening or debilitating episodes, and a course of long-term maintenance blood transfusions to prevent recurrent sickling is indicated in such cases. Such a program should probably be associated with phlebotomies prior to transfusion and/or the institution of an iron chelation program in order to prevent or delay the complications of iron overload (see Ch. 141). Pregnant women with sickle cell syndromes should be transfused through the latter half of pregnancy, primarily to prevent fetal wastage owing to infarction of the placenta but also to prevent the occurrence of postpartum maternal cardiovascular complications. Finally, any patient with a clinically significant sickle cell syndrome should receive a partial exchange transfusion to lower the Hb S value to less than 50 per cent prior to general anesthesia for surgical procedures because of the risk of a fatal or incapacitating sickling episode in the event of an anesthetic accident or transient hypoxia. With the exception of the hypoplastic crises and acute sequestration crises, blood transfusions are not usually required to maintain hemoglobin levels above 6.5 to 7 grams per deciliter, and transfusions are not required on a chronic basis simply to treat the anemia.

Because of the high risk of septicemia and other serious infections caused by *Diplococcus pneumoniae*, persons with sickle cell anemia, especially children over the age of two years, should be vaccinated with the newer pneumococcal vaccines. Although vaccination does not provide absolute protection against infection, it may significantly decrease the incidence of fatal pneumococcal infections in patients with sickle cell anemia.

PROGNOSIS. The prognosis of patients with sickle cell syndromes is variable. A significant number of infants with sickle cell anemia and Hb SC disease may die in the first two to three years because of overwhelming sepsis and/or acute splenic sequestration crises. Cord blood screening programs and identification of affected individuals with subsequent close medical follow-up should prevent or decrease the incidence of these early fatalities. For the group of patients who survive the early years, improved general medical care has substantially prolonged survival in the last two decades. There are reports of patients surviving to the fifth and sixth decades, although the mean survival is probably to the fourth decade, with death resulting from cardiopulmonary complications and/or renal insufficiency. Other causes of death include sepsis and cerebrovascular accidents. In general patients with Hb S–β thalassemia and Hb SC disease have a longer survival than patients with sickle cell disease, although there are unexplained cases of relatively mild disease with homozygous inheritance of Hb S.

*Investigational agent available from the National Cancer Institute.

PREVENTION. Sickle cell disease and other clinically significant sickle syndromes can be prevented in two general ways. First, genetic counseling of identified heterozygotes can alert couples at risk about the possibility of having affected offspring. However, no matter how good the program of genetic counseling and education, it rarely significantly affects the reproductive behavior of identified carriers and generally has little impact on the overall incidence of the disease.

An alternative approach is the availability of prenatal diagnostic services for pregnancies at risk for sickle cell anemia and other sickle hemoglobinopathies. Prenatal diagnosis for sickle cell anemia has gone through many stages in recent years, including fetal blood sampling by fetoscopy for assays of hemoglobin synthesis and analysis by gene mapping techniques of DNA from amniotic fluid cells, obtained after amniocentesis, for restriction fragment length polymorphisms shown to be linked to the sickle gene by prior study of DNA from family members. A restriction endonuclease enzyme (Mst II) has been identified that can distinguish between a sickle and a nonsickle β globin gene because the recognition site for this enzyme is specifically abolished by the nucleotide base substitution that is associated with the sickle mutation. Thus, the most reliable and acceptable method for the prenatal diagnosis of sickle cell anemia is the analysis of fetal DNA by the enzyme Mst II. Although amniotic fluid cells obtained after 14 weeks of gestation are currently the source of DNA, it is likely that biopsy of trophoblastic villi in the first trimester will eventually be proved safe and replace amniocentesis.

HOMOZYGOUS Hb C DISEASE. Individuals homozygous for Hb C usually have a mild to moderate hemolytic anemia characterized by splenomegaly and large numbers of target cells on peripheral blood smear. Occasionally intraerythrocytic crystals of Hb C can be visualized in fixed blood smears. The clinical manifestations and general laboratory findings are those of any mild chronic hemolytic anemia. Diagnosis is established by hemoglobin electrophoresis.

Bunn HF, Forget BG: Sickle cell disease—clinical and epidemiological aspects; and molecular basis of sickle cell disease. *In* Hemoglobin: Molecular, Genetic and Clinical Aspects. Philadelphia, W. B. Saunders Company, 1984 (in press). Platt O, Nathan DG: Sickle cell disease. *In* Nathan DG, Oski FA (eds.): Hematology of Infancy and Childhood. 2nd ed. Philadelphia, W. B. Saunders Company, 1981, pp 687–725. *Up-to-date comprehensive chapters in hematology textbooks covering the pathophysiology as well as the clinical manifestations and therapy of sickle cell disease.*

Dean J, Schecter AN: Sickle-cell anemia: Molecular and cellular bases of therapeutic approaches. N Engl J Med 299:752, 804, 863, 1978. *A detailed review of the physical chemistry and pathophysiology of sickling as well as the rationale and biochemical basis for antisickling compounds.*

Fleming AF (ed.): Sickle Cell Disease: A Handbook for the General Clinician. New York, Churchill Livingstone, 1982. *Comprehensive and detailed clinical description of the manifestations of sickle cell anemia.*

Klotz IM, Haney DN, King LC: Rational approaches to chemotherapy: Antisickling agents. Science 213:724, 1981. *A sophisticated review of chemical approaches to developing antisickling agents.*

143. UNSTABLE HEMOGLOBINS

Ronald F. Rieder

DEFINITION. The abnormal human hemoglobins manifest their presence by a variety of clinical syndromes of differing severity. One class of mutants, the unstable hemoglobins, is characterized by an increased tendency of the hemoglobin molecule to undergo denaturation. This increased rate of denaturation results in congenital Heinz body hemolytic disease of varying severity.

PATHOGENESIS. The complex three-dimensional arrangement of the four polypeptide subunits of the hemoglobin molecule is maintained primarily by hydrogen bonding and hydrophobic interactions between different amino acids (see Ch. 139). Amino acid substitutions that weaken these forces holding the molecule together result in decreased thermal stability and an increased tendency for hemoglobin to precipitate, especially when exposed to oxidant compounds. Approximately 100 hemoglobin variants have now been described with such amino acid substitutions (Table 143–1). The largest group of unstable hemoglobins are those with structural alterations that affect the strength of binding of the heme group to the protein by eliminating a specific heme-globin bond or by altering the configuration of the hydrophobic heme pocket. In some of these hemoglobins the binding of the heme group is so weakened that spontaneous loss of heme groups occurs. Hemoglobin Gun Hill has a deletion of a stretch of five amino acids, including the proximal histidine (β92), which normally forms a covalent bond with the heme iron atom; as a result the β chains of hemoglobin Gun Hill lack heme groups. In other unstable hemoglobins there is interference with the helical structure that provides rigidity to the polypeptide chains. Finally, the structural stability and the physiologic function of hemoglobin depend upon the tetrameric arrangement. In several abnormal hemoglobins an amino acid substitution results in the loss of a hydrogen bond that normally serves to stabilize and reinforce an interchain linkage. In unstable hemoglobin Philly the replacement of tyrosine by phenylalanine results in the loss of a single interchain hydrogen bond, permitting greater ease of separation of the α and β chains and denaturation of the hemoglobin. Hemolysis caused by an unstable hemoglobin is a direct result of the intracellular precipitation of hemoglobin to form multiple insoluble aggregates (Heinz bodies), which attach to the red cell membrane. Clearance from the circulation of erythrocytes containing such inclusion bodies by the reticuloendothelial system or removal of inclusions from the cells by pinching off ("pitting") with reduction in red cell membrane and resultant increased fragility is responsible for decreased red cell life span.

TABLE 143–1. SOME REPRESENTATIVE UNSTABLE HEMOGLOBINS

Designation	Amino Acid Change	Structural Alteration
Hammersmith	β42 Phe → Ser	Heme group contact lost, opening heme pocket to H_2O
Zürich	β63 His → Arg	Arg cannot fit in heme pocket and side chain swings to surface, leaving heme pocket open
Sydney	β67 Val → Ala	Heme contact lost, weakening the binding to globin
Philly	β35 Tyr → Phe	Loss of OH group removes H-bond, weakening $\alpha_1\beta_1$ contact
Genova	α28 Leu → Pro	Proline disrupts helical structure of chain
Sabine	β91 Leu → Pro	Heme contact lost and helix disrupted
Bushwick	β74 Gly → Val	Replacement of small amino acid by large one forces apart the sides of heme pocket

CLINICAL MANIFESTATIONS. These disorders are inherited as autosomal dominant traits. Only heterozygotes have been found. The severity of the clinical presentation of patients with unstable hemoglobins is quite varied; some subjects have chronic hemolytic anemia, whereas others with less labile hemoglobins exhibit only mild compensated hemolysis with normal hemoglobin levels. However, exposure of even such mildly affected subjects to a variety of oxidant drugs and chemicals, many of which in large doses can cause methemoglobinemia in normal persons (see Table 145–1), can result in an acute severe hemolysis with the development of pronounced anemia, striking reticulocytosis, and sudden jaundice. Bouts of acute hemolysis may also occur spontaneously during bacterial and viral infections. Some affected subjects exhibit dark urine (pigmenturia) during periods of hemolysis owing to the presence of poorly characterized heme breakdown compounds called dipyrroles.

DIAGNOSIS. Diagnosis of an unstable hemoglobin depends upon the demonstration of a mutant hemoglobin with an increased tendency to precipitate. Intraerythrocytic inclusion bodies (Heinz bodies) can frequently be demonstrated during periods of hemolysis by staining the peripheral blood with a vital dye such as new methylene blue or brilliant cresyl blue. If absent from the circulating red cells, Heinz bodies may appear after incubation of the blood in vitro for two hours at 37° C in the presence of the dye. Instability of the hemoglobin can be demonstrated in hemolysates by formation of a large precipitate with a decrease in the concentration of soluble hemoglobin after heating to 50° C, or to 37° C in the presence of 17 per cent isopropanol. Since similar hemolytic episodes can occur after drug administration in subjects with glucose-6-phosphate dehydrogenase deficiency, this condition should be considered in the differential diagnosis. Hemoglobin electrophoresis may show an abnormal hemoglobin band frequently amounting to less than 25 per cent of the total hemoglobin. Occasionally because of marked preferential destruction of the abnormal molecular species, the unstable hemoglobin may be present in the peripheral blood as only a small percentage of the circulating hemoglobin. Some of the reported unstable hemoglobins are the result of the exchange of one uncharged amino acid for another. Since no alteration in total charge occurs, such mutant hemoglobins may migrate in the same electrophoretic position as hemoglobin A and are therefore difficult to detect by electrophoresis.

TREATMENT. Treatment of subjects with unstable hemoglobins mainly consists of the avoidance of drugs capable of inducing hemolysis (see Table 145–1). Subjects with chronic compensated hemolysis may benefit from prophylactic folic acid administration. Transfusions are required only during periods of profound acute hemolytic anemia. Splenectomy has been helpful when hypersplenism has developed. Special attention should be paid to the possible development of serious hemolytic anemia during episodes of infection.

Rieder RF: Human hemoglobin stability and instability: Molecular mechanisms and some clinical considerations. Semin Hematol 11:423, 1974. *Correlates structural alterations with clinical manifestations. Emphasis on protein structure.*

White JM: The unstable haemoglobin disorders. Clin Haematol 3:333, 1974. *Provides details of clinical manifestations.*

Winslow RM, Anderson WF: The hemoglobinopathies. *In* Stanbury JB, Wyngaarden JB, Fredrickson DS, Goldstein JL, Brown MS (eds.): The Metabolic Basis of Inherited Disease. New York, McGraw-Hill Book Company, 1983, pp 1666–1710. *This is an up-to-date, comprehensive treatment of the genetics, structure, function, and clinical properties of the various types of abnormal hemoglobins.*

144. ABNORMAL HEMOGLOBINS WITH ALTERED OXYGEN AFFINITY

Ronald F. Rieder

DEFINITION. The ability of hemoglobin to function as a useful means of transporting oxygen depends upon its becoming fully loaded with oxygen in the lungs and unloading a proportion of this oxygen in the tissues at partial pressures of oxygen which are compatible with cell function and viability. A change in the structure of the hemoglobin molecule can affect this respiratory function. An increase in oxygen affinity can impair the ability of the pigment to donate its oxygen to the cells, whereas a decrease in affinity can prevent it from picking up enough oxygen as it passes through the pulmonary circulation. This affinity for oxygen is frequently expressed as the partial pressure of oxygen at which hemoglobin is half-saturated (P_{50}). Over 80 mutant hemoglobins have been discovered which have some degree of alteration of oxygen-binding properties, but only a few have clinically significant defects. Some of these hemoglobins have increased oxygen affinity (decreased P_{50}), whereas others have a decreased capacity for binding oxygen (increased P_{50}).

PATHOGENESIS. During the process of oxygenation and deoxygenation, hemoglobin undergoes reversible structural changes which involve alterations in the three-dimensional configuration of the individual polypeptide chains, as well as shifts in the way the four chains are arranged in the $\alpha_2\beta_2$ tetramer. When fully deoxygenated, hemoglobin is said to be in the T or tense state and has a relatively low affinity for oxygen. Conversely, when hemoglobin is fully oxygenated, it is in the R or relaxed state and has a high affinity for oxygen. This intramolecular reorganization with its resultant change in oxygen affinity is reflected in the physiologically important sigmoidal shape of the hemoglobin-oxygen dissociation curve (see Ch. 139).

The complex stereochemical changes in molecular structure are accomplished by considerable relative movement of the α and β globin chains along the $\alpha_1\beta_2$ interface and of the C-terminal regions of the β chains. Hydrogen bonds, hydrophobic interactions, and salt bridges between amino acids are broken and new ones are formed during these R-T transitions.

Genetic mutations which affect amino acids situated at the $\alpha_1\beta_2$ interface or which otherwise alter molecular structure to interfere with the R-T equilibrium may affect the respiratory function of hemoglobin. Thus an amino acid substitution which destabilizes the T or low O_2 affinity state would tend to favor the R state and increase the oxygen affinity of a mutant hemoglobin. In abnormal hemoglobin Kempsey, asparagine replaces aspartic acid at position β99. Asparagine, unlike aspartic acid, cannot form the hydrogen bond with tyrosine at α42 that normally stabilizes the deoxyhemoglobin conformation. As a result hemoglobin Kempsey has a high oxygen affinity. In contrast in hemoglobin Kansas, threonine replaces asparagine at position β102. Threonine cannot form the hydrogen bond with aspartic acid at α94 that normally stabilizes the R or high affinity state. Therefore hemoglobin Kansas is shifted toward the T state and has a low oxygen affinity.

2,3-Diphosphoglycerate (2,3-DPG) acts as a physiologic modulator of hemoglobin oxygen affinity and binds to specific amino acid sites on the protein. 2,3-DPG increases the P_{50} (lowers the oxygen affinity), and mutations which inhibit binding of this small molecular weight effector result in hemoglobin with increased oxygen affinity.

CLINICAL MANIFESTATIONS. Most of the abnormal hemoglobins with detectable alterations in oxygen binding characteristics are only minimally affected and of no physiologic significance. However, mutant hemoglobins with greatly increased oxygen affinity tend to unload much less oxygen to the tissues, and this results in relative tissue hypoxia. As a result erythropoietin secretion is increased and erythropoiesis is stimulated with a rise in hematocrit value. Thus subjects with high-affinity hemoglobins may have *erythrocytosis*. The disorder is frequently familial and is inherited as an autosomal dominant. No increase in white blood cell or platelet counts occurs. Plasma concentrations of erythropoietin are normal when the subject is polycythemic, but if the hematocrit level is lowered to normal by phlebotomy, an increase in erythropoietin production can be detected.

In subjects with mutant hemoglobins having moderately lowered oxygen affinity, the increased tendency of the hemoglobin to unload oxygen results in enhanced delivery to the tissues. Such persons therefore require less hemoglobin to provide the same volume of oxygen and as a consequence frequently have decreased hematocrit values. In this situation the usually *mild anemia* is not a pathologic condition but is a physiologic response to the increased availability of oxygen at the tissue level.

In some subjects with a hemoglobin with greatly decreased oxygen affinity, *cyanosis* has been present owing to the marked inability of the mutant hemoglobin to bind oxygen. Hematocrit values in such cases have been normal.

Even in the presence of markedly abnormal hemoglobin function, subjects with hemoglobins with altered oxygen affinity have usually been asymptomatic.

DIAGNOSIS. The presence of a hemoglobin with high oxygen affinity should be considered in any patient who has isolated erythrocytosis unaccompanied by increased leukocyte and platelet proliferation (see Ch. 153). After eliminating causes such as the presence of hypoxemia with secondary erythrocytosis as well as other causes of increased erythropoietin secretion, evidence for an abnormal hemoglobin should be sought. Hemoglobin electrophoresis may reveal an abnormal hemoglobin band, but several of the high affinity hemoglobins have electrophoretic mobilities identical to hemoglobin A. An oxygen-hemoglobin dissociation curve performed on whole blood and especially on isolated hemoglobin should be obtained. The latter can eliminate any contribution of diminished or increased 2,3-DPG levels. By adding back 2,3-DPG to the purified hemoglobin, evidence for diminished 2,3-DPG binding can be detected. A low-affinity hemoglobin should be considered in instances of unexplained cyanosis with normal arterial oxygen tension.

TREATMENT. Aside from either erythrocytosis or mild anemia, subjects having these functionally defective hemoglobins are usually asymptomatic and no treatment is indicated. Cyanosis accompanying the rare hemoglobins having very low affinity for oxygen is only a cosmetic problem.

Jensen M, Oski FA, Nathan DG, Bunn HF: Hemoglobin Syracuse ($\alpha_2\beta_2$ $^{143(H21)His \rightarrow Pro}$), a high affinity variant detected by special electrophoretic methods. Observations on the auto-oxidation of normal and variant hemoglobins. J Clin Invest 55:469, 1975. *The detection and analysis of a mutant hemoglobin with high oxygen affinity.*

Nagel RL, Lynfield J, Johnson J, Landau L, Bookchin RM, Harris MB: Hemoglobin Beth Israel. A mutant causing clinically apparent cyanosis. N Engl J Med 295:125, 1976. *The detection and analysis of an interesting mutant hemoglobin with markedly diminished oxygen affinity.*

145. METHEMOGLOBINEMIA AND SULFHEMOGLOBINEMIA

Ronald F. Rieder

METHEMOGLOBINEMIA

DEFINITION. The reversible oxygenation and deoxygenation of hemoglobin at physiologic partial pressures of oxygen require that the heme iron of deoxyhemoglobin remain in the ferrous (Fe^{+2}) form. In methemoglobin the iron atom is oxidized to the ferric (Fe^{+3}) form, rendering the molecule incapable of binding oxygen. When hemoglobin is oxygenated during the process of respiration, an electron is partially transferred from the ferrous iron atom to the bound oxygen molecule. Thus in oxyhemoglobin iron possesses some of the characteristics of the ferric (Fe^{+3}) state, whereas the oxygen takes on the characteristics of the superoxide (O_2^-) anion. Under normal circumstances upon deoxygenation of the hemoglobin molecule the electron is returned to the iron atom and the O_2 molecule is released. Interference with the return of the electron to the iron atom results in the formation of methemoglobin. Normally approximately 3 per cent of the hemoglobin is spontaneously oxidized to methemoglobin each day, but the concentration is maintained below 1 per cent by its reconversion to hemoglobin by metabolic processes. A shift in this equilibrium can result in increased amounts of methemoglobin in the peripheral blood and the development of cyanosis. Enzymatic reducing systems in the red cells are responsible for the maintenance of the heme iron of hemoglobin in the ferrous state. An enzyme variously termed NADH–methemoglobin reductase, NADH-dehydrogenase, NADH-diaphorase, or erythrocyte cytochrome b_5 reductase is responsible for over 90 per cent of the hemoglobin reducing capacity of the erythrocyte under physiologic conditions, catalyzing the transfer of an electron from NADH to oxidized cytochrome b_5:

$$\text{NADH} + \text{Fe}^{+3}-\text{cytochrome } b_5 \xrightarrow{\text{reductase}} \text{NAD}^+ + \text{Fe}^{+2}-\text{cytochrome } b_5$$

Flavine adenine dinucleotide may participate as a prosthetic group on the reductase. Reduced cytochrome b_5 then directly interacts with methemoglobin to result in its reduction to ferrous hemoglobin:

$$\text{Fe}^{+2}-\text{cytochrome } b_5 + \text{Fe}^{+3}-\text{hemoglobin} \longrightarrow \text{Fe}^{+3}-\text{cytochrome } b_5 + \text{Fe}^{+2}-\text{hemoglobin}$$

The reconversion of NAD to NADH depends upon the Embden-Meyerhof glycolytic pathway, primarily at the reaction in which glyceraldehyde-3-phosphate is converted to 1,3-diphosphoglycerate by the enzyme glyceraldehyde phosphate dehydrogenase. An NADPH-dependent methemoglobin reductase is present within the erythrocyte, but normally there is no linked physiologic electron carrier available which is capable of directly donating an electron to reduce methemoglobin. However, when provided with an artificial electron carrier such as methylene blue, this enzyme is of great importance in the therapy of acute toxic methemoglobinemia (see below). Ascorbic acid and reduced glutathione are capable of directly reducing methemoglobin, but these reactions occur quite slowly.

CLASSIFICATION. Methemoglobinemia may be hereditary or acquired. Hereditary methemoglobinemia may result from an abnormality in the metabolic processes which normally reconvert methemoglobin to hemoglobin (see above) or from an inherited abnormality of the hemoglobin molecule conducive to methemoglobin formation. Acquired methemoglobinemia results from exposure to certain chemical agents which increase the formation of methemoglobin.

Hereditary Methemoglobinemia Caused by Defective Reduction of Methemoglobin

Over one hundred subjects with hereditary methemoglobinemia resulting from NADH–methemoglobin reductase deficiency have been described, and several abnormal variant enzymes differing in catalytic activity, structural stability, and electrophoretic mobility are known. The disorder is inherited as an autosomal recessive trait. It occurs with unusually high frequency in Alaskan Eskimos and Indians, Navajo Indians, and Puerto Ricans. In certain families with this disorder there has been an associated mental deficiency with neurologic defects, but the relationship of these problems to the methemoglobinemia is not clear; a more generalized deficiency of the enzyme involving nervous tissue may be responsible. Patients with methemoglobinemia have persistent slate-gray cyanosis. In contrast to deoxyhemoglobin, which produces cyanosis only when present at levels above 5 grams per deciliter, methemoglobin at a concentration of only 1.5 to 2 grams per deciliter produces significant cyanosis. Homozygotes usually have methemoglobin levels of 15 to 25 per cent, but no deleterious effect at this concentration is apparent. At concentrations of methemoglobin up to 40 per cent, some symptoms of fatigability and malaise have been described. The patients have been characterized as being more blue than sick. No clubbing or cardiopulmonary disease is present, and mild compensatory erythrocytosis has been noted only occasionally. Heterozygotes for the enzyme deficiency have normal concentrations of methemoglobin but manifest an increased susceptibility to the methemoglobin-producing properties of various oxidant drugs and chemicals. (Table 145–1).

DIAGNOSIS. Persistent cyanosis without hypoxia should suggest the possibility of methemoglobinemia. The peripheral blood is reddish brown and does not become bright red when exposed to oxygen. Methemoglobin has a characteristic absorption peak at 630 nm, which disappears upon addition of cyanide. Several assays are available to quantitate the level of NADH–methemoglobin reductase in erythrocytes, and staining procedures can reveal an abnormal enzyme with altered electrophoretic mobility.

TREATMENT. Treatment of congenital methemoglobinemia caused by reductase deficiency is generally not required, but cosmetic improvement of the cyanosis can be achieved by treatment with methylene blue, 100 to 300 mg per day orally, or ascorbic acid, 500 mg per day orally. Riboflavin, 20 mg per day orally, is also effective. Methylene blue has the disadvan-

TABLE 145–1. DRUGS AND CHEMICALS HAVING TOXIC EFFECT ON HEMOGLOBIN MOLECULE

Agent	Hemoglobin Derivative Observed	
	Methemoglobin	*Sulfhemoglobin*
Acetanilid, phenacetin	+	+
Nitrites (amyl, sodium, potassium, nitroglycerin)	+	+
Trinitrotoluene, nitrobenzene	+	+
Aniline, hydroxylamine, dimethylamine	+	+
Sulfanilamide	+	+
Para-aminosalicylic acid	+	
Dapsone	+	
Primaquine, chloroquine	+	
Prilocaine, benzocaine, lidocaine	+	
Menadione, naphthoquinone	+	
Naphthalene	+	
Resorcinol	+	
Phenylhydrazine	+	+

tage of producing blue urine. Large doses of ascorbate may lead to oxalate stone production.

Hereditary Methemoglobinemia Due to Abnormal (M) Hemoglobins

Several variant hemoglobins have been discovered with substitutions in the amino acids which line the heme crevice of the globin chain and contact the porphyrin group or the iron atom. These mutations affect the configuration of the polypeptide chain surrounding the heme group, alter the hydrophobic environment, and often weaken the binding of the porphyrin to the protein. Some of these variant hemoglobins are unstable and lose heme (see Ch. 143), and others are permanently fixed in the methemoglobin state (M hemoglobins). The five M hemoglobins are listed in Table 145–2. In normal hemoglobin the so-called proximal histidine at position 92 in the β chain and position 87 in the α chain is covalently linked to the heme iron atom. On the opposite side of the heme disc the iron atom also faces a "distal" histidine located at positions β63 and α58. In four of the M hemoglobins (Table 145–2) one of these histidines is replaced by a tyrosine whose hydroxyl group forms a stable complex with iron in the ferric state. The hemoglobin is thus fixed in the oxidized form. The methemoglobin reductase system of the erythrocyte is ineffective in reducing these abnormal methemoglobins.

CLINICAL MANIFESTATIONS. Subjects inheriting an M hemoglobin are cyanotic but are usually otherwise unaffected by the trait.

Mild chronic hemolysis has been observed in association with hemoglobin M Hyde Park, which has a tendency to lose heme and is slightly unstable. The disorder is inherited in a dominant pattern, and families have been reported in which the condition has been noted in several generations.

DIAGNOSIS. The blood has a brown appearance and does not become bright red upon agitation in air. Neither does the addition of cyanide produce the change to the red color that occurs upon such treatment of normal methemoglobin. In subjects with β chain mutations approximately 50 per cent of the hemoglobin is affected, whereas 20 to 25 per cent of the circulating hemoglobin is methemoglobin in persons with an α Hb M. The presence of an abnormal methemoglobin can be detected by spectrophotometric analysis. The normal absorption peaks of methemoglobin at 630 and 502 nm are shifted to slightly lower wavelengths in the M hemoglobins. In addition, the M hemoglobins have an altered electrophoretic migration; separation from Hb A is most easily demonstrated if first the hemolysate is completely converted to methemoglobin with ferricyanide. No treatment is required for this condition, and methylene blue and ascorbic acid administration are ineffective for significant conversion to reduced hemoglobin.

TABLE 145–2. M HEMOGLOBINS

Designation	Amino Acid Change
M—Boston	α58 Histidine → tyrosine
M—Iwate	α87 Histidine → tyrosine
M—Saskatoon	β63 Histidine → tyrosine
M—Hyde Park	β92 Histidine → tyrosine
M—Milwaukee-1	β67 Valine → glutamic acid

Acquired or Toxic Methemoglobinemia

A variety of chemical agents and drugs are able to accelerate the oxidation of hemoglobin and produce a significant methemoglobinemia in otherwise normal individuals (Table 145–1). Many of these agents occasionally induce sulfhemoglobinemia and can cause hemolysis in subjects with unstable hemoglobins or glucose-6-phosphate dehydrogenase deficiency. Often these compounds are unable directly to induce the oxidation of hemoglobin in vitro, and thus their toxicity in vivo is probably a result of conversion to intermediate forms which are direct oxidants. Nitrates, which have been implicated in methemoglobinemia in infants as a result of the use of contaminated well water in the preparation of feeding formulas, must be converted to nitrite to produce methemoglobinemia. Such conversion may occur as a result of the action of bacteria in the gastrointestinal tract. The ability of drugs to produce large amounts of methemoglobin depends upon overwhelming the normal pathway in the red cell responsible for maintenance of hemoglobin iron in the ferrous state. In normal subjects large doses of drugs are generally necessary. When the activity of the methemoglobin-reducing system is depressed, susceptibility to these agents is increased. Thus heterozygotes for NADH–methemoglobin reductase variants and newborn infants who normally have low levels of the enzyme until about four months of age are very susceptible to the development of methemoglobinemia. Normal doses of primaquine and dapsone have caused methemoglobinemia in enzyme-deficient adults. Menadione, naphthalene, and aniline dyes used by laundries to mark diapers have been implicated in the induction of methemoglobinemia in very young infants. On the other hand, such agents as prilocaine and sulfanilamide have commonly been reported to cause methemoglobinemia in normal persons.

CLINICAL MANIFESTATIONS. Methemoglobinemia induced by drugs is usually an asymptomatic condition, and any associated ill effects are generally due to other actions of these chemicals. However, severe acute methemoglobinemia with levels of methemoglobin greater than 60 to 70 per cent have been associated with collapse, coma, and death. Affected patients develop severe cyanosis, and upon examination the blood is chocolate brown.

DIAGNOSIS. Diagnosis depends upon demonstration of the presence of methemoglobin (see above) and identification of the causative agent. Erythrocyte reductase levels should be measured to rule out enzyme deficiency.

TREATMENT. With mildly affected patients treatment, aside from discontinuing the offending agent, is not required, and the methemoglobin will be reduced spontaneously to ferrous hemoglobin over a period of two to three days. For severely affected patients therapy with methylene blue is effective. One to 2 mg per kilogram of a 1 per cent solution of methylene blue in saline is administered intravenously over ten minutes. If there is no adequate response within an hour, a second dose may be administered. This treatment generally results in the prompt conversion of methemoglobin to hemoglobin. Such therapy is not effective in subjects with glucose-6-phosphate dehydrogenase deficiency resulting from the inactivity of the hexose monophosphate shunt pathway for the production of NADPH, which is required for the reconversion of oxidized methylene blue to reduced or leuko-methylene blue. Exchange transfusion may be required in severely symptomatic patients. Oral ascorbic acid should not be used in the treatment of acute toxic methemoglobinemia, since its speed of action is slow.

Bunn HF, Forget BG, Ranney HM: Human Hemoglobins. Philadelphia, W.B. Saunders Company, 1977. *Has an excellent chapter on M hemoglobins.*

Jaffé ER: Methaemoglobinemia. Clin Haematol 10:99, 1981. *Review emphasizing enzyme deficiency.*

Schwartz JM, Reiss AL, Jaffé ER: Hereditary methemoglobinemia with deficiency of NADH cytochrome b_5 reductase. *In* Stanbury JB, Wyngaarden JB, Fredrickson DS, Goldstein JL, Brown MS (eds.): The Metabolic Basis of Inherited Disease. 5th ed. New York, McGraw-Hill Book Company, 1983, p 1654. *Authoritative, detailed review of all aspects of the inherited enzyme deficiency.*

Smith RP, Olson MV: Drug-induced methemoglobinemia. Semin Hematol 10:253, 1973. *A good review of acute toxic methemoglobinemia.*

SULFHEMOGLOBINEMIA

DEFINITION. Sulfhemoglobin is an incompletely characterized greenish-brown hemoglobin derivative found in the blood of some subjects after exposure to large amounts of various drugs or organic chemicals. The pigment causes cyanosis, imparts a reddish-brown color to blood, and has a characteristic optical absorption spectrum with a peak at 620 nm which is not abolished by the addition of cyanide. Seemingly pure preparations have been made by reacting methemoglobin with hydrogen peroxide in the presence of ammonium sulfide. The precise structure of the abnormal pigment is not known.

PATHOGENESIS. Abnormal pigments with similar optical absorption characteristics have been noted in the blood of patients after ingestion of toxic doses of acetanilid, phenacetin, and other drugs, as well as after exposure to large amounts of aromatic amino and nitro compounds. The mechanism for the production of sulfhemoglobin in vivo is not understood. Many of the same compounds which have been noted to cause methemoglobinemia in some patients have been implicated in the appearance of sulfhemoglobin in others (see Table 145–1). Neither the reason for the appearance of one hemoglobin derivative rather than the other nor the relationship in vivo to sulfur is clear. Chronic constipation with the production of excess hydrogen sulfide in the gut has been postulated but never proved to be a contributing factor.

CLINICAL MANIFESTATIONS. Cyanosis is the characteristic feature of subjects with sulfhemoglobinemia. As little as 0.5 gram per deciliter produces a slate-gray discoloration of the skin and mucous membranes. This amount of sulfhemoglobin is much less than the 1.5 and 5 grams per deciliter required for methemoglobin and reduced hemoglobin to cause cyanosis. Patients generally experience no ill effects from the condition, and asymptomatic persons with as much as 10 grams per deciliter have been described.

DIAGNOSIS. Positive identification of sulfhemoglobin as the cause of cyanosis in a patient can be made by observing the characteristic optical absorption spectrum of an hemolysate before and after the addition of a small amount of potassium cyanide.

TREATMENT. Treatment consists primarily of identifying the causative agent and eliminating further contact. Reconversion of sulfhemoglobin to hemoglobin is not possible, and there is no useful acute medical therapy for sulfhemoglobinemia. After cessation of contact with the offending agent, production of sulfhemoglobin ceases and the compound is eliminated from the blood over a period of weeks during the normal course of erythrocyte aging and clearance from the circulation.

Kneezel LD, Kitchens CS: Phenacetin-induced sulfhemoglobinemia: Report of a case and review of the literature. Johns Hopkins Med J 139:175, 1976. *Describes an interesting case and discusses the disorder in detail.*

Salvati AM, Tentori L: Determination of aberrant hemoglobin derivatives in human blood. Methods Enzymol 76:715, 1981. *Details methods of measuring sulfhemoglobin levels.*

146. BLOOD TRANSFUSION

Herbert A. Perkins

A standard unit of blood donated for transfusion consists of 450 ml of blood mixed with 63 ml of a solution that contains citrate to prevent clotting and glucose, phosphate, and adenine for optimal preservation of red cell viability. Without adenine, storage of red cells is limited to 21 days; with adenine, 35 days is acceptable. Nonviable cells are quickly removed from the circulation of the recipient; the remainder are restored to biochemical normality and live out the rest of their usual life span (up to 120 days).

INDICATIONS FOR BLOOD TRANSFUSION

Blood transfusions have the potential for many harmful side effects. Therefore, blood should never be transfused when the risks to the patient outweigh the expected benefit, or when more specific and safer therapy (e.g., iron, B_{12}) is available. When blood transfusions are indicated, only that fraction of the blood that the patient requires should be administered. Most blood donations are separated into components after collection: red blood cells, platelet concentrates, and/or cryoprecipitates and plasma. The plasma may be subsequently fractionated to provide albumin, gamma globulin, and coagulation factor concentrates.

Separation of whole blood into components has several advantages: (1) Each component is provided in a concentrated form which will result in greater increments of that component in the recipient's circulation as compared with administration of an equal volume of whole blood. (2) Overexpansion of the recipient's circulation with resulting heart failure is less likely. (3) Transfusion of potentially harmful materials which the patient does not need (e.g., citrate, potassium) is minimized. (4) Maximal use is made of every blood donation. Blood is always in short supply.

This discussion will be restricted to the use of red blood cell concentrates and whole blood. The indications for transfusion of platelet concentrates are discussed in Ch. 166, for leukocytes in Ch. 150, and for cryoprecipitates and coagulation factor concentrates in Ch. 167.

Demands for platelets and coagulation factor concentrates have increased, and therefore whole blood has become less available. This serves to promote the more appropriate red blood cell therapy. The patient who is anemic but has a normal blood volume should receive only red blood cells; therefore whole blood transfusions are rarely justifiable on a medical service. Acute hemorrhage is more common on the surgical services, but even here whole blood is inappropriate in most situations. Patients with acute hemorrhage often have a relatively greater deficit of red cells than of plasma. Transfusing red cells until the blood volume is normalized will result in a higher hematocrit and, in turn, greater oxygen-carrying capacity than would an equal volume of whole blood. Moreover, the usual bleeding patient who loses less than 20 to 25 per cent of his blood volume (1000 to 1500 ml in an adult) can be transfused with red cells supplemented by electrolytes instead of whole blood with no impairment of his recovery. It is common practice in many hospitals to provide red cells, not whole blood, for the first three units crossmatched for routine surgery. Whole blood is of greatest value when there has been massive acute blood loss creating need for large-scale red cell and volume replacement. Even in this situation, whole blood is not a necessity but a convenience, since it can be replaced by red cells plus electrolytes or colloid, supplemented as necessary by platelet and coagulation factor concentrates.

RED BLOOD CELLS. A variety of red blood cell components can be prepared. These are listed in Table 146–1, together with their usual packed cell volume (PCV) and the proportion of red blood cells (RBC), white blood cells (WBC), and plasma of the original whole blood that remains in the final product.

Red blood cells, often called packed red blood cells, should be the primary component for the treatment of chronic anemia or hemorrhage. This component contains all the red cells of the original unit with enough plasma so that it will flow reasonably rapidly through an intravenous needle.

Leukocyte-poor red blood cells are prepared by centrifugation and are given to patients who have had prior febrile reactions to transfusions caused by recipient alloantibodies reacting with

TABLE 146–1. RED BLOOD CELL COMPONENTS

Component	PVC	RBC	WBC	Plasma
Red blood cells	70–80%	100%	100%	20%
Leukocyte-poor red blood cells	80–95%	80%	10–15%	5–10%
Washed red blood cells	80%	95%	50%	0
Washed leukocyte-poor red blood cells	80%	80–90%	10%	0
Frozen red blood cells	80%	85%	5–10%	0

donor leukocytes. Eighty-five to 90 per cent of the donor leukocytes have been removed, and this is sufficient to prevent febrile reactions in at least 90 per cent of alloimmunized patients. Twenty per cent of the red cells must be discarded to achieve this level of leukocyte depletion, and the final hematocrit varies with the exact procedure.

Washed red blood cells are rarely indicated. They are required only when a recipient has had prior severe reactions to donor plasma proteins. Although they have often been recommended for patients with paroxysmal nocturnal hemoglobinuria, recent evidence indicates that they are rarely necessary. Washed red blood cells should not be considered to be leukocyte poor unless the washing process was modified to remove the buffy coat.

Washed leukocyte-poor red blood cells are easily prepared by blood banks with a currently available automated centrifuge system. These have advantages over leukocyte-poor red cells prepared by differential centrifugation: red cell recovery is higher, leukocyte removal is somewhat better, and almost all of the plasma has been removed.

Frozen red blood cells are also washed and leukocyte poor by the time they have been readied for transfusion. Red cell loss is greater than with washed red blood cells and the procedures involved are considerably more time consuming and expensive. Red blood cells, when prepared with glycerol, can be stored in the frozen state for as long as three years; therefore the most important reason to freeze red cells is for preservation of a type so rare that it would otherwise be unavailable for the patient who must receive it. Frozen red cells are also useful for the patient with antibodies to donor leukocytes so strong that he has an uncomfortable febrile reaction to leukocyte-poor red cells.

Other suggested indications for frozen red cells are more controversial. Clearly, the process does not prevent post-transfusion hepatitis. Frozen red cells have been most widely used for patients waiting for a kidney transplant. Frozen red cells have less tendency to induce formation of lymphocytotoxic alloantibodies than red blood cells or even leukocyte-poor red blood cells, and thus recipients of frozen red cells are less likely to have transplantation contraindicated by a positive lymphocytotoxic crossmatch with the cells of their intended kidney donor. However, renal allograft recipients with no prior blood transfusions have very poor graft survival compared with those who have received red blood cells or leukocyte-poor red blood cells. The evidence that frozen red blood cells can provide this protective effect is conflicting.

PROVIDING COMPATIBLE BLOOD FOR TRANSFUSION

BLOOD GROUPS. The external surfaces of all blood cells and plasma proteins contain very large numbers of antigenic determinants whose structures are programmed by genes. Many of these genetic loci have multiple possible alleles, with the result that all blood transfusions expose the recipient to a large number of foreign immunogens. Fortunately, most of these antigenic determinants are poor immunogens or result in antibodies that have no notable clinical effect. In routine transfusions, it is usually sufficient to avoid incompatibility for only three antigens (A, B, and D), all on the red blood cells.

The red blood cell antigenic determinants are divided into blood groups, each blood group consisting of the alleles of a single genetic locus. The most important red blood cell group is the ABO group, with two antigens: A and B. The primary importance of the ABO blood group in transfusion therapy is based on two facts: (1) Anti-A and anti-B are regularly present ("naturally occurring") in the plasma of persons who lack the corresponding antigen on their red cells (Table 146–2), presumably because of previous immunization to crossreacting antigens in bacteria and foods. (2) Anti-A and anti-B are almost always present in high concentration, activate the full complement cascade, and are capable of intravascular destruction of an almost unlimited number of incompatible red blood cells.

The second important red cell blood group is Rh. This is important because one of the antigenic determinants in this group (D) is an unusually potent immunogen, and 15 per cent of Caucasoids lack the D antigen. The term "Rh-positive" indicates the presence of D; "Rh-negative" indicates its absence. There are a large number of additional Rh gene products, but only a few of these commonly stimulate production of alloantibodies: C, E, c, and e. C and c resemble alleles, as do E and e, in that one—but not both—is the product of each normal Rh gene. There is no allele for D, but the symbol "d" may be used to indicate its absence.

Altogether, more than 300 different antigenic determinants have been identified on human red blood cells. Some of these have been assigned to blood groups; others have not. In addition to the Rh antigens mentioned, additional important red cell immunogens are found in the Kell, Duffy, and Kidd systems. Antibodies to the Rh, Kell, Duffy, and Kidd antigens are not "naturally occurring" and are found after prior transfusions or pregnancies. Typing donors for these antigens (other than D) is necessary only when the recipient has formed the corresponding antibody. Antibodies to certain other red cell antigens (e.g., M, Lewis, P, I) are relatively common and often naturally occurring, but since these antibodies are generally inactive at body temperature, they are rarely of clinical significance.

COMPATIBILITY TESTING. A hospital transfusion service must type the red blood cells of the patient for A, B, and D and confirm the typing of the donor. Further tests are performed to ensure that the patient has not formed "unexpected" antibodies, i.e., antibodies other than the expected anti-A or B. The search for unexpected antibodies is carried out in two ways: (1) Antibody screening involves testing the serum of the patient with a small number of red cells selected to contain among them all of the antigens which commonly cause trouble. (2) Compatibility testing, or crossmatching, tests the patient's serum with red blood cells from the units intended for transfusion. If unexpected antibodies are detected which appear likely by their specificity and characteristics to impair the survival of transfused red cells containing the corresponding antigen, red cells to be transfused must lack that antigen. In general, a positive crossmatch contraindicates transfusion; exceptions should be approved by someone thoroughly knowledgeable about the possible effects of the antibodies detected.

EMERGENCY TRANSFUSIONS. Under normal circumstances, transfused red cells are of the same ABO type as those of the recipient; but in urgent situations when ABO-identical red cells are not available, ABO-compatible red cells may be transfused. For example, type O red cells can be given to a recipient of any ABO type, and the type AB recipient can receive red cells of any ABO type. Whole blood should be avoided in these circumstances, since the anti-A and/or anti-B of the donor plasma may destroy recipient red cells.

TABLE 146–2. THE ABO GROUP

Red cell type	O	A	B	AB
Possible genotypes	OO	AA or AO	BB or BO	AB
Antibodies in serum	Anti-A and B	Anti-B	Anti-A	None
Frequency in Caucasoids	45%	40%	10%	5%

If Rh-negative red cells are not available for an Rh-negative recipient, Rh-positive cells may be transfused in an emergency, but only if the recipient has no anti-D in his or her serum. Special effort should be made to avoid transfusion of Rh-positive cells into Rh-negative recipients who are females and not yet past the childbearing age. The recipient has approximately a 70 per cent chance of being immunized to D, and a subsequent pregnancy with an Rh-positive fetus is very likely to result in severe hemolytic disease of the newborn. If Rh-positive red cells must be transfused into an Rh-negative female of reproductive age, Rh immunoglobulin treatment may prevent immunization.

With sudden massive hemorrhage, it may be necessary to transfuse blood without all of the usual preliminary tests. Type O Rh-negative blood is often reserved for such situations on the grounds that it is likely to be compatible with all recipients. Such blood is in limited supply, however, and it takes only a few minutes to determine the ABO and Rh types of the recipient. Meanwhile, electrolytes or colloid (e.g., albumin) can be used to maintain the patient's circulation. The usual in vitro compatibility tests can be waived if the emergency is sufficiently great, but there must be written documentation of the urgency.

HAZARDS OF BLOOD TRANSFUSIONS

The many potential complications of blood transfusion are listed in Table 146–3.

HEMOLYTIC REACTIONS. Hemolytic reactions correctly attract the most attention, since they can result in serious morbidity or death and commonly result from negligence. Almost all immediate hemolytic transfusion reactions are caused by ABO mismatches. The cause of the error is almost always clerical. The most common error is incorrect labeling of the patient sample taken for compatibility testing. The patient must be identified without error at the time of sampling, and the correct label must be applied to the crossmatch tube before leaving the patient's side. The other major source of trouble is transfusion of a unit other than the one intended for that patient. The donor blood label, crossmatch slip, and patient identification must be crosschecked carefully before the transfusion is started.

The most dangerous antibodies are those which activate the complete complement cascade, resulting in intravascular hemolysis. Other antibodies (e.g., Rh, Kell) merely become attached to the red cell, in some instances with subsequent attachment of complement components C3 and C4. The coated red cells may then be destroyed in the reticuloendothelial system by macrophages, which have receptors for the Fc portion of IgG molecules and the C3 and C4.

Intravascular hemolysis (such as that caused by anti-A or anti-B) results in release of free hemoglobin into the plasma, binding of hemoglobin to haptoglobin with subsequent removal of the complex, hemoglobinuria once haptoglobin has been saturated, and later rise of serum bilirubin and possibly methemalbumin. Extravascular hemolysis (typical of Rh antibodies) occurs primarily in the spleen, takes place more slowly, and may be limited by saturation of the reticuloendothelial system. Hyperbilirubinemia is the major laboratory abnormality.

TABLE 146–3. HAZARDS OF BLOOD TRANSFUSION

1. Hemolytic reactions
2. Chill-fever reactions
3. Contaminated blood
4. Noncardiac pulmonary edema
5. Post-transfusion thrombocytopenic purpura
6. Transmission of disease
   a. Hepatitis
   b. Malaria
   c. Syphilis
   d. Cytomegalovirus
   e. Acquired immune deficiency syndrome (AIDS) (?)
7. Allergic reactions
   a. Urticaria
   b. Anaphylaxis
8. Circulatory overload
9. Air embolism
10. Hemosiderosis (see Ch. 141)
11. Massive transfusion problems
12. Graft-versus-host disease

The clinical symptoms associated with hemolytic transfusion reactions are highly variable and range in severity from death to shortened survival of the transfused cells unaccompanied by symptoms. The most frequent complaints are chills, fever, and aching in various parts of the body. Oliguria or anuria caused by acute renal failure may follow these symptoms or in some cases may be the first recognized sign that a hemolytic transfusion reaction has occurred. If the patient is under anesthesia, incompatible red cells may continue to be infused until the magnitude of the intravascular antigen-antibody reaction activates disseminated intravascular coagulation. Under anesthesia, then, generalized bleeding and an unexpected drop in blood pressure may be the first evidence of a hemolytic reaction.

Delayed hemolytic reactions may be recognized when the recipient receives a large volume of red cells containing an antigen to which he was previously immunized. The antibody may have become undetectable by the time of the current crossmatch and too weak to cause a reaction at the time of transfusion. Anamnestic increase in antibody concentration to high levels occurs with obvious effects five to ten days after transfusion. The recipient's hemoglobin falls rapidly and he becomes jaundiced. At this point, the alloantibody is usually easily detectable.

When a hemolytic transfusion reaction is suspected, the transfusion must be stopped and the blood container and attached tubing returned to the laboratory accompanied by a new blood and urine sample from the patient. The laboratory will test for evidence that hemolysis has occurred, recheck the identity of all samples, and retest samples obtained before and after the reaction for evidence of incompatibility. If an antibody is identified, blood lacking the corresponding antigen may then be transfused.

The patient's fluid intake and output must be monitored and he should be well hydrated, avoiding circulatory overload. If oliguria occurs, diuretics may be prescribed. The primary danger comes from rising serum potassium; therefore serial monitoring of electrolytes and electrocardiograms is mandatory. Dangerous levels of potassium may be combated by methods described in Ch. 76. Acute renal failure in these cases is self-limited, and full recovery can be expected, barring complications, if electrolytes remain under control at all points.

NONHEMOLYTIC FEBRILE TRANSFUSION REACTIONS. Febrile reactions to blood transfusions are far more likely to have been caused by recipient alloantibodies to donor leukocytes than to donor red cells. Alloantibodies to leukocytes develop at some time in at least 20 per cent of women as a result of pregnancy and in 70 to 90 per cent of multitransfused persons. Donor white cells reacting with recipient antibodies will cause a febrile response in proportion to the number of incompatible cells and the rate at which they are transfused.

Mild reactions cause fever alone. If the fever rises rapidly, shaking chills may occur. Severe reactions may be associated with vomiting and collapse. These reactions can be very uncomfortable but are unlikely to cause prolonged morbidity or mortality per se. The febrile response is completed within 12 hours.

If red cell incompatibility has been eliminated as the cause of the reaction, confirmation that white cells were responsible can be obtained by demonstrating antibodies to leukocytes in the serum of the recipient or by showing that the reactions can be prevented by transfusing leukocyte-poor red cells. If leukocyte-poor red cells fail to reduce symptoms adequately, frozen red cells should be tried.

CONTAMINATED BLOOD. Some bacteria are almost inevitably introduced into a small proportion of blood units collected for transfusion, but most fail to multiply at 4° C storage or are killed through the bactericidal effect of blood leukocytes and antibodies. The dangerous organisms are those which grow preferentially at 4° C. These are gram-negative rods which produce endotoxin. If blood heavily contaminated with endotoxin is transfused, shock, generalized bleeding, and death are almost inevitable. Confirmation of the diagnosis is accomplished by a Gram stain of the donor blood.

These contaminated blood reactions are extremely rare, and published reports suggest that many of them could have been prevented by inspection of the blood before transfusion. Contamination of a unit of blood should be suspected if the blood is of abnormal color, if there is evidence of excessive hemolysis, or if clots are readily demonstrable.

NONCARDIAC PULMONARY EDEMA. Rarely blood transfusion has been associated with sudden onset of dyspnea with radiologic evidence of pulmonary opacities. In many of these cases donor antibodies reacting with recipient leukocytes have been detected.

POST-TRANSFUSION THROMBOCYTOPENIC PURPURA. Thrombocytopenic purpura may occur suddenly seven to ten days after transfusion in association with recipient antibodies to donor platelets. In most cases the antibody has been anti-$P1^{A1}$, and the recipient has been a female with a history of pregnancies. Destruction of the patient's own platelets is assumed to be secondary to the intravascular reaction with donor platelets (the "innocent bystander" reaction), but it is not clear why the thrombocytopenia may last for a number of weeks. The most effective treatment has been plasma exchange, presumably through removal of the alloantibody to platelets.

TRANSMISSION OF DISEASE. *Hepatitis* remains the most serious unsolved problem in blood transfusion therapy. It is probable that clinically evident hepatitis follows at least 1 per cent of all transfusions and that ten times as many subclinical cases may occur. Hepatitis B has been greatly reduced by eliminating blood donors who are positive for HB_sAg, but it still accounts for at least 10 per cent of post-transfusion cases. Unsuspected hepatitis A is unlikely in a healthy blood donor, because infection with this virus does not result in a carrier state. Non-A non-B hepatitis accounts for almost all of the remaining 90 per cent of cases. Cytomegalovirus explains a minute percentage, and EB virus almost none.

Until the non-A non-B virus(es) is identified and tests to detect it are available, post-transfusion hepatitis is best prevented by elimination of paid blood donors and other high-risk groups and by a six-month deferral of prospective donors after an intimate contact with a potential source of hepatitis.

The relative hepatitis risks of various blood components are indicated in Table 146–4.

Malaria remains a rare but definite problem despite deferral of blood donors for three years if they have had malaria or have taken prophylaxis. A six-month deferral appears adequate if the donor had exposure to a malaria area but did not take prophylaxis. (Prophylaxis may only prolong the incubation period.)

Syphilis is rarely transmitted at present because of early detection and treatment of infected cases. Regulations still require a serologic test for syphilis on all blood donations, although it serves little purpose and unnecessarily excludes donors with biologic false-positive tests and with previous adequately treated syphilis.

Cytomegalovirus is responsible for the heterophil-negative, infectious mononucleosis–like syndrome which may occur approximately 40 days after transfusion of large amounts of fresh blood. Cytomegalovirus infection may be transmitted to newborn infants, especially if premature, and to other immunosuppressed patients.

Acquired immune deficiency syndrome (AIDS) is probably transmitted by blood components or derivatives, with recipients of commercial clotting factor concentrates at highest risk. The probability of acquiring AIDS from a standard blood component is extremely low, being in the range of 1/1,000,000 before blood banks eliminated high-risk donors. If AIDS is caused by an infectious agent, the few patients developing transfusion-associated cases must have had unusual susceptibility.

ALLERGIC REACTIONS. Urticaria may occur in as many as 3 to 5 per cent of transfusions but is rarely of serious concern and can usually be controlled or prevented by antihistamines. The very rare anaphylactoid reactions are characterized by flushing, tachycardia, wheezing, dyspnea, fall in blood pressure, and unconsciousness. One death has been reported. Most if not all such reactions are caused by recipient antibody to donor IgA globulin. Almost all of the involved recipients have no detectable IgA in their sera and have formed antibodies reacting with all IgA preparations (class-specific). Rare persons with normal IgA have produced alloantibodies to an IgA allotype. IgA is absent from the serum of 1 in 900 blood donors; 25 to 50 per cent of these donors have antibodies to IgA. Anaphylactoid reactions are so rare in comparison as to suggest that most of the detected antibodies are not of clinical significance.

Patients with previous anaphylactoid reactions associated with anti-IgA should receive only blood products which lack IgA. Red blood cells can be washed free of plasma proteins. Plasma products should be from donors who lack IgA.

If an anaphylactoid reaction occurs, transfusion should be stopped and intravenous antihistamine given. In most cases, epinephrine and corticosteroids will also be required.

CIRCULATORY OVERLOAD. This is a common side effect of transfusion, especially serious if the patient is in danger of heart failure. The risk is minimized by the use of concentrated components. If the need for red cells is great but the patient is in heart failure, it may be advisable to remove blood from the recipient, discarding the plasma and returning the red cells supplemented with red cells from other donors.

AIR EMBOLISM. This is rarely a problem but if a large amount of air enters the bag as the transfusion set spike is inserted, subsequent external pressure on the bag can embolize air.

MASSIVE TRANSFUSION PROBLEMS. Transfused blood has been altered during collection and storage, and additional problems occur when the volume and rate of blood transfusion introduce abnormalities faster than they can be corrected by the recipient.

Bleeding tendency: Blood stored more than 24 hours is essentially devoid of viable platelets, and dilutional thrombocytopenia becomes possible after transfusion of a volume of blood more than 1.5 to 2 times the blood volume of the recipient. Disseminated intravascular coagulation (DIC) is a frequent complication of conditions requiring massive transfusion. Restoration and maintenance of normal blood volume are essential prerequisites to control of DIC. It will usually be necessary to replace platelets (concentrates), fibrinogen (cryoprecipitates), and possible other plasma coagulation factors (fresh-frozen plasma).

Citrate intoxication: Although depression of ionized calcium is inevitable when large amounts of citrated blood are rapidly transfused, the recipient has a number of compensating mechanisms. Correction of the hypocalcemia with intermittent intra-

TABLE 146–4. RELATIVE RISK OF HEPATITIS FROM BLOOD AND PLASMA COMPONENTS AND DERIVATIVES

Very high risk
Commercial coagulation factor concentrates
Intermediate risk
Whole blood
Plasma
Cryoprecipitate
Platelet concentrate
Granulocyte concentrate
Relatively low risk (possible but not proved)
Frozen red cells
Washed red cells
Leukocyte-poor red cells
No risk
Albumin
Plasma protein fraction
Gamma globulin

venous calcium solutions is almost never necessary and may be dangerous.

Hypothermia is a serious risk when large volumes of cold blood are rapidly transfused. Ventricular fibrillation may result. This should be prevented by warming the blood either immediately prior to or during transfusion.

Microaggregates in stored blood can be removed during transfusion using special filters. However, there is no evidence that these filters are required for the usual small volume transfusions, and there is no agreement that microaggregates are harmful during massive transfusion.

Hyperkalemia and *acidosis* are primarily of concern in the transfusion of newborn infants. In fact, the massively transfused adult usually has a low plasma potassium despite the increased levels of potassium in the plasma of the transfused blood.

GRAFT-VERSUS-HOST DISEASE (GVHD). This is a rare but increasingly recognized complication of blood transfusion. Engraftment of stem cells in the donor blood can result if the immunologic responses of the recipient are sufficiently impaired. Immunocompetent donor lymphoid cells are responsible for GVHD. Recipients with congenital deficiencies of T lymphocytes and those prepared for a marrow transplant are at greatest risk. Others at risk include some patients whose immune apparatus has been suppressed to more than the usual degree by antineoplastic therapy. The risk of engraftment increases with the number of mononuclear cells in the transfused blood component. Granulocyte concentrates appear to carry the highest risk.

The clinical signs of GVHD are nonspecific: dermatitis, gastrointestinal disturbances, and liver dysfunction. The best supportive evidence for GVHD is obtained by demonstrating that the recipient's blood carries genetic markers other than his own. HLA typing is most useful for this purpose.

Engraftment can be prevented by irradiating blood prior to transfusion. Doses of 1500 to 5000 rads are used and have no demonstrable effect on red cell viability or on platelet and granulocyte function. Except for patients with severe combined immunodeficiency disease and those prepared for marrow transplantation, the indications for irradiation of blood prior to transfusion are not well established.

Blood transfusion is a very effective form of therapy but with potential serious side effects. Decisions to transfuse must always consider the risk-benefit ratio. The components prescribed must be appropriate for the indications and selected, when necessary, to avoid repetition of previous transfusion reactions.

Mollison PL: Blood Transfusion in Clinical Medicine. 6th ed. Oxford, Blackwell Scientific Publications, 1972. *This is the "bible" of transfusion medicine, emphasizing the laboratory aspects. The answers to most of your questions can be found here; if you need more detailed information, Mollison has probably provided the references.*

Petz LD, Swisher SN: Clinical Practice of Blood Transfusion. New York, Churchill Livingstone, 1981. *This text addresses transfusion problems from the point of view of the clinician, providing not only the necessary background but also addressing specific clinical situations.*

147. DEVELOPMENT AND MORPHOLOGY OF GRANULOCYTES AND MACROPHAGES

David W. Golde

STEM CELLS AND THE REGULATION OF MYELOPOIESIS. All of the circulating cellular elements of blood are ultimately derived from a pluripotent hematopoietic stem cell in the bone marrow with the capacity to give rise to granulocytes, monocytes, erythrocytes, thrombocytes, and immunocytes. An overall review of hematopoiesis is provided in Ch. 130.

A stem cell is a cell with extensive capacity for self-renewal (production of identical daughter cells) and the ability to give rise to more differentiated cells of several lineages (see Fig. 130–5). The stem cells cannot be identified morphologically, and there is no definitive assay for pluripotent stem cells in man. Multipotent stem cells give rise to "committed" precursor cells that have extensive capacity for replication but are restricted with respect to their subsequent maturational potential. Thus, at some point in stem cell development, a cell becomes committed to development along the erythroid, megakaryocytic, or granulocyte-monocyte pathway. Committed precursor cells will form colonies of differentiated cells under appropriate stimulation in in vitro bone marrow culture systems.

There is a common committed progenitor cell for the neutrophilic and monocyte-macrophage pathway. This cell is referred to as CFU-G,M (colony-forming unit—granulocyte, monocyte) because of its ability to give rise to colonies of granulocytes and monocytes-macrophages in bone marrow cultures. The common precursor (CFU-G,M) for the neutrophil and the monocyte-macrophage requires the presence of *colony-stimulating factor (CSF)* for its development. Colony-stimulating factor is necessary for the in vitro growth of granulocytes and monocytes, and it is probably the physiologic regulator of granulopoiesis and monocytopoiesis in vivo, as is erythropoietin for erythropoiesis. The CSFs, a family of glycoproteins with molecular weights between 20,000 and 50,000, circulate in the blood and can be assayed there as well as in the urine. Human CSF has not been completely characterized.

The CFU-G,M must "decide" at some point whether to differentiate along the monocytic or granulocytic pathway, but the factors in this decision are not known. There may be different CSFs for monocytic and granulocytic development, and other stimuli may affect their development. It is also possible that cells at the promyelocyte stage may switch to the monocyte-macrophage pathway. CSF, the putative granulopoietin, is produced by many cells in the body, but most prominently by cells of the monocyte-macrophage series and activated T lymphocytes. Certain immunologic reactions and the presence of microorganisms increase the production of CSF and therefore of neutrophils and monocytes. Negative feedback from the mature neutrophil or macrophage may serve to limit excessive myelopoiesis after inflammatory stimuli have been removed. The cells of the eosinophil and basophil pathways appear to be regulated by specific hormones related to, but not identical with, the CSF for neutrophil and monocyte-macrophage development.

MORPHOLOGY. ***Granulocytes.*** The earliest morphologically identifiable cell of the granulocyte series is the *myeloblast.* Myeloblasts are between 15 and 20 μm in diameter and constitute about 1 to 3 per cent of the bone marrow population. The myeloblast has a relatively large nucleus with evenly distributed chromatin and one or more prominent nucleoli. The scant cytoplasm is basophilic (blue) owing to the high concentration of ribonucleoprotein, and normally contains few cytoplasmic granules. The *promyelocyte,* next in the maturation sequence, has a nucleus similar to that of the myeloblast but also has prominent azurophilic or nonspecific granules (Fig. 147–1). These azurophilic granules, which are distinct from the specific granules that appear later in maturation, contain myeloperoxidase, an abundant and important enzyme of granulocytes. They also contain lysosomal enzymes such as acid phosphatase and β-glucuronidase.

The *myelocyte,* which derives from the promyelocyte, shows evidence of chromatin clumping in its nucleus and indistinct or absent nucleoli. There is abundant cytoplasmic granulation, including the "specific granules" which contain the alkaline phosphatase characteristic of mature neutrophils. The specific granules also contain lysozyme and various proteases. The myelocyte retains the capacity to proliferate and is the last cell in the "proliferative compartment" of the marrow (see below). The *metamyelocyte* has an eccentric nucleus with extensive

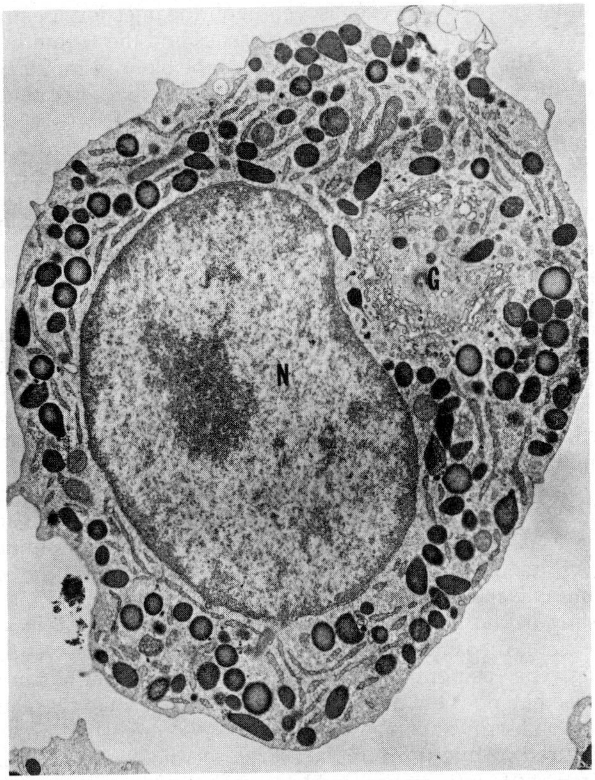

Figure 147–1. Transmission electron micrograph of a neutrophilic promyelocyte reacted for peroxidase. Note the prominent Golgi region (G), nucleus (N) with single nucleolus, and peroxidase-containing primary or azurophil granules. × 15,000. (Reproduced with permission from Bainton DF, Ullyot JL, Farquhar MG: J Exp Med 134:907, 1971.)

chromatin clumping and early evidence of nuclear segmentation. The cytoplasm contains both azurophilic (nonspecific) and "specific" granules. It has lost the ability to replicate, but matures to the *"band" form,* an incompletely segmented neutrophil that normally constitutes 3 to 5 per cent of the circulating leukocyte pool.

The *polymorphonuclear neutrophil* ("poly") is the final stage of cellular maturation (see Fig. 148–1). The nucleus is dense and has assumed its characteristic lobulated appearance. The neutrophil is of uniform size (12 to 15 μm), and there are usually three nuclear lobes. In females, about 1 to 3 per cent of the polymorphonuclear leukocytes contain a "drumstick," a small nuclear appendage correlated with the presence of a Barr body representing the XX genotype. The mature poly functions most importantly in host defense against bacterial invasion (see Ch. 148). The process of cellular maturation in the neutrophil series equips these cells with the properties of motility, phagocytosis, and killing of ingested organisms.

Eosinophils. The eosinophil is a specialized granulocyte that generally undergoes the same maturational sequence as the neutrophil. Only one granule type is formed, however; this is substantially larger than those found in neutrophils and stains bright orange or red with Wright's stain. The eosinophilic granules contain a type of myeloperoxidase but no alkaline phosphatase or lysozyme. The granules of the mature eosinophil have a crystalline core demonstrable by electron microscopy. In the eosinophilic promyelocyte the few homogeneously dense granules lack the crystalloid characteristic of the mature eosinophil. Eosinophilic myelocytes are easily identifiable because of their characteristic granulation. The mature cell normally does not contain more than two lobes. Despite the well-documented association of the eosinophil with allergic disorders and certain parasitic diseases (e.g., trichinosis), the specific function of the eosinophil in human physiology and pathology is largely unknown.

Basophils. Basophils, constituting 1 per cent or less of the total circulating leukocytes, are distinguished by their large, blue-black granules revealed by Romanowsky stains. They are believed to originate in the bone marrow from a promyelocyte. The basophil granules have a crystalline or fibrillar substructure and abundant acid mucopolysaccharides, which are probably responsible for their affinity for basic dyes. They also have a characteristic tinctorial quality known as metachromasia, i.e., a change in the expected coloring after staining with a specific dye. Thus, the basophil granules stain violet with basic aniline dyes that normally stain blue. Circulating basophils and tissue mast cells are similar in many respects, and possibly have a progeny-progenitor relationship. The granules of basophils are believed to contain heparin and uniquely large amounts of histamine. Mast cell granules contain histamine, heparin, and in some species 5-hydroxytryptophan. Human mast cells also contain alkaline phosphatase, peroxidase, and β-glucuronidase.

Monocytes and Tissue Macrophages. Circulating blood monocytes and tissue macrophages belong to the family of mononuclear phagocytic cells. Although mononuclear phagocytes are widely distributed throughout the body, the monocyte-macrophage system in man may be viewed as a continuum of progressively more mature cells beginning with progenitors in the bone marrow. The *promonocyte,* the earliest morphologically identifiable cell of the mononuclear phagocyte series, has a well-developed Golgi complex and contains peroxidase-positive granules. It is about 10 to 18 μm in diameter and has poorly

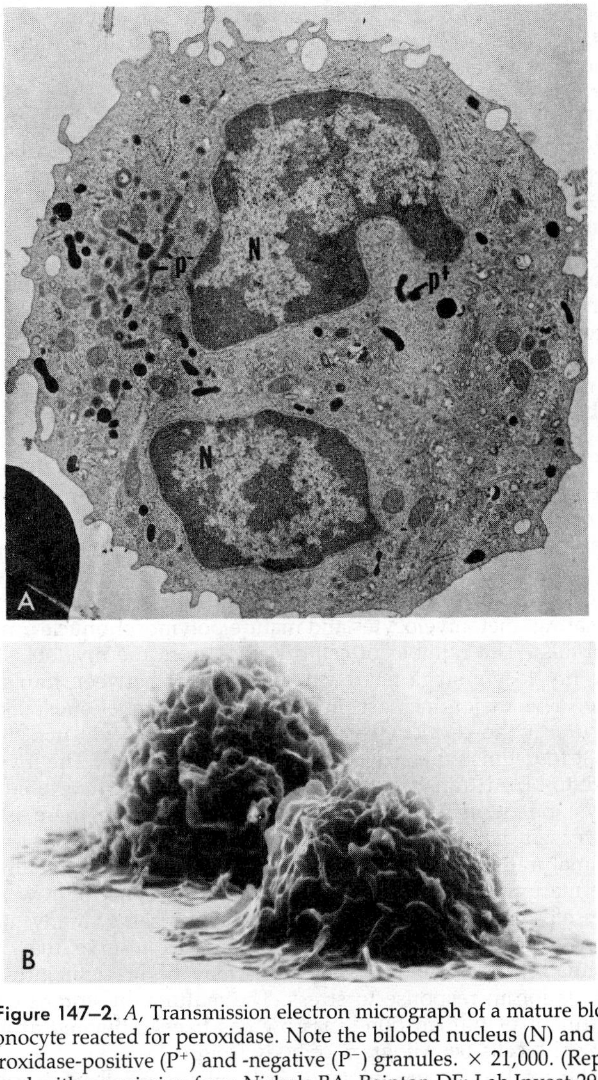

Figure 147–2. *A,* Transmission electron micrograph of a mature blood monocyte reacted for peroxidase. Note the bilobed nucleus (N) and the peroxidase-positive (P^+) and -negative (P^-) granules. × 21,000. (Reproduced with permission from Nichols BA, Bainton DF: Lab Invest 29:27, 1973.) *B,* Scanning electron micrograph of two alveolar macrophages obtained by bronchopulmonary lavage from a normal volunteer. Note extensive ruffled membrane and attachment of cells to the substrate by lamellipodia. × 4000.

developed phagocytic capacity. The *mature monocyte* is about 12 to 20 μm in diameter and has an oval, notched, or horseshoe-shaped nucleus. The chromatin is reticulated, and there are no nucleoli. The cytoplasm is abundant and gray or bluish, and has occasional vacuoles and numerous granules (Fig. 147–2*A*). Most but not all of the monocyte granules stain for peroxidase.

The monocyte leaves the circulation and enters the tissues, where, if it remains viable, it will mature into a macrophage. The *tissue macrophages* exist in protean forms, including the hepatic Kupffer cell, alveolar macrophage of the lung, giant cell of granuloma, dermal Langerhans cell, peritoneal and pleural macrophage, and osteoclast. The bone marrow origin of the human alveolar and hepatic macrophages has been substantiated, and similar studies in animals have shown that the dermal Langerhans cell also has a bone marrow origin. The human osteoclast has been demonstrated to originate in the bone marrow, as shown dramatically by the cure of osteopetrosis by allogeneic bone marrow transplantation. The tissue macrophages (also referred to as *histiocytes*) lose their peroxidase activity. They are highly motile and have extensive phagocytic capability. The surface morphology shows extensive cell membrane ruffling (Fig. 147–2*B*), and motility is evidenced by pseudopod formation. The macrophages in the various tissues may acquire specialized functions. Thus, the alveolar macrophage uniquely resides at an air-tissue surface and has developed an appropriate aerobic metabolism. The alveolar macrophage defends against inhaled particulate matter, airborne microorganisms, and environmental toxins to which it is directly exposed.

Tissue macrophages are able to proliferate in situ. The alveolar and hepatic macrophage populations may not be critically dependent on the influx of monocytes to sustain their numbers. Tissue macrophages defend against microbial invasion, remove senescent cells, sequestrate toxic particulate matter, and synthesize various biologically important compounds such as complement, prostaglandins, lymphocyte activators, plasminogen activator, and colony-stimulating factor. Monocytes and tissue macrophages characteristically stain heavily for α-naphthyl acetate (or butyrate) esterase; this provides a useful cytochemical marker for their presence.

LEUKOCYTE KINETICS. ***Granulocytes.*** The kinetics of granulopoiesis and of the resulting granulocytes are best understood by following the movement of these specialized cells through the interconnections and subsets of three major compartments: bone marrow, blood, and tissue. Bone marrow granulocytes may be divided into (1) the proliferative compartment capable of replication (myeloblasts, promyelocytes, and myelocytes), and (2) the maturation-storage compartment, which is nonreplicating (metamyelocytes and mature polymorphonuclear neutrophils). The number of cell divisions from the myeloblast to the myelocyte stage has been estimated at between four and five. The major increase in granulocyte number most likely occurs at the myelocyte level, since the myelocyte pool is at least four times the size of the promyelocyte pool. The myelocyte-to-blood transit time has been estimated at five to seven days, but it may be as short as 48 hours when there is an increased demand, such as during infection. With completion of maturation, the polymorphonuclear leukocytes remain in the maturation-storage compartment of the bone marrow and are referred to as the mature granulocyte reserve. Many more leukocytes are normally contained in this reserve than are circulating in the blood; these cells may be brought into the circulation in response to stress. The maturation storage compartment of human bone marrow has been estimated at 6 to 13×10^9 cells per kilogram of body weight.

The total blood granulocyte pool consists of all neutrophils in the vascular spaces. Some of these granulocytes do not circulate freely but adhere to the endothelium of small vessels, constituting the *"marginated granulocyte pool."* Cells readily move from the marginated granulocyte pool to the circulating granulocyte pool with exercise, epinephrine injection, or stress. Granulocytes ultimately enter the tissues and die within hours to days. They do not normally return to the blood. Granulocytes leave the circulation in a random manner with a half-time of approximately seven hours. Thus, granulocytes newly released from the marrow are as likely to leave the blood as neutrophils that have been circulating for several hours. Certain senescent neutrophils, however, may be removed in a nonrandom fashion and are probably disposed of by macrophages in the reticuloendothelial system. In man, the circulating granulocyte pool has been estimated at 31×10^7 cells per kilogram of body weight, with the marginated pool being approximately the same. The mean production of granulocytes in the steady state in man is believed to be about 0.9 to 1.6×10^9 cells per kilogram of body weight per day. This enormous production rate is necessary because of the cell's short half-life. Neutrophil production can increase dramatically in response to inflammatory stimuli.

Eosinophils. Less is known about eosinophilic granulocyte kinetics. The mean transit time of the eosinophil in the bone marrow is thought to be about nine days with a postmitotic transit time of about 2.5 days. Less than 1 per cent of the total eosinophils in the body are found in the peripheral blood, most existing in the bone marrow and tissues. The half-disappearance time of eosinophils from the blood is probably five to six hours. The eosinophil likely survives for longer periods in the tissues than does the neutrophil. The normal human circulating eosinophil count averages 150 per μl. Peripheral eosinopenia is induced by injections of glucocorticosteroids or epinephrine. There is little information available regarding basophil production in man.

Monocytes. Monocytes normally account for 3 to 11 per cent of the circulating leukocytes. The earliest monocytic precursor in the bone marrow must undergo at least three generations before the mature circulating monocyte is produced. This process probably takes about six days. In the adult man, the total number of monocytes in the bone marrow is estimated at 7.3×10^9 cells. The monocytes normally leave the marrow space within 24 hours after completing their last division. Thus, there is no marrow reserve pool analogous to the granulocyte reserve. The total number of circulating monocytes is estimated at 1.7×10^9 for an adult, with a half-life of 71 hours in the circulation. Like the neutrophils, monocytes leave the peripheral blood in a random fashion. Once in the tissues, the monocytes are not thought to re-enter the circulation.

Bainton DF: Neutrophil granules. Br J Haematol 29:17, 1975. *A succinct review of granulocyte maturation and granule development.*

Brennan JK, Lichtman MA, DiPersio JF, Abboud CN: Chemical mediators of granulopoiesis: A review. Exp Hematol 8:441, 1980. *Excellent review of the regulation of granulopoiesis.*

Cline MJ, Golde DW: Cellular interactions in haematopoiesis. Nature 277:177, 1979. *Review of interaction between hematopoietic cells and their regulatory functions.*

Golde DW, Takaku F (eds.): Hematopoietic Stem Cells. New York, Marcel Dekker, Inc., 1984. *Multi-author text on normal and abnormal hematopoiesis.*

Groopman JE, Golde DW: The histiocytic disorders: A pathophysiologic analysis. Ann Intern Med 94:95, 1981. *Review of macrophage physiology and pathology.*

Hocking WG, Golde DW: The pulmonary-alveolar macrophage. N Engl J Med 301:580, 639, 1979. *Review of the lung macrophage with emphasis on human physiology.*

148. FUNCTION OF NEUTROPHILS AND MONONUCLEAR PHAGOCYTES

Bernard M. Babior

Neutrophils and mononuclear phagocytes are essential components of the host defense system. Both are made in the bone marrow, and both accomplish most of their purposes through the act of eating (Gr. *phagein,* to eat). Mononuclear phagocytes are versatile cells whose functions include the destruction of invading pathogens, the elimination of debris from the bloodstream and from sites of tissue damage, the remodeling of normal tissues, and the assignment of targets to lymphocytes.

Neutrophils, on the other hand, are singlemindedly dedicated to the destruction of invading pathogens.

THE NEUTROPHIL

STRUCTURE. The neutrophil is a terminally differentiated, nondividing cell that is well equipped to perform its function of killing microorganisms. Figure 148–1 shows a neutrophil as it appears under an electron microscope. The cell is packed with granules whose contents are used for the destruction and degradation of target microorganisms. These granules are of two types: *azurophil,* which contains proteases and other hydrolytic enzymes as well as a Cl^--oxidizing enzyme known as myeloperoxidase, and *specific,* which contains among other things a collagenase and an enzyme that releases C5a from the complement component C5. The granules arise from the Golgi apparatus, which appears as a stack of flattened vesicles near the center of the cell. Also seen is the nucleus, in this cell a vestigial structure that can no longer replicate its DNA, and the plasma membrane, which contains an element of the neutrophil's killing apparatus as well as sensors that locate and identify the microorganisms against which the neutrophil acts. Not shown is the cytoskeleton, a complex system of tubes and fibers that is responsible for the orderly movement of this highly motile cell.

FUNCTION. Neutrophils undergo radical and abrupt changes in behavior in response to external stimuli. These changes include aggregation, degranulation (i.e., the discharge of granule contents through the plasma membrane), and the initiation of oxidant production. They are provoked by many stimuli, the most important of which are target microorganisms and chemotactic factors at high concentration (see below). These behavioral changes convert the neutrophil from a placid resident of the bloodstream to a powerful and dangerous weapon. A cell that has undergone these changes is known as an *activated neutrophil.* The destruction of a microorganism by a neutrophil

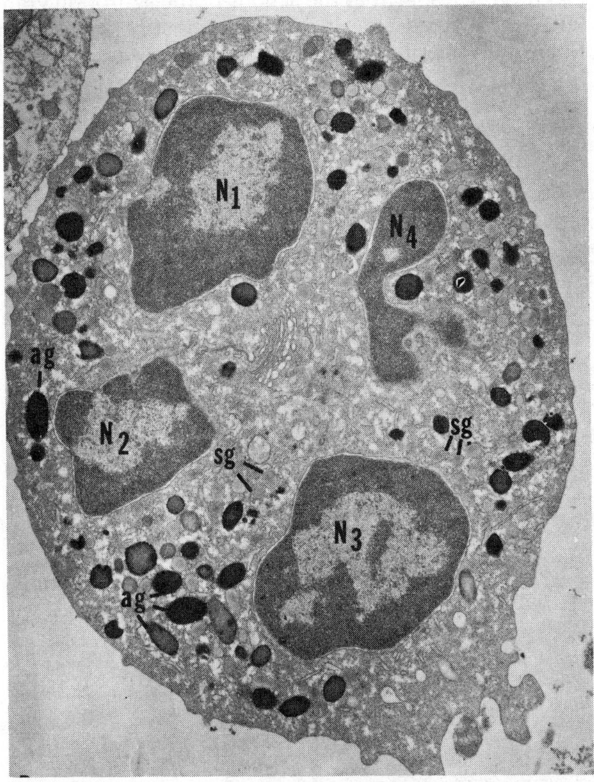

Figure 148–1. Neutrophil. Transmission electron micrograph of a mature neutrophil reacted for peroxidase. Note the multilobed nucleus (N_1–N_4), the peroxidase-positive azurophilic granules (ag) and the peroxidase-negative secondary or specific granules (sg). ×21,000. (Reproduced with permission from Bainton DF, Ullyot JL, Farquhar MG: J Exp Med 134:907, 1971.)

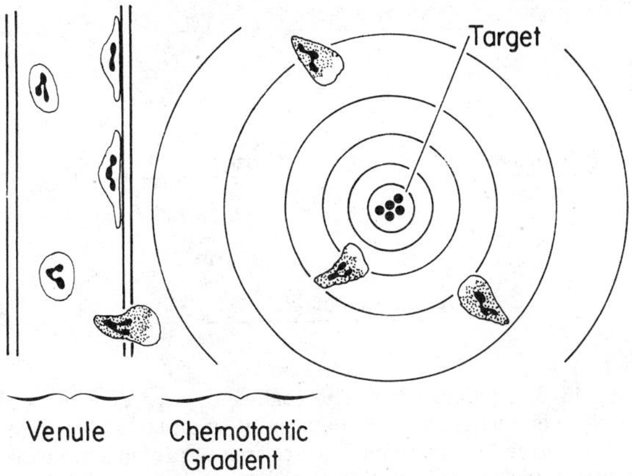

Figure 148–2. Chemotaxis. Neutrophils in the venule undergo margination in response to chemotactic factor, then leave the vessel by migrating between the endothelial cells (diapedesis) and travel up the chemotactic gradient towards the target.

can be divided into three stages: finding the microorganism, ingesting it, and finally killing it and disposing of its remains.

Chemotaxis. The neutrophil finds its target through a chemical sense that enables the cell to detect certain substances known as *chemotactic factors.* These chemotactic factors are continuously released and diffuse away from sites where microorganisms have invaded tissues, setting up a concentration gradient. Neutrophils in the circulation are able to sense this gradient and travel toward its source. They begin their journey by attaching themselves to the capillary and postcapillary endothelium, a process known as *margination.* They then migrate outward between the endothelial cells into the extravascular tissues, penetrating the subendothelial basement membrane by local digestion, presumably with collagenase. Once outside the capillaries, they continue their directed migration, eventually reaching the site of origin of chemotactic factors—that is, the region of tissue that has been invaded by microorganisms. This process of migrating up a chemical gradient toward the source of the chemical is known as *chemotaxis* (Fig. 148–2).

Neutrophils are able to respond to a very large number of chemotactic factors, but three appear to be of primary importance: (1) *N-formylated oligopeptides,* (2) the complement fragment *C5a,* and (3) a product of arachidonate oxidation known as *leukotriene* B_4 *(LTB_4).* These chemotactic factors are produced both by the invading microorganisms (N-formylated oligopeptides and C5a) and by the neutrophils themselves (C5a and LTB_4). N-formylated oligopeptides are intermediates in bacterial protein synthesis and are released from bacteria that have been damaged or killed. C5a is produced by the complement system when it interacts with microorganisms and also by activated neutrophils through the release of the C5-splitting enzyme of the specific granules. LTB_4 is also produced by activated neutrophils, which manufacture it by liberating and oxidizing arachidonic acid from endogenous phospholipids. The production of C5a and LTB_4 by activated neutrophils lends a self-reinforcing character to the process of chemotaxis, since neutrophils that have arrived at a site of inflammation are activated to generate chemotactic factors that attract more neutrophils to the inflamed region.

Bacteria in the circulation are thought to be handled primarily by the mononuclear phagocytes (see below). Neutrophils, however, may play a role in clearing the circulation of microorganisms that enter the bloodstream suddenly and in large numbers. During such episodes of bacteremia, the complement system is activated, releasing C5a into the circulation. Neutrophils react to this pulse of C5a by marginating in the pulmonary capillaries where they may act temporarily (15 to 30 minutes)

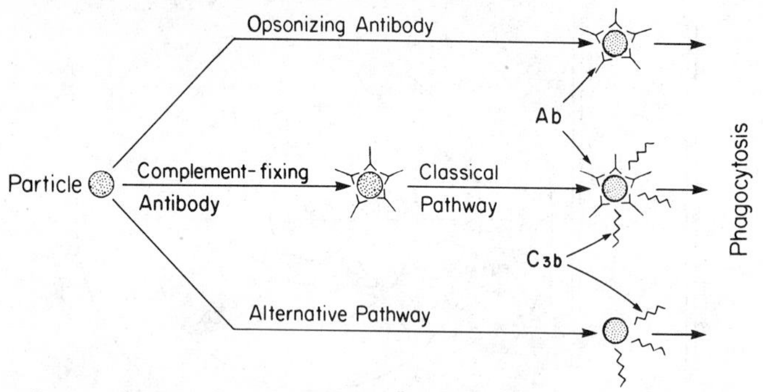

Figure 148–3. Opsonization. The coating of a particle by a plasma protein that is recognized by neutrophil receptors as a signal for ingestion is termed *opsonization*. Two classes of proteins are capable of opsonizing particles for ingestion by neutrophils: opsonizing antibodies, and complement component C3b.

as a filtration system, removing microorganisms from the blood as they pass through the pulmonary circulation. In this special situation, chemotaxis is not needed to help the neutrophils find their targets, because the targets are brought directly to the phagocytes by the flow of blood.

Ingestion. Once the neutrophil has come into contact with the microorganism, the stage is set for ingestion. For this to occur, the cell has to recognize the microorganism as an edible target, not just a piece of random debris. Generally it is not the microorganism itself that the cell recognizes, but certain plasma proteins that coat the microorganism once it has entered the bloodstream or tissues. These proteins are called *opsonins* (Gr. *opson*, seasoning), and their attachment to the surface of the microorganism is called *opsonization* (Fig. 148–3).

The proteins that are able to opsonize targets for ingestion by neutrophils include antibodies belonging to certain of the IgG subclasses (opsonizing antibodies), and the complement component C3b. Opsonizing antibodies bind to the microbial surface by means of a simple antigen-antibody reaction. C3b binds to the microbial surface by a more complex process that involves the activation of the complement system through either the classical pathway (initiated by an antigen-antibody complex) or the alternative pathway (initiated by certain complex carbohydrates such as are found on microbial surfaces) (see Ch. 428). One of the steps in complement activation by either of these pathways is the cleavage of component C3 into two pieces: C3a, a small fragment that induces capillaries and venules to dilate and become leaky, and C3b, the large opsonizing fragment. Immediately upon release, this opsonizing fragment locks onto the target through a covalent bond. The opsonized targets then attach to the neutrophil surface by means of these opsonins, which are recognized and bound by receptors in the neutrophil membrane: the Fc receptors, which recognize complexes between antigen and opsonizing antibody, and the C3 receptors, which recognize particle-associated C3b.

The attachment of the target to the neutrophil surface is the signal for ingestion (Fig. 148–4). The membrane in the region of the attached particle invaginates into the cell, carrying the particle in with it. When the particle is fully internalized, the invagination closes at its neck to form a vesicle, which detaches from the inner surface of the cell membrane and is released into the cytoplasm of the neutrophil. The end result of the phagocytic event is that a particle initially attached to the surface of the neutrophil is translocated to the cell's interior enclosed in a vesicle lined with what was originally a portion of the neutrophil plasma membrane. This vesicle, known as the *phagocytic vesicle,* is the site of killing of the ingested organism.

Killing. Killing involves two separate actions on the part of the neutrophils: *degranulation* and the *activation of the respiratory burst.* Degranulation refers to a process whereby the granule membrane fuses with another cellular membrane, releasing the granule contents into the compartment on the opposite side of the other membrane (Fig. 148–5). In the case of the azurophil granules, degranulation occurs almost exclusively into the phagocytic vesicles, so that the actions of the azurophil granule contents are directed almost entirely against the ingested microorganisms. Specific granules degranulate into both the

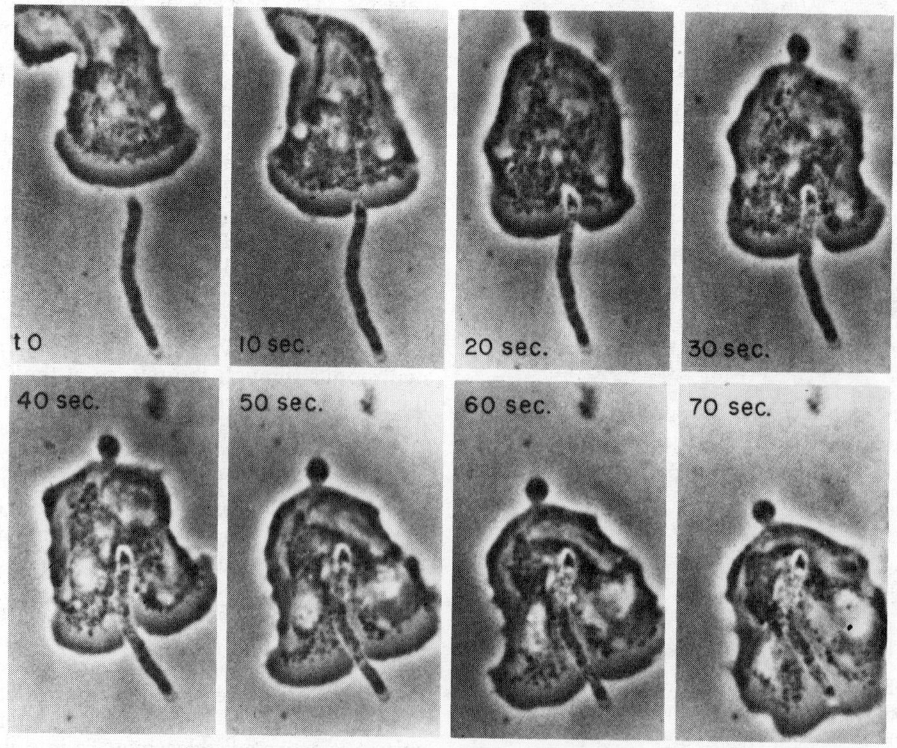

Figure 148–4. Ingestion of a target microorganism by a neutrophil. (Reproduced from Hirsch JG: Cinemicrophotographic observations of granule lysis in polymorphonuclear leucocytes during phagocytosis. J Exp Med 116:827, 1962, by copyright permission of the Rockefeller University Press.)

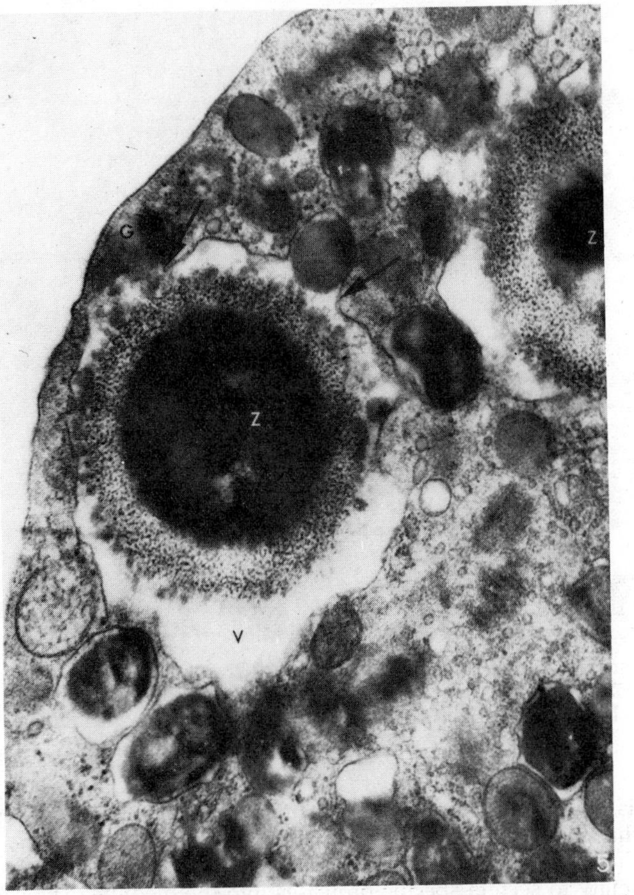

Figure 148–5. Degranulation. V, phagocytic vesicle; Z, zymosan (a yeast cell wall particle). Arrows show granules in the act of discharging their contents into the phagocytic vesicle. (Reproduced from Zucken-Franklin D, Hirsch JG: Electron microscope studies on the degranulation of rabbit peritoneal leukocytes during phagocytosis. J Exp Med 120:569, 1964, by copyright permission of the Rockefeller University Press.)

phagocytic vesicles and the external environment, so their contents exert effects exterior to the neutrophils as well as on the ingested microorganisms. Some of the constituents of each of these granules are listed in Table 148–1, together with their actions.

The *respiratory burst* refers to a sequence of metabolic events the purpose of which is the production of potent microbicidal oxidants through the partial reduction of oxygen. The burst is

TABLE 148–1. CONTENTS OF NEUTROPHIL GRANULES

Component	Function
Azurophil granules	
Acid hydrolyases (glycosidases, phospholipases, acid proteases)	Degradation of ingested material
Neutral proteases (cathepsin G, elastase)	Destruction of inflamed tissue?
Lysozyme	Digestion of bacterial cell wall
"Catonic proteins"	Bacterial killing?
Myeloperoxidase	Oxygen-dependent bacterial killing
Specific granules	
Lysozyme	Digestion of bacterial cell wall
Cobalamin-binding protein	Binding of bacterial cobalamin analogs
Apolactoferrin	Binding of free iron, control of granulopoiesis
Collagenase	Digestion of connective tissue
C5-splitting enzyme	Release of C5a
Indeterminate	
Bactericidal/permeability-increasing protein	Killing of gram-negative bacteria

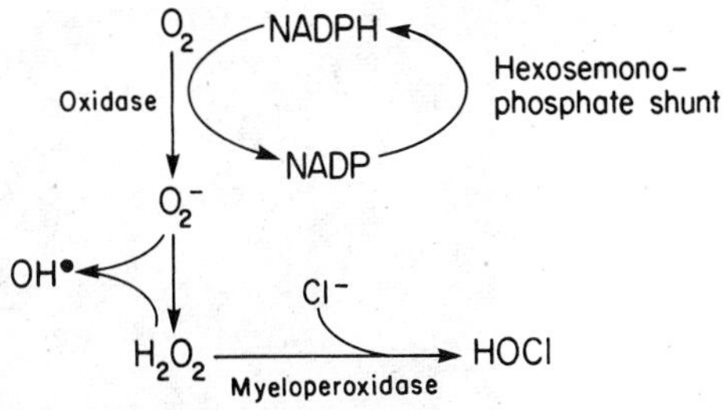

Figure 148–6. The respiratory burst.

activated by the same stimuli that provoke degranulation of the specific granules—primarily contact with ingestible particles, and exposure to chemotactic factors at high concentrations. These stimuli activate a plasma membrane–bound oxidase dormant in resting cells that catalyzes the one-electron reduction of oxygen to superoxide ($O_2^{\cdot}$) at the expense of NADPH (Fig. 148–6). Most of the $O_2^{\cdot}$reacts with itself to yield H_2O_2, while at the same time NADPH is regenerated by way of the hexosemonophosphate shunt. These events have nothing to do with respiration as it is usually understood, but they acquired the name "respiratory burst", because of the large increase in neutrophil oxygen uptake that is associated with their onset.

The microbicidal oxidants are derived from the H_2O_2: (1) A portion of the H_2O_2 is used to oxidize Cl^- to the highly microbicidal hypochlorite ion (OCl^-), a reaction catalyzed by myeloperoxidase, an enzyme delivered into the phagocytic vesicle from the azurophil granules. (2) Another portion of the H_2O_2 is converted to the exceedingly reactive hydroxyl radical ($OH^{\cdot}$) in a metal-catalyzed reaction with $O_2^{\cdot}$. These and related oxidants attack and kill ingested microorganisms by oxidizing their cellular constituents.

MONONUCLEAR PHAGOCYTES

Mononuclear phagocytes and neutrophils are closely related. Both are derived from the same ancestor, a dually committed marrow stem cell that gives rise in culture to mixed colonies of the two kinds of phagocytes (Ch. 147) and both share many functions, including the unusual ability to ingest particles as large as half or more their own diameter. There is, however, only one type of neutrophil, whereas there are many varieties of mononuclear phagocytes.

STRUCTURE AND DIFFERENTIATION. All mononuclear phagocytes are derived from a single juvenile precursor: the monocyte (see Fig. 147–2). Larger than the neutrophil and with a larger, less deformed nucleus, the monocyte has a cytoplasm that is filled with granules whose contents include hydrolytic enzymes and other proteins necessary for the cell's activities. Unlike the neutrophil, the monocyte seems to have retained a limited capacity to divide and in addition is able to undergo considerable further differentiation.

Monocytes are able to diversify into the many types of cells that constitute the mononuclear phagocyte system. Monocytes circulate in the bloodstream for a period of time ($t\frac{1}{2} \sim 12$ hours) and then enter the tissues, where they differentiate into mature macrophages that live for weeks to months. The properties of these macrophages are characteristic for the tissues in which they reside. Those in the liver, for example, are the Kupffer cells, spidery phagocytes that straddle the sinusoids separating adjacent plates of hepatocytes (Fig. 148–7*A*). Those in the lungs are the large ellipsoidal alveolar macrophages (Fig. 148–7*B*). These and other tissue macrophages are listed in Table 148–2. Little is known about the factors responsible for the various patterns of mononuclear phagocyte differentiation seen in different tissues.

Macrophages are important components of the inflammatory reactions elicited by the noxious agents (e.g., microorganisms

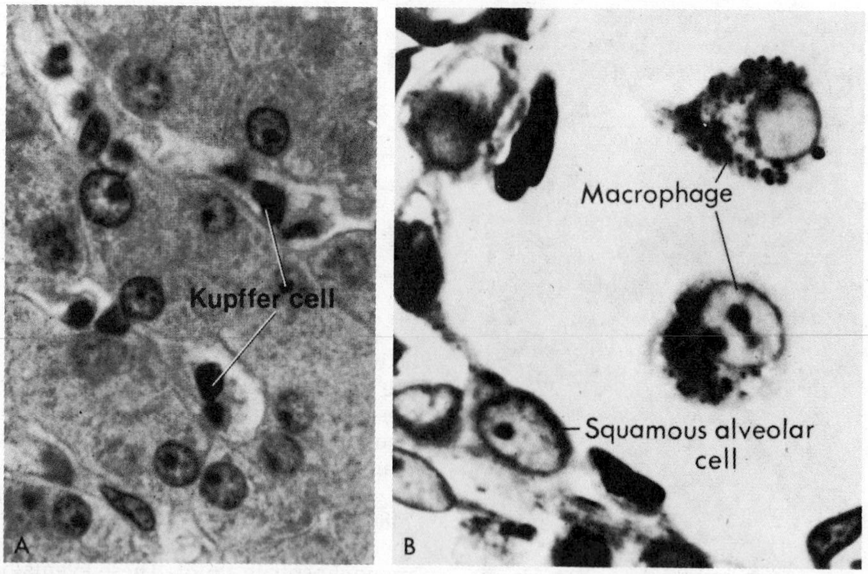

Figure 148–7. Some tissue macrophages. *A*, Kupffer cell. (Reprinted with permission from Popper H: Liver Structure and Function. New York, McGraw-Hill Book Company, 1957, p 97.) *B*, Alveolar macrophage. (Reprinted with permission from Sorokin SP: The respiratory system. *In* Weiss L, Greep RO: Histology. 4th ed. New York, McGraw-Hill Book Company, 1977, p 765.)

or foreign bodies). Some of the macrophages that appear at a site of inflammation have been recruited from the surrounding tissues, while others are derived from monocytes that have migrated there from the bloodstream. Once at the inflamed site, the macrophages undergo a sequence of functional and morphologic changes whose purpose appears to be to enable them to deal more effectively with the inciting agent (Fig. 148–8). Initially, the cells increase in size, accumulate many new granules, and begin to secrete large quantities of certain specific proteases, including collagenase, elastase, and plasminogen activator, a component of the fibrinolytic system (see Ch. 167). Their capacity for phagocytosis is increased, as is their ability to degrade ingested material. They have developed into what might be termed "augmented" macrophages (Fig. 148–8*B*). If the inciting agent has not been eliminated within the first few days, the phagocytes begin to aggregate into a granuloma. Further stimulation results in additional growth of the aggregated cells and a further augmentation in secretory capacity; the phagocytes have now turned into epithelioid cells, the characteristic constituents of mature granulomas (Fig. 148–8*C*). Eventually, giant cells appear, arising through the fusion of epithelioid cells with each other and with newly arrived macrophages (Fig. 148–8*D*). With the elimination of the inciting agent, the inflammatory process resolves and the macrophages disappear. What becomes of them is not known.

THE "ACTIVATED" MACROPHAGE. When mononuclear phagocytes in culture are exposed to a T lymphocyte product known as *macrophage activating factor* (this may actually be γ-interferon) or to *lipopolysaccharide* from the cell walls of gram-negative organisms, they undergo a series of changes that seem quite similar to those occurring during the conversion of a resident tissue macrophage to an "augmented" macrophage. These changes include increases in size and granule numbers, a sharply increased phagocytic capacity, and a newly acquired ability to secrete specific proteases into the medium. The cells become stickier and more motile and develop the ability to manufacture lethal oxidizing agents. Most important, their microbicidal power is greatly increased, so they become capable of killing pathogens that they were unable to deal with in their former state. Cells that have attained this heightened degree of microbicidal potency are known as "activated" macrophages.

Activation of macrophages occurs in vivo as well as in vitro, since animals treated in such a way as to release macrophage-activating factor from their lymphocytes are resistant to macrophage-controlled infections (e.g., listeriosis) that kill their untreated counterparts. It is likely that in whole animals activated macrophages are members of the class referred to previously as "augmented."

FUNCTIONS. Mononuclear phagocytes carry out three basic functions: secretion, ingestion, and interaction with lymphocytes.

Secretion. Mononuclear phagocytes secrete a large number of substances, some protein and others nonprotein in nature, into the extracellular environment (Table 148–3). Lysozyme is secreted by mononuclear phagocytes regardless of their state of activation, whereas proteases active at neutral pH ("neutral proteases") are secreted only by activated cells. Other substances such as $O_2^{\overline{\cdot}}$ (superoxide) and leukotrienes are secreted under even more specialized circumstances.

Ingestion. Mononuclear phagocytes received their name from their ability to ingest. These cells use this ability for two separate purposes: to eliminate waste and debris (scavenging) and to kill invading pathogens.

SCAVENGING. Mononuclear phagocytes play a highly important role as general scavengers. They dispose of effete or worn out cells, remove foreign material from the bloodstream, and clean up debris at sites of infection or tissue damage.

Cell disposal by mononuclear phagocytes is best exemplified by their role in the elimination of outdated erythrocytes. These are recognized in some fashion by the phagocytes, which internalize and degrade them by a process of phagocytosis, degranulation, and digestion similar to that described for neutrophils. The hemoglobin is converted to bilirubin, iron, and amino acids by lysosomal proteases and other enzymes as

TABLE 148–2. TISSUE MACROPHAGES

Fixed
Kupffer cells
Microglial cells (central nervous system)
Macrophages of spleen, lymph nodes, and bone marrow sinusoids
Mesangial cells (kidney)
Osteoclasts
Wandering
Macrophages of serosal cavities (pleural, peritoneal, pericardial)
Alveolar macrophages

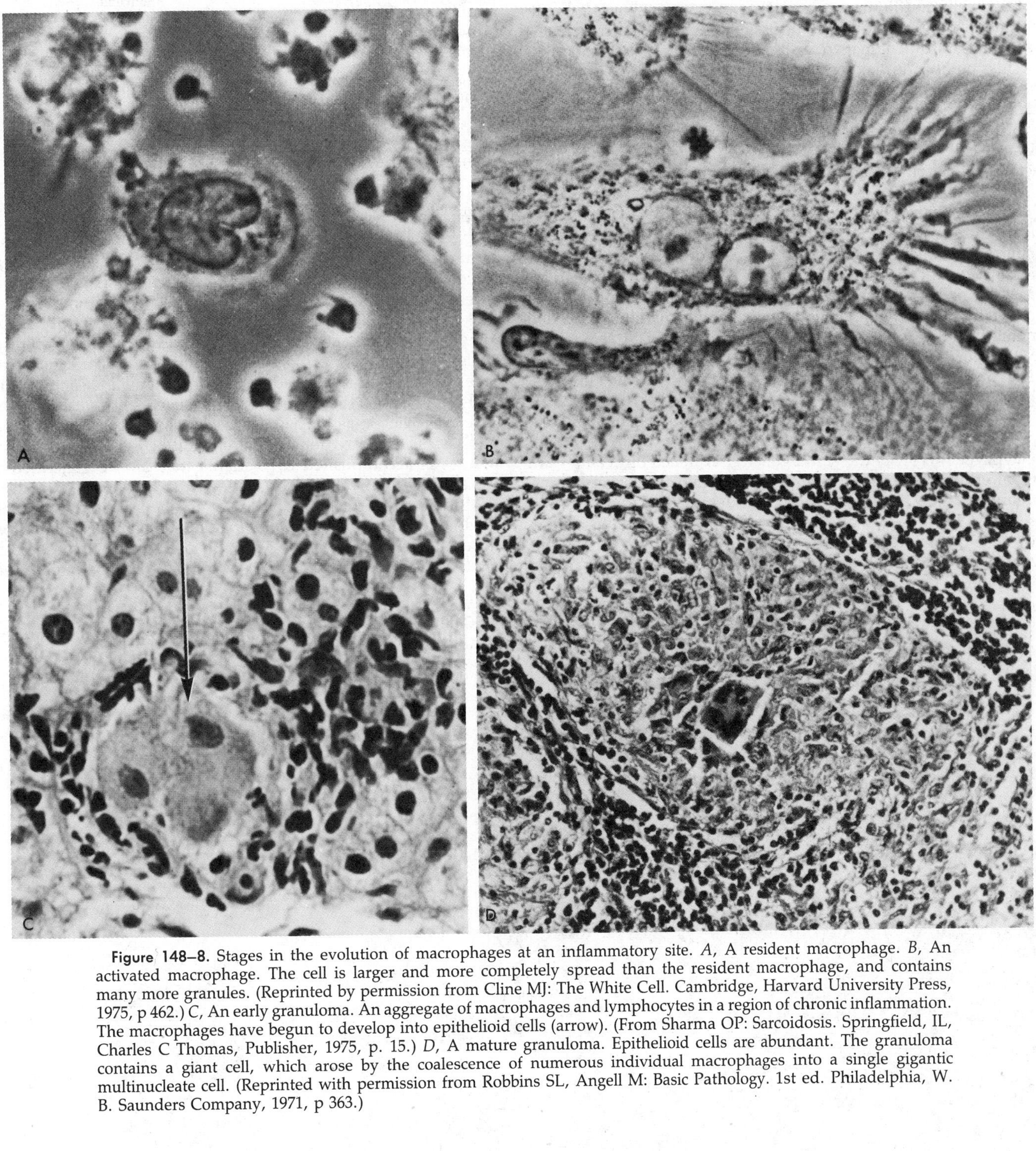

Figure 148–8. Stages in the evolution of macrophages at an inflammatory site. *A*, A resident macrophage. *B*, An activated macrophage. The cell is larger and more completely spread than the resident macrophage, and contains many more granules. (Reprinted by permission from Cline MJ: The White Cell. Cambridge, Harvard University Press, 1975, p 462.) *C*, An early granuloma. An aggregate of macrophages and lymphocytes in a region of chronic inflammation. The macrophages have begun to develop into epithelioid cells (arrow). (From Sharma OP: Sarcoidosis. Springfield, IL, Charles C Thomas, Publisher, 1975, p. 15.) *D*, A mature granuloma. Epithelioid cells are abundant. The granuloma contains a giant cell, which arose by the coalescence of numerous individual macrophages into a single gigantic multinucleate cell. (Reprinted with permission from Robbins SL, Angell M: Basic Pathology. 1st ed. Philadelphia, W. B. Saunders Company, 1971, p 363.)

TABLE 148–3. SUBSTANCES SECRETED BY MACROPHAGES

Substance	State of Macrophage	Additional Stimulus Needed
Lysozyme	Resident, activated	None
Neutral proteases	Activated	None
Collagenase		
Elastase		
Plasminogen activator		
Interleukin 1	Resident, activated	Lymphokine, endotoxin, others
Superoxide	Activated	Contact with particles or appropriate solubles stimulus
Leukotrienes	Resident, activated	(same as above)
Complement components		

described in Ch. 117, while the lipids and complex carbohydrates of the red cell membrane are degraded by lysosomal lipases and glycosidases. Other effete cells are presumably dealt with in a similar manner.

Foreign material is removed from the bloodstream primarily by mononuclear phagocytes in the liver and spleen. In these two organs, the blood is forced to flow past a meshwork of mononuclear phagocytes, which ingest foreign matter encountered in the stream. Bacteria and bacterial breakdown products (e.g., lipopolysaccharide) that enter the bloodstream from the large intestine are removed primarily by the Kupffer cells of the liver, because these are the first mononuclear phagocytes encountered by the gastrointestinal venous drainage.

Dead cells and tissue fragments are presumably ingested and degraded at sites of infection or tissue damage by macrophages recruited to the damaged area. Ingestion may be aided by circulating fibronectin, a plasma protein that is able to opsonize denatured collagen for phagocytosis by macrophages. The activated macrophages secrete into the environment neutral proteases that are able to break down damaged connective tissue (collagenase, elastase) and fibrin mesh (plasminogen activator), clearing the way for the reconstruction of the injured tissues.

Mononuclear phagocytes also eliminate from the circulation denatured proteins, protein fragments, and certain native proteins (for example, activated clotting factors). Protein elimination is accomplished through *pinocytosis*, a process in which the material to be eliminated is taken into the cell along with a miniscule quantity of plasma via a tiny invagination of the cell membrane that buds off and enters the cytoplasm as a pinocytotic vesicle. Pinocytosis is constantly going on in mononuclear phagocytes; these cells take in and process several times their own volume of plasma during the course of a day.

KILLING. Like neutrophils, mononuclear phagocytes are able to kill invading microorganisms. Killing by both types of phagocytes involves the same general sequence of events—an initial encounter between the phagocyte and the target microorganism, ingestion, and finally the destruction of the target (see Fig. 148–4)—but the events differ in detail between the two cell types. Neutrophils, for example, generally find their targets by migrating up a chemotactic gradient, while many mononuclear phagocytes (the fixed tissue varieties such as Kupffer cells and splenic macrophages) have their targets brought to them by the bloodstream. Those mononuclear phagocytes that find their targets by chemotaxis (e.g., monocytes) respond to a wider variety of attractants than neutrophils do. Monocytes, for instance, are attracted by lymphocyte-generated chemotactic factors that have no effect on neutrophils. With respect to ingestion, mononuclear phagocytes can take up particles opsonized by IgE as well as IgG; neutrophils will only take up the latter. Mononuclear phagocytes lose their myeloperoxidase as they develop from monocytes into macrophages, so that oxygen-dependent killing by mature macrophages is accomplished by oxidants that can be generated in the absence of myeloperoxidase (e.g., hydroxyl radical).

TABLE 148–4. INTRACELLULAR PATHOGENS AGAINST WHICH MACROPHAGES PLAY A SPECIAL ROLE

Bacteria	Chlamydiae
Salmonella	Rickettsiae
Brucella	Protozoan parasites
Listeria	Leishmania
Legionella	Trypanosoma
Mycobacteria and systemic fungi	Toxoplasma
M. tuberculosis	
Coccidioides immitis	
Histoplasma capsulatum	
Others	

Mononuclear phagocytes play a particularly important role in defending against nonviral pathogens that live and grow intracellularly (Table 148–4). For the destruction of these pathogens, macrophage activation is critical. The pathogens are

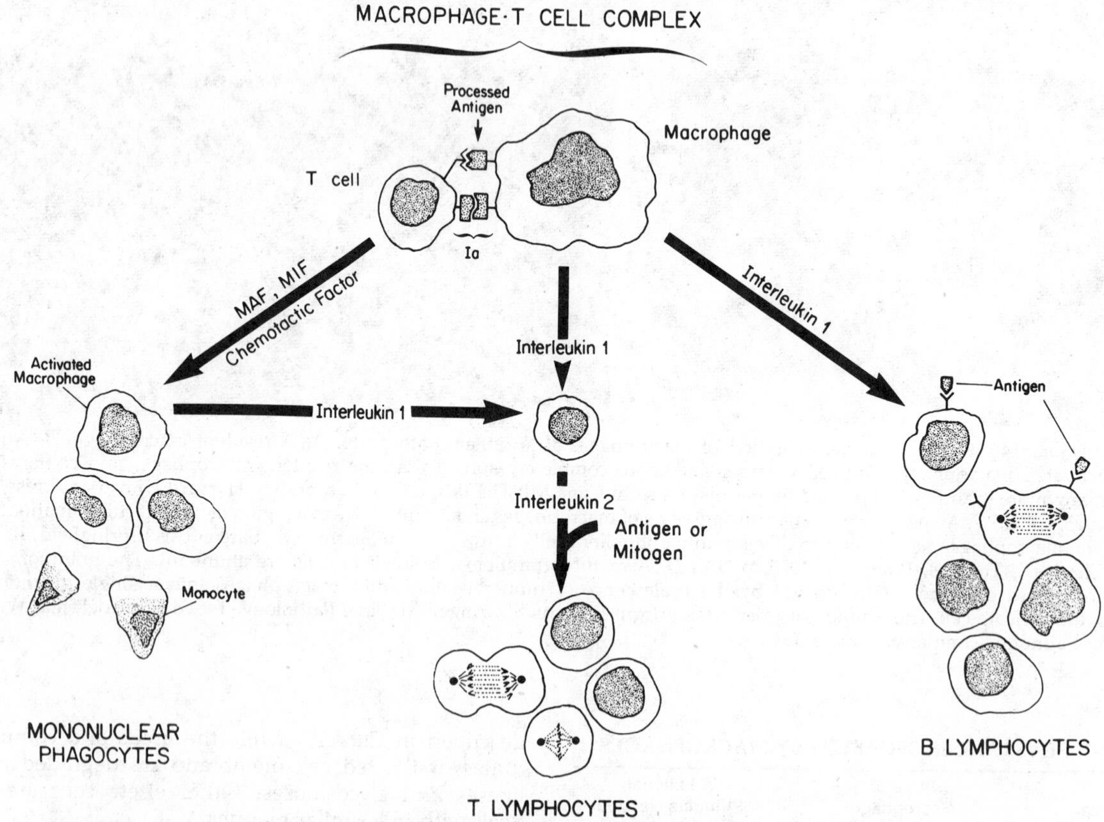

Figure 148–9. Macrophage-lymphocyte interactions. The macrophage, acting in its capacity as an "accessory cell," presents antigen to an Ia-identical T cell that is equipped with specific receptors for the antigen being presented. The T cell to which the antigen has been presented undergoes activation, and begins to secrete lymphokines. These lymphokines include monocyte chemotactic factor, macrophage-immobilizing factor (MIF) and macrophage-activating factor (MAF; ? γ-interferon); they cause macrophages to accumulate and undergo activation at the site of the initial macrophage-T cell interaction. Macrophages so activated secrete interleukin 1, a potent mediator capable among other things of inducing the proliferation of both B and T lymphocytes. B cells are directly stimulated by interleukin 1 to proliferate and to differentiate into antibody-secreting plasma cells. T cells, however, proliferate under the influence of a mediator known as interleukin 2 (T cell growth factor), itself a T cell product; interleukin 1 promotes the proliferation of T lymphocytes indirectly by inducing them to secrete interleukin 2.

readily killed by activated macrophages, but they are able to infect and multiply within unactivated macrophages, eventually killing them and spreading to infect fresh macrophages. Little is known about how the pathogens evade the microbicidal systems of the unactivated macrophages.

Mononuclear phagocytes, particularly activated macrophages, are also able to kill malignant cells in vitro. The extent to which they perform this anti-tumor function in vivo is unknown.

Interactions Between Mononuclear Phagocytes and Lymphocytes. The activation of mononuclear phagocytes by macrophage-activating factor is one of a series of mutually potentiating interactions between mononuclear phagocytes and lymphocytes that take place at sites of inflammation (Fig. 148–9). Both T cells and B cells participate in these interactions.

The interactions with T lymphocytes begin with a particular type of physical encounter between a T cell and a mononuclear phagocyte. When an antigen-bearing particle is ingested by a mononuclear phagocyte, the antigen is for the most part completely destroyed. A small portion of the antigen, however, is retained by the phagocyte, having been processed to a form suitable for "presentation" to a lymphocyte. The state and location of this "presentable" antigen is currently unknown; for purposes of conceptualization, however, it might be regarded as consisting of a few antigen molecules embedded in the outer membrane of the phagocyte with their antigenic determinants projecting outward into the extracellular environment. If a T lymphocyte programmed to respond to these particular antigenic determinants should encounter this antigen-primed mononuclear phagocyte, it will recognize the presence of the antigen on the phagocyte; the phagocyte is said to have "presented" the antigen to the lymphocyte. If in addition the T lymphocyte recognizes that the phagocyte is one of those that carries on its surface the immune response antigen known as "Ia" (the Ia antigen is one of the products of the major histocompatibility complex [see Ch. 436] that controls immune responses to such challenges as foreign proteins, virally infected cells, and tissue allografts), it binds to the phagocyte, and both cells begin to secrete immunologic mediators. Those secreted by the T lymphocytes are called *lymphokines.* They include macrophage activating factor, macrophage inhibitory factor, and monocyte chemotactic factor. Their net effect is to cause the accumulation and activation of mononuclear phagocytes in the region where the initial interaction took place between the antigen-bearing phagocyte and its complementary T lymphocyte. Those secreted by mononuclear phagocytes are known as *monokines.* One of these is called *interleukin 1;* among other effects (for a list, see Table 148–5), it stimulates the proliferation of T lymphocytes indirectly by causing them to secrete *interleukin 2* (also known as *T cell growth factor*), a substance that promotes their own growth.

Macrophages also act upon B lymphocytes. The macrophages are not needed to present antigen to the B lymphocytes, because these lymphocytes carry surface immunoglobulins that directly recognize the antigens against which the cells are programmed. Rather, they exert their effects after the antigen-recognition step. They operate through interleukin 1, which they secrete and which causes the antigen-primed B cells to proliferate and to differentiate into antibody-secreting plasma cells.

The interactions between lymphocytes and mononuclear phagocytes may be summarized as follows:

1. Mononuclear phagocytes activate T lymphocytes by presenting antigen to them. This interaction is highly immunospecific: activation can take place only under two specific circumstances: (1) if the T cell is preprogrammed to respond to the antigen being presented by the mononuclear phagocyte, and (2) if the T cell and the mononuclear phagocyte carry identical Ia antigens on their surfaces. Mononuclear phagocytes acting in this capacity are referred to as *accessory cells.*

2. Activated T lymphocytes cause the accumulation and activation of mononuclear phagocytes. These effects are mediated through lymphokines that are secreted by the activated T cells. In contrast to antigen presentation, this interaction has no immunologic restrictions; lymphokines from a given T cell are able to exert these effects on every mononuclear phagocyte in their vicinity.

3. Macrophages stimulate the proliferation and differentiation of B lymphocytes. This interaction, also immunologically unrestricted, is mediated through the action of interleukin 1.

Antigens also appear to be presented by a newly identified class of cells known as *dendritic cells.* These cells are widely distributed, being found in the follicles of the lymph nodes and spleen, in the thymus, and perhaps in other tissues. Like the antigen-presenting class of mononuclear phagocytes, they carry the Ia antigen on their surfaces. Their role in antigen presentation is not fully worked out; in particular, it is not clear whether they present new antigens or participate only in anamnestic responses and immunologic memory.

TABLE 148–5. SOME ACTIONS OF INTERLEUKIN 1

Site of Action	Effect
T lymphocytes	Secretion of interleukin 2 (T cell growth factor)
B lymphocytes	Proliferation, secretion of immunoglobulins
Hepatocytes	Production of acute-phase reactants
Hypothalamus	Fever
Muscle	Catabolism of protein

Gallin JI, Fauci AS (eds.): Advances in Host Defense Mechanisms, Vol 1. Phagocytic cells. New York, Raven Press, 1982. *An up-to-date compilation of authoritative articles on many aspects of phagocyte function. Neutrophils, eosinophils, and mononuclear phagocytes are discussed.*

Klebanoff SJ, Clark RA: The neutrophil: Function and clinical disorders. Amsterdam, Elsevier/North-Holland Biochemical Press, 1978. *A comprehensive treatise on the neutrophil, containing a detailed discussion of all topics related to neutrophil function. Exhaustively referenced.*

Nathan CF, Murray HW, Cohn ZA: The macrophage as an effector cell. N Engl J Med 303:622, 1980. *A short, well-referenced article on the secretory and killing functions of macrophages.*

Unanue ER: Cooperation between mononuclear phagocytes and lymphocytes in immunity. N Engl J Med 303:977, 1980. *A lucid and concise discussion of the interactions between macrophages and lymphocytes.*

Unanue ER, Beller DI, Lu CY, Allen PM: Antigen presentation: Comments on its regulation and mechanism. J Immunol 132:1, 1984. *A brief but thorough analysis of the current state of the problem.*

Williams GT, Williams WJ: Granulomatous inflammation: A review. J Clin Pathol 36:723, 1983. *An excellent review of the development and function of granulomas.*

149. DISORDERS OF NEUTROPHIL FUNCTION

Bernard M. Babior

Disorders of neutrophil function are relatively common. For the most part, they are minor manifestations of systemic diseases, rarely diagnosed and of little clinical significance. There are a few disorders, however, in which neutrophil function is defective enough to lead to serious clinical problems. Most of these are inherited disorders in which particular elements of neutrophil function are almost totally deficient.

The principal clinical manifestation of a serious disorder of neutrophil function is the repeated occurrence of major bacterial infections in the affected patient. Such recurrent bacterial infections are most commonly associated with severe neutropenia (<500 neutrophils per cu mm) or an abnormality affecting the immunoglobulins or complement components. In an occasional patient, however, repeated bacterial infections cannot be accounted for by abnormalities in the neutrophil count, the immunoglobulins, or the complement system. In such a patient, a qualitative abnormality in neutrophil function is likely to be at the root of the problem.

Evaluating Neutrophil Function

A complete evaluation of neutrophil function, including motility, granule content and function, respiratory burst activity, and bacterial killing, requires the services of a specialized

TABLE 149–1. SCREENING FOR ABNORMALITIES OF NEUTROPHIL FUNCTION

Examination of blood film
Rebuck skin window
NBT test
Special stains: myeloperoxidase, alkaline phosphatase

laboratory. Screening for functional abnormalities, however, can be carried out relatively simply (Table 149–1). Morphologic abnormalities such as the large malformed granules of Chediak-Higashi disease can be detected by *examination of a blood film* under the microscope. Chemotaxis and locomotion can be estimated by means of a *Rebuck skin window*, a test in which the migration of phagocytes onto a glass coverslip applied to a superficial abrasion is measured over time. The respiratory burst is evaluated by the *NBT test*, in which cells attached to a glass slide are activated in the presence of nitroblue tetrazolium (NBT), a dye that precipitates as a mass of deep blue granules onto any cell that is engaged in the production of $O_2^{\overline{\cdot}}$. Neutrophil enzymes can be detected by *special stains for myeloperoxidase and alkaline phosphatase*. One or more of these tests will be abnormal in most symptomatic disorders of neutrophil function.

ACQUIRED DISORDERS

In acquired disorders of neutrophils, functional abnormalities are generally incomplete. Accordingly, signs and symptoms due to neutrophil dysfunction are uncommon in these conditions.

ADHESION (Table 149–2). In the normal course of events, neutrophils undergo frequent alterations in their adhesiveness. These alterations are often expressed as changes in the size of the marginated pool. (Neutrophils in the circulation are found in two separate pools: the *circulating pool*, composed of cells that are suspended in the bloodstream, and the *marginated pool*, containing cells that have settled onto the endothelium of the capillaries and postcapillary venules. Neutrophils exchange freely between these two pools.) *Corticosteroids* and *epinephrine* reduce neutrophil adhesiveness, releasing the cells from the marginated pool into the circulating pool. Conversely, *C5a* or agents that cause the release of C5a (e.g., an episode of gram-negative bacteremia) increase neutrophil adhesiveness, causing cells in the circulation to marginate. C5a also causes neutrophils to aggregate into clumps. These tend to be trapped in small vessels, particularly in the lungs.

Besides corticosteroids and epinephrine, certain drugs, notably *aspirin* and *alcohol*, cause decreased adhesiveness of neutrophils. With these agents, the drop in adhesiveness is apparent on testing in vitro but is not associated with demargination. Evidently, neutrophil adhesiveness covers a broader range of functions than merely the ability to attach to an endothelial cell.

In patients undergoing *hemodialysis*, neutrophil counts fall sharply, rising a few minutes later to values that exceed the predialysis counts. Pulmonary symptoms may accompany these changes in neutrophil counts. The fall in the neutrophil count and the accompanying pulmonary symptoms occur because C5a is released when the complement system is activated by the passage of blood over the dialysis membrane, causing neutrophils to marginate and be trapped in the lungs. The subsequent neutrophilia reflects the release of cells from the marrow storage pool, possibly another effect of complement activation.

TABLE 149–2. ACQUIRED ALTERATIONS OF NEUTROPHIL ADHESIVENESS

Decreased adhesiveness
With demargination
Corticosteroids
Epinephrine
Without demargination
Aspirin
Alcohol
Increased adhesiveness
Bacteremia
Hemodialysis

TABLE 149–3. CONDITIONS ASSOCIATED WITH DEPRESSED NEUTROPHIL CHEMOTAXIS

Diabetes mellitus
Uremia
Cirrhosis of liver
Severe burns
Bacterial infections
Anergy
Hodgkin's disease
Leprosy
Sarcoidosis
Hypophosphatemia
Neonates

CHEMOTAXIS. Depressed neutrophil chemotaxis is seen in a large number of conditions (Table 149–3). In some of these conditions, chemotactic depression is caused by a circulating inhibitor, while in others the neutrophils themselves are defective. These chemotactic abnormalities contribute in only a minor way to the decreased resistance to bacterial infections characteristic of many of these disorders.

MYELOGENOUS LEUKEMIA AND MYELODYSPLASIA. Variable functional abnormalities are seen in neutrophils from patients with these conditions. Cells in *chronic myelogenous leukemia* are very sluggish, showing markedly reduced motility and chemotaxis. Granules are often abnormal in number and type (specific granules, for example, may be absent), the respiratory burst is frequently attenuated, and bacterial killing may be depressed. These cells, however, make up in numbers what they lack in function, so infections are unusual in patients with chronic myelogenous leukemia.

In patients with *acute myelogenous leukemia*, neutrophils may arise from residual normal stem cells or by differentiation of the leukemic clone; in the latter case, the neutrophils may show abnormalities similar to those seen in chronic myelogenous leukemia. *Myelodysplasia* is a disease in which hematopoiesis is taken over by a nonmalignant but defective stem cell that gives rise to inadequate numbers of functionally abnormal blood cells. Bilobed nuclei (pseudo–Pelger-Huët anomaly) and abnormal granulation are typical of myelodysplastic neutrophils. In both acute myelogenous leukemia and myelodysplasia, bacterial infections are frequent, but their frequency is due more to neutropenia than to functional abnormalities of the phagocytes.

CONGENITAL DISORDERS

CHRONIC GRANULOMATOUS DISEASE. Chronic granulomatous disease (CGD) is the name given to a family of inherited disorders in which phagocytes are unable to express a respiratory burst (Ch. 148). Most cases of the disease are transmitted in an X-linked fashion, but a substantial minority have an autosomal recessive pattern of inheritance. The disorder is caused by a gross impairment in the function of the $O_2^{\overline{\cdot}}$-forming NADPH oxidase, whose activity is profoundly reduced in cells from patients with CGD. In some patients, the biochemical lesion responsible for the impairment in oxidase activity is in the enzyme itself, while in other patients the lesion affects the system that activates the enzyme. It has not yet been possible to correlate the biochemical lesion with the mode of inheritance of the disorder.

The clinical picture of CGD is one of recurrent severe bacterial infections that are slow to heal and difficult to treat. The infections include sinusitis, pneumonia, and abscesses that usually involve the deep subcutaneous tissues, lymph nodes, or liver. Infections generally begin in infancy or early childhood, although the disease is occasionally detected only in adolescence or later. In its unmodified form, the course of CGD is characterized by frequent hospitalizations for repeated and protracted infections caused by bacteria that the defective phagocytes are unable to kill (mostly *S. aureus* and enterobacteria), with death from infection occurring in the first or second decade. With chronic antibiotic prophylaxis, however, the course of the disease has changed. Hospitalization is much less frequent and survival seems to be prolonged, but the patients develop serious complications due to imperfectly suppressed infections—strictures of the bladder and GI tract, for example, and chronic lung disease with fibrosis and bronchiectasis. Death often results from infections by fungi, particularly *Aspergillus*.

The diagnosis is made by neutrophil function studies. Most of these are normal, but those that measure the respiratory burst are severely deranged: the NBT test is negative (i.e., few if any cells are stained by formazan precipitates) (Fig. 149–1), and $O_2^{\bar{\cdot}}$ production and other manifestations of the respiratory burst are greatly reduced or absent. Many microorganisms are handled in a normal fashion by CGD neutrophils (including pneumococci and streptococci, accounting for the rarity of pneumococcal and streptococcal infections in CGD patients), but those such as *S. aureus* whose destruction is particularly dependent on oxidant production by phagocytes are poorly killed by these defective cells. In CGD carriers, the size of the respiratory burst is decreased by about half, so suspected carriers can often be diagnosed by quantitation of the burst. Female carriers of X-linked CGD are particularly easy to detect: because these carriers are mosaics, only a fraction of their neutrophils are able to make $O_2^{\bar{\cdot}}$; the NBT test stains only that fraction, leaving the rest of the cells unstained.

Management of CGD consists of chronic prophylaxis (trimethoprim-sulfamethoxazole at a trimethoprim dose of 5 to 10 mg per kilogram per day is satisfactory) and vigorous treatment of acute infections with antibiotics in adequate doses plus surgery if indicated. Leukocyte transfusions may be helpful. Complications should be treated as conservatively as possible, although surgery may be required. Bone marrow transplantation has been performed in a few instances, but with its widely known hazards and the improvement in the outlook of CGD resulting from the use of chronic prophylaxis, marrow transplantation must be regarded as a last resort. Families of CGD patients should be investigated to ascertain the mode of transmission of the disease, and genetic counseling should be offered to them. In pregnant carriers, CGD may be diagnosed prenatally through NBT tests of fetal blood.

A picture similar to CGD has been seen in a few patients with exceptionally severe *glucose-6-phosphate dehydrogenase (G-6-PD) deficiency*. G-6-PD is essential for the production of NADPH, the reducing agent used by the $O_2^{\bar{\cdot}}$-forming oxidase. In neutrophils that are severely deficient in G-6-PD, the levels of NADPH may be so low that the $O_2^{\bar{\cdot}}$-forming oxidase is starved for substrate, so the cells cannot express an adequate respiratory burst.

CHEDIAK-HIGASHI DISEASE. Chediak-Higashi disease is an autosomally inherited defect in the production of lysosomes, the membrane-enclosed granular organelles that are found in almost every type of cell. Normally, these organelles are oval bodies of relatively uniform size, but in Chediak-Higashi disease they are very irregular both in size and shape, ranging from tiny spheres to huge malformed bodies many times larger than normal. The molecular lesion responsible for Chediak-Higashi disease is unknown, although there is some evidence that the condition may result from an abnormality in microtubule function.

The clinical features of Chediak-Higashi disease result from the malfunction of three types of lysosome-containing cells: the melanocytes, the platelets, and the phagocytes. Melanocyte dysfunction leads to *partial albinism*, a uniform but incomplete loss of pigment from the irises, skin, and hair that can be detected even at birth. The platelet defect causes a *mild bleeding disorder* associated with a prolonged bleeding time. The most serious clinical problems, however, are caused by the abnormalities in the phagocytes. These lead to a *marked lowering of resistance to bacterial infections*, so that Chediak-Higashi patients suffer from frequent deep tissue abscesses as well as recurrent attacks of severe bacterial sinusitis and pneumonia. These infections are difficult to treat and often lead to death in the first or second decade.

Chediak-Higashi patients who survive into their teens or later are confronted with a further clinical problem, probably the most serious of all. In most of these patients, the disease

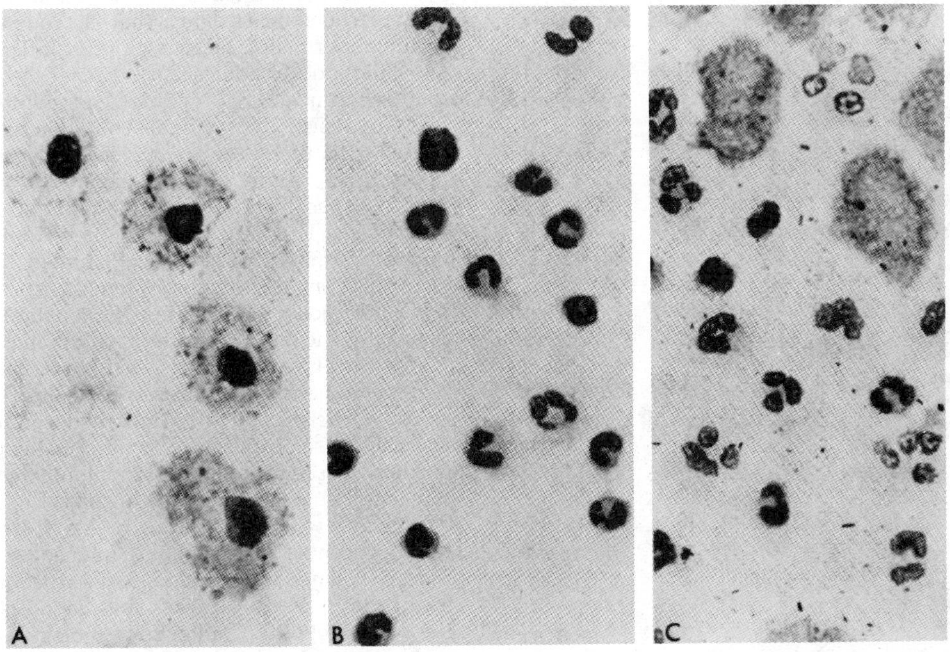

Figure 149–1. The NBT test in CGD. Left, normal; center, CGD; right, carrier of x-linked CGD, showing an NBT positive and an NBT negative population of neutrophils. (Reprinted with permission from Babior BM, Crawley CA: Chronic granulomatous disease and other disorders of oxidative killing by phagocytes. *In* Stanbury JB, Wyngaarden JB, Frederickson DS, Goldstein JL, Brown MS [eds.]: The Metabolic Basis of Inherited Disease. 5th ed. New York, McGraw-Hill Book Company, p 1956.)

ultimately evolves into a fatal form known as the "accelerated phase." This is a peculiar lymphoma-like illness in which the lymph nodes, liver, spleen, and bone marrow become infiltrated with small lymphocytes recently identified as T cells. The lymphocytes look perfectly benign but they behave in a malignant fashion, causing the infiltrated organs to enlarge and producing through marrow infiltration and splenomegaly a rapid, relentless, and ultimately fatal progression of the mild pancytopenia seen in the stable phase of the disease. Death from pancytopenia generally occurs within a few months after the onset of the accelerated phase.

In Chediak-Higashi disease, the WBC count is typically low (2,000 to 3,000 per cubic millimeter), a result of ineffective granulopoiesis (destruction of granulocytes before they leave the marrow). The low white count is an important factor in the low resistance to infection that characterizes this condition. Neutrophil chemotaxis and degranulation are depressed, but phagocytosis and the respiratory burst are normal. Bacterial killing is defective, probably because the abnormality in degranulation impedes the delivery of microbicidal substances into the phagocytic vesicles. The *diagnosis* is made by demonstrating under the microscope the presence of giant granules (lysosomes) in neutrophils and eosinophils, a feature that is virtually pathognomonic of Chediak-Higashi disease (Fig. 149–2). The diagnosis of the accelerated phase depends on finding the characteristic lymphocytic infiltrate in a biopsy of the involved tissue.

The management of the early stage of Chediak-Higashi disease amounts to the management of the infectious complications. Prophylactic antibiotics (trimethoprim-sulfamethoxazole at the dose given previously) should be used, and infections should be treated vigorously with appropriate antibiotic therapy. Ascorbic acid (20 mg per kilogram per day) has corrected the microbicidal defect in some but not all patients with Chediak-Higashi disease. Treatment of the accelerated phase is unsatisfactory; splenectomy has been tried, as has chemotherapy with a variety of agents, but neither has proved to be of any benefit. Marrow transplantation has also been used in Chediak-Higashi disease, though the indications for transplantation (for example, the question of transplantation in early childhood as opposed to transplantation for the accelerated phase) are not yet clearly established.

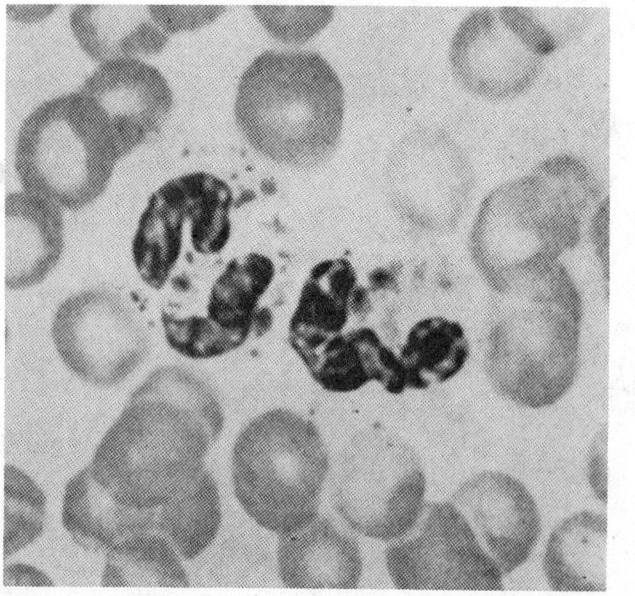

Figure 149–2. Neutrophils in Chediak-Higashi disease, showing the giant granules that are the hallmark of the disease. (Reprinted with permission from Windhorst DB, Zelickson AS, Good RA: Chediak-Higashi syndrome hereditary gigantism of cytoplasmic organelles. Science 151:81–83, 1966.)

TABLE 149–4. DISORDERS OF NEUTROPHIL MOBILITY

Disorder	Distinguishing Features
Job's syndrome	Cold abscesses Eosinophilia Greatly increased IgE
Juvenile periodontitis	Early severe gingival inflammation Systemic infections only in occasional patients
Mo1 deficiency	Omphalitis or other infections in newborn Leukemoid reactions
Congenital absence of specific granules	Abnormal segmentation of nucleus Alkaline phosphatase decreased or absent

DISORDERS OF NEUTROPHIL MOBILITY (Table 149–4). There are a number of conditions in which recurrent abscesses or other bacterial infections occur because of a severe impairment in neutrophil mobility. Neutrophils from affected patients migrate poorly onto a glass coverslip in the Rebuck skin window test and show grossly impaired chemotaxis when tested in vitro. These disorders are thought to be inherited, although evidence for their heritability is often weak. For most of them (e.g., congenital actin dysfunction, congenitally increased microtubule assembly), only one or two cases have been reported. A few, however, have been seen in several patients. These will be discussed here.

Job's Syndrome. This is a condition in which reduced neutrophil motility is associated with bacterial respiratory tract infections and cold staphylococcal abscesses (i.e., abscesses lacking much of the swelling and redness associated with inflammation), eosinophilia, and greatly increased levels of IgE. Patients characteristically have very high blood levels of an antistaphylococcal IgE antibody. Neutrophils from these patients show greatly reduced chemotaxis if assayed immediately after isolation, but chemotaxis returns to normal if the cells are stored for a few hours in the absence of serum prior to assay. This finding suggests that the abnormality lies in the serum, not the cells. The nature of the abnormality is unknown, although a monocyte-derived chemotactic inhibitor has been suggested as the cause of the condition.

Juvenile Periodontitis. In this familial disease neutrophils show a chemotactic defect that is thought to be caused by a serum abnormality. Serious gingival inflammation develops in late childhood or adolescence, similar to but more severe than that seen in normal middle-aged adults with poor dental hygiene. Affected individuals will often have lost many of their teeth by the time they are 30 years old. Among the organisms infecting the gums of such patients is Capnocytophaga, an anaerobic bacillus that secretes a potent inhibitor of neutrophil chemotaxis. This antichemotactic agent enters the bloodstream, where in a few patients with juvenile periodontitis it reaches concentrations that impair systemic host defenses and result in repeated bacterial infections. Elimination of the Capnocytophaga by means of long-term antibiotics and vigorous local therapy will correct the impairment in host defenses and normalize the patient's resistance against bacterial infections.

Mo1 Deficiency. In this inherited condition, a chemotactic defect is caused by absence or abnormality of Mo1, a membrane glycoprotein required for a normal interaction between neutrophils and surfaces. Patients are subject to recurrent infections, particularly with *Pseudomonas*. The first infection may occur in the newborn as an omphalitis. Infections are generally accompanied by a neutrophilic leukemoid reaction in which the white count may exceed 100,000. The diagnosis can be made with the Mo1 antibody (Coulter Immunology), which binds to normal but not Mo1-deficient white cells. Vigorous and prolonged therapy is necessary for successful treatment of infections in Mo1 deficiency. Prophylactic antibodies are indicated in this condition; they maintain the patient's health and keep the white count at normal or near normal levels.

Congenital Absence of Specific Granules. In this disorder a chemotactic defect results in recurrent severe bacterial infections. The neutrophils show abnormalities in nuclear segmentation, most frequently a bilobed nucleus (the Pelger-Huët anomaly), and stain poorly or not at all for alkaline phosphatase. Proteins located in the specific granules (e.g., cobalamin-binding protein) are absent from the neutrophils, and bacterial killing is impaired. Under the electron microscope, the neutrophils show normal numbers of azurophil granules, but specific granules are rare or absent.

MYELOPEROXIDASE DEFICIENCY. Deficiency of myeloperoxidase (MPO) is the commonest of the inherited disorders of neutrophil function. Transmitted as an autosomal recessive trait, it is estimated to affect one person in 500, indicating that nearly one person in ten is a heterozygous carrier. Once thought to be quite rare, its true incidence was revealed through the use of automated white cell differential counters that rely on the peroxidase stain to identify neutrophils. Investigations of blood samples reported by these counters to contain high percentages of "large unidentified white blood cells" revealed that most were from patients with unsuspected MPO deficiency.

Clinically, MPO deficiency is almost completely silent. The only problem that can be attributed to it is an increase in the severity of *Candida* infections seen in a few MPO-deficient patients with coincident diabetes mellitus. The original misconception about the incidence of MPO deficiency can probably be explained by the very low incidence of clinical disease in patients with this condition.

MPO-deficient neutrophils show characteristic functional abnormalities. Chemotaxis, phagocytosis, and degranulation are normal, but the respiratory burst is prolonged because of an increase in the survival of the $O_2^{\bar{}}$-forming oxidase, which is normally destroyed by a myeloperoxidase-dependent process during the course of the respiratory burst. Bacterial killing by MPO-deficient cells is delayed, but eventually reaches completion, indicating that the myeloperoxidase-independent oxidants generated by the deficient cells kill more slowly but just as effectively as the myeloperoxidase-dependent oxidants of normal cells. The completeness of bacterial killing by MPO-deficient cells contrasts with the extensive failure of bacterial killing in CGD, and explains why bacterial infections are such a serious problem in the latter but not the former condition.

The diagnosis is made from a peroxidase stain of the blood film. This stain normally shows activity in three types of cells: neutrophils, monocytes, and eosinophils. In MPO deficiency, the activity is missing from neutrophils and monocytes. Eosinophils, however, stain normally, since their peroxidase is different from the myeloperoxidase found in neutrophils and monocytes and is not affected in myeloperoxidase deficiency. Peroxidase levels can be quantitated spectrophotometrically if desired, but this is usually unnecessary.

No treatment is required for MPO deficiency.

Babior BM, Crowley CA: Chronic granulomatous disease and other disorders of oxidative killing by phagocytes. *In* Stanbury JB, et al. (eds.): The Metabolic Basis of Inherited Disease. 5th ed. New York, McGraw-Hill Book Company, 1983, pp 1956–1985. *A recent review on disorders of oxygen-dependent killing by neutrophils, including CGD, MPO deficiency, and others.*

Boogaerts MA, Nelissen V, Roelant C, Goossens W: Blood neutrophil function in primary myelodysplastic syndromes. Br J Haematol 55:217, 1983. *A thorough study of neutrophil dysfunction in myelodysplasia.*

Dana N, Todd RF III, Pitt J, Springer TA, Arnaout MA: Deficiency of a surface membrane glycoprotein (Mo1) in man. J Clin Invest 73:153, 1984. *An important study of this newly recognized disease.*

Donabedian H, Gallin JI: The hyperimmunoglobulin E recurrent infection (Job's) syndrome. A review of the NIH experience and the literature. Medicine 62:195, 1983. *A detailed clinical study of Job's syndrome.*

Gallin JI, Wright DG, Malech HL, David JM, Klempner MS, Kirkpatrick CH: Disorders of phagocyte chemotaxis. Ann Intern Med 92:520, 1980. *A brief survey of conditions associated with defective neutrophil chemotaxis and motility.*

Gallin JI, Fauci AS (eds.): Advances in Host Defense Mechanisms. Vol 1. Phagocytic Cells. New York, Raven Press, 1982. *A multiauthor volume containing several chapters on various abnormalities of neutrophil function.*

Goldman JM, Catovsky D: The function of phagocytic leucocytes in leukemia. Br J Haematol 23 (Suppl):223, 1972. *A description of the functional abnormalities in neutrophils from patients with acute and chronic myelogenous leukemia.*

Klebanoff SJ, Clark RA: The Neutrophil: Function and Clinical Disorders. Amsterdam, Elsevier/North-Holland Biochemical Press, 1978. *This comprehensive treatise includes detailed discussions on many abnormalities of neutrophil function. Separate chapters are devoted to CGD, MPO deficiency, and Chediak-Higashi disease. Exhaustively referenced.*

Rebuck JW, Crowley JH: A method for studying leukocyte function in vivo. Ann NY Acad Sci 59:759, 1955. *How to perform and interpret the Rebuck skin window test.*

Wolff SM, Dale DC, Clark RA, Root RK, Kimball HR: The Chediak-Higashi syndrome: Studies of host defenses. Ann Intern Med 76:293, 1972. *A discussion of Chediak-Higashi disease emphasizing the abnormalities in neutrophil function seen in this condition.*

150. THE LEUKOPENIC STATE

Dane R. Boggs

Leukopenia is a reduction in the total number of leukocytes in the blood, usually to less than 4.0×10^9 per liter. It is a laboratory observation of little diagnostic significance unless absolute numbers of specific types of cells are calculated from an accompanying differential cell count. Each of the leukocytes (neutrophils, lymphocytes, monocytes, eosinophils, and basophils) constitutes a separate and distinct system (systems, in the case of lymphocytes) with respect to function and to control of production and distribution. Since neutrophils are the most common blood leukocyte, leukopenia usually reflects neutropenia. Neutropenia may be an isolated finding or may be accompanied by lymphopenia and/or decreased numbers of other leukocytes, particularly in patients with aplastic anemia. Lymphopenia may occur as an isolated finding but usually does not result in leukopenia. Reduced numbers of monocytes, eosinophils, or basophils may be observed in certain conditions, but such reduction usually is not detected in "routine" laboratory examination, for when the usual 100-cell differential count is employed, failure to observe one of any of these cells is within the normal distributional error of the count.

NEUTROPENIA

The lower normal limit for neutrophil concentration in the blood of whites is approximately 2.0×10^9 per liter. In blacks it is somewhat lower, approximately 1.5×10^9 per liter. Normal values for other leukocytes as well as for red cells and platelets apparently are similar in the two groups.

KINETICS OF NEUTROPHILS. The production of neutrophils is limited to the bone marrow of normal postnatal man. They are released into the blood for a brief sojourn from which they enter tissues and body cavities or areas of inflammation.

The *marrow compartment* can be divided into a proliferative (mitotic) compartment and a postmitotic compartment. As with any cellular system in which cells are regularly lost, a stem cell is a necessary component of cell renewal. Normal hematopoietic stem cells (HSC) must have two essential characteristics: ability to divide and reproduce themselves (self-replication), and ability to differentiate into mature blood cells. The ultimate HSC is totipotent for all blood cells, including lymphocytes (see Ch. 130). Leukocytes are ordinarily produced from stem cells that are descendants of the totipotent cell but of more restricted pluripotency. The cell that produces colonies of neutrophils and monocytes in vitro in semisolid media (CFUnm) is the prime candidate for the immediate HSC for neutrophils. This is probably a true stem cell, although evidence for self-replication is indirect. The CFUnm requires colony-stimulating factor (see below) to initiate and sustain growth of the colony.

The morphologically recognized mitotic compartment is divided into myeloblasts, promyelocytes, and myelocytes. The promyelocyte stage is defined by the synthesis of primary granules, peroxidase-positive lysosomes. The myelocyte stage is recognized by the synthesis of secondary granules and by the nucleolus becoming inapparent under light microscopy. Cells in the mitotic compartment undergo approximately five multiplicative divisions over five days. Thus for each myeloblast produced from the stem cell compartment, approximately 32 maturing cells emerge five days later.

When the metamyelocyte stage is reached, cell division ceases and maturation proceeds through the band stage, culminating in the segmented neutrophil (seg). Bands and segs are released readily to the blood, although segs are released preferentially. Release of more than an occasional cell less mature than bands is unusual unless there is intrinsic disease of the bone marrow. Therefore the compartment of bands and segs constitutes the marrow neutrophil reserve, which is called upon to supply an increased demand for blood neutrophils prior to an increase in neutrophil production. The transit time through the postmitotic compartment normally is six to ten days, so that the time from the myeloblast stage to emergence into the blood of a segmented neutrophil is about two weeks. However, under conditions of extreme demand for neutrophils, this transit time can be reduced to four to five days.

The *blood compartment* is a rapid-transit, one-way street for neutrophils. The average time spent in the blood is but ten hours, and loss from the blood is in a random fashion; that is, a neutrophil that has just entered the blood from the marrow is as likely to leave it as one that has been in circulation for some time. The major site for egress from the blood is unknown. Approximately half the neutrophils in the blood are not circulating freely but are stuck to or rolling along the walls of capillaries or postcapillary venules (marginated neutrophils). Thus the blood compartment is divided into two pools, the circulating and the marginal pool, but exchange between the two can be almost instantaneous.

Systems regulating the rate of production and the distribution of neutrophils are incompletely understood. The prime candidate for a major regulator of production is the family of glycoproteins called *colony-stimulating factor* (Ch. 151). These are necessary for the growth of neutrophil colonies in vitro in semisolid media and for their growth in liquid culture. A role for an inhibitor in controlling production has been suggested in certain studies and excessive numbers of mature neutrophils can be shown to be inhibitory in certain in vitro circumstances. If neutropenia is induced in man or in other experimental animals, the rate of release of mature cells from the marrow storage pool to the blood is rapidly accelerated. This is mediated by an increase in the concentration of *neutrophil-releasing factor* in plasma. Releasing factor probably has no direct effect upon the rate of production. Thus it seems likely that regulation of this system is more complex than erythroid regulation by erythropoietin.

Etiology. Neutropenia can accompany many diseases, can be produced by a variety of drugs, or can occur as a congenital or an idiopathic acquired syndrome (Table 150–1). It can result from one or a combination of four kinetic mechanisms: (1) decrease in the size of the production pool; (2) ineffective production with cell death in the marrow; (3) shift or "pseudo" neutropenia, in which the circulating pool is depleted but the marginal pool is within normal limits, giving a total blood pool within the lower limits of normal; or (4) an increased rate of loss of blood neutrophils, to the point that the marrow cannot compensate by an increase in production (Fig. 150–1).

Neutropenia Induced by Drugs or Physical Agents. This is the most common cause of neutropenia. It is predictably produced by certain drugs (or physical agents such as x-irradiation), most notably those used in cancer chemotherapy, and occurs unpredictably and idiosyncratically in occasional patients exposed to any of more than 100 different drugs. The dose-related marrow toxins interfere with cell production in general, so in many instances neutropenia is accompanied by other cytopenias.

Idiosyncratic neutropenic reactions to drugs may be the result of decreased production or increased destruction. *Chlorpromazine* and related compounds decrease production; amidopyrine* can be considered the index drug producing increased destruction of blood neutrophils. Two different forms of production defects may be induced in occasional (perhaps 1 in 1200) patients exposed to chlorpromazine. In one form blood neutrophils suddenly disappear, and examination of the marrow reveals an absence of recognizable precursors. When the drug is stopped, neutrophil production is resumed within a day or two, suggesting that the stem cell system was not affected. Reexposure to the drug results in almost immediate loss of cell production, but in most instances closely related phenothiazines do not produce the syndrome. In other patients, a mild degree of neutropenia develops, and examination of bone marrow in such patients indicates that production is decreased but not abolished. If the drug is continued at the same dosage, neutropenia persists but usually does not worsen. If the dosage is increased, neutropenia may become more severe, and when the drug is stopped many weeks may pass before blood neutrophils gradually return to normal. In many instances closely related phenothiazines also produce neutropenia. If the use of chlorpromazine or related compounds is clearly indicated, the latter form of neutropenia is not a contraindication for their use, although blood counts should be monitored frequently after neutropenia is detected. There is evidence to suggest that patients who develop neutropenia in response to chlorpromazine have an innate abnormality in DNA synthesis in neutrophil precursors.

*Amidopyrine** (and other drugs such as sulfonamides) may act

*Not commercially available in the United States.

TABLE 150–1. CAUSES OF NEUTROPENIA

Decreased production
1. Congenital
   a. Dominantly inherited—reduced feed-in from stem cells
   b. Recessively inherited (Kostmann's syndrome)—increased feed-in from stem cells but either cell death or "maturation arrest" beyond the promyelocytic stage
   c. Cyclic—cyclic variation in feed-in from stem cells, so that blood neutrophils "cycle" from normal to ± zero levels every 21 days
2. Drug induced
   a. Cytotoxic therapy or accidental exposure—all dividing cells or even resting stem cells may be damaged and/or killed
   b. Idiosyncratic—an occasional patient develops neutropenia (often severe) due to loss of neutrophil precursors at doses that have no effect in most patients
3. Associated with other diseases
   a. Acute leukemias—(?) leukemic stem cell is recognized by the normal control mechanisms as if it were a normal cell, and stem cell output declines (?)
   b. Vitamin B_{12} and folate deficiency—number of neutrophil precursors in the marrow is actually increased, but they die in the marrow (ineffective hematopoiesis)

Increased destruction (loss of neutrophils from blood)
1. Immune mediated
   a. Idiopathic—antineutrophil antibody coats the neutrophil so that it is phagocytosed by macrophages
   b. Drug induced
      (1) Hapten type—drug as antigen induces antibody that crossreacts with neutrophils
      (2) "Accidental passenger"—antibody is to drug but drug binds to neutrophil so antibody also affects neutrophil
   c. Associated with other diseases
      (1) Felty's syndrome—antibody develops that may also react with marrow precursors as well as with blood neutrophils, so production is highly variable
2. Severe pyogenic infection

Pseudoneutropenia (shift from circulating to marginal pool)

Reduced release from marrow (production and size of the storage pool are normal or increased)

Congenital diseases in which the mature neutrophil seems functionally abnormal, termed "myelokathexis" and "lazy leukocyte syndrome"; the latter has also been reported as an acquired disease

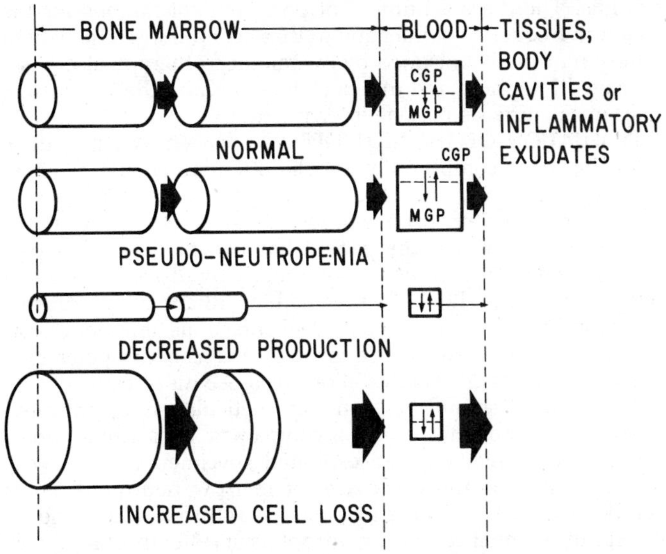

Figure 150–1. Kinetic mechanisms of neutropenia. The bone marrow is illustrated as two tubes, indicating first in, first out cellular systems. The first tube is the mitotic compartment (myeloblasts, promyelocytes and myelocytes) which is fed by a stem cell compartment and in turn feeds into a second tube, the nonmitotic maturation (metamyelocytes and bands) and storage (bands and segmented neutrophils) compartment. The blood is a square, indicating a random cell loss system, and is divided into circulating (CGP) and marginated (MGP) pools. Decreased production is illustrated as an actual decrease in size of the mitotic pool but may also be the result of "ineffective granulocytopoiesis" in which case the production pool may be increased in size but intramedullary cell death occurs.

as a hapten and its use lead to formation of antineutrophil antibodies. When such patients recover, a single dose of amidopyrine eliminates blood neutrophils in a few hours and the plasma of such neutropenic patients produces neutropenia when infused into normal subjects. An antibody may be active against the drug and the drug may attach to the neutrophil, which is then attacked as an "innocent bystander." Marrow examination in patients with antibody-induced neutropenia may or may not reveal an increased production pool.

Sudden and transient increase in the ratio of marginated to circulating neutrophils resulting in "pseudo" neutropenia develops during the early phase of hemodialysis as well as in other instances in which blood is exposed to cellophane or various plastics. This is the result of activation of the C5a des-Arg component of complement, which in turn produces reversible aggregation and increased adhesion of neutrophils. Affected neutrophils marginate in the lungs, the site of the first capillary bed that they encounter, and neutropenia is the result. The neutropenia persists for less than an hour.

Neutropenia Associated with Various Diseases. A wide spectrum of diseases result in neutropenia, but only a few will be discussed as examples of various mechanisms: the acute leukemias, infections, rheumatoid arthritis, vitamin B_{12} deficiency, and congestive splenomegaly with cirrhosis of the liver.

Acute leukemias are almost always associated with neutropenia at diagnosis, as well as with anemia and thrombocytopenia, and this represents decreased normal cell production. It seems likely that production from the stem cell compartment is reduced owing to faulty recognition of the leukemic compartment as if it were an expanded normal stem cell compartment. In acute myeloblastic or promyelocytic leukemia there is increased production of those precursors by the leukemic stem cell clone, but only a few are able to mature into segs, and even these are functionally abnormal.

Infections may induce neutropenia by several different mechanisms. While neutrophilia is anticipated with pneumococcal pneumonia, otherwise normal patients with extensive disease may develop neutropenia. This represents utilization of so many neutrophils in the pneumonic exudate that the marrow reserve is exhausted, and this has long been recognized as a grave prognostic sign. Neutropenia secondary to loss of cells in infected areas obviously is much more common in patients with underlying disease of the marrow and a reduced marrow neutrophil reserve than in otherwise normal patients. Mild neutropenia is a common finding in typhoid fever but is not indicative of a poor prognosis. Mild neutropenia is common with malaria, dengue, yellow fever, and a variety of viral infections such as measles, influenza, and infectious mononucleosis. The kinetic mechanism has not been studied in most circumstances, but in malaria it is a "pseudo" neutropenia resulting from an increase in the marginal–circulating pool ratio.

Rheumatoid arthritis may occasionally be associated with splenomegaly and severe neutropenia (*Felty's syndrome*). Antineutrophil antibodies are demonstrable in most such patients. The kinetic pattern leading to neutropenia is highly variable. Rate of loss of blood neutrophils is accelerated but the marrow mitotic pool size varies from less than normal to 10 times normal. Splenectomy may or may not be beneficial but can be tried, especially if the patient has experienced a severe infection, and may be more likely to prove of benefit if normal or increased neutrophil production is present as compared to decreased production.

Deficiency of vitamin B_{12} *or folic acid* often is associated with neutropenia. This is due to ineffective neutrophil production in which the marrow production pool is increased in size but intramedullary cell death is occurring. The mature cells produced are abnormally large and hypersegmented, and in B_{12} (not in folic acid) deficiency they have defective bactericidal capacity.

Congestive splenomegaly, as occurs secondary to cirrhosis of the liver, may produce neutropenia as well as anemia and thrombocytopenia. This appears to be secondary to neutrophil sequestration or destruction in the abnormal spleen. Blood neutrophil turnover rate is markedly accelerated, and the marrow mitotic pool is increased in size. Splenectomy eliminates neutropenia but is almost never indicated for this purpose. Under ordinary circumstances the spleen is not an important site of neutrophil destruction, so why it should become so when congested is unclear. The congested spleen produces anemia and thrombocytopenia primarily by sequestering the cells without much increase in their rate of destruction.

Congenital Neutropenia. More than 12 separate types of congenital neutropenia can be distinguished. Probably the most common is a transient neonatal neutropenia caused by placental passage of maternal antibody directed against fetal neutrophils. This occurs when the mother has been exposed to neutrophils of the antigenic type of the fetus (different from her own) during a previous pregnancy or by transfusion. There are at least three forms of dominantly inherited neutropenia, but all three are usually benign and rarely lead to life-threatening infection.

Kostmann's neutropenia, possibly inherited as a recessive trait in some patients, is a severe disorder with neutrophils virtually absent from the blood. Marrow CFUnm is increased, as are myeloblasts and promyelocytes, but more mature cells are reduced markedly. Some but not all patients can transiently produce mature cells in response to severe infection. Whether the defect is one of true maturation arrest at the promyelocyte stage or of intramedullary destruction of maturing neutrophils is unknown. Most patients die of infection before reaching adulthood. This probably is a disease of hematopoietic stem cells, since one patient has been cured by allogeneic marrow transplantation.

Chronic benign neutropenia is a seemingly nonfamilial, congenital neutropenia. It may be due to increased peripheral destruction of neutrophils, since marrow production pools and CFUnm are increased. Neutropenia with excessive numbers of segmented neutrophils in the marrow but with a defect in release of cells has been termed *myelocathexis* when the mature neutrophils in the marrow were morphologically abnormal and *lazy leukocyte syndrome* when they appeared normal.

Cyclic neutropenia has been present at birth as a familial or sporadic occurrence. Neutrophils decline to near 0 in the blood every three weeks, and then return to normal levels within a few days. Monocytes, platelets, and reticulocytes cycle also, although not in phase with the neutrophils, and the cycling of blood cells reflects cyclical changes in production. Severe infections may accompany the neutrophil nadir, but most patients survive these if vigorously treated until the neutrophils reappear. Such cyclic hematopoiesis probably is due to a defective stem cell; the disease has been transmitted by allogeneic marrow transplantation in humans and dogs. Very rarely congenital neutropenia may be a "pseudo" neutropenia. Congenital neutropenia in association with pancreatic insufficiency has been reported, as has severe neutropenia associated with severe combined immunologic deficiency.

Other Forms of Neutropenia. Neutropenia can develop at any age as an isolated blood abnormality unassociated with any apparent underlying disease or toxic exposure. In certain patients isolated neutropenia is due to decreased production and mimics the most common form of dominantly inherited neutropenia almost exactly. In some of these it may be inherited but not detected before adulthood. In other patients, the production pool is expanded and CFU nm is increased, suggesting that neutropenia might be due to increased destruction of cells. Antineutrophil autoantibodies have been detected in some patients with neutropenia associated with increased destruction.

CLINICAL MANIFESTATIONS. *Infections* and *oral ulceration* are the only manifestations that can be attributed to neutropenia in most instances. However, when neutropenia is of very sudden onset and due to rapid destruction of cells, as with amidopyrine sensitivity, severe but transient chills, fever, and malaise may be present in the absence of infection. The most commonly infected sites are the *lungs*, the *oropharyngeal cavity*, and the *perianal area*. In general, the infecting organisms are those that commonly produce acute bacterial infections, but there are certain special features of infection in neutropenic patients. Infection is often more virulent once it begins in patients with neutropenia than in normal persons. The absence of infection-localizing properties of the neutrophil may result in septicemia within a few hours of the onset of a seemingly minor infection. Furthermore, septicemia in which there is no demonstrable portal of entry is not uncommon. Poor localization can change the characteristic appearance of infections so that staphylococcal skin infections may mimic erysipelas rather than appearing as furuncles. Pneumonic infiltrates may not appear as dense as usual owing to reduced neutrophil exudation. Pyelonephritis may not be recognized, because the usual clue of increased urinary neutrophils may be absent. Mouth ulcers are somewhat mysterious as to their cause. In most instances culture of these lesions does not suggest an infectious cause, and they are much more common with some syndromes such as cyclic neutropenia than with others such as Felty's syndrome.

The frequency and severity of infection vary remarkably among the various types of neutropenia and correlate poorly at best with the severity of neutropenia. However, within any type of neutropenia, life-threatening infections usually are found in patients with less than 0.5×10^9 neutrophils per liter. Ancillary abnormalities undoubtedly contribute to the liability to infections associated with neutropenia. For example, when blood neutrophils are virtually absent secondary to vigorous cancer chemotherapy, the majority of patients will become infected unless neutrophils recover within two weeks. On the other hand, it is not unusual for a patient with Felty's syndrome or with severe congenital neutropenia to remain uninfected for months and sometimes for years with virtually no blood neutrophils. There are a number of possible explanations for the different frequency of infection in these conditions. The patient whose marrow is poisoned by cancer chemotherapy also has a damaged lymphoid and monocyte system, and the integrity of his serosal surfaces may be interrupted.

EVALUATION OF THE NEUTROPENIC PATIENT. When neutropenia has been confirmed, particular attention should be given to determining any and all drugs or potential toxins to which the patient may have been exposed, a history of any infections, and when and where the patient has had blood studies performed previously. Clues to any underlying disease associated with neutropenia should be searched for. Rheumatoid arthritis, systemic lupus erythematosus, and infectious mononucleosis should be considered, since on rare occasions neutropenia may precede other overt manifestations of those diseases.

The marrow should be examined meticulously by the physician. If neutropenia is not accompanied by anemia and/or thrombocytopenia, then an aspirated specimen of marrow is entirely sufficient since the size of marrow neutrophil pools can be estimated from the myeloid to erythroid (M:E) ratio. A careful differential count of neutrophils and neutrophil precursors (neutrophil compartment) should be done. Normally, the mean percentage of different cells in that compartment (as a percentage of the compartment, not of all marrow cells) is myeloblasts, 2; promyelocytes, 6; myelocytes, 24; metamyelocytes, 30; bands, 24; and segs, 14. A marked shift in cell ratio toward a predominance of myeloblasts and promyelocytes raises the question of (1) acute myeloid leukemia, (2) observation of the precursor compartment at an opportune time when regeneration from an insult is occurring, or (3) Kostmann's neutropenia (in infants or young children). The percentage of bands and segs provides a visual estimate of the size of the marrow neutrophil reserve (MNR). If these constitute less than 25 per cent of the neutrophil compartment, one can be confident that the MNR is decreased, as might be expected with neutropenia of any cause in which control of cell release is normal. With neutropenia, cell release should be demanded and the MNR should decline. This morphologic appearance, abundant precursors through the metamyelocyte stage with a decreased percentage of bands and segs, has often been referred to by the term "maturation arrest," a kinetic misconception. If anemia is not present, normal, decreased, or increased production can be estimated from the M:E ratio, correcting for the reduced percentage of bands and segs. If other blood cells are present in abnormal concentration, or if there is reason to suspect tumor, granuloma, or fibrosis in the marrow, a section of a needle biopsy specimen should also be examined. From this, overall marrow cellularity can be estimated as an aid in subsequently determining the significance of the M:E ratio.

If bands and segs are in excess of 25 per cent of the neutrophil compartment in marrow, two possibilities should be raised and tested: (1) marrow release is abnormal, or (2) the neutropenia is due to an intravascular shift from circulating to marginal pools. Injection of endotoxin, etiocholanolone, or an adrenal glucocorticosteroid will transiently accelerate release. Following intravenous injection of 8 μg of endotoxin, a peak response is observed in two to six hours with circulating neutrophils increasing by at least 2×10^9 per liter and the band to seg ratio at least doubling. An early peak or a reduced peak response but with a normal or exaggerated band to seg change may be seen in conditions associated with rapid blood neutrophil turnover such as congestive splenomegaly. Failure to release with a visually normal-sized MNR implies defective neutrophils or defective release mechanisms. The release response merely tells one if there is or is not a "functionally adequate" MNR; it does not measure the size of the MNR.

With normal release in a neutropenic patient, the possibility of a shift from circulating to marginal pools but with a normal total sized blood pool ("pseudoneutropenia") should be considered. Infusion of epinephrine, 1 mg intravenously in an adult, normally mobilizes marginated neutrophils and results in at least a 40 per cent increase in circulating neutrophils within a few minutes. In "pseudoneutropenia," which is very unusual, an absolute increase in neutrophils in excess of 1 × 10^9 per liter should be observed following epinephrine, as well as a distinct exaggeration of the normal, relative percentage increase.

With a decreased M:E ratio (corrected for percentage of bands and segs) in a normal or hypocellular marrow, one can be reasonably assured that decreased neutrophil production is present. Estimates of total neutrophil precursors per kilogram of body weight can be obtained by isotopic techniques, but these are available only in specialized research laboratories. If facilities are available to study the in vitro growth of neutrophils (CFUnm), values for their concentration from blood and marrow may reflect "stem cell" status and be a useful adjunct in understanding the mechanisms of neutropenia.

If neutropenia is mild (~>1 × 10^9 per liter), then the possibility that this is a "normal value" for that patient should be considered. The infectious history is very helpful in regard to the "seriousness" of neutropenia. As a test for "functional neutropenia," a small skin abrasion can be made and covered with a plastic cap filled with 2 ml of autologous serum. The number of neutrophils entering this "exudate" is measured for 24 hours. If a mildly neutropenic patient has a normal exudate response (more than 40 × 10^6 neutrophils), one can be reasonably assured that this "neutropenia" should be of little concern to physician or patient.

When no explanation for neutropenia is uncovered, the possibility of one of the familial neutropenias or of autoimmune neutropenia must be considered. Parents, siblings, and particularly children should be tested; failure to uncover any historical evidence of familial neutropenia is inadequate. With at least one form of dominantly inherited, mild neutropenia, affected adults may no longer be neutropenic, so as many family members as possible should be studied.

Serum for detection of antineutrophil antibodies should be sent to a highly specialized laboratory, as there is no satisfactory, easily available, "routine" test for these. It is possible that antibodies affect precursors as well as mature neutrophils so antibodies should be studied in any patient with unexplained, chronic neutropenia.

When the aforementioned studies have been completed, a significant number of patients with unexplained neutropenia will remain. Our understanding of the causes and classification of neutropenia is still decades behind that of anemia.

TREATMENT. Little can be done to alter neutropenia unless a treatable underlying disease is present or unless there is a causative drug or toxin which can be withdrawn. Obviously a prompt and correct diagnosis followed by proper antimicrobial treatment of an infection is mandatory. Therapy designed to affect the neutrophil count directly must be considered experimental.

Lithium increases the rate of neutrophil production in normal humans and increases platelets to a modest degree as well. With intensive cancer chemotherapy, lithium, given either before or after, may lessen the severity and duration of iatrogenic neutropenia. Lithium is effective in this setting in at least some patients with relatively normal marrow function (i.e., with carcinoma) but has not been effective in the acute leukemias. There are anecdotal reports of lessening of neutropenia with lithium therapy in hairy cell leukemia and both favorable and unfavorable reports in Felty's syndrome, aplastic anemia, preleukemia and early acute myeloid leukemia, and in various congenital and idiopathic forms of neutropenia. For the present, a trial of lithium may be advisable in any patient with severe symptomatic neutropenia. Lithium carbonate* is given orally, 300 mg 3 times daily, and blood levels must be maintained with adjustment of dose to maintain 0.5 to 1.8 mEq per liter of lithium. Therapy should be given for six weeks before a conclusion that lithium is ineffective is reached, but toxicity often precludes continued therapy.

Cyclic hematopoiesis in the dog can be abolished by lithium, but has not been effective in cyclic disease in man. *Prednisone* abolished cycles in patients with acquired cyclic hematopoiesis but has failed to influence the congenital form of disease. Therapy with adrenal glucocorticosteroids may lead to an improvement in many types of neutropenia, but this is the result of reducing the rate of egress from the blood, potentially making the patient more susceptible to infection than he was initially. Therefore steroids are contraindicated unless an antineutrophil antibody is present. There are only anecdotal reports of benefit from prednisone and/or cyclophosphamide in neutropenic patients with antineutrophil antibodies.

Splenectomy has been tried in virtually all types of neutropenia (except drug-induced neutropenia), but it has rarely proved beneficial except in some patients with Felty's syndrome. If medically feasible, all drugs should be discontinued. Reduction in the use of household cleansers, solvents, and paints, as well as cosmetics, is advised, although there is no proof that most of these products will produce neutropenia. However, any compound could be toxic to a rare patient. For instance, if chloramphenicol produced aplastic anemia in 1 of 200,000 persons so treated instead of 1 in 20,000 to 60,000, it would never have been recognized as causative.

Allogeneic *marrow transplantation* is an accepted form of therapy for patients with severe aplastic anemia. Mortality from the allogeneic transplant procedure may approach 50 per cent, so this is acceptable therapy only if death from the disease being treated is anticipated. Therefore, of the idiopathic acquired and congenital forms of neutropenia, allogeneic transplantation would be clearly indicated only in patients with congenital neutropenia plus severe immune deficiency or in those with Kostmann's syndrome. If a patient with severe acquired neutropenia, apparently caused by decreased production, were fortunate enough to have a normal identical twin, then infusion of the twin's marrow would represent a reasonable therapeutic trial. Autologous marrow transplantation is under study as a potential means of reducing the duration of neutropenia (pancytopenia) induced by vigorous chemotherapy of certain cancers.

Treatment of the Infected Neutropenic Patient. Neutropenia per se is not an indication for hospitalization. If a patient is going to become infected, microorganisms in the general environment are preferable to those found in hospitals. However, the patient should be instructed to call with any fever or any evidence of infection and should immediately see the physician if any signs and symptoms of infection develop. Emphasis should be placed on scrupulous hygiene, particularly of oral and anal areas. Prophylactic antimicrobial agents, with the probable exception of trimethoprim sulfamethoxazole, should not be used.

If there is evidence of infection, culture of blood and urine and any visible lesion should be obtained, and a combination of antimicrobial drugs with a broad spectrum of activity should immediately be started, using the intravenous route of administration. If a causative organism is isolated, therapy should be altered to the agent with the narrowest spectrum to which the organism is sensitive. Superinfections are common in neutropenic patients, and it is desirable to change their bacterial flora as little as possible. If the patient is no better after three days of therapy and the cause of infection has not been found but the patient does not appear critically ill, it probably is advisable to stop therapy and reculture. However, if the patient is no better in two to three days and does appear critically ill, a program of neutrophil transfusion should be begun. Addition of amphotericin B should also be considered, especially in patients with acute leukemia, since *Candida* infections are common and most are not diagnosed during life. In patients with any chronic form of neutropenia, neutrophil transfusion should be limited to intractable life-threatening infections, since development of alloantibodies may limit their subsequent usefulness. If the patient has an HLA identical sibling as an available donor, a more liberal attitude toward transfusion might be taken.

Neutrophil transfusion is of benefit as ancillary therapy of the

*This use is not listed in the manufacturer's directive.

infected, neutropenic patient. Most controlled clinical trials have demonstrated superior survival from infection in neutropenic patients, primarily patients with acute leukemia, who were given such transfusions. Neutrophil transfusions given on a daily basis during the period of severe pancytopenia following allogeneic marrow transplantation also have been shown to provide prophylactic protection against infection in a controlled trial. However, despite the modest benefit provided by this procedure, it is attended by multiple problems and as yet is far from being a "routine" part of the expected activity of most blood banks. The short blood half-time of normal neutrophils and their relatively small numbers in the blood of normal donors presently preclude "replacing" neutrophils in a neutropenic patient as is done with red cell and is possible with platelet transfusion. In many instances there is no detectable increase in circulating neutrophils following infusion of 10^{10} allogeneic neutrophils, the minimal number considered of possible benefit to an adult. Collection requires processing of approximately the equivalent of the total blood volume of the donor by use of either the continuous or discontinuous centrifugation technique. The donor must be connected to the collecting apparatus for two to four hours, and most consider at least five consecutive days of transfusion as minimal acceptable therapy. Consequently the procedure is very expensive in time and money for personnel, as well as in equipment cost. Recipients should be tested for the presence of preformed antibodies against the potential donor's leukocytes, since their presence probably not only negates the usefulness of the transfusion but also increases the likelihood of transfusion reaction, consisting of fever, chills, malaise, and sometimes dyspnea. The major histocompatibility loci (HLA) match of donor and recipient may be important, as there is evidence to suggest that the post-transfusion increment in neutrophil concentration is higher when donor and recipient are matched at two or more of the four HLA sites than when they are completely mismatched.

Sterile environments markedly reduce the probability of infection in neutropenic patients. In many instances all detectable bacteria and fungi can be eliminated by vigorous skin and mucous membrane antisepsis and by administration of nonabsorbable antimicrobials, with the patient either in complete barrier isolation ("life island") or in a room with a laminar flow filtration system. The psychologic stress of such isolation is considerable, and usually a constantly visible attendant is needed. Expense of maintaining patients in such environments is considerable but may be financially balanced by reduced antibiotic and neutrophil transfusion requirements.

DECREASE IN OTHER TYPES OF LEUKOCYTES

LYMPHOPENIA. Acute, transient decrease in blood lymphocytes to less than 1.5×10^9 per liter is very common, occurring with almost any form of stress, be it an acute bacterial infection or a traumatic injury. This type of lymphopenia may be mediated by increased secretion of adrenal glucocorticosteroids. Lymphocytes recirculate from blood to lymphoid tissue to blood, and steroids change the recirculatory pattern, redistributing lymphocytes but having no apparent effect on rates of production or destruction of normal lymphocytes, at least when given in moderate doses for relatively brief periods. When normal subjects are given steroids, blood lymphocytes are reduced within two hours, but even if the drug is continued, they return to normal within two days.

Chronic lymphocytopenia is less common. It is observed in patients with diseases characterized by defective cellular immunity such as Hodgkin's disease or congenital immune deficiency syndromes, and it presumably reflects a reduction in the total number of thymic-derived (T) lymphocytes in the body. Vigorous cancer chemotherapy and particularly radiotherapy may lead to lymphopenia. Blood lymphocytes may remain reduced for a year or more after completion of a course of radiotherapy.

MONOCYTOPENIA. Monocytopenia is occasionally observed as the only abnormality in the blood of a subject, but nothing is known of its cause or its consequences. Similarly, patients have been observed in whom a scan of several smears failed to reveal either any *eosinophils* or *basophils*, but whose blood was otherwise unremarkable. Acute eosinopenia is a well known accompaniment of a wide variety of acute stresses. All three of these blood cells are affected by the same dose-related toxins which affect the neutrophil system.

Boggs DR, Joyce RA: The hematopoietic effects of lithium. Sem Hematol 20:129, 1983. Joyce RA, Boggs DR, Chervenick PA: Neutrophil kinetics in hereditary and congenital neutropenias. N Engl J Med 295:1385, 1976. Joyce RA, Boggs DR, Hasiba U, Srodes CH: Marginal neutrophil pool size in normal subjects and neutropenic patients as measured by epinephrine infusion. J Lab Clin Med 88:614, 1976. Joyce RA, Boggs DR: Visualizing the marrow granulocyte reserve. J Lab Clin Med 93:101, 1979. Joyce RA, Boggs DR, Chervenick PA, Lalezari P: Neutrophil kinetics in Felty's syndrome. Am J Med 69:695, 1980. *These references represent an interrelated series of studies by the author and/or his colleagues relative to the kinetics and causes of neutropenia.*

Gross R, Hellriegel KP: Drug induced agranulocytosis. Blut 32:409, 1976. *This represents in-depth discussion of drug-induced neutropenias (see also the Wintrobe et al. and Williams et al. references, below).*

Krance RA, Spruce WE, Forman SJ, Rosen RB, Hecht T, Hammond WP, Blume KG: Human cyclic neutropenia transferred by allogeneic bone marrow grafting. Blood 60:1263, 1982. *Donor marrow from a person with congenital cyclic hematopoiesis was used in an attempt to cure a sibling with acute leukemia. Cyclic hematopoiesis was induced in the recipient, as shown previously in the inherited cyclic hematopoiesis of the dog.*

Lalezari P, Jiang A-F, Yegen L, Santorineou M: Chronic autoimmune neutropenia due to anti-NA2 antibody. N Engl J Med 293:744, 1975. *A convincing report of neutropenia due to the presence of an idiopathic, autoimmune, antineutrophil antibody.*

Pizzo PA, Robichaud KJ, Edwards BK: Oral antibiotic prophylaxis in patients with cancer—A double-blind randomized placebo-controlled trial. J Pediatr 102:125, 1983. *Compromised hosts treated prophylactically with trimethoprim sulfamethoxazole had a lesser frequency of infection than those treated with a placebo. However, the favorable effect was only demonstrable in patients with excellent compliance in taking drugs.*

Pizzo PA, Schimpff SC: Strategies for the prevention of infection in the myelosuppressed or immunosuppressed cancer patient. Cancer Treat Rep 67:223, 1983. *An in-depth discussion of possible means of preventing infection in neutropenic patients.*

Rappeport JM, Parkman R, Newburger P, Comitter BM, Chusid MJ: Correction of infantile agranulocytosis (Kostmann's syndrome) by allogeneic bone marrow transplantation. Am J Med 68:605, 1980. *This paper reports successful marrow transplantation in Kostmann's syndrome, suggesting strongly that it is due to a stem cell defect rather than to an abnormal hematopoietic microenvironment.*

Skubitz KM, Craddock PR: Reversal of hemodialysis granulocytopenia and pulmonary leukostasis. A clinical manifestation of selective Down-regulation of granulocyte responses to C5a des-Arg. J Clin Invest 67:1383, 1981. *The in vivo effect of activation of C5a des-Arg on neutrophil aggregation and adhesiveness.*

Wintrobe MM, Lee RE, Boggs DR, Bithel T, Athens JW, Foerster J: Clinical Hematology. 8th ed. Philadelphia, Lea & Febiger, 1981. Williams WJ, Beutler E, Erslev AJ, Lichtman MA: Hematology. 3rd ed. New York, McGraw-Hill Book Company, 1983. *These are two reasonably definitive textbooks of hematology and as such have highly pertinent information on various types of neutropenia and other leukopenias in many chapters. In Wintrobe, in Appendix C, page 1815, drugs that have been incriminated as a cause of neutropenia are listed.*

151. LEUKEMOID REACTIONS

Dane R. Boggs

A leukemoid reaction is defined as a change in the blood or in the bone marrow of such magnitude that serious consideration is given to a diagnosis of one of the forms of leukemia, but this diagnosis proves not to be correct. Three types of laboratory abnormality, singly or as a group, are concerned: (1) leukocytosis of a greater degree than expected with the underlying disease (a leukocyte count > 30 to 50×10^9 per liter is sometimes defined); (2) abnormal and usually immature-appearing cells in the blood irrespective of leukocyte concentration; and (3) an abnormally high concentration of immature cells in bone marrow and/or abnormal-appearing cells in bone marrow.

A correct diagnosis of leukemoid reaction rather than leukemia is extraordinarily important. Even a hint that leukemia is present may profoundly alarm the patient. The treatment of most forms of leukemia involves measures that of themselves are life threatening; therefore, the use of such treatment in what proves to be a leukemoid reaction must be avoided. Sometimes the only way in which the dilemma can be resolved is to treat the underlying disease, or suspected underlying disease, and see if the blood and/or marrow permanently returns to normal. The diagnostic criteria for certain forms of leukemia are far from exact; at times the only means of making a firm diagnosis of leukemia is to exclude a leukemoid reaction. Fortunately, the differential diagnosis is usually made with ease. In most patients, the underlying disease producing the leukemoid reaction is flagrantly obvious and the question is not one of leukemia explaining the entire picture but one of leukemia also being present. Leukemoid reactions mimicking any of the many types of leukemia may be seen.

REACTIONS MIMICKING CHRONIC MYELOID LEUKEMIA

The hallmark of chronic myeloid leukemia (CML) is neutrophilia, which is also very commonly observed with many types of disease or even following various physiologic stimuli. Extreme neutrophilia ($> 30 \times 10^9$ per liter) occasionally accompanies infections or carcinomas or may be seen with other neoplastic diseases of the myeloid hematopoietic stem cell system—principally idiopathic myelofibrosis (IMF) and polycythemia vera (PV).

CLONAL MYELOID NEOPLASMS AND NEUTROPHILIA. CML, IMF, and PV, as well as acute myeloid leukemia (AML), are clonal neoplasms originating in a hematopoietic stem cell that is pluripotent for all or most of the hematopoietic cells (see Ch. 152). Since the neutrophil system is part of the neoplastic clone in these disorders, extreme neutrophilia seen with IMF or less frequently with PV may be difficult to differentiate from CML. Certain examinations that may be of use in making this differentiation are summarized in Table 151–1.

The *Ph¹ chromosome defect* is identified as the loss of a portion of the long arms of chromosome 22. The lost chromatin usually is found on 9, but other translocations may be seen. This defect is found in approximately 90 per cent of patients with CML; some physicians are very reluctant to make a diagnosis of CML in its absence. The Ph^1 is not specific for CML, being occasionally seen in IMF, AML, acute lymphoblastic leukemia (ALL), or still other neoplasms of the hematopoietic stem cell (HSC). However, it has *not* been described with leukemoid reactions due to non-HSC neoplasms. Its presence or absence is of obvious diagnostic importance.

Myelofibrosis is not particularly helpful whether present or absent in the differential diagnosis of CML from IMF, or for that matter of IMF from PV or leukemia from leukemoid reaction. Increased fibroblasts and fibroblastic activity in marrow is a very common finding in many diseases and presumably represents an idiopathic response to injury.

The presence or absence of *immature neutrophils* in the blood is of but modest help in distinguishing CML from leukemoid reactions. In the early phase of CML virtually all blood neutrophils may be mature. In the rare disorder chronic neutrophilic leukemia, circulating neutrophils are generally mature even when they exceed 100×10^9 per liter. The presence of immature blood neutrophils with normal or only modest leukocytosis is more characteristic of IMF than of CML. Neutrophilia, secondary to diseases other than HSC neoplasms, is usually limited to the presence of mature neutrophils. Cells less mature than a metamyelocyte usually are not prominent in the blood of patients with infection or carcinoma.

More than 50×10^9 per liter mature neutrophils have also been reported in a variety of other diseases such as rheumatoid arthritis, acute glomerulonephritis, and dermatitis herpetiformis.

TUMOR-ASSOCIATED NEUTROPHILIA. Extreme and persistent neutrophilia, unrelated to any other hematologic disease, is probably seen most frequently in patients with various types of carcinoma, including a variety of fibrosarcomas and liposarcomas as well as more common cancers such as carcinoma of the lung, breast, and kidney. The cancer may not be particularly widespread or even be metastatic to marrow. Surgical excision of the principal bulk of these cancers usually has been associated with reduction or loss of the neutrophilia, which has usually recurred as the tumor regrew. These observations, together with studies of transplantable murine tumors associated with neutrophilia, suggest that the tumor secretes some humoral substance that induces neutrophilia. The principal candidate for physiologic, humoral stimulation of neutrophil production is the family of glycoproteins termed *colony-stimulating factor(s)* (CSF). CSF is necessary for the growth of colonies of neutrophils and monocyte-macrophages in semisolid in vitro cultures (see below). Some but not all neutrophilia-producing tumors have been shown to produce large amounts of CSF when incubated in vitro or to be associated with elevated CSF levels in serum or urine. It is possible that the humoral substance and the kinetic mechanism of neutrophilia induction may differ from tumor to tumor.

NEUTROPHILIA OF CHRONIC INFECTION. A number of chronic

TABLE 151–1. CERTAIN COMPARATIVE FEATURES OF "LEUKEMOID REACTIONS,"* CHRONIC MYELOID LEUKEMIA,† POLYCYTHEMIA VERA,† AND IDIOPATHIC MYELOFIBROSIS

	Leukemoid Reactions	Chronic Myeloid Leukemia	Polycythemia Vera	Idiopathic Myelofibrosis
Physical findings				
Enlarged spleen	Rare‡	Expected	Expected	Expected
Enlarged liver	Rare‡	Common	Rare	Common
Sternal tenderness	Rare	Common	Rare	Rare
"Routine" laboratory				
Neutrophils	[↑ by definition]*	↑↑↑↑	↑–N	↑–N–↓
Red cells	↓–N	↓–(N)§	↑↑	↓–(↑)
Platelets	N–↑–↓	↑–N	↑–N	↑–N–↓
Basophils	N	↑–(N)	↑–(N)	↑–(N)
Eosinophils	↓–N	↑–(N)	↑–N	↑–N
Monocytes	N–↑–↓	↑–(N)	N–↑	↑–N
Lymphocytes	↓–N	↑–N	N	N–↓
Uric acid	N	↑–N	↑–N	↑–N
Chromosomal abnormality	None	Ph^1–90%	Various (50%)	Various (50%)
Leukocyte alkaline phosphatase	↑–(N)	↓–90%	↑–(N)	↑–(N)–(↓)
Growth of granulocytic colonies in vitro (CFUnm)	Normal	Normal	Normal	Normal
CFUnm in blood	N–↑	↑	N	↑↑–(N)

*Those reactions mimicking chronic myeloid leukemia, not applicable to those mimicking acute or chronic lymphoid leukemias.

†Excludes patients who have developed secondary myelofibrosis and those entering a blastic phase of the disease.

‡Rare, unless the finding is a part of the underlying disease producing the leukemoid reaction; e.g., with visceral tuberculosis, hepatosplenomegaly would be common.

§Parentheses indicate an uncommon finding.

CFUnm, colony-forming units for neutrophil monocytes.

infections, particularly tuberculosis and various fungal infections, are often considered to cause neutrophilia sufficient to suggest CML. However, reports of cure of the infection with subsequent disappearance of the leukemoid reaction are difficult to find. Many of these reports may represent patients with leukemia and an infection. Patients in an early stage of CML with only minimally elevated blood neutrophils may develop striking degrees of neutrophilia when infected or in the presence of noninfectious diseases such as myocardial infarction or pulmonary embolization.

REACTIONS MIMICKING THE ACUTE LEUKEMIAS

In most instances AML will be the diagnosis under consideration, since blood pictures mimicking ALL are virtually nonexistent if the "leukolymphosarcomas" are excluded (see below). Rarely the activated T lymphocytes of diseases such as infectious mononucleosis may be confused with the lymphoblasts of ALL, particularly when they are present in very large numbers in the blood.

Circulating myeloblasts and promyelocytes suggestive of AML may be seen with IMF and do not necessarily indicate an imminent conversion to acute leukemia. Such "blasts" may be present for many years in patients with fairly stable IMF in numbers insufficient to produce leukocytosis. Appreciable numbers of circulating neutrophil precursors less mature than metamyelocytes are rarely seen in neutropenic patients except in AML or IMF. With exceedingly vigorous cancer chemotherapy, the normal barrier to release of immature cells may be damaged and, as the myeloid system regenerates, immature cells may occasionally appear in the blood in large numbers. This leukemoid reaction usually subsides within a few days.

Auer rods are the single most useful finding for distinguishing AML from a leukemoid reaction. These rod-shaped, oval, fusiform, or filamentous granules are seen only in AML, excepting the blastic phase of CML and related diseases and possibly fetal promyelocytes (Ch. 156). Other helpful findings are the presence of acquired chromosomal abnormalities and abnormal growth in vitro of "leukemic" as compared to "leukemoid" cells. Patients with "preleukemia" (see below) may have either or both of these findings.

Down's syndrome (Ch. 35) may rarely be associated with a unique leukemoid reaction that is indistinguishable from AML in terms of physical findings and blood and marrow changes, including leukocytosis with large numbers of blasts in the blood. In many of these patients the "AML" has resolved spontaneously. Whether this is a leukemoid reaction or a form of AML with a high incidence of very long-lasting spontaneous remission is unclear. In addition, there is an unusually high incidence of both classical AML and ALL in Down's syndrome.

The *question of acute leukemia may be falsely raised upon examining the marrow* because (1) other types of tumor cells are mistaken for blasts of acute leukemia; (2) the marrow is obtained just as the myeloid cells are regenerating from a toxic insult and normal but very immature types of cells predominate; (3) in rare types of congenital neutropenia, including the recessively inherited Kostmann's syndrome, maturation appears to be blocked at the promyelocyte stage; and (4) the syndrome known as "preleukemia" or the "myelodysplastic syndrome" may be present.

Carcinoma cells in marrow are usually but not always easily distinguished from leukemic cells. They usually are seen in clumps, as a syncytium or a rosette and are larger and contain more cytoplasm than leukemic cells. Cells of non-Hodgkin's lymphoma in the bone marrow may be morphologically identical to cells of ALL (or CLL), making the differential diagnosis impossible on the basis of marrow examination in isolation. Rarely large numbers of these lymphoid tumor cells may appear in blood to produce leukolymphosarcoma that may resemble either ALL or CLL or be rather unique in appearance. On very rare occasions, carcinoma cells may be in the blood in large numbers ("carcinocythemia") but only as a preterminal event with widespread cancer.

Neutropenia, or pancytopenia, may be induced by some agent that virtually eliminates morphologically identifiable precursors from the bone marrow, but recovery may quickly occur when the agent is withdrawn. This is seen with most drugs used in cancer chemotherapy and also as an idiosyncratic reaction to other drugs. A wave of blasts and promyelocytes may be the predominant marrow cells during the recovery interval and together with the pancytopenia may be falsely attributed to AML. If this picture is seen in a patient who is neutropenic but not anemic, AML probably should not be considered. In any event, this wave of recovery in the marrow will be followed within a few days by a rising blood neutrophil count to clarify the situation. With many blasts in the blood, there is some urgency in starting antileukemic therapy but this is not the case when a patient with AML is leukopenic.

Kostmann's syndrome and related forms of congenital neutropenia present a marrow dominated by myeloblasts and promyelocytes that, in isolation, is morphologically indistinguishable from AML. This syndrome is discussed in Ch. 150 Observation rather than antileukemic therapy is indicated and will clarify the diagnosis, as will the study of in vitro growth of granulocyte-macrophage colonies (see below).

A discussion of the *preleukemic syndromes* is beyond the scope of this chapter (see Ch. 156). This syndrome is suspected when a very careful evaluation fails to disclose any cause for anemia (which may or may not be accompanied by other hematologic abnormalities). The diagnosis is confirmed only when the patient goes on to develop AML (or rarely, CML or IMF). The presence of chromosomal abnormalities, and particularly of abnormal growth of granulocyte colonies in culture, strengthens the suspicion that preleukemia is present. This may, in fact, simply represent an early phase of already present AML and in some patients it is difficult to decide if one should or should not make a diagnosis of AML and treat accordingly. In such a patient, the term preleukemia seems more appropriate than leukemoid reaction.

REACTIONS MIMICKING CHRONIC LYMPHOCYTIC LEUKEMIA (CLL)

This type of reaction is exceedingly rare. CLL, a disease of the middle aged and elderly, requires the presence of persistent lymphocytosis for its diagnosis (see Ch. 155). Diseases routinely associated with lymphocytosis due to normal-appearing small lymphocytes, such as pertussis and infectious lymphocytosis, are primarily seen in children. Recovery phases of infections such as tuberculosis may be associated with modest lymphocytosis. A CLL-like blood picture with marked lymphocytosis has been reported in a variety of metastatic cancers (stomach, breast, melanoma) but in no such reports can one exclude the possibility that CLL and another disease coexisted.

The differential diagnosis of CLL from a "leukemoid lymphocytosis" is simple and fairly definitive. CLL is a clonal lymphoid neoplasm and the cells express B type lymphocyte characteristics in approximately 90 per cent of patients. One simply tests the blood lymphocytes for type of light chain in the surface immunoglobulin on the B lymphocytes, using a fluorescent-labeled antibody. If the cells are part of a clonal neoplasm (CLL), most will have only a monoclonal immunoglobulin, detected by finding only κ or only λ light chains. If the lymphocytosis is "reactive," the cells will have polyclonal surface immunoglobulins and about half will have κ chains and half λ chains. There is no urgency in making a diagnosis of CLL, particularly in a relatively asymptomatic patient, since antileukemic therapy does not appreciably prolong life. Thus, simply observing the patient over a period of time will clarify the situation.

EOSINOPHILIC LEUKEMOID REACTIONS

There are no generally agreed upon criteria for the diagnosis of eosinophilic leukemia. The so-called "hypereosinophilic syndrome," characterized by a marked increase in eosinophils in blood and their precursors in marrow and by a proliferative endocardial fibroelastosis, thrombophlebitis, and pulmonary infiltration, may be termed a "leukemia" or a "leukemoid reaction," depending upon one's point of view (see Ch. 162 for a detailed discussion). There are no data that allow one to determine if the eosinophilia represents a clonal tumor. Certainly eosinophilic leukemias exist—one that mimics CML even to the extent of the presence of the Ph[1] chromosome and another that appears to be an AML variant with eosinophilic "promyelocytes" as the predominant cell. Eosinophilic "leukemoid reactions" occur secondary to various cancers. Very marked eosinophilia may rarely precede or be concurrent with ALL. The eosinophils have been shown *not* to be a part of the clone of ALL cells in such patients. Elevated serum IgE is strong evidence that eosinophilia is a reactive part of an allergic response rather than leukemic.

NEW DIRECTIONS

Colonies of neutrophils, monocyte-macrophages, eosinophils, basophils, erythrocytes, megakaryocytes, and T and B lymphocytes or various combinations of these cells can be grown in vitro from cells found in normal blood, bone marrow, and spleen. While these techniques are still limited to research laboratories, the colony growth pattern is assuming increasing importance as a diagnostic technique. For example, a normal neutrophil-monocyte colony is defined as one containing more than 50 cells and the cells mature in the colony. In the acute myeloid leukemias, one of three abnormal patterns is seen: (1) no growth, (2) growth of clusters instead of colonies (a cluster contains less than 50 cells by definition), or occasionally (3) growth of colonies that contain only immature cells. This type of in vitro approach will find many uses in the future.

A large number of *monoclonal antibodies* that react with specific antigens found on some blood cells but not on others or with antigens that are present at certain stages in cell maturation but not at others are being developed. It is hoped that these specific markers will prove useful in distinguishing leukemia from leukemoid reactions. Unfortunately, however, virtually all currently known tumor cell antigens are tumor associated but not tumor specific.

Andres TL, Kadin ME: Immunologic markers in the differential diagnosis of small round cell tumors from lymphocytic lymphoma and leukemia. Am J Clin Pathol 79:546, 1983. *An example of the growing literature on the use of monoclonal antibodies in the differential diagnosis of leukemia.*

Shah I, Mirchandani I, Khilanani P, Zafar RS: Comparison of circulating colony-forming cells in chronic granulocytic leukemia and leukemoid reaction. Acta Haematol 69:340, 1983 and Strife A, Lambek C, Wisniewski D, Arlin Z, Thaler H, Clarkson B: Proliferative potential of subpopulations of granulocyte-macrophage progenitor cells in normal subjects and chronic myelogenous leukemia patients. Blood 62:389, 1983. *Examples of how the growth pattern of hematopoietic colonies grown in semisolid media is becoming a useful technique in diagnosis.*

Slungaard A, Ascensao J, Zanjani E, Jacob HS: Pulmonary carcinoma with eosinophilia. N Engl J Med 13:778, 1983. *An extract of the tumor as well as the patients' sera stimulated the growth of colonies of eosinophils when added to cultures of normal human marrow. No such activity was seen in extracts from normal tissue, tumors not associated with eosinophilia, or normal sera. An excellent editorial on this subject by Paul Brown is in the same issue.*

Wintrobe MM, Lee RE, Boggs DR, Bithell T, Athens JW, Foerster J, Lukens J: Clinical Hematology. 8th ed. Philadelphia, Lea and Febiger, 1981. *A more detailed discussion of leukemoid reactions is found in this general textbook of hematology.*

152. CLONAL DEVELOPMENT AND STEM CELL ORIGIN OF PROLIFERATIVE DISORDERS

Philip J. Fialkow

Determination of whether a tumor arises from one or many cells can provide important clues about how it develops. For example, a neoplasm resulting from a rare event like mutation in a single somatic cell would by definition have a unicellular (clonal) origin. On the other hand, multicellular origin would be represented by a proliferative process caused by horizontal cell-to-cell spread of some agent such as a virus.

The number of cells from which tumors arise can be conveniently investigated in a person who has at least two genetically distinct types of cells. The normal tissues contain cells of both types, but if the tumor is of clonal origin, it contains only one cell type.

One example of such a model system is the cellular mosaicism present in females heterozygous for the gene on the X chromosome that determines glucose-6-phosphate dehydrogenase (G-6-PD). In accordance with X chromosome inactivation, only one of the two G-6-PD genes is active in a given somatic cell. Thus, women who carry a gene for the usual type of G-6-PD (Gd^B) on one X chromosome and the common variant Gd^A on the other have two cell populations, one producing A-type and the other B-type G-6-PD. Since the two enzymes have different electrophoretic mobility, they are easily distinguishable. Cell proliferations with a clonal origin should exhibit only one type of enzyme (A *or* B), whereas those arising from many cells would usually have both A *and* B types. Once it has been determined that a proliferation is clonal, hierarchal relationships of stem cells can be investigated. For example, if both the granulocytes and erythrocytes of a heterozygous female with leukemia have only one and the same G-6-PD type, it can be inferred that the disease involves a stem cell multipotent for granulocytes and erythrocytes.

MYELOPROLIFERATIVE DISORDERS

Included in this group of diseases are chronic myelogenous leukemia, agnogenic myeloid metaplasia, polycythemia vera, and "essential" thrombocythemia. Although each disorder is characterized by predominance of one cell type (i.e., white cells, red cells, or platelets), there is often evidence of proliferation of other marrow-cell types (e.g., in polycythemia vera erythrocytes predominate, but granulocytes and megakaryocytes also often are increased).

CHRONIC MYELOGENOUS LEUKEMIA. This disorder is of particular interest, since about 90 per cent of patients have a very specific and characteristic cytogenetic abnormality, the Philadelphia chromosome rearrangement (Ph[1]) (see Ch. 155). Because Ph[1] is so specific and when present is generally found in over 90 per cent of dividing marrow cells, it is most easily inferred that the disease develops from a single cell containing Ph[1]. However, the leukemia could have a multicellular origin if, for example, an agent inducing Ph[1] had a specific affinity for regions on the two involved chromosomes: 22 and 9.

Strong support for the clonal theory of Ph[1]-positive chronic myelogenous leukemia was provided by the finding of only A *or* B G-6-PD in granulocytes from 26 patients with the disease, whereas both enzyme types were detected in the patients' normal tissues. Conversely, in Gd^B/Gd^A heterozygotes without blood-cell abnormalities, the granulocytes show both B and A enzymes. The conclusion based on these and other observations that chronic myelogenous leukemia is a clonal disease obviously applies only to the stage at which the disorder is studied. Conceivably, many cells could be affected at an early phase, but when leukemia is clinically evident, only one clone is detected.

Ph[1] has been found in erythroid precursors, suggesting that chronic myelogenous leukemia involves pluripotent stem cells. This postulate has been confirmed with G-6-PD: the same single-enzyme type found in the leukemic granulocytes was found in erythrocytes, eosinophils, monocytes, platelets, and B lymphocytes. These marker studies in chronic myelogenous leukemia provide definitive evidence for the existence in man of a stem cell pluripotent for lymphoid as well as myeloid cells.

OTHER MYELOPROLIFERATIVE DISORDERS. Although only a few patients have been evaluated with G-6-PD, the results suggest that the other chronic marrow cell proliferations—

agnogenic myeloid metaplasia, polycythemia vera, essential thrombocythemia, and Ph[1]-negative chronic myelogenous leukemia—are also clonal. Furthermore, in each instance, circulating red cells, granulocytes, and platelets displayed only one G-6-PD type, indicating that pluripotent stem cells were involved.

PATHOGENETIC IMPLICATIONS. It is generally agreed that the defect in chronic myelogenous leukemia is intrinsic to the leukemic cells, but some workers have proposed that other myeloproliferations such as polycythemia vera or myeloid metaplasia result from proliferation of normal stem cells in response to abnormal stimuli. The G-6-PD studies suggest that the proliferating cells are very probably clonal and by inference that they are neoplastic in origin. Other points that have emerged from these studies are as follows:

Chromosomal Abnormalities. Specific cytogenetic abnormalities have been described in some patients with polycythemia vera (see Ch. 153). However, in the two studied Gd^B/Gd^A women with this disease, no chromosomal abnormalities were detected, indicating that at least in some patients these aberrations are not a prerequisite for the characteristic clonal proliferation of marrow stem cells. Accordingly, when a chromosomal abnormality occurs, it probably represents emergence of a subclone not required for the initial development of the disease.

Myelofibrosis. Ph[1] has not been detected in most studies of cultured marrow fibroblasts from patients with chronic myelogenous leukemia. It could be argued that the chromosomal abnormality arose in myeloid but not fibroblastic cells after the inception of the disease; however, the finding of normal double-enzyme G-6-PD types in the cultured fibroblasts indicates that they are not part of the neoplastic process. Similar observations suggest that the myelofibrosis that occurs in polycythemia vera and myeloid metaplasia is secondary. This is especially noteworthy for agnogenic myeloid metaplasia in which myelofibrosis is often the predominant clinical manifestation.

Remission. In clinical remission of chronic myelogenous leukemia or polycythemia vera achieved with conventional therapy, there is persistence of abnormal single-enzyme G-6-PD types in blood cells and the percentage of Ph[1]-positive marrow cells generally does not decline. Thus, even though these remissions may be prolonged, they are not accompanied by repopulation of the marrow with normal stem cells.

Residual Normal Stem Cells. In contrast to the results achieved with conventional therapy, about a third of patients with chronic myelogenous leukemia treated with intensive combination chemotherapy have reappearance in their marrows of large populations of Ph[1]-negative cells. Studies of G-6-PD in one such patient indicated that the Ph[1]-negative cells arose from nonclonal, presumably normal stem cells. Findings in patients with polycythemia vera also suggest the presence of residual normal stem cells. When erythroid or granulocytic progenitors of normal heterozygotes are plated at low density for colony growth in vitro, each colony exhibits only one or the other of the two enzyme types, indicating that the colony arose from a single progenitor. Under similar conditions, but in the absence of erythroid stimulating factors, erythroid colonies from patients with polycythemia vera show only the enzyme type of the abnormal blood cells. However, when grown in the presence of stimulating factors, a notable portion of erythroid (and granulocytic) colonies show the G-6-PD type not characteristic of the abnormal clone. Thus, residual normal stem cells are present in patients with polycythemia vera, and their expression is suppressed in vivo.

Summary. Studies with G-6-PD suggest that the myeloproliferative disorders are clonal proliferations of pluripotent marrow stem cells and, by inference, that they are neoplasms with varying rates of progression. Myelofibrosis occurs in all of the disorders, but it is apparently "reactive" and not part of the abnormal clone. Normal stem cells are present in these patients, and in some cases their expression is suppressed in vivo. Finally, since the clinical manifestations in each disorder are different despite the fact that the diseases all arise in pluripotent stem cells, the clinical variability presumably reflects differences in the responses of cells in the abnormal clones to certain regulatory factors. Determining the nature of these regulatory interactions may permit development of more efficient therapeutic modalities than are currently available.

ACUTE NONLYMPHOCYTIC LEUKEMIA

Many patients with acute nonlymphocytic leukemia have chromosomal abnormalities in marrow cells (see Ch. 156). These aberrations are not as specific as Ph[1] in chronic myelogenous leukemia, but the data suggest that within a given patient the chromosomally abnormal cells are members of a single clone. Findings of single-enzyme G-6-PD types in 14 heterozygotes with acute nonlymphocytic leukemia indicate that their diseases were clonal.

Stem cell relationships have been evaluated with G-6-PD in 11 patients with this leukemia. The observations in seven young patients that erythroid cells did not arise from the leukemic clone indicate that the clone did not prevent erythroid differentiation from normal progenitors. Conversely, in four elderly patients the leukemia involved stem cells pluripotent for at least granulocytes, erythrocytes, and platelets. These results indicate that acute nonlymphocytic leukemia is heterogeneous. In some patients it is expressed in cells with restricted differentiative expression; in others it involves stem cells with multipotent differentiative expression. Perhaps these differences underlie variations in cause and clinical features, including prognosis.

Chromosomal studies suggest that during clinical remission of this malignancy the marrow is repopulated by normal stem cells. This supposition is supported by the return to normal double-enzyme blood-cell G-6-PD types observed during remission in six patients whose leukemia showed restricted differentiative expression. Thus, normal stem cells must have been present but their proliferation was suppressed during the acute phase of the disease. Another type of clinical remission, one that was associated with persistence of clonally derived stem cells, was found in two patients whose leukemia involved multipotent stem cells.

LYMPHOPROLIFERATIVE DISORDERS

Ig MOSAICISM. Immunoglobulin (Ig), as well as G-6-PD, is a useful marker in lymphoproliferative neoplasms. Since each Ig-synthesizing cell is committed to producing antibody molecules having only one variable region (idiotypic specificity) and only one light chain class (κ or λ) and there are thousands of different antibodies, the immune system has extensive cellular mosaicism. Cells in a tumor with a clonal origin synthesize only one type of Ig molecule. B lymphocytes, the precursors of plasma cells which secrete antibody, synthesize Ig which can be detected in the cytoplasm or on the cell's surface.

CHRONIC LYMPHOCYTIC LEUKEMIA. The proliferating cells in about 95 per cent of patients with this leukemia are B lymphocytes. The supposition that the disease is clonal based on Ig markers has been confirmed with G-6-PD. The G-6-PD studies also indicate that chronic lymphocytic leukemia is expressed in progenitors with differentiative expression restricted to the B-lymphocyte pathway and not to myeloid cells or at least to most blood T lymphocytes.

MULTIPLE MYELOMA. With rare exceptions, all the plasma cells in a given myeloma patient secrete Ig with the same light chain and idiotype, indicating clonal development. The total blood-lymphocyte count is usually not increased in this disease. However, the fact that the surfaces of many circulating B lymphocytes and the cytoplasm of some pre-B cells have the same Ig molecules as those in the plasma indicates proliferation of a clone of early lymphocytes that ultimately differentiates into Ig-secreting plasma cells. This situation differs from that in chronic lymphocytic leukemia, in which maturation of the clone is restricted; i.e., most such patients do not have high levels of monospecific Ig in their serum.

WALDENSTRÖM'S MACROGLOBULINEMIA. This disease has features in common with chronic lymphocytic leukemia and multiple myeloma (see Ch. 163). As in myeloma, the same monospecific Ig found in the plasma is present on many marrow and circulating lymphocytes. In this sense Waldenström's macroglobulinemia and multiple myeloma might be regarded as forms of chronic lymphocytic leukemia in which the lymphocyte clone continues to mature from the small B cell to the mature plasma cell.

ACUTE LYMPHOCYTIC LEUKEMIA. In those few studied patients whose acute leukemia cells synthesize Ig, the data suggest clonal origin. Studies with G-6-PD in untreated patients with the common form of this disease have not been reported, but results of chromosomal investigations are compatible with clonal development. G-6-PD data in treated patients whose disease has relapsed indicate that the disease is clonal at that stage and involves progenitors with differentiative expression limited to the lymphoid pathway. Cells in the common form of acute lymphocytic leukemia do not have T cell surface markers or Ig synthesis. However, they do have rearranged Ig genes, indicating that they have B-cell lineage differentiation potential. In each patient, the Ig gene rearrangement is of a single type in all of the blast cells, suggesting that the common type of acute lymphocytic leukemia develops clonally.

NON-HODGKIN'S LYMPHOMA. Ig markers in almost all studied B-cell lymphomas indicate clonal origin. Burkitt's lymphoma, a disease for which there is much circumstantial evidence of a viral cause, has been evaluated extensively with G-6-PD and Ig. The results indicate clonal development. Thus, if a virus causes the lymphoma, it either does so by inducing a rare change or constitutes but one of several factors necessary for tumorigenesis.

Burkitt's Tumor Relapses. Although the majority of patients with Burkitt's lymphoma have therapeutically induced clinical remissions, tumors reappear in over half the cases. Clinical and cell marker studies indicate that there are important biologic differences between early and late relapses. Thus, the G-6-PD and Ig types of early (<5 months) recurrent tumors were the same as those detected in the tumors on initial presentation, indicating re-emergence of the malignant clones. In contrast, the markers in some late (>5 months) Burkitt's tumor relapses were discordant with those originally found, indicating emergence of newly malignant cells or of neoplastic cells present but undetected when the patients were initially studied.

Fialkow PJ: Clonal and stem cell origin of blood cell neoplasms. *In* Lobue J, Gordon AS, Silber R, Muggia FM (eds.): Contemporary Hematology/Oncology. New York, Plenum Press Publishing Corporation, Vol I, 1980, pp 1–46. *A detailed review of studies of blood cell neoplasms with glucose-6-phosphate dehydrogenase and immunoglobulin markers; 184 references.*

Fialkow PJ, Singer JW, Adamson JW, Vaidya K, Dow LW, Moohr JW: Acute nonlymphocytic leukemia: Heterogeneity of stem cell origin. Blood 57:1068, 1981.

Korsmeyer AJ, Arnold A, Bakhsi A, Ravetch JV, Siebenlist U, Hieter PA, Sharrow SO, LeBien TW, Kersey JH, Poplack DG, Leder P, Waldmann TA: Immunoglobulin gene rearrangement and cell surface antigen expression in acute lymphocytic leukemias of T cell and B cell precursor origins. J Clin Invest 71:301, 1983.

153. ERYTHROCYTOSIS AND POLYCYTHEMIA

Paul D. Berk

Erythrocytosis, manifested by elevations of the red blood cell count, hematocrit, and hemoglobin concentration, represents a complex problem in differential diagnosis. Accurate diagnosis is crucial to appropriate management, particularly because therapy for certain diagnostic categories would be contraindicated in others.

Early in the evaluation of erythrocytosis it is important to differentiate an increase in the total red cell mass (absolute erythrocytosis) from a decrease in plasma volume (relative erythrocytosis). Patients with absolute erythrocytosis must be further categorized into those in whom excessive production of red cells results from a disorder intrinsic to the erythroid progenitor cells of the bone marrow (primary) or from excessive stimulation of an otherwise normal marrow by substances such as erythropoietin (secondary).

RELATIVE POLYCYTHEMIA

The hemoglobin concentration, hematocrit, and red blood cell count are usually interpreted as indicators of the circulating red blood cell or hemoglobin masses. In fact, these variables are merely measures of the extent to which the red cell mass is diluted in the plasma volume. Both the red cell mass and the plasma volume are regulated by separate and to a considerable extent independent physiologic controls. Hence, a patient with an elevated hemoglobin concentration, hematocrit, or red cell count may have (1) an elevated red cell mass, i.e., an absolute erythrocytosis; (2) a reduction in the plasma volume; or (3) a combination of a red cell mass at the upper end of the normal range and plasma volume at the lower end of the normal range. These latter two situations have been termed "relative" or "spurious" polycythemia, since the elevated hemoglobin concentration, hematocrit, and red cell count do not reflect an absolute increase in the mass of circulating erythrocytes. Strictly speaking, the designation polycythemia should be reserved for conditions involving increased levels of other formed elements (granulocytes, platelets) in addition to erythrocytes; in fact, the term polycythemia is generally applied to disorders characterized solely by abnormalities in erythroid parameters and will therefore be employed in this chapter.

The most frequent cause of relative polycythemia is dehydration. In settings in which dehydration is likely, fluid balance should be corrected before a hematologic evaluation of an elevated hematocrit is done. As an important first step, after dehydration is ruled out, patients with absolute polycythemia can be accurately distinguished from those with relative polycythemia by measurement of both the red cell mass and plasma volume, using ^{51}Cr-labeled erythrocytes and ^{125}I-albumin, respectively. This is especially important because, in the absence of conditions associated with arterial hypoxemia (cyanotic congenital heart disease, chronic pulmonary disease), cases of relative polycythemia are at least as common as cases of absolute polycythemia but need not be subjected to the extensive and expensive investigations that may be required to determine the cause of an absolute increase in the circulating red cell mass.

The normal red cell mass averages 30 ± 3 (SD) ml per kilogram in men and 27 ± 2 ml per kilogram in women. Although some studies indicate that hematocrits as high as 54 per cent in men or 48 per cent in women may be normal, increased red cell masses will be found in a small proportion of individuals of either sex with hematocrits in the upper 40's. As the hematocrit increases into the 50's, the proportion of patients with an increased red cell mass also increases, but does not reach 100 per cent until the hematocrit is in excess of 60. Since approximately half of patients with polycythemia vera and other forms of true erythrocytosis and a large majority of those with spurious erythrocytosis present with hematocrits between 50 and 60, the need for direct measurement of the red cell mass to distinguish true polycythemia from spurious erythrocytosis is apparent.

Relative erythrocytosis, also called spurious polycythemia, stress polycythemia, and Gaisböck's syndrome, typically occurs in hypertensive obese middle-aged men, and especially in those who are heavy smokers. The male:female ratio is at least 5:1. Its underlying pathophysiology remains obscure. Both hypertension and its frequent therapy with diuretics may lead to reduction in the plasma volume. Smoking may contribute by two mechanisms. Both nicotine and carboxyhemoglobin, which circulates in smokers due to inhalation of carbon monoxide, may have mild diuretic effects. In addition, the presence of carboxyhemoglobin causes a shift to the left in the oxygen dissociation curve of the remaining hemoglobin, leading to mildly impaired tissue oxygenation. Normal compensatory mechanisms, in turn, lead to a modest increase in the red cell mass that may not always exceed the normal range, particularly when expressed per kilogram of body weight in an obese patient. In some smokers discontinuation of smoking results in cure of the erythrocytosis.

Relative erythrocytosis is not always a benign condition, the prevalence of thromboembolic events reaching almost 30 per cent in some series, especially in patients with an absolute reduction in plasma volume. Treatment remains controversial, but maintenance of the hematocrit at no more than 50 per cent by a judicious phlebotomy regimen is often recommended and may be beneficial.

Brown SM, Gilbert HS, Krauss S, Wasserman LR: Relative polycythemia: A nonexistent disease. Am J Med 50:200, 1971. *An attempt to show that in many cases relative polycythemia is not a disease but an overinterpretation of a borderline low plasma volume combined with a borderline high red cell mass.*

Burge PS, Johnson WS, Prankard TAJ: Morbidity and mortality in pseudo polycythemia. Lancet 1:1266, 1975. *Follow-up study documenting an excess morbidity and mortality in patients with relative erythrocytosis.*

Smith JR, Landaw SA: Smokers' polycythemia. N Engl J Med 293:6, 1978. *A report convincingly linking smoking to polycythemia and suggesting that chain smoking is the link that ties stress to polycythemia.*

ABSOLUTE POLYCYTHEMIA: PATHOPHYSIOLOGY AND CLINICAL EVALUATION

Regulation of the Red Cell Mass

The circulating red cell mass is determined by a balance between the rate at which new erythrocytes are produced and released from the bone marrow and the rate of peripheral red cell destruction. The latter, as measured by studies of the red cell life span, is ordinarily fixed, with a normal mean value of about 100 days. While red cell life span may be reduced in pathologic states, there are no mechanisms by which it may be increased. Hence, physiologic regulation of the red cell mass occurs entirely by changes in the rate of red cell production.

Alterations in the red cell mass are effected so as to provide for a critical level of tissue oxygenation (Fig. 153–1). The principal sensors of the state of tissue oxygenation in adults are probably located in the kidney, although the existence of extrarenal oxygen sensors has also been proposed. The kidney responds to the perceived adequacy of oxygen delivery by modulating the output of the hormone erythropoietin, a carbohydrate-rich glycoprotein with a molecular weight of 39,000 daltons.

The initial commitment of pluripotent bone marrow stem cells to differentiate to the earliest erythroid-committed progenitors, the *erythroid burst-forming units* (BFU_E), depends principally on a poorly characterized growth regulator called *burst-promoting activity*. By contrast, erythropoietin, the principal regulator of the subsequent stages of erythropoiesis, appears to stimulate proliferation of the *erythroid colony–forming units* (CFU_E), the more differentiated but still morphologically unrecognizable progeny of the BFU_E. Since further differentiation of the CFU_E to early, recognizable proerythroblasts is a stochastic process, expansion of the pool of CFU_E results in an increase in the production of recognizable erythroid precursors in the marrow. Erythropoietin also shortens the overall maturation time of developing erythroid precursors and accelerates the release of reticulocytes into the circulation. Hence, its net effect is to increase the output of red cells from the marrow and ultimately to expand the circulating red cell mass.

Mechanisms Producing Erythrocytosis

Erythrocytosis or "polycythemia" reflects an increase in marrow red-cell production caused by increased proliferation of erythroid progenitors. This proliferation could be either "autonomous" as a result of an intrinsic cellular defect permitting escape from normal regulatory mechanisms or secondary to an external stimulus.

AUTONOMOUS PROLIFERATION. The increased erythroid activity in the primary polycythemias, including polycythemia rubra vera and the recently described entity of "primary erythrocytosis," is autonomous in that increased red cell production occurs despite low or undetectable levels of erythropoietin as measured by in vivo bioassay techniques. Moreover, "endogenous colonies" of erythroid progenitors from such patients may be successfully grown in various in vitro tissue culture systems without added erythropoietin, which is otherwise essential for erythroid progenitor growth in vitro. Finally, phlebotomy to low normal or anemic levels produces an increase in erythropoietin production, indicating that the "servomechanism" relating erythropoietin output to tissue oxygen delivery is intact.

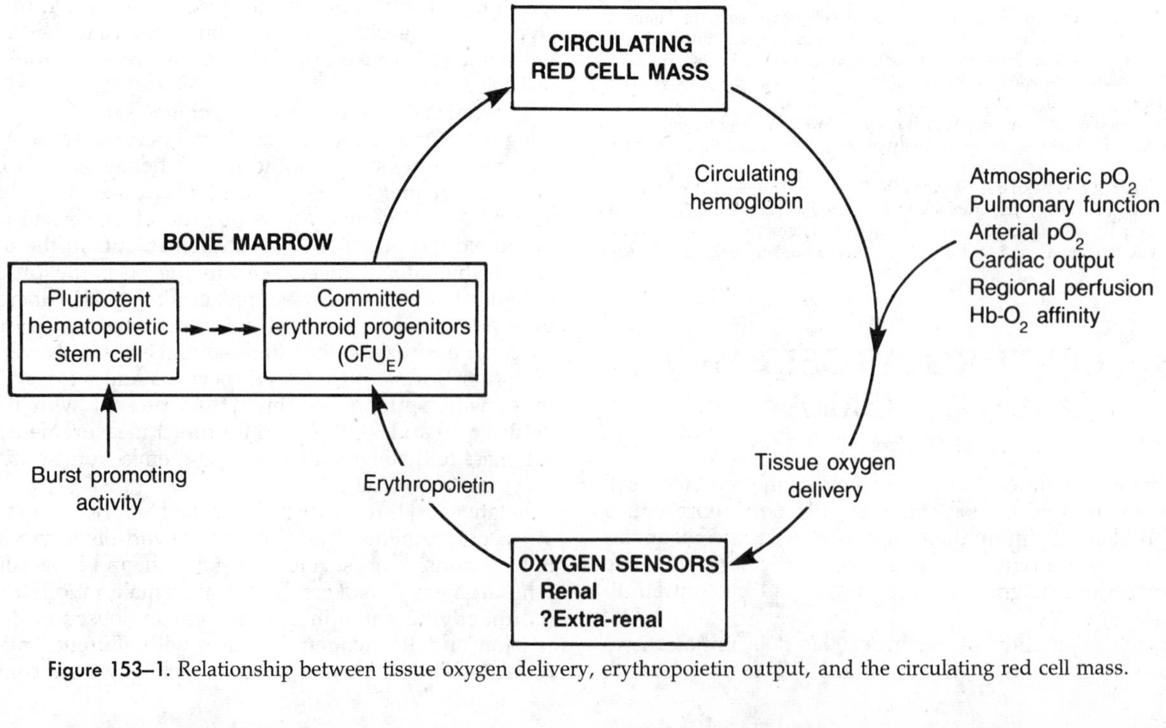

Figure 153–1. Relationship between tissue oxygen delivery, erythropoietin output, and the circulating red cell mass.

SECONDARY PROLIFERATION. Alternatively, the proliferation could result from abnormalities in the erythropoietic regulatory mechanism extrinsic to the erythroid progenitors themselves. The increased red cell production in these circumstances is driven by increased levels of erythropoietin or other erythroid stimulatory substances, and erythroid progenitors require exogenous erythropoietin to grow successfully in vitro. These features characterize the various secondary polycythemias.

The secondary polycythemias can be further subdivided into three categories. The *first* is disorders in which the signal resulting in erythrocytosis, most often an increase in erythropoietin production, represents a physiologically appropriate response to poor tissue oxygenation caused by arterial hypoxemia, genetically determined or "acquired" high affinity hemoglobins that release oxygen to tissue inadequately, or reduced tissue perfusion. For these conditions, reduction of the red cell mass by phlebotomy, even to values still substantially greater than normal, may reduce tissue oxygen delivery and result in a further increase in erythropoietin output. The *second* category is disorders characterized by excessive autonomous production of erythropoietic stimulatory substances (erythropoietin, androgens, adrenal corticosteroids). Increased, autonomous erythropoietin production may occur in certain neoplasms, as a result of non-neoplastic lesions in the kidney (hydronephrosis, cysts, tumors, vascular lesions) that produce local ischemia involving the renal oxygen sensing mechanism, or in certain rare, familial syndromes, without a demonstrable anatomic lesion. For the disorders in this category, erythropoietin production is not influenced by phlebotomy-induced changes in the red cell mass. The *third* category is the recently reported entity in which erythropoietin secretion remains under physiologic control in that it responds to phlebotomy, but at a level of production inappropriately high for the level of tissue oxygenation. A classification of the various absolute polycythemias, based on underlying mechanisms, is presented in Table 153–1.

Pathophysiology of Absolute Erythrocytosis

Irrespective of underlying etiology, all disorders characterized by an absolute erythrocytosis share certain common clinical manifestations resulting from the expanded blood volume and increased blood viscosity. The increased blood volume leads to generalized vascular expansion and venous engorgement, which are reflected by the characteristic ruddy cyanosis of the skin and mucous membranes. These factors are magnified by the marked decrease in cerebral blood flow that accompanies elevation of the hematocrit and in turn contributes to headaches, tinnitus, a frequently described feeling of fullness in the head and neck, and light-headedness. There appears to be an increase in thrombotic complications, particularly involving the cerebrovascular circulation, in patients with markedly elevated hematocrit and expanded blood volume. Epistaxis and upper gastrointestinal hemorrhage are also more frequent in the hypervolemic patient. The increase in viscosity accompanying hypervolemia and erythrocytosis may result in a decrease in cardiac output, reduction in regional blood flow, and ultimately in an impairment of tissue oxygenation, even in cases in which the underlying initial stimulus was poor oxygen delivery.

TABLE 153–1. CAUSES OF ERYTHROCYTOSIS

I. Relative erythrocytosis (stress, spurious, or pseudopolycythemia; Gaisböck's syndrome)
II. Absolute erythrocytosis
  A. Primary (proliferative bone marrow disorder)
    1. Polycythemia vera
    2. Primary erythrocytosis
  B. Secondary (increased marrow stimulation by erythropoietin, etc)
    1. Physiologically appropriate increased erythropoietin production
      a. Arterial hypoxemia
        i. High altitude
        ii. Chronic pulmonary disease
        iii. Cardiovascular shunt (right-to-left)
        iv. Massive obesity (Pickwickian syndrome)
        v. Postural hypoxemia
      b. Abnormal release of oxygen from hemoglobin
        i. Hereditary high oxygen affinity hemoglobin
        ii. Congenitally decreased red cell 2,3-DPG
        iii. Smoker's polycythemia (carboxyhemoglobinemia)
      c. Interference with tissue oxygen metabolism
        i. Cobalt
    2. Physiologically inappropriate erythropoietin production
      a. Neoplasms
        i. Renal, adrenal, hepatocellular, and ovarian carcinomas
        ii. Cerebellar hemangioblastomas (e.g., von Hippel-Lindau syndrome)
        iii. Adrenal cortical adenoma and/or hyperplasia
        iv. Pheochromocytoma
        v. Large uterine fibroids (rare)
      b. Non-neoplastic renal diseases
        i. Cysts, hydronephrosis
        ii. Bartter's syndrome
        iii. Post-transplantation
      c. Autonomous, fixed increased erythropoietic production without demonstrable anatomic lesion (familial)
      d. Recessive basal erythropoietin output with further augmentation following phlebotomy (familial)
    3. Therapeutic administration or excess production of androgens or certain other corticosteroids

In contrast to the consequences of expanded blood volume and blood viscosity, the consequences of bone marrow hyperactivity and of increased red cell destruction are minimal. Because expansion of the red cell mass often occurs very slowly, increases in bone marrow volume, alterations in the myeloid:erythroid ratio, and changes in reticulocyte count or plasma iron turnover may be difficult to appreciate. Similarly, although a doubling of the red cell mass results in a doubling of bilirubin production, this may be insufficient to drive the plasma unconjugated bilirubin concentration outside of its relatively wide normal range.

Clinical Evaluation of the Patient with Erythrocytosis

ROLE OF CONVENTIONAL DIAGNOSTIC MODALITIES. A systematic approach to the evaluation of the patient with erythrocytosis is illustrated in Figure 153–2. This algorithm ensures the correct classification of patients with relative as opposed to absolute erythrocytosis. In the majority of instances, patients with absolute erythrocytosis can also be appropriately classified as having primary or secondary erythrocytosis, and in the latter case, the specific underlying cause can be identified on the basis of conventional, widely available diagnostic studies. The diagnosis of polycythemia vera is discussed later in this chapter.

SPECIAL STUDIES: ASSAY OF ERYTHROPOIETIN AND ENDOGENOUS COLONY FORMATION. Erythropoietin is most commonly estimated by an in vivo bioassay in polycythemic mice. Injection of patient plasma or urine preparations into such animals stimulates the incorporation of ^{59}Fe into newly produced erythrocytes, to a degree proportional to the erythropoietin content of the injected material. When this assay is applied to urine samples, normal individuals have basal levels of erythropoietin excretion within a well-defined normal range. After phlebotomy urinary erythropoietin excretion increases, and an inverse logarithmic relationship is observed between the hematocrit and the erythropoietin excretion rate. Patients with hypoxic secondary erythrocytosis have variable basal values ranging from normal to increased, but all have increased values following phlebotomy to a normal hematocrit. In contrast, basal urinary erythropoietin excretion is very low in patients with polycythemia vera. Normal human plasma appears to contain 10 to 20 mU of erythropoietin per milliliter. The lower limit of sensitivity of the polycythemic mouse assay is approximately 50 mU per milliliter. Hence, when applied to plasma, this assay cannot distinguish normal subjects from those with polycythemia vera, since both groups fall below this sensitivity limit. The assay can detect the elevated levels seen in some cases of secondary polycythemia. Procedures to concentrate the plasma 40-fold may increase the sensitivity of this technique to approximately 5 mU per milliliter. Using this procedure, patients with polycythemia vera still had undetectable plasma levels of erythropoietin by bioassay, whereas most (but not all) normal subjects had detectable values averaging 7.8 ± 1.1 (SD) mU per milliliter. Unfortunately, the concentration procedure is

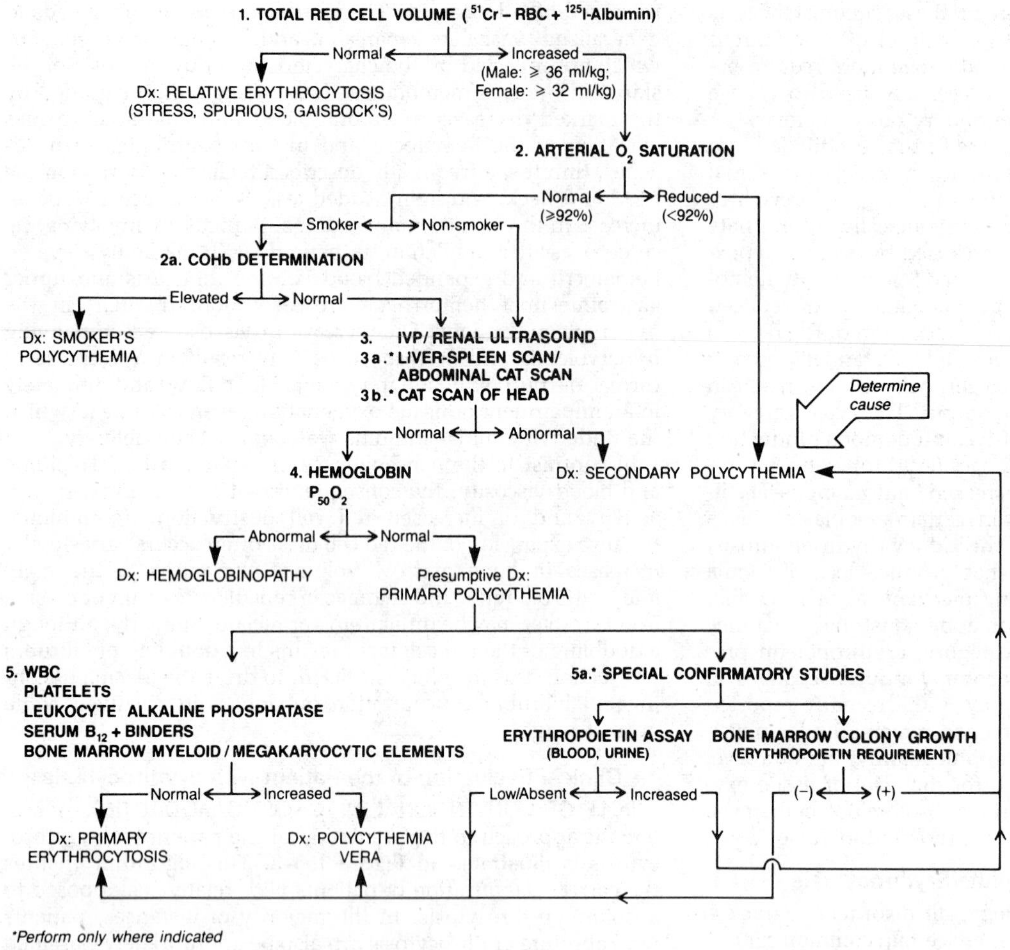

Figure 153–2. Algorithm for evaluation of an elevated hematocrit.

cumbersome and may introduce artifacts into the in vivo bioassay. Of various alternative techniques for measuring erythropoietin, only a hemagglutination inhibition assay is commercially available, but it suffers from considerable variability between different kits and not infrequent divergence of the results from those obtained with the in vivo bioassay. Similarly, recently introduced radioimmunoassay procedures report elevated erythropoietin levels in many cases of secondary polycythemia but equivalent levels in normal subjects and patients with polycythemia vera, possibly reflecting immunoreactive but biologically inert erythropoietin fractions or other materials.

The ability to grow erythroid progenitors from bone marrow or peripheral blood in vitro without added erythropoietin strongly supports the diagnosis of a primary bone marrow disorder of erythroid regulation.

As indicated in the foregoing discussion and in Figure 153–2, when erythropoietin assays and/or studies of in vitro endogenous colony formation are available, they may help to distinguish patients with primary polycythemias from those with secondary polycythemias. In addition, the influence of phlebotomy on erythropoietin output may separate the physiologically appropriate secondary polycythemias from those in which erythropoietin output is autonomous. In the majority of cases, these distinctions can be made on the basis of conventional diagnostic investigations.

Adamson JW: The erythropoietin-hematocrit relationship in normal and polycythemic man: Implications for marrow regulation. Blood 32:597, 1968. *A classic study demonstrating the feedback regulation of erythropoietin production by phlebotomy-induced alterations in the red cell mass.*

Erslev AJ, Caro J, Kansu E, Miller O, Cobbs E: Plasma erythropoietin in polycythemia. Am J Med 66:243, 1979. *Clearest demonstration of the role of erythropoietin in the pathophysiology and diagnosis of polycythemic states.*

Finch CA, Lenfant C: Oxygen transport in man. N Engl J Med 286:407, 1972. *An outstanding review of the many factors that assure an adequate oxygen supply to all tissues.*

Golde DW, Hocking WG, Koeffler HP, Adamson JW: Polycythemia: Mechanisms and management. Ann Intern Med 95:71, 1981. *An outstanding review of the pathophysiology, diagnosis, and management of the various polycythemias, with a comprehensive bibliography.*

Prchal JF, Adamson JW, Murphy S, Steinman L, Fialkow PJ: Polycythemia vera: The in vitro responses of normal and abnormal stem cell line to erythropoietin. J Clin Invest 61:1044, 1978. *An important milestone demonstrating the apparently erythropoietin-independent growth in vitro of erythroid progenitors from patients with polycythemia vera.*

SECONDARY POLYCYTHEMIAS

In the secondary polycythemias a normal bone marrow is stimulated to produce increased numbers of red blood cells, leading to an increase in the circulating red cell mass, as a result of increased production of erythropoietin or of other erythrostimulatory substances. These disorders all have in common the diverse symptomatic consequences of hypervolemia and increased blood viscosity described earlier. The secondary polycythemias may be classified into those in which the polycythemia is an appropriate physiologic response to inadequate tissue oxygenation and those in which the development of erythrocytosis is inappropriate to the oxygen balance of the patient (Table 153–1).

Physiologically Appropriate Polycythemias

HIGH ALTITUDE. In the presence of normal hemoglobin A and appropriate intraerythrocytic levels of 2,3-diphosphoglyceric acid (DPG), the partial pressure of oxygen pressure in capillaries must be maintained close to 40 mm Hg to ensure adequate off-loading of oxygen to tissues. At sea level, where the atmospheric partial pressure of oxygen is approximately 160 mm Hg, oxygen is readily loaded onto the hemoglobin molecule, and the steep oxygen pressure gradient from the alveoli to the tissue capillaries ensures an adequate driving force for tissue oxygenation. In contrast, at elevated altitudes the atmospheric oxygen tension diminishes, and at approximately 5400 meters, the altitude of the highest permanent human settlement, atmospheric oxygen pressure is only 80 mm Hg, providing a much smaller alveolar:capillary oxygen pressure gradient. To provide adequate tissue oxygenation in the face of this reduced driving force, individuals chronically exposed to high altitude are acclimatized by two principal mechanisms, hyperventilation and the development of erythrocytosis. Hyperventilation causes a reduction in the pulmonary dead space and an increase in the surface area of adequately perfused alveoli. Erythrocytosis increases the oxygen-carrying capacity of circulating blood. Together, these two alterations permit acclimatization to occur without the need for a significant increase in cardiac output. In general, although a shift in the oxygen hemoglobin dissociation curve to the right would also increase tissue oxygenation at a given capillary oxygen tension, such a change would also impair the on-loading of oxygen in the lungs at high altitudes. The latter appears to take precedence in that direct measurement of oxygen dissociation curves among individuals who live at high altitudes generally reveals patterns within the normal range.

Approximately 25,000,000 people live at altitudes between 3000 and 5400 meters. The latter, with an atmospheric pressure of approximately one half normal, appears to represent the extreme limit of human chronic physiologic adaptation. Transient adaptation to higher levels is possible, as demonstrated by the successful 1978 scaling of Mount Everest (8848 meters), where atmospheric pressure is approximately one third of normal, without the use of administered oxygen.

Those who dwell for long periods at high altitudes typically develop an increased anteroposterior thoracic diameter, and a ruddy cyanosis secondary to hypervolemia. The increased blood volume is manifested in the engorged capillaries of the conjunctivae, skin, and mucous membranes, and may contribute to all of the classic symptoms of hypervolemia. The hematocrit is elevated, reflecting an increased red cell mass in the presence of a normal plasma volume. White blood cells and platelets are normal and bone marrow aspirates may appear to be normal or to show modest erythroid hyperplasia. The acute and chronic effects of living at high altitude are further described in Ch. 560.

CARDIOPULMONARY DISEASE. Arterial hypoxemia, resulting from right-to-left shunts in congenital heart disease (see Ch. 44) or from chronic obstructive pulmonary disease (see Ch. 60), results in expansion of the red cell mass. This may be masked in part in both settings by a concomitant increase in plasma volume.

ALVEOLAR HYPOVENTILATION. Arterial hypoxemia, cyanosis, and secondary erythrocytosis may also result from either centrally mediated or peripheral impairment of alveolar ventilation. One of the settings in which this occurs, Monge's disease (chronic mountain sickness), is described in Ch. 560. Another is the so-called Pickwickian syndrome, in which the work load of ventilation in a severely obese individual is aggravated by central hyporesponsiveness to hypoxemia and hypercapnia. In a third group of patients postural hypoxemia occurs during sleep. All of these conditions may be associated with increased erythropoietin production and secondary erythrocytosis.

ABNORMALITIES OF THE OXYGEN-HEMOGLOBIN DISSOCIATION CURVE. Abnormalities in the ability of hemoglobin to release oxygen to tissues, manifested by a shift in the oxyhemoglobin dissociation curve to the left, may occur on either a congenital or an acquired basis. At least 25 such hemoglobins have been described (Ch. 143). In most an amino acid substitution occurring in the contact area between the alpha and beta chains interferes with the normal conformational changes that facilitate oxygen release from the molecule. The resulting high affinity hemoglobin results in noncyanotic tissue hypo-oxygenation and ultimately in secondary erythrocytosis. High affinity variants involving both alpha chain substitutions (hemoglobin Capetown, hemoglobin Chesapeake) and beta chain substitutions (hemoglobin Ranier, hemoglobin Yakima) have been described. Most of these high affinity mutations are electrophoretically silent because there is no charge difference between the normal and variant hemoglobin. Hence, determination of an oxygen hemoglobin dissociation curve or determination of the P_{50} is essential in the evaluation of patients suspected of having a high oxygen affinity hemoglobin. This suspicion particularly should be directed toward individuals in whom familial erythrocytosis is observed.

Secondary erythrocytosis may also occur in the presence of certain hereditary methemoglobinemias, disorders in which amino acid substitutions occur in the regions of the heme pockets. Most of these conditions are associated with hemolysis, but, in the few in which the rate of red cell destruction is near normal, compensatory mechanisms may result in a secondary erythrocytosis. Several different congenital disorders involving a decreased ability to synthesize 2,3-DPG have been described. Since reductions in red cell 2,3-DPG content are associated with an increased oxygen affinity for hemoglobin, such patients may behave clinically as if they had a high affinity hemoglobin disorder with resulting secondary erythrocytosis, even though they in fact have hemoglobin A. Finally, chronic exposure to carbon monoxide, occasionally on an industrial basis but more frequently in chain smokers, results in erythrocytosis because carboxyhemoglobin has the effect of increasing the oxygen affinity of the remaining heme prosthetic groups. The hematocrit is often increased out of proportion to the red cell mass because of secondary effects of carboxy hemoglobin or nicotine or both in reducing the plasma volume.

Physiologically Inappropriate Erythrocytosis

NEOPLASMS AND NON-NEOPLASTIC RENAL DISEASES. Physiologically inappropriate erythrocytosis is seen in a variety of neoplasms, including renal and adrenal carcinoma, cerebellar hemangioblastoma, hepatocellular carcinoma, ovarian carcinoma, pheochromocytoma, and massive uterine fibroids (Ch. 173). The proportion of each of these tumors in which erythrocytosis develops is highly variable. It seems to be particularly high in cases of hepatocellular carcinoma. In most instances, increased erythropoietin production by the tumor is believed to be the underlying mechanism leading to erythrocytosis.

Secondary erythrocytosis also occurs in a variety of nonmalignant disorders of the kidney, including cystic disease and hydronephrosis, and following renal transplantation. Production of increased erythropoietin levels in the presence of renal cystic disease appears likely in view of the frequent documentation of high titers of the hormone in aspirated cyst fluid. Local intrarenal ischemia resulting from various types of renal pathology is believed to mediate an increased erythropoietin output in these disorders. Recent reports have also described familial syndromes in which autonomous production of increased quantities of erythropoietin has been observed without a demonstrable anatomic lesion. Erythropoietin output in these syndromes does not vary in response to phlebotomy. A single report also describes an inappropriately high level of basal erythropoietin output in an individual in whom phlebotomy resulted in a further increase in hormone production. The nature of the underlying defect in these two syndromes is unclear.

DRUG-INDUCED. Testosterone and its various derivatives, and a variety of adrenal corticosteroids, may stimulate red cell production. Testosterone-like compounds are often used therapeutically for this purpose in patients with renal failure who are on dialysis or in patients with aregenerative anemia. In some instances, androgens will also stimulate granulocyte and platelet production. Occasionally, increased levels of steroid hormones, whether administered therapeutically or produced in the course of adrenal disorders, may result in secondary erythrocytosis.

Treatment of the Secondary Polycythemias

Hypervolemia and increased blood viscosity accompany the development of erythrocytosis. Accordingly, when a secondary erythrocytosis is not in response to an appropriate physiologic stimulus, phlebotomy to a hematocrit of less than 50 per cent is an appropriate part of the treatment regimen, which should also address itself to the underlying disorder.

The issue is more complex in those secondary erythrocytoses that represent a physiologic response to poor tissue oxygenation. The beneficial effect of expansion of the red cell mass may ultimately be offset by the detrimental effect of increasing blood viscosity on cardiac output, systemic oxygen transport, and local tissue oxygen delivery. In a normovolemic state, oxygen transport is optimal at a hematocrit of 40 to 45 per cent. In the presence of hypervolemia, optimal oxygen delivery may occur at hematocrits close to 60 per cent. However, hematocrits higher than this inevitably impair oxygen delivery. Nevertheless, in a given patient, if an increase in the hematocrit to the region of 60 per cent does not achieve normal tissue oxygenation, a continued increase in erythropoietin output may result in overcompensation. This overcompensation may not only decrease net tissue oxygen delivery but may also impair regional blood flow in a number of organs, particularly within the cerebral circulation. In summary, in the physiologic secondary polycythemias, there is a balance between the beneficial effects of an increasing hematocrit and the negative consequences of an excessive increase in blood viscosity. In general, hematocrits in excess of 60 per cent are detrimental and should be reduced by phlebotomy. In patients with arterial hypoxemia resulting from pulmonary disease or right-to-left cardiac shunts, the optimal level of hemoglobin and hematocrit may be difficult to determine except by trial and error. In some cases, improvement in cerebral function and decrease in congestive heart failure may follow a reduction in blood volume to hematocrits in the mid 50's or even lower.

Balcerzak SP, Bromberg PA: Secondary polycythemia. Semin Hematol 12:353, 1975. *A comprehensive review, with bibliography to match.*

Distelhorst CW, Wagner DS, Goldwasser E, Adamson JW: Autosomal dominant familial erythrocytosis due to autonomous erythropoietin production. Blood 58:1155, 1981. *A well-described family with this rare syndrome. Bibliography includes references to cases with the slightly more common recessive variant.*

Erslev AJ: Blood and mountains. *In* Wintrobe MM (ed.): Blood, Pure and Eloquent. New York, McGraw-Hill Book Company, 1980, pp 257–280. *A lucid and fascinating review of the evolution of current concepts of human adaptation to the hypoxemia of high altitudes. Excellent bibliography.*

Smith JR, Landaw SA: Smokers' polycythemia. N Engl J Med 298:6, 1978. *Lucid description of secondary polycythemia in chain smokers.*

Stephens AD: Polycythemia and high affinity haemoglobins. Br J Haematol 36:1543, 1977. *A description of the effect of oxygen dissociation curve on the delivery of oxygen in the tissues and of the fact that a shift to the left owing to high oxygen affinity of hemoglobin will cause hypoxia and secondary polycythemia.*

Whitcomb WH, Peschle C, Moore M, Nitschke R, Adamson JW: Congenital erythrocytosis: A new form associated with an erythropoietin-dependent mechanism. Br J Haematol 44:17, 1980. *An unusual syndrome characterized by inappropriately high basal erythropoietin output that increased further after phlebotomy.*

York EL, Jones RL, Menon D, Sproule BJ: Effects of secondary polycythemia on cerebral blood flow in chronic obstructive pulmonary disease. Am Rev Respir Dis 121:813, 1980. *Provides a physiologic basis for the mental deterioration observed with excessive compensation to hypoxemia. Complete bibliography.*

POLYCYTHEMIA VERA: A CLONAL STEM CELL DISORDER

Nature of the Defect in Polycythemia Vera

Polycythemia vera is a hematologic malignancy characterized by excessive proliferation of erythroid, myeloid, and megakaryocytic elements within the bone marrow, resulting in an elevated red blood cell mass and, frequently, elevated peripheral granulocyte and platelet counts. Several lines of evidence, including cytogenetic observations and isoenzyme marker studies in G-6-PD heterozygotes, indicate that the increased proliferation of all three hematopoietic cell lines can trace its origin to a single abnormal clone, which has presumably developed at the level of the pluripotent stem cell (Ch. 152). Studies of the growth of both erythroid progenitors and granulocyte/macrophage progenitors (CFU_C) in vitro have demonstrated the presence of residual normal stem cells in the marrow early in the disease but a steady decline in the proportion of the normal elements as the duration of the illness lengthens.

Thrombotic episodes that are usually attributed to increased blood viscosity and/or thrombocytosis, hemorrhagic episodes associated with thrombopathy and/or the elevated platelet and erythrocyte counts, the development of a "spent" phase characterized by cytopenias, myelofibrosis, and myeloid metaplasia, and the transformation to acute leukemia are among the principal complications of this disorder. Polycythemia vera shares several clinical, pathophysiologic, and histologic features with agnogenic myeloid metaplasia, chronic myelogenous leukemia, and primary (essential) thrombocythemia, which are collectively classified as the myeloproliferative disorders (Ch. 154).

The excessive rate of erythropoiesis in polycythemia vera occurs despite low or absent bioassayable erythropoietin levels; endogenous erythroid colonies in this disorder can grow in vitro without added erythropoietin. These observations led to the concept that erythropoiesis in polycythemia vera was "autonomous." The growth of endogenous colonies from patients with polycythemia vera can be markedly reduced or eliminated by adding antierythropoietin antibody to the culture, however, and can be restored by the re-addition of minute quantities of the hormone. This suggests that erythroid progenitors in polycythemia vera, rather than being independent of the hormone, may be uniquely sensitive to trace levels of erythropoietin. The reason for the exquisite sensitivity is unclear but may reflect increased numbers of erythropoietin receptors on the membranes of erythroid progenitors. Increased numbers of Fc receptors have been shown to occur on granulocytes and platelets in polycythemia vera. Since these receptors are normally found in young cells but undergo involution with cell maturation, these observations have led to the hypothesis that failure of membrane maturation occurs during the development of both the myeloid and megakaryocytic cell lines in polycythemia vera. The increased erythropoietic sensitivity in polycythemia may possibly reflect a failure of membrane maturation and receptor involution at the CFU_E level similar to that observed in the myeloid and megakaryocytic lineages.

The mechanism of malignant transformation in polycythemia vera is unknown. The familial occurrence of documented polycythemia vera has been reported only rarely, and neither toxic chemicals nor exposure to radiation are established etiologic factors. The incidence of polycythemia vera has not been appreciably increased in survivors of the Hiroshima atomic bomb explosion. The disease is typically one of later life, with the median age at presentation being close to 60 years. Nevertheless, patients in their second through fourth decades are not rare. The disorder is characterized by a slight preponderance in males and a propensity to occur with somewhat increased frequency in patients of Jewish ancestry.

Clinical Manifestations

Multiphasic screening is currently resulting in an increasing percentage of cases being detected prior to the development of symptoms. Alternatively, a routine blood count may demonstrate an elevated hematocrit and other abnormalities in patients who present with only mild headaches and plethoric facies. Further symptoms as they develop usually will be referrable to the combination of hypervolemia and hyperviscosity resulting from the increased red cell mass and blood volume, frequently aggravated by thrombocytosis and platelet dysfunction; to the local consequences of panhyperplasia of the bone marrow; or to the metabolic consequences of increased cell turnover.

SYMPTOMS. Headaches, tinnitus, light-headedness and vertigo, and blurred vision appear to result principally from increased blood viscosity and hypervolemia. Thrombotic complications, which may involve both arterial and venous occlusive events, are usually attributed to a combination of hyperviscosity, thrombocytosis, and platelet dysfunction. An increased incidence of epistaxis, spontaneous bruising, and upper gastrointestinal hemorrhage is also ascribed to the effects of hypervolemia and platelet dysfunction. Peptic ulcer disease seems to occur with increased frequency in patients with polycythemia vera as does pruritus, sometimes aggravated after a hot bath or shower, and occasionally so severe as to be disabling. The increased frequency of both peptic ulcer and pruritus may be related to the increased histamine release caused by excessive turnover of granulocytes and, more specifically, basophils. Approximately one third of patients complain of sweating and weight loss, presumed to be on the basis of a hypermetabolic state. Patients with polycythemia vera often complain of severe pain in their feet, which is characteristically relieved by very low doses of aspirin or nonsteroidal anti-inflammatory agents.

PHYSICAL FINDINGS. In established cases, physical examination typically reveals plethora or dusky cyanosis of the face, hands, feet, and mucous membranes. Engorgement of the conjunctivae and retinal veins is frequently present and, in patients with markedly elevated hematocrit, retinal hemorrhages are occasionally seen. Mild hypertension is noted in approximately one third of patients. Ecchymoses are not infrequently observed. The most useful physical finding in terms of differential diagnosis is splenomegaly, which is present in approximately 75 per cent of patients with polycythemia vera and tends to exclude the diagnosis of most of the secondary polycythemias. Procedures such as abdominal computed tomographic scanning will demonstrate splenomegaly in a percentage of those patients in whom the spleen is not palpably enlarged. Splenic enlargement appears to reflect principally the development of extramedullary hematopoiesis. Hepatomegaly is present in approximately 40 per cent of patients.

Symptomatic bone pain and tenderness on physical examination, particularly in the ribs and sternum, are occasionally severe and reflect intense panhyperplasia of the bone marrow. In addition to hyperhistaminemia, the cellular proliferation of polycythemia vera results in overproduction of uric acid leading, not infrequently, to either uric acid stone diathesis or overt secondary gout.

Laboratory Data

The characteristic laboratory findings in polycythemia vera reflect the various consequences of increased bone marrow activity.

ERYTHROCYTES. Patients with this disorder typically present with an elevation of the hemoglobin concentration, hematocrit, and red blood cell count. Red blood cell morphology usually reveals hypochromic microcytic cells with a reduced mean corpuscular volume, suggestive of iron deficient erythropoiesis. This suggestion is frequently confirmed by a low serum iron and an absence of bone marrow iron stores. These features may occur prior to the onset of therapeutic phlebotomy and without any history of gastrointestinal blood loss, and result from the shift of iron from various body storage pools into the circulating erythron as the red cell mass is expanded. This phenomenon may of course be exaggerated in patients who have gastrointestinal bleeding or in whom therapeutic phlebotomies have been initiated. Of the three conventional parameters reflecting the red cell mass, the red blood count is often most strikingly elevated, and red cell counts of 10×10^6 per microliter may be seen in the newly diagnosed patient. In contrast, the hematocrit probably provides the best, although imperfect, simple guide to the size of the circulating red cell mass and to blood viscosity. It is difficult to define the precise upper limit for the normal hematocrit. As noted earlier, elevated red cell masses may be found in a small percentage of patients with hematocrits of 48 per cent or above, and an increase in the hematocrit to greater than 60 per cent is required before the hematocrit alone can be taken positively as evidence for an absolute erythrocytosis. The plasma volume in polycythemia vera has variously been reported to be normal, reduced, or increased, and thus has no direct correlation with the red cell mass. The red cell life span is normal in the early phases of polycythemia vera, even in the presence of moderate splenomegaly. As the disease evolves, the development of increasingly ineffective erythropoiesis, and a larger element of extramedullary hematopoiesis with hepatomegaly and splenomegaly, result in a progressive shortening of the red cell life span in some patients. This development is usually associated with the appearance of anisocytosis and poikilocytosis, nucleated red blood cells, and teardrop cells in the peripheral blood. When such studies are available, patients with untreated polycythemia vera will invariably demonstrate very low levels of plasma and urine erythropoietin, and the ability to grow endogenous, erythropoietin-independent colonies of erythroid progenitors in vitro from either peripheral blood or bone marrow samples.

LEUKOCYTES. Sixty per cent of patients with polycthemia vera will have an increased granulocyte count in the peripheral blood at the time of diagnosis. Early in the disease, elevations are usually modest and involve the presence of only normal granulocytes and bands. Subsequently, striking elevations in total white count may achieve leukemoid proportions, associated with the appearance of early myeloid forms, particularly myelocytes and metamyelocytes. When the appearance of these cells is accompanied by increasing splenomegaly and the appearance of abnormal erythroid elements in the periphery, a significant element of myeloid metaplasia is likely. The alkaline phosphatase activity of circulating granulocytes is increased in polycythemia vera, in contrast to the reduction observed in chronic granulocytic leukemia. Increased granulocyte turnover is reflected by high serum and urine muramidase (lysozyme) levels, and by an increase in serum B_{12} and unbound B_{12} binding capacity that results from high levels of transcobalamins 1 and 3. The basophil count and, to a lesser extent, the eosinophil count may also be increased in polycythemia vera. Increased excretion of histamine metabolites reflects increased turnover of the former cell line.

PLATELETS. At diagnosis, the platelet count exceeds 500,000 per microliter in approximately half of patients with polycythemia vera, and striking elevations into the millions have been recorded. There is a tendency for the platelet count to increase with time, particularly in patients who are treated principally with phlebotomy. The platelets in polycythemia vera frequently appear morphologically abnormal, with megathrombocytes and megakaryocytic fragments being observed in the peripheral blood smear. An appreciable fraction of patients with polycythemia vera also have abnormalities of conventional studies of platelet function, including aggregation; a prolonged bleeding time may be present. Studies of prostaglandin metabolism also demonstrate abnormalities in the platelets of patients with polycythemia vera and other myeloproliferative diseases. However, it has not been possible to correlate either the height of the platelet count or the presence of platelet functional abnormalities with the propensity to thrombosis in these patients. In contrast, there seems to be a crude association between the extent of the elevation of the platelet count and the propensity to hemorrhagic complications.

BONE MARROW. The bone marrow in polycythemia vera is typically hyperplastic and reveals a panmyelosis. Because of the parallel increase in all three cell lines, the myeloid:erythroid ratio may be normal. Megakaryocytes are not merely increased but typically are seen in sheets or clumps, a finding strongly supportive of the diagnosis of a myeloproliferative disease. Bone marrow biopsy as well as aspirate is useful in the assessment of a patient with polycythemia vera, both because it gives a better indication of the extent of hypercellularity and because connective tissue staining will illustrate the extent of myelofibrosis. Serum levels of the procollagen III amino terminal peptide, now measurable by commercially available radioimmunoassay, also reflect the extent of myelofibrosis. Cytogenetic studies reveal various abnormalities in as many as 50 per cent of patients with polycythemia vera. Aneuploidy, particularly involving either loss or trisomy of a C group chromosome, is the most frequent abnormality observed, but no abnormality is either specific for or diagnostic of polycythemia vera. Interestingly, the presence of cytogenetic abnormalities at the time of diagnosis appears to be of no prognostic significance.

MISCELLANEOUS. Low serum cholesterol concentrations are frequently observed in patients with polycythemia vera; these reflect accelerated catabolism of low density lipoproteins, presumably by the spleen. Hyperuricemia, reflecting a general increase in cell turnover, and an increase in lactic dehydrogenase and the indirect serum bilirubin concentration, reflecting accelerated erythroid turnover, are other commonly found abnormalities.

Diagnosis and Differential Diagnosis

Diagnosis of polycythemia vera is based on the demonstration of an increased red cell mass that is not associated with excessive erythropoietin production, as well as evidence of a concomitant increase in bone marrow production of granulocytes and thrombocytes. Polycythemia is one of two disorders characterized by "autonomous" erythropoiesis. It differs from the entity recently described and designated as *primary erythrocytosis* in its associated increase in granulocyte and megakaryocytic proliferation, and the presence of related abnormalities such as elevated levels of leukocyte alkaline phosphatase and serum B_{12} binding proteins. The abnormalities in primary erythrocytosis are limited to the erythroid series, but within this sphere the low bioassayable erythropoietin levels and the presence of endogenous colonies are similar to those seen in polycythemia vera. Some argue that primary erythrocytosis represents a disorder arising in the committed erythroid stem cell compartment, i.e., at a later stage than the pluripotent stem cell affected in polycythemia vera, but primary erythrocytosis has not yet been demonstrated to be a clonal disorder. Others believe that these patients represent a forme fruste of typical polycythemia vera and that granulocytic or thrombocytic abnormalities will be revealed if patients are followed for sufficient periods.

The diagnosis of a primary bone marrow disorder with autonomous erythropoiesis may be made in accordance with the algorithm illustrated in Figure 153–2 by systematically excluding the various secondary causes of an absolute erythrocytosis. Patients appearing to have increased erythroid proliferation due to a primary bone marrow defect would be classified as having polycythemia vera if they have concomitant granulocytic or platelet abnormalities in the peripheral blood, evidence of a panmyelosis in the bone marrow, or splenomegaly. In the absence of these features, when abnormalities are restricted solely to the erythroid series, the diagnosis of primary erythrocytosis would be made.

The Polycythemia Vera Study Group has developed a set of empirical criteria that permit the diagnosis of polycythemia vera to be established in many patients within one to two office visits (Table 153–2). In patients who meet these criteria, the diagnosis of polycythemia vera is highly likely, the false-positive rate having been found to be less than 0.5 per cent.

TABLE 153–2. PARAMETERS FOR THE DIAGNOSIS OF POLYCYTHEMIA VERA

A1 ↑ Red cell mass Male: ≥ 36 ml/kg Female: ≥ 32 ml/kg	B1 Thrombocytosis: Platelet count > 400,000/μl
A2 Normal art. O_2 sat. (≥ 92%)	B2 Leukocytosis: > 12,000/μl (no fever or infection)
A3 Splenomegaly	B3 ↑ Leuk. alk. p'tase (LAP) (> 100)
	B4 ↑ Serum B_{12} (> 900 pg/ml) or ↑ $UB_{12}BC$ (> 2200 pg/ml)*

Dx. acceptable if following combinations are present:
A1 + A2 + A3
A1 + A2 + any two from category B
*$UB_{12}BC$ = unbound serum B_{12} binding capacity

False-positive results are most likely in patients who are excessive users of both alcohol and tobacco. In this setting, excessive erythroid proliferation associated with carboxyhemoglobinemia and splenomegaly, leukocytosis, and an elevated leukocyte alkaline phosphatase activity and elevated serum B_{12} associated with alcoholic liver disease may confound the diagnosis. The false-negative rate for the Polycythemia Vera Study Group criteria is unknown. Patients with early disease who do not yet meet these criteria may ultimately prove to have polycythemia vera, or at least a form of primary erythrocytosis, when evaluated more extensively in accordance with the criteria of Figure 153–2.

Course

In the absence of treatment, polycythemia vera is a serious disease in which a high incidence of fatal thrombotic or hemorrhagic complications historically has led to a median survival of 6 to 18 months from diagnosis. Current treatment programs designed to maintain peripheral blood counts and the red cell mass at close to normal levels have achieved median survivals approximating ten years, during the course of which aspects of the natural history of the disease have become more evident. In many patients, polycythemia vera is a readily managed disorder that remains asymptomatic for long periods of time. However, inadequate control of the red cell mass predisposes to both thrombotic and hemorrhagic complications, of which cerebrovascular, coronary, and abdominal vascular occlusions involving both arterial (e.g., mesenteric artery) and venous (Budd-Chiari syndrome) thromboses are most frequent. Thrombosis is the major cause of death in polycythemia vera, accounting for approximately one third of all fatalities. Transformation to acute leukemia, the development of other neoplasms, hemorrhage, and myelofibrosis are other major causes of fatality and collectively, along with thrombosis, account for 75 per cent of all deaths. Acute leukemia is clearly a part of the natural history of polycythemia vera, occurring with an incidence of up to 2 to 4 per cent even in patients who have not been exposed either to radiotherapy or to radiomimetic drugs.

Upper gastrointestinal hemorrhage, particularly from bleeding peptic ulcers, occurs with an increased incidence in patients with polycythemia vera. Underlying etiologic factors are believed to be increased acid secretion stimulated by hyperhistaminemia and vascular mucosal ischemia caused by increased blood viscosity and poor regional perfusion.

The complete natural history of polycythemia vera involves the ultimate transition from the proliferative phase, during which therapy is aimed at reducing peripheral blood counts, to a stable phase in which relatively normal blood counts may be maintained without therapy, to the so-called *burned out* or *spent phase*. Transition results predominantly from the gradual development of progressive myelofibrosis and, possibly, from a gradual reduction in the proliferative capacity of the abnormal hematopoietic clone. That myelofibrosis is a complication of polycythemia vera has long been recognized, but the nature of the association has been uncertain. The bulk of current evidence suggests that bone marrow fibroblasts in this setting are not part of the hematopoietic malignant clone. Similar conclusions have been reached in studies of the bone marrow fibroblast following transplantation. Hence, the increasing proliferation of fibroblasts and increased collagen deposition leading to myelofibrosis appear to be reactive phenomena rather than an intrinsic component of the neoplastic process. The clinical features and the management of postpolycythemic myelofibrosis do not differ appreciably from those of idiopathic myelofibrosis with myeloid metaplasia (see Ch. 154).

Treatment

The initial treatment for any newly diagnosed patient with polycythemia vera is phlebotomy. Efforts should be made to reduce the hematocrit to approximately 45 per cent, a level at which the complications of hypervolemia and hyperviscosity will be minimized. In patients with appreciable splenomegaly, the hematocrit no longer reliably reflects the red cell mass, which may continue to be significantly elevated despite hematocrits in the upper 40's. The initial phlebotomy regimen may involve removal of 500 ml aliquots of whole blood as often as every two to three days until a normal hematocrit is achieved. Subsequent phlebotomies should be carried out as frequently as necessary to maintain the hematocrit at or below 45 per cent. As iron deficiency supervenes, red cell production will be retarded such that patients managed by phlebotomy alone may require as few as two or three phlebotomies per year.

Some investigators believe that phlebotomy alone, at rates sufficient to maintain a normal hematocrit and blood viscosity, is adequate to prevent the thrombotic complications of the disease and provides a minimal incidence of leukemic transformation. Others argue that some form of myelosuppression is preferable, in part because this offers an approach to the control of the thrombocytosis that is often a major clinical feature of the illness. Myelosuppression in this disorder has most often been carried out with radioactive phosphorus, with alkylating agents such as chlorambucil or busulfan and more recently with the nonalkylating myelosuppressive agent hydroxyurea.

A median survival of at least ten years can be achieved equally well with phlebotomy alone or with the use of radioactive phosphorus or chlorambucil, according to recent studies. Although chlorambucil-treated patients had a slightly poorer survival than those in the other two treatment groups, the difference had not achieved statistical significance after ten years of study. Despite the lack of major differences in overall survival, the causes of death varied appreciably as a function of the treatment administered. Thus, patients treated with phlebotomy alone had a significant excess incidence of severe and often fatal thrombotic complications, particularly in the first two to four years of treatment. Thrombotic complications were particularly frequent in more elderly patients (e.g., older than 70), in those with a high phlebotomy requirement (more than 4 to 6 per year), and in those who had had a prior history of a thrombotic event. Beyond three years, the incidence of thrombotic complications became the same in patients treated with phlebotomy alone as in those treated with myelosuppression, suggesting that a subset of patients particularly susceptible to thrombosis had been selected out by this time.

Radioactive phosphorus (^{32}P), preferably given as an intravenous dose of 3 to 5 mCi, reliably produces a reduction in bone marrow proliferation with few immediate side effects. Chlorambucil,* at initial daily doses of 4 to 8 mg per day, or busulfan,* administered either continuously or intermittently, also successfully controls peripheral counts in a high proportion of patients. In contrast to ^{32}P, an appreciable incidence of cytopenias, which in the case of busulfan may be prolonged and troublesome, indicates the need for judicious monitoring of patients on chemotherapy. Myelosuppression with either ^{32}P or alkylating agents effectively decreases the risk of thrombotic complications in thrombosis-prone patients early in the disease. However, both chlorambucil and ^{32}P are associated with a statistically significant increased risk of acute leukemia, which becomes particularly prominent after five to seven years of treatment, and a somewhat later increased incidence of carcinomas of the skin and gastrointestinal tract. Thus, long-term myelosuppression with either of these agents is associated with an increased propensity for malignant transformation of the three rapidly proliferating tissues of the body: bone marrow, skin, and gastrointestinal mucosa.

Hydroxyurea,* administered at a dose of 0.5 to 1.5 grams per day, has recently been shown to be an effective nonalkylating chemotherapeutic agent in the management of polycythemia vera. To date, this regimen has not been associated with an increased incidence of malignant transformation. However, the maximal follow-up with this agent, approximately four years, is too short for its full mutagenic potential to have been realized.

Since no form of treatment for polycythemia vera is without some risks, the following recommendations would appear to provide the best control of the disease with the fewest treat-

*This use is not listed in the manufacturer's directive.

ment-related complications. Because of the increased risk of thrombosis associated with age, patients over 70 are most effectively treated with a combination of ^{32}P and supplemental phlebotomy. Patients below the age of 50, and particularly those in the childbearing years, should be treated with phlebotomy alone whenever possible. Myelosuppression with hydroxyurea would seem advisable in such younger patients if they are particularly at risk for thrombotic complications because of a high phlebotomy requirement or a history of prior thrombotic events. The role of myelosuppression is most uncertain in the age group between 50 and 70. In the absence of thrombosis-associated risk factors, it is probably preferable to attempt to manage such patients by phlebotomy alone. If chemotherapy is deemed advisable, hydroxyurea would appear to be the agent of choice. Chlorambucil would now seem to be contraindicated for long-term therapy of polycythemia vera in view of its unacceptably high risk of leukemic transformation, which may apply as well to other alkylating agents.

Although conclusive data are lacking, any physicians believe that a substantial increase in platelet count (i.e., in excess of 10^6 per microliter) is an indication for myelosuppressive therapy. Excessive splenic enlargement with local symptoms, bony tenderness, intractable pruritus, and poor veins may be other indications for the addition of myelosuppression to the treatment regimen. H_1 (cyproheptadine, 4 mg by mouth three times daily) and H_2 blockers (cimetidine, 300 mg by mouth three times daily), alone or in combination, provide relief from pruritus in some patients.

Recent attempts to reduce the incidence of thrombotic complications with the use of platelet antiaggregating agents, including aspirin and dipyridamole, have been unsuccessful. Indeed, not only has no significant benefit been achieved in terms of a reduction in thrombosis, but these agents have been associated with a statistically significant increase in the incidence of gastrointestinal hemorrhage, particularly when administered to patients with platelet counts greater than one million. Hence, the continued use of this group of agents cannot be recommended at this time.

Treatment of the burned-out myelofibrotic stage of polycythemia vera can be extremely difficult, but does not differ from that described for idiopathic myelofibrosis. The acute leukemias that develop in polycythemia vera, either spontaneously or following myelosuppressive therapy, may be myeloid, myelomonocytic, lymphoid, or biphenotypic in morphology. In those patients with lymphoid morphology and/or increased levels of terminal deoxyribonucleotidyl transferase (TdT), a trial of vincristine and prednisone is indicated. Nevertheless, response to any form of treatment in these patients is infrequent, and median survival in a recent series of postpolycythemic acute leukemias was approximately 30 days.

Meticulous control of blood volume and viscosity with the use of phlebotomy, supplemented when specifically indicated by judicious use of myelosuppression, can ensure most patients with polycythemia vera a prolonged period of relatively symptom-free survival. Median survival in recent series has exceeded ten years, and symptom-free survival of 15 to 20 years is no longer uncommon. The longest documented survival following a well-founded diagnosis is 34 years.

Adamson JW, Fialkow PJ, Murphy S, Prchal JF, Steinmann L: Polycythemia vera: Stem cell and probably clonal origin of the disease. N Engl J Med 295:913, 1976. *The fundamental studies leading to our current concepts of this disorder.*

Berk PD, Goldberg JD, Silverstein MN, Balcerzak SP, Berlin NI, Brubaker LH, et al.: Increased incidence of acute leukemia in polycythemia vera associated with chlorambucil therapy. N Engl J Med 304:441, 1981. *Incontrovertible evidence, based on a large, randomized study of 431 patients. Extensive bibliography on leukemia and polycythemia.*

Wasserman LR, Balcerzak SP, Berk PD, Dresch C, Ellis JT, Goldberg JD, et al.: Influence of therapy on causes of death in polycythemia vera. Trans Assoc Am Physicians 94:30, 1981. *A detailed analysis by the Polycythemia Vera Study Group of the largest and longest prospective study in this disorder.*

Zanjani ED, Lutton JD, Hoffman R, Wasserman LR: Erythroid colony formation by polycythemia vera bone marrow in vitro: Dependence on erythropoietin. J Clin Invest 59:841, 1979. *Use of antierythropoietin antibodies to demonstrate that endogenous erythroid colonies are not truly independent of erythropoietin.*

154. MYELOPROLIFERATIVE DISORDERS

Paul D. Berk

The normal bone marrow contains self-replicating pools of morphologically undifferentiated stem cells, recognizable hematopoietic cells undergoing differentiation and maturation, and connective tissue stromal elements. There is a hierarchy of stem cell populations: (1) a pluripotent stem cell capable under appropriate conditions of producing erythroid, myeloid, megakaryocytic, macrophage, and B lymphocyte progeny; (2) intermediate stem cells capable of producing several but not all of these lineages; and (3) committed, unipotent stem cells giving rise exclusively to erythroid, myeloid, or megakaryocytic offspring. The rate of proliferation, pool size, and rate of transition from less restricted to more restricted potential are carefully regulated so that the bone marrow can respond to the body's need for blood elements in a manner that is both selective in terms of the cell types produced and restricted or self-limited in duration (Fig. 130–2). Thus in hemolysis, pyogenic infection, and immune platelet destruction, specific needs for increased production of erythrocytes, granulocytes, and platelets, respectively, are met ordinarily by selective erythroid, myeloid, or megakaryocytic hyperplasia of the marrow. Stromal cells such as fibroblasts do not appear to play a significant role in these responses.

In the myeloproliferative disorders, in contrast, each of the three major marrow cell lines proliferates in an unregulated, essentially autonomous and self-perpetuating manner. Four disorders—polycythemia vera, agnogenic myeloid metaplasia, chronic myelogenous leukemia, and essential thrombocythemia—can usefully be classified under this heading. Although the proliferation of one particular cell line may dominate the clinical picture, each of these disorders is a clonal hematopoietic malignancy arising at the level of the pluripotent stem cell (Ch. 152). In each disorder erythroid, myeloid, and megakaryocytic elements proliferate excessively, but to varying degrees, in the bone marrow and in sites of extramedullary hematopoiesis (often resulting in splenomegaly). In each disorder there is a variable tendency for reactive proliferation of the otherwise normal bone marrow fibroblast—which is not a part of the malignant clone—with the development of myelofibrosis, and for termination in an acute blastic leukemia. Despite differences in the predominant cell line released into the periphery, bone marrows at the time of presentation show many similarities and may be indistinguishable, with clumps or sheets of abnormal megakaryocytes being common to all. Hyperuricemia secondary to increased cell turnover and abnormal levels of serum B_{12} and its binding proteins and of leukocyte alkaline phosphatase activity are also common to this group. Some investigators include acute leukemias of various types (notably erythroleukemia) and paroxysmal nocturnal hemoglobinuria within the myeloproliferative syndromes; others consider these disorders sufficiently different from the basic four to warrant their exclusion.

The myeloproliferative syndromes have long been considered to exhibit transitions between the various entities. The evolution of polycythemia vera into a disorder characterized by myelofibrosis with myeloid metaplasia is well documented, as is the transition of all entities—albeit with varying frequency—to acute leukemia. Other transitions have been harder to document. Thus, Philadelphia chromosome–positive chronic myelogenous leukemia may present transiently with elevated red cell and platelet counts but does not at this stage represent polycythemia vera. Similarly, a patient with polycythemia vera who has suffered a gastrointestinal hemorrhage may at initial examination have only an elevated platelet count, resembling essential thrombocythemia. Repletion of iron stores with resulting erythrocytosis does not represent a true transition from essential thrombocythemia to polycythemia vera.

Despite the failure to confirm true transitions among several of these disorders, the concept of a myeloproliferative syndrome involving the four basic entities just listed is now firmly supported by their clonal, morphologic, pathophysiologic, and clinical similarities. Various nonspecific cytogenetic abnormalities are also observed in each of these entities. The appearance of the Philadelphia (Ph^1) chromosome, characteristic of chronic myelogenous leukemia, is a late event in the pathogenetic evolution of the disorder and follows the initial development of the malignant clone of pluripotent stem cells.

Adamson JW, Fialkow PJ: The pathogenesis of myeloproliferative syndromes. Br J Haematol 38:299, 1978. *A concise review of cell biologic, cytogenetic, and enzymatic evidence for an analogous clonal origin of the major myeloproliferative disorders.*

Dameshek W: Some speculations on the myeloproliferative syndrome. Blood 6:372, 1951. *A classic article in which the concept of related myeloproliferative syndromes was first developed.*

Gilbert HS: The spectrum of myeloproliferative disorders. Med Clin N Am 57:355, 1973. *A reassessment of the myeloproliferative disorder concept after 20 years of critical clinical experience.*

MYELOFIBROSIS WITH MYELOID METAPLASIA

Definition and Pathogenesis

Myelofibrosis with myeloid metaplasia is a syndrome in which morphologic evidence of excessive fibroblast proliferation and collagen deposition in the bone marrow is accompanied by myeloid metaplasia of organs such as the liver, spleen, and lymph nodes. These organs, involved normally in fetal but not adult erythropoiesis, become active sites of extramedullary hematopoiesis. Similar clinical syndromes may be seen in three distinct settings. The first of these is progressive hepatosplenomegaly and the evolution of a leukoerythroblastic peripheral blood picture indicative of myeloid metaplasia occurring in the absence of an apparent inciting cause. This disorder, termed *agnogenic myeloid metaplasia,* is a clonal stem cell hemopathy constituting one of the primary myeloproliferative syndromes. Second, a similar picture of myelofibrosis with myeloid metaplasia may evolve in the course of polycythemia vera or chronic granulocytic leukemia, either as a part of the natural history of the illness or as a consequence of the myelosuppressive therapies administered. The third setting is myeloid metaplasia with varying degrees of reactive myelofibrosis that may occur secondary to a wide spectrum of clinical disorders including, among others, severe hemolytic anemia, Hodgkin's disease, various nonhematopoietic neoplasms metastatic to the bone marrow, and infections such as tuberculosis, or following bone marrow injury caused by radiation, benzol, fluorine, phosphorus, or strontium.

In myelofibrosis with myeloid metaplasia, the extent of extramedullary hematopoiesis tends to parallel the extent of bone marrow fibrosis. Indeed, it was previously believed that the mesenchymal cells in the liver, spleen, and lymph nodes resumed their embryonic potential for hematopoiesis in an attempt to compensate for myelophthisis. However, in some cases there is a dissociation between the degree of marrow fibrosis and extramedullary hematopoiesis resulting in: (1) marrow fibrosis without evidence of significant myeloid metaplasia, or (2) progressive hepatosplenomegaly with a leukoerythroblastic peripheral blood picture in the absence of significant fibrosis. Pluripotent hematopoietic stem cells, presumably of bone marrow origin, are constantly present in the circulation of normal individuals and appear in increased numbers in the peripheral blood of patients with myelofibrosis. It is more likely that these circulating stem cells take up residence in organs such as the liver and spleen to produce extramedullary hematopoiesis than that this represents the reactivation of hematopoietic capabilities in local mesenchymal cells. Except in the secondary settings noted above, the primary pathogenetic event is believed to be a mutation leading to a malignant hematopoietic clone at the level of a pluripotent stem cell. The development of myelofibrosis appears to be a reaction to the presence of this proliferating clone. The release of increased megakaryocyte- and platelet-derived growth factor from the markedly expanded bone marrow megakaryocyte pool of the myeloproliferative syndromes may be in part responsible for the secondary fibroblast proliferation and collagen deposition. Colonization of the liver, spleen, and lymph nodes may, in this setting, represent a form of metastasis of abnormal stem cells to organs that retain an intrinsic potential to support erythropoiesis.

Clinical Features

Myelofibrosis with myeloid metaplasia, whether agnogenic or secondary to another myeloproliferative syndrome, is primarily a disorder of the middle-aged or older adult. At least 60 per cent of cases occur between the ages of 50 and 70, with no predilection for either sex. The onset of symptoms is usually insidious over several years and in most cases disease progression is slow. Most commonly presenting symptoms are referable to anemia with its consequent cardiovascular consequences, or to increased abdominal girth or discomfort resulting from splenic and hepatic enlargement. Bone pain, often migratory, and gouty arthritis occasionally bring the patient to medical attention. Deafness resulting from otosclerosis occurs in a small minority of cases. Increasing numbers of asymptomatic patients are being detected today in the course of routine screening laboratory or physical examinations.

On physical examination, splenomegaly is an almost universal finding. In approximately 85 per cent of cases, the spleen extends $\geq$ 8 cm below the left costal margin, and in one third of cases is enlarged more than 16 cm. Occasional patients without palpable splenomegaly will be demonstrated to have splenic enlargement by means of an isotopic or computerized tomographic imaging study. Rarely significant myelofibrosis with cytopenia occurs, at least initially, without myeloid metaplasia and with no evidence of splenic enlargement. Hepatomegaly occurs in approximately 50 per cent of cases, frequently with mild abnormalities of liver function tests—especially elevation of alkaline phosphatase. Hepatomegaly in the absence of splenomegaly is extremely rare in agnogenic myeloid metaplasia or when the syndrome occurs secondary to another myeloproliferative disease, and points to a diagnosis of secondary myeloid metaplasia. Extramedullary hematopoiesis is frequently demonstrable histologically in lymph nodes, but clinically significant lymph node enlargement occurs in only 10 per cent of cases. Petechiae, caused by both thrombocytopenia and platelet dysfunction, have been reported in up to 25 per cent of patients, and jaundice, edema, and ascites are found in 10 to 20 per cent of cases.

Laboratory Data

At diagnosis, a mild to moderate degree of anemia is typical with the hemoglobin ranging between 9 and 13 grams per 100 ml. Red cells are initially normocytic and normochromic with mild poikilocytosis. Polychromatophilia, a modest reticulocytosis of 2 to 5 per cent, and occasional teardrop erythrocytes are seen (Color plate *3D*). The presence of at least a few normoblasts and occasionally even earlier erythroid precursors is extremely common. As the disease progresses and the spleen enlarges, more severe anisocytosis, poikilocytosis, polychromasia, basophilic stippling, and normoblastosis may be sufficiently characteristic to indicate the diagnosis. The white blood cell count is initially normal in about one third of patients, elevated in approximately one half, and low in the remaining 15 per cent. Most typically, the count is in the range of 15,000 to 30,000 per cubic millimeter but counts as high as 70,000 per cubic millimeter are observed. The white count tends to fluctuate with time and often does not show the downward trend observed for the hemoglobin concentration and platelet count. A degree of granulocyte immaturity in the peripheral blood is typical, including the presence of as many as 10 per cent blasts. This does not necessarily suggest the evolution of acute leukemia, particularly when there are proportionate numbers of promyelocytes, myelocytes, and metamyelocytes as well. Basophilia and an acquired Pelger-Hüet anomaly are other typical features of the peripheral blood smear. The leukocyte alkaline phosphatase score is variable but is most often normal or increased. The platelet count initially is most often normal, although reduced or elevated counts are not uncommon. Exceedingly high counts in excess of 10^6 per microliter may cause this condition to be confused with the entity of primary thrombocytosis. Morphologically, megathrombocytes and megakaryocytic fragments are extremely common. Over a period of time, the platelet count gradually tends to decrease, and thrombocytopenia is common late in the disorder. Overall, a peripheral blood smear demonstrating striking teardrop poikilocytosis, leukoerythroblastic nucleated cells, and megathrombocytes and megakaryocytic fragments is highly suggestive of the syndrome of myelofibrosis with myeloid metaplasia. Erythrocyte survival is almost invariably reduced and splenic sequestration often is present. Platelet production is usually increased even in patients with thrombocytopenia, associated with a marked increase in splenic pooling.

Normal or slightly elevated serum levels of vitamin B_{12} and B_{12} binding proteins occur both in agnogenic myeloid metaplasia and postpolycythemia myelofibrosis, but the values are not as striking in those seen in chronic granulocytic leukemia. Hyperuricemia, due to increased uric acid production, is common. Miscellaneous laboratory abnormalities include high levels of LDH, modest elevations of serum transaminase and bilirubin levels, increased serum alkaline phosphatase activity caused by both hepatic and bone isoenzyme fractions, and modest increases in muramidase (lysozyme).

Cytogenetic abnormalities occur in up to 50 per cent of patients with agnogenic myeloid metaplasia with trisomy for a C group chromosome being probably the most common consistent alteration. The Ph^1 chromosome is not present.

Osteosclerosis distributed primarily in the flat bones of the axial skeleton and in the metaphyseal ends of the femur and humerus may be recognized radiographically in up to 70 per cent of patients. Osteosclerosis involving the ear ossicles may result in deafness. The typical radiographic finding is the loss of definition of individual bony trabeculae, leading to a ground glass appearance.

Attempts to aspirate bone marrow almost invariably lead to a dry tap, even when the marrow is very cellular. Accordingly, bone marrow biopsy, either percutaneous or surgical, is usually required for diagnosis. Demonstration of bone marrow fibrosis, often with accompanying osteosclerosis, is the sine qua non. The bone marrow may sometimes be hypercellular, frequently demonstrating a panhyperplasia, in residual focal areas. Even in these areas, in which mature collagen may not be evident, an increase in reticulin fibers can usually be demonstrated by silver impregnation. Extramedullary hematopoiesis is demonstrable in both liver and spleen, but because of the risks involved in percutaneous biopsy of these organs, its diagnosis usually is based on the typical leukoerythroblastic blood picture and occasionally on isotopic erythrokinetic studies. The increase of bone marrow collagen content in myelofibrosis is principally the result of excessive collagen deposition and is reflected in an increase in the serum level of procollagen III amino terminal peptide.

Course of the Disease

The course of both agnogenic and postpolycythemic myelofibrosis is characterized by progressive splenic enlargement and, typically, by slightly less striking enlargement of the liver. The spleen will often fill the entire left side of the abdomen, extending beyond the midline to the right and down into the pelvis. The resulting early satiety, associated with a hypermetabolic state from increased cell turnover, may result in appreciable weight loss. Painful splenic infarcts may also complicate the disease. The marked splenic enlargement and consequent increase in splenic blood flow, coupled with increased resistance to flow within the liver caused by extramedullary hematopoiesis, lead to portal hypertension and its various complications including ascites, edema, and variceal hemorrhage in a small proportion of patients. Hepatic vein thrombosis with Budd-Chiari syndrome is another recognized complication. The progressive splenomegaly is accompanied almost inevitably by progressive anemia and thrombocytopenia, the former occasionally complicated by iron deficiency of blood loss or, less frequently, by folic acid deficiency. Although granulocyte counts are usually better maintained than those of other blood cellular elements, eventually granulocytopenia may develop. In this setting bacterial infections occur with increased frequency and may be a major factor leading to death. The association of myelofibrosis with tuberculosis is well documented, and this infection should be excluded by histologic and bacteriologic examination. When the two disorders coincide it is not clear whether myelofibrosis is always secondary to tuberculous infection of the marrow, or whether, conversely, tuberculosis has supervened in a patient with an underlying clonal hemopathy. Because of the almost inevitable hyperuricemia, attacks of gouty arthritis may develop in untreated patients.

Treatment and Prognosis

No agreement has been reached as to the optimal treatment of agnogenic myeloid metaplasia or of postpolycythemic myelofibrosis. There is thus far no effective treatment that inhibits the fibrotic process. Moreover, none of the conventional forms of treatment, including androgen therapy to stimulate erythropoiesis, chemotherapy, or splenectomy, has been shown to prolong life. Because of the relatively indolent progression of the disorder in most patients, a majority of hematologists undertake no specific treatment in the asymptomatic patient except for the administration of allopurinol at doses of 200 to 400 mg per day to avoid the complications of hyperuricemia.

In the presence of symptomatic anemia, androgens may be employed: testosterone enanthate, 200 to 600 mg weekly intramuscularly, or oxymetholone, 50 to 150 mg daily by mouth. Treatment must be continued for at least three months to establish whether a particular preparation is effective, and some hematologists argue that patients who fail to respond to one androgen preparation may ultimately respond to another. Androgens seem most effective in women who have been splenectomized previously or who have never had massive splenomegaly. The doses employed inevitably lead to excessive fluid accumulation and, in female patients, to significant masculinization. The hemolytic anemia almost never responds to corticosteroids; these drugs may, however, increase the risk of infection in granulocytopenic patients. In patients with marked thrombocytosis, busulfan, in an initial dose of 4 mg per day followed by lower doses as the platelet count normalizes, or hydroxyurea at a dose of 500 to 1500 mg per day, is often effective in obtaining control of the platelet count. Although busulfan is widely used in this setting, its potential mutagenic risks are a cause for concern. These agents may occasionally produce a beneficial reduction in spleen size and/or increase the hemoglobin concentration but equally frequently will result in suppression of erythropoiesis and thrombopoiesis. Radiation therapy to the spleen has largely been abandoned because the doses required to produce a meaningful reduction in spleen size often cause severe leukopenia and thrombocytopenia.

The role of splenectomy in patients with agnogenic myeloid metaplasia or postpolycythemic myelofibrosis is highly controversial. As a high risk procedure, it should probably be reserved for patients with severe hemolytic anemia, thrombocytopenia sufficient to produce bleeding, portal hypertension, or severe discomfort secondary to pressure symptoms or infarction. Striking thrombocytosis with thrombosis or hemorrhage or both may develop postoperatively and may require aggressive myelosuppression. In some patients splenectomy is followed by progressive enlargement of the liver, with recurrent hemolysis and thrombocytopenia. The diagnosis of acute leukemia is often difficult to make in these patients in whom the percentage of blasts in the peripheral blood may increase slowly and progressively for years.

Survival in agnogenic myeloid metaplasia and in postpolycythemic myelofibrosis is difficult to define with certainty. Several authors suggest that median survival in agnogenic myeloid metaplasia is approximately ten years from the onset of the disease and five years from the time of diagnosis. However, there is considerable heterogeneity, with both shorter and longer survival frequently observed. The syndrome of acute myelofibrosis, which is a rapidly progressive and fatal variant, has been shown by various cytologic marker studies to represent an acute megakaryocytic leukemia.

Bone marrow transplantation has been attempted both by conventional techniques and after surgical manipulation of bone marrow cavity spaces in attempts to provide an improved microenvironment for the transplanted marrow. Only occasional successes have been reported, and this procedure must be considered highly experimental.

Berk PD, Castro-Malaspina H, Wasserman LR (eds.): Myelofibrosis and the Biology of Connective Tissue. New York, Alan R. Liss, Inc., 1984. *This book contains 29 concise chapters by multiple authors who review the available information about the regulation of fibroblast proliferation, collagen biosynthesis, cell biology of marrow stromal cells, and other aspects of basic biologic science believed to be of relevance to the pathogenesis of myelofibrosis.*

Kroopman JE: The pathogenesis of myelofibrosis in myeloproliferative disorders. Ann Intern Med 92:858, 1980. *Excellent brief summary of recent speculations on the pathogenesis of myelofibrosis.*

Silverstein MN: The evolution and treatment of late stage polycythemia vera. Semin Hematol 13:79, 1976. *An excellent description of post-polycythemic myelofibrosis or the "spent phase" of polycythemia vera with emphasis on practical management.*

Varki A, Lottenberg R, Griffith R, Reinhard E: The syndrome of idiopathic myelofibrosis. Clinicopathologic review with emphasis on the prognostic variables predicting survival. Medicine 62:53, 1983. *This is a useful recent review of 88 consecutive patients with bone marrow fibrosis seen at Barnes Hospital. As noted in the title, there is considerable emphasis on prognostic features.*

Ward HP, Block MH: The natural history of agnogenic myeloid metaplasia (AMM) and a critical evaluation of its relationship with the myeloproliferative syndrome. Medicine 50:357, 1971. *A classic encyclopedic description of this disorder.*

ESSENTIAL THROMBOCYTHEMIA

Essential thrombocythemia, also known as a hemorrhagic thrombocythemia or essential thrombocytosis, is a primary myeloproliferative disorder in which the predominant laboratory feature is a persistent, striking elevation of the platelet count to values in excess of 1×10^6 per microliter. The disorder shows many features of polycythemia vera including an almost identical distribution of patient ages at the time of diagnosis, similar degrees of leukocytosis, and morphologically similar bone marrow abnormalities. Splenomegaly has been reported to occur in from 30 to 75 per cent of cases. The criteria outlined in the following paragraph would restrict the diagnosis to patients who have either normal or reduced hemoglobin concentrations, those with concomitant erythrocytosis being classified as having polycythemia vera.

The Polycythemia Vera Study Group has recently proposed the following diagnostic criteria for essential thrombocythemia: (1) platelet count persistently greater than 1×10^6 per microliter in the absence of an identifiable cause such as malignancy, infection, chronic inflammatory disease, or previous splenectomy; (2) normal total red cell volume, the measurement of which may be omitted if the hemoglobin concentration is less than 13 grams per 100 ml; (3) presence of iron in the bone marrow; if iron is absent, failure of the hemoglobin concentration to increase by more than 1 gram per 100 ml after a one-month trial of oral iron therapy; (4) absence of collagen fibrosis in bone marrow biopsy; and (5) absence of the Philadelphia chromosome from unstimulated metaphases obtained from a bone marrow aspirate. Because of both morphologic and clinical similarities, criteria 2 and 3 are necessary to exclude a diagnosis of polycythemia vera, whereas criteria 4 and 5 distinguish the disorder from agnogenic myeloid metaplasia and chronic myelogenous leukemia, respectively.

Clinical Features

The predominant clinical manifestations of essential thrombocythemia result from hemorrhagic and/or thrombotic events. Some patients have easy bruising, epistaxis, unexplained gastrointestinal bleeding, and an excessive tendency to postoperative hemorrhage. Conversely, other patients present evidence for microvascular occlusion in sites such as the extremities, the central nervous system, and the coronary circulation. The commonest manifestation of microvascular occlusion is burning pain in the feet, hands, and digits, which may progress to frank gangrene. Although these symptoms are striking when they occur, large numbers of patients, particularly younger patients, may be asymptomatic for long periods. Hence, the precise incidence of these complications is unknown. Similarly, transition to acute leukemia has been clearly documented, but there is no accurate estimate of its frequency, particularly in patients not previously exposed to mutagenic agents.

Course and Prognosis

The natural history of this disease is poorly appreciated, and most reports in the literature describe very small series of patients with a focus on a particular complication. Descriptions emphasizing hemorrhagic, thrombotic, and embolic episodes and a high fatality rate are directly contradicted by others emphasizing prolonged periods without complications. The largest series suggest a life expectancy perhaps analogous to that of polycythemia vera.

Therapy

Because of uncertainties about its natural history, there is a substantial lack of agreement about appropriate therapy for essential thrombocythemia. Despite strikingly high platelet counts, many hematologists recommend expectant management in asymptomatic patients under the age of 60, while others recommend the use only of platelet antiaggregating agents (e.g., aspirin 300 mg per day with or without dipyridamole 50 mg three times daily).* However, the experience in polycythemia vera suggests that chronic administration of platelet antiaggregating agents may increase the risk of gastrointestinal hemorrhage. Chronic myelosuppression should be attempted in older patients and those who have a history of significant thrombotic episodes. In these cases, prevention of neurologic damage takes precedence over concern about long-term mutagenic effects of myelosuppression. Control of the thrombocytosis can be achieved with melphalan* 6 to 10 mg per day by mouth for one week followed by 4 to 6 mg per day until the platelet count is in the normal range. Subsequent maintenance with 2 to 6 mg per week is continued indefinitely. Alternatively, hydroxyurea* at an initial dose of 500 to 1500 mg per day, tapered to an individualized maintenance dose as the platelet count falls, or radioactive phosphorus 2.9 mCi per square meter of body surface area intravenously, repeated as necessary at intervals of not less than three months, is highly effective in achieving normalization of the platelet count. Patients presenting with serious thrombotic or hemorrhagic manifestations and uncontrolled thrombocytosis should be treated with platelet antiaggregating agents, urgent platelet phoresis, and the initiation of a myelosuppressive regimen. Every effort should be made to avoid splenectomy in patients with essential thrombocythemia because of the extreme thrombocytosis and serious complications that often follow this procedure.

---

*This use is not listed in the manufacturer's directive.

Murphy S: Thrombocytosis and thrombocythaemia. Clin Hematol 12:89, 1983. *A detailed review of the pathogenesis, pathophysiology, and management of this puzzling disorder. Excellent bibliography.*

Kessler CM, Klein HG, Havlik RJ: Uncontrolled thrombocytosis in chronic myeloproliferative disorders. Br J Haematol 50:157, 1982. *A retrospective study suggesting that, at least in the younger patient, severe thrombocytosis in myeloproliferative disease may have fewer complications than previously believed.*

Jabaily J, Iland HJ, Laszlo J, Massey EW, Faguet GB, Briere J, Landaw SA: Neurologic manifestations of essential thrombocythemia. Ann Intern Med 99:513, 1983. *A contrary report on the largest series of patients with essential thrombocythemia yet assembled, suggesting that approximately two thirds have evidence of at least transient neurologic dysfunction.*

155. THE CHRONIC LEUKEMIAS

Bayard Clarkson

Chronic Myelogenous Leukemia (Chronic Myeloid Leukemia [CML], Chronic Myelocytic Leukemia, Chronic Granulocytic Leukemia)

DEFINITION. Chronic myelogenous leukemia (CML) is a chronic form of leukemia originating in a primitive myeloid stem cell in which the leukemic cells retain the capacity for differentiation and are able to perform the essential functions of normal hematopoietic cells that they replace in the marrow. The leukemic cells have a pronounced tendency to undergo further malignant transformation with loss of ability to differentiate in later stages of the disease. Although commonly included among other myeloproliferative disorders (see Ch. 154), CML is a distinct entity that is easily recognized because the leukemic cells have a distinctive cytogenetic abnormality, the Philadelphia (Ph^1) chromosome.

ETIOLOGY. The etiology is unknown. The majority of patients with CML have no history of excessive exposure to ionizing radiation or chemical leukemogens, but the incidence increases greatly with exposure to high doses of radiation. This may occur following chronic exposure in radiologists who practice without adequate shielding, in patients who have received radiation treatments for ankylosing spondylitis or other chronic diseases, and in subjects exposed to a single massive dose of radiation as in the atomic bomb explosions in Hiroshima and Nagasaki in 1945. After subacute or acute exposure to large radiation doses as in the last two instances, there is a latent period of several years after which the incidence of both acute myeloid leukemia and CML increases in an approximately linear relationship to the radiation dose. In the atomic bomb survivors the peak incidence occurred about seven years after the explosion and was about 50 times that of nonexposed subjects. The rate then declined but still exceeded the national average 15 years later. Radiation hazards are more extensively discussed in Ch. 562.

The contribution of chemicals to the causation of CML is hard to assess. Any chemical capable of causing myelotoxicity or chromosome damage is suspect. However, persons in industrialized societies are exposed to such a wide variety of chemicals with these properties, including solvents, insecticides, hair dyes, and various drugs, that their very prevalence makes it difficult to incriminate specific candidates. Heavy occupational exposure to benzene is commonly cited as having an etiologic role, but here, too, it is difficult to exclude other contributory factors. Cytotoxic drugs, especially alkylating agents and when used in combination with radiation in the treatment of other neoplastic diseases (such as Hodgkin's disease), are known to increase the incidence of leukemia, usually after a latent period of several years. The most common type of leukemia is one of the variants of acute myeloid leukemia, but CML may also occur rarely. The minimal leukemogenic dose has not been established for any chemical or drug in humans, but it is only prudent to try to minimize unnecessary exposure to any potential leukemogens.

INCIDENCE AND PREVALENCE. The incidence of CML in the United States and most Western countries is about 1.5 per 100,000 population per year and accounts for about 15 per cent of all cases of leukemia. CML is slightly more frequent in men than women, but the course of the disease is the same. The median age is about 45 and the disease is uncommon below the age of 20. In children with CML in whom the Ph^1 chromosome is present, the course of the disease is similar to that of adults. A juvenile form of CML, described in very young children, has a more rapidly progressive course and the leukemic cells lack the Philadelphia (Ph^1) chromosome.

Although a few instances have been noted of CML occurring in multiple family members, familial occurrence is uncommon, and children born to mothers who have the disease are normal.

PATHOGENESIS AND MECHANISMS. Chronic myelogenous leukemia is a uniclonal neoplastic proliferation of hematopoietic stem cells (see Ch. 152). In about 90 per cent of cases the leukemic cells have a unique chromosomal abnormality, the Philadelphia (Ph¹) chromosome. The Ph¹ anomaly results from a reciprocal translocation of a portion of the long arm of chromosome 22 to another chromosome, usually the long arm of chromosome 9, although sometimes to another chromosome. Both deletion of the long arm of number 22 and translocation to another chromosome must be demonstrated by appropriate banding studies in order to confirm Ph¹ positivity. Although no specific phenotypic change has yet been identified that is linked to this unique genetic alteration, the anomaly is so consistent that it appears likely with further application of modern molecular genetic techniques that it will soon be possible to demonstrate the genetic lesion is in some way related to the leukemic cells' abnormal proliferation. For example, the cellular oncogenes c-abl and c-sis (so called because of their associations with Abelson leukemia and simian sarcoma viruses) are normally located on chromosomes 9 and 22, respectively. C-abl is located on the long arm of chromosome 9 at band q34, which is the breakpoint in the 9;22 translocation in CML. The c-abl oncogene is consistently translocated to chromosome 22 in Ph¹-positive CML, and c-sis also undergoes reciprocal translocation to chromosome 9. It has been proposed that the former translocation may result in activation of the c-abl oncogene, or perhaps alter the transcriptional activity at some nearby regulatory gene (as yet unidentified), but it is not yet understood how the genetic rearrangements are related to the transformed cells' altered behavior.

About 10 per cent of patients who present with the clinical features of CML do not have the Ph¹ chromosome in their marrow cells. The course of the disease is atypical in these Ph¹-negative patients in that they generally have a poor response to treatment and shorter survival than Ph¹-positive patients.

There is good evidence, based on the occurrence of CML in patients with chromosome mosaicism and in those heterozygous for the enzyme glucose-6-phosphate dehydrogenase, that the leukemic population arises from a single cell because the Ph¹ anomaly has been found to be restricted to just one of their dual cell lines. The defect is an acquired one, since the Ph¹ marker is not present in nonhematopoietic cells and monozygous twins of patients with CML do not have the Ph¹ chromosome in their myeloid cells. The presence of the Ph¹ genetic marker in erythrocyte, granulocyte, monocyte, and megakaryocyte precursors indicates that the original transformation occurred in an ancestral cell common to these myeloid cell types, but the exact location of the transforming event within the progenitor cell lineages is still uncertain.

The Ph¹ chromosome is absent in the majority of mature lymphocytes, although in some patients some of the B cells and more rarely T cells have been found to contain the Ph¹ marker. When one or more of the chronic phase leukemic cells undergo blastic transformation, in about 25 per cent of such cases the blasts have been found to have phenotypic properties associated with lymphocyte precursors, including high levels of terminal deoxynucleotidyl transferase and reactivity with specific antisera prepared against the common type of acute lymphoblastic leukemic cells. Some cases of CML blastic transformation have been reported in which the blasts contain intracellular IgM, a characteristic of pre-B cells. While in most cases of lymphoid blastic transformation detectable cytoplasmic and surface immunoglobulin are lacking, in the majority of cases there is rearrangement of the immunoglobulin heavy chain genes, and in some there is also progression to light chain–gene rearrangements. Since these gene rearrangements are a mandatory early step in B cell development and rarely occur within other human hematopoietic lineages, the findings provide strong evidence that the lymphoid blasts are early B cell precursors.

On the basis of serial hematologic examinations of atomic bomb survivors who developed CML, it has been estimated that about eight years elapse between the original mutational event that results in the first Ph¹-positive leukemic cell in the marrow and the development of clinical symptoms when the diagnosis is ordinarily made. Since the average survival after diagnosis is three years, the total course of the disease is thus about 11 years. At the time of diagnosis 85 to 100 per cent of the dividing marrow cells contain the Ph¹ marker in the majority of patients. A few patients have lesser degrees of replacement of normal marrow cells by leukemic cells at diagnosis, and in such cases the leukemic and normal populations may coexist in nearly equal balance for a year or more before the leukemic cells eventually replace the normal cells. Cells containing the Ph¹ chromosome have not been found in normal subjects.

The reason why the leukemic cells have a proliferative advantage is not known. In the chronic stage of the disease the leukemic cells retain the capacity to differentiate almost normally, and the enzymatic and functional defects exhibited by the leukemic cells are not of sufficient severity to prevent them from carrying out their essential functions in supporting life in the absence of normal cells. Many of the defects somehow appear to be related to the increased mass of the leukemic population because such abnormalities as deficient neutrophil alkaline phosphatase, impaired phagocytic capacity of neutrophils, and various platelet and red cell abnormalities return toward normal after the cell density has been reduced by treatment.

There is characteristically a marked shift toward granulocyte differentiation at the expense of erythroid differentiation in untreated CML, but the myeloid:erythroid ratio usually returns toward normal after treatment. In most cases, neutrophilic granulocytes predominate, but eosinophilia and/or basophilia and monocytosis also occur frequently. Increased numbers of megakaryocytes and thrombocytosis frequently accompany the increased granulocyte production, but thrombocytopenia may also be observed. Some degree of anemia is common, and rarely erythrocytosis may occur.

The mass of myeloid tissue is usually greatly increased in CML at the time of diagnosis, sometimes ten-fold or more. The leukemic granulocytic precursors in the marrow and spleen divide less rapidly than the corresponding cells in normal marrow, although their rate of proliferation may be nearly normal very early in the disease or after the myeloid mass has been reduced by treatment. In the chronic phase the percentage of myeloblasts is usually not increased compared to normal marrow, but their absolute number is greatly increased because of the expanded mass of myeloid tissue in the marrow, spleen, blood, and sometimes other extramedullary sites. There is also a greatly increased incidence of earlier committed granulocyte-monocyte precursors that form colonies and clusters in semisolid culture systems and that show nearly normal in vitro maturation and growth. The primary reason for the expanded myeloid mass is that the leukemic stem cells continue to proliferate after exceeding the cell density limit in the marrow at which normal stem cells arrest cell production. The specific biochemical abnormalities responsible for the failure of the multipotent leukemic stem cells to respond normally to feedback regulation are not yet well understood, although the CML precursors have been shown to be relatively insensitive to several naturally occurring physiologic inhibitors (e.g., lactoferrin).

The leukemic cells in chronic phase CML have a striking propensity for further malignant transformation. After a variable duration of the chronic phase, averaging about three years, the disease enters an accelerated or blastic phase. Such malignant progression occurs in about 80 per cent of patients and probably would eventually occur in all of them if they did not die of other complications of the disease or of unrelated causes. The Ph¹ chromosome is preserved, but the transformed cells may acquire additional chromosomal abnormalities such as an additional Ph^1 chromosome, trisomy of chromosome 8 or 17, or trisomy of the long arm of 17. The rapidity with which the transition occurs depends on the degree of further transformation and on the comparative proliferative properties of the chronic and acute phase stem cells. In the accelerated phase the cells retain their capacity for partial differentiation, whereas in the blastic phase they are arrested at the blastic level of differentiation. The direction of differentiation in the accelerated phase is variable as in the chronic phase. Transitional forms may occur between the chronic, accelerated, and blastic phases.

CLINICAL MANIFESTATIONS. ***Symptoms.*** Occasionally CML is diagnosed in an asymptomatic patient after incidental detection of splenomegaly or unexplained leukocytosis, basophilia, or thrombocytosis. Common early symptoms are *fatigue* and reduced exercise tolerance resulting from anemia, anorexia, reduction in food capacity, weight loss, and a sense of fullness in the left upper quadrant as a result of progressive splenic enlargement. Headaches, sweating, fever, and bone pain or tenderness may also occur, especially if the leukocyte count is very elevated. *Hemorrhagic manifestations* such as ecchymoses after minor trauma, petechiae, retinal hemorrhages, or hematuria may occur in patients in whom there is severe thrombocytopenia or in those with thrombocytosis with abnormal platelets. *Thrombotic episodes* such as splenic or myocardial infarction and thrombophlebitis are common, and priapism or severe headaches may result from leukostasis in patients with extreme leukocytosis. Acute *gouty arthritis* or *nephrolithiasis* is sometimes associated with elevated uric acid levels. Infections are uncommon in the chronic phase, but occasional patients may have unusual and persistent infections which are difficult to diagnose. Low grade *fever* in the absence of infection is not unusual in the chronic phase when there is extreme leukocytosis, and the temperature returns to normal when the WBC is lowered by treatment.

PHYSICAL EXAMINATION. The most common finding on physical examination at diagnosis is *splenomegaly*. The spleen may be enormous and fill most of the abdomen, or only minimally enlarged; in less than 10 per cent of cases the spleen is not palpable or enlarged on splenic scan. Slight hepatomegaly is common, but when extreme liver enlargement occurs as a result of leukemic infiltration or there is infiltration of lymph nodes, skin, or other tissues, these are usually indications that the disease will have a rapidly progressive course. Patients who present with the disease already in blastic transformation or in whom this event occurs later in the course of the disease may exhibit any of the clinical findings associated with acute leukemia. Unlike in acute leukemia, persistent fever unrelated to infection is common in the blastic phase of CML.

LABORATORY ABNORMALITIES. The most consistent laboratory abnormality at diagnosis is *leukocytosis*. The white blood cell count (WBC) may range from a minimal elevation to over a million leukocytes per cubic millimeter. The marrow is hypercellular, and differential counts of both marrow and blood show a spectrum of mature and immature granulocytes similar to that found in normal marrow. Increased numbers of eosinophils and/or basophils are often present, and sometimes monocytosis is seen. Increased megakaryocytes are often found in the marrow, and sometimes fragments of megakaryocyte nuclei are present in the blood, especially when the platelet count is very high. The percentage of lymphocytes is reduced in both the marrow and blood in comparison to normal subjects, but the absolute lymphocyte count is usually normal or increased with normal proportions of B and T cells. The myeloid:erythroid ratio in the marrow is usually greatly elevated. The percentage of blasts in the marrow and blood is usually less than 3 per cent in the chronic phase at diagnosis and less than 1 per cent after the WBC has been reduced by treatment; a persistent elevation of greater than 10 per cent usually indicates impending transformation. About half of patients present with some degree of *thrombocytosis* at diagnosis; thrombocytopenia is much less frequent. Extreme degrees of thrombocytopenia or thrombocytosis may develop as the disease progresses. In some patients, cyclic fluctuations of the leukocytes and platelets have been observed that are unrelated to treatment.

There may be no anemia at presentation, but variable degrees of *anemia* are common when the WBC exceeds 50,000 per cubic millimeter. The anemia is normocytic and normochromic, unless complications such as bleeding occur, resulting in iron deficiency. Some patients, especially those with greatly enlarged spleens, have circulating nucleated erythrocyte precursors, but this finding is not usually prominent. There may be shortened red cell survival in patients with severe splenomegaly and/or hepatomegaly, but autoimmune hemolysis is not seen in uncomplicated CML. The reticulocyte count is normal or only slightly increased.

The mature granulocytes in CML usually have markedly diminished neutrophil alkaline phosphatase activity and their content of myeloperoxidase and lactoferrin may also be decreased. Plasma and leukocyte levels of histamine and histamine metabolites are usually elevated. Other common laboratory abnormalities in CML that are associated with the increased rates of cell production and turnover are elevated levels of serum uric acid, lactic dehydrogenase, vitamin B_{12}, the B_{12} binding protein transcobalamin I, and serum urinary lysozyme. Hyperkalemia resulting from leakage of potassium from leukocytes occurs rarely. Hypercalcemia may also occur, usually in patients with blastic transformation or in those who are entering an accelerated phase and have lytic bone lesions.

Myelofibrosis, demonstrated by special stains of marrow biopsy specimens, may develop in the course of CML. Significant myelofibrosis is more often seen late in the course of disease, but rarely severe acute myelofibrosis is seen prior to treatment in patients with prominent megakaryocytic proliferation. The marrow histiocytes sometimes display prominent phagocytic activity and become engorged with glycolipids, resembling Gaucher cells.

Transition from the chronic phase to the accelerated or blastic phase may occur gradually over a year or longer or abruptly ("blast crisis"). The disease becomes progressively less responsive to previously effective treatment. Common signs and symptoms heralding such a change are progressive leukocytosis, thrombocytosis or thrombocytopenia, anemia, increasing and painful splenomegaly, lymphadenopathy, hepatomegaly, or infiltration of other organs, fever, bone pain, development of destructive bone lesions, and thrombotic or bleeding complications. In the accelerated phase, the cells are still completely or partially differentiated, although they usually show increasing morphologic abnormalities. There are no standardized criteria for distinguishing between the accelerated and blastic phases, but most authorities use a persistent elevation of greater than 20 or 30 per cent blasts in the blood and/or marrow or of blasts plus promyelocytes of 30 per cent in blood or 50 per cent in marrow to define the blastic phase. When the spleen is the primary source of the transformed cells, the percentage of blasts in the blood may be higher than in the marrow. The blasts have the morphologic appearance of lymphoblasts in about 25 per cent of cases and contain terminal deoxynucleotidyl transferase, whereas in the remainder they are recognized as primitive myeloid precursors.

DIAGNOSIS. Persistent unexplained leukocytosis with circulating immature granulocytes and an enlarged spleen suggests the diagnosis of CML; some degree of splenomegaly is present at diagnosis in over 90 per cent of patients. A bone marrow aspiration and biopsy should always be done if the diagnosis of CML is suspected. Demonstration of the Ph^1 chromosome in dividing marrow cells provides confirmation of the diagnosis in Ph^1-positive CML. The 10 per cent or so of patients with Ph^1-negative CML are often older males, usually have a lesser degree of leukocytosis and more pronounced thrombocytopenia and/or anemia than the Ph^1-positive cases, and often have greatly elevated levels of serum and urinary muramidase.

Leukemoid reactions associated with infections are usually distinguishable in most cases because prominent splenomegaly is absent, neutrophil alkaline phosphatase activity is elevated instead of low, and the Ph[1] chromosome is not present (see Ch. 151). Leukemoid or leukoerythroblastic reactions also occur with certain neoplasms, especially when there is involvement of the bone marrow, but sometimes even in the absence of marrow metastases. Experienced morphologists are usually able to distinguish metastatic tumor cells from immature hematopoietic cells, although repeated aspirations and/or biopsies may sometimes be necessary if the distribution of the tumor cells is patchy. Leukoerythroblastic reactions may also be associated with hemorrhagic shock or hemolysis or as a rebound phenomenon following cytotoxic or infectious depression of the marrow; but a careful history, appropriate diagnostic tests, and a short period of observation should avoid confusion with CML.

Myelofibrosis, polycythemia vera, and other myeloproliferative variants may present with splenomegaly, leukocytosis, and immature granulocytes in the blood, but the neutrophil alkaline phosphatase activity is usually high in these disorders, and the Ph[1] chromosome is absent. The hematocrit is elevated in polycythemia vera (unless bleeding occurs), whereas it is normal or decreased in CML. Bone marrow biopsy and appropriate stains may reveal some increase in reticulin fibers or fibrosis in CML, but these findings are less prominent than in myelofibrosis. Patients who have the clinical manifestations of CML but without the Ph[1] chromosome may have mixed features of CML and other myeloproliferative disorders. Chronic monocytic or chronic myelomonocytic leukemia and the chronic form of erythroleukemia are more properly regarded as variants of acute leukemia. Splenomegaly may occur in these latter conditions, but leukocytosis is seldom as prominent as in CML, and pancytopenia is more common. The Ph[1] chromosome is not present, although other chromosomal abnormalities may occur.

Basophilic leukemia and eosinophilic leukemia may rarely occur as variants of CML or other myeloproliferative diseases and are usually associated with a poor prognosis. Basophilic leukemia should be distinguished from mast cell leukemia, in which urticaria pigmentosa is usually seen concomitantly. Thrombocythemia and megakaryocytic leukemia occur fairly commonly as variants of CML or other myeloproliferative disorders. Infrequently unexplained "essential" thrombocythemia and megakaryocytic hyperplasia are observed as isolated findings without Ph[1]-positive cells in the marrow or other abnormalities of the myeloid elements. Such patients often later develop other manifestations of one of the myeloproliferative diseases.

Chronic neutrophilic leukemia is a rare disease, occurring mostly in older patients, which is characterized by marked splenomegaly, leukocytosis with 90 per cent or more mature neutrophils in the blood, elevated neutrophil alkaline phosphatase, and a chronic course. The absence of immature granulocytes in the blood and of the Ph[1] chromosome in the marrow distinguish this type of leukemia from CML.

The first clinical manifestations of blastic transformation may occur in extramedullary sites such as the spleen, lymph nodes, meninges, or other tissues, while the marrow and blood are still filled with chronic phase leukemic cells. If immature granulocytes are the predominant cell type, the extramedullary tumors may have a green hue owing to myeloperoxidase and are sometimes diagnosed as chloromas or granulocytic sarcomas. If the transformed cells resemble lymphoblasts, an erroneous diagnosis of lymphoma is sometimes made. Demonstration of the Ph[1] chromosome in the blasts will lead to the correct diagnosis. Since localized blastic lesions invariably become disseminated, usually within several months, systemic treatment, sometimes in addition to local irradiation, is justified once the diagnosis is made.

The leukemic cells in CML sometimes undergo early blastic transformation without recognition of the chronic phase, and patients may present with what appears to be acute leukemia, either lymphoblastic or one of the myeloid variants. A very large spleen, extreme leukocytosis (>400,000 per cubic millimeter), prominent eosinophilia and/or basophilia, and a normal or elevated platelet count should alert the physician to this possible diagnostic dilemma. However, all of these features may be absent in patients with CML presenting in blastic crisis de novo, and cytogenetic examination of the marrow is necessary to confirm the presence or absence of the Ph[1] chromosome. Patients presenting with the lymphoblastic type of blastic transformation of CML without a preceding chronic phase are being diagnosed more frequently when cytogenetic analysis of the marrow is performed in patients with a clinical diagnosis of lymphoblastic leukemia (ALL). Whenever possible, all patients with this suspected diagnosis should have cytogenetic analyses performed prior to treatment because there are important prognostic differences between ALL and lymphoblastic CML (Ph[1] + ALL). The incidence of Ph[1] + ALL is about 20 per cent and 2 per cent in adults and children, respectively, in patients with a suspected diagnosis of ALL.

TREATMENT. Asymptomatic patients in the chronic phase in whom the WBC is below 50,000 per cubic millimeter can be observed without treatment until the disease progresses and symptoms develop. When clinical manifestations appear they can usually be controlled with cytotoxic drugs or splenic irradiation, but unlike in acute leukemia, true remissions are very rare and the marrow remains largely populated with leukemic cells containing the Ph[1] marker.

Chemotherapy. The most common conventional drug used is *busulfan*, but other alkylating agents such as cyclophosphamide and antimetabolites are also effective. One must be careful to avoid overtreatment of CML, as severe myelosuppression can occur. The usual starting oral dose of busulfan is 4 to 8 mg per day, but doses of 12 to 16 mg or higher may be required initially if the blood leukocyte and/or platelet counts are very high and rapid reduction is necessary. The dose should be reduced as the WBC falls and the spleen shrinks during the first several weeks, roughly in proportion to halving of the WBC. For example, if the initial WBC is 100,000 per cubic millimeter and the initial dose of busulfan is 8 mg per day, when the WBC reaches 50,000 per cubic millimeter the dose should be lowered to 4 mg per day. The drug should be stopped when the WBC reaches about 25,000 per cubic millimeter, as it may continue to fall after stopping and overtreatment can cause prolonged marrow hypoplasia. Other manifestations of chronic busulfan toxicity include sterility, hyperpigmentation, adrenal insufficiency, and, rarely, severe pulmonary fibrosis. In some patients the WBC and spleen size may remain nearly normal without further treatment for months after initial control has been achieved, whereas others require continuous treatment. There is considerable variability in responsiveness, and the exact dose must be titrated individually. The dose of busulfan required to maintain control of the chronic phase is usually between 2 mg every other day and 4 mg per day. Some authorities prefer intermittent therapy rather than continuous treatment. The amount of drug needed for control does not appear to be related to prognosis.

Purine and pyrimidine antagonists and hydroxyurea, a ribonucleotide reductase inhibitor, are also effective in controlling chronic phase CML. The usual initial oral dose of *hydroxyurea* is between 1 and 3 grams per day, depending on the height of the WBC and the body surface area. Hydroxyurea should be taken as a single dose at least an hour before eating. After the WBC and spleen size are reduced to normal, the dose required for maintenance is usually between 0.5 gram every other day and 2.0 grams per day and must be titrated individually. Continuous treatment and close monitoring of the WBC are necessary with hydroxyurea, as its inhibitory effects on myeloproliferation are much more transient than with busulfan and the WBC may rise rapidly when it is discontinued. Hydroxyurea is generally well tolerated, but it may cause nausea, vomiting, diarrhea, stomatitis, dermatitis, and megaloblastosis.

Treatment of Acute Leukostatic or Thrombotic Complications. Some patients with CML may present with acute leukostatic or thrombotic complications (e.g., priapism, thrombophlebitis, infarctions of the spleen or other organs, sagittal sinus thrombosis, or other complications affecting the central nervous system), and in such cases it is mandatory to lower the WBC and/or platelet count rapidly with cytotoxic drugs. A continuous intravenous infusion of cytosine arabinoside, 200 mg per square meter of body surface area per 24 hours, or of hydroxyurea, 2 to 3 grams per square meter per day for four or five days, will usually lower the WBC and platelet count rapidly, relieve the acute symptoms, and prevent additional complications. Leukapheresis and/or plateletpheresis is also effective in rapidly reducing the counts if a continuous flow centrifuge is available. The reduction is usually very transient, however, and chemotherapy should also be begun immediately for sustained control. Thrombocytosis sometimes persists after the WBC has been reduced by chemotherapy, and in such cases melphalan and/or thiotepa may be useful in controlling the platelets.

Tumor Lysis Syndrome. The patient should be well hydrated and allopurinol administered before beginning cytotoxic therapy when rapid cell lysis is anticipated in order to prevent exacerbation of hyperuricemia and development of uric acid nephropathy or acute arthritis. Hyperkalemia, hyperphosphatemia, elevation of lactic dehydrogenase, and other biochemical abnormalities may also occur during sudden massive leukemic cell destruction ("tumor lysis syndrome"), but with adequate hydration to maintain a good urinary output and close monitoring, serious complications resulting from these biochemical alterations can usually be avoided.

Splenic Radiation. Splenic radiation is also effective in reducing the size of the spleen and WBC. The radiation treatments should be given cautiously in fractionated doses over several weeks because the WBC may continue to fall after stopping, and, as with busulfan, overtreatment can cause prolonged marrow hypoplasia. The total splenic dose needed for control is usually between 300 and 1200 rads, depending on the size of the spleen and radiation port, but the splenomegaly in some patients may be refractory to even larger doses. Splenectomy performed early in the chronic phase does not significantly affect survival, although in patients who are prone to develop massive splenomegaly it prevents later complications which become difficult to manage (e.g., hypersplenism, inanition, repeated infarctions).

Aggressive Combination Chemotherapy. Some centers have recently taken a more aggressive therapeutic approach in chronic phase CML with the use of combination chemotherapeutic regimens effective in acute myeloid leukemia. Complete remissions with marked reduction or disappearance of Ph^1-positive leukemic cells in the marrow have been obtained in 20 to 50 per cent of patients, but most of the remissions have been of short duration. Patients having remissions live longer than nonresponders, but overall survival does not appear to be significantly prolonged by the intensive treatment regimens employed to date.

Marrow Transplantation. It has only been possible to eradicate the leukemic clone by administering very high doses of alkylating agents in combination with a supralethal dose of total body irradiation, followed by rescue with transplantation of marrow from a histocompatible donor. Over a dozen patients with CML with identical twins have been so treated during the last few years, of whom the majority remain free of disease without further treatment with no detectable Ph^1-positive cells in the marrow for periods of up to five years. The hazards associated with allogeneic marrow transplantation using histocompatible nonidentical sibling donors are still formidable, especially in older patients, but in the last several years over a hundred patients with chronic phase CML, mostly under the age of 40, have received allogeneic transplants. It is too soon to evaluate the long-term results, but it appears that 60 to 70 per cent of patients are surviving the procedure; the others have usually died within a few months of complications related to the transplantation procedure, most often of interstitial pneumonia or graft-versus-host disease. The majority of the survivors have had either acute or chronic graft-versus-host disease, but so far there have been relatively few relapses and most of the patients have remained Ph^1 negative (see Ch. 165).

Treatment of the Accelerated or Blastic Phase. When CML enters an accelerated phase it becomes increasingly refractory to therapy that was previously effective. Increasing doses of busulfan or hydroxyurea are required to control the WBC and spleen size and, in some cases, progressive thrombocytosis. In some cases, severe anemia and/or thrombocytopenia develop, either because of the disease or as a result of drug toxicity.

Therapy of the blastic phase is generally unsatisfactory, and most patients die within a few months after blastic transformation occurs. Hydroxyurea is most commonly used to control myeloid blastic transformation, but multidrug regimens designed for acute nonlymphoblastic leukemia are also used. In the 25 per cent of patients with lymphoblastic transformation, remission can often be achieved with prednisone and vincristine with reversion to the chronic phase, but these are usually of short duration and the average survival in different series was three to eight months. Complete remissions with disappearance of the Ph^1-positive cells in the marrow have rarely been achieved with intensive combinations of regimens designed for acute lymphoblastic leukemia, but these have all been only temporary and no cures have resulted. The average survival of patients with lymphoblastic transformation who are treated with modern intensive programs designed for ALL is about a year. The response is not significantly different in patients who initially present in blastic phase (Ph^1 + ALL) compared with those who develop lymphoblastic transformation after a recognized chronic phase. Any of the myriad complications seen in acute leukemia can be encountered during the blastic phase of CML. Meningeal leukemia should be treated with intrathecal methotrexate or arabinosylcytosine and/or cranial irradiation as in acute leukemia.

Since few patients respond satisfactorily to any treatment after myeloid blastic transformation is fully developed, there have been recent attempts to treat such patients aggressively with combination regimens designed for acute myeloid leukemia as soon as early evidence of impending blastic transformation can be detected, such as by appearance of additional chromosomal abnormalities or by a change in the growth pattern of the marrow colony forming cells in vitro. Although this approach may delay overt blastic transformation, it is not clear that survival is significantly affected. Previous trials of aggressive treatment followed by allogeneic marrow transplantation in the blastic phase were largely unsuccessful, but the results of more recent trials in earlier stages of accelerated or blastic disease have been more favorable. There are now an appreciable number of disease-free survivors, although longer follow-up will be required to be certain these patients have been cured. Intensive treatment of the blastic phase followed by transplantation of stored autologous stem cells obtained from the marrow or blood during the chronic phase has been successful in temporarily restoring the disease to the chronic phase in some patients, but the mortality has been high and it has not been demonstrated that overall survival is increased.

PROGNOSIS. The median survival of patients with Ph^1-positive CML from diagnosis is about three years, with a range of less than a year to over ten years. Although the clinical manifestations of the chronic phase can usually be readily controlled by appropriate treatment and most patients are able to lead normal lives, treatment has not substantially improved survival. Survival after development of an accelerated phase is usually less than a year and after blastic transformation only a few months, although patients with lymphoblastic transformation may live longer with appropriate treatment. The median survival of Ph^1-negative patients is usually about a year, and after blastic transformation only a few months. However, occasionally Ph^1-negative patients may have an indolent course and long survival.

Until recently there has been no generally accepted staging system for chronic phase Ph^1-positive CML at diagnosis that allows one to reliably predict prognosis. In a recent multi-institutional study of disease features at diagnosis in over 800 patients with Ph^1 + nonblastic CML, the most important predictors of survival were the percentage of circulating blasts and spleen size. These features, together with age, behaved as continuous variables with progressively worse prognosis at higher values. The platelet count did not influence survival at values below 700,000 per cubic millimeter but was increasingly unfavorable above this level. Basophils plus eosinophils over 15 per cent, more than 5 per cent marrow blasts, and karyotypic abnormalities in addition to the Ph^1 chromosome were also significant unfavorable features. The use of four variables representing percentage of circulating blasts, spleen size, platelet count, and age allowed the identification of a lower-risk group with a two-year survival of 90 per cent and a median survival of five years, an intermediate group, and a high-risk group with a two-year survival of 65 per cent and a median survival of two and one half years. Other features, such as liver size, hematocrit, and WBC count, appeared to be secondary prognostic indicators. If this staging system proves valid and reliable, it should be helpful in advising patients when they should consider alternate forms of treatment, such as bone marrow transplantation.

Bakhshi A, Minowada J, Arnold A, Cossman J, Jensen JP, Whang-Peng J, Waldmann TA, Korsmeyer ST: Lymphoid blast crises of chronic myelogenous leukemia represent stages in the development of B-cell precursors. N Engl J Med 309:826, 1983. *In eight of nine episodes of lymphoid blast crisis in CML, rearrangements of immunoglobulin heavy-chain genes were found, and in three, there were also rearrangements in light-chain genes. These findings provide strong evidence that the lymphoid blasts are early B cell precursors.*

Broxmeyer HE, Bognacki J, Dorner MH, de Sousa M: Identification of leukemia-associated inhibitory activity as acidic isoferritins. J Exp Med 153:1426, 1981. *A concise summary of recent studies directed toward elucidation of the regulatory disturbances in acute leukemia and chronic myelogenous leukemia which may be responsible for suppression of normal hematopoiesis and for the proliferative abnormalities of the leukemic populations. References are given to more detailed reports of the original investigations.*

Clarkson B, Rubinow SI: Growth kinetics in human leukemia. *In* Drewinko B, Humphrey RM (eds.): Growth Kinetics and Biochemical Regulation of Normal and Malignant Cells. The University of Texas System Cancer Center, M.D. Anderson Hospital and Tumor Institute. 29th Annual Symposium on Fundamental Cancer Research, 1976. Baltimore, Williams & Wilkins Company, 1977, p 591. *A review of experimental and theoretical considerations of disturbances in the growth kinetics of normal cells and leukemic cells in acute leukemia and chronic myelogenous leukemia. Appropriate references are given.*

Fefer A, Cheever MA, Greenberg PD, Applebaum FR, Boyd CN, Buckner CD, Kaplan HG, Ramberg R, Sanders JE, Storb R, Thomas ED: Treatment of chronic granulocytic leukemia with chemoradiotherapy and transplantation of marrow from identical twins. N Engl J Med 306:63, 1982. *A recent update of results of patients with CML treated with intensive chemotherapy and total body irradiation followed by rescue with marrow transplantation from their identical twins. The results appear promising; the earliest patients treated have now remained well without evidence of leukemic relapse for over four years.*

Goldman JM, Kearney L, Worsley A, Baughan A, Catovsky E, Gordon-Smith EC, Goolden AWG, Galton DAG: Bone marrow transplantation for patients with chronic granulocytic leukemia. Exp Hematol 10:18, 1982. *A recent report of the results of allogeneic bone marrow transplantation in patients with CML.*

Goto T, Nishikori M, Arlin Z, Gee T, Kempin S, Burchenal J, Strife A, Wisniewski D, Lambek C, Little C, Jhanwar S, Chaganti R, Clarkson B: Growth characteristics of leukemic and normal hematopoietic cells in Ph^1+ chronic myelogenous leukemia and effects of intensive treatment. Blood 59:793, 1982. *Report of a clinical trial in which patients in the chronic phase of CML were treated with a moderately intensive regimen consisting of splenectomy and combination chemotherapy. Although some complete remissions were achieved these were usually of short duration. The results of other recent trials of splenectomy and intensive treatment are reviewed.*

Heisterkamp N, Stephenson JR, Groffen J: Localization of the c-abl oncogene adjacent to a translocation breakpoint in chronic myelocytic leukemia. Nature 306:239, 1983. *A description of recent studies demonstrating that the human c-abl oncogene, normally located on chromosome 9, is translocated to chromosome 22 in CML. The possible significance of this finding is discussed.*

Jain K, Arlin Z, Mertelsmann R, Gee T, Kempin S, Koziner B, Middleton A, Jhanwar S, Chaganti R, Clarkson B: Philadelphia chromosome and terminal transferase positive acute leukemia: Similarity of terminal phase of chronic myelogenous leukemia and de novo acute presentation. J Clin Onc 1:669, 1983. *A review of the clinical and laboratory features and results of intensive treatment of patients with CML with lymphoblastic transformation, either presenting de novo as "Ph^1 + ALL" or as the terminal event after a chronic phase.*

Kamada N, Uchino H: Chronologic sequence in appearance of clinical and laboratory findings characteristic of chronic myelocytic leukemia. Blood 51:843, 1978. *A significant study which demonstrates the evolution of CML in survivors of the atomic bomb explosion in Hiroshima in 1945. The findings indicate that the original mutation resulting in the first leukemic cell probably occurs about eight years prior to development of clinical symptoms.*

Koeffler HP, Golde DW: Chronic myelogenous leukemia: New concepts. N Engl J Med 304:1201, 1269, 1981. *Recent, authoritative review that summarizes current knowledge of CML, with emphasis on pathogenesis and treatment; 204 references.*

McGlave PB, Hurd DD, Kim AD, Kersey J: Successful treatment of chronic myelogenous leukemia with allogeneic bone marrow transplantation. Exp Hematol 10:18, 1982. *Another recent report of results of allogeneic bone marrow transplantation in the chronic phase of CML.*

Sandberg AA: The Chromosomes in Human Cancer and Leukemia. New York, Amsterdam, Elsevier–North Holland, 1980. *Included in this volume is an excellent chapter which comprehensively reviews the cytogenetic abnormalities occurring in CML.*

Sokal JE, Cox EB, Baccarani M, Tura S, Gomez GA, Robertson JE, Tso CY, Braun TJ, Clarkson BD, Cervantes F, Rozman C, The Italian Cooperative CML Study Group: Prognostic discrimination in "good-risk" chronic granulocytic leukemia. Blood April, 1984. *A multivariate regression analysis of the prognostic significance of disease features at the time of diagnosis in 813 patients with Ph^1+ nonblastic CML collected from six American and European series. Using the Cox model, four key variables were found that enabled identification of low, intermediate, and high risk groups of patients.*

Chronic Lymphocytic Leukemia

DEFINITION. Chronic lymphocytic leukemia (CLL) is a monoclonal neoplasm of slowly proliferating long-lived lymphocytes, usually B lymphocytes, which are immunologically defective.

ETIOLOGY. The etiology is unknown. Unlike the situation in acute and chronic myelogenous leukemia, exposure to ionizing radiation and cytotoxic drugs or chemicals does not result in an increased incidence of CLL. There does appear to be some genetic predisposition, since CLL is the most frequent type of leukemia occurring in multiple family members. There is no clear inheritance pattern, but siblings, especially brothers, appear to have the highest concordance of CLL. Except in rare high incidence families, the incidence of CLL among close relatives is probably about three times that in the general population. Patients with CLL have a high incidence of second malignancies, and their family members also have a higher incidence of cancer than expected.

INCIDENCE. The incidence of CLL in the United States is about 3 per 100,000 population, or about 25 per cent of all leukemias. The incidence in most Western countries is similar, with CLL being slightly more common than CML. CLL is twice as common in males as in females. The mean age is about 60, and the incidence increases with age. It is rare before age 30 and almost never occurs in children. In Japan and several other Asian countries where reliable statistics exist, B cell CLL is very uncommon. This may be due to genetic factors; Japanese living in the United States have a slightly higher incidence than native Japanese, but still lower than the rest of the US population. On the other hand, T cell variants of CLL and related lymphoproliferative diseases are not uncommon and appear to be endemic in certain areas of Japan. A human T cell leukemia virus (HTLV) has recently been described that is strongly suspected of having an etiologic role in these T cell neoplasms in Japan, as well as in patients from the Caribbean and less often in the United States and other countries.

PATHOGENESIS AND MECHANISMS. In the great majority of cases, CLL results from a monoclonal proliferation of B lymphocytes, although a few cases of T cell CLL have been observed. The leukemic B cells have monoclonal surface immunoglobulin (although in lower density than normal B lymphocytes), exhibit Ia-like cell surface antigens, carry receptors for the Fc fragment of IgG (as recognized by the binding of heat-aggregated IgG and several rosetting techniques) and for the C3d and occasionally the C3b complement components, and form spontaneous rosettes with mouse red blood cells. Intracellular crystalline inclusions containing IgM and λ light chains have been observed in the leukemic cells of some patients. Recently a murine monoclonal antibody has been described that recognizes a 65,000 to 67,000 dalton antigen

(Leu-1) present on B-CLL cells, but not on cells from other types of B cell leukemias or lymphomas. This surface antigen is also expressed by human thymocytes and peripheral T cells, but is absent on normal B cells.

The leukemic lymphocytes in CLL proliferate very slowly, as is also true of normal B lymphocytes and several other low growth fraction B cell neoplasms such as multiple myeloma and most nodular lymphomas. The great majority of CLL lymphocytes are small cells that are in a quiescent state (G_0). In most cases, only a small fraction of the population consists of intermediate-sized or large lymphocytes, of which some are in various stages of the cell cycle preparing to divide. Although only a small fraction of the total leukemic population is proliferating at any time, because the leukemic cells have a very long life span they accumulate and continue to recirculate through the blood, marrow, lymph nodes, spleen, and other tissues. The leukemic lymphocytes in CLL inhibit normal hematopoiesis to a much lesser extent than the leukemic cells in acute leukemia or CML.

The leukemic lymphocytes in CLL are immunologically defective. They respond sluggishly to mitogens or immunologic stimuli and usually fail to proliferate or differentiate into plasma cells. Severe immunologic abnormalities such as hypogammaglobulinemia are frequently associated with CLL. Although normal B cells are present in the lymph nodes and in the blood mixed with the leukemic cells, they are often unable to respond appropriately to antigenic stimulation. In the early stages of CLL, T lymphocytes are present in the blood in normal or elevated absolute numbers, although in reduced proportions. Purified T cells from CLL patients respond normally to mitogens but form fewer T cell colonies in vitro compared to T cells from normal subjects, and are defective in natural killer and antibody-dependent cell-mediated cytotoxicity. Normal T cells can be divided into subpopulations according to their type of Fc receptor for immunoglobulin: Tμ (IgM), Tα (IgA), and Tγ (IgG), or their reactivities with monoclonal antibodies. In CLL, the proportion of T cells with receptors for IgG (Tγ) is markedly increased resulting in an abnormal helper (Tμ) to suppressor (Tγ) ratio. Patients with B-CLL have abnormal T cell subsets resulting in a decreased helper (OKT4) to suppressor (OKT8) ratio. Similarly, using the Leu monoclonal antibodies, a decreased ratio of helper to inducer ($Leu\text{-}3a^+$) to cytotoxic-suppressor ($Leu\text{-}2a^+$) has been found in most patients with CLL; the decrease is more pronounced in later stages of CLL, suggesting its causal relationship to the immunosuppression commonly observed in advanced disease.

CLINICAL MANIFESTATIONS. ***Staging.*** About 25 per cent of patients with CLL are asymptomatic when first seen, and the diagnosis is made following detection of lymphocytosis on an incidental blood count or in the course of investigating the cause of enlarged lymph nodes or splenomegaly. Some patients may have a very benign course and remain asymptomatic for many years, whereas in others the disease can progress rapidly. The average survival in CLL is about four to five years. A simple clinical staging system for CLL (see Table 155–1) has proved of prognostic value in several large series. Median survival decreases with advancing stage: Stage 0 = 14 (range 12 to 15) years; Stage I = 8 (5 to 11) years; Stage II = 6 (4 to 9) years; and Stages III and IV = 2 (1 to 3½) years. A diagnosis of CLL may be made in some patients with a lesser degree of absolute lymphocytosis than 15,000 per cubic millimeter (i.e., earlier than Stage 0) if cell marker studies demonstrate a monoclonal B cell population characteristic of CLL in the blood and marrow. The rate at which the disease progresses from early to late stages is quite variable in individual patients. Recently, a revised prognostic staging system was proposed by an international workshop on CLL that is based on the number of lymphoid areas involved and the degree of bone marrow failure (Table 155–2). Clinical enlargement of the spleen, liver, and of lymph nodes in the cervical, axillary, and inguinal regions constitute five separate areas of involvement, each of which is considered one area irrespective of whether the lymphadenopathy is unilateral or bilateral. The advantages of the revised system are that it has fewer stages (which should simplify design and evaluation of comparative therapeutic trials), it recognizes that anemia and thrombocytopenia have a similar prognosis and do not require separate stages, and it recognizes a predominantly splenic form of the disease that may have a relatively favorable prognosis. Survival curves have so far shown distinct differences between the three groups: the median survivals for Groups A, B, and C were >10, 7, and 2 years, respectively.

TABLE 155–1. RAI'S STAGING SYSTEM FOR CLL*

Stage 0	Absolute lymphocytosis in blood of >15,000 per cubic millimeter
Stage I	Absolute lymphocytosis plus enlarged lymph nodes
Stage II	Absolute lymphocytosis plus enlarged liver and/or spleen (with or without lymph node enlargement)
Stage III†	Absolute lymphocytosis plus anemia (hemoglobin <11 grams per deciliter in males and <10 grams per deciliter in females)
Stage IV†	Absolute lymphocytosis plus thrombocytopenia (platelets <100,000 per cubic millimeter)

*From Rai KR, et al.: Blood 46:219, 1975.
†Stage III and IV patients may or may not have enlarged lymph nodes, liver, and/or spleen.

TABLE 155–2. PROPOSED INTERNATIONAL STAGING SYSTEM FOR CLL*

Clinical Stage†		
A A(0), A(I), or A(II)	No anemia or thrombocytopenia	Less than three areas of lymphoid enlargement
B B(I) or B(II)	No anemia or thrombocytopenia	Three or more involved areas
C C(III) or C(IV)	Anemia and/or thrombocytopenia	Regardless of the number of areas of lymphoid enlargement

*From Binet JL, et al.: Br J Haematol 48:356, 1981.
†It was recommended that the revised classification be integrated with the Rai system by using Roman numerals in parenthesis to represent the latter.

Symptoms. Patients with early stage disease are often asymptomatic, but increasing symptoms develop with advancing stage and include malaise, easy fatigability, anorexia, weight loss, low grade fever, and night sweats. Bacterial infections, such as sinusitis, pneumonia, or cutaneous infections, are common and should be treated promptly with appropriate antibiotics. Patients in advanced stages become progressively more immunodeficient, anemic, and neutropenic and are unable to mobilize a normal response to infections. Viral infections such as herpes zoster are also common. Vaccinations for smallpox and other viral illnesses should be avoided because of the danger of generalized vaccinia or other severe reactions. Hyperreactivity to insect bites is common.

Physical Findings. Physical examination in Stage 0 CLL (Rai classification) reveals no abnormalities, but in later stages the lymph nodes, spleen, and liver may become progressively enlarged, and there may also be extensive leukemic infiltration of other tissues, including the skin, orbit, conjunctivae, pharynx, lungs, pleura, heart, and gastrointestinal tract. Obstructive jaundice may occur from periportal infiltration or from nodes compressing the bile duct, and venous compression by enlarged nodes may cause edema and/or thrombophlebitis. Pronounced inanition is common late in the disease, and ascites and/or anasarca may develop in association with severe hypoalbuminemia. Leukostasis may cause priapism or infarctions of various organs. Bleeding manifestations such as bruising and epistaxis are common in advanced stages with severe thrombocytopenia. Leukemic involvement of the meninges is rare, but leukoencephalopathy may occur, probably owing to a viral infection.

Laboratory Abnormalities. The WBC may range from a slight elevation to over a million per cubic millimeter. The *percentage of lymphocytes is always increased* and may be over 98 per cent. *Anemia, thrombocytopenia,* and *neutropenia* develop in advanced stages owing to impairment of normal hematopoiesis. The anemia is usually normochromic and normocytic, and the reticulocyte count is normal or reduced. Patients also frequently develop shortened red cell and/or platelet survival resulting from hypersplenism in advanced disease. Autoimmune hemolytic anemia, usually caused by warm reacting IgG antibodies, is common and may be accompanied by reticulocytosis, erythroid hyperplasia in the marrow, a positive direct Coombs' antiglobulin test, and hyperbilirubinemia. Autoimmune thrombocytopenia or cold hemagglutinin disease may also occur, and occasionally such autoimmune phenomena may precede other clinical manifestations of CLL or develop shortly after beginning treatment.

Hypogammaglobulinemia is present at diagnosis in about half of patients and eventually develops in almost all of them as the disease advances. Any or all classes of immunoglobulins may be reduced. A small percentage of patients have monoclonal immunoglobulins or light chains demonstrable on electrophoresis or immunoelectrophoresis of the blood or urine. Rarely the abnormal proteins may cause hyperviscosity or cryoprecipitation. Angioneurotic edema may also occur rarely owing to formation of immune complexes.

Unlike CML, until recently no characteristic cytogenetic abnormality was described in CLL and most studies showed normal karyotypes. More recently, trisomy of chromosome 12 has been reported in the leukemic lymphocytes in about one third of patients with CLL. The Kirsten sarcoma oncogene (ras^K) is located on chromosome 12, but its possible role in the pathogenesis of CLL is not yet known.

Blastic transformation analogous to that commonly seen in CML is infrequent in CLL, although instances of transformation to a more rapidly growing cell type have been reported. In the past, such tumors have usually been diagnosed as diffuse histiocytic lymphoma or reticulum cell sarcoma (Richter's syndrome) or Hodgkin's disease when the tumor is pleomorphic and contains multinucleated cells which can be mistaken for Reed-Sternberg cells. It is impossible to tell from the earlier reports whether they were new neoplasms or malignant evolution of the original leukemic cells, but recent studies have clearly demonstrated in some instances that the more malignant cells retain the same phenotypic expression as the original CLL lymphocytes.

DIAGNOSIS. The diagnosis of CLL depends on the demonstration of a persistent absolute lymphocytosis in the blood and an increased percentage (usually >50 per cent) of small lymphocytes with round nuclei in the marrow. Pertussis and infectious lymphocytosis and other viral infections can sometimes cause striking lymphocytosis, but these illnesses usually occur in children or young adults, are usually accompanied by fever and other acute symptoms, and are of transient duration. Chronic infections such as tuberculosis may be accompanied by lymphocytosis, but this is usually less prominent than in CLL and appropriate workup should lead to the correct diagnosis. If there is any question about the diagnosis, appropriate cell marker studies as described under Pathogenesis should be performed to establish the monoclonality of the lymphocytic population and to distinguish CLL from other lymphoproliferative diseases.

If the lymph nodes are involved in CLL, the histologic pattern and immunologic markers characteristic of the cells are identical to those of diffuse well-differentiated lymphocytic lymphoma (DWDL), and these two diagnostic entities appear to be merely different variants of the same type of B cell neoplasia. DWDL may initially be localized in lymph nodes without involvement of the blood or marrow, but in more advanced stages it may be indistinguishable from CLL. Other types of disseminated lymphomas such as diffuse poorly differentiated lymphocytic lymphoma (DPDL), which may involve the blood and marrow, can be distinguished from CLL by differences in morphologic appearance of the tumor cells and appropriate cell marker analysis.

Waldenström's macroglobulinemia may be confused with CLL, but the neoplastic lymphocytes in the former usually have a plasmacytoid appearance, more prominent surface, as well as cytoplasmic immunoglobulin, and they usually do not invade the blood to the same extent as CLL lymphocytes. There is invariably a prominent monoclonal IgM spike in the serum, whereas this is rare in CLL. A few cases may exhibit mixed features of the two entities.

Prolymphocytic leukemia is a rare disease occurring mostly in males in the sixth or seventh decade characterized by prominent splenomegaly, minimal adenopathy, and a poor prognosis. The prolymphocytes differ from CLL lymphocytes in that they are larger and have more cytoplasm, a more prominent nucleolus, and a greater density of surface immunoglobulin, which, again in contrast to CLL cells, exhibits polar migration ("capping") after incubation at 37° C.

Hairy cell leukemia is sometimes misdiagnosed as CLL. In the former, the leukocyte count is usually low rather than elevated, and although hairy cells may resemble CLL lymphocytes on Romanowsky-stained smears, close scrutiny will reveal hair-like projections. If there is any doubt, special morphologic and cell marker studies should be done as described in Ch. 155.

Sézary's syndrome, a cutaneous lymphoma of helper T cell origin closely related to mycosis fungoides, is characterized by a chronic exfoliative erythrodermatitis and circulating atypical lymphocytes with cerebriform nuclei and acid phosphatase activity limited to the cytoplasmic granules instead of the Golgi zone. The prominent skin manifestations and the lesser degree of involvement of the marrow and lymph nodes usually suffice to differentiate Sézary's syndrome from the rare cases of T cell CLL.

TREATMENT. Since CLL is a disease mainly affecting older persons, many of whom have a remarkably benign and prolonged course, and since there is no good evidence that early treatment will cure the disease or improve survival, most authorities recommend merely observing asymptomatic patients with early stage disease until the disease progresses and symptoms develop. Indications for treatment include development of symptomatic or cosmetically disfiguring lymphadenopathy, progressive splenomegaly and/or hepatomegaly, recurrent infections, persistent unexplained fever, weight loss, and development of significant anemia, thrombocytopenia, and/or neutropenia resulting from progressive marrow infiltration, hypersplenism, or autoimmune complications. The rate at which the disease progresses from an early asymptomatic stage to an advanced stage requiring treatment is quite variable, and patients should be observed closely every few months until it can be determined whether their disease is going to remain indolent or become symptomatic. Some patients remain asymptomatic for many years without treatment, and such patients require re-examination only about every six months.

Treatment should be begun when troublesome symptoms develop. *Chlorambucil* (Leukeran) is the most commonly employed drug, but other alkylating agents such as cyclophosphamide are also effective. Because of the slow proliferative rate of the neoplastic cells, antimetabolites are generally ineffective. The usual starting dose of chlorambucil is 6 to 12 mg (0.1 to 0.2 mg per kilogram of body weight) daily for three to six weeks, followed by a maintenance dose of 2 to 6 mg daily, the exact dose depending on the extent of disease, the severity of symptoms, and the patient's weight. The dose should be titrated individually according to the therapeutic response. The drug should be taken at least one hour prior to eating so as not to interfere with its absorption. About 70 per cent of previously untreated patients will show a satisfactory response to chlorambucil with reduction in the WBC and shrinkage of the enlarged lymph nodes and organomegaly when present. Maintenance treatment is usually continued for six months to a year until a maximal response has been achieved. In some patients the disease may then remain asymptomatic for many months without further treatment, whereas others require continuous treatment for control.

Intermittent administration of chlorambucil has been recommended by some investigators. Various dosage schedules have been employed, usually 0.4 to 0.8 mg per kilogram as a single dose every two weeks or 0.4 to 2.0 mg per kilogram once a month. These high intermittent doses sometimes cause gastrointestinal toxicity, which may be partly alleviated by antiemetics. There is no unanimity of opinion as to whether continuous or intermittent treatment is superior in terms of antileukemic activity. Myelosuppression is the usual dose-limiting toxicity with chlorambucil. Immunosuppression, sterility, alveolar dysplasia, pulmonary fibrosis, chromosomal damage, and secondary acute myeloid leukemia may occur following chronic chlorambucil administration.

Corticosteroids are effective in controlling acute symptoms, especially autoimmune complications such as hemolytic anemia or thrombocytopenia. Corticosteroids may also have a pronounced cytolytic effect on the leukemic cells; the WBC may fall rapidly, or it may rise temporarily concomitantly with regression of the enlarged lymph nodes and spleen. Prednisone is the corticosteroid most commonly prescribed, usually in doses of 10 to 20 mg daily, but larger doses of 50 to 100 mg may be necessary to control hemolytic anemia. Large doses of corticosteroids given over a prolonged period are inadvisable because they may cause severe cushingoid symptoms and increase the risk of infections. Some investigators recommend that short courses of prednisone in relatively high doses (e.g., 80 mg daily for five days) be given as adjuvant therapy with intermittent chlorambucil, since intermittent steroid therapy produces the desired lymphocytolytic effect and improves the therapeutic response compared to chlorambucil alone while reducing the toxicity associated with continuous steroid administration. Long-term control of autoimmune complications associated with CLL such as hemolytic anemia, thrombocytopenia, or angioneurotic edema is dependent on adequate control of the leukemia. When the leukemic mass has been reduced sufficiently, the autoimmune manifestations usually subside. However, splenectomy is sometimes indicated to control hemolytic anemia, thrombocytopenia, or progressive splenomegaly refractory to drug treatment.

Local radiotherapy is often useful in the treatment of splenomegaly or greatly enlarged lymph nodes resistant to chemotherapy. Whole body external radiation given cautiously in fractionated doses over several months has been reported to increase the incidence of remissions and prolong survival, and thymic radiation has also been reported to have a good therapeutic effect. However, both thymic and whole body irradiation have also caused prolonged myelosuppression and fatalities in CLL and must be regarded as experimental forms of treatment that cannot be generally recommended until more experience clearly validates their therapeutic value.

Extracorporeal irradiation of the blood has also been shown to be effective in reducing the WBC and organomegaly, but facilities for this procedure are not available in most centers and leukapheresis is more commonly employed. Leukapheresis is particularly useful in reducing very high lymphocyte counts and organomegaly in advanced disease in the presence of severe thrombocytopenia that limits additional cytotoxic drug therapy. Repeated leukapheresis may reduce the extent of leukemic infiltration of the marrow sufficiently to allow the platelet count to rise and permit resumption of chemotherapy.

Several clinical trials have been reported in which patients with CLL have been treated more aggressively with various combinations of alkylating agents and other cytotoxic drugs in an attempt to increase the incidence of remissions and improve survival. With conventional doses of chlorambucil either alone or with prednisone, the frequency of remissions has usually been about 10 per cent (range, 0 to 20 per cent in different series), whereas with more intensive treatment higher remission rates have been reported (18 to 45 per cent). The relative effectiveness of the different regimens is difficult to compare, however, because of differing criteria for completeness of remission and durations of observations. Eradication of the leukemic clone has not been possible with any regimen yet tried, because leukemic cells have reappeared after treatment has been discontinued in all patients who have been observed long enough. Patients having remissions live longer than nonresponders, but there is as yet no convincing evidence that overall survival is significantly improved compared to patients treated with conventional doses of chlorambucil. It is not yet known whether the more intensive regimens will result in a higher incidence of myeloid leukemia or other secondary malignancies in CLL.

Hypogammaglobulinemia when present usually persists even after the leukemic mass has been reduced by treatment. Administration of gamma globulin intramuscularly is of little value; clinical trials of various preparations of gamma globulin for intravenous use are currently under way to determine if it is possible to significantly correct the deficiency and reduce the incidence of infections and autoimmune cytopenias. In the rare patient who develops hyperviscosity or circulating autoantibodies, plasmapheresis with replacement by normal plasma is effective in temporarily lowering the abnormal proteins and relieving symptoms. When infections occur, every effort should be made to identify the offending organism and to begin specific antimicrobial treatment promptly.

PROGNOSIS. Median survival times of four to five years from diagnosis of CLL have been reported in several recent series, with a range of three to nine years. Since CLL has an extremely variable natural history, ranging from less than a year to over 20 years, the differences are probably due to inclusion of differing proportions of patients with early or advanced disease rather than to differences in treatment. The utility of the proposed clinical staging systems in predicting prognosis has been mentioned earlier. There have also been attempts to correlate prognosis with various morphologic, immunologic, or proliferative characteristics of the leukemic cells, but these studies require extension and confirmation before their prognostic value can be accepted. Attempts to eradicate the disease with aggressive treatment have so far been unsuccessful, and there is as yet no convincing evidence that intensive treatment is preferable to more conservative treatment in prolonging overall survival.

Common causes of death in CLL are intercurrent infections, uncontrollable progressive leukemic infiltration of vital organs, extreme inanition, and bleeding. Since CLL occurs mainly in older persons, some patients also die as a result of unrelated diseases. Patients with CLL have a high incidence of second malignancies (3 to 34 per cent in different series), both cutaneous and nondermatologic tumors. Many of the tumors were diagnosed prior to treatment of CLL and cannot be causally related to treatment. The incidence of acute myeloid leukemia is higher than expected in CLL following treatment and is probably related to administration of alkylating agents and/or radiation therapy, as has been reported in Hodgkin's disease and other neoplastic diseases.

Binet JL, Auguier A, Dighiero G: A new prognostic classification of chronic lymphocytic leukemia derived from a multivariate survival analysis. Cancer 48:198, 1981. *A report describing the recently proposed international prognostic staging system for CLL.*

Byhardt RW, Brace KC, Wiernik PH: The role of splenic irradiation in chronic lymphocytic leukemia. Cancer 35:1621, 1975. *A good review of the indications for splenic irradiation in control of CLL.*

Chiorazzi N, Fu SM, Montazen G, Kunkel HG, Rai N, Gee T: T cell helper defect in patients with chronic lymphocytic leukemia. J Immunol 122:1087, 1979. *This paper reports the results of studies in two patients with CLL demonstrating a defect in T helper cell activity.*

Huguley CM Jr: Treatment of chronic lymphocytic leukemia. Cancer Treat Rev 4:261, 1977. *A good review of conventional management of CLL.*

Hurley JN, Fu SM, Kunkel HG, Chaganti RSK, German J: Chromosome abnormalities of leukemic B lymphocytes in chronic lymphocytic leukemia. Nature 283:76, 1980. *A brief report describing aneuploid karyotypes of the leukemic lymphocytes from two patients with CLL. In distinction to prior reports, in which it was not possible to establish whether the metaphases analyzed were in normal or leukemic cells, in this study the abnormalities were clearly demonstrated to be in the leukemic cells.*

Kempin SJ, Lee BJ, Thaler HT, et al.: Combination chemotherapy of advanced chronic lymphocytic leukemia: The M-2 protocol (vincristine, BCNU, cyclophosphamide, melphalan and prednisone). Blood 60:1110, 1982. *The results of intensive treatment of a series of patients with advanced stages of CLL with a combination chemotherapy protocol are described; a comprehensive review of other attempts of intensive treatment is included.*

Koziner B, Gebhard D, Denny T, Evans RL: Characterization of B cell type chronic lymphocytic leukemia cells by surface markers and a monoclonal antibody. Am J Med 73:802, 1982. *An original report showing expression of the Leu-1 surface antigen on the neoplastic lymphocytes of most patients with CLL; this antigen, recognized by the Leu-1 mouse monoclonal antibody, is normally expressed on thymocytes and peripheral T cells, but not B cells. The recent literature on other surface antigens in CLL is reviewed.*

Koziner B, Kempin S, Passe S, Gee T, Good RA, Clarkson BD: Characterization of B-cell leukemias: A tentative immunomorphological scheme. Blood 56:815, 1980. *A recent summary of the morphologic features and immunologic markers of the B-cell leukemias, including CLL and hairy cell leukemia. References are given to most of the important original work in this area.*

Mittelman A, Denny T, Gebhard D, Cirrincione C, Kurland E, Koziner B: Analysis of T-cell subsets in B-cell chronic lymphocytic leukemia: A correlation with the stage of disease. Am J Hematol (In Press), 1984. *A report of recent analysis of T cell abnormalities in CLL using Leu monoclonal antibodies, including a review of the literature.*

Rai KR, Sawitsky A, Cronkite EP, Chanana A, Levy RN, Pasternak BS: Clinical staging of chronic lymphocytic leukemia. Blood 46:219, 1975. *Original description of Rai's clinical staging system for CLL. The utility of this simple system for prognosis has since been amply confirmed, although minor modifications have been proposed to improve its accuracy.*

Sawitsky A, Rai KR, Glidwell O, Silver RT, and participating members of CALGB (Cancer and Leukemia Group B): Comparison of daily versus intermittent chlorambucil and prednisone therapy in the treatment of patients with chronic lymphocytic leukemia. Blood 50:1049, 1977. *Report of a clinical trial in CLL by a cooperative group in which the efficacy of intermittent chlorambucil in combination with prednisone was compared with chlorambucil administered continuously and with prednisone alone. The complete and partial remission rate and duration of survival were best with the intermittent chlorambucil arm, but there was no significant difference in survival time between the three treatment schedules.*

Hairy Cell Leukemia
(Leukemic Reticuloendotheliosis)

DEFINITION. Hairy cell leukemia (HCL) is a chronic form of leukemia involving an unusual type of cell, probably a B lymphocyte. HCL accounts for approximately 2 per cent of all the leukemias. The etiology is unknown.

PATHOGENESIS AND MECHANISMS. There has been much controversy concerning the origin of the hairy cell, and its normal counterpart within the hematopoietic cell lineages has not yet been identified. Most recent studies support the view that it is an unusual type of neoplastic B lymphocyte that may have variable phagocytic capability.

The hairy cell appears on Wright-Giemsa–stained smears as an intermediate-sized or large lymphocyte (10 to 18 μ in diameter), with fine cytoplasmic projections that give the cell its name. The nucleus may be round, oval, horseshoe shaped, or slightly folded, and it is often eccentrically located. The chromatin can be evenly distributed, moderately coarse, or stippled, and one or more small nucleoli may be present. The cells usually have moderate amounts of pale blue-gray cytoplasm with irregular serrated edges and sometimes pseudopodial extensions. The cytoplasmic surface projections are best recognized under the phase-contrast microscope or the scanning electron microscope (Fig. 155–1). The latter reveals a characteristic surface pattern with prominent folds or ruffles that are similar to those present on monocytes but more conspicuous.

Cytochemical reactions are helpful in identifying hairy cells, but show variability in different cases and within the cells of any one population. Hairy cells are almost always positive for *acid phosphatase*, which is commonly, but not invariably, completely or partially resistant to addition of tartaric acid. However a negative reaction does not exclude the diagnosis of

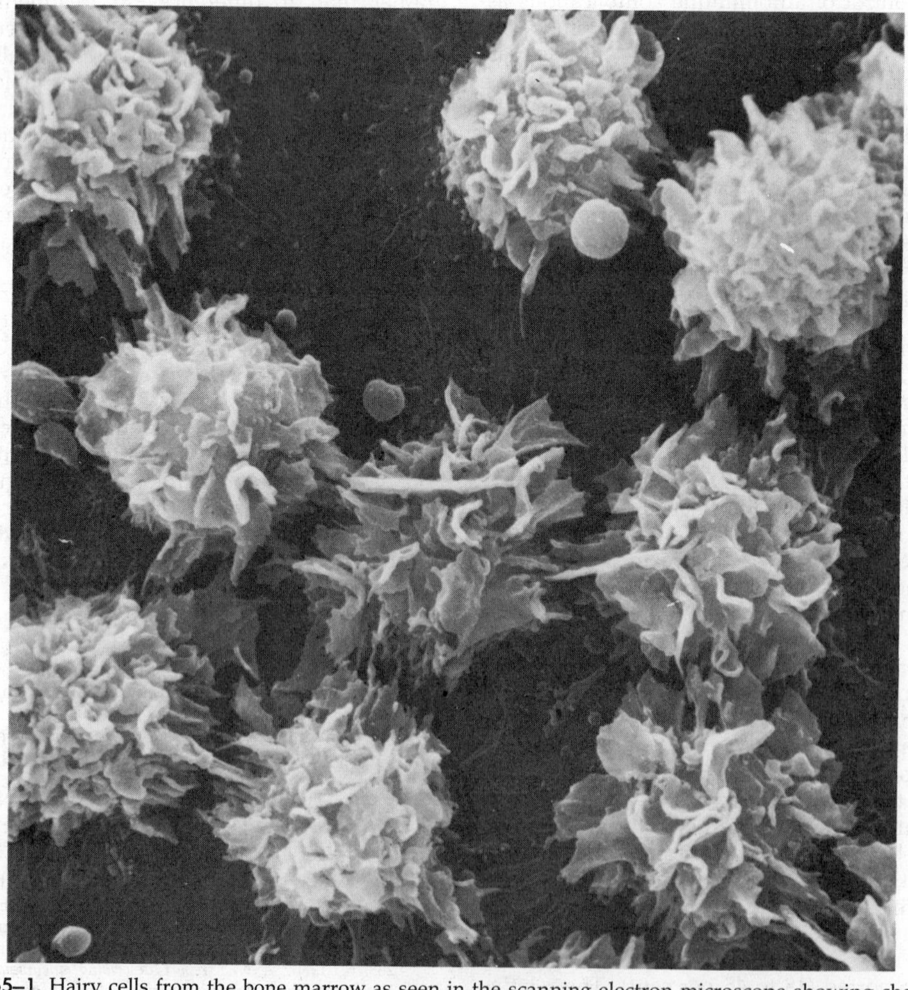

Figure 155–1. Hairy cells from the bone marrow as seen in the scanning electron microscope showing characteristic prominent surface ruffles. Magnification ×8750. (Courtesy of Dr. Etienne deHarven and Nina Lampen.)

HCL, and a positive reaction is not necessarily diagnostic. Hairy cells in the great majority of patients show varying degrees of positivity for alpha naphthyl acetate or butyrate esterase and this reaction is usually completely inhibited by sodium fluoride. Cytochemical reactions associated with the granulocytic differentiation pathway (e.g., myeloperoxidase) are invariably negative in hairy cells. Lysozyme activity is absent in hairy cells, which helps to distinguish them from normal or leukemic monocytes.

Surface immunoglobulin (Ig) is present on hairy cells in the great majority of cases. The Ig is usually monoclonal, although in a few cases two different immunoglobulins have been reported. Hairy cells are capable of resynthesizing surface Ig, usually IgM and/or IgD, thus providing strong evidence for their B cell derivation. Hairy cells usually do not form rosettes with sheep red blood cells, a characteristic of T lymphocytes, although a few cases of HCL have been reported in which the hairy cells have T cell properties. Hairy cells generally lack receptors for the third component of complement (C3), thus providing a helpful diagnostic distinction from monocytes and CLL cells which carry the C3 receptor. A number of monoclonal antibodies have been prepared with varying degrees of specificity for hairy cells. Most support the B cell lineage of hairy cells but show the presence of multiple phenotypes reflecting different stages of maturity; maturation is more advanced than in CLL.

The capacity of hairy cells to phagocytize bacteria, fungi, and particulate matter varies from case to case as well as in the percentage of cells within any one population showing phagocytic capability. The phagocytic activity of hairy cells has been taken as evidence that they are derived from the monocyte lineage or from a hybrid cell with composite lymphocyte and monocyte features. However, normal lymphocytes have been reported to acquire phagocytic potential under certain conditions without transforming morphologically into macrophages. It appears likely that the phagocytic capability of some hairy cells is a function that may be acquired or accentuated during neoplastic transformation of B lymphocyte precursors. In some patients with HCL, abnormal platelet aggregating properties and erythrocyte abnormalities have been described, but their significance is uncertain. It has been suggested that these abnormalities in other cell lines might reflect neoplastic involvement of a very early common precursor, but it is also quite possible that they are merely acquired secondary defects, possibly related to hypersplenism.

Hairy cells usually have a very low proliferative activity; the percentage of hairy cells in the marrow or blood in DNA synthesis is almost invariably less than 1 per cent. Hairy cells also usually respond poorly in vitro to stimulation with mitogens. Chromosome abnormalities have been difficult to demonstrate because of the low incidence of mitoses, but trisomy of chromosome 12 (similar to CLL) has been reported in a few cases of HCL.

CLINICAL MANIFESTATIONS AND DIAGNOSIS. HCL occurs mainly in adults, the majority of whom are over 50 years old. Males are affected about four times more frequently than females. Clinical manifestations are usually attributable to hairy cell infiltration of the bone marrow, which can cause suppression of normal hematopoiesis, and of the red pulp of the spleen, which can result in hypersplenism. The onset is usually insidious, and the most common symptoms are weakness caused by *anemia*, development of infections as a result of *neutropenia*, and pain or discomfort in the left hypochondrium owing to *progressive splenic enlargement*.

The liver is enlarged owing to hairy cell infiltration in about 40 per cent of cases, but prominent involvement of the lymph nodes is infrequent. Systemic vasculitis and lytic bone lesions associated with pain and sometimes pathologic fractures may occur. Infiltration of the skin or lungs occurs only rarely, and meningeal involvement is almost never seen.

The majority of patients have *pancytopenia*, but sometimes only one or two of the myeloid cell lines are depressed, most commonly the platelets and neutrophils. Monocytopenia is also frequent and may contribute to the increased susceptibility to infections. In most cases, hairy cells can be identified in smears of the blood or buffy coat, but in some patients they are very rare in the blood. Occasional patients have leukocytosis with numerous circulating hairy cells instead of leukopenia. The bone marrow is always diffusely infiltrated by hairy cells, but it may be difficult to aspirate the marrow in about half of the patients (i.e., "dry tap"). If the diagnosis of HCL is suspected but hairy cells cannot be demonstrated in the blood and bone marrow aspiration is unsuccessful, a marrow biopsy should be performed and imprint preparations made of the freshly obtained biopsy specimen so that the appropriate confirmatory cytologic and cytochemical tests can be done. Reticulin fibers are often increased in the marrow as well as in the spleen, and the marrow may also contain increased numbers of plasma cells. If a splenectomy is performed, experienced pathologists can usually make a definitive diagnosis because involvement of the red pulp by hairy cells and the presence of pseudosinuses are uniquely characteristic of HCL. Sections of liver biopsies show hairy cell infiltration largely confined to the portal areas without destruction of parenchymal hepatic cells. Liver function tests are often normal; the most common abnormality is an elevated serum alkaline phosphatase that is related to the degree of periportal infiltration.

Other disease entities with which HCL may be confused are CLL, Waldenström's macroglobulinemia, some of the diffuse varieties of non-Hodgkin's lymphomas, histiocytic medullary reticulosis, and monocytic leukemia. The leukocyte count in HCL is usually low instead of elevated as in CLL. The serum immunoglobulins are usually normal or show a polyclonal increase in HCL in contrast to CLL, in which they are often depressed, or to Waldenström's macroglobulinemia, in which there is a monoclonal IgM spike. Histiocytic medullary reticulosis (HMR, malignant histiocytosis, histiocytic leukemia) is a rare, rapidly progressive fatal disease characterized by fever, wasting, jaundice, generalized lymphadenopathy, and hepatosplenomegaly. The involved organs are infiltrated with abnormal histiocytes that commonly show intense erythrophagocytosis, a functional characteristic rarely exhibited by hairy cells. Acute or chronic monocytic leukemia can also be confused with HCL, but the serum or urinary lysozyme levels in HCL are normal or low in contrast to the high levels found in monocytic leukemia.

Although the aforementioned clinical and laboratory features are useful in distinguishing HCL from other disease entities, the essential requirement for the diagnosis is positive identification of the characteristic hairy cells. Their unique features can readily be demonstrated by appropriate morphologic, cytochemical, and immunologic tests, as described under Pathogenesis. Although occasional cells closely resembling or identical to hairy cells have been observed in some varieties of non-Hodgkin's lymphomas, in none of these conditions or in any of the other lymphoproliferative or histiocytic-monocytic neoplasias mentioned earlier is the marrow diffusely infiltrated by characteristic hairy cells.

Not uncommonly, the diagnosis of HCL is not suspected prior to performing a splenectomy for some ill-defined condition such as "chronic anemia" or "primary splenic lymphoma." However, experienced hematopathologists can usually readily diagnose HCL on examination of histologic sections of the spleen and distinguish this entity from lymphomas and other conditions causing splenic enlargement.

PROGNOSIS AND TREATMENT. HCL generally has a chronic course, with a median survival of three to five years and with some patients surviving many years. Rarely the disease is rapidly progressive and may be accompanied by massive infiltration of the skin and multiple internal organs, leading to death within a year. However, early death is most commonly due to infection as a consequence of neutropenia. A large variety of bacteria, fungi, viruses, and mycobacteria have been reported to cause terminal infections.

There is no consistently satisfactory treatment for HCL, and because it is not presently possible to cure the disease most authorities recommend a conservative approach to treatment. Patients who are relatively asymptomatic at the time of diagnosis should merely be observed, since the disease may progress very slowly and not require treatment for long periods.

Splenectomy. If there is progressive worsening of the anemia, thrombocytopenia, or neutropenia, splenectomy should be considered, as this has proved to be beneficial in about two thirds of cases and to improve survival in patients who respond favorably. A good response to splenectomy with improvement in one or more of the blood elements is not well correlated with spleen size, but patients with only patchy marrow involvement are more likely to have a favorable response than those whose marrows are densely infiltrated with hairy cells. When in doubt as to whether to perform a splenectomy, appropriate red cell and/or platelet survival measurements or ferrokinetic studies should be performed in order to assess the relative contribution of hypersplenism as opposed to impaired marrow production in causing depression of the blood elements. Improvements in surgical techniques and in prevention of serious infections have greatly reduced the complications of splenectomy in recent years. The majority of patients with HCL will have some hematologic improvement after splenectomy, but the degree and duration of improvement are quite variable. In most cases the improvement will be noted within a few weeks after the operation. About 40 per cent of patients have no response or only a partial response, and the latter usually have relapsed within a few months. Forty to 60 per cent of patients in different series have a significant rise in the blood cell counts following splenectomy, with an average duration of response of over a year and with some patients remaining well for several years.

Chemotherapy. The results of treatment with chemotherapeutic agents in HCL have been disappointing. Treatment with corticosteroids sometimes results in hematologic improvement and reduction in the size of the spleen, but even in patients who respond the effect is usually short lived. Some hematologists recommend pretreatment with corticosteroids for several weeks in preparation for splenectomy, but others believe the potential benefit is outweighed by an increased risk of infection. Splenic irradiation has also been used preoperatively to reduce the size of the spleen, but the results have been variable, and again there is no universal agreement as to its value.

Antimetabolites and other cytotoxic drugs that only affect actively proliferating cells are ineffective and may be harmful in HCL, because the slowly proliferating hairy cells are less sensitive than the residual normal hematopoietic cells to such drugs. Patients with progressive disease who fail to respond to splenectomy or who later relapse frequently benefit from treatment with low doses of alkylating agents (e.g., chlorambucil or cyclophosphamide) with a decrease in hairy cell infiltration of the marrow and improvement in their blood cell counts. Since alkylating agents may also be deleterious by causing further myelosuppression, such therapy should be limited to patients whose disease is clearly progressing following splenectomy. Some patients who fail to respond to chlorambucil or who have relapsed show significant hematologic improvement with androgens (e.g., Halotestin* 10 mg three times a day or oxymetholone* 150 mg four times a day), and sometimes the responses are prolonged. However, it is not yet clear what proportion of patients can be expected to have a significant response to androgens and further trials are indicated. Patients with leukocytosis and large numbers of circulating hairy cells may benefit from intensive leukapheresis, but no significant improvement can be expected in the majority of patients who are leukopenic. A few patients with refractory disease and severe neutropenia and thrombocytopenia secondary to bone marrow replacement by hairy cells have had good durable remissions following intensive chemotherapy with an anthracycline or cyclophosphamide, sometimes in combination with other cytotoxic drugs. However, such therapy is extremely hazardous and requires intensive supportive treatment, including repeated granulocyte and platelet transfusions during the period of prolonged marrow aplasia. Elderly patients with HCL tolerate intensive chemotherapy poorly, and this approach should probably be restricted to younger patients with clearly progressive disease who have failed to respond or who have relapsed after splenectomy and treatment with alkylating agents in low doses.

Recently, it has been reported that patients with hairy cell leukemia may respond favorably to treatment with human leukocyte interferon, and its usefulness in this disease is being evaluated.

*This use is not listed in the manufacturer's directive.

Bouroncle BA: Leukemic reticuloendotheliosis (hairy cell leukemia). Blood 53:412, 1979. *A review of the manifestations of hairy cell leukemia by the physician who first recognized this disease as a clinical entity.*

Catovsky D: Hairy-cell leukemia and prolymphocytic leukemia. Clin Haematol 6:245, 1977. *A good review of the criteria for diagnosis of hairy cell leukemia and of techniques for identification of hairy cells. Dr. Catovsky also reviews and appraises the methods of treatment which have been employed for hairy cell leukemia.*

Golomb HM: Hairy cell leukemia: Lessons learned in 25 years. J Clin Oncol 1:652, 1983. *Good recent review of the clinical features, therapeutic options, and biology of HCL with an up-to-date list of pertinent references.*

Jansen J, LeBien TW, Kersey JH: The phenotype of the neoplastic cells of hairy cell leukemia studied with monoclonal antibodies. Blood 59:609, 1982. *Eighteen cases of hairy cell leukemia were studied with a battery of polyclonal anti-Ig and monoclonal antibodies. The results support the B cell origin of HCL and suggest that the maturation arrest in HCL is at a more mature stage than in CLL.*

Posnett DN, Chiorazzi N, Kunkel HG: Monoclonal antibodies with specificity for hairy cell leukemia cells. J Clin Invest 70:254, 1982. *Recent studies of three monoclonal antibodies prepared against hairy cells are described, one of which was found to be specific for some (but not all) hairy cells and which did not react with any other cells tested. A review of the recent literature is included.*

Quesada JR, Reuben J, Manning JT, Heuh EM, Gutterman JU: Alpha interferon for induction of remission in hairy-cell leukemia. N Engl J Med 310:15, 1984. *The beneficial therapeutic effects of human leukocyte interferon in HCL are described for the first time.*

Stewart DJ, Benjamin RS, McCredie KB, Murphy S, Keating M: The effectiveness of rubidazone in hairy cell leukemia (leukemic reticuloendotheliosis). Blood 54:298, 1979. *Two patients with progressive hairy cell leukemia are reported who had an excellent response to intensive treatment with an anthracycline (rubidazone). It is emphasized that both patients were relatively young and that they required intensive supportive care during the prolonged period of myelosuppression that followed treatment.*

156. THE ACUTE LEUKEMIAS

Howard J. Weinstein

DEFINITION. The acute leukemias are primary malignant diseases of the blood-forming organs characterized by a predominance of immature myeloid or lymphoid precursors ("blasts"). The blasts progressively replace normal bone marrow, migrate, and invade other tissues. There is diminished production of normal erythrocytes, granulocytes, and platelets in acute leukemia, and this leads to the most important complications of this disease—anemia, infection, and hemorrhage.

The acute leukemias are classified morphologically by reference to the predominant cell line involved as lymphoblastic (ALL) and myelogenous (AML) forms. If untreated, both forms are universally fatal within a period of months to one year. Therapy has markedly altered prognosis, and many patients with acute leukemia remain free of disease for prolonged periods.

ETIOLOGY. The mechanism of leukemogenesis in humans is unknown, but inciting agents are well established.

Ionizing Radiation. Physicians and scientists exposed to excessive amounts of radiation during the early years of research on medical application of x-rays, patients given low-dose radiation for rheumatoid spondylitis, and persons exposed acutely to radiation during the nuclear attacks on Hiroshima and Nagasaki have all been found to have an increased incidence of leukemia. The incidence of leukemia in survivors of the atomic bombings was dose related, being high in those who were less than 1500 meters from the hypocenter of the explosion and virtually normal for those beyond 2000 meters. The first cases of leukemia were noted two years after irradiation. A peak was reached after five to seven years, but 20 years later there was still an increased incidence. Studies of the effects of exposure to low-dose irradiation in utero have not consistently shown an increased incidence of leukemia.

Oncogenic Viruses (see also Ch. 169). Horizontally transmissible *RNA viruses* (retroviruses) are clearly capable of inducing acute leukemia in mice, domestic cats, cattle, chickens, and gibbon apes. Unequivocal evidence for either an endogenous or a horizontally transmitted human leukemia virus is still lacking. A naturally occurring human type C retrovirus, human T cell leukemia virus (HTLV), has recently been isolated from tumor cells of adults with leukemia and lymphomas of mature T lymphocytes. HTLV-associated leukemia is prevalent in certain geographic regions such as Southwestern Japan and the West Indies. In Southern Japan, where clustering of adult T cell leukemia occurs, most patients and 10 per cent of healthy individuals have natural antibodies to HTLV, suggesting that HTLV is a common infection. The molecular mechanism of neoplastic transformation of human T cells by HTLV is currently not known.

Genetic and Congenital Factors. The strongest evidence for a genetic predisposition to acute leukemia is the occurrence of this disease in identical twins. If one of a set of identical twins develops leukemia before six years of age, the risk of disease in the other twin is 20 per cent. Leukemia usually develops in a co-twin within months of the first case. Concordant leukemia in monozygotic infant twins may reflect a common prezygotic determinant, shared intrauterine insult, or blood-borne metastases from one twin to the other. For fraternal twins and siblings, the risk of developing leukemia is between two- and four-fold higher than for children in the general population.

Congenital conditions associated with chromosomal instability and a predisposition to acute leukemia include three autosomal recessive disorders: Bloom's syndrome, Fanconi's anemia, and ataxia telangiectasia. Ataxia telangiectasia is commonly accompanied by rearrangement of the long arm of chromosome 14, and is one of the inborn immunodeficiency syndromes that predispose to lymphoreticular neoplasms, including acute lymphoblastic leukemia.

Down's syndrome (trisomy 21) is associated with a 10- to 20-fold increased risk of leukemia during the first decade of life. The cell types of leukemia follow the usual distribution, but the age peak is nearly three years earlier than expected. Newborns with Down's syndrome may show a transient proliferation of blast cells (usually myeloblasts) that is often clinically and hematologically indistinguishable from congenital leukemia. In contrast to congenital leukemia, complete permanent recovery occurs within weeks to months without specific antileukemia therapy.

Chemical Agents. Many chemicals have been associated with leukemia. Benzene exposure increases the risk of AML, with bone marrow hypoplasia and/or pancytopenia often preceding the diagnosis of leukemia. Less convincing reports have implicated chloramphenicol and phenylbutazone as leukemogenic agents.

The use of alkylating agents for neoplastic and non-neoplastic diseases has resulted in development of AML or some variant, although the precise incidence of this complication is not known. These leukemias have developed in the absence of radiation or underlying diseases that produce immunologic deficiency.

INCIDENCE. The incidence of ALL increases rapidly after birth, peaks before five years of age, and subsequently declines. The peak incidence before age five reaches 50 per million annually, falling to 20 or less by age eight. At puberty, the rate declines to about 10 per million. The incidence remains below 10 per million until age 65, when it again climbs to about 15 per million at age 75. In contrast to ALL, the annual incidence of AML is quite constant from birth throughout the first 10 years at about 10 cases per million. A slight peak in late adolescence occurs and the incidence remains at a nearly constant 15 per million until age 55, after which the incidence progressively rises to 50 per million at age 75.

The overall incidence in males as compared with that in females is 1.3:1. Approximately 80 per cent of children with acute leukemia have the lymphoblastic type, and over 80 per cent of adults with acute leukemia have the myelogenous subtypes.

PATHOPHYSIOLOGY. The molecular basis of leukemic transformation in man is unknown. The fundamental defect in acute leukemia appears to be an unregulated proliferation of early precursor cells that have lost their capacity to differentiate in response to normal hormonal signals and cellular interactions. Previously, the accumulation of the leukemic cell population was attributed only to rapid and uncontrolled proliferation.

A leukemic aberration may arise at any point during the differentiation of the hematopoietic pluripotential stem cell. Chromosome and glucose-6-phosphate dehydrogenase studies show that the cellular level of origin of AML is heterogeneous. In some patients, the leukemia is expressed in the erythrocytic and granulocytic pathways, suggesting involvement of the CFU-S (myeloid stem cell). In other patients, the leukemia is expressed in cells restricted to granulocytic and macrophage lineage, suggesting involvement of CFU-GM (committed granulocyte-macrophage progenitor). Acute lymphoblastic leukemia is superimposed on normal hematopoietic cells that are products of normal CFU-S because committed myeloid progenitors in ALL do not contain chromosomal markers that are found in the leukemic lymphoblasts.

Both ALL and AML are of unicellular or monoclonal origin (Ch. 152). The disappearance of the nonrandom chromosome abnormalities during remission and their subsequent reappearance at the time of relapse also support the clonal nature of these diseases.

In acute leukemia normal and malignant cells coexist and compete for ascendancy within the bone marrow. For example, a normal karyotype may appear in remission or normal and abnormal karyotypes may coexist in relapse. This is in contrast to chronic myelogenous leukemia, in which few normal myeloid stem cells are detectable at the time of diagnosis.

Certain in vitro investigations and clinical studies provide some evidence that acute leukemia, although clonal, can be influenced by extracellular leukemogenic factors or deficiencies of differentiation factors. Acute leukemia has appeared in the engrafted cells of a leukemic patient who received a marrow transplant from a histocompatible sibling, for example, suggesting that leukemogenesis may result from unidentified factors that persist in certain susceptible hosts.

CLASSIFICATION. The acute leukemias are extraordinarily heterogeneous, reflecting the complexities of hematopoietic differentiation. The various types of acute leukemia are characterized by multiple methods that include morphology and histochemistry, cell surface and cytoplasmic markers, and chromosomal changes.

Morphology and Histochemistry. Blast cells are immature precursors, lacking many of the features for differentiating a lymphoid from a myeloid origin. The capacity to distinguish these blasts is of marked therapeutic and prognostic importance; various cytologic criteria have been established to differentiate between them.

Using the French-American-British (FAB) international morphologic classification, ALL has been divided into subgroups L1 to L3 and AML into subgroups M1 to M6. In L1, the common type of ALL, lymphoblasts treated with Wright's stain have smooth, homogeneous nuclear chromatin with indistinct nucleoli and only a small rim of light-blue staining cytoplasm. L2 is a lymphoid leukemia variant sometimes referred to as *undifferentiated leukemia*. L3 is characterized by deeply basophilic cytoplasm and prominent cytoplasmic vacuolization and is indistinguishable from the Burkitt type of leukemia. The ma-

TABLE 156–1. FAB CLASSIFICATION OF ACUTE MYELOGENOUS LEUKEMIA

FAB Class	Common Name	Morphology	Histochemistry	Common Consistent Chromosomal Defects
M1	Acute myelocytic leukemia without differentiation	Myeloblasts predominate; distinct nucleoli; few granules	MP+	t(9;22), +8, del 5 or 7
M2	Acute myelocytic leukemia with differentiation	Myeloblasts and promyelocytes predominate; further maturation abnormal	MP+	t(8;21), +8, del 5 or 7
M3	Acute promyelocytic leukemia	Promyelocytes predominate; hypergranular	MP+	t(15;17)
M4	Acute myelomonocytic leukemia	Myelocytic and monocytic maturation evident; may be peripheral monocytosis	MP+ NSE+	t(9;11), +8, inv 16
M5	Acute monocytic leukemia with differentiation	Promonocytes predominate; large cerebriform nuclei	NSE+	t(9;11), +8 (M5 and M5A)
M5A	Acute monoblastic leukemia without differentiation	Completely undifferentiated blast cells	NSE+	
M6	Erythroleukemia	Bizarre, multinucleated, megaloblastoid erythroblasts predominate; myeloblasts also present	MP+ (myeloblasts) PAS+ (erythroblasts)	+8, del 5 or 7

FAB = French-American-British classification
MP = Myeloperoxidase
NSE = Nonspecific esterase
PAS = Periodic acid-schiff
t = Translocation
del = Deletion (loss of entire chromosome or part of the long arm)
inv = Inversion

jority of L1 and L2 types of lymphoblasts are reactive with periodic acid-Schiff (PAS), and they are nonreactive with myeloperoxidase.

A summary of the AML subtypes and their histochemical reactivity is listed in Table 156–1. *Auer rods,* which are azurophilic granular cytoplasmic inclusion bodies, are thought to be pathognomonic of AML and are most commonly seen in the M2 and M3 subtypes. Acute leukemias derived from eosinophilic, basophilic, and megakaryocytic precursors, although uncommon, display unique characteristics as well as many features in common with other acute myelogenous leukemias.

Surface Markers. Three broad subclasses of ALL are defined by leukemic cell surface markers and have prognostic and therapeutic significance. This classification of ALL and the approximate percentage of patients in each subclass is shown in Table 156–2.

The common acute lymphoblastic leukemia antigen, or CALLA, is a glycosylated polypeptide that is expressed on the cell surface in approximately 65 and 50 per cent of cases of childhood and adult ALL, respectively. CALLA is also detected in some of the non-Hodgkin's lymphomas, in one third of cases of blast crisis of Ph^1 chromosome–positive CML, on a small percentage of normal bone marrow cells, and on some nonhematopoietic tissues. Common ALL blasts and some unclassified ALL blasts have undergone immunoglobulin gene rearrangements, indicating a commitment to B cell differentiation. This suggests that most cases of non-T ALL may be of B cell lineage.

TABLE 156–2. IMMUNOLOGIC SUBCLASSIFICATION OF ACUTE LYMPHOBLASTIC LEUKEMIA

	Common	T Cell	B Cell	Unclassified
Frequency (per cent)	65	15–20	<5	10–15
Surface markers				
Ia	+	−	+	+
E-rosette	−	+[1]	−	−
CALLA	+	−[2]	−	−
T antigens	−	+	−	−
sIg	−	−	+	−
cIg	+/−[3]	−	−	−

The antigens are as follows:

Ia = immune response antigen
E-rosette = receptor on T lymphocytes that spontaneously binds sheep erythrocytes
CALLA = common acute lymphoblastic leukemia antigen
T antigens = defined by reactivity with monoclonal anti-T antibodies
sIg = surface immunoglobulin
cIg = cytoplasmic immunoglobulin (M)

1. A small per cent of cases of T ALL are E-rosette negative.
2. A small per cent of cases of T ALL are CALLA positive.
3. 30 per cent of common ALL is further characterized by cIg (called "pre-B cell").

T cell ALL is the only immunologic subclass that has a characteristic clinical presentation—that is, adolescent males who present with a high white blood cell count and a mediastinal mass. Using monoclonal hybridoma antibodies, distinct stages of T cell differentiation have been defined; these identify the heterogeneity of T cell leukemia in humans.

Blast cells from patients with AML react with many monoclonal antibodies that define antigens at various stages of erythroid, granulocytic, monocytic, and megakaryocytic differentiation. Myeloid leukemic blasts in most instances have Ia antigens but lack T cell, B cell, and CALLA antigens. A few instructive cases of ALL and AML express lineage nonspecific markers (e.g., rearranged immunoglobulin genes in a myeloblast).

Cytoplasmic Markers. At least five cytoplasmic marker enzymes have been used in the classification of acute leukemias: terminal deoxynucleotidyl transferase, hexosaminidase, N-alkaline phosphatase, 5′-nucleotidase, and adenosine deaminase. T lymphoblasts have diminished 5′-nucleotidase and increased adenosine deaminase activity as useful distinguishing characteristics. For example, an inhibitor of adenosine deaminase, deoxycoformycin, has induced remission in T cell ALL. Terminal deoxynucleotidyl transferase activity provides an excellent diagnostic differentiation between ALL and AML, as it is present in 95 per cent of cases of ALL and is mostly absent in AML. It has also correctly defined the lymphoblastic crisis in CML and predicted the efficacy of ALL therapy in its management.

Chromosome Changes. A detectable nonrandom chromosome change is usually present in leukemic cells in AML. Moreover, specific chromosomal abnormalities correlate with particular subtypes of AML (Table 156–2). Loss of chromosomes 5 or 7 or trisomy 8 has been most consistently observed in patients with preleukemia or secondary AML (previous history of radiation, cytotoxic drugs, or exposure to strong mutagenic agents).

The leukemic blasts in most patients with ALL have an abnormal karyotype, and the modal chromosome numbers appear to be much higher than in AML. Two interesting subgroups of patients have been identified: those with a Ph^1 chromosome and those with B cell ALL. It is unclear whether Ph^1-positive ALL is a variable expression of chronic myelogenous leukemia (presentation in lymphoid blast crisis) or a different disease process. Patients with B cell ALL (L3) have translocations between chromosomes 2;8, 14;8, and 22;8 as in Burkitt's lymphoma.

The mechanism by which cells carrying chromosome abnormalities gain selective advantage is beginning to be understood. The chromosome position of several cellular oncogenes is now known. The cellular oncogenes are homologous to recognized transforming genes of the acute retroviruses. Little is known about their function in the human genome, but they may be in part responsible for control of cellular proliferation and differentiation. These cellular oncogenes may be perturbed or activated by several mechanisms, including chromosome rearrangement, alteration in gene dosage (gain or loss of a chromosome), or small mutations. Activation or altered expression of cellular oncogenes may turn out to be one of several key steps in neoplastic transformation (see Ch. 169 for a more detailed discussion).

CLINICAL MANIFESTATIONS. The signs and symptoms of acute leukemia relate to decreased numbers of normal hematopoietic cells and invasion of other organs by leukemic cells. Why normal hematopoiesis is suppressed in leukemia is not known. It may result in part from the release of suppressor substances by leukemic blasts.

Anemia. Asthenia, pallor, headache, tinnitus, dyspnea, angina, edema, and congestive heart failure may all indicate anemia. The anemia generally results from decreased erythropoiesis and blood loss. Evidence of specific antibody-mediated hemolysis is uncommon.

Hemorrhage. Hemorrhagic manifestations in newly diagnosed acute leukemia are usually caused by thrombocytopenia. Oozing gums, epistaxis, petechiae, ecchymoses, menorrhagia, melena, and excessive bleeding after tooth extraction are common initial manifestations. Retinal hemorrhages and subarachnoid bleeding are rare. Most thrombocytopenic bleeding occurs when the platelet count is less than 20,000 per microliter.

Intracranial hemorrhages may result from leukostasis, i.e., intravascular clumping of blasts, especially within small vessels of the brain, leading to infarction and hemorrhage. Leukostasis occurs most frequently in acute myelogenous leukemia when the peripheral leukocyte count is in excess of 150,000 per microliter.

In acute promyelocytic leukemia, the abnormal granules in the blast appear to contain tissue thromboplastin activity or fibrinolysins that initiate disseminated intravascular coagulation or fibrinolysis. Massive hemorrhage can occur in this setting (see Ch. 167).

Infection. Most early infections in acute leukemia are presumably bacterial, but specific etiologic agents are often not found. Leukemia may first be recognized by the occurrence of an infection (respiratory, dental sinus, perirectal abscess, urinary tract, and skin) that never fully clears. These early infections appear to be attributable to granulocytopenia, with the risk of infection being greatest when the absolute granulocyte count is less than 200 cells per microliter. Repeated search for an infectious source of fever is required in all patients, because "leukemic fever" is extremely rare.

Leukemic Infiltration. Although leukemia is primarily a disease of bone marrow and peripheral blood, other tissues may also become infiltrated by the blast cells. The organs most commonly showing initial clinical involvement are the liver, spleen, and superficial lymph nodes. Bone pain is one of the initial symptoms in 25 per cent of patients with acute leukemia, and children with ALL may present with migratory joint pain accompanied by swelling and tenderness that may be confused with juvenile rheumatoid arthritis. These symptoms may be the result of direct leukemic infiltration of the periosteum, periosteal elevation by underlying cortical disease, bone infarction, or expansion of the marrow cavity by leukemic cells.

Central nervous system leukemia (leptomeningeal involvement) is clinically present at the time of diagnosis in about 2 per cent of patients. The most common signs and symptoms include vomiting, headache, papilledema, nuchal rigidity, and cranial nerve palsies. Spinal fluid pleocytosis with the presence of blasts usually makes the diagnosis a simple one, but even with cytocentrifugation techniques between 5 and 15 per cent of patients with arachnoid infiltration will not have identifiable leukemic cells in the spinal fluid.

Thymic or mediastinal infiltration, most commonly seen in T cell ALL, may cause life-threatening airway or cardiovascular compression. Patients with the monocytic variants of AML have a high frequency of skin and gum infiltration. These extramedullary involvements are probably caused by the specific properties of monoblasts.

Chloromas, unique clinical variants of acute myelogenous leukemia, are tumors that often appear green on the cut surface because of the presence of large amounts of the enzyme myeloperoxidase. These tumors may arise in bones or soft tissues and are frequently seen around the orbits or in other areas of the skull, ribs, and proximal long bones. Chloromas may develop before the onset of detectable bone marrow disease.

LABORATORY MANIFESTATIONS. Clinical laboratory data often provide a broad spectrum of abnormal findings in the patient with newly diagnosed acute leukemia. Anemia, abnormal white cell and differential blood counts, and thrombocytopenia are common, but as many as 10 per cent of patients may have normal routine blood counts at the time of diagnosis even when the bone marrow is replaced by leukemic cells. Pancytopenia without recognizably abnormal leukocytes is found in a small percentage of patients and has been called "aleukemic leukemia."

Blast cells are usually easily detectable in the peripheral blood when the white count exceeds 5000 per microliter. The morphology of peripheral blasts may not accurately reflect the status of the bone marrow. For example, normal myeloblasts may be detected in the circulation when lymphoblasts invade the marrow as part of the so-called leukoerythroblastic response to marrow invasion. The definitive diagnosis of leukemia should be made only from a bone marrow aspiration. The marrow specimen is usually hypercellular, and contains from 50 to 100 per cent blast cells. Occasionally, bone marrow aspiration results in a "dry tap." This may be attributed to a very packed marrow, reticulum fibrosis, or bone marrow necrosis within the marrow cavity. Marrow needle biopsy will usually produce an adequate specimen. The sample obtained by this technique should be touched to glass slides before it is placed in a fixative, because such touch preparations are very useful in assessing morphology.

Muramidase or lysozyme is a hydrolytic enzyme that is present in the primary granules of primitive granulocyte and monocyte precursor cells. Elevated serum and urine levels of this enzyme are present in acute myelogenous leukemia, with the highest levels in the monocytic and myelomonocytic subtypes. Renal tubular dysfunction and hypokalemia have been reported with increased blood and urine lysozyme.

DIFFERENTIAL DIAGNOSIS. The diagnosis of acute leukemia is seldom difficult. Infections, neoplasms, and other marrow infiltrations may lead to leukocytosis and to immature cells in the peripheral blood. These leukemoid reactions generally mimic chronic myelogenous leukemia (Ch. 155). Neutropenia induced by drugs, toxins, or infection may result in a bone marrow that is left shifted (filled with myeloblasts and promyelocytes). This normal, early myeloid population can be confused with AML, but it will mature in a few days, thus establishing the diagnosis.

Infectious mononucleosis and other viral illnesses can masquerade as leukemia. This differential diagnosis is particularly difficult in the rare patient whose viral illness is complicated by thrombocytopenic purpura or immunohemolytic anemia. Patients with both acute leukemia and aplastic anemia may present with pancytopenia. The bone marrow aspirate in aplastic anemia will be hypocellular, but rarely the two diseases cannot be differentiated initially because a small number of patients with acute leukemia present with a hypocellular bone marrow.

THERAPY. The possibility of cure for both acute lymphoblastic and acute myelogenous leukemia has become realistic. A complete remission is required in order to provide a significant prolongation of survival. Such a remission is commonly defined as the reduction of leukemic cells to undetectable levels and the restoration of normal bone marrow function. This includes a return to less than 5 per cent blasts in the bone marrow; normalization of hemoglobin, granulocyte, and platelet counts; resolution of organomegaly; and return of the patient to normal life style.

Initial treatment is directed toward correcting metabolic abnormalities, anemia and thrombocytopenia, and toward controlling infection and preventing hyperuricemia. This may require up to 48 hours but can usually be achieved in 24 hours. Allopurinol is started at diagnosis to decrease the formation of relatively insoluble uric acid from the catabolic products of leukemia cells. Hyperuricemia may occur prior to antileukemic treatment and occasionally may be severe enough to produce impaired renal function before therapy can be started. In this setting, alkalinization and high urine flow should be established before cytotoxic therapy is initiated.

Acute Lymphoblastic Leukemia. Once the patient's condition is stabilized, antileukemic chemotherapy should begin without delay. Therapy is divided into three phases: remission induction, central nervous system prophylaxis, and treatment in remission (maintenance or continuation therapy).

REMISSION INDUCTION. Combinations of two agents have been consistently superior to single agents for inducing complete remission of patients with ALL. The most effective combination has been vincristine and prednisone, which produces complete remission in more than 90 per cent of pediatric patients and 50 per cent of adults with ALL. For patients over 15 years of age, the addition of a third drug (L-asparaginase, methotrexate, doxorubicin, or daunorubicin) increases the remission rate to over 80 per cent.

CENTRAL NERVOUS SYSTEM PROPHYLAXIS. The single most important advance in the recent treatment of childhood ALL has been central nervous system (CNS) prophylaxis. As more patients experienced longer bone marrow remission, the central nervous system became the first site of relapse in over 50 per cent of patients. The risk of relapse in the CNS can be markedly reduced by treatment with irradiation, 2400 rads to the cranial-spinal axis or 2400 rads to the cranium, combined with five doses of methotrexate given intrathecally. Intrathecal methotrexate alone is effective CNS prophylaxis in selected patients with ALL. Treatment of the CNS sanctuary reduces the frequency of subsequent bone marrow relapse and increases the percentage of children remaining in continuous complete remission. CNS prophylaxis is usually administered following completion of the induction regimen, and is now routinely used in all childhood and most adult ALL treatment programs. In the adult age group, CNS leukemia is significantly reduced by similar prophylaxis, but this has not resulted in longer bone marrow remissions.

Cranial irradiation combined with intrathecal methotrexate is very effective CNS prophylaxis, but carries some risk of CNS damage. For example, irradiation alters vascular permeability to methotrexate, such that subsequent administration of parenteral methotrexate in large doses may result in a demyelinating leukoencephalopathy.

MAINTENANCE OR CONTINUATION THERAPY. After remission induction and CNS prophylaxis, continued therapy is necessary to prevent bone marrow relapse. Combinations of drugs not used in the induction regimen are most effective in maintaining a remission, of which 6-mercaptopurine and methotrexate are the most effective. In some studies, multiple cell cycle–specific and nonspecific agents are used during maintenance therapy to prevent the emergence of drug-resistant leukemic cells.

How long maintenance therapy should be continued is unclear, in part because of the inability to assess minimal residual disease (less than 10^9 leukemic cells). In the absence of objective evidence some patients have been treated for 2.5 to 5 years. If a continuous complete remission has been maintained for 2.5 to 3 years, the overall frequency of relapse following cessation of treatment is about 25 per cent. The most common site of relapse is in the bone marrow, with the risk highest during the first year after treatment has been stopped. Patients who have been in remission for 4 years after completing 2.5 to 3 years of treatment have a negligible risk of relapse. These data apply to children only.

RELAPSE. CNS relapse has dramatically declined with the routine use of CNS prophylactic therapy; however, the testes are an important extramedullary site of relapse. The risk period for testicular relapse is bimodal. Males with T cell disease are at early risk (within one year from diagnosis) and males with common ALL are at risk for testicular relapse after cessation of therapy. If testicular relapse occurs during or following cessation of therapy, irradiation in a dose of 2400 rads should be given to both testes. As when CNS relapse occurs, systemic spread must be assumed, and therefore a systemic chemotherapy regimen should be given. The prognosis for males with late testicular relapse appears to be favorable.

The majority of patients who have relapse during treatment will achieve second remissions with chemotherapy, but these are short-lived. Bone marrow transplantation, however, is a potentially useful therapy for these patients (Ch. 165). A few centers have reported 20 to 30 per cent five-year survival in patients with ALL who were treated by allogeneic bone marrow transplantation in second or subsequent remission. Autologous bone marrow transplantation is an experimental procedure for patients who lack HLA-identical donors. Bone marrow is obtained in second remission, treated in vitro by physical, immunologic (e.g., anti-CALLA antibody), or pharmacologic techniques to remove residual leukemia cells and cryopreserved. The patient receives supralethal chemoradiotherapy and reinfusion of autologous "treated" bone marrow.

PROGNOSTIC FEATURES. Prognostic factors are most helpful for identifying subsets of patients, but the relative importance of a given factor varies among treatment programs. Clinical and laboratory findings at the time of diagnosis such as age, race, sex, amount of organ infiltration, white blood count, lymphoblast morphology, immunologic markers, and chromosome aberrations have been correlated with prognosis. In childhood studies, relatively favorable factors include age of two to ten years, white race, female sex, a white blood count less than 20,000 per microliter, L1 morphology, and CALLA positivity. Over 60 per cent of patients in this group remain in continuous complete remission for five or more years after diagnosis. Less favorable prognostic factors include age less than two or greater than ten years, male sex, a mediastinal mass, L3 or Burkitt-type leukemia, Ph^1 chromosome, and an extremely elevated white blood cell count. The presence of T cell disease has a strong correlation with some high risk clinical features but is not an independent prognostic variable. Only 30 per cent of patients over 15 years of age remain in remission for five or more years. The poorer prognosis observed in the older age group may in part be due to a different distribution of biologic subsets of ALL between adults and children. The intensive use of cytotoxic drugs including adriamycin, L-asparaginase, cyclophosphamide, and cytosine arabinoside following remission induction appears to have improved durations of remission for high risk patients (adolescents and adults) with ALL.

Acute Myelogenous Leukemia. Progress in the treatment of acute myelogenous leukemia has not equaled that in the management of acute lymphoblastic leukemia. More effective antileukemic chemotherapy and more sophisticated supportive care have recently increased the complete remission rate and the duration of remission, however.

Remission Induction. Remission induction is now successful in 50 to 85 per cent of patients (adults and children) with acute myelogenous leukemia. The drug dosages necessary to kill myeloblasts come dangerously close to destroying normal marrow cells and cause prolonged bone marrow aplasia until normal hematopoietic progenitors can repopulate the marrow. Therefore, effective remission induction programs are associated with considerable morbidity and mortality. The introduction of cytosine arabinoside (ara-C) and the anthracyclines (daunorubicin and doxorubicin) represented a major advance in the therapy of AML. Remission can be achieved in the majority of patients under 60 years of age with a single course of seven days of cytosine arabinoside and three days of daunorubicin or doxorubicin. In the past, only about one third of patients over age 60 achieved complete remission, but recent results are more encouraging.

Postremission Induction. As in ALL, remission induction therapy reduces but does not eradicate the leukemic clone of cells. Therefore, additional therapy is necessary to achieve prolonged remission durations in patients with AML. With different chemotherapy treatment programs, median durations of remission have been 12 to 18 months, but with only 10 to 20 per cent of patients remaining in remission at five or more years. Factors potentially responsible for treatment failure during remission include inadequate chemotherapy-induced reduction of residual leukemic cells and the development of drug resistance by such residual tumor cells.

In an effort to increase leukemic cell kill during remission, patients have been treated with intensification or consolidation chemotherapy for periods of a few months to one year after induction of remission. This has been based on the steep dose response curve for most chemotherapeutic agents. In some studies, sequential "noncross-resistant" drug combinations have been administered to circumvent the problem of acquired drug resistance. The chemotherapeutic strategies used (i.e., VAPA study) have resulted in marked improvements in remission durations for patients of less than 18 years with AML (life table estimates of 50 per cent leukemia-free survival at five years). For similarly treated adults (18 to 60 years), median durations of remission were longer compared to other reported chemotherapy regimens, but a higher plateau of five-year leukemia-free survival was not achieved.

An alternative form of treatment is bone marrow transplantation in selected patients when an appropriate donor is available (see Ch. 165). Transplantation is ideally performed as soon as patients enter complete remission. The outcome of bone marrow transplantation for patients with AML in first remission is also encouraging. Leukemia-free survival estimates are as high as 50 to 60 per cent for young patients (less than 20 years) but decrease in older adults (greater than 30 years). Relapse of leukemia after marrow transplantation has not been a major obstacle to success. Graft versus host disease and interstitial pneumonitis account for the major mortality and morbidity in these patients. Bone marrow transplantation is the current treatment of choice for the patient with AML who has had relapse after an initial course of chemotherapy.

Central Nervous System Leukemia. CNS relapse is substantially less common than in acute lymphoblastic leukemia, in part because of earlier death from systemic disease. Patients with myelomonocytic or monocytic leukemia are at increased risk for CNS disease. CNS prophylaxis has reduced the incidence of meningeal relapse, but this has not translated into longer hematologic remissions. The major thrust of treatment should be directed toward the most frequent site of relapse, the bone marrow.

PROGNOSTIC FACTORS. Correlations between age, sex, performance status, morphologic classification, blast cytokinetics, platelet count, splenomegaly, and the response to therapy have been described but are controversial. There is a correlation between the chromosomal karyotypic abnormality in pretreatment bone marrow samples and response to initial therapy. Patients with only abnormal metaphases in their bone marrow at diagnosis or those with deletions of chromosomes 5 or 7 represent a group of patients who are unlikely to achieve complete remission with drug therapy.

The terms "preleukemia" and "smoldering leukemia" have been applied to a spectrum of abnormalities of bone marrow function characterized by normal to increased marrow cellularity and ineffective hematopoiesis. These patients often have a panmyelopathy, and chromosomal abnormalities are present in up to 50 per cent of cases. Many of these patients will develop acute myelogenous leukemia. The response to chemotherapy is poor and is comparable to that of patients with de novo AML who have only abnormal metaphases at diagnosis.

Acute myelogenous leukemia has been reported in patients who received chemotherapy (alkylating agents and nitrosoureas) for neoplastic diseases, including malignant lymphoma, ovarian carcinoma, and gastrointestinal carcinoma. The response of these patients to chemotherapy is poor, with remission rates of less than 50 per cent in most series.

IMMUNOTHERAPY. For immunotherapy to be effective, one must hypothesize that leukemia-specific or leukemia-associated antigens exist, that the host can mount an immune response against these antigens, and that this immune response will favorably affect the course of the patient's disease. Most studies find immunotherapy to be effective against only relatively small numbers of tumor cells, usually less than 10^5. Because of this limitation, the majority of immunotherapy trials have been performed in patients in remission. A variety of immunotherapeutic agents have been examined, including BCG, *Corynebacterium parvum* and irradiated allogeneic leukemic blast cells with BCG. In most trials patients have been randomized to receive chemotherapy alone, immunotherapy alone, or both chemotherapy and immunotherapy. Immunotherapy has failed to increase remission durations in AML, but several trials have indicated substantial increase in survival of patients receiving immunotherapy and chemotherapy, as compared with chemotherapy alone. This effect appears to be related to an increase in postrelapse survival and may be due to a higher rate of second remissions.

SUPPORTIVE CARE. Advances in the treatment of acute leukemia, especially AML, have depended on progress in the control of infection and bleeding. Infection is a major complication of induction chemotherapy for AML, with mortality rates of 20 to 50 per cent. Neutropenia, impaired immunity, and toxicity to nonhematopoietic tissues (gastrointestinal tract) are predisposing factors. Virtually all patients with AML become febrile while receiving induction chemotherapy. Although infection is usually suspected, it is documented in only 50 to 70 per cent of cases. Nevertheless, febrile neutropenic patients should immediately receive broad-spectrum antibiotics after appropriate cultures have been obtained. A semisynthetic penicillin and an aminoglycoside are generally included.

The roles of oral nonabsorbable antibiotics, protected environments (laminar airflow), and granulocyte transfusions during induction of remission in patients with AML are not yet clear. Oral nonabsorbable antibiotics reduce enteric colonization and have been shown to reduce systemic infection. Several studies indicate a decreased incidence of infections in protected environments, but overall remission rates remain unchanged. Therapeutic granulocyte transfusions in some studies have improved survival in patients with gram-negative bacteremia. The prophylactic use of granulocyte transfusions in the setting of prolonged granulocytopenia is currently under investigation (see Ch. 150). Although these efforts to improve infection control are reasonable in a research setting, they are clearly not required for successful remission induction chemotherapy.

In addition to bacteria, a variety of opportunistic organisms invade the immunosuppressed host. Patients on "broad-spectrum" antibiotics who remain febrile and granulocytopenic should be carefully evaluated for fungal infections. *Pneumocystis carinii* threatens the immunosuppressed host and causes severe interstitial pneumonitis. Infection with this organism can be markedly reduced by prophylactic therapy with trimethoprim-sulfamethoxazole.

Platelet transfusions from HLA mismatched donors are successful in restoring hemostasis in thrombocytopenic patients, but result in alloimmunization in 30 to 50 per cent of patients (see Ch. 166). The alloimmunized patient may be managed by the use of HLA-matched platelets, single donor platelets obtained by plateletpheresis, or autologous cryopreserved platelets. There is controversy as to whether platelets should be transfused prophylactically (i.e., platelet count less than 20,000 per microliter) or whether they should be used only for active bleeding. In making this decision the patient's overall clinical status, platelet responsiveness, the availability of HLA-matched and single-donor platelets, and whether bone marrow transplant is a future consideration are factors to be taken into consideration. The hemorrhagic complications of acute promyelocytic leukemia can be prevented and controlled by administration of heparin.

Transfusion of blood products from normal donors has been associated with graft versus host disease in the immunosuppressed and myelosuppressed patient with acute leukemia. Irradiation of blood products at dosages sufficient to destroy T lymphocytes prevents the development of graft versus host disease.

Bennett JM, Catovsky D, Daniel MT, et al.: Proposals for the classification of the acute leukemias. Br J Haematol 33:451, 1976. *Detailed description of the French-American-British (FAB) classification of acute leukemia.*

Casciato DA, Scott JL: Acute leukemia following prolonged cytotoxic agent therapy. Medicine 58:32, 1979. *Includes a complete review of drug-induced leukemia and a complete bibliography.*

Foon KA, Schroff RW, Gale RP: Surface markers on leukemia and lymphoma cells: Recent advances. Blood 60:1, 1982. *Detailed review of the cell surface phenotypes defined by monoclonal antibodies in the leukemias and lymphomas.*

Gale RP: Advances in the treatment of acute myelogenous leukemia. N Engl J Med 300:1189, 1979. *Excellent clinical review of current therapies and supportive care for patients with AML. Includes a complete bibliography.*

Gallo RC, Wong-Staal F: Retroviruses as etiologic agents of some animal and human leukemias and lymphomas and as tools for elucidating the molecular mechanism of leukemogenesis. Blood 60:545, 1982. *Review of viral etiology of leukemias including the HTLV retrovirus.*

Levine AS, Deisseroth AB: Recent developments in the supportive therapy of acute myelogenous leukemia. Cancer 42:883, 1978. *Good review of transfusion support, protective isolation, and management of infection in patients with AML.*

Lister TA, Rohatiner AZS: The treatment of acute myelogenous leukemia in adults. Semin Hematol 19:172, 1982. *Detailed review of clinical chemotherapy trials in acute myelogenous leukemia.*

Mauer AM: Therapy of acute lymphoblastic leukemia in childhood. Blood 56:1, 1980. *Complete clinical review of the phases of treatment for ALL. Bibliography is complete and includes references on bone marrow transplantation and immunotherapy.*

McCulloch EA: Stem cells in normal and leukemic hemopoiesis (Henry Stratton Lecture, 1982). Blood 62:1, 1983. *Good review and bibliography of the nature of differentiation in normal and leukemic processes.*

Sallan SE, Ritz J, Pesando J, et al.: Cell surface antigens: Prognostic implications in childhood acute lymphoblastic leukemia. Blood 55:395, 1980. *The relative importance of cell surface markers as compared to clinical prognostic factors are explored. Includes the CALLA subset of ALL.*

Schiffer CA: Granulocyte transfusion therapy. Cancer Treatment Reports 67:113, 1983. *State of the art review of granulocyte transfusion therapy.*

Thomas ED: Marrow transplantation for malignant diseases. J Clin Oncol 1:517, 1983. *Overview of marrow transplantation for acute leukemia.*

Weinstein HJ, Mayer RJ, Rosenthal DS, et al.: Chemotherapy for acute myelogenous leukemia in children and adults: VAPA update. Blood 62:315, 1983. *Results of intensive sequential chemotherapy for patients with AML and references to other chemotherapy and transplant studies.*

Yunis JJ: The chromosomal basis of human neoplasia. Science 221:227, 1983. *Complete review of consistent chromosome lesions in the leukemias and oncogene mapping.*

157. INTRODUCTION TO NEOPLASMS OF THE IMMUNE SYSTEM

Carol S. Portlock

Neoplasms of the immune system are a heterogeneous group of tumors whose cells of origin may be the lymphocyte, the histiocyte, or other cell components of the immune system. Each neoplasm is thought to be a monoclonal expansion of malignant cells, although this has only been conclusively demonstrated for lymphocytic tumors. Interestingly, these neoplasms often retain many morphologic, functional, and migratory characteristics common to their normal cell counterparts.

With increasing understanding of the normal immune system, it has become possible to classify malignant immune disorders according to their cell of origin. Table 157–1 lists these neoplasms, utilizing current immunologic concepts. Tumors of B lymphocyte lineage are identified by the presence of cell surface immunoglobulin, utilizing fluorescent anti-immunoglobulin antibodies. Each B lymphocytic neoplasm can be immunotyped according to its heavy chain and light chain classes and can be shown to be a monoclonal process. Such immunologic phenotyping may identify distinct groups of patients with different clinical presentations and prognoses. In addition to membrane-bound immunoglobulin, malignant B lymphocytes may have Ia antigen and Fc receptors, as well as receptors for complement.

Tumors of T lymphocyte lineage are identified in vitro by the formation of E rosettes after incubation with sheep erythrocytes. Moreover, monoclonal antibodies that react with normal T cell differentiation antigens can be used to detect distinct malignant T cell subsets. Enzyme determination of terminal deoxynucleotidyl transferase (TdT) may also identify a T cell lineage, as well as pre-B and lymphoid stem cells.

Utilizing current immunologic techniques, however, some tumors that are of lymphocyte origin morphologically cannot be shown to contain B or T cell surface markers and consequently are termed "null" cell. Nevertheless, immunoglobulin gene rearrangements may be detected in such "null" cells, suggesting a pre-B cell origin. Tumors of histiocytic lineage

TABLE 157–1. LYMPHOMAS AS NEOPLASMS OF SPECIFIC CELL CLASSES OF THE IMMUNE SYSTEM

Cell Class	Neoplasm
B cell	
Medullary B cell	Chronic lymphocytic leukemia
	Diffuse small lymphocytic cell lymphomas
Follicular B cell	Follicular lymphomas
	Diffuse small and large cleaved cell lymphomas
	Burkitt's lymphoma
Immunoblastic B cell	Diffuse large cell immunoblastic lymphoma
T cell	
Thymic T cell	Lymphoblastic lymphoma
Mature T cell	Chronic lymphocytic leukemia (rare)
	HTLV-associated lymphoma
	Mycosis fungoides
	Sézary's syndrome
Immunoblastic T cell	Diffuse large cell lymphoma (rare)
Histiocytic	
Histiocyte	Malignant histiocytosis
	Diffuse large cell lymphoma (uncommon)
Unknown	Hodgkin's disease

Modified from Strauchen JA: West J Med 135:276, 1981.

have not yet been identified by monoclonal antibody techniques. These cells lack endogenous immunoglobulin but may acquire exogenous immunoglobulin on their cell surface. They may be rich in lysozyme or muramidase and as phagocytic cells, they can be shown to ingest latex particles or sensitized erythrocytes. The cell lineage of the Reed-Sternberg cell in Hodgkin's disease is not known with certainty. It has in vitro characteristics in common with both histiocytes and lymphocytes. Recent work suggests that it may derive from a dendritic cell or lymphocyte.

In addition to a specific immunologic phenotype, chromosomal abnormalities can be detected in the majority of immune system neoplasms. In many, the karyotype appears to be specific (follicular lymphomas, Burkitt's lymphoma, mycosis fungoides). Another marker that appears to be specific is the presence of antibodies to HTLV (human T cell lymphoma virus) found in patients with mature T cell lymphoma. These and other in vitro methods may provide additional information for defining prognostically important patient subsets.

Each neoplasm of the immune system is a distinct clinicopathologic entity. However, these disorders tend to share some common clinical features. For example, systemic symptoms of fever, night sweats, and weight loss may be present and tend to correlate with advanced stage of disease. The neoplasm usually arises in one or more organs of the hematopoietic system (lymph nodes, spleen, liver, bone marrow) and if untreated or ineffectively treated, it tends to disseminate to all those organs, as well as to other sites. Bone marrow involvement with or without peripheral blood manifestation is common in certain disorders and may be the predominant feature. Meningeal infiltration is often present when aggressive neoplasms involve the bone marrow.

PATHOLOGY AND CLASSIFICATION

Neoplasms of B or T lymphocytic lineage are termed non-Hodgkin's lymphomas. They are a diverse group of diseases with varying clinical presentations, responses to therapy, and prognoses. The Rappaport histopathologic classification of the non-Hodgkin's lymphomas (Table 157–2) has been used successfully in clinical trials and practice. It has permitted the identification of specific clinicopathologic entities and of favorable and unfavorable prognostic groups since 1966. Nevertheless, the Rappaport classification, based exclusively upon morphologic concepts, does not take into account recent information regarding the immune system. For example, the term, "histiocytic" lymphoma is generally incorrect because virtually all of the non-Hodgkin's lymphomas are of lymphocytic origin.

Recently the National Cancer Institute sponsored an inter-

TABLE 157–2. CLASSIFICATION OF THE NON-HODGKIN'S LYMPHOMAS

NCI Working Formulation (1982)	Rappaport Classification (1966)
Low grade	
Small lymphocytic cell	Diffuse lymphocytic, well differentiated
Follicular, small cleaved cell	Nodular lymphocytic, poorly differentiated
Follicular, mixed small cleaved and large cell	Nodular mixed lymphocytic-histiocytic
Intermediate grade	
Follicular, large cell	Nodular histiocytic
Diffuse, small cleaved cell	Diffuse lymphocytic, poorly differentiated
Diffuse, mixed small cleaved and large cell	Diffuse mixed lymphocytic-histiocytic
Diffuse, large cell (cleaved and noncleaved)	Diffuse histiocytic
High grade	
Diffuse, large cell (immunoblastic)	Diffuse histiocytic
Small noncleaved cell (Burkitt and non-Burkitt)	Diffuse undifferentiated
Lymphoblastic (convoluted and nonconvoluted)	

national multi-institutional study to determine the clinical relevance of six major pathologic classifications of the non-Hodgkin's lymphomas. Table 157–2 juxtaposes the working formulation developed in that study with the Rappaport classification. Tumor architecture is an important feature in both: Rappaport's "nodular" is replaced by the more immunologically accurate term "follicular." Cell morphology is more descriptive in the working formulation and "histiocytic" is replaced by "large cell." Prognostically favorable and unfavorable groups are termed low, intermediate, and high grade, respectively. The low grade category includes small lymphocytic consistent with chronic lymphocytic leukemia; a miscellaneous category includes mycosis fungoides and true histiocytic lymphoma.

Many non-Hodgkin's lymphomas may exhibit two distinct histologic subtypes. Both the architecture and the cell type may change, usually evolving from a low grade lymphoma to an intermediate or high grade lymphoma. Rarely, two histologies may be present at diagnosis in the same lymph node (composite lymphoma). More often, two histologies may be seen at diagnosis in two separate biopsy specimens; most frequently, one histology is seen at diagnosis and a second at relapse or autopsy. It is thought that such "transformation" represents clonal expansion of a more aggressive cell line. Its clinical importance is that both therapy and prognosis may be dramatically altered by its emergence.

DIAGNOSIS AND STAGING

The diagnosis of a neoplasm of the immune system is based upon pathologic classification of biopsy material. This requires adequate tissue (preferably lymph node, so that both architecture and cell type may be assessed), proper handling, and excellent hematopathologic interpretation. Special studies such as imprints, immunotyping, karyotyping, TdT determination, and electron microscopy may provide additional information for classification. Since these latter studies require fresh tissue and special handling, it is important that the pathologist be involved *before* biopsy. Likewise, it is important that each patient be evaluated jointly by a medical oncologist, radiation therapist, surgeon, and radiologist from the outset.

With the diagnosis established, the extent of disease should be completely defined. Since each neoplasm has distinct clinicopathologic features, the choice of staging studies will be based on that information. All patients should have a complete history, particularly assessing the presence or absence of systemic symptoms, and physical examination. All nodal areas should be examined, including Waldeyer's ring and preauricular, epitrochlear, and popliteal lymph nodes. In addition to liver and spleen, epigastric or other abdominal masses may be found. The lungs, skin, breasts, testicles, and central nervous system should be carefully examined for extranodal involvement. Blood counts and liver and renal function tests are necessary in all patients. In addition to chest x-ray, tomography or CT scanning may be indicated in an abnormal chest. Abdominal CT and lymphography are often complementary and not mutally exclusive. Gallium-67 scanning may be useful but is not a diagnostic method. Liver and spleen scans are of minimal value. Studies of bone or GI tract should be performed only when symptoms are present. Bone marrow biopsy is often indicated, particularly if advanced clinical disease is present or the patient has a low grade lymphoma. CSF cytology should be performed in all patients with intermediate and high grade lymphomas who have bone marrow involvement and in all patients with Burkitt's lymphoma, lymphoblastic lymphoma, or malignant histiocytosis.

Several different staging systems are applied to neoplasms of the immune system. Their purpose is to define disease extent, to assist in treatment strategies, to evaluate therapeutic results, and to determine prognosis. In Hodgkin's disease the utility of staging has been elegantly demonstrated, and excellent clinical care demands careful clinical and pathologic staging. Staging laparotomy with splenectomy and biopsy of liver, lymph nodes, and bone marrow was developed for adequate intra-abdominal assessment of Hodgkin's disease. It accurately identifies pathologic stage and its results often dictate treatment strategy. The Ann Arbor staging system for Hodgkin's disease has also been applied to the non-Hodgkin's lymphomas. In this setting it has less value in determining therapy but remains an important prognostic variable. Modified staging systems are used in pediatric lymphomas, chronic lymphocytic leukemia, Burkitt's and lymphoblastic lymphomas, and mycosis fungoides. Since pathologic intra-abdominal assessment is rarely needed to determine treatment in the non-Hodgkin's lymphomas, staging laparotomy is usually unnecessary. Nonetheless, careful clinical staging is imperative in all cases.

DIFFERENTIAL DIAGNOSIS

The differential diagnosis of neoplasms of the immune system is usually that of lymphadenopathy. Reactive processes, infections, other malignancies, and collagen-vascular disorders may all cause enlarged lymph nodes or hepatosplenomegaly or both. The location(s) of the lymph nodes, their size, shape, consistency, rapidity of onset, and other characteristics may aid in determining etiology.

Regional lymph node hyperplasia may be seen with acute or chronic infections of the extremities and with vaccinations or insect bites. Diffuse lymphadenopathy may occur following ingestion of phenytoin. Other diffuse reactive processes such as acquired immunodeficiency syndrome, angioimmunoblastic lymphadenopathy, and collagen-vascular disorders may be associated with an increased likelihood of developing lymphoma. Consequently, a single lymph node biopsy may not solve the diagnostic dilemma. That is why pathologic consultation before biopsy is recommended.

Among infectious etiologies, viral illnesses predominate and often produce bizarre pathologic material. Infectious mononucleosis may present with features common to Hodgkin's disease. Cytomegalovirus, cat scratch disease, toxoplasmosis, tuberculosis, and syphilis are other considerations. Other malignancies usually involve lymph nodes by regional spread. For example, cervical lymphadenopathy may be the first symptom of a malignancy involving the oropharynx or nasopharynx. Likewise, breast cancer may present with axillary adenopathy and a microscopic primary tumor.

In virtually all instances, the only way to determine conclusively the cause of lymphadenopathy is by pathologic tissue examination. Low cervical and supraclavicular lymph nodes are more likely to yield diagnostic material than axillary and inguinal nodes. When only intrathoracic or abdominal disease is present, bone marrow biopsy may provide diagnostic information and obviate the need for surgery. Fine needle aspiration is of lesser value in neoplasms of the immune system than in solid tumors, because cell morphology and architecture are both important diagnostic parameters.

Berard CW: A multidisciplinary approach to non-Hodgkin's lymphomas. Ann Intern Med 94:218, 1980. *A discussion moderated by Berard of the immunologic concepts pertinent to an understanding of the non-Hodgkin's lymphomas.*

Non-Hodgkin's lymphoma pathologic classification project. National Cancer Institute sponsored study of classifications of non-Hodgkin's lymphomas: Summary and description of a working formulation for clinical usage. Cancer 49:2112, 1982. *The working formulation is presented and six pathologic classifications are compared.*

Rudders RA: Surface markers in non-Hodgkin's lymphomas. Hosp Pract 18:161, 1983. *A review of marker studies and recent analysis of prognostic subsets.*

Warnke RA, Link MP: Identification and significance of cell markers in leukemia and lymphoma. Annu Rev Med 34:117, 1983. *A review of methodology and the diagnostic use of monoclonal antibody reagents.*

158. NON-HODGKIN'S LYMPHOMAS

Thomas E. Davis

The non-Hodgkin's lymphomas are a heterogeneous group of malignant neoplasms that arise from lymphoid components of the immune system. These disorders are histopathologically distinct from Hodgkin's disease and include the following subtypes: lymphocytic, histiocytic, mixed histiocytic and lymphocytic, pleomorphic (or stem cell type), lymphoblastic, and Burkitt's tumor (Burkitt's tumor is described in Ch. 159).

ETIOLOGY. In most cases, the cause of non-Hodgkin's lymphoma is unknown. Although viruses are associated with the development of lymphoid neoplasia in several animal species, specific viruses have been identified as etiologic agents in only two rare subtypes of human lymphoid malignancy. The Epstein-Barr virus (EBV) has been causally linked to the development of Burkitt's tumor, and the human T cell leukemia/lymphoma virus (HTLV) has more recently been isolated from patients with T cell lymphoid malignancies. An increased frequency of lymphocytic lymphomas and Hodgkin's disease has been reported in survivors of the atomic bomb explosions in Japan. Patients with genetic or acquired disorders associated with immune deficiency are known to be predisposed to lymphoid malignancy. The genetic disorders include ataxia telangiectasia, the Wiskott-Aldrich syndrome, congenital sex-linked agammaglobulinemia, and the Chédiak-Higashi syndrome. The acquired disorders associated with an increased frequency of lymphoid malignancy include the acquired immune deficiency syndrome (AIDS), acquired hypogammaglobulinemia, Sjögren's syndrome, and certain of the autoimmune syndromes. In addition, patients with renal allografts and others receiving long-term immunosuppressive therapy have an increased incidence of malignant lymphoid neoplasms.

EPIDEMIOLOGY. In the United States, the non-Hodgkin's lymphomas are approximately three times as common as Hodgkin's disease. There will be an estimated 24,000 new cases in 1984, representing 3 per cent of all new cancer diagnoses. The non-Hodgkin's lymphomas can occur in individuals of any age, although they are rare in children younger than two years and become increasingly frequent with advancing age. Worldwide there are striking variations in the incidence of certain types of non-Hodgkin's lymphoma. There is a high incidence of Burkitt's tumor among children in central Africa. Intestinal lymphoma is associated with immunoglobulin abnormalities among individuals in the Middle East.

PATHOLOGY. The diagnosis and classification of a lymphoma must be based on careful evaluation of biopsy material. However, in certain instances it may be difficult to distinguish benign from malignant disorders. Misinterpretations with respect to histopathologic subclassification are also common. Frequently the distinction between leukemia and lymphoma cannot be made on the basis of biopsy alone. For these reasons, it is important in each case to integrate the biopsy findings with clinical information obtained from the patient's history, physical examination, peripheral blood, bone marrow, and other laboratory studies.

The non-Hodgkin's lymphomas have traditionally been classified according to their morphology under the light microscope. Most of the terminologies used to describe and classify these disorders were proposed long before the remarkable developments in immunology of recent years. The immune system can be subdivided into several distinct populations of cells with varied physiologic functions distinguished on the basis of electron microscopy, cytochemistry, cell surface receptors, and functional characteristics. As newer techniques in immunology have been applied to the study of the non-Hodgkin's lymphomas, several new classification systems have been suggested. However, the ultimate value of these remains to be demonstrated. The ideal classification system should have three characteristics: (1) it should provide information that is clinically relevant in terms of predicting response or prognosis; (2) it should establish criteria sufficiently distinctive to yield reproducible results when applied by expert pathologists; and (3) it should be consistent with modern concepts of immunobiology.

In the United States, the most widely utilized classification is the one originally proposed by Rappaport in 1966 (Table 157–1). This has been found by many investigators to be both clinically relevant and reproducible, although it does not incorporate some of the newer concepts regarding lymphocytic differentiation. The Rappaport classification is based upon two morphologic features: the cytologic characteristics of the malignant cell populations and the histologic pattern of lymph node involvement. Patients with a nodular pattern of involvement generally have a more favorable prognosis than those with a diffuse histologic pattern.

In 1982, an expert panel assembled by the National Cancer Institute (NCI) reported the results of an international multi-institutional clinicopathologic study involving 1175 cases of non-Hodgkin's lymphoma. The study was designed to test both the reproducibility and the clinical relevance of six major classifications for the non-Hodgkin's lymphomas. The principal conclusion of the study was that the six classifications were comparable in terms of reproducibility and clinical relevance. On the basis of this study, the NCI expert panel proposed a working formulation that separates the non-Hodgkin's lymphomas into ten major histopathologic subtypes utilizing morphologic criteria only. This working formulation was proposed not as a new classification to supersede all others but as a means of translation among the various classifications in order to facilitate comparisons of case reports and therapeutic clinical trials.

The working formulation proposed by the NCI expert panel in 1982 is presented in Table 157–2. The individual histopathologic subtypes within the older Rappaport classification have been arranged to correspond to those of the new working formulation. Because the majority of studies published within the past two decades concerning the staging and treatment of the non-Hodgkin's lymphomas have utilized the Rappaport classification, we shall rely upon the terminology of the Rappaport classification while inviting the reader to refer to Table 157–2 for the corresponding terminology of the new working formulation.

Lymphocytic, Well Differentiated Type. This variety of non-Hodgkin's lymphoma is characterized by a diffuse and relatively homogeneous infiltrate of small, normal-appearing lymphocytes. The histologic pattern is identical to that of chronic lymphocytic leukemia. Well differentiated lymphocytic lymphoma may present either with focal lymph node enlargement or with generalized lymphadenopathy and splenomegaly. The bone marrow is usually involved. A monoclonal gammopathy may occur without appreciable numbers of plasmacytoid lymphocytes in the histologic sections. The disease most commonly occurs after the fifth decade and tends to be slowly progressive.

Chronic lymphocytic leukemia, Waldenström's macroglobulinemia, and well differentiated lymphocytic lymphoma appear to represent different manifestations of a fundamentally similar disorder, namely, the proliferation of well differentiated B lymphocytes. Nevertheless, these entities differ sufficiently from each other in terms of laboratory features, natural history, prognosis, and other clinical aspects to justify their continued separation as distinct clinicopathologic entities. In young persons, these diseases are uncommon and a proliferation of normal-appearing lymphocytes is more frequently associated with a reactive process or occasionally with Hodgkin's disease of the lymphocyte predominant type.

Lymphocytic, Poorly Differentiated Type. In adults, these tumors arise primarily in the lymph nodes and are composed of cells which exhibit considerable variation in size, configuration, and degree of differentiation. The histologic pattern may be nodular or diffuse. Patients with a nodular pattern have few symptoms at the time of presentation. They generally have a more favorable prognosis than patients with a diffuse histologic pattern. Although the bone marrow is frequently involved, only 5 to 10 per cent of adults with poorly differentiated lymphocytic lymphoma develop frank leukemia.

Children most commonly present with abdominal, retroperitoneal, or mediastinal disease. A nodular histologic pattern is exceedingly rare. Progression to acute leukemia is very common in children, and involvement of the central nervous system occurs frequently.

Histiocytic Type. Although the malignant cells in histiocytic lymphoma resemble histiocytes morphologically, they are presently considered to be derived from lymphoid elements. These malignant cells tend to be large and irregular with relatively abundant cytoplasm which is frequently acidophilic. In certain instances, the cells may be multinucleated and difficult to distinguish from Reed-Sternberg cells. There may be increased reticulin associated with individual cells, but this feature is not a diagnostic criterion. The histologic pattern is usually diffuse. The uncommon nodular histiocytic subtype frequently evolves to a diffuse pattern and has the least favorable prognosis among the nodular lymphomas.

Histiocytic lymphoma occurs predominantly in adults, with increased frequency in the older age groups. Patients may present with either localized or widespread lymphadenopathy. However, extranodal presentations are more common with this disease than with the lymphocytic lymphomas. On the other hand, the bone marrow is involved in less than 10 per cent of the patients at the time of presentation, and progression to frank leukemia is rare.

Mixed Histiocytic-Lymphocytic Type. This variety of non-Hodgkin's lymphoma is characterized by a mixed population of malignant cells, with the larger cells resembling histiocytes and the smaller ones appearing more like poorly differentiated lymphocytes. The histologic pattern is usually nodular at the time of presentation. In some cases, there is evolution with time and treatment to a pattern of diffuse histiocytic lymphoma. This disease occurs predominantly in older adults who typically seek medical attention because of generalized lymphadenopathy.

Undifferentiated or Pleomorphic Type. These tumors are composed of undifferentiated cells which vary widely in size and may include bizarre giant forms. Subsequent differentiation to lymphocytic or histiocytic types may occur. These should not be confused with Burkitt's tumor, in which the malignant cells also lack evidence of cytologic differentiation but have a uniform and characteristic appearance in tissue sections and imprints.

Lymphoblastic Type. Lymphoblastic lymphoma has recently been delineated as a distinct clinicopathologic entity. These tumors are composed of a diffuse, relatively uniform proliferation of cells with round or convoluted nuclei and scanty cytoplasm. Cytologically, the cells are similar to those of acute lymphoblastic leukemia. In the majority of cases, the cells form rosettes with sheep erythrocytes and react with antisera directed against T cell antigens.

Lymphoblastic lymphoma is seen most commonly in older children and young adults, but may also occur in elderly patients. Approximately 50 per cent of patients present with mediastinal lymphadenopathy. Although the disease may appear to be localized at the time of diagnosis, there is usually rapid dissemination to the bone marrow, peripheral blood, and meninges. Historically, the prognosis has been grim, with a median survival of less than one year in the larger published series. However, recent studies have demonstrated the efficacy of intensive systemic chemotherapy in conjunction with prophylactic treatment of the central nervous system.

Two disorders which share certain clinical and pathologic features with the non-Hodgkin's lymphomas deserve brief mention, although their position in the classification of lymphoid neoplasia remains to be clarified. *Angioimmunoblastic lymphadenopathy* is a systemic disease characterized by lymphadenopathy, hepatosplenomegaly, and constitutional symptoms. Anemia, lymphocytopenia, and polyclonal hypergammaglobulinemia are frequently present. The histologic picture is benign, consisting of immunoblasts, plasma cells, and proliferation of small vessels. Although the disease is responsive to therapy with prednisone or cytotoxic agents, the median survival is only three years. In about one third of the patients, transformation to a malignant lymphoma may be observed on repeated biopsies or at autopsy. *Malignant lymphoma with a high content of epithelioid histiocytes* ("Lennert's lymphoma") resembles the diffuse, mixed cell lymphoma of the Rappaport classification. However, this entity can be distinguished morphologically by the presence of epithelioid cell clusters scattered throughout the stroma. Constitutional symptoms and bone marrow involvement are common. Patients respond poorly to chemotherapy, and the median survival is short.

CLINICAL MANIFESTATIONS. The most common clinical manifestation of non-Hodgkin's lymphoma is painless enlargement of one or more peripheral lymph nodes. The average patient has been aware of the enlarged lymph nodes for several months before consulting a physician. Systemic symptoms of fever, night sweats, or weight loss are usually not prominent. Anterior mediastinal adenopathy occurs infrequently as contrasted with Hodgkin's disease, in which 50 to 70 per cent of patients manifest mediastinal involvement. Lymphoid structures throughout the body may be involved, including the tissue within Waldeyer's ring and preauricular, epitrochlear, or mesenteric lymph nodes. Palpable *splenomegaly* occurs in about 20 per cent of the patients and is more frequently observed in the lymphocytic varieties.

Approximately one third of the patients with non-Hodgkin's lymphoma initially present with extranodal disease. This is most common in patients with diffuse histiocytic lymphoma and occurs infrequently in patients with nodular lymphocytic lymphoma. The *gastrointestinal tract* may be the primary site of disease or may be involved as part of a more generalized process. The stomach and small intestine are most often involved, although the pancreas is frequently found to be infiltrated at autopsy. Primary histiocytic lymphoma of the stomach may be confused with carcinoma. Symptoms and signs of gastrointestinal involvement include malabsorption, obstruction, perforation, and bleeding.

Hepatic enlargement and jaundice are uncommon presenting manifestations, but percutaneous biopsy will demonstrate liver involvement in about 20 per cent of patients. Further diagnostic procedures to evaluate the liver, including peritoneoscopy and laparotomy, increase the yield of positives to about 50 per cent. Jaundice, when it occurs, is usually caused by tumor infiltration of the liver, but in certain cases it may be due to extrahepatic biliary obstruction.

Although *impaired renal function* may rarely occur secondary to direct parenchymal infiltration, it is more often due to obstruction of the urinary outflow. Other causes of renal dysfunction in patients with non-Hodgkin's lymphoma include compression of the renal vascular supply, hypercalcemia, hyperuricemia, amyloidosis, and radiation nephritis. Cardiac involvement is frequently noted at autopsy, but clinical manifestations are unusual. Primary lymphomas of the lung are rare, whereas secondary spread to the lungs is more common. Primary lymphomas also have been reported to occur in the bone, thyroid, testes, female genital organs, and salivary glands. Diffuse histiocytic lymphoma is the most commonly observed histologic pattern in patients with these extranodal presentations. Primary lymphomas of bone usually appear as lytic lesions and most frequently involve the femur, tibia, humerus, scapula, or pelvis.

The most common *neurologic manifestation* of lymphoma is spinal cord compression resulting from extradural tumor. Meningeal involvement is unusual in adults, generally a late manifestation of the disease. In children, central nervous system involvement is much more common, occurring in about 25 per cent of patients. Parenchymal brain involvement is rare, but has been noted to occur in patients with renal allografts.

The non-Hodgkin's lymphomas may occur as primary *skin* tumors. More frequently the skin is involved as part of a generalized disease process. *Sézary's syndrome,* a T cell variant of the non-Hodgkin's lymphomas, is characterized by chronic erythroderma with diffuse infiltration of the dermis and characteristic abnormal lymphocytes in the peripheral blood.

Bone marrow is invaded in about one third of the patients with non-Hodgkin's lymphoma, but the incidence of marrow involvement varies considerably among the different histologic types. The bone marrow biopsy may be positive at the time of presentation in more than half the patients with diffuse well differentiated lymphocytic lymphoma or nodular poorly differentiated lymphocytic disease.

Most patients with lymphoma have normal peripheral blood counts early in their clinical course. However, nearly 50 per cent will develop *anemia* as their disease progresses. The causes of anemia include marrow replacement, hypersplenism, autoimmune hemolytic anemia, hemorrhage, and marrow hypoplasia resulting from chemotherapy or irradiation. The peripheral white blood counts are usually normal, but lymphocytosis may occur, particularly in association with well differentiated lymphocytic lymphoma. A small number of characteristic notched or cleft cells may be seen in the peripheral blood of patients with nodular, poorly differentiated lymphocytic lymphoma. The conversion to a frank *leukemic phase* is uncommon in adults, but may occur with any of the histologic varieties of lymphoma. In children, leukemic conversion is observed in about 25 per cent of the patients.

STAGING. After establishing the diagnosis of non-Hodgkin's lymphoma, the next responsibility of the physician is to obtain an adequate assessment of the extent of disease. Careful staging prior to the initiation of therapy is important for several reasons: (1) to provide an estimate of prognosis, (2) to aid in the selection of an appropriate treatment program, and (3) to establish a precise point of reference which will later permit accurate assessment of the response to therapy. A standardized system of diagnostic procedures and descriptive terminology is also important in facilitating the comparison of therapeutic results among patients treated in different medical centers.

The continuing evolution in the staging of Hodgkin's disease over a period of 40 years culminated in the adoption of the Ann Arbor staging classification in 1971. This classification system, shown in Table 158–1, has also been widely applied to the staging of the non-Hodgkin's lymphomas. The Ann Arbor system has proved to be of exceptional value in the management of patients with Hodgkin's disease. However, the prognosis of patients with non-Hodgkin's lymphomas is influenced to such an important degree by the histologic classification that the Ann Arbor staging sytem is of limited clinical value. As an example, certain patients who present with what appears to be a localized form of diffuse histiocytic lymphoma may develop rapidly fatal disease progression in spite of intensive treatment. Conversely, many patients with nodular lymphocytic lym-

TABLE 158–1. ANN ARBOR STAGING CLASSIFICATION

Stage I:	Involvement of a single lymph node region (I) or a single extralymphatic site (IE)
Stage II:	Involvement of two or more lymph node regions on the same side of the diaphragm (II) or a solitary extralymphatic site and one or more of lymph node areas on the same side of the diaphragm (IIE)
Stage III:	Involvement of lymph node regions on both sides of the diaphragm (III), accompanied by spleen involvement (IIIS), or by solitary involvement of an extralymphatic organ or site (IIIE) or both (IIISE)
Stage IV:	Diffuse involvement of extralymphatic sites with or without lymph node enlargement

Clinical stage and pathologic stage defined for each patient; extranodal sites are designated by specific denominators; presence or absence of symptoms is designated B or A, respectively phoma that is widespread at the time of initial presentation may experience a very indolent clinical course for several years with only a minimum of therapy. Despite these limitations, the Ann Arbor classification does provide a standardized system of terminology which has facilitated the comparison of therapeutic results among patients treated in different medical centers.

The staging evaluation of any patient with one of the non-Hodgkin's lymphomas must begin with a careful clinical history and a thorough physical examination, including a description of all superficial lymph nodes and of the lymphoid structures within Waldeyer's ring. It is also important to obtain a chest x-ray, complete blood count, and serum chemistry determinations. In recent years, the use of more invasive staging procedures has become increasingly common. These procedures include lymphangiography, bone marrow biopsy, percutaneous liver biopsy, peritoneoscopy, and exploratory laparotomy. Widespread use of these techniques has demonstrated that the likelihood of detecting occult lesions increases in proportion to the diagnostic effort employed. The incidence of Stage I or II disease may be about 20 to 30 per cent in patients with a diffuse histologic pattern and as low as 10 per cent in patients with nodular lymphoma.

The *retroperitoneal lymphangiogram* is a major tool in the evaluation of patients with non-Hodgkin's lymphoma. In this procedure, a radiopaque dye is injected into the small lymphatics of the foot under pressure. The dye is taken up by the abdominal lymph nodes and can then be seen in roentgenograms of the abdomen for several months afterward, permitting assessment of treatment response. False-negative studies occur in only 15 per cent of the patients with non-Hodgkin's lymphoma, and false-positive findings are even less common. The lymphangiogram is positive at the time of presentation in 75 to 90 per cent of patients with a nodular histologic pattern. At staging laparotomy, most of these patients will have additional sites of subdiaphragmatic involvement. A normal lymphangiogram does not exclude subdiaphragmatic disease. Involvement of the spleen and mesenteric lymph nodes occurs in about half the patients with nodular lymphoma who have a normal lymphangiogram. The lymphangiogram is initially positive in approximately 50 per cent of the patients with a diffuse histologic pattern. At laparotomy, most of these patients will also have additional foci of disease in the spleen, mesenteric lymph nodes, or liver. However, patients with diffuse histology and negative lymphangiogram rarely have subdiaphragmatic involvement.

Exploratory laparotomy and splenectomy have been widely employed in the staging evaluation of patients with Hodgkin's disease. Hodgkin's disease usually presents with an orderly pattern of involvement. Data obtained from meticulous surgical staging can serve as an important guide to therapy, particularly in the selection of appropriate radiotherapy fields. In patients with non-Hodgkin's lymphoma, the indications for exploratory laparotomy are far less certain and the routine use of this staging technique cannot be recommended. A sequential approach to staging would appear to be the most reasonable strategy in these patients. In the majority of patients with nodular lymphoma, biopsy of the bone marrow along with percutaneous liver biopsy or peritoneoscopy will yield evidence of disseminated disease. In patients with either nodular or diffuse lymphoma, a positive lymphangiogram is so frequently associated with involvement outside the usual nodal irradiation fields that a decision to employ systemic therapy may be based upon the positive lymphangiogram alone. Exploratory laparotomy would appear to be of value in the selection of therapy only for patients with Stage I or II disease in whom the bone marrow biopsy, lymphangiogram, and closed liver biopsy are negative. The potential clinical benefits of laparotomy must also be weighed against the expected complications of this procedure, which may be increased in elderly patients or in patients with associated medical illnesses. If the treatment program will not be influenced by laparotomy regardless of the findings, then surgical exploration is not justified.

TREATMENT. The most effective modalities for the treatment of non-Hodgkin's lymphoma are irradiation and chemotherapy. Historically, surgery was employed not only to establish the diagnosis but also to remove localized tumor masses. However, surgery alone rarely resulted in long-term control of the disease.

Radiotherapy. The non-Hodgkin's lymphomas are generally considered to be among the most radiosensitive human neoplasms. It is frequently possible to achieve permanent control of individual tumors with doses of irradiation in the range of 3500 to 5000 rads. However, the curative potential of radiotherapy is severely limited by the fact that the vast majority of patients present with widely disseminated disease. Radiotherapy alone is the treatment of choice only for carefully staged patients with localized disease. Approximately 60 per cent of patients with Stage I disease and 30 per cent with Stage II disease will be relapse-free at five years following radiotherapy. The use of total nodal radiotherapy does not appear to have improved these figures.

Extralymphatic structures are involved in about one third of the relapses which occur following radiotherapy. It is also common for relapses to occur in lymph nodes located outside the fields normally used for total nodal radiotherapy. These patterns of relapse have suggested that it may not be possible to improve cure rates through the refinement of conventional radiotherapy methods. An alternative approach utilizing *total body irradiation* has been proposed by several investigators. With this technique, about 15 rads is administered to the entire body twice a week until a total of approximately 150 rads is delivered or until severe hematopoietic depression occurs. This total dose of 150 rads is far below the doses of 3500 to 5000 rads delivered within conventional radiotherapy fields. However, the total body technique has the advantage of reaching sites of occult disease which must be excluded from conventional fields. Total body irradiation has most frequently been employed in patients with advanced lymphocytic lymphoma whose potential for cure with either chemotherapy or conventional radiotherapy is very low. Nevertheless, about 80 per cent of previously untreated patients have achieved a complete remission. This technique is now being compared with chemotherapy or conventional radiotherapy in prospective clinical trials.

Palliative radiotherapy continues to play an important role in the management of bulky masses and in the control of specific symptoms. In patients with advanced disease, lymphomatous masses may encroach on vital structures, resulting in serious morbidity. Obstruction of the ureters, bowel, or upper airway and extradural compression of the spinal cord represent medical emergencies. In these clinical situations, radiotherapy may be very effective in relieving symptoms and preventing irreversible damage. Radiotherapy to the brain combined with intrathecal chemotherapy is useful in controlling meningeal involvement.

Chemotherapy. The non-Hodgkin's lymphomas are highly responsive to a wide variety of chemotherapeutic agents. In the past, most patients with advanced disease were treated with single agents. A high percentage of these patients exhibited an objective response to chemotherapy, but complete responses were uncommon. Patients who achieved only a partial response to treatment with a single drug generally relapsed within six months, in spite of maintenance therapy. Patients with nodular lymphomas exhibited a higher rate of complete response, as well as a longer duration of remission and survival, when compared to patients with diffuse lymphomas.

Combination chemotherapy was introduced into the treatment of patients with non-Hodgkin's lymphomas in the late 1960's. The goal of combination drug treatment was to improve the complete response rate without increasing the degree of bone marrow suppression. Several of the more effective drug combinations developed over the past ten years are shown in

Table 158–2. Each of these combinations incorporates at least three of the most active single agents. The use of combination chemotherapy has increased the rate of complete remission to between 40 and 80 per cent, depending on the histologic subtype. In general, patients who achieve a complete response experience a longer median survival than nonresponding patients or those who achieve only a partial response. The long-term results of several chemotherapy trials have suggested that some patients with diffuse histiocytic, diffuse mixed, pleomorphic, nodular histiocytic, or nodular mixed cell lymphomas may be cured with drug combinations. In one series, for example, 10 of 11 complete responders with diffuse histiocytic lymphoma were alive and free of disease from 26 to 105 months following the completion of treatment. The impact of combination chemotherapy on the survival of patients with lymphocytic lymphomas is not as clear. Although 80 per cent of these patients may achieve complete remission with drug combination, relapses continue to occur as late as five years after completion of treatment. Several more years of observation will be required to determine whether a small fraction of patients with lymphocytic lymphoma might have been cured as a result of combination chemotherapy.

Combined Radiotherapy and Chemotherapy. The most common sites of relapse following chemotherapy are the documented sites of initial involvement. Conversely, the most likely sites of relapse following radiotherapy are unirradiated nodal and extranodal sites remote from the area of initial involvement. Therefore it would appear reasonable to manage patients with Stage I, II, or III disease by treating the sites of documented involvement with irradiation and the sites of clinically occult disease with chemotherapy. Several controlled clinical trials designed to test this hypothesis are now in progress. At present, none of these has provided evidence that the combination of radiotherapy and chemotherapy is superior to either modality alone. However, judgment regarding the ultimate value of combined therapy should be reserved until more information becomes available.

Recommended Therapy. The proper management of any patient with non-Hodgkin's lymphoma generally requires close collaboration between the attending physician, a medical oncologist, an experienced pathologist, a radiation therapist, and, frequently, a skilled surgeon. The final therapeutic decision must take into account the histologic type of lymphoma, the pattern of lymph node involvement, the stage of disease, and the general medical condition of the patient.

Although the therapy of patients with non-Hodgkin's lymphoma is presently undergoing rapid evolution, certain basic recommendations appear to be valid. Patients with Stage I or II diffuse, well differentiated lymphocytic lymphoma may be treated with involved-field radiotherapy alone, although most will ultimately relapse after a long disease-free interval. Since their clinical course is usually quite indolent, patients with this histologic subtype who present with Stage III or IV disease should probably be treated with chlorambucil alone or with a well-tolerated drug combination such as cyclophosphamide, vincristine, and prednisone.

Patients with Stage I or IE disease of the other histologic varieties should be treated with radiotherapy alone. When the primary site of involvement is in the peripheral lymph nodes or in extranodal sites outside the abdomen, radiotherapy is generally given to the involved fields and to adjacent normal lymph nodes. For patients with localized disease in the abdomen, consideration should be given to techniques which can deliver irradiation to the whole abdomen. The use of total nodal radiotherapy has not been shown to enhance the cure rates in patients with Stage I or IE disease.

Patients with Stage II poorly differentiated lymphocytic or nodular mixed cell lymphoma are uncommon. Since these tumors tend to be very radiosensitive, irradiation frequently results in the control of local disease for many years. Patients with Stage II histiocytic, pleomorphic, or diffuse mixed cell lymphoma pose a more difficult management problem. Despite careful staging, no more than a third of these patients will achieve durable remissions with radiation therapy alone. Recent studies involving a limited number of patients have suggested that intensive chemotherapy may be superior to radiation therapy alone. However, it is by no means clear at this time that radiation therapy should be abandoned entirely in the initial management of these patients with prognostically unfavorable histologic subtypes.

Patients with Stage III or IV diffuse histiocytic, nodular histiocytic, pleomorphic, diffuse mixed, or nodular mixed lymphoma should be treated aggressively with a drug combination of the type listed in Table 158–2. These patients are potentially curable if they achieve a complete remission with their initial chemotherapeutic program.

There is considerable variation of opinion regarding the

TABLE 158–2. REPRESENTATIVE DRUG COMBINATIONS

Reference	Drug Regimen			Response (%)	Complete Response (%)
Bagley (1972)	Cyclophosphamide Vincristine Prednisone	400 mg/M² PO days 1–5 1.4 mg/M² IV day 1 100 mg/M² PO days 1–5	Repeat q 3 wks	91	57
McKelvey (1976)	Adriamycin Vincristine Prednisone	80 mg/M² IV day 1 1.4 mg/M² IV day 1 100 mg PO days 1–5	Repeat q 3 wks	88	61
Stein (1974)	Cyclophosphamide Vincristine Procarbazine Prednisone	600 mg/M² IV days 1 and 8 1.4 mg/M² IV days 1 and 8 100 mg/M² PO days 1–10 40 mg/M² PO days 1–14	Repeat q 4 wks	82	68
McKelvey (1976)	Cyclophosphamide Adriamycin Vincristine Prednisone	750 mg/M² IV day 1 50 mg/M² IV day 1 1.4 mg/M² IV day 1 100 mg PO days 1–5	Repeat q 3 wks	92	71
Sweet (1980)	Cyclophosphamide Vincristine Methotrexate Cytosine arabinoside	1500 mg/M² IV day 1 1.4 mg/M² IV days 1,8,15 120 mg/M² PO + Leucovorin weekly × 8 (days 22–71) 300 mg/M² IV weekly × 8 (days 22–71)	Repeat q 12 wks	74	55
Rodriguez (1977)	Cyclophosphamide* Adriamycin* Vincristine Prednisone Bleomycin†	750 mg/M² IV day 1 50 mg/M² IV day 1 1.2 mg/M² IV days 1 and 5 100 mg PO days 1–5 15 units IV days 1 and 5	Repeat q 3 wks	92	66

*Starting dose to be reduced by 20 per cent for patients with prior extensive radiotherapy or hypocellular bone marrow (<20 per cent).
†Dose to be reduced to 4 units per square meter on days 1 and 5 for patients older than 60 years.

optimal therapy for patients with Stage III or IV nodular lymphocytic lymphoma. Certain highly selected patients whose disease was asymptomatic at the time of initial presentation have been followed without any treatment for periods up to several years. Although complete response rates are reported to be higher with combination chemotherapy, the use of sequential single agent therapy appears to yield equivalent median survival figures. Long-term remissions have also been reported with total body irradiation, although, again, median survival does not seem to have been improved with this technique.

Patients with Stage III or IV diffuse, poorly differentiated lymphocytic lymphoma should probably be treated aggressively with combination chemotherapy. The average clinical course of these is not as indolent as that of patients with nodular lymphocytic disease. On the other hand, it has not yet been demonstrated that a significant percentage will be cured as a result of combination chemotherapy.

SELECTED CLINICAL PROBLEMS. The rapid turnover of tumor cells in patients with non-Hodgkin's lymphoma may result in the production of increased quantities of uric acid. Treatment with either chemotherapy or irradiation may further increase the size of the uric acid pool owing to metabolism of nucleic acids released during rapid tumor cell destruction. *Acute uric acid nephropathy* was once a relatively common complication of initial therapy. For this reason, it is currently recommended that allopurinol, a metabolic inhibitor of xanthine oxidase, be administered routinely at the start of therapy, along with enough fluids to ensure an adequate urine output. Patients with non-Hodgkin's lymphoma are also at *increased risk of infection* because of immune disturbances resulting from therapy or induced by the disease itself. Infectious complications must be adequately diagnosed prior to the initiation of antimicrobial therapy, since they are frequently caused by unusual organisms. These include herpes zoster, cytomegalovirus, *Cryptococcus, Candida, Listeria, Nocardia, Pneumocystis,* and *Toxoplasma.* Most of the modern chemotherapy and radiotherapy regimens are safe enough for administration to outpatients and are not designed to produce severe bone marrow depression. However, platelet and white cell transfusions should be available for the occasional patient who develops severe pancytopenia during the course of treatment.

PROGNOSIS. The outlook for many patients with non-Hodgkin's lymphoma has improved in recent years. This improvement has not resulted from the introduction of new treatment methods. It has occurred gradually as our understanding of lymphoid neoplasia has increased, and as the available treatment methods have been refined and applied with greater precision. It is now possible to identify a group of patients with localized disease who can be cured with radiotherapy alone. It is also possible to define a group of patients with advanced disease who can be cured with chemotherapy alone. The challenge for the future is to integrate the best available radiotherapy techniques and chemotherapy regimens to improve the management of patients who presently cannot be cured with either modality. This will require effective collaboration between medical oncologists and radiotherapists in the implementation of well-designed, prospective clinical trials.

Blayney DW, Jaffe ES, Blattner WA, Cossman J, Robert-Guroff M, Longo DL, Bunn PA Jr, Gallo RC: The human T-cell leukemia/lymphoma virus associated with American adult T-cell leukemia/lymphoma. Blood 62:401, 1983. *A detailed description of the clinical features observed in 13 cases of HTLV-associated lymphoid malignancy from medical centers in the United States.*

Golomb HM (ed.): Non-Hodgkin lymphoma. Semin Oncol 7:221, 1980. *A collection of 11 review articles dealing with the pathogenesis, histopathologic classification, staging, and treatment of the non-Hodgkin's lymphomas.*

Mann RB, Jaffe ES, Berard CW: Malignant lymphomas: A conceptual understanding of morphologic diversity. Am J Pathol 94:105, 1979. *In this excellent review, the morphologic diversity of the malignant lymphomas is examined in the light of recent information concerning the normal anatomic and functional components of the immune system.*

Miller TP, Jones SE: Initial chemotherapy for clinically localized lymphomas of unfavorable histology. Blood 62:413, 1983. *Describes a series of 45 patients with Stage I or Stage II non-Hodgkin's lymphoma of unfavorable histologic type (41 patients with diffuse histiocytic lymphoma) who received initial treatment with intensive combination chemotherapy. An impressive 98 per cent of the patients in this series achieved a complete response, and 84 per cent remain continuously free of disease with a median follow-up time of 41 months.*

Portlock CS, Rosenberg SA: No initial therapy for Stage III and IV non-Hodgkin's lymphomas of favorable histologic types. Ann Intern Med 90:10, 1979. *A provocative article which describes the Stanford experience with a "hands-off" approach to the management of selected patients with prognostically favorable histologic types of non-Hodgkin's lymphoma.*

Sweet DL, Kinzie J, Gaeke ME, Golomb HM, Ferguson DL, Ultmann JE: Survival of patients with localized diffuse histiocytic lymphoma. Blood 58:1218, 1981. *Describes a series of 28 meticulously staged patients with localized diffuse histocytic lymphoma (Stage I or Stage II) who received initial treatment with radiotherapy. Although 93 per cent of the patients in this series achieved a complete remission, 10 of 14 patients (71 per cent) with Stage II disease relapsed or died whereas only 1 of 14 patients (7 per cent) with Stage I disease relapsed.*

The Non-Hodgkin's Lymphoma Pathologic Classification Project: National Cancer Institute Sponsored Study of Classifications of Non-Hodgkin's Lymphomas. Cancer 49:2112, 1982. *Presents a working formulation separating non-Hodgkin's lymphomas into 10 major types utilizing morphologic criteria only. This formulation is proposed not as a new classification but as a means of translation among various classification systems to facilitate comparisons of case reports and therapeutic clinical trials.*

Weinstein HJ, Cassady JR, Levey R: Long-term results of the APO protocol (vincristine, doxorubicin [Adriamycin], and prednisone) for treatment of mediastinal lymphoblastic lymphoma. J Clin Oncol 1:537, 1983. *The results of this study demonstrate the efficacy of treating patients with mediastinal lymphoblastic lymphoma as a disseminated lymphoid malignancy.*

159. BURKITT'S LYMPHOMA

Carol S. Portlock

Burkitt's lymphoma is a rare monoclonal B cell neoplasm of great biologic importance. It was first described in 1958 by Dr. Denis Burkitt, who reported rapidly growing jaw tumors and abdominal masses in Ugandan children. Over the next 25 years, the elucidation of its unique epidemiologic, pathologic, clinical, and laboratory features has pioneered research into the etiology, pathogenesis, and therapy of lymphoma.

EPIDEMIOLOGY

Burkitt's lymphoma is the most common childhood malignancy in Uganda. The disease is found along a "lymphoma belt" lying approximately 10° north and 10° south of the African equator. Within the belt there are altitude, temperature, and rainfall restrictions; these climactic conditions are similar to those of Papua, New Guinea, where Burkitt's lymphoma is also commonly identified. Holoendemic or hyperendemic malaria follows the geographic distribution of the lymphoma belt, and originally suggested to Burkitt a mosquito-borne vector and/or associated host immune dysfunction.

In addition to its geographic restrictions, endemic Burkitt's lymphoma is associated with time-space clustering. Nonendemic Burkitt's lymphoma, a similar disease occurring rarely and sporadically in other areas of the world (less than one case per million annually in the United States), has also been reported to occur in time-space clusters. Moreover, nonendemic Burkitt's lymphomas may be associated with preceding immune dysfunction (e.g., organ transplantation and acquired immunodeficiency syndrome).

ETIOLOGY AND PATHOGENESIS

The Epstein-Barr virus (EBV) is present in almost 90 per cent of African Burkitt's lymphoma but less than half of nonendemic cases. Whether the virus plays an etiologic role or is merely a passenger in Burkitt's lymphoma remains controversial. Typically, primary EBV infection precedes the development of Burkitt's lymphoma by at least seven or more months. Ugandan children with high EBV capsid antigen titers have a 30-fold greater risk of developing Burkitt's lymphoma as compared with controls. Elevated EBV/VCA titers are also associated with a favorable prognosis in both African and nonendemic tumors.

Specific chromosomal translocations have been identified in Burkitt's lymphoma (with or without the concurrent detection of EBV) and involve chromosomes 2, 8, 14, and 22. The most frequent translocation is t(8;14) (q24;q32) and less commonly t(2;8) (p12;q24) and t(8;22) (q24;q11). The immunoglobulin heavy chain maps to chromosome 14, κ light chain to chromosome 2, and λ light chain to 22. In cell culture, there is a direct correlation between the kind of light chain expressed and the type of chromosomal translocation. Moreover, the cellular oncogene *c-myc* maps to chromosome 8 and is involved in each of the three translocations specific to Burkitt's lymphoma. When *c-myc* is translocated to chromosome 14 within the immunoglobulin heavy-chain gene, the break may occur at different nucleotide sequences, e.g., the variable or switch regions, in different Burkitt's cell lines. It is proposed that this transposition of the oncogene to a transcriptionally active site may thus lead to oncogene activation and ultimately, lymphomagenesis. The delineation of the role of *c-myc* and/or other oncogenes in the etiology of Burkitt's lymphoma and the interrelationship of *c-myc* (if any) with EBV awaits future research.

PATHOLOGY

According to the working formulation of non-Hodgkin's lymphomas developed in a National Cancer Institute international multi-institutional study, Burkitt's lymphoma is classified as a high grade small noncleaved cell malignant lymphoma. It is composed of intermediate size lymphoid cells containing round nuclei of uniform size and shape, with coarse chromatin and one or more distinct nucleoli. A rim of basophilic cytoplasm is usually present. Large numbers of mitotic figures are invariably seen and a "starry sky" pattern is characteristic. The cells are of monoclonal B cell lineage, expressing IgM of a single light chain class on their cell surface.

CLINICAL FEATURES

Although similar histologically, African and nonendemic Burkitt's lymphomas are clinically distinct. The African disease affects children aged 2 to 16, average 7 years, with a 2:1 male predominance. Bulky extranodal tumors of the jaw (70 per cent), abdominal viscera (50 per cent), particularly kidneys, ovaries, and retroperitoneum, and meninges (30 per cent) predominate. Nonendemic Burkitt's affects children primarily, average 11 years, but has been documented in adults as old as 70 years. Male predominance is only evident in patients younger than 15 years. Jaw tumors are rare, abdominal disease involves mesenteric lymph nodes rather than viscera, and bone marrow involvement is frequent.

Burkitt's lymphoma has a growth fraction approaching 100 per cent, and a tumor doubling time in vivo of less than 3 days. Patients present with dramatic enlargement of tumors and these rapidly enlarging masses may obstruct the GI tract or ureters, or compress nerve roots or spinal cord. Metabolic consequences of rapid tumor growth include excess urate and lactic acid production as well as acute renal failure.

DIAGNOSIS AND STAGING

The diagnosis must be established by biopsy, since the clinical features are not specific. Diseases that may present similarly include other non-Hodgkin's lymphomas, acute myelogenous leukemia with chloromas, plasmacytoma, fibrous dysplasia of bone, disseminated fungal infection, and several pediatric solid tumors (rhabdomyosarcoma, neuroblastoma, retinoblastoma, and Wilms' tumor). In addition to pathologic sections, touch imprints, immunotyping, and tumor karyotype may be of value.

Rigorous staging is of less therapeutic and prognostic importance in Burkitt's lymphoma than in other lymphomas because all patients receive chemotherapy and the rapidity of disease progression demands treatment within 48 hours of presentation. Nevertheless, it is important to document disease extent in order to evaluate therapeutic efficacy. Studies should include a careful history and physical examination, blood counts, chemistries (including lactate dehydrogenase), chest x-ray, abdominal CT scan, gallium-67 scan, bone marrow biopsy or aspirate, and CSF cytology.

MANAGEMENT AND PROGNOSIS

The most important prognostic variable in Burkitt's lymphoma is total tumor volume at initiation of chemotherapy. Surgical debulking prior to chemotherapy is clearly of value in those patients with localized disease. On the other hand, radiation therapy does not offer the same benefit. Combination chemotherapy is used in all patients and may be highly effective. High dose cyclophosphamide may be curative as a single agent; however, the complete response rates and remission durability of combination regimens are superior.

Prior to initiation of any systemic therapy it is necessary to stabilize the patient's condition metabolically, with particular attention to renal function. acid-base balance, and electrolytes. Anticipatory therapy of uric acid nephropathy and acute tumor-lysis syndrome (rapid rises in serum potassium, phosphate, uric acid, xanthine, and LDH with reciprocal fall in serum calcium) with initiation of chemotherapy is mandatory.

With current combination chemotherapy programs (which include cyclophosphamide, Adriamycin, vincristine, and methotrexate) virtually all patients achieve complete remission, while approximately half will have relapse. In spite of CNS prophylaxis, meningeal relapse is common. Nevertheless, aggressive second-line approaches, including high dose regimens with bone marrow transplantation, may be curative. Most relapses after discontinuing initial treatment occur during the first three to six months and are unaffected by maintenance therapy. However, in African Burkitt's lymphoma, very late relapses (occurring 12 to 79 months after discontinuation of treatment) have been reported. Whether some of these relapses represent second neoplasms is not known.

Burkitt DP: The discovery of Burkitt's lymphoma. Cancer 51:1777, 1983. *A personal account.*

Ziegler JL: Burkitt's lymphoma. N Engl J Med 305:735, 1981. *A complete review of laboratory and clinical data, as well as recommendations for management.*

160. HODGKIN'S DISEASE

John H. Glick

DEFINITION. Hodgkin's disease is a unique malignant disorder, usually arising in lymph nodes, with a characteristic histopathologic appearance. It is defined by the presence of the virtually pathognomonic Reed-Sternberg giant cell in an appropriate cellular background. The disease was first recognized as a distinct clinicopathologic entity in 1832 by Thomas Hodgkin, who described seven patients with a fatal illness involving "hypertrophy of the lymphatic system." Although the etiology is unknown, definitive evidence has emerged that Hodgkin's disease is indeed a malignant neoplasm and not a granulomatous infection or a chronic immunologic disorder. Advances in the pathology, staging, and treatment of Hodgkin's disease during the past two decades have provided a dramatic improvement in the prognosis and potential for cure of all patients with this disease.

ETIOLOGY AND PATHOGENESIS. The cause of Hodgkin's disease is unknown, and the nature of the Reed-Sternberg cell remains an enigma. There is now clear evidence that the Reed-Sternberg giant cell as well as its mononuclear variants is malignant. The neoplastic character of these cells is established by their sustained proliferation in vitro, aneuploidy, and heterotransplantability when inoculated intracerebrally into nude mice. Spleen cells taken from Hodgkin's patients have been grown in tissue culture, with the demonstration of macrophage characteristics including phagocytic activity and surface receptors for the Fc fragment of immunoglobulins and for the C3b component of complement. Some investigators have suggested that Reed-Sternberg cells more closely resemble interdigitating reticulum cells found in the interfollicular or T cell region of lymph nodes. Reed-Sternberg cells and interdigitating reticulum cells both demonstrate strong expression of human Ia-like antigens, a close physical association with helper/inducer T cells, and a lack of at least two common macrophage antigens. Malignant transformation of the interdigitating reticulum cell to a Reed-Sternberg cell could result in diminished antigen-presenting capacity and could contribute to the known defect in T cell–mediated immunity commonly observed in Hodgkin's disease patients.

The controversy pertaining to the cell of origin is far from resolved. A mouse monoclonal antibody against the Hodgkin cell line L428 has been noted to be specific for both Reed-Sternberg cells and their mononuclear variants, and for a minute and distinct new cell population in normal tonsils and lymph nodes. This observation suggests that a previously unrecognized early myeloid-monocytoid cell may be the progenitor of the Reed-Sternberg cell.

No confirmation of a suggested bacterial, viral, or fungal cause has been obtained. The problem of frequent secondary infections in the immunocompromised patient with advanced Hodgkin's disease continues to thwart investigators searching for an infectious origin. Any theory of the cause of Hodgkin's disease must account for the wide panorama of histopathologic and clinical presentations, the variety of neoplastic giant cells, the signs of an inflammatory reaction and infectious-like symptoms, the characteristic immunologic defects, and the specific epidemiologic patterns.

EPIDEMIOLOGY. Only 7100 new cases of Hodgkin's disease are diagnosed each year in the United States, with approximately 1600 deaths. These patients average 32 years of age and are more commonly male (incidence rate of 36 per million) than female (26 per million). The age-specific distribution curve is an unusual bimodal pattern for both sexes, with the first peak at ages 15 to 35 and the second after age 50. Hodgkin's disease is distributed throughout the world, but the age-specific rates differ markedly in different countries. The developed areas of the United States and Northern Europe have a prominent young adult peak, which is lower in less developed countries and absent in Japan.

There is an inverse risk with family size, with a rate 2.5 times greater among persons without siblings than those with four or more siblings. There is up to a seven-fold increased risk among siblings of young adults with Hodgkin's disease. Increased risk also occurs with early birth order position and improved living conditions. All these factors tend to decrease and delay exposure to infectious agents. It has been suggested that Hodgkin's disease may be an age-dependent host response to a common infection. Population-based studies have failed to document significant "clustering" of cases. No increased risk in medical personnel exposed to large numbers of Hodgkin's patients has been observed. Thus, at the present time, there is no firm evidence for a contagious etiology.

PATHOLOGY. Histologic diagnosis of Hodgkin's disease requires the presence of characteristic Reed-Sternberg giant cells in association with an appropriate stromal background or cellular milieu. The classic Reed-Sternberg cell (Fig. 160–1*A*) is a large, bilobed cell with prominent eosinophilic nucleoli, perinucleolar clearing, thick nuclear membrane, and relatively abundant cytoplasm. Distinctive multinuclear giant cells in lacunar-like spaces (Fig. 160–1*B*) are associated with the nodular sclerosis subtype and are considered Reed-Sternberg variants. Mononuclear variants are also found on biopsy but cannot be considered as reliably diagnostic. Although the diagnosis of Hodgkin's disease is rarely made in the absence of Reed-Sternberg cells, the presence of such a cell is not pathognomonic of the disease. Cells indistinguishable from or closely resembling Reed-Sternberg cells may be found in reactive conditions such as infectious mononucleosis in which immunoblasts, or transformed lymphocytes, may mimic Reed-Sternberg cells. The character of the stromal background is as important for the diagnosis of Hodgkin's disease as is the Reed-Sternberg cell. This background consists of a mixed population of cytologically benign cells, including reactive lymphocytes, benign histiocytes, plasma cells, and eosinophils.

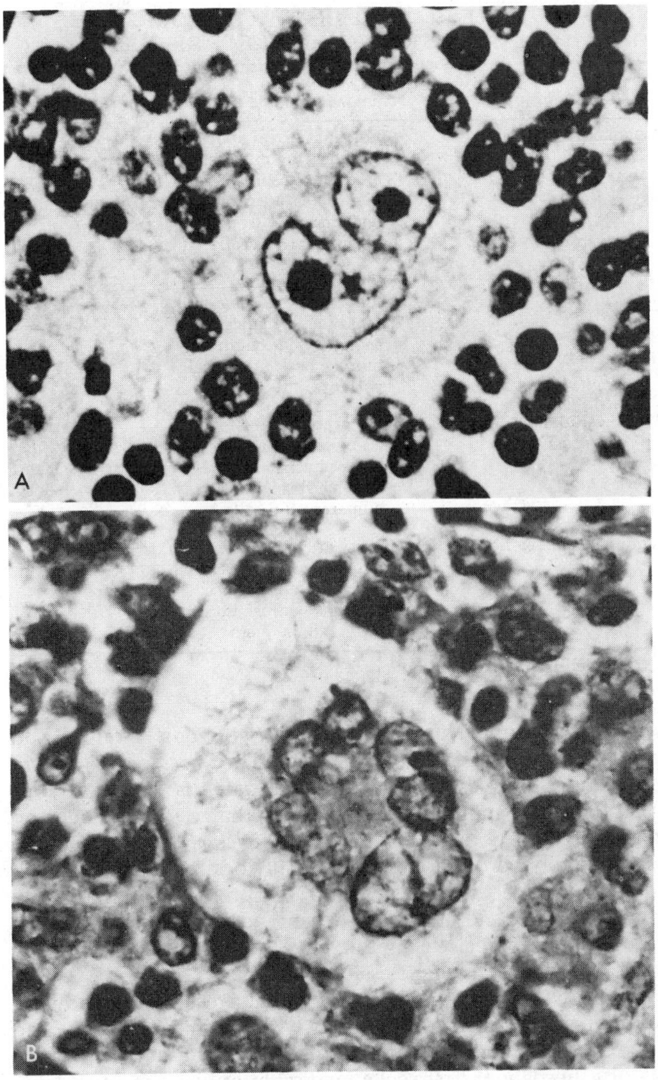

Figure 160–1. Pathologic diagnosis. *A*, Diagnostic Reed-Sternberg cell with large inclusion-like nucleoli, high power. *B*, Reed-Sternberg cell variant, lacunar cell type, high power. (Reprinted by permission from Tindle BH: Pathology of Lymphomas. *In* Bennett JM (ed.): Lymphomas I. The Hague, Martinus Nijhoff, 1981, p 70.)

Problems in identifying Reed-Sternberg cells and in appreciating the appropriate cellular background frequently relate to poor histologic fixation or to inadequate sectioning and staining procedures. Frozen section material should not be used to make a definitive diagnosis when Hodgkin's disease is suspected because of the presence of artifacts. Formalin-fixed tissue is required for careful histologic review. If any uncertainty of diagnosis exists, consultation with an experienced hematopathologist is required. Needle aspiration of lymph nodes for diagnostic purposes is generally not reliable because insufficient tissue is obtained for accurate evaluation.

Hodgkin's disease is subclassified histopathologically into four subtypes according to the Rye classification (Table 160–1). The relative frequency of the four groups is variable in different series, depending on epidemiologic and patient referral factors. The natural history of Hodgkin's disease correlates well with the histopathologic group. The *lymphocyte predominance type* is the most favorable and is associated with early stage disease in asymptomatic patients with nodal presentations. The *nodular sclerosis variety* has a relatively favorable prognosis, usually

TABLE 160–1. RYE HISTOPATHOLOGIC CLASSIFICATION OF HODGKIN'S DISEASE*

Subgroup	Major Histologic Features	Relative Frequency
Lymphocyte predominance	Abundant normal-appearing lymphocyte infiltrate with or without benign histiocytes; occasionally nodular; rare Reed-Sternberg (R-S) cells	5–15%
Nodular sclerosis	Nodules of lymphoid infiltrate of varying size, separated by bands of collagen and containing numerous "lacunar" cell variants of R-S cells	40–75%
Mixed cellularity	Pleomorphic infiltrate of eosinophils, plasma cells, histiocytes, and lymphocytes with numerous R-S cells	20–40%
Lymphocyte depletion	Paucity of lymphocytes with numerous R-S cells, often bizarre in appearance; may have diffuse fibrosis or reticulum fibers	5–15%

*Modified from Lukes and Butler.

occurs in young women with multiple node groups, and frequently involves the mediastinum. The *mixed cellularity pattern* tends to occur in middle-aged patients with systemic symptoms and more extensive disease than is first evident on initial presentation. The *lymphocyte depletion subtype* has the least favorable prognosis, as it generally occurs in patients with advanced stage disease, systemic symptoms, and frequently involves the bone marrow. Recent advances in aggressive therapy, after precise staging, have obscured the prognostic value of histopathologic classification.

CLINICAL MANIFESTATIONS. The initial presentation and subsequent clinical course of patients with Hodgkin's disease can be extremely variable, depending on when in the natural history the patient first seeks medical attention.

Adenopathy. The majority of patients present with a painless and enlarging mass, most commonly in the neck, but occasionally in the axilla or inguinal-femoral region. This lymphadenopathy is usually discovered accidentally by the patient and is often the only manifestation of the disease at the time of diagnosis. Upon examination, this mass is found to be a discrete rubbery usually nontender lymph node or group of surrounding enlarged and matted lymph nodes. Asymptomatic lymphadenopathy also may be noted by the physician on a routine physical examination. In other instances, a chest x-ray, taken for either a routine purpose or because of a persistent dry nonproductive cough, may demonstrate a mediastinal mass. Physical examination may then disclose lymphadenopathy of which the patient had been unaware. Although these typical presentations may occur at any age with any histopathologic type, they are more common in young patients, usually between 15 and 35 years of age with the nodular sclerosis histologic pattern.

The duration of lymphadenopathy prior to diagnosis is extremely variable. Typically, several weeks to several months elapse between the time of the patient's first observation of an asymptomatic mass and the diagnostic biopsy. However, some patients report that a particular mass has been present for many months to several years, with intermittent waxing and waning in size.

Fever and Systemic Symptoms. Although the asymptomatic presentation is most common, one quarter to one third of patients will present with unexplained and persistent fever and/or night sweats as initial symptoms. Fatigue and weight loss may be associated complaints. Patients with these symptoms tend to be in the older age group, are more often men than women, and are generally discovered to have more widespread disease than the usual patient presenting without symptoms. Although superficial lymphadenopathy is present in most such patients, occasionally palpable lymphadenopathy is absent in the patient past the age of 40 with severe systemic symptoms. These patients present with fever of undetermined origin. Extensive diagnostic efforts may be required to discover the presence of Hodgkin's disease, including lymphangiography, abdominal CT scanning, bone marrow biopsies, or even exploratory laparotomy.

The presence of fever, drenching night sweats requiring the changing of bed clothing, or weight loss exceeding 10 per cent of baseline body weight during the six months preceding diagnosis constitute systemic or B symptoms for staging purposes, and confer an adverse prognosis.

Although fever secondary to Hodgkin's disease is usually low grade, occasional patients have intermittent evening fever lasting several days, alternating with afebrile periods lasting days or weeks. This cyclic fever has been labeled the *Pel-Ebstein type* but is rarely the presenting manifestation of the disease.

Pruritus. Pruritus is another characteristic systemic symptom of Hodgkin's disease. It may be mild and localized, but usually progresses and becomes generalized. Severe pruritus may result in extensive excoriations and inability to sleep. It is rarely relieved by topical medications or antihistamines. The prognostic significance of pruritus itself is unclear. It rarely occurs in the absence of fever and/or night sweats but is no longer considered as a B symptom because its presence does not correlate with an adverse prognosis. Generalized severe pruritus may occur in patients with non-Hodgkin's lymphomas and in other medical and dermatologic conditions, but its presence should always suggest Hodgkin's disease. Its cause is unknown.

Rarely, patients complain of pain in the sites of Hodgkin's disease within a few minutes after drinking alcoholic beverages. The pain ranges from sharp and severe to a mild, dull ache and is of no prognostic significance. If this syndrome occurs, it is very suggestive of Hodgkin's disease and may point to an area for potential biopsy. However, it is not a diagnostic symptom of Hodgkin's disease and its mechanism is unknown.

SELECTED CLINICAL PROBLEMS. A wide variety of other symptoms may initially call the attention of patients and their physicians to the disease. These same problems occur more commonly as the course of Hodgkin's disease progresses. In addition, almost all patients receive treatment that profoundly affects the natural history of their illness, resulting in either apparent cure or persistent relapsing Hodgkin's disease, or frequently in complications that become difficult to separate from the manifestations of the disease itself.

Pulmonary involvement occurs in only 10 to 20 per cent of patients at presentation. It appears to arise by spread along lymphatics from ipsilateral hilar lymph nodes. Hodgkin's disease frequently involves the lungs with a patchy pulmonary infiltrate without circumscribed borders. Its appearance is variable and must be distinguished from radiation effects, drug reactions, and the wide variety of pulmonary infections that occur in these immunocompromised patients. In a severely ill patient in whom the diagnosis is uncertain, the therapeutic significance of these lesions is so great that a diagnostic thoracotomy may be justified. Bronchoscopy is rarely of value in defining the etiology of a pulmonary infiltrate in this population. Pleural effusions, either transudates, exudates, or chylous, are most frequently caused by central lymphatic and venous obstruction resulting from Hodgkin's disease in the mediastinum or obstruction of the thoracic duct. These effusions are rarely caused by direct pleural involvement, and cytologic examination of the fluid or pleural biopsy infrequently reveals diagnostic Reed-Sternberg cells.

Superior vena caval obstruction or compression of the upper airway by mediastinal Hodgkin's disease may be the initial presentation or a complication in the course of the disease.

This represents a medical emergency that must be treated promptly and that frequently requires immediate radiotherapy. Myocardial involvement is extremely unusual, but pericardial effusions may occur from direct invasion by adjacent mediastinal Hodgkin's disease. Effusions rarely produce cardiac tamponade, and this complication is more often a consequence of radiation-induced pericarditis.

Spinal cord compression, usually caused by epidural spread of tumor from paravertebral lymph nodes through intervertebral foramina in the thoracic or lumbar regions, may be a devastating acute complication. This syndrome may be seen in patients with an otherwise favorable prognosis, although it usually occurs in patients with progressive tumor in whom primary treatment has failed. Back or neck pain, either directly over the vertebral body or occurring in a radicular pattern, should promptly raise the suspicion of cord compression. Symptoms suggestive of more advanced cord compression include numbness, tingling or weakness of an extremity, motor weakness, and bladder or bowel dysfunction. Prompt diagnostic evaluation, including myelography and/or CT scanning, are mandatory, as is prompt therapeutic intervention with immediate radiotherapy to prevent permanent neurologic damage. Surgical decompression is rarely indicated.

Bone involvement may occur from hematogenous spread in advanced disease or by local nodal spread to adjacent bone. Bone involvement often produces pain but rarely fracture, since the bone lesion is generally osteoblastic or mixed osteoblastic and osteolytic. Multiple osseous lesions may occur with a predilection for the axial skeleton.

Hepatic involvement is present in less than 5 per cent of patients at the time of diagnosis and is generally focal in nature. Liver involvement in Hodgkin's disease is almost always associated with splenic involvement. Massive hepatomegaly or jaundice is rarely seen at the time of initial presentation. However, as the liver becomes progressively involved, diffuse infiltration of the portal spaces may be associated with serious hepatic dysfunction and laboratory features of intrahepatic biliary obstruction. Rarely, enlarged lymph nodes in the porta hepatis may produce extrahepatic biliary obstruction. Direct *renal involvement* is rarely a clinically significant problem, but ureteral obstruction and hydronephrosis, secondary to massive retroperitoneal lymphadenopathy, may be seen in far-advanced disease. The nephrotic syndrome, presenting as lipoid nephrosis, is a rare manifestation of Hodgkin's disease and is occasionally accompanied by evidence of glomerular immune complex deposition.

Infectious complications are common in patients with Hodgkin's disease and may or may not be temporarily related to concurrent treatment. Virtually all patients with uncontrolled Hodgkin's disease who succumb to this disorder will have episodes of serious infections at some point in the course of their disease. Localized or disseminated herpes zoster is the most frequently diagnosed serious viral infection, while cryptococcosis, especially of the lungs and meninges, is the most virulent of the fungal complications. *Pneumocystis carinii* pneumonia causes diffuse pulmonary infiltrates and may appear in patients who are in remission between cycles of chemotherapy, as well as in the patient in relapse. Toxoplasmosis is being recognized with increasing frequency, while tuberculosis has become distinctly uncommon in this population. Children who have undergone splenectomy are particularly predisposed to overwhelming pneumococcal infections unless prophylactic antibiotics or pneumococcal vaccine is administered.

Immunologic abnormalities are common in patients with Hodgkin's disease even at the time of initial diagnosis and prior to initiation of any treatment. A significantly higher frequency of cutaneous anergy is observed than in a control population. The presence or absence of anergy, however, has been shown to have no influence on the prognosis within a specific stage, given the effectiveness of modern therapy. Thus, there is no role for the routine anergy panel. With refined immunologic techniques, a defect in delayed hypersensitivity and T lymphocyte transformation can be detected even in early stage I disease. These deficits are aggravated by therapy and persist for many years even after successful curative treatment. A serum factor, probably an immune complex, has been identified that interferes with T cell function. This factor can be removed in vitro, can block the usual T cell reactions of normal cells, and is probably different from prostaglandins, which are also increased in the serum of some patients. Therapy for Hodgkin's disease undoubtedly accentuates the T cell abnormality. However, it is still unknown whether the observed immunologic abnormalities contribute to the pathogenesis of the disease or are merely secondary phenomena.

STAGING. The progress achieved in the treatment of Hodgkin's disease has paralleled the improvement in techniques for identifying the extent or stage of disease in the untreated patient. In view of the current choices of therapy, it is essential that all patients with Hodgkin's disease be completely evaluated before therapeutic decisions are made. The primary goals of staging are to assess the extent of disease, facilitate the selection of an appropriate treatment program, provide an accurate determination of prognosis, and establish a baseline for re-evaluation following completion of therapy.

The staging classification in current use is outlined in Table 160–2. Patients are assigned a *clinical stage* (CS) on the basis of their initial symptoms, physical examination, laboratory results, and radiologic procedures. However, treatment decisions are generally based on a *pathologic stage* (PS), after the extent of involvement has been documented with appropriate biopsies. The basic staging classification is modified by the poor prognostic significance of systemic symptoms (B disease) and by the realization that localized contiguous extranodal extension (E disease) generally does not carry the same poor prognosis as hematogeneous extranodal involvement (stage IV disease).

Within each stage of Hodgkin's disease there is a spectrum of patients who have a more or less favorable prognosis, depending on the site or sites of disease, size of the tumor masses, and degree of symptoms. The importance of these prognostic factors and substages within the Ann Arbor classification has become increasingly recognized, because treatment methods are now tailored to individual clinical situations. Controversy exists about the prognostic and therapeutic significance of the E lesion, the size of a mediastinal mass, and the substaging of IIIA patients. PS IIIA disease, for example, may

TABLE 160–2. MODIFIED ANN ARBOR STAGING CLASSIFICATION

Stage	
I	Involvement of a single lymph node region (I) or of a single extralymphatic organ or site (I_E)
II	Involvement of two or more lymph node regions on the same side of the diaphragm (II) or localized involvement of an extralymphatic organ or site and of one or more lymph node regions on the same side of the diaphgram (II_E)
III	Involvement of lymph node regions on both sides of the diaphragm (III), which may also be accompanied by involvement of the spleen (III_S) or by localized involvement of an extralymphatic organ or site (III_E) or both (III_{SE})
III_1	Involvement limited to the lymphatic structures in the upper abdomen; that is, spleen, or splenic, celiac, or hepatic portal nodes, or any combination of these
III_2	Involvement of lower abdominal nodes; that is, para-aortic, iliac, inguinal or mesenteric nodes, with or without involvement of the splenic, celiac, or hepatic portal nodes
IV	Diffuse or disseminated involvement of one or more extralymphatic organs or tissues, with or without associated lymph node involvement

Note: E = extralymphatic site; S = splenic involvement. The presence of fever, night sweats, and/or unexplained loss of 10 per cent or more of body weight in the 6 months preceding admission is denoted by the suffix letter B. The letter A indicates the absence of these symptoms. Each patient is assigned a clinical stage (CS) on the basis of physical examination, laboratory and radiologic results, and a pathologic stage (PS) on the basis of biopsy results.

TABLE 160–3. DIAGNOSTIC EVALUATION

A. Required procedures
1. Histologic confirmation by biopsy
2. Detailed history for unexplained fever, weight loss, night sweats, and pruritus
3. Physical examination to document all areas of lymphadenopathy, including Waldeyer's ring; size of liver and spleen; bony tenderness and neurologic evaluation
4. Laboratory studies
   a. CBC and platelet count, ESR
   b. Serum alkaline phosphatase, LDH
   c. Evaluation of renal function, including uric acid
   d. Liver function tests
5. Radiologic studies
   a. Chest roentgenogram
   b. Bipedal lymphangiogram
   c. CT scan of the whole abdomen including the pelvis

B. Frequently performed procedures under specific clinical conditions
1. CT scan of the chest
2. Bone marrow biopsy (needle or open surgical technique)
3. Bone x-rays and scan for areas of bone pain or tenderness
4. Staging laparotomy and splenectomy, if therapeutic decisions will depend on the identification of subdiaphragmatic disease

be subdivided into a prognostically favorable III_1 group, in which abdominal disease is confined to the upper abdominal nodes and/or the spleen, and a less favorable III_2 group with disease extending to the lower abdomen, including the para-aortic, iliac, or inguinal lymph nodes. A thorough knowledge of staging is vital to guide an efficient but thorough diagnostic evaluation. The tests performed as part of a staging evaluation must be individualized rather than obtained automatically.

DIAGNOSTIC EVALUATION. Recommended staging procedures are outlined in Table 160–3. This evaluation should commence promptly after the initial biopsy establishes the diagnosis.

History and Physical Examination. A careful history and physical examination are essential to discover characteristic systemic symptoms and to describe all the lymph node areas of the body. Enlarged lymph nodes are not necessarily involved by disease; reactive lymphoid hyperplasia occasionally occurs in some patients with Hodgkin's disease. If confirmation of Hodgkin's disease in suspicious lymph nodes will change the therapeutic approach, then additional biopsies should be obtained. Although Waldeyer's ring involvement is uncommon in Hodgkin's disease, the lymphoid tissues in the oral cavity should be evaluated by physical examination. The size of the liver and spleen should be carefully determined, although mild enlargement of either organ may merely be a sign of nonspecific hypertrophy rather than involvement by Hodgkin's disease. A palpable abdominal mass caused by enlarged mesenteric or para-aortic lymph nodes is a rare initial finding. The bones should be examined for areas of tenderness, and a careful baseline neurologic examination performed.

Laboratory Studies. Routine laboratory tests include a complete blood count, erythrocyte sedimentation rate (ESR), urine analysis, renal and liver function tests, and serum alkaline phosphatase. Mild to moderate anemia may be found in patients with widespread disease and is often associated with systemic symptoms. The anemia is usually associated with normal indices, normal or low reticulocyte count, and a negative Coombs' test. Anemia in a patient with Hodgkin's disease is usually caused by the typical chronic anemia of malignancy, and rarely is secondary to hypersplenism, marrow involvement, or a Coombs-positive hemolytic anemia. A moderate to marked neutrophilic leukocytosis and thrombocytosis are characteristic of active, symptomatic Hodgkin's disease. Occasionally, the granulocytosis may be so marked as to suggest chronic granulocytic leukemia, but more careful evaluation usually demonstrates that this represents a "leukemoid" reaction. Eosinophilia of a mild degree is common. In patients with severe and longstanding pruritus, moderate or marked eosinophilia frequently occurs. Absolute lymphopenia ($<$ 1000 per cubic millimeter) may be seen in a small percentage of patients with more advanced disease, and is usually a poor prognostic sign.

The ESR is commonly elevated in patients with active disease; it has limited sensitivity, however, and extensive radiation therapy may cause the ESR to remain elevated for more than one year after treatment without evidence of relapsing tumor. Other nonspecific laboratory abnormalities include increased levels of serum alpha-2-globulin, fibrinogen, haptoglobin, copper, and zinc; depression of serum iron and iron-binding capacity; and elevation of leukocyte alkaline phosphatase. An elevated serum alkaline phosphatase may be a nonspecific finding or secondary to involvement of bone, bone marrow, or liver with Hodgkin's disease. Elevation of the serum uric acid is rare at the time of initial presentation, except in advanced stages of disease with massive nodal or bone marrow involvement.

Radiologic Studies. Radiologic examinations should include routine chest x-rays, which will demonstrate mediastinal involvement in 50 to 60 per cent of patients (Fig. 160–2). In contrast, hilar disease is seen at presentation in less than 20 per cent of cases. In the absence of mediastinal involvement, hilar disease is unusual. Whole lung tomography is of marginal clinical value. Computed tomography (CT scan) of the chest allows better definition of mediastinal, hilar, and paravertebral

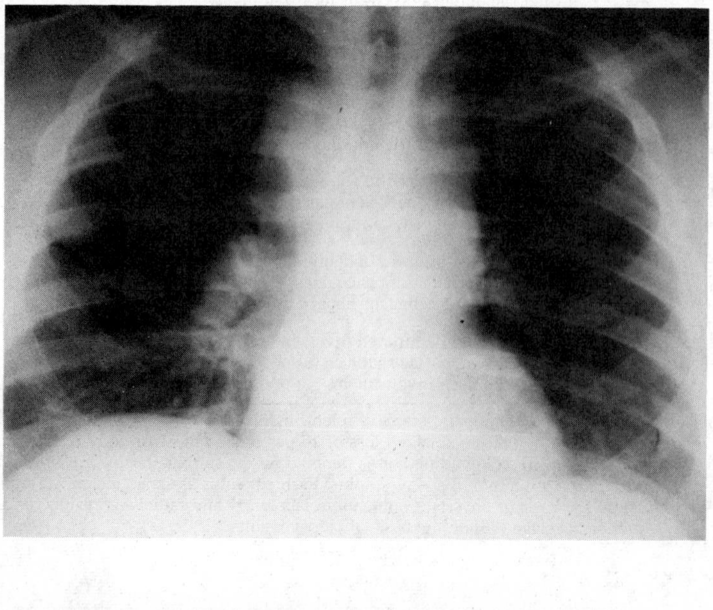

Figure 160–2. Typical mediastinal and right hilar lymphadenopathy in a patient with Hodgkin's disease prior to therapy.

adenopathy, and pulmonary involvement. CT scanning of the chest is indicated when hilar or mediastinal disease is present or suspected. Its role is to define more precisely the extent of disease, including possible localized extension into the pulmonary parenchyma, as well as to assist in radiation treatment planning. The presence of a small pleural effusion in the patient with a mediastinal mass does not necessarily indicate malignant involvement of the pleura. Thoracentesis or pleural biopsy are rarely diagnostic of Hodgkin's disease in these situations.

Subdiaphragmatic sites are best evaluated by performing both bipedal lymphangiography and abdominal-pelvic CT scanning. These examinations are complementary, and neither procedure should replace the other. The lymphangiogram is the most reliable means of assessing involvement of retroperitoneal or pelvic lymph nodes, in that abnormalities of intranodal architecture can be demonstrated in up to 25 per cent of cases at presentation (Fig. 160–3). The overall accuracy of this procedure is 80 to 90 per cent. Lymphangiography is also valuable in preparation for exploratory laparotomy, in that it directs the surgeon to potentially abnormal areas for lymph node biopsy. Lymphangiography is also helpful for planning radiotherapy fields, and especially for assessing the degree of response to therapy during serial follow-up evaluation of the involved retroperitoneal lymph nodes.

Abdominal CT scanning can complement the lymphangiogram by demonstrating lymphadenopathy in the mesentery, porta hepatis, celiac nodes, and para-aortic nodes above the level of those opacified by the lymphangiogram. CT scanning can only assess nodal involvement when there is an increase in lymph node size. In contrast, lymphangiography provides information on abnormal architecture even in unenlarged nodes. Thus, reliance on CT scanning alone may lead to understaging.

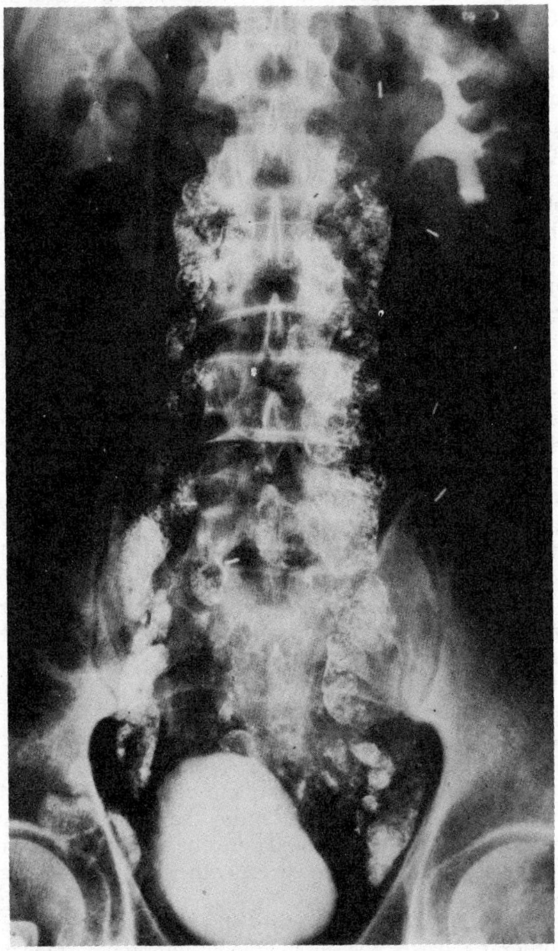

Figure 160–3. Abnormal lymphangiogram with enlargement and distortion of the internal architecture in the pelvic, iliac, and para-aortic lymph nodes. Despite the extensive lymphadenopathy, little displacement of the ureters and no obstruction of the upper urinary tracts were seen. (Reprinted by permission from Kaplan HS: Hodgkin's Disease. 2nd ed. Cambridge, Harvard University Press, 1980, p 194.)

Routine bone scans or skeletal x-rays are not indicated in the asymptomatic patient with a normal alkaline phosphatase. However, in those patients with areas of bone pain or tenderness, bone scans complemented by selective x-rays are indicated to detect osseous lesions. Unless the patient has significant hepatomegaly or marked elevations of the liver function tests, liver-spleen scan is not indicated. A single percutaneous needle biopsy of the liver is rarely diagnostic, because of the focal nature of hepatic involvement.

Bone Marrow Biopsy. This procedure should be performed in all patients with either systemic symptoms and/or clinical stage III disease. It is also useful in patients with significant peripheral blood count abnormalities, elevated serum alkaline phosphatase of bony origin, and in those patients with positive bone x-rays or scans. Hodgkin's disease in the bone marrow is rarely demonstrable by simple marrow aspiration. Involvement is usually focal, often associated with fibrosis, and is diagnosed more readily by either a unilateral or bilateral bone marrow biopsy.

Staging Laparotomy. In the absence of medical contraindications, an exploratory laparotomy with splenectomy is widely employed as part of the routine staging evaluation to identify and confirm the presence of Hodgkin's disease below the diaphragm. The purpose of the laparotomy is diagnostic, the results of which may alter treatment selection significantly. Laparotomy findings that frequently influence both the staging and subsequent treatment include detection of Hodgkin's disease in the spleen, detection of the extent of splenic involvement, and detection of presence of disease in the celiac or retroperitoneal lymph nodes. Secondary benefits from the laparotomy include attempting to preserve ovarian function by means of an oophoropexy when pelvic irradiation is to be utilized in young women, reducing required irradiation fields when the spleen is treated, and improving the peripheral blood counts in the occasional patient with hypersplenism. In one third of patients with normal-sized spleens on physical examination, Hodgkin's disease will be found in the spleen removed at surgery. Conversely, approximately 25 per cent of patients with clinical enlargement of the spleen do not have histologic involvement. The identification of Hodgkin's disease in the liver is especially difficult. Physical examination, routine liver function tests, and liver scans correlate poorly, if at all, with histologic verification. Liver involvement can be demonstrated at laparotomy on wedge or needle biopsy, and is more often found in patients with significant splenomegaly and/or positive lymphangiograms.

Staging laparotomy is not a routine diagnostic procedure and should be performed only in those patients in whom the results will potentially modify treatment selection. Discussion of potential treatment options with the radiotherapist or medical oncologist for each stage of Hodgkin's disease should be held prior to the decision to perform a laparotomy. Thus, staging laparotomy with splenectomy is generally recommended for patients with clinical stage I to IIA/B or IIIA disease. Patients with stage IIIB or IV disease are not candidates for laparotomy because combination chemotherapy will be used as their primary treatment modality.

In some clinical situations the yield from laparotomy is too low to warrant its routine use. Patients with clinical stage IA disease limited to the high neck (above the thyroid cartilage) or patients with lymphadenopathy limited to the mediastinum (no palpable lymph nodes in the neck or axilla and a negative lymphangiogram) may be staged reliably by clinical studies alone without laparotomy. In other cases, staging laparotomy must be deferred or omitted. The patient who presents with massive mediastinal lymphadenopathy should not undergo laparatomy because of the dangers of anesthesia in these patients. In addition, combination chemotherapy is frequently employed in patients with large mediastinal masses, thus eliminating the need for precise staging below the diaphragm.

As a result of staging laparotomy and splenectomy, approximately one third of patients with clinical stages I and II are found to have either subdiaphragmatic lymph node disease or splenic involvement, necessitating extension of the subdiaphragmatic radiation portals. If extensive splenic involvement (> four nodules) is documented, either combination chemotherapy alone or a combined modality program is required. Approximately one quarter of clinical stage IIIA patients (i.e., those with suspicious lymphangiograms or abdominal CT scans) have a negative staging laparotomy that allows their pathologic stage to be downgraded to I or II. Although the results of the laparotomy allow change in the stage in as many as 35 per cent of patients, this change modifies the treatment plan in only approximately 20 per cent, depending on the extent of disease found below the diaphragm. Even in the hands of experienced surgeons, staging laparotomy is associated with a small risk of perioperative morbidity, including infection, fever, and phlebitis. Rare fatalities have been reported. Because of occasional severe bacterial infections occurring after splenectomy, pneumococcal vaccine should be administered preoperatively.

MODE OF SPREAD. Careful mapping of initial sites of involvement of Hodgkin's disease and the use of lymphangiography, staging laparotomy, and splenectomy provide evidence that involvement of various lymph node groups is distinctly nonrandom. Two different theories have been proposed to account for the nonrandom patterns of spread: (1) The *contiguity theory* (Rosenberg and Kaplan) postulates that the disease is unifocal in origin, beginning in an initial focus within the lymphatic system and spreading via lymphatic channels to contiguous lymphatic structures. The contiguity theory has been challenged because of the frequency of cervical, supraclavicular, and retroperitoneal lymph node involvement without intervening mediastinal disease, as well as the common involvement of the spleen, which has no afferent lymphatics. (2) The *susceptibility theory* (Smithers) postulates that the disease is multifocal in origin. The giant cells of Hodgkin's disease are thought to migrate in and out of lymph nodes from the bloodstream but are thought to grow only in preferential sites, presenting an appearance of contiguous spread. Noncontiguous spread is more common in the mixed cellularity and lymphocyte depletion subtypes, when multiple sites are present and when vascular invasion is present. However, the role of vascular invasion in the spread of Hodgkin's disease is not fully understood. Vascular invasion in the spleen may lead to hematogenous dissemination, since the spleen is almost invariably involved when Hodgkin's disease is present in the liver or bone marrow.

TREATMENT. The prognosis for patients with Hodgkin's disease has improved dramatically during the past three decades because of (1) the advances in precise staging and an awareness of the important prognostic factors previously described, (2) the development of supervoltage radiotherapeutic techniques, and (3) the use of effective combination chemotherapy programs.

Radiotherapy. Important factors in determining the success of radiation therapy include the radiation dose per field, the extent of the fields employed, the beam energy, and precision of treatment planning. A tumoricidal dose of 3600 to 4400 rads is required to eradicate the lesions of Hodgkin's disease. Lymphoid regions adjacent to areas of known disease or those that are contiguous via lymphatic channels are usually treated to full dose. Apparently uninvolved areas are treated prophylactically for subclinical disease with dosages of 3600 rads. Large fields, shaped to conform to the patient's anatomy, are designed to treat multiple contiguous lymph node regions. A *mantle* port covers the cervical, supraclavicular, infraclavicular, axillary, mediastinal, and hilar lymph nodes. The *para-aortic* field includes the para-aortic lymph nodes from the level of the diaphragm down to the aortic bifurcation but omits the pelvis and treats the splenic hilar lymph nodes in a patient with a prior splenectomy. An *inverted Y* port includes in one field not only the para-aortic and splenic hilar lymph nodes but also extends into the pelvis to encompass the iliac and inguinal-femoral lymph nodes. The combination of a mantle and para-aortic field is also referred to as subtotal nodal or extended field irradiation. *Total lymphoid irradiation* implies sequential treatment to both a mantle and an inverted Y field.

The use of sequential large field irradiation minimizes the risk of either overlap or underdosage, which could result in either undue normal tissue toxicity or inadequate therapy. Treatment of these large fields requires supervoltage radiation. This capability is available primarily with contemporary linear accelerators, which have the advantages over cobalt of skin sparing, increased depth dose, and sharp beam edges with reduced lateral scatter. The use of a treatment simulator to plan the radiotherapy fields and proper field verification (portal films) during the treatment process is essential.

Definitive radiation therapy alone is appropriate initial management for the majority of patients with pathologic stage I and II Hodgkin's disease. Mantle and para-aortic radiation is the treatment of choice for stages IA and IIA disease, providing a 75 to 90 per cent chance of cure with irradiation alone. Patients with stage IB and IIB disease are treated with mantle and para-aortic or total lymphoid irradiation and have a 70 per cent chance of cure with such treatment. Controversy exists about the indications for using both radiotherapy and chemotherapy with stage I or II patients who present with either large mediastinal masses, limited contiguous extranodal disease (the E lesion of the Ann Arbor system), or systemic symptoms. In each of these disease settings, the use of radiation alone results in lower disease-free survival than when a combined modality program is employed as the initial treatment, although the use of chemotherapy at relapse may provide an equivalent chance of cure. Patients with $III_{S}A$ or $III_{1}A$ Hodgkin's disease and minimal splenic involvement are usually treated with total lymphoid irradiation alone. Controversy exists as to whether prophylactic hepatic radiation should be delivered to those patients with splenic involvement.

Complications of radiation are related to the technique employed, dosage administered, and irradiated volume. Acute side effects of radiotherapy include transient nausea and vomiting, dysphagia, and marrow suppression. These effects subside shortly after radiation therapy is completed. Late potential side effects of radiation include hypothyroidism, pneumonitis, transient myelitis (generally manifested as electric-like shocks in limbs on neck flexion known as *Lhermitte's sign*), and rarely pericarditis. Persistent myelosuppression is a rare late complication. Radiation-induced decreased bone growth has been noted in children.

Chemotherapy. The major advance in the treatment of stage IIIB and IV Hodgkin's disease was the development of curative combination chemotherapy. The initial studies from the National Cancer Institute demonstrated that a four-drug combination known as MOPP (nitrogen mustard, vincristine, procarbazine, and prednisone) was capable of producing documented complete remissions in 70 to 80 per cent of patients with advanced Hodgkin's disease. At least one half to two thirds of the patients who achieved complete remission with MOPP have not had recurrence after more than 10 to 15 years of observation. Thus, more than 50 per cent of all patients treated with stage IIIB and IV were cured with MOPP chemotherapy alone.

The potential for clinical cure of Hodgkin's disease with chemotherapy exists for all histologic subtypes, stages, and extranodal sites of disease. Patients who have received prior radiotherapy and subsequently relapse have an equivalent chance of being cured with "salvage" chemotherapy. Older patients and those with bone marrow involvement, systemic symptoms, and poor performance status have a less favorable long-term response with chemotherapy. The best results have been reported for asymptomatic patients with disease limited to the lymph nodes and/or lung.

It is essential to administer the drugs in the MOPP regimen at full doses and in a timely fashion. Therapy is repeated every four weeks for a minimum of six cycles. An additional two cycles are administered after a complete clinical remission is obtained. At that time chemotherapy is discontinued only when repeat restaging studies document that a true complete remission has been obtained. The restaging diagnostic evaluation includes repeat radiologic procedures and biopsies as indicated to verify the complete response status. Maintenance chemotherapy beyond the documentation of a restaged complete remission is of no advantage in improving either disease-free or overall survival.

No alternative four- or five-drug combinations have been demonstrated conclusively to be superior to MOPP, considering differences in patient selection, prognostic factors, restaging evaluation, and adequate follow-up. However, comparable results to MOPP have been achieved with a variety of alternative chemotherapy programs that offer significantly less toxicity than MOPP. Combinations that contain cyclophosphamide or chlorambucil instead of nitrogen mustard, vinblastine in place of vincristine, and/or the addition of a nitrosourea appear to be as efficacious as MOPP in producing durable complete responses but have substantially fewer side effects. The BCVPP (BCNU, cyclophosphamide, vinblastine, procarbazine, and prednisone) regimen is one example of an equally effective and less toxic alternative to MOPP.

Patients who have relapse after definitive irradiation for early stage disease are often salvaged and cured with chemotherapy. Patients who have relapse after initial chemotherapy have a poorer but not hopeless outlook. Patients who have recurrence after a MOPP-induced complete remission of at least one year may benefit from a second course of the same therapy and achieve a second long-term complete remission, but cure is unlikely. Patients who are definitely MOPP-resistant should be treated with chemotherapy regimens that contain different or noncross-resistant drugs. The ABVD program (Adriamycin, bleomycin, vinblastine, and DTIC) is a widely used second-line regimen that results in complete remission in up to 60 per cent of patients. However, the follow-up is still too limited to place confidence in the curative potential of these second-line chemotherapy programs.

The identification of an active noncross-resistant combination in the relapsed patient led to the investigation of sequential alternating chemotherapy regimens (i.e., MOPP alternating monthly with ABVD) as primary induction therapy. By exposing tumor cells to more drugs early in the course of disease, drug-resistant clones might be eradicated before growing too large to be cured. The objective is to increase the complete remission rates over that which has been demonstrated with MOPP and, more importantly, to improve relapse-free and overall survival. This approach shows considerable promise, especially for patients with stage IV disease, but longer follow-up will be required before this strategy can be adopted as standard practice for advanced Hodgkin's disease.

The major complication of chemotherapy is bone marrow suppression with increased risk of infection and, rarely, hemorrhage. The peripheral blood counts are monitored carefully during chemotherapy and drug doses are adjusted depending on the degree of myelosuppression. However, drug dose reductions made simply for the purpose of decreasing subjective toxicity are inappropriate because the opportunity for cure is also reduced. Sterility, more commonly seen in males, is a permanent side effect of chemotherapy. Significant nausea and vomiting are seen with the MOPP and ABVD regimens. These drug programs often produce serious psychological problems that require effective counseling, as well as antiemetic agents. Mild peripheral neuropathy is commonly seen with vincristine, but paresthesias are not an indication to reduce drug dosage. Acute leukemia as a late effect of chemotherapy alone is a recognized but unusual complication.

Combined Modality Therapy. Combinations of irradiation and chemotherapy in the treatment of Hodgkin's disease have been utilized during the past 15 years with the goal of increasing the cure rate. It is logical to assume that combination chemotherapy, effective in curing a significant percentage of patients with advanced disease, should be even more effective for occult disease that might be present after radiation therapy. Patients who have recurrence after receiving MOPP chemotherapy nearly always have relapse involving sites of major pretreatment involvement, including bulky lymph node areas. Additional rationale for combined modality therapy includes improved management of childhood Hodgkin's disease by reduction of radiation fields that may cause bone growth retardation, decreased requirement for staging laparatomy, and reduced complications from newer radiotherapy techniques involving larger treatment fields.

Adjuvant chemotherapy can substitute effectively for prophylactic irradiation of apparently uninvolved sites, but to date there is no clear justification for the routine use of a combined modality approach for the overwhelming majority of patients with pathologic stage I or II disease. However, there are certain subsets of patients with early stage Hodgkin's disease for whom combined modality treatment may be indicated because of an unacceptably high relapse rate; that is, patients with large mediastinal masses or contiguous extranodal involvement.

The treatment of pathologic stage IIIA Hodgkin's disease remains controversial. Retrospective studies have concentrated on identifying prognostic subgroups in which there is an unacceptably low disease-free survival with radiotherapy alone. At the present time, it would be premature for radiation therapists to abandon total nodal irradiation in III_1A patients in whom the prognosis is favorable and who at laparotomy are found to have minimal involvement of the spleen or upper abdominal nodes. In this subgroup, only those who have relapse after primary radiotherapy should receive combination chemotherapy. For patients with clinical stage IIIA/pathologic III_2A disease, and for those with extensive splenic involvement, no one management strategy has been proved superior. Acceptable treatment alternatives for this subgroup include total nodal irradiation utilizing the Stanford technique (including prophylactic liver radiation when the spleen is involved), combined modality therapy with total nodal or subtotal nodal radiotherapy plus MOPP, initial chemotherapy followed by low-dose irradiation to sites of pretreatment involvement, and chemotherapy alone.

Although combination chemotherapy remains the mainstay for stage IIIB disease, recent results have suggested both improved disease-free and overall survival for these patients in whom initial MOPP chemotherapy followed by total nodal irradiation is utilized. An alternative approach for stage IIIB and even IV disease has been to obtain a complete remission with combination chemotherapy, followed by low-dose radiotherapy (1500 to 2000 rads) to areas of major pretreatment involvement. The preliminary results of this combined modality strategy for advanced disease are encouraging, but the results of confirmatory trials are not available as of this writing.

Significant improvement in survival rates as a result of combined modality programs has not yet been clearly demonstrated. In part, this is because of the long period of time (ten or more years) required to establish an overall survival benefit. Combined modality programs generally demonstrate improved disease-free survival, but interpretation of current clinical trials must be tempered by the observation that patients who relapse after radiation alone are frequently salvaged or cured with chemotherapy administered only at the time of relapse. It may be more acceptable to treat patients conservatively at the onset of their disease with one modality, reserving the more complicated combined modality programs for those patients with poor prognostic factors and an unacceptably high relapse rate after primary irradiation alone.

TABLE 160–4. THE TREATMENT OF HODGKIN'S DISEASE

Ann Arbor Pathologic Stage	Recommended Therapy	Estimated Five-Year Disease-Free Survival (%)	Investigational Therapy
IA, I_EA, IIA, II_EA*	Mantle and para-aortic radiotherapy	85	Limited radiotherapy ± combination chemotherapy
IB, I_EB, IIB, II_EB*	Mantle and para-aortic or total lymphoid radiotherapy	70	Limited or total lymphoid radiotherapy + combination chemotherapy; chemotherapy alone
III_1A, III_SA, III_EA*†	Total lymphoid radiotherapy	65	Combination chemotherapy ± total lymphoid radiotherapy; total lymphoid radiotherapy, including hepatic irradiation
III_2A	Combination chemotherapy (i.e., MOPP) ± total lymphoid radiotherapy	65	Combination chemotherapy + limited radiotherapy to areas of pretreatment involvement
IIIB, III_SB, III_EB	Combination chemotherapy (i.e., MOPP)	60	Combination chemotherapy + either total lymphoid radiotherapy or low-dose radiotherapy to areas of pretreatment involvement
IVA, IVB	Combination chemotherapy (i.e., MOPP)	50	Alternating noncross-resistant chemotherapy (i.e., MOPP-ABVD); combination chemotherapy followed by low-dose radiotherapy to areas of pretreatment involvement

*The disease in patients with large mediastinal masses (>0.3 of the transverse diameter of the chest) will be controlled by irradiation alone in only approximately 40 to 50 per cent of cases. These patients could appropriately receive combined modality therapy (chemotherapy and irradiation) as primary management.

†The disease in patients with extensive involvement of the spleen (>4 nodules) will be controlled by irradiation alone in only approximately 40 per cent of cases. They could appropriately receive combined modality therapy (chemotherapy and irradiation) or chemotherapy alone as primary management.

The complications and morbidity of combined modality programs are significant. The potential risk of acute complications, including profound and prolonged myelosuppression, sterility of both men and women, and demonstrated risk of second malignancies, has modified the enthusiasm for a combined modality approach. The incidence of acute myelomonocytic leukemia is approximately 5 per cent for patients at risk for seven to ten years following combined modality treatment. Paradoxically, this incidence is greatest in patients over the age of 40 years, the group most likely to have an unfavorable prognosis.

Recommended Therapy. The recommended therapy for a patient with Hodgkin's disease must be individualized. Important management considerations include stage of disease, age, prior therapy, medical complications, and availability of modern skills in radiotherapy and chemotherapy. The improved results of aggressive therapy after accurate clinical evaluation and pathologic staging are achievable only by experienced teams of physicians working closely together to achieve the excellent cure rates now possible while avoiding the risks of excesses in treatment. The recommended therapeutic approaches for the previously untreated patient with various stages of Hodgkin's disease are listed in Table 160–4. Estimated results are expressed as the percentage of patients likely to achieve a disease-free interval of five years. Careful evaluation and observation of a high proportion of patients, perhaps 90 or 95 per cent, who have survived free from relapse for five years demonstrate that they are cured of their disease.

An early stage patient who has relapse after radiation therapy alone may be cured with salvage chemotherapy. Thus, freedom from first or even second relapse must be considered in the evaluation of both disease-free and overall survival when the results of current clinical trials are analyzed. With dramatically improved treatment results, the challenge facing physicians and investigators caring for patients with all stages of Hodgkin's disease is to weigh carefully the toxicity-benefit ratio for each new recommended regimen.

PROGNOSIS. Hodgkin's disease is a curable malignancy. Advances in histopathologic classification, precise diagnostic evaluation, and selection of appropriate aggressive therapy have led to continuous improvement in both disease-free and overall survival. Survival figures and prognostic factors that were acceptable 10 or even 20 years ago are not acceptable today. The five-year survival rate has increased from approximately 25 to 50 per cent 20 years ago to at least 75 per cent today.

The success of modern radiotherapy, chemotherapy, or combined modality programs has obscured the significance of such important prognostic factors as histologic subtype, stage of disease, and the presence of systemic symptoms. In recent years, newer prognostic factors have been identified, including anatomic substage III_2A, five or more sites of lymph node involvement, extensive splenic disease, bulky mediastinal lymphadenopathy, and contiguous extranodal extension. The significance of these more recently described prognostic factors remains controversial. Although an unacceptably high relapse rate is noted in many of these situations after primary radiotherapy, the efficacy of salvage chemotherapy must be recognized. Combined modality treatment programs frequently have been recommended for patients with these unfavorable prognostic factors. Any potential disease-free survival advantage seen after combined modality therapy must be balanced by the potential risk of late complications, particularly second malignancies, and must be translated into an overall survival benefit before general acceptance.

Table 160–4 presents a reasonable estimate of prognosis, recommended therapy, and current appropriate investigative approaches for the various stages of Hodgkin's disease. These treatment recommendations provide only the broadest of guidelines. Therapy must be individualized, depending on the specific clinical situation and the skill and experience of physicians treating the patient. Any treatment recommendations and estimates of cure must be viewed with the understanding that the management of Hodgkin's disease is dynamic, constantly undergoing change and refinement, and is designed to provide each patient with the best probability of cure and the least possibility of long-term toxicity.

Canellos GP, Come SE, Skarin AT: Chemotherapy in the treatment of Hodgkin's disease. Semin Hemat 20:1, 1983. *A complete review of the current status of chemotherapy for both early and advanced stages of disease.*

DeVita VT Jr, Simon RH, Hubbard SM, Young RC, Berard CB, Moxley JH III, Frei E III, Carbone PP, Canellos GP: Curability of advanced Hodgkin's disease with chemotherapy: Long-term follow-up of MOPP-treated patients at the National Cancer Institute. Ann Intern Med 92:587, 1980. *A classic review of the development and experience with the MOPP program as seen by the National Cancer Institute group.*

Farber LR, Prosnitz LR, Cadman EC, et al.: Curative potential of combined modality therapy for advanced Hodgkin's disease. Cancer 46:1509, 1980. *A report of the use of adjuvant radiotherapy for patients with stage III and IV disease who have been treated with chemotherapy; an uncontrolled but provocative study.*

Glick JH: Chemotherapy of Hodgkin's and non-Hodgkin's lymphoma. *In* Bennett JM (ed.): Lymphoma I. The Hague, Martinus Nijhoff, 1981, pp 343–446. *A comprehensive, well-referenced review of the role of chemotherapy for all stages of disease.*

Hoppe RT: Stage I-II Hodgkin's disease: Current therapeutic options and recommendations. Blood 62:32, 1983. *A concise and thoughtful review emphasizing the Stanford radiotherapy experience.*

Kaplan HS: Hodgkin's Disease. 2nd ed. Cambridge, Harvard University Press, 1980. *A detailed, extensively illustrated and referenced volume covering every aspect of the disease as seen by one of the acknowledged experts in the field.*

Proceedings of the Symposium on Contemporary Issues in Hodgkin's Disease: Biology, staging, and treatment. Cancer Treat Rep 66:601, 1982. *The most up-to-date collection of important papers covering all aspects of Hodgkin's disease. The papers on biology, staging, treatment, and complications are especially worthwhile.*

Rosenberg SA, Kaplan HS, Hoppe RT, Kushlan P, Horning S: The Stanford randomized trials of the treatment of Hodgkin's disease: 1967–1980. *In* Rosenberg SA, Kaplan HS (eds.): Malignant Lymphomas: Etiology, Immunology, Pathology, Treatment. New York, Academic Press, 1982, pp 513–522. *An update on a large controlled trial of the use of MOPP as an adjuvant to radiotherapy for stages I, II, and III. This is the major study with the longest follow-up on this subject.*

Santoro A, Bonadonna G, Bonfante V, Valagussa P: Alternating drug combinations in the treatment of advanced Hodgkin's disease. N Engl J Med 306:770, 1982. *A preliminary report of MOPP-ABVD alternating chemotherapy for stage IV. The patient numbers are small and the follow-up too short to allow a firm conclusion as to the superiority of MOPP-ABVD.*

Santoro A, Bonfante V, Bonadonna G: Salvage chemotherapy with ABVD in MOPP-resistant Hodgkin's disease. Ann Intern Med 96:139, 1982. *A description of the ABVD regimen used as second line chemotherapy. Most other groups have not been able to do as well with this combination.*

Schwab U, Stein H, Gerdes J, Lemke H, Kirchner H, Schaadt, Diehl V: Production of a monoclonal antibody specific for Hodgkin and Sternberg-Reed cells of Hodgkin's disease and a subset of normal lymphoid cells. Nature 299:65, 1982. *The authors describe the production of mouse monoclonal antibodies against a Hodgkin cell line. One antibody was found to be specific for Reed-Sternberg cells and for a new, so far unidentified cell population in normal lymphoid tissue.*

Twomey JJ, Rice L: Impact of Hodgkin's disease upon the immune system. Semin Oncol 7:26, 1980. *A comprehensive review of the immunologic abnormalities associated with Hodgkin's disease, including 175 references.*

161. LANGERHANS CELL (EOSINOPHILIC) GRANULOMATOSIS

Jerome E. Groopman

The numerous and sometimes confusing classifications of clinical disorders associated with Langerhans cell proliferation reflect our ignorance of both the cause and pathophysiology of many of these diseases. The Langerhans cell belongs to the larger family of cells termed *histiocytes.* Histiocytes are tissue macrophages and include the hepatic Kupffer cell, the alveolar macrophage of the lung, the giant cell of granulomas and the osteoclast in addition to the dermal Langerhans cell. The microglial cell of the brain is probably of macrophage origin as well. All of these tissue macrophages derive from precursor cells that normally reside in bone marrow, mature into circulating blood monocytes, and then egress into tissues and differentiate into a particular type of histiocyte.

A number of benign disorders are associated with proliferation of histiocytes and their fusion into multinucleated giant cells that form granulomas (Table 67–3). Langerhans cell (eosinophilic) granulomatosis is an idiopathic benign disease characterized by proliferation and infiltration of tissue by histiocytes and eosinophils. Although this disorder was previously termed "eosinophilic granuloma," the proliferating cell that appears primarily responsible for the clinical manifestations of the disorder is the Langerhans cell. The eosinophils may take residence in the lesion because of potent eosinophilic chemotactic factors released secondarily by the histiocytes. Langerhans cell granulomatosis is a distinct disorder unrelated to the eosinophilic syndromes (Ch. 162).

The interaction of "activated macrophages" with surrounding normal tissues may form the pathophysiologic substructure of many of the clinical features of Langerhans cell granulomatosis. The structure and function of macrophages are described in Ch. 147.

Clinical conditions of unknown cause characterized pathologically by proliferation of tissue macrophages in sheetlike masses with interspersed eosinophils have been difficult to define as specific disease entities. There is great histologic variability within these disorders, and lesions taken from different sites in the same patient may differ pathologically. The clinical course and prognosis do not correlate with histopathologic findings. The concept of Langerhans cell granulomatosis, Hand-Schuller-Christian disease (the classic triad of exophthalmos, diabetes insipidus, and bone destruction) and Letterer-Siwe disease as elements of a continuum termed *histiocytosis X* fails to recognize important differences in clinical course, organ involvement, and therapeutic response. This chapter will discuss unifocal Langerhans cell granulomatosis, multifocal Langerhans cell granulomatosis, and Letterer-Siwe disease. These are the best characterized idiopathic histiocytoses, yet in clinical practice many cases do not readily fit into these categories.

UNIFOCAL LANGERHANS CELL (EOSINOPHILIC) GRANULOMATOSIS

Unifocal Langerhans cell granulomatosis is a benign disorder generally occurring in males during childhood or early adult life. It may occur as late as the sixth or seventh decade of life.

CLINICAL MANIFESTATIONS. The most common presentation of the disorder is a single osteolytic lesion in a long or flat bone, most frequently in the calvarium or femur in children and in a rib in adults. The predilection for skull, femur, rib, pelvis, vertebra, and mandible is not understood. The small bones of the distal extremities are not generally involved. Although the lesions are usually purely lytic, mixed blastic and lytic lesions occur. Pain and swelling over the affected area are common presenting symptoms, although disruption of teeth with mandibular disease, fracture, and otitis media due to mastoid involvement are not infrequent. Many lesions are asymptomatic and diagnosed serendipitously during radiologic evaluation for unrelated problems. Unifocal Langerhans cell granulomatosis of lymph nodes, thymus, or salivary glands is very rare and has the same benign course as that of the more frequent bony lesions. Unifocal Langerhans cell granulomatosis is rarely associated with systemic symptoms and there are no characteristic laboratory findings. Diagnosis is established by biopsy.

DIAGNOSIS. The bone scan is very useful in determining that the lesion is indeed unifocal and in following patients over time for development of new osteolytic lesions. An open biopsy should be performed for diagnosis. Pathologically, an infiltrate with foamy macrophages and admixed eosinophils favors the diagnosis of Langerhans cell granulomatosis. Langerhans histiocytes contain a cytoplasmic inclusion of unknown composition but with constant thickness and striation termed an X *body*.

TREATMENT. At the time of biopsy, curettage, with or without bone chip packing, should be carried out. This simple surgical approach is almost uniformly successful as definitive therapy for an individual lesion. Lesions in anatomic sites that are difficult to approach surgically, such as weight-bearing bones or cervical vertebrae, are best treated by low-dose (300 to 600 rads fractioned total dose) local supervoltage irradiation. This low-dose radiotherapy generally eradicates the proliferating histiocytes and allows for normal bone repair, while high-dose radiotherapy leads to tissue damage and resultant poor healing. Surgical decompression followed by low-dose irradiation is sometimes indicated for lesions requiring emergency intervention, such as those compressing the spinal cord. Patients should be carefully followed after therapy for the development of new lesions, which generally arise within the first year after diagnosis. Individuals with a lesion in the bones of the head, neck, or pelvis are more likely to have subsequent disease. Bone scans to detect new lesions and plain films to follow the known site of involvement should be obtained every six months for one to two years after therapy. Extraosseous Langerhans cell granulomatosis involving soft tissue is generally successfully managed by complete surgical excision if possible, or by low-dose irradiation.

MULTIFOCAL LANGERHANS CELL (EOSINOPHILIC) GRANULOMATOSIS

CLINICAL MANIFESTATIONS. Similar to the unifocal form, multifocal Langerhans cell granulomatosis generally presents in children, predominantly in males, and often with *bone lesions.* In addition to the calvarium, the sphenoid bone, sella turcica, mandible, and long bones of the upper extremities may be involved. This tropism for the head is unexplained but may indicate local reaction to an inciting agent that enters via the nasopharynx or oropharynx. Complications of this disorder include chronic otitis media caused by destruction of temporal and mastoid bones, proptosis with orbital masses, loose teeth with infiltration of maxilla or mandible, and both anterior and posterior pituitary dysfunction with involvement of the sella turcica. This last complication may occur with focal disease of hypothalamus or pituitary without bone involvement, and growth retardation of the patient may occur. Diabetes insipidus is caused by granulomatous involvement of the hypothalamus or pituitary and may be either transient or permanent. The classic triad of lytic skull lesions, exophthalmos, and diabetes insipidus called *Hand-Schuller-Christian disease* is best viewed as a subset of multifocal Langerhans cell (eosinophilic) granulomatosis. Dermal lesions may appear papulosquamous, seborrheic, eczematous, and rarely xanthomatosis. Vulvar lesions with ulceration are not uncommon. Hepatosplenomegaly and lymphadenopathy are unusual in multifocal Langerhans cell granulomatosis.

In *Langerhans cell granulomatosis* the lung is an important extraosseous site of involvement. The disorder mainly affects young adult men and often presents with a chronic cough, pneumothorax, and constitutional symptoms. The chest radiograph usually shows a diffuse micronodular and interstitial infiltrate involving the mid-zones and bases of the lungs with relative sparing of the costophrenic angles. Ultimately a honeycomb appearance may occur; it is caused by coalescence of small parenchymal pulmonary cysts. Fibrosis is a late finding that may lead to chronic cor pulmonale. Pulmonary function tests may show restrictive impairment. Diagnosis is best made by biopsy that shows the mixed histiocytic-eosinophilic infiltrate with a variable degree of fibrosis. Pulmonary Langerhans cell granulomatosis has a highly variable natural history. Spontaneous remissions are not infrequent, but prognosis is poorer at the extremes of age and with involvement of extrapulmonary organs.

DIAGNOSIS. There are no distinctive laboratory abnormalities in multifocal Langerhans cell granulomatosis. The leukocyte count is generally normal and eosinophilia is not present unless it is from another cause. Hypercalcemia generally does not result from bone lesions.

The diagnosis of multifocal Langerhans cell granulomatosis is definitively made by biopsy, usually of a bone lesion. The extent of multifocal involvement is established by physical examination, chest x-ray, bone scan, and if indicated, computerized tomographic scan of the brain. This last test is useful for hypothalamic or pituitary lesions associated with diabetes insipidus.

TREATMENT. The natural history of multifocal Langerhans cell granulomatosis is relatively favorable when cases best diagnosed as Letterer-Siwe disease (see below) are excluded. Destructive lesions of bone when present early in the clinical course may predict a better outcome. The therapy is guided by the particular organs involved. Diabetes insipidus and growth retardation should be treated by hormonal replacement with vasopressin (Ch. 226) and human growth hormone, respectively. Low-dose irradiation to the suprasellar area may restore endocrine function in certain individuals. The seborrheic dermal eruption is responsive to tar treatments. X-irradiation using doses generally below 600 rads to symptomatic bony lesions is nearly always effective. Surgery may be necessary to relieve spinal cord compression and mastoid problems and to excise skull lesions eroding through skin. Oral granulomatosis can be treated with dexamethasone elixir used as a mouth rinse three times a day. Similarly, topical steroid creams may accelerate the healing of vulvar lesions.

Systemic therapy is indicated when either radiation fails or multiple sites demand treatment. Corticosteroids alone may achieve dramatic results. Prednisone at a single dose of 0.5 to 1.0 mg per kilogram can be used in the acute phase. Alternate day corticosteroid therapy can be initiated after remission is achieved. Use of cytotoxic agents, such as vinblastine or methotrexate, is generally reserved for aggressive and refractory disease.

There is insufficient experience to recommend a single first-line chemotherapeutic regimen. Addition of vinblastine at a dose of 0.1 mg per kilogram intravenously every week for four to eight weeks is generally successful in achieving remission. It is unclear whether maintenance chemotherapy with weekly vinblastine or prednisone is required to sustain remission. Should disease recur within several months after discontinuation of therapy for the acute phase, the patient should be retreated with the initially successful regimen and placed on maintenance therapy. The striking variability in clinical course makes it difficult to generalize with regard to therapeutic guidelines.

LETTERER-SIWE SYNDROME

In 1924 Letterer described a six-month-old child with diffuse purpura, fever, otitis media, lymphadenopathy, and hepatosplenomegaly. Nine years later, Siwe included this case in a series of six similar cases. In all instances, there was diffuse tissue infiltration by histiocytes. The histiocytes of Letterer-Siwe disease have abundant acidophilic cytoplasm and are often vacuolated. There may be prominent hemophagocytosis. Generally there is a relative paucity of eosinophils in the histiocytic infiltrates.

CLINICAL MANIFESTATIONS. Children are usually affected in the first years of life, although an adult form of the syndrome may exist. Liver, spleen, lymph nodes, lung, and bone are the most commonly affected areas. Laboratory evaluation often demonstrates leukocytosis, although pancytopenia caused by hypersplenism or bone marrow infiltration may be seen. The dermal lesion of Letterer-Siwe disease is generally a brown-red, scaly eczematoid or seborrheic eruption, and purpura secondary to thrombocytopenia may be present. Hepatosplenomegaly may occur with or without jaundice or elevated levels of hepatic parenchymal enzymes. There is no familial or hereditary predisposition and that distinguishes Letterer-Siwe disease from another histiocytic disorder of infants, familial erythrophagocytic lymphohistiocytosis. A clinical pathologic syndrome nearly identical to Letterer-Siwe disease has recently been described in immunologically compromised children infected with a variety of viruses. In addition, certain cases termed Letterer-Siwe disease may actually be unusual forms of malignant lymphoma.

TREATMENT. The course of Letterer-Siwe disease is commonly fulminant and fatal. Spontaneous remissions are rare. It is important to distinguish Letterer-Siwe disease from disorders of infectious or clearly neoplastic origin before initiating therapy. Systemic symptoms of Letterer-Siwe disease often improve with corticosteroids and focal lesions may be palliated with radiotherapy. Occasionally, clinical remission has been achieved with chemotherapy, particularly vinblastine and prednisone. If this regimen fails, methotrexate and 6-mercaptopurine may be used.

Greenberger JS, Crocker AC, Vawter G, Jaffe N, Cassady JR: Results of treatment of 27 patients with systemic histiocytosis (Letterer-Siwe syndrome, Schuller-Christian syndrome and multifocal eosinophilic granuloma). Medicine 60:311, 1981. *A detailed analysis of therapy of histiocytic disorders at a single academic medical center.*

Groopman JE, Golde DW: The histiocytic disorder: A pathophysiologic analysis. Ann Intern Med 94:95, 1981. *Comprehensive review of the histiocytic disorders with emphasis on pathophysiologic mechanisms; extensive bibliography.*
Risdall RJ, McKenna RW, Nesbit ME, et al.: Virus-associated hemophagocytic syndrome. A benign histiocytic proliferation distinct from malignant histiocytosis. Cancer 44:993, 1979. *Importance of considering infectious causes of clinicopathologic syndromes easily misdiagnosed as histiocytic disorders.*
Sims DG: Histiocytosis X: Follow-up of 43 cases. Arch Dis Child 52:433, 1977. *A large series followed over a long period; illustrates the striking variability in clinical course.*
Zinkham WH: Multifocal eosinophilic granuloma: Natural history, etiology and management. Am J Med 60:457, 1976. *A comprehensive and well-written clinical paper; of great assistance in clinical management.*

162. EOSINOPHILIC SYNDROMES

David A. Bass

Many diseases which cause eosinophilia, such as parasitic infestations, allergies, and drug reactions, are discussed elsewhere in this book. This chapter provides a brief summary of the distinctive qualities of eosinophils and the types of disease that may be associated with eosinophilia in the peripheral blood.

Eosinophils are granulocytic leukocytes and share with neutrophils similar life cycles, morphology, lysosomal enzymes, potent oxidative metabolism, and phagocytic ability. The distinctive qualities of eosinophils become apparent in their responses during specific immunologic and inflammatory processes. Acute inflammation causes stimulation of neutrophil production, inhibition of eosinophil production, and eosinopenia in the peripheral blood. Administration of glucocorticosteroids causes eosinopenia and neutrophilia. Moreover, unlike neutrophils, eosinophils appear closely linked to the immune system. Eosinophil stimulation most commonly follows repeated or prolonged antigenic exposure, especially when the antigens are deposited in tissues and elicit hypersensitivity reactions. Stimulation of eosinophilia in delayed hypersensitivity reactions is T lymphocyte dependent. During immune responses to metazoan parasites, lymphocytes release substances that stimulate eosinopoiesis.

The functions of eosinophils remain a subject of debate. The two currently favored hypotheses appear contrasting, if not contradictory. One hypothesis views the eosinophil as a protective killer cell, similar to the neutrophil, but specifically involved in defense against metazoan parasites. The alternative theory views the eosinophil as an anti-inflammatory modulator of hypersensitivity reactions, serving to constrain the immune response and minimize its unnecessary spread. There are experimental data to support both hypotheses, and the role of eosinophils in immunologic reactions is a field of active study.

Eosinophils may on occasion be harmful rather than beneficial. Prolonged, marked eosinophilia may be associated with Löffler's endomyocardial disease, discussed below. Eosinophils may also contribute to localized tissue damage in specific syndromes. For example, a component of eosinophil granules, the major basic protein, causes cytopathic changes in tracheal epithelium in vitro that are similar to the changes observed in patients with asthma.

EOSINOPHILIC SYNDROMES AFFECTING ORGAN SYSTEMS

HYPEREOSINOPHILIC SYNDROME. This is a myeloproliferative syndrome with persistent, marked eosinophilia (above 1500 per cubic millimeter) and evidence of organ involvement. Eosinophilic infiltrates may cause dysfunction of diverse tissues, including the following: The heart may reveal the changes of Löffler's endomyocardial disease. Most patients have hepatosplenomegaly, although laboratory studies of hepatic functions demonstrate minimal abnormalities, usually limited to a modest elevation of serum alkaline phosphatase. Central nervous system complications may present as diffuse changes (confusion, delusion, psychosis, coma) or localized problems, including peripheral neuropathies or hemiparesis. Gastrointestinal involvement may cause diarrhea, nonspecific abdominal pains, and occasionally malabsorption syndromes. Pulmonary involvement may present as interstitial infiltrates that contain large numbers of eosinophils on biopsy. Pleural effusions may occur. Rashes occur in 25 to 50 per cent of the patients and are usually nonspecific, urticarial, or maculopapular. The presence of angioedema has been suggested to be a favorable indicator of therapeutic responses. Patients often have a mild normochromic normocytic anemia, but severe anemia or thrombocytopenia is rare. Once organ involvement is demonstrated, the prognosis of these patients, if they are left untreated, is not good. Of the patients reported in the literature, half had died by nine months of observation. However, about one third of the patients with this syndrome may respond to corticosteroid therapy; moreover, the majority of the remainder may have a favorable response to hydroxyurea. Death is often due to cardiac involvement with endomyocarditis and congestive failure. Death caused by infections or thrombocytopenia with bleeding is unusual. However, rare cases have terminated in a blastic crisis, even following "successful" treatment with hydroxyurea.

EOSINOPHILIC LEUKEMIA. Eosinophilic leukemia is rare. A number of patients have been described with immature eosinophils in the peripheral blood, thrombocytopenia, and severe anemia. In some patients chromosomal aberrations, including the Philadelphia chromosome, have been described.

LÖFFLER'S ENDOMYOCARDIAL DISEASE. This involves a thickening of the endocardium with subendocardial myocardial degeneration and infiltration by eosinophils. Either or both ventricles may be involved; atria are usually minimally affected. It may present as a restrictive cardiomyopathy and/or valvular dysfunction, usually mitral regurgitation, leading to right- or left-sided congestive heart failure. Mural thrombi may further compromise cardiac function or cause embolic events. Over 90 per cent of the patients are males. This disease may be due to the release of some component of eosinophil leukocytes, since it has been observed during diverse illnesses characterized by high and prolonged blood eosinophilia, i.e., an eosinophil count higher than 2000 per cubic millimeter for longer than 12 months, including solid tumors, metazoan parasites, hypersensitivity vasculitis, the hypereosinophilic syndrome, and eosinophilic leukemia.

DISEASES ASSOCIATED WITH EOSINOPHILIA (Table 162–1)

ALLERGIES AND DRUG REACTIONS. These are discussed in other chapters. Although acute allergic reactions may cause leukemoid eosinophilic responses (eosinophils above 20,000 per cubic millimeter), chronic allergy is rarely associated with eosinophil counts above 2000 per cubic millimeter.

INFECTIONS. Infestations by *invasive metazoan parasites* almost always cause eosinophilia. Noninvasive helminths (e.g., pinworm, whipworm) or encysted parasites (e.g., echinococcus) are less regularly associated with peripheral eosinophilia. Protozoa do not usually cause eosinophilia. Mycobacterial and fungal infections are not usually associated with eosinophilia; however, about 10 per cent of patients with afebrile *tuberculosis* may have a modest increase in blood eosinophils. Acute *coccidioidomycosis* often causes immunologic manifestations, including erythema nodosum, erythema multiforme, urticaria, polyarthritis, and eosinophilia. Acute bacterial and viral infections are usually associated with eosinopenia in the peripheral blood. Exceptions to this rule include the eosinophilias of *chlamydial pneumonia of infancy, cat scratch disease, infectious lymphocytosis,* and occasional cases of *infectious mononucleosis.* During the convalescent phase of acute infections, occasional patients will develop a transient, usually mild eosinophilia. In scarlet fever, eosinophilia regularly appears coincidentally with the characteristic rash.

SKIN DISEASES. Diverse skin diseases may be associated with

TABLE 162–1. DISORDERS ASSOCIATED WITH EOSINOPHILIA

- I. Allergy
  - A. Allergic rhinitis
  - B. Asthma
  - C. Atopic dermatitis
  - D. Acute urticaria
  - E. Drug reactions
- II. Infectious diseases
  - A. Tissue-invasive helminths
    - 1. Major tropical
      - a. Filariasis
      - b. Schistosomiasis
    - 2. North America
      - a. Strongyloides
      - b. Trichinosis
      - c. Toxocariasis
      - d. Ascaris
      - e. Occasional in hookworm, echinococcus, cysticercosis
  - B. Other infections
    - 1. Acute coccidioidomycosis
    - 2. Afebrile tuberculosis
    - 3. Cat scratch disease
    - 4. Chlamydial pneumonia of infancy
    - 5. Convalescent phase of many infections, especially scarlet fever
- III. Other cutaneous diseases
  - A. Bullous pemphigoid
  - B. Herpes gestationis
  - C. Recurrent granulomatous dermatitis
  - D. Scabies
- IV. Other pulmonary diseases
  - A. Transient pulmonary eosinophilic infiltrates (Löffler's syndrome)
  - B. Hypersensitivity pneumonitis
  - C. Allergic bronchopulmonary aspergillosis
  - D. Tropical eosinophilia
  - E. Chronic eosinophilic pneumonia
- V. Connective tissue diseases
  - A. Polyarteritis group
    - 1. Allergic granulomatosis (Churg/Strauss type)
    - 2. Angiitis with hepatitis B antigenemia
  - B. Rheumatoid arthritis (severe)
  - C. Eosinophilic fasciitis
  - D. Sjögren's syndrome
- VI. Neoplastic and myeloproliferative diseases
  - A. Solid tumors, especially mucin-secreting, epithelial cell origin especially when metastatic to serosa or bone
  - B. Lymphoid
    - 1. Lymphomas, especially T cell type and Hodgkin's disease
    - 2. T cell and acute lymphoblastic leukemias
    - 3. Occasional with myeloma (heavy chain disease)
  - C. Hypereosinophilic syndrome
  - D. Other
    - 1. Histiocytosis with cutaneous involvement
    - 2. Angiolymphoid hyperplasia (Kimura's disease)
- VII. Immunodeficiency diseases
  - A. Selective IgA deficiency
  - B. Swiss-type and sex-linked combined immunodeficiency
  - C. Nezelof syndrome
  - D. Wiskott-Aldrich syndrome
  - E. Hyper-IgE syndrome
  - F. Graft versus host reactions
- VIII. Occasional causes of eosinophilia
  - A. Eosinophilic gastroenteritis
  - B. Inflammatory bowel disease
  - C. Chronic active hepatitis
  - D. Chronic dialysis
  - E. Acute pancreatitis
  - F. Postirradiation
  - G. Hypopituitarism
  - H. Other localized disorders with occasional blood eosinophilia
    - 1. Eosinophilic lymphadenitis
    - 2. Eosinophilic cystitis
    - 3. Eosinophilic cholecystitis
    - 4. Eosinophilic meningitis

eosinophilia. Best documented are the eosinophilias of *atopic dermatitis, eczema, acute urticaria* (but not chronic urticaria or angioneurotic edema), *pemphigus, bullous pemphigoid,* and *herpes gestationis. Well's syndrome* is a recurrent, usually itchy, occasionally painful, papulovesicular eruption which in severe cases may be associated with fever, arthralgias, and malaise. This might be mistaken for bacterial cellulitis or a viral exanthem, except that it is often accompanied by systemic eosinophilia. Eosinophil counts may also be useful in the evaluation of *toxic epidermal necrolysis*. Eosinophil counts are usually elevated when this entity is due to a drug reaction but are usually reduced when staphylococci are the cause.

PULMONARY EOSINOPHILIAS. See Ch. 62.

EOSINOPHILIC GASTROENTERITIS. See Ch. 162.

NEOPLASTIC DISORDERS. A small proportion, about 5 per cent, of patients with *carcinomas* and *sarcomas* may have eosinophilia. Eosinophilia with solid tumors may be indicative of metastatic dissemination. A mild eosinophilia accompanies *Hodgkin's disease* in roughly one fifth of patients; however, in occasional cases, marked eosinophilia (up to 98 per cent) has occurred. *Immunoblastic lymphadenopathy* is associated with eosinophilia in about one third of cases. Cutaneous involvement with neoplastic disorders, including histiocytic medullary reticulosis, mycosis fungoides, and Sézary's syndrome, may have an associated eosinophilia.

IMMUNE DISEASES. In the absence of pulmonary involvement, polyarteritis is rarely associated with eosinophilia. By contrast, *polyarteritis with pulmonary involvement* (asthma) and the *allergic granulomatosis of Churg and Strauss* are associated with eosinophilia in a great majority of cases. The syndrome of *polyarteritis in association with hepatitis antigenemia* may also be accompanied by eosinophilia. A mild eosinophilia occurs in about 10 per cent of patients with *rheumatoid arthritis* at some time during their disease. Occasional cases, usually those of long standing with nodules and pleuropulmonary involvement, may have a marked peripheral blood eosinophilia. The syndrome of *eosinophilic fasciitis* is discussed in Ch. 448. In one large series, about two thirds of patients with *Sjögren's syndrome* had eosinophilia. Mild eosinophilia is often noted in *immune deficiency syndromes,* whether involving the T or B lymphocyte series, and in certain defects of neutrophil production or function. Such patients may respond to pulmonary infection by *Pneumocystis carinii* with a marked eosinophilia. The syndrome of *eosinophilic lymphadenitis* is characterized by peripheral blood eosinophilia associated with localized, usually inguinal or axillary, lymphadenopathy. The response appears to follow repeated local exposures to an antigen, such as an insect sting, on a peripheral extremity. Involved lymph nodes may be densely infiltrated with eosinophils.

Many other diseases of presumed immunologic etiology are not associated with eosinophilia; these include systemic lupus erythematosus, systemic sclerosis, glomerulonephritis, acute rheumatic fever, serum sickness, autoimmune hemolytic anemia, thrombocytopenic purpura, Hashimoto's thyroiditis, pernicious anemia, and myasthenia gravis.

RADIATION-RELATED EOSINOPHILIA. About 40 per cent of patients with an intra-abdominal neoplasm exhibit eosinophilia during the first few weeks of radiation therapy. Such patients may also develop proctitis with a marked local infiltration of eosinophils.

INFLAMMATORY BOWEL DISEASE. Local inflammatory lesions of *ulcerative colitis* may be rich in eosinophils, and a slight elevation of blood eosinophils may occur in this disease. Some observers have also reported modest eosinophilia during symptomatic phases of *Crohn's disease,* and this may be a helpful guide in differentiating Crohn's disease from acute appendicitis.

CHRONIC ACTIVE HEPATITIS. About one third of patients with chronic hepatitis have eosinophilia in excess of 5 per cent.

DRESSLER'S SYNDROME. Although not mentioned in recent reviews, 20 per cent of the patients in Dressler's original series had eosinophilia.

PANCREATIC DISEASES. A distinctive clinical syndrome associated with acinar cell carcinoma of the pancreas includes polyarthritis, subcutaneous panniculitis, and blood eosinophilia. Although the arthritis and panniculitis are thought to be caused by pancreatic lipase, the cause of the eosinophilia is unknown. Similar symptoms and signs may be observed two to six weeks following acute pancreatitis.

DIALYSIS. About one third of patients undergoing chronic hemodialysis develop blood and bone marrow eosinophilia without apparent cause. Similarly, chronic peritoneal dialysis may evoke an eosinophilic peritoneal effusion and occasionally elevated numbers of eosinophils in the blood. This eosinophilic peritonitis may be associated with abdominal pain and fever, and may be mistaken for a bacterial infection unless a differential count of the exudate is obtained.

ADDISON'S DISEASE. Although occasional patients with Addison's disease and eosinophilia have been observed, this is not typical. In one series, the only patients with eosinophilia had hypopituitarism.

Beeson PB, Bass DA: The Eosinophil. Philadelphia, W. B. Saunders Company, 1977. *This monograph is equally divided between an analysis of current knowledge of eosinophil structure, physiology, and biochemistry and a comprehensive review of altered eosinophil responses (either eosinophilia or eosinopenia) in human diseases.*

Fauci AS, Harley JB, Roberts WC, Ferrans VJ, Gralnick HR, Bjornson BH: The idiopathic hypereosinophilic syndrome: Clinical, pathophysiologic, and therapeutic considerations. Ann Intern Med 97:78, 1982. *An excellent up-to-date summary of the esoinophil and hypereosinophilia from the National Institutes of Health.*

Weller PF, Goetzl EJ: Dermatological conditions associated with eosinophilia and eosinophilic diseases. *In* Kay AB, Goetzl EJ (eds.): Contemporary Issues in Clinical Immunology and Allergy: Immunodermatology. Edinburgh, Churchill Livingstone, in press, 1984. *A general review of the disorders associated with eosinophilia and how they should be approached clinically.*

163. PLASMA CELL DISORDERS

Sydney E. Salmon

The plasma cell disorders are a group of related neoplastic diseases associated with proliferation of a single clone of immunoglobulin-secreting plasma cells derived from the B cell series of immunocytes. This group of disorders has variously been referred to with a series of synonymous terms: monoclonal gammopathies, plasma cell dyscrasias, gammopathies, immunoglobulinopathies, paraproteinemias, and dysproteinemias.

The plasma cell disorders to be discussed here are monoclonal neoplasms; their secreted immunoglobulin products are electrophoretically and immunologically homogeneous and therefore readily distinguished from the heterogeneous populations of immunoglobulin-antibody molecules secreted by the numerous clones of normal B cells. There are five major classes of immunoglobulins synthesized by B lymphocytes and plasma cells: IgG, IgA, IgM, IgD, and IgE (see Ch. 427). Immunoglobulins are antibody protein molecules that all have a basic monomeric unit structure of two heavy (H) chains and two light (L) chains, which each have "constant" and "variable" regions with respect to amino acid sequence. IgG, IgA, IgD, and IgE are synthesized and secreted as monomers with molecular weights in the range of 150,000 to 190,000; IgM is secreted as a pentameric structure with a molecular weight of 900,000. Class specificity of each immunoglobulin is defined in terms of a series of antigenic determinants on the constant regions of the H chains (γ, α, μ, δ, ε). There are also two major types of L chains (κ and λ) defined by antigenic determinants on the constant regions of the L chains. The amino sequence in the variable regions of immunoglobulin molecules corresponds to the zone of the active antigen combining site of the antibody, whereas the constant regions convey other biologic properties. (Structural and functional properties of immunoglobulins are summarized in Table 427–1 and Figure 427–1.)

A homogeneous immunoglobulin, as a sharp peak or "spike" in the beta or gamma globulin zone on electrophoresis, is referred to as an M-component. Electrophoresis and immunoelectrophoresis, respectively, are used to quantitate and qualitatively identify M-components. Definition of an M-component as monoclonal (having a single H chain and a single L chain type) requires immunoelectrophoretic analysis. A comparison of a normal serum and an M-component on serum electrophoresis is depicted in Figure 163–1.

Plasma cells represent the most well-differentiated progeny in the B cell series of immunocytes. They contain substantial quantities of rough-surfaced endoplasmic reticulum that is rich in RNA, and are specialized for production of antibody molecules at a rapid rate. In the normal immune response, individual plasma cells can synthesize and secrete immunoglobulin at rates up to 100,000 molecules per minute. Immunoglobulin secretion rates of neoplastic plasma cells are generally somewhat lower than those for normal plasma cells. Additionally, in neoplastic clones, H and L chain biosynthesis is sometimes "unbalanced" with excessive synthesis of free L chains, which are usually secreted by the cell as L chain dimers of molecular weight 60,000. The relatively low molecular weight of secreted L chains permits them to undergo renal glomerular filtration. While limited amounts of free L chains can be reabsorbed and catabolized by the renal tubule, excessive amounts are excreted in the urine. Monoclonal L chains in the urine in association with B cell neoplasms are referred to as *Bence Jones proteins* in tribute to the clinical chemist who discovered the differential solubilization on boiling and precipitation on cooling of the urinary protein in the case of multiple myeloma first reported in the mid-1800's by McIntyre. Electrophoretic and immunologic techniques are now used to assess urinary L chain excretion. The B lymphoid cell precursors of plasma cells have somewhat more limited capability for immunoglobulin synthesis; the immunoglobulin they produce is more frequently displayed on the cell membrane than secreted by the cell. In some instances, individual lymphoid cells may display more than one immunoglobulin on their surfaces (particularly IgD plus IgM). In such instances, both molecules express the identical L

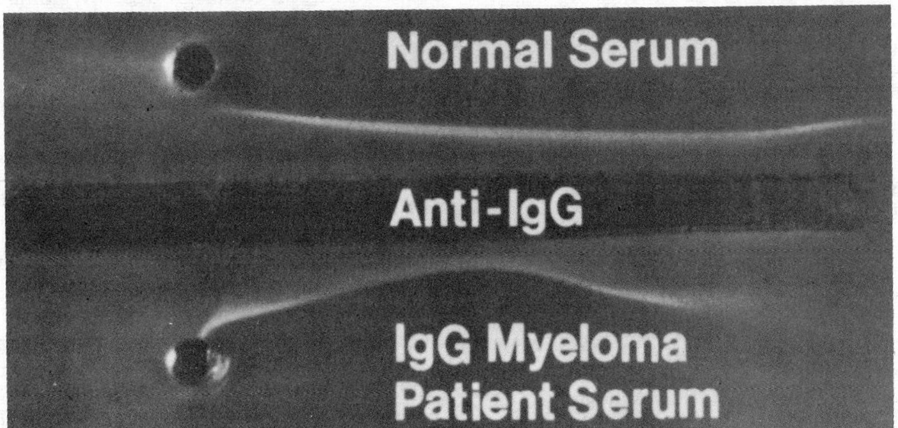

Figure 163–1. Agar gel immunoelectrophoresis of serum from a patient with IgG multiple myeloma and a normal control. The bowing of the IgG precipitation arc reflects the presence of an M-component. Confirmation that this arc is a monoclonal immunoglobulin is obtained by simultaneously running additional similar gels with anti-kappa or anti-lambda antisera in the central trough. In this case, the patient had an IgG-kappa M-component. Immunoelectrophoresis of the patient's urine revealed free kappa light chains ("Bence Jones protein").

chain type and apparent antibody specificity, and the immunoglobulin class expressed is in the course of being "switched" in association with clonal proliferation and differentiation. A number of the B cell neoplasms discussed in this text are manifest as if frozen at various points along this differentiation pathway. Most cases of chronic lymphocytic leukemia, non-Hodgkin's lymphomas, multiple myeloma, macroglobulinemia, and related disorders appear to originate from monoclonal B cell progenitors and are expressed as immunoglobulin-synthesizing neoplasms with either surface membrane or secreted monoclonal immunoglobulin (see Ch. 152). Despite the apparently common origin of these neoplasms, the clinical manifestations, response to treatment, and prognosis of these neoplasms differ substantially. In most instances, the tumor stem cells for one of these neoplasms (those progenitor cells responsible for the metastatic spread and self-renewal of the tumor) give rise to cells that express the original differentiation state and clinical features of the particular neoplasm (e.g., multiple myeloma). In occasional instances of plasma cell neoplasia (and chronic lymphocytic leukemia and follicular lymphoma) apparent "subcloning" occurs during the patient's clinical course, and the pattern of histology and tumor growth takes on a less differentiated form—e.g., as a poorly differentiated large cell lymphoma. Such transformations are often associated with some change in immunoglobulin synthesis or secretion. Immunologic commonality with the original clone can usually be found, however, by the use of sophisticated techniques. A classification of B cell disorders associated with secretion of an M-component appears in Table 163–1.

TABLE 163–1. CLASSIFICATION OF DISORDERS ASSOCIATED WITH MONOCLONAL IMMUNOGLOBULIN (M-COMPONENT SECRETION)

Disorder	M-Component	
1. Plasma cell neoplasms		
A. Multiple myeloma	IgG>IgA>IgD>IgE ±free L chain or L chain alone (κ>λ) rarely biclonal or without detectable Ig abnormality	
B. Macroglobulinemia	IgM±free L chain (κ>λ)	
C. H chain diseases	γ, α, or μ chain or fragment; ?, δ, or ε	
D. Primary amyloidosis	Free L chain (λ>κ) or L chain fragment alone or plus IgG, IgA, IgM, or IgD	
E. Monoclonal gammopathy of unknown significance	IgG, IgM, IgA, or IgD without L chain secretion	
2. Other B cell neoplasms	*M-component* (occasionally secreted)	
A. Chronic lymphocytic leukemia	IgM>IgG	
B. B cell non-Hodgkin's lymphomas (any morphologic pattern or lymphoid cell types)		
3. Nonlymphoid neoplasms—Chronic myelogenous leukemia; carcinoma of colon, breast, prostate, or other sites	No consistent patterns	
4. "Autoimmune" or autoreactive disorders	*M-component*	*Antibody activity of M-component*
A. Cold agglutinin disease (some characteristics of Waldenström's macroglobulinemia)	IgMκ most common	Anti-I antigen of RBC membrane
B. Mixed cryoglobulinemia	IgM	Anti-IgG
C. Hypergammaglobulinemia	IgG	Anti-IgG
D. Sjögren's syndrome	IgM	?
5. Miscellaneous inflammatory, storage, or infectious disorders		
Lichen myxedematosus	IgGλ	
Gaucher's disease	IgG	
Cirrhosis, sarcoid, parasitic diseases, renal acidosis	No consistent pattern	

Stites DP, Stobo JD, Fudenberg HH, Wells JV: Basic and Clinical Immunology. 4th ed. Los Altos, Lange Medical Publications, 1982. *An excellent and reasonably priced text on immunology for students, house staff, and physicians.*
Salmon SE, Seligman M: B-cell neoplasia in man. Lancet 2:1230, 1974. *A generalized hypothesis relating the stages of proliferation and differentiation of normal B cell clones to neoplastic transformation and the manifestations and classification of the various B cell neoplasias, including chronic lymphocytic leukemia, B cell lymphomas, macroglobulinemia, and myeloma. The scheme accounts for various intermediate forms, and is consistent with available data on cell surface and secreted monoclonal Ig.*
Schedel I, Peest D, Stunkel K, et al: Idiotype-bearing peripheral lymphocytes in human multiple myeloma and Waldenström's macroglobulinemia. Scand J Immunol 11:437, 1980. *Study of immunologic characteristics of circulating tumor cells in monoclonal plasma cell disorders.*

MULTIPLE MYELOMA

DEFINITION. Multiple myeloma (plasma cell myeloma, myelomatosis) is a disseminated malignant disease in which a clone of transformed plasma cells proliferates in the bone marrow, disrupting its normal functions as well as invading the adjacent bone. The disease is frequently associated with extensive skeletal destruction, hypercalcemia, anemia, impaired renal function, immunodeficiency, and increased susceptibility to infection. Amyloidosis, clotting disorders, and other protein abnormalities are occasional associations. The neoplastic plasma cells usually produce and secrete M-component immunoglobulin, the amount of which in any given case varies proportionally with the total body tumor burden.

ETIOLOGY. The etiology of human myeloma is unknown; however, genetic predisposition, oncogenic viruses, inflammatory stimuli, and chronic antigenic stimulation have all been implicated.

A mouse model of myeloma has provided some basis for the aforementioned hypotheses. Myeloma can be readily induced in the inbred BALB-C strain of mice by intraperitoneal injection of mineral oil. Such mice are known to harbor oncogenic type C RNA viruses. Of interest, BALB-C mice raised in a germ-free environment fail to develop myeloma after oil injection (although other lymphoid neoplasms may arise). This suggests that bacterial antigenic exposure may be required to increase sufficiently the proliferation of populations of immunoglobulin producing B cells to render them susceptible to myeloma induction. Myeloma appears to be epizootic, having been reported in rats, dogs, cats, horses, and other mammalian species.

INCIDENCE AND PREVALENCE. Multiple myeloma is a disease most frequently observed in the middle-aged and elderly (median age 60), with an incidence that increases with age. Rare cases have been reported in younger persons, including a few teenagers. The annual incidence of myeloma is 3 per 100,000 population (about as common as Hodgkin's disease). It is slightly more common in males than females, and has been reported in all racial groups. Myeloma accounts for about 10 per cent of hematologic malignancies and 1 per cent of all forms of cancer.

PATHOPHYSIOLOGY. The symptoms and signs of multiple myeloma and its consequences on the patient are related primarily to (1) the growth kinetics of the neoplastic plasma cells and the total body tumor burden and (2) secreted products of the tumor cells which have physiochemical, immunologic, or humoral effects. The various secreted products can induce a wide variety of clinical syndromes in patients with myeloma.

MYELOMA CELL MASS. Once transformed plasma cells begin to proliferate in a malignant fashion, the clone appears to grow relatively rapidly with a tumor stem cell doubling time of 24 to 48 hours. Although the neoplasm appears to originate from a single transformed cell (10^0 cells) at a single location, progressive myeloma growth is associated with hematogenous spread of the neoplastic cells to various skeletal sites, leading to widespread involvement of the bone marrow with nodules or sheets of plasma cells (Fig. 163–2). Marrow involvement leads to development of a normochromic normocytic anemia that is apparent in virtually all patients with myeloma. This appears to be the consequence of tumor-related inhibition of erythropoiesis as well as the disturbance of marrow architecture. A

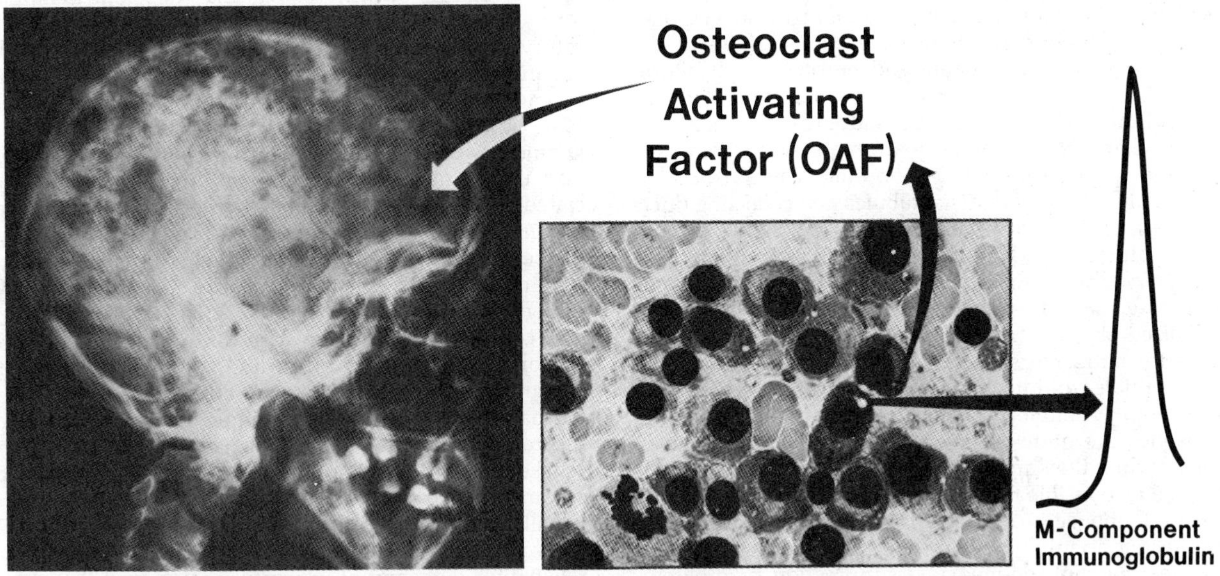

Figure 163–2. Clinicopathologic features of multiple myeloma. The type of extensive skeletal destruction ("Swiss cheese"-like lesions) observed in Stage III myeloma patients is represented by the skull at the left of the figure. The patient's bone marrow (center) contains an infiltrate of neoplastic plasma cells which can synthesize and secrete both an osteoclast activating factor (OAF), and a monoclonal immunoglobulin, which appears as a "spike" on protein electrophoresis. Serial measurements of the M-component provide a useful quantitative marker for growth or regression of the neoplasm, as the M-component production rate per myeloma cell remains relatively constant in most cases.

slight shortening in red cell survival, iron deficiency, and blood loss may also contribute to the anemia. High concentrations of a serum M-component may lead to blood sludging and hyperviscosity. Rouleaux formation observed on the peripheral blood smear and an increase in the sedimentation rate are also due to high concentrations of myeloma globulins in the plasma. In addition to monoclonal immunoglobulin, myeloma cells also secrete a calcium-mobilizing substance, "osteoclast activating factor" (OAF), which stimulates local bone resorption by osteoclasts in the vicinity of foci of myeloma in the bone marrow. Simultaneously, local osteoblastic activity is inhibited. Radiographically, this may result in osteopenia resembling osteoporosis and in discrete osteolytic bone lesions as well as hypercalcemia and hypercalciuria (Fig. 163–2). Secretion of the M-component immunoglobulin appears to occur at a relatively constant rate per myeloma cell in approximately 90 per cent of myeloma patients. Availability of this tumor marker permits quantitation of the total body tumor burden because both the cellular synthetic rate of the M-component and its total body synthetic rate can be determined. "Early myeloma" is associated with a substantial tumor burden $\approx 5 \times 10^{12}$ myeloma cells (about 0.5 kg). As the total body tumor mass reaches the clinical level of detection, its growth rate slows substantially (to a doubling time of two to six months) following a typical gompertzian growth curve (see Ch. 168). Cytokinetically, this slowing of growth is associated with a fall in the fraction of tumor cells traversing the cell cycle as determined with tritiated thymidine autoradiography. Patients with extensive myeloma who are close to death generally have $>3 \times 10^{12}$ myeloma cells in the body (3.0 kg) as well as extensive lytic bone lesions and fractures and other findings characteristic of myeloma.

M-Components in Myeloma. The monoclonal immunoglobulin types that are secreted as M-component are usually IgG, IgA, or free L chains of Ig. Occasionally, the M-component will be IgD and extremely rarely, IgE. (IgM secretion is characteristically associated with macroglobulinemia.) The frequency of these different immunologic types of plasma cell disorders is roughly proportional to the serum concentration (see Table 427–1) and total body synthetic rate for the various immunoglobulins. When L chains are secreted (as dimers) into the plasma, they are rapidly extracted and metabolized by the kidney and thus are not usually detected on serum electrophoresis. When the renal threshold is exceeded, L chains appear in the urine (Bence Jones proteins). If the patient has renal failure (sometimes induced by L dimers), a serum M-component composed only of L chains may appear. L chains or L chain fragments with high tissue affinity are sometimes deposited as a characteristic infiltrative deposit ("amyloid") in certain tissues (see Immunocytic [Primary] Amyloidosis, below).

If an IgG or IgA M-component has a high intrinsic viscosity (related to molecular aggregation or asymmetry) and is present in high concentrations, hyperviscosity and bleeding disorders may develop. These complications are less common in myeloma than in macroglobulinemia. Serum M-components can induce bleeding disorders by complexing or binding immunologically with coagulation factors I, II, V, VII, or VIII. Occasionally, M-components will have narrow thermal amplitude and form cryoglobulins (including mixed cryoglobulin) and lead to Raynaud's phenomenon, impaired circulation, and potential gangrene after cold exposure. Some of these bleeding and circulatory syndromes and other immunologically predicated syndromes (e.g., hemolytic anemia, hyperlipidemia) can now be defined as being due to the M-component's having specific antibody function. These antibodies may have a low binding affinity for a normal antigenic determinant in blood or other tissue, but this may suffice for an interaction in the presence of the large amount of M-component present. Virtually all myeloma immunoglobulins are thought to have some antigen-binding specificity (as the neoplasm arises from a normal committed antibody-producing clone), but in most instances the antibody specificity of any given patient's M-protein remains unknown. Only in the exceptional clinical syndromes (such as those mentioned above) is it likely to be discovered or characterized.

Renal Failure. Renal failure is observed in at least 20 per cent of patients with myeloma and is frequently of mixed pathogenesis. Hypercalcemia produced by OAF-stimulated osteolytic bone resorption leads to calcium nephropathy and is the most common cause of renal failure in myeloma. Second in importance is the presence of heavy Bence Jones proteinuria, which also leads to tubular injury. Additional factors that may also contribute to renal failure in myeloma include hyperuricemia (in association with increased tumor cell DNA turnover), pyelonephritis, and amyloidosis. Functional abnormalities of the kidney in myeloma include acute and chronic renal failure, defects in urine concentration and acidification, and acquired Fanconi syndrome. Histologically the kidneys are usually enlarged; the glomeruli are usually normal. A characteristic "blocked pipe" appearance with eosinophilic casts surrounded by an epithelial syncytium in distal tubules and collecting ducts is the hallmark of "myeloma kidney." This is somewhat more common in patients with lambda L chain excretion.

Immunodeficiency. Patients with myeloma usually have severely depressed serum levels of normal immunoglobulins and a compromised ability to manifest a normal humoral immune response after antigenic stimulation. Consequently, they are highly susceptible to infection from common encapsulated organisms (e.g., pneumococcus), and pneumonia and other septic episodes are quite common in patients at the time of diagnosis or when they are in relapse. A series of mechanisms appears to be responsible for this immunodeficiency syndrome. In the BALB-C mouse model (and presumably in man), myeloma cells secrete an inhibitory substance (not immunoglobulin) that activates macrophage-mediated suppression of proliferation of normal antibody producing B-cell clones. Such macrophage-induced suppression of normal immunoglobulin synthesis has been observed in patients with myeloma. Additionally, in IgG myeloma the secreted IgG M-component accelerates the catabolism of the patient's normal IgG. This is because the IgG fractional catabolic rate increases as the total serum IgG concentration rises, resulting in a shorter half-life for both myeloma and normal IgG. These defects in humoral immunity are often compounded by faulty granulocyte function wherein opsonization and phagocytosis of bacteria may be impaired by the large quantities of M-protein. Finally, the number of available circulating granulocytes may be significantly reduced as a consequence of the disease or myelosuppression secondary to chemotherapy.

CLINICAL MANIFESTATIONS (Table 163–2). Presenting symptoms and signs of myeloma include bone pain (often associated with pathologic fractures of the spine or ribs), weakness resulting from anemia, recurrent infection, hypercalcemia (associated with confusion, polyuria, and constipation), and azotemia, occasionally with paralysis secondary to spinal cord compression or with bleeding disorders. Asymptomatic patients are sometimes identified by the presence of proteinuria in the absence of hypertension, or the presence of an elevated total serum protein on a multichemistry profile. Not infrequently the presentation is that of back pain, anemia, and a very high sedimentation rate in an older patient. Some patients present with acute renal failure with oliguria, especially following dehydration.

DIAGNOSIS. Patients with one or more of the aforementioned symptoms and signs require laboratory confirmation of the diagnosis of multiple myeloma. Patients may have pallor or focal bone tenderness on examination, but there are no characteristic physical findings. In advanced stages of myeloma, soft tissue plasmacytomas (usually as direct extensions from underlying ribs or other bones) may develop. Lymphadenopathy or splenomegaly are only occasional findings. The laboratory diagnosis of myeloma includes serum electrophoresis, electrophoresis of a 24-hour urine specimen (with immunologic typing of any serum and/or urine M-components found), and bone marrow aspiration. A complete skeletal x-ray survey should be carried out. Radionuclide bone scans are of little or no value because the suppression of osteoblastic activity associated with myeloma inhibits radionuclide uptake into the lesions. This is also the presumed explanation of the fact that the serum alkaline phosphatase level is usually normal despite severe bony involvement. Typical skeletal x-ray findings appear in Figure 163–2.

A complete blood count with differential, a serum calcium, one or more tests of renal function, and measurement of serum immunoglobulin levels are also useful. These tests aid in staging the patient's condition and distinguishing myeloma from other disorders. Patients suspected of having myeloma on the basis of skeletal and/or bone marrow involvement but lacking a serum M-component generally have L chain myeloma. This is usually identifiable on protein electrophoresis of a 24-hour urine concentrate. Dipsticks for detecting proteinuria are unreliable for detection of urinary L chains, and the heat test for Bence Jones proteins is positive in only about one half of cases of L chain myeloma. Urinary L chains also occur in some patients with primary amyloidosis and about 20 per cent of patients with macroglobulinemia. The rare patients with H chain disease also have urinary or serum M-components on electrophoresis. However, the clinical presentation and immunologic findings are otherwise quite different in those entities.

The definitive diagnosis of multiple myeloma requires the demonstration of plasmacytosis in the marrow or a soft tissue lesion and the presence of significant M-component production plus some evidence of invasiveness. The presence of lytic bone lesions is the best sign of invasiveness. The suppression of normal immunoglobulins, as well as anemia, hypercalcemia, azotemia, bone demineralization, compression fractures, and disease progression, is supportive in making the diagnosis when the major criteria are not all present. Other disorders that must be distinguished from myeloma include monoclonal gammopathy of unknown significance (see under Monoclonal Gammopathies of Undetermined Significance) and metastatic carcinomas. Additionally, indolent myeloma and the occasional case of solitary plasmacytoma (soft tissue) must be distinguished from myeloma because these patients do not require systemic chemotherapy. In patients with myeloma approximately 53 per cent of M-components are IgG, 25 per cent IgA, and 1 per cent IgD. About 20 per cent have apparent pure Bence Jones (L chain) myeloma, with only urinary L chain excretion. Two thirds of patients who have a serum M-component (IgG or IgA) also have concomitant Bence Jones proteinuria. Fewer than 1 per cent of patients have no definable M-component in the serum or urine. Such patients usually have L chain myeloma also, but this is masked by the ability of the kidney to completely catabolize the presented L chains. Immunofluorescent studies of the bone marrow plasma cells with anti–L chain antisera generally identify such patients. One relatively uncommon presentation of myeloma is with plasma cell leukemia. Such patients often have hepatosplenomegaly and occasionally lymphadenopathy as well as an M-component, bone lesions, and a circulating plasma cell count of greater than 2000 per cubic millimeter.

CLINICAL STAGING. As is the case in other neoplasms, quantitative staging information is useful in projecting the prognosis for individual patients and for deciding on the approach and intensity of treatment. A prognostically useful staging system has been developed for myeloma by correlating various pretreatment prognostic factors (hemoglobin, calcium, quantity of M-component secretion, and degree of skeletal involvement on x-rays) with the total body tumor cell number as measured immunologically (Table 163–3). Thus, myeloma patients can be

TABLE 163–2. CLINICAL MANIFESTATIONS OF MULTIPLE MYELOMA

Bone involvement—osteolysis due to OAF; pain; pathologic fractures; hypercalcemia
Anemia—decreased RBC production plus mild hemolysis
Renal failure—due to calcium nephropathy, L chains, uric acid, amyloid, infection, proteinuria (hypertension is rare), uremia; occasionally acute, oliguric renal failure
Recurrent infections—especially respiratory
Amyloidosis (develops in about 15 per cent)
Plasmacytomas
Rare paraprotein-associated syndromes—hyperviscosity syndrome, cryoglobulinemia, hyperlipoproteinemia
Hemorrhagic diatheses
Very high erythrocyte sedimentation rate and rouleaux formation on blood smear (with serum M-component)

TABLE 163–3. MYELOMA STAGING SYSTEM*

Stage	Criteria	Measured Myeloma Cell Mass (Cells × 10^{12} per Square Meter)
I.	*All* of the following:	<0.6 (low)
	1. Hemoglobin value >10 grams/dl	
	2. Serum calcium value (≤12 mg/dl)	
	3. On x-ray, normal bone structure (scale 0) or solitary bone plasmacytoma only	
	4. Low M-component production rates	
	a. IgG value <5 grams/dl	
	b. IgA value <3 grams/dl	
	c. Urine L chain M-component on electrophoresis <4 grams/24 hours	
II.	Fitting neither Stage I nor Stage III	0.6–1.20 (intermediate)
III.	One or more of the following:	>1.20 (high)
	1. Hemoglobin value <8.5 grams/dl	
	2. Serum calcium value >12 mg/dl	
	3. Advanced lytic bone lesions (scale 3)	
	4. High M-component production rates	
	a. IgG value >7 grams/dl	
	b. IgA value >5 grams/dl	
	c. Urine L chain M-component on electrophoresis >12 grams/24 hours	

Subclassification:
A = Relatively normal renal function (serum creatinine value <2.0 mg/dl)
B = Abnormal renal function (serum creatinine value ≥2.0 mg/dl)
Examples:
Stage IA = Low cell mass with normal renal function
Stage IIIB = High cell mass with abnormal renal function

*From Durie BGM, Salmon SE: Cancer 36:842, 1975.

categorized as being Stage I (low), II (intermediate), or III (high) with respect to tumor burden.

Impairment of renal function has an adverse effect on survival. Patients with a serum creatinine >2.0 mg per deciliter are thus staged with the additional designation B, whereas those with more normal renal function are classed as A. The effect of stage on prognosis is depicted in Figure 163–3. Patients with Stage IA disease sometimes require observation without treatment or, if available, cell kinetic studies to establish whether they actually do have progressive myeloma rather than indolent myeloma or a monoclonal gammopathy of undetermined significance. Active myeloma is associated with progressive symptoms and increasing M-component production. In vitro flash labeling of the marrow myeloma cells with tritiated thymidine reveals a significantly higher proportion of the tumor cells in DNA synthesis in myeloma than in either indolent myeloma or monoclonal gammopathy of unknown significance. Urinary L chain excretion also serves as a signal of an aggressive tumor.

TREATMENT AND PROGNOSIS. Some patients with myeloma have relatively indolent disease that, in Stage I cases, is sometimes confused with "monoclonal gammopathies of unknown significance." The overwhelming majority of patients have more advanced disease and require active systemic treatment. Two areas of treatment are important: (1) systemic chemotherapy for multiple myeloma, and (2) supportive care for treatment of complications of the disorder (e.g., spinal cord compression, bone pain, hypercalcemia, sepsis, anemia, and renal failure).

Systemic Chemotherapy. Improvements in systemic chemotherapy for multiple myeloma (in the 1960's) resulted in an increased life expectancy for these patients. Prior to this era, the median life expectancy of untreated myeloma patients was less than one year (3.5 to 8.5 months), whereas at present, with optimal chemotherapy, it is about three years on average, and up to five years or more for patients who respond to chemotherapy. Survival is also influenced by the presenting clinical stage and renal function.

Cell cycle nonspecific cytotoxic drugs (alkylating agents, nitrosoureas, and anthracycline antibiotics) have proved to be the most useful agents in the chemotherapy of myeloma. Vinca alkaloids and corticosteroids appear to potentiate the efficacy of the other cytotoxic drugs. Agents currently classed as investigational for the treatment of myeloma include human leukocyte interferon, cis-platinum, and hexamethylmelamine. Systemic chemotherapy for myeloma traditionally has employed single agent chemotherapy with an oral alkylating agent plus prednisone. To prevent complications of hypercalcemia, hyperuricemia, and azotemia, patients should be well hydrated before treatment is initiated and ambulated if at all possible. Prevention of treatment-associated hyperuricemia with allopurinol is also of value during the first few months of treatment. (Management of other complications of myeloma is described under Supportive Care.)

The single agents most widely used for the treatment of myeloma are melphalan (Alkeran, L-phenylalanine mustard) and cyclophosphamide (Cytoxan). Either can be given on a chronic low dose daily basis or in intermittent pulsed courses of therapy. Although equivalent therapeutic results appear to obtain with either of these schedules, the intermittent course approach necessitates fewer physician visits and may be associated with less late failure of hematopoietic stem cells. For the intermittent pulse schedules, melphalan is generally administered in a total dose of 8 mg per square meter per day orally for four days and repeated every three to four weeks. Alternatively, higher doses may be given with longer intervals between treatments. Cyclophosphamide is given in a dose of 0.8 gram per square meter either intravenously as a single dose or in divided daily oral doses over four days, every three to four weeks. Both of these alkylating agent schedules usually incorporate a course of 60 mg per square meter of prednisone per day for four days. The amounts given of both of the alkylating agents must be monitored closely with regard to the magnitude and duration of toxic side effects, particularly myelosuppression. Oral melphalan seems to vary significantly in

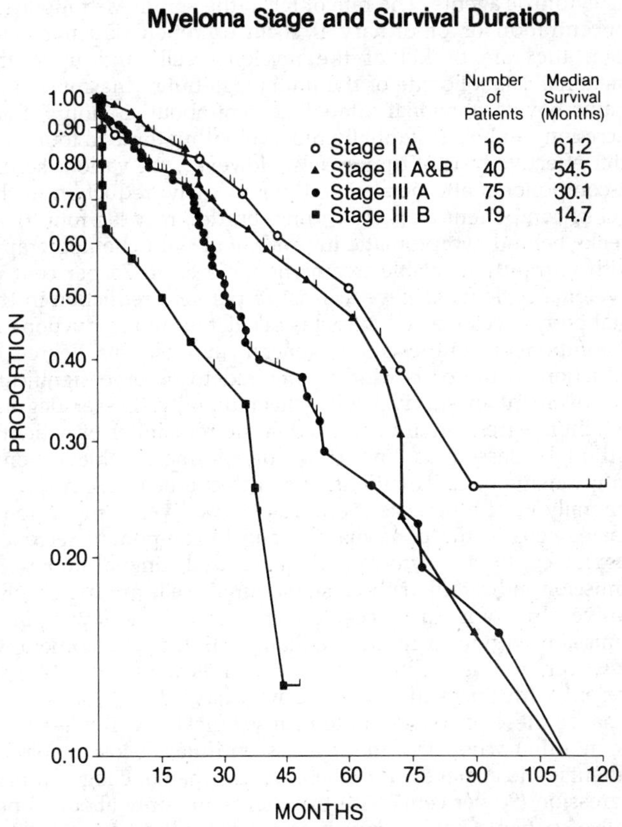

Figure 163–3. Life table survival curves for 150 patients with multiple myeloma categorized by stage. (O) Stage IA, (▲) Stages IIA and B, (●) Stage IIIA, and (■) Stage IIIB. Stage IA survival is significantly better than that of Stages IIIA and IIIB. Stages IIA and B are significantly better than Stages IIIA and IIIB. Stages IIIA and IIIB are significantly different from one another. (From Durie BGM, Salmon SE, Moon TE: Blood 55:364, 1980. With permission of the authors and publisher.)

bioavailability from patient to patient. In lieu of an assay for its plasma level, it is important to use a sufficient dose to induce some myelosuppression. Both melphalan and cyclophosphamide dosages are generally reduced if the total white blood count at the time of the next treatment is less than 3000 and the granulocyte count less than 2000 or the platelet count less than 100,000. Addition of vincristine (Oncovin) to the alkylating agent combination has produced a modest (10 to 15 per cent) improvement in responsiveness. Recently, melphalan, cyclophosphamide, and the nitrosourea carmustine (BCNU) have been combined in various ways, often with the addition of vincristine and sometimes doxorubicin (Adriamycin). Results with these more intensive regimens, including alternations of a number of active agents, appear better in high tumor burden patients (Stage III) than simple alkylating agent prednisone combinations. Whether such intensive therapy is warranted for Stage I patients remains to be defined, as the combined approaches often cause more toxicity than the simpler regimens, including more frequent and profound myelosuppression and gastrointestinal side effects.

After systemic chemotherapy is initiated, patients with responsive myeloma generally have prompt relief of bone pain and reversal of symptoms and signs of hypercalcemia, anemia, and recurrent infection. Other symptoms frequently improve, and there is often a feeling of general well-being. However, major healing of osteolytic lesions or improvement in the depressed levels of normal immunoglobulins is distinctly uncommon, suggesting some persisting cellular or humoral defect in the recovery from these two myeloma-induced abnormalities. Associated with such symptomatic and general improvement, the quantity of the M-component produced falls progressively as the myeloma cells responsible for its synthesis are killed by the cytotoxic agents. The rate of fall in the serum M-component concentration or of urinary L chain excretion depends both upon the rate of kill of the myeloma cells and upon the fractional catabolic rate of the immunoglobulin. Inasmuch as L chains have a fractional catabolic rate of about six hours, their excretion can be substantially reduced within three to four days after effective lysis of tumor cells. However, the various serum M-components are metabolized more slowly; reduction in the IgG M-component marker of tumor burden may lag four to six weeks behind symptomatic improvement with chemotherapy. With currently available treatment some 60 to 75 per cent of myeloma patients achieve at least 75 per cent reduction in the total body myeloma cell mass (as calculated from reductions in M-component synthesis). In general, at least this degree of reduction in tumor burden is required to observe significant improvement in survival with chemotherapy. Lesser degrees of tumor regression are observed in the remainder of patients. Although classed as "nonresponders," most achieve some symptomatic benefit. Patients who achieve objective response generally have a persistent and stable low level of monoclonal plasma cells in the bone marrow and M-component secretion despite continued cytotoxic therapy. Cell kinetic studies in remission indicate that the residual tumor cells are hypoproliferative. In some instances, patients can be followed in a remission without continued administration of chemotherapy. However, this is a difficult course to follow in patients who present with Stage III disease or who have Bence Jones myeloma, as these patients tend to relapse quickly (within less than six months) when treatment is discontinued. Most myeloma patients who achieve remission have less than one log of tumor regression (90 per cent) with treatment, and only about 10 per cent of patients have as much as a two log regression (99 per cent). Thus, even in remission, there is a large subclinical residue of tumor cells (greater than 10^{10} tumor cells). Even though many of these cells may not be in the tumor stem cell compartment, there is still a sufficient number of malignant cells present to lead to eventual relapse in virtually all patients with multiple myeloma. Cures will require development of more effective therapy in the future. Patients who present with renal failure and those whose tumor clones produce only L chains (particularly of the λ type) tend to have a poorer response to treatment with more frequent early relapse and shorter survival than those who present with a serum M-component. Outcome in IgG cases also tends to be somewhat better than that in IgA cases. Among Stage III patients, the fraction of the tumor cells in DNA synthesis (growth fraction) also affects prognosis, with the patients with a high growth fraction having relatively brief responses to treatment and short survival. Patients presenting with plasma cell leukemia also have a high growth fraction, poor response to treatment, and short survival.

Patients with tumors exhibiting a high growth fraction tend to respond very quickly to chemotherapy, with a rapid fall in the M-component to remission levels (e.g., within six weeks), but then relapse quickly. More durable responses require three to eight months to achieve. For patients who achieve objective remission, serial monitoring of the quantity of serum and/or urinary M-component on electrophoresis or with nephelometry provides an excellent means for assessing the stability of the remission and for detecting relapse at its earliest stages, often before the patient develops recurrent hypercalcemia or new lytic lesions.

Most patients with myeloma who achieve 75 per cent tumor regression remain in remission for at least three years before they relapse, as manifested by a rising M-component or new symptoms. Only occasional Stage III patients are still in remission beyond six years after the diagnosis (Fig. 163–3). Some useful approaches to secondary chemotherapy have been devised that are beneficial to patients who relapse from primary treatment. For example, there is not complete cross-resistance between melphalan and cyclophosphamide, and patients relapsing after treatment with one of these agents will occasionally respond to the other. A more useful approach has been that of the intravenous combination of carmustine (BCNU) and doxorubicin (Adriamycin) with each drug administered at a dosage of 30 mg per square meter every three weeks. Vincristine (Oncovin) and prednisone can be administered along with these drugs in an attempt to potentiate their effect. About one half of patients who initially respond to alkylating agents can achieve second remissions with these agents. Second remissions rarely last longer than one year. The terminal phase of myeloma is characterized by symptoms and signs of progressive growth of the drug-resistant tumor (e.g., bone pain, hypercalcemia, fractures, rising M-component, anemia, and renal failure). A late complication of treatment of myeloma (particularly with melphalan) is injury of normal bone marrow stem cells. This injury can result in development of a chronic refractory sideroblastic anemia or acute myelogenous leukemia. It has been projected that well over 5 per cent of myeloma patients may eventually develop leukemia as a result of treatment. However, the risk-benefit ratio for myeloma patients still favors use of systemic chemotherapy. The immediate cause of death is frequently sepsis or renal failure. Recent advances in chemotherapy have resulted in some improvement in the prognosis for patients with myeloma. Better results will require the identification of new drugs with significant antimyeloma activity.

Supportive Care. Patients with newly diagnosed myeloma and those in relapse often have problems that require immediate or emergency management that may have to be carried out concomitantly with initiation of chemotherapy.

HYPERCALCEMIA AND OSTEOLYSIS. Hypercalcemia as a metabolic complication of osteolysis is common in myeloma; the serum calcium should be determined initially even in patients lacking the characteristic symptoms of confusion, irritability, and constipation. The effects of hypercalcemia relate to the ionized fraction, which is greater when the serum albumin is low. When serum calcium is only modestly elevated (e.g., 11.5 to 12 mg per deciliter), hydration with several liters of intravenous saline, alone or with furosemide, will often suffice until the effect of systemic chemotherapy can induce a more sustained reduction in the calcium. Ambulation should be encouraged, as it also reduces bone resorption. Oral phosphate solutions (Fleet's phosphosoda enemas) may also prove useful for mild hypercalcemia if renal function is not impaired and the serum phosphate is not elevated. Greater degrees of hypercalcemia (serum calcium >12 mg per deciliter) represent a medical emergency because of both cardiac and renal effects, and often require the addition of more aggressive measures, including large doses of corticosteroids. Injections of calcitonin or mithramycin are also indicated if serum calcium is very high (e.g., >14 mg per deciliter) or if the response to steroids is not rapid. Mithramycin (25 μg per kilogram of body weight) can often normalize the serum calcium in less than 24 hours, but frequently repeated injections are undesirable, as they can induce thrombocytopenia, which may compromise the ability to administer systemic chemotherapy for myeloma. (See Ch. 246 for a further discussion of the treatment of hypercalcemia.)

SPINAL CORD COMPRESSION. Developing neurologic symptoms in the lower extremities plus focal back pain in a patient with myeloma should lead to an emergency evaluation for the possibility of cord compression secondary to an extradural plasmacytoma. Consultations involving neurology, radiation therapy, and neurosurgery should be obtained promptly. If the diagnosis is established with myelography before paralysis develops, the chance for recovery of neurologic function with high dose steroids and emergency radiotherapy (with or without laminectomy) is excellent. Delays in diagnosis or therapy (even 12 hours) can leave the patient with irreversible paraplegia.

BONE PAIN. Bone pain caused by expanding plasmacytomas can usually be managed with analgesics and systemic chemotherapy. In some instances a single bone lesion will be responsible for the patient's pain. Such focal lesions can usually be palliated effectively and quickly with moderate doses of local radiotherapy (2000 to 3000 rads). Radiotherapy generally should be used only if pain is not relieved promptly with chemotherapy, and it should be limited to a relatively small field, as it impairs normal bone marrow function. Long delays in systemic chemotherapy for administration of radiotherapy should be avoided, as new bone lesions often develop during such intervals.

ANEMIA. Transfusion of packed red blood cells is often required in the initial management of Stage III myeloma patients. Occasionally, normal hematopoiesis can be stimulated with androgens. Other hematinics (iron, folic acid, vitamin B_{12}) are not of value. Patients experiencing an objective response to myeloma chemotherapy generally have a rise in hemoglobin of several grams during the first year after initiation of treatment.

INFECTION. Because of the known increased incidence of bacterial infection in myeloma (particularly pneumococcal), various efforts have been made to prevent infection. Immunization with polyvalent pneumococcal vaccine would not be anticipated to be worthwhile because of the profound defect that myeloma patients have in responding to carbohydrate antigens. Prophylactic administration of large doses of gamma globulin has been tried, but has proved ineffective, in part because of the hypercatabolism of all IgG in patients with IgG myeloma. Prophylactic use of antibiotics (penicillin, ampicillin) is of some benefit in infection-prone patients. If the patient can be depended upon to recognize the earliest signs of infection, then prompt treatment at the time of fever or sputum production will usually suffice. When a patient with myeloma has a major septic episode, bactericidal antibiotics must be administered in adequate dosage. Nephrotoxic antibiotics (e.g., aminoglycosides) should be avoided in view of the frequency of overt or subclinical renal impairment in myeloma.

RENAL INSUFFICIENCY. Renal failure is a major cause of death in multiple myeloma. The major causes of renal failure are hypercalcemia and Bence Jones proteinuria. Both are potentially treatable. The patient should be kept well hydrated, and treated promptly for hypercalcemia when it is present. Allopurinol should also be used to prevent hyperuricemia and hyperuricosuria. Intravenous pyelography can precipitate renal failure in myeloma patients (perhaps because of dehydration) and should be approached with caution and with maintenance of hydration. Acute renal failure should be treated aggressively with standard measures, including hemodialysis, with the understanding that it may no longer be required if the injury is not too severe and if a good response is seen to chemotherapy. Some patients in remission have been supported with long-term hemodialysis. Chronic dialysis is clearly not indicated if the patient fails to achieve clinical remission with systemic chemotherapy.

VARIANT FORMS OF MYELOMA. ***Indolent Myeloma.*** About 5 per cent of patients under evaluation for multiple myeloma have a more indolent form of the disease with a life expectancy of up to ten years. Such patients are currently difficult to identify prospectively without specialized testing or a period of observation without treatment. Some are asymptomatic patients diagnosed after routine biochemical studies. One or two lytic bone lesions may be present. Most such patients are in Stage I, and significant bone pain, hypercalcemia, azotemia, and Bence Jones proteinuria are absent. The tumor cells in indolent myeloma are hypoproliferative with a tumor cell tritiated thymidine labeling index of less than 0.5 per cent. Patients with indolent myeloma can be followed symptomatically without initiation of systemic chemotherapy. This group is relatively rare, however, and it is probably better to err on the side of treatment if the evidence for indolence is equivocal.

Solitary Myeloma. Occasional patients present with an apparently solitary myeloma. Bilateral core bone marrow biopsies from the iliac spine and a sternal aspirate, as well as electrophoretic studies of the blood and urine, should be performed in all cases thought to involve a solitary lesion. Only about half of patients with solitary myeloma have a demonstrable M-component, and even then a relatively small one. The normal immunoglobulins should also not be depressed in patients with a solitary lesion. Those involving soft tissues (particularly in the head and neck region) have a relatively high probability of being solitary and can often be managed with local surgery and radiation therapy. After effective local treatment of a soft tissue plasmacytoma, myeloma proteins in the blood or urine should disappear promptly. If they do not, occult dissemination can be predicted. In general, patients with solitary soft tissue plasmacytoma will not require chemotherapy.

In contrast, patients with apparently solitary myeloma of bone generally do have additional occult disease. They also frequently respond unusually well to systemic chemotherapy after the original local focus is treated with about 4000 rads of radiotherapy. In the author's experience, patients with apparently solitary myeloma of bone can often be followed in unmaintained remission after the initial year of treatment with radiation and chemotherapy.

Alexanian R: Localized and indolent myeloma. Blood 56:521, 1980. *Criteria are defined for recognizing patients with localized myeloma of bone or solitary plasmacytoma, and evidence given favoring delay of chemotherapy.*

Bergsagel DE, Bailey AJ, Langley GR, et al.: The chemotherapy of plasma cell myeloma and the incidence of acute leukemia. N Engl J Med 301:743, 1979. *Report of a recent large scale chemotherapy trial which places the incidence of acute leukemia in perspective.*

Broder SB, Humphrey R, Durn M, Blackman M, Meade B, Goldman C, Strober W, Waldmann T: Impaired synthesis of polyclonal (non-paraprotein) immunoglobulins by circulating lymphocytes from patients with multiple myeloma. N Engl J Med 293:887, 1975. *This clinical investigation clearly implicates the circulating peripheral blood monocyte in the suppression of immunoglobulin synthesis by normal B cells in multiple myeloma.*

Durie BGM, Salmon SE, Moon TE: Pretreatment tumor mass, cell kinetics and prognosis in multiple myeloma. Blood 55:364, 1980. *A detailed analysis of tumor cell burden, thymidine labeling, response to treatment, and survival in myeloma which identifies kinetically unfavorable patient groups.*

Kyle RA, Bayrd ED: The Monoclonal Gammopathies. Springfield, Ill., Charles C Thomas, 1976. *A very good summary text on multiple myeloma and related plasma cell disorders. Historical perspectives, clinical features, and laboratory diagnostic procedures are particularly well delineated.*

Salmon SE (ed.): Myeloma and Related Disorders. Clin Haematol Vol II, 1982. *An up-to-date review by leading clinical investigators of major clinical and research advances that pertain to multiple myeloma and related entities.*

Salmon SE, Hamburger AW, Soehnlen BJ, et al.: Quantitation of differential sensitivity of human tumor stem cells to anticancer drugs. N Engl J Med 298:1321, 1978. *This paper describes an in vitro technique for measuring drug sensitivity and predicting response to treatment in multiple myeloma and other disorders.*

Salmon SE, Haut A, Bonnet JD et al.: Alternating combination chemotherapy improves survival in multiple myeloma: A Southwest Oncology Group Study. J Clin Oncol 1:453, 1983. *Recent evidence supporting the use of aggressive combination chemotherapy for advanced stage myeloma patients.*

MACROGLOBULINEMIA OF WALDENSTRÖM

DEFINITION. Waldenström's macroglobulinemia is characterized by the proliferation and accumulation of malignant cells with lymphoplasmacytic morphology that secrete IgM M-components. Sites of B cell development, including the bone marrow, lymph nodes, and spleen, are usually involved. Major clinical manifestations of the disorder are related to hyperviscosity of the circulating intravascular macroglobulin. The disease has some similarities with myeloma, lymphoma, and chronic lymphocytic leukemia.

ETIOLOGY AND PATHOPHYSIOLOGY. Waldenström's macroglobulinemia is of unknown etiology, but appears to have a slightly increased familial incidence. It has a slight male predominance and increases in incidence with age, usually beginning in the fifth or sixth decade. The neoplasm appears to originate in a plasmacytic lymphocyte in the B cell series, which proliferates in the bone marrow and/or lymph nodes and spleen. Cytogenetic markers are sometimes found but are nonspecific. IgM M-components frequently have physiochemical properties that lead to hyperviscosity, cryoprecipitation, or bleeding phenomena. In contrast to myeloma, osteolysis, renal impairment, and amyloidosis are all quite rare in macroglobulinemia.

CLINICAL FEATURES. The clinical onset of macroglobulinemia is often gradual and associated with increasing weakness, fatigue, epistaxis, or other bleeding manifestations. Recurrent infection, visual difficulties, weight loss, or neurologic symptoms are also common. Bone pain is not a symptom of macroglobulinemia, and skeletal x-rays are usually unremarkable. On physical examination, patients often exhibit pallor, lymphadenopathy, and hepatosplenomegaly. Ophthalmoscopic examination usually reveals marked dilatation and vascular segmentation of the retinal veins ("sausage links") secondary to hyperviscosity, and occasional retinal hemorrhages and exudates. About one fourth of macroglobulinemic patients present with neurologic signs secondary to slow blood flow or sludging, including peripheral neuropathy, transient paresis, abnormal reflexes, headache, dizziness, deafness, and/or impaired state of consciousness or coma. Hyperviscosity also leads to bleeding and oozing from mucous membranes. Such symptoms and signs of hyperviscosity are uncommon when the serum viscosity is less than 4 units (normal, 1.4 to 1.8) and increase dramatically in frequency with values above 6 units.

Laboratory findings include a normochromic normocytic anemia, which is partially due to a reduced red cell mass and partially to an expanded plasma volume as a result of hyperviscosity. Rouleaux formation is quite prominent, and the sedimentation rate is increased markedly unless plasma gelation occurs. Plasmacytic lymphocytes are often present on the blood smear and are sometimes present in leukemic proportions. Coombs-positive hemolytic anemia or cold hemagglutinins are occasional findings. (The cold hemagglutinin syndrome is a variant of macroglobulinemia.) An M-component is present on serum electrophoresis in macroglobulinemia and can be shown to be monoclonal IgM with immunoelectrophoresis. Eighty per cent of IgM M-components have κ L chains, and the remaining 20 per cent are λ. Most macroglobulins will precipitate in distilled water (Sia test); however, this test is nonspecific. About 10 per cent of macroglobulins have cryoglobulin properties; some will form gels as the patient's blood is drawn unless a prewarmed syringe is used and subsequent separative procedures are carried out at 37° C. Bence Jones (L chain) proteinuria is also present in 10 per cent of patients with macroglobulinemia. The serum viscosity is usually elevated. Normal immunoglobulins (IgG or IgA) are commonly reduced. The bone marrow aspirate usually reveals a substantial infiltrate with plasmacytic lymphocytes and plasma cells.

DIAGNOSIS. The diagnosis of Waldenström's macroglobulinemia requires the presence of typical symptoms and signs, the presence of an IgM M-component of greater than 3 grams per deciliter, and histologic evidence on bone marrow aspirate or biopsy. The differential diagnosis from chronic lymphocytic leukemia, lymphoma, multiple myeloma, and monoclonal gammopathies of undetermined significance depends upon the presence of characteristic immunologic and clinical features. Intermediate forms with characteristics of several of these related B cell disorders occasionally occur. IgM elevations of smaller magnitude are also seen in a variety of infectious and inflammatory disease, including those listed in Table 163–1.

TREATMENT AND PROGNOSIS. Patients with macroglobulinemia who present with a severe hyperviscosity syndrome and marked neurologic findings (e.g., impending coma or paresis) or serious bleeding should be treated by intensive emergency plasmapheresis. This is best accomplished with an intermittent or continuous flow blood cell separator, although standard centrifuge techniques with plasmapheresis packs can also be used. Red cell transfusion and/or volume replacement are generally required, as 6 to 8 liters of plasma may have to be removed during the first two to four days. Plasmapheresis is quite effective in macroglobulinemia because 90 per cent of the M-component remains in the intravascular compartment as a result of its high molecular weight.

Inasmuch as plasmapheresis removes only a troublesome tumor product and does not alter the underlying tumor, specific therapy requires the suppression of the neoplasm with systemic chemotherapy.

Chlorambucil (Leukeran) is usually administered orally at a dosage of 6 to 8 mg per day, with dosage adjustments made in accord with the WBC and platelet count. Although chlorambucil is well tolerated, the various drug regimens used in the treatment of multiple myeloma are useful in macroglobulinemia and are quite acceptable alternatives. Once patients achieve remission with chemotherapy (at least 80 per cent of cases), intermittent plasmapheresis can usually be discontinued. Systemic treatment is usually continued indefinitely in macroglobulinemia, since treatment, although suppressive, does not eradicate the IgM producing clone.

The median survival in macroglobulinemia is about three years; however, many patients may have an indolent disease and may survive for ten years or more.

MacKenzie MR, Fudenberg HH: Macroglobulinemia: An analysis of 40 patients. Blood 39:874, 1972. *Useful review of clinical and laboratory features of macroglobulinemia of Waldenström.*

Waldenström J: Studies on conditions associated with disturbed gamma globulin formation (gammopathies). Harvey Lect Series 56:211, 1961. *A lengthy and stimulating discussion of macroglobulinemia and related plasma cell disorders by the clinical investigator who first described macroglobulinemia.*

HEAVY CHAIN DISEASES

The heavy chain diseases are a group of rare lymphoplasmacytic neoplasms associated with secretion of a monoclonal heavy chain or heavy chain fragment by the neoplastic cells. Thus far, H chain diseases related to the three major immunoglobulin classes have been reported (γ, α, μ). The clinical syndromes vary with H chain type but have some similarities with other B cell neoplasms.

GAMMA (γ) CHAIN DISEASE. This syndrome was the first heavy chain disease to be recognized. More than 40 cases have been reported. The symptoms and clinical presentation are similar to those of malignant lymphomas; the patients frequently have recurrent infections, lymphadenopathy, and hepatosplenomegaly. Characteristically, edema of the soft palate and uvula associated with Waldeyer's ring involvement has been observed in γ heavy chain diseases. Normochromic normocytic anemia is typical, and many patients are pancytopenic save for an eosinophilia. Several patients have also manifested plasma cell leukemia, but skeletal lesions are uncommon.

Histologic studies of the lymph nodes and bone marrow usually reveal a pleomorphic infiltrate of lymphoplasmacytic and large lymphoid cells and eosinophils, abnormalities reminiscent of Hodgkin's disease.

All patients have free γ heavy chains present in the serum and urine determined by immunologic and electrophoretic techniques. The urinary protein lacks the heat properties of L chains. Immunoelectrophoresis shows the monoclonal peak to have γ chain determinants but to lack κ or λ L chains. Of interest, there is a large deletion (200 amino acids) in the variable region of the γ chain. As in myeloma and macroglobulinemia, normal immunoglobulins are reduced. Although some patients have pursued a rapid downhill course, use of intensive combination chemotherapy (as in diffuse lymphomas) has resulted in long survival in some patients.

ALPHA (α) CHAIN DISEASE. This rare and interesting syndrome has a characteristic genetic and geographic distribution and is about twice as common as γ chain disease. It has been observed predominantly in young Arabs and non-Ashkenazic Jews living in the Middle East ("Mediterranean lymphoma"). However, the disease does occur in patients of other ethnic backgrounds. Patients usually present with abdominal discomfort and weight loss owing to malabsorption and diarrhea and have extensive mesenteric and small intestinal lymphatic involvement with lymphoma (see Ch. 103). The lamina propria is extensively infiltrated with neoplastic plasma cells. Cellular morphology is similar to that in γ chain disease; however, marrow involvement is rare. Pulmonary involvement has been observed in two children with α chain disease.

Immunodiagnosis of α chain disease is relatively difficult, as a sharp M-component spike is usually not observed in the serum or urine, and the entity must be thought of in patients with intestinal lymphoma. α Chains have a tendency to polymerize and thereby become heterodisperse on electrophoresis, giving the appearance of either a normal serum electrophoresis or diffuse hypergammaglobulinemia. Immunoelectrophoresis, however, demonstrates that only the α chain is present and that L chains are absent. More detailed structural studies have proved the α chains to be monoclonal. Only about half of the patients have had free α chain in the urine, presumably because of the tendency for formation of large complexes which do not pass the glomerulus. Although most cases of α chain disease have been fatal, some patients have achieved remissions with chemotherapy. A few patients have achieved remission with antimicrobial therapy, suggesting that an infectious agent may underlie this unusual monoclonal B cell proliferation.

MU (μ) CHAIN DISEASE. Secretion of free μ heavy chains into the plasma is a rare occurrence in chronic lymphocytic leukemia. The seven patients reported have had longstanding CLL with retroperitoneal adenopathy and hepatosplenomegaly. Bone marrow aspiration has shown vacuolated lymphoplasmacytic cells. Hypogammaglobulinemia was seen on serum electrophoresis, and immunoelectrophoresis was required to detect the small amount of free μ chains. Most of the patients also had substantial amounts of κ L chain in the urine. The monoclonal lymphoid cells of the neoplasm appear to have a defect in H-L chain assembly, as intracellular L chains are detectable but do not assemble normally into IgM prior to secretion.

Franklin EC, Lowenstein J, Bigelow B, Meltzer M: Heavy chain disease—a new disorder of serum γ-globulins: Report of the first case. Am J Med 37:332, 1964. *Excellent immunologic analysis of the first reported patient with γ-heavy chain disease.*

Franklin EC: μ-Chain disease. Arch Intern Med 135:71, 1975. *The major clinical features of μ-chain disease are summarized.*

Seligman M: Immunochemical, clinical and pathological features of α chain disease. Arch Intern Med 135:71, 1975. *A clinically relevant immunologic description of α-chain disease.*

IMMUNOCYTIC (PRIMARY) AMYLOIDOSIS (see also Ch. 210)

DEFINITION. Amyloidosis is not a single disease entity but a term applied to a complex of disorders associated with deposition of insoluble fibrillar proteins in virtually pure form in various tissues of the body. The disease complex was first designated "amyloid" in the 1850's by Virchow, who considered the "waxy, eosinophilic" homogeneous and amorphous tissue deposits to be composed of polysaccharide or starch-like substances. Amyloid stains pink with hematoxylin and eosin and metachromatically with methyl or crystal violet. Congo red stain produces green birefringence under polarized light and is the most specific light microscopic stain for amyloid. Under the electron microscope, amyloid has a characteristic fibrillar B-pleated sheet structure. This structure is not found in normal mammalian tissues.

A complete description of the various forms of amyloidosis is contained in Chapter 210 and a classification based on the chemistry of the amyloid fibrils is presented in Table 210–1. Since immunocytic (primary or AL) amyloidosis may shade into the plasma cell disorders, a further brief summary is given here.

PATHOPHYSIOLOGY. Amyloid fibrils from primary amyloidosis are homogeneous and homologous to the variable region fragment of either κ or λ L chains (Ig-V_L) and thus have been defined as immunoglobulin amyloid-fibril proteins (AL). There is a clear relationship between amyloid-fibril deposits and Bence Jones proteins, which are related to multiple myeloma and related plasma cell disorders. Furthermore, AL appear to be produced in these disorders through a proteolytic mechanism to which only certain free L chains (and not intact Ig components) are susceptible. Such "amyloidogenic" L chains are more frequently of λ than κ L chain type. The characteristic "B-pleated sheet" amyloid fibrils can be produced in vitro by treating certain Bence Jones proteins with proteolytic enzymes. As a result of these studies and the finding of AL type amyloid fibrils in association with virtually all monoclonal gammopathies (including myeloma, macroglobulinemia, H chain diseases, B cell lymphoid neoplasms, and gammopathies of unknown significance) as well as agammaglobulinemia, Glenner proposed that primary amyloidosis be designated *immunocytic amyloid*. This designation clearly has a recognizable relationship to the pathophysiology of amyloid formation in monoclonal B cell disorders.

CLINICAL FEATURES. Patients with immunocytic amyloid present with complaints of weakness, weight loss, ankle swelling, paresthesias, and lightheadedness. Symptoms of multiple myeloma may also be present when the amyloid is associated with that disorder (about 15 per cent of myeloma cases). Major physical findings of immunocytic amyloid include enlargement

TABLE 163–4. CLASSIFICATION OF THE ACQUIRED SYSTEMIC AMYLOIDOSES (β-Fibrilloses)

Classification	Major Protein Component
A. Immunocytic amyloidosis	
1. No evidence of coexisting disease	AL
2. Multiple myeloma	AL
3. Other monoclonal gammopathy	AL
4. Agammaglobulinemia	AL
B. Reactive systemic amyloidosis	AA
1. Acute recurrent and chronic infections	AA
2. Chronic inflammatory conditions (e.g., rheumatoid arthritis)	AA
C. Localized amyloid (involvement of a single organ without generalized involvement)	AL
D. Familial amyloidosis	AA, PA

AL = Amyloid light chain.
AA = Amyloid A (protein A).
PA = Prealbumin amyloid.

of the tongue, purpura, hepatomegaly, and occasional splenomegaly. Skin manifestations can include plaques, papules, or nodules. Involvement of periarticular regions can give an appearance similar to that of rheumatoid arthritis. Involvement of the glenohumoral joint leads to a characteristic "shoulder pad sign." Periorbital purpura may appear spontaneously or after straining ("raccoon eyes"). Purpuric bleeding is sometimes associated with an acquired deficiency of factor X. Ankle edema in amyloidosis is often associated with congestive heart failure or the nephrotic syndrome. Heart failure occurs in about 30 per cent of patients, and renal involvement is a leading cause of death. The carpal tunnel syndrome, peripheral neuropathy, and orthostatic hypotension are additional associations with amyloid infiltration.

Laboratory findings include evidence of anemia and/or renal failure in about half of the patients. Ninety per cent have proteinuria. Serum immunoelectrophoresis reveals an M-component in about half of the patients with amyloidosis and in three quarters of those with amyloid associated with myeloma. Addition of urinary immunoelectrophoresis permits detection of an M-component in almost 90 per cent of cases. λ L chain excretion is more common than κ (2 to 1) in amyloidosis. Some increase in marrow plasma cells is common.

Diagnosis of amyloidosis requires tissue biopsy and demonstration of amyloid deposition by the green birefringence of the Congo red stain by polarization microscopy. If easily obtained, the initial biopsy should be of the organ suspected of being infiltrated with amyloid. Alternatively, the first biopsy may be taken from the rectal mucosa, as it is relatively safe and easy to obtain, and with adequate tissue is positive in more than 75 per cent of cases. Other useful biopsy sites include the gingiva, skin, kidney, and carpal ligament (in patients with the carpal tunnel syndrome). Endomyocardial biopsy via catheter has led to the detection of amyloid in unexplained cases of cardiac failure.

TREATMENT. Because of the relationship of AL amyloid to monoclonal plasma cell proliferation, systemic chemotherapy with alkylating agent–prednisone combinations has been tried with some evidence of improvement or halting in progression of amyloid deposition. Therefore, a trial of therapy similar to that used for myeloma is warranted. Unfortunately, treatment has not yet significantly improved survival, and new approaches are needed. Colchicine has been tried in AL amyloid without proven success. Supportive measures in systemic amyloidosis include management of cardiac and renal failure. Congestive heart failure caused by amyloid does not usually respond to cardiac glycosides, and sudden deaths from arrhythmia have been reported. Diuretics have been useful for relief of edema.

The prognosis in systemic immunocytic amyloidosis is poor. In one recent review of 236 cases, the average survival was 14.7 months for patients without underlying myeloma (about 50 to 60 per cent of cases) and four months for those with amyloidosis and myeloma (about 20 per cent of cases).

Buxbaum JN, Hurley ME, Chuba J, Spira T: Amyloidosis of the AL type: Clinical, morphologic, and biochemical aspects of the response to therapy with alkylating agents and prednisone. Am J Med 67:867, 1979.

Durie BGM, Persky B, Soehnlen BJ, Grogan TM, Salmon SE: Amyloid production in human myeloma stem-cell culture, with morphologic evidence of amyloid secretion by associated macrophages. N Engl J Med 307:1689, 1982.

Kyle RA, Greipp PR: Amyloidosis (AL), clinical and laboratory features in 229 cases. Mayo Clin Proc 58:665, 1983. *The best current review of this entity drawing upon the extensive Mayo experience.*

MONOCLONAL GAMMOPATHIES OF UNDETERMINED SIGNIFICANCE

If a patient has an M-component in the serum but lacks other diagnostic findings for myeloma, macroglobulinemia, or one of the other plasma cell neoplasms, the disorder is best classified as monoclonal gammopathy of unknown significance (MGUS). Formerly, the term "benign monoclonal gammopathy" was applied; however, this term is misleading, as some patients in this category do, in fact, develop myeloma or macroglobulinemia after a period of follow-up. Serum M-components without other signs of myeloma or macroglobulinemia occur in about 1 per cent of the population above age 50 and 3 per cent above age 70. Most of these persons never develop signs of a malignant plasma cell disorder. A number of patients have been followed for 15 years or more without developing myeloma.

Patients with monoclonal gammopathy of unknown significance have relatively small M-components present in the serum (usually less than 2 grams per deciliter) and do not excrete urinary L chains (Bence Jones protein). The bone marrow plasma cell percentage is generally less than 5 per cent. Marrow plasma cells from patients with MGUS have an extremely low tritiated thymidine labeling index (less than 0.5 per cent). When anemia, osteolytic lesions, hypercalcemia, Bence Jones proteinuria, or renal failure is present, the patient does not fall in the category of having a monoclonal gammopathy of undetermined significance and should be considered to have a malignant disorder. The levels of nonmonoclonal immunoglobulins are sometimes normal in monoclonal gammopathy of unknown significance, but this does not provide significant differentiation between benign and malignant plasma cell disorders. If there is only a serum M-component and no clear associated disease demonstrable by baseline observations, the patient should be followed without any treatment for the monoclonal gammopathy. In general, the patient should be seen at least every three months during the first year and at intervals of six months thereafter. If the monoclonal protein increases by 50 per cent on repeated serum electrophoresis, then a complete re-evaluation is warranted. In Kyle's five-year study of the natural history of 241 cases of monoclonal gammopathy of unknown significance, 57 per cent of patients retained stable protein levels; 9 per cent had a 50 per cent increase in the serum M-component or developed Bence Jones proteinuria; 23 per cent died without five-year serum studies; and 11 per cent developed myeloma, macroglobulinemia, or amyloidosis.

OTHER DISEASES ASSOCIATED WITH MONOCLONAL GAMMOPATHY. Patients with a variety of diseases have also been observed to have a monoclonal gammopathy of unknown significance. Among neoplastic diseases, monoclonal gammopathy has been observed in association with colonic cancer and certain other carcinomas, as well as with several B cell neoplasms (chronic lymphocytic leukemia and various lymphomas). Although M-components in lymphoid neoplasia may relate to their B cell origin and function, the explanation in nonlymphoid neoplasms remains obscure and could be coincidental. Several surveys of nonlymphoid neoplasms suggest that the incidence of monoclonal gammopathy in this patient group is no greater than for the general population of that age range.

Among non-neoplastic disorders, a monoclonal gammopathy is regularly associated with the rare skin disorder lichen myxedematosus (papular mucinosis). Patients with this disorder have diffuse progressive deposition of protein in the dermis in association with the presence of a highly cationic IgG M-component, which usually has λ L chains. Monoclonal gammopathies are occasionally associated with other disorders, including Gaucher's disease, hepatitis and other liver diseases, collagen vascular diseases, and myasthenia gravis. Transient monoclonal gammopathies are sometimes observed after bone marrow transplantation, particularly in children with immunodeficiency syndrome.

Kyle RA: Monoclonal gammopathy of undetermined significance. Natural history in 241 cases. Am J Med 64:814, 1978. *An excellent and detailed analysis of the Mayo Clinic experience.*

Miglione PJ, Alexanian R: Monoclonal gammopathy in human neoplasia. Cancer 21:1127, 1968. *These authors analyze the experience at M.D. Anderson Hospital in Houston and suggest that monoclonal gammopathy associated with neoplasms other than myeloma or macroglobulinemia is only coincidental.*

Talerman A, Haije WG: The frequency of M-components in sera of patients with solid malignant neoplasms. Br J Cancer 27:276, 1973.

164. DISEASES OF THE SPLEEN

Richard A. Rifkind

Confusion has existed since earliest times over the role of the spleen, Galen's "organ of mystery," with respect to normal physiology and disease. The spleen is responsible for at least four major physiologic functions, calling into play its unique cellular and anatomic characteristics: (1) *A hemoclastic function,* concerned with sequestration, pooling, remodeling, and destruction of normal and pathologic blood cells. (2) *A role as an organ of the immune system,* although not an indispensable immunologic organ, because its immunologic functions are shared with the other lymphoreticular organs. Nevertheless, the spleen serves an important function in protection from blood-borne microorganisms. (3) *A hematopoietic function.* During normal embryogenesis and under conditions when the marrow is invaded or is stimulated to expand beyond its capacity to respond, the spleen may become a major site of extramedullary hematopoiesis. (4) *A role in the regulation of portal blood flow.* The splenic vasculature plays a contributory role in the *regulation of portal blood flow* and, by mechanisms not as yet fully established, has an effect on salt and water metabolism and total plasma volume. The discussion will describe these several functional properties of the spleen in relationship to *hyposplenism,* resulting most commonly from surgical ablation or vascular accidents; to *splenomegaly;* and to that particular hematologic syndrome termed *hypersplenism,* which sometimes, but by no means invariably, accompanies splenomegaly.

NORMAL ANATOMY AND FUNCTIONS. The principal anatomic components of the spleen are (1) its capsule, composed of a fibrous connective tissue, and extensions of the capsule in the form of trabeculae that course throughout the organ carrying blood vessels, efferent lymphatics, and nerves; (2) a complex and unique branching arterial tree and its venous return; (3) a cordal and sinusoidal system forming the *red pulp;* and (4) lymphoid tissues, which constitute the *white pulp* (see accompanying figure). The splenic artery divides to form trabecular arteries, which in turn divide to form central arteries, each surrounded by a sheath of thymus-dependent or T lymphocytes, as well as lymph follicles composed principally of non-thymus-dependent B lymphocytes and their plasma cell progeny. Follicular arteries come off each central artery in a manner creating a skimming effect of the blood, sending a cell-poor, plasma-rich fraction to the white pulp. These follicular arteries serve as the afferent lymphatics for the splenic white pulp; no traditional afferent lymphatic vessels have been detected in this organ. This unique feature of the splenic lymphoid tissues provides the organ with its special ability to clear blood-borne microorganisms.

Leaving the white pulp, the central arteries divide into small penicillar arteries that deliver a plasma-poor, cell-rich blood to the cords and sinusoids of the red pulp. Although there are, perhaps, direct connections between the terminal penicillar arterioles and the splenic sinusoids, achieving a closed circulation from the arterial to the venous vasculature, a significant portion of this terminal splenic blood flow enters directly into the splenic cords and must navigate this anatomic filtration system in order to reach the venous circulation. The ultrastructural anatomy of splenic cords and sinusoids is particularly critical to the hemoclastic functions of the spleen.

The splenic (Billroth) cords constitute a true vascular sieve, in the form of a feltwork of loose reticular connective tissue containing macrophages and monocytes and separated by a fenestrated basement membrane from the splenic sinusoids. The sinusoidal basement membrane and endothelial cells together provide a final filtration barrier in the splenic red pulp. Only about 5 per cent of the blood that enters the normal spleen must pass through this vascular filter. Nevertheless, the red pulp is capable of exercising a profound regulatory function with regard to the quality and life span of both normal and injured blood cells. This capability depends on several features: the unique anatomic characteristics of the splenic cord–sinusoid complex, the biologic properties of the macrophages residing there, and the capacity of the spleen to increase blood flow to the cordal circulation and to undergo reticuloendothelial cell hyperplasia in response to a filtration load. The splenic red pulp provides an effective physical filtration system that can retain blood cells, particularly erythrocytes, which have lost their normal deformability. Entrapment in the splenic cords, even transiently, is in itself deleterious to both normal and injured red blood cells. They are subjected to hypoxia, hypoglycemia, and acidosis, which deteriorate their physical properties. This effect, termed *conditioning,* leads to more efficient entrapment on subsequent passages through the spleen and finally to erythrophagocytosis of the senescent cells by the cordal macrophages. Classic examples of the sieving effect of the splenic cords on pathologic red cells are the *Heinz body anemias.* Red cells containing rigid precipitates of denatured hemoglobin (owing to enzymatic or globin chain disorders) are trapped in the cordal filter where macrophages ingest them whole (*culling* function) or selectively ingest the inclusions (*pitting* function). Rigid microspherocytes, as in hereditary spherocytosis, are likewise retarded owing to their deformity, *conditioned* by the severe cordal environment, and destroyed by macrophages. Cordal sequestration is not only responsive to changes in the physical properties of erythrocytes; red cells sensitized by immunoglobulins or complement may also be

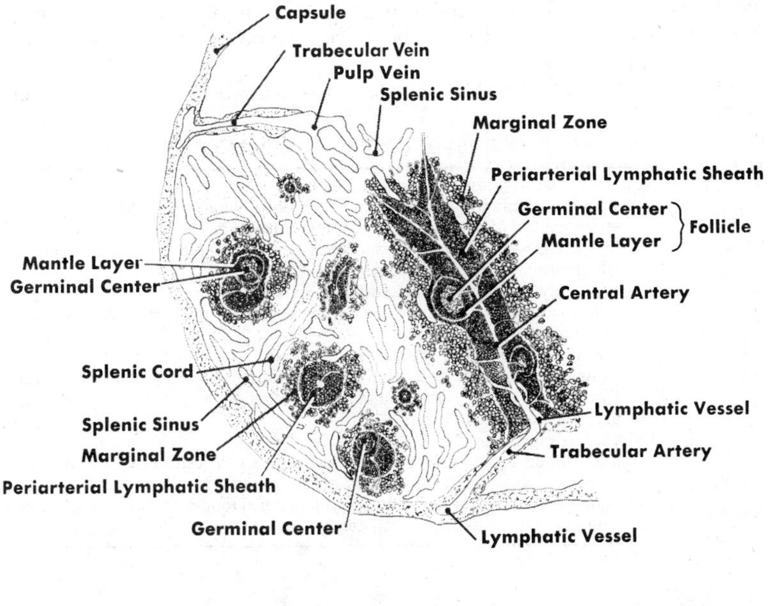

Figure 164–1. Diagrammatic representation of the structure of the spleen. (From Weiss L: Semin Hematol, October 1970, p 373.)

retarded within the splenic cords by virtue of specific receptors on cordal macrophages. The role of the spleen in the removal of normal senescent or injured platelets and granulocytes remains less clear than that outlined for erythrocytes. It must be assumed, at least in the case of immunologically injured platelets and granulocytes, that mechanisms similar to those trapping sensitized erythrocytes are effective.

HYPOSPLENISM

DEFINITION. Surgical excision, vascular accidents such as the splenic infarctions that occur during the natural history of sickle cell anemia, and congenital asplenia account for most instances of absent or reduced splenic function. Although absence of the spleen is not regularly accompanied by significant signs of disease, both laboratory and clinical features result from loss or suppression of specific splenic functions. These features may, under certain circumstances, be responsible for serious illness.

PATHOPHYSIOLOGY. The consequences of splenectomy relate to each of the specific functional properties of the spleen described earlier. The spleen is responsible for the sequestration and *pitting* of inclusion-bearing red blood cells. Such inclusions, e.g., *siderosomes* and *Howell-Jolly bodies,* which are intracorpuscular residua of erythroid cell maturation, are removed from intact red blood cells by cordal macrophages. In the absence of the spleen, erythrocytes containing such inclusion bodies may be detected in the peripheral circulation. The presence of Howell-Jolly bodies is a useful criterion for functional or anatomic asplenia. Nucleated red blood cells, which are trapped and enucleated in the normal spleen, may be found in small numbers in the peripheral blood following splenectomy or splenic vascular accidents. The splenic cords are also responsible for the normal maturation of the red cell plasma membrane. Young reticulocytes are delivered to the circulation with a relatively high membrane to cytoplasm ratio; during their brief sojourn in the spleen reticulocytes lose membrane and mature to the normal erythrocyte. *Target cells,* displaying a high membrane to cytoplasm ratio, are a common consequence of hyposplenic states.

The normal spleen contains a platelet pool constituting approximately 30 per cent of total circulating platelets. There may, as well, be a small pool of splenic granulocytes. Following splenectomy, a transient modest leukocytosis lasting up to one to two weeks is not uncommon, and should not be mistaken for a sign of infection. A transient thrombocytosis is quite regularly observed, with platelet counts between 500,000 and 1,000,000 per cubic millimeter, lasting generally for not longer than two to four weeks. Persistent, severe thrombocytosis, which may be associated with thrombotic complications, is particularly likely to occur when hemolytic disease persists following splenectomy. The management of such patients generally dictates the use of anticoagulants. The use of specific platelet functional antagonists, such as aspirin, under these circumstances is presently the subject of clinical evaluation. The risk of overwhelming septicemic infection by encapsulated pathogens, most commonly *Diplococcus pneumoniae* and *Hemophilus influenzae,* in the asplenic patient is now well established. The spleen plays a critical role in such infections, especially under conditions of inadequate immune response as in the very young and the immune suppressed, but the risk is not confined to these populations. Depression of a number of immunologic functions, including phagocytosis, serum IgM levels, cell-mediated immune reactivity, and complement-mediated opsonization of microorganisms, may contribute to this predisposition. It appears reasonable to consider partial splenectomy or splenic repair as an alternative to splenectomy for traumatic rupture and to postpone splenectomy when possible during infancy. Likewise, the indications for diagnostic staging splenectomy in lymphomatous disease must include this risk factor in the analysis. In general, splenectomized patients should be vaccinated with pneumococcal vaccine. At least those in the high risk categories, and perhaps all patients, should receive prophylactic penicillin for several years after splenectomy. All splenectomized patients and their families must be warned of the need to seek prompt medical assistance for febrile illness, including blood cultures and early antibiotic treatment.

SPLENOMEGALY AND HYPERSPLENISM

DEFINITIONS. Palpable *splenomegaly* can be detected in small numbers of patients (fewer than 1 per cent in the Western world) without *apparent* pathophysiologic significance, but the presence of a palpably enlarged spleen is best considered a physical finding that demands diagnostic evaluation. Splenomegaly may be accompanied by *hypersplenism,* a term used to describe the blood cytopenia-producing effects of overactivity of the hemoclastic functions of the spleen.

ETIOLOGY AND PATHOGENESIS. The spleen is a functionally complex organ, and the causes of splenomegaly emcompass a wide variety of primary illnesses (Table 164–1). The relative incidence of these illnesses associated with splenomegaly depends largely upon geographic and ethnic epidemiologic patterns. Because the spleen is a major reticuloendothelial organ, many *acute and chronic infectious processes* as well as noninfectious *inflammatory disorders* are accompanied by splenomegaly. *Splenic abscess* is a rare cause of splenomegaly, accompanied most commonly by tenderness in the left upper quadrant, fever, and findings of pleural reaction. The principal causes and predisposing factors are metastatic infections (endocarditis, for example), splenic infarction (sickle cell disease and its variants), splenic trauma, and disease in a contiguous area (ruptured viscus or neoplasm, for example). Septicemia, tuberculosis, typhoid fever, subacute bacterial endocarditis, and infectious mononucleosis may manifest splenomegaly, most commonly without abscess formation. In non-Western societies, other infectious agents, malaria, leishmaniasis, trypanosomes, and echinococcosis make a significant contribution to the incidence of infectious splenomegaly. Noninfectious inflammatory states such as Felty's syndrome (rheumatoid arthritis with splenomegaly), sarcoidosis, and beryllium disease are also associated with splenomegaly.

Splenomegaly Due to Reticuloendothelial Hyperplasia. The volume of splenic tissue is sensitive to the demand for clearance of normal and injured blood cells. Splenomegaly is a frequent finding in hematologic conditions characterized by accelerated clearance of blood cells bearing congenital or acquired defects. Many hemolytic anemias (hereditary spherocytosis, certain hemoglobin disorders, autoimmune hemolytic anemias) as well as other anemias with a significant hemolytic component (the megaloblastic anemias and thalassemias, for example) are associated with splenomegaly. Immune thrombocytopenias (as in lupus erythematosus and, less commonly, idiopathic thrombocytopenia) may also be accompanied by varying degrees of splenomegaly.

Congestive Splenomegaly. An enlarged spleen, with its en-

TABLE 164–1. CAUSES OF SPLENOMEGALY

Infectious and inflammatory splenomegaly
- Septicemia, typhoid, infectious mononucleosis, subacute bacterial endocarditis, disseminated tuberculosis, malaria, leishmaniasis, trypanosomes, echinococcosis, sarcoidosis, beryllium, Felty's syndrome (rheumatoid arthritis), splenic abscess

Splenomegaly due to reticuloendothelial hyperplasia
- Hemolytic anemias, immune thrombocytopenias, lupus erythematosus, thyrotoxicosis

Congestive splenomegaly
- Laennec's and postnecrotic cirrhosis; hepatic schistosomiasis; hepatic vein thrombosis; portal vein thrombosis, stenosis, cavernous transformation, or occlusion by neoplasm

Infiltrative splenomegaly
- Benign conditions: Gaucher's disease, Niemann-Pick disease, amyloidosis, diabetic lipemia, extramedullary hematopoiesis
- Neoplastic conditions: leukemias, lymphomas, Hodgkin's disease, primary tumors, metastatic neoplasm, polycythemia vera, myeloid metaplasia

larged vascular bed, may make a significant contribution to increased portal blood flow and portal pressures. More commonly, however, splenomegaly is a consequence of portal hypertension caused by any one of a number of obstructive portal vascular diseases, including Laennec's and postnecrotic cirrhosis, hepatic schistosomiasis, and hepatic vein thrombosis, as well as thrombosis, stenosis, cavernous transformation, or tumor compression of the portal vein. Under these circumstances splenomegaly is usually overshadowed by other manifestations of the primary disease such as hepatic failure, ascites, or bleeding esophageal varices. Hypersplenism, manifested most commonly by granulocytopenia and thrombocytopenia, is a common accompaniment of congestive splenomegaly.

Infiltrative Splenomegaly. Both benign and malignant infiltrative diseases may cause splenomegaly and the hypersplenic syndrome. Metabolic disorders, such as Gaucher's disease, Niemann-Pick disease, and diabetic lipemia, are characterized by accumulation in splenic macrophages of the metabolic product characteristic of each disease. Myelophthisic replacement of the bone marrow by fibrous tissue (myelofibrosis), granulomas or tumor tissue, and chronic medullary stimulation, as in congenital hemolytic anemias, is associated with extramedullary splenic hematopoiesis and splenomegaly resulting from proliferating blood precursors. Alternatively, splenomegaly may result from involvement of the spleen by truly neoplastic infiltrations such as the acute leukemias, chronic myelogenous leukemia, and the lymphoproliferative disorders, including chronic lymphocytic leukemia and Hodgkin's and non-Hodgkin's lymphomas. The spleen is an uncommon site for metastasis by nonhematologic malignancies. Primary tumors and cysts of the spleen are also uncommon causes of splenomegaly. These include hemangiomas, lymphangiomas, sarcomas, and hamartomas.

The Hypersplenic Syndrome. The cardinal features of hypersplenism are (1) splenomegaly, (2) some reduction in the number of circulating blood cells, affecting granulocytes, erythrocytes, or platelets in any combination, (3) a compensatory proliferative response in the bone marrow, and (4) the potential for correction of these hematologic abnormalities by splenectomy. Since the functional compartments of the spleen are intimately interconnected, virtually all causes of splenomegaly may be associated with varying degrees of hypersplenism. Both infiltrative and congestive forms of splenomegaly are not uncommonly associated with hypersplenism. The hyperplastic response of splenic reticuloendothelial cells in a hemolytic anemia may initiate nonspecific sequestration of other blood cells, increase the conditioning of both injured and transfused erythrocytes, and accelerate the anemia. The concept of primary or idiopathic hypersplenism is questionable at best. As the relationship between systemic disease, splenomegaly, and the several splenic functions becomes better understood, the number of cases that fall in this wastebasket category is gradually decreasing. In this era of world travel the differential diagnosis of splenomegaly and hypersplenism must include worldwide disease patterns.

The mechanisms whereby splenomegaly results in hypersplenism are best understood with respect to erythrocyte sequestration. Whether such mechanisms apply to platelets and granulocytes has yet to be determined. There is normally a large pool of sequestered platelets within the spleen, and with splenomegaly the volume of pooled platelets, transiently withdrawn from the general circulation, increases strikingly. Pooling of otherwise normal platelets may play a significant role in some instances of thrombocytopenia attributable to hypersplenism. Whether such a mechanism is a factor in hypersplenic leukopenia has yet to be documented. Finally, splenomegaly itself makes a contribution, by mechanisms not fully understood, to an expanded total plasma volume. An apparent peripheral blood cytopenia may at times be the result of an expanded plasma volume and be independent of specific splenic sequestration and hemoclastic functions.

DIAGNOSIS. Additional studies may be required to confirm that a palpable abdominal left upper quadrant mass represents splenomegaly. The principal noninvasive technique for determining spleen size is the radionuclide spleen scan. Several techniques are available, including colloidal suspensions of radionuclides such as technetium (^{99m}Tc), as well as the use of mildly heat-injured erythrocytes labeled with ^{55}Cr. Quantitative evaluation of the distribution of chromium-labeled erythrocytes also provides information concerning the relative importance of the spleen, as compared with other reticuloendothelial organs such as the liver, in a hemolytic anemia. Such information may be useful as part of the evidence adduced to determine the advisability of splenectomy. Selective splenic angiography may also be a useful preoperative procedure in the evaluation of splenomegaly. The further diagnostic approach to the patient with splenomegaly is dictated by the accompanying features, such as hematologic findings, lymphadenopathy, portal hypertension, liver dysfunction, or systemic infection.

INDICATIONS FOR SPLENECTOMY. Because there are potential serious risks inherent in splenectomy, including (1) operative and anesthetic morbidity, (2) postsplenectomy thrombosis and thromboembolic complications, and (3) the risk of overwhelming bacterial infection, the indications for splenectomy should be strictly and carefully applied to the individual patient. These include (1) hemolytic syndromes, in which the selective role of the spleen in red cell sequestration and destruction can be documented or is an established aspect of the disease; (2) acute splenic vascular accidents or traumatic rupture requiring immediate surgical intervention; in this context, splenectomy may be indicated prophylactically for massive splenomegaly if there is severe discomfort or a threat of traumatic rupture; (3) immunologically mediated thrombocytopenias (see Ch. 166); (4) myeloid metaplasia and other instances of extramedullary hematopoiesis, when clinical evidence suggests that the hematopoietic functions of the enlarged spleen are outweighed by accelerated sequestration and blood cell destruction; (5) the staging of Hodgkin's disease or other lymphomas when a therapeutic decision rests upon the presence or absence of splenic disease; and (6) splenic abscess (accompanied by suitable antibiotics). In the case of congestive splenomegaly, the factors that determine prognosis are rarely the hypersplenic functions of the enlarged spleen; most commonly these are liver failure and the vascular consequences of portal hypertension. Rectification of these defects must regularly take precedence over hypersplenism. In the face of severe hypersplenism resulting from infiltrative or hyperplastic splenomegaly (such as Gaucher's disease or severe Felty's syndrome) and when required for the diagnosis of splenomegaly of undetermined etiology, splenectomy may also be entertained after due consideration of the benefits and risks. When splenectomy is needed in the face of unacceptable surgical risk, transcatheter splenic embolization by an experienced angiographer may be a potentially helpful preoperative procedure.

Chun CH, Raff MJ, Contreras L, Varghese R, Waterman N, Daffner R, Melo JC: Splenic abscess. Medicine 59:50, 1980. *A thorough review of the clinical manifestations of this infrequent condition, stressing early recognition and intervention to avoid high mortality.*

Francke EL, Nev HC: Postsplenectomy infection. Surg Clin North Am 61:135, 1981.

Hess CE, Ayers CR, Sandusky WR, Carpenter MA, Wetzel RA, Mohler DN: Mechanism of dilutional anemia in massive splenomegaly. Blood 47:629, 1976. *A clinical and physiologic study of the effects of portal vascular volume on plasma volume expansion.*

Jacob HS: Hypersplenism: Mechanisms and management. Br J Haematol 27:1, 1974. *Reviews the clinical manifestations and indications for intervention.*

165. BONE MARROW TRANSPLANTATION

Rainer Storb

MARROW TRANSPLANT PRINCIPLES. Transplantation of marrow from a donor identical with the recipient at the major histocompatibility complex reduces graft-versus-host disease

(GVHD) and improves survival of the recipient. This seminal demonstration in experimental animals prepared the stage for human transplantation using allogeneic, HLA identical sib donors. Successful transplants were carried out first in children with immunodeficiency diseases (reviewed in Ch. 429) and subsequently in patients with severe aplastic anemia and leukemia.

Marrow transplantation differs in several aspects from transplantation of solid organs, in particular kidney (see Ch. 79): (1) the host-versus-graft reaction can generally be abrogated by a single short course of high-dose immunosuppressive therapy given immediately before transplantation; (2) preceding blood transfusions are not beneficial but rather can interfere with subsequent marrow engraftment, particularly in patients with aplastic anemia; (3) donors have mostly been HLA-identical family members; (4) donors do not suffer a permanent organ loss, since the removed marrow is replaced within weeks; and (5) post-grafting immunosuppression of recipients can generally be terminated after 3 to 12 months.

To prepare for marrow transplantation the recipient's immune system must first be destroyed. This is effectively accomplished by use of cyclophosphamide (CY), at 50 mg per kilogram per day for four days, or total body irradiation (TBI), at 800 to 1500 rad midline tissue doses (4 to 25 rad per minute) either alone or combined with CY or other chemotherapeutic agents. This program not only sets the stage for establishment of the allogeneic graft but also serves to kill leukemic cells if that is the patient's basic disease.

After the conditioning regimen, 2 to 6 $\times$ 10^8 donor marrow cells per kilogram are infused intravenously. Most grafts are initially successful such that within two to four weeks marrow cellularity increases and peripheral blood counts of donor origin rise. Over time all hematopoietic and immune cells of the recipient are replaced by those from the marrow donor, including plasma cells and tissue macrophages.

Among the serious problems that may develop in patients with successful grafts is *graft-versus-host disease (GVHD)*. Methotrexate or cyclosporine is given within the first 3 to 12 months after grafting as perhaps the most effective immunosuppressive agents to prevent GVHD. Once the drugs are discontinued, many patients do well with persisting graft-host tolerance. However, acute GVHD occurs in approximately 35 to 60 per cent of the patients, and as many as 40 per cent of afflicted patients die. Xenogeneic antihuman thymocyte globulin (ATG), prednisone, or cyclosporine have been used to treat acute GVHD with some success. Better approaches to prevent or treat acute GVHD are necessary, such as the more imaginative use of known immunosuppressive agents, the use of "germ-free" isolation, or the removal of T cells from the marrow inoculum by antibodies to human T lymphocytes.

More recently, *chronic GVHD* has been recognized as a problem affecting approximately 25 to 45 per cent of patients surviving more than 180 days. It is most frequent in older patients and those who had acute GVHD. It resembles collagen vascular diseases and is characterized by severe immune deficiency, impaired granulocyte chemotaxis, and recurrent, sometimes life-threatening bacterial infections. Combination therapy with prednisone and either azathioprine, CY, or procarbazine has proved to be effective in most patients with chronic GVHD.

Interstitial pneumonias, either of unknown etiology or associated with infectious agents such as cytomegalovirus, are a cause of morbidity and fatality during the first four months after grafting. They are a major problem in patients treated with TBI and then transplanted for leukemia and a minor problem in CY-treated patients transplanted for aplastic anemia. Probably these infections are the result of deficient immune reactivity of the compromised host (see Ch. 257) although radiation effects may also play a role. Effective methods of accelerating the immune reconstitution and/or the use of antiviral agents or hyperimmune globulin might be of value in obviating the problem of interstitial pneumonia.

CLINICAL RESULTS

SEVERE APLASTIC ANEMIA. Aplastic anemia is most frequently attributable to a stem cell defect (see Ch. 132). In many cases infusion of marrow from a monozygotic twin (syngeneic transplant) has been successful in reconstituting the marrow without immunosuppression of the recipient. Some syngeneic grafts have been successful only after preparation with CY and a second transplant, suggesting that these cases may involve other mechanisms, perhaps an autoimmune etiology, which can be overcome by CY.

Allogeneic marrow transplantation (donors are HLA-identical family members) is often effective therapy for severe aplastic anemia. A prospective cooperative study has shown significantly better survival for patients treated by transplantation than for those who did not receive transplants.

One frequent problem associated with high mortality in aplastic anemia has been marrow graft rejection, seen until 1975 with a frequency of 30 to 60 per cent. Accordingly, long-term survival was on the order of only 45 per cent. Two factors have predicted graft rejection: (1) positive in vitro tests of cell-mediated immunity, indicating reaction of recipient lymphocytes against donor cells before transplantation; and (2) a low number of transplanted marrow cells ($<3 \times 10^8$ per kilogram). Transfusion-induced sensitization is the major cause of graft rejection. Unfortunately most patients with aplastic anemia who have received marrow transplants in the past had had previous blood transfusions. We have now carried out transplants in 43 patients who had not received transfusions before transplantation. Graft failure was the exception, and 83 per cent of the patients are alive between 1 and 11½ (median 4) years after grafting (Fig. 165–1). We believe that the immunologic mechanisms involved in graft failure are, for the most part, iatrogenic (i.e., induced by previous blood transfusion).

Many programs are being carried out to avoid rejection in multiply transfused patients by using more intensive immunosuppressive conditioning regimens. In all programs cyclophosphamide is used, but other features of the conditioning regimens vary. In Seattle either methotrexate or cyclosporine is used after grafting and viable donor buffy-coat cells are

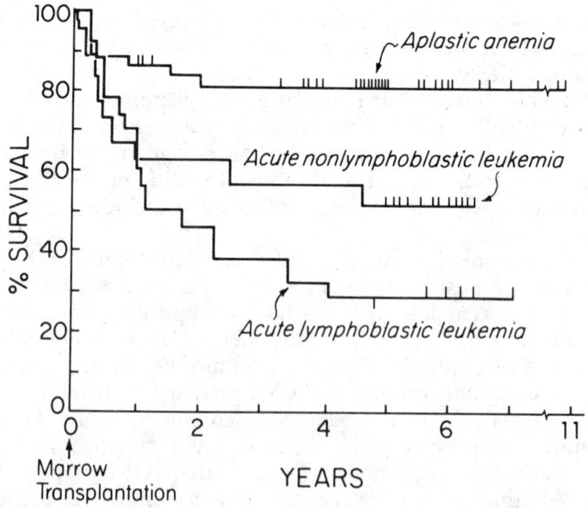

Figure 165–1. The survival of 43 untransfused patients with aplastic anemia, 22 patients with acute nonlymphoblastic leukemia having transplants in first remission, and 22 patients with acute lymphoblastic leukemia having transplants in second or subsequent remission after marrow grafts from HLA-identical family members. The surviving patients with leukemia remain in unmaintained remission. Day "0" is the day of marrow transplantation. The tick marks indicate living patients. Survival is as of June 1983.

infused together with the marrow inoculum. Graft rejection seems to be less likely when a larger number of marrow cells is infused. The donor's peripheral blood is a potential source of additional pluripotent hematopoietic stem cells and/or lymphoid cells capable of overcoming rejection. It is possible that pluripotent stem cells circulate in humans, as they have been shown to do in certain experimental animals. Also, peripheral blood and thoracic duct lymphoid cells enhance allogeneic marrow engraftment in vivo in mice and dogs and erythropoiesis in vitro in dogs and humans. As a rule, the rejection rates have decreased and survival has increased. Of the last 65 Seattle patients with aplastic anemia who received marrow grafts from HLA-identical siblings following multiple transfusions, 71 per cent are alive after follow-up periods of 1 to 7½ years.

Most of the regimens have associated risks. The addition of buffy-coat cells may lead to an increased risk of chronic GVHD. A major problem with radiation regimens is that of a potential risk for late malignancies. Because of these problems and the still-existing mortality from rejection, emphasis should be placed on measures to prevent rather than overcome sensitization by blood transfusions. For this the physician should be aware of the possibility of marrow transplantation when aplastic anemia is first diagnosed in a patient. If an HLA-identical family member is available, early transplantation before transfusions is the therapy of choice.

LEUKEMIA. Marrow grafting for leukemia presents the same general transplantation problems encountered for aplastic anemia. However, graft rejection is rare. The unique problem is recurrence of leukemia. Until 1975 marrow transplantation was carried out only after failure of all other therapy when patients were in advanced relapse. A survival curve of the first 100 patients with acute leukemia grafted in Seattle after CY and TBI shows that 12 per cent of these patients with otherwise *refractory leukemia* are alive in remission between 8 and 13 years without any maintenance therapy. Statistical analysis of the data indicates that, if no patient died of other causes, 75 per cent of all patients could be expected to have recurrent leukemia within two years of transplantation. Leukemic recurrence usually originated from host-type cells indicating that it is difficult to kill every leukemic cell once the patient has reached the end-stage of the disease. Current attempts to reduce the rate of leukemic relapse and increase long-term survival in patients with leukemia transplanted in the end-stage of their disease involve the use of higher doses of TBI by means of fractionating the radiation and the use of additional chemotherapeutic agents. Perhaps these attempts are doomed to failure since, in an exponential cell kill process, it is difficult to kill the last leukemic cell. Some of the apparent cures may have occurred because of leukemic cell kill by immune mechanisms directed at non-HLA antigens expressed on leukemic cells. This is suggested by the observation of a graft-versus-leukemia effect in man.

It is attractive to carry out marrow transplantation earlier in the course of the disease while the patient is in remission. The advantages of this approach include treatment when the number of leukemic cells in the body is small and before the cells become resistant to therapy, and while the patient is in good clinical condition and therefore better able to tolerate the therapy. Accordingly, the group in Seattle began in 1976 to treat patients with acute nonlymphoblastic leukemia by marrow grafting in first or subsequent remission and those with acute lymphoblastic leukemia in second or subsequent remission after conditioning with CY and TBI.

Patients with acute nonlymphoblastic leukemia treated by chemotherapy have an approximate median duration of survival of 2 years (see Ch. 156). Only 15 to 20 per cent of chemotherapy-treated patients are alive at five years. Of the first 22 patients with *acute nonlymphoblastic leukemia* treated by marrow transplantation in *first remission*, 12 are alive in unmaintained remission between five and seven years after transplantation (Fig. 165–1). The survival curve shows a plateau at

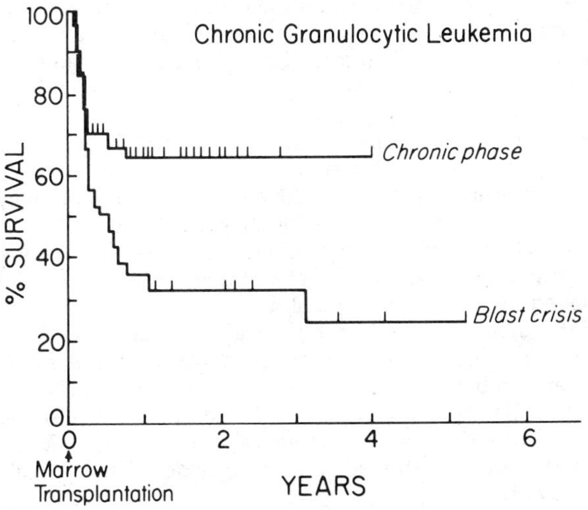

Figure 165–2. Survival after marrow grafting on patients with chronic granulocytic leukemia having transplants either in blast crisis (n = 29) or in chronic phase (n = 35). The tick marks indicate living patients. Survival is as of May 1983.

55 per cent. Only 23 of the first 171 patients in Seattle now transplanted have had a recurrence of leukemia. Evidently the CY-TBI regimen is capable of destroying residual leukemic cells in most patients with acute nonlymphoblastic leukemia in first remission. These encouraging results have recently been confirmed by other groups.

Approximately 50 per cent of patients with acute lymphoblastic leukemia, especially children, can be cured by chemotherapy (see Ch. 156). Once a patient has relapsed, another remission can often be induced with chemotherapy, but long-term survival is poor with very few of the patients alive at two years. Treatment of patients with acute lymphoblastic leukemia in second or subsequent remission by marrow transplantation seems justified in an attempt to change the otherwise grim outlook and perhaps "cure" some of these patients of their disease.

The survival curve of the first 22 patients with *acute lymphoblastic leukemia in second or subsequent remission* receiving marrow grafts in Seattle shows a plateau at 27 per cent 5½ to 7 years after transplantation (Fig. 165–1). A prospective study showed marrow grafting to be superior to chemotherapy. Recurrent leukemia in cells of host type has been the major problem. Apparently the current conditioning regimen was ineffective in eradicating residual leukemic cells in approximately 60 per cent of the patients.

The results of marrow transplantation for the treatment of patients with *chronic granulocytic leukemia* in blast crisis have been similar to those in patients with leukemia in relapse. The projected survival is approximately 20 per cent (Fig. 165–2). The patients' marrows show absence of the Philadelphia chromosome, a unique result.

Transplantation during the *chronic phase of chronic granulocytic leukemia* promised to improve these results. Although follow-up is still short, it appears that long-term disease-free survival will be on the order of 60 per cent (Fig. 165–2).

Marrow transplantation has now also been successfully applied to the treatment of patients with non-Hodgkin's lymphoma, myelofibrosis, multiple myeloma, preleukemia, and hairy cell leukemia.

CONCLUSIONS

Marrow transplantation, once considered a desperate form of therapy in end-stage patients, has now become increasingly successful when used early in the course of aplastic anemia or leukemia. The current success now obliges the physician to identify, soon after diagnosis, those patients who have suitable donors and who may be candidates for transplantation. Marrow grafting has now been extended to the therapy of patients with other hematologic malignancies and genetic disorders of hematopoiesis. The longest survivor with malignant non-Hodgkin's lymphoma is now in unmaintained remission 14 years after marrow grafting. Cures of congenital Fanconi's anemia, paroxysmal nocturnal hemoglobinuria, thalassemia major, osteopetrosis, and certain genetic storage diseases have been achieved by marrow transplantation.

Many patients do not have HLA-identical sibs, and very few have monozygotic twins. To extend marrow transplantation to a larger number of patients, the use of less well matched family members has been explored with success. Recently, successful human transplants from unrelated donors for the treatment of patients with acute leukemia and aplastic anemia have been carried out.

Storb R, Thomas ED: Current state of marrow transplantation. *In* Silker R, Gordon AS, Lobue J (eds.): Contemporary Hematology/Oncology. Vol 3. New York, Plenum Medical, 1984, pp 235–266. *General review with emphasis on GVHD, immunological aspects, opportunistic infections, and recurrence of leukemia.*

Storb, R, Thomas ED, Buckner CD, Appelbaum FR, Clift R, Deeg HJ, Doney K, Hansen JA, Prentice RL, Sanders JE, Stewart P, Sullivan KM, Witherspoon RP: Marrow transplantation for aplastic anemia. Semin Hematol 21:27, 1984. *Analysis of past and current clinical results of marrow transplantation for aplastic anemia.*

Thomas ED, Clift RA, Storb R: Indications for marrow transplantation. Annu Rev Med (In press). *General review with emphasis on clinical results.*

Thomas ED, Storb R, Clift RA, Fefer A, Johnson FL, Neiman PE, Lerner KG, Glucksberg H, Buckner CD: Bone-marrow transplantation. N Engl J Med 292:832, 895, 1975. *Review of basic principles and clinical applications of marrow transplant biology.*

166. HEMORRHAGIC DISORDERS: ABNORMALITIES OF PLATELET AND VASCULAR FUNCTION

Aaron J. Marcus

Introduction

NORMAL HEMOSTASIS

In hemostasis a series of events culminates in spontaneous arrest of bleeding from a damaged blood vessel. At least three closely linked biologic systems are involved: *blood vessels, platelets,* and proteins of the *coagulation system*. The initial physiologic response to interruption of continuity of a vascular surface is a platelet-vascular interaction known as primary hemostasis. It is essentially independent of the coagulation mechanism. Within seconds of vascular injury, blood vessels constrict owing to contraction of their smooth muscle, and platelets adhere to exposed subendothelial factor VIII–related von Willebrand factor (factor VIII: vWF) polymers and collagen in connective tissue beneath the endothelial layer to initiate plug formation. Adherence of platelets induces configurational changes in their plasma membranes that are accompanied by (1) secretion of components of intracellular granules (release reaction), (2) synthesis of thromboxane A_2 and hydroxy acids, (3) the capacity to bind and thereby catalyze interactions between plasma coagulation proteins, leading to thrombin formation, and (4) recruitment and aggregation of more platelets.

Platelet secretion, especially that of adenosine diphosphate (ADP), causes aggregation of other platelets and augments formation of the platelet plug. ADP induces exposure of platelet fibrinogen-binding sites. Bound fibrinogen then serves to enhance platelet-platelet adhesion, possibly by formation of molecular bridges. A complex of platelet glycoproteins IIb and IIIa may be an integral component of the fibrinogen receptor. The aggregation process itself will stimulate further release of ADP from other platelets (recruitment) (Fig. 166–1). Other compounds released by stimulated platelets include serotonin (5-HT, a potent vasoconstrictor), platelet factor 4 (a protein capable of neutralizing heparin), beta-thromboglobulin (a platelet-specific protein of unknown function), lysosomal enzymes, and a platelet-derived growth factor that stimulates proliferation of smooth muscle and fibroblasts. Platelet adherence to collagen also liberates the essential fatty acid arachidonic acid and thereby initiates a series of reactions, culminating in thromboxane and hydroxy acid synthesis (see Ch. 223). Arachidonate is oxygenated by cyclo-oxygenase (an enzymatic reaction irreversibly inhibited by aspirin and therefore of clinical interest) and cyclized to form endoperoxides PGG_2 and PGH_2 (Fig. 166–1). In platelets the endoperoxides are converted by thromboxane synthetase to thromboxane A_2, which is itself released into the surrounding medium to induce further platelet aggregation and vasoconstriction. Thromboxane A_2 inhibits platelet adenylate cyclase, resulting in a fall in cyclic AMP levels. The latter is associated with calcium mobilization and promotion of aggregation. Thrombin or collagen in appropriate quantities can induce intracellular calcium mobilization independently of thromboxane A_2. In endothelial cells endoperoxides are largely converted to prostacyclin (PGI_2), which inhibits platelet aggregation and release by increasing platelet cyclic AMP levels (Fig. 166–1).

Primary hemostasis represents a complex sequence of events, but its clinical assessment is relatively simple. The bleeding time provides a sensitive and reliable index of platelet function in primary hemostasis. A prolonged bleeding time indicates pathologic impairment of platelet plug formation, which may be due to poor adhesion, poor cohesion (aggregation), or insufficient quantities of platelets.

In secondary hemostasis the platelet membrane–catalyzed coagulation sequence converts plasma prothrombin into the serine protease thrombin (see Ch. 167). Thrombin plays a complex role in hemostasis: (1) It directly and irreversibly aggregates platelets and stimulates release. (2) It initiates thromboxane A_2 production and thereby indirectly augments aggregation and release. (3) It converts fibrinogen to fibrin strands that consolidate the platelet mass. (4) It enhances prothrombin conversion by stimulating the binding of coagulation factors Va and Xa to the platelet membrane. (5) It activates coagulation factor XIII, which catalyzes formation of covalent amide bonds between fibrin polymers to produce clot stabilization. The coagulation cascade is summarized in Ch. 167.

BLOOD PLATELETS

Platelets are anucleate cytoplasmic fragments derived from marrow megakaryocytes by extension of cytoplasmic processes that undergo attenuation, develop constrictions at their distal ends, and then rupture in the form of free platelets. Production and release of platelets from the marrow may be controlled by two "thrombopoietins"—one regulating the quantity of megakaryocyte-committed stem cells and another modulating megakaryocyte maturation. The presence of large platelets (megathrombocytes) in the circulation may be directly related to the degree of thrombopoietic stimulation. Platelets, which normally circulate for about ten days, are 2 to 3 μm in diameter. The normal platelet count is 150,000 to 400,000 per cubic millimeter. On a stained blood smear one can visualize about three to ten platelets per oil-immersion field. At any given time approximately 70 per cent of platelets are circulating and 30 per cent are in the spleen.

Despite its comparatively simple structure the platelet is functionally complex. Stimulated platelets adhere to damaged vessel surfaces (adhesion) as well as to each other (cohesion or aggregation). Stimulation is also a prerequisite for the release reaction and transformation of arachidonic acid to thromboxane A_2, which reinforces hemostatic function. Platelets maintain "vascular integrity" through obscure mechanisms. Rapid onset of thrombocytopenia is often associated with spontaneous

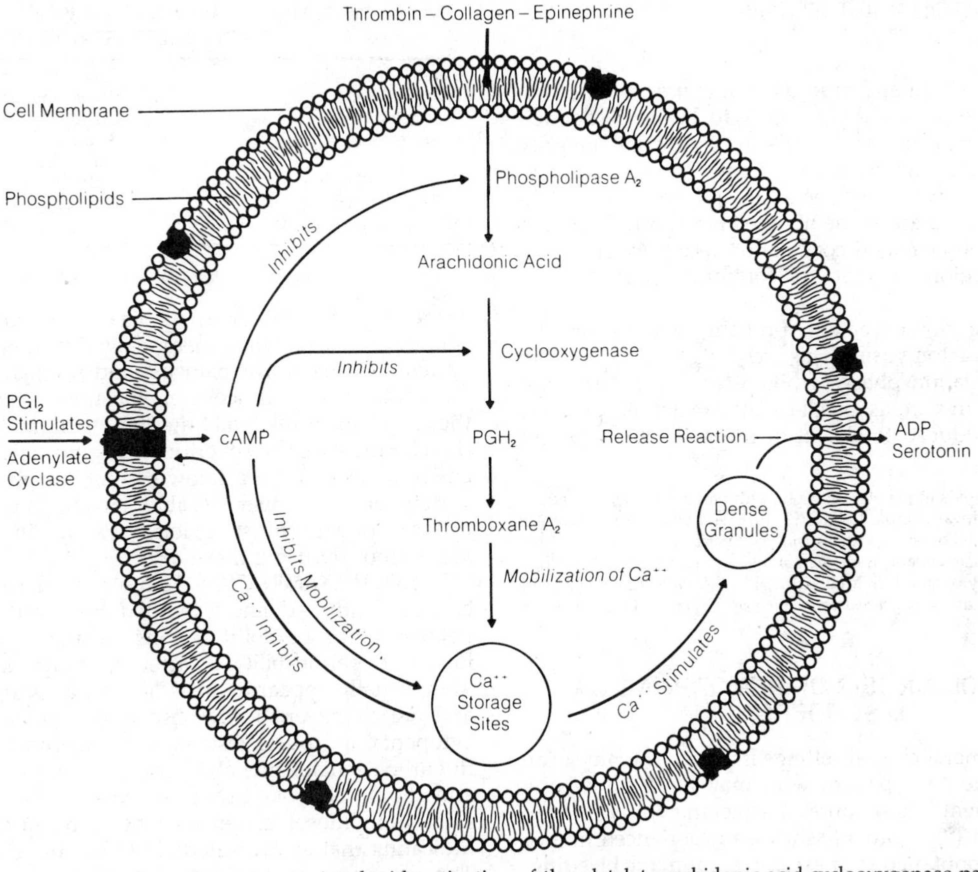

Figure 166–1. Diagram of events associated with activation of the platelet arachidonic acid cyclooxygenase pathway. The end product, thromboxane A_2, induces intracellular calcium mobilization and is also released into the microenvironment where it acts as a direct agonist for additional platelet aggregation and vasoconstriction. Mobilized calcium is the major stimulus for initiation of dense granule secretion. ADP and serotonin are among the most important products of the platelet release reaction. The increase in intracellular calcium also inhibits adenylate cyclase, thus lowering cyclic AMP levels, which further promotes aggregation and release. In contrast, PGI_2, the major cyclooxygenase product of endothelial cells, stimulates adenylate cyclase, thus elevating platelet cyclic AMP and blocking calcium mobilization and its consequences. In this manner PGI_2 attenuates platelet responsiveness. Platelets also contain a lipoxygenase pathway of arachidonate metabolism, the function of which is currently under study. (Courtesy of the Upjohn Co.)

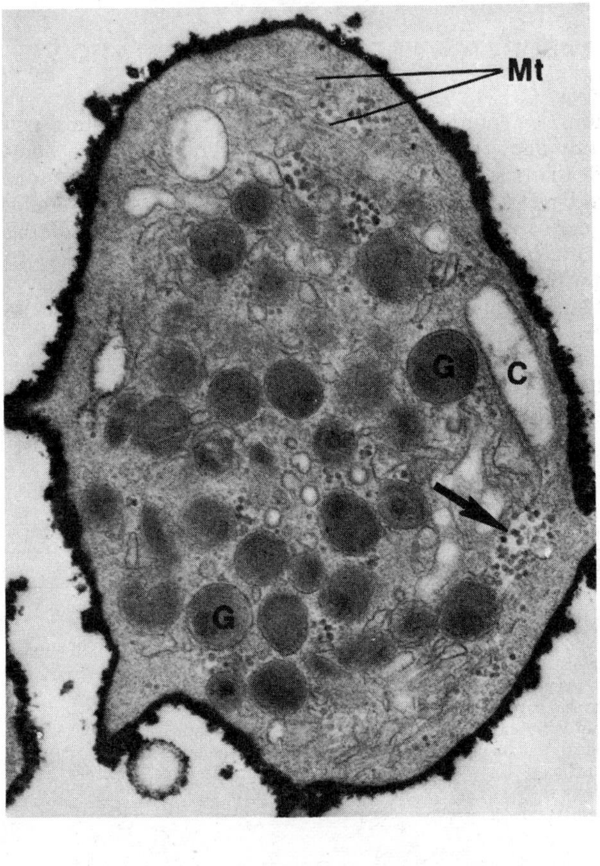

Figure 166–2. Electron micrograph of human platelet. Glutaraldehyde fixation in the presence of ruthenium red has enhanced the electron density of the platelet coat. The coat averages 20 nm in thickness and is composed of sulfated acid mucopolysaccharides derived from the megakaryocyte. It is associated with both the surface membranes and those that compose the open canalicular system. G = granule; glycogen (arrow); Mt = microtubules; C = canalicular system. (× 29,000.) (From Zucker-Franklin D: *In* Collagen-Platelet Interaction. Proceedings of the First Munich Symposium on the Biology of Connective Tissue. Stuttgart, F. K. Schattauer Verlag, 1978.)

hemorrhage into the skin and mucous membranes, whereas in chronic thrombocytopenias there seems to be an ill-defined compensatory mechanism for the missing "vascular integrity factor(s)" and hemorrhage is less frequent. Platelets function in the intrinsic coagulation system. The phospholipoprotein surface of stimulated platelet membranes binds and catalyzes interactions between activated coagulation factors culminating in thrombin formation, a property formerly referred to as platelet factor 3.

Platelets mediate clot retraction, probably via the platelet contractile protein actomyosin. This may play a role in vivo during the consolidation phase of hemostatic plug formation and can be studied in vitro as a well-defined metabolic process. Clot retraction is reduced to absent in thrombocytopenia and thrombasthenia.

Marcus AJ: The role of lipids in platelet function, with particular reference to the arachidonic acid pathway. J Lipid Res 19:793, 1978. *Arachidonic acid metabolism in platelets as related to hemostasis, coagulation, and thrombosis.*

Shattil SJ, Bennett JS: Platelets and their membranes in hemostasis: Physiology and pathophysiology. Ann Intern Med 94:108, 1980. *Recent advances in platelet research are correlated with new developments in our understanding of the pathogenesis of platelet disorders.*

CLINICAL DIAGNOSIS OF HEMORRHAGIC DISORDERS

There are two general clinical settings in which the physician is required to evaluate a patient who may have a bleeding tendency: (1) a patient who requires a screening study prior to major surgery, and (2) a patient who has experienced one or more episodes of spontaneous or excessive traumatic bleeding. In both instances a careful personal and family history and physical examination, together with judiciously selected laboratory screening tests, should establish (1) whether a hemorrhagic tendency is present; (2) whether it is an abnormality of coagulation, a vascular defect, or platelet disorder; and (3) whether the disorder is congenital or acquired (Table 166–1).

HISTORY. A history of bleeding or bruising occurring spontaneously or after minor trauma is significant, especially if the bruise is 3 cm or larger. Such episodes are usually associated with vascular abnormalities, but they can occur in coagulation and platelet disorders as well. A previous history of bleeding following dental extraction or surgery should be sought. In platelet diseases bleeding is usually immediate and transient. If a coagulation disorder is present, postoperative hemorrhage is usually delayed and prolonged. Mucous membrane bleeding, as exemplified by epistaxis, is a common presenting symptom, although it is of less concern if of short duration, especially in children. A family history is important, especially in males, because deficiencies of factor VIII and of factor IX are X-linked. Approximately 85 per cent of congenital coagulation abnormalities are due to factor VIII deficiency. An additional 10 per cent are due to factor IX deficiency. All the other disorders, which are autosomal recessive, constitute approximately 5 per cent of the total. In 30 per cent of hemophilic patients a family history cannot be elicited. Several systemic diseases may be accompanied by acquired abnormalities of platelets, blood vessels, coagulation factors, or a combination of these (including circulating anticoagulants)—especially liver disease, malignancies, systemic lupus erythematosus, and uremia. A very important facet of the history concerns medication. *Aspirin ingestion* during the previous week will interfere with platelet function and thereby increase the severity of a hemostatic disorder. A number of other drugs are known to inhibit platelet function by a variety of mechanisms (Table 166–2). Patients on coumarin drugs or heparin must obviously be identified, including those surreptitiously using these drugs.

TABLE 166–2. DRUGS ASSOCIATED WITH ABNORMALITIES IN PLATELET FUNCTION

Aspirin	Low molecular weight dextran
Chlorpromazine	Meclofenamic acid
Clofibrate	Nitrofurantoin
Dipyridamole	Penicillins
Ethanol	Phenylbutazone
Glyceryl guaiacolate	Sulfinpyrazone
Hydroxychloroquine	Tricyclic antidepressants
Indomethacin	

PHYSICAL EXAMINATION. Knowledge gained from the history can be confirmed and extended by a physical examination. Petechiae are pinpoint lesions, resulting from breakage or increased permeability of arterioles, capillaries, and venules. They usually appear in areas of the skin subjected to pressure, and are characteristically observed in patients with thrombocytopenia. Purpuric lesions, which probably represent confluent petechiae, are also associated with thrombocytopenia and should be looked for in mucosal surfaces as well as in the skin. Ecchymoses are extensions of purpuric lesions, usually indicating that extravasated blood has traversed fascial planes. The presence of spontaneous ecchymoses is of concern and suggests a defect in blood coagulation. Hemarthroses or ankylosed joints strongly suggest hemophilia or factor IX deficiency. The physical examination may reveal evidence for a systemic disease complicated by hemorrhage, or the telangiectasia of Osler-Weber-Rendu disease.

Moake JL, Funicella T: Common Bleeding Problems. Clinical Symposia 35. West Caldwell, NJ, Ciba Pharmaceutical Company, 1983, pp 1–32. *A succinct, well organized and illustrated monograph containing a logical approach to diagnosis and treatment of hemorrhagic disorders.*

LABORATORY STUDIES OF HEMOSTATIC FUNCTION

Although a complete history and physical examination will frequently allow the physician to tentatively diagnose a hemorrhagic diathesis, final diagnosis requires definitive laboratory studies. Basic screening tests should be ordered first to examine the integrity of platelet and coagulation components of the hemostatic process. More sophisticated and expensive assays should await results of these initial tests (Table 166–3).

An estimate of *platelet numbers and gross morphology* can be made from the blood smear. In addition, visualization of other formed elements may suggest systemic or hematologic disease. The platelet count will document whether or not thrombocytopenia (<100,000 per cubic millimeter) is present.

The *bleeding time* is usually carried out by a modified Ivy

TABLE 166–1. DIFFERENTIAL CLINICAL DIAGNOSIS OF COAGULATION, PLATELET, AND VASCULAR DISORDERS

	Coagulation Defect	Platelet Disorder	Vascular Abnormality
Family history	Usually positive	Negative	Usually negative
Sex predominance	Males	Frequently females	Mainly females
Nature of symptoms and signs	Visceral, intramuscular and joint hemorrhage; spontaneous and post-mild trauma	Cutaneous, mucous membrane, and CNS hemorrhage; petechiae, purpura, hematuria; hemarthroses rare	Ecchymoses, purpura, frequently spontaneous; melena; no hemarthroses
Time sequence of hemorrhage	Post-traumatic delay followed by persistent oozing	Concomitant with and immediately following trauma; usually of short duration	Post-traumatic or spontaneous localized ecchymoses; generalized bleeding rare
Response to local pressure	Usually ineffective	Usually effective	Effective

TABLE 166–3. SCREENING TESTS FOR PRIMARY AND SECONDARY HEMOSTASIS

Disorder	Platelet Count (~300 × 10^3/cu mm)	Bleeding time (<9 minutes)	Clot Retraction	Prothrombin Time (12 seconds)	Activated Partial Thromboplastin Time (33–45 Seconds)	Thrombin Time (3–5 Seconds Above Control)
Thrombocytopenia	Low	Prolonged	Poor to absent	Normal	Normal	Normal
Vascular defects	Normal	Prolonged (tourniquet test positive)	Normal	Normal	Normal	Normal
Qualitative platelet defect	Normal	Prolonged	Normal (poor to absent in thrombasthenia)	Normal	Normal	Normal
Extrinsic coagulation system						
Factor VII deficiency	Normal	Normal	Normal	Prolonged	Normal	Normal
Factor II, V, or X deficiency	Normal	Normal	Normal	Prolonged	Prolonged	Normal
Intrinsic coagulation system						
Factor VIII and IX deficiency	Normal	Normal	Normal	Normal	Prolonged	Normal
von Willebrand's disease	Normal	Prolonged	Normal	Normal	Variable—usually prolonged	Normal
Afibrinogenemia, dysfibrinogenemia	Normal	Variable	Normal	Normal	Normal	Prolonged
DIC, liver failure	Usually low	Variable, often prolonged	Sometimes poor	Prolonged	Prolonged	Prolonged

method in which an incision approximately 1 cm long and 1 mm deep is made on the volar surface of the forearm while 40 mm Hg of pressure is maintained on the upper arm with a blood pressure cuff. In thrombocytopenia, qualitative platelet defects, and rarely vessel disorders the bleeding time usually exceeds nine minutes. *Clot retraction* will be absent in thrombocytopenia and usually defective in thrombasthenia. The *one-stage prothrombin time* provides an overall assessment of the extrinsic coagulation system. The *activated partial thromboplastin time* test is an excellent screening procedure for the intrinsic clotting mechanism. Even slight prolongation of this test may be significant and must be further evaluated. Prolongation of the *thrombin time* indicates that the fibrinogen level is below 100 mg per deciliter, that the fibrinogen is structurally abnormal, or that an inhibitor is present. The thrombin time is also a good screening test for the presence of fibrinogen-fibrin degradation products, as occurs in disseminated intravascular coagulation (DIC).

Not uncommonly routine screening procedures reveal a combination of a slightly prolonged bleeding time and a normal platelet count. This is frequently due to ingestion of aspirin during the week prior to testing or occasionally to glyceryl guaiacolate, a component of cough remedies. A prolonged bleeding time in a patient with a normal platelet count is indicative of a qualitative platelet defect—especially in the absence of drug ingestion (Table 166–2). Platelet aggregometry can furnish additional information concerning the platelet defect. Platelet aggregation is measured by an increase in light transmission through platelet-rich plasma, which is stirred while a specific aggregating agent is being added—usually ADP, collagen, thrombin, epinephrine, sodium arachidonate, or ristocetin. A normal platelet count in the setting of an abnormal bleeding time and a prolonged partial thromboplastin time mandate a ristocetin agglutination study for von Willebrand's disease, which will be abnormal in this disorder. Platelets from patients with thrombasthenia do not respond to any aggregation stimulus. Persons with acquired defects in the platelet release reaction (drug ingestion, uremia) or those with congenital release abnormalities will demonstrate a single, reversible wave of platelet aggregation. Platelets from patients who have recently ingested aspirin are unresponsive to arachidonate. Platelet aggregometry requires laboratory expertise, and abnormalities of platelet aggregation do not consistently correlate with clinically significant disease.

In general, the patient whose coagulation and platelet screening tests are completely normal does not require further evaluation. However, there are instances in which very mild coagulation or platelet disturbances might be further elucidated by specific assays for coagulation factors, or by platelet aggregation studies using a more extended group of stimuli. A re-evaluation may also be indicated when results do not correlate with clinical findings or fall within the borderline range.

Harker LA, Zimmerman TS (eds.): Measurements of Platelet Function. Methods in Hematology Series. Vol 8. New York, Churchill Livingstone, 1983. *This book is an up-to-date compilation of recommended methodology for evaluating platelet function.*

Quantitative Platelet Disorders

THROMBOCYTOPENIA

Thrombocytopenia may be defined as a platelet count below 100,000 per cubic millimeter. With the exception of chronic, longstanding thrombocytopenia, correlations can be made between the platelet count and hemorrhage. Platelet counts in

TABLE 166–4. CAUSES OF THROMBOCYTOPENIA

I. Decreased platelet production
  - Reduced megakaryocytes in marrow
    - Marrow infiltration—malignancy; myelofibrosis, chemicals and drugs
    - Marrow hypoplasia—radiation, chemicals, insecticides, drugs, viruses, idiopathic, alcohol
    - Congenital—Fanconi's pancytopenia, thrombocytopenia with absent radius, autosomal recessive thrombocytopenia, cyclic thrombocytopenia, infection (congenital rubella)
  - Ineffective thrombocytopoiesis (normal or increased marrow megakaryocytes)
    - Hereditary
      - Autosomal dominant thrombocytopenia
      - May-Hegglin anomaly
      - Wiskott-Aldrich syndrome
    - Megaloblastic anemias
      - Di Guglielmo's syndrome
      - Preleukemia

II. Decreased platelet survival
  - Increased destruction
    - Drug-induced thrombocytopenic purpura
    - Idiopathic thrombocytopenic purpura
    - Post-transfusion purpura
    - Isoimmune neonatal purpura
    - Secondary immunologic purpura
  - Increased consumption
    - Thrombotic thrombocytopenic purpura
    - Disseminated intravascular coagulation
    - Cavernous hemangioma
    - Hemolytic-uremic syndrome
    - Acute infections
    - Cardiopulmonary bypass

III. Sequestration (hypersplenism)

IV. Dilutional thrombocytopenia

the range of 40,000 to 60,000 per cubic millimeter may lead to post-traumatic bleeding. Spontaneous bleeding may occur with counts below 20,000 per cubic millimeter, and at these levels central nervous system or gastrointestinal hemorrhage constitutes a major hazard. Thrombocytopenic patients with fever and anemia are particularly susceptible to the development of bleeding, and respond poorly to platelet transfusions.

Thrombocytopenias result from four basic mechanisms (Table 166–4): (1) decreased or ineffective platelet production, (2) a short platelet survival time in the circulation based on increased destruction and/or consumption, (3) sequestration (in the spleen), or (4) intravascular dilution of circulating platelets.

Decreased Platelet Production

REDUCED MEGAKARYOCYTES. Decreased production of platelets by megakaryocytes may occur as a result of marrow replacement, chemical damage, or congenital disorders. The erythroid or myeloid marrow elements may also be compromised to various degrees. Platelet survival is normal or slightly decreased, the basic defect being that of the rate at which platelets enter the circulation. Lesions in the marrow that mechanically displace megakaryocytes and that may be associated with thrombocytopenia include metastatic carcinoma, myeloma, leukemias or lymphomas, xanthomatoses, myelofibrosis, and, occasionally, granulomas. Decreased megakaryocytopoiesis may follow injury by radiation, chemicals, drugs, or infectious agents. Cancer chemotherapeutic agents predictably induce megakaryocyte damage, but drugs such as chloramphenicol and phenylbutazone do so less consistently. Other drugs that have been implicated include alcohol, anticonvulsants, tranquilizers, thiazides, solvents, and insecticides. Megakaryocytic hypoplasia may occur in congenital or genetic disorders, as exemplified by pancytopenia associated with Fanconi's syndrome—a rare, fatal childhood illness in which there are multiple congenital and skeletal abnormalities. Another disorder, known as congenital hypoplastic thrombocytopenia, is associated with absent radii. Megakaryocytic hypoplasia also occurs as an autosomal recessive trait in the absence of other somatic abnormalities and following intrauterine infection with rubella virus.

INEFFECTIVE THROMBOCYTOPOIESIS. In this instance megakaryocytes may be increased in number but the rate at which platelets appear in the circulation is reduced. This may be due to (1) poor platelet formation, (2) defective release of platelets from the marrow, or (3) intramedullary platelet destruction. An autosomal dominant form of this type of thrombocytopenia has been reported, sometimes in association with elevations in serum IgA, nephritis, deafness, and "giant" platelets. Ineffective platelet production is also characteristic of patients with the May-Hegglin anomaly as well as the Wiskott-Aldrich syndrome. In vitamin B_{12} and folate deficiencies the marrow megakaryocyte cytoplasmic mass is increased, but with relatively ineffective platelet production. Alcohol-induced thrombocytopenia is complex and may relate to associated folate deficiency, megakaryocytic hypoplasia, increased platelet splenic pooling, and a shortening of the platelet survival time.

Decreased Platelet Survival Due to Increased Destruction

Drug-Induced Thrombocytopenic Purpura

Approximately 70 drugs have been implicated in or have been proved to induce thrombocytopenic purpura. In adults presenting with thrombocytopenic purpura, a drug cause should be the first consideration—even in the setting of prolonged use of a medication without previous ill effects. In a typical episode the sensitized patient may become symptomatic, with flushing and chills a few minutes after ingesting an offending agent. Petechiae and purpuric lesions occur in dependent areas, although the palms and soles are usually unaffected. Hemorrhagic bullae may appear in the oral mucosa, a finding virtually pathognomonic of the thrombocytopenic state. Hemorrhage from the gastrointestinal and urinary tracts typically occurs several hours later. The petechiae are nontender and nonpruritic and do not have an erythematous border; this distinguishes them from other allergic skin reactions.

PATHOGENESIS. A drug can induce thrombocytopenia by direct action on the circulating platelets—as in the case of ristocetin, an antibiotic no longer in clinical use. Intravenous or subcutaneous heparin occasionally lowers circulating platelet levels through mechanisms not fully clarified. Thiazides and alcohol may block megakaryocyte number and function. The most frequent mechanism underlying drug-induced purpura, however, is immunologic platelet destruction. Common offending drugs are quinidine, quinine, sulfonamides, and thiazide derivatives. Other widely used compounds, such as aspirin, penicillin, digitoxin, and phenobarbital, have also been implicated. Table 166–5 summarizes some of the agents currently thought to produce thrombocytopenic purpura.

The immunologic reaction terminating in platelet destruction occurs as follows: the drug (or one of its derivatives) acts as a hapten and forms a complex with a plasma protein ("carrier"). This complex is antigenic and induces production of high

TABLE 166–5. THERAPEUTIC AND CHEMICAL AGENTS THAT MAY PRODUCE THROMBOCYTOPENIC PURPURA

I. Direct marrow suppressants	
Generalized marrow hypoplasia or aplasia	
Antimetabolites	
Antimitotic agents	
Anti-tumor antibiotics	
Benzene and derivatives	
Ionizing radiation	
Nitrogen mustard and congeners	
Occasional association with marrow hypoplasia or aplasia	
Chloramphenicol	
Gold compounds	
Methylphenylethyl hydantoin (Mesantoin), trimethadione (Tridione)	
Phenylbutazone	
Quinacrine	
Selective suppression of megakaryocytes	
Chlorothiazides	
Estrogenic hormones	
Ethanol	
Tolbutamide	
II. Production of thrombocytopenia by an immunologic mechanism	
Acetazolamide (Diamox)	p-Aminosalicylic acid (PAS)
Carbamazepine	Phenytoin (Dilantin)
Chlorothiazides	Quinidine
Chlorpropamide	Quinine
Desipramine	Rifampin
Digitoxin	Stibophen (Fuadin)
Gold salts	Sulfamethazine
Hydroxychloroquin	Sulfathiazole
Methyldopa	
III. Direct damage to circulating platelets	
Heparin	
Ristocetin	
IV. Probable immunologic mechanism; antibodies not always demonstrated	
Acetaminophen	Organic hair dyes
Aminopyrine	Nitroglycerin
Aspirin and sodium salicylate	Paramethadione
	Penicillin
Barbiturates	Phenacetin
Bismuth	Phenylbutazone
Carbutamide	Potassium iodide
Cephalothin	Prednisone
Chloroquine	Prochlorperazine
Chlorpheniramine maleate	Promethazine
Chlorpromazine	Propylthiouracil
Codeine	Pyrazinamide
Dextroamphetamine sulfate	Reserpine
Diazoxide	Spironolactone
Digitalis and digoxin	Streptomycin
Disulfiram (Antabuse)	Sulfonamides (sulfadiazine, sulfadimetine, sulfamerazine, sulfamethoxazole, sulfisoxazole)
Ergot	
Erythromycin	
Insecticides	Tetracycline
Iopanoic acid (Telepaque)	Tetraethylammonium (TEA)
Isoniazid	Thiourea
Meperidine	Trimethadione
Meprobamate	Turpentine
Mercurial diuretics	

affinity antibodies. The antibodies bind to the drug, and the antigen-antibody complex adsorbs to platelet membranes via their Fc receptor. Adsorption of the antigen-antibody complex by platelets is therefore nonspecific: i.e., the platelets are "innocent bystanders" in the reaction. The coated platelets are rapidly removed from the circulation by the reticuloendothelial system.

DIAGNOSIS. In all thrombocytopenic patients a detailed history of drug ingestion or unusual environmental exposure is mandatory. The patient should even be questioned concerning intake of beverages such as tonic water, since it contains quinine, which in small amounts can induce thrombocytopenia ("cocktail purpura"). All medications should be stopped in thrombocytopenic patients until a diagnosis has been made. This also serves as a diagnostic test, since the purpura may begin to clear within a few days following removal of the offending drug.

In vitro tests for identifying circulating antibodies in drug-induced thrombocytopenia are difficult to perform in routine laboratories. No single test (e.g., complement fixation, "immunoinjury" tests) will detect all cases. Direct binding assays for IgG or complement on the platelet surface are useful but difficult to perform. Readministration of the drug to confirm an etiologic diagnosis is not recommended. If the other hematologic parameters are normal, a bone marrow examination may not be necessary. However, if thrombocytopenia persists for more than two weeks following abstinence from the drug, another diagnosis should be considered and a bone marrow examination is indicated. Exceptions include slowly excreted drugs such as gold salts and arsenicals.

TREATMENT. Frequently no treatment will be necessary, since withdrawal of the offending agent should result in recovery. If the purpura increases in severity or spontaneous bleeding occurs from mucous membranes, corticosteroid therapy is recommended for its effect on vascular integrity and interference with phagocytosis of antibody-coated or complement-coated platelets by macrophages in the spleen. If platelet counts are below 30,000 per cubic millimeter, corticosteroids should be administered initially. Life-threatening hemorrhage should be managed with platelet transfusions or, as a last resort, exchange transfusions. The latter would lower plasma concentrations of the drug as well as of antibody. Since the antibodies in drug-induced thrombocytopenia are specific, alternative compounds that are pharmacologically equivalent can be used. Future use of the offending drug is contraindicated.

Idiopathic Thrombocytopenic Purpura

DEFINITION. Idiopathic thrombocytopenic purpura (ITP) refers to thrombocytopenia in the absence of toxic exposure or of a disease associated with low platelet levels. An immunologic process involving an IgG-type antibody can be demonstrated in about 85 per cent of patients with ITP. There are two forms of ITP, acute and chronic. In both types there are normal or increased numbers of megakaryocytes in the marrow, a shortened platelet survival time, and an absence of splenomegaly.

ACUTE ITP. Acute ITP is mainly a disorder of childhood, most common between the ages of two and six and affecting both sexes equally. There is usually a history of an antecedent upper respiratory infection one to three weeks prior to onset. (The peak seasonal incidence of acute ITP during fall and winter may parallel the prevalence of viral infections and respiratory illnesses.) Petechial hemorrhages and purpura occur abruptly and may be accompanied by hemorrhagic bullae in the oral cavity, along with gastrointestinal and genitourinary bleeding. Platelet counts of 20,000 per cubic millimeter or below are commonly observed; therefore, the patient is at risk for intracranial hemorrhage. The peripheral smear commonly shows eosinophilia and lymphocytosis. In 80 per cent of cases spontaneous remissions occur in two to six weeks. However, spontaneous recovery in adults is less common.

Therapy is not required unless spontaneous mucous membrane hemorrhage occurs or ecchymoses continue to develop. Many physicians elect to treat all patients, especially adults, with prednisone (1 to 2 mg per kilogram of body weight) at least during the first four weeks of illness when the risk of hemorrhage is maximal. Platelet transfusions should be reserved for the rare life-threatening situation, because survival of transfused platelets in ITP may be as short as a few minutes.

About 10 to 15 per cent of patients with acute ITP will not recover in a six-month period. Such patients will rarely undergo a subsequent spontaneous remission and may require treatment with corticosteroids. Children who do not respond within six to twelve months should be considered for splenectomy. Permanent remission follows splenectomy in 85 per cent of cases.

CHRONIC ITP. Chronic ITP usually begins insidiously in adults between the ages of 20 and 40, although it can occur at any age. Women are affected three times more commonly than men. In contrast to acute ITP, a history of antecedent infection is highly unusual. Typically the patient notices occasional petechiae, a bruising tendency, or moderate bleeding immediately after trauma or surgical procedures such as dental extractions. Women may develop menorrhagia. Skin hemorrhages are most common on the distal portions of the upper and lower extremities. If the spleen is palpable, the primary diagnosis is probably not ITP. Platelet counts are in the range of 30,000 to 80,000 per cubic millimeter, and marrow megakaryocytes are normal or increased in number.

Chronic ITP is usually characterized by remissions and relapses alternating over long periods of time. In some patients exacerbations are cyclical and can be correlated with such events as menstruation. The evaluation of treatment is therefore difficult. Life-threatening hemorrhage is unusual. Although the acute form of ITP in children is not associated with other immune-type disorders, adults with chronic ITP require periodic evaluation for the coexistence of diseases such as systemic lupus erythematosus, lymphoproliferative disorders, and the development of autoimmune hemolytic anemia (Evans' syndrome).

Recently, development of ITP has been reported in the homosexual male population. The patients were all sexually active and therefore presumably exposed to viral antigens and multiple drugs. Management of these patients is the same as that for classical ITP. The thrombocytopenic purpura does not seem to be related to the ultimate prognosis in these patients, with regard to development of Kaposi's sarcoma or opportunistic infections.

PATHOGENESIS OF ITP. The concept of an immune mechanism in ITP originated with two observations: (1) Fifty per cent of infants born to mothers with ITP were thrombocytopenic, presumably owing to transplacental transfer of an antiplatelet antibody. (2) Infusion of plasma from patients with ITP produced transient thrombocytopenia with platelet destruction in normal subjects. The ITP factor is an immunoglobulin of the IgG class (7S, subclasses 3 and 1), which is species specific, fixes complement (C3), and can be absorbed from serum with normal platelets. The antibody can also be formed in vitro by cultured splenic cells.

In vitro test systems for qualitative and quantitative analysis of antibody on the platelet surface are technically difficult. These tests, an antiglobulin consumption assay, a competitive binding radioimmunoassay, and a fluorescent anti-IgG assay, quantitate the amount of autoantibody coating the platelet surface. Normal subjects have less than 0.3 pg of IgG per platelet, but patients with ITP have 0.5 to 3.4 pg. Platelet counts are lower when there is more IgG on the platelet surface. The quantity of complement (C3) fixed is usually proportional to the amount of antibody on the surface. Some IgG may be associated with the platelet surface in a nonspecific manner. Thus the direct relationship of platelet IgG measurements to immunologically-mediated ITP may require reassessment.

DIAGNOSIS OF CHRONIC ITP. Immunogenic thrombocytopenia induced by drugs is frequently indistinguishable from ITP; thus an exogenous cause should be ruled out initially. If possible, all medications should be eliminated (or replaced) during the diagnostic study. A bone marrow examination may be helpful if other conditions with which ITP can be confused are under consideration. Antiplatelet antibodies on the platelet surface (IgG) or C3 should be determined if these techniques are available, as positive results are helpful. Measurements of membrane-bound IgG and C3 are much more valuable than those of antibodies in serum. In 50 to 75 per cent of patients a serum antibody is demonstrable.

TREATMENT. There are three major therapeutic modalities for chronic ITP: corticosteroids, splenectomy, and immunosuppressive agents. The clinical course of chronic ITP is variable, but spontaneous recovery occurs in less than 10 per cent of patients. Patients whose platelet counts are in the range of 100,000 with hemorrhagic manifestations limited to scattered petechiae and occasional bruising may be followed at bimonthly intervals, with treatment reserved for any downward trend in platelet count or lengthening of the bleeding time.

Corticosteroids. Therapy is usually initiated with prednisone, approximately 60 mg or 1 mg per kilogram daily, to which 70 to 90 per cent of patients will respond with a rise in platelet count and decrease in bleeding tendency. There are several possible but no precise explanations for the beneficial effect of corticosteroids in ITP: an increase in platelet production, inhibition of the antibody-platelet interaction, impairment of immunoglobulin synthesis, suppression of phagocytic activity in the reticuloendothelial system, and a reduction in capillary fragility. Frequently the hemorrhagic disorder disappears before the platelet count returns to normal levels. Complete normalization of the platelet count with total reversal of the bleeding diathesis occurs in 50 to 60 per cent of patients. Clinical response to corticosteroids becomes evident in one to three weeks, although rarely a beneficial effect may not be observed for up to eight weeks. After approximately four to six weeks the dose of corticosteroids should be tapered gradually and finally discontinued if the bleeding time is normal, even if the platelet count is below 50,000. The clinical status of the patient with regard to hemostasis is more important than the platelet count. About 20 per cent of patients will respond satisfactorily to corticosteroids alone; if a relapse occurs later, readministration of corticosteroids will induce another remission. Approximately 80 per cent of patients who respond to corticosteroids initially will relapse within weeks to months following discontinuation of therapy. The subsequent course of these patients is often an unfortunate one of corticosteroid refractoriness or prohibitive toxicity.

Splenectomy. When the platelet count cannot be maintained above 50,000 with a nontoxic dose of corticosteroid therapy, splenectomy should be performed. About 70 to 80 per cent of patients will improve after splenectomy, and in 60 per cent the platelet count returns to normal. Frequently those who have previously responded to corticosteroid therapy will benefit from splenectomy. In some patients (about 10 per cent) remission may be delayed for weeks to months following splenectomy. Patients who relapse after splenectomy may then respond to steroid therapy.

Refractory ITP. About 5 to 20 per cent of patients with chronic ITP eventually fail to respond to corticosteroid therapy or splenectomy. Immunosuppressive drugs (cyclophosphamide, azathioprine, and vincristine) have been beneficial in such persons, despite a lag period between administration and signs of improvement. Of these agents, vincristine is preferred since it does not simultaneously suppress platelet production in the marrow and may also exert an inhibitory effect on phagocytosis of coated platelets by the reticuloendothelial system. How long responses to immunosuppressive agents can be sustained is not fully known. Two new experimental approaches are promising—intravenous gamma globulin and danazol.

Platelet transfusions are much less effective in ITP than in nonimmune thrombocytopenias because the platelets are rapidly destroyed upon administration. However, they may be required in life-threatening complications such as intracranial hemorrhage or during major surgical procedures, including splenectomy. Prophylactic use of platelet concentrates in ITP patients should be avoided. Women with ITP who become symptomatic during menses have been shown to benefit from anovulatory medications.

McMillan R: Chronic idiopathic thrombocytopenic purpura. N Engl J Med 304:1135, 1981. *This review thoroughly encompasses current clinical, laboratory, and therapeutic aspects of chronic ITP.*

Morris L, Distenfeld A, Amorosi E, Karpatkin S: Autoimmune thrombocytopenic purpura in homosexual men. Ann Intern Med 96:714, 1982. *These 11 patients did not have Kaposi's sarcoma or opportunistic infections. Thus an abnormality of immune regulation rather than immunosuppression may have been present.*

Picozzi VJ, Roeske WR, Creger WP: Fate of therapy failures in adult idiopathic thrombocytopenic purpura. Am. J Med 69:690, 1980. *An interesting retrospective study in which spontaneous recovery in patients with ITP was surprisingly frequent.*

Post-Transfusion Purpura

Post-transfusion purpura is an acute form of thrombocytopenic purpura, clinically indistinguishable from ITP or drug-induced thrombocytopenia. Typically a fulminant episode of thrombocytopenic purpura occurs five to eight days following transfusion of whole blood. These patients, usually women, have developed an antibody to a genetically determined platelet antigen known as Pl^{A1}, which is present in 98 per cent of the population. Although 1 in 50 recipients is mismatched with respect to Pl^{A1} antigen, post-transfusion purpura is fortunately very rare and production of the antibody is transient. Platelet counts are usually less than 10,000, and thrombocytopenia may persist for up to seven weeks. Corticosteroids have been employed for treatment, but the severity of the thrombocytopenia and risk of hemorrhage have prompted use of exchange transfusions and plasmapheresis, which are of definite benefit. Platelet transfusions are ineffective. The anti-Pl^{A1} antibody can be detected in most patients by agglutination and complement fixation techniques, rendering the diagnosis definitive. Post-transfusion purpura may be heterogeneous and is not limited to females or Pl^{A1} negative persons.

Isoimmune Neonatal Purpura

Rarely thrombocytopenic purpura occurs in the neonate owing to fetal-maternal platelet incompatibility. The thrombocytopenia is presumably due to transplacental passage of platelet isoantibodies produced by the mother against antigens on the platelets of the infant, most commonly the Pl^{A1} system (50 per cent). Shortly after delivery the infants develop petechiae, ecchymoses, and hematomas, with platelet counts usually below 35,000 per cubic millimeter. Therapy has included exchange transfusions, platelet transfusions, and corticosteroids, Usually recovery is uneventful, and platelet counts return to normal in 21 days.

Secondary Immunologic Thrombocytopenia

Immunologic platelet injury can also occur as a complication of systemic diseases associated with abnormal immune responses. About 10 per cent of patients with systemic lupus erythematosus will develop a syndrome quite similar to chronic ITP. In some instances patients with early lupus will present with an ITP-like disorder. For this reason, immunologic tests for lupus erythematosus should be performed in all new cases of ITP. In Evans' syndrome ITP is associated with Coombs-positive autoimmune hemolytic anemia. In chronic lymphocytic leukemia and in malignant lymphoma an ITP-like syndrome also occurs, although in most cases thrombocytopenia is due to marrow involvement. Mild forms of immunologic thrombocytopenia have been described in rheumatoid arthritis, hyperthyroidism, and sarcoid.

In allergic reactions to insect bites, tetanus toxoid, foods, and vaccines, platelets damaged by antigen-antibody complexes may be sequestered in the reticuloendothelial system resulting in thrombocytopenia. A comparable mechanism may occur during recovery from viral infections such as rubella or infectious mononucleosis. In some patients with infectious mononucleosis, cold antibodies against the "i" antigen coat the platelets, which are then removed by the reticuloendothelial system.

Decreased Platelet Survival Due to Increased Consumption

Thrombotic Thrombocytopenia Purpura (Moschcowitz's Syndrome)

Thrombotic thrombocytopenic purpura (TTP) is an acute, diffuse disorder of the microcirculation characterized by thrombocytopenic purpura, microangiopathic hemolytic anemia, transient and fluctuating neurologic signs, renal dysfunction, and a febrile course. More than 400 cases have been reported, of which approximately two thirds have been women with a mean age of 39. The hemorrhagic disorder is widespread and includes petechiae and ecchymoses, gastrointestinal bleeding, hematuria, and retinal hemorrhage. The neurologic findings are quite variable and frequently include an organic mental syndrome, paresis, headache, aphasia, slurred speech, vertigo, and seizures. The renal disease is progressive and manifested by proteinuria, hematuria, and a rising blood urea nitrogen.

Almost all patients are thrombocytopenic with an initial platelet count of less than 50,000 per cubic millimeter. Examination of the peripheral blood smear reveals the characteristic abnormalities of microangiopathic hemolytic anemia—fragmented red cells (schistocytes), burr cells, helmet-shaped erythrocyte forms, and normoblasts. The Coombs' test is negative, and there is usually a marked reticulocytosis. In early stages of the disease laboratory tests do not suggest DIC. However, as the syndrome progresses to the point of hepatic and renal decompensation or onset of sepsis, frank DIC occurs.

The characteristic pathologic lesion of TTP is the hyaline thrombus that occludes arterioles and capillaries of virtually every tissue in the body. Although endothelial proliferation may be seen near the lesions, inflammatory reactions and vasculitis do not occur. The hyaline material is thought to consist of dense platelet aggregates rimmed with thin layers of fibrin.

The cause of the diffuse occlusive lesions of the microcirculation in TTP is unknown. In about one third of patients a history of previous upper respiratory tract infection can be elicited. The disorder has been linked with oral contraceptives, antibiotics, surgery, pregnancy, meningococcal infections, coxsackievirus B, vaccines, and mycoplasmas. An abnormal immune response may be involved in the pathogenesis of TTP, since the syndrome has been reported in association with disseminated lupus erythematosus, low levels of serum complement, and the presence of complement components in the vascular lesions. The recent successful therapeutic use of exchange transfusions and plasmapheresis has been cited as evidence to support the concept that vascular injury, platelet sequestration, and microvascular thrombosis in TTP could be due to deposition of immune complexes in arterioles and capillaries. However, to date circulating immune complexes have not been identified in TTP.

In a typical case the presence of thrombocytopenia, hemolytic anemia, neurologic abnormalities, fever, and renal dysfunction will suggest the appropriate diagnosis. If patients are seen late in the course, disseminated intravascular coagulation may be difficult to rule out, although the hemolysis in DIC is not as severe as in TTP. The hemolytic-uremic syndrome of infants and children may resemble TTP, although neurologic symptoms are rare and TTP involves more organ systems than does the hemolytic-uremic syndrome. In some cases skin, muscle, gingival, lymph node, and marrow biopsies have been employed with moderate success. A TTP-like syndrome can occur in patients with malignancies following chemotherapy.

TTP is a rare disease and frequently fatal (50 to 80 per cent). Therapy has been difficult to evaluate. Splenectomy, massive corticosteroids, and inhibitors of platelet function—such as dipyridamole, aspirin, and dextran—have all been used with varied success. Recently exchange transfusions, plasmapheresis, and plasma infusions have been used with encouraging results. Some patients have obtained complete remissions of long duration, whereas others have required continued plasma infusions. Plasma infusions or plasmapheresis or both are currently the treatment of choice and should be employed as soon as the diagnosis is made.

Marcus AJ: Moschcowitz revisited. N Engl J Med 307:1447, 1982. *Discussion of a new approach to the pathogenesis and treatment of chronic TTP.*

Lian EC-Y, Mui PTK, Siddiqui FA, Chiu AYY, Chiu LLS: Inhibition of platelet-aggregating activity in thrombotic thrombocytopenic purpura plasma by normal adult immunoglobulin G. J Clin Invest 73:548, 1984. *Normal IgG inhibits platelet-aggregating activity present in TTP plasma.*

Disseminated Intravascular Coagulation (DIC)

The syndrome of disseminated intravascular coagulation encompasses a number of clinical situations in which thrombin gains access to the general circulation. It occurs in patients in whom there is no previous history of a hemorrhagic disorder and who may be undergoing treatment for conditions unassociated with hemorrhage. The primary features are discussed in Ch. 167; DIC is mentioned here because thrombocytopenia may occur out of proportion to the coagulation abnormality. Thrombin is a strong stimulus for platelet aggregation and release, which results in enhanced platelet consumption. In addition, platelet adhesion to damaged tissues and blood vessels will increase the degree of thrombocytopenia.

Diagnosis of DIC must be based on clinical evidence of hemorrhage (or thrombosis) and positive laboratory parameters. Treatment of the underlying pathogenesis is more important than heparin therapy, which should only be used as a last resort—especially in thrombocytopenic patients.

Cavernous Hemangioma (Kasabach-Merritt Syndrome)

Approximately 0.3 per cent of infants with hemangiomas, either subcutaneous or visceral, have thrombocytopenia. Since the lesions are congenital, bleeding may occur during the first few days of life. Thrombocytopenia does not directly correlate with the size of the lesion. Microangiopathic hemolytic anemia and DIC may occur in some patients. Most capillary and cavernous hemangiomas spontaneously regress, but lesions in vital areas such as the neck and thorax require radiotherapy or surgical removal.

Hemolytic-Uremic Syndrome (Gasser's Syndrome)

The hemolytic-uremic syndrome (HUS) usually occurs in infants and young children, and is characterized by microangiopathic hemolytic anemia, thrombocytopenia, and acute renal failure. Occasional cases have been reported in adolescents and young adults. In infants a typical episode is heralded by abdominal pain, vomiting, and diarrhea. There is evidence of anemia, hemorrhage, renal insufficiency, and cardiac decompensation. In contrast to TTP, neurologic signs and symptoms are rare. Severe thrombocytopenia (in 85 per cent of cases) occurs with Coombs-negative microangiopathic hemolytic anemia. Laboratory features of DIC may be present early in the course, but subsequently coagulation factor levels can increase as a "rebound" phenomenon. Thus, it is not conclusive that HUS is an instance of DIC. A disorder similar to HUS has been reported in women in association with pregnancy, the postpartum period, and ingestion of oral contraceptives. This appears to be a variant of HUS and leads to nephrosclerosis.

The major pathologic lesion consists of occlusive hyaline deposits in the renal microcirculation. Fibrin and platelets have also been identified in the vessels. HUS is thought to result from an incomplete response to a primary antigenic stimulus with subsequent formation of circulating immune complexes and accompanying fibrin deposition in the renal microvasculature.

The major therapeutic objective is management of renal failure with peritoneal dialysis. The combination of erythrocyte transfusions, dialysis, and other vigorous supportive measures has reduced the overall mortality from 30 to 35 per cent to about 5 per cent. Corticosteroids, heparin, and fibrinolytic therapy have not been consistently beneficial. Agents that interfere with platelet aggregation, such as aspirin and dipyridamole, have been successfully used in a small number of patients. Plasma and plasmapheresis for treatment of HUS may prove to be of value.

Kaplan BS, Drummond KN: The hemolytic-uremic syndrome is a syndrome. N Engl J Med 298:964, 1978. *This discussion considers the definition and pathogenesis of the hemolytic-uremic syndrome. The central feature is damage to the vascular endothelium in glomerular capillaries and renal arterioles. Differentiation of this disorder from thrombotic thrombocytopenic purpura is discussed.*

Thrombocytopenia in Acute Infections

Bacterial, viral, fungal, rickettsial, and protozoan infections have all been associated with thrombocytopenia. Febrile patients with platelet counts below 200,000 per cubic millimeter should be evaluated for gram-negative sepsis or, less commonly, gram-positive sepsis. In some cases platelet production may be suppressed, and in others direct platelet destruction by viruses and bacteria has been demonstrated in vitro. Development of DIC as a complication of infection would further contribute to thrombocytopenia. Toxins produced by microorganisms can bind to platelets with resulting aggregation and release, and circulating immune complexes may adsorb to the platelet surface. Only a small percentage of patients develop a hemorrhagic diathesis, with platelet levels returning to normal during recovery.

Thrombocytopenia in Cardiopulmonary Bypass

Thrombocytopenia is one of several hemostatic complications that may occur during cardiopulmonary bypass. Contact of platelets with surfaces of oxygenators may serve as a stimulus for aggregation and release. Traces of thrombin may form in the pump and at surgical sites. Thus DIC can accompany and complicate the thrombocytopenia. Platelet transfusions are the treatment of choice, although more recently prostacyclin (PGI_2) has been used to block platelet aggregation and release in extracorporeal circulatory equipment. Thus, "post-pump" thrombocytopenia may be preventable with the use of prostacyclin, which will increase platelet cyclic AMP.

Thrombocytopenia Due to Sequestration

Moderate splenomegaly is frequently accompanied by platelet counts in the range of 50,000 to 100,000 per cubic millimeter (see Ch. 164). A hemorrhagic diathesis per se is rare, but trauma or major surgery in such patients can be accompanied by excessive bleeding. Bone marrow megakaryocytes are normal or increased, and anemia and leukopenia may also occur. Normally about 30 per cent of the platelets are in the spleen, but in hypersplenic patients this quantity may approach 90 per cent. Platelet pooling in hypersplenism must be distinguished from actual platelet destruction, which occurs in the reticuloendothelial system of the spleen in the immune thrombocytopenias. Platelet survival curves in hypersplenism indicate low recovery in the peripheral blood but an essentially normal life span—i.e., delayed transit time through the spleen. Splenectomy is followed by restoration of the platelet count to normal but is rarely required for the thrombocytopenia.

Dilutional Thrombocytopenia

In addition to effects of dilution, at least three hemostatic deficits can occur in patients having massive transfusion: thrombocytopenia, platelet functional abnormalities, and a coagulation disorder. Platelet counts may fall to 50,000 but rarely below this level. Platelet transfusions may be necessary, but this should be governed by clinical evaluation of the patient rather than use of the platelet counts per se. The thrombocytopenia is usually reversible within three to five days.

THROMBOCYTOSIS AND THROMBOCYTHEMIA

Thrombocytosis, an elevation of the platelet count above 400,000 per cubic millimeter, occurs in three forms: (1) transitory or "physiologic," (2) reactive or "secondary," and (3) autonomous or "primary" (thrombocythemia).

Transitory thrombocytosis can occur following exercise and stress, and may reflect release of platelets from the lung, since it occurs in splenectomized persons. Epinephrine administration produces a 20 to 50 per cent rise in platelet count, which originates from the splenic pool since it does not occur in asplenic individuals. Transitory thrombocytosis results from mobilization of preformed platelets rather than from accelerated platelet production.

Secondary or reactive thrombocytosis does result from accelerated platelet production, although the stimulus is not known. Reactive thrombocytosis occurs in response to hemorrhage, hemolysis, infectious and inflammatory diseases, carcinomas, and lymphomas. If the underlying disorder is successfully treated, platelet counts return to normal levels. It is rarely necessary to lower platelet counts by therapeutic means. The reactive thrombocytosis following splenectomy occurs during the first few days and may reach 1,000,000 per cubic millimeter during the next three weeks. Platelet counts may not return to normal for two months, but during this time a thrombotic or hemorrhagic disorder rarely occurs and therapy is not necessary.

In *primary thrombocythemia* the elevated platelet production is sustained and independent of normal regulatory processes. Megakaryocytes are markedly increased in number and mass, and platelet production correspondingly elevated as much as 15-fold. Paradoxically, platelet counts in the range of 1 to 2 million per cubic millimeter may be associated with either hemorrhage or thrombosis. The hemorrhage is usually from mucosal surfaces and may be due to a functional platelet abnormality. Platelets from these patients respond poorly, if at all, to epinephrine in vitro. The thrombotic lesions may be related to an increased circulating platelet mass per se, or there may be a disturbance in the balance between thromboxane A_2 production in platelets and prostacyclin production by vascular endothelium. Endothelial cells can utilize endoperoxides produced by stimulated platelets for prostacyclin synthesis. When platelets are present in excess, they may preferentially use their own endoperoxides for thromboxane production, which would then result in more platelet aggregation and vasoconstriction.

Essential or hemorrhagic thrombocythemia is encountered mainly in myeloproliferative disorders (see Ch. 154 for a more definitive description of this entity) and may accompany or evolve into chronic myelogenous leukemia, polycythemia vera, or agnogenic myeloid metaplasia. Eighty per cent of the patients have splenomegaly. In addition to mucous membrane bleeding, hemorrhage may complicate trauma and/or surgery. Although there are alternating episodes of hemorrhage and thrombosis, thromboembolic phenomena are the most common cause of death. Marked abnormalities of platelet size and shape are seen on blood smears, together with aggregates of platelets and occasional fragments of megakaryocytes. The bone marrow shows megakaryocytic hyperplasia.

The presence of thrombocytosis gives rise to spurious laboratory values for substances in the circulation that are normal platelet components released into serum in excessive amounts. Thus, a patient may demonstrate pseudohyperkalemia as well as increases in serum acid phosphatase, lactic dehydrogenase, and zinc. In contrast to serum, these measurements are normal in the patient's plasma. With automated counting devices the large platelets seen in thrombocytosis may be estimated as erythrocytes, resulting in a spuriously low platelet count.

The incidence of clinical bleeding or thrombosis does not correlate with in vitro tests of platelet function, but lowering platelet production will reduce or eliminate hemorrhagic and/or thrombotic complications. Alkylating agents such as melphalan or busulfan are useful. The drug is discontinued as platelet counts approach normal levels. The alkylating agent will not reach therapeutic effectiveness for four to six weeks, so that plateletpheresis is recommended for an immediate although transient result. Indications for plateletpheresis would include brisk spontaneous hemorrhage, repeated thrombotic episodes, or preparation for surgery. Results of treatment with anticoagulants such as heparin and coumarins have not been consistent. The use of aspirin (325 mg daily) and dipyridamole* (75 mg three times daily) to interfere with platelet function is recommended on theoretical grounds.

Qualitative Platelet Disorders

Patients with a prolonged bleeding time and normal platelet count are considered to have a qualitative platelet disorder. The cause of the abnormality could be intrinsic to the platelet itself or due to deficiency of a plasma factor required for normal platelet function. Usually one of three aspects of platelet function is abnormal in congenital or acquired platelet disorders: adhesion, aggregation, or the release reaction. Congenital platelet diseases are quite rare, but their investigation has provided new insights into basic mechanisms of platelet function.

Weiss HJ: Disorders of hemostasis-qualitative platelet disorders. *In* Williams WJ, Beutler E, Erslev AJ, Lichtman MA (eds.): Hematology. 3rd ed. New York, McGraw-Hill, 1983, pp 1346-1362. *Congenital and acquired platelet diseases are classified in an orderly fashion. Emphasis is placed on recently elucidated functional and biochemical aspects of these disorders.*

BERNARD-SOULIER (GIANT PLATELET) SYNDROME

The Bernard-Soulier syndrome is a rare inherited bleeding disorder of unusual severity, transmitted as an autosomal recessive trait and characterized by the presence of platelets with an unusually wide variation in size and morphology. Cutaneous, mucous membrane, and visceral hemorrhages have been reported, and fatalities have occurred. The bleeding time is markedly prolonged, probably because of impaired adhesion of defective platelets to subendothelial tissues. Abnormal prothrombin consumption, reported in most patients, reflects poor coagulation-promoting properties of the platelets, probably owing to impaired binding of coagulation factors. Platelet aggregation by collagen, epinephrine, and ADP is normal, but ristocetin agglutination is absent. In contrast to patients with von Willebrand's disease, the ristocetin agglutination reaction cannot be corrected by addition of normal plasma or the moiety of the factor VIII molecule known as von Willebrand factor. A complex on the platelet membrane, glycoprotein I, probably mediates ristocetin-induced, von Willebrand factor–dependent agglutination. Platelet glycoprotein Ib is deficient in patients with the Bernard-Soulier syndrome. The only available treatment is platelet transfusions.

PLATELETS IN VON WILLEBRAND'S DISEASE

Adhesion of platelets to subendothelium is defective in von Willebrand's disease as it is in the Bernard-Soulier syndrome. However, in contrast to Bernard-Soulier disease, the adhesion defect is based on a plasma abnormality rather than a platelet abnormality. Thus, infusion of cryoprecipitate preparations will usually correct the bleeding time in patients with von Willebrand's disease but does not do so in the Bernard-Soulier patient. Standard platelet aggregation tests are normal in von Willebrand's disease, but the platelets will not agglutinate to ristocetin. However, the ristocetin response is corrected by addition of normal plasma or a source of plasma von Willebrand factor. Von Willebrand's disease is discussed in greater detail in Ch. 167.

THROMBASTHENIA (GLANZMANN'S DISEASE)

Thrombasthenia is a moderately severe platelet disorder with autosomal recessive inheritance. Most bleeding manifestations are mucosal, with menorrhagia and epistaxis predominating. However, the severity of hemorrhage is variable and many patients have minimal symptoms. The syndrome is characterized by a prolonged bleeding time, normal platelet count, poor to absent clot retraction, and normal agglutination with ristocetin. Platelets from thrombasthenic patients do not aggregate in response to ADP, collagen, thrombin, epinephrine, arachidonate, and endoperoxide PGH_2. Nevertheless, thrombasthenic platelets will undergo a normal shape change and release reaction in response to aggregating agents. Platelet adhesion to rabbit aorta subendothelium and to collagen is normal in thrombasthenia, but no aggregates appear on the adherent monolayer. Thus, platelet-platelet interactions (cohesion) are defective. Platelet glycoproteins IIb and IIIa are deficient in thrombasthenia. This may be related to the defect in ADP aggregation because an IgG antibody from the plasma of a patient with thrombasthenia will inhibit aggregation of normal platelets by ADP. Platelets from some thrombasthenic patients are deficient in the alloantigen Pl^{A1}, and it is possible that glycoprotein IIb or IIIa carries the Pl^{A1} antigenic determinant. Fibrinogen binding to the platelet surface following ADP stimulation is also defective in thrombasthenia. These patients are usually responsive to platelet transfusions if local measures fail to control bleeding.

*This use is not listed in the manufacturer's directive.

ABNORMALITIES OF THE PLATELET RELEASE REACTION

A syndrome characterized by a mild bleeding tendency and menorrhagia may result from defects in the platelet release reaction. The bleeding time is slightly prolonged, but platelet counts and levels of coagulation factors are normal. The aggregation response to ADP occurs in a single reversible wave, and collagen-induced aggregation is markedly reduced—presumably because of lack of ADP release. One group of patients with release reaction defects has a storage pool disorder in that their platelets are deficient in a specific pool of ADP normally stored in dense granules. Normally, this released ADP is responsible for the second, or irreversible, phase of platelet aggregation. Storage pool deficiency also accompanies several other hereditary disorders, including the Hermansky-Pudlak, Wiskott-Aldrich, and Chédiak-Higashi syndromes.

Another group of patients demonstrates normal ADP content in dense granules, but the mechanism for its release is deficient. This has also been termed an "aspirin-like" disorder and must be differentiated from that observed in patients who surreptitiously ingest aspirin or aspirin-like drugs. Reports of cyclooxygenase and thromboxane synthetase deficiencies are also beginning to appear. Such lesions will require biochemical verification.

Patients with glycogen storage disease, Type I (glucose-6-phosphatase deficiency), may have a mild hemorrhagic tendency characterized by a long bleeding time. There is a defect in ADP release resulting from failure of nucleotide synthesis secondary to hypoglycemia. This is correctable by intravenous glucose administration.

In general, patients with release reaction abnormalities require only local therapeutic measures. Aspirin should be avoided, since it may exaggerate the defect. Serious hemorrhage may require platelet transfusions.

ACQUIRED DISORDERS OF PLATELET FUNCTION—SYSTEMIC DISEASES

UREMIA. Uremia may be associated with a hemorrhagic diathesis manifested by ecchymoses, epistaxis, and bleeding from the gastrointestinal tract, frequently secondary to defective platelet function. Prolongation of the bleeding time may also correlate with thrombocytopenia as well as with defects in platelet aggregation, prothrombin consumption, and clot retraction. Both the bleeding tendency and laboratory abnormalities are corrected following hemodialysis. This suggests that platelet dysfunction in uremia is induced by a dialyzable substance(s), of which most interest has centered on urea, guanidinosuccinic acid, and various phenols. Possibly many of the metabolites that accumulate in uremia collectively interfere with platelet function. In addition, patients with chronic renal disease receive a large number of medications, many of which can induce platelet dysfunction. Thus the pathogenesis of the "uremic platelet defect" is probably three-fold—thrombocytopenia, the adverse effect of accumulated metabolites, and a drug-induced, qualitative platelet abnormality. Bleeding in uremia is also discussed in Ch. 167 in relation to abnormalities in coagulation.

PARAPROTEINEMIAS. The hemorrhagic diathesis that complicates paraproteinemias is usually multifactorial: thus, coagulation disorders, thrombocytopenia, qualitative platelet defects, plasma hyperviscosity, and vascular disturbances related to coating of vessel walls by abnormal proteins have all been reported. Paraproteins may adsorb to the platelet surface, thereby interfering with function. Platelet dysfunction has been demonstrated in macroglobulinemia, and in IgA and IgG myeloma. The clinical and laboratory abnormalities can be directly correlated with paraprotein concentrations and are corrected by plasmapheresis. Therapeutic plasma expanders such as dextran can induce a similar defect in platelet function.

OTHER SYSTEMIC DISEASES. Prolonged bleeding times and in vitro platelet functional abnormalities have been reported in many systemic diseases. These include the acute and chronic leukemias, systemic lupus erythematosus, pernicious anemia, scurvy, homocystinuria, and hepatic cirrhosis. In DIC, fibrinogen-fibrin degradation products interfere with platelet function in vivo and in vitro. This accounts at least in part for the prolonged bleeding time observed in DIC. The disorders of platelet function described in the aforementioned conditions are inconsistent and not a major pathologic feature of the disease. In retrospect, many of the qualitative defects described in early reports may have been medication induced.

Platelet Transfusions

Platelet transfusions are employed to arrest bleeding in thrombocytopenic patients or in persons with severe qualitative platelet defects. They are generally indicated in thrombocytopenias caused by decreased platelet production. Platelet counts below 40,000 per cubic millimeter carry an increased risk of hemorrhage, and platelet numbers less than 10,000 per cubic millimeter are associated with morbidity from spontaneous and traumatic bleeding. Platelet transfusions have been exceedingly helpful in the management of acute leukemias—especially during treatment with chemotherapeutic agents. In the latter instance, prophylactic use of platelet concentrates when levels are 20,000 per cubic millimeter or below has resulted in substantial reduction in death from bleeding. In such patients bleeding also occurs in the setting of fever, infection, and mucosal ulcerations. In these instances transfusions are indicated at even higher platelet levels, since they are less effective in these circumstances. Patients eventually become alloimmunized to platelets from random donors in proportion to the number of units received. At that point platelets from histocompatible siblings or HLA-matched platelets are required for therapeutic effectiveness. The isoimmunization process may be somewhat retarded in leukemic patients, because chemotherapeutic agents are immunosuppressive.

In aplastic anemia platelet transfusions are also effective for correction of bleeding, but isoimmunization occurs more rapidly than in leukemic patients. Thus, prophylactic use of platelets should be avoided. This is especially important if marrow transplantation is anticipated. In patients with aplastic anemia or leukemia, splenectomy may result in improved platelet survival and a decrease in transfusion requirements.

When thrombocytopenic bleeding results from increased platelet destruction or consumption, platelet transfusions are much less effective. For example, in acute and chronic ITP, the drug-induced purpuras, or TTP, transfused platelets are rapidly destroyed. In DIC transfused platelets may serve to further enhance the coagulation process. However, in all of these instances use of massive platelet transfusions as a life-saving measure for intractable hemorrhage is justified.

Platelet transfusions are effective in patients with congenital qualitative platelet abnormalities. These may be required in preparation for or during surgical procedures. Patients with excessive surgical oozing attributable to aspirin or aspirin-like drugs will also respond to platelet transfusions if required. If necessary, platelet-related bleeding in uremic patients should be treated by dialysis, since the transfused platelets will acquire the same defect from the uremic plasma.

Platelet concentrates are the preferred form of therapy. To obtain 1 unit of platelet concentrate, platelet-rich plasma from a standard blood donation is centrifuged and the resulting pellet resuspended in 50 ml of residual plasma. The concentrate will contain approximately 7×10^{10} platelets, which is 70 per cent of the platelets present in the original unit of whole blood. With an appropriate cell separator, 4 to 7 units can be prepared from a single donor. The number of units of platelet concentrate required by an individual recipient can be calculated by dividing the patient's weight in kilograms by 10. Theoretically this estimated dose should increase the platelet count by 70,000 per cubic millimeter. Therapy is considered satisfactory if the platelet count can be maintained above 20,000 per cubic millimeter daily. This may necessitate administration of approximately 5 units of concentrate every other day. In an average adult, 5 units should increase the platelet count from 20,000 to 50,000 per cubic millimeter. However, these increments will be lower in febrile and infected patients. Following multiple platelet transfusions over a six- to twelve-week period, patients become alloimmunized. Platelet counts are then no longer an accurate guide for therapeutic requirements. Thus platelet concentrates must be used in quantities sufficient to arrest bleeding as evaluated clinically. Refractoriness to platelet transfusions can be delayed if HLA-matched donors can be obtained.

Daly PA, Schiffer CA, Aisner J, Wiernik PH: Platelet transfusion therapy: One-hour posttransfusion increments are valuable in predicting the need for HLA-match preparations. JAMA 243:435, 1980. *A very useful guide to the therapeutic use of platelet concentrates in oncology patients.*

Vascular Purpuras

When blood vessels are severed or damaged they constrict; other mechanisms by which they participate in hemostasis are not known. Tests of hemostasis currently in use are designed mainly to evaluate coagulation and platelet function. There are no accurate methods to assess contributions of vessels to hemostasis, and therefore it is difficult to classify vascular purpuras.

In these disorders bleeding occurs from the skin and mucous membranes (petechiae and/or ecchymoses) in the absence of demonstrable abnormalities of platelet function or coagulation (Table 166–6). A positive Rumpel-Leede vascular fragility test in the setting of a prolonged bleeding time, normal platelet count, and normal platelet function points to vascular purpura.

ALLERGIC PURPURA (HENOCH-SCHÖNLEIN OR ANAPHYLACTOID PURPURA). Henoch-Schönlein purpura, a disease mainly of children from two to seven years of age with male predominance, usually begins with urticaria, which fades and is replaced by red maculopapular lesions. The latter gradually coalesce to form symmetrical ecchymoses, especially over the extensor aspects of the lower extremities and buttocks. Two thirds of children have periarticular joint involvement characterized by nonmigratory polyarthralgias in the ankles and knees. Colicky abdominal pain with melena occurs due to hemorrhage and edema in the small intestine, and may also lead to intussusception. Many patients develop acute glomerulonephritis with gross or microscopic hematuria, proteinuria, and edema, especially in the second or third week. Occasionally renal involvement is accompanied by hypertension with a

TABLE 166–6. VASCULAR PURPURAS

Allergic purpura (Henoch-Schönlein)
Dysproteinemias
Macroglobulinemia
Cryoglobulinemia
Primary hyperglobulinemic (benign) purpura
Multiple myeloma
Amyloidosis
Purpura simplex
Drug-induced vascular purpura
Senile purpura
Hereditary disorders of connective tissue
Ehlers-Danlos syndrome
Pseudoxanthoma elasticum
Marfan's syndrome
Osteogenesis imperfecta
Cushing's syndrome
Scurvy
Autoerythrocyte and DNA sensitivity

transient decrease in renal function, which rarely may progress to chronic renal failure (less than 15 per cent). Biopsy of skin lesions reveals aseptic vasculitis with perivascular cuffing, fibrinoid necrosis, platelet plugging, and interstitial edema. Among the substances identified at the site of the inflammatory lesions are IgA, IgM, C3-C5, and properdin. Similar lesions have been seen in the bowel, and renal biopsies have shown segmental or rarely diffuse glomerular proliferation with occlusion of capillaries by fibrinoid material. A discussion of the relationship of Henoch-Schönlein purpura to Berger's disease and other forms of IgA nephropathy is found in Ch. 80. The histopathologic lesions resemble those induced experimentally in immune complex disease, but no antigen has been identified in association with Henoch-Shönlein purpura.

Children with abdominal and joint involvement have been treated with prednisone to reduce edema, but steroids have no effect on the renal lesion, nor do they modify skin manifestations. There is a 50 per cent recurrence rate in the initial weeks of recovery, but long-term prognosis is good in the absence of chronic renal disease.

PARAPROTEINEMIAS. Vascular purpuras occur in the paraproteinemias, but the hemostatic defect usually represents a combination of abnormalities, including thrombocytopenia, a qualitative platelet disorder, and coagulation disturbances. Several factors contribute to the vascular purpura per se. These include hyperviscosity, "sludging" of erythrocytes and leukocytes leading to capillary anoxia, and direct damage to endothelial cell surfaces by precipitated paraproteins.

In cryoglobulinemia as well as cryofibrinogenemia exposure of extremities and other body surfaces to cold may induce purpuric lesions that can subsequently ulcerate. The lesions are probably caused by precipitation of cryoglobulins on intravascular surfaces which then interfere with vessel integrity.

In macroglobulinemia mucosal bleeding is more common than cutaneous hemorrhage. Patients with primary hyperglobulinemic purpura develop recurrent episodes of purpura, especially in relation to exertion or mechanical trauma. The lower extremities are affected most commonly, and the purpuric episode may be preceded by a prodrome of itching and erythema. Progressive pigment deposition at the site of lesions is common. The hyperglobulinemia is of the monoclonal type and is due to the presence of large quantities of IgM. Benign hyperglobulinemic purpura occurs in association with other systemic diseases such as Sjögren's syndrome, disseminated lupus erythematosus, or rheumatoid arthritis.

In myeloma the most common cause of bleeding is thrombocytopenia. This is followed in frequency by a coagulation disorder, a qualitative platelet abnormality, and, finally, vascular purpura (see Ch. 163). The purpura seen in amyloidosis results from deposition of amyloid in the skin and subcutaneous tissues with a resultant defect in vascular integrity (see Ch. 163), especially around the orbital area (a sign called "raccoon eyes").

PURPURA SIMPLEX. This is a mild disorder, most frequent in women, in which lesions are limited to the skin. Ecchymoses or purpura frequently occurs in the lower extremities, with exacerbations during menstrual periods. The syndrome has also been referred to as "devil's pinches." Although a hereditary form of purpura simplex has been reported, some cases may represent drug-induced purpura or platelet-release defects caused by aspirin and/or aspirin-like drugs. The effects of the abnormality are mainly cosmetic and do not require treatment.

DRUG-INDUCED VASCULAR PURPURA. Many drugs are capable of producing generalized purpura in the absence of thrombocytopenia or a qualitative platelet defect. Typical examples are iodides, quinine, procaine penicillin, chlorothiazides, various sulfa drugs, and coumarin anticoagulants. Although an autoimmune reaction involving vascular endothelium has been suggested, no antibodies have been demonstrated to date. Upon discontinuance of the drug, the purpura subsides.

SENILE PURPURA. This disorder results from degeneration and loss of collagen, elastin, and subcutaneous fat in dermal tissues. Location of the purpura also correlates with areas having received most exposure to actinic irradiation. The lesions, usually consisting of red to purple ecchymoses, may arise spontaneously or as a result of pressure on the face, neck, dorsum of the hands, forearms, and legs. The lesions usually persist for weeks and may leave residual brownish pigment deposits, resulting from poor phagocytic function in the area. There is currently no therapy of proven value.

HEREDITARY DISORDERS OF CONNECTIVE TISSUE. In these mesenchymal dysplasias there are abnormalities of connective tissue and perivascular supporting structures of vessel walls. They may account for structural defects in major arteries that result in increased vascular fragility and abnormal platelet adhesiveness. Bleeding varies from easy bruisability to serious hemorrhage from viscera and major blood vessels.

CUSHING'S SYNDROME. Vascular purpura on the trunk and extremities is a common complication of prolonged administration of relatively high doses of corticosteroids or Cushing's disease. Bruising occurs spontaneously and after minor trauma. The pathogenesis of this vascular purpura may be due to a catabolic effect of steroids on perivascular supporting tissues. The disorder is reversible upon cessation of steroid therapy or treatment of Cushing's disease.

SCURVY. In scurvy, collagen synthesis is defective, as is deposition of "intercellular cement" along the endothelial lining and perivascular supporting tissues of small blood vessels. Patients present with gingival bleeding and hemorrhage into subcutaneous tissues and muscles. Bleeding is conspicuous around hair follicles. Subperiosteal hemorrhages are common in children but rare in adults, who more often develop intramuscular hematomas. Other vitamin and nutritional deficiencies frequently coexist and complicate the clinical picture. In adults 1 gram of ascorbic acid per day will terminate the hemorrhagic disorder of scurvy.

AUTOERYTHROCYTE AND DNA SENSITIVITY. "Autoerythrocyte sensitivity" is a rare disorder characterized by formation of painful ecchymoses on the extremities that are frequently preceded by sensations of stinging, itching, or burning. The fully formed lesions usually have an erythematous border and may progressively enlarge. Coincident with the onset of bruising there is frequently a history of severe emotional stress. In addition, patients may have accompanying headache, nausea, and vomiting along with gastrointestinal, genitourinary, or intracranial bleeding. Approximately 100 such patients have been described, 95 of whom are women. Intradermal injection of autologous erythrocytes or erythrocyte stroma usually results in appearance of similar ecchymotic lesions at the injection site. This has led to speculation that the purpura results from autosensitization to a component of the erythrocyte membrane. Remissions and exacerbations over long periods of time are characteristic, and supportive psychotherapy may be useful.

The syndrome of DNA autosensitivity resembles autoerythrocyte sensitization. The lesions begin as painful wheals or nodules on the extremities that enlarge and become indurated. Twenty-four hours later ecchymoses are seen, which may then become bullous. Spontaneous resolution occurs over a period of days to weeks. Intradermal injection of the patient's leukocytes or a solution of DNA into the skin of an extremity will induce formation of ecchymoses. Although the mechanism of action is unknown, administration of chloroquine has been thought to be therapeutically effective. It is not clear whether autosensitivity to DNA is the same syndrome as autoerythrocyte sensitivity.

Bleeding disorders caused by vascular abnormalities. *In* Wintrobe MM, Lee GR, Boggs DR, Bithell TC, Foerster J, Athens JW, Lukens JN (eds.): Clinical Hematology. Philadelphia, Lea & Febiger, 1981, pp 1072–1089. *In this chapter the vascular purpuras are classified and described in an orderly and comprehensive manner. In addition, it contains an excellent bibliography.*

Ratnoff OD: The psychogenic purpuras: A review of autoerythrocyte sensitization, autosensitization to DNA, 'hysterical' and factitial bleeding, and the religious stigmata. Semin Hematol 17:192, 1980. *This is a scholarly summary of the latest information concerning autoerythrocyte sensitization and sensitization to DNA. It also discusses the controversial relationship between emotional stress and the development of hemorrhagic symptomatology.*

Hereditary Hemorrhagic Telangiectasia (Osler-Weber-Rendu Disease)

Hereditary hemorrhagic telangiectasia is an inherited disease resulting from a developmental abnormality of the vasculature. Dilatation and convolution of venules and capillaries give rise to telangiectatic lesions in the skin and mucous membranes. Vessel walls are thinned out to the level of a single layer of endothelium which is lacking in support and contractility. This fragile angiomatous mass of vascular components is known as a telangiectasis. Bleeding may result from minor trauma or occur spontaneously. The abnormality is inherited as an autosomal dominant trait of high penetrance. Although both sexes are affected equally, bleeding seems to be less severe in women. This disease is probably the most common hereditary vascular disorder associated with a hemorrhagic diathesis.

Visible lesions can be as large as 3 mm in diameter and are commonly found on the nasal mucous membranes, lips, gingiva, buccal mucosa, palate, both sides of the tongue, face, trunk, and palmar and plantar surfaces. The telangiectases are violaceous and flat, blanch on pressure exerted by a glass slide, and may vary in shape form pinpoint to nodular or "spider-like." Although the lesions may be seen in children, their appearance increases with age and reaches a peak between the fourth and fifth decades. At that time the hemorrhagic diathesis may increase in frequency and severity. Visceral telangiectases are found in the gastrointestinal, respiratory, and genitourinary tracts.

The most common clinical problem is mucous membrane bleeding—especially epistaxis. However, telangiectases in any location may become a troublesome source of recurrent hemorrhage. Fortunately hemostasis and coagulation are normal, and the patients can tolerate surgical procedures when necessary. Iron deficiency anemia eventually becomes a clinical problem in many patients.

Pulmonary arteriovenous fistulas can be demonstrated radiographically in about 15 per cent of patients with hereditary telangiectasia. These malformations, which increase with age, are usually multiple and may be a source of hemoptysis as well as loci for infection. In addition, shunting of blood may induce hypoxemia, clubbing, and polycythemia. Arteriovenous fistulas in the cerebral, hepatic, and splenic arteries have also been reported, as have hemangiomas of the liver and polycystic kidneys. Infected arteriovenous fistulas may also be a source of metastatic brain abscesses.

The diagnosis is readily made if the classic triad is present: (1) repeated episodes of hemorrhage, (2) presence of multiple telangiectasia, and (3) characteristic family history. The diagnosis is more difficult when the bleeding is very mild and telangiectases are absent from the skin or not readily visible, in the setting of an unclear family history. Fiberoptic endoscopy has been helpful as a diagnostic procedure. Pulmonary arteriovenous fistulas may be demonstrated by pulmonary angiography.

Treatment is mainly supportive and symptomatic. An associated iron deficiency should be treated by replacement therapy (see Ch. 134). Whenever possible, hemorrhage should be controlled by local therapy only. Topical hemostatic agents are useful when the site is accessible. Cautery of bleeding sites is not recommended. Estrogenic hormone preparations have been used to induce squamous metaplasia of the nasal mucosa, but the results have been controversial. Surgical intervention for uncontrollable lesions or arteriovenous fistulas must be considered on an individual basis. Despite the lack of therapeutic measures and the potential hazard of spontaneous hemorrhage, the prognosis for these patients is relatively good. Oral contraceptives should be avoided.

167. DISORDERS OF BLOOD COAGULATION

Patrick A. McKee

Introduction

Normal hemostasis depends upon the interaction of blood vessels, platelets, and blood coagulation. The general biology of hemostasis and the approach to the patient suspected of having a hemorrhagic diathesis have been discussed in Ch. 166. In this chapter attention is focused on hemorrhagic disorders that occur as a consequence of abnormalities in blood coagulation: (1) inherited diseases manifested by a clotting factor being deficient in amount or defective in function; (2) acquired deficiency states; (3) depletion of clotting factors by consumption during the formation of intravascular thrombi; (4) abnormal increases in fibrinolysis; and (5) the abnormal development of circulating inhibitors of blood clotting factors.

BLOOD CLOTTING REVIEWED. Normal blood coagulation proceeds as a highly organized sequence of rapid, progressively amplified chemical reactions, beginning with the activation of only a few molecules and culminating in the formation of an insoluble protein (fibrin) that stops bleeding. This complex cascade of reactions involves 20 or so substances, most of which are plasma proteins. The majority of these have been assigned Roman numerals (Table 167–1); however, some are occasionally referred to by the surnames of the patients in whom they were first discovered, e.g., factor IX (Christmas factor); factor X (Stuart-Prower factor); factor XII (Hageman factor).

Figure 167–1 depicts the amplification scheme of blood coagulation. All of the blood clotting factors circulate in blood in precursive forms, or zymogens, or as cofactor proteins that have somewhat different structures until activated or altered during the clotting process. Traditionally the blood coagulation scheme has been divided into two pathways, *extrinsic* and *intrinsic*, both of which converge into a final common pathway for the production of thrombin. Although it is operationally convenient to think of these as separate, many of their reactions result in "crosstalk" between the two pathways. The term *extrinsic* implies that an extravascular substance(s) is required to initiate blood coagulation; *intrinsic* indicates that all components required to trigger blood clotting are contained within the vascular system.

The precise mechanism by which blood coagulation is initiated continues to cause much debate. Many of the reactions that are described probably occur on the membrane surfaces of an aggregated mass of platelets that is adherent to sites of intimal injury. In the instance of the extrinsic pathway, it is generally believed that contact of blood with a lipoprotein (tissue thromboplastin; tissue factor), which is contained in virtually all tissues, allows the formation of a complex between this lipoprotein and the plasma protein factor VII (proconvertin). Either as a result of a change in shape or because of a proteolytic cleavage while complexed to tissue factor, factor VII becomes activated. (Henceforth the enzymatically active form of clotting factors will be designated by a subscript "a," e.g., factor VII_a.) Factor VII_a binds to tissue factor, and this complex cleaves factor X to give rise to another proteolytic enzyme, which forms a complex with factor V, calcium, and phospholipid. The activation of factor X plus the formation of the factor X_a–Ca^{++}–phospholipid–factor V complex, which seems to occur on the platelet membrane, converts prothrombin by a series of proteolytic cleavages to the active enzyme thrombin.

The initiation of blood clotting via the intrinsic pathway is complex. When blood comes in contact with an abnormal surface (glass, various negatively charged surfaces, an abnormal endothelium, collagen, or other subendothelial components), factor XII zymogen (Hageman factor) adheres and becomes altered in shape so that its active site is exposed. Simultaneously, prekallikrein (Fletcher factor), factor XI, and high molecular weight kininogen (Fitzgerald factor) bind to the abnormal or damaged surface and form a surface-localized complex. High molecular weight kininogen serves as a surface cofactor to assemble prekallikrein or factor XI in proximity to the surface-bound factor XII (Hageman factor). Reciprocal proteolytic activation between factor XII and prekallikrein may be the very first reaction in the intrinsic pathway. Hageman factor can become activated in the absence of prekallikrein or high molecular weight kininogen, but the rate is 50 to 100 times slower. Once activated, factor XII_a then converts factor XI in the juxtaposed factor XI–high molecular weight kininogen complex to factor XI_a. The fact that the extrinsic and intrinsic pathways are probably intertwined at some points is supported by factor XII_a being able to activate factor VII, the latter ordinarily considered unique to the extrinsic system. In short, the outcome of these initial series of reactions, which constitute the contact phase of blood coagulation, can be summarized as follows: (1) surface bound Hageman factor, which has its active site exposed, converts plasma prekallikrein to kallikrein; (2) kallikrein proteolytically cleaves the zymogen form of Hageman factor to give rise to activated Hageman factor; (3) kallikrein cleaves high molecular weight kininogen to produce the peptide bradykinin, which has the properties of dilating blood vessels, contracting smooth muscle, producing pain, and promoting leukocyte migration; (4) activated factor XII activates factor XI and may activate factor VII; and (5) under certain conditions, activated factor XII may convert plasminogen to plasmin.

Once generated, activated factor XI_a converts the proenzyme factor IX (Christmas factor) to its activated form, provided that calcium ion is present. Unlike the activation of other vitamin K–dependent proenzymes, phospholipid is not required for the generation of factor IX_a. Another example of interaction between the extrinsic and intrinsic pathways is the observation that the tissue thromboplastin–calcium ion–factor VII complex can activate factor IX directly and independently of activated factor XI. Although the interaction of factor IX_a with factor VIII (antihemophilic factor) is unclear at this time, most studies indicate that activated factor IX becomes bound to factor VIII, phospholipid, and calcium ion to form a complex that then converts the proenzyme factor X (Stuart-Prower factor) to factor X_a.

The precise structural and functional features of factor VIII, or the antihemophilic factor, remain elusive. It circulates in a complex with von Willebrand factor and appears to require cleavage by a thrombin-like enzyme to develop the procoagulant activity that interacts with factor IX_a, Ca^{++}, and phospholipid to form an activator of factor X. The factor VIII–von Willebrand–glycoprotein complex also possesses an activity, not affected by thrombin, that is important to platelet function (*von Willebrand activity*). Von Willebrand activity is necessary for platelets to adhere to the severed edges of a blood vessel or to foreign surfaces, and in addition serves as a cofactor with the antibiotic ristocetin to cause platelet aggregation in laboratory assays. To date, the physiologic equivalent for this latter phenomenon has not been identified. The two diverse activities of the factor VIII–von Willebrand factor complex, i.e., procoagulant activity and platelet adhesion effects, are tightly associated in vivo and can be separated in vitro only under unusual physicochemical conditions. Hence, the moiety traditionally referred to as factor VIII in the past literature should now be termed the factor VIII–von Willebrand complex.

Phospholipid is required as a cofactor in several steps of blood coagulation. For the extrinsic pathway, it is supplied in the form of thromboplastin (tissue factor), and for the intrinsic pathway, from platelet membranes and to a much lesser extent from plasma phospholipids. There are no known hemorrhagic or thrombotic disorders caused by a deficiency or excess of phospholipids. Calcium ion is also needed in most of the same blood clotting reactions requiring phospholipid. The vitamin K–dependent blood clotting factors—prothrombin and factors VII, IX, and X—are synthesized in the hepatocyte where vitamin K serves as a cofactor in the carboxylation of specific glutamic acid groups located in their amino terminal regions. These modified glutamic acids, now containing a second carboxyl group and termed γ-carboxyglutamic acids, form calcium binding sites that are important for the attachment of vitamin K factors to phospholipid surfaces. For example, the conversion

TABLE 167–1. BLOOD COAGULATION FACTORS

Roman Numeral	Substance	Normal Plasma Concentration (μg/ml)	Functional Groupings
I*	Fibrinogen	2500	*Contact phase:*
II*	Prothrombin	150	Factor XII
III*	Tissue thromboplastin; tissue factor	—	Factor XI
IV*	Calcium ion	—	Prekallikrein
V	Proaccelerin; labile factor	10	High molecular weight kininogen
(VI)	Not assigned	—	
VII	Proconvertin; stable factor	<1	*Vitamin K-dependent coagulation factors:*
VIII	Antihemophilic factor	?	Prothrombin Factor X
IX	Christmas factor; plasma thromboplastin component (PTC)	3	Factor VII Protein C
X	Stuart factor or Stuart-Prower factor	<5	Factor IX Protein S
XI	Plasma thromboplastin antecedent (PTA)	<5	*Consumed during clotting (in plasma but not in serum):*
XII	Hageman factor	<5	Prothrombin
XIII	Fibrin-stabilizing factor	10	Fibrinogen
—*	Prekallikrein (Fletcher factor)	30	Antihemophilic factor
—*	High molecular weight kininogen (Fitzgerald, Williams, or Flaujeac factor)	80	Factor V
—*	von Willebrand factor	15	Factor XIII
—*	Protein C	<5	
—*	Protein S	<5	

*Not usually referred to by Roman numeral or has not been assigned a number.

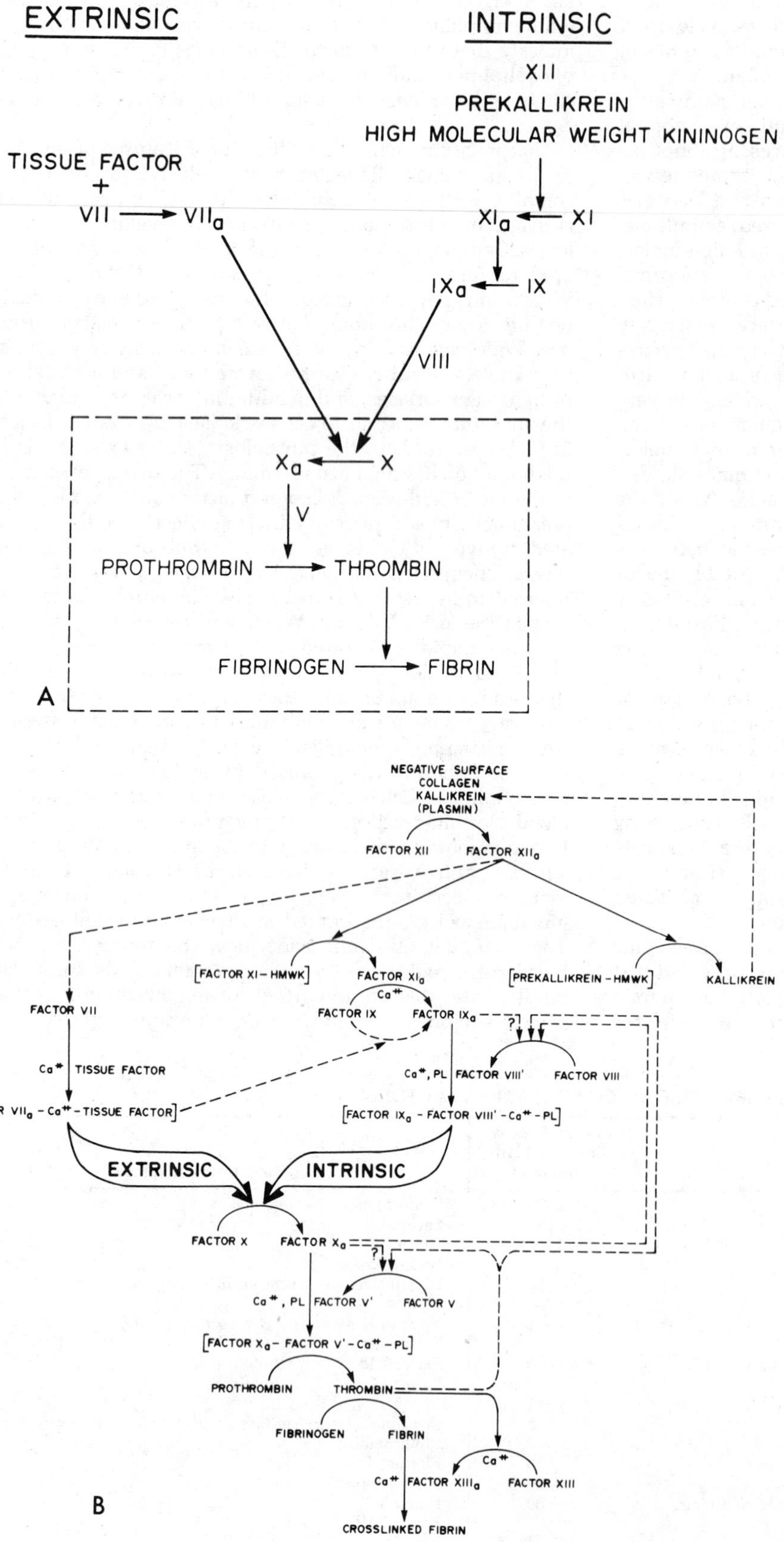

Figure 167–1. *A,* Simplified version of blood clotting. Activated clotting factor serine proteases are indicated by the subscript *a.* The prothrombin time test assesses the *extrinsic* pathway, whereas the partial thromboplastin time reflects deficiencies in the *intrinsic* pathway. The reactions common to both the intrinsic and extrinsic systems are enclosed by the dashed box. *B,* Blood coagulation scheme as modified from previous diagrams by Davie and Ratnoff. High molecular weight kininogen is abbreviated HMWK. Active complexes of enzyme-phospholipid (PL)-calcium are enclosed by brackets. The subscript *a* designates the activated or enzymatic form of the clotting factor. The dashed lines indicate pathways that are probably important in vivo but continue somewhat uncertain. Both factors V and VIII, which are believed to be cofactors rather than enzymes, are cleaved by thrombin to produce species which have enhanced activity indicated by the superscript *prime.*

of prothrombin to thrombin can occur much more efficiently if both prothrombin and factor X_a are bound to a negatively charged phospholipid surface in the presence of factor V.

The common pathway of blood coagulation, in which the extrinsic and intrinsic systems converge in a series of steps leading to the production of thrombin, begins with the generation of factor X_a. Thrombin is a highly specific serine protease that may participate in several blood coagulation reactions: (1) it specifically binds to platelets and promotes the release of certain platelet constituents, one being ADP, which causes platelet aggregation; (2) thrombin also causes the activation of platelet membrane phospholipase C that initiates prostaglandin synthesis to generate thromboxane A_2, which stimulates platelet aggregation (see Ch. 166); (3) it has a proteolytic effect on both factors V and VIII that may be requisite for either factor V or factor VIII to manifest procoagulant activity; (4) thrombin cleaves fibrinogen to initiate its conversion to fibrin; and (5) thrombin initiates the activation of factor XIII (fibrin-stabilizing factor) by proteolytic cleavage.

Human fibrinogen is present in plasma in a concentration range of 150 to 400 mg per deciliter. It has a molecular weight of about 340,000 and is composed of three pairs of unique polypeptides. The subunit chain formula for fibrinogen is written as $(A\alpha B\beta\gamma)_2$, where A and B denote the fibrinopeptides A and B, each about 2000 daltons, that are cleaved by thrombin from the amino terminal portions of the α and β chains to form fibrin monomer $(\alpha\beta\gamma)_2$. Fibrin monomers align with one another through noncovalent bonds to form a visible fibrin clot. Such fibrin is termed soluble, or noncrosslinked, since it is readily soluble in dilute acids or various dispersing agents. Thrombin starts the activation of factor XIII by cleaving an amino terminal peptide. In the presence of the mid-portion of either α chain of a fibrin monomer, physiologic concentrations of calcium promote the completion of factor XIII activation by dissociating the thrombin-cleaved factor XIII into its dimeric halves, one pair being the enzymatically active subunits that catalyze the formation of covalent ε-(γ-glutamyl)-lysine crosslink bonds in soluble fibrin. These crosslinks not only stabilize fibrin and add to its tensile strength, but also cause fibrin to become insoluble in dilute acids and other strong solvents.

Two recently discovered plasma proteins, protein C and protein S, also have important functions in human blood coagulation. Both are vitamin K dependent, containing γ-carboxyglutamic acid residues. Protein C exists in zymogen form and is activated by thrombin to form a serine protease, which rapidly cleaves and destroys the procoagulant functions of activated factor V and factor VIII. As a consequence factor X_a and thrombin formation is diminished. Protein S, which is probably not a serine protease, seems to act as a cofactor in these reactions. The activation of protein C occurs most rapidly when thrombin binds to an endothelial surface cofactor protein, thrombomodulin. Interestingly, this also provides an anticoagulant effect because the ability of thrombin to clot fibrinogen or to activate factor V is then impaired. Besides functioning as an anticoagulant, activated protein C also appears to stimulate fibrinolysis.

Plasmin is a proteolytically active enzyme that is liberated from its zymogen plasminogen through the action of several substances (Fig. 167–2). Plasmin readily digests fibrin, which many investigators believe to be its prime function. It also hydrolyzes and inactivates other coagulation factors, most notably factor V, factor VIII, and fibrinogen. In addition to the negative effects of plasmin on blood coagulation, there are other plasma proteins that serve as potent inhibitors of certain blood coagulation enzymes. These are α_2-macroglobulin, α_2-antiplasmin, antithrombin III, α_1-antitrypsin, and C1 inactivator, the last-named being a component of the complement system. Of these, the first three have major importance to the coagulation system, with α_2-antiplasmin and antithrombin III probably having the greatest physiologic significance. In some circumstances, these normally occurring inhibitors may modulate the expression of activity of certain blood coagulation proteases. In other situations they may serve as virtually absolute inhibitors. α_2-Macroglobulin suppresses most if not all the activity of bound thrombin or plasmin. Whether it is also important as an in vivo inhibitor of other blood clotting proteases is not certain. α_2-Antiplasmin is a very rapid and potent inhibitor of plasmin, forming an irreversible one-to-one stoichiometric complex. Antithrombin III is a particularly effective inhibitor of activated factor X and thrombin, but it also blocks the activity of the other blood clotting serine proteases except

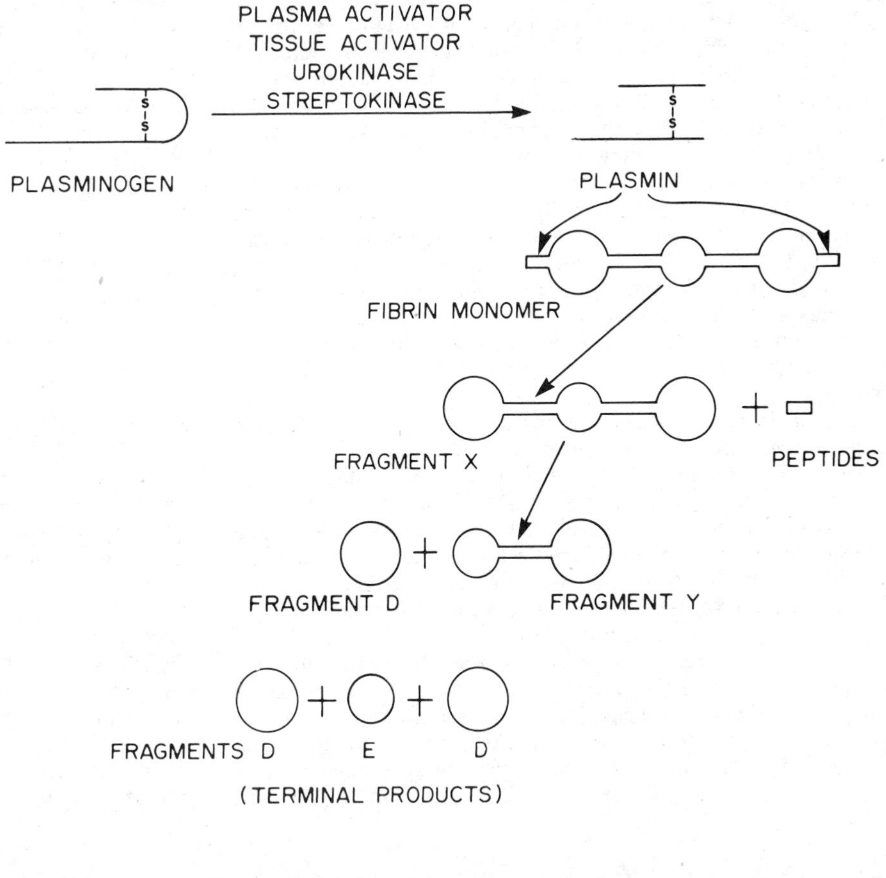

Figure 167–2. Plasminogen activation and sequential cleavage of fibrin by plasmin to produce fibrin degradation products (fragments X, Y, D, and E). Fragments X and Y are the ones that contribute most to defective fibrin polymerization.

for activated factor VII. Theoretically, interactions between antithrombin III and those serine protease clotting factors formed in the earliest stages of clot formation may be more important in preventing thrombosis than the interactions of antithrombin III with activated factor X or thrombin. Heparin dramatically potentiates the rate at which antithrombin III participates in these interactions. In the presence of heparin, antithrombin III may also inhibit activated factor VII. The inhibition of proteases by any of these plasma inhibitors is thought to be essentially complete and irreversible. The inhibitor-protease complexes are cleared very rapidly, probably by the liver and reticuloendothelial systems.

CLINICAL FEATURES. The medical history can provide helpful clues about the cause of bleeding disorders. The age of onset and whether bleeding is strictly localized and due to a specific lesion (e.g., carcinoma), or whether a bleeding tendency has become unmasked (e.g., by mild trauma), or whether the patient suffers from generalized bleeding are important facts to elicit from the history. In the instance of generalized bleeding it should be determined if the patient bleeds from multiple sites, if the bleeding is spontaneous, and whether the bleeding occurs as petechiae, purpura, mucous membrane bleeding, hematomas, gastrointestinal hemorrhage, or hemarthroses. Petechiae, purpura, and mucous membrane bleeding usually suggest decreased platelet number or function. Gastrointestinal and genitourinary bleeding may be due to deficiencies of platelet number or function or of certain clotting factors. Hemarthroses occur with severely decreased function of certain plasma clotting factors. When the bleeding tendency is inherited, the defect is usually noted in infancy, e.g., prolonged bleeding from the umbilical cord or at circumcision; there may be a history of significant bleeding after relatively unimpressive trauma. A carefully obtained, detailed family history may suggest or define an inheritance pattern. The physical examination allows an evaluation of the type and extent of bleeding if petechiae, purpura, hematomas, or hemarthroses are present.

LABORATORY ASSESSMENT. The initial laboratory tests are intended to segregate the clotting defect to one of three areas in the blood coagulation scheme. First, the level and function of fibrinogen must be above 50 mg per deciliter to give a fibrin gel end-point in subsequent coagulation assays to be performed on the patient's plasma. All of the usual survey tests ultimately measure the rate or amount of fibrin formation as an end-point. The adequacy of the fibrinogen level can be crudely screened by observing the clotting time and quality of clots formed when thrombin is added to whole plasma.

The *prothrombin time* is a screening test for plasma deficiencies in the extrinsic system (factor VII) as well as for deficiencies of those factors common to the extrinsic and intrinsic systems, namely, factor X, factor V, prothrombin, and fibrinogen. If the fibrinogen level is normal, a prolonged prothrombin time signifies a deficiency of one of the factors mentioned above, the presence of a specific inhibitor to one of those factors, or a level of fibrin split products sufficiently high to delay fibrin formation.

The *partial thromboplastin time,* assuming a normal fibrinogen level, screens for plasma deficiencies of factors in the intrinsic system (XII, XI, IX, VIII) or deficiencies of clotting factors common to the intrinsic and extrinsic systems. Specific inhibitors to any of these clotting factors will also cause a prolonged partial thromboplastin time. The test is often performed as an "activated" partial thromboplastin time, which indicates that kaolin or some other surface-active substance was added to maximize the contact activation of factors XII and XI and consequently decrease the possibility that the activation rates of these two factors will affect the rate of thrombin generation and subsequent fibrin formation. If suggested by the history or physical examination, a screening test for fibrin-stabilizing factor may be included. It is performed by observing the rate at which a plasma fibrin clot will dissolve in 1 per cent monochloroacetic acid or 5M urea. Normal clots should be essentially insoluble at 24 hours.

The presence of circulating inhibitors to various clotting factors must be considered in the event of a prolonged prothrombin time or activated partial thromboplastin time. Depending on which is prolonged, the failure of an equal volume of normal plasma to correct the defect in the patient's plasma indicates the presence of such an inhibitor. (See p. 1057 for discussion of lupus anticoagulant.) Then the identity of the clotting factor toward which the inhibitor is directed can be established by specific assays.

These screening tests provide a great deal of diagnostic information. If the fibrinogen level is normal, then various combinations of test results from the prothrombin time and partial thromboplastin time assays will limit the diagnostic possibilities in a patient with a bleeding diathesis. For example, if there is a defect in the reactions common to both the extrinsic and intrinsic systems, then both the prothrombin time and partial thromboplastin time will be prolonged. If the prothrombin time is normal and the partial thromboplastin time is prolonged, then deficiencies of factors XII, XI, IX, or VIII are possible. When the clotting factor deficiency has been localized, it usually can be specifically identified by knowing that barium sulfate adsorbs the vitamin K–dependent clotting factors and that normal serum contains activated factors IX, X, XI, and XII but *not* factors V or VIII. For example, complete correction of a prolonged partial thromboplastin time by adsorbed normal plasma, but not by normal serum, identifies factor VIII deficiency (classic hemophilia). On the other hand, were the partial thromboplastin time to have been corrected by normal serum but not by adsorbed normal plasma, then a diagnosis of factor IX deficiency would have been made. If both a prolonged prothrombin time and partial thromboplastin time are corrected by adsorbed plasma but not serum, then factor V deficiency is suggested. A correction of both tests by normal serum, but not by adsorbed plasma suggests factor X deficiency. Most clinical laboratories now identify specific clotting factor deficiencies by testing the patient's plasma against plasmas with known, well-established deficiencies. Using the format of the prothrombin time or partial thromboplastin time assay, dilutions of the patient's plasma can be compared to those of normal control plasma for the ability to correct the clotting time of plasma known to have the suspected factor deficiency. The patient's values are expressed as a percentage of normal control values to give an estimation of the level of clotting factor activity.

Jackson CM, Nemerson Y: Blood coagulation. Ann Rev Biochem 49:765, 1980. *Best summary of the biochemistry of blood clotting; helpful to those wanting more information about structure-function relationships of the clotting factors.*

McKee PA: Hereditary disorders of hemostasis. *In* Stanbury JB, Wyngaarden JB, Fredrickson DS, Goldstein JL, Brown MS (eds.): The Metabolic Basis of Inherited Disease. 5th ed. New York, McGraw-Hill Book Company, 1983, pp 1531–1560. *Excellent, comprehensive coverage, emphasizing genetic aspects.*

Owen CA Jr, Bowie EJW, Thompson JH Jr: The Diagnosis of Bleeding Disorders. 2nd ed. Boston, Little, Brown & Company, 1975. *Gives concise explanations of all laboratory tests. Numerous clinical examples are provided. The section on the history of blood clotting may interest some.*

Thompson AR, Harker LA: Manual of Hemostasis and Thrombosis. 3rd ed. Philadelphia, F.A. Davis Company, 1983. *A quick, helpful review especially useful to students and house staff. Contains many practical bits of information.*

Inherited Disorders of Blood Coagulation

Most of the plasma protein clotting factors have been identified as a consequence of patients presenting with unknown bleeding disorders, eventually recognized as unique and familial. Bleeding may be due to a structural defect in a clotting factor (crossreacting material positive; CRM+) or to a lack of its synthesis (CRM−). Table 167–2 lists the inheritance pattern and approximate frequency of the clotting factor deficiencies. Deficiencies of factor VIII and factor IX are the only two coagulation diseases inherited as X-linked traits with bleeding occurring in the male hemizygotes. Von Willebrand's disease appears to be an autosomal codominant disorder. Deficiencies of all the other clotting factors are transmitted as autosomal recessive traits, with clinically significant bleeding usually man-

TABLE 167–2. CHARACTERISTICS OF INHERITABLE COAGULATION DISORDERS

Coagulation Factor	Inheritance Pattern of Deficiency	Estimated Frequency per Million	Usual Hemorrhagic Symptoms	Laboratory Assessment: Thrombin Time	Prothrombin Time	Partial Thromboplastin Time	Bleeding Time	Selected Tests
Intrinsic system								
Prekallikrein	Autosomal recessive	<0.5	None	N	N	↑	N	Specific assay*
High molecular weight kininogen	Autosomal recessive	<0.5	None	N	N	↑	N	Specific assay*
Factor XII	Autosomal recessive	1.0	None	N	N	↑	N	Specific assay*
Factor XI	Autosomal recessive	1.0	Mild	N	N	↑	N(↑)	Specific assay*
Factor IX	X-linked recessive	10	Mild to severe	N	N	↑	N	Specific assay*
Factor VIII	X-linked recessive	50	Mild to severe	N	N	↑	N	Normal ristocetin-induced platelet aggregation
von Willebrand's Disease	Autosomal codominant	5–10	Mild to severe	N	N	↑	↑	Usually low plasma level of von Willebrand protein by immunologic testing; ristocetin-induced platelet aggregation decreased
Extrinsic system								
Factor VII	Autosomal recessive	<0.5	Mild to moderate	N		N(↑)	N	Specific assay*
Common pathway								
Prothrombin	Autosomal recessive	<0.5	Mild to severe	N		↑	N	Specific assay*
Factor X	Autosomal recessive	<0.5	Severe	N		↑	N	Specific assay*
Factor V	Autosomal recessive	<0.5	Moderate	N	↑		N	Specific assay*
Fibrin formation								
Afibrinogenemia	Autosomal recessive	<0.5	Severe	∞	∞	∞	N(↑)	Fibrinogen absent immunologically
Dysfibrinogenemia	Autosomal recessive	<0.5	None to mild	± ↑	± ↑	± ↑	N	Delayed fibrinopeptide release or impaired fibrin monomer aggregation
Factor XIII	Autosomal recessive	<0.5	Severe	N	N	N	N	Plasma clots are soluble in 5M urea or 1 per cent monochloroacetic acid
Fibrinolytic system								
Plasminogen	Autosomal recessive	<0.5	Mild; no bleeding tendency; frequent thromboses	N	N	N	N	Euglobulin lysis time prolonged
Protein C	Autosomal	<0.5	Thromboses; no bleeding tendency	N	N	N	N	Low plasma level by immunologic assay

N = normal.
↑ = prolonged. (↑) = only occasionally prolonged.
*Specific assay using plasma from a person with known deficiency of the clotting factor in question in the patient's plasma.

ifested only by the homozygote. Heterozygous carriers may have reduced plasma levels of a clotting factor activity, but the deficiency seldom affects hemostasis. Inherited combined deficiencies have been reported, but their basis is not understood. Most frequently cited are patients with combined factor V and factor VIII deficiencies that appear to be familial. Repeated hemorrhagic episodes caused by combined deficiencies in the function of prothrombin and factors VII, IX, and X have been observed in patients found to have congenitally defective vitamin K–induced γ-carboxylation.

Soff GA, Levin J: Familial multiple coagulation deficiencies. Semin Thromb Hemostas 7:112, 1981. *Good coverage of rarely encountered disorders, reports of which are usually scattered separately in the literature.*

CLASSIC HEMOPHILIA

Classic hemophilia, or factor VIII deficiency, is the most frequently encountered disorder of blood coagulation, occurring in 1 in 10,000 of the male population. Some patients with this disorder lack plasma antihemophilic factor; others have a nonfunctional factor VIII molecule present in normal concentrations. About 70 per cent of hemophiliacs give a positive family history, the pedigree of which indicates an X-linked inheritance pattern. Hence, the disorder occurs only in males, except in the remote event that a homozygous female results from the mating of a hemophilic male and a female carrier. The hemophilic patient's daughters will all be carriers, but all his sons will be normal. A carrier woman has a 50 per cent chance of producing a hemophilic son and a 50 per cent chance of producing a female carrier. She is a true genetic mosaic, since her cells will consist of two populations with respect to either containing a normal X chromosome or an abnormal X chromosome (bearing the hemophilic gene). Since one of the X chromosomes is randomly and irreversibly inactivated in each cell, usually prior to implantation of the embryo, most carrier women will have about 50 per cent of the normal level of factor VIII activity. The broad range of observed factor VIII levels in carriers, however, supports the speculation that inactivation of one of the X chromosomes is often disproportionate. Hence more than the expected 50 per cent of cells may contain either a functioning normal or a functioning abnormal X chromosome. If extreme "lyonization" (see under Introduction) occurs so that the preponderance of cells in the carrier female contains the X chromosome with the hemophilic gene, the woman may have clinical and laboratory phenotypic features of hemophilia.

CLINICAL MANIFESTATIONS. In general, the level of factor VIII activity tends to correlate with the frequency of clinically significant bleeding; however, the relationship may not be as reliable as the observation that bleeding severity tends to be fairly similar in members of a given family. Bleeding is rare at birth, even from the umbilical cord, since platelet function and the extrinsic limb of the coagulation system are intact. Depending on the severity of the defect, soft tissue hematomas may develop during early infancy. Most difficulties begin when the child becomes physically active. Bleeding occurs frequently in joints, most notably in large joints such as the elbows, knees, and ankles. Although involved less frequently, the joints of the wrist and hands may also become severely deformed by hemarthroses. About half of all hemophiliacs have severe, spontaneous hemorrhages into joints that result in eventual deformity and crippling. Such patients have factor VIII activity levels well below 5 per cent of normal, usually being <1 per cent of normal. The patient experiences considerable pain with bleeding into joints, since the joint capsule becomes so markedly distended. Movement is severely limited. Pressure erodes the ends of long bones, causing periosteal pain, eventual necrosis, and pseudocyst formation.

Extensive bleeding with hematoma formation often occurs in muscles and soft tissues. Considerable blood loss may occur in the thigh muscles or retroperitoneally; the amount of blood loss in these areas may be difficult to discern clinically and is frequently underestimated. The bleeding of hemophilia can involve virtually any anatomic area and give rise to secondary symptoms and signs of depressed organ function caused by compression. Nosebleeds are uncommon; however, if bleeding occurs in the pharynx or neck, airway obstruction can result. Gastrointestinal hemorrhage may be a major problem. Bleeding may occur from peptic ulcerations, partial intestinal obstruction may result from hemorrhage into the bowel wall, and mesenteric bleeding has led to the development of bowel ischemia and necrosis. Hematuria can present as ureteral colic caused by bleeding and formation of clots that obstruct the ureter. Subdural hematomas and other central nervous system hemorrhages are uncommon, but do represent a major cause of death and disability. Most bleeding in the hemophiliac appears to develop spontaneously, the patient being unable to remember trauma or other provoking causes. Many times spontaneous bleeding occurs during periods of stress such as before school examinations or following family dissension. When bleeding follows trauma, it may be delayed since the primary hemostasis furnished by vessels and platelets is intact (see Ch. 166).

Major or minor surgery, including dental extractions, can result in marked blood loss in the hemophiliac and therefore must be carried out in conjunction with factor VIII replacement therapy. Even those patients with mild hemophilia, i.e., factor VIII levels of 5 to 25 per cent, may develop clinically significant bleeding with surgery or trauma because (1) their rate of factor X activation occurs far too slowly with respect to their rate of blood loss and (2) their submarginal levels of factor VIII are depleted by the clotting that does occur. Hence, at such times, even mild hemophiliacs will require replacement therapy.

DIAGNOSIS. The bleeding pattern of the patient, the family history, and the physical examination may provide important clues to the diagnosis of hemophilia. Laboratory tests show the fibrinogen level and prothrombin time to be normal but the partial thromboplastin time prolonged. Adsorbed plasma, but not normal serum, will correct the patient's partial thromboplastin time, thereby indicating that the most likely diagnosis is factor VIII deficiency. Usually dilutions of the patient's plasma are then tested for the ability to correct the defect in the plasma of another person who is known to specifically lack factor VIII activity and who has not developed an inhibitor to factor VIII. The values from this assay are compared to those of normal control plasma, and the level of factor VIII activity in the patient's plasma is expressed as a percentage of normal. Hemophilia can be confused with von Willebrand's disease; however, unlike hemophilia, von Willebrand's disease usually presents with a prolonged bleeding time and defective platelet aggregation when the antibiotic ristocetin is added to platelet-rich plasma. When the diagnosis of hemophilia is suspected, it may be helpful to perform laboratory tests on family members to determine if an inheritance pattern is present. Finally, even at the time of diagnosis, it is important to exclude the presence of an inhibitor as the basis for the deficient factor VIII function.

TREATMENT. The patient and family must be educated about the severity of the disease, the immediate management of various types of bleeding episodes, the difference the disorder may make in the patient's future life style, and the genetics of its transmission. The patient, family and physician share in the major goal of having the patient lead as normal a life as possible. Depending on the medical history, the degree of physical impairment, the severity of bleeding given by the family history, and the plasma level of factor VIII, the patient can be guided into activities commensurate with the severity of the disease. As children, these patients should be reared in an environment that initially is more protective than will be required when they themselves better understand the consequences of hemophilia.

It is important for the physician to recognize the denial mechanisms sometimes constructed by the patient and the parents about the disease. For example, the patient may develop a willingness and receive unconscious encouragement from the parents to participate in dangerous activities. Usually as adults, these patients recognize the constraints imposed by the disease. They should be encouraged to develop their education and interests as fully as possible. Any career that does not expose the patient to undue hazard can be allowed. In short, the goal is to keep patients as functional as possible as they develop a normal life within their capacity. To accomplish this, they must become knowledgeable about the disease and participate in their own care.

Bleeding episodes are managed primarily by administering factor VIII, usually as a commercially prepared lyophilized concentrate or sometimes in the form of cryoprecipitate. Blood banks prepare cryoprecipitate by freezing fresh normal plasma (assumed to contain 1 unit of factor VIII activity per milliliter) at −90° C and then thawing at 4° C. Approximately 50 per cent of the factor VIII contained in the plasma remains as a precipitate, which is then stored frozen. The cryoprecipitate, now containing factor VIII concentrated five- to ten-fold with respect to plasma, is thawed at 37° C and administered intravenously as soon as possible to the patient. The use of cryoprecipitate or other forms of factor VIII concentrate avoids the potential complication of overtransfusing with the large volume of plasma necessary to attain acceptable levels of factor VIII activity. The guidelines for replacement therapy depend on (1) the severity and site of hemorrhage, (2) the plasma level of factor VIII estimated to be required to halt the bleeding, (3) the amount of factor VIII contained in the concentrate to be administered, (4) the disappearance rate of the infused factor VIII, and (5) whether the patient has an inhibitor to factor VIII. The latter is particularly important to determine before administering replacement therapy, since a circulating inhibitor may initially appear at almost any time in the life of a hemophiliac and need not be associated with any obvious change in the clinical severity of the disorder. Early hemarthrosis or hematuria can be managed by raising and maintaining the plasma factor VIII level at 25 to 50 per cent of normal for two to three days. Muscle hematomas, however, require a longer period of sustained factor VIII levels, usually about 40 per cent of normal for four to six days. Major trauma requires that the factor VIII level be maintained in excess of 40 per cent for about two weeks. If bleeding persists despite replacement therapy, it may be that simply not enough factor VIII is being given, or the factor VIII concentrates contain less activity than usual, or the patient has developed an inhibitor.

The amount of cryoprecipitate needed to achieve a desired level of factor VIII activity can be estimated by knowing (1) that the patient's plasma volume is about 40 ml per kilogram of body weight, (2) that each bag of cryoprecipitate contains approximately 100 units of factor VIII activity, and (3) that factor VIII has a half-life of about ten to twelve hours in the circulation. Therefore replacement therapy is ordinarily administered twice a day, and calculations are made to ensure the presence of an adequate plasma level of factor VIII before the next infusion. If commercial glycine-precipitated factor VIII concentrates are to be given, the activity unitage on each vial can be used to guide therapy. Major surgery should be performed on patients only after administering sufficient lyophilized factor VIII concentrate to attain a level of 70 per cent of normal. Postoperatively a level of 25 to 50 per cent of normal is maintained for about two weeks. Exactly when factor VIII therapy can be stopped in the management of spontaneous bleeding episodes is difficult to define. As a rule of thumb, factor VIII infusions are usually continued for two days after the cessation of any symptoms or signs of bleeding.

Home treatment programs for hemophiliacs have been successful in allowing the patient a fuller life with fewer hospitalizations and less acute medical care. The family and the patient are taught how to give intravenous infusions of lyophilized factor VIII concentrates on any suspicion or evidence of bleeding, especially recurrent hemarthroses.

Joint bleeding is initially managed by immobilization of the affected limb and application of ice packs to diminish swelling and discomfort of the joint. An immediate infusion of concentrate to raise plasma factor VIII levels to 10 per cent of normal is often sufficient to stop bleeding; depending on the clinical findings and the patient's past history, however, higher factor VIII levels may be required. Because the risk of introducing infection or causing additional bleeding is considered too high, hemarthroses are not aspirated unless such acute pain and tension are present that pressure necrosis becomes a major possibility. Then an aspiration is performed only after giving factor VIII concentrate as noted above. Splinting or using elastic bandages over a hemarthrosis may be done to make the patient more comfortable and to ensure that a position of joint function is maintained during the acute stage. With a physician who is expert in managing replacement therapy, some highly skilled orthopedists are now performing synovectomies and artifical joint replacements in hemophiliacs who have severe chronic joint deformities. In many instances these have been very successful in improving the usefulness of a joint.

The patient must be instructed about the importance of dental hygiene and advised to have frequent examinations by a dentist familiar with the care of hemophilic patients in cooperation with physicians. The use of a local anesthetic by needle puncture should be done only after giving prophylactic cryoprecipitate; hence, dental fillings of caries as well as extractions require the prior administration of factor VIII concentrate. Administration of ϵ-aminocaproic acid by mouth is also useful in controlling bleeding following dental procedures.

Bleeding may cause extraordinary pain, especially in joints. The injudicious use of narcotics can lead to addiction in hemophilic patients. Aspirin should be avoided by the hemophiliac because it decreases platelet aggregation and may accentuate bleeding. Hence acetaminophen and codeine are recommended as the first choices of analgesics.

PROGNOSIS. The major long-term complications of moderately severe and severe hemophilia are (1) progressive joint deformity and crippling, (2) development of inhibitors to factor VIII activity, (3) hepatitis, and (4) acquired immune deficiency syndrome (Ch. 430). The chances of developing either of the latter three complications correlate somewhat with the frequency of replacement therapy. Other mechanisms may be operative in the case of inhibitor development, since most of the 15 per cent of hemophiliacs who develop an inhibitor to factor VIII activity do so in childhood. Some propose that the tendency to develop antibodies may be genetic. Patients with mild to moderate hemophilia should lead reasonably normal lives, being at risk for bleeding only with major trauma, surgery, and dental extractions. Even patients with severe hemophilia can now expect a fairly bright future with respect to their disease, especially if they willingly join in their care by a knowlegeable physician. Life expectancy has been prolonged as a consequence of easy access to improved forms of replacement therapy. Unfortunately, however, many hemophiliacs still become severely crippled and, ultimately, chronic invalids. Hemorrhage continues to be the major cause of death.

CARRIER DETECTION. Women who have relatives with hemophilia frequently seek help in determining whether they may pass the disorder to their children. Daughters of men with the disorder, mothers of more than one hemophiliac, and mothers who have a hemophilic son and another hemophilic male relative in their pedigree are obligate carriers of the hemophilic gene. Only about 15 per cent of the instances of hemophilia arise because of spontaneous mutation. Merely determining the level of factor VIII procoagulant activity is inadequate to identify carrier women, because low normal levels overlap to a great extent with factor VIII levels found in obligate heterozygotes. In the carrier state, the level of factor VIII procoagulant activity is disproportionately lower than the concentration of factor VIII–like antigen relative to normal women. Therefore, women who are suspected of possibly carrying the trait can be identified by simultaneously performed determinations of (1) factor VIII procoagulant level and (2) the concentration of factor VIII–like protein measured by an enzyme-linked immunosorbent assay. When these values are analyzed by logarithmic discriminant analysis, greater than 95 per cent of carriers can be identified.

Buchanan GR: Hemophilia. Pediatr Clin North Am 27:309, 1980. *Thorough, succinct review. Contains practical advice for diagnosis and treatment. Well referenced.*

Graham JB, Barrow ES, Reisner HM, Edgell C-JS: The genetics of blood coagulation. *In* Harris H, Hirschhorn K (eds.): Advances in Human Genetics. Vol. 13. New York, Plenum Publishing Corporation, 1983, pp 1–81. *Excellent section on the biochemistry and genetics of the factor VIII—von Willebrand complex. Cites all relevant literature.*

Ratnoff OD: Antihemophilic factor (factor VIII). Ann Intern Med 88:403, 1978. *Excellent, succinct review for students, house staff, and experienced clinicians. Gives details of clinical management. Well referenced.*

VON WILLEBRAND'S DISEASE

This disorder, named for the physician who described it in 1926, is due to a deficiency of a plasma protein required for the normal adherence of platelets to sites of vascular injury and possibly for the formation of platelet aggregates. It is inherited as an autosomal codominant defect, but for unknown reasons it is observed more often in women than men.

PATHOGENESIS. Structural relationships exist between factor VIII and von Willebrand factor that cause these two activities to circulate in normal plasma as a complex protein, frequently denoted as factor VIII–von Willebrand protein. About 75 per cent of von Willebrand patients have a prolonged bleeding time, abnormal platelet aggregation in response to the antibiotic ristocetin, low levels of factor VIII procoagulant activity, and decreased amounts of factor VIII–von Willebrand protein. Interestingly, intravenous infusions of small amounts of normal plasma, hemophilic plasma, or normal serum cause a delayed increase in factor VIII procoagulant activity that is out of proportion to the content of factor VIII in the transfused plasma or serum. The transfused factor VIII–von Willebrand protein disappears with the usual half-life of 10 to 14 hours. Despite the prolonged elevation in the level of factor VIII procoagulant activity that follows, there is not a concomitant increase in the level of factor VIII–von Willebrand protein. The explanation for these observations remains unclear. Many investigators interpret them as suggesting the presence of a tropin-like substance in the transfused plasma or serum that stimulates the production or release of factor VIII procoagulant activity independently from the von Willebrand entity. In those forms of the disease in which von Willebrand factor antigen levels are near normal, incomplete or abnormal sugar sequences in the carbohydrate side chains of the factor VIII–von Willebrand protein have been suggested as the molecular defects that decrease or abolish its cofactor activity in platelet adhesion and aggregation interactions.

CLINICAL MANIFESTATIONS. Von Willebrand's disease has a broad spectrum of clinical and laboratory features, many of which relate to low levels of factor VIII activity. Hence, it must be considered in the differential diagnosis of classic hemophilia and vice versa. Unlike other disorders of blood coagulation, in von Willebrand's disease the severity of symptoms varies considerably among afflicted family members. Usually only those homozygous for the disorder manifest severe bleeding. In heterozygotes the hemorrhagic tendency is usually asymptomatic or mild and becomes evident or troublesome only with trauma, surgery, or dental extractions. Women with the disorder commonly experience excessive menses and postpartum bleeding. Gastrointestinal bleeding is common, whereas joint hemorrhage occurs rarely. For reasons not understood, the frequency and severity of bleeding in patients with this disorder tend to lessen with age.

DIAGNOSIS. The diagnosis of von Willebrand's disease is usually established by observing a prolonged bleeding time and a low level of factor VIII procoagulant activity by specific assay. About three fourths of patients with von Willebrand's disease have a prolonged bleeding time, decreased factor VIII procoagulant activity, abnormally low levels of factor VIII–von Willebrand protein by immunologic assays, and diminished to absent platelet aggregation when ristocetin is added to their platelet-rich plasma (Type I von Willebrand's disease). Approximately 15 per cent of patients classified as having von Willebrand's disease present with the usual bleeding problems and have a prolonged bleeding time and impaired ristocetin-induced platelet aggregation; however, they have a normal level of the factor VIII–von Willebrand protein by immunologic assays and normal to slightly decreased factor VIII procoagulant activity (Type IIA). Even more rarely encountered are those patients whose plasma is hypersensitive to the effects of lower amounts of ristocetin than normally used in the ristocetin-induced platelet aggregation assay. In these patients, the higher molecular weight multimers are depleted, presumably as a consequence of spontaneous binding to platelets and subsequent clearance (Type IIB). Other combinations of abnormal laboratory assays are less frequently encountered in patients who present with bleeding, and these are believed to represent either variability in the natural history of the disorder or still other variant forms in a spectrum of von Willebrand's disease.

TREATMENT. Cryoprecipitate concentrates of factor VIII–von Willebrand protein are used to treat clinically severe bleeding. Unlike cryoprecipitate, more highly purified factor concentrates, such as commercially available glycine-precipitated preparations, may not correct the bleeding time defect. Hence, despite the fact that the lyophilized concentrates will correct the factor VIII procoagulant deficiency, bleeding may persist. Although the main goal of therapy should be a normal bleeding time, in practice the ability to actually achieve this is highly variable. For the most part, the amount of cryoprecipitate to be given (usually about 5 to 10 bags twice daily) is based on the restoration of acceptable levels of factor VIII procoagulant activity in the patient's plasma as well as the correction of the patient's Duke bleeding time. In general, the regimen outlined for replacement therapy in classic hemophilia is suitable for managing the bleeding of von Willebrand's disease. In contrast to hemophilia, the patient with von Willebrand's disease who is to have surgery should receive cryoprecipitate several hours before operation so that a maximal effect is achieved. Although very rare, the development of antibodies to the platelet cofactor activity of von Willebrand protein has been reported. In women with von Willebrand's disease, excessive menstrual blood loss can be managed with hormonal suppression. Levels of factor VIII procoagulant activity, von Willebrand platelet cofactor activity, and factor VIII–von Willebrand antigen may become essentially normal during pregnancy in women with this disorder. Obstetric delivery may occur without excessive hemorrhage despite the bleeding time remaining long. However, postpartum blood loss is frequently severe enough to require replacement infusions of cryoprecipitate.

Zimmerman TS, Ruggeri ZM: Von Willebrand's disease. Prog Hemostasis Thromb 6:203, 1982. *Thorough review that covers almost all aspects of this disorder; cites all relevant literature. For those who truly want to understand the disease.*

OTHER HERITABLE DISORDERS OF BLOOD COAGULATION

Table 167–2 lists the inherited blood clotting disorders and their approximate frequencies in the general population. These deficiencies will be discussed according to their approximate position in the sequence of blood coagulation reactions leading to fibrin formation.

Contact Factor Deficiencies

FACTOR XII (HAGEMAN FACTOR) DEFICIENCY. This is an autosomal recessive disorder, virtually always asymptomatic and usually identified as a result of delayed clotting times in routine laboratory assays. On rare occasions factor XII deficiency has been incriminated in mild bleeding. The diagnosis is suspected when the whole blood glass clotting time or partial thromboplastin time is prolonged in a patient who does not have a history of any bleeding tendency. The clotting defect can be identified by the inability of the patient's plasma to correct the partial thromboplastin time of plasma from a patient known to have factor XII deficiency. Plasma from patients with other known clotting factor deficiencies will correct the Hageman factor deficient plasma. Of interest, the man in whom factor XII deficiency was first discovered, John Hageman, died of pulmonary embolism after a fracture of the pelvis.

PREKALLIKREIN DEFICIENCY (FLETCHER TRAIT). This disorder often goes by the surname of the family members in whom first discovered. Fletcher trait is a rare defect in blood coagulation that is not accompanied by bleeding tendencies; hence in this respect the history and physical examination are not helpful. Fletcher trait might be suspected by a prolonged partial thromboplastin time in an asymptomatic patient. Fletcher factor, or prekallikrein, is believed to circulate in a complex with high molecular weight kininogen. Hageman factor that has been activated as a consequence of sticking to an abnormal surface converts prekallikrein to the proteolytic enzyme kallikrein. Kallikrein can then activate additional zymogen Hageman factor to its activated form, factor XII_a, that proteolytically activates factor XI. Hence, it is believed that reciprocal activation occurs between Hageman factor and prekallikrein. Deficient concentrations of otherwise normal prekallikrein and normal levels of subfunctional forms of prekallikrein have been described. Since patients with this defect do not bleed, no therapy is needed.

HIGH MOLECULAR WEIGHT KININOGEN DEFICIENCY (FITZGERALD, WILLIAMS, OR FLAUJEAC TRAIT). This disorder, which also often bears the surname of one of the three families in whom it was first reported, is not accompanied by bleeding problems and so far does not seem to be associated with any disease. It also might be initially suspected because of a prolonged partial thromboplastin time in an otherwise normal person. The clotting defect is due to a deficiency of high molecular weight kininogen which serves as a nonenzymatic cofactor in the activation of prekallikrein by factor XII as well as a cofactor in the activation of factor XI by activated Hageman factor. Persons with this disorder have no clinical symptoms, and no therapy is needed.

Although deficiencies of factor XII, prekallikrein, or high molecular weight kininogen are clinically benign, patients with these abnormalities may be told that they have a clotting disorder on the basis of prolonged whole blood clotting times or prolonged partial thromboplastin times. Therefore it is important to establish the correct diagnosis and relieve the patient of any concerns about a laboratory abnormality that carries no risk for bleeding.

FACTOR XI DEFICIENCY. This deficiency is seldom encountered. Usually those affected are of Jewish or Japanese descent. It is not rare in Jews of European descent, and therefore patients with factor XI deficiency are usually clustered in large cities, where its prevalence may be comparable to that of classic hemophilia. The defect is usually asymptomatic, but it does occasionally cause spontaneous bleeding. Bleeding that becomes clinically significant usually occurs in association with trauma, surgery, or dental extractions. Major bleeding into muscles or joints is rare. The inheritance pattern is autosomal recessive so that the defect can be found with about equal frequency in men and women. The partial thromboplastin time is prolonged and the prothrombin time is normal. The bleeding time is normal. Normal serum or barium sulfate–adsorbed plasma will partially correct the partial thromboplastin time. Specific assays for factors VIII and IX are normal. The diagnosis is established by demonstrating that the patient's plasma does not correct the partial thromboplastin time of plasma known to be deficient in factor XI. Fresh-frozen plasma is used for treatment of bleeding; ordinarily this need not be repeated, since factor XI has a half-life of about three days. Some patients with this disorder may also require transfusion of fresh-frozen plasma before certain surgical or dental procedures.

Cochrane CG, Griffin JH: Molecular assembly in the contact phase of the Hageman factor system. Am J Med 67:657, 1979. *Good explanation of the details of interactions between factors XII and XI, prekallikrein, and high molecular weight kininogen. Fairly short; easy to understand and recommended for all levels.*

Cochrane CG, Griffin JH: The biochemistry and pathophysiology of the contact system of plasma. Adv Immunol 33:241, 1982. *Detailed presentation of the early stages of clotting; only for readers wanting very specific information; numerous references.*

Vitamin K–Dependent Clotting Factor Deficiencies

FACTOR IX DEFICIENCY. This disorder, sometimes termed hemophilia B, is inherited as an X-linked recessive defect that presents with essentially the same historical and clinical features of classic hemophilia (hemophilia A). The deficiency is usually quantitative, but several families have now been described in whom qualitative defects of factor IX structure have been found. Ordinarily the severity of bleeding is similar in members of the same family, but differs considerably among different families. Although many patients with low levels of factor IX are asymptomatic, the tendency to hemorrhage spontaneously correlates fairly well with the plasma level of factor IX activity. Bleeding into large joints, muscle hematomas, and gastrointestinal hemorrhage are encountered frequently in factor IX–deficient patients. Central nervous system bleeding often results in death. Epistaxis and mucous membrane bleeding are unusual. Just as in classic hemophilia, patients having factor IX deficiency may develop crippling joint deformities.

This disorder is suspected with the finding of a normal prothrombin time and a prolonged partial thromboplastin time that can be corrected by normal serum, but not by barium sulfate–adsorbed plasma. The inability of the patient's plasma to correct the prolonged partial thromboplastin time of plasma from a patient with known factor IX deficiency establishes the diagnosis. Fresh-frozen plasma is used to treat mild to moderate bleeding, especially in those patients who only infrequently have hemorrhagic episodes. For moderate to severe hemorrhage, such as large hemarthrosis or muscle hematomas, treatment with commercially prepared factor IX concentrates is indicated. Ordinarily transfusions of 500 ml of plasma twice daily are sufficient to maintain an acceptable level of factor IX activity in view of its 20-hour half-life. The length of therapy with either plasma or factor IX concentrates is dependent on the severity of the hemorrhage and the patient's response and is generally continued for two days after bleeding and related symptoms have subsided. Potential complications of repeated plasma therapy include the rare development of an antibody inhibitor to factor IX procoagulant activity. Commercial, lyophilized concentrates of factor IX remain relatively crude and carry a risk for development of hepatitis or thromboembolism especially when used in high dosage or in patients with liver disease. It is advisable to reserve their use for patients with antibody to hepatitis B surface antigen or for instances in which overtransfusion with plasma is a major risk. The care and long-term goals of therapy for the patient with factor IX deficiency are essentially identical to those for the patient with classic hemophilia. Women who are carriers of this disorder may have factor IX levels that are sufficiently low to cause mild bleeding, especially after trauma or surgery. Although a low factor IX activity may be helpful, laboratory definition of the carrier state is still unreliable. Those carriers of an abnormal structural gene may have about twice the level of crossreacting material in plasma with respect to activity, depending on the extent of lyonization.

FACTOR VII DEFICIENCY. This is a rare abnormality, having been reported in fewer than 100 patients. The disorder is inherited as an autosomal recessive defect and is found with equal frequency in men and women. Both qualitative and quantitative congenital deficiencies of factor VII have been reported. Patients present with a history of bleeding, usually beginning in infancy or early childhood. Bleeding is frequently mild even in those patients who are homozygous. Persons heterozygous for the disorder have no bleeding tendency. Mucous membrane bleeding, epistaxis, intramuscular hemorrhage, hemarthroses, and menorrhagia are common. Gastrointestinal bleeding occurs in about 20 per cent of factor VII–deficient patients; hematuria is observed only occasionally. Central nervous system bleeding occurs infrequently. Over time, clinical manifestations of bleeding may range from very mild to severe in the same patient. In fact, patients with impressive bleeding histories have undergone major surgery without accompanying hemorrhage. Presently this phenomenon remains unexplained. Also of interest are the observations of thromboembolism in factor VII–deficient patients. A diagnosis of factor VII deficiency may be initially considered if the prothrombin time is prolonged and the partial thromboplastin time is normal. The failure of barium sulfate–adsorbed plasma to correct the patient's prothrombin time indicates that the patient has a normal level of factor V. The clotting time of the patient's plasma in response to Russell's viper venom (Stypven time), which directly activates factor X, is normal and therefore excludes factor X deficiency, except in the presence of the rare factor X Friuli variant, which is activated by Russell's viper venom. The diagnosis is established by the inability to correct the patient's prothrombin time by plasma from a person known to have factor VII deficiency. The treatment of bleeding is with normal plasma, not necessarily stored frozen, since factor VII activity is very stable. Commercially available "prothrombin complex" concentrates, which contain factors VII, IX, X, and prothrombin, can be used if it is essential to avoid any possibility of intravascular volume overload, keeping in mind the attendant risks for thromboembolism or hepatitis. The half-life of factor VII is short, being around two to six hours, and therefore frequent treatment is needed during a bleeding episode. Excessive blood loss during menses may be controlled with oral contraceptive agents.

FACTOR X (STUART-PROWER) DEFICIENCY. This rare autosomal recessive disorder was studied intensively in the Stuart and Prower families. Deficiencies are secondary to reduced or absent synthesis of a normal molecule or to production of a normal amount of antigen that has little or no function. Clinical symptoms include epistaxis, occasional mucous membrane, joint, and muscle hemorrhages, and gastrointestinal bleeding. Women with this deficiency may have severe, life-threatening menses and postpartum hemorrhage. The diagnosis is suspected when both the prothrombin time and partial thromboplastin time are prolonged. A normal thrombin time indicates that the level and function of the patient's fibrinogen are normal. The prothrombin time and partial thromboplastin time will correct with normal serum, but not with barium sulfate–adsorbed plasma. The latter observation excludes factor V deficiency. In the Stypven clotting time, Russell's viper venom, which specifically activates factor X, will clot normal plasma more quickly than factor X–deficient plasma. This result eliminates a possible deficiency of factor VII, with the exception that the factor X Friuli variant will show normal activation by Russell's viper venom but not by the intrinsic or extrinsic systems of blood coagulation. Prothrombin deficiency must also be considered; however, if the patient's prothrombin time does not become normal with addition of plasma known to be specifically deficient in factor X, the diagnosis of factor X deficiency is established. Bleeding episodes are treated with fresh plasma, remembering that the plasma half-life of factor X ranges from 32 to 48 hours.

PROTHROMBIN DEFICIENCY. Usually referred to as hypoprothrombinemia, this disorder has an autosomal recessive inheritance and is among the rarest of the congenital clotting abnormalities. In the 20 or so patients reported, decreased to nondetectable levels of immunoreactive prothrombin have been observed in some, whereas others have crossreacting material in the expected amount but without biologic activity. The disorder occurs with equal frequency in men and women. Bleeding ranges from mild to severe and generally occurs only if the prothrombin activity level is below 20 per cent of normal. Symptoms include umbilical bleeding at birth, epistaxis, menorrhagia, postpartum hemorrhage, and bleeding after trauma or minor surgical procedures. Intracranial hemorrhage has been reported. The diagnosis is suspected if the prothrombin time and partial thromboplastin time are prolonged and the thrombin time is normal. Given those results, deficiencies of factor V, VII and X also have to be considered. If permutations of different assays or specific assays for those three factors indicate normal levels, then a specific assay for prothrombin is done. The diagnosis can be proved by showing that dilute solutions of purified normal prothrombin will correct the patient's abnormal laboratory assays. Bleeding in these patients is treated with infusions of fresh frozen plasma, which are necessary only every two days since the half-life of prothrombin is about three days.

PROTEIN C DEFICIENCY. This vitamin K–dependent clotting factor circulates in zymogen form and is converted to its active, enzymatic form by thrombin that is complexed to the endothelial surface bound protein, thrombomodulin. Activated protein C inhibits coagulation by proteolytically cleaving factors V and VIII and, in addition, enhances fibrinolysis by stimulating increased circulating plasminogen activator levels. Patients with decreased levels of protein C appear to be at risk for thromboses. Deficiencies of 40 per cent of normal or less have been associated with a propensity for thrombotic disease. Patients with a combined congenital deficiency of factor V and factor VIII are no longer believed to lack a naturally occurring plasma inhibitor of activated protein C, which, if the initial hypothesis were valid as proposed, would allow the unopposed destruction of factor V and factor VIII.

Esmon CT: Protein-C biochemistry, physiology and clinical implications. Blood 62:1155, 1983. *Short, succinct review of a new and exciting area of blood coagulation. Contains all pertinent references.*

Mariani G, Mazzucconi MG: Factor VII congenital deficiency. Clinical picture and classification of the variants. Haemostasis 13:169, 1983. *Excellent, detailed review. Complete list of references.*

Roberts HR, Zeitler KD: Inherited disorders of prothrombin conversion. *In* Colman RW, Marder VJ, Salzman EW (eds.): Hemostasis and Thrombosis: Basic Principles and Clinical Practice. 1st ed. Philadelphia, J. B. Lippincott Company, 1982. *Good review; thoroughly referenced. For students, house officers, and clinicians desiring more detailed information about the diagnosis and management of patients with deficiencies of factors VII, IX, or X.*

Shapiro SS, McCord S: Prothrombin. Prog Hemostasis Thromb 4:177, 1978. *Comprehensive; gives a thorough review of all aspects of this clotting factor.*

van Dam Mieras MC, Hemker HC: Half-life time and control frequency of vitamin K–dependent coagulation factors. Theoretical considerations on the place of factor VII in the control of oral anticoagulation therapy. Haemostasis 13:201, 1983. *For those wanting details about the circulatory survival of these clotting factors. Highly specific information that is difficult to find in other literature.*

Factor V Deficiency

This disorder is due to a deficiency of the plasma protein factor V and in the past was termed parahemophilia, since it mimics certain clinical features of classic hemophilia. Factor V is not an enzyme, but instead a cofactor in the conversion of prothrombin to thrombin by factor X_a. The cofactor activity of factor V is substantially increased if factor V is initially treated with thrombin to form factor V_a. Plasma factor V is adsorbed by platelets and, once converted to V_a, serves as a specific binding site for factor X_a; consequently the final clotting reactions in the generation of thrombin are concentrated on the platelet membrane. This phenomenon may account for the observation that some patients, despite very low plasma factor V levels, have infrequent hemorrhage.

Factor V deficiency is most likely inherited as an autosomal recessive trait, but suggestions of an autosomal dominant transmission have been made. Immunologic results are consistent with decreased or absent synthesis of factor V protein. Males and females are affected with about equal frequency. As with other clotting factor deficiencies, hemorrhage may occur in almost any anatomic area. Bleeding may vary from mild to severe; death from hemorrhage is known to occur. Skin hemorrhages and bleeding from the mucous membranes of the nose and oral cavity are common. Unlike classic hemophilia, hemarthroses are unusual. Menorrhagia may be particularly troublesome, and women have bled to death during their first menstrual period. Some women with this deficiency, however, have normal menses or only mild menorrhagia. Obstetric deliveries may occur with little or no bleeding, but postpartum hemorrhage is frequent and requires replacement therapy.

For unknown reasons, some patients have a prolonged bleeding time. The diagnosis is made by noting that the partial thromboplastin time and prothrombin time are both prolonged. The prothrombin time can be corrected by barium sulfate–adsorbed fresh plasma, but not by serum. Because of the extreme lability of factor V, stored plasma is not effective. Definitive diagnosis is established if the patient's plasma does not correct the deficiency of a patient known to lack factor V activity. The treatment of this disorder is with freshly frozen plasma, the therapeutic goal being to achieve factor V activity levels at least 25 per cent of normal. The plasma half-life of factor V activity varies from 12 to 36 hours. Fresh-frozen plasma retains adequate levels of factor V activity for several months. At this time there are no concentrates of factor V; cryoprecipitate and concentrates of antihemophilic factor are not useful in treating this disorder. A few patients with this deficiency have developed antibodies to normal factor V, presumably as a result of frequent transfusions.

Graham JB, Barrow ES, Reisner HM, Edgell C-JS: The genetics of blood coagulation. *In* Harris H, Hirschhorn K (eds.): Advances in Human Genetics. Vol. 13. New York, Plenum Publishing Corporation, 1983, pp 1–81.

McKee PA: Hemostasis and disorders of blood coagulation. *In* Stanbury JB, Wyngaarden JB, Fredrickson DS, Goldstein JL, Brown MS (eds.): The Metabolic Basis of Inherited Disease. 5th ed. New York, McGraw-Hill Book Company, 1983, pp 1531–1560. *Both of these sources contain good sections on Factor V deficiency and are exceptionally well referenced.*

Conversion of Fibrinogen to Fibrin

FIBRINOGEN DISORDERS. These are clearly divided into two categories of autosomal recessive abnormalities. First are those patients who have absent or very low plasma fibrinogen concentrations and are therefore termed *afibrinogenemic* or *hypofibrinogenemic*. A bleeding tendency may be noted or suspected at birth, often because of continued oozing from the umbilical stump. The tendency and frequency of bleeding vary from mild to severe and are probably directly related to the severity of trauma or the extensiveness of surgery. Death from intracranial hemorrhage is frequent in infancy and early childhood. It is not completely understood why some patients with no fibrinogen manifest little or no bleeding tendency. Presumably most bleeding secondary to traumatic vascular injury is controlled by platelet adhesion and aggregation interactions. The diagnosis is established by the lack of fibrin end-points in any clotting assay, this observation being most useful in the thrombin time. Plasma fibrinogen cannot be detected by direct assays, including immunologic testing, which show an absolute lack of fibrinogen. Treatment of bleeding episodes consists of giving cryoprecipitate, the protein content of which is approximately 70 per cent fibrinogen, or by giving infusions of purified human fibrinogen concentrates. Fibrinogen levels in excess of about 100 mg per deciliter will generally control most occurrences of bleeding. Commercially prepared fibrinogen concentrates carry a very high risk of hepatitis and are to be avoided since adequate levels of fibrinogen can be achieved with cryoprecipitate.

The second major category of fibrinogen disorders includes those patients who have an abnormally functioning fibrinogen, usually termed *dysfibrinogenemia*. The current policy is to name these disorders after the city in which discovered. The clinical features are unusually variable. Most of these patients are asymptomatic; however, some have mild to moderate bleeding tendencies, usually becoming manifest only after surgical procedures or trauma. Wound dehiscence has been a clinical problem in some; a few patients have a tendency for thromboses. Unique structural defects have now been identified in several instances of dysfibrinogenemia. Examples are fibrinogens Detroit and Petoskey, which have different amino acid substitutions in the fibrinopeptide *A* region, and fibrinogen Paris, which has an extended γ-chain carboxyl terminal sequence. Several of the abnormal fibrinogens show a very slow release of fibrinopeptide(s) by thrombin. Others, once converted to fibrin monomer by thrombin, may display an impaired aggregation into a fibrin gel. In some instances the abnormal fibrinogen has been proved to have a shortened half-life in both the patients and a normal person, whereas normal fibrinogen had a normal half-life in both. The diagnosis of these disorders may be suspected when delayed or poorly formed fibrin end-points are observed in prothrombin time, partial thromboplastin time, and thrombin time assays. The fibrinogen level is normal to low normal, sometimes being less than 100 mg per deciliter. The majority of these patients do not require treatment. In instances of bleeding or before surgical procedures in a patient known to have a propensity to bleed, the goal of replacement therapy is to attain a plasma fibrinogen level of 150 mg per deciliter by infusions of cryoprecipitate or human fibrinogen concentrates, appreciating that the half-life of plasma fibrinogen is about four days. There are no absolute guidelines for how long therapy must be continued, but infusions of cryoprecipitate should be administered for two days after bleeding stops.

Gralnick HR: Congenital disorders of fibrinogen. *In* Williams WJ, Beutler E, Erslev AJ, Lichtman MA (eds.): Hematology. New York, McGraw-Hill Book Company, 1983, pp 1399–1410. *For students and clinicians who want detailed information about inherited fibrinogen abnormalities. All pertinent literature cited.*

FACTOR XIII (FIBRIN-STABILIZING FACTOR) DEFICIENCY. Analyses of several kindreds indicate that factor XIII deficiency is an autosomal recessive disease. Approximately 100 patients have now been reported. The homozygote has an immunologic absence of the enzymatically active subunit of the factor XIII molecule. Only the homozygote bleeds abnormally, having a factor XIII level almost always less than 1 per cent of normal. The heterozygote is asymptomatic. Bleeding, which usually starts in infancy and continues lifelong, frequently begins a few days after trauma and characteristically continues to ooze slowly. Umbilical stump hemorrhage, soft tissue hematomas, central nervous system bleeding, and impaired wound healing are commonly encountered. The impressive scar formation that may follow relatively minor trauma may reflect a requirement for factor XIII catalysis of crosslinks between the cell surface protein, fibronectin, and fibrin. Male homozygotes appear to be sterile, and women with the disorder have a high incidence of fetal wastage. There is no impairment of thrombin formation or the conversion of fibrinogen to a fibrin gel. Consequently all routine tests of blood coagulation are normal. Platelet function tests will also be normal. The laboratory diagnosis consists of demonstrating that a fibrin clot, made by recalcifying a plasma sample from the patient, dissolves overnight at room temperature in 5M urea or 1 per cent monochloroacetic acid. Normal fibrin clots remain intact indefinitely in these solvents. The finding of clot solubility is compatible with a factor XIII level of less than 1 per cent and therefore indicates a propensity to hemorrhage. Treatment is simple and consists of giving fresh-frozen normal plasma or cryoprecipitate. One unit of cryoprecipitate contains about 15 to 30 per cent of the factor XIII activity in the starting plasma volume. Achieving a plasma factor XIII level of about 10 per cent will provide normal hemostasis. The half-life of factor XIII is biphasic, the second phase being about 12 days. Hence prophylactic management of this disorder is easy and inexpensive. Because central nervous system hemorrhage is a major risk, factor XIII–deficient patients are given 500 ml of fresh-frozen plasma or four to six bags of cryoprecipitate every three weeks. In only one instance has an antibody to factor XIII developed as a consequence of transfusion therapy.

Kitchens CS, Newcomb TF: Factor XIII. Medicine 58:413, 1979. *Superb comprehensive review for all levels of students and physicians. All pertinent literature cited. Enjoyable to read.*

Acquired Disorders of Blood Coagulation

VITAMIN K DEFICIENCY

NORMAL METABOLISM AND FUNCTION. Vitamin K is required for the synthesis of normally functioning prothrombin, factor VII, factor IX, and factor X. These clotting factors are made exclusively by the liver, and although the precise chemical reactions remain undefined, vitamin K clearly promotes the post-translational attachment of a second carboxyl group on certain glutamic acids. These residues, now termed γ-carboxyglutamic acid, are present in the amino terminal regions of the vitamin K–dependent clotting factors and form calcium binding sites. Currently it is believed that calcium is involved in the attachment of the zymogen form of the clotting factor to platelet phospholipid, thereby helping to concentrate, approximate, and ultimately convert these clotting factors to active serine proteases. In vitamin K–deficient states, immunologic testing shows that levels of prothrombin and factors VII, IX, and X are normal; however, their function is severely impaired. As vitamin K deficiency develops, factor VII activity decreases fairly rapidly and is then followed by diminishing levels of factors IX, X, and prothrombin activity in that order.

There are no body stores of vitamin K. A normal diet containing sufficient green leafy vegetables will provide the adult daily requirement of vitamin K, which is approximately 0.03 μg per kilogram of body weight. In addition, vitamin K is synthesized by normal gastrointestinal bacterial flora. Vitamin K also promotes the post-translational γ-carboxylation of glutamic acid during the synthesis of certain other proteins, an example being osteocalcin, which constitutes 1 per cent of total bone protein. Vitamin K is one of the fat-soluble vitamins, and consequently the solubilization of fat must occur before vitamin K can be absorbed (see Ch. 103). Hence, vitamin K deficiency may occur in bile salt–deficient states, in malabsorption disorders, or with an inadequate dietary intake combined with gastrointestinal sterilization by orally administered antibiotics. Vitamin K occurs naturally in two forms, vitamin K_1 (phylloquinone) and vitamin K_2 (menaquinone), both of which require lipid for absorption. A synthetic water-soluble form, vitamin K_3 (menadione), is commercially available. Despite its ready absorption from the intestine, menadione must be converted to vitamin K_2 by the liver and therefore is not as rapidly effective as vitamin K_1 in promoting the γ-carboxylation reaction.

CAUSES OF VITAMIN K DEFICIENCY. There are three frequently encountered vitamin K–deficient states: (1) vitamin K deficiency of the newborn; (2) malabsorption syndromes including biliary disease; and (3) oral anticoagulation.

Vitamin K Deficiency of the Newborn. At birth vitamin K levels are low, and its production by intestinal bacteria is insufficient to meet the infant's requirements (estimated to be 1 μg per kilogram per day) for production of normally functioning clotting factors. The vitamin K–deficient state lasts for three to five days and may be the reason why Israelites did not circumcise their babies until the eighth day (Leviticus 12:3). Unlike cow's milk, human milk contains essentially no vitamin K. The physiologic state of neonatal hypoprothrombinemia can lead to hemorrhagic disease of the newborn unless vitamin K is given. Serious bleeding, with central nervous system hemorrhage being feared most, occurs most frequently in premature infants. Bleeding from the umbilicus may be severe. Ecchymoses, hematomas, and hematuria are commonly encountered. The prophylactic administration of vitamin K at delivery, a 1-mg dose of vitamin K_1 given intramuscularly, virtually eliminates the risk of subsequent hemorrhage. Excessive administration of vitamin K (usually 5 mg or more) causes hemolytic anemia and kernicterus in the newborn.

Malabsorption Syndromes. Dietary vitamin K is soluble only in lipids; its absorption is dependent on the ability of the gastrointestinal tract to absorb fat. Malabsorption states (see Ch. 103), such as adult celiac disease, regional enteritis, those caused by drugs such as cholestyramine or neomycin, or those associated with deficient intraluminal bile salts (obstruction of biliary ducts, cholestatic liver disease), impair fat absorption and may lead to vitamin K deficiency. Similarly, various chronic diarrheas can cause vitamin K deficiency, presumably owing to decreased transit time and a relative malabsorption of fats. Vitamin K deficiency is manifested by impaired synthesis of its dependent clotting factors. Ecchymoses, gingival bleeding, hematomas, hematuria, and melena often develop. Daily oral administration of 2.5 to 10.0 mg of vitamin K_1 will correct and prevent the deficiency. The bleeding tendency is easily corrected by giving 10 to 25 mg of vitamin K_1 intramuscularly. In instances of clinically important bleeding, up to 20 to 40 mg of vitamin K_1 may be infused intravenously at a very slow rate. If this dose does not correct the prothrombin time, it is unlikely that additional vitamin K will have any effect. Bleeding secondary to malabsorption states should be virtually nonexistent, since the physician should anticipate it as a potential problem and administer vitamin K early in the course of the illness.

Coumarin Anticoagulants. Coumarin and its analogues appear to competitively inhibit the effects of vitamin K in the post-translational γ-carboxylation of factors VII, IX, X, and prothrombin. The polypeptide chain structure of each of these clotting factors is synthesized normally and is present in normal or even increased concentration in plasma but lacks the additional carboxyl groups on certain glutamic acids necessary for normal procoagulant activity. The coumarins suppress the vitamin K–dependent factors in the following order: factors VII, IX, X, and prothrombin. Coumarin and its derivatives are administered frequently on a chronic basis for the prevention of thromboembolism in disorders such as deep vein thromboses, pulmonary embolism (see Ch. 65), or myocardial infarction (see Ch. 49). The laboratory goal of coumarin administration is to maintain the prothrombin time about one and one-half times prolonged with respect to a normal control. Ratios below this are not believed effective in preventing thromboses, whereas values twice normal carry a high risk for hemorrhage. It is not uncommon for patients to experience slight gingival bleeding, purpura with insignificant trauma, or minimal hematuria while adequately anticoagulated. More extensive ecchymoses commonly follow slight trauma when the patient is overanticoagulated. Hemorrhage from severe trauma can be life threatening; cerebral bleeding is a potential fatal complication with minimal head injuries. There is an ever expanding list of drugs that either *enhance* (e.g., allopurinol, chloral hydrate, cimetidine, clofibrate, indomethacin, phenylbutazone, chloramphenicol, phenytoin, tolbutamide) or *depress* (e.g., barbiturates, ethanol, glutethimide, estrogens) the effects of what otherwise would be considered acceptable therapeutic doses of coumarins. (See references following for full listing of such drugs as well as the mechanisms by which they interfere.)

The diagnosis of bleeding secondary to anticoagulation seldom presents a problem, since it is virtually always evident from the patient's medical history. If only the prothrombin time is prolonged and clinically significant bleeding is not a problem, a dose or two of the coumarin can be omitted until the desired prothrombin time is obtained. When clinical evidence of bleeding accompanies overanticoagulation, 5 to 25 mg of vitamin K_1 may be given orally or intramuscularly with the expectation that the prothrombin time will be appreciably shortened in 8 to 24 hours. If bleeding is considered serious, and more rapid correction is desired, 20 to 40 mg of vitamin K_1 given intravenously should significantly correct the prothrombin time in four to six hours. Whenever possible, vitamin K_1 should be used orally or intramuscularly, since serious adverse reactions occasionally occur with intravenous administration. If the latter route is necessary, the vitamin K should be given at a rate of about 1 mg per minute. Patients who develop life-threatening hemorrhage while on coumarin drugs can be given fresh frozen plasma that will rapidly correct the multiple clotting deficiencies; however, because of the short half-lives of the clotting factors in the infused plasma, the correction does not last long. The use of "prothrombin complex" or factor IX concentrates is seldom warranted owing to the occasional thrombotic complication and high risk of hepatitis associated with its use.

Besides those patients being given coumarin anticoagulants for prevention of thromboembolism, patients with severe psychiatric disturbances occasionally present with various bleeding complications after surreptitiously ingesting a coumarin compound. These patients, who are usually depressed and receive gain from medical attention, frequently belong to the health professions.

Anticoagulants (Systemic). *In* Drug Information for the Health Care Provider. Vol. 1. USPDI. Rockville, MD, United States Pharmacopeial Convention, Inc., 1984, pp 117–125. *Practical guide to use of oral anticoagulant drugs, their interaction with other drugs, and management of bleeding complications.*

Gallop PM, Lian JB, Hauschka PV: Carboxylated calcium-binding proteins and vitamin K. N Engl J Med 302:1460, 1980. *Excellent, succinct review for students, house officers, and clinicians. Makes a difficult subject understandable.*

O'Reilly RA: The pharmacodynamics of the oral anticoagulant drugs. Prog Hemostasis Thromb 2:175, 1974. *Lucid presentation for those wanting more basic information than usual.*

Suttie JW: Mechanism of action of vitamin K: Synthesis of gamma-carboxyglutamic acid. *In* Fasman GD (ed.): CRC Handbook in Critical Reviews in Biochemistry. Vol. 8. Boca Raton, CRC Press, Inc., 1980, pp 191–223. *Complete review of what is known about the biochemistry of vitamin K action. Only for readers wanting a most advanced knowledge. Cites essentially all the important work to that date.*

LIVER DISEASE

The liver synthesizes the four vitamin K–dependent clotting factors (II, VII, IX, X), factor V, fibrinogen, plasminogen, and probably factors XI and XII. Patients with various liver diseases occasionally develop petechiae, ecchymoses, prolonged bleeding from venipunctures, or gastrointestinal hemorrhage. Clinically significant bleeding may occur with minor trauma, biopsies, and other surgical manipulations. Neither the frequency nor the severity of bleeding necessarily correlates with the extent or duration of the patient's liver disease. Thrombocytopenia is common but does not regularly cause bleeding. In many patients with alcoholic liver disease, bleeding is secondary to vitamin K deficiency and will respond promptly to parenteral vitamin K. With progressive hepatocellular disease and diminished protein synthesis, some patients may also be vitamin K deficient, presumably because of poor nutrition and some degree of malabsorption. In more advanced liver disease, the synthesis of the four vitamin K–dependent factors as well as factor V may be severely impaired; however, except in fulminant hepatocellular disease, plasma fibrinogen levels are seldom depressed sufficiently to be considered the cause of bleeding. Generally a poor prognosis is associated with prolonged prothrombin times (greater than 1.5 times normal) that do not become correct with intravenous vitamin K. If the patient no longer responds to parenteral vitamin K, abnormal bleeding must be managed by transfusions of fresh-frozen plasma or commercial factor IX concentrates.

Acquired dysfibrinogenemia, manifested by abnormal fibrin polymerization, has been observed in several patients having hepatic diseases such as alcoholic cirrhosis, postnecrotic cirrhosis of unknown cause, drug-induced hepatic failure, and hepatoma. The fibrinogen in these patients has about twice the normal content of sialic acid, indicating an overall increase in the amount of attached carbohydrate. The clotting of these fibrinogens by thrombin is delayed in proportion to the increase of sialic acid. If the liver disease improves, the defect may disappear.

Patients with liver disease commonly have increased fibrinolytic activity because of an inability to maintain normal levels of plasmin inhibitors or because of decreased hepatic clearance of plasminogen activators, or both. However, enhanced fibrinolysis is rarely the primary cause of bleeding. Occasionally chronic, smoldering diffuse intravascular coagulation may develop, in which case the platelet count is somewhat decreased and levels of several clotting factors are low owing to their consumption during microthrombi formation. These patients do not require therapy unless they exhibit clinically significant bleeding. Then their management is the same as for patients with other causes of diffuse intravascular coagulation (see below).

Efforts should be made to correct the coagulation defects in patients with liver disease prior to surgery, biopsies, or other invasive procedures that may allow bleeding to go unrecognized for a significant time. Fresh-frozen plasma is the replacement therapy of choice, having the potential to correct multiple deficiencies. In these situations factor IX concentrates are not recommended for prophylaxis because of the risk they carry for causing thromboembolism. Platelet concentrates may be necessary if thrombocytopenia is likely to cause hemorrhage with surgical manipulations; however, should hypersplenism be present, achieving a satisfactory platelet count may be difficult.

Blanchard RA, Furie BC, Jorgensen M, Kruger SF, Furie B: Acquired vitamin K–dependent carboxylation deficiency in liver disease. N Engl J Med 305:242, 1981. *Interesting clinical study of circulating levels of normal and abnormal prothrombin.*

Martinez J, Palascak JE, Kwasniak D: Abnormal sialic acid content of the dysfibrinogenemia associated with liver disease. J Clin Invest 61:535, 1978. *Well documented clinical study.*

Poller L: Coagulation abnormalities in liver disease. Rec Adv Blood Coagulation 2:267, 1977. *Easy readable general reference.*

RENAL DISEASE

Patients with uremia occasionally develop purpura, mucous membrane bleeding, gastrointestinal hemorrhage, and prolonged bleeding from venous and arterial needle puncture sites. In addition to occasional thrombocytopenia, platelet adhesion to glass beads, and platelet aggregation in response to adenosine diphosphate, collagen, thrombin, and ristocetin are often impaired. In addition to the platelet abnormalities of uremia, discussed in Ch. 166, certain coagulation factors, primarily the vitamin K–dependent factors and factor V, tend to be low in chronic renal disease. Their levels are seldom decreased enough to explain bleeding in these patients. Some of these deficiencies probably result from varying degrees of hepatic insufficiency or vitamin K deficiency secondary to oral antibiotic therapy, malabsorption caused by uremic enteritis, and diminished dietary intake. Very low plasma factor IX levels (10 per cent of normal activity) have been observed in patients with the nephrotic syndrome, especially when urinary protein loss exceeds 10 grams per day. With that degree of proteinuria, factor IX is found in the urine; however, other clotting factors are not, which suggests a preferential loss of factor IX. Subclinical diffuse intravascular coagulation occasionally occurs in chronic renal disease patients, as evidenced by elevated amounts of fibrin split products in their serum and urine. In general, the bleeding tendency in patients with chronic renal disease is complex and is most likely always due to platelet abnormalities and to multiple clotting defects. Renal dialysis usually corrects the patient's tendency to bleed within 48 hours. There is no specific replacement therapy for the bleeding of renal disease. Fresh-frozen plasma is given in order to correct the greatest number of possible clotting deficiencies that could be causing the patient's bleeding. Infusion of ten bags of cryoprecipitate approximately every 24 hours has been useful in correcting the bleeding tendency in uremia. Although uncertain, the correction may be related to the high molecular weight von Willebrand factor multimers contained in the cryoprecipitate; these are also increased endogeneously by the drug deamino-8-D-arginine vasopressin, which, when given intravenously, has been shown to correct temporarily the bleeding time in patients with uremia.

Rabiner SF: Uremic bleeding. Prog Hemostasis Thromb 1:233, 1972. *Addresses all possible causes of uremic bleeding; contains results of fairly conclusive studies. Extensive list of references.*

Janson PA, Jubelirer SJ, Weinstein MJ, Deykin D: Treatment of the bleeding tendency in uremia with cryoprecipitate. N Engl J Med 303:1318, 1980. *Good clinical study demonstrating a new approach to uremic bleeding.*

Mannuci PM, Remuzzi G, Pusineri F, Lombardi R, Valsecchi C, Mecca G, Zimmerman TS: Deamino-8-D-arginine vasopressin shortens the bleeding time in uremia. N Engl J Med 308:8, 1983. *Explains why cryoprecipitates sometimes correct bleeding related to uremia.*

ACQUIRED FACTOR X (STUART-PROWER) DEFICIENCY

Several patients with amyloidoses have been reported to develop factor X deficiency. This occurs as a consequence of an affinity between zymogen factor X and the amyloid protein, which results in factor X being removed from the circulation. These patients do not have circulating inhibitors of blood coagulation, and vitamin K has no effect on the deficiency. Patients may present with mild to severe bleeding just as seen in the inherited form of factor X deficiency. Replacement therapy consists of plasma or "prothrombin complex" concentrates. The in vivo disappearance time of factor X in this disorder is markedly shortened.

Greipp PR, Kyle RA, Bowie EJ: Factor X deficiency in amyloidosis: A critical review. Am J Hematol 11:443, 1981. *Well documented description of the cause of this deficiency.*

DISSEMINATED INTRAVASCULAR COAGULATION (DIC)

The syndrome of disseminated (also termed "diffuse") intravascular coagulation is characterized by the slow formation of fibrin in the microcirculation and the development of concomitant fibrinolysis. The net result of these processes is the consumption of platelets and clotting factors in the *thrombotic process* and the proteolytic digestion of several clotting factors by the *fibrinolytic process;* hence the coagulability of the patient's blood becomes decreased. Diffuse intravascular coagulation is always secondary to another disorder; it never occurs as a primary disease. Many illnesses have been described in association with diffuse intravascular coagulation. These fall into three general categories, with many of the pathophysiologic features obviously overlapping: (1) *Release of procoagulant substances into the blood,* as may occur in amniotic fluid embolism, abruptio placentae, certain snake bites, and various malignancies. (2) *Contact of blood with an injured or abnormal surface,* as may occur in extensive burns, infections, heat stroke, organ grafts, and during extracorporeal circulation. Any instance in which blood becomes exposed to the tissue thromboplastin as a result of damage to large segments of the microcirculation can initiate coagulation via the extrinsic pathway. In addition, the contact of blood with subendothelial components such as collagen may activate factor XII (Hageman factor) and trigger coagulation through the intrinsic pathway. (3) *Generation of procoagulant-active substances within the blood* may occur if red cell, white cell (e.g., treatment of promyelocytic leukemia), or platelet membranes become damaged and release thromboplastic substances. Hence diffuse intravascular coagulation may complicate hemolytic transfusion reactions and microangiopathic hemolytic anemia. Bacterial endotoxins present in gram-negative sepsis also have thromboplastin-like properties that initiate clotting.

As microthrombi form, plasminogen binds to fibrin and is converted to the fibrinolytically active enzyme plasmin by activators that are either bound to the fibrin or diffuse into the microthrombi. The degree of plasminogen activation is roughly proportional to the extent of fibrin formation. Plasminogen activation probably also occurs as a consequence of activator release from damaged endothelial cells as well as by the generation of activated factor XII. In severe diffuse intravascular coagulation, the formation of plasmin may exceed the capacity of its naturally occurring inhibitors, α_2-antiplasmin or α_2-macroglobulin, to bind and inactivate it. Then hyperplasminemia develops and factor V, factor VIII, and fibrinogen may become digested by plasmin. Both fibrin and fibrinogen are cleaved into a family of fragments termed fibrinogen-fibrin degradation products, the major ones being fragments X, Y, D, and E as shown in Figure 167–2. Since the fibrinogen-fibrin split products have structural features in common with the parent molecule, certain ones, usually fragments X and Y, become bound to intact fibrin monomer during the polymerization process. Because the fragments lack other critical binding sites needed for rapid polymerization, fibrin gel formation is delayed. Hence the fibrinogen-fibrin split products act as inhibitors and delay the appearance of fibrin end-points in routine clotting assays such as the thrombin time, prothrombin time, and partial thromboplastin time.

DIAGNOSIS. Intravascular clotting occurs most frequently with shock, sepsis, cancer, obstetric complications, burns, and liver disease. There are no specific symptoms or signs unique to diffuse intravascular coagulation, its clinical presentation being almost as diverse as the number of diseases in which it is seen. Bleeding, however, is much more common than thrombosis. The rate and extent of clotting factor activation and consumption, the concentration of naturally occurring inhibitors, and the level of fibrinolytic activity determine the severity of the bleeding tendency. In some patients there is no clinical evidence of bleeding or thrombosis, the syndrome becoming apparent only as a consequence of deranged blood coagulation tests. Many patients develop only a few petechiae and ecchymotic areas and bleed a little more than usual from venipuncture sites. More pronounced forms of diffuse intravascular clotting may become evident as a result of severe gastrointestinal hemorrhage or genitourinary bleeding. In some instances bleeding may cause death. Hemorrhaging caused by the diffuse intravascular coagulation syndromes can be especially life threatening in association with obstetric complications or in conjunction with surgery. It is worth noting that thromboses, with or without embolism, may occur with little or no bleeding and be the prime manifestation of diffuse intravascular coagulation. Conversely, fibrinolysis may dominate and cause extensive hemorrhaging.

LABORATORY TESTS. The laboratory diagnosis of diffuse intravascular coagulation depends on the results of a group of tests, none of which alone is specific for the diagnosis. The platelet count is often decreased but can be normal and at times even elevated. Evaluation of the blood smear is helpful if schistocytes (red cells damaged by passage through a partially thrombosed microvasculature) are seen. Most notably, abnormally low levels of those blood clotting factors known to be consumed during coagulation should be found. The fibrinogen level is usually decreased from its normal level, which varies between 150 and 400 mg per deciliter. Since fibrinogen is an acute phase reactant and frequently becomes elevated in inflammatory, infectious, and neoplastic conditions, intravascular coagulation may be accompanied by fibrinogen levels that are within normal limits while actually being relatively depleted. Often the thrombin clotting time, performed by adding bovine thrombin to whole plasma, is prolonged because of lowered fibrinogen levels and inhibition of fibrin formation by fibrinogen-fibrin degradation products. Factors V, VII, and VIII and prothrombin are often consumed during intravascular clotting, and as a consequence the prothrombin time and partial thromboplastin time may be prolonged. Single or combined deficiencies of factor VII, factor V, prothrombin, or fibrinogen, as well as interference by fibrinogen-fibrin degradation products, may account for the prolonged prothrombin time. The partial thromboplastin time may be abnormally long because of decreased levels of factor VIII, factor V, prothrombin, or fibrinogen; in addition, the presence of fibrinogen-fibrin degradation products may delay the fibrin endpoint of the assay. Specific assays of factors V, VII, and VIII do not provide useful clinical information in this disorder. In general, if a patient has consistent clinical findings in the presence of thrombocytopenia, hypofibrinogenemia, and prolongations of the prothrombin time, partial thromboplastin time, and thrombin time, diffuse intravascular coagulation is almost certainly present.

The detection of fibrinogen-fibrin degradation products is also helpful, since their presence signifies that fibrin has been deposited in vessels and increased fibrinolytic activity is present. Depending on their level, the degradation products may inhibit the appearance of fibrin end-points in any routine coagulation assay by competing for the action of thrombin and by interfering with fibrin polymerization to cause defective fibrin formation. Normal serum contains few or no detectable levels of fibrinogen-fibrin degradation products, since essentially all of the plasma fibrinogen will have been polymerized into fibrin. In contrast, patients with disseminated intravascular coagulation usually have significant increases of degradation products in the serum as a result of not being incorporated into fibrin. The agglutination of latex particles coated with an antibody to fibrinogen-fibrin degradation products is a reliable method for the semiquantitative measurement of degradation products in serum. In vivo, certain of the degradation products may become bound to fibrinogen and circulate as complexes that precipitate when protamine is added to the patient's plasma. If in high concentration, these same complexes also precipitate spontaneously to form "cryofibrinogen" when a sample of the patient's plasma is chilled to 4° C.

Antithrombin III may be depleted as a result of its accelerated involvement in the inhibition of pathologic levels of activated factor X, thrombin, and perhaps other blood clotting serine proteases as well.

TREATMENT. Therapy should be aimed primarily at eradicating the disease believed to have triggered intravascular clotting (e.g., treating infection or, in some obstetric situations, emptying the uterus). If bleeding is manifested only by prolonged oozing at venipuncture sites and perhaps accompanied by a few petechiae and bruises, no specific therapy is necessary, provided that the patient's main disease can be controlled. If, however, bleeding is more significant and improvement in the patient's primary disease is unlikely to occur soon, replacement of platelets and coagulation factors is done to control bleeding, and the use of heparin to inhibit the intravascular clotting process must be considered.

Coagulation Factors. In the patient with significant bleeding secondary to diffuse intravascular coagulation, fresh-frozen plasma is given to replace depleted clotting factors while emphasizing efforts to control the underlying disorder. There are no specific guidelines for its use, but ordinarily an adult patient will require 2 to 10 units per day. Fresh-frozen plasma may also replace plasma levels of the various plasma serine protease inhibitors such as antithrombin III, α_2-macroglobulin, and α_2-antiplasmin. Having an adequate level of antithrombin III is particularly important if benefit from heparin anticoagulation is expected; hence infusion of antithrombin III concentrates may be useful in those instances in which heparin is to be given. Cryoprecipitate, which contains a high concentration of fibrinogen, is used to elevate plasma fibrinogen levels that are below 100 mg per deciliter. Since fibrinogen survives in the circulation for three to six days, repeated infusions may be necessary. As a rule of thumb, one bag of cryoprecipitate will usually raise the plasma fibrinogen level by 2 to 5 mg per deciliter.

Platelets. If a patient has clinically important hemorrhage, a prolonged bleeding time, and a platelet count less than 50,000 per microliter, platelet transfusions should be given. Although the patient's platelet count does not increase very much following such transfusions, 6 to 10 platelet packs given on one or two occasions will often correct the bleeding time and help to control hemorrhage. Arguments have been advanced that replacing platelets or clotting factors is hazardous because this form of therapy may fuel the intravascular clotting process and ultimately cause organ impairment. However, most investigators now conclude that the possible consequences of continuing hemorrhage outweigh the chance that replacement therapy will perpetuate the diffuse intravascular coagulation syndrome and cause additional fibrin deposition.

Heparin. Considerable controversy continues to surround the use of heparin in DIC. Some favor its use early in the course of intravascular clotting, believing that the dominant problem is the generation of very high levels of activated factor X and thrombin. Others advocate the use of heparin only in fulminant, explosive forms of diffuse intravascular clotting. Agreement does exist, however, that heparin should *not* be used in patients who have major bleeding from a localized site, a possible central nervous system hemorrhage, or uncontrolled hypertension with diastolic blood pressure greater than 110 mm Hg, or in those who have undergone surgery in the past five days.

The current trend is to reserve heparin anticoagulation for situations in which massive defibrination is accompanied by fibrinogen levels of less than 100 mg per deciliter and replacement therapy is not controlling hemorrhage. In this instance, intravascular clotting is continuing unabated and heparin may potentiate the ability of antithrombin III to bind and inhibit activated factor X and thrombin. Examples of settings in which this approach may be necessary include various malignancies, particularly promyelocytic leukemia; certain infections; purpura fulminans; heat stroke; venous thromboembolism; giant hemangioma with excessive bleeding; and before induction of labor in obstetric patients with retained dead fetus and hypofibrinogenemia. Heparin is given as a continuous intravenous infusion at a rate of 10 to 15 units per kilogram per hour. The duration of the infusion depends on (1) whether the patient continues to bleed, (2) how soon the fibrinogen level returns to normal, (3) whether the platelet count increases, and (4) whether the underlying disease is under control. The plasma fibrinogen level should usually return to normal one to three days after the heparin infusion is started. Simultaneously the titer of fibrinogen-fibrin degradation products should return toward normal. The platelet count does not respond as quickly and may remain somewhat low for several weeks. Heparin therapy is guided by the following approximations: If bleeding worsens while the platelet counts and blood coagulation laboratory values improve, heparin is decreased or stopped because heparin itself may now be causing the clotting defect. On the other hand, if bleeding and the coagulation test values worsen, heparin is increased. Similarly if bleeding stabilizes but the blood coagulation values worsen, heparin is increased. In diffuse intravascular bleeding syndromes in which the patient is in immediate danger of dying from hemorrhage, 5000 to 10,000 units of heparin are given intravenously as a bolus and heparin is then continued at an infusion rate of 1000 units per hour. Purpura fulminans should be treated with large doses of heparin that are continued for at least one week after bleeding stops and all clotting tests have become normal. Patients have been known to relapse if treatment is stopped before this.

Bick RL: Disseminated intravascular coagulation and related syndromes. Boca Raton, CRC Press, Inc., 1983. *Exhaustive, detailed, but lucid coverage of this topic.*

Feinstein DI: Diagnosis and management of disseminated intravascular coagulation: the role of heparin therapy. Blood 60:284, 1982. *Very good review, especially the management of DIC. Recommended for students, house officers, and clinicians.*

Marder VJ: Consumptive thrombohemorrhagic disorders. *In* Williams WJ, Beutler E, Erslev AJ, Lichtman MA (eds): Hematology. New York, McGraw-Hill Book Company, 1983, pp 1433–1461. *Excellent comprehensive review of pathogenesis and associated disorders. Good discussion about the different features and management of diffuse intravascular coagulation in the major diseases in which it is encountered.*

Talbert LM, Blatt PM: Disseminated intravascular coagulation in obstetrics. Clin Obstet Gynecol 2:889, 1979. *Gives succinct overview of pathogenesis and treatment; excellent for students and house staff.*

FIBRINOLYSIS

Plasminogen is the circulating precursor of the plasma protease that degrades fibrinogen and fibrin. Its usual plasma concentration ranges from 12 to 25 mg per deciliter; free plasmin is not detectable except in certain disease states. A variety of substances, termed activators, promote the conversion of plasminogen to plasmin. These include urokinase, which circulates as a trace plasma protein and is found in high concentration in human urine; other plasma proteins and proteins unique to certain tissues, referred to as plasma activators or tissue activators; and the bacterial enzymes, streptokinase and staphylokinase. Plasma activator, which may be produced and released by endothelial cells, is known to be increased in response to exercise, hypoxia, traumatic shock, anxiety, electroconvulsive therapy, localized ischemia, and drugs such as epinephrine or nicotinic acid. None of these instances, however, are usually associated with pathologic primary fibrinolysis. Plasminogen has a high affinity for fibrin, probably becoming bound during the fibrin polymerization process. This serves as a concentrating mechanism, placing the zymogen protein proximate to either the plasma activator or the tissue activator, which also bind to fibrin. Hence, under normal conditions the conversion of plasminogen to plasmin is thought to occur on the fibrin substrate. These series of interactions also maximize the ability of plasmin to digest fibrin by placing it in an environment relatively free of the naturally occurring serine protease inhibitors. For example, the plasma protein α_2-antiplasmin is a very potent, essentially instantaneous inhibitor of plasmin; other, less rapid inhibitors of plasmin include α_2-macroglobulin and α_1-antitrypsin.

Inherited disorders of fibrinolysis have been reported only recently. Abnormal forms of plasminogen have been described in patients who exhibited a propensity for thrombosis. These patients tend to have normal levels of immunoreactive plasminogen, but when converted to plasmin, little or no proteolytic activity develops. The inheritance pattern is probably autosomal recessive. In rare instances a thrombotic tendency has been suggested due to decreased plasmin activator activity. Conversely, prolonged bleeding after trauma or dental procedures has been described in one patient who appeared to have congenitally elevated levels of the plasma activator of plasminogen.

SECONDARY FIBRINOLYSIS. The occurrence of fibrinolysis in association with diffuse intravascular coagulation has been covered under the preceding heading. Secondary fibrinolysis accompanying diffuse intravascular coagulation may become so dominant and out of proportion to intravascular thrombi deposition that massive hemorrhaging occurs. This is most frequently associated with obstetric complications such as amniotic fluid embolism, premature separation of the placenta, profound hemorrhagic shock, or neoplasms such as metastatic carcinoma of the prostate, carcinoma of the pancreas, or acute myelogenous leukemia. In these patients the secondary fibrinolysis may be so severe that clotted blood dissolves literally in minutes. These conditions are managed as described for diffuse intravascular coagulation.

PRIMARY FIBRINOLYSIS. A few patients have been described who suddenly developed overwhelming hemorrhage clearly resulting from fibrinolysis. These patients have sometimes had an accompanying malignancy (which presumably synthesized and released activator) or were undergoing major surgery (e.g., cardiopulmonary bypass) at which time bleeding suddenly could not be controlled, with little or no clot formation in the wound site. Occasionally fibrinolysis is considered a major factor in bleeding that may accompany liver disease. These conditions are defined as primary fibrinolysis. Except for the platelet count remaining normal, laboratory results do not distinguish primary fibrinolysis from diffuse intravascular clotting. Some investigators consider these instances to be merely an extreme polarization of the fibrinolysis that ordinarily accompanies diffuse intravascular coagulation. One must be as confident as possible about the diagnosis of primary fibrinolysis, since its therapy is very different from that for fibrinolysis secondary to diffuse intravascular coagulation. In primary fibrinolysis, ε-aminocaproic acid, which inhibits the conversion of plasminogen to plasmin and, perhaps more importantly, the binding of plasminogen or plasmin to fibrin, is administered to decrease fibrinolytic activity. In situations in which intravascular clotting is occurring, however, ε-aminocaproic acid therapy will allow the formation of fully stabilized fibrin clots in a milieu free of any fibrinolytic activity. Hence it is critical to exclude the presence of disseminated intravascular thrombosis, because ε-aminocaproic acid carries the serious risk of promoting additional thrombosis. Where hematuria is present, a potential complication associated with the use of ε-aminocaproic acid is formation and lodgment of blood clots in the genitourinary tract.

LOCALIZED FIBRINOLYSIS. Considerable hematuria may follow prostatectomy, whether for cancer or benign hypertrophy or other procedures within the urinary bladder. The increased fibrinolysis in the operated site results either from urinary urokinase activation of plasminogen or from the release of tissue activator from the bladder epithelial tissue or from the prostate. If the clinical situation warrants, the hematuria can be managed by administration of ε-aminocaproic acid, since the bleeding originates in the urinary bladder and a catheter is in place through which irrigations can be done. In this situation, the upper genitourinary tract is unlikely to become involved with thrombi as a complication of antifibrinolytic therapy. Localized fibrinolysis is also thought to be a cause of rebleeding after subarachnoid hemorrhage, and some physicians use ε-aminocaproic acid in the management of these patients (see Ch. 495).

THERAPEUTIC FIBRINOLYSIS (THROMBOLYSIS). The intravenous administration of either streptokinase or urokinase has now been accepted as useful therapy in the management of deep vein thromboses (see Ch. 54), pulmonary embolism (see Ch. 65), acute myocardial infarction (see Ch. 49), and peripheral arterial thromboembolism (see Ch. 54). Large scale studies have indicated that either agent provides potential benefit by reestablishing patency of vessels more quickly than heparin. For each of these disorders, the dosage and method of administration of streptokinase or urokinase are specific. In some instances the administration of streptokinase or urokinase is by selective catheterization of the involved vessel, e.g., intracoronary infusion of streptokinase for myocardial infarction. When given systemically rather than locally, a therapeutic effect is evident if the thrombin time is greater than twice normal. Following thrombolytic therapy and before the thrombin time has returned to its normal range, heparin is given to fully anticoagulate the patient for five to ten days. Coumarin may be started before the heparin is stopped, depending on whether prolonged anticoagulation will be required in the management of the patient's disorder.

The main complication of fibrinolytic therapy is hemorrhage, usually in the form of continuous, slow oozing at sites of invasive procedures. Most often this can be controlled by pressure dressings. If bleeding is more significant, streptokinase or urokinase must be stopped. Because these agents have very short half-lives, fibrinolytic activity usually subsides in a few hours. Severe bleeding requires the discontinuance of fibrinolytic therapy and blood replacement with fresh whole blood to restore levels of factors V and VIII and fibrinogen that become digested by plasmin during the hyperplasminemic state. The intravenous infusion of ε-aminocaproic acid in a typical dose of 4 grams every four hours may control hemorrhaging within 12 to 24 hours.

Aoki N, Moroi M, Sakata Y, Yoshida N, Matsuda M: Abnormal plasminogen. A hereditary molecular abnormality found in a patient with recurrent thrombosis. J Clin Invest 61:1186, 1978. *First unequivocal demonstration of an inherited plasminogen defect. Excellent clinical study.*

Bick RL: Disseminated intravascular coagulation and related syndromes. Boca Raton, CRC Press, Inc., 1983. *Easily readable, complete section on primary fibrinolysis.*

Kennedy JW, Ritchie JL, Davis KB, Fritz JK: Western Washington randomized trial of intracoronary streptokinase in acute myocardial infarction. N Engl J Med 309:1477, 1983. *Excellent, well-constructed large clinical trial of fibrinolytic treatment for acute myocardial infarction.*

Kline DL, Reddy KNN: Fibrinolysis. Boca Raton, CRC Press, Inc., 1980. *Encyclopedic; contains details of all aspects of fibrinolysis; primarily for those wanting advanced knowledge; very current with what is known about fibrinolysis.*

Sharma GV, Cella G, Parisi AF, Sasahara AA: Thrombolytic therapy. N Engl J Med 306:1268, 1982. *Excellent general review for all levels of learners; contains important practical information.*

PHYSIOLOGIC INHIBITORS OF BLOOD COAGULATION AND FIBRINOLYSIS

ANTITHROMBIN III. Deficiencies of 50 per cent or greater of this plasma protein may predispose to thromboses. The frequency, severity, and duration of acquired antithrombin III deficiencies are still uncertain. An inherited deficiency occurs as a dominant trait in about 0.02 per cent of the population and is expressed equally in both sexes as a quantitative (Type I; decreased antigen) or qualitative (Type II; altered forms) defect. In the Type II deficiency, decreased and increased heparin affinity, reduced thrombin binding, and diminished heparin cofactor activity have each been described. Anticoagulation with coumarin has been associated with an increase in the level of functional antithrombin III and decreased thrombotic episodes.

α_2-ANTIPLASMIN. This plasma protease inhibitor is virtually specific for plasmin, which it inhibits extremely rapidly and irreversibly. Acquired deficiencies occur in diffuse intravascular coagulation and during the infusion of streptokinase or urokinase. Recurrent moderate to severe hemorrhage has been reported in patients with inherited deficiencies of this inhibitor, presumably from unopposed fibrinolysis.

α_2-MACROGLOBULIN. In the single report of an inherited deficiency of this inhibitor, circulating levels of 25 per cent of normal were clinically silent.

α_1-ANTITRYPSIN. This plasma protease inhibitor probably has little or no function in blood coagulation or fibrinolysis; however, a single amino acid substitution in a genetic variant caused it to function as a very potent antithrombin-like inhibitor with clinical manifestations of severe hemorrhage.

Bauer KA, Ashenhurst JB, Chediak J, Rosenberg RD: Antithrombin "Chicago": A functionally abnormal molecule with increased heparin affinity causing familial thrombophilia. Blood 62:1242, 1983. *Besides being an excellent clinical study of a family with a high incidence of thromboembolism, this is a quick review of all forms of antithrombin III deficiency. Recommended for students, house officers, and clinicians. Contains all pertinent references.*

Collen D, Wiman B, Verstraete M: The Physiological Inhibitors of Blood Coagulation and Fibrinolysis. New York, Elsevier/North Holland Biomedical Press, 1979. *Extensive review with exhaustive referencing. Only for those wanting highly specific information.*

Owen MC, Brennan SO, Lewis JH, Carrell RW: Mutation of antitrypsin to antithrombin: α_1-Antitrypsin Pittsburgh (358 Met → Arg), a fatal bleeding disorder. N Engl J Med 309:694, 1983. *Superb clinical study of a case in which sophisticated basic science methods were used.*

ANTICOAGULANTS

An anticoagulant is any substance which, when added to blood, decreases the ability of the blood to clot. The mechanisms by which anticoagulants achieve their effects are extraordinarily diverse. In the strictest sense, the coumarin antagonists of vitamin K are not anticoagulants, since their effect is mediated by interference with the hepatic synthesis of normal clotting factors. The four general categories of anticoagulation important to human clinical disease are (1) heparin and heparin-like substances, (2) factor VIII inhibitors, (3) anticoagulants associated with lupus erythematosus (so-called "lupus anticoagulant"), and (4) miscellaneous rare inhibitors of other clotting factors.

HEPARIN. Heparin is used commonly for its anticoagulant properties in the prevention and therapy of thromboembolism and to keep blood fluid during extracorporeal circulation, such as with renal hemodialysis or during cardiopulmonary bypass. When bleeding occurs secondary to heparin, it is virtually always known that the patient has been receiving heparin. Only rarely is heparin used surreptitiously to self-induce bleeding. When used therapeutically, bleeding develops because larger heparin doses than necessary are unintentionally administered to a patient. Commonly, underlying factors such as concomitant use of aspirin, inadvertent intramuscular injections, uremia, thrombocytopenia, or advanced age of the patient may contribute to the development of hemorrhagic complications secondary to heparin. Purpura, ecchymoses, hematomas, gastrointestinal hemorrhage, hematuria, and retroperitoneal bleeding are regularly encountered complications of heparin therapy. Frequently bleeding is most pronounced at sites of invasive procedures. Heparin appears to bind to certain lysine residues and a single tryptophan in the plasma protein antithrombin III, thereby altering the shape of antithrombin III and dramatically accelerating its inhibition of thrombin and activated factors IX, X, XI, and XII. Interestingly, activated factor VII is inhibited by antithrombin III only in the presence of heparin. Heparin prolongs the whole blood clotting time, the prothrombin time, the partial thromboplastin time, and the thrombin time. The diagnosis of bleeding secondary to heparin can be made by observing that the patient's plasma is readily clotted by the snake venom enzyme reptilase, which is unaffected by heparin. Heparin is cleared from the circulation fairly rapidly so that if bleeding is minimal and can be controlled by local measures, discontinuing heparin may be all that is necessary. If bleeding is severe, the effects of heparin can be counteracted by giving 1 mg of protamine sulfate for each 100 units of heparin. After about one week of heparin therapy, thrombocytopenia is occasionally observed, but subsides when heparin is discontinued. The cause of the thrombocytopenia may be immunologically mediated or it may be due to a heparin-related platelet aggregating factor.

Two patients, both with neoplastic plasma cell disorders, have manifested clinical bleeding secondary to a circulating heparin-like proteoglycan that also required antithrombin III for its function and that could be neutralized by protamine sulfate.

FACTOR VIII INHIBITORS. Endogenously produced anticoagulants, usually referred to as *circulating anticoagulants,* are not normally synthesized by the body. Their production is pathologic and often results in hemorrhage. Factor VIII inhibitors have been observed in classic hemophilia (factor VIII deficiency), the postpartum state, certain chronic diseases with associated immunologic abnormalities, and in elderly persons having no obvious illnesses. The factor VIII inhibitors which occur in about 15 per cent of patients with *severe* hemophilia (less than 1 per cent of normal factor VIII activity) have no known cause. In most instances these patients have received considerable transfusion therapy and have manifested the inhibitor since childhood. The proposal has been made that the tendency to develop an inhibitor is inherited. Once developed, the inhibitor usually continues as a periodic problem throughout the hemophiliac's life, so that replacement therapy may be made so ineffective that catastrophic hemorrhage results. Factor VIII inhibitors are IgG immunoglobulins that do not fix complement.

Factor VIII inhibitors develop much more rarely in nonhemophiliacs. Depending on the inhibitor titer, clinically significant bleeding resembling that of classic hemophilia can occur and on occasion can result in death. These inhibitors, also IgG antibodies, have been reported following obstetric delivery (for up to one year); in rheumatoid arthritis, systemic lupus erythematosus, regional enteritis, bronchial asthma, and penicillin allergy; and in geriatric patients without evident disease.

When a factor VIII inhibitor is present, the prothrombin time is normal but the partial thromboplastin time is prolonged. If the patient's plasma is mixed with an equal quantity of normal plasma, the partial thromboplastin time will continue to be prolonged. Therapy, especially in the situation of the hemophiliac with an inhibitor, consists of managing bleeding episodes which are not life threatening by means other than factor VIII replacement, since the inhibitor titer will rise sharply if any factor VIII protein is given. With major bleeding episodes, replacement therapy will be necessary and large amounts of cryoprecipitate must be given to overcome the inhibitor. Alternatively, hemarthroses and other major bleeding episodes may respond to the commercial "prothrombin-complex" concentrates, which contain factors VII, IX, X and prothrombin. Theoretically these products bypass the need for factor VIII. In recent studies, about 50 per cent of hemarthroses responded to a single dose of "prothrombin-complex" concentrate. The "prothrombin complex" concentrates are possibly associated with an increased risk of thromboembolism, especially in high doses, and just as with factor VIII concentrates, hepatitis may follow their use. If the inhibitor level is so high that the amount of replacement therapy is prohibitive, then plasmapheresis or exchange transfusion may lower the inhibitor to a level that can be more easily neutralized by factor VIII replacement therapy. In countries where approved for use, bovine or porcine factor VIII concentrates have been given as a last resort, since some human inhibitors have no activity toward them. Immunosuppressive therapy to diminish the production of factor VIII inhibitors has not been very successful.

ANTICOAGULANTS ASSOCIATED WITH LUPUS ERYTHEMATOSUS. Patients with systemic lupus erythematosus sometimes develop a circulating anticoagulant unrelated to the severity or duration of disease. Only rarely does this circulating inhibitor cause clinically significant bleeding; usually, an accompanying thrombocytopenia or a moderate reduction in prothrombin, or both, is the more frequent basis for bleeding. Paradoxically, patients with the lupus anticoagulant have a significantly increased risk for thromboembolic events. Patients having the lupus anticoagulant but adequate platelet numbers and a normal prothrombin time have undergone major surgery without excessive postoperative hemorrhage. The lupus anticoagulant appears directed toward certain acidic phospholipids and as a consequence probably inhibits the thromboplastic phospholipid used in the prothrombin time and partial thromboplastin time to cause impressive prolongations of both assays. Presumably platelet membranes, rather than phospholipid micelles, provide the surface for activation of factor X and prothrombin, thus accounting for the fact that clinically significant bleeding does not occur. Consequently, despite deranged laboratory tests of coagulation, no therapy is required for the lupus anticoagulant.

MISCELLANEOUS INHIBITORS OF CLOTTING FACTORS. Approximately 2 to 5 per cent of patients with factor IX deficiency (hemophilia B, Christmas disease) develop inhibitors to factor IX after repeated transfusion. Inhibitors to factor V have been reported in about eight patients, only one of these being a factor V–deficient patient. Acquired inhibitors to von Willebrand factor activity have developed in a very few patients. An IgG inhibitor has been noted in only one factor XIII–deficient patient following transfusion. There are a few instances of patients receiving isoniazid who have developed an inhibitor directed toward the fibrin crosslinking sites; this results in defective fibrin polymerization. On rare occasion myeloma or other paraproteinemias may give rise to defective fibrin polymerization as a result of interference by high concentrations of gamma globulin. If overt bleeding occurs, plasmapheresis may restore adequate hemostasis by reducing serum protein concentration.

Furie B: Acquired anticoagulants. *In* Williams WJ, Beutler E, Erslev AJ, Lichtman MA (eds.): Hematology. New York, McGraw-Hill Book Company, 1983, pp 1424–1432. *For all levels, including students through hematologists. Good discussion of factor VIII inhibitors.*

Lusher JM, Blatt PM, Penner JA, Aledort LM, Levine PH, White GC, Warrier AI, Whitehurst DA: Autoplex versus proplex: A controlled, double-blind study of effectiveness in acute hemarthroses in hemophiliacs with inhibitors to factor VIII. Blood 62:1135, 1983. *Presents data from important, ongoing superbly designed clinical trial to determine usefulness of prothrombin-complex concentrates. Contains all important references. For anyone involved in care of hemophilic patients.*

Shapiro SS: Antibodies to blood coagulation factors. Clin Haematol 8:207, 1979. *Good general review of this topic. Well referenced.*

Shapiro SS, Thiagarajan P: Lupus anticoagulants. Prog Hemostasis Thromb 6:263, 1982. *Excellent, thorough review of an interesting phenomenon.*

Wessler S, Gitel SN: Heparin: New concepts relevant to clinical use. Blood 53:525, 1979. *Excellent review for students, house officers, and clinicians. Scholarly treatment of subject; gives practical guidelines for use of heparin.*

Part XIV
ONCOLOGY

168. INTRODUCTION

John Laszlo

HISTORICAL BACKGROUND AND DEFINITIONS

The name cancer is an English term derived from the Greek word for crab, Karkinos, which was believed to be first used by Hippocrates, in the names carcinos and carcinoma. He attributed this affliction to an excess of black bile. Cancer was known in antiquity, being described in the early writings of Greeks and Romans. Tumors in Egyptian mummies dating back 5000 years represent the first known human malignant growths, although there is pathologic evidence of bone tumors occurring in dinosaurs and other prehistoric animals.

Kipling wrote, "Cancer the Crab lies so still that you might think he was asleep if you did not see the ceaseless play and winnowing motion of the feathery branches round his mouth. That movement never ceases. It is like the eating of a smothering fire into a rotten timber in that it is noiseless and without haste." And Peyton Rous, a Nobel laureate for his pioneering work on viral causes of animal tumors, wrote: "Tumors destroy man in an unique and appalling way, as flesh of his own flesh, which had somehow been rendered proliferative, rampant, predatory and ungovernable.

Cancer is a prevalent group of diseases, with about 800,000 new cases diagnosed annually in the United States alone and over 400,000 deaths. Trends in the cancer death rates for males and females are shown in Figures 168–1 and 168–2. There are more than 3 million Americans who have survived cancer; in more than 2 million of these the diagnosis was established five or more years ago.

Cancer is difficult to define, but any definition must consider (1) the property of an uncontrollable growth of cells originating from normal tissues and (2) the property of killing the host by means of local extension or distant spread (metastasis). Cancer has been defined in terms of an autonomous growth which is unresponsive to normal regulatory factors; in terms of the irreversibility with which cancer cells progressively lose the differentiated characteristics and functions of the normal tissue of origin; on the basis of morphologic or cytogenetic features; and on the basis of a reversion to growth and antigenic properties characteristic of fetal cells. All of these qualities are typical of most cancer cells, but they are not universally characteristic. The exceptions make any single definition suspect. Some endocrine-related tumors, for example, not only closely resemble the morphologic features of the tissue of origin but also mimic its functions. They may even be at least partially responsive to hormonal control.

Certain animal and human tumors are capable of differentiation and even spontaneous remission. The embryonal cell carcinoma, for example, may begin with a single type of undifferentiated cell and give rise to highly differentiated teratoid tumors containing tissues such as cartilage and hair. Human leukemic cells can be stimulated to undergo terminal differentiation in vitro, and there is the potential to accomplish this by pharmacologic means in patients. Even the property of rapid growth is not characteristic of most tumors, nor does it distinguish a tumor from rapidly growing fetal tissues or certain normal adult tissues such as bone marrow cells or gastrointestinal epithelium. For example, chronic lymphocytic leukemia results from the accumulation of a slowly proliferating clone of small (B) lymphocytes that are identifiable because they share characteristic enzymatic and cell membrane properties. Etiology is not useful as a means of separating cancers from normal tissues, since the etiology is usually unknown. Indeed, different etiologies of a single type of malignancy may give rise to varying behavior. For example, acute myelogenous leukemia arising de novo differs in its behavior from a morphologically similar leukemia caused by exposure to ionizing radiation.

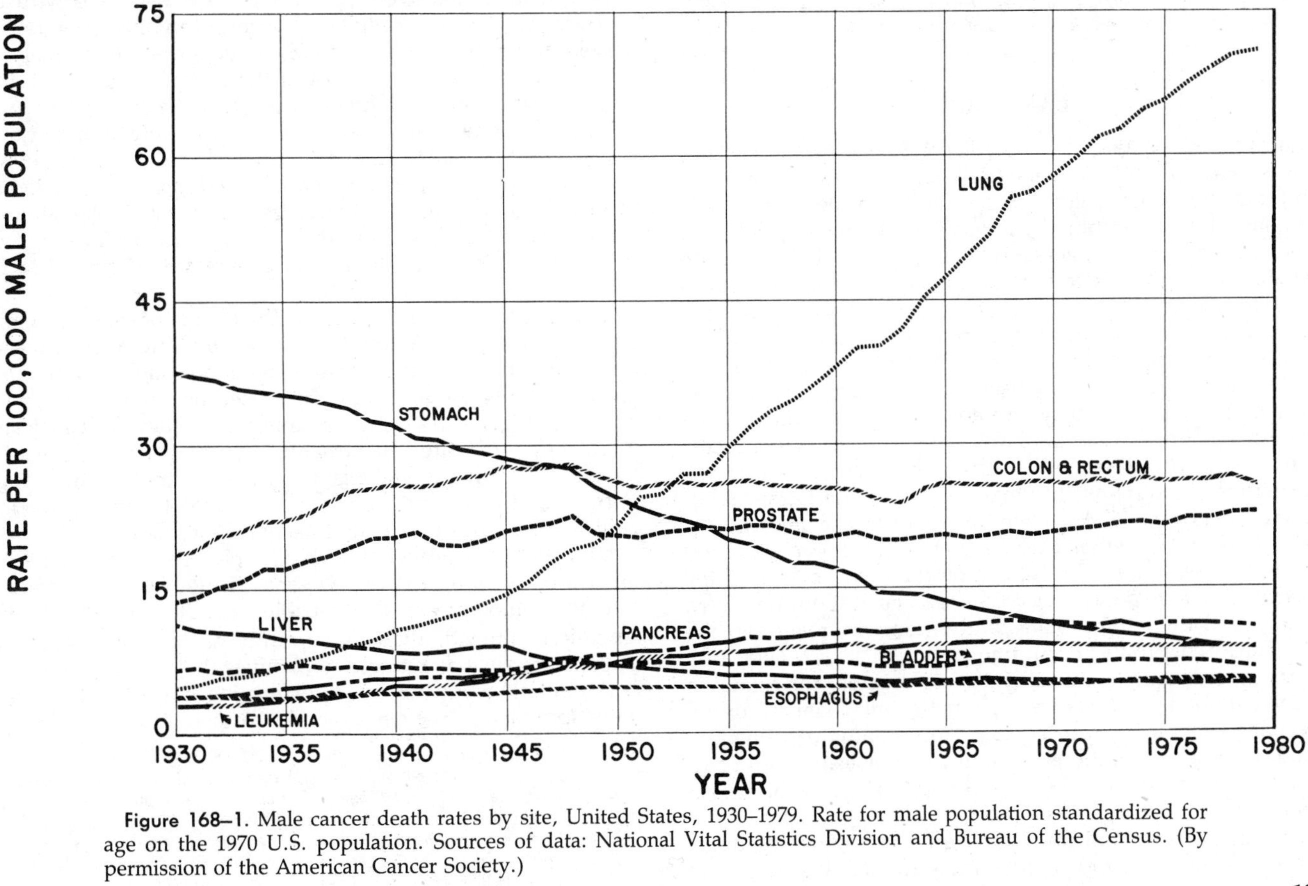

Figure 168–1. Male cancer death rates by site, United States, 1930–1979. Rate for male population standardized for age on the 1970 U.S. population. Sources of data: National Vital Statistics Division and Bureau of the Census. (By permission of the American Cancer Society.)

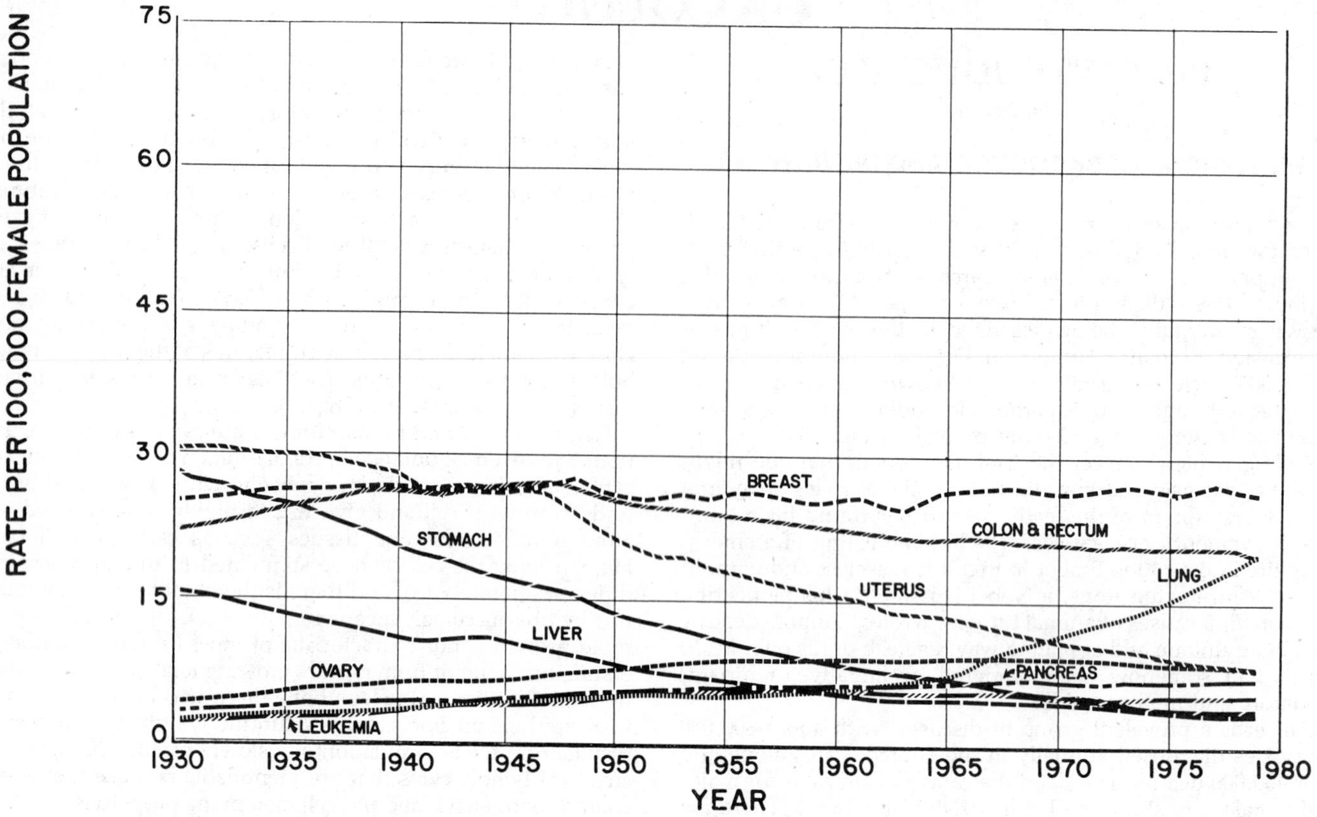

Figure 168–2. Female cancer death rates by site, United States, 1930–1979. Rate for female population standardized for age on the 1970 U.S. population. Sources of data: National Vital Statistics Division and Bureau of the Census. (By permission of the American Cancer Society.)

Shimkin MB: Contrary to Nature. Washington, D.C., US Department of Health, Education and Welfare, 1977. *An outstanding and eminently readable work on the development of knowledge about cancer from earliest records to present-day therapy. This well-illustrated book traces the impact of the scientists and institutions that have contributed to cancer research throughout the world.*

ETIOLOGY

Many chemicals (benzpyrene, aflatoxin, arsenicals, asbestos), viruses, and physical agents (ionizing radiation, ultraviolet light) can serve as carcinogenic stimuli capable of inducing malignant transformation in animals or humans (Ch. 170). Some cancers are iatrogenic in origin, as in patients who develop acute leukemia or other cancers years after being cured of systemic cancer by the use of cytotoxic chemotherapeutic drugs, or in patients who receive prolonged immunosuppressive therapy as part of their renal transplantation program.

Substances that are not themselves carcinogens may serve as co-carcinogens in that they promote tumor formation when given in conjunction with or following exposure to specific carcinogens. This phenomenon has been clearly demonstrated in experimental systems. The major public health hazard relating to cancer in the USA is from the use of *tobacco products. The incidence, time to occurrence, and site of cancer depends upon the frequency and mode of use (smoking, chewing), as well as on exposure to potentiating factors such as alcohol or asbestos.* About one third of cancers in the United States and Europe are related to the use of tobacco products. Additionally, *host susceptibility* is a critical determinant in the carcinogenic process, for a known carcinogen may cause cancer, premalignant changes, or no detectable effect in a given person. This is partly explained by genetic (or acquired) differences in the metabolism of a precursor to the proximate carcinogen, and by differences in hormonal milieu and immunologic resistance.

Fundamental mechanisms that govern the etiology of human cancer, a subject devoid of new ideas for many years, have recently become enormously exciting as new information about cancer genes, viruses, carcinogens, cell growth, and differentiation is being discovered. Retroviruses (RNA tumor viruses), oncogenes (pieces of cellular DNA found in oncogenic retroviruses) and proto-oncogenes (DNA sequences in normal cells related to oncogenes) are part of the lexicon of this molecular biology that seeks to explain these essential regulatory processes. The genetic information encoded by retroviruses can be integrated into mammalian cells near proto-oncogenes and can activate them by a variety of means to produce malignant transformation. There is recent evidence for similar viral oncogenesis in humans, as in the case of a unique form of T cell lymphoma. This exciting area of progress is discussed in Ch. 169.

In addition to that associated with viral oncogenesis, chemical modification of DNA could take place by a number of mechanisms. Agents that cause hypomethylation could activate cancer genes, with or without retrovirus insertion. In order for chemical carcinogens to cause heritable neoplastic cell transformation, they must alter the structure and function of DNA. This generally involves metabolism of the substance by the liver to form the ultimate carcinogen. For their part tumor promotors will interact with cell membranes and internalize and activate a critical effector reaction, such as a protein kinase in the case of the potent phorbol carcinogens. Curiously, some of these tumor promotors are also capable of inducing cellular differ entiation—indeed, there is currently an intensive search for substances such as retinoid derivatives that might produce the differentiating but not the transforming effects, as a possible new approach to prevention and treatment of cancer.

Bishop JM: Cancer genes come of age. Cell 32:1018, 1983. *A current minireview of this field by one of its foremost experts takes a broad view of the phylogenetic, neoplastic, and growth control implications of the oncogene story.*
Farber E: Chemical carcinogenesis. N Engl J Med 305:1379, 1981. *The multiple and sometimes seemingly disparate components of the carcinogenic process are analyzed individually and collectively. This article provides a good review of the origins of thinking as well as the present status of this important field.*

Sporn MP, Roberts AB: Role of retinoids in differentiation and carcinogenesis. Cancer Res 43:3034, 1983. *This selected review provides a perspective on the subject of how control of gene expression might be accomplished and the process of carcinogenesis prevented or reversed.*

HISTOLOGY, METASTASIS, AND GROWTH

For practical purposes a diagnosis of cancer is made on the basis of abnormal histologic features and an abnormal pattern of growth. Cancer cells in variable measure bear some of the morphologic features both of the tissue of origin and of its embryologic progenitor cell. Cancer cells tend to have large and sometimes irregular nuclear outlines that reflect the abnormalities in cell division and in the polyploid DNA content. Nuclei are larger and often more numerous than normal, and mitotic cells are more common in malignant tumors than in either benign tumors or normal tissue. The frequency of mitotic cells in a tumor mass is roughly proportional to its rate of growth. Sometimes qualitative changes in the process of cell division lead to multinucleated and variably sized giant cells. The cytoplasm generally stains deeply with basophilic dyes and may be both scanty and vacuolated. Special histochemical and immunologic stains and procedures may be particularly useful in classifying leukemias and lymphomas, and for identifying unique structures such as melanin, myofibrils, and immunoglobulin markers.

Even in well-differentiated tumors, the pattern of growth of tumor cells is abnormal compared to the tissue of origin. Benign tumors are composed of cells that resemble normal tissue; their pattern of growth is usually circumferential and rounded in gross appearance, and often the tumor is encapsulated by surrounding fibrous tissue. These slow-growing tumors do not become necrotic and hemorrhagic, in contrast to malignant tumors, which more readily outgrow their vascular supply. Benign tumors may show a spectrum of variation from normal, and on occasion the differentiation of a benign from a malignant lesion on the basis of histology alone may be subtle. Malignant tumors are more deviant in their cellular and organizational characteristics, and the cells adhere less to one another. Aided also by the elaboration of proteases, they thus tend to spread locally and replace normal stromal and parenchymal cells, and also to metastasize. As they grow they develop their own blood vessels, presumably in response to a tumor angiogenesis factor. The associated unique vascular pattern can often be demonstrated angiographically as a "tumor blush." Although tumors may be surrounded by varying amounts of fibrous tissue and lymphoid cells, they tend to invade lymphatics and capillaries. When tumors metastasize to distant sites, most commonly to lungs, liver, and bone marrow, they are often rounded in appearance, growing out from a presumed single clone of cells. To the extent that the histologic pattern of the parent tumor varies, metastases may differ in their morphologic characteristics. This divergence may be extreme at times, causing the pathologist to question whether a given metastasis represents a separate primary tumor.

A clinically recognizable tumor includes (1) a small but variable fraction of proliferating cells, only some of which are clonigenic in that they can give rise to additional tumors, and (2) nonproliferating cells, some of which are potentially clonigenic if properly stimulated, and the remainder of which lack the capacity for cell division and are themselves programmed for death. A spectrum of morphologic findings may reflect stages in neoplastic transformation. Dysplastic changes of bronchial epithelium or of the cervix are considered to be premalignant, although not necessarily destined to become cancerous, particularly if the inciting stimulus is removed. As cells become more anaplastic in appearance, they may begin to show microscopic invasion, progressing from carcinoma in situ to microscopic invasion to overt invasive disease. *Dysplastic* changes in other organs also precede frank carcinomatous changes, but once the tumors are established they are programmed for continuing survival and growth, save in rare cases of spontaneous regression. Malignant transformation may possibly be considerably more frequent than is clinically apparent, but be held in check by mechanisms of immune surveillance. This hypothesis is attractive but controversial and certainly has not as yet been proved.

Tumors are named for the cell type from which they originate. For example, they are termed carcinoma if epithelial in origin, or sarcoma if mesenchymal in origin. Carcinomas are designated as "squamous cell" or "adeno" in type depending on whether they show microscopic evidence of keratin or glandular formation. If the growth pattern of tumors is clearly malignant, then the term carcinoma or sarcoma should be included in the name. When the carcinoma has lost its differentiated features and no longer resembles a recognizable cell of origin, then it is called undifferentiated or poorly differentiated, as the case may be. Careful morphologic classification of some malignancies can be critical in predicting their biologic behavior and response to treatment.

METASTASIS AND CELL HETEROGENEITY. The lack of adherence of tumor cells to one another accounts in part for their ability to migrate and invade adjacent tissues and also to spread to distant sites. Tumor masses are not homogeneous; their biologic properties vary from one subpopulation of cells to another. Many cancer cells may be shed from a tumor; fewer may invade and erode a blood vessel to be disseminated by the circulation; and only a rare cell may have the capacity to lodge successfully in a supportive site and begin to grow into a discrete metastasis. One subpopulation of cancer cells may be more successful in growing in lung, whereas another may grow better in liver or bone marrow, for reasons that are not currently understood. Curiously, extensive selective pressures make metastasis an unlikely event for any given cell. The mere presence of tumor cells in the venous drainage of a tumor specimen does not necessarily presage the development of a metastasis. Metastases, like the primary tumor, may cause pressure symptoms or replace normal tissues to damage the host further. The phenotypic heterogeneity of tumors may explain the emergence of resistant lines following chemotherapy, radiation therapy, or hormonal therapy. The emergence of resistant lines is based on chromosomal instability, clonal selection, and the capacity for gene amplification.

CYTOGENETICS. Many types of cytogenetic abnormalities have been observed in leukemias and other cancers by study of metaphase preparations, by high resolution banding with the use of fluorescent acridine stains, and by other new techniques that make it possible to visualize previously undetectable chromosomal defects that could be important to the carcinogenic process. The most common of the recurring defects is either a band deletion or a reciprocal translocation between two chromosomes in which one breaks at a specific site. Although there has long been evidence of aneuploidy, additions, deletions, and translocations for leukemias and for many other tumors, unique chromosomal abnormalities characteristic for particular tumors are only now being recognized. The best known among the latter group is the Philadelphia chromosome (Ph^1) in chronic myelogenous leukemia, a translocation abnormality of the long arm of the G22 to the C9 chromosome. Present in some 85 per cent or more of CML patients, it curiously has been correlated with a better prognosis than is noted for patients with CML who lack this marker chromosome (see Ch. 155). Studies with the Ph^1 chromosome, and selected isoenzymes such as glucose-6-phosphate dehydrogenase in heterozygotes, have shown clonal abnormalities in myeloid, erythroid, and megakaryocytic cells that point to an earlier common progenitor cell as the source of this clonal malignancy (see Ch. 152). Other interesting chromosomal abnormalities have been reported for specific tumor types, such as a missing G group chromosome in meningiomas, the frequent occurrence of a 14 q^+ translocation in malignant lymphomas, and the aneuploid cytogenetic characteristics of adult leukemia. A series of chromosomal abnor-

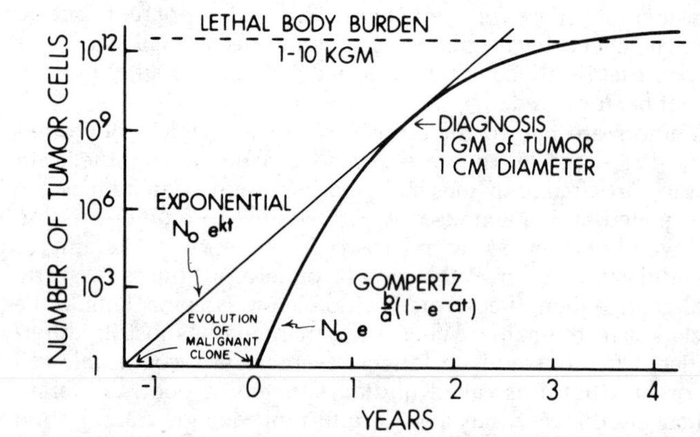

Figure 168–3. A schematic log-linear plot to describe models of exponential and gompertzian growth curves. Over any short span of observation it is not possible to distinguish between the two, but conclusions drawn about the latent period, prognosis, and susceptibility to treatment may be quite different between the two models. (Kindly prepared by Dr. Edwin Cox.)

malities are found in Burkitt's lymphoma, Wilms' tumor, neuroblastoma, and small cell lung cancer.

Pierce GB, Fennell RH: Pathogenesis of cancer: Pathology. *In* Holland JF, Frei E III (eds.): Cancer Medicine. Philadelphia, Lea & Febiger, 1982, p 149. *A lively discussion of the properties of cancer cells and how they relate in histology and growth to the normal cells of origin. Subsequent chapters on tumor invasion, metastases, cell kinetics, and cytogenetics also give details to supplement this introductory chapter.*

Yunis JJ: The chromosomal basis of human neoplasia. Science 221:227, 1983. *Summarizes recent evidence obtained by newer techniques that chromosomal abnormalities exist in most malignancies. It integrates the emerging oncogene story with findings of consistent morphologic evidence of chromosomal deletion, translocation, and so on.*

GROWTH KINETICS. Oncologists endeavor to quantify the growth rate of tumors as objectively as possible and to avoid loose terms such as slow- and fast-growing tumors. The growth kinetics most frequently measured are the growth fraction of tumors, the duration of the cell cycle, the number of cells in the resting (G_0) phase, and the rate of cell death and removal (Fig. 168–4). The size of a tumor mass is increased by the presence of stromal cells and water, or decreased by tumor necrosis owing to nutritional and oxygen deprivation. In turn, these factors vary for different tumors, for different sites of growth, and during the course of advancing growth. The kinetics of tumor growth are crucial in determining prognosis and are also factors in determining response to chemotherapy. "Doubling time" tends to be characteristic of particular tumors. *A tumor that has reached the size of clinical detectability (ca. 1 cm) has already undergone approximately 30 doublings to reach 10^9 cells. Only 10 further doubling cycles are required to produce a tumor burden of approximately 1 kg, which is usually lethal.*

The simple exponential growth curve is a useful first approximation to the growth of tumors (Fig. 168–3). Deviation of the growth rate from a simple exponential expression has important implications for early diagnosis and for explaining difficulties in curing bulky tumors. As most tumors grow, the generation time of dividing cells remains fairly constant, but an ever-increasing percentage of daughter cells enters a nonproliferating state, G_0, from which they may (potentially) be recruited back into cell cycle if the tumor cell population is reduced (Fig. 168–4). In many instances, less than 10 per cent of the cells constituting the tumor mass are actively proliferating by the time the tumor is detected; thus the remaining 90 per cent of cells are not susceptible to most antimetabolites because they are not engaged in DNA synthesis. The progressive movement of cells into G_0 and the increasing relative death rate of cells as the tumor grows larger combine to produce a slowing of the relative growth rate, reflected in a deviation of the growth curve away from a simple exponential function.

Tumor growth curves are often better described by the Gompertz equation, first reported by Benjamin Gompertz in 1825 to express his "law of human mortality." Since that time the Gompertz function has also been found useful to describe biologic growth, such as the growth of the human fetus, of individual organs, and of transplantable tumors. Tumors described by the Gompertz curve appear to be growing exponentially over any short span of observation, up to three or four doublings. Observation over a longer time span reveals the gradual slowing of relative growth rate (Fig. 168–3), to an eventual plateau level at which the rate of new cell production just equals the rate of cell loss. Fitting an exponential curve to tumors that show a Gompertz growth characteristic is somewhat misleading in that it underestimates the underlying growth rate, overestimates the latent period between evolution and diagnosis of the malignant cell line, and predicts more rapid progression and death than are observed.

A number of concepts for cancer treatment based on this kinetic model have been suggested (see Ch. 176). One of these is surgical "debulking" of tumors to reduce them to a small size at which their growth rate increases and the cells are more susceptible to chemotherapy as a function of increased cell division. The availability of more potent and potentially curative chemotherapy programs has given this added importance. A second and related notion is that of deriving comparable equations for expressing cell killing by drugs, in order to predict how many courses of treatment would be required to achieve a total cell kill. The reader will find additional information in the sources listed below.

Collins VP, Loeffler RK, Tivey H: Observation on growth rates of human tumors. Am J Roentgenol 76:988, 1956. *This classic article deals with growth of tumors and emphasizes the relationship of growth to the size of tumor, the time to achieve clinical detectability, and lethal burden.*

Cox EB, Woodbury MA, Myers LE: A new tumor model based on a postulated inhibitory substance. Comput Biomed Res 13:437, 1980. *This article addresses the issue that the Gompertz growth model is not based on biologic factors in growth regulation. The authors derive new equations believed to be more relevant to in vivo determinants of tumor growth. Interesting reading for those who are mathematically inclined.*

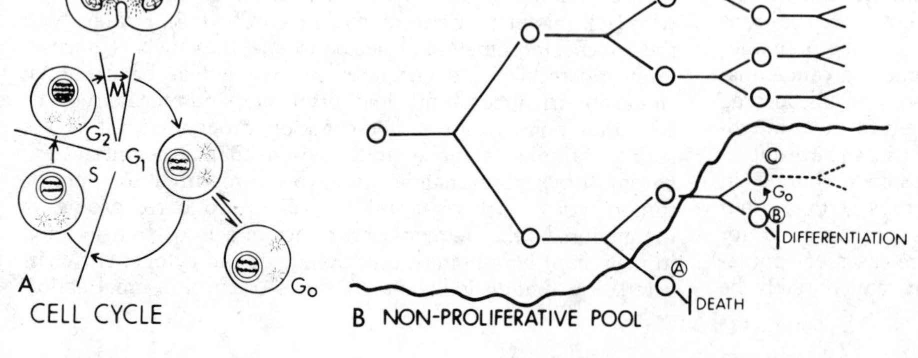

Figure 168–4. *A*, A diagrammatic representation of the events during the cell cycle. M is the period of mitosis—ca. one hour from prophase to cell division. G_1 reflects normal cell metabolism prior to DNA synthesis and usually constitutes more than half of the total cell generation time. Cells not actively undergoing replication are described as being G_0; here they may remain indefinitely or be recruited back into the cycle. The DNA synthetic (S) phase is generally six to 24 hours. *B*, A schematic representation of tumor growth. As the cell population expands, a progressively higher percentage of cells leave the proliferative pool by death (A), by differentiation (B), or by entering resting phase G_0 (C) from which they may be recruited back into the proliferative pool if the population size is reduced.

Lloyd HH: Estimation of tumor cell kill from Gompertz growth curves. Cancer Chemother Rep 59:267, 1975. *Illustrates Gompertz growth curves for experimental tumors and applies theories on tumor growth rates to estimate tumor cell killing due to treatment.*

Rai KR, Sawitsky A, Cronkite EP, et al.: Clinical staging of chronic lymphocytic leukemia. Blood 46:219, 1975. *Tumor burden and prognosis can be predicted for some malignancies by statistical analysis of simple descriptors. More complex and sophisticated systems for multiple myeloma have also been developed which depend upon estimating the mass of malignant cells by its immunoglobulin products* (e.g., Durie et al.: Blood 55:364, 1980).

STAGING, CLASSIFICATION, MARKERS, AND PROGNOSIS

Quantitative means for staging and classification of the clinical features of patients with cancer are important to provide prognostic information, guide therapy, design clinical trials, and communicate information among physicians. Major emphasis has been given to staging or classification of the anatomic extent of the tumor at the time of initial treatment. The complex TNM system, the three elements of which are the primary *t*umor, regional *n*odes, and *m*etastasis, was designed to be applicable to all types of cancer. TNM staging is particularly useful in cancers of the head and neck, breast, and most types of lung cancer, in which the clinical course is often reproducible and described by progression of disease as a local growth, followed by increasing regional node involvement, and finally by distant metastasis (Table 168–1). By contrast, it is less useful for tumors, such as small cell lung cancer, which tend to metastasize early. The size of the primary tumor ranges up to 2 cm for T_1 lesions, 2 to 4 cm for T_2, and larger than 4 cm for T_3 (these criteria vary slightly for some other tumors). Progressive involvement of regional nodes is clinically assessed from the nondemonstrable N_0 to the large and fixed nodes of an N_3 lesion. Metastases are either clinically unsuspected, M_0, or are present beyond the cervical lymph nodes, M_1, in the case of head and neck cancer. Related staging systems based on anatomic extent of disease are also useful for tumors such as cervical cancer and Hodgkin's disease. Indeed, the combined contribution of careful morphologic classification, clinical staging, and substaging together with systematic treatment is best demonstrated in Hodgkin's disease, in which these concerted studies have raised the overall curability from 10 per cent to over 80 per cent during the past 25 years.

Although for many years the TNM system has been standard for some sites, use of the system by practicing physicians is still the exception rather than the rule. In addition to anatomic extent of disease, there are other determinants of prognosis, response to treatment, and quality of life (Table 168–2). Table 168–3 relates the general factors listed in Table 168–2 to specific prognostic factors in breast cancer, and is designed to include almost all factors potentially relevant to outcome. Not all of these are equally important, or even comparable for different tumors. In breast cancer the most commonly used information includes the characteristics of the local lesion (size, location, fixation, skin or nipple involvement), extent of regional node involvement, presence of metastases, and type of hormonal receptors on the tumor. The Karnofsky scale (Table 168–4) is the most widely used shorthand measure of a patient's performance status.

There are other types of tumor markers that may be useful in diagnosing or in following the response to treatment of various cancers (see Ch. 172). Some of these are relatively specific markers such as the beta subunit of HCG, α-fetoprotein, thyrocalcitonin, breast cyst antigen, serum acid phosphatase, monoclonal immunoglobulins, and urinary lysozyme. Others such as carcinoembryonic antigen (CEA) and serum LDH are quite nonspecific but may nevertheless be useful in charting the progress of treatment. Although some of the clinical and

TABLE 168–1. THE TNM SYSTEM

Primary Tumor (T)	
T_0	No evidence of primary tumor
T_{1b}	Carcinoma in situ
T_1,T_2,T_3,T_4	Progressive increase in tumor size and involvement, e.g., for breast cancer, 0–2 cm, 2–5, >5, any size plus skin or chest wall
Regional Lymph Nodes (N)	
N_0	Regional nodes not demonstrable
N_{1a},N_{1b}	Homolateral regional nodes (breast): metastases not suspected (a), suspected (b)
N_2,N_3	Homolateral regional nodes: fixed axillary (N_2), homolateral supraclavicular (N_3), or edema of arm; metastases suspected
N_x	Regional lymph nodes cannot be assessed clinically
Distant metastasis (M)	
M_0	No known distant metastasis
M_1	Distant metastasis present
Specific site ______________	

The Manual for Staging of Cancer may be obtained free of charge from the American Joint Committee, 55 East Erie Street, Chicago, Ill. 60611.

TABLE 168–2. POSSIBLE DETERMINANTS OF RESPONSE TO TREATMENT AND LENGTH AND QUALITY OF SURVIVAL

I. Biologic characteristics of tumor
  a. Growth fraction
  b. Generation time
  c. Rate of spontaneous cell loss
  d. Degree of differentiation, cell-cell interaction
  e. Propensity to metastasis
II. Host resistance
  a. Status of immune competency
  b. Nutrition
  c. Co-morbid medical conditions
III. Host-tumor interaction
  a. Microenvironment, invasiveness
  b. Location of tumor
    (1) Interference with function of vital organs
    (2) Extirpation without harm to vital functions
  c. Systemic effects of tumor, paraneoplastic syndromes
  d. Occurrence of metastasis (regional node involvement)
  e. Site of metastasis, multiple versus single
  f. Endocrine and other metabolic modulation of tumor growth
IV. Effect of treatment on the tumor versus effect on host
  a. Completeness of extirpation of primary tumor
  b. Timing of primary extirpation with respect to occurrence of metastasis
  c. Dose-response relationship to tumor cell killing
  d. Toxicity, therapeutic ratio
  e. Reinforcement of normal host defense mechanisms (immunostimulation, fibrosis in irradiated area)

TABLE 168–3. POTENTIAL PROGNOSTIC FACTORS IN BREAST CANCER*

Primary disease
  Epidemiology
    Familial occurrence (I, II, III)
    Endocrine milieu (menstrual history, hormone administration) (IIIf)
  Primary lesion
    Size (IVb)
    Location (IIIb, IIId, IVa)
    Histologic type and grade (Ia, Id, IIIa)
    Ulceration, invasion, fixation (IIIa, IIIb)
    Kinetic analysis, thymidine labeling (Ia, Ib, Ic)
    Pathology description of surgical specimen (IVa)
  Extraprimary
    Involvement of regional lymph nodes (Ie, IIId, IIIe, IVb)
    Metastatic involvement—history and physical examination, screening and selected special studies (Ie, IIId, IIIe, IVb)
Recurrent disease
  Time to first recurrence (Ia, Ib, Ic, IIIf, IVa)
  Site(s) of metastasis (Ie, IIIa, IIIb, IIIf)
  Hormone receptors and hormonal responsiveness (IIIf, IVd)
  Doubling time, kinetic studies (Ia, Ib, Ic)
  Response to chemotherapy (IVc, IVd)
  Response to radiation therapy (IVc, IVd, IVe)
  Serum calcium (IIIc)
General
  Skin testing, immunoglobulin levels, macrophage chemotaxis (IIa)
  General medical history and physical (IIb, IIc)

*Numerals refer to Table 168–2.

TABLE 168–4. "PERFORMANCE STATUS" (KARNOFSKY SCALE)

Criteria of Performance Status (PS)		
Able to carry on normal activity; no special care is needed	100	Normal; no complaints; no evidence of disease
	90	Able to carry on normal activity; minor signs or symptoms of disease
	80	Normal activity with effort; some signs or symptoms of disease
Unable to work; able to live at home and care for most personal needs; a varying amount of assistance is needed	70	Cares for self; unable to carry on normal activity or to do active work
	60	Requires occasional assistance but is able to care for most of his needs
	50	Requires considerable assistance and frequent medical care
Unable to care for self; requires equivalent of institutional or hospital care; disease may be progressing rapidly	40	Disabled; requires special care and assistance
	30	Severely disabled; hospitalization is indicated although death not imminent
	20	Very sick; hospitalization necessary; active supportive treatment is necessary
	10	Moribund, fatal processes progressing rapidly
	0	Dead

laboratory descriptors are not routinely available for all patients, many of the elements are measured during the usual course of patient care. Systematization of data collection would permit comparison of data between institutions and prognostic assessment of the individual patient over time. Although such systems are just beginning to be developed, they hold future promise in predicting the outcome of therapeutic interventions.

American Joint Committee for Cancer Staging and End-Results Reporting: Manual for Staging of Cancer. Chicago, American Joint Committee, 1978. *This manual is available free of charge from the American Joint Committee, 55 East Erie St., Chicago, Ill. 60611.*

Berry WR, Laszlo J, Cox E, Walker A, Paulson D: Prognostic factors in metastatic and hormonally unresponsive carcinoma of the prostate. Cancer 44:763, 1979. *Illustrates how simple clinical data on even small numbers of patients can provide important prognostic information.*

Coltman CA (ed.): Hodgkin's disease. Semin Oncol Vol 7, June 1980. *This monograph contains succinct summaries of the importance of histopathologic classification, clinical staging, and substaging on the selection of treatment, determination of survival, and complications.*

Cox EB, Laszlo J, Freiman A: Classification of cancer patients: Beyond TNM. JAMA 242:2691, 1979. *A critical review of the elements of classification systems, with a discussion of how computers can help to expand clinicians' ability to assess individual patients.*

DIAGNOSIS OF CANCER AND ITS COMPLICATIONS

GENERAL EVALUATION. The diagnosis of cancer can be simple or it can tax all of the skills of clinical investigation, depending on the site and extent of the disease. The challenge is to detect cancer as early as possible, when it is most likely to be curable. (In large cancer centers one third of new patients are found to have in situ or localized cancer, one quarter to have regional disease, and one third to have distant disease. The rest are unknown or unstaged.) Early detection of localized, malignant disease is aided by an awareness of risk factors in the family history, personal habits (tobacco, alcohol, sun exposure) and occupational exposure (e.g., asbestos, chromium, plastic factory). It also requires attention to subtle and nonspecific symptoms of fatigue, weakness, weight loss, depression, headache, pain, changes in bowel habits, persistent cough or hoarseness, and other clues from the history. The frequency with which the diagnosis of cancer results from attention to such nonspecific manifestations is obviously much less than if the patient presents with physical evidence such as masses in the skin or abdomen, enlargement of nodes or organs, evidence of lymphatic or venous obstruction, or pleural or ascitic effusions.

The physician should carefully examine the nose, oral cavity, pelvis, and rectum for masses or ulcerated lesions as part of any complete evaluation, and these should not be "deferred." More subtle clues may be seen in the skin with petechiae, with hyperpigmentation of skin folds (acanthosis nigricans), rarely with herpes zoster that can antedate the finding of certain cancers such as lymphoproliferative malignancies, or with peculiar types of neuromyopathies (see Ch. 174 and 175). Leads from laboratory testing may be found in unexplained anemia, thrombocytopenia, hypercalcemia, or elevation of serum LDH and alkaline phosphatase, or by specific search for tumor markers.

INITIAL DIAGNOSIS. There are two major categories of diagnostic problems: obtaining the original diagnosis, and correctly identifying the many types of complications or intercurrent illnesses which may arise during the course of the disease. The former is usually the simpler of the two, requiring a tissue diagnosis, for example, in a patient who has a signal lesion in the lung, an enlarging lymph node, or a skin lesion. Intra-abdominal disease is more difficult to find—for example, in the patient with anorexia and extensive weight loss who has a pancreatic neoplasm. Fortunately, advances in imaging techniques (ultrasound, CT scanning, liver and spleen scanning) frequently help to demonstrate pancreatic tumor tissue when it exists (see Ch. 108). Radionuclide bone scanning is a powerful tool for detecting metastases that are not yet visible on standard bone radiographs, although bone scans may also be abnormal owing to arthritis or previous trauma. *Indirect diagnostic techniques are not a substitute for a histologic or cytologic diagnosis of cancer.* Occasionally it may not be possible to obtain tissue for histologic diagnosis, e.g., when there is a deep-seated brain tumor.

Physicians often face the diagnostic dilemma posed by the discovery of a metastatic lesion when the primary site of tumor is unknown. For example, a mass on the arm is excised and found to be an adenocarcinoma, but radiographic studies of lung, bowel, and kidneys are normal. The most common sources of such lesions are tumors of the lung and pancreas. Even so, the majority of primary sites are never found. It is of dubious value to perform blind and invasive diagnostic procedures in the absence of some directive clues.

DETECTION AND SCREENING. How can the presence of cancer be detected at a curable stage in asymptomatic people? One needs to consider that it is not sufficient to make an earlier diagnosis unless that knowledge prolongs life. Detailed discussion of the cost-benefit factors of various screening techniques is beyond the scope of this chapter, and the reader is referred to a thoughtful analysis by Eddy. It is almost impossible to prove that a detection test decreases mortality. Clearly, simple and inexpensive measures such as self-examination of the breasts or testes, routine cervical cytology, and examination of stools for occult blood seem more likely to be of value, particularly in high-risk groups, than frequent chest x-rays, routine proctoscopies, and widespread mammography. The latter procedures are better advised for specific high-risk groups. Some of the old adages about cancer detection are having to be revised in order to make more efficient use of current knowledge in curability of cancers. For example, even the effectiveness of routine screening for occult blood in the stool has recently been called into question. (The American Cancer Society is a good source of guidelines for various screening procedures.)

Diagnostic approaches taken for the *symptomatic patient* are relatively direct compared to the question of cost-effectiveness of mass screening, which is more difficult and controversial. Perhaps the most unheralded and practical problem for the doctor is how much testing is advisable for a concerned asymptomatic patient who can afford noninvasive procedures even if they have a lower yield than would seem appropriate for mass screening. There are no good sources or valid generalizations about this subject, and the answer will depend on the information and attitude of the doctor and his relationship with his patient.

DIAGNOSTIC PROBLEMS DURING CONTINUING CARE OF THE PATIENT WITH CANCER. The physician who undertakes the continuing care of a patient with cancer must be vigilant in promptly identifying complications arising from the progression of tumor, and in detecting curable intercurrent illness which may be mistaken for manifestations of cancer itself. The patient with a known tumor who develops anorexia, weight loss, and jaundice may have cholecystitis and biliary obstruction, rather than metastatic cancer, and may die from that disorder unless the correct diagnosis is established. Furthermore, some potentially treatable conditions are actually caused by the cancer therapy—as in postoperative adhesions or radiation-induced strictures leading to bowel obstruction, or chemotherapy-induced immunosuppression leading to an opportunistic fungal infection. Certain drugs may even produce complications which simulate paraneoplastic syndromes, such as inappropriate secretion of ADH, neuromyopathy, or cerebellar degeneration. Although errors in diagnosis of intercurrent medical and surgical illness sometimes seem almost inevitable, the best way to minimize these problems is to *assume that each new condition is due to a nonmalignant process, until it is proven otherwise.*

Eddy DM: Finding cancer in asymptomatic people. Cancer 51:2440, 1983. *The author reviews the degrees of evidence that early detection tests are effective in reducing mortality, with emphasis on the two areas (breast, lung) in which randomized controlled studies exist.*

PRINCIPLES OF MANAGEMENT OF THE PATIENT WITH CANCER

APPROACHES TO TREATMENT. A therapeutic strategy should be clearly defined for each patient with cancer, once the diagnosis has been firmly established, staging of the tumor has been carried out, and careful assessment has been made of the patient's overall physical, psychologic, and social situation. Such a strategy is often best devised by a multidisciplinary team, including medical, surgical, and radiation oncologists who will weigh the possibilities of cure or significant palliation, consider the various treatment options and their expected untoward effects, and then embark on a therapeutic trial. Fortunately the therapeutic horizons are constantly changing. For example, patients with disseminated testicular cancer, acute lymphocytic leukemia, Ewing's sarcoma, Wilms' tumor, ovarian carcinoma, Hodgkin's disease, and histiocytic lymphoma now have an excellent chance for a cure, whereas this would have been impossible even in the recent past. Since the outcome for an individual patient cannot be precisely predicted, the initial treatment plan must often be updated on the basis of changing circumstances or after restaging procedures, in order to provide the broadest chance of response to therapy. Obviously surgery or localized radiation therapy with the aim of cure is a desirable option if the clinical circumstances are appropriate. Surgery is used as the sole initial treatment for over 50 per cent of patients with *all* types of localized cancer, the remainder being treated either with radiation alone or in various combinations with or without chemotherapy. Local or regional recurrences may still permit localized radiotherapy with the intent of cure, but systemic disease requires chemotherapy if all tumor cells are to be reached. The difficulty of attempting to predict tumor response to chemotherapy may one day be overcome through in vitro sensitivity tests, but for the present the selection process depends upon prior reports of clinical trials for particular types of cancer.

Forty to fifty per cent of all patients with cancer are potentially curable at the time of diagnosis. It is more important to understand the principles underlying the various types of treatment, the order in which they are used, and how aggressively they are to be applied than to remember their dosage schedules. The risk of serious side effects may be much more acceptable to a patient who stands a good chance for a cure than to one who does not. A limited trial of therapy in patients who have tumors that are unlikely to respond may be warranted, with a careful look for changes in tumor size or tumor markers. At least such an approach gives patients an opportunity for palliation, without committing them to many months of ineffective treatment. These judgmental decisions must bridge the gap between careful assessment of the individual patient and knowledge concerning current therapeutic modalities.

SUPPORTIVE CARE. In its broadest sense, "supportive care" refers to all types of medical care required to provide for the needs of the patient with cancer. Certain specific supportive care programs for patients receiving aggressive chemotherapy for leukemia and other conditions have led to gratifying improvements in cure rates by anticipating and/or counteracting potentially fatal complications such as *infection and bleeding.* Early detection and vigorous treatment with newer antibiotics can be lifesaving for infected patients during periods of severe granulocytopenia. It has become unusual to see a fatal infection during the first few such episodes in the treatment of cancer. Similarly, platelet transfusions can minimize the risk of hemorrhage during periods of profound thrombocytopenia. These two advances, together with aggressive systemic and intrathecal chemotherapy, are responsible for the 50 per cent cure rate that can now be achieved in childhood leukemia, for example.

Severe *nausea and vomiting* induced by combination chemotherapy may be major, even limiting, factors in patient compliance because of the serious deterioration in the quality of life induced by these potent drugs. The woman receiving adjuvant chemotherapy for breast cancer or the man being treated for testicular cancer may endure a year or more of these exhausting side effects unless an effective antiemetic program is administered. Many patients fail to respond to conventional antiemetics, such as large doses of phenothiazines, but may respond very well to the active ingredient of marijuana, delta-9-tetrahydrocannabinol (THC). Synthetic cannabinoid derivatives, high dose metoclopramide and steroids, haloperidol and other antiemetics may further alleviate this very troublesome problem. The effectiveness of antiemetic drugs varies, depending on the type of chemotherapy, with high dose cis-platinum therapy being the most potent and difficult emetic stimulus to control.

General supportive care also involves meeting nutritional, rehabilitative, psychosocial, and analgesic requirements (see below). Anorexia and weight loss are almost invariably associated with advanced cancer; occasionally profound *cachexia* may occur in a patient with only a small and apparently localized lesion such as lung cancer. There are several potential explanations for the varying *nutritional problems*—anatomic causes such as abdominal pressure or head and neck surgery, liver disease, paraneoplastic syndromes, effects of chemotherapy, and depression. In the individual patient it is often difficult to sort out the factors that contribute to anorexia and hypercatabolism, and frequently they occur together. Regardless of etiology it is important to reverse this catabolic trend, since malnourished patients tolerate the usual courses of chemotherapy or radiation therapy very poorly and may die prematurely of complications related to treatment toxicity. Thus, in the case of a patient with recurrent cancer of the head and neck, improvement in nutrition is often a necessary prerequisite to the use of chemotherapeutic drugs. Increasingly, oncologists are using parenteral or tube feedings prior to major cancer surgery, radiation therapy, or chemotherapy. The dietitian familiar with the practical problems faced by these patients is an essential member of the team working with the patient and family.

Hyperuricemia and *hyperuricosuria* have the potential of producing acute urate nephropathy in patients in whom tumors are rapidly destroyed by chemotherapy. This complication can be effectively prevented by the use of allopurinol to block urate synthesis and by vigorous hydration prior to and during administration of cytotoxic therapy of lymphocytic leukemia or lymphoma, for example.

Every physician caring for patients with cancer must appreciate the cumulative debilitating effects of bed rest, continuous intravenous infusions, weight loss, and cytotoxic chemotherapy. Losses of muscle mass and bone structure are predictable in patients with advanced cancer, and they predispose to further immobility, hypercalcemia, and fractures. A simple and useful exercise program developed by Rosenbaum and associates can be done at home or in the hospital. The program also contributes to a feeling of well-being and preservation of body image.

The *psychosocial problems* that may be encountered by patients with cancer are profound and varied. Many of these are not unique to cancer and occur in age-matched patients with other types of chronic illness and shortened life expectancy. Shock, bereavement, anger, denial, withdrawal, and depression are common responses of people faced with such overwhelming problems. Disfigurement, feelings of shame and disgrace, loss of sexual activity, and job discrimination are problems that are more prevalent in patients with cancer than in those with many other illnesses. *The attitude of the physician and staff* is of key importance in helping the patient make the best possible adjustment, given all of the premorbid factors and limitations imposed by the illness. The physician who (verbally or nonverbally) conveys the impression that "There is nothing further that I can do" is sentencing his patient to untold misery or forcing him into the waiting arms of enthusiastic cancer quacks. All patients need help. Most patients respond positively to it, and they appreciate a gently supportive role that stresses honesty, trust, and a willingness simply to be available to help both patient and family with their fears and needs.

The *care of the patient who is dying of cancer* is the most sensitive issue for both patient and family. This is also commonly the period in which patients feel abandoned by physicians who themselves are frustrated by their inability to cure or cause remission of the illness and by the tragic human circumstances that often accompany such illnesses. Indeed, these take their toll on doctors and nurses as well as on relatives and friends, and busy cancer clinics recognize the need for support groups for their staff. The physician must be sensitive to these problems and prepare a reassuring setting so that when specific therapy is no longer warranted, patient comfort will be attended to in just as considerate and thoughtful a manner. In the final weeks of the illness, family members may require even more attention than the patient, and the team of doctor, nurse, social worker, and chaplain should provide the necessary support for all concerned, including staff.

Adequate techniques are available to control *pain* in most patients, if these are used in a timely and appropriate fashion. Here again a carefully obtained history is an important initial step in diagnosis, for a patient with pain may have anything from cord compression or bone metastasis to a benign condition such as arthritis. The complaint of pain may even reflect the fear of abandonment. Relatively simple radiotherapy or neurosurgical procedures employed sufficiently early for localized pain and the liberal use of narcotics for generalized pain are usually successful in alleviating cancer-related pain. One need not be concerned with potential narcotic addiction in dying patients. Patients themselves are often reluctant to take adequate doses of analgesics and should be encouraged to take them with sufficient frequency to alleviate pain *before* it becomes very severe.

Depending on the wishes of the family, it is often preferable to provide for the care of the dying patient in his own home. This can be done with a home care program supplemented by visiting nurses and volunteers. *Hospice programs* are rapidly developing in the United States, and these can provide the supportive ingredients for both the patient and family that others cannot supply. The patient is often much more comfortable in familiar surroundings and near to his loved ones. Family and friends usually respond cheerfully to their duties when properly directed. Finally, the savings in costly hospitalizations can conserve already depleted financial resources.

Clark RL, Howe C (eds.): Cancer Patient Care. Chicago, Year Book Medical Publishers, 1976. *Written by the excellent staff of the M. D. Anderson Hospital and Tumor Institute, this book has practical chapters on the supportive care, nutritional needs, and emotional aspects of the patient with cancer.*

DeVita VT, Hellman S, Rosenberg SA (eds.): The Principles and Practice of Oncology. Philadelphia, J. B. Lippincott Company, 1982. *A major new text of oncology that is particularly useful for looking up specific tumors and treatment.*

Holland JF, Frei E III (eds.): Cancer Medicine. Philadelphia, Lea & Febiger, 1981. *Excellent textbook with resource materials for all levels of study. It is an oncology textbook with general articles on diagnostic procedures and principles of treatment, as well as hard-to-find highly technical and basic articles related to various aspects of cancer research.*

Laszlo J: Antiemetics and Cancer Chemotherapy. Baltimore, Williams & Wilkins Company, 1983. *The first detailed study of the neurophysiology, fluid balance, drug therapies, and behavioral therapy of the nausea and vomiting produced by chemotherapeutic drugs.*

Rosenbaum EH, Rosenbaum IR: A Comprehensive Guide for Cancer Patients and Their Families. Palo Alto, Calif., Bull Publishing Co., 1980. *A sensitive and practical new manual describing the attitudes, stresses, and losses of the patient who has cancer, and a helpful guide to rehabilitative services, nutrition, and bed care management. Encompasses the range of personal support services to patients in a book which is suitable for the entire health team.*

169. ONCOGENES

J. Michael Bishop

CANCER AS A GENETIC DISEASE

Astute observers have long nurtured the thought that cancer might be at its heart a genetic disease. The thought was at first vague and arose from seemingly disparate discoveries that included the existence of heritable diatheses to cancer, the presence of abnormal chromosomes in cancer cells, and the remarkable stability of cancerous growth once it has appeared as a phenotypic property of cells. Medical geneticists and epidemiologists first conceived the possibility of "cancer genes," prompted by occasional examples of human tumors whose occurrence seemed dictated by recessive or dominant inherited traits. Now the long-imagined cancer genes have been brought to view, unearthed by two experimental strategies: the use of viruses that cause tumors in animals and the search for tumorigenic genes in the DNA of cancer cells. From these studies we have learned that the human genome contains a set of genes (more than 20 loci but perhaps less than 100) that may lie at the heart of every cancer. These genes are called *proto-oncogenes* (to designate them as precursors to oncogenic determinants) or *cellular oncogenes* (to designate them as potentially oncogenic determinants that are part of the genetic dowry of all normal cells), and their value to cancer research is beyond measure. They are our present best hope of achieving an understanding of the molecular mechanisms by which cancer arises, a keyboard on which many different carcinogens may play, the possible components of a final common pathway to neoplastic growth.

FIRST DESCRIPTIONS: VIRAL ONCOGENES

Documentation that specific genes can elicit cancerous growth emerged first from the study of viruses that cause tumors in animals. By the use of formal genetic analyses, and later of recombinant DNA, investigators were able to show that the tumorigenicity of many viruses can be attributed to domains within the genomes of the viruses. In time, these domains became known as "oncogenes" because they are oncogenic and are coincident with active viral genes that encode proteins produced in infected cells.

Oncogenes were first found in viruses with DNA genomes (the papovaviruses and adenoviruses), but in this form proved to be so intricately involved with viral replication that the significance of their tumorigenic properties was difficult to realize. DNA tumor viruses kill cells that sustain the full viral life cycle, obviating any tumorigenic potential of viral genes. The oncogenes of DNA viruses therefore became apparent only when experimentalists deployed tumor viruses in animals and cells that do not permit viral replication.

The frankly artificial setting in which these discoveries were made cast doubts on viral tumorigenesis that for a while overshadowed the immense importance of what had been found. The oncogenes of DNA tumor viruses were in reality the first embodiment of "cancer genes," and their properties heralded two major themes that now pervade all research on oncogenes: cells can be converted to cancerous growth by dominant genetic traits, but the conversion is nevertheless a multistep process like that first envisioned by students of tumor progression. Ironically, there is as yet no persuasive evidence for oncogenes in the one group of DNA viruses acknowledged to cause tumors in their natural hosts (the herpesviruses).

THE ONCOGENES OF RETROVIRUSES

A more decisive paradigm for the genetic origins of cancer emerged from the study of retroviruses, whose genes are carried in RNA but are copied into DNA by reverse transcriptase early in viral replication. The life cycle of retroviruses provides a microcosm of carcinogenesis. The viral DNA produced by reverse transcriptase is inserted (or "integrated") into the chromosomal DNA of the host cell. Thereafter, the cell uses its own machinery to express the integrated viral genes. These events hold two possibilities for carcinogenesis. First, the integration of viral DNA is potentially mutagenic: it can damage vital cellular genes, and it can influence their expression by bringing them under the sway of powerful viral signals. Virologists call this *insertional mutagenesis;* it may indeed be tumorigenic (see below), and the cellular genes perverted by viral DNA are candidate "proto-oncogenes." Second, some (but not all) retroviruses carry oncogenes whose expression is sufficient to give rise to cancerous growth. The oncogenes of retroviruses make no apparent contribution to viral replication; therefore, their presence in viral genomes posed a puzzle. The puzzle was solved with the discovery that retroviral oncogenes are not viral genes at all, but wayward copies of cellular genes, acquired during the course of viral replication by a process known formally as "transduction" and carried as mere passengers in the viral genome. It is likely that transduction by retroviruses is a rare accident of nature, without design for the virus, and attributable to details of the curious means by which retroviruses replicate. There is no reason to believe that the transduction is limited to genes with tumorigenic potential. However, transduction by retroviruses is of profound consequence because it has brought to view cellular genes whose activities may be central to all forms of carcinogenesis. Many decades might have been necessary to find these genes in the morass of the mammalian genome; instead, the genes were manifested in viruses, excerpted and made available for close scrutiny.

THE PATHOGENIC MECHANISMS OF RETROVIRAL ONCOGENES

The study of viral oncogenes began with the hope that the mechanisms by which these genes act might help to reveal the inner workings of the cancer cell, to elucidate the biochemical abnormalities that prompt cancerous growth. This is now a burgeoning prospect because the number of retroviral oncogenes has grown to almost 20, each inducing specific forms of malignancy, each encoding a protein whose action apparently causes harm (Table 169–1). The first hint of how informative these genes might be came with the discovery that several retroviral oncogenes encode protein kinases, located on the plasma membrane of the cell and possessing a previously unencountered substrate specificity for tyrosine. It would be difficult to envision a better explanation for neoplastic transformation: by phosphorylating numerous cellular proteins, a single enzyme could rapidly change myriad aspects of cellular structure and function. If the phosphorylated proteins can be found (only a few have been, to date), a door will be opened on the secrets of neoplastic growth.

Protein phosphorylation is not the only means by which retroviral oncogenes may act (Table 169–1). As more and more of the proteins encoded by oncogenes came into view, a provocative diversity emerged: some of the proteins are protein kinases, others are not (one is a component of the growth factor normally released by platelets); some attack in the nucleus of the cell, some in the cytoplasm, some at the plasma membrane, at least one in the cytoskeleton; and there is little correlation between what we now know of how oncogenes function and the character of their tumorigenicities. What does this diversity signify? The growth of cells is regulated by an interdigitating network that spans from the surface of the plasma membrane to the depths of the nucleus. If that network were to be touched at any point by an adverse influence and tilted out of balance, cancerous growth might ensue. Perhaps the diverse means by which different oncogenes act may mirror various components of the regulatory network, revealing how the network performs its task. By studying oncogenes, we are likely to be learning of both cancerous and normal growth at

TABLE 169–1. THE PROTEINS ENCODED BY RETROVIRAL ONCOGENES

Oncogenes	Tumorigenicity	Biochemical Properties	Subcellular Location
abl	Lymphoma	Protein kinase	Plasma membrane
*erb-A**	?	?	?
erb-B	Erythroleukemia	Glycosylated	Intracellular and plasma membranes
*ets**	?	?	?
fgr	Sarcoma	Protein kinase	Plasma membrane
fms	Sarcoma	Glycosylated	Cytoskeleton
fos	Osteosarcoma	?	Nucleus
fps/fes†	Sarcoma	Protein kinase	Plasma membrane
mos	Sarcoma	?	Cytoplasm
myb	Myelomonocytic leukemia	?	Nucleus
myc	Carcinomas, leukemia and sarcoma	Binds to DNA	Nucleus
raf/mht†	Sarcoma	Glycosylated	Membranes
ras	Sarcoma and erythroleukemia	Binds GTP	Plasma membrane
rel	Lymphoma	?	?
ros	Sarcoma	Protein kinase	Plasma membrane
sis	Sarcoma	Growth factor	Cytoplasm
ski	Sarcoma	?	Nucleus
src	Sarcoma	Protein kinase	Plasma membrane
yes	Sarcoma	Protein kinase	Plasma membrane

*The exact contribution of *erb-A* and *ets* to tumorigenesis by the viruses in which they occur is not yet apparent.
†Double names denote genes isolated from different species but later proved to be homologous.

one and the same time. It is an old adage of medical science that study of the abnormal can reveal the normal.

PROTO-ONCOGENES AND ONCOGENES

The cellular genes whose transduction engenders retroviral oncogenes provided the first glimpse and the first definition of proto-oncogenes, or cellular oncogenes. By all available criteria, these are cellular genes, not viral genes in disguise. They can be found in every member of every vertebrate species examined, probably in all metazoan organisms, and perhaps even in simple eukaryotes such as yeast. Evolutionary conservation of this magnitude signifies that the proto-oncogenes serve essential functions for the species in which they are harbored. We have little evidence as to what those functions might be, although it is clear that each proto-oncogene and its progeny viral oncogene encode proteins that are very similar in structure and biochemical activity. Proto-oncogenes are expressed in normal cells and tissues, and their expression can vary from one tissue to another, from one embryologic lineage to another, from one time in embryogenesis to another. It is widely assumed that, in their normal guise, proto-oncogenes help to control the growth and development of cells and organisms. Testing this assumption will not be easy, but it is well worth the effort because scientists presently have little access to the molecular genetics of mammalian differentiation and embryogenesis.

Why are the transduced forms of proto-oncogenes tumorigenic? What converts a proto-oncogene, a compliant member of the cellular citizenry, to an oncogene—an unruly and potentially lethal enemy? The possible answers to these questions have taken two general forms: transduction may have unleashed the genes from their usual controls and outlandish or inappropriate expression of otherwise normal genes might be the fatal flaw; alternatively, mutation during or after transduction could change the structure of the genes and the proteins they encode, giving rise to abnormal function. For the moment, it appears that either explanation may on occasion apply. There is no question but that transduction by retroviruses mandates relatively vigorous gene expression. Comparisons of retroviral oncogenes to their cellular progenitors have revealed a variety of structural changes sufficient to evoke anomalous function. These issues are not arcane: they prefigure the debate over whether, and if so how, proto-oncogenes might be the intrinsic "cancer genes" of human cells.

PROTO-ONCOGENES AS CANCER GENES

Do proto-oncogenes participate in many or all forms of tumorigenesis? Are they a common keyboard for all the players in carcinogenesis? Since these questions were first raised, the pertinent evidence has grown from a thin thread to a rich and provocative fabric of experimental observation.

1. Direct manipulation of proto-oncogenes isolated by molecular cloning has revealed that some (but not all) of these ostensibly normal genes can elicit neoplastic growth if they are first attached to viral signals that command vigorous gene expression and then inserted into cells in culture.

2. There is evidence that retroviruses without oncogenes of their own initiate tumorigenesis by the mutation of proto-oncogenes in the manner just described. The mutations may be of two sorts: those that enhance expression of a gene and those that change the structure of the protein(s) encoded by a gene.

3. Some human tumors (the exact number is not yet clear) display karyotypic evidence of gene amplification (double-minute chromosomes and homogeneously staining regions in marker chromosomes) and contain one or another proto-oncogene whose number has been multiplied as much as 200-fold over normal. As a consequence of amplification, the proto-oncogene is expressed in inordinately large amounts.

4. At least several of the chromosomal translocations that typify a substantial variety of human tumors move a proto-oncogene from one chromosome to another. As a consequence, expression of the proto-oncogene may be altered, or the gene may sustain mutations within the domain that encodes a protein. Present examples include Burkitt's lymphoma and chronic myelogenous leukemia, in which the Philadelphia chromosome (Ph^1) raised the possibility many years ago that consistent forms of chromosomal damage might figure in tumorigenesis.

ONCOGENES IN THE DNA OF HUMAN TUMORS

The frequency with which proto-oncogenes first identified through the use of retroviruses have been implicated in the genesis of human tumors is not easy to dismiss as coincidence. The incriminating evidence remained entirely circumstantial, however, until a direct assault revealed biologically active oncogenes in human tumors. Application of DNA from a large number of human tumors to cells in culture can elicit neoplastic growth, as if the DNA contained oncogenes of the sort once found only in viruses. Approximately 20 per cent of all human tumors demonstrate activity of this type, no matter what their histopathology. The responsible genes have now been identified for a substantial variety of tumors. With remarkable frequency, they have proved to be one or another member of a family of proto-oncogenes known as *ras* genes and already familiar to us from the study of retroviruses. The activity of the isolated oncogenes has been attributed to single mutations that change single amino acids in the protein products of the genes. By all available accounts, these solitary changes convert harmless proto-oncogenes to authentic oncogenes. So far, there appear to be but two positions in the proteins encoded by *ras* genes (amino acid residues 12 and 61) where mutations can confer tumorigenic potential. At either position, more than one form of amino acid substitution can accomplish this. These findings provide direct evidence that proto-oncogenes are involved in tumorigenesis, embody mutational carcinogenesis in a dramatic fashion, and offer great promise for learning how damage to DNA contributes to tumorigenesis and how the structure of proteins determines their function.

ONCOGENES AND THE MULTIPLE STEPS IN CARCINOGENESIS

The attribution of tumorigenesis to oncogenes seemed at first glance simplistic, since the genesis of tumors has long been described as a protracted and complex sequence of events. However, the identification of oncogenes and the proto-oncogenes from which they are derived has given us a tool with which to recognize several separate steps in tumorigenesis. In a remarkable variety of human and animal tumors, it is possible to point to at least two coexistent genetic lesions afflicting proto-oncogenes in various ways. For example, two oncogenes have been incriminated in the genesis of Burkitt's lymphoma: a proto-oncogene that has been relocated and possibly activated by chromosomal translocation; and another gene, whose action transforms rodent cells in culture, apparently because a mutation has altered the protein encoded by the gene.

The manner in which such pairings might exemplify distinct steps in carcinogenesis has been demonstrated by experiment. Oncogenes from two mutually exclusive groups can be combined to elicit a tumorigenic phenotype in cultures of embryonic rodent cells that could not be rendered tumorigenic by any single oncogene. The cooperating oncogenes appear to supply complementary functions that together convert cells to neoplastic growth. Medical geneticists have in the past suggested that at least some tumors may owe their origins to no more than two genetic lesions. These suggestions now appear more credible than ever before.

By one means or another, at least 11 proto-oncogenes have been implicated in different types of tumorigenesis. In some instances, expression of the gene is enhanced; in other instances, the structure of the protein encoded by the gene has been changed. In a few instances, both of these events may have occurred. These are remarkable conclusions, reached within a decade of the discovery of proto-oncogenes. However, the unknown still outweighs the known. How extensive is the role of proto-oncogenes in tumorigenesis? How are we to explain the majority of human tumors that as yet offer no evidence of genetic lesions? How important are recessive genetic traits in tumorigenesis, how are they to be identified, and by what means do they act? What is the nature of heritable susceptibility to carcinogenesis and does this diathesis ever originate from proto-oncogenes? How do the proteins encoded by oncogenes conduct their nefarious business? Above all, will we be able to parlay the growing information about oncogenes into devices for the prevention, diagnosis, and treatment of human cancer? It is too early to foretell how quickly the answers to these questions may come, but there now seems little reason to doubt that we have laid hold of cancer with a grip that should eventually extract the deadly secrets of the disease.

Bishop JM: The molecular biology of RNA tumor viruses: A physician's guide. N Engl J Med 303:675, 1980.
Bishop JM: Oncogenes. Sci Am 246(3):80, 1982.
Weinberg R: A molecular basis of cancer. Sci Am 249(5):126, 1983.
Bishop JM: Viruses, genes and cancer. Harvey Lectures, 1983–1984.
Bishop JM: Cellular oncogenes and retroviruses. Ann Rev Biochem 52:301, 1983.
All of these references offer general reviews of this rapidly expanding area of medical research; the first four references in particular are suitable for the student or physician who wants an overview.

170. EPIDEMIOLOGY OF CANCER

Joseph F. Fraumeni, Jr.

INTRODUCTION

Epidemiology has contributed substantially to knowledge about the origins of human cancer, and provides the foundation for measures designed to prevent cancer. The approach dates from the eighteenth century, when the occupational physician Bernardino Ramazzini reported that nuns were at high risk of breast cancer, and the surgeon Percivall Pott observed that chimney sweeps exposed to soot were prone to scrotal cancer. The initial leads to epidemiologic investigation have often come from astute clinicians who noted an excessive number of patients with the same tumor and traced the "cluster" to a particular cultural, occupational, or iatrogenic exposure. Major insights into cancer etiology are provided also by experimental approaches to detect carcinogens in laboratory animals or mutagens in short-term test assays, and to clarify basic mechanisms of carcinogenesis. In recent years the pace of epidemiologic and experimental research in cancer etiology has accelerated, including efforts to identify environmental factors, which are generally held responsible for a large proportion of cancers in the general population.

PATTERNS OF CANCER OCCURRENCE

Cancer is second only to heart disease as a cause of death in the United States, and accounts for 20 per cent of all deaths. It is estimated that in 1984 about 870,000 Americans will develop cancer, excluding in situ carcinomas and nonmelanoma skin cancer, and that about 450,000 will die from the disease. The most common cancers occur in the lung in males, the breast in females, and the colon and rectum in both sexes combined.

It has been widely reported that 80 to 90 per cent of all cancer is related to environmental influences, particularly those related to life style practices. These estimates are derived from the substantial international variation in cancer incidence, in which rates for the lowest risk countries are subtracted from the rates prevailing in the United States. The resulting difference is attributed to environmental causes, and the lowest risk is assumed to represent the baseline level for tumors that develop "spontaneously" and cannot be prevented. Around the world the reported age-adjusted incidence rates for total cancer vary by a factor of about three, whereas the rates for certain anatomic sites, particularly the esophagus and liver, is greater than 100-fold. Even the risks for the more common tumors in Western countries differ by factors of about 8 to 40. Although some of this variation may have a genetic basis, evidence supporting a major role for environmental factors can be found in the experience of migrant populations, such as the Japanese who moved to Hawaii and California. Generally, as migrant groups adopt customs of the new land, their risk of various cancers shifts away from the rate prevailing in the country of origin to approximate that of the host country. The change in incidence for some cancers, notably cancer of the colon, is evident within two to three decades of migration, whereas the change for other cancers, notably cancer of the breast, requires more than one generation. Although variations within countries are not as great as those seen internationally, the recent mapping of cancer death rates in the United States at the county level has revealed geographic clustering that provides leads to the investigation of environmental exposures.

Variations in cancer incidence and mortality over time may also reflect environmental factors, although some fluctuations can be explained by changing medical practices and reporting procedures. Most dramatic has been the increase in lung cancer rates in the United States and other countries; in the 1950's several studies established that cigarette smoking was responsible. Upward trends have been noted also for thyroid cancer resulting from x-ray exposures to the head and neck during childhood, malignant melanoma from changing clothing styles and recreational exposures to sunlight, and endometrial cancer from the use of menopausal estrogens. The increases in prostatic cancer and multiple myeloma, however, are at least partly due to improvements in diagnostic measures. In the black population of the United States, sharp increases over time have been reported for cancers of the lung, esophagus, prostate, and pancreas and multiple myeloma, so that these tumors are now more common in blacks than whites. Several cancers have shown little change, while a few have displayed downward trends, including cancers of the stomach, cervix, and liver.

THE CAUSES OF CANCER

Although much remains to be learned about the factors responsible for variations of cancer in the general population, several environmental exposures have been identified as causes of cancer (Table 170–1). The evidence is based primarily on case-control studies (comparing the past experience of persons with and without a particular cancer) or cohort studies (following-up individuals whose experiences and characteristics are already defined). There is a growing recognition, however, that most cancers result from the combined effects of multiple exposures and susceptibility states. This is consistent with multistage models in which different risk factors accelerate the transition rates at various stages of carcinogenesis. Some affect early stages as initiators, others act at late stages as promoters, and still others influence both early and late stages. It is generally thought that cumulative environmental exposures, long latency periods, and multistage processes account for the increasing risk of most cancers with advancing age.

TOBACCO. The principal carcinogenic hazard is tobacco smoking, which produces cancers of the lung, larynx, mouth, pharynx, esophagus, bladder, pancreas, and kidney. It is estimated that smoking, especially cigarettes, contributes to about 25 to 30 per cent of all cancer in men and 5 to 10 per cent in women. The greatest impact is on lung cancer, with the risk

TABLE 170–1. ENVIRONMENTAL CAUSES OF HUMAN CANCER

Agent	Type of Exposure	Site of Cancer
Alcoholic beverages	Drinking	Mouth, pharynx, esophagus, larynx, liver
Alkylating agents (melphalan, cyclophosphamide, chlorambucil, semustine)	Medication	Leukemia
Androgen-anabolic steroids	Medication	Liver
Aromatic amines (benzidine, 2-naphthylamine, 4-aminobiphenyl)	Manufacture of chemicals	Bladder
Arsenic (inorganic)	Mining and smelting of certain ores, pesticide manufacturing and application, medication and contaminated drinking water	Lung, skin, liver (angiosarcoma)
Asbestos	Manufacturing and application	Lung, pleura, peritoneum, gastrointestinal cancers
Benzene	Leather, petroleum, and other industries	Leukemia
Bis(chloromethyl)ether	Manufacture of ion exchange resins	Lung
Chlornaphazine	Medication	Bladder
Chromium compounds	Manufacturing	Lung
Estrogens	Medication	
Synthetic (DES)		Vagina, cervix (adenocarcinoma)
Conjugated (Premarin)		Endometrium
Steroid contraceptives		Liver (benign)
Immunosuppressants (azathioprine, cyclosporin)	Medication	Lymphoma (histiocytic), skin (squamous carcinoma), soft tissue sarcoma
Ionizing radiation	Atomic blasts, medical use, radium dial painting, uranium and metal mining	Nearly all sites
Isopropyl alcohol production	Manufacturing by strong acid process	Nasal sinuses
Mustard gas	Manufacturing	Lung, larynx, nasal sinuses
Nickel dust	Refining	Lung, nasal sinuses
Phenacetin-containing analgesics	Medication	Renal pelvis
Polycyclic hydrocarbons	Coal carbonization products and some mineral oils	Lung, skin (squamous carcinoma)
Tobacco chews and powder	Snuff dipping and chewing of tobacco, betel, lime	Mouth
Tobacco smoke	Smoking, especially cigarettes	Lung, larynx, mouth, pharynx, esophagus, bladder, pancreas, kidney
Ultraviolet radiation	Sunlight	Skin, including melanoma
Vinyl chloride	Manufacture of polyvinyl chloride	Liver (angiosarcoma)
Wood dusts	Furniture manufacturing	Nasal sinuses

for male smokers of two or more packs per day being about 20 times that of nonsmokers. However, the rates for lung cancer are now rising more sharply in women than in men, reflecting the growing popularity of cigarettes among women in the past 20 to 30 years. Smokers of filter-tipped cigarettes with reduced tar and nicotine have a lower risk of lung cancer than do smokers of nonfilter cigarettes, but still a much higher risk than do nonsmokers. Smokeless tobacco products are also of concern, since oral cancer has been linked with snuff dipping, a common practice in rural southern areas of the United States. In parts of Asia, oral cancer is very common in people exposed to various tobacco chews, which are often mixed with betel, lime, and other agents that may enhance the risks.

ALCOHOL. Consumption of alcoholic beverages has been shown to multiply the effects of tobacco smoking on cancers of the mouth, pharynx, esophagus, and larynx. The risk for heavy drinkers who do not smoke appears only slightly elevated. Heavy drinking also increases the risk of liver cancer, particularly among cirrhotic patients. Ethanol is not carcinogenic in laboratory animals, so the mechanism by which alcohol promotes carcinogenesis is not clear. Under suspicion are nutritional deficiencies associated with heavy drinking, the effects of congeners or contaminants (e.g., nitrosamines, hydrocarbons) in alcoholic beverages, and the capacity of alcohol to solubilize carcinogens or enhance their penetration into tissue.

SOLAR RADIATION. The dominant risk factor for nonmelanoma skin cancer (squamous and basal cell carcinomas) and for malignant melanoma is ultraviolet (UV) radiation from the sun. The evidence is based on the tendency for skin cancers to arise on sun-exposed surfaces, the high rates among outdoor workers, the inverse correlation between skin cancer incidence and distance from the equator, the predisposition of light-skinned and especially fair-complexioned populations who sunburn easily, the resistance of dark-skinned populations with protective melanin pigment, the exceptional risks of skin cancer among persons with genetic diseases exacerbated by sunlight (e.g., xeroderma pigmentosum, albinism), and the capacity of UV radiation in repeated doses to induce skin cancer in experimental animals.

IONIZING RADIATION. Although ionizing radiation probably accounts for less than 3 per cent of all cancer, it appears that virtually no site of the body is spared from its carcinogenic effects. It is difficult to measure directly the effects of low doses of sparsely ionizing radiation, such as x- or gamma rays, but extrapolations are possible by studying populations who have been exposed to high and moderate doses for medical, occupational, or military reasons. In general, the breast, thyroid, and bone marrow are the most radiosensitive organs. Radiogenic leukemia shows a wave-like pattern with the excess risks starting about two to four years after exposure, peaking at six to eight years, and declining to normal within 25 years. In contrast, radiogenic carcinomas have a minimal latent period of five years and a temporal distribution that resembles the natural incidence curve, suggesting that age-dependent factors influence tumor expression. Surveys of medically irradiated populations have revealed an excess risk of leukemia and other cancers among patients treated for ankylosing spondylitis, benign gynecologic diseases, and various neoplasms; breast cancer among women treated for postpartum mastitis or who received fluoroscopies to monitor pneumothorax treatment of tuberculosis; thyroid cancer among children treated for thymus enlargement, benign head and neck disease, or tinea capitis; leukemia and other childhood cancers following prenatal x-rays; and various cancers following use of radioactive compounds (osteosarcoma with radium-224, leukemia with phosphorus-32, and leukemia and liver angiosarcoma with Thorotrast).

OCCUPATIONAL HAZARDS. Occupational exposures are usually reported to account for less than 5 per cent of all cancer in men, but the percentage is higher for certain tumors, such as the bladder. Most occupational carcinogens have been first detected through clinical and epidemiologic observations with subsequent confirmation by laboratory studies. However, inorganic arsenic has not been shown to be carcinogenic in laboratory animals. In the case of mustard gas and vinyl chloride, the risks were detected in humans after the substances had been shown to induce tumors in laboratory animals, although little attention was given to the experimental studies when first reported. The effects of some agents, particularly asbestos and radon, are greatly potentiated by cigarette smoking, so that programs to reduce either the workplace exposure or smoking would significantly lower but not eliminate the occupational risk. A number of manufacturing industries (e.g., furniture, leather, rubber) are associated with cancer risk, although the specific carcinogens have not been identified. Industrial hazards and their detection have important implications beyond the work force, since most agents are not confined to the plant but ultimately become part of the general environment to which large segments of the population may be inadvertently exposed.

ENVIRONMENTAL POLLUTION. Pollutants in the urban air have long been suspected in the etiology of lung cancer, with fossil fuel combustion products, especially polycyclic hydrocarbons, being of special concern. In several studies the rates for lung cancer have shown correlations with measurement of benzo(*a*)pyrene in the ambient air, yet the available evidence suggests that the urban excess of lung cancer is mainly due to cigarette smoking and partly to occupational exposures. In the large-scale survey of the American Cancer Society, age- and smoking-standardized rates for lung cancer were computed among men not occupationally exposed to dust, fumes, or vapors. No major differences in mortality were seen between urban and rural areas, or between cities characterized by indices of pollution. Another approach has been to extrapolate from studies of workers heavily exposed to hydrocarbons, with the results suggesting only small effects from urban air pollutants. In some studies the effects of smoking a particular amount were greater in urban than rural areas, suggesting that tobacco smoke may interact with carcinogens in the ambient atmosphere.

Asbestos bodies and calcified pleural plaques have been reported in large segments of the urban population, but the carcinogenic effects following nonoccupational exposures are uncertain. It is clear, however, that mesotheliomas may result from neighborhood exposures to asbestos industries and from household contact with asbestos dust, particularly through laundering of work clothing. Another hazard may result from airborne levels of arsenic, since high mortality rates for lung cancer have been reported among male and female residents in communities with arsenic-emitting smelters.

Recent interest has centered on contaminants in drinking water, since several halogenated organic compounds produced during chlorination are carcinogenic and mutagenic in laboratory tests. Levels of these compounds in drinking water have shown correlations with the rates for cancers of the bladder, colon, and rectum in the same area.

MEDICATIONS. Several carcinogens have been detected by studies of patients exposed to medicinal agents. Some drugs have been withdrawn from clinical practice, while others are retained since risk-benefit considerations may warrant their use in certain conditions. A major impetus to research in this area was the discovery in 1971 that synthetic estrogens given during pregnancy produced adenocarcinomas of the vagina and cervix several years later in daughters exposed in utero. This was the first demonstration of transplacental carcinogenesis in humans. A series of studies then firmly linked endometrial cancer to the use of conjugated estrogens for menopausal symptoms. Oral contraceptives have been related to benign liver tumors, to endometrial cancer among users of the sequential type of contraceptives, and possibly to breast cancer among some high-risk women (e.g., with benign breast disease or familial predisposition).

An excess risk of acute nonlymphocytic leukemia, and perhaps other cancers, has been seen among patients receiving certain alkylating agents. These risks may be acceptable when treating conditions with a poor prognosis such as metastatic cancer, but for conditions with a favorable long-term prognosis the benefits of treatments should be carefully weighed against the risks. These drugs may exert their action in part by breaking chromosomes, since other leukemogens (radiation, benzene) have a similar effect.

Immunosuppressive agents have been assessed primarily by studies of renal transplant recipients, most of whom have had azathioprine and corticosteroids. The risk of histiocytic lymphoma is very high, and first appears within months of transplantation. This explosive onset has suggested that a latent oncogenic virus may be activated by immunologic mechanisms. For all other cancers combined, the excess risk is about twofold and first becomes evident about two years after transplantation. It has not affected all forms of cancer, as might be predicted by the hypothesis of "immunologic surveillance," but increased risks have been noted for cancers of the liver, biliary system, and bladder, and for soft-tissue sarcomas, adenocarcinoma of the lung, squamous carcinoma of the skin, and malignant melanoma. Recently, other groups of patients receiving immunosuppressants have shown an excess of lymphomas, squamous carcinoma of the skin, and soft-tissue sarcomas, but at lower rates than those seen in transplant patients. It is noteworthy that the predominance of lymphomas with drug-induced immunosuppression is seen also among patients with primary immunodeficiency syndromes.

INFECTIOUS AGENTS. Viruses have not been causally tied to the origins of any human cancer, although several candidate agents are under active study. The epidemiologic patterns of cervical cancer have long suggested venereal transmission of an infectious agent, with herpes simplex virus type 2 being a chief suspect. The Epstein-Barr virus (EBV) is linked to nasopharyngeal cancer and Burkitt's lymphoma, particularly in areas of the world where these tumors are highly prevalent. Hepatitis B infection is related to hepatocellular carcinoma, especially in endemic regions of Africa and Asia. Outbreaks of adult T cell leukemia in certain areas, especially in Japan and the Caribbean, have been linked to infection with the human T cell leukemia virus (HTLV). This newly discovered retrovirus has been isolated also from some patients with Kaposi's sarcoma and opportunistic infections associated with the acquired immune deficiency syndrome (AIDS), which has clustered since 1981 among male homosexuals, illicit-drug users, hemophiliacs, and Haitian immigrants to the United States. In addition, a viral origin for Hodgkin's disease has been suggested by the association with childhood environments, such as small family size, that tend to reduce or delay early life exposures to infections in a manner resembling the pattern for paralytic poliomyelitis. EBV may be involved, since an increased risk of Hodgkin's disease has been reported among persons with infectious mononucleosis.

If viruses are oncogenic in humans, it seems likely that predisposing factors are operating. Thus, EBV may interact with certain histocompatibility antigens to produce the high rate of nasopharyngeal cancer in Chinese populations, with persistent malarial infections to induce African Burkitt's lymphoma, or with a genetic immunodeficiency trait to cause family clusters of lymphoma. Hepatitis B infection may combine with dietary aflatoxin to produce liver cancer in endemic regions. In animal models the production of immunodeficiency enhances viral carcinogenesis, so that the narrow range of tumors complicating immunodeficiency states of humans suggests that viruses play only a limited role in human cancer.

Parasitic infections affect the risk of cancer in certain areas of the world. In Africa and Papua New Guinea, the geographic patterns of malaria and Burkitt's lymphoma are closely correlated; in the Middle East and north Africa schistosomiasis produces squamous carcinoma of the bladder; and in Asia infestation with liver flukes (clonorchiasis and opisthorciasis) predisposes to cholangiocarcinoma.

NUTRITION. International correlations and migrant studies have suggested that certain features of the affluent Western diet contribute to a sizable proportion of all cancers. Various nutritional hypotheses are under study, although the mechanisms appear complex and difficult to unravel. For example, high dietary fat may affect the risk of colonic cancer by increasing the concentration of bile acids in the bowel, which are then metabolized by bacterial flora into carcinogens or co-carcino-

TABLE 170–2. HEREDITARY NEOPLASMS

	Inheritance*	Features
Retinoblastoma	AD	Susceptibility to second primary tumors, including osteosarcoma of leg and radiogenic sarcoma of orbit; chromosome deletion (13q 13 −) in some cases
Nevoid basal cell carcinoma syndrome	AD	Basal cell cancers of skin increased by UV and ionizing radiation; medulloblastoma, ovarian fibromas, and developmental defects in some cases
Multiple endocrine neoplasia I (Wermer's syndrome)	AD	Adenomas of anterior pituitary, parathyroid, pancreatic islet cells, thyroid, and adrenal cortex; carcinoid tumors of intestine and bronchus in some cases
Multiple endocrine neoplasia II (Sipple's syndrome)	AD	Pheochromocytoma and medullary thyroid carcinoma; parathyroid tumors and neurofibromas in some cases
Chemodectomas	AD	Paragangliomas from chemoreceptor system
Polyposis coli	AD	Multiple adenomatous polyps and adenocarcinomas of large bowel; some families feature osteomas, fibromas, lipomas, and epidermal cysts (Gardner's syndrome)
Tylosis with esophageal carcinoma	AD	Squamous cell carcinoma of esophagus with keratoses of palms and soles
Dyplasic nevus syndrome	AD	Hereditary melanomas derived from nevi, especially after sun exposure

*AD = autosomal dominant.

gens, and it may promote the development of breast cancer by increasing estrogen production and prolactin release. Dietary fat and caloric excess may also contribute to endometrial cancer and the associated manifestations of obesity, diabetes, and hypertension.

It appears also that a low intake of certain food classes may predispose to cancer. In several studies, the risk of colonic cancer has been inversely related to the consumption of fiber, which may protect against intestinal carcinogens or precursors by dilutional or other effects. Micronutrients and trace metals may also have a protective influence, since cancers of the lung and other sites have been associated with a low intake of vitamin A, carotene, and selenium. The risk of stomach cancer has been related to a deficiency of fruits and vegetables containing vitamin C, which may act by inhibiting the formation of carcinogenic nitrosamines in the stomach. In one study of colonic cancer, patients ingested smaller than usual amounts of cruciferous vegetables (e.g., cabbage, Brussels sprouts, cauliflower), containing indole compounds, which can inhibit carcinogenesis in laboratory animals. In a study of esophageal cancer, the high rate among black males was attributed to heavy alcohol consumption and generalized poor nutrition.

A variety of other dietary factors, including additives and contaminants, have fallen under suspicion. The consumption of aflatoxin, a carcinogenic metabolite of the fungus *Aspergillus flavus,* correlates closely with the distribution of liver cancer in Africa. Coffee intake has been associated with bladder and pancreatic cancers in some studies, but causal relationships have not been established. The artificial sweeteners saccharin and cyclamate are weak bladder carcinogens or co-carcinogens in laboratory animals, but a recent large-scale study of bladder cancer indicated that the risk in humans is very small if present

TABLE 170–3. HEREDITARY PRENEOPLASTIC SYNDROMES

	Inheritance*	Neoplasms
Phacomatoses		
Neurofibromatosis	AD	Sarcomatous change in 10% of cases; gliomas of brain and optic nerve, acoustic neuromas, meningiomas, and acute leukemia
Tuberous sclerosis	AD	Hamartomatous growths in several organs; brain tumors, chiefly giant-cell astrocytoma, in 1–3% of patients
von Hippel-Lindau syndrome	AD	Angiomatosis of retina and cerebellum; renal adenocarcinoma, pheochromocytoma, and ependymoma in some cases
Multiple exostoses (diaphyseal aclasis)	AD	Chondrosarcoma in 5–11% of patients
Peutz-Jeghers syndrome	AD	Rare malignant change in hamartomatous polyps of gastrointestinal tract; ovarian neoplasms in 5% of female patients
Cowden's multiple hamartoma syndrome	AD	Oral papillomas, cystic mastopathy and breast cancer, thyroid and colonic neoplasms
Genodermatoses		
Xeroderma pigmentosum	AR	Various skin cancers in all patients exposed to sunlight; defective cellular repair of DNA damage induced by UV light
Albinism	AR	Skin cancers, chiefly squamous, in sun-exposed areas
Epidermodysplasia verruciformis	AR	Skin cancers, chiefly squamous, in multiple warts induced by papillomavirus
Polydysplastic epidermolysis bullosa	AR	Skin cancers, chiefly squamous, in scars
Dyskeratosis congenita	AR	Squamous carcinomas of skin and mucous membranes; features of Fanconi's anemia in several cases
Werner's syndrome (adult progeria)	AR	Soft tissue sarcoma, other tumors
Chromosome instability		
Bloom's syndrome	AR	Acute leukemia, lymphoma, other cancers
Fanconi's anemia	AR	Acute myelomonocytic leukemia and squamous carcinoma of mucous membranes; hepatoma reported after androgen-anabolic steroids
Immune deficiency		
Ataxia telangiectasia	AR	Lymphoma, lymphocytic leukemia, stomach cancer, other tumors; chromosome fragility and ineffective DNA repair reported; heterozygous carriers prone to leukemia, lymphoma, and carcinomas of biliary tract, stomach and ovary
Common variable immunodeficiency	?AR	Lymphoma, stomach cancer
Wiskott-Aldrich syndrome	XR	Lymphoma, acute leukemia
X-linked (Bruton's) agammaglobulinemia	XR	Lymphoma, acute leukemia
X-linked lymphoproliferative syndrome	XR	Abnormal response to infection by Epstein-Barr virus, resulting in severe infectious mononucleosis, immunoblastic sarcoma, B cell lymphoma, or plasmacytoma

*AD = autosomal dominant; AR = autosomal recessive; XR = X-linked recessive.

at all. Cooking practices may release hydrocarbons or other carcinogens in food, although no epidemiologic observations are available.

GENETIC SUSCEPTIBILITY. Compared to environmental factors in cancer, genetic determinants are less conspicuous and more difficult to identify by clinical and epidemiologic means. Although the racial and ethnic differentials for most cancers appear largely modulated by environmental influences, genetic factors appear to contribute to some high rates (e.g., nasopharyngeal cancer among Chinese and gallbladder cancer among American Indians and certain Hispanic groups) and some low rates (e.g., testicular cancer and Ewing's sarcoma among blacks in Africa and the United States). Genetic susceptibility is most evident for skin cancer, since ethnic variations correspond to the degree of protective skin pigmentation.

Although only a small percentage of cancer is inherited in a mendelian fashion, over 200 single-gene disorders have been linked to neoplasia. Table 170–2 lists some cancers that occur as an inherited trait (hereditary neoplasms), and Table 170–3 presents those arising as a complication of inherited precursor lesions (preneoplastic states). In some syndromes environmental factors contribute to the development of cancer. Neoplasms of a hereditary nature tend to occur earlier in life than do nonfamilial occurrences of the same tumor, and usually arise from multiple foci within the affected organ.

In contrast to the hereditary syndromes, the common human cancers show small familial risks, on the order of two- to threefold. However, the familial risks for breast and colonic cancers are as high as 20- to 30-fold among subgroups of patients with early onset and bilateral or multifocal origin. Familial susceptibility also appears to enhance the effects of environmental exposures, such as smoking in lung cancer, and sunlight exposure in melanomas derived from dysplastic nevi. In some families there are remarkable aggregations of cancer consistent with an autosomal dominant mode of inheritance. These "cancer families" may display either a single type of cancer or a constellation of multiple cancers, especially adenocarcinomas of the colon and endometrium, or the breast and ovary. Other families are prone to diverse cell types of childhood and adult cancers, particularly soft-tissue and bone sarcomas, breast carcinoma, brain tumors, adrenocortical neoplasms, and leukemia. The delineation of genetic and familial syndromes is helpful in applying laboratory probes to clarify the heritable component of carcinogenesis, and in targeting screening and prevention programs designed to protect high risk individuals.

Doll R: The epidemiology of cancer. Cancer 45:2475, 1980. *A clear, succinct presentation of the methodologic approaches and current state of knowledge in cancer epidemiology.*

Doll R, Peto R: The causes of cancer: Quantitative estimates of avoidable risks of cancer in the United States today. J Natl Cancer Inst 66:1191, 1981. *A critical review of carcinogenic hazards with emphasis on quantitative risk assessment and the preventable nature of most forms of cancer.*

Schottenfeld D, Fraumeni JF Jr (eds.): Cancer Epidemiology and Prevention. Philadelphia, W. B. Saunders Company, 1982. *A detailed and current survey of cancer epidemiology, with 70 chapters covering virtually all aspects of the field. The contribution of epidemiology to the development and evaluation of preventive measures is emphasized.*

171. BIOLOGIC EFFECTS OF TUMORS

Philip S. Schein

The symptoms produced by cancer are commonly viewed as manifestations of direct or metastatic involvement of an organ or of specific neural and vascular structures. Tumors can also produce important nonmetastatic alterations of the metabolism and function of virtually all body systems (Table 171–1). These systemic effects of cancer, or "paraneoplastic syndromes," may be entirely unrelated to the normal physiologic activities of the mature tissue from which the tumor originated. Importantly, paraneoplastic syndromes may cause greater morbidity than the actual physical presence of the malignant mass. Even small tumors can produce devastating remote effects.

Approximately 75 per cent of patients with cancer will develop at least one paraneoplastic syndrome during the course of their illness, not infrequently as the first symptom or sign of an occult malignancy. The putative biochemical and immunologic mediators of these syndromes, in most instances, remain to be identified. The isolation and characterization of these tumor products might allow for a better understanding of the processes of ontogeny and cellular differentiation, as well as providing a means for earlier detection of cancer.

TABLE 171–1. PARANEOPLASTIC SYNDROMES

1. Cachexia of malignancy—wasting of the host
2. Cutaneous manifestations of malignancy (see Table 175–1)
3. Neuromyopathies (see Table 174–1)
   - Dementia
   - Cerebellar degeneration
   - Sensorimotor neuropathy
   - Dermatomyositis
   - Myasthenic syndrome (Eaton-Lambert syndrome)
   - Subacute sensory neuropathy
   - Polyneuritis
   - Autonomic neuropathy
   - Polymyositis
4. Ectopic hormone production (see Table 173–1)
   - ACTH
   - PTH
   - Erythropoietin
   - Growth hormone
   - Chorionic gonadotropin
   - Hypoglycemia-producing factors
   - Vasopressin (ADH)
   - Calcitonin
5. Tumor markers
6. Hypertrophic osteoarthropathy
7. Hematologic-hemostatic abnormalities
   - Anemia—simple, microangiopathic, or autoimmune hemolytic
   - Erythrocytosis (erythropoietin secretion)
   - Leukemoid reactions, eosinophilia, thrombocytosis
   - Disseminated intravascular coagulation (DIC)
   - Migratory thrombophlebitis (Trousseau's syndrome)
   - Nonbacterial thrombotic ("marantic") endocarditis
   - Thrombotic thrombocytopenic purpura syndrome (TTP)
8. Renal manifestations
   - Nephrotic syndrome
   - Renal disease secondary to hyperuricemia, hypercalcemia, amyloid, or paraproteins
9. Fever (see Ch. 255)

This chapter will consider the association of malignancy with wasting of the host, hematologic abnormalities, and renal manifestations. The other syndromes listed in the table and the secretion of tumor markers unassociated with clinical syndromes are discussed in other chapters of Part XIV.

ANOREXIA AND CACHEXIA. A profound state of malnutrition and wasting is a frequent and important systemic effect of cancer. Anorexia and weight loss may present as the first manifestation of cancer, often grossly out of proportion to the tumor burden. Anorexia is often compounded by a decreased acuity or by a perverted sense of taste and smell with an acquired abhorrence of specific foods. The principal example is an aversion to meat, a phenomenon which has been correlated with a lowered taste threshold for urea. In other patients a hypercatabolic state results from rapid tumor growth or infection. Malabsorption may be a consequence of tumor involvement or surgical resection of specific regions of the gastrointestinal tract. Radiation therapy to the head and neck region may produce a loss of taste and salivation, whereas irradiation of the abdomen may result in endarteritis, fibrosis, or ulceration of the bowel with the loss of motility and absorptive function. Chemotherapy often induces anorexia, nausea, and vomiting.

In many cases, however, a specific etiology for the wasting is not found, and the patient is said to exhibit the syndrome of *"cachexia of malignancy."* This poorly understood manifestation of cancer has been correlated with several important alterations in metabolism: (1) a resistance to endogenous and exogenous insulin, while insulin receptors on monocytes remain normal; (2) an increased oxidation of free fatty acids, whereas utilization of glucose as a metabolic fuel is reduced; and (3) an increase in Cori cycle activity. The last-named phenomenon, with the attendant enhanced gluconeogenesis from amino acids and lactate, results in an increased and inappropriate expenditure of high energy phosphates (ATP), which may contribute to the wasting state. Successful treatment of the underlying tumor may produce a complete reversal of the cachexia syndrome, suggesting that the neoplasm had elaborated an as yet unidentified metabolic toxin. Nutritional management is essential to sustain the patient until such time as anticancer treatment has controlled the underlying malignancy.

HEMATOLOGIC COMPLICATIONS. *Anemia* is found in more than 50 per cent of patients with advanced cancer. The mechanism is often multifactorial and attributed to chronic disease, blood loss, bone marrow involvement by tumor, or suppression of erythropoiesis by chemotherapy. *Autoimmune hemolytic anemia* is found in association with chronic lymphocyte leukemia and lymphomas, as well as with ovarian carcinoma. *Microangiopathic hemolytic anemia* is a rare complication of gastric or breast cancer (see Ch. 138). Hemolysis in such cases is usually abrupt in onset and often severe. In many patients there is an associated thrombocytopenia or laboratory evidence of *disseminated intravascular coagulation (DIC)*. The mechanism for carcinomatosis-associated microangiopathic hemolytic anemia remains to be fully determined. It had been assumed that erthrocyte fragmentation resulted from shearing on fibrin strands produced by intravascular coagulation. Many cases of this syndrome, however, have not exhibited the clinical and laboratory evidence of DIC or have been found to have only a few fibrin thrombi noted at postmortem examination. An alternative explanation is red blood cell shearing secondary to direct contact with intraluminal embolic tumor cells.

Erythrocytosis in patients with kidney tumors, hepatoma, or cerebellar hemangioblastoma may result from an inappropriate production of erythropoietin. *Leukemoid reactions* occur in patients with carcinomas of the lung, stomach, and pancreas; hepatoma and lymphomas; neutrophilia postulated to be due to marrow stimulation by metastases within it, tumor necrosis, or tumor elaboration of a granulopoietic factor. Eosinophilia is largely confined to lymphomas, especially Hodgkin's disease, whereas thrombocytosis is an occasional manifestation of renal cell carcinoma or disseminated gastrointestinal neoplasms.

DIC in a patient with a malignancy may have many possible causes such as sepsis and hemolytic transfusion reactions. This syndrome may also result from the release of thromboplastins from malignant cells, as is the case in acute promyelocytic leukemia. Mucus from mucin-producing adenocarcinomas can initiate coagulation by the nonenzymatic activation of factor X to X_a, and a glycoprotein has been isolated which induces intravascular coagulation when infused into rabbits. Cancer-associated DIC may be chronic and mild or acute and fulminant. The treatment of DIC is discussed in Ch. 167. In patients with myeloma and Waldenström's macroglobulinemia, a paraprotein may interfere with coagulation proteins or induce abnormalities of platelet function.

Malignant tumors may be associated with a state of hypercoagulability, which often antedates the discovery of the underlying disease by many months. A clinical picture of either *superficial migratory thrombophlebitis (Trousseau's syndrome)* or *deep vein thrombosis* may ensue with an unusual distribution which may include the upper extremities as well as the intra-abdominal, cerebral, jugular, corpora caverosa, and chest wall veins. Pulmonary embolization has occurred in as many as half of the patients. Carcinoma of the pancreas and of the lung are the two most frequently reported neoplasms that produce this syndrome. Treatment consists of effective management of the underlying cancer as well as the initiation of heparin or streptokinase, since the condition is frequently resistant to oral forms of anticoagulation. Mucin-producing adenocarcinomas may be associated with the development of *nonbacterial thrombotic endocarditis* (marantic endocarditis) with vegetations on the mitral and/or aortic heart valves. The syndrome usually presents with embolic disease to the brain, to the coronary arteries with myocardial infarction, or to the spleen and kidneys.

A syndrome with the clinical features of *thrombotic thrombocytopenic purpura (TTP)* or hemolytic uremia has been recognized in patients with gastric cancer. The patients are frequently in remission following effective treatment with mitomycin-C based chemotherapy when microangiopathic hemolytic anemia, symptomatic thrombocytopenia, and abnormalities of renal function abruptly begin. There is no evidence of disseminated intravascular coagulation, but an increased concentration of circulating immune complexes has been found. Treatment has been empirical, but cases involving circulating immune complexes have been successfully managed with plasmapheresis, inhibitors of platelet aggregation, and immunosuppressive therapy.

RENAL MANIFESTATIONS. Deterioration of kidney function in association with cancer may result from many causes, including direct infiltration by lymphoma and leukemia, obstruction of the ureters, hyperuricemia, hypercalcemia, or the deposition of paraprotein or amyloid.

Nephrotic syndrome in association with carcinoma has been correlated with the development of a membranous glomerulopathy. There is deposition of immunoglobulins and complement along the glomerulocapillary loop, and electron microscopy demonstrates immune deposits along the subepithelial side of the glomerular basement membrane. Carcinoma-related glomerulopathy may be the result of tumor or oncofetal antigen-antibody complexes as a manifestation of the presence of tumor antigens recognized as foreign by the host's immune system. The prognosis of patients with carcinoma-related nephrotic syndrome is grave. The reported median survival of three months has been attributed to both the advanced stage of the tumor and the renal complications.

Nephrotic syndrome occurring as a consequence of Hodgkin's disease presents with several distinguishing characteristics: (1) the syndrome is early in onset, occurring several months before or after the diagnosis of the lymphoma; (2) in most cases the syndrome results from minimal change glomerulopathy, although membranous and proliferative glomerulonephritides have also been described; (3) the attainment of a tumor response with chemotherapy or radiation therapy almost uniformly causes a remission of the nephrotic syndrome, whereas proteinuria may return during periods of reactivation of Hodgkin's disease. The pathogenesis of nephrotic syndrome with this lymphoma remains speculative.

Antman KH, Skarin AT, Mayer RJ, Hargraves HK, Canellos GP: Microangiopathic hemolytic anemia and cancer: A review. Medicine 58:377, 1979. *A fully documented presentation of this syndrome with a critical discussion of the past concepts of pathogenesis.*

Brennan MF: Total parenteral nutrition in the cancer patient. N Engl J Med 305:375, 1981. *A comprehensive analysis of the rationale and indications for intensive nutritional supportive care in the management of patients with cancer.*

Eagen JW, Lewis EJ: Glomerulopathies of neoplasia. Kidney Int 11:297, 1977. *A lucid discussion of the distinguishing forms of nephrotic syndrome found in association with carcinoma and lymphoma.*

Kressel BR, Ryan KP, Duong ATT, Berenberg J, Schein PS: Microangiopathic hemolytic anemia, thrombocytopenia and renal failure in patients treated for adenocarcinoma. Cancer 48:1738, 1981. *A comprehensive review of the clinical and pathologic features of a syndrome resembling thrombotic thrombocytopenic purpura in patients with successfully treated adenocarcinoma. This syndrome may become very important as treatment for gastric carcinoma becomes more effective.*

Macdonald JS, Schein PS: Mechanisms and management of malnutrition states in patients with cancer. Clin Gastroenterol 5:809, 1976. *This fully referenced chapter serves as a general guide to the many factors that contribute to the state of malnutrition associated with cancer. The nutritional complications resulting from cancer treatment are reviewed.*

Pascal RR: Renal manifestations of extrarenal neoplasms. Hum Pathol 11:7, 1980. *A review of the spectrum of paraneoplastic phenomenon that influences renal function.*

Sack G, Levin J, Bell W: Trousseau's syndrome and other manifestations of chronic disseminated coagulopathy in patients with neoplasms. Medicine 56:1, 1977. Rickles FR, Edwards RL: Activation of blood coagulation in cancer: Trousseau's syndrome revisted. Blood 62:14, 1983. *Authoritative review of the interrelated syndromes of hypercoagulation found in association with adenocarcinomas.*

Schein PS, Kisner DL, Haller DG, Blecher M, Hamosh M: Cachexia of malignancy: Potential role of insulin in nutritional management. Cancer 43:2070, 1979. *The phenomenon of selective resistance of glucose mobilization to endogenous and exogenous insulin is presented, and the probable importance of this phenomenon is reviewed.*

172. TUMOR MARKERS

Philip S. Schein

INTRODUCTION. The physical examination and standard diagnostic radiologic procedures have serious limitations in the early detection and localization of small tumor masses. A neoplasm of 1 cubic centimeter, a realistic limit of clinical screening, has already completed approximately 30 doublings or two thirds of its growth. It contains 1 billion cancer cells, and viable cells are likely to have been shed into the bloodstream or lymphatic system. Despite an "early" diagnosis and surgical removal, the patient may have many undetected microscopic metastases. In patients with advanced stages of disease, particularly with intra-abdominal malignancy, it is often difficult to assess disease progression and response to treatment.

Research has therefore been directed toward the identification of tumor-specific products in body fluids that might have three potential applications in clinical practice: (1) early diagnosis of malignancy, (2) the pre- or postoperative assessment of prognosis, and (3) a chemical assay of changing tumor cell burden. An ideal tumor marker not only should signal the presence of microscopic tumor but also should define the site and morphologic type of the malignancy. Unfortunately, the available markers have not attained such a high degree of sensitivity and specificity. The problem of sensitivity has been addressed by the use of radioimmunoassays that can measure nanogram quantities of antigen. The problem of specificity has been more difficult to resolve. The use of normally occurring hormones, enzymes, proteins, or oncofetal antigens requires that the blood concentration of these materials be present in excess of the established normal range. Attention has more recently been directed toward the placental hormones, which are not normally found in the blood of adult males and nonpregnant females.

ONCOFETAL ANTIGENS. Oncofetal antigens are products of genes that are expressed during differentiation of fetal tissue, but that are partially or completely repressed in adult life. With a state of dedifferentiation there may be a reactivation of dormant genomes and consequently a reappearance of embryonic antigens as an index of neoplastic transformation.

Carcinoembryonic antigen (CEA) was first described as a specific antigen for adenocarcinoma of the colon and for the digestive organs of the two- to six-month human fetus. A glycoprotein with a molecular weight of 200,000 daltons, CEA is secreted into the glycocalyx surface of gastrointestinal cells. More recently CEA-like material, measured by radioimmunoassay, has been detected in normal adult colonic mucosae, secretions, and feces, and in the normal secretion of the pancreaticobiliary system. With invasion of the subepithelial tissues by a malignancy there is a disintegration of the basement membrane. The neoplastic glycocalyx is then absorbed into vascular and lymphatic channels. Radioimmunoassays of CEA allow for the quantitative measurement of plasma concentrations less than 1.0 ng per milliliter; CEA levels above 2.5 ng per milliliter are considered abnormal in healthy nonsmoking subjects.

Abnormal serum CEA levels occur in a wide range of malignancies, particularly the entodermally derived tumors of the gastrointestinal tract and lung, and in association with several nonmalignant conditions, including alcoholic cirrhosis and pancreatitis, inflammatory bowel disease, and rectal polyps, as well as cigarette smoking. There is no clear threshold difference in CEA concentration in patients with malignant versus nonmalignant disease, but elevations are rare in normal persons and when observed are relatively modest (<20 ng per milliliter). Patients with early stages of colonic cancer may also have a normal plasma CEA concentration. Because of this overall lack of specificity and sensitivity, the CEA should not be regarded as a diagnostic test for cancer. Plasma concentrations of CEA in excess of 2.5 ng per milliliter have been reported in 60 to 95 per cent of patients with colonic cancer, largely dependent upon three factors: (1) the extent of disease: patients with tumor confined to the wall of the colon have an abnormal plasma value in 20 to 40 per cent of cases, compared to 85 to 95 per cent with advanced metastatic disease; (2) the differentiation of the tumor: anaplastic lesions have a lower incidence of positive CEA; and (3) the presence or absence of liver metastases: the onset of hepatic involvement with tumor is frequently associated with a marked elevation of CEA. Elevations of plasma CEA have also been associated with advanced stages of pancreatic cancer (90 per cent), gastric cancer (60 per cent), lung cancer (75 per cent), breast cancer (50 per cent), and malignancies of many other organs.

^{131}I-labeled anti-CEA antibody is now being evaluated as a means of *in vivo* immunodetection and radioimmunologic localization of colon carcinoma. In initial studies, 83 per cent of primary colorectal cancers were demonstrated preoperatively, as well as 90 per cent of metastatic tumors. The false-positive rate was less than 4 per cent and sites of tumor were identified that were not detected by other clinical methods in 20 per cent of patients.

The principal clinical use of plasma CEA is as a monitor of disease progression and response to treatment. Following the complete resection of a tumor, an elevated preoperative CEA should return to a normal concentration by one month following surgery. A persistent elevation or increasing concentration on serial testing is strongly correlated with residual or metastatic tumor. In patients with documented tumor recurrence, a rising CEA may occur months prior to clinical detection of relapse.

Several clinical trials are evaluating the use of a rising CEA as an indication for re-exploration, to identify an early tumor relapse. In early analyses, a local resectable recurrence has been found in only 30 per cent of patients, and the impact of such salvage procedures on survival remains to be determined.

Alpha-fetoprotein (AFP), a 70,000 molecular weight protein with an alpha electrophoretic mobility, is synthesized by the liver, yolk sac, and gastrointestinal tract of the human fetus. The peak AFP concentration occurs during the twelfth to fifteenth weeks of gestation, following which it declines to reach the normal adult level (less than 40 ng per milliliter) by the sixth to twelfth month following birth.

Abnormal serum levels of AFP have been reported in 30 to 95 per cent of patients with hepatocellular carcinoma. The wide range is partly explained by differences in the sensitivity of the assay systems employed and the patient population studied. A higher incidence of positive AFP has been reported for patients from regions in which hepatoma is endemic, such as the Bantu of South Africa. With the current use of radioimmunoassay, 70 to 95 per cent of all cases have a level in excess of 50 ng per milliliter. Elevated serum AFP is also found in association with teratocarcinomas (75 per cent) and embryonal cell carcinoma of testis, ovary, and extragonadal sites. In contrast, patients with seminomas, or the corresponding dysgerminomas of the female, have normal blood levels. Abnormal levels of AFP have been reported with pancreatic cancer, gastric cancer, and colonic or lung cancer.

Like CEA, the AFP is not a specific marker for malignancy. The measurement of amniotic fluid AFP is used for the early diagnosis of fetal neural tube defects such as anencephaly and spina bifida. During pregnancy, AFP produced by the fetus crosses the placenta, resulting in an increased maternal concentration. Virtually all patients with ataxia telangiectasia have elevated AFP levels. The principal source of "false-positive" elevations of AFP has been benign forms of liver disease. In large series, 15 to 75 per cent of patients with cirrhosis and alcoholic hepatitis have demonstrated abnormal serum levels. Viral hepatitis is also accompanied by a transient elevation in AFP in 30 to 60 per cent of cases.

The serum concentration of AFP in benign disease is usually less than 500 ng per milliliter, whereas the majority of patients with hepatoma have levels greatly in excess of this value. Nevertheless, the AFP should not be considered a diagnostic test for cancer. The principal clinical application is a monitor for the effectiveness of surgical and chemotherapeutic management of hepatoma and germ cell neoplasms.

Pancreatic oncofetal antigen (POA) is a glycoprotein found in fetal pancreas and pancreatic cancer tissue, but not in the normal adult pancreas. This substance has now been detected in serum of normal adults, and in elevated concentration in some patients with lung, gastric, colonic, and breast cancer. However, the highest absolute levels and greatest frequency of abnormality have been found for patients with pancreatic cancer, particularly those with well differentiated tumors. There appears to be no concordance between the POA and CEA.

PLACENTAL PROTEINS. *Human chorionic gonadotropin (hCG)*, a glycoprotein hormone that is normally secreted by the trophoblastic epithelium of the placenta, is composed of dissimilar alpha and beta subunits. The alpha subunit shares similarities in primary structure with the comparable alpha subunit of human luteinizing hormone (hLH), whereas there are major differences in their respective beta subunits. Sensitive radioimmunoassays have been developed that utilize antisera produced to the beta subunit, hCG-B, which allow for discrimination between hCG and hLH. hCG can be measured in both fetal and maternal serum during pregnancy and in the immediate postpartum period; however, the presence of hCG in the plasma of a male or nonpregnant female is indicative of underlying neoplasm.

Until recently the principal clinical application of hCG measurements has been for the diagnosis and management of trophoblastic tumors. It enables the chemotherapist to assay chemically for the presence of retained trophoblastic or neoplastic cells, and also furnishes a sensitive guide for follow-up of treated cases. hCG may also be secreted by germ cell neoplasms of the testes or ovary, or by extragonadal sites such as the mediastinum or retroperitoneum and be present in the plasma of 50 to 60 per cent of patients with embryonal and teratocarcinoma of the testis, 40 per cent of patients with seminoma, and virtually all patients with testicular choriocarcinoma. Detectable hCG has also been demonstrated in the plasma of patients with adenocarcinoma of the ovary (42 per cent), pancreatic cancer (33 per cent), gastric cancer (22 per cent), and hepatomas (17 per cent).

Human placental lactogen (hPL) is normally found in the serum of pregnant women. Post partum, hPL rapidly disappears and is essentially undetectable within 48 hours. This hormone is secreted by the majority of trophoblastic neoplasms and has been demonstrated in a small percentage of patients with hepatoma, leukemia and lymphomas, endocrine tumors, and lung cancer.

Placental alkaline phosphatase (PAP), or Regan isoenzyme, is synthesized in the trophoblast, where it is located on the macrovilli membranes of the plasma membrane. It is readily distinguished from other isoenzymes of alkaline phosphatase by its heat stability, electrophoretic mobility, and immunochemical specificity. Elevated PAP activity is present in the serum of 5 to 15 per cent of patients with cancer of the female reproductive organs, breast, and lung.

ECTOPIC POLYPEPTIDES. Many tumors produce augmented quantities of hormones or proteins that are normally secreted by the cell origin. Examples include the hypersecretion of insulin and gastrin by islet cell tumors, the M spike of multiple myeloma, and the elevated serum acid phosphatase activity associated with metastatic cancer of the prostate. The abnormal plasma concentration of these markers must be distinguished from the phenomenon of ectopic secretion.

The concept of ectopic secretion has rested upon the basic assumption that all somatic cells contain a complete genetic complement. In association with malignant transformation there may be selective derepression of a previously dormant genome responsible for the production of a specific polypeptide that can be used as a tumor marker. As an example, small cell carcinoma of the lung may produce ACTH, antidiuretic hormone, or calcitonin. This is covered in greater detail in Ch. 173.

MISCELLANEOUS. Putrescine, spermidine, and spermine are members of a class of small hydrocarbon polycationic amine substances known as *polyamines*. They are found in highest concentrations in rapidly proliferating tissues, where they have been linked to the control of RNA metabolism. Elevated urinary excretion of polyamines has been demonstrated in approximately two thirds of patients with metastatic cancer of the large intestine, breast, and lung. Urinary polyamines are not specific markers for malignancy; increased urinary excretion has also been documented in association with benign prostatic hypertrophy, bronchial adenomas, pernicious anemia, and acromegaly.

Methylated nucleosides and pseudouridine are found in transfer RNA and, to a lesser extent, in ribosomal RNA. Increased transfer RNA methylase activity is a common characteristic of malignancy, and elevated concentrations of methylated bases have been demonstrated in the tRNA of human and animal tumors. Catabolism of these macromolecules results in the excretion of these nucleosides in the urine as free bases, where they can be measured as an index of tRNA methylation and turnover. Methylated nucleoside and pseudouridine have been found in abnormal amounts in the urine of patients with a wide range of hematologic and solid tumors, including 60 per cent of patients with advanced breast cancer.

EDCI is a glycoprotein that has been isolated in the urine of patients with acute myelogenous leukemia and adenocarcinoma of the ovary and colon. The cellular origin of this material is not known, but the close correlation between urinary excretion of this antigen and response of the neoplasm to treatment suggests that it is produced by neoplastic cells.

The prostatic acinar epithelium elaborates a specific *tartrate-inhibitable acid phosphatase*, which has been used as a serum marker for metastatic cancer of the prostate. However, the standard enzymatic assays have not had sufficient sensitivity to diagnose patients with localized tumors. A solid-phase radioimmunoassay for acid phosphatase has been developed that combines increased specificity with a high degree of sensitivity. Approximately one third of patients with occult neoplasms and 75 per cent of those with palpable tumors confined within, or locally extending beyond, the prostatic capsule (Stages II and III) can now be detected. A small number of patients with benign prostatic hypertrophy have also been demonstrated to have an elevated serum concentration. This assay for prostatic acid phosphatase may have a future application for mass screening.

A distinct form of *serum galactosyltransferase (GT-II)* has been reported in patients with neoplastic disease. This isoenzyme is present in the serum of 75 per cent of patients with gastrointestinal carcinomas and 78 per cent with breast cancer, as well as in prostatic cancer and lymphoproliferative disorders. Although the presence and concentration of GT-II correlates with the extent of disease, the majority of patients with Dukes' B colonic cancer are reported to have detectable levels. False-positive tests are uncommon, but have occurred in association with severe alcoholic hepatitis and celiac disease.

Gelder FB, Reese CJ, Moossa AR, Hall T, Hunter R: Purification, partial characterization, and clinical evaluation of a pancreatic oncofetal antigen. Cancer Res 38:313, 1978. *The clinical usefulness of a new oncofetal antigen, initially thought to be specific for pancreatic cancer, is presented in detail. The problem of selectivity, which plagues this field of investigation, is addressed.*

Goldenberg DM, Kin EE, Bennett SJ, Nelson MO and Deland FA: Carcinoembryonic antigen radioimmunodetection in the evaluation of colorectal cancer and in the detection of occult neoplasms. Gastroenterology 84:524, 1983. *The use of radiolabeled anti-CEA antibody allowed for the detection of a very high percentage of primary and metastatic colon cancers with a low false-negative index.*

Podolsky DK, McPhee MS, Alpert E, Warshaw AL, Isselbacher KJ: Galactosyl–transferase isoenzyme II in the detection of pancreatic cancer. N Engl J Med 304:1313, 1981. *An apparently successful attempt to define a tumor-specific isoenzyme that serves as a marker for the diagnosis of pancreatic carcinoma.*

Rosen SW, Weintraub BD, Vaitukaitus JL, Sussman HH, Hershman JM, Muggia FM: Placental proteins and their subunits as tumor markers. Ann Intern Med

82:71, 1975. *A useful guide to the rationale and clinical application of several proteins specific to the normal placenta, which are expressed by tumors of both germ and somatic cell origin.*

Wanebo HJ, Rao B, Pinsky CM, Hoffman RG, Stearns M, Schwartz M, Oettgen HF: Preoperative carcinoembryonic antigen level as a prognostic indicator in colorectal cancer. N Engl J Med 299:448, 1978. *The authors propose that the preoperative CEA level serves as an independent prognostic determinant for tumor recurrence after colonic cancer surgery with curative intent.*

173. ENDOCRINE MANIFESTATIONS OF TUMORS: "ECTOPIC" HORMONE PRODUCTION

William D. Odell

Cancers often produce symptoms by means of the elaboration of humoral or hormonal substances in addition to those symptoms produced directly by tumor mass or invasion. These humoral or hormonal substances seem always to be protein or peptide in nature. The single exception to this rule is that of the prostaglandins, but they are so ubiquitously distributed that it is difficult to determine whether they are ectopic or entopic. Furthermore, as is discussed later, it is questionable whether they are responsible for producing symptoms in patients with cancer. It appears very likely that *all* cancers are associated with ectopic or abnormal elaboration of proteins. In most instances these proteins are biologically inactive, or weakly bioactive and produce no recognizable clinical symptoms. When biologically active substances are produced, clinical symptoms result. The number of proteins produced by cancers is enormous. The syndromes listed in Table 171–1 are believed to be humoral in origin. Table 173–1 lists the hormones or hormone precursors that have been reported to be produced by cancers. Steroids or thyronines have not been reported as part of ectopic endocrine syndromes, although rarely a cancer may convert a bioinactive steroid such as dehydroepiandrosterone to a bioactive one. Some of the hormones listed in the accompanying table will be discussed here in more detail.

ECTOPIC ACTH PRODUCTION. The association of Cushing's syndrome with carcinoma, first described over 50 years ago, remains the most common ectopic endocrine syndrome. Fifty per cent of reported patients have carcinoma of the lung (predominantly oat cell or small round cell), 10 per cent have carcinoma of the thymus, 10 per cent have carcinoma of the pancreas (including carcinoids and islet cell tumors), 5 per cent have medullary carcinoma of the thyroid (which also produces calcitonin), and 5 per cent have neoplasms derived from the neural crest (pheochromocytoma, neuroblastoma, paraganglioma, and ganglioma). Considered conversely, about 3 per cent of patients with oat cell carcinoma of the lung have clinical or laboratory evidence of Cushing's syndrome—often extremely subtly manifested. Although other carcinomas are associated with Cushing's syndrome less frequently, numerous isolated case reports suggest that any carcinoma may show this association.

Furthermore, immunoactive ACTH can be detected universally in extracts prepared from carcinomas of the lung, colon, stomach, pancreas, or esophagus. In fact, a large glycoprotein containing immunoactivities of both ACTH and beta-melanocyte stimulating hormone may be extracted from all normal nonendocrine tissues of both the rat and the human. This material, present in small quantities in normal tissues, is present in large quantities in extracts of carcinomas, regardless of histologic type. It has no biological activity in sensitive dispersed adrenal cell assays in vitro, but is converted to a 4500 MW bioactive ACTH by exposure to trypsin. Presumably, this material in both normal tissue extracts, as well as in carcinomas, is *proopiomelanocortin* (POMC). An identical material is detectable in the blood of 70 per cent of patients with carcinoma of the lung, regardless of histologic type, using immunoassays. However, only some carcinomas enzymatically convert this biologically inactive POMC to biologically active ACTH. This conversion process is preferentially associated with the histologic types of neoplasms previously listed as being associated with clinical Cushing's syndrome.

POMC, in addition to the ACTH sequence, also contains the sequence of the endorphins, lipotropin, and beta-melanocyte stimulating hormone. Previous reports of MSH and lipotropin production by cancers are best explained by detection of circulating POMC per se or its cleavage products, lipotropin and/or MSH.

The symptoms produced by the ectopic production of *bioactive* ACTH are varied, ranging from none—simply the laboratory data of elevated cortisol—to full features of Cushing's syndrome. Often they are subtle, consisting only of mild weakness or the laboratory finding of hypokalemia without physical abnormalities. The classic Cushing's syndrome is not commonly associated with cancer, for such physical changes usually require from months to years to be produced and often the neoplasm is present but a short while. The occurrence of psychosis, weakness, hypokalemia, or an abnormal glucose tolerance curve in a patient with known cancer suggests ectopic bioactive ACTH production. Hypokalemia is uncommon in Cushing's disease of pituitary origin. Plasma ACTH concentrations are often extremely high, unlike those in Cushing's disease, which are usually "normal" but in association with an elevated cortisol. In addition, suppression with high doses of oral dexamethasone (8 mg per day) usually does not occur in ectopic ACTH syndrome, but does occur in Cushing's disease (of pituitary origin). Adrenal carcinomas or adenomas producing excess cortisol are associated with undetectable or very low plasma ACTH in conjunction with elevated plasma cortisols (see Ch. 229).

Approximately 50 to 60 per cent of patients with bronchial adenoma and ectopic Cushing's syndrome show cortisol or ACTH suppression with administration of large doses of dexamethasone. The most likely explanation at present is that these neoplasms produce corticotropin-releasing hormone (CRH) (a 41 amino acid peptide normally produced by the hypothalamus to control pituitary ACTH secretion). The tumor CRH stimulates secretion of ACTH by the normal pituitary. In such patients dexamethasone inhibits CRH action directly at the pituitary gland. Although this hypothesis is untested with respect to bronchial adenoma–ACTH syndrome, the production of CRH-like material by tumors has been described.

Treatment of Cushing's syndrome caused by cancer depends upon resection of the tumor or effective chemotherapy. If this is not possible, treatment with drugs that interfere with adrenal steroid synthesis prevents the continued ACTH production from stimulating excess adrenal secretion of cortisol—e.g., metyrapone or aminoglutethimide.

In summary, POMC is probably produced in small quantities by all normal nonendocrine tissues. It may be an autocrine or paracrine substance. Cancers produce increased quantities of POMC that can often be detected by immunoassay in increased quantities in the blood of patients with cancer. Selected carci-

TABLE 173–1. HORMONES REPORTED TO BE SECRETED BY CANCERS

Proopiomelanocortin (POMC)	Calcitonin
ACTH	Growth hormone
Chorionic gonadotropin (CG)	Prolactin
Alpha peptide chain of CG	Gastrin
Beta peptide chain of CG	Secretin
Vasopressin	Glucagon
Somatomedins	Corticotropin releasing hormone
Hypoglycemia producing factors	Growth hormone releasing hormone
Parathyroid hormone	Gastrin-releasing peptide
Osteoclast activating factor	Somatostatin
Prostaglandins	Chorionic somatotropin
Erythropoietin	Neurophysins
Hypophosphatemia producing factor	Eosinophilopoietin

nomas, related to histologic type, metabolize POMC to biologically active ACTH and occasionally MSH or lipotropin, producing the so-called "ectopic" ACTH-MSH syndrome. These and similar data concerning chorionic gonadotropin (CG) have led to the belief that "ectopic" humoral syndromes are not ectopic. Why some cancers metabolize POMC and most do not remains an important unanswered question.

HYPERCALCEMIA AND CANCER. Hypercalcemia is a common finding in patients with cancer. In a large series of patients with bronchogenic carcinoma, 12.5 per cent were hypercalcemic. The frequency of hypercalcemia varied with histologic type: 23 per cent with epidermoid carcinoma, 12.5 per cent with anaplastic carcinoma, and 2.5 per cent with adenocarcinoma. When carcinoma-associated hypercalcemia occurs, the tumors most frequently found are carcinoma of the lung (approximately 35 per cent), carcinoma of the kidney (24 per cent), and carcinoma of the ovary (8 per cent). Any carcinoma may produce hypercalcemia. The cause of hypercalcemia in the majority of patients remains controversial. Production by the tumor of a protein, structurally different from parathormone (and hence poorly active in PTH immunoassays) but with biological properties similar to PTH, appears most likely. In addition to this postulated PTH-like substance, three other substances have been suggested to cause hypercalcemia in patients with cancer: *parathormone, prostaglandins,* and *osteoclast activating factor* (OAF).

Parathormone (PTH). Albright was the first to postulate (in 1941) tumor production of a parathormone-like material as an explanation for the hypercalcemia and hypophosphatemia found in certain patients with malignant disease. Subsequently, immunoactive parathormone was identified in tumor extracts of patients with carcinomas and hypercalcemia. One report described an arteriovenous gradient of immunoactive parathormone across a renal carcinoma associated with hypercalcemia. After removal of the tumor, serum parathormone and calcium fell to normal and extracts of the tumor contained extremely large amounts of parathormone. Similarly, a patient with acute myeloblastic leukemia exhibited hypercalcemia that relapsed and remitted repeatedly in parallel with the leukemic process. On two of these occasions serum parathormone was elevated. In vitro studies showed that the myeloblasts released immunoactive parathormone into medium; normal cells did not.

This type of observation and many other data not reviewed here led to the conclusion that cancer elaboration of parathormone was the usual cause of hypercalcemia associated with cancer. (See also Ch. 246 for a discussion of PTH and malignancy.)

Subsequent studies have cast great doubt that PTH per se is the responsible agent for tumor-associated hypercalcemia. The immunoassays used in most of the studies reviewed were so-called carboxyl terminus-directed assays, which give unreliable results in patients with hypercalcemia and cancer. When amino terminal assays are used, such patients rarely show elevated immunoactive PTH; values are "normal" or below detection limits. In an important study 11 patients with hypercalcemia and hypophosphatemia associated with cancer without known bony metastases were investigated. In nine patients treatment of the tumor with surgical ablation or with chemotherapy restored serum calcium to normal. Parathormone was quantified with several radioimmunoassays designed to react with the intact hormone as well as hormone fragments, but none was detectable in either tumor extracts or in blood. However, using an in vitro bioassay (based on calcium resorption from mouse calvarium), a substance that stimulated bony reabsorption was detected in tumor extracts from all 11 patients. Recently, a cytochemical assay for PTH has been developed and used to study patients with tumor-associated hypercalcemia. About 50 per cent of patients in a small series had elevated cytochemically active PTH but not immunoactive PTH. Histologically, the bones of patients with tumor-associated hypercalcemia appear as if a substance with biological properties of PTH were acting. In addition, a recent careful study using a specific hybridization assay has shown that the messenger RNA of parathormone is not detectable in tumor-producing hypercalcemia.

In summary, PTH per se (identical to parathormone secreted by the normal parathyroids) does not appear to be produced by cancers. Instead, a substance with similar biological properties, but which is immunologically different, appears to be produced. Several laboratories are attempting to isolate and characterize this material. A more complete discussion of the variables in the immunoassay of PTH is contained in Ch. 246.

Prostaglandins. There are at least two animal models of tumor-associated hypercalcemia: a fibrosarcoma in mice and a carcinoma in rabbits. In both instances, the hypercalcemia has been shown to be caused by elaboration of prostaglandins, predominantly PGE_2. The hypercalcemia was treatable with indomethacin, an inhibitor of prostaglandin synthesis. Subsequently several human carcinomas have been described in which hypercalcemia was associated with increased prostaglandin excretion or production. In a few patients, treatment with indomethacin returned elevated serum calcium levels to normal. However, as large numbers of patients were studied, no investigators have reported success with routine use of indomethacin as treatment for hypercalcemia caused by cancer. At the time of this writing, it is generally believed that cancer production of prostaglandins with release systemically is not commonly a cause of hypercalcemia in patients.

Osteoclast Activating Factor. A third cause of hypercalcemia in certain patients with malignancies is the elaboration of osteoclast activating factor (OAF), a protein with a molecular weight of 20,000 daltons, that is normally produced by white blood cells. It stimulates bone resorption very actively in in vitro assay systems. OAF is extractable from myeloma cells and is thus implicated as the cause of the osteolysis and resulting hypercalcemia in multiple myeloma and in at least some rare instances of other hematologic malignancies producing hypercalcemia (see Fig. 163–2).

Concurrent Primary Hyperparathyroidism. Hyperparathyroidism per se is a common disorder and has repeatedly been described in patients with known cancers. The presence of hyperparathyroidism in a patient with cancer may be suggested by high plasma parathormone (which is very rare in cancer), using amino terminal PTH immunoassays.

In summary, hypercalcemia is a common abnormality produced by cancer. Since hypercalcemia may itself produce considerable morbidity or even death, recognition and prompt treatment are essential, and the diagnosis should be considered in any patient with cancer who develops polyuria, constipation, lethargy, or personality change. Patients with known carcinomas may be eucalcemic when active and ambulatory, but may rapidly develop dangerous hypercalcemia when immobilized. The nonspecific treatment of severe hypercalcemia is described in Ch. 243. It generally depends on infusions of saline, diuresis with furosemide, and ambulation. If this does not suffice, treatment with mithramycin, which inhibits bone resorption, may be necessary as an emergency procedure. The administration of calcitonin and glucocorticoids has been used for short-term treatment. Diphosphonate or phosphate, given orally, has been used for long-term treatment. Obviously therapy directed toward the tumor itself should be concomitantly employed, but this is much more slowly effective, if at all.

HYPOPHOSPHATEMIA. A rare syndrome of profound hypophosphatemia, with normal serum calcium, in association with an unusual variety of neoplasms, has been described in perhaps 20 patients. The neoplasms producing this syndrome include pleomorphic sarcomas, hemangiomas, giant cell tumors of bone, or benign osteoblastomas. This syndrome may be more common than previously recognized, being sometimes erroneously reported as adult onset vitamin D–resistant rickets. Recently, patients with prostatic carcinoma were reported to have hypophosphatemia. The syndrome is associated with dramatic phosphaturia, normal or undetectable plasma parathormone, normal serum calcium, and, often, severe muscle spasms. There is severe osteomalacia with bone pain and fractures that occur with minimal trauma. In some (perhaps all) patients, the profound phosphaturia is also associated with aminoaciduria and glucosuria. Blood concentrations of 25-hydroxy vitamin D are normal; 1,25-dihydroxy D concentrations are low. The serum phosphorus returns to normal following resection of the tumor or following treatment with 1,25-dihydroxy vitamin D. These tumors apparently elaborate a material which inhibits 1-hydroxylation of vitamin D by the kidney.

CHORIONIC GONADOTROPIN. Chorionic gonadotropin (CG) as secreted by normal trophoblastic cells is a glycoprotein with a molecular weight of approximately 40,000 daltons. A similar, but probably not identical, substance is elaborated by all normal human tissues and is extractable from all carcinomas. In about 5 to 15 per cent of patients with carcinomas of all kinds, this gonadotropin is detectable in blood. The difference between chorionic gonadotropin secreted by the trophoblast and that contained in normal tissues lies in the carbohydrate composition. Carbohydrate constitutes about a third of the molecular weight of trophoblast CG. Normal tissue CG contains little or no carbohydrate. The degradation rate or metabolic clearance rate from plasma of chorionic gondotropin is inversely related to its carbohydrate content. Thus, presumably, carbohydrate-free CG has extremely little biologic activity in vivo and is cleared from plasma with a half-life in minutes. Carbohydrate-rich CG is cleared slowly with a half-life of hours. All carcinomas also secrete CG. However, those associated with detectable blood concentrations also glycosylate this material, increasing biologic activity and slowing metabolic clearance sufficiently to reach detectable blood concentrations. Approximately 10 per cent of patients with a wide variety of carcinomas have elevated blood CG (e.g., carcinoma of the lung, stomach, pancreas, colon). Men with such tumors often have mild gynecomastia. A rare syndrome produced by CG is precocious puberty in boys with hepatoblastoma.

HYPOGLYCEMIA AND CANCER. Tumor-associated hypoglycemia occurs most frequently with neoplasms that can be loosely termed mesotheliomas. They include more specifically fibrosarcomas, neurofibromas, neurofibrosarcomas, spindle cell carcinomas, rhabdomyosarcomas, and leiomyosarcomas. Such tumors are usually large when hypoglycemia is noted, ranging in size from 800 to 10,000 grams, and are found mainly in the abdomen. They may also develop within the thorax. In the remaining one third, the most frequent tumors are hepatic carcinomas (21 per cent), adrenal cortical carcinomas (6 per cent) and a variety of anaplastic adenocarcinomas, pseudomyxomas, and cholangiomas. The hypoglycemia produced by hepatic carcinomas is not simply a mass effect owing to tumor replacement of hepatic parenchyma with consequent decrease in hepatic glucose output. Studies utilizing both tumor extracts and blood samples can be summarized as follows: (1) a hypoglycemic factor that mimics insulin activity by in vitro bioassay is often demonstrable; (2) insulin itself is usually not demonstrable by insulin radioimmunoassay; and (3) a substance is often detectable in increased concentrations as measured by radioreceptor assays that quantify somatomedins and so-called nonsuppressible insulin-like activity (NSILA) or insulin-like growth factors (IFG-I and IGF-II). Thus, hypoglycemia associated with cancer may be caused by one or more of the somatomedins, a family of protein substances normally elaborated by the liver that differ structurally from insulin but that have many of its biologic properties. Using current assay systems, such substances are increased in blood and tumor extracts from some (perhaps 50 per cent), but not all, of the patients with this syndrome.

GROWTH HORMONE AND GROWTH HORMONE RELEASING HORMONE. Acromegaly associated with bronchial carcinoid or pancreatic islet cell tumor has been described in a small number of patients. In at least five of these patients, growth hormone (GH) secretion was restored to normal or the clinical signs of acromegaly subsided after the extrapituitary tumor was removed without any therapy being directed toward the pituitary gland. Extracts from such an adenoma were found to contain a potent substance capable of releasing GH from dispersed pituitary cells in culture. This GH releasing hormone (GHRH) has been shown to be a 44 amino acid peptide, probably identical to that produced by the hypothalamus normally to control secretion of GH. Elaboration of GHRH by a peripheral tumor may therefore have the potential of leading to a pituitary tumor. The presence of an extrapituitary tumor should be excluded in any patient with acromegaly.

In addition to elaboration of GHRH, tumors could elaborate GH per se. High concentrations of GH have been found in extracts of ovarian carcinomas in patients without acromegaly. There is one report of extractable GH in a lung tumor. However, it is apparent that cancer elaboration of GH per se could not produce a pituitary tumor and acromegaly.

CALCITONIN. Calcitonin is normally secreted by the parafollicular cells of the thyroid gland and serves as an excellent hormonal marker of tumors developing from these cells—medullary carcinomas (Ch. 243). Calcitonin is also secreted ectopically by a variety of carcinomas, but since this hormone has little or no biologic effect in normal adults, no symptoms are produced. Elevated plasma concentrations of calcitonin have been described by several groups of investigators in patients with carcinomas of the lung (regardless of histologic type), colon, breast, and pancreas. Direct synthesis of calcitonin by the tumor or an arteriovenous gradient of the hormone across a tumor has not been reported. In fact, in one patient with lung carcinoma and elevated plasma calcitonin the source appeared to be the normal thyroid and not the tumor. If this is commonly the case, it would have to be postulated that the neoplasm elaborated a material that stimulates thyroid production of calcitonin. Too few data exist now to clarify this point.

VASOPRESSIN. Schwartz and Bartter first described the syndrome of cancer associated with hyponatremia, hypervolemia, renal sodium loss, and inappropriately high urine osmolality to which their name is sometimes attached (see Ch. 76). The associated symptoms are those of decrease in mental acuity, confusion, or even seizures. This syndrome, which is most frequently associated with carcinoma of the lung, has been attributed to secretion of arginine vasopressin (AVP) by the tumor; vasopressin has been demonstrated by bioassay and radioimmunoassay in extracts of such neoplasms, and synthesis of AVP (incorporation of tritiated amino acids) by extracts of lung cancer has been found in vitro. Ectopic production of vasopressin is very common in patients with carcinoma of the lung (found in 42 per cent in one series). Excess vasopressin produces no symptoms unless the patient continues to drink "excess" water. In normal persons thirst is suppressed by a fall in plasma osmolality. Possibly the smaller percentage of patients with excess vasopressin who develop symptoms of water intoxication and hyponatremia have both a sustained hypersecretion of vasopressin and a defect in thirst control. The treatment of the syndrome of inappropriate secretion of antidiuretic hormone, sometimes called SIADH, is considered in Ch. 76. Treatment usually consists only of restricting water intake to less than insensible loss (exhaled water vapor plus sweat loss). Under these conditions plasma osmolality rises. In severe cases cautious use of diuretics with or without infusion of hypertonic saline may be warranted.

A single larger precursor molecule contains the amino acid sequence of both neurophysin II and arginine vasopressin (see Ch. 226). Normally enzymatic cleavage releases neurophysin II and vasopressin on a mole-for-mole basis. Elevation of plasma neurophysin has been found in approximately 40 per cent of unselected patients with lung carcinoma, a value similar to that found for vasopressin.

ERYTHROPOIETIN. This glycoprotein hormone is normally secreted by the kidney and stimulates differentiation of early red cell stages, resulting in increased red cell production (see

Ch. 153). A variety of benign and malignant conditions involving the kidney have been described to be associated with erythrocytosis. About 63 per cent of patients have hypernephroma, renal cysts, or hydronephrosis. These are not examples of ectopic hormonal syndromes, but represent retained properties of a neoplasm derived from the tissue normally producing the hormone. About 37 per cent of patients have neoplasms derived from tissues not known to produce erythropoietin normally. These include hemangioblastomas (21 per cent), uterine fibromas (6 per cent), adrenal cortical neoplasms (3 per cent), ovarian neoplasms (3 per cent), hepatomas (3 per cent), and pheochromocytomas (1 per cent). The biochemical characteristics of the tumor-produced erythropoietin are indistinguishable from erythropoietin produced by the normal kidney.

EOSINOPHILOPOIETIN. The concurrent appearance of eosinophilia with various malignancies has been observed in the occasional patient over the past 30 years. Eosinophilia, irrespective of cause, is in turn often associated with endocardial fibrosis, mural thrombus development, and embolic phenomenon. An undifferentiated lung carcinoma that produced this syndrome was found to contain large amounts of an eosinophilopoietin-like material, measured by an in vitro eosinophil colony growth assay. In close proximity to fibrotic cardiac endothelium were masses of aggregated eosinophils. These eosinophils were shown to generate large amounts of toxic oxygen species, demonstrated to be toxic to cultured endothelial cells in vitro.

SUMMARY. A large variety of protein hormones or protein hormone-like materials are produced by cancers. Most are biologically inert or weakly bioactive. Similar or identical substances are often produced by most or all normal tissues (e.g., POMC, CG) or by a selected group of normal tissues (e.g., erythropoietin, IGF-I and II). Selected carcinomas, correlated with histologic type, metabolize some of these substances into bioactive forms, producing humoral syndromes. It may presently be hypothesized that ectopic hormone production is not ectopic. Detection and quantification of the biologically inactive or weakly bioactive proteins have been useful in early tumor diagnosis and in following response to therapy.

General References

Frohman LA: Ectopic hormone production. Am J Med 70:995, 1981. *A recent editorial overview of current concepts concerning production of hormones by tumors. There is a short but useful list of recent references.*

Odell WD: Humoral manifestations of cancer. *In* Williams RH (ed.): Textbook of Endocrinology. 7th ed. 1984, Philadelphia, W.B. Saunders Company, 1984, Chapter 31.

Odell WD, Wolfsen A, Yoshimoto Y, et al.: Ectopic peptide synthesis—a universal concomitant of neoplasia. Trans Assoc Am Physicians 90:204, 1977. *This paper offers the hypothesis that ectopic peptide synthesis is always present when a neoplasm develops. Data supporting this hypothesis include studies of ACTH-ProACTH, kipotropin, vasopressin, the free alpha chain of hCG, and Hcg per se.*

Proopiomelanocortin, Lipotropin, MSH

Gewirtz G, Yalow, RS: Ectopic ACTH production in carcinoma of the lung. J Clin Invest 53:1022, 1974. *This paper describes for the first time that extracts of all carcinomas of the lung contain immunoreactive ACTH. This ACTH was shown to have little biologic activity in in vitro bioassays, but to be convertible to bioactive ACTH by trypsin action.*

Saito E, Odell WD: Corticotropin/lipotropin common precursor-like material in normal rat extrapituitary tissues. Proc Natl Acad Sci USA 80:3792, 1983.

Saito E, Iwasa S, Odell WD: Widespread presence of large molecular weight adrenocorticotropin-like substances in normal rat extrapituitary tissues. Endocrinology 113:1010, 1983. *These two papers show for the first time that proopiomelanocortin is extractable from all normal nonendocrine tissues.*

Wolfsen AR, Odell WD: ProACTH—use for early detection of lung cancer. Am J Med 66:765, 1979. *This manuscript describes that immunoactive ACTH is detectable, and usually present in large amounts in extracts of all carcinomas of the lung, colon, stomach, pancreas, and breast. This ACTH did not react in a radioreceptor assay and had a larger molecular weight than bioactive ACTH.*

Hypercalcemia

Bender RA, Hansen H: Hypercalcemia in bronchogenic carcinoma. A prospective study of 200 patients. Ann Intern Med 80:205, 1974. *An analysis of the frequency of hypercalcemia in patients with various histologic types of lung cancer.*

Brereton HD, Halushka PV, Alexander RW, et al.: Indomethacin responsive hypercalcemia in a patient with renal cell carcinoma. N Engl J Med 291:83, 1975. *This is the first publication to demonstrate that prostaglandin elaboration may be a cause of hypercalcemia in patients with cancer.*

Breslau NA, McGuire JL, Zerwekh JE, Frenkel EP, Pak CYC: Hypercalcemia associated with increased serum calcitriol levels in three patients with lymphoma. Ann Intern Med 100:1, 1984. *An interesting study that suggests that certain lymphomas may synthesize calcitriol and therefore produce hypercalcemia.*

Buckle RM, McMillan M, Mallinson C: Ectopic secretion of parathyroid hormone by a renal adenocarcinoma in a patient with hypercalcemia. Br Med J 4:724, 1970. *This paper offers perhaps the only incontrovertible data that renal carcinoma may elaborate parathormone. Artial venous difference of this hormone existed across the kidney containing the tumor, and tumor extracts contained parathormone.*

Goltzman D, Stewart AF, Broadus AE: Malignancy-associated hypercalcemia: Evaluation with a cytochemical bioassay for parathyroid hormone. J Clin Endocrinol Metab 53:899, 1981.

Powell D, Singer FR, Murray TM, et al.: Nonparathyroid hypercalcemia in patients with neoplastic disease. N Engl J Med 289:176, 1973. *This pivotal publication offers solid data to challenge the concept that parathyroid elaboration is a common cause of hypercalcemia in patients with cancer. It suggests even that the elaboration of parathormone may not occur at all.*

Simpson EL, Mundy GR, D'Souza SM, Ibbotson KJ, Bockman R, Jacobs JW: Absence of parathyroid hormone messenger RNA in nonparathyroid tumors associated with hypercalcemia. N Engl J Med 309:325, 1983.

Tashjian AH: Prostaglandins, hypercalcemia and cancer. N Engl J Med 293:1317, 1975. *This editorial gives good perspective to the hypothesis that prostaglandin elaboration is a common cause of hypercalcemia in cancer.*

Hypophosphatemia

Daniels RA, Weisenfeld I: Tumorous phosphaturic osteomalacia. Am J Med 67:155, 1979. *A single case report and excellent review of the literature. This study confirms that 1,25-dihydroxy-cholecalciferol deficiency is present, and that treatment with this substance abolishes the biochemical abnormalities. In addition to phosphaturia, glycosuria was present in this patient.*

Chorionic Gonadotropin

Braunstein GD, Vaitukaitis JL, Carbone PP, et al.: Ectopic production of human chorionic gonadotropin by neoplasms. Ann Intern Med 78:39, 1973. *This frequently cited paper presents data to indicate that hCG is ectopically produced by a wide variety of nontrophoblastic carcinomas, e.g., about 5 to 15 per cent of carcinomas of the colon, stomach, pancreas, and lung.*

Yoshimoto Y, Wolfsen AR, Odell WD: Glycosylation, a variable in the production of hCG by cancers. Am J Med 67:414, 1979. *This study demonstrates that hCG-like material is present in extracts of all carcinomas and of all normal human tissues. The hCG in most carcinomas and in all normal tissues except the placenta is very low or free of carbohydrate. The hCG extracted from placenta or present in cancers or blood of patients with cancer associated with detectable hCG is carbohydrate rich.*

Hypoglycemia

Plovink H, Ruderman NB, Aoki T, et al.: Non-beta-cell tumor hypoglycemia associated with increased nonsuppressible insulin-like protein (NSILP). Am J Med 66:154, 1979. *A thoroughly studied patient with hypoglycemia attributed to a tumor producing NSILP. The discussion gives a good perspective for the view that somatomedins are always the cause of hypoglycemia in this syndrome.*

Growth Hormone and Growth Hormone Releasing Hormone (GHRH)

Frohman LA, Szabo M, Berelowitz M, et al.: Partial purification and characterization of a peptide with growth hormone-releasing activity from extrapituitary tumors in patients with acromegaly. J Clin Invest 65:43, 1980. *This manuscript is a good source of reference for this syndrome. In addition, this offers the first chemical characterization of GHRH extracted from extrapituitary tumors causing pituitary tumors and acromegaly.*

Calcitonin

Schwartz KE, Wolfsen AR, Forster B, Odell WD: Calcitonin in nonthyroidal cancer. J Clin Endocrinol Metab 49:438, 1979. *This report offers a good review of earlier publications and itself indicates the frequency of elevated blood calcitonin in patients with a wide variety of carcinomas. Fluctuations in calcitonin in parallel with removal and relapse of the tumor are shown.*

Silva OL, Becker KL, Primack A, et al.: Hypercalcitonemia in bronchogenic cancer. Evidence for thyroid origin of the hormone. JAMA 234:183, 1975. *This study shows that the elevated calcitonin in a patient with lung cancer was derived from the thyroid.*

Vasopressin

George JM, Capen CC, Phillips AS: Biosynthesis of vasopressin in vitro and ultrastructure of a bronchogenic carcinoma in a patient with the syndrome of inappropriate secretion of antidiuretic hormone (SIADH). J Clin Invest 51:141, 1972. *The demonstration of synthesis of ADH by a neoplasm from a patient with SIADH.*

Erythropoietin

Hammond D, Winnick S: Paraneoplastic erythrocytosis and ectopic erythropoietins. Ann NY Acad Sci 230:219, 1974. *A thorough review and discussion of the ectopic production of erythropoietin.*

Eosinophilopoietin

Slungaard A, Ascensao J, Zanjani E, Jacob HS: Pulmonary carcinoma with eosinophilia: demonstration of a tumor-derived eosinophilopoietic factor. N Engl J Med 309:778, 1983.

174. NONMETASTATIC EFFECTS OF CANCER ON THE NERVOUS SYSTEM

Jerome B. Posner

When patients with systemic cancer develop nervous system dysfunction, metastasis is usually the cause. However, cancer also exerts deleterious effects on the nervous system in the absence of direct metastatic involvement. Recognition of these nonmetastatic neurologic complications can prevent inappropriate and perhaps harmful therapy directed at a nonexistent metastasis. Since at times the nervous system symptoms precede the discovery of the cancer, they can also lead the physician to the diagnosis of an otherwise occult neoplasm.

An almost bewildering variety of neurologic disorders have been ascribed to effects of systemic cancer (Table 174–1). Most patients with nervous system dysfunction not caused by metastases are eventually found to be suffering from systemic infections, from vascular or metabolic disorders that affect the nervous system secondarily, or from unwanted side effects of cancer therapy. This chapter discusses two types of nervous system damage related to cancer and not described elsewhere in this book: "remote effects," or paraneoplastic syndromes, and radiation injury.

TABLE 174–1. NONMETASTATIC EFFECTS OF CANCER ON THE NERVOUS SYSTEM

I. "Remote effects"
- A. Brain and cranial nerves
  1. Dementia
  2. Bulbar encephalitis
  3. Subacute cerebellar degeneration—opsoclonus*
  4. Optic neuritis—retinal degeneration
- B. Spinal cord
  1. Gray matter myelopathy
     - a. Subacute motor neuropathy
     - b. "Autonomic insufficiency"
  2. Subacute necrotic myelopathy
- C. Peripheral nerves and roots
  1. Subacute sensory neuronopathy (dorsal root ganglionitis)*
  2. Sensorimotor peripheral neuropathy
  3. Acute polyneuropathy, "Guillain-Barré" type
  4. Autonomic neuropathy
- D. Neuromuscular junction and muscle
  1. Polymyositis and dermatomyositis (dermatomyositis in older men*)
  2. "Myasthenic" syndrome*
  3. Myasthenia gravis (thymoma)
  4. Neuromyotonia

II. Metabolic encephalopathy
- A. Destruction of vital organs
  1. Liver (hepatic coma)
  2. Lung (pulmonary encephalopathy)
  3. Kidney (uremia)
  4. Bone (hypercalcemia)
- B. Elaboration of hormonal substances by tumor
  1. "Parathormone" (hypercalcemia)
  2. "Corticotropin" (Cushing's syndrome)
  3. Antidiuretic hormone (water intoxication)
- C. Competition between tumor and brain for essential substrates
  1. Hypoglycemia (large retroperitoneal tumors)
  2. Tryptophan (carcinoid)
- D. Malnutrition

III. Infections (usually associated with lymphomas)
- A. Parasites
  1. Toxoplasma cerebral abscess
- B. Fungi
  1. Meningitis (cryptococcosis)
  2. Encephalitis (aspergillosis, mucormycosis)
- C. Bacteria
  1. Meningitis *(Listeria monocytogenes)*
- D. Viruses
  1. Herpes zoster (radiculitis, myelitis, encephalitis, granulomatous vasculitis)
  2. Progressive multifocal leukoencephalopathy

IV. Vascular disease
- A. Intracranial hemorrhage
  1. Subdural hematoma
  2. Subarachnoid hemorrhage
  3. Intracerebral hemorrhage
- B. Cerebral infarction
  1. Thrombotic (due to "hypercoagulability")
  2. Embolic nonbacterial thrombotic endocarditis

V. Side effects of therapy
- A. Chemotherapy
  1. Central nervous system
  2. Peripheral nervous system
- B. Radiation therapy
  See Table 174–2

*Neurologic disorders which may precede diagnosis of cancer and strongly suggest its presence.

REMOTE EFFECTS

Remote effects of cancer on the nervous system is a term used to describe nervous system dysfunction of unknown cause occurring exclusively or at higher frequency in patients with cancer. Paraneoplastic syndromes is a term also used.

Remote effects are not common. In a series of 1465 patients with cancer, they were found in only about 7 per cent, and a rather ill-defined weakness and wasting of proximal muscles associated with diminished deep tendon reflexes accounted for two thirds of these patients. The incidence varied by the type of cancer, with ovary (16 per cent) and lung (15 per cent) leading the list. Since carcinoma of the lung is much more common than ovarian carcinoma, about half of all the patients in this large series with remote effects had lung cancer, usually of the oat cell type. My experience is that remote effects are even less common than the 7 per cent reported, and the diagnosis should never be accepted until a thorough evaluation has excluded metastatic or other nonmetastatic causes of neurologic dysfunction. In particular, infiltration of nerve roots by tumor in the leptomeninges (meningeal carcinomatosis) may mimic a "remote" peripheral neuropathy.

The etiology of "remote effects" is unknown. Circulating antibodies against the target nervous system organ can be found in some patients suffering remote effects. In a few instances, injection of the antibody or extracts of tumor into experimental animals has reproduced portions of the clinical syndrome, suggesting an autoimmune mechanism, with the antigen originating in the tumor. Patients with remote effects appear to survive longer than those with the same cancer but no remote effect. Not all patients harbor such antibodies, and other suggestions for etiology have included viral infections, toxins secreted by the tumor, and nutritional deprivation. The neurologic disorders described later are separated by their clinical signs into anatomic categories. However, more than one clinical syndrome may be present in a given patient, and similar clinical syndromes may be associated with slightly different pathologic changes. This is particularly true of the dementias, which are often lumped together with brainstem, cerebellar, and spinal cord lesions as "carcinomatous encephalomyelitis," and of myopathy and peripheral neuropathy associated with cancer, often called "carcinomatous neuromyopathy."

Brain and Cranial Nerves

CEREBRUM. Cerebral remote effects are usually characterized by dementia with or without other neurologic findings. Dementia is usually insidious in onset and progressive. Loss of recent memory and an alteration of the affect, either anxiety or depression, characterize the disorder. Generally seizures are prominent in some patients, and others have a fluctuating confusional state mimicking metabolic encephalopathy. When other abnormal neurologic signs are present, they usually point to brainstem, cerebellar, or peripheral nerve involvement (see below). The electroencephalogram in the demented patient is diffusely slow, and the cerebrospinal fluid sometimes contains 10 to 40 lymphocytes per cubic milliliter and a slight elevation of the protein concentration.

Pathologically, there are two main groups. In some patients, no significant pathologic changes are found in the cerebrum despite unequivocal clinical dementia. Other patients demonstrate widespread cerebral neuronal loss with perivascular collections of lymphocytes, particularly in the medial temporal lobes (limbic encephalitis) or the thalamus.

The etiology of the dementing illness is unknown, but the inflammatory changes have led some to propose that a virus is responsible. The differential diagnosis includes metastatic disease of the brain or meninges, fungal or parasitic infections of the brain, metabolic encephalopathy, and multifocal leukoencephalopathy. In the first three disorders, focal cerebral signs other than dementia are present, and CT scans (Ch. 471) and cerebrospinal fluid studies support the diagnosis of infectious or metastatic disease of the brain. Metabolic encephalopathy can usually be diagnosed by appropriate laboratory tests, as indicated in Ch. 472. The presence of a progressive dementia in middle age accompanied by cerebellar, brainstem, or peripheral nerve dysfunction but no other focal cerebral signs suggests dementia as a remote effect of cancer. There is no specific treatment for these dementias, but they may improve with successful therapy of the cancer.

BULBAR ENCEPHALITIS. Brainstem dysfunction associated with dementia, which develops insidiously or subacutely and is progressive, may be a remote effect of the cancer. The brainstem signs include vertigo, nystagmus, dysphagia, ophthalmoplegia, and at times ataxia and extensor plantar reflexes. The pathologic changes, predominantly in the lower pons and medulla, are those of neuronal loss and perivascular lymphocytic cuffing. The lymphocytic infiltration is responsible for the term encephalitis. The cause is unknown, and there is no effective treatment.

CEREBELLUM. Subacute cerebellar degeneration caused by cancer has a clinical picture sufficiently characteristic to suggest strongly that cancer is present even if the neurologic symptoms predate the appearance of the tumor. There is usually subacute onset of bilateral and symmetrical cerebellar dysfunction, the patient being equally ataxic in arms and legs. Severe dysarthria is usually present, and vertigo and diplopia are common, but nystagmus may be absent. Many patients have neurologic signs pointing to disease outside the cerebellum: extensor plantar responses are common; tendon reflexes may be either diminished or exaggerated; and dementia occurs in about half. The cerebrospinal fluid is usually normal, but there may be as many as 40 lymphocytes per cubic milliliter and an elevated protein content. The disease, which may be associated with any cancer, precedes the discovery of the neoplasm by periods of from weeks to three years in more than half the patients, and it tends to run a progressive course over weeks to months, rendering the patient severely disabled. Cerebellar atrophy may be seen on a CT scan, particularly if done late in the course of the illness. Characteristic pathologic changes consist of diffuse or patchy loss of Purkinje cells in all areas of the cerebellum. There may be lymphocytic cuffs around blood vessels, particularly in the deep nuclei. This illness can be distinguished from cerebellar metastases by the symmetry of its signs and the absence of increased intracranial pressure, and from alcoholic-nutritional cerebellar degeneration because dysarthria and ataxia in the upper extremities are prominent in the carcinomatous cerebellar degenerations, and are usually mild or absent in the alcoholic variety. The hereditary cerebellar degenerations rarely run so rapid a course. At times the disorder stabilizes or improves with successful treatment of the tumor. Antibodies to cerebellar Purkinje cells have been found in the serum of a few patients.

Another, less common cerebellar syndrome is that of opsoclonus (spontaneous, conjugate, chaotic eye movements most severe when voluntary eye movements are attempted). Opsoclonus is frequently associated with cerebellar ataxia and myoclonus of the trunk and extremities. It is most common in children as a remote effect of neuroblastoma. In children, the neurologic symptoms respond to adrenocorticosteroid therapy and to therapy of the tumor.

Spinal Cord

Two rare but distinct myelopathies complicate cancer: the first, *subacute motor neuropathy,* involves spinal gray matter (particularly anterior horn cells), and usually affects patients with Hodgkin's disease or other lymphomas. The course is subacute, with progressive painless asymmetric lower motor neuron weakness of the legs and arms. Some patients complain of sensory symptoms, but sensory loss is mild or absent despite profound weakness. The major pathologic finding is neuronal degeneration of anterior horn cells of the spinal cord. Sometimes there is inflammation in the anterior horns and demyelination in the white matter of the spinal cord. The clinical course is different from most remote effects in that many patients improve spontaneously, independent of the course of the underlying lymphoma. The etiology is unknown, but a similar disorder in mice harboring lymphomas appears to be caused by a virus. Rarely, gray matter myelopathies with clinical courses resembling syringomyelia or autonomic insufficiency (q.v.) complicate systemic cancer.

The second complicating condition is *subacute necrotic destruction of the spinal cord,* a myelopathy in which both gray and white matter are affected to an equal degree. Clinically, there is rapidly ascending sensory and motor loss, usually to mid-thoracic levels, the patient becoming paraplegic and incontinent within hours or days of the onset of symptoms. The neurologic symptoms often precede the discovery of the neoplasm, and the illness is clinically and pathologically indistinguishable from idiopathic subacute necrotic myelopathy. Since epidural spinal cord compression from metastatic tumor or arteriovenous spinal cord anomalies may present similar clinical signs, a myelogram is essential to the diagnosis. In addition to the two aforementioned entities, many patients with carcinomatous cerebellar degeneration develop extensor plantar responses, mild sensory changes, and reflex asymmetries and weakness associated with degenerations of long tracts and anterior horn cells of the spinal cord. However, spinal cord symptoms do not predominate in these patients. Amyotrophic lateral sclerosis has been reported as a remote effect of cancer, but it is doubtful that it occurs in patients with cancer more often than in the general population.

Peripheral Nerves

Four clinical peripheral nerve disorders occur in association with cancer. Characteristic of carcinoma is a *subacute sensory* neuronopathy marked by loss of sensation with relative preservation of motor power. The illness sometimes precedes the appearance of the carcinoma and progresses over a few months, leaving the patient with a moderate or severe disability. The cerebrospinal fluid protein is usually elevated. Pathologically, there is destruction of posterior root ganglia with perivascular lymphocytic cuffing and wallerian degeneration of sensory nerves. Many of the patients have inflammatory and degenerative changes in brain and spinal cord as well. The entity is rare and there is no treatment.

More common than sensory neuropathy is a *distal sensorimotor polyneuropathy* characterized by motor weakness, sensory loss, and distal reflex absence in the extremities. The illness is pathologically characterized by either segmental demyelination or wallerian degeneration (or both) of sensory and motor peripheral nerves. Dorsal root ganglia are never involved to the same degree that they are in the purely sensory neuropathy. Pathologically and clinically, the sensorimotor neuropathy is indistinguishable from polyneuropathies not associated with cancer. Indeed, some have suggested that the late or terminal polyneuropathy may be due to nutritional deprivation associated with cancer. Its etiology, however, is not clear, and it does not respond to treatment with vitamins and other nutritional supplements. In one patient with progressive sensorimotor neuropathy associated with plasma cell dyscrasia producing a monoclonal IgM protein, the IgM was found to bind to peripheral myelin, and the patient improved after plasmapheresis and immune suppression.

A *polyneuritis* clinically and pathologically indistinguishable from acute postinfectious polyneuropathy (Guillain-Barré syndrome) also complicates cancer, particularly Hodgkin's disease, with impaired immunity. A few patients with *neuropathy limited to the autonomic nervous system* have been reported.

Neuromuscular Junction and Muscles

NEUROMUSCULAR JUNCTION. *Myasthenia gravis* is associated with thymomas but usually not other systemic tumors. However, a *"myasthenic syndrome"* occurs predominantly in men over 40 and is associated with intrathoracic tumors in 70 per cent of the patients (sometimes called the Eaton-Lambert syndrome). The patients complain of weakness and fatigability of proximal muscles, particularly of the pelvic girdle and thighs. The cranial nerves and respiratory muscles are involved less. In addition, patients complain of dryness of the mouth, impotence, pain in the thighs, and peripheral paresthesias. On examination there is weakness of the proximal muscles, but strength increases over several seconds of a sustained contraction. The deep tendon reflexes are diminished or absent. The diagnosis is made by electromyographic studies in which repeated nerve stimulations at rates above ten per second cause a progressive *increase* in the size of the muscle action potential (the opposite of myasthenia gravis). The neuromuscular defect in this illness is believed to be deficient release of acetylcholine. Similar findings have been produced in experimental animals by injection of either serum IgG or extract of tumor in patients with the disorder, suggesting an autoimmune etiology. Plasmapheresis and immune-suppressant drugs may relieve symptoms. The illness responds poorly to anticholinesterase drugs, but does respond to guanidine hydrochloride given in doses of 15 to 40 mg* per kilogram per day.

MUSCLE. Typical *dermatomyositis* or *polymyositis* may occur as a remote effect of cancer (Ch. 454). Fewer than 10 per cent of patients with this disorder have cancer, but the figure is higher in older patients. The clinical picture of polymyositis associated with cancer (i.e., subacute development of weakness, particularly involving proximal muscles and sometimes bulbar muscles) is indistinguishable from that of dermatomyositis or polymyositis not associated with cancer. Pathologically, however, there may be two groups: one with the typical inflammatory lesions of polymyositis, and one with little inflammation but severe muscle necrosis. The latter group may suffer an explosive clinical course. The patients respond somewhat less well to corticosteroid therapy than do those with dermatomyositis unaccompanied by cancer, although substantial improvement with steroid treatment does occur in some.

Muscle Weakness

Some patients with cancer complain of *weakness* and *fatigability* that seems worse than can be accounted for by their cancer alone. Cachexia and weight loss alone do not usually cause measurable muscle weakness. The weakness is usually proximal and produces particular difficulty climbing stairs or getting out of low chairs. Ankle reflexes may be diminished or absent. Further neurologic evaluation does not yield findings diagnostic of one of the remote effects of cancer described above. Brain and his colleagues have labeled this entity a "neuromyopathy" because its exact anatomic locus is unclear, but others have suggested that it is a nonspecific accompaniment of cachexia and systemic illness. Specific (type II) muscle fiber atrophy develops early in patients with systemic cancer. The cause and treatment of the weakness are unknown.

Henson RA, Urich H: Cancer and the Nervous System. Oxford, Blackwell Scientific Publications, Ltd., 1982. *Comprehensive and up-to-date descriptions of all of the paraneoplastic disorders affecting the nervous system.*

Vinken PJ, Bruyn GW (eds.): Handbook of Clinical Neurology, Vol 38, Neurological Manifestations of Systemic Disease, Part I. New York, Elsevier–North Holland, 1979. Chapters 26–28: *Reviews of encephalopathy, spinal cord, and peripheral nerve remote effects of cancer.* Chapters 3, 11: *Reviews on remote effects of cancer on the neuromuscular system.*

NERVOUS SYSTEM INJURY FROM THERAPEUTIC RADIATION

When parts of the nervous system are included within an ionizing irradiation portal, adverse effects may result (Table 174–2). The likelihood of adverse effects is related to the total dose of radiation, the size of each fraction, the total duration over which the dose is received, and the volume of nervous system tissue irradiated. Other factors, such as underlying nervous system disease (e.g. brain tumor, cerebral edema), previous surgery, concomitant use of chemotherapeutic agents, and individual susceptibility make it impossible to define precisely a safe dose for any given individual. However, general guidelines allow the radiation therapist to calculate generally safe nervous system doses. Adverse effects may involve any portion of the central or peripheral nervous system and may occur acutely or be delayed weeks to years following irradiation.

*May exceed manufacturer's recommended maximum dosage.

TABLE 174–2. RADIATION INJURY TO THE NERVOUS SYSTEM

Time After RT	Organ Affected	Clinical Findings
Primary injury		
Immediate (min to hrs)	Brain	Acute encephalopathy
Early-delayed (6–16 wks)	Brain	Somnolence, focal signs
	Spinal cord	Lhermitte's sign
Late-delayed (mos to yrs)	Brain	Dementia, focal signs
	Spinal cord	Transverse myelopathy
	Peripheral nerves	Paralysis, sensory loss
Secondary injury (years)	Several	Brain, cranial and/or peripheral nerve sheath tumors
	Arteries (atherosclerosis)	Cerebral infarction
	Endocrine organs	Metabolic encephalopathy

CLINICAL MANIFESTATIONS. *Acute encephalopathy* may follow large radiation doses to patients with increased intracranial pressure, particularly in the absence of corticosteroid prophylaxis. Immediately following treatment, susceptible patients develop headache, nausea and vomiting, somnolence, fever, and occasionally worsening of neurologic signs, rarely culminating in cerebral herniation and death. Acute encephalopathy usually follows the first radiation fraction and becomes progressively less severe with each ensuing fraction. This disorder is believed to result from increased intracranial pressure and/or brain edema from radiation-induced alteration of the blood-brain barrier. It responds to corticosteroids. Acute worsening of neurologic symptoms does not occur after spinal cord irradiation.

Early-delayed encephalopathy or myelopathy appears 6 to 16 weeks after therapy and persists for days to weeks. In children, the encephalopathy commonly follows prophylactic irradiation of the brain for leukemia and is called the "radiation somnolence syndrome." The disorder is characterized by somnolence, often associated with headache, nausea, vomiting, and sometimes fever. The electroencephalogram may be slow, but there are no focal signs. In adults, the syndrome usually follows whole-brain irradiation for brain tumors and is characterized by lethargy and worsening of focal neurologic signs. Both disorders usually respond to steroids but if untreated will resolve spontaneously. In adults, the syndrome may be distinguished from recurrent brain tumor by CT scan. In children, lumbar puncture rules out the potential diagnosis of meningeal leukemia. *Early-delayed myelopathy* follows radiation therapy to the neck or upper thorax and is characterized by Lhermitte's sign (an electric shock–like sensation radiating into various parts of the body when the neck is flexed). The symptoms resolve spontaneously. Early-delayed radiation syndromes are believed to result from demyelination, possibly due to radiation-induced damage to oligodendroglia.

Late-delayed radiation injury appears months to years following radiation and may affect any part of the nervous system. In the brain, there are two clinical syndromes. The first follows whole-brain irradiation either to patients without brain tumors (prophylactic irradiation for oat cell carcinoma) or in some patients with primary and metastatic brain tumors. The disorder is characterized by dementia without focal signs. There is cerebral atrophy on CT scan, pathologic changes are nonspecific, and there is no treatment. The second disorder affects patients who receive either focal brain irradiation during therapy of extracranial neoplasms or whole-brain irradiation for intracranial neoplasms. Neurologic signs suggest a mass and include headache, focal or generalized seizures, and hemiparesis. Brain CT scans reveal a hypodense mass, sometimes with contrast enhancement. Neuropathologic features include coagulative necrosis of white matter, telangiectasia, fibrinoid necrosis and thrombus formation, and glial proliferation and bizarre multinucleated astrocytes. The clinical and CT findings cannot be distinguished from brain tumor, and the diagnosis can be made only by biopsy. Corticosteroids sometimes ameliorate symptoms. The treatment, if the disorder is focal, is surgical removal. *Late-delayed myelopathy* is characterized by progressive paralysis, sensory changes, and sometimes pain. A Brown-Sequard syndrome (weakness and loss of proprioception in the extremities of one side with loss of pain and temperature sensation on the other) is often present at onset. Patients occasionally respond transiently to steroids, and the disorder may stop progressing, but generally patients become paraplegic or quadriplegic. Pathologic changes include necrosis of the spinal cord. *Late-delayed neuropathy* may affect any cranial or peripheral nerve. Common disorders are blindness from optic neuropathy and paralysis of an upper extremity from brachial plexopathy after therapy for lung or breast cancer. The pathogenesis is probably fibrosis and ischemia of the plexus. There is no treatment.

Radiation-induced tumors, including meningiomas, sarcomas, or, less commonly, gliomas, may appear years to decades after cranial irradiation and may follow even low-dose radiation therapy. Malignant or atypical nerve sheath tumors may follow irradiation of the brachial, cervical, and lumbar plexuses. The central nervous system may also be damaged when radiation alters extraneural structures. Radiation therapy accelerates *atherosclerosis*, and cerebral infarction associated with carotid artery occlusion in the neck may occur many years after neck irradiation. *Endocrine* (pituitary, thyroid, parathyroid) dysfunction from radiation may be associated with neurologic signs. Hypothyroidism often presents as a neurologic disorder, and hyperthyroidism or hyperparathyroidism from radiation may also cause an encephalopathy.

Gilbert HA, Kagan AR (eds.): Radiation Damage to the Nervous System. A Delayed Therapeutic Hazard. New York, Raven Press, 1980. *A comprehensive description of all of the nervous system side effects of therapeutic irradiation.*

175. CUTANEOUS MANIFESTATIONS OF INTERNAL MALIGNANCY

Marie-Louise Johnson

Many changes in the skin are associated with malignancy and with a variety of other pathologic processes as well. The skin shares in the array of predispositions, interactions, and disruptions peculiar to the malignant process. It has the clear advantage of being easily observed and easily biopsied. The disadvantage is variability in the strength of the association of cutaneous signs with malignant diseases. Some skin changes are clear indicators of tumor; others merely arouse grave suspicion. But one successful correlation of a skin sign as a benign surface indicator of a previously unsuspected internal malignancy, curable because of early discovery, reinforces the value of a thorough knowledge of these associations. A better understanding of the pathogenetic mechanisms linking skin changes to internal malignancy might also enhance our understanding of the biology of neoplasia.

Skin signs of internal malignancy are remarkably diverse. They may range from pruritus to diffuse pigmentation; they may be an extension of the tumor itself, or a common dermatosis in an uncommon presentation. For some signs the pathogenicity is clear, but for many it is not. For several the association is merely suspected because of concurrent start, a parallel course, or a uniformity of the type of associated neoplasm. Those skin changes that result from the obstructive aspects of tumor as with jaundice, or from hormone excess or deficiency as with endocrine tumors, will be left to the chapters concerned with those malignancies.

TUMOR. Internal malignancy may extend or metastasize to the skin. Primary lesions in lung or bone can appear by direct lymphatic extension but usually not until the primary is of considerable size. Metastatic lesions, however, may be the first sign of tumor. As solitary papules or nodules, firm or hard, and often of innocent appearance, they are found freely movable in the skin or just beneath it. One notable exception is the inflammatory sclerosing breastplate of cutaneous metastases, the carcinoma en cuirasse, that occurs with malignancy of the breast. Another is the pulsatile nodule of carcinoma of the kidney or thyroid.

Of all patients with metastatic disease, 3 to 5 per cent have metastases to the skin. In order of decreasing frequency, the metastatic tumors will originate from breast, stomach, lung, uterus, kidney, and, less often, colon, prostate, ovary, or testicle. The location of a skin metastasis is important. If the metastasis is to the abdominal wall, the most common primary site is lung, stomach, or kidney in men, and ovary in women; if to the scalp—lung, kidney, or breast; if to the thorax—lung or breast; if to the face—carcinoma of the oropharynx; if to the extremities—melanoma.

With myelomonocytic leukemia, cellular infiltrates of the skin develop into pink to purple papules, which later grow into nodules that ulcerate. In acute granulocytic leukemia the myeloperoxidase in the infiltrating leukemic cells can lend a pathognomonic greenish color, the so-called chloroma. Dermal or subcutaneous nodules can occur secondary to an internal lymphoma, most often with histiocytic lymphoma and lymphoblastic lymphoma. In Hodgkin's disease, cutaneous papules and nodules are rare. Mycosis fungoides, the T cell lymphoma most common in the skin, has plaques and tumefactions as a hallmark (Ch. 557).

Clearly, any skin nodule or plaque of obscure origin and uncertain diagnosis should be biopsied, especially if there are reasons to suspect malignancy.

NONTUMOR. Within the space available it is impossible to discuss individually the broad array of cutaneous lesions associated with internal malignancy. The purpose of Table 175–1 is to assemble in a readily retrievable form the many cutaneous signs and syndromes that have an association with internal malignancy. Distinction is made between those of frequent association and those less frequent, with further separation of those inherited disorders that have cutaneous manifestations and a propensity toward the development of internal malignancy. Only a few selected examples will be discussed in the text.

Intense pruritus may be associated with lymphoma or Hodgkin's disease. It is often refractory to all therapy except the successful treatment, at least to remission, of the underlying disorder. The pruritus can be intolerable and unremitting. It may begin with the feet or legs, often associated with burning sensations, and then become generalized. Initially the skin may appear normal except for excoriations and the occasional papules or nodules that are the cutaneous response to the trauma of scratching. With leukemia, the normal-appearing skin may become erythematous until there is a generalized erythroderma or even exfoliation. The intensity and persistence of the pruritus are the strongest indicators of malignancy. Milder, intermittent itching can also occur with tumor, or herald it (as for example with malignancies of the gastrointestinal tract, bronchus, ovaries, and prostate), but the variability in severity and localization of the itching makes it a weaker signal. In the older patient, the most common cause of pruritus is dry skin. If the skin

TABLE 175–1. CUTANEOUS LESIONS ASSOCIATED WITH MALIGNANCY*

Lesion or Syndrome	Description and Distribution	Malignancy
	I. Malignancy Evident	
Stewart-Treves syndrome	Edematous upper extremity following radical mastectomy; livid or dusky red blebs exuding fluid with lymph chemistries	Lymphangiosarcoma
Paget's disease	Marginated scaling of the nipple and areola	Breast
Bowen's disease (carcinoma in situ)	Circumscribed erythematous scaling plaque (if multiple on covered areas of body, arsenical ingestion?)	Urinary tract, bronchus, with arsenical ingestion
	II. Frequent Association	
Dermatomyositis (>40 yrs)	Heliotrope erythema on eyelids, upper cheeks, forehead, temples; edema of hands and arms; scaly bluish-red plaques over knuckles; erythema of scalp and alopecia; cutaneous calcification	Breast, lung, gastrointestinal tract, genitourinary system, lymphoma
Leser-Trélat sign	Sudden development of a large number of seborrheic keratoses	Carcinoma of stomach
Extramammary Paget's disease	Erythematous to gray-white plaque which may be scaly, crusted, ulcerated, or papillary in appearance on vulva or perianal area	Rectum, cutaneous adnexal tumors
Urticaria pigmentosa	Multiple reddish-brown or yellow macules, papules, or nodules; heavily pigmented macules or erythroderma; macules urticate	Mast cell leukemia, systemic mastocytosis
Acquired hypertrichosis lanuginosa	Long, fine, silky hair on face and other sites normally clinically hairless (does not involve palms and soles)	Bronchus, gallbladder, rectum, bladder
Acquired pachydermoperiostosis	Skin of forehead and scalp thickened and thrown into folds; skin of hands and feet thickened; increased sebaceous activity on face and scalp	Bronchus, stomach, esophagus, thymus, mesothelioma
von Hippel-Lindau syndrome	Angiomas	Hypernephroma, pheochromocytoma
Carcinoid	Telangiectasias on face and upper trunk; hyperpigmentation (gray-black) on legs, forearms, trunk with hyperkeratosis; yellow-brown pigmentation on forehead, back, wrists, and thighs	Metastatic carcinoids
Necrolytic migratory erythema	Dermatitis of two forms: (1) generalized symmetrical dermatitis initially eczematous over perineum, buttocks, and extremities; (2) erythematous areas with central blister formation progressing to central crusting and healing, followed by hyperpigmentation of perineum, buttocks, groin, lower abdomen, and lower extremities	Glucagonoma
Erythema gyratum repens	Irregular wavy bands with peculiar gyrate or serpiginous outline, with marginal desquamation on trunk, neck, and extremities	Breast, lung, tongue
Acanthosis nigricans	Confluent hyperpigmented, hyperkeratotic verrucosities in body folds, especially axillae, nipples, and umbilicus; diffuse keratoderma of palms and soles (Pachydermatoglyphy)	Adenocarcinoma of stomach, pancreas, colon, lung, breast, uterus, ovary, rectum, cystic and hepatic ducts
Acrokeratosis paraneoplastica (Bazex syndrome)	Erythematous, psoriasiform scaling fingers, toes, often symmetrical; then aural helices; violaceous scaling dermatitis over bridge of nose; may extend to extremities	Pharyngolaryngeal region, esophagus, tongue, lower lip, apical segment of lungs
Vinyl chloride disease	Acrosclerosis with or without osteolysis and papular skin lesions	Angiosarcoma
Torre's syndrome	Multiple sebaceous adenomas of trunk	Gastrointestinal
Dominant inheritance:	*Recognized as Inherited Disorders:*	
Gardner's syndrome	Epidermal inclusion cysts and sebaceous cysts on scalp and face (trunk)	Colon
Cowden's syndrome	Warty papules and nodules on central face, oral mucosa, hands, and dorsal forearms	Breast, thyroid, female reproductive
Multiple endocrine neoplasia, Type III	Multiple neuromas of lips, eyelids, nares, and anterior two thirds of tongue (pink nodules)	Thryoid, pheochromocytoma
Autosomal recessive:		
Ataxia telangiectasia	Telangiectasia on bulbar conjunctiva → ears, eyelids, cheeks, limbs; hair may be prematurely gray	Reticulum cell sarcoma, lymphosarcoma, Hodgkin's disease, gastric
Sex-linked recessive:		
Wiskott-Aldrich syndrome	Eczematous lesions on scalp, face, flexures, and buttocks; purpura on skin and mucous membranes	Reticuloendothelial
	III. Occasional Association	
Congenital nevi	Sebaceous nevus—circumscribed, slightly raised hairless plaques of orange-yellow which become verrucous and nodular in puberty; bathing trunk nevus or other congenital pigmented nevus—dark brown and raised surface which is irregular with small mammillary projections (may have hair, well defined margins); nevus verrucosus and nevus unius lateris—skin colored or yellow-brown with rough warty surface, more often on limbs and trunk	Melanoma, basal cell epithelioma, squamous cell carcinoma
Alopecia mucinosa	Well demarcated, slightly raised plaque which is erythematous and indurated; may have fine scale—face, neck, head	Mycosis fungoides, lymphomas
Nodular liquefying panniculitis (with pancreatitis)	Tender subcutaneous erythematous nodules, lower legs and thighs occasionally	Pancreatic carcinoma
Erythroderma	Generalized erythematous skin with scaling	Lymphoma, lung, rectum, leukemia
Erythema annulare centrifugum	Small pink papule slowly enlarges to form a ring; as the central area flattens and fades, may attain diameter of 6 to 8 cm; buttocks, thighs, upper arms	Variable; skin lesions reported to disappear with excision of malignancy and to reappear with recurrence or metastases
Thrombophlebitis migrans	Successive crops of tender, linear, and oval nodules affecting large and small vessels throughout the body	Lung, pancreas, breast, colon, stomach
Systemic amyloidosis	Small, glistening papules on eyelids, central area of face, lips, and tongue; macroglossia; nodules in auditory meatus and body flexures; small hemorrhages induced by stroking skin; may have leonine facies due to plaques	Multiple myeloma
Reticulohistiocytoma	Small, firm, pink, moderately pruritic papules or nodules on dorsa of hands, forearms, scalp, face, ears, trunk, and mucosa of lip; fluctuates in severity	Sarcoma, gastric, colon, lung
Cushing's syndrome	Redistribution of subcutaneous fat, vascular fragility, moon face, striae, hirsutism, obese trunk and slender limbs	Oat cell of lung, pituitary, hypothalamus, adrenal
Acquired ichthyosis	Usually starts at the legs; generalized dry, cracking skin; hyperkeratotic palms and soles; alopecia	Hodgkin's disease
Acanthosis palmaris	Late onset, noninherited hyperkeratosis and acanthosis of palms, fingers ("tripe palms")	Bronchogenic carcinoma

TABLE 175–1. CUTANEOUS LESIONS ASSOCIATED WITH MALIGNANCY* (*Continued*)

Lesion or Syndrome	Description and Distribution	Malignancy
	III. Occasional Association (Continued)	
	Recognized as Inherited Disorders:	
Dominant inheritance:		
Tylosis	Late onset keratosis palmaris et plantaris; diffuse palmar and plantar hyperkeratoses with hyperhidrosis	Esophageal
Neurofibromatosis (von Recklinghausen)	Café-au-lait spots; axillary freckles; white macular areas; multiple tumors which may be small to large, soft to firm, most numerous on trunk and limbs—rare (elephantiasis neuromatosa—wrinkled and pendulous skin with overgrowth of subcutaneous tissue along nerve trunk with diffuse neurofibromatosis)	Sarcomas, pheochromocytomas, astrocytomas, gliomas
Peutz-Jeghers-Touraine syndrome	Discrete mucocutaneous pigmentation, including lips, face, buccal mucosa, and hands; brown-black, discrete macular lesion 2 to 5 mm	Malignancy proximal to ligament of Treitz
Tuberous sclerosis	Adenoma sebaceum—firm discrete, yellow or telangiectatic papules 1 to 10 mm extend from nasolabial fold, occasionally in the ear; periungual fibroma and smooth firm, flesh-colored excrescences emerging from nailbeds (5 to 10 mm); shagreen patch—irregular soft, elevated plaque in lumbosacral area; ash leaf spots; poliosis	Brain, rhabdomyoma
Nevoid basal cell carcinoma syndrome	Multiple basal cell carcinomas, epidermoid cysts, "pits" of palms and soles	Medulloblastoma, fibrosarcoma of jaw
Autosomal recessive:		
Bloom's syndrome	Erythema of face most pronounced in butterfly area—may involve margins of eyelids, forehead, and ears; sunlight may provoke bullae, bleeding, and crusting	Leukemia
Chédiak-Higashi syndrome	Lightened color of skin, hair—pyodermas, giant melanosomes	Lymphoma
Werner's syndrome	Premature aging, early graying, balding, scleroderma-like changes, leg ulcers	Sarcoma, meningioma
Sex-linked recessive:		
Dyskeratosis congenita	Dystrophic nails, suppurative paronychia, fine reticulate gray-brown pigment on neck, thighs, and involving greater part of trunk with telangiectasias; face is red and atrophic with irregular macular pigmentation; mucous membranes—bullae, erosions, and leukoplakia; hands and feet—atrophic shiny skin; palms and soles may be hypohidrotic and form bullae with trauma	Carcinoma develops in area of leukoplakia (squamous cell)

*Compiled with Dr. Virginia Fallon-Pellicci.

appears normal, however, and there is no underlying thyroid disease or diabetes, and if the pruritus is new and unresponsive to simple measures, then malignancy should be suspected.

Paget's disease of the breast is almost invariably associated with underlying intraductal adenocarcinoma (see Ch. 556). Dusky papules arising on a persistently edematous upper extremity following radical mastectomy are lymphangiosarcoma until proved otherwise *(Stewart-Treves syndrome)*. Nodules arising in a *giant pigmented hairy nevus*, or under a skin graft in an area where a nevus was removed, are almost certainly melanoma (see Ch. 557).

A number of other skin lesions exhibit frequent association with malignancy when they appear in previously normal persons. They are distinct from those cutaneous markers that identify an antecedent syndrome or inherited diathesis that places a patient at greater risk of malignancy. The pathogenesis of malignancy with concomitant or antecedent cutaneous change can have a perplexing relationship, as in the onset of weakness with the heliotrope erythema of *dermatomyositis* (see Ch. 454). Associated with malignancy in those over 40 years of age, and slightly more often in men, the dermatomyositis often precedes the appearance of the tumor by as much as six months, but they may appear together.

The circumscribed scaling erythematous lesion of *Bowen's disease* is itself a squamous cell carcinoma in situ (see Ch. 556), but at the same time it is an example of an indicator of underlying malignancy. If evoked by arsenical exposure, the lesion indicates a patient at risk of malignant change of the respiratory, genitourinary, or gastrointestinal tracts. Here an exogenous carcinogen has endangered multiple organs, but it is in the skin where the change is most visible. The average latent period for the development of the visceral malignancy is eight years. The signal is stronger when the cutaneous lesion occurs on a sun-protected area where there can be no supplemental actinic effect.

The stigmata of ionizing radiation in the skin suggest the possibility of underlying malignant change: carcinoma of the thyroid if there is a nodule under x-ray–damaged skin of the neck, or an increased risk of lymphoma if the radiation changes are of the back and the treatment was for ankylosing spondylitis.

Acanthosis nigricans in the epidermotrophic form is another important sign of malignancy. The clinical and histologic appearance of the verrucous velvety change of the body folds are the same in the adult-onset, malignancy-linked form as in that induced by genetodevelopmental defects or friction maceration (see Ch. 556). The appearance of acanthosis nigricans may precede the malignancy (20 per cent), follow it (20 per cent), or be noted simultaneously (60 per cent). Regression of the skin sign has been observed following therapy for the malignancy, and reappearance with reactivation of the tumor. The stomach is the most common site of malignancy (two thirds), but it may appear elsewhere in the gastrointestinal tract and less often in the ovaries, prostate, breast, or lung. There are rare reports of association of acanthosis nigricans with lymphomas and squamous cell carcinoma. The cause of the skin change is unknown, but a circulating epidermotrophic factor is suspected.

Color changes of the skin are nonspecific indicators of malignant diseases. The pallor of anemia, the flush of carcinoid, the dusky erythema of polycythemia, and the hyperpigmentation secondary to excessive MSH or MSH-like peptides all can be associated with malignancy, but they may not be. The same holds true for the altered keratinization limited to the palms and soles or generalized, and for the erythemas: generalized exfoliative erythroderma, erythema nodosum, and urticaria. The reader is referred to the table for a summary of these interesting and often clinically useful associations.

Braverman IM: Skin Signs of Systemic Disease. 2nd ed. Philadelphia, W. B. Saunders Company, 1981. *Excellent focus on skin signs of malignancy.*

176. PRINCIPLES OF CANCER THERAPY

Bruce A. Chabner

During the past two decades, fundamental changes have taken place in the treatment of cancer. Once an undertaking with limited therapeutic goals and expectations, the treatment of cancer is now increasingly effective on the basis of a clearer understanding of the biology of malignant cells and the development of new drugs and more effective radiotherapy and surgery. Many advanced malignancies affecting younger age groups, such as the lymphomas, choriocarcinoma, testicular cancer, and childhood leukemia, can often be cured by drug therapy with or without irradiation. The solid neoplasms of later life, particularly the adenocarcinomas originating in the gastrointestinal tract and lung, remain a formidable therapeutic challenge in which the potent toxicities and risks of aggressive therapy must be carefully weighed against the limited benefits likely to result. This chapter will consider the basic biologic and pharmacologic principles that govern the selection of a therapeutic plan for patients with cancer. The treatment of patients with specific tumors will be discussed elsewhere.

The objectives of cancer treatment are not the same for all patients and all diseases. They are conditioned by an appreciation of the potential for cure or palliation and an assessment of the patient's tolerance to the side effects of possible treatments. For example, although curative chemotherapy exists for a substantial fraction of patients with diffuse histiocytic lymphoma, not all patients with this diagnosis are appropriate candidates for intensive therapy. Some patients have serious underlying medical problems, such as heart disease, or a pattern of tumor involvement, such as diffuse gastrointestinal metastasis, that precludes effective treatment. In such cases, the physician must weigh the chances of successful treatment against the probability of life-threatening side effects, and must discuss these conditions frankly with the patient and family. At times, less intensive treatment or only supportive care with pain control and psychologic support may be the wisest therapeutic choice.

Palliation of symptoms and attention to the details of good medical care are often neglected in patients who have reached an incurable phase of their illness. Detection and treatment of complications such as intestinal obstruction, brain metastases, and hypercalcemia, although not affecting the ultimate outcome of disease, may allow the patient extended periods of functional and pain-free life. Thus, it is vital for the physician to listen to his patient's complaints, to conduct periodic physical examinations, and to maintain a concerned and supportive relationship, despite his knowledge of the likely eventual outcome.

DETERMINANTS OF TREATMENT PLAN

The primary determinants in the choice of treatment are (1) the histologic diagnosis of the malignancy, (2) the stage or extent of disease (including specific sites of organ involvement), and (3) an assessment of the biologic features or specific growth characteristics of the individual tumor.

DIAGNOSIS AND CLASSIFICATION. Accurate pathologic diagnosis and classification of a tumor are obviously crucial. Correct histologic subtyping of tumors is similarly important for many tumors, such as the lymphomas, carcinoma of the lung, and testicular carcinoma. These general categories encompass disease types with variant patterns of clinical progression and response to treatment. *Histologic grading* is also required for an accurate prognosis and as a guide to therapy in some tumors. Biochemical characterization may be required to identify tumors, e.g., mediastinal malignant teratomas which contain marker proteins (β-subunits of human chorionic gonadotropin or α-fetoprotein); these features assist in distinguishing these from other undifferentiated carcinomas. Similarly, histiocytic lymphoma may be difficult to distinguish from an unusual primary occurrence of acute myeloid leukemia arising in lymph node or bone, unless appropriate touch preps and histochemical stains are examined. The distinction between various forms of lymphoid leukemias, such as B cell chronic lymphocytic leukemia (CLL), T cell CLL, and hairy cell leukemia, may require the use of cell-surface immunologic typing and histochemical staining for tartrate-resistant acid phosphatase, in addition to the usual histologic evaluation. The prognosis and treatment of each of these disorders are distinct and different. *The internist must always consider the possibility of alternative, treatable diagnoses, and must seek expert pathologic clarification before committing the patient to a plan of treatment.*

STAGING. In general, knowledge of the extent of a malignant disease *(staging)* is essential in order to plan effective treatment. In selected cases, staging procedures may pose inappropriate risks to the patient, and should never take precedence over necessary therapeutic intervention. For patients with life-threatening local complications of disease, such as upper airway obstruction, superior vena cava obstruction, or biliary obstruction, definitive staging should be delayed in order to administer surgical or local radiation therapy or chemotherapy.

Staging strategies are based on a knowledge of the natural history of disease, specifically its likely patterns of dissemination to regional and distant sites. In developing a staging plan, the morbidity of a given procedure must be balanced against its probable yield of positive information (the "risk-benefit ratio"). The procedure should be performed only if the results obtained would affect the treatment decision. For example, a procedure such as lymphangiography, which has a low morbidity in the absence of compromised pulmonary function, has great usefulness in lymphomas because of its high yield of positive results and the major impact of these results on treatment choice. In contrast, the staging laparotomy frequently employed to define intra-abdominal disease in Hodgkin's disease has only limited utility in non-Hodgkin's lymphomas. The latter diseases are usually disseminated at presentation and in advanced stages are not appropriately treated for cure with local therapeutic measures such as radiation therapy. For patients with solid tumors of epithelial origin (carcinomas), an orderly progression of disease occurs, first with involvement of local lymph nodes, and then dissemination to distant sites such as lung, bone, and liver. In such patients, the initial diagnostic workup usually includes bone and liver scans and chest x-ray; if these sites are free of tumor, a definitive surgical procedure is undertaken, with removal of the primary mass and adjacent lymph nodes. In general, the physician should resist the temptation to order batteries of duplicative tests, such as CT scans and ultrasound evaluations, or tests that have low yield in the absence of localizing symptoms, such as bone scans in asymptomatic patients with clinically localized breast cancer.

BIOLOGIC CHARACTERISTICS OF THE TUMOR. In planning a treatment program, the physician must also take into account the biologic characteristics of the tumor, and in particular its growth rate. Aggressive treatment is likely to be least beneficial and effective in tumors that contain a small fraction of actively dividing cells. Thus, certain patients with nodular forms of non-Hodgkin's lymphoma may give a clinical history indicating extremely indolent clinical behavior of the tumor over a period of several years. These patients are unlikely to be cured by aggressive treatment, and many can be safely followed without treatment. In contrast, other patients with the same diagnosis may have a more aggressive clinical course indicating a need for early aggressive combination chemotherapy. In summary, although the clinical impression of tumor growth rate is not frequently used as a determinant of a therapeutic choice, it may be an important criterion in determining when to begin chemotherapy in patients with nodular lymphomas, chronic lymphocytic leukemia, and other "indolent" types of malignancy.

The foregoing information concerning pathology, stage, and clinical progression must then be synthesized to yield a clear understanding of the clinical circumstances at the time of making a decision about treatment. At this point, certain questions must be faced: (1) Is cure possible and, if so, by what therapies? What are the possible short-term and long-term side effects of the various alternative therapies? (2) If cure is impossible, is significant prolongation of survival possible and, if so, at what cost to the patient's sense of well-being and his or her ability to derive satisfaction from daily life? (3) Is palliation of

TABLE 176–1. COMBINED MODALITY THERAPY OF SOFT TISSUE SARCOMA*

Aim	Therapeutic Procedure	Rationale
Control of primary tumor	1. Wide local excision	Removal of bulk tumor and preservation of limb function
	2. High-dose local radiation	Sterilization of residual microscopic tumor implants of moderately radiosensitive tumor
Prevention of distant recurrence	Adjuvant chemotherapy with doxorubicin, cyclophosphamide, methotrexate	Metastases are most sensitive to treatment at low tumor burden

*From Rosenberg SA, Kent H, Costa J, et al.: Surgery 84:62, 1978.

symptoms a more reasonable objective than undertaking high-risk, life-threatening treatment? In no other specialty of medicine is the treatment decision more influenced by the personal philosophies of physician and patient and their assessment of potential risks and benefits. Increasingly, conclusions from prospective clinical trials are providing a rational basis for making these decisions, but there is no single simple answer for all patients with the same diagnosis.

MANAGEMENT OF LOCAL-REGIONAL DISEASE

CANCER SURGERY. Prior to the advent of radiotherapy in the 1920's and chemotherapy in the 1950's, cancer treatment was the exclusive province of the surgeon. Cancer surgery for localized tumors was and still is based on the principle of establishing tumor-free surgical margins whenever possible. Current treatment often calls for integration of surgery with radiotherapy or chemotherapy in order to preserve bodily function and to prevent distant metastases. As examples, limited, limb-sparing surgery with high-dose irradiation may be used for soft tissue sarcomas of the extremities (Table 176–1) and surgical biopsy followed by local irradiation for breast cancer primary tumors that are small. Evidence now indicates that simple mastectomy or "lumpectomy" with irradiation is as effective as radical mastectomy in local control of breast lesions less than 5 cm in diameter (see Ch. 138). The internist and radiotherapist should participate in treatment planning before definitive surgical procedures are undertaken.

Surgical resection of regional lymph nodes is performed for both diagnostic and, less frequently, therapeutic reasons. In some instances—e.g., testicular carcinoma with occult retroperitoneal lymph node metastases and in carcinomas of the head and neck—radical lymphadenectomy may be curative. In most other carcinomas (breast carcinoma, malignant melanoma, and colonic carcinoma), lymph node dissection provides important staging information, but, if lymph nodes are positive, the operation is usually not curative because of the strong association between nodal metastases and later relapse in distant sites. This prognostic information is of particular benefit for diseases in which effective adjuvant therapy is available. In breast cancer, gastric carcinoma, and rectal carcinoma, lymph node dissection has become a staging, rather than a purely therapeutic, procedure. Its findings are critical in making the decision of whether to use adjuvant chemotherapy

While the role of surgery for treatment of local and regional disease has been modified to accommodate multimodality strategies, its employment in patients with disseminated disease has expanded. Early and aggressive resection of pulmonary metastases in patients with osteogenic sarcoma or soft tissue sarcoma has led to improved survival rates and occasional cures. Surgical resection of solitary intracranial metastases is clearly indicated for patients with breast cancer or malignant melanoma if this lesion is the sole site of metastatic disease. Reduction of tumor bulk by surgery, while not curative in its own right, may increase recruitment of previously dormant cells into active DNA synthesis and thereby render the residual tumor more susceptible to chemotherapy. It may also remove a source of tumor antigen and allow improved host immune response to the remaining neoplasm.

In summary, the specific indications for surgery clearly vary with clinical diagnosis and overall circumstances and need not be restricted to primary curative treatment of nonmetastatic disease.

RADIATION THERAPY. As an alternative to surgery, radiation therapy possesses significant advantages for locoregional treatment of malignancy, because it produces less acute morbidity and loss of function of the affected body part. Radiotherapy causes its biologic effect through the formation of ion pairs or reactive oxygen metabolites such as superoxide, H_2O_2, or hydroxyl radicals. These products cause breaks in DNA, which, if not repaired, may lead to cell death. Mutagenesis and carcinogenesis, resulting from sublethal effects of radiation on DNA, are other recognized late effects of radiation therapy. Radiation therapy may be delivered in the form of electromagnetic waves, such as x-rays or gamma rays, or as particle streams, such as heavy ions, protons, neutrons, pi mesons, or electrons. The characteristics of these forms of radiation, given in Table 176–2, have important implications for their clinical use. Low energy x-rays, or *kilovoltage* x-rays, yield their energy readily as they pass through tissue, and consequently cause considerable damage to skin and normal tissues overlying deep-seated tumors. Higher energy x-rays, generated by linear accelerators, and gamma radiation generated by a ^{60}Co-machine, cause less skin damage, a significant advantage in the treatment of visceral tumors such as gastrointestinal carcinomas, brain tumors, or carcinoma of the lung. Particle beams, particularly neutrons, heavy ions, and pi mesons, have the further advantage of depositing their energy in a sharply focused peak below the skin surface (Fig. 176–1).

The biologic effects of conventional x-ray therapy in both the kilovoltage and megavoltage energy range are greatly enhanced by the presence of oxygen. Hypoxic cells, as found in the poorly vascularized centers of large tumors, are relatively insensitive to x-rays. In contrast, charged particle beams, such as heavy ions and protons, are less dependent on oxygen in their cytotoxic action. Thus, with respect to biologic action and dose distribution characteristics, particle therapy has significant theoretical advantages for treating large, poorly vascularized

TABLE 176–2. SOURCES AND CHARACTERISTICS OF RADIATION THERAPY BEAMS

Source	Energy Range (Volts)	Beam Character	Tissue Effect* Surface	Tissue Effect* Penetration	Tissue Effect* Scatter
Kilovolt†	$200–250 \times 10^3$	Electromagnetic	4^+	2^+	4^+
Cobalt-60†	1.5×10^6	γ-Particles	3^+	3^+	3^+
Linear accelerator†	$4–35 \times 10^6$	Electromagnetic	3^+	3^+	2^+
		Electron beam	4^+	1^+	1^+
Cyclotron or fast‡ neutron generator	14×10^6	Fast neutron	3^+	3^+	3^+
Proton accelerator‡	—	Negative pi meson	1^+	4^+	1^+
Implanted isotopes† (^{60}Co, ^{192}Ir, ^{137}Cs)	—	β-Particles or γ-particles	1^+	4^+	1^+
Heavy ion linear accelerator	—	α-Particles, neon, argon ions	1^+	4^+	1^+

*Relative tissue effect expressed on a scale of 1^+ (minimal) to 4^+ (maximal).
†In common clinical use.
‡Under experimental evaluation.

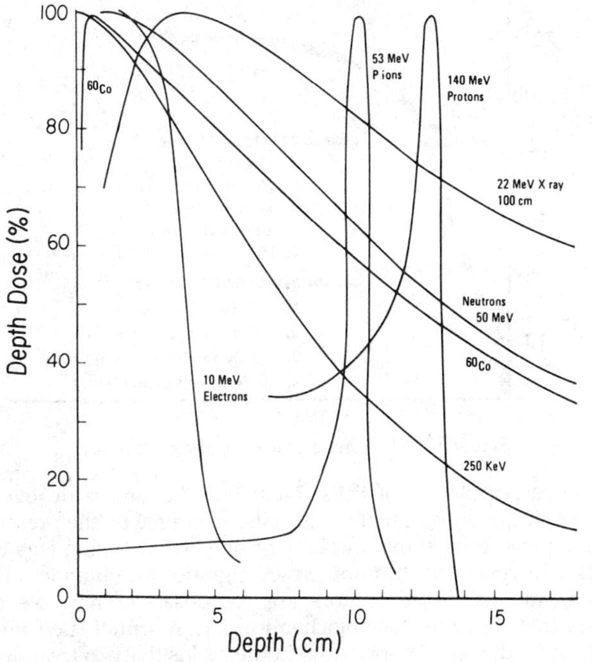

Figure 176–1. Penetration of various types of x-rays. Percentage of radiation dose absorbed at indicated depth below skin surface. MeV = million electron volts, KeV = thousand electron volts. (From Becker FF [ed.]: Cancer, A Comprehensive Treatise, Vol VI. New York, Plenum Press, 1977.)

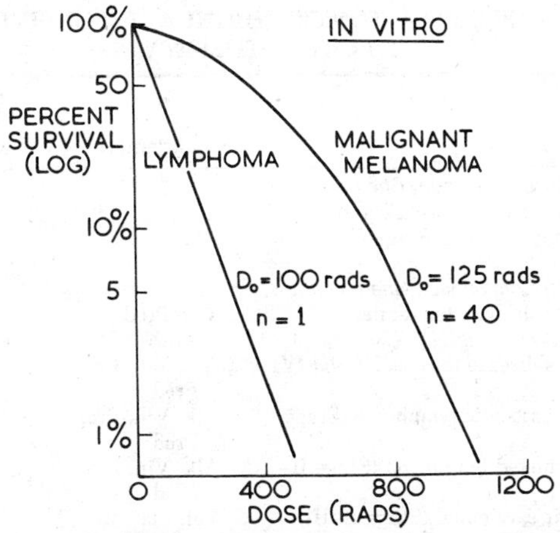

Figure 176–2. Curves demonstrating the sensitivity of lymphoma and malignant melanoma cells to radiation to tissue culture. D_0 refers to the slope of the cell kill curve, and is an index of the efficiency of cell kill; "n" is the extrapolation number, a rough measure of the shoulder of the killing curve. A high n value indicates an increased ability to repair radiation damage. The D_0 values for the two cell lines are approximately equal, but the more resistant melanoma cells have an increased repair capability, as reflected in the prominent shoulder and high "n" value. (From Becker FF [ed.]: Cancer, A Comprehensive treatise, Vol VI. New York, Plenum Press, 1977.)

visceral tumors. Clinical evaluation of the various types of particle therapy is incomplete at this time.

Radiotherapy is typically administered in fractionated doses of 150 to 250 rads per day, four or five days per week, for four to seven weeks. Fractionation produces an improved therapeutic index as compared with single large doses, possibly because of differences in the ability of normal and malignant cells to repair radiation-induced damage. All tissues are capable of repairing limited amounts of irradiation, although this tolerance varies considerably among normal tissues (Table 176–3). For single doses of radiation, a shoulder is observed in the curve that relates dose to cell kill (Fig. 176–2). The width of this shoulder is believed to reflect the ability of the cell to repair DNA breaks. In general normal cells have a broader radiation dose-response shoulder and therefore tolerate individual doses of radiation with less damage than do malignant cells. Fractionation of doses has the further advantage of allowing time for death of tumor cells in the interval between fractions; the reduction in tumor size is associated with improved oxygenation of formerly hypoxic tumor cells, rendering them more sensitive to subsequent radiation. The choice of fraction size is determined by the relative radiosensitivity of the tumor. Less sensitive tumors, such as malignant melanoma or sarcomas, are usually treated with larger individual fractions. Fraction size may also be determined by the rapidity with which a therapeutic effect is required.

Attempts have been made to identify drugs that enhance radiation effect (radiosensitizers) or selectively protect normal tissues (radioprotectors). The nitroimidazole class of compounds, including the common antitrichomonal drug metronidazole (Flagyl), sensitizes hypoxic cells in tissue culture by accepting free electrons and forming toxic free-radicals in a manner similar to oxygen. These compounds have little effect on the toxicity of radiotherapy for oxygenated cells, and thus do not appreciably increase toxicity to normal tissues. A second class of radiosensitizers, the halopyrimidines such as bromodeoxyuridine, is incorporated into DNA, which sensitizes the nucleic acid to strand breakage by irradiation. Clinical trials of such compounds have not been completed at this writing. An alternative approach is the use of protective compounds such as sulfhydryl compounds that interact with and detoxify the free-radicals produced by irradiation. These compounds would have to be selectively taken up by normal tissues to create a therapeutic advantage. Their use is still in the experimental stage.

Nonpharmacologic measures may also enhance radiation effects; these measures include hyperbaric oxygenation, which decreases the proportion of anoxic, and thus radioresistant, cells; and hyperthermia, which enhances toxicity to both normal and malignant cells. Neither of these ancillary measures has received thorough clinical trial.

TABLE 176–3. NORMAL TISSUE TOLERANCE TO RADIOTHERAPY

Tissue	Toxic Effect	Dose Limit (Rads)*
Bone marrow	Aplasia	250
Liver	Hepatitis	3000
Intestine	Ulceration, perforation, fibrosis	4500
Brain	Infarction, necrosis	6000
Spinal cord	Infarction, necrosis	4500
Heart	Pericarditis	4500
Lung	Pneumonitis, fibrosis	2500
Kidney	Nephrosclerosis	2000
Skin	Sclerosis, dermatitis	5500

*Radiation delivered in 200-rad fractions, five days per week, will produce a 5 per cent incidence of toxicity.

THE MANAGEMENT OF METASTATIC CANCER

Fewer than 25 per cent of patients with cancer are cured by local or regional forms of treatment. For the remainder, systemic therapy is used at some time during their illness, and in selected diseases and selected clinical situations this therapy may be curative (Table 176–4). In other diseases (Table 176–5), drug therapy produces a partial or complete regression in the majority of patients, and treatment is associated with a prolongation of survival. However, few of these patients are cured by chemotherapy, and relapse eventually leads to death. It has been estimated that approximately 50,000 cancer patients each year are cured by chemotherapy, either by treatment of clinically apparent metastatic disease or by adjuvant chemotherapy. The therapeutic index, or margin of safety between therapeutic and toxic drug doses, is extremely narrow for many of the effective compounds; thus, small changes in pharmacokinetics or increased patient sensitivity to drug action may lead to

TABLE 176–4. TUMORS HIGHLY RESPONSIVE TO CHEMOTHERAPY

	Agent(s)	Long-Term Disease-Free Survival (%)
Curable with Single-Agent Chemotherapy		
Choriocarcinoma (low-risk patients)	MTX	90
Burkitt's lymphoma (Stage I)	Alk	90
Curable with Combination Chemotherapy		
Acute lymphocytic leukemia	Vin, Pred, Anth	50
Hodgkin's disease (Stages III and IV)	Alk, Vin, Pro, Pred	50
Diffuse histiocytic lymphoma (Stage II–IV)	Alk, Vin, Pro, Pred	50
Nodular mixed lymphoma (Stage II–IV)	Alk, Vin, Pro, Pred	75
Testicular carcinoma (Stage II–III)	Vel, Plat, Bl	70–90
Childhood sarcomas (with radiation and surgery)	Act-D, Alk, Vin	70–90
Childhood lymphomas	Alk, Vin, Pred, Anth	75

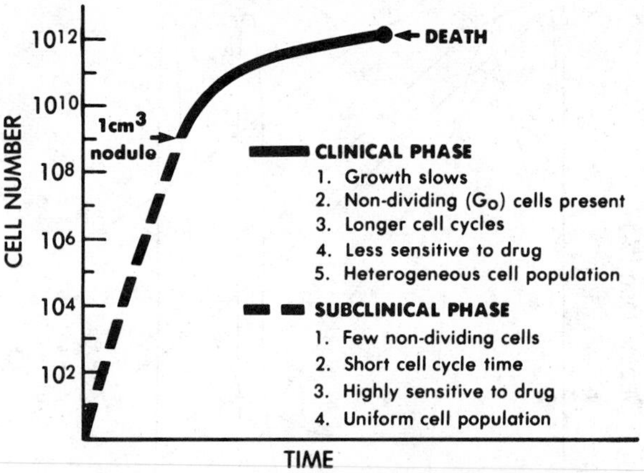

Figure 176–3. Kinetic phases of tumor growth.

unacceptable toxicity or death. In this setting, the clinician requires as much information as possible concerning the determinants of tumor cell kill, prediction of antitumor effects, pharmacokinetics, and drug interactions in order to maximize the effectiveness of therapy and to avoid needless toxicity.

The Kinetic Basis of Drug Therapy

FRACTIONAL KILL HYPOTHESIS. The kinetics, or growth cycle, of mammalian cells have been summarized in Ch. 168. In treating experimental tumors, a constant fraction of the total cell population is killed by a given dose of drug. Since each treatment cycle kills a specific fraction of the remaining cells, the results of treatment are a direct function of the dose of drug administered and the frequency with which treatment is repeated. However, because tumors in man are large and are composed of heterogeneous cell populations, the "fractional kill" hypothesis does not apply as well in this situation because the initial treatment will eliminate sensitive cells, leaving behind the more drug-resistant population. Most human neoplasms are diagnosed at an advanced stage when they contain a large fraction of slowly dividing or nondividing cells (termed G_0 cells) (Fig. 176–3). Since many antineoplastic agents are most effective against rapidly dividing cells, the initial kinetic stage is unfavorable for drug treatment. However, if the number of tumor cells can be reduced by surgical treatment or radiotherapy, the remaining cells are recruited into active proliferation and become increasingly susceptible to therapy with drugs. Through this mechanism, an initially slowly responding tumor may actually become more responsive to therapy as its size is reduced by treatment.

HETEROGENEITY OF HUMAN TUMORS. The fractional kill hypothesis assumes that tumors are composed of a uniformly sensitive population of cells. Most human tumors do evolve from a single clone of malignant cells, as judged by the presence of unique chromosomal markers or by G-6-PD typing (see Ch. 152). However, as tumors grow, significant mutation takes place, and advanced tumors are composed of multiple cell types that differ in their biochemical and morphologic characteristics and, most importantly, in their sensitivity to treatment. Drug-resistant cells are believed to arise from a parent-sensitive population by random mutation. The probability that a drug-resistant cell exists in a tumor is a function of the mutation rate for the drug-resistance gene and the absolute number of tumor cells. Thus, the chances for cure are greatest when the tumor population is smallest and least likely to contain treatment-resistant mutants. Also, combination therapies employing drugs with differing mechanisms of action are more likely to eradicate a tumor population than single-agent treatment, since a given cell is less likely to be simultaneously resistant to more than one agent.

CELL CYCLE IN TUMORS. Although precise information on the growth kinetics of human tumors is difficult to obtain, there appears to be a general correlation of sensitivity to drug treatment and the rate of tumor growth—i.e., the faster a tumor is growing, the greater is its sensitivity to drug therapy. In the past, the cell proliferation kinetics of tumor cells in individual patients could be determined only by laborious studies utilizing ^{3}H-thymidine labeling of tumor cells. A new experimental device, the flow microfluorometer, is able to determine the DNA content of individual cells, and translates this information into a profile of fraction of cells in each phase of the cell cycle. It is possible to obtain precise information on the fraction of dividing cells and the changes in cell cycle induced by treatment. Such measurement might be utilized in the future to select advantageous schedules for drug administration, and might provide important information on the likelihood of response to treatment.

PREDICTION OF DRUG RESPONSE. The selection of drugs for treating individual patients is primarily based on past experience in treating patients with the same histologic diagnosis and

TABLE 176–5. TUMORS RESPONSIVE TO CHEMOTHERAPY

	Agents	Partial or Complete Response (%)	Long-Term Disease-Free Survival (%)
Breast carcinoma (Stage III–IV)	MTX, FU, Alk, Anth	75	rare
Small cell carcinoma of the lung	Alk, MTX, Pro, Anth	90	10
Gastric carcinoma	FU, Anth, Mit	50	rare
Ovarian carcinoma	MTX, FU, Alk, Plat, Hex	75	10
Multiple myeloma	Alk, Pred, Vin, Anth	75	rare
Acute nonlymphocytic leukemia	Ara-C, Anth, Alk	75	10
Chronic lymphocytic leukemia	Alk, Pred	75	rare
Prostate cancer	H T	75	rare
Head and neck cancer	Bl, MTX, Plat	75	rare
Mycosis fungoides	Alk, MTX	75	rare

Combination therapy yields responses in majority of patients, but less than 25% have long-term disease-free survival. Median survival of treated patients is prolonged.

Agents: Act-D = actinomycin D; Anth = anthracycline (adriamycin or daunomycin); Alk = alkylating agents; Ara-C = cytosine arabinoside; Bl = bleomycin; H T = hormonal therapy; FU = 5-fluorouracil; Hex = hexamethylmelamine (investigational drug available from National Cancer Institute); MTX = methotrexate; Mit = mitomycin C; Plat = cis-platinum; Pred = prednisone; Pro = procarbazine; Vel = vinblastine (Velban); Vin = vincristine.

stage of disease. It would be highly desirable to be able to predict the sensitivity of individual tumors to treatment, and thus avoid needless toxicity of ineffective agents. It is now possible to grow certain types of malignant cells in culture in semisolid media, and to conduct drug sensitivity tests prior to treatment. Human ovarian cancer, breast cancer, renal cell carcinoma, malignant melanoma, and multiple myeloma all can be grown consistently. As presently performed, the human tumor stem cell assay has significant technical drawbacks, including: (1) a minority of solid tumor samples produces enough colonies to allow meaningful testing in vitro; (2) drugs requiring hepatic microsomal activation (cyclophosphamide, DTIC, mitomycin, hexamethylmelamine) cannot be tested in routine assay systems; and (3) the drug concentrations and durations of exposure used in vitro only roughly approximate clinical conditions. In practice, despite these shortcomings, in vitro tests demonstrating drug resistance are associated with a clinical lack of response in 96 per cent of such tests for patients with ovarian cancer, myeloma, and melanoma. However, predictions of sensitivity are associated with clinical response only 60 per cent of the time. Thus, in vitro sensitivity tests are more accurate in predicting tumor resistance than in predicting response. It is quite likely that in vitro test systems, with technical improvement, will become important future aids in the selection of cancer treatments.

BIOCHEMICAL TESTS. Biochemical tests based on the mechanism of drug action or mechanisms of tumor resistance are able to predict response in animal tumors, but have not been used extensively in clinical trials. A notable exception is the treatment of acute myeloblastic leukemia with cytosine arabinoside. The duration of complete remission in this disease may be predicted prior to treatment by the ability of leukemic cells to activate this drug to its triphosphate form. The response of leukemic cells to methotrexate is influenced by the intracellular concentration of the target enzyme dihydrofolate reductase. However, these biochemical tests have not been studied prospectively in a large patient population in order to prove their value in routine treatment. Thus, biochemical testing for drug sensitivity has made little impact on clinical chemotherapy, but offers a rational future approach.

HORMONE RECEPTORS. The most successful laboratory aid for predicting response is the measurement of hormone receptors as a guide for hormonal therapy of breast cancer. This topic will be considered in detail later in this chapter.

PHARMACOKINETIC DETERMINANTS OF RESPONSE

The outcome of cancer chemotherapy depends in large part on the inherent sensitivity of the tumor under treatment to the agents being used. However, pharmacokinetic factors such as drug absorption, metabolism, and elimination also influence response and are extremely variable from one patient to the next. Up to 10-fold variability in the bioavailability of orally administered 6-mercaptopurine, methotrexate, hexamethylmelamine,* and melphalan has been reported. In addition, elimination rates for commonly used agents may vary considerably, are not always predictable on the basis of abnormalities in renal or hepatic function, and may well account for the lack of response of tumors that are "sensitive" in vitro. Measurement of the plasma concentrations of a drug provides the best guide for dosage adjustment when reliable assays are available.

ASSESSMENT OF RESPONSE

An objective assessment of the response of a tumor to treatment is of central importance. Too often subjective impressions of improvement based on a patient's sense of well-being or performance status are not borne out by objective criteria. The standard criterion for partial response is a 50 per cent or greater reduction in the product of perpendicular diameters of all lesions measurable by physical examination or by radiologic techniques. A complete response denotes complete disappearance of disease, and in most diseases *should be documented by pathologic restaging if possible.* Pathologic restaging requires rebiopsy of previously involved organ sites. For tumors which secrete quantifiable marker proteins, such as gestational choriocarcinoma or germinal cell tumors of the testis, a fall of these markers to normal levels and a persistence at this level for two to three months is necessary for a judgment of complete remission. Even in the presence of normal markers, persistent abnormalities on chest film or computed scanning may still require biopsy. Partial responses rarely lead to significantly improved survival.

*Investigational drug available from National Cancer Institute.

STRATEGIES OF CLINICAL CHEMOTHERAPY

COMBINATION CHEMOTHERAPY. ***Background.*** The first effective drugs for treating cancer were introduced in the mid and late 1940's, but initial therapeutic results were disappointing. Although impressive regressions of acute lymphocytic leukemia and adult lymphomas were obtained with nitrogen mustard, antifolates, corticosteroids, and the vinca alkaloids, responses were only partial in degree and of short duration. Attempts at retreatment usually met with a diminished response or frank resistance to further therapy. Increased doses could not be given because of prohibitive bone marrow toxicity or neurotoxicity, and few patients derived lasting benefit. The introduction of combination chemotherapy for acute lymphocytic leukemia of childhood in the early 1960's marked a turning point in the effective treatment of neoplastic disease. Such combinations of chemotherapeutic agents are now the standard for the treatment of most advanced cancers.

Rationale. The principal rationale for combination chemotherapy derives from an appreciation of the reasons for failure of single-agent treatment: (1) Initial resistance to any given single agent is frequent, even in the most responsive tumors. (2) Initially responsive tumors rapidly acquire resistance after drug exposure. Drugs either induce resistance or select resistant mutants from an initially heterogeneous tumor cell population. Multiple agents with different mechanisms of action kill cells independently. Cells resistant to one agent might still be sensitive to the several other drugs in the regimen. If drugs have different, nonoverlapping toxicities, each can be used in full dosage in a combination regimen. For example, drugs such as vincristine, prednisone, bleomycin, and hexamethylmelamine, which lack bone marrow toxicity, are particularly valuable for combination with myelosuppressive agents. On the basis of these principles, curative combinations have been devised for acute lymphocytic leukemia (vincristine-prednisone ± Adriamycin and L-asparaginase), Hodgkin's disease (nitrogen *m*ustard–vincristine [*O*ncovin]–*p*rednisone–*p*rocarbazine; called MOPP), histiocytic lymphoma (C-MOPP), and testicular carcinoma (bleomycin–vinblastine–cis-platinum).

Scheduling. The scheduling of drugs in combinations was initially based on convenience and empirical experience. Intermittent cycles of therapy allow for periods of recovery of host bone marrow and immune function. More recent combinations have incorporated nonmyelosuppressive agents in the "off period" between doses of myelotoxic drugs. High-dose methotrexate with leucovorin rescue has proved to be particularly useful in this capacity in the "off period" because of its minimal effect on white blood cell and platelet counts. Logic dictates the initial use of cycle-nonspecific drugs, such as the alkylating agents or nitrosoureas (if active against the disease in question), in order to reduce tumor bulk and recruit slowly dividing cells into active DNA synthesis, then to be followed by cell cycle–dependent agents (such as methotrexate or the fluoropyrimidines). An example of such a regimen in which cycle-nonspecific drugs are followed by cycle-specific agents is shown in Table 176–6.

Drug Interactions. Drug interactions, both favorable and

TABLE 176–6. EXAMPLE OF DRUG SEQUENCES IN COMBINATION CHEMOTHERAPY—CAMF PROTOCOL FOR BREAST CANCER (UNDER EVALUATION AT NATIONAL CANCER INSTITUTE)

		Day		
	(mg/m²)	*1*	*8*	*9*
Cyclophosphamide	750	×		
Adriamycin	30	×		
Methotrexate	40		×	
5-Fluorouracil	500			×
Repeat every 21 days until disease becomes progressive				

Notable features:
1. Cytoreduction with cycle nonspecific agents on day 1
2. Cycle-specific drugs on day 8,9
3. Methotrexate precedes 5-fluorouracil to enhance 5-FdUMP and 5-FUTP formation

TABLE 176–7. EXAMPLE OF AN ALTERNATING CYCLE STRATEGY FOR COMBINATION CHEMOTHERAPY

Regimen (ProMACE)* For Diffuse Histiocytic Lymphoma	Day *1*	*8*	*14*	*15*	*16*	
Adriamycin, 25 mg/m²	×	×				Repeat cycles every four weeks for a maximum of 3 cycles or until maximal response; then MOPP (see Ch. 158) chemotherapy for an equal number of cycles; and finally "consolidation" with ProMACE, 2–3 cycles
Cyclophosphamide, 650 mg/m²	×	×				
VP-16, 120 mg/m²	×	×				
Prednisone, 60 mg/m²	daily	daily	daily			
Methotrexate, 1.5 grams/m² over 12 hours			×			
Leucovorin rescue				×	×	

Notable features:
1. Noncross-resistant drugs with independent actions
2. Intermittent, intensive cycles of therapy
3. Nonmyelosuppressive drugs in "off" period (day 14)
4. Treat to maximal response with ProMACE, then switch to noncross-resistant combination (MOPP)

*Fisher RI, DeVita V, Hubbard S, et al.: Ann Intern Med 98:304, 1983.

unfavorable, must be considered in developing combination regimens. Drugs such as cis-platinum and methotrexate, which cause renal toxicity, must be used with caution in combination since their excretion depends on normal renal function. The sequence of methotrexate with 5-fluorouracil is critical in determining the cytotoxicity of this combination in experimental systems. In cell culture, synergistic results are obtained when methotrexate precedes 5-fluorouracil by at least one hour, probably owing to increased activation of 5-fluorouracil to its nucleotide form. The opposite sequence (fluoropyrimidine, then methotrexate) leads to antagonistic results because of fluoropyrimidine block of the thymidylate synthetase pathway, which prevents accumulation of intracellular folates in the dihydrofolate form, and negates the effect of inhibition of dihydrofolate reductase by methotrexate (Fig. 176–4).

Adjustments within Combinations. All drug combination regimens require dose adjustment scales to allow increases or decreases of dose according to toxicity. It becomes difficult to determine which of the several agents is responsible if overlapping toxicity patterns are present. In this setting, arbitrary scales of dose adjustment according to bone marrow toxicity or other readily identifiable and quantifiable toxicity are usually provided with protocols.

New Strategies. In the first combination chemotherapy trials, such as MOPP chemotherapy of Hodgkin's disease, the overall strategy was to deliver intensive therapy over a finite time period and then to restage the patient to rule out the presence of occult residual disease. Treatment was discontinued in those having complete remission. The duration of unmaintained complete remission then served as an index of the completeness of response. In an effort to improve the long-term disease-free survival rate associated with cyclic chemotherapy, this basic strategy has been modified in the following ways:

1. Alternative combinations to the primary regimen have been identified by trials in patients resistant to the primary treatment. An example is the ABVD regimen for Hodgkin's disease, which incorporates four agents (Adriamycin, bleomycin, vinblastine, and DTIC) that are noncross-resistant with the MOPP drugs. The second regimen can then be used in alternating cycles of treatment with the primary combination, or one set of drugs can be used on day 1 and a second set on day 8 of a 28-day cycle.

2. A variant of the alternating cycle strategy is to treat patients with the primary regimen until a maximal response is obtained, and then to switch to a second combination. An example is shown in Table 176–7.

3. A third alternative is to use noncross-resistant agents for maintenance therapy, after induction of complete remission with the standard combinations.

COMBINED RADIATION AND CHEMOTHERAPY. Chemotherapy can often be usefully combined with other forms of treatment, such as irradiation or surgery. As an example, surgical resection of residual testicular carcinoma following chemotherapy leads to cure of a fraction of patients who would otherwise be only partial responders. There is evidence that the combination of irradiation and chemotherapy may improve the complete response rate and survival in patients with early Hodgkin's disease and in solid tumors of children.

Unfortunately, chemotherapy and radiotherapy have synergistic actions on *both* normal and malignant tissue, and this may lead to problems in their integrated use. The normal tissue of greatest concern is the bone marrow. Radiation given to the pelvic or midline abdominal areas produces a decline in blood counts and a decrease in bone marrow reserve. Appropriate shielding of the pelvic structures and the use of megavoltage radiation with limited scatter can preserve a significant portion of this marrow-bearing tissue. The sequence of administration may be of crucial importance. For example, chemotherapy followed by total nodal irradiation is less well tolerated because of severe myelosuppression in the radiation phase of treatment. One must anticipate cumulative effects of both chemotherapy and irradiation on bone marrow reserve.

Other examples of interactions between chemotherapeutic agents and irradiation are as follows: (1) Adriamycin and concurrent mediastinal irradiation enhance toxicity for the heart, esophagus, and lung. (2) Bleomycin enhances x-ray damage to pulmonary tissue. (3) Methotrexate may produce recall reactions in previously irradiated skin. (4) Prednisone suppresses the immediate reaction to pulmonary irradiation, but withdrawal of steroids may be associated with a serious flare in radiation-induced pneumonitis. Reduction of radiation dose or an alteration in drug dose or schedule may be necessary to avoid untoward effects.

The *carcinogenicity* of both radiotherapy and chemotherapy is

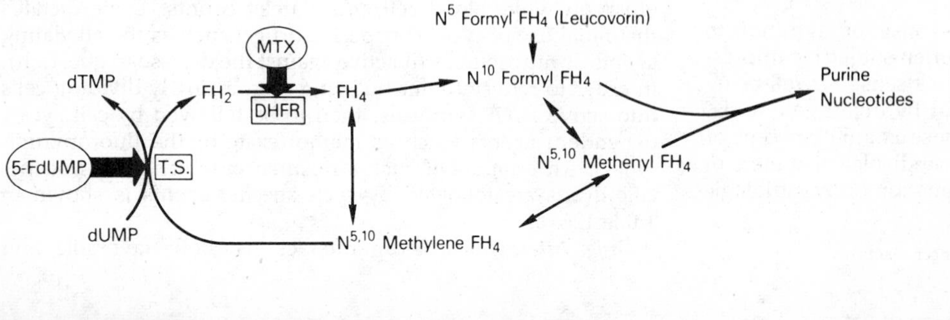

Figure 176–4. Sites of action of methotrexate (MTX) and 5-fluorodeoxyuridylate (5-FdUMP). DHFR = dihydrofolate reductase; T.S. = thymidylate synthetase; FH_2 = dihydrofolic acid; FH_4 = tetrahydrofolic acid. Note that MTX inhibition of DHFR affects the supply of FH_4-derived cofactors needed for both thymidylate (dTMP) and purine synthesis.

another negative consideration in their combined use. Agents listed in Table 176–8 are strongly suspected of being carcinogenic, based on (1) association with a high incidence of second malignancies in man, (2) proven carcinogenicity in animals, or (3) strongly positive mutagenicity in bacterial assays. Alkylating agents and procarbazine are highly carcinogenic in animals, and are strongly suspected of causing tumors in man. Irradiation is also strongly mutagenic and carcinogenic. The combination of alkylating agents and procarbazine with irradiation has led to an estimated 5 per cent incidence of second malignancies (most frequently acute myelocytic leukemia) in patients with Hodgkin's disease. The carcinogenic potential of specific regimens is difficult to quantitate because of the brief survival of many patients undergoing such treatment and uncertainty as to the number of patients at risk in retrospective studies. Nonetheless, there is sufficient evidence of irradiation-drug synergy to warrant caution in accepting combinations of irradiation and carcinogenic drugs, particularly for patients who have an excellent chance of cure or long-term survival by single modality treatment.

Both irradiation and chemotherapy are capable of producing *infertility.* Cyclophosphamide, chlorambucil, busulfan, melphalan, and procarbazine, as well as combination regimens, cause infertility in both males and females, often with permanent sterility. Adriamycin, cis-platinum, the vinca alkaloids, the antimetabolites, and the nitrosoureas have not been carefully studied in this respect. Drugs induce menopause most frequently in premenopausal women of the 40- to 49-year-old age group, as compared with younger women in whom the cessation of menses may be only temporary. In men, the development of azoospermia is usually but not always irreversible.

ADJUVANT THERAPY. Adjuvant therapy is treatment given after surgical resection of a primary tumor in an effort to prevent recurrence at distant sites. The need for adjuvant therapy arises from two sources: (1) the high recurrence rate of certain tumors following surgery for apparently localized disease (e.g., breast cancer, soft tissue sarcoma, osteogenic sarcoma, Dukes' B and C colonic cancer, level 3 to 5 malignant melanoma, and various solid neoplasms of childhood), and (2) the failure of chemotherapy or combined modality treatment to cure patients after recurrence of disease. Neoplastic cells are generally most susceptible to chemotherapy at their earliest stages of growth. This increased sensitivity of small tumors is based on a higher growth fraction and a shorter cell cycle time, and allows for a greater fractional cell kill for a given drug. As the same tumors enlarge, their growth fraction falls, the cell cycle time lengthens, and tumor cells become much less sensitive to treatment. In addition, patients are able to accept adjuvant chemotherapy with fewer complications because they are not debilitated by metastatic disease.

There are disadvantages of adjuvant therapy related to both short-term and long-term risks. An unidentifiable fraction of patients receiving adjuvant treatment will have been cured by the primary surgical procedure and therefore will be experiencing needless risks and toxicity. In considering adjuvant therapy, late complications such as carcinogenicity (Table 176–8) and sterility assume greater importance.

TABLE 176–8. CARCINOGENICITY OF ANTINEOPLASTIC AGENTS

	Second Tumors in Man	Carcinogen in Animals	Mutagen*
High risk:			
Cyclophosphamide	+	+	+
Melphalan	+	+	+
Chlorambucil	+	+	NR
Procarbazine	+	+	–
Methyl CCNU	+	+	NR
6-Mercaptopurine	+	+	+
Adriamycin	NR	+	+
Low risk:			
Methotrexate	–	–	–
Cytosine arabinoside	–	–	–
5-Fluorouracil	–	NR	–
Risk unknown:			
Bleomycin	NR	–	–
Cis-platinum	NR	NR	+
Actinomycin D	NR	–	+
Vincristine	NR	–	–
Vinblastine	NR	+	–

*Mutagen in Ames assay using *Salmonella typhimurium* testor strain and rat liver microsomes.

NR = not reported.

ANTINEOPLASTIC DRUGS

The effective and safe use of cancer chemotherapeutic agents requires a fundamental understanding of their action, pharmacokinetics, and toxicity in man. Primary reviews of antineoplastic drugs should be consulted for more detailed information.

ANTIMETABOLITES. ***Antifolates.*** Antimetabolites act as fraudulent substrates for vital biochemical reactions. The first antimetabolite to be used clinically was aminopterin, which has since been replaced by another folate analogue, *methotrexate,* which has more predictable clinical toxicity and at least equal clinical activity. Tetrahydrofolates, among other functions, carry one-carbon groups used in the synthesis of the purine nucleotides and thymidylate, which are precursors of DNA (Fig. 176–4). In the synthesis of thymidylate, N^{5-10} methylenetetrahydrofolate donates its one-carbon methylene group and at the same time is oxidized to dihydrofolate, an inactive form of folic acid. Methotrexate and its polyglutamate metabolites inhibit dihydrofolate reductase (Fig. 176–4), the enzyme responsible for reducing inactive dihydrofolate back to the active tetrahydrofolate form. The resulting deficiency of tetrahydrofolate (FH_4) blocks synthesis of thymidylate; at higher drug concentrations purine nucleotide synthesis ceases. The polyglutamate forms of methotrexate, particularly those with three or four additional glutamates, are preferentially retained within tumor cells and are potent inhibitors of a number of folate-dependent enzymes in addition to dihydrofolate reductase.

The biochemical effects of methotrexate can be reversed by administration of the reduced folate leucovorin (D,L-N^5-formyltetrahydrofolic acid). This leucovorin "rescue" prevents methotrexate toxicity to bone marrow and gastrointestinal epithelium if administered in sufficient doses within 36 hours after infusions of high doses of methotrexate. Methotrexate infusions of 6 to 36 hours in duration, and in total doses of 1500 mg per square meter* or greater, can be given safely if followed by leucovorin rescue. The dose of leucovorin required (usually 15 to 50 mg per square meter every 6 hours for 48 hours) depends on the methotrexate concentration at the time of rescue, and may have to be increased in patients with inadequate renal function and delayed drug elimination.

Tumor cells acquire resistance to antifolates by several different biochemical mechanisms. It is unclear which mechanism accounts for resistance in the clinical setting: (1) deletion of a high-affinity, carrier-mediated transport system for reduced folates, shared by methotrexate; (2) an increase in the concentration of dihydrofolate reductase; or (3) an altered reductase that fails to bind methotrexate. An increase in enzyme concentration owing to amplification of the reductase gene is readily induced by exposure of cells to gradually increasing drug concentration and then becomes a heritable characteristic of the resistant cell line. In attempts to overcome resistance, high doses of methotrexate (1500 mg per square meter* or greater) are given in 6- to 36-hour infusions, followed by repeat doses of the rescue agent leucovorin. This therapy is designed to provide sufficiently high drug concentrations to penetrate the cell membrane by passive diffusion and to saturate increased concentrations of enzyme. Methotrexate is usually administered intravenously in doses ranging from 25 to 7500 mg per square meter.* Its primary plasma half-life is approximately two to

*Exceeds manufacturer's recommended maximum dose.

three hours with excretion largely by the kidney (90 per cent). In patients with abnormal renal function or in those receiving doses above 1000 mg per square meter, monitoring of drug concentration in plasma is recommended to avoid serious toxicity. Methotrexate concentrations in plasma can be measured accurately with a competitive binding assay and are useful for detecting patients at high risk of toxicity, who should then receive leucovorin rescue doses.

Methotrexate distributes slowly into "third spaces" such as ascites, pleural effusions, or cerebrospinal fluid. The slow reentry of drug into the systemic circulation from ascites has been associated with a prolonged terminal half-life and unexpected toxicity. Systemic methotrexate enters spinal fluid poorly with concentrations only 3 per cent of those simultaneously in plasma. Only with high-dose methotrexate therapy are cytotoxic concentrations achieved in the spinal fluid. Alternatively, methotrexate may be injected directly into the lumbar intrathecal space or, directly into the ventricle through an indwelling reservoir.

Acute methotrexate toxicity results from its effects on rapidly proliferating tissues (bone marrow and intestinal and oral epithelium). Drug concentrations of 1×10^{-8} M or greater in plasma produce myelosuppression and mucositis, which peak 5 to 14 days following a bolus dose or short-term infusion, with rapid recovery. More prolonged toxicity may be observed in patients who fail to eliminate the drug normally. High-dose therapy with methotrexate may lead to acute renal injury, believed to result from intrarenal precipitation of methotrexate or methotrexate-derived material. This can be prevented by vigorous pretreatment hydration, urine alkalinization ($pH \geq 7$), and, in patients with underlying renal disease, a dose reduction proportional to the decrease in renal function. Both acute and chronic hepatotoxicity may be caused by methotrexate with acute elevation of hepatic enzymes and, in patients receiving long-term oral treatment, hepatic fibrosis and cirrhosis. An acute pneumonitis, possibly of hypersensitivity origin, and rare episodes of anaphylaxis have been described.

Various manifestations of neurotoxicity are observed in up to 30 per cent of patients receiving intrathecal methotrexate, including motor dysfunction, cranial nerve palsies, coma, or seizures. Symptoms are accompanied by increased spinal fluid pressure and protein concentration and a reactive pleocytosis. Continued methotrexate treatment may be fatal.

Fluoropyrimidines. 5-Fluorouracil (5-FU), an analogue of thymine, inhibits thymidylate synthesis. 5-FU has antitumor activity against many solid tumors, including breast, colon, and ovarian carcinoma, and is now commonly used in combination therapy. Two biochemical actions may account for its cytotoxicity. 5-FU is converted to its corresponding ribose-triphosphate (5-FUTP) which, in turn, is incorporated in RNA and inhibits RNA processing and function. A second metabolite, 5-FdUMP, binds tightly to thymidylate synthetase and inhibits the eventual formation of dTTP, one of the four necessary precursors of DNA. In experimental tumors, resistance to 5-FU develops through deletion of one of the several key enzymes required for its activation (uridine kinase, nucleoside phosphorylase, and orotic acid phosphoribosyl transferase). Increased thymidylate synthetase has also been found in resistant cells. It is not known which of these changes is responsible for clinical resistance.

5-FU is usually given intravenously or intra-arterially because of erratic oral absorption and rapid first-pass metabolism in the liver. After intravenous administration of 10 to 15 mg per kilogram, peak plasma concentrations reach 0.1 to 1 mM, but rapid metabolism to dihydrofluorouracil in the liver and other tissues leads to an abrupt fall in plasma concentrations with a half-time of about ten minutes. By six hours after injection, plasma concentrations of 5-FU are below 1 μM, the threshold for cytotoxic effects in tissue culture.

5-FU can be infused into the hepatic artery or portal vein for treatment of hepatic metastases, and only small amounts of drug will reach the systemic circulation. Greater than 80 per cent of administered 5-FU is inactivated by metabolism, the remainder being excreted in the urine. Doses do not have to be modified in the presence of hepatic dysfunction, since significant metabolism occurs in extrahepatic tissues.

The primary toxicities of *bolus* intravenous 5-FU are myelosuppression and mucositis. *Continuous intravenous infusion* of 5-FU at doses of 30 mg per kilogram per day* for five days gives equivalent therapeutic results, but different toxicity. Myelosuppression is mild, but gastrointestinal symptoms predominate (again, stomatitis and diarrhea). Other less common toxicities of 5-FU include acute neurologic symptoms in patients receiving intracarotid infusions, a syndrome of chest pain and serum enzyme elevations consistent with myocardial ischemia, and acute and chronic conjunctivitis.

Cytosine Arabinoside. Cytosine arabinoside (ara-C, cytarabine) is an analogue of deoxycytidine, differing only in the substitution of the sugar arabinose for deoxyribose. Ara-C readily penetrates cells by a carrier-mediated process and then is converted by salvage pathway enzymes to its active form, ara-CTP (Fig. 176–5), an inhibitor of DNA polymerase in competition with dCTP. Ara-C is also incorporated into DNA, and causes premature termination of the growing strand of newly synthesized DNA. Two inactivating enzymes, cytidine deaminase and dCMP deaminase (which degrade ara-C and ara-CMP, respectively), are present in high concentration relative to the activating enzymes and are thought to exert an important negative influence on drug action (Fig. 176–5). Ara-C kills cells selectively during the S phase of the cell cycle, and has little activity against slowly growing solid tumors.

Resistance to ara-C is not well understood, but may relate to (1) deletion of deoxycytidine kinase, a necessary enzyme for activation, (2) an increased intracellular pool of dCTP (the nucleotide that competes with ara-CTP), (3) increased cytidine deaminase, or (4) a deficiency of the membrane transport process. Clinical response to ara-C may be predicted by the ability of leukemic cells to form and to retain ara-CTP after exposure to ara-C in vitro.

Ara-C is administered intravenously and is distributed rapidly into total body water, including cerebrospinal fluid. Owing to rapid inactivation (half-time of seven to twenty minutes) and its S-phase specificity, ara-C is given by continuous infusion or in bolus doses of 50 to 100 mg every eight to twelve hours for five to ten days. More than 70 per cent of administered ara-C is excreted in the urine as its inactive metabolite ara-U, which

*Exceeds manufacturer's recommended maximum dose.

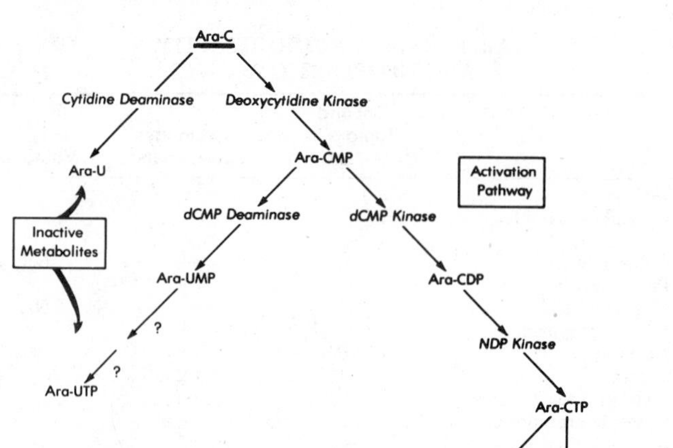

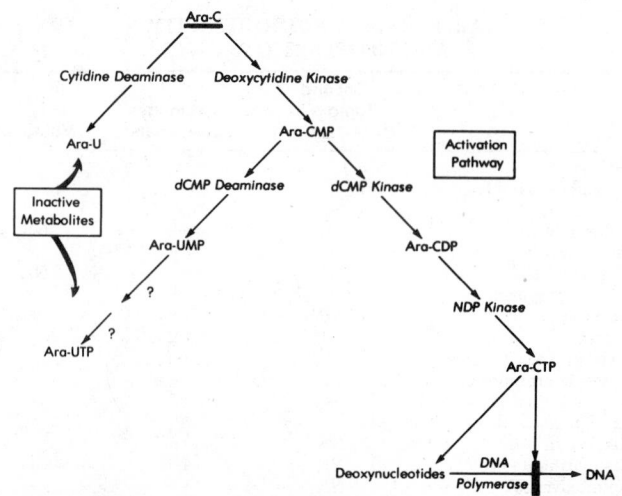

Figure 176–5. Pathways for metabolism of cytosine arabinoside (ara-C) in human leukemic myeloblasts. Enzyme names are indicated in italics. Ara-CTP inhibits DNA polymerase and is itself incorporated into DNA. Uracil arabinoside (ara-U) and its nucleotides have no known cytotoxic effects.

is formed in liver, plasma, granulocytes, and other sites (Fig. 176–5). Alternatively, ara-C has been given in very high doses (up to 3 grams per square meter*) every 12 hours for six days, a regimen that appears to improve the response rate in refractory types of acute myelocytic leukemia.

Ara-C may also be administered intrathecally for treatment of meningeal leukemia or carcinomatosis. Because spinal fluid contains little cytidine deaminase, intrathecal doses of 50 mg per square meter yield high peak levels (1 mM), which decline with a half-time of two hours.

The primary side effects of ara-C are myelosuppression and gastrointestinal epithelial injury (nausea, vomiting, diarrhea). Patients frequently develop mild serum enzyme elevations consistent with hepatocellular damage, but these changes rarely necessitate a discontinuation of treatment. High-dose ara-C treatment causes cerebral dysfunction, ataxia, and conjunctivitis, toxicities not seen with conventional doses.

Ara-C has shown synergistic biochemical interaction with many other antitumor agents, including alkylating agents, cisplatinum, thiopurines, uridine analogues, and antifolates. Ara-C enhances cyclophosphamide and BCNU activity by inhibiting repair of strand breaks caused by the alkylating agents. Methotrexate given three to six hours prior to ara-C enhances ara-CTP formation in experimental tumors by undefined mechanisms.

A second cytidine analogue, *5-azacytidine (5-azaC),* is activated to 5-azaCTP, which is incorporated into RNA and causes defective protein synthesis and degradation of polyribosomes. It also inhibits methylation of DNA, and thus can activate genes, such as those for fetal hemoglobin, which are normally inactivated during differentiation. In addition to its antileukemic activity, 5-azaC has the unique action of increasing fetal hemoglobin synthesis in patients with β thalassemia (Ch. 141). The rapid decomposition of 5-azacytidine in alkaline or neutral solution necessitates either fresh mixing prior to administration or formulation at a slightly acid pH in Ringer's lactate (pH 6.2). The drug undergoes rapid removal from the plasma, either through metabolism or chemical decomposition. Less than 2 per cent of an administered dose remains in plasma as parent compound 30 minutes after administration. The primary toxicities of 5-azacytidine are myelosuppression and severe and prolonged nausea and vomiting. The latter symptoms are lessened by a prolonged or continuous infusion, with no apparent change in its therapeutic efficacy.

Purine Analogues. 6-Mercaptopurine (6-MP) and 6-thioguanine (6-TG) have the single substitution of a thiol group in place of the 6-hydroxyl group found in the basic purine nucleus. Both require activation to the nucleotide level by hypoxanthine–guanine phosphoribosyltransferase (HGPRT'ase) in order to inhibit de novo purine biosynthesis and block the conversion of the purine precursor inosinic acid to adenylic acid or to guanylic acid (Fig. 176–6). The triphosphate nucleotides of 6-TG and 6-MP are incorporated into DNA and produce a delayed toxicity after several cell divisions. Biochemical resistance to these agents in human leukemic cells is commonly associated with increased concentrations of a degrading enzyme, a membrane-bound alkaline phosphatase, or decreased concentrations of the activating enzyme HGPRT'ase. 6-MP is not reliably absorbed orally; 6-TG is erratically absorbed, and is thus administered by intravenous infusion. 6-MP is rapidly eliminated (plasma half-time 20 to 45 minutes) by oxidation to 6-thiouric acid catalyzed by xanthine oxidase. This reaction is inhibited by allopurinol; thus, the dose of orally administered 6-MP must be reduced 75 per cent in the presence of the xanthine oxidase inhibitor. 6-TG is degraded by desulfuration and by oxidation with a plasma half-time of 80 to 90 minutes. No reduction in 6-TG dosage is required for patients who are also receiving allopurinol. Both agents are well tolerated in doses of approximately 100 mg per square meter for at least five days. 6-MP is used at reduced doses for maintenance of remission.

*Exceeds manufacturer's recommended maximum dose.

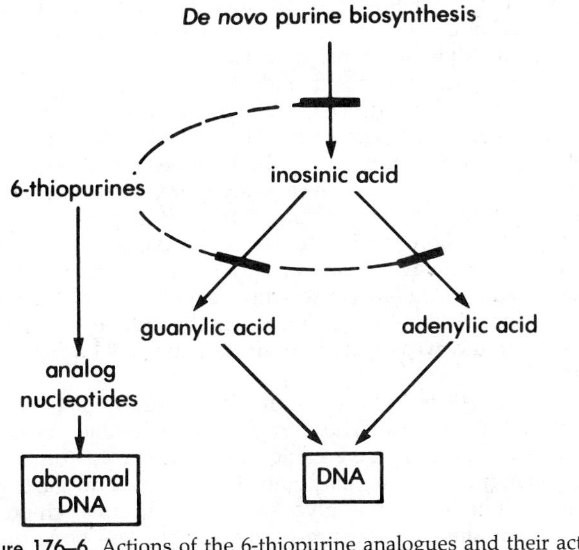

Figure 176–6. Actions of the 6-thiopurine analogues and their active metabolites. These analogues are also incorporated into DNA in place of guanine, an action which may contribute to their cytotoxicity.

The primary toxicity of both thiopurines is myelosuppression and epithelial injury. Myelosuppression is maximal within seven days of drug administration, and recovery occurs in one to two weeks. Both drugs produce a reversible hepatotoxicity with enzyme and bilirubin elevation in a pattern suggesting cholestatic jaundice. Mucositis, esophagitis, and gastrointestinal complaints are usually mild.

The 6-thiopurines and the related compound azathioprine, which is metabolized to 6-mercaptopurine by the liver, are potent suppressors of cell-mediated immunity, and thus find numerous applications for treating autoimmune diseases and preventing transplant rejection. Immunosuppression with these agents can be achieved at doses that produce little decrease in the white blood cell count. Long-term immunosuppressive therapy with azathioprine, prednisone, and other immunosuppressive agents in renal transplantation is associated with an increased risk of squamous carcinomas of skin and histiocytic lymphoma, and predisposes patients to bacterial and opportunistic infections (see Ch. 79).

ALKYLATING AGENTS. Alkylating agents kill tumor cells and normal dividing tissues by forming covalent bonds with nucleic acids. The alkyl groups attach to DNA, interfere with its integrity, and thereby produce significant cytotoxic, mutagenic, and carcinogenic effects.

Alkylating agents spontaneously form positively charged carbonium ions in aqueous solution. In the case of chloroethyl derivatives, the alkylating intermediate is $R\text{-}CH_2CH_2^+$, which attacks nucleophilic (electron-rich) sites on nucleic acids, proteins, sulfhydryls (glutathione), and amino acids. It is likely that the primary cytotoxic and mutagenic effects of alkylating agents result from binding to guanine (which accounts for about 90 per cent of alkylated sites), adenine, and cytosine. Base alkylation leads to misreading of the DNA code, but also single-strand breakage. Crosslinkage of DNA occurs when bifunctional alkylating agents are employed. These agents, such as nitrogen mustard, possess two chloroethyl groups, each capable of forming a carbonium ion. The formation of crosslinks correlates closely with the lethality of alkylating agents and nitrosourea derivatives in cell culture. Alkylating agents such as nitrogen mustard and cyclophosphamide kill cells in all phases of the cell cycle, but have quantitatively greater activity against rapidly dividing cells.

Alkylating agents share a common mechanism of action, but they differ in their pharmacokinetic features, lipid solubility, chemical reactivity, metabolism, and membrane transport properties (Table 176–9). Tumors may, therefore, differ in their response or resistance to agents in this class. The structures of commonly used alkylating agents are shown in Figure 176–7.

Nitrogen mustard (mechlorethamine), the first alkylating agent

TABLE 176–9. ALKYLATING AGENTS

Agent	Route (IV/PO)	Schedule	Dose (mg/m²)	Plasma t½ (hrs)	Elimination*
Cyclophosphamide	IV	q.d. × 5	400	6–12	M
	PO	q.d.	50–100		
Chlorambucil	PO	q.d.	1–2	1.5	SCD
Melphalan	IV	q.d. × 5	4	1.8	SCD
	IV	q. 4 w.	8		
	PO	q.d. × 5	8		
Nitrosoureas					
BCNU	IV	q. 6 w.	150–225		SCD
CCNU	PO	q. 6 w.	100–150		SCD
Methyl CCNU	PO	q. 6 w.	150–200		SCD

*M = metabolic.
SCD = spontaneous chemical degradation.

to receive clinical trial, is used primarily for treatment of malignant lymphomas and as a topical solution for treatment of mycosis fungoides. Nitrogen mustard enters cells through an active transport mechanism shared with the physiologic amine choline. Resistance is believed to result from enhanced repair of DNA alkylation. The primary clinical toxicities of nitrogen mustard consist of myelosuppression and gastrointestinal symptoms (nausea and vomiting). Minor cholinergic side effects occur at high doses, and include lacrimation, diarrhea, and diaphoresis. The high chemical reactivity of this compound causes severe local tissue injury when infiltrated into the skin. It is used to ablate the pleural space in patients with chronic pleural effusion (0.2 to 0.4 mg per kilogram into the pleural space after draining the effusion).

Cyclophosphamide (Cytoxan) has largely replaced nitrogen mustard in clinical use. The drug requires hepatic activation in a multi-step process to yield the active compound, phosphoramide mustard, and a side product, acrolein. Acrolein may be responsible for the common side effect of hemorrhagic cystitis, a complication that can be reduced by orally administered thiols. Cyclophosphamide is well absorbed orally but is usually

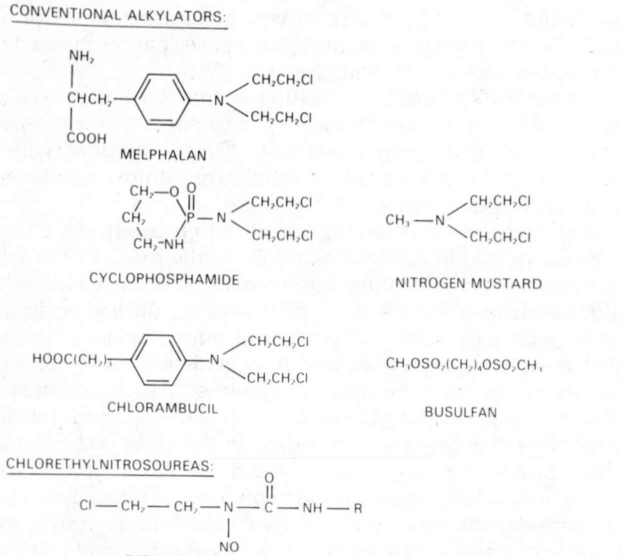

Figure 176–7. Chemical structure of clinically useful alkylating agents and the related class of nitrosourea compounds.

given by intravenous infusion. It produces only mild thrombocytopenia in comparison with leukopenia. Nausea, vomiting, and alopecia are common side effects. Attempts to prevent cystitis by hydration of such patients carry the risk of inducing symptomatic hyponatremia, since in high-dose infusion regimens (50 mg per kilogram doses) cyclophosphamide causes a syndrome of inappropriate water retention owing to direct effects on the renal tubule. Hyponatremia, seizures, and death have occurred as a consequence of water retention. Other toxicities associated with cyclophosphamide treatment include suppression of humoral and delayed immunity, acute myocardial necrosis (after high-dose administration), and, after prolonged courses of treatment, acute myeloblastic leukemia and pulmonary fibrosis.

Melphalan (L-phenylalanine mustard, Alkeran) has activity similar to that of cyclophosphamide (lymphomas, breast and ovarian cancer, multiple myeloma) but does not cause hemorrhagic cystitis. The drug has variable bioavailability by the oral route; thus, the average dose of 0.1 to 0.2 mg per kilogram must be adjusted according to bone marrow tolerance. Melphalan enters cells by active transport, utilizing amino acid transport systems. After intravenous administration, the parent compound disappears from plasma with a half-life of approximately two hours. Less than 15 per cent of the drug is excreted in the urine intact.

Chlorambucil (Leukeran), a close structural congener of melphalan, is also stable in aqueous solution and is given orally. Thus, it is a convenient alkylating agent for treating chronic lymphocytic leukemia, nodular lymphomas, or multiple myeloma, which require long-term management. It has suppressive effects on both granulocytes and platelets, but few other side effects. Like cyclophosphamide and melphalan, chlorambucil therapy has been linked to late occurrences of acute myeloblastic leukemia.

Busulfan (Myleran) consists of two labile methane-sulfonate groups attached at opposite ends of a four-carbon alkyl chain. This compound is sufficiently stable for oral administration, but it rapidly forms carbonium ions leading to alkylation of DNA. It is primarily used for the treatment of chronic granulocytic leukemia, in which its myelosuppressive action provides effective, long-term regulation of the white blood cell count. Myelosuppression is not quickly reversible and may be permanent if excessive doses are used. In addition to myelosuppression, busulfan causes diffuse pulmonary fibrosis and an addisonian-like state characterized by cutaneous hyperpigmentation and weakness, but without abnormal adrenal function.

The *chloroethylnitrosoureas* form a structurally distinct group of alkylating agents. These highly lipid-soluble, chemically reactive compounds have clinical activity against the lymphomas, malignant melanoma, brain neoplasms, and gastrointestinal carcinomas. A new glycosylated nitrosourea, chlorozotocin,* has a similar spectrum of activity but less bone marrow

*Investigational drug.

toxicity. Chemical decomposition of these agents yields a reactive chloroethyl carbonium ion ($ClCH_2CH_2^+$) that alkylates DNA. Decomposition of nitrosoureas also yields isocyanates of differing reactivity that may attack NH_2 groups in a carbamylation reaction and are believed to inhibit DNA repair and to alter maturation of RNA. Because of the extreme clinical reactivity of these compounds in aqueous solution, intact parent compounds (BCNU, CCNU, or methylCCNU) have not been detected in plasma, and little is known about their disposition in man. The high lipid solubility of the nitrosoureas may account for their excellent activity against intracranial tumors, in which the chloroethyl portion of CCNU reaches concentrations 30 per cent of those found simultaneously in plasma. The primary toxicity of the nitrosoureas is delayed and cumulative myelosuppression. Nadir leukopenia and thrombocytopenia occur six to eight weeks after dosage. These compounds are strongly carcinogenic in animal test systems, and methylCCNU has been associated with cases of acute myeloplastic leukemia in humans. Pulmonary fibrosis and renal failure are observed in patients after prolonged courses of treatment (greater than 1500 mg per square meter of BCNU or its congeners).

CIS-PLATINUM. Cis (II) platinum diamminedichloride (cis-DDP), the only heavy metal compound used as a cancer chemotherapeutic agent, has a unique mechanism of action and spectrum of biologic effects. It possesses important therapeutic activity against testicular tumors, ovarian carcinoma, and head and neck cancer. The cis-dichloro complex structure has cytotoxic activity by virtue of its ability to form covalent bonds and crosslinks with DNA. Both chloride ions of this coordinate complex are slowly displaced by water, generating a positively charged platinum complex. This activated complex then interacts with a nucleophilic site on DNA, RNA, or protein to form covalent crosslinks in a manner similar to alkylating reactions. The formation of crosslinks continues for hours after drug exposure, and is opposed by repair processes which excise and rebuild damaged segments of DNA. It is likely that the ability to repair DNA is an important determinant of sensitivity to this drug, as is the intracellular glutathione content.

Cis-platinum is usually administered after a four- to six-hour period of hydration and diuresis with 1 liter of a sodium chloride solution. The total dose administered is 40 to 75 mg per square meter and varies according to frequency of administration and individual patient tolerance. An alternative schedule is 20 mg per square meter per day for five days, a regimen that causes less nephrotoxicity and nausea. The clearance of total platinum from plasma proceeds rapidly during the first few hours after injection (half-time, 20 to 60 minutes), but slowly thereafter owing to covalent binding of drug to serum proteins. Between 20 and 75 per cent of administered drug is excreted in the urine in the 24 hours after administration. The remainder is probably bound to tissues or plasma protein. Cis-DDP penetrates poorly into the central nervous system, the plasma–cerebrospinal fluid ratio being 21:1 or greater.

Cis-platinum causes nephrotoxicity in 30 per cent of patients treated with 50 to 75 mg per square meter per course unless preventive pretreatment hydration is undertaken. The primary pathologic findings are coagulative necrosis of the distal tubular epithelium and collecting ducts. In patients with platinum nephrotoxicity, changes in tubular function include magnesium wasting and the excretion of high molecular weight proteins. Hypomagnesemia, a common finding in patients treated with cis-DDP, is usually asymptomatic but may lead to tetany. Nausea and vomiting are distressing symptoms in patients taking cis-DDP, and are poorly relieved by standard antiemetics. These symptoms may be lessened by giving smaller doses once daily for five days. Cis-DDP causes only moderate myelosuppression. Leukopenia, thrombocytopenia, and anemia may develop in patients after extended treatment. Other toxicities include a distal, sensory neuropathy after prolonged treatment; hypersensitivity reactions such as urticaria, wheezing, and hypotension (which can be prevented in some patients by pretreatment with antihistamines and corticosteroids); and a progressive loss of high frequency hearing, particularly in older patients.

ANTITUMOR ANTIBIOTICS. ***Bleomycin.*** Bleomycin, a mixture of antibiotic peptides, is widely used for treating lymphomas, testicular cancer, and head and neck cancer. Bleomycin produces single and double strand breaks in DNA through a complex sequence of reactions, beginning with its binding to DNA. Ferrous ion (Fe^{2+}), which is intimately bound to bleomycin, then undergoes spontaneous oxidation to the Fe^{3+} state, liberating an electron that is accepted by oxygen to form reactive oxygen species such as the superoxide or hydroxyl radicals. These radicals in turn attack the phosphodiester bonds between DNA bases. Free bases are released from DNA, leading to strand breaks.

Bleomycin kills cells preferentially during the premitotic, or G_2, phase or in the mitotic phase of the cell cycle. The possibility of increasing cell kill by exposing cells during the G_2 phase or mitosis has led to continuous infusion of bleomycin. The determinants of bleomycin sensitivity are poorly understood. There is indirect evidence that the same processes required to repair radiation damage to DNA also repair bleomycin-induced lesions.

Bleomycin is administered by subcutaneous, intramuscular, or intravenous injection with no obvious differences in clinical response rates. Following an intravenous bolus injection of 15 units per square meter, bleomycin has a biphasic plasma disappearance with half-times of 24 minutes and two to four hours. The drug is primarily excreted unchanged in the urine. Bleomycin pharmacokinetics are therefore markedly altered in patients with abnormal renal function. A half-time of 21 hours has been reported in a patient with a creatinine clearance of 11 ml per minute; a decreased dosage of bleomycin (25 to 50 per cent of normal) is indicated for patients with severely compromised renal function.

Bleomycin has myelosuppressive toxicity only at high doses (above 25 units per square meter) or in patients with hypoplastic bone marrow. The most important toxicity of bleomycin is a progressive interstitial pulmonary fibrosis, manifested first by cough, dyspnea, and bibasilar pulmonary infiltrates on a chest radiograph. The diffusion capacity of the lung progressively decreases with increased total doses of the drug. The decline becomes more rapid above doses of 250 units, and the incidence of significant pulmonary toxicity is 10 per cent at total doses above 450 units. Toxicity is more likely to occur in patients over 70 years of age, in patients with underlying lung disease, and in those previously treated with pulmonary irradiation. Anti-inflammatory agents such as corticosteroids have not been proved to prevent or effectively treat this fibrosis. The clinical symptoms and x-ray findings of bleomycin pulmonary toxicity are difficult to distinguish from other pulmonary syndromes observed in cancer patients, such as progressive tumor, infectious processes such as *Pneumocystis carinii* or cytomegalovirus, or radiation pneumonitis. Open lung biopsy, often required to rule out these other processes, reveals an acute inflammatory infiltrate, interstitial and intra-alveolar edema, pulmonary hyaline membrane formation, and interstitial fibrosis.

Bleomycin also causes cutaneous toxicity with erythema, induration, thickening, and eventual peeling of skin over the fingers, palms, and extremity joints. Many patients develop hyperpigmentation of skin creases and a general skin darkening. Raynaud's phenomenon has also been reported during bleomycin therapy. Other less frequent toxicities include acute hypertension (at doses greater than 25 units per day), hyperbilirubinemia, fever, and hypersensitivity reactions with urticaria and bronchospasm.

Anthracyclines. Daunomycin and doxorubicin (Adriamycin) belong to the anthracycline class of antibiotics produced by *Streptomyces* species. Anthracyclines have a wide spectrum of clinical activity, including breast cancer, leukemia, and sarcomas. Anthracyclines have many biologic and biochemical effects, including (1) chelation of divalent cations, especially Fe^{2+}, with production of oxygen radicals and superoxide, (2) cyclic oxidation-reduction of the quinone-hydroquinone functional group; and (3) intercalation between strands of the DNA double helix. Intercalation results in inhibition of DNA, RNA, and ultimately protein synthesis. It is not known which of these actions is responsible for cytotoxicity.

The anthracyclines induce single-stranded DNA breaks. These breaks are believed to result either from distortions in the double helix caused by intercalation or from free radicals initiated by reduction of the anthracyclines. Tocopherol (vitamin E), a known free-radical scavenger, lessens oxygen radical generation by doxorubicin in vitro and in animals lessens the cardiac toxicity of Adriamycin without diminishing its antitumor activity. The reason for the particular susceptibility of the heart to doxorubicin action is not clear but may be due to the lack of free-radical detoxifying enzymes, particularly glutathione peroxidase.

Assay methods for the anthracyclines have been developed but are not routinely available. The pharmacokinetics of the parent drug include half-lives of 11 minutes, 3 hours, and 25 to 28 hours. The liver is the main site of metabolism of both doxorubicin and daunorubicin. As a result, drug dosages are often modified in the face of abnormal liver function, but precise guidelines based on pharmacokinetics are not available. A 75 per cent reduction for bilirubin greater than 3 mg per deciliter has been recommended.

Myelosuppression and mucositis are the dose-limiting acute toxicities of the anthracyclines. Alopecia is also common. Extravasation of these agents leads to severe local reaction, beginning as erythema and pain which progress over weeks to deep ulcerative lesions.

Cardiac damage is the most serious toxicity caused by these agents. In rare instances, an acute syndrome develops hours to days after a dose of doxorubicin or daunorubicin and consists of arrhythmias or pump failure, but clinically significant acute effects are unusual (supraventricular arrhythmias, heart block, and ventricular tachycardia). A more serious toxicity is cumulative, dose-dependent cardiomyopathy, which leads to congestive heart failure in 1 to 10 per cent of the patients who receive more than 550 mg per square meter of doxorubicin or daunomycin. A progressive decrease in cardiac contractility is observed with increasing total dose, and is associated with progressive pathologic changes on endocardial biopsy. Congestive heart failure may not appear until up to nine months after cessation of anthracycline therapy. There are no proven methods for preventing acute or chronic anthracycline-induced cardiac damage. Vitamin E and other free-radical scavengers are undergoing clinical trial but have uncertain effectiveness.

Mitomycin. Mitomycin C is an antibiotic with clinical activity in gastrointestinal tumors, breast cancer, and ovarian cancer. Its mechanism of action is unclear, but may be the result of free radical generation by its quinone group, or alkylation by its urethane or azuridine groups. Only when metabolically activated does the drug alkylate DNA, producing intrastrand and interstrand crosslinks, inhibition of DNA synthesis, and cell death.

There is little information on the pharmacokinetics and disposition of this agent. Bolus intravenous doses of 22.5 to 45 mg per square meter produce plasma levels of 0.4 μg per milliliter. Metabolic activation occurs in many tissues and may account for its rapid clearance from the plasma. The liver plays an uncertain role in metabolism of mitomycin C, so there are no guidelines for dose modification in the presence of liver disease.

The major dose-limiting toxicity of mitomycin C is myelosuppression, which is delayed in onset and cumulative with successive cycles of therapy. Leukocyte and platelet counts usually reach a nadir four to six weeks after treatment. Doses often require modification by the third course of treatment. This drug has been implicated in unusual instances of interstitial pneumonitis, nephrotoxicity, and a syndrome resembling thrombotic thrombocytopenic purpura. It may accelerate the development of anthracycline-induced cardiomyopathy.

Actinomycin D. Actinomycin D has activity in the treatment of Wilms' tumor, Ewing's sarcoma, embryonal rhabdomyosarcoma, and gestational choriocarcinoma. This antibiotic intercalates with DNA by virtue of a specific interaction between its cyclic polypeptide chains and deoxyguanosine, causing inhibition of RNA and DNA synthesis. At low concentrations, actinomycin D inhibits RNA synthesis predominantly, whereas at higher concentrations both RNA and DNA synthesis are blocked. Actinomycin D also causes single-stranded DNA breaks. As with doxorubicin and other intercalators, these breaks are believed to result from torsion on the DNA helix, and may be mediated by an enzyme which produces the break and becomes covalently linked to DNA in the process.

Actinomycin D is primarily excreted unchanged in bile and urine. Clearance of the drug from plasma is rapid initially, but a slow phase (half-time of 36 hours) of drug disappearance predominates, corresponding to slow release of drug from tissues. Human pharmacologic data are inadequate to allow rational dose modification in the face of liver or renal failure. The dose-limiting toxicity of this agent is myelosuppression, but gastrointestinal side effects are also prominent, and include abdominal pain, cramps, diarrhea, and mucositis. Actinomycin D also enhances x-irradiation toxicity to skin, the gastrointestinal tract, and other sites. A cutaneous recall reaction may occur in patients treated with actinomycin D several months after x-irradiation.

PLANT PRODUCTS. The vinca alkaloids vincristine and vinblastine, derived from the ornamental shrub *vinca rosea* (periwinkle), and the epipodophyllotoxins VM-26* and VP-16, derived by modification of a product of the mandrake plant, are among the few plant products with clinically useful cytotoxic activity.

Vinca Alkaloids. The vinca alkaloids bind to tubulin, an intracellular protein that polymerizes to form the microtubular apparatus. Microtubules are components of the mitotic spindle, but also play an important role in maintaining cell structure and in providing channels for movement of cellular secretions and neurotransmitters. The vinca alkaloids inhibit the assembly of microtubules and cause dissolution of the mitotic spindle. Vincristine and vinblastine are poorly absorbed orally and therefore are usually given intravenously in doses of 1.0 to 1.4 mg per square meter and 2 to 4 mg per square meter, respectively, at weekly intervals. Only minute concentrations of these alkaloids (less than 0.01 μM) are required to kill sensitive cells. Mechanisms of resistance to the vinca alkaloids are not well understood, although patterns of cross-resistance with the anthracyclines and actinomycin D suggest that these agents share a common transport pathway. Both alkaloids undergo hepatic metabolism and biliary excretion with very little excreted in the urine. A 50 per cent reduction in dose of either vinca alkaloid is recommended for patients with hepatic dysfunction and a serum bilirubin above 3 mg per deciliter; no dose adjustment is necessary for patients with altered renal function.

Total doses of vincristine greater than 2 mg often cause a progressive neurotoxicity, particularly in older patients and in those receiving weekly treatment. Patients experience a decrease in deep tendon reflexes, paresthesias of the fingers and lower extremities, and, at more advanced stages, cranial nerve palsies, and profound weakness of the dorsiflexors of the foot and extensors of the wrist. The sensory changes may improve with discontinuation of vincristine, but motor deficits usually show little improvement. Vincristine causes little myelosuppression. The platelet count may actually rise during treatment as a result of endoreduplication of megakaryocytes. In

*Investigational drug.

contrast, vinblastine is highly toxic to bone marrow, producing leukopenia and thrombocytopenia. Mucositis is also a frequent side effect, but neurotoxicity is rare. Vindesine,* another vinca alkaloid, causes both myelosuppression and moderately severe neurotoxicity. Vincristine promotes release of antidiuretic hormone and may rarely cause symptomatic dilutional hyponatremia. This syndrome is easily treated by simple fluid restriction.

Podophyllotoxins. Two glycosidic derivatives of podophyllotoxin, VP-16 and VM-26, have important clinical activity in the treatment of lymphomas, small cell carcinoma of the lung, and testicular cancer. Their mechanism of action is poorly understood. In contrast to podophyllotoxin, VP-16 and VM-26 have no effect on microtubular assembly and arrest cells in G_2 rather than in mitosis. VP-16 is administered in a drinking ampule or intravenously, whereas VM-26 is given only intravenously. VP-16 has a shorter terminal half-life, less metabolic alteration, and greater renal excretion (30 per cent unchanged in urine) than VM-26. Both drugs penetrate poorly into the cerebrospinal fluid despite their high lipid solubility. The primary route of elimination for VM-26 is metabolic.

Typical well-tolerated intravenous doses of VP-16 are 45 mg per square meter per day for seven days, 86 mg per square meter per day for twice-weekly doses, and 290 mg per square meter once weekly; oral doses are two-fold higher. VM-26 is usually given in weekly doses of 67 mg per square meter. The dose-limiting toxicity for both drugs is leukopenia. Nausea, vomiting, and neurotoxicity (paresthesias or tendon reflex depression) occasionally occur in patients receiving these drugs.

OTHER AGENTS. ***Hexamethylmelamine.*** Hexamethylmelamine (HMM) exhibits significant activity against ovarian cancer, breast cancer, the lymphomas, and small cell carcinoma of the lung. HMM consists of a symmetrical 6-member triazene ring to which are attached three dimethylamine groups (Fig. 176–8). The 6 methyl side groups are removed sequentially by hepatic microsomal metabolism to yield various methylmelamine derivatives plus formaldehyde, which is itself a weakly cytotoxic compound. The methylmelamine metabolites are noncytotoxic in vitro but can be converted by enzymatic hydroxylation to methylol ($R\text{-}CH_2OH$) analogues, which are cytotoxic in tissue culture and may be the active alkylating form of the drug. Because of its limited aqueous solubility, HMM can be given only by the oral route. Usual doses of 4 to 12 mg per kilogram per day are given for courses of 14 to 21 days. However, the bioavailability of HMM by this route is highly variable. The parent compound has a half-time of 4.7 to 10.2 hours in plasma. HMM produces nausea and vomiting as its dose-limiting toxicity. HMM also produces neurotoxic symptoms, such as mood alterations, hallucinations, and peripheral neuropathy. These effects gradually increase in severity during a protracted course of treatment and disappear upon drug withdrawal.

Dacarbazine (DTIC). DTIC, an imidazole-4-carboxamide derivative, was first synthesized as an inhibitor of purine biosynthesis but, in fact, functions as an alkylating agent. It is active against Hodgkin's disease, malignant melanoma, and soft tissue sarcomas. The metabolic activation of this agent by hepatic microsomes leads to production of an active methyl cation (CH_3^+), which binds to nucleic acid bases. This alkylation is believed to be responsible for the cytotoxic action of DTIC. Schedules of intravenous administration vary from 150 to 300 mg per square meter per day for five to ten days, depending on prior treatment history, concurrent therapy, and patient tolerance. There is no accurate information on its pharmacokinetics or metabolism in man. Severe nausea and vomiting occur during the first days of treatment but may be lessened by reducing the initial dose and gradually increasing the dose during the course of treatment. Mild myelosuppression may occur two to three weeks following treatment. Other toxicities include a flu-like syndrome and a possible enhancement of Adriamycin cardiac toxicity.

Procarbazine. Procarbazine has become an important agent in the treatment of Hodgkin's disease, brain tumors, and lung cancer. It undergoes metabolic activation, yielding several potential alkylating products, including a methyldiazonium ion ($^+CH_2-N=NH$), which become bound to nucleic acids, phospholipids, and protein in vivo. The pharmacokinetics of procarbazine in humans have been incompletely characterized. The parent drug disappears from plasma with a rapid half-time of seven minutes following intravenous administration. Procarbazine is usually administered orally in daily doses of 100 mg per square meter per day for 10 to 14 days.

Procarbazine may produce a number of adverse reactions. It causes moderate nausea and decreased appetite, mild to moderate leukopenia and thrombocytopenia, and, less frequently, neurotoxicity (paresthesias of the extremities, drowsiness, or depression). These mental status changes may be related to inhibition of monoamine oxidase; therefore, patients taking procarbazine should avoid foods containing tyramine, such as wine, bananas, yogurt, and ripe cheese, since these may provoke a hypertensive crisis. Other monoamine oxidase inhibitors should not be used with this drug. Procarbazine has an Antabuse-like action, which may lead to sweating, flushing, and headache upon ingestion of alcohol. It also causes hypersensitivity reactions, most prominently a maculopapular rash or pulmonary infiltrates. In addition to its cytotoxic action, procarbazine is a potent immunosuppressant, teratogen, and carcinogen. The compound is highly mutagenic in bacterial assays and produces both adenocarcinomas and acute myelocytic leukemia in rodents and monkeys. An increased incidence of both sarcomas and acute leukemia has been observed in patients receiving MOPP combination chemotherapy with irradiation for Hodgkin's disease, and procarbazine is suspected of being the responsible carcinogen in this combination. Thus, its use for non-neoplastic diseases should be carefully weighed with these late toxicities in mind.

L-Asparaginase. L-Asparagine is a nonessential amino acid synthesized by transfer of an amine group to L-aspartic acid (Fig. 176–9). The synthetic reaction is catalyzed by the enzyme L-asparagine synthetase, which is found in many tissues but is lacking in certain human malignancies, particularly those of lymphocyte origin. In tumor cells lacking L-asparagine synthetase, the amino acid can be obtained only from the plasma pool of amino acids. The enzyme L-asparaginase, obtained from *E. coli* or *Erwinia carotovora,* degrades asparagine and has potent activity against childhood acute lymphocytic leukemia. Resistance to L-asparaginase arises through an increase in L-asparagine synthetase activity in tumor cells. Preparations of L-asparaginase from different bacterial strains have slightly different properties and are not cross-reactive in immunologically sensitized patients. Thus, preparations from *Erwinia* may be used in patients who are hypersensitive to the *E. coli* L-asparaginase. Most L-asparaginase preparations contain L-glutaminase activity, which is 3 to 5 per cent of the L-asparaginase

*Investigational drug that has been recommended for approval by FDA Oncologic Drug Advisory Committee.

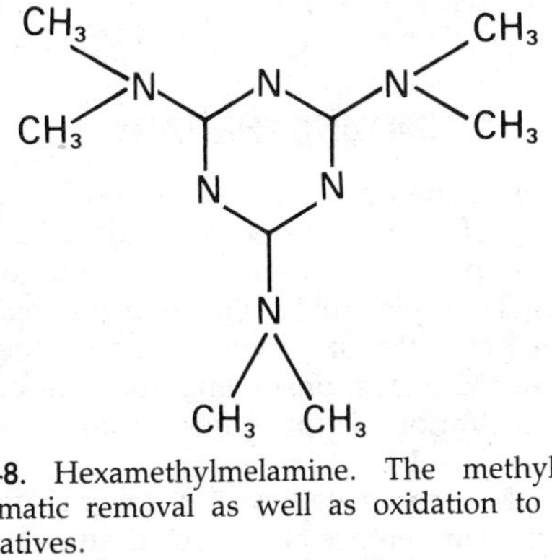

Figure 176–8. Hexamethylmelamine. The methyl side groups undergo enzymatic removal as well as oxidation to form cytotoxic methylol derivatives.

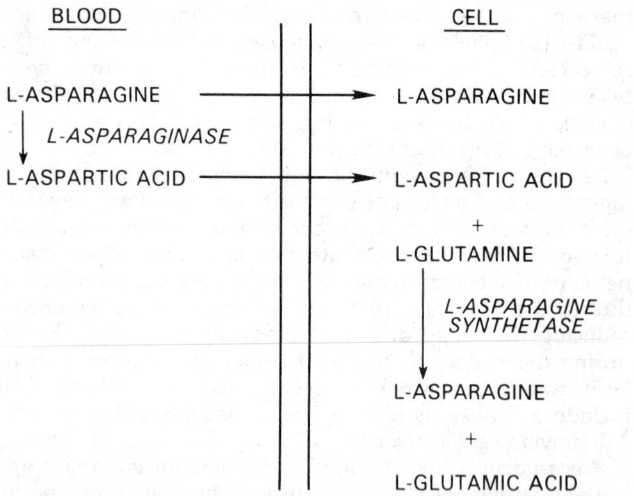

Figure 176–9. Pathways of L-asparagine metabolism, and site of action of L-asparaginase.

activity. The usual doses are 6000 international units (IU) per square meter every other day for three to four weeks, or 1000 to 2000 IU per square meter daily for ten to twenty days.

The half-life of L-asparaginase in plasma is 14 to 22 hours, but there is considerable variation among different preparations. Plasma clearance is greatly accelerated in hypersensitive patients, and enzyme activity may disappear from plasma within four hours. The enzyme distributes primarily within the intravascular space. However, the cerebrospinal fluid concentration of asparagine falls rapidly, and an antileukemic effect is exerted in this sanctuary. The primary toxicities of L-asparaginase are related to immunologic sensitization or result from decreased protein synthesis. Positive skin tests to L-asparaginase are rarely observed in untreated persons, but anaphylaxis may occur with the first dose of drug. Allergic reactions, such as urticaria, laryngeal edema, bronchospasm, or hypotension, occur following multiple courses of the enzyme. Passive hemagglutinating antibodies are observed in patients who subsequently develop anaphylaxis, and complement-fixing antibodies are found in serum after an anaphylactic episode. Toxic effects resulting from inhibition of protein synthesis include hypoalbuminemia and decreased serum fibrinogen, prothrombin, and other clotting factors; decreased serum insulin with hyperglycemia; decreased serum lipoproteins; and, in 25 per cent of patients, cerebral dysfunction with confusion, stupor, or frank coma. Improvement in cerebral dysfunction has been reported in patients treated with L-asparaginase 1 to 2 mmoles per kilogram per day for up to 44 days. Other toxicities not explained by inhibition of protein synthesis include acute pancreatitis and abnormal liver function tests (increased serum bilirubin, SGOT, and alkaline phosphatase). Approximately 65 per cent of patients receiving L-asparaginase experience nausea, vomiting, and chills as an immediate reaction, but these side effects are controlled by antiemetics, antihistamines, or corticosteroids. L-Asparaginase has no known toxicity to gastrointestinal mucosa or bone marrow, and thus is easily used in combination chemotherapy. The only well-established drug interactions are its ability to terminate methotrexate action and its enhancement of ara-C cytotoxicity. Large doses of the antifolate are well tolerated if followed by L-asparaginase rescue because the duration of effective exposure of the bone marrow and gastrointestinal mucosa to methotrexate is limited. The combination of methotrexate and L-asparaginase may have value in the treatment of acute lymphocytic leukemia.

HORMONAL THERAPY

Steroid hormones, like the polypeptide hormones, initiate their action at the cellular level by their binding to discrete intracellular proteins called receptors. These receptors are present in tumors derived from steroid-responsive normal tissues, such as endometrium, prostate, or breast, and can be assayed in cytosol supernatants of tumor homogenates by competitive binding methods. The correlations between estrogen steroid receptor content and clinical response is high. For example, the response rate to hormonal manipulation in estrogen receptor positive (ER^+) patients with breast cancer is approximately 65 per cent, whereas it is less than 10 per cent in ER^- patients. Thus ER^- patients can safely be excluded from consideration for endocrine therapy on the basis of the assay. At least three factors must be kept in mind in assessing the value of the steroid receptor assay: (1) The laboratory performing the test should conform in its methods to nationally established standards. (2) Repeat evaluation of receptor status should be undertaken with each change in therapy, if possible. Receptor status may evolve with time and with intervening treatment. For example, changes from ER^+ to ER^- status clearly occur in approximately 20 per cent of patients having sequential analyses of metastatic breast cancer. (3) Multiple sites should be evaluated if accessible, since biopsy results will differ in receptor content in 10 to 20 per cent of patients with metastatic breast cancer.

The general mechanism of action of steroid hormones is described in Ch. 221. In brief, this action is initiated by binding of the hormone to cytoplasmic receptor, followed by an incompletely understood transformation of the steroid-receptor complex to an "active" form, translocation of the receptor-steroid complex to the nucleus, and binding of the complex to an acceptor site on chromatin. Nuclear binding then affects the transcription of messenger RNA coding for specific protein, and in poorly understood ways causes changes in cell kinetics and, ultimately, cell death (see Fig. 221–5). In experimental systems, many possible mechanisms of steroid resistance, in addition to absence of the receptor protein, have been identified involving defects in receptor binding, complex transformation and translocation, and nuclear binding. Steroid antagonists, such as the anti-estrogen tamoxifen, bind to receptor and undergo translocation but fail to initiate the transcriptional changes produced by the native steroids. A list of commonly used steroid hormones and antagonists, as well as their major pharmacologic properties, is provided in Table 176–10.

Surgical or radiotherapeutic ablation of an endocrine gland presents an alternative to hormonal therapy in some cases, but has the obvious disadvantage of the ablative procedure itself, and produces in some cases undesirable hormonal deficiencies. For example, adrenalectomy for metastatic breast cancer leads to glucocorticoid and mineralocorticoid deficiency which necessitates replacement therapy. Ablative procedures currently represent first-line therapy only in prostatic cancer, male breast cancer, and premenopausal female breast cancer. As an alternative to adrenalectomy, the production of estrogenic steroids by the adrenal may be inhibited by aminoglutethimide, plus a glucocorticoid (added to suppress pituitary ACTH production).

Analogs of luteinizing hormone-releasing hormone (LHRH) have received preliminary clinical evaluation and are capable of inducing a fall in plasma testosterone levels to castration values. These analogs are effective in producing a remission of symptoms in patients with prostatic cancer, although clinical experience with their use is limited at this time.

IMMUNOTHERAPY

Cytotoxic chemotherapy, irradiation, and surgery are the principal forms of cancer treatment but have the inherent disadvantage of producing damage and loss of function to normal tissues. Therapies that utilize immunologic reactions to destroy tumor cells are of growing interest because of the specificity of immune responses and their lack of toxicity to normal organs. Various approaches to immunotherapy are shown in Figure 176–10.

Tumor growth is associated with a progressive impairment of immunologic competence. In selected animal models, aug-

TABLE 176–10. HORMONES AND HORMONE ANTAGONISTS IN CANCER TREATMENT

Agent	Route	Dose and Schedule	Acute Toxicity	Late Complications	Uses
Estrogen:					
Diethylstilbestrol	PO	5 mg t.i.d. (breast) 1–3 mg q.d. (prostate)	Nausea, vomiting, sodium and fluid retention, uterine bleeding, hypercalcemia (in patients with bone metastases)	Feminization, risk of death from cardiovascular disease	Prostate cancer, postmenopausal breast cancer
Estrogen antagonist:					
Tamoxifen	PO	10 mg b.i.d.	Hypercalcemia, nausea, thrombocytopenia (transient), mild estrogenic action, hot flashes	Retinal degeneration, cataracts	Breast cancer
Progestins:					
Hydroxypro-gesterone	IM	1 gram b.i.w.	Fluid retention, hypercalcemia, cholestatic jaundice		Breast, endometrial, renal cancer
6-Methyl hydroxy-progesterone	IM PO	200–600 mg b.i.w. 100–200 mg q.d.			
Megestrolacetate	PO	160 mg q.d.			
Androgens:					
Fluoxymesterone	PO	10–20 mg q.d.	Cholestatic jaundice (fluoxymesterone), virilization, fluid retention, ureteral obstruction (males), hypercalcemia (in patients with bone metastases)	Hepatic adenomas, hepatoma	Breast carcinoma in ER⁺ patients who have prior response to estrogen or anti-estrogen therapy
Glucocorticoids:					
Prednisone Hydroxycortisone hemisuccinate	PO IV	40 mg/m² q.d. 200 mg/m² q.d.	Fluid retention, hyperglycemia, euphoric state, hypokalemia	Osteoporosis, immunosuppression, cushingoid habitus, gastrointestinal ulcers, hypertension, suppression of pituitary-adrenal axis	Lymphomas, leukemia, multiple myeloma, breast cancer
Dexamethasone	PO	2–10 mg/m² q.d. in divided doses		Same as above	Cerebral edema

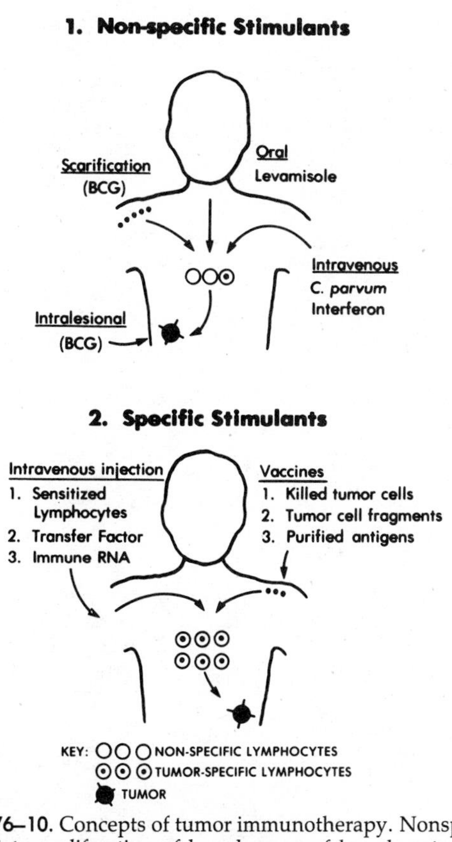

Figure 176–10. Concepts of tumor immunotherapy. Nonspecific stimulants initiate proliferation of broad range of lymphocytes, including previously sensitized tumor-specific cells. Specific immune stimulants promote selective proliferation of tumor-specific immune cells.

mentation of immunity can lead to tumor regression. In clinical studies, cell-mediated immunity may be enhanced by *nonspecific stimulants:* (1) BCG (bacillus Calmette-Guérin), *C. parvum,* or extracts of these bacteria; (2) chemicals such as levamisole; (3) plant extracts; and (4) animal products such as lymphokines and interferon, the latter a class of proteins produced by lymphocytes, fibroblasts, and other tissues. Interferons possess antiviral and antitumor activity. In preliminary clinical trials, leukocyte interferon produced by recominant DNA technology has produced brief responses in patients with non-Hodgkin's lymphoma, breast cancer, and multiple myeloma, but as yet the mode of action of interferons is not clear, although they stimulate the antitumor activity of natural killer cells (lymphocytes that have nonspecific tumoricidal action). *Specific immunotherapies* have also been devised, and include vaccines composed of killed or inactivated tumor cells from the patient (autochthonous cells) or from a patient with a similar type of tumor (allogeneic cells), or composed of partially purified cell fragments. Lymphocytes sensitized in vitro to a tumor, or extracts of sensitized lymphocytes such as RNA or so-called transfer factor, can produce antitumor effects in animals. Finally, monoclonal antibodies highly specific for individual tumors have been produced by the hybridoma technique, have produced a remission in one well-studied case of non-Hodgkin's lymphoma, and offer great promise for both diagnostic and therapeutic purposes. However, none of these therapies has yet made a significant impact on the treatment of any type of human malignancy. Such treatments must be refined and enhanced in potency before they will replace standard measures.

CONCLUSION

This description of tumor growth and principles of cancer treatment has provided a framework for developing rational therapies. However, these principles must be complemented by a clear understanding of the characteristics of specific tumor types, and an appreciation for the needs and expectations of the individual patient. In this endeavor, the internist can be given no simple remedies or uniform prescriptions for what must be a complex and prolonged treatment experience. The internist must be guided by knowledge of the disease, its potential treatments, and the patient's capacity to tolerate the side effects of these treatments.

Chabner BA: The Pharmacologic Basis of Cancer Treatment. Philadelphia, W. B. Saunders Company, 1982. *A text covering both the clinical and experimental pharmacology of anticancer drugs, with particular emphasis on clinical pharmacokinetics, cell kinetics, and drug interactions.*

De Vita VT Jr, Hellman S, Rosenberg SA: Cancer: Principles and Practice of Oncology. Philadelphia, J. B. Lippincott Co., 1982. *A detailed consideration of three treatment methods of cancer: surgery, irradiation, and chemotherapy.*

Goldie JH, Coldman AJ: A mathematic model for relating the drug sensitivity of tumors to their spontaneous mutation rate. Cancer Treat Rep 63:1727, 1979. *The most useful and illuminating analysis of the relationship of spontaneous mutation rate to drug resistance.*

Pinedo HM, Chabner BA: Cancer Chemotherapy 1984. Amsterdam, Elsevier–North Holland, 1984. *A yearly update of drug research and clinical chemotherapy, with detailed and critical evaluation of important new papers.*

Shackney SE, McCormack GW, Cuchural GJ: Growth rate patterns of solid tumors and their relation to responsiveness to therapy: An analytical review. Ann Intern Med 89:107, 1978. *Describes the relationship between tumor growth rate and responsiveness to chemotherapy, emphasizing the kinetic reasons for success and failure of cancer treatment.*

Tannock I: A presentation of classical cell kinetics and its application to cancer chemotherapy: A critical review. Cancer Treat Rep 62:1117, 1978. *A lucid discussion of the basic principles of cellular kinetics and their application, or lack thereof, in the design of current clinical chemotherapy regimens.*

Part XV
METABOLIC DISEASES

177. INTRODUCTION

James B. Wyngaarden

The term *metabolism* encompasses the numerous chemical transformations that occur within living organisms. These are often divided into two large categories. Those reactions or processes that are synthetic, and in general result in a larger molecule than any of the reactants, are called *anabolic*. Such reactions are usually energy requiring. Those reactions that are degradative and involve the breakdown of large molecules into smaller products are termed *catabolic*. Such processes are essentially energy yielding. The term *intermediary metabolism* refers to all changes that take place between the moment of entry of a nutrient into the organism and the discharge of all of the chemical products into the environment. It is customary to consider separately the intermediary metabolism of carbohydrates, lipids, and proteins, although no sharp lines can be drawn among these three areas of knowledge. The term *basal metabolism* refers to energy requirements for maintenance and conduct of cellular and tissue processes under conditions in which the effects of muscular activity and the work of digestion and metabolism of foodstuffs are minimal.

Part XV of this textbook is concerned with Metabolic Diseases. A disorder is classified as a metabolic disease when the fundamental pathogenetic mechanism involves a chemical transformation or process. Many diseases of metabolism involve specific enzyme or other protein abnormalities. When these can be attributed to an underlying genetic abnormality, they are termed *inborn errors of metabolism* (see Ch. 32). Disorders associated with specific enzyme defects have been described for more than 100 individual enzymes. Most of these are described somewhere in this textbook, but not all have been collected into Part XV. For example, hemolytic anemias attributable to specific enzyme defects are included with the other hemolytic anemias in Part XIII, Hematologic and Hematopoietic Diseases, and adrenal hyperplasia attributable to specific enzyme defects is discussed in Part XVII, Endocrine and Reproductive Diseases. The disorders included in this Part are chiefly those whose manifestations are multisystemic or in which the biochemical and genetic factors dominate the description.

PATHOGENESIS OF HEREDITARY METABOLIC DISEASES. The etiology of an inborn error of metabolism is a mutant gene. The alteration in DNA structure produces a disturbance in protein structure and function, which in turn affects cell and organ function. Hereditary metabolic diseases can be considered in terms of these three sequential levels.

Altered DNA Structure. The nature of mutations can be deduced from changes in amino acid sequences in the mutant proteins and the genetic codes (see Ch. 31 and 32). This approach has been applied most extensively in studies of variant hemoglobins and glucose-6-phosphate dehydrogenases. DNA restriction enzyme analyses and DNA sequencing techniques now permit direct analysis of alterations in DNA structure. By these methods, point mutations, deletions, and insertions are now readily identified, and hybrid proteins or prematurely terminated or aberrantly extended proteins or totally deleted proteins explained in terms of genetic mechanisms. Restriction endonucleases identify variations in gene structure as fragment-length polymorphisms. The latter approach has provided a first clue to the genetic abnormality in Huntington's disease. With the availability of DNA cloning techniques it is now possible to study directly the altered DNA sequence in many human mutations, even those that involve genes that code for quantitatively minor proteins such as enzymes. These techniques also disclose mutations in noncoding regions of DNA that affect rate of synthesis, processing, or stability of specific messenger RNAs.

Altered Protein Function. Abnormalities in the synthesis or structure of a specific enzyme protein result in absent, reduced, or (occasionally) enhanced rates of a specific enzyme-catalyzed reactions. In most genetic enzyme deficiency states, a reduced but detectable level of enzymatic activity can be measured by sensitive assays. The residual enzyme activity can frequently be shown to be due to a catalytically abnormal enzyme, which may exhibit decreased affinity for substrates, cofactors, or inhibitors. In the most extensively studied series of enzyme defects, those involving glucose-6-phosphate dehydrogenase, most of the enzyme deficiencies reflect unstable enzymes whose activities decay as the erythrocyte ages. This is a common mechanism of enzyme deficiency in the anucleated red blood cell, but has not been demonstrated to be an important cause of enzyme deficiency in disorders that affect primarily nucleated cells. The most interesting example of mutations leading to increased enzyme activites involves phosphoribosylpyrophosphate synthetase. Different mutations in an X-linked structural gene lead to four discrete subtypes exhibiting (1) reduced sensitivity to nucleotide regulators, (2) increased affinity for substrate, (3) increased specific activity per enzyme molecule, or (4) combination of (1) and (3). Relatively few lesions, other than hemoglobinopathies, have been shown to be due to mutations in genes coding for nonenzymic proteins. One example is the ZZ variant of α_1-antitrypsin deficiency, in which an altered protein is not susceptible to normal post-translational processing (glycosylation), with the result that the defective glycoprotein cannot be secreted by the liver. In some nonenzymic proteins, a structural abnormality leads to aggregation (e.g., sickle cell hemoglobin). In others, the mutation affects the affinity of a receptor for a specific ligand (e.g., the LDL receptor in familial hypercholesterolemia; the cytoplasmic androgen receptor in complete testicular feminization).

Disrupted Cell and Organ Function. Most genetic diseases first come to clinical attention because of disturbances at the level of cell and organ function. Several types of derangements occur:

1. Altered flux through metabolic pathways. This is the most frequent basis of recognition of an inborn error of metabolism. The product may be missing (albinism), or a precursor may accumulate (mucopolysaccharidoses) or be shunted into a toxic metabolite (phenylketonuria).

2. Disordered feedback regulation of synthetic pathways. Decreased synthesis of a regulatory end-product may result in faulty control of an early step of the pathway with excessive production of intermediates. The classic example is acute intermittent porphyria, in which a deficiency of uroporphyrinogen synthetase leads to diminished production of heme, a normal feedback inhibitor of porphyrin synthesis. Decreased production of heme leads to overactivity of δ-aminolevulinic acid synthetase, overproduction of nonheme porphyrins, and acute intermittent porphyria.

3. Disordered membrane function. This is the basis for a large group of genetic diseases in which there is impairment of a specific function of a plasma membrane protein. In one type, transmembrane transport of specific small molecules is defective, apparently because a membrane carrier protein is nonfunctional. The affected substrates can be amino acids (cystinuria), carbohydrates (renal glycosuria), or ions (renal tubular acidosis). In another type, receptor-mediated endocytosis of a macromolecule is defective. In familial hypercholesterolemia a mutation in the gene that codes for a receptor results in defective uptake and degradation of low density lipoproteins by body cells, resulting in accumulation of LDL and its cholesterol in plasma and arterial walls. Still another type involves a defect in a plasma membrane protein whose action is required for hormone action. In pseudohypoparathyroidism, the GTP-sensitive N protein is defective, and parathyroid hormone cannot stimulate adenylate cyclase in the target cell. The latter

two types of defects are inherited as dominant traits, in contrast to those that involve transmembrane transport of small molecules which behave as recessive traits.

4. Disordered intracellular compartmentation. A few examples of primary genetic defects in cell compartmentation are known. The ZZ variant of α_1-antitrypsin deficiency, discussed above, is one. Another is I-cell disease, in which there is a deficiency of a processing enzyme that is normally responsible for the occurrence of mannose-6-phosphate residues in lysosomal enzymes. In the absence of mannose-6-phosphate residues, enzymes do not bind to a specific receptor that directs them to the lysosome, and these enzymes pass through the cell into the plasma like a secretory protein. An additional example is a rare form of familial hypercholesterolemia in which there is an abnormal cell surface receptor that can bind LDL but cannot transport it into the cell.

5. Distorted cell or tissue architecture. The distorted shapes of erythrocytes in sickle cell diseases and in hereditary spherocytosis are an example of this type. A second example is illustrated by the immotile cilia syndrome (Kartagener's syndrome), in which a structural protein of cilia, dynein, is defective. In consequence the "dynein arms" that cross-link microtubules are missing, they cannot slide properly, and cilia cannot undulate. A third type is exemplified by Type VI Ehlers-Danlos syndrome, in which collagen is deficient in hydroxylysine and does not cross-link normally.

ACQUIRED METABOLIC DISEASES. There are many examples of metabolic diseases which are acquired rather than hereditary. Gout exists in primary and secondary varieties. The secondary types occur because of excessive nucleic acid turnover in myeloproliferative diseases or chronic hemolytic anemias, or because of impaired renal excretion of uric acid resulting from drug effects upon the kidney or acquired renal disease. Certain varieties of porphyria can be attributed to acquired intoxications. Hyperlipoproteinurias are common accompaniments of other diseases: hypothyroidism, the nephrotic syndrome, acute and chronic alcoholism, biliary obstruction. In many conditions there is a prominent interaction between hereditary and environmental factors: obesity and diabetes mellitus, ingestion of phenylalanine-containing proteins in phenylketonuria, ingestion of milk in galactosemia. Without the environmental stress these conditions would remain silent.

Some of the diseases of metabolism are very common, such as diabetes, with a prevalence in the United States of about 2.5 per cent, and the hyperlipidemias. Others are quite rare, and a few are perhaps more properly regarded as biochemical anomalies rather than diseases—pentosuria, for example. The study of rare metabolic disorders has provided a better understanding of normal metabolic processes, and in some instances has allowed early recognition of a disorder whose manifestations are preventable simply by adjustment of diet (galactosemia, phenylketonuria). The identification of specific enzyme defects has led to attempts at replacement therapy with inklings of success following enzyme infusion (Gaucher's disease, Fabry's disease) or organ transplantation (bone marrow in immunologic deficiency states; kidney in cystinosis, Fabry's disease, Gaucher's disease).

Bondy PK, Rosenberg LE (eds.): Metabolic Control and Disease. 8th ed. Philadelphia, W. B. Saunders Company, 1980. *An excellent general text.*

Garrod AE: Inborn errors of metabolism (Croonian Lectures). Lancet 2:1, 73, 142, 214, 1908. *A classic! The original exposition of the concept of inborn errors of metabolism.*

Stanbury JB, Wyngaarden JB, Fredrickson DC, Goldstein JL, Brown MS (eds.): The Metabolic Basis of Inherited Disease. 5th ed. New York, McGraw-Hill Book Company, 1983. *An authoritative text that presents detailed discussions of various hereditary diseases of metabolism by recognized experts on each topic.*

178. GALACTOSEMIA

Ernest Beutler

The galactosemias are characterized by inability to metabolize galactose normally. When patients with galactosemia ingest galactose, either in its free form or as the galactose-containing disaccharide lactose, galactose and some of the products of its incomplete metabolism accumulate in the blood, tissues, and usually the urine. Three types of galactosemia exist, each the result of a specific enzyme deficiency. The classic form of the disorder, galactose-1-phosphate uridyl transferase deficiency, is to be distinguished from galactokinase deficiency and from deficiency of the other enzyme of galactose metabolism, UDP glucose-4-epimerase.

CLASSIC GALACTOSEMIA

ETIOLOGY. Classic galactosemia is an autosomal recessive disorder due to a marked deficiency of the enzyme galactose-1-phosphate uridyl transferase.

PREVALENCE. The prevalence of classic galactosemia is approximately 1 per 60,000 births.

PATHOGENESIS. The galactose molecule is identical to the glucose molecule except for the relative position of the hydroxyl and hydrogen groups attached to the fourth carbon. The body is unable to utilize this sugar until it has been converted to glucose. Galactose is phosphorylated in the 1-position by ATP through the mediation of the enzyme galactokinase:

$$\text{Galactose} + \text{ATP} \xrightarrow{\text{galactokinase}} \text{galactose-1-P}$$

Next, galactose-1-P exchanges with the glucose-1-P moiety attached to a uridine diphosphate carrier. This reaction is catalyzed by galactose-1-phosphate uridyl transferase:

$$\text{Galactose-1-P} + \text{UDPG} \xrightleftharpoons{\text{transferase}} \text{glucose-1-P} + \text{UDPGal}$$

Finally, uridine diphosphogalactose (UDPGal) may be converted to uridine diphosphoglucose (UDPG) through the action of UDP glucose-4-epimerase:

$$\text{UDPGal} \xrightleftharpoons{\text{epimerase}} \text{UDPG}$$

In classic galactosemia the absence of galactose-1-phosphate uridyl transferase activity results in accumulation of both galactose and galactose-1-P. Galactose may serve as a substrate for aldose reductase and for L-hexonate dehydrogenase. These enzymes oxidize NADPH, reducing galactose to its polyol derivative, dulcitol, to which cell membranes are relatively impermeable. In the lens of the eye this creates an unbalanced osmotic force resulting in excessive hydration. At the same time it may deplete the lens of its supply of NADPH. The result of these changes is the irreversible precipitation of the lens protein with the formation of cataracts.

Cirrhosis of the liver and mental retardation are also characteristic of classic galactosemia. Since these changes do not occur in galactokinase deficiency (see below), it may be presumed that they are the result of galactose-1-phosphate accumulation.

CLINICAL MANIFESTATIONS. Occasionally infants with galactosemia have cataracts at birth. More typically the symptoms of galactosemia begin within a few days or weeks of birth. The infant takes feeding poorly, vomits frequently, and may have diarrhea. Many galactosemic infants die in the first few weeks of life. Progressive hepatomegaly and ascites may enlarge the abdomen. Jaundice usually appears quite early, hemolytic anemia may occur, and the disorder has at times been mistaken for hemolytic disease of the newborn. Proteinuria and generalized aminoaciduria are constant findings. If cataracts are not present at birth, they may develop within a few weeks, or in some instances not for many months. Mental retardation becomes evident as the infant matures. Administration of large galactose loads, as in the performance of galactose tolerance tests, may produce dangerous hypoglycemia.

DIAGNOSIS. The diagnosis of galactosemia is often first suspected when a reducing sugar not reacting in the glucose oxidase system is found in the urine. Diagnosis depends on the demonstration that galactose-1-P uridyl transferase activity is absent or nearly absent from the erythrocytes.

TREATMENT. The treatment of galactosemia consists of immediate institution of a diet with a very low galactose content. Known carriers of galactosemia should avoid milk during pregnancy to prevent prenatal damage to a galactosemic fetus. Because milk contains a high concentration of lactose, a disaccharide of glucose and galactose, a milk substitute such as Nutramigen must be fed during infancy. Although the effectiveness of the low-galactose diet in infants is established, no data are available regarding the necessity for maintaining strict dietary control after the first few years of life. It is likely that the ingestion of small amounts of galactose is relatively harmless after the fifth or sixth year of life. However, it is probably wise to continue a moderate degree of dietary restriction throughout life.

PROGNOSIS. Untreated infants with classic galactosemia rarely survive more than a few months, and may succumb within a few days. A few cases first diagnosed in later childhood or early adult life are known. With the prompt institution of a low-galactose diet, the development of galactosemic children appears to be normal or nearly so. If treatment is delayed, however, some degree of permanent mental retardation and irreversible cataracts are often present. Signs of liver failure and growth retardation appear to respond promptly to therapy in most instances, and patients who are treated generally survive into adult life.

PREVENTION. Heterozygotes for classic galactosemia have one half normal galactose-1-P uridyl transferase activity in their red cells. However, not all persons with this level of enzyme activity are carriers of galactosemia. Persons homozygous for the gene for the Duarte variant also have one half normal transferase activity, but may be differentiated from those heterozygous for galactosemia on the basis of the electrophoretic properties of the red cell enzyme. Prenatal diagnosis can be achieved by assaying cultured amniotic cells for galactose-1-P uridyl transferase.

Prevention of the clinical sequelae of galactosemia by early diagnosis and prompt institution of treatment is the most practical means of control.

GALACTOKINASE DEFICIENCY

ETIOLOGY. Galactokinase deficiency is a hereditary disorder caused by an autosomally inherited enzyme deficiency.

PREVALENCE. Only about 25 families with galactokinase deficiency have been described. The prevalence may be of the order of 1 in 500,000 births. As many as 1 in 100 patients developing cataracts of unknown origin during the first year of life may have this defect.

PATHOGENESIS. Galactokinase catalyzes the first step of galactose metabolism (see above). A deficiency of galactokinase results in the accumulation of galactose in the body, and in the formation of cataracts through the same mechanism outlined under Classic Galactosemia.

It is uncertain whether only galactokinase-deficient individuals with virtually total absence of the enzyme develop cataracts. An increased incidence of cataracts has been noted among heterozygotes in some families of galactokinase-deficient persons. However, most heterozygotes do not develop cataracts, and the link between partial galactokinase deficiency and cataracts is not firmly established.

CLINICAL MANIFESTATIONS. The only well-established clinical manifestation of galactokinase deficiency is the development of cataracts.

DIAGNOSIS. The diagnosis of galactokinase deficiency should be considered in any person developing cataracts of unknown cause during early childhood. The diagnosis is established by measuring red blood cell galactokinase activity.

TREATMENT. The treatment of galactokinase deficiency consists of institution of a low-galactose diet (see above).

PROGNOSIS. If a low-galactose diet is initiated at the time of birth or shortly thereafter, cataract formation is prevented. When cataracts are already present, improvement, if any, seems to be very limited.

PREVENTION. The effects of galactokinase deficiency can be prevented by early detection and institution of a low-galactose diet. The heterozygote may be identified by measuring the galactokinase activity in red cells. However, one half normal levels of galactokinase are also commonly encountered as an apparently harmless polymorphism in the black population. Genetic counseling is potentially useful with families in which a case of galactokinase deficiency has been found. Screening of the blood of neonates by methods which detect increased blood galactose levels makes possible early detection so that treatment can be instituted promptly.

UDPG-4-EPIMERASE DEFICIENCY

A deficiency of UDPG-4-epimerase (epimerase) has been described only a few times. In all but one of the reported cases the defect was entirely benign, the deficiency apparently being limited to the erythrocytes. One patient, a product of a consanguineous marriage, manifested the deficiency not only in red cells but also in cultured skin fibroblast and presumably in other tissues. Vomiting, jaundice, hepatomegaly, and abnormal liver function test results occurring in the neonatal period ameliorated in response to low galactose diet.

Beutler E, Matsumoto F, Kuhl W, Krill A, Levy N, Sparkes R, Degnan M: Galactokinase deficiency as a cause of cataracts. N Engl J Med 288:1203, 1973. *Galactokinase determinations performed on 210 patients under the age of 40 who had developed cataracts revealed a significantly increased incidence of low galactokinase activities in the 92 patients who developed cataracts in the first year of life.*

Holton JB, Gillett MG, Macfaul R, Young R: Galactosaemia: A new severe variant due to uridine diphosphate galactose-4-epimerase deficiency. Acta Biol Med Ger 40:885, 1981. *The only reported case of clinically significant epimerase deficiency.*

Kalckar HM, Kinoshita JH, Donnelly GN: Galactosemia: Biochemistry, genetics, pathophysiology, and developmental aspects. Biol Brain Dysfunct 1:31, 1972. *A detailed review of clinical manifestations and biochemical pathophysiology of galactosemia.*

Levy HL, Hammersen G: Newborn screening for galactosemia and other galactose metabolic defects. J Pediatr 92:871, 1978. *An evaluation of screening methods for various forms of galactosemia. Includes prevalence data based on nearly 6,000,000 infants.*

Segal S: Disorders of galactose metabolism. *In* Stanbury JB, Wyngaarden JB, Fredrickson DS, Goldstein JL, Brown MS (eds.): The Metabolic Basis of Inherited Disease. 5th ed. New York, McGraw-Hill Book Company, 1982. *A comprehensive review of biochemical genetics of galactokinase deficiency.*

179. THE GLYCOGEN STORAGE DISEASES

R. Rodney Howell

Glycogen is the principal storage form of carbohydrate in man and is found in varying concentrations in virtually all cells. Glycogen is composed exclusively of glucose molecules, and differs from starch in having a highly branched structure that greatly enhances its solubility.

In the glycogen storage diseases the tissue concentration of glycogen is most commonly elevated, but in certain of these disorders the significant abnormality is in the structure of glycogen. Although liver glycogen content reflects to some extent the nutritional status of the subject, excessive alimentation does not lead to abnormal accumulation of hepatic glycogen in the normal subject in the absence of corticosteroid treatment.

The glycogen storage diseases are of historic importance in that the first direct demonstration of a liver enzyme deficiency in man was carried out in Type I glycogen storage disease by the Coris over 30 years ago.

As new specific enzyme defects were recognized, the Coris began a numbering system for the glycogen storage diseases that is still in wide use. We will refer to the numbering system here; however, its use is to be discouraged, because the numbers beyond VI vary considerably from author to author and the existence of some of the conditions defined by recent numbers is in doubt.

Although most of the glycogen storage diseases produce fairly widespread accumulation of glycogen, in large part the diseases present clinically as either hepatic or muscular forms.

THE HEPATIC FORMS OF GLYCOGEN STORAGE DISEASE. *Type I glycogen storage disease* or hepatorenal glycogen storage disease (von Gierke's disease) is the prototype of the hepatic forms of glycogen storage disease. Children with this disorder have proportionately short stature with very prominent abdomens and massive enlargement of the liver. The hepatic enlargement is due to both glycogen and lipid accumulation. Although the kidneys are enlarged because of the deposition of glycogen, this cannot be appreciated clinically except by radiographic examination. The eyes reveal multiple bilateral, symmetric, yellowish, discrete, paramacular lesions, which are specific for Type I glycogen storage disease. Xanthomas are common over the extensor surfaces of the arms and legs; bleeding may present major clinical problems.

Prominent hypoglycemia on fasting and a reduced rise of blood sugar after subcutaneous injection of epinephrine or glucagon are typical. The response to glucagon and epinephrine is rarely "flat" because the degradation of branch points of glycogen leads to free glucose even in the absence of glucose-6-phosphatase. Dramatic elevations of blood lactate, pyruvate, triglycerides, cholesterol, and uric acid are usual.

After puberty the hyperuricemia with complicating clinical gouty arthritis and the occurrence of multiple benign hepatic adenomas (and very rarely hepatic carcinoma) become the main clinical problems. Death from renal disease, possibly related to uric acid, has occurred in several adult patients.

The precise diagnosis must be routinely established by a liver biopsy and the demonstration of a deficient activity of the enzyme glucose-6-phosphatase. Patients are recognized (termed Type Ib glycogen storage disease) who demonstrate no glucose-6-phosphatase activity on a fresh biopsy sample, but demonstrate completely normal activity on the frozen sample. This condition represents a defect in glucose-6-phosphate translocase, a specific protein that shuttles glucose-6-phosphate across the membrane. Glucose-6-phosphatase activity is normal.

Other prominent forms of hepatic glycogen storage disease appear clinically similar to Type I glycogen storage disease except that they are milder. In *Type III glycogen storage disease,* the deficiency of the debrancher enzyme leads to excessive accumulation of glycogen of abnormal structure. The stored glycogen has short outer branches. These patients generally have much milder hypoglycemia and much milder growth retardation and do not present with hyperuricemia or the severe lipid problems that are seen in Type I glycogen storage disease. Hepatic adenomas are not known to occur.

The typical patient with Type III glycogen storage disease tends to achieve a more normal height, and following puberty the liver will frequently appear normal in size. Because of the generalized nature of the enzyme defect in these patients (including liver as well as muscle), some of these patients have had significant myopathy in adulthood related to the storage of the abnormally structured glycogen. This muscle weakness and wasting can be the predominant finding in the older patient. At least six subtypes of Type III glycogen storage disease are recognized, depending on variations of the tissue distribution of the enzyme defect. The diagnosis in this condition is usually established by assaying liver, muscle, white cells, or red cells for the specific debranching enzyme. Direct liver assay is often required.

In *Type IV disease,* a genetic deficiency of the branching enzyme presents as liver failure in early infancy. These children display the usual hallmarks of liver failure (jaundice, ascites), usually by age two. Muscle weakness can be prominent. A deficiency of the branching enzyme can be demonstrated in leukocytes and in fibroblasts as well as in liver tissue. The glycogen content of the liver is usually normal or below normal, but the structure demonstrates very long outer branches secondary to the genetic deficiency of the branching enzyme.

A group of patients has been recognized with very mild clinical symptoms of hypoglycemia and growth retardation but with substantial hepatomegaly. Some lack clinical symptoms. On biochemical examination they have a significant increase of normally structured liver glycogen and a deficiency of the enzyme phosphorylase. These patients have traditionally been classified as having *Type VI storage disease.* The deficiency in all instances has been a partial enzyme deficiency (perhaps a total deficiency would be lethal). The outlook in these phosphorylase-deficient patients is good, and ordinarily no specific treatment is required.

Further study of patients with defects in the phosphorylase system has demonstrated a substantial number of males who are genetically deficient in the enzyme phosphorylase b kinase. This glycogen storage disease is different from all of the rest (which are inherited in all instances as autosomal recessive traits), in that phosphorylase b kinase activity is inherited in an X-linked recessive manner. Females who carry this gene (heterozygotes) may have modest hepatomegaly, whereas affected males (hemizygotes) have substantial hepatomegaly but not the other major symptoms of hypoglycemia or hyperlipidemia. Their response to epinephrine and glucagon is variable, but they routinely have significant plasma elevations of liver enzymes such as SGOT and SGPT. The liver shows inflammatory changes on biopsy. The phosphorylase b kinase patients have traditionally been categorized as having *Type VIII glycogen storage disease.*

Treatment of the Hepatic Forms of Glycogen Storage Disease. A variety of hormonal treatments, such as thyroxine and glucagon administration, have been ineffective in the hepatic forms of glycogen storage disease. Surgical portacaval shunting has been performed on a number of occasions. Some patients have benefited substantially, most specifically in restoration of growth. Most of these shunting procedures have been carried out in Type I patients, but an occasional patient with Type III (debrancher deficiency) has been treated. Because of substantial morbidity this treatment is no longer recommended.

At present, the most appropriate treatment for the symptomatic forms of hepatic glycogen storage disease is nasogastric infusion of a high carbohydrate diet. Continuous nasogastric feeding overnight with either carbohydrate alone or carbohydrate plus protein is of great benefit not only by restoring growth toward normal but also, importantly, by restoring the lipid and carbohydrate abnormalities toward normal. This treatment, currently in wide use, is safe and has its clearest benefit on growth.

The adult patient with hyperuricemia and gout is effectively treated with allopurinol and is usually not responsive to uricosuric drugs.

THE MUSCULAR FORMS OF GLYCOGEN STORAGE DISEASE. The most dramatic of the muscular forms of the glycogen storage diseases is Type II glycogen storage disease or generalized glycogen storage disease. There is prominent deposition of glycogen in all muscular tissues and a genetic deficiency of the lysosomal enzyme alpha-1,4-glucosidase.

This condition was originally described in infants as *Type II glycogen storage disease* (Pompe's disease), with the typical child dying of cardiorespiratory disease in the first two years of life. In recent years, additional patients with muscular glycogen storage disease, secondary to deficiency of alpha-1,4-glucosidase, have presented with muscular weakness in late childhood or in adulthood. Respiratory failure has been the presenting symptom in certain adults. Cardiac involvement has been either minimal or absent in the older patients.

The diagnosis of Type II glycogen storage disease depends on a muscle biopsy that demonstrates an increased concentration of glycogen, which on electron microscopy is within the lysosome. Alpha-1,4-glucosidase deficiency is transmitted in an autosomal recessive manner. Specific enzyme analyses of leukocytes can demonstrate an absence of an acid alpha-1,4-glucosidase, but such studies are not always reliable. The presence in white cells of a neutral maltase that has considerable activity in the range of pH 4 can lead to relatively normal white cell activities for alpha-1,4-glucosidase, although the acid maltase characteristic of the lysosome is deficient. There is a consistent deficiency of alpha-1,4-glucosidase activity in cultured skin fibroblasts. Patients with myopathy appearing in late adulthood must be considered as potential candidates for Type II glycogen storage disease, as well as for debrancher deficiency glycogen storage disease, as mentioned above.

Muscle phosphorylase deficiency or McArdle's disease *(Type V glycogen storage disease)* is perhaps the rarest of the glycogen storage diseases. Patients with this disorder are probably underrecognized, for their symptoms appear functional. Patients are usually asymptomatic until adolescence or early adulthood when they develop painful muscle cramps after exercise. If exercise is continued, myoglobinuria and renal failure may ensue.

These patients demonstrate an absence of the rise in venous lactate which follows anaerobic exercise. The condition should be suspected in healthy, well-developed adults who present with painful muscle cramps after exercise and who demonstrate no rise in lactate after exercise. A specific diagnosis is made on muscle biopsy which demonstrates an increased concentration of structurally normal glycogen and a deficiency of phosphorylase activity. This condition is inherited as an autosomal recessive trait. Patients with a genetic deficiency of muscle phosphofructokinase activity *(Type VII glycogen storage disease)* appear clinically identical to patients with an absence of muscle phosphorylase activity. The diagnosis is established in a similar fashion; they have painful muscle cramps after exercise, demonstrate no rise in venous lactate after anaerobic exercise, but on biopsy show an increased concentration of glycogen in the muscle and an absence of muscle phosphofructokinase activity.

Treatment of the Muscular Glycogen Storage Diseases. Patients with deficiencies of phosphofructokinase or of phosphorylase in muscle can be benefited by avoiding strenuous exercise. There is some suggestion that isoproterenol (which increases blood flow to the muscle) may be helpful by making more glucose available for direct utilization by muscle.

At present there is no specific treatment for Pompe's disease or Type II glycogen storage disease. A strain of cattle in Australia affected with a condition identical to Pompe's disease in man is proving valuable as an experimental model.

Isolated patients have been reported in whom activities of phosphohexoisomerase, phosphoglucomutase, or cyclic 3′,5′-AMP–dependent kinase have been deficient, but these conditions need further clarification. Reported deficiencies of UDP-8-glycogen transferase activity probably represent defects in gluconeogenesis; the low enzyme activity is likely due to the well-known instability of the enzyme when tissue glycogen content is low.

PRENATAL DIAGNOSIS OF THE GLYCOGEN STORAGE DISEASES. Type I glycogen storage disease cannot be diagnosed prenatally because the enzyme deficient in this condition (glucose-6-phosphatase) is not present in normal cultured human fibroblasts. New techniques of molecular genetics (e.g., restriction mapping) should permit prenatal diagnosis in the near future. However, the enzyme alpha-1,4-glucosidase is active in normal cultured skin fibroblasts, and Pompe's disease can be reliably diagnosed in utero. Debrancher deficiency glycogen storage (Type III) disease is difficult to establish in utero. Although the debranching enzyme is present in normal fibroblasts, widespread tissue variability of the inherited deficiency makes the prenatal diagnosis of Type III difficult. Brancher deficiency glycogen storage disease can be diagnosed in utero.

Phosphorylase b kinase deficiency (Type VIII glycogen storage disease) can be diagnosed in cultured human fibroblasts. The mildness of this condition, however, makes prenatal diagnosis inappropriate.

Bosch EP, Munsat TL: Metabolic myopathies. Med Clin North Am 63:759, 1979. *The disorders of glycogen as they affect muscles are reviewed in detail from both a clinical and a biochemical standpoint.*

DiMauro S, Hartwig GB, Hays A, Eastwood AB, Franco R, Olarte M, Chang M, Roses A, Fetell M, Schoenfeldt RS, Stern LZ: Debrancher deficiency: Neuromuscular disorder in 5 adults. Ann Neurol 5:122, 1979. *This article presents a detailed review of the muscular problems in adults with debrancher deficiency.*

Howell RR, Williams JC: The glycogen storage diseases. *In* Stanbury JB, Wyngaarden JB, Fredrickson DS, Goldstein JL, Brown MS (eds.): The Metabolic Basis of Inherited Disease. 5th ed. New York, McGraw-Hill Book Company, 1983. *This is a thorough coverage of the clinical and biochemical aspects of the glycogen storage diseases. This article is extensively referenced.*

Narisawa K, Otomo H, Igarashi Y, Arai N, Otake M, Tada K, Kuzuya T: Glycogen storage disease type Ib: Microsomal glucose-6-phosphatase system in two patients with different clinical findings. Pediatr Res 17:545, 1983. *This article summarizes current information about the microsomal glucose-6-phosphatase system and the glucose-6-phosphate translocase.*

Slonim AE, Lacy WW, Terry A, Greene HL, Burr IM: Nocturnal intragastric therapy in Type I glycogen storage disease: Effect on hormonal and amino acid metabolism. Metabolism 28:707, 1979. *This group reviews their extensive experience in the nocturnal intragastric therapy of Type I glycogen storage disease and the effects on hormonal and amino acid abnormalities. They review and reference the experience of others.*

180. PENTOSURIA

(Essential Pentosuria)

R. Rodney Howell

Pentosuria is an innocuous, rather common heritable abnormality of carbohydrate metabolism that occurs almost exclusively in Jews and Lebanese. It is transmitted in an autosomal recessive fashion with an estimated prevalence of 1:2000 to 1:5000 in these populations. Affected persons excrete between 1 and 4 grams of the pentose L-xylulose in the urine daily. Loading of the glucuronic acid cycle by the oral administration of glucuronolactone will cause an increase in urinary L-xylulose excretion in the homozygote and a lesser response in the heterozygote. Assay of the erythrocytes of affected individuals demonstrates a deficiency of the specific NADP-linked enzyme xylitol dehydrogenase, which converts L-xylulose to xylitol. The affinity of the mutant enzyme for NADP is significantly less than that of the normal enzyme. The presence in the urine of L-xylulose, a reducing sugar, has in the past led to false diagnoses of diabetes. The sugar can easily be distinguished from others by paper or thin-layer chromatography. Glucose oxidase, which is the reagent in the commonly used dipstick type of urine test, does not react with this sugar, whereas reducing agents will.

Hiatt HH: Pentosuria. *In* Stanbury JB, Wyngaarden JB, Fredrickson DS (eds.): The Metabolic Basis of Inherited Disease. 4th ed. New York, McGraw-Hill Book Company, 1978, p 110. *This is a detailed review of the history and biochemistry of essential pentosuria.*

Wang YM, VanEys J: The enzymatic defect in essential pentosuria. N Engl J Med 282:892, 1970. *This paper first describes the specific defect in essential pentosuria.*

181. ESSENTIAL FRUCTOSURIA AND HEREDITARY FRUCTOSE INTOLERANCE

R. Rodney Howell

ESSENTIAL FRUCTOSURIA (FRUCTOSURIA). Fructosuria is a rare asymptomatic condition caused by a deficiency of the enzyme fructokinase. It is inherited in an autosomal recessive manner and has a recognized prevalence of 1:130,000. Fructokinase activity is normally present only in liver, kidney, and intestinal mucosa, and catalyzes the first reaction in the major pathway of fructose utilization in man. The diagnosis of fructosuria is established indirectly by a fructose loading test. Following such a load, an excessive rise in fructose concentration in the blood and the chromatographic identification of significant amounts of fructose in the urine are diagnostic. In normal persons after fructose loading the blood fructose concentration will peak at one hour and not exceed 25 mg per deciliter, with no significant concentration of fructose in the urine. Hepatic fructokinase activity is undetectable in tissue from patients with essential fructosuria. Fructose is a reducing sugar and does react with Clinitest tablets and other reducing agents, so confusion with diabetes must be avoided. Since fructose does not react with glucose oxidase in the urine dipstick utilized in most clinical laboratories, the confusion of this benign condition with diabetes is less of a problem now than in the past.

HEREDITARY FRUCTOSE INTOLERANCE. Unlike fructosuria, hereditary fructose intolerance produces major clinical symptoms. This condition is due to a structural mutation of the liver enzyme fructose-1-phosphate aldolase (aldolase B) and is transmitted in an autosomal recessive fashion. The largest documented family demonstrated considerable consanguinity. In humans there are three types of aldolases (A, B, and C) that are tetrameric molecules that may form hybrids. They differ in their tissue distribution and in their activity ratios toward the two substrates fructose-1,6-diphosphate (FDP) and fructose-1-phosphate (F1P). Aldolase B is characterized by an activity ratio of 1 and is present in large amounts in liver, renal cortex, and small intestine. Tissue from patients with hereditary fructose intolerance exhibits a profound deficiency of activity against fructose-1-phosphate and a modest reduction in activity against fructose-1,6-diphosphate. The FDP/F1P ratios have ranged from 2.5 to 20 instead of from 1.0 to 1.3 as in normal liver.

Symptoms are present only after the ingestion of fructose. Immediately after fructose ingestion there is a brisk reduction in blood glucose and serum phosphorus concentrations and a marked increase in serum uric acid concentration. There is a striking deterioration of renal tubular function as manifested by the inability to acidify the urine, bicarbonaturia, aminoaciduria, and phosphaturia in the presence of a falling serum phosphorus concentration. Hypokalemia may occur. The infant who continues to ingest fructose will exhibit vomiting, failure to thrive, hypotonia, jaundice, hepatosplenomegaly, ascites, bleeding disorders, abnormal liver function test results, hypoglycemia, acidosis, proteinuria, and fructosuria. The differential diagnosis includes galactosemia and tyrosinemia, and diagnosis can be difficult.

The acidosis is due primarily to excess lactic acid and to a lesser extent to proximal renal tubular dysfunction. The fructosemia and fructosuria are secondary to the inhibition of fructokinase by its accumulated reaction product fructose-1-phosphate. The hypoglycemia following ingestion of fructose results from a defect in the phosphorolysis of glycogen to glucose-1-phosphate.

Liver biopsies show early stages of cirrhosis. The brain has been reported to show diminished neurons. In spite of the recurrent hypoglycemia in infancy, affected adults have normal intelligence.

The dose dependent reduction of ATP and the accumulation of fructose-1-phosphate within the renal cortex have been thought to explain the Fanconi-like syndrome observed in these patients. The reduction of phosphate is, however, of greatest importance. The hyperuricemia results from the increased conversion of adenine nucleotides to urate induced by fructose and from a decreased renal clearance of urate in the presence of elevated blood lactate concentrations.

Older affected children and adults are protected by the development of an aversion to sweets and a self-imposed fructose-free diet. This results in beautiful teeth without caries. Intravenous fructose has been life threatening when administered to an undiagnosed adult in an emergency. In such a situation the patient shows acute icterus, severe gastrointestinal hemorrhage, hypoglycemia, pronounced proximal tubular acidosis, disseminated intravascular coagulation, and Fanconi's syndrome.

The diagnosis can be reliably established by monitoring serum concentrations of glucose, phosphorus, urate, magnesium, and fructose after the intravenous infusion of fructose. In all cases studied at the tissue level, the presence of cross-reacting material indicates a structural defect in the enzyme.

The treatment is the exclusion of fructose from the diet. On a fructose-free diet the outlook is favorable.

Gitzelmann R, Steinmann B, van den Berghe G: Essential fructosuria, hereditary fructose intolerance, and fructose-1,6-diphosphate deficiency. *In* Stanbury JB, Wyngaarden JB, Fredrickson DS, Goldstein JL, Brown MS (eds.): The Metabolic Basis of Inherited Disease. 5th ed. New York, McGraw-Hill Book Company, 1983. *This review covers in detail the clinical and biochemical aspects of hereditary fructose intolerance and essential fructosuria.*

Gregori C, Schapira F, Kahn A, Delpech M, Dreyfus JC: Molecular studies of liver aldolase B in hereditary fructose intolerance using blotting and immunological techniques. Ann Hum Genet 46:281, 1982. *This paper summarizes enzymatic studies in 15 liver biopsies from patients with hereditary fructose intolerance. Good discussion of various aldolases and substrate specificity.*

Lameire N, Mussche M, Baele G, Kint J, Ringoir S: Hereditary fructose intolerance: A difficult diagnosis in the adult. Am J Med 65:416, 1978. *This article reviews the clinical features and presentation of hereditary fructose intolerance in the adult.*

Morris RC, McInnes RR, Epstein CJ, Sebastian A, Scriver CR: Genetic and metabolic injury of the kidney. *In* Brenner BM, Rector FC (eds.): The Kidney. Philadelphia, W. B. Saunders Company, 1976, pp 1214-1218. *This chapter details the mechanism of renal injury in hereditary fructose intolerance.*

Richardson RM, Little JA, Patten RL, Goldstein MB, Halperin ML: Pathogenesis of acidosis in hereditary fructose intolerance. Metabolism 28:1133, 1979. *This article reviews the etiology of the metabolic acidosis and hypokalemia in patients with hereditary fructose intolerance.*

Steinmann B, Gitzelmann R: The diagnosis of hereditary fructose intolerance. Helv Paedit Acta 36:297, 1981. *Excellent review of diagnostic tests for hereditary fructose intolerance.*

182. PRIMARY HYPEROXALURIA

Lloyd H. Smith, Jr.

Primary hyperoxaluria is a general term for two rare genetic disorders of glyoxylate metabolism productive of excessive synthesis and urinary excretion of oxalic acid. Both disorders are transmitted as autosomal recessive traits. The diseases are characterized by the onset in childhood of recurrent calcium oxalate nephrolithiasis or nephrocalcinosis, or both, usually leading to early death secondary to renal failure. In addition to the usual clinical features of uremia, severe peripheral vascular insufficiency may complicate the course of the disease. At postmortem examination calcium oxalate may be found widely deposited in extrarenal sites, a condition known as *oxalosis*. More rarely, milder forms of the disease may be found in adults. Although oxalate is an important constituent in approximately two thirds of all kidney stones, most adult patients with calcium oxalate nephrolithiasis excrete normal amounts of urinary oxalate (Ch. 89).

Primary hyperoxaluria Type I (glycolic aciduria) represents a genetic defect in the soluble enzyme α-ketoglutarate: glyoxylate carboligase. The resulting accumulation of glyoxylate leads to its excessive oxidation to oxalate and its reduction to glycolate, both of which are excreted in increased amounts in the urine (more than 60 mg per 1.73 square meters per 24 hours each). In *primary hyperoxaluria Type II* (L-glyceric aciduria) there is a defect in the enzyme D-glyceric dehydrogenase. Hydroxypyruvate accumulates and is reduced by lactic dehydrogenase

(LDH) to L-glyceric acid, a compound that is undetectable in normal urine. The reduction of hydroxypyruvate to L-glycerate is probably coupled to the oxidation of glyoxylate to oxalate, both catalyzed by LDH. Each disease can be diagnosed by the characteristic pattern of metabolites in urine: Type I, oxalate and glycolate; Type II, oxalate and L-glycerate. Pyridoxine deficiency in laboratory animals and man also leads to hyperoxaluria and even oxalosis with a urinary pattern similar to that of the genetic disease Type I. With the onset of renal failure the clearance of oxalate is reduced (its clearance is normally about 1.2 times that of creatinine) so that its urinary excretion may return to normal. The diagnosis may then be difficult to establish because of the unreliability of current methods for measuring serum oxalate.

No specific methods of treatment are now available. Efforts are directed toward reducing the amount of oxalate excreted and increasing its solubility. Large amounts of pyridoxine (200 to 400 mg per 24 hours) may decrease oxalate excretion in the Type I disease. Dilute urine should be maintained by forcing fluids, and a phosphate or magnesium oxide supplement may offer partial protection against stone formation. Renal homotransplantation has been disappointing because of rapid deposition of calcium oxalate in the transplanted kidney, but a few reports of success have recently appeared. Chronic dialysis and pyridoxine are therefore indicated when renal failure is severe. Nitroglycerin has been reported to be effective in treatment of

the peripheral vascular insufficiency associated with oxalosis. A search for an inhibitor of oxalate synthesis is being conducted.

Increased urinary excretion of oxalate and stone diathesis (in the absence of glycolic aciduria or L-glyceric aciduria) occur in many patients who have small bowel disease and malabsorption. Normally oxalate and fatty acids of the small intestine compete for available calcium ion, and calcium oxalate is poorly absorbed. This important form of acquired hyperoxaluria results from excessive absorption of dietary oxalate in the presence of significant steatorrhea. It can be controlled by a low oxalate diet.

Earnest DL: Enteric hyperoxaluria. Adv Intern Med 24:407, 1979. *An excellent general review of the clinical features, pathogenesis, and treatment of the most frequent cause of hyperoxaluria, that associated with its excessive absorption from dietary sources.*

Whelchel JD, Alison DV, Luke RG, et al.: Successful renal transplantation in hyperoxaluria. Transplantation 35:161, 1983. *Although the general experience in renal transplantation in primary hyperoxaluria has been adverse, there are now a few reports, as in this article, of success.*

Williams HE, Smith LH Jr: Primary hyperoxaluria. *In* Stanbury JB, Wyngaarden JB, Fredrickson DS, Goldstein JL, Brown MS (eds.): The Metabolic Basis of Inherited Disease. 5th ed. New York, McGraw-Hill Book Company, 1983, p 204. *This general review of oxalate metabolism in man emphasizes the enzyme defects and the resulting metabolic derangements associated with the two recognized variants of the genetic disorder primary hyperoxaluria.*

Disorders of Lipoprotein Metabolism

183. THE HYPERLIPOPROTEINEMIAS

John D. Brunzell

Disorders of lipoprotein metabolism are related to abnormalities in the synthesis and degradation of plasma lipoproteins. These abnormalities may result from primary inborn errors of metabolism or may be secondary to a variety of other disease states. Hyperlipidemia, the elevation of plasma cholesterol and/or triglyceride concentrations, is the hallmark of the lipoprotein disorders. Clinical delineation of these disorders is important because of the association of some with premature coronary artery disease and others with recurrent pancreatitis.

The classification of disorders of lipoprotein metabolism was first based on the varieties of xanthomas that occur and the appearance of plasma turbidity due to the accumulation of large, light scattering lipoprotein particles in plasma. With the discovery of relatively discrete lipoprotein species, classification of these disorders was done on the basis of the separation of lipoproteins by ultracentrifugation or by electrophoresis. Recent understanding of lipoprotein physiology has allowed classification of lipoprotein disorders according to pathophysiologic defects, with specific discrete apoprotein, enzyme, or receptor abnormalities identified in some disorders.

PHYSIOLOGY OF LIPOPROTEIN TRANSPORT

Structure and Function of Lipoproteins

The structure of the lipoprotein macromolecule is well-suited for the solubilization of lipids in plasma. The nonpolar lipids—cholesteryl ester and triglyceride—are present in the lipoprotein core surrounded by a monolayer composed of specific proteins and the polar lipids, unesterified cholesterol and phospholipid. This monolayer allows the lipoprotein to remain miscible in plasma.

The lipoproteins function as an efficient vehicle for site-to-site transport of triglyceride and cholesterol of both exogenous and endogenous origin. Although caloric need is fairly constant throughout the day, food is ingested only periodically. The excess calories that enter the circulation with each meal are transported mainly as triglyceride to be stored in adipose tissue for future utilization between meals as free fatty acids. Ingested and synthesized cholesterol also needs to be transported to extrahepatic tissues to serve as a source of membrane cholesterol and as substrate for steroid hormone synthesis. The transport of triglyceride and cholesterol is accomplished by a spectrum of lipoproteins that have been classified by arbitrary operational boundaries according to either their density by ultracentrifugation or mobility by electrophoresis (Table 183–1). Fortunately, the lipoproteins, as separated by ultracentrifuga-

TABLE 183–1. PHYSICAL CHARACTERISTICS OF LIPOPROTEIN FRACTIONS

	Triglyceride-Rich				Cholesterol-Rich
Density (g/ml)	0.95	1.006	1.006–1.019	1.019–1.063	1.063–1.21
Electrophoretic mobility	Origin	Prebeta	Beta	Beta	Alpha
Flotation rate (Sf)	400	20–400	12–20	0–12	—
Chylomicron	———	→			
Chylomicron remnant	———	———	→		
Endogenous VLDL	———	→			
Endogenous VLDL remnant		———	→		
Low density lipoprotein			———	→	
High density lipoprotein			———	———	→
Lipid phenotype when fraction increased*	I	IV	III	IIA	

*Based on World Health Organization recommendations.

tion or electrophoresis, are so similar that the synonyms based on each of these methods of separation are essentially interchangeable (Table 183–1).

The triglyceride-rich lipoproteins can enter the plasma as chylomicrons derived from dietary fat adsorbed from the gut or endogenously as triglyceride-rich very low density lipoprotein synthesized from glucose or circulating free fatty acids in the liver. After removal of some of their triglycerides and surface components, the remaining lipoprotein remnant of the chylomicron is taken up by the liver and degraded. The remnant of endogenous triglyceride-rich lipoprotein probably also requires the liver for further processing. In contrast to the chylomicron, however, only some components of VLDL are removed, resulting in formation of the low density cholesterol-rich lipoprotein.

This is likely to be an oversimplification, as it is apparent that there is a continual spectrum of particles, and lipoproteins enter and exit at many sites along this spectrum of varying lipoprotein sizes. High density lipoproteins interact with this system for transport of triglyceride and cholesteryl ester, as will be noted later.

Both the physiology and the pathophysiology of lipoproteins can be evaluated by examining the sites of lipoprotein production and the multiple steps in lipoprotein catabolism. Most pathophysiologic abnormalities leading to hyperlipidemic states can be understood by examining four sites of regulation of plasma lipoprotein transport: (1) triglyceride-rich lipoprotein input, (2) lipoprotein lipase–mediated triglyceride catabolism, (3) remnant catabolism, and (4) cholesterol-rich lipoprotein catabolism (Fig. 183–1).

Production of Triglyceride-Rich Lipoproteins

After hydrolysis of dietary triglycerides in the small intestine, the resulting fatty acids and monoglycerides are taken up by the absorptive cells of the small intestine and incorporated into large triglyceride-rich lipoproteins with a specific form of apoprotein B (apo B-48), phospholipid, and a small amount of cholesterol. These chylomicrons are secreted from the absorptive cells into the lymphatics and subsequently enter the plasma via the thoracic duct. Chylomicron secretion and transport represent a system of high capacity energy flux allowing calories ingested at one time, over and above immediate needs, to be transferred to sites of storage for use between meals. The chylomicron remnant taken up and degraded by the liver suppresses synthesis of components of endogenous triglyceride-rich lipoproteins.

Input into plasma of triglyceride-rich lipoproteins also occurs from endogenous sources. During meals plasma free fatty acids enter the liver, where they may be esterified with glycerol to form triglyceride. Between meals, free fatty acids are mobilized from adipose tissue triglyceride stores. These serve as a potential source for hepatic triglyceride synthesis. Lipogenesis, synthesis of fatty acids de novo from carbohydrate, also occurs in the liver. Fatty acids in the cytosol of the hepatocyte can either enter mitochondria, where oxidation occurs, or can remain in the cytosol, where they are esterified to form triglyceride. These processes appear to be regulated by changes in insulin and glucagon levels that occur with feeding: glucagon enhances and insulin prevents mitochondrial fatty acid uptake by regulating long chain acyl carnitine transferase. Insulin also induces lipogenic enzymes in the hepatocytes that regulate the synthesis of fatty acids.

Triglyceride synthesized in the liver, together with cholesteryl ester, is combined with the lipoprotein monolayer composed of phospholipid, unesterified cholesterol, and apoprotein B, and secreted into the hepatic venous outflow as triglyceride-rich very low density lipoprotein. Hepatic apoprotein B (apo B-100) in VLDL appears to have a larger molecular weight than intestinal apoprotein B (apo B-48) found in chylomicrons.

In normal individuals, the majority of triglyceride input into the plasma is of dietary origin. While the average American diet contains about 100 grams of triglyceride per day, it appears that less than 30 grams of triglyceride are secreted endogenously.

Lipoprotein Lipase–Mediated Triglyceride Catabolism

The triglyceride that enters the plasma in chylomicrons and endogenously synthesized triglyceride-rich lipoproteins is transported to adipose tissue for storage or to muscle for utilization. The enzyme in adipose tissue and muscle that catalyzes this triglyceride uptake is lipoprotein lipase. In adipose tissue the enzyme is synthesized in the fat cell, and following secretion and transport to the capillary endothelial cell, hydrolyzes the triglyceride in these lipoproteins at the endothelial surface. At least two of the three fatty acids potentially releasable from triglyceride hydrolysis are then transported to the fat cell where they are re-esterified with glycerol and stored as intracellular adipocyte triglyceride. The vast majority of the triglyceride in the adipocyte enters by this mechanism; little lipogenesis de novo from glucose occurs in adipose tissue in man. The functional activity of lipoprotein lipase in adipose tissue is increased during and after meals. In humans, most of this increase in function is due to the increase in triglyceride-rich lipoproteins that serve as enzyme substrate. Although insulin is required to maintain lipoprotein lipase

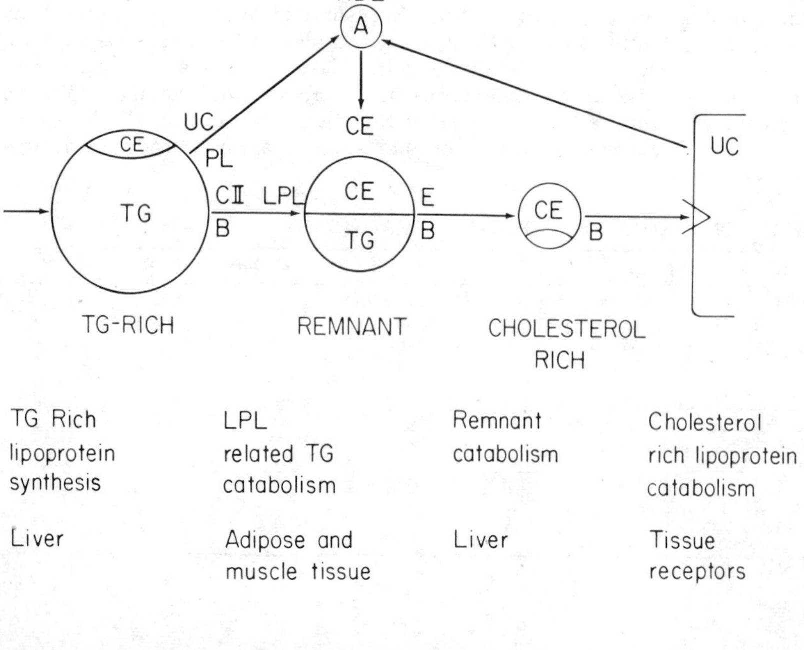

Figure 183–1. The triglyceride-rich lipoprotein is synthesized in the liver and contains apo-B, which remains with the particle through its subsequent catabolism. The triglyceride-rich lipoprotein core contains triglyceride (TG) and cholesteryl ester (CE) and surface unesterified cholesterol (UC) and phospholipid (PL). Upon entering plasma, acquired apo CII activates lipoprotein lipase (LPL) to catabolize TG core. The resulting remnant acquires apo-E, which interacts with hepatic receptors to catabolize remnant to cholesterol-rich low density lipoprotein (LDL). The LDL binds to high affinity receptor, with subsequent intracellular degradation of the lipoprotein. High density lipoproteins with apoproteins AI and AII (A) acquire surface components of lipoproteins and plasma membranes of cells and forms cholesteryl esters. These cholesteryl esters exchange with other lipoproteins or are delivered directly to the liver and may be the primary source of biliary cholesterol and bile acids.

levels in adipose tissue, little change in enzyme levels occurs with normal meals. Between meals calories stored as triglyceride are released from the adipocyte as free fatty acids. This hydrolysis of intracellular adipocyte triglyceride is mediated by "hormone sensitive" lipase of the fat cells. Between meals, when insulin levels are low and glucagon is rising, "hormone sensitive" lipase activity increases, and free fatty acids are released to be used for energy utilization by most tissues of the body.

The interaction of lipoprotein lipase with triglyceride in triglyceride-rich lipoproteins requires a cofactor, apoprotein CII, which is a component of these lipoproteins. When secreted from the absorptive cell of the gut and from the liver, chylomicrons and VLDL do not contain this activator. Shortly after entering plasma these lipoproteins pick up apoprotein CII from a reservoir in circulating high density lipoprotein. Thus, the triglyceride-rich lipoproteins contain both substrate and activator for their hydrolysis by lipoprotein lipase. Following hydrolysis of the triglyceride in these lipoproteins, the apoprotein CII is released and again picked up by the high density lipoproteins (HDL). Thus, HDL appears to serve as a shuttle for apoprotein CII (as well as other lipoprotein components) (see below). Other apoproteins (CI and CIII) are transferred bidirectionally between triglyceride-rich lipoproteins and HDL and may play an as yet not clearly defined role in lipoprotein lipase triglyceride hydrolysis, as well as other lipoprotein interactions.

Remnant Lipoprotein Catabolism

Following hydrolysis of the triglyceride in triglyceride-rich lipoproteins and the simultaneous removal of surface components, "remnant" lipoproteins are formed from chylomicrons and endogenous triglyceride-rich lipoproteins. The intermediate density lipoprotein fraction isolated by ultracentrifugation consists largely of remnant particles of VLDL. Those remnants formed from chylomicrons and large endogenous VLDL often distribute, however, in the density range of small VLDL. Thus, remnants and endogenously synthesized triglyceride-rich lipoproteins cannot be separated completely by ultracentrifugation. Once formed, the remnant has a short half-life in plasma and appears to be taken up by the liver. The endogenous triglyceride-rich lipoprotein remnant is further processed into the cholesterol-rich low density lipoprotein. During this catabolic process, further triglyceride and cholesterol as well as some surface proteins are removed. The remnant lipoprotein contains apoprotein B, and several forms of apoprotein C and apoprotein E. The apoprotein E that accumulates as the remnant lipoproteins are formed appears to be important for hepatic uptake of those remnants. There is a complex interaction of hepatic receptors specific for apoprotein E and other receptors that bind both apoprotein B and apoprotein E, with the apoproteins in the remnant lipoproteins regulating their hepatic uptake. By the time the cholesterol-rich low density lipoprotein has been formed, apoprotein B is the only apoprotein of the triglyceride-rich lipoproteins remaining.

Cholesterol-Rich Low Density Lipoprotein Catabolism

As the cholesterol-rich low density lipoprotein normally arises from the remnant lipoprotein of VLDL, it contains the same amount of apoprotein B per lipoprotein particle as endogenous triglyceride-rich VLDL, while other apoproteins have been almost entirely removed, together with much of the phospholipid and some cholesterol. The cholesterol-rich lipoprotein appears to be removed from plasma by extrahepatic tissues where it functions as the chief source of cholesterol for membrane synthesis or steroid hormone synthesis by these tissues. Alternatively, the lipoprotein may be taken up by the liver and degraded if not utilized peripherally. Apoprotein B in the cholesterol-rich lipoprotein appears to be recognized by a specific, high affinity binding site in tissues. Once bound, the lipoprotein is internalized by the cell in an endocytotic vesicle that fuses with a primary or pre-existing secondary lysosome. The protein moiety is degraded and the cholesteryl ester hydrolyzed to unesterified cholesterol by a lysosomal acid cholesteryl ester hydrolase. Hydrolysis of the triglyceride and phospholipid may also occur in the lysosome. The cell is able to regulate its own cholesterol content through a feedback control system in which intracellular free cholesterol suppresses endogenous cholesterol production by inhibiting the rate-limiting enzyme in cholesterol synthesis (HMG CoA reductase). Furthermore, accumulation of intracellular free cholesterol limits the further uptake of cholesterol-rich lipoproteins by inhibiting synthesis of the lipoprotein receptor itself and stimulates its own re-esterification to cholesteryl ester by activating an acyl CoA:cholesterol transferase in the cytosol. Cholesterol content in the cell may also be regulated by a removal system involving high density lipoproteins as a vehicle for cholesterol.

Apoprotein B containing lipoproteins may also be degraded by a scavenger system other than the high affinity LDL receptor. This scavenger pathway involves the macrophage system and assumes greater importance in lipoprotein catabolism when defects in the LDL receptor or other abnormalities in lipoprotein catabolism exist.

Lipoprotein Surface Catabolism

Newly synthesized lipoproteins with their hydrophobic triglyceride and cholesteryl ester core are surrounded by a monolayer composed of protein, unesterified cholesterol, and phospholipid. As the core is removed and the lipoprotein decreases in size, several mechanisms process the resulting "excess" surface. The catabolism of these surface components involves high density lipoprotein (HDL) and the enzyme lecithin-cholesterol-acyl-transferase (LCAT). HDL, synthesized by the liver and the intestine, is composed of phospholipid and two major structural apoproteins, apoprotein AI and apoprotein AII. This HDL serves as an acceptor for the phospholipid (mainly lecithin) and unesterified cholesterol from the triglyceride-rich lipoprotein surface. LCAT associated with HDL then removes a fatty acid from lecithin and transfers it to cholesterol, producing cholesteryl ester and lysolecithin. The cholesteryl ester is transferred from HDL to the liver directly or after transfer to other lipoproteins, making the HDL available to shuttle more lipoprotein surface components. HDL, LCAT, and transfer proteins may also play a role in the regulation of intracellular cholesterol content by enhancing the efflux of free cholesterol from extrahepatic tissues. Thus, HDL may play a role in the transport of cholesterol from cells to liver where it is ultimately excreted. In addition, HDL serves as the shuttle for apoprotein CII and apoprotein E to and from triglyceride-rich lipoproteins as part of their catabolism.

Cholesterol Excretion

Cholesterol and phospholipids are excreted as such in the bile, or after conversion of cholesterol into bile acid. A large proportion of the secreted bile acids are reabsorbed in the enterohepatic circulation and are recycled. However, a net loss of bile acid, cholesterol, and phospholipid in the stool occurs by this pathway.

The definitive source of the cholesterol for output in the bile and for bile acid formation has not been determined. Cholesterol excreted into the bile may be synthesized directly in the liver. Alternatively, cholesterol may be secreted from the liver and gut in triglyceride-rich lipoproteins and may be esterified by the LCAT-HDL system, and may reenter the liver directly with HDL or via remnant lipoproteins.

INBORN ERRORS OF LIPOPROTEIN METABOLISM

The primary, or inborn, errors of lipoprotein metabolism leading to hyperlipidemia generally can be grouped into disorders associated with overproduction of triglyceride-rich lipoproteins or disorders due to defects in one of three catabolic steps in lipoprotein degradation (Fig. 183–1). Much more is

TABLE 183–2. INBORN ERRORS OF LIPOPROTEIN METABOLISM

Name	Prevalence	Physiologic Abnormality	Protein Abnormality	Lipoprotein Phenotype	Lipoproteins that Accumulate
Familial hypercholesterolemia	1/500	↓ LDL catabolism	Abnormal LDL receptor	IIA (IIB)	LDL ± VLDL
Familial dysbetalipoproteinemia	1/10,000	↓ Remnant catabolism	Abnormal apoprotein E	III	β VLDL
Lipoprotein lipase or Apo CII deficiency	Very Rare	↓ TG catabolism	Absent LPL or apoprotein CII	I (V)	Chylo ± VLDL
Familial hypertriglyceridemia	?1/100	? ↑ VLDL-TG synthesis	?	IV (V)	VLDL ± Chylo
Familial combined hyperlipidemia	?1/100	↑ Apoprotein B synthesis	Apoprotein B and apoprotein AI	IIA, IIB, IV	LDL and/or VLDL

Phenotypes based on World Health Organization recommendations.
Chylo = chylomicron.

known about defects in lipoprotein catabolism than about defects leading to lipoprotein overproduction (Table 183–2).

Defective Low Density Lipoprotein Catabolism: Familial Hypercholesterolemia

DEFINITION. Familial hypercholesterolemia is an autosomal dominant trait with defective receptors for plasma low density lipoproteins. An increase in LDL cholesterol is associated with characteristic xanthomas in the Achilles tendons, the patellar tendons, and the extensor tendons of the hands, and early coronary artery disease.

ETIOLOGY AND PATHOGENESIS. This disorder in LDL catabolism is caused by one of several alleles producing an abnormal high affinity LDL receptor. One of these alleles is associated with absent LDL receptor synthesis and the others with the production of receptors of abnormal composition. These nonfunctional receptors are associated with decreased LDL catabolism and, in the heterozygote, with an approximate two-fold increase in LDL levels. In the very rare homozygote, no high affinity receptor degradation occurs and LDL is removed by a lower affinity "scavenger" pathway with a six-fold or greater increase of cholesterol-rich lipoproteins in plasma.

CLINICAL MANIFESTATIONS. This disorder often manifests as coronary artery disease in a young male, who then is noted to have elevated cholesterol levels. The mean age of the first myocardial infarction in males with familial hypercholesterolemia who develop atherosclerosis is about 41 years. Affected women often go through life without clinical manifestations of atherosclerosis. Low HDL cholesterol levels and cigarette smoking have marked effects on accelerating coronary artery disease and may be the major determinant of clinical disease in females. Peripheral vascular disease and cerebrovascular disease do not seem to be increased as much as coronary artery disease in this disorder. Lipid deposits in tendons are pathognomonic for this disorder. These xanthomas, which are usually bilateral, may be nodular irregularities in the Achilles tendons or extensor tendons of the hands, but can extend to diffuse, generalized thickening. Corneal arcus and xanthalasma may occur but are found with other lipoprotein abnormalities as well.

DIAGNOSIS. Plasma cholesterol levels in familial hypercholesterolemia are in the upper 1 per cent of levels seen in the general population (e.g., 300 to 500 mg per deciliter). Since this disease seems to be present in one in 500 individuals, at least one person in five with such plasma cholesterol levels would be expected to have this disease. Patients with defective remnant removal and those with chylomicronemia may also have markedly elevated cholesterol levels, but they can be distinguished by the degree of coincident hypertriglyceridemia. Hypothyroidism and the nephrotic syndrome are also associated with elevated cholesterol levels. The increase in LDL in familial hypercholesterolemia uniquely is persistent, is almost always present in a parent, and is detectable at birth. The coexistence of tendon xanthomas and hypercholesterolemia is diagnostic of this disorder. Unilateral Achilles tendon thickening may be the result of injury.

TREATMENT. Discontinuation of smoking should be the first consideration for those who smoke. A low saturated fat, low cholesterol diet should be initiated in all affected individuals with this disorder, even though only a 5 to 15 per cent reduction in LDL levels occurs. Normalization of LDL levels occurs with the combination of a bile acid–binding resin (15 to 30 grams per day in divided doses with meals) and very high dose nicotinic acid with meals and at bedtime (2 to 7.5 grams per day). Compliance with each drug regimen has been poor. Fat-soluble vitamins should be given at bedtime, since the resins (colestipol or cholestyramine) prevent their absorption. Some recommend therapy with nicotinic acid and resins for all affected individuals. More conservatively, treatment can be restricted to postadolescent males and cigarette-smoking women. Drugs that suppress hepatic HMG-CoA reductase and hepatic cholesterol synthesis may be available soon and should simplify the treatment of this disorder.

Remnant Removal Disease: Dysbetalipoproteinemia

DEFINITION. This disorder is due to the interaction between (1) an autosomal recessive defect in apoprotein E with abnormal remnant catabolism and (2) independent overproduction of triglyceride-rich lipoproteins. This results in the accumulation of postlipoprotein lipase remnants from both chylomicrons and endogenously synthesized VLDL that cause xanthomas and coronary artery and peripheral vascular disease.

ETIOLOGY AND PATHOGENESIS. About 1 per cent of individuals have two genes leading to an abnormal apoprotein E. Multiple alleles exist for apoprotein E; those producing amino acid substitutions in a critical region of the apoprotein have abnormal apoprotein E binding to hepatic membranes. Homozygous individuals either have two identical abnormal genes or are compound heterozygotes with two different abnormal genes. Most of these individuals do not have hyperlipidemia but rather have low plasma cholesterol and LDL levels, presumably because of defective conversion of VLDL remnants to LDL. VLDL remnants that are cholesteryl ester enriched are present, but plasma triglyceride levels are usually normal. About one in 100 individuals with this abnormal apoprotein E has hyperlipidemia with remnant removal disease. These individuals appear to have an independent abnormality leading to hypertriglyceridemia in addition to the defect in apoprotein E, and accumulate significant levels of chylomicron and VLDL remnants. Much rarer forms of remnant removal disease are caused by total absence of apoprotein E or an absence of postheparin plasma hepatic triglyceride lipase.

CLINICAL MANIFESTATIONS. This disorder may present initially as premature clinical atherosclerosis or as planar or tuberous xanthomata, or it may be detected as hyperlipidemia on routine laboratory screen. This disorder is usually not manifested as an abnormality in triglyceride or cholesterol levels in men until the third or fourth decade or in women until after menopause. The coexistent apoprotein E abnormality can be detected at birth. The onset of the xanthomas also is late. Planar xanthomas of the palmar crease and tuberous or tuberoeruptive xanthomas are highly suggestive of this disorder, although both can occur in severe, chronic obstructive liver disease with residual hepatocellular function. Atherosclerosis often is first noted in men around age 50 years. Peripheral vascular disease often predominates, but coronary artery disease is increased as well. In females, development of peripheral vascular and coronary artery disease after menopause is rapid as compared with nonaffected females. The presence of estrogen in the premenopausal state seems to minimize the defect in remnant catabolism.

DIAGNOSIS. The presence of palmar or tuberous xanthomas in the absence of liver disease is diagnostic. Plasma cholesterol and triglyceride are increased to similar levels. A method for separation of VLDL from the remainder of the more dense lipoproteins is necessary to demonstrate that these VLDL are cholesteryl ester enriched, have beta mobility on electrophoresis ("beta VLDL") rather than the typical prebeta mobility of VLDL. An abnormal apoprotein E can usually be demonstrated by isoelectric focusing. The concentration of LDL is typically low, and HDL is often normal or slightly depressed. Hypothyroidism can aggravate this disorder or rarely can lead to remnant accumulation by itself.

TREATMENT. In obese individuals with this disorder, weight loss should be considered in lowering triglyceride and cholesterol levels. In postmenopausal females, low dose ethinyl estradiol seems to normalize the defect in remnant removal and to correct the hypercholesterolemia. Clofibrate (1 gram twice a day) or gemfibrosil (0.8 gram twice a day) also are effective in decreasing lipid levels. Alternatively, high dose nicotinic acid is considered by some investigators as the drug of choice for treatment of this disorder. There is evidence that the form of atherosclerosis occurring with this disorder might be partially reversible with treatment.

Defective Lipoprotein Lipase–Related Triglyceride Catabolism

DEFINITION. Familial LPL deficiency is a rare autosomal recessive trait characterized by complete absence of active enzyme protein in all tissues leading to massive hypertriglyceridemia from birth and recurrent episodes of pancreatitis. Similar syndromes also are caused by inborn defects in other aspects of the LPL system.

ETIOLOGY AND PATHOGENESIS. Hydrolysis of triglyceride from chylomicrons and endogenous VLDL in vivo requires both lipoprotein lipase and its activator apo CII. The absence of either of these proteins is associated with severely decreased triglyceride removal and massive hypertriglyceridemia. In infants and young children, the triglyceride accumulates primarily as chylomicron triglyceride of dietary origin. As the patient gets older, a defect in VLDL triglyceride removal becomes more apparent as well. Both LPL and apoprotein CII deficiency are autosomal recessive; often consanguinity can be documented. Individuals may also exist who have lipoprotein lipase activity missing from only selected tissues, or other individuals may have a familial inhibitor of LPL activity. These latter groups of individuals usually have less severe hypertriglyceridemia and become symptomatic later in life than in the classical form of LPL deficiency.

CLINICAL MANIFESTATIONS. Infants with LPL deficiency rapidly manifest intolerance to fatty foods. As these children grow, they learn to avoid certain high fat foods such as whole milk. Abdominal pain, often with pancreatitis, occurs in association with the high levels of chylomicron triglyceride. Eruptive xanthomas of extensor surfaces, notably the elbows, knees, and the buttocks occur, and are pathognomonic for chronic chylomicronemia. Hepatomegaly and occasionally splenomegaly occur due to the accumulation of lipid-laden foam cells. The hepatosplenomegaly rapidly diminishes on a fat-free diet, which clears the chylomicronemia. Eruptive xanthomas also disappear with time after lowering chylomicron levels. Other signs and symptoms seen with chronic chylomicronemia may also occur (see below).

DIAGNOSIS. A young child with abdominal pain and milky, lactescent plasma should be evaluated for a genetic abnormality in lipoprotein lipase. Other causes of chylomicronemia before adulthood relate to the occurrence of a common form of hypertriglyceridemia with diabetes or glucocorticoid therapy. Absent or diminished activity of lipoprotein lipase can be demonstrated in adipose tissue or muscle tissue, or in plasma after intravenous heparin. Apoprotein CII deficiency can be detected by radioimmunoassay or by gel electrophoresis of the protein components of lipoproteins.

TREATMENT. In all the inborn errors of the LPL-related triglyceride removal system associated with chylomicronemia, a decrease in total dietary fat is absolutely indicated. A total of polyunsaturated and saturated fat as low as 10 to 20 per cent of calories is often required. Medium-chain triglycerides can be used to prepare some foods, since their fatty acids leave the gut unesterified via the portal vein rather than via the thoracic duct as chylomicron triglyceride. The goal is to decrease the amount of dietary fat to a level low enough to eliminate the occurrence of abdominal pain. These individuals can also be sensitive to agents that raise endogenous VLDL levels, such as alcohol or glucocorticoids, and to the effects of pregnancy.

Other Genetic Disorders with Mild to Moderate Hypertriglyceridemia

A number of less well characterized disorders associated with persistent or intermittent elevated VLDL levels exist. Some may be associated with increased hepatic secretion of VLDL, others with defective VLDL catabolism. It has been useful to classify those conditions into several relatively homogenous groups on the basis of the existence of large, fairly well-characterized families for each.

FAMILIAL HYPERTRIGLYCERIDEMIA. This apparently autosomal dominant trait may be quite common. Individuals with familial hypertriglyceridemia appear to have a defect leading to enhanced hepatic triglyceride synthesis with subsequent secretion of triglyceride-enriched, large VLDL. These individuals may also have increased cholesterol synthesis and cholic acid synthesis. Lipoprotein lipase–related triglyceride removal and remnant lipoprotein catabolism appear to be normal. LDL levels are normal, while HDL are triglyceride-enriched with depletion of HDL cholesterol.

Most individuals with this disorder do not have an increased predisposition for coronary artery disease, remain asymptomatic, and are detected by routine lipid screen. Occasionally with the onset of another disorder associated with elevated triglyceride levels, they will develop the chylomicronemia syndrome (see below). These individuals develop no characteristic xanthomas. There is no increase in obesity in this disorder, and no increase in the frequency of diabetes.

Individuals with this disorder have persistent hypertriglyceridemia once they become adults. Below the age of 20, the abnormality is not manifest. Some of the increase in VLDL may persist after weight loss. Increased levels of low density lipoprotein do not occur. One parent is characteristically affected, as are half of the siblings. These individuals appear to be quite sensitive to other factors that cause only mild hypertriglyceridemia in normal adults: obesity, alcohol, estrogen, and glucocorticoid therapy.

Treatment with clofibrate or gemfibrosil usually leads to significant decreases in VLDL levels. In families without evidence of increased atherosclerosis, no known benefit accrues from this therapy, and it should be discouraged. Drugs causing elevation of triglyceride levels should be avoided because they may precipitate massive chylomicronemia and pancreatitis.

FAMILIAL COMBINED HYPERLIPIDEMIA. This disorder was first suggested in 1973 to be very common in those with premature coronary heart disease, to be inherited as an autosomal dominant trait, and to be characterized by different "combinations" of hyperlipidemia: elevated cholesterol alone, elevated triglyceride alone, or elevations in both lipids (familial multiple lipoprotein-type hyperlipidemia). It now appears that this disorder is better characterized as one with elevated plasma apoprotein B levels with variable lipid phenotype even in the same individual at different times, in contrast with familial hypercholesterolemia. The increase in apoprotein B, whether in VLDL or in LDL, appears to be caused by increased hepatic synthesis of the apoprotein. These individuals also have abnormalities in HDL with a mild decrease in HDL cholesterol and apoprotein AI.

Males with this disorder have premature coronary artery disease with mean age of infarct at about 40 years. Smoking has a marked effect on the prevalence of clinical heart disease. Individuals with this disorder are slightly more obese and usually have more systemic hypertension. They have no characteristic xanthomas but occasionally have nonspecific xanthalasma.

OTHER FORMS OF HYPERTRIGLYCERIDEMIA. Individuals with chylomicronemia and triglyceride levels between 1000 and 2000 are said to aggregate in families. In addition, some individuals with marked hypertriglyceridemia and a particular isoform of apoprotein E (apo E_4) have been reported. Finally, there are individuals with primary hypertriglyceridemia noted to have a defect in VLDL removal not characterized by one of the above defects in the lipoprotein lipase system.

APPROACH TO THE PATIENT WITH MILD TO MODERATE HYPERTRIGLYCERIDEMIA. The major concern with the individual with hypertriglyceridemia relates to the possible increase in risk for atherosclerosis that potentially might be present. When an individual is identified with elevated plasma triglyceride levels, acquired forms of hyperlipidemia should be identified and treated, and the primary forms of hypertriglyceridemia associated with defective remnant catabolism or lipoprotein lipase deficiency should be ruled out.

Elevations in plasma triglyceride levels often serve as a marker for associated abnormalities potentially related to atherosclerosis. A strong family history of early coronary artery disease in the father or mother's male relatives helps to identify such a hypertriglyceridemic individual at risk for early atherosclerosis.

The hypertriglyceridemic individual who intermittently develops hypercholesterolemia caused by increased LDL levels as well as those who can be demonstrated to have elevated LDL apoprotein B levels with normal LDL cholesterol also seem to be ones with increased risk for atherosclerosis.

HDL cholesterol is often low in the presence of hypertriglyceridemia. This can occur with familial lipoprotein lipase deficiency and with familial hypertriglyceridemia and does not seem to be associated with the increase in coronary risk seen with low HDL cholesterol in the absence of hypertriglyceridemia. However, a decrease in the level of the major apoprotein of HDL, apoprotein AI, seems to be a good predictor of risk, even in the presence of hypertriglyceridemia.

The aforementioned abnormalities characteristic of the hypertriglyceridemic subject at risk for atherosclerosis are similar to those seen in familial combined hyperlipidemia, but the relationship between these groups is not understood.

While weight loss and clofibrate (or gemfibrosil) therapy lower VLDL levels, those at risk for early coronary disease may respond with an increase in LDL levels. Preferred therapy for the hypertriglyceridemic individual at risk, in particular the one with familial combined hyperlipidemia, may be like that used to treat elevated LDL levels in familial hypercholesterolemia: combined bile acid resin and high dose nicotinic acid therapy, in addition to a diet low in saturated fat and cholesterol. Because of the uncertainty of the significance of elevated triglyceride levels and the unknown risks of lifelong drug therapy, many authorities have recommended diet therapy alone for hypertriglyceridemia.

TABLE 183–3. ACQUIRED DISORDERS OF LIPOPROTEIN METABOLISM

A. Hypertriglyceridemia
  1. Mild to moderate hypertriglyceridemia
    a. Diabetes mellitus*
    b. Uremia and/or dialysis*
  2. Minimal hypertriglyceridemia alone
    a. Obesity
    b. Estrogen*
    c. Alcohol*
    d. Diuretics*
    e. Beta-adrenergic blocking agents*
  3. Rare forms of moderate to marked hypertriglyceridemia
    a. Systemic lupus erythematosus
    b. Dysgammaglobulinemias
    c. Glycogenosis Type I
    d. Lipodystrophy
B. Combined hyperlipidemia
  1. Hypothyroidism*
  2. Nephrotic syndrome
  3. Glucocorticoid excess*
C. Hypercholesterolemia
  1. Acute intermittent porphyria
  2. Anorexia nervosa

*Can be associated with chylomicronemia syndrome when it occurs with the familial forms of hypertriglyceridemia.

ACQUIRED DISORDERS OF LIPOPROTEIN METABOLISM

Some disease states are associated with mild to moderate hyperlipidemia in the absence of primary forms of hyperlipidemia, while others seem to have a significant effect only in the presence of a familial form of hyperlipidemia. In general, these can be divided into conditions associated with increased levels of triglyceride-rich lipoproteins and those associated with multiple lipoprotein-type expression (acquired combined hyperlipidemia) (Table 183–3).

Hypertriglyceridemia

DIABETES MELLITUS. Persons with untreated insulin-dependent diabetes and untreated symptomatic noninsulin-dependent diabetes have low adipose tissue or muscle lipoprotein lipase with a mild to moderate increase in triglyceride levels and decreased HDL cholesterol levels. With insulin resistance and milder degrees of insulin deficiency, hypertriglyceridemia is caused by excess free fatty acids mobilized from adipose tissue that are re-esterified in the liver and secreted as endogenous VLDL. Treatment with insulin or oral sulfonylurea agents will correct the abnormality in lipoprotein lipase over a period of weeks. In the treated diabetic variability in free fatty acid mobilization and hepatic triglyceride synthesis, related to the degree of diabetic control, account for most of the variation in triglyceride levels.

CHRONIC UREMIA AND DIALYSIS. Many individuals with chronic uremia have elevated VLDL levels with hypertriglyceridemia and low HDL cholesterol levels. This persists after initiation of maintenance hemodialysis or peritoneal dialysis. These lipoprotein abnormalities appear to be related to defects in lipoprotein lipase–mediated triglyceride removal, and, with smoking and hypertension, account for the marked atherosclerosis in the dialysis population.

OTHER. Obesity, estrogen use, and alcohol are associated with minimal to mild increases in triglyceride levels, usually not to levels considered abnormal, and appear to be caused by modest increases in hepatic VLDL secretion. Diuretic agents and beta-adrenergic blocking agents are also associated with small increases in triglyceride levels.

Moderate to marked hypertriglyceridemia occurs extremely rarely in systemic lupus erythematosus or dysgammaglobulinemia caused by an immunoglobulin lipoprotein interaction. Moderate hypertriglyceridemia can also occur in very rare disorders such as glycogenosis (Type I), lipodystrophy, and carnitine-palmitoyl transferase deficiency.

Combined Hyperlipidemia

HYPOTHYROIDISM. Thyroid hormone appears to be necessary for proper functioning of most steps in lipoprotein metabolism. Thyroxin is necessary for maintenance of the LDL receptor; in hypothyroidism LDL levels are elevated because of defective catabolism. Remnant removal is impaired resulting in the accumulation of chylomicron and VLDL remnants, and finally lipoprotein lipase is low, resulting in hypertriglyceridemia. Thyroxin replacement corrects all of these defects.

NEPHROTIC SYNDROME. With urinary loss of albumin and the development of hypoalbuminemia, increases in levels of VLDL or LDL or both occur. These lipoprotein abnormalities are associated with increased hepatic lipid synthesis and defective catabolism of triglyceride-rich lipoproteins. The latter defect may be related to the loss in the urine of cofactors required for lipoprotein lipase function.

GLUCOCORTICOID EXCESS. Excess glucocorticoid levels caused by Cushing's syndrome or exogenous steroid therapy are associated with elevated VLDL and/or LDL levels. The best studied situation is in the glucocorticoid-treated renal transplant subject, who in the absence of uremia or proteinuria has combined hyperlipidemia.

Hypercholesterolemia

Elevated LDL levels might occur in occasional individuals in response to high saturated fat and cholesterol feeding. Much of the hypercholesterolemia in the population has remained unexplained and has been termed multifactorial, suggesting that it is due to interaction of multiple genes (polygenic) with the environment. Elevated LDL levels will occur in acute intermittent porphyria and have been reported with hepatomas and in anorexia nervosa.

CHYLOMICRONEMIA SYNDROME

DEFINITION. Marked chylomicronemia with plasma triglyceride levels in excess of 2000 mg per deciliter is associated with a constellation of signs and symptoms called the chylomicronemia syndrome.

ETIOLOGY AND PATHOGENESIS. This syndrome can occur because of one of several inborn errors in the lipoprotein lipase system for plasma triglyceride removal as noted earlier. Much more commonly, the marked hypertriglyceridemia occurs as a result of the interaction of two common forms of hypertriglyceridemia, usually one genetic and one acquired. Untreated, symptomatic diabetes mellitus in the presence of familial hypertriglyceridemia, familial combined hyperlipidemia, or, less commonly, remnant removal disease, is a frequent cause of chylomicronemia. Commonly used drugs that interact with these inborn errors are the estrogens, diuretics, beta-adrenergic blocking agents, alcohol, and glucocorticoids. Hypothyroidism and uremia may also occasionally contribute.

CLINICAL MANIFESTATIONS. For unexplained reasons, some individuals are asymptomatic with plasma triglyceride levels as high as 29,000 mg per deciliter. More commonly, abdominal pain and/or pancreatitis or even chest pain is present. Impairment of recent memory can often be detected and the patient may complain of paresthesias of the extremities, similar to the carpal tunnel syndrome. Lipemia retinalis can often be observed, hepatomegaly is common, splenomegaly can occur, and eruptive xanthomas are evidence of chronic chylomicronemia. All of these symptoms and signs clear when triglyceride levels are decreased below 1000 or 2000 mg per deciliter. Marked hypertriglyceridemia may cause insulin resistance and impair control of diabetes. Also, many routine laboratory tests are invalid in the presence of milky plasma. Simple removal of chylomicrons from plasma by short-term ultracentrifugation helps to avoid this problem.

DIAGNOSIS. It is very simple to make a presumptive diagnosis of chylomicronemia syndrome by visual examination of the patient's plasma. Milky plasma always indicates the presence of chylomicrons, as does a plasma triglyceride level above 1000 mg per deciliter. In the presence of symptoms and signs of the chylomicron syndrome, a definitive diagnosis is made if these clear when the triglyceride level is lowered.

TREATMENT. With pancreatitis, the discontinuation of oral intake will rapidly decrease triglyceride levels. With refeeding, fat must be avoided initially and replaced slowly. Often, mild to moderate abdominal pain can be treated by lowering dietary fat content and avoiding alcohol. The mainstay of treatment is to identify the causes of the elevation in triglyceride levels. A genetic form of hypertriglyceridemia is invariably present and may need to be treated with clofibrate, gemfibrosil, or nicotinic acid. The latter drug is difficult to use in diabetic patients because it impairs insulin sensitivity. The acquired disease or agent contributing to the hypertriglyceridemia should be treated or removed. Slowly, the patient can be refed while the plasma is watched for turbidity and the patient's symptoms and signs are observed. With appropriate therapy, the chylomicronemia syndrome should rarely recur.

HYPERLIPIDEMIA AND ATHEROSCLEROTIC VASCULAR DISEASE

Although the etiology of atherosclerosis is multifactorial, the development of premature coronary artery disease and peripheral vascular disease is strongly dependent on abnormalities in plasma lipoprotein metabolism. Thus, coronary artery disease in men under the age of 50 years and in women of any age is more likely to occur in the presence of one of the inborn errors or acquired forms of hyperlipidemia. Independently high density lipoproteins may protect against atherosclerosis. Differences in HDL cholesterol levels between men and women may explain a large part of the sex difference in development of atherosclerosis.

Familial hypercholesterolemia unequivocally is associated with premature coronary artery disease and aggravated by cigarette smoking and low HDL cholesterol levels. Remnant removal disease is also associated with peripheral vascular disease and coronary artery disease. Familial hypertriglyceridemia may impose some increased risk for atherosclerosis in a few families, but atherosclerosis is generally not increased in this form of hypertriglyceridemia. The increased atherosclerosis seen in diabetics and in patients on chronic hemodialysis may also be related in part to abnormalities in lipoprotein metabolism.

Nonetheless, all of these factors still only account for a minor part of premature atherosclerosis. Elevated levels of LDL, apoprotein B, or triglyceride, and low levels of HDL cholesterol and apoprotein AI, have been suggested to be present in the majority of patients with premature coronary artery disease. The frequency of familial combined hyperlipidemia in this undefined heterogenous group of individuals has yet to be determined.

The goal of therapy aimed at correcting hyperlipidemia is to prevent the progression of atherosclerosis. Although indirect evidence suggests this might be possible in some individuals with specific lipoprotein abnormalities, general proof is still lacking.

RARE DISORDERS OF LIPOPROTEIN METABOLISM

Several rare inherited disorders of lipoprotein metabolism are of considerable theoretical importance because they assist in understanding normal lipoprotein physiology. Each of these disorders is an autosomal recessive trait.

Abetalipoproteinemia presents in early childhood and is associated with absence of apoprotein B containing lipoproteins due to defective synthesis. Intestinal fat malabsorption, ataxia, neuropathy, retinitis pigmentosa, and acanthocytosis result. *Tangier disease* presents in childhood with absence of HDL and extremely low levels of apoproteins AI and AII. Cholesteryl esters deposit in tonsils and other lymphoid tissues and corneal opacitites develop. *Lecithin-cholesterol acyltransferase deficiency* presents in the young adult as hemolytic anemia and renal failure. Although the free cholesterol level in plasma is variable, the cholesteryl ester level is very low. Other even rarer disorders are described in recent reviews.

Havel RJ: Symposium on lipid disorders. Med Clin North Am 66:317, 1982. *Contains 12 review articles by experts in the field concerning basic biochemistry and physiology of lipoproteins, pathophysiology of specific diseases, and therapy of these disorders.*

Disorders of lipoprotein and lipid metabolism. *In* Stanbury JB, Wyngaarden JB, Fredrickson DS, Goldstein JL, Brown MS (eds.): The Metabolic Basis of Inherited Disease. 5th ed., 1983, pp 589–747. *Seven extensive reviews in great detail about the inborn errors leading to abnormalities in plasma lipoproteins.*

184. FABRY'S DISEASE (Glycosphingolipidosis)

James B. Wyngaarden

DEFINITION. Fabry's disease is an inborn error of glycosphingolipid metabolism characterized by telangiectatic skin lesions, hypohidrosis, corneal opacities, acral pain and paresthesias, intermittent fevers, renal failure, and cardiovascular, gastrointestinal, and central nervous system disturbances.

PREVALENCE. The disease has an estimated prevalence of 1:40,000 births.

ETIOLOGY AND PATHOGENESIS. Fabry's disease is an X-linked condition, fully manifest in the hemizygous male. Heterozygous females may exhibit the disease in an attenuated form, and usually show corneal clouding; occasionally a female may have most of the features of the full syndrome, including renal failure.

The biochemical defect is a deficiency of the lysosomal enzyme, α-galactosidase-A. The enzymatic defect leads to a progressive deposition of neutral glycosphingolipids with terminal α-galactosyl moieties in most visceral tissues and fluids of the body. The most prominent of these is a trihexosylceramide called globotriaosylceramide, a product of globoside that is a constituent of membranes. The majority of anatomic and physiologic abnormalities observed in Fabry's disease can be related to the cumulative deposition of glycosphingolipid, particularly in the lysosomes of the cardiovascular-renal system.

PATHOLOGY. Morphologically, Fabry's disease is characterized by widespread tissue deposits of a crystalline glycosphingolipid that shows birefringence with typical Maltese crosses. The glycosphingolipid is deposited in all areas of the body, predominantly in the lysosomes of endothelial, perithelial, and smooth muscle cells of blood vessels. Lipid deposits are also prominent in epithelial cells of the cornea, in glomeruli and tubules of the kidney, in muscle fibers of the heart, and in ganglion cells of the autonomic nervous system. The skin lesions are telangiectases or small superficial angiomas. Capillaries, venules, and arterioles show pathologic lipid storage, and there is marked dilatation of the capillaries of the dermal papillae just below the epidermis. The larger lesions are usually located in the upper dermis, where they may produce elevation, flattening, or hypertrophy of the epithelium, with keratosis; hence the term *angiokeratoma*. On electron microscopy lipid inclusions show a concentrically arranged lamellar structure with alternating light- and dark-staining bands. Peripheral nerves show densely stained inclusions in the cytoplasm of perineurial fibroblasts and the endothelial cells of the endoneurial blood vessels. There is loss of unmyelinated neurons but not of myelinated neurons. Some neurons contain ceramide trihexoside.

CLINICAL MANIFESTATIONS. *Telangiectases* may occur in childhood and lead to early diagnosis. They increase in size and number with age, and range from barely visible to several millimeters in diameter. The lesions are punctate, dark red to blue-black, and flat or slightly raised. They do not blanch with pressure, and the larger ones may show slight hyperkeratosis. The lesions tend to occur in the "bathing trunk area," but may occur anywhere, including the oral mucosa. The hips, thighs, buttocks, umbilicus, lower abdomen, scrotum, and glans penis are common sites, and there is a tendency toward bilateral symmetry. In some patients skin lesions are absent and lesions are entirely visceral. Sweating is often decreased, and hair may be sparse; shaving may be required only infrequently. Ocular lesions may be present in all elements of the eye. The most prominent are in the cornea, conjunctiva, and retina. Corneal opacities, observed by slit lamp examination, are present in most heterozygotes. The early lesion is a diffuse haziness of the epithelial layer. Later there may be whorled streaks extending from a central vortex to the periphery. The conjunctival and retinal vessels may show mild to marked tortuosity, with aneurysmal dilatations of thin-walled venules, as well as angulation and segmental, sausage-like dilatation of veins.

Pain is the most debilitating symptom. Fabry's crises, lasting from minutes to several days, consist of agonizing, burning pain in palms, soles, and proximal extremities, associated with fever. The pain may become more severe with age, or may disappear. Attacks of abdominal or flank pain may simulate appendicitis or renal colic. In addition, there may be chronic troublesome paresthesias of hands and feet.

With increasing age progressive infiltration of the cardiovascular-renal system with glycosphingolipid gives rise to anginal chest pain, myocardial infarction, cardiomegaly, or congestive heart failure. Involvement of renal parenchymal vessels leads to hypertension. During childhood and adolescence protein, red cells, casts, and desquamated kidney and urinary tract cells appear in the urine. Azotemia is common in the second to fourth decade. Birefringent lipid globules with characteristic Maltese crosses within and without cells can be observed in the urine sediment by polarized light microscopy. Other features may include chronic bronchitis and dyspnea, lymphedema of the legs without hypoproteinemia, episodic diarrhea, osteoporosis, retarded growth, and delayed puberty. The mean age at death is 41 years, but survival may extend into the sixties.

DIAGNOSIS AND DIFFERENTIAL DIAGNOSIS. The diagnosis in hemizygous males is most readily made from the history of painful paresthesias and episodic crises with fever, and the observation of characteristic skin lesions, corneal opacities, and conjunctival lesions. The disorder is often misdiagnosed as rheumatic fever, erythromelalgia, or neurosis. The skin lesions must be differentiated from the benign angiokeratomas of the scrotum of older men (Fordyce's disease), or from angiokeratoma circumscripta. Angiokeratomas identical to those of Fabry's disease have been reported in alpha-1-fucosidase deficiency. The diagnosis is confirmed biochemically by demonstration of markedly deficient α-galactosidase-A activity in plasma or serum, leukocytes, tears, biopsied tissue, or cultured skin fibroblasts. Increased levels of globotriaosylceramide are found in urinary sediment, plasma, or cultured fibroblasts.

Suspect heterozygotes may show corneal opacities, isolated skin lesions, and lipid-laden cells in skin or other tissues or in urinary sediment. Intermediate activities of α-galactosidase A can usually be demonstrated.

Prenatal diagnosis of Fabry's disease may be made by amniocentesis at approximately 14 weeks of gestation and demonstration of deficient α-galactosidase-A activity and XY karyotype in cultured amniotic cells, and accumulated trihexosylceramide in amniotic fluid.

TREATMENT. Pain may be relieved with phenoxybenzamine or phenytoin in some patients. Phenytoin combined with carbamazepine and maintenance corticosteroid therapy have also provided symptomatic relief. Renal insufficiency is treated with chronic hemodialysis or renal transplantation. In some recipients biochemical and clinical regression, with relief of pain, has followed placement of renal allografts. α-Galactosidase-A purified from human placenta has been administered to several hemizygotes. The enzyme was rapidly cleared from plasma and taken up by liver. There was a reduction in level of circulating trihexosylceramide. Current research centers on target delivery of enzyme and methods of protecting it from rapid inactivation.

Case Records of the Massachusetts General Hospital: Case 2–1984 (Fabry's Disease). N Engl J Med 310:106, 1984. *Excellent presentation of nervous system involvement in Fabry's disease.*

Desnick RJ, Klionsky B, Sweeley CC: Fabry's disease (α-galactosidase A deficiency). *In* Stanbury JB, Wyngaarden JB, Fredrickson DS, Goldstein JL, Brown MN (eds.): The Metabolic Basis of Inherited Disease. 5th ed. New York, McGraw-Hill Book Company, 1983. *A definitive chapter describing clinical, pathologic, and biochemical manifestations of Fabry's disease; 400 references.*

185. GAUCHER'S DISEASE (Glucosyl Ceramide Lipidosis)

Edwin H. Kolodny

DEFINITION. This disease was first described in 1882 by Philippe C. E. Gaucher, who believed it to be a primary epithelioma of the spleen. It is a relatively common familial disorder that results from progressive accumulation of glucocerebroside within phagocytic cells of the monocyte-macrophage system involving the liver, spleen, bone marrow, and lymph nodes. Three clinical types have been differentiated: Type 1, a chronic non-neuronopathic or "adult" form that may appear at any age and is associated with hypersplenism and bone lesions; Type 2, an acute neuronopathic or "infantile" form that presents in infancy with bulbar involvement; and Type 3, a "juvenile" subacute neuronopathic form that starts in childhood and causes seizures and mental deterioration. The activity of glucocerebrosidase is deficient in all three types but each is due to a different mutation. Treatment is directed toward the hematologic and orthopedic complications.

PATHOLOGIC PHYSIOLOGY AND PATHOGENESIS. Glucocerebroside contains equimolar amounts of sphingosine, fatty acid, and glucose. Considerable quantities of this compound are generated daily by the turnover of senescent red and white blood cells. In the central nervous system, glucocerebroside is produced in the course of ganglioside metabolism. A deacylated derivative, glucosylsphingosine, also accumulates in Gaucher's disease. This highly cytotoxic compound is believed responsible for the nerve cell destruction that occurs in the neuropathic forms of the disease. Both of these glycolipids are degraded by acidic glucosylceramide-β-D-glucosidase (glucocerebrosidase; E.C. 3.5.1.2.1), a lysosomal enzyme with multiple molecular forms that has been mapped to chromosome 1.

A distinctive morphologic feature is the *Gaucher cell*, a large round or polyhedral phagocyte, 20 to 100 μ in diameter, containing one or more small eccentrically placed nuclei and a pale striated cytoplasm resembling wrinkled tissue paper or crumpled silk (Fig. 185–1A). Under the electron microscope, this fibrillary network consists of numerous dilated saclike structures resembling lysosomes containing tubules; these are similar to the twisted bilayers characteristic of glucocerebroside deposits. The reaction of the Gaucher cell cytoplasm with the periodic acid–Schiff stain is strongly positive. Stains for iron and acid phosphatase are also positive but the reaction with lipid stains is weak. The bone marrow of patients with chronic myelogenous leukemia often contains cells with a similar appearance; the deposits in these "pseudo-Gaucher" cells are linear rather than twisted.

Glucosylceramide is increased two-fold to three-fold in plasma and more than 200-fold in the spleen and liver. Gaucher cells are present in virtually all organs surrounding small blood vessels and as sheets infiltrating their parenchyma. The spleen may become massively enlarged and develop multiple infarcts and fibrosis. The red pulp of the spleen appears white because of lipid infiltration by Gaucher cells; foci of extramedullary hematopoiesis can occur. In most patients the liver is also enlarged, the Kupffer cells of their sinusoids transformed into

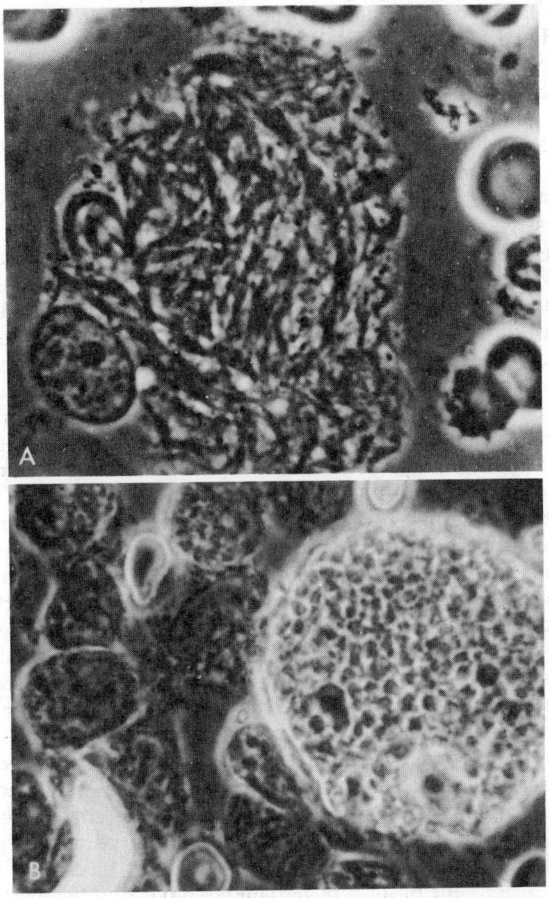

Figure 185–1. Appearance of the typical Gaucher cell *(A)* and a foam cell seen in Niemann-Pick disease *(B)*. Both are viewed under phase microscopy in unstained smears of aspirated bone marrow. Magnification can be estimated from adjacent red cells.

Gaucher cells. Fibrosis is present but there is no proliferation of the bile ducts and liver failure is rare. Excretion of glucosylceramide into the bile probably prevents more massive accumulation within the liver. In some cases, portal hypertension develops.

Gaucher cells may completely fill the medullary cavity of bone, causing thinning of the cortex, loss of its normal trabeculation, patchy myelosclerosis, bone infarcts, and osteonecrosis. An *Erlenmeyer flask deformity* of the distal femur is an early radiographic sign of bone involvement. With progression of the disease, spontaneous fractures and painful lytic lesions are found. Diffuse pulmonary infiltration can occur with direct involvement of the alveoli, pleura, and interstitium resulting in dyspnea and cor pulmonale. Renal involvement with severe proteinuric nephropathy and glomerulonephritis occurs in a few cases.

Central nervous system pathology has been found in all three types. Perivascular collections of Gaucher cells, nerve cell loss, neuronophagia, and infiltration of microglia are the principal changes observed. The most affected areas in type 2 are the deeper layers of the frontal cortex and the nuclei of the basal ganglia, midbrain, and brainstem. The high concentrations of glucosylsphingosine, a cytotoxic compound, present in the brain, liver, and spleen of type 2 patients probably contributes to the necrosis that occurs in these tissues.

The activity of tartrate-resistant acid phosphatase and angiotensin converting enzyme and concentrations of several serum proteins, including the immunoglobulins, are increased, especially in type 1 patients. Some older patients develop a monoclonal gammopathy with multiple myeloma. Leukemias and other forms of malignant neoplasm are also more frequent in elderly patients wth type 1 disease.

CLINICAL MANIFESTATIONS. *Chronic Non-neuropathic Type.* This disease is transmitted as an autosomal recessive trait and affects both sexes equally. It has been observed in whites, blacks, and Asians, but more than half of all cases are found in Ashkenazic Jews. Since one in 20 of this population is a carrier, it is not unusual for the disease to appear in two successive generations of the same family. Clinical symptoms in this so-called "adult" form may appear at any age, from the first year of life to the ninth decade. One third of all cases are diagnosed in the first decade. The majority of these children are not of Jewish ancestry. They develop massive enlargement of the spleen and evidence a delay in somatic growth that severely hampers their intellectual and social development. The condition in another 25 per cent of patients is not diagnosed until after age 30. These patients have a much more benign course. Only rarely do these individuals have serious hematologic or osseous complications.

The most common presenting symptom is excessive fatigue associated with a hypochromic anemia and splenomegaly. Frequently there is a long history of bleeding tendency such as repeated epistaxis and ecchymoses but this rarely attracts medical attention unless it is associated with a major hemorrhage such as splenic rupture, bleeding from esophageal varices, subdural hematoma, or hemopericardium. The first indication in some patients may be the appearance of bone or joint pain or a pathologic fracture. Lytic lesions develop in the shafts of the long bones, vertebrae, ribs and pelvis. This produces osteosclerosis and, in the most virulent cases, osteonecrosis and eventually collapse of bone. In the acute crises affecting bone or joints there is severe incapacitating pain, erythema, swelling, tenderness, and occasionally joint effusion. While only 20 per cent of all type 1 patients have significant clinical involvement of bone, more than half have radiologic evidence of the Erlenmeyer flask deformity with tapering of the midshaft of the femur and failure of normal trabeculation causing a widening of the distal end.

The clinical course is variable. In response to an acute infection, the size of the spleen may increase dramatically and then regress, but slowly progressive splenomegaly is the usual pattern. Anemia, thrombocytopenia, and leukemia are frequent but rarely cause significant morbidity. Bleeding may occur if the platelet count falls below 50,000 to 70,000 per cu mm; however, the count usually rises again spontaneously within a few weeks. Hepatomegaly with a hard firm liver edge is common and in a few severe cases there is liver failure and portal hypertension. Older type 1 patients are prone to malignancy.

Acute Neuronopathic Type. This form of the disease is much rarer than the adult type 1 variety. It is observed in infants of different ethnic groups and does not show any predilection for Jews. The disease may present in utero as hydrops fetalis, at birth with failure to thrive, or after a few months with a fixed strabismus and marked increase in the size of the liver and spleen. In some cases, developmental milestones are normal until the second or third year. The major central nervous system signs reflect brainstem and cranial nerve involvement. These include extreme arching of the neck, retraction of the lips, trismus, laryngeal spasm with a chronic cough and stridor, and rigid spastic extremities. Seizures and psychomotor retardation also occur. Death results from respiratory infection within a few months to two years after signs appear.

Juvenile Type. This includes a heterogenous group of patients with signs of the chronic adult type combined with progressive neurologic disease that begins in childhood or adolescence. Swedish patients with this disease are referred to as having the *Norrbotten type.* Their growth is retarded and there is hypersplenism and skeletal changes of the type that occurs in the chronic non-neuropathic form. In addition, they develop oculomotor apraxia, convergent squint, seizures, and a delay in motor development. In splenectomized patients, the accumulation of glucosylceramide is greater and the mental deterioration faster than in nonsplenectomized patients. In other patients with the juvenile type, the principal manifestations are medication-resistant myoclonic seizures and slow intellectual decline.

DIAGNOSIS. Gaucher's disease should be suspected in any patient with unexplained splenomegaly and a bleeding tendency, bone or joint pains, or pathologic fractures. A radioisotope scan of the liver and spleen will reveal the extent of the hepatosplenomegaly and the presence of infarcts. A bone scan is useful to locate recent lytic changes. The bone marrow may demonstrate Gaucher cells. The diagnosis is established by assaying the activity of glucosylceramide-β-D-glucosidase in leukocytes or cultured fibroblasts. The artificial fluorogenic substrate, 4-methylumbelliferyl-β-glucoside, is commonly employed as a substitute for the natural lipid substrate. The enzyme deficiency is similar in all three clinical subtypes of Gaucher's disease. However, they can be distinguished by immunologic detection of the three molecular forms of the enzymes after their separation by polyacrylamide gel electrophoresis. Within the same family, expression of the disease may vary considerably so that enzyme assays should be done on all close relatives of the patient, whether or not they are symptomatic. Heterozygotes have approximately one half the normal enzyme activity; however, with current methods the range of values overlaps with the normal range. Therefore, carrier detection cannot be done with 100 per cent certainty. Prenatal diagnosis is possible using cultured amniotic cells.

TREATMENT AND PROGNOSIS. Iron therapy may partially correct the anemia but the persistent use of iron in the presence of adequate iron stores increases the risk of hemochromatosis. Splenectomy is performed for severe and persistent thrombocytopenia or when mechanical factors cause massive swelling, abdominal pain, or gastrointestinal dysfunction. Correction of the pancytopenia occurs immediately after the operation. However, splenectomy may hasten the pace of lipid deposition into the liver and bones. Therefore, to preserve spleen tissue as a potential reservoir for the storage of glucosylceramide, the surgeon may elect to leave in place any accessory spleen tissue that is present or to perform a partial splenectomy. Acute lesions in bone and joints are initially treated with immobilization and the prevention of weight bearing. However, as soon as possible a graduated program of exercises is introduced to maintain joint mobility and prevent further loss of bone. Fractures of the head and neck of the femur are usually treated by prosthetic hip replacement. Enzyme replacement therapy with intravenous injections of purified placental β-glucosidase has shown promising results in a few patients with non-neuronopathic Gaucher's disease. Bone marrow transplantation has been tried in patients with type 1 and type 3 disease with correction of the enzyme defect in circulating leukocytes and reduction in the amount of stored lipid. Further trials and long-term follow-up are needed to assess the effectiveness of this potentially useful therapy. The prognosis in children with the early onset form of the type 1 disease is poor because of the severe lung, liver, and bone involvement in these cases. In milder cases of later onset, longevity is normal. Children with the infantile neuronopathic form do not survive beyond age two to three years, whereas those with the juvenile subacute neuronopathic variant may live into their third decade.

Brady RO, Barranger JA: Glucosylceramide lipidosis: Gaucher's disease. *In* Stanbury JB, Wyngaarden JB, Fredrickson DS, Goldstein JL, Brown MS (eds.): The Metabolic Basis of Inherited Disease. 5th ed. New York, McGraw-Hill Book Company, 1983. *A complete and up-to-date review of the clinical and metabolic abnormalities in Gaucher's disease.*

Desnick RJ, Gatt S, Grabowski GA (eds): Gaucher Disease: A Century of Delineation and Research. New York, Alan R. Liss, 1982. *A complete review of all aspects of Gaucher's disease based on reports presented at the First International Symposium on Gaucher Disease held in July, 1981.*

Ginns EI, Tegelaers FPW, Barneveld R, Galjaard H, Reuser AJJ, Brady RO, Tager JM, Barranger JA: Determination of Gaucher's disease phenotypes with monoclonal antibody. Clin Chim Acta 131:283, 1983. *A short description of the molecular forms of β-glucocerebrosidase and their differences in the three subtypes of Gaucher's disease.*

186. NIEMANN-PICK DISEASE (Sphingomyelin Lipidosis)

Edwin H. Kolodny

DEFINITION. The eponym Neimann-Pick disease originally referred to the classic infantile form of lipid storage disease described more than a half century ago. The lysosomal enzyme sphingomyelinase is absent in this disease; this causes widespread deposition of sphingomyelin, a ceramide phospholipid. Foam cells proliferate within the liver, spleen, and bone marrow and there is nerve cell loss within the central nervous system. This acute neuronopathic form was subsequently designated as Type A to distinguish it from other variants of sphingomyelin lipidosis that have since been described. These variants are distinguished by their age of onset, degree of central nervous system involvement, and sphingomyelinase activity (Table 186–1).

PATHOLOGY. ***Foam Cell.*** The cytoplasm of this large histiocyte contains numerous uniform-sized lipid-staining droplets that create a fine reticulated web resembling a honeycomb or mulberry (Fig. 185–1*B*). Under the electron microscope these cytosomes consist of both concentrically laminated membranous arrays and dense homogeneous bodies. Foam cells are present in the tissues of the reticuloendothelial system.

Sphingomyelin. The ceramide and phosphorylcholine portions of this lipid are linked by a phosphodiester bond that under normal circumstances is cleaved by sphingomyelinase. Sphingomyelin is increased 15- to 45-fold in the liver and spleen of patients with Type A Niemann-Pick disease, and about half as much in Type B patients. The organs of Type C patients exhibit a 3- to 6-fold increase in sphingomyelin, but it is not the major accumulating lipid in this variant. Sphingomyelin storage occurs in the brain of Type A but not Type B patients. Patients with every variety of Niemann-Pick disease also accumulate bis (monoacylglycero) phosphate, unesterified cholesterol, glucosylceramide, and other neutral glycolipids.

Sphingomyelinase. Patients with Type A and Type B Niemann-Pick disease are totally deficient in sphingomyelinase, the acid hydrolase that removes the phosphorylcholine moiety from sphingomyelin. The absence of this phosphodiesterase probably explains the simultaneous increase of bis (monoacylglycero) phosphate. The sphingomyelinase deficiency in Type C patients is incomplete and demonstrable only after isoelectric focusing of enzyme extracts from cultured fibroblasts.

CLINICAL MANIFESTATIONS. ***Type A.*** Hepatosplenomegaly, diffuse pulmonary infiltration, and developmental delay are noticeable as early as one to two months of age. Weight gain is poor due in part to vomiting associated with feedings. Lymphadenopathy, opisthotonic posturing, and seizures develop. Eye signs include periorbital puffiness, clouding of the corneas, yellowish discoloration of the lens, and cherry-red maculae. The skin becomes brownish-yellow and xanthomata may appear. The affected child becomes emaciated with very thin extremities, a protuberant abdomen, and ascites. Developmental milestones normal for a one-year-old are never attained, and after the child lingers in a vegetative state for many months, death occurs usually before the fourth year. Postmortem studies reveal a large yellow liver and atrophic brain with widespread nerve cell loss and gliosis. The cytoplasm of remaining neurons and of the glial cells is ballooned with lipid inclusions. A high percentage of patients with this rare autosomal recessive disorder are of Ashkenazi Jewish ancestry.

Type B. Severe early involvement of the lungs, liver, and spleen also characterizes Type B Niemann-Pick disease, but mental development in this variant is normal. The chest radiograph reveals nodular densities throughout the lung fields and thickening of the interlobar fissures. Signs of hypersplenism such as mild anemia, leukopenia, and thrombocytopenia with easy bruising often occur. A few patients have been described with a brownish-red spot in the macula, and sea-blue histiocytes are sometimes found in the bone marrow. These cells contain ceroid that confers on them a bluish cast when stained with Giemsa. Normal longevity is possible but may be limited by chronic pulmonary insufficiency and the mechanical effects of the enlarged spleen and liver on other abdominal organs.

Type C. This diagnosis has been applied to a heterogeneous group of patients with a variable age of onset. In some cases, jaundice is present during the first three months but this subsides despite the progression of the disease. A liver biopsy in these instances may show chronic hepatitis with giant cells. One group of Type C patients, between ages 1½ and 3 years, exhibits slowing of speech and motor development and then develops blindness and spasticity. The condition of these children deteriorates rapidly over a two-year period and they die at age five to six years. Other Type C patients may not develop overt neurologic symptoms until after age five years. These consist of a decline in intellect, progressive impairment of vertical gaze, dysarthria, dysphagia, incoordination, seizures, and involuntary movements. A few have also developed cataplexy. These patients usually survive into adult life.

Type D. This designation is used for cases similar to Type C occurring in descendents of an Acadian couple born in Yarmouth, Nova Scotia, in the 1600's. No sphingomyelinase deficiency has been reported in these cases.

DIAGNOSIS. Niemann-Pick disease should be suspected whenever foam cells are present in the bone marrow of a patient with hepatosplenomegaly. The infant of Ashkenazi-Jewish heritage who develops slowly would suggest the Type A variant. Early jaundice and a subsequent period of normal development might stimulate a workup for Type C Neimann-Pick disease. The foam cell, a lipid-laden histiocyte, should not be confused with the Gaucher cell, which also contains lipid, but of a different morphologic appearance. Foam cells also occur in hypertriglyceridemia and certain other lysosomal storage diseases such as fucosidosis, mannosidosis, G_{M1} gangliosidosis, Sandhoff's disease, Wolman's disease, and I-cell disease. In longstanding cases of Type B disease, sea-blue histiocytes containing a ceroid-like material are also observed in the bone marrow. The definitive diagnosis of Niemann-Pick disease

TABLE 186–1. THE SPHINGOMYELIN LIPIDOSES

Type	Descriptive Name	Racial and/or Geographic Predilection	Affects Brain	Sphingomyelinase Deficiency
A	Acute neuronopathic	Ashkenazi Jewish	Yes	Yes
B	Chronic non-neuronopathic	No	No	Yes
C	Subacute neuronopathic or juvenile dystonic lipidosis	No	Yes	Single fibroblast isozyme missing
D	Nova Scotian	Yarmouth County, Nova Scotia	Yes	No
E	Adult non-neuronopathic	No	No	No

Types A and B is based upon the assay of sphingomyelinase activity. Homogenates of cultured skin fibroblasts or leukocytes from these patients, when incubated with sphingomyelin labeled with ^{14}C in the choline portion of the molecule, have <5 percent of control activity. Two artificial substrates, N-ω-trinitrophenylaminolaurylsphingosylphosphorylcholine and 2-n(hexadecanoyl)-amino-4-nitrophenylphosphorylcholine, may also be used. All three are commercially available. Intermediate values are obtained for Type A and Type B heterozygotes. Type C homozygotes may exhibit a partial deficiency but Type C heterozygotes cannot be diagnosed enzymatically. Prenatal diagnosis of Type A and Type B Neimann-Pick disease is accomplished by determining the enzyme activity of cultured amniotic fluid cells.

Indeterminate Forms of Sphingomyelin Storage. The patient with unexplained hepatosplenomegaly, bone marrow foam cells, and sphingomyelinase activity that is normal or only mildly deficient should have an open liver biopsy. The tissue should be divided so that some can be frozen for subsequent chemical and enzymatic analyses, some prepared for light microscopy and histochemical staining, and some submitted for electron microscopy. The paraffin-embedding process generally used to prepare tissue slices for light microscopy may remove the stored lipid, producing a negative result when special stains for lipid are employed. To circumvent this difficulty, fresh frozen sections cut from formalin-fixed material are used for lipid histochemistry. Fresh or frozen unfixed tissue is also analyzed for its content of phospholipids, glycolipids, and neutral lipids and is used for assays of appropriate lysosomal enzymes.

TREATMENT. There is no specific treatment available for any of the sphingomyelin storage diseases. In Type B patients splenectomy may be done to relieve mechanical pressure within the abdomen or to correct a thrombocytopenia with hemorrhagic diathesis. Neither replacement with exogenous enzyme nor organ transplants have been successful, but it is possible that bone marrow transplantation will in the future prove beneficial to patients without central nervous system involvement. Animal models of Niemann-Pick disease are available for laboratory trials of potential new therapies.

Besley GTN, Moss SE: Studies on sphingomyelinase and β-glucosidase activities in Niemann-Pick disease varients. Phosphodiesterase activities measured with natural and artificial substrates. Biochim Biophys Acta 752:54, 1983. *Sphingomyelinase activity in cultured skin fibroblasts and liver is characterized and the deficiency in Types A, B and C Neimann-Pick disease described.*

Brady RO: Sphingomyelin Lipidosis: Neimann-Pick Disease. *In* Stanbury JB, Wyngaarden JB, Fredrickson DS, Goldstein JL, Brown MS (eds.): The Metabolic Basis of Inherited Disease. 5th ed. New York, McGraw-Hill Book Company, 1983. *A comprehensive review of the different clinical forms of sphingomyelin lipidoses. Details of their pathology, metabolic disturbance, and enzymatic aspects are provided, as well as a complete bibliography.*

Breen L, Morris HH, Alperin JB, Schochet SS: Juvenile Niemann-Pick disease with vertical supranuclear ophthalmoplegia. Arch Neurol 38:388, 1981. *A comprehensive review of the clinical features in the later onset form of Type C. References to the sea blue histiocyte syndrome are included.*

Winsor EJ, Welch JP: Genetic and demographic aspects of Nova Scotia Niemann-Pick disease. Am J Hum Genet 30:530, 1978. *A useful source of references to Type D Niemann-Pick disease.*

Inborn Errors of Amino Acid Metabolism

187. HYPERAMINOACIDURIA (With a Classification of the Inborn and Developmental Errors of Amino Acid Metabolism)

Charles R. Scriver

Study of the inborn errors of amino acid metabolism has improved our knowledge of metabolism, and in several instances has improved diagnosis and treatment of specific diseases. The inborn errors of transport are important "probes" of the mechanisms dedicated to amino acid reabsorption. They identify either the carriers or the metabolic processes that are coupled to the transcellular flux that achieves net reabsorption.

A certain amount of L-aminoaciduria, representing less than 2 to 3 per cent of the total urinary nitrogen, is a normal phenomenon. A small fraction, usually less than 5 per cent, of the filtered load of the amino acids in plasma is not reabsorbed completely by the proximal portion of the renal tubule and is excreted in the urine. In the healthy person, the efficiency of renal tubular transport of the individual amino acids is related to their chemical and steric structure, the amount in the glomerular filtrate, and the sex, age, and physiologic state of the subject.

Abnormal aminoaciduria will result when there is an acquired or hereditary disturbance of cellular metabolism or transport of amino acids. The known hyperaminoacidurias (see Table 187–1, which also includes several inborn errors of amino acid metabolism not necessarily associated with hyperaminoaciduria per se) can be classified according to four basic mechanisms (Fig. 187–1):

1. *Saturation*: Amino acid is at elevated concentration and approaches or exceeds the capacity of the system to reabsorb it ("overflow" aminoaciduria).
2. *Competition*: One amino acid at elevated concentration competes with others sharing access to a transport system ("combined" aminoaciduria).
3. *Modification of reactive site(s)*: Amino acid(s) is (are) not transported efficiently because access to the system is impaired ("renal" aminoaciduria).
4. *Inhibition of substrate transfer*: Energy-dependent processes coupled to the carrier and transfer of substrates across membranes are impaired ("renal" aminoaciduria).

The individual mechanisms required for transport of each amino acid can be grouped into at least five major gene-controlled and non-overlapping systems, each having a preference for a particular group of amino acids normally found in plasma and revealed by a mendelian phenotype (see Table 187–1, Group III). Another series of carriers appears able to recognize individual free amino acids, with perhaps one site for each of the protein amino acids. (Yet another series permits transepithelial absorption of oligopeptides, with hydrolysis following uptake of the peptides.)

The *group-specific sites* are classified into the β-amino system and the α-amino systems. Within the following list, the representative inborn error of amino acid metabolism that reveals the system is also indicated.

1. *The β-amino system*: β-alanine, β-aminoisobutyric acid, and taurine (viz., hyper-β-alaninemia)
2. *The α-amino systems*:
   a. "Dibasic" systems
      i. System I: lysine, arginine, ornithine, and cystine in brush border membrane (viz., cystinuria)
      ii. System II: lysine, arginine, ornithine in basal-lateral membrane (viz., lysine protein intolerance)
   b. "Acidic" system: aspartic, glutamic (viz., dicarboxylic aminoaciduria)
   c. "Neutral" systems
      i. System I: proline, hydroxyproline, and glycine (viz., hyperprolinemia and renal iminoglycinuria)
      ii. System II: the remaining neutral α-amino acids (viz., Hartnup disorder)

It is usually possible to classify the aminoaciduria and its pathogenesis by analyzing the amino acid content of plasma

Text continued on page 1126

TABLE 187–1. HEREDITARY AND ACQUIRED AMINOACIDOPATHIES

The aminoacidurias presented in this table are divided into acquired and inherited types. Disturbances related to perinatal adaptive phenomena of multifactorial origin are included. The classification recognizes physiologic factors affecting amino acid distribution between plasma and urine, and whether the disorder primarily affects catabolism or membrane transport of the amino acid(s). Thus the disorders are grouped according to mechanism and preferred fluid for detection. The data refer to those conditions associated with perturbation of the normal content of ninhydrin-reactive metabolites in plasma or urine; some exceptions have been made to include ninhydrin-negative metabolites.

GROUP IA

The primary defect is in catabolism. There is a low renal clearance of amino acid but a hyperaminoaciduria by saturation of transepithelial transport. Detection in the plasma is preferable unless otherwise indicated, but the use of urine for screening (or diagnosis) is not precluded; assignment to this group implies primarily that diagnosis (or screening) of the condition is feasible by virtue of significant metabolite accumulation in blood (or plasma). *Amino Acid Affected:* ↓ = decreased; ↑ = increased. Source of enzyme number is *Enzyme Commission.* IP: Apparent inheritance pattern; AR = autosomal recessive; AD = autosomal dominant; (AR) = probably autosomal recessive; XL = X-linked. *Remarks:* CNS = central nervous system; CoA = coenzyme A; CSF = cerebrospinal fluid.

Condition or Disease	Amino Acid Affected	Enzyme Affected (Synonym) *In Group A*	IP	Remarks
		*Common Perinatal (Adaptive) Traits**		
1. Neonatal hyperphenylalaninemia	Phenylalanine	Phenylalanine 4-monooxygenase (phenylalanine-hydroxylating system) [1.14.16.1]	—	Benign; may respond to folic acid; often occurs with tyrosinemia
2. Neonatal tyrosinemia	Tyrosine	4-Hydroxyphenylpyruvate dioxygenase (*p*-hydroxyphenyl pyruvic acid hydroxylase) [1.13.11.27]	—	Benign; responds to ascorbic acid and reduced protein intake
3. Hypermethioninemia	Methionine	? Methionine adenosyltransferase (ATP:L-methionine *S*-adenosyltransferase) [2.5.1.6]	—	Benign; usually found with high protein intake
4. Hyperhistidinemia	Histidine	? L-Histidine ammonia-lyase [4.3.1.3]	—	Benign; related to high protein intake
		Inherited Traits		
Hyperphenylalaninemia				
5. Classic phenylketonuria	Phenylalanine	Phenylalanine 4-monooxygenase (L-phenylalanine, tetrahydropteridine:oxygen oxidoreductase [4-hydroxylating]) [1.14.16.1]	AR	Plasma phenylalanine > 16 mg/100 ml; causes mental retardation; when untreated, L-phenylalanine tolerance in diet is 250–500 mg/day
6. Atypical phenylketonuria	Phenylalanine	Same as for entry 5	(AR)	Plasma phenylalanine > 16 mg/100 ml; similar to entry 5, but dietary tolerance for L-phenylalanine is > 500 mg/day
7. Transient phenylketonuria	Phenylalanine	Same as for entry 5	(AR)	Plasma phenylalanine > 16 mg/100 ml; change in status to that for entry 8, or normal, several months or years after birth
8. Benign hyperphenylalaninemia	Phenylalanine	Same as for entry 5	AR	Plasma phenylalanine < 16 mg/100 ml on normal diet; benign trait
9. Phenylketonuria (dihydropteridine reductase deficiency)	Phenylalanine	Dihydropteridine reductase [1.6.99.7]	—	Resembles classic phenylketonuria, but no CNS response to diet; enzyme can be assayed in cultured skin fibroblasts
Hypertyrosinemias				
10. Tyrosinosis (Medes)	Tyrosine	? Tyrosine aminotransferase (L-tyrosine:α-ketoglutarate aminotransferase) [2.6.1.5]	(AR)	One case known; myasthenia gravis probably incidental finding
11. Hypertyrosinemia	Tyrosine	Soluble (cytosol) tyrosine aminotransferase [2.6.1.5]	(AR)	Associated with developmental retardation; Richner-Hanhart syndrome in some patients
12. a. Hereditary tryosinemia	Tyrosine (and methionine in acute stage)	Fumarylacetoacetase [3.7.1.2]	AR	Hepatic cirrhosis and renal tubular failure; usually fatal in absence of tyrosine restriction
b. Hawkinsinuria	Tyrosine, 4-hydroxyphenylpyruvate, 4-hydroxycyclo-hexylacetate and "hawkinsin"	4-Hydroxyphenyl pyruvate dioxygenase [1.13.11.27]	AD	Variable phenotype; failure to thrive, acidosis, without liver disease (vs. entry 12a)
Hyperhistidinemias†				
13. Classic form	Histidine (alanine in some cases)	L-Histidine ammonia-lyase [4.3.1.3]; liver, epidermis	AR	Occasionally associated with mental retardation and speech defect
14. Variant form	Histidine	L-Histidine ammonia-lyase [4.3.1.3]; liver only	(AR)	Same as for entry 13
Branched-chain hyperaminoacidemia‡				
15. Classic "maple syrup urine disease"	Leucine, isoleucine, valine, alloisoleucine	Branched-chain α-ketoacid lipoate oxidoreductase (probably decarboxylase component) [1.2.4.3(4)]	AR	Postnatal collapse; mental retardation in survivors; diet therapy can be effective
16. Intermittent form	Leucine, isoleucine, valine, alloisoleucine	Branched-chain α-ketoacid oxidase(s)§ [1.2.4.3(4)]	(AR)	Intermittent symptoms; development may be otherwise normal
17. Mild form	Same as for entry 16	Same as for entry 16	(AR)	Unremittent; milder than for entry 15
18. Thiamin-responsive form	Same as for entry 16	Same as for entry 16	(AR)	Mild form; responsive to thiamin (vitamin B_1)

Table continues on following page. See page 1123 for footnotes.

TABLE 187–1. HEREDITARY AND ACQUIRED AMINOACIDOPATHIES (*Continued*)

Condition or Disease	Amino Acid Affected	Enzyme Affected (Synonym) *In Group A*	IP	Remarks
		Inherited Traits (Continued)		
19. Multiple dehydrogenase form	Same as for entry 16 (plus pyruvate and α-ketoglutarate)	Dihydrolipoyl dehydrogenase (E_3) [1.6.4.3]	(AR)	Congenital lactic acidosis plus branched-chain amino–keto acid disorder
20. Hypervalinemia	Valine	Branched-chain amino-acid aminotransferase (valine aminotransferase) [2.6.1.42]	AR	Retarded development and vomiting; responds to diet
21. Hyperleucinemia	Leucine or isoleucine	Branched-chain amino-acid aminotransferase (leucine/isoleucine aminotransferase) [2.6.1.42]	(AR)	Retarded development
22. Homocyst(e)inuria† (cystathionine β-synthase deficiency)	Methionine and homocyst(e)ine	Cystathionine β-synthase (L-serine hydrolyase [adding homocysteine]) [4.2.1.22]	AR	Usually associated with thromboembolic disease, mental retardation, and Marfan-like phenotype
23. Homocyst(e)inuria (methylene THF reductase deficiency)	Methionine (low) and homocyst(e)ine (high)	5,10-Methylenetetrahydrofolate reductase [1.1.1.68]	AR	Defective remethylation of homocysteine to methionine; neurologic and behavioral symptoms associated
24. Homocyst(e)inuria (with methylmalonic aciduria)	Homocyst(e)ine (high), methionine (low); plus methylmalonate	Defective cobalamin coenzyme biosynthesis	(AR)	Defective remethylation of homocysteine and methylmalonyl-CoA mutase (MMA mutase) activity; severe neurologic signs and acidosis after birth
25. Cystathioninuria†	Cystathionine	Cystathionine γ-lyase [4.4.1.1]	AR	Probably benign trait; vitamin B_6 corrects biochemical trait in most patients
Hyperglycinemias				
26. Ketotic form	Glycine and other glucogenic amino acids	Propionyl-CoA carboxylase (ATP-hydrolyzing) (propionyl-CoA:carbon-dioxide ligase [ADP-forming]) [6.4.1.3]	AR	Ketosis, neutropenia, mental retardation; often fatal; detectable in skin fibroblasts
27. Ibid.		Methylmalonyl-CoA racemase [5.1.99.1] or methylmalonyl-CoA mutase [5.4.99.2]	(AR)	Symptoms are those of methylmalonic aciduria with acidosis (some mutase-affected patients are responsive to vitamin B_{12})
28. Ibid.		Acetyl-CoA acyltransferase (β-ketothiolase) [2.3.1.16] deficiency¶	(AR)	Symptoms are those of α-methyl-β-hydroxybutyric aciduria (with or without tiglic aciduria) and acidosis
29. Nonketotic form	Glycine	Glycine cleavage reaction (CO_2, NH_3, and hydroxymethyltetrahydrofolate formed)	AR	Severe CNS depression soon after birth; high CSF:plasma glycine ratio; benzoate decreases plasma glycine; no effect on CNS prognosis; strychnine improves seizures
30. Sarcosinemia†	Sarcosine	Sarcosine oxidase (sarcosine:oxygen oxidoreductase [demethylating]) [1.5.3.1]	AR	Benign trait (probably)
31. "Sarcosinemia" (glutaric aciduria, type II)	Sarcosine (glutaric acid and multiple fatty acids)	? Electron transfer flavoprotein (affecting multiple aryl-CoA dehydrogenases)	(AR)	Postnatal lethargy, vomiting, coma, and acidosis; odor; multiple abnormalities of fatty acid oxidation
Hyperprolinemias				
32. Type I	Proline	L-Proline dehydrogenase (oxidase) (EC number not assigned)	AR	Benign trait
33. Type II	Proline	1-Pyrroline dehydrogenase (Δ^1-pyrroline-5-carboxylate:NAD^+ oxidoreductase) [1.5.1.12]	AR	Benign trait; Δ^1-pyrroline-5-carboxylate and 3-hydroxy-1-pyrroline-5-carboxylate excreted in urine; proline concentration > type I
34. Hydroxyprolinemia	Hydroxyproline	4-Hydroxy-L-proline dehydrogenase (oxidase) (EC number not assigned)	AR	Benign trait
Hyperlysinemias				
35. Type I	Lysine (and glutamine)	Saccharopine dehydrogenase ($NADP^+$, lysine-forming) [1.5.1.8]	AR	Associated with mental retardation and hypotonia
36. Type II	Lysine, arginine (sometimes NH_3)	? Partial defect of enzyme in entry 35 or different enyzme	(AR)	Hyperammonemia symptoms, related to protein intake
37. Saccharopinuria†	Lysine, saccharopine, citruline	? Saccharopine dehydrogenase ($NADP^+$, L-glutamate-forming) (saccharopine dehydrogenase) [1.5.1.10]	(AR)	Two cases; associated with mental retardation
38. Pipecolic acidemia†	Pipecolic acid	? L-Pipecolate dehydrogenase (pipecolate oxidase) [1.5.99.3]	(AR)	Hepatomegaly and mental retardation
39. a. α-Aminoadipic aciduria	α-Aminoadipic acid	a. ? Mitochondrial α-aminoadipate amino transferase [EC2.6.1-]	(AR)	Variable clinical features
b. α-Ketoadipic aciduria	α-Aminoadipic and α-ketoadipic acids	b. ? Unknown	(AR)	Mental retardation
40. a. Glutaric aciduria Type I	Glutaric acid	? Glutaryl-CoA dehydrogenase	(AR)	Mental retardation

Table continues on opposite page.

TABLE 187–1. HEREDITARY AND ACQUIRED AMINOACIDOPATHIES (*Continued*)

Condition or Disease	Amino Acid Affected	Enyzme Affected (Synonym) *In Group A*	IP	Remarks
		Inherited Traits (Continued)		
b. Glutaric aciduria Type II (multiple acyl-CoA dehydrogenase deficiency)	Glutaric acid, complex organic aciduria, sarcosine	? Electron transport flavoprotein	(AR)	Severe form, neonatal metabolic disease; adult form, recurrent hypoglycemia
c. Hydroxylysinemia	Free hydroxylysine	? Hydroxylysine kinase [2.7.1.81]	(AR)	Mental retardation
d. Tryptophanemia	Tryptophan (with indoleketonuria)	? Formamidase [EC3.5.1.9]	(AR)	Variable
*Hyperammonemias***				
41. Carbamyl phosphate synthetase (CPS) deficiency	Glycine, glutamine	Carbamate kinase (ATP:carbamate phosphotransferase) [2.7.2.2]	AR	Group of diseases with ammonia intoxication, protein intolerance, hepatomegaly, vomiting, etc.; argininosuccinic aciduria also has trichorrhexis nodosa
42. Ornithine transcarbamylase (OTC) deficiency	Glutamine	Ornithine carbamoyltransferase (carbamoylphosphate:L-ornithine carbamoyltransferase [2.1.3.3.]	XL	Same as above
43. Citrullinemia	Citrulline	Argininosuccinate synthetase (L-citrulline:L-aspartate ligase [AMP-forming]) [6.3.4.5]	AR	See entry 41
44. Argininosuccinicaciduria†	Argininosuccinic acid	Argininosuccinate lyase (L-argininosuccinate arginine-lyase) [4.3.2.1]	AR	See entry 41
45. Hyperargininemia	Arginine	Arginase (L-arginine amidinohydrolase) [3.5.3.1]	(AR)	Deterioration of CNS function and I.Q. in childhood; hyperammonemia (inconstant) aggravated by protein
46. Hyperornithinemia	Ornithine	a. L-Ornithine; 2-oxoacid aminotransferase [2.6.1.13]	AR	a. Associated with gyrate atrophy of choroid and retina but no hyperammonemia (HOGA syndrome)
		b. Unknown (mitochondrial ornithine transport system?)	—	b. Associated with hyperammonemia and homocitrullinemia (HHH syndrome)
47. Hyperalaninemias	Alanine	Pyruvate dehydrogenase (lipoate) (pyruvate dehydrogenase) [1.2.4.1] deficiency	(AR)	Lactic acidosis, intermittent ataxia, mental retardation
48. Ibid.		Pyruvate carboxylase [6.4.1.1] deficiency	(AR)	Intermittent lactic acidosis, intermittent hypoglycemia
49. Aspartylglucosaminuria	Glycoasparagines	Aspartylglucosylaminase (2-acetamido-1-[β^1-L-aspartamido]-1,2-dideoxyglucose amidohydrolase) [3.5.1.26]	AR	? Lysosomal disease; mental retardation
50. "Glutathionemia"	Glutathione or related peptide	γ-Glutamyltransferase (γ-glutamyltranspeptidase) [2.3.2.2]	(AR)	Mental retardation associated with finding
51. Hyperthreoninemia	Threonine	Unknown	(AR)	One case; seizures
		Other Conditions Which May Affect Amino Acids in Plasma		
52. Protein-calorie malnutrition	Tryptophan/ leucine/isoleucine/valine ↓; tyrosine/glycine/proline ↑	—	—	Severity of change related to severity of malnutrition
53. Prolonged fasting	Alanine ↓ ;threonine, glycine ↑	—	—	Early fasting does not show same pattern
54. Obesity	Leucine/isoleucine/ valine/phenylalanine/ tyrosine ↑; glycine ↓	—	—	Reflects insulin insensitivity
55. Hepatitis	Methionine/tyrosine ↑	—	—	Reflects severity of liver disease

*These conditions have been detected by screening methods applied in the newborn period of life. They should not be misdiagnosed as permanent disorders of amino and metabolism also identifiable by screening.

†Urine screening is as efficient as, or even more reliable than, blood screening in these conditions.

‡A number of disorders of branched-chain amino acid catabolism cause accumulation of substances which are ninhydrin negative. These compounds can usually be detected by gas-liquid chromatographic methods (see Goodman SI: Am J Hum Genet 32:781, 1980).

§Partial activity; more than 2 per cent of normal.

¶Hyperglycemia observed only in some patients with this enzyme deficiency.

**See also entry 36.

GROUP IB

The primary defect is in catabolism. There is a high renal clearance of amino acid and a hyperaminoaciduria by saturation of transepithelial transport. Detection in the urine is preferable. See also entries 22, 25, and 44 in Group IA.

Source of enzyme number is *Enzyme Commission*. IP: Apparent inheritance pattern; AR = autosomal recessive; (AR) = probably autosomal recessive; AD = autosomal dominant.

Condition or Disease	Substance Affected (Synonym)	Enzyme Affected (Synonym) [Enzyme Commission No.]	IP	Remarks
1. Hypophosphatasia	Phosphoethanolamine	? Deficiency of ethanolaminephosphate phospho-lyase (*O*-phosphorylethanolamine phospho-lyase) [4.2.99.7]	AR	"Rickets" unresponsive to vitamin D; craniosynostosis; hypercalcemia
2. Pseudohypophosphatasia	Phosphoethanolamine	"Alkaline phosphatase" activity present but altered (K_m mutant)	(AR)	Same as for entry 1
3. β-Aminoisobutyric-aciduria	β-Aminoisobutyric acid	?	AD/AR	Benign polymorphic trait

Table continues on following page.

TABLE 187–1. HEREDITARY AND ACQUIRED AMINOACIDOPATHIES (*Continued*)

Condition or Disease	Substance Affected (Synonym)	Enyzme Affected (Synonym) *In Group A*	IP	Remarks
4. Hyper-β-alaninemia	β-Alanine	? β-Alanine-pyruvate aminotransferase (β-alanine transaminase) [2.6.1.18]	(AR)	Seizures; somnolence; mental retardation
5. Carnosinemia	Carnosine	Aminoacyl-histidine dipeptidase (carnosinase) [3.4.13.3]	AR	Seizure and mental retardation; or benign possibly
6. Pyroglutamic aciduria*	L-Pyroglutamic acid (5-oxo-L-proline; pyrrolidone-2-carboxylic acid)	Glutathione synthetase [6.3.2.3]	(AR)	L-Pyroglutamic acid (5-oxo-L-proline) results from overproduction via modified γ-glutamyl cycle

*Urine screening is as efficient as, or even more reliable than, blood screening in these conditions.

GROUP II

There is a primary defect in catabolism and a secondary defect in transport. Hyperaminoaciduria is of combined origin—saturation and competition. Detection is possible in both plasma and urine.

Disease	Amino Acids: Affected in Plasma	Amino Acids: Present in Urine	Remarks
1. Hyperprolinemia, types I and II	Proline	Proline, + hydroxyproline and glycine	See entries 32 and 33 in Group IA; competition occurs on iminoglycine transport system (see Group III)
2. Hyper-β-alaninemia	β-Alanine	β-Alanine, + β-aminoisobutyric acid and taurine	See entry 4 in Group IB; competition occurs on β-amino transport system
3. Hyperlysinemia	Lysine	Lysine, + ornithine and arginine	See entries 35–38 in Group IA; competition occurs on "dibasic" transport system (see Group III)
4. Hyperargininemia	Arginine	Ornithine and lysine, and sometimes generalized hyperaminoaciduria	See entry 45 in Group IA; competition occurs on "dibasic" transport system (see Group III); pathogenesis of generalized aminoaciduria unknown

GROUP III

The primary defect is in the renal membrane transport site. There is a high renal clearance of amino acid, and detection is possible only in the urine. *Activity Affected:* Presumed gene product activity affected by mutant gene. IP: Apparent inheritance pattern; AD = autosomal dominant; (AD) = probably autosomal dominant; AR = autosomal recessive; (AR) = probably autosomal recessive; XL = X-linked. *Remarks:* hetz = heterozygote; homoz = homozygote. PTH = parathyroid hormone.

Trait	Substance Affected	Activity Affected	Other Tissues Affected	IP	Remarks
		Common Perinatal (Adaptive) Trait			
1. Neonatal iminoglycinuria	Proline, hydroxyproline, glycine	Specific proline and specific glycine transport (probably)	—	—	Benign adaptive trait; prolinuria subsides at ~100 days, glycinuria at ~200 days after full-term birth
2. Neonatal cystine-lysinuria	Cystine and dibasic amino acids (lysine, ornithine, and arginine)	Specific dibasic transport system	—	—	Transient; evident in newborn period in some but not all infants
		Inherited Hyperaminoacidurias			
Selective					
3. Hyperdibasic aminoaciduria	Lysine, ornithine, arginine ("dibasic" group)	Shared "dibasic" amino acid transport system in basolateral membrane	Intestine and kidney (basolateral membrane in Type I); ? liver; ? brain	AD/AR	Two alleles (? different loci); type I associated with protein intolerance, failure to thrive, hyperammonemia basolateral membrane defect; hetz silent; type II associated with mental retardation in recently discovered homoz; hetz have modest dibasic aminoaciduria
4. Cystinuria	Lysine, ornithine, arginine, and cyst(e)ine	Shared membrane system in brush-border membrane	Intestine and kidney (brush border membrane); ? brain (skin fibroblasts are normal)	AR	"Negative" reabsorption of affected amino acid can occur; three alleles (? same locus), each causing different phenotypes: in type I hetz (vs. types II and III) no excess of amino acids in urine ("silent"); in type III homoz, intestinal transport intact (or partial defect)
5. Hypercystinuria	Cystine	Specific system for cyst(e)ine	?	(AR)	One pedigree only
6. Iminoglycinuria	Proline; hydroxyproline; glycine	Shared system for imino acids, glycine (and sarcosine)	Intestine	AR	Four alleles (? same locus); I and II are silent hetz; III and IV are hyperglycinuric hetz; I associated with intestinal defect; IV with K_m mutant
7. Hartnup syndrome	Neutral amino acids (excluding imino acids and glycine)	Shared system for large neutral amino acid group (luminal membrane)	Intestine (skin fibroblasts are normal)	AR	Two alleles (? same locus); I, intestine affected; II, intestine normal; hetz "silent" in both
8. Histidinuria	Histidine	? Specific histidine system	Intestine	(AR)	Associated with mental retardation in siblings

Table continues on opposite page.

TABLE 187–1. HEREDITARY AND ACQUIRED AMINOACIDOPATHIES (*Continued*)

Trait	Substance Affected	Activity Affected	Other Tissues Affected	IP	Remarks
		Inherited Hyperaminoacidurias (Continued)			
9. Dicarboxylic aminoaciduria (glutamate-aspartate transport defect)	Glutamic acid, aspartic acid	? Shared dicarboxylic acid transport system	? Intestine	(AR)	Hypoglycemia (occasional)
Generalized					
10. Idiopathic Fanconi's syndrome	Generalized effect on all solutes and water	? Coupling of energy; ? tight junction integrity	Secondary to renal phenotype	AR (and ?AD)	Adult onset and infantile-childhood forms are differentiated; basic defect unknown; probably several alleles
Symptomatic forms of Fanconi syndromes					
11. Cystinosis: type I, type II	Same as for entry 10 (secondary response)	Cystine storage (lysosomal defect), with secondary damage to tubule and glomerulus (later)	Secondary to renal phenotype	AR*	Several alleles; infantile (type I) and adolescent (type II) forms have differing rates for onset of nephropathy; "adult" form (type III) has no nephropathy
12. Hereditary fructose intolerance	Same as for entry 10, + fructose	Fructose-1-phosphate aldolase (fructose bisphosphate aldolase) (with secondary effects on cellular ATP)	Secondary to renal phenotype (hepatic cirrhosis)	AR	Nephropathy dependent on intact PTH-cAMP axis in kidney; responds to fructose withdrawal
13. Galactosemia	Same as for entry 10, + galactose	Galactose-1-phosphate uridylyltransferase (with secondary effects on cellular ATP)	Secondary to renal phenotype (cataracts, CNS effects)	AR	"Galactosemia" due to galactokinase deficiency does *not* have Fanconi's syndrome; Fanconi's syndrome responds to galactose withdrawal
14. Hereditary tyrosinemia	Same as for entry 10, + tyrosine metabolites	Unknown (with secondary effects on cellular ATP)	Secondary to renal phenotype (hepatic cirrhosis)	(AR)	Fanconi's syndrome responds to tyrosine restriction
15. Wilson's disease	Same as for entry 10, with proximal and distal renal tubular acidosis	Unknown (? secondary effects on cytochrome oxidase system)	Hepatolenticular degeneration	(AR)	Fanconi's syndrome responds to depletion of copper storage
16. Lowe's oculocerebrorenal syndrome	Generalized dysfunction with defective urinary NH_3 production	Unknown	An oculocerebro-intestinal-renal syndrome (? involving tissues with high γ-glutamyl cycle activity)	XL†	Basic defect still unknown: treatment for tubular reclamation defects does not improve mental retardation or the cataracts and hydrophthalmia
17. Vitamin D dependency (Type I) (pseudodeficiency rickets)	Generalized defect (secondary response)	Type I: 25-Hydroxy-vitamin D-1-α-hydroxylase Type II: Defective binding of hormone	Vitamin D hormone synthesis occurs in kidney mitochondria; deficiency of synthesis or binding affects intestinal absorption of calcium and initiates PTH response	AR	Nephropathy dependent on PTH excess and hypocalcemia (phenocopy occurs in vitamin D deficiency)
Miscellaneous					
18. Glucoglycinuria	Glucose and glycine	Unknown (the two solutes do *not* share a common carrier)	—	(AD)	Asymptomatic; normal-Tm (type B) glucosuria; possibility that this is a heterozygous manifestation of a Fanconi-like tubulopathy merits consideration
19. Luder-Sheldon syndrome	Generalized amino acids, glucose, and phosphate	Unknown	—	(AD)	Same as for entry 18; symptoms of Fanconi's syndrome have occurred in probands
20. Rowley-Rosenberg syndrome	Generalized aminoaciduria	Unknown	—	(AR)	Associated components of syndrome: growth retardation, muscular hypoplasia, pulmonary involvement, and right ventricular hypertrophy

*For each type.
†Recessive.

General References:

1. Scriver CR, et al.: Kidney Int 9:149, 1976.
2. Scriver CR: Table 75, Biological Handbook II: Human Health and Disease. Bethesda, MD., FASEB, 1977.

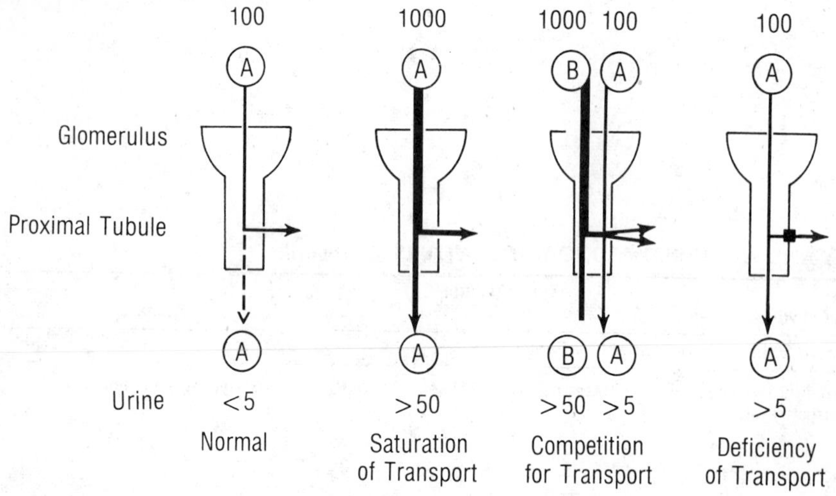

Figure 187–1. Mechanisms of hyperaminoaciduria. *Panel 1*: Normal reabsorption reclaims > 95% of filtered amino acid molecules. Hyperaminoaciduria can occur if *(Panel 2)* filtered load increases (10× increase shown) and transport mechanism is saturated, or *(Panel 3)* amino acid in excess competes with another on a shared carrier, or *(Panel 4)* carrier is modified (mutant) or coupling of energy to carrier is impaired.

and urine collected conjointly (see Table 187–1 and Fig. 187–1). Elution chromatography and gas chromatography–mass spectrometry will reveal the details of hyperaminoaciduria and any related organic aciduria. The recognition of a specific disorder of amino acid metabolism may provide an opportunity for treatment and, by genetic counseling, could prevent disease in relatives.

Scriver CR, Rosenberg LE: Amino Acid Metabolism and Its Disorders. Philadelphia, W. B. Saunders Company, 1973.
Rosenberg LE, Scriver CR: Disorders of amino acid metabolism. *In* Bondy PK, Rosenberg, LE (eds.): Metabolic Control and Disease. Philadelphia, W. B. Saunders Company, 1980, pp 583–776.
Wellner D, Meister A: A survey of inborn errors of amino acid metabolism and transport in man. Annu Rev Biochem 50:911, 1981.

188. THE HYPERPHENYLALANINEMIAS

Lloyd H. Smith, Jr.

Phenylalanine is an essential amino acid. In its main metabolic pathway phenylalanine is irreversibly hydroxylated in the 4 position of its phenyl ring to form tyrosine, a reaction catalyzed by phenylalanine hydroxylase (Fig. 188–1). In addition to its role in protein synthesis, tyrosine is necessary as a precursor of the biogenic amines dopamine and norepinephrine in the central nervous system, of thyroxine and triiodothyronine in the thyroid gland, and of melanin in melanocytes. The hydroxylation of phenylalanine to form tyrosine is a complex reaction that requires the apoenzyme phenylalanine hydroxylase, oxygen, and a specific cofactor, tetrahydrobiopterin, as an electron donor. In the process of the reaction tetrahydrobiopterin is oxidized to dihydroquinone and must be regenerated by dihydropteridine reductase (and NADH) before it is again functional in phenylalanine metabolism (Fig. 188–1). In this system there are several sites for possible metabolic errors, and in fact a number of disorders have been described characterized by hyperphenylalaninemia (greater than 1.2 mg per deciliter of plasma). When phenylalanine accumulates there is increased shunting into its minor metabolites: phenylpyruvate, phenyllactate, phenylacetate, and phenylacetylglutamine.

CLASSIC PHENYLKETONURIA

Phenylketonuria was one of the first metabolic abnormalities to be established as a cause of mental deficiency, being discovered in 1934 by Følling with the use of the ferric chloride test (for phenylpyruvate). Phenylketonuria is an autosomal recessive disorder, which in the homozygote results in a severe deficiency of phenylalanine hydroxylase activity secondary to an abnormality of the apoenzyme. Heterozygotes have partial activity, which is sufficient to maintain normal plasma levels of phenylalanine in most circumstances. Phenylketonuria occurs with a prevalence of approximately 1 in each 10,000 to 12,000 births in whites and Orientals with a carrier rate of 2 per 100, but much less frequently in blacks.

CLINICAL MANIFESTATIONS. Patients with phenylketonuria

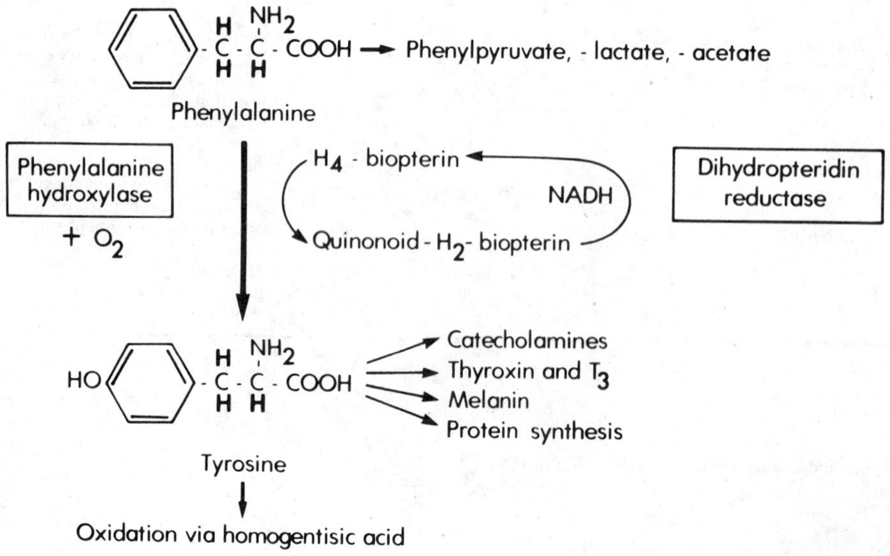

Figure 188–1. Pathways of phenylalanine and tyrosine metabolism.

are usually normal at birth. If the disease is unrecognized and untreated, however, the infant during the first year of life gradually develops mental retardation, delayed psychomotor maturation, tremors, seizures, eczema, a tendency to hypopigmentation, and hyperactivity. Impairment of mental function is usually severe, with I.Q. scores less than 50, and this taken with the other neurologic problems leads to the need for the majority of untreated patients to be institutionalized. There may be a "mousy odor" to the patient, and especially to the urine, which has been attributed to phenylacetic acid. Early diagnosis and treatment of phenylketonuria, within the first month of life, will prevent the development of these clinical complications.

PATHOGENESIS. The marked reduction in phenylalanine hydroxylase activity in classic phenylketonuria results in hyperphenylalaninemia with concentrations usually exceeding 16 mg per deciliter of plasma (approximately 1 mM). In addition, the shunting of phenylalanine into its transamination pathway leads to the excessive production and urinary excretion of phenylpyruvate and the other metabolites listed earlier. The mechanism of the neurologic deficit in phenylketonuria has not been established, but it is clearly related to the accumulation of phenylalanine (or its metabolites) rather than to a deficiency of tyrosine or its metabolites, since control of the hyperphenylalaninemia by diet prevents complications. Phenylalanine may inhibit the transport and therefore the availability of other amino acids to the brain during a critical time in its growth and maturation. Phenylalanine has been shown to be a competitive inhibitor of tyrosinase in the pathway of melanin synthesis, which is the probable explanation for the pigment dilution seen in untreated patients. In phenylketonuria tyrosine becomes an essential amino acid, but this requirement for tyrosine is usually adequately met from dietary sources.

DIAGNOSIS. The diagnosis of phenylketonuria is now usually made by screening techniques during the neonatal period. These techniques depend upon the demonstration of hyperphenylalaninemia rather than urinary phenylketonuria, since the transaminase necessary for the formation of phenylpyruvate may not be fully active in the neonatal period. The most widely used test is the Guthrie bacterial inhibition assay, which can detect excess levels of phenylalanine from a single drop of capillary blood collected from a heel prick onto a special type of filter paper. An abnormal result must be followed up with more specific determinations of plasma phenylalanine, which is usually found to be >16 mg per deciliter when there is normal protein ingestion after the first few days of life. The differentiation of phenylketonuria from the other forms of the hyperphenylalaninemias depends upon the level of amino acid measured, whether it is sustained with time, and the biochemical and clinical response to dietary therapy. The recent cloning of the human phenylalanine hydroxylase gene now allows for the prenatal detection of about 75 per cent of either the carrier state or the homozygous disease in white families and the localization of this gene on chromosome 12.

TREATMENT. In the absence of any method to replace the missing phenylalanine hydroxylase apoenzyme, treatment is dependent upon dietary restriction of phenylalanine. By the use of special semisynthetic diets, such as Lofenalac or PKUaid in the United States, it is possible to reduce phenylalanine intake to 250 to 500 mg per day while maintaining good nutrition for all other dietary requirements. Phenylalanine ingestion is monitored to maintain its plasma level in the range of 3 to 12 mg per deciliter. This regimen has been found to be highly successful in preventing the clinical manifestations of the disease. Scrupulous adherence to such a dietary regimen is of particular importance during the early months of life. In the absence of clearly established guidelines, it is probably wise to continue dietary therapy at least through the first decade and perhaps indefinitely. It is particularly important that a woman with phenylketonuria maintain careful dietary control of her plasma levels of phenylalanine during pregnancy in order that the developing central nervous system of the fetus may not be damaged during intrauterine life.

HYPERPHENYLALANINEMIC VARIANTS

A number of variants from classic phenylketonuria may also be associated with increased concentrations of plasma phenylalanine in newborns. This is not surprising in view of the usual heterogeneity of genetic disorders and also the number of factors in the complex reaction catalyzed by phenylalanine hydroxylase (Fig. 188–1). It is important to distinguish these variants from classic phenylketonuria because they may have different prognoses and require different treatment programs. The benign disorders must also be carefully distinguished from "malignant hyperphenylalanemia," as noted below.

TRANSIENT PHENYLKETONURIA. A number of patients have been described who exhibited the chemical findings of phenylketonuria at birth but in whom these abnormalities disappeared over the following few weeks. It has been assumed that this syndrome represents a maturational delay in the development of some component of the phenylalanine hydroxylase system, although this has not been established. Dietary control of hyperphenylalaninemia is indicated during the initial phases of this syndrome (when it may not be distinguishable from classic phenylketonuria), but can later be discontinued.

PERSISTENT HYPERPHENYLALANINEMIA. Some patients exhibit milder forms of phenylketonuria and probably represent variants with higher residual activities of phenylalanine hydroxylase. Even in the absence of dietary control, their plasma levels of phenylalanine may be in the range of 4 to 16 mg per deciliter, levels not ordinarily associated with mental deficiency. Many of these patients do not require therapy and would never have come to attention were it not for mass screening programs for newborns. This is a heterogeneous group of patients with varying degrees of impairment in the metabolism of phenylalanine.

MALIGNANT HYPERPHENYLALANINEMIA. A small number of patients diagnosed as having phenylketonuria by the criteria just outlined fail to respond clinically to dietary restriction of phenylalanine. The hyperphenylalaninemia responds to diet as anticipated, but despite this chemical response they develop progressive neurologic deficits and seizures and usually die in the first few years of life. These patients, who represent between 1 and 3 per cent of all infants with a positive Guthrie test, are missing dihydropteridine reductase, necessary for the regeneration of the tetrahydrobiopterin cofactor of phenylalanine hydroxylase (Fig. 188–1). Activity of dihydropteridine reductase can be assayed in skin fibroblasts and in peripheral blood cells (lymphocytes, granulocytes, and platelets). More rarely they may retain the reductase but exhibit a block in the biosynthesis of the cofactor. Although the adverse effects of the resulting defect in phenylalanine metabolism can be largely circumvented by diet, tetrahydrobiopterin is also a cofactor for at least two other hydroxylations important in the production of neurotransmitters in the central nervous system: the hydroxylation of tryptophan to 5-hydroxytryptophan and of tyrosine to L-dopa. It is assumed that these deficits, or deficits of other reactions not yet demonstrated that require the cofactor, explain the progressive neurologic abnormalities. A rapid test for malignant hyperphenylalaninemia is available in that a single oral dose of tetrahydrobiopterin* (2 mg per kilogram) will reduce the plasma phenylalanine to normal in six hours in these patients. Classic phenylketonuria, as expected, shows no response. Treatment of these patients is being attempted with 5-hydroxytryptophan and L-dopa as well as with a low phenylalanine diet. These patients can be treated with tetrahydrobiopterin and neurotransmitters without dietary restriction of phenylalanine. Tetrahydrobiopterin is not transported in significant amounts into the brain, so treatment with it alone does not suffice as replacement in malignant hyperphenylalaninemia.

---

*Investigational drug.

Danks DM, Schlesinger P, Firgaira F, et al.: Malignant hyperphenylalaninemia—clinical features, biochemical findings and experience with administration of biopterins. Pediatr Res 13:1150, 1979. *This report presents four patients with this most recently described variant of hyperphenylalaninemia and summarizes current clinical and biochemical knowledge concerning the effects of biopterin deficiency.*

Scriver CR, Clow CL: Phenylketonuria: epitome of human biochemical genetics. N Engl J Med 303:1336, 1394, 1980. *This scholarly review is probably the single best and most up-to-date compendium of information concerning our current knowledge of phenylketonuria, including its genetics, pathogenesis, clinical manifestations, and treatment.*

Tourian AY, Sidbury JB: Phenylketonuria. *In* Stanbury JB, Wyngaarden, JB, Fredrickson DS, Goldstein JL, Brown MS (eds.): The Metabolic Basis of Inherited Disease. 5th ed. New York, McGraw-Hill Book Company, 1983, p 270. *Although the emphasis in this review is on the pathogenesis of the various forms of the hyperphenylalaninemias, there is a reasonable clinical description and an extensive and useful bibliography.*

Woo SLC, Lidsky AS, Güttler F, Chandra T, Robson KJH: Clonal human phenylalanine hydroxylase gene allows prenatal diagnosis and carrier detection of classical phenylketonuria. Nature 306:151, 1983. *The human gene for phenylalanine hydroxylase was cloned and used to study the gene locus in the human genome. The gene is present in classical PKU, showing that this is not a deletion mutation. The detection of polymorphism at this locus, using restriction enzymes, allows for prenatal diagnosis of classic phenylketonuria and identification of carriers in approximately 75 per cent of white PKU families.*

See also General References following Ch. 193.

189. ALCAPTONURIA

James B. Wyngaarden

DEFINITION. Alcaptonuria is a rare hereditary disease in which homogentisic acid oxidase activity is missing. Homogentisic acid produced during the metabolism of phenylalanine and tyrosine accumulates and is excreted in the urine. It causes pigmentation of cartilage and other connective tissue (ochronosis) and in later years a degenerative arthritis of the spine and the larger peripheral joints. The disease has historic significance, for it was chiefly on the basis of study of families with alcaptonuria that Sir Archibald Garrod developed the concept of inborn errors of metabolism.

INCIDENCE AND PREVALENCE. At least 600 cases have been reported, including one in an Egyptian mummy 3500 years old. A prevalence of 3 to 5 per million individuals was found in Northern Ireland.

ETIOLOGY. The disease is inherited as an autosomal recessive trait. In a family in which alcaptonuria in five successive generations at first suggested a dominant form of the disease, further study disclosed three instances of consanguinity and pedigree analysis confirmed a recessive pattern of inheritance. No method of detection of heterozygotes has been found.

PATHOGENESIS. The activity of homogentisic acid oxidase in the normal adult human liver is sufficient to metabolize over 1600 grams of homogentisic acid per day. Normally, no homogentisic acid can be detected in plasma or urine. In alcaptonuric individuals there is no detectable activity of this enzyme in liver or kidney tissue. Plasma levels of homogentisic acid rise to about 3 mg per deciliter, and the urinary excretion ranges from 4 to 8 grams per day. Mammalian tissue contains an enzyme called homogentisic acid polyphenol oxidase that catalyzes the oxidation of homogentisic acid to an ochronotic pigment, but pigment can also be produced nonenzymatically in the presence of oxygen and alkali, as for example in urine. The homogentisic acid polymer has a high affinity for cartilage and connective tissue macromolecules. The stained tissue is fragile and eventually may break down, leading to degenerative intervertebral disc or joint disease. Homogentisic acid may also have a direct effect upon collagen synthesis through inhibition of lysyl hydroxylase.

PATHOLOGY. In an adult alcaptonuric patient cartilage in many areas, particularly the costal, laryngeal, and tracheal cartilage, is densely pigmented, sometimes being coal-black in appearance. Pigmentation is also present throughout the body in fibrous tissue, fibrocartilage, tendons and ligaments. To a lesser degree it is also found in the endocardium, in the intima of larger vessels, in various organs such as kidney and lung, and in the epidermis. The pigment is deposited both intracellularly and intercellularly, and may be granular or homogeneous.

CLINICAL MANIFESTATIONS. Homogentisic acid is present in urine from birth, but urine is colorless when passed. Before the days of disposable napkins the diagnosis was sometimes made when diapers turned brown in alkaline soaps. Homogentisic acid reduces Benedict's reagent to give a yellow-orange-brown precipitate, and this reaction has given rise to false-positive diagnoses for diabetes. Pigment may appear in perspiration and stain clothing in the axillary and genital regions. Generally, the earliest change that can be detected externally is a slight pigmentation of the sclerae or the ears, beginning at 20 or 30 years of age. The cartilage of the ears may be slate blue or gray and feel irregular and thickened. Sometimes dusky discolorations of underlying tendons can be seen through the skin over the hands. In many patients, however, pigment is scarcely evident. The arthritis usually presents with limitation of motion of the hips, knee joints, or shoulders. There may be periods of acute inflammation, and later there is usually rather marked limitation of motion and ankylosis in the lumbosacral region. The arthritic complications are often severe and painful and may lead to extensive crippling. In addition, alcaptonuric patients appear to have a high incidence of cardiovascular disease, including generalized arteriosclerosis and chronic mitral and aortic valvulitis, with calcification of valves and annulus. At least one degenerated pigmented aortic valve has been replaced with a prosthesis. Myocardial infarction is a common cause of death. Other reported complications include ruptured intervertebral discs, prostatitis, or renal stones.

X-RAY CHANGES. These may be almost pathognomonic of alcaptonuria. The vertebral bodies of the lumbar spine show degeneration of the intervertebral discs with narrowing of the space and dense calcification of remaining disc material. There is variable fusion of vertebral bodies, but little osteophyte formation and minimal calcification of intervertebral ligaments. The degenerative changes of ochronotic arthritis are most severe in the hip, shoulder, and knee, and there may be calcific deposits in the tendons. The sacroiliac joints and smaller joints of the extremities usually show little or no abnormality. Ear cartilage may be calcified.

DIAGNOSIS AND DIFFERENTIAL DIAGNOSIS. The diagnosis is suggested by the history of pigmentary changes of urine, the presence of nonglucose reducing substance, the pigmentation of sclerae or cartilage, the arthritic episodes, and especially the typical x-ray changes of the lumbar spine. Specific identification of homogentisic acid in urine can be accomplished by chromotographic or enzymatic assays.

The ochronotic changes of skin and cartilage may be confused with pigmentary changes resulting from prolonged use of Atabrine, or use of carbolic acid dressings for chronic cutaneous ulcers. The arthritis must be differentiated chiefly from rheumatoid arthritis, osteoarthritis, and gout.

TREATMENT. There is no effective treatment. Dietary restriction of phenylalanine and tyrosine of the degree necessary to reduce homogentisic aciduria is impractical and potentially deleterious. Large amounts of ascorbic acid have been given in an effort to reduce pigment formation. Ascorbic acid protects lysyl hydroxylase from inhibition by homogentisic acid in vitro. It does not alter the metabolic defect.

La Du BN: Alcaptonuria. *In* Stanbury JB, Wyngaarden JB, Fredrickson DS (eds.): The Metabolic Basis of Inherited Disease. 4th ed. New York, McGraw-Hill Book Company, 1978, p 268. *A detailed discussion of the history, clinical features, and biochemical derangements of alcaptonuria and ochronosis.*

Lee SL, Stenn FF: Characterization of mummy bone ochronotic pigment. JAMA 240:136, 1978. *Radiologic examination of an Egyptian mummy showed typical changes of ochronosis. Pigment of bone was characterized as a homogentisic acid-derived polymer.*

Pinnell SR: Disorders of collagen. *In* Stanbury JB, Wyngaarden JB, Fredrickson DS, Goldstein JL, Brown MN (eds.): The Metabolic Basis of Inherited Disease. 5th ed. New York, McGraw-Hill Book Company, 1983. *Included in this chapter is a discussion of the effects of homogentisic acid on collagen biosynthesis.*

190. HISTIDINEMIA

Lloyd H. Smith, Jr.

Histidinemia is a rare genetic disorder, probably transmitted as an autosomal recessive trait, in which the activity of histidase is markedly diminished. As a result there is a block in the conversion of histidine to urocanic acid. Histidine accumulates in the blood and is transaminated in increased amounts to imidazolepyruvic acid. In a screening program of urine specimens from newborns in Massachusetts, a prevalence of 1 in 14,190 was found for histidinemia. The diagnosis is established by demonstrating fasting hyperhistidinemia (4 to 10 times increased over the normal of approximately 1 mg per deciliter), histidinuria, and urinary imidazolepyruvic acid (which will give a positive ferric chloride test or Phenistix test for phenylketonuria). The enzyme defect can be demonstrated in biopsy specimens from skin and liver. In several patients low levels of platelet serotonin have been noted. In the past, varying degrees of mental retardation and of speech defects have been attributed to this genetic disorder. More recent evidence suggests that these represented the bias of ascertainment and that histidinemia has no demonstrated biological disadvantage.

191. THE HYPERPROLINEMIAS AND HYDROXYPROLINEMIA

Lloyd H. Smith, Jr.

The imino acids proline and hydroxyproline are nonessential; proline is readily synthesized in the body from glutamate and ornithine and hydroxyproline from proline. The synthesis of hydroxyproline occurs uniquely in peptide linkage largely as a constituent of collagen. Three rare genetic disorders of the degradative pathways of the imino acids have been described.

HYPERPROLINEMIAS. Two distinct disorders of proline metabolism, both transmitted as autosomal recessive traits, are associated with hyperprolinemia. In Type I hyperprolinemia there is a block in the metabolism of proline to Δ' pyrroline-5-carboxylate because of decreased activity of the enzyme proline oxidase. In Type II hyperprolinemia there is a block at the second step in the degradative pathway, the conversion of Δ'-pyrroline-5-carboxylate to L-glutamate, because of decreased activity of Δ'-pyrroline-5-carboxylate dehydrogenase. In both disorders the accumulation of proline in the blood leads to prolinuria and, through competition for a common renal tubular transport mechanism, to hydroxyprolinuria and glycinuria as well. In the Type II disorder there is also excessive urinary Δ'-pyrroline-5-carboxylate. The disorders can be diagnosed by finding the characteristic changes of hyperprolinemia and iminoaciduria as noted above. Although various forms of renal disease have been described with the Type I disorder and neurologic abnormalities and seizures in some patients with either Type I or Type II hyperprolinemia, these may represent the bias of ascertainment. Since no clinical entity has been clearly established, there is no indicated therapy for either form of hyperprolinemia.

HYDROXYPROLINEMIA. An increased plasma level of free hydroxyproline associated with hydroxyprolinuria has been described in members of several families, but this disorder has not resulted in prolinuria or glycinuria. The disorder is assumed to be an autosomal recessive trait in which the homozygote has deficient activity of hydroxyproline oxidase. There is no associated abnormality of collagen metabolism, and the urinary excretion of peptide-bound hydroxyproline is normal. As in the case of the hyperprolinemias, no clinical entity has been demonstrated and no treatment is indicated.

192. DISEASES OF THE UREA CYCLE

Lloyd H. Smith, Jr.

Humans are ureotelic; they are dependent upon the synthesis of urea for nitrogen excretion. The only source of net urea formation is through the urea cycle (Figure 192–1), which consists of five enzymes necessary for the sequential synthesis of carbamyl phosphate, citrulline, argininosuccinate, arginine, and urea. When the function of this pathway is impaired, ammonia tends to accumulate. The associated clinical abnormalities show certain common features such as mental retardation and severe neurologic dysfunction. Genetic diseases associated with blocks at each of these five steps have been discovered and will be described briefly below. In addition, one patient has been described with deficiency of N-acetylglutamate synthetase, which catalyzes the formation of acetylglutate, which is required for the activation of carbamyl phosphate synthetase in step 1, as shown in Figure 192–1.

CARBAMYL PHOSPHATE SYNTHETASE (CPS) DEFICIENCY. Carbamyl phosphate (CAP) channeled for urea synthesis, in contrast to pyrimidine-channeled CAP, is synthesized in mitochondria from ammonia, bicarbonate, and ATP in a reaction

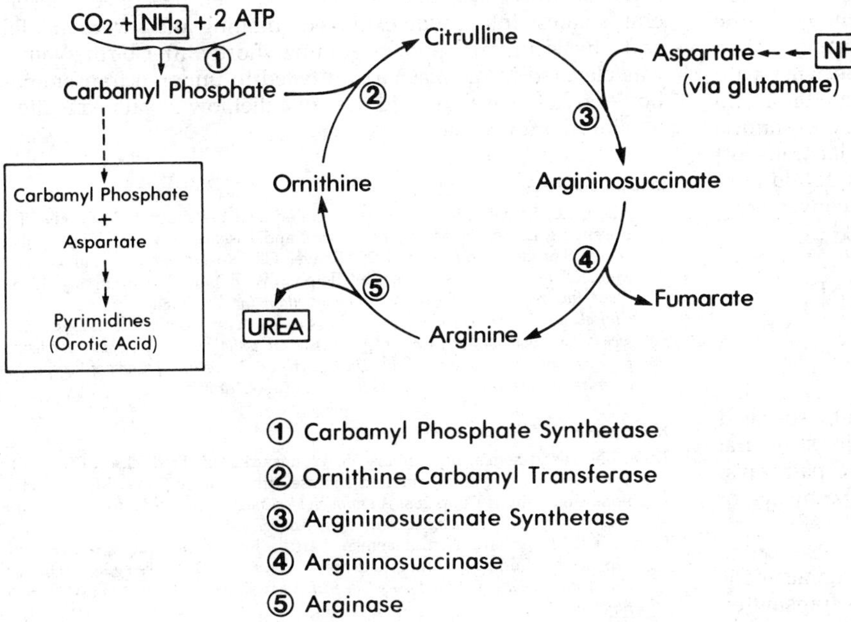

Figure 192–1. The urea cycle.

catalyzed by CPS in the presence of N-acetylglutamate as an enzyme activator. Approximately 19 patients with deficiency of CPS have been discovered, usually presenting with hyperammonemia, protein intolerance, and neurologic symptoms during the neonatal period. The diagnosis is established by measuring carbamyl phosphate synthetase in a liver biopsy or in peripheral leukocytes. There are no characteristic changes in amino acids in blood or urine.

ORNITHINE CARBAMYL TRANSFERASE (OCT) DEFICIENCY. OCT catalyzes the mitochondrial carbamylation of ornithine by CAP to form citrulline. Approximately 40 to 50 patients have been described with hyperammonemia and neurologic abnormalities secondary to deficient activity of OCT. The disorder seems to be transmitted as a sex-linked dominant trait with hemizygous males rarely surviving the neonatal period; females manifest varying degrees of protein intolerance. As in the case of CPS deficiency, there are no detectable abnormalities of amino acid metabolism. Mitochondrial CAP accumulates, however, and spills over into the cytosol to drive pyrimidine synthesis (Fig. 192–1). This results in orotic aciduria as a constant finding. The enzyme defect can be shown in biopsy specimens from liver or intestinal mucosa or in leukocytes.

ARGININOSUCCINATE (ASA) SYNTHETASE DEFICIENCY (CITRULLINEMIA). Citrulline synthesized in mitochondria normally diffuses into the cytosol, where it is condensed with L-aspartic acid in the presence of ATP to form argininosuccinic acid. This reaction is catalyzed by ASA synthetase. Approximately 20 patients who have been documented as having neonatal citrullinemia have exhibited marked heterogeneity in the severity of their clinical and chemical manifestations. The associated hyperammonemia is in general less severe than in deficiency of CPS or OCT but does occur after protein ingestion. Citrulline is elevated in blood and urine, and secondary orotic aciduria has been noted, presumably reflecting excess CAP. Patients with a late onset form of presentation have been described, especially from Japan.

ARGININOSUCCINASE (ASase) DEFICIENCY (ARGININOSUCCINIC ACIDURIA). Cytosolic argininosuccinic acid undergoes reversible cleavage to arginine and fumarate catalyzed by ASase. Approximately 60 patients have been described with argininosuccinic aciduria. Clinical findings, which vary widely in severity, have included mental retardation, seizures, ataxia, hepatomegaly, and friable hair (trichorrhexis nodosa). In addition to large amounts of ASA in blood, urine, and cerebrospinal fluid (readily demonstrable by chromatography), patients with ASase deficiency may have citrullinemia.

ARGINASE DEFICIENCY (HYPERARGININEMIA). Arginine is hydrolyzed to urea and ornithine, catalyzed by arginase, in the last step of the urea cycle. Only 13 patients have been described with deficiency of arginase, which has been associated with mental retardation and spasticity. Arginine is elevated in blood and urine and may occasionally cause secondary cystinuria owing to competitive inhibition of the renal tubular transport of dibasic amino acids. Hyperammonemia may be found after protein ingestion. The absence of arginase can be conveniently demonstrated in circulating erythrocytes.

193. BRANCHED-CHAIN AMINOACIDURIA

Lloyd H. Smith, Jr.

Leucine, isoleucine, and valine are essential, so-called branched-chain amino acids, which have certain structural resemblances and share some common metabolic pathways. Three rare genetic disorders in the degradative pathways of the branched-chain amino acids will be described briefly.

MAPLE SYRUP URINE DISEASE. This disorder, also called *branched-chain ketonuria,* derives its name from the characteristic odor of the urine of affected infants. The disease is transmitted as a rare (1 in 120,000 to 290,000 births) autosomal recessive trait in which the affected homozygote exhibits deficient activity in the oxidative decarboxylation pathway of leucine, isoleucine, and valine. As a consequence these three amino acids and their corresponding keto acids accumulate in excess in blood and urine and presumably throughout the body. A few patients have a variant disorder that responds to treatment with large amounts of thiamin (20 times the normal daily requirement). These patients have recently been found to have a dehydrogenase enzyme with a decreased affinity for α-ketoisovalerate and thiamin pyrophosphate. The pathogenesis of the deleterious effects in maple syrup urine disease has not been firmly established and may be complex, but probably relates mostly to the accumulation of leucine.

Severe hypotonia, lethargy, feeding difficulties, and hypoglycemia develop in the first week in an infant who seemed normal at birth. Convulsions and decorticate rigidity may develop, and most patients die, often of intercurrent infection, within the first year of life (often within the first few weeks). The diagnosis can usually be suspected from the characteristic odor of the urine and is confirmed by the abnormal pattern of amino acids and keto acids in blood and urine. The enzyme defect is demonstrable in leukocytes and fibroblasts. Treatment—by careful dietary control of leucine, isoleucine, and valine—is simple in theory but difficult in practice because of the necessity to balance three individual essential amino acids that are not easily analyzed. In those few cases in which rigid dietary control with careful monitoring of plasma levels has been instituted early, the results have been gratifying. A few patients have been described with milder variants of maple syrup urine disease. Thiamin therapy should be tried, as noted.

ISOVALERIC ACIDEMIA. This is a rare genetic disorder in the degradative pathway of leucine presumed to be due to a block in the conversion of isovaleric acid to β-methylcrotonic acid, which is catalyzed by isovaleryl-CoA dehydrogenase. Isovaleric acid accumulates in blood and urine and gives rise to an odor that has been described as "like sweaty feet." The pathogenesis of the associated clinical features has not been established. Symptoms, which usually begin in the first week of life, consist of attacks of vomiting, acidosis, tremors, lethargy, or even coma. Leukopenia, anemia, and thrombocytopenia have been observed during acute attacks. Patients who survive have generally exhibited mental retardation. As in the case of maple syrup urine disease, which it may clinically resemble, isovaleric acidemia may be suspected from the associated odor. The diagnosis is established by the demonstration of excess isovaleric acid in the serum by gas-liquid chromatography or of isovalerylglycine in the urine. Treatment is by strict control of dietary leucine.

HYPERVALINEMIA. This disorder has been described only in one Japanese infant who exhibited vomiting and severe mental and physical retardation, beginning shortly after birth. Valine was elevated in his plasma and failed to undergo transamination to α-ketoisovaleric acid. Use of a diet low in valine resulted in clinical improvement.

General References

Rosenberg LE, Scriver CR: Disorders of amino acid metabolism. *In* Bondy PK, Rosenberg LE (eds.): Metabolic Control and Disease. 8th ed. Philadelphia, W. B. Saunders Company, 1979. Scriver CR, Rosenberg LE: Amino Acid Metabolism and Its Disorders. Philadelphia, W. B. Saunders Company, 1973. *These two reviews by the same authors contain the best overall treatment of the clinical and metabolic abnormalities associated with disorders of amino acid metabolism. Both authors, who are geneticists and pediatricians, have made extensive personal contributions to this field. These references can be used for any of the specific disorders for which other references have been suggested below.*

Histidinemia

LaDu BN: Histidinemia. *In* Stanbury JB, Wyngaarden JB, Fredrickson DS (eds.): The Metabolic Basis of Inherited Disease. 4th ed. New York, McGraw-Hill Book Company, 1978, p 268. *A thorough biochemically oriented review of this rare disorder, especially valuable concerning its pathogenesis.*

Scriver CR, Levy HL: Histidinaemia. Part I: Reconciling retrospective and prospective findings. J. Inherited Metab Dis 6:51, 1983. *The authors conclude that histidinemia is not "a disease" in that it has not been shown to impair cerebral function.*

Hyperprolinemia and Hydroxyprolinemia

Scriver CR, Smith RJ, Phang JM: Disorders of proline and hydroxyproline metabolism. *In* Stanbury JB, Wyngaarden JB, Fredrickson DS, Goldstein JL, Brown MS (eds.): The Metabolic Basis of Inherited Disease. 5th ed. New York, McGraw-Hill Book Company, 1983, p 360. *An extensive analysis of the chemical derangements in these rare disorders.*

Diseases of the Urea Cycle

Brusilow SW, Danney M, Waber LJ, et al.: Treatment of episodic hyperammonemia in children with inborn errors of urea synthesis. N Engl J Med 310:1630, 1984. *A recent review of interesting new therapeutic approaches.*

Walser M: Urea cycle disorders and other hereditary hyperammonemic syndromes. *In* Stanbury JB, Wyngaarden JB, Fredrickson DS, Goldstein JL, Brown MS (eds.): The Metabolic Basis of Inherited Disease. 5th ed. New York, McGraw-Hill Book Company, 1983, p 402. *A large number of disorders are associated with derangements in urea synthesis. This chapter gives a lucid summary of the biochemistry of urea synthesis and the pathogenesis of the various disorders associated with that pathway. As always in* The Metabolic Basis of Inherited Disease, *there is a large and useful bibliography.*

Branched-Chain Aminoaciduria

Chuang DT, Ku LS, Cox RP: Thiamin-responsive maple syrup urine disease: Decreased affinity of the mutant branched-chain α-keto acid dehydrogenase for α-ketoisovalerate and thiamin pyrophosphate. Proc Natl Acad Sci 79:3300, 1982. *An in vitro demonstration of the biochemical basis for thiamin responsivity in this variant disorder.*

Tanaka K, Rosenberg LE: Disorders of branched chain amino acid and organic acid metabolism. *In* Stanbury JB, Wyngaarden JB, Fredrickson DS, Goldstein JL, Brown MS (eds.): The Metabolic Basis of Inherited Disease. 5th ed. New York, McGraw-Hill Book Company, 1983, p 440. *This is the most sophisticated general presentation of the pathogenesis of this group of disorders. Although the emphasis is on the biochemical basis, there is a useful clinical discussion and an extensive bibliography.*

194. HOMOCYSTINURIA

S. Harvey Mudd

DEFINITION. The term *homocystinuria* designates a biochemical abnormality, not a specific disease entity. Several known genetic disorders lead to homocystinuria. Most common is cystathionine β-synthase deficiency. In this condition ectopia lentis, mental retardation, bony abnormalities, osteoporosis, and thromboembolic phenomena are frequent.

PREVALENCE. More than 350 adequately documented cases of cystathionine β-synthase deficiency have been reported. Screening of newborn infants indicates a *minimal* prevalence of 1 in 200,000 worldwide.

ETIOLOGY AND PATHOGENESIS. Cystathionine β-synthase deficiency is inherited as an autosomal recessive trait. Deficient activity of this enzyme has been demonstrated in liver extracts, in brain, and in cultured skin fibroblasts and lymphocytes. The enzyme deficiency results in a failure of homocysteine to react with serine to form cystathionine on the pathway to cysteine. Homocystine is the disulfide oxidation product formed from two molecules of homocysteine. Normally, homocystine is not detected in human plasma by methods of the usual sensitivity. In cystathionine β-synthase–deficient patients fasting plasma concentrations of up to 0.2 μmol per milliliter of homocystine have been reported. The urine may contain up to 1 mmol of homocystine per day. Plasma methionine levels are also raised, and plasma cystine is low. Detailed studies, chiefly of cultured fibroblasts, suggest extensive heterogeneity in the genetic lesions producing deficient activity of cystathionine β-synthase. An important manifestation of such genetic heterogeneity is pyridoxine responsiveness. In 40 to 50 per cent of cystathionine β-synthase–deficient patients, administration of relatively large amounts of pyridoxine markedly reduces or eliminates homocystinuria, homocystinemia, hypermethioninemia, and hypocystinemia. Within any one sibship, all affected sibs are either B_6-responsive or B_6-nonresponsive.

Many of the manifestations of homocystinuria are related to abnormal connective tissue, probably secondary to defective crosslinking of collagen. Outwardly the condition in these patients may resemble that in those with Marfan's syndrome, but the joints are not hyperextensible. The pathogenesis of the thrombotic tendency is not clearly understood. Elevation of plasma homocyst(e)ine, rather than plasma methionine, is likely to underlie the thrombotic tendency.

PATHOLOGY. There is fraying and disruption of the zonular fibers of the lens, with resulting subluxation. The skeleton is markedly osteoporotic, and the vertebrae show rarefaction of spongy bone with biconcave (codfish) compression. Thrombi and emboli have been reported in almost every artery or vein, even in many smaller vessels. These result in brain infarcts, coronary occlusion and myocardial infarction, pulmonary infarcts, renal infarcts, and thrombophlebitis with pulmonary emboli. The liver shows fat accumulation, largely in the centrilobular hepatocytes.

CLINICAL MANIFESTATIONS. The clinical abnormalities in this disorder develop after birth. *Ectopia lentis* is rare before age two, but eventually occurs in 95 per cent or more of patients. Acute glaucoma and reduced visual acuity may occur. The osteoporosis is rare in early childhood but may be present by age six and becomes progressively more frequent and severe. The spine is the most common site, followed by the long bones. Scoliosis occurs in many individuals, although kyphosis is infrequent. Vertebral collapse and pathologic fractures of long bones may occur. The long bones are generally thin and excessively lengthened. Pectus carinatum or excavatum is common. Mental retardation is frequent, and may present as a developmental delay within the first weeks of life, but more commonly becomes manifest in the first or second year. However, at least 20 per cent of patients have average or above average intelligence. The life-threatening complication of cystathionine β-synthase deficiency is *thromboembolism.* Large and small arteries and veins may be affected. Vascular occlusions may occur at any age. Major cerebral vascular thrombosis may occur in infancy. Sudden death from coronary occlusion may occur in early childhood or young adult years. Venous thrombosis with pulmonary emboli is common. The number and severity of clinical complications vary markedly. At the mild end of the spectrum are those who seek medical help as adults with only ectopia lentis or with an early thromboembolic episode. Most such patients are B_6-responsive.

DIAGNOSIS AND DIFFERENTIAL DIAGNOSIS. The diagnosis is suggested by ectopia lentis and thromboembolic phenomena, together with other aforementioned features. The urinary cyanide-nitroprusside reaction is positive. Other disulfidurias, for example cystinuria, also produce a positive cyanide-nitroprusside reaction, so homocystinuria should be confirmed by column chromatography or other means. Hypermethioninemia accompanying homocystinemia and homocystinuria distinguishes cystathionine β-synthase deficiency from alternative forms of homocystinuria. Cystathionine β-synthase deficiency is confirmed by demonstration of markedly reduced enzyme activity with cultured skin fibroblasts, phytohemagglutinin-stimulated lymphocytes, or in a liver biopsy specimen.

Heterozygotes may be tentatively identified by assay of cystathionine β-synthase activity in liver biopsy tissue, cultured fibroblasts, or phytohemagglutinin-stimulated lymphocytes. In most instances values for obligate heterozygotes fall below the control range, but there is some overlap.

Rarer forms of homocystinuria are caused by decreased 5-methyltetrahydrofolate–dependent homocysteine methylation, owing to (1) inability to form or accumulate methylcobalamin; (2) decreased 5, 10-methylenetetrahydrofolate reductase activity; or (3) Imerslund's syndrome (defective absorption of vitamin B_{12} in the presence of intrinsic factor). In all of these, plasma methionine levels are low. The patients present in childhood. Homocystinuria also occurs following 6-azauridine triacetate administration, because of inhibition of cystathionine β-synthase.

TREATMENT. Management is directed toward the biochemical abnormality with the aim of preventing or ameliorating clinical manifestations, and toward the clinical treatment of complications.

A low methionine diet (with cystine supplementation) results in some degree of control of biochemical abnormalities. Begun in infancy, such dietary control may prevent severe mental retardation. Pyridoxine in doses as high as 500 to 1000 mg per day, accompanied by folate repletion, is often given to responsive patients to alleviate biochemical abnormalities. Late treatment with diet or B_6 often produces behavioral improvement, suggesting a reversible component to the mental disturbance, although correction of I.Q. impairment is usually minimal. The long-term effects of these therapies in preventing lens dislocation, thromboembolic episodes, or osteoporosis have not been fully established. Recently betaine, which lowers homocysteine by accelerating its methylation, has appeared useful in early studies in patients not responsive to pyridoxine. Antithrombotic therapy with aspirin and dipyridamole has also been advocated.

Drayer, JIM, Cleophas AHM, Trijbels JMF, Smals AGH, Klopperborg PWC: Symptoms, diagnostic pitfalls, and treatment of homocystinuria in seven adult patients. Neth J Med 23:89, 1980. *Cystathionine β-synthase deficient patients presenting as adults.*

Mudd SH, Levy HL: Disorders of transsulfuration. *In* Stanbury JB, Wyngaarden JB, Fredrickson DS, Goldstein JL, Brown MS (eds.): The Metabolic Basis of Inherited Disease. 5th ed. New York, McGraw-Hill Book Company, 1982. *A detailed review of the clinical features of 350 confirmed cases of cystathionine β-synthase deficiency, with a discussion of metabolic factors in homocystinuria.*

Pullon DHH: Homocystinuria and other methioninemias. *In* Bickel H, Guthrie R, Hammersen G (eds.): Neonatal screening for inborn errors of metabolism. Heidelberg, Springer-Verlag, 1980. *An evaluation of the effect of therapy started in the newborn period.*

Wilcken DEL, Wilcken B, Dudman NPB, Tyrrell PA: Homocystinuria—the effects of betaine in the treatment of patients not responsive to pyridoxine. N Engl J Med 309:448, 1983. *Eleven patients responded with a substantial decrease in plasma homocysteine levels and an increase in total cysteine levels. In six there was prompt clinical improvement, such as darkening of new hair and improvement in behavior.*

Disorders of Purine and Pyrimidine Metabolism

195. GOUT

James B. Wyngaarden

Gout is a term representing a heterogeneous group of genetic and acquired diseases manifested by *hyperuricemia* and a characteristic *acute inflammatory arthritis* which tends to be recurrent. The arthritis is induced by *crystals* of monosodium urate monohydrate which are demonstrable in the leukocytes of the synovial fluid. Some patients develop aggregated deposits of these crystals *(tophi)* in and around the joints of the extremities that can lead to joint destruction and severe crippling. Many patients with gout develop a *chronic interstitial nephropathy,* which is usually only slowly progressive and without noticeable effect upon life expectancy. In addition, *urolithiasis* resulting from uric acid stones is particularly common in patients with gout.

Some gouty patients develop all of the features of the disease described above, but these manifestations can occur in different combinations. However, essential hyperuricemia alone, even when complicated by uric acid lithiasis, should not be called gout; the term gout signifies inflammatory arthritis or tophaceous disease.

A classification emphasizing the heterogeneity of gout is presented in Table 195–1.

HISTORY. Gout has been known for at least 2500 years. In the fifth century B.C., Hippocrates devoted six of his aphorisms to this disease: VI-28, Eunuchs do not take the gout, nor become bald; VI-29, A woman does not take the gout, unless her menses be stopped; VI-30, A youth does not get gout before sexual intercourse; VI-40, In gouty affections, inflammation subsides within 40 days; X-25, Swellings and pains in the joints, without sores, whether from gout or from sprains, in most cases are relieved by a copious affusion of cold water . . .; XI-55, Gouty affections become active in spring and in autumn. References to inheritance of gout can be traced to the first century A.D. (Seneca; Pliny the Elder). Tophi were first described by Galen, who attributed gout to "debauchery, intemperance, and a hereditary trait." The term gout, derived from the Latin word *gutta,* a drop, was first used in the thirteenth century and reflected the Hippocratic belief that the disease was caused by a noxa, a poison, falling drop by drop into the joint. The modern clinical history of gout began in 1683 with Thomas Sydenham, whose descriptions of the disease, based on 34 years of personal affliction ("I am at a loss to know whether the stone or the gout be more severe"), have yet to be surpassed. Crystals were first described in a gouty tophus in 1679, by Antonj van Leeuwenhoek, the Dutch inventor of the microscope. Uric acid was discovered as a component of stones by Scheele in 1776, followed two decades later by its identification in tophi by Wallaston (1797). In 1848, Alfred Baring Garrod discovered the hyperuricemia of gout by an ingenious technique (crystallization of uric acid on a linen fiber suspended in acidified serum). In 1931, his son Archibald Garrod included gout as one of the inborn errors of metabolism. The first specific enzymatic defect responsible for one rare subtype of hereditary gout, partial hypoxanthine-guanine phosphoribosyltransferase (HGPRT) deficiency, was discovered by Seegmiller and associates in 1967. A second, phosphoribosylpyrophosphate synthetase overactivity, was discovered by Sperling and co-workers in 1972.

A drug probably identical with colchicine (white hellebore) was described in the Ebers papyrus (1500 B.C.) and recommended by Hippocrates as a "sovereign purge" for gout. Probenecid, the first effective and well tolerated uricosuric agent, was introduced in 1950, followed by the xanthine oxidase inhibitor allopurinol in 1963.

PREVALENCE AND INCIDENCE. The prevalence of gout varies from about 0.13 to 0.37 per cent of the populations of Europe and the United States to 10 per cent of adult male Maori of New Zealand. Exceptionally high prevalences are also found in Filipinos (in the United States, but not in the Philippines) and in the natives of the Mariana Islands. During World Wars I and II acute gouty arthritis was uncommon in Europe. When dietary protein again became plentiful, its frequency returned

TABLE 195–1. CLASSIFICATION OF HYPERURICEMIA AND GOUT

Type	Disturbance in Uric Acid Metabolism	Inheritance
Primary		
I. Idiopathic (> 99% of primary gout)		
A. Normal urinary excretion (80–90% of primary gout)	Overproduction and/or decreased renal clearance	Polygenic
B. Increased urinary excretion (10–20% of primary gout)	Overproduction ± decreased renal clearance	Polygenic
II. Associated with specific enzyme or metabolic defects (< 1% of primary gout)		
A. Increased activity of PP-ribose-P synthetase	Overproduction; increased synthesis of PP-ribose-P	X-linked
B. "Partial" deficiency of hypoxanthine-guanine phosphoribosyl-transferase	Overproduction; increased PP-ribose-P concentration	X-linked
Secondary		
I. Associated with increased purine biosynthesis de novo		
A. "Complete" deficiency of hypoxanthine-guanine phosphoribosyltransferase	Overproduction; Lesch-Nyhan syndrome	X-linked
B. Glucose-6-phosphatase deficiency	Overproduction and decreased renal clearance; glycogen storage disease, Type I (von Gierke)	Autosomal recessive
II. Associated with increased nucleic acid turnover	Overproduction, e.g., chronic hemolysis; polycythemia; myeloid metaplasia	—
III. Associated with decreased renal clearance of uric acid	Reduced renal functional mass; inhibition of secretion and/or enhanced reabsorption by drugs, toxins, or endogenous metabolic products	—

to prewar levels. Although formerly rare in Japan, gout has now become common in parallel with the increase in protein consumption in that country.

Primary gout is chiefly a disease of the adult male; only about 5 per cent of cases are found in women, largely in the postmenopausal group. The frequency of gout is increased in patients taking diuretics, especially of the thiazide group, in those with lead nephropathy from consumption of bootleg whiskey, and in patients with polycythemia vera, myeloid metaplasia, or chronic hemolysis. Gout in all of its forms makes up about 5 per cent of arthritis cases.

GENETICS OF GOUT. A family history for clinical gout is generally found in 6 to 18 per cent of patients in the United States and Denmark. Figures of 40 to 80 per cent have been reported from England, and also from the United States following tenacious family studies. About 25 per cent of first-degree relatives of gouty subjects are hyperuricemic, and about 20 per cent of these have symptomatic gout. Familial hyperuricemia is polygenic and multifactorial. Hyperuricemia is correlated with maleness, surface area, obesity, "ponderal index," protein intake, social status, and educational level. Thus many variables affect the phenotypic expression of hyperuricemia. In primary gout associated with HGPRT deficiency and PP-ribose-P synthetase variants, the genetic transmissions are X-linked. Glycogen storage disease Type I, which is associated with a specific form of secondary gout, is an autosomal recessive trait. Further progress in determining the patterns of inheritance of gout must await the definition of additional specific subtypes in pathogenetic terms.

PATHOGENESIS AND PATHOLOGY. The hallmark of gout is hyperuricemia. The risk of development of gout increases with the degree of hyperuricemia and also with age (Table 195–2). Virtually all patients with gout have serum urate values above 7.0 mg per deciliter. An occasional patient with gout will have a lower value at the time of attack, perhaps attributable to the urate diuresis that sometimes accompanies the inflammatory response. Repeat analyses will almost always show hyperuricemia during quiescent periods.

In normal prepubertal children, serum urate values average 3.6 mg per deciliter in both sexes. At puberty these levels increase, and thereafter mean values are 5.1 mg per deciliter in males and 4.1 mg per deciliter in females. After the menopause, mean values in females increase to approximate levels in males. Serum urate values in normal subjects do not fit a gaussian distribution; hence it is not appropriate to define a normal range as the mean value ±2 standard deviation. In the United States the central 95 per cent segment of the distributions encompasses values of 2.2 to 7.5 mg per deciliter in adult males and 2.1 to 6.6 mg per deciliter in adult premenopausal females. Definitions of hyperuricemia based on distributions of serum urate are useful for epidemiologic studies. Arbitrary limits of 7.0 in males and 6.0 in females have often been selected for such purposes. But statistical expressions are not adequate definitions of the pathophysiologic significance of hyperuricemia, for it is the *solubility* of urate in plasma and body fluids that is important. There is no evidence that urate in solution is toxic; all of the features of gout derive from responses to the urate crystal.

The solubility of urate in body fluids is strongly influenced by pH and temperature (Table 195–3). At pH 7.4 and 37° C,

TABLE 195–2. PREVALENCE OF GOUTY ARTHRITIS IN MEN IN RELATION TO SERUM URATE CONCENTRATION AND AGE

Serum Urate Level (mg/dl)	Mean Age 49 Years* (%)	Mean Age 58 Years† (%)
6.0–6.9	2	2
7.0–7.9	4	17
8.0–8.9	11	25
9.0–9.9	30	90
10 +	48	90

*Zalokar et al.: Chron Dis 25:305, 1972.
†Hall et al.: Am J Med 42:27, 1967.

TABLE 195–3. SOLUBILITY OF URATE ION AS A FUNCTION OF TEMPERATURE IN THE PRESENCE OF 140 mM Na^+ *

Temperature (° C)	Maximal Equilibrium Concentration of Urate in the Presence of 140 mM Na^+ (mg/dl)
37	6.8
35	6.0
30	4.5
25	3.3
20	2.5
15	1.8
10	1.2

*From Loeb: Arthritis Rheum 15:189, 1972.

the solubility of urate in fluid having the sodium composition of plasma is 6.4 to 6.8 mg per deciliter. An additional 0.4 mg per deciliter is protein bound, chiefly to an α_1-α_2 globulin. Thus 7.0 mg per deciliter may be taken as the solubility limit of urate in plasma at 37° C, the normal central body temperature. But solubility is considerably less at the temperature of peripheral joints, which may be 32° C in the knee, and 29° C in the ankle (Hollander, 1949). Concentrations of plasma urate above 7 mg per deciliter at 37° C define hyperuricemia in a physicochemical sense. Urate forms stable supersaturated solutions, but such solutions are poised for crystal formation when perturbed.

Mechanisms of Hyperuricemia. The concentration of urate in plasma is determined by the balance between absorption and production of purines on the one hand, and destruction and excretion on the other. Exogenous purines contribute substantially to body uric acid stores, unless the individual is on a highly artificial purine-free formula diet. Purine restriction leads to a reduction of serum urate of 0.6 to 1.8 mg per deciliter in normal subjects. Similar regimens have little effect on hyperuricemia of gouty subjects who greatly overproduce purines, but exhibit comparable effects in gouty subjects with reduced renal urate clearances. Although dietary purines may modify plasma urate levels, abnormalities of absorption have not been implicated as a cause of hyperuricemia.

In animals, urate is converted by uricase to soluble allantoin. In human beings, who lack uricase, uric acid is the end-product of purine metabolism. Uric acid is secreted into the gut in bile and intestinal juices where uricolysis is carried out by bacterial enzymes. In normal subjects approximately one third of the uric acid disposed of each day is degraded in the gut, and two thirds is excreted unchanged by the kidney. Studies in gout have not implicated decreased uricolysis as a mechanism for hyperuricemia. In fact, with high urate concentrations in body fluids enteric uricolysis is enhanced; with the onset of renal insufficiency intestinal uricolysis assumes increased importance and in extreme instances may account for 80 per cent of daily urate disposition. By contrast, both increased purine biosynthesis and decreased renal excretion of uric acid play important roles in the pathogenesis of primary hyperuricemia.

Since urinary uric acid represents a variable fraction of the daily turnover of urate even when dietary purines are restricted, its measurement does not precisely assess the rate of purine production. Random samples in normal men commonly contain 500 to 1000 mg per 24 hours. On a purine-restricted diet these values average 418±70 mg per 24 hours. Gouty subjects show slightly higher average values, 497 mg per 24 hours, but the overlap with the normal range is extensive. From 10 to 20 per cent of gouty subjects show basal values above the upper limits of normal. Because of the insensitivity of urinary urate measurements in the assessment of purine production, isotopic tracer studies have been employed for this purpose. With labeled uric acid the miscible pool of uric acid in normal man averages 1200 mg, and the daily rate of production averages 750 mg. From one half to three fourths of the pool turns over each day. The difference between the rate of production and the rate of excretion of urate ranges from 100 to 365 mg per day, and represents the amount of intestinal uricolysis. A second method of study involves measurement of the magnitude and time course of incorporation of a purine precursor, usually glycine, into urinary uric acid. The incorporation can be corrected for extrarenal disposal to give total incorporation values. By use of these methods, evidence of some degree of excessive production of uric acid has been obtained in about two thirds of patients with primary gout. The most extreme values are found in subjects with HGPRT deficiency or PP-ribose-P synthetase variants, but these represent fewer than 1 per cent of gouty subjects. Many gouty subjects whose 24-hour urinary uric acid values fall within the normal range show modest increases in the rate of turnover of an enlarged uric acid pool, and (or) overincorporation of glycine into urate. Studies of the intramolecular distribution of ^{15}N in uric acid, following administration of ^{15}N-glycine, show excessive labeling of position 9, which is derived from the amide-N of glutamine and from ammonia. Thus many more gouty subjects show evidence for mild overproduction of purine than would have been deduced from urinary uric acid measurements alone.

The first unique reaction of purine biosynthesis and the site of metabolic regulation by purine ribonucleotide inhibitors is that which synthesizes phosphoribosylamine, catalyzed by amidophosphoribosyltransferase (Fig. 195–1):

$$\text{Glutamine} + \text{PP-ribose-P} + H_2O \xleftrightarrow{Mg^{2+}} \text{phosphoribosylamine} + \text{glutamic acid} + \text{PPi}$$

There are several possible mechanisms for loss of rate control at this site, and resulting acceleration of purine biosynthesis. These include (1) excessive concentrations of the substrates PP-ribose-P, glutamine, or both; (2) a structural alteration in the enzyme, rendering it more active or less sensitive to normal feedback control by purine ribonucleotides, or alternatively, an increased amount of normally active enzyme; or (3) a reduced concentration of one of the regulatory nucleotides (AMP or GMP) which exert cooperative allosteric modulation of enzyme activity. Intracellular levels of PP-ribose-P are strikingly raised in HGPRT deficiency and also in PP-ribose-P synthetase overactivity. The increased concentration of PP-ribose-P drives purine biosynthesis both by furnishing more of the rate-limiting substrate and by allosteric activation of amidophosphoribosyltransferase. PP-ribose-P turnover is accelerated in gouty patients who overproduce uric acid. However, erythrocyte PP-ribose-P levels are normal in gouty patients without specific enzyme defects. Plasma glutamate values are slightly raised in gouty subjects, both in the fasting state and after oral glutamate loads, but plasma glutamine levels are normal. Although reduced activities of glutaminase and of glutamic dehydrogenase have been postulated in gout, no direct evidence for such enzyme deficiencies exists. The hyperuricemia of glycogen storage disease, and also that which follows fructose infusion, has been attributed to nucleotide breakdown to free purines, release of feedback inhibition of amidophosphoribosyltransferase, and secondary acceleration of purine biosynthesis de novo. Any process that results in accelerated breakdown of intracellular adenyl nucleotides may lead to hyperuricemia by prompt degradation of daughter purine compounds to uric acid, and an ensuing secondary acceleration of purine synthesis de novo through release of feedback inhibition of amidophosphoribosyltransferase. This biphasic mechanism has been implicated in glycogen storage disease type I (see below), following fructose infusion, following alcohol ingestion, and in a gouty patient with a variant AMP deaminase that showed reduced sensitivity to GTP, its normal regulator. The last example has been proposed as a possible general mechanism in idiopathic gout. There are no examples of gout attributable to intrinsic alterations of the amidophosphoribosyltransferase itself.

In the normal turnover of nucleic acids and nucleotides some are degraded to free purine bases, chiefly hypoxanthine and guanine. Nucleotides synthesized de novo in excess of nucleotide and nucleic acid requirements are promptly degraded to hypoxanthine. Guanine is deaminated to xanthine by guanase. Hypoxanthine and xanthine are oxidized to uric acid by xanthine oxidase (Fig. 195–2). Hepatic xanthine oxidase activity is increased in gouty overproducers, but this appears to be an induced rather than a primary change. Nevertheless, this is an additional factor contributing to accelerated uric acid synthesis in these patients.

In a substantial fraction of gouty subjects current techniques do not disclose excessive production of uric acid. In this group the immediate pathogenetic mechanism of hyperuricemia appears to be a decreased renal tubular clearance of urate. Renal excretion of urate is a complex function of glomerular filtration, tubular reabsorption, and tubular secretion. Filtration of plasma urate is assumed to be complete, on the basis of micropuncture studies in animals and ultrafiltration studies of human plasma in vitro. Less than 5 per cent of plasma urate is protein bound in man under physiologic conditions at 37° C. Filtered urate appears to be almost completely reabsorbed in the proximal tubule (presecretory reabsorption). Some of the secreted urate is also reabsorbed in the distal portion of the proximal tubule, and to a lesser extent in the ascending portion of the loop of Henle and in the collecting ducts (postsecretory reabsorption). The urate that is excreted is thought to arise almost entirely by tubular secretion. These conclusions are tentative; they rest on clearance studies with and without inhibitors of reabsorption, such as probenecid, or of secretion, such as pyrazinamide, which have major limitations that cannot be detailed here.

Many gouty patients show reduced renal clearance of urate. Studies with pyrazinamide have been interpreted as indicating reduced secretion of urate per nephron, but enhanced postsecretory reabsorption would also explain the data. The difference in renal tubular handling of urate in gout is small, and conclu-

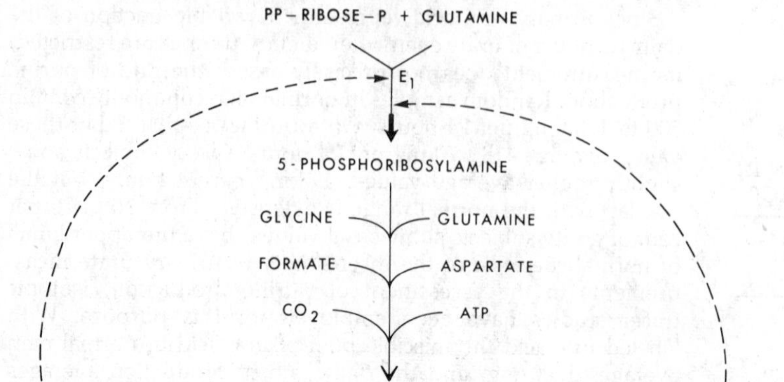

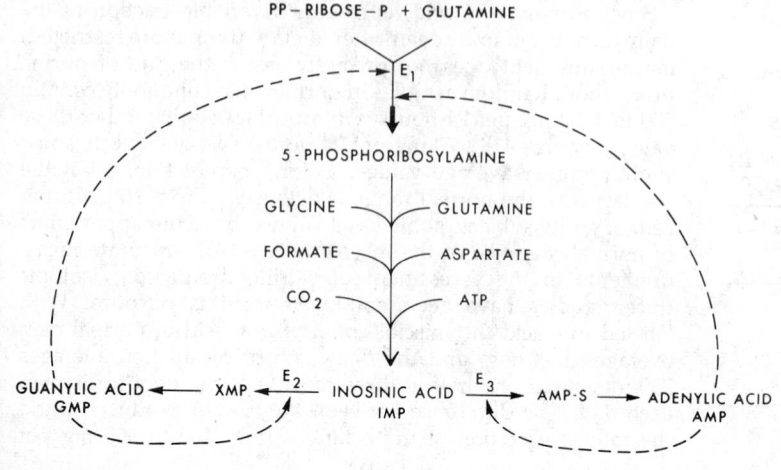

Figure 195–1. De novo pathway of purine nucleotide biosynthesis and the feedback control mechanisms (— — — →). E_1, Amidophosphoribosyltransferase; E_2, inosine 5′-phosphate dehydrogenase; E_3, adenylsuccinic acid (AMP-S) synthetase; XMP, xanthosine 5′-phosphate.

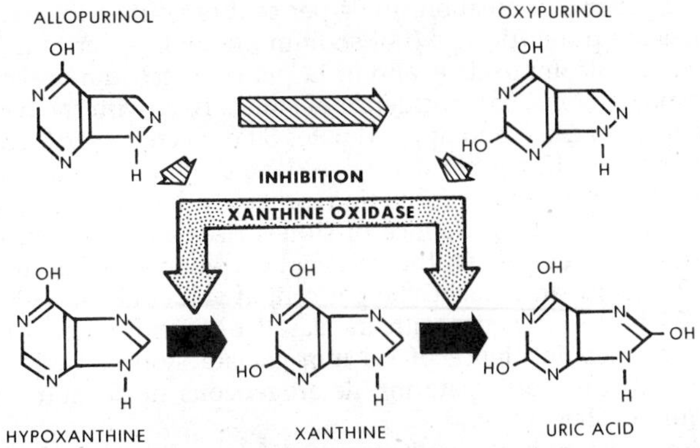

Figure 195–2. Pathway of uric acid synthesis catalyzed by xanthine oxidase and the site of action of allopurinol.

sions rest upon statistical analysis of clearance data on groups of patients. On this basis the renal contribution to hyperuricemia is most marked in patients with normal 24-hour excretion values of urate, normal turnover values of the uric acid pool, and normal values of glycine incorporation into uric acid. But reduced renal urate clearances per nephron are not restricted to this group. With the exception of patients with HGPRT deficiency or PP-ribose-P synthetase variants, overproducer gouty subjects as a group also show reduced renal urate clearances (Simkin). Thus, although some investigators have separated the large group of patients with an undefined biochemical lesion, *idiopathic gout,* into two discrete subgroups, termed metabolic (overproducer) and renal gout, the evidence does not support this categorical distinction. There is extensive sharing of these manifestations, and they appear to be arrayed as two overlapping spectrums, with many subjects showing both defects.

There is a prototype of a dual pathogenesis of hyperuricemia in the case of glycogen storage disease Type I, in which marked overproduction and reduced clearance of uric acid coexist. Both abnormalities appear to be secondary to hypoglycemia, which leads to glycogenolysis with excessive production of lactate, to nucleotide consumption with a compensatory increase in purine biosynthesis, and to lipolysis. Hyperlactic acidemia inhibits renal urate secretion. However, these particular mechanisms have been excluded in the common forms of gout.

The complexity of the pathogenesis of hyperuricemia is further illustrated by two additional observations. The first is that asymptomatic hyperuricemia begins at puberty in the male as an exaggeration of the modest increase in serum urate concentration that normally occurs at that age. Asymptomatic hyperuricemics resemble their older gouty counterparts in showing both overproduction and reduced clearance of urate, often simultaneously. The second is that both of these pathogenetic mechanisms may be reversible. Subjects with primary (idiopathic) gout are on average 15 to 30 per cent overweight, and 75 per cent or more show fasting hypertriglyceridemia. Hyperuricemia is present in over 80 per cent of all patients with hypertriglyceridemia. The association of hyperuricemia resulting from reduced renal urate clearance and hypertriglyceridemia is strong, both in primary gout and other conditions, but the relationship is not explained. In some gouty patients, weight reduction reverses hypertriglyceridemia, hyperuricemia, excessive urate excretion, and evidence of overproduction by isotopic studies, as well as evidence of impaired renal urate clearance. Additional studies may determine whether the renal defect in urate handling is secondary to an induced metabolic disturbance in a genetically predisposed individual, or whether those patients without manifest overproduction of urate have a genetically distinct form of gout expressed as an intrinsic tubular defect, as some investigators propose.

The Acute Gouty Attack. In 1859, A. B. Garrod, in the second and fourth of his ten propositions on "The True Nature of Essence of Gout," wrote: "Investigations recently made in the morbid anatomy of gout, prove incontestably that true gouty inflammation is *always* accompanied with a deposition of urate of soda in the inflamed part. . . . The deposited urate of soda may be looked upon as the cause, and not the effect, of the gouty inflammation." This hypothesis received strong support from the experimental work of Freudweiler (1899), who reproduced acute gouty attacks by the injection of microcrystals of sodium urate. For many years this work was overlooked, and other observations seemed to cast doubt on a specific role for uric acid in the acute gouty attack. The urate crystal was restored to its central position in the pathogenesis of the acute attack in 1961 when McCarty and Hollander observed sodium urate crystals, both free and within leukocytes, in synovial fluid of gouty effusions during acute inflammation. Acute attacks of colchicine-responsive arthritis were reproduced experimentally by the injection of microcrystals of urate. Aspiration of these joints revealed phagocytosis of some of these crystals by leukocytes; no experimental gouty arthritis could be produced in laboratory animals in the absence of leukocytes. The crystal-induced synovitis is not a specific response to urate microcrystals; it can be reproduced experimentally by other crystals of similar size and shape, such as sodium orotate or calcium oxalate, and also occurs in pseudogout caused by calcium pyrophosphate dihydrate crystals, and in xanthine oxidase deficiency (xanthinuria) presumably caused by xanthine crystals.

Although a number of cellular mechanisms are activated by the urate crystal, the exact sequence by which inflammation is initiated is uncertain. Hageman factor, kallikrein, kinin-like peptides, and the complement system have all been shown to participate in the response to the crystal, but each has also been excluded as an obligatory factor in the inflammatory reaction. Urate crystals are leukotactic. Leukocytes and synovial lining cells ingest the urate crystals. Within minutes leukocytes release a glycoprotein chemotactic factor (mw = 11,500) that attracts additional leukocytes into the joint space. Production of this glycoprotein is specifically suppressed by colchicine. The acute inflammatory response to injected urate crystals is prevented by prior treatment with colchicine, but the inflammatory response to purified crystal-induced chemotactic factor is not. Thus this factor may be an important mediator of the inflammatory reaction in gout. Another substance present in greatly increased concentrations in inflammatory exudates induced by the urate crystal (chickens) is prostaglandin D_2. Macrophages and platelets are also stimulated by urate crystals in vitro, but little is known about their roles in gout.

Phagocytosis of the crystal leads to rapid destruction of the phagolysosome membrane with release of hydrolytic enzymes into the cell. This results in cell necrosis and release of the original crystal and lysosomal and cytoplasmic enzymes into the surrounding tissue. The interactions between crystals and phagolysosomal membranes are thought to involve hydrogen bonding, leading to breaks in continuity. In a simulated system (liposomes) phospholipid membranes are susceptible to urate-induced lysis if they contain cholesterol or testosterone, and refractory if they contain β-estradiol. These observations suggest obvious interpretations, based upon the relative preference of gout for men and postmenopausal women.

The events leading to the putative burst of microcrystals of urate that initiates the acute attack are largely speculative. Three major theories have been advanced. The first draws upon the demonstration that synovial and cartilaginous tophi may precede a gouty attack, and postulates that trauma may result in shedding of crystals into the synovial fluid. The second emphasizes the well known affinity of cartilage for urate, and the ability of organized proteoglycans to absorb (solubilize) urate. With trauma, disruption and increased turnover of proteoglycans are postulated, with release of additional urate into the already supersaturated synovial fluid, and resulting crystallization. The third postulates a joint effusion with trauma, followed by a more rapid rate of reabsorption of water than of solute, resulting in further supersaturation of synovial fluid with urate, and precipitation of crystals. The first metatarsophalangeal joint is exposed to the greatest pressure per unit area of any joint in the body during walking, and it and other lower extremity joints are susceptible to trauma. In addition, the low temperature of peripheral leg joints will favor crystallization of urate from supersaturated synovial fluid. Thus each of these theories, which are not mutually exclusive, has merit.

Tophi. The pathognomic lesion of gout is the *tophus*, a deposit of fine acicular crystals of monosodium urate monohydrate often radially arranged, surrounded by a mononuclear reaction and a foreign body granuloma of epithelial and giant cells, some of which may be multinucleate. Urate crystals are water soluble, but when tissues are treated with nonaqueous fixatives (e.g., absolute alcohol) the crystals are preserved and are brilliantly anisotropic and negatively birefringent in compensated polarized light. Tophi are commonly found in articular and other cartilage, synovia, tendon sheaths and other periarticular structures, epiphyseal bone, the subcutaneous layers of the skin, and the interstitial areas of the kidney. The articular cartilages are the most common and at times the exclusive sites of urate deposition. The deposits, although superficial, are actually embedded in the intercellular matrix. In the joint, cartilaginous degeneration, synovial proliferation and pannus, destruction of subchondral bone, proliferation of marginal bone, and sometimes fibrous or bony ankylosis develop. The punched-out lesions of bone commonly seen on roentgenograms represent marrow tophus deposits, which may communicate with the urate crust on the articular surface through defects in the cartilage. In vertebral bodies, urate deposits involve the marrow spaces adjacent to the intervertebral discs, as well as the discs themselves.

All of these sites of urate deposition are rich in proteoglycans, and the postulated role of these substances in attracting and solubilizing urate when organized, and of releasing urate during metabolic turnover, cited above, may serve to explain both localization and occurrence of tophi. Curiously, the process in the tissues evokes only a minimal inflammatory response in comparison with the violence of the acute gouty attack brought about by crystals within the synovial space. Urate crystals stimulate mesenchymal cells of joints to produce collagenase and prostaglandin E_2, both of which may play roles in articular destruction.

The Gouty Kidney. The only distinctive histologic feature of the gouty kidney is the presence of sodium urate crystals in the medulla or pyramids and surrounding round cell and giant cell reaction. These are found in a high percentage of gouty patients at autopsy and are associated with acute and chronic interstitial inflammatory changes, fibrosis, tubular atrophy, glomerular sclerosis, and arteriolar nephrosclerosis. The earliest change in the kidney is an interstitial reaction, maximal near the loops of Henle, associated with tubular damage. In kidneys without tophi the interstitial reaction tends to spare the medulla and juxtamedullary cortex. Although renal disease is common in gout, it is generally mild and only slowly progressive. The origin of the interstitial nephropathy is not known. It is not even certain that in the absence of crystalline deposits it is related to hyperuricemia. Other possibilities include hypertension, uric acid stone disease, urinary infection, aging, and lead poisoning. Crystalline deposits may occur within the distal tubules and collecting ducts, and are probably composed of uric acid and related to the intratubular concentration of uric acid and the acid pH of the urine; they lead to dilatation and atrophy of the more proximal tubules. Deposits within the interstitium are composed of sodium urate, and are believed to be related to the elevated urate concentration of plasma and interstitial fluid.

Uric Acid Urolithiasis. The overall incidence of renal stones in gout is about 20 per cent, several hundred-fold higher than in the general population. In 84 per cent of gouty subjects, the stones are pure uric acid (not sodium urate); in 4 per cent, uric acid and calcium oxalate; and in 12 per cent, calcium oxalate or phosphate alone. The incidence of stones rises with the degree of hyperuricemia, and approximates 50 per cent at serum urate values above 12 mg per deciliter. Marked hyperuricemia probably influences stone formation primarily by increasing uric acid *excretion*. The incidence of stones rises above 20 per cent of gouty subjects when the uric acid excretion exceeds 700 mg per 24 hours, and reaches 50 per cent at values above 1100 mg per 24 hours. Patients with increased uric aciduria also have an increased incidence of calcium oxalate stones. Urate (not uric acid) can participate in "heterogeneous nucleation" with calcium oxalate.

Other factors in the pathogenesis of uric acid stones include the *concentration* of uric acid in urine, the *acidity* of urine, and possibly the availability of stone *matrix* and the level of *solubilizing substances* in the urine. The solubility of urate decreases with fall of pH because of the shift to free uric acid. The pKa of uric acid is 5.75. In plasma at pH 7.4 over 99 per cent is present in ionized form (urate), whereas in urine at pH 5.0 about 85 per cent is un-ionized (uric acid). At this pH only 15 mg of uric acid is soluble per deciliter of urine at 37° C, so supersaturation is required to excrete an average uric acid load in a normal urine volume. The solubility increases more than ten-fold at pH 7.0 and more than 100-fold at pH 8.0 over pH 5.0.

Both gouty and nongouty uric acid stone formers exhibit unusually low urinary pH values both when fasting and throughout the day. The persistently acid urine has been attributed to subnormal ammonium production with a compensatory increase in titratable acidity. There is debate whether these data reflect occult or measurable renal damage (e.g., interstitial nephropathy), aging, or an intrinsic renal defect. Regardless of the explanation, the tendency toward persistently acid urine favors uric acid stone formation. Studies in search of a deficit of putative solubilizing substances have shown no differences in uric acid solubility in urine of gouty and normal subjects at equivalent pH values.

CLINICAL MANIFESTATIONS. The clinical manifestations of gout are conveniently described in four categories: acute gouty arthritis, tophaceous gout, gouty nephropathy, and uric acid urolithiasis. In primary gout, even though the genetic determinants have been present since conception, clinical gout is extraordinarily rare before puberty, when males at risk for the usual form of gout first develop hyperuricemia. Exceptions occur in the juvenile gout of the Lesch-Nyhan syndrome or glycogen storage disease Type I, in which marked hyperuricemia is present from infancy. Only about 20 per cent of hyperuricemic subjects ever develop acute gout, although this figure rises as the degree of hyperuricemia increases (Table 195–2). Gout is uncommon before the third decade; its peak age of onset in men is about 45 years. Thus the usual gouty male is exposed to 30 years of hyperuricemia before the disease declares itself. In women the onset of primary gout is usually some years after the menopause, when serum urate values rise to hyperuricemic levels in those genetically at risk for gout.

Acute Gouty Arthritis. When acute gouty arthritis develops, it often appears as a fulminating attack of incapacitating severity. The description of the acute attack provided by Sydenham in 1683 remains a classic:

> "The victim goes to bed and sleeps in good health. About two o'clock in the morning he is awakened by a severe pain in the great toe; more rarely in the heel, ankle or instep. This pain is like that of a dislocation, and yet the parts feel as if cold water were poured over them. Then follows chills and shivers, and a little fever. The pain, which was at first moderate, becomes more intense. With its intensity the chills and shivers increase. After a time this comes to its height, accommodating itself to the bones and ligaments of the tarsus and metatarsus. Now it is a violent stretching and tearing of the ligament—now it

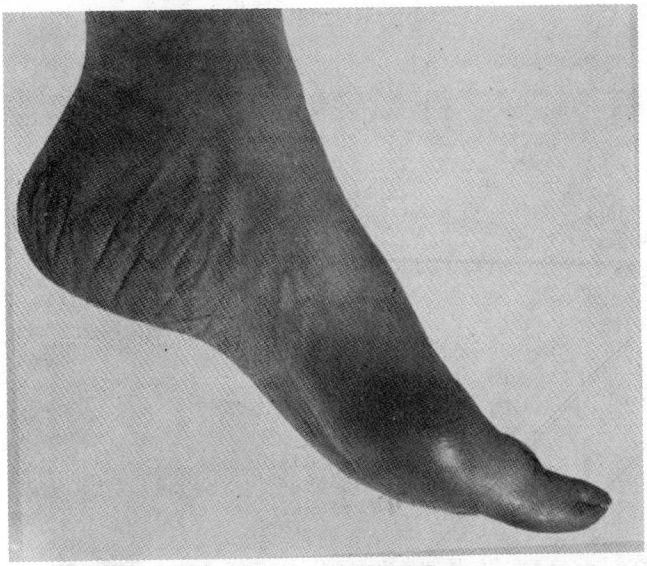

Figure 195–3. Acute gouty arthritis of great toe (podagra).

is a gnawing pain and now a pressure and tightening. So exquisite and lively meanwhile is the feeling of the part affected, that it cannot bear the weight of the bedclothes nor the jar of a person walking in the room. The night is passed in torture, sleeplessness, turning of the part affected, and perpetual change of posture; the tossing about of the body being worse as the fit comes on. Hence the vain effort, by change of posture, both in the body and the limb affected, to obtain an abatement of the pain."

Acute gout is predominantly a disease of the lower extremity. Seventy-five to 90 per cent of initial attacks are monoarticular, and at least half of first attacks involve the metatarsophalangeal joint of the great toe (podagra) (Fig. 195–3). Next in order of frequency as sites of initial involvement are the instep, ankle, heel, knee, wrist, finger, and elbow. Later attacks are more often polyarticular, and may include the shoulder or hip, or rarely such joints as the sacroiliac, sternoclavicular, mandibular, or even the spine. The more distal the site of involvement, the more typical are the attacks.

Some patients report short trivial episodes of "ankle sprains" or sore heels or twinges of pain in the great toe prior to the first attack, sometimes going back over several years. More often the first attack occurs with explosive suddenness during apparent excellent health, often at night. Within minutes to hours the affected joint becomes hot, dusky red, and exquisitely painful. Lymphangitis may be evident. Systemic signs of inflammation may include fever, leukocytosis, and elevation of the erythrocyte sedimentation rate. The inflammatory reaction may suggest a cellulitis or septic joint, and on occasion a joint is erroneously incised by an unwary physician.

Acute gouty arthritis often follows a precipitating event, such as trauma, surgery, alcohol ingestion, dietary overindulgence, starvation, or infection. Attacks may follow a long walk, golf, or hunting trip (e.g., "pheasant hunter's toe"). Postoperative gout usually occurs on the third to the fifth day, and has been attributed to the subsidence of the adrenal alarm by analogy with the recrudescence of acute gout that may follow cessation of steroid therapy. Alcohol ingestion and starvation increase serum urate levels by inhibition of renal excretion through the accompanying lactic acidosis and ketosis, respectively. Alcohol also increases urate production. Thus the legendary association of gout with imbibition may rest upon demonstrable effects on urate dynamics. Experimentally, urate crystals coated with endotoxin are particularly inflammatory; a subthreshold dose of injected uncoated crystals becomes violently inflammatory when endotoxin is given intravenously. Perhaps these observations bear upon the role of infection in precipitating attacks. It is postulated that uricosuric agents and allopurinol may induce acute attacks by lowering synovial fluid urate and favoring shedding of synovial crystals during dissolution.

The course of an untreated attack is highly variable. Initial attacks are usually self-limited. Mild attacks may subside in several hours or a few days. Severe attacks may last many days to several weeks. "With age and impaired habits gout may last two months" (Sydenham). As the attack subsides, the inflamed skin may desquamate. Once the attack has broken, recovery is generally rapid and complete. The patient then re-enters an asymptomatic phase, often termed *intercritical* gout in recognition of the tendency of acute attacks to recur. The subsequent course of gout is difficult to predict. Some patients never have a second attack. Others never fully recover from the first episode and suffer a series of exacerbations leading directly to chronic gouty arthritis. More commonly a pattern of recurrences develops. In Gutman's extensive series, 62 per cent of patients had recurrences within the first year, 16 per cent in one to two years, 11 per cent in two to five years, and 4 per cent in five to ten years; 7 per cent had no recurrence during prolonged follow-up. In the untreated patient the frequency of attacks often increases, and they may become more severe, last longer, and eventually resolve less completely. The patient may reach a state in which he is rarely free of gouty inflammation, and in which residual swelling, stiffness, and joint pain give permanent disability not responsive to measures usually effective in acute attacks.

Tophaceous Gout. Before effective control of hyperuricemia became possible, more than one half of gouty patients developed visible tophi. The incidence now ranges from 13 to 25 per cent. In noncompliant patients it still exceeds 50 per cent. Development of tophi is correlated with the degree of hyperuricemia, severity of renal involvement, and duration of disease. The time from initial attack to visible tophaceous involvement ranged from 3 to 42 years in one large series, with an average of 11.6 years (Hench, 1936). In 0.5 per cent of patients, tophi are present at the time of the initial attack; virtually all such patients have gout secondary to a myeloproliferative disease. Destruction of tissue is particularly evident in cartilage and bone, leading to radiolucent "punched-out" lesions, and to cortical erosions with characteristic "overhanging margins" (Fig. 195–4).

Chronic gouty arthritis is a consequence of the progressive inability to dispose of urate as rapidly as it is produced. The urate pool expands and crystalline deposits of urate appear in and around joints in cartilage, bone, synovial membranes, tendons, and bursae. A frequent site of tophaceous deposits is the external ear, especially in the helix and antihelix. Subcutaneous deposits, especially of fingertips, palms, and soles, may be visible as yellowish-white infiltrates. Tophaceous deposits may produce irregular asymmetric tumescences over joints, requiring patients to wear larger shoes or gloves. The classic gouty shoe has a window cut to accommodate a tender prominent joint, usually the first metatarsophalangeal. At later stages, fusiform or nodular enlargements of Achilles tendons, or saccular distentions of olecranon bursae, are common and characteristic.

The process of tophaceous deposition advances insidiously, and although the tophi themselves are relatively painless, often progressive stiffness and persistent aching limit the use of affected joints. Eventually extensive destruction of joints and large subcutaneous tophi may lead to grotesque deformities, particularly of hands and feet, and to progressive crippling (Fig. 195–4). The tense, shiny, thin skin overlying the tophus may ulcerate and extrude white chalky or pasty material composed of myriads of fine, needle-like crystals. The olecranon bursa may be massively distended with "urate milk." Rarely tophi may involve the tongue, epiglottis, vocal cords, arytenoid cartilage, corpus cavernosum and prepuce of the penis, aorta, aortic or mitral valves, and cardiac conducting system causing

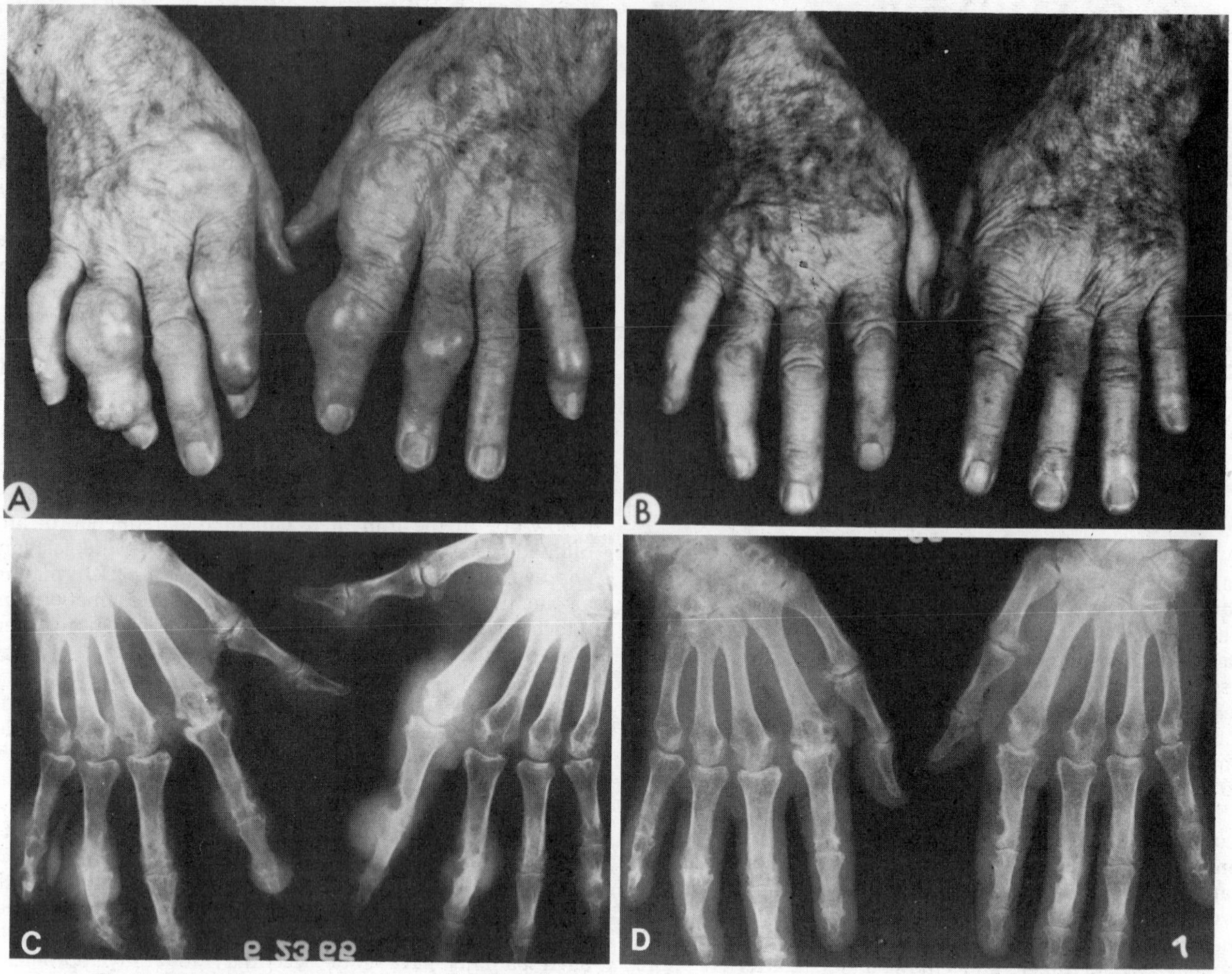

Figure 195–4. Chronic gouty arthritis *(A)* with tophaceous destruction of bone and joints *(C)*, and improvement after three years of treatment with allopurinol, prophylactic colchicine, and a moderately low purine diet *(B* and *D)*. (Courtesy of R. Wayne Rundles, Duke University Medical Center.)

rhythm disturbances. They do not involve the liver, spleen, lungs, or central nervous system.

As chronic gouty changes and renal disease advance, acute attacks occur less frequently and are milder; those that appear may be superimposed upon the indolent soreness of an involved joint, or may seek out previously uninvolved sites. No joint is exempt from chronic gouty involvement, although those of the lower extremity and hand are most commonly involved. The hip and spinal joints are rarely affected by tophaceous changes in the absence of extensive disease elsewhere. Radiographic changes of the sacroiliac joint and aseptic necrosis of the hip are sometimes attributable to gout.

Gouty Nephropathy. Renal disease is common in gout. One third of patients show isosthenuria and moderate albuminuria, which may be intermittent. The glomerular filtration rate is well preserved in many gouty subjects, but in others it gradually falls. Decline in renal function appears to be correlated with aging, renal vascular disease and hypertension, renal calculi, pyelonephritis, or independently occurring nephropathy, including that of lead poisoning. Only occasionally is it ascribable to gout alone. Hyperuricemia alone had no deleterious effect upon renal function during follow-up studies of gouty subjects ranging up to 12 years (Berger and Yu). Renal dysfunction does not shorten life expectancy in the average gouty subject, even though uremia is the eventual cause of death in 17 to 25 per cent of subjects. The majority of gouty patients die of cardiac or cerebral vascular disease (60 per cent) or malignancies, which occur in about the same incidence and at about the same time of life as in nongouty American males.

Hypertension is present in one third to one half of patients, and may be severe (diastolic pressure >130 mm Hg) in 10 per cent. Arterial and arteriolar nephrosclerosis are frequently prominent post mortem. There are no characteristic clinical or laboratory features to distinguish gouty kidney from other causes of chronic renal failure, except for the association of gout with the former. Renal failure from gouty nephropathy in the absence of gouty arthritis, tophi, or stones is extraordinarily rare; indeed, the entity is open to question.

Gouty nephropathy, sometimes referred to as *urate nephropathy* to emphasize the identity of the interstitial crystals, must be distinguished from *uric acid nephropathy*, an entirely different entity leading to acute renal failure from tubular obstruction by uric acid crystals. With sudden exceptionally high levels of uric acid excretion, seen most commonly following overly aggressive chemotherapy or radiation therapy of leukemia or lymphoma, crystals may occlude the distal collecting ducts and ureters. The crystals form in the distal tubule at the site of maximal concentration and acidification. Gouty patients with extremely high 24-hour uric acid excretion values, such as may occur in subjects with HGPRT deficiency or PP-ribose-P synthetase variants, are also at risk for uric acid nephropathy. This condition, and its treatment, are discussed in Ch. 81.

Urolithiasis. The incidence of urolithiasis in gout is correlated with both the degree of hyperuricemia and the magnitude of the 24-hour uric acid excretion. Above serum levels of 12 to 13 mg per deciliter or excretion values of 1100 mg per 24 hours, the incidence is 50 per cent. Many of these subjects will have secondary gout, with overproduction of uric acid caused by a myeloproliferative disease such as polycythemia vera or myeloid metaplasia. The incidence of stones in such patients is 35 to 40 per cent. Of gouty subjects who pass stones, about one third have their first episode of urolithiasis before the onset of gouty arthritis, sometimes more than a decade earlier. As pointed out above, in 84 per cent of subjects the stones are pure uric acid, but in 12 per cent they are calcium oxalate or calcium phosphate alone. These apparently uric acid–free stones may represent concretions that form about a tiny nidus of urate crystals. The fact that even these stones are reduced in frequency in patients given allopurinol supports this hypothesis. The overall prevalence of urolithiasis in the United States is about 0.1 per cent, and 5 to 10 per cent of all kidney stones in adults are composed of pure uric acid. However, only about 20 per cent of uric acid stone formers are hyperuricemic. Uric acid stones are radiolucent, being demonstrable only by the use of contrast media. Other radiolucent stones, so-called matrix stones which are predominantly proteinaceous, xanthine stones, and 2,8-dihydroxyadenine stones, are extremely rare.

GOUT ASSOCIATED WITH SPECIFIC ENZYME DEFECTS. Gout occurring on the basis of specific enzyme defects has special clinical features. These forms of gout are rare, accounting for fewer than 1 per cent of cases.

Glycogen Storage Disease Type I (see Ch. 179). Over 50 cases of von Gierke's glycogen storage disease (glucose-6-phosphatase deficiency) and gout have been recorded. Gout does not complicate other forms of glycogen storage disease. Affected subjects have hyperuricemia, hypertriglyceridemia, hyperlacticacidemia, and acidosis from infancy, and may develop gouty arthritis by the end of the first decade of life, sometimes of disabling severity. Chronic tophaceous gout and gouty nephropathy may account for a major portion of morbidity when these patients become adults. The sexes are involved equally. Avoidance of nocturnal hypoglycemia by a diet high in starch or by continuous intragastric feeding may markedly reduce or even correct hyperuricemia, and ameliorate gout. The hyperuricemia also responds to allopurinol, less well to uricosuric agents because of renal disease.

Hypoxanthine–Guanine Phosphoribosyltransferase Deficiency. Deficiency of HGPRT gives rise to two different X-linked syndromes. A complete deficiency is associated with the Lesch-Nyhan syndrome characterized by choreoathetosis, spasticity, growth and mental retardation, self-mutilation, and marked hyperuricemia (see Ch. 196). There is extreme exaggeration of uric acid production, and the greatly elevated excretion leads to crystalluria, renal stones with ureteral colic, and sometimes uric acid nephropathy. Death from renal failure usually occurs by age ten; if allopurinol therapy is begun early, the patients may live into their 20's. The kidneys are small with striking deposits of sodium urate and uric acid. A few of the more than 100 reported patients, all males, have had typical attacks of gouty arthritis.

An incomplete deficiency of HGPRT is associated with renal stones and recurrent acute gouty arthritis. Erythrocytes show from 0.2 to 50 per cent of normal HGPRT activity; the disorder is heterogeneous. Fifteen per cent of patients show minimal to moderate neurologic dysfunction resembling spinocerebellar ataxia or cerebral palsy. A few have survived neonatal episodes of uric acid nephropathy. Gout usually begins in the second or third decades; tophi develop early. Three quarters of patients have formed renal stones, half of these before age ten. These subjects have more marked hyperuricemia (usually >10 mg per deciliter) and uricaciduria (usually >1 gram per 24 hours) than most gouty subjects. Fewer than 100 cases—again, all males—have been described. HGPRT normally catalyzes a reaction between hypoxanthine or guanine and PP-ribose-P in reconstituting ribonucleotides, often called a "salvage" reaction. In HGPRT deficiency intracellular PP-ribose-P levels are raised and drive the first reaction of purine biosynthesis to excess. The female heterozygous carriers of complete HGPRT deficiency are not hyperuricemic, and their erythrocytes show normal HGPRT assay values. Carriers of the partial defect may be hyperuricemic and may show intermediate levels of HGPRT activity. Presumably, only cells possessing at least minimal HGPRT activity survive lyonization. Heterozygotes for the partial defect may develop uric acid stones or typical gout, which may occur before the menopause. Partial HGPRT deficiency should be considered in all females with gout or uric acid stones who exhibit raised urinary uric acid excretion values.

Phosphoribosylpyrophosphate Synthetase Variants. These patients resemble those with partial HGPRT deficiency in showing marked hyperuricemia and uricaciduria, and in developing uric acid stones or gout, and sometimes uric acid nephropathy, at an early age. They do not have neurologic abnormalities. Purine overproduction is prodigious. The enzyme abnormality, of which there are four different types leading to increased activity, results in increased intracellular concentrations of PP-ribose-P and excessive purine biosynthesis. The surplus of purine ribonucleotides is promptly degraded to uric acid. This, too, is an X-linked disorder, and all gouty patients are males. Fewer than 20 families have been identified with this disorder. Two females, first-degree relatives of gouty males, have shown hyperuricaciduria and may be manifesting heterozygotes.

SECONDARY GOUT. Any acquired hyperuricemic state may be complicated by secondary gout. This disorder occurs in 5 to 10 per cent of patients with polycythemia vera, especially those cases merging into the phase of myeloid metaplasia, occasionally in secondary polycythemia complicating congenital heart disease or chronic pulmonary disease, in chronic myelogenous leukemia, in multiple myeloma, or in chronic hemolytic anemias. In such instances the mean age of onset is later (59 years), women are more commonly involved (16 per cent), and both serum and urinary uric acid values tend to be higher than in idiopathic primary gout. Acute gouty arthritis may occasionally antedate evidence of the myeloproliferative disorder by many months, or even by several years. A syndrome of coexisting sarcoidosis, psoriasis, and gout has been described but may represent fortuitous concurrence of common diseases. Recently, gout associated with marked hyperuricaciduria has been attributed in a number of instances to a compensated hemolytic state *without* anemia.

In all the instances mentioned above, hyperuricemia appears to result from an increased tissue synthesis and breakdown and the resulting increase in turnover of nucleic acid. Hyperuricemia may also result from reduced renal excretion of urate, either because of chemical interference with tubular secretion of urate or because of reduced glomerular filtration resulting from parenchymal disease.

Hyperuricemia frequently follows the use of potent diuretic agents. Mean increases in serum urate concentrations are less than 2 mg per deciliter, but some subjects exhibit rises of 4 to 5 mg per deciliter. The hyperuricemic effect of diuretic agents results from salt and water loss, volume contraction, and avid solute reabsorption (including urate) in the proximal tubule. Typical gouty attacks may occur in patients receiving such drugs as hydrochlorothiazide, ethacrynic acid, or furosemide. In the 14-year study of the adult population of Framingham, Massachusetts, one half of the new cases of gout occurred in subjects taking potent diuretics. Three to five per cent of patients with gout have diabetes, but this incidence is not far from that of diabetes in the population of equivalent age. In markedly obese patients, total caloric restriction may result in extreme hyperuricemia, which is correlated with serum levels of β-hydroxybutyric acid and is not infrequently associated with severe attacks of acute gouty arthritis, especially of knees and ankles.

Chronic renal disease is a frequent cause of hyperuricemia,

but only about one patient per thousand develops gout. Uremia appears to interfere in some way with the inflammatory response to urate crystals. Garrod commented on the association of gout with lead poisoning in his treatise of 1876. Gout continues to be found in patients who survive lead exposure early in life and go on to develop slowly progressive lead nephropathy. In addition, "saturnine gout" is particularly prevalent in the southeastern United States, where it is attributed to the chronic ingestion of moonshine whiskey of high lead content with resulting renal tubular damage. Lead nephropathy and polycystic renal disease predispose to gout more often than do other forms of chronic renal disease.

DIAGNOSIS. The diagnosis of acute gouty arthritis is not difficult to suspect when there is an explosive onset of a typical inflammatory attack of characteristic severity in a peripheral joint, especially of the lower extremity. The diagnosis is established by the demonstration of typical negatively birefringent needle-shaped crystals of sodium urate in the leukocytes of synovial fluid (Fig. 195–5). With proper technique, including the use of a polarizing microscope, intraleukocytic sodium urate crystals are found in over 95 per cent of aspirates from joints in acute gout. The leukocyte count may range from 1000 to over 50,000, depending on the acuteness of the inflammation. A Gram stain should always be done to evaluate infection, which may coexist. In the rare event of failure to find crystals on the first attempt, a second aspirate obtained some hours later is usually positive. Urate crystals must be distinguished from calcium pyrophosphate dihydrate crystals of pseudogout. The latter are weakly positively birefringent under polarized light, and usually more rectangular in shape than urate crystals. Every patient suspected of having gout should have the diagnosis confirmed by crystal demonstration. It is not necessary to repeat the procedure in later attacks, unless they are atypical and other diagnoses (trauma, infection) are also under consideration. A rapid response of pain and inflammation to the administration of colchicine is so characteristic as also to be of diagnostic value. Responses of rheumatoid arthritis and sarcoid arthritis to colchicine are not so dramatic or complete as those in gout. The finding of hyperuricemia is anticipated and helpful, but since hyperuricemia is common (13 per cent of hospitalized male patients), it may coexist with other acute arthropathies. The presence of tophi or of typical roentgenographic findings of punched-out, destructive bony lesions will help

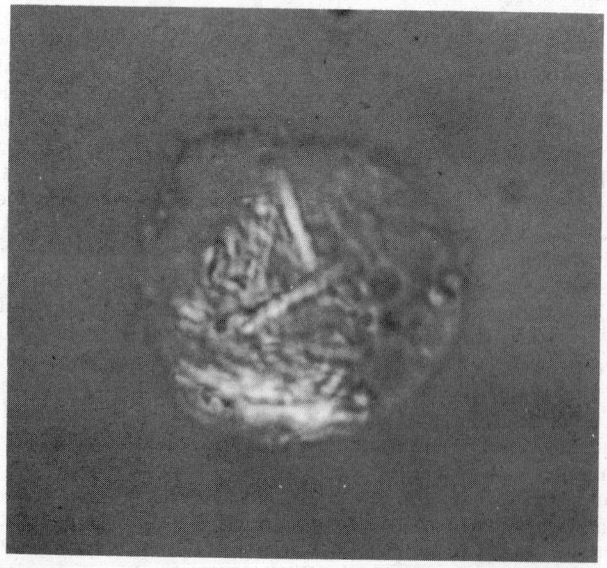

Figure 195–5. Sodium urate monohydrate crystals phagocytized by leukocyte in synovial fluid from acute gouty arthritis, examined by polarized light. (Courtesy of Edward W. Holmes, Duke University Medical Center.)

establish the diagnosis of chronic tophaceous gout but does not prove that the current event is acute gout. Only the demonstration of a large proportion of intraleukocytic crystals of sodium urate in the synovial fluid of the involved joint will do that. In 70 per cent of patients with crystal-proven gout, extracellular urate crystals are demonstrable in asymptomatic first metatarsophalangeal joints. Such crystals are rare (5 per cent) in hyperuricemic subjects who have never had clinical gout.

Each gouty patient should also have a determination of the 24-hour urinary excretion value of uric acid. The sample should be collected after three days of moderate purine restriction, during an intercritical period. Values of greater than 600 mg per 1.72 square meters per day under these conditions probably indicate overproduction, and those of over 800 mg per day warrant additional studies for a specific subtype of primary gout, such as HGPRT deficiency or PP-ribose-P synthetase overactivity, or of secondary gout, such as a myeloproliferative disorder or compensated hemolysis. Elevated urinary uric acid values may thus be a clue to a coexisting disorder. They also signify that the patient is at higher risk for renal stone and represent an indication for allopurinol rather than uricosuric drug therapy for gout.

Chronic gouty arthritis may be diagnosed by the presence of urate deposits in or near the affected joints or bursae or of soft-tissue deposits in the helix of the ear, the fingertips, the Achilles tendon, or other locations. The diagnosis may be confirmed by removal of the chalky contents of a tophus, by microscopic identification of sodium urate crystals by optical means, by chemical identification by the murexide test, or, preferably, by ultraviolet spectrophotometry and degradation by uricase.

DIFFERENTIAL DIAGNOSIS. Acute gout must be differentiated from acute rheumatic fever, rheumatoid arthritis, traumatic arthritis, osteoarthritis, pyogenic arthritis, sarcoid arthritis, cellulitis, bursitis, tendinitis, and thrombophlebitis. All patients with monoarticular arthritis should have synovial fluid aspiration in search of crystals, infection, or both. Podagra, the most common initial presentation of gout, can be mimicked by trauma, degenerative arthritis, acute sarcoidosis, psoriatic arthritis, pseudogout, palindromic rheumatism, Reiter's syndrome, or infection. Acute monoarticular arthritis of the great toe in the immediate postoperative period following parathyroidectomy can be caused by hydroxyapatite crystals. These various forms of "pseudopodagra" may be suggested by a negative examination of synovial fluid for urate crystals. Pseudogout (see Ch. 455), which is manifested by acute attacks of arthritis of knees and other joints, is usually accompanied by calcification of joint cartilage; the synovial fluid contains non-urate crystals of calcium pyrophosphate. However, gout and pseudogout may coexist, and both types of crystals will then be found in synovial fluid leukocytes.

Chronic gouty arthritis must chiefly be differentiated from rheumatoid arthritis, osteoarthritis, traumatic arthritis, and residua of pyogenic arthritis. The history of onset, progression, response to colchicine, and demonstration of hyperuricemia, asymmetric tumescences, typical roentgenographic changes, and tophi or crystals of urate in synovial fluid and leukocytes should establish the diagnosis.

TREATMENT. The therapeutic aims in gout are (1) to terminate the acute gouty attack as promptly and gently as possible, (2) to prevent recurrences of acute gouty arthritis, (3) to prevent or reverse complications of the disease resulting from deposition of sodium urate in joints and kidneys, and (4) to prevent formation of uric acid kidney stones. The therapeutic program differs according to the stage of the disease and the complications present. In the majority of patients it is possible to abort or prevent acute attacks, to control hyperuricemia, and to prevent chronic gouty arthritis, nephropathy, and stones.

Acute Attack. The affected joint should be placed at rest, and an anti-inflammatory agent administered promptly. Three types of agents are available for treatment of the acute gouty attack: colchicine, nonsteroidal anti-inflammatory agents, and glucocorticoids (or ACTH). *Colchicine* is the only therapeutic agent of specific diagnostic value in acute gout. It should be given as soon as the diagnosis is suspected. The initial dose of 0.6 to 1.2 mg of colchicine is followed by 0.6 mg every hour for eight hours and then every two hours until pain is relieved or until nausea, vomiting, cramping, or diarrhea develops. Maximum tolerated doses range from 4 to 8 mg. In many patients dramatic relief of pain and gastrointestinal side effects occur simultaneously. The diarrhea may be treated with paregoric, 4 ml, or Kaopectate, 30 ml, after each loose stool. Colchicine should be discontinued until gastrointestinal symptoms subside. Since the effective dose of colchicine varies, each patient should learn his own tolerance dose and stop just short of this in treatment of subsequent attacks. If started promptly, colchicine affords relief over 90 per cent of the time; if treatment is delayed beyond 12 hours, only 75 per cent of patients will respond within 24 to 48 hours. Since colchicine is concentrated within cells and turns over with a half-life of about 30 hours, repeated courses of colchicine carry a higher risk of toxicity; treatment failures should be treated with indomethacin or phenylbutazone.

Colchicine may also be given intravenously (subcutaneous infiltration may result in tissue necrosis). The usual initial dose is 1 to 2 mg in 20 ml saline solution given slowly, and if a single dose is not effective, the injection may be repeated once in four to five hours (maximum intravenous dose, 3 to 5 mg). Gastrointestinal symptoms are uncommon with intravenous administration, although occasionally nausea will occur.

Dose-related toxic responses to colchicine include alopecia (reversible), bone marrow suppression (leukopenia, thrombocytopenia, anemia), and hepatocellular damage. The drug should not be used in patients with advanced hepatic or renal disease.

Indomethacin is equally effective in acute gout. It is given orally in initial doses of 50 mg three or four times a day. When pain is relieved, doses are tapered over another 48 to 72 hours. Larger doses may cause severe headache, gastric distress, or a transient depersonalization reaction in some patients, but these side effects have been noted only rarely in gouty patients receiving short courses of the drug. *Phenylbutazone* and *oxyphenbutazone* (Tandearil) are also effective in acute gouty arthritis, and may be preferred when the gouty attack has proceeded for some time, or when the attack does not abate completely with colchicine or indomethacin. The initial dose is 400 mg orally, followed by 100 mg every four to eight hours for two to three days. Bone marrow suppression may rarely occur, even after a short course of either drug. Other nonsteroidal anti-inflammatory agents, such as *naproxen* and *ibuprofen*, can also be used, especially in patients with a history of peptic ulcer.

If full doses of colchicine, indomethacin, or phenylbutazone are contraindicated (e.g., in postoperative gout) or ineffective, *ACTH* may be employed by intravenous drip (40 units per day) or as intramuscular gel (40 to 80 units per day), or systemic glucocorticoids may be given for two to three days, rarely longer, following which the doses are reduced in stepwise fashion and discontinued. Unfortunately, rebound attacks of gout are rather common after such therapy. *Triamcinolone hexacetonide* in a dose of 5 to 20 mg injected intra-articularly into the involved joint is useful in treating acute gout limited to a single joint or bursa, particularly in patients in whom the standard drugs cannot be used, and relief from pain is usually prompt and complete within 24 to 36 hours. Steroid hormones are not recommended for parenteral use in acute gout, as the effects are inconsistent and rebound attacks frequent.

Uricosuric agents and allopurinol are of no value in treatment of the acute attack.

Interval Phase. The patient with gout should avoid high purine foods so as to lessen the burden of uric acid excretion. A severe limitation of purine-containing foods is rarely indicated, unless renal function is poor. Gradual weight reduction is indicated if the patient is overweight, and may of itself reduce hyperuricemia and the tendency to develop attacks of gout. Sudden weight reduction may precipitate gouty attacks and should be avoided. In general, diets of moderate protein content, somewhat low in fat, are preferred. Hypertension should be treated vigorously, even if antihypertensive agents worsen hyperuricemia; that result can be countered with appropriate antihyperuricemic drug therapy.

A high fluid intake is advisable to maintain a urinary output of 2000 ml per day. Uric acid excretion is thus promoted, and the dangers of crystal formation in the kidney or ureter are reduced. Beer, ale, and wine should be avoided, as they may precipitate attacks. Distilled alcoholic beverages in moderation generally have little influence on the gouty process. Illicit liquor (moonshine) should be prohibited. Excessive alcohol in any form should be avoided, particularly in patients with hypertriglyceridemia.

Patients who recognize prodromal symptoms may abort acute attacks by prompt institution of colchicine, phenylbutazone, or indomethacin therapy; they frequently require only a few tablets to achieve success. The daily ingestion of 0.6 to 1.8 mg of colchicine is generally effective in reducing the number of acute gouty attacks in patients who are subject to frequent episodes. Toxicity is rare, but may include alopecia, bone marrow suppression, and hepatocellular damage. Maintenance colchicine therapy is particularly important during the first months or year after institution of uricosuric drugs, or of allopurinol. Daily ingestion of indomethacin, 25 or 50 mg, has also been employed for this purpose and appears to be effective. The risks of renal and gastrointestinal toxicity make use of indomethacin undesirable as a prophylactic agent or as therapy for chronic gouty arthritis.

Chronic Gouty Arthritis. Use of a drug to lower the serum level of uric acid to 6 mg per 100 ml or less is indicated in all gouty patients with visible tophi, with roentgenographic evidence of urate deposits, or with a history of two or more major attacks of acute gouty arthritis. Either uricosuric agents or allopurinol may be used. With either type of agent the number of acute gouty attacks may be increased during the first few months unless maintenance colchicine therapy is given, whereas after 12 to 18 months the number may be decidedly reduced. Uricosuric drugs block tubular reabsorption of filtered urate. Those of use in gout are probenecid and sulfinpyrazone. These agents begin to lose effectiveness when the creatinine clearance falls below 80 ml per minute and are completely ineffective when the clearance falls below 30 ml per minute.

Probenecid is given in doses of 0.5 to 3 grams daily in two or three evenly spaced doses (average dose, 1 to 1.5 grams). This drug may produce gastrointestinal upsets, headaches, or skin rash. *Sulfinpyrazone* may be given in doses of 100 to 600 mg daily in three or four divided doses (average dose, 300 mg). This drug is related to phenylbutazone and may cause untoward reactions, but is generally somewhat better tolerated than probenecid. *Salicylates* block the uricosuric action of both probenecid and sulfinpyrazone and must not be used concurrently. Salicylates are uricosuric when given in high doses (4 to 6 grams daily), but few patients can tolerate these quantities.

With all uricosuric agents the doses should be low initially, so as to avoid sudden excretion of large quantities of urate, and increased at weekly intervals to maintenance levels. Fluids should be forced so as to prevent formation of concentrated urine, especially during the late hours of the night. During the first days or weeks of therapy the urine should be kept at pH 6 or above, by administration of sodium bicarbonate or sodium citrate–citric acid (Shohl's solution); this may be difficult to achieve, as gouty patients tend to produce acid urine. In patients who are mobilizing urate, and especially those who form uric acid gravel, alkalinization during the night, when fluid intake is reduced, is important. A single 250-mg tablet of acetazolamide (Diamox) taken at bedtime will serve to keep the urine alkaline and dilute throughout the night.

A second approach toward controlling serum urate levels is that of regulating production of uric acid, rather than (or in addition to) augmenting its excretion. This is achieved by use of allopurinol, a potent inhibitor of xanthine oxidase. Allopurinol is converted to oxipurinol in the body, and the latter compound has a longer biologic half-life (28 hours), ultimately being largely excreted in the urine. Inhibition of conversion of hypoxanthine and xanthine to uric acid permits these precursors to be excreted instead. In gouty subjects other than those with HGPRT deficiency, the increment in hypoxanthine plus xanthine excretion is only about two thirds of the decrement in uric acid excretion, presumably because of enhanced feedback inhibition of purine synthesis de novo by nucleotides reconstituted from hypoxanthine. The induced xanthinuria has not resulted in xanthine stone formation in the usual gouty subjects, but has done so in a rare patient with HGPRT deficiency and in patients being treated with antineoplastic agents. Use of allopurinol results in reduction of levels of uric acid in serum *and in urine.* The drug is effective even in the presence of renal failure, when uricosuric agents generally are not. Its action is not blocked by salicylates. The usual dose is 300 mg, given orally once a day. In the presence of moderate nitrogen retention the dose of allopurinol should be reduced, as the biologic half-life of the active metabolite, oxipurinol, is prolonged. Allopurinol is usually well tolerated, but may cause gastric irritation, diarrhea, or skin rash, or induce an attack of gout. Toxic hepatitis, epidermal necrolysis, and vasculitis may occasionally be severe, even fatal. Toxic effects are more frequent and more severe in the presence of renal failure. Intramuscular crystals of xanthine and oxipurinol have been described in patients receiving allopurinol, but their significance in terms of toxicity is not clear. Uricosuric agents may be used concurrently with allopurinol to hasten mobilization of urate deposits, but combined therapy may require larger doses of allopurinol because uricosuric drugs also enhance the excretion of oxipurinol. Since allopurinol decreases uric acid excretion, it is also very useful in controlling uric acid stone formation, especially in patients who are overproducers of uric acid. If the serum urate values can be controlled at levels below saturation of urate in body fluids, extensive resolution of soft tissue tophi and modest reduction in size of bony erosions may be achieved, together with some recalcification of bony lesions (Fig. 195–4). Joint mobility and comfort may be greatly improved.

In selected patients surgical removal of large extra-articular urate deposits, such as those in olecranon bursae, may be advisable. Occasionally amputation of irreparably damaged digits, especially those containing draining sinuses, is indicated. Physical therapy and appropriate self-help devices are valuable in patients who are partially disabled.

Asymptomatic Hyperuricemia. Asymptomatic hyperuricemia is frequent in family members of patients with gout and in the general population. It usually requires no therapy, as only about one fifth of patients will ever develop articular attacks, and adequate therapy can be instituted when these supervene. Exceptions may exist in patients with markedly elevated serum levels of uric acid, especially if urinary urate excretion is low and there is a family history of tophaceous disease. In such circumstances the asymptomatic subject should be treated with allopurinol before articular or renal complications develop. It is essential that the physician maintain frequent close observation of the patient.

Berger L, Yu T-F: Renal function in gout. IV. An analysis of 524 gouty subjects including long-term follow-up studies. Am J Med 59:605, 1975. *An important study showing that deterioration of renal function in gout is largely associated with aging, renal vascular disease, hypertension, renal calculi with pyelonephritis, or independently occurring nephropathy. Hyperuricemia alone had no deleterious effect on renal function over periods up to 12 years.*

Gutman AB, Yu T-F: Uric acid nephrolithiasis. Am J Med 45:756, 1968. *A thorough discussion of incidence, pathogenesis, and management.*

Rieselbach RE, Steele TH: Influence of the kidney upon urate homeostasis in health and disease. Am J Med 56:665, 1974. *A review of mechanisms of renal excretion of urate, and of evidence for diminished excretion of urate per nephron in many patients with gout.*

Simkin PA: Uric acid excretion in patients with gout. Arthritis Rheum 22:98, 1979. *An analysis of six published studies relating the rate of urate excretion to plasma urate levels in normal and gouty subjects. The kidneys of the average gouty person lag significantly behind the normal in their response to any concentration of plasma urate. The kidneys of overproducers (38 of 73 gouty subjects) were no less handicapped than those of other gouty subjects.*

Spilberg I, Mandell B, Mehta J, Simchowitz L, Rosenberg D: Mechanism of action of colchicine in acute urate crystal-induced arthritis. J Clin Invest 64:775, 1979. *Phagocytosis of urate crystals by neutrophils induces the synthesis and release of a glycoprotein which is chemotactic both in vitro and in vivo. Colchicine decreases production and release of this factor. Colchicine abrogates the acute arthritis produced by urate crystals in rabbits but has no effect upon the arthritis induced by injection of purified cell-derived chemotactic factor.*

Wyngaarden JB, Kelley WN: Gout. *In* Stanbury JB, Wyngaarden JB, Fredrickson DS, Goldstein JL, Brown MS (eds): The Metabolic Basis of Inherited Disease. 5th ed. New York, McGraw-Hill Book Company, 1983. *A detailed account of purine metabolism and the pathogenesis of primary gout.*

Wyngaarden JB, Kelley WN: Gout and Hyperuricemia. New York, Grune & Stratton, 1976. *Everything you have always wanted to know about gout but never dared to ask, condensed into 500 pages.*

196. OTHER DISORDERS OF PURINE METABOLISM

Edward W. Holmes

XANTHINURIA

Classical xanthinuria, which is inherited as an autosomal recessive trait, is the consequence of an isolated deficiency of xanthine oxidase. As a result of this enzyme deficiency, uric acid is replaced by xanthine and hypoxanthine as the end products of purine metabolism. Serum urate concentrations in these patients range from 0 to 1.4 mg per deciliter and urinary uric acid excretion ranges from 0 to 8 mg per day; serum oxypurine (xanthine plus hypoxanthine) concentrations and urine oxypurine excretion are increased in this disorder.

About 45 patients with classical xanthinuria have been described, and the prevalence of this disorder is estimated to be approximately 1:45,000. Over 50 per cent of individuals with classical xanthinuria are asymptomatic, the diagnosis being suspected by the incidental finding of a very low serum urate concentration during evaluation of presumably unrelated medical problems. The diagnosis is virtually established by the demonstration of low serum and urinary uric acid levels in association with increased urinary oxypurine excretion, and it is confirmed by assaying liver or intestinal mucosa for xanthine oxidase activity. One third of patients develop radiolucent renal calculi composed of xanthine. Four adult patients have had myopathic symptoms characterized by muscle cramps following exercise, and crystalline deposits of xanthine and hypoxanthine have been found in skeletal muscle. Recurrent polyarthritis has been described in three patients, and it has been suggested but not established that this symptom may represent crystal-induced synovitis.

A new subtype of xanthinuria has been described in which the deficiency of xanthine oxidase is associated with a deficiency of sulfite oxidase. Both of these enzymes require a molybdenum cofactor for catalytic activity, and absence of this cofactor has been demonstrated in the liver of a patient with this combined enzyme defect. Four patients have been reported with an inherited deficiency of these two enzymes, and all four presented in the first weeks of life with a severe neurologic disorder characteristic of isolated sulfite oxidase deficiency. Symptoms include feeding difficulties from birth, tonic-clonic seizures, nystagmus, enophthalmus, ocular lens dislocation, and Brushfield spots. As in isolated sulfite oxidase deficiency, urinary excretion of sulfate is low while that of sulfite, thiosulfate, S-sulfocysteine, and taurine is increased. Characteristic biochemical findings of xanthinuria are also present.

An acquired phenocopy of the combined defect has been described in a 20-year-old male with short bowel syndrome maintained for 18 months on total parenteral nutrition. In addition to hypouricemia and hypouricosuria, urinary excretion of sulfite and thiosulfate was increased while excretion of sulfate was decreased. Following infusion of commercially available amino acid solutions the patient experienced headaches, night blindness, irritability, lethargy, and then coma.

The prognosis in classical xanthinuria is excellent, as shown by the high percentage of patients who are asymptomatic. Therapy for xanthine calculi includes high fluid intake, and on occasion allopurinol has been used in patients with residual xanthine oxidase activity to increase the excretion of hypoxanthine relative to xanthine, the former being more soluble than the latter. In patients with the inherited form of combined xanthine oxidase and sulfite oxidase deficiency, the neurologic symptoms have been refractory to therapy with a number of agents, including oral ammonium molybdate. With the acquired form of this combined disorder, treatment with ammonium molybdate reversed the biochemical abnormalities and the neurologic symptoms were markedly ameliorated.

Holmes EW, Wyngaarden JB: Hereditary xanthinuria. *In* Stanbury JB, Wyngaarden JB, Fredrickson DS, Goldstein JL, Brown MS (eds.): The Metabolic Basis of Inherited Disease. 5th ed. New York, McGraw-Hill Book Company, 1983, pp 1192–1201. *A thorough coverage of the clinical and biochemical abnormalities found in classical xanthinuria, as well as the inherited and acquired forms of the combined deficiency of xanthine oxidase and sulfite oxidase.*

Johnson JL, Waud WR, Rajagopalan KV, Duran M, Beemer FA, Wadman SK: Inborn error of molybdenum metabolism: Combined deficiencies of sulfite oxidase and xanthine dehydrogenase in a patient lacking the molybdenum cofactor. Proc Natl Acad Sci USA 77:3715, 1980. *Extensive metabolic observations on the initial case of this new disorder.*

THE LESCH-NYHAN SYNDROME AND PARTIAL DEFICIENCY OF HYPOXANTHINE-GUANINE PHOSPHORIBOSYLTRANSFERASE

The Lesch-Nyhan syndrome, caused by a virtually complete deficiency of hypoxanthine-guanine phosphoribosyltransferase (HPRT) activity, is manifested clinically by hyperuricemia, excessive production of uric acid, and neurologic features including self-mutilation, choreoathetosis, spasticity, and mental retardation. Partial deficiency of HPRT activity is associated with uric acid overproduction, severe gout, and occasionally neurologic abnormalities, but self-mutilation is absent. The Lesch-Nyhan syndrome occurs in about 1:100,000 births, and partial deficiency of HPRT is noted in less than 1 per cent of the gouty population.

ETIOLOGY AND PATHOGENESIS. Recent studies have demonstrated a single but different amino acid substitution in several mutant forms of HPRT. Failure to reutilize hypoxanthine in the salvage pathway as a result of HPRT deficiency leads to increased oxidation of this purine base to uric acid. An increase in the intracellular concentration of phosphoribosylpyrophosphate, which also results from reduction in hypoxanthine reutilization, leads to an increase in the rate of purine biosynthesis de novo. The combined effect of these abnormalities is increased uric acid production resulting in hyperuricosuria, which predisposes to uric acid crystal and stone formation, and hyperuricemia, which leads to gouty arthritis and tophaceous deposits. The biochemical basis for the unusual and devastating neurologic abnormalities seen in the Lesch-Nyhan syndrome remains unexplained.

CLINICAL MANIFESTATIONS. The gene for HPRT is located on the X chromosome, and consequently the deficiency of HPRT activity is fully expressed only in affected males. Females heterozygous for HPRT deficiency may have subtle abnormalities in purine metabolism, but they are generally asymptomatic.

Infants with the Lesch-Nyhan syndrome are normal at birth, and the earliest consistent abnormality is a delay in motor development noted at three to four months of age. Between eight and twelve months extrapyramidal signs develop leading to choreoathetosis, and at about one year of age signs of pyramidal tract involvement, such as hyper-reflexia, clonus, and scissoring of the legs, appear. Compulsive self-destructive behavior appears any time between early childhood and adolescence. This is the most distinctive neurologic feature of the syndrome, and is manifested by biting of the fingers, lips, and buccal mucosa. Repeated attempts at self-injury, such as placing extremities in dangerous areas and self-inflicted head trauma, are also common. Sensation is intact in these children. Mental retardation is noted in most cases, but it is unclear whether the enzyme deficiency per se causes this or whether it is the result of poor performance on formal testing in children with dysarthria and choreoathetosis. Growth retardation is also a prominent feature of the syndrome. Uric acid crystalluria may be noted as orange crystals on the diaper during the first weeks of life, and in untreated patients progresses to uric acid nephrolithiasis, obstructive uropathy, and azotemia. Hyperuricemia is usually present and may attain levels of 18 mg per deciliter, but the serum urate concentration may be normal, especially before puberty. Gout is unusual in the Lesch-Nyhan syndrome before 12 to 15 years of age. Death usually occurs in the second or third decade from infection or renal failure.

Patients with partial deficiency of HPRT develop uric acid crystalluria and renal calculi in childhood, and gouty arthritis often occurs before 20 years of age. Neurologic manifestations, including mental retardation, mild spastic quadriplegia, dysarthria, cerebellar ataxia, and seizures, are noted in 20 per cent of patients with partial HPRT deficiency, but self-mutilation does not develop. Patients with partial HPRT deficiency may seek medical attention with the only symptom being the passage of a renal calculus or an attack of gouty arthritis. Life expectancy is normal in these patients.

DIAGNOSIS. Self-destructive behavior is the most distinguishing clinical feature of the Lesch-Nyhan syndrome; whereas retarded children with other disorders will bite their fingers, mutilation to the point of tissue destruction is rare in any disorder other than the Lesch-Nyhan syndrome. Severe self-biting in other neurologic disorders is usually associated with a loss of pain sensation. As pointed out, hyperuricemia is usually present but this is not an invariable finding. The diagnosis is established by demonstrating a virtual absence of HPRT activity in readily accessible tissues such as erythrocytes. Analyses of erythrocyte lysates are not useful in identifying heterozygous female carriers, but this can be accomplished with cell culture of skin fibroblasts or through analysis of hair follicles.

Partial deficiency of HPRT should be suspected in male patients with the onset of gouty arthritis before 20 years of age and in young males with uric acid crystalluria or uric acid nephrolithiasis. Uric acid overexcretion is found invariably in patients with normal renal function, and the diagnosis is confirmed by enzyme assay. Patients with partial HPRT activity will have erythrocyte lysate values that are usually in the range of 0.1 to 5 per cent of control values, rarely up 30 to 50 per cent of control values, while Lesch-Nyhan patients will have values less than 0.01 per cent of control values.

TREATMENT. Uric acid stone formation, tophi, and gouty arthritis can be controlled in both the Lesch-Nyhan syndrome and partial deficiency of HPRT with drugs that inhibit xanthine oxidase activity. However, a few patients have developed xanthine stones on this therapy. No drugs have been found that correct the neurologic deficits, but supportive measures such as restraints that reduce the tendency to self-mutilation are well accepted by the patient. Drugs such as diazepam help control the movement disorder. Given the devastating neurologic complications of the Lesch-Nyhan syndrome, therapeutic abortion has been used as a preventive measure following heterozygote identification and intrauterine diagnosis.

Edwards NL, Recker D, Fox IH: Overproduction of uric acid in hypoxanthine-guanine phosphoribosyltransferase deficiency. J Clin Invest 63:922, 1979. *A careful analysis of the basis for uric acid overproduction in patients with HPRT deficiency.*

Kelley WN, Wyngaarden JB: Clinical syndromes associated with hypoxanthine-guanine phosphoribosyltransferase deficiency. *In* Stanbury JB, Wyngaarden JB, Fredrickson DS, Goldstein JL, Brown MS (eds.): The Metabolic Basis of Inherited Disease. 5th ed. New York, McGraw-Hill Book Company, 1983, pp 1115–1143. *A detailed description of the clinical and biochemical consequences of HPRT deficiency.*

Wilson JM, Young AB, Kelley WN: Hypoxanthine-guanine phosphoribosyltransferase deficiency: The molecular basis for the clinical syndromes. N Engl J Med 309:900, 1983. *A description of specific mutations at the molecular level in patients with HPRT deficiency.*

2,8-DIHYDROXYADENINE RENAL STONES

Deficiency of adenine phosphoribosyltransferase, an enzyme in the salvage pathway of purine nucleotide synthesis, leads to the accumulation and increased urinary excretion of 2,8-dihydroxyadenine, the product of adenine oxidation by xanthine oxidase. Because of the insolubility of this purine, patients with this autosomal recessive disorder are predisposed to development of renal calculi composed of 2,8-dihydroxyadenine. Six individuals homozygous for this enzyme deficiency have presented with acute renal failure, and three of these patients suffered permanent renal damage. Renal colic may occur within the first months of life, as late as 40 years of age, or individuals with this disorder may be asymptomatic. 2,8-Dihydroxyadenine stones are usually radiolucent and have been confused with uric acid because of the structural similarity of these two purines. The diagnosis is confirmed by analysis of the stone with ultraviolet, infrared, or mass spectrometry or x-ray crystallography, or by demonstrating the absence of adenine phosphoribosyltransferase activity in erythrocyte lysates. Except for the excessive excretion of adenine and its metabolites with the consequent development of renal calculi, no other biochemical or clinical abnormalities have been reported in individuals homozygous for this enzyme deficiency.

The prevalence of the homozygous state is not documented, but it is calculated to occur once in 35,000 to 250,000 births, since the frequency of heterozygosity for adenine phosphoribosyltransferase deficiency varies from 0.4 to 1.0 per 100. Individuals heterozygous for the enzyme deficiency have no recognized clinical abnormalities.

Prognosis depends on renal function at the time of diagnosis. Therapy with dietary purine restriction, high fluid intake, and allopurinol—to prevent oxidation of adenine to 2,8-dihydroxyadenine—is effective in reducing stone formation and preserving renal function.

Simmonds A, Van Acker KL: Adenine phosphoribosyltransferase deficiency. *In* Stanbury JB, Wyngaarden JB, Fredrickson DS, Goldstein JL, Brown MS (eds.): The Metabolic Basis of Inherited Disease. 5th ed. New York, McGraw-Hill Book Company, 1983. *A detailed review of all known cases of complete APRT deficiency and discussion of the metabolic defect.*

Van Acker KJ, Simmonds A, Potter C, Cameron JS: Complete deficiency of adenine phosphoribosyltransferase. Report of a family. N Engl J Med 297:127, 1977. *Adenine, 8-hydroxyadenine and 2,8-dihydroxyadenine amounted to 25 per cent of urinary purines in two homozygous male children, one of whom had "pure uric acid stones" later correctly identified as 2,8-dihydroxyadenine.*

MYOPATHY ASSOCIATED WITH MYOADENYLATE DEAMINASE DEFICIENCY

Deficiency of myoadenylate deaminase has been noted in approximately 2 per cent of muscle biopsies submitted for routine investigation in some centers. This isozyme of AMP deaminase is found only in skeletal muscle, and this is the only organ affected by this enzyme deficiency. Three quarters of patients with myoadenylate deaminase deficiency report exercise-related symptoms of easy fatigability, cramps, and myalgias, usually beginning in childhood or young adulthood. Weakness without exercise is noted in less than one third of patients. Hypotonia has been described in two patients. Reduced AMP deaminase activity has occasionally been reported in patients with other neuromuscular disorders, but no definite association of this enzyme deficiency has been established with any symptom complex other than easy fatigability, cramps, and myalgias. Since a few individuals with myoadenylate deaminase deficiency have been reported to be asymptomatic, factors in addition to AMP deaminase deficiency may contribute to the exercise-related manifestations described above.

Serum creatine kinase activity is mildly and variably increased in about one half of patients with this disorder, and routine laboratory studies including electromyography and histochemistry of muscle are not diagnostic. In the patient with exercise-related symptoms the specific diagnosis of myoadenylate deaminase deficiency is suggested by the finding of reduced NH_3 production in a forearm ischemic exercise test. NH_3 is a product of AMP deamination, a normal consequence of ATP catabolism in skeletal muscle. However, not all patients with reduced NH_3 production following ischemic forearm exercise will have myoadenylate deaminase deficiency, and the diagnosis needs to be confirmed by direct assay of AMP deaminase activity in skeletal muscle.

AMP deaminase is one of the components of the purine nucleotide cycle, a series of reactions that is potentially important in energy production and utilization in skeletal muscle. Deficiency of myoadenylate deaminase activity may impair energy generation through diminished production of citric acid cycle intermediates, and it may adversely affect energy utilization through a reduction in the rate of ATP hydrolysis by myofibrillar ATPase.

Prognosis in myoadenylate deaminase deficiency is not known because the disorder has been described only recently. Present experience suggests the symptoms are slowly progressive and the disorder leads to mild disability in most cases, although there have been exceptions to these generalizations. No effective therapy is available at this time.

Fishbein WN, Armbrustmacher VM, Griffin JL: Myoadenylate deaminase deficiency: A new disease of muscle. Science 200:545, 1978. *The original description of five patients with AMP deaminase deficiency.*

Sabina RL, Swain JL, Olanow CW, Bradley WG, Fishbein WN, DiMauro S, Holmes EW: Myoadenylate deaminase deficiency: Functional and metabolic abnormalities associated with disruption of the purine nucleotide cycle. J Clin Invest 73:720, 1984.

Swain JL, Sabina RL, Holmes EW: Myoadenylate Deaminase Deficiency. *In* Stanbury JB, Wyngaarden JK, Fredrickson DS, Goldstein JL, Brown MS (eds.): The Metabolic Basis of Inherited Disease. 5th ed. New York, McGraw-Hill Book Company, 1983, pp 1184–1191. *Discussion of the clinical and biochemical findings in 26 patients with myoadenylate deaminase deficiency, as well as a review of the role of the purine nucleotide cycle in skeletal muscle function.*

IMMUNE DYSFUNCTION ASSOCIATED WITH PURINE ENZYME DEFICIENCIES

Adenosine deaminase deficiency is an uncommon disorder, approximately 50 families having been identified, which leads to a clinical syndrome of severe combined immunodeficiency, i.e., a defect in both T cell and B cell function. About one third of patients with severe combined immunodeficiency, in which the disorder is inherited as an autosomal recessive condition, will have this enzyme deficiency. Approximately 85 per cent of patients with adenosine deaminase deficiency come to medical attention at one to two months of age with recurrent infections of the skin and the gastrointestinal and respiratory systems. Both ordinary and opportunistic pathogens are encountered, and candidiasis is almost invariably present. Diarrhea is common, as well as delayed physical growth and development. Physical findings are for the most part unremarkable except for the absence of lymph nodes and pharyngeal lymphoid tissue. A rachitic rosary, or prominence of the costochondrial junctions, has been noted in some patients. Laboratory tests show absence of a thymic shadow, lymphopenia, negative skin test results for delayed hypersensitivity, attenuated lymphocyte responses to lectins and antigens in vitro, and hypogammaglobulinemia. The diagnosis is established by documenting adenosine deaminase deficiency in erythrocyte lysates or other cell extracts. Approximately 15 per cent of individuals with this disorder have a milder disease with later age of onset and relative sparing of humoral immunity. In the severe form of this disorder, if untreated, overwhelming infection and sepsis lead to death before two years of age.

Current mechanisms favored to explain the immune defects observed in adenosine deaminase deficiency are deoxy ATP accumulation leading to inhibition of ribonucleotide reductase with resultant decrease in DNA replication, and S-adenyosylhomocysteine accumulation leading to inhibition of transmethylation reactions. Either or both of these proposed mechanisms could reduce lymphocyte proliferation and function.

Treatment of adenosine deaminase deficiency by bone marrow transplantation has resulted in virtually complete immune reconstitution in some patients, and at present this is the preferred therapy if compatible donors are available. Enzyme replacement with repeated transfusions has improved immune function in some patients.

Purine nucleoside phosphorylase deficiency is less common than adenosine deaminase deficiency, approximately 10 patients having been recognized with this disorder. Purine nucleoside phosphorylase deficiency is also inherited as an autosomal recessive disorder, but it leads to a defect in cell-mediated immunity with little if any abnormality in humoral immunity. Patients with this disorder have been diagnosed as early as four months and as late as nine years of age with infections involving skin, lung, middle ear, mastoids, and urinary tract. Infections with nonbacterial agents have been most common, reflecting the primary defect in cellular immunity. Laboratory tests show lymphopenia, diminished number of circulating T cells, reduced lymphocyte response to antigens, and negative skin test results for delayed hypersensitivity. Immunoglobulin levels are normal, but several patients have exhibited signs of immunoregulatory abnormalities as shown by autoimmune hemolytic anemia, antinuclear antibodies, and rheumatoid factor. In addition, patients with purine nucleoside phosphorylase deficiency have hypouricemia, a finding of no clinical consequence in itself but one that suggests the diagnosis of this enzyme deficiency in a child with recurrent infections.

Confirmation of the diagnosis is obtained by assay of erythrocyte lysate or other cell extracts for purine nucleoside phosphorylase activity. It has been proposed that accumulation of deoxy GTP in T lymphocytes with resultant inhibition of ribonucleotide reductase and DNA replication is responsible for the immune defect in this disorder. Prognosis in purine nucleoside phosphorylase deficiency is generally better than that for adenosine deaminase deficiency, but therapy with bone marrow transplantation and erythrocyte transfusion has been less successful.

Enzyme Defects and Immune Dysfunction. Ciba Foundation Symposium 68 (new series). Amsterdam, Excerpta Medica, 1979. *A collection of papers dealing with clinical, metabolic, and immunologic aspects of ADA and PNP deficiencies.*

Giblett ER: Adenosine deaminase and purine nucleoside phosphorylase deficiency: How they were discovered and what they may mean. *In* Elliot K, Whelan J (eds.): Enzyme Defects and Immune Dysfunction. CIBA Foundation Symposium 68 (new series). New York, Excerpta Medica, 1979, p 3. *An interesting story about scientific serendipity and discovery of a new group of clinical disorders.*

Kredich N, Hershfield MS: Immunodeficiency diseases caused by adenosine deaminase deficiency and purine nucleoside phosphorylase deficiency. *In* Stanbury JB, Wyngaarden JB, Fredrickson DS, Goldstein JL, Brown MS (eds.): The Metabolic Basis of Inherited Disease. 5th ed. New York, McGraw-Hill Book Company, 1983, pp 1157. *An authoritative review of the clinical, laboratory and biochemical abnormalities in these disorders. This chapter also includes a detailed discussion of purine nucleoside metabolism in normal and pathological situations.*

197. DISORDERS OF PYRIMIDINE METABOLISM

Lloyd H. Smith, Jr.

Pyrimidine nucleotides share equally with purine nucleotides the chemical chore of transmitting genetic information for reproduction or for phenotypic expression within the cell. They also function in the intermediary metabolism of lipids and carbohydrates. Only a few disorders of pyrimidine metabolism have been recognized.

Hereditary orotic aciduria is a rare genetic disorder of pyrimidine metabolism characterized by megaloblastic anemia resistant to the usual hematinic agents, leukopenia, failure of normal growth and development, and the continued excessive urinary

excretion of orotic acid. Patients also have impaired cellular immunity with intact humoral immunity. Orotic acid is highly insoluble and often forms a heavy sediment of urinary crystals that may on occasion result in ureteral or urethral obstruction. The disorder, which is transmitted as an autosomal recessive trait, is usually characterized by reduced activities of two consecutive enzymes in pyrimidine biosynthesis, orotate phosphoribosyltransferase (OPRT) and orotidine 5′-phosphate decarboxylase (ODC). A single patient has been described with isolated deficiency of ODC. There is a prompt and sustained hematologic and general clinical response to oral uridine (2 to 4 grams per day), which must be continued indefinitely as replacement therapy. The disease has attracted special attention because it represents a block in the de novo pathway of pyrimidine synthesis, is an example of a double enzyme defect, and produces a requirement for replacement of a normal metabolic intermediate, uridine.

Orotic aciduria, without the characteristic hematologic abnormalities, also occurs in *ornithine transcarbamylase deficiency*. It is presumed that this results from the overflow of carbamyl phosphate from urea synthesis (partially blocked in this disease) to pyrimidine synthesis. Orotic aciduria has also been found in purine nucleoside phosphorylase deficiency and in PP-ribose-P synthetase deficiency (see Ch. 429).

Excessive urinary excretion of orotic acid and orotidine occurs during treatment with *allopurinol* or *6-azauridine*.* Metabolic products of both compounds inhibit orotidine 5′-decarboxylase activity.

Beta-aminoisobutyricaciduria is a benign hereditary disorder of thymine catabolism that occurs in 5 to 10 per cent of Caucasians and in a much higher percentage of Asians. The defect presumably lies in the transamination of beta-aminoisobutyric acid to methylmalonic acid semialdehyde. The aminoaciduria that results, representing the only known disorder of pyrimidine catabolism, has no known biologic disadvantage.

Pyrimidine 5′-nucleotidase deficiency is a rare form of hereditary hemolytic anemia, transmitted as an autosomal recessive trait. The erythrocytes exhibit prominent basophilic stippling owing to aggregates of undegraded ribosomes and on analysis contain very high concentrations of cytidine and uridine nucleotides. The mechanism by which the nucleotidase deficiency leads to hemolysis is unclear. Lead inhibits pyrimidine 5′-nucleotidase activity and leads to a similar anemia with basophilic stippling, possibly through this mechanism.

Girot R, Hamet M, Perignon J-L, et al.: Cellular immune deficiency in two siblings with hereditary orotic aciduria. N Engl J Med 308:700, 1983. *Two children with orotic aciduria exhibited impaired cellular immunity but normal humoral immunity, analogous to that seen with purine nucleoside phosphorylase deficiency.*

Kelley, WN: Hereditary orotic aciduria. *In* Stanbury JB, Wyngaarden JB, Fredrickson DS, Goldstein JL, Brown MS (eds.): The Metabolic Basis of Inherited Disease. 5th ed. New York, McGraw-Hill Book Company, 1983, p 1202. *This is the most complete description of normal pyrimidine metabolism in man and the derangements that occur in hereditary orotic aciduria.*

Smith LH Jr: Purine and pyrimidine metabolism in man. *In* Smith LH Jr, Thier SO (eds.): Pathophysiology: The Biological Principles of Disease, 2nd ed. International Textbook of Medicine, Vol 1. Philadelphia, W. B. Saunders Company, 1985. *This chapter in the companion textbook of pathophysiology gives a classification and general survey of the currently recognized diseases involving the synthesis or degradation of pyrimidines.*

Valentine WN, Fink K, Paglia DE, et al.: Hereditary hemolytic anemia with human erythrocyte pyrimidine 5′-nucleotidase deficiency. J Clin Invest 54:866, 1974. *This is the original and still the best description of the altered pyrimidine metabolism leading to hemolytic anemia in this rare but interesting genetic disease.*

*Investigational drug.

INHERITED DISORDERS OF CONNECTIVE TISSUE

198. THE MUCOPOLYSACCHARIDOSES

William S. Sly

The mucopolysaccharidoses are a group of lysosomal storage diseases, each of which is produced by an inherited deficiency of an enzyme involved in degradation of acid mucopolysaccharides (now called glycosaminoglycans and abbreviated GAGs). They are clinically progressive and have many common features that result from accumulation of partially degraded GAGs in various tissues. They produce disability primarily from storage-related abnormalities of the connective tissue, the heart, the bony skeleton, and the central nervous system.

Delineation of this group of diseases on the basis of clinical features, radiologic findings, and biochemistry of the urinary GAGs led to the famous classification of McKusick into MPS I to VI in 1966. Over the next six years, an exciting series of investigations from the laboratories of Neufeld and co-workers led to the discoveries that fibroblasts from patients with these disorders show storage abnormalities in culture, that fibroblasts from genetically different patients could "cross-correct" each other in culture, and that this "cross-correction" was due to secretion and recapture of lysosomal enzymes by the complementing fibroblast cell lines, each of which could secrete the enzyme the other was missing and take up the "corrective factor" for which it was deficient. These complementation studies served for nearly a decade as means for clinical diagnosis, for segregation of the disease into complementation groups (e.g., segregation of Hurler's and Scheie's syndromes into one complementation group, and separation of Sanfilippo's syndrome into several complementing groups), and also guided the purification of the corrective factors, each of which was eventually identified as a specific GAG degradative enzyme. Although still useful in certain situations, the complementation assays have largely been replaced by direct assays for the enzymes listed in Table 198–1 as deficient for each of the disorders.

ETIOLOGY OF GLYCOSAMINOGLYCAN STORAGE. The GAGs are long linear polysaccharide molecules composed of repeating dimers, each of which contains a hexuronic acid (or galactose in the case of keratan sulfate) and an amino sugar. They are usually found in covalent linkage to a core protein on which they are synthesized and from which they branch like bristles from a brush. The individual GAGs differ from each other in the hexuronic acid–amino sugar combinations in the repeating dimers, in the linkages between these components, in the linkages between repeating dimers, and in the degree to which individual sugar components are N-acetylated or sulfated. The major GAGs and their respective repeating dimers are chondroitin sulfate (glucuronic acid β1-3 N-acetylgalactosamine-4/6-sulfate); dermatan sulfate (iduronic acid α1-3 N-acetylgalactosamine-4-sulfate); heparan sulfate, which has both glucuronic acid and iduronic acid linked β1-4 and α1-3, respectively, to either N-acetylglucosamine or glucosamine N-sulfate; and keratan sulfate (galactose β1-4 N-acetylglucosamine-6-sulfate). The large proteoglycan molecules made up of protein cores and their GAG branches are secreted by cells and make up a significant fraction of the extracellular matrix of connective tissue. Their turnover depends on their subsequent internalization by endocytosis, their delivery to lysosomes, and their digestion by lysosomal enzymes. Lysosomal proteases digest the core protein, endoglycosidases reduce the size of the GAGs to oligosaccharides of varying length, and many exoglycosidases act sequentially to degrade the GAGs to their monosaccharide components. Each lysosomal enzyme is specific for a specific linkage. An inherited deficiency for any enzyme involved will disrupt the sequential degradative process and lead to accumulation in lysosomes of partially degraded GAG. The accumulation is progressive and eventually disrupts cellular architecture and disturbs cell function. The tissues and organs most affected and the severity depend on the degree of enzyme deficiency, i.e., whether partial or complete. Severity also depends on which enzyme is missing, since individual GAGs vary in their tissue distribution and their rate of turnover.

The enzyme deficiencies, the major storage products, and the clinical features for the mucopolysaccharidoses are summarized in Table 198–1. There is marked genetic heterogeneity within this group of disorders, with many different clinical phenotypes resulting from the different enzyme deficiencies (see MPS I–VII, Table 198–1). It is now clear also that quite different phenotypes can result from the same enzyme deficiency, depending on whether it is partial or complete (see MPS I-H, MPS I-S, and MPS I-H/S in Table 198–1).

GENETICS OF THE MUCOPOLYSACCHARIDOSES. Except for Hunter's syndrome (MPS II), in which the missing enzyme is specified by a gene on the X chromosome and the inheritance is X-linked, all of the mucopolysaccharidoses result from deficiencies of enzymes specified by autosomal genes. Thus, the inheritance pattern is autosomal recessive. In most cases, affected offspring can be shown to be the products of heterozygous carrier parents, both of whom have about half normal levels of the enzyme for which the affected patient is deficient. Even though the enzymes can now be measured for most of these disorders, the disorders are too rare to make screening for carriers practical. However, carrier status can be determined by enzyme assays in high-risk individuals, and prenatal diagnosis for most of these disorders is available to high-risk mothers, such as mothers of an affected offspring, who face a 25 per cent chance of another affected offspring in a subsequent pregnancy.

CLINICAL AND PATHOLOGIC CONSEQUENCES OF GLYCOSAMINOGLYCAN STORAGE. Connective tissue storage produces connective tissue laxity in most of these disorders, manifest by inguinal and umbilical hernias. Connective tissue thickening also occurs, owing in part to GAG storage and in part to excessive collagen deposition. This combination leads to coarse facial features, peripheral nerve entrapments, thickened meninges that may lead to cord compression and hydrocephalus, and thickened joint capsules. Connective tissue deposition in valve leaflets, the endocardium, and the myocardium produces symptomatic heart disease, a common cause of death in these patients to which coronary vascular insufficiency also contributes. Most of these disorders produce short stature, partly because of impaired long bone growth and partly because of vertebral abnormalities. These and many other changes in the bony skeleton are collectively referred to as *dysostosis multiplex*. Central nervous system storage may produce progressive mental retardation, especially in disorders involving impaired degradation of heparan sulfate (MPS I, II, and III). Corneal clouding and visual handicap result from storage of the partially degraded GAGs in the corneal stroma, especially in disorders involving impaired degradation of dermatan sulfate and keratan sulfate (MPS I, IV, and VI). Hepatomegaly is common and may be massive, but rarely is important clinically. Excessive urinary excretion of incompletely degraded GAGs (mucopolysacchariduria) is a constant finding of considerable diagnostic significance (Table 198–1) but has little pathologic significance.

HURLER'S SYNDROME (MPS I-H). ***Pathology.*** The basic defect is a deficiency of α-L-iduronidase, an enzyme that participates in degradation of dermatan sulfate and heparan sulfate. Accumulation of membrane bound storage material in parenchymal and mesenchymal cells is the chief pathologic finding. It affects every organ. Vacuolated cells distended with storage material distort normal cell and tissue architecture. In most cells this storage material is granular and composed of GAGs. In neurons, lipids are also present, presumably because stored GAGs inhibit sphingolipid degradation.

Clinical Features. Although patients are thought to be normal until six months of age, they develop persistent nasal discharge, noisy breathing, frequent upper respiratory infections, stiff joints, a thoracolumbar gibbus, and some degree of chest deformity in the last half of the first year of life. Over the second year, the classic syndrome develops with large head, coarse features, corneal clouding, hypertelorism, prominent eyebrows, thick lips, and broad flat nose with depressed nasal bridge. The hands are short and stubby, and joint limitation produces a claw hand deformity. Abdominal protuberance results from hepatosplenomegaly and lax abdominal musculature, often with inguinal and umbilical hernias. Dwarfism is obvious by the end of the second year, by which time cardiac murmurs are present.

Developmental delay is obvious before 18 months of age, and mental retardation progresses slowly. Limitation of joint movement leads to contractures of the hands, the elbows, and the knees. Death usually occurs by the age of ten from pneumonia or heart failure, after about five years of steady regression and near total loss of acquired skills. Hearing loss is usually moderate to severe, and coronary and peripheral vascular insufficiency are important late findings.

Radiologic abnormalities of dysostosis multiplex are striking. The skull is large and scaphycephalic, and the calvarium is thickened. The sinuses are poorly developed. The sella is enlarged anteriorly and referred to as J-shaped. The ribs are oar-shaped, being narrow posteriorly and greatly expanded anteriorly. The medial third of the clavicle is thickened. The vertebrae are initially rounded and appear ovoid. One or two lower thoracic and upper lumbar vertebrae are often hypoplastic and wedge shaped, producing the gibbus deformity. The

TABLE 198–1. THE MUCOPOLYSACCHARIDOSES (MPS STORAGE DISEASES I TO VII)

Abbreviation	Eponym	Enzyme Deficiency	Major Storage Product	Urinary GAGs	Clinical Features
MPS I-H	Hurler's	α-L-Iduronidase	DS + HS	↑ 5–25X DS > HS	Onset 6–12 months, coarse features, rhinorrhea, grunting respiration, corneal clouding, cardiac disease, visceromegaly, dwarfism, dysostosis multiplex, progressive mental retardation after the first year; death by 5–10 years
MPS I-S (formerly MPS V)	Scheie's	α-L-Iduronidase	DS + HS	↑ 5–25X DS > HS	Onset 5–15 years, corneal clouding, stiff joints, claw hand, genu valgum, dysostosis multiplex, aortic valve disease; however, normal height, normal intelligence, and long survival (difficult to distinguish clinically from mild MPS VI)
MPS I-H/S	Hurler-Scheie	α-L-Iduronidase	DS + HS	↑ 5–25X DS > HS	Onset 2–4 years, all findings of MPS-H but milder, slower progression, and survival into 20's
MPS II, severe	Hunter's severe form	L-Sulfoiduronate sulfatase	HS + DS	↑ 5–25X DS = HS	Onset 2–4 years, clear corneas, deafness, all other features of MPS I-H, but milder; mental retardation progresses to profound state; death by 10–15 years
MPS II, mild	Hunter's mild form	L-Sulfoiduronate sulfatase	HS + DS	↑ 5–25X DS = HS	Onset in first decade, short stature, clear corneas, joint stiffness, dysostosis multiplex, visceromegaly, cardiac disease, nerve entrapments, near-normal intelligence; survival to 30's–60's, depending on heart involvement
MPS III-A	Sanfilippo's, type A	Heparan sulfate sulfamidase	HS	↑ 5–20X 85% HS	Onset 2–6 years, large head, normal height; Hurler-like features, dysostosis multiplex, hepatomegaly, are all mild; mental retardation is rapidly progressive and severe; death at end of puberty
MPS III-B	Sanfilippo's, type B	N-acetyl-α-D-glucosaminidase	HS	↑ 5–20X 85% HS	Clinically indistinguishable from MPS III, type A
MPS III-C	Sanfilippo's, type C	Acetyl CoA: α-glucosamide N-acetyltransferase	HS	↑ 5–20X 85% HS	Clinically indistinguishable from MPS III, type A
MPS III-D	Sanfilippo, type D	N-acetyl-α-D-glucosaminide-6-sulfatase	HS	↑ 5–20X 85% HS	Clinically indistinguishable from MPS type III A
MPS IV-A	Morquio's, classic form	N-acetylgalactosamine-6-sulfatase (gal-6-sulfatase)	KS + Ch 6-S	↑ 3–5X KS + Ch-S	Characteristic facies, short trunk dwarfism, deformed thorax, corneal clouding, hearing deficit, aortic valve disease, unstable neck, spinal cord transection; intelligence is normal; death usually in 20's from cardiorespiratory problems
MPS IV-B	Morquio-like syndrome	β-Galactosidase deficiency	KS + Ch 4-S	↑ 2–5X KS = Ch-S	Short stature, corneal clouding, mild dysostosis multiplex, prominence of lower face, pectus carinatum, hip deformity, normal intelligence
MPS VI	Maroteaux-Lamy, severe	N-acetylgalactosamine-4-sulfatase (arylsulfatase B)	DS + ?Ch 4-S	↑ 4–20X 70–90% DS	Onset age 2–4 years, growth failure from age 4 slowly progressive, joint stiffness, corneal clouding, aortic valve disease, and severe hip deformity; dysostosis multiplex, striking white cell inclusions; intelligence normal; death in 20's
	Maroteaux-Lamy, mild	N-acetylgalactosamine-4-sulfatase (arylsulfatase B)	DS + ?Ch 4-S	↑ 4–20X 70–90% DS	Onset 5–7 years, short stature, severe osseous changes, especially in the hips; nerve entrapment, corneal clouding, aortic valve disease; normal intelligence, long survival; difficult to distinguish from MPS I-S
MPS VII	Sly	β-Glucuronidase	HS, DS, Ch-S	↑ 6–8X HS, DS Ch 4/6-S	Onset 1–2 years, mild to moderate Hurler-like features, dysostosis multiplex, pectus carinatum, visceromegaly, cardiac murmurs, short stature, moderate mental retardation; slowly progressive after infancy; striking granulocyte inclusions; milder forms exist.

Abbreviations: DS = dermatan sulfate; HS = heparan sulfate; Ch-S = chondroitin sulfate; KS = keratan sulfate.

pelvis shows flared iliac wings, a small body of the ilium, and shallow oblique acetabula. The hips show coxa valga deformities. The metatarsals and phalanges are short and wide; the proximal ends of the metacarpals taper sharply, a classic finding called proximal pointing. The long tubular bones have expanded diaphyses. There is loss of normal angulation of the humerus at the shoulder. The radiologic changes are progressive, but the changes vary considerably from patient to patient at a given age. The lower extremities are generally more mildly affected than the upper extremities, except for the hips, which often show changes resembling aseptic necrosis of the femoral heads that correlate with severe hip disability clinically.

Diagnosis. The diagnosis can be suspected on clinical and radiologic grounds, supported by demonstration of mucopolysacchariduria (DS>HS), and established definitively by demonstration of the enzyme deficiency, using the commercially available phenyl-L-iduronide substrate. Enzyme activity can be measured in extracts of leukocytes or cultured fibroblasts.

Treatment. Only supportive and symptomatic treatment can be offered to patients, as no effective treatment for the storage abnormality is available.

SCHEIE'S SYNDROME. This rare disorder is also due to a deficiency of α-L-iduronidase and is characterized by severe corneal clouding, deformity of the hands, and aortic valve disease. Symptoms appear between the ages of five and twenty. The height is normal, as is the intelligence. The striking joint stiffness of the hands is similar to that seen in Hurler's syndrome, but is complicated by the carpal tunnel syndrome with median nerve entrapment. Aortic stenosis, regurgitation, or both are present, but are usually not symptomatic in early life. Life expectancy may be nearly normal. Diagnosis depends on the same criteria as for Hurler's syndrome.Corneal transplant and aortic valve replacement are reasonable, since intelligence is normal.

THE HURLER-SCHEIE COMPOUND. Some patients with a phenotype that is intermediate between that of Hurler's and Scheie's syndromes are thought to represent compound heterozygotes, having inherited one Hurler and one Scheie gene from each parent.

HUNTER'S SYNDROME. Hunter's syndrome is distinguished from Hurler's syndrome by three features: (1) slower progression with longer survival, (2) lack of corneal clouding, and (3) X-linked rather than autosomal recessive inheritance. A severe and a mild form exist. The severe form has most of the features of Hurler's syndrome, but they are slightly milder except for hearing impairment, which is more severe. The patients usually die by age 15. A much milder form has been reported with near normal intelligence and near normal survival. Diagnosis is made on the basis of the clinical findings, radiologic evidence of dysostosis multiplex, elevated urinary GAGs, and demonstration of sulfoiduronate sulfatase deficiency on serum, or on extracts of leukocytes or cultured fibroblasts. Carrier detection is still imperfect, but prenatal diagnostic tests are reliable.

SANFILIPPO'S SYNDROME (MPS III). This syndrome can be produced by a deficiency of at least four different enzymes, all of which participate in degradation of heparan sulfate (Table 198–1). Early development is normal, but slows or halts between the ages of two and six years, after which mental deterioration is often rapid. Gait becomes unsteady, muscles atrophy, and the patient becames bedridden. Death usually occurs by puberty. The head is large, the hair coarse, and hirsutism common. Visceromegaly is mild to absent. Cardiac involvement is rare. Height may be normal through the first decade and then falls behind. Skeletal findings of dysostosis multiplex are mild and include thickened calvarium, ovoid vertebral bodies, mild dysplasia of the pelvis, and mild rib changes. The clinical diagnosis may be suspected from the severe mental retardation, which appears disproportionate with relatively mild somatic and radiologic abnormalities, supported by the presence of heparan sulfaturia, and established definitively by demonstration of the specific enzyme deficiency.

MORQUIO'S SYNDROME, CLASSIC FORM (MPS IV-A). The predominant clinical features relate to skeletal abnormalities and to symptoms of spinal cord compression resulting from instability of the neck. Intelligence is normal. By the age of two years, pigeon chest deformity, genu valgum, and gait disturbance appear. Knees and wrists enlarge. The neck appears short, and the head seems to sit on the deformed thorax. Universal platyspondyly, evident on x-ray, kyphoscoliosis, and contractures at the knees and hips all contribute to dwarfism. The face is unusual because of mid-face hypoplasia, depressed nasal bridge, flared nares, and prominence of the lower third of the face on side view. The teeth are wide spaced and the dental enamel thin. Corneal clouding is mild but slowly progressive. Aortic regurgitation is common. Long survival is rare, with death between the ages of 20 and 40 from cardiopulmonary complications. The cardiac disease is valvular. The respiratory problems arise from thoracic deformities, and from neurotrophic myelopathy caused by atlantoaxial subluxation. Diagnosis depends on the clinical and radiologic features, which are characteristic, the finding of keratan sulfaturia (which may disappear in adolescence), and the deficiency for N-acetylgalactosamine-6-sulfatase, which is active on both GalNAc 6-S in chondroitin sulfate and Gal 6-S in keratan sulfate. The enzymatic assay is available in only a few laboratories. Treatment is symptomatic. Posterior cervical fusion should be done early in the disease to prevent spinal cord damage. Correction of the genu valgum requires a single operation at about six years.

THE MORQUIO-LIKE SYNDROME WITH β-GALACTOSIDASE DEFICIENCY (MPS IV-B). Short stature, mild pectus carinatum, corneal clouding, odontoid hypoplasia with cervical instability, mild dysostosis multiplex, moderate lumbar kyphosis, and mild genu valgum are all features that are found in this Morquio-like disease resulting from β-galactosidase deficiency. Absent are hearing deficit, dental abnormalitites, cardiac murmurs, hepatomegaly, and joint laxity. Keratan sulfaturia is present. The diagnosis is based on normal N-acetylgalactosamine-6-sulfatase levels and reduced β-galactosidase levels. Presumably, this disorder reflects a mutation which impairs the activity of the enzyme on galactose linkages in keratan sulfate but spares its activity on GM_1 ganglioside. Thus, the findings of chondrodystrophy predominate and the neurologic manifestations of GM_1 gangliosidosis are absent.

THE MAROTEAUX-LAMY SYNDROME, SEVERE AND MILD TYPES (MPS VI). Maroteaux and colleagues recognized a new form of mucopolysaccharidosis in 1963 that resembled Hurler's syndrome but differed in that intelligence of the dwarfed, deformed patients was spared, the urinary GAG was almost exclusively dermatan sulfate, and the leukocytes exhibited striking metachromatic inclusions. Affected patients often die in their 20's with cardiac failure. Many suffer cervical cord compression and hydrocephalus resulting from thickened meninges. Since specific enzymatic assays have become available both for arylsulfatase B, missing in ML VI, and α-L-iduronidase, missing in ML I, it has become clear that many patients with milder forms of ML VI exist who might previously have been thought to have Scheie's syndrome. No specific treatment is available for the storage abnormality. However, shunting for hydrocephalus, spinal fusion for atlantoaxial subluxation, corneal transplants for visual handicap, and cardiac valve and hip replacement are all reasonable when required, because intelligence is preserved and patients with milder forms of the abnormalitiy have the potential for long survival.

MPS VII β-GLUCURONIDASE DEFICIENCY MUCOPOLYSACCHARIDOSES. Most patients present by age three with a Hurler-like illness manifest by frequent upper respiratory infections, chest deformities, cardiac murmurs, hepatosplenomegaly, hernias, dysostosis multiplex, and mild to moderate mental retardation. Many develop corneal clouding. About twenty patients, showing a wide range of clinical severity, have been recognized. Most of the patients have shown slow progression in clinical abnormalities after the age of six. The natural history beyond the teens is yet to be determined. Urinary GAGs have been elevated, and heparan sulfate, dermatan sulfate, and chondroitin sulfate have all been reported to be elevated in urine. Striking inclusions in leukocytes are typical, as in MPS VI. The diagnosis depends on the demonstration of the enzyme deficiency. Carrier detection and prenatal diagnosis are available.

OTHER DISORDERS RELATED TO THE MUCOPOLYSACCHARIDOSES. Mucolipidosis II (also called I-cell disease) and mucolipidosis III (also called pseudo-Hurler polydystrophy) are severe and milder forms, respectively, of a Hurler-like disease with many features in common with the mucopolysaccharidoses. However, these patients do not have mucopolysacchariduria.

These disorders result, not from a deficiency for a single lysosomal enzyme like the mucopolysaccharidoses, but from a defect in the processing N-acetylglucosaminyl phosphotransferase that normally targets acid hydrolases to lysosomes. Failure to add the phosphomannosyl-recognition marker that normally directs their segregation into lysosomes allows acid hydrolases to be secreted instead. As a consequence, there is an intracellular deficiency of most of the enzymes involved in the degradation of GAGs (and an extracellular excess), which is part of a general pattern of deficiency involving nearly all lysosomal enzymes. The absence of mucopolysacchariduria, and the 10- to 50-fold elevations of acid hydrolases in serum, distinguish these two disorders from the single enzyme deficiency mucopolysaccharidoses.

Another group of disorders, not classified with the mucopolysaccharidoses, may produce a Hurler-like picture, including mental retardation, visceromegaly, and dysostosis multiplex. These disorders result from single enzyme deficiencies for enzymes involved in the catabolism of the oligosaccharide components of glycoproteins. Included are mannosidosis, fucosidosis, and the recently delineated group of sialidoses (one of which has been described under the name mucolipidosis I). The sialidoses result from a deficiency of oligosaccharide N-acetyl-neuraminidase. The primary storage products in these disorders are oligosaccharides derived from glycoproteins. However, there is some storage of keratan sulfate as well. It appears that these enzymes are required for degradation of some oligosaccharide side chains on keratan sulfate. Impaired degradation of keratan sulfate may explain the dysostosis multiplex that mimics the skeletal findings of the mucopolysaccharidoses in these disorders.

Kelly TE: The mucopolysaccharidoses and mucolipidoses. Clin Orthop Rel Res, 114:116, 1976 *A nice summary of clinically relevant information.*

McKusick VA, Neufeld EF, Kelly TE: The mucopolysaccharide storage diseases. *In* Stanbury JB, Wyngaarden JB, Fredrickson DS, Goldstein JL, Brown MS (eds.): The Metabolic Basis of Inherited Disease. 5th ed. New York, McGraw-Hill Book Company, 1983. *An excellent and comprehensive chapter with good historical perspective.*

Sly WS: The mucopolysaccharidoses. *In* Bondy PK, Rosenberg LE (eds.): Metabolic Control and Disease. 8th ed. Philadelphia, W. B. Saunders Company, 1980, pp 545–581. *A blend of the biochemical and clinical data, the excellence of which the author is too modest to discuss.*

199. MARFAN'S SYNDROME

Sheldon R. Pinnell

Marfan's syndrome is a generalized disorder of connective tissue with skeletal, ocular, and cardiovascular manifestations. The syndrome is inherited as an autosomal dominant. Approximately 15 per cent of cases are apparently new mutations. Paternal age averages seven years older in these sporadic cases. A large amount of clinical variability may occur among affected members of a family. The diagnosis in a sporadic case may be difficult. The prevalence is estimated to be four to six per 100,000 births. There is neither sexual nor racial predilection. Although the nature of the molecular defect is unknown, diminished type I collagen synthesis has been reported in tissue culture of a Marfan's aorta. In addition, a structural abnormality in the α_2 chain of type I collagen has been detected in a sporadic case.

MANIFESTATIONS. ***Skeletal and Connective Tissue.*** Characteristically the affected person is tall and thin with long extremities. The arm span is greater than the height, and the floor-to-pubis measurement (lower segment) exceeds the pubis-to-crown measurement (upper segment). Fingers are long, thin, and hyperextensible. The palate is arched, and the anterior teeth may be crowded. Kyphoscoliosis, asymmetry of the thoracic cage, and sternal deformity (pectus excavatum or pectus carinatum) are common. Musculature may be poorly developed and hypotonic. Inguinal hernias are common and often recur after repair. Lungs may be emphysematous, and spontaneous pneumothorax occasionally occurs. Atrophic striae occur symmetrically on the skin.

Ocular. Subluxed lenses occur in 50 to 80 per cent; they are bilateral, are displaced upward, and usually occur in utero. Vision may be relatively normal in the presence of ectopia lentis. Myopia, spontaneous retinal detachment, and flattened corneas are frequent.

Cardiovascular. Aortic involvement occurs in 80 per cent and is the usual cause of death. Degenerative changes in the media may lead to aneurysm and subsequent rupture. Dilation of the aortic ring results in regurgitation and cardiac decompensation. Mitral valve prolapse is common. Echocardiography is a sensitive diagnostic procedure for cardiovascular involvement and a good way to follow progression of aortic root enlargement prior to surgical intervention. Bacterial endocarditis may be superimposed on the cardiac lesion.

DIFFERENTIAL DIAGNOSIS. Several marfanoid syndromes have been described. A marfanoid hypermobility syndrome has crossover features with the Ehlers-Danlos syndrome. The syndrome includes generalized joint hypermobility, hyperextensible skin, marfanoid habitus, muscular hypotonia, and aortic regurgitation. Contractural arachnodactyly is a dominantly inherited syndrome with arachnodactyly, kyphoscoliosis, congenital contractures, abnormally shaped ears, and osteopenia. Cardiovascular or eye involvement is absent. Homocystinuria is inherited as an autosomal recessive and results from a deficiency of cystathionine synthetase. Patients characteristically have a marfanoid habitus, kyphoscoliosis, ectopia lentis (usually dislocated downward), and sternal deformity. In addition they may have osteoporosis, mental deficiency, accelerated arteriosclerosis, vascular occlusion, and a malar flush. They excrete excessive homocystine in the urine. A marfanoid syndrome also occurs with mucosal neuromas, pheochromocytoma, and medullary carcinoma of the thyroid.

TREATMENT. Surgical repair of aortic lesions has been increasingly successful in Marfan's syndrome. The decision to operate can optimally be made by serially monitoring aortic dilation by echocardiography. Propranolol has been recommended for retarding aortic dilation, but results have not been encouraging. Replacement of the mitral valve with a prosthesis is occasionally required. Weight lifting, contact sports, isometric exercises, and pregnancy increase the risk of cardiovascular catastrophy. Prophylactic antibiotics to prevent endocarditis should be taken for dental procedures. Regular ocular examinations should be undertaken at an early age to prevent amblyopia. Spinal curvature should be corrected with bracing and spinal fusion if necessary. Hormonal induction of puberty is sometimes helpful in management of the skeletal disorder.

PROGNOSIS. The average age at death of 72 patients was 32 years. Essentially all deaths have a cardiovascular cause.

McKusick VA: Heritable Disorders of Connective Tissue. 4th ed. St. Louis, C. V. Mosby Company, 1972, pp 61–200. *Extensive clinical description of the manifestations of Marfan's syndrome.*

Pyeritz RE, McKusick VA: The Marfan syndrome: Diagnosis and management. N Engl J Med 300:772, 1979. *Up-to-date review of a large ongoing clinical experience at the Johns Hopkins Hospital. Frequency data on 50 patients.*

200. EHLERS-DANLOS SYNDROME

Sheldon R. Pinnell

DEFINITION. The Ehlers-Danlos syndrome is a group of inherited disorders of connective tissue sharing phenotypic expressions, including hyperextensible skin and joints, easy bruisability, and friability of tissues with poor wound healing. Eleven forms of the condition are recognized on the basis of clinical, genetic, and biochemical evidence. Life-threatening complications, including spontaneous arterial rupture and gastrointestinal perforation, occur especially in the ecchymotic form (type IV).

ETIOLOGY. Biochemical abnormalities in collagen biosynthesis have been described in four of the varieties of the syndrome. Fragility and hyperelasticity of tissues would seem to be consistent with altered collagen structure, since strength and limited extensibility are characteristics of normal collagen.

PREVALENCE. Ehlers-Danlos syndrome has been reported most often in persons of European ancestry, but dark-skinned races may be involved. Prevalence is estimated at 1:200,000, although mild forms of the disease are undoubtedly common and unrecognized.

PATHOLOGY. No diagnostic abnormality is ordinarily apparent in skin and connective tissues by routine histologic techniques. Electron microscopic studies have revealed abnormal collagen fiber diameters.

PATHOGENESIS. Patients with type IV (ecchymotic) Ehlers-Danlos syndrome have been reported with diminished levels of type III collagen. This species of collagen molecule is present in most tissues of the body, but is predominant in blood vessels and the gastrointestinal tract—tissues most severely involved in this form of the disease. Type VI (hydroxylysine-deficient collagen disease) is associated with diminished hydroxylysine levels in tissue collagens resulting from a deficiency of lysyl hydroxylase. Hydroxylysine is necessary for collagen crosslinking, and its lack results in structural weakness. In type VII (procollagen peptidase deficiency) an enlarged form of collagen accumulates. Collagen is synthesized in precursor form (procollagen), which is converted to collagen by enzymes (procollagen peptidases) that cleave nonhelical extension polypeptides from both ends of the molecule. Defective cleavage of the aminoterminal extension peptide results in an enlarged, incompletely processed collagen molecule that is incapable of entering into normal collagen fibril formation and subsequent crosslinking. A subtype has been recognized with a structural mutation of Pro α_2(I) resulting in defective procollagen cleavage. In type IX (occipital horn), lysyl oxidase activity is diminished as a result of defective copper metabolism. This copper-dependent enzyme is essential for collagen and elastin crosslinking.

CLINICAL MANIFESTATIONS. Clinical features are variable and many are shared among the different forms of the disorder. Common facial features include epicanthal folds, a flat nasal bridge, and ears which stick out from the side of the head and point downward.

The skin is unusually soft and feels like chamois. It may be thin and is often strikingly hyperextensible; its response to stretching is usually rubber-like, although with aging, skin may sag, particularly over the elbows. In contrast to the rest of the body, skin over the palms and soles is often wrinkly and redundant. Fragile skin may split with blunt trauma, and gaping wounds may result which often require taping to repair because the tissue is too friable to hold stitches. Wound healing is prolonged and scar tissue is of poor quality. Wide "fish mouth" scars result from poor retraction of atrophic scar tissue. So-called molluscoid pseudotumors are common over elbows and knees and apparently result from repeated trauma, hemorrhage, connective tissue organization, fatty degeneration, and calcification. Pea-sized, freely movable calcified spherules can often be palpated subcutaneously over the arms and legs.

Easy bruisability may be the most striking clinical manifestation of the disease and may result in extensive hematologic evaluation. Since results of clotting studies are ordinarily normal, ecchymoses are thought to be related to friable blood vessels and dissection of blood through planes of tissue that are poorly held together. Varicosities are often prominent under the thin skin.

Joints may be remarkably hyperextensible. Chronic dislocations of patellae, shoulders, hips, clavicles, and temporomandibular joints may require surgical intervention. Hypermobile joints make motor control difficult during early life. Repeated falls coupled with friable skin and poor wound healing often result in appreciable cosmetic disfigurement. In time, joint hypermobility may lead to "wear and tear" arthritis and joint effusion. Although there is notable lack of bony fragility in Ehlers-Danlos syndrome, kyphoscoliosis is frequent; joint looseness and hypotonic musculature may contribute to this complication. Pes planus is common. Teeth may be carious, and periodontitis is occasionally severe.

Ophthalmologic involvement, including blue sclerae, microcornea, and myopia, is common. Ocular fragility may occur, and keratoconus, keratoglobus, dislocated lens and retinal detachment have been described.

Rupture of large arteries is a dramatic and often catastrophic manifestation of type IV (ecchymotic). Angiography is risky and should ordinarily be avoided. Mitral valve prolapse can often be demonstrated by echocardiography, but functional insufficiency is unusual. Many congenital cardiac defects, including atrial septal defect, tetralogy of Fallot, heart block, and aortic arch anomalies, have been described. Emphysema, as well as lung rupture and pneumothorax, can occur.

Inguinal, hiatal, and umbilical hernias occur at all ages, and recurrence after repair is frequent. Cryptorchidism as well as diverticula of the gastrointestinal and genitourinary tract are common. Visceral perforation may be life threatening and is most often associated with type IV (ecchymotic). Surgery must be undertaken with caution; serious bleeding as well as persistent oozing, hematoma formation, difficulty in working with friable tissue, and poor healing leading to wound dehiscence may prove disastrous.

Pregnancy is likewise risky; perineal lacerations and hemorrhage occur regularly. Forceps delivery should be avoided so that fragile tissues are not unnecessarily torn. Premature birth is common and is often associated with premature rupture of fetal membranes. Since the membranes are mostly derived from the fetus, they share its poorly made connective tissue. Uterine rupture is a risk in type IV (ecchymotic).

Type I (gravis) is characterized by striking hyperextensibility of skin and joints, fragile skin that bruises easily, poor wound healing, hernias, and premature birth associated with premature rupture of fetal membranes. The inheritance is autosomal dominant.

Type II (mitis) has only mild manifestations and often goes undiagnosed. Joint hypermobility is usually limited to hands and feet; skin hyperextensibility and bruisability are mild. Inheritance is autosomal dominant.

Type III (benign hypermobile) has as its major manifestation marked hyperextensibility of joints which occasionally become arthritic. Skin hyperextensibility is variable, and inheritance is autosomal dominant.

Type IV (ecchymotic) is associated with thin transparent skin and impressive bruising. Joint and skin hyperextensibility are minimal. Serious internal manifestations, including arterial rupture, uterine rupture, and intestinal perforation, are often life threatening. Both autosomal dominant and autosomal recessive forms occur.

Type V (X-linked) has only moderate involvement of skin and joints. Bruising may be prominent. Inheritance is X-linked recessive.

In type VI (hydroxylysine-deficient collagen disease) joint hypermobility is extreme, and dislocated joints and kyphoscoliosis are common. Skin hyperextensibility, easy bruisability, and poor wound healing are usual, and ocular fragility has been described. Inheritance is autosomal recessive.

Type VII (procollagen peptidase deficiency) patients have short stature; their joints are lax, and hip dislocation is frequent. Inheritance is autosomal recessive.

Type VIII (periodontitis) is characterized by severe, generalized periodontal disease with premature loss of teeth, associated with pretibial skin fragility and moderate joint hypermobility. Inheritance is autosomal dominant.

Type IX (occipital horn) is characterized by cranial spurs, mild skin and joint hypermobility, bladder diverticula, osteoporosis, and reduced serum levels of copper and ceruloplasmin. Inheritance is X-linked recessive.

Type X (fibronectin deficient) is associated with moderate skin and joint laxity. Bruising, which is associated with abnormal platelet aggregation, is partially corrected with fibronectin. Inheritance is autosomal recessive.

Type XI (familial joint laxity) is associated with marked joint hypermobility and recurrent joint dislocation. Skin is normal. Inheritance is autosomal dominant.

DIAGNOSIS. The combination of hyperextensible skin and hypermobile joints usually suggests the diagnosis. Involvement of other family members helps establish the genetic type. Biochemical studies to document abnormalities in collagen biosynthesis are research procedures of limited availability.

In *cutis laxa,* the skin may be hyperextensible, but in contrast to Ehlers-Danlos syndrome it is loose, inelastic, and hangs in folds. Joint hypermobility is not usually present. Hypermobile joints and blue sclerae are associated with *osteogenesis imperfecta,* but prominent bony fragility and lack of skin hyperelasticity usually suggest this diagnosis. Hypermobile joints and skeletal deformities are found in *Marfan's syndrome,* but prominence of lens dislocation and disproportionate long bone growth usually make this diagnosis apparent. Hyperelastic joints and skin may be found in *Bonnevie-Ullrich-Turner syndrome,* but other features of this disorder, including dwarfism, webbing of the neck, gonadal dysgenesis, and XO chromosome pattern, establish this diagnosis.

TREATMENT. Ascorbic acid, 2 to 4 grams per day, has been effective in some forms of Ehlers-Danlos syndrome. Protection from trauma to skin and joints is helpful. As children learn to walk on unstable joints, environmental protection is particularly important. Proper repair of lacerations is necessary to prevent cosmetic disfigurement. Taping is often helpful, and because wound healing is delayed, support from sutures and tape must remain for as long as needed. An exercise program to strengthen muscles around hypermobile joints may improve function. Surgical procedures are risky, as fragile tissues may unexpectedly tear, suturing may be difficult or impossible, and massive bleeding is often impossible to control. Genetic counseling can be expected to become more precise as the biochemical nature of the different forms of the disease is better understood.

PROGNOSIS. Prognosis for life is good except in the ecchymotic form of the disease, in which arterial rupture or visceral perforation may be catastrophic. Connective tissue strength improves with age, and most clinical problems lessen as the patient gets older.

Hollister D, Byers PH, Holbrook KA: Genetic disorders of collagen metabolism. Adv Hum Genet 12:1, 1982. *Review of genetic collagen disorders.*

McKusick VA: Heritable Disorders of Connective Tissue. 4th ed. St. Louis, C. V. Mosby Company, 1972. *Clinical description in classic textbook of connective tissue disease.*

Pinnell SR: Disorders of collagen. *In* Stanbury JB, Wyngaarden JB, Fredrickson DS, Goldstein JL, Brown MN (eds.): The Metabolic Basis of Inherited Disease. 5th ed. New York, McGraw-Hill Book Company, 1983. *Review of collagen biochemistry with discussion of abnormalities in connective tissue disorders.*

201. OSTEOGENESIS IMPERFECTA

David W. Rowe

Osteogenesis imperfecta is a heritable disorder of connective tissue that results primarily in fragile bones that break with minimal trauma. The disease may be limited to a few fractures in childhood, cause 50 to 100 fractures by adulthood with severe long bone deformity, or cause death in the newborn. The prevalence rate is 5 per 100,000 live births and there is no known racial or ethnic predilection. Interest in this disease has increased recently with the recognition that individual variants result from a structural or regulatory abnormality of the alpha 1 or alpha 2 chain of type I collagen. Recent advances in the molecular biology of collagen now permit definition of these abnormalities at the level of type I collegen gene.

PATHOGENESIS. The tissues that are abnormal in osteogenesis imperfecta are composed primarily of type I collagen and demonstrate either a deficiency or a structural abnormality of this collagen type. The mildest form (type I—see below) appears to result from an underproduction of a normal type I collagen. Thus, multiple fractures occur during childhood when bone cellular turnover is high; the tendency toward breakage appears to diminish after puberty slows growth. The more severe forms of osteogenesis imperfecta (types II to IV) are associated with a defective molecule that does not provide adequate structural support because of a mutation that interferes with the normal triple helical orientation of the collagen chains. The severity of the clinical defect is probably related to the qualitative nature of the mutation and the accumulation of abnormal chains in specific tissues.

TYPES AND CLINICAL MANIFESTATIONS. The terms osteogenesis imperfecta tarda or congenita have been replaced by a classification scheme based on relatively distinct syndromes that reflect fundamentally different defects in type I collagen biosynthesis. Type I is the mildest form and is associated with nondeforming fractures during childhood that cease after puberty. In most cases a dominant family history can be elicited having the associated features that diminish with age of blue sclera, joint laxity, and thin skin. More variable are hearing abnormalities, short stature, and dentinogenesis imperfecta. Sporadic cases occur and presumably reflect a new mutation. Fractures can reappear with trauma and in postmenopausal women. In contrast, the most severe form of osteogenesis imperfecta (type II) results in infants that do not survive the newborn period. Their bones have a crumpled appearance on x-ray and are so weak that dismemberment may occur. The disorder is inherited either as a recessive trait or a new dominant mutation. Intrauterine diagnosis in this form of osteogenesis imperfecta has been accomplished with the use of ultrasound. In osteogenesis imperfecta type III, there are severe deformities of long bones, marked short stature, and moderate joint laxity. More variable are the blue sclera, hearing difficulties, and dentinogenesis imperfecta. Fractures and deformity are usually present at birth such that ambulation is never possible. Severe scoliosis can progress to cause respiratory failure. The inheritance is recessive. Osteogenesis imperfecta type IV is less severe but usually results in moderate long bone deformity. Ambulation is possible but may require external bracing or internal fixation of the long bones. Blue sclera, lax joints, and hearing impairment are less common, while dentinogenesis imperfecta is more frequently found. Both dominant and recessive modes of inheritance occur. This is the most heterogeneous group and is often difficult to distinguish from groups I and III.

DIAGNOSIS. The diagnosis of each form of osteogenesis imperfecta is based on the history, physical examination, family pedigree, and x-ray features. The bone biopsy is not usually of diagnostic aid. Only the milder forms of this disease should pose a diagnostic problem from other disorders that cause minimal bone deformity or fractures. The bowing and fractures associated with osteomalacia or rickets are differentiated by x-ray and the biochemical measures of calcium, phosphorus, PTH, and vitamin D. Juvenile osteoporosis, disuse and steroid-induced osteoporosis can be distinguished by history. Other rare diagnoses to be considered are infantile cortical hyperketosis (Caffey's disease) and hypophosphatasia. Studies of collagen synthesis in cultured fibroblasts are beginning to provide the means for a specific diagnosis for the various forms of osteogenesis imperfecta but at present they remain experimental.

TREATMENT. The use of supplemental calcium, vitamin D, fluoride, anabolic steroids, calcitonin, and pyrophosphate has not been shown to provide a satisfactory response. Since many of these drugs were used in heterogeneous groups of patients with osteogenesis imperfecta, there may be subgroups of patients who could benefit from certain medical regimens. At present therapy is primarily orthopedic with external bracing, and surgical straightening with intramedullary splinting (rodding) of the long bone deformities. Use of lightweight plastic bracing will assume a greater role in promoting ambulation. However, attempts to halt the progression of scoliosis in osteogenesis imperfecta have not been successful. In all forms of osteogenesis imperfecta maintenance of good muscle tone and range of motion is crucial for the optimal use of the extremities. Creative use of physical therapy, especially in the form of swimming, may be the most useful preventive measure in this disorder.

Akeson WH, Bornstein P, Glimcher MJ: Symposium on Heritable Disorders of Connective Tissue. St. Louis, C. V. Mosby Company, 1982. *See Chapters 20–23 for a general review of clinical, morphologic, and biochemical aspects of osteogenesis imperfecta.*

Albright JA, Millar EA: Osteogenesis imperfecta. Clin Orthoped Rel Res 159:2, 1981. *A collection of numerous articles on the pathology and treatment of this disease.*

Shapiro JR, Rowe DW: Collagen genes and brittle bones. Ann Intern Med 99:700, 1983. *The author's personal views on the pathogenesis of osteogenesis imperfecta.*

Smith R, Francis MJO, Houghton GP: The Brittle Bone Syndrome. London, Butterworth Co., 1982. *A comprehensive review by one group of investigators having a large experience with osteogenesis imperfecta. Chapter 7 has a good differential diagnosis.*

202. PSEUDOXANTHOMA ELASTICUM

Jouni Uitto

Pseudoxanthoma elasticum (PXE) (synonyms: Grönblad-Strandberg syndrome, systemic elastorrhexis) is a generalized progressive connective tissue disorder primarily affecting the elastic fibers. Clinically, PXE manifests as characteristic cutaneous lesions, ocular changes, and widespread vascular abnormalities. The relative severity of these changes results in the presentation of a variety of clinical pictures. The onset of the disease may be in early childhood, and in most cases the cutaneous changes are evident before the age of 30. The exact prevalence of PXE is not known, although estimates are about 1 in 160,000 persons. The male to female ratio is probably 1:1.

CLINICAL MANIFESTATIONS. ***Skin.*** The primary cutaneous lesions are relatively small (1 to 3 mm) yellowish papules that give the affected area a pebbly, "plucked chicken skin" appearance. The primary lesions tend to coalesce into larger plaques, and the skin of the involved areas becomes thickened and leathery (Fig. 202–1). Gradually, the affected skin becomes redundant, lax, and inelastic. The predilection sites are the

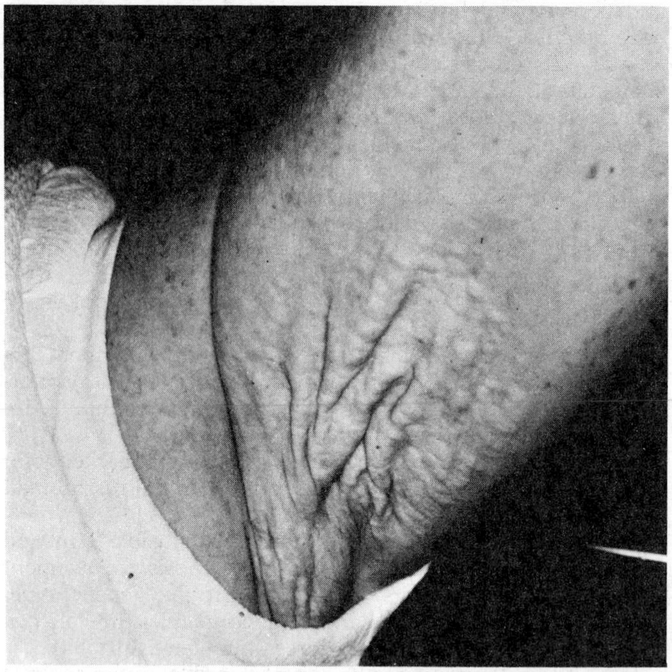

Figure 202–1. Typical cutaneous manifestations of pseudoxanthoma elasticum. The lesion demonstrates redundant and inelastic skin in the axillary fold.

face, neck, axillary folds, lower abdomen, and thighs. The nasolabial folds and chin creases may be strikingly accentuated. Yellowish lesions similar to those noted on the skin can also be seen on the mucous membranes.

Eye. The ocular changes are characterized by angioid streaks, i.e., grayish or brownish-red, poorly defined streaks radiating across the fundus of the eye. Their development usually starts later than that of the cutaneous lesions, often during the third or fourth decade of life. The ocular changes are commonly bilateral and include hemorrhages and exudates in Bruch's membrane, an elastin-rich structure located between the retina and the choroid. The degenerative changes of the eye frequently lead to impaired vision, and complete blindness, although rare, is one of the major complications of PXE. Angioid streaks may be present without noticeable cutaneous changes, but other accompanying observations, such as vascular changes, may lead to correct diagnosis of PXE. Angioid streaks are not specific for PXE but can also be associated with other diseases—for example, Paget's disease of bone, sickle cell anemia, tumoral calcinosis, lead poisoning, and idiopathic thrombocytopenia.

Vascular Manifestations. The early manifestations of arterial involvement include hypertension, weak peripheral pulses, and, occasionally, intermittent claudication. The most devastating complications develop as a result of coronary occlusion or cerebral hemorrhage; the most frequent complication is recurrent bleeding from the gastrointestinal tract. A common site of the gastrointestinal bleeding is the gastric mucosa, where the elastic fibers of the arteries are particularly affected. Bleeding from the urinary tract can also occur.

INHERITANCE. Most cases of PXE are inherited as an autosomal recessive disease. However, autosomal dominant inheritance has been documented in a few families. The classification proposed by Pope divides the dominantly inherited form of PXE into two categories. The type I dominant form is characterized by classic cutaneous changes associated with severe vascular complications. The type II dominant form, which is more frequent than the type I, is characterized by focal cutaneous involvement associated with hyperextensible skin, blue sclerae, high arched palate, and loose-jointedness. The type I recessively inherited form of the disease is the classic, most frequently encountered type of pseudoxanthoma elasticum, characterized by typical cutaneous, vascular, and ocular manifestations. The type II recessively inherited disease, characterized by generalized cutaneous involvement and by the absence of vascular and ocular manifestations, is very rare.

In addition to the inherited forms, several cases with cutaneous findings consistent with pseudoxanthoma elasticum but without family history and without vascular or ocular involvement have been reported. In some of these cases, the development of skin lesions is related to external trauma, such as exposure to Norwegian saltpeter. Recently, patients with an unusual perforating variant of cutaneous pseudoxanthoma elasticum have been described. In these patients, the lesions are confined to the abdomen, most often in a periumbilical distribution. Periumbilical perforating pseudoxanthoma elasticum appears to be a distinct acquired form of the disease.

PATHOLOGY. Histopathologic examination of the involved skin demonstrates an accumulation of structures in the middle or lower dermis that stain positively with stains specific for elastic fibers, e.g., Verhoeff stain. In contrast to the elastic fibers in normal skin, the elastic material in pseudoxanthoma elasticum appears irregularly clumped and fragmented. The accumulation of elastic fibers has also been quantitated by computerized morphometric analyses and by assay of desmosine, an elastin-specific crosslink compound. Characteristically, the fragmented elastic fibers contain calcium that appears bluish on routine hematoxylin-eosin stain and that can be demonstrated by calcium-specific stains. Electron microscopy of affected skin demonstrates that the amorphous elastin component has been replaced by bundles of granular material with staining properties different from normal elastin. Also, foci containing calcium hydroxyapatite crystals can be detected in the elastic fibers. These morphologic findings thus provide evidence for derangement in the organization of the elastic structures in pseudoxanthoma elasticum. Biochemical proof of the exact molecular defect in the structure or metabolism of elastin is, however, lacking, and it is unclear whether the calcification of elastic fibers is a primary or secondary event. Studies employing cultured skin fibroblasts have suggested that the cells from patients with pseudoxanthoma elasticum synthesize an abnormal polyionic substance, probably a glycosaminoglycan, which is deposited on the surface of the elastic fibers. This material might bind calcium salts, a process that causes the calcification of the elastic fibers, followed by subsequent fiber degeneration. Alternatively, an aberration in the primary structure of elastin or in the enzymes participating in the synthesis and degradation of elastic fibers may be the primary underlying molecular defect in the condition.

THERAPY. No specific treatment is available, and the primary prevention entails genetic counseling. Although treatment with vitamin E, vitamin C, or with a low calcium diet has been advocated in isolated case reports, no clinical proof of their efficacy is available in the form of controlled clinical trials. In selected cases, plastic surgery may be helpful in improving the cosmetic appearance of the skin.

Neldner KH, Martinez-Hernandez A: Localized acquired cutaneous pseudoxanthoma elasticum. J Am Acad Dermatol 1:523, 1979. *Clinical description of a distinct acquired form of pseudoxanthoma elasticum.*

Pope FM: Two types of autosomal recessive pseudoxanthoma elasticum. Arch Dermatol 110:219, 1974. *A clinical study establishing the genetic heterogeneity of this condition.*

Sandberg LB, Soskel NT, Leslie JG: Elastin structure, biosynthesis and its relationship to disease states. N Engl J Med 304:566, 1981. *A comprehensive review on elastin structure and metabolism.*

Uitto J, Paul JL, Brockley K, Pearce RH, Clark JG: Elastic fibers in human skin: Quantitation of elastic fibers by computerized digital image analyses and determination of elastin by a radioimmunoassay of desmosine. Lab Invest 49:499, 1983. *Demonstration of increased elastin concentrations in the lesional skin in pseudoxanthoma elasticum.*

Uitto J, Ryhänen L, Abraham PA, Perejda AJ: Elastin in diseases. J Invest Dermatol 79 (Suppl 1):160s, 1982. *A review on the molecular defects of elastin in heritable connective tissue diseases, including pseudoxanthoma elasticum.*

Disorders of Porphyrins or Metals

203. PORPHYRIA

D. Montgomery Bissell

Porphyrias are characterized clinically by neurologic and/or cutaneous manifestations and chemically by overproduction of porphyrins or the porphyrin precursors, δ-aminolevulinic acid (ALA) and porphobilinogen (PBG). The most important members of this group of diseases are hereditary, but acquired porphyria occurs also; in all instances, porphyria must be distinguished from simple porphyrinuria, which accompanies a variety of common conditions and is without clinical significance.

BIOSYNTHESIS OF HEME. Heme is a metalloporphyrin, a member of a group that includes chlorophyll and vitamin B_{12}. These have been termed the molecules of life, in view of their importance to aerobic metabolism. Heme is formed from succinyl CoA and glycine in a series of enzyme-catalyzed steps (Figure 203–1). The initial enzyme of the pathway, ALA synthetase, is rate-determining for the overall synthesis. Its activity is regulated in a "feedback" manner, so that it responds rapidly to the changing needs of the tissue for heme. When a relative deficiency of heme occurs—from increased heme-protein formation or impaired heme synthesis or both—ALA synthetase is stimulated, and the flow of heme precursors into the pathway increases. With formation of the initial porphyrin-like intermediate uroporphyrinogen, a branch point occurs involving different porphyrin isomers. While there are four possible isomers of uroporphyrinogen, only I and III occur in nature, isomer III being the physiologic intermediate. The isomer I pathway is abortive, proceeding only as far as coproporphyrin I, and normally is inconsequential. Metabolism of uroporphyrinogen III involves modifications of porphyrin side chains that render the molecule progressively more lipophilic and redirect its excretion from the body. Whereas the water-soluble ALA, PBG, and uroporphyrin are excreted entirely or very largely in urine, coproporphyrin is excreted in both urine and feces and protoporphyrin solely in feces. It should be noted that porphyrinogens constitute the true intermediates of heme synthesis. The porphyrins—with the exception of protoporphyrin—are side products of the pathway that are irreversibly oxidized and must be excreted. Although loss of heme precursors from the pathway occurs and is measurable in urine or stool, it normally represents less than 1 per cent of heme synthesis. Increased excretion of these compounds implies an underlying disturbance of heme formation, either hereditary or acquired.

TISSUE SITES OF PORPHYRIN PRODUCTION. Heme serves as the prosthetic group for mitochondrial cytochromes as well as for other heme-proteins and therefore is required by all cells in the body; presumably, each tissue provides its own heme by endogenous synthesis. This requirement, however, varies widely among individual tissues, reflecting large differences in the concentration and turnover of specific heme-proteins. Relatively high rates of heme synthesis are characteristic of both bone marrow and liver. In bone marrow, heme synthesis is devoted very largely to formation of hemoglobin; in liver, heme is required for several relatively short-lived heme-proteins, in particular a group of microsomal cytochromes known as P-450. In rat liver, turnover of these cytochromes appears to account for 60 to 70 per cent of heme utilization. Synthesis of hepatic cytochrome P-450 is inducible by numerous drugs and possibly also by endogenous lipophilic substances, and administration of an inducing drug results in stimulation of ALA synthetase and a consequent increase in the rate of heme formation. In extrahepatic tissues (including bone marrow), the regulatory role of ALA synthetase remains poorly defined, and inducing effects of administered drugs have not been documented.

CLASSIFICATION, GENETICS, AND PREVALENCE. In the hereditary porphyrias, the specific genetic defect presumably is pres-

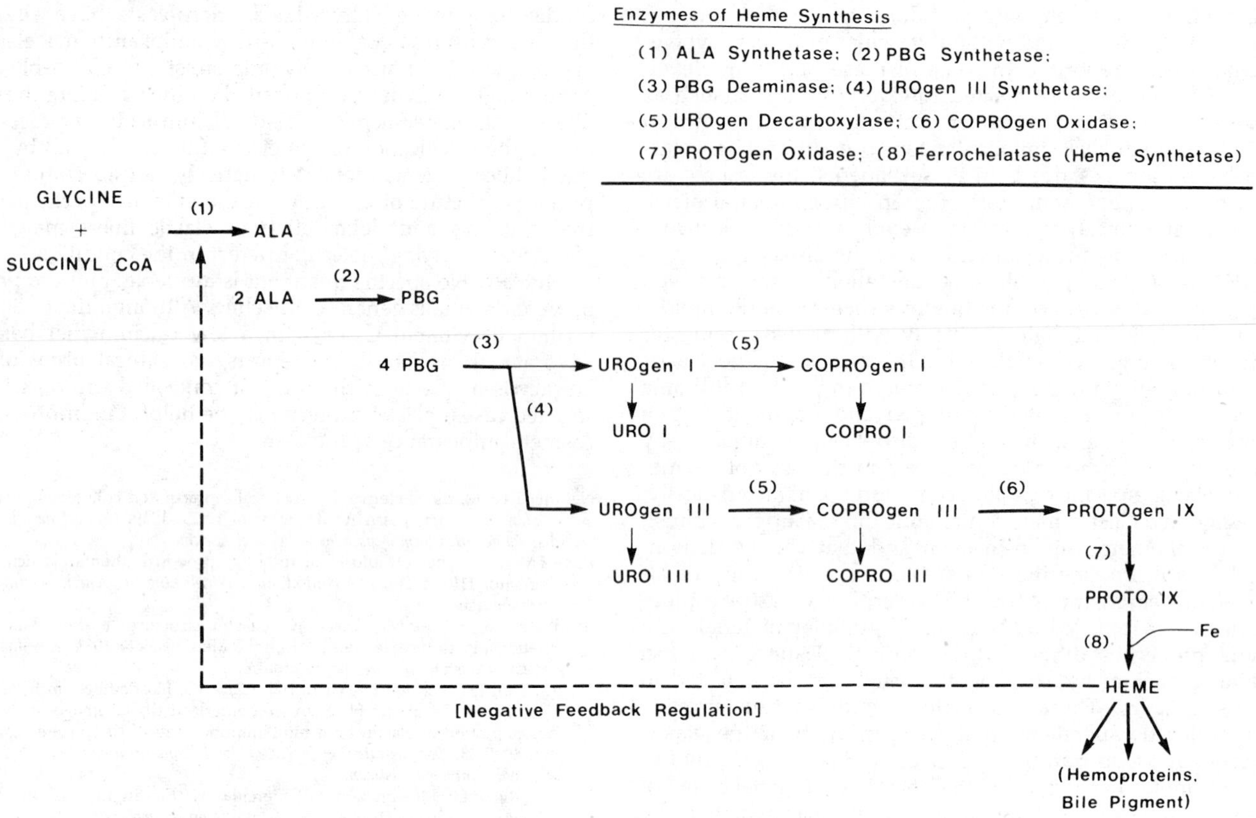

Figure 203–1. Pathway of heme biosynthesis (ALA = δ-aminolevulinic acid; PBG = porphobilinogen; URO = uroporphyrin; COPRO = coproporphyrin; PROTO = protoporphyrin).

ent in all cells of the body. However, for reasons as yet unclear, abnormal porphyrinogenesis is confined largely to either bone marrow or liver, with the possible exception of protoporphyria, which may involve both tissues. Accordingly, the classification presented in Table 203–1 separates the porphyrias into erythropoietic and hepatic types. Other tissues may be affected by the porphyria-producing lesion, but their contribution to total body production of heme precursors is small. Congenital erythropoietic porphyria is a rare autosomal recessive disease; all of the other hereditary porphyrias are dominant disorders, and the sexes are equally affected. Although their distribution appears to be worldwide, accurate prevalence figures are not available because many carriers in the general population are asymptomatic. Clinically manifest hepatic porphyria appears to be much more common in whites than in blacks or Asians; whether this reflects differences in carrier rates or only variable clinical expression of the defect among these populations is unknown.

BIOCHEMICAL CHARACTERIZATION. While the porphyrias as a group represent disturbances of heme synthesis, they may be differentiated on the basis of the specific enzymatic defect in each type and the unique pattern of excretion of heme precursors (ALA, PBG, or porphyrins) associated with each defect (Table 203–2). This pattern is determined with quantitative tests; qualitative tests such as the Watson-Schwartz test for PBG are best reserved for urgent circumstances or when quantitative determinations are unavailable. With examination of the entire array of heme precursors in urine and feces, true porphyrias are readily differentiated from asymptomatic porphyrinuria, which may accompany acute liver disease, various tumors (hepatoma, Hodgkin's disease), and neurologic diseases. Porphyrinuria in these instances generally involves an isolated increase in urine coproporphyrin, with or without a modest increase in uroporphyrin. In lead poisoning, urine exhibits a significant increase in ALA with a lesser increase in coproporphyrin; PBG and fecal porphyrins are normal. None of these patterns resemble those associated with porphyria (Table 203–2).

Overproduction, with excess excretion, of ALA and PBG or porphyrins is associated with specific clinical manifestations. Increased circulating ALA and PBG are linked to a variety of neurologic problems that may include psychosis, seizures, and paresis. A neuropathic effect of ALA or PBG has been postulated. By contrast, overproduction of porphyrins is associated predominantly with cutaneous photosensitivity; no effect on neurologic function has been observed. The dermatologic effects of porphyrins are proportional to their approximate concentration in subcutaneous tissues and depend on excitation of porphyrins by visible light (peak effective wavelength, ca. 400 nm).

TABLE 203–1. CLASSIFICATION OF THE PORPHYRIAS

Erythropoietic
Congenital erythropoietic porphyria (Günther's disease)
Protoporphyria (erythropoietic or erythrohepatic protoporphyria)
Hepatic
Acute intermittent porphyria (pyrroloporphyria)
Hereditary coproporphyria
Variegate porphyria (South African porphyria)
Porphyria cutanea tarda (symptomatic porphyria)
Toxic porphyria

CONGENITAL ERYTHROPOIETIC PORPHYRIA

Fewer than 100 patients with this condition have been described. Pink urine and cutaneous photosensitivity are the principal manifestations and, classically, are present from early childhood. While the diagnosis usually is made at this time, a first presentation has been described also in adults, whose clinical state resembled that of relatively severe porphyria cutanea tarda (see below). Acute attacks of abdominal pain with neurologic manifestations do not occur. Cutaneous lesions

TABLE 203–2. PATTERNS OF OVERPRODUCTION OF HEME PRECURSORS IN THE HEREDITARY PORPHYRIAS

Type of Porphyria	Heme Precursors Present in Abnormal Amounts				Enzyme Defect
	Urine	*Feces*	*RBC*	*Plasma*	
Acute intermittent porphyria	ALA < **PBG*** > > URO	—	—	ALA, PBG	PBG deaminase (3)†
Congenital erythropoietic porphyria	URO > > COPRO	URO > COPRO	**URO**	URO	?UROgen III cosynthetase (4)
Porphyria cutanea tarda	**URO** > > COPRO	URO	—	URO	UROgen decarboxylase (5)
Hereditary coproporphyria	ALA < PBG < URO < COPRO	**COPRO** > > PROTO	—	COPRO	COPROgen oxidase (6)
Variegate porphyria	ALA < PBG < URO < COPRO	COPRO < **PROTO**	—	COPRO, PROTO	PROTOgen oxidase (7)
Protoporphyria	—	PROTO	**PROTO**	PROTO	Ferrochelatase (8)

*The diagnostic abnormality for each type is in boldface type.
†Numbers in parentheses denote the position of the enzyme defect in the heme synthetic pathway (see Fig. 203–1).
ALA = δ-aminolevulinic acid; PBG = porphobilinogen; URO = uroporphyrin; COPRO = coproporphyrin; PROTO = protoporphyrin.

consist of bullae, vesicles, and shallow ulcers on light-exposed skin. Repeated injuries are accompanied by hypertrichosis and, in patients surviving beyond childhood, may cause disfiguring scars with loss of portions of the nose, ears, eyelids, and digits. Erythrodontia, reflecting accumulation of porphyrins in teeth and bones, and splenomegaly also have been present in a high proportion of cases, associated with a compensated hemolytic anemia, which may be intermittent. The chemical abnormality that characterizes this disease is overproduction of uroporphyrin and also of coproporphyrin, predominantly of the isomer I type; this is consistent with a defect in the formation of uroporphyrinogen III, although the inherited enzymatic lesion remains to be defined. Blood and urine both exhibit striking—and often massive—increases in these porphyrins, whereas urinary ALA and PBG are present in normal amounts. Circulating normoblasts and, to a lesser extent, reticulocytes exhibit intense fluorescence owing to their high content of uroporphyrin. The feces also contain excess uroporphyrin and coproporphyrin with a minimal increase in protoporphyrin. Treatment relies on avoidance of sunlight; topical sunscreens and β-carotene (the latter useful in protoporphyria) are of no proven value. In patients with hemolysis, splenectomy may lead to prolongation of red cell life span and diminished porphyrin excretion.

PROTOPORPHYRIA

This is a relatively common condition, which in most patients is manifest solely as cutaneous photosensitivity. Within minutes of exposure, sunlight causes a burning, stinging sensation or pruritus of unprotected skin, followed by erythema and/or edema ("solar urticaria"). Attacks subside over a period of hours, often without sequelae; in some patients, repeated episodes lead to thickening of the skin ("solar eczema"). The cutaneous manifestations associated with other types of porphyria (bulla formation, mechanical fragility, or hypertrichosis) are absent in protoporphyria. The disease is characterized chemically by excess protoporphyrin IX in erythrocytes, plasma, and feces. Excretion of ALA, PBG, and uroporphyrin is normal, whereas fecal coproporphyrin may be moderately elevated in some patients. Diffusion of protoporphyrin from red cells to plasma and cutaneous tissues appears to be responsible for the observed photosensitivity and distinguishes protoporphyria from other, acquired conditions with elevation of red cell porphyrin. In iron deficiency, lead intoxication, and certain refractory chronic anemias, excess protoporphyrin is present in erythrocytes but is bound within the cell; plasma protoporphyrin levels invariably are normal, and cutaneous symptoms are absent.

The hereditary defect is a partial deficiency of ferrochelatase, which is the final enzyme of the heme synthetic pathway, catalyzing the conversion of protoporphyrin to heme. In some patients, the excess protoporphyrin appears to be derived entirely from the bone marrow, whereas in others the liver has been implicated as well. The clinically latent carrier state is frequent. About 10 per cent of patients form protoporphyrin-containing gallstones, and subclinical liver disease also appears to be relatively common, presumably because of deposition of protoporphyrin in the liver. In rare instances, the presenting manifestation is cholestasis, with inflammation, fibrosis, and crystalline protoporphyrin inclusions in bile canaliculi and liver cells. Progression to portal hypertension and death may be rapid. Fatal hepatic involvement has been associated with markedly elevated plasma protoporphyrin concentrations (>1000 μg per deciliter).

Treatment of cutaneous manifestations includes administration of β-carotene, which increases the patient's tolerance for sunlight apparently by quenching light- and porphyrin-induced active intermediates that cause cutaneous injury. As a screening measure for possible hepatic involvement, all patients should receive routine evaluation of liver function, those with abnormalities undergoing liver biopsy.

There is no established prophylaxis or therapy for the liver disease of protoporphyria. Individual case reports suggest that cholestyramine or activated charcoal may be beneficial by binding protoporphyrin within the intestinal lumen, interrupting its enterohepatic circulation and thereby reducing the amount of protoporphyrin presented to the liver.

HEPATIC PORPHYRIA WITH NEUROLOGIC MANIFESTATIONS

DEFINITIONS. ***Acute Intermittent Porphyria.*** This disease is due to a hereditary partial deficiency of PBG deaminase and is characterized by excretion of excess ALA and PBG in urine. Acute neurologic attacks occur; cutaneous symptoms are not a feature of this type of porphyria.

Hereditary Coproporphyria. A partial deficiency of coproporphyrinogen oxidase is present, leading to excretion of excess ALA, PBG, uroporphyrin, and coproporphyrin in urine and excess coproporphyrin in feces. In addition to acute neurologic attacks, approximately 30 per cent of patients experience cutaneous manifestations consistent with overproduction of porphyrins.

Variegate Porphyria. This type is due to a partial deficiency of protoporphyrinogen oxidase and is characterized by excess excretion of the entire series of heme precursors; excretion of protoporphyrin in feces is characteristically high. Erythrocyte porphyrin levels are normal. Cutaneous photosensitivity or unusual fragility of sun-exposed skin is present in a majority of affected individuals and may be a chronic manifestation; the lesions are similar to those present in porphyria cutanea tarda (see below). However, as in the two preceding types, the occurrence of acute neurologic attacks is the most important clinical feature.

PATHOGENESIS. The individual genetic defect in each type appears to limit the flow of heme precursors and to be responsible for potential or actual heme deficiency in the liver. Circumstances that increase the demand for heme synthesis—the classic example being induction of cytochrome P-450 by barbiturates—cause the deficiency to be expressed, leading to derepression of ALA synthetase, overproduction of heme precursors preceding the genetic defect, and clinical symptoms. In addition to drugs, changes in endogenous factors have also been implicated in precipitating acute attacks. Involvement of steroid hormones is suggested by the fact that symptoms are rare prior to puberty, and disease is expressed clinically in women more often than in men. Estrogens (including oral contraceptives) are among the drugs that precipitate attacks; and cyclical, premenstrual exacerbations occur in some women, resolving with onset of menstruation. The effect of pregnancy on disease activity is unpredictable. Infection or fasting (deliberate or as a result of concurrent illness) also predisposes carriers to acute attacks.

CLINICAL PRESENTATION. Acute neurologic attacks are common to all three of the porphyrias cited above, and their identical presentations and management justify treating these types as a group. An acute attack consists of abdominal, back, or extremity pain, initially subacute but increasingly intense over a period of 24 to 48 hours until it may suggest acute cholecystitis, appendicitis, or other surgical diagnosis. Anorexia, nausea, and vomiting are frequent. Constipation typically is longstanding and worsens at the onset of an attack. In evaluating pain, the examiner may be impressed that the severity of the symptoms is out of proportion to the abdominal findings; rebound tenderness is seldom present. Tachycardia is a frequent finding and a useful parameter of disease activity. Fever is unusual and suggests a concurrent infectious process. X-ray examination of the abdomen may show dilated loops of small bowel consistent with paralytic ileus. In general, the abdominal manifestations are believed to represent a neurogenic motility disturbance of the bowel. They often occur in association with frank neurologic dysfunction: generalized seizures or mental abnormalities that range from confusion to psychosis may be presenting features of an acute attack. With prolonged attacks, motor and sensory deficits appear and may progress to quadriplegia, respiratory paralysis, and death. The neuropathic changes are variable; patchy demyelination of peripheral nerves and focal degeneration of the autonomic nervous system have been described. Routine laboratory tests generally are unremarkable. Anemia is not a feature of the hepatic porphyrias, and blood loss does not precipitate acute attacks. Liver function test results similarly are normal, apart from slight elevation of serum transaminase activity. Hyponatremia occurs in a minority of patients but occasionally is striking; it may reflect inappropriate secretion of antidiuretic hormone, complicated in some instances by aggressive intravenous fluid therapy with glucose and water.

Apart from acute episodes, in which the diagnosis is obvious, carriers of these genetic defects may complain of mood swings and bodily pains, which fail to suggest a specific diagnosis and may be without associated physical findings. The porphyric nature of such symptoms often is difficult to resolve; although excretion of heme precursors is uniformly increased in acute attacks, it varies widely among asymptomatic carriers and thus does not provide a secure basis for differentiating porphyric from nonspecific manifestations. Treatment is empiric, with due regard for those drugs that may induce acute attacks (see below). There is no evidence that dietary manipulations (e.g., excess carbohydrate) are useful.

DIAGNOSIS. Urinary PBG is elevated in these porphyrias during acute attacks and remains elevated while symptoms persist. This may be documented by rapid qualitative methods (Watson-Schwartz or Hoesch tests) in which PBG reacts with Ehrlich's reagent (dimethylaminobenzaldehyde in HCl) to form a red complex that is not extractable with *n*-butanol. Positive test results should be confirmed by quantitation of urinary PBG by ion-exchange column chromatography. With quantitation of urinary and fecal porphyrins, the specific type of porphyria usually can be established. Uroporphyrin often is reported as elevated in acute intermittent porphyria, despite the fact that its formation theoretically is compromised by the genetic defect of this type. This apparently is due to nonenzymatic conversion of PBG to a dark uroporphyrin-like compound ("porphobilin"), which may occur in the urinary bladder. The conversion is accelerated by exposure of urine to light, accounting for the visible darkening of voided urine from patients with acute intermittent porphyria. A "urine porphyrin screen" does not measure PBG and therefore could be misleading in the evaluation of patients with acute abdominal pain.

In the absence of clinical symptoms, elevation of urinary PBG is inconstant. In 20 to 30 per cent of asymptomatic carriers of acute intermittent porphyria, PBG in urine is within the normal range. In these cases, assay of erythrocyte PBG deaminase may be used to identify carriers. This activity is significantly reduced in affected persons and is abnormal regardless of the age or clinical state of the person. Many asymptomatic carriers with hereditary coproporphyria or variegate porphyria excrete PBG in normal amounts. Identification of carriers requires measurement of fecal coproporphyrin in the case of hereditary coproporphyria and fecal protoporphyrin for variegate porphyria. While the inherited defects in these types of porphyria are known, the enzymes are intramitochondrial; therefore, their assay requires nucleated cells (leukocytes or cultured skin fibroblasts) and at present is a research procedure.

MANAGEMENT. Emphasis is on the prevention of acute neurologic attacks. In families with a known case of porphyria, identification of carriers is mandatory, using the appropriate screening procedure for the type of porphyria involved (see above). Carriers should be instructed as to the hazards of fasting and of taking drugs that may precipitate acute attacks (Table 203–3). Carriers of hereditary coproporphyria or variegate porphyria who experience cutaneous manifestations in the absence of a porphyrogenic drug should minimize their exposure to sunlight and wear protective clothing.

The management of neurologic exacerbations includes immediate withdrawal of possible offending drugs, administration of carbohydrate, correction of electrolyte abnormalities, and general supportive care. Carbohydrate is given to reverse the fasting state, usually as intravenous dextrose because of nausea or vomiting, and in amounts approaching 400 grams per day. To avoid administration of a water load, hypertonic solutions infused by a central line may be used. Seizures, when present, generally occur early in the course of an attack and respond to parenteral diazepam. For analgesia, chlorpromazine may be used, although the specificity of its action is uncertain; excessive sedation is a troublesome side effect. In many patients, meperidine will be required despite the danger of addiction. Propranolol counters the tachycardia of acute attacks; it should be introduced at very low doses (e.g., 10 mg twice daily).

If acute manifestations fail to respond to these measures within 48 hours, treatment with hematin (hydroxyheme) is

TABLE 203–3. HAZARDOUS AND SAFE DRUGS IN PORPHYRIA WITH NEUROLOGIC MANIFESTATIONS

May Precipitate Acute Attacks	Believed To Be Safe
Apronalid	Aspirin
Barbiturates	Bromides
Chlordiazepoxide	Chlorpromazine
Chloroquine	Corticosteroids
Chlorpropamide	Diazepam
Dichloralphenazone	Dicumarol
Ergot preparations	Digoxin
Estrogens	Diphenhydramine
Ethanol	Ether
Glutethimide	Guanethidine
Griseofulvin	Meperidine
Hydantoins	Morphine
Imipramine	Neostigmine
Meprobamate	Nitrous oxide
Methsuximide	Penicillins
Methyldopa	Propranolol
Methyprylon	Tetracyclines
Novonal	
Sulfonamides	

indicated with the rationale that it compensates for the genetic impairment of endogenous heme synthesis. The solution consists of pyrogen-free hemin (ferriprotoporphyrin IX chloride) dissolved in aqueous sodium carbonate (10 grams per liter), adjusted to pH 8.0 with HCl and sterilized by membrane filtration. It is infused slowly (over 10 to 15 minutes) into the largest available vein. The maximal recommended dose is 3 mg per kilogram body weight at 12-hour intervals. Smaller doses (1 to 2 mg per kilogram) at daily intervals may be equally effective, particularly if freshly prepared hematin is available. The hematin solution is unstable and should be administered as soon as is practicable after its preparation or reconstitution from lyophilized powder. Solutions may be refrigerated for up to 12 hours but then should be discarded. The principal complications of hematin administration are a chemical phlebitis at the site of infusion (4 per cent of cases) and reduced clotting activity. Abnormal coagulation tests and reduced platelets have been observed in several patients receiving hematin. These abnormalities appear to depend on the dose of hematin administered and are transient, being maximal 10 minutes after injection of hematin, diminished at 5 hours and undetectable at 48 hours. Clinically significant bleeding has not occurred except in patients also receiving another anticoagulant. The findings suggest that hematin should not be used in patients with impaired coagulation or in those undergoing surgical procedures. At doses substantially in excess of the recommended maximum, hematin has caused renal toxicity, which was reversible. Similar problems have not been observed with the usual doses, despite the fact that patients with acute hepatic porphyria may exhibit reduced renal function. A clinical and biochemical response (decreased excretion of PBG) may be expected within 72 to 96 hours after starting hematin treatment, and maximal benefit after a total of 10 to 12 doses. With cessation of hematin treatment, a rise in urinary PBG may occur, although the patient's clinical condition usually remains stable (Fig. 203–2).

PROGNOSIS. The vast majority of carriers remain asymptomatic, provided that they avoid drugs associated with exacerbations, and their longevity appears to be unaffected. Acute neurologic attacks formerly carried a substantial mortality. However, as a result of hematin therapy and modern intensive care for complications such as respiratory failure, the outlook for these patients is much improved. Neurologic deficits may require months or years to resolve, but complete recovery is observed in many instances. Although mental abnormalities occur in acute attacks, these are neither persistent nor progressive.

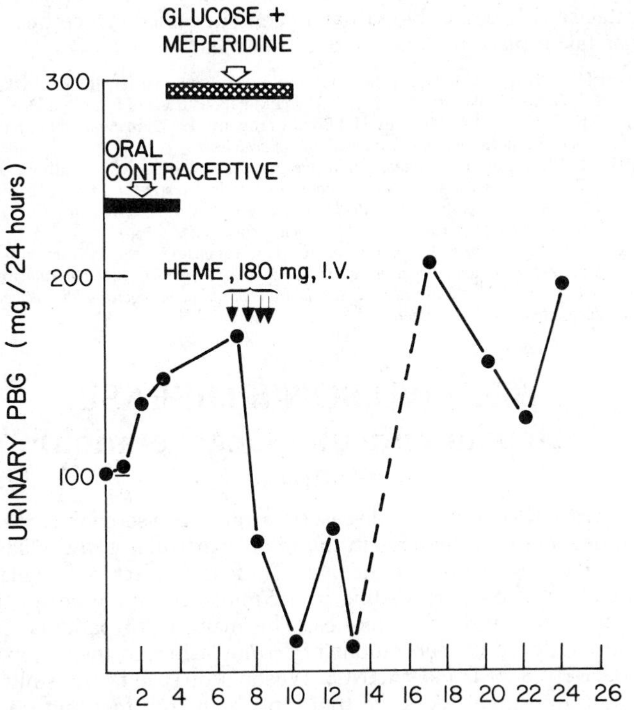

Figure 203–2. Acute intermittent porphyria in a patient taking oral contraceptive medication: response of urinary PBG (porphobilinogen) to administered heme (hematin). Normal PBG less than 2 mg per 24 hours.

PORPHYRIA CUTANEA TARDA

This relatively common condition is characterized by mechanical fragility and blistering of light-exposed skin. Acute neurologic attacks do not occur. The onset of manifestations is insidious, patients often failing to associate cutaneous lesions with sun exposure. Seemingly trivial trauma to the dorsa of the hands, arms, face, or feet leads to vesicles that rupture to an open sore, eventually healing with scar formation. Sclerodermoid changes and hypertrichosis may occur. A history of ethanol abuse and/or chronic liver disease can be obtained from a majority of patients with this type of porphyria. The pathologic changes seen in liver biopsies are nonspecific and do not correlate with the severity of the porphyria. In a few patients, hepatomas containing a high concentration of porphyrin have been diagnosed and presumably were the cause of cutaneous manifestations. Almost all liver biopsy specimens exhibit an increase in stainable iron, and freshly obtained tissue is fluorescent under ultraviolet light because of its high content of uroporphyrin. Associations of this disease with systemic lupus erythematosus, diabetes mellitus, and hemochromatosis (heterozygous state) have been reported.

Urine from patients is red-orange or brown. Its uroporphyrin content (predominantly isomer I) is strikingly elevated; cutaneous manifestations are associated with levels greater than 800 μg per 24 hours (normal, <50 μg per 24 hours). Urinary coproporphyrin excretion is moderately increased, whereas fecal coproporphyrin and protoporphyrin are normal. This pattern clearly distinguishes patients with porphyria cutanea tarda from those with variegate porphyria who exhibit cutaneous manifestations (Table 203–2).

The *pathogenesis* of porphyria cutanea tarda is incompletely understood. The pattern of porphyrin excretion, with predominance of isomer I compounds, suggests a partial defect at the level of uroporphyrinogen III synthetase; on the other hand, excretion of uroporphyrin is greater than that of coproporphyrin, consistent with deficient activity of uroporphyrinogen decarboxylase. A partial deficiency of the latter activity appears to be present in the liver of all patients with porphyria cutanea tarda. Whether or not this represents a hereditary abnormality in all cases is controversial at present. In some patients, the defect is expressed not only in liver but also in erythrocytes; first-degree relatives of these patients also exhibit the defect in a pattern consistent with autosomal dominant inheritance. On the other hand, in some patients the defect is detectable solely in liver tissue. The erythrocyte enzyme of the patient and family members is normal. The latter has been termed *sporadic* porphyria cutanea tarda. The available data are insufficient for determining whether this is an acquired disease or a hereditary variant of porphyria cutanea tarda. Regardless of the genetic component, it is clear that environmental or purely acquired factors play a central role in the pathogenesis of symptoms. Increased hepatic iron, ethanol ingestion, and certain drugs (notably, estrogens) all may provoke increased porphyrin production, apparently acting in concert with the underlying genetic defect to compromise heme synthesis at the level of uroporphyrinogen III formation. The cutaneous manifestations of porphyria cutanea tarda have been observed in a few patients with renal failure receiving hemodialysis, and elevation of plasma uroporphyrin has been noted; the pathogenesis is obscure.

Management involves attention to possible aggravating factors: administered iron, estrogen, ethanol, or occupational exposure to noxious chemicals should be eliminated, and this alone may lead to a reduction in porphyrin excretion and remission of cutaneous manifestations. However, phlebotomy, to remove iron from the liver and accelerate resolution of the disease, usually is indicated. With monitoring of the patient's hemoglobin level, 500 to 1000 ml of blood may be removed once or twice monthly, until urine porphyrin levels begin to decline. The time-course of the response varies widely among patients, averaging six months. For patients with disabling cutaneous disease and unable to tolerate phlebotomy, chloroquine* at low doses may be introduced. However, this carries a definite risk of a hepatotoxic reaction, and close monitoring of liver function is required. Plasmapheresis also may be useful for directly reducing the concentration of circulating uroporphyrin. Topical sunscreens and β-carotene offer little or no protection against light-induced damage in this disease. When pathogenic environmental factors have been eliminated, a clinical response is observed in virtually all patients treated with serial phlebotomies and usually is long lasting.

TOXIC PORPHYRIA

Cutaneous porphyria on a large scale occurred in Turkey in 1959, when several thousand persons consumed grain that had been treated with a fungicide (hexachlorobenzene). Other cases have resulted from accidental or industrial exposure to hepatotoxins, epidemiologic considerations indicating that the disease is acquired rather than hereditary. The clinical manifestations and laboratory abnormalities are indistinguishable from those of porphyria cutanea tarda.

Bissell DM: Heme metabolism and the porphyrias. *In* Wright R, Alberti KGMM, Karran S, Millward-Sadler GH (eds.): Liver and Biliary Disease. London, W. B. Saunders Company, 1984. *The hepatic porphyrias, with emphasis on the clinical aspects.*

Dean G: The Porphyrias. A Story of Heredity and Environment. 2nd ed. London, Pitman Medical, 1971. *Studies of a very large kindred with variegate porphyria in South Africa.*

Kappas A, Sassa S, Anderson KE: The porphyrias. *In* Stanbury JB, Wyngaarden JB, Fredrickson DS, Goldstein JL, Brown MS (eds.): The Metabolic Basis of Inherited Disease. 5th ed. New York, McGraw-Hill Book Company, 1983. *A detailed review of genetic and biochemical aspects of the porphyrias.*

Ridley A: The neuropathy of acute intermittent porphyria. Quart J Med 38:307, 1969. *Neurologic manifestations in 25 patients.*

Stein JA, Tschudy DP: Acute intermittent porphyria. A clinical and biochemical study of 46 patients. Medicine 49:1, 1970. *A tabulation of clinical features in a large series.*

Watson CJ, Pierach CA, Bossenmaier I, Cardinal R: Use of hematin in the acute attack of the "inducible" hepatic porphyrias. Adv Intern Med 23:265, 1978. *Summary of an experience with 160 hematin infusions in 26 patients.*

204. ACATALASIA

James B. Wyngaarden

DEFINITION AND SYNONYMS. Acatalasia is a rare inherited deficiency of catalase in erythrocytes (acatalasemia) and other tissues. In some subjects acatalasia is associated with severe gangrenous lesions of the oral cavity and destruction of alveolar bone (Takahara's disease).

EPIDEMIOLOGY. Acatalasia was discovered in Japan in 1946. Takahara's disease occurs chiefly among Japanese and Koreans but has also occurred in Peru. Asymptomatic acatalasemia has been reported from Japan, Korea, Switzerland, Israel, Mexico, and Peru, and hypocatalasemia from several additional countries, including the United States.

ETIOLOGY AND PATHOGENESIS. Acatalasia is inherited as an autosomal recessive condition and is often associated with consanguinity. In Japan the estimated frequencies of homozygotes and heterozygotes are 4×10^{-6} and 1.7×10^{-3}, respectively. The distribution of blood catalase values among homozygous affected, heterozygous, and normal subjects is triphasic, without overlap. Residual catalase activity among Japanese with acatalasia is very low; the enzyme is electrophoretically normal, of normal stability and low specific activity. Among Swiss homozygotes, residual catalase activity is higher, and the enzyme is electrophoretically abnormal and heat labile. Swiss heterozygotes have normal blood catalase levels.

Takahara's disease results from oral sepsis with hydrogen peroxide–producing bacteria and appears to be restricted to subjects with very low catalase activities. Acatalasemic Japanese with Takahara's disease have 0.23 per cent of normal catalase activity; those without have 0.57 per cent. Homozygotes from Switzerland, Israel, and Mexico have higher values and are clinically normal. Homozygotes have been classified into five subtypes by Aebi and Wyss, on the basis of genetic and clinical heterogeneity.

CLINICAL MANIFESTATIONS. About half of acatalasemic subjects remain asymptomatic throughout life. Takahara's disease usually begins before age ten, sometimes during infancy. Over 50 cases have been reported. Mild disease consists of ulcers in the dental alveoli or in tonsillar crypts. In moderate disease (the most common) there is alveolar gangrene, recession of alveolar bone, and loss of teeth. In severe cases there is widespread destruction with gangrene of the maxilla and soft tissue, similar to "noma." After healing, extensive scarring may limit opening of the mouth. Gangrenous lesions of the oral cavity are rare after puberty.

DIAGNOSIS. The disease should be suspected in any child with shaggy discolored ulcers of dental alveoli or gangrenous lesions of the mouth. A presumptive diagnostic test is easily performed as follows: when hydrogen peroxide is added to acatalasemic blood, it turns brown-black because of formation of methemoglobin, whereas normal blood bubbles vigorously and remains pink. Asymptomatic acatalasemic and hypocatalasemic subjects have been diagnosed in family studies or in population surveys by quantitative assays of blood catalase activity.

TREATMENT. Curettage and excision of granulating tissue, drainage, irrigation of septic areas, extraction of teeth, and antibiotic therapy have been employed. Reconstructive surgery and bone grafts have been required. Direct application of crystalline catalase suspensions and transfusions of normal catalase-rich whole blood have been suggested. Once healing has taken place the disease does not recur.

Aebi HE, Wyss SR: Acatalasemia. *In* Stanbury JB, Wyngaarden JB, Fredrickson DS, Goldstein JL, Brown MN (eds.): The Metabolic Basis of Inherited Disease, 5th ed. New York, McGraw-Hill Book Company, 1983. *An authoritative review of genetic, metabolic, and clinical features of acatalasia.*

Delgado W, Calderon P: Acatalasia in two Peruvian siblings. J Oral Pathol 8:358, 1979. *Takahara's disease was diagnosed in two brothers, ages 10 and 11 years. Thirteen hypocatalasemic individuals, including both parents, were found among 29 relatives of the probands examined from four generations.*

Ogata M, Mizugaki J: Properties of residual catalase in the erythrocytes of Japanese-type acatalasemia. Hum Genet 48:329, 1979. *Residual catalase is stable, electrophoretically normal. Levels are lower in homozygotes with Takahara's disease than in those without.*

205. WILSON'S DISEASE (Hepatolenticular Degeneration)

Ara Tourian

DEFINITION. Wilson's disease is a rare disease characterized by degenerative changes in the brain, particularly in the basal ganglia, and cirrhosis of the liver. There is a defect in the biliary excretion of copper, leading to accumulation of copper in the liver, brain, and other tissues. The majority of patients also show reduced concentrations of ceruloplasmin in the serum.

GENETICS AND PREVALENCE. Wilson's disease is transmitted as an autosomal recessive trait, and high consanguinity rates are found among parents of affected individuals. The estimated gene frequency is 0.006, with a disease prevalence of 0.0001.

ETIOLOGY AND PATHOGENESIS. The primary genetic defect is unknown. One hypothesis, first advanced by Uzman et al., is that the product of the mutant gene of Wilson's disease is

*This use is not listed in the manufacturer's directive.

an abnormal intracellular protein that has increased affinity for copper. This hypothesis has received support from evidence presented by Evans and colleagues for an abnormal hepatic copper-binding protein. Increased binding of copper, but not cadmium, by cellular proteins of secondary skin fibroblasts in culture has been observed by Chan and colleagues.

Copper homeostasis in the body is in part maintained by a high capacity excretory mechanism in the liver. The biliary excretion of copper is impaired in Wilson's disease, and the copper content of liver, brain, kidney, and cornea is markedly increased. The earliest site of accumulation is the cytoplasm of the liver parenchymal cell. Late in advanced cases the copper is concentrated in pericanalicular lysosomes. As the disease progresses, hepatocellular changes result in release of copper from within the hepatocyte. The released copper is deposited in various tissues of the body such as brain and kidney, giving rise to cellular and organ damage.

PATHOLOGY. The brain usually shows no external abnormality. The corpus striatum and sometimes the subthalamic nuclei have a brownish or brick-red coloring, depending on the duration of formalin fixation. The central white matter of cerebral or cerebellar hemispheres may also show spongy softening or cavitation, and the overlying cortex may then be atrophic. The putamen shows increased cellularity resulting chiefly from proliferation of astrocytic nuclei, but there is a reduction in the number of both large and small neurons.

Hepatomegaly may be present in the early stages of the disease, although there is usually atrophy at the terminal stage. Multilobular cirrhosis is indistinguishable from postnecrotic cirrhosis. The color of the nodules varies in different cases, and the individual lobules may also vary, some being yellow, others brick red, greenish, or brown, depending on the amount of copper storage, fatty degeneration, or bile staining. There is fibrosis of degenerating lobules with increase in connective tissue. The fibrous septa may contain perivascular collections of lymphocytes and numerous small bile ducts. There is also marked glycogen infiltration of nuclei. The Kupffer cells are normal. Copper and iron pigment are present in the liver parenchyma.

CLINICAL MANIFESTATIONS. The age of onset and clinical manifestations of Wilson's disease are quite variable. Symptoms may appear as early as four years of age or as late as the fifth decade. The mean age of onset for both males and females is 23.2 years in the United States but is 12 to 16 years in most other countries; this indicates that important genetic and environmental variables modulate the clinical expression of this disease. There is no racial or geographic predilection.

The clinical presentation and natural history of Wilson's disease fall into two distinct categories: an acute hepatic form and a subacute or chronic central nervous system form.

Hepatic Manifestations. Approximately 40 per cent of patients present with symptoms of hepatic disease. The disease commonly presents in children as atypical or prolonged hepatitis, which may be indistinguishable from juvenile cirrhosis. These patients may develop increasing hepatic failure with coma and die within weeks of onset, but more often die after several years. Rarely, esophageal variceal bleeding may herald the disease. Signs of brain dysfunction are minimal.

In adults, clinical signs of severe hepatic insufficiency are uncommon. Hepatomegaly occurs in one out of three patients and jaundice and ascites in one out of five. The liver function tests most likely to show abnormal results are prothrombin time and sulfobromophthalein retention.

The liver is enlarged and firm and may be accompanied by splenomegaly. The liver disease may progress to subacute hepatitis and cirrhosis. Neurologic symptoms may supervene at any stage of the disease.

Neurologic Manifestations. This group is characterized by a symptom complex the chief features of which are tremor exaggerated on movement, difficulty of speech and swallowing, incoordination, personality changes, and dementia. Deteriorating handwriting, poor school performance, and emotional lability may be the earliest changes observed. The dystonic form of the disease occurs predominantly in young adults. Uncontrollable increases in hand, head, and body tremors, periodic in nature, may occur. Muscular rigidity, contractures, and mental deterioration dominate the clinical picture and the patient becomes completely bedridden. Drooling of saliva and fever of unexplained origin occur in one third of patients. Jacksonian seizures have been observed in occasional patients. Death may occur within two to seven years.

Pigmentary Changes. Kayser-Fleischer rings occur in patients with overt neurologic symptoms but not in children with hepatic manifestations alone. The rings are caused by copper deposits at the margins of the cornea near the limbus, resulting in golden brown or green discoloration. They are best visualized from above with a slit lamp, with light directed from the side of the eye. The copper deposits are at the inner surface of the cornea in Descemet's membrane, and the intensity is reduced medially and laterally. Kayser-Fleischer rings disappear upon treatment with penicillamine or hepatic transplantation. In a few patients, careful examination of the eye will reveal a sunflower cataract. Azure lunulae of the nails are occasionally present.

Hemolytic Anemia. Acute episodes of hemolytic anemia without precipitating cause may occur years before the onset of neurologic or hepatic disease and may clear spontaneously. Such episodes occur only in untreated patients or in those whose treatment is interrupted. Sudden release of copper into the circulation from overloaded tissues is the postulated mechanism of the hemolysis. Copper excretion in the urine is markedly increased up to 6000 μg per day, and serum copper is acutely elevated.

Renal Involvement. Renal glomerular and tubular function is reduced, as manifested by decreased filtration and by proteinuria, aminoaciduria, glycosuria, uricaciduria, hyperphosphaturia, and hypercalciuria. A decrease in the normal capacity of the kidney to acidify the urine also occurs. The renal impairment is presumed to result from the toxic effect of copper, and renal function may return to normal on treatment with penicillamine.

Bone Lesions. A wide variety of bone lesions has been described in Wilson's disease, including osteoporosis, subarticular cysts, and fragmentation of bone about wrists, ankles, and feet. Most of these changes can be attributed to severe tubular dysfunction with concomitant hyperphosphaturia and hypophosphatemia (renal rickets).

DIAGNOSIS. A large majority of patients with Wilson's disease present with neurologic dysfunction, Kayser-Fleischer rings, and ceruloplasmin concentrations below 20 mg per deciliter, in addition to other biochemical abnormalities characteristic of the hepatic and renal components of the disease. However, in problem cases, none of these criteria is sufficient by itself to make an unequivocal diagnosis of Wilson's disease.

The mean total serum copper concentration in normal individuals is 108 ± 10 mg per deciliter, of which 90 to 95 per cent is bound to ceruloplasmin. The level of direct reacting (nonceruloplasmin-bound) copper in the serum of patients with Wilson's disease is elevated. The normal ceruloplasmin values are 20 to 40 mg per deciliter (95 per cent confidence limits). At the time of diagnosis 60 per cent of patients with Wilson's disease have less than 5 mg per deciliter, and 80 per cent have serum ceruloplasmin levels below 10 mg per deciliter. Sixteen per cent of patients have values between 10 and 20 mg per deciliter, but 4 per cent have ceruloplasmin levels within 95 per cent confidence limits of normals. In otherwise normal persons pregnancy, the administration of estrogens, and inflammatory diseases (including hepatitis) can result in a pronounced increase in the concentration of serum ceruloplasmin. Pregnancy and estrogens can also elevate ceruloplasmin in Wilson's disease. Hepatic parenchymal dysfunction has been shown to impair degradation of estrogens. A combination of these factors may explain why some Wilson's disease patients have normal ceruloplasmin levels. At present there is no convincing evidence in favor of structural or functional differences between the ceruloplasmin synthesized by normal persons and that of persons with Wilson's disease. Ten per cent of heterozygote carriers of the Wilson's disease gene have reduced ceruloplasmin levels. Kayser-Fleischer rings are no longer thought to be pathognomonic of Wilson's disease, since they have been observed also in rare cases of biliary cirrhosis or in intrahepatic cholestasis. However, in such cases the serum ceruloplasmin concentration is elevated. Hepatic copper elevations in the same range as in Wilson's disease, above 50 μg per gram dry weight, also occur in Laennec's, postnecrotic, and biliary cirrhosis; cholestatic syndromes; and biliary atresia; but such patients do not have hypoceruloplasminemia.

Urinary excretion of copper is usually above 100 μg per 24 hours in patients with symptomatic Wilson's disease, but it is similarly high in patients with biliary cirrhosis. Fecal copper is low in Wilson's disease, reflecting diminished biliary excretion of copper.

Radiocopper studies with ^{64}Cu and ^{67}Cu can help differentiate normal persons and patients with other liver diseases from patients with Wilson's disease. In the first two groups, the absorbed copper loosely complexes to albumin and peaks in the serum between one and two hours, followed by a fall and then by a slow secondary rise of radioactivity beginning at four to six hours when the isotope is incorporated into freshly synthesized ceruloplasmin secreted by the liver. In patients with Wilson's disease, this secondary rise is absent owing to impaired ceruloplasmin synthesis.

A definitive diagnosis of Wilson's disease should lead to screening of siblings and other relatives for asymptomatic Wilson's disease.

TREATMENT. The aim of treatment is to prevent the accumulation of copper in tissues and to remove the excessive amounts that have already been deposited. The drug of choice is D-penicillamine, a copper-binding agent which promotes the urinary excretion of copper. The recommended dose is 1 to 2 grams per day for adults and 0.5 to 0.75 gram per day for children under the age of ten years. Potassium sulfide, 20 mg three times daily, and a diet low in copper are also recommended. The effectiveness of treatment can be followed by monitoring the enhanced urinary excretion of copper, 3000 to 5000 μg copper per day, and the drop in serum copper as the nonceruloplasmin bound fraction of serum copper returns toward normal.

Toxic reactions to penicillamine include febrile hypersensitivity, mild leukopenia, the nephrotic syndrome, and optic neuritis (see Ch. 194). Desensitization with steroids should be undertaken and penicillamine therapy slowly reinstituted. Pyridoxine (50 mg per day) will prevent optic neuritis. An alternative decoppering agent is triethylene tetramine dihydrochloride, 1.0 gram per day. During the first six to eight weeks of treatment with penicillamine the symptoms and signs may worsen. Two to five years of uninterrupted therapy may be required to achieve the maximal benefit in reversal of central nervous system dysfunction. Similarly, clinical signs and symptoms of liver disease improve, abnormal liver function test results gradually return to normal, and portal hypertension decreases. Treatment is less satisfactory in the acute juvenile hepatic and advanced neurologic forms. When the treatment is started during the presymptomatic phase the development of clinical Wilson's disease is completely prevented, underscoring the extreme importance of early diagnosis and treatment.

Camakaris J, Ackland L, Danks DM: Abnormal copper metabolism in cultured fibroblasts from patients with Wilson's disease. J Inherited Metab Dis 3:155, 1980.

Chan WY, Cushing W, Coffman MA, Rennert DM: Genetic expression of Wilson's disease in cell culture: A diagnostic marker. Science 208:299, 1980. *The Wilson's disease phenotype can be detected by abnormal copper binding of cellular proteins, using skin fibroblasts in culture.*

Danks DM: Hereditary disorders of copper metabolism in Wilson's disease and Menkes' disease. *In* Stanbury JB, Wyngaarden JB, Fredrickson DS, Goldstein JB, Brown MS (eds.): The Metabolic Basis of Inherited Disease. 5th ed. New York, McGraw-Hill Book Company, 1983, pp 1251–1268. *An authoritative review of clinical, metabolic, and genetic aspects of Wilson's disease, with 132 references.*

Evans GW, Dubois RS, Hambidge KM: Wilson's disease: Identification of an abnormal copper-binding protein. Science 181:1175, 1973. *The copper-binding constant for the protein metallothionein of liver from patients with Wilson's disease was found to be four times as great as that of control subjects.*

Sternlieb I: Diagnosis of Wilson's disease. Gastroenterology 74:787, 1978. *An excellent article reviewing the criteria for the diagnosis of Wilson's disease.*

Strickland T, Len M-L: Wilson's disease: Clinical and laboratory manifestations in 40 patients. Medicine 54:113, 1975. *A large series of patients, with excellent quantitative analysis of clinical and laboratory findings in Wilson's disease.*

Uzman LL, Iber FL, Chalmers TC, Knowlton M: The mechanism of copper deposition in the liver in hepatolenticular degeneration (Wilson's disease). Am J Med Sci 231:511, 1956. *Increased binding of copper by liver cellular protein, measured by the method of equilibrium dialysis, was shown in a case of Wilson's disease.*

206. HEMOCHROMATOSIS (Iron Storage Disease)

Arno G. Motulsky

DEFINITION. The most common generalized iron storage disease in the United States and in persons of European origin is a genetic disorder known as idiopathic hemochromatosis that is linked to the HLA locus. Massive iron deposits in parenchymal cells may develop after many years of increased iron absorption, and functional organ impairment of the liver, heart, and other organs ensues. Hemochromatosis with parenchymal cell involvement also occurs in a variety of anemias associated with both ineffective erythropoiesis and increased iron absorption—most commonly in homozygous beta thalassemia. Blood transfusions contribute further to the pathologic iron overload. In these patients, clinical signs and symptoms of excessive iron storage develop in adolescence or even earlier.

Hemochromatosis affecting parenchymal tissues needs to be differentiated from iron loading of macrophages of the reticuloendothelial system that is relatively benign. If severe and generalized, the latter condition is known as hemosiderosis and typically occurs after multiple blood transfusions in patients with aplastic anemia in whom iron absorption is not increased. Iron overload of parenchymal liver cells is rarely observed under such conditions and occurs only with massive iron deposits after considerable time has elapsed to permit redistribution of iron.

ETIOLOGY, GENETICS, AND PATHOGENESIS. "Idiopathic" hemochromatosis is caused by an autosomal recessive gene that causes increased iron absorption in the gut. The nature of the metabolic abnormality remains unknown but may relate to failure of iron storage in gastrointestinal and reticuloendothelial cells. Thus, instead of being stored normally in such cells, iron enters the bloodstream to be deposited in parenchymal cells of the liver and other organs. Clinical signs and symptoms will develop after many years of excessive iron absorption when total body iron stores have reached levels of 15 to 40 grams as compared with normal iron stores of 0.2 to 2.0 grams.

The gene for hemochromatosis is located on the short arm of chromosome 6 and is linked to the HLA locus. The hemochromatosis gene is physically close to the HLA A allele of the HLA complex. About 70 per cent of hemochromatosis patients carry the HLA A_3 allele as compared to 25 to 30 per cent of the general population. Among HLA A_3 positive patients, more than two thirds are heterozygotes (A_3/A_x), while the rest are homozygotes (A_3/A_3).

Recombination between the hemochromatosis gene and the HLA A allele is very rare, suggesting very tight genetic linkage. An increased frequency of HLA B_7 and HLA B_{14} is also observed and is caused by "hitchhiking" of each of these determinants on the chromosome carrying the hemochromatosis gene (linkage disequilibrium). Whether the hemochromatosis gene is located between the HLA A and HLA B genes, or is distal to the HLA A gene is unknown. The development of clinical hemochromatosis in the vast majority of cases requires the "double dose" of the mutant gene, and affected patients are homozygotes. Among families that include at least one affected homozygote patient with hemochromatosis, additional homozygotes as well as heterozygote carriers can often be defined by HLA testing using the principles of genetic linkage. Thus, the HLA status of the affected patient who has inherited a single hemochromatosis gene from each parent is determined (Fig. 206–1). Sibs with both HLA haplotypes identical to that of the affected patient will carry the linked hemochromatosis allele on the maternal as well as the paternal chromosome 6 and are at high risk to develop iron overload. Such persons are homozygous and may already be affected. Sibs who share only one HLA allele are heterozygotes and sibs who share no HLA type are normal, not having inherited any hemochromatosis gene. Tests to detect heterozygotes in the general population do not exist. Screening for homozygotes in the population at large must utilize nonspecific and indirect measures of iron storage (transferrin saturation, serum ferritin) and nonspecific indices of liver damage (e.g., transaminase). HLA testing is not useful for detection in the population.

Homozygotes for hemochromatosis absorb increased iron. The actual amount of stored iron at a given time depends upon several additional factors such as age, sex, iron content of food, caloric intake, and degree of alcohol ingestion. Not enough iron to produce clinical findings will have been absorbed in younger persons. Countries that fortify their flour with iron, such as Sweden, may have more patients with clinical manifestations of hemochromatosis than those that do not follow this practice. Males generally eat larger quantities of food than females and therefore absorb more iron. Most importantly, females lose iron periodically during menstruation and occasionally during pregnancy. Therefore, while the incidence of homozygotes for the hemochromatosis gene is identical in both sexes, the frequency of clinically apparent hemochromatosis is about 10 times higher in males. Excessive alcohol intake further contributes to liver damage and about one third of patients with the clinical disease give a history of excessive alcohol intake. Alcohol and iron interact in an as yet unknown manner to impair the liver. Furthermore, alcohol may stimulate iron absorption and certain alcoholic beverages such as red wines contain increased amounts of iron. Ingestion of iron-containing medications—particularly over prolonged periods—would cause additional iron absorption.

Prolonged storage of excessive iron in various parenchymal organs, particularly the liver and the heart, is required before clinical manifestations develop. There is a fairly good correlation between the quantity of iron stored and the development of clinical signs and symptoms. Heterozygotes for the hemochromatosis gene may absorb somewhat increased amounts of iron, and minor abnormalities of iron loading have sometimes been detected. Test results of iron status in heterozygotes are closer to those found in normals than to those in homozygotes for hemochromatosis; clinical manifestations rarely if ever occur. However, it is conceivable that heterozygotes are at higher risk to develop iron overload under conditions at which normal persons would not be affected. Iron overload in alcoholic liver disease appears not to be associated with the heterozygote state for hemochromatosis. Not all homozygotes develop clinical disease. The fraction of those who do so depends upon the various cricumstances affecting iron balance already discussed. It is clear that full-blown clinical findings are the "tip of the iceberg" and that many homozygotes may have no symptoms or exhibit only mild clinical findings that are not recognized as being related to the underlying iron storage disease. As in other hereditary diseases, our understanding of the clinical spectrum of the disease has changed with earlier and more complete ascertainment.

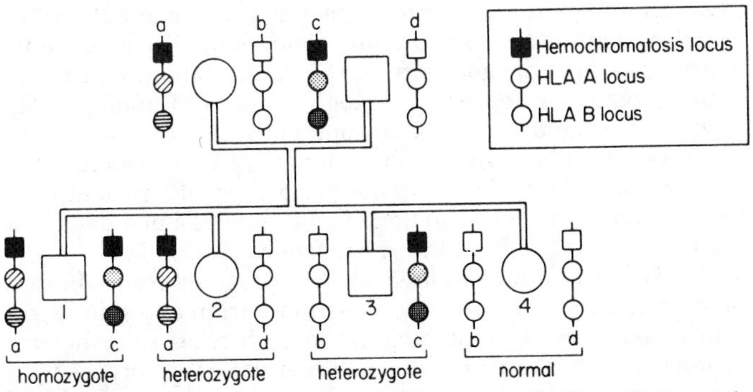

Figure 206–1. Hypothetical distribution of iron-loading alleles, each designated by an HLA haplotype, among family members of a patient (1) with fully developed idiopathic hemochromatosis. The "topographic" relationships between the gene (■) and the HLA loci (○) are diagrammatic approximations. The mother of the patient has two number 6 chromosomes, designated a and b, of which chromosome a carries the mutant allele of the hemochromatosis locus. In the father the mutant allele occurs on the sixth chromosome that is designated c. The patient inherited both mutant genes and is a homozygote. (From Bothwell TH, Charlton RW, Motulsky AG: Idiopathic hemochromatosis. *In* Stanbury JB, Wyngaarden JB, Fredrickson DS, Goldstein JL, Brown MS (eds.): The Metabolic Basis of Inherited Disease, 5th ed. New York, McGraw-Hill Book Company, 1983.)

PATHOLOGY. Although iron in reticuloendothelial cells is relatively harmless, parenchymal cell deposits are noxious to tissues. Iron in hemochromatosis is stored mostly in parenchymal cells as insoluble granular gold-brown aggregates known as *hemosiderin.* Normally, most iron is stored as ferritin but with increasing iron overload the proportion of hemosiderin increases and the liver enlarges. With advancing hemosiderosis, fibrosis increases and cirrhosis is the rule in fully developed cases. In such patients wide fibrotic bands characteristically separate liver lobules to cause monolobular cirrhosis.

Skin pigmentation is caused by melanin in the deeper epidermis while the slate-gray appearance in some cases is caused by hemosiderin. Pancreatic iron deposits are more marked in exocrine than in endocrine cells and fibrosis is the rule. The heart is usually enlarged. Iron pigment is deposited in myocardial fibers. Synovial linings as well as various endocrine glands, including thyroid, parathyroid, and anterior pituitary, are heavily infiltrated with hemosiderin. Testicular atrophy without hemosiderin deposits is frequent. These descriptions refer to fully developed cases. Early cases exhibit significantly fewer pathologic findings.

PREVALENCE. Studies in Utah, Brittany (France), and Sweden suggest homozygote frequencies varying between 1/200 to 1/600. This implies a high frequency of the heterozygote state for the disease, ranging from 8 to 13 per cent. Such frequencies make hemochromatosis one of the most common genetic diseases. Since only a certain portion of homozygotes will develop overt clinical findings, the frequency of the clinical disease will usually be lower and was estimated to be roughly 1/5000 in the Pacific Northwest of the United States. More prevalence studies in random populations are required.

CLINICAL MANIFESTATIONS IN THE FULL-BLOWN DISEASE. Because of the long time required to produce organ damage, the onset of clinical disease is usually delayed to the age of 40 to 60. Males are more frequently and earlier affected than menstruating females. The most important clinical signs and symptoms in the fully developed disease include hepatomegaly, skin pigmentation, weakness and malaise, chronic abdominal pain, diabetes, arthropathy, impotence, loss of libido, and nonspecific neurologic symptoms. However, more and more patients in the early stages of the disease with only few or no clinical findings are being discovered.

The *skin pigmentation* causes browning of the skin that is most pronounced in exposed areas and scars. Conjunctival and lid margin pigmentation is seen occasionally and oral pigmentation is more rarely observed. With increasing hemosiderin deposits, the skin takes on a slate-gray appearance.

Hepatomegaly is the most common physical finding and may occur without symptoms and with normal liver function test results. Portal hypertension and esophageal varices are seen less frequently than in Laennec's cirrhosis. Episodes of hepatic failure are rare but may be precipitated by blood loss or surgical procedures. *Splenomegaly* is frequent. Chronic aching *abdominal pain* is common and may be the presenting symptom. Carcinoma of the liver is a relatively frequent late complication. Unfortunately, once cirrhosis has developed, the risk of a malignant hepatoma appears undiminished by iron removal and emphasizes the importance of early case detection and initiation of iron-removing therapy (see below). Dysrhythmia and refractory cardiac failure occur in more than one third of patients and present clinically as *congestive cardiomyopathy.*

Insulin-dependent diabetes is often seen. A family history of diabetes unrelated to iron storage is more common among patients with hemochromatosis than among controls, suggesting expression of a genetic predisposition to diabetes in persons with liver and pancreatic injury. *Arthropathy* different from rheumatoid arthritis and osteoarthritis is common. The second and third metacarpophalangeal joints are usually first involved. Knees, hips, shoulders, and lower back may be affected and acute synovitis with pseudogout of the knees is frequent. X-rays show chondrocalcinosis with small cysts characteristically affecting the second or third metacarpophalangeal joints. Osteoporosis is sometimes observed. *Loss of libido* and sexual impotence with testicular atrophy are common. Scanty body hair may be present long before significant hepatic impairment. Clinically manifest *hypogonadism* is usually of hypogonadotrophic origin. Marked lethargy, increased sleep requirements, and inability to think clearly are frequent complaints. Some patients with severe iron overload are said to have set off metal detection devices used at airports.

DIAGNOSIS. The clinical diagnosis of hemochromatosis requires a high index of suspicion and may be difficult in early cases. Many patients are being detected fortuitously after discovery of saturated transferrin levels performed as part of general workups. Iron overload should be carefully considered among patients (particularly males) who present with any one or a combination of the following: hepatomegaly, idiopathic cardiomyopathy, abnormal skin pigmentation, atypical arthritis, diabetes, impotence, and unexplained chronic abdominal pain. Excessive alcohol intake increases the diagnostic probability. A careful family history should be obtained and diagnostic suspicions should be particularly high when the family history is positive for the various clinical findings that might suggest this disease.

The diagnosis requires several laboratory tests of iron status. The most practical screening test for iron overload is the determination of serum iron and of transferrin saturation. Serum iron is characteristically elevated in patients with hemochromatosis and there is increased saturation of transferrin with iron ranging between 80 and 100 per cent (normal: less than 50 per cent). However, abnormally high transferrin saturation can occur as a result of sample contamination, physiologic plasma iron fluctuation, iron therapy, liver disease, and red cell disorders. A saturated transferrin value is seen early in the course of the disease and does not reflect the extent of iron storage. A valuable noninvasive test to assess iron stores is the measurement of serum ferritin, which correlates reasonably well with the extent of iron storage in the absence of excessive alcohol consumption, inflammation, neoplasia, and liver disease such as that induced by drugs or viral hepatitis. Without such complications, a level above 300 μg/l in males and above 200 μg/l in females indicates increased iron stores and requires further investigation. Patients with fully developed hemochromatosis have levels ranging between 700 and several thousand μg/l. However, rare families with significant iron overload and normal ferritin values have been described. Iron stores can also be assessed by measuring the amount of urinary iron excreted following intramuscular administration of the chelator desferrioxamine (10 mg per kilogram). The amount of urinary iron excreted in 24 hours following this agent is normally less than 3 mg. The quantity of iron excreted is proportional to the amount of stored iron in parenchymal tissues, but the test is not reliable for assessment of relatively early disease.

The definitive test for hemochromatosis is a *liver biopsy.* Parenchymal hemosiderin deposits can be demonstrated histochemically and the actual concentration of iron should be estimated biochemically. The extent of liver damage and cirrhosis can be determined by histologic examination.

DIFFERENTIAL DIAGNOSIS. The most common differential diagnostic problem is raised by alcoholic liver disease not associated with HLA-linked hemochromatosis. Many such patients have an increased amount of stainable liver iron but no increased iron stores. Unlike in genetic hemochromatosis, the iron in such patients is mostly located in reticuloendothelial cells. Liver function abnormalities are more severe than in hemochromatosis. Appropriate tests (including serum ferritin, red cell ferritin, iron excretion following desferrioxamine) can often establish whether there is increased generalized iron storage. HLA testing and studies of iron status in family members may be helpful since familial aggregation and the HLA linkage of idiopathic hemochromatosis are not seen in patients with alcoholic liver disease. Iron overload due to chronic anemias (see below) such as beta thalassemia major rarely raises diagnostic problems, although occasional patients with thalassemia intermedia or sideroblastic anemia with only slightly depressed hematocrits may give diagnostic difficulties. Iron overload (siderosis) caused by ingestion of fermented beverages brewed in iron containers is seen in South African blacks but seldom causes full-blown hemochromatosis.

FAMILY DETECTION FOR PREVENTION. Early treatment can remove increased iron stores that ultimately cause disease. Most importantly, treatment before the onset of cirrhosis probably prevents the high frequency of hepatoma observed in hemochromatosis. All efforts should therefore be made to detect the disease as early as possible. Since the disease is an autosomal recessive trait, there is a 25 per cent chance that sibs of a patient will be similarly affected. All sibs should therefore be tested for HLA status, transferrin saturation, and serum ferritin. If the characteristic iron metabolism abnormalities and full identity in HLA status are found, a liver biopsy should be performed to assess the extent of iron storage. With iron overload, phlebotomies to remove iron should be initiated. Sib testing should be initiated at about puberty for males and after the age of 20 years for females. HLA identical male sibs found to have a normal iron load should be restudied every two to three years, females somewhat less frequently. Frequent blood donations (three times a year) will prevent potentially toxic iron accumulation and are recommended by some authorities for HLA identical sibs. Parents and children of affected patients are obligate heterozygote carriers. Since the gene frequency of hemochromatosis appears to be high, matings of homozygotes with heterozygotes are not uncommon and one half of the offspring of such couples will be homozygotes (pseudodominant transmission). Thus, a parent or a child of a patient with hemochromatosis may also be a homozygote. Family detection therefore should include the entire family.

Occasionally, differentiation of heterozygotes from affected homozygotes may be difficult by serum ferritin and transferrin testing alone. HLA status will aid in such cases since heterozygotes usually share only one half their HLA haplotypes with their homozygote sibs. Treatment to remove iron is rarely if ever required in heterozygotes.

TREATMENT. Excess iron can usually be removed by periodic venesections. The removal of one unit (approximately 500 ml) of blood depletes the body of 200 to 250 mg of iron. Weekly venesections are required for about two to three years to return iron stores to normal levels in patients with the full-blown disease and for lesser periods for those with early disease. Even though there is no scientific or medical contraindication to using blood from hemochromatic patients for blood transfusions, many blood banks do not use such blood. Myocardial irritability may be an occasional problem during the initial venesections. Beta-adrenergic blocking agents and continuous infusion of desferrioxamine during venesection may aid in counteracting these effects. After several months, cardiac function usually improves.

Treatment should be monitored by frequent hematocrit determinations and plasma iron and ferritin levels six to ten times per year (Fig. 206–2). After an initial fall, hematocrit levels stabilize at approximately 90 per cent of pretreatment levels. Indicators of iron status do not change until significant depletion of iron stores has occurred. After iron stores have been normalized as shown by ferritin and transferrin levels, venesections are required at two to three month intervals to prevent reaccumulation of iron. An iron-free diet is not necessary at any time during treatment. Treatment of hepatic, cardiac, endocrinologic, and metabolic complications is along conventional lines. Many manifestations of hemochromatosis *except* for hypogonadism, arthropathy, portal hypertension, cirrhosis, and hepatoma are dramatically improved by phlebotomy therapy.

PROGNOSIS. The five-year survival rate after diagnosis in untreated patients with the fully developed disease is 18 per cent and the ten-year survival rate 6 per cent. The principal cause of death in such patients relates to liver complications: hepatic failure and portal hypertension (30 per cent) and malignant hepatoma (30 per cent). An additional one third of patients die of cardiac failure.

With removal of iron, the five-year survival is 66 per cent and ten-year survival 32 per cent. Results are poorer in alcoholic patients. The prognosis is likely to improve as patients in the early stages of iron overload are treated. It is noteworthy that hepatoma has never been reported in individuals with hemochromatosis who had not developed cirrhosis.

SECONDARY HEMOCHROMATOSIS. Classic hemochromatosis with iron deposits of parenchymal cells of the liver and other organs is observed in a variety of anemias associated with erythroid hyperplasia of the bone marrow when delivery of viable red cells to the circulation is defective (ineffective erythropoiesis). Beta thalassemia major (or beta thalassemia/Hb E disease in Southeast Asia) is the most common anemia of this type. Severe iron loading secondary to ineffective erythropoiesis and increased iron absorption occurs already before transfusion therapy. Repeated blood transfusions produce further iron overload. In contrast to the HLA-linked hemochromatosis, iron overload in beta thalassemia major is relatively rapid and

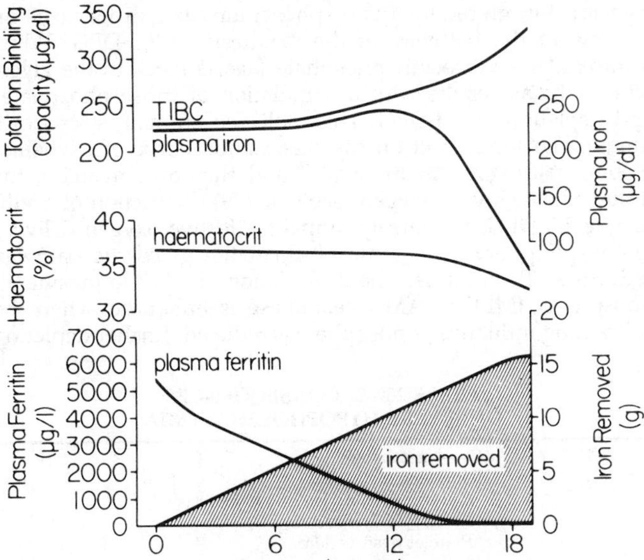

Figure 206–2. Serial changes in the hematocrit, plasma iron concentration, total iron-binding capacity, and plasma ferritin concentration in a subject with idiopathic hemochromatosis on repeated venesection therapy. (From Bothwell TH, Charlton RW, Cook JD, Finch CA: Idiopathic haemochromatosis. *In* Iron Metabolism in Man. Oxford, Blackwell Scientific Publications, 1979.)

causes clinical symptoms early in life. Hepatic fibrosis is already common in children as is retarded growth and delayed puberty. Cardiac death usually occurs in adolescence or early adulthood unless iron removal is carried out.

Phlebotomies cannot be done since these patients are severely anemic. Desferrioxamine therapy together with frequent transfusions has improved the prognosis markedly. While the long-term consequences of prolonged parenteral chelation therapy remain unknown, it is likely that death due to complications of iron storage can be prevented if iron removal can be initiated before clinical signs and symptoms of iron overload appear. Since effective chelation therapy is expensive and complex, there is urgent need for the development of oral chelating agents.

Patients with hypoplastic anemias do not absorb increased amounts of iron but often require blood transfusions over prolonged periods of time. The transfused iron is largely stored in macrophages. No clinical signs or symptoms occur with storage of iron in macrophages. Redistribution to parenchymal cells with development of hepatic cirrhosis and/or other typical organ involvement occurs rarely.

Bothwell TH, Charlton RW, Cook JD, Finch CA: Idiopathic haemochromatosis. *In* Iron Metabolism in Man. Oxford, Blackwell Scientific Publications, Ltd., 1979, pp 121–155. *A detailed discussion with special attention to iron metabolism.*

Bothwell TH, Charlton RW, Motulsky AG: Idiopathic hemochromatosis. *In* Stanbury JB, Wyngaarden JB, Fredrickson DS, Goldstein JL, Brown MS (eds.): The Metabolic Basis of Inherited Disease. 5th ed. New York, McGraw-Hill Book Company, 1983, pp 1269–1298. *A full discussion of all aspects of iron metabolism and genetics in HLA-linked and secondary hemochromatosis.*

Edwards CO, Cartwright GE, Skolnick MH, Amos DB: Homozygosity for hemochromatosis: Clinical manifestations. Ann Intern Med 93:519, 1980. *The widening spectrum of hemochromatosis after family detection.*

Finch CA, Huebers H: Perspectives in iron metabolism. N Engl J Med 306:1520, 1982. *Excellent overview of the pathophysiology of iron metabolism providing the rationale for pathogenesis and treatment.*

Halliday JW, Powell LW: Iron overload. Semin Hematol 19:42, 1982. *A balanced discussion of all aspects of idiopathic and secondary hemochromatosis.*

Milder MS, Cook JD, Stray S, Finch CA: Idiopathic hemochromatosis, an interim report. Medicine 59:34, 1980. *Clinical features and treatment of idiopathic hemochromatosis based on 34 cases.*

Olsson KS, Ritter B, Rosen U, Heedman PA, Staugard F: Prevalence of iron overload in Central Sweden. Acta Med Scand 213:145, 1983. *Random population survey by ferritin and transferrin saturation levels in a country with iron fortification. Three of 623 males aged 32 to 39 had genetic hemochromatosis.*

Simon M, Bourel M, Genetet B, Fauchet R: Idiopathic hemochromatosis. Demonstration of recessive transmission and early detection by family HLA typing. N Engl J Med 297:1017, 1977. *Data to support HLA linkage and review of the inheritance of hemochromatosis with practical recommendations.*

207. PHOSPHORUS DEFICIENCY AND HYPOPHOSPHATEMIA

Lloyd H. Smith, Jr.

Phosphorus is necessary for the structural and functional integrity of all living things. In hydroxyapatite it is a key constituent of bone; as a part of phospholipids (lecithin, sphingomyelin) it is necessary for the structure of all cell membranes, both external and internal (endoplasmic reticulum, lysosomes, nuclear membranes). It furnishes the backbone of nucleic acids, captures and stores metabolic energy (~P), serves as a second messenger in endocrinology (cAMP, cGMP), regulates the release of O_2 by hemoglobin (2,3-diphosphoglycerate), and buffers urine. Even this partial list indicates that a severe deficiency of phosphorus would lead to widespread and serious consequences.

In an adult of average size there are approximately 700 to 800 grams (25 moles) of phosphorus, of which 80 to 85 per cent is in the skeleton and 10 per cent in muscle. Phosphate is the major anion of intracellular fluid (about 100 mM), where it is found mostly as phosphoproteins, phospholipids, or phosphosugars rather than as free orthophosphate. In extracellular fluid the normal concentration of phosphorus in adults is 2.7 to 4.5 mg per deciliter (0.9 to 1.5 mM), of which most is free; perhaps

10 per cent is protein bound. Serum phosphorus is normally higher in children (4.0 to 7.0 mg per deciliter). (It is conventional to express serum phosphate as the amount of elemental P, since pH influences the relative amounts of $H_2PO_4^-$ and $HPO_4^=$ present.) The average American diet contains about 1000 mg P, most of which is absorbed by active transport, increased by 1,25-dihydroxycholecalciferol. Approximately 90 per cent of that absorbed from the diet is excreted in the urine by a process involving filtration and partial renal tubular reabsorption. The tubular reabsorption of phosphate is diminished by parathyroid hormone (PTH), acting with cAMP as a second messenger. Through vitamin D, PTH, calcitonin, and the mineralization of osteoid, phosphate metabolism is closely linked with that of calcium. These interrelationships are discussed more completely in Ch. 243.

Hyperphosphatemia occurs almost exclusively in three clinical conditions: (1) renal insufficiency (see Ch. 77), (2) hypoparathyroidism (including various types of pseudohypoparathyroidism) (see Ch. 246) and (3) acromegaly or gigantism (see Ch. 225). When severe, hyperphosphatemia may contribute to the acidosis of uremia, further reduce the extracellular fluid concentration of ionized calcium, or lead to metastatic calcification in extraosseous sites.

CAUSES OF HYPOPHOSPHATEMIA. Hypophosphatemia (serum P <2.7 mg per deciliter) may be associated with a normal total body phosphate (representing a transient intracellular shift) or with phosphate deficiency. The two most common causes of transient hypophosphatemia are (1) ingestion of carbohydrates, which deplete phosphate in ECF in the process of their intracellular transport and metabolism, and (2) acute respiratory alkalosis, which leads to an intracellular shift of phosphate through mechanisms not fully explained.

It is convenient to summarize the causes of hypophosphatemia as those that usually result in only moderate reductions in serum P (1.0 to 2.5 mg per deciliter) and those that may result in severe hypophosphatemia (P <1.0 mg per deciliter) (Table 207–1). The latter may also be associated with lesser degrees of phosphate depletion as well.

Moderate hypophosphatemia may occur transiently during carbohydrate metabolism or alkalosis, as noted above, in the absence of phosphate depletion. Increased PTH, associated with either primary or secondary hyperparathyroidism, reduces the renal tubular reabsorption of phosphate and leads to renal phosphate wasting. In familial hypophosphatemic rickets there may be a primary defect in the renal tubular reabsorption of phosphate. The association of hypophosphatemia with hyperparathyroidism and the various types of osteomalacia or rickets is discussed more fully in Ch. 245 and 246. Hypomagnesemia and ECF volume expansion may result in reduced renal tubular reabsorption of phosphate and mild hypophosphatemia. Hemodialysis with equilibration against a dialysate deficient in phosphate may lead to overshoot hypophosphatemia. There are no well defined acute metabolic consequences of moderate hypophosphatemia. Prolonged hypophosphatemia in this range may result in the defective mineralization of bone characteristic of osteomalacia or rickets.

Severe hypophosphatemia may cause serious metabolic consequences as described below. The most frequent cause of severe hypophosphatemia in clinical practice is *alcoholism,* especially during the withdrawal phase. The causes of phosphate depletion in alcoholics are complex and may include (1) poor dietary intake, (2) vomiting, (3) diarrhea, (4) the use of antacids which bind phosphate and reduce its absorption, (5) a possible phosphaturic effect of ethanol itself, (6) magnesium deficiency with phosphaturia, and (7) calcium deficiency with secondary hyperparathyroidism. The serum P level may be further reduced by the hyperventilation characteristic of alcohol withdrawal and by the therapeutic infusion of glucose. Patients with *uncontrolled diabetes mellitus* often become phosphate depleted through catabolism of intracellular organic phosphates and phosphaturia secondary to osmotic diuresis. Initial serum P levels are often normal or even high during diabetic ketoacidosis, but rapidly fall to hypophosphatemic levels during the first six to twelve hours of treatment with volume expansion, glucose, and insulin. Hyperventilation with *marked respiratory alkalosis* can cause profound hypophosphatemia within minutes; metabolic alkalosis of the same degree causes only moderate hypophosphatemia. Excessive ingestion of *phosphate binding antacids,* such as aluminum hydroxide, may inhibit phosphate absorption from the intestine sufficiently to cause chronic depletion, especially when combined with reduced dietary ingestion of phosphate. Excessive utilization of phosphate during tissue repletion may occasionally result in severe hypophosphatemia during *hyperalimentation* (without adequate supplementary P) and during the *nutritional recovery syndrome* of refeeding patients with protein-calorie malnutrition or starvation. Whatever its cause, severe hypophosphatemia requires early attention because of its potential consequences.

CONSEQUENCES OF SEVERE HYPOPHOSPHATEMIA (Table 207–2). The long-term consequences of severe hypophosphatemia are largely structural, those of metabolic bone disease (see Ch. 245). The acute consequences may be considered to be metabolic, although the distinction is an arbitrary one.

Red cell dysfunction in severe hypophosphatemia may result from two biochemical abnormalities, depletion of intracellular 2,3-diphosphoglycerate (2,3-DPG) and of ATP. Phosphate is a cofactor for glyceraldehyde-3-phosphate dehydrogenase, an enzyme in the pathway of the synthesis of 2,3-DPG. When intracellular erythrocytic phosphate falls, a block in the glycolytic pathway results with accumulation of triose phosphates and depletion of 2,3-DPG. This molecule normally exercises a unique allosteric effect on the dissociation curve of oxyhemoglobin, shifting it "to the right" and thereby enhancing the tissue availability of oxygen (see Ch. 139). Reduction of erythrocytic 2,3-DPG, conversely, impairs effective oxygen delivery to the periphery. The same block in the glycolytic pathway reduces ATP synthesis. The degradation of AMP to inosine 5′-phosphate (IMP) by AMP deaminase is enhanced when the restraining influence of phosphate is reduced, further depleting

TABLE 207–1. CAUSES OF HYPOPHOSPHATEMIA*

Moderate hypophosphatemia (P 1.0 to 2.5 mg per deciliter)
- Hyperparathyroidism
- Osteomalacia (usually with hyperparathyroidism), malabsorption, deficiency of vitamin D, familial hypophosphatemic rickets, vitamin D dependent rickets, oncogenic rickets
- Carbohydrate administration or ingestion or enhanced metabolism—glucose, fructose, glycerol, lactate, insulin administration
- Hypomagnesemia
- ECF volume expansion
- Acute alkalosis—bicarbonate infusion or moderate hyperventilation
- Hemodialysis

Severe hypophosphatemia (P less than 1.0 mg per deciliter)
- Chronic alcoholism and alcoholic withdrawal
- Diabetic ketoacidosis, recovery phase
- Enteric phosphate binding—excessive use of agents binding phosphate in the gut
- Hyperalimentation
- Nutritional recovery syndrome

*Modified from Knochel JP: West J Med 134:15, 1981.

TABLE 207–2. CONSEQUENCES OF SEVERE HYPOPHOSPHATEMIA

Acute—"metabolic"
- Hematologic
  - Red cell dysfunction and hemolysis
  - Leukocyte dysfunction
  - Platelet dysfunction
- Muscle
  - Weakness
  - Rhabdomyolysis
  - Myocardial dysfunction
- Central nervous system dysfunction
- Hepatic dysfunction

Chronic—"structural"
- Osteomalacia or rickets

the intracellular concentration of adenine nucleotides. As a result the concentration of erythrocytic ATP tends to fall in parallel with the reduction of serum phosphorus. At a critical level of ATP (usually with serum P <0.5 mg per deciliter), the energy metabolism of the erythrocyte may become inadequate to maintain the integrity of its membrane and *hemolysis* may occur.

Leukocyte dysfunction has been demonstrated during phosphate depletion in experimental animals, characterized by impaired chemotaxis, phagocytosis, and bactericidal function. These defects presumably result from inadequate ATP for normal cellular functions, possibly including the synthesis of phospholipids in membranes. Similarly *platelet dysfunction* occurs in experimental phosphate depletion, but no hemorrhagic diathesis has been attributed to phosphate deficiency in man.

Many patients with severe hypophosphatemia complain of *weakness*, but this is nonspecific and difficult to delineate from that caused by the associated disorder. *Rhabdomyolysis* is an occasional complication of severe hypophosphatemia, perhaps being somewhat analogous to hemolytic anemia in its pathogenesis, i.e., related to deficiency of ATP. The severity of rhabdomyolysis varies from that manifested solely by an elevated serum level of "muscle enzymes" (aldolase and creatine phosphokinase) to a full-fledged syndrome of muscle weakness, pain, tenderness, and stiffness associated with myoglobinuria (see Ch. 539). Interestingly, the release of phosphate from the necrosis of muscle may suffice to return the serum P level to normal. A few patients with severe phosphate depletion have exhibited congestive cardiomyopathy, which has seemed to respond to phosphate repletion. These clinical observations are strengthened by the demonstration of decreased myocardial contractility during experimental phosphate depletion in dogs.

Severe hypophosphatemia may result in *central nervous system dysfunction* with a constellation of symptoms and signs designated as metabolic brain disease or metabolic encephalopathy (see Ch. 472). These abnormalities may vary from irritability, weakness, and paresthesias to obtundation, seizures, and coma. It is presumed that this CNS dysfunction results from deranged energy metabolism of the brain secondary to ATP depletion. Observations have suggested that hepatic function is further impaired in alcoholics with severe hypophosphatemia, with early improvement during replacement therapy, but a clinical entity of *hypophosphatemic hepatic dysfunction* has not yet been well established.

TREATMENT OF HYPOPHOSPHATEMIA. The treatment of hypophosphatemia depends upon its cause, its acuteness, and its severity. Hypophosphatemia caused by acute respiratory alkalosis or the infusion of carbohydrates does not require replacement therapy. Chronic hypophosphatemia associated with aluminum hydroxide therapy, for example, may require reduction of the antacid and an oral source of supplemental phosphate such as milk (1 gram of P or 30 to 35 mmole per quart) or a balanced solution of phosphate salts (sodium or potassium salts as in Fleet's enema solution or Neutraphos). It is rare that hypophosphatemia is so acute and severe as to require parenteral replacement therapy. When such treatment is undertaken it is well to remember that (1) it is unusual for hypophosphatemia to cause metabolic disturbances at concentrations >1.0 mg per deciliter, so full parenteral replacement is neither necessary nor desirable; and (2) if hyperphosphatemia results, there is a danger of producing a fall in ionized calcium (with tetany or convulsions) and/or metastatic calcification of soft tissues. It is usually safe and sufficient to administer intravenously 1 mmole of phosphate per kilogram of body weight evenly over a 24-hour period in the treatment of acute, severe hypophosphatemia associated with phosphate depletion. Since potassium depletion is so frequently associated with phosphate depletion both in alcoholics and in patients with diabetic ketoacidosis, it may be useful as a guideline to give half of parenterally administered potassium as its phosphate salt. Obviously parenteral phosphate should not be given in the face of hyperphosphatemia.

DeFronzo RA, Lang R: Hypophosphatemia and glucose intolerance: Evidence for tissue insensitivity to insulin. N Engl J Med 303:1259, 1980. *In an interesting clinical study hypophosphatemia was found to cause glucose intolerance and insulin resistance in six nondiabetic subjects. This observation further enhances the importance of treating hypophosphatemia in the management of diabetic ketoacidosis.*

Fitzgerald FT: Hypophosphatemia. Adv Intern Med 23:137, 1978. Janson C, Birnbaum G, Baker FJ: Hypophosphatemia. Ann Emerg Med 12:107, 1983. Knochel JP: Hypophosphatemia. West J Med 134:15, 1981. *These three articles give excellent general reviews of the clinical and pathophysiologic aspects of phosphate deficiency syndromes in man and related disorders produced in experimental animals. They have useful bibliographies that allow the reader to pursue in depth the available information about each specific syndrome described above.*

208. DISORDERS OF MAGNESIUM METABOLISM

Lloyd H. Smith, Jr.

Magnesium is the fourth most common cation in the human body (after sodium, potassium, and calcium) and the cation in second highest concentration intracellularly. The average adult body contains about 25 grams (1000 mmole) of magnesium, of which 50 to 60 per cent is in bone. The normal serum magnesium concentration is 1.6 to 2.1 mEq per liter, approximately one fourth to one third being protein bound. The average American diet contains approximately 500 mg (20 mmole) of magnesium, much of this in chlorophyll. It has been estimated that about 0.15 mmole (3.5 to 4.5 mg) of dietary magnesium per kilogram per day is necessary to maintain a positive balance in adults. More is required in children. Magnesium is actively absorbed in the small intestine by a process that is enhanced by 1,25-dihydroxycholecalciferol, resulting in a net absorption of about 30 to 40 per cent of that ingested. This net absorption is balanced at equilibrium by renal excretion, which reflects filtration of the 65 to 75 per cent not protein bound followed by net renal tubular reabsorption of approximately 95 per cent. The kidney can control the excretion of magnesium over a wide range—from more than 250 mmole to less than 1 mmole per day. The factors that control the renal tubular reabsorption of magnesium are not completely understood but include sodium excretion, calcium excretion, parathyroid hormone, and ECF volume. Excretion is also increased by ethanol and by many diuretic agents.

Magnesium has a structural role in bone crystal. It also serves as an activator of a large number of specific enzymes. Of particular importance it is a cofactor in all transphosphorylation reactions involving ATP, so that it is intimately involved in energy metabolism and the synthesis of macromolecules, for example. Perhaps even more basic in biology is its obligate role in the function of chlorophyll. By and large it has not been possible to correlate the signs or symptoms of magnesium deficiency or excess with any one of its specific biochemical functions.

HYPERMAGNESEMIA. Because of the ability of the normal kidney to excrete a magnesium load, significant hypermagnesemia is rarely seen in clinical practice. In the past magnesium ion was occasionally infused as a hypotensive agent in the treatment of acute hypertension with the secondary production of symptomatic hypermagnesemia. In patients with renal insufficiency the excessive use of magnesium, as in magnesium-containing antacids, may cause hypermagnesemia. The manifestations of hypermagnesemia are largely in the central nervous system and the cardiovascular system. Ionized magnesium is a sedative which depresses the function of the central nervous system and exerts a curare-like effect on the neuromuscular junction at high concentrations (>10 mEq per liter). The cardiovascular effects of hypermagnesemia are those of peripheral vasodilatation resulting in hypotension, generalized depression of the cardiac conduction system, bradyrhythmias, and asystole with cardiac arrest in diastole. The cardiac effects of Mg^{++} are usually manifested at serum concentration >10 mEq per liter with asystole at levels >25 mEq per liter, but a few patients have exhibited exceptional sensitivity with cardiotoxicity at levels of 4.5 to 5.5 mEq per liter. Factors which augment the cardiotoxicity of Mg^{++} include hypocalcemia, hyperkalemia, acidosis, digitalis therapy, and renal insufficiency (beyond its effect on the serum Mg^{++} level). Treatment of hypermagnesemia is usually limited to discontinuing its exogenous source. In severe hypermagnesemia, intravenous treatment with calcium may temporarily reverse many of the toxic effects because of the pharmacologic antagonism of ionized calcium and magnesium in the central nervous system.

HYPOMAGNESEMIA. Hypomagnesemia is a much more frequent metabolic derangement than hypermagnesemia, and usually occurs as one component of a complex deficiency state, affecting many minerals, vitamins, and nutrients.

Causes of Hypomagnesemia. Magnesium deficiency and hypomagnesemia result from decreased absorption or from increased excretion (Table 208–1). Very rarely it may result from "loss" into bone during excessive osteogenesis, the "hungry bone syndrome," during the repair of osteitis fibrosa generalisata following the removal of a parathyroid tumor (see Ch. 246). In general, decreased absorption of magnesium occurs in the same circumstances as does decreased calcium absorption, especially caused by dietary deficiency and malabsorption syndromes of whatever origin. Decreased absorption in uremia may result from deficiency of 1,25-dihydroxycholecalciferol. A few infants have been described with convulsions associated with hypocalcemia and hypomagnesemia in the absence of renal magnesium wasting. They have responded to continued high ingestion of magnesium, but not of calcium, and are thought to have a selective defect in gut absorption of magnesium. It is not clear whether ethanol diminishes magnesium absorption directly or only through diminished ingestion or vitamin D deficiency.

Increased loss of magnesium can occur from excessive vomiting, from diarrhea, or via the kidney. Rarely patients may exhibit what appears to be an inherited renal tubular defect in magnesium reabsorption. These patients have tended to have potassium wasting as well and to present with hypokalemia, hypomagnesemia, and hypocalcemia (secondary to hypomagnesemia). In general magnesium clearance tends to parallel that of sodium and calcium, and may be increased by diuretics (osmotic, thiazides, ethacrynic acid, furosemide), by ionized calcium, and possibly by ethanol. Renal magnesium wasting has been described during therapy with gentamicin and cisplatinum. The magnesium wasting of uncontrolled diabetes mellitus probably results from tissue catabolism and osmotic diuresis. Lactation hypomagnesemia is well described in cattle and has been documented in one woman whose serum Mg^{++} fell to 0.4 mEq per liter.

Consequences of Hypomagnesemia. Hypomagnesemia rarely occurs as a single deficiency so that it is not always possible to distinguish its signs and symptoms from those of associated deficiency states. Selective magnesium deficiency has been produced experimentally in man, however, and it is based on these observations together with clinical correlations on patients that the spectrum of manifestations listed in Table 208–2 has been described. Patients with magnesium deficiency are lethargic, weak, and irritable with decreased attention span. They may have tetany with positive Chvostek and Trousseau signs because of associated hypocalcemia (see below). In experimental magnesium deficiency, muscles are weak and may show hyaline and vacuolar degeneration of myofibers, sometimes followed by leukocytic infiltration, segmental necrosis, and early calcification. Patients with hypomagnesemia are generally anorectic and may have nausea, vomiting, and poor intestinal mobility. Hypomagnesemia may occur in congestive heart failure because of anorexia, malabsorption, and the excessive use of diuretic agents. Magnesium deficiency increases the sensitivity of the heart to digitalis glycosides so that digitalis toxicity occurs at a lower serum level and also tends to persist longer. Some believe that hypomagnesemia also causes tachyrhythmias, but this has been difficult to establish because other abnormalities generally coexist, especially hypokalemia.

TABLE 208–1. CAUSES OF HYPOMAGNESEMIA (SEEN MOST FREQUENTLY CLINICALLY IN ALCOHOLISM AND MALABSORPTION)

Decreased absorption from dietary sources
Diet poor in magnesium
Parenteral feeding without magnesium
Ethanol effect on absorption
Malabsorption syndromes
Uremia
Selective intestinal defect for magnesium absorption (rare)
Increased loss of magnesium from the body
Gastrointestinal tract
Kidney
Primary renal tubular defects
Secondary—diuretics, Ca^{++}, ethanol, expansion of ECF, diabetes mellitus, treatment with gentamicin, cis-platinum, or amphotericin
Breast—lactation hypomagnesemia (mostly in cattle, rarely in humans)
Increased loss into bone ("hungry bone syndrome")

TABLE 208–2. CONSEQUENCES OF MAGNESIUM DEFICIENCY

Neuromuscular
Lethargy, weakness, fatigue, decreased mentation
Neuromuscular irritability, in part due to associated hypocalcemia
Hyaline and vacuolar degeneration of myofibers with segmental necrosis
Gastrointestinal
Anorexia, nausea, vomiting
Paralytic ileus
Cardiovascular
Increased sensitivity to digitalis glycosides
Possible cause of tachyarrhythmias
Metabolic
Hypocalcemia—probably due to the combined result of decreased PTH secretion and decreased end organ responsiveness to PTH
Hypokalemia—tendency toward renal potassium wasting

Magnesium metabolism has a number of interesting interrelationships with that of calcium: (1) both are absorbed by the gut through mechanisms enhanced by vitamin D; (2) excess magnesium may inhibit calcium absorption, but not vice versa; (3) calcium and magnesium may compete for renal tubular reabsorption; (4) calcium and magnesium are physiologic antagonists in the central nervous system; and (5) magnesium is necessary for the normal secretion of parathyroid hormone (PTH) in response to hypocalcemia and also for the activity of PTH as a hormone at the site of its target organs. *Hypocalcemia* is one of the most consistent and important findings in magnesium deficiency with hypomagnesemia. Hypocalcemia responds promptly to magnesium replacement and is accompanied by a rise in plasma PTH. A burst of PTH secretion occurs within minutes after the infusion of magnesium intravenously into patients with combined hypocalcemia and hypomagnesemia. Many of these patients show evidence of resistance to exogenous PTH as well. Hypomagnesemia therefore results in a complex combination of hypoparathyroidism and acquired pseudohypoparathyroidism. This entity should be suspected especially in alcoholics or patients with malabsorption who present with hypocalcemia. *Hypokalemia* is frequently found with hypomagnesemia. Although some of the conditions that cause magnesium depletion also produce potassium depletion, there is evidence that magnesium deficiency itself enhances renal excretion of potassium. This associated hypokalemia is usually resistant to potassium replacement unless magnesium is replaced first.

Treatment of Hypomagnesemia. The treatment of hypomagnesemia is rarely an acute emergency. When rapid replacement therapy is judged to be vital (convulsions, tachyrhythmias), 2 grams of $MgSO_4$ (16.3 mEq) can be given intravenously over several minutes. This can be followed by a constant intravenous infusion of approximately 1 mEq of magnesium per kilogram per 24 hours, which usually suffices for initial replacement therapy. Ampules often contain 1.0 gram of $MgSO_4 \cdot 7H_2O$ which is 8.1 mEq Mg, so that initial replacement therapy usually requires 8 to 10 grams of $MgSO_4$ given either intravenously as above or intramuscularly as 2.0 grams every four hours for five doses. After the first day approximately 0.5 mEq of Mg per kilogram per 24 hours should be given intravenously or intramuscularly for two to five days, based on the return of the serum magnesium level to normal. Parenteral replacement therapy is often preferable to oral therapy because of the tendency of magnesium salts to cause diarrhea. When renal function is impaired, the aforementioned schedules for magnesium replacement must be followed with extra caution and with careful monitoring of serum levels. When there is chronic loss of magnesium (renal wasting, for example) oral therapy is preferred and can be carried out with various preparations as tolerated without diarrhea—magnesium hydroxide tablets, magnesium acetate solution, or liquid milk of magnesia.

Cronin RE, Knochel JP: Magnesium deficiency. Adv Intern Med 28:509, 1983. *An excellent recent general review of magnesium metabolism and the pathophysiology of magnesium deficiency (102 references).*

Dirko JH: The kidney and magnesium regulation. Kidney Int 23:771, 1983. *A succinct review of the role of the kidney in magnesium metabolism and of the causes of hypomagnesemia (36 references).*

Levine BS, Coburn JW: Magnesium, the mimac/antagonist of calcium. N Engl J Med 310:1253, 1984. *A recent editorial about the complex interactions of these important cations.*

Shils ME: Experimental production of magnesium deficiency in man. Ann NY Acad Sci 162:847, 1969. *This classic paper describes the experimental production of magnesium deficiency in human subjects by rigid control of dietary intake (0.7 mEq Mg per day). It is still the standard reference for the chemical and clinical abnormalities of magnesium deficiency, with careful documentation of the symptoms which developed over one and a half to nine months of dietary deficiency.*

Wacker WEC: Magnesium and Man. Cambridge, Mass., Harvard University Press, 1980. *A short monograph (171 pages) that is the most complete summary of normal and abnormal Mg metabolism in man.*

Other Hereditary Disorders

209. FAMILIAL MEDITERRANEAN FEVER

Anthony S. Fauci

DEFINITION. Familial Mediterranean fever, also called *paroxysmal polyserositis, familial recurrent polyserositis,* or *periodic fever,* is an inherited disease characterized by acute self-limited attacks of fever accompanied by peritonitis, pleuritis, and arthritis. The attacks recur at irregular, unpredictable intervals and do not manifest true periodicity.

ETIOLOGY. The etiology of familial Mediterranean fever remains unknown. Because psychologic stress may precipitate attacks and because many patients have secondary psychologic abnormalities, it has been suggested that psychologic factors may play a primary role in the etiology of the disease. There is no good evidence for this concept.

INCIDENCE, PREVALENCE, AND GENETICS. The disease occurs predominantly in patients of Mediterranean or Middle East origin, particularly Sephardic or non-Ashkenazic Jews, Armenians, Arabs, and Turks. It is also seen less commonly in other parts of the world and in Italians, Greeks, Anglo-Saxons, and others.

The disease appears to be inherited as a single autosomal recessive trait. There is a male:female predominance of 3:2.

PATHOLOGY. The pathologic findings related to the acute attack are nonspecific. Serosal exudates from peritoneum, pleura, and joint spaces contain predominantly polymorphonuclear leukocytes. In addition, biopsy specimens of serosal surfaces such as peritoneum show acute inflammation. Inflammatory attacks may result in secondary adhesions. In particular, intra-abdominal adhesions may result in mechanical obstruction of bowel.

The most striking and serious histopathologic findings relate to the amyloidosis which accompanies certain cases of familial Mediterranean fever. Amyloid is deposited in the intima and media of arterioles, as well as the subendothelial region of venules in all organs. In addition, there is a characteristic pattern of parenchymal distribution of amyloid, including extensive involvement of renal glomeruli, adrenals, spleen, and pulmonary alveolar septa, with remarkable sparing of the liver sinusoids and heart muscle.

CLINICAL MANIFESTATIONS. Characteristically, patients appear and feel quite normal until their first attack, which in most cases is during the first or second decade. Rarely, onset may be in infancy or as late as the fifth or sixth decade. The acute attacks are of short duration, usually lasting from 24 to 48 hours but occasionally for several days. Between attacks, patients are normal. The duration and particularly the frequency of attacks vary considerably among patients and in the same patient. Attacks usually occur once or twice a month. However, some patients have attacks as frequently as one to two per week or as infrequently as one per year. Rarely, some patients have no attacks for years and then resume the more frequent pattern. Freedom from attacks is characteristic during pregnancy, with resumption of episodes post partum.

The acute attack is characterized in most cases by fever, which may reach as high as 39 to 40° C. Rarely, the fever may occur without symptoms of serositis, but it usually occurs with other classic findings of peritonitis, pleuritis, or arthritis. The peritoneal attack is the most common, occurring in more than 95 per cent of patients. The intensity of symptoms is quite variable, but in its severe form the attack is characterized by pain that begins locally and then spreads over the entire abdomen, gaining in intensity. It may be associated with abdominal distention, rigidity, rebound tenderness, and ileus. Abdominal x-rays may reveal small fluid levels and bowel wall edema. Nausea and vomiting sometimes occur. Because this pattern is indistinguishable from an acute abdominal catastrophe, many patients have undergone laparotomy, some more than once.

Approximately 75 to 85 per cent of patients develop attacks resembling acute febrile pleuritis with pleuritic pain (usually unilateral), diminished breath sounds, and small pleural effusions.

Acute arthritis during one or more attacks is seen in up to 75 per cent of Israeli patients. However, frank arthritis is much less common in the United States. When arthritis occurs, it usually involves a single large joint, particularly the knee. Arthritic attacks usually last a few days but may assume a protracted course of weeks or, rarely, months. Radiologic findings are nonspecific, including reversible soft tissue swelling, mild osteoporosis, and occasionally osteoarthritic changes (in chronic attacks).

Erysipelas-like skin lesions occur in approximately 25 per cent of patients. They are characterized by painful, rather sharply circumscribed, patchy areas of erythema and swelling, usually on the lower extremity below the knee.

The most serious and dreaded complication of this disease is amyloidosis, which is progressive and usually leads to death in renal failure. A high proportion of Turkish and Israeli patients develop amyloidosis. In Israel, this complication has caused death in adolescence and even earlier. More than 90 per cent of patients in Israel are of phenotype I, in which the acute attacks precede amyloidosis. In phenotype II, amyloidosis precedes the acute attacks, negating the concept that recurrent febrile or inflammatory episodes lead to amyloidosis in this disease.

Amyloidosis is rarely seen in the United States as a complication of familial Mediterranean fever, although there are many Jews of different ethnic subgroups, Armenians, and others with the disease in this country. The explanation for this difference is unknown, but it strongly suggests the interrelationship of environmental or other factors with genetic factors in the development of amyloidosis in this disease.

Laboratory findings are nonspecific. During acute attacks, these include an elevated erythrocyte sedimentation rate, leukocytosis (up to 30,000 per cubic millimeter), and elevated acute phase reactants. Laboratory findings with amyloidosis reflect the resulting nephrotic syndrome and renal failure.

DIAGNOSIS. When characteristic recurrent self-limited attacks occur in a person of appropriate ethnic background, the diagnosis is not difficult. However, because of frequent failure to think of the diagnosis, patients still go undiagnosed for substantial periods of time, and may be subjected to one or more laparotomies.

An abdominal attack must be differentiated from the spectrum of acute abdominal disorders, particularly appendicitis, pancreatitis, cholecystitis, and intestinal obstruction. Porphyria and hyperlipidemias with acute abdominal symptoms must also be considered.

Pleural attacks may closely mimic acute infections or pulmonary emboli with infarction, whereas joint manifestations may resemble the acute infectious and noninfectious arthritides.

Patients with this disease who present with fever alone are quite rare, and all ultimately manifest serositis. In such a patient, an orderly approach to a fever of unknown origin should be undertaken.

TREATMENT. During acute attacks symptomatic and supportive measures are indicated. Because of the recurrent nature of the disease, narcotics should be avoided except in unusual circumstances.

Colchicine* should be started at the first prodromal indication of an attack. Such a regimen has been shown to abort attacks in some patients. The dosage is 0.6 mg every hour for four hours, then every two hours for four hours, and then every 12 hours for two days. The mechanism of colchicine effect in this disease is uncertain, although it is speculated that this drug interferes with the cellular phase of the inflammatory response.

Prophylactic use of colchicine will reduce the number of acute attacks in most but not all patients. A dose of 0.6 mg three times a day by mouth is most effective; if patients develop gastrointestinal symptoms on this dose, it may be reduced to 0.6 mg twice a day. Since familial Mediterranean fever is a lifelong disease and since colchicine therapy may cause azoospermia and chromosomal abnormalities, patients who respond to prophylactic therapy should have their maintenance dosage tapered to the lowest effective schedule. Of particular interest is the possibility, based on data from Israel, that long-term colchicine therapy may prevent the development of amyloidosis in susceptible patients with familial Mediterranean fever.

PROGNOSIS. The prognosis for normal longevity with this disease in the United States is excellent. Patients are usually normal between attacks without residua or debilitation. However, psychologic difficulties related to the chronic and recurrent nature of the disease may occur. In addition, drug addiction may result from the inappropriate administration of narcotics.

The prognosis in patients in the Middle East who develop amyloidosis is quite poor. Death, usually from renal failure, almost always occurs. Renal transplantation has been attempted, but several patients have developed amyloidosis in the donor kidney.

Dinarello CA, Wolff SM, Goldfinger SE, Dale DC, Alling, DW: Colchicine therapy for familial Mediterranean fever. A double-blind trial. N Engl J Med 291:934, 1974. *One of the original studies that firmly established the efficacy of prophylactic colchicine in the prevention of attacks of familial Mediterranean fever.*

Meyerhoff J: Familial Mediterranean fever: Report of a large family, review of the literature, and discussion of the frequency of amyloidosis. Medicine 59:66, 1980. *Up-to-date review article concerning multiple aspects of the epidemiologic, clinical, and pathologic manifestations of familial Mediterranean fever. Places particular emphasis on the frequency of amyloidosis in this disease, as well as the approach toward this complication from a preventive and possibly therapeutic standpoint.*

Schwabe AD, Peters RS: Familial Mediterranean fever in Armenians. Analysis of 100 cases. Medicine 53:453, 1974. *A well-written article describing the clinicopathologic manifestations of familial Mediterranean fever in 100 Armenian patients. Findings are compared and contrasted with those of previous reports. The longevity and absence of amyloidosis in this group is contrasted with the series reported from Israel.*

Sohar E, Gafni J, Pras M, Heller H: Familial Mediterranean fever. A survey of 470 cases and review of the literature. Am J Med 43:227, 1967. *One of the original extensive review articles documenting 470 cases of familial Mediterranean fever studied in Israel. A genetic analysis is presented, as well as a description of the different phenotypes of this disease with regard to the development of amyloidosis.*

Wright DG, Wolff SM, Fauci AS, Alling DW: Efficacy of intermittent colchicine therapy in familial Mediterranean fever. Ann Intern Med 86:162, 1977. *Important study which established the efficacy of intermittent cochicine therapy in aborting attacks in certain patients with familial Mediterranean fever. Of particular importance in this disease, since chronic long-term therapy is clearly effective but potentially dangerous.*

*Investigational drug for this purpose.

210. THE AMYLOID DISEASES

Joel N. Buxbaum

DEFINITION. The amyloid diseases comprise a group of conditions of diverse etiologies that is characterized by the accumulation of fibrillar material in various tissues such that vital organ function is compromised. The associated disease states may be inflammatory, hereditary, or neoplastic and the deposition can be local or systemic. The clinical outcome may be benign or as malignant as the most aggressive of neoplasms. In many senses, amyloid deposition is a symptom of an underlying disorder much as anemia is a symptom of a variety of pathologic states. Like anemia, which can produce secondary symptoms on the basis of the extent of the reduced oxygen-carrying capacity of the blood or diminished intravascular volume, the symptoms of amyloidosis depend upon the amount and localization of its deposition.

Amyloid substances of all types share certain properties. In tissue sections with conventional staining techniques, all amyloid appears homogeneous and eosinophilic. All types bind Congo red and under polarized light emit an apple-green fluorescence when stained with this dye. Viewed with the electron microscope, all amyloid contains two discrete structures, a major fibrillar component with a characteristic periodicity and a minor rodlike component that, viewed on end, has the appearance of a pentamer with a hollow core (the P component). The P component appears to be physically and chemically identical in all amyloids and normally circulates as a soluble serum protein that, in the mouse but not in humans, behaves as an acute phase reactant. Its role in the process of tissue infiltration has not been established.

The deposited fibril, regardless of its chemical nature, when isolated and analyzed has the x-ray diffraction pattern characteristic of a β-pleated sheet. It is insoluble at physiologic salt concentrations but can be released from tissue deposits by extraction with distilled water. The latter observation, made in the early 1970's, allowed the chemical analysis of fibrils obtained from many preparations of amyloid from tissues of individuals with different diseases. These studies have, in turn, permitted a more precise, chemically based, classification of the various amyloid syndromes (Table 210–1).

The ability to analyze the deposited proteins has also allowed the identification of circulating precursors of the insoluble fibrils and given general insight into processes that may be common to all types of amyloid deposition. It appears that all amyloid fibrils have a soluble precursor. In those individuals with pathologic deposition, either the amount of precursor is increased or the precursor is processed in such a way as to render it insoluble under physiologic conditions. It is not clear when or how processing takes place vis-à-vis deposition. In some instances, it appears that structurally normal proteins, e.g., some intact Ig light chains, may be amyloidogenic even without extensive processing, and it is excessive production that leads to tissue deposition. It is also not certain what controls the site and rate of deposition. While some molecules undergo the entire process of synthesis, processing and deposition in a confined locale, other equally amyloidogenic substances are deposited far from the site of synthesis.

Over the years, numerous attempts have been made to classify the amyloidoses. Histologic distribution, specific organ involvement, and the presence or absence of other overt disease have served as distinguishing parameters. Each of these classifications had some merit but none of them was without overlap or inconsistencies. The currently utilized chemically based scheme is the result of the analysis of the structure of proteins making up the deposited fibrils (Table 210–1). What has become obvious, as well as confusing, is that the same protein may constitute the fibril in diseases of apparently different etiologies. While this seeming paradox will eventually be resolved with greater understanding of the pathogenesis of the various forms, for the moment it remains a vexation.

PATHOGENESIS

AA AMYLOIDOSIS. AA amyloid is most frequently found when deposition takes place in the course of chronic inflammatory disease. In the past, chronic infectious processes, such as tuberculosis and osteomyelitis, were the usual precipitating diseases. In recent years, the most commonly associated conditions have been the chronic noninfectious inflammatory diseases. Rheumatoid arthritis has a reported incidence of up to 20 per cent in autopsy series with somewhat lower incidence clinically (5 to 7 per cent). The incidence in juvenile rheumatoid disease varies considerably in different countries (e.g., 0.14 per cent in the United States to 10 per cent in Poland). Other inflammatory joint diseases including the seronegative spondyloarthropathies, gout, and psoriasis as well as inflammatory bowel disease, even without arthritis, have been associated with amyloid deposition. Also at high risk for the development of AA disease are those individuals who inject foreign substances intra- or subcutaneously. The chronic or recurrent skin inflammation found in these patients seems to be particularly effective in the induction of amyloidosis.

Renal deposition of the AA protein has been the ultimately fatal event in the course of some groups of patients with *familial Mediterranean fever* (FMF) (Ch. 209). In the past, approximately 90 per cent of North African patients with this disease succumbed to renal failure by the age of 40.

AA deposition is also seen with a variety of nonlymphoid tumors and some nonimmunoglobulin producing lymphomas. Renal and gastric carcinomas and Hodgkin's disease have been the tumors most frequently associated with AA amyloid.

Kidneys, liver, and spleen are the most important sites of AA deposition. The renal disease is characterized initially by proteinuria of the glomerular type. Early in the disease, the kidneys may be enlarged but with time they shrink and the ultimate course is one of progressive renal failure. A variety of tubular disorders have also been described, including renal tubular acidosis, because of impaired bicarbonate reabsorption, nephrogenic diabetes insipidus, glycosuria, and hyperkalemia caused by decreased potassium exchange. The liver disease is relatively nonspecific, usually resulting in only moderate hepatomegaly and liver function test abnormalities.

In the past, when chronic infections were the most frequent stimuli to amyloid deposition, a small number of cases was reported in which eradication of the infection resulted in arrest of the progression or actual regression of the amyloidosis as documented by biopsy. In general, even without treatment the course of AA disease is more chronic than that of AL amyloid.

The deposited AA protein appears to be a discrete proteolytic product of the serum AA protein (SAA) that has a monomer molecular weight of 12,500 but circulates as a molecule of 220,000 to 235,000 molecular weight complexed to high density lipoprotein. It has also been found complexed to albumin. It behaves as an acute phase protein, rising rapidly in the course of inflammation (infectious or noninfectious) and peaking and falling to normal levels with resolution of the inflammation. SAA levels are generally higher in the elderly, and high levels have also been noted in patients with myeloma. In experimental animals, its production in the liver can be induced by the administration of bacterial lipopolysaccharide, which causes the production of *interleukin I* by macrophages. This substance,

TABLE 210–1. CHEMICAL CLASSIFICATION OF THE AMYLOID DISEASES

Clinical Syndrome	Fibril Precursor	Fibril	Common Term	Chemical Description
Primary myeloma with amyloid	Ig L-chain	L chain or V_L fragment	AL	A_λ $(_{1-n})$ or A_κ $(_{1-n})$
Secondary (inflammation associated)	SAA	AA	AA	$AA_{prototype}$ $AA(_{trp})$ var†
Localized				
Endocrine			AE	
Thyroid medullary carcinoma*	Procalcitonin	? Procalcitonin	AE_t	$A_{procalcitonin}$
Pancreatic islet	—	—	AE_i	—
Skin–Papular, macular, nodular	—	—	AD	—
Senile				
Cardiac	Prealbumin	Prealbumin	AS_{c1} AS_{c2}	$A_{prealbumin}$ —
Brain	—	—	AS_b	—
Pancreas	—	—	AS_p	—
Familial				
Neuropathic				
Portuguese	Prealbumin	Prealbumin	AF_p	$A_{prealbumin}$;
Swedish	Prealbumin	Prealbumin	AF_{sw}	$A_{prealbumin}$ (var)
Is	Prealbumin	Prealbumin	AF_{Is}	$A_{prealbumin}$ (var)
Japanese	—	—	AF_j	—
Indiana-Maryland	—	—	AF_{i-m}	—
Iowa	—	—	AF_i	—
Nephropathic				
FMF (North African)	SAA	AA	AF_{FMF}	AA
Irish-American	SAA	AA	AF_{IR}	AA
Urticaria, deafness (England)	—	—	AF_d	—
Polish (hypertensive)	—	—	AF_p	—
German (renal failure)	—	—	AF_g	—
Vascular				
HCHWA (Iceland)§	Gamma trace‡	Gamma trace fragment polymer	AF_{HCHWA}	$A_{\gamma\ trace}$

*Also found in other APUD tumors.

†This designation is used to denote amino acids that depart from the prototype sequences.

§Hereditary cerebral hemorrhage with amyloidosis.

‡Gastroenteropancreatic neuroendocrine protein is a hormonelike peptide with no known function to date found in peptidergic CNS neurons, the anterior pituitary, and pancreas. Its concentration is high in cerebrospinal fluid.

in turn, causes an increase in the production of an mRNA coding for the serum precursor. The actual steps in the processing of SAA to AA have not been identified, although it has been shown that human monocyte ectoproteases as well as serum enzymes when presented with SAA in vitro can digest it into either small fragments or AA-sized polypeptides. SAA production is necessary, but not sufficient, for AA deposition, since some mouse strains that are resistant to experimental AA amyloid induction make normal amounts of SAA. It is also likely that the liver is not the only site of SAA synthesis. It is probable, although not proven, that prolonged SAA production in individuals in whom the ability to degrade the molecule is deficient, either genetically or otherwise, is associated with AA deposition.

AL AMYLOIDOSIS. AL (or light chain–related) deposition is the most common form of amyloidosis seen in current clinical practice. The proportion of the total number of cases that represent multiple myeloma or primary amyloid is difficult to judge, since marrow plasmacytosis may be significant in both and the diagnostic distinctions between the primary disease and myeloma blurred (Ch. 163). Functionally, both diseases are malignant. In the case of myeloma, the outcome is related primarily to the proliferative capacity of the neoplastic clone. When AL deposition is present, it contributes to the poor prognosis. In primary amyloid disease the growth of a dominant plasma cell clone appears to be limited, but the amyloidogenicity of its homogeneous product results in the ultimately fatal compromise of organ function, most commonly renal or cardiac.

AL deposition is more likely to occur in tongue, heart, lymph nodes, spleen, carpal ligaments, joints, peripheral nerves, and skin than the AA type. Hence, cardiac failure, arrhythmias, carpal tunnel syndrome, peripheral neuropathy, and ecchymoses are more frequent in AL disease. A deficiency of clotting factor X has been reported with an attendant bleeding diathesis. There is evidence to suggest that some AL proteins may have affinity for the clotting factor with resultant lowering of the plasma levels. Removal of an amyloid-laden spleen has reversed the deficiency in some patients. Blood vessels tend to be fragile in AL patients, since the amyloid is deposited in vessel walls. When vessel walls become rigid, not only are they sensitive to trauma but also they do not respond well in the reflex-mediated changes in body position. When this occurs, orthostatic hypotension may become a major clinical problem. Coronary artery amyloid deposition can result in clinical angina pectoris or myocardial infarction.

Many investigators have now documented that the deposited fibrillar protein is related to the excess monoclonal light chain produced by the expanded plasma cell clone and found in the patient's serum, urine, or both. The actual tissue protein may represent the whole light chain or a fragment thereof, usually containing at least the variable region. Amino acid sequence analyses of tissue AL protein and the isolated light chain obtained from the same patient have demonstrated chemical identity.

Despite several detailed analyses, it is still not clear what makes a given light chain amyloidogenic. Of light chain types associated with either primary amyloid or myeloma-associated amyloid, it appears that lambda chains are more frequent than kappa, and that the $V\lambda_{VI}$ light chain subgroup is overly represented. It has been suggested that tissue affinity could be charge related or that the interaction between light chain and tissues could represent an autoantibody antigen interaction. Neither of these hypotheses has conclusive experimental support. Further, it has not been established whether amyloidogenesis involves only the processing of intact light chains to fragments or if some of the molecules are synthetic fragments that are predisposed to deposition. It is possible that both phenomena occur.

Most AL patients, even those with primary amyloid, have a detectable M component, usually free light chains of a single class, found in the serum or urine. However, 5 to 10 per cent have not had such proteins detectable. Analyses of a small number of these patients indicate that in tissue culture their bone marrow cells synthesize an excess of free monoclonal light chains. Because of their low concentration in the serum and their presumed high affinity for tissues they cannot be detected by conventional immunochemical techniques. In no instance yet reported has an immunoglobulin heavy chain been found to make up the fibril isolated from human amyloid tissue.

Recently, a number of patients has been reported in whom organ compromise has taken place because of infiltration with monoclonal light chains without discrete fibril formation. Some of these patients have had clinical multiple myeloma; others have not. It is likely that this condition is analogous to AL amyloid but that the deposited proteins do not have the intrinsic properties necessary to form β-pleated sheets of sufficient size and stability to make fibrils. While these proteins have been identified in tissue deposits by immunofluorescence, chemical studies of the circulatory and tissue forms have not yet been carried out; therefore, formal proof of their identity is lacking.

SENILE AMYLOIDOSIS. The term senile amyloid has been used to describe Congo red binding material found at autopsy in the tissues of elderly individuals. The material is most commonly found in the heart but has also been noted in the pancreas and brain. The cerebral plaques identified in Alzheimer's disease are congophilic. The clinical import of these deposits has not yet been fully established. While many individuals in their eighth and ninth decades have scattered atrial deposits, clinically significant cardiac disease, characterized by either congestive heart failure or arrhythmia, appears to occur rarely. Once it does, the prognosis is poor. The presence of a chronic inflammatory disease (e.g., rheumatoid arthritis) or multiple myeloma does not increase the incidence of senile cardiac amyloid (SCA) deposition; this suggests an independent pathogenesis for all three diseases.

It has been theorized that the atrial, pancreatic, and cerebral deposits may be related to each other and independent of the clinically significant ventricular form that occurs in a much smaller proportion of the elderly.

The fibril of SCA isolated from ventricular myocardium has an amino acid sequence identical with serum *prealbumin* (up to residue 26). It has been suggested, but not yet established, that the deposited prealbumin has been proteolytically processed. Since prealbumin is not normally synthesized by myocardial cells, SCA suggests that the precursor is produced at a remote site and localizes in its target organ by some unknown mechanism. Clinical studies have suggested that pulmonary involvement may also be associated with cardiac deposition, implying that deposition of the SCA protein may be more systemic than previously appreciated.

AL, AA, and SCA make up the bulk of the amyloid diseases encountered in clinical practice; however, there are additional, less common forms, the analysis of which has yielded insight into the genesis of these deposits. Localized forms have been noted in cases of medullary carcinoma of the thyroid in which the fibrillar protein is related to procalcitonin and in insulinomas, in which the material appears to be antigenically related to insulin.

FAMILIAL AMYLOIDOSIS. A series of genetically transmitted amyloid deposition diseases with characteristic clinical syndromes has been described. Several of these are primarily neuropathic with autosomal dominant inheritance. The *Portuguese-Japanese* type initially affects the lower limbs, usually in the third and fourth decades. Gastrointestinal neuropathy is common, while other viscera may become mildly involved later. In contrast, the *Maryland* or *Indiana* type affects the upper extremities, occurs somewhat later in life, and manifests itself as carpal tunnel syndrome with little visceral involvement. In the *Swedish* and *Iowa* forms, both upper and lower extremities are involved, renal disease is significant, and both show pupillary abnormalities. The Swedish form also shows autonomic and central nervous system involvement.

Recently, fibrils from the Portuguese, the Swedish, and a similar polyneuropathic amyloidotic syndrome of Ashkenazic Jews have been isolated and analyzed. In each instance, the monomer molecular weight of the fibril was approximately 14,000 and shared either antigenic determinants or amino acid homology with prealbumin. In two instances, there were amino acid differences between the fibril sequences and that previously determined for normal serum prealbumin. It has not yet been determined if these differences are pathogenetically significant.

Hence, for reasons that are not yet clear, prealbumin appears to be the fibril precursor in two types of disease, one with both a clear-cut genetic component and a relatively early onset and another (SCA) occurring late with little evidence to date of anything other than sporadic occurrence.

The fibril from an additional hereditary form of central nervous system amyloidosis, hereditary cerebral hemorrhage with amyloidosis, has been found to be related to a neuroendocrine hormone-like material, *gamma trace*.

Other hereditary forms of primarily nephropathic, cardiopathic, or cutaneous nature have also been described. The best studied of the renal forms is FMF, which has been discussed elsewhere. Other kindreds have exhibited deafness, urticaria, and febrile episodes (Derbyshire), splenic involvement and hypertension with negative rectal biopsies (Polish), and lung involvement (Irish-American) in addition to the progressive renal disease. In the last syndrome the fibril was found to be of the AA type. Only a single Danish family exhibiting a pure cardiomyopathy has been reported, while seven instances of familial primary cutaneous amyloidosis with no evidence of visceral involvement have been studied. The fibrils in the latter two conditions have not been analyzed.

CLINICAL MANIFESTATIONS. Regardless of the type of protein, the clinical manifestations of amyloid deposition in a given organ are similar. The renal disease is primarily manifested by proteinuria, reflecting the glomerular localization of the deposition. Renal tubular defects have also been reported. Azotemia and renal failure usually occur late. The latter may be associated with vascular involvement. There is a 5 to 15 per cent incidence of renal vein thrombosis, particularly in patients with AA disease and the nephrotic syndrome. Amyloid renal disease may be associated with hypertension. The kidneys may be small, normal sized, or enlarged. Contraction of kidneys usually occurs late in the disease.

The most characteristic cardiac presentation is that of a restrictive cardiomyopathy with congestive heart failure. Supraventricular arrhythmias are common, as are varying degrees of A-V block. Echocardiographic studies usually show a thickened ventricular wall without a dilated ventricle and a characteristic "glitter" or sparkling of the myocardial echoes. Patients with myocardial amyloidosis tend to be sensitive to digitalis glycoside toxicity, and these drugs are generally not used. Pulmonary involvement tends to mirror cardiac involvement both in frequency and extent, but rarely it becomes a dominant clinical syndrome with impairment of both the mechanics of respiration and gas exchange. Localized upper and lower airway amyloid infiltration can present major mechanical problems requiring surgical intervention.

Gastrointestinal involvement is most frequently manifested by bleeding, although diarrhea and malabsorption due to either submucosal infiltration or autonomic neuropathy have been reported.

DIAGNOSIS. The diagnosis of amyloidosis is made by the demonstration of the characteristic tissue deposits. Over the years the choice of appropriate tissue for biopsy has become wider. In patients in whom the diagnosis is suspected on clinical grounds recent data suggest that subcutaneous fat aspiration will yield Congo red–positive material in 90 to 95 per cent of cases of AL disease and two thirds of patients with AA deposition. Rectal biopsy in similar patients yields positive results in 75 to 85 per cent, if adequate mucosal and submucosal tissue is obtained. Gingival tissue will be positive in approximately one half of cases. Bone marrow biopsies have been positive in 40 to 50 per cent of patients with AL disease. These sites can be sampled with little chance of serious complications.

When there is evidence of involvement of a particular organ, diagnostic yields improve considerably. Operative specimens from carpal tunnel releases performed on patients with AL or hereditary neuropathic disease may show 95 per cent positivity. Renal biopsies in individuals with proteinuria have been reported to be positive in more than 90 per cent of patients. Liver biopsies also have a high yield, however; as with closed renal biopsies, significant, even fatal bleeding has occurred. Hence these procedures are performed only after evaluation of bleeding tendencies and clotting factors. Liver biopsy is generally not carried out if there is substantial hepatomegaly.

In recent years it has become possible to distinguish the chemical types of amyloid from biopsy material. In the past a diagnosis of the AL type of disease could be inferred by the presence in the serum and urine of monoclonal Ig's or light chains. With the use of potassium permanganate to bleach Congo red staining it is now possible to distinguish AA from AL in about two thirds of cases, AA staining being permanganate sensitive and the AL type resistant. More recently, antisera to the different light chain classes, AA proteins, and prealbumin have been utilized either in the immunofluorescent or immunoperoxidase staining of biopsy samples. Since each of the deposited proteins arises from a different precursor, presumably in response to a different stimulus, it is reasonable to assume that these distinctions will eventually have therapeutic implications.

TREATMENT AND PROGNOSIS. AL deposition associated with multiple myeloma has been treated in the course of treating the neoplastic process. While 50 to 60 per cent of patients with myeloma will respond to treament with alkylating agents and prednisone with an extension of survival, the disease has not yet been cured nor has the amyloid deposition been reversed.

A number of patients with AL disease but without overt myeloma have been reported to show prolonged survival after therapy with myeloma-like protocols. However, these are anecdotal results at best and a single attempt at a randomized trial of alkylating agent therapy did not provide convincing evidence of prolonged survival. Nonetheless, it appears that some patients may respond to these regimens. There have also been occasional reports of improvement in AL disease during administration of the organic solvent dimethyl sulfoxide, usually with concurrent alkylating agent therapy.

The most successful therapy of amyloid to date has been the prophylactic use of colchicine in patients with North African FMF. Administration of 0.6 mg of colchicine* three times daily to newly diagnosed patients has prevented the previously uniform occurrence of fatal renal disease. The therapy should be instituted before significant AA deposition to be most effective, although reductions in proteinuria have been reported in patients with clinically evident disease. As a result of this experience and the observation that colchicine will also prevent experimental casein-induced murine AA deposition, several groups have instituted large-scale trials of colchicine in both AA and AL disease. Apart from the FMF experience, to date no regimen has been uniformly successful in the treatment of any form of amyloid deposition once it has become established.

*This use is not listed in the manufacturer's directive.

Glenner GG: The β-fibrilloses. N Engl J Med 302:1283;1333, 1980. *A comprehensive review of the amyloidogenic proteins and the pathology of the disease in the context of newer information concerning the chemical structure of the fibrils.*

Gorevic PD: The amyloid diseases: Clinicopathologic and biochemical correlations. In Franklin EC (ed.): Clinical Immunology Update 1981, pp 1–30. *Describes experimental and clinical amyloidosis with a particularly good summary of the heredofamilial forms and the histologic techniques used in diagnosis.*

Kushner I, Volanakis JE, and Gewurz H (eds.): C-Reactive Protein and the Plasma Protein Response to Tissue Injury. Ann NY Acad Sci Vol 389, 1982. *The proceedings of a meeting in which several papers describe the biology of SAA and P component with respect to structure, biosynthesis, and the response to inflammation.*

Kyle RA: Amyloidosis: Review of 236 cases. Medicine 54:271, 1975. *The Mayo Clinic experience from 1960 to 1972 is described retrospectively. This is a very good review of the clinical features of the major syndromes seen in a large referred population.*

Kyle RA, Greipp PR: Amyloidosis (AL), clinical and laboratory features in 229 cases. Mayo Clin Proc 58:665, 1983. *This more recent reference extends the Mayo Clinic experience with an excellent description of the relevant features of this type of amyloidosis (117 references).*

Wegelius O, Pasternack A (eds.): Amyloidosis, Proceedings of the Fifth Sigrid Juselius Symposium 1976. New York, Academic Press. *A watershed meeting in which the new nomenclature based on the chemical structure of the fibril was first proposed. It contains papers on every aspect of amyloid disease. Some of the data have never been reported elsewhere.*

211. HEREDITARY SYNDROMES INVOLVING MULTIPLE ORGAN SYSTEMS

Arno G. Motulsky

The emergence of clinical genetics as a specialty has led to the definition of a large number of previously undifferentiated birth defects and syndromes. In some of these diseases the origin is monogenic, and multiple organ involvement is caused by the action of the mutant gene in various tissues. In other cases, a detectable chromosomal error or a known teratogen (such as Dilantin) causes multiorgan birth defects. Most frequently, neither a specific genetic nor environmental cause can be identified. Clinical genetics has grown rapidly, and most physicians are unable to keep abreast of the many newly described syndromes. While most of these conditions become manifest in infancy or childhood, adolescent and adult patients with such conditions often initially come to internists and primary care physicians, who should be aware of the various diagnostic, genetic, and management problems. A vague diagnosis of "multiple birth defects" or "genetic syndrome" usually is not sufficient. Appropriate genetic counseling ideally must be based on a definite diagnosis; optimal care often requires knowledge of the specific diagnosis and natural history of a given syndrome. The reader is referred to various textbooks and compendia for orientation and diagnostic approaches. Because of phenotypic variability in most syndromes, diagnosis may be difficult and new syndromes continue to be described. In this chapter a few selected syndromes are discussed briefly.

Bergsma D: Birth Defects Compendium. 2nd ed. New York, Alan R. Liss, 1979. *An encyclopedic guide to birth defects.*

Cohen MM Jr: The Child with Multiple Birth Defects. New York, Random Press, 1982. *An excellent analytical introduction of approaches to syndromes and multiple birth defects.*

de Grouchy J, Turlean J: Clinical Atlas of Human Chromosomes. New York, John Wiley & Sons, 1977. *A good reference volume for syndromes associated with cytogenetic abnormalities.*

McKusick V: Mendelian Inheritance in Man. 6th ed. Baltimore, Johns Hopkins University Press, 1983. *Standard reference book listing definite and possible monogenic disease, traits, and syndromes with short descriptions and literature citations.*

Smith D: Recognizable Patterns of Human Malformation. 3rd ed. Philadelphia, W. B. Saunders Company, 1982. *The "bible" for description of malformation syndromes. Many photographs and short accounts of many different types of defects. Practically useful.*

WERNER'S SYNDROME

Werner's syndrome is a rare disorder with some clinical features that resemble early aging. Onset of clinical findings is usually in the second or third decade. Affected patients are short because of absence of the adolescent growth spurt and have slender limbs. There is premature graying and then loss of hair. Atrophy and hyperkeratosis of the skin with ulcerations around the feet are often seen. A characteristic squeaky voice and atrophy of muscle, fat, and bone of the extremities are the rule. Soft tissue calcifications usually develop. Atherosclerosis is premature with coronary heart disease and medial calcification of peripheral vessels. Juvenile cataracts and osteoporosis are typical. Hypogonadism occurs in both sexes, and mild diabetes is common. Malignancies occur in about 10 per cent of cases, with an unusually high occurrence of meningiomas and sarcomas. Mean age of death is in the early 40's. The phenotype of Werner's syndrome has been considered as a "caricature" of senescence rather than as a model of the normal aging process. The condition is inherited as an autosomal recessive trait. Altered glycosaminoglycan turnover in various tissues with increased excretion of hyaluronic acid in the urine has been frequently noted and suggests a fundamental abnormality affecting connective tissue. However, hyaluronicaciduria is not specific for Werner's syndrome. Fibroblasts from skin biopsies of patients with Werner's syndrome are difficult to culture. They grow more slowly, assume a senescent morphology more rapidly, and demonstrate a markedly reduced lifespan in vitro. DNA repair is normal. Karyotype preparations show a normal number of chromosomes, but variable stable chromosomal rearrangements such as translocations involving several chromosomes (variegated translocation mosaicism) are seen in over 90 per cent of cells (fibroblasts or lymphocytes). Werner's syndrome therefore can be classified among the group of chromosomal instability syndromes. No single enzymatic defect has been discovered yet to explain the multiple clinical, biochemical, and cytogenetic manifestations. Werner's syndrome is sometimes termed adult progeria but it is entirely unrelated to the pediatric syndrome of progeria (Hutchison-Gilford), in which death occurs in early adolescence from cardiac or cerebrovascular disease.

Epstein CJ, Martin GM, Schultz AL, Motulsky AG: The Werner's syndrome. Medicine 45:177, 1966. *A detailed summary of clinical and laboratory characteristics of 125 patients with Werner's syndrome.*

Salk W: Werner's syndrome. A review of recent research with an analysis of connective tissue metabolism, growth control of cultured cells, and chromosomal aberrations. Hum Genet 62:1, 1982. *A review of the current status of Werner's disease.*

SYNDROMES ASSOCIATED WITH HYPOGONADISM AND VARIOUS CONGENITAL ANOMALIES

LAWRENCE-MOON-BARDET-BIEDL SYNDROME AND RELATED DISORDERS. The Lawrence-Moon-Bardet-Biedl syndrome clinically exhibits the pentad of retinal dystrophy (usually pigmentary retinopathy), truncal obesity, mild to severe mental retardation, polydactyly, and hypogonadism. When not all of the five cardinal findings are seen, the diagnosis may be difficult. Electroretinography is useful for early diagnosis of the retinal dystrophy. Loss of central vision is gradual and total blindness usually occurs after the age of 30 years. Although primary and secondary hypogonadism have been reported, hypogonadism is less frequently found in females. Interstitial nephritis may lead to renal failure.

Some investigators (the "splitters") distinguish between the Bardet-Biedl and the Lawrence-Moon syndrome by the presence of spastic paraplegia and the absence of polydactyly and obesity in the latter condition. However, others (the "lumpers") believe that these distinctions relate to variable expression of a single disorder.

Alstrom's syndrome appears distinct and is also associated with retinal dystrophy and obesity. Affected patients are usually blind in early childhood and develop moderately severe deafness before age 10. Diabetes mellitus and slowly progressive chronic nephropathy in young adults are seen. Mental retardation and digital anomalies are not encountered.

Carpenter's syndrome (acrocephalopolysyndactyly) is a syndrome characterized by acrocephaly, syndactyly, and a characteristic facial appearance associated with polydactyly of the feet, obesity, mental retardation, and hypogonadism. The various characteristic skeletal findings should cause few diagnostic difficulties.

All these conditions (the syndromes of Lawrence-Moon-Bardet-Biedl, Alstrom, Carpenter) are inherited as autosomal recessive traits.

PRADER-WILLI SYNDROME. In this not uncommon condition, infants are born with severe hypotonia and feeding difficulties;

boys exhibit a small penis and cryptorchidism, and hypoplastic labia are seen in girls. The feeding difficulties of infancy give way to compulsive hyperphagia with development of severe obesity in later childhood. The hands and feet are characteristically small (acromicria). Affected patients are short and there is hypogonadotrophic hypogonadism with sterility. Mild to severe mental retardation with behavioral and personality problems are the rule. Mild diabetes mellitus is often seen. Retinal abnormalities and polydactyly do not occur. In about 50 per cent of cases a chromosome abnormality affecting band q11-12 of the long arm of chromosome 15 has been detected by high resolution methods. The defect usually is a small deletion, but more complex rearrangements affecting the relevant chromosomal segment have also been seen. Although the syndrome usually occurs as a sporadic event, rare familial cases have been reported. Parental chromosomes are usually normal. It is likely that an as yet undetectable chromosomal defect exists in those cases in which no visible chromosomal abnormality has been found. The relationship of the unique and specific chromosomal deletion to the pathogenesis of the syndrome remains unknown.

NOONAN'S SYNDROME. This syndrome is often diagnosed; however, its boundaries are not sharply defined. Its frequency has been estimated to range between 1/1000 to 1/8000. It is likely that there is etiologic heterogeneity with several unrelated conditions lumped under the category of Noonan's syndrome. Because girls with this syndrome had clinical resemblance to girls with Turner's syndrome, the syndrome was first described as the male Turner's syndrome; however, females can be affected as well. There are no chromosomal abnormalities. Affected patients are often but not always short and have a somewhat characteristic facial appearance with hypertelorism, low-set ears, epicanthal folds, ptosis, antimongoloid slant of eyes, and micrognathia. Webbing of the neck or a short neck and a low posterior hair line are common. Cubitus valgus and chest deformities such as the simultaneous presence of proximal pectus carinatum and distal pectus excavatum are frequent. Congenital heart disease, usually pulmonic stenosis, and mild mental retardation are often seen. Peripheral lymphedema may occur. While hypogonadism in both sexes may be encountered, some patients have been fertile.

The condition is sometimes transmitted as an autosomal dominant trait, but most cases are sporadic. Many cases represent new mutations. Since there is marked clinical variability, relatives occasionally show minor signs of the condition.

Turner's syndrome in female patients can easily be excluded by the chromosome findings. The autosomal dominant Leopard's syndrome (a mnemonic for multiple *l*entigines, *E*CG abnormalities, *o*cular hypertelorism, *p*ulmonary stenosis, growth *r*etardation, and *d*eafness) needs to be differentiated from Noonan's syndrome. Differential diagnosis is simple if there are multiple lentigines and deafness but these findings may be missing.

Goldstein J, Fialkow PJ: The Alstrom syndrome. Medicine 52:53, 1973. *Classic summary of the clinical, genetic, and pathophysiologic aspects of the syndrome.*

Holm VA, Sulzbacher SJ, Pipes PL (eds.): Prader-Willi Syndrome. Baltimore, Baltimore University Press, 1982. *A multiauthored symposium volume dealing with all aspects of Prader-Willi syndrome.*

Klein D, Amman F: The syndrome of Lawrence-Moon-Bardet-Biedl and allied disorders. J Neurol Sci 9:470, 1969. *Clinical description and differential diagnosis.*

Ledbetter DH, Mascarello JT, Riccardi VM, Harper VD, Airhart SD, Strobel RJ: Chromosome 15 abnormalities and the Prader-Willi syndrome: A follow-up report of 40 cases. Am J Hum Genet 34:278, 1982. *Current status of the chromosomal defect affecting chromosome 15 q11-12.*

Mendez H: Noonan syndrome. Review of the literature and report on association with neurofibromatosis. Am J Med Genet, in press. *Recent review of various manifestations.*

Shechat A, Maumenee IH: The Bardet-Biedl syndrome and related disorders. Arch Ophthalmol 100:285, 1982. *Diagnostic classification using "splitting" criteria.*

Part XVI
NUTRITIONAL DISEASES

212. NUTRIENT REQUIREMENTS

Robert M. Russell

RECOMMENDED DIETARY ALLOWANCES

Recommended Dietary Allowances (RDAs) have been established for most essential nutrients by the Food and Nutrition Board of the National Academy of Sciences (NAS). These dietary allowances (Table 212–1) do not represent nutrient requirements for individuals; they are designed as guidelines for the daily intake of nutrients sufficient to ensure that almost all members of the population are not at risk of developing nutrient deficits. Thus, the RDAs exceed the nutrient requirements for most healthy individuals. Recommendations for energy intakes are an exception in that they represent averages ± 1 SD for particular age and sex groups.

RDAs have been determined by balance studies, measurement of the amount of a nutrient needed to result in tissue saturation, examination of the food supplies of healthy populations, examination of minimum nutrient intakes required to prevent or correct either a naturally occurring deficit or an experimentally produced deficit, epidemiologic observations, and animal studies. Precise RDAs have not been established for some nutrients (e.g., vitamin K, selenium, etc.) because of limited experimental data. However, ranges of safe intakes of these nutrients have been determined by the National Academy of Sciences and are provided in Table 212–2. Continued consumption of trace minerals above the upper limit of the recommended ranges can lead to toxic effects.

The RDAs should be met by a variety of foods for two major reasons. First, certain dietary components (e.g., carotene, fiber, and possibly others as yet undefined), which are not considered "required," may nevertheless have a beneficial effect on body functioning. For example, if an individual is limited to a diet containing only preformed vitamin A, he or she could be deprived of the alleged beneficial effects of carotene (a vitamin A precursor). Second, a monotonous diet over a prolonged period may not supply a beneficial ratio of individual nutrients (e.g., a diet of very high carbohydrate content may increase the body's need for thiamin). Many such nutrient-nutrient interactions are not fully known at present.

Body growth, body size, pregnancy, and lactation alter the RDAs. Other factors that result in an alteration of dietary needs include environmental temperature, fever, menstruation (an increased requirement for iron), malabsorptive diseases, and medications. The RDAs are not applicable to sick or traumatized patients or to individuals with metabolic disorders such as hyperthyroidism. Table 212–3 provides a guide to the possible effects of medication on nutrient requirements and the mechanisms by which these interactions occur.

Nutrient requirements and dietary recommendations for adults are defined in broad age classes in Table 212–1, namely 19 to 22 years, 23 to 50 years, and 51 years and older (76 years and older for energy). In the absence of adequate information, the present recommendations used for the elderly are the same as for the young adult population with few exceptions. However, age-related changes affect the absorption, metabolism, and excretion of many nutrients so that age-specific standards for the elderly are needed. In addition, chronic disability, illness, and the increased use of medications in the elderly introduce other variables. Despite all of these caveats, the RDAs do serve as useful guidelines for the practitioner when judging the adequacy of an individual's diet.

ENERGY

Energy needs vary with body size, growth phase, age, sex, and activity. Factors that increase energy requirements are cold exposure, pregnancy, lactation, infection, fever, hyperthyroidism, and trauma. Recommended energy allowances for all ages are presented in Table 212–4. The energy allowances for children are based on median heights of American children at different ages. The allowances for young adults are based on so-called "desirable" weights of American men and women engaged in light work (e.g., walking, shopping, playing golf, etc.). In addition to the age groups 19 to 22 and 23 to 50 years, energy recommendations for older people are divided into 57 to 75 and 75+ years. The aging process normally results in a progressive decrease in energy needs primarily as a result of a decrease in energy expenditure.

Protein and carbohydrate supply approximately four calories per gram, alcohol seven calories per gram, and fat nine calories per gram. Basal energy expenditure (BEE) may be estimated for healthy individuals using the Harris Benedict equations:

$$\text{Men: BEE} = 66 \pm (13.7 \times \text{weight in kg}) + (5 \times \text{height in cm}) - 6.8\ (\text{age in years})$$

$$\text{Women: BEE} = 65.5 + (9.6 \times \text{weight in kg}) + (1.7 \times \text{height in cm}) - 4.7\ (\text{age in years})$$

Depending on factors such as activity level or illness, energy needs may be increased many times over the basal level. For example, the energy expenditure of a 70-kg man at rest is approximately 70 kcal per hour. However, heavy labor may increase this expenditure to 600 kcal per hour. For each Celsius degree of fever, a 13 per cent increase in calories is required. In catabolic patients, 150 to 200 per cent of the BEE may be necessary to prevent further tissue breakdown. Malnutrition caused primarily by insufficient energy in the diet is known as marasmus, named from the Greek word meaning "to waste away" (Ch. 214).

PROTEIN

A constant supply of protein is needed to maintain body function and structure. On a protein-free diet, the average net loss of body protein by males is about 0.34 gram per kilogram of body weight. However, when allowance is made for incomplete utilization of dietary protein and for variability in needs, the allowance recommended for adults rises to 0.8 gram of protein per kilogram. Protein needs in part are dependent on energy intakes. Increased energy intakes result in protein conservation and decreased energy intakes result in the diversion of protein to meet energy needs. Pregnancy and lactation increase the body's protein requirement.

Dietary proteins differ in their digestibility and in their amino acid composition. Nine essential amino acids must be provided in the diet, since the human body lacks the ability to synthesize them. These proteins are lysine, leucine, isoleucine, valine, methionine, phenylalanine, tryptophan, threonine, and possibily histidine, especially for infants. The condition of malnutrition caused by inadequate protein intake is known as kwashiorkor (Ch. 214) and is seen mainly in infancy.

High-quality proteins have a high degree of bioavailability (i.e., they are easily digested and absorbed) and have a high biologic value (a measure of the efficiency of utilization of absorbed protein, which in turn is dependent on adequate amounts and proportions of essential amino acids). The highest-quality proteins are found in eggs and milk. Seeds and nuts, rice, corn, and grain proteins are of lesser quality. It is recommended that 10 to 15 per cent of caloric intake should be derived from protein. Amino acids supplied in excess of the body's requirement are not stored but are degraded to metabolic products (urea, uric acid), and the carbon skeleton is converted to carbohydrate and fat or oxidized for energy. It is important that a mixed diet be consumed so that adequate amounts of each essential amino acid are received. Some amino acids are

TABLE 212–1. FOOD AND NUTRITION BOARD, NATIONAL ACADEMY OF SCIENCES—NATIONAL RESEARCH COUNCIL RECOMMENDED DAILY DIETARY ALLOWANCES,* Revised 1980

Designed for the maintenance of good nutrition of practically all healthy people in the U.S.A.

	Age (years)	Weight (kg)	Weight (lb)	Height (cm)	Height (in)	Protein (g)	Fat-Soluble Vitamins: Vitamin A (μg RE)†	Vitamin D (μg)‡	Vitamin E (mg α-TE)§	Water-Soluble Vitamins: Vitamin C (mg)	Thiamin (mg)	Riboflavin (mg)	Niacin (mg NE)¶	Vitamin B_6 (mg)	Folacin** (μg)	Vitamin B_{12} (μg)	Minerals: Calcium (mg)	Phosphorus (mg)	Magnesium (mg)	Iron (mg)	Zinc (mg)	Iodine (μg)
Infants	0.0–0.5	6	13	60	24	kg × 2.2	420	10	3	35	0.3	0.4	6	0.3	30	0.5††	360	240	50	10	3	40
	0.5–1.0	9	20	71	28	kg × 2.0	400	10	4	35	0.5	0.6	8	0.6	45	1.5	540	360	70	15	5	50
Children	1–3	13	29	90	35	23	400	10	5	45	0.7	0.8	9	0.9	100	2.0	800	800	150	15	10	70
	4–6	20	44	112	44	30	500	10	6	45	0.9	1.0	11	1.3	200	2.5	800	800	200	10	10	90
	7–10	28	62	132	52	34	700	10	7	45	1.2	1.4	16	1.6	300	3.0	800	800	250	10	10	120
Males	11–14	45	99	157	62	45	1000	10	8	50	1.4	1.6	18	1.8	400	3.0	1200	1200	350	18	15	150
	15–18	66	145	176	69	56	1000	10	10	60	1.4	1.7	18	2.0	400	3.0	1200	1200	400	18	15	150
	19–22	70	154	177	70	56	1000	7.5	10	60	1.5	1.7	19	2.2	400	3.0	800	800	350	10	15	150
	23–50	70	154	178	70	56	1000	5	10	60	1.4	1.6	18	2.2	400	3.0	800	800	350	10	15	150
	51+	70	154	178	70	56	1000	5	10	60	1.2	1.4	16	2.2	400	3.0	800	800	350	10	15	150
Females	11–14	46	101	157	62	46	800	10	8	50	1.1	1.3	15	1.8	400	3.0	1200	1200	300	18	15	150
	15–18	55	120	163	64	46	800	10	8	60	1.1	1.3	14	2.0	400	3.0	1200	1200	300	18	15	150
	19–22	55	120	163	64	44	800	7.5	8	60	1.1	1.3	14	2.0	400	3.0	800	800	300	18	15	150
	23–50	55	120	163	64	44	800	5	8	60	1.0	1.2	13	2.0	400	3.0	800	800	300	18	15	150
	51+	55	120	163	64	44	800	5	8	60	1.0	1.2	13	2.0	400	3.0	800	800	300	10	15	150
Pregnancy						+30	+200	+5	+2	+20	+0.4	+0.3	+2	+0.6	+400	+1.0	+400	+400	+150	‡‡	+5	+25
Lactation						+20	+400	+5	+3	+40	+0.5	+0.5	+5	+0.5	+100	+1.0	+400	+400	+150	‡‡	+10	+50

*The allowances are intended to provide for individual variations among most normal persons as they live in the United States under usual environmental stresses. Diets should be based on a variety of common foods in order to provide other nutrients for which human requirements have been less well defined.

†Retinol equivalents. 1 retinol equivalent = 1 μg retinol or 6 μg β-carotene.

‡As cholecalciferol. 10 μg cholecalciferol = 400 IU of vitamin D.

§α-tocopherol equivalents. 1 mg d-α-tocopherol = 1 α-TE.

¶1 NE (niacin equivalent) is equal to 1 mg of niacin or 60 mg of dietary tryptophan.

**The folacin allowances refer to dietary sources as determined by *Lactobacillus casei* assay after treatment with enzymes (conjugases) to make polyglutamyl forms of the vitamin available to the test organism.

††The recommended dietary allowance for vitamin B_{12} in infants is based on average concentration of the vitamin in human milk. The allowances after weaning are based on energy intake (as recommended by the American Academy of Pediatrics) and consideration of other factors, such as intestinal absorption.

‡‡The increased requirement during pregnancy cannot be met by the iron content of habitual American diets nor by the existing iron stores of many women; therefore the use of 30 to 60 mg of supplemental iron is recommended. Iron needs during lactation are not substantially different from those of nonpregnant women, but continued supplementation of the mother for two to three months after parturition is advisable in order to replenish stores depleted by pregnancy.

TABLE 212–2. ESTIMATED SAFE AND ADEQUATE DAILY DIETARY INTAKES OF SELECTED VITAMINS AND MINERALS*

		Vitamins			Trace Elements†						Electrolytes		
	Age (years)	*Vitamin K (μg)*	*Biotin (μg)*	*Panthothenic Acid (mg)*	*Copper (mg)*	*Manganese (mg)*	*Fluoride (mg)*	*Chromium (mg)*	*Selenium (mg)*	*Molybdenum (mg)*	*Sodium (mg)*	*Potassium (mg)*	*Chloride (mg)*
Infants	0–0.5	12	35	2	0.5–0.7	0.5–0.7	0.1–0.5	0.01–0.04	0.01–0.04	0.03–0.06	115–350	350–925	275–700
	0.5–1	10–20	50	3	0.7–1.0	0.7–1.0	0.2–1.0	0.02–0.06	0.02–0.06	0.04–0.08	250–750	425–1275	400–1200
Children	1–3	15–30	65	3	1.0–1.5	1.0–1.5	0.5–1.5	0.02–0.08	0.02–0.08	0.05–0.1	325–975	550–1650	500–1500
and	4–6	20–40	85	3–4	1.5–2.0	1.5–2.0	1.0–2.5	0.03–0.12	0.03–0.12	0.06–0.15	450–1350	775–2325	700–2100
Adolescents	7–10	30–60	120	4–5	2.0–2.5	2.0–3.0	1.5–2.5	0.05–0.2	0.05–0.2	0.10–0.3	600–1800	1000–3000	925–2775
	11 +	50–100	100–200	4–7	2.0–3.0	2.5–5.0	1.5–2.5	0.05–0.2	0.05–0.2	0.15–0.5	900–2700	1525–4575	1400–4200
Adults	—	70–140	100–200	4–7	2.0–3.0	2.5–5.0	1.5–4.0	0.05–0.2	0.05–0.2	0.15–0.5	1100–3300	1875–5625	1700–5100

*Because there is less information on which to base allowances, these figures are not given in the main table of RDA and are provided here in the form of ranges of recommended intakes.

†Since the toxic levels for many trace elements may be only several times usual intakes, the upper levels for the trace elements given in this table should not be habitually exceeded.

From National Research Council: Recommended Dietary Allowances. 9th ed. Washington, DC, National Academy of Sciences, 1980.

TABLE 212–3. EXAMPLES OF DRUG-NUTRIENT INTERACTIONS

Drug	Increased Requirement	Potential Mechanism	Deficiency Symptoms
Antacids (aluminum and magnesium hydroxides)	Phosphate	Formation of insoluble salts	Malaise, paresthesias, anorexia
Anticonvulsants (phenobarbital, phenytoin)	Vitamin D	Induction of hepatic microsmal enzymes resulting in inactive vitamin D metabolites	Rickets, osteomalacia
Oral contraceptives (norethindrone/mestranol)	Folic acid	Inhibition of polyglutamic folate absorption	Megaloblastic anemia
Antituberculous drugs (isoniazid, cycloserine)	Vitamin B_6	Excretion of pyridoxal hydrazone complex	Peripheral neuropathy
Anticoagulants (coumarin, warfarin)	Vitamin K	Inhibition of vitamin K recycling	Hypoprothombinemia
Diuretics (benzothiadiazides)	Potassium	Enhancement of renal excretion	Hypokalemia

TABLE 212–4. MEAN HEIGHTS AND WEIGHTS AND RECOMMENDED ENERGY INTAKE*

Category	Age (years)	Weight (kg)	Weight (lb)	Height (cm)	Height (in)	Energy Needs (kcal)
Infants	0.0–0.5	6	13	60	24	kg × 115
	0.5–1.0	9	20	71	28	kg × 105
Children	1–3	13	29	90	35	1300 ± 400
	4–6	20	44	112	44	1700 ± 400
	7–10	28	62	132	52	2400 ± 400
Males	11–14	45	99	157	62	2700 ± 400
	15–18	66	145	176	69	2800 ± 400
	19–22	70	154	177	70	2900 ± 400
	23–50	70	154	178	70	2700 ± 400
	51–75	70	154	178	70	2400 ± 400
	76+	70	154	178	70	2050 ± 400
Females	11–14	46	101	157	62	2200 ± 400
	15–18	55	120	163	64	2100 ± 400
	19–22	55	120	163	64	2100 ± 400
	23–50	55	120	163	64	2000 ± 400
	51–75	55	120	163	64	1800 ± 400
	76+	55	120	163	64	1600 ± 400
Pregnancy						+300
Lactation						+500

*Adapted from National Research Council: Recommended Dietary Allowances. 9th ed. Washington DC, National Academy of Sciences, 1980.

complementary; for example, tyrosine may in part meet the body's requirement for phenylalanine, and cystine may in part meet the body's requirement for methionine. The ability of the body to utilize protein is impaired if one essential amino acid is missing, underscoring the need for mixed sources of dietary proteins.

In parenterally fed patients, zero nitrogen balance may be achieved with as little as 0.5 gram per kilogram per day of mixed amino acids (including all essential amino acids). However, patients with abnormal losses or increased demands (burns, trauma, wound repair) may require 1.5 to 2.5 grams per kilogram of amino acids per day.

In the clinical setting, the state of nitrogen balance can be crudely estimated by measuring the 24-hour urinary urea nitrogen level:

$$\text{Nitrogen balance} = \frac{\text{protein intake}}{6.25} - (\text{urinary urea nitrogen} + 4)$$

CARBOHYDRATE AND FAT

Because protein and fat alone can provide all the energy needs of the body, there is no fixed requirement for carbohydrate in the diet. However, carbohydrates help to make the diet palatable and comprise the main energy source for most people in the world. Further, a diet devoid of carbohydrate would be likely to result in ketosis. Fiber is an unabsorbed carbohydrate. Primarily because of epidemiologic disease patterns (e.g., for colon cancer and diverticulitis), an increase of dietary fiber to approximately 40 grams per day has been suggested.

Fat, a source of concentrated calories, serves as a carrier for fat-soluble vitamins. All body cells with the exception of the central nervous system and erythrocytes can directly utilize fatty acids as a source of energy. Deficiency of linoleic acid results in the syndrome of essential fatty acid deficiency, consisting of scaling skin and impaired growth in children. Linoleic acid deficiency has also been recognized among patients on prolonged parenteral feedings not containing fat. Three per cent of calories in the form of linoleic acid is recommended for the average daily diet.

FAT-SOLUBLE VITAMINS
(see Ch. 217 for more complete discussion)

VITAMIN A. High concentrations of preformed vitamin A are found in dairy products, fish oils, and liver. Good carotene sources include both yellow and green vegetables. The overall utilization of the provitamin, β carotene, as vitamin A is approximately one sixth that of retinol (the alcohol form of vitamin A) because of inefficient carotene absorption and hydrolysis. The vitamin A value of diets is expressed in retinol equivalents, where 1 retinol equivalent is equal to the following: 1 μg retinol, 6 μg β carotene, 12 μg of other provitamin A carotenoids, 3.33 IU of vitamin A activity from retinol, and 10 IU vitamin A activity from β carotene.

Vitamin A is essential for the integrity of epithelial tissues and for retinal function. Night blindness is one of the earliest symptoms of vitamin A deficiency, followed by follicular hyperkeratosis, xerosis, Bitot spots, corneal ulceration, and scleromalacia. Fat malabsorption increases the requirement for vitamin A and for all fat-soluble vitamins. When used regularly over prolonged periods, mineral oil may increase the dietary requirement for all fat-soluble vitamins. Acute toxicity from vitamin A may result in pseudotumor cerebri and exfoliative dermatitis. Chronic ingestion of excess vitamin A may result in a myriad of problems, the most serious of which are hepatic fibrosis and portal hypertension. The lowest reported dose of vitamin A to cause chronic intoxication is 25,000 IU over a period of 7 years.

VITAMIN D (Ch. 244). With normal exposure to ultraviolet light, the skin forms vitamin D_3 (cholecalciferol) from 7-dehydrocholesterol in amounts that are probably sufficient to meet the body's requirement. The vitamin D requirement can also be readily satisfied by diets containing vitamin D–fortified foods. Vitamin D deficiency may result in people who have little or no sunlight exposure and diets containing low amounts of animal tissue or milk that has been fortified with either vitamin D_2 (ergocalciferol) or vitamin D_3 (cholecalciferol). Vitamin D deficiency results in rickets and growth failure in children and osteomalacia in adults. Active metabolites of vitamin D are formed in the liver (25-hyroxyvitamin D) and kidney (1,25-dihydroxyvitamin D).

VITAMIN E. Vitamin E appears to play a role as an intracellular antioxidant. Although the biochemical mechanism is unclear, vitamin E also prevents cell membrane damage. Vitamin E-deficient red blood cells undergo excessive hemolysis when exposed to dilute hydrogen peroxide. Infants who are vitamin E-deficient have been reported to develop hemolytic anemia and muscle damage. Vitamin E deficiency has been described in adults undergoing prolonged parenteral nutrition, and the resulting neuropathy and retinopathy have been found to respond to the administration of vitamin E. Some of the better food sources of vitamin E include vegetable shortenings and oils, margarine, seeds, whole grains, and liver. Since other isomers of tocopherol are not necessarily as well utilized, the vitamin E content of the diet is expressed in α-tocopherol equivalents (αTE) (1α-tocopherol equivalent = 1 mg dl-α-tocopherol or 1.1 IU). Although oils in general are rich sources of vitamin E, the ingestion of a diet high in polyunsaturated fats increases the requirement for vitamin E. Vitamin E toxicity has not been described, although there is evidence that high doses of vitamin E may antagonize the vitamin K-dependent carboxylation of proteins.

VITAMIN K. The synthesis of coagulation factors prothrombin VII, IX, and X by the liver is dependent on vitamin K (Ch. 217). Vitamin K acts as a catalyst to gamma carboxylate glutamic acid residues in the precursor of prothrombin as well as other vitamin K-dependent proteins. Warfarin-type anticoagulants interfere with vitamin K recycling. Phylloquinone (vitamin K_1) is found in green leafy vegetables, and menaquinone (vitamin K_2) is found in bacteria and animals. It is uncertain whether intestinal bacterial synthesis of menaquinones alone is sufficient to meet the human requirement for this vitamin. Deficiency of vitamin K results in hemorrhage and may be seen in infants with immature gut colonization or in adults with malabsorption who are receiving antibiotics or who are on diets lacking in vitamin K. Administration of synthetic vitamin K (menadione) may cause hemolytic anemia.

WATER-SOLUBLE VITAMINS
(see Ch. 217 for more complete discussion)

THIAMIN (VITAMIN B_1). Thiamin functions in the utilization of pentose sugars in the hexose monophosphate shunt and serves as a coenzyme (thiamine pyrophosphate) in the metabolism of alpha keto acid and 2-keto sugars. Beriberi is the deficiency disease state, which involves the cardiovascular and nervous systems and is seen largely in populations subsisting on unenriched rice and wheat flour and in chronic alcoholics (as a result of poor diet, decreased absorption, and altered metabolism). Wernicke's encephalopathy and Korsakoff's psychosis among alcoholics (Ch. 17) may respond to therapeutic doses of thiamin (50 mg thiamin per day until there is stabilization). A clinical test for thiamin deficiency is the measurement of red blood cell transketolase activity.

Thiamin is easily destroyed by cooking and food processing. The best sources of thiamin include whole grains, organ meats, pork, and legumes. The dietary requirement for thiamin increases in diets high in carbohydrate and caloric content and appears to be slightly reduced in diets in which a high proportion of calories is achieved from fat.

RIBOFLAVIN (VITAMIN B_2). Dietary riboflavin sources include milk, meat and poultry, fish, and leafy green vegetables. The vitamin is very sensitive to sunlight and high cooking temperatures. Deficiency of riboflavin is accompanied by mouth lesions, angular stomatitis, cheilosis, glossitis, skin lesions (seborrhea, scrotal or vulval dermatitis), and conjunctivitis. Riboflavin functions as the active component of coenzymes (e.g., flavin mononucleotide, flavin-adenine dinucleotide) for flavo proteins involved in tissue oxidation and reduction reactions (e.g., glutathione reductase, cyclochrome c reductase, succinic dehydrogenase, amino oxidases).

NIACIN. Pellagra is caused by niacin deficiency and is manifested by dermatitis, diarrhea, and dementia, some or all of which may be present in any one patient. The deficiency state is not uncommon among peoples subsisting on corn. It is also found quite regularly among alcoholics. Niacin is needed for fat synthesis, glycolysis, and tissue respiration and is a component of nicotinamide adenine dinucleotide and nicotinamide adenine dinucleotide phosphate. Good food sources for niacin include meat, poultry, fish, whole grains, and legumes. Tryptophan is converted in the body to niacin, and the niacin requirement is inversely related to tryptophan intake. However, tryptophan cannot in practicality meet the niacin requirement since one niacin equivalent (1 mg of niacin) is equal to 60 mg of tryptophan. Ingestion of pharmacologic doses of nicotinic acid may result in dilation of blood vessels, gastrointestinal symptoms, and alterations in lipid metabolism.

PYRIDOXINE (VITAMIN B_6). Pyridoxine is one of several active forms of vitamin B_6 (pyridoxine, pyridoxamine, pyridoxal) that are involved in protein, fat, and carbohydrate metabolism. Pyridoxal phosphate and pyridoxamine act as coenzymes in decarboxylation and deamination reactions of amino acids. Convulsions have been reported among infants who are deficient in pyridoxine, and pyridoxine-responsive anemias and calcium oxalate kidney stones have been reported in adults who are deficient. Paradoxically, the neuropathy caused by isoniazid, which binds to pyridoxine, may be prevented by concurrent administration of extra pyridoxine. Neurologic damage caused by pyridoxine has been described recently among individuals ingesting large doses of this vitamin over prolonged periods. Biochemical deficiency may be diagnosed by decreased red blood cell transaminase levels.

Good food sources of vitamin B_6 include meats (particularly liver), wheat germ, potatoes, bran, and whole grain cereals. The requirement appears to be increased by high-protein diets and ingestion of oral contraceptive agents.

FOLIC ACID. Folates are a group of molecules that are metabolically interrelated and function as coenzymes for one-carbon transfers in the synthesis of DNA and the interconversions of amino acids (Ch. 135). Folate deficiency is common during pregnancy and among alcoholics and institutionalized elderly patients. Megaloblastic anemia caused by folate deficiency is also common among patients with proximal small intestinal disease (e.g., celiac sprue) or resection. Azulfidine appears to interfere with the absorption of folate from the gastrointestinal tract. Alcohol appears to directly interfere with folate metabolism. In one human study of a low-folate diet, megaloblastic anemia occurred at approximately 16 weeks.

Rich food sources of folate include liver, yeast, and green leafy vegetables. Estimates of body stores of folate range from 10 to 50 mg.

VITAMIN B_{12}. Vitamin B_{12} has essential coenzyme activity for the methylation of homocysteine to methionine and for the conversion of methyl malonyl coenzyme A to succinyl coenzyme A. Vitamin B_{12} is also essential for the regeneration of tetrahydrofolate from 5-methyl tetrahydrofolate, a link in the synthesis of DNA. The megaloblastic anemia caused by vitamin B_{12} deficiency responds to the administration of folate (Ch. 135). However, the nerve degeneration caused by vitamin B_{12} deficiency continues unabated despite folate therapy. In the absence of vitamin B_{12} enterohepatic circulation, the storage of the vitamin appears to last for two to five years. Primary dietary sources of vitamin B_{12} are animal products.

VITAMIN C. Specific biochemical reactions dependent on vitamin C activity have not been well defined. However, the vitamin appears to play a role in biological oxidation-reduction reactions, collagen formation, and iron absorption. Deficiency of vitamin C may lead to the clinical syndrome called scurvy, consisting of perifollicular hemorrhage, subperiostal hemorrhage, petechiae, ecchymosis, and bleeding gums. Smoking and oral contraceptives have been reported to decrease plasma levels of vitamin C, but the significance of these observations remains uncertain. There is no convincing evidence that large doses of vitamin C provide any benefits to humans. Hyperoxaluria has been noted occasionally as a side effect of excessive vitamin C intake.

BIOTIN. Biotin is widely distributed among many foodstuffs. Biotin is essential for the activity of many enzyme systems involved in the metabolism of fat and carbohydrate (e.g., pyruvate carboxylase, acetyl coenzyme A carboxylase). Deficiency in adults has only been produced by feeding large amounts of a biotin binder (avidin) and in patients on total parenteral nutrition. Symptoms and signs of deficiency include dermatitis, glossitis, anemia, and depression.

PANTOTHENIC ACID. Pantothenic acid is a component of acetyl coenzyme A that plays a key role in the intermediary metabolism of fats, carbohydrates, and protein. Pantothenic acid is also required for the synthesis of sterols, steroid hormones, and acetyl choline. In the absence of complicating medical conditions, dietary deficiency in man has not been recognized in populations eating a variety of foods, since pantothenic acid appears to be ubiquitous. No formal RDA has been established.

MINERALS

CALCIUM. Calcium is a major mineral constituent of the body and makes up about 2 per cent of body weight (see Ch. 243). Ninety-nine per cent of body calcium is contained in the skeleton, and the small amount of calcium that is present in intracellular and extracellular fluids plays an important role in membrane and muscle function and in blood coagulation. Milk and cheese are rich in calcium, as are shellfish and egg yolk.

Dietary constituents that decrease calcium availability include phytate, liver, oxalate, and malabsorbed fatty acids. Increased dietary protein appears to augment losses of calcium of skeletal origin in the urine. The intestine is able to increase the efficiency of calcium absorption when chronically presented with food that is low in calcium content. Vitamin D is necessary for efficient calcium absorption. There is evidence that the present RDA for calcium for adults (800 mg) is too low.

PHOSPHORUS. Dietary deficiency of phosphorus is unlikely, since nearly all foods contain phosphorus. Prolonged use of nonabsorbable antacids may result in phosphorus deficiency. Phosphorus is important for bone mineralization and for a variety of biochemical reactions in the body (e.g., energy transfer, buffering activity, oxygen transfer from hemoglobin). See Ch. 207 for more details.

MAGNESIUM. Regulation of electrical potential across nerve and muscle membranes is dependent on magnesium. The magnesium deficiency syndrome is similar to hypocalcemic tetany (see Ch. 208). In addition, many enzyme systems are magnesium-dependent. Malabsorptive diseases, alcoholism, kwashiorkor, and diabetes mellitus may all contribute to magnesium deficiency. Phytate decreases the absorption of magnesium, and diuretics promote urinary loss. Magnesium is plentiful in most foods.

IRON. Hemoglobin, myoglobin, and a number of enzymes contain iron. Gastric acidity and reducing and chelating substances such as ascorbic acid promote the absorption of iron from the gastrointestinal tract, whereas calcium and phosphate salts, tannic acid (tea), phytates, and antacids decrease iron availability. Further, heme iron has a greater bioavailability than nonheme iron. Although the normal intestine is somewhat able to adapt its efficiency in absorbing iron to low or high dietary intakes of iron, iron overload may result in hemosiderosis and hemochromatosis. Thirty per cent of body iron is in a nonfunctional storage pool that must be depleted before a reduction in hemoglobin occurs. Microcytic anemia is therefore an insensitive indicator of iron status; rather serum ferritin appears to be a more sensitive clinical indicator of body iron stores.

Trace Minerals
(see Ch. 218 for more details)

ZINC. Zinc deficiency syndrome in humans was first described in Iran and Egypt with growth stunting and hypogonadism recognized as pronounced features. Zinc is an integral part of many enzyme systems (e.g., both DNA and RNA polymerases). Functions such as taste and smell and dark adaptation may also, in part, depend on the state of zinc nutriture. Acrodermatitis enterohepatica is a childhood syndrome caused by an impaired ability of the intestine to absorb zinc. Acute zinc toxicity has been described following ingestion of lemonade mixed in galvanized containers. The syndrome includes nausea, vomiting, and diarrhea. Chronic zinc ingestion in doses of 625 mg has resulted in hypochromic anemia due to copper deficiency. Phytate and fiber are known to impair zinc absorption from the gastrointestinal tract.

COPPER. Copper is a component of numerous metalloenzymes that are critical in mitochondrial energy generation (e.g., cytochrome C oxidase), melanin synthesis, and the cross-linking of collagen. Sources of dietary copper are shellfish, organ meats, and nuts, while dietary factors that decrease the bioavailability of copper include liver, phytate, zinc, calcium, molybdenum, and sulfates. Deficiency of copper is manifested by hypochromic anemia (due to impaired iron absorption and utilization), leukopenia, and hypotonia. Inherited disorders of copper metabolism include albinism and Menkes kinky hair syndrome, wherein impaired copper absorption results in neurological degeneration, growth retardation, and brittle, sparse hair. Copper toxicity is manifested by nausea, vomiting, myalagia, and hemolysis and may occur when dietary intakes of copper exceed 10 to 12 mg per day.

IODINE, FLUORIDE, MANGANESE, SELENIUM, COBALT, CHROMIUM, MOLYBDENUM. For a discussion of iodine, fluoride metabolism, and electrolytes, see Chapters 228, 218, and 76, respectively.

In many animal species *manganese* is a component of enzymes involved in energy and protein metabolism and in mucopolysaccharide synthesis. *Chromium* (as glucose tolerance factor) may promote the action of insulin at the cell membrane level. Meat products and cheese are good dietary sources of chromium. Selenium is needed for glutathione peroxidase activity,

which protects the cell against oxidative damage. A fatal cardiomyopathy seen in Chinese children (Keshan disease) may result from *selenium* deficiency. The requirement for selenium may be higher when dietary vitamin E levels are low. A single patient with *molybdenum* deficiency has been described who, after a course of prolonged total parenteral nutrition, developed neurologic and metabolic abnormalities related to a defect in sulfur amino acid metabolism.

U.S. DIETARY GOALS
(see Ch. 13 concerning the judicious diet)

The U.S. dietary goals, prepared and published in 1977, attempt to outline a prudent diet for the relatively affluent United States public in order to avoid diseases and disabilities that appear to have a relation to diet. These goals recommend a reduction in the percent of calories ingested as fat by the U.S public from 42 per cent to 30 per cent (10 per cent saturated, 20 per cent mono- or polyunsaturated). At least 12 per cent of total calories should be ingested as protein. It further recommends that total calories ingested as carbohydrate be increased from 40 per cent to 58 per cent with an increase in complex carbohydrates (e.g., fiber) and naturally occurring sugars from 28 per cent to 48 per cent. Refined and processed sugar ingestion should be decreased to 10 per cent of the total caloric intake. As more knowledge becomes available, these guidelines may be altered in the future.

Goodhart RS, Shils ME (ed.): Modern Nutrition in Health and Disease. Philadelphia, Lea and Febiger, 1980.
National Research Council: Recommended Dietary Allowances. 9th ed. Washington DC, National Academy of Sciences, 1980.
Roe DA: Drug Induced Nutritional Deficiencies. Westport, AVI Publishing Company Inc. 1976.
Select Committee on Nutrition and Human Studies, United States Senate: Dietary Goals for the United States. US Government Printing Office, 1977.

All of the above are general references that give a broad overview of human nutrition and of recommended dietary allowances. As such they provide excellent background information as well as references concerning more specific topics.

213. NUTRITIONAL ASSESSMENT

Robert M. Russell

The recognition and treatment of malnutrition that accompanies illness plays an important role in optimizing patient care. New modes of delivering nutrients to sick patients by both the parenteral and enteral routes have reduced morbidity and mortality and have shortened the length of hospitalization for both medical and surgical patients.

Methods of nutritional assessment that have been used for some time to judge the severity of malnutrition in lesser developed countries (e.g., anthropometric measures) are now being applied to hospitalized patients in North America and Western Europe. An unexpectedly high prevalence (up to 40 per cent) of protein energy malnutrition has been identified among Western patients. Some of the reasons for the lack of recognition of malnutrition in hospitalized patients include preoccupation with the treatment of the disease process, neglect of the overall nutritional status of the patient, lack of sensitivity of casual observation in the recognition of protein energy malnutrition, absence of a single indicator for diagnosis of malnutrition, and latent onset of clinical signs of malnutrition and relative lack of specificity of these signs. A single nutrient deficiency rarely occurs in a patient; rather, a complex and confusing array of deficiencies are most often present at the same time.

The diagnosis of malnutrition should be made on the basis of dietary information, anthropometric and laboratory measurements, and clinical examination. By using all of this information, a more accurate diagnosis of the malnourished can be achieved, and an effective plan of treatment can be instituted.

DIET

It is not expected that the physician will interpret dietary records of a patient in detail. However, he or she should be aware of the key questions to ask patients, which provide clues about whether or not the patient's dietary intake requires adjustment (Table 213–1). A detailed medical and social history can alert the physician to an existing dietary problem or the likelihood of a dietary problem occurring in the future. For example, poverty, physical or mental disability, complaints of dysphagia, anorexia, nausea, abdominal pain while eating, or ill fitting dentures, and alcoholism may all be factors that prevent adequate dietary intake. Increased nutritional requirements can result from diarrhea, fever, open wounds or burns, malabsorption, diabetes, and hyperthyroidism. The physician should be able to counsel patients regarding general dietary guidelines and recognize cases for referral to a dietitian for more detailed counseling.

The elderly are a group with an increased risk of malnutrition. The reasons for this include poverty, the inability to move around easily, the accumulation of chronic disease necessitating multiple medications, social isolation, and the lack of knowledge for adequate preparation of meals (particularly among elderly men). Problems often arise when interviewing the elderly person for dietary habits if the individual is senile or has impaired short-term memory. A family member may therefore be of great assistance when obtaining dietary information. Finally, appropriate standards for judging the elderly person's diet are not currently available. The Recommended Dietary Allowances (see Table 212–1) were developed as population standards (not individual requirements) and are set to meet the needs of most healthy individuals. The standards for adults are based only on young adults. As a result, they may not be appropriate for meeting the needs of the elderly patient, who has an array of chronic diseases or aging disorders or both.

ANTHROPOMETRIC MEASUREMENTS

Sophisticated and specialized methods to assess body composition are available, e.g., underwater weighing for body density, CT scanning, neutron activation analysis, and K^{40} counting. However, none of these methods is available for widespread clinical use. Anthropometric measurements are inexpensive, quick, and convenient ways of estimating the patient's nutritional status in terms of protein and fat reserves. The most useful anthropometric measures include height, weight, triceps skinfold (actually fatfold) thickness, and midarm circumference. Accurate measurements require only three simple pieces of equipment: a beam or lever balance scale with a vertical measuring rod and a headpiece, a constant tension skinfold caliper, and a flexible measuring tape, preferably with an insertion.

TABLE 213–1. KEY QUESTIONS TO ASK AS PART OF THE NUTRITIONAL ASSESSMENT OF THE ADULT

1. Is there recent weight gain or weight loss? How much?
2. Are there alterations in appetite, sense of smell, or taste?
3. Are there problems with chewing or swallowing? Does the patient have poor dentition or poorly fitting dentures?
4. Are there symptoms of gastrointestinal disorders: diarrhea, constipation, nausea, vomiting, early satiety?
5. Does the patient live alone? If not, who prepares meals? Does he/she know how to cook?
6. What type of cooking facilities and refrigeration are in the patient's home?
7. Does the patient purchase a variety of food? If not, is it due to financial difficulties?
8. How many meals are eaten per day? How many snacks? Are one or more meals eaten outside of the home? If so, where?
9. Is the patient physically or mentally handicapped? Does this prevent the individual from shopping, cooking, or feeding herself or himself?
10. Does the patient take any dietary supplements (e.g., vitamins)?
11. How much alcohol does the patient consume?
12. Does the patient use prescription or nonprescription drugs?
13. Are there any religious or ethnic beliefs or food intolerances that prevent adequate food intake?
14. Does the patient follow a dietary restriction? Is it prescribed or self-imposed?
15. Is the patient depressed?

TABLE 213–2. REFERENCE WEIGHT/HEIGHT FIGURES DERIVED FROM ACTUARIAL (MORTALITY EXPERIENCE) DATA OF THE 1979 BUILD AND BLOOD PRESSURE STUDY*

Height		Weight			
		Male		Female	
(in)	(cm)	(lb)	(kg)	(lb)	(kg)
58	147.3	—	—	114	51.7
59	149.9	—	—	116.5	52.8
60	152.4	—	—	119	53.9
61	154.9	—	—	122	55.3
62	157.5	133	60.3	125	56.7
63	160.0	135	61.2	128	58.0
64	162.6	137.5	62.4	131	59.4
65	165.1	140	63.5	134	60.8
66	167.6	143	64.9	137	62.1
67	170.2	146	66.2	140	63.5
68	172.7	149	67.6	143	64.9
69	175.3	152	68.9	146	66.2
70	177.8	155	70.3	149	67.6
71	180.3	158.5	71.9	152	69.0
72	182.9	162	73.9	—	—
73	185.4	166	75.3	—	—
74	188.0	169.5	76.9	—	—
75	190.5	174	78.9	—	—

*Weights represent the midpoint of the middle frame for each height. These values correct the 1983 Metropolitan Tables to nude weights and heights.

WEIGHT FOR HEIGHT. Single reference weights for each inch of height have been derived from United States life insurance actuarial data on longevity and have been termed "ideal" or "optimal" by some investigators. However, these single weights should not be interpreted as "ideal," since they represent the midpoint of an acceptable range for a person of medium frame and were derived from the mortality experience of only those men and women between the ages of 20 to 59 years who could afford life insurance. These weights are neither age nor race specific and do not represent all cultural groups. Further, these reference weights cannot be applied to patients with peripheral edema or ascites. Despite the recognized flaws in using such single reference weights as standards, clinicians have found the 1983 Metropolitan Life Insurance Reference Weights for height useful for judging a patient's nutritional status reflecting caloric sufficiency. These reference weights (corrected to the nude state) are provided in Table 213–2. Using these weights for heights as a reference, 20 per cent above each weight places approximately 25 per cent of the United States population in the overweight for height or obese category, and 20 per cent below places less than 5 per cent of the population in the underweight category. Although these values were derived from a younger population, it appears that these reference values can be applied cautiously to the elderly based on data indicating that mean weights of healthy men and women from ages 70 to 90 years old closely approximate the Metropolitan weights. In children, weight and height are often used as separate measures to indicate malnutrition and are expressed as percentiles of a cross-section of American children. Weight and height tables for children can be found in most pediatric textbooks.

The amount of weight lost and the rate at which it was lost by a patient are also important for judging an individual's nutritional status. A history of weight loss of 10 per cent or greater (6 per cent in an overweight patient) over a six-month period can be indicative of malnutrition.

TRICEPS SKINFOLD THICKNESS. This measurement provides an estimate of the body's fat reserves. The measurement should be taken at a marked point on the right arm, halfway between the acromial process of the scapula and the olecranon process of the elbow. The patient's arm should be relaxed when the fatfold is grasped posteriorly between the thumb and forefinger of the examiner. The fold should be raised, allowing underlying

TABLE 213–3. RECOMMENDED ANTHROPOMETRIC MEASUREMENT STANDARDS FOR THE UNITED STATES ADULT POPULATION

	Triceps Skinfold (mm)		Mid-Arm Muscle Circumference (cm)	
	25–64 yr	*>65 yr*	*25–64 yr*	*>65 yr*
Male	12	11	27.9	26.8
Female	21	24	21.2	22.5

muscle to fall back to the bone, and the calipers applied. The measurement is useless if arm edema or paralysis is present. Age- and sex-specific standards for triceps skinfold (TSF) thickness have been published by Frisancho (1981) for all ages through 75 years (summarized in Table 213–3). A range of 40 to 190 per cent of the standard is considered an acceptable TSF measure, since large variances are found for fatfold thicknesses in the normal population. A patient whose TSF thickness is

TABLE 213–4. SUGGESTED CRITERIA TO JUDGE MALNUTRITION AND OBESITY IN THE UNITED STATES ADULT POPULATION

	Malnutrition		Obesity	
	Per Cent of Standard	*Corresponding Percentile*	*Per Cent of Standard*	*Corresponding Percentile*
WT/HT	<80	5th	>120	<5*
Triceps Skinfold	<40	5th	>190	>90th
Midarm Muscle Circumference	<80	5th	NA	NA

*Weight for height percentiles are based on the Health and Nutrition Examination Survey (HANES) of 1971–1974 comparison to Metropolitan 1983 standards. Triceps skinfold and midarm muscle circumference percentiles are derived from HANES data.

TABLE 213–5. CLINICAL SIGNS AND SYMPTOMS OF NUTRITIONAL INADEQUACY IN ADULT PATIENTS

	Clinical Sign or Symptom	Nutrient
General	Wasted, skinny	Calorie
	Loss of appetite	Protein-energy
Skin	Psoriasiform rash, eczematous scaling	Zinc
	Pallor	Folate, iron, vitamin B_{12}, copper
	Follicular hyperkeratosis	Vitamin A
	Perifollicular petechiae	Vitamin C
	Flaking dermatitis	Protein-energy, niacin, riboflavin, zinc
	Bruising	Vitamin C, vitamin K
	Pigmentation changes	Niacin, protein-energy
	Scrotal dermatosis	Riboflavin
	Thickening and dryness of skin	Linoleic acid
Head	Temporal muscle wasting	Protein-energy
Hair	Sparse and thin, dyspigmentation Easy to pull out	Protein
Eyes	History of night blindness (also impaired visual recovery after glare)	Vitamin A, zinc
	Photophobia, blurring, conjunctival inflammation	Riboflavin, vitamin A
	Corneal vascularization	Riboflavin
	Xerosis, Bitot spots, keratomalacia	Vitamin A
Mouth	Glossitis	Riboflavin, niacin, folic acid, vitamin B_{12}, pyridoxine
	Bleeding gums	Vitamin C, riboflavin
	Cheilosis	Riboflavin
	Angular stomatitis	Riboflavin, iron
	Hypogeusia	Zinc
	Tongue fissuring	Niacin
	Tongue atrophy	Riboflavin, niacin, iron
	Scarlet and raw tongue	Niacin
	Nasolabial seborrhea	Pyridoxine
Neck	Goiter	Iodine
	Parotid enlargement	Protein
Thorax	Thoracic rosary	Vitamin D
Abdomen	Diarrhea	Niacin, folate, vitamin B_{12}
	Distention	Protein-energy
	Hepatomegaly	Protein-energy
Extremities	Edema	Protein, thiamin
	Softening of bone	Vitamin D, calcium, phosphorus
	Bone tenderness	Vitamin D
	Bone ache, joint pain	Vitamin C
	Muscle wasting and weakness	Protein, calorie, vitamin D, selenium, sodium chloride
	Muscle tenderness, muscle pain	Thiamin
	Hyporeflexia	Thiamin
	Ataxia	Vitamin B_{12}
Nails	Spooning	Iron
	Transverse lines	Protein
Neurologic	Tetany	Calcium, magnesium
	Paresthesias	Thiamin, vitamin B_{12}
	Loss of reflexes, wrist drop, foot drop	Thiamin
	Loss of vibratory and position sense	Vitamin B_{12}
	Dementia, disorientation	Niacin
Blood	Anemia	Vitamin E, B_{12}, folate, iron, pyridoxine
	Hemolysis	Phosphorus

less than 40 per cent of the HANES standard is considered to have depleted body fat stores, while the patient whose TSF thickness is more than 190 per cent of standard is considered obese.

MIDARM MUSCLE CIRCUMFERENCE. This derived value is used to estimate lean body or skeletal muscle mass. To calculate this value, the midarm circumference must first be measured at the same site as the triceps fatfold with the patient's right arm in a relaxed posture. The formula to calculate midarm muscle circumference (MAMC) is:

$$\text{MAMC (cm)} = \text{midarm circumference (cm)} - (0.314 \times \text{TSF (mm)})$$

Median values are summarized in Table 213–3. Twenty per cent below this standard is indicative of a depletion of lean body mass. Neither TSF nor MAMC standards have been derived for the very elderly (i.e., older than 75 years). A summary of criteria to judge malnutrition and obesity by anthropometric measurements is presented in Table 213–4.

CLINICAL ASSESSMENT

Early clinical symptoms and signs of malnutrition are rather vague and often include weakness, lethargy, irritability, and lightheadedness. Many of the symptoms and signs are nonspecific for a single nutrient deficit and may be caused by insufficiency of one of several nutrients. For example, flaking dermatitis may accompany deficiencies of protein, riboflavin, or linoleic acid. On the other hand, when certain clinical signs appear, the nutrient deficit may be very severe (e.g., scleromalacia, a leading and rapidly progressive cause of blindness due to vitamin A deficiency). Table 213–5 contains a listing of clinical presentations and the associated nutrient deficits that may cause them.

Functional and end organ testing have been advocated for diagnosis of specific nutrient deficits (e.g., dark adaptation for vitamin A, taste and smell for zinc, bone density for vitamin D, and so on). However, functional tests are not available to assess the status of most nutrients, and, as with clinical signs, the functional tests are often nonspecific. For example, impairment of dark adaptation may be caused by zinc deficiency as well as vitamin A deficiency. Taste and smell may be affected by age, smoking, and drugs as well as by zinc nutriture. Bone density is diminished in both osteoporosis and osteomalacia due to vitamin D deficiency.

As with dietary assessment, the elderly present a particular problem when evaluated for the presence or absence of clinical signs or symptoms of malnutrition. Some of the changes associated with malnutrition may also be a function of normal aging (e.g., hypogeusia, dry skin, sparse hair, atrophy of the tongue, bleeding gums from ill fitting dentures). Nevertheless, as with younger patients, clinical signs should be assessed for possible nutritional implications.

LABORATORY ASSESSMENT

Laboratory measurements are another tool that can aid the physician in making a diagnosis of malnutrition. Modern analytical instruments (e.g., high-performance liquid chromatography), techniques (e.g., radio or enzyme immunoassays), and computerization have greatly increased the capability of nutritional biochemical testing. Currently available biochemical tests for assessing nutritional status include the direct measurement of a nutrient or nutrient metabolite in blood, other body fluid (e.g., urine, saliva), or tissues (e.g., white blood cells, hair, liver) and the measurement of a biochemical function that is nutrient specific. For example, laboratory tests for pyridoxine status may include the direct measurement of pyridoxal 5′-phosphate in plasma or the enzymatic activity of erythrocyte transaminase, for which pyridoxal 5′-phosphate is a cofactor. The latter test involves the calculation of an activity coefficient whereby red blood cell transaminase activity is determined before and after the addition of pyridoxal 5′-phosphate. An activity coefficient of greater than 1 is indicative of pyridoxine deficiency.

The establishment of normal nutrient values in body fluids or tissues for each sex varies from laboratory to laboratory, and the normal range usually represents a mean ± 2 SD of a normal population. Optimally, a low biochemical nutrient value in body fluids or tissue should be coupled with a specific functional abnormality before making the diagnosis of a nutrient deficiency. However, in practice this is rarely done. One guide for interpretation of laboratory values that reflects the status of various nutrients in the blood or serum of adults is presented in Table 213–6. For some nutrients (e.g., vitamin A) children have a different normal range than adults. The reader is referred to a pediatric or nutrition text for detailed information on age-specific normal values. Normal biochemical ranges have not been established for the very old (i.e., over 75 years). The physician must rely upon values derived from younger populations to judge the nutritional biochemical parameters for this group.

TABLE 213–6. GUIDE FOR INTERPRETATION OF BIOCHEMICAL INDICES FOR SELECTED NUTRIENTS

Nutrient	Normal*	Deficient	Marginal
Albumin	3.5–5.5 g/dl	2.8–3.2	3.2–3.5
Transferrin	200–400 mg/dl	< 200	
Prealbumin	10–40 mg/dl	<10	
Ferritin	12–300 ng/ml	< 12	
Retinol	30–90 μg/dl	< 15	15–30
Carotene	40–240 μg/dl	< 40	
Vitamin E	0.5–1.8 mg/dl	< 0.5	0.5–0.7
Vitamin D (25-OH-D_3)	15–40 ng/ml		
Thiamin (erythrocyte)	0.9–1.25†	> 1.25	1.25–1.20
Riboflavin	0.9–1.39†	> 1.40	1.30–1.40
Pyridoxine	0.9–2.2†	> 2.2	
Niacin (urine 2-pyridone/N′-methyl nicotinamide—metabolite ratio)	1.0–4.0	< 1.0	
Serum Folate	6–20 ng/ml	≤ 3.0	3–6
Red Cell Folate	150–450 ng/ml	< 150	
Vitamin B_{12}	> 200 pg/ml	< 150	150–200
Vitamin C	0.3–2.0 mg/dl	< 0.2	0.2–0.3
Calcium	8.5–10.5 mg/dl	< 8.5	
Phosphorus	2.5–4.5 mg/dl	< 2.5	
Iron	50–170 μg/dl		
Zinc	70–130 μg/dl	≤ 65	65–70
Copper	70–160 μg/dl	< 70	
Magnesium	1.4–2.5 mg/dl	≤ 1.4	

*These normal values will vary with the method used and in different laboratories.
†An enzymatic assay. Values represent an activity coefficient.

Many nutrient biochemical diagnostic tests are not readily available in a hospital clinical chemistry laboratory. Nevertheless, there are several laboratory tests that are routinely performed (e.g., hemoglobin level, serum protein level) that may aid the physician in assessing the nutritional status of his or her patients. In the absence of liver disease, a low serum albumin may be used as an indicator of protein nutriture. In sick patients who are obese, silent kwashiorkor (protein malnutrition) may develop, as reflected by low serum protein values, although the patient may continue to look overnourished and anthropometric measures may be normal or exceed the normal range. Other proteins that are synthesized in the liver and that have a more rapid turnover than albumin (e.g., transferrin, prealbumin) may also be used to diagnose protein malnutrition at an earlier stage. The transferrin in serum, if not directly measured, may be estimated from the total iron binding capacity (TIBC) according to the formula: $(0.8 \times \text{TIBC}) - 43$. Protein values that are more than 20 per cent below the lower limit of the normal range are generally regarded as severely substandard. It has been suggested that elderly people have a somewhat lower normal serum albumin value and that age-specific standards for serum protein values are needed.

Muscle protein can be estimated from urinary creatinine excretion; this complements the anthropometric indicator MAMC. The amount of creatinine appearing in the urine over 24 hours is proportional to muscle mass. A crude standard for creatinine excretion can be derived by multiplying an individual's reference weight-for-height by 23 or 18 (for males and females respectively). Twenty per cent below these derived values may represent muscle protein depletion. However, several factors are known to affect creatinine excretion (e.g., kidney disease, diet, fever, strenous exercise, menstrual cycle), and the interpretation, therefore, must be carried out cautiously.

In protein energy malnutrition, the number of circulating lymphocytes diminish, and the patient demonstrates impaired delayed hypersensitivity to common skin antigens (e.g., mumps, *Candida* tuberculin). Thus, these tests also may be used in assessing the patient's nutritional status. A lymphocyte count of less than 1200 per cubic millimeter is regarded as severely substandard. The effect of advanced age on these parameters is uncertain.

Frisancho AR: New norms of upper limb fat and muscle areas for assessment of nutritional status. Am J Clin Nutr 34:2540, 1981. *This article presents American standards for athropometric measures for ages 1 to 75 years, derived from the HANES survey of 1971–1974.*

Goodhart RS, Shils ME (eds.): Modern Nutrition in Health and Disease. Philadelphia, Lea and Febiger, 1980. *This nutrition textbook provides detailed discussion of signs and symptoms of nutritional disorders.*

Jelliffe DB: The Assessment of Nutritional Status. Oxford University Press (in press). *An updated version of the World Health Organization's Manual for Nutritional Assessment of Populations.*

Paige DM (ed.): Manual of Clinical Nutrition. Pleasantville, Nutrition Publications, Inc., 1983. *This manual provides most tables and information for clinical assessment of nutritional status for pediatric and adult patients.*

Sauberlich HE, Dowdy RP, Skala JH: Laboratory Tests for the Assessment of Nutritional Status. Boca Raton, CRC Press, 1979. *This volume provides descriptions and some evaluation measures for laboratory tests used for the assessment of nutritional status.*

214. PROTEIN-CALORIE UNDERNUTRITION

Errol B. Marliss

The syndromes of protein-calorie malnutrition (PCM) were defined in the 1920's in areas where food was deficient in quantity and/or quality. The terms kwashiorkor and marasmus have retained an "exotic" ring in developed countries and rarely if ever appear in the diagnostic categories on discharge summaries, despite the fact that between 450 million and one billion humans suffer from chronic hunger and malnutrition. However, these syndromes are anything but curiosities. With a resurgence of interest in the role of nutrition in health and disease, a veritable "epidemic" has been recognized in a number of patient populations. In particular, hospitalized adult medical and surgical patients have been shown to develop signs of PCM in 25 to 50 per cent of cases within two weeks of admission. Thus PCM is not only a problem of postweaning third-world children, but is an almost ubiquitous problem that can be readily treated, but preferably prevented. This chapter emphasizes the forms most likely to be encountered in developed countries.

DEFINITION AND ETIOLOGY

Precise definitions require quantitative reference to appropriate control populations and depend upon the anthropomorphic and laboratory measures referred to in Ch. 213. "Undernutrition" is the state produced by inadequate intake of food and may have as its only manifestation retarded growth in children or loss of weight in adults. While "malnutrition" can refer to over- or undernutrition, it most commonly connotes a dietary lack of one or more nutrients, which markedly retards development in children and causes the appearance of specific, clinically recognizable deficiency states at all ages. Marasmus is the clinical syndrome resulting from prolonged limitation of intake of both protein and energy, whereas kwashiorkor results from deficiency of protein relative to energy. Caloric intake may be adequate or even excessive, and kwashiorkor may occur concurrently with marasmus. PCM is classified as primary, due to limited food supply, and secondary, due to the presence of disease(s) that prevents access to or absorption of food, causes excessive caloric loss, or increases demand for energy, or combinations of these. However, since primary PCM is often complicated, as by infection, this distinction may be difficult to make.

INCIDENCE, PREVALENCE, AND EPIDEMIOLOGY

Undernutrition is encountered with different frequencies in different age and population groups, and prevalence data vary according to diagnostic criteria. In children, decreased weight for height is taken as the diagnostic criterion but is criticized because stunting is not thereby ascertained. Similarly, mortality rates in infancy are a crude index of undernutrition because all causes are grouped together. Although in this age group diarrheal diseases are still the commonest cause of mortality world wide, they are highly correlated to poor nutritional status. Furthermore, early childhood mortality rates increase, especially with decrease below 80 per cent of normal weight for height. Thus figures of 25 per cent (in 28 developing countries) to 64 per cent (in Central America) of children with malnutrition gives indication of the enormous magnitude of this problem. In developing countries, it must be considered to be a social "disease," affecting families, communities, and geographic areas: undernourished adults show poor work performance, perhaps lower intellectual performance, suceptibility to infection, and poor reproduction performance in terms of weight gain in pregnancy, small-for-dates babies, and inadequate milk production. Thus, although fewer adults show overt clinical signs of malnutrition themselves (e.g., 8 per cent of hospital admissions in Guatemala), they are index cases of a more widespread problem. This is referred to as the "microenvironment," i.e., the family and individual level, compared to the "macroenvironment," i.e., the regional or national level. Factors in the microenvironment that lead to poor nutrition include restricted purchasing power, poor nutrition education leading to poor consumption practices, and inappropriate distribution of nutrients among family members. One distressing feature of the macroenvironment is that production on a worldwide basis is in fact adequate to feed the population, and this also applies to many individual countries with high prevalence of malnutrition. This situation is explicable by losses of food between production and utilization (30 per cent in some countries), by problems of distribution between areas of production and consumption, and by economic and political factors. Improvements especially in the "macroenvironment" had led to decreases in infant mortality over the two decades preceding the recent recession, but international economic factors have reversed this trend in recent years.

The microenvironmental factors also occur in developed countries. As improbable as it might seem, kwashiorkor has been reported in several United States centers. Some cases are due to peculiar dietary habits imposed by parents on children (e.g., unbalanced vegetarian diets), almost total elimination of protein in children considered (often incorrectly) to have sensitivity to cow's milk, and replacement of milk by low-protein nondairy creamers, as well as extreme poverty, parental alcoholism, and other social disruptions. The incidence of such cases is probably higher than reported.

Furthermore, nutritional surveys even in pediatric teaching hospitals have also revealed a striking prevalence of PCM, e.g., 37 per cent in one study. Several such surveys in hospitalized adults in the past ten years have shown both anthropomorphic and biochemical evidence for PCM; Bistrian and colleagues' data suggested 44 per cent of general medical patients and 50 per cent of surgical patients were afflicted. In patients in a medical service for two or more weeks, 79 per cent showed decreases in arm muscle circumference, 74 per cent lost weight (average 4.5 kg), 64 per cent had decreases in hematocrit, and 47 per cent had declining serum albumin (Butterworth et al). Patients at greatest risk for PCM in hospital were found to have the following: (1) gross underweight (less than 80 per cent weight for height), (2) gross overweight (because their requirements are often overlooked), (3) recent loss of more than 10 per cent body weight, (4) alcoholism, (5) "nil per os" orders for more than ten days on 5 per cent dextrose in water solutions intravenously, (6) protracted nutrient losses (gut, fistulas, dialysis), (7) increased metabolic needs, and (8) therapies with catabolic, anorexogenic, or antinutrient drugs (steroids, chemotherapy, immunosuppressants). Aged patients are likely at greatest risk because of poor premorbid nutrition, polypharmacy, and concurrent illnesses. Certain psychiatric patients in hospitals and the community are probably malnourished. Much hospital PCM is the direct result of spectacular therapeutic advances that prolong the lives of patients, while their concurrent nutrient requirements are not attended to. Other groups at risk are those who self-administer nutritionally inadequate reducing diets with the primary aim of fat mobilization. Those at all parts of the weight spectrum—the obese, those with normal weight who wish to lose weight for cosmetic reasons, and those with anorexia nervosa—may suffer PCM of variable severity and duration during such diets. The prevalence of these subsets of PCM is particularly difficult to ascertain, as are potential long-term consequences (see Ch. 215 and 216). They are likely to be common, however, given the widespread use of reducing regimens and the large numbers of individuals in these categories.

PATHOPHYSIOLOGY

METABOLIC FACTORS. Maintenance of normal body composition and energy fuel homeostasis requires regular intake of energy substrates, protein, water and electrolytes, vitamins, and other essential micronutrients. Reference values are given in Ch. 212. Specific quantitative and qualitative increments are required for growth, pregnancy, muscular exercise, severe environmental conditions, and disease. In the case of the undernourished adult, deficits in energy and protein are made up from endogenous sources, via an elegantly orchestrated set of hormonal, neural, and local tissue enzymatic responses. These appear to operate in a hierarchial fashion with highest priority on sparing protein (of which there is no known "storage" form) by use of endogenous fat stores for energy. Early in undernutrition, liver and possibly muscle glycogen are depleted but appear to be at least partly restored later—possibly constituting a short-term "emergency" energy supply. The mobilization of protein stores beyond a critical limit presumably results in death. This may well be the case in kwashiorkor, in which some fat stores remain, but in other forms of starvation, exhaustion of fat stores may be the critical step, even with some protein theoretically still available.

The best controlled data in such states are from experimental studies of total fasting. This, however, is a state rarely encountered clinically; either the individual has maintained some level of oral energy and protein intake, or some level has been provided parenterally. In total fasting increased ketogenesis provides the brain with a fuel that displaces its glucose requirement and thereby allows for sparing of the protein (which would otherwise be used for glucose synthesis). This response is not directly applicable to the starved individual, since very little carbohydrate is required to suppress ketogenesis (e.g., 50 grams per day, or a sum of protein plus carbohydrate of 100 grams per day), and the undernourished individual is not typically ketotic or even ketonuric (a highly sensitive index). Exceptions are in therapeutic hypocaloric "protein-sparing modified fasts" (see Ch. 216) with increased energy requirement and in diabetics.

Although carbohydrate alone is "protein sparing" (vis-à-vis total fasting), the fundamental law of protein homeostasis is that it requires exogenous protein. At any given protein intake, added calories either as carbohydrate or fat enhance the availability for maintenance of protein synthesis of the constituent amino acids, which would otherwise be oxidized as an energy source. Thus the protein requirement varies with concurrent energy intake, being higher in both relative (protein-energy ratio) and absolute terms when energy intake is below requirement. Furthermore, the protein quality (in terms of essential amino acid composition) is a factor. The higher the quality (animal proteins), the lower the relative requirement. Unfortunately, where malnutrition is rampant, not only quantity but quality of protein is often poor—being mainly from vegetable sources. Of protein consumed in North America, 70 per cent is from animal sources, whereas it is as low as 14 to 20 per cent in developing countries. Thus the diet most likely to be associated with malnutrition is one based on cereal grains, starchy roots, cornstarch, possibly with overdiluted milk, snack foods, and alcohol and without animal protein. Such a diet is low in animal and separated vegetable fats, with less than 10 per cent of energy from the naturally occurring vegetable fat in developing countries, but it may have a substantial fat intake in developed countries if it is based on processed foods.

In energy-balance terms such diets, even if adequate in calories, are often very low in protein of good biologic value. When total calories are restricted further, the protein inadequacy assumes even greater importance. In either case in the adult, body protein is mobilized, and in the energy-starved individual both protein and fat are depleted, the latter generally more rapidly. The body progressively adapts to this situation by decreased energy expenditure (metabolic rate) overall and per unit of lean body mass, decreased physical activity, and decreased rates of body protein turnover. If such changes result in equilibrium with intake, a fragile state of "maximal adaptation" occurs that may persist over long periods. However, once the caloric deficit is severe, basal energy expenditure may be normal or increased relative to lead body mass, which then decreases at a faster rate.

In childhood, the energy and protein deficiencies occur when requirements are high per unit of body weight. Pathophysiology of the deficits varies with age. If they occur before weaning, they are in both protein and energy, leading to retarded growth with decreased or absent fat stores. If after weaning, the replacement nutrients determine the course in one of three usual patterns: (1) Marginal protein and calories, a pattern that perpetuates undernutrition. The adapted state continues with slower than normal physical growth, but with frequent infections (e.g., measles, pertussis, parasitic infestations, diarrheal diseases) that may precipitate severe PCM. (2) Severe restriction, which results in marasmus. (3) High calorie but protein-deficient diets, which lead to the typical edematous PCM of the "sugar-baby" type. In all cases brain growth and development may well be retarded, and irreversible deficits may occur. Concurrently, head circumference may remain small, and muscle mass and muscle cell size are subnormal. Tissues with rapid cell turnover also develop impaired size and possibly impaired function. Atrophy of the gut, and deficiency of intestinal, pancreatic, and biliary secretions may compound PCM by reducing absorption of what is ingested. Those who survive to adulthood then may remain in this precariously adapted state, although with smaller body size than had the malnutrition started in adulthood.

ENDOCRINE FACTORS. The changes in endocrine and neuroendocrine function in PCM are complex and some remain controversial. Insulin is the principal hormone of anabolism, and catabolism is enhanced when its levels fall. Both postabsorptive and postchallenge (glucose, amino acids) insulin levels are lowered in PCM. These levels allow net mobilization of fatty acids from adipose tissue triglyceride and of amino acids from protein (subsequently oxidized, recycled into protein synthesis, or converted to glucose by gluconeogenesis), as well as decreased protein synthesis in many tissues. However, a stimulation of insulin secretion by carbohydrate administration during protein deficiency in PCM has been considered partly responsible for the kwashiorkor-like syndrome in malnourished hospital patients. The resulting "high" insulin levels have been postulated to restrict fat mobilization, to limit use of muscle-derived amino acids for synthesis of "visceral" proteins, and to result in more amino acid oxidation. (This hypothetical sequence could equally well be interpreted to implicate the lack of exogenous protein and ongoing caloric deficits as responsible.) Insulin responses are certainly related to the sum of carbohydrate and protein intake, but other mechanisms not as yet defined remain capable of assuring that caloric deficits are filled from endogenous fat (when present), at widely varying insulin levels. Thus, strategies of nutrient replacement should not be aimed at achieving the lowest theoretical insulin response, but must take account of the other mechanisms, as well as the impairment of insulin responsiveness, that are clearly characteristic of PCM. Insulin secretion returns to normal after recovery from PCM. Increase in glucagon levels occurs in total fasting but not necessarily in PCM, and the role of this hormone is not likely to be central.

Hypothalamic-pituitary function is also altered in a complex manner. Growth hormone levels are generally increased in PCM, although plasma somatomedins are low, especially with severe protein deficiency. The pituitary-thyroid axis may well be an important factor in the decrease in metabolic rate. Carbohydrate intake appears to play an important role in this response. When intake is decreased, although TSH and its responses to TRH are unaltered, thyroxine levels are often normal (but may be low), but its peripheral conversion to triiodothyronine is altered, in favor of the inactivating pathway to reverse triiodothyronine (Ch. 228). Interpretation of thyroid hormone values must take account of decreases in binding proteins in PCM, and of decreased synthesis of triiodothyronine receptors.

The pituitary-adrenal axis has been the focus of hypotheses to explain differences between kwashiorkor and marasmus: An increase in activity (hypercortisolemia) in marasmus was postulated to sustain flux of amino acids from muscle (increasing the wasting) to liver to support albumin synthesis, whereas the calories provided in kwashiorkor were supposed sufficient not to result in hypercortisolemia, and therefore to restrict such flux, with consequent hypoalbuminemia. While a coherent hypothesis, the data have not so far proven this to be the case. When hypercortisolemia occurs, it appears more related to impaired catabolism than to increased production, and its pathophysiologic significance is not clear.

A variety of abnormalities in pituitary-gonadal function has been reputed, including low testosterone accompanied by high FSH and LH in adult males and many reproductive disorders in females, most of which return toward or to normal after treatment.

ELECTROLYTE, MINERAL, AND MICRONUTRIENT CHANGES. The tissue loss leads to concomitant losses of body nitrogen, potassium, and phosphorus. Fluid shifts may further lead to changes of sodium and chloride and to exchange of sodium intracellularly for potassium and magnesium. In kwashiorkor, the frequent diarrhea further exacerbates losses. Extrarenal fluid and electrolyte losses are an important factor in hospital PCM, with the acid-base alterations that accompany them. The most prominent, clinically important depletions are of potassium and magnesium. Total and extracellular water and sodium are increased in kwashiorkor, related to the hypoproteinemia, and associated with increased plasma aldosterone. In severe cases, renal plasma flow, glomerular filtration rate, urine concentrating ability, and acidification are impaired. Zinc and chromium deficiencies are recognized in certain geographic regions and during prolonged parenteral nutrition, and their role in PCM is currently the subject of active study. The manifestations of vitamin deficiencies will vary with local dietary patterns or the inpatient population considered. Although clinical signs of water-soluble vitamin deficiencies may be uncommon, and serum levels normal, inadequate intake of thiamin, riboflavin, ascorbic acid, niacin, and folate may have taken place. In kwashiorkor, serum vitamin A is consistently low and may be accompanied by ocular lesions. This is often accounted for not only by poor intake of vitamin A, but also by abnormal absorption and transport. Vitamin E shows similar decreased levels and kinetic defects. Some reports have indicated elevated levels of vitamin B_{12}.

IMMUNE RESPONSES. Almost all aspects of the immune response have been shown to be impaired in PCM, with the degree of impairment related to severity. Concurrent infection, especially with loss of nutrients, exacerbates this state. Some resistance to infection is conferred during breast feeding, but this depends on the adequacy of maternal nutrition and is lost on weaning. When PCM begins at or before birth, the infant is generally immunocompromised, with decreases in IgG, IgA, IgM, and IgE, whereas in older children immunoglobulins are usually normal, or elevated when infection is present. Often a single class may be increased, e.g., IgA, perhaps reflecting the frequency of respiratory and gastrointestinal infections. Specific antibody production to many antigens is subnormal, and this causes poor responses to immunization programs, although responses to different agents vary. Not only the quantity of the antibody response, but affinities and binding capacities are reduced. In vivo and in vitro tests of cell-mediated immunity are impaired, and skin tests for delayed-type hypersensitivity give subnormal responses. The thymus is atrophic. Typically, peripheral blood lymphocyte counts are decreased, especially thymus-derived lymphocytes, with values commonly less than 1200 per cu mm. Some of the cellular immune abnormalities may be related to trace metal deficiencies, including zinc. Nonspecific defenses are abnormal, including opsonization, interferon production, bacterial killing by phagocytes (although phagocytosis itself may be normal), and neutrophil and plasma lysozyme levels. Complement components other than C_4 may be decreased. Iron deficiency may contribute to the impaired bacterial killing after phagocytosis. Frequently acute phase protein levels are elevated, including C-reactive proteins, alpha-2-macroglobulin, alpha-1-antitrypsin, and haptoglobin, related to the protein loss and infection. The critical factors that decrease resistance to infection in PCM have not been fully elucidated but are of obvious importance. Introduction of nutrients seems to reverse most if not all the abnormalities; in fact, in the hospital setting, they are largely preventable. Even in previously normal adults, immune deficits appear to develop sufficiently rapidly that preventive measures appear mandatory.

OTHER PHYSIOLOGIC CHANGES. The adrenergic limb of the sympathetic nervous system is highly responsive to both energy and protein intake, with decreased norepinephrine turnover in many tissues (as long as salt intake is maintained), possibly responsible in part for the fall in metabolic rate. Dietary amino acids have a precursor role in neurotransmitter synthesis (tyrosine for norepinephrine, tryptophan for serotonin), such that their levels and turnover decrease with protein deficiency. Electroencephalograms may show diminished voltage and excessively slow rhythmic activity. The decreases in triiodothyronine, adrenergic tone, insulin, and possibly the lack of "insulation" by subcutaneous fat are associated with decreased body temperature and decreased febrile response to infection.

Many aspects of cardiovascular function change in PCM via complex mechanisms related to serum proteins, extracellular and vascular volume, adrenergic activity, and cardiac muscle size and performance. Cardiac output declines in parallel to metabolic rate; blood pressure is reduced, although pulse rate may increase; and electrocardiograms show low voltage. Postural hypotension occurs. Renal function decreases, but usually remains adequate because of the decrease in requirements, unless an additional metabolic or infective burden is superimposed. Blood volume, the hematocrit, and erythrocyte counts decrease, producing a normochromic, normocytic anemia whose pathogenesis relates to multiple deficiencies.

Despite marked fatty changes in the liver, beginning in the periportal of the lobule and extending toward the portal vein, common tests for liver function are usually normal in the absence of hepatitis. The exocrine pancreas decreases in size and its secretions diminish, and indices of small intestinal mucosal turnover and function do likewise. These can result secondarily in malabsorption and lactose intolerance, even without bacterial overgrowth or other infections. Epidermal atrophy with varying degrees of hyperkeratosis and parakeratosis is found in the skin.

CLINICAL MANIFESTATIONS AND DIAGNOSIS

(Table 214–1)

The classic syndromes of kwashiorkor and marasmus are not encountered frequently in clinical practice in developed areas. Even in developing countries in Asia, Africa, and Latin America, intermediate syndromes are in fact more common. In both settings chronic mild to moderate malnutrition is the form that predominates, and while not difficult to diagnose it is less flagrant than the "textbook" PCM usually described. In children, longstanding restriction is apparent from retardation in height and weight gain; when adapted to PCM the stunted child may even have adequate weight for height. This is not "normal but small," because immaturity in biologic development is present: deficits in lean body mass and adiposity, with relative overhydration, reduced physical activity, apathy, frequent episodes of ill-defined sickness, anorexia, diarrhea, and a higher mortality rate from common infectious diseases. Furthermore, psychomotor and mental development are retarded, although it is uncertain what contribution is from the social versus the nutritional deprivations so common in such individuals. In adults, similar body compositional changes occur, but physically the appearance is of leanness that may merge into cachexia. Since protein requirements are lower per unit of lean body mass in children, the manifestations are most often those of caloric deficits. In the aging population, especially the disadvantaged, prevalence of such changes may be very high. Symptoms are nonspecific, but the complex of weight loss (irrespective of whether prior weight was normal or elevated), decreased effort tolerance, lethargy, cold intolerance, ankle swelling, and dry flaking skin should arouse concern for nutritional status. The physical examination is similarly not diagnostic—especially if weight is still at or above normal—and is based on height, weight, midarm muscle circumference, and skinfold thickness measurements (see Ch. 213) with reference to norms and previous data from the individual. In addition, one may find easily pluckable hair, edema, and delayed wound healing. Often the clinical picture is dominated by the underlying cause in cases of secondary undernutrition. Laboratory studies in such individuals demonstrate low excretion of urea nitrogen per gram creatinine, decreased plasma levels of branched-chain amino acids, decreased hydroxyproline excretion, and small decreases in serum transferrin and albumin. With significant protein depletion the creatinine/height index is decreased. When PCM is severe it tends to follow the patterns of the two classic forms.

KWASHIORKOR. This form of PCM is typically found in the hospitalized adult unable to eat and/or under the stress of an acute illness or major surgery. In this setting, symptoms and signs of prior lesser degrees of malnutrition are as noted in the

TABLE 214–1. INDICES OF UNDERNUTRITION*

Variable	Abnormal Status Suggested by
MINIMAL ASSESSMENT (ROUTINE CLINICAL USE)	
Anthropomorphic	
Adults	
loss of weight in 1 month	⩾5%
loss of weight in 6 months	⩾10%
Children	
body weight for height,	<80% standard
or percentile drop in weight from growth chart over 6-month period	⩾20 percentiles
Laboratory	
Serum albumin	⩽2.8 g/dl
Serum transferrin	⩽150 mg/dl
Lymphocyte count	⩽1200 cells/mm^3
COMPREHENSIVE ASSESSMENT (DETAILED FOLLOW-UP AND RESEARCH)	
Anthropomorphic	
Skinfold thickness	
Midarm muscle circumference	
Creatinine—height index	
Body composition	
underwater weighing	
multiple isotope dilution	
neutron activation analysis	
Immunologic	
Delayed cutaneous hypersensitivity	
T-cell subsets	
Immunoglobulins	
Fat Metabolism	
Cholesterol, total and fractions	
Triglycerides	
Ketone bodies	
Protein Metabolism	
Plasma individual free amino acids	
Urine total nitrogen, urea, ammonium	
Urine hydroxyproline	
Labeled amino acid turnover	
Hormones	
Insulin	
Catecholamines	
Growth hormone	
ACTH, cortisol	
TSH, thyroxine, triiodothyronine, reverse triiodothyronine	
Reproductive hormones	
Vitamins	
Vitamin A	
Vitamin E	
Folates	
Vitamin B_{12}	
Vitamin C	
Muscle Function	
Force, relaxation, fatigability	
Respiratory muscle function	
Other Circulating Proteins	
Retinol-binding protein	
Thyroxine-binding proteins	
Acute phase proteins	

*Modified from Alpers et al., 1983.

previous paragraph, or may be absent if the time course has been short. Hepatomegaly may be present. The child with severe kwashiorkor will have marked edema or anasarca, decreased movement of the extremities, and extreme apathy; will cry only weakly if disturbed; and will show severe anorexia and diarrhea. The "flaky-paint" lesions of the skin are pigmented, dry, hyperkeratotic, sometimes excoriated, and commonly located in the perineum, extremities, and face. They may involve the trunk. Hair becomes dry, fine, brittle, straight, and reddish or yellowish. The abdomen is distended due to flaccid muscles, ascites, and hepatomegaly. Blood pressure is decreased and the pulse may be slow. Hypothermia is common. The laboratory diagnosis is based on a sharp decline in serum albumin to less than 2.8 grams per deciliter, lymphocyte count to less than 1200 cells per cu mm, serum transferrin less than 150 mg per deciliter, and nonreactive skin tests. Those abnormalities listed above under mild malnutrition are present but are more marked. Other findings are variably present. Anemia is common, most frequently normochromic and normocytic, but varies according to other deficiencies. Liver function is not usually impaired, and enzyme levels may be below normal. The alterations in immunoglobulins, lymphocytes, neutrophils, vitamins, and other micronutrients may be as referred to earlier, and plasma glucose and lipids tend to be low. Other transport proteins, like ceruloplasmin, retinol-binding protein, and hormone-binding proteins are decreased. The hormonal changes have been described earlier. Urea nitrogen in serum and urine is low, and urine creatinine is decreased. Hypokalemia and hypomagnesemia are common, and metabolic acidosis may be present. Hypocalcemia is due to the decreased albumin. The heart is usually small and exhibits a decreased cardiac output. All of these laboratory studies are by no means necessary to establish the diagnosis or even to serve as a baseline for therapy, but when they are done for other reasons, the effect of PCM must be considered in their interpretation.

MARASMUS. The clinical picture of marasmus is dominated by growth arrest, emaciation, loss of muscle and fat, and atrophy of most organs, resulting in a "skin and bones" appearance. The sky is dry, "baggy," and decreased in turgor, although without the lesions of kwashiorkor. Hair is sparse, thin and dry, and dull in appearance. Edema is absent; appetite is adequate or increased; and while the patient is irritable, the apathy of the kwashiorkor victim is not present, although weakness may be profound. Bowel action is usually decreased, but bouts of diarrhea are not rare. Pulse, blood pressure, and temperature may be low. In contrast to kwashiorkor, fewer laboratory values are abnormal, with serum albumin greater than 2.8 grams per deciliter. Except in the severest cases, the other "visceral" proteins may be unaffected. While any of the other changes described above may be found, especially where a mixed picture of the two types is present, they may be absent. Where available, objective studies of muscle function show altered force of contraction and an increased fatigability and slowed relaxation rates in all types of malnutrition.

TREATMENT

In the case of mild to moderate PCM, the strategy is to treat the precipitating event and increase protein and energy intake calculated on the basis of actual height in children and ideal weight in adults. This will give a relatively greater intake of both than if intake is based on actual age or weight and will allow for the extra requirement for "catch-up" in children or "regrowth" in the adult. Specific supplementation of individual nutrients is indicated by the presence of signs of their deficiency.

In severe PCM, rehabilitation is pursued in two phases. The first is the resuscitation from the acute infection, water and electrolyte imbalances, or other factors that caused decompensation. The second phase is devoted to repletion of depleted protein and energy. Specific issues requiring attention in the first phase are the total body potassium depletion; the metabolic acidosis; and the risks of hypocalcemia and hypomagnesemia while correcting acidosis and hypoalbuminemia, if calcium and magnesium replacement are insufficient. When indicated, all nutrients can be given parenterally (see Ch. 220). Introduction of nutrients into the gut of the malnourished individual can itself generate diarrhea because of the atrophy of the mucosa and the deficiency of digestive enzymes. Lipids and lactose are given sparingly for the first week, then in gradually increasing amounts. Starting at 0.8 gram of protein and 80 kcal per kilogram per day in children, the goal is to provide 4 grams of protein and 150 kcal per kilogram once tolerated and until recovery is complete. These calculations are based on actual weight. In the adult, daily initial intakes of 0.6 gram of protein and 50 kcal per kilogram are increased to 3 to 4 grams of protein and 80 to 100 kcal per kilogram. Vitamins, including folate, should be administered from the outset, including a large initial loading dose of vitamin A. When the oral or enteral route can be used but elemental formulations are preferred because of bowel disease, preparations are selected accordingly (see Ch. 219). Care must be taken in conversion from total parenteral nutrition to oral feeding, and in the introduction of normal nutrients after elemental diets.

The course of children is toward complete nutritional recovery within three to four months, with clearly measurable laboratory changes present within two to three weeks and anthropomorphic changes from three weeks onward. The changes may be slower in adults, unless the PCM was acute and of short duration. Comprehensive programs of nutrition education, psychosocial stimulation, and progressive increments in physical activity should be undertaken.

PREVENTION

In the hospitalized population, physicians should be aware of the patients who are at risk of developing PCM, as listed above. A checklist of use in assuring adequate nutrition of all patients to prevent PCM, as well as to monitor treatment of it, is presented in Table 214–2. These are easily incorporated into the nursing, dietetic, laboratory and pharmaceutical monitoring that accompanies standard medical practices. There is good evidence that both morbidity and mortality can be reduced in a cost-effective manner by such approaches. The prevention of childhood PCM, especially in developing countries, is oriented first toward prevention of severe cases, and second toward improvement of the nutrition of populations. Direct actions to achieve the first include encouragement of breast feeding and adequate supplementation of the diet of infants, together with supplements for women while pregnant and lactating and for children up to school age. Improvements of sanitary conditions and specific nutrition education are critical measures. However,

TABLE 214–2. CHECKLIST OF PROCEDURES TO PREVENT AND TREAT HOSPITAL MALNUTRITION*

1. Make an accurate record of admission height and weight and weekly follow-up weights.
2. Record specific orders regarding diet, and monitor ability to eat and amounts consumed.
3. Obtain consultation with dietician and assure follow-up collaboration on oral and tube feeding regimens.
4. Ascertain regularly whether the composition of nutrients consumed or infused is sufficient to cover basal and stress-related needs.
5. Be informed as to composition of standard nutrient preparations and supplements used in your hospital.
6. Do not wait longer than 3 to 5 days before adding protein, calories, and other nutrients to intravenous regimens. Avoid prolonged used of D5W and saline alone.
7. Use the simple anthropometric and available laboratory tests to assess and to monitor nutritional state.
8. Be cognizant that "hospital food," witholding meals for tests, and anorexia from medication can cumulatively contribute to malnutrition.
9. Consult the nutrition support service when indicated and monitor its recommended regimen.
10. Be especially vigilant with patients at high risk (see text).

*Inspired by Butterworth et al., 1980.

the solution to these problems also presupposes more effective means of distribution of available food to needy populations.

Alpers DH, Clouse RE, Stenson WF: Manual of Nutritional Therapeutics. Boston, Little, Brown and Company. 1983. *Well organized, readable, and contemporary, well-referenced how-to-do-it manual.*

Bistrian BR, Blackburn GL, Vitale J, Cochran D, Naylor J: Prevalence of malnutrition in general medical patients. JAMA 235:1567, 1976. *One of a series of studies establishing the high incidence of malnutrition in teaching hospitals.*

Butterworth CE, Jr, Weinsier RL: Malnutrition in hospital patients: Assessment and treatment. *In* Goodhart RS, Shils ME (eds.): Modern Nutrition in Health and Disease. 6th ed. Philadelphia, Lea and Febiger, 1980, p 667. *Contains more detail of the nutritional examination, strategy of therapy, and comprehensive list of effects of drugs on nutritional status.*

Chase HP, Kumar V, Caldwell RT, O'Brien D: Kwashiorkor in the United States. Pediatrics 66:972, 1980. *Occurrence and causes of the classic syndrome in the United States brought into focus.*

Crim MC, Munro HN: Protein-energy malnutrition and endocrine function. *In* DeGroot LJ (ed.): Endocrinology. New York, Grune and Stratton, 1979, p 1987. *This chapter reviews major hormones and their responses and roles in PCM and raises questions of relevance of changes found to PCM pathophysiology.*

Suskind RM (ed.): Malnutrition and the Immune Response. Kroc Foundation Series, Volume 7. New York, Raven Press, 1977. *A symposium report that covers all relevant aspects of immune response in PCM, the central issue in infection susceptibility.*

Viteri FE, Torun B: Protein-calorie malnutrition. *In* Goodhart RS, Shils ME (eds.): Modern Nutrition in Health and Disease. 6th ed. Philadelphia, Lea and Febiger, 1980, p 697. *Well-balanced review of classic syndromes of PCM.*

Waterlow JC: Childhood malnutrition—the global problem. Proc Nutr Soc 38:1, 1979. *The perspective of a renowned investigator on the world-wide impact of PCM, in a symposium on this topic.*

215. ANOREXIA NERVOSA

Gerald F. M. Russell

DEFINITION. Anorexia nervosa is a prolonged illness principally affecting young girls after puberty. It is characterized by severe weight loss which is self-induced, amenorrhea, and a specific psychopathology.

HISTORICAL NOTE. Sir William Gull described anorexia nervosa in 1868 and 1874. For a long time, confusion resulted from the concept of "Simmonds' cachexia," which embodied the mistaken view that panhypopituitarism caused loss of weight and wasting. Much needless effort was spent on the differential diagnosis of these two disorders which do not resemble each other.

ETIOLOGY. The cause of anorexia nervosa is unknown. A partial genetic contribution is favored by the finding of a significantly higher concordance of anorexia nervosa among monozygous than dizygous twins. Morbidity is also higher among sisters of patients (6.6 per cent). Anorexia nervosa used to be considered a rare illness. However, a five-fold increase in incidence was noted in Malmö, Sweden, between the 1930's and 1950's. Similar observations in Britain and the United States favor the view that culturally determined attitudes might lead to the illness. In recent years the upper social class bias for anorexia nervosa has diminished. The incidence of new cases ranges from 0.6 to 1.6 per 100,000 of the whole population, but the prevalence may be high in groups at special risk: 1 in 250 among schoolgirls aged 16 or over in England, 7 per cent of ballet students in Canada.

PSYCHOPATHOLOGY AND PATHOGENESIS. Anorexia nervosa is usually thought to be a disorder of psychogenic origin. The illness can also be viewed as a disorder of the feeding and endocrine functions normally controlled by the hypothalamus. It is important to consider simultaneously the mental and bodily disturbances in anorexia nervosa so as to comprehend their interaction as far as is possible.

The evidence for a psychogenic origin of anorexia nervosa is strong. Patients explain that they cannot eat because they feel guilty after eating, or are fearful that they will be unable to stop and hence will become unbearably fat. Disturbed family relationships or the conflicts of puberty and adolescence often play an important role. A disturbance of body image underlies the illness; for example, patients tend to overestimate the width of their own body. Food intake becomes determined by the patient's impression of the size of her own body. Because this impression is a distorted one and she imagines herself to be already too fat, she starves herself so as to acquire what she considers to be more desirable proportions.

Anorexia nervosa was originally considered to be a hypothalamic disorder on the grounds that destruction of the "feeding centers" in animals causes refusal of food. The strongest evidence for a primary hypothalamic disorder is the failure in the function of the hypothalamic–anterior pituitary–gonadal axis. Gonadotropins (FSH and LH) are not released from the anterior pituitary, the ovarian production of estrogens ceases, and ovulation fails to occur. There is a reversible hypothalamic disturbance interfering with the secretion of gonadotropin-releasing hormone and hence a diminished release of FSH and LH. As the patient regains weight, the recovery of endocrine function follows a definite sequence. First, there is a gradual increase in the levels of gonadotropins; the anterior pituitary also responds to administered LH-releasing hormones by releasing FSH and LH. Next, a return of the negative feedback effect of estrogens can be shown indirectly with clomiphene (blocking the negative feedback action), which causes a rise in basal plasma LH levels. The positive feedback effect of estrogens is last to return and can be demonstrated directly with a three-day course of ethinyl estradiol, which is followed by a peak rise in plasma LH. This final stage of recovery may be delayed, even after the patient's weight has returned to normal, but is necessary for the resumption of cyclical menstruation and ovulation. The persistence of abnormal endocrine function in anorexia nervosa is probably also dependent in part on the patient's abnormal mental state: a complete response to administered estrogens (with a positive feedback effect) is less likely to occur if there is a persistence in the psychologic disorder. These findings, together with the early onset of amenorrhea which may precede weight loss, indicate that the endocrine disorder is not wholly due to malnutrition.

A simplified diagram (Fig. 215–1) serves to emphasize the complexity of the interactions between the psychologic disorder, the endocrine disturbances, and the malnutrition in anorexia nervosa. The thickness of the lines reflects the strength of the evidence in support of each interaction. The best established pathways are those of the mental disorder causing a reduced food intake and weight loss (a), which in turn cause the endocrine disturbance and amenorrhea (b). It is also probable that weight loss and malnutrition worsen the mental disorder (c). The adverse effects of the patient's abnormal mental state on her endocrine and menstrual function support

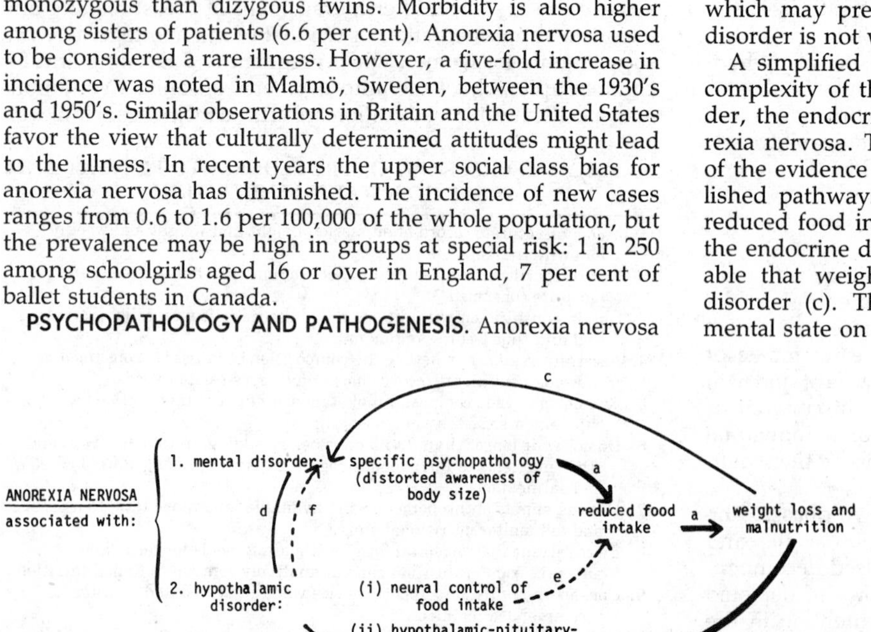

Figure 215–1. Psychologic, endocrine, and nutritional factors in anorexia nervosa. (Modified from Psychol Med 7:365, 1977.)

pathway (d). The original postulate that a disorder in the hypothalamic control of food intake might underlie the food refusal of anorexia nervosa is represented by the dotted line (e). There is no direct evidence in support of this mechanism or for the postulated link (f), representing the neural effects of a hypothalamic disorder in molding mental function so as to give rise to faulty attitudes to eating and body size. Nevertheless, it is clear that self-perpetuating disturbances play an important part in anorexia nervosa.

CLINICAL MANIFESTATIONS. The illness usually begins in a girl aged 14 to 17 years, but it can be earlier (9 to 13 years) or up to the age of the menopause. The patient's previous personality may have been normal, or there may be a preceding history of food fads or difficulty in making friendships; other signs of maladjustment are excessive tidiness or fears of meeting strangers or of taking school examinations. Loss of weight may be the first feature noticed by the parents, who draw the patient's attention to it. She is likely to explain the weight loss as the result of "dieting" for the purpose of improving her figure. Menstruation will have ceased by the time there has been a significant loss of weight, or this may happen as the first feature of the illness. There is often a change in the girl's temperament, consisting of impatience, irritability, and depression. She may become preoccupied with schoolwork or indulge in solitary exercises, thus withdrawing from her customary social life. The loss of weight can be very rapid, with a fall from 55 kg (121 pounds) to 35 kg (77 pounds) within two to three months. This is achieved mainly by avoiding carbohydrate-containing foods, but self-induced vomiting, the abuse of purgatives, and excessive exercising, in various combinations, may accelerate the loss of weight. The patient's life becomes unhappy and constricted. If she has a boyfriend, she loses interest in him and avoids any sexual contact. Relations with members of the family become strained. Parents react to their daughter's food refusal by a passive acceptance of her behavior for fear of making her condition worse. Food refusal leads to malnutrition which may persist for months or even years. The patient subsists on a diet of vegetables, fruit, and cheese, and avoids bread, potatoes, cakes, and sugar. On some days she may take only black coffee. In severe cases the patient presents a pitiable sight of emaciation, apathy, weakness, and severe depression. There is a risk of death from suicide or complications of malnutrition—especially potassium depletion or hypothermia.

In spite of progressive malnutrition, the patient may reject her parents' entreaties to see a doctor, and she minimizes the extent of her food avoidance. When she does agree to seek help, she is likely to deny that she is unwell or admit only to insomnia, constipation, sensitivity to cold, or some depression of mood.

Mental Examination. Examination of the patient's mental state may reveal a variety of disturbances. There may be depression and agitation; compulsive features may be prominent, such as elaborate feeding rituals and the counting of calories eaten daily; hysterical mechanisms may account for her assertion that she is eating well at the same time that she is hiding food or vomiting in secret. In addition, however, more specific psychologic abnormalities will be present. Their central theme is the patient's fear of becoming fat as a result of "losing control over eating." To play safe she resolves to remain thin and sets herself a sharply defined weight threshold above which she is unwilling to rise, defending her chosen weight as "right" for her. She may betray an abnormal sensitivity about the shape and size of her body, saying that fat would go to her stomach (hips, thighs, or some other part of the body). She may overestimate her weight and maintain, with all sincerity, that she eats large amounts of food. In an extreme case she may deny that she is thin, or even assert that she is fat in spite of obvious emaciation. The patient's distorted awareness of her size can be tested by getting her to estimate the width of her body. Her estimate is liable to exceed her actual measurements by as much as 50 per cent.

Physical Examination. Physical examination will reveal the signs of severe malnutrition in a young girl who has usually developed secondary sex characteristics. The malnutrition is of a calorie-deficiency type. The disappearance of subcutaneous fat leads to gaunt, hollow facial features; bony prominences stand out sharply, the limbs are reduced to sticks, the belly is flat, the breasts shrunken, and the buttocks wasted. The hands and feet remain cold and blue, even when the room temperature is warm. The central body temperature may be reduced by 1° C. The blood pressure is low (e.g., 90/60), and the heart rate is slow (50 to 60). The skin is dry, and there is an excessive growth of dry, downy hair over the nape of the neck, cheeks, forearms, and legs (lanugo hair), changes attributed to a follicular keratosis. In older patients purpuric patches resembling senile purpura may appear over the dorsum of the hands, the forearms, and the legs after minor knocks.

In patients who vomit, dehydration ensues, together with a marked fall in the level of serum potassium, but this finding and associated complications are more frequent in bulimia nervosa (see below). Serum cholesterol levels may be raised. Carotenemia may follow a high intake of carrots or spinach, and causes a yellow pigmentation of the palms and soles. Vitamin deficiencies (e.g. thiamin) occur rarely.

Endocrine Changes. Patients who are wasted show a fall in the plasma levels of LH, FSH, and estrogens. A course of clomiphene fails to raise the low plasma LH levels. Specific measures of thyroid function fall within the normal range. Plasma levels of growth hormone and cortisol are normal or elevated and can be raised further by the administration of insulin. Most of the physical abnormalities disappear when the malnutrition is corrected. An exception to this recovery is the disorder of gonadotropin activity, as described above.

Side Effects of Refeeding. Peripheral edema may occur, especially when the diet has a high content of salt, water, and carbohydrates which cause water retention. A moderate normochromic normocytic anemia may result from hemodilution, or a more severe anemia may result from hemolysis or temporary hypoplasia of the bone marrow; occasionally, moderate iron deficiency anemia may occur. Acute dilatation of the stomach is a rare but dangerous complication of too rapid refeeding.

Delayed Puberty. If the illness occurs before the menarche (e.g., 9 to 14 years), the sequence of pubertal events will probably be delayed by several years. Thus the patient has primary amenorrhea, together with a short stature and undeveloped breasts. When malnutrition is corrected and weight is adequately maintained, a full recovery often ensues with growth in height, development of breasts, and establishment of menstruation. If malnutrition is prolonged, however, there may be permanent sequelae such as a shortness in height (e.g., 152 cm) or underdeveloped breasts. Menstruation may be delayed until 21 years or later. It is therefore essential to treat these very young patients vigorously and effectively.

Anorexia Nervosa in the Male. The illness in the male closely resembles that in the female but is 10 to 20 times less common. The age of onset is usually a few years after puberty. The young boy rapidly loses weight as a result of avoiding carbohydrate-containing foods. Like the female, he expresses a fear of becoming fat and resorts to a similar abnormal behavior of food refusal, possibly with vomiting, purgation, or exercising to excess. The malnutrition in the male is more likely to be of a type combining a deficiency of calories and proteins. The endocrine disorder is analogous to that in the female. Urinary gonadotropins and blood LH levels are low; the urinary output of testosterone is reduced. Questioning will elicit loss of recently acquired sexual interest and potency. As in the female, these hormonal abnormalities can be slowly reversed by treatment resulting in weight gain.

TREATMENT. The general management of patients is empirically based but nevertheless highly rewarding: the treatments used are those which have been found to be effective in

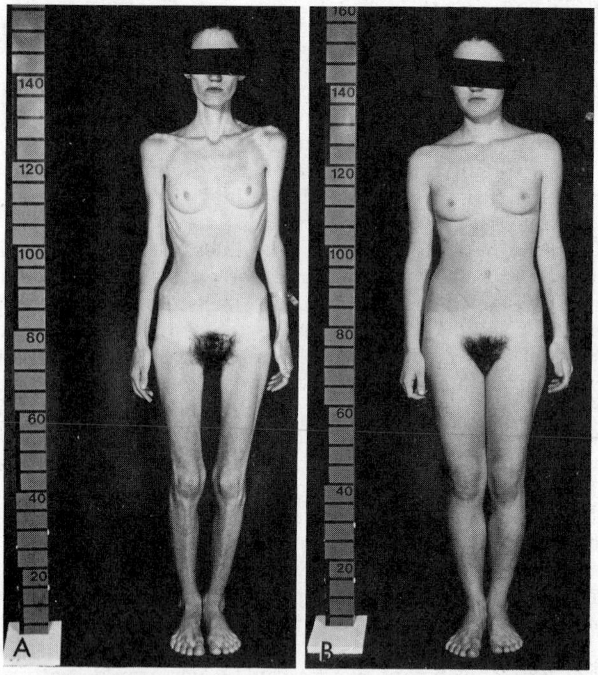

Figure 215–2. Photographs of the same patient on admission *(A)* and at the completion of treatment, nine weeks later *(B)* when she had gained 18.3 kg.

practice. The immediate aim is to treat the patient's malnutrition, which can become severe and dangerous. Even during the early stages of treatment it is desirable to try altering abnormal attitudes, for the course of the illness is much affected by the psychologic state. Thus treatment is best administered in a psychiatric unit, but it is essential that there be good nursing facilities. The long-term aim of treatment is to reduce the duration of the illness and prevent relapses.

Short-Term Treatment. Securing the Patient's Cooperation. The first need is to obtain as much cooperation from the patient as possible. By the time there has been severe loss of weight, admission to hospital is the only certain way of restoring her nutrition to normal. The doctor's skills must therefore be focused on persuading the patient to come into hospital. Compulsory admission, although occasionally indicated, is best avoided because the patient's continued cooperation is essential throughout the course of the illness, which may last for a few years.

Nursing Treatment. The refeeding of the patient is best achieved by skilled nurses. The nurse should establish a trusting relationship with the patient, but one which is not dependent on giving way to requests to avoid food and weight gain. The patient is asked to put her trust in the nurse as someone who, for the time being, takes over decisions regarding the necessary daily food intake. She is frankly told that because of her illness she will be tempted to be deceitful about eating, vomiting, or taking purgatives, so that close supervision is necessary. The nurse sits with the patient during each meal and cajoles her to finish all the food put on her plate. When the patient has regained her weight, she is complimented on her improved appearance and is encouraged to buy new clothes to fit her healthier size. In the course of treatment the nurse decides on a judicious balance of restrictions and privileges: the balance is gradually altered in favor of added privileges as rewards for continued progress.

Diet. No special diets are needed. The patient is given her own choice of food so long as she does not exclude carbohydrate-containing foods. To begin with, the food intake should be 1500 calories daily; within seven to ten days she should be persuaded to accept full meals totaling 3000 to 5000 calories daily. Concentrated foods may be used (e.g., Complan, Metrecal, or Carnation breakfast food) by adding them to milk.

Additional Measures. The nursing care described should be viewed as a form of *psychologic treatment* embodying the principles of psychotherapy and behavior therapy.

Large doses of chlorpromazine used to be advocated to reduce the patient's resistance to eating, but they can be dangerous in undernourished patients, and are not necessary. In very agitated patients the nursing task can be facilitated by administering moderate, divided doses of chlorpromazine up to a total of 300 mg daily. There is no place for tube feeding nor for leukotomy: weight gain can be achieved by conservative treatment, and the risk of suicide is increased after leukotomy.

Assessment of Progress. The patient is weighed daily before breakfast, and this provides the best check on her progress. A weight gain of up to 28 pounds (12.7 kg) in eight weeks should be possible. Figure 215–2 shows an 18-year-old patient before treatment and nine weeks later when she had gained 18.3 kg. The patient should maintain a healthy weight for about two weeks before being discharged from hospital.

Long-Term Treatment. There is less known about the efficacy of long-term treatments. After discharge from hospital, it is necessary to provide outpatient supervision. Psychotherapy should be directed to whatever emotional problems have been identified in the patient. Family therapy which involves therapeutic interviews with the whole family may be rewarding when there is evidence of disturbed relationships between its members. Even when a normal weight is maintained, amenorrhea may persist for months or years. When the patient is eager to resume normal menstruation, one or two courses of clomiphene (50 to 100 mg daily for seven days) may be effective, but only when body weight has been restored to a normal level. In the event of a serious relapse, readmission to hospital will be necessary.

PROGNOSIS. The short-term prognosis is usually excellent. Treatment should lead to a return to a normal weight; at the same time, the majority of patients show a marked improvement in their mental state. Deaths from malnutrition should not occur.

The long-term prognosis is more problematical. Relapses requiring readmissions occur in about half the patients. The illness often lasts two to three years or even longer. In a follow-up of severely ill patients who had been treated at least four years previously, 40 per cent had recovered, 27 per cent had menstrual irregularity or a moderately low body weight, 29 per cent had serious weight loss with amenorrhea, and 5 per cent had died. A proportion of the patients who fail to recover enter the chronic phase of bulimia nervosa. Poor prognostic signs are a later age of onset (early twenties as opposed to early teens) or an illness which has lasted more than five years. Even in these patients, however, good results can still be obtained from energetic treatment. In many patients the prognosis is good—their health returns to normal, and they may marry and can bear children.

BULIMIA NERVOSA

Bulimia nervosa is so called because it represents a chronic phase of anorexia nervosa, and its primary symptom consists of recurrent gorging with food. The psychopathology is the same as in typical anorexia nervosa: the patient has an exaggerated dread of becoming fat. It is this fear which leads her to get rid of the food each time she overeats. She makes herself vomit by pushing her fingers or a toothbrush down her throat. Abuse of purgatives is often combined with self-induced vomiting or may occur on its own. The resulting loss of body fluids and electrolytes leads to hypokalemia, hyponatremia, and hypochloremic alkalosis. Physical complications include erosion of dental enamel, muscular weakness, electrocardiographic abnormalities, tetany, and epileptic seizures; chronic potassium depletion may lead to urinary infections and renal failure. In contrast with typical anorexia nervosa, body weight may reach a relatively normal level, menstruation may be resumed, and fertility restored.

MENTAL EXAMINATION. The patient's morbid dread of fatness can be assessed from the weight threshold which she has set for herself, usually several kilograms below her original "healthy" weight. Signs of depression may be present.

PHYSICAL EXAMINATION. Physical examination may reveal injury to the skin over the back of the hand from rubbing against the upper incisors when inducing vomiting. Swelling of the salivary glands or signs of tetany are occasionally present. Serum potassium levels may be low (e.g., to 1.4 mEq per liter). Renal function may be impaired.

TREATMENT. Intractable self-induced vomiting and purging require admission to hospital. The nurse conveys to the patient sympathy for her preoccupation with food and controls the overeating by limiting food intake to mealtimes. This usually suffices to control vomiting; but if not, closer supervision, especially after meals, will have the desired effect. The use of purgatives must also be stopped. Potassium supplements are ineffective unless vomiting ceases, and are then unnecessary. The patient is persuaded to accept a higher body weight, which reduces the craving for food and improves the chances of maintained control over gorging and vomiting after leaving hospital. Long-term supportive psychotherapy is indicated to help the patient with interpersonal and social problems. Good results have been reported with cognitive behavioral therapy. The value of antidepressants is often limited to the relief of depressive symptoms. Prognosis for a full recovery is seldom good, and there is a risk of suicide.

Crisp AH, Palmer RL, Kalucy RS: How common is anorexia nervosa? A prevalence study. Br J Psychiat 128:549, 1976. Garner DM, Garfinkel PE: Sociocultural factors in the development of anorexia nervosa. Psychol Med 10:647, 1980. *These two references provide recent evidence supporting the relatively high prevalence of anorexia nervosa and the effects of sociocultural pressures on its incidence.*

Darby PL, Garfinkel PE, Garner DM, Coscina DV (eds.): Anorexia Nervosa: Recent Developments and Research. Neurology and Neurobiology. Vol 3. New York, Alan R. Liss, Inc., 1984. *Recent reports on psychosocial and biologic factors in anorexia nervosa and a section on treatment. There is also an article on delayed puberty.*

Garfinkel PE, Garner DM: Anorexia Nervosa: A Multidimensional Perspective. New York, Brunner/Mazel, 1982. *This is the best book for a comprehensive account of anorexia nervosa. It includes an extensive bibliography.*

Harris RT: Bulimarexia and related serious eating disorders with medical complications. Ann Intern Med 99:800, 1983. *An up-to-date review article with 44 references, better from the medical than the psychiatric point of view.*

Minuchin S, Rosman B, Baker L: Psychosomatic Families: Anorexia Nervosa in Context. Cambridge, Harvard University Press, 1978. *An account of family therapy in anorexia nervosa, including the theoretical models which have led to its introduction.*

Russell GFM: Bulimia nervosa: An ominous variant of anorexia nervosa. Psychol Med 9:429, 1979. *A detailed clinical account of a newly identified disorder closely related to anorexia nervosa.*

216. OBESITY

Edwin L. Bierman

Obesity is the most common disorder of metabolism in man and is also one of the oldest documented metabolic disturbances in recorded history. A limestone statuette dating from the Stone Age has been unearthed which appears to be the most ancient example of obesity, antedating the development of agriculture by about 10,000 years. Similar historical evidence for obesity is found in Egyptian mummies and Greek sculpture. This abnormality has persisted throughout the centuries, which have been characterized by markedly different environmental stresses and dietary habits. However, the problem of obesity has dramatically increased since the evolutionary advantage of the ability to efficiently store energy as fat has been dissipated in modern affluent societies. Thus caloric excess and sedentary habits have led to an increased prevalence of obesity and its life-shortening consequences, including cardiovascular disease, diabetes, and hypertension.

DEFINITION AND MEASUREMENT. Obesity can be defined as excess adipose tissue. However, it is still not clear whether obesity represents a "disease" or a common clinical manifestation of a group of disorders like anemia or hypertension. The definition of obesity is necessarily arbitrary, since body weight (or more accurately, quantity of body fat) is continuously distributed in populations with no clear dividing line between individuals who are obese and those who are thin. A definition of obesity could be made more easily if there were a distinct point at which a clear influence of obesity on morbidity and mortality begins. This is not the case, however, since there is a continually progressive excess mortality for increasing degrees of overweight beyond about 30 per cent. Moreover, the metabolic, physiologic, and pathophysiologic consequences appear to increase continuously with the degree of deviation above average weight.

Although it is the simplest index of obesity, body weight is not always the best reflection of the relative proportion of adipose tissue in the body or of total adipose mass that needs to be determined or estimated if exact knowledge of the degree of excess adiposity is desirable. Weight adjusted to body size gives a better indication than body weight alone. For clinical purposes, per cent ideal body weight (relative weight) based on the readily available Metropolitan Life Insurance Company tables usually gives a close approximation of the degree of adiposity (Table 216–1). Although modifications of the guide-

TABLE 216–1. GUIDELINES FOR BODY WEIGHT*

Metric Height (m)†	Men (Weight in kg) Average	Men Acceptable Weight Range		Women (Weight in kg) Average	Women Acceptable Weight Range	
1.45				46.0	42	53
1.48				46.5	42	54
1.50				47.0	43	55
1.52				48.5	44	57
1.54				49.5	44	58
1.56				50.4	45	58
1.58	55.8	51	64	51.3	46	59
1.60	57.6	52	65	52.6	48	61
1.62	58.6	53	66	54.0	49	62
1.64	59.6	54	67	55.4	50	64
1.66	60.0	55	69	56.8	51	65
1.68	61.7	56	71	56.8	52	66
1.70	63.5	58	73	60.0	53	67
1.72	65.0	59	74	61.3	55	69
1.74	66.5	60	75	62.6	56	70
1.76	68.0	62	77	64.0	58	72
1.78	69.4	64	79	65.3	59	74
1.80	71.0	65	80			
1.82	72.6	66	82			
1.84	74.2	67	84			
1.86	75.8	69	86			
1.88	77.6	71	88			
1.90	79.3	73	90			
1.92	81.0	75	93			

Nonmetric Height† (Ft	in)	Men (Weight in lbs) Average	Men Acceptable Weight Range		Women (Weight in lbs) Average	Women Acceptable Weight Range	
4	10				102	92	119
4	11				104	94	122
5	0				107	96	125
5	1				110	99	128
5	2	123	112	141	113	102	131
5	3	127	115	144	116	105	134
5	4	130	118	148	120	108	138
5	5	133	121	152	123	111	142
5	6	136	124	156	128	114	146
5	7	140	128	161	132	118	150
5	8	145	132	166	136	122	154
5	9	149	136	170	140	126	158
5	10	153	140	174	144	130	163
5	11	158	144	179	148	134	168
6	0	162	148	184	152	138	173
6	1	166	152	189			
6	2	171	156	194			
6	3	176	160	199			
6	4	181	164	204			

*Adapted from the recommendations of the Fogarty Center Conference 1973. Data from the Metropolitan Life Insurance Company tables.

†Height without shoes, weight without clothes.

lines have recently been made, the effect of age on average or ideal weight is not considered. Nevertheless, for common use, obesity can be defined as that body weight over 20 per cent above mean average body weight.

A variety of methods for assessment of total body fat, such as body density, x-ray, distribution of fat-soluble gases, total body water, and total body potassium-40, have been used for research purposes. In addition, a variety of anthropometric measurements (limb and trunk diameters and circumferences, skin-fold thicknesses) have been used to derive regression equations that correlate closely with per cent fat.

However, elaborate techniques are usually not necessary to quantify body fat for clinical purposes. The weight/height^2 index (body mass index) is one of the most useful anthropometric measurements and the simplest to obtain; it de-emphasizes the effect of stature on body weight and also correlates closely with adiposity. Obesity can be defined as a body mass index of greater than 27 (kilograms per square meter) for men and 25 for women (approximately equivalent to 120 per cent of ideal body weight). Subscapular and triceps skin-fold thickness measurements using inexpensive skin-fold calipers also provide an accurate and simple guide. On the basis of population studies, it has been suggested that triceps skin-fold thickness greater than 23 mm in men and 30 mm in women should be defined as obesity.

PREVALENCE AND EPIDEMIOLOGY. A large proportion of Western populations is obese. In the United States, using a definition of obesity based on triceps skin-fold thickness, approximately 20 per cent of middle-aged males and 40 per cent of middle-aged females are obese. In cross-sectional population surveys, the prevalence of obesity increases with age, reaching a peak by age 50 in males and somewhat later in females. The lower prevalence of obesity in older age groups may reflect the higher mortality at earlier ages associated with obesity-related diseases.

Cultural influences and socioeconomic status have a strong influence on the prevalence of obesity. Every social factor studied has been correlated with obesity, and thus there are many determinants. Socioeconomic status, based on occupation, education, and income, shows a particularly strong inverse correlation with obesity among women, i.e., the lower the socioeconomic status, the higher the prevalence of obesity.

PATHOGENESIS. ***Clinical Types.*** Although it has been clear for some time that there are two clinical types of obesity, there has been little metabolic or physiologic evidence until recently to support such a concept. In one type *(lifelong obesity)*, patients give a characteristic history. Although generally of normal birth weight, they tend to have been heavier as children, to have had a large spurt in weight gain during puberty, and (in females) to give a history of gaining weight with each successive pregnancy. These individuals usually have tried all available methods and fads promoted for caloric restriction and weight reduction to no permanent avail. After successful weight loss regardless of the program, they usually return gradually to approximately their prereduction level of overweight as though it were preset. These individuals also tend to be grossly obese (more than 175 per cent of ideal body weight) adults.

The other clinical type *(adult-onset obesity)* is much more common and represents "middle-age spread." These individuals give a history of being thin or of average weight until age 20 to 40, when weight gain associated with a more sedentary existence begins. This type of weight gain in adult life is extremely common and is seen in most affluent populations.

A possible explanation for weight gain during adult life that does not appear to be tenable is a decrease in basal energy utilization with aging. Basal oxygen consumption decreases only slightly during adult life. Body composition is changing, however, even at constant body weight. There is a larger proportion of body fat and a smaller proportion of lean body mass with age, so that basal oxygen consumption in terms of lean body mass (predominantly muscle and bone) may actually be constant with age. Although basal energy utilization may be constant, it has been suggested that obesity occurs in concert with a decline in energy utilization associated with food intake ("dietary-induced thermogenesis") and with exercise. Alternatively, adult-onset obesity simply may reflect an imbalance between caloric intake and utilization because such individuals do not reduce their caloric intake with age appropriately for their change in body composition. Ahrens has calculated that the daily caloric requirement for weight maintenance of adults decreases 43 calories per decade per square meter of surface area for males and 27 calories per decade per square meter for females.

These two broad clinical types of obesity were recognized early by Albrink, who proposed that adult-onset obesity is mainly central in location (the "middle-age spread"), whereas lifelong obesity might be peripheral as well as central. For peripheral localization of adiposity, skin-fold thickness of the forearm or the triceps is measured and compared with skin-fold thickness over the tip of the scapula. Weight gain during adult life is significantly correlated with costal, scapular, and, to a lesser extent, triceps skin-fold thickness but not with ulnar skin-fold thickness. Thus forearm fat is minimally influenced by adult-onset obesity, whereas adipose tissue of the trunk is most influenced by weight gain during adult life.

Pathophysiology. A possible pathophysiologic basis for these clinical observations was first proposed by Bjurulf, who suggested that some forms of obesity might be due to increased numbers of cells. Proof of this hypothesis was provided by the elegant experiments of Hirsch and his coworkers, who measured the cellularity of adipose tissue sampled by needle aspiration biopsy. They demonstrated that grossly obese humans (lifelong) characteristically have an increase in adipose cell number as well as adipose cell size. After weight reduction, adipose cell size shrinks, but hypercellularity remains fixed.

Adult-onset obesity (after age 20) appears to be characterized predominantly by adipose cell hypertrophy with no increase in cell number. Thus all human obesity is accompanied by cellular enlargement. Adipocyte hyperplasia becomes increasingly marked beyond body weights greater than 175 per cent of ideal. Adipose cell number appears to be determined very early in life. In studies with rats, animals subjected to overnutrition before weaning maintained larger numbers of adipose cells throughout life than did litter mates subjected to undernutrition prior to weaning. Weight changes during adult life did not influence the cell number of these animals. Studies in man also have shown that adipose cell number is determined early in life. In the nonobese, two periods of adipose cell proliferation have been identified: in the first two years and again just prior to puberty. In obese children, adipose cell number increases throughout childhood.

Experimental Obesity. Support for the concept of two types of obesity also comes from studies of experimental obesity in man by Sims and coworkers. They force-fed volunteers to produce 20 to 30 per cent increments in weights associated with central distribution of excess fat, which was predominantly due to an increase in adipose cell size without a change in adipose cell number. Prompt, spontaneous reversal of excess fat and cell size was achieved at the end of the experimental forced feeding. Thus there appears to be no change in adipose cell number during temporary overfeeding in adulthood despite changes in body weight.

Studies of experimental obesity in animals also lend some support to these concepts. Genetically transmitted obesity in rodents is characterized by adipose cell hyperplasia as well as hypertrophy, whereas experimentally induced obesity, such as that obtained by destruction of the ventromedial nucleus of the hypothalamus, is associated with hypertrophy alone. A summary of these two broad general categories of obesity is given in Table 216–2. All obesity is hypertrophic because the adipose cells are enlarged, but only certain individuals have adipose hyperplasia. Massive obesity is usually of the juvenile onset, lifelong hyperplastic type.

TABLE 216–2. TYPES OF OBESITY

	Hyperplastic	Hypertrophic
Severity	Marked	Moderate
History	Lifelong	Adult-onset
Fat distribution	Peripheral and central	Central ("middle-age spread")
Adipose cellularity	Increase in cell number and cell size	Increase in cell size only
Insulin resistance	Related to cell size	Related to cell size
Metabolic consequences	Related to cell size	Related to cell size

ETIOLOGY. Possible factors in the pathogenesis of adipose cell hypertrophy are listed in Table 216–3. No primary biochemical lesion of adipose tissue has ever been firmly documented as a cause of generalized obesity in man. Also, little is known of the etiologic basis for adipose cell hyperplasia. Genetic factors play a role, but their mechanism remains unknown. Estrogen-androgen balance also appears to influence the site and amount of adipose tissue deposition, since women and prepubertal children have a higher proportion and different distribution of subcutaneous fat than men.

Only in rare instances of hypothalamic obesity in man, in which damage to the ventromedial hypothalamic nucleus occurs as a result of tumor or trauma, can an etiology be defined and, with surgical removal of the tumor, obesity cured. This hypothalamic center appears to regulate the deposition of adipose tissue triglyceride. Formerly its role as an appetite or satiety center was emphasized, and when it was destroyed its role was related to obesity in man because inappropriate hyperphagia sometimes occurred. Recent studies, however, have shown that experimentally induced hypothalamic lesions alter insulin levels and lipogenesis independent of changes in food intake. Anomalous insulin secretion after hypothalamic injury in man has also been observed. Possibly it can be linked to the development of obesity in such individuals. In any event, the relevance to the common types of human obesity of experimental animal models whose obesity has been produced by injuring the hypothalamus is open to serious question.

Cerebral and emotional influences on eating patterns as well as cultural influences and socioeconomic status surely play a role in obesity, but, aside from overt psychiatric disturbances, the general role of altered behavioral patterns in the etiology of obesity has been difficult to define, and a specific type of personality associated with obesity has not been distinguished. No less important, habit and environment also appear to influence appetite regulation. Presumably because of decreased spontaneous activity, an obese individual will actually consume fewer calories than will his thin control counterpart.

Fatty acid mobilization from adipose tissue appears to be normal in simple obesity. There is little evidence that decreased lipolysis, or resistance to normal fat-mobilizing stimuli (hormonal, neuronal), plays an etiologic role in the usual forms of obesity (Table 216–3).

Lipoprotein lipase (the enzyme in adipose tissue responsible for assimilation of fatty acids contained in circulating triglyceride-rich lipoproteins) is increased in hypertrophic adipose cells. Increased lipoprotein lipase activity could lead to further increased deposition of dietary and endogenous fat in adipose tissue in obesity. A possible primary role for this enzyme in the etiology of obesity in some individuals is suggested by the finding that obese individuals maintain high levels of lipoprotein lipase in adipocytes after weight reduction. Also in the genetically obese rat, adipose tissue lipoprotein lipase is increased even before the animals become obese, and this increase is maintained despite food restriction. These recent findings are consistent with the idea that fat mass is regulated by as yet unknown neurohumoral factors that modulate adipose tissue lipoprotein lipase activity and provide a biochemical basis for the difficulty some obese individuals have in maintaining a weight-reduced state. Although overall basal energy utilization may be normal in obesity, subtle defects have been described in red cell sodium-potassium pump activity which correlate with the degree of obesity. The possible role of this biochemical energy-utilizing system in the etiology of obesity remains to be clarified.

TABLE 216–3. POSSIBLE FACTORS IN THE PATHOGENESIS OF OBESITY (ADIPOCYTE HYPERTROPHY)

- Excessive lipid deposition
  - Increased food intake
  - Hypothalamic lesions
  - Adipose cell hyperplasia
  - Hyperlipogenesis
  - Increased lipoprotein lipase activity
- Diminished lipid mobilization
  - Decrease in lipolytic hormones
  - Defective adipose-cell lipolysis
  - Abnormality of autonomic innervation
- Diminished lipid utilization
  - Aging
  - Defective lipid oxidation
  - Defective thermogenesis
  - Inactivity

Metabolic Abnormalities. Regardless of the cause or type of obesity, the metabolic consequences are predictable. They appear to relate directly to fat cell size, and virtually all metabolic disturbances that have been observed are inducible with weight gain and reversible with weight reduction. Thus, although numerous hormonal imbalances have been described in obesity, they are likely to be consequences of rather than causes of the obese state (Table 216–4).

The metabolic alteration with the most profound influence is the acquired resistance to the action of insulin on glucose utilization by fat and muscle cells. A predominance of abdominal adiposity in premenopausal women, similar to fat distribution in adult men, is particularly associated with insulin resistance. Insulin resistance associated with adiposity or experimental weight gain has been demonstrated both in vivo and in isolated fat cell systems. Muscle metabolism also presumably plays an important role in the insulin resistance of obesity. One of the consequences of this resistance to the action of insulin appears to be a feedback compensatory hyperinsulinism. The beta cells of the pancreatic islets are stimulated by an unknown mechanism to produce more insulin, and beta-cell hypertrophy eventually results. The signal is as yet unknown but may be neuronal or hormonal, or may involve small changes in glucose, fatty acids, or specific amino acids. In any case, the result is an increase in circulating insulin levels (both basal and in response to a variety of stimuli), which is directly related to the degree of adiposity and is reversible with weight reduction. It is not simply a matter of body weight or lean body mass that is associated with hyperinsulinemia, since very muscular individuals who are heavy do not appear to have hyperinsulinism. Circulating levels of insulin regulate their own receptors on cell surfaces. Thus obesity has been associated with fewer numbers of insulin receptors on muscle, liver, and adipose cell surfaces, thereby further contributing to insulin resistance and impaired glucose utilization by cells. However, decreased postreceptor insulin responsiveness of adipose tissue appears to be the major contributor to the insulin resistance of obesity.

TABLE 216–4. METABOLIC AND ENDOCRINE CONSEQUENCES OF OBESITY

- Decreased sensitivity to insulin (muscle, adipose tissue)
- Hyperinsulinemia
- Decreased glucose tolerance, hyperglycemia
- Hyperaminoacidemia
- Hypertriglyceridemia
- Hypercholesterolemia
- Decreased growth hormone responses
- Decreased prolactin responses
- "Resistance" to ketosis
- Increased glucocorticoid secretion

The emergence of adult-onset (non-insulin-dependent) diabetes mellitus in the population is profoundly influenced by the degree and duration of obesity. One concept is that prolonged hyperinsulinism might lead to beta-cell "exhaustion" in those individuals who are genetically susceptible. As is well known, when the pressure is off after successful weight reduction, glucose intolerance is reversed. Thus glucose intolerance in the obese adult may represent "high-output failure," in which the beta cell has failed to compensate fully for the degree of peripheral insulin resistance associated with adiposity. Abnormal regulation of growth hormone and prolactin secretion has been associated with obesity, but the significance of these findings and their relation to the glucose intolerance of obesity is not understood. These changes in insulin and growth hormone regulation in obesity can be found even in early childhood.

Another metabolic consequence of obesity is hypertriglyceridemia, which may result in part from the associated hyperinsulinism. Triglyceride levels in populations are correlated with relative body weight, with skin-fold thickness, and particularly with weight gain in adult life. In a variety of studies circulating insulin levels are consistently correlated with triglyceride levels, and insulin is one of the factors involved in endogenous triglyceride-rich lipoprotein secretion by the liver. In obese individuals, both hyperinsulinism and hypertriglyceridemia are reversible with weight reduction. The role of obesity in determining serum lipid levels is suggested by the finding that age-related curves of relative body weight, plasma triglyceride, and plasma cholesterol in comparable population groups are superimposable.

Serum cholesterol levels are less closely linked with obesity, but a significant relationship exists. This could be explained in part by the observation that the cholesterol production rate appears to be related to the degree of adiposity. This relationship may be linked to the increased propensity of obese individuals to develop gallstones. Elevated triglyceride-rich lipoprotein levels are associated with reduced levels of high density lipoprotein (HDL) cholesterol, characteristic of obesity.

The influence of obesity on glucose, lipid, and lipoprotein levels also may be related to the increased tendency of the obese to develop all the complications of atherosclerosis. Thus obesity, altered carbohydrate and fat metabolism, and atherosclerosis appear to be linked.

CLINICAL MANIFESTATIONS. The pathophysiologic consequences of obesity lead to a variety of clinical manifestations and aggravate or predispose to a number of common diseases (Table 216–5). For many of these diseases obese individuals have higher death rates than their thin counterparts affected by the same disorder.

Every major organ system appears to be involved. In the *cardiovascular system,* obesity is associated with five major risk factors for atherosclerosis, i.e., hypertension, diabetes, hypercholesterolemia, hypertriglyceridemia, and low HDL cholesterol. Therefore it is not surprising that obese individuals have more atherosclerotic manifestations and are more prone to sudden death. The effect of obesity in predisposing to atherosclerosis may be mediated by these factors rather than by more direct mechanisms related to nonspecific myocardial lesions or hemodynamic factors (increased oxygen consumption, blood volume, cardiac output, stroke volume, and cardiac work).

TABLE 216–5. DISEASES ASSOCIATED WITH OBESITY

Cardiovascular disease	Arthritis
Atherosclerotic	Osteoarthritis
Hypertensive	Gout
Cor pulmonale	Varicose veins and thromboembolism
Hypertension	Intertriginous dermatitis
Pulmonary disease	Hernias, ventral and diaphragmatic
Diabetes mellitus, adult-onset	Endometrial carcinoma
Fatty liver	Toxemia of pregnancy
Cholelithiasis and cholecystitis	Amenorrhea and oligomenorrhea

There is a close correlation between blood pressure levels and obesity in most populations. (In the markedly obese individual with large subcutaneous fat deposits in the arm, blood pressure measurements should be made with a large leg cuff which more accurately reflects arterial levels.) A large portion of the increased death rate of moderate or markedly obese individuals may be a direct or indirect consequence of hypertension (e.g., cerebrovascular accidents). Several factors have been implicated in the association between obesity and hypertension, including hemodynamic alterations resulting from increased blood volume and the need for increased perfusion of excess adipose tissue and lean body mass, and increased salt intake accompanying increased food consumption. Increased stroke volume and left ventricular hypertrophy often result. Obese individuals appear to respond to antihypertensive management as do their nonobese hypertensive counterparts with an improvement in morbidity and mortality from cerebrovascular complications.

In the *respiratory system,* alveolar hypoventilation associated with massive obesity eventually leads to carbon dioxide retention (P_{CO_2} values consistently above 48 mm Hg), daytime somnolence, chronic fatigue, dyspnea, and personality changes (the obesity-hypoventilation syndrome or pickwickian syndrome, named after a character in Dickens' *Pickwick Papers,* Fat Joe, who fell asleep at the most inopportune moments). The syndrome is initiated by the increased work of respiration necessary to move the ponderous thoracic wall and abdomen and is associated with decreased compliance of the thorax. Hypoxia, secondary polycythemia, pulmonary hypertension, and eventually cor pulmonale with cardiopulmonary failure ensue. Occasionally, sleep apnea (see Ch. 472.5) may be an associated feature. Many of these abnormalities can be partly reversed by weight loss. Although the full-blown syndrome is seen in only grossly obese adults, milder pulmonary functional abnormalities can be detected with lesser degrees of obesity, including reduction in vital capacity and expiratory reserve volume, and ventilation-perfusion disturbances resulting in mild decreases in arterial oxygenation. All these abnormalities contribute to the increased surgical risk in obesity associated with use of general anesthetics.

Obesity is the single important factor associated with the emergence of *diabetes mellitus* in populations throughout the world. In the United States more than 80 per cent of adult-onset diabetics are obese. The duration rather than the degree of obesity in individuals is more closely correlated with glucose intolerance. As indicated, certain genetically prone individuals may not be able to sustain the chronic oversecretion of insulin necessary to overcome the insulin resistance of obesity, and although absolute circulating insulin levels after carbohydrate intake may be higher than in thin individuals, they may not be high enough to compensate for the extra demand resulting from adiposity. Again, weight reduction may be dramatically successful in reducing the hyperglycemia of the adult diabetic and is the treatment of choice; however, the influence of weight gain and loss on the associated microangiopathy of diabetes is unknown.

Gastrointestinal symptoms are frequent in the obese and are usually nonspecific (bloating, dyspepsia). Diaphragmatic hernias may become symptomatic. Fatty liver is common, with associated abnormalities of liver function being detectable in as many as 85 per cent of obese patients (mild abnormalities of SGPT and LDH that become normal with weight reduction). The incidence of cholesterol-rich gallstones is strikingly related to the degree of obesity, particularly among women. Women below the age of 50 with cholelithiasis average 25 pounds heavier than women without gallstones. The mechanism presumably relates to the supersaturation of bile with cholesterol resulting from the overproduction and increased excretion of cholesterol in obesity. Weight reduction will reduce the saturation of bile with cholesterol after a new stable lower weight is achieved. However, during the period of active weight loss, bile remains supersaturated, apparently because of increased mobilization of cholesterol from large adipose tissue stores.

Thus continuous weight loss–weight gain cycles characteristic of many obese patients during their lifetime may be a potent predisposing condition for gallstone formation.

The incidence of several types of *arthritis* is increased among the obese. In populations, uric acid levels are directly related to the degree of overweight, and the prevalence of gouty arthritis is increased in obesity. Gouty arthritis may also be precipitated during treatment of obesity with carbohydrate-deficient ("ketogenic") fad diets (see Treatment) presumably related to the hyperuricemia resulting from the competition between ketone acids and uric acid for renal excretion. Osteoarthritis is also more common and severe, particularly in the spine and other joints that bear the brunt of excess weight bearing.

In addition to the arterial lesions of atherosclerosis, *varicose veins* are common, as is venous stasis and edema. This contributes to the increased postoperative morbidity caused by thrombophlebitis and pulmonary embolism in obesity.

Flabby and redundant *skin* associated with excessive subcutaneous fat produces moist folds, resulting in a propensity to fungal and yeast skin lesions (intertriginous dermatitis, particularly in the axillae, in the perineal region, and under the breasts).

Women who are obese tend to have irregular *menses* and increased morbidity associated with *pregnancy* and again after childbearing ceases. The incidence of toxemia of pregnancy and hypertension is increased. Obstetric risk is higher due to longer duration of labor, larger babies, more cesarean sections, and higher anesthetic risk. Later in life, there are more uterine fibroids and an increased risk of development of endometrial cancer directly related to the degree of obesity. The large adipose mass is associated with both increased estrogen storage and increased conversion of adrenal androgens to estrone, which may result in increased chronic hormonal stimulation of the uterus.

Surgical risk is in general greater in obesity. Mortality figures for a variety of surgical procedures may be two- to three-fold higher for the obese than for the nonobese. Contributing factors include increased anesthetic risk, technical difficulties and longer duration of procedures, and increased atelectasis, wound infection, and thrombophlebitis postoperatively.

DIFFERENTIAL DIAGNOSIS. Less than 1 per cent of obesity can be ascribed to an identifiable cause or aggravating factor (Table 216–6). There is no rationale for the use of the popular diagnostic term "exogenous" obesity, which has no pathophysiologic meaning.

Endocrine lesions as specific primary causes of adiposity are uncommon. It is clear, however, that hormones influence fat deposition. This may involve a general effect on adipocyte metabolism throughout the body (e.g., insulin, thyroid hormone) or characteristic regional effects (e.g., glucocorticoids, estrogen). Hyperinsulinism can lead to adiposity, as exemplified by patients with insulinoma. However, individuals with this tumor are rarely markedly obese.

Although much attention has been given to hypothyroidism and milder degrees of "hypometabolism" as a cause of obesity, and vast quantities of thyroid extract have been administered for treatment, there is little evidence for deficiency of thyroid hormone secretion or action as a primary cause in most cases. Most of the weight gain associated with the development of myxedema is due to the accumulation of fluid rather than to adipose mass. Furthermore, the administration of thyroid hormone to obese patients may result in a loss of lean body mass exceeding the loss of fat and in increased appetite. Circulating thyroid hormone levels, thyroidal radioiodine uptake, and Achilles reflex time are usually normal.

TABLE 216–6. DIFFERENTIAL DIAGNOSIS OF OBESITY*

Endocrine syndromes	Inflammatory disease
Hypothyroidism	Increased intracranial pressure
Hyperadrenocorticism	Pseudotumor cerebri
Hypogonadism	Empty sella syndrome
Insulinoma	Adiposogenital dystrophy
Polycystic ovaries (Stein-Leventhal)	Prader-Willi syndrome
Pseudohypoparathyroidism	Laurence-Moon-Biedl syndrome
Hypothalamic syndromes	Multiple lipomatosis
Tumors	Partial lipodystrophy
Craniopharyngioma	Drugs
Others	Cyproheptadine
Trauma	Phenothiazine

*An identifiable cause such as any of those listed above is present in less than 1 per cent of cases.

The fat deposition associated with hyperadrenocorticism (Cushing's syndrome) is characteristic. Helpful diagnostic clinical features, in addition to fat distribution, that distinguish the much more common obese individual with mild hypertension and glucose intolerance from obesity secondary to adrenal hypersecretion include thick rather than thin skin, pale rather than purplish striae, absence of plethora and polycythemia, preservation of muscle strength, and absence of osteoporosis. Laboratory tests are also helpful. Higher than normal urinary excretion rates of hydroxycorticoids and an increase in cortisol turnover may be present, but these changes correlate with the increase in lean body mass associated with obesity. Blood and urine cortisol levels tend to be normal in obesity and are usually suppressible, and the diurnal rhythm in adrenal steroid secretion appears to be maintained.

Gonadal deficiency certainly is not a common cause of obesity. Although in animals it has been shown that castration is often followed by obesity, this association has been much less prominent in humans. Nevertheless, it has been observed, particularly when the castration is performed after puberty. Moreover, some eunuchoid males are found to be somewhat obese and tend to lose some of the obesity after the administration of testosterone. Women with the Stein-Leventhal syndrome tend to be obese. Presumably the obesity results from the secretion by the ovary of steroids with actions similar to those of some of the adrenal steroids.

Hypothalamic syndromes are rare causes of obesity in man. Bray has collected a series of these patients and found that they were of the hypertrophic type but were characterized by unusually high insulin levels. In the case of gross lesions found in the vicinity of the hypothalamus, e.g., craniopharyngioma or lesions caused by trauma, obesity associated with hypogonadotropic hypogonadism, and in some instances with diabetes insipidus, is part of the syndrome. It is not clear to what extent impairment of the secretion of hypothalamic pituitary–releasing factors might contribute to the obesity.

Obesity rarely may be present in early childhood as part of a variety of congenital syndromes such as adiposogenital dystrophy (Fröhlich's syndrome), Prader-Willi syndrome, Laurence-Moon-Biedl syndrome, Alström's syndrome, and pseudohypoparathyroidism. The cause of the obesity in these syndromes remains unknown, although structural or functional hypothalamic defects have been postulated.

Unusual distributions of adiposity can occur. Partial lipodystrophy is a rare variation of congenital lipodystrophy (lipoatrophy), in which subcutaneous fat is totally absent from a portion of the body and hypertrophied in the remainder. In multiple lipomatosis, a familial disorder characterized by localized, discrete, subcutaneous fat deposits throughout the body, stored triglyceride in lipoma cells (indistinguishable from the more usual adipose tissue cells) appears to be unavailable for mobilization even during starvation.

TREATMENT. In general, obesity can be treated by reduction of caloric intake or increase of caloric expenditure, or both. In special circumstances, particularly as applied to lifelong obesity, surgical techniques to decrease gastrointestinal adsorption of food and to decrease fat storage capacity by resection of large amounts of tissues have been used. Weight loss can be achieved by caloric restriction, regardless of the nature of the diet. The amount of weight loss depends largely on the degree of negative energy balance that is attained. Unfortunately, oxygen consumption declines in parallel with weight loss, making it more difficult to maintain a steady degree of weight loss over the long term.

Diet. Although there have been many suggestions that the macronutrient composition of the calorically restricted diet is important for successful weight reduction, there is no firm evidence that a calorie is anything more or less than a calorie, regardless of the food source from which it is derived, despite the popularity of many calorically unbalanced "fad" diets. The rate of weight loss on low calorie diets high in protein is the same as the rate on diets high in fat or high in carbohydrate. Previous observations that indicated less rapid weight loss with high-carbohydrate, low-calorie diets have been attributed to short-term treatment in which changes in salt and water balance obscure changes in weight. It is apparent that an obese individual has a marked propensity to retain sodium during weight reduction and that this tendency is transiently exaggerated by carbohydrate in the diet. Carbohydrate-depleted ("ketogenic") diets increase weight loss solely by affecting water excretion, and their long-term use associated with mild ketosis and acidosis may cause decreased bone mineralization and amenorrhea. Meal frequency may play a role in the degree of success; frequent feedings may be more likely to prompt weight loss than less frequent consumption of larger loads which may lead to abnormal eating patterns, such as the night-eating syndrome. Although obesity may be more common in individuals who eat less frequently, there is no evidence of an effect of feeding frequency on the rate of weight loss in obese subjects studied in a metabolic ward. Total starvation has been promoted as a rapid route to achieve or start weight loss. However, the additional metabolic and other consequences of prolonged total starvation, such as unexplained anemia, body potassium depletion, hyperuricemia, gout, ketosis, lactic acidosis, liver function abnormalities, arrhythmias, hypotension, and, rarely, sudden death, have limited the utility of this form of treatment. Furthermore, it has been shown that the additional weight loss achieved by total starvation or carbohydrate-deprived diets over that achieved by a 600 to 800 mixed calorie diet is achieved by a selective loss in lean body mass rather than by additional loss of fat mass. The protein-modified fast may minimize this loss, but does not influence the other side effects of starvation. Thus a minimal quantity of protein and carbohydrate in weight reduction diets appears necessary, although the body has an unusual capacity to conserve nitrogen. In principle, it is clear that the aim of a weight reduction diet should be to keep normal body composition as well as to attain normal weight or to prevent further weight gain. There is no evidence to support the superiority of any form of low-calorie diet over that of any other. Thus a practical dietary recommendation for long-term management of obesity would be 15 to 20 cal per kilogram of ideal body weight, containing 20 per cent protein, 45 per cent carbohydrate, and 35 per cent fat calories. Substitution of one or more meals each day by fixed composition liquid formulas appears to have contributed to successful initiation of weight loss in many individuals. However, unbalanced formulations, such as the high protein, "protein-sparing" formula, appear to be associated with the same untoward consequences as seen with total starvation and other carbohydrate-deprived regimens, and the use of liquid protein hydrolysates to supplement total fasting has been associated with increased mortality. When psychologic problems appear prominent, emotional support may be necessary. The success of weight reduction groups for many individuals indicates that support of the "group therapy" type may be a useful adjunct.

Exercise. The most common method for promoting caloric expenditure in obese individuals is increased exercise. Obese patients, particularly adolescent females, are consistently less active than are thin individuals. In practice, obese individuals on weight reduction diets tend spontaneously to decrease their activity further, perhaps to compensate for decreased caloric intake in an attempt to preserve their fat mass. Exercising animals appear to gain less weight than do free-eating sedentary controls as a result of both an increase in caloric expenditure and a decrease in food intake. Exercise results in a significant decrease in the percentage of body fat, with a proportional increase in lean body mass. Thus exercise does appear to influence both body composition and food intake and should be part of reducing regimens. Exercise alone, however, does not appear to be an effective means of weight reduction, since the caloric equivalent of most activities is easily nullified by small amounts of food intake.

Drugs. Appetite suppressants (usually amphetamine derivatives) are of limited utility, because their effect is transient and rarely leads to more than a 10 per cent weight reduction. Inasmuch as the treatment of obesity is lifelong, such drugs have no demonstrable role in the long-term management of obesity. However, since neural regulation of adipose mass appears likely, future development of drugs altering such mechanisms holds promise. Thyroid hormone has been widely used to increase oxygen consumption of obese patients regardless of whether they suffer from hypothyroidism or "hypometabolism." Studies of body composition have shown that the accelerated weight loss from superimposition of thyroid extract on a low-calorie diet is due to a differential loss of lean body mass rather than to loss of fat tissue. Numerous other medications have been promoted for ability to achieve weight loss in obese individuals. Evaluation of these becomes a problem, because the routine of frequent physician visits, weight measurement, emotional support, medication, and diet itself promotes weight loss, and it is difficult to ascribe success to a particular medication. Furthermore, weight loss may result predominantly from loss of fluid, as with the widely dispensed diuretics, rather than from loss of adipose mass.

Surgery. A jejunoileal bypass operation has been used as a radical form of treatment of severe and refractory obesity in an attempt to lessen morbidity and early mortality. This procedure was devised to eliminate the function of a sufficient length of jejunum and ileum to cause weight loss without producing clinical steatorrhea. The distal ileum is essentially bypassed. Unfortunately, bypass surgery has, in several instances, caused massive fatty changes in the liver, cholestasis, fibrosis, interstitial inflammation, and fatal hepatic necrosis. Other complications include high operative mortality, severe crippling diarrhea, electrolyte imbalance, arthritis, and oxalate renal stones. Because of fewer reported complications, gastric partitioning procedures have been used more recently as the preferable surgical treatment. At present, caution in use of these experimental procedures is warranted, since complications such as peripheral neuropathy are being reported. There is no rationale for adipectomy in the management of lifelong obesity, although the disorder is characterized by adipose cell hyperplasia. Experimental studies in animals lead to little optimism, because excision of large adipose deposits has been followed by compensatory hypertrophy of remaining fat cell mass.

Behavior Modification. Since there are differences in feeding behavior between lean and some obese individuals, the newer methods of behavioral control have been applied to overeating. Short-term success in small groups of patients has been reported, and this approach appears to have promise, particularly as an adjunct to other forms of therapy, but long-term success does not appear to be enhanced.

PROGNOSIS. Overall mortality rates are higher in untreated moderate or severe obesity beyond about 30 per cent overweight. Insurance company figures suggest that for 45-year-old men averaging about 30 per cent overweight, death rates are 40 per cent higher than those for all insured men. For any degree of obesity, the mortality risk is higher for males than females and is greater for obesity occurring at a younger rather than an older age. These higher mortality rates can be reversed with weight reduction.

Unfortunately, successful weight reduction over the long term is difficult to achieve. The prognosis for treatment of obesity appears to vary with the clinical type. Lifelong obesity is frustrating to treat and leads to grief on the part of both physician and patient. In view of the poor results after long-term follow-up of a variety of dietary weight reduction schemes (which may be very successful in the short term), this form of obesity may be virtually irreversible. It is a common experience in obesity clinics that less than 5 per cent of the grossly (presumably lifelong) obese patients ever attain normal weight, and few can maintain a short-term weight loss in excess of 40 pounds. The long-term prognosis after gastrointestinal surgery is as yet unknown. Reduced caloric intake in childhood may lead to short stature and delayed puberty.

On the other hand, the more common adult-onset obesity should be amenable to treatment, so that most of the metabolic and pathophysiologic consequences of enlarged adipose cell mass and its associated diseases can be reversed.

PREVENTION. As with hypertension, most obesity is "essential," because definable, preventable, and treatable causes rarely can be identified. However, focus on the most refractory form of obesity, hyperplastic or juvenile-onset, should produce additional insights leading to more effective prevention. It is premature to suggest to physicians that obesity must be prevented in childhood if there is to be an impact on obesity in the adult.

Thus it can no longer be assumed that most obesity is simply the result of overeating and that every fat person is an overfed normal one. Most slightly overweight adults are fundamentally normal, but have eaten a little too much and exercised much too little. The grossly overweight patient who has had the problem from early childhood suffers from a disorder that is not well understood and is unsuccessfully treated. Nevertheless some of the complications of obesity can be managed, and the obese individual who has experienced multiple failures in weight reduction needs sympathetic attention rather than admonition.

Alexander JK, Peterson KL: Cardiovascular effects of weight reduction. Circulation 45:310, 1972. *A study of hemodynamic variables in markedly obese patients before and after significant weight reduction, indicating that the circulatory effects of gross obesity are largely reversible with weight loss.*

Alpers DH: Surgical therapy for obesity. N Engl J Med 308:1026, 1983. *A brief review of the present status of surgical approaches with an editorial comment on the companion article concluding, on the basis of late follow-up, that jejunoileal bypass surgery is no longer justified.*

Bray GA (ed.): The Obese Patient. Philadelphia, W. B. Saunders Company, 1976. *A compendium of information about the epidemiology, pathogenesis, and metabolic and physiologic effects and treatments of obesity. A valuable source of references.*

Bray GA, Gallagher TF Jr: Manifestations of hypothalamic obesity in man. A comprehensive investigation of eight patients and a review of the literature. Medicine 54:301, 1975. *An in-depth review of one of the known causes of human obesity.*

Czech MP, Richardson DK, Smith CJ: Biochemical basis of fat cell insulin resistance in obese rodents and man. Metabolism 26:1057, 1977. *The mechanisms of impaired glucose utilization in response to insulin in fat cells isolated from obese individuals is reviewed. Emphasis is on altered metabolic activities rather than insulin receptors or the hormone effector system.*

Glass AR, Burman KD, Dahms WT, Boehm TM: Endocrine function in human obesity. Metabolism 30:89, 1981. *A comprehensive review of abnormalities of endocrine function in obesity.*

Hirsch J, Batchelor B: Adipose tissue cellularity in human obesity. Clin Endocrinol Metab 5:299, 1976. *A review of the current status of the role of adipose cell hyperplasia in obesity.*

Hubert HB, Feinleib M, McNamara PM, Castelli WP: Obesity as an independent risk factor for cardiovascular disease: A 26-year follow-up of participants in the Framingham Heart Study. Circulation 67:968, 1983. *A reexamination of the relationship of degree of obesity and the incidence of cardiovascular disease over 26 years in more than 5200 men and women indicates that obesity was a significant independent predictor, particularly among women.*

Knittle JL, Timmer K, Ginsberg-Fellner F, Brown RE, Katz DP: The growth of adipose tissue in children and adolescents. Cross-sectional and longitudinal studies of adipose cell number and size. J Clin Invest 63:239, 1979. *A detailed cross-sectional and longitudinal study of adipose cell number as a function of age in obese and nonobese children from ages 4 months to 19 years, documenting continuing hyperplasia in the obese throughout childhood.*

Lew EA, Garfinkel L: Variations in mortality by weight among 750,000 men and women. J Chron Dis 32:563, 1979. *A description of the mortality experience of 750,000 men and women in a long-term prospective study by the American Cancer Society, documenting that individuals 30 to 40 per cent heavier than average had a mortality rate 50 per cent higher than those of average weight. Mortality comparisons as a function of weight for all the common diseases are included.*

Schwartz RS, Brunzell JD: Increase of adipose tissue lipoprotein lipase activity with weight loss. J Clin Invest 67:1425, 1981. *Evidence that increased adipose tissue lipoprotein lipase activity in obesity is a metabolic abnormality not corrected by weight reduction and thus might be a primary abnormality leading to enhanced fat deposition.*

Sims EAH, Danforth E Jr, Horton ES, Bray GA, Glennon JA, Salans LB: Endocrine and metabolic effects of experimental obesity in man. Recent Prog Horm Res 29:457, 1973. *A summary of the results of a comprehensive study of the metabolic effects of experimental overfeeding in man.*

Stunkard AJ: The Pain of Obesity. Palo Alto, The Bull Publishing Company, 1976. *A review of the psychosocial aspects of obesity and the possible role of psychiatry in therapy.*

Van Itallie TB: Obesity: Adverse effects on health and longevity. Am J Clin Nutr 32:2723, 1979. *A summary of the health implications of obesity and the variety of disorders thought to be caused or aggravated by obesity.*

Van Itallie TB, Yang MU: Diet and weight loss. N Engl J Med 297:1158, 1977. *A review and a careful metabolic study of the effects of macronutrient composition of low calorie reducing diets on body composition. Carbohydrate depleted (ketogenic) diets increase weight loss solely by affecting water excretion.*

217. DISORDERS OF VITAMIN METABOLISM: DEFICIENCIES, METABOLIC ABNORMALITIES, AND EXCESSES

Richard S. Rivlin

In approaching disorders of vitamin metabolism, several considerations should be kept in mind about the properties of vitamins, their roles in biochemistry, and the shifting nature of their deficiencies that have evolved over a period of years. In general most vitamins must be acquired from dietary sources because they cannot be synthesized in the body. There are several exceptions to this rule in that certain vitamins can be synthesized in the body but in very small amounts. An example is niacin, which is formed in vivo from an essential amino acid, tryptophan. A tryptophan-poor diet cannot provide sufficient precursor to meet the metabolic needs for niacin, and niacin would have to be obtained from dietary sources in order to avoid deficiency. Other examples of vitamins synthesized by the body, or more correctly by the intestinal microflora, are vitamin K and biotin. Deficiency of these vitamins may result from long-term antibiotic therapy, which eliminates the bacterial sources. Under normal circumstances, however, endogenous supplies are not sufficient, and some must be obtained from food sources. Another example is vitamin D, which can be synthesized in the skin after exposure to light (Ch. 244).

Many vitamins, particularly the B vitamins, function as essential coenzymes required in intermediary metabolism. The dietary form of the vitamin is first converted into its active derivatives before it can serve as a coenzyme. Examples include dietary thiamin and its coenzyme derivative thiamin pyrophosphate, pyridoxine and pyridoxal phosphate, and riboflavin and flavin adenine dinucleotide. Vitamin deficiencies may arise not only because of dietary deficiencies but also because conversion of the dietary form of the vitamin to its coenzyme derivatives is diminished by drugs, diseases, or other factors. Vitamin deficiencies may also be caused by abnormalities of intestinal absorption, plasma transport, tissue storage, binding to proteins, or excretion. Assuring adequate vitamin status involves *exogenous* factors, such as dietary adequacy and food processing, preparation, and storage, as well as *endogenous* factors, that is, those that control vitamin utilization by the body.

Overt vitamin deficiencies caused by diet are seldom isolated. Although generations of students are familiar with scurvy caused by vitamin C deficiency and pellagra resulting from niacin deficiency, in common clinical practice in the United States these classical syndromes are encountered only rarely. Rather, the typical picture one encounters in hospitalized patients with protein-calorie malnutrition is that of multiple deficiencies, because a diet poor in one vitamin is usually poor in several others. Furthermore, one vitamin is often required for the metabolism of another. An example is riboflavin, which is involved in the metabolism of folic acid, pyridoxine, vitamin K, and niacin.

The clinical development of vitamin deficiencies is generally gradual; the physical examination is usually not useful in detecting deficiencies of specific vitamins early in their course. For example, by the time that perifollicular hemorrhages characteristic of scurvy have developed, vitamin C deficiency is already far advanced. Even the abnormalities detected by physical examination late in the course of the deficiency state are often not pathognomonic. Cheilosis and glossitis, typically attributed to deficiency of riboflavin, can be observed with deficiencies of a number of other B vitamins. Finding an abnormality of this kind on physical examination helps to establish the diagnosis of malnutrition but does not identify a specific nutrient as missing from the diet.

Increasing attention is now being paid to drugs and alcohol as significant causes of specific vitamin deficiencies. Drug-induced vitamin deficiencies often are poorly recognized and become evident most frequently in chronically ill long-term drug users on a marginally adequate diet. The elderly are particularly vulnerable to the deleterious effects of ethanol. This commonly used and abused substance is now established as the major cause of deficiencies of folate and thiamin among individuals 65 years of age and older, and this is probably true in younger age groups as well.

The rate at which vitamin stores are depleted following restriction of dietary intake varies widely among vitamins. The body stores of some vitamins, such as B_{12}, may not be depleted for years, whereas folic acid, thiamin, and niacin may be depleted within weeks or months. In general, the body's capacity for storage of water-soluble vitamins is limited, and when the storage capacity is exceeded, the excess is usually excreted rapidly; their tissue concentrations often cannot be increased even by massive doses given parenterally. By contrast, body stores of fat-soluble vitamins may become very great, and toxicity often develops with prolonged administration of doses greatly exceeding the recommended dietary allowances (RDA).

At present, many individuals are consuming vitamins in doses far in excess of the RDA. More than one third of individuals 65 years of age and older in the United States are estimated to be taking some kind of nutritional supplement. Toxicity frequently develops with prolonged use of megadoses of vitamins A and D. Individuals vary considerably in the rate at which they develop toxicity with prolonged use of megadoses of vitamins. Certain conditions predispose to early symptomatology. For example, individuals with a gouty diathesis may be at increased risk for renal toxicity caused by megadoses of vitamin C, and the onset of acute liver disease may precipitate vitamin A toxicity in a previously stable patient who has taken megadoses of this vitamin.

Under certain circumstances vitamins may be used appropriately as drugs. For example, ascorbic acid is widely employed to acidify the urine in cases of refractory urinary tract infections. Certain derivatives of vitamin A, in particular the 13-cis isomer of retinoic acid, have potent antikeratinizing effects that have been applied to the treatment of cystic acne. Nicotinic acid is utilized in the management of severe hyperlipoproteinemia. Thus, the therapeutic applications of vitamins extend far beyond their roles in correcting dietary deficiency.

VITAMIN B_1 (THIAMIN)

Structure and Biochemical Function

The thiamin molecule is composed of pyrimidine and thiazole moieties joined by a methylene bridge, as shown in Figure 217–1. The principal biochemical role of thiamin is that of precursor of thiamin pyrophosphate, a coenzyme required for oxidative decarboxylation of α-ketoacids to aldehydes. These reactions are widely distributed and are an important source of energy generation. In addition, thiamin pyrophosphate serves as the coenzyme for transketolase, which catalyzes the conver-

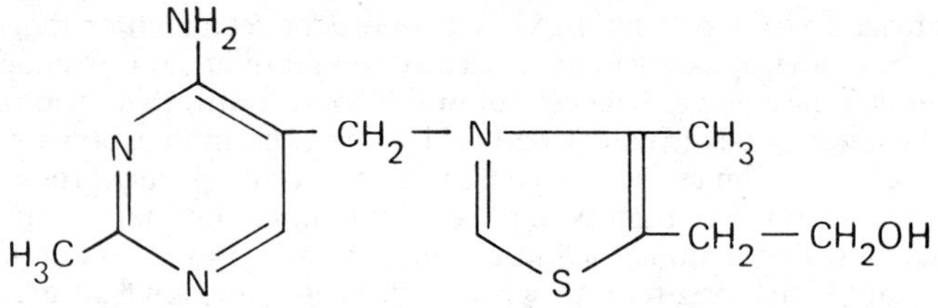

Figure 217–1. Structural formula of thiamin.

sion of the two 5-carbon sugars, xylulose-5-PO_4 and ribose-5-PO_4, to the 7-carbon sugar, sedoheptulose-7-PO_4, and the 3-carbon sugar glyceraldehyde-3-PO_4. This reaction is used as a functional index of thiamin nutritional status, as discussed later in this chapter.

In addition to serving as a coenzyme, thiamin may have a role in the neurophysiology of facilitating conduction in peripheral nerves. The initiation of nerve impulses is associated with hydrolysis of thiamin pyrophosphate or thiamin triphosphate or both.

Normal Physiology

Dietary thiamin is absorbed from the intestinal tract both by passive diffusion (high concentrations) and by active transport (low concentrations). The absorptive process is associated with phosphorylation of the thiamin molecule within the mucosal cell. In folate deficiency the absorption of thiamin is diminished. Muscle serves as the major storage organ for thiamin; most of the body stores are in the form of thiamin pyrophosphate, with lesser amounts stored as thiamin triphosphate, thiamin monophosphate, and thiamin itself. The degradation and excretion pathways of thiamin are not known with certainty, and more than 25 metabolites of the vitamin have been recovered from urine.

Requirements and Dietary Sources

The RDA for thiamin in adult males is 1.2 to 1.5 mg per day and in adult women, 1.0 to 1.1 mg per day, depending upon age, with a 50 per cent increase during pregnancy and lactation. The allowance is generally related to caloric intake as 0.5 mg per 1000 Kcals, although it is recommended that thiamin intake not go below 1.0 mg per day even with a caloric intake reduced below 2000 Kcal. The best dietary sources of thiamin are beef, pork, whole grains, enriched cereal grains, peas, beans, and nuts. Thiamin is rapidly destroyed at alkaline pH and is also heat-sensitive when not under strongly acid conditions. Some food items, particularly raw fish and seafood, are believed to contain thiaminases, which destroy the dietary supply of thiamin. A number of antithiamin factors have been identified from both plant and animal sources.

Deficiency

PATHOGENESIS. In addition to being caused by a poor diet, thiamin deficiency in the United States most commonly occurs as a result of alcoholism. Thiamin absorption is exquisitely sensitive to ingested ethanol, which significantly interferes with thiamin absorption even in healthy individuals. Repeated drinking throughout the day prevents most of the dietary thiamin from being absorbed, particularly in alcoholics, in whom some degree of malabsorption is quite common. Approximately 25 per cent of alcoholics admitted to general hospitals in the United States have evidence of thiamin deficiency either by clinical or biochemical criteria. Alcoholism is clearly the most important cause of thiamin deficiency in older age groups and probably in younger age groups as well. There is some evidence that alcohol also adversely affects the intermediary metabolism of thiamin, and chronic liver disease secondary to alcoholism may diminish the conversion of thiamin to thiamin pyrophosphate. Refeeding an alcoholic patient without thiamin may precipitate thiamin deficiency. It is likely that other factors, such as heavy coffee consumption, possibly may diminish the intestinal absorption of thiamin. Thiamin deficiency is also observed with diabetes, cancer, other chronic illnesses, and with long-term parenteral nutrition or use of intravenous fluids not containing thiamin.

CLINICAL FEATURES. Early thiamin deficiency is characterized by anorexia, irritability, and weight loss. Later, individuals experience weakness, peripheral neuropathy, headache, and tachycardia. Advanced thiamin deficiency presents with involvement of two major organ systems predominantly: the cardiovascular system (the syndrome known as "wet beriberi", i.e., beriberi heart disease) and the nervous system, both central and peripheral (known as "dry beriberi").

The following criteria are generally accepted for the diagnosis of beriberi heart disease: absence of other known etiologic factors, history of at least three months of documented dietary thiamin deficiency, associated peripheral neuritis, enlarged heart with normal sinus rhythm (usually tachycardia), peripheral edema, nonspecific ST- and T-wave changes, and rapid therapeutic response to thiamin administration. Beriberi heart disease is well recognized as a cause of high output failure, which is a consequence of the profound peripheral vasodilatation. Resting tachycardia, weakness, and weight loss often resemble the clinical features of apathetic hyperthyroidism, with which it is frequently confused.

The central nervous system manifestations of thiamin deficiency consist primarily of the Wernicke-Korsakoff syndrome (Ch. 482). The Wernicke's component is an acute disorder consisting of variable degrees of vomiting, horizontal nystagmus, ophthalmoplegia caused by weakness of the rectus muscles, fever, ataxic gait, and progressive mental impairment. Patients have died when the disease has been unrecognized and allowed to progress. The Korsakoff syndrome typically has loss of memory and confabulation as prominent features.

The peripheral nervous system abnormalities of thiamin deficiency typically consist of a symmetrical lesion that involves motor, sensory, and reflex responses. The legs are usually involved earlier and more completely than the arms. Pain and paresthesias may be particularly disabling to afflicted patients. It is possible that there is genetic variation in the susceptibility to dietary thiamin deficiency associated with differences in the binding affinity of transketolase for thiamin.

DIAGNOSIS. Thiamin status can be evaluated using bioassays, microbiologic technique, chemical analyses, and functional enzyme assays. In actual practice, the two most widely used assays are urinary thiamin excretion and the transketolase activity coefficient. Urinary thiamin can be determined accurately, but the results may be misleading if there has been recent thiamin intake in a previously deficient patient or if the patient has recently taken diuretics, which promote thiamin excretion. The results obtained under those circumstances would not yield the expected low value. Transketolase, as noted previously, requires thiamin pyrophosphate as its cofactor. In vitamin deficiency, the erythrocyte apoenzyme is not fully saturated with its cofactor, and addition of the cofactor in vitro to an erythrocyte hemolysate results in an increase in measured enzyme activity. The degree of increase in the activity coefficient (i.e., enzyme activity after incubation with the cofactor in vitro compared to that before incubation in vitro, expressed as a per cent) is an indication of the degree of unsaturation of the apoenzyme with thiamin pyrophosphate. The degree of unsaturation, in turn, is indicative of the magnitude of depletion of body stores of thiamin. An activity coefficient of 15 to 20 per cent or greater is generally regarded as reflecting significant thiamin deficiency. If these assays are unavailable, a therapeutic trial of thiamin, which provides rapid improvement (in 12 hours or less) in cardiovascular function and in ophthalmoplegia, may be regarded as supportive evidence for the diagnosis of thiamin deficiency. Cardiac output may diminish and vascular resistance increase within 30 minutes of intravenous administration of a single 100 mg dose of thiamin given to a patient with beriberi.

TREATMENT. If thiamin deficiency is suspected, rapid treatment with large doses of the vitamin is essential. Generally, 50 to 100 mg are administered intramuscularly or intravenously every day for the first few days, after which lower doses in the range of 5 to 10 mg may be given orally. Other therapeutic applications for which pharmacologic doses of thiamin are required include several rare inborn errors of metabolism: thiamin-responsive megaloblastic anemia, thiamin-responsive lactic acidosis, and thiamin-responsive branched-chain ketoaciduria, as well as subacute necrotizing encephalomyelopathy (Leigh's syndrome), a condition in which thiamin triphosphate is deficient in the brain.

Toxicity

Thiamin can be given safely by mouth in very large amounts without fear of toxicity, although the intestinal absorptive capacity is limited. When given by the intravenous route, large doses of thiamin on very rare occasions have been associated with poorly understood reactions resembling anaphylactic shock. Fortunately, these reactions occur so rarely that intravenous therapy with thiamin should not be withheld from a seriously ill thiamin-deficient patient.

Iber FL, Blass JP, Brin M, Leevy CM: Thiamin in the elderly—Relation to alcoholism and to neurological degenerative disease. Am J Clin Nutr 36:1067 (Suppl), 1982. *Discussion of effects of alcohol and drugs upon thiamin bioavailability.*

Neal RA, Sauberlich HE: Thiamin. *In* Goodhart RS, Shills ME (eds.): Modern Nutrition in Health and Disease. 6th ed. Philadelphia, Lea & Febiger, 1980. pp 191–197. *Discussion of structure, functions, requirements, and toxicity of thiamin.*

VITAMIN B_2 (RIBOFLAVIN)

Structure and Biochemical Functions

Riboflavin must be converted to its coenzyme derivatives, flavin mononucleotide (riboflavin-5′-phosphate, FMN) and flavin adenine dinucleotide (FAD), in order to be metabolically active (Fig. 217–2). These coenzymes are formed sequentially from dietary riboflavin after reacting with ATP and function as cofactors for a wide variety of enzymes in intermediary metabolism, particularly those involving oxidation-reduction reactions. FAD-dependent enzymes include α-glycerophosphate dehydrogenase, xanthine oxidase, and NADPH-cytochrome c reductase. A small fraction of tissue flavin is found in covalent linkage with protein and includes the enzymes monoamine oxidase (MAO), succinic dehydrogenase, and sarcosine dehydrogenase.

Normal Physiology

Riboflavin and FMN are absorbed from the upper gastrointestinal tract by a specific and saturable transport process. FAD, the predominant form in foods such as meat, must first be degraded to riboflavin and FMN prior to being absorbed. Covalently-bound flavins are largely unavailable as nutritional sources of riboflavin. A number of metals and drugs form complexes or chelates with dietary riboflavin and may influence the bioavailability of this vitamin. Such agents include copper, zinc, iron, saccharin, tryptophan, and ascorbic acid. After absorption, riboflavin is bound to several serum proteins and particularly to IgG during normal pregnancy. The renal tubule transports riboflavin in both directions, and in urine the predominant form detected is riboflavin rather than the coenzyme derivatives. Recently, several new metabolites of riboflavin have been identified in human urine, including 7α- and 8α-hydroxyriboflavin. The precise metabolic pathways are unknown.

Thyroid and adrenal hormones regulate the conversion of riboflavin to FMN, FAD, and covalently-bound flavins. Analogues of riboflavin interfere with certain actions of aldosterone and may possibly have potential as antihypertensive agents.

Requirements and Dietary Sources

The RDA for riboflavin in adult males is 1.4 to 1.7 mg per day and in adult females, 1.2 to 1.3 mg per day, depending upon age. Allowances are increased during pregnancy and lactation and probably should be increased with heavy exercise.

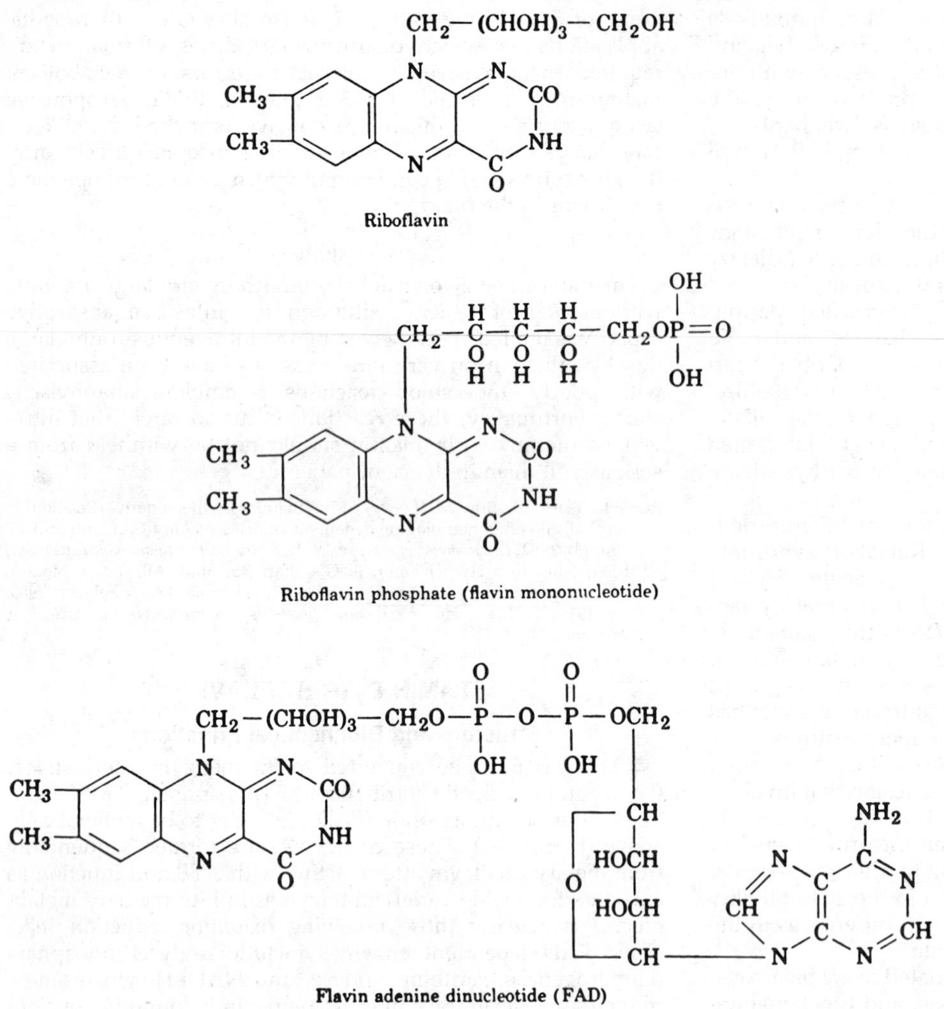

Figure 217–2. Structural formulae of riboflavin (vitamin B_2) and its coenzyme derivatives.

When riboflavin is consumed in amounts greater than the RDA, increased urinary excretion occurs promptly. In the United States, milk and milk products supply close to half the daily intake of riboflavin, with meat, fish, poultry, eggs, and legumes providing another 30 per cent; the remainder comes largely from fruits, vegetables, and grain products. In developing countries, the principal sources are cereals, roots, and tubers. Riboflavin is light-, acid-, and alkali-sensitive and rapidly loses biological activity when exposed to sunlight or when treated with sodium bicarbonate, a common but unfortunate practice used to retain the color of green vegetables.

Deficiency

PATHOGENESIS. Riboflavin deficiency arises not only because of an inadequate diet, but also when hormones, drugs, or diseases impair the absorption, utilization, metabolic transformations, binding, or excretion of this vitamin. In experimental animals, hypothyroidism and the psychotropic drugs, chlorpromazine, imipramine, and amitriptyline, diminish the conversion of riboflavin to its active coenzyme derivatives, FMN and FAD. The underlying mechanism of this effect appears to be inhibition of flavokinase, the enzyme that converts riboflavin to FMN, the first of two steps in the biosynthesis of FAD. Phototherapy of newborn infants with hyperbilirubinemia may lead to some decomposition of riboflavin because of its light sensitivity. Boric acid forms a complex with riboflavin and leads to massive riboflavinuria. Ethanol may diminish both the intestinal absorption of riboflavin and its bioavailability from food sources. Deficiency of riboflavin likely results also after severe trauma, burns, surgery, chronic debilitating diseases, and severe and prolonged diarrhea. Increased riboflavin excretion may occur under conditions of negative nitrogen balance, including diabetes after withdrawal of insulin.

CLINICAL FEATURES. Early symptoms of riboflavin deficiency include soreness of the mouth, burning and itching of the eyes, and personality deterioration. Advanced riboflavin deficiency produces a constellation of findings that include cheilosis, angular stomatitis, seborrheic dermatitis, glossitis, corneal vascularization, reticulocytopenia and anemia, and retarded intellectual development. Cheilosis and angular stomatitis, once thought to be specific for riboflavin deficiency, are now known to occur frequently in other nutritional deficiencies. The clinical picture of riboflavin deficiency isolated from other deficiencies is rarely observed. Riboflavin deficiency is a major cause of congenital malformations in experimental animals, but it is unclear at present whether malformations result from human maternal riboflavin deficiency. The rate of metabolism of a number of drugs is altered in riboflavin deficiency, at least in part because the microsomal hydroxylase system requires a flavin cofactor.

DIAGNOSIS. In riboflavin deficiency, there is a reduction in urinary excretion of riboflavin as well as a reduction in the concentrations of various flavins in plasma and in erythrocytes. A functional test of riboflavin status is the activity coefficient of erythrocyte glutathione reductase, an FAD-requiring enzyme. When FAD is added in vitro to an erythrocyte hemolysate the increase in activity produced is much greater in erythrocytes from riboflavin-deficient than from riboflavin-replete individuals. As with transketolase and thiamin pyrophosphate (referred to above), this assay reflects the lesser degree of saturation of the apoenzyme with its cofactor in deficient compared with normal individuals. Results are expressed as the activity coefficient, i.e., the ratio of enzyme activity after incubation with FAD in vitro to that before incubation. Activity coefficients greater than 1.2 to 1.3 are generally considered to be indicative of a riboflavin-deficient state.

TREATMENT. Riboflavin deficiency can be treated satisfactorily with food sources high in riboflavin, such as milk, liver, meat, eggs, and certain vegetables, or with the vitamin itself. Deficient patients treated with 10 to 15 mg per day of riboflavin undergo healing of skin lesions within days to weeks of initiation of therapy. The intravenous administration of riboflavin, which may be needed in debilitated patients or in those with serious disorders of the gastrointestinal tract, is greatly restricted by its limited solubility in aqueous solution.

Toxicity

Riboflavin, FMN, and FAD are completely free of any known toxicity.

Massey V, Williams CH (eds.): Flavins and Flavoproteins. Seventh International Symposium. North Holland, NY, Elsevier, 1983. *Volume covering the latest conference proceedings of subjects related to biochemistry, chemistry, and medical aspects of riboflavin and its coenzyme derivatives.*

Merrill AH, Lambeth JD, Edmondson DE, McCormick DB: Formation and mode of action of flavoproteins. *In* Darby WJ, Broquist HP, Olson RE (eds.): Annual Review of Nutrition. Vol. 1. Palo Alto, Annual Reviews Inc., 1981, pp 281–317. *Review of the basic biochemistry of riboflavin and its derivatives and flavin enzymes.*

Rivlin RS: Riboflavin. *In* Olson RE (ed.): Present Knowledge in Nutrition. 5th ed. Washington DC, The Nutrition Foundation, 1984, pp 285–302. *Discussion of the physiology, sources, functions, and metabolic roles of riboflavin.*

NIACIN

Structure and Biochemical Function

The term niacin is used in this review to refer to two compounds, nicotinic acid and nicotinamide, and other biologically active pyridine derivatives, as shown in Figure 217–3. The term niacin is sometimes restricted to nicotinic acid only. Although niacin was formerly referred to as "vitamin B_3," this term is no longer used as an official designation. Niacin is a precursor of two coenzymes, nicotinamide adenine dinucleotide (NAD) and nicotinamide adenine dinucleotide phosphate (NADP), which function in a wide number of oxidation and reduction reactions. NAD and NADP are involved in glycolysis, pyruvate metabolism, pentose biosynthesis, and lipid, amino acid, protein, and purine metabolism. These coenzymes also have other functions, some of which are discussed in the following paragraphs. Niacin is stable both to light and to heat.

Normal Physiology

Niacin given by itself appears to be nearly completely absorbed by diffusion from the stomach and small intestine in amounts as high as 3 grams. When present in a bound form in certain foods such as corn, however, niacin has only limited bioavailability. A portion of dietary niacin occurs in a bound form (as niacinogen) in cereal grains but remains biologically available. As noted previously, niacin can be synthesized from the essential amino acid tryptophan. Under normal circumstances approximately 1.5 per cent of dietary tryptophan is converted to niacin. The efficiency of this conversion is regulated by a number of hormonal and nutritional factors and is greater under conditions of niacin deficiency. Vitamins B_2 and B_6 are required for this conversion. Niacin is present in all cells, and only small amounts can be stored in the body. Both nicotinic acid and nicotinamide, as well as certain of their metabolites, particularly N-methylnicotinamide and 2-pyridone, are excreted in urine.

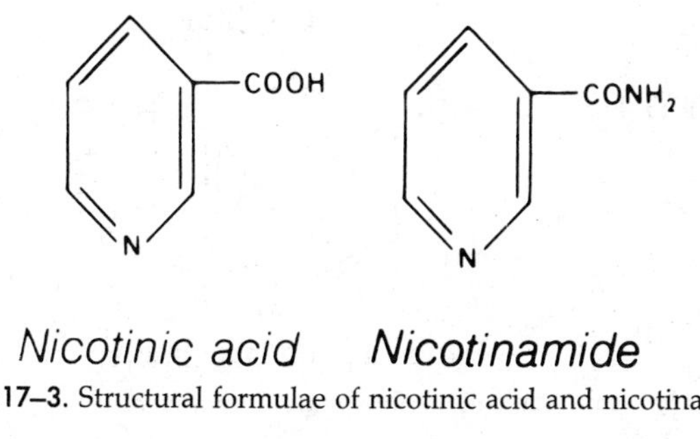

Figure 217–3. Structural formulae of nicotinic acid and nicotinamide.

Requirements and Dietary Sources

The RDA for niacin in adult males is 16 to 19 mg and in adult females, 13 to 14 mg, depending upon age, with an additional 2 mg recommended for pregnancy and 5 mg for lactation. The allowance is expressed in terms of niacin equivalents, because approximately 60 mg of dietary tryptophan are needed to form 1 mg of niacin. Proteins of animal origin such as meat, milk, and eggs have a relatively high tryptophan content and therefore are good sources of endogenously generated niacin. Vegetable proteins also supply tryptophan, but the concentration is lower than in animal proteins. Diets dependent heavily upon corn are a particular problem because not only is the tryptophan content low but also the niacin is poorly available. Niacin from wheat sources also has limited bioavailability. Pyridoxine and riboflavin deficiencies increase the dietary requirement for niacin, because these vitamins are required for the biosynthesis of niacin from tryptophan.

PATHOGENESIS. Niacin deficiency may develop because of a number of factors. First, dietary deficiency develops when corn is the major staple of the diet. Pellagra caused by consumption of corn was once very common in parts of the United States but fortunately has largely disappeared at the present time. Secondly, niacin deficiency may arise as a result of alcoholism, a condition in which diet is often poor and erratic. It is likely that in prolonged alcoholism, particularly in the presence of other nutrient deficiencies, the absorption and metabolism of niacin may be impaired. In addition, certain drugs interfere with niacin metabolism to a clinically significant degree, the best known of which is isonicotinic acid hydrazide (INH). The neurologic symptoms occurring with INH treatment can be ameliorated by administration of pyridoxine. Certain anticancer drugs, particularly 6-mercaptopurine, may produce niacin deficiency. In the rare inborn error of Hartnup's disease, pellagra may develop because of a defect in the intestinal and renal tubular transport of tryptophan and of several other amino acids (Ch. 83.3). Malnourished patients with the malignant carcinoid syndrome have been known rarely to exhibit manifestations of pellegra; under these circumstances, dietary tryptophan is diverted from niacin to serotonin (Ch. 242). Under certain conditions, excess leucine in the diet produces a deficiency by inhibiting the conversion of tryptophan to niacin.

CLINICAL FEATURES. In the early stages of niacin deficiency, clinical findings may be vague and nondiagnostic. Patients often complain of decreased appetite, loss of weight, abdominal aching and discomfort, weakness, irritability, inability to concentrate, and other nonspecific indications of illness. As the deficiency progresses, there may be epithelial changes that include glossitis, stomatitis, soreness and pain in the mouth (particularly the tongue), and eventually development of the characteristic skin lesions. These lesions, when well established, are dark, scaling, and cracking and occur over the areas of skin that are exposed to sunlight, frequently leaving a sharp line of demarcation at the unexposed skin surfaces. The lesion may resemble a necklace and is described as Casal's necklace.

In addition to the dermatitis, patients with the advanced form of niacin deficiency, that is, pellegra, have diarrhea and dementia. The diarrhea is often severe and intractable and may have a component of malabsorption that appears to be related to villous atrophy. The latter likely results from the long period of minimal food intake. Neuropsychiatric manifestations are mild at first but in advanced cases may progress to confusion, disorientation, seizures, hallucinations, and frank psychosis. Death may result in very advanced cases, usually preceded by major confusional states. Pellagra is popularly known for the four D's: dermatitis, diarrhea, dementia, and death.

Niacin deficiency secondary to drugs is generally mild and often unrecognized by clinicians. The consequences of drug-induced deficiencies of niacin and of other vitamins are much greater in the presence of a marginal or frankly deficient diet.

DIAGNOSIS. The diagnosis of advanced deficiency can often be made on clinical grounds alone if the patient exhibits the classic findings. Such patients are very unusual, however. In the early stages of the illness or in the absence of all the classic features, diagnosis may be difficult and is often missed without a high index of suspicion. Blood concentrations of NAD and NADP are reduced but may not be indicative of niacin deficiency, because reduced levels also occur in other severe, constitutional illnesses that are unrelated to niacin status. Attention has therefore turned to assay of urinary metabolites of niacin as indices of niacin nutriture. The most widely used is N-methylnicotinamide. Low urinary levels are interpreted as indicative of niacin deficiency. The excretion of another metabolite, 2-pyridone, is less widely used and requires a cumbersome assay. Some investigators have considered the ratio of these two metabolites in urine to be the most accurate index of niacin nutriture.

TREATMENT. The treatment of advanced pellagra has been accomplished satisfactorily by administering large oral doses (approximately 50 to 150 mg) of niacin as nicotinamide (the form present in most commercial vitamin formulations). The exact dose given is somewhat empirical. The therapeutic response is often dramatic, and patients may show marked improvement within several days after the start of therapy. Maintenance levels are then given together with dietary repletion. Nicotinamide is usually well tolerated under these circumstances.

Other therapeutic applications of niacin include its use as nicotinic acid in the control of elevated serum cholesterol and triglyceride levels in daily doses of 3 grams or more (Ch. 183–186). Nicotinic acid may be useful in treating patients of types II, IV, and V hyperlipoproteinemia. The mechanism of the therapeutic effect on lipid metabolism is not known, and this property is not shared by nicotinamide. With nicotinic acid treatment, HDL levels rise because of a slight decrease in synthetic rate with a large decrease in degradative rate. Because of the toxicity of nicotinic acid at high doses, treatment with this agent is generally reserved for patients with extreme lipid abnormalities. At the present time, nicotinic acid is believed to reduce the recurrence rate of nonfatal myocardial infarction but not to influence overall mortality rate.

Doses in the range of those used to treat pellagra are also needed to treat niacin deficiency in Hartnup's disease and in the carcinoid syndrome. Massive doses of niacin have not proven useful in the treatment of schizophrenia and other psychiatric disorders, despite the claims of food faddists and so-called "orthomolecular" therapists.

Toxicity

At the doses of nicotinamide used to treat niacin deficiency (described previously) there is little if any toxicity. When nicotinic acid in doses of 3 grams or more is used in the treatment of a lipid disorder, the most common side effect observed is flushing of the face due to vascular dilatation. Other common side effects of nicotinic acid may include dryness, itching and increased pigmentation of the skin, and abdominal pain. Rarely, hepatotoxicity, hyperuricemia, and worsening of peptic ulcer and glucose tolerance have been observed. The abnormalities in liver function may be severe, but both biochemical and histologic findings regress with discontinuation of nicotinic acid.

Henderson LaVM: Niacin. *In* Darby WJ, Broquist HP, Olson RE (eds.): Annual Review of Nutrition. Vol. 3. Palo Alto, Annual Reviews Inc, 1983, pp 289–307. *This review covers transport, metabolism, and physiologic and pharmacologic effects of niacin.*

Moran JR, Greene HL: The B vitamins and vitamin C in human nutrition. II. "Conditional" B vitamins and vitamin C. Am J Dis Child 133:308, 1979. *Discussion of physiology, metabolic disorders, and toxicity of niacin.*

Narasinga Rao BS, Gopalan C: Niacin. *In* Olson RE (ed.): Present Knowledge in Nutrition. 5th ed. Washington DC, The Nutrition Foundation, 1984, pp 318–331. *Review stressing metabolism, function, pathogenesis of deficiency, and therapeutic uses of niacin.*

VITAMIN B_6 (PYRIDOXINE)

Structure and Biochemical Function

The term vitamin B_6, or pyridoxine, is used to refer to three closely interrelated compounds, pyridoxine, pyridoxamine, and pyridoxal, together with their phosphate derivatives (Fig. 217–4). Of all these compounds, pyridoxal-5-phosphate is the most important, because it constitutes the major coenzyme involved in the intermediary metabolism of amino acids, in-

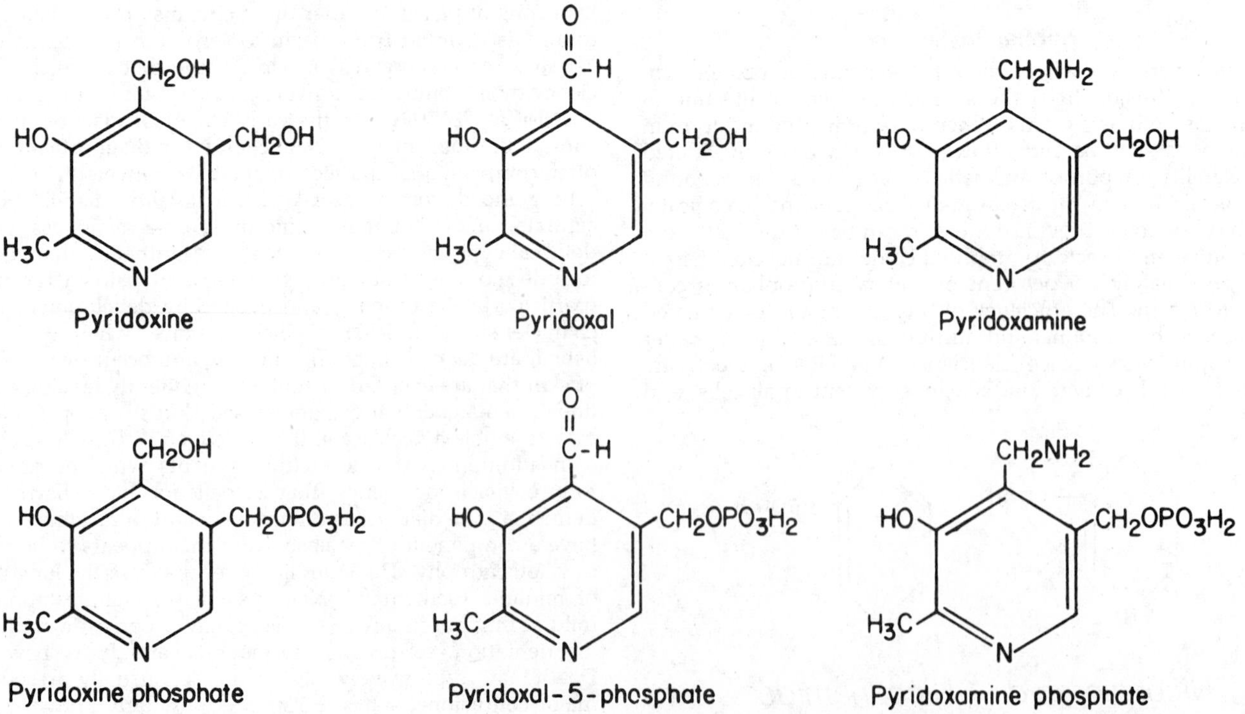

Figure 217–4. Structural formulae of pyridoxine, pyridoxal and pyridoxamine, and their phosphate derivatives.

cluding aminotransferases, decarboxylases, racemases, and synthetases. Pyridoxal phosphate is also involved in biosynthesis of heme and sphingosine. Under certain circumstances, pyridoxamine phosphate can also fulfill a coenzyme function. Pyridoxine is the major dietary source found in plants, whereas pyridoxal and pyridoxamine constitute the major forms in foods from animal sources. Pyridoxine is stable in acid solutions, but is highly light-sensitive in acid or neutral solutions. Pyridoxal and pyridoxamine are destroyed at high temperatures, particularly by autoclaving.

Normal Physiology

Dietary pyridoxine and related compounds are absorbed from the upper gastrointestinal tract probably by simple diffusion. The vitamin is widely distributed in the body; muscle constitutes an important storage organ, in which it is bound to phosphorylase, thus serving to stabilize the enzyme molecule. The various forms of pyridoxine are readily interconverted to one another by the liver under normal circumstances. Only very small amounts of dietary pyridoxine are converted to pyridoxal phosphate. In urine, pyridoxine, pyridoxal, and pyridoxamine can all be detected but at low concentrations; the major metabolite of pyridoxine, 4-pyridoxic acid, is found in urine in high concentrations.

Thyroid hormones reduce the concentrations of vitamin B_6 in various tissues, and increased sensitivity to insulin is demonstrable during B_6 deficiency.

Requirements and Dietary Sources

The RDA for vitamin B_6 is 2.2 mg per day for adult males and 2.0 mg per day for adult females, regardless of age, with a 0.5 to 0.6 mg per day increase during pregnancy and lactation. The requirement for vitamin B_6 is greater with a higher protein intake.

Vitamin B_6 is widely distributed in the food supply and can be derived from both plants and animals. Sources of vitamin B_6 are similar to those of other B vitamins and include liver, meat, wheat, nuts, beans and other vegetables, fruits, and cereals. Considerable losses occur during prolonged cooking, particularly pressure cooking. The bioavailability of vitamin B_6 from dietary sources varies widely depending upon storage, processing, and composition of food.

Deficiency

PATHOGENESIS. Dietary deficiency of pyridoxine is unusual, perhaps because of its widespread sources in the food supply. Rather, deficiency of pyridoxine is recognized increasingly as a consequence of prolonged therapy with certain medications. Foremost among these drugs is isoniazid, which complexes with pyridoxal phosphate to a clinically significant degree. Individuals with the genetic trait of inactivating isoniazid at a slow rate are particularly susceptible to B_6 deficiency from this drug. Isoniazid induces peripheral neuritis and diarrhea in adult patients; in children it produces anemia and seizures that can be prevented by coincident administration of pyridoxine. Cycloserine, another drug widely used for tuberculosis, is also a vitamin B_6 antagonist. With the widespread use of penicillamine for the treatment of rheumatoid arthritis, its B_6-antagonistic properties are of increasing clinical importance. Pyridoxine deficiency occurs frequently in alcoholism in association with other deficiencies, particularly folic acid deficiency. The increased urinary excretion of certain tryptophan metabolites, particularly xanthurenic acid, in women treated with oral contraceptives has been interpreted as indicating vitamin B_6 deficiency because B_6 is needed for conversion of tryptophan to niacin. L-DOPA, used for Parkinson's disease, may also cause B_6 deficiency over a prolonged period of time.

CLINICAL FEATURES. Deficiency of vitamin B_6 is not thought to produce a characteristic syndrome. As with deficiencies of other B vitamins, dermatitis, glossitis, cheilosis, and stomatitis may be manifestations of pyridoxine deficiency. Markedly deficient patients may have irritability, weakness, depression, dizziness, peripheral neuropathy, and seizures. As noted previously, deficiency in infants and children is typically characterized by diarrhea, anemia, and seizures. The rapidity with which drug-induced deficiency of B_6 occurs depends upon the adequacy of the patient's diet as well as the dosage and duration of drug therapy. Chronic vitamin B_6 deficiency also leads to secondary hyperoxaluria, increasing the risk of kidney stone formation (Ch. 89).

In addition to the deficiency syndromes of vitamin B_6 caused by diet or drugs or both, there is a group of disorders in which the affected patients do not display manifestations of deficiency, either clinically or biochemically, and yet require massive doses of this vitamin for adequate treatment. These disorders are known as dependency syndromes and include such diverse entities as pyridoxine-dependent convulsions, pyridoxine-responsive anemia, homocystinuria caused by cystathionine synthetase deficiency, cystathioninuria, and xanthurenic aciduria. Of these, pyridoxine-responsive anemia requires special mention because it is often confused with iron-deficient anemia; both disorders are characterized by hypochromic, microcytic red cells. In the pyridoxine-responsive anemia, however, serum iron is elevated with an increase in saturation of transferrin and an increase in iron absorption from the intestinal tract. There is evidence of iron overload, with hemosiderin deposits in bone marrow, liver, and other organs. Many patients have hepatosplenomegaly, and a hemolytic component may contribute to the anemia. It is important to differentiate this syndrome from iron-deficient anemia, because in the former inadvertent administration of iron worsens pyridoxine-responsive anemia. The blood count rises satisfactorily in response to pharmacologic doses of vitamin B_6.

DIAGNOSIS. The diagnosis of pyridoxine deficiency can be made by direct assay of vitamin B_6 in blood (normal levels generally are greater than 50 ng per milliliter) or by determining the urinary excretion of the main metabolite of pyridoxine, 4-pyridoxic acid. The excretion of less than 1.0 mg per day of this compound is generally considered suggestive of deficiency. Less frequently, the excretion of pyridoxine in urine is also determined. Functional enzyme assays, similar to those in use for diagnosing thiamin and riboflavin deficiencies, have also been developed for vitamin B_6 using aspartate aminotransferase or alanine aminotransferase in erythrocyte hemolysates. Enzyme activity is determined with and without the addition of pyridoxal phosphate in vitro. When activity coefficients (as defined previously) are greater than 1.5 for aspartate aminotransferase and 1.2 for alanine amino transferase, they are considered to be indicative of pyridoxine deficiency. These procedures have generally supplanted the tryptophan load test, in which the increased excretion of xanthurenic acid is taken as an index of B_6 nutriture.

TREATMENT. Dietary deficiency of pyridoxine can be treated satisfactorily with oral doses in the general range of 2 to 10 mg per day; doses of 10 to 20 mg per day may be needed in pregnancy. Pyridoxine deficiency occurring in association with specific drugs that inhibit pyridoxine metabolism, such as isoniazid, cycloserine, and penicillamine, requires higher doses, perhaps up to 100 mg per day, to ameliorate peripheral neuropathy. Rather than administer B_6 when symptoms develop, it is much more effective to prevent these side effects by administering vitamin B_6 when therapy with a B_6-antagonizing drug is initiated and particularly when a prolonged course of treatment is anticipated. Since iatrogenic vitamin B_6 deficiency is entirely preventable, B_6 is now routinely prescribed for patients receiving INH. Treatment with high doses of vitamin B_6 is contraindicated in patients receiving L-DOPA, however, as it may interfere with the efficacy of the drug.

Treatment of a pyridoxine-dependency syndrome requires much higher doses of B_6, and up to 1500 mg per day have been prescribed. The possible effectiveness of pyridoxine in the management of the carpal-tunnel syndrome and premenstrual tension is controversial. In some women on contraceptive steroids, vitamin B_6 has appeared to benefit depression. Pyridoxine is regarded as ineffective in treating schizophrenia, autism, and childhood hyperactivity, as well as peripheral neuropathies in which there is no known B_6 deficiency, such as in diabetes.

Toxicity

Pyridoxine has generally been considered to be safe and without toxicity. Recently, a sensory neuropathy was described in a small number of patients receiving 2 grams or more of pyridoxine per day. This potentially important finding requires confirmation and extension. At the present time, there are no indications for treatment of any disorder, even a pyridoxine-dependency syndrome, with doses of this magnitude. Thus, pyridoxine appears to be safe when prescribed in the appropriate milligram amounts needed to correct deficiency and to treat dependency states.

Henderson LM: Vitamin B_6. *In* Olson RE (ed.): Present Knowledge in Nutrition. 5th ed. Washington DC, The Nutrition Foundation, 1984, pp 303–317. *Review of B_6 stressing absorption, transport, and human requirements.*

Schaumburg H, Kaplan J, Winderbank A, et al.: Sensory neuropathy from pyridoxine abuse. A new megavitamin syndrome. N Engl J Med 309:445, 1983.

Sturman JA, Rivlin RS: Pathogenesis of brain dysfunction in deficiency of thiamine, riboflavin, pantothenic acid, or vitamin B_6. *In* Gaull GE (ed.): Biology of Brain Dysfunction. Vol. 3. New York, Plenum Press, 1975, pp 425–475. *Discussion of the pyridoxine-dependent syndromes.*

VITAMIN B_{12} (COBALAMIN)

The structure, function, pathophysiology, and therapeutic use of vitamin B_{12} are discussed in Ch. 135 in association with the megaloblastic anemias.

VITAMIN C (ASCORBIC ACID)

Structure and Biochemical Function

Ascorbic acid, a 6-carbon α-keto-lactone, resembles glucose in having several polyhydroxyl groups adjacent to one another (Fig. 217–5). Ascorbic acid can be oxidized to dehydro-L-ascorbic acid, which is also biologically active, and can be generated from the latter by reacting with reduced glutathione.

Ascorbic acid participates in oxidation-reduction reactions and in hydrogen ion transfer. This vitamin is a powerful reducing agent or anti-oxidant, particularly in lipid and vitamin metabolism, and is especially important in preventing oxidation of tetrahydrofolate. In addition, ascorbic acid enhances the intestinal absorption of nonheme iron. This vitamin is required in collagen metabolism, specifically for the synthesis of chondroitin sulfate and of hydroxyproline from proline. Defects in collagen biosynthesis are believed to be the basis for much of the symptomatology of scurvy. In the absence of vitamin C, dopamine-β-hydroxylase activity is reduced, impairing the biosynthesis of neurotransmitters. Ascorbic acid is also involved in carnitine biosynthesis, tyrosine metabolism, cholesterol metabolism, wound healing, and immune function and is a component of drug-metabolizing enzyme systems.

Prolonged storage or excessive cooking diminishes the biological activity of ascorbic acid. This highly water-soluble vitamin is also destroyed by oxidation, particularly by exposure to air in the presence of copper ion and an alkaline medium.

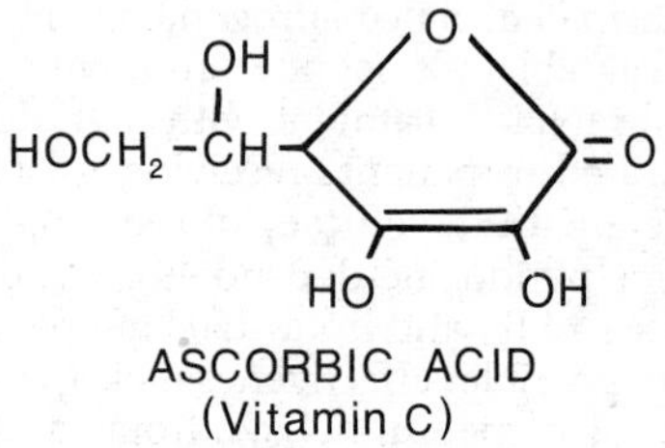

Figure 217–5. Structural formula of ascorbic acid.

Normal Physiology

Ascorbic acid is absorbed by a limited-capacity mechanism in the distal small intestine. As dietary intake of ascorbic acid increases, a progressively smaller proportion is absorbed, that is, about 95 per cent at 100 mg, 75 per cent at 1 gram, but only 20 per cent at 5 grams. Within the usual range of dietary ascorbic acid intake of 10 to 130 mg per day, the plasma level is proportional to the amount ingested. As the dietary intake increases further, however, the low renal threshold for excretion assures that excess plasma levels of ascorbic acid are promptly excreted. Another mechanism protecting against excessive accumulation of ascorbic acid is the microsomal enzyme, NADPH monodehydro-ascorbate transhydrogenase, which is induced by its substrate, ascorbic acid; in response to a large dietary load of ascorbic acid, degradative capacity is rapidly and substantially increased.

The body pool of ascorbic acid in adult males consuming about 80 mg per day is estimated to be approximately 1500 mg, and the rate of catabolism is about 3 per cent of the pool size per day. Increasing the dietary intake of ascorbic acid to more than 80 mg per day seems not to increase significantly the saturation of tissues with this vitamin. As with most B vitamins, the storage capacity for vitamin C is limited. Urinary excretion is in the form of ascorbic acid and dehydro-L-ascorbic acid, as well as several metabolites, including a sulfated derivative, ascorbate-2-sulfate, and oxalic acid.

Requirements and Dietary Sources

The RDA for ascorbic acid is 60 mg per day for all healthy adult males and females regardless of age. This allowance is generally regarded as quite generous inasmuch as 10 mg per day prevents scurvy. As noted, amounts greatly in excess of the RDA do not increase tissue stores significantly. The dietary allowance is increased by 20 mg per day during pregnancy and 40 mg per day during lactation. Human milk contains 30 to 55 mg per liter. It is especially important to maintain an adequate intake of ascorbic acid during lactation, because the vitamin concentration in milk is closely dependent upon dietary intake.

Serum ascorbic acid levels are lowered in smokers, possibly as a result of accelerated metabolism, and in users of oral contraceptive drugs, but the implications of these findings are unclear. The decreases are quantitatively small and can be corrected with a modest increase in consumption of ascorbic acid from dietary sources (about 40 mg for smokers). Patients who are exposed to cold or heat stress or who are febrile, undergoing surgery, or subjected to trauma have increased requirements for vitamin C. Patients receiving parenteral nutrition have higher requirements because of urinary losses.

The best dietary sources of ascorbic acid appear to be citrus fruits and green vegetables, especially broccoli, green peppers, tomatoes, cabbage, oranges, grapefruits, and lemons. Care must be taken during food preparation in order to avoid losses of the vitamin. Much smaller amounts are contained in milk, meats, and cereals. As noted above, ascorbic acid is heat-sensitive and is destroyed by alkali. Some decreased vitamin content is also observed with prolonged storage.

Deficiency

PATHOGENESIS. Urban poor, particularly the elderly, are at increased risk for dietary deficiency of ascorbic acid, in large measure because economic deprivation prevents them from obtaining the richest sources, namely citrus fruits, leafy vegetables, and tomatoes.

An increasingly important cause of ascorbic acid deficiency is food faddism and bizarre nutritional practices. The strict macrobiotic diet may lead to scurvy, particularly with pressure cooking of food items that have little ascorbic acid to begin with. Elderly individuals following a "tea and toast" diet are vulnerable to a number of deficiencies, particularly of ascorbic acid, as these sources are grossly inadequate. Children develop scurvy when fed unsupplemented cow's milk for the first year of life. Vitamin C deficiency progressing to scurvy is common in chronic alcoholics, probably because the diet is notably deficient in vitamin C-containing food items. Vitamin C deficiency, however, is not generally as prevalent as deficiencies of B vitamins in chronic alcoholism.

CLINICAL FEATURES. In the early stages of deficiency, symptoms and signs may be fairly nonspecific and include general malaise, lethargy, and weakness. As the disease progresses, probably one to three months after onset, patients may complain of dyspnea and pain in bones and joints, due predominantly to hemorrhages below the periosteum. Perifollicular hemorrhages, particularly about hair follicles, are indicative of advanced deficiency. Petechiae often are prominent and may appear over the arms after application of a sphygmomanometer. This finding is known as the Rumpel-Leed test. With progressive vitamin C depletion, there are ecchymoses and purpura initially at areas of trauma irritation, or pressure points. Joints, muscles, and subcutaneous tissues may become sites of hemorrhage. Swollen, bleeding gums are characteristic manifestations of advanced deficiency. Pallor and anemia may be the result of prolonged bleeding or to associated folic acid deficiency, with which scurvy commonly occurs. In children, disturbances of growth occur, and teeth, bones, blood vessels, and other collagen-rich structures develop abnormally. Preformed teeth may become loose and fall out because of alveolar bone resorption.

Wounds heal poorly, and previously healed wounds may open up again. In very advanced deficiency, edema, oliguria, and neuropathy are prominent. Should intracerebral bleeding occur, serious neurologic sequelae and even death may result.

DIAGNOSIS. The diagnosis of advanced scurvy is often made on clinical grounds alone because the skin changes may be quite characteristic. Capillary fragility is commonly abnormal. X-rays are useful in demonstrating subperiosteal elevation, disturbances of calcification of the cartilage matrix, fractures and dislocations, ground glass appearance of the cortex, alveolar bone resorption, and other findings.

Plasma ascorbic acid levels are greatly reduced in scurvy, usually to 0.1 mg per deciliter or lower. Some depression of plasma ascorbic acid levels occurs, however, in a variety of other conditions, including cigarette smoking, tuberculosis, rheumatic fever, many chronic disorders, and in some women using oral contraceptive drugs. These conditions must be considered when a low ascorbic acid level is detected.

The assay of ascorbic acid in serum or plasma can be accomplished with titrimetric, spectrophotometric, or fluorometric methods. Some laboratories prefer to make the diagnosis of scurvy by assay of platelet ascorbic acid.

TREATMENT. As little as 10 mg per day of ascorbic acid can completely prevent the clinical manifestations of scurvy. Even far-advanced cases of scurvy respond rapidly to ascorbic acid in the range of 100 to 200 mg per day. Marked improvement is to be expected within several days. Patients should also be instructed in the importance of a proper diet to prevent further recurrences.

Patients with rare inborn errors of metabolism, including tyrosinemia, osteogenesis imperfecta, and Chédiak-Higashi syndrome, have had some apparent benefit from the use of ascorbic acid in the range of 50 to 200 mg per day. Certain forms of the Ehlers-Danlos syndrome are the only disorders in which pharmacologic doses (4 grams) were reported to be effective.

Special mention must be made of two conditions in which the use of megadoses of ascorbic acid has attracted wide attention: the common cold and advanced cancer. Many studies have been performed on the possible benefits of 2 grams and higher per day of ascorbic acid on the prevention of colds and on the alleviation of symptoms once they develop. On balance, the predominance of evidence favors the view that while some individuals may receive slight benefit in terms of symptoms, probably as a result of a mild antihistamine action of ascorbic acid, no consistent, reproducible improvement occurs in the frequency, duration, or severity of illness in the great majority of cases.

With respect to advanced cancer, there is some theoretical basis for the view that maintenance of immune function may depend upon the adequacy of vitamin C nutriture, as may wound healing and collagen formation. Nevertheless, treatment of cancer patients with megadoses of vitamin C after chemotherapy and radiation has been ineffective when evaluated in an objective manner. The use of vitamin C under no circumstances should replace established methods of treating cancer with chemotherapy, surgery, or radiation.

Vitamin C at a dose level of approximately 0.5 to 3 grams per day has been used to acidify the urine in cases of refractory urinary tract infections. Ascorbic acid is only a weak acidifying agent, and its efficacy under these circumstances is difficult to evaluate.

Ascorbic acid in amounts ordinarily contained in food may be useful in facilitating the intestinal absorption of nonheme iron. To be effective, the ascorbic acid and the iron sources must be consumed together. As little as 100 ml of orange juice, which contains 40 to 50 mg of ascorbic acid, has been reported to increase the absorption of nonheme iron more than threefold.

A potentially useful application of ascorbic acid lies in its ability to inhibit in vitro the conversion of nitrites and secondary amines to the carcinogenic nitrosoamines. Whether ascorbic acid can achieve this effect in vivo under ordinary circumstances of food consumption is important to determine.

Toxicity

At the dose range of approximately 1 gram per day and higher there is potential for toxicity. There is great variability among individuals in regard to susceptibility to the side effects of megadoses of ascorbic acid and the doses necessary to cause toxicity. In the intestinal tract, large doses (2 grams and higher) of ascorbic acid may produce pain, discomfort, and an osmotic diarrhea. Such doses of ascorbic acid give a false-negative guaiac test for blood, thereby obscuring recognition of occult bleeding. Urine tests for glucose also may be misleading when large doses of ascorbic acid are ingested, producing a false-negative Testape and false-positive Clinitest.

As oxalate is a degradative product of ascorbic acid, large amounts of this vitamin will be expected to increase the delivery of oxalate to the renal tubule, posing the potential risk of oxalate stones in susceptible individuals. The increase in oxalate excretion is small in magnitude, however, and in most cases still falls within the normal range. Uricosuria and uric acid stones are also believed to occur with increased frequency because uric acid has less solubility in an acid medium. Nevertheless, the frequency of kidney stone formation in megadose users of ascorbic acid is not known precisely at present.

There is a likelihood of exacerbating systemic acidosis in those disorders with failure of urinary acidification, such as chronic renal disease and renal tubular acidosis. Certain patients with diminished glucose-6-phosphate dehydrogenase activity may be at increased risk for hemolytic episodes with megadose ascorbic acid therapy. Scurvy has been reported in several infants of mothers who consumed large amounts of ascorbic acid during pregnancy, presumably as a result of a dependency state developing in the infant. Therefore, it is probably not advisable to treat pregnant women with large doses of vitamin C. There is some concern that ascorbic acid, which increases intestinal absorption of iron, may also increase absorption of heavy metals such as lead and mercury and accelerate the development of toxicity from these metals.

Sauberlich HE: Ascorbic acid. *In* Olson RE (ed.): Present Knowledge in Nutrition. 5th ed. Washington DC, The Nutrition Foundation, 1984, pp 260–272.

Vitler RW: Nutritional aspects of ascorbic acid: Uses and abuses. West J Med 133:485, 1980. *Useful discussion of clinical features of ascorbic acid deficiency and treatment, including risks of megadoses.*

Wooliscroft JO: Megavitamins: Fact and fancy. Disease-a-Month 29:1, 1983.
Discussion of the hazards of misuse of large doses of vitamin C and other vitamins.

VITAMIN A

Structure and Biochemical Function

The structure of vitamin A and its major derivatives is shown in Figure 217–6. Vitamin A refers to retinol, although the term is often used loosely to indicate all of these compounds. Recently, the term retinoids has been used to designate all the natural and synthetic isomers and derivatives of vitamin A. Retinol is oxidized to vitamin A aldehyde (retinal), which is critical to vision. Retinoic acid (vitamin A acid) is the major oxidative metabolite of retinol. Retinoic acid can fulfill the growth-promoting and epithelial-differentiating roles of retinol but cannot fully maintain its function in reproduction, nor can retinoic acid fulfill the functions of retinal in vision. Carotenoids are larger precursor molecules that undergo cleavage to yield retinal. The most important of the more than 30 carotenoids with pro-vitamin A activity is β-carotene (Fig. 217–6).

Of the various metabolic roles of vitamin A, the best understood is the visual process. Retinal is the prosthetic group of all the visual pigments that capture light. The human retina contains four kinds of visual pigments: rhodopsin in rods and three iodopsins in cones. In the dark-adapted retina, rhodopsin is activated by photons of light. This event initiates the visual cycle, during which retinal changes its conformation from a cis to a trans isomer, and other conformational changes occur in the protein. During dark adaptation, these processes are reversed and rhodopsin is regenerated. In view of the absolute requirement for retinal, it is not surprising that loss of highly sensitive night vision is an early symptom of vitamin A deficiency. Vitamin A probably serves additional roles in the normal functioning of the retina.

The mechanism of action of vitamin A in growth and differentiation is not known. One hypothesis is that vitamin A is similar to steroid hormones in influencing events in the genome following attachment to specific cellular binding proteins. An alternative hypothesis is that vitamin A participates in the synthesis of glycoproteins, which in turn mediate metabolic events. The striking effects of vitamin A upon differentiation, particularly of epithelial tissues, underlie the current concept that this vitamin and its derivatives may possibly have a role in the prevention of certain cancers, particularly of epithelial origin.

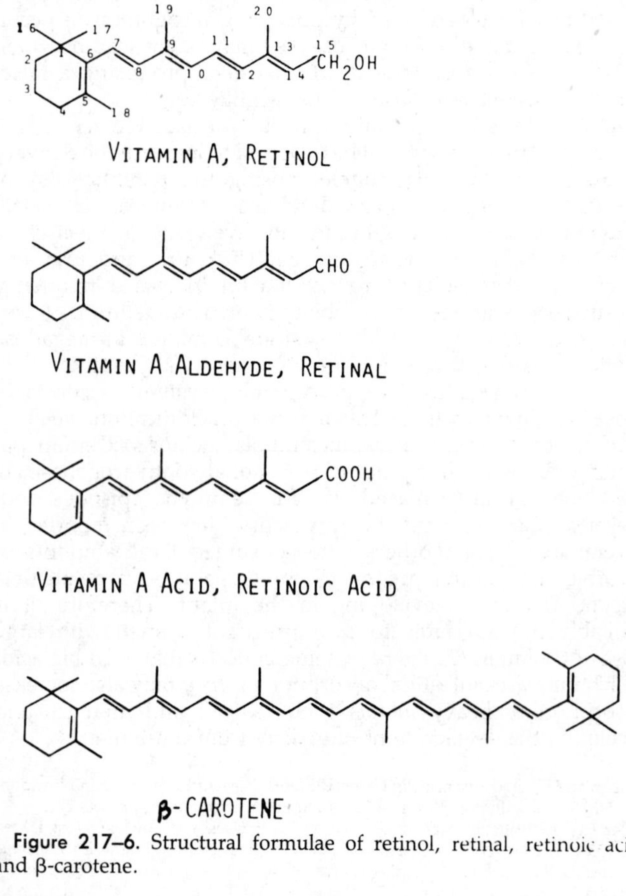

Figure 217–6. Structural formulae of retinol, retinal, retinoic acid, and β-carotene.

Retinol is fat soluble, sensitive to acid and heat, and is rapidly oxidized upon exposure to light and oxygen. β-carotene is relatively less heat-sensitive than retinol.

Normal Physiology

Foods containing retinol or carotenoids are digested by gastric pepsin and intestinal enzymes, and then both forms are absorbed by the intestinal mucosa. About 80 to 90 per cent of dietary vitamin A is absorbed. The rate of absorption of dietary β-carotene is much slower, and only 40 to 60 per cent is absorbed. Within the intestinal mucosa, β-carotene is cleaved to two molecules of retinal, which are then reduced to retinol. The retinol generated from β-carotene, as well as that absorbed directly, is esterified with palmitic acid. The retinyl esters formed are incorporated into chylomicra and transported via lymph to the general circulation, where the triglycerides in the chylomicra are degraded by lipoprotein lipase. The smaller chylomicra remnants remaining are then cleared by the liver, the major storage organ for vitamin A, which contains approximately 90 per cent of the total body reserves. Retinyl esters, mostly in the form of retinyl palmitate, are stored in the liver as a complex; hydrolysis of the retinyl esters in the liver generates retinol, which binds to a specific apo-retinol binding protein (RBP). The holo-RBP is secreted into the plasma, where it forms a 1:1 molar complex with prealbumin, a tetrameric serum protein that also binds thyroxine and triiodothyronine.

Cell surfaces recognize the RBP-retinol complex rather than retinol, and once inside the cell, retinol binds to a specific binding protein, cellular retinol binding protein (CRBP). A cellular retinoic acid binding protein (CRABP) has also been detected in a number of neonatal tissues and epithelial tumors that are sensitive to retinoic acid therapeutically.

In vitamin A deficiency, total plasma RBP levels fall to about half their normal levels and consist primarily of apo-RBP. At the same time, the liver concentration of apo-RBP is greatly increased. With vitamin A repletion, the liver apo-RBP becomes saturated, and levels of holo-RBP begin to rise in blood.

The degradative metabolism of retinol and its derivatives proceeds by a series of chain-shortening steps to yield a group of compounds of little if any intrinsic biological activity. These compounds can be detected in urine but have not been generally utilized diagnostically to characterize vitamin A nutriture.

Requirements and Dietary Sources

The RDA for vitamin A is currently 1000 μg of retinol equivalents (RE) for adult males and 800 μg for adult females. One RE is defined as 1 μg retinol or 6 μg β-carotene. The allowances are calculated in this fashion because the overall utilization of β-carotene is only about one sixth that of retinol, as a result of the relative inefficiency with which β-carotene is absorbed and converted to vitamin A.

Vitamin A allowances were formerly expressed in terms of international units (IU), and this nomenclature still appears on most commercial vitamin bottles. One retinol equivalent is equal to 3.33 IU retinol and 10 IU β-carotene. The RDA for vitamin A expressed in terms of IU is 5000 for adult males and 4000 for adult females. These figures are based upon the estimate that the U.S. diet contains approximately equal amounts of β-carotene (2500 IU = 250 RE, for males) and retinol (2500 IU = 750 RE, for males).

β-carotene is derived predominantly from plant sources, including vegetables such as carrots and sweet potatoes, leafy green vegetables, and some fruits. Palm oil is a particularly rich source of carotenes. Preformed vitamin A is derived almost exclusively from animal sources. Liver obviously is the richest source, followed by kidney, milk and milk products, and eggs. Fish liver oils have unusually high concentrations of vitamin A.

Deficiency

PATHOGENESIS. Vitamin A deficiency is a very common problem world wide, particularly in developing countries, as a consequence of famine or shortages of vitamin A-rich foods. The ocular manifestations of vitamin A deficiency are such a serious problem that they now constitute the leading cause of blindness in young children throughout the world. In such situations, a diet high in rice, wheat, maize, and tubers contain little if any β-carotene. Breast and cow's milk do not provide enough vitamin A to meet the needs of the growing child.

In the United States, vitamin A deficiency is encountered among the urban poor, the elderly, alcoholics, patients with malabsorption, and those individuals on a marginal diet. Individuals chronically using laxatives, particularly mineral oil, and certain other drugs are vulnerable to vitamin A deficiency. In alcoholism, vitamin A deficiency may develop for several reasons. Zinc deficiency, which frequently occurs in alcoholism, impairs the release of RBP from liver and probably interferes with the conversion of retinol to retinal needed in vision. Thus, alcoholism-associated zinc deficiency may intensify night blindness and other sequelae of dietary vitamin A deficiency. Also, in alcoholism the degradative enzyme, alcohol dehydrogenase, which converts retinol to retinal in the retina, may be so saturated with ethanol that retinal production is sharply diminished. Furthermore, as malabsorption develops in chronic alcoholism, dietary carotenes and vitamin A may be lost in increasing amounts in the stool.

Vitamin A deficiency may occur after long term use of mineral oil because this fat-soluble vitamin is dissolved in the oil. Other laxatives may result in vitamin A deficiency because of rapid intestinal transit and diminished intestinal absorption. Vitamin A deficiency may result also after prolonged use of drugs, such as cholestyramine, colestipol, neomycin and colchicine.

CLINICAL FEATURES. Night blindness, as noted previously, may be an early manifestation of vitamin A deficiency. It has been suggested that the frequent episodes of falling and of traffic accidents involving chronic alcoholics at night may be due to some degree to underlying night blindness. In addition, dryness or xerosis of the conjunctivae and later of the cornea may develop, leading to softening and perforation of the cornea and development of Bitot's spots (small, white patches) on the sclerae. Because of the role of vitamin A in maintaining differentiated epithelium, deficiency leads to abnormal development of epithelial tissue and keratinization, particularly in the eye, lung, sweat glands, and gastrointestinal tract. Loss of taste may also occur.

It has been suggested that decreased intake of β-carotene or vitamin A-rich foods or both may be associated with an increased prevalence of epithelial cancers, particularly lung cancers, among smokers. Also, vitamin A-deficient animals have an increased risk of chemical carcinogenesis; administration of retinoids can prevent chemically induced cancers in animals.

DIAGNOSIS. The demonstration of abnormal dark adaptation is important evidence for the diagnosis of vitamin A deficiency. Techniques are being developed that can be carried out under field conditions without expensive equipment. Retinol can be detected directly in serum by immunoassay. Normal levels are in the approximate range of 30 to 65 μg per deciliters. Serum levels may be increased by hypothyroidism, nephrotic syndrome, oral contraceptives, and other disorders of lipid metabolism. By the time serum levels of retinol begin to decrease in dietary deficiency, liver reserves are already seriously depleted.

TREATMENT. The extensive eye problems of vitamin A deficiency encountered in developing countries are best approached through a systematic plan of prevention. Such programs are increasing in scope and magnitude. Injections of vitamin A in large doses (50,000 to 100,000 IU), every four to six months are highly effective and are tolerated remarkably well. In the United States, when dietary deficiency is advanced, it should be treated with doses similar to these but for several days only, and then maintenance doses should be administered. Water-soluble forms of vitamin A under development should provide great assistance in patient management.

Derivatives of vitamin A (referred to as retinoids), particularly 13-cis-retinoic acid (isotretinoin), have been applied recently to the treatment of cystic acne with considerable success. Investigations are continuing in other dermatologic disorders, including psoriasis, actinic keratosis, leukoplakia, and pityriasis rosea. The mechanism of action of this derivative may lie in its inhibition of keratinization, suppression of sebaceous gland secretion, or possibly to a direct anti-inflammatory effect.

The use of β-carotene or retinoids or both, especially the less toxic forms, for the possible prevention of epithelial cancers is under intense study. Smokers should be expected to benefit particularly by increasing their intake of vitamin A and/or carotenoids. The exact doses necessary to achieve preventive effects are not known, and it is possible that major benefits can be obtained simply by increasing the intake of foods rich in carotenoids or vitamin A without additional supplementation. Further research is needed to clarify these vital issues.

Toxicity

The carotenoids are generally without toxicity. Consumption of β-carotene in large amounts from foods, for example, carrots, may stain the skin a curious yellow-orange color, but this phenomenon is believed to be entirely benign. The sclerae remain white in carotenemia; thus the condition can easily be differentiated from jaundice.

Vitamin A (retinol), on the other hand, is quite toxic when taken continuously in large amounts, particularly at the level of 50,000 IU and higher, for periods of three months or more. The skin may become dry, pruritic, coarse, and scaly with fissures; hair loss may occur. It is of interest that both vitamin A excess and deficiency have adverse effects upon the skin. Sore mouth, anorexia, and vomiting may ensue. The most serious side effects of vitamin A overdosage pertain to the central nervous system: patients may develop serious headaches, drowsiness, irritability, failure to concentrate, increased intracranial pressure, and papilledema. The liver may enlarge, rarely progressing to fibrosis and cirrhosis. Generalized lymph node enlargement may become evident. There may be painful hyperostoses, and there are preliminary indications that long-term use of vitamin A in large amounts possibly may accelerate the bone loss of aging. Congenital malformations have occurred in the infants of several women consuming 50,000 IU per day during pregnancy.

In cases of vitamin A toxicity, serum vitamin A levels are increased, particularly in the form of retinyl esters. In an asymptomatic patient receiving megadoses of vitamin A, the onset of liver disease such as hepatitis may precipitate overt clinical toxicity, presumably by releasing stored retinol into the general circulation. With discontinuation of megadoses of vitamin A, the symptoms will gradually recede.

The development of synthetic retinoids with lower toxicities and greater uptake in target organs is expected to facilitate the application of these agents in the possible chemoprevention of cancer.

Goodman DS: Vitamin A and retinoids in health and disease. N Engl J Med 310:1023, 1984. *This comprehensive review highlights recent advances relating vitamin A and retinoids to clinical medicine and public health, particularly ophthalmology, nutrition, dermatology, and cancer.*

Olson JA: Vitamin A. *In* Olson RE (ed.): Present Knowledge in Nutrition. 5th ed. Washington DC, The Nutrition Foundation, 1984, pp 176–191. *Recent review of physiology, binding proteins, metabolism, and function of vitamin A.*

Olson JA, Bridges CDB, Packer L, Chytil F, Wolf G: The function of vitamin A. Fed Proc 42:2740, 1983. *Succinct review of biochemical functions of vitamin A in the retina, in differentiation, and at nuclear and extranuclear sites.*

Sporn MB, Roberts AB: The role of retinoids in differentiation and carcinogenesis. Cancer Res 43:3134, 1983. *Discussion of the recent application of vitamin A and its related compounds to the chemoprevention of certain forms of cancer.*

VITAMIN D

Vitamin D is discussed in Chapter 244 in association with calcium metabolism and metabolic bone diseases.

VITAMIN E

Vitamin E activity is derived from a series of dietary tocopherols and tocotrienols, the most potent of which is d-α-tocopherol. This vitamin serves as an antioxidant, protecting polyunsaturated fatty acids in membranes and possibly also in tissues from attack by free radicals. Vitamin E deficiency in animals increases the likelihood of membrane and cellular damage from ozone, nitrogen dioxide, and hyperbaric oxygen. Dietary selenium is a precursor of selenide, a cofactor for glutathione peroxidase, which also provides important protection against lipid peroxidation in vivo. Dietary selenium under certain circumstances may spare the requirement for vitamin E.

Intestinal absorption of tocopherols requires normal mechanisms of digestion and absorption of fat, particularly bile formation. Tocopherols are transported to the general circulation in chylomicra. Levels of tocopherols in blood correlate with those of plasma lipoproteins to which they are bound both normally and in various disease states. In contrast to vitamin A, there does not appear to be a specific carrier protein in blood for vitamin E, nor a specific organ in which it is stored. Since dietary deficiency occurs only under very unusual circumstances, cases of E deficiency have usually been identified with prolonged and severe fat malabsorption. Vitamin E deficiency has also been detected in patients receiving parenteral nutrition.

The dietary allowance for vitamin E is expressed in terms of mg α-tocopherol equivalents (α-TE), and is 10 mg per day (15 IU) for adult males and 8 mg per day (12 IU) for adult females, with increases of 2 mg per day for pregnancy and 3 mg per day for lactation. The increased requirement for vitamin E with diets high in polyunsaturated fatty acids, previously shown in experimental animals, is thought not to be clinically relevant, since the items highest in vitamin E content—soybean, corn, cottonseed, wheat germ, and safflower oils and their derivatives—are also high in polyunsaturated fatty acids.

Deficiency of vitamin E has generally not been recognized as a clearly definable syndrome. The red cell half-life may be shortened, although anemia is uncommon in the absence of other precipitating causes. Clinical and neuropathologic evidence of posterior column abnormalities have been described, with disturbances of gait, proprioception, and vibration. In premature infants, vitamin E deficiency is associated with hemolytic anemia, thrombocytosis, and edema. Diagnosis of vitamin E deficiency is usually made by measurement of plasma E levels; normal levels are generally 0.50 to 0.70 mg per deciliter and higher. In several of the hemolytic anemias, such as sickle cell anemia and G-6-PD deficiency, serum vitamin E levels tend to be low.

The therapeutic role of vitamin E remains controversial at the present time. Although vitamin E has been advocated by food faddists as an "anti-aging" vitamin, there is no evidence that it prolongs life in man. This vitamin has been claimed to enhance sexual performance, an attribute that also has not been substantiated. Some patients with intermittent claudication appear to have improved after therapy with vitamin E. Hemolytic anemia in the premature newborn is generally benefited by vitamin E therapy, and the severity but not the incidence of retrolental fibroplasia may be reduced. Large doses may prevent the neurologic complications from developing in abetalipoproteinemia and cholestatic liver disease.

There are a number of other effects of vitamin E demonstrable, in vitro, in experimental animals and in some instances in man, but their clinical relevance remains unresolved. These effects include reducing platelet aggregation, inhibiting conversion of nitrites to nitrosoamines, inhibiting prostaglandin synthesis, improving erythrocyte formation, and protecting against environmental toxicants and pollutants. Further research is needed on these important issues.

Vitamin E is certainly far less toxic than the other fat-soluble vitamins, and a daily intake in the range of 200 to 600 mg per day (20 to 60 times the RDA) is generally considered safe. Nausea, flatulence, and diarrhea have been reported at doses in excess of 600 mg. The intestinal absorption of vitamins A and K is reduced at high doses, which may be clinically significant in patients on marginal diets. Vitamin E appears to increase the vitamin K requirement, and megadoses of vitamin E administered together with the anticoagulant drug warfarin may result in overt bleeding.

Bieri JG, Corash L, Hubbard VS: Medical uses of vitamin E. N Engl J Med 308:1063, 1983. *This article reviews the rationale for treatment with vitamin E in various clinical disorders, limitations of treatment, and toxicities encountered.*

Horwitt MK: Therapeutic uses of vitamin E in medicine. Nutr Rev 38:105, 1980. *Current status of the medical uses of vitamin E.*

Lubin B, Macklin LJ (eds.): Vitamin E: Biochemical, Hematological and Clinical Aspects. New York, New York Academy of Sciences, 1982. *This volume covers the proceedings of a conference dealing with cellular biochemistry, relation to human diseases, deficiencies and therapeutic doses of vitamin E.*

VITAMIN K

Vitamin K occurs naturally in two forms, both of which are naphthoquinone derivatives, differing from one another only in their side chains. Vitamin K_1 is made by plant sources: vitamin K_2 is synthesized by normal intestinal flora. It is also contained in some foods. Vitamin K_3 (menadione) is an artificial provitamin that can be converted to menoquinone (K_2) by the liver.

The intestinal absorption of various forms of vitamin K resembles that of vitamin E in requiring bile and other normal mechanisms of fat absorption. There are differences in the absorption of vitamin K_1 and vitamin K_2: vitamin K_1 is absorbed principally in the proximal segment via a saturable energy-dependent process, whereas vitamin K_2 is absorbed by the small intestine and by the colon via a noncarrier-mediated, nonenergy-dependent process. The efficiency of absorption varies greatly and is markedly diminished by mineral oil, other fat solvents, and laxatives. In patients who have fat malabsorption that is severe and prolonged, as in sprue, regional ileitis, and other disorders, or in patients with obstruction to bile flow, vitamin K deficiency commonly develops. Deficiency also may occur after prolonged antibiotic therapy, destroying the intestinal synthesis of vitamin K.

After absorption, vitamin K is transported in plasma chylomicrons. The main excretory products of vitamin K in urine are derivatives that have undergone chain shortening and oxidation.

Vitamin K deficiency occurs frequently in newborn infants for several reasons. First, fetal stores tend to be low because very little of this vitamin is transported across the placenta. In addition, the fetal gut is sterile, and therefore the newborn lacks the supply of vitamin K that can be provided by normal intestinal flora. As the intestinal tract becomes colonized postnatally, the synthesis of vitamin K becomes appreciable.

The best sources of vitamin K are green, leafy vegetables, particularly turnip greens, broccoli, and brussels sprouts. There are moderate amounts in liver, bacon, cheese, butter, and coffee. No single recommended dietary allowance is made for vitamin K because of the important and variable contribution made by intestinal bacteria. It is recommended only that normal adults consume 70 to 140 μg per day. Dietary deficiency based upon consuming less than this amount is uncommon at the present time in the United States, because the usual diet contains ample amounts of vitamin K.

The mechanism of action of vitamin K consists of a post-translational γ-carboxylation of glutamic acid moieties in inactive precursor proteins, which confers calcium-binding properties to the proteins. The most widely known of these proteins are involved in blood coagulation. Four clotting factors are dependent upon vitamin K for this important action: prothrombin (factor II), proconvertin (factor VII), Christmas factor (factor IX), and Stuart-Prower factor (factor X). Lack of vitamin K may result in death from uncontrolled hemorrhage.

The anticoagulant drugs, warfarin and dicoumarol, inhibit the vitamin K-dependent γ-carboxylation by interfering with activation of vitamin K to its metabolically active hydroquinone form. As a result of this inhibition, the synthesis of the four clotting factors is greatly reduced.

A recent advance in the field of vitamin K research has been the identification of proteins that are involved in the mineralization of bone (osteocalcin) and possibly also in calcium resorption from the renal tubule. The vitamin K antagonists, warfarin and dicoumarol, cause a marked decrease in formation of osteocalcin, presumably by interfering with γ-carboxylation.

Vitamin K deficiency responds rapidly to the administration of vitamin K, provided that liver function is normal. A number of preparations of vitamin K are available, some of which are water soluble, for example, menadiol sodium diphosphate. These forms are more toxic than the lipid-soluble phylloquinone form. In patients with advanced liver disease, the serum prothrombin is decreased and responds poorly if at all to administration of vitamin K. Patients with low serum prothrombin caused by vitamin K deficiency can be distinguished from those with low prothrombin caused by liver disease because in vitamin K deficiency the prothrombin precursor in blood is not γ-carboxylated; normally γ-carboxylated prothrombin is found in patients with liver disease.

Olson RE: Vitamin K. *In* Goodhart RS, Shils ME (eds.): Modern Nutrition in Health and Disease. 6th ed. Philadelphia, Lea & Febiger, 1980, pp 170–180. *Thorough discussion of nutritional aspects of vitamin K, with emphasis upon biochemical mechanisms.*

Suttie JW: Current concepts of the mechanism of action of vitamin K and its antagonists. *In* Lindenbaum J (ed.): Nutrition in Hematology. Contemporary Issues in Clinical Nutrition. Vol. 5. New York, Churchill Livingstone, 1983, pp 245–270. *Discussion of the basic biochemistry of vitamin K and its relation to clotting factors.*

Suttie JW: Vitamin K Metabolism and Vitamin K-Dependent Proteins. Baltimore, University Park Press, 1980. *Comprehensive volume dealing with biochemical, nutritional, and functional aspects of vitamin K.*

218. DISTURBANCES OF TRACE MINERAL METABOLISM

Clifford Tasman-Jones

The bulk of living matter is formed by eleven elements, all of which are from the lowest part of the periodic table (H, C, N, O, Na, Mg, P, S, Cl, K, and Ca). In addition to these, there are essential minerals that are present in trace amounts. These latter include F, Si, V, Cr, Mn, Fe, Co, Ni, Cu, Zn, Se, Mo, Sn, and I.

While deficiencies of trace minerals and vitamins are uncommon in humans eating a normal diet, there is a likelihood of trace mineral deficiencies developing with the use of enteral and parenteral feeding. Deficiencies developing during parenteral nutrition have focused attention on trace mineral function in human metabolism.

Trace minerals essential for life act as essential cofactors of enzymes and as organizers of the molecular structures of the cell (e.g., mitochondria) and its cellular membrane. There is an optimal tissue concentration for trace minerals; excess can be toxic and insufficiency leads to metabolic failure.

Trace minerals are absorbed through the intestine; their bioavailability is dependent on the processing that occurs within the intestinal mucosa. In plasma, trace minerals are bound either to a specific protein or to albumin for transportation. There may be a small amount of unbound trace mineral. The excretory path varies but most are excreted into the gastrointestinal tract, many by way of bile; some are excreted in the urine and some by the sweat glands. Not all trace minerals have been shown to be clinically important. Some, such as iron and iodine, are so important in specific disorders that they are covered separately in this volume.

ZINC

METABOLISM. Although zinc represents only 0.003 per cent (1.4 to 2.3 grams) of the human body, it is an intrinsic part of at least 70 metalloenzymes and other cellular components and is essential for the synthesis of protein, DNA, and RNA.

Zinc is absorbed from the small intestine, although the exact mechanism for this remains uncertain. A low-molecular-weight zinc-binding ligand possibly secreted from the pancreas is a postulated mechanism for absorption.

In the human body, zinc has a nonuniform distribution with the highest concentrations occurring in the prostate, the skin and its appendages, the brain choroid, the liver, the pancreas, bone, and blood. In blood approximately 80 per cent of zinc is in erythrocytes, 16 per cent in plasma, 3 per cent in leukocytes, and the remaining 1 per cent in platelets. Plasma zinc is normally 12 to 20 μmol per liter, but this amount may not truly reflect tissue store. Zinc is excreted mainly in the feces, but small amounts (between 4.0 and 12.0 μmol per 24 hours) are secreted in the urine.

DEFICIENCY SYNDROMES. In man zinc deficiency has been described in a chronic form and in an acute form. In Iran and Egypt hypogonadal dwarfism in males is associated with zinc deficiency and a deficiency of dietary protein. Additionally, these children usually eat clay, which may bind zinc, making it unavailable for absorption.

Acrodermatitis enterohepatica, a rare autosomal recessive inherited disorder of zinc metabolism, represents a chronic form of pure zinc deficiency. This entity is characterized by diarrhea; an unpleasant skin rash of the extremities, face, and perineum; alopecia; mental irritability; muscle wasting; and depression. Although the nature of the disease remains in doubt, it may be caused by an absence of the ligand essential for zinc absorption. This ligand is present in human milk but not in cow's milk.

Acute zinc deficiency has been described in patients receiving parenteral nutrition. This syndrome is characterized by diarrhea; disturbance of the central nervous system with mental irritability and depression; skin lesions of the face, perineum, limbs, and skin folds; alopecia; loss of taste; and defects in the immunologic mechanisms. Treatment with zinc supplementation, usually in the form of zinc sulfate, results in a dramatic response.

Zinc deficiency may occur in inflammatory bowel disease, malabsorption, cirrhosis, and high alcohol intake, probably because of an increased excretion of zinc in the urine. In Crohn's disease, when there is severe catabolism, zincuria may be severe, depleting body stores that are needed during anabolism. Although the alcoholic has increased zinc loss, there appears to be increased absorption to compensate.

Zinc taken in excess may cause gastrointestinal upset with nausea and vomiting.

COPPER

METABOLISM. An average healthy adult has 12.6 to 18 mmol of body copper. Copper is absorbed from the stomach and proximal duodenum by complexing with amino acids. In the presence of excess intraluminal micronutrients such as zinc or cadmium, copper absorption may be reduced. Absorbed copper is bound to albumin, and after circulating through the liver, it is complexed to ceruloplasmin for distribution to body tissues. The plasma concentration of copper is 13 to 22 μmol per liter, 90 per cent of which is bound to ceruloplasmin. Plasma copper may not adequately reflect copper stores but rather reflect plasma ceruloplasmin concentrations.

The best known function of copper is its effect on erythropoiesis. It is essential for hemoglobin formation. There are many copper enzymes known. Copper is necessary for collagen formation, the functioning of the central nervous system, and skin pigmentation.

Usually copper is excreted in the bile as a form of metallocomplex. There is an additional copper loss in the urine (0.16 to 0.95 μmol per day) and saliva (0.006 to 0.008 μmol per day).

The highest concentrations of copper occur in the liver, brain, heart, spleen, kidneys, and blood. The mean daily requirement of copper is estimated to be between 5 and 15 μmol when given intravenously and between 30 and 40 μmol when given orally.

DEFICIENCY SYNDROMES. Hypocupremia occurs in a number of inherited disorders such as Wilson's disease (a disease of copper excess), Menkes' kinky hair syndrome, a syndrome of neurologic disorder with hypocupremia, and familial hypoceruloplasminemia. It may also be found with decreased copper intake, as in parenteral nutrition, or with the poor absorption or increased loss associated with protein-losing enteropathy, the nephrotic syndrome, cystic fibrosis, and other malabsorptive disorders such as coeliac disease and sprue.

Menkes' kinky hair disease is a rare X-linked genetic disorder in which there is defective connective tissue formation, gross mental retardation, imperfect keratinization of the skin, and depigmentation of the hair. Serum copper and ceruloplasmin levels are very low and return to normal when parenteral but not when oral copper is given. This therapy has no demonstrated benefit in the disease, however.

Chronic copper deficiency causes anemia, usually of a microcytic type, but sometimes it is associated with megaloblastic changes in the marrow, leukopenia, and neutropenia.

EXCESS. Hypercupremia occurs in response to inflammation and has been described in rheumatoid arthritis. The rise in copper is most probably caused by the rise in ceruloplasmin—an acute-phase reactant protein. Copper in excess may produce nausea, vomiting, myalgia, and hemolysis. *Wilson's disease,* the most important human disorder of excess copper, is described in detail in Ch. 205.

MANGANESE

METABOLISM. Manganese, a trace element essential for life, is present in an amount of approximately 12 to 20 mg in the average adult. Maximally absorbed in the duodenum by an unknown transport mechanism, magnesium is bound to transmanganin, a specific β_1 globulin transport protein. Manganese is concentrated in tissues rich in mitochondria and is widely distributed in the body with maximum concentrations in the brain, kidneys, pancreas, and liver. The blood and serum levels vary widely. Excretion of manganese is principally by the bile.

Manganese is an activator of many enzymes, but only one manganese metalloenzyme is known—pyruvate carboxylase. It appears to be intimately involved in the synthesis of DNA, RNA, and protein.

DEFICIENCY. The syndrome associated with deficiency of manganese includes the following features: impaired growth, skeletal abnormalities, abnormal reproductive function, ataxia, convulsions, and anomalies of fat metabolism. In the best described patient with manganese deficiency there were weight loss, a transient dermatitis, nausea and vomiting with changes in the color and growth of hair, and hypocholesterolemia.

EXCESS. Manganese poisoning, which usually occurs after industrial exposure, induces a syndrome that closely resembles Parkinson's disease.

CHROMIUM

METABOLISM. Chromium is an essential micronutrient required for the maintenance of normal blood glucose levels. The recommended daily intake is 50 to 200 μg, and the normal serum level is 0.5 to 9.0 μg per liter. Chromium is present in yeast, meat, and grain. Chromium complexes with nicotinamide to form the glucose tolerance factor. This factor acts as a facilitator for insulin to react at receptor sites on insulin-sensitive tissues.

DEFICIENCY. Chromium deficiency is characterized by impaired glucose tolerance, encephalopathy, and neuropathy. Because of impaired insulin activity, patients may develop hyperglycemia with hyperosmolar nonketotic coma. Chromium deficiency may give a confusional state similar to hepatic encephalopathy with ataxia and peripheral neuropathy. A suggested association between chromium deficiency and coronary artery disease awaits confirmation.

EXCESS. If too much chromium is given, symptoms of nausea, vomiting, gastrointestinal ulceration, liver damage, kidney damage, and central nervous system abnormalities with convulsions may occur.

SELENIUM

METABOLISM. Selenium has a significant biological role believed to be due to selenocysteine in the enzyme glutathionine peroxidase. This enzyme is important in protecting the lipids of the cell membrane, proteins, and nucleic acids against oxidant damage. There are significant regional differences in serum selenium concentrations in the United States, but the mean level is about 0.135 μg per milliliter. A low blood selenium concentration reflecting a low soil content has been noted in three areas: Finland, China, and New Zealand.

The daily requirement for selenium is not known. It is probably dependent on the supply of other trace minerals, including zinc, copper, magnesium, and iron and also the supply of other antioxidant substances, such as vitamin E and vitamin C. In the United States the intake is above 150 μg per day.

DEFICIENCY. *Keshan disease* is a syndrome of endemic cardiomyopathy in the People's Republic of China which is alleviated by giving oral sodium selenite. In the areas of China where Keshan disease is prevalent the dietary intake is estimated at approximately 11 μg per day. A New Zealand woman on intravenous feeding developed muscle pains and tenderness and a very low blood selenium level. The symptoms were alleviated by giving selomethionine. In Finland a reduced serum selenium concentration has been shown to correlate with cardiovascular death and acute coronary heart disease. In a prospective study the selenium level in the serum of those patients who subsequently developed malignancy was found to be significantly lower than that of controls.

EXCESS. Excess selenium is a cell toxin, and as such, selenium should be given with considerable care.

MAGNESIUM

METABOLISM. The amount of magnesium in the human body is about 1000 mmol of which about 50 per cent is contained in the skeleton and only 1 per cent is extracellular. Intracellular magnesium is the second most common cation in the human body, but the serum levels justify its inclusion in a section on trace minerals.

The recommended intake is about 15 mmol, and this comes largely from green vegetables, meat, and fish. Magnesium is absorbed in the entire small bowel but mainly from the distal part of the ileum.

Magnesium is an essential part of some 300 different enzymes and is necessary for cell membrane permeability; neuromuscular excitability; protein, nucleic acid, and fat synthesis; muscle contraction, and so on. While there is no laboratory test which unequivocally reveals magnesium deficiency, the serum magnesium level is not without value. Normal values for serum magnesium are 0.8 to 1.0 mmol per liter. Magnesium deficiency is often present without low serum magnesium levels. Urinary magnesium analysis may be of some value and is usually 3 to 5 mmol per day.

Disorders of magnesium metabolism are described in detail in Ch. 208.

VANADIUM

Analysis of vanadium is difficult. The total body vanadium is about 100 μg. Blood levels are very low and are between 0.005 and 8.4 μmol per liter.

Vanadium depresses plasma cholesterol levels, Na^+/K^+ ATPase, myosin, Ca^{++} ATPase, adenylate kinase, and phosphofructokinase, and it stimulates adenyl cyclase. Vanadium deficiency has been postulated to play a role in nutritional edema, and vanadium excess has been postulated to be a factor in manic-depressive illness. Neither of these suggestions has been confirmed.

COBALT

Cobalt in human metabolism is related to vitamin B_{12}, a topic which is covered in Ch. 135 on pernicious anemia.

NICKEL

For a long time nickel was not believed to have any biologic function. Recently, it has been shown to be a component of urease in plant cells and to be present in some bacterial hydrogenases. Its importance in normal human metabolism is not yet established.

Its importance in human medicine relates to the contact dermatitis that frequently has been associated with it.

SILICON

Silicon is found in high concentrations in tendons, aorta, and eye tissues. It is necessary for mammalian bone growth and calcification. In experimental animals, silicon appears to inhibit atheroma development. Chronic inhalation of silicon as silica (SiO_2) produces lung disease, as described in Ch. 559.

Burch RE, Sullivan JE: Symposium on trace metals. Med Clin North Am 60:653, 1976. *A general review of trace mineral metabolism in the human.*

Chan X, Yang G, Chen J, Chen X, Wen Z, Go K: Studies on the relations of selenium and Keshan Disease. Biol Trace Element Res 2:91, 1980. *An interesting study relating selenium deficiency as a major factor in a specific form of cardiomyopathy.*

Jeejeebhoy KN, Chu RC, Marliss et al.: Chromium deficiency, glucose intolerance and neuropathy reversed by chromium supplementation in a patient receiving long term total parenteral nutrition. Am J Clin Nutr 30:531, 1977. *Parenteral nutrition afforded the opportunity to identify the important role of chromium in glucose metabolism.*

Mills PR, Fell GS, Bessent TG, et al.: A study of zinc metabolism in alcoholic cirrhosis. Clin Sci 64:527, 1983. *A careful study indicating the nature of altered zinc metabolism in alcoholic liver disease.*

Salonca JT, Alfthan G, Nuttunen JK, et al: Association between cardiovascular death and myocardial infarction and serum selenium in a match-pair longitudinal study. Lancet 2:175, 1982. *Selenium deficiency appears to be one correlate with myocardial infarction in Finland.*

Tasman-Jones C: Zinc deficiency states. Adv Intern Med 26:97, 1980. *A review of zinc deficiency with particular emphasis on the acute zinc deficiency syndrome.*

Ulmer DD: Trace Elements. N Engl J Med 297:318, 1977. *A general review of the major trace minerals.*

Williams DM: Copper deficiency in humans. Semin Hematol 20:118, 1983. *Major features of normal copper metabolism and copper deficiency are summarized in a very readable form.*

219. ENTERAL NUTRITIONAL THERAPY

David H. Alpers

Enteral nutrition therapy implies modification of the usual diet and is used for two major general indications. The first is supplementation of protein and calories in a wide variety of situations with the intention of providing part or all of the daily requirements. This use is not disease-specific. The second and more traditional indication involves the use of diets for specific diseases or pathophysiologic situations. The diets used involve restricting a particular element of the diet (e.g., fat, lactose), adding a nutrient that may be required in larger amounts than are available from a well-balanced diet (e.g., calcium, potassium), or altering the consistency of the diet (e.g., high-fiber, full-liquid). These two major indications will be discussed in this chapter. Also included is a discussion about formulating a plan for calorie and protein supplementation, which will place this and the following chapter on parenteral nutrition in proper perspective.

PROTEIN AND CALORIE SUPPLEMENTATION

Initial Decisions: Completeness of Nutrient Provision and Route of Administration

The range of methods for providing protein and calorie supplements has expanded greatly beyond table foods in recent years, and likewise the range of available products for this use is very great. For many patients all that may be needed is a careful history of dietary intake, estimation of protein and caloric requirements, and adjustment of the diet to provide the needed nutrients. Whether table foods or commercial supplements are used, there are two major considerations for the physician in order to provide the most appropriate therapy for each patient: (1) Is the supplement intended as a partial fulfillment of daily needs (incomplete provision) or a total replacement of calories and protein (complete provision)? (2) Are the nutrients to be delivered by the enteral or the parenteral route? Table 219–1 summarizes these major choices. Forced enteral feeding refers to the delivery of nutrients to the small intestine via a small (7 to 8 French) polyurethane or silicone catheter (e.g., Dobbhoff, Duo-tube, Keofeed or by a surgically placed feeding tube). Parenteral supplementation by peripheral or central vein will be discussed in Ch. 220. The options listed in Table 219–1 are not mutally exclusive. For example, sometimes forced enteral feeding can be used together with peripheral vein feeding; nutritionally complete commercial supplements can be used orally in some patients to supply total macronutrient requirements; central vein feeding can be supplemented by oral intake. The choices made in formulating a support plan will depend upon a number of considerations as discussed in the following paragraph.

Formulating a Protein-Calorie Support Plan

Figure 219–1 illustrates a flow diagram useful for selecting patients in negative protein and calorie balance for intensive nutritional support. The correct choice for nutritional support (enteral vs. parenteral, oral vs. forced enteral) depends largely upon the four key questions outlined in the figure. The physician should estimate protein and caloric requirements for the individual patient. Methods for making these estimates are available in a number of handbooks. While the estimates are fairly crude, they are clinically useful, since they provide some quantitative guidelines for deciding the magnitude of supplementation needed. If the diet is meeting requirements (question 1), no further therapy is needed. If the diet is inadequate, an assessment of the patient's present nutritional status is then obtained. Caloric reserves are monitored most easily by body weight and protein reserves by serum albumin levels. Other available methods are discussed in Chapter 213. If the degree of depletion (question 2) as assessed by body weight is mild (about 5 per cent decreased) and the gastrointestinal tract is intact, oral supplements may be used. If the degree of depletion is moderate (5 to 10 per cent decreased) to severe (over 10 per cent decreased) and the anticipated duration of support is long (question 3), intensive therapy may be needed. Whether forced enteral feeding or total parenteral nutrition (TPN) via a central vein is chosen depends on the availability or adequacy of the gastrointestinal tract (question 4). The gastrointestinal tract is usually evaluated by history (the presence or absence of diarrhea or malabsorption), physical exam (normal motility or ileus), and barium radiographs. Some patients are selected for TPN because of the need for complete bowel rest. Data to support the use of this therapy have been obtained in Crohn's disease, ulcerative colitis, the postoperative adaptive period of

TABLE 219–1. STRATEGY FOR CALORIC AND PROTEIN SUPPLEMENTATION

Route of Delivery	Incomplete Provision	Complete Provision
Enteral	Oral supplementation Table foods e.g., milk, peanut butter, egg Commercial supplements Individual macronutrients (e.g., protein, fat, carbohydrate) Nutritionally complete supplement	Forced enteral feeding Nutritionally complete commercial diets Blenderized formulas
Parenteral	Peripheral (e.g., 3 per cent amino acids, 5 to 10 per cent dextrose, 10 per cent lipid emulsion)	Central (e.g., 4.25 per cent amino acid, 25 per cent dextrose, vitamins, minerals, fatty acids)

the short bowel syndrome, and severe pancreatitis (see Ch. 200). Some patients with these disorders can be treated with forced enteral feeding. Often, however, bowel rest will control symptoms more rapidly. Other considerations (social, economic) may play a role in the final choice of therapy for a given patient. The patient may be unwilling to maintain a nasal feeding tube, or hospitalization may not be possible because of cost restrictions. Finally, an occasional patient may need to be fed via gastrostomy or jejunostomy.

The following categories of patients are commonly considered for enteral nutrition therapy: (1) chronically ill patients with anorexia, (2) patients with chronic inflammatory illnesses who have increased requirements but a usual caloric intake for their size, (3) poorly or marginally nourished patients preparing for tests or intestinal surgery, and (4) patients with specific dietary needs that benefit from the special characteristics of some commercial supplements (e.g., low residue, lactose-free). Forced enteral feeding typically is used for those patients who have moderate to severe anorexia, those who cannot maintain a calorie and protein intake commensurate with their needs (e.g., burn patients), or those whose illnesses prevent them from satisfactory oral feeding (e.g., patients with neck fractures or swallowing disorders).

Choice of Supplements

Table Foods

If requirements are not great and appetite is good, table foods can be recommended as protein and calorie supplements. Each ounce of meat, fish, poultry, or cheese contains about 7 grams of protein, an egg 6 to 7 grams and one cup of milk 8 grams. One-half cup of dried beans, peas, or nuts contains 5 grams or more of protein, but these sources contain protein of a lower biologic value (sustains growth less well) and are not usually recommended for "catch up" therapy. Milk products are very useful, provided that lactose intolerance is not a problem. Meat and fish are helpful if fat is well tolerated. Otherwise, poultry without skin or tuna canned in water should be selected. Peanut butter contains 8 grams of fat and 4.2 grams of protein per tablespoon and is a good source of concentrated calories and protein. Table foods remain an excellent choice for oral supplementation, since they are tasty, esthetically and socially appealing, reasonable in cost, easily obtained, and

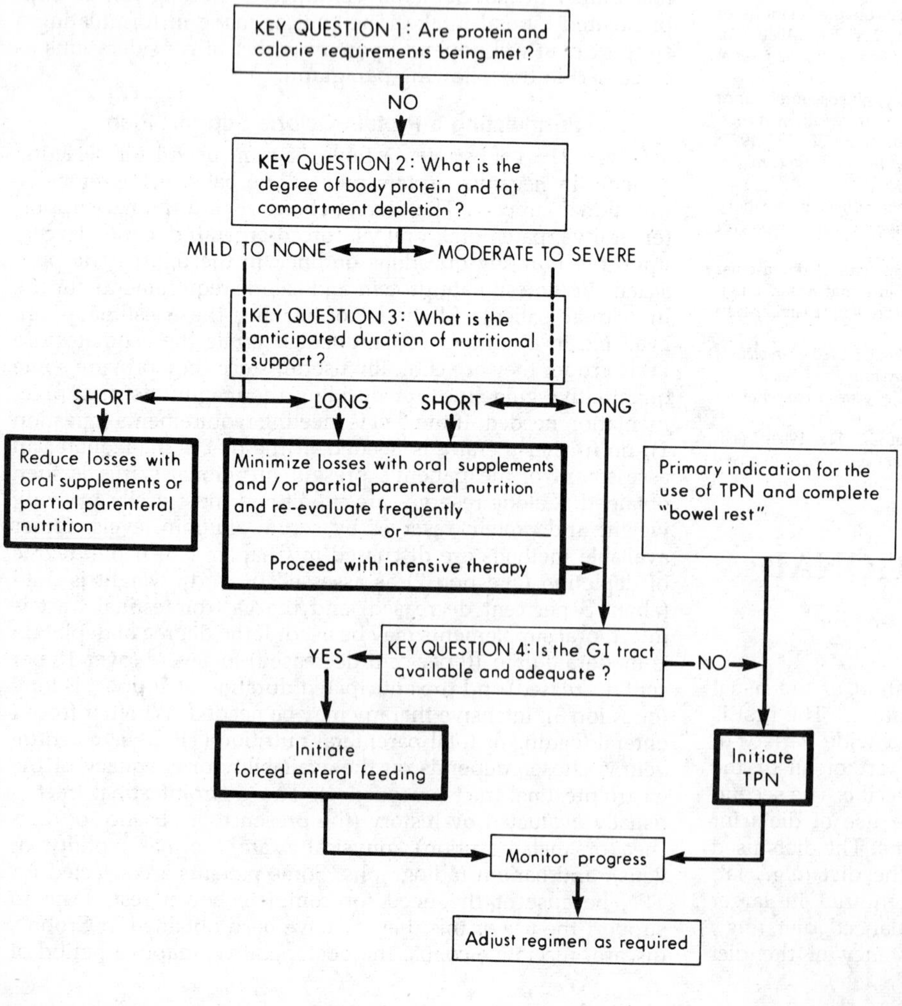

Figure 219–1. Flow diagram useful for selecting patients in negative protein and calorie balance for intensive nutritional support. TPN = total parenteral nutrition; GI = gastrointestinal.

available in a wide variety of choices. They should not be supplemented by commercial supplements unless the supplements exhibit specific properties that make them preferable.

Commercial Supplements

Commerical supplements, like table foods, display a diversity of characteristics that help the physician determine the choice for each patient (Table 219–2). These products are of high caloric density and precisely defined nutrient composition but have the disadvantages of limited esthetic and taste appeal, taste fatigue with constant use, frequent occurrence of diarrhea, and higher cost than table foods. The nutritionally incomplete supplements can be used when the deficiency is specific (protein or calorie) or the deficiency is only anticipated for a short time, as in preparation for surgery. Protein is not wisely provided without another source of calories, since about 25 to 40 nonprotein kcal per gram of protein are needed to maintain positive nitrogen balance. Otherwise, a portion of the amino acids in the protein is converted to carbohydrate to provide the energy needed for assimilation.

The nutritionally complete supplements are largely distinguished by four major characteristics: (1) the presence or absence of lactose, (2) the use of intact protein or hydrolyzed protein (or amino acids), (3) the presence of small or large amounts of fat as caloric sources, and (4) isotonic or hypertonic osmolality. Supplements that are isotonic or nearly so contain less available carbohydrate and more lipid, which is osmotically less active. This characteristic is of greatest importance when forced enteral feeding is used, but any of the hypertonic solutions may be diluted or infused at a slower rate. The other three characteristics are more important for patients with abnormal intestinal absorption. Hydrolyzed protein may be useful for patients with pancreatic insufficiency, lactose-free supplements for patients with lactose intolerance, and low-fat supplements for those with limited intestinal fat absorption. The nutritionally complete supplements just described are designed to be the sole source of daily nutrients and thus contain all needed micronutrients in adequate quantities, if deficiencies are not present and if requirements are usual. Nonprescription milk-based products also provide good sources of protein and calories in a wide variety of flavors (e.g., Metrical, Sego, and Carnation Instant Breakfast). If the patient is lactose tolerant, they may be used very successfully.

COMPLICATIONS OF ENTERAL FEEDING USING COMMERCIAL SUPPLEMENTS. The use of enteral feeding with highly concentrated supplements can be limited by side effects. The most common is diarrhea, which can be due to intolerance to one of the macronutrients (fat, lactose) or intolerance to the osmotic load. Altering the rate of delivery or the concentration of the supplement is often helpful. Complications of forced enteral feeding alone include esophagitis and tracheobronchial aspiration. Volume or sodium overload can occur, especially in the edema-prone patient.

TABLE 219–2. GENERAL CLASSIFICATION OF COMMERCIALLY AVAILABLE SUPPLEMENTS

Classification	Examples
Macronutrient specific	
Protein	Gevral, Casec
Carbohydrate	Polycose, Hy-Cal
Lipid	Lipomul-Oral, Microlipid
Protein + carbohydrate	Citrotein
Nutritionally complete	
Intact protein	
Not fat restricted	Meritene, Ensure, Precision Isotonic
Low fat (≤ 15 grams fat/1000 kcal)	Precision LR, Sustagen
Hydrolyzed protein or amino acids	Vivonex Standard, Vital
Lactose free	Most products
Isotonic	Isocal, Precision Isotonic

THERAPEUTIC DIETS FOR SPECIFIC DISORDERS OR PATHOPHYSIOLOGIC STATES

Restrictive Diets

The diets most commonly used to control symptoms are those that restrict one or another element in the diet. Diets restricted for each of the major macronutrients (fat, carbohydrate, and protein) have their individual uses (Table 219–3). As expected, these diets are helpful in altering pathophysiologic states and are not specific for any disease. Any condition causing steatorrhea can be improved symptomatically by limiting fat intake. Care must be taken with any restrictive diet to supplement any nutrients that have been secondarily limited. Thus, a fat-restricted diet must be made isocaloric by increasing carbohydrate intake. In order for this diet to be successful the patient must not have any generalized carbohydrate intolerance. Similarly, the low lactose or low available carbohydrate diet is low in calcium. Most restrictive diets do not eliminate the nutrient whose content is altered. A low-lactose diet is much easier to achieve than a truly lactose-free one and is usually sufficient to relieve symptoms. Control of symptoms is the usual goal of dietary management, and restriction of the appropriate nutrient to the point at which symptoms are altered is an acceptable goal. Thus, a low-protein diet for hepatic encephalopathy should still deliver the estimated daily protein requirement (0.5 to 0.8 gram per kilogram of body weight) to avoid protein deficiency. This concept is especially important in the management of chronic renal failure, a situation in which the protein requirement may be actually increased. When the glomerular filtration rate (GFR) falls below 25 ml per minute, the protein allowance should be not more than 1.3 grams per kilogram per day (referring to ideal body weight), and falls to 0.6 gram per kilogram per day for a GFR of 4 to 10 ml per minute. Over 50 per cent of the protein intake should be of high biologic value (with high essential amino acid content). Requirements actually increase with dialysis because of the loss of amino acids in the dialysate. The allowance rises with hemodialysis to 1 gram per kilogram per day, and to 1.2 to 1.5 grams per kilogram per day with chronic peritoneal dialysis.

Some of the diets used for therapy actually control or modify the content of macronutrients rather than restrict them. The diet for diabetes mellitus is a good example of this principle (Ch. 230). Successful management of the obese diabetic combines a weight reduction diet with regulation of the carbohydrate content. The prudent diet recommended by the American Diabetes Association still contains 40 to 50 per cent of calories as carbohydrates, but there is much less simple sugar (requiring no pancreatic digestion) and more starch than in normal diets. There is also less cholesterol and saturated fats to reduce blood lipids. These latest recommendations contain relaxed restrictions on carbohydrate intake. High starch diets are well tolerated by diabetics as long as total caloric intake is controlled. Many patients require diets that may utilize elements from diets designed specifically for weight reduction, diabetes mellitus, hyperlipidemias, and chronic renal failure.

TABLE 219–3. THERAPEUTIC DIETS CHARACTERIZED BY RESTRICTION OF DIETARY COMPONENTS

Diet	Typical Indication
Low fat (60–75 grams/day)	Steatorrhea, mild
Low fat (40–60 grams/day)	Steatorrhea, severe
Low oxalate	Enteric hyperoxaluria
Low lactose	Lactose intolerance
Low available carbohydrate	Reactive hypoglycemia
Gluten free	Celiac sprue (see Ch. 103)
Low fiber	Acute diarrhea, bowel prep
Low protein	Hepatic encephalopathy (see Ch. 127) Chronic renal failure (see Ch. 78)
Elimination	Food allergies
Controlled carbohydrate	Diabetes mellitus (see Ch. 230)
Calorie restricted	Obesity
Low sodium	Edematous states
Low fat, cholesterol, or carbohydrate according to type	Hyperlipidemia (see Ch. 183)
Low copper	Wilson's disease
Low phosphate	Chronic renal failure (see Ch. 78)

TABLE 219–4. THERAPEUTIC DIETS CHARACTERIZED BY SUPPLEMENTATION OF DIETARY COMPONENTS

Diet	Typical Indication
High fiber	Irritable bowel, prevention of recurrent diverticulitis
High calcium (milk products, $CaCO_3$, or combination)	Postmenopausal osteoporosis
High protein (high biologic value)	Chronic hemo- or peritoneal dialysis
High protein	Malabsorption
Supplemental potassium	Diuretic use

Diets That Supplement Dietary Components

Although less commonly required, diets that add a component to the normal diet are often employed. A high fiber intake has not been clearly shown to have a beneficial effect on the symptoms of the irritable bowel syndrome and on the recurrence of attacks of acute diverticulitis, although supplementation with fiber is now commonly used for these disorders. The reasons for the uncertainty are that (1) these disorders are identified mostly by clinical criteria, (2) the irritable bowel syndrome is probably a heterogeneous group of motility disorders, (3) the definition of fiber and estimation of its intake are imperfectly developed, and (4) many types of fiber supplements are used, containing different components of dietary fiber. There are limited data on the food content of the major components of dietary fiber, i.e., cellulose, hemicelluloses, pectin, mucilage and gums, and lignins. Thus, it is not always clear when an individual patient is ingesting a low-fiber diet. Most often fiber is supplemented by ingestion of commercial preparations containing psyllium seed or by the use of bran. Psyllium is rich in hemicelluloses, while bran contains more cellulose. Present practice recommends the addition of 6 to 10 grams of fiber per day (2 teaspoons of psyllium seed or one-half cup of bran) for the irritable bowel syndrome (characterized by alternating diarrhea and constipation) and for recurrent diverticulitis. Benefits of high-fiber intake (type and amount variable) have been reported for diabetes mellitus, maintenance of lower calorie intake, and lowering of serum cholesterol. At present the data do not clearly support a role for a fiber-supplemented diet in any of these disorders.

A diet low in fiber (Table 219–3) is useful in acute diarrheal illness and as a preparation for barium enema, colonoscopy, and intestinal surgery. The diet is then additionally modified in the form of a clear liquid diet (Table 219–4) for further reduction in ileal residue.

The best treatment for postmenopausal osteoporosis is still debatable, but it is generally agreed that increased calcium intake is a necessary component of the treatment plan (Ch. 249). Milk products serve this role best, as they provide protein as well as calcium. In the patient who is lactose-intolerant or who does not like milk, calcium carbonate (40 per cent calcium by weight) may be used. If achlorhydria is present, a more water-soluble form of organic calcium (e.g., glubionate or gluconate) should be used, since the carbonate salt requires an acid pH to be solubilized.

Protein supplements are needed for conditions characterized by excessive protein loss, such as protein-losing enteropathy, dialysis, and burns. These supplements can be supplied as table food or as commercial supplements. For each 10 grams of protein added, another 250 kcal from nonprotein sources must also be ingested to ensure that the amino acids will be converted into body protein.

When diuretics and low-sodium diets are used, potassium is frequently replaced as an inorganic salt, but dietary supplementation can often be used and would be more palatable. For instance, the salt substitutes often used with low-sodium diets contain about 12 mEq of potassium per gram and potassium is present in fairly high concentration in most fruits and vegetables and their juices (Table 219–5). Eight ounces of frozen orange or tomato juice contains 12 mEq of potassium, one medium orange or banana 6 to 8 mEq, and one 6 × 2 inch watermelon slice 16 mEq. Milk is also a good source of potassium, but because of its high sodium content would be an inappropriate supplement for a patient taking diuretics.

Diets That Alter the Consistency of Food

One of the most common dietary manipulations used in hospitalized patients is the *liquid diet.* The clear liquid diet provides the daily requirement for water and requires minimal digestion and intestinal motility, but it does not provide adequate amounts of protein or calories. It is also a low-fiber diet. If the patient who requires such a diet is already protein and calorie malnourished, the diet needs to be supplemented with carbohydrate, protein, or both (see Table 219–2). Even so, it is difficult to provide much more than 1000 kcal per day. For chronic use the full liquid diet is more often prescribed. If table foods from all food groups are used or the diet is enriched with commercial supplements, the diet can be nutritionally complete. Care should be given to determining the actual food ingested, however, since a full liquid diet is often used for a patient who has some difficulty in swallowing table food. Thus, the ingested food may not equal what is ordered. This precaution of course should be exercised when any diet is used for therapy, but it is particularly important when impaired food ingestion or anorexia is the cause of the prescribed diet.

The *bland diet* is often combined with a mechanical soft diet for the treatment of peptic ulcer disease. Despite this widespread use, there are no data that clearly support the value of such a diet for any clinical condition, and present practice does not favor its use (Ch. 99). Restriction of seasonings makes the food less palatable and discourages the successful use of whichever diet is being presented.

Alpers DH, Clouse RE, Stenson WF: Manual of Nutritional Therapeutics. Boston, Little, Brown and Co, 1983. *A detailed practical account of the use of diets and enteral therapy. Includes nutritional characteristics of most commercial supplements and diets.*

American Dietetic Association: Handbook of Clinical Dietetics. New Haven, Yale University Press, 1982. *A comprehensive and carefully outlined source for obtaining the details of most diets.*

Connor WE, Connor SL: The dietary treatment of hyperlipidemias. Med Clin North Am 66:485–518, 1982. *A current summary of the use of diets in five types of hyperlipidemia.*

Friedman GR: Diet in treatment of diabetes mellitus. *In* Goodhart RS, Shils MR, (eds.): Modern Nutrition in Health and Disease. Philadelphia, Lea and Febiger, 1980, pp 977–997. *A good summary of the current dietary recommendations.*

Garrow JS: Treat Obesity Seriously. London, Churchill Livingstone, 1981. *A sensible and multifaceted approach to the therapy of obesity, especially the use of diet.*

Paige DM (ed.): Lactose Digestion. Baltimore, Johns Hopkins Unitersity Press, 1981. *An up-to-date symposium covering all aspects of lactose intolerance.*

Spiller GA, Kay RP (eds.): Medical Aspects of Dietary Fiber. New York, Plenum Press, 1980. *Summarizes the evidence for the role of dietary fiber in human disease.*

TABLE 219–5. SODIUM AND POTASSIUM CONTENT OF COMMON FOODS

Food	Portion	Sodium Content (mg)	Potassium Content (mg)
Milk	cup	120	350
Meat, fish, poultry	ounce	25	100–180
Most fruits and their juices	cup	4–10	300–490
Most vegetables	½ cup	5–9	300–500

220. PARENTERAL NUTRITION

Ray E. Clouse

Parenteral nutrition includes delivery of micro- and macronutrients. Those nutrients that can rapidly become depleted in disease, such as water and major minerals (e.g., sodium, potassium), are administered routinely by vein in the hospitalized patient. In the last decade the technical feasibility of providing nutrients that become depleted more slowly, such as amino acids, calorie sources, and the essential fatty acid linoleic acid, has resulted in the ability to deliver total parenteral nutritional support not only in the hospital but also at home. The most obvious long-term usefulness of these advances has been for patients who have irreversibly inadequate small bowel absorptive capabilities either from advanced disease (such as scleroderma) or because of intestinal resection (as from mesenteric infarction). The application of short-term total parenteral nutrition (TPN), however, far exceeds the use in this small number of patients. In fact, concern has been expressed regarding the possible excessive use of this technique in patients for whom some form of enteral therapy would suffice or for whom the expected nutritional losses from acute illness would be adequately tolerated without intensive support.

Parenteral delivery of protein and calories can serve either to partially meet the daily requirement (for instance in combination with an otherwise inadequate enteral plan) or to totally meet or exceed the requirements. Thus, parenteral nutrition can be utilized in much the same way as enteral supplements or forced enteral feeding when designing an appropriate nutritional support plan (Ch. 219). The technique of delivery and the morbidity (physical, psychological, financial) of such methods are more important considerations in the choice of parenteral or enteral nutrition routes than are differences in basic concepts of energy or specific nutrient requirements.

PARENTERAL ENERGY AND PROTEIN DELIVERY

Basic Considerations

Protein and calorie requirements are closely linked. Positive nitrogen balance, reflecting net positive endogenous protein synthesis, cannot be accomplished without positive energy balance. Thus, amino acids alone, even if provided in excessive quantities, will not be adequate to promote sustained net protein synthesis. Additional caloric sources in the form of carbohydrate or fat must be provided to prevent the use of amino acids (delivered or from catabolism) as energy substrates. If nonprotein calories are provided for the average hospitalized patient in a ratio of calories to amino acid nitrogen (in grams) of $\geq$ 150:1, delivered amino acids are likely to be utilized for protein synthesis. The ratio decreases in more intense catabolic states (e.g., major burns), in which protein requirements are higher, and increases in less stressed situations. This fact is not unique to parenteral nutrition; similar energy-to-nitrogen ratios apply to enteral nutrition techniques.

Protein balance can be approximated by measuring nitrogen losses in urine and other fluids and by estimating the relatively small fecal and skin losses. Achieving positive protein (nitrogen) balance is a goal in long-term parenteral nutrition therapy for several reasons: (1) A positive nitrogen balance indirectly implies adequate energy delivery. (2) The body's proteins are all functional; there are no excess stores. Continued losses from both the visceral (metabolic proteins of the organs and circulating proteins) and somatic (largely skeletal muscle) protein compartments will eventually be detrimental to recovery from disease. (3) Many patients already have moderate to severe depletion of these protein compartments. Thus the need to begin restoration, as well as prevent further depletion, is often already present (see Ch. 219 for patient selection).

Some short-term beneficial effect is gained by providing nitrogen as amino acids without additional calories. The degree of negative nitrogen balance may be reduced, but positive balance is not achieved with this approach. Since endogenous protein catabolism is reduced, the effect is termed "protein sparing." Energy requirements are met under these circumstances from endogenous fat stores and from any additional caloric sources provided. This approach as well as the parenteral delivery of small amounts of carbohydrates in combination with amino acids can be useful in short-term management in that the degree of negative nitrogen balance will be diminished.

Practical Applications

A combination of dextrose, amino acids, and water provides the base solution for parenteral protein and calorie delivery (Table 220–1). Major and minor minerals as well as vitamins can be added to this solution. The monohydrate form of dextrose used in most commercial intravenous solutions provides 3.4 kcal per gram in contrast to 4 kcal per gram for the carbohydrate alone. When a peripheral vein is used as the access route, osmolarity limitations prevent the use of concentrated solutions that provide all the daily energy and protein requirements as dextrose and amino acids. For example, a formulation made from 800 ml of a 3 per cent amino acid solution and 200 ml of 50 per cent dextrose will provide only 340 nonprotein kcal with 24 grams of amino acids, but the osmolarity will exceed 800 mOsm per liter. Solutions with osmolarities in excess of 600 mOsm per liter often produce thrombophlebitis when continuously infused into the peripheral veins. Co-infusion of a lipid emulsion will reduce the osmolarity, since lipid emulsions are isotonic (280 to 340 mOsm per liter). Typical solutions for total parenteral nutrition have final osmolarities in excess of 2000 mOsm per liter and therefore must be infused into central veins (e.g., superior vena cava).

Lipid emulsions contain a source of calories in the form of emulsified droplets of soybean or safflower oil, which provide 9 kcal per gram, supplemented slightly by the caloric contribution of the emulsifiers (Table 220–1). Until recently, lipid emulsions were used mainly to supply the essential fatty acid linoleic acid in biweekly infusions or were co-administered with base solutions in peripheral veins to boost daily caloric delivery while reducing infusate osmolarity. Fat calories in the daily nutrition plan were not considered necessary, especially during total parenteral nutrition given by central vein where concentrated dextrose readily meets usual daily energy requirements. More recently, lipid emulsions have been utilized daily to provide 20 to 40 per cent of the total nonprotein calorie requirement, despite the knowledge that positive nitrogen and energy balance had routinely been accomplished with dextrose as the only nonprotein calorie source.

Parenteral nutrition with concentrated glucose as the calorie source results in greater CO_2 production than similar energy provided by a glucose-lipid combination. Theoretically, this could be clinically detrimental to patients with CO_2 retention or those being weaned from ventilators. Patients given calories as the lipid-dextrose combination are also less likely to develop symptomatic fatty liver than those given the same amount of calories from the carbohydrate alone. However, this can be avoided by keeping the energy provision close to the daily

TABLE 220–1. PROTEIN AND CALORIE SOURCES UTILIZED IN PARENTERAL NUTRITION

Macronutrient Category		Parenteral Form of Macronutrient	Nonprotein Caloric Value
Protein		Crystalline amino acids	
Calories	Carbohydrate	Dextrose monohydrate	3.4 kcal/g
	Fat	Lipid emulsion	10% emulsion—1.1 kcal/ml
			20% emulsion—2.0 kcal/ml

requirement. The use of lipids daily also provides a parenteral "diet" with a macronutrient composition that approximates that of the average oral diet. Resistance to the routine use of lipids is based on (1) the expense of lipid emulsions compared to dextrose; (2) the cumbersome need to piggy-back the emulsions into the parenteral nutrition line, thereby enhancing the likelihood of contamination; and (3) the risk of morbidity, albeit small, of lipid infusion. All in all, the actual superiority in the average patient of either a combination of fat and carbohydrate or carbohydrate alone as the parenteral energy source remains unresolved.

TOTAL PARENTERAL NUTRITION

Besides amino acids and calorie sources, all other recognized nutrients can be provided by a parenteral route. Total parenteral nutrition (TPN) is required for short or long periods of time by patients who either temporarily or permanently have an unusable or an inadequate small intestine. The techniques of TPN beyond the scope of this textbook are described in many monographs and handbooks. The most successful TPN programs involve the direction of a knowledgeable physician and the cooperation of informed and interested colleagues in the pharmacy, nursing, and dietetics departments.

Indications

A small number of patients require lifelong TPN because of extensive resection (e.g., from mesenteric vascular accidents, Crohn's disease, trauma) or advanced small bowel disease (e.g., scleroderma, radiation enteritis). The majority of patients with short bowel syndrome from resection, however, can eventually be managed with oral feeding after an initial adaptation period. TPN is indicated as a temporary nutritional therapy mainly for two patient groups: (1) those selected for intensive nutritional support in whom the intestinal tract is not usable for forced enteral feeding (see Ch. 219) and (2) those in whom a nothing-by-mouth regimen ("bowel rest") would be beneficial to the primary gastrointestinal disease. The majority of patients placed on TPN are those with the first indication. Figure 219–1 gives a flow diagram incorporating the various questions used in deciding which patients are indeed candidates for intensive nutritional support. In general, this group has moderate to severe protein compartment depletion at the initial evaluation and is expected to suffer significant additional losses with the current illness.

In the nothing-by-mouth regimen TPN is used for both *parenteral nutrition* and *bowel rest* in an attempt to actually assist in disease regression. Prior to the availability of TPN, regression had been observed in some patients who were not allowed to eat or who minimized input for brief periods, especially those with Crohn's disease, ulcerative colitis, enterocutaneous fistulas, and pancreatitis (Table 220–2). With TPN, regression of disease is variable but is most frequent in patients with uncomplicated Crohn's disease of the small bowel who have failed usual regimens (Table 220–2). In a prospective randomized trial, patients with acute ulcerative colitis who were managed with TPN and bowel rest in addition to usual medical measures did no better than those given oral feedings and standard intravenous fluids as the nutritional adjuvants, as judged by the number requiring colectomy or the induction of remission. However, nutritional benefits that are gained by the severely malnourished patient or nutritional deterioration that is prevented by initiating TPN in the healthier patient preoperatively will not be reflected in a small number of patients if colectomy is the only end point. In all of these diseases, the best gauge of the success of TPN is its effect on nutritional parameters (Ch. 213). TPN allows total bowel rest to be carried on for longer periods of time without the fear of nutritional deterioration, possibly improving the chances that bowel rest will be successful in aiding disease regression. An adequate TPN plan will also uniformly replete the malnourished patient in the process; any additional beneficial effects of nutritional repletion on the primary disease are difficult to assess.

TABLE 220–2. SUMMARY OF THE EFFECTS OF TOTAL PARENTERAL NUTRITION (TPN) WITH BOWEL REST IN VARIOUS DISEASES

Disease	Nutritional Maintenance or Repletion Achieved	Short-term (In-hospital) Disease Regression	Long-term Disease Regression
Ulcerative colitis*	Majority	30–50%	20–30%
Crohn's disease*	Yes	60–80%	50–60%
Subgroup with fistulas†	Yes	30–40%	10–30%
Subgroup with colitis†	Yes	60%	NA‡
Enterocutaneous fistulas (not Crohn's disease)	Yes	30–70% closure§	NA
Severe pancreatitis	Yes¶	NA	NA

*Many patients in reported series are treated with corticosteroids as well as TPN and bowel rest.
†Small patient series; subgroups not always designated.
‡Adequate data not available.
§Many patients eventually managed with surgical therapy; wide range of reported success rates.
¶Parenteral nutrition is successful and does not contribute to morbidity of pancreatitis despite theoretical concern regarding pancreatic stimulatory effects.

In patients with cancer nutritional status can be maintained or improved with an adequate TPN program, but this has not proved to be of overall benefit in enhancing tumor responsiveness to antineoplastic agents. The best candidates for intensive nutritional support are those who have tumors potentially responsive to anticancer therapy but who could not receive optimal management because of the combined detrimental effects of the planned therapy and malnutrition. Some of these patients can be managed with forced enteral nutrition rather than TPN.

Nutrients Provided During TPN (Table 220–3)

Protein requirements (as described in Ch. 212) are met with crystalline amino acids in commercially available solutions. Nonprotein calories are provided by concentrated dextrose and by lipid emulsions. Two liters of a base solution composed of equal amounts of 8.5 per cent amino acids and 50 per cent dextrose in conjunction with 500 ml of a 10 per cent lipid emulsion is a feasible daily protein-calorie prescription. This would provide approximately 80 grams of protein as amino acids, 1680 carbohydrate calories, and 550 fat calories. The resultant nonprotein calorie-to-nitrogen ratio is 170:1, with 25 per cent of the daily calories provided by fat. An alternate regimen would provide all the nonprotein calories as dextrose. The daily protein and calorie prescription should be tailored to a patient's requirements or exceed them by 20 to 40 grams of protein and 500 to 1000 kcal if restoration of depleted compartments is a goal.

Major mineral requirements vary considerably from patient to patient and during any one patient's course of TPN. In particular, potassium requirements may be initially large because of extra- to intracellular fluxes with glucose (and possibly insulin) infusion and because of reversal of the catabolic state. The ranges of major mineral requirements listed in Table 220–3 are typical for the average adult patient, but careful monitoring of serum levels is always necessary to determine the correct provision, especially in the first few weeks of TPN.

Deficiencies of trace minerals are rarely observed in patients on oral feedings because these nutrients are widely distributed among foods and the requirements are low. Deficiencies of zinc, chrominum, copper, and selenium may occur during long courses of TPN, however. Such deficiencies are now prevented

TABLE 220–3. TYPICAL DAILY NUTRIENT PROVISIONS DURING TOTAL PARENTERAL NUTRITION (TPN) FOR STABLE ADULT PATIENTS WITHOUT CARDIAC, HEPATIC, OR RENAL FAILURE

Calories	Dextrose	60–80% of requirement (see Ch. 212)
	Lipid emulsion*	20–40% of requirement
Protein	Crystalline amino acids	100% of requirement (see Ch. 212)
Minerals	Sodium	90–120 mEq
	Potassium	90–150 mEq
	Chloride	90–150 mEq
	Calcium	12–16 mEq
	Phosphorus	20–40 mmole
	Magnesium	12–16 mEq
	Iron†	
	Zinc‡	2–8 mg
	Copper	1–1.6 mg
	Chromium	10–16 μg
	Manganese	0.4–0.8 mg
	Selenium§	120 μg
	Iodine§	50–80 μg
Vitamins¶	A	3300 IU
	D	200 IU
	E	10 IU
	B_1 (thiamin)	3.0 mg
	B_2 (riboflavin)	3.6 mg
	B_3 (pantothenic acid)	15.0 mg
	B_5 (niacin)	40.0 mg
	B_6 (pyridoxine)	4.0 mg
	B_7 (biotin)	60.0 μg
	B_9 (folic acid)	400.0 μg
	B_{12} (cobalamin)**	5.0 μg
	C (ascorbic acid)	100.0 mg††
	K	5 mg/wk§§
Essential Fatty Acid¶¶	Linoleic acid	4% of total calories

*See text for a discussion of the use of lipid emulsion as a daily calorie source. May be co-administered with the base solution.

†The daily requirement (not taking phlebotomy losses into consideration) is about 1.5 mg and can be met by giving 1 ml (50 mg Fe) of iron-dextran solution intramuscularly per month. Replacement is usually dictated by indices of iron stores.

‡Requirements are increased if intestinal fluid losses are great (see Ch. 218).

§Additive usually reserved for patients on long courses of TPN.

¶Based on guidelines from the American Medical Association/Nutrition Advisory Group, 1975. These guidelines do not take into account increased requirements during metabolic stress.

**May be given by monthly intramuscular injection.

††Daily provision often increased to 50 mg or more during periods of catabolic stress.

§§Not provided by multivitamin preparation; given by separate injection.

¶¶Provided by lipid emulsions on a biweekly or triweekly basis. Linolenic acid is also present in some emulsions and may be required during long term TPN (see text).

by supplementing TPN fluid with trace minerals from the outset. Zinc, copper, chromium, and manganese are commonly provided; selenium and iodine are usually given only to patients on very long courses of TPN, such as during home TPN. See Ch. 218 for further discussion of the trace minerals.

Recommendations for vitamin supplementation are given in Table 220–3; few detrimental effects have appeared when these guidelines have been followed. More commonly, vitamin deficiency results from the inadvertent omission of folate or cobalamin, which may not be included in the multivitamin preparation used, or from omission of vitamin K, which is not included in any parenteral multivitamin formulation.

Linoleic, linolenic, and arachidonic acids cannot be synthesized by humans. However, essential fatty acid (EFA) deficiency can usually be prevented by supplying adequate quantities of linoleic acid alone. EFA deficiency is rarely observed as an isolated deficiency except during TPN. A large amount (8 to 10 per cent) of the fat in adipose tissue contains the EFAs. However, the high insulin levels observed during TPN with concentrated dextrose are believed to impair access to this store through inhibition of lipolysis. Manifestations of EFA deficiency include dry, cracked skin, coarsening of the hair, hair loss, and impaired wound healing. It is estimated that 2 to 4 per cent of the daily energy requirement should be provided by linoleic acid to prevent deficiency, and lipid emulsions (500 ml of 10 per cent emulsion triweekly) will satisfy this requirement. A report of linolenic acid deficiency in a child receiving a lipid emulsion low in this fatty acid during long-term TPN suggests that linoleic acid alone may not always be adequate to prevent essential fatty acid deficiency in humans. Use of a lipid emulsion with both linoleic and linolenic acid is currently recommended to avoid EFA deficiency during long courses of TPN.

COMPLICATIONS OF PARENTERAL NUTRITION

Both nonmetabolic and metabolic complications may occur with parenteral nutrition. Thrombophlebitis from hyperosmolar solutions is the most frequent nonmetabolic complication when a peripheral vein is used. The complications related to a central vein intravenous catheter or to its insertion include pneumothorax, hemothorax, air embolus, arterial laceration, brachial plexus injury, inappropriate tip placement, venous thrombosis, and catheter-related sepsis. Some of these complications will be detected by a chest radiograph after catheter insertion, a practice that should always be followed. Others may appear later during the course of TPN. Some degree of clinically inapparent catheter-related thrombosis may occur in as many as 50 per cent of patients. At present, only symptomatic patients (certainly < 5 per cent of those with subclavian vein catheters) are evaluated and treated for noninfected thrombosis along the catheter path. Catheter-related sepsis should also occur in no more than 5 per cent of patients treated with TPN of varying

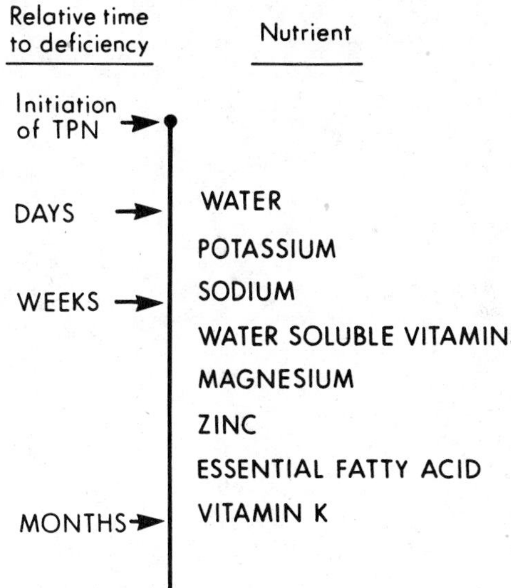

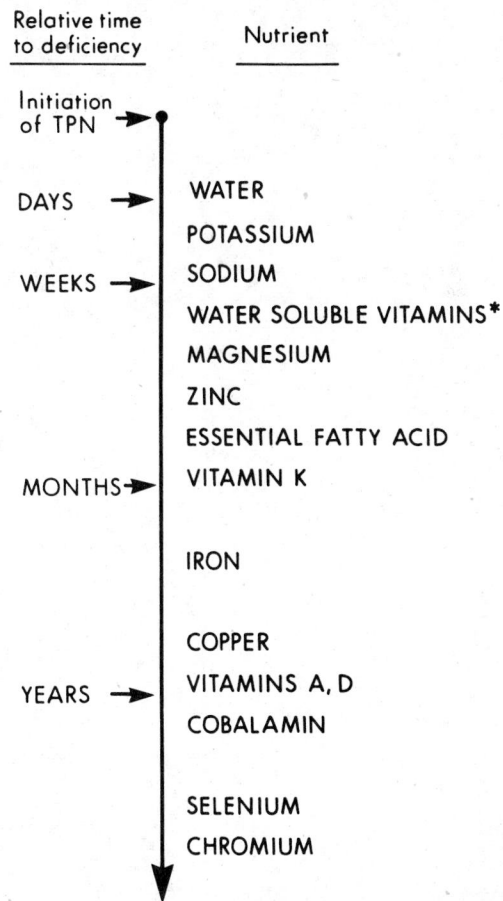

Figure 220–1. Relative time to the development of nutrient deficiencies during inadequately supplemented total parenteral nutrition (TPN). The time is proportional to body stores and inversely related to the fractional catabolic rate of the nutrient in an individual patient. Thus, the relative times given are only estimates. (*Excluding cobalamin.)

course length in a typical hospital-based program if maximal efforts are being made to prevent infection. Culturing of removed catheter tips often reveals that the source of fever was not actually an infected catheter.

Metabolic complications include the appearance of nutritional deficiencies resulting from inadequately prescribed TPN. Figure 220–1 shows the relative time to appearance of deficiencies under these circumstances. Each deficiency of course will become more quickly apparent if body stores of that nutrient were originally depleted.

Hyperglycemia is common in patients given concentrated dextrose by central vein. Regular insulin added to the base solution should be used to keep serum glucose below 200 mg per deciliter. Hypoglycemia is not likely to occur if (1) exogenous insulin is added to the base solution rather than given subcutaneously, (2) the base solution is never interrupted abruptly, and (3) termination of TPN is performed slowly over 24 hours or more with a stepwise reduction of glucose delivery rate. Incorrect provisions of major minerals can also be detected by regular laboratory monitoring, especially during the first two weeks of TPN.

Other metabolic complications include alterations in liver enzymes (usually transient and inconsequential); fatty liver; periarticular, long bone, and back pain; and gallbladder disease. The cause of the bone pain, which usually appears months into a course of TPN, remains unclear, but is likely related to altered vitamin D metabolism. Patients respond to discontinuation of TPN and to removal of vitamin D from the TPN fluid. As many as one third of patients treated with TPN for a period of two years have detectable gallstones. The prevalance is even higher (50 per cent) in the subset with ileal disease (Crohn's disease or prior resection or both). Gallbladder stasis and an increase in bile saturation with fasting are possible explanations for these higher than expected prevalences. Other metabolic complications resulting from alteration of normal physiology are likely to be recognized as more patients with potentially catastrophic small bowel resections or diseases are maintained with long courses of TPN both in the hospital and at home.

Alpers DH, Clouse RE, Stenson WF: Manual of Nutritional Therapeutics. Boston, Little, Brown and Company, 1983. *This manual outlines parenteral nutrient requirements and describes techniques of parenteral nutrition in a chapter devoted to the subject. It is also a reference source for nutrient composition of proprietary products.*

Bengoa JM, Rosenberg IH: Parenteral nutritional therapy in gastrointestinal disease. Adv Intern Med 28:363, 1983. *Provides a critical review and summary of the use of these techniques in patients with inflammatory bowel disease and other gastrointestinal disorders.*

Brennan MF: Total parenteral nutrition in the cancer patient. N Engl J Med 305:375, 1981. *The many studies examining various effects of parenteral nutrition on cancer management are reviewed. The author summarizes reasonable expectations of the use of this form of nutritional support in cancer patients. Correspondence regarding this review should also be read (N Engl J Med 305:1589, 1981).*

Grant JP: Handbook of Total Parenteral Nutrition. Philadelphia, W. B. Saunders Company, 1980. *A well-referenced monograph with a detailed review particularly of uses and complications of parenteral nutrition.*

Part XVII
ENDOCRINE AND REPRODUCTIVE DISEASES

221. PRINCIPLES OF ENDOCRINOLOGY

John D. Baxter

Multicellular organisms must communicate among their cells to maintain homeostasis, to carry out normal growth and development, and to allow for effective adaptations to stress. The endocrine system and the nervous system, both separately and through their interactions, have evolved to meet that need. In general the nervous system, of ectodermal origin, informs by the local release of neurotransmitters in the immediate vicinity of the target cell. By contrast, the endocrine glands, usually of mesodermal or entodermal origin, release hormones into the systemic circulation for a more universal distribution. However, hormones may have more restricted pathways of effective distribution; this occurs, for instance, in the portal systems of the abdomen and of the hypothalamic-hypophyseal region. Finally, both hormones and neurotransmitters can migrate to target cells through the interstitial fluid without entering the circulation (paracrine communication).

In the nervous system there is physical continuity with complex arcades of integration; the endocrine system is multifocal in form and function. Strictly speaking, it is not one "system" but a series of systems for intercellular chemical communication. There can be integration among glands in the flow of information, as illustrated by the sequential responses that follow the release of corticotropin releasing factor (CRF) by the hypothalamus. CRF triggers corticotropin (ACTH) release from the adenohypophysis (anterior pituitary gland), which stimulates cortisol release from the adrenal cortex to effect physiologic responses in the target tissues. Other endocrine glands are more freestanding. The parathyroid glands and their hormone, parathyroid hormone (PTH), function in a closed circuit to maintain extracellular calcium homeostasis independent of the nervous system, and have no known direct interactions with the pituitary gland, although they are indirectly linked to the endocrine systems of calcitonin and of vitamin D and its products.

In spite of these distinctions, the endocrine and nervous systems overlap in their functions and are closely interrelated. Thus, the ectodermal posterior pituitary gland (neurohypophysis) and adrenal medulla are arguably parts of the nervous system, although they release vasopressin and epinephrine, respectively, for systemic distribution. Further, nervous impulses can trigger hormone release and vice versa. Neurotransmitters and hormones also share common mechanisms in eliciting their actions.

Neuroendocrinology has emerged as a discipline that focuses on the interrelationships between the nervous and endocrine systems. The central role of the hypothalamus as a neuroendocrine organ has long been known, as summarized in Ch. 224. Several of its secretory products that trigger the release of hormones (e.g., ACTH, gonadotropins) from the anterior pituitary gland have been characterized and synthesized for clinical use. The peptides with opiate activity found in both the pituitary and central nervous system are discussed in Ch. 222. Even hormones previously thought to be strictly gastrointestinal (gastrin, cholecystokinin) are now known to be abundant in the central nervous system. Thus it is clear that the two major systems for communication are interrelated directly and in more subtle ways. Perhaps it is more appropriate to think instead of a single neuroendocrine integrating system with subspecialization of delivery systems into neurons, gland cells, and various mixed forms in between.

The *target cell* for hormone action must possess special mechanisms for recognizing and responding to these particular chemical signals, accepting those which are appropriate and rejecting those which are inappropriate from among the jumble of substances to which it is exposed. This specificity of recognition exists in the three-dimensional structure of unique macromolecules termed *receptors* that bind the hormone selectively and with high affinity. The target cell must also contain a mechanism to couple the hormone-receptor interaction with the subsequent steps in the cellular response to the information received.

A *hormone* therefore is a substance that is released in one tissue and travels through the circulation (usually) to the target tissue, where it elicits a particular response. There are interesting variations in this simple schema. A precursor to a hormone may be released, for example, with the final effector molecule being formed in the circulation, in the target tissue, or even in another organ. Renin substrate (angiotensinogen) is synthesized in the liver as a prohormone to be subsequently converted in the plasma to the effector substance angiotensin II by two successive modifications catalyzed by renin (kidney) and angiotensin-converting enzyme (lung and other tissues), respectively. Testosterone is converted to dihydrotestosterone, which is responsible for many androgenic actions, by 5α-reductase in the target tissue. The endogenous biosynthesis of the most active form of vitamin D_3, 1,25-dihydroxycholecalciferol, requires steps that are sequentially carried out in the skin, liver, and kidney. Also, in some cases, hormones may act in cells in which they are produced; estradiol, for instance, can affect ovarian granulosa cells.

What then are the limits of endocrinology? They are not always easy to define. Are the brain (endorphins, gastrin, releasing factors) and liver (renin substrate, 25-hydroxycholecalciferol) endocrine glands? Should the kidney be so classified based on erythropoietin, renin, prostaglandins, and 1,25-dihydroxycholecalciferol? The definitions become arbitrary and conventional. The prostaglandins are important intercellular regulators, although they are not often considered to be hormones in the strict sense, since they may serve more for local transfer of information. They are discussed together with other arachidonate metabolites in Ch. 223. By convention the major islet cell hormones have been translocated into "metabolism" and the extensive gastrointestinal hormone system has been woven into gastroenterology. Various polypeptide growth factors (nerve, epidermal, platelet derived) for specific target tissues have been identified, but are not yet generally sanctified as hormones. Further, whereas oncology is not generally considered a discipline of endocrinology, certain products of cancer genes now appear to be similar to growth factors. The thymus has emerged more into immunology than endocrinology, but thymosin might properly be considered a hormone, and, more remotely, the various lymphokines are recognized as chemical messengers as well. Since "hormone" derives from a Greek verb meaning "to set in motion" or "to spur on," what better candidate can there be than a chemotactic factor? Armed with powerful new tools for separating, purifying, and chemically defining "factors" and the cells and genes that produce them, and with exquisitely sensitive assay systems of increasing specificity, the endocrinologist has greatly enhanced means now to better understand molecule-mediated communication systems and their interrelations.

A communication system must be coupled for both emission (signal) and reception. Beyond that it should allow for an appropriate response. Classic endocrinology has been signal oriented. Attention has been devoted mostly to the release and transport of hormones and the arcades of control which govern those phenomena. This has been enormously productive in the study of normal physiology and of the pathophysiology, diagnosis, and treatment of human endocrine diseases. It seemed at one time that endocrinology, almost by definition quantifiable by measurements of hormone levels in the circulation, could be reduced to a Mendeleev-type periodic table of syndromes representing all possible combinations of "too much" or "too little" of the known hormones. As such it might be considered largely a laboratory endeavor. More recently attention has been increasingly shifted to the reception-response domain of the discipline. Pseudohypoparathyroidism was recognized as a syndrome of resistance to hormone action as early as 1942 in the classic clinical investigation carried out by Fuller Albright and his colleagues. Many examples of such resistance, both genetic and acquired, are now known, as will be described below and in specific detail in other chapters of Part XVII. The structures of hormone receptors and how they are linked to cellular responses are now becoming understood. The mechanisms that have been detected and the experimental approaches merge into molecular biology without sharp distinction. Endocrinology *within the cell* increasingly is being pursued through receptor and postreceptor mechanisms to the point of response generation. Perhaps Albright with his whimsy would have called this "endoendocrinology."

HORMONE SYNTHESIS AND RELEASE

Over 50 different hormones are produced by the body. As usually defined, these are represented by several types of molecules: (1) amino acid analogues and derivatives (thyroid hormones, catecholamines), (2) polypeptides, and (3) steroids. The arachidonic acid system (prostaglandins, leukotrienes) will not be discussed here, but is presented in Ch. 223. Endocrine glands synthesize and to some extent store their hormones for subsequent release into the circulation. This function is similar whether it is found in an anatomically separate gland (pituitary, thyroid, adrenal, parathyroids) or in specialized cells or cell clusters within other host tissues (islets of Langerhans, testis, ovary, small intestine, kidney). In some cases the endocrine function has not been found to be isolated to cells specialized for that function—e.g., the production of somatomedins or renin substrate by liver, or of erythropoietin or 1,25-dihydroxycholecalciferol by the kidney.

AMINO ACID ANALOGUES AND DERIVATIVES. Tyrosine is the unique amino acid precursor of these hormones. In the thyroid gland, tyrosine moieties within the large protein thyroglobulin are iodinated to form monoiodotyrosine (MIT) and diiodotyrosine (DIT) while still in peptide linkage. These iodotyrosines undergo oxidative condensation, which couples the respective phenolic groups through ether linkage to form the iodinated thyronines, thyroxine (T_4), and triiodothyronine (T_3). The thyroglobulin of colloid is then taken up by the cuboidal cells of the thyroid follicle in which the action of proteases and peptidases release T_3 and T_4 to be delivered into the circulation. The major secretory product, T_4, serves largely as a prohormone, since it is then further converted to the more active T_3 in the peripheral tissues by the removal of an outer ring iodine. These steps are detailed in Ch. 228 (see Fig. 228–1).

Catecholamines and dopamine, in contrast, are synthesized from free tyrosine in a series of reactions that enzymatically hydroxylate and decarboxylate the parent molecule. These reactions are summarized in Ch. 241.

POLYPEPTIDE HORMONES. Most of the polypeptide hormones are the products of particular genes and are synthesized by the steps outlined in Figure 221–1. The polypeptide gene contains sequences whose transcripts code for the hormones; these are flanked by DNA sequences important for directing the initiation and termination of transcription and in many cases the level of expression of the gene. Between the flanking sequences are "exon" sequences in the DNA whose transcripts contain the RNA sequences that are contained in the mature mRNA product of the gene. The exon sequences are usually interrupted in one or more places in the gene by intervening sequences termed "introns." When the gene is transcribed, a large precursor messenger RNA (pre-mRNA) is made. This is then processed by polyadenylation, the removal of the sequences transcribed from the introns, and splicing together of the exon sequences in the RNA to form the mature mRNA that is transported to the cytoplasm. The polypeptide hormones, like other secreted proteins, are synthesized in a larger precursor form termed a "prehormone" as the direct product translated from the mRNA. In addition to the amino acids of the hormone (or "prohormone"; see below), the prehormone contains a "signal peptide" sequence at the amino terminus that is important for transfer of the protein from the surface of the endoplasmic reticulum in the cytoplasm, where it is synthesized, into the endoplasmic reticulum. The signal peptide sequence is responsible for binding of the polyribosome complexes, containing mRNA, ribosomes, and nascent protein chains being synthesized, to the rough endoplasmic reticulum. The signal peptide sequence is subsequently removed by proteolysis, leaving either the hormone (e.g., growth hormone, prolactin) or a prohormone (e.g., proinsulin, proparathyroid hormone, proopiomelanocortin, procalcitonin). Further proteolysis of the prohormone in the endoplasmic reticulum is required to yield the hormone itself. Insulin is formed, for example, by the excision of a "C" peptide that connects the "A" and "B" chains in the nascent molecule. In the mature molecule, the latter chains are linked through disulfide bonds. ACTH is cleaved from the center of a much larger protein (proopiomelanocortin) that contains several other hormones, including β-endorphin and α- and β-melanocyte-stimulating hormone. Some hormones are further modified by glycosylation prior to their release; these include thyroid-stimulating hormone (TSH), luteinizing hormone (LH), chorionic gonadotropin (HCG), and follicle stimulating hormone (FSH). These hormones consist of two subunits, each encoded by a separate gene. The subunits bind together following their synthesis.

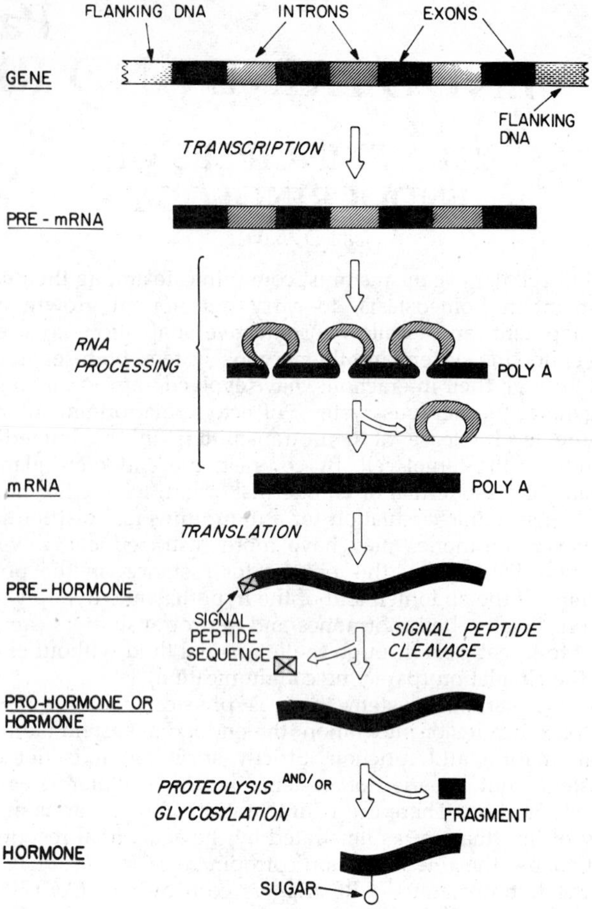

Figure 221–1. Steps in polypeptide hormone biosynthesis.

Variations in this scheme can sometimes result in different hormones arising from the same gene. For instance, growth hormone pre-mRNA is processed in two ways that differ in the size of one of the intervening sequences that is removed.

These differences result in two growth hormone mRNAs and consequent protein forms that differ somewhat in their biologic activities. The pre-mRNA that yields mRNA coding for preprocalcitonin is alternatively processed primarily in the brain to yield an mRNA that codes for a different peptide. At the post-translational level, proopiomelanocortin can be processed to yield in some cases predominantly ACTH and β-lipotropin (β-LPH) and in other cases predominantly corticotropin-like intermediate lobe peptide (CLIP) and β-endorphin.

The hormones within the cisternae of the endoplasmic reticulum are transported to the Golgi complex. This occurs either by direct transfer through the cisternae, which are in continuity with the membrane channels of the Golgi complex, or by the formation of vesicles (transition elements). Secretory vesicles (and/or secretory granules) with more condensed protein contents are formed in the Golgi complex. The hormones are then released into the extracellular fluid by exocytosis, which involves a fusion of the membrane of the granules with the plasma membrane.

STEROIDAL HORMONES. The steroid hormones are derived from cholesterol, and 7-dehydrocholesterol is the precursor to vitamin D. In a series of modification reactions, the side chain of cholesterol is cleaved to yield the 21-carbon steroid pregnenolone. The functioning steroidal hormones are then derived through a series of specific hydroxylations and other modification reactions. For example, there is placement of a 4-5 double bond in the A ring with progesterone, testosterone, cortisol, and aldosterone and aromatization of the A ring in the case of estrogens. Most of these reactions take place in the specific endocrine gland, although in some cases final modifications occur in the target tissue (testosterone→dihydrotestosterone) or in other peripheral tissues (testosterone in the female; estradiol in the male). As an example, the biosynthetic pathway for the glucocorticoids is shown in Ch. 229. Specificity in the production of steroidal hormones depends upon the presence of the appropriate enzymes. Through this mechanism almost all of the aldosterone is produced in the adrenal glomerulosa, most cortisol in the adrenal fasciculata-reticularis, and most estradiol in women in the ovary.

HORMONE STORAGE AND RELEASE. Endocrine cells store hormones to a varied extent. For example, the steroid hormones, although predominantly hydrophobic in nature, still are polar enough not to accumulate in large supply in lipid stores. By contrast, vitamin D and its metabolites accumulate in appreciable quantities in lipid stores. With many of the polypeptide hormones, the glands can store substantial quantities of the hormones. For example, a five-day supply of insulin can be stored in the pancreatic islets. Although the thyroid gland does not store thyroxine per se in appreciable quantities, the gland can have about a two-week supply of this hormone stored as a precusor in thyroglobulin. Also, nerve endings usually contain several days' supply of norepinephrine.

The stimuli to hormone production can trigger both the release of stored hormone and the synthesis of new hormone. The various mechanisms for hormone release have received relatively little attention in comparison with the extensive studies on hormone synthesis (with which it is closely linked). Some of the polypeptide hormones (insulin, glucagon, growth hormone) are released by active exocytosis of granules in which they are stored. Thyroid hormones are released by proteolysis of thyroglobulin derived from follicular stores by pinocytosis. Steroidal hormones seem only to diffuse down concentration gradients.

The pattern of release of hormones shows marked variations. The release of some hormones (ACTH, cortisol) is predominantly pulsatile in nature. The mechanisms by which this occurs are not clear; nor is it established whether these irregular bursts of secretion reflect predominantly changes in synthesis promoting release or in secretion alone. It is especially important to be aware of such episodic changes in evaluating the significance of random blood samples assayed for hormones released in this way. By contrast, the release of other hormones (PTH, prolactin) is more steady. Some hormones (e.g., insulin) display both pulsatile and steady release characteristics. Finally, a few hormones also have an overall pattern of release that is circadian (e.g., ACTH and cortisol).

REGULATION OF HORMONE PRODUCTION
(Fig. 221–2)

For the endocrine system to serve effectively its function of communicating information among cells, it must have mechanisms for regulating the release of hormones. These include not only mechanisms that affect basal and circadian release of hormones but also those that allow hormone levels to increase or decrease in response to physiologic or pathologic stimuli. The system also makes use of mechanisms that monitor whether the hormonal signal has been appropriate to attain its goals of maintenance of homeostasis, stimulation of growth and development, and response to stress.

For the most part, three types of influences govern hormone release: (1) There can be spontaneous release of hormone from the gland at a relatively constant rate (e.g., thyroxine) or in a circadian rhythm (e.g., cortisol). These patterns may be due to intrinsic activity of the gland, or to extrinsic factors that affect hormone release. (2) Hormone release can be affected by a variety of physiologic or pathologic influences that act through the same mechanisms that affect the basal release or through separate pathways. (3) "Sensor" mechanisms monitor the appropriateness of the hormonal levels or responses and provide further regulation. Three major modulators of hormone release that can act at any of the levels discussed above are other hormones, the central nervous system, and the physiologic responses produced.

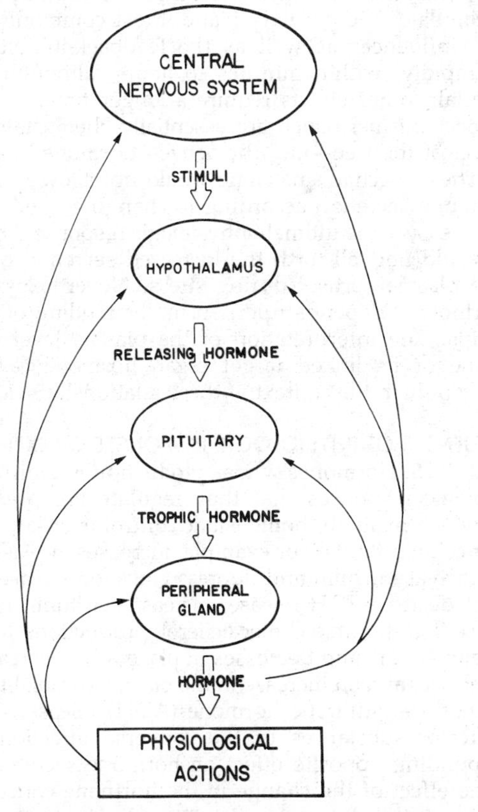

Figure 221–2. Organization of a set of endocrine glands, with interrelated regulatory elements. Shown is the flow of information from the central nervous system through the hypothalamus to the pituitary and then to the peripheral glands. Also indicated is that either the hormone product of the peripheral gland or the physiologic actions induced by the hormone can feedback-inhibit the stimuli to hormone release at any of several loci. As a rule, all of the potential regulatory influences do not operate with respect to a given set of glands, nor do all of the components shown operate for all endocrine glands.

HORMONES THAT STIMULATE THE RELEASE OF OTHER HORMONES. The primary function of several hormones is to stimulate or inhibit the release of other hormones. This is the case with the "tropic" hormones of the anterior pituitary gland (ACTH, TSH, LH) and the hypothalamic releasing factors (CRF, thyrotropin releasing hormone [TRH], gonadotropin releasing hormone [GnRH]). Some of these factors are essential for the release of the respective hormones under their control. For instance, with TSH or ACTH deficiency, thyroxine and cortisol production, respectively, drop to negligible levels and there is atrophy of the corresponding glands. By contrast, with chronic excess of these hormones there can be hyperplasia and hypertrophy of the target gland that, in addition, increases its capacity to produce hormones. Other factors are inhibitory of hormone release; their disappearance leads to an increased production of hormone by the gland. Lesions of the pituitary stalk can block the inhibitory influence of dopamine on the prolactin-producing cells of the anterior pituitary gland, resulting in an increase in the secretion of this hormone. The production of tropic hormones is usually modulated by the hormones whose production they stimulate; thus these hormones themselves measure the appropriateness of the response to the tropic hormone. For instance, feedback inhibition of ACTH release occurs in response to cortisol, inhibition of TSH release occurs in response to thyroxine, and inhibition of LH release occurs in response to testosterone. Conversely, during the menstrual cycle, the rising concentration of estradiol triggers the surge of LH and FSH release prior to ovulation (see Ch. 225). The feedback influences can be exerted either directly at the level of the pituitary or more indirectly at the level of the hypothalamus to block production of the releasing factor that stimulates the pituitary gland. Most commonly, the stimulatory influences as well as the feedback-inhibitory effects occur rapidly, within minutes to hours, although the tropic and certain other effects require a longer time. These simple servomechanisms, which are essentially chemostats, maintain the level of the free—i.e., the active—hormone at a "normal" level. These mechanisms alone would not allow for alterations in hormone secretion according to changing need, since they do not measure the ultimate physiologic response. For example, they would not call forth the increased secretion of ACTH to elevate plasma cortisol during stress. Nevertheless, much of endocrinology depends upon an understanding of these relationships. The interpretation of the plasma level of a tropic hormone or its linked target organ hormone can be made logically only in the context of these relationships, as described below.

INFLUENCES OF PHYSIOLOGIC RESPONSES OR EXTRACELLULAR SUBSTANCES. Hormones whose production is controlled by the physiologic responses that they regulate are predominantly those which maintain homeostatic control over key substances in extracellular fluids. For example, increases in plasma glucose levels increase insulin and depress glucagon release. Increases in Ca^{++} decrease PTH release, increase calcitonin release, and decrease 1,25-hydroxycholecalciferol production. Increases in extracellular Na^{+} and decreases in plasma K^{+} decrease aldosterone release, and an increase in the plasma osmolality increases vasopressin antidiuretic hormone (ADH) release. Changes in the effector substances in the converse direction have the corresponding opposite effect on hormone secretion. In each case the effect of the change in the hormone concentration is to "correct" the changes in the extracellular substance toward "normal." These mechanisms most often operate rapidly (minutes to hours), and they provide an exquisitely sensitive system for the maintenance of homeostasis. The regulation by the effector substance can occur directly on the hormone-producing cell, as with the effect of glucose on insulin or glucagon release or of K^{+} on aldosterone release, or it can occur indirectly. As an example of the latter, an increase in plasma sodium (probably through its associated Cl^{-}) depresses the release of renin by the kidney. The decreased renin level results in less angiotensin production, which in turn results in lower aldosterone production.

CENTRAL NERVOUS SYSTEM. The central nervous system (CNS) participates in the regulation of hormone release in several ways. It not only directs the spontaneous patterns of hormone secretion, but also mediates stress-stimulated secretion and other responses that interrupt the spontaneous (basal) rhythms. These influences occur through effects on the hypothalamus with consequent changes in the delivery of releasing factors to the pituitary, and they also occur through influences on the sympathetic nervous system. The influences of the CNS on the hypothalamus govern the circadian release of CRF that stimulates ACTH release, the surges in growth hormone during REM sleep, events surrounding the onset of puberty, the release of prolactin during suckling, and the release of growth hormone and ACTH with "stress." Little is known about how the spontaneous patterns are determined, although in some cases they may be due to the influences of extrinsic factors on the CNS. The circadian rhythm of ACTH release in rodents appears to be "set" predominantly by the feeding cycle. Events influenced by the CNS through the sympathetic nervous system include the release of insulin by the pancreas, of renin by the kidney, and of epinephrine by the adrenal medulla. These can be considered as part of "fight or flight" responses. Thus, the CNS is able to determine the needs of the organism for normal physiology and development, to sense when there is a need for intervention for specific purposes, and to dictate the appropriate response.

There are many aspects of the regulation of hormone synthesis and release that remain poorly understood in terms of both the mechanisms involved and why certain stimuli are effective. For instance, the release of growth hormone is influenced by the level of blood sugar or certain amino acids, but these may not be the most important physiologic determinants for its secretion. What is the function and the control of prolactin secretion in the male? What are the physiologic roles of intestinal vasoactive peptide and somatostatin?

HORMONE TRANSPORT

The polypeptide hormones circulate largely as free entities. By contrast, the steroid and thyroid hormones circulate largely bound by plasma proteins. For most of these (aldosterone is an exception), specific plasma proteins bind the hormones with high affinity such that only a small amount of the hormone (<1 to 10 per cent) is free. Thyroxine-binding globulin (TBG), thyroid hormone–binding prealbumin (TBPA), and corticosteroid-binding globulin (CBG) are examples of such specific proteins. The hormones rapidly equilibrate with their protein carriers and also rapidly dissociate from them when the free hormone concentration is lowered. The function of these proteins is unknown. They do not appear to have an obligatory role in hormone action, and genetic disorders in which the binding proteins are markedly reduced or increased are not associated with abnormal endocrine function. They do not appear to be required to "transport" the hormones, which are soluble enough at concentrations at which they are active. The plasma proteins serve to some extent as a reservoir that "buffers" the plasma against rapid fluctuations in hormone release and also tend to decrease the clearance of the circulating hormones, making them less accessible to degradative enzymes and to loss through glomerular filtration. CBG-like proteins also exist within some cell types; in the kidney, these may serve to sequester cortisol and prevent it from occupying mineralocorticoid receptors that mostly bind aldosterone (Ch. 73). In addition to the association with high-affinity plasma-binding proteins, hormones also bind with lower affinity to other proteins, particularly to albumin.

Free hormone rather than the plasma-bound hormone appears to be responsible for eliciting hormone action. Furthermore, the physiologic regulatory mechanisms that are sensitive to the concentration of hormones in plasma respond to the free rather than to the total hormone concentration.

The concentrations of the plasma binders of hormones vary both on a genetic basis and as the result of the effects of certain drugs or other factors. For instance, estrogens increase CBG and TBG. In contrast, the synthesis of these binding proteins tends to be diminished by androgens and in patients with severe liver disease, and they may be lost in the urine in the nephrotic syndrome. As noted, there are rare persons who have a genetic deficiency of a specific binding protein.

It is particularly important to be aware of plasma binding in the clinical evaluation of endocrine excess and deficiency states. Since the free hormone is biologically active and is maintained by homeostatic mechanisms, this fraction rather than the total hormone concentration reflects the state of endocrine function. Plasma assays of free hormone concentrations have been developed but are not commonly available; instead, the total plasma hormone concentration is usually measured. The total plasma concentration of a hormone will be elevated or depressed in parallel with any change in the level of its binding protein, even though the free hormone concentration will usually be maintained normal by homeostatic control mechanisms. Conversely, a patient with low binding protein levels could have a high free hormone level and endocrine hyperfunction in the face of a low total hormone concentration, and a patient with a high binding protein level could have an elevated total but a low free hormone concentration and therefore endocrine hypofunction.

METABOLISM OF HORMONES

In order for the endocrine system to be able to adapt to physiologic needs, there must be a turnover of the circulating hormones. This requires mechanisms for removal of active hormones, which may be very rapid (a few minutes for most protein hormones) or comparatively prolonged (over a week for thyroxine). As might be expected, the rapidity of removal tends to parallel the rapidity with which the specific endocrine gland is called upon to adapt its secretion to normal stimuli.

The polypeptide hormones are broken down to their component amino acids in the plasma and by tissue proteases and peptidases. To some extent this occurs intracellularly after the hormone is taken up (internalized). Inactive fragments of polypeptide hormones may circulate (e.g., fragments of PTH) and thereby constitute a problem in radioimmunoassay procedures (see Ch. 246). At present, there are no known endocrine syndromes caused by abnormalities in the metabolism of polypeptide hormones, although sometimes insulin resistance in diabetes can be due to excessive subcutaneous destruction of the injected hormone.

Thyroid hormones are metabolized largely by deiodination in peripheral tissues and to a lesser degree by the oxidative deamination and decarboxylation of the alanine side chain. Part of the metabolism of T_4 is its conversion, as a prohormone, to the more potent T_3. Some T_4 and T_3 are excreted in the bile and undergo an enterohepatic circulation. In a number of disease states (Ch. 228) the metabolism of T_4 is altered to favor initial deiodination in the inner ring to form more reverse T_3, and less T_3 is formed. This may represent part of the body's adaptation to disease by creating a state of relative hypothyroidism that reduces the metabolic demands elicited by the actions of these hormones. The metabolism of catecholamines, by O-methylation and oxidative deamination (see Ch. 241), leads to end-products (vanillylmandelic acid, metanephrine, normetanephrine) which can be readily identified in the urine and measured for diagnostic purposes.

Steroidal hormones are hydrophobic. Thus, although the free hormones are filtered by the kidney, they are mostly reabsorbed and are therefore poorly excreted. To facilitate their removal, they are metabolized to more polar forms through the reduction of double bonds, further hydroxylations, and conjugation with glucuronide or sulfate prior to excretion into the urine and to a lesser extent into the gut. As an example, the metabolic pathway for inactivation of cortisol is described in Ch. 229. An important step in this pathway, the reduction of ring A by specific hepatic enzymes, may be impaired in severe liver disease such that the half-life of cortisol and of estradiol, for instance, is significantly prolonged. Whereas plasma cortisol is maintained at a normal level, in this case by appropriate reduction in its rate of secretion by the adrenal cortex, the abnormality results in elevated estradiol levels. The obverse obtains in thyrotoxicosis: cortisol is more rapidly metabolized; however, the plasma cortisol level is maintained normal by enhanced secretion. Sometimes drugs can increase the rate of steroid metabolism.

Again, homeostatic mechanisms may operate to normalize the hormone concentration by compensatory changes in output. Such variations can be important when hormones are used in therapy either for replacement of an endocrine deficiency or for treating nonendocrine diseases with pharmacologic doses (see Ch. 229).

MECHANISMS OF HORMONE ACTION

The action of a hormone is initiated by its binding to a specific receptor protein. The polypeptide and catecholamine hormones bind to receptors that are located on the cell surface; the steroid and thyroid hormones bind to receptors within the cell. The polypeptide or catecholamine hormone-receptor interaction usually triggers changes in the production of or in the levels of intracellular mediators, which in turn are responsible for eliciting the hormone effect. The steroid and thyroid hormone-receptor interactions appear to stimulate or inhibit the transcription of particular genes. The translation products of the resulting mRNAs then mediate the hormonal effect. There are exceptions to these generalities. Certain actions of thyroid and steroid hormones may not be mediated through nuclear events, for example. Furthermore, the possibility that polypeptide hormones may act by binding to receptors inside the cell is a subject of active inquiry.

HORMONE RECEPTORS. Hormone-receptor proteins bind hormones specifically and with high affinity; this binding then triggers subsequent reactions that result in the hormone response. The binding is noncovalent in nature, is driven predominantly by hydrophobic interactions, and is facilitated by electrostatic and other ionic interactions between the hormone and the receptor. Since the hormone-receptor interaction is reversible, the laws of mass action may be applied to its study. The initial binding reaction can conform to the relationship:

$$\text{Hormone (H)} + \text{receptor (R)} \rightleftharpoons \text{[HR] complex}$$

Thus, the equilibrium dissociation constant (K_d), which is the reciprocal of the equilibrium association constant (K_a), conforms to:

$$K_d = \frac{[H]\,[R]}{[HR]} = \frac{[H]\,[R_{TOTAL} - HR]}{HR}.$$

Rearrangement of this and substituting bound (B) for HR, free (F) for H, and R_T for R_{TOTAL} yields the Scatchard equation:

$$\frac{B}{F} = \left(-\frac{1}{K_d}\right) B + \frac{R_T}{K_d}.$$

This is the equation of a straight line of which the slope is $-1/K_d$ and the intercept on the abscissa equals R_T. Thus, in a plot of B/F as a function of B, the finding of a straight line indicates that the reaction is bimolecular, and the slope and intercept of that line indicate, respectively, the affinity (K_d) and the total concentration of binding sites.

For most hormone-receptor interactions a straight line is obtained. There are exceptions, however, and these generally indicate either the presence of several independent classes of sites or of negative cooperativity. For example, with insulin and aldosterone binding, concave Scatchard plots can be generated. With insulin (especially at temperatures below physiologic), there is negative cooperativity whereby binding of the first molecule of insulin lowers the affinity of other unoccupied receptor units for binding subsequent molecules. By contrast, aldosterone binds to two molecular species, exhibiting a higher affinity binding to "mineralocorticoid" receptors that mediate sodium-retaining actions, and lower affinity binding to "glucocorticoid" receptors that mediate glucocorticoid actions.

The structure of the binding site on the receptor is such that it exhibits a high specificity for binding the major hormones that act through it. For example, glucagon receptors have a high affinity for glucagon but not insulin, and vice versa. However, there are several circumstances in which different "classes" of hormones are similar enough in structure to lead to overlapping association. This is illustrated by the weak binding of aldosterone to glucocorticoid receptors; this is probably of little consequence physiologically, since the concentration of aldosterone relative to its affinity for these receptors is too low to result in appreciable occupancy. Conversely, cortisol can bind significantly to mineralocorticoid receptors that are the primary mediators of aldosterone action. Even though cortisol has only 1 to 2 per cent of the affinity of aldosterone for these receptors, it circulates at concentrations much higher than aldosterone, and consequently cortisol probably does play some role as a salt-retaining hormone. As another example, epinephrine as a catecholamine binds to and acts through both α- and β-adrenergic receptors.

In most, if not all, cases the hormone-receptor interaction results in conformational changes in the receptor that lead to the cascade of events in the hormone response. Thus, hormone receptors are generally considered to be allosteric proteins. These properties of receptors distinguish them from other hormone-binding proteins such as the plasma hormone–binding proteins. The specific post-receptor-binding responses are described in the following sections.

The structures of the hormone receptors are beginning to be elucidated. For instance, the glucocorticoid receptor is a single polypeptide chain of about 90,000 molecular weight that contains steroid-binding, DNA-binding and "effector" domains. The insulin receptor contains four polypeptide chains linked by disulfide bonds. This receptor also is glycosylated, and these sugar moieties are critical for receptor function. This receptor can be autophosphorylated in response to insulin and phosphorylated in response to other stimuli; these phosphorylations can affect receptor-binding activity.

HORMONE AGONISTS AND ANTAGONISTS. A hormone agonist is a compound that is capable of eliciting the actions of the hormone; a hormone antagonist is a compound that can directly block agonist actions. Antagonists bind to receptors, but they do not (in contrast to agonists) trigger the subsequent steps in the hormonal response. If present in sufficient concentrations, antagonists occupy sufficient sites to block the binding of agonists by the receptors and therefore prevent agonist action. Some compounds are partial agonists in that they bind to receptors and elicit a response, but one that is not as great as that of a full agonist. If the partial agonist is present in sufficient concentration, it can block the binding and actions of an agonist, but in this case it serves as a "partial antagonist" since its partial agonist response will be observed. Hormone antagonists (e.g., the antimineralocorticoid spironolactone and the β-adrenergic blocker propranolol) can have important clinical uses.

POLYPEPTIDE AND CATECHOLAMINE HORMONES. The cell surface receptors that mediate polypeptide and catecholamine hormone action have their binding sites exposed to the outside surface of the cell. Binding of the specific hormone by the receptor alters the conformation of the receptor in a manner such that intracellular mediators are affected; these in turn are responsible for eliciting the hormonal responses. These mediators include cyclic AMP that activates serine and threonine kinases, tyrosine kinases, phospholipids, calcium ion, and possible protein mediators. Examples of hormones that appear to act through particular mechanisms are shown in Table 221–1. In numerous instances hormones utilize more than one mechanism, and as described below, these effector systems have extensive interrelations. Knowledge in this area is evolving rapidly, and the list in Table 221–1 will probably be modified. Often the tabulation reflects prevalent thinking rather than established fact.

In many cases, occupancy of only a small proportion of the receptors for polypeptide and catecholamine hormones results in a full hormonal response. In these cases, "spare receptors" are said to be present. This situation arises because the limiting factor in determining the magnitude of the hormonal response resides in some step distal to the initial hormone-receptor interaction. The spare receptors are hardly spare, however, as they are functional and allow for a greater receptor occupancy (and, as a consequence, a greater hormonal response) at lower concentrations of the hormone. This derives from the fact that the quantity of hormone-receptor complexes is proportional not only to the hormone but also to the receptor concentration.

Cyclic AMP (cAMP) and Kinase Activation. cAMP is the intracellular mediator for the actions of many hormones. These can increase or decrease cAMP levels and do so by affecting the production or, rarely, the degradation of the nucleotide. cAMP is formed from ATP by adenylate cyclase (Fig. 221–3).

At least three components are necessary for the activation or inactivation of adenylate cyclase (Fig. 221–3): the hormone receptor, a guanine nucleotide–binding regulatory protein (N protein), and a catalytic unit of the cyclase enzyme itself. There are two regulatory proteins. One stimulates and the other inhibits the activity of the enzyme in response to the hormone-receptor complex (Fig. 221–3). For activation of the cyclase the hormone binds to the membrane receptor, and the resulting receptor-hormone complex associates with N protein. This stimulates N protein to bind GTP and also activates a GTPase activity of the protein. GTP binding promotes the association

TABLE 221–1. MEDIATORS OF POLYPEPTIDE AND CATECHOLAMINE HORMONE ACTIONS

Elevate cAMP	Stimulate Phospholipid Turnover and/or Synthesis
ACTH	ACTH
β-adrenergic agonists	Angiotensin II
Calcitonin	α-adrenergic agents
HCG	HCG
CRF	EGF
FSH	FSH
GHRF	GnRH
LH	LH
PTH	Muscarinic agents
Prostaglandin E_1	PTH
TSH	TRH
Vasopressin	TSH
	Vasopressin
Lower cAMP	**Increase Intracellular Ca^{++}**
α_2-adrenergic agents	ACTH
Angiotensin II	α-adrenergic agents
Insulin	Angiotensin II
Muscarinic agents	HCG
Opiates	EGF
Oxytocin	FSH
Somatostatin	GnRH
	LH
Stimulate Tyrosine Kinase	TSH
EGF	Vasopressin
Insulin	
Platelet-derived growth factor	
Insulin-like growth factor 1	

ACTH, corticotropin; HCG, chorionic gonadotropin; CRF, corticotropin releasing factor; EGF, epidermal growth factor; FSH, follicle-stimulating hormone; GHRF, growth hormone releasing factor; GnRH, gonadotropin releasing hormone; LH, luteinizing hormone; PTH, parathyroid hormone; TRH, thyrotropin releasing hormone; and TSH, thyroid-stimulating hormone. The classification in this table is meant to reflect current thinking rather than established fact.

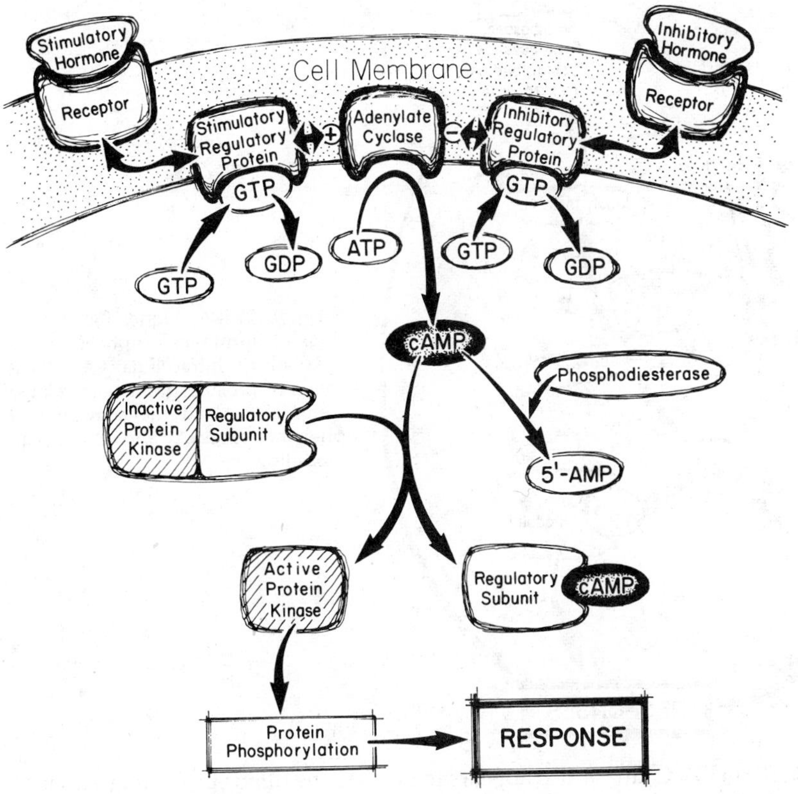

Figure 221–3. Steps in the hormonal activation or inactivation of adenylate cyclase and in the actions of cAMP.

of the N-GTP complex with the catalytic moiety of adenylate cyclase in such a way that the latter is activated to convert ATP to cAMP. The GTPase activity of N protein then converts GTP to GDP. This results in a loss of activity of the regulatory proteins, which terminates the activation. Analogous steps occur when hormones inhibit adenylate cyclase; in these cases the hormone-receptor complex binds to the inhibitory protein that in turn inhibits the activity of the cyclase.

cAMP is formed inside the cell and acts intracellularly. Some cAMP may leak into the extracellular fluid, but there is no evidence that it has any extracellular function. This extracellular cAMP can occasionally be of diagnostic usefulness; urinary cAMP measurements can provide an index of the actions of PTH on the kidney (see Ch. 246).

Most if not all of the actions of intracellular cAMP appear to be mediated through its activation of intracellular protein kinases (Fig. 221–3). These cAMP-activated protein kinases (only a small subset of the total cellular kinases) exist in an inactive basal state in association with two regulatory subunits. cAMP binds to and promotes dissociation of the regulatory subunits from the catalytic subunit, thereby activating it to stimulate the phosphorylation of specific serine and, to a lesser extent, threonine residues on proteins. Some of these phosphorylations alter the conformation and thus the enzymatic activities of proteins that in turn affect metabolic events in the cell.

cAMP is degraded by phosphodiesterases (Fig. 221–3). Since the concentration of intracellular cAMP represents a balance between its synthesis and degradation, regulation could occur at either step. Although it appears that regulation of cAMP synthesis is the predominant mechanism, there are circumstances in which phosphodiesterase is regulated; for example insulin in some cases can increase phosphodiesterase. Certain pharmacologic agents, such as the methylxanthines (caffeine, theophylline) can inhibit phosphodiesterase (although they may also have other actions) and thereby elevate cAMP levels.

Calcium as a Second Messenger. Ionized calcium also plays a role in mediating the actions of many hormones. The hormone-receptor interaction in some way affects the cellular distribution of calcium either by promoting its uptake through the cell membrane or else by stimulating its release from intracellular organelles (e.g., mitochondria or sarcoplasmic reticulum) into the cytoplasm (Fig. 221–4). In the case of cell membrane–stimulated uptake, the hormone-receptor complex may directly, or indirectly, open calcium channels, permitting the influx of ionized calcium into the cell from the extracellular space. A major stimulant for such release appears to be inositol-1,4,5-triphosphate, generated from hormone-receptor complex activation of phospholipase C, as discussed in the following section.

The actions of calcium as a hormonal second messenger are often mediated through an intracellular calcium receptor termed calmodulin (Fig. 221–4). When calmodulin binds calcium, the protein changes to a configuration in which it activates a number of enzymes, including glycogen phosphorylase kinase, Na^+/K^+ ATPase, calcium-dependent protein kinase, myosin light chain kinase, adenylate cyclase, and cAMP phosphodiesterase.

One of the best-studied actions of Ca^{++} is the activation of glycogen phosphorylase that catalyzes the breakdown of glycogen to glucose 1-phosphate. Catecholamines bind to α-adrenergic receptors in cell membranes of hepatocytes and thereby stimulate an increase in intracellular Ca^{++}. In this case, calmodulin is an integral part of the glycogen phosphorylase kinase enzyme complex, binds calcium, and is induced to activate the enzyme.

Although most hormone actions mediated by calcium appear to involve calmodulin, several other Ca^{++}-binding proteins also participate in metabolic control. For example, troponin C is a calcium-binding protein that influences the contraction of smooth muscle. In this case, acetylcholine stimulates smooth muscle contraction by increasing intracellular Ca^{++} and therefore the concentration of the troponin C-Ca^{++} complex, whereas catecholamines produce relaxation by decreasing the intracellular Ca^{++} levels.

Phospholipids. Recent work suggests that membrane phospholipids and their metabolic products appear to participate in hormone action in at least two ways: (1) as a source of arachidonic acid precursors for synthesis of prostaglandins and

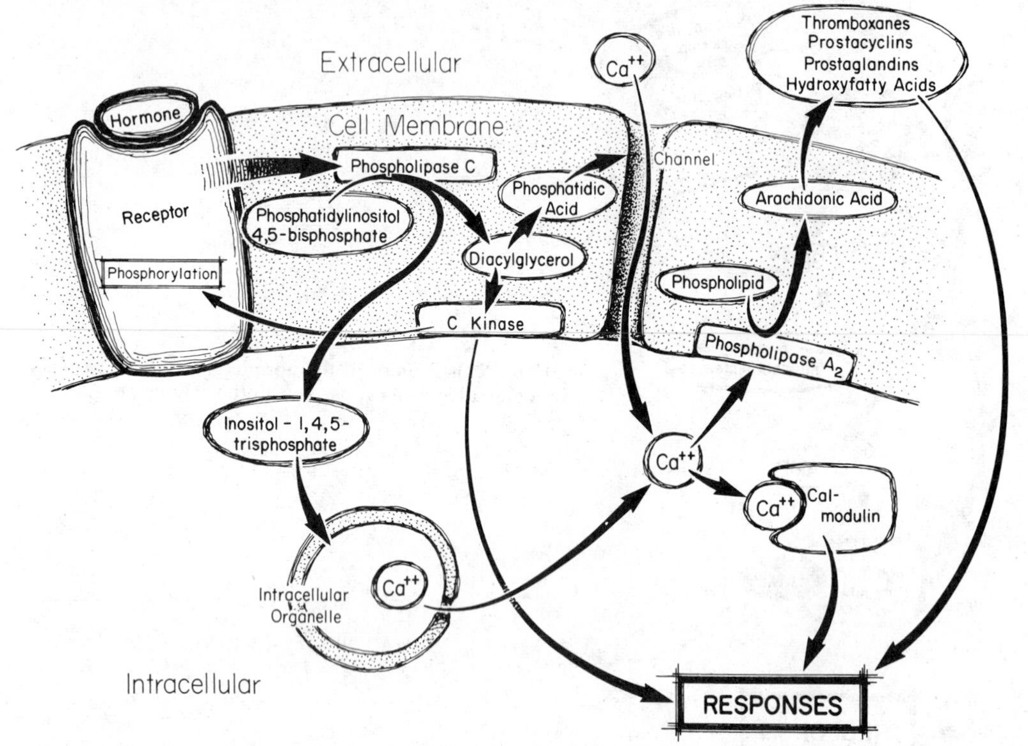

Figure 221–4. Model for the actions of hormones on phospholipid metabolism, intracellular Ca^{++}, synthesis of prostaglandins and related compounds, and the activation of phospholipases A_2 and C and calmodulin.

related compounds that secondarily have target-tissue effects and (2) by stimulating an increased turnover and/or synthesis of phosphoinositides that influence target-cell metabolism.

STIMULATION OF ARACHIDONIC ACID AND OTHER PRECURSORS OF PROSTAGLANDINS AND RELATED COMPOUNDS. Arachidonic acid—a precursor to the prostaglandins, prostacyclins, thromboxanes and hydroxy fatty acids—is released from phospholipids by phospholipase A_2 (Fig. 221–4). Several hormones (ACTH, hypothalamic releasing factors) have been shown to activate such membrane-associated phospholipases that catalyze arachidonic acid release, leading to an increase in the synthesis of the products listed above. These compounds can then elicit other actions on target cell metabolism to form important links between hormone action and prostaglandin, prostacyclin, thromboxane, and hydroxyfatty acid action (see Ch. 223). The mechanisms by which phospholipase A_2 is activated are not clear, although they may be indirect. The activation in many cases is Ca^{++} dependent, and as Figure 221–4 shows, it may be the result of hormone-induced changes in intracellular Ca^{++}. Other sites in the pathway of phospholipid metabolism may also be activated. In ovarian granulosa cells, for example, prostaglandin production is increased by LH, not by increasing arachidonic acid formation but by increasing prostaglandin synthetase activity.

STIMULATION OF PHOSPHOINOSITIDE TURNOVER (Fig. 221–4). Phosphoinositides make up a minor proportion of the membrane phospholipids. The breakdown and resynthesis and/or the synthesis of these phospholipids is enhanced by a number of hormones (Table 221–1). Phosphatidylinositol is converted to phosphatidylinositol 4-phosphate that is converted to phosphatidylinositol 4,5-bisphosphate. The latter can be converted into diacylglycerol plus inositol 1,4,5-trisphosphate catalyzed by phospholipase C (Fig. 221–4). Hormones such as vasopressin and angiotensin II may activate this reaction through influences on the enzyme or its substrates. Diacylglycerol can activate a serine and threonine kinase, termed C kinase, that differs from the cAMP-activated kinase. C kinase can phosphorylate epidermal growth factor (EGF) receptors with a consequent decrease in their affinity for EGF binding and capacity for EGF stimulation of tyrosine kinase activity (discussed below). Thus, this pathway may be involved in heterologous and homologous down-regulation of hormone responsiveness (discussed below). C kinase also appears to mediate the tumor-promoting activities of certain agents such as phorbol esters and may mediate the actions of hormones that stimulate phospholipid turnover. Inositol 1,4,5-trisphosphate appears to be capable of increasing intracellular Ca^{++} by stimulating the release of the ion from intracellular organelles, and may therefore be responsible for many of the effects of hormones that increase intracellular Ca^{++} (Fig. 221–4). Diacylglycerol can also be converted to phosphatidic acid that has been proposed to have calcium ionophore activity (Fig. 221–4). Hormones can also stimulate phosphoinositide synthesis. As is the case with effects on phospholipase A_2, these actions appear to be Ca^{++} dependent and may be secondary to other hormone effects such as those that elevate intracellular Ca^{++}. For example, actions of trophic hormones in steroidogenic tissues on phosphoinositide synthesis may participate in subsequent stimulation of steroidogenesis. Changes in phospholipid synthesis may also be stimulated by cAMP through Ca^{++}-dependent mechanisms, providing a link between adenylate cyclase activation and effects on Ca^{++}.

Activation of Tyrosine Kinase. The binding of at least four classes of hormones (Table 221–1) to their receptors results in activation of tyrosine kinase activity of the receptor. This results in phosphorylation of tyrosine moieties on the receptors and other cellular proteins. These phosphorylations may mediate subsequent events in the actions of these hormones, although the specific steps are not known. The products of certain oncogenes also have similar tyrosine kinase activity; this suggests possible similarities in the actions of growth factors and oncogene products.

Other Possible "Second Messengers." A number of other factors are currently under consideration as possible second messengers for hormones. These include cyclic GMP, changes in phospholipid methylation, other ions (K^+, Cl^-), certain other enzymes that may modify protein structure by other phosphorylations, acetylation, or methylation, for example, and peptide mediators, as for instance with insulin or prolactin action.

INTERNALIZATION OF SURFACE RECEPTORS FOR HORMONES (Fig. 221–5). Cell surface receptors and their complexes are internalized by invagination of the cell membrane into vesicles, particularly at specialized regions of the cell membrane termed coated pits. At these distinctive regions the protein clathryn accumulates on the inside portion of the membrane. Vesicles

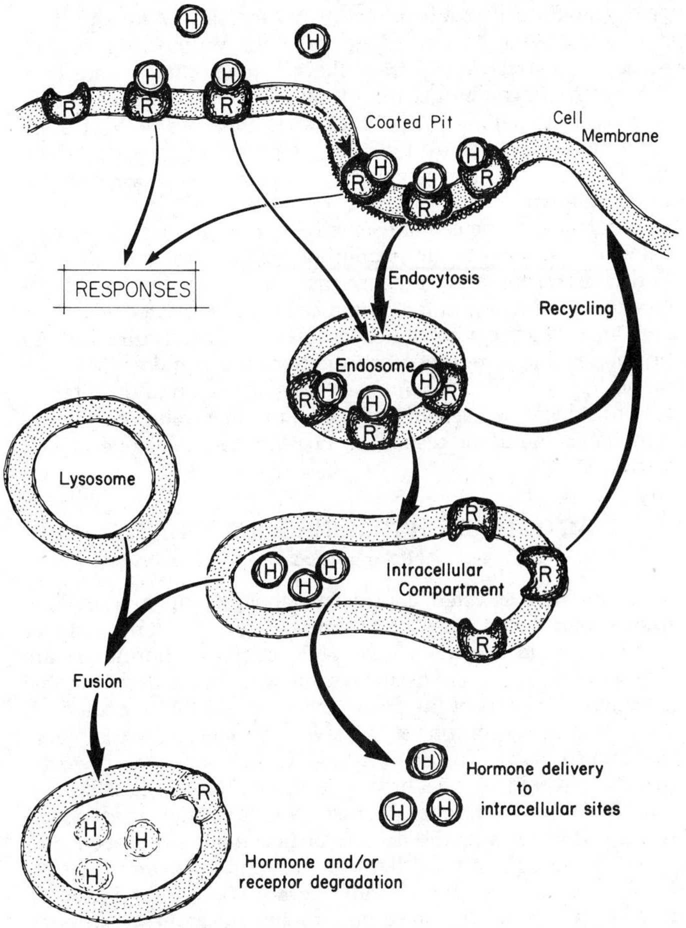

Figure 221–5. Internalization of hormone-receptor complexes and intracellular trafficking and metabolism of hormones and receptors. H = hormone; R = receptor.

from coated pits, termed endosomes, can then have a variety of fates. The endosome appears to have specialized functions such as a proton pump that can decrease the intraendosomal pH. This promotes in some cases the dissociation of the hormone from the receptor. The endosome can be returned to the cell membrane or can differentiate into other cellular compartments where the hormones and receptors can be separated. Membranes of these compartments can then pinch off and either be returned to the membrane to deliver the receptor and sometimes the hormone-receptor complex back to the cell surface or can be fused with the lysosome wherein the hormone or the receptor or both can be degraded.

The quantitative aspects of these pathways vary considerably with different hormones. For instance, most of the internalized insulin is degraded whereas most of the receptors are returned to the membrane. With EGF, most of the receptors and hormone are degraded. This provides one of the mechanisms whereby hormones can down-regulate the levels of their receptors. With iron bound to transferrin, the metal is released inside the cell and both transferrin and its receptor are returned to the membrane. With the lipoprotein receptor, cholesterol bound to lipoprotein is released inside the cell where its metabolic products feedback-inhibit cholesterol biosynthesis.

STEROID HORMONES (Fig. 221–6). Steroid hormones penetrate cells readily. The existence of transport systems has not been excluded, but if they exist, they do not appear appreciably to affect the accessibility of the hormone to the soluble intracellular receptors. In some cases (estrogens), the hormone-free receptors appear to be concentrated in the nucleus, whereas in other cases (glucocorticoids) at least some of the free receptors may be in the cytoplasm. Binding of the active steroid induces conformational changes in these receptors termed activation or transformation that stimulate their binding to the nuclear chromatin. This binding then influences the rates of transcription of specific genes. The translation products of the resulting mRNAs then mediate the response to the steroid hormone. For instance, glucocorticoids increase the synthesis of certain hepatic enzymes involved in gluconeogenesis and decrease the synthesis of proopiomelanocortin. Mineralocorticoids induce proteins that facilitate Na^+ reabsorption in the cortical collecting tubules of the kidney.

Steroid hormone–responsive genes contain specific DNA sequences on which receptor-steroid complexes act. These regulatory sequences are distinct from the promoter sequences where DNA transcription is initiated by RNA polymerase, and they can be located either fairly close to or at least up to several hundred nucleotides away from the promoter (Fig. 221–6). The regulatory sequences bind the receptor-steroid complexes (alone or in conjunction with other factors) with a much higher affinity than does random DNA. This DNA binding then results in an increased rate of initiation of transcription at the promoter of the steroid-responsive gene. The mechanisms by which the stimulation occurs are not known, but may involve a receptor-induced perturbation of chromatin structure that increases RNA polymerase accessibility to the promoter.

In some cases, steroid hormones can regulate mRNA levels through influences on mRNA stability. The mechanisms by which this occurs are not understood, but the steroids could, through transcriptional mechanisms, regulate other proteins that secondarily have effects on mRNA stability.

There is usually a close correlation between steroid binding by the receptor and the relative magnitude of the hormone

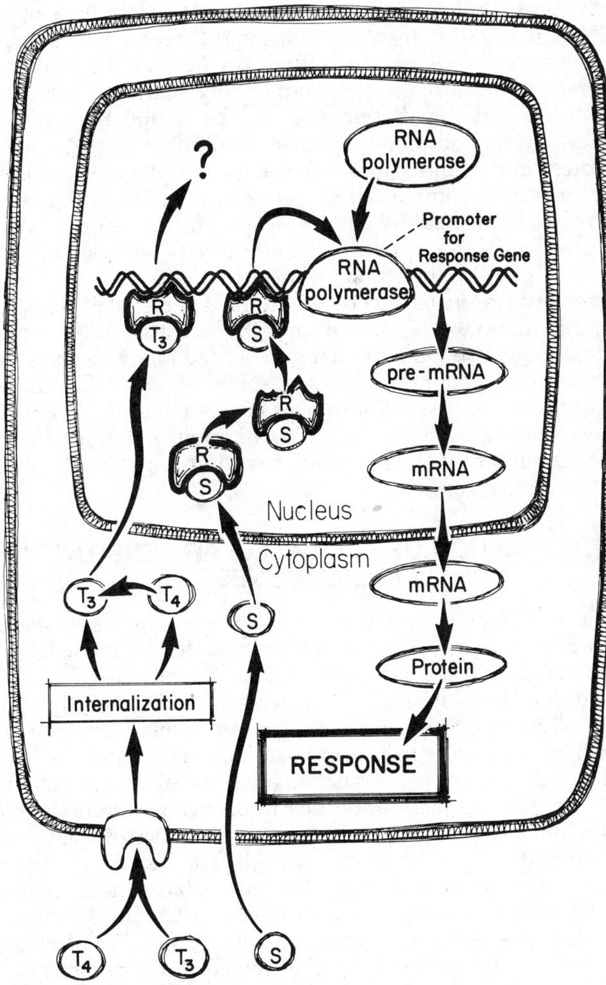

Figure 221–6. Steps in steroid and thyroid hormone action. (S = steroid; T_3 = triiodothyronine; T_4 = thyroxine; R = receptor.) The arrow between the steroid-receptor complex and the RNA polymerase depicts that the complex in some way increases RNA polymerase entry or activity.

response. This implies that the receptor rather than other elements of the response is limiting in determining the magnitude of the response.

Responses to steroid hormones are ordinarily observed several hours after administration of the hormone. This latent period represents the time required for the steroid-induced mRNAs and proteins to accumulate. Similarly, following removal of the steroid, the effect may last for a considerable period of time (hours to days). Again, this prolonged effect probably reflects the time required for degradation of the induced mRNAs and proteins. There are exceptions to these general mechanisms, but they are probably rare. Glucocorticoids inhibit ACTH release within a very few minutes, too rapidly for the effect to be due to an influence of the hormones on the transcription of DNA and its ultimate phenotypic expression. Even in this system, however, the hormone elicits other slower actions on ACTH mRNA that probably are mediated through nuclear mechanisms similar to those discussed above.

THYROID HORMONES (Fig. 221–6). Thyroid hormone receptors are found on the nuclear chromatin whether or not they are bound by the hormone. Thyroxine (T_4) and triiodothyronine (T_3) bind to sites on the cell surface and these protein-hormone complexes are internalized. This mechanism probably accounts for thyroid hormone uptake. Once inside the cell, T_4, which largely serves as a prohormone, is converted to T_3, and this newly formed T_3 plus that which had entered the cell then binds to the chromatin receptors.

The chromatin receptor–T_3 interaction stimulates the transcription of specific genes, and the translation products of the mRNAs that result then account for the hormone response. For instance, the hormones induce Na^+/K^+ ATPase that may generate heat through its ion-pumping activity. This may explain in part the thermogenic actions of the thyroid hormones. Thyroid hormones increase the number of β-adrenergic receptors in certain tissues, which enhances the cellular sensitivity to catecholamines. It is not known how the hormone-receptor complex stimulates transcription. Thyroid hormone–receptor complexes appear to bind to DNA and could act in a way analogous to the steroid hormones.

There appear to be exceptions to this overall scheme. Some of the influences of T_3 on blocking TSH release and on amino acid transport are too rapid to be accounted for by mechanisms involving transcription. Possibly some of the cell surface–binding sites for thyroid hormones mediate these rapid effects. Cytosolic and mitochondrial thyroid hormone–binding proteins have been reported, but there are no convincing data that these are hormone receptors.

REGULATION OF THE CELLULAR SENSITIVITY TO HORMONES

The sensitivity of target cells to hormones can show striking variations. These can occur in disease states (discussed later) or as normal physiologic or developmental events.

The number of hormone receptors can be extensively regulated with a resulting distinct effect on cellular sensitivity to that hormone. Polypeptide and catecholamine hormones generally induce a down-regulation (desensitization, tachyphylaxis, negative regulation) of their respective receptors (homologous down-regulation) and this can occur occasionally with steroid and thyroid hormones as well. For instance, hyperinsulinism associated with hyperglycemia reduces the number of insulin receptors and lowers sensitivity to insulin. Hormones can also increase or decrease the affinity or number of sites of receptors for other hormones (heterologous down-regulation). For example, estrogens can increase progesterone levels.

Several different mechanisms account for such down-regulation. The degradation of hormone receptors induced by internalization discussed above is operative in some cases. In other circumstances, hormones can influence receptor synthesis or degradation through different mechanisms. With catecholamine receptors, hormone binding either can induce receptors to be sequestered away from the cell membrane where they are inactive or can induce receptor phosphorylation by a cAMP-dependent mechanism that inactivates them; in both of these cases, the receptors are ultimately recycled to an active state. Homologous or heterologous hormones can induce receptor phosphorylations that can alter hormone affinity.

Regulation of the cellular sensitivity to hormones also occurs extensively owing to modulation of postreceptor mechanisms. Both synergisms and antagonisms exist. As examples, glucocorticoids are required for certain actions of the catecholamines and vice versa; certain glucocorticoid actions require thyroid hormone; glucagon, glucocorticoid hormones, and growth hormone have actions that oppose those of insulin and therefore lead to a decreased sensitivity to insulin. Magnesium deficiency diminishes the tissue response to parathyroid hormone as well as its secretion.

ACTIONS OF HORMONES: INTEGRATED RESPONSES

The endocrine system controls metabolic events in individual tissues and coordinates effects that occur simultaneously or sequentially in many tissues. The actions of hormones are diverse, affecting every tissue in some way, but with substantial selectivity in terms of the particular functions that are affected. Some tissues respond to only a few hormones, whereas others respond to many. The actions of some hormones are predominantly directed at one or a few tissues (e.g., aldosterone), whereas other hormones (cortisol, epinephrine) affect many tissues. Examples of the actions of hormones have been provided previously in this chapter, with particular emphasis on trophic hormones and on how certain hormones influence cellular sensitivity to the same or other hormones. Although any attempt to list the actions of hormones represents an oversimplification, some of the more prominent types of influences deserve emphasis.

Hormones exert major control of intermediary metabolism. Many of the responses are due to coordinated influences on several tissues and can involve several different hormones. The actions of hormones on carbohydrate metabolism are illustrative. In liver, glucagon and epinephrine promote glycogen breakdown and inhibit glycogen synthesis. These hormones and cortisol stimulate glucose production by enhancing gluconeogenesis. In fat cells, epinephrine, cortisol, and growth hormone stimulate lipolysis, providing free fatty acids (an alternative to glucose as an energy source) and glycerol, which may be converted to glucose. Epinephrine and cortisol inhibit glucose uptake by fat cells, and epinephrine stimulates glycogenolysis in muscle. Cortisol inhibits glucose uptake in lymphoid and fibroblastic tissues, and inhibits protein synthesis and stimulates protein breakdown in several tissues. The amino acids released increase the substrate available for gluconeogenesis. All of these responses tend to elevate the blood sugar and can make glucose available, for instance, during fasting. By contrast, insulin lowers the blood sugar by stimulating glycogen synthesis, by inhibiting lipolysis and stimulating lipogenesis, and by promoting protein synthesis. Thus, through its ability to recruit several different hormones and to affect multiple tissues in an integrated way, the endocrine system can be highly effective in the maintenance of homeostasis. Such an integrated system may reduce dependency on only one hormone or tissue, a feature that can facilitate compensation in disease states.

Many hormones affect growth. Prominent among these is growth hormone, which stimulates the production of yet other growth factors termed somatomedins. Epidermal growth factor, fibroblast growth factor, multiplication-stimulating activity (MSA), nonsuppressible insulin-like activity (NSILA), sex steroids, thyroid hormones, erythropoietin, and the "tropic" hormones that affect endocrine glands are also growth factors. Although in some cases the physiologic roles of these hormones are understood, in other circumstances considerable additional clarification is needed.

Hormones affect water and mineral metabolism. Thus, aldosterone regulates sodium, potassium, and hydrogen ions; vasopressin regulates water; PTH, vitamin D, and calcitonin affect calcium and phosphate ions; and prolactin affects milk production.

Hormones, especially the catecholamines, affect the cardiovascular and respiratory systems. Glucocorticoids can promote bronchodilatation in asthma. Angiotensin and vasopressin cause vasoconstriction; bradykinin produces vasodilation. Some hormonal actions on the cardiovascular system are indirect. For instance, sodium retention induced by an excess of aldosterone can cause hypertension.

Hormones are important in development and differentiation. Deficiency of thyroid hormone in childhood results in the serious and irreversible intellectual impairment of cretinism. Abnormalities in sexual maturation result from deficient androgenic effects during development. In fact, most classes of hormones have some developmental actions.

Hormones vary considerably in the rapidity with which they act. Some hormones act quickly and are more important in the minute-to-minute control of metabolism. Epinephrine, glucagon, and other "surface-active" hormones are representative of this type of hormone. Other classes of hormones regulate more long-term responses and thus tend to provide more chronic types of adaptations. Steroid and thyroid hormones generally fall into this latter category. These patterns may not be surprising based on the molecular mechanisms of action of these hormones. The surface-active hormones commonly activate enzymes by mechanisms that do not require macromolecular synthesis, whereas the slower responses to the steroid and thyroid hormones reflect the time required to change the levels of the mRNAs and proteins whose synthesis they regulate. Exceptions to these generalities occur. Thyroid and steroid hormones can have rapid actions (discussed above), and hormones that bind to surface receptors can have influences on gene transcription.

DISORDERS OF THE ENDOCRINE SYSTEM
(Fig. 221–7)

Endocrinology has traditionally been signal oriented, concerning itself largely with whether hormones are secreted appropriately or inappropriately (in excess or deficit). Indeed, most recognizable disorders of the endocrine system are due to an excess or a deficiency of particular hormones, whether caused by abnormalities of endocrine glands, ectopic production of hormones, abnormal conversion of prehormones to their active forms, or iatrogenic factors. Endocrine abnormalities can also be due to changes in the responses (either enhanced or diminished) of target tissues to hormones. These disorders can occur by a variety of mechanisms.

HORMONE DEFICIENCY SYNDROMES. ***Hypofunction of Endocrine Glands.*** Endocrine glands may be injured or destroyed by neoplasia, infections, hemorrhage, autoimmune disorders, and other causes. The destruction can be acute, but commonly it is chronic with normal basal hormone production until late in the disease. The gland is usually compromised in its reserve capacity before the basal level of secretion falls and cannot respond normally in circumstances in which an increase in hormone production is needed. Such partial defects may therefore not be detected by measurement of basal hormone levels, but require other testing of the reserve function of the gland. Since many manifestations of endocrine disease require weeks or even months to develop, there can be considerable differences in the clinical presentation, depending on the rapidity of glandular destruction. In acute endocrine deficiency, chronic manifestations of the disease may not be present.

As would be expected, a deficiency of a hormone that controls the synthesis and release of another hormone may result in a syndrome which simulates a primary deficiency of that target organ. Thus, hypothalamic lesions resulting in impaired secretion of releasing hormones can be manifested by pituitary dysfunction, and the latter can result in abnormalities in the function of its various target organs (gonads, thyroid, adrenal).

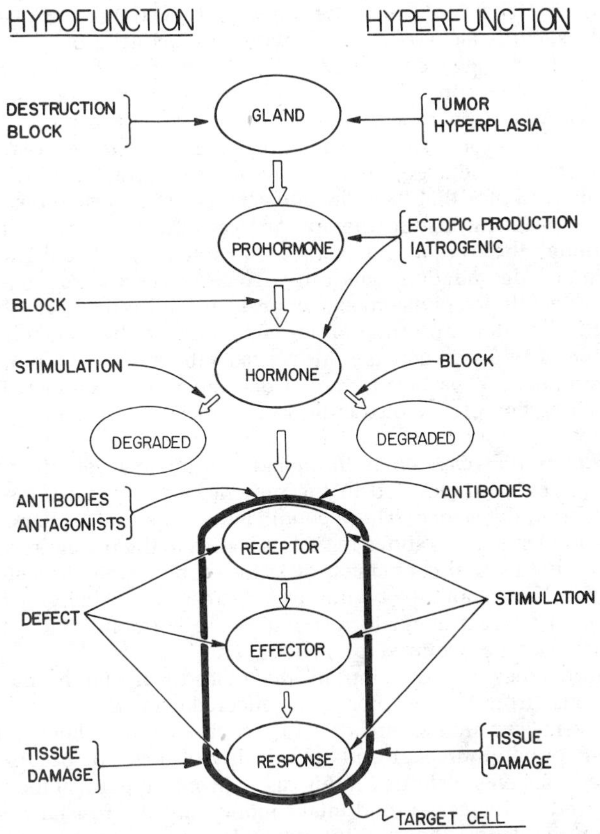

Figure 221–7. Causes of hypofunction or hyperfunction of the endocrine system.

Genetic defects can cause endocrine hypofunction, usually because of abnormalities in hormone synthesis but rarely because of the production of an abnormal hormone (as documented for insulin in a rare form of diabetes melitus). These genetic defects in hormone synthesis can be partial or complete. For example a rare form of growth hormone deficiency is due to deletion of the growth hormone gene. A partial defect may be somewhat analogous to incomplete destruction of the gland—i.e., basal hormone production may be normal, but reserve may be inadequate. In fact, sometimes genetic defects present not with the problems of hormone deficiency but with manifestations of a compensatory adaptation. For instance, partial blocks in thyroid hormone biosynthesis may result in an enlarged thyroid gland (goiter) that is due to the TSH hypersecretion that results from low levels of thyroid hormone. With the 17α-hydroxylase syndrome, there is defective cortisol production and consequent ACTH hypersecretion with an excessive production of adrenocorticosteroids that are not 17α-hydroxylated (see Ch. 229). One of these (corticosterone) substitutes for cortisol such that manifestations of cortisol deficiency are not observed. On the other hand, excessive compensatory synthesis of corticosterone and deoxycorticosterone leads to a mineralocorticoid excess syndrome with hypertension and hypokalemia.

Hormone Deficiency Secondary to Extraglandular Disorders. In principle, a number of types of extraglandular disorders could result in hormone deficiency. These could involve defective conversion of prohormones to active forms, enhanced degradation of hormones or the production of substances (antibodies, hormone antagonists) that block the actions of hormones. Impaired conversion of a prohormone to a hormone occurs in chronic renal disease and in pseudo–vitamin D resistant rickets in which there is defective conversion of 25-hydroxycholecalciferol to 1,25-hydroxycholecalciferol. A rare form of androgen deficiency is due to an abnormality in 5α-reductase that converts testosterone to dihydrotestosterone. In this condition, there is only a partial loss of androgenic effects since testosterone itself is weakly active in some target tissues. Rare forms of diabetes mellitus result from antibodies to the insulin receptor that block insulin action. Antibodies to insulin develop during insulin therapy and can affect its availability. Although there are no syndromes known to be due to enhanced hormone degradation, this can vary as discussed earlier and can affect the response to exogenously administered hormones (e.g., phenytoin and thyroid hormone increase the metabolism of certain glucocorticoids). Also, such influences can unmask or aggravate a partial hormonal deficiency; for example, the development of thyrotoxicosis can unmask latent Addison's disease.

Hyporesponsiveness to Hormones. Hormone levels may be normal or even elevated in the presence of manifestations of endocrine deficiency. These conditions can be due to some of the problems listed above (e.g., antibodies to the insulin receptor and abnormal conversion of testosterone to dihydrotestosterone). They can also be due to a decreased capability of the endocrine target gland to respond to the hormone. Such disorders can be acquired or genetic, and they can be due to abnormalities at any step in the cascade of the hormone response from the receptor to the effect generated.

Several syndromes are due to receptor abnormalities. The most commonly recognized abnormality of this type occurs in type II diabetes mellitus. In this case, chronic hyperinsulinemia induced by increased food intake induces insulin resistance by down-regulating the concentration of insulin receptors. Recognition of this problem also affects the therapy, since treatment is directed not only at correcting the hyperglycemia with insulin or other drugs but also at decreasing insulin need by dietary maneuvers. This form of diabetes also exhibits the additional and perhaps primary abnormality whereby the pancreatic islets do not release insulin normally in response to glucose, but can respond normally to other agents. In the testicular feminization syndrome there is unresponsiveness to androgens. As a consequence, a female phenotype occurs in a person with a male genotype. Most persons with this X-linked disorder have a defect in the androgen receptor.

At least one disorder is due to an abnormality in the coupling of hormone-receptor complexes to effector mechanisms. In pseudohypoparathyroidism there are symptoms and chemical derangements of hypoparathyroidism associated with elevated PTH levels and insensitivity to this hormone (see Ch. 246). In some such patients this insensitivity can be shown to be due to decreased levels of the guanyl nucleotide–binding regulatory protein that couples the PTH-receptor complex to adenylate cyclase.

Overall damage to the hormone target tissue can result in insensitivity to hormones. For instance, renal disease can lead to insensitivity to vasopressin, and liver disease can lead to insensitivity to glucagon.

There are several forms of target organ insensitivity in which the molecular mechanisms have not been elucidated. One form of dwarfism (Laron) is due to an impaired ability of growth hormone to generate somatomedin production. Vasopressin-resistant diabetes insipidus is not associated with frank renal disease. There is a syndrome of hypercortisolism with decreased sensitivity to glucocorticoids. In this case, the hypercortisolism compensates for the hyposensitivity, but the mineralocorticoid actions of the steroid also cause hypertension with hypokalemia.

Abnormal Production or Administration of Antagonists. Rarely, endogenously produced or exogenously administered substances can produce a hormone-deficient state. Antibodies to the insulin receptor can produce insulin resistance with functional insulinopenia. Cimetidine given for peptic ulcer disease can act as an androgen antagonist and produce an androgen-deficient state.

HORMONE EXCESS SYNDROMES. Hormone excess syndromes can result from hyperfunctioning endocrine glands, "ectopic" hormone production by tumors, less commonly from influences on target tissues that enhance hormone sensitivity, autoimmune disease in which antibodies cause hypersecretion of hormones or act as hormone agonists, defects in hormone biosynthesis in which precursor hormones produced in excess have deleterious consequences, and iatrogenic or therapeutic administration of hormones or substances that act like hormones.

Hyperfunction of Endocrine Glands. The most common cause of hormone excess syndromes is hyperfunction of endocrine glands secondary to tumors of the glands or to hyperplasia of several causes. Hyperfunctioning tumors of endocrine glands are usually well-differentiated adenomas (although carcinomas also occur) so that the prognosis is usually favorable with an early diagnosis. In addition to the manifestations of hormone excess, local extension of the tumor can produce symptoms. For instance, pituitary tumors can destroy the normal gland or extend into the suprasellar region to cause headaches or visual impairment.

Hyperplasia is a cause of hyperfunction of several of the endocrine glands (thyroid, adrenals, parathyroids). The most common form of thyroid hyperplasia appears to be due to an immunologic abnormality in which antibodies stimulate the gland in a manner similar to TSH. Hyperplasia of the zonae fasciculata and reticularis of the adrenal with consequent cortisol hypersecretion is usually due to ACTH hypersecretion by a pituitary tumor or an ectopic hormone-secreting tumor. The etiology in other cases of endocrine gland hyperplasia is less clear, as with hyperplasia of the adrenal zona glomerulosa with excessive aldosterone production, or of chief cell hyperplasia of parathyroid glands with PTH hypersecretion.

Ectopic Hormone Production by Tumors (see Ch. 173). Sometimes hormones are produced in excess by cells of endocrine or nonendocrine origin that are not normally the primary source of the hormone. In most cases, hormones produced ectopically by tumors are those that arise from a single gene (e.g., ACTH, growth hormone, prolactin, PTH, calcitonin, gastrin, erythropoietin), or two genes (HCG, LH, FSH). This may be due to the fact that for other hormones (e.g., steroids, thyroid hormones, catecholamines) a large number of genes not ordinarily expressed by the tumor but whose products participate in hormone biosynthesis would need to be activated to produce the hormone. Although a large number of different types of tumors can produce hormones, specific cell types are more commonly associated with certain tumors (see Ch. 173). For instance, certain cells of entodermal origin, termed *a*mine *p*recursor *u*ptake and *d*ecarboxylation (APUD) cells, are more commonly associated with ectopic hormone production. These cells are found in oat cell carcinoma of the lung, carcinoid tumors, thymomas, and others. Although a number of molecular mechanisms are now understood that could explain how genes that are ordinarily not expressed are activated in tumors, those actually causing ectopic hormone production are not understood.

Iatrogenic Causes. When hormones are used to treat nonendocrine diseases, when hormone replacement therapy is excessive, and sometimes when patients self-administer hormones (or their analogues), iatrogenic endocrine disease may occur. Patients will sometimes take excessive doses of glucocorticoids or thyroxine because these hormones produce a feeling of well-being. Rarely, administration of nonhormonal substances can cause hormone-like effects. Licorice ingestion can produce a syndrome mimicking primary aldosteronism, for example.

Tissue Hypersensitivity. Endocrine excess syndromes caused by hypersensitivity of target tissues are uncommon. Thyroid hormones increase the catecholamine receptors in certain tissues and thereby lead to excessive β-adrenergic stimulation. In this case the hyperresponsiveness is actually part of the syndrome of hyperthyroidism. Many of the manifestations of primary aldosteronism are simulated in a rare syndrome with low plasma renin and aldosterone levels in which the kidney responds as if it is excessively stimulated by aldosterone. Finally, disease of the target tissue itself can render it excessively sensitive to a hormone. For instance, cardiac arrhythmias, such as atrial fibrillation in thyrotoxicosis, probably occur most frequently in an already damaged heart.

A lingering question is whether subtle abnormalities in the sensitivity to hormones contribute to the pathogenesis of disease more than is generally perceived. With more refined methods for measuring alterations in sensitivity to hormones, it may be possible to detect more subtle abnormalities. For instance, are some forms of essential hypertension due to increased sensitivity to pressor substances or decreased sensitivity to vasodilator substances? Are some forms of osteoporosis due to abnormalities in sensitivity to estrogens or to calcium-regulating hormones? Why do glucocorticoids increase the intraocular pressure (and even precipitate glaucoma) in some persons but not in others?

Autoimmune Disease. Autoimmune disease can result in the production of antibodies that act as hormones. The most frequent situation in which this occurs is with Graves' disease, discussed in Ch. 228. Rarely, antibodies to the insulin receptor are formed that have insulin-like actions.

Hormone Biosynthetic Defects. Certain adrenal steroid biosynthetic defects (the 21α- and 11β-hydroxylase syndromes) result in overproduction of hormones proximal to the block; these syndromes are discussed in Ch. 229.

Secondary Causes of Hormone Hypersecretion. Hypersecretion of hormones may be due to excessive physiologic stimulation of glands that are basically normal. The secondary hyperaldosteronism of hepatic disease and ascites, congestive heart failure, the nephrotic syndrome, and other conditions is illustrative. The excess aldosterone can aggravate the tendency to edema in these conditions. Secondary hyperparathyroidism occurs in azotemia (see Ch. 248).

MULTIPLE ENDOCRINE SYNDROMES (see also Ch. 240). Simultaneous involvement of more than one endocrine gland can result in syndromes of hyper- or hypofunction. The most common syndrome of multiple endocrine deficiencies, sometimes termed Schmidt's syndrome, can involve the pancreatic islets, thyroid, adrenals, parathyroid glands, and gonads. The disease appears to be caused by immunologic destruction of the glands. This may result from common antigenic determinants, caused possibly by a common developmental origin of the glands.

At least three syndromes of multiple endocrine hyperfunction result from hyperplasia, adenomas, or carcinomas of endocrine tissues, termed multiple endocrine neoplasia (MEN) types 1, 2, and 3. Type 1 is associated with hyperfunction of the parathyroids, pancreatic islets, pituitary, adrenal cortex, and thyroid. In some cases more than one hormone may be produced by the tumor; islet cell tumors can produce insulin, glucagon, gastrin, vasoactive intestinal peptide (VIP), prostaglandins, ACTH, PTH, ADH, somatostatin, and serotonin. MEN type 2 is associated with pheochromocytoma (sometimes bilateral and extra-adrenal), medullary carcinoma of the thyroid, and parathyroid hyperplasia. MEN type 3 is associated with medullary thyroid carcinoma, pheochromocytoma, and other features such as neuromas. These syndromes are often familial with a dominant transmission, but the basic pathogenesis is unknown.

ABNORMALITIES OF ENDOCRINE GLANDS NOT ASSOCIATED WITH HORMONAL IMBALANCE. Tumors, nodules, cysts, infiltrative diseases, and other abnormalities may involve endocrine glands without impairing their secretory functions significantly. For instance, nodules of the thyroid gland are common but usually nonfunctioning. The major problem is that malignancy may develop in them. Sometimes particular processes have a propensity for affecting an endocrine tissue. This is the case with tuberculosis and the adrenals.

CLINICAL ASSESSMENT OF ENDOCRINE STATUS

The assessment of the endocrine status of a patient relies on findings from the history and physical examination and on laboratory testing. The latter can involve measurements of levels of hormones or their metabolites in plasma or urine either in the basal state or in response to provocative testing. Laboratory tests may also be used to measure abnormalities that result from derangements in hormonal secretion and to evaluate the patient's sensitivity to hormones.

HISTORY AND PHYSICAL EXAMINATION. Many syndromes of hormonal excess or deficiency display manifestations that are readily apparent at the time of the initial presentation, e.g., severe thyrotoxicosis or Cushing's syndrome. In other instances, the clinical presentation can be more subtle and the physician must rely on laboratory testing to establish a diagnosis. This is especially true in the early stages of most endocrine problems, in elderly persons (e.g., with thyrotoxicosis or myxedema), or when the disease presents acutely and has not been present long enough for chronic manifestations to develop. Since it is beneficial to treat these diseases early, it is important for the physician to consider endocrine diseases in patients without full-blown manifestations, despite the fact that in the early stages of many of these disorders (e.g., adrenal insufficiency, hypothyroidism, Cushing's syndrome, hyperparathyroidism) the presenting symptoms and signs are sufficiently vague to suggest more common problems. Thus, endocrine diseases should be considered in the differential diagnosis of many common problems, such as weakness, tiredness, vague gastrointestinal discomfort, hypertension, or weight loss or gain. Once the diagnosis is considered, it is usually relatively easy to establish whether or not the disorder is present. Since endocrine diseases can be caused by primary processes external to the endocrine systems, the physician should consider these in taking the history and performing the physical examination. Sometimes, the primary process (e.g., carcinoma of the lung producing ACTH, tuberculosis causing adrenal insufficiency) will dominate the clinical presentation such that hormonal abnormalities are more difficult to detect clinically.

LABORATORY TESTING. *Hormone Levels.* Over the past few decades, assays have been developed to measure the levels of most of the hormones in body fluids. These vary in the ease with which they can be performed and their overall reliability; some assays are generally available, whereas others are performed only in certain research institutions.

RADIOIMMUNOASSAY. The advent of radioimmunoassay, first developed for measuring plasma insulin levels, was a major breakthrough in endocrinology. Antibodies that are relatively specific for certain chemical groups or conformations on the hormone can be developed for the polypeptide hormones and also for the smaller ligands such as thyroid and steroid hormones. The success of the assay depends on the specificity of the antibody as well as its affinity for binding the hormone.

In the radioimmunoassay, the plasma or urine sample or an extract of it is incubated with the antibody to the hormone along with a tracer of radiolabeled hormone. Then the antibody-tracer complexes are quantified in a variety of ways. For instance, charcoal can be used to adsorb and thereby remove the hormone that is not bound by the antibody, and the remaining radiolabeled hormone–antibody complexes can then be assessed. The extent to which the hormones in the sample block the binding of the radiolabeled hormone by the antibody is then related to a standard curve prepared from reactions in which known quantities of the hormone are present to yield the concentration of the hormone in the sample.

In most cases, radioimmunoassay yields extremely accurate information. However, there are problems that the physician should consider in interpreting the results. The antibody may cross-react with related hormones or with precursors or metabolites of the hormone. If these compounds are present in sufficient concentration, they can give spuriously high values. For instance, some antibodies are specific for the carboxyterminal portion of PTH. This part of the molecule is present in certain circulating fragments of PTH that are biologically inactive. This is especially true in chronic renal disease, in which PTH levels by radioimmunoassay are extremely high. This problem can be obviated by the use of antibodies that are specific for other parts of the PTH molecule (see Ch. 246).

COMPETITIVE PROTEIN-BINDING AND RADIORECEPTOR ASSAYS. These assays depend on the availability of a protein that binds the hormone with high affinity and specificity. The protein can be the normal receptor for the hormone, or it can be another protein, usually a plasma hormone–binding protein (CBG, TBG, sex hormone–binding globulin [SHBG]). The assay is performed in a manner analogous to that of the radioimmunoassay.

These assays provide an indication of summed products of the affinities times the concentrations of all compounds in the sample that bind to the protein. Typically, however, only one hormone accounts for most or all of the activity that is present. Radioreceptor assays are not widely used currently, in part because it is difficult to work with receptor preparations. By contrast, several competitive protein-binding assays have come into general use. Noteworthy are the CBG-isotope and TBG assays for cortisol and thyroxine, respectively, that depend on the fact that the major chemical species in plasma that binds to CBG is cortisol and to TBG is thyroxine.

CHEMICAL ASSAYS. Many hormones can be assayed by chemical means. For example, the fluorimetric assay for cortisol depends on the fluorescence of steroids with Δ^4-3-ketone, 20-ketone, and 11β- and 21-hydroxyl groups. Ordinarily, cortisol is the only steroid present in the circulation at sufficient concentration to react significantly in this way, although in certain congenital adrenal biosynthetic defects and adrenal carcinomas, other steroids produced can contribute substantially to the assay results.

HIGH-PERFORMANCE LIQUID CHROMATOGRAPHY (HPLC). The development of more sophisticated HPLC techniques has increased their capability for routine measurements. Although these methods are not commonly used for hormone measurements, they will probably be used increasingly for the measurement of smaller molecules such as steroids, catecholamines, and small peptides.

LEVELS OF FREE HORMONE. Free hormone, rather than that which is protein bound, is usually the best index of its effective concentration in plasma. The problems with assessment of total hormone concentrations due to potential variations in the concentrations of plasma steroid and thyroid hormone–binding proteins have been emphasized earlier in this chapter.

Levels of free hormone can be assessed in several ways: (1) The free hormone can be physically separated from that which is plasma bound and measured directly, although these methods have not yet come into general use. (2) The plasma concentration of the binding protein can be measured directly. Again this approach has not been applied widely. (3) The saturation of the binding protein can be assessed. When plasma levels of binding proteins are high, the protein will be undersaturated and less of the total hormone is free, whereas the converse occurs when plasma levels are low. This approach is now used in the case of TBG. Thus, the T_3 uptake assay measures the capacity in plasma for T_3 binding, which mostly reflects the extent of saturation of TBG. By combining knowledge of the total T_4 levels with the extent of saturation of TBG, a reasonable estimate of the effective plasma hormone concentration can be obtained (see Ch. 228). (4) An index of the free hormone concentration can sometimes be obtained by measuring its urinary excretion (or that of one of its metabolites). For instance, a small fraction (less than 1 per cent) of the secreted cortisol is excreted unchanged into the urine. A measurement of the 24-hour urine free cortisol usually provides a reasonable estimate of the integrated levels of free plasma hormone. In essence this method uses the glomerular basement membrane to separate hormone that is bound from that which is free.

SECRETION AND PRODUCTION RATES. Hormone production can be assessed by more complicated assays that involve either the injection of radioactive tracers or a combined assessment of plasma levels and hormone excretion. These techniques can circumvent many of the problems in interpretation associated with sole measurements of plasma or urinary hormones. Unfortunately, these procedures are cumbersome and not generally available.

SELECTIVE SAMPLING. Sometimes more accurate indications of a hormone-excess state and the site of hormone hypersecretion can be obtained by assaying the venous effluent from a given gland or organ. For example, in renovascular hypertension, peripheral renin levels may be normal, but sampling from a catheter inserted into the renal veins may reveal renin hypersecretion from one side and hyposecretion from the other side. Pituitary venous effluent sampling from the petrosal sinuses can be useful to determine whether ACTH hypersecretion results from a pituitary adenoma or from ectopic sites.

CLINICAL INTERPRETATION. With marked hormone excess or deficiency states, plasma or urinary hormone measurements commonly provide a clear indication of the abnormality. Nevertheless, it is important to be aware of the limitations of such tests. Hormone levels increase and decrease owing to physiologic stimuli, the presence of which must be considered when evaluating the significance of a hormone determination. For instance, plasma insulin levels should be evaluated in relation to the plasma glucose concentration, and PTH levels should be considered in relation to the serum calcium levels. Basal hormone secretion may not reflect the functional capacity of the gland, as considered in more detail under Dynamic Testing, below. Hormone levels should be evaluated in relation to target cell sensitivity. For example, in maturity onset diabetes of the obese, plasma insulin levels are often elevated but may still be inappropriately low in view of the associated insulin resistance. Since the release of many hormones is not constant, random readings can be particularly misleading. Cortisol, for example, is released episodically. In Cushing's syndrome the number of these releases is increased. Although this commonly results in an elevation of the plasma cortisol throughout the day, the morning plasma levels of this steroid may be normal. Since cortisol production integrated over a 24-hour period is increased in Cushing's syndrome, the 24-hour urine free cortisol will provide a more accurate index of whether there is cortisol hypersecretion.

Although urinary measurements can sometimes be more useful than plasma assays for obtaining an integrated assessment of the production of certain hormones (especially steroids), they cannot be used in this way for other hormones (e.g., thyroid hormones) whose metabolites are not predominantly secreted into the urine. Further, urinary metabolites of steroids can sometimes be derived from several sources (e.g., 17-ketosteroids from the adrenal and gonads), and hormone excretion can be influenced by changes in renal function. There are also circumstances in which the quantities of metabolites (e.g., of aldosterone) can be primarily affected by factors that do not affect the production of the hormone.

Sometimes the significance of hormone levels can be evaluated only by the simultaneous measurement of more than one hormone. For instance, with progressive damage to the thyroid gland and impaired release of thyroid hormones, secretion of TSH increases in a compensatory fashion such that normal plasma levels of the thyroid hormones may be maintained. By simultaneously measuring thyroid hormone levels and TSH, an indication of the compensatory response can be obtained. Such a simultaneous assessment of linked hormones can also provide an indication of the site of a primary defect. Plasma estrogens are low in ovarian failure. If ovarian failure is due to disease of the ovary, plasma gonadotropins will be elevated. If ovarian failure is secondary to pituitary or hypothalamic disease, plasma gonadotropin levels will be decreased.

Dynamic Testing. Provocative testing assesses the ability of a gland to respond to stimuli as an index of its reserve capacity. This is especially useful when plasma or urinary hormone measurements are borderline. It can also yield information about the site of the endocrine defect. In some cases, a hormone is given that stimulates the release of another hormone(s). For example, the administration of gonadotropin releasing hormone (GnRH) stimulates LH and FSH release, and TRH stimulates TSH and prolactin release. In other cases hormone production is blocked to interrupt normal feedback inhibition. Metyrapone blocks cortisol production by inhibiting 11β-hydroxylation, thereby stimulating ACTH release. The elevated ACTH levels increase the release of adrenal steroids proximal to the block (e.g., 11-deoxycortisol). A normal increase in 11-deoxycortisol signifies not only a normal adrenal but also a normal hypothalamic-pituitary axis. Sometimes a physiologic stimulus to hormone release is given. Insulin-induced hypoglycemia is used to assess the ability of cells that produce ACTH and growth hormone to respond. With endocrine hyperfunction, provocative tests can assess the extent to which the normal physiologic mechanisms that control hormone release are suppressed or the degree of autonomy of the hormone-producing tumor or hyperplastic gland. In primary aldosteronism resulting from an aldosterone-producing adenoma, the plasma renin levels that are suppressed by excessive sodium retention will not rise with acute postural, salt restriction, or diuretic stimuli. In Cushing's syndrome resulting from ectopic secretion of ACTH by a tumor, the glucocorticoid dexamethasone will not ordinarily suppress the elevated ACTH levels.

Tests That Provide Indirect Information. Useful information can frequently be obtained from laboratory tests that provide an index of the actions of the hormones (or a lack of them) or else an indication of the primary process causing the endocrine disease. Thus, it is helpful to follow the blood sugar levels in diabetes, the serum calcium levels in hyperparathyroidism, and the serum potassium levels in primary aldosteronism. Such tests often provide indices of the severity of the condition even more important than the hormone level. In conditions in which immunologic processes are important, assessment of antibody levels can be particularly helpful. Other tests provide information that is more of a corroborative nature, but which nonetheless can be useful. For instance, the serum sodium is almost always greater than 139 mEq per liter in patients with an aldosterone-producing adenoma; the plasma cholesterol tends to be high in hypothyroidism and low in hyperthyroidism; the serum potassium tends to be high in Addison's disease; the alkaline phosphatase tends to be elevated in osteomalacia; and the serum phosphate levels tend to be elevated in acromegaly.

Evaluation of the Sensitivity of Target Cells to Hormones. Suspicion of hyposensitivity to a hormone is raised when manifestations of deficiency of the hormone occur in the presence of elevated hormone levels. In type II diabetes mellitus there is hyperglycemia with hyperinsulinism; in pseudohypoparathyroidism, hypocalcemia and symptoms resulting from this with elevated PTH levels; and in pseudohermaphroditism caused by the testicular feminization syndrome, decreased androgenicity with elevated plasma testosterone levels. The existence of hyposensitivity can be confirmed by administering the hormone in question and determining the presence or extent of response, although commonly it is not necessary to do this. In some cases, such as with insulin or androgen resistance, it is possible to obtain further confirmation of the hyposensitivity state by isolating cells from the patient and measuring receptors or responses, although these techniques are not generally available. Conversely, hypersensitivity to hormones is characterized by low hormone levels relative to the response. In low-renin "essential" hypertension the adrenal glomerulosa is excessively sensitive to angiotensin II. This is reflected by normal to elevated plasma aldosterone levels in the presence of low angiotensin II levels. This sensitivity can be documented by measuring the plasma aldosterone levels following an infusion of angiotensin.

TREATMENT OF ENDOCRINE DISEASES

For endocrine deficiency syndromes, hormones are generally administered to replace the deficiency. In general the hormone that is deficient is replaced. In some cases this is not possible or expedient, and other hormones are given that help compensate for the defect. For instance, vitamin D is given instead of PTH to treat hypoparathyroidism since it can increase the extracellular Ca^{++}. In cases in which hormone resistance is present, steps are taken when possible to alleviate this, as through diet restriction in diabetes.

In hormone-excess syndromes, a variety of approaches is used. Hyperfunctioning tumors are removed when possible, and sometimes hyperplastic glands are removed. In other cases drugs are given to block hormone production (propylthiouracil in thyrotoxicosis and bromocriptine for prolactin-producing adenomas). Antagonists such as spironolactone in primary aldosteronism due to hyperplasia can sometimes be useful.

For both excess and deficiency syndromes adjunctive therapy is frequently important. Thus multiple measures are used to treat the complicatons to diabetes mellitus, and patients with Addison's disease are cautioned to avoid stress.

SUMMARY

Endocrinology in the 1980's is an open-ended discipline for the study of molecule-mediated communication and response. New systems are still being elaborated (opioids, prostaglandins, leukotrienes, vitamin D, cell growth factors); older systems are increasingly being defined in molecular terms. In addition, the clinical abnormalities that occur are being understood and the means to evaluate them are being refined to allow more rational, accurate, and beneficial approaches to diagnosis and treatment. This introductory chapter has presented a general overview of this discipline as a background for the following chapters, which will be devoted to its specific components and the disorders that occur in human endocrine diseases.

Alberts B, Bray D, Lewis J, Raff M, Roberts K, Watson JD: Molecular Biology of the Cell. New York, Garland Publishing, Inc., 1983. *Reviews in detail recent advances in cell and molecular biology, including information on gene structure and function, protein synthesis, internalization, and hormone action.*

Cohen P: The role of protein phosphorylation in neural and hormonal control of cellular activity. Nature 296:613–620, 1982. *An overview of the role of phosphorylation in hormone action.*

Felig P, Baxter JD, Broadus AE, Frohman LA (eds.): Endocrinology and Metabolism. New York, McGraw-Hill Book Company, 1981. *Provides an extensive analysis of the topics included in this chapter. The chapters by Vaitukaitis on hormone assays, by Habner on hormone biosynthesis and secretion, and by Catt and Dufau on hormone action provide much detailed information.*

Ganong WF: The brain as an endocrine organ. Acta Physiol Lat Am 32:31–44, 1982. *Provides an excellent discussion of neuroendocrine relationships.*

Greenspan FS, Forsham PH (eds.): Basic and Clinical Endocrinology. Los Altos, Lange Medical Publications, 1983. *An excellent general reference on endocrinology and metabolism.*

Hopkins CR: The importance of the endosome in intracellular traffic. Nature 304:684–685, 1983. *A concise update of the events in hormone and receptor internalization, recycling, and degradation.*

Karin M, Haslinger A, Holtgreve H, Cathala G, Slater E, Baxter JD: Activation of a heterologous promoter in response to dexamethasone and cadmium by metallothionein gene 5′-flanking DNA. Cell 36:371–379, 1984. *Discusses recent advances in understanding the mechanisms of steroid receptor function.*

Lieberman S, Greenfield NJ, Wolfson A: A heuristic proposal for understanding steroidogenetic processes. Endocr Rev 5:128–148, 1984. *A comprehensive account of the mechanisms of steroid biosynthesis.*

Verhoven GFM, Wilson JD: The syndromes of primary hormone resistance. Metabolism 28:253, 1979. *An extensive discussion of the problems of hyposensitivity to hormones and of the clinical approaches to the diagnosis of these disorders.*

Williams RH (ed.): Textbook of Endocrinology. 6th ed. Philadelphia, W. B. Saunders Company, 1981. *An excellent general reference on endocrinology and metabolism.*

222. ENDORPHINS, ENKEPHALINS, AND OTHER OPIOID PEPTIDES: THEIR SIGNIFICANCE IN PHYSIOLOGY AND MEDICINE

Roger Guillemin

INTRODUCTION. The word *endorphin,* from (end)ogenous and m(orphin)e, was originally coined to define peptides of brain origin with biologic activities similar to those of the alkaloids of opium (morphine). The word *enkephalin* (from the Greek roots for "inside the head") will be used exclusively to define two specific pentapeptides also with morphine-like activities. The word *dynorphin* (from the Greek dyna, power) refers to a family of peptides with unusually potent opiate-like activity. The necessity and significance of this nomenclature will become evident as this chapter unfolds. All these substances are also referred to as *endogenous opioid peptides.*

The hypothesis that there should be *endogenous* opioid peptides involved in the normal biochemistry and physiology of the brain evolved from the pharmacologic concept of opiate receptors in the brain. In the early 1970's, the alkaloids of opium were shown to bind specifically to so-called opiate receptors, which have the following characteristics: (1) they are protein molecules on synaptosomes from various parts of the brain; (2) binding of the opiate molecules on these receptors is stereospecific; i.e., only those stereoisomers of the opiate series that have biologic (analgesic) activity bind to the receptor; (3) the binding of the opiates is competed for by synthetic analogue antagonists such as naloxone or naltrexone; and (4) opiate receptors exist in higher concentrations in those regions of the brain where opiates are known to exert their biologic effects as analgesic agents. It seemed clear in this early conceptualization that these opiate receptors in the brain of vertebrates did not exist solely for the binding of the alkaloids of opium. It seemed more likely that they served to recognize and bind endogenous molecules, with or without structural similarities to the opiate alkaloids, which would normally be involved in the control of pain in the central nervous system. In early studies such endogenous molecules, peptidic in nature, could indeed be demonstrated in crude extracts of the brain. The original characterization of the endogenous opioid peptides did not use the receptor affinity as an assay system, but a simple pharmacologic bioassay. It had been known for years that opiate alkaloids could affect the electrically induced contraction of the smooth muscles of thin strips of guinea pig ileum (or of mouse vas deferens) kept in a simple in vitro perfusion system, and that synthetic analogues of some of these opiate alkaloids were active in this in vitro system as antagonists in roughly the same ratios as they were antagonists of the in vivo analgesic effects of opiates. In 1975, two groups, taking advantage of such simple bioassays, isolated and characterized the first endogenous opioid peptides from brain extracts and pituitary extracts. From extracts of porcine brains, Hughes, Kosterlitz, and their colleagues characterized two pentapeptides, differing by only one amino acid at the C-terminus, and which were called Met^5-enkephalin and Leu^5-enkephalin. From extracts of the neurohypophysis plus hypothalamus, Ling, Burgus, and I characterized a hexadecapeptide which was called α-endorphin, labeled α since there was evidence in the last stages of purification that several peptides with opiate-like activity were present and would eventually have to be characterized. The remarkable observation was made that the complete amino acid sequence of the pentapeptide Met^5-enkephalin was contained as the N-terminal pentapeptide of the amino acid sequence of α-endorphin. Perhaps even more remarkably, both Met^5-enkephalin and α-endorphin were found to be fragments of *β-lipotropin,* a larger 91 amino acid polypeptide which had been found in extracts of the pituitary gland by C. H. Li and collaborators in 1964. No major biologic activity had ever been found for β-lipotropin except for a minor fat-mobilizing effect in some in vitro systems, from which its name was derived. An extraordinary flurry of excitement followed these early reports. It became very rapidly obvious that a series of fragments of the 61–91 C-terminal region of β-lipotropin would show opiate-like activity in the in vitro system and also in binding assays to synaptosomes. The most potent of all of these peptides, on a molar basis, was shown to be the complete 61–91 peptide, which had been isolated from pituitary extracts and named *β-endorphin* by C. H. Li. Figure 222–1 shows the amino acid sequences of the various endorphins which have been isolated and characterized as α, β, γ, and δ, all related fragments of the C-terminal region of β-lipotropin.

BIOSYNTHESIS. *Endorphins* are located in all cells of the intermediate lobe of the pituitary gland and also in scattered cells of the adenohypophysis, as shown by immunocytochemical techniques. These same regions also contain ACTH and β-lipotropin. It is now known that the endorphins, β-lipotropin, and ACTH are synthesized as parts of a common larger glycoprotein prohormone with a molecular weight of approximately 31,000 daltons for which a complete amino acid sequence has been proposed from DNA-recombinant studies. There is now satisfactory evidence that all endorphins are actually part of this biosynthetic pathway and that they are enzymatically processed in the pituitary cells from that common precursor (Fig. 222–1).

Immunocytochemistry (Fig. 222–2*A*) and early biochemistry have shown that endorphins are also present in some neurons in a well-defined system of the brain; their biosynthesis in

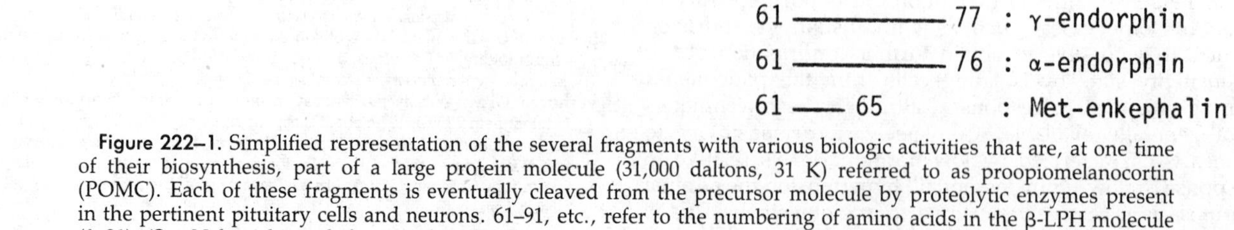

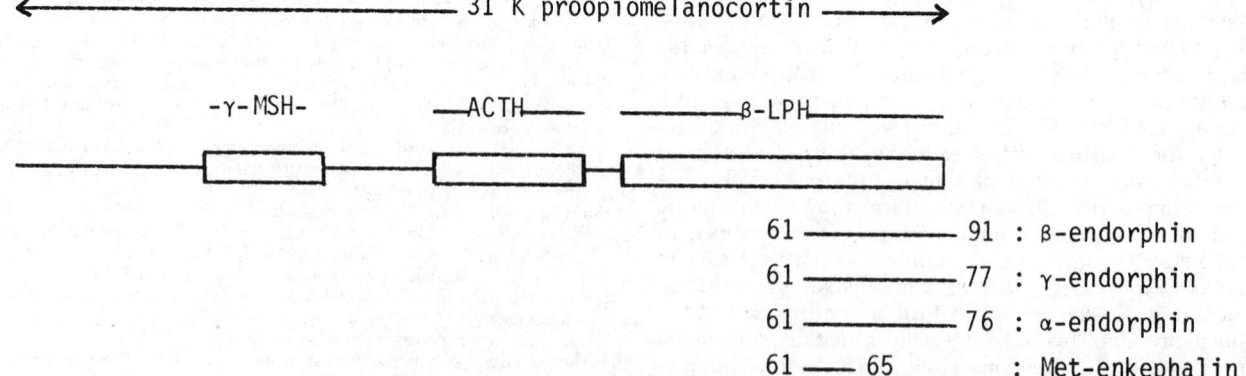

Figure 222–1. Simplified representation of the several fragments with various biologic activities that are, at one time of their biosynthesis, part of a large protein molecule (31,000 daltons, 31 K) referred to as proopiomelanocortin (POMC). Each of these fragments is eventually cleaved from the precursor molecule by proteolytic enzymes present in the pertinent pituitary cells and neurons. 61–91, etc., refer to the numbering of amino acids in the β-LPH molecule (1–91). (See Nakanishi et al. for complete details.)

these neurons is known to be identical to that in the cells of the intermediate lobe of the pituitary.

ENKEPHALINS. The biosynthetic pathway for the enkephalins is totally different. It was originally assumed that the pentapeptide enkephalins would come from the larger endorphins by enzymatic cleavage. The first evidence that enkephalins and endorphins come from different biosynthetic pathways was suggested from immunocytochemical studies showing that immunoreactive β-endorphin and enkephalins have a vastly different anatomic distribution in the brain. Further discrepancies in the biosynthetic pathways for the endorphins and the enkephalins have become evident. Immunoreactive enkephalins, not endorphins, have been observed in the gut and the adrenal medulla, in addition to the locations in the brain and spinal cord mentioned above (Fig. 222–2*B*). The adrenal medulla in particular contains several polypeptides of molecular weights ranging from 5,000 to 25,000 daltons and which, from partial amino acid sequencing, contain one or several replicates of the amino acid sequences of both Met^5-enkephalin and Leu^5-enkephalin. The enkephalin sequences in the large adrenomedullary polypeptides are usually found between pairs of basic amino acids, such as Arg-Arg or Lys-Arg, which are now recognized as the hallmark of enzymatic processing by intracellular enzymes, as in the case of proinsulin to insulin, proopiomelanocortin to ACTH, β-lipotropin, β-endorphin, etc. Moreover, several groups have now shown the presence of small peptides containing the sequence of one of the enkephalins preceded and/or followed by amino acid sequences with no relation to those of β-lipotropin. Such is the case for the recently characterized peptides *α-neoendorphin* and *dynorphin*, both of which, particularly dynorphin, appear to be endowed with extremely high opiate-like activity. They are several times more potent than β-endorphin on a molar basis, which is itself 10 to 100 times more potent than morphine on a molar basis, depending on the type of assay used. The complete nucleotide sequence of the cDNA coding for the precursor protein of each of these opioid peptides has now been established from cloning mRNA of either adrenal medulla or brain origin.

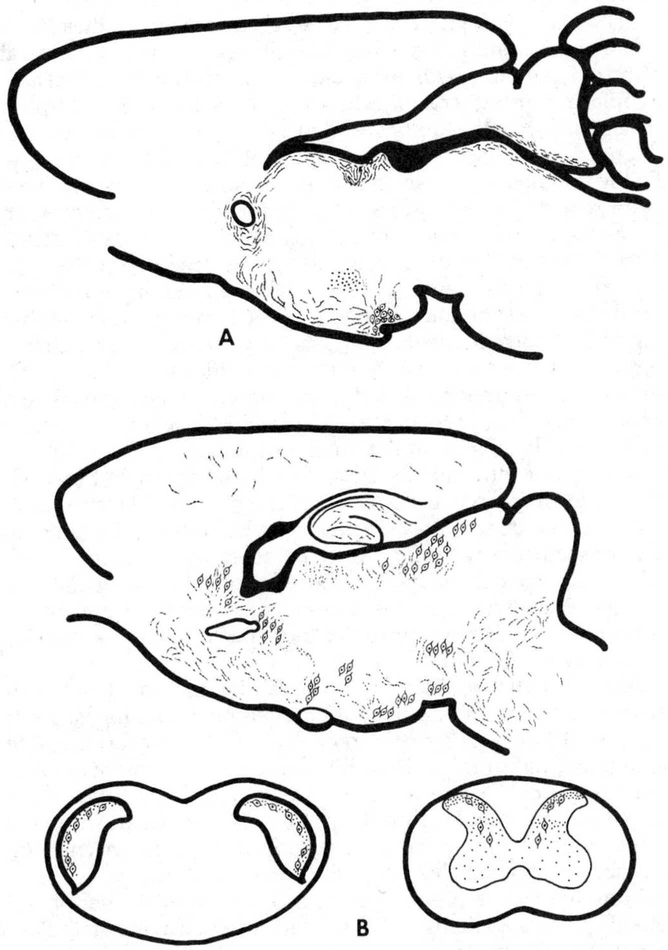

Figure 222–2. *A*, Schematic sagittal view of β-endorphin-reactive neurons and fibers in the rat brain. The neuronal perikarya in the basal hypothalamic region give rise to fibers that sweep forward along the routes indicated to enter the preoptic area and then to course within the periaqueductal region of the diencephalon and pons. *B*, Diagram of the distribution of enkephalin-containing neurons and fibers (sagittal section of the rat brain). Note also the presence of enkephalin-containing neurons in mid-brain and spinal cord.

MAPPING OF RECEPTORS FOR THE OPIOID PEPTIDES. Assays based on competition of displacement of tritiated ligands, such as tritiated morphine or normorphine, have permitted the mapping of opiate receptors in the central nervous system and other organs, while radioimmunoassays are being used to measure quantitatively the endogenous opioid peptides. Receptors for endogenous opioid peptides are mostly present in those anatomic areas of the central nervous system in which opiates have been known to exert their biologic activity as analgesic agents. These same regions correspond to those with the highest concentrations of immunoreactive endorphins or enkephalins.

Opiate receptors, as well as opioid peptides, have been found primarily in (1) the ventral hypothalamus, which is known to integrate visceral pain, a type which responds best to opiates; (2) the substantia gelatinosa of the spinal cord, also known to participate in the transmission of sensory inputs (only enkephalins, not β-endorphin, are found in the spinal cord); (3) the mid-brain nuclei corresponding to the vagus and glossopharyngeal nerves—these are known to be involved in the coughing reflex and gastric motility and secretion, events known to be affected by opiates (enkephalins and dynorphin are reported to be present in these nuclei); (4) the amygdala of the limbic system, where opiate receptors are located on nerve endings (immunocytochemistry shows the presence of β-endorphin on these nerve endings, but not in any neurons—an anatomic distribution which may be related to the participation of the limbic system in emotional behavior); and (5) the area postrema of the fourth ventricle and the periaqueductal gray matter, two regions in which electrical stimulation as well as stereotaxic placement of opiates will produce, respectively, nausea or relief from visceral pain, or both. There are also opiate receptors in the gut, and likely in the endocrine pancreas. Binding of endorphins has also been reported for some leukocytes.

In the pituitary gland the neural lobe has opiate receptors; it does not contain endorphins but appears to contain enkephalins, whereas endorphins are found in the pars intermedia and the anterior lobe, as pointed out above. The presence of opiate receptors and enkephalins in the neural lobe has been related to an enkephalinergic mechanism involved in the control of vasopressin (antidiuretic hormone) secretion.

PHYSIOLOGIC AND PATHOPHYSIOLOGIC EFFECTS OF THE OPIOID PEPTIDES. Peripheral injection of relatively high doses of enkephalins (up to 1 mg per 100 grams of body weight in laboratory animals) produces practically no observable systemic effect. This is best explained by the very short half-life of the enkephalins (a matter of seconds), owing to enzymatic degradation. A specific *enkephalinase* has been isolated and characterized. Similarly, peripheral injection of large amounts of synthetic β-endorphin does not lead to any obvious major effects in terms of analgesia. This is best explained by proposing that β-endorphin does not readily cross the blood-brain barrier, although it appears to have a rather long half-life (up to 30 minutes). Following peripheral administration of β-endorphin, there is evidence of decreased motility of the gut, with slowing of the gut transit. β-Endorphin also acutely releases growth hormone, as well as prolactin and antidiuretic hormone, probably by acting at the level of the median eminence, which is somewhat outside the blood-brain barrier. The effects on the secretion of growth hormone, prolactin, and antidiuretic hormone are not directly at the level of pituitary tissues, since β-endorphin has no such activity when added to pituitary tissues in in vitro systems.

The injection of β-endorphin directly into the cerebrospinal fluid, bypassing the blood-brain barrier (e.g., as by injection into the cisterna magna, or the lateral or third ventricle of the brain), produces far more striking biologic effects. In nanomolar quantities β-endorphin will produce, in laboratory animals, profound and complete analgesia lasting for several hours, depending on the dose administered. In rodents (rats, mice, rabbits), but not in monkeys, the same doses of β-endorphin produce an unusual state of rigid muscular immobility highly reminiscent of the clinical syndrome of catatonia. Laboratory animals also show profound hypothermia after a central administration of β-endorphin. All these effects are removed in a matter of seconds following the intravenous administration of an opiate antagonist such as naloxone. When injected intrathecally, enkephalins produce minor analgesia which is not as marked as that produced by β-endorphin and is of very short duration. The enkephalins behave more like true synaptic transmitters, which can be promptly inactivated by enzymatic mechanisms. There is no evidence of a reuptake mechanism by neurons of either enkephalins or endorphins.

SECRETION BY THE PITUITARY. β-Endorphin is secreted by the adenohypophysis simultaneously with ACTH and roughly in equimolar ratios in all acute or chronic circumstances, such as stress, which have been known to be accompanied by the classic pituitary and adrenal secretions of ACTH and glucocorticoids. This is of course best explained by the evidence presented above of the common precursor of biosynthetic origin for β-endorphin and ACTH (Fig. 222–1). Pituitary secretory granules have been shown to contain both endorphins and corticotropin, and all stimuli or secretagogues, including the hypothalamic releasing factor CRF (corticotropin-releasing factor), known to stimulate the secretion of ACTH in vivo or in vitro have been shown also to stimulate the concomitant secretion of β-endorphin. This holds true also for perturbations in the adrenal-pituitary feedback system: adrenalectomy is accompanied by chronic elevation of plasma levels of ACTH and β-endorphin, whereas acute or chronic administration of a glucocorticoid such as dexamethasone will suppress the plasma concentrations of ACTH and β-endorphin. It is of course tempting to propose, on that basis, some sort of unified theory of pituitary involvement in response to acute stress—ACTH and glucocorticoids being involved in the metabolic, somatic, stress-induced response, and the endorphins being involved with the response of the central nervous system to painful or emotionally disturbing stimuli. This would explain the age-old observation of nonresponse to, or lack of awareness of, painful stimuli at times of acute stress or emergency. If this is the case, we have to assume that pituitary endorphins, secreted during stress, somehow pass directly into the central nervous system, since intravenous injection of large amounts of synthetic β-endorphin produces no evidence of major analgesia. Pituitary endorphins could enter the third ventricle by upward flow in the hypothalamohypophyseal portal vessels. The matter is far from being settled.

In animal studies relatively small concentrations of β-endorphin injected directly into the arterial circulation of the pancreas stimulate the secretion of insulin and glucagon and concomitantly inhibit the secretion of somatostatin. These results must be mediated by opiate receptors, since they are sensitive to the administration of the antagonist naloxone.

The enkephalins are probably true neurotransmitters, particularly in the afferent systems for pain in the spinal cord. Evidence for this role is based on their size, the short duration of their biologic activity, and their location, as observed by refined immunocytochemistry. The role of the endorphins in the brain appears to be far more complex. The long duration of the effects of a single administration of β-endorphin in the central nervous system is completely different from the brief effects of classic synaptic transmitters, and is reminiscent of the role and effects of hormones.

An important question for pharmacologists, physiologists, and clinicians has been whether chronic administration of β-endorphin and/or enkephalins would lead to tolerance regarding their analgesic effects as well as to addiction, in analogy with the opiate alkaloids. The biologic half-life of the enkephalins is so short and their specific activity so limited that the question has little significance in their case. In the case of β-endorphin, which is far more potent on a molar basis than the enkephalins (approximately 100-fold), the original question must be modified by the additional requisite that it pertain to β-endorphin injected directly into the brain tissue or into cerebrospinal fluid. Studies both in laboratory animals and in a few clinical cases in which β-endorphin was injected intravenously have led to no reliable results, most likely because of the fact that β-endorphin does not readily cross the blood-brain barrier. When β-endorphin is injected repeatedly every 24 hours into the cisterna of laboratory rats for as long as ten days, there is no obvious decrease in the profound analgesic activity of the same dose of the peptide. This would imply that tolerance to the analgesic effect of endorphin, when it is injected into the cerebrospinal fluid in these relatively short studies, is absent or minimal. Reports are conflicting regarding addiction of laboratory animals to chronic doses of β-endorphin.

CLINICAL STUDIES. There have been a few studies with endorphins administered intrathecally in patients. In several hundred patients with intractable pain caused by metastatic neoplasms, intrathecal injection of 1 to 3 mg of β-endorphin (by spinal tap in the lumbar region) led in all cases to remarkable degrees of analgesia in the absence of any additive therapy. Following one of these intrathecal injections, patients have been reported as being free of pain for up to five days, with an average effectiveness of approximately 72 hours. Patients injected up to five times with the same dose of synthetic β-endorphin by the same spinal intrathecal route have reported no decrease of the pain-relieving effect of the peptide. With 3 mg of β-endorphin injected intrathecally, several of the patients reported a sense of euphoria. It is difficult to distinguish whether this euphoria was due to complete relief from severe and chronic pain or to a true euphorigenic effect of the peptide that would be similar to the "high" of opiates.

In cases of intractable pain caused by disseminated carcinomas, neurosurgeons have occasionally implanted electrodes in the periaqueductal gray matter which, upon delivering an electrical current with the proper parameters, will relieve pain, usually for up to 24 hours. It has been shown that such effective central electric analgesia is accompanied by elevation of the concentration of immunoreactive β-endorphin in the ventricular cerebrospinal fluid.

Some diabetics receiving chlorpropamide therapy develop an acute and intense facial flush after even moderate ingestion of alcohol. It has recently been reported that the powerful opiate antagonist naloxone will inhibit or prevent this vascular reaction. Also some synthetic analogues of enkephalin which are active peripherally will produce the typical facial flush in the same subjects. It appears that an enkephalinergic mechanism may be involved in this particular clinical feature.

Immunoreactive β-endorphin has been found in peripheral blood of some patients with pituitary tumors, with medullary carcinoma of the thyroid, or with oat-cell carcinomas of the lung. In all cases the immunoreactive β-endorphin was detected along with immunoreactive ACTH and usually other peptides, such as calcitonin or somatostatin. It has been proposed that the measurement of plasma immunoreactive β-endorphin could serve as a marker of the presence of neoplastic tissues.

There have been reports that peripheral administration of β-endorphin in large amounts (milligrams) has led to dramatic improvements in psychiatric patients with schizophrenia or manic-depressive psychosis. These reports, occasionally marked by sensationalism, have not been confirmed by other investigators. First of all, as noted above, β-endorphin given peripherally enters the central nervous system to a very limited degree, if at all. Furthermore, the experimental administration of the powerful opiate antagonist naloxone, which readily passes into the central nervous system, has led to conflicting reported results in schizophrenia. There have also been reports that levels of immunoreactive endorphins in the cerebrospinal fluid of schizophrenics in acute exacerbation or remission phases vary in relation to the clinical status.

None of these provocative and preliminary observations has led to any consensus. There are first of all major methodologic problems; there are also major problems in the clinical interpretations. The concept, however, that molecules such as the opioid peptides could be involved in the maintenance of normal behavior and that alterations in the normal metabolism of these opioid peptides could be accompanied by abnormalities in behavior is of such heuristic significance that it should not be discarded on the basis of preliminary conflicting evidence. One of the major requisites for such studies will, in my opinion, be a much larger number and variety of studies in man than have actually been available so far.

CONCLUSIONS. There is little doubt that endogenous opioid peptides are involved in the normal neurophysiologic processing of painful stimuli, particularly those known to be processed by the visceral system. It is possible that endorphins and/or enkephalins are involved in the normal processing of other sensory stimuli: immunoreactive enkephalins have recently been reported in some amacrine cells of the retina, and immunoreactive endorphins have been measured in extracts of peripheral nerves such as the vagus or the sciatic nerve. The role, if any, of endorphins of pituitary origin is not clear and remains to be investigated further.

Proposed roles of the brain endorphins in the central nervous system biochemistry of normal, hence also abnormal, behavior remain to be demonstrated. Interrelationships between the opioid peptides and the classic neurotransmitters (acetylcholine, dopamine, catecholamines) are just beginning to be explored. There is no dearth of working hypotheses, many of profound heuristic significance, to approach and carry out these studies.

Bloom F, Battenberg E, Rossier J, Ling N, Guillemin R: Neurons containing β-endorphin in rat brain exist separately from those containing enkephalin: Immunocytochemical studies. Proc Natl Acad Sci (USA) 75:1591, 1978. *Immunocytochemistry with the peroxidase method using antisera against β-endorphin and enkephalin, with several plates.*

Bradbury AF, Smith DG, Snell CR, Birdsall NJM, Hulme EC: C-fragment of lipotropin has a high affinity for brain opiate receptors. Nature 260:793, 1976. *Technical report on the opiate-like activity, assessed by binding to synaptosomes, of the C-terminal fragment 61–91 of the ovine pituitary β-lipotropin.*

Goldstein A: Opioid peptides (endorphins) in the pituitary and brain. Science 193:1081, 1976. *A general review by one of the earliest pharmacologists to have proposed the existence of specific opiate receptors. Covers that concept and the recent isolation of enkephalins and endorphins.*

Gubler U, Seeburg P, Hoffman BJ, Gage LP, Udenfriend S: Molecular cloning establishes proenkephalin as precursor of enkephalin-containing peptides. Nature 295:206, 1982. *The complete primary structure of the precursor protein for both Met- and Leu-enkephalins deduced from the nucleotide sequence of the corresponding cDNA of bovine adrenal origin.*

Hökfelt T, Johansson O, Ljungdahl A, Lundberg M, Schultsberg M: Peptidergic neurones. Nature 284:515, 1980. *An elegant and comprehensive review by one of the best groups of immunocytologists in the world. Includes discussions of anatomic localizations, relations between various "networks" of peptides containing neurons, and relations with the classic catecholaminergic systems. Discusses peptidergic neurons in the brain, the spinal cord, the gastrointestinal tract, and other non-central nervous system locations.*

Hughes J, Smith T, Kosterlitz H, Fothergill L, Morgan B, Morris H: Identification of two related pentapeptides from the brain with potent opiate agonist activity. Nature 258:577, 1975. *The original technical report on the isolation and characterization (amino acid sequence) of the two enkephalins, with the statement about the relationship between their amino acid sequence and that of a region of pituitary β-lipotropin.*

Kakidani H, Furutani Y, Takahashi H, Noda M, Morimoto Y, Hirose T, Asai M, Inayama S, Numa S: Cloning and sequence analysis of cDNA for porcine β-neo-endorphin/dynorphin precursor. Nature 298:245, 1982. *A technical report describing how the primary structure of a precursor protein that contains β-neo-endorphin, dynorphin, and a third leu-enkephalin sequence with a carboxyl extension*

was deduced from the nucleotide sequence of cloned DNA to the porcine hypothalamic mRNA encoding it.

Leslie RDG, Pyke DA: Chlorpropamide-alcohol flushing: A dominantly inherited trait associated with diabetes. Br Med J 2:1519, 1978. *Case reports and proposal of the hypothesis.*

Lewis RV, Stern AS, Kimura S, Rossier J, Stein S, Udenfriend S: An about 50,000-dalton protein in adrenal medulla: A common precursor of [Met]- and [Leu]-enkephalin. Science 208:1459, 1980. *The first technical report on the presence in the adrenal medulla of a large protein (50,000 daltons), which, upon partial tryptic digestion, generates peptide-fragments with the (characterized) amino acid sequence of Met- and Leu-enkephalin, and also has opiate-like biologic activities.*

Li CH, Chung D: Isolation and structure of an untriakontapeptide with opiate activity from camel pituitary glands. Proc Natl Acad Sci (USA) 73:1145, 1976. *Technical report of the isolation and characterization (amino acid sequence) of a peptide from camel pituitary glands corresponding to the fragment 61–91 of β-lipotropin, with bioassay data showing its opiate-like activity.*

Ling N, Burgus R, Guillemin R: Isolation, primary structure and synthesis of α-endorphin and γ-endorphin, two peptides of hypothalamic-hypophysial origin with morphinomimetic activity. Proc Natl Acad Sci (USA) 73:3942, 1976. *The original technical report on the isolation and characterization (amino acid sequence) of the first two molecules of hypothalamic and pituitary origin, isolated on the basis of their opiate-like activity in a bioassay, and different from the enkephalins.*

Mains RE, Eipper BA, Ling N: Common precursor to corticotropins and endorphins. Proc Natl Acad Sci (USA) 74:3014, 1977. *The original technical description of the existence of multiple sizes of immunoreactive ACTH (adrenocorticotropin) and lipotropin, with the evidence that the largest molecule (31,000 daltons) is immunoreactive with both antisera to ACTH and lipotropin (more exactly β-endorphin) from a tumoral cell line of mouse pituitary origin.*

Nakanishi S, Inoue A, Kita T, Nakamura M, Chang ACY, Cohen SN, Numa S: Nucleotide sequence of cloned c-DNA for bovine corticotropin-β-lipotropin precursor. Nature 278:423, 1979. *The first report of the nucleotide sequence of cloned c-DNA for bovine corticotropin-β-lipotropin precursor, accompanied by the proposed amino acid sequence of the whole protein precursor (now called pro-opio-melano-cortin)—includes the proposal of the existence of a new form of melanotropin-γ-MSHs.*

223. PROSTAGLANDINS, THROMBOXANE A_2, AND LEUKOTRIENES

John A. Oates

Thromboxane A_2, prostacyclin, prostaglandin D_2, prostaglandin E_2, and the leukotrienes are potent compounds which participate in pathologic processes as diverse as platelet aggregation and asthma. They have in common a biosynthesis that originates with the oxygenation of arachidonic acid, but their structures and their actions differ markedly. Although there is considerable variety in the possible metabolic pathways for arachidonic acid within the body, specific cells are highly selective in the biotransformation of this fatty acid. This selectivity in arachidonic acid metabolism usually can be linked to a function of the cell.

THE CYCLOOXYGENASE PATHWAY (Fig. 223–1). The biotransformation of arachidonic acid into thromboxane A_2, prostacyclin, prostaglandin D_2, (PGD_2), PGE_2, and $PGF_{2\alpha}$ is initiated by a common enzyme, the *fatty acid cyclooxygenase* (Fig. 223–1). This enzyme catalyzes the attachment of molecular oxygen at C_{11} of arachidonic acid. There is subsequent rearrangement to a cyclic endoperoxide in which a dioxygen bridge links C_9 and C_{11}. The formation of the endoperoxide is closely coupled to the introduction of a second oxygen molecule at C_{15} to yield a 15-hydroperoxy cyclic endoperoxide (PGG_2). The subscript 2 in this and other prostaglandin nomenclature refers to the two double bonds in the structure. The cyclooxygenase enzyme is inhibited by aspirin, indomethacin, and the other nonsteroidal anti-inflammatory drugs (see Fig. 223–3). A hydroperoxidase converts the 15-hydroperoxy group of PGG_2 to a hydroxyl, yielding the 15-hydroxy-endoperoxide PGH_2 in a reaction that liberates a free radical as a byproduct. PGH_2 is the common precursor of PGD_2, PGE_2, $PGF_{2\alpha}$, thromboxane A_2, and prostacyclin (PGI_2). The enzymes which catalyze the metabolism of PGH_2 to these active products confer cellular specificity. PGH_2 is a labile intermediate which undergoes nonenzymatic breakdown in water. However, in cells which contain an appropriate

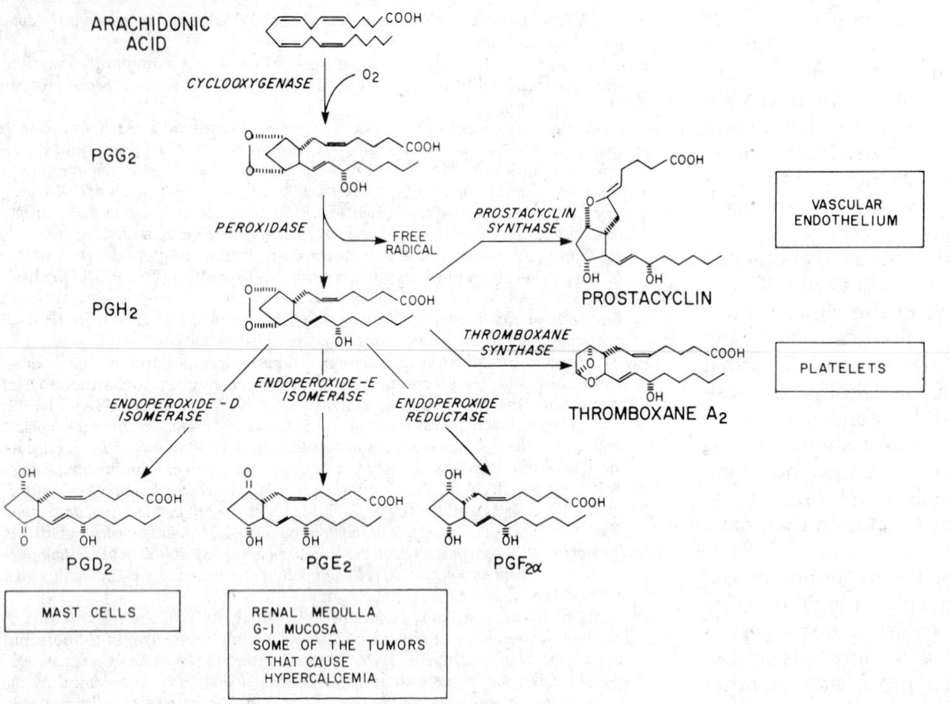

Figure 223–1. The cyclooxygenase pathway of arachidonic acid metabolism leading to the synthesis of prostaglandins.

enzyme for metabolizing PGH_2, it is rapidly converted to a specific prostaglandin, as noted below.

Thromboxane A_2. Thromboxane A_2 is the predominant product of arachidonic acid in the platelet and is formed from PGH_2 in a reaction catalyzed by thromboxane synthase (Fig. 223–1). Thromboxane A_2 is a potent aggregating agent which is released in a burst at the initiation of platelet aggregation (see Ch. 166). The inhibition of platelet aggregation by aspirin results from blockade of thromboxane A_2 biosynthesis. Thromboxane A_2 is quite labile, undergoing nonenzymatic hydrolysis to a relatively inactive product, thromboxane B_2, with a half-life of 30 seconds.

In addition to causing platelet aggregation, thromboxane A_2 contracts arterial smooth muscle, including that of the coronary and cerebral arteries.

Prostacyclin. Disruption of the vascular endothelium leads to the adherence of platelets, which release thromboxane A_2 locally to signal neighboring platelets to join in the aggregation process. Clearly some mechanism is required to restrain the further recruitment of platelets short of aggregation of the total body pool. One restraint that normal vascular endothelium imposes on the aggregation process is the release of prostacyclin, which is a potent inhibitor of aggregation. Prostacyclin is the essentially exclusive product of PGH_2 metabolism in the vascular endothelium and is produced in far smaller quantities by other cells, such as macrophages. It also is labile in aqueous solution, with a half-life of about three minutes, undergoing nonenzymatic degradation to 6-keto-$PGF_{1\alpha}$.

The inhibition of platelet aggregation by prostacyclin is accompanied by a marked rise in the concentration of cyclic AMP in the platelet. Current evidence suggests that this cyclic nucleotide mediates the inhibition of aggregation. Prostacyclin is a general inhibitor of platelet aggregation, blocking aggregation evoked by a variety of stimuli, including thrombin, ADP, and epinephrine. This is in contrast to cyclooxygenase inhibitors, such as aspirin, which inhibit the aggregation evoked by only a subset of specific stimuli. Thus, aspirin will block the aggregation evoked by collagen and will shift the dose response curve to ADP, but its effect is readily overridden by thrombin. Thrombin-induced aggregation can take place by a mechanism that is independent of thromboxane A_2.

The inhibition of aggregation by prostacyclin is illustrated by its ability to prevent almost completely the adhesion and aggregation of platelets in extracorporeal circuits such as pump oxygenators and hemodialysis units. In contrast, heparin and aspirin are relatively ineffective in preventing the trapping of platelets in extracorporeal circuits and the release of platelet aggregates from their surfaces. Prostacyclin also will prevent the formation of platelet aggregates evoked by vascular trauma or marked vascular stenosis.

In addition to inhibiting platelet aggregation, prostacyclin is a vasodilator. Its actions on platelets as well as any vasodilator role that it may have are local phenomena, for the production of prostacyclin under normal circumstances is not great enough to exert vasodilator or antiplatelet effects by acting as a circulating hormone.

Prostaglandin D_2. Prostaglandin D_2 is the principal cyclooxygenase product of arachidonic acid produced by the *mast cell* (see Fig. 438–1). Its formation from PGH_2 is catalyzed by the endoperoxide D_2 isomerase. It is released from the mast cell along with histamine when antigens bind to IgE on the mast cell surface. Like histamine, PGD_2 is a vasodilator. Its precise role in the normal immunologic responses mediated by the mast cell is unknown. Patients with systemic mastocytosis have mast cell infiltration in multiple body organs (see Ch. 438). Massive overproduction of prostaglandin D_2 participates along with histamine in the episodes of flushing, hypotension, and even shock that some patients with mastocytosis experience.

Prostaglandin E_2. The metabolism of PGH_2 to PGE_2 is catalyzed by the endoperoxide E_2 isomerase in several tissues, including the renal medulla and gastrointestinal mucosa. PGE_2 is a vasodilator. Its other actions include inhibition of gastric acid secretion and inhibition of renal tubular sodium reabsorption.

A number of solid tumors are known to produce hypercalcemia by an endocrine mechanism (see Ch. 173). In a subset of these, the hypercalcemia is evoked by an overproduction of PGE_2 by the tumor. PGE_2 evokes hypercalcemia in these patients by stimulating osteoclastic activity. The excessive production of PGE_2 can be quantified by measuring one of the urinary metabolites of this prostaglandin. Administration of aspirin or indomethacin in doses sufficient to reduce PGE_2 metabolite excretion will lower serum calcium substantially in these patients. Such a beneficial effect on serum calcium is seen only when the tumor is acting through a humoral mechanism and not after extensive metastases to bone, in which case local mechanisms for hypercalcemia supervene.

Prostaglandin $F_{2\alpha}$. $PGF_{2\alpha}$ is formed from PGH_2 via the action of endoperoxide reductase. It also is formed as a metabolite of PGD_2. $PGF_{2\alpha}$ stimulates uterine and bronchial smooth muscle and is a vasoconstrictor in some vascular beds. Neither a unique site of its formation nor a clearly defined pathophysiologic role for $PGF_{2\alpha}$ has been found. The administration of this prostaglandin is employed therapeutically to induce labor.

Additional Products. In addition to initiating the oxygenation of arachidonic acid to thromboxane A_2 and the prostaglandins, the cyclooxygenase enzyme also initiates conversion of other polyunsaturated fatty acids to corresponding oxygenated metabolites. Eicosatrienoic acid (20:3ω6) undergoes cyclooxygenation to metabolites with structures corresponding to those formed from arachidonic acid, with the exception that they have only one double bond (Δ^{13}) and are designated PGE_1, $PGE_{1\alpha}$, and so forth. Eicosapentaenoic acid (20:5ω3), a polyunsaturated fatty acid prevalent in the marine food chain, is transformed by the cyclooxygenase to corresponding metabolites with three double bonds ($\Delta^{5,13,17}$), e.g., PGI_3. When dietary arachidonic acid is substituted with 20:5ω3, the biosynthesis of proaggregatory thromboxanes is reduced, in part because 20:5ω3 is not efficiently converted to thromboxane A_3. This leads to reduced aggregation of platelets and prolongation of bleeding time.

FUNCTIONS OF ARACHIDONIC ACID METABOLITES. The effects of cyclooxygenase inhibitors that can be replicated by several of the drugs in this class are assumed to result from blocking the formation of one or more of the cyclooxygenase metabolites. By this approach, the functions of the metabolites of arachidonic acid, whose formation is catalyzed by cyclooxygenase, can be inferred even though the specific metabolite mediating the function is not known with certainty.

Fever. Salicylates were introduced to medicine as antipyretics, and all cyclooxygenase inhibitors will attenuate fever. The cyclooxygenase metabolite that mediates pyrexia is not known.

Inflammation. The major use of aspirin and the nonsteroidal anti-inflammatory drugs is for the treatment of noninfectious inflammatory disorders such as arthritis. The specific inflammatory mediator has not been ascertained.

The Gastric Mucosa. Certain prostaglandins, particularly PGE_2, will increase gastric mucosal blood flow and block pentagastrin-evoked acid secretion. In addition, they seem to exert a "protective" effect on the gastric mucosa through mechanisms that are unclear. When these prostaglandin-mediated effects are abolished by cyclooxygenase inhibitors, gastric erosion and ulceration may result as major adverse effects of this class of drugs. There is evidence that their deleterious effect on the gastric mucosa is enhanced if the gastric mucosa is directly exposed to large concentrations of cyclooxygenase inhibitor in addition to the lesser concentrations delivered via the circulation.

The Release of Renin. The adrenergic nervous system is a major regulator of the release of renin. An additional nonadrenergic mechanism also contributes to the control of the release of renin, as for example in renal artery stenosis. Most if not all of the nonadrenergic regulation of renin release is mediated by a cyclooxygenase metabolite of arachidonic acid. As such, the release of renin may be partially blocked by cyclooxygenase inhibitors such as indomethacin. The reduction of renin by cyclooxygenase inhibition has obvious implications in the diagnostic application of renin measurements. Furthermore, the associated decrease in aldosterone production may be deleterious for patients who are prone to hyperkalemia.

Renal Function. Inhibition of cyclooxygenase has little effect on the glomerular filtration rate in normal persons. In various disease states associated with impaired renal function, inhibition of cyclooxygenase will decrease glomerular filtration rate. Substantial diminution in glomerular filtration may be seen after the administration of cyclooxygenase inhibitors to patients with the nephropathy of systemic lupus erythematosus, Bartter's syndrome, cardiac failure, and cirrhosis. In patients with cardiac failure, the reduction in glomerular filtration rate together with inhibition of renin-mediated aldosterone production can lead to hyperkalemia.

Prostaglandin E_2, the predominant prostaglandin produced in the renal medulla, is natriuretic. In part its natriuretic action may be due to inhibition of sodium reabsorption in the distal tubule. Administration of a cyclooxygenase inhibitor will cause sodium retention for a day or two, following which sodium balance is restored despite continued treatment with the agent. This is of little consequence in normal persons, but may be of importance in those in whom sodium retention has deleterious hemodynamic effects.

Indomethacin and other cyclooxygenase inhibitors enhance the antidiuretic action of vasopressin, implicating an arachidonic acid metabolite in the elimination of water. The extent to which this is a primary action of the cyclooxygenase metabolite on water transport versus an increase in the medullary sodium content (driving force for sodium reabsorption) is not clear. Indomethacin will diminish the excessive water elimination in nephrogenic diabetes insipidus and in lithium-induced diabetes insipidus.

Patent Ductus Arteriosus. In the neonatal period, closure of a persistently patent ductus arteriosus can be achieved by inhibition of the cyclooxygenase with indomethacin. This implies that some (unknown) cyclooxygenase metabolite contributes to ductal patency. The E prostaglandins dilate the ductus, and infusion of PGE_1 has been used to maintain an open ductus in infants with pulmonary atresia and other disorders in which ductal patency is advantageous until operative intervention can be accomplished.

Asthma and Anaphylaxis Evoked by Aspirin. In some patients with bronchial asthma (about 10 per cent) aspirin will provoke attacks of bronchoconstriction. These attacks may be very severe and can be induced with small doses of aspirin, as well as with all of the nonsteroidal anti-inflammatory drugs. The bronchoconstriction therefore does not result from an allergy to aspirin, but from some consequence of cyclooxygenase inhibition. This could be the reduced formation of a prostaglandin that normally restrains the release of mediators that cause bronchoconstriction, or the shunting of arachidonic acid into other pathways such as that leading to the leukotrienes (see below).

In a subset of patients with recurrent anaphylaxis, aspirin and other cyclooxygenase inhibitors also act as triggers for the episodes of hypotension, flushing, tachycardia, and dyspnea. Some of these patients have systemic mastocytosis as an underlying disorder. Anaphylaxis provoked by cyclooxygenase inhibitors may be severe and even fatal.

THE LIPOXYGENASE PATHWAY (Fig. 223–2). In addition to the cyclooxygenase pathway described above, oxygenation of arachidonic acid also can proceed via lipoxygenation. The lipoxygenation reactions result in the insertion of an oxygen molecule at a carbon adjacent to one of the double bonds, yielding a hydroperoxy-arachidonic acid. These oxygenations are not blocked by aspirin or indomethacin. The important biologic implications of lipoxygenation emerged from studies of this pathway in leukocytes, in which a major route of arachidonic acid metabolism is 5-lipoxygenation (Fig. 223–2). The initial reaction product is 5-hydroperoxy-eicosatetraenoic acid (5-HPETE) which undergoes further transformation to either 5-hydroxy-eicosatetraenoic acid (5-HETE) or to a 5,6 epoxide which is termed leukotriene A_4 because of the conjugated triene structure that results from the formation of the 5,6 epoxide. The subscript 4 refers to the four double bonds in the structure. Leukotriene A_4 is a precursor for several other compounds with a conjugated triene structure. One of these is leukotriene B_4 (5,12-dihydroxy-eicosatetraenoic acid). Leukotriene B_4 is a potent chemotactic agent for leukocytes. Leukotriene A_4 also undergoes biotransformation to a series of compounds which constitute the mixture previously known as the "slow-reacting

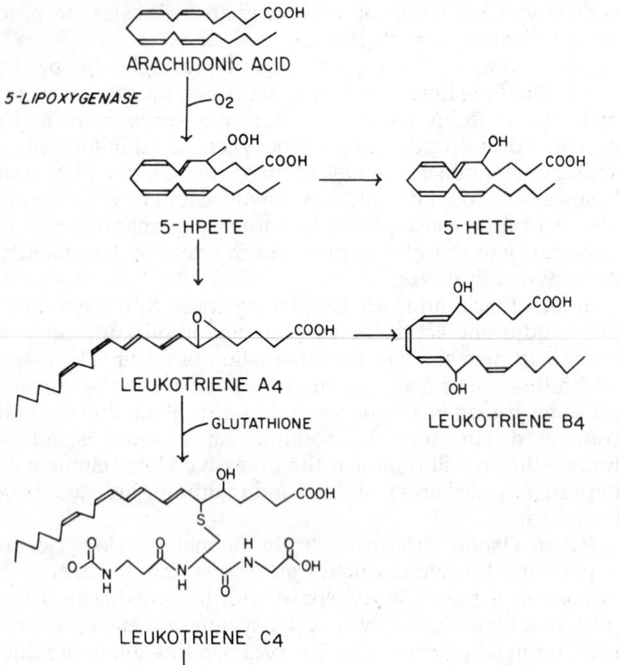

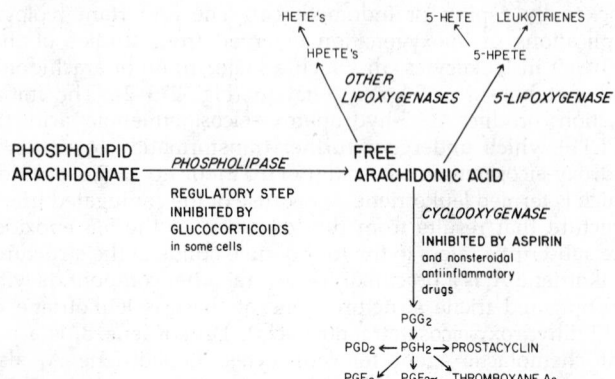

Figure 223–2. The lipoxygenase pathway of arachidonic acid metabolism leading to the formation of the leukotrienes.

substances of anaphylaxis" (SRS-A). Biosynthesis of SRS-A results from reaction of leukotriene A_4 with glutathione to form the glutathionyl adduct leukotriene C_4. Leukotriene C_4 undergoes further biotransformation by γ-glutamyl transpeptidase to yield the cysteinyl-glycine adduct, which is termed leukotriene D_4. Leukotriene D_4 is an extremely potent bronchoconstrictor, having an action approximately 1000 times the molar potency of histamine. In addition, leukotriene D_4 evokes increased vascular permeability. Leukotriene C_4 is a somewhat less potent bronchoconstrictor. Leukotriene C_4 also is a pulmonary vasoconstrictor, an action blocked by indomethacin, suggesting that this vasoconstriction may be mediated via the release of thromboxane A_2 by leukotriene C_4. There is considerable evidence that leukotrienes C_4 and D_4 contribute to antigen-evoked bronchoconstriction.

REGULATION OF BIOSYNTHESIS. None of the arachidonic acid oxygenation products described above are stored for subsequent release from cells; rather, their release is equivalent to biosynthesis. The controlling step for biosynthesis is the liberation of free arachidonic acid from lipid esters (Fig. 223–3). This has been elucidated most clearly in the platelet, where arachidonic acid is liberated from phosphatidyl inositol by an initial reaction with phospholipase C followed by diglyceride lipase to yield free arachidonic acid. In conjunction with the liberation of arachidonic acid during platelet aggregation, phosphatidyl inositol stores are depleted. It is likely that there are cells in which acyl hydrolases other than phospholipase C regulate the release of free arachidonic acid. In most instances, the liberation of arachidonic acid from phospholipids is calcium dependent.

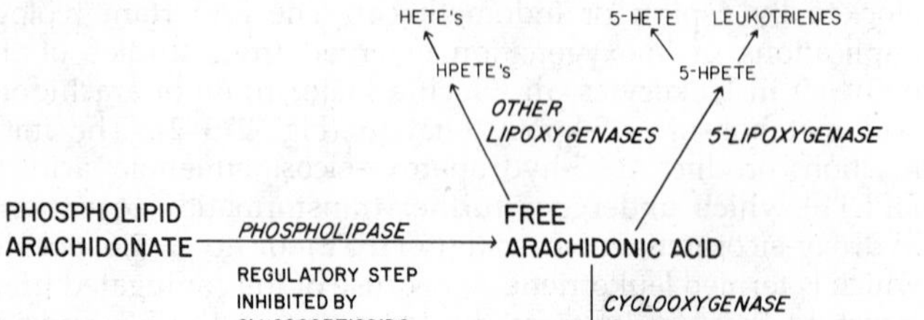

Figure 223–3. Sites of inhibition of arachidonic acid release and metabolism by pharmacologic agents.

PHARMACOLOGIC INHIBITION OF BIOSYNTHESIS. It is possible to inhibit the fatty acid cyclooxygenase clinically with a number of drugs, including aspirin, salicylic acid, indomethacin, phenylbutazone, oxyphenbutazone, ibuprofen, fenoprofen, tolmetin, piroxicam, sulfinpyrazone, and sulindac. There are important differences among these drugs, however. Whereas indomethacin and the other nonsteroidal anti-inflammatory drugs are competitive inhibitors of the cyclooxygenase in vivo and therefore inhibit for a limited duration, aspirin covalently acetylates the enzyme, producing irreversible inhibition. As the platelet is incapable of synthesizing new enzymes, the irreversible inhibition of platelet cyclooxygenase by aspirin persists throughout the life span of the circulating platelet. Because small doses of aspirin (approximately 300 mg) almost completely inhibit the platelet cyclooxygenase, a daily dose in this range is sufficient to maintain a high degree of cyclooxygenase inhibition. Other tissues, including the vascular endothelium, can synthesize new cyclooxygenase, and the effect of low dose aspirin on these nonplatelet sites is more transient. Thus it seems likely that a low dose of aspirin would be preferable if the aim is to inhibit platelet thromboxane A_2 production with a less protracted effect on prostacyclin synthesis by the endothelium, and indeed, 324 mg of aspirin daily has been shown to reduce the incidence of myocardial infarction and death in men with unstable angina. Another tissue that may be selectively affected by the irreversible inhibition of cyclooxygenase by aspirin is the mucosa of the stomach and duodenum. If aspirin is given in a pharmaceutical preparation that undergoes dissolution in the stomach, the mucosa is exposed briefly to larger concentrations of aspirin and thereby to a higher degree of irreversible inhibition of the cyclooxygenase than are tissues which receive the drug through the systemic circulation. In contrast, salicylic acid and other competitive inhibitors of cyclooxygenase exert a greater inhibition on the gastric mucosa for only the brief period in which they are present in the stomach. Sulfinpyrazone and sulindac are prodrugs that inhibit the cyclooxygenase only slightly, but undergo metabolic transformation by the intestinal flora to potent cyclooxygenase inhibitors. Effects of these prodrugs on gastric mucosa are equivalent to those at other tissue sites.

Sharing the common action of inhibiting cyclooxygenase, this class of drugs is composed of a diverse array of chemical structures, and their therapeutic actions and adverse effects are not all identical.

In some cells, the liberation of arachidonic acid from phospholipids is inhibited by glucocorticoids, but this is not the universal effect of glucocorticoids in all cell types. Release of arachidonic acid during platelet aggregation, for example, is not inhibited by glucocorticoids. In those cells in which glucocorticoids do inhibit arachidonic acid mobilization, the formation of both cyclooxygenase and lipoxygenase products is inhibited, whereas the effects of aspirin-like drugs are limited to blocking the cyclooxygenase pathway. This provides an attractive hypothesis for the broader range of anti-inflammatory effects of glucocorticoids, the proof of which is still forthcoming.

Kuehl FA Jr, Egan RW: Prostaglandins, arachidonic acid and inflammation. Science 210:978, 1980. *A review of the metabolism of arachidonic acid as it relates to inflammation, including information on the action of anti-inflammatory drugs. The references provide an excellent entrée to the original articles in this area.*

Moncada S, Vane JR: Mode of action of aspirin-like drugs. Adv Intern Med 24:1, 1979.
Moncada S, Vane JR: Prostacyclin and the cardiovascular system. Adv Prostaglandin Thromboxane Res 6:43, 1980. *Overviews of the biosynthesis and pharmacology of prostacyclin by the discoverers of this prostaglandin.*
Samuelsson B: Leukotrienes: Mediators of immediate hypersensitivity and inflammation. Science 220:568, 1983. *A review describing the structure and biosynthesis of the leukotrienes (slow-reacting substances of anaphylaxis).*

224. NEUROENDOCRINE REGULATION AND ITS DISORDERS

Lawrence A. Frohman

NEUROENDOCRINE REGULATION

The central nervous system exerts profound regulatory control over hormonal secretion and metabolic events. The integration of this control is focused in the region of the ventral hypothalamus and consists of three major systems:

1. A classic neuronal pathway traveling through the base of the brain, through the autonomic nervous system pathways of the spinal cord, and terminating in the liver, gastrointestinal tract, pancreas, adrenal medullae, and adipose tissue. The pathway, which consists of bidirectional fibers, is involved in neurometabolic regulation, and its greatest effects are on blood glucose and fatty acid regulation and on metabolic homeostasis, i.e., appetite control (satiety), temperature control (thermoregulation), and body fat stores.

2. A neurosecretory pathway from the anterior hypothalamus that traverses the floor of the ventral hypothalmus and pituitary stalk and terminates in specialized neuronal elements called pituicytes, located in the posterior pituitary. The system is involved in osmoregulation, through the production of vasopressin, and in parturition and nursing, through the secretion of oxytocin. A detailed discussion of this system is provided in Ch. 226.

3. A neuroendocrine system involving clusters of peptide- and monoamine-secreting cells in the anterior and mid-portion of the ventral hypothalamus whose products are transported along nerve fibers to terminals in the outer layer of the median eminence, from where they are released into the capillary vessels of the hypothalamic-hypophyseal portal system and transported to the pituitary to regulate the secretion of the hormones of the anterior pituitary.

Neuroendocrine Anatomy

In contrast to tissues outside the central nervous system and even within many portions of the brain, much of the functional morphology of the hypothalamus cannot be precisely defined in terms of its anatomic structure. The neurometabolic function of the hypothalamus can be divided into those components associated with the sympathetic or the parasympathetic branches of the autonomic nervous system. Medial sympathetic and lateral parasympathetic zones of the hypothalamus have been defined on the basis of extensive studies in laboratory animals and pathologic findings in patients with anatomically defined diseases of the hypothalamus who exhibit disorders of neurometabolic regulation (i.e., temperature control and nutrient homeostasis). However, the cellular elements (neuronal perikarya) involved in a particular function cannot be precisely localized to one specific nuclear region. Neurons involved in the inhibitory control of food intake (satiety) are located more medially, and those responsible for appetite stimulation are located more laterally. This distinction probably explains why destructive lesions of the hypothalamus, which frequently occur in the midline, are more likely to result in obesity than in starvation. A second reason is that fibers from the hypothalamic controlling centers cross the midline, and thus bilateral hypothalamic destruction is necessary for interruption of normal regulatory control.

Neurons of the neurohypophyseal system represent a more anatomically distinct entity with cell bodies located in the paraventricular and supraoptic hypothalamic nuclei. Within these areas there are also neurons producing a variety of other neuropeptides. The posterior pituitary hormones, oxytocin and vasopressin, are synthesized in the cell bodies as part of a precursor molecule, which also contains a specific carrier protein (neurophysin), and transported along axonal fibers through the ventral hypothalamus and pituitary stalk, during which time the hormones are cleaved from the precursor. In the pituicytes of the posterior pituitary they are packaged into storage granules to be released in response to stimulation (e.g., osmotic, barometric) of receptors on the cell bodies in the hypothalamus. The posterior pituitary is therefore functionally an integral part of the brain.

The cell bodies of the neuroendocrine system are diffusely distributed throughout the mediobasal hypothalamus in an area known as the hypophysiotropic region. Although the releasing hormone–secreting neurons receive input from other brain regions in response to changes in the external environment, they continue to function even in the absence of extrahypothalamic input, indicating that their most important homeostatic stimuli are blood borne. Thyrotropin releasing hormone (TRH)- and somatotropin release inhibiting factor (SRIF)-secreting cells that regulate pituitary function are located in the anterior hypothalamus, while those secreting growth hormone releasing factor (GRF) are concentrated in the region of the ventromedial and arcuate nuclei. Gonadotropin releasing hormone (GnRH)-secreting cells are more widely distributed with cell bodies in both the anterior hypothalamus and the arcuate nuclei. Cell bodies of corticotropin releasing factor (CRF) neurons terminating in the median eminence are located predominantly in the paraventricular nucleus.

The releasing and inhibiting hormones are stored in nerve terminals in the median eminence where their concentrations are 10 to 100 times as great as elsewhere in the hypothalamus. Since the portal blood flow to the pituitary is not compartmentalized, i.e., various cells types in the pituitary are distributed throughout the gland, releasing and inhibiting factors secreted into the portal system have access to all cell types of the anterior pituitary. Specificity of action is achieved not by anatomic segregation but by the presence of specific receptors on individual pituitary cell types.

The cells of both the neuroendocrine and neurohypophyseal systems have been called transducer cells, containing both neuronal and endocrine characteristics. They respond to classic neurotransmitter-mediated signals, yet they respond by releasing peptide hormones into a regional or systemic circulation.

PORTAL VASCULAR SYSTEM. The vascular supply of the anterior pituitary is unique in that there are no direct connections with the arterial system. All of the arterial blood flows through the hypothalamic arteries and forms a capillary plexus within the outer layer of the median eminence in juxtaposition to nerve terminals of the hypophysiotropic neurons. In contrast to most other brain regions, the blood-brain barrier in the area of the median eminence is incomplete, permitting protein and peptide hormones as well as other charged particles access to the intercapillary spaces and the nerve terminals contained therein. These terminals respond to changes in concentrations of circulating hormones and metabolic signals as well as to classic neuronal stimuli by secreting releasing and inhibiting factors into the portal system.

The portal capillaries coalesce into a series of veins that descend through the pituitary stalk and form a second capillary plexus that bathes the cells of the anterior pituitary. Venous drainage from the anterior pituitary passes through the posterior pituitary and from there into systemic veins. Some reverse blood flow occurs from the posterior pituitary to a variable length up the pituitary stalk but does not reach the median eminence, and thus its physiologic significance is uncertain.

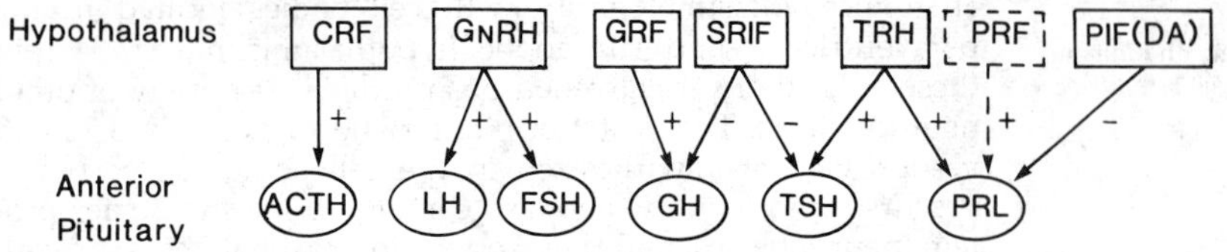

Figure 224–1. Interrelationships between hypothalamic and pituitary hormones. Solid lines denote hormones, the structures of which have been determined. Interrupted lines indicate factors, the identity of which is still unknown.

Releasing and Inhibiting Hormones

The hypothalamic hormones that control the secretion of anterior pituitary hormones and their effects on pituitary hormone secretion are shown in Figure 224–1. Several different patterns of control exist: (1) a single hypothalamic hormone stimulating release of a single pituitary hormone (CRF: ACTH), (2) a single hypothalamic hormone stimulating release of several pituitary hormones (GnRH: luteinizing hormone [LH] and follicle-stimulating hormone [FSH], TRH: thyroid-stimulating hormone [TSH] and prolactin), and (3) several hypothalamic hormones affecting a single pituitary hormone (GRF and SRIF: growth hormone [GH]).

With one exception, the predominant influence of the hypothalamic hormones on the pituitary is stimulatory. Interference with the integrity of the hypothalamic-pituitary connection results in decreased secretion of pituitary hormones. The exception is prolactin, the secretion of which is increased when hypothalamic influence is removed.

All of the hypothalamic hormones whose structures have been determined are, again with one exception, peptides with sequence length ranging from 3 to 44 amino acids. Their structures, shown in Figure 224–2, were identified over a 14-year period, beginning in 1969, and resulted in awarding of a Nobel Prize to the two pioneers in the field: Roger Guillemin and Andrew Schally. As the complexity of the structures increases, both multiple forms of the peptide (see section on somatostatin and GRF) and marked species variation in sequence occur. Whereas the structures of TRH, GnRH, and SRIF are identical in all mammalian species studied to date, and for TRH, in amphibia as well, those of GRF and CRF exhibit marked species specificity. The structures of rat GRF and CRF differ from their human and ovine counterparts by 14 and 7 amino acids respectively. The structure of human CRF has been determined from its gene sequence and is identical in structure to rat CRF. The existence of a separate PRF is still controversial, though a candidate for this title is vasoactive intestinal polypeptide (VIP). The one nonpeptide hypophysiotropic hormone is dopamine. In addition to its major role as a neurotransmitter, dopamine is the most important physiologic inhibitor of prolactin.

ROLE OF BIOGENIC AMINES AND NEUROPEPTIDES IN THE REGULATION OF HYPOTHALAMIC HORMONE SECRETION. The major neurotransmitter systems utilized for intercellular communication within the central nervous system consist of monoamines and peptides. Neurotransmitters can influence the hypothalamic hormone-secreting neurons at several sites (Fig. 224–3). These include axodendritic connections (site 1) and axoaxonic connections involving presynaptic receptors on the hormone-containing nerve terminals (site 3). Multiple neurotransmitters may also participate in the regulation of hormone secretion through intermediary neurons (site 2), and neurotransmitters may be released directly into the portal system to modify the effect of hypothalamic hormones on the pituitary (site 4). Major advances in the understanding of hypothalamic-pituitary function have occurred as a consequence of the availability of neuropharmacologic compounds that selectively alter neuro-

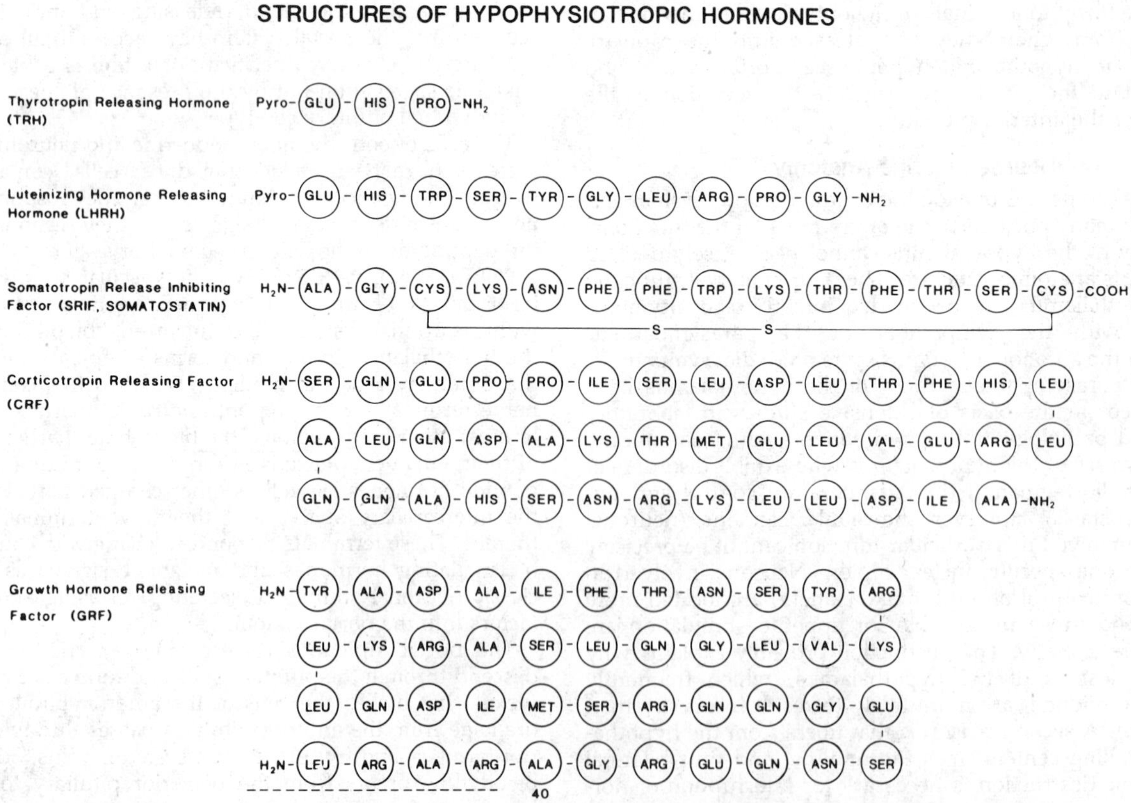

Figure 224–2. Structures of hypothalamic hormones. The sequences of TRH, GnRH, and somatostatin are believed to be similar in all mammalian species, whereas those of CRF (shown as ovine) and GRF (shown as the human sequence derived from a pancreatic tumor) exhibit considerable variability.

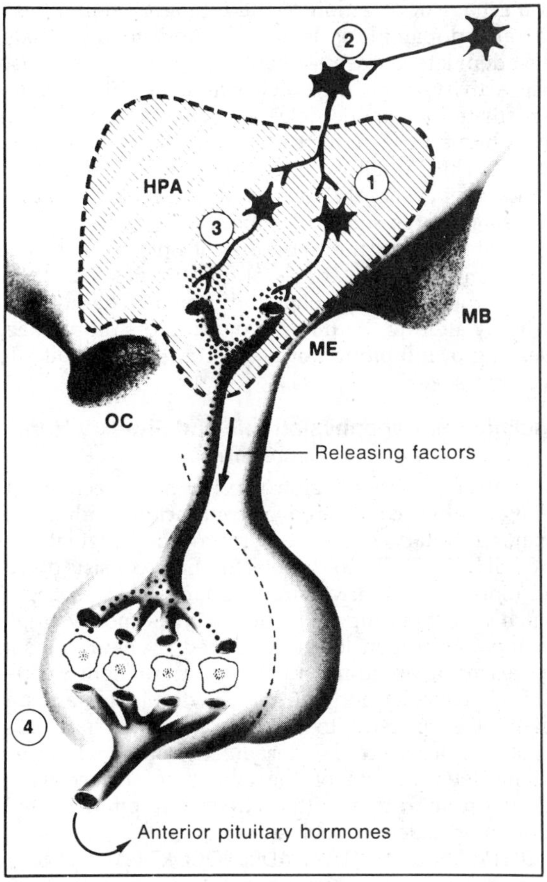

Figure 224–3. Sites of potential neurotransmitter effects on hypothalamic releasing and inhibiting hormone secretion and function. HPA = hypophysiotropic area; OC = optic chiasm; ME = median eminence; MB = mamillary body. Refer to text for description of effects at each site. (Reprinted with permission from Frohman LA: Clinical neuropharmacology of hypothalamic releasing factors. N Engl J Med 286:1391, 1972.)

transmitter function. Information resulting from techniques with only limited application to human investigation has been supplemented by the use of the neuropharmacologic probes that can be safely studied in man. A brief review of biogenic amine neurotransmitters is provided to indicate where selective neuropharmacologic agents can be used to alter neurotransmitter effects, and in turn, hypophysiotropic hormone function.

Catecholamines (Dopamine, Norepinephrine, Epinephrine). The common precursor for the catecholamines is tyrosine, which is actively transported from the blood into catecholaminergic neurons in the CNS. Tyrosine is converted to dihydroxyphenylalanine (L-dopa) by tyrosine hydroxylase, which, because of its low concentration, represents the rate-limiting step in catecholamine biosynthesis. It is therefore the enzyme most susceptible to pharmacologic blockage by tyrosine analogues such as α-methylparatyrosine. L-dopa is rapidly decarboxylated by aromatic L-amino acid decarboxylase to dopamine (5-hydroxytryptamine). This enzyme can be inhibited by L-dopa analogues such as α-methyldopa and α-methyldopahydrazine (carbidopa). In dopaminergic neurons, dopamine is stored in secretory granules and released as a neurotransmitter, while in noradrenergic and adrenergic neurons it is further hydroxylated by dopamine β-hydroxylase to form norepinephrine. Copper-chelating agents such as disulfiram are potent inhibitors of this step and impair the conversion of dopamine to norepinephrine. In noradrenergic neurons, this transmitter is packaged similarly to that of dopamine, whereas in selective neurons it is converted to epinephrine by phenylethanolamine-N-methyltransferase. See Ch. 241 also for a discussion of catecholamine metabolism.

In nerve endings, newly synthesized catecholamines are stored in secretory granules that protect them from enzymatic degradation. There are at least two distinct pools of neurotransmitters that are differentially susceptible to releasing stimuli. A long-lasting depletion of catecholamines can be produced by reserpine, which causes a slow but constant release of the monoamines and inhibits reuptake. Catecholamine release occurs in response to nerve stimulation by fusion of the secretion vesicle membrane with the cell membrane and extrusion of the amine directly into the intercellular space. Once released, catecholamines bind to postsynaptic receptors that appear to be similar in the hypophysiotropic neurons to those demonstrated in other neural sites. In addition, they bind to presynaptic receptors on the nerve terminals to effect a feedback regulation. Alterations in presynaptic and postsynaptic receptor activity are accomplished by the use of receptor agonists and antagonists. The specificity of most of the available agents, however, is not absolute. Catecholamine action terminates by reuptake of the neurotransmitter into the presynaptic neuron, removal into circulation, or by metabolic degradation. The first mechanism is the most important one. Drugs such as cocaine, tricyclic antidepressants, or nomifensine inhibit reuptake, resulting in enhancement of catecholamine effects. Metabolic degradation occurs by two enzymes: monoamine oxidase (MAO) and catechol-O-methyltransferase. Catecholamine action is therefore enhanced by MAO inhibitors such as pargyline and tranylcypromine.

Indolamines (Serotonin, Melatonin). Tryptophan, the precursor of serotonin, is actively transported from blood to brain. Since tryptophan hydroxylase activity is not saturated at physiologic concentrations, fluctuations in plasma tryptophan levels determine the rate of brain serotonin synthesis. After hydroxylation, 5-hydroxytryptophan is converted to serotonin by aromatic L-amino acid decarboxylase. Serotonin functions as a neurotransmitter and, in the pineal, also serves as a precursor of melatonin. Serotonin synthesis can be inhibited by p-chlorophenylalanine, which inhibits tryptophan hydroxylase, and by L-dopa, which competes with 5-hydroxytryptophan for decarboxylation. The storage, release, and uptake of serotonin are similar to that of norepinephrine with many of the same agents (i.e., amphetamine) releasing both compounds. Tricyclic antidepressants inhibit serotonin uptake, though in contrast to norepinephrine, imipramine and amitriptyline are more potent than their desmethyl derivatives (desmethylimipramine and nortriptyline). Alteration of serotonin receptor activity can be produced by agonists such as quipazine and LSD and by antagonists (methysergide and cyproheptadine). Termination of serotonin effects occurs by pre-synaptic reuptake and metabolic degradation involving MAO. Drugs interfering with MAO activity also enhance serotonin effects.

Acetylcholine. Acetylcholine is synthesized from acetyl-CoA and choline. The source of choline is probably phosphatidylcholine which, after crossing the blood-brain barrier, is partially degraded to choline. Choline is then converted to acetylcholine by choline acetyltransferase. There are two types of acetylcholine receptors, muscarinic and nicotinic, which have different anatomic distribution and physiologic function. Arecoline and atropine, a muscarinic agonist and antagonist, respectively, cross the blood-brain barrier and modify acetylcholine receptor activity.

Gamma-Aminobutyric Acid (GABA). In the mammalian hypothalamus GABA is an inhibitory neurotransmitter. It is formed by the decarboxylation of L-glutamate and is metabolized by transamination. Numerous agents inhibit GABA synthesis and degradation, but none is specific or useful clinically in altering neuroendocrine function.

Histamine. Histamine is synthesized within the CNS from histidine by a specific decarboxylase and the nonspecific aromatic L-amino acid decarboxylase. Alteration of histamine effects is brought about primarily by histamine receptor antagonists. There are two classes of histamine receptors: H_1 and H_2. Drugs such as diphenhydramine and cyproheptadine inhibit

TABLE 224–1. NEUROPEPTIDES WITH POTENTIAL EFFECTS ON HYPOTHALAMIC RELEASING HORMONES

Somatostatin
Thyrotropin releasing hormone
Vasoactive intestinal polypeptide
Cholecystokinin
Gastrin
Substance P
Neurotensin
Bombesin/gastrin releasing peptide
Secretin
Motilin
Insulin
Glucagon
Pancreatic polypeptide
Methionine-leucine-enkephalin
Beta-endorphin
Alpha-melanocyte–stimulating hormone
Neuropeptide PYY
Neuropeptide PHI
Calcitonin
Angiotensin
Bradykinin

H_1 receptors, while cimetidine and ranitidine inhibit H_2 receptors.

Neuropeptides. A large number of neuropeptides have been identified in the hypothalamus, and their role in the regulation of neuroendocrine function is, at present, only incompletely understood. A list of neuropeptides with potential effects on releasing and inhibiting hormones is provided in Table 224–1. Many of these peptides are widely distributed in extrahypothalamic CNS and function as neurotransmitters or neuromodulators in other pathways. Of particular significance is a group of peptides common to both the CNS and the gastrointestinal tract. Although the function of these peptides within the CNS remains to be determined, they may have a role in a number of integrative systems relating to homeostatic mechanisms. Their presence throughout evolution and as far back as unicellular organisms underscores their essential role in intercellular communication. With the exception of analogues of enkephalin capable of crossing the blood-brain barrier and of TRH, neuroendocrine effects of peptides other than hypophysiotropic hormones have not been documented in man. Limited information is available concerning biosynthesis, storage, secretion, and metabolism of hypothalamic neuropeptides. Peptidases capable of degrading neuropeptides have been demonstrated, though their specificity and physiologic importance are not yet known.

MECHANISM OF ACTION OF HYPOTHALAMIC HORMONES. Hypophysiotropic hormones affect pituitary hormone secretion by several mechanisms. Specific, high-affinity receptors are present on the anterior pituitary target cells, and cyclic AMP stimulation occurs as a consequence of releasing hormone–receptor interaction. Releasing hormone action is also calcium dependent, and a convincing role now exists for Ca^{++} as a second messenger. In addition, releasing hormones stimulate RNA and protein synthesis, and excessive stimulation can lead to cellular hyperplasia and even tumor formation.

The mechanism of action of the inhibitory hormones somatostatin and dopamine is less well understood. Somatostatin inhibits adenylate cyclase formation and enhances phosphodiesterase activity, both of which actions would impair cyclic AMP–mediated hormone release. Somatostatin also inhibits transmembrane Ca^{++} transport and may have other effects on exocytosis. The inhibitory effects of dopamine appear to be independent of cyclic AMP levels, but, like somatostatin, occur at a late stage in the secretory process.

The effects of all of the hypophysiotropic hormones studied to date are modified by target gland hormones, i.e., thyroxine, cortisol, estrogens, androgens, and inhibin. The hormones act primarily by altering the number of receptors on pituitary cells for releasing or inhibiting hormones, but also exhibit effects at postreceptor sites.

Regulation of Hypophysiotropic and Pituitary Hormone Secretion

The control of hypophysiotropic hormone secretion is best appreciated when considered in conjunction with that of the five major pituitary hormone systems they regulate: ACTH, LH and FSH, TSH, GH, and prolactin. Each consists of feedback (closed loop) systems involving primarily blood-borne signals on which are superimposed other signals mostly originating within the CNS (open loop), mediated by neurotransmitters, and representing environment (temperature, light-dark), stress (pain, fear, psychic) and intrinsic rhythmicity (ranging from ultradian or short-term to diurnal, monthly, and seasonal). Thus, both internal and external environmental factors are important determinants of the activity of these systems. A summary of neurotransmitter effects on pituitary hormone secretion is provided in Table 224–2.

HYPOTHALAMIC-PITUITARY-ADRENOCORTICAL AXIS. Nearly all of the monoamine neurotransmitters have effects on CRF release. Acetylcholine stimulates CRF release predominantly through nicotinic receptors and appears to be the primary neurotransmitter mediating stress-induced CRF release. Serotonin also stimulates CRF release, but the effect is likely mediated through a cholinergic interneuron, since it can be blocked by atropine. Norepinephrine inhibits the cholinergic effects on CRF release through an α-adrenergic receptor, and GABA exerts a similar effect. Melatonin inhibits CRF release and may be responsible for the circadian pattern of CRF release that is entrained to the light-dark cycle. Enkephalins exert inhibitory effects on the pituitary-adrenal axis. This effect is believed to occur within the hypothalamus at the level of CRF release, though an additional action on the pituitary has not been excluded.

CRF stimulates ACTH release, which in turn stimulates the secretion of glucocorticoids and mineralocorticoids from the adrenal cortex. Glucocorticoids inhibit ACTH secretion by a concentration–dependent rapid feedback (minutes) and a concentration–independent delayed feedback (hours). The rapid feedback occurs primarily at the pituitary by inhibiting the response to CRF but also by inhibiting CRF release. The delayed feedback also occurs at both pituitary and hypothalamic levels and appears to reflect inhibitory effects on CRF and ACTH synthesis. In addition, ACTH exerts a "short-loop feedback" on CRF release.

TABLE 224–2. EFFECTS OF AMINERGIC AND PEPTIDERGIC NEUROTRANSMITTERS ON ANTERIOR PITUITARY HORMONE SECRETION

	Norepinephrine	Dopamine	Serotonin	Acetylcholine	Histamine	GABA	Other
ACTH	α ↑	–	↑	↑	–	–	Enkephalins ↓
LH and FSH	(↑)	↓	–	–	–	–	–
TSH	↑	↓	↑	–	–	–	Neurotensin ↓
GH	α ↑ β ↓	↑	↑	↑	–	(↑)	Neurotensin ↓ Substance P ↓ Enkephalins ↑
Prolactin	–	↓	↑	–	↑	↑	Neurotensin ↓ Enkephalins ↑ VIP ↑

NOTE: ↑ = stimulates; ↓ = inhibits; – = no effect or insufficient data; ( ) = conflicting data exist. All effects reflect CNS rather than peripheral sites of action (with the exception of dopamine). The data are derived (whenever possible) from studies in humans.

Plasma ACTH secretion exhibits a diurnal pattern, with lowest levels occurring between 6 and 11 P.M. followed by a rise in the early morning, peaking between 6 and 8 A.M. The pattern appears independent of sleep stage. Superimposed on this regulatory system are the stimulatory effects of stress, including severe trauma, pyrogens, hypoglycemia, and anxiety. Considerable interaction exists between the feedback influence of circulating corticosteroids and neurotransmitters. Phenytoin administration, for example, decreases CNS sensitivity to steroid feedback, thereby diminishing the ACTH response to metyrapone (which reduces circulating glucocorticoid levels) but also enhances pulsatile ACTH secretion while not affecting the ACTH response to stress and vasopressin. Vasopressin, once believed to be CRF, stimulates ACTH release directly as well as through a CNS-mediated mechanism and potentiates the effects of CRF.

HYPOTHALAMIC-PITUITARY-GONADAL AXIS. The major neurotransmitter effects on GnRH identified to date involve dopamine and serotonin. Dopamine stimulates the release of GnRH, though it is not clear whether this involves the tonic or cyclic release of GnRH. Serotonin exerts an inhibitory effect on both cyclic and tonic GnRH secretion. Norepinephrine may also stimulate GnRH release.

The regulation of the hypothalamic-pituitary-gonadal axis is complex, varying with age and sex. LH and FSH are present in circulation from birth, and through the early stages of puberty FSH levels gradually increase to a greater degree than do LH levels. During this period, FSH responses to GnRH are greater than LH responses, a pattern opposite to that seen following puberty, and the hypothalamus is exceedingly sensitive to the suppressive effects of gonadal steroids. In the later prepubertal period (seven to nine years) sleep-related pulsatile LH secretion begins, and synchronization occurs between LH and FSH pulses, particularly in girls. These pulses stimulate the secretion of testosterone in boys and estradiol in girls that initiates the clinical characteristics of puberty. At the same time, evidence for lessening sensitivity of hypothalamic GnRH secretion in response to steroid feedback can be demonstrated. In women, development of positive LH and FSH feedback to gonadal steroids permits the cyclic preovulatory gonadotropin surge resulting in the establishment of cyclic ovulation by the mid teens. In adult males the LH secretory pattern is characterized by 8 to 10 spikes occurring randomly through the day, and the teenage relationship to the sleep-wake pattern disappears. Similar pulsatile secretion of LH and FSH occurs in mature women, the frequency in magnitude of the pulses varying with the phase of the menstrual cycle. When ovarian follicles disappear at menopause, secretion of the major ovarian hormones stops, and the loss of negative feedback of these hormones enhances secretion of FSH and, to a lesser extent, LH. A similar increase in LH and FSH is observed in men in the seventh and eighth decade in response to decreasing testicular function.

In men, surgical stress results in a transitory rise in the level of LH followed by a prolonged fall, accompanied by a fall in testosterone levels. No changes have been observed in women, although hypothalamic anovulation is frequently seen during periods of stress. Pheromones or other environmental factors have been implicated as the cause for the synchronization of menstrual cycles seen in women living in close association.

Steroid hormones regulate LH and FSH secretion by two major mechanisms. Gonadal steroids regulate tonic secretion by a negative feedback mechanism. Testosterone appears to be more potent than estrogen in this negative feedback effect, while progesterone has an intermediate effect. Inhibin, a peptide produced by germinal epithelium, has a selective action in inhibiting FSH release, possibly by impairing the effects of GnRH. Cyclic release of LH and FSH is stimulated by a positive feedback effect of ovarian steroids during the final phases of follicular growth prior to ovulation. The preovulatory surge of LH is preceded by an increase in circulating estrogen levels in the presence of low or decreasing progesterone levels. The positive effects occur at both the hypothalamic and pituitary levels, though the latter appear to be more important. GnRH is released in a tonic pulsatile manner by the hypothalamus every 60 to 90 minutes, and this pattern of secretion is critical for its effects on the pituitary. In an individual deficient in GnRH secretion, pulsatile administration of GnRH allows restoration of normal cyclic ovulation. In contrast, constant infusion of GnRH leads to down-regulation of pituitary GnRH receptors and a loss of gonadotropin secretion. This observation has enormous implications in terms of therapy aimed at enhancing or preventing fertility. In contrast to its effects on GnRH, dopamine inhibits tonic LH secretion. The physiologic significance of this observation is unclear, since inhibitory effects on the midcycle LH surge can also be blocked by dopamine receptor blockers.

HYPOTHALAMIC-PITUITARY-THYROID AXIS. TSH secretion by the pituitary is regulated by TRH and somatostatin. For a discussion of the control of somatostatin secretion, the reader is referred to the section on the regulation of GH secretion. TRH secretion is stimulated by norepinephrine and dopamine and is inhibited by serotonin. TRH stimulates TSH secretion, which in turn enhances the release of thyroxine and triiodothyronine by the thyroid. The feedback effects of these hormones, primarily triiodothyronine, occur principally in the pituitary where they inhibit the TSH response to TRH. A reduction in circulating thyroid hormone levels leads to a prompt rise in TSH levels. TRH is not required for this acute response, though it is necessary for the full expression of TSH hypersecretion over a long time. In addition, TRH is required for maintaining basal TSH secretion. In contrast to its effects on the pituitary, triiodothyronine exerts a stimulatory effect on TRH secretion from the hypothalamus.

Acute changes in environmental conditions requiring increased metabolic activity, such as cold exposure, lead to a TRH-mediated increase in TSH secretion. This effect is readily demonstrable in infants but not in adults, in whom other mechanisms of thermogenesis (mediated by the autonomic nervous system and resulting in shivering and free fatty acid mobilization) are more important. Agents inhibiting adrenergic neurotransmission block the TSH response to cold.

Dopaminergic agents exert an inhibitory effect on TSH release by the pituitary that is most pronounced in patients with elevated TSH levels but also seen in normals. A role of endogenous dopamine in suppressing TSH secretion has also been demonstrated.

Somatostatin inhibition of TSH secretion exerts a relatively minor physiologic role under normal circumstances, but increases in hypothalamic somatostatin release as a result of elevated GH levels can suppress TSH secretion to subnormal levels.

HYPOTHALAMIC-PITUITARY-SOMATOTROPH AXIS. GH secretion is regulated by releasing and inhibiting hormones: GRF and SRIF (somatostatin). Many physiologic stimuli affect GH secretion. Intrinsic GH rhythmicity involves a diurnal pattern with stable basal patterns superimposed on which are occasional surges of GH unrelated to any known signals, the most consistent of which occurs about one hour after the onset of sleep and is associated with sleep stages 3 and 4. With age, GH secretion changes dramatically, both qualitatively and quantitatively. Extremely high levels seen in the first few days of life decrease by two weeks of age. During the pubertal period levels indistinguishable from those of adults are seen, though the GH surges occur more frequently. By the fifth and sixth decade, GH surges, both during the day and in association with sleep, are diminished. Similarly, responses to GH releasing stimuli decrease with age. Neurotransmitter regulation of GH secretion has been extensively defined. Dopamine, norepinephrine (through the alpha receptor), epinephrine, serotonin, GABA, and acetylcholine have all been shown to stimulate GH secretion. Melatonin has both stimulatory and inhibitory effects, TRH and neurotensin exhibit inhibitory effects, and endorphins/enkephalins have stimulatory effects, all mediated within the CNS. The mechanism by which these neurotransmitters affect the secretion of GRF and SRIF is not completely understood, though dopamine, norepinephrine, acetylcholine, GABA, neurotensin, substance P, and bombesin have all been reported to stimulate SRIF release.

GH secretion is profoundly affected by nutrients. Elevations of amino acid levels, decreases in free fatty acids, and hypoglycemia all stimulate GH secretion, while hyperglycemia inhibits GH release. GH secretion is increased by exercise, anxiety, and emotional or physical stress. Many hormones affect GH responsiveness. Estrogen administration increases GH responsiveness, while excesses of corticosteroid and thyroid hormone decrease responsivity. GH secretion is also decreased in states of thyroid hormone deficiency. In pubertal and prepubertal males, androgen administration also enhances GH responses.

In addition to these "open loop" stimuli, a closed loop feedback system also exists. GH stimulates the production of somatomedins (insulin-like growth factors [IGF] I and II) by the liver, and both GH and IGF-I exhibit feedback effects. IGF-I stimulates the release of somatostatin and also inhibits basal and GRF-stimulated GH release by the pituitary. GH itself stimulates somatostatin secretion at concentrations that are reached during secretory bursts. It is not yet known whether GH and IGF-I exhibit effects on GRF secretion.

HYPOTHALAMIC-LACTOTROPH-BREAST AXIS. Prolactin secretion is predominantly controlled by inhibitory CNS influences, with dopamine being the major prolactin inhibiting factor. Two peptides, TRH and vasoactive intestinal polypeptide (VIP), appear to have physiologic prolactin releasing factor (PRF) activity, though their relative importance is not yet clear. Neurotransmitter influences on prolactin secretion are extensive. Serotonin stimulates prolactin release by effects on PRF. Melatonin and histamine have stimulatory effects within the CNS as do opioid peptides and GABA. The effect of the latter two agents appears due to their inhibitory effects on the tuberoinfundibular dopaminergic system.

Prolactin secretion is increased by tactile stimulation of the breast via receptors in the nipple and areola that reach the spinal cord by the intercostal nerves. During pregnancy, prolactin levels increase as a result of estrogen stimulation. Following parturition, the rapid decline in estrogen and progesterone levels allows the unopposed action of prolactin to stimulate lactation from the estrogen-primed breast. The suckling stimulation of prolactin secretion is in part controlled by VIP. Prolactin levels return to normal after several months even during continual lactation. Prolactin is a stress-responsive hormone, and increased secretion is observed after surgical stress, exercise, and insulin hypoglycemia. Prolactin secretion is increased in states of thyroid hormone deficiency and decreased in the presence of thyroid hormone excess.

del Pozo E, Lancranjan I: Clinical use of drugs modifying the release of anterior pituitary hormones. *In* Ganong WF, Martini L (eds.): Frontiers in Neuroendocrinology. Vol 5. New York, Raven Press, 1978, pp 207–248. *A detailed review of the neuropharmacologic agents that have been used to modify pituitary hormone secretion. Both diagnostic and therapeutic uses are covered, with particular emphasis on drugs affecting dopaminergic systems.*

Epstein A: Neuroendocrinology of thirst and salt appetite. *In* Ganong WF, Martini L (eds.): Frontiers in Neuroendocrinology. Vol 5. New York, Raven Press, 1978, pp 101–134. *An extremely well-written review of neural regulation of salt and water metabolism. The studies are primarily in laboratory animals, though the principles apply to human physiology.*

Krieger DT: Neuroendocrine physiology. *In* Felig P, Baxter JD, Broadus AE, Frohman LA (eds.): Endocrinology and Metabolism. New York, McGraw Hill Book Company, 1981, pp 125–250. *A systematic in-depth presentation of the anatomy and physiology of human neuroendocrinology. Designed for the advanced medical student and clinical trainee.*

Krieger DT: Brain peptides: What, where and why? Science 222:975, 1983. *An excellent and comprehensive review of the recent developments in neural peptide research, their implications, and an attempt to explain their presence throughout evolution. Interesting for clinicians, though not of immediate use.*

Krieger DT, Brownstein M, Martin JB (eds.): Brain Peptides. New York, John Wiley & Sons, 1983. *A comprehensive collection of monographs on the role of brain peptides as transmitters, hypophyseotropic hormones, and messengers throughout the nervous system. This will be a definitive reference volume for years. Of interest to the medical student, neurobiologist, and clinical trainee.*

Krieger DT, Hughes JC (eds.): Neuroendocrinology. Sunderland, Sinauer Associates, Inc., 1980. *A collection of reviews on hypothalamic function involving normal physiology and organic and behavioral disease states. Articles are very readable and beautifully illustrated, although they do not provide in-depth coverage of subject material.*

McCann SM: The role of brain peptides in the control of anterior pituitary hormone secretion. *In* Muller EE, MacLeod RM (eds.): Neuroendocrine Perspectives. Vol 1. Amsterdam, Elsevier Biomedical Press, 1982, pp 1–22. *An up-to-date review of releasing and inhibiting factors and of other neural peptides that regulate hormone secretion by the pituitary. Results are derived from animals but form the basis for evaluating human neuroendocrine regulation as well.*

Morley JE: The endocrinology of the opiates and opioid peptides. Metabolism 30:195, 1981. *A well-documented, current review of the role of opiates and the endorphin/enkephalin family of peptides in relation to neuroendocrine function and the regulation of neurometabolic control. Both human and animal studies are discussed.*

Rivier J, Spiess J, Thorner M, Vale W: Characterization of a growth hormone releasing factor from a human pancreatic islet tumor. Nature 300:276, 1982. Guillemin R, Brazeau P, Bohlen P, Esch F, Ling N, Wehrenberg WB: Growth hormone releasing factor from a pancreatic tumor that caused acromegaly. Science 218:585, 1982. *Two papers describing the isolation and characterization of growth hormone releasing factor from pancreatic islet adenomas. The culmination of a 20-year search, with an unexpected tissue source leading to the solution.*

DISEASES OF THE CENTRAL NERVOUS SYSTEM WITH ALTERED NEUROENDOCRINE AND NEUROMETABOLIC FUNCTION

The frequent association of altered hormone secretion with disorders of the CNS has been recognized for many decades. The hypothalamus was the initial focus of attention because of its crucial role in neuroendocrine regulation. However, it is now recognized that diseases localized to extrahypothalamic brain regions as well as nonlocalized CNS disorders can also produce disturbances in neuroendocrine function. The clinical and laboratory manifestations of these disorders are frequently indistinguishable from those of hypothalamic origin, since their mediation is usually via the hypothalamus. Similarly the distinction between hypothalamic and pituitary causes of certain pituitary hormone secretory disorders may be difficult for other reasons.

Because of the reticular organization of the anatomic structure of the hypothalamus, some functions can be localized to a precise anatomic locus, whereas others require the participation of diffuse areas. In addition, neurons within a specific hypothalamic locus may be involved in several separate regulatory functions. Consequently the extent of endocrine or metabolic disturbance is more dependent on the location than the size of the hypothalamic lesion. Furthermore, slowly growing lesions tend to be silent until they have reached considerable size, whereas rapidly enlarging lesions, depending on location, can cause dramatic clinical and laboratory manifestations even when quite small.

Acute hypothalamic damage is associated with impairment of consciousness, sustained hyperthermia, and severe disturbances of cardiovascular, gastrointestinal, or respiratory function. In contrast, persistent disease in the hypothalamus results in alterations in cognition and complex homeostatic functions. Although disorders of neuroendocrine regulation can be produced by acute lesions destroying the median eminence or the pituitary stalk, they generally tend to be seen with chronic disorders and often result in inability of the endocrine system to adapt to environmental changes rather than in alteration of basal hormone secretion. Because hypothalamic neuronal projections, in contrast to those involving sensory and motor function, are generally not lateralized, unilateral damage seldom results in significant or prolonged symptoms. Thus disturbances of hypothalamic function are most commonly seen with infiltrative or inflammatory diseases that affect the region diffusely, with tumors of the midline that expand bilaterally, or with disorders affecting the median eminence, the final common effector pathway to the pituitary.

Etiology of Hypothalamic Disease

Defined anatomic disorders of the hypothalamus vary in frequency with different age groups and are summarized in

Table 224–3. In addition, disturbances of neuroendocrine or neurometabolic function are frequently unassociated with anatomic evidence of hypothalamic disease. Many have been attributed to disorders of neurochemical function, though it is currently not known whether they represent defects in receptor binding, postreceptor mechanisms, biosynthetic defects, or other disorders.

TUMORS. Hypothalamic tumors are frequently located in the region of the third ventricle. Those tumors located in the inferior portion of the third ventricle or the anterior mediobasal hypothalamus frequently produce disturbances in neuroendocrine and neurometabolic regulation. The most frequent hypothalamic tumors are craniopharyngiomas (see next section) and their variants (ependymomas and epidermoid cysts), followed by astrocytomas and dysgerminomas. Two other tumor types, hypothalamic pinealomas and hamartomas, will be considered separately because of their association with specific neuroendocrine disorders. Since they are frequently of developmental origin, the majority of hypothalamic tumors occur in patients under 25 years of age. Endocrine disturbances generally result from destruction of those neuronal elements required for normal pituitary function. The most frequently occurring manifestations are diabetes insipidus, hypogonadism, and growth retardation. Disturbances in thyroid and adrenal function are less common. The diagnosis of a hypothalamic tumor is made by standard neuroradiologic and neuro-ophthalmologic procedures, using computed tomography, visual field measurement, and visual evoked responses. The combination of an atypical visual field defect (i.e., loss of inferior visual fields), normal sellar anatomy, and intact responses to releasing hormones in a patient with hypopituitarism points to primary hypothalamic disease. The surgical treatment of hypothalamic tumors generally precludes complete removal without destruction of normal tissue critical for maintaining homeostasis. Many of these tumors, because of their developmental origin, tend to be slow growing and may even undergo spontaneous growth arrest or regression. Cystic tumors can be aspirated or marsupialized into the cerebroventricular system. Radiotherapy is also effective in many of these tumors. The loss of endocrine function is, however, rarely reversible, and replacement hormone therapy is required.

TABLE 224–3. ETIOLOGY OF HYPOTHALAMIC DISEASE

Neonates	
	Intraventricular hemorrhage
	Meningitis: bacterial
	Tumors: glioma, hemangioma
	Trauma
	Hydrocephalus, hydranencephaly, kernicterus
1 Month–2 Years	
	Tumors: glioma, especially optic glioma, histiocytosis X, hemangiomas
	Hydrocephalus, meningitis
	"Familial" disorders: Laurence-Moon, Bardet-Biedl, Prader-Labhart-Willi, etc.
2–10 Years	
	Tumors: craniopharyngioma, glioma, dysgerminoma, hamartoma, histiocytosis X, leukemia, ganglioneuroma, ependymoma, medulloblastoma
	Meningitis: bacterial, tuberculous
	Encephalitis: viral and demyelinating, various viral encephalitides and exanthematous demyelinating encephalitides, disseminated encephalomyelitis
	"Familial" disorders: diabetes insipidus, etc.
	Damage from nasopharyngeal radiation therapy
10–25 Years	
	Tumors: craniopharyngioma, pituitary tumors, glioma, hamartoma, dysgerminoma, histiocytosis X, leukemia, dermoid, lipoma, neuroblastoma
	Trauma
	Subarachnoid hemorrhage, vascular aneurysm, arteriovenous malformation
	Inflammatory diseases: meningitis, encephalitis, sarcoidosis, tuberculosis
	Associated with midline brain defects: agenesis of corpus callosum
	Chronic hydrocephalus or increased intracranial pressure
25–50 Years	
	Nutritional: Wernicke's disease
	Tumors: glioma, lymphoma, meningioma, craniopharyngioma, pituitary tumors, angioma, plasmacytoma, colloid cysts, ependymoma, sarcoma, histiocytosis X
	Inflammatory: sarcoidosis, tuberculosis, viral encephalitis
	Subarachnoid hemorrhage, vascular aneurysms, arteriovenous malformation
	Damage from pituitary radiation therapy
50 Years and older	
	Nutritional: Wernicke's disease
	Tumors: sarcoma, gliobastoma, lymphoma, meningioma, colloid cysts, ependymoma, pituitary tumors
	Vascular: infarct, subarachnoid hemorrhage, pituitary apoplexy
	Infectious: encephalitis, sarcoidosis, meningitis

Adapted from Plum F, Van Uitert R: Non-endocrine diseases of the hypothalamus. *In* Reichlin S, Baldessarini RJ, Martin JB (eds.): The Hypothalamus. New York, Raven Press, 1978, p 415.

Hamartomas. One type of hypothalamic tumor, the hamartoma, has been associated with increased, rather than decreased, hypothalamic function. Hamartomas consist of masses of redundant, partially disoriented glial and neuronal cells or an abnormally lodged collection of normal nerve tissue. Hamartomas associated with precocious puberty consist of encapsulated nodules in the posterior hypothalamus containing membrane-bound secretion granules similar to those in hypothalamic neurosecretory cells. Vessels in the hamartoma have fenestrations characteristic of those in the median eminence, suggesting a secretory process similar to that in the median eminence. These vessels are presumed to connect to the pituitary portal system. The secretion granules contain GnRH, which is found in high concentrations in CSF from patients with this disorder. Hamartomatous cells are believed to secrete GnRH in a pulsatile manner, but are not under normal prepubertal inhibitory influences. The resultant hormonal effects produce pubertal changes that in girls lead to menarche and cyclic ovulatory menses as early as the second year of life.

Harmartomas are present in one third of all children with this form of precocious puberty. Specific therapy aimed at the hamartoma appears unnecessary, since its course is benign with no other neuroendocrine disturbances and no loss of nonendocrine hypothalamic structure or function. Therapy of the precocious puberty, however, is of great importance both for psychologic reasons and for prevention of premature epiphyseal fusion and stunted growth. Current therapy consists of monthly injections of a long-acting progesterone that inhibits the gonadotropin response to GnRH and effectively inhibits vaginal bleeding but is only partially effective in slowing bone growth. A GnRH analogue, currently in investigational status, acts by down-regulating the pituitary GnRH receptor, resulting in diminished gonadotropin secretion, and is capable of suppressing the accelerated bone growth. The use of GnRH analogues should become standard therapy in the future.

Hypothalamic hamartomas have also been associated with acromegaly and GH-secreting pituitary tumors. They have been shown to contain GRF, which is secreted into the portal system, resulting in GH hypersecretion and somatotroph tumor formation.

Gangliocytomas. A closely related tumor, the gangliocytoma, consists of randomly oriented large ganglion cells similar to those in the hypothalamic magnocellular (large cell) nuclei. Intrapituitary gangliocytomas are also seen in association with acromegaly and GH-secreting tumors of the pituitary and contain GRF. In contrast to hypothalamic hamartomas, the axons of the intrapituitary tumors directly contact the somatotropic cells.

Pineal Tumors. Pineal tumors constitute less than 1 per cent of all intracranial neoplasms and consist of three separate tumor types: pinealomas (pineal parenchymal tissue tumor [20 per cent]), glial tumors (25 per cent), and germinomas (also called ectopic pinealomas or teratomas [55 per cent]). The neuroendocrine effects (precocious puberty) of the first two types are most likely a consequence of destruction of the normal pineal by tumor, leading to loss of pineal secretory products (possibly melatonin, arginine vasotocin, or another factor) that normally inhibit the initiation of sexual maturation. Only a small percentage of pineal tumors cause sexual precocity and usually not until they extend beyond the pineal region. Some pineal tumors are associated with delayed puberty, which may be mediated by production of an antigonadotropic factor. Precocious puberty associated with germinomas, which are similar both histologically and functionally to ovarian and testicular germ cell tumors, is caused by the production of chorionic gonadotropin. Levels as high as those seen during the first month of pregnancy are often present. Many of the "ectopic" pinealomas occur in the midline of the ventral hypothalamus and result in loss of other endocrine functions. Surgical treatment of pinealomas is generally unsatisfactory though the tumors consisting of germinal elements are exquisitely radiosensitive. The tumors frequently contain nongerminal elements (teratomas) that are relatively radioresistant.

INFILTRATIVE AND INFLAMMATORY DISEASES

Histiocytosis X (see also Ch. 161). This granulomatous disease of the histiocytic type, with eosinophilic elements, involves the ventromedial hypothalamus and is associated with diabetes insipidus, anterior hypopituitarism due to destruction of releasing hormone–secreting neurons, or both. The three clinical subgroups of the disease are Hand-Schüller-Christian disease, the most common type characterized by polyuria, exophthalmos, and skull defects; Letterer-Siwe disease, a more rapidly progressive form; and eosinophilic granuloma, in which similar pathologic findings are present in isolated bone lesions. The disease may begin with diabetes insipidus, which is present in nearly 50 per cent of patients with Hand-Schüller-Christian disease. Less commonly, growth failure, hypogonadism, and panhypopituitarism are seen. The diagnosis is established by bone or intracranial biopsy. The CNS forms of the disease may respond to high-dose glucocorticoid therapy or chemotherapy, but the impairment in neuroendocrine function appears irreversible.

Sarcoidosis (see Ch. 67). Involvement of the CNS by sarcoidosis in uncommon. When it is present, however, the hypothalamus and pituitary are frequently involved with infiltrating granulomatous nodules. Patients may develop diabetes insipidus, galactorrhea due to hyperprolactinemia, partial or total anterior pituitary insufficiency, and neurometabolic and neurovegetative symptoms such as somnolence or hyperphagia. In general, the usual treatment with glucocorticoids does not improve the endocrine dysfunction.

TRAUMA. Basal skull fractures are frequently accompanied by shearing of the pituitary stalk, leading to panhypopituitarism and diabetes insipidus. In patients who become comatose following skull fractures, impairment in the pituitary-thyroid and pituitary-gonadal axes have been reported in the absence of stalk damage. Gonadal and thyroid hormones generally return to normal upon recovery.

RADIATION-INDUCED HYPOTHALAMIC DYSFUNCTION. Radiation therapy for intracranial neoplasms, including pituitary tumors, and for nasopharyngeal and maxillary sinus carcinomas frequently leads to hypopituitarism. The interval between therapy and appearance of hormone deficiencies ranges from one to ten years or possibly longer. Children appear more susceptible than adults, and the critical dose is believed to be about 4000 rads. In children, growth failure associated with reduced GH secretion, hypogonadotropic hypogonadism, and hypothyroidism is seen. The site of the defect appears to be variable, with some patients exhibiting hypothalamic and others pituitary damage.

FUNCTIONAL DISEASES OF THE CENTRAL NERVOUS SYSTEM WITH NEUROENDOCRINE DISTURBANCES

Disturbances in neuroendocrine function manifested by both decreased and increased pituitary hormone secretion can occur in the absence of structurally detectable disease in the pituitary or CNS. With the aid of releasing hormones to test specifically the pituitary component and other stimuli to test the hypothalamic-pituitary unit, some degree of discrimination can be made as to the source of the disordered hormone secretion. The following are recognized functional disturbances that have been attributed to hypothalamic (or possibly other CNS) disease. The specific biochemical defect responsible remains to be determined.

HYPOTHALAMIC HYPOGONADISM. This disorder is defined as an impairment in pituitary-gonadal function caused by deficient or disordered secretion of GnRH. The manifestations vary according to the age of presentation.

Prepubertal. The presence of hypothalamic hypogonadism prior to puberty results in failure of normal sexual maturation. Other pituitary hormone deficiencies, also attributed to hypothalamic dysfunction, may coexist. A major subgroup of this disorder, most frequently seen in boys, includes anosmia or hyposmia (*Kallmann's syndrome* or olfactory-genital dysplasia). This syndrome may be associated with other neurologic defects such as color blindness and nerve deafness. The disorder is frequently familial, though sporadic cases have also been reported. Midline developmental defects occasionally occur, and hypoplasia in the region of the anterior commissure, olfactory bulb, and hypothalamus has been found. In some patients there is an additional defect characterized by decreased testicular response to LH. The gonadotropin responses to a single injection of GnRH are markedly impaired or absent, indicating a lack of prior GnRH function. Repeated administration of GnRH, given to prime the gonadotrophs, eventually produces a normal or supranormal gonadotropin response and serves to differentiate this disorder from that of primary gonadotroph failure. Standard therapy consists of the use of gonadal steroids for the development and maintenance of secondary sexual characteristics and gonadotropins for promoting fertility. The administration of GnRH analogues can produce both effects, provided pulsatile administration is used, by means of an intermittent infusion pump, to simulate endogenous secretion.

Postpubertal. Postpubertal hypothalamic hypogonadism affects primarily women. It is manifested clinically by secondary amenorrhea or oligomenorrhea and occasionally by infertility associated with anovulatory cycles. The terms *functional* or *psychogenic amenorrhea* and *infertility* have also been used for this disorder. Patients may exhibit normal tonic levels of gonadotropins and estradiol, resulting in maintenance of normal secondary sexual characteristics, although pulsatile secretion of LH, seen in normal women, is absent and the cyclic ovulatory surge of gonadotropins does not occur. The gonadotropin responses to a single injection of GnRH reveal enhancement of the FSH rather than the LH response. These women respond normally to clomiphene, an estrogen receptor antagonist, suggesting the defect is related to a functional derangement in the positive estrogen feedback mechanism. The disorder is usually self-limited.

Hyperprolactinemia exerts an inhibitory effect on the positive feedback effect of estradiol on GnRH secretion that has been attributed to enhanced tuberoinfundibular dopamine secretion. The negative estrogen feedback mechanism appears intact, since elevated FSH and LH levels are maintained in postmenopausal women with hyperprolactinemia. In men, hyperprolactinemia produces hypogonadism, manifested most frequently by diminished libido and potency.

In severe cases, basal estradiol levels and serum gonadotropin responses to GnRH are reduced, implying a defect in tonic as well as cyclic GnRH secretion. Similar physiologic disturbances are seen in some patients with hyperprolactinemia irrespective of cause. Marked increases and decreases in body weight are often accompanied by amenorrhea, as occurs in professional ballet dancers and female athletes; anorexia nervosa (see details later in this section); and severe obesity.

Treatment of this disorder depends on the extent of hypogonadism and the patient's desire for fertility. Restoration of ovulatory menses may be accomplished by cycles of clomiphene administration, cyclic estrogen-progestin (oral contraceptive) therapy, gonadotropin administration, or GnRH infusions, depending on the desired goal. In hypoestrogenemic women, decreased vaginal secretions, leading to dyspareunia and decreased libido, and the long-term consequences of osteopenia and metabolic bone disease warrant replacement therapy. In men, testosterone replacement therapy is indicated if endogenous hormone levels are subnormal.

Polycystic Ovary Syndrome (See also Ch. 236). The polycystic ovary (Stein-Leventhal) syndrome is characterized by amenorrhea, obesity, hirsutism, and consistently elevated LH levels. It is occasionally associated with a history of childhood CNS injury or "encephalitis." The altered hormonal secretory pattern of polycystic ovaries appears to be secondary to the increased LH secretion. This syndrome is occasionally seen in patients with hyperprolactinemia, but the causal relationship remains to be established (see Ch. 236.)

HYPOTHALAMIC HYPOTHYROIDISM. This is an uncommon disorder manifested by hypothyroidism, a low plasma TSH level, and an exaggerated and delayed response of TSH to TRH. In patients with this disorder, peak TSH responses occur at 90 to 120 minutes, in contrast to the 15- to 30-minute peak response time seen in normal subjects. Children of one subgroup have shown elevated basal TSH levels, but in most subjects basal levels are normal. Hypothalamic hypothyroidism can occur as an isolated defect or, more commonly, is seen in association with deficiencies of gonadotropin, GH, or ACTH secretion. Treatment of this disorder is with thyroxine.

HYPOTHALAMIC-ADRENAL DYSFUNCTION. Decreased ACTH secretion on the basis of hypothalamic or other CNS disorders is relatively rare. It is seen most commonly in association with other pituitary hormone dificiencies during childhood and, by inference, has been attributed to a CNS cause. Disturbances of ACTH diurnal rhythm and suppressibility of ACTH are common in patients with a variety of intracranial diseases and reflect disturbances in neuroendocrine control mechanisms. They do not have major clinical significance, but subtle effects on behavior cannot be excluded. In particular, patients with affective disorders (unipolar depression) or experiencing bereavement exhibit a lack of normal glucocorticoid suppressibility similar to that seen in Cushing's disease.

IDIOPATHIC HYPERPROLACTINEMIA. Idiopathic hyperprolactinemia (IH) is a disorder in which prolactin levels are elevated in the absence of demonstrable pituitary or CNS disease and of any other recognized cause of increased prolactin secretion. The clinical manifestations of IH consist of galactorrhea and amenorrhea. In some patients, oligomenorrhea is present, and in a few, sporadic ovulation persists. Prolactin levels are elevated but rarely exceed 150 ng per milliliter. The disease is confined to women of the childbearing age. The diagnosis remains inferential and based on exclusion of a pituitary microadenoma.

Many patients in whom IH was previously diagnosed have subsequently been found by computed tomography to harbor microadenomas. Extensive testing using neuropharmacologic probes has failed to distinguish patients with IH from those with microadenomas, suggesting that the same pathophysiologic mechanism underlies both disorders. IH has been attributed to a CNS neurotransmitter defect related to dopamine metabolism, based on the observations that drugs impairing dopaminergic neurotransmission (i.e., neuroleptic dopamine receptor antagonists) increase prolactin secretion. The major action of these drugs in elevating prolactin levels, however, appears to be at the pituitary rather than within the CNS. IH is a rather benign condition, since only a small percentage of patients followed over a period of years will subsequently show evidence of a pituitary tumor.

Therapy depends on the level of symptoms and the degree of inconvenience they produce. Bromocriptine, (2.5 mg two or three times a day) is a dopamine receptor agonist that suppresses prolactin levels, eliminates galactorrhea, and restores cyclic menses and fertility. Nearly 80 per cent of patients will experience menses within two months of initiating therapy, and 65 per cent will become fertile. The effect of the drug is of short duration, however, and hyperprolactinemia recurs following its discontinuation. In some patients, hyperprolactinemia may remit spontaneously or following a pregnancy subsequent to bromocriptine administration. There is no evidence that long-term bromocriptine therapy per se restores prolactin secretory dynamics to normal.

HYPOTHALAMIC DISORDERS OF GROWTH HORMONE SECRETION. ***Idiopathic Growth Hormone Deficiency.*** Idiopathic GH deficiency (IGHD) occurs as either an isolated hormone deficiency or in association with other anterior pituitary hormone deficiencies and as both a familial and sporadic disorder. It is a disease of childhood, the diagnosis frequently being made because of impaired linear growth when the child is between two and three years of age. Impairment in GH secretion may be complete, with basal levels barely detectable, or partial, with subnormal responses to stimuli. The absence of radiologic abnormalities of the pituitary and the frequent coexistence of TRH- and GnRH-responsive deficiencies of TSH and gonadotropins suggest the defect is located in the hypothalamus. No histologic studies of the pituitary or hypothalamus are available because of the generally benign nature of the disease. It is assumed to be due to a deficiency of GRF secretion, most likely on the basis of a neurotransmitter or biosynthetic abnormality, rather than to a structural defect in the hypothalamus. Preliminary studies with synthetic GRF have indicated subnormal GH responsiveness. The significance of these findings, however, remains to be determined. Several subgroups of GH deficiency are now recognized, including one in which partial deletion of the GH gene results in complete absence of the hormone and another in which there is spontaneous recovery of GH secretion. Therapy of IGHD is limited to the prepubertal period and consists of human GH. Hypothyroidism, if present, must also be treated. If gonadotropin deficiency is present, therapy with gonadal steroids is postponed as long as possible to avoid accelerating bone growth and producing epiphyseal closure before acceptable linear bone growth is achieved by GH.

Psychosocial Dwarfism. A pattern indistinguishable from IGHD is seen occasionally in children reared in environments with deficient maternal care and affection. Children with this disorder, also termed the emotional deprivation syndrome, exhibit impaired GH responses to stimuli when studied. Within a short time in an improved environment, however, GH secretion returns to normal, and linear growth is restored. It is presumed that the impaired GH secretion is secondary to a behaviorly associated alteration in neurotransmitter metabolism.

Cerebral Gigantism. This childhood disease is characterized by rapid growth, accelerated bone age, and mental retardation. Ventricular enlargement is present, although no focal CNS lesions have been detected. GH secretion has been normal in the few patients described with this disorder. A variant of the syndrome is associated with lipodystrophy, hyperpigmentation, hypertrichosis, hepatosplenomegaly, increased adrenal steroid production, and hyperlipemia.

CENTRAL NERVOUS SYSTEM DISORDERS OF WATER REGULATION. Organic lesions of the CNS and drug therapy can lead to "cerebral hyponatremia" or "cerebral hypernatremia," which are entities distinct from diabetes insipidus (see Ch. 226, Posterior Pituitary).

Hyponatremia. The syndrome of inappropriate secretion of antidiuretic hormone (ADH) results from the autonomous secretion of vasopressin, resulting in hyponatremia, renal sodium loss, and inability to excrete dilute urine in the presence of normal renal, pituitary, adrenal, and thyroid function; resistance to correction by hypertonic saline; and reversibility following restriction of water (see Ch. 76). The increased renal sodium excretion occurs secondary to expanded extracellular volume, resulting in suppression of aldosterone secretion. When measured, vasopressin levels in the circulation have been increased.

This syndrome has been reported in patients with carcinoma metastatic to the brain, primary brain tumors, cerebral infarction, basal skull fracture, subarachnoid hemorrhage, meningoencephalitis, and acute intermittent porphyria, but it may also occur in the absence of any underlying structural disease. Certain hypoglycemic and antineoplastic drugs can produce the same syndrome. The former, including chlorpropamide and tolbutamide, augment ADH action on the renal tubule and also stimulate ADH release. Vincristine and cyclophosphamide have direct neurotoxic effects on neurohypophyseal tissue. Other agents such as carbamazepine (Tegretol), amitriptyline (Elavil), thioridazine (Mellaril), and clofibrate also produce the syndrome, presumably by affecting endogenous vasopressin release.

Hypernatremia. Patients with intracranial lesions with or without disturbances of consciousness may exhibit hypernatremia in the presence of normal renal function, adequate fluid intake, absence of thirst, and failure of forced fluid intake to correct the hyperosmolality. This syndrome has been attributed to impaired regulation of thirst as well as vasopressin secretion, and has been described in association with histiocytosis, craniopharyngioma, optic nerve glioma, pineal tumor, encephalitis, and ruptured intracranial aneurysm. The treatment of this disorder, above and beyond that of the specific causative lesion, is similar to that for diabetes insipidus.

DISORDERS OF NEUROMETABOLIC REGULATION

Acute Disorders. Acute disturbances of metabolic regulation occur most commonly in states of stress that activate the sympathetic nervous system. Thus, patients with hypothermia, trauma, sepsis, and burns, and in the presence of general anesthesia, may exhibit hyperglycemia and hyperglucagonemia along with impaired insulin secretion. In most instances these changes represent merely an extension of normal physiologic processes, do not result in significant clinical problems, and resolve spontaneously when the stress disappears. However, when stress is prolonged, as in severe burns, the responses can produce a severe catabolic state that can be life threatening.

Stress diabetes, seen frequently in the same clinical disorders, may have several causes. Some patients may manifest true diabetes mellitus for the first time under circumstances in which there is enhanced secretion of cortisol, glucagon, catecholamines, and GH, but in other patients the marked hyperglycemia may be unrelated to true diabetes. A syndrome indistinguishable from nonketotic hyperglycemia with or without coma is associated with severe head injury, cerebral thrombosis, encephalitis, and heat stroke. The severity of the hyperglycemia and its duration predict the probability of survival following head injury. Treatment consists of hydration and small doses of insulin. Beta adrenergic blockade has been used in some patients, but should not be considered standard therapy.

Hypoglycemia is seen only rarely with hypothalamic disease. It has been reported in association with subdural hemorrhage.

Chronic Disorders. Destruction of the ventromedial hypothalamus leads to a syndrome of obesity, but damage to the ventrolateral hypothalamus results in anorexia and inanition. Because bilateral destruction is necessary, inanition is infrequently observed, since the concomitant loss of other important homeostatic mechanisms is usually incompatible with prolonged survival. An anatomically identifiable hypothalamic lesion is present in only a small percentage of patients with extensive obesity or inanition. However, the remarkable similarity of clinical and biochemical features in patients with and without definable lesions suggests that many "functional" disorders of caloric homeostasis ("essential" obesity and anorexia nervosa) are caused by biochemical disturbances in hypothalamic function that are presently undefined.

HYPOTHALAMIC OBESITY. Ventromedial hypothalamic destruction resulting from encephalitis, infiltrative diseases (leukemia or histiocytosis X), trauma, vascular accidents, and tumors has been associated with obesity. Oxygen consumption, insulin secretion, body composition, and adipose metabolism are similar in patients with hypothalamic obesity and in those with "essential" obesity. Adipose tissue mass increases primarily as the result of hypertrophy rather than hyperplasia. Marked insulin resistance is present, and diabetes may develop in some patients. GH secretion is impaired, and hypogonadism is common.

A number of familial disorders (Laurence-Moon, Bardet-Biedl, Alstrom-Hallgren, Prader-Willi) are associated with extreme obesity and evidence of other hypothalamic disturbances, including hypogonadism, temperature intolerance, and loss of diurnal rhythms; and of extrahypothalamic disturbances, such as deafness, pigmentary retinopathy, hypotonia, and mental retardation.

Therapy of hypothalamic obesity is not very successful. Once true destruction has occurred, the functional alterations are almost always irreversible. In children with hypothalamic leukemic infiltrates, successful chemotherapy can lead to cessation of hyperphagia and reduction of weight to normal. In general, therapeutic measures are aimed at treatment of the morbidly obese patient.

ANOREXIA NERVOSA. This disorder has been recognized for more than 300 years, is seen almost exclusively in young women, and consists of weight loss, amenorrhea, and behavioral disturbances. See Ch. 215 for a detailed description.

Almost every neuroendocrine system is affected by the disorder. Gonadotropin secretion "regresses" to a prepubertal stage characterized by absence of pulsatile secretion of LH and altered FSH-LH responses to GnRH. GH levels are normal or, at times, elevated, particularly in the presence of severe malnutrition, in which a paradoxic response to glucose may be observed. TSH responses to TRH are reduced, but thyroid function tends to be normal. Plasma cortisol levels are elevated, but diurnal variation is generally preserved. Patients tend to be poikilothermic, exhibiting difficulty in maintaining body temperature in response to changes in the environment. Impaired vasopressin secretion can be demonstrated, but is rarely of clinical importance.

Most of the endocrine metabolic disturbances can be attributed to the severe malnutrition, and successful therapy resulting in weight gain is usually accompanied by restoration of normal neuroendocrine responses. One exception is gonadotropin secretion, which frequently remains abnormal and results in persistence of amenorrhea in up to one third of patients. Another appears to be osmoregulation, which remains discoordinated, with vasopressin being secreted for prolonged periods.

Prognosis for the reversal of cachexia and weight loss is reasonably good. Mortality is currently less than 5 per cent, and the majority of patients return to within 10 per cent of original body weight. Only 40 per cent of patients maintain their weight over a long term; the remainder exhibit moderate to severe weight loss with time.

CENTRAL NERVOUS SYSTEM BEHAVIORAL DISORDERS AFFECTING NEUROENDOCRINE FUNCTION. Disturbances of endocrine function have been observed in patients with a variety of psychiatric illnesses. The association is presumably through disordered neurotransmitter metabolism, although it is still unclear whether the same defect underlies both the behavioral and neuroendocrine dysfunction or whether altered behavior itself secondarily affects neuroendocrine function.

Of all the conditions studied, depressive affective behavior and the manic-depressive state have been most clearly shown to exhibit endocrine changes. Cortisol secretion in depressed patients is enhanced, and they are relatively resistant to dexamethasone suppression. This abnormality reverts to normal with successful treatment. In manic-depressive patients, cortisol secretion tends to be decreased during manic states and elevated during depressive periods.

Brown GM, Garfinkel PE, Grof E, Grof P, Cleghorn JM, Brown P: A critical appraisal of neuroendocrine approaches to psychiatric disorders. *In* Muller EE, MacLeod RM (eds.): Neuroendocirne Perspectives. Vol 2. Amsterdam, Elsevier Biomedical Press, 1983, pp 329–364. *A review of the recent flurry of excitement concerning the use of neuroendocrine testing to obtain indirect evidence for neurotransmitter disorders in patients with psychiatric disease. The linkage of* selective neuroendocrine defects to specific diagnostic entities may provide new insights into their pathophysiology.*

Comite F, Cutler GB, Rivier J, Vale WW, Loriaux DL, Crowley WF: Short-term treatment of idiopathic precocious puberty with a long-acting analogue of luteinizing hormone-releasing hormone. N Engl J Med 305:1546, 1981. *The use of an agonist of GnRH paradoxically decreases pituitary gonadotropin secretion when given continuously, as a result of down-regulation of the pituitary GnRH receptor. This approach to treatment is the basis for future use of GnRH analogues as contraceptive agents.*

Frohman LA: Clinical aspects of hypothalamic disease. *In* Motta M (ed.): The Endocrine Functions of the Brain. New York, Raven Press, 1980, pp 419–446. *A comprehensive review of neuroendocrine and neurometabolic disorders in man. Emphasis is on the overall integration of homeostatic systems.*

Frohman LA, Krieger DT: Endocrine disorders due to central nervous system disease. *In* Felig P, Baxter JD, Broadus AE, Frohman LA (eds.): Endocrinology and Metabolism. New York, McGraw-Hill Book Company, 1981, pp 233–252. *A systematic review of neuroendocrine pathophysiology and anatomic and functional disorders. Designed for the medical student, clinical trainee, and practicing physician.*

Gold PW, Kaye W, Robertson GL, Ebert M: Abnormalities in plasma and cerebrospinal fluid arginine vasopressin in patients with anorexia nervosa. N Engl J Med 38:1117, 1983. *A careful investigation of the disturbances in water regulation in patients with anorexia nervosa. Insight is provided into some of the previously recognized features of a mild diabetes insipidus-like state.*

Hoffman AR, Crowley WF Jr: Induction of puberty in men by long-term pulsatile administration of low-dose gonadotropin-releasing hormone. N Engl J Med 307:1237, 1982. *Description of the use of pulsatile administration of GnRH to stimulate gonadotropin secretion in subjects with hypogonadotropic hypogonadism. A classic example of the transfer of information from animal physiologic studies to treat human disease.*

Jeffcoate WJ, Laurance BM, Edwards CRW, Besser GM: Endocrine function in the Prader-Willi syndrome. Clin Endocrinol 12:81, 1980. *A human model of hypothalamic obesity with careful neuroendocrine studies that provide an important characterization of the disorder.*

Lieblich JM, Rogol AD, White BJ, Rosen SW: Syndrome of anosmia with hypogonadism (Kallmann's syndrome). Clinical and laboratory studies in 23 cases. Am J Med 73:506, 1982. *An excellent clinical study of Kallmann's syndrome with detailed endocrine studies very lucidly presented.*

Scherbaum WA, Bottazzo GF: Autoantibodies to vasopressin cells in idiopathic diabetes insipidus: Evidence for an autoimmune variant. Lancet 1:897, 1983. *Circulating antibodies to hypothalamic vasopressin-secreting cells but not to vasopressin are demonstrated in one third of patients with idiopathic diabetes insipidus, suggesting the existence of a new entity.*

225. THE ANTERIOR PITUITARY

Lawrence A. Frohman

ANATOMY

The pituitary is located in a saddle-shaped cavity, the *sella turcica,* which is an integral portion of the sphenoid bone. Its anterior boundary is the midline *tuberculum sella* and the anterior clinoid processes that project posteriorly from the sphenoid wings. The posterior limit is the *dorsum sella,* which projects laterally to form the posterior clinoid processes. The lateral boundaries of the sella are nonosseous and consist of the medial wall of the cavernous sinus, in which is contained the internal carotid artery. The *diaphragma sella,* a thickened reflection of the *dura mater,* forms the roof of the sella and is attached to the clinoid processes. Only the external layer of the dura extends into the sella as a periosteal lining, and thus the pituitary is normally extradural and not in direct communication with cerebrospinal fluid. The pituitary stalk and its blood vessels pass through a foramen in this membrane that may be incomplete or fenestrated.

The shape of the sella varies from ovoid to spheroid, resulting in considerable variation in normal pituitary dimensions. The average dimensions of the pituitary are 10 mm (anterior-posterior) by 13 mm (transverse) by 6 mm (height). Pituitary weight varies from 0.5 to 0.7 grams, being slightly greater in women. The anterior lobe constitutes about 75 per cent of the total pituitary weight and during pregnancy can increase up to two-fold in size.

The arterial blood supply of the pituitary originates from the internal carotid artery via branches from the circle of Willis and hypophyseal arteries. Whereas the posterior lobe is supplied directly by the inferior hypophyseal artery, the blood supply of the anterior lobe is derived entirely from the portal vascular system (see Ch. 224). Venous drainage from the anterior lobe enters the posterior pituitary capillary bed and then the cavernous sinus. The nerve supply of the anterior pituitary consists almost exclusively of postganglionic sympathetic fibers that accompany and terminate on arteriolar vessels. The importance of these fibers in regulating pituitary blood flow is unknown. There are also nerve fibers connecting the posterior and anterior lobes, and their function is also unknown.

EMBRYOLOGY

The glandular portion of the pituitary *(adenohypophysis)* is derived from Rathke's pouch, an ectodermal evagination of the oropharynx that fuses with an outpouching of the region of the third ventricle in the developing embryo. This portion of the diencephalon eventually differentiates into the *neurohypophysis,* or posterior lobe. That portion of Rathke's pouch not in contact with the diencephalon differentiates to form the *pars anterior,* or anterior lobe. Two lateral outgrowths from the anterior lobes fuse in the midline and extend forward along the hypophyseal stalk to form the *pars tuberalis,* which in humans is limited to a small group of cells along the anterior region of the stalk. The portion of Rathke's pouch contiguous with the neurohypophysis develops less extensively and forms the *pars intermedia,* or intermediate lobe. This structure is not well defined in humans and tends to become intermingled with the anterior lobe. This combined structure has been called the *pars distalis.*

Cells of the pars anterior differentiate into cells that secrete growth hormone (GH), prolactin, corticotropin (ACTH), thyroid-stimulating hormone (TSH), luteinizing hormone (LH), and follicle-stimulating hormone (FSH). Cells of the pars intermedia secrete ACTH, lipotropin, and endorphins. Pituitary tumors developing in various regions of the pars distalis tend to reflect the predominant cell types in each region.

The lumen of Rathke's pouch is obliterated during development, although remnants may persist at the boundary of the neurohypophysis as either a cleft or small colloid-filled cysts. The connection with the oropharynx disappears early in development, because of growth of the sphenoid bone, although a few cells in the lower portion of the pouch may persist along the tract, occasionally within the sphenoid bone, and are known as the pharyngeal pituitary. These cells contain secretory granules for GH and prolactin, can be a source of "ectopic" pituitary tumor development, and conceivably could exhibit significant endocrine function subsequent to destruction or removal of the pars distalis.

The fetal pituitary anlage is first recognizable at four to five weeks of gestation, and cellular cytologic differentiation occurs between the seventh and tenth weeks. Monoamine fluorescence in the median eminence occurs by 13 weeks and is followed shortly thereafter by development of the portal vascular system. The hypothalamic-pituitary unit appears anatomically mature by 20 weeks. Pituitary hormones are detected immunochemically as early as the seventh week, and CNS control of anterior pituitary hormone secretion occurs early in gestation. In contrast, true functional maturation, including aspects of feedback regulation, do not develop until well into postnatal life.

CELL TYPES

The anterior pituitary contains many cell types, the predominant function of which is the synthesis, storage, and release of a specific hormone(s). Immunohistochemical stains have permitted distinction of specific hormone-containing granules, leading to identification of individual cell types. Secretory granules and the structure of certain cellular organelles, vary greatly between cell types. The secretion granule size within a single cell type varies considerably, depending on the functional state of the cell. The recognized anterior pituitary cell types are as follows:

SOMATOTROPHS. Originally identified as acidophilic cells, these cells secrete GH. Tumors of the cell type predominate in patients with acromegaly. The cells are located predominantly in the lateral portions of the anterior lobe.

LACTOTROPHS. Lactotrophs are also acidophilic and secrete prolactin. They tend to be located more peripherally than somatotrophs, and their secretion granules are smaller. During pregnancy and fetal life, lactotrophs are increased in number, reflecting the effects of increased estrogen levels. Virtually all of the increase in pituitary size during pregnancy can be accounted for by lactotroph proliferation. Both lactotrophs and somatotrophs appear to be derived from a common stem cell, tumors of which may secrete both GH and prolactin.

THYROTROPHS. The basophilic staining cells that secrete TSH occur most frequently at the anterior edge of the pituitary near the midline, although they are also present in deeper portions of the gland. Their secretion granules are smaller than GH and prolactin granules and exhibit considerable heterogeneity. Under normal conditions, thyrotrophs constitute only about 6 per cent of anterior lobe cells. In primary hypothyroidism, they undergo marked hypertrophy, exhibit changes indicative of increased secretory activity, and can eventually undergo neoplastic transformation.

GONADOTROPHS. These cells are located deep in the lateral portion of the gland in association with lactotrophs and secrete both LH and FHS. Although constituting only 3 to 4 per cent of anterior pituitary cells normally, they increase in number following castration and decrease during pregnancy as a result of placental gonadotropin production.

CORTICOTROPHS. This cell type, which can exhibit chromophobic or basophilic characteristics, is found in two separate locations. One group of cells resides most commonly in the medial mucoid region of the anterior lobe. A second group migrates during development to the junctional region of the anterior and posterior lobes and also to the pars tuberalis. Anterior lobe corticotrophs exhibit sparse granulation, whereas those in the pars tuberalis–posterior lobe region contain large and electron-dense granules. The same precursor molecule is present in both cell types, although processing enzyme activity varies, resulting in different ratios of hormones derived from the precursor (ACTH, melanocyte-stimulating hormone [MSH], endorphin) in the two different regions. Increases in glucocorticoid levels produce degranulation and microtubular hyalinization of corticotrophs (Crooke's changes). Anterior lobe corticotrophs increase in number with glucocorticoid deficiency, while those in the intermediate-posterior lobe region decrease, suggesting that only the former are physiologically important ACTH-secreting cells.

OTHER CELL TYPES. As many as 15 to 20 per cent of anterior pituitary cells cannot be stained by antibodies to any of the recognized anterior pituitary hormones. Some of these may represent resting degranulated cells or undifferentiated primitive secretory cells. However, some may be responsible for the secretion of other as yet uncharacterized pituitary hormones such as ovarian growth factor or exophthalmos-producing substance. In addition, a few cells are stellate, with cellular processes extending into the perivascular spaces in a manner suggestive of primitive follicle formation. These cells generally do not contain secretory granules, and their function is unknown.

ANTERIOR PITUITARY HORMONES

The anterior pituitary secretes six well-recognized hormones for which specific and sensitive radioimmunoassays are available. They can be divided into three general categories: corticotropin and related peptides, glycoprotein hormones, and somatomammotropin hormones. The chemical characteristics of these hormones are given in Table 225–1.

CORTICOTROPIN-RELATED PEPTIDES. ACTH and its related family of peptides are synthesized as a single precursor molecule, preopiomelanocortin, with a molecular weight of approximately 29,000. Following glycosylation, the molecule is differentially cleaved into an N-terminal fragment, the biologic activity of which remains uncertain; a midportion, which contains ACTH; and a C-terminal portion, β-lipotropin (LPH). Subsequent processing, which varies in the different groups of corticotrophs and also in the brain, may also cleave ACTH into α-MSH and corticotropin-like intermediate lobe peptide. β-LPH is also differentially processed further to β-endorphin and other endorphin-related peptides (Ch. 222). Although the structures of β-MSH and met-enkephalin are contained within the β-LPH sequence, the former is not synthesized in human pituitaries, and the biosynthesis of the latter occurs through a separate precursor.

ACTH. The primary effects of ACTH are stimulation of secretion of glucocorticoid, mineralocorticoid, and androgenic steroids by the adrenal cortex. ACTH binds to specific receptors on adrenocortical cell membranes and stimulates steroidogenesis by enhancing cholesterol conversion to pregnenolone. ACTH also stimulates adrenal protein synthesis, leading to cellular growth and hyperplasia.

A number of extra-adrenal effects of ACTH have also been described, including stimulation of lipolysis in adipose tissue, insulin-releasing effects on the pancreatic B cell, stimulation of GH secretion, enhancement of glucose and amino acid transport into muscles, and prolongation of cortisol half-life in plasma. Except in patients with ACTH-secreting tumors, it is unlikely that plasma ACTH levels sufficient to produce these

TABLE 225–1. ANTERIOR PITUITARY HORMONES IN HUMANS

Class	Members	Molecular Weight	Amino Acids	Carbohydrate	Other Features
Corticotropin-lipotropin	ACTH	4,500	39		All members of class derived from a single precursor
	α-MSH	1,800	13		N-terminal 13 amino acids of ACTH. In humans, found only in fetal life
	β-Lipotropin	11,200	91		
	β-Endorphin	4,000	31		C-terminal (amino acids 61–91) portion of β-LPH
Glycoprotein	LH	29,000	α subunit: 89 β subunit: 115	1% sialic acid	All have two subunits, with the α subunit being identical or nearly identical and the β subunit conferring biologic specificity
	FSH	29,000	α subunit: 89 β subunit: 115	5% sialic acid	
	TSH	29,000	α subunit: 89 β subunit: 112	1% sialic acid	
	Chorionic gonadotropin*	46,000	α subunit: 92 β subunit: 139	12% sialic acid	
Somatomammotropin	Growth hormone	21,800	191		All single-chain proteins with two or three disulfide bridges
	Prolactin	22,500	198		
	Placental lactogen*	21,800	191		

Adapted from Frohman, LA: Diseases of the anterior pituitary. *In* Felig P, Baxter JD, Broadus AE, Frohman LA (eds.): Endocrinology and Metabolism. New York, McGraw-Hill Book Company, 1981.

*Of placental origin and included for comparison purposes.

effects are ever achieved. Although ACTH has less potent pigmenting effects than α-MSH or β-MSH, it has long been considered the major pigmenting hormone in man. Recent studies, however, have indicated control of pigmentation to be a complex process, and the importance of ACTH has come under question.

ACTH is the most difficult of the pituitary hormones to measure and exhibits the greatest variability, in part because of its episodic secretion. Plasma ACTH levels in normal adults range from undetectable to 80 pg per milliliter (the lower limit of detection in most assays is approximately 10 pg per milliliter. In addition to its episodic secretion, a diurnal rhythm can be detected with lowest levels in the evening and peak levels in the early morning. Changes in plasma ACTH levels can be shown to precede those of plasma cortisol with a short lag period. With stress, plasma ACTH levels can reach several hundred picograms per milliliter. In patients with ectopic ACTH production, immunoreactive ACTH levels may be exceedingly high and consist in part of larger molecular sized forms ("big" ACTH) believed to represent partially processed precursor molecules. ACTH is rapidly eliminated from plasma; its half-life is 3 to 9 minutes, leading to an estimated secretion rate of 25 μg per day, which represents approximately 5 per cent of pituitary hormone content.

β-LPH, Endorphins, and Related Peptides. β-LPH and β-endorphin are secreted in an equimolar ratio to ACTH in response to all types of stimulation. The presence of both molecules in the same precursor as ACTH, with enzymatic cleavage immediately prior to or concomitant with the secretory process, offers an attractive explanation for this observation. The plasma levels of β-LPH and β-endorphin, however, do not necessarily parallel those of ACTH because of a slower metabolic clearance rate. β-LPH is cleared primarily by the kidneys, and its levels rise disproportionately to those of ACTH in renal failure. Since ACTH secretion is normal in this disorder, β-LPH must exert relatively little feedback effect on its own secretion or that of ACTH. The relative ease of measuring β-LPH, in contrast to ACTH, has prompted its use as a marker for the diagnosis of ACTH-secreting tumors, much as C peptide is used in the diagnosis of insulinomas. (β-LPH and β-endorphin have not been shown to have any effects peripherally at the levels normally seen in plasma).

GLYCOPROTEIN HORMONES. The pituitary glycoprotein hormones consist of an α and β subunit, each containing a peptide core with branched carbohydrate side chains that are required for biologic activity and for stability in plasma. The α subunits of the glycoprotein hormones are identical, whereas the β subunits vary, thereby providing the biologic specificity of each hormone. There is considerable homology between β subunits of the different hormones as well as cross-species homology of both α and β subunits, which explains why bovine or ovine glycoprotein hormones are active in humans. The isolated subunits have no intrinsic biologic activity. Evidence of hormone heterogeneity, related to the degree of glycosylation, has been detected and may explain the reported variations in glycoprotein bioactivity at different times in the menstrual cycle. The individual subunits are synthesized separately, and the rate-limiting step in glycoprotein hormone secretion is controlled by β subunit production. Elevations in plasma α subunit levels can be seen after both TRH and GnRH stimulation and also in occasional pituitary tumors.

TSH. TSH effects on the thyroid cells are largely analogous to those of ACTH on the adrenal cortex. High-affinity receptors are present on cell membranes, and TSH binding leads to activation of adenylate cyclase, enhanced iodine transport and binding to protein, increased thyroglobulin and thyroid hormone synthesis, and increased thyroglobulin proteolysis with release of thyroid hormones. RNA and protein synthesis are also stimulated, leading to an increase in thyroid size and vascularity.

TSH is measured by a specific assay utilizing an antibody directed to antigenic determinants on the β subunit that exhibit little or no cross-reactivity with other glycoprotein hormones. Normal levels of plasma TSH are generally reported as under 6 μU per milliliter, with most assays being unable to detect levels less than 1 μU per milliliter. Some of the more recently developed assays appear to have greater sensitivity and specificity, resulting in an upper limit of 3 μU per milliliter and the ability to discriminate normal from low levels. In primary hypothyroidism, TSH levels may increase to greater than 100 μU per milliliter. A few patients have been described with hypothyroidism and slightly elevated TSH levels in whom administration of thyrotropin releasing hormone (TRH) results in an exaggerated TSH increase and a concomitant increase in thyroxine. Evidence for a biologically less potent TSH has been found in such individuals. TSH is cleared from circulation with a half-life of 75 to 80 minutes, and the secretion rate of the hormone is 100 to 200 mU per day. In hypothyroidism, secretion rates may be increased 10 to 15 times that in normals.

LH and FSH. Gonadal function is regulated by two pituitary hormones: (1) FSH, which stimulates ovarian follicular growth, testicular growth, and spermatogenesis, and (2) LH, which promotes ovulation and follicular luteinization, stimulates testicular interstitial cell function, and enhances production of steroids in both ovary and testis. Both gonadotropins bind to receptors in the ovary and testis. In the ovary, FSH promotes growth and maturation of the primordial follicle cell, and LH stimulates progesterone production by the corpus luteum by enhancing the conversion of cholesterol to pregnenolone. In the testis, FSH acts on the Sertoli cell, where, in conjunction with testosterone, the production of an androgen-binding protein is stimulated. The target cell of LH is the Leydig cell, leading to enhanced testosterone production. The androgen-binding protein serves to transport testosterone in high concentrations into the tubular cells to stimulate spermatogenesis. (See also discussion in Ch. 234.)

The gonadotropin assays exhibit some degree of cross-reactivity between the hormone and its subunits, though this is not a practical problem. Of importance, however, is the cross-reactivity due to the great similarity between LH and chorionic gonadotropin. Most LH assays do not discriminate between the two hormones.

Plasma levels of FSH and LH in women vary with the menstrual cycle. FSH levels rise slightly and then decline progressively during the early follicular phase of the cycle, during which time LH levels are generally stable or rise slightly. An abrupt rise in LH at midcycle, initiated by increasing estrogen secretion by the developing follicle and accompanied by an FSH rise, triggers ovulation. Both hormone levels decline during the luteal phase. Levels of FSH and LH in males are similar to those in females during the follicular phase. FSH and LH levels increase in response to age-related decreases in gonadal function in both sexes. In women this occurs at menopause, and in men a gradual increase is seen during the sixth to eighth decades. The half-life of LH in circulation is approximately 30 minutes, whereas that of FSH is twice as long, the difference being attributed to the varying sialic acid content of the hormones.

SOMATOMAMMOTROPIC HORMONES. This hormonal class consists of GH, prolactin, and a structurally similar placental hormone, chorionic somatomammotropin, or placental lactogen. Extensive interspecies homology exists for both GH and prolactin, suggesting relatively limited changes in gene duplication during evolution. Despite the similarity, subprimate growth hormones are biologically inactive in humans. GH and placental lactogen exhibit 83 per cent homology in contrast to only 16 per cent homology between GH and prolactin. Despite these differences, each hormone has both intrinsic lactogenic and growth-promoting activity. The biosynthetic precursor molecules for both GH and prolactin contain an N-terminal extension of approximately 30 amino acids that is cleaved during processing and packaging in the endoplasmic reticulum. Large, molecular weight-sized hormones ("big" GH and pro-en identified in both pituitary and plasma. The appear to be dimers connected by interchain disulfide linkages. They are secreted by the pituitary, bind to the hormone target cell receptors, and exhibit reduced biologic activity as compared to the monomer. There are four or five additional GH variants, including proteolytically modified forms, electrophoretic variants, and a smaller molecule ("20K variant") lacking amino acids 32 to 46, which is encoded by a separate mRNA species derived from the authentic GH gene and formed by differential splicing of pre-mRNA to mRNA. This variant, while representing 10 to 20 per cent of pituitary GH, constitutes less than 5 per cent of secreted GH, and levels in circulation do not change in response to GH secretagogues. It is of potential clinical interest because it possesses the same growth-promoting and lactogenic activity as the normal 22K GH but lacks the hyperglycemic or diabetogenic activity.

Growth Hormone. GH exhibits an important role in production of linear growth and regulation of metabolic processes. GH administration to GH-deficient patients results in positive nitrogen balance, decreased urea production, decreased body fat stores, and enhanced carbohydrate utilization. Biphasic effects on circulating glucose, amino acid, and free fatty acid levels occur in response to GH with an initial decrease and subsequent return to normal or an increase. The acute effects of GH in isolated tissues resemble those of insulin and include increased amino acid uptake and incorporation into protein, stimulation of new RNA synthesis, and enhanced glucose utilization. GH also antagonizes the lipolytic effect of catecholamines in adipose tissue. These acute effects disappear within three to four hours, by which time a series of delayed effects appears. These include enhanced triglyceride lipolysis, increased sensitivity to catecholamine-mediated lipolysis, and inhibition of glucose uptake and utilization secondary to impaired pyruvate decarboxylation. These effects form the basis of the diabetogenic action of the hormone. GH also exhibits multiphasic effects on insulin secretion. There is an acute direct stimulatory effect on the beta cell, a subsequent inhibitory effect, and a late and persistent stimulation of insulin release that occurs secondary to the impairment of carbohydrate utilization. The last effect has the greatest pathophysiologic significance in the development of diabetes secondary to GH hypersecretion.

Many GH effects cannot be produced by exposure of tissues to the hormone and are mediated by a group of GH-dependent growth factors, most of which are synthesized in the liver. GH binds to specific receptors on hepatocyte membranes to stimulate their production. The most important of these factors is somatomedin C or insulin-like growth factor I (IGF I), a peptide of about 7500 daltons that has many similarities to insulin, including structural resemblance to proinsulin and binding to insulin receptors. Somatomedin C receptors are present in many tissues, including cartilage, where sulfate incorporation into proteoglycan and amino acid uptake incorporation are stimulated. A closely related peptide, somatomedin A (IGF II), and a platelet–derived growth factor are also GH dependent, though they are less important in both mediating the growth-stimulating effects of GH and peripheral feedback of GH secretion. GH also stimulates cardiac and renal hypertrophy and production of specific hormones such as renin and aldosterone and conversion of thyroxine to triiodothyronine.

Immunoreactive measurements of GH are considered valid indicators of GH bioactivity. Mean GH levels during adolescence and adult life are generally less than 3 ng per milliliter, although the spontaneous secretory pulses of GH can produce elevations as great as 30 to 50 ng per milliliter in young adult subjects. Levels in women during the childbearing age are generally greater than in men, particularly in response to exercise or other stimuli. GH is cleared from plasma primarily by the liver and to a lesser extent by the kidney. The half-time of GH disappearance from circulation is 20 to 25 minutes, and the overall secretion in normal adults ranges from 300 to 500 μg per square meter per day.

Prolactin. The major effect of prolactin is to stimulate the synthesis of milk constituents, including lactalbumin, lipids, and carbohydrates (Ch. 238). Prolactin receptors are present on alveolar surfaces of mammary cells and, in addition, have been identified in liver and kidney. Prolactin is not required for normal breast development in humans, and pathologic elevations of the hormone are not associated with an increase in breast size. During pregnancy, prolactin, in conjunction with estrogen, progesterone, and placental lactogen, results in further breast development and milk formation. Following parturition, the abrupt decrease in estrogen and progesterone derived from the placenta permits initiation of lactation. This effect underlies the use of estrogens to inhibit lactation in the postpartum period and explains the frequent development of galactorrhea in hyperprolactinemic women after discontinuance of oral contraceptives. Continued prolactin secretion is required to maintain lactation once it is initiated, and the return of prolactin to normal levels in the postpartum period is delayed in women who nurse for prolonged periods. The actual milk let-down reflex is mediated by the release of oxytocin in the posterior pituitary rather than by prolactin. Oxytocin stimulates contraction of myoepithelial cells surrounding the terminal acinar lobules that expel their milk into the lobular ducts. Although prolactin has numerous effects on behavior and on fluid and electrolyte metabolism in lower species, no such effects have been convincingly demonstrated in humans.

Normal prolactin levels do not exceed 15 ng per milliliter in men or 20 ng per milliliter in women. There are no significant changes during the menstrual cycle, but levels decrease at menopause. During pregnancy, prolactin levels rise continuously from early gestation to values of 150 to 200 ng per milliliter at term. Prolactin is cleared from circulation with a half-time of approximately 50 minutes. The liver and, to a lesser extent, the kidney are the major sites of prolactin removal.

TESTS OF ANTERIOR PITUITARY HORMONE FUNCTION

ACTH. Since ACTH levels in normal subjects may be undetectable at times, random measurements of the hormone are of limited value. In a patient with signs and symptoms of adrenocortical insufficiency and low plasma cortisol levels, a low or even normal ACTH level is suggestive of hypothalamic-pituitary disease. The most useful test for evaluating ACTH function is that of insulin hypoglycemia. A dose of insulin calculated to decrease the fasting blood glucose to 40 mg per deciliter is administered, and plasma cortisol levels are measured over a two-hour period. A rise greater than 10 μg per deciliter or a peak level greater than 20 μg per deciliter is indicative of a normal hypothalamic-pituitary-adrenal axis. The standard dose of insulin is 0.1 U per kilogram (intravenously), although the dose should be decreased by 50 per cent when the diagnosis of hypopituitarism is strongly suspected and increased by 50 per cent in patients with anticipated insulin resistance (i.e., obesity). No treatment is necessary for mild symptoms of hypoglycemia (catecholamine-mediated phenomena), but symptoms of central glucopenia (impaired mentation or altered states of consciousness) require immediate therapy. This test must not be performed in patients with suspected primary adrenal insufficiency.

Corticotropin releasing factor (CRF) is currently being evaluated as a diagnostic agent for assessing ACTH function and, when available for general use, is expected to provide a valuable adjunct. A normal response to CRF and an impaired response to insulin hypoglycemia, for example, would suggest hypothalamic rather than pituitary disease. Impairment of normal cortisol feedback using metyrapone, an 11β-hydroxylase inhibitor, at a dose of 750 mg orally every four hours for six doses, with measurement of plasma 11-desoxycortisol or urinary 17-hydroxycorticoids, is an alternative way to test the entire hypothalamic-pituitary-adrenal axis. This test is less useful than insulin hypoglycemia in predicting normal responsiveness of the axis to stress.

The best test of suspected excessive ACTH and cortisol secretion is by dexamethasone suppression. The rapid dexamethasone suppression test involves administration of 1 mg dexamethasone orally at 11 P.M. and measurement of plasma cortisol at 8 o'clock the following morning. A level of less than 5 μg per deciliter indicates normal suppressibility. In patients in whom normal suppression is not demonstrated, a standard low-dose dexamethasone suppression test (0.5 mg orally every six hours for 48 hours) is performed. Plasma cortisol will be suppressed to less than 5 μg per deciliter, and urinary free cortisol levels will be suppressed to within the normal range in normal subjects but not in patients with pituitary ACTH hypersecretion or primary adrenocortical hypersecretion. In patients in whom suppression fails, a high-dose dexamethasone suppression test (2 mg orally every six hours for 48 hours) is then used to distinguish between pituitary and adrenal causes.

TSH. Impairment of TSH secretion should be suspected in patients with hypothyroidism in whom plasma TSH levels are not elevated. Differentiation of pituitary from hypothalamic causes of TSH deficiency can usually, but not always, be accomplished by administering TRH, 500 μg (intravenously), and measuring plasma TSH levels. In normal persons, plasma TSH increases to at least 8 μU per milliliter after TRH administration, and peak levels usually occur at 15 to 30 minutes. In patients with hypothalamic hypothyroidism, the response may be exaggerated and is frequently prolonged, with peak values occurring at 90 to 180 minutes. Since thyroxine impairs the TSH response to TRH, it is not possible to assess TSH function in patients receiving thyroid hormone replacement therapy until at least a month after discontinuation of medication.

LH AND FSH. LH and FSH deficiency should be suspected in patients with clinical evidence of hypogonadism and subnormal testosterone or estradiol levels in whom gonadotropin levels are not elevated. Gonadotropin releasing hormone (GnRH) (100 μg, intravenously) can be administered and gonadotropin responses measured. An increase of at least three- to five-fold in LH is seen in normal subjects. A single injection, however, may not distinguish between hypothalamic and hypopituitary causes, since impaired responses may be seen in both disorders and only after repeated injections does a response occur in patients with hypothalamic hypogonadism. Clomiphene, an estrogen antagonist, will stimulate gonadotropin levels in some patients with hypothalamic hypogonadism.

GROWTH HORMONE. The most frequently employed stimulus for GH secretion is the insulin hypoglycemia test. The details of testing and the cautions required are as described under ACTH testing. Peak growth hormone levels usually occur at 60 or 90 minutes, and a peak level of 9 ng per milliliter or greater is required for a normal response. Up to 30 per cent of normal subjects may not respond to insulin hypoglycemia. L-arginine (0.5 gram per kilogram intravenously during a 30-minute period), L-dopa (0.5 gram orally), and clonidine (25 μg orally) are other effective stimuli used to test GH secretory reserve. The responses are comparable in magnitude to those after insulin. Although other stimuli have been used (glucagon plus propranolol, endotoxin, vasopressin, ACTH), none has any advantage over those described. There is currently insufficient information to know whether growth hormone releasing factor (GRF) will be useful as a diagnostic test in distinguishing pituitary from hypothalamic causes of GH deficiency.

Suppressibility of GH secretion in patients with elevated GH levels is evaluated with a standard glucose tolerance test. A decrease in GH levels to less than 2 ng per milliliter is seen in normal subjects. TRH is also used in distinguishing between types of suspected GH hypersecretion. TRH has no effect on GH levels in normal subjects, whereas in 80 to 90 per cent of patients with acromegaly a rapid increase in GH levels occurs.

PROLACTIN. Impaired prolactin secretion is rarely a clinical problem. Prolactin deficiency can be suspected in patients with levels of less than 2 ng per milliliter, and the diagnosis is confirmed by the absence of a response to TRH. Elevated prolactin levels in nearly all patients, with the exception of occasional patients with prolactin-secreting tumors and patients with chronic renal failure, can be suppressed by dopamine infusions, L-dopa, or other dopaminergic agents. These tests have limited usefulness in determining the cause of hyperprolactinemia and are generally not used.

Ezrin C, Horvath E, Kovacs K: Anatomy and cytology of the normal and abnormal pituitary gland. *In* DeGroot LJ, Cahill GF Jr, Martini L, et al (eds.): Endocrinology. Vol. 1. New York, Grune & Stratton, 1979, pp 103–121. *A well-organized and referenced presentation of pituitary structure with emphasis on the changes in human disease.*

Frohman LA: Diseases of the anterior pituitary. *In* Felig P, Baxter JD, Broadus E, Frohman LA (eds.): Endocrinology and Metabolism. New York, McGraw-Hill Book Company, 1981, pp 151–231. *A detailed systematic description of the chemistry, physiology, and pathophysiology of the pituitary. Of particular use to the clinical trainee and practicing physician.*

Frohman LA: Growth hormone releasing factor: A neuroendocrine perspective. J Lab Clin Med 103:819, 1984. *A review of the clinical studies leading to the isolation and characterization of GRF and the initial results of its use in normal human subjects and patients with GH secretory disorders.*

Jaffe RB, Monroe SE: Hormone interaction and regulation during the menstrual cycle. *In* Ganong WF, Martini L (eds.): Frontiers in Neuroendocrinology. Vol. 6. New York, Raven Press, 1980, pp 219–248. *A comprehensive review of the hormonal interactions responsible for the cyclical reproductive cycle in women. Provides a firm basis with which to understand pathophysiologic conditions.*

Lufkin EG, Kao PC, O'Fallon WM, Mangan MA: Combined testing of anterior pituitary gland with insulin, thyrotropin-releasing hormone, and luteinizing hormone-releasing hormone. Am J Med 75:471, 1983. *A clearly presented study confirming that the combined use of the three standard agents used in testing pituitary hormone function is more efficient than individual testing protocols.*

Miller WL, Eberhardt NL: Structure and evolution of the growth hormone gene family. Endocr Rev 4:97, 1983. *This review documents in great detail the recent exciting developments in molecular biology related to GH gene expression. Although of limited practical use to the clinician, this work describes concepts important for understanding recombinant DNA technology as applied to the production of human hormones.*

Orth DN, Jackson RV, DeCherney CS, DeBold CR, Alexander AN, Island DP, Rivier J, Rivier C, Spiess J, Vale W: Effect of synthetic ovine corticotropin-releasing factor. Dose response to plasma adrenocorticotropin and cortisol. J Clin Invest 71:587, 1983. *Classic study of the use of a new releasing hormone to evaluate ACTH secretion. When available for clinical use, this peptide should permit differential assessment of hypothalamic and pituitary components of the regulation of ACTH secretion.*

Scanlon MF, Lewis M, Weightman DR, Chan V, Hall R: The neuroregulation of human thyrotropin secretion. *In* Ganong WF, Martini L (eds.): Frontiers in Neuroendocrinology. Vol. 6. New York, Raven Press, 1980, pp 333–380. *An excellent review of mechanisms by which the CNS influences the secretion of TSH. The interaction of neurotransmitters, TRH, and thyroid hormones is clearly described.*

Tolis G, Stefanis C, Mountokalakis, T, Labrie F (eds.): Prolactin and Prolactinomas. New York, Raven Press, 1983. *A series of monographs on various aspects of prolactin physiology and pathophysiology with particular emphasis on hyperprolactinemic states with and without pituitary tumors.*

HYPOPITUITARISM

DISEASE STATES ASSOCIATED WITH HYPOPITUITARISM (Table 225–2). The subject's age, rapidity of onset of the disorder, and the extent of impaired hormone secretion as well as the specific pathologic process all influence the clinical manifestations. When acute and complete the disease can be life threatening, but in a mild form it can remain undetected for many years. Hypopituitarism can occur as a result of a *primary* disorder due to absence or destruction of anterior pituitary cells or *secondary* to CNS disease. In the latter, pituitary hormone deficiency occurs because of a lack of appropriate releasing factors.

The classic example of *primary hypopituitarism* is ischemic postpartum pituitary necrosis, first associated with the clinical features of hypopituitarism by Simmonds and characterized by Sheehan. The mechanism of acute ischemic necrosis is believed to relate to vasospasm of hypophyseal vessels, possibly influenced by estrogen-induced sensitivity to the vasoconstrictive stimulus of hypoxia. This disorder occurs most frequently in the immediate postpartum period and is associated with severe hemorrhage and hypotension. Some degree of hypopituitarism occurs in up to one third of women experiencing severe hemorrhage during delivery. The disorder is recognized by absence of lactation in the postpartum period and failure of normal cyclic menstruation to resume. Because of the slowly progressive nature of this disease the presence of postpartum

TABLE 225–2. ETIOLOGY OF HYPOPITUITARISM

A. Primary
- Ischemic necrosis of the pituitary
  - Postpartum (Sheehan's syndrome)
  - Diabetes mellitus
  - Other systemic diseases (temporal arteritis, sickle-cell disease and trait, arteriosclerosis, eclampsia)
- Pituitary tumors
  - Primary intrasellar (chromophobe adenoma, craniopharyngioma)
  - Parasellar (meningioma, optic nerve glioma)
- Aneurysm of intracranial internal carotid artery
- Pituitary apoplexy (almost always related to a primary pituitary tumor)
- Cavernous sinus thrombosis
- Infectious disease (tuberculosis, syphilis, malaria, meningitis, fungal disease)
- Infiltrative disease (hemochromatosis)
- Immunologic (lymphocytic hypophysitis)
- Iatrogenic
  - Irradiation to nasopharynx
  - Irradiation to sella
  - Surgical destruction
- Primary empty sella syndrome
- Metabolic disorders (chronic renal failure)
- Idiopathic (frequently monohormonal and occasionally familial)

B. Secondary
- Destruction of pituitary stalk
  - Trauma
  - Compression by tumor or aneurysm
  - Iatrogenic (surgical)
- Hypothalamic or other central nervous system disease
  - Inflammatory (sarcoidosis)
  - Infiltrative (lipid storage diseases)
  - Trauma
  - Toxic (vincristine)
  - Hormone induced (glucocorticoids, gonadal steroids)
  - Tumors (primary, metastatic, lymphomas, leukemia)
  - Idiopathic (frequently congenital or familial, often restricted to one or two hormones, and may be reversible)
  - Nutritional (starvation, obesity)
  - Anorexia nervosa
  - Psychosocial dwarfism

Adapted from Frohman LA: Diseases of the anterior pituitary. *In* Felig P, Baxter JD, Broadus AE, Frohman LA (eds.): Endocrinology and Metabolism. New York, McGraw-Hill Book Company, 1981.

lactation does not preclude development of the disorder at a later time. Since complete hypopituitarism requires at least 90 per cent destruction of the pituitary, the diagnosis may never be made in many patients with pituitary necrosis and minimal evidence of hypopituitarism. The disease is currently much less common than previously, because of the marked improvement in obstetric care during the past half century. Ischemic pituitary necrosis can be seen with other disorders, though much less commonly.

The most common cause of hypopituitarism is a pituitary tumor (discussed in the following section). Other parasellar mass lesions, including CNS tumors and internal carotid aneurysms, can also invade the sella and destroy the pituitary. Intrapituitary hemorrhage *(pituitary apoplexy)* associated with pituitary tumors may produce varying degrees of hypopituitarism. If bleeding occurs gradually, the pituitary is compressed and symptoms of hypopituitarism predominate. If the hemorrhage is sudden, presenting symptoms include headache, visual field defects or blindness, ophthalmoplegia, and subarachnoid irritation. Furthermore, a pre-existing pituitary tumor may suddenly expand. Immediate glucocorticoid therapy is essential in such patients. Most will recover without the need for surgical intervention, but it may be necessary in some to restore visual function.

Radiation therapy for treatment of malignant tumors of the head and neck frequently causes primary or secondary hypopituitarism. Growth disturbances are the most common manifestations in children, whereas hypogonadism is more common in adults. Hypopituitarism may occur within 6 to 12 months after a dose of 3000 rads or greater, and children appear to be more susceptible than adults. The disorder may not appear until several years following irradiation. Lymphocytic hypopituitarism, a recently recognized disorder, tends to occur in the postpartum period and may present as an expanding pituitary mass lesion associated with hypopituitarism (and occasionally hyperprolactinemia). Destruction of pituitary tissue with round cell infiltration has been found histologically, but the cause is unknown. Hypopituitarism may occur without detectable underlying disease and may be limited to one or two hormones rather than involving all of them. There are reports of both autosomal and X-linked recessive varieties of the disease. Partial hypopituitarism also occurs in patients with chronic renal failure and is reversible after renal transplantation.

Secondary hypopituitarism can be caused by diverse CNS disorders, all of which disrupt the delivery of releasing factors to the pituitary. The distinction between CNS and pituitary causes can frequently, but not always, be made on the basis of responses to the hypothalamic releasing hormones. Diseases of the pituitary stalk are most frequently due to trauma. Basilar skull fractures often shear the stalk, rupturing both neural and vascular connections. Parasellar tumors and aneurysms can compress the stalk sufficiently to impair blood flow to portal vessels. Disorders of the CNS, primarily the hypothalamus, that impair releasing factor secretion are described in Ch. 224.

CLINICAL FEATURES. In the most dramatic form of hypopituitarism, panhypopituitarism occurring after surgical hypophysectomy, severe pituitary apoplexy, or withdrawal of hormone therapy, clinical features are noted within a few hours (diabetes insipidus) to a few days (adrenal insufficiency). In partial hypopituitarism the signs and symptoms develop slowly and may be vague and nonspecific. The clinical features are best considered in terms of the deficiencies of individual pituitary hormones.

Hormone-specific Features

ACTH. Manifestations of ACTH deficiency are similar to those of adrenocortical deficiency. Weakness, postural hypotension, malaise, dehydration, and cold intolerance are common, though a true addisonian crisis is infrequent because some aldosterone secretion is maintained through the renin-angiotensin mechanism, which is independent of ACTH. Nausea, vomiting, and severe hypothermia can occur, and hypoglycemia associated with prolonged fasting or alcohol ingestion may be seen as a result of impaired gluconeogenesis. In contrast to Addison's disease, in which hyperpigmentation occurs, patients with ACTH deficiency frequently exhibit depigmentation and decreased tanning after exposure to sunlight. If ACTH secretion is only partially impaired, symptoms may be experienced only during periods of stress. Adrenal androgen deficiency occurs and contributes to decreased libido and to loss of axillary and pubic hair in women. In men the deficiency is of little consequence if testicular function is preserved.

TSH. The features of primary and secondary TSH deficiency are quite similar with the exception of severity. Patients experience cold intolerance, dry skin, pallor, mental slowing, bradycardia, hoarseness and constipation. True myxedema and hypercholesterolemia are seen only infrequently. Menstrual flow may be increased or more likely decreased because of associated gonadotropin deficiency. During childhood, TSH deficiency results in growth retardation which is unresponsive to GH treatment.

LH AND FSH. In women, gonadotropin deficiency results in amenorrhea and signs of estrogen deficiency, including breast atrophy, skin dryness, decreased vaginal secretions, and, occasionally, decreased libido. In males, the testes decrease in size and become softened. Decreased androgen production results in a loss of libido and potency, decreased rate of growth of secondary sexual hair, and reduced muscular strength. If the deficiency occurs prior to puberty there is total or partial impairment of secondary sexual development. If GH secretion is unaltered, failure of sex steroid–induced epiphyseal closure of the long bones produces excessive growth of limbs, leading to a eunuchoid appearance.

GROWTH HORMONE. GH deficiency in the adult is unassociated with significant clinical symptoms. Carbohydrate tolerance is impaired in GH-deficient subjects, but this disorder is distinct from diabetes mellitus and is not associated with microangiopathy. In children, GH deficiency results in growth retardation. Fasting hypoglycemia is often seen, particularly when ACTH deficiency is also present.

PROLACTIN. Prolactin deficiency results only in the absence of postpartum lactation.

VASOPRESSIN. Deficiency of vasopressin results in diabetes insipidus, described in detail in Ch. 226. The impairment of water reabsorption by the kidneys results in polyuria and polydipsia, and, if fluid intake is not maintained, severe dehydration. Extreme thirst may be present that is preferentially relieved by ice water. Polyuria may not be present when ACTH deficiency coexists because of the requirement of cortisol for free water excretion. The appearance of polyuria during ACTH or glucocorticoid administration is highly suggestive of a combined vasopressin and ACTH deficiency.

OXYTOCIN. Oxytocin deficiency is unassociated with any clinically apparent disease in humans. In particular, in women with panhypopituitarism who become pregnant, initiation of labor is normal, as is parturition.

General Clinical Features. The skin of hypopituitary patients often exhibits decreased turgor and a waxy character. Perioral and periorbital wrinkling is common, giving the appearance of premature aging. Nutrition, in general, is quite well preserved. Moderate anemia commonly occurs that is usually normochromic and normocytic, but it may be hypochromic or macrocytic and is attributed to a combination of thyroid, testosterone, and erythropoietin deficiencies. Mental slowing and apathy are quite common, as are other psychiatric symptoms, including delusions and occasionally paranoid psychosis. Carbohydrate metabolism is generally intact in nondiabetics, but in insulin-requiring diabetics, hypopituitarism necessitates reduction in insulin dosage, frequently to less than half of the original level; there is also an increased tendency for hypoglycemic reactions. These changes may persist even with full glucocorticoid replacement therapy.

The sequence of pituitary hormone loss varies among patients with hypopituitarism. In general, deficiencies of GH and gonadotropins are the earliest to occur and, thus, the most frequently observed. ACTH and TSH deficiencies are less common and are seen at a later stage in the natural history of the disease. The pattern, however, is not predictable in individual patients, thus precluding the usefulness of evaluating pituitary function by measurement of only one or two hormones.

DIFFERENTIAL DIAGNOSIS. The major categories of diseases with which hypopituitarism can be confused include (1) disorders of multiple target glands or of the CNS and (2) diseases that share the generalized features of hypopituitarism that are unassociated with endocrine dysfunction.

While measurement of pituitary hormones is indispensable in the differential diagnosis, certain clinical features have discriminatory value. Primary adrenal insufficiency is associated with hyperkalemia, hyperpigmentation, and salt craving, all of which are absent in hypopituitarism. Some patients with primary gonadal failure exhibit a discrepancy between the loss of gonadal steroid production and the loss of spermatogenesis or ovulation. Both components of gonadal function are diminished to the same extent in hypopituitarism. Primary ovarian failure often results in characteristic symptoms (hot flashes) that are usually not seen when ovarian failure is secondary to gonadotropin deficiency.

Patients with chronic malnutrition or liver disease exhibit weakness, lethargy, cold intolerance, and decreased libido, frequently raising the possibility of hypopituitarism. The presence of cachexia is important in suggesting a nonpituitary disease. Although anorexia nervosa may often be confused with hypopituitarism, the severe weight loss, psychiatric symptoms, and preservation of axillary and pubic hair are all useful discriminating factors (Ch. 215).

DIAGNOSIS. The diagnosis of hypopituitarism should be carefully and appropriately established since therapeutic decisions imply lifelong hormonal replacement therapy. In addition, studies directed at determining the etiology of the hypopituitarism (neuroanatomic studies) are an integral part of the workup and are discussed in the section on pituitary tumors.

Functional studies of each of the anterior pituitary hormones have been described in the previous section, where the specific testing details are provided. Certain general concepts used in testing are described here.

In evaluation of ACTH secretion, it is important to consider the practical implications. Testing is performed to identify patients with suspected partial adrenal insufficiency in whom an inadequate response to stress may occur. The best stimulus for this purpose is insulin hypoglycemia, in which the response to cortisol correlates well with that to surgical stress. The same test can also be used to evaluate GH responsiveness. Recent administration of glucocorticoid therapy can complicate the workup of a patient with suspected hypopituitarism. The suppressive effects of glucocorticoids on the hypothalamic-pituitary-adrenal axis can result in a subnormal response or absence of response to any of the stimuli used. Glucocorticoids should be discontinued for at least one month, if possible, prior to definitive testing.

A similar problem occurs in evaluating TSH function in patients who have been receiving long-term thyroid hormone therapy, which can impair the TSH response to TRH for at least one month.

In patients with gonadotropin deficiency, distinguishing between hypothalamic and pituitary causes is often difficult. A single GnRH challenge is frequently of little help in making this distinction and is useful primarily when neuroanatomic evidence of pituitary disease is present and the status of the gonadotrophs is being questioned.

Documentation of GH deficiency is important primarily in children of short stature when therapy with exogenous GH is being considered. Decisions concerning GH therapy require careful assessment because of the effort and expense involved. Failure of response to at least two stimuli, usually insulin hypoglycemia and arginine, is generally required before institution of GH therapy. In addition, hypothyroidism, if present, must be corrected prior to GH testing. In adults, GH deficiency serves as a marker for acquired hypopituitarism, particularly with pituitary tumors. In children and adults with obesity, GH responses to all stimuli tested are impaired, even in the presence of seemingly normal growth.

THERAPY. Hormonal replacement therapy must be determined individually, and treatment goals specifically defined. The therapeutic use of pituitary hormones is restricted to GH for correcting growth retardation and gonadotropins for inducing fertility. Potential uses of hypothalamic hormones or their synthetic analogues are at present limited to GnRH for the treatment of hypothalamic hypogonadism, though current research in this field may shortly result in other potential uses. For the most part, target organ hormones are used because of their cost advantage, ease of administration, and prolonged action.

ACTH. ACTH deficiency is treated with glucocorticoids. Cortisone (25 mg orally), hydrocortisone (20 mg orally), or prednisone (5 mg orally) given as a divided dose provides adequate therapy for most patients under normal conditions. Supplemental mineralocorticoid therapy is unnecessary because of the partial preservation of aldosterone secretion. The use of prednisone is preferred because of its reduced cost. Occasional patients may require full glucocorticoid replacement therapy (a dose 50 per cent greater than those listed), but in most patients this dose is excessive. During stress, the dose should be increased two- to three-fold and then gradually tapered. If oral medication cannot be retained, injectable steroids (hydrocortisone hemisuccinate [Solu-Cortef] for initial emergency use, 100 mg intramuscularly or intravenously), or cortisone acetate for long-term use (50 to 100 mg intramuscularly every 12 hours) is indicated. Treatment of the acutely ill hypopituitary patient requires the same dosage of hydrocortisone (100 to 300 mg per day) as used in primary adrenal insufficiency. Preoperatively, patients should receive hydrocortisone hemisuccinate 50 mg intramuscularly every 6 hours beginning the evening prior to surgery and continuing through the immediate postoperative period, followed by gradual tapering to maintenance dosage. Treatment of patients with partial ACTH deficiency without symptoms in the nonstressed state is more controversial. With adequate education, many patients will not need maintenance replacement therapy except in times of stress. Such patients in particular should wear appropriate medical identification bracelets.

TSH. TSH deficiency is treated with L-thyroxine 0.15 to 0.2 mg per day, though a lower dose may suffice in occasional patients. Clinical assessment of the patient and serum thyroxine levels during initiation of therapy are used to establish the appropriate dose. Adrenal insufficiency must be corrected prior to instituting thyroid hormone replacement therapy, and patients with partial adrenal insufficiency may require glucocorticoid replacement only after thyroid hormone replacement is started. In the presence of severe or longstanding hypothyroidism a small dose of thyroxine (0.025 mg per day) should be used initially and increased slowly to a maintenance dose. The use of triiodothyronine, particularly as long-term therapy, is not recommended, because its shorter biologic half-life results in more rapid appearance of thyroid deficiency in the event therapy is omitted.

LH and FSH. Treatment of gonadotropin deficiency requires consideration of both gonadal steroid replacement and treatment of infertility. The subjects are considered in greater detail in Ch. 234 and 236.

WOMEN. Estrogen replacement therapy is indicated in premenopausal women to maintain secondary sex characteristics and to prevent osteoporosis and possibly coronary artery disease. This can be accomplished with ethinyl estradiol 5 to 20 μg per day or conjugated estrogens (Premarin) 0.6 to 1.25 mg per day. The lowest possible dose that produces the desired clinical effects should be used. To induce cyclic bleeding, estrogen should be given for 25 days each month, accompanied on the last five days by a progestinic agent such as medroxyprogesterone 5 to 10 mg per day. Alternatively, an oral contraceptive preparation containing no more than the equivalent of 25 μg estradiol per day can be used. The advantage of replacement therapy after the menopause is still controversial, and the potential risks and benefits should be discussed with the patient to help make an appropriate decision. Estrogen therapy usually corrects the dyspareunia attributable to local estrogen deficiency in women with hypopituitarism, but decreased libido due to the absence of adrenal androgens often persists. This can be corrected by injection of a small dose of long-acting androgen such as testosterone enanthate 50 mg every one to two months or by oral administration of fluoxymesterone 5 to 10 mg once or twice weekly.

Restoration of fertility is possible in a large percentage of women with clomiphene or GnRH therapy if the cause of the disorder is hypothalamic or with combined FSH/LH preparations if pituitary disease is present. An FSH-rich preparation from postmenopausal urine is used to initiate follicular growth and maturation; it is monitored by measurement of plasma estradiol levels. Human chorionic gonadotropin is then injected to induce ovulation. This therapy is expensive, entails the risk of superovulation and multiple pregnancy, and should be undertaken only under the direction of an experienced physician.

MEN. Testosterone replacement therapy in adult males is accomplished by intramuscular injection of a long-acting testosterone preparation (testosterone enanthate or cypionate, 200 mg every three to four weeks). The endpoints are restoration of full androgenization, including beard growth, improvement in muscular strength, libido and potency. Androgen therapy should be withheld as long as possible in the adolescent with growth retardation to avoid premature epiphyseal closure, which limits the potential for future linear growth. Testosterone therapy may be required for many months before full restoration of libido and performance. If gonadotropin deficiency has developed before puberty, full androgenization may never occur. In patients with longstanding hypogonadism, psychosocial behavorial changes affecting the patient's entire lifestyle may be disrupted by initiation of testosterone therapy, leading to major adjustment problems with both sexual and nonsexual relationships.

Infertility in men with hypopituitarism can be corrected with a combination of FSH and human chorionic gonadotropin (HCG), though therapy is required for several months, and the success rate is less than 50 per cent. Current studies indicate that, in the future, GnRH analogues may provide a convenient and less expensive form of therapy for individuals with hypothalamic hypogonadism.

Growth Hormone. GH therapy is indicated for the correction of impaired linear growth, and its use is thus confined almost exclusively to childhood and adolescent years. Early establishment of the diagnosis is critical, since the probability of successful long-term therapy is inversely related to the extent of growth retardation. Treatment requires the use of human GH, which has traditionally been extracted and purified from pituitaries obtained at autopsy. Preliminary studies with GH produced by recombinant DNA technology have indicated comparable hormone biopotency, and this source should provide an unlimited supply of GH in the near future. GH is administered intramuscularly or subcutaneously in a dosage of 0.1 to 0.2 U per kilogram three times weekly; its use is continued until the final height is achieved, coincident with long-bone epiphyseal closure. A goal of 5 feet 4 inches is generally pursued but not always achieved. Careful attention must be given to concomitant hormone deficiencies, particularly thyroid. Glucocorticoids should be used sparingly because of their interference with growth-promoting effects of GH. Some physicians have proposed that small doses of oral androgens be used simultaneously to increase growth velocity, though this has not gained widespread acceptance. Estrogens are to be avoided because of their greater effect on epiphyseal closure. Gonadal steroid therapy is usually initiated during the years of puberty to avoid psychosocial problems. However, if significant catch-up growth is required, its use should be delayed. GH therapy increases height age more rapidly than bone age, may initially be associated with a decrease in body fat, and also corrects the fasting hypoglycemia of GH-deficient children.

Asa SL, Bilbao JM, Kovacs K, Josse RG, Kreines K: Lymphocytic hypophysitis of pregnancy resulting in hypopituitarism: A distinct clinicopathological entity. Ann Intern Med 95:166, 1981. Baskin DS, Townsend JJ, Wilson CB: Lymphocytic adenohypophysitis of pregnancy simulating a pituitary adenoma: A distinct pathological entity. Report of two cases. J. Neurosurg 56:148, 1982. *Two reports of a newly recognized pregnancy-related syndrome diagnosed by histological examination of pituitary tissue. Clinical differentiation from pituitary tumors is difficult, and the pathogenesis is unclear.*

Frasier SD: Human pituitary growth hormone (hGH) therapy in growth hormone deficiency. Endocr Rev 4:155, 1983. *An up-to-date assessment of the use of human GH as therapy in children with GH deficiency. Critical evaluation of various treatment protocols, necessitated because of the limited supply of GH, has resulted in effective means of assessing the responses to the hormone.*

Gharib H, Frey HM, Laws ER Jr, Randall RV, Scheithauer BW: Coexistent primary empty sella syndrome and hyperprolactinemia. Report of 11 cases. Arch Intern Med 143:1383, 1983. *The empty sella syndrome is being recognized with greater frequency, and coexisting hyperprolactinemia does not necessarily imply the presence of a pituitary microadenoma.*

Phillips JA, Parks JS, Hjelle BL, Herd JE, Plotnick LP, Migeon CJ, Seeburg PH: Genetic analysis of familial isolated growth hormone deficiency type I. J Clin Invest 70:489, 1982. *Analysis of nuclear DNA from patients with familial isolated GH deficiency has suggested the presence of genetic mutations. Similar studies can be expected in the future that may explain the pathogenesis of many isolated hormonal deficiencies.*

Sheehan HL, Summers VK: The syndrome of hypopituitarism. Quart J Med 42:319, 1949. *The classic monograph describing the clinical-pathologic correlations of hypopituitarism. Its lucid and detailed presentation make it worthwhile reading even after three decades.*

Stackpoole PW, Interlandi JW, Nicholson WE, Rabin D: Isolated ACTH deficiency: A heterologous disorder. Critical review and report of four new cases.

Medicine 61:13, 1982. *The pathogenesis of this disorder is heterologous despite similar clinical manifestations. Detailed endocrine testing is required to differentiate the various causes.*

PITUITARY TUMORS

CLASSIFICATION. Pituitary tumors are subdivided by their histologic characteristics and also by their functional activity. Specific considerations of hormone-secreting pituitary tumors will be found in the next section. The two major histologic types of primary pituitary tumors are the adenoma and the craniopharyngioma. In addition, parasellar tumors such as optic nerve glioma, meningioma, sphenoid wing sarcoma, as well as metastatic tumors can also be present within the sella turcica.

Pituitary Adenomas. This cell type constitutes greater than 90 per cent of all pituitary tumors. The classic subdivision into chromophobic and chromophilic tumors has given way to more specific identification on the basis of immunohistochemical stains for individual hormones. Using these techniques, only 10 to 20 per cent of pituitary adenomas appear to be nonfunctioning. Pituitary tumors account for 6 to 18 per cent of all brain tumors, and small adenomas, many of which are functioning, have been detected in up to 30 per cent of unselected autopsy series. The growth pattern of pituitary adenomas appears unrelated to hormone secretion. Rapidly enlarging tumors are generally recognized because of their mass lesion effects, whereas slowly growing tumors tend to allow for expression of their hormone hypersecretory effects. The peak incidence of nonfunctioning pituitary adenomas is between 40 and 50 years, and the frequency is uninfluenced by sex. Although pituitary adenomas are almost always histologically benign, they may exhibit aggressive growth behavior with invasion of surrounding structures, making their surgical removal impossible. Adenomas are generally solid with a well-defined capsule, although they may on occasion be cystic and hemorrhagic. Calcification, if present, results from organization of a previous hemorrhage.

Craniopharyngiomas. These tumors are of congenital origin, may be partly or entirely cystic, and are always benign. The cysts may contain an oily fluid with a high cholesterol content. Calcification, generally concentric, is present in 50 per cent. The tumors grow at variable rates and may remain dormant for many years. Although half of the tumors are seen during childhood, they may appear at any time during life. The site of origin of most tumors is in the midline at the upper portion of the pituitary stalk, and approximately 15 per cent involve the upper portion of the anterior lobe and are therefore intrasellar. Variations of craniopharyngiomas include ependymomas and epidermoid cysts.

CLINICAL FEATURES. The manifestations of pituitary tumors are neuroanatomic, endocrinologic, and radiologic. Presenting symptoms of pituitary tumors have changed in frequency over the years with refinements in diagnostic procedures. Whereas in nearly 90 per cent of cases diagnosed 30 years ago, patients exhibited visual disturbances, only 25 per cent do so at present. In contrast, the most common presentation today relates to impaired gonadal function, frequently associated with prolactin-secreting pituitary tumors. A small percentage of patients (less than 5 per cent) are discovered accidentally on review of skull films obtained for other purposes as a result of bony destruction of the sella turcica.

Neuroanatomic manifestations occur secondary to tumor growth causing pressure on the overlying dura and the diaphragma sellae. This results in headaches that are variable in nature, imprecisely located, generally of dull quality, unassociated with nausea or visual symptoms, unrelated to position, and inconsistently relieved by analgesics. Disappearance of headache is frequently a sign of rupture of the dura. With continued expansion the tumor exerts pressure on the optic chiasm, leading to the classic findings of bitemporal hemianopsia. At earlier stages the field defects may be asymmetric and involve only the superior temporal fields. Eventually, blindness and optic atrophy will occur. Anterior growth of the tumor may cause symptoms limited only to one eye. Papilledema occurs in one fourth of craniopharyngiomas but rarely in pituitary adenomas. Further growth results in hypothalamic compression leading to temperature instability, hyperphagia, altered sleep patterns, and emotional disturbances. Pressure on the third ventricle results in internal hydrocephalus. Rarely, temporal or frontal lobe compression may cause behavioral changes and seizures, and midbrain compression may produce long-tract signs. Lateral extension is more common and leads to compression of the third, fourth, and sixth cranial nerves in the cavernous sinus, resulting in ophthalmoplegia and diplopia. Expansion inferiorly into the sphenoid sinus may result in cerebrospinal fluid rhinorrhea. Hemorrhage into the tumor, *pituitary apoplexy,* may result in rapid expansion of the tumor and lead to the sudden appearance of headache of varying intensity that subsides after a few days. If the tumor is intrasellar, hypopituitarism often results; if extrasellar, there may be rapid deterioration of vision. "Spontaneous" cures of hormone-secreting pituitary tumors may also occur as the result of hemorrhagic tumor necrosis.

Neuroradiologic presentations consist of a deformed or enlarged sella seen on standard skull roentgenography or a mass lesion seen on computed tomography (CT) performed for unrelated reasons. In the absence of endocrine symptoms a low-density lesion suggests an empty sella (discussed below).

Endocrine symptoms include diminished function secondary to destruction of normal pituitary tissue by tumor or interference with portal blood supply and hyperfunction due to tumor or hyperplasia. The two may be combined. In addition, diminished function may occur secondary to the effects of hormone hypersecretion (i.e., hypogonadism secondary to hyperprolactinemia). The frequency of presentation and the manifestations have been described in the previous section.

DIAGNOSTIC PROCEDURES. Diagnosis of a pituitary tumor necessitates differentiation from other parasellar disorders, determination of the tumor size and extent of sellar and extrasellar destruction, and assessment of the extent of hormone deficiencies. Endocrine evaluation should be performed prior to definitive therapy, if possible, since the extent of hypopituitarism may influence the type and extent of therapy. When this is not possible, because of rapidly deteriorating vision or progressive neurologic symptoms, the patient must be considered to have panhypopituitarism and immediate treatment with glucocorticoids must be initiated.

Neuroradiologic procedures have improved remarkably during the past decade, and the definitive study is currently the CT scan, performed with intravenous contrast media, using a third or fourth generation scanner (Fig. 225–1). The best views

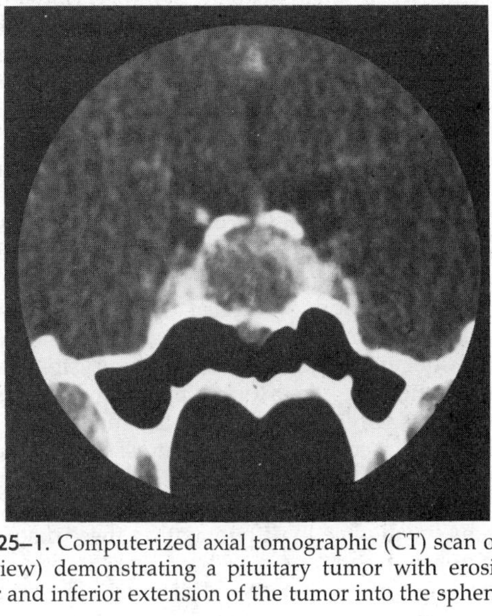

Figure 225–1. Computerized axial tomographic (CT) scan of pituitary (coronal view) demonstrating a pituitary tumor with erosion of the sellar floor and inferior extension of the tumor into the sphenoid sinus.

are obtained using coronal sections. This technique permits evaluation of the contents of the sella as well as the surrounding bony structures, which provide the only clues on routine x-ray studies. CT can also indicate the degree of extension of pituitary tumors in all directions and has precluded the need for invasive procedures such as pneumoencephalography. Digital vascular imaging is also useful as an adjunct in determining the position of the carotid arteries in relation to the tumor prior to surgical intervention and has almost entirely replaced carotid angiography.

The most important neuro-ophthalmologic study is evaluation of visual fields using Goldmann perimetry. Test objects of varying sizes and colors can provide an excellent assessment of both central and peripheral fields. The technique is reproducible and sensitive and useful in observing patients for serial changes. Bitemporal field defects are, however, not specific for pituitary tumors; they may occur with parasellar tumors, vascular abnormalities, arachnoiditis, or rarely with chiasmal prolapse into the sella associated with the empty sella syndrome. Atypical field defects may also occur, even those suggesting superior rather than inferior pressure. The visual evoked response (VER) is an even more sensitive technique for detecting early chiasmal compression by pituitary tumors. The VER measures the pattern and latency of the response from the occipital cortex produced by photic stimulation. Chiasmal pressure produces a delayed or reduced response in the crossed pathways as compared with uncrossed pathways and may provide evidence of abnormalities before they are evident on visual field examination.

DIFFERENTIAL DIAGNOSIS. Disorders that must be differentiated from pituitary tumors include the empty sella syndrome, parasellar diseases, and pituitary enlargement associated with other endocrine disorders.

The *empty sella* is partly or nearly completely filled with CSF and results from extension of the subarachnoid space into the intrasellar region. The pituitary gland is flattened along the posterior portion of the floor and the dorsum. Primary empty sella syndrome is unassociated with prior surgical or irradiation therapy and has been found in up to one quarter of autopsy series, usually unassociated with endocrine disease. The etiology is unknown, but the syndrome has been postulated to be due to incomplete formation of the diaphragma sella, permitting CSF pressure to be transmitted to the sella and gradually leading to herniation of the arachnoid and remodeling of the sella. Nearly all patients are asymptomatic, though some may have nonspecific headaches. The syndrome is seen commonly in obese women and in association with systemic hypertension, benign intracranial hypertension (pseudotumor cerebri), and CSF rhinorrhea. The sella is usually symmetrically enlarged or ballooned and may be deformed. Results of testing of endocrine function are generally normal, though patients may exhibit diminished TSH and gonadotropin secretion, hyperprolactinemia, and rarely panhypopituitarism or diabetes insipidus. The diagnosis is established by CT, which on occasion may need to be performed in conjunction with metrizamide cisternography. The empty sella may coexist with a pituitary tumor, which is usually hyperfunctional. The secondary empty sella syndrome is seen in patients following pituitary surgery or irradiation.

The signs and symptoms of parasellar disorders may mimic those of pituitary tumors. Parasellar disorders include inflammatory and granulomatous diseases (sarcoidosis, eosinophilic granuloma), degenerative disorders (aneurysms), and neoplasms (meningiomas, hamartomas, metastatic tumors). Suprasellar tumors usually present with the neurologic manifestations of increased intracranial pressure, hypothalamic symptoms, and internal hydrocephalus. Endocrine manifestations tend to follow rather than precede neurologic symptoms. CT is extremely valuable in differentiating these disorders from primary pituitary tumors.

Longstanding primary hypothyroidism or hypogonadism can result in sellar enlargement, increased TSH or gonadotropin secretion, hyperplasia of tropic hormone–producing cells, and in some patients, hormone-secreting tumors. Institution of appropriate replacement hormone therapy can reverse the hypersecretory and hyperplastic changes in their early stages.

THERAPY. Treatment of pituitary tumors is required to prevent or limit the loss of pituitary function and the consequences of extrasellar extension. The two therapeutic methods include surgery and radiation therapy.

Pituitary surgery, established as a safe and effective procedure by Cushing, is the conventional therapy for pituitary tumors. The transsphenoidal approach is currently used for all tumors except those with extensive suprasellar extension, particularly when separated from the intrasellar portion by a narrow neck. Tumors encircling optic nerves can be removed only by a transfrontal approach. Currently the operative mortality is less than 1 per cent. The transsphenoidal approach includes the use of modern fluoroscopic aids and microsurgical techniques. It provides better visualization of the sellar contents and has been instrumental in permitting selective adenomectomy to be performed. If preoperative evaluation reveals preservation of anterior pituitary function, a more conservative approach is indicated to preserve remaining pituitary hormone secretion. A small rim of adenohypophyseal tissue is often sufficient to maintain adequate pituitary function. Glucocorticoid coverage is essential for the perioperative period even for patients with intact pituitary-adrenal function and is accomplished with parenteral administration of hydrocortisone, 50 mg intramuscularly every six hours. Postoperatively the patient must be carefully observed for the development of diabetes insipidus, particularly since an obtunded patient may not perceive thirst. Transient polyuria and increased plasma osmolality commonly occur in the immediate postoperative period as a result of mild trauma to the pituitary stalk. Persistence of these findings beyond the first 48 hours usually indicates significant destruction of the stalk or posterior pituitary and permanent impairment of function. However, fluctuations in posterior pituitary function may occur for a period of several weeks, and recovery has been observed as late as several months postoperatively. Initially the patient should be treated with aqueous vasopressin (5 U subcutaneously) rather than with a long-acting preparation so the natural history of the process can be observed.

Radiation therapy can be used as an alternative to surgical excision of the pituitary tumor or as adjunct therapy. Although less popular as primary therapy, because of its delayed effects, radiation therapy using conventional high-energy sources (supravoltage) or heavy-particle (proton beam) sources is an effective method of treatment. Radiation therapy is to be avoided in patients with significant suprasellar extension or in the presence of marked visual field defects.

The recurrence rate of pituitary tumors following surgical treatment alone ranges from 25 to nearly 100 per cent in different series. Since postoperative radiographic and endocrine studies indicate that intraoperative assessment of the extent of pituitary tumor removal is often inaccurate, postoperative irradiation is indicated in all patients with pituitary adenomas unless specifically contraindicated. The dose currently employed is 4500 to 5000 rads, which can be given with minimal side effects. Some late loss of pituitary function occurs in 15 to 25 per cent of patients.

Burrow GN, Wortzman G, Rewcastle NB, Holgate RC, Kovacs K: Microadenomas of the pituitary and abnormal sellar tomograms in unselected autopsy series. N Engl J Med 304:156, 1981. *Clinically unrecognized microadenomas were found in one third of an autopsy series. Many were hormone containing but without manifestations of hypersecretion.*

Carbezudo JM, Vaquero J, Areitio E, Martinez R, De Sola RG, Bravo G: Craniopharyngiomas: A critical approach to treatment. J Neurosurg 55:371, 1981. *Increasing experience with this tumor indicates the importance of radiation therapy in addition to surgery in preventing tumor recurrence. In most patients total excision is not recommended.*

Cook DM: Pituitary tumors: Diagnosis and therapy. CA 33:215, 1983. *An excellent, well-referenced review of the recent literature that compares therapeutic effectiveness of methods as reported by others. Very readable.*

Crane TB, Yee RD, Hepler RS, Hallinan JM: Clinical manifestations and radiologic findings in craniopharyngiomas in adults. Am J Ophthalmol 94:220, 1982. *A comprehensive review of the clinical features in 51 patients emphasizing the predominance of visual findings.*

Daniels DL, Williams AL, Thornton RS, Meyer GA, Cusick JF, Haughton VM: Differential diagnosis of intrasellar tumors by computed tomography. Radiology 141:697, 1981. Chambers EF, Turski PA, LaMasters D, Newton TH: Regions of low density in the contrast enhanced pituitary gland: Normal and pathologic processes. Radiology 144:109, 1982. *The use of CT in diagnosis of pituitary tumors is now well established. Subtleties in interpretation of the results, however, must be carefully assessed.*

Max MB, Deck MD, Rottenberg DA: Pituitary metastasis: Incidence in cancer patients and clinical differentiation from pituitary adenoma. Neurology 31:998, 1981. *A careful analysis of both autopsy and clinical series in which differentiation was facilitated by the clinical rather than the radiologic characteristics.*

Valenta LJ, Sostrin RD, Eisenberg H, Tamkin JA, Elias AN: Diagnosis of pituitary tumors by hormone assays and computerized tomography. Am J Med 72:861, 1982. *Analysis of 170 patients with endocrine abnormalities by dynamic testing and CT examination demonstrating the value of each in the diagnosis or exclusion of tumors.*

Zull DN, Falko JM: Metrizamide cisternography in the investigation of the empty sella syndrome. Arch Intern Med 141:487, 1981. *This enhancement of the standard CT has simplified the diagnosis of the empty sella and has eliminated the need for invasive radiologic techniques previously used.*

PITUITARY HYPERFUNCTION: HORMONE-SECRETING PITUITARY TUMORS

Except in the case of certain hormone-secreting tumors, pituitary hormone hypersecretion generally involves overproduction of only a single hormone. Physiologically, hormone overproduction occurs in response to altered feedback signals (i.e., hyperprolactinemia due to increased estrogen secretion in pregnancy; ACTH, TSH, and gonadotropin hypersecretion in response to diminished target organ feedback in primary hypofunction of the adrenal, thyroid, and gonads; and GH hypersecretion associated with chronic and severe caloric malnutrition). Whereas these changes begin as functional alterations, prolonged stimulation can result in hyperplastic as well as hypersecretory changes. Pathologic hyperfunction occurs in association with pituitary hyperplasia or tumor unrelated to regulatory feedback mechanisms. These disorders involve, almost exclusively, somatotrophic, lactotrophic, and corticotrophic cells.

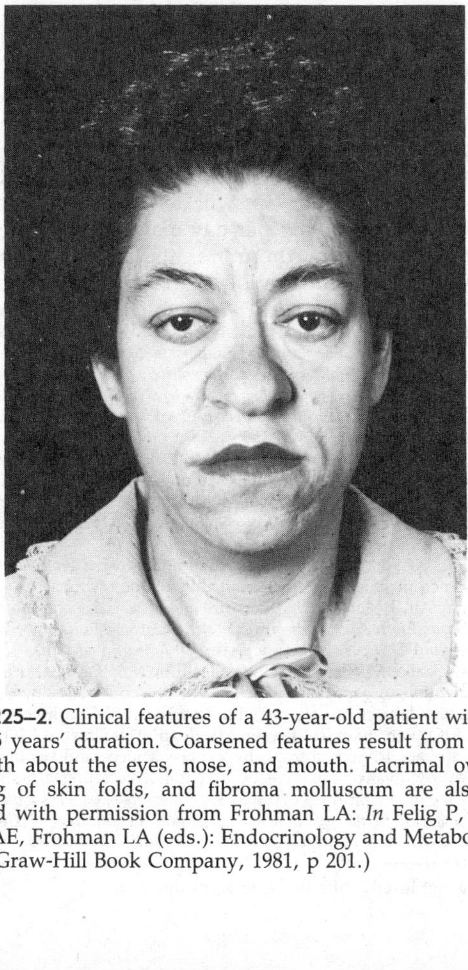

Figure 225–2. Clinical features of a 43-year-old patient with acromegaly of 15 years' duration. Coarsened features result from soft tissue overgrowth about the eyes, nose, and mouth. Lacrimal overgrowth, thickening of skin folds, and fibroma molluscum are also present. (Reprinted with permission from Frohman LA: *In* Felig P, Baxter JD, Broadus AE, Frohman LA (eds.): Endocrinology and Metabolism. New York, McGraw-Hill Book Company, 1981, p 201.)

Growth Hormone–Secreting Tumors: Acromegaly

GH hypersecretion is most commonly associated with a pituitary somatotroph tumor or rarely somatotroph hyperplasia. These tumors previously were considered eosinophilic (due to GH storage granules) or chromophobic (when little hormone was stored). Tumors with abundant hormone storage tend to be better differentiated and more slowly growing, resulting in more pronounced clinical features of GH hypersecretion, whereas the less differentiated non–hormone-storing tumors tend to grow more rapidly, leading to more pronounced effects of an expanding tumor mass.

CLINICAL FEATURES. The clinical manifestations of GH hypersecretion depend on the age at which the disorder begins. During childhood and prior to epiphyseal fusion, GH hypersecretion produces proportional skeletal growth leading to gigantism. Hypogonadism is frequently present, leading to delayed epiphyseal closure and thus a more prolonged growth period. The tallest reported patient with gigantism reached a height of nearly 9 feet. It is more common for patients to exhibit features of both gigantism and acromegaly, reflecting persistence of GH hypersecretion into adult life.

Signs and symptoms of GH hypersecretion beginning during adult life develop slowly. Soft tissue swelling and hypertrophy involving the extremities and face are the earliest findings (Fig. 225–2). These changes are usually best documented by comparing photographs taken over a one- or two-decade span. Spadelike changes develop in the fingers, and increased soft tissue volume necessitates ring enlargement and increases in glove and shoe sizes. The skin becomes thickened and leathery, and skin folds increase in prominence. A generalized increase in hair growth and pigmentation often occurs. Fibroma molluscum (pedunculated epithelial tags) and acanthosis nigricans are common. The skin becomes oily, and sebaceous cyst formation is common. Increased sweating occurs in most patients and is a sensitive biologic indicator of disease activity.

Bony changes occur more slowly and include cortical thickening, tufting of terminal phalanges, and osteophyte proliferation. Degenerated articular cartilages and ligamentous hypertrophy produce a hypertrophic arthropathy that eventually leads to deforming and crippling arthritis. Prognathism results from mandibular enlargement and causes a significant overbite of the lower incisors and increased spacing of the teeth. Bony overgrowth of the frontal, malar, and nasal bones occurs; increase in size of the paranasal sinuses together with vocal cord hypertrophy leads to deepening of the voice. Eustachian tube mucosal hypertrophy often produces obstruction and serous otitis media.

Peripheral neuropathy commonly occurs because of nerve entrapment by surrounding tissue overgrowth, most commonly affecting the median nerve and producing the carpal tunnel syndrome. Axonal demyelinization of peripheral nerves associated with perineurial and subepineurial proliferation results in palpable nerve fibers. Paresthesias, sensory losses, and proximal muscle weakness occur frequently.

Prolonged hypersecretion leads to generalized visceromegaly involving salivary glands, liver, spleen, and kidneys. Salivary gland enlargement is detectable clinically whereas that of the other organs is not, and significant hepatosplenomegaly usually implies the presence of a coexisting disease. Both secretory and reabsorptive functions of the kidney are increased in acromegaly.

Thyroid enlargement with nodule formation is common, but true hyperfunction is infrequent. Parathyroid hyperplasia and adenoma are frequently associated, explaining the hypercalciuria and nephrolithiasis often observed. Mild elevations of prolactin levels may also occur, resulting in galactorrhea, amenorrhea, and decreased libido.

The effects of GH on the cardiovascular system are controversial. Hypertension is common but generally mild and responsive to drug therapy. Cardiomegaly is routinely found, but there is no characteristic form of acromegalic heart disease. Cardiac failure, when it occurs, appears related to hypertension and not to the effects of GH hypersecretion. Yet the incidence of cardiovascular disease is increased in acromegalics, as is mortality. Weight gain is uncommon, but carbohydrate intolerance and diabetes are seen in 25 per cent of acromegalics, primarily in those with a family history of diabetes. Insulin resistance is common and the development of ketosis is occasionally noted. Diabetic microangiopathy, however, is extremely uncommon, even in longstanding disease.

LABORATORY STUDIES. The diagnosis of acromegaly is established by the finding of elevated plasma GH levels that do not respond normally to physiologic suppression and stimulation; in adults, a GH value greater than 2 ng per milliliter in males or 5 ng per milliliter in females after oral glucose administration is confirmatory. Randomly obtained samples with markedly elevated levels are also diagnostic. However, in normal children and young adults, GH levels as high as 50 ng per milliliter are sporadically exhibited, thereby necessitating dynamic studies of GH secretion in many patients. TRH stimulates GH secretion in 70 to 80 per cent of acromegalics but not in normal subjects, and this procedure is useful in following the patient after therapy as well. Plasma GH levels are paradoxically suppressed by dopaminergic agents and frequently stimulated by GnRH, but these tests are of limited clinical use. GH secretion in acromegalics differs in other ways from that in normal persons, including absence of a sleep-associated increase in GH and a tendency for wide spontaneous fluctuations in GH levels, indicating intermittent secretory activity.

Plasma somatomedin C (IGF-I) levels are also increased in acromegaly and provide good correlation with the clinical manifestations of GH hypersecretion. Determination of somatomedin C levels for assessing disease activity has been proposed, but at present its value remains as a supportive measurement.

DIFFERENTIAL DIAGNOSIS. The clinical features of acromegaly are not confused with other diseases. The question commonly raised is whether features suggestive of the disease are associated with active disease, inactive disease, or no disease. Dynamic studies of GH secretion are required to differentiate these possibilities. Gigantism during childhood occasionally occurs in the absence of GH hypersecretion (cerebral gigantism) through a yet to be determined mechanism. GH levels are elevated in patients with renal failure, cirrhosis, protein calorie malnutrition and anorexia nervosa and in the Laron dwarf (a dwarf with a defect in somatomedin generation), but in these conditions the clinical features of acromegaly are absent.

PATHOGENESIS. Acromegaly can occur as a primary disorder due to neoplastic transformation of somatotrophs within the pituitary or secondary to excessive stimulation by an ectopic GH- or GRF-secreting tumor. The vast majority of patients with acromegaly have primary pituitary disease. Selective removal of the GH-secreting adenoma is followed in most patients not only by restoration of normal GH values but by normal responses to dynamic testing. In some patients, however, GH-secreting pituitary tumors have been associated with carcinoid tumors of the bronchus and foregut, pancreatic islet tumors, and small cell carcinoma of the lung. Removal of the extrapituitary tumor has resulted in a return of GH levels to normal and regression of the pituitary tumor. GRF has been isolated from several of these tumors; in fact, its sequence was first determined from a pancreatic islet tumor rather than from the hypothalamus. Pituitary histology in patients with secondary acromegaly ranges from local or generalized somatotroph hyperplasia to actual tumor formation. In addition, neuronal tumors present in the hypothalamus (hamartomas) or in the pituitary, contiguous with the somatotroph adenoma (gangliocytoma or choristoma), may also be the source of GRF production in a few patients with acromegaly. Since excessive stimulation by GRF is capable of inducing adenomas as well as hyperplasia, it is possible that some patients now considered to have primary pituitary disease actually have a hypothalamic disorder characterized by excessive GRF production from nontumorous tissue.

Comparison of the limited numbers of reported patients with secondary acromegaly does not provide any evidence of differences in either clinical manifestations or responses to dynamic studies of GH secretion. In patients with ectopic GRF production, immunoreactive plasma GRF levels are readily detectable, in contrast to patients presumed to have primary pituitary disease in whom levels are near or beneath the limits of detectability.

THERAPY. Therapy for patients with acromegaly involves three potential methods: surgery, irradiation, and medical (pharmacologic). Considerations of the space-occupying mass and of hypopituitarism are similar to those described for nonfunctioning pituitary tumors. Prior to initiation of therapy to the pituitary itself, consideration should be given to the possibility of an extrapituitary tumor, removal of which may reverse the GH hypersecretion.

Surgical treatment of GH-secreting pituitary tumors is currently the most commonly used method. Transsphenoidal or, if necessary, transfrontal adenomectomy is indicated once the presence of the disease has been established, even though the radiologic findings are minimal. The results in published series vary, some reports indicating up to 90 per cent cure rates with small tumors. The success in returning GH levels to normal is inversely related to the size of the tumor; less favorable results occur with tumors greater than 2 cm in diameter or plasma GH levels greater than 100 ng per milliliter. The clinical features of GH, however, are frequently improved dramatically even without complete restoration of GH values to normal. In patients whose GH levels return to the normal range, tumor recurrence is infrequent (approximately 5 per cent), but with incomplete removal the recurrence rate is greater than 50 per cent if no further therapy is administered.

Radiation therapy, using methods similar to those for nonfunctioning tumors, is effective as a primary means of treatment of acromegaly. The reduction in GH hypersecretion is, however, slow, and return to normal levels may require five or even ten years, although 70 to 80 per cent of patients will exhibit normal GH levels after two years. Postoperative irradiation is indicated when GH levels remain elevated and, used in conjunction with surgery, offers the best prognosis.

Pharmacologic therapy in acromegaly is of very limited value. The only useful agent for long-term use is the dopamine agonist bromocriptine,* but it is effective in lowering GH levels to normal in only 25 per cent of patients. In approximately 5 per cent of patients the tumor size will decrease during therapy as well. Doses of up to 60 mg per day may be required, and side effects are frequent. Furthermore, therapy is effective only during continued administration of the drug.

Arosio M, Giovanelli MA, Riva E, Nava C, Ambosi B, Faglia G: Clinical uses of pre- and postsurgical evaluation of abnormal GH responses in acromegaly. J Neurosurg 59:402, 1983. *Responses to dynamic testing of GH secretion indicate that persistence of abnormal responses postoperatively even when the basal GH levels are within the normal range should be considered evidence of residual neoplastic tissue. The studies may help distinguish between reactivation of disease and true recurrence.*

Baskin DS, Boggan JE, Wilson CB: Transsphenoidal microsurgical removal of growth hormone-secreting pituitary adenomas. A review of 137 cases. J Neurosurg 56:634, 1982. *The largest published series of GH-secreting tumors to date indicating that the greatest success occurs in patients with tumors confined to the sella and with GH levels less than 40 ng per milliliter.*

Dons RF, Rieth KG, Gorden P, Roth J: Size and erosive features of the sella turcica in acromegaly as predictors of therapeutic response to supervoltage irradiation. Am J Med 74:69, 1983. *Size and basal GH levels tended to parallel one another and formed a rough predictor of the response to therapy. In all patients the decrease in GH levels occurred in proportion to the initial value.*

Frohman LA, Szabo M, Berelowitz M, Stachura ME: Partial purification and characterization of a peptide with growth hormone-releasing activity from extrapituitary tumors in patients with acromegaly. J Clin Invest 65:43, 1980. Thorner MO, Perryman RL, Cronin MJ, Rogol AD, Draznin M, Johanson A, Vale W, Kovacs K: Somatotroph hyperplasia. Successful treatment of acromegaly by removal of a pancreatic islet tumor secreting growth hormone-releasing factor. J Clin Invest 70:965, 1982. *Reports of patients with ectopic GRF secretion that led to the isolation and structural identification of GRF, the only hypothalamic releasing factor to be sequenced first from human tissue.*

*This use is not listed in the manufacturer's directive.

Melmed S, Braunstein GD, Horvath E, Ezrin C, Kovacs K: Pathophysiology of acromegaly. Endocr Rev 4:271, 1982. *Thoughtful analysis of the various characteristics of GH-secreting pituitary tumors, together with a thorough discussion of the multiple pathogenetic mechanisms resulting in acromegaly. The disease clearly has more than one cause, and the numerous possibilities are presented.*

Moses AC, Molitch ME, Sawin CT, Jackson IM, Biller BJ, Furlanetto R, Reichlin S: Bromocriptine therapy in acromegaly: Use in patients resistant to conventional therapy and effect on serum levels of somatomedin C. J Clin Endocrinol Metab 53:772, 1981. *Although this agent is not nearly as effective as in the treatment of hyperprolactinemia, most patients with acromegaly exhibit clinical improvement along with reduction of GH levels. Its use is advocated only as an adjunct in patients inadequately treated by other means.*

Schuster LD, Bantle JP, Oppenheimer JH, Seljeskog EL: Acromegaly: Reassessment of the long-term therapeutic effectiveness of transsphenoidal pituitary surgery. Ann Intern Med 95:172, 1981. *The recurrence of disease prompted a critical review of hormone measurements after surgery, leading to the conclusion that GH suppression to levels seen in normal individuals is required if the patient is to be considered cured.*

Prolactin-Secreting Tumors: Amenorrhea-Galactorrhea Syndrome

Hyperprolactinemia is the most common form of pituitary hyperfunction. It is present in as many as 25 per cent of infertile women. The incidence in men is much lower. In patients with pituitary tumors the incidence of elevated prolactin levels ranges from 60 to 80 per cent and is greater than that of any other pituitary hormone. The distinction between patients with *idiopathic hyperprolactinemia* and those with *prolactin-secreting tumors* is currently made on the basis of CT examination of the pituitary. Thus, changes in the relative frequency of the two diseases reflect primarily recent improvements in radiologic technology.

CLINICAL FEATURES. In women, hyperprolactinemia causes galactorrhea, oligomenorrhea or amenorrhea, and infertility (see Ch. 238 for a discussion of galactorrhea). Galactorrhea requires near-normal levels of ovarian steroids and is therefore not seen in all patients. It frequently occurs in association with oral contraceptive use, usually following their discontinuation. The reported incidence of galactorrhea in patients with prolactin-secreting tumors varies from 50 to 90 per cent. Oligomenorrhea or amenorrhea occurs in a similar percentage of patients and in nearly all with radiographic evidence of a pituitary tumor. The development of amenorrhea and the development of galactorrhea are not necessarily related to one another and are of no diagnostic importance. The cause of amenorrhea is related to effects of altered CNS neurotransmitters, principally dopamine, as a result of hyperprolactinemia, which interferes with a normal positive feedback effect of estradiol on GnRH secretion. The effects of anovulation include hypoestrogenemia, which results in decreased vaginal secretion, and dyspareunia, which may be responsible for diminished libido. Mild hirsutism may also occur in association with increased dehydroepiandrosterone sulfate production by the adrenals. Longstanding hyperprolactinemia has, in some women, been associated with decreased bone density, only part of which may be attributed to the hypoestrogenemia.

In men, hyperprolactinemia results in impotence and diminished libido. A defect in endogenous GnRH secretion is present, along with diminished testosterone secretion. The decreased libido is, however, not explained entirely on this basis, since it often persists despite testosterone replacement therapy. In some men oligospermia is also present.

LABORATORY STUDIES. Plasma prolactin levels in patients with prolactin-secreting tumors vary from slightly above normal (15 to 20 ng per milliliter) to values greater than 10,000 ng per milliliter. Levels less than 200 ng per milliliter are of little use in distinguishing between the various causes of the disorder, whereas levels greater than 200 ng per milliliter are invariably associated with prolactin-secreting tumors. Since prolactin is a stress-responsive hormone and levels fluctuate in normal subjects, repeated sampling in patients with moderate degrees of hyperprolactinemia is essential.

A large number of dynamic studies of prolactin secretion reveal differences between normals and pathologic hyperprolactinemics, but none is reliable in distinguishing between idiopathic hyperprolactinemia and prolactin-secreting tumors. Prolactin responses to submaximally suppressive infusions of dopamine are impaired in such patients, as compared to those with known extrapituitary disorders causing hyperprolactinemia, though the latter can usually be distinguished on clinical grounds. Patients with prolactin-secreting tumors and idiopathic hyperprolactinemia have impaired responses to dopamine receptor–blocking agents, to stimulation with TRH, to a combination of L-dopa plus the dopa decarboxylase inhibitor, carbidopa, and to cimetidine, a histamine H_2-receptor blocker.

In some patients with pituitary tumors and mild hyperprolactinemia (i.e., less than 100 ng per milliliter) the tumor does not secrete prolactin, but rather appears to interrupt hypothalamic-pituitary portal blood flow, resulting in increased prolactin secretion by normal lactotrophs.

DIFFERENTIAL DIAGNOSIS. Consideration should be given to an extrapituitary cause for hyperprolactinemia in all patients, since subtle changes on CT studies may not always indicate the presence of a pituitary tumor. This is particularly true in patients with prolactin levels less than 200 ng per milliliter. The differential diagnosis of hyperprolactinemia is given in Table 225–3. If none of the disorders listed is present and there is no history of drug ingestion, the patient with a normal radiographic examination is considered to have idiopathic hyperprolactinemia.

The many similarities between patients with idiopathic hyperprolactinemia and those with small prolactin-secreting pituitary tumors (microadenomas) have led to the belief that these entities represent different stages of the same disorder. Follow-up evaluation of idiopathic hyperprolactinemia suggests that only a small percentage of patients (under 5 per cent) progress to demonstrable pituitary tumor formation and that among cases of microadenoma, the vast majority remain stable for years with respect to both prolactin levels and tumor size.

Some patients with galactorrhea have normal or borderline elevation of prolactin levels, normal dynamic studies of prolactin secretion and ovulatory menses, and normal fertility. These patients represent the most common type of nonpuerperal galactorrhea, termed *normoprolactinemic galactorrhea,* which is attributed to enhanced sensitivity of the breast to prolactin. It can be seen as persistence of postpartum galactorrhea or following discontinuation of oral contraceptives.

PATHOGENESIS. As with GH-secreting tumors, a controversy currently exists whether prolactin-secreting tumors represent a primary pituitary disease or are secondary to altered hypotha-

TABLE 225–3. DIFFERENTIAL DIAGNOSIS OF NONPHYSIOLOGIC HYPERPROLACTINEMIA

A. Pharmacologic Agents
- Monoamine synthesis inhibitors (alpha-methyldopa)
- Monoamine depletors (reserpine)
- Dopamine receptor antagonists (phenothiazines, butyrophenones, thioxanthines)
- Estrogens (oral contraceptives)
- Narcotics (morphine, heroin)

B. Central Nervous System Disorders
- Inflammatory/infiltrative (sarcoidosis, histiocytosis)
- Traumatic (stalk section)
- Neoplastic (hypothalamic or parasellar tumors)

C. Pituitary Disorders
- Prolactin-secreting tumors
  - Macroadenomas
  - Microadenomas
- Empty sella syndrome

D. Idiopathic Hyperprolactinemia

E. Other
- Hypothyroidism
- Renal failure
- Cirrhosis
- Chest wall/breast disease or surgery
- Thoracic spinal lesions
- Nonendocrine tumors with ectopic hormone production (rare)

lamic influence. Prolactin-secreting tumors also occur in association with other tumors, in particular pancreatic islet tumors and parathyroid tumors/hyperplasia as part of the multiple endocrine neoplasia syndrome type I (Ch. 232).

A hypothalamic etiology is supported by a large number of pharmacologic studies suggesting impaired CNS dopaminergic tone. However, evidence for prolactin resistance to dopamine has also been demonstrated, though this appears to be unrelated to altered dopamine receptors. A possible role of oral contraceptives has been suggested, since idiopathic hyperprolactinemia and prolactin-secreting tumors are primarily diseases of women of childbearing age. Most studies, however, have failed to support this hypothesis.

THERAPY. The therapy for prolactin-secreting tumors has undergone considerable change in the past decade. Surgery remains the primary form of therapy for large prolactin-secreting tumors (macroadenomas). The timing of surgery in relation to pharmacotherapy is discussed below. The overall management of large tumors that either secrete prolactin or are nonfunctioning is similar, i.e., removal of the tumor mass and preservation of pituitary function. Primary therapy of small tumors (microadenomas) has also been surgical, and cure rates of 90 per cent, as judged by restoration of cyclic menses and fertility, are achieved. However, growth of microadenomas is infrequently observed, and this, plus their detection in up to one third of unselected autopsies, raises the question whether their removal is indeed necessary in all patients. In addition, long-term follow-up of presumably cured patients indicates recurrence of hyperprolactinemia in at least 25 per cent.

A frequent reason for treatment of microadenomas is infertility. The most rapid and effective means of reducing prolactin levels to normal in such patients is by use of the dopamine agonist bromocriptine, which suppresses prolactin secretion in all forms of hyperprolactinemia by an action directly on the lactotroph. Prolactin levels are decreased by more than 90 per cent and galactorrhea is improved or eliminated in most patients, even if prolactin levels remain slightly elevated. Similarly, cyclic menses and fertility may return without complete normalization of prolactin levels. The dosage required for most patients is 2.5 to 7.5 mg per day in divided doses. Some patients may require up to 15 mg per day. Side effects consist primarily of nausea and vomiting due to stimulation of the emesis center and occasionally of hypotension due to a CNS-mediated mechanism and mood changes. The side effects may be minimized by initiating therapy with a small dose and gradually increasing it, though 5 to 10 per cent of patients are unable to tolerate the drug. The incidence of congenital abnormalities in infants of women who have conceived while taking bromocriptine does not appear to be increased, and even when given throughout pregnancy the drug appears to be safe. It is, in fact, the recommended therapy for women who develop signs and symptoms of a prolactin-secreting tumor during pregnancy. Bromocriptine is effective in males with hyperprolactinemia; restoration of serum testosterone levels and of libido follows institution of therapy.

Bromocriptine also decreases the size of prolactin-secreting adenomas, most dramatically of very large tumors. In approximately two thirds of patients bromocriptine will reduce tumor size by 50 to 75 per cent. The effects are usually quite rapid, occurring within days, but in some patients tumor shrinkage may require several months. The reduction in size continues as long as the patient takes the drug, even as long as eight to ten years. Following discontinuance of bromocriptine, however, there is rapid regrowth of the tumor, and symptoms may recur within days. The drug is useful in reducing the size of very large tumors prior to surgery, in postoperative treatment of patients in whom partial tumor removal was accomplished, and in patients who are not candidates for surgery.

Bonneville JF, Poulignot D, Cattin F, Couturier M, Mollet E, Dietemann JL: Computed tomographic demonstration of the effects of bromocriptine on pituitary microadenoma size. Radiology 143:451, 1982. *Careful radiographic examinations reveal that bromocriptine shrinks microadenomas as well as macroadenomas, and in some patients the tumor can no longer be demonstrated radiographically.*

Chiodini P, Liuzzi A, Cozzi R, Verde G, Oppizzi G, Dallabonzana D, Spelta B, Silvestrini F, Borghi G, Luccarelli G, Rainer E, Horoski R: Size reduction of macroprolactinomas by bromocriptine or lisuride treatment. J Clin Endocrinol Metab 53:737, 1981. *Two thirds of macroprolactinomas are decreased in size by these dopaminergic agonists, though in none did the tumor disappear completely. The drugs are proposed as a first-stage treatment for all macroprolactinomas prior to surgery or irradiation.*

Glickman SP, Rosenfield RL, Bergenstal RM, Helke J: Multiple androgenic abnormalities, including free testosterone, in hyperprolactinemic women. J Clin Endocrinol Metab 55:251, 1982. *Adrenal androgens are increased in women with hyperprolactinemia, and an increase in free testosterone is also present, related to decreased testosterone-binding globulin. These alterations explain the increased androgenization seen in some hyperprolactinemic patients.*

Herman V, Kalk WJ, de Moor NG, Levin J: Serum prolactin after chest wall surgery: Elevated levels after mastectomy. J Clin Endocrinol Metab 52:148, 1981. *Mastectomy stimulates prolactin secretion in most subjects, with levels remaining elevated for months and explaining the frequently observed galactorrhea on the basis of neurogenic stimulation via the sucking reflex.*

Randall RV, Laws ER Jr, Abboud CE, Ebersold MJ, Kao PC, Scheithauer BW: Transsphenoidal microsurgical treatment of prolactin producing adenomas. Results in 100 patients. Mayo Clin Proc 58:108, 1983. Wilson CB, Dempsey LC: Transsphenoidal microsurgical removal of 250 pituitary adenomas. J Neurosurg 48:13, 1978. *Two large series of patients with prolactinomas treated surgically show similar results in that the cure rate is highest in microadenomas and considerably lower in large tumors and in patients with prolactin levels above 200 ng per milliliter.*

Schlechte JA, Sherman B, Martin R: Bone density in amenorrheic women with and without hyperprolactinemia. J Clin Endocrinol Metab 56:1120, 1983. *Hyperprolactinemic women have decreased bone density that is unexplained by their amenorrhea and hypoestrogenemia. The mechanism remains to be clarified.*

Serri O, Rasio E, Beauregard H, Hardy J, Somma M: Recurrence of hyperprolactinemia after selective transsphenoidal adenomectomy in women with prolactinoma. N Engl J Med 309:280, 1983. *Despite return of prolactin levels to normal following surgery, 80 per cent of patients with macroadenomas and 25 per cent of patients with microadenomas exhibit recurrent hyperprolactinemia within a few years. These results require reevaluation of the currently used methods for treating these disorders.*

Spark RF, Willia CA, O'Reilly G, Ransil BJ, Bergland R: Hyperprolactinemia in males with and without pituitary macroadenomas. Lancet 2:129, 1982. *The major clinical manifestation of hyperprolactinemia in males is impotence. Bromocriptine is effective in restoring normal testosterone levels and potency in most subjects with or without tumors.*

von Werder K, Eversmann T, Rjosk H-K, Fahlbusch R: Treatment of hyperprolactinemia. *In* Ganong WF, Martini L (eds.): Frontiers in Neuroendocrinology. Vol 7. New York, Raven Press, 1982, pp 123–160. March CM, Kletzky OA, Davajan V, Teal J, Weiss M, Apuzzo MLJ, Marrs RP, Mishell DR: Longitudinal evaluation of patients with untreated prolactin-secreting pituitary adenomas. Am J Obstet Gynecol 139:835, 1981. *These two studies report on the natural history of idiopathic hyperprolactinemia and microadenomas, followed without specific treatment. They indicate that in the vast majority (> 90 per cent) size and prolactin levels remain relatively stationary for many years, concluding that immediate surgical intervention is not required in many patients.*

Wollesen F, Anderson T, Karle A: Size reduction of extrasellar pituitary tumors during bromocriptine treatment. Ann Intern Med 96:281, 1982. *Bromocriptine treatment reduces the size of prolactin-secreting tumors, and when large doses are used, even other tumors (including nonsecreting tumors) exhibit a response, though of lesser magnitude.*

ACTH-Secreting Tumors: Cushing's Disease

Basophilic adenomas of the pituitary associated with bilateral adrenocortical hyperplasia and the features of hypercortisolism constitute a disorder first described by Cushing. The tumors, which tend to be located in the midline or near the anterior-posterior pituitary junction, are usually benign, but in contrast to other pituitary tumors, often exhibit more aggressive growth behavior, may have true malignant potential, and on rare occasions metastasize within and without the CNS. Corticotroph tumors may first become clinically apparent following bilateral adrenalectomy in patients with Cushing's disease (Nelson's syndrome). Corticotroph tumors may also be chromophobic and are found in 5 to 7 per cent of pituitaries at autopsy in patients without evidence of ACTH hypersecretion during life. Defects in the hormone secretory process may be responsible for these nonfunctioning tumors.

CLINICAL FEATURES. The clinical features of corticotroph tumors consist of those related to hypercortisolism and those caused by hypersecretion of ACTH and related peptides. The signs and symptoms of hypercortisolism are indistinguishable from those associated with adrenocortical adenomas or exogenous hormone administration and include centripetal obesity, hypertension, diabetes, amenorrhea, hirsutism, acne, osteoporosis and compression fractures, muscle atrophy, violaceous striae, capillary fragility, impaired wound healing, decreased resistance to infection, and behavorial changes. These are discussed in greater detail in Ch. 229. Increased secretion of ACTH and β-LPH produces pigmentation similar to that seen in Addison's disease. In addition to generalized pigmentation, the pressure points (knuckles, elbows, knees, belt or brassiere strap regions), areolae, genitalia, mucous membranes, and recently healed scars are particularly affected. Because ACTH production is only partially autonomous in this disease, hyperpigmentation is mild or moderate in the early stages and becomes more pronounced after adrenalectomy or in very large tumors.

LABORATORY STUDIES. Plasma cortisol levels are elevated in only about half of the patients with Cushing's disease. The 24-hour urinary free cortisol is the most reliable measurement for distinguishing patients with increased adrenocortical function. Normal values are less than 100 μg per 24 hours. Of the dynamic tests, dexamethasone suppressibility is the most reliable and widely used. In normal subjects, low-dose dexamethasone decreases urinary free cortisol to less than 20 μg per 24 hours and plasma cortisol to less than 5 μg per deciliter. Patients with corticotroph tumors exhibit impaired suppression with the low dose but at least 50 per cent suppression with the high dose. In some patients, however, larger doses may be required to demonstrate suppression. Dexamethasone does not suppress cortisol secretion fully at any dose in patients with adrenal adenomas or ectopic ACTH secretion. These conditions can be distinguished by measurement of plasma ACTH levels, which are absent in the former and exceedingly high in the latter. Patients with Cushing's disease exhibit ACTH hyperresponsiveness to CRF; those with adrenal adenomas or ectopic ACTH production do not exhibit a response. High-quality CT scanning of the pituitary will demonstrate the presence of a tumor in only 60 per cent of patients with Cushing's disease.

DIFFERENTIAL DIAGNOSIS. ACTH-secreting tumors are responsible for approximately 80 per cent of cases of endogenous hypercortisolemia. Adrenal tumors are present in about 15 per cent, and the remainder are caused by ectopic ACTH-secreting tumors. The differential diagnosis of these disorders is discussed in greater detail in Ch. 229. Ectopic ACTH production can occur in a variety of tumors, most commonly small-cell lung carcinomas, carcinoids, and pancreatic islet tumors (Ch. 173). The disease can mimic that of corticotroph tumors, though in patients with malignant diseases, weight gain is often absent and severe hypokalemia is a prominent feature. Some of these tumors have been shown to secrete CRF alone or in combination with ACTH, explaining the occasional similarity in responses to dynamic hormone testing to those in patients with corticotroph tumors. Ectopic ACTH secretion should be suspected when the clinical and biochemical features of hypercortisolism occur on a periodic or intermittent basis.

Mild elevations of plasma cortisol, loss of diurnal variation, and absence of dexamethasone suppressibility are seen in patients under stress, during periods of bereavement, and in patients with depressive illness. Biochemically it is frequently impossible to distinguish these patients from those with ACTH-secreting tumors, though the clinical features of hypercortisolism are generally absent.

PATHOGENESIS. Arguments have been made for both a hypothalamic and a pituitary cause of ACTH-secreting tumors. Hypothalamic tumors have been identified in association with Cushing's disease, suggesting tumorous overproduction of CRF. Patients with ACTH-secreting tumors generally respond to CRF, as does tumor tissue tested in vitro. Basophilic hyperplasia, rather than tumor, is occasionally found in patients with Cushing's disease. In addition, cyproheptadine, a serotonin-receptor blocker, suppresses ACTH secretion in some patients with the disorder, providing strong support for a primary CNS role. The major argument for a primary pituitary disorder is based on the successful treatment by transsphenoidal adenomectomy, which includes reestablishment not only of normal quantitative cortisol secretion but of diurnal periodicity and glucocorticoid suppressibility. It is possible that two subgroups of the disease exist that are not readily distinguishable by clinical or laboratory methods currently available.

THERAPY. Definitive treatment of ACTH-secreting pituitary tumors is indicated as soon as the diagnosis has been established. Once ectopic ACTH or CRF production has been excluded, surgical removal of the pituitary ACTH-secreting tumor is indicated. Tumors may be extremely small and difficult to identify. If the tumor cannot be located or if the patient remains hypercortisolemic following surgery, anterior hypophysectomy or bilateral total adrenalectomy is necessary, the decision being influenced by the patient's age, desire for subsequent pregnancy, and overall general health. Following pituitary adenomectomy, adrenocortical hypofunction requiring glucocorticoid replacement therapy may persist for as long as two years. A success rate of up to 85 per cent has been reported in patients with small ACTH-secreting tumors, although in those with large tumors this figure is reduced to about 30 per cent.

Radiation is also effective as primary therapy in ACTH-secreting tumors. Cure rates have been reported of 80 per cent in children and 60 per cent in adults with either conventional radiotherapy or proton beam therapy. Some long-term loss of other pituitary function has been noted after radiotherapy.

Pharmacologic therapy of Cushing's disease is directed at suppression of cortisol biosynthesis by the adrenals, using aminoglutethimide, metyrapone, or mitotane (o,p'-DDD); at neurotransmitter metabolism within the CNS; or at the pituitary directly. Detailed discussion of drugs acting on the adrenal is provided in Ch. 229. They have been used, together with radiotherapy, as an alternative to surgical treatment in selected patients. The combination of metyrapone, aminoglutethimide, and dexamethasone has been advocated for restoring cortisol secretion to normal prior to pituitary adenomectomy. This is unnecessary in most patients, but in some with severe disease it may be of use. The serotonin-receptor blocker cyproheptadine and the GABA agonist sodium valproate have been successful in a small number of patients with Cushing's disease in restoring both ACTH and cortisol secretion to normal. Responses have also been seen in patients with Nelson's disease. A few patients will also exhibit decreases in ACTH secretion during bromocriptine therapy. There is no evidence for regression of tumor size by these agents to date.

Dornhorst A, Jenkins JS, Lamberts SW, Abraham RR, Wynn V, Beckford U, Gillham B, Jones MT: The evaluation of sodium valproate in the treatment of Nelson's syndrome. J Clin Endocrinol Metab 56:985, 1983. *This GABA agonist reduced ACTH levels, produced clinical improvement, and in one patient decreased pituitary tumor size. The site of action is believed to be the hypothalamus, where it increases GABA activity, thereby inhibiting CRF release.*

Findling JW, Aron DC, Tyrrell JB, Shinsako JH, Fitzgerald PA, Norman D, Wilson CB, Forsham PH: Selective venous sampling for ACTH in Cushing's syndrome: Differentiation between Cushing's disease and the ectopic ACTH syndrome. Ann Intern Med 94:647, 1981. *The selective sampling procedure used was capable of identifying the source of elevated ACTH levels when other procedures failed to differentiate between pituitary and extrapituitary sources.*

Fitzgerald PA, Aron DC, Findling JW, Brooks RM, Wilson CB, Forsham PH, Tyrrell JB: Cushing's disease: Transient secondary adrenal insufficiency after selective removal of pituitary microadenomas: Evidence for a pituitary origin. J Clin Endocrinol Metab 54:413, 1982. *Temporary adrenal insufficiency is observed after successful removal of an ACTH-secreting tumor, providing evidence for suppression of residual pituitary corticotrophs.*

Krieger DT: Physiopathology of Cushing's disease. Endocr Rev 4:22, 1983. *A detailed review presenting the arguments pro and con for both pituitary and CNS causes of Cushing's disease. Evidence for multiple causes are supported by the author's arguments.*

Lamberts SW, de Lange SA, Stefanko SZ: Adrenocorticotropin-secreting pituitary adenomas originate from the anterior or the intermediate lobe in Cushing's disease: Differences in the regulation of hormone secretion. J Clin Endocrinol Metab 54:286, 1982. *ACTH-secreting tumors can be subdivided into two subgroups with different sites of origin, responses to dynamic testing, and probabilities of surgical cure.*

Lankford HV, Tucker HTS, Blackard WG: A cyproheptadine-reversible defect in ACTH control presenting after removal of the pituitary tumor in Cushing's disease. N Engl J Med 305:1244, 1981. *Relative resistance of cortisol feedback suppression in Cushing's disease persists after removal of the pituitary tumor and is correctable by a serotonin-receptor blocker, providing evidence for a CNS role in the pathophysiology of the disease.*

Muller OA, Stalla GK, von Werder K: Corticotropin releasing factor: A new tool for the differential diagnosis of Cushing's syndrome. J Clin Endocrinol Metab 57:227, 1983. *Patients with pituitary ACTH-secreting tumors exhibit hyper-responsiveness to CRF, while those with adrenal adenomas and ectopic ACTH-secreting tumors do not respond, providing a diagnostic test of considerable clinical importance.*

Other Hormone-Secreting Tumors

TSH and gonadotropin secretion by pituitary tumors is extremely rare. TSH-secreting tumors are detected during the workup of hyperthyroid patients with elevated rather than suppressed TSH levels. The clinical manifestations consist of hyperthyroidism and a pituitary tumor mass. Occasionally mixed pituitary cell types are present with coexisting GH or prolactin hypersecretion. TSH secretion is not completely autonomous, since suppression of thyroxine production by methimazole frequently results in an increase of TSH secretion. Treatment must be directed to removal of the tumor mass, though medical therapy to suppress the elevated thyroxine levels is required preoperatively.

FSH and FSH/LH-secreting pituitary tumors are very rare and often associated with longstanding hypogonadism. Occasionally tumors otherwise considered to be nonfunctioning may produce the isolated glycoprotein alpha subunit that is devoid of any clinical manifestations and serves primarily as a tumor marker.

Harris RI, Schatz NJ, Gennarelli T, Savino PJ, Cobbs WH, Snyder PJ: Follicle-stimulating hormone–secreting pituitary adenomas: Correlation of reduction of adenoma size with reduction of hormonal hypersecretion after transsphenoidal surgery. J Clin Endocrinol Metab 56:1288, 1983. *Convincing evidence is presented for production of FSH by pituitary tumors with concomitant reduction in serum testosterone levels presumably caused by impairment of LH secretion from normal gonadotrophs.*

Klibanski A, Ridgway EC, Zervas NT: Pure alpha subunit-secreting pituitary tumors. J Neurosurg 59:585, 1983. *Six patients with otherwise "nonfunctioning" pituitary tumors are described with elevated glycoprotein alpha subunit levels that can be used as a marker for monitoring the effects of therapy. No clinical manifestations of the secretory product have yet been recognized.*

Smallridge RC, Smith CE: Hyperthyroidism due to thyrotropin-secreting pituitary tumors. Diagnostic and therapeutic considerations. Arch Intern Med 143:503, 1983. *In a review of 33 reported cases the authors describe the characteristic laboratory findings and provide recommendations for therapy.*

226. THE POSTERIOR PITUITARY

*Thomas E. Andreoli**

ANTIDIURETIC HORMONE

The neurohypophysis of man elaborates two hormones: *arginine vasopressin* (AVP), which exhibits vasopressor and antidiuretic activity, and *oxytocin*, which is galactobolic and uterotonic. Both hormones are octapeptides of approximately 1100 daltons, with a 20-member ring structure created by disulfide bonds. The antidiuretic and vasopressor activities of AVP are each approximately 100 times as great as those of oxytocin, a difference that is related to the different tertiary conformations of the two peptides.

The posterior pituitary gland contains terminal axons whose cell bodies lie in hypothalamic cell clusters known as the *supraoptic* and *paraventricular nuclei*. Synthesis of posterior pituitary hormones occurs in these hypothalamic nuclei rather than in the posterior pituitary gland: (1) AVP can be demonstrated immunochemically in cells of both the supraoptic and the paraventricular nuclei; and (2) neurosecretory granules accumulate only on the hypothalamic side of a sectioned hypophyseal stalk.

*The author acknowledges the dialogue and constructive suggestions provided by R. Michael Culpepper, M.D., Assistant Professor of Internal Medicine, University of Texas Medical School at Houston, and Attending Physician, Hermann Hospital, for his assistance in the preparation of this chapter. T.E.A.

Vasopressin is synthesized as a prohormone in conjunction with a specific carrier protein, neurophysin II, and then is transported to the posterior pituitary gland in discrete neurosecretory granules by axonal streaming within the cytoplasm of pituicytes (see Fig. 226–1). In the posterior pituitary gland, these granules rest in terminal projections of axonal plasma membranes, which are juxtaposed to capillaries of the systemic circulation. Other pituicyte nerve fibers terminate in the median eminence and along the third ventricle, thus allowing access of vasopressin to cerebrospinal fluid.

There are two pools of AVP-containing neurosecretory granules in pituicytes: one adjacent to the cell membrane and therefore available for immediate release, and a second storage pool removed from immediate contact with the plasma membrane. Release of hormone occurs by an exocytotic process involving fusion of neurosecretory granules with pituicyte plasma membranes. In other words, AVP release is quantal. A stimulus to the hypothalamic pituicyte cell body is transmitted to the site of granule storage, where it causes cell membrane depolarization, an associated increase in calcium permeability, and rapid calcium entry into the pituicytes. This influx of calcium activates the exocytosis of AVP-containing neurosecretory granules.

RELEVANT PHYSIOLOGY. Detailed accounts of the renal and pituitary processes resulting in the formation of a dilute or concentrated urine are presented in Ch. 73 and 76. Antidiuretic hormone (ADH) exerts major physiologic effects on discrete regions of the nephron and also affects vascular smooth muscle tone. In all epithelia which respond to ADH, the hormone binds to specific receptors on the basolateral plasma membrane of the cell and, in so doing, activates the enzyme adenylate cyclase. Adenylate cyclase increases the production of 3′,5′-cyclic adenosine monophosphate (cAMP) from its substrate adenosine triphosphate (ATP). Cyclic AMP then acts as a second messenger to activate a cell-specific protein kinase, which induces the final cellular response to the hormone (see Ch. 221). ADH-stimulated adenylate cyclase is present in the collecting duct and in the medullary, but not cortical, thick ascending limb of Henle (mTALH) of mammalian kidneys.

The *cardinal* physiologic effect of ADH is to promote the formation of a hypertonic urine. The formation of a hypertonic urine depends particularly on two sets of events operating in parallel within the renal medulla. First, in the thick ascending limb of Henle, approximately 15 to 20 per cent of the filtered load of sodium chloride is absorbed. Since the mTALH is water impermeable, this process contributes simultaneously to the maintenance of a hypertonic medullary interstitium and to the formation of a dilute urine. Under normal circumstances, the osmolality of the renal medullary interstitium rises from isotonic, at the corticomedullary junction, to very hypertonic, approximately 1200 mOsm per kilogram of H_2O, at the papillary tip; and approximately 10 per cent of fluid filtered at the

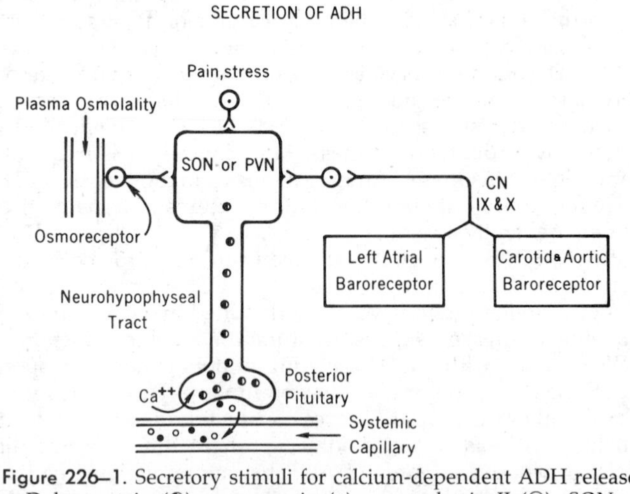

Figure 226–1. Secretory stimuli for calcium-dependent ADH release: van Dyke protein (◐), vasopressin (●), neurophysin II (○). SON = supraoptic neuron, PVN = paraventricular neuron.

glomerulus, or about 18 liters daily, reaches the early distal tubule with an osmolality of approximately 50 mOsm per kilogram of H_2O. Since the enrichment of medullary interstitial osmolality and dilution of tubular fluid both depend on sodium chloride absorption by the water-impermeable mTALH, the latter region of the nephron is commonly termed the medullary diluting segment.

When ADH is absent, the water permeability of collecting ducts is at a minimum. Thus there is reduced osmotic equilibration of fluid passing through collecting ducts with the medullary interstitium, and most of the fluid escapes unchanged as hypotonic urine. Since only 10 per cent of filtered water normally reaches the collecting duct system, the maximal degree of polyuria in a patient with complete pituitary diabetes insipidus (or complete nephrogenic diabetes insipidus) is therefore approximately 18 liters daily. During normal antidiuresis, ADH, acting through the second messenger cAMP, increases the water permeability of luminal (urinary) cell membranes of cortical and outer medullary collecting ducts. Thus in the presence of ADH, there is osmotic equilibration of hypotonic luminal fluid in collecting ducts with the hypertonic medullary interstitium and, consequently, water absorption, a reduction in urine volume, concentration of urine, and conservation of body water.

The ADH-dependent increase in the water permeability of collecting ducts is due to a hormone-dependent increase in the number of water-specific channels available for water transport through luminal membranes. These channels are rather narrow, approximately 2 Å in radius, and therefore exclude urea and NaCl. As a consequence, the luminal fluid concentrations of these two solutes increase when water is abstracted from cortical and outer medullary collecting ducts during antidiuresis. In turn, the increase in luminal urea concentration creates a favorable gradient for passive urea diffusion out of inner medullary (papillary) collecting ducts into the interstitium, thereby maintaining interstitial hypertonicity. ADH also causes a slight increase in papillary duct urea permeability, thus favoring passive movement of urea down its concentration gradient for recirculation through the medullary interstitium.

A *second ADH-mediated* event in the antidiuretic response is to increase the rate of NaCl transport in medullary, but not cortical, thick ascending limbs of Henle (mTALH). This process involves a furosemide-sensitive electroneutral cotransport of $Na^+:K^+:2Cl^-$ from luminal fluid into cells; virtually all of the potassium entering cells through this process is recycled back into luminal fluid via potassium-specific channels in luminal membranes. This potassium recycling contributes to the establishment of a lumen-positive voltage, which in turn drives the reabsorption of additional sodium through the paracellular pathway. Thus there occurs net absorption of sodium chloride by net transcellular absorption of chloride and net sodium absorption through both cellular and paracellular routes. Ultimately the energy source for this process depends on the maintenance of low concentrations of sodium and high concentrations of potassium within renal tubular cells; both of these conditions are met by the $(Na^+ + K^+)$-ATPase situated in basolateral membranes.

The action of ADH on increasing the rate of salt absorption in the mTALH appears to involve a hormone-dependent increase in both the functional number of $Na^+:K^+:2Cl^-$ cotransport units and potassium-specific channels in apical membranes of medullary diluting segments. Consequently, the action of ADH on the medullary diluting segment provides a means for enriching medullary interstitial osmolality.

This effect of ADH is opposed, however, by at least three other factors. First, as interstitial NaCl concentrations increase, the backleak of NaCl into the tubular lumen of the mTALH also increases, and thereby tends to reduce net NaCl absorption by the mTALH. Second, increases in interstitial osmolality down-regulate the ADH stimulation of NaCl cotransport. Finally, prostaglandins of the E series, which are produced in abundance in the renal medullary interstitium, inhibit competitively the ADH-mediated increases in the rate of intracellular cAMP formation.

Thus these latter three processes have a negative feedback on ADH enhancement of active NaCl transport in the mTALH. Consequently, the diluting power of the mTALH remains constant during either antidiuresis or water diuresis.

At levels of hormone that exceed those necessary for antidiuresis, ADH also has pressor activity (this was the first known effect of posterior pituitary extract, and provided the basis for the name vasopressin) that is the result of a direct constricting effect on vascular smooth muscle. At all but high pharmacologic doses, this pressor effect is easily overcome by compensatory vasodilatory reflexes, so that hypertension is not routinely seen during AVP replacement therapy. Lesser doses may, however, cause significant vasoconstriction of coronary arteries. Another effect of vasopressin, seen at levels that supersede those necessary for antidiuresis, is stimulation of intestinal motility. Finally, some evidence suggests that AVP released into the CSF and thalamic centers may play a role in such diverse processes as memory and regulation of corticotropin release.

OSMOTIC REGULATION OF ADH RELEASE. Verney's elegant studies demonstrated a strong antidiuretic response to perfusion of carotid vessels with hypertonic solutions of various solutes, including sodium salts and glucose; hypertonic urea solutions elicited no such response. Therefore he concluded that specific cells that acted as osmoreceptors were present within the distribution of the carotid circulation and that the plasma membranes of these cells were impermeable to sodium salts and glucose, but permeable to urea. In the presence of extracellular hyperosmolality induced by impermeable species, these osmosensing cells reached osmotic equilibrium by losing water to the hypertonic plasma. In other words, Verney deduced that osmoreceptor shrinkage, produced by raising plasma osmolality with solutes restricted to the extracellular compartment, was the stimulus for ADH release.

When the anterior wall of the third ventricle is exposed to hypertonic saline, neurons in both the anterior hypothalamus and the preoptic area have increased rates of depolarization. Concomitantly, about half of the pituicytes in hypothalamic nuclei show a characteristic depolarization pattern, and plasma antidiuretic activity increases. Therefore it is probable that the neurons in the anterior hypothalamus and preoptic areas, which depolarize in response to hypertonic saline, represent Verney's osmoreceptors.

In normal man, plasma AVP levels are undetectable below a plasma osmolality of 280 mOsm per kilogram of H_2O. Since the usual plasma osmolality in man is approximately 287 mOsm per kilogram of H_2O, secretion of AVP is tonic; the average circulating hormone levels are between 2.0 and 2.5 pg per milliliter. Vasopressin levels increase in a linear fashion with increasing plasma osmolality, such that a rise in plasma osmolality of only 1 per cent (2.9 mOsm per kilogram of H_2O) evokes a 1 pg per milliliter rise in AVP. Parallel examinations of plasma AVP and urine osmolality indicate that each unit increase in AVP allows an increase of 250 mOsm per kilogram of H_2O in urinary concentration. Since the maximal concentrating ability of the human kidney is approximately 1200 mOsm per kilogram of H_2O, maximal water conservation is therefore achieved at a plasma AVP level of 5.0 pg per milliliter.

Combining these relations yields a measure of the efficiency of the water homeostatic mechanism: for each 1 mOsm per kilogram of H_2O change in plasma osmolality there is a change in urinary concentration of 95 mOsm per kilogram of H_2O, which represents a gain of almost 100-fold. The ingestion of water sufficient to decrease plasma osmolality by only 1 mOsm per kilogram of H_2O will reduce urinary concentration by 95 mOsm per kilogram of H_2O, thus allowing the water to be excreted and osmotic balance to be restored. The opposite effect, water loss, results in stimulation of ADH release, increase in urinary concentration and conservation of body water by the same magnification phenomenon.

NONOSMOTIC REGULATION OF ADH RELEASE. Isotonic or hypotonic volume depletion of man or experimental animals results in an antidiuretic state. Evidence now exists for stretch receptors, or baroreceptors, that sense changes in vascular wall tension in both the venous (low pressure) and arterial (high pressure) circulations. Immersion and negative pressure breathing, i.e., maneuvers that augment intrathoracic blood volume, as well as balloon distention of the left atrium, all produce a water diuresis which can be overcome by administering ADH. Conversely, positive pressure breathing and upright posture, which reduce intrathoracic blood volume, or left atrial collapse, produce antidiuresis. These observations indicate that the left atrium and the pulmonary vasculature are the major loci for low pressure baroreceptors which modulate ADH release.

Hypotension, or selective clamping of major systemic arterial vessels, also produces a profound antidiuresis. These data indicate the presence of a baroreceptor system in the arterial circulation, localized to the carotid bifurcations and aortic arch, which also modulates ADH release. This type of nonosmotic ADH release is modulated by stimulatory or inhibitory signals arriving from the baroreceptors via parasympathetic pathways in the vagus and glossopharyngeal nerves. The low pressure baroreceptors are more sensitive regulators of ADH release than those in high pressure regions of the circulation. These relations are summarized in Figure 226–1.

Circulating levels of ADH rise with vascular volume depletion. However, volume-mediated, nonosmotic ADH release has a "threshold" requiring more than 7 per cent blood volume depletion, with greater degrees of blood volume contraction eliciting exponential rises in circulating ADH levels. Thus nonosmotic ADH release differs strikingly from osmotically mediated ADH release, which occurs with only a 1 to 2 per cent increase in plasma osmolality and rises linearly with further increases in plasma osmolality. With less than a 7 per cent decrease in blood volume, ADH release is governed wholly by plasma osmolality. At greater reductions in blood volume, ADH release is increasingly dominated by nonosmotic, volume-dependent stimuli. This observation explains the finding of progressive fluid dilution in patients with hypovolemia or states of decreased cardiac output.

Input from higher cortical functions also appears to influence ADH release. Pain, emotion, stress, and some psychotic states are associated with ADH stimulation or inhibition. Most common is the transient antidiuresis that occurs postoperatively.

PATHOLOGIC ALTERATION OF ADH RELEASE. A wide variety of drugs are known to affect ADH activity (Table 226–1). Nicotine, as a stimulant of ADH release, and acute alcohol ingestion, as an inhibitor of ADH release, have figured prominently in devising means to assess neurohypophyseal integrity. Stimulatory drugs such as clofibrate and chlorpropamide have been utilized to treat states of partial ADH insufficiency. Other drugs, such as lithium and demethylchlortetracycline, are prominent for their effect on the renal collecting duct, making it unresponsive to ADH, and thereby producing nephrogenic diabetes insipidus.

TABLE 226–1. DRUGS THAT ALTER ANTIDIURETIC HORMONE ACTIVITY

Drugs That Modify Release of ADH	
Enhance	*Suppress*
Vincristine	Phenytoin
Cyclophosphamide	Alcohol
Clofibrate	Narcotic antagonists
Carbamazepine	α-Adrenergic agents
Barbiturates	
Morphine and narcotic analogues	
Chlorpropamide	
Nicotine	
β-Adrenergic agents	
Drugs That Modify the ADH Effect on Collecting Ducts	
Enhance	*Suppress*
Chlorpropamide	Lithium
Biguanides	Methoxyflurane
Indomethacin	Demeclocycline

The syndrome of inappropriate antidiuretic hormone secretion (SIADH) is characterized by persistent hyponatremia, an inappropriately elevated urine osmolality, and no discernible stimulus for ADH release. A common cause for this condition is neoplastic, most notably oat cell carcinoma of lung; SIADH is due to ectopic production of ADH by the tumor, with persistent release of hormone independent of regulatory influences. Inflammatory disorders of the lung, such as pneumonia or cavitary tuberculosis, provide other sites for ectopic ADH production. The syndrome also occurs in patients with head trauma or with other diseases of the central nervous system and often terminates with recovery of neurologic function. The SIADH syndrome is discussed in detail in Ch. 76.

THIRST REGULATION. Body water content is governed not only by ADH modulation of renal water excretion but also by regulation of water intake through thirst. Both systems operate in parallel under the influence of osmotic and volume mediators. Thirst also requires an intact cerebral cortex, which transforms the urge to drink into appropriate behavior to secure water.

Hyperosmolality, and presumably shrinkage of thirst receptors, is the primary stimulus for thirst, and requires only a 2 per cent rise in plasma osmolality. The thirst "threshold" in conscious man is about 294 mOsm per kilogram, the same osmolality at which maximal urinary concentration under ADH is achieved. Hypovolemia also stimulates thirst via an angiotensin II–mediated mechanism. Indeed, hyperreninemic states such as malignant hypertension are often accompanied by pathological thirst. Phenothiazines enhance thirst and contribute to the hyponatremia seen in some patients treated with these drugs for affective disorders. Finally, prostaglandin E also stimulates thirst. The polydipsia which accompanies hypokalemia probably depends on increased production of prostaglandin E.

WATER REPLETION REACTION. It is evident from the preceding description that hyperosmolality and blood volume contraction simultaneously stimulate ADH release and thirst. The integrated activity of ADH and thirst has been termed the water repletion reaction, and may be viewed as shown in Figure 4 of Chapter 76.

Because the afferent, or positive, limbs of this system respond to 1 to 2 per cent changes in plasma osmolality, the day-to-day regulation of body water osmolality is remarkably constant, and variations in a given normal person's osmolality are negligible. The serum sodium concentration, which reflects body fluid osmolality, is therefore also constant in normal individuals. Finally, both ADH release and thirst give preference to volume maintenance at the expense of body fluid osmolality when vascular volume is reduced by more than 7 per cent. Consequently, profound volume contraction is accompanied by antidiuresis, increased thirst, and hyponatremia.

Culpepper RM, Andreoli TE: Interactions among prostaglandin E_2, antidiuretic hormone and cyclic adenosine monophosphate in modulating Cl^- absorption in single mouse medullary thick limbs of Henle. J Clin Invest 71:1588–1601, 1983. *An analysis of the interactions between prostaglandins and ADH in modulating NaCl transport in the medullary diluting segments.*

Culpepper RM, Hebert SC, Andreoli TE: Nephrogenic diabetes insipidus. *In* Stanbury JB, Wyngaarden JB, Fredrickson DS, Goldstein JL, Brown MS (eds.): The Metabolic Basis of Inherited Disease. New York, McGraw-Hill Book Company, 1982, pp 1867–1888. *A comprehensive review of the physiology of vasopressin and the renal concentrating mechanism; extensively referenced.*

Robertson GL, Shelton RL, Athar S: The osmoregulation of vasopressin. Kidney Int 10:25, 1976. *A quantitative examination of the relationships among plasma osmolality, vasopressin secretion, and urinary concentration.*

Verney EB: The antidiuretic hormone and the factors which determine its release. Proc R Soc Lond (Biol) 135:25, 1947. *A classic treatise describing a series of elegant studies which led to the notion of a central nervous system osmoreceptor for ADH secretion.*

DIABETES INSIPIDUS

Pituitary Diabetes Insipidus

DEFINITION. Pituitary diabetes insipidus is a polyuric syndrome that results from a lack of sufficient ADH to effect appropriate concentration of the urine for water conservation. The disease is identified by the persistence of an inappropriately dilute urine in the presence of strong osmotic or nonosmotic stimuli to ADH secretion, and in the absence of renal concentrating defects, and a rise in urine osmolality upon the administration of vasopressin. Pituitary diabetes insipidus may result either from destruction of the centers of ADH synthesis or from failure of the mechanisms effecting ADH release.

ETIOLOGY. Trauma to the neurohypophysis, either accidental or as a result of hypophysectomy, is the major identifiable cause of diabetes insipidus. A second major cause for pituitary diabetes insipidus is an intracranial tumor, which may be primary, as in craniopharyngioma, or metastatic, among which breast carcinoma is the most likely cause. Less frequent causes of pituitary diabetes insipidus are granulomatous lesions of the central nervous system, including tuberculosis and sarcoidosis, the histiocytoses, encephalomeningitis, or vascular lesions. There is a rare familial form of pituitary diabetes insipidus which affects either sex, occurs at any age, and is associated with extensive gliosis of neurohypophyseal nuclei. Finally, 30 to 40 per cent of all patients with pituitary diabetes insipidus have no identifiable cause for the disorder.

PATHOGENESIS. Pituitary diabetes insipidus depends on one of two different pathogenic mechanisms. Most commonly, the disorder occurs when there is atrophy or destruction of the hypothalamic centers responsible for hormone production. Neither removal of the posterior pituitary gland alone nor low section of the neurohypophyseal tract with preservation of hypothalamic nuclei is sufficient to produce a permanent polyuric state. Rather, direct trauma to the pituitary gland or low section of the neurohypophyseal tract results in a transient diabetes insipidus; for example, the polyuric state following low stalk section lasts for only one to two weeks postsurgery. Since the anterior and posterior lobes of the pituitary gland have totally separate blood supplies, infarction of the anterior pituitary gland does not disrupt posterior pituitary function.

A second group of patients has been identified, often classed under the heading "essential hypernatremia," in which osmotic stimuli fail to elicit ADH release, while nonosmotic stimuli result in antidiuresis. Although euvolemic, these patients are polyuric and excrete a hypotonic urine, and water deprivation alone fails to elicit an antidiuretic response. However, when these patients are volume contracted, a significant antidiuresis ensues. Thus in this disorder, there is selective failure of osmoreceptors to stimulate ADH release. The intact response of ADH release to nonosmotic stimulation verifies the integrity of the hypothalamic centers that produce ADH.

Nephrogenic Diabetes Insipidus

DEFINITION. The term *nephrogenic diabetes insipidus* should be applied to disorders in which renal tubular unresponsiveness to ADH, without disturbances either in solute delivery to the loop of Henle or in countercurrent multiplication or exchange processes, is responsible for polyuria and hyposthenuria. Thus nephrogenic diabetes insipidus may be due to inability of ADH to raise cellular cAMP concentrations, to inability of cAMP to increase the water permeability of luminal membranes of collecting ducts, or to a combination of these two disorders.

FAMILIAL NEPHROGENIC DIABETES INSIPIDUS. This familial disorder occurs primarily in males and exhibits a hereditary pattern of X-linked transmission with variable penetrance in females. In normal individuals or patients with pituitary diabetes insipidus, exogenous ADH can increase the rate of urinary cAMP excretion. In some patients with familial nephrogenic diabetes insipidus, comparable doses of ADH do not increase rates of urinary cAMP excretion. However, in two groups of children with nephrogenic diabetes insipidus, both basal and ADH-stimulated rates of urinary cAMP excretion exceeded those of normal children. These disparate results led to the postulate that familial nephrogenic diabetes insipidus is a heterogeneous disorder produced by either a defect in hormone receptor adenylate cyclase stimulation or a defect beyond the generation of cAMP. In patients with familial nephrogenic diabetes insipidus, however, plasma cortisol concentrations can rise in response to ADH, a finding interpreted to indicate that vasopressin stimulation of extrarenal, i.e., pituitary, cAMP formation is intact in the disease.

ACQUIRED NEPHROGENIC DIABETES INSIPIDUS. Vasopressin-resistant hyposthenuria associated with otherwise normal or nearly normal renal function may occur as a complication of drug therapy or in association with systemic diseases. Appropriately termed acquired nephrogenic diabetes insipidus, this condition is to be distinguished from the rare familial disorder described earlier.

Vasopressin-unresponsive hyposthenuria occurs in patients receiving demeclocycline; both the concentrating defect and vasopressin-unresponsiveness are reversible and disappear shortly after discontinuance of antibiotic therapy. The glomerular filtration rate in these patients is generally normal, as is the ability for maximal urinary dilution (positive free water formation), indicating that solute abstraction from the loop of Henle is probably unimpaired.

In human renal medulla, demeclocycline noncompetitively inhibits basal adenylate cyclase activity, ADH-stimulated adenylate cyclase activity, and cAMP-dependent protein kinase activity. Thus demeclocycline-induced nephrogenic diabetes insipidus may be due in part to inhibition of cAMP accumulation in collecting duct cells.

Nephrogenic diabetes insipidus may also be produced by volatile fluorocarbon anesthetics. Methoxyflurane anesthesia is complicated by a full spectrum of renal injury, ranging from vasopressin-resistant polyuria and hyposthenuria to acute tubular necrosis. Both fluoride and oxalic acid, which are metabolic products of methoxyflurane, contribute to the nephrotoxicity of the anesthetic. However, the polyuric state is related to the markedly increased serum concentration and urinary excretion of inorganic fluoride. Sodium fluoride causes vasopressin-resistant polyuria in dogs, and in rats inorganic fluoride seems to reduce collecting duct water permeability without affecting salt transport in the ascending limb.

Serum lithium concentrations of 0.5 to 1.5 mEq per liter, which are generally regarded as being in the therapeutic range for affective disorders, produce vasopressin-resistant diabetes insipidus. Nephrogenic diabetes insipidus has been observed in 12 to 30 per cent of patients receiving lithium therapy; the defect is usually reversible, and urinary concentrating ability returns toward normal when lithium is discontinued. Finally, nephrogenic diabetes insipidus characterized by persistent, vasopressin-resistant hyposthenuria and polyuria occurs rarely in certain systemic diseases, including most notably sarcoidosis and Sjögren's syndrome.

ACQUIRED POLYURIC STATES. There are also sets of disorders that may present with polyuria and relative vasopressin resistance, although not necessarily with profound hyposthenuria. Rather, these polyuric disturbances are generally characterized by inability to concentrate urine maximally in response to vasopressin, either stimulated endogenously or administered exogenously; random urine samples are ordinarily not profoundly hypotonic but are usually only slightly hypotonic or modestly hypertonic.

In general, such polyuric disorders occur most commonly in association with hypokalemic nephropathy (Ch. 76) or hypercalcemic nephropathy (Ch. 246), or as a consequence of diseases that disrupt medullary architecture and consequently impair the generation and maintenance of a hypertonic medullary interstitium. The latter disorders include those diseases that affect particularly the renal interstitium, such as sickle cell disease, pyelonephritis, analgesic nephropathy, and multiple myeloma. These diseases are considered in Ch. 81.

Finally, states characterized by osmotic, or solute, diuresis, for example, in diabetic ketoacidosis and hyperglycemic nonketotic states, may result in polyuria with isotonic urine formation and unresponsiveness to vasopressin. In these disorders, the fraction of isotonic glomerular filtrate delivered to the loop of Henle is greatly increased because of failure to absorb solute, for example, glucose, in the proximal nephron. Thus the amount of solute and water reaching the loop of Henle becomes large with regard to the diluting or concentrating ability of the loop of Henle and collecting ducts, respectively, and vasopressin-resistant polyuria and isosthenuria ensue. Consequently the polyuric state in osmotic diuresis differs from that in nephrogenic diabetes insipidus in two respects: urinary solute excretion is dramatically increased in osmotic diuresis but not in nephrogenic diabetes insipidus; and the urine osmolality is nearly isotonic in solute diuresis but rather hypotonic in nephrogenic diabetes insipidus.

PITUITARY OR NEPHROGENIC DIABETES INSIPIDUS

CLINICAL MANIFESTATIONS. The foremost clinical feature of either pituitary or nephrogenic diabetes insipidus is *polyuria*, with urine volumes ranging from 3 to 15 liters per day. Along with polyuria there is near-continuous *thirst*, often with a preference for ice cold water. The disease is almost always accompanied by *nocturia*, in contrast to persons with primary polydipsia (compulsive water drinking), in whom nocturia is usually absent. The onset of polyuria in pituitary diabetes insipidus is most often abrupt, with peak urine flow reached in one or two days. Therefore, polyuria developing over weeks or months suggests a disease other than pituitary diabetes insipidus. The polyuria of familial nephrogenic diabetes insipidus is present from birth.

The polyuria in complete diabetes insipidus, either pituitary or nephrogenic, has an upper limit of approximately 18 liters daily, or about 10 per cent of filtered water, since 90 per cent of the glomerular filtrate is normally absorbed by the nephron prior to reaching the collecting system. In partial pituitary diabetes insipidus, the daily urine volume may be considerably smaller. In contrast, persons afflicted with compulsive water drinking, often referred to as primary or psychogenic polydipsia, not infrequently ingest more than 20 liters of fluid daily. Therefore, the daily urine volume in these patients may also exceed 20 liters.

Modest degrees of volume depletion may curtail polyuria, even in complete diabetes insipidus, for two reasons. First, volume contraction will increase the fraction of glomerular filtrate absorbed by the proximal nephron, so that a smaller volume of hypotonic fluid reaches the collecting duct system. Second, even in the absence of ADH, or when collecting ducts are unresponsive to ADH, collecting ducts have a slight permeability to water; consequently, a small fraction of the water reaching the collecting duct system can be absorbed even without ADH. Since the volume of glomerular filtrate reaching the collecting duct system is reduced during volume contraction, the further absorption of relatively small volumes of water by collecting ducts during the volume-contracted state can result in dramatic reductions in polyuria.

Aside from the discomfort and inconvenience of polyuria and polydipsia, patients with pituitary or nephrogenic diabetes insipidus suffer no ill effects unless they are *deprived of access to water*. When this happens, *circulatory collapse* or *hypertonic encephalopathy* may occur. Because of the high rates of urine flow in some patients with diabetes insipidus, these complications may develop in a period of hours. For example, a patient with pituitary diabetes insipidus might excrete 5 per cent of his glomerular filtrate daily, or about 9 liters of urine. In a 70-kg man having 42 kg of body water, this loss, if not continuously replenished, would result in a 20 per cent reduction in body water in only 24 hours.

Hypertonic Encephalopathy. Both in man and in experimental animals, acute increases in extracellular fluid osmolality to levels exceeding 350 mOsm per kilogram of H_2O produced by solutes such as NaCl or glucose (in diabetes), which cross cell membranes poorly, result in central nervous system dysfunction ranging from lethargy to frank coma. Since comparable elevations of plasma osmolality produced by urea, which permeates cell membranes freely, do not produce the disorder, it is evident that hyperosmolality per se is not the basis for the disturbance. Rather, acute hypertonic encephalopathy occurs because cell membranes, being freely permeable to water, are in virtually constant osmotic equilibrium with extracellular fluid. When hypernatremia develops acutely, cellular water loss produces brain shrinkage; and the increase in brain solute content is accounted for entirely by a rise in intracellular Na^+, K^+, and Cl^- concentrations.

In children who develop acute hypernatremia and attain a serum sodium concentration above 160 mEq per liter in 24 hours, the mortality rate exceeds 40 per cent; about two thirds of the survivors have permanent neurologic sequelae. The autopsy results in these circumstances reveal widespread damage in cerebral vasculature. Vessels are markedly congested and engorged, hemorrhages are evident both in subcortical brain parenchyma and subarachnoid spaces, and venous thrombosis occurs.

When hypernatremia develops gradually, the incidence of hypertonic encephalopathy is greatly reduced, both in man and in experimental animals. This occurs because brain cells adapt to gradually developing hypernatremia by accumulating solutes intracellularly. The sum of brain Na^+, K^+, and Cl^- accounts for approximately 75 per cent of intracellular solutes; the remaining solutes, as yet unidentified, are commonly referred to as "idiogenic osmoles." Thus in chronic hypernatremia, brain accumulation of "idiogenic osmoles" minimizes the extent of water loss and consequently brain shrinkage. This in turn reduces the frequency with which encephalopathy develops.

Posthypophysectomy Course. The acute diabetes insipidus following hypophysectomy has a characteristic triphasic response. For a few hours to days following the insult, there exists a polyuric, hyposthenuric phase which depends on inhibition of ADH release. Next, there follows a period with reduced urine volume and a rise in urine osmolality. During this phase, there is persistent release of ADH from atrophying neurons, an inability to excrete a water load, and the risk of progressive hypotonicity with continued parenteral adminstration of large volumes of hypotonic fluids. The final phase, if the diabetes insipidus becomes permanent, is marked by recurrence of polyuria and hyposthenuria.

Laboratory Manifestations. Persistent hyposthenuria, with a urine specific gravity of 1.005 or less and urine osmolality less than 200 mOsm per kilogram of H_2O, is the hallmark of the diabetes insipidus syndromes. In euvolemic patients, the glomerular filtration rate (GFR) is normal. Since patients with diabetes insipidus ingest water in response to plasma hypertonicity, random plasma osmolality determinations in these patients will be, on the average, above the usual norm of 287 mOsm per kilogram of H_2O. The serum sodium concentrations are also elevated and account quantitatively for the increases in plasma osmolality. In contrast, persons with primary polydipsia have a primary aberration of the thirst mechanism and ingest water independent of physiologic stimuli. These patients often have a mild dilutional hyponatremia.

In patients whose diabetes insipidus, either pituitary or nephrogenic in origin, begins in childhood, considerable dilation of the urinary bladder, ureters, and renal pelvis may occur. This dilation has led to a reduction in GFR in some patients.

DIAGNOSIS. Based on the underlying pathophysiology, the polyuric syndromes may be grouped into the following general categories: (1) pituitary diabetes insipidus, in which there is absence or diminished production and secretion of ADH; (2)

solute diuresis, in which excessively high rates of solute delivery to the loop of Henle overwhelm quantitatively the ability of distal nephron segments to dissociate solute and water absorption; (3) nephrogenic diabetes insipidus, either familial or acquired, in which collecting duct cells are partially or completely unresponsive to ADH; (4) renal concentrating disorders, in which there is impaired generation of a hypertonic medullary interstitium by renal countercurrent multiplication and exchange processes; and (5) primary polydipsia, in which the ingestion of unusually large volumes of water results in polyuria, the appropriate physiologic response.

Disorders such as diabetes mellitus, which produces a solute diuresis, are characterized by an isotonic urine and by glycosuria. The history and laboratory data are adequate to identify disorders such as sickle cell disease or interstitial nephritis, both of which impair the ability to generate a hypertonic medullary interstitium. Routine laboratory screening readily identifies the presence of hypercalcemia or hypokalemia. Finally, congenital nephrogenic diabetes insipidus is identified by a history of having been present since birth, generally in males, and by *persistent* unresponsiveness to exogenous ADH. Acquired nephrogenic diabetes insipidus is recognized by ADH unresponsiveness combined with a history of exposure to agents, such as lithium, demeclocycline, or methoxyflurane anesthesia, which antagonize the action of ADH on collecting ducts.

The more difficult diagnostic problem is the differentiation of patients with partial or complete deficiency of ADH from those with primary polydipsia. Certain factors may point toward the most likely diagnosis. For example, a 24-hour urine volume greater than 18 liters, a random plasma osmolality determination below 285 mOsm per kilogram of H_2O, and a history of episodic polyuria all suggest compulsive water drinking as the underlying disorder. A history of head trauma or neoplasm, a history of sudden onset of unrelenting polyuria, and a random plasma osmolality determination greater than 290 mOsm per kilogram of H_2O all suggest pituitary diabetes insipidus.

The basis of all tests for pituitary diabetes insipidus rests on the ability of the kidney to excrete a hypertonic urine after an osmotic stimulus. The simplest maneuver is to produce hypertonicity of body fluids by water deprivation. The absolute level of urine concentration achieved with water deprivation is nondiagnostic, since maximal concentrating ability depends on the degree of medullary hypertonicity as well as the presence of adequate amounts of ADH. For example, Miller et al. found the maximal urine osmolality produced by water deprivation in a group of randomly selected hospitalized patients to be 764 mOsm per kilogram of H_2O as compared with 1067 mOsm per kilogram of H_2O in healthy volunteers. Presumably, the lower value for maximal urine concentrating ability in hospitalized patients reflects a reduction in medullary interstitial hypertonicity with respect to that present in normal volunteers.

However, even in patients with a reduced medullary interstitial tonicity, the maximal urine osmolality achieved with water deprivation depends on maximal degrees of endogenous ADH release in response to dehydration. Therefore, in those with intact mechanisms for ADH production and release, the administration of exogenous ADH will not produce an increase in the maximal urine osmolality achieved via water deprivation. This rationale forms the framework for a test scheme, illustrated in Figure 226–2, for distinguishing complete or partial pituitary diabetes insipidus from other polyuric syndromes.

In patients with mild polyuria, water deprivation may begin the night preceding the test; patients with severe polyuria should have water restricted during the day, to allow for close observation. The test begins with paired measurements of urine and plasma osmolality. All water intake is then withheld and hourly measurements of urine osmolality and body weight are made. When two sequential urine osmolalities vary by less than 30 mOsm per kilogram of H_2O, or when 3 to 5 per cent body weight is lost, 5 units of aqueous vasopressin is injected subcutaneously. A final urine osmolality is measured 60 minutes later.

The time required to achieve a maximal urine concentration varies from 4 to 18 hours. In normal persons, water deprivation results in a urine osmolality two to four times greater than that of plasma. More important, the subsequent administration of exogenous ADH results in a less than 5 per cent further increase in urine osmolality. Patients with primary polydipsia, who have a reduced medullary interstitial tonicity as a result of prolonged water diuresis, may concentrate the urine only slightly after water deprivation. However, they too will have stimulated endogenous ADH release maximally and will exhibit a less than 5 per cent rise in urine osmolality with supplemental ADH.

Patients with complete pituitary diabetes insipidus will not raise urine osmolality above that of plasma in response to water deprivation, but will show a greater than 50 per cent increase in urine osmolality in response to injection of ADH. Patients with partial pituitary diabetes insipidus may concentrate the urine to some degree in response to water deprivation, but they will also increase urine osmolality by at least 10 per cent after ADH injection. An interesting observation is that patients with partial pituitary diabetes insipidus often show a peak urine osmolality that decreases with further water restriction. This suggests a limited reserve of neurohypophyseal hormone

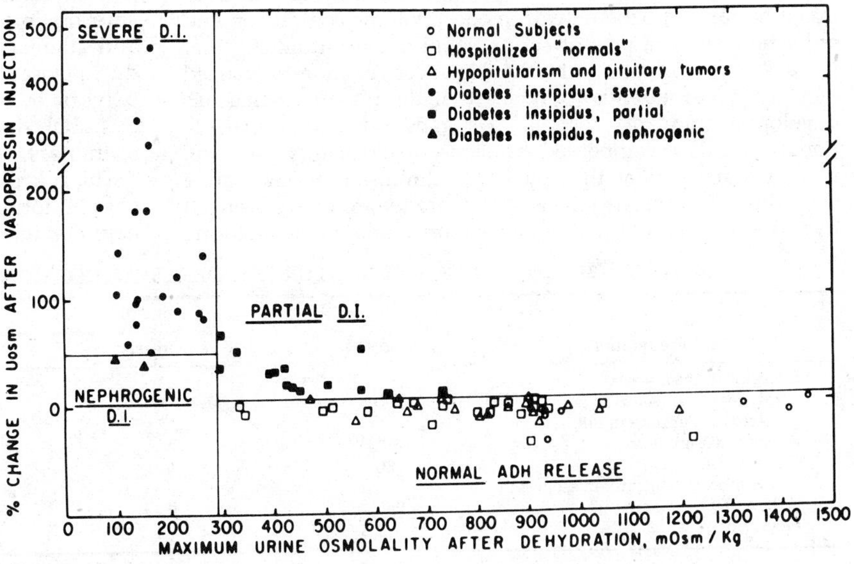

Figure 226–2. Maximal urine osmolality after dehydration versus the percentage change in urine osmolality induced by subsequent vasopressin injection. D.I. = diabetes insipidus; ADH = antidiuretic hormone. (From Miller M, et al.: Ann Intern Med 73:721, 1970. Reprinted with permission of the publisher.)

which is depleted after an initial secretory burst. Finally, patients with nephrogenic diabetes insipidus deprived of water fail to raise the urine osmolality above that of plasma even when given exogenous ADH. When a diagnosis of pituitary diabetes insipidus is made, a careful evaluation for neoplasm involving the hypothalamus or neurohypophyseal tract is mandatory.

Levels of circulating vasopressin measured by radioimmunoassay have heretofore been available only for research purposes. A commercial assay is now marketed for clinical use, but its utility is, as of now, undefined. Hypertonic saline infusions have also been utilized to test for release of antidiuretic hormone. This procedure is hazardous in patients with limited cardiac reserve, in whom volume expansion may precipitate cardiac decompensation. Moreover, the results of the test are uninterpretable if the patient develops a salt diuresis, thus fixing urine osmolality near isotonicity.

Nicotine, a nonosmotic stimulus to ADH secretion, has been used to elicit antidiuresis in those patients who have "essential hypernatremia," i.e., ADH release in response to volume contraction but not to hypertonicity. A more preferable diagnostic approach in these patients is to assess the antidiuretic response to mild volume contraction.

TREATMENT. Patients with diabetes insipidus, either pituitary or nephrogenic, may require emergency treatment of hypertonic encephalopathy or maintenance therapy for polyuria.

Hypertonic Encephalopathy. The goal in treating this medical emergency is to replenish body water, thereby restoring osmotic balance and repleting cell volume, at a rate that avoids significant complications. Since the brain adjusts to hypertonicity, at least in part, by increasing intracellular osmolar content via accumulation of "idiogenic osmoles," rapid repletion of body water with extracellular fluid dilution will cause translocation of water into cells to achieve osmotic equilibrium. The result of this water movement is cell swelling and cerebral edema. Seizures occur in up to 40 per cent of patients treated for severe hypernatremia by rapid infusions of hypotonic solutions. If water repletion is undertaken at a slower rate, brain cells lose the accumulated intracellular solutes and osmotic equilibration can occur without cell swelling. Consequently, a good rule of thumb is to adminster fluids at a rate which reduces the serum sodium concentration to normal over a 36- to 48-hour period, or to reduce the serum sodium concentration by about 1 mEq per liter every two hours.

The choice of fluid to be administered in the diabetes insipidus syndromes depends in large part on three factors: the extent to which circulatory collapse may be present; the rate at which hypernatremia has developed; and the magnitude of hypernatremia. Hypotonic NaCl solutions are best used as initial therapy in patients with modest volume contraction and only modest elevations of serum sodium concentrations, that is, less than 160 mEq per liter. However, in more advanced cases of hypernatremia, particularly if the hypernatremia has developed gradually, that is, over a period greater than 24 hours, and is accompanied by signs of circulatory collapse, more prudent initial therapy is to administer normal saline solutions. The reasons for this choice are two-fold: in advanced hypernatremia, a normal saline solution is dilute relative to the patient's body fluid osmolality and thus will dilute the latter while minimizing the risk of iatrogenic cerebral swelling; at the same time, the normal saline solution provides an effective means of volume expansion. Finally, 5 per cent glucose solutions may be used to replenish body water in acute hypernatremia without significant circulatory collapse. However, the glucose infusion rate must be less than the rate of glucose metabolism to avoid glycosuria. Otherwise, the resulting osmotic diuresis will thwart attempts to replenish body free water. The treatment of drug-induced nephrogenic diabetes insipidus consists of removal of the offending agent.

Polyuria. Patients with partial hormonal deficiency and volumes of urine output between 2 and 6 liters daily may require no treatment as long as they are assured access to water. Specific therapy for pituitary diabetes insipidus is some form of ADH replacement. A variety of hormone preparations are available which differ in the ratio of antidiuretic to vasopressor activity and the duration of biologic effect. These relations are depicted in Table 226–2.

Early preparations of dried posterior pituitary extract, termed "pituitary snuff," were given by nasal insufflation, had an effective biologic life of only a few hours, and inevitably produced chronic rhinitis, which often led to inadequate absorption of hormone. Aqueous vasopressin injections, having an activity span of only a few hours, are not practical, although nasal sprays of aqueous lysine vasopressin may provide intermittent relief of polyuria. Rhinitis, although not so severe as with dried extract, is also a frequent concomitant to this form of therapy.

The most widely used preparation has been Pitressin Tannate in oil, which is given intramuscularly. As little as 0.5 ml per day may provide adequate hormone for 24 to 48 hours. Great care must be exercised in preparing the injection by careful warming and mixing of the ampule so as to suspend the pellet of hormone in the oil. Failure to do so may result in injection of the oil vehicle alone and apparent "vasopressin resistance." Pain at injection sites and sterile abscesses are frequent complaints with this preparation. Persistent abdominal pain from the effect of ADH on intestinal motility is a not uncommon problem.

A synthetic analogue of vasopressin, dDAVP (1-deamino,8-D-arginine vasopressin), provides antidiuretic activity for 8 to 20 hours with negligible pressor effect, can be taken as a nasal spray, and is the current drug of choice. The drug is best started at night to find the lowest dose that will prevent nocturia. This dose, usually 5 to 10 μg, can be given twice daily or doubled as a single morning dose. A nasal catheter is provided, which is measured for convenient dosing in the 5 to 20 μg range. Headache may be a troublesome side effect with large doses but usually disappears with a reduction of dosage.

For patients having some residual ADH production, the oral hypoglycemic agent chlorpropamide may provide adequate amelioration of symptoms. This drug stimulates ADH secretion and augments the activity of residual ADH on the collecting duct. Doses of 250 to 500 mg daily are sufficient to reduce polyuria in most patients with partial pituitary diabetes insipidus, but the side effect of hypoglycemia limits the drug's usefulness.

Thiazide diuretics may reduce the volume of urine in patients with all forms of diabetes insipidus, that is, either pituitary or nephrogenic, by causing a state of mild salt depletion. This

TABLE 226–2. COMPARISON OF NEUROHYPOPHYSEAL HORMONES AND SYNTHETIC ANALOGUES

Preparation	Activity					Duration of Activity	Route of Administration
	Antidiuretic	:	Vasopressor	:	Oxytocic		
8-Arginine vasopressin							
Pitressin, Aqueous	100	:	100	:	5	2–6 hours	Intravenous
Pitressin Tannate in oil						24–48 hours	Intramuscular
8-Lysine vasopressin							
Lypressin	60	:	70	:	1	2–6 hours	Nasal insufflation
1-Deamino, 8 D-arginine vasopressin							
dDAVP, Desmopressin	290	:	0.14			6–20 hours	Nasal insufflation
Oxytocin	1	:	1	:	100		

results in a secondary increase in isotonic proximal tubular fluid absorption and a decrease in the volume of fluid delivered to the collecting duct. The effect is produced by 50 to 100 mg of hydrochlorothiazide daily, is sustained even in the absence of diuretics by salt restriction, and can be abolished by salt loading even with continued diuretic administration.

Vasopressin infusions have also been used to treat bleeding esophageal varices by reducing splanchnic blood flow. Desmopressin, a synthetic analogue of arginine vasopressin, stimulates the production of clotting factor VIII. These other actions are discussed elsewhere in this textbook.

Nephrogenic Diabetes Insipidus. The therapeutic considerations outlined above, particularly with respect to the treatment of hypertonic encephalopathy and to the value of a chronic mild salt-depleted state in minimizing polyuria, apply equally well to the care of patients with pituitary or nephrogenic diabetes insipidus. In patients with nephrogenic diabetes insipidus acquired as a consequence of drug therapy (for example, lithium or demeclocycline), the offending agent should be discontinued.

Finally, it is important to stress the need to minimize the extent of polyuria in children with congenital nephrogenic diabetes insipidus, since there is a close correlation between repeated bouts of dehydration during childhood and mental dullness in adulthood. Alternatively, in patients in whom episodes of dehydration have been minimal, both mental and physical growth retardation can be avoided.

Andreoli TE: The polyuric syndromes. *In* Andreoli TE, Hoffman JF, Fanestil DD (eds.): Physiology of Membrane Disorders. New York, Plenum Medical Book Company, 1978, pp 1063-1091. *A discussion of the physiology of the polyuric states, their differentiation one from another, and therapeutic approaches; extensively referenced.*

Arieff AI, Schmidt RW: Fluid and electrolyte disorders and the central nervous system. *In* Maxwell MH, Kleeman CR (eds.): Clinical Disorders of Fluid and Electrolyte Metabolism. New York, McGraw-Hill Book Company, 1980, pp 1409-1480. *This chapter is a superb review of the pathophysiology, manifestations, and treatment of the hyperosmolar syndrome; thoroughly referenced.*

Barlow ED, De Wardener HE: Compulsive water drinking. Quart J Med 28:235, 1959. *A thorough examination of the clinical course and pathophysiology of urinary concentration in a group of patients with primary polydipsia.*

DeRubertis FR, Michelis MF, Beck N, Field JB, David, BB: "Essential" hypernatremia due to ineffective osmotic and intact volume regulation of vasopressin secretion. J Clin Invest 50:97, 1971. *A description of patients having intact neurohypophyseal function but lacking normal regulation of ADH because of a specific defect in osmoregulation.*

Miller M, Dalakos T, Moses AM, Fellerman H, Streeten DHP: Recognition of partial defects in antidiuretic hormone secretion. Ann Intern Med 73:721, 1970. *A concise guide to testing procedures for states of ADH insufficiency and a rational scheme for interpreting the test results.*

Robertson GL: Thirst and vasopressin function in normal and disordered states of water balance. J Lab Clin Med 101:351, 1983. *A detailed account of the physiology and pathophysiology of ADH secretion and thirst in normal patients and those with polyuric disorders.*

Zerbe RL, Robertson GL: Osmoregulation of thirst and vasopressin secretion in human subjects: Effect of various solutes. Am J Physiol 244:E607, 1983. *The role of various ECF solutes on ADH release.*

THE SYNDROME OF INAPPROPRIATE ADH PRODUCTION (SIADH)

For convenience SIADH has been discussed in Ch. 76 as a major disorder producing hyponatremia.

OXYTOCIN

Oxytocin is produced in the same hypothalamic nuclei and by the same synthetic mechanism as vasopressin. AVP and oxytocin are produced in both the paraventricular and the supraoptic nuclei of the hypothalamus. However, a given neuron in these nuclei produces only one hormone. Neurophysin I is the specific carrier protein synthesized with oxytocin and has been used as a marker for oxytocin release.

PHYSIOLOGY. The primary stimuli for oxytocin secretion are nipple stimulation (suckling) and deformation of the reproductive tract (especially the vagina) in females, and muscular contraction of the reproductive organs in the male. The neural arcs serving these stimuli are not well defined, but some evidence suggests that the final synaptic transmitter is dopamine. Estrogens appear to influence secretion directly, based on observations of increased neurophysin I in blood during estrogen peaks of the menstrual cycle, or permissively, based on findings of a graded response to vaginal distention over the period of a menstrual cycle and an enhanced response with exogenous estradiol. Progesterones inhibit response to mechanical stimuli. Hypertonicity of body fluids also appears to cause oxytocin secretion, and congenitally vasopressin-deficient rats (Brattleboro strain) show little neurohypophyseal oxytocin until given vasopressin, suggesting that these animals attempt to compensate for AVP insufficiency with the weaker antidiuretic hormone, oxytocin.

BIOLOGIC ACTIVITY. In females, oxytocin initiates its primary effect by binding to specific myometrial receptors, the affinity of which increases strikingly in the presence of estrogen. Exogenously administered oxytocin elicits contractions of the fundus indistinguishable from those of labor. However, the initiation of labor is apparently oxytocin independent, with increasing secretions seen only with dilation of the birth canal. Oxytocin may play a key role in final expulsion of the fetus and placenta. The total absence of oxytocin does not prevent parturition, although prolonged labor is seen in such women. The cellular events leading to uterine contraction are unknown, but parallel an oxytocin-induced increase in ion permeability with depolarization of the myometrial cell membrane.

The milk-ejection reflex is also mediated via oxytocin. Contraction of mammary myoepithelium is stimulated, leading to a rise in intramammary pressure and expulsion of milk from alveolar channels to large sinuses, where it is accessible to the suckling infant. A true galactogenic effect of oxytocin leading to increased milk production has not been convincingly demonstrated. Absence of oxytocin abolishes the milk-ejection reflex.

In the male, oxytocin increases ejection of sperm into the semen in response to stimulation of the reproductive organs. Oxytocin retains some antidiuretic activity, about 1 per cent that of AVP, but exerts no significant antidiuretic effect at physiologic levels of secretion. Vascular smooth muscle is relaxed by oxytocin, causing a decrease in blood pressure, cutaneous flushing, and increased limb blood flow. Reflex tachycardia and sympathetic responses quickly restore hemodynamics to normal except when such reflexes are rendered inactive as in deep anesthesia.

THERAPEUTIC USE. The primary use of oxytocin (Pitocin) is to induce or to improve the quality of labor. The uterus is relatively resistant to oxytocin in early pregnancy, but infusions given with hypertonic saline injections may speed abortions of later pregnancy.

With long-term infusion of oxytocin, patients may experience sufficient antidiuretic effects to be at risk of water intoxication. Antidiuresis may be detected at oxytocin infusion rates of 15 mU per minute, and maximal urinary concentration is usually attained at rates of 45 mU per minute. Infusions for delivery and control of postpartum uterine hemorrhage may reach 20 to 40 mU per minute, and infusions for therapeutic abortions range from 20 to 100 mU per minute.

Roberts JS: Oxytocin, Vol I. Montreal, Eden Press, 1977. *This review covers the extensive work in oxytocin physiology and chemistry; very readable and fully referenced.*

227. THE PINEAL

Seymour Reichlin

The pineal gland was discovered more than 20 centuries ago, and its function has long been a matter of scientific and philosophic speculation. Arising embryologically from ependyma lining the roof of the third ventricle, the pineal consists of parenchymal cells supported by a meshwork of neuroglia.

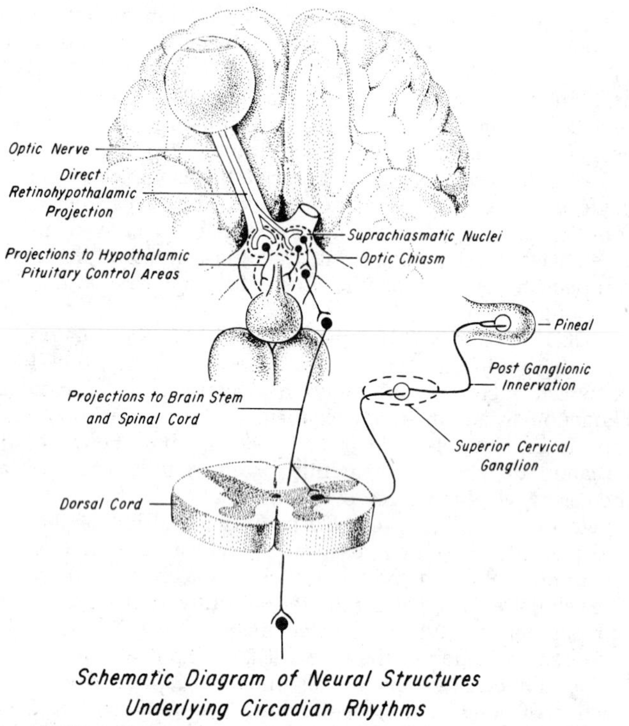

Figure 227–1. Control system for pineal regulation. Light impinging upon the retina is transduced into neural signals that reach the brain, giving both visual and nonvisual responses. This diagram outlines the nonvisual component. Those involved in endocrine regulation are mainly conducted by the direct retinohypothalamic projection to the suprachiasmatic nuclei (located in the hypothalamus). From the suprachiasmatic nuclei, nerve pathways project to the hypophysiotropic control areas of the hypothalamus and also to the spinal cord, where they influence the primary neurons of the sympathetic nerve outflow tract that terminate in the superior cervical ganglia. From the superior cervical ganglia, postganglionic sympathetic nerves (noradrenergic in function), accompanying the venous drainage of the pineal gland, enter the gland to innervate the pineal parenchymal cells. Suprachiasmatic nuclei are responsible for endogenous rhythms as well as those influenced by external lighting (see text). (Redrawn from Moore RY: *In* Yen SSC, Jaffe RB [eds.]: Reproductive Endocrinology: Physiology, Pathophysiology and Clinical Management. Philadelphia, W. B. Saunders Company, 1978, pp 3–33.)

In the adult, the gland weighs between 100 and 180 mg and is a cone-shaped organ lying in the groove formed by the superior colliculi. Although connected to the epithalamus by a peduncle, the pineal does not receive a direct nerve supply from this source. Rather, it is innervated by postganglionic nerve fibers that arise in the cervical sympathetic ganglia and travel along the great vein of Galen, the blood vessel into which pineal secretions drain. The sympathetic inflow to the pineal is in turn regulated by impulses arising in the suprachiasmatic nuclei, paired structures lying just above the optic chiasm (Fig. 227–1). This nucleus is innervated by a direct nerve pathway from the retina termed the retinohypothalamic tract. Changes in external lighting influence pineal activity (and other endocrine functions) via this pathway even when pathways mediating conscious light perception have been severed. The suprachiasmatic nucleus is also believed to serve as an internal "clock" (or biologic oscillator), regulating a number of endogenous endocrine rhythms. Circadian changes can occur even in the absence of external sensory cues, including light changes, thus indicating that there is a mechanism for determination of intrinsic rhythms. The rhythm of the endogenous oscillator can be modified by external signals such as normal light-dark cycles.

SECRETIONS OF THE PINEAL

Many different neurotransmitter substances, including norepinephrine, serotonin, histamine, melatonin, dopamine, octopamine, and gamma-aminobutyric acid, are found in the pineal. It also contains the hypothalamic peptides somatostatin and TRH. Of all these biologically active substances, only melatonin has been shown to be secreted into the blood and can be looked upon as a true hormonal secretion of the pineal. Melatonin is present in blood, cerebrospinal fluid, and urine of many species of animals, including man. Hormone levels show a marked diurnal rhythm, with night values up to ten times higher than day values. Turning lights off is a potent stimulus to melatonin release. Melatonin is believed to exert suppressive effects on a number of endocrine functions in experimental animals, the most important of which is on the release of gonadotropic hormones. When given to man in high dosage, melatonin suppresses plasma LH levels and stress-induced growth hormone secretion. Important effects of melatonin injection in man are the production of sleepiness and changes in the electroencephalogram, mainly an increase of alpha waves. Melatonin is formed by a series of enzymatic steps from tryptophan in which one of the intermediates is serotonin (Fig. 227–2). Enzymic activity of the pineal gland and its secretory function are regulated by noradrenergic nerve endings on pinealocytes. Beta-catecholamine receptors activate adenyl cyclase with the formation of cyclic AMP through the classic second messenger mechanism. The activated ATP-protein kinase is believed to promote the formation of the melatonin-synthesizing enzymes. Norepinephrine also stimulates pineal uptake of the precursor tryptophan.

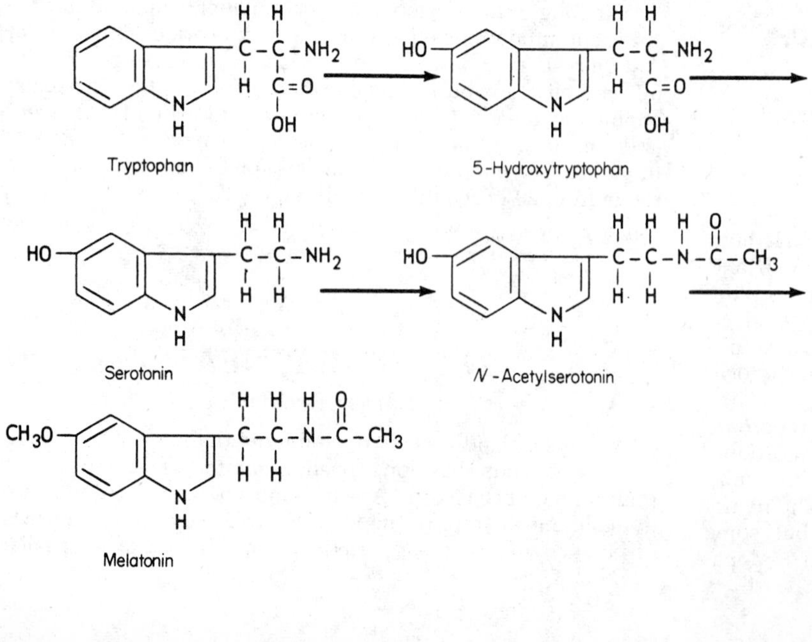

Figure 227–2. Biosynthesis of melatonin from tryptophan in the pineal gland. Step 1 is catalyzed by tryptophan hydroxylase; Step 2 by L-aromatic amino acid decarboxylase; Step 3 by N-acetylating enzyme; and Step 4 by HIOMT. (From Wurtman RJ, Axelrod J, Kelly D: The Pineal. New York, Academic Press, 1968, p 60.)

ABNORMALITIES OF THE PINEAL

The pineal gland has no known function in man but becomes of clinical significance because of the occurrence of calcification and of tumor formation. Calcific nodules termed *acervuli* form in a matrix of ground substance secreted by pinealocytes. This process begins in early childhood and becomes increasingly evident by roentgenography beginning in the second decade of life. Calcification has no known effect on pineal function.

Diseases of the pineal are rare. A few cases of hypoplasia and aplasia have been reported, and these have been associated in a relatively high proportion with genital precocity. Less than 1 per cent of intracranial neoplasms are tumors of the pineal gland, and they are seen almost exclusively in young males. The term *pinealoma* refers to a tumor of the pineal parenchymal cell, called pineoblastoma or pineocytoma according to its degree of differentiation. In one series of pineal tumor cases, only 9 of 53 fitted this category and there were 13 glial tumors, including astrocytomas and glioblastomas. The most common tumor (approximately 50 per cent) is best termed *germinoma* because it apparently arises from germ cells and not from pineal parenchymal cells. They are believed to be due to embryologic rests of germ cells. Identical tumors are found in the testis and anterior mediastinum. Approximately 10 per cent of intracranial germinomas metastasize to the spinal cord. Germinomas arising in the pineal gland may infiltrate the third ventricle and the floor of the hypothalamus, producing a characteristic triad: *diabetes insipidus, hypogonadism,* and *optic atrophy*. An identical clinical presentation can be due to germinomas arising from midline tissues at the base of the brain. X-ray of the skull rarely shows abnormality even when hypothalamic functions are grossly deranged. *Teratomas* may also arise in the pineal region, and rarely give rise to choriocarcinomas. Several cases of precocious puberty have been reported to be caused by gonadotropin-secreting choriocarcinomas of the pineal, an abnormality associated with detectable HCG in the spinal fluid.

Pineal tumors also cause sexual precocity by hypothalamic damage which destroys structures normally inhibitory to the development of puberty. Pinealomas cause precocious puberty almost exclusively in males. The most important local manifestations of pineal neoplasms are due to pressure on the quadrigeminal plate of the midbrain. An enlarging mass in the pineal region compresses the aqueduct of Sylvius and distorts the upper brainstem. Internal hydrocephalus gives rise to characteristic headache, vomiting, papilledema, and disturbed consciousness. Pressure on the superior colliculi causes paralysis of conjugate upward gaze (Parinaud's syndrome). The characteristic wide-based gait may be due to pressure on the cerebellum or brainstem.

Although a number of surgical cures have been reported, pineal tumors are rarely resectable by the time that clinical signs appear. Fortunately, the germinoma type is radiosensitive, and prolonged survival has been observed. Most workers recommend that craniotomy be carried out for diagnostic purposes, but that removal be attempted only if the lesion is favorably localized, or if it is a radioresistant lesion. Supervoltage roentgen therapy is usually given. There is little experience with chemotherapy of these tumors. In emergency situations presenting with hydrocephalus, it is usually necessary to decompress by shunting the third ventricle prior to definitive therapy.

Reichlin S: Neuroendocrinology. *In* Williams R (ed.): Textbook of Endocrinology. 6th ed. Philadelphia, W. B. Saunders. Company, 1981. *Comprehensive and systematic review of pineal function. Detailed account of clinical aspects, including diagnosis and management. Designed for medical students and fellows.*

Relkin R: The Pineal Gland. New York, Elsevier Biomedical, 1983. *A detailed basic and clinical text of greatest value because of its complete bibliography.*

Reppert SM, Klein DC (eds.): Mammalian pineal gland: Basic and clinical aspects. *In* Motta M (ed.): The Endocrine Functions of the Brain. New York, Raven Press, 1980, pp 327–371. *Detailed, authoritative review of chemistry and physiologic functions of the pineal gland.*

Schmidek HH: Pineal Tumors. New York, Masson U.S.A., 1977. *Includes excellent account of anatomy and physiology of the pineal, diseases, diagnosis, and treatment. The definitive monograph for the clinician responsible for patient care. Schmidek's views represent a comparatively conservative surgical approach.*

Wurtman RJ, Moskowitz MA: The pineal organ. N Engl J Med 296:1329, 1977. *Medical Progress review of the pineal brings the field up to date circa 1976.*

228. THE THYROID

P. Reed Larsen

Introduction

The thyroid gland secretes thyroxine, 3,5,3′,5′-tetraiodothyronine (abbreviated T_4) and small amounts of 3,5,3′-triiodothyronine (abbreviated T_3). The principal role of these substances is to regulate tissue metabolism. In infants, adequate supplies of thyroid hormone are necessary for the development of the normal central nervous system in the first one to two years of life. The absence of thyroid hormone during this period results in irreversible mental retardation, a syndrome known as *cretinism*. The hormone is also required for normal growth and bone maturation in children. Despite these important functions, the body can withstand marked reductions in thyroid hormone for long periods, although at the cost of abnormal operation of many organ systems.

EMBRYOLOGY AND ANATOMY

The thyroid develops from a combination of pharyngeal midline and bilateral primitive tissues from the fourth branchial pouch. These primitive thyroid cells migrate from the pharyngeal floor, leaving behind a residual thyroglossal duct which normally becomes obliterated. The major portion of the thyroid cell mass is derived from the median mid-pharyngeal tissue. The lateral thyroid anlagen migrate medially to fuse with median thyroid but primarily contribute the *parafollicular* or *C-cells*. The C-cells secrete thyrocalcitonin, not thyroid hormone, and do not play a role in thyroid physiology (see Ch. 228). The evolution of thyroid function occurs over the first 10 to 12 weeks of fetal life, with definite appearance of T_4 in the gland by 10 to 11 weeks. The placenta is impermeable to T_3 and T_4; the fetus depends on its own thyroid for its supply of these hormones. The adult size (15 to 20 grams) of the thyroid is reached at about age 15. The thyroid gland has the configuration of a butterfly, with the two lobes measuring about 5 × 2 cm. The lobes are composed of spherical structures called *follicles,* consisting of *colloid* surrounded by a single layer of epithelial cells enclosed by a basement membrane. Colloid consists predominantly of the protein *thyroglobulin,* which is the storage form of T_4 and T_3.

THYROID PHYSIOLOGY

The structures of the thyroid hormones and their precursors, mono-and diiodotyrosine (MIT and DIT), are shown in Figure 228–1. Iodine accounts for 65 per cent of the weight of T_4. Since this is a relatively scarce element in the earth's crust, mechanisms are present in the thyroid cell to allow it to concentrate and conserve iodine.

IODINE METABOLISM. The daily intake of iodine in man varies markedly in different areas of the world. It ranges from extremely low levels (20 μg or less per day) to as high as 600 or 700 μg per day in certain areas of the United States. The optimal iodine intake for adults is thought to be 150 to 300 μg per day. Levels appreciably below this lead to the condition known as *endemic goiter*, which is discussed later in this chapter. The high level of iodine intake in the United States is, in part, due to iodination of salt. Iodine in all forms is reduced to iodide

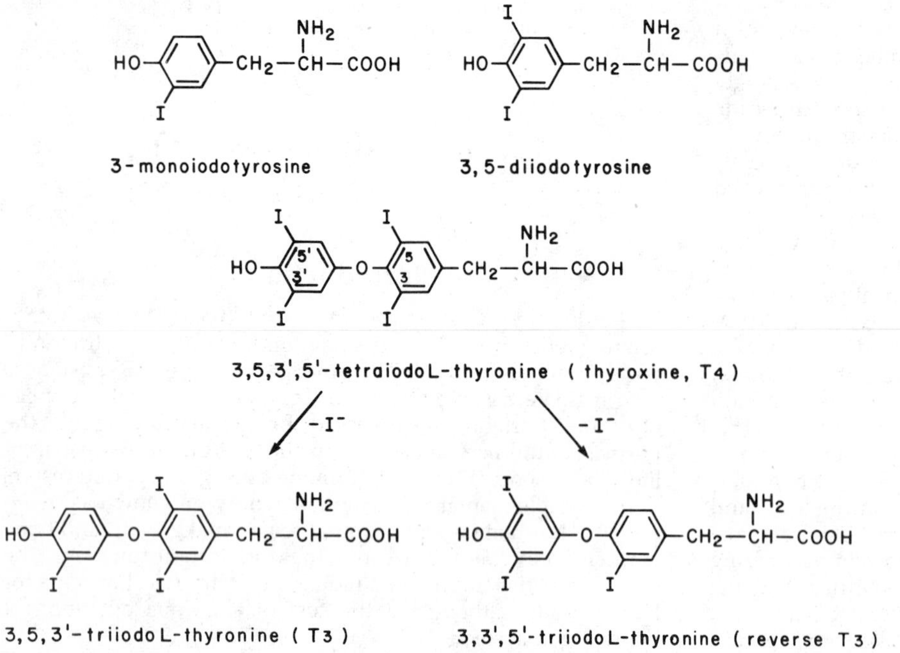

Figure 228–1. Structure of the thyroid hormones and their precursors.

(I^-) in the gastrointestinal tract and absorbed within 30 minutes of ingestion. I^- leaves the blood via two mechanisms. It is concentrated by the thyroid or excreted in the urine.

The plasma I^- concentration in man depends to a great extent on iodine intake but usually is 0.1 to 1 μg per deciliter. The thyroid clearance varies inversely with the plasma I^- and ranges from 10 to 30 ml per minute, while the urinary clearance is about 30 ml per minute. There is a wide variation in the fraction of I^- concentrated by the thyroid per 24 hours, again depending on iodine uptake. In the United States, iodine uptake by the thyroid varies from about 5 to 30 per cent.

INTRATHYROIDAL IODIDE METABOLISM. In Figure 228–2 are shown the steps involved in the synthesis of the thyroid hormones. Because the concentrations of I^- in the plasma are so low, the thyroid cell concentrates I^-, the cell:plasma ratio being about 20 to 40:1. The trapped I^- is rapidly oxidized and incorporated into protein. As a consequence, there is little I^- per se in the thyroid gland. The process of I^- oxidation and its incorporation into tyrosine is known as *organification*. The substrate for iodine is the 660,000 molecular weight glycoprotein thyroglobulin. Only about 25 per cent of the tyrosine residues of this specialized protein are available for iodination. Both mono- and diiodotyrosine are formed (MIT and DIT). In a typical molecule of fully iodinated human thyroglobulin, there are approximately 6 to 7 residues of MIT, 4 to 5 of DIT, 3 to 4 of T_4 and 0.2 to 0.3 of T_3. The T_4 and T_3 arise from the coupling of either 2 DIT residues or 1 MIT and 1 DIT residue, a reaction that requires thyroid peroxidase. This process is known as *coupling*. Both organification and coupling are inhibited by *thiourea compounds*, which are used in the treatment of patients with hyperthyroidism (see below). The thyroglobulin is iodinated at the apical border of the cell and is then exocytosed into the colloid. Under normal circumstances, T_4 and T_3 secretion occurs from this pool. The thyroid secretory process starts with phagocytosis of thyroglobulin by the apical cell membrane, leading to the formation of a *colloid droplet*. This is combined with a lysosome, and, as the colloid droplet traverses the thyroid cell, proteolysis occurs with eventual release of T_4 and T_3 at the basal cell border. Deiodination of T_4 to T_3 also occurs during this process, resulting in a ratio of T_4 to T_3 in thyroid secretion which is somewhat less than the 15:1 value found in the thyroglobulin itself. In order to conserve iodine for reuse in the thyroid cell, a *deiodinase* is present which removes the iodine from MIT and DIT, allowing it to recycle.

CIRCULATING T_4 AND T_3. Thyroid hormones in plasma exist in two forms, free and protein-bound. Although only about 0.02 per cent of total plasma T_4 and 0.3 per cent of plasma T_3 are free, it is the free hormone concentration which is maintained constant by the feedback regulatory system and which appears to parallel the rate of cellular uptake of these hormones. It is, therefore, the free hormone concentration which determines the thyroid status irrespective of the total plasma concentration. In the euthyroid person, the total hormone is determined by the quantity and affinity of certain thyroid hormone–binding proteins, which are *thyroxine-binding globulin* (TBG), *thyroxine-binding prealbumin* (TBPA), and albumin. TBG is by far the most important of these, transporting about 75 per cent of serum T_4 and T_3. It is a glycoprotein, with a

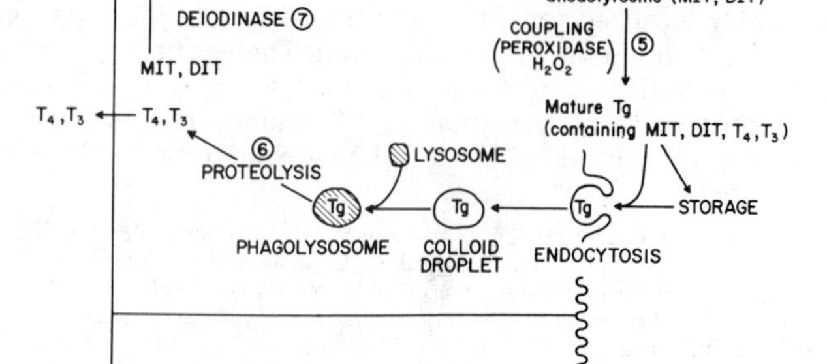

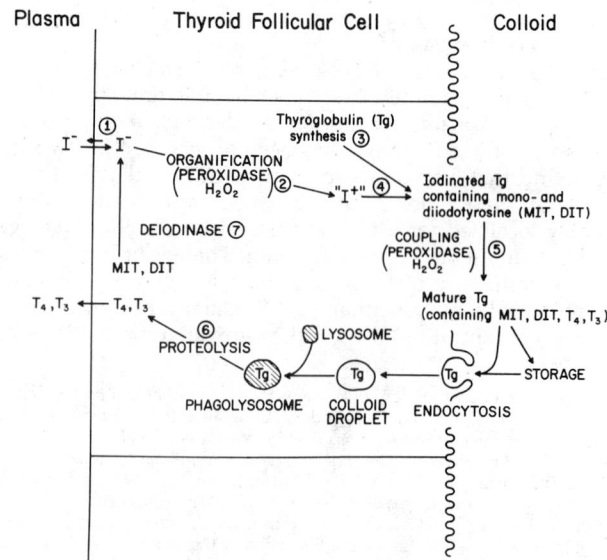

Figure 228–2. Principal steps in the synthesis and secretion of thyroid hormones. MIT = monoiodotyrosine; DIT = diiodotyrosine. The steps denoted by the numbers are those in which defects have been identified in patients with inherited abnormalities in thyroid hormone biosynthesis (see Sporadic and Endemic Goiter, below).

TABLE 228–1. CIRCUMSTANCES ASSOCIATED WITH CHANGES IN THE CIRCULATING CONCENTRATION OF THYROXINE-BINDING GLOBULIN (TBG)

Increased TBG
1. Pregnancy
2. Treatment with supraphysiologic amounts of estrogens, including oral contraceptives
3. In some patients with cirrhosis or acute hepatitis
4. As a congenital abnormality
5. In acute intermittent porphyria

Decreased TBG
1. Protein malnutrition
2. Nephrotic syndrome
3. Severe hepatic failure
4. After L-asparaginase
5. As a congenital abnormality (usually X-linked)
6. During treatment with androgenic steroids or pharmacologic doses of glucocorticoids.

molecular weight of 55,000, which is synthesized in the liver. TBG has a high affinity for both T_4 and T_3, although the affinity for T_4 is about 10- to 15-fold higher than that for T_3. There is normally sufficient TBG in serum to bind approximately 20 μg of T_4 per deciliter at a molar ratio of 1:1. The serum TBG concentrations change under many circumstances, which are listed in Table 228–1. It is important to recognize these conditions, since the resultant changes in total T_4 and T_3 may duplicate abnormalities which are found in patients with thyroid dysfunction. For example, during pregnancy, serum total T_4 and T_3 are increased but serum free T_4 and T_3 concentrations remain constant. The relationships are described in the following equation:

$$[\text{TH}] \text{ is proportional to } \frac{[\text{TH}\text{——}\text{TBG}]}{[\text{TBG}]}$$

where TH = free T_4 or T_3, [TH——TBG] = TBG-bound T_4 or T_3, and TBG = unoccupied TBG. When [TBG] increases, the bound hormone also increases until a new steady state is achieved at which [TH] is again normal. This occurs through both decreased metabolism and increased secretion of T_4 and T_3. To interpret a total serum T_4 or T_3 measurement accurately it is necessary to know the fraction of the hormone which is free; alternatively the free hormone can be measured directly or estimated (see Direct Tests of Thyroid Function later in this chapter). Certain compounds compete with T_4 and T_3 for binding to TBG. Two such drugs are salicylates and phenytoin. About a 20 to 30 per cent reduction in serum T_4 and T_3 is observed when 300 mg of phenytoin or salicylates in excess of 2.4 grams per day are given.

KINETICS OF T_4 AND T_3. Deiodination of the iodothyronines is the most significant metabolic transformation of the thyroid hormones. In the case of T_4, deiodination of the distal ring, occurring predominantly in liver and kidney, gives rise to T_3, which has approximately three to four times the metabolic potency of the parent hormone (Fig. 228–1). About 30 to 40 per cent of the 80 μg of T_4 produced per day is metabolized via this pathway (Table 228–2), giving rise to about 80 per cent of the T_3 produced daily. Loss of an iodine in the proximal ring of T_4 leads to formation of *reverse* T_3 (3,3′,5′-triiodothyronine), a compound which appears to have no metabolic effect. About 40 per cent of T_4 is metabolized via this pathway, the remainder being excreted via the biliary tract into the feces following conjugation with glucuronide. T_3 and reverse T_3 are, in turn, deiodinated in both proximal and distal rings, giving rise to the predicted mono- and diiodothyronines, none of which have physiologic effects. T_4 to T_3 conversion and reverse T_3 deiodination appear to be catalyzed by the same enzyme. If this reaction is inhibited, as it is under diverse circumstances, a reduction in serum T_3 and an increase in the serum reverse T_3 concentration occur.

The differences between T_3 and T_4 in terms of distribution volume, the intracellular fraction, and half-life can be attributed principally to the differences in the affinities of these two hormones for the plasma binding proteins (Table 228–2). The higher intracellular T_3 content explains in part its higher potency relative to T_4. Given the 3 to 4:1 ratio of metabolic potency of T_3 and T_4 and the fact that approximately one third of T_4 is converted to T_3, it appears that T_4 has little intrinsic metabolic activity in man.

TABLE 228–2. COMPARISON OF T_3 AND T_4 IN MAN

	T_3	T_4
Serum concentration		
Total (μg/dl)	0.14	8
Free (ng/dl)	0.4	1.6
Fraction of total serum hormone which is in the free form (%)	0.3	0.02
Distribution volume (liters)	35	10
Fraction intracellular (%)	64	10–20
Half-life (days)	1	7
Production rate (μg/day)	33	80
Fraction directly from thyroid (%)	20	100
Relative metabolic potency	1	0.3

REGULATION OF T_4 TO T_3 CONVERSION. The liver and kidney are the most active tissues in converting T_4 to T_3 based on in vitro studies. This enzyme, 5′-iodothyronine deiodinase, requires a sulfhydryl (SH)-containing cofactor which may be reduced glutathione. The T_3 produced by liver and kidney enters the T_3 pool. Thus, the liver and kidney are activators of T_4, producing T_3 for other tissues such as skeletal and heart muscle where this conversion occurs much more slowly. A number of factors influence the peripheral monodeiodination of T_4 to T_3 (Table 228–3). The first group includes pharmacologic agents which either are competitive inhibitors of the enzyme or interact with the SH-containing cofactor. Propylthiouracil appears to act via the latter mechanism, whereas the iodinated contrast agents used for oral cholecystography, iopanoic acid and sodium ipodate, act by the former. The latter drugs also inhibit T_4 uptake by the liver. In addition, there are significant reductions in T_4 to T_3 conversion during stress which occur because of decreased hepatic T_4 uptake, reduced SH-cofactor, and decreased enzyme content. T_4 to T_3 conversion in most tissues of the fetus is markedly reduced, probably owing to low endogenous concentrations of reduced glutathione. Many of these physiologic reductions in T_4 activation can be thought of as teleologically sound, conserving body resources in times of stress, but proof that this is so is lacking. However, reduction in the serum T_3 concentration relative to that of T_4 in all these circumstances is important when interpreting measurements of serum thyroid hormone concentrations in sick patients.

MECHANISM OF ACTION OF THYROID HORMONE. The mechanism by which thyroid hormone produces its protean effects remains obscure. In animal studies, thyroid hormone–responsive tissues contain nucleoproteins which have an extremely high affinity for thyroid hormones. These proteins, unlike those in the serum, have approximately ten-fold higher affinity for T_3 than T_4, further explaining why T_3 is the more potent hormone. Both in tissue culture and in animals, the occupancy

TABLE 228–3. PHYSIOLOGIC AND PHARMACOLOGIC INFLUENCES ON PERIPHERAL MONODEIODINATION OF T_4 TO T_3

Pharmacologic Inhibitors of T_4 to T_3 conversion
1. Propylthiouracil (not methimazole [Tapazole])
2. Iopanoic acid (Telepaque) and sodium ipodate (Oragrafin)
3. Amiodarone* (an antiarrhythmic agent)
4. Propranolol
5. Pharmacologic quantities of glucocorticoids

Physiologic situations in which T_4 to T_3 conversion is reduced
1. Fasting (particularly carbohydrate deprivation)
2. Severe acute or chronic illness of any sort or after surgery
3. In the presence of significant hepatic disease
4. In the human fetus

*Investigational drug.

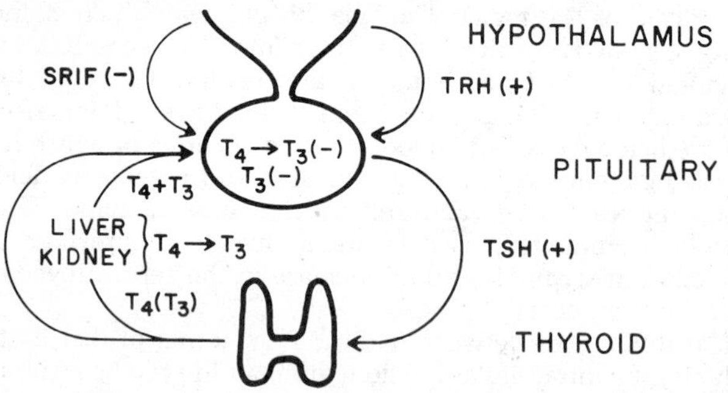

Figure 228–3. Current concepts of hypothalamic-pituitary-thyroid inter-relationships.

of these receptors by thyroid hormone can be related to changes in the rate of messenger RNA synthesis for various thyroid hormone–dependent proteins. At present, it would appear that these changes can explain virtually all the effects of thyroid hormone, although additional independent effects at the cell membrane or mitochondrion have not yet been completely excluded. The thyroid hormone nuclear receptor present in human tissues bears a close resemblance to that found in animals and appears to have the same physiologic relevance.

REGULATION OF THYROID FUNCTION. At least two tissues, anterior pituitary and cerebral cortex, are unique with respect to deiodination. In these two tissues, T_4 is monodeiodinated to T_3, but a substantial portion of the T_3 is then immediately bound to nuclear receptors without re-entering the plasma. Based on studies in the rat, at least 50 per cent of the intracellular T_3 in these two tissues originates from this source. When serum T_4 is reduced but T_3 remains constant, intracellular T_3 in these tissues will be reduced. Accordingly, the pituitary and, presumably, the cerebral cortex can recognize a decrease in serum T_4, per se, independent of changes in serum T_3.

The feedback loop for regulation of thyroid function is presented in Figure 228–3. *Thyrotropin-releasing hormone* (TRH) is secreted by hypothalamic cells and stimulates synthesis and release of thyrotropin (TSH). This hormone in turn stimulates all of the steps involved in thyroid hormone synthesis and release through activation of adenylate cyclase. T_4 and smaller amounts of T_3 are released from the gland with monodeiodination of T_4 to T_3 in liver and kidney. Both serum T_3 and T_4 (via its intrapituitary conversion to T_3) suppress the synthesis and release of TSH competing with TRH to complete the feedback loop. *Somatostatin* (SRIF) and possibly other substances such as neuropeptides and dopamine also inhibit TSH release (see Ch. 224). The role of thyroid hormones in feedback suppression at the level of the brain is poorly defined at present.

DeGroot LJ, Larsen PR, Refetoff S, Stanbury JB: The Thyroid and Its Diseases. 5th ed. New York, John Wiley & Sons, 1984. *An up-to-date revision of a classic text.*

Larsen, PR: Feedback regulation of thyrotropin secretion by hormones. N Engl J Med 306:23, 1982. *A more detailed, but clinically oriented, discussion of recent studies on the feedback regulation of TSH secretion by thyroid hormones.*

Larsen PR, Silva JE, Kaplan MM: Relationships between circulating and intracellular thyroid hormones: Physiological and clinical implications. Endocr Rev 2:87, 1981. *A recent review of the physiologic significance of intracellular T_4 to T_3 conversion and nuclear binding in various tissues.*

Oppenheimer JH: Samuels HH (eds.): Molecular basis of Thyroid Hormone Action. New York, Academic Press, 1983. *A thorough review of the evidence supporting the currently accepted mechanism for thyroid hormone action.*

Refetoff S: Thyroid hormone transport. *In* DeGroot LJ, et al. (eds.): Endocrinology, Vol I. New York, Grune & Stratton, 1979. *A comprehensive discussion of the serum thyroid hormone binding proteins.*

Werner SC, Ingbar SH: The Thyroid. 4th ed. Hagerstown, Harper & Row, 1978. *A basic text.*

Testing for Suspected Thyroid Dysfunction

The thyroid gland is unique among the endocrine organs in that symptoms may arise from two general types of problems. Hyperfunction of the thyroid (*hyperthyroidism* or *thyrotoxicosis*) or decreased secretion of thyroid hormone (*hypothyroidism* or *myxedema*) may cause the patient to seek medical help. Alternatively, physical enlargement of the thyroid (*goiter*) may cause respiratory embarassment or dysphagia or, more commonly, cosmetic abnormalities. The last-named condition may exist in the absence of any functional abnormality. Although the most severe forms are dramatic and unmistakable, milder degrees of thyroid dysfunction lead to many symptoms which are nonspecific, requiring biochemical tests for confirmation of the diagnosis.

PHYSICAL EXAMINATION OF THE THYROID

The high incidence of thyroid disease, particularly in the female (5 to 10 per cent), makes a careful examination of the thyroid gland an important part of the general physical examination. Thyroid enlargement may be the first clue to thyroid functional abnormalities in a patient with otherwise nonspecific symptoms. A cup of water is a necessity, and the patient should first be asked to swallow with the neck moderately extended while the anterior neck is inspected. Significant thyroid enlargement and thyroid nodules can often be discerned by this maneuver. The position of the trachea should then be determined, followed by palpation of the thyroid. Using the author's approach, the isthmus of the thyroid is first identified and is usually found just inferior to the cricoid cartilage. The left and right thumbs are then employed in turn to palpate the left and right lobe of the gland as the patient swallows. The normal thyroid gland is palpable in a large proportion of younger persons, although in the elderly patient it is not surprising to find the cricoid cartilage at or below the sternal notch. The pyramidal lobe, a small ridge of tissue extending vertically from the isthmus to the thyroid cartilage to the left or right of the midline, can often be palpated as well.

DIRECT TESTS OF THYROID FUNCTION

MEASUREMENT OF TOTAL SERUM THYROID HORMONE CONCENTRATIONS. Serum T_4 and T_3 are both readily quantitated by specific radioimmunoassays which require 200 μl or less of serum. Typical normal ranges for the total T_4 and T_3 concentrations are presented in Table 228–4, as well as the values in patients with alterations in TBG and in those with thyroid dysfunction.

SERUM FREE T_4 AND T_3 AND THE FREE T_4 INDEX. Since it is the concentration of free, rather than total, thyroid hormones which parallels the thyroid status, the ideal thyroid function test would be the direct determination of free thyroid hormones. The absolute serum free T_4 and T_3 can be measured either by immunoassay of a dialysate of human serum or by estimating the dialyzable (free) fraction of T_3 and T_4, multiplying this by the total hormone concentration (see Table 228–2). In patients who have abnormal total T_4 and T_3 concentrations caused by changes in serum TBG concentration but who are euthyroid, the free hormone concentrations are normal. Unfortunately, such determinations are time consuming and expensive, and an excellent indirect estimate of the free fraction of T_4 and T_3

TABLE 228–4. SERUM THYROID HORMONE CONCENTRATIONS IN NORMAL PERSONS AND PATIENTS WITH THYROID DISEASE

	Serum T_4 (μg/dl)		Serum T_3 (ng/dl)	
	Mean	*Range*	*Mean*	*Range*
Euthyroid				
Normal TBG	8	5–11	140	80–220
Increased TBG	12	8–20	190	120–320
Reduced TBG	2	<1–5	60	20–100
Infants				
Cord serum	11	8–15	48	20–80
Age six weeks	10	7–14	163	120–220
Hyperthyroidism	21	8–35	480	200–1600
Hypothyroidism	2	<1–5	50	<20–150

can be obtained from a T_3 (or T_4) *resin or charcoal uptake* test. In this test, tracer T_3 (or rarely T_4) is added to a diluted sample of unknown serum. After a brief incubation, resin or charcoal is added and the tubes centrifuged. The fraction of the tracer thyroid hormone bound to the resin or charcoal is then determined. In some tests this is expressed directly as a fraction of the total tracer added, e.g., a typical normal range is 25 to 35 per cent. In some methods anti-T_3 or T_4 antibody immobilized on a solid phase is used to bind the T_3, but the principle is identical. The result may also be normalized to those in standard samples with normal quantities of T_4 and TBG (normal range generally 0.85 to 1.15). The fraction of the tracer thyroid hormone bound to the resin or charcoal is directly proportional to the free fraction of the thyroid hormones. Since T_3 is usually bound to the same proteins as is T_4, the free fraction of T_4 can also be predicted from a test in which T_3 is used as the tracer. The similarity between the free fraction of thyroid hormones and the resin or charcoal uptake can be formalized by calculating the *free T_4 (or T_3)* index. This is the product of the normalized value for the T_3 uptake and the total serum T_4 (or T_3) concentration. The normal range for these indices in units is approximately the same as the total thyroid hormone concentrations. In the author's laboratory, the normal free T_4 index is 4.7 to 10.5. The free T_4 index is an excellent approximation of the free T_4. An alternative estimate of the free T_4 may be obtained by using one of several commercial kits. In one such method, a labeled analogue of T_4 is employed to compete with the endogenous free T_4 for binding to an antibody. The higher the concentration of free T_4, the lower is the analogue binding, and vice versa. While there are some technical advantages to these tests, they do not measure the free T_4 directly, but provide only an estimate of its concentration, as does the free T_4 index. One notable clinical situation in which both methods provide falsely high estimates of the free T_4 is in the hereditary syndrome *euthyroid dysalbuminemic hyperthyroxinemia*. In patients with this syndrome large quantities are synthesized of an albumin that binds T_4, but not T_3, with abnormally high affinity. The total T_4 value is elevated, but the free fraction of T_4 by dialysis is reduced; therefore the endogenous free T_4 concentration is normal. Neither the T_3 resin uptake nor the analogue methods reflect the reduced free T_4 fraction, since, on the one hand, T_3 does not bind to the abnormal albumin with increased avidity and, on the other, the abnormal albumin apparently competes with the antibody for the T_4 analogue. Thus, a high concentration of free T_4 is estimated and a mistaken diagnosis of hyperthyroidism is made. A T_4 uptake test would give a proper result in this syndrome. It should be noted that a "T_3 uptake test" or "T_3 resin" is *not* a measure of the serum T_3 concentration.

COMPARISON OF THE UTILITY OF T_4 AND T_3 DETERMINATIONS. The free T_4 index is the best screening test for thyroid dysfunction. It is superior to the free T_3 index by virtue of the fact that the principal thyroid secretory product is T_4. About 80 per cent of circulating T_3 derives from T_4 to T_3 conversion. Therefore, in patients who are sick or who have received any of the drugs listed in Table 228–3, the serum T_3 will invariably be reduced relative to the serum T_4, but this does not imply thyroid disease. In hypothyroidism, serum T_3 may be normal despite significant impairment of thyroid function. On the other hand, in hyperthyroidism there is a small fraction of patients in whom serum T_4 is not elevated but the concentration of serum T_3 is. This condition is called *T_3 thyrotoxicosis* (below).

SERUM REVERSE T_3 AND OTHER IODOTHYRONINES. The normal concentration of reverse T_3 is 15 to 50 ng per deciliter. It derives virtually exclusively from peripheral metabolism of T_4, and its concentration in the blood reflects a combination of that process and the rate of reverse T_3 degradation. It is not generally useful clinically, although it is an excellent barometer of the rate of T_4 to T_3 conversion. Immunoassays have been developed for both mono- and diiodinated thyronines, but these measurements do not have clinical applicability at present.

SERUM THYROID HORMONE–BINDING PROTEIN CONCENTRATIONS. The normal concentration of circulating TBG and TBPA can be measured by immunoassay or by determination of the binding capacity. The normal concentration of TBG is 1.5 mg per deciliter. This quantity of protein will bind approximately 20 μg of T_4 (1 mole T_4 per 1 mole TBG). The binding capacity of TBPA is approximately 250 μg T_4 per deciliter. These measurements are rarely necessary for clinical purposes. Virtually all of the necessary information regarding binding can be obtained from a T_3 uptake test.

RADIOACTIVE IODINE UPTAKE (RAI UPTAKE). The normal 24-hour thyroidal uptake of radioiodine ranges from 5 to 30 per cent. All the radioiodine in the thyroid at this time is in the organified form. Because of the broad normal range for this test, it is not a valid method for determining thyroid status. Its major diagnostic use is in separating patients who have hyperthyroidism caused by subacute thyroiditis from those with Graves' disease (see next section). It is contraindicated in pregnancy.

TESTS OF THYROID REGULATION

SERUM THYROTROPIN (TSH). The normal range for serum TSH by radioimmunoassay is from 1.5 to 3.5 μU per milliliter. However, for many clinical assays a normal range of up to 5 or even 10 μU per milliliter is accepted owing to the technical difficulties in attaining precise measurements. Virtually all patients with clinical symptoms attributible to primary hypothyroidism will have serum TSH concentrations >20 μU per milliliter, and many subjects with minimal symptoms or goiter alone will have results between 10 and 20 μU per milliliter. An elevation of the serum TSH concentration almost always indicates that thyroid function is impaired. It is also the critical test for separating patients with primary thyroid disease from those with hypothyroidism resulting from hypothalamic or pituitary dysfunction.

THYROTROPIN-RELEASING HORMONE (TRH) INFUSION TEST. TRH can be infused intravenously to determine the pituitary TSH reserve. This is reduced in patients with hyperthyroidism and in those with autonomous thyroid hormone production or with hypothalamic or pituitary disease. Typical normal and pathologic responses are shown in Figure 228–4. In practice, a basal serum sample is obtained, followed by intravenous infusion of 400 μg of TRH over 1 minute. A second serum sample is obtained 30 minutes after the infusion, and both are assayed for TSH. In normals, the minimal TSH increment is 2 μU per milliliter except in males over the age of 40, in the seriously ill or in patients with depression or exogenous or endogenous glucocorticoid excess in whom the normal response can be lower. The response is amplified (30-minute value >25 μU per milliliter) in patients with primary hypothyroidism. A significant increment in TSH eliminates the diagnosis of hyperthyroidism except in the extremely rare patient with the TSH-induced form of this disease.

T_3 SUPPRESSION TEST. Prior to the availability of TRH, the "T_3 suppression test" was used to determine if thyroid function was autonomous. A 24-hour RAI uptake is determined before and after the patient receives 75 to 100 μg of triiodothyronine (Cytomel) per day for one week. In normal patients, a reduction in the RAI uptake to less than 50 per cent of the original value occurs owing to suppression of endogenous TSH. In patients with hyperthyroidism or autonomous thyroid function, negligible suppression of radioactive uptake is seen. A second RAI uptake can also be determined one week after a single thyroxine dose of 3 mg. This has been reported to cause fewer symptoms and result in smaller elevations of serum T_3 in patients who have autonomous thyroid function. Neither test should be used in patients with complicating illnesses (especially of the cardiovascular system), and both have generally been superseded by the TRH test. Suppression tests can also be used in conjunction with a thyroid scan to document autonomy in thyroid nodules (see below).

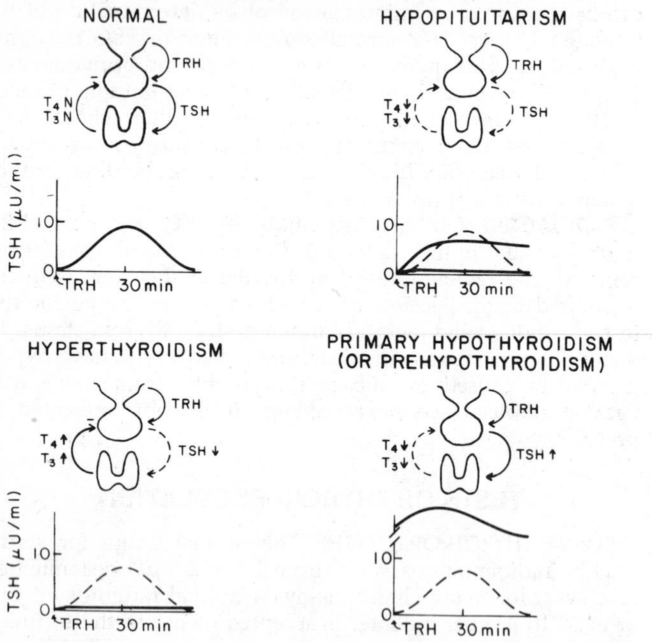

Figure 228–4. Typical responses to the infusion of TRH in patients with hyperthyroidism and primary and secondary hypothyroidism. In patients with hypopituitarism or hypothalamic disease virtually any TRH response pattern can be seen. The most pertinent diagnostic information is that serum TSH is not increased in a patient with a reduced serum free T_4 index.

METABOLIC INDICES OF THYROID STATUS

BASAL METABOLIC RATE (BMR). Since thyroid hormone is an important factor in the regulation of the rate of oxygen consumption, this test should theoretically be useful in evaluating thyroid status. However, it has given way to serum measurements, since these are more specific and usually more accurate. The normal range for the BMR is usually from −15 to +5 per cent.

DEEP TENDON REFLEX CONTRACTION AND RELAXATION TIMES. Thyroid status is reflected in the rate (not amplitude) of contraction and relaxation of skeletal muscle. These rates are more rapid in hyperthyroidism and slowed in hypothyroidism. Some clinicians have employed a kinemometer tracing to quantitate these events and have observed as high as 70 per cent diagnostic accuracy with this test. Like the BMR, it is less specific than serum hormone measurements, since hypothermia, peripheral neuropathy, gross edema, and many other conditions may slow the rate of relaxation. However, a clinically apparent delay in the relaxation phase of the deep tendon reflexes is almost invariably present in patients with significant hypothyroidism, although the more rapid relaxation in hyperthyroidism is difficult to appreciate visually.

ANATOMIC EVALUATION OF THE THYROID GLAND

THE THYROID SCAN. The capacity of the thyroid gland to trap ions such as I^- or molecules with a similar charge and configuration has provided a useful method for correlating structure and function. Of the iodine isotopes either ^{123}I or ^{131}I can be used. ^{123}I, although more expensive, is to be preferred for scanning, particularly in younger persons, since the radiation dose to the thyroid is 7.5 mrads per microcurie administered, as opposed to 800 mrads per microcurie for ^{131}I. Another isotope which gives a low radiation dose is $^{99}mTcO_4^-$ (pertechnetate), which is trapped, but not organified, by the thyroid. Because of this, a scan is performed 30 minutes after intravenous injection of this isotope. The thyroid scan is usually used to determine the functional state of a palpable thyroid nodule (see later in chapter) or in evaluating masses in the neck or upper chest to see if thyroid tissue is present.

THYROID ULTRASOUND. A determination of whether a given thyroid mass is solid or cystic can be made by ultrasonography.

NEEDLE BIOPSY OR ASPIRATION. Either a fine (21 to 26 gauge) or cutting needle (Vim-Silverman) can be used to obtain a sample of thyroid tissue for histologic examination. These techniques have received increased attention in recent years as a method for evaluation of thyroid nodules. Accurate interpretation of a fine needle aspirate requires an experienced cytologist, which has limited the experience with this simple technique to date.

OTHER TESTS SPECIFICALLY RELATED TO THYROID FUNCTION OR DISEASE

ANTITHYROID ANTIBODIES. In autoimmune thyroid disease (Hashimoto's thyroiditis or Graves' disease), antibodies which bind to various antigens of thyroid tissue are present in the serum. The most important of these is the *thyroid antimicrosomal antibody*. This antibody is found in approximately 95 per cent of patients with Hashimoto's thyroiditis and in only about 10 per cent of adults with no apparent thyroid disease. The test is generally performed by a tanned red cell hemagglutination technique, and the results are reported as the highest titer causing agglutination. Titers in excess of 1:100 are significant. About 55 per cent of patients with Graves' disease also have circulating antibodies to thyroid microsomes. *Antithyroglobulin antibodies* are also present in the serum of about 60 per cent of patients with Hashimoto's disease. Antibodies directed against the thyroid TSH receptor, present in the sera of patients with Graves' disease, can be measured either by incubation of IgG with fresh thyroid slices, quantitating the increase in cyclic AMP, or with thyroid membranes and tracer TSH in a competition technique. The result of the former method is denoted the *thyroid stimulating immunoglobulin* (TSI), and it is somewhat more specific than is the latter, called the *thyrotropin displacing activity* (TDA) (see Graves' Disease and Other Causes of Hyperthyroidism).

SERUM THYROGLOBULIN. The normal serum thyroglobulin (Tg) concentration is 2 to 20 ng per milliliter. Serum Tg may be elevated in any patient with an enlarged thyroid or following acute trauma to the thyroid whether this be a consequence of inflammation, surgery, or radiation. Thyroglobulin determinations are most useful in the follow-up of patients with metastatic thyroid carcinoma following thyroidectomy. An increase in serum Tg indicates the presence of tumor tissue, although a normal value does not eliminate this possibility.

THE EFFECTS OF NONTHYROIDAL ILLNESS ON THYROID FUNCTION TESTS

Patients with nonthyroidal illnesses can have abnormalities in serum T_4 and T_3 concentrations that may suggest underlying thyroid dysfunction. All patients will have impaired T_4 to T_3 conversion and, accordingly, have low or subnormal serum T_3 and raised serum reverse-T_3 concentrations. Most will also have slight reduction in total serum T_4 concentrations. A portion of this decrease is a result of a reduced serum TBG, especially if severe liver disease or proteinuria is present. However, about 10 per cent of patients with typical medical illnesses will have a subnormal free T_4 index. This may be due to the release of a substance that inhibits the binding of T_4 to TBG. The fracture of free T_4, as measured by equilibrium dialysis, is usually increased in such patients. Thus, the free T_4 is normal, indicating that hypothyroidism is not present. Occasionally a patient may have severe illness and an elevated level of serum T_4. Such patients should be suscepted of having underlying autonomous thyroid function and often must be treated for hyperthyroidism. This phenomenon may also occur in patients with *acute psychiatric illness* and *hyperemesis gravidarum*. Strategies for dealing with these potentially confusing situations are presented later in the chapter.

Buergi H, Wimpfheimer C, Burger A, Zaumbauer W, Rosler H, Lemarchand-Beraud T: Changes of circulating thyroxine, triiodothyronine and reverse triiodothyronine after radiographic contrast agents. J Clin Endocrinol Metab 43:1203, 1976. *The changes which occur in serum thyroid hormones and TSH following oral cholecystographic agents provide an excellent model for the effects of inhibition of T_4 to T_3 conversion on thyroid function.*

Chopra IJ, Hershman JM, Pardridge WM, Nicoloff JT: Thyroid function in nonthyroidal illnesses. Ann Intern Med 98:946–957, 1983. *A review of many of the effects of systemic illness on thyroid function.*

Docter R, Bos G, Krenning, EP, Fekkes D, Visser TJ, Hennemann G: Inherited thyroxine excess: A serum abnormality due to an increased affinity for modified albumin. Clin Endocrinol 15:363–371, 1981. *An explanation of the thyroid hormone–binding abnormalities in families with euthyroid dysalbuminemic hyperthyroxinemia.*

Kaplan MM, Larsen PR, Crantz FR, Dzau VJ, Rossing TH, Haddow JE: Prevalence of abnormal thyroid function test results in patients with acute medical illnesses. Am J Med 72:9–16, 1982. *This is a prospective study of thyroid function test abnormalities in unselected patients with acute medical illnesses.*

Schimmel M, Utiger RD: Thyroidal and peripheral production of thyroid hormones: Review of recent findings and their clinical implications. Ann Intern Med 87:760, 1977. *A discussion of the relationships between serum T_4, T_3, and reverse T_3 in the clinical setting.*

Graves' Disease and Other Causes of Hyperthyroidism

DEFINITION. The clinical syndrome of hyperthyroidism is one of the most dramatic in clinical medicine. The major symptoms associated with this syndrome are predominantly a reflection of the hypermetabolism resulting from excessive quantities of circulating thyroid hormone. The many disorders that can be associated with this syndrome are listed in Table 228–5 in their approximate order of frequency. Graves' disease accounts for over 85 per cent of such patients. Toxic nodular goiters, both multinodular *(Plummer's disease)* and uninodular, and subacute thyroiditis account for the bulk of the remainder.

GRAVES' DISEASE

In 1835, Robert Graves described a clinical syndrome including hypermetabolism, diffuse enlargement of the thyroid gland, and *exophthalmos* (forward displacement of the eyes). In continental Europe, the same condition is known as Basedow's disease after von Basedow's description in 1840. In addition to thyroid involvement and ophthalmopathy, patients may have a dermatologic condition, *pretibial myxedema.* As presently defined, patients with Graves' disease may have only one of these three major clinical manifestations, and the only common denominator is likely to be the presence of thyroid-stimulating antibodies in the serum.

ETIOLOGY AND PATHOGENESIS. The precise etiology of Graves' disease is still not known, but it seems likely that it is an autoimmune disorder. Hyperthyroidism is its principal manifestation, yet TSH is suppressed and no intrinsic regulatory abnormalities in the thyroid have been identified. Thus the thyroid stimulation seems likely to be a consequence of a circulating, non-TSH, thyroid stimulator. In 1956, Adams and Purves identified a substance in the serum of many patients with Graves' disease which caused thyroid stimulation in a mouse bioassay. Because the thyroid stimulation from this substance lasted longer than did TSH-induced stimulation, it was called *long-acting thyroid stimulator (LATS).* LATS is now known to be a 7-S gamma globulin. The LATS hypothesis was initially received with enthusiasm, but soon lost popularity as patients were found with hyperthyroidism who did not have detectable LATS. In addition, some LATS-positive patients were not hyperthyroid. Many of the latter cases may be explained by the coexistence of thyroid destruction caused by a chronic thyroiditis (Hashimoto's disease; see Thyroiditis). Recent studies have provided a more inclusive hypothesis. Serum LATS activity is decreased on exposure to thyroid tissue, suggesting that the antibody binds to a thyroid antigen. In sera from certain hyperthyroid patients who were LATS negative, a gamma globulin was found that neutralized the capacity of thyroid tissue to bind the LATS in positive sera. This antibody, called *LATS protector,* stimulated human thyroid tissue in vivo or thyroid tissue from chicks even though it did not stimulate the mouse thyroid. This observation suggested that one of the limitations in previous studies was a restriction of the bioassay to the mouse, which could well have different, albeit overlapping, antigenic sites from human thyroid tissue. In subsequent studies it has been found that LATS, LATS protector, and similar proteins present in Graves' disease patients' sera interfere with the binding of TSH to the human thyroid cell membrane, suggesting that these proteins are antibodies to the TSH receptor. These substances activate adenylate cyclase in human thyroid cell membranes, providing a plausible mechanism for thyroid stimulation in this condition. Several assays are now available to quantitate what are termed *thyroid-stimulating immunoglobulins* (TSI) or *thyrotropin-displacing activity* (TDA) (see Testing for Suspected Thyroid Function). TSI or TDA is found in 85 to 90 per cent of patients with Graves' disease. The negative sera may be explained by residual difficulties in the assay technique. The stimulus for the antibody production in these subjects remains obscure.

The etiology of Graves' exophthalmopathy is not known. Patients with exophthalmos and particularly those with dermopathy almost invariably have high titers of circulating TSI, suggesting that these two clinical manifestations represent the most severe form of this disease. Antibodies to soluble human eye muscle antigens were found in 17 of 23 patients with Graves' ophthalmopathy, but not in Graves' patients without this manifestation and rarely in those with Hashimoto's thyroiditis. This suggests a similar autoimmune etiology for ophthalmopathy and for hyperthyroidism. It has also been proposed that Tg–anti-Tg circulating immune complexes may bind to eye muscles and play a pathogenic role. Further studies will be required to resolve this question.

Emotional Factors in the Etiology of Hyperthyroidism. The emotional lability of the patient with hyperthyroidism has led many clinicians to question the role of psychologic trauma in the pathogenesis of this disease. Numerous anecdotes have been cited to suggest that emotional trauma may somehow trigger the onset of overt hyperthyroidism. If this is so, it would still appear to require participation of the immune system, since circulating TSI is such a constant feature of the clinical picture. In the author's mind, it seems more likely that an episode of physical or emotional trauma brings the patient to medical attention, at which time preexisting hyperthyroidism is recognized.

INCIDENCE. Graves' disease is common, affecting as many as 1.9 per cent of the female population and about a tenth that number of males, according to a population survey in northern England. It reaches its peak incidence in the third and fourth decades. The reason for the female predominance in this as in all thyroid diseases is not known. There is a strong familial component to Graves' disease with a family history of autoimmune thyroid disease (Graves' disease, Hashimoto's thyroiditis, or "goiter") in a significant fraction of patients. The importance of genetic inheritance in the predisposition to this syndrome has been confirmed by finding a higher relative risk of this

TABLE 228–5. DISEASES OR CLINICAL SYNDROMES ASSOCIATED WITH THYROTOXICOSIS

Graves' disease
Toxic multinodular goiter
Toxic adenoma
Iodide-induced hyperthyroidism
Subacute thyroiditis
Factitious (exogenous) thyrotoxicosis
Neonatal thyrotoxicosis (mother with Graves' disease)
TSH-secreting pituitary tumor
Nontumorigenic pituitary-induced hyperthyroidism
Choriocarcinoma (uterine or testicular origin) or hydatidiform mole
Struma ovarii
Hyperfunctioning thyroid carcinoma (usually metastatic)

TABLE 228–6. COMMON SYMPTOMS AND SIGNS OF HYPERTHYROIDISM (THYROTOXICOSIS)

Symptoms	Signs
Nervousness and/or tremor	Tachycardia or atrial fibrillation
Weight loss (usually with increased appetite)	Widened pulse pressure with increased systolic and decreased diastolic pressures
Palpitations	Hyperdynamic precordium and accentuated S1
Heat intolerance and excessive perspiration	Warm, smooth skin
Emotional lability	Tremor
Muscle weakness	Proximal muscle weakness
Hyperdefecation	Thyroid enlargement or abnormality

condition in patients with the histocompatibility antigens HLA-B8 and in Caucasians with HLA-DR3 and in Japanese and Chinese populations with HLA-B35 and HLA-Bw46, respectively.

PATHOLOGY. The thyroid of the patient with Graves' disease is diffusely enlarged and hypercellular. In patients undergoing thyroidectomy without prior treatment with antithyroid drugs or iodine, a diffusely hyperplastic epithelium is noted with little or no colloid present and often with lymphocytic infiltration, varying from minimal to extensive. In some specimens it is impossible to distinguish the microscopic picture from Hashimoto's thyroiditis (a condition sometimes called hashitoxicosis). If the patient receives iodide preoperatively, the gland contains large amounts of colloid, cells are of normal height, and the vascularity is markedly reduced. Other tissues show no specific changes except in severely hyperthyroid patients. In those situations there may be edema and focal necrosis in the liver with cellular infiltration.

In hyperthyroid patients with mild eye manifestations of Graves' disease such as lid retraction and stare, no significant orbital pathology is found, and these changes probably are due to the hyperthyroidism per se. In more severe cases, edema of the extraocular muscles occurs in association with infiltration with lymphocytes, plasma cells, and neutrophils. In addition, hydrophilic mucopolysaccharide collects in the orbital tissues. The conjuctivae may show perivascular lymphocytic infiltration and edema *(chemosis).* The end-stage of these processes is fibrosis, which most often involves the inferior eye muscles, causing restriction of upward globe movement.

CLINICAL PICTURE. The common clinical symptoms of thyrotoxicosis are listed in Table 228–6. These occur in any patient with excessive thyroid hormone secretion whether this be due to Graves' disease or some other cause. They are a consequence of the stimulatory effect of thyroid hormone on the metabolic rate and on many other tissues, especially the heart and central nervous system. The typical patient with Graves' disease is in her mid-20's with symptoms that can often be dated to six to twelve months previously. The patient is nervous, anxious, and fidgeting, and speaks rapidly. She will complain of her agitated fatigue, palpitations, and, in warmer climates, heat intolerance. There may be weight loss despite increased appetite, or the patient may merely report success in her efforts at weight control. An increased frequency of bowel movements and, rarely, diarrhea, may be noted. Emotional lability is often apparent during the interview, and a history of deteriorating domestic or occupational relationships may be obtained. A history of neck swelling (often not noted first by the patient) may be present. Amenorrhea or oligomenorrhea is not uncommon. Rarer manifestations of hyperthyroidism include pruritus and urticaria. About 5 per cent of males may experience gynecomastia, and even less commonly *hypokalemic periodic paralysis* may occur. For unknown reasons, this condition is much more common in males of Oriental extraction.

Apathetic or Masked Hyperthyroidism. The symptoms given in Table 228–6 are those generally found in the younger patient. The clinician should be aware that in some patients, particularly the elderly, the clinical symptoms and signs of hypermetabolism may not be so dramatic. Rather than appearing agitated, the elderly patient with hyperthyroidism may be depressed. Weight loss and symptoms of congestive heart failure can be the predominant manifestations of the hypermetabolic syndrome. Often this is complicated by atrial fibrillation or other supraventricular tachyarrhythmia, leading to suspicion that the heart, rather than the thyroid, is the source of the problem. Because of the subtlety of this clinical form of hyperthyroidism it is recommended that any patient with the recent onset of atrial fibrillation have tests of thyroid function. In this way a reversible cause of congestive heart failure and/or recurrent arrhythmias may be recognized and appropriate treatment instituted.

Graves' Ophthalmopathy. Eye symptoms are present in more than 50 per cent of patients with Graves' disease but, except for modest lid lag and stare, are rare in patients with other causes of hyperthyroidism. This is a useful point in establishing the diagnosis. Common complaints are protruding eyes, easy tearing, especially on exposure to wind or cold, photophobia, a gritty foreign body sensation in the eyes, and, less commonly, diplopia. (Fig. 228–5). The patient with significant *proptosis* (exophthalmos) may complain of irritation, particularly on arising, since the eyelids do not completely cover the sclera when the patient is sleeping *(lagophthalmos).* Rarely, severe chemosis, inflammation, and periorbital edema occur (malignant exophthalmos). Eye complaints are usually bilateral but may be unilateral, and Graves' disease is one of the most common causes of unilateral exophthalmos.

Pretibial Myxedema. In a few patients with Graves' disease (1 to 2 per cent) a brawny, nonpitting swelling of the pretibial area, ankles, and/or feet is present. This can appear in plaques. It has an orange-skin appearance and is usually not tender. This dermopathy, found exclusively in Graves' disease, is termed *pretibial myxedema.* The name derives from the histologic similarity of the mucopolysaccharide infiltration of the subcutaneous tissues to that found in advanced hypothyroidism (myxedema).

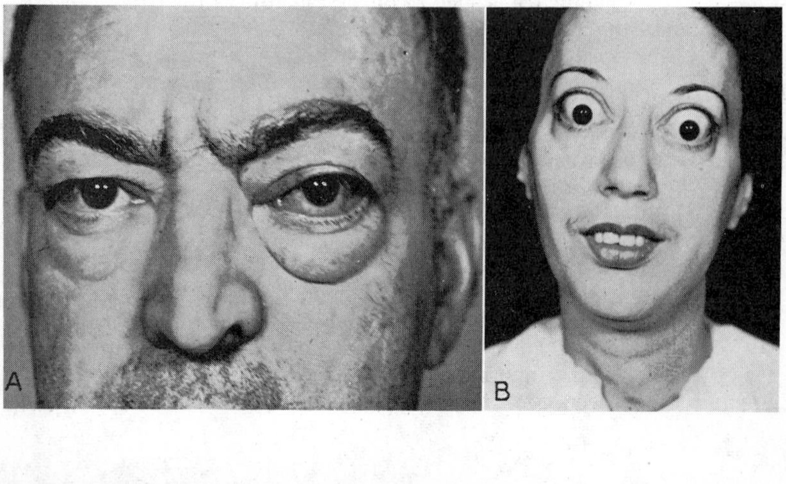

Figure 228–5. Two patients showing the typical ophthalmopathy characteristic of Graves' disease. Patient A demonstrates marked periorbital swelling, exophthalmos, chemosis, and conjunctival injection. The proptosis, limitation of extraocular movements, and other manifestations of ophthalmopathy are much more severe in Patient A than in Patient B. Patient B has marked widening of the palpebral fissures owing to lid retraction and also has significant proptosis. Patient A is euthyroid; Patient B is mildly hyperthyroid. (From Williams RH (ed.): Textbook of Endocrinology. 6th ed. Philadelphia, W. B. Saunders Company, 1981, p 189.)

Euthyroid Graves' Disease. In a small fraction of patients with Graves' disease, eye manifestations (unilateral or bilateral) with or without pretibial myxedema appear but hyperthyroidism is not present. This can arise because of destruction of the thyroid as a result of coexistent Hashimoto's disease or hyperthyroidism may be delayed in its appearance for months or years after the first eye symptoms. In many such patients, appropriate testing will often reveal subtle evidence of thyroid dysfunction.

PHYSICAL SIGNS. In younger patients, tachycardia is almost universal. The systolic blood pressure is elevated primarily because of the increased inotropic effect of thyroid hormone on the heart. The diastolic pressure is reduced owing to a decrease in peripheral vascular resistance associated with increased skin capillary blood flow. Body temperature is usually normal. The skin is smooth, warm, and moist, and the patient may radiate heat. A fine tremor of the outstretched hands and occasionally *onycholysis* of the fourth and fifth fingers or clubbing *(thyroid acropachy)* are observed. The thyroid is almost always diffusely enlarged from 1.5 to 5 to 6 times normal. One third of elderly patients will not have a detectable goiter. The gland may be soft or firm, depending on the degree of hyperthyroidism and the level of iodine intake. Auscultation of the neck may reveal a multitude of sounds. In the younger patient a *venous hum* may be heard over the external jugular vein, particularly with the patient in the sitting position. Third or fourth heart sounds are heard easily in the neck, and a carotid bruit is not uncommon. In addition, a bruit over the thyroid gland is present in some patients, a manifestation of the high blood flow to this organ. A diffuse lymphadenopathy may be present in hyperthyroidism, and splenomegaly is found in 10 per cent of patients. The liver is not enlarged except in elderly patients with congestive failure. The neurologic examination shows tremor and proximal muscle weakness. Eye signs include lid lag, a failure of the upper lid to cover the upper margin of the iris as the globe traverses from upward to downward gaze, a widened palpebral fissure so that the sclera is visible above and/or below the iris, conjunctival injection and chemosis, periorbital swelling, and proptosis. The last-named finding is determined by measuring the distance from the lateral portion of the bony orbit to the cornea, using the *exophthalmometer*. In whites this distance is 17 mm or less, with an upper limit of normal of 20 mm (22 mm for blacks). The difference between the two eye measurements should not be more than 3 mm. In addition to these moderate abnormalities, there may be impairment of globe movement. The most common restriction is in upward and/or outward gaze. This is due not to weakness of the superior eye muscles but to swelling and fibrosis of the inferior rectus and inferior oblique muscles beneath the globe. In addition, abduction and convergence may also be affected. Eye signs may be absent or mild, are usually bilateral when present, but may be asymmetric.

LABORATORY DIAGNOSIS OF HYPERTHYROIDISM. The various steps to be followed in establishing the laboratory diagnosis of hyperthyroidism are outlined in Figure 228–6. The initial screening test is to determine the free T_4 index. In virtually all patients an elevation in the free T_4 index is present. In the hospitalized patient the diagnosis may be somewhat more complicated if the patient is severely ill or has received any of the agents, listed in Table 228–3, which cause inhibition of T_4 to T_3 conversion. In these patients an impairment of T_4 clearance or inhibition of T_4 to T_3 conversion may lead to an elevation in the serum free T_4 index without hyperthyroidism. Other causes of an elevated free T_4 index, not necessarily indicating hyperthyroidism, are *euthyroid dysalbuminemic hyperthyroxinemia* (see Testing for Suspected Thyroid Dysfunction), hyperemesis gravidarium and acute psychosis. In the last two conditions, the increase in the free T_4 index is usually transient.

In such patients and in patients in whom the clinical suspicion of hyperthyroidism is present but the free T_4 index is normal or equivocal, a serum T_3 determination should be performed. The ratio of T_3 to T_4 is increased in the thyroid gland in patients with Graves' disease. As a consequence, the T_3 production rate and the fraction of T_3 coming directly from the thyroid are increased. Thus, the serum T_3 is elevated to a greater extent than is the serum T_4 (see Table 228–4). Patients in whom serum T_3 is elevated but the serum free T_4 index is

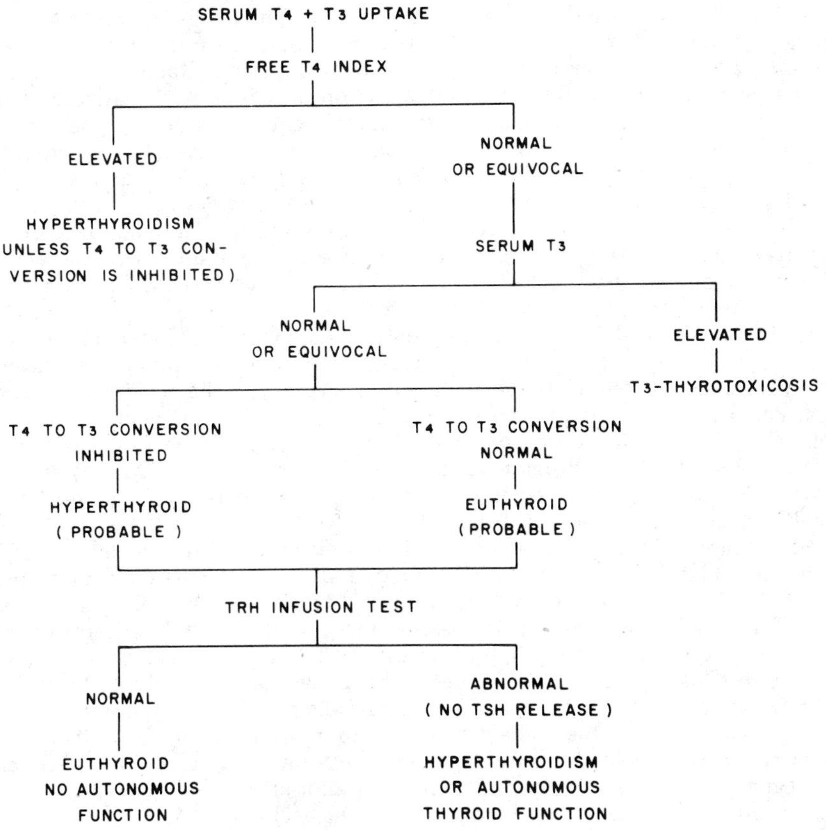

Figure 228–6. Laboratory diagnosis of hyperthyroidism.

not have T_3 *thyrotoxicosis,* which occurs in 3 to 5 per cent of patients in the United States but more commonly in areas where dietary iodine is lower. The diagnosis of hyperthyroidism cannot be eliminated until the free T_3 index (as well as the free T_4 index) has been found to be normal. Even in hyperthyroidism, a substantial fraction of T_3 derives from peripheral T_4 to T_3 conversion. Impairment of this process from any of the causes listed in Table 228–3 can lead to a reduction in serum T_3. However, in hyperthyroidism, even with severe illness, the serum T_3 is rarely depressed to less than 100 ng per deciliter.

In equivocal situations, it may be necessary to perform a TRH infusion test, (see Testing for Suspected Thyroid Dysfunction). A normal increase in TSH unequivocally eliminates all forms of hyperthyroidism except those associated with increased TSH secretion, which are extremely rare (see below). Since patients with fixed or autonomous, but not supranormal, thyroid hormone production may also have pituitary TSH depletion, an abnormal test does not indicate the presence of hypermetabolism and the need for treatment. However, particularly in patients who have only eye manifestations, the discovery of abnormalities in pituitary-thyroid regulation is consistent with the diagnosis of Graves' disease as the cause of the eye symptoms. A T_3 or T_4 suppression test (see Testing for Suspected Thyroid Dysfunction) will provide similar information.

In patients with a classic history and laboratory abnormalities, an RAI uptake and thyroid scan are not necessary to establish the diagnosis. However, if the hyperthyroidism is of brief (less than three months') duration, if the thyroid is not enlarged or palpable, or if it is tender, subacute thyroiditis must be considered, and an uptake and scan should be performed after pregnancy has been excluded. These tests are also required when nodular goiter is suspected or when factitious thyrotoxicosis is to be considered (Table 228–5).

Unilateral Ophthalmopathy. Since Graves' ophthalmopathy may be unilateral and not associated with frank hyperthyroidism, local pathology such as orbital tumor, pseudotumor of the orbit, cavernous sinus–carotid aneurysm, and sphenoid ridge meningioma must be considered. In addition to the free T_4 index, serum T_3, and TRH test, such patients require orbital x-rays, ultrasound, and CT scan. In almost all patients with Graves' ophthalmopathy, bilateral involvement of the extraocular muscles will be found even though clinically the process appears unilateral. Positive serum tests for TSI or antithyroid microsomal antibodies will provide further support for this diagnosis.

Other Chemical Abnormalities Associated with Hyperthyroidism. In 5 to 20 per cent of patients with hyperthyroidism any of the following may be found: modest hypercalcemia, increased alkaline phosphatase (bone or hepatic isozyme), increased direct bilirubin, and a mild anemia of "chronic disease." Modest neutropenia may occur (1000 to 2000 per cubic millimeter).

DIFFERENTIAL DIAGNOSIS. There are few clinical syndromes which mimic hyperthyroidism. Pheochromocytoma and neurocirculatory asthenia may cause some clinical confusion, but appropriate laboratory testing will eliminate these from consideration. Differentiation of patients with Graves' disease from those with other forms of hyperthyroidism is rarely difficult based solely on the history and physical examination (Table 228–5). The use of the RAI uptake and scan to identify patients with subacute thyroiditis or nodular disease has been discussed. Iodine-induced hyperthyroidism is due to either multinodular goiter or Graves' disease (Jod-Basedow). Factitious thyrotoxicosis, the ingestion of excess thyroid hormone, should be considered particularly in paramedical personnel in whom symptoms and laboratory manifestations are associated with a nonpalpable thyroid gland. TSH-induced hyperthyroidism is often diagnosed retrospectively after treatment has begun. It is so rare that it is not cost-effective to screen all hyperthyroid patients for this disease. Chorionic gonadotropin–induced hyperthyroidism is confirmed by the elevation in serum HCG in association with molar pregnancy or choriocarcinoma.

TREATMENT. The treatment of patients with Graves' disease must be considered in the context of its natural history. From 10 to 50 per cent of patients, depending on the series, return to normal thyroid function (remission) in association with (but probably not because of) drug treatment directed at the thyroid, not at the apparent primary defect in the immune system. If the patient destined to remit could be identified, a rational treatment approach for this disease could be developed. At present this is difficult, though some studies have suggested that patients with HLA-B8 and HLA-DR-3 antigens are less likely to have spontaneous remission than are those with other genetic backgrounds. Reduction in circulating TSI or TDA generally accompanies remission, and it may be possible to employ such assays in the future to guide definitive therapy. Currently TSI and TDA assays are available primarily as a research tool. Early studies suggested that if patients were given antithyroid drugs for 12 to 18 months, approximately 50 per cent would remain euthyroid after their discontinuation. More recently that fraction may have decreased to 10 to 20 per cent. The reason for the apparent change in the natural history of hyperthyroidism in the United States is not clear. One possible explanation is the recent increase in iodine intake. Since antithyroid drugs markedly deplete thyroidal iodine, the capacity to re-establish excessive secretion of thyroid hormone could be influenced by the iodine supply. In patients with Graves' disease who undergo a remission, hypothyroidism may occur some 20 to 30 years later. This is presumably autoimmune in origin, further emphasizing the similarities between Graves' disease and Hashimoto's thyroiditis. Lastly, patients in remission may have a relapse months to years later.

As the underlying cause for Graves' disease is not known, no specific therapy for this condition is available. There are two phases of the treatment of the hyperthyroidism of Graves' disease. The first is acute therapy with the goal of re-establishing euthyroidism. The second phase is definitive therapy, the induction of a permanent alteration in thyroid function.

Acute Treatment of Hyperthyroidism. ANTITHYROID DRUGS. In a typical patient with hyperthyroidism caused by Graves' disease, the first step in management is to suppress the elevated thyroid hormone secretion rate. The drugs of choice for this purpose are derivatives of thiourea. In the United States, propylthiouracil (PTU) and methimazole (Tapazole) are used. Both inhibit the organification of iodine by the thyroid gland as their major mechanism of action. Neither drug affects I^- trapping, nor does either inhibit the release of preformed thyroid hormone. PTU, but not methimazole, is an inhibitor of T_4 to T_3 conversion. Since this reaction appears to be necessary for the full effect of T_4, this drug has special importance in the acute treatment of hyperthyroidism. Carbimazole, rapidly converted to methimazole in the body, is used in Europe and is equally potent to methimazole.

PTU and methimazole are rapidly absorbed and are probably concentrated by the hyperactive thyroid. Although the plasma half-life is relatively short, suggesting the need for frequent dosage, in practice it is often possible to maintain satisfactory suppression of thyroid hormone synthesis by administration of these drugs twice or even only once per day. Methimazole is approximately 15 times as potent as PTU. Initial treatment consists of 300 to 450 mg of PTU per day (or the equivalent of methimazole) divided into three doses. Rarely as much as 1600 mg per day of PTU is required, but problems with compliance are common at such dosages. Since there is a five- to ten-day half-time for the disappearance of the metabolic effects induced by excess thyroid hormone, it is not unusual for the serum level of T_4 to fall before the patient begins to obtain relief from the symptoms of hyperthyroidism. It is the author's practice to see the patient three to four weeks after the initial visit, obtaining a free T_4 index and serum T_3 at that point to ascertain the progress of therapy. If clinical improvement has not occurred, the serum T_4 has not decreased and compliance has been maintained, the dose of antithyroid drug should be increased. After the first months of treatment, the dose of antithyroid drug can be reduced to a level of 100 to 300 mg per day of PTU, and the patient seen at two- to three-month intervals. In patients to be treated for six to eighteen months, therapy can be monitored by both clinical and laboratory parameters. The serum T_3:T_4 ratio will be increased because of intrathyroidal iodine deficiency and the increased thyroidal T_3:T_4 ratio in Graves' disease. Therefore both serum T_3 and the free T_4 index should be monitored. Serum TSH may increase if the serum T_4 falls below normal even if serum T_3 is normal. This is undesirable since it can lead to further thyroid enlargement and possibly an exacerbation of eye symptoms.

Thiourea derivatives have several side effects. A maculopapular rash occurs in 2 to 8 per cent of patients but does not usually require discontinuation of the drug. Both agents can rarely cause hepatocellular damage, and PTU can cause vasculitis. The most serious side effect of both agents is agranulocytosis. This occurs in 2 to 5 of 1000 patients and can be fatal if not recognized. Since this reaction may be abrupt in onset and is so rare, it is not, in the opinion of many experts, necessary to monitor the white blood count at frequent intervals. Instead, a baseline WBC and differential are obtained, and the patient is cautioned on each visit about the symptoms and significance of agranulocytosis. The patient is instructed to report immediately if infection occurs and to stop the medication. If this happens, the WBC and differential are repeated and the drug discontinued permanently if necessary. The reaction may appear at any time during therapy and does not appear to be dose related (except at extremely high doses). It is seen most commonly in the first few months of therapy. If such a reaction occurs, the drug should be withdrawn and appropriate supportive care provided. Recovery occurs in almost all patients, and an alternative treatment modality should then be used. Special precautions about the use of antithyroid drugs in pregnancy are discussed below.

The benefits of bed rest, adequate diet, and the extrication of the patient from the usual occupational or domestic pressures cannot be overemphasized. Remarkable clinical improvement is often noted within one to two days simply as a result of hospitalization. The acute treatment of severe hyperthyroidism is discussed below under Thyroid Storm.

β-ADRENERGIC BLOCKING AGENTS. The similarity of the symptoms of hyperthyroidism to those of catecholamine excess is striking. The molecular basis for this similarity is not clearly established. Although animal studies have shown thyroid hormone–induced increases in β-adrenergic receptors in cardiac tissue, the receptor number is normal in lymphocytes from patients with thyrotoxicosis. Plasma catecholamine concentrations are normal in hyperthyroidism. Nevertheless, blockade of β-adrenergic receptors by propranolol may result in symptomatic improvement prior to a decrease in serum thyroid hormones. A dose of 20 to 40 mg of propranolol every four to six hours may be used, but patients with congestive heart failure or bronchial asthma should not receive this therapy. In most patients with mild to moderate hyperthyroidism this adjunctive therapy is not necessary and may complicate the therapeutic regimen. In patients with more profound tachycardia or with thyroid storm (see below), it may have an important beneficial effect. Propranolol, although decreasing pulse rate and cardiac output in patients with hyperthyroidism, does not alter the elevated basal metabolic rate. Therefore, the tissues continue to consume oxygen at a high rate in the presence of decreased blood supply.

The Second Phase of Hyperthyroidism Treatment. If the symptoms of hyperthyroidism are not severe or after the acute treatment of symptoms with thiourea drugs, a decision must be made as to long-term therapy. There are three choices: further antithyroid drugs with hopes of a spontaneous remission, surgery, or radioiodine. None of these is ideal, and the choice for each patient must be made individually.

CHRONIC ANTITHYROID DRUG THERAPY. If chronic antithyroid drug therapy is undertaken in anticipation of a remission, it should be continued for six to eighteen months. If the quantities of drug required to maintain euthyroidism remain relatively large (e.g., 200 mg of PTU or greater) and serum T_3 and T_4 rise when the dosage is reduced, then a remission has not occurred. If the thyroid becomes smaller and the required amount of antithyroid drug lower, then a remission is probable. Some authorities recommend a TRH test at this juncture, but the author prefers to obtain a serum T_3 and T_4, to discontinue the treatment, and to repeat these tests in four weeks. The serum T_3 is especially important, since it may become elevated prior to the T_4 when a relapse occurs. If thyroid hormones remain normal, the patient should be seen at bimonthly intervals for one year, at which time the visits can be reduced in frequency.

SURGERY. Surgical removal of a portion of the thyroid gland to regulate hyperthyroidism is a time-honored and effective treatment in the hands of expert surgeons. Hyperthyroidism rarely recurs, although roughly 50 to 60 per cent of patients will eventually become hypothyroid. In most patients, hyperthyroidism is controlled by antithyroid drugs for one to two months prior to surgery. About seven to ten days before the operation, saturated solution of potassium iodide (1 gram of potassium iodide per milliliter), 2 drops three times a day, or Lugol's solution (≈ 125 mg iodide per milliliter), 10 drops three times a day, is begun to reduce the vascularity of the thyroid gland. Iodide alone can be used in patients with allergies to thiourea drugs to suppress thyroid function for periods of 10 to 28 days, as this will inhibit preformed hormone release. In addition, the elevated intracellular I^- content will block organification (Wolff-Chaikoff effect). Treatment with I^- alone should not be given beyond two to three weeks, since the hormone release rate will often increase again (escape phenomenon).

Alternatively, propranolol alone may be used to prepare the patient, or it may be combined with $I-$. One to two weeks of pretreatment with 40 mg of propranolol every six hours has been given. This approach is still experimental and should not be employed for patients who can undertake standard preoperative therapy with thiourea drugs. Aside from hypothyroidism, other potential complications of surgery include neck hemorrhage, recurrent laryngeal nerve damage, and hypoparathyroidism. In highly experienced clinics, such complications are quite rare (<1 per cent).

RADIOIODINE. Treatment of hyperthyroidism with ^{131}I has been used since the late 1940's. The principal complication of this treatment is hypothyroidism, which occurs in about 10 per cent of patients in the first year and increases about 5 per cent per year thereafter over 20 years. Depending on the dose given, about 20 per cent of patients require a second treatment. No increased risk of thyroid carcinoma or leukemia occurs after such treatment. For many years, there was a reluctance to employ ^{131}I in the treatment of women in the childbearing age group, but the ovarian dose from a typical 10 mCi treatment is approximately 2 to 4 rads, which is in the same range as that from hysterosalpingography or a barium enema. Although any unnecessary radiation is to be avoided, the calculated increase in the gamete mutation rate from exposure in this range is only a small fraction of the spontaneous mutation rate. Thus ^{131}I therapy does not appear to offer a significant risk of fetal malformation, although it is recommended that pregnancy not be undertaken for six months after this therapy to avoid transient radiation-induced changes in the gametes.

The author will generally pretreat patients who are to have ^{131}I therapy with thiourea derivatives to provide symptomatic relief and avoid the remote chance of an exacerbation of hyperthyroidism from radiation thyroiditis. These are discontinued four days prior to determining the 24-hour ^{131}I uptake. The author's practice is to administer orally an amount of ^{131}I, which when multiplied by the RAI uptake will result in thyroidal accumulation of 5 mCi ^{131}I. This will result in an average dose of 80 to 90 μCi per gram or 6000 to 7000 rads, which is associated with resolution of hyperthyroidism in about 80 per cent of patients within six months. Therapy with thiourea drugs may be restarted after one week, although it is not usually required. Patients are seen monthly thereafter with appropriate diagnostic and therapeutic measures to maintain the euthyroid state. At least six months is allowed to elapse before considering a second treatment. Since radioiodine crosses the placenta and would be concentrated by the thyroid of the fetus at 12 weeks and older, it is imperative that possibility of pregnancy be eliminated before radioiodine is administered.

The therapist administering radioiodine is committed to the planning of adequate follow-up. This consists of thoroughly informing the patient about the risks of delayed hypothyroidism (occurring in 80 to 100 per cent), providing written documentation of the treatment and its complications, and maintaining proper communication with referring physicians as to the need for indefinite follow-up. Patients are alerted to the symptoms of hypothyroidism and instructed that after the acute phase of treatment they should be seen at least every four to six months for appropriate thyroid function testing until hypothyroidism appears and treatment is initiated.

Choice of Therapy. None of the three long-term therapies for hyperthyroidism is ideal. Some thyroidologists will not use radioiodine in patients under the age of 35 or 40 because of the fear of long-term complications, whereas others employ radioiodine routinely in the treatment of hyperthyroidism in children. The author follows an intermediate position and will employ ^{131}I in patients as young as 18 years of age. In patients under the age of 18, one to two years of therapy with antithyroid drugs are given in hopes of observing a spontaneous remission. In women with this disease, the desire to raise a family will often require a decision for definitive therapy, especially if PTU requirements are high. In those patients who are over 18 at this point, ^{131}I is given, whereas for those who do not desire ^{131}I or who are under 18, surgery is recommended. Surgery is also recommended for patients with extreme thyroid enlargement or who have coexisting nonfunctioning thyroid nodules. The physician advising patients regarding this decision must consider not only these theoretical considerations and the patient's preferences but also the availability of a skilled surgeon.

Hyperthyroidism in Pregnancy. The peak incidence of Graves' disease occurs in women during the reproductive period. Therefore, it is not uncommon to find hyperthyroidism in a pregnant patient or for pregnancy to occur during therapy with antithyroid drugs. Both PTU and methimazole cross the placenta, whereas thyroid hormones do not. Excessive quantities of antithyroid drugs may cause impairment of fetal thyroid hormone synthesis. Depending on the dose, the consequence may be a compensatory hypertrophy of the thyroid gland resulting from increased TSH or frank fetal hypothyroidism with potential impairment of normal central nervous system development. I^- crosses the placenta, and the fetal thyroid is not able to adapt to high plasma I^- levels. Therefore, I^- therapy may result in iodide-induced fetal hypothyroidism. A congenital lesion, *aplasia cutis* (a 1 to 4 cm circular lesion on the scalp in which no hair follicles or accessory skin structures are present), has been found with increased frequency in infants of mothers receiving methimazole but not PTU. Uncontrolled hyperthyroidism in pregnancy is associated with an increased risk of spontaneous abortion and may lead to thyroid storm at the time of delivery.

With these facts in mind, pregnant patients with hyperthyroidism should be seen at monthly intervals, with careful clinical examination supplemented by measurements of serum T_3, T_4, and T_3 uptake. It should be recalled that the normal range for both serum T_4 and T_3 is higher during pregnancy (see Table 228–4). PTU should be given at the lowest dosage which maintains the patient at an acceptable euthyroid state. The author does not employ supplemental thyroid hormones in the treatment of the pregnant hyperthyroid patient, as has been recommended by some. If the patient's hyperthyroid symptoms cannot be controlled on less than 300 mg of PTU per day, then subtotal thyroidectomy is recommended during the second trimester. Iodides can be given for seven to ten days in preparation for surgery.

The newborn infant of the mother with Graves' disease should be examined carefully for either hypothyroidism as a consequence of excessive antithyroid drug or hyperthyroidism resulting from transplacental passage of TSI. In either situation goiter may be present, which may lead to respiratory embarrassment. Even the most meticulously managed patients will often have infants with modest reductions in serum T_4 that quickly normalize in the first week of life. Neonatal hyperthyroidism is transient but occasionally must be treated with antithyroid drugs and digitalis for tachycardia. An exacerbation of hyperthyroidism may occur following delivery and should be anticipated. The quantities of PTU in the milk of mothers receiving 200 to 300 mg PTU per day are not great enough to cause impairment of an infant's thyroid function. It seems likely that nursing mothers could take PTU at low doses, though the infant could still be at risk for nonthyroidal complications of this drug. Methimazole (and presumably carbimazole) is present in milk in significant amounts and should not be given to nursing mothers.

Lithium. Lithium has an effect on thyroid secretion quite similar to that of I^- in that it inhibits release of preformed thyroid hormone from the thyroid, probably by inhibiting thyroglobulin hydrolysis. It may also inhibit peripheral degradation of T_4. In patients with allergies to both antithyroid drugs and iodide, lithium carbonate, 0.9 to 1.5 grams per day (serum lithium concentrations of 0.5 to 1.0 mEq per liter), may be of value in the treatment of acute thyrotoxicosis. Serum lithium levels must be closely monitored, as some of the toxic effects of lithium are similar to those of hyperthyroidism.

Thyroid Storm. Some patients with hyperthyroidism develop severe manifestations which are exaggerations of many of the symptoms listed in Table 228–6. Often these occur because of superimposed stress or infection. The patient may be febrile, have abdominal pain, and become delirious, obtunded, or psychotic. This condition, called *thyroid storm*, has a mortality of 20 to 40 per cent. Such patients should be hospitalized and treated with a protocol such as is outlined in Table 228–7. I^- is

TABLE 228–7. MANAGEMENT OF PATIENTS WITH THYROID STORM

Diagnostic

1. Serum T_3 and T_4 concentrations, resin or charcoal T_3 uptake
2. Appropriate evaluation for underlying precipitating causes such as infection, acute surgical abdomen, central nervous system lesions, or psychologic trauma
3. Baseline WBC and differential, electrolytes, Ca, P
4. Plasma cortisol

Therapeutic

1. Intravenous fluids—dextrose with or without electrolytes as indicated, multivitamins
2. Propylthiouracil, 400 mg every six hours (by nasogastric tube, if necessary), to inhibit thyroid hormone synthesis and block T_4 to T_3 conversion
3. Sodium iodide, 250 mg every six hours (orally or intravenously)
4. Hydrocortisone, 50 to 100 mg every six hours intravenously
5. External cooling and acetaminophen (300 to 600 mg) every four to six hours for severe hyperpyrexia (do not use salicylates, which increase free thyroid hormones and oxygen consumption)
6. Propranolol—in patients without asthma, chronic bronchitis, or non-arrhythmia-related, congestive heart failure, 10–40 mg may be given every four to six hours orally; a slow intravenous infusion of 1 mg per minute for two to ten minutes with careful monitoring of blood pressure and ECG may be used if oral therapy is not feasible; propranolol may precipitate pulmonary edema in a few patients with hyperthyroidism; reserpine or guanethidine would not appear to have any advantages over propranolol in this situation
7. Oxygen may be helpful
8. Digitalis glycosides should be employed for therapy of congestive failure and for blockade of a rapid ventricular response to an atrial tachyrhythmia
9. Appropriate treatment of precipitating event if any

the most effective agent for inhibiting release of preformed thyroid hormone. If it is felt that the patient has a surgical abdomen, intravenous propranolol may be used intraoperatively to control tachycardia, assuming that there are no contraindications. The line between severe hyperthyroidism and thyroid storm is nebulous. In patients with severe symptoms but without fever, I^- should be added to PTU therapy to achieve a more rapid decrease in thyroid hormones. The I^- can be discontinued after one week.

Treatment of Ophthalmopathy. In most patients with ophthalmopathy no specific therapy is needed. Return of the hyperthyroid patient to euthyroidism will often result in amelioration of many of the minor symptoms, including stare and lid lag. It is important to avoid hypothyroidism, as anecdotal data suggest that this may be associated with an exacerbation of eye symptoms. The patient may note periorbital edema, especially on arising in the morning. An extra pillow or elevation of the head of the bed will relieve this. Alternatively, a diuretic can be administered at bedtime. In patients with more severe symptoms, artificial tears (1 per cent methylcellulose) are prescribed.

A small fraction of patients with Graves' disease will have more severe problems than can be relieved by these minor therapeutic measures. In patients with severe proptosis, desiccation of the sclera or even cornea may occur at night because of lagophthalmos. Taping the lids closed at night may alleviate this symptom, although lateral tarsorrhaphy is a more permanent solution. Diplopia may be treated by prisms or, if permanent, by muscle repositioning or relief of fibrous adhesions. This procedure should not be performed until the eye disease has stabilized, often a matter of two to three years. In the patient with severe inflammation and chemosis *(malignant exophthalmos)*, prednisone is required. Although 15 to 20 mg per day may be sufficient, in many patients as much as 100 mg per day is necessary with the attendant complications of treatment. Such patients should have frequent measurements of visual acuity and visual fields. Deterioration of either test is an emergency requiring steroid treatment and ophthalmologic consultation. In the case of optic compression or persistent corneal ulceration, surgical decompression may be required. Fortunately, in most patients, the severity of the eye manifestations will abate after 12 to 18 months, although in many the proptosis will never revert to normal.

Pretibial Myxedema. The lesions of pretibial myxedema are not generally incapacitating but may be cosmetically disfiguring. They may be treated with topical application of glucocorticoids, with enhancement of absorption by occlusive dressings if necessary.

PROGNOSIS. In most patients, Graves' disease is an extremely benign disorder in which the physician can play an important role in providing considerable relief to the patient. Because of the complications of treatment and the possibility of hypothyroidism even in patients with a spontaneous remission, patients with Graves' disease require lifelong observation.

TREATMENT OF OTHER CAUSES OF HYPERTHYROIDISM

The acute treatment of hyperthyroidism associated with toxic multinodular goiter or toxic adenoma does not differ from that of patients with Graves' disease. These entities are discussed in detail later in the chapter. The hyperthyroidism associated with subacute thyroiditis (particularly the lymphocytic variety) has been a subject of great interest in the past five years. This is discussed in the section Thyroiditis.

TSH-secreting pituitary tumor must be treated by surgery or x-ray. Patients with this condition are identified and separated from the group with nontumorigenic TSH–induced hyperthyroidism by finding elevation of the value of the serum α-TSH subunit as well as elevation of the value of TSH. Nontumorigenic hypersecretion of TSH is thought to be due to a reduction in feedback sensitivity to T_3 and T_4 at the pituitary level. Such patients are treated with antithyroid drugs. In patients with choriocarcinoma or hydatidiform mole, removal of the tumor will relieve these symptoms. Extremely rare is the ovarian teratoma containing thyroid tissue, *struma ovarii.* This should be treated surgically. In general, thyroid carcinoma does not function well enough to lead to hyperthyroidism. Hyperthyroidism can occur if extensive metastases are present which retain a significant degree of function, as may be seen occasionally in follicular carcinoma. This condition is readily diagnosed and is treated with ^{131}I.

Borst GC, Eil C, Burman KD: Euthyroid hyperthyroxinemia. Ann Intern Med 98:366–378, 1983. *The differential diagnosis of individuals with an elevated serum T_4.*

Cheron RG, Kaplan MM, Larsen PR, Selenkow HA, Crigler JF, Jr: Neonatal thyroid function after propylthiouracil therapy for maternal Graves' disease. N Engl J Med 304:525–528, 1981. *A prospective study of the effects of maternal antithyroid drug treatment on newborn thyroid function.*

Dallow RL: Reliability of orbital diagnostic tests: Ultrasonography, computerized tomography and radiography. Ophthalmology 85:1218, 1978. *The author describes results of these various diagnostic techniques in 342 patients with unilateral exophthalmus.*

Davis PJ, Davis FB: Hyperthyroidism in patients over the age of 60 years. Medicine 53:161, 1974. *An excellent summary of the clinical syndrome of hyperthyroidism in the elderly patient.*

Fradkin JE, Wolff J: Iodide-induced thyrotoxicosis. Medicine 62:1,1–20, 1983. *Iodide, or drugs containing this element, can cause many confusing syndromes especially in patients with underlying thyroid disease. The spectrum of these problems is reviewed in this article.*

Holm LE, Dahlquist I, Israelsson A, Lundell G: Malignant thyroid tumors after *^{131}I therapy. N Engl J Med 303:188, 1980. In a group of 3000 patients, the authors found no increased incidence of malignant thyroid tumors after ^{131}I therapy an average of 13 years earlier.*

Morley JE, Jacobson RJ, Melamed J, Hershman JM: Choriocarcinoma as a cause of thyrotoxicosis. Am J Med 60:1036, 1976. *Three typical cases of this syndrome are presented with complete thyroid evaluation.*

Weintraub BD, Gershengorn MC, Kourides IA, Fein H: Inappropriate secretion of thyroid-stimulating hormone. Ann Intern Med 95:339–351, 1981. *A review of the pathophysiology, diagnosis and treatment of TSH-induced hyperthyroidism.*

Zakarija M, McKenzie JM, Banovac K: Clinical significance of assay of thyroid-stimulating antibody in Graves' disease. Ann Intern Med 93:28–32 (part 1), 1980. *A careful study of the correlation between remission and TSI in patients with Graves' Disease.*

Hypothyroidism and Myxedema

DEFINITION. *Hypothyroidism* is the clinical syndrome which results from a deficiency of thyroid hormone. In severe hypothyroidism a hydrophilic mucopolysaccharide substance accumulates in subcutaneous tissues, causing a nonpitting edema referred to as *myxedema.* Some authorities use the terms hypothyroidism and myxedema interchangeably, whereas others reserve the latter term for the severe form of this syndrome.

ETIOLOGY. A list of causes to be considered in patients with hypothyroidism is given in Table 228–8. *Primary hypothyroidism,* that caused by thyroid gland malfunction, accounts for over 95 per cent of such cases, of which Hashimoto's thyroiditis, idiopathic myxedema (probably a variant of Hashimoto's thyroiditis), and thyroid destruction resulting from ^{131}I therapy or surgery for hyperthyroidism account for the greatest proportion. Hashimoto's and subacute thyroiditis are discussed in the next section. Hypothyroidism after therapeutic irradiation to the thyroid area for lymphoma or Hodgkin's disease is found in from 10 to 30 per cent of these patients, usually within one to two years of treatment.

Hypothyroidism can also occur with normal or near-normal thyroid tissue when there is a superimposed stress on thyroid cell function. Hypothyroidism may be caused either by severe iodine deficiency (<25 μg iodine per day) or by naturally occurring goitrogens such as have been found in Colombia or are generated by eating the cassava plant in Africa (see Sporadic and Endemic Goiter). In patients with Graves' disease, especially after RAI treatment, or in those with mild Hashimoto's thyroiditis, iodine excess may cause hypothyroidism through the Wolff-Chaikoff effect (I^- induced inhibition of organification). These glands are unable to reduce I^- uptake in the presence of an elevated plasma I^- as normally occurs. The

TABLE 228–8. CAUSES OF HYPOTHYROIDISM

I. Primary hypothyroidism
  A. Acquired
    1. Destructive lesions
      a. Hashimoto's thyroiditis
      b. Idiopathic myxedema (probably the end-stage of Hashimoto's thyroiditis)
      c. ^{131}I therapy for hyperthyroidism
      d. Subtotal thyroidectomy, especially for Graves' disease
      e. Therapeutic external x-ray treatment to the neck for other diseases
      f. After subacute thyroiditis (may be transient)
      g. Cystinosis
    2. Impaired function of a normal or near-normal gland
      a. Endemic goiter—iodine deficiency or naturally occurring goitrogens
      b. Iodine excess (>6 mg per day) in patients with underlying thyroid disease
      c. Drug-induced; lithium carbonate, para-aminosalicylic acid, thiourea drugs, sulfonamides, phenylbutazone, and others
  B. Congenital
    1. Defects in enzymes required for thyroid hormone synthesis (congenital goiter)
    2. Thyroid agenesis
    3. Thyroid dysgenesis or ectopy
    4. Maternal iodide or antithyroid drugs
II. Secondary hypothyroidism
  A. Hypothalamic dysfunction
    1. Neoplasms
    2. Eosinophilic granuloma
    3. Therapeutic irradiation
  B. Pituitary dysfunction
    1. Neoplasms
    2. Pituitary surgery or irradiation
    3. Idiopathic hypopituitarism
    4. Sheehan's syndrome (postpartum pituitary necrosis)
    5. Dopamine infusion and/or severe illness(?)
III. Tissue resistance to thyroid hormone

drugs listed in Table 228–8 all inhibit organification of thyroidal I^-. In most cases the hypothyroidism associated with these drugs is mild.

Screening of newborns for hypothyroidism is now widely practiced, and the incidence of this condition is about 1 in 4000 births. About 65 per cent of infants with congenital hypothyroidism in North America have thyroid agenesis or hypoplasia, 25 per cent have ectopic thyroid glands, and about 10 per cent have defects in one of the steps required for thyroid hormone synthesis (see Sporadic and Endemic Goiter).

Secondary hypothyroidism occurs as a result of hypothalamic or pituitary dysfunction. Dopamine infusion and/or severe illness may suppress TSH release sufficiently to cause a modest, transient hypothyroidism. A rare cause of hypothyroidism is tissue resistance to thyroid hormones, which may be due to an abnormality in the nuclear receptor for these hormones.

INCIDENCE. Hypothyroidism is common in adults. In one recent epidemiologic survey, 1.4 per cent of adult females and about 0.1 per cent of adult males were affected. Autoimmune destruction of the thyroid gland is the most common cause of thyroid gland failure in adults. This generally affects women over the age of 40 but can occur at any age. Hypothyroidism is also a common congenital disease, occurring in about 1 of 4000 neonates in North America and Western Europe and more frequently in areas of iodine deficiency.

PATHOLOGY. The pathology of the thyroid gland in hypothyroidism depends on the etiology of the syndrome. In "idiopathic myxedema," the thyroid tissue is generally replaced by fat with few intact follicles and lymphocytic infiltration (see also Thyroiditis). When the thyroid cells remain partly functional, the elevated serum TSH leads to hyperplasia and hypertrophy. In secondary hypothyroidism, the follicular cells are low and considerable colloid is present. The gland is small in contrast to the goiter found when thyroid cell dysfunction is present and TSH secretion is elevated.

The nonthyroidal pathology of the hypothyroid state is the same regardless of its etiology. The longer the duration and the more severe the deficiency, the greater are the changes. The accumulation of mucopolysaccharide in connective tissues has already been mentioned. This material may also appear in muscle. Effusions, which often have a high protein content, occur in various serous cavities.

CLINICAL MANIFESTATIONS. The common clinical manifestations of this syndrome in the adult are summarized in Table 228–9. These symptoms and signs can be attributed to either deceleration of cellular metabolic processes or the accumulation of the hygroscopic mucopolysaccharide in the vocal cords or oropharynx, as well as the more obvious changes in the subcutaneous tissues. The symptoms are nonspecific, particularly in the early phases, and may either pass unnoticed by the patient or be attributed to advancing age. Characteristically, the patient becomes aware of their multiplicity and severity only after thyroid hormone replacement leads to a return of normal function. This is particularly true of younger patients. In the elderly, hearing impairment, somnolence, and decreased memory and ability to calculate may occur. These may lead to an apparent psychologic withdrawal and paranoia at times requiring hospitalization. The term *myxedema madness* has been used to describe this syndrome, which can be mistaken for cerebrovascular insufficiency or senile dementia. Alternatively, the patient may confabulate or respond with humorous non sequiturs to draw the interviewer's attention from his or her limited recall of recent events. This behavior has been termed *myxedema wit.* A variety of menstrual disorders may be present, although menorrhagia is said to be the most common pattern. Pregnancy may occur in patients with hypothyroidism, and the increased hormone requirements of that condition may cause a previously borderline functioning thyroid to decompensate. Despite the developmental abnormalities associated with congenital hypothyroidism, the symptoms of hypothyroidism in infants are few. Severe thyroid hormone deficiency is associated with growth retardation in the older infant and child. In the adolescent, thyroid enlargement, *adolescent goiter,* may be the only manifestation and is usually seen in the pubertal female. In some patients in whom the hypothyroidism is of rapid onset, cramps in large muscle groups may be a prominent symptom. Such symptoms usually occur after a rapid change from a hyperthyroid to a hypothyroid state, such as after surgery for Graves' disease, a second RAI treatment for hyperthyroidism, or even vigorous antithyroid drug therapy.

Many of the common signs of hypothyroidism are the opposite of those seen in the hyperthyroid patient. Bradycardia is common and is sometimes associated with hypothermia. Systolic pressure is generally reduced and diastolic pressure increased, the latter resulting from increased peripheral vascular resistance. Myxedema is manifested by a puffy, nonpitting swelling of the subcutaneous tissue, which may particularly collect in the periorbital area. Body and scalp hair is reduced; the skin may be coarse, may have a sandpaper texture, and is usually cool and sallow. The yellow complexion is due to the accumulation of carotene in the serum in patients with significant hypothyroidism. The thyroid may be enlarged, of normal size, or not palpable, depending on the cause. The heart sounds are distant, and the heart shadow is often enlarged. The latter can be a manifestation of pericardial effusion, which is common but rarely leads to tamponade. In addition to the cortical dysfunction previously mentioned, cerebellar ataxia may be

TABLE 228–9. COMMON SYMPTOMS OF HYPOTHYROIDISM

Weakness, fatigue, lethargy
Dry, coarse skin
Swelling of the hands, face, and extremities
Cold intolerance, decreased sweating
Coarsening or huskiness of the voice
Modest weight gain (~10 lbs) with anorexia
Decreased memory, hearing impairment
Arthralgia, paresthesias
Constipation
Muscle cramps

present. Other neurologic signs, including delayed relaxation of the deep tendon reflexes, peripheral neuropathy, and carpal tunnel syndrome, can completely resolve with treatment. There may be few signs of hypothyroidism in the newborn, hence the need for routine screening. The most common signs are hypotonia, umbilical hernia, and skin mottling, but none is present in more than one third of infants with confirmed hypothyroidism in the first three months of life.

Certain physiologic abnormalities are characteristic of hypothyroidism. Cardiac output is reduced, although not out of proportion to the decrease in O_2 consumption. Glomerular filtration is also subnormal, leading to an impairment of the capacity to excrete free water. In addition there is evidence supporting inappropriate ADH secretion in primary hypothyroidism, which may lead to hyponatremia. Gastrointestinal motility is reduced, and occasionally the patient may develop an apparent obstruction, *myxedema megacolon*. There are important abnormalities in the medulla. The sensitivity to both hypercarbia and hypoxia is reduced, and such patients may readily develop CO_2 narcosis or cardiac arrhythmias associated with hypoxia. This is one of the chief causes of death in the severe form of myxedema, *myxedema coma*. Pituitary function is impaired in severe hypothyroidism even of the primary variety. Hypoglycemic stress does not elicit normal growth hormone or cortisol responses in such patients, so that testing pituitary function must be delayed until the hypothyroid state has been corrected. Serum prolactin is elevated in moderate to severe primary hypothyroidism, and this may lead to galactorrhea in a small percentage of patients.

LABORATORY DIAGNOSIS. The diagnosis of hypothyroidism can be easily confirmed by using the scheme outlined in Figure 228–7. When the diagnosis is not made, it is usually because the nonspecificity of signs and symptoms does not immediately suggest this cause. This disease is one of the "great imitators," and a high index of suspicion should be maintained as the condition is so readily diagnosed and treated. In all patients with hypothyroidism, the free T_4 index will be reduced. It is unlikely that significant symptoms will be present in patients with an equivocal reduction in this hormone. Once a reduced free T_4 index has been found, it is imperative to determine whether the cause of the disease is primary, i.e., owing to thyroid disease, or secondary, involving the hypothalamic-pituitary axis. An elevation in serum TSH establishes the diagnosis of primary hypothyroidism. If the serum TSH concentration is normal or borderline, then the diagnosis of pituitary or hypothalamic hypothyroidism is made and further steps are taken to evaluate the possibility of a deficiency of other pituitary hormones. It is extremely important that this be done prior to the onset of therapy, since thyroid replacement will exacerbate mild ACTH insufficiency associated with hypothalamic or pituitary disease. *If unrecognized, such patients may have an addisonian crisis provoked by thyroid hormone replacement.* There are two situations recognized in which primary hypothyroidism is not associated with an elevated serum TSH. This may occur when hypothyroidism follows shortly after a period of hyperthyroidism which causes a suppression of pituitary TSH synthesis and release lasting four to five weeks. Dopamine infusion may also cause suppression of an elevated TSH into the normal range. In the patient whose symptoms are nonspecific or borderline and in whom an equivocally reduced free T_4 index is obtained, the serum TSH may be significantly elevated. An elevated TSH is the most sensitive index of impairment of thyroid gland function. Whether or not such patients are actually metabolically hypothyroid cannot be determined by using present tests. In the case of early primary thyroid disease, an exaggerated TSH response to TRH will occur (see Fig. 228–4), the TSH being greater than 25 μU per milliliter 20 minutes after TRH infusion.

There are a few clinical situations in which the free T_4 index is reduced but serum TSH is not elevated in the absence of hypothalamic or pituitary disease. This occurs in patients receiving 2 to 3 grams per day of salicylate-containing compounds, in those receiving phenytoin (300 mg per day), and in those ingesting replacement quantities (25 μg or more) of triiodothyronine (Cytomel). Occasionally, the severely ill patient without primary thyroid disease may have a reduced free T_4 index with or without dopamine infusion. Such patients presumably have transient mild hypothyroidism, although in individual cases it may be extremely difficult to determine whether permanent hypothalamic-pituitary hypothyroidism is also present. A serum cortisol determination is indicated in these patients to eliminate the possibility of ACTH deficiency before initiating therapy with both thyroxine and glucocorti-

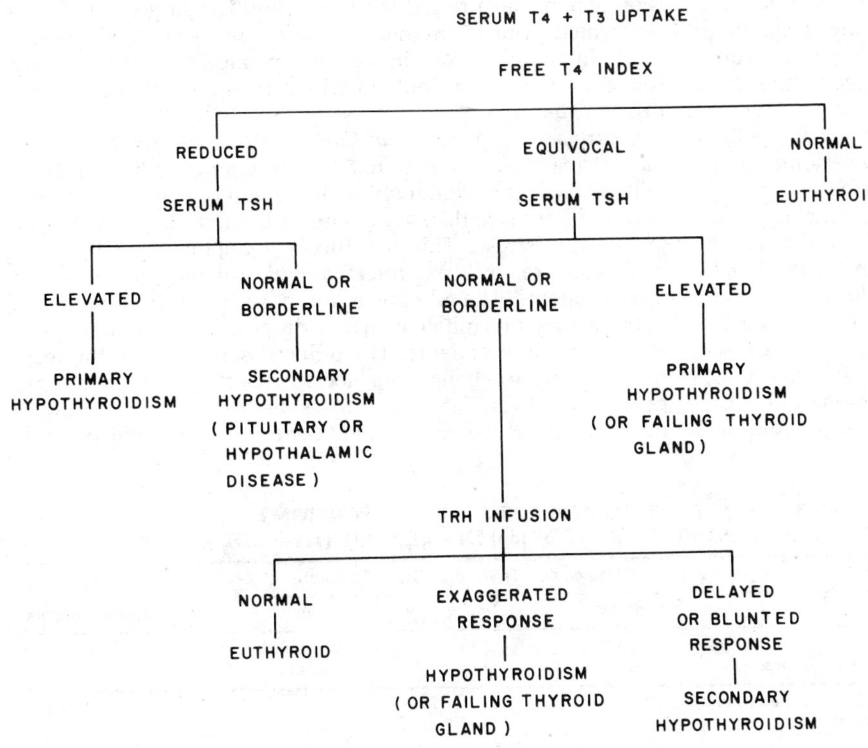

Figure 228–7. Laboratory diagnosis of hypothyroidism.

coid. A 24-hour RAI uptake test does not separate hypothyroidism from the euthyroid state, and serum T_3 concentrations may be in the normal range even in patients with significant hypothyroidism (see Table 228–4).

Other Biochemical Abnormalities and Associated Diseases in Patients with Hypothyroidism. Serum cholesterol and triglycerides, creatine phosphokinase (MM isozyme), aldolase, LDH, and SGOT may all be elevated in the patient with moderate to severe hypothyroidism. Hyponatremia with or without the inappropriate ADH syndrome is seen. There is often a modest anemia of chronic disease which may be macrocytic. Serum vitamin B_{12} should be measured in these patients because of the 3 to 6 per cent coexistence of pernicious anemia with Hashimoto's thyroiditis. Other conditions found with increased frequency in patients with autoimmune thyroid disease include idiopathic adrenocortical deficiency, diabetes mellitus, hypoparathyroidism, myasthenia gravis, and vitiligo. (Ch. 240).

DIFFERENTIAL DIAGNOSIS. There are few conditions which can masquerade as hypothyroidism in its classic form. However, patients with nephrotic syndrome or hypoalbuminemia and associated peripheral edema may be suspected of this diagnosis. Although the serum T_4 in these conditions is reduced because of hypoproteinemia, the T_3 uptake is generally quite elevated with a consequent normal free T_4 index. Patients with chronic renal disease may have symptoms entirely similar to those of hypothyroidism (including hypothermia), and laboratory tests are required to evaluate the possible coexistence of these two diseases. In patients with spontaneous primary hypothyroidism, the tests for autoantibodies to either thyroglobulin or microsomal components of the thyroid cell are generally positive. This is true even if the typical thyroid enlargement of Hashimoto's thyroiditis is not present. The other causes of hypothyroidism have already been discussed (Table 228–8), and reversible causes should be eliminated.

THERAPY. Hypothyroidism is a readily treatable disease. The preparations available for thyroid replacement are listed in Table 228–10. For many years desiccated thyroid was used quite satisfactorily, and it continues to be prescribed for about 40 per cent of the hypothyroid patients in the United States today. Although any of these substances given in the appropriate amounts are adequate to treat the major symptoms of hypothyroidism, the serum hormone results in patients receiving replacement doses of thyroxine appear to be most similar to those in normal persons. In patients receiving desiccated thyroid or the combination T_4-T_3 products, the ratio of serum T_3 to T_4 is usually higher than it is in normal subjects, since the ratio in these preparations (4:1) is higher than that in thyroid secretion. In addition, transient serum T_3 elevations above the physiologic normal range are found two to four hours after administration of desiccated thyroid and may be associated with symptoms. As noted, some tissues (e.g., pituitary and cerebral cortex) depend on serum T_4 for a significant portion of their intracellular T_3, whereas others derive most intracellular T_3 directly from the serum. Therefore, it would appear that both serum T_3 and T_4 concentrations should be normalized to fulfill the intracellular T_3 concentrations of all tissues. Because the USP standard for thyroid replacement preparations does not require specific measurement of thyroid hormones, only of organic iodine, some preparations of desiccated thyroid or thyroxine may meet these criteria without containing adequate quantities of biologically active thyroid hormone. Modifications of USP standards have been proposed to deal with this issue. The author prefers to use a brand name L-thyroxine as replacement. A dose of approximately 2.25 μg of T_4 per kilogram (1 μg of T_4 per pound), given once a day, achieves a satisfactory symptomatic and biochemical replacement in most patients. The difference between this dosage and the thyroxine production rate (≃80 to 90 μg per day) is due to the 50 to 70 per cent absorption of orally administered L-thyroxine. In patients who are in good health otherwise or whose hypothyroidism is very modest, therapy can be initiated with half-replacement doses immediately on establishing the diagnosis. This can be increased to full replacement after one month. In patients with more severe hypothyroidism, elderly patients, or those with a history of cardiovascular disease, the author prefers to begin therapy with smaller amounts (25 μg of thyroxine per day) and to increase these by 25-μg increments at four-week intervals (with due attention to symptoms) until a replacement dose is achieved. In patients with primary hypothyroidism there may rarely be an associated primary autoimmune hypoadrenalism *(Schmidt's syndrome).* Such patients will require adequate replacement of glucocorticoid prior to institution of thyroid hormone replacement. A similar procedure must be employed in patients who have hypothalamic-pituitary disease as a cause of hypothyroidism. Biochemical evaluation of the progress of treatment of primary hypothyroidism consists of quantitation of the serum free T_4 index and TSH. The dose should be increased (symptoms permitting) until the serum TSH and free T_4 index have reached the normal range. The replacement dose of T_4 may be 20 to 40 per cent lower in elderly patients.

Hypothyroidism and Coronary Artery Disease. The patient who presents simultaneously with angina and hypothyroidism poses a serious therapeutic problem. In some patients with coronary artery disease, reintroduction of thyroid hormones results in increased myocardial oxygen demands without an adequate increase in myocardial blood flow. A trial of propranolol with small increments of thyroxine may reduce myocardial oxygen consumption without decreasing the pulse rate to unacceptably low levels. If an exacerbation of angina occurs during thyroxine therapy, T_4 to T_3 conversion may be acutely reduced in peripheral tissues with propylthiouracil (see Graves' Disease and Other Causes of Hyperthyroidism). In patients with localized coronary artery disease in whom bypass graft surgery is indicated, the frequent adverse effects of thyroxine replacement have raised the possibility that surgery should be performed prior to thyroid hormone replacement. The overall morbidity may be lower in patients operated on in the hypothyroid state than in patients in whom replacement is attempted prior to surgery.

Treatment of Myxedema Coma. In severe myxedema the patient may lapse into coma. This serious complication (mortality, 20 to 50 per cent) occurs most commonly in patients with severe hypothyroidism who are subjected to an additional physiologic stress. This may occur spontaneously, following cold exposure, or during infection, but in all too many instances it is iatrogenic. The administration of sedatives to hypothyroid patients may precipitate coma, as drugs are not metabolized as rapidly in these patients. The reduced sensitivity of the respiratory center to changes in blood gases may lead to inappropriately small ventilatory responses. In other situations, surgery may be performed in a patient who is not recognized to be

TABLE 228–10. HORMONE CONTENT OF THYROID REPLACEMENT PREPARATIONS (AMOUNTS APPROXIMATELY EQUIVALENT TO 1 GRAIN (65 mg) DESICCATED THYROID)

		Liotrix		Desiccated Thyroid (1-Grain Tablets)			
	L-Thyroxine	*Euthroid-1*	*Thyrolar-1*	*Armour*	*Proloid*	*Generics*	L-Triiodothyronine
T_4 (μg)	100	60	50	63	55	Variable*	0
T_3 (μg)	0	15	12.5	12	16	Variable*	25

*Eight generic preparations contained 9 to 59 μg T_4 and 8 to 18 μg T_3 per 1-grain tablet.
Data from Rees-Jones RW, Rolla AR, Larsen PR: JAMA 243:459, 1980.

TABLE 228–11. MANAGEMENT OF PATIENTS WITH MYXEDEMA COMA

Diagnostic
1. Serum T_4, T_3 uptake (or equivalent), TSH
2. CBC, glucose, electrolytes, blood gases, BUN, creatinine, CPK
3. Plasma cortisol before and 30 and 60 minutes after Cortrosyn, 0.25 mg, intravenous bolus
4. Careful evaluation for concomitant disease; continuous ECG and temperature monitoring

Therapeutic
1. L-Thyroxine, 2 μg per kilogram intravenously over five to ten minutes initially, and 100 μg intravenously every 24 hours thereafter
2. Cover to conserve body heat; do not rewarm externally
3. Tracheal intubation and mechanical ventilation as required
4. Intravenous fluids as determined by initial blood glucose and electrolytes and by the state of hydration; watch for water retention
5. Hydrocortisone, 100 mg by intravenous bolus, then 25 mg every six hours as a continuous intravenous drip
6. Vigorous treatment of associated and precipitating conditions such as infection

severely hypothyroid, and postoperative opiates or sedatives lead to clinical deterioration. In Table 228–11 are shown the important steps in management of patients with myxedema coma. In these emergent situations it is important to institute treatment immediately. If the serum free T_4 index is reduced, treatment is begun even if the cause of the hypothyroidism (primary versus secondary) has not been identified. Accordingly, testing for adrenal function is carried out immediately, followed by institution of glucocorticoid replacement. Because of the irregularities of either intramuscular or gastrointestinal absorption in hypothyroidism, medications should be given intravenously. Glucocorticoid replacement should not be given in pharmacologic quantities, since this will impair T_4 to T_3 conversion.

PROGNOSIS. The prognosis of hypothyroidism is excellent, provided that thyroid hormone replacement is maintained.

Withdrawal of Thyroid Hormone After Prolonged Replacement. The question sometimes arises as to whether thyroid hormone therapy is indicated in a patient already receiving it. If, based on the history, the physician is skeptical of the need for replacement, such a patient is instructed to discontinue the medication completely and return for serum free T_4 index and TSH determinations in three weeks. The patient is advised that there may be mild manifestations of low thyroid function and to notify the physician sooner if these become severe. Three weeks after cessation of treatment, a patient with normal thyroid function will have a low normal serum free T_4 index, but the serum TSH will not be elevated. If this correlates with the clinical symptomatology, the patient is instructed to return after a further three-week interval for repeat testing. The results after six weeks can be used as a reliable index of the underlying thyroid functional capacity. If the free T_4 index and TSH are normal at that time, one can exclude the diagnosis of significant hypothyroidism.

Bigos ST, Ridgway EC, Kourides IA, Maloof F: Spectrum of pituitary alterations with mild and severe thyroid impairment. J Clin Endocrinol Metab 46:317, 1978. *Mild decreases in serum T_4 with no changes in serum T_3 can be associated with significant increases in serum TSH in patients with modest impairment of thyroid function.*

Dussault JH, Walker P (eds.): Congenital Hypothyroidism. New York, Marcel Dekker, Inc., 1983. *A comprehensive discussion of the diagnosis and treatment of congenital hypothyroidism.*

Rees-Jones RW, Rolla AR, Larsen PR: Hormonal content of thyroid replacement preparations. JAMA 243:459, 1980. *Analyses of desiccated thyroid tablets show that some generic preparations have reduced quantities of T_4 and T_3 relative to those contained in brand-name products.*

Refetoff S: Syndromes of thyroid hormone resistance. Am J Physiol 243 (Endocrinol Metab 6):88–98, 1982. *A review of the various ways in which thyroid hormone-resistance may present and of the pathophysiology of these disorders.*

Sawin CT, Surks MI, London M, Ranganathan C, Larsen PR: Oral thyroxine: Variation in biologic action and tablet content. Ann Intern Med 100:641, 1984. *An example of one of the problems that may be encountered in the treatment of hypothyroid patients.*

Weinberg AD, Brennan MD, Gorman CA, Marsh HM, O'Fallon WM: Outcome of anesthesia and surgery in hypothyroid patients. Arch Intern Med 143:893–897, 1983. *Results of this experience at the Mayo Clinic suggest that patients with mild to moderate primary hypothyroidism withstand nonelective general surgery as well as do euthyroid patients.*

Thyroiditis

Thyroiditis is classified into three types: acute, subacute, and chronic. Despite the common factor of inflammation in all of these entities, there are marked differences in their clinical presentations and etiology.

ACUTE THYROIDITIS

Acute thyroiditis results from a bacterial infection of the thyroid gland with typical symptoms of such involvement, including a fever, local tenderness, and swelling. This condition is quite rare. The infection may involve the whole gland or only a portion of it. Laboratory studies generally show normal thyroid function, but there is an elevated leukocyte count with a polymorphonuclear predominance. The thyroid scan may show an area of decreased uptake corresponding to the involved portion, but the 24-hour RAI uptake is usually normal. Treatment of this condition requires proper identification of the causative agent and appropriate antimicrobial drugs. This may require a needle aspiration. If localized abscess formation occurs, it should be drained. The process usually responds rapidly to these measures.

SUBACUTE (NONSUPPURATIVE) THYROIDITIS

This condition is also referred to as *giant cell thyroiditis*, *granulomatous thyroiditis*, or *de Quervain's thyroiditis*. In the classic form of this disease the patient presents with an exquisitely tender thyroid, which is pathologically characterized by follicular cell destruction and by a lymphocytic and polymorphonuclear leukocyte infiltration, together with multinucleate giant cells. In recent years, a different type of subacute thyroiditis has appeared, which is often painless and associated with hyperthyroidism. It shares some pathologic features with Hashimoto's thyroiditis (see below). This condition, which will be denoted *subacute lymphocytic thyroiditis*, is discussed separately below because of its unique features. The disease described by de Quervain will be referred to as *subacute granulomatous thyroiditis*.

INCIDENCE. The incidence of subacute granulomatous thyroiditis is not known, but it is not rare. It is most common in the third to fifth decades, and females are affected about three to four times more commonly than males. It occurs with increased frequency in HLA-B35 positive individuals.

ETIOLOGY. The granulomatous form of subacute thyroiditis often follows a viral infection by several weeks. At the time of the acute illness, elevated titers of antibody to influenza virus, coxsackievirus, or adenovirus can be found. Over the next few months these fall in many patients, suggesting that an acute infection has recently occurred. In only two cases has a virus been cultured from thyroid tissue, which in both cases was mumps. Some authorities interpret the thyroiditis as being a consequence of a process set in motion by the viral illness but not representing a direct infection of the gland. The precise etiology is unknown.

PATHOLOGY. The classic pathologic picture includes the cellular infiltrate described above, along with severe destruction of the normal follicular architecture. Fibrosis appears in the latter phases. Despite the extensive destruction, complete restoration of the normal thyroid structure generally occurs.

CLINICAL MANIFESTATIONS. Subacute granulomatous thyroiditis is characterized by an often exquisitely painful two- to three-fold enlargement of the thyroid gland together with systemic symptoms, including fever, chills, and malaise. Patients often complain of neck or ear pain or dysphagia and may have had evaluation for pharyngeal infection. Symptoms of hyperthyroidism may also be present. The patient may report a prior viral illness. If symptoms of hyperthyroidism are present, they are generally of very short duration (less than two months) and are due to the release of thyroid hormones resulting from thyroid destruction. Physical examination may show fever, tachycardia, and exquisite tenderness of the slightly enlarged thyroid gland. This generally involves the whole gland but may be asymmetric.

DIAGNOSIS. The leukocyte count is mildly elevated, but there is characteristically a marked elevation of the erythrocyte sedimentation rate (ESR). This has been one of the hallmarks of this disease. The free T_4 index may be normal or increased. As would be expected from the pathology, the RAI uptake is low and the thyroid is poorly visualized on scan. The RAI uptake is the principal test for separating patients with this disease from those with hyperthyroidism resulting from Graves' disease. There may be an asymmetric involvement of the thyroid with decreased function in that area. Antimicrosomal and antithyroglobulin antibodies are absent or low in titer, although the serum thyroglobulin may be elevated, reflecting the destructive process.

TREATMENT. Since this is a self-limited disease, treatment is symptomatic. Mild analgesics such as aspirin (2 to 4 grams per day) should be given for neck discomfort. In a significant fraction of patients, this will not be sufficient, and prednisone, 20 to 40 mg per day, is required. The immediate relief associated with this therapy is almost diagnostic. The glucocorticoid should be continued for two to three weeks and then tapered over the next three weeks. There may be an exacerbation of the original symptoms during discontinuation of glucocorticoid requiring reinstitution of this therapy. Eventually this will not occur. The hyperthyroidism is usually mild but may require propranolol. Antithyroid drugs are of no use, as the serum T_4 and T_3 will decrease when the glandular supply is exhausted.

There may be transient hypothyroidism following subacute granulomatous thyroiditis, and this may be severe enough to require treatment in some patients. Therefore it is important for these patients to be followed closely during the recovery period to ascertain whether or not this complication has occurred. Replacement thyroxine can be discontinued after three to six months with appropriate biochemical monitoring to establish that thyroid function has returned to normal. In 5 to 10 per cent of patients, permanent hypothyroidism supervenes. Occasionally a patient will be seen initially in the hypothyroid phase of this illness. An elevation in serum TSH and low thyroid hormones in the absence of antimicrosomal or antithyroglobulin antibodies should alert the physician to this possibility.

SUBACUTE LYMPHOCYTIC THYROIDITIS

This disease has been referred to by a variety of descriptive terms, including *painless thyroiditis, lymphocytic thyroiditis, lymphocytic thyroiditis with spontaneously resolving hyperthyroidism, hyperthyroiditis*, and *atypical subacute thyroiditis*. This confused nomenclature reflects the principal clinical and pathologic features of the disease: hyperthyroidism which is self-limited, and lymphocytic infiltration of the thyroid.

ETIOLOGY. The etiology of the disease is unknown. There is little suggestion of a prior viral illness in these patients. The pathologic features are much closer to those of Hashimoto's disease than to those of granulomatous thyroiditis, suggesting an autoimmune etiology.

INCIDENCE. The precise incidence is not known, but one suspects that it has been increasing over the last five to ten years. This condition may account for 5 to 20 per cent of patients with hyperthyroidism. About two thirds of reported cases are in women, with patients ranging from 13 to over 80 years of age.

PATHOLOGY. Lymphocytic infiltration is the common feature in all specimens studied. Destruction of follicular architecture and fibrosis similar to that of subacute granulomatous thyroiditis is seen, but foreign body giant cells are rare. Germinal centers characteristic of Hashimoto's disease are rarely seen.

CLINICAL MANIFESTATIONS. The principal symptoms of this form of subacute thyroiditis are those of hyperthyroidism, as described in the section Graves' Disease and Other Causes of Hyperthyroidism. Nonthyroidal stigmata of Graves' disease, exophthalmos and pretibial myxedema, are not present, although a stare and widened palpebral fissure may occur as a consequence of the hyperthyroidism per se. The duration of the hyperthyroid phase is short (usually less than three months), and it is generally modest in severity. Physical signs include those typical of hyperthyroidism and a normal or slightly enlarged thyroid gland which is not tender. The gland may be firm.

The natural history of thyroid function in a patient who had a typical episode of this disease is presented in Figure 228–8.

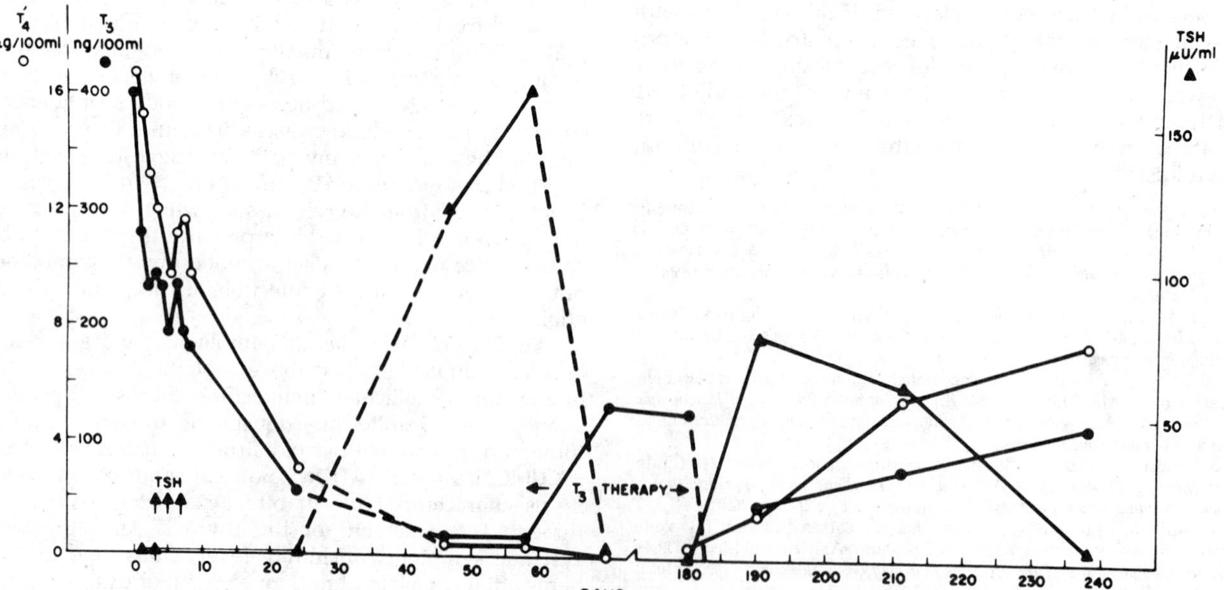

Figure 228–8. Changes in serum T_3, T_4, and TSH in a patient with subacute lymphocytic thyroiditis. The rapid decrease in serum T_3 and T_4 in the first five days is due to exhaustion of thyroidal stores as a consequence of the destructive process. Transient T_3 replacement was employed because of prolonged hypothyroidism. Normal thyroid function had returned by eight months after the initial episode. (From Larsen PR: Metabolism 23:467, 1974.)

The acute phase of hyperthyroidism resolved rapidly and spontaneously and was followed by a period of transient hypothyroidism requiring treatment. This was discontinued after three months, and, after an initial period of thyroidal resistance to TSH, normal function returned. A phase of significant hypothyroidism such as this follows the hyperthyroidism in about one third of patients. For obscure reasons, this form of thyroiditis occurs with increased frequency in the first few months postpartum.

LABORATORY DIAGNOSIS. Serum T_4 and T_3 concentrations are generally elevated, the leukocyte count normal, and the ESR normal or only slightly elevated (<50 mm at 1 hour, Westergren). This is in marked contrast to the results in the granulomatous form of the disease. The 24-hour RAI uptake is reduced and will not increase even after TSH injections. Serum thyroglobulin is elevated in the acute phase of the disease, and antimicrosomal and antithyroglobulin antibodies are usually negative or low in titer in the usual assays.

This disease must be separated from other causes of hyperthyroidism, notably Graves' disease. The best test for this is the 24-hour RAI uptake. A low uptake may occasionally also be observed in a patient with Graves' disease who has received excess iodide. This may be obvious from the history or can be eliminated by measuring the urinary iodide, which must be considerably elevated (>2 mg per 24 hours) to suppress the uptake in hyperthyroidism associated with thyroid hyperfunction. A needle biopsy will also be diagnostic. It should also be separated from Hashimoto's thyroiditis because of the difference in the natural history of these two diseases. The low antimicrosomal antibody titer will usually accomplish this, as well as the fact that hyperthyroidism is rarely seen in Hashimoto's disease. To distinguish this condition from factitious hyperthyroidism, 10 units of bovine TSH can be injected, followed in one day by a 24-hour RAI uptake. No change in the uptake is found in patients with subacute lymphocytic thyroiditis.

TREATMENT. As with subacute granulomatous thyroiditis, treatment is symptomatic. Beta-adrenergic blockade may be required for the hyperthyroid phase, but propylthiouracil is of no value except to inhibit T_4 to T_3 conversion. Glucocorticoid is not required since there is no tenderness, but more rapid resolution of the hyperthyroidism has been reported in patients given a four-week course of prednisone starting at 40 mg per day. A hypothyroid phase should be treated for three to six months, followed by withdrawal of the therapy.

PROGNOSIS. The hyperthyroid phase usually remits within a few months, and the entire history of this disease lasts less than a year. However, the potential for subsequent hypothyroidism indicates the need for annual examination of thyroid function in these patients.

CHRONIC THYROIDITIS

There are two types of chronic thyroiditis: Hashimoto's and Riedel's thyroiditis *(Riedel's struma).*

Hashimoto's Thyroiditis

This is an apparently autoimmune disease of the thyroid gland. It appears to be closely related to Graves' disease. Synonyms for this condition are *chronic lymphocytic thyroiditis* and *lymphadenoid goiter*.

ETIOLOGY. The sera of patients with this condition contain antibodies to one or more thyroid antigens, including thyroid microsomes, thyroglobulin, or a colloid antigen which can be separated from thyroglobulin. At present it is not certain whether these antibodies are the cause or the result of this disease. The pathologic features of the condition can be reproduced in laboratory animals by immunization with thyroid tissue. However, the experimental disease is not sustained once immunizations have been discontinued, nor can the injury be induced by serum from immunized animals. Since the disease can be transferred by sensitized lymphocytes, it has been proposed that the destruction is produced by cell-mediated processes. On exposure to thyroid tissue antigens in vitro, lymphocytes of patients with Hashimoto's thyroiditis (and Graves' disease) will produce substances causing inhibition of leukocyte migration. This response is not found in patients with other forms of thyroid disease or by exposure to extracts of other tissues. Similar observations have been made in patients with idiopathic myxedema, suggesting that the atrophic thyroid found in this condition is affected by a similar process. Other evidence supporting the autoimmune hypothesis is the increased prevalence of many of the so-called autoimmune diseases in patients with Hashimoto's thyroiditis. These include Sjögren's syndrome, lupus erythematosus, idiopathic thrombocytopenic purpura, and pernicious anemia. As many as 6 per cent of patients with Hashimoto's disease have been reported to have pernicious anemia. Although rare, involvement of endocrine glands by this immunopathologic process may occur. Idiopathic Addison's disease and Hashimoto's disease may appear in the same patients. This combination is called Schmidt's syndrome (see Ch. 240). The parathyroids, the β cells of the pancreatic islets, the pituitary, and the gonads may also be involved. There are a few reports of transplacental passage of maternal thyroid antibodies leading to transient impairment of thyroid function in neonates, but such cases are the exception rather than the rule. An increased risk of the atrophic form of Hashimoto's thyroiditis is present in patients who are HLA-DR3 or HLA-B8 antigen positive.

INCIDENCE. Women are affected four to five times more frequently than men. The incidence increases with increasing age. Antimicrosomal thyroid antibodies have been found in about 10 per cent and 3 per cent of adult females and males, respectively. Ten to 20 per cent of these persons can be expected to have chemical or biochemical evidence of thyroid disease. This disease is probably the most common cause of goiter in adolescents, although the incidence is not as high as in older women.

PATHOLOGIC FINDINGS. The thyroid gland is normal or may be enlarged twofold to fivefold, depending on the degree of fibrosis. Microscopic examination reveals that varying degrees of infiltration with lymphocytes and plasma cells, fibrosis, and, in many cases, germinal centers are present. An oxyphilic change may be present in the cytoplasm of the residual thyroid follicular cells. It may be occasionally difficult to differentiate Hashimoto's disease from primary lymphoma of the thyroid gland.

CLINICAL MANIFESTATIONS. Two clinical forms of thyroid involvement are described. In the so-called atrophic form the gland is normal or reduced in size, and hypothyroidism is the prominent symptom (Table 228–9). This may well be the same syndrome as idiopathic myxedema. In other patients, variable degrees of thyroid enlargement and hypothyroidism occur, but goiter is the most common chief complaint. The gland is generally symmetrically enlarged, and often the pyramidal lobe is quite prominent, suggesting generalized hypertrophy. The thyroid is firm and may feel lobular or diffusely enlarged. Occasionally Hashimoto's disease presents as a single nodule in the thyroid gland, which represents the residual functioning thyroid tissue in a gland the remainder of which has been destroyed by this disease. The patient may have a family history of Graves' or Hashimoto's disease, pernicious anemia, or other autoimmune phenomena.

LABORATORY DIAGNOSIS. The serum free T_4 index is reduced and serum TSH elevated in many patients with this syndrome. Approximately 95 per cent of patients have positive antimicrosomal antibodies, and about 50 to 60 per cent are positive for antithyroglobulin antibodies. The PBI may be normal or elevated even in the presence of a reduced free T_4 index as a result of the presence of iodoproteins circulating in the blood. The RAI uptake may be reduced, normal, or even increased, depending on the residual thyroid cell function and the serum TSH. The thyroid scan generally reveals a heterogeneous uptake of the isotope. Occasionally a single island of functioning tissue remains. This can be differentiated from a functioning adenoma of the thyroid only by appropriate tests of thyroid function. If the diagnosis remains in doubt, a needle biopsy can be performed which will reveal the characteristic changes of lymphocytic infiltration in the majority of cases.

TREATMENT. In the early phases of Hashimoto's thyroiditis, goiter may be present, the serum TSH mildly elevated, but the free T_4 index in the lower normal range. Nevertheless, the presence of an elevated serum TSH suggests substantial decompensation of the thyroid, since in the presence of normally responsive thyroid tissue such TSH levels are quite stimulatory. Accordingly, even though the patient may have few symptoms of hypothyroidism, it is the author's practice to initiate treatment in the patient with thyroid enlargement once a secure serologic diagnosis has been established. In this way it is hoped that further thyroid enlargement and possibly surgery can be avoided. Untreated patients are also susceptible to iodide-induced myxedema and may have spontaneous fluctuation in thyroid function. Transient hypothyroidism has been noted, especially in the first few months after delivery, in women with Hashimoto's thyroiditis. More severe degrees of hypothyroidism are treated as described in the section, Hypothyroidism and Myxedema. If obstructive symptoms appear and they do not respond to TSH suppression, then surgery is required. Occasionally, the firm nature of the thyroid gland can suggest the presence of malignancy. If thyroid function is normal and there is no serologic evidence for Hashimoto's thyroiditis, then needle biopsy or surgery is required. In the younger patient, TSH suppression may cause the thyroid gland to decrease in size. On the other hand, in older subjects, particularly when fibrosis is present, little if any reduction will occur. Occasionally, Hashimoto's thyroiditis may present with hyperthyroidism ("hashitoxicosis"), which should be treated as is Graves' disease. Appropriate evaluation of the patient for the involvement of other tissues by autoimmune disease should be performed as indicated.

PROGNOSIS. The prognosis of this condition is excellent as long as thyroid hormone therapy is provided when indicated. In patients with serologic evidence of Hashimoto's thyroiditis but normal thyroid function, an annual evaluation for hypothyroidism is indicated.

Riedel's Thyroiditis

This is a rare disorder of unknown cause in which a sclerosing fibrous infiltration of the thyroid gland occurs, causing the gland to become extremely firm. As the disease progresses, local muscles in the neck and the trachea are infiltrated and hypothyroidism appears. This condition may be difficult to differentiate from carcinoma of the thyroid. It is clinically associated with both retroperitoneal fibrosis and sclerosing cholangitis. Obstruction of the trachea may occur as the fibrosis proceeds, and a surgical approach is the only satisfactory method of treatment to relieve tracheal obstruction. Glucocorticoid therapy can be beneficial to some patients.

Amino N, Mori H, Iwatani Y, Tanizawa O, Kawashima M, Tsuge I, Ibaragi K, Kumahara Y, Miyai K: High prevalence of transient post-partum thyrotoxicosis and hypothyroidism. N Engl J Med 306:14, 849–852, 1982. *A prospective survey showing a 5.5 per cent incidence of transient thyrotoxicosis or hypothyroidism post partum.*

Bartholomew LC, Cain JC, Woolner LB, et al.: Sclerosing cholangitis. Its possible association with Riedel's struma and fibrous retroperitonitis; report of two cases. N Engl J Med 269:8, 1973. *The clinical spectrum of this unusual form of thyroiditis is described.*

Nikolai TF, Brosseau J, Kettrick MA, Roberts R, Beltaos E: Lymphocytic thyroiditis with spontaneously resolving hyperthyroidism (silent thyroiditis). Arch Intern Med 140:478, 1980. *Clinical and laboratory results in 62 episodes of subacute lymphocytic thyroiditis, which these authors estimate is the cause of hyperthyroidism in 10 to 20 per cent of their patients.*

Strakosch CR, Wenzel BE, Row VV, Volpe R: Immunology of autoimmune thyroid diseases. Seminars in Medicine of the Beth Israel Hospital, Boston, N Engl J Med 307:24, 1499–1507, 1982.

Tunbridge WMG, Evered DC, Hall R, Appleton D, Brewis M, Clark F, Grimley-Evans J, Young E, Bird T, Smith PA: The spectrum of thyroid disease in a community: The Whickham survey. Clin Endocrinol 7:481, 1977. *The epidemiology of thyroid disease in an English community; this study provides a firm basis for estimates of the prevalence of Hashimoto's and Graves' disease as well as nodular goiter.*

Benign and Malignant Tumors of the Thyroid: The Solitary Thyroid Nodule

In this section are discussed those benign and malignant tumors that usually present as a solitary thyroid nodule. Multinodular goiter is discussed in the next section, Sporadic and Endemic Goiter. Virtually all tumors of the thyroid arise from glandular cells and are therefore adenomas or carcinomas. A scheme for evaluation of the patient with a solitary thyroid nodule is presented at the end of this chapter.

ETIOLOGY. The fundamental cause of thyroid tumors is unknown. However, two factors, exposure to ionizing radiation and the presence of TSH, have been found to be important for inducing thyroid tumors in animals. Similar data are available with respect to radiation exposure in man, which is responsible for an increased incidence of both benign and malignant thyroid neoplasms. A large proportion of patients presenting with thyroid carcinoma have a history of radiation delivered to the upper thorax 10 to 15 years earlier for treatment of "status thymolymphaticus," enlarged tonsils and adenoids, acne, eustachian tube dysfunction, facial hemangiomas, pertussis, and tinea capitis. In patients who receive at least 300 to 400 rads of thyroidal irradiation at less than five years of age, the incidence of thyroid carcinoma is approximately 6 per cent 10 to 20 years later. Benign thyroid tumors are about three to four times as prevalent in the same patients. For doses of external thyroid irradiation in this range, the expected incidence of carcinoma is three cases per rad per year per 1 million persons exposed. TSH stimulation per se does not appear to cause thyroid carcinoma, as this disease is not increased in areas of iodine deficiency; however, it plays a permissive role.

There are two types of familial thyroid carcinoma. The first is medullary carcinoma occurring in families with the syndrome of multiple endocrine neoplasia Type II (pheochromocytoma, parathyroid hyperplasia) or Type III (pheochromocytoma, mucosal neuroma) (Ch. 240). Papillary or follicular carcinoma may occur as part of the familial multiple hamartoma syndrome (Cowden's disease).

INCIDENCE AND PREVALENCE. Solitary thyroid nodules are common. The estimated incidence is about 1 to 3 per cent of the adult population, with a 2 to 1 preponderance of females. There is some difficulty in obtaining precise figures in this area, since a significant number of nodules which seem to be solitary by palpation are found to be dominant nodules in multinodular goiters at surgery or autopsy. Such nodules are rarely true neoplasms. The estimated incidence of thyroid nodules is 0.1 per cent per year, but since many nodules are found at autopsy that were not suspected clinically the true incidence may be higher. The incidence of thyroid carcinoma is estimated to be 36 new patients per year per 1 million persons. These two estimates would suggest that about 3 or 4 per cent of patients who develop solitary thyroid nodules have thyroid carcinoma. Many surgical series report thyroid carcinoma in from 10 to 30 per cent of resected solitary nodules, which indicates that the screening procedures employed to identify high risk patients are effective. Various autopsy series have reported an incidence of thyroid carcinoma ranging from 0.1 to 6 per cent. The higher figures are from studies in which an extremely careful search was made for microscopic carcinomas, virtually all being less than 5 mm in diameter. The clinical significance of such lesions is negligible, and this "background" of asymptomatic microscopic lesions should be kept in mind when evaluating this literature.

BENIGN NEOPLASMS

PATHOLOGY. The *follicular adenoma* is by far the most common benign thyroid tumor. It varies from microscopic to 8 to 10 cm in size and is composed of a normal-appearing thyroid epithelium arranged in a follicular structure. An intact capsule surrounds these tumors, and there is often evidence of compression of surrounding normal thyroid tissue. The follicles may range from extremely small with little colloid (*fetal adenoma* or *microfollicular adenoma*) to large distended structures (*macrofollicular adenoma*). The *embryonal* adenoma is an even more primitive-appearing structure possessing very little colloid. On occasion, the tumors may be composed of oxyphils (*oxyphil adenoma* or *Hürthle cell adenoma*). None of these differences in microscopic picture appear to bear on the functional characteristics of these nodules, nor do such nodules appear to become malignant. The hypercellular adenomas may be extremely difficult to differentiate from follicular carcinomas, especially when only a needle biopsy sample is available. Follicular adenomas have specific receptors for TSH, and these cells respond to TSH normally. However, many of these tumors do not possess the capacity for concentrating iodide or other similar substances. Since such nodules do not concentrate isotopes, they are referred to as *nonfunctioning* or *cold*.

CLINICAL MANIFESTATIONS. Thyroid adenomas fall into two categories: those that produce significant quantities of thyroid hormones, and those that do not. The latter are the more common (90 to 95 per cent). Patients with these tumors present with an asymptomatic mass in the neck. The patient may be discovered to have this tumor on routine physical examination and often is completely unaware of its existence. The tumor usually becomes palpable by the time it reaches 1 cm in diameter, but it may reach 5 to 10 cm without being noticed by the patient. Thyroid function studies in patients with nonfunctioning follicular adenomas are normal, and the thyroid scan will generally reveal an area of decreased or absent uptake of $^{123}I^-$ or $^{99m}TcO_4^-$ (a "cold" nodule). The precise diagnosis can be made only by obtaining a tissue specimen by aspiration biopsy, cutting needle biopsy (Vim-Silverman needle or its equivalent), or excision of the nodule. As these nodules may outgrow their blood supply, cystic degeneration may occur. Ultrasonography of such a lesion will reveal a cystic cavity within the nodule.

Functioning follicular adenomas may present with or without symptoms of hyperthyroidism, largely depending on their size. Lesions over 3 cm in diameter tend to cause thyrotoxicity and constitute about 50 per cent of these adenomas in patients 60 years and older. T_3 thyrotoxicosis was found in 46 per cent of such patients in one large series. More commonly, the patient is asymptomatic and a thyroid scan shows that the only area concentrating radioactivity is the nodule itself. Such patients generally have normal or high-normal serum thyroid hormone levels, and TRH infusion will not cause TSH release. Such nodules are functioning autonomously at a rate sufficient to suppress TSH synthesis in the pituitary (hence the lack of function in the remainder of the thyroid) but not at a sufficiently high level as to cause metabolic hyperthyroidism. It is the author's practice to categorize functional lesions which have suppressed TSH synthesis but not caused hyperthyroidism as *warm* nodules, whereas those associated with hyperthyroidism are called *hot* nodules. Assessment of the thyroid functional state is necessary for proper evaluation of these lesions since the thyroid scan is identical. This is especially important since Hashimoto's disease may present as a solitary focus of functioning thyroid tissue, as may congenital absence of one lobe of the thyroid. The presence of potentially functioning thyroid tissue can be demonstrated by injection of 10 units of bovine TSH, followed in 24 hours by a thyroid scan. Unlike multinodular goiters, follicular adenomas of the thyroid rarely grow large enough to cause significant physical encroachment on the trachea or esophagus.

TREATMENT. The finding of an autonomously functioning nodule virtually eliminates the diagnosis of thyroid carcinoma. Treatment at that point depends on the thyroid status. If the patient is euthyroid (a warm thyroid nodule), nothing more than an annual follow-up with appropriate thyroid function tests (including a serum T_3) need be performed. In the hyperthyroid patient, surgery or ^{131}I is available for definitive treatment, although antithyroid drugs may be necessary to control symptomatic hyperthyroidism prior to definitive therapy. The choice of treatment depends on the age of the patient and the size of the nodule. In patients under the age of 20, surgical resection should be performed, as the radiation delivered to extranodular tissue after radioiodine therapy may reach a level which is considered carcinogenic. In older patients with cosmetically disfiguring lesions or those which are compressing vital structures in the neck, surgery is also preferred. For the rest, ^{131}I is indicated. The author attempts to deliver 10 mCi of ^{131}I into the nodule. Following either surgery or radioactive iodine treatment, a period of four to six weeks is required for re-establishment of pituitary TSH secretion, following which function of the previously suppressed normal thyroid tissue should occur. The patient may need to receive thyroxine supplementation during this interim period but may not require indefinite replacement. The approach to the *nonfunctioning thyroid nodule* is described below under The Solitary Nodule.

MALIGNANT THYROID TUMORS

There are four common malignancies of thyroid tissue. About 50 per cent of thyroid carcinomas are pure papillary or mixed papillary-follicular carcinoma, 25 per cent follicular carcinoma, 15 per cent undifferentiated carcinoma, and 10 per cent medullary carcinoma. The last-named disorder is a tumor of the thyrocalcitonin-producing C cells and has no relationship to thyroid follicular epithelium.

PATHOLOGY AND NATURAL HISTORY. *Papillary carcinoma* is the most benign and the most common form of thyroid carcinoma. It is two to three times more common in women than in men and occurs with equal frequency in the third to seventh decades. Since the less well-differentiated forms of carcinoma increase with age, papillary carcinoma is the most common thyroid malignancy in younger patients. The size of these tumors varies from microscopic to several centimeters in diameter. Of the clinically apparent variety, the *occult* tumors (defined as those less than 1.5 cm in diameter) are differentiated from the *intrathyroidal* tumors, which are larger but do not extend through the thyroid surface. The tumor is classified as *extrathyroidal* if it extends through the thyroid capsule and involves surrounding tissues. Microscopically, papillary carcinoma consists of well-differentiated thyroid epithelium covering papillary fibrovascular stalks. The nuclei are frequently clear, as opposed to the denser appearance of normal nuclei. A virtually pathognomonic feature in about 40 per cent of papillary thyroid carcinomas is the so-called *psammoma body*. These calcific globules are 5 to 100 microns in diameter and are often present in the tips of the papillary projections. Their etiology is unknown, but their presence in the thyroid tumor raises the high likelihood of its carcinomatous nature. Cervical lymphatic involvement even with occult thyroid tumors is common, occurring in as many as 50 per cent. Blood-borne metastases are uncommon. The presence or absence of lymph node metastases does not seem to alter the prognosis. In a large series studied at the Mayo Clinic, the 20-year survival of patients with occult or intrathyroid papillary carcinoma was not significantly different from that of a control group. However, the 20-year survival for patients with extrathyroidal carcinoma was about 40 per cent, and this dropped to 20 per cent over the next ten years. Many thyroid cancers have areas of follicular as well as papillary structure, and blood-borne metastases may appear which have a follicular pattern even though the primary tumor is papillary. Thus, many predominantly papillary tumors have follicular elements, but the biologic behavior of these lesions seems to be a function of the predominant microscopic appearance.

Follicular carcinomas also are more common in women than in men but tend to increase in incidence with increasing age.

The tumors vary from well-differentiated, virtually normal appearing thyroid tissue to nearly solid sheets of follicular epithelium with little evidence of follicle formation. The former are differentiated from follicular adenomas only by demonstration of capsular and vascular invasion. Such a diagnosis generally cannot be made without the entire nodule for examination, and even at frozen section the carcinomatous nature of the lesion may not be recognized. Cyst formation may occur as it does in benign follicular tumors, and calcification may occur centrally. Follicular carcinomas tend to metastasize via blood vessel invasion and not, in general, via lymphatics. Metastases may not be evident at the time of initial evaluation but may appear years later despite apparent complete excision of the tumor. It is not unusual for the follicular carcinoma to concentrate radioiodine, although it does so considerably less well than does normal thyroid tissue. Thus, it is only in the absence of normal thyroid tissue and in the presence of an elevated TSH that this potential is appreciated. However, it is useful in treatment in some of these tumors (see below). Patients who have had removal of well-encapsulated, noninvasive follicular carcinomas appear to have a normal life span. On the other hand, patients with tumors which show extensive local involvement and angioinvasion at the time of initial surgery have an approximately 30 per cent ten-year survival, which is decreased to less than 20 per cent at 20 years.

The most aggressive form of thyroid carcinoma, *anaplastic carcinoma,* may appear in either small cell or giant cell varieties. The small cell carcinoma may resemble a lymphoma. The cells have a uniform appearance, often having a fibrous stroma but no amyloid. The giant-cell variety, also called a spindle-cell or carcinosarcoma, is the most highly malignant tumor of the thyroid gland. It is found almost exclusively in patients over the age of 60. The average prognosis from diagnosis to death in the giant cell tumors is less than six months, whereas patients with small cell carcinoma may have five-year survival of 20 to 25 per cent. Both tend to extend locally and often cause tracheal obstruction. Distant metastases may occur with either type.

Medullary carcinoma of the thyroid is a malignant tumor of the C cell and produces thyrocalcitonin. Its occurrence in association with multiple endocrine neoplasia syndromes has been mentioned. It may also occur spontaneously. These tumors are characterized by sheets of tumor cells separated by a hyaline-amyloid–containing stroma. The amyloid is formed by the tumor cells and deposited in the stroma. The tumors may also produce ACTH, prostaglandin, or carcinoembryonic antigen. In familial syndromes, the penetrance of this tumor is complete, so that screening of family members is indicated by use of calcium and/or pentagastrin infusions to stimulate thyrocalcitonin release from pathologic cells (see Ch. 247).

CLINICAL MANIFESTATIONS AND DIAGNOSIS OF THYROID CARCINOMA—THE SOLITARY NODULE. The approach to the patient with a solitary thyroid nodule is a matter of considerable disagreement among clinicians. For some, thyroid carcinoma is sufficiently serious to require a surgical approach to all potentially carcinomatous lesions; others feel that considerable selection should be used prior to surgery. The benign nature of the common forms of thyroid carcinoma and the relatively large number of benign nodules make a conservative approach rational. There are several clinical characteristics which dictate an open surgical approach to a nonfunctioning thyroid nodule. This includes a history of prior irradiation. Nodules in such patients carry a 20 to 25 per cent risk of carcinoma. A history of rapid growth, evidence of recurrent nerve paresis, obvious involvement of lymph nodes, or fixation of the nodule to surrounding tissues should also lead to serious consideration of immediate surgery. Statistically, the risk of a solitary cold nodule being malignant is higher in a male than in a female, since benign disease of the thyroid is much more common in females. Thyroid nodules in children are more likely to be carcinoma than those in adults.

In the absence of specific signs pointing to a diagnosis of thyroid carcinoma, there are two avenues of approach (Fig. 228–9*A* and 9*B*). If there is no obvious thyroid dysfunction (either hyperthyroidism or hypothyroidism) and an experienced cytopathologist is available, a needle aspiration can be performed (Fig. 228–9*A*). If the lesion is a simple cyst this will be curative; otherwise the cytologic report guides therapy. If carcinoma is found, then surgical exploration is indicated. If a cellular follicular aspirate is obtained that is consistent with a benign or a malignant lesion, then a ^{123}I (or ^{131}I) scan is performed. If the lesion is hypofunctional, again surgical exploration is advised. If it is warm or hot, then management is as discussed earlier under autonomous nodules. If the aspirate is benign, thyroxine replacement is given and the patient followed at six-month intervals. The need for surgery is then determined by the natural history of the individual case. Much experience with aspiration biopsy cytology has shown that false-positive results are very rare, and false-negative results, that is, a benign diagnosis in a patient with a malignant lesion, should occur in only 2 to 3 per cent of patients. This figure, however, may be higher during the early experience with this technique in a given center. In most clinics, aspiration cytology has reduced the apparent need for surgical exploration by 50 to 60 per cent. In other words, approximately 40 per cent of patients with solitary nodules will require surgical exploration because of frankly or suspiciously malignant lesions.

If a trained cytopathologist is not available, then a thyroid scan is performed followed by ultrasonography if the nodule is not hyperfunctioning (Fig. 228–9*B*). Rarely a malignant nodule will be warm by $^{99m}TcO_4^-$ but cold by iodine scan. This should be suspected and tested for when warm lesions do not suppress function in the remainder of the gland. Ultrasonography of hypofunctioning nodules is performed. A cystic lesion can be treated by aspiration and the procedure repeated twice more if the fluid reaccumulates before surgery is indicated. In the nonfunctioning solid nodule, needle aspiration cytology, cutting needle biopsy, or surgical exploration is advised. The author recommends surgical excision for patients under 20, for all males, and for those high risk patients with familial carcinoma and radiation exposure. The availability of experienced thyroid surgeons plays an important role in this approach, since serious morbidity attends inadvertent resection of the parathyroid glands or recurrent laryngeal nerve paresis. In older women and men in whom other illnesses make surgery less desirable, a diagnosis may be obtained by needle biopsy or aspiration cytology.

If these techniques are not available, the patient may be given a trial of thyroxine replacement for a period of three to six months and any change in the size of the nodule noted. Continuing enlargement in the presence of TSH suppression is an indication for surgical intervention or at least a biopsy, whereas reduction of the nodule size, although rare, is gratifying. Maintenance of the same nodule size usually justifies a continued conservative approach. If needle biopsy confirms a benign lesion, then thyroxine suppression is provided and surgery employed only if the nodule becomes physically symptomatic. Patients who have had a lobectomy should receive thyroxine replacement. The prognosis of these lesions is excellent with no evidence of malignant degeneration.

A frozen section should be performed on all solitary thyroid nodules and an attempt made to provide definitive treatment at the time of initial surgery. A reasonable approach to intrathyroidal papillary carcinoma is to perform a lobectomy with isthmectomy and explore for and remove any involved lymph nodes. An examination of the other lobe should be made for tumor, but, except in the irradiated patient, bilateral lobectomy is not required. With extrathyroidal extension of papillary carcinoma and bilateral lymph node metastases, a total thyroidectomy is performed with great care to preserve the recurrent laryngeal nerves and parathyroid glands. A follicular carcinoma is approached as are the papillary lesions, with the exception that the presence of distant lymph node metastases or extensive capsular and vascular invasion in the initial frozen section

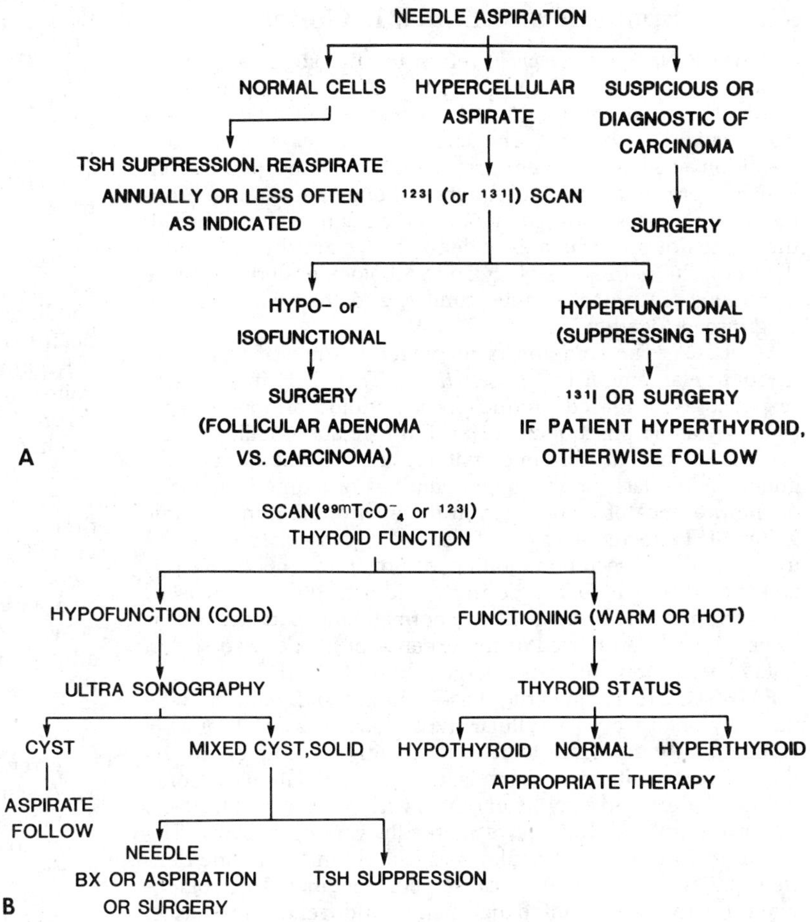

Figure 228–9. Panel *A* shows a schema for the diagnostic evaluation of a patient with a solitary thyroid nodule based on aspiration biopsy cytology. Panel *B* presents an alternative solution to the same problem starting with a thyroid scintiscan.

should lead to consideration of bilateral thyroidectomy. This is done to remove residual normal tissue to facilitate radioiodine therapy (see below). Radical neck dissection does not offer any advantage over the less-mutilating procedures described above. Medullary carcinoma of the sporadic variety may be treated as papillary carcinoma, but the familial form requires bilateral lobectomy. It is, of course, important to determine that pheochromocytoma and hyperparathyroidism are not present before undertaking surgery. Anaplastic carcinoma is rarely restricted enough to lend itself to surgical therapy with the exception of palliation to prevent tracheal compression.

RADIATION THERAPY. I^- may be concentrated to a sufficient degree as to be useful by as many as 50 to 60 per cent of well-differentiated thyroid tumors. This can be demonstrated only after the establishment of hypothyroidism with an elevation of serum TSH. In general, prophylactic therapy with radioiodine in patients with papillary carcinoma does not appear to be beneficial, although metastases may respond to this modality. In follicular carcinoma with evidence of vascular invasion or in patients with follicular metastases, particularly to the lungs, significant amelioration of symptoms and dramatic changes in the x-ray picture may be associated with this therapy. It does not appear to be as useful for patients with bone metastases. To be weighed against these beneficial effects is the increased incidence of leukemia in patients treated with large doses of ^{131}I (300 mCi and more).

The usual approach to evaluation of the feasibility of this therapeutic modality is to remove residual functioning thyroid tissue surgically or by ^{131}I administration. After this, the patient is switched to triiodothyronine (50 μg per day) for a period of approximately three weeks, following which the hormone is discontinued. Within two to three weeks, most patients will show the maximal uptake in metastatic tissue. At that time, a tracer dose of ^{131}I should be given with appropriate dosimetry of the tumor mass, bone marrow, and lungs. Following this, the maximal tolerable ^{131}I dose should be given and the patient started on TSH-suppressive therapy with thyroxine one day later. Local recurrences of papillary carcinoma can often be treated surgically by removal of involved lymph nodes. In such patients this is preferable to ^{131}I, which should be reserved for a nonresectable lesion.

Despite the poor function of thyroid tumors in terms of radioiodine trapping, carcinomatous thyroid cells have TSH receptors and respond to TSH in vitro. Accordingly, considerable effort should be made to suppress TSH to undetectable levels. A useful technique for verification that this has occurred is to perform a TRH stimulation test periodically. There should be no response. In patients who have had total thyroidectomy, serum thyroglobulin measurements may be a useful parameter of recurrence and activity of the tumor tissue.

Favus NJ, Schneider AB, Stachura ME, Arnold JE, Ryo UY, Pinsky SM, Colman M, Arnold MJ, Frohman LA: Thyroid cancer occurring as a late consequence of head and neck irradiation. N Engl J Med 294:1019, 1976. *Evaluation of roughly 1000 patients who received tonsillar or pharyngeal irradiation in childhood. The data demonstrate the increased prevalence of thyroid carcinoma in this group.*

Kaplan MM, Garnick MB, Gelber R, Li FP, Cassady JR, Sallan SE, Fine WE, Sack MJ: Risk factors for thyroid abnormalities after neck irradiation for childhood cancer. Am J Med 74:272–280, 1983. *This study shows that both benign and malignant thyroid nodules, as well as hypothyroidism, may appear 5 to 35 years after therapeutic irradiation to the neck.*

Lowhagen T, Granberg PO, Lundell G, Skinnari P, Sundblad R, Willems JS: Aspiration biopsy cytology (ABC) in nodules of the thyroid gland suspected to be malignant. Surg Clin North Am 59:3–18, 1979. *A study of the correlation between surgical and aspiration biopsy cytology diagnoses in more than 400 patients with solitary thyroid nodules.*

Mazzaferri EL, Young RL: Papillary thyroid carcinoma: A 10 year follow-up report of the impact of therapy in 576 patients. Am J Med 70:511–518, 1981. *An update of a large retrospective evaluation of the results of various treatment modalities in patients with well-differentiated thyroid carcinoma.*

Van Herle AJ, Rich P, Ljung, BME, Ashcraft MW, Solomon DH, Keeler EB: The thyroid nodule. Ann Intern Med 96:221–232, 1982. *A critical evaluation of the various approaches that can be used for patients with thyroid nodules.*

Sporadic and Endemic Goiter

DEFINITION. *Sporadic goiter* refers to thyroid enlargement, which is found in a relatively small fraction of a given population. The cause for the thyroid enlargement may be different from patient to patient. The term *endemic goiter* refers to a condition seen in a much larger fraction of the population, which is presumably a consequence of one or several environmental influences, most commonly iodine deficiency. Although the causes of sporadic and endemic goiter are, by definition, different, the pathophysiology and pathology underlying these conditions are probably quite similar, and they will therefore be grouped together.

ETIOLOGY. The common factor which is thought to lead to thyroid enlargement is *hypersecretion of TSH.* TSH increases in response to decreased production of thyroid hormones, especially T_4, as a consequence of an intrinsic abnormality in the process of thyroid hormone synthesis in the case of sporadic goiter, or the lack of adequate quantities of iodine in the diet or the presence of a goitrogen in the environment in endemic goiter. TSH increases as T_4 falls. As a consequence of the increased TSH secretion, iodine turnover by the thyroid is accelerated, the T_3 to T_4 ratio in thyroid secretion is increased, and serum T_3 may remain entirely normal. Such patients appear to be clinically euthyroid at the expense of an elevated serum TSH concentration and an enlarged thyroid gland.

PATHOLOGY. In the early phases, the thyroid gland may be diffusely enlarged with cellular hyperplasia as a result of TSH stimulation. Later, large follicles form with low epithelium. As the process continues, there is further stimulation of some thyroidal areas and atrophy of others with concomitant fibrosis. These multiple nodules have markedly varying activity. The accumulation of thyroglobulin, particularly in the iodine-deficient patients, may occur because poorly iodinated thyroglobulin is relatively resistant to digestion by endogenous proteases. To some extent, the same phenomenon may be occurring in the multinodular goiters which are sporadic and in which a specific cause has not been identified.

SPORADIC GOITER

Sporadic goiter affects about 5 per cent of the population in the United States. Females outnumber males by a 3:1 ratio. In some patients an enzymatic defect in one of the steps in thyroid hormone synthesis can be identified (see Fig. 228–2). However, in most patients no specific cause can be isolated, but it is possible that milder forms of similar enzymatic deficiencies may be present.

CONGENITAL GOITER. This condition is sometimes referred to as *sporadic cretinism.* This term refers to the syndrome of infantile myxedema characterized by growth failure, mental retardation, diffuse myxedema, and many of the signs and symptoms of hypothyroidism outlined in the section Hypothyroidism and Myxedema. Goitrous hypothyroidism can be due to a defect in any of the steps leading to the formation of thyroid hormone synthesis already discussed in the Introduction. Defects have been identified in (1) iodide transport; (2) organification of iodide due to reduction in or absence of peroxidase, to an abnormal enzyme, or to diminished peroxide generation; (3) synthesis of an abnormal thyroglobulin molecule; (4) a structural abnormality in peroxidase, impairing its function as an iodine acceptor; (5) abnormal interrelationships of iodotyrosine; (6) impaired thyroglobulin proteolysis; and, lastly, (7) a defect in iodotyrosine deiodination. The numbers given refer to the specific steps shown in Fig. 228–2. In some disorders of thyroglobulin synthesis the formation of an iodinated albumin-like protein has been described. All of these defects are rare. In North America and Europe, they constitute less than 10 per cent of the approximately 1 in 4000 infants with congenital hypothyroidism.

A detailed description of each of these various defects is beyond the scope of this general text. The most common defect is the inability to organify iodine. (defects in steps 2, 3, or 4). Such patients accumulate large amounts of I^- in the thyroid. This can be demonstrated by performance of a *perchlorate* (ClO_4^-) *discharge test.* If organification of I^- is defective, it is only the I^- trapping mechanism which keeps I^- in the thyroid cell. The ClO_4^- ion is concentrated by the same mechanism as is I^-, and in large quantities it will completely block the I^- trap. Therefore, if 500 mg of $NaClO_4$ is given one to two hours after tracer I^-, a marked decrease in thyroidal radioactivity will occur as the trapped I^- leaves the thyroid. In normal persons there will be no change in this parameter, since the tracer I^- has already been incorporated into protein. In some patients this condition has been found in association with eighth nerve deafness and has the eponym *Pendred's syndrome.*

Regardless of the specific defect, these patients present with goiter and hypothyroidism, the serum T_4 index is reduced, and serum TSH is elevated. Further evaluation for the type of biochemical defect requires careful laboratory investigation. The treatment of such patients is with exogenous thyroid hormone. Thyroxine treatment will cause regression of the enlarged thyroid, and mental retardation may be ameliorated or prevented if treatment is started before three months of age. Genetic counseling is desirable so that these patients will be aware of the risk of hypothyroidism in subsequent offspring.

MULTINODULAR GOITER IN THE ADULT. The hypothesis that adults with multinodular goiter have mild defects in thyroid hormone synthesis similar to the more complete forms found in infants remains to be proved. If this is the case, then the goiter could be explained by modest increases in TSH, which is secreted by the pituitary in response to the reduced serum T_4. A significant physiologic increase in TSH may be as little as 2 to 3 μU per milliliter, often below the sensitivity of the TSH immunoassay which is clinically available. The compensatory increase in the size of the thyroid gland under these circumstances results in adequate rates of thyroid hormone formation, so that the vast majority of patients with this abnormality are euthyroid.

CLINICAL MANIFESTATIONS. Patients with multinodular goiter may come to the physician because of respiratory obstruction or dysphagia. More often, the patient is asymptomatic and the enlarged multinodular thyroid is discovered on a routine physical examination. Such patients should be questioned carefully for symptoms of respiratory obstruction. The goiter often extends retrosternally; this may be demonstrated by having the patient extend the arms directly over the head. If a significant substernal goiter is present, jugular venous distention and suffusion of the face occurs *(Pemberton's sign).* Aside from physical obstruction, the most significant clinical aspect of the multinodular goiter is the tendency for hyperthyroidism to develop late in life *(Plummer's disease).* It is postulated that after decades of stimulation by TSH one or more of the nodular hyperplastic areas become autonomous. Since this condition generally appears in the elderly patient, the resulting hyperthyroidism may be of the apathetic variety (see the section Graves' Disease and Other Causes of Hyperthyroidism). In one series, administration of 50 to 100 mg of KI per day to eight patients with multinodular goiter resulted in hyperthyroidism in four patients, which required definitive treatment. The etiology of this form of iodide-induced thyrotoxicosis (probably not Jod-Basedow) is not clear, but caution is needed in administration of iodides to patients with multinodular goiter.

LABORATORY DIAGNOSIS. The physician must investigate both the anatomic and the functional nature of the thyroid pathology. Anatomic information is gained predominantly by chest and esophageal radiography and by scintiscan. ^{131}I is recommended for thyroid scanning of these patients since the γ rays emitted by $^{99m}TcO_4^-$ and $^{123}I^-$ may not be strong enough to penetrate the sternum. The scintiscan image shows patchy focal uptake of radioactivity in an enlarged thyroid gland. The significance of the nonfunctioning areas in such scintiscans is discussed below. Measurements of serum free T_4 index, T_3, TSH, and antimicrosomal and antithyroglobulin antibodies should be obtained, expecially since Hashimoto's thyroiditis may present as a multinodular goiter. A TRH test is indicated if Plummer's disease is suspected.

TREATMENT. The proper treatment depends on the clinical manifestations in the individual patient. Hyperthyroidism associated with multinodular goiter is best treated with radioactive iodine. However, because of the heterogeneity of the tissue uptake of radioiodine, a larger dose of radioiodine will be necessary (180 μCi per gram) or 10 mCi in a typical gland. The not uncommon coexistence of cardiac or pulmonary disease in this age group, together with the large size of the thyroid gland and the possibility of radiation thyroiditis, has led the author to pretreat most elderly hyperthyroid patients with antithyroid drugs prior to radiotherapy. The antithyroid drugs are discontinued approximately four to five days prior to treatment. If a high plasma I^- (low RAI uptake) does not permit the use of radioiodine, then surgical treatment must be undertaken after appropriate preparation with antithyroid drugs.

Hypothyroid patients require treatment with thyroxine as described in the section Hypothyroidism and Myxedema. Young euthyroid patients with diffuse thyroid enlargement may be started on thyroxine replacement therapy to suppress TSH, particularly if this is slightly elevated. One may block further thyroid enlargement by this treatment as well as cause regression of goiter in some. In patients over the age of 40, it is unlikely that a significant amelioration in physical symptoms will occur with TSH suppression, but this hormone may be administered on a trial basis. Great care must be exercised, particularly in the elderly, since one or more of the hyperplastic thyroid nodules may be functioning autonomously. In such circumstances, well-meaning attempts to suppress TSH can cause iatrogenic hyperthyroidism. If physical symptoms of obstruction are present or there is evidence of recurrent laryngeal nerve dysfunction, then surgical treatment is generally in order.

The Multinodular Goiter and Thyroid Carcinoma. Nodular disease of the thyroid is common and thyroid carcinoma is relatively rare. Poorly functioning areas may be present in the thyroid scintiscans of multinodular goiters, but this is not an indication for surgery for malignant disease. As heterogeneity of function is the rule, other criteria must be employed for recognition of malignancy in the multinodular goiter. Factors which raise this possibility include previous exposure to therapeutic thyroidal irradiation in childhood, a family history of thyroid carcinoma or enlargement of cervical lymph nodes, recurrent laryngeal nerve palsy, or the continuing enlargement of a single "cold" nodule in an otherwise stable gland. In situations in which doubt exists, needle biopsy may provide the requisite microscopic diagnosis to reassure the patient and the physician that conservative therapy is the appropriate course of action.

PROGNOSIS. Patients with euthyroid multinodular goiter should have thyroid function and physical findings evaluated at annual intervals. Most do not require surgery.

ENDEMIC GOITER

Iodine deficiency is the most common cause of thyroid disease in the world population, although iodination of salt has eliminated this problem in North America. Areas in which iodine intake remains low include mountainous regions such as the Andes and Himalayas. In addition, there are areas of endemic goiter in Central Africa, New Guinea, and Indonesia. Iodine prophylaxis, either in foodstuffs or in the form of iodized oil injection, has been successful in many of these countries, but iodine deficiency remains a considerable public health problem. In a few geographical locations, ingestion of a goitrogen has been implicated in the high incidence of goiter. Examples include a thiocyanate derivative from the cassava, which is eaten in large quantities in central Africa, and a goitrogenic hydrocarbon found in the water supply in parts of Colombia and in Chile.

CLINICAL MANIFESTATIONS IN ADULTS. The minimal quantity of iodine required for normal thyroid function is approximately 100 μg per day. As the level of iodine in the diet decreases below this level, there is a progressive fall in serum T_4 and a progressive rise in serum TSH. Serum T_3 concentrations remain normal or slightly elevated, a persistently elevated TSH being required for this compensation. Serum TSH concentrations may exceed 100 μU per milliliter. In the presence of lifelong stimulation of this degree, enormous hypertrophy and hyperplasia of the thyroid gland can occur. Such glands may weigh 1 to 5 kg, producing considerable physical impairment.

EFFECTS OF IODINE DEFICIENCY IN INFANTS. In areas of endemic goiter, cretinism is not uncommon. Despite the capacity of the placenta to transport I^-, in areas where iodine intake is severely reduced (25 μg per day or less) the 24-hour maternal RAI uptake is virtually 100 per cent. Infants in these areas may be born with congenital hypothyroidism as a consequence of iodine deficiency. The central nervous system may obtain a considerable portion of intracellular T_3 via conversion of T_4 to T_3 within this tissue rather than from the circulating T_3 in the serum. Although a normal serum T_3 may provide adequate levels of intracellular T_3 to tissues such as the muscles, liver, and kidney, the central nervous system, like the pituitary gland, may not be replete if T_4 is reduced and serum T_3 normal.

In areas such as the Andes or New Guinea where iodine intake may be less than 20 μg per day, a different form of *endemic cretinism* may be seen. As opposed to dwarfism and mental retardation, some children in these areas have spastic diplegia, squint, and deafness. The etiology of this syndrome is still not clarified. It may be a manifestation of the effect of iodine deficiency per se on the embryologic development of the central nervous system. Fetal or maternal hypothyroidism as a consequence of severe iodine deficiency may also contribute to this problem.

TREATMENT. The treatment of iodine deficiency is to supply this element either as a food additive or by direct injections of iodinated oil. This has often been difficult because of the inaccessibility and restricted governmental resources of those countries in which iodine deficiency is a problem. The *Jod-Basedow phenomenon* (iodine-induced hyperthyroidism) will occur in some patients receiving iodine supplementation. These presumably are individual patients with underlying Graves' (Basedow's) disease who are suddenly given adequate supplies of the substrate for thyroid hormone synthesis.

Lever EG, Medeiros-Neto GA, DeGroot LJ: Inherited disorders of thyroid metabolism. Endocr Rev 4:213–239, 1983. *A modern comprehensive review of this topic.*

Stanbury JB, Dumont JE: Familial goiter and related disorders. *In* Stanbury JB, Wyngaarden JB, Fredrickson DS, Goldstein JG, Brown MS (eds.): The Metabolic Basis of Inherited Disease. 5th ed. New York, McGraw-Hill Book Company, 1983, pp. 231–269. *A thorough review of the literature in this area with 327 references. The emphasis is on the emzymology of pathogenesis.*

Stanbury JB, Hetzel BS (eds.): Endemic goiter and endemic cretinism. New York, John Wiley & Sons, 1980. *A detailed discussion of the current state of this worldwide problem by many authorities.*

Thilly CH, Delange F, Lagasse R, Bourdoux P, Ramioul L, Berquist H, Ermans AM: Fetal hypothyroidism and maternal thyroid status in severe endemic goiter. J Clin Endocrinol Metab 47:354, 1978. *The effects of iodine deficiency on mother and newborn are described, comparing treated and untreated patients.*

Wolff J: Congenital goiter with defective iodide transport. Endocr Rev 4:240–254, 1983. *The clinical, pathophysiological and biochemical findings in patients with this form of sporadic goiter.*

229. DISORDERS OF THE ADRENAL CORTEX

J. Blake Tyrrell and John D. Baxter

Structure and Development of the Adrenal Cortex

John D. Baxter

The major function of the adrenal cortex is to provide glucocorticoid and mineralocorticoid hormones, of which cortisol and aldosterone, respectively, are the most important in man. The glucocorticoids, named for their carbohydrate-regulating properties, are essential for survival, at least in times of stress, and regulate intermediary metabolism, hemodynamic functions, and developmental processes. The mineralocorticoids regulate sodium, potassium, and hydrogen ion balance, and secondarily affect the blood pressure. Either an excess or deficiency of these steroids can have deleterious effects. Glucocorticoid excess and deficiency are termed Cushing's syndrome and Addison's disease, respectively. Aldosterone excess and deficiency are referred to as aldosteronism and hypoaldosteronism, respectively. Whereas diseases of the adrenal cortex are relatively uncommon, their clinical stigmata are part of the differential diagnosis of common problems. In addition, iatrogenic glucocorticoid excess is a common clinical problem due to the widespread usage of glucocorticoids in therapy. Secondary hyperaldosteronism is also a common problem requiring antimineralocorticoid therapy.

In addition to these two steroids the human adrenal cortex produces at least 50 other steroids. This gland is a major source of androgenic steroids in the female (Ch. 236), although in the male (Ch. 234) the importance of androgens produced by the adrenal is trivial compared to those produced by the testes. The adrenal produces only minute quantities of estrogens and progestins. Some of these steroids ordinarily produced in physiologically insignificant quantities can result in clinical abnormalities when they are produced in excess in certain pathologic states.

STRUCTURE. There are two adrenal glands, located extraperitoneally at the upper poles of each kidney lateral to the eleventh thoracic to first lumbar vertebrae. The right gland tends to be higher and more lateral than the left. The average gland weighs 4 grams and is 2 to 3 cm wide and 4 to 6 cm long. A series of small arteries arising from the abdominal aorta, renal and phrenic arteries, and occasionally from ovarian or spermatic arteries, feed the gland. Because of this, arterial infarction is unusual. The venous drainage of the gland on the left is ordinarily into the renal vein and on the right into the inferior vena cava. The gland is innervated by autonomic fibers whose roles in regulation are not understood.

The adrenal cortex comprises about 90 per cent of the gland and surrounds the centrally located medulla that produces catecholamines. The cortex has three zones. The zona glomerulosa, about 15 per cent of the cortex, is ill defined and present in foci under the capsule, contains cells with a small cytoplasmic volume and lipid content, and produces aldosterone. The remainder of the cortex, the zonae reticularis and fasciculata, can be considered as a single unit involved predominantly in cortisol and androgen production. Cells of the zona fasciculata, about 25 per cent of the cortex, appear vacuolated or clear on stained sections because of their high cholesterol content. By contrast, cells of the inner zone, the zona reticularis, are more compact with less lipid, and are responsible for basal cortisol production.

The morphology of the gland can be influenced by ACTH, angiotensin II, and potassium. Elevations of ACTH levels increase adrenal blood flow within minutes and combined weight within hours; the clear fasciculata cells lose their fat, attain the compact morphology and ultrastructural features of reticularis cells, and produce cortisol. With prolonged stimulation there is hyperplasia and hypertrophy that can double the adrenal weight. Similar increases in angiotensin II and potassium result in hypertrophy and hyperplasia of the glomerulosa cells and increased aldosterone production. With deficiency of angiotensin II there is atrophy of the zona glomerulosa and with deficiency of ACTH there is atrophy of the zonae fasciculata-reticularis; this is reversible upon restimulation. Occasionally, accessory adrenal glands may be present in a variety of locations in the abdomen or pelvis and can assume significant function in states of ACTH excess.

DEVELOPMENT. The adrenal cortex is derived from mesenchymal tissue. Cortical cells emerge to form a primitive fetal cortex around the sixth week of development. This then evolves into a fetal zone that is involved predominantly in the synthesis of androgen and estrogen precursors, and a definitive zone destined to become the adult gland. The fetal zone constitutes the major bulk of the adrenal cortex at birth; it begins to recede by the last intrauterine month and disappears around the end of the first year. The permanent cortex is formed from cells of the outer portion of the fetal gland and is not developed completely until around 3 years of age.

Synthesis, Circulation, and Metabolism of Adrenal Steroids

John D. Baxter

SYNTHESIS

The structures and steps in biosynthesis of a number of steroid hormones are shown in Figure 229–1. The letter designation for the carbon rings and the number designation of the carbon atoms are shown for pregnenolone, a key biosynthetic intermediate. α- and β- are used to designate the positions of the side groups above (β) or below (α) the plane of the molecule. The various steroids differ in the saturation of the A ring; hydroxyl and ketone groups at positions 3, 11, 17, and 21; the presence of a 3-carbon side chain at position 17; and an aldehyde group at position 18. Since the chemical nomenclature is cumbersome, trivial names for the steroids are most frequently used.

All steroids are derived from cholesterol that is either synthesized by the gland or obtained from the plasma lipoproteins. The gland is enriched in receptors that internalize low- and high-density lipoproteins. This uptake mechanism is increased when the adrenal is stimulated and provides the major cholesterol source.

Subsequent steps occur in the mitochondrion or endoplasmic reticulum. The first step is the conversion of cholesterol to pregnenolone. This step is rate limiting and is regulated by the major factors (ACTH, angiotensin II, and potassium) that stimulate steroid biosynthesis. This conversion involves several steps, catalyzed by the enzyme 20,22-desmolase (cholesterol side chain cleavage enzyme). Pregnenolone is then modified either (1) by converting its 5,6 to a 4,5 double bond with the use of 3β-hydroxysteroid dehydrogenase and Δ^5-oxysteroid isomerase, resulting in progesterone; or (2) by addition of a 17α-hydroxyl group with the use of 17α-hydroxylase, resulting in 17α-hydroxypregnenolone. The former pathway occurs in the glomerulosa, which lacks 17α-hydroxylase activity; although controversial, the latter pathway probably predominates in the fasciculata-reticularis, with subsequent conversion of 17α-hydroxypregnenolone to 17α-hydroxyprogesterone.

CORTISOL. Cortisol is synthesized by two successive hydroxylations. The first is at the 21 position, catalyzed by 21-hydroxylase, and results in 11-deoxycortisol (also called compound S). The second, at the 11 position of 11-deoxycortisol, is catalyzed by another hydroxylase and yields cortisol (also

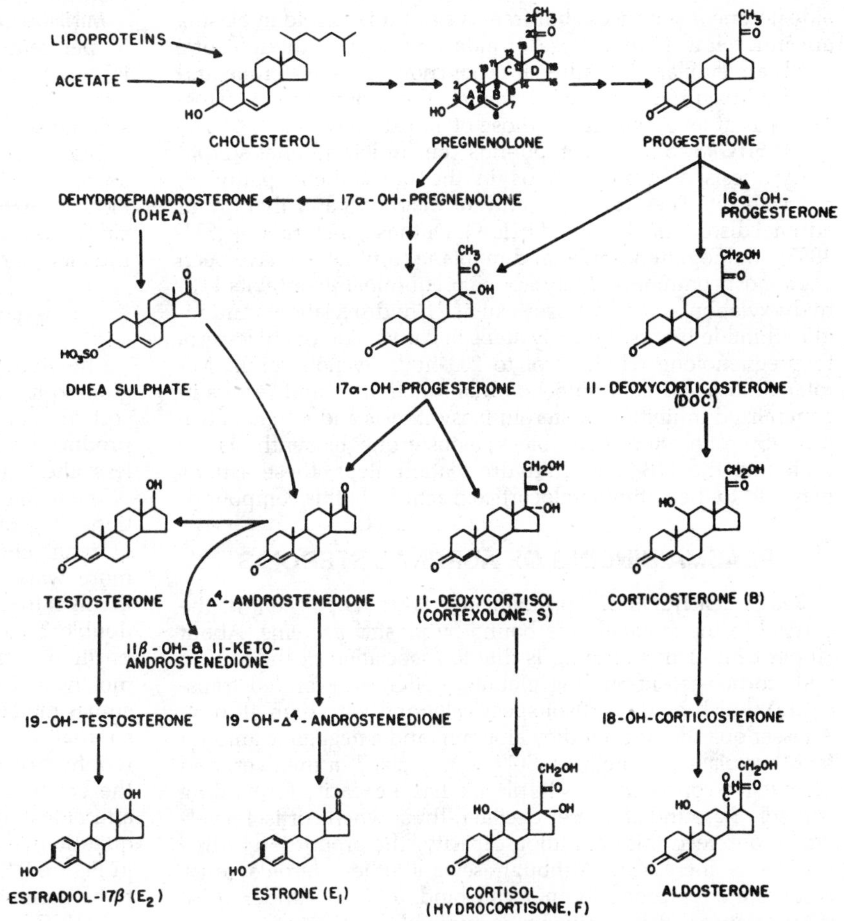

Figure 229–1. Steps in adrenal steroid biosynthesis. The numbers for the carbon atoms and the letters designating the rings of the steroid molecule are shown for pregnenolone. Arrows indicate the conversion pathways; the use of two arrows between intermediates indicates that more than one step is involved in the interconversion. (Reprinted from Baxter JD, Tyrrell JB: *In* Felig P, Baxter JD, Broadus AE, Frohman LA (eds.): Endocrinology and Metabolism. New York, McGraw-Hill Book Company, 1981, p 390.)

called hydrocortisone or compound F). These hydroxylations also require a flavoprotein dehydrogenase and cytochrome P450.

ALDOSTERONE. Aldosterone is produced by 21-hydroxylation of progesterone to form deoxycorticosterone (DOC); 11β-hydroxylation of DOC to form corticosterone; 18-hydroxylation of the latter to form 18-hydroxycorticosterone; and oxidation of the 18 CH_2OH group to an aldehyde to form aldosterone with the use of 18-hydroxycorticosteroid hydroxylase. This step is unique to the glomerulosa, explaining why aldosterone is not made by the zonae fasciculata and reticularis.

ANDROGENS. The adrenal androgens have 19 carbon atoms (C-19 steroids) and mostly serve as precursors for more potent androgens produced in peripheral tissues. These are dehydroepiandrosterone (DHEA) and its sulfate (DHEA-S), androstenedione and testosterone. DHEA is derived from 17α-hydroxypregnenolone by removal of its C-17 side chain, that leaves a keto group, with the use of C-17,20-lyase, and 17β-hydroxysteroid dehydrogenase. The sulfation of DHEA at the 3 position to DHEA-S is catalyzed by a sulfokinase. Androstenedione can be derived from either 17α-hydroxyprogesterone by removal of the C-17 side chain or from DHEA by conversion of the 5,6 to a 4,5 double bond and formation of the 3-keto group as described above. The adrenal can synthesize the C-18 steroids estradiol (from testosterone via 19-hydroxytestosterone) and estrone (from androstenedione via 19-hydroxy Δ^4-androstenedione) as outlined in Figure 229–1, but the quantities produced are minute. However, DHEA and DHEA-S synthesized by the fetal adrenal account for about 90 per cent of maternal estriol, 50 per cent of estradiol and estrone, and a substantial amount of testosterone and androstenedione production.

PRODUCTION RATES. The production rates and the blood levels under basal conditions of the major adrenal steroids are shown in Table 229–1. More cortisol is produced than any other steroid; much less aldosterone is produced. The production of DHEA plus DHEA-S is nearly as high as cortisol, although the plasma levels of DHEA are only a fraction of those of cortisol; however, plasma levels of DHEA-S are several-fold higher than those of cortisol because of the slow metabolism of DHEA-S. Corticosterone has substantial glucocorticoid activity, but is produced at much lower levels than cortisol. Similarly, DOC has substantial mineralocorticoid activity, and more DOC than

TABLE 229–1. SECRETION RATES AND PLASMA CONCENTRATIONS OF ADRENAL STEROIDS*

Steroid	24-hr Secretion (mg)	Mean Plasma Concentration (ng/ml)
Aldosterone	0.15	0.16
Androstenedione	2.4	1.5
Corticosterone	2.5	3
Cortisol	16	100
11-Deoxycorticosterone (DOC)	0.6	0.16
11-Deoxycortisol	0.4	1.7
DHEA	0.7(F), 3.0(M)	5.4
DHEA-S	7	1200
Progesterone	nil	0.2(M,F), 12(F)†
17α-Hydroxyprogesterone	nil	0.2(M), 0.6(F),2.0(F)†
Testosterone	0.2	5.6(M), 0.5(F)

*Mean values are reported for adults. Individual female (F) and male (M) values are reported only when these differ by more than two-fold. (Modified from Baxter JD, Tyrrell JB: The adrenal cortex. *In* Felig P, Baxter JD, Broadus AH, Frohman LA. (eds.): Endocrinology and Metabolism. New York, McGraw-Hill Book Company, 1981, p 394, where references to primary source material can be found.)

†Refers to the luteal phase of the menstrual cycle.

aldosterone is produced, but free levels of this steroid in plasma are much lower than those of aldosterone even though total levels are similar. The adrenal production of progesterone and 17α-hydroxyprogesterone is minimal. The production of testosterone is at levels similar to those of aldosterone.

INHIBITORS. Several compounds can inhibit adrenal steroid biosynthesis at various steps in the biosynthetic pathway, respectively. They can be useful for diagnosis and therapy of adrenal disorders (discussed below). Of these, metyrapone (SU-4885), aminoglutethimide, and mitotane (o,p′-DDD) have been used most commonly. Metyrapone predominantly inhibits 11β-hydroxylation and to a lesser extent 21-hydroxylation. Aminoglutethimide blocks the early steps in conversion of cholesterol to pregnenolone (cholesterol to 20α-hydroxycholesterol). Mitotane blocks adrenal mitochondrial functioning and results in generalized inhibition of steroid biosynthesis and adrenal atrophy. Spironolactone can block aldosterone biosynthesis by inhibiting the 11β- and 18-hydroxylation steps; these actions may add to the antimineralocorticoid actions of this compound.

PLASMA BINDING OF ADRENAL STEROIDS

GLUCOCORTICOIDS. Approximately 90 to 93 per cent of the cortisol in the circulation is bound by plasma proteins. About 80 per cent of this binding is due to association of the steroid with corticosteroid-binding globulin (CBG, also termed transcortin) which binds cortisol specifically and with high affinity. A lesser quantity is bound by albumin, and a negligible amount by other plasma proteins. CBG is synthesized in the liver, and at its usual concentrations in plasma has a capacity for binding cortisol of around 25μg per deciliter; thus, when cortisol levels begin to exceed this saturation capacity, the proportion of free cortisol is increased. Although several other steroids (e.g., corticosterone, progesterone) can bind to CBG, under most circumstances such occupancy is minimal.

CBG concentrations in plasma can vary among individuals on a genetic basis and can also be regulated by hormones and other factors. Estrogens, thyroid hormones, diabetes, and certain hematologic disorders increase CBG levels. Thus, CBG is increased in pregnancy (by almost two-fold during the third trimester), in hyperthyroidism, and by estrogens and oral contraceptives. Such effects can be maximal in three to five days and reversed by two to three weeks after cessation of therapy. CBG levels can be low congenitally and in liver disease (decreased protein production), multiple myeloma, obesity, and the nephrotic syndrome (through urinary loss).

The physiologic role of the plasma steroid–binding proteins such as CBG has not been determined. Although these have been called transport proteins, there is no obligatory need for this as cortisol is soluble at concentrations spanning its physiologic effectiveness. Similarly there appears to be no obligatory role for CBG in glucocorticoid hormone action. For instance, tissue culture cells respond to cortisol in the absence of detectable CBG. Further, the free rather than the plasma-bound steroid is physiologically active, and physiologic stimuli that regulate cortisol levels respond to the free rather than the total steroid concentration. Thus, when the CBG levels are primarily elevated or depressed, there are elevations or depressions, respectively, of the total cortisol in plasma, but the free cortisol concentration remains the same. This point is critical for evaluation of states of glucocorticoid excess or deficiency.

That CBG may have some importance is suggested by its ubiquity in mammals, even though plasma levels vary enormously, and the fact that congenital absence of CBG in man has never been found in spite of extensive screening. Recent evidence suggests that CBG or CBG-like proteins are located intracellularly, and in the kidney may sequester and therefore prevent cortisol from occupying the mineralocorticoid receptors. This would preserve the latter for the action of aldosterone as the major salt-regulating hormone. Furthermore, the protein binding of steroids in the blood may buffer rapid changes in plasma free cortisol levels that would otherwise occur as a result of episodic release of cortisol from the adrenal gland.

MINERALOCORTICOIDS. Under physiologic conditions, about 55 per cent of the total plasma aldosterone is protein bound, largely to albumin. The binding is weaker than that of cortisol with CBG, and the free rather than the plasma-bound aldosterone seems to be physiologically active.

DOC has potent mineralocorticoid activity, and its plasma levels are similar to those of aldosterone. However, DOC is not normally a physiologically important mineralocorticoid since over 95 per cent of it is bound to plasma proteins and thus its free levels are much lower than those of aldosterone.

METABOLISM OF ADRENAL STEROIDS

The hydrophobic steroids, although filtered by the renal glomerulus and excreted into the intestine, are mostly reabsorbed. For example, only about 1 per cent of the cortisol produced daily is excreted unchanged in the urine. Nevertheless, the kidneys account for over 90 per cent of the excretion of the metabolized steroids (DOC and corticosterone are exceptions); the remainder is lost in the gut. To render them capable of renal elimination, the steroids are inactivated and made more water soluble through enzymatic modifications. These involve hydroxylation of the keto groups, reduction of the double bond in the A ring, and conjugation at the 3 or 21 position with glucuronide or sulfate. These conversions occur mostly in liver, although during pregnancy the placenta assumes metabolic importance. The conversions alter the steroids so that the renal clearance of a major cortisol metabolite, tetrahydrocortisone glucuronide, is around 75 per cent that of the creatinine clearance. More than 50 metabolites of cortisol and aldosterone have been detected in humans. Although the quantitative aspects are still being refined, the pathways shown in Figure 229–2, and best studied for cortisol, appear generally to be dominant.

GLUCOCORTICOIDS. Cortisol is cleared from the plasma with a half-life of 70 to 120 minutes. About 70 per cent of infused cortisol, and presumably of that secreted, will be eliminated within 24 hours. The 11β-hydroxyl group of cortisol can be oxidized to the ketone, forming cortisone. The reaction is reversible, and in general the equilibrium is shifted to favor the 11β-hydroxyl group. However, because the adrenal produces much more cortisol than cortisone, there is substantial cortisol to cortisone conversion. These two steroids have similar subsequent metabolic fates, and roughly equivalent quantities of metabolites of these steroids are produced. Quantitatively the most important subsequent modification involves reduction of the 3-keto moiety to form dihydrocortisol and dihydrocortisone, followed by a reduction of the 4,5 double bond to form tetrahydrocortisol and tetrahydrocortisone. When the 3-hydroxyl group is formed, over 95 per cent of the products are conjugated at this position to form the glucuronide and to a lesser extent the sulfate derivatives. Conjugates of these two steroids make up around 30 per cent of the urinary cortisol metabolites. The second major site for modification involves the reduction of the 20-ketone to a hydroxyl, with subsequent reduction of the A ring, resulting in cortol (11-OH) or cortolone (11-keto). These account for approximately 25 per cent of the cortisol metabolites. Alternatively, there can be conversion of the 21-hydroxyl to a COOH; cortoic (11-hydroxyl) or cortolonic (11-keto) acid results when the A ring is reduced and the C-20-hydroxyl is formed, and they account for about 10 per cent of the cortisol metabolites. Other minor pathways involve the C-17 modifications discussed above without A-ring reduction, removal of the C-17 side chain with formation of 17-keto or 17-COOH moieties, formation of the C-21 COOH (without C-20-keto) and 6β-hydroxylation. The latter modifications constitute a major pathway in infants in whom the esterification mechanism has not been developed and for the synthetic glucocorticoids used in therapy.

MINERALOCORTICOIDS. Aldosterone is cleared with a half-

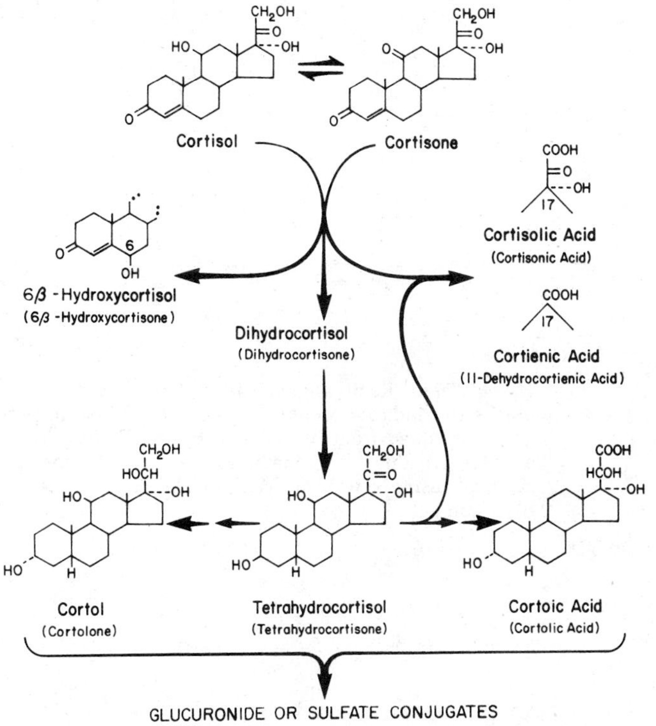

Figure 229–2. Metabolism of cortisol. See text. The interconversion of cortisol to cortisone is shown. The other steroid metabolites can be derivatives of either cortisol or cortisone. Structures shown and names are for the cortisol derivative. The names of the cortisone derivatives are shown in parentheses. In some cases, only part of the steroid molecule is shown; in these cases numbers refer to the steroid carbons for orientation. For tetrahydrocortisol, tetrahydrocortisone, and their derivatives, the 3-hydroxyl and 5-hydrogen are shown in the α and β configurations, respectively, but both α- and β-orientations occur at both positions. For a more extensive discussion and references, see Baxter JD, Tyrrell JB: *In* Felig P, Baxter JD, Broadus AE, Frohman LE (eds.): Endocrinology and Metabolism. New York, McGraw-Hill Book Company, 1981, pp 411–415.

life of around 15 minutes. Its conversion to metabolites is so effective that very little aldosterone survives passage through the liver. Less than 0.5 per cent of the aldosterone appears in the urine in the free state. The metabolism of aldosterone is similar to that of cortisol. About 35 per cent of the steroid appears as tetrahydroaldosterone glucuronide (3 position). However, two major differences are that there is much less 11β-hydroxy to 11-keto conversion, and 15 to 20 per cent of the aldosterone appears as a C-18 glucuronide that is acid labile; measurements of the urinary "aldosterone" usually reflect this metabolite.

ANDROGENS. The metabolism of androgens is discussed in Ch. 234.

VARIABLES IN RATES OF METABOLISM. The rate of steroid metabolism can be altered in certain clinical states and by various drugs. Agents that affect plasma steroid–binding proteins secondarily affect metabolism because of inhibitory influences of plasma binding on clearance. In chronic liver disease, hypothyroidism, infancy, very old age, anorexia nervosa, and protein calorie malnutrition, the rate of steroid metabolism is decreased. The converse occurs in hyperthyroidism. These states are in general not associated with abnormal free steroid levels (anorexia nervosa is an exception) because the regulatory systems tend to compensate by altering steroid production. Also, there is no major effect of renal disease (even though it does affect the clearance of some metabolites) or of most chronic diseases, obesity, and stress.

Drugs that affect steroid metabolism usually have the greatest influence on 6β-hydroxylation. Since this pathway in adults is relatively minor in terms of cortisol, these drugs do not have a major effect on endogenous cortisol. However, they can have a substantial influence on the clearance of synthetic glucocorticoids such as dexamethasone and prednisone, and this is therefore an important consideration with steroid therapy or with the use of glucocorticoids to assess the hypothalamic-pituitary-adrenal axis. These drugs include mitotane, phenytoin, rifampicin, aminoglutethimide, and barbiturates.

Regulation of Adrenal Steroid Production

John D. Baxter

Adrenal cortisol and androgen production is regulated by the hypothalamic-pituitary-adrenal axis, whereas aldosterone production is regulated predominantly by the renin-angiotensin system and by potassium (Fig. 229–3). These systems allow for basal and circadian steroid production, regulation of plasma steroid levels in normal circumstances, and increased or decreased steroid production in response to a number of specific stimuli.

REGULATION OF GLUCOCORTICOID PRODUCTION

The hypothalamus, pituitary, and adrenal comprise a neuroendocrine axis concerned with regulation of cortisol production. This axis is discussed in Ch. 224. Corticotropin releasing factor (CRF), elaborated by the hypothalamus, travels through its portal system to the anterior pituitary where it stimulates corticotropin (ACTH) release. The latter travels in the circulation to the adrenal where it stimulates cortisol production.

Three types of mechanisms are involved in regulating cortisol release: (1) circadian rhythms of secretion are established by the brain, (2) a number of types of excitatory factors can increase cortisol production, and (3) production of CRF and ACTH are regulated negatively by glucocorticoids.

ACTH AND RELATED PEPTIDES. ACTH circulates in the plasma largely as a free peptide with a half-life of around 10 minutes. It is derived from the proteolysis of proopiomelanocortin, a larger precursor pituitary protein of about 290 amino acids that also contains the sequences of several other proteins, including β-endorphin, α-, β-, and γ-melanocyte-stimulating hormones (MSH), β-lipotropin and an amino-terminal fragment (Ch. 221). Although MSH itself has the greatest pigment-stimulating activity, this activity in man is due predominantly to MSH sequences contained within ACTH (α-MSH), β-lipotropin (β-MSH) and the amino-terminal fragment (γ-MSH), as there appears to be very little MSH per se in the circulation. ACTH stimulates cortisol release by the adrenal within two to three minutes. This is due to increased cortisol synthesis primarily through stimulation of cholesterol to pregnenolone conversion, rather than through effects on secretion of stored hormone. More prolonged stimulation results in increased protein, RNA, and DNA synthesis with both hypertrophy and hyperplasia. ACTH binds to surface receptors and activates adenylate cyclase and phospholipase A_2 by a Ca^{++}-dependent mechanism. This results in increased Ca^{++} uptake, cyclic AMP generation, and phospholipid turnover. These effects increase cholesterol esterase, block cholesterol ester synthesis, increase lipoprotein uptake and stimulate cholesterol to pregnenolone conversion.

SPONTANEOUS RHYTHMS. The circadian rhythm of ACTH and cortisol results in decreasing release through the afternoon and evening. Secretion begins to increase around 3 to 4 A.M., peaks by around 8 A.M., and then begins to decline. This release occurs in pulses with intervals between them of 40 minutes to 8 hours; the changes in overall cortisol production are due to influences in the number of pulses that occur. These result in cortisol levels that vary enormously within minutes; thus, single plasma cortisol determinations may not give an adequate integrated assessment of overall cortisol production.

The spontaneous rhythm of cortisol secretion can be inter-

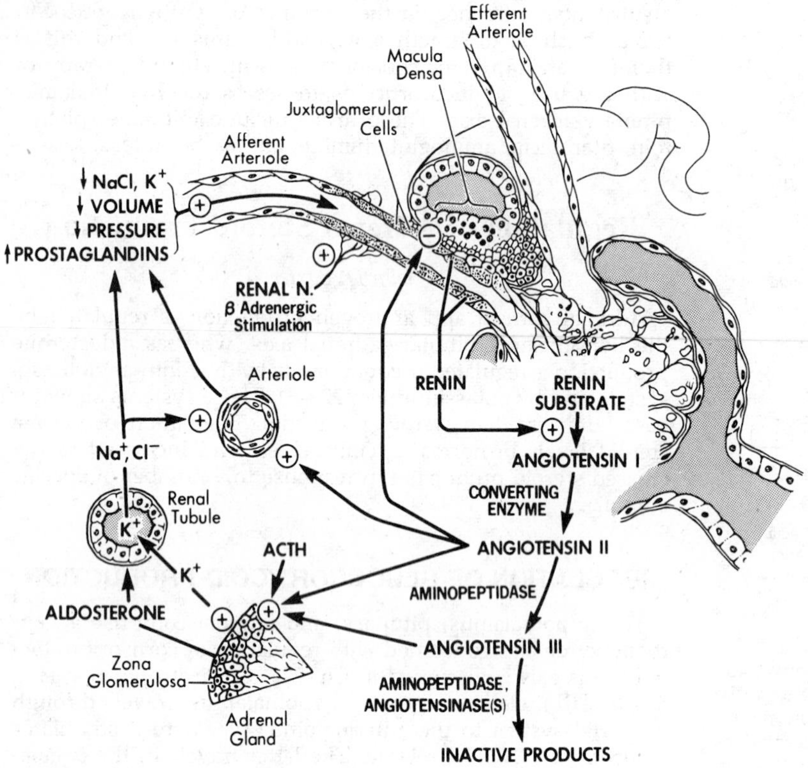

Figure 229–3. Renin-angiotensin system. The plus and minus signs indicate stimulation and inhibition, respectively. (Reprinted from Biglieri EG, Baxter JD: *In* Felig P, Baxter JD, Broadus AE, Frohman LA (eds.): Endocrinology and Metabolism. New York, McGraw-Hill Book Company, 1981, p 556.)

rupted acutely by a variety of psychologic and physical factors. These can vary from seemingly mild stresses such as the confrontation for venesection to more severe ones such as the preparation for cardiac surgery or severe anxiety. However, there are major individual variations. Major trauma or surgery, severe illness, hypoglycemia, fever, burns, and intensive exercise are illustrative of physical stresses that increase cortisol production by up to six-fold of normal. Minor illnesses such as upper respiratory infections or minor surgery can have minimal or no influence. Variations in cortisol levels can be blunted by chronic diseases such as congestive heart failure with hepatic congestion due to delayed cortisol clearance and with central nervous system disease and pituitary tumors even when they do not affect basal ACTH release. In depression, there is a circadian rhythm, but there can be increased cortisol secretion and impaired suppression by glucocorticoids. Although a number of drugs do not affect ACTH release, serotonin antagonists such as cyproheptadine inhibit both spontaneous and stimulated changes in ACTH release.

FEEDBACK INHIBITION OF ACTH RELEASE. Glucocorticoids feedback-inhibit the release of both CRF and ACTH (Ch. 221). Thus endogenous levels and stress-induced increases of cortisol and ACTH are depressed with exogenous glucocorticoid administration. ACTH levels are increased up to 10-fold to 20-fold in primary adrenal insufficiency. The feedback inhibition in response to glucocorticoids occurs within a few minutes, is progressive with continual exposure in a dose- and time-dependent fashion, affects both basal and stress-stimulated release, and is reversible. Although there are considerable individual variations, administration of a large dose of glucocorticoids for a few days does not, in general, result in suppression of pituitary function for more than a few hours; more prolonged exposure is accompanied by substantial suppression. Thus after several years of glucocorticoid therapy and then withdrawal of steroid administration, up to one year may be required for the hypothalamic-pituitary-adrenal axis to return to normal functioning. Although significant suppression occurs at both the hypothalamic and pituitary levels, the quantitative contribution of each of them has not been clarified.

REGULATION OF MINERALOCORTICOID PRODUCTION

Aldosterone production is controlled predominantly by the renin-angiotensin system and potassium, although other factors such as sodium, ACTH, and serotonin can also affect aldosterone secretion (Fig. 229–3). The renin-angiotensin system is important for adaptive blood pressure changes and is involved in the pathogenesis of some forms of hypertension.

RENIN. Renin, a glycoprotein of 340 amino acids, is produced in the juxtaglomerular cells of the afferent renal arteriole as a precursor protein (prorenin) that is cleaved to yield active renin. These cells release renin into the circulation where it has a half-life of around 15 minutes. Although renin may also be made in other tissues, the biologic role for this is uncertain, and extrarenal renin does not contribute to the plasma renin. Renin release is stimulated by lowering the blood pressure, assumption of the erect posture, salt depletion, β-adrenergic or central nervous system stimulation, and certain prostaglandins. It is inhibited by increases in blood pressure (except with malignant hypertension), salt loading, angiotensin II, vasopressin, potassium, calcium, β-adrenergic antagonists, α-methyldopa, clonidine, and by inhibitors of prostaglandin synthesis such as indomethacin.

Three types of influences mediate changes in renin release: (1) Changes in renal tubular sodium chloride concentration are detected by the macula densa, a specialized segment of the distal tubule that makes contact with the afferent arteriole just before it enters the glomerulus. This information is transmitted to the juxtaglomerular cells so that factors that reduce volume or lower the plasma sodium and chloride levels (e.g., dehydration, fluid or blood loss) increase renin release. (2) Renal baroreceptors stimulate renin release in response to decreases in renal perfusion pressure as with fluid loss or decreases in blood pressure. These receptors can function independently of innervation and salt delivery and respond more to changes in pressure than to the absolute pressure. (3) Renal sympathetic nerves that terminate in the juxtaglomerular cells and smooth muscle cells of the renal afferent arterioles secrete norepinephrine, which in turn stimulates renin release through β-adrenergic receptors. Blockage of this mechanism by agents such as propranolol probably explains how they decrease renin release. However, catecholamines can have other indirect effects on renin release through influences on renal blood flow and glomerular filtration.

Renin acts in the plasma proteolytically on renin substrate (angiotensinogen) to yield the decapeptide angiotensin I. Angiotensinogen contains over 400 amino acids and is secreted by the liver. Although its levels can be increased by estrogens and glucocorticoids, this does not appear to be an important normal mechanism of regulation. Angiotensin I is not known to have physiologically important actions; instead it serves as a substrate for production of angiotensin II.

CONVERTING ENZYME. The conversion of angiotensin I to the octapeptide angiotensin II is catalyzed by converting enzyme. Although a number of tissues have this enzyme, the lung contains much of the activity, perhaps around 50 per cent. In certain pulmonary diseases there can be decreases or increases in the plasma levels of the enzyme, although these changes do not appear to have a physiologically important effect on angiotensin II generation. Converting enzyme also catalyzes other reactions; important among these is the inactivation of bradykinin. Clinically useful inhibitors of converting enzyme are available; of these captopril has been used the most extensively. Normally, except when this enzyme is blocked pharmacologically, the rate-limiting step for angiotensin II generation is the production of angiotensin I.

ANGIOTENSIN II. Angiotensin II is the most potent vasoconstrictor known and has direct effects on arterioles. It also inhibits directly the release of renin by the juxtaglomerular cells. Finally it is a potent stimulator of aldosterone release. The hormone also has other complex effects on the kidney that affect salt balance, possibly through influences on kallikreins and prostaglandins. Plasma concentrations of angiotensin II can vary by 10-fold to 25-fold; the hormone has a half-life of only one to two minutes. There are several breakdown products of angiotensin II. One of these, angiotensin III, a polypeptide of seven amino acids, has angiotensin II activity, but its biologic importance is probably much less than that of angiotensin II.

Angiotensin II stimulates both early and late steps in aldosterone biosynthesis, resulting in increased conversion of cholesterol to pregnenolene and of corticosterone to 18-hydroxycorticosterone. Angiotensin II binds to cell surface receptors, but unlike ACTH it does not activate adenylate cyclase. It probably affects Ca^{++} influx and phospholipid turnover. Angiotensin II also has a tropic influence on the adrenal zona glomerulosa.

POTASSIUM. Increased potassium stimulates and decreased potassium inhibits aldosterone production. These effects are elicited by changes in potassium of as little as 0.1 mEq per liter in the physiologic range and are independent of sodium or angiotensin II. Prolonged hyperkalemia, like excess angiotensin II, has a tropic influence on the adrenal.

OTHER FACTORS. Other factors of lesser importance also affect aldosterone release. ACTH has a transient effect, and, rarely, aldosterone production can be blunted with chronic ACTH deficiency. Sodium deficiency decreases and sodium loading increases aldosterone release, but these influences are probably mediated through effects on renin. Dopamine agonists can inhibit and dopamine antagonists can increase plasma aldosterone. Aldosterone release is episodic and shows a tendency to a circadian rhythm that is similar to but much less prominent than that of cortisol; the mechanisms for this periodicity are not understood.

REGULATION OF ADRENAL ANDROGEN PRODUCTION

Adrenal androgen production is regulated by ACTH in a manner similar to that of cortisol. Thus plasma androgen levels tend to show the same circadian periodicity as cortisol. However, this is not the case with DHEA-S as a result of its slow turnover that tends to blunt the magnitude of increases due to episodic steroid release. Adrenal androgen release may also be affected by other factors such as during prepuberty (adrenarche); however, these are poorly understood. Finally, it should be remembered that androgens released by the testes and ovaries contribute to plasma androgen levels.

Actions of Adrenal Steroids

John D. Baxter

GLUCOCORTICOIDS

Glucocorticoids have diverse actions that in some way affect most mammalian tissues. They are also essential for survival, at least in times of stress.

INTERMEDIARY METABOLISM. Named for their carbohydrate-regulating activities, glucocorticoids have multiple influences on glucose metabolism with diverse secondary effects (Fig. 229–4). In most tissues these steroids inhibit glucose uptake. Liver, heart, brain, and erythrocytes are exceptions. In many of these tissues the steroids also block protein and nucleic acid synthesis and stimulate turnover of these macromolecules. In adipose tissue the steroids inhibit lipolysis and block lipogenesis. In liver the steroids stimulate glycogen deposition, gluconeogenesis, and the ability of other hormones to stimulate gluconeogenesis. The latter is further facilitated because of increased availability of glycerol and amino acid substrate due to the effects in peripheral tissues. The steroids also tend to stimulate the appetite, and in adrenal insufficiency there is anorexia. Finally the steroids tend to blunt the actions of insulin and decrease the affinity for insulin binding to its receptors.

The net effect of these influences is a glucocorticoid-induced tendency to hyperglycemia. This can be seen as early as 1 hour following glucocorticoid administration. However, in normal subjects the elevated levels of glucose increase insulin release that in turn tends to blunt the effects of the steroid. However,

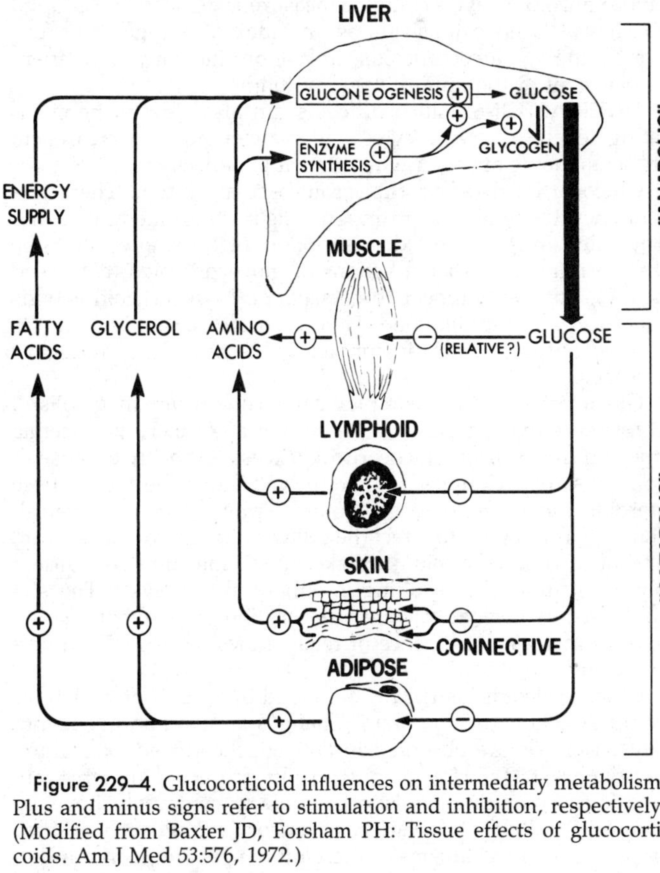

Figure 229–4. Glucocorticoid influences on intermediary metabolism. Plus and minus signs refer to stimulation and inhibition, respectively. (Modified from Baxter JD, Forsham PH: Tissue effects of glucocorticoids. Am J Med *53*:576, 1972.)

in diabetes or latent diabetes, significant hyperglycemia and insulin resistance can ensue. Similarly, secondary hyperinsulinism may explain why there is a lack of fat wasting in Cushing's syndrome; lipogenesis induced by secondary increases in plasma insulin levels along with the increased food intake due to appetite stimulation may explain the truncal and sometimes generalized obesity seen in the syndrome. Conversely, in adrenal insufficiency there is a tendency to hypoglycemia; usually this is not marked, but it can be significant if there is concomitant fasting. Many of the actions of glucocorticoids on intermediary metabolism can be perceived as a protection against fasting; there is peripheral catabolism with sparing of essential tissues (heart, brain, blood cells) to make available substrate for maintenance of the blood sugar levels.

These actions of glucocorticoids on intermediary metabolism also explain many other effects of glucocorticoid excess. Thus inhibition of tissue metabolic functions may explain glucocorticoid-induced myopathy, inhibition of immunologic and inflammatory responses, and poor wound healing, thinning of the skin, striae, and osteoporosis.

INFLAMMATORY AND IMMUNOLOGIC RESPONSES. In excess, glucocorticoids suppress a number of inflammatory and immunologic responses, but it is not clear whether they normally modulate immunologic systems. In excess, glucocorticoids inhibit antigen processing, T cell function, synthesis of cellular mediators of the inflammatory response such as interleukins, plasminogen activator, lymphokines, and other active peptides, cellular migration and action at sites of inflammation, and inflammatory reactions themselves. In general they do not affect most antibody responses, although there are a few exceptions. Some populations of lymphocytes are killed by glucocorticoids; this explains the efficacy of these steroids in certain leukemias such as acute lymphoblastic leukemia of childhood. The steroids also affect mononuclear cell trafficking and tend to decrease blood monocyte, lymphocyte, and eosinophil levels and increase polymorphonuclear leukocytes; there are reciprocal changes during adrenal insufficiency. In the era before hormone levels could be measured, the blood eosinophil count was used extensively as an index of adrenal function. Interestingly, glucocorticoids do not produce any permanent impairment of the immunologic system.

OTHER ACTIONS. Glucocorticoids can also elevate the circulating levels of erythrocytes and platelets, and decreases in these elements are seen with adrenal insufficiency.

Glucocorticoids affect the cardiovascular system. There is a tendency to hypertension in Cushing's syndrome and to hypotension in Addison's disease. Some of these effects can be due to mineralocorticoid actions of glucocorticoids (discussed below), but there appear to be separate glucocorticoid actions that are poorly understood. Glucocorticoids also stimulate the cardiac output, which is conversely decreased in Addison's disease.

Glucocorticoids have complex actions on calcium metabolism. Hypercalcemia can occur in Addison's disease. Hypocalcemia does not result from glucocorticoid excess (probably because of compensatory changes in parathyroid hormone), but these steroids can be used to ameliorate certain types of hypercalcemia. They appear to affect the cellular distribution of calcium, and also to block calcium uptake by the intestine and certain bone cell functions resulting in enhanced osteolysis. The steroids decrease renal calcium reabsorption, and hypercalciuria and an increased incidence of renal stones occur in Cushing's syndrome.

Glucocorticoids penetrate the blood-brain barrier and have complex actions on the brain. Changes in mood and occasionally psychosis are observed in both glucocorticoid excess and deficiency states. However, with glucocorticoid therapy, euphoria is common. Addisonian subjects commonly have increased sensitivity to a variety of sensory stimuli such as smell or taste. The mechanisms of these influences are poorly understood. Glucocorticoids increase the intraocular pressure, probably by blocking fluid uptake by the trabecular meshwork. In susceptible individuals they can precipitate glaucoma and more rarely may result in cataract formation.

In the gastrointestinal tract glucocorticoids can inhibit DNA synthesis and tend to enhance stimuli to gastric acid secretion. They probably also enhance the tendency to form duodenal ulcers and, in high doses, the tendency to develop gastritis, although these side effects are controversial.

In excess, glucocorticoids inhibit linear growth, possibly as a result of their inhibitory influences on a number of tissues. However, glucocorticoid action appears to be required for a number of developmental processes. One particularly important process is the synthesis of surfactant in the lung. Lack of glucocorticoid induction of this factor in premature birth contributes to the respiratory distress syndrome of the newborn.

Complex interrelationships exist between glucocorticoids and other hormones. Glucocorticoids can inhibit vasopressin release; conversely, ACTH deficiency can lead to hyponatremia with water intoxication. Glucocorticoids secondarily increase insulin and parathyroid hormone (PTH) levels, and in some cases blunt the production of growth hormone, prolactin, insulin, glucagon, thyroid-stimulating hormone (TSH), and testosterone. Multiple synergisms and antagonisms between glucocorticoids and other hormones also exist at the cellular level. For example, they are synergistic with epinephrine and glucagon in stimulating hepatic gluconeogenesis. These effects are sometimes termed permissive glucocorticoid actions.

STRESS. Why glucocorticoids are essential for survival in times of stress is poorly understood. Two factors are probably operative. First, stress increases the production of a number of biologically active substances such as catecholamines, prostaglandins and other arachidonic acid metabolites, proteinases, and kinins. Glucocorticoids, by contrast, tend to blunt the production and actions of these substances, which, if left unchecked during stress, would lead to shock and vascular decompensation. Second, the stimulation of cardiovascular functions by glucocorticoids may be critical in times of stress when other compensatory systems may be less effective.

MOLECULAR MECHANISMS OF ACTION. Glucocorticoids penetrate cells and bind to intracellular receptors; the resulting hormone-receptor complexes then bind to specific sites on the DNA where they enhance the ability of RNA polymerase to stimulate transcription of glucocorticoid-responsive genes (Ch. 221). The protein products of the resulting mRNAs then mediate the glucocorticoid responses. In some circumstances the steroids probably block transcription by similar mechanisms. Also, some glucocorticoid effects occur by mechanisms that do not involve stimulation of transcription.

MINERALOCORTICOIDS

Mineralocorticoid hormones act on kidney, gut, salivary glands, and sweat glands to affect the balance of electrolytes. Direct actions on other tissues have been proposed but not clearly documented. Thus the spectrum of mineralocorticoid action is more restricted than that of glucocorticoid action.

In the kidney, the most important target organ, mineralocorticoids promote the linked reabsorption of sodium and secretion of potassium in the cortical collecting tubules of the nephron, and stimulate the secretion of hydrogen ion in the medullary collecting tubules. Thus, with mineralocorticoid excess, there is sodium retention, hypokalemia, and a tendency to alkalosis. In primary mineralocorticoid excess, hypertension develops with time. With mineralocorticoid deficiency there is sodium loss and a tendency to hyperkalemia and acidosis. The overall effects of mineralocorticoids on both sodium and potassium also depend on the level of salt intake. Increased sodium intake results in more tubular sodium for reabsorption; this enhances potassium secretion. Conversely, sodium restriction diminishes aldosterone-induced kaliuresis. In most circumstances with persistent mineralocorticoid excess, the sodium retention that occurs reaches a limit such that the body "escapes" from further sodium retention. This may be due to the secretion of other factors or hormones, or to changes in renal hemodynamics with secondary and compensating influences on sodium excretion, or to both. Exceptions are the secondary hyperaldosteronism of heart failure and of cirrhosis with ascites where sodium retention is progressive. As noted, hyperkalemia directly stimulates aldosterone secretion, which in turn enhances renal potassium excretion. This servomechanism forms an important component of the body's defense against hyperkalemia.

Mineralocorticoid actions are probably mediated through molecular mechanisms similar to those described above for cortisol, and in Ch. 221. The mineralocorticoid receptors bind aldosterone and DOC with high affinity; they also bind cortisol with 1 to 2 per cent of the affinity for aldosterone. Since plasma free cortisol concentrations are around 100-fold higher than those of aldosterone, there is probably some occupancy of mineralocorticoid receptors by cortisol, although this may be blunted by other cellular proteins that sequester cortisol. The synthetic steroid 9α-fluorocortisol binds tightly to mineralocorticoid receptors and is used for mineralocorticoid replacement therapy, since it is more stable than aldosterone after oral administration. Mineralocorticoid antagonists such as spironolactone bind to these receptors and in this way block aldosterone action.

Aldosterone stimulates the synthesis of several renal proteins that result in increases in (1) sodium permeability in the apical membrane exposed to the tubular lumen; (2) various mitochondrial enzymes that increase cellular ATP and thereby enhance the actions of the Na^+-K^+ ATPase; (3) possibly the Na^+-K^+ ATPase itself; and (4) probably other as yet unidentified factors that influence fatty acid and phospholipid metabolism. Of these the effects on the sodium channel are probably the most important. Potassium ion secretion increases secondarily to a rise in the electrochemical gradient for potassium entry into the tubular lumen, a gradient that is enhanced by the Na^+-K^+ ATPase-dependent pumping of sodium ion into the cell, thereby increasing lumen negativity.

Renal tubular transport of hydrogen ion, about which little is known, has been postulated to result from an hormonal influence on an H^+ ATPase. The mineralocorticoid-induced tendency to extracellular alkalosis is also promoted in part by hydrogen ion movement into cells in exchange for losses in potassium, leading to the dichotomy of extracellular acidosis in the presence of extracellular alkalosis. Potassium ion deficiency increases hydrogen ion excretion by decreasing Na^+-K^+ exange, which in turn increases the Na^+-H^+ exchange. As in the case of potassium, hydrogen ion loss can be blunted with sodium restriction.

The major known extrarenal targets for aldosterone are the sweat and salivary glands, ileum, and colon where the steroid promotes potassium loss and sodium retention. These actions are ordinarily minor in terms of overall salt balance. However, the aldosterone-induced changes in the salivary sodium-potassium ratio and the potential difference across the colonic epithelium have been used as diagnostic indices of mineralocorticoid activity.

Laboratory Evaluation of Adrenocortical Function

J. Blake Tyrrell

Most functions of the adrenal cortex can now be assessed by using plasma assays. Certain urinary assays remain useful, however, despite the disadvantage of 24-hour collections. Trophic hormones, e.g., ACTH, and related peptides, renin and angiotensin, can also be precisely measured and compared to adrenal secretion. The following considerations must be remembered when using these assays. (1) Current assays measure total hormone concentration, not bioactive free hormone. (2) Plasma levels of cortisol and ACTH vary greatly because of episodic secretion and many other factors (see below); thus single levels cannot always be relied upon for a definitive diagnosis. (3) In assessing adrenal function, stimulation and suppression testing provide the most definitive information.

GLUCOCORTICOID FUNCTION

ACTH AND RELATED PEPTIDES. Immunoassays for ACTH, although not always available, are extremely useful. ACTH is unstable in plasma and adheres to glass; specimens should be collected in anticoagulated plastic or silicon-coated tubes on ice, centrifuged in the cold without delay, and frozen until assayed. The normal range of plasma ACTH in the morning (8 to 9 A.M.) is 20 to 100 pg per milliliter in most current clinical assays. Values at other times of the day are lower, and consideration of this episodic secretion is important in interpretation.

Plasma ACTH levels are primarily used to differentiate pituitary, adrenal, and other causes of adrenal dysfunction. Thus, in patients with primary adrenal insufficiency (Addison's disease) elevated ACTH levels (generally greater than 250 pg per milliliter) confirm the diagnosis. Conversely, with secondary adrenal insufficiency due to hypothalamic or pituitary disease, or steroid therapy, ACTH levels will be low normal or subnormal (<50 pg per milliliter). In states of cortisol excess (Cushing's syndrome), a suppressed or undetectable ACTH level (<20 pg per milliliter) is diagnostic of an adrenal tumor hypersecreting cortisol (or of exogenous glucocorticoids). With ACTH–producing pituitary tumors (Cushing's disease), plasma ACTH levels are normal to modestly elevated (40 to 200 pg per milliliter), whereas in the ectopic ACTH syndrome they are usually elevated markedly (100 to >1000 pg per milliliter). ACTH levels in the two latter conditions may overlap, but very high (>300 pg per milliliter) values point to an ectopic tumor. Plasma ACTH levels are also elevated in congenital adrenal hyperplasia proportional to the extent of cortisol deficiency, and are markedly elevated in pituitary tumors that arise following bilateral adrenalectomy (Nelson's syndrome).

Immunoassays for other peptides derived from proopiomelanocortin are also becoming available. The available antisera usually measure both β-LPH and β-endorphin, and many reports of "beta endorphin levels" reflect in fact predominantly β-LPH that is present in the circulation in higher concentrations than β-endorphin. Reported normal morning values of immunoreactive β-LPH/β-endorphin are 20 to 200 pg per milliliter. Levels of these peptides vary similarily to those of ACTH, but because of its longer plasma half-life, β-LPH peptide levels show less episodic variability than ACTH. Also β-LPH is considerably more stable than ACTH in plasma and when frozen prior to assay. As a result, elevated β-LPH levels are seen more consistently than are elevated ACTH levels in patients with pituitary-dependent hypercortisolism. Whether measurement of β-LPH or β-endorphin will supplant measurement of ACTH levels in clinical disorders of pituitary and adrenal dysfunction remains to be determined.

PLASMA CORTISOL AND RELATED STEROIDS. Plasma cortisol is most frequently measured by radioimmunoassay; current antisera show little cross-reactivity with other natural or synthetic steroids. Competitive protein binding, fluorimetric, and high–performance liquid chromatography assays are also in use. Normal values of plasma cortisol vary with the circadian rhythm of ACTH. Mean levels at 8 A.M. are 10 to 12 μg per deciliter with a range of 3 to 20 μg per deciliter. Values at 4 to 6 P.M. are approximately 50 per cent of the morning levels, although there is great variability. Values obtained between 10 P.M. and 2 A.M. are less than 3 μg per deciliter and may be unmeasurable. (In all cases, values are 2 to 3 μg per deciliter higher than those given above when the fluorimetric assay is used.) Episodic variability and the numerous conditions increasing cortisol secretion or CBG concentrations (Table 229–2) limit the utility of single cortisol determinations; as a result, unless marked elevations are present, these values are rarely diagnostic per se.

Measurement of plasma 11-deoxycortisol (compound S) is generally available and has been used extensively in metyrapone testing of pituitary-adrenal reserve (see below).

URINARY CORTICOSTEROIDS. Measurements of urinary steroids have been traditionally used to evaluate adrenal function and provide an integrated assessment of steroid production and excretion. With the exception of urinary free cortisol, however, which is essential in the evaluation of cortisol excess, other methods are less advantageous and are being supplanted by measurements of plasma cortisol or ACTH levels.

Urine free cortisol, although less than 1 per cent of total adrenal cortisol secretion, is a useful measurement in the diagnosis of hypercortisolism. The urine is first extracted and the steroid is then measured by radioimmunoassay or competitive protein binding. Normal values range from 20 to 100 μg per 24 hours. Elevated levels are almost always present in Cushing's syndrome but not in simple obesity; this ability to separate these conditions is a major advantage. Urinary cortisol excretion is increased by any condition that increases adrenal cortisol secretion (Table 229–2) and is decreased in renal failure. Current clinical assays are insensitive at the lower range; this method is not reliable in the diagnosis of decreased cortisol production.

Urinary 17-hydroxycorticosteroids (17-OHCS) and 17-ketogenic steroids (17-KGS) measure steroid metabolites, predominantly those of cortisol and 11-deoxycortisol. These methods are currently not recommended in most situations, since the levels are altered in many disease states and the assays are subject to interference by commonly used drugs and medications.

SUPPRESSION TESTS. Suppression tests use dexamethasone, a potent synthetic glucocorticoid not measured in current cortisol assays, to inhibit ACTH and cortisol secretion. In Cushing's syndrome there is abnormal feedback by glucocorticoids, and this abnormality is diagnostic. There are two types of dexamethasone suppression tests: (1) Low-dose tests are used to document the presence of Cushing's syndrome. (2) High-dose tests are used to distinguish the various causes of Cushing's syndrome. The techniques for performing these tests and the expected responses are summarized in Table 229–3.

Low-Dose Dexamethasone Tests. The overnight 1 mg dexamethasone suppression test is an excellent screening procedure for detecting the presence of Cushing's syndrome. The test can be used on an ambulatory basis, and in this setting false-negative and false-positive responses are rare. The test is much less useful in hospitalized and chronically ill patients, of whom 25 per cent have false-positive responses. False-positive responses also occur in 15 per cent of obese patients and in a number of other conditions, including acute illness, anxiety, depression, alcoholism, estrogen therapy, and uremia. Drugs that accelerate dexamethasone metabolism, especially phenytoin and phenobarbital, also cause false-positive results. The two-day low-dose test provides the same information as the 1 mg overnight test but is more time consuming. Abnormal responses occur in about 95 per cent of patients with Cushing's syndrome. False-positive responses occur rarely in obesity or with estrogen therapy, but are seen more commonly with acute illness, depression, alcoholism, and anticonvulsant therapy.

TABLE 229–2. CONDITIONS CAUSING ELEVATED CORTISOL LEVELS

Increased CBG	Increased Secretion
Estrogen therapy	Exercise
Pregnancy	Meals
Hyperthyroidism	Physical stress
Diabetes mellitus	Anxiety
Hematologic disorders	Depression
Congenital	Starvation
	Anorexia nervosa
	Alcoholism
	Chronic renal failure

TABLE 229–3. DEXAMETHASONE SUPPRESSION TESTS

Low-dose tests

Overnight test
Dexamethasone, 1 mg p.o. at 11 P.M.; plasma cortisol at 8 to 9 A.M.
Normal response—plasma cortisol <5 μg/dl

Two-day test
Dexamethasone 0.5 mg p.o. q6h for 8 doses; plasma cortisol 6 hours after last dose and 24-hr urine free cortisol and/or 17-OHCS during second day of dexamethasone

Normal response—plasma cortisol <5 μg/dl; urine free cortisol <25 μg/24 hr; urine 17-OHCS <4 mg/24 hr or <1 mg/gram urine creatinine

High-Dose Tests

Overnight test
Dexamethasone 8 mg p.o. at 11 P.M.; plasma cortisol before and at 8 to 9 A.M. after dexamethasone

Response—Cushing's disease; suppression of cortisol to <50% of baseline; ectopic ACTH/adrenal tumors: no cortisol suppression

Two-day test
Dexamethasone 2.0 mg p.o. q6h for 8 doses; plasma cortisol before dexamethasone and after last dose; 24-hr urine free cortisol and/or 17-OHCS before dexamethasone and during second day
Response—Cushing's disease; suppression of plasma or urine steroids to <50% of baseline; ectopic ACTH/adrenal tumors: no steroid suppression

High-Dose Dexamethasone Tests. Glucocorticoids in pharmacologic doses suppress ACTH and cortisol secretion in most patients with pituitary ACTH-producing tumors, but not in patients with adrenal and ectopic tumors. Two tests are available (Table 229–3). The overnight high-dose test is simpler and more accurate than the two-day high-dose test. Approximately 90 per cent of patients with Cushing's disease have suppression of cortisol levels to less than 50 per cent of baseline levels, whereas about 95 per cent of those with adrenal tumors or the ectopic ACTH syndrome do not achieve this degree of suppression. The two-day high-dose test is more time consuming and less reliable in that 15 to 30 per cent of patients with Cushing's disease fail to achieve greater than 50 per cent suppression of urine 17-OHCS, urine free cortisol, or plasma cortisol.

STIMULATION TESTS. These procedures assess the reserve capacity of the hypothalamic-pituitary-adrenal axis and its ability to respond appropriately to stressful situations. These tests act at different sites of the axis and thus can be used to assess its different functions.

CRF Testing. Corticotropin releasing factor (CRF), currently being studied, should soon be available for the investigation of pituitary-adrenal disorders. CRF may be useful in the diagnosis of secondary adrenocortical insufficiency due to both hypothalamic-pituitary disorders and glucocorticoid therapy. However, data comparing this procedure with metyrapone stimulation or insulin-induced hypoglycemia are not yet available. CRF has already proven to be useful in the differential diagnosis of Cushing's syndrome. In states of hypercortisolism, CRF elicits responses of both ACTH and cortisol when Cushing's disease is present; in the ectopic ACTH syndrome or adrenal tumors no response is observed. Again, only limited data are thus far available, and one exception has been reported in which an ectopic tumor responded to CRF. In current protocols, CRF is generally administered intravenously in a dose of 1 μg per kilogram of body weight. ACTH and cortisol secretion peak at 30 to 60 minutes and may be sustained for several hours. Flushing and occasionally hypotension have been observed, and thus the test should be performed with the patient supine.

ACTH Testing. The administration of ACTH, which allows direct assessment of adrenal glucocorticoid reserve, is most useful in the diagnosis of adrenal insufficiency, both primary and secondary. The rapid ACTH stimulation test is best carried out with synthetic human ACTH (α1–24 ACTH), which has full biologic potency and a lesser incidence of allergic reactions than previously used ACTH preparations. The test is performed by administering 250 μg of synthetic ACTH (Cortrosyn) intravenously or intramuscularly; plasma cortisol levels are obtained prior to and at 30 or 60 minutes after ACTH administration. Normally the plasma cortisol level will be greater than 15 to 18 μg per deciliter and will have increased by at least 5 μg per deciliter. Subnormal responses to ACTH stimulation establish the diagnosis of adrenal insufficiency.

By contrast, a normal response excludes primary adrenal failure and complete secondary insufficiency, but it does not exclude partial secondary adrenal insufficiency. A normal response to ACTH in the latter case occurs when there is sufficient basal ACTH secretion to prevent adrenal atrophy but not enough pituitary reserve to respond to stress. When this infrequent situation is suspected, the issue can be resolved with the use of metyrapone or insulin hypoglycemia testing. Performance of the rapid ACTH stimulation test will delay therapy of suspected acute adrenal insufficiency by only 30 minutes, following which therapy can be administered while awaiting the results.

The rapid ACTH stimulation test gives no information regarding the cause of demonstrated adrenal dysfunction. This distinction can be made by measuring either the basal plasma ACTH level or the aldosterone response to ACTH stimulation (normally an increment in the plasma aldosterone of at least 4 ng per deciliter above baseline). The latter test is based on the fact that the zona glomerulosa responds acutely to ACTH and that this response is preserved in secondary adrenal insufficiency, but is deficient in the primary form in which the entire adrenal cortex is destroyed.

In secondary but not primary adrenal insufficiency, cortisol secretion will increase after three days of ACTH administration. Although previously useful, these tests are rarely used at present because of the availability of plasma ACTH and aldosterone measurements.

Metyrapone Testing. Metyrapone inhibits the synthesis of cortisol by blocking 11β-hydroxylation. As a result, ACTH secretion increases and drives the production of steroids proximal to the site of the block. Plasma 11-deoxycortisol is measured in response to the metyrapone test. The overnight test is most commonly used because of its rapidity and simplicity; because of the short duration of inhibition of cortisol synthesis there is little risk of precipitating acute adrenal insufficiency. In this procedure metyrapone is given at midnight with food, and plasma for 11-deoxycortisol and cortisol determinations is obtained at 8 A.M. The dose of metyrapone* is 2 grams for patients less than 70 kg; 2.5 grams for those 70 to 90 kg and 3 grams for patients weighing more than 90 kg. A plasma cortisol value <10 μg per deciliter indicates adequate 11β-hydroxylase inhibition, and in normal persons plasma 11-deoxycortisol increases to greater than 7 μg per deciliter. If assays for 11-deoxycortisol are unavailable, a three-day test can be performed in which urinary 17-OH corticosteroids, which include 11-deoxycortisol metabolites, are measured. A normal response to metyrapone requires function of both the pituitary and adrenals. A subnormal response establishes the diagnosis of adrenal insufficiency and correlates well with deficient responses to stress and hypoglycemia. The test per se does not differentiate primary and secondary causes. Since a normal response to the rapid ACTH stimulation test is usually found prior to performance of the metyrapone test, a subnormal response then indicates secondary adrenal insufficiency.

Insulin Hypoglycemia Testing (Ch. 231). Hypoglycemia elicits a central nevous system stress response that in turn stimulates CRF and ACTH secretion and, as a consequence, cortisol release. A normal cortisol response to hypoglycemia indicates a normal hypothalamic-pituitary-adrenal axis and rules out adrenal insufficiency or decreased pituitary ACTH reserve. This test is most often utilized in the evaluation of suspected hypothalamic or pituitary disorders, since growth hormone reserve can be assessed simultaneously with that of ACTH.

*This dosage is not listed in the manufacturer's directive.

OTHER PROCEDURES. Other agents such as pyrogens or vasopressin have also been used to stimulate pituitary ACTH secretion, but have achieved less acceptance. Synthetic CRF is currently being evaluated to determine if it will stimulate ACTH and cortisol release more effectively in pituitary tumors than in ectopic or adrenal tumors and can be useful to distinguish hypothalamic pituitary causes of impaired ACTH release.

MINERALOCORTICOID FUNCTION

PLASMA RENIN. Assessment of plasma renin is essential in the diagnosis of states of excess and deficient mineralocorticoid secretion; it is also helpful in the evaluation of other types of hypertension (Ch. 47). Currently used assays do not measure the plasma renin concentration directly, but instead measure the plasma renin activity (PRA) by quantifying the amount of angiotensin I generated over time in the patient's plasma. The normal values of PRA depend on the salt intake and postural status. In subjects with moderate salt intake (around 110 mEq Na^+ per day) and in the seated position, the plasma renin activity ranges from 1.5 to 5 ng of angiotensin I generated per milliliter per hour (ng A_I per milliliter per hour). In individuals in whom salt has been restricted (20 mEq Na^+ per day) for four days and who have been in the upright posture for two hours the values range from 5 to 10 ng A_I per milliliter per hour. Factors that affect renin release have been described above, since they are those that regulate mineralocorticoid production. Of those seen in clinical practice, diuretic therapy is the most commonly observed factor that increases the PRA. In patients with primary hyperaldosteronism the PRA is characteristically suppressed. With aldosterone-producing adenomas, the PRA is unresponsive or only weakly responsive to provocative stimuli, whereas in those with primary aldosteronism with bilateral hyperplasia, the PRA does respond to such stimuli.

In patients with only borderline low PRA in whom primary aldosterone excess is suspected, stimulation tests with measurement of PRA may be necessary. Patients can be subjected to salt restriction (20 mEq of sodium per day for five days) or given 40 mg of furosemide the evening and morning before sampling; blood samples are then taken after two hours in the upright posture. If the plasma renin does not increase under these conditions it is likely that primary aldosteronism is present. Caution should be exercised in performing these tests since severe and life-threatening volume depletion or hypokalemia could ensue; these risks must be weighed before the test is performed.

ALDOSTERONE MEASUREMENTS. These measurements are most often utilized in the diagnosis of primary aldosteronism and in the differentiation of its subtypes of adenoma and hyperplasia. Plasma measurements ordinarily involve extraction and chromatography of the steroid followed by radioimmunoassay. The urine measurements ordinarily quantify by radioimmunoassay the 18-glucuronide metabolite of aldosterone (about 15 per cent of the total aldosterone production). Alternatively, urinary tetrahydroaldosterone can be measured.

These measurements should be made after adequate sodium repletion (a sodium intake of at least 120 mEq per 24 hours for four days) and withdrawal of diuretics for at least two to three weeks, and in the case of plasma measurements after at least 6 hours of recumbency. Normal values for aldosterone excretion are 5 to 20 μg per 24 hours; basal plasma values in the supine patient are usually 5 to 15 ng per deciliter. Although problems with episodic steroid release are less with aldosterone than with cortisol, these may explain why measurements of plasma aldosterone levels are less reliable than are urinary assays in the diagnosis of mild aldosterone hypersecretion. Plasma aldosterone values are of greater utility in the differential diagnosis of hyperaldosteronism, as discussed under primary aldosteronism. A simple and reliable method of differentiating primary aldosteronism due to an adenoma from that due to hyperplasia is to measure the plasma aldosterone response to posture. Plasma aldosterone levels in hyperplasia, but not adenoma, are still under control of the renin-angiotensin system. Thus, the plasma aldosterone is initially measured in the supine position at 8 A.M. after four days of a sodium intake of at least 120 mEq per 24 hours and then subsequently after two to four hours in the upright posture. In patients with an adenoma there is either no increase or an actual decrease in plasma aldosterone in the upright position, whereas with hyperplasia, there is an increase in plasma aldosterone concentrations after two to four hours in the upright position.

If there is still uncertainty, additional tests can be employed. Deoxycorticosterone acetate (DOCA), 10 mg intramuscularly every 12 hours, can be given for three days to patients whose intake is 120 mEq of sodium per 24 hours and plasma or urinary aldosterone measured in relation to pretreatment values. Aldosterone is minimally or not at all suppressed in patients with an aldosterone-producing adenoma and in most patients with hyperplasia. Although some groups have given 0.3 mg of 9α-fluorocortisol orally twice for three days instead of DOCA, others have found this test to be less reliable, presumably because 9α-fluorocortisol suppresses ACTH and aldosterone production in some patients with primary aldosteronism. Saline infusion is also used; 0.5 to 2 liters of normal saline is administered over four hours and in normal persons plasma aldosterone suppresses to less than 5 ng per deciliter.

ADRENAL ANDROGENS

Plasma levels of the predominant adrenal androgens, DHEA, DHEA-S, and androstenedione, can be measured. These assays plus that of testosterone are most frequently used for the evaluation of hirsutism. Stimulation and supression tests have not been as useful as in other pituitary and adrenal disorders. Plasma free testosterone measurements usually provide a better index of total androgenicity than total levels of the hormone, since androgen excess decreases sex hormone–binding globulin and can result in a normal total level in the presence of an elevated free testosterone concentration. Measurement of androstanediol and its glucuronide, metabolic products of dihydrotestosterone, provides an index of peripheral androgen production, and may provide the best index of androgen excess.

Urinary 17-ketosteroids were traditionally measured to assess adrenal androgen production. This procedure measures mainly DHEA and DHEA-S metabolites. However, this test has limited utility since the more potent androgens such as testosterone and dihydrotestosterone contribute less than 1 per cent of the total urinary 17-ketosteroids and thus are not assessed. Furthermore, 17-ketosteroids are increased in obesity without androgen excess, and there is interference by multiple drugs and medications.

Adrenocortical Hypofunction

John D. Baxter

Adrenal insufficiency is defined by deficient production of glucocorticoids or mineralocorticoids or both. Primary adrenocortical insufficiency (Addison's disease) is due to destruction of the adrenal cortex, whereas in secondary adrenocortical insufficiency impaired cortisol production is due to deficient ACTH production. Hyporeninemia causes selective aldosterone deficiency. Selective adrenal defects due to congenital enzyme deficiencies also occur (Ch. 233).

PRIMARY ADRENOCORTICAL INSUFFICIENCY

ETIOLOGY. Primary adrenocortical insufficiency has multiple causes. In the United States over 80 per cent of the cases are due to autoimmune destruction of the adrenal. Tuberculosis is the second most frequent cause and remains a common cause of the disease in underdeveloped countries with a higher incidence of tuberculosis. Other rare causes include hemorrhage due to sepsis, anticoagulation, coagulopathies, trauma, surgery, and pregnancy; bilateral infarction, e.g., due to thrombosis or arteritis; fungal infection; invasive disorders such as lymphoma, metastatic tumors, amyloidosis, sarcoidosis, and hemochromatosis; surgery; cytotoxic agents such as mitotane; and congenital hypoplasia and hyporesponsiveness to ACTH. Nonetheless, primary adrenocortical insufficiency due to any cause is a rare disease with an estimated incidence in Western countries of around 50 per million population.

The idiopathic, presumed autoimmune form of adrenal insufficiency is 2-fold to 3-fold more common in females and is usually diagnosed in the third to fifth decades of life. Early in the disease there is lymphocytic infiltration of the gland, and there is a high association (40 to 53 per cent of patients) with disorders of other endocrine glands or with pernicious anemia or vitiligo. Antibodies to the gland are commonly present, and there is evidence for abnormal cell-mediated immunity.

The association of Addison's disease with the other disorders has been referred to as *Schmidt's syndrome*, autoimmune endocrine failure, and the polyglandular failure syndrome. Approximate associations are ovarian failure, 25 per cent of female patients (testicular failure in males is unusual); hyperthyroidism, 7 per cent (mostly female); hypothyroidism or Hashimoto's thyroiditis with goiter, 9 per cent; subclinical thyroiditis, up to 80 per cent; diabetes mellitus (type I), 12 per cent; vitiligo, 9 per cent, presumably due to immunologic destruction of melanocytes; hypoparathyroidism, 6 per cent; and, pernicious anemia, 4 per cent. Whereas these problems are common with adrenal insufficiency, patients with more common problems such as diabetes or thyroid disease only rarely develop Addison's disease. The development of autoimmune adrenocortical insufficiency shows some hereditary predisposition, and an autosomal recessive pattern of inheritance has been suggested. About 40 per cent of patients have first- or second-degree relatives with one of the associated disorders. Further, there is an increased incidence of histocompatibility antigen (HLA) types B8, Dw3 and of the haplotype HLA-A1,B8.

CLINICAL MANIFESTATIONS. The development of clinical manifestations of adrenocortical insufficiency requires loss of more than 90 per cent of the adrenal cortices. The rate of destruction varies, depending on the cause, but with the idiopathic variety this usually (but not always) requires several months. With gradual destruction, increases in ACTH secondary to the lower cortisol levels tends to stimulate the gland maximally. Thus there is a period when the gland can produce normal levels of cortisol, but when responses to stress are impaired. These patients may experience minimal symptoms unless exposed to some stressful event. In fact, in about 25 per cent of the patients symptoms first appear in a crisis or impending crisis. However, in the majority of cases destruction becomes more complete, and the patient experiences symptoms that lead to medical evaluation before a crisis occurs. The destruction of the gland results in loss of both glucocorticoid and mineralocorticoid functions and secondary increases in ACTH and in renin.

The clinical presentation depends on the rate and degree of adrenal destruction, the presence of stressful influences, and the pathology of associated or causative conditions. For these reasons it is convenient to discuss separately the chronic and acute presentations.

Chronic primary adrenocortical insufficiency may go unnoticed for some time, because of its gradual development, although retrospectively the patients frequently recall symptoms beginning months to years earlier. The major clinical features, as noted in Table 229–4, are weakness and fatigue, weight loss, anorexia, hyperpigmentation, hypotension, gastrointestinal upset (including nausea, vomiting, and less commonly diarrhea), salt craving, and postural dizziness. Weakness is generalized and not restricted to particular muscle groups. Weight loss is due both to dehydration secondary to salt loss, and to anorexia. Mild hypoglycemia is common in adults, but it is unusual for it to be severe enough to be symptomatic; however, clinically symptomatic hypoglycemia is more common in children. Fe-

TABLE 229–4. CLINICAL FEATURES OF CHRONIC PRIMARY ADRENOCORTICAL INSUFFICIENCY

	%
Weakness and fatigue	100
Weight loss	100
Anorexia	100
Hyperpigmentation	92
Hypotension	88
Gastrointestinal symptoms	56
Salt craving	19
Postural symptoms	12

From Baxter JD, Tyrrell JB: The adrenal cortex. *In* Felig P, Baxter JD, Broadus AH, Frohman LA (eds.): Endocrinology and Metabolism. New York, McGraw-Hill Book Company, 1981, p 453.

male patients can also have amenorrhea and loss of axillary hair, the latter due to decrease of adrenal androgens. Although dehydration can be significant, this is typically compensated for by increased salt intake. Hyponatremia is present in most patients, although it may be masked somewhat if there is dehydration. Mild hyperkalemia is also usually present; the presence of severe hyperkalemia should suggest concomitant renal or other disease. A normocytic, normochromic anemia is common, but can also be masked by dehydration and hemoconcentration. There tends to be neutropenia, lymphocytosis, and eosinophilia. Dehydration when present leads to increases in blood urea nitrogen and creatinine, and there may be mild acidosis. The heart tends to be small and vertical on x-ray examination; the abdominal radiograph is usually normal, but can show adrenal calcification in about 50 per cent of those cases due to tuberculosis. Calcification of the ear lobes sometimes occurs in longstanding cases.

Hyperpigmentation is an important diagnostic feature and may precede other manifestations. It is generalized, but is accentuated in sun-exposed areas, pressure points such as the elbows, knees, knuckles, and toes, and on palmar creases, nail beds, buccal mucosa, tongue, nipples, aerolae, and perivaginal or perianal mucosa, and in recent surgical scars. In blacks, pigmentation of the tongue is of diagnostic helpfulness. Hyperpigmentation is commonly misinterpreted as an excessive sun tan and the "healthy" appearance of the patient may lead to a dismissal of other symptoms.

Acute adrenocortical insufficiency is seen most commonly in a patient with either undiagnosed or diagnosed adrenocortical insufficiency who is exposed to one of the stresses discussed earlier and who therefore has an increased requirement for glucocorticoids. It can also be seen with acute adrenal destruction secondary to hemorrhage, most commonly associated with septicemia or anticoagulant therapy (adrenal apoplexy). In these cases, anorexia is often profound with nausea and vomiting that exaggerates volume depletion and dehydration. Abdominal pain is frequent and may mimic a surgical condition of the abdomen; however, these symptoms are usually vague. The blood pressure falls, and hypovolemic shock develops that is incompletely responsive to fluid replacement. Fever is common and may or may not be due to the precipitating event. Hyperpigmentation will be present or absent, depending on the duration of the disease; when present it is an important diagnostic sign. The presence of hyperkalemia, lymphocytosis, and eosinophilia should also suggest the diagnosis. Severe hypoglycemia is uncommon and is more likely to occur in children or in adults with secondary adrenal insufficiency with both ACTH and growth hormone deficiency. The diagnosis of acute adrenocortical insufficiency should be considered in any patient with unexplained shock, and the consideration of this should not be diverted by the presence of an accompanying disorder such as infection or diabetic ketoacidosis.

SECONDARY ADRENOCORTICAL INSUFFICIENCY. Secondary adrenocortical insufficiency results from inadequate ACTH production. The causes are discussed in Ch. 225. For spontaneous disease, pituitary and hypothalamic tumors are the most common cause. In these cases there is progressive loss of ACTH such that cortisol production and responses to stress are decreased, but mineralocorticoid production is almost always normal. In addition to spontaneous causes, chronic suppression of ACTH production with exogenous glucocorticoids followed by their withdrawal also causes the syndrome and is by far the most frequent cause.

The development of clinical manifestations is usually chronic but like primary adrenocortical insufficiency can be acute. The presenting features are similar to those of primary adrenocortical insufficiency with three exceptions: (1) Since hypersecretion of ACTH and related peptides is absent, there is no hyperpigmentation; in fact, patients with hypopituitarism commonly exhibit pallor of the skin. (2) The electrolyte abnormalities of hyponatremia, hyperkalemia, and mild acidosis are absent because of preservation of aldosterone secretion. Hyponatremia, if present, is due to decreased glomerular filtration rate, hypothyroidism, or increased vasopression release. (3) Other features of hypopituitarism (Ch. 225) may be present.

DIAGNOSIS. The clinical suspicion of Addison's disease should be confirmed by definitive laboratory testing. In seriously ill patients, however, therapy should not be delayed by prolonged diagnostic measures; if means for a rapid diagnosis are unavailable, therapy should be initiated if the clinical suspicion of adrenal insufficiency is significant. The diagnosis can be established or ruled out later. Diagnostic reliance on basal urine or plasma measurements is dangerous. Although an elevated plasma cortisol level (e.g., greater than 25 μg per deciliter) makes the diagnosis unlikely, normal basal cortisol levels can be present with impaired adrenal responsiveness to stress. Thus the adrenal reserve should be tested.

Figure 229–5 shows a plan of approach. If adrenocortical insufficiency is suspected, the rapid ACTH stimulation test should be performed. This test requires only 30 minutes and can be done even in most acute situations. A normal response excludes the diagnosis of primary adrenocortical insufficiency; an abnormal response establishes the presence of adrenocortical insufficiency. Only rare patients with secondary adrenocortical insufficiency will respond normally because of partial ACTH deficiency that still allows the adrenal to respond. The basal plasma ACTH level, determined prior to ACTH administration, is measured to distinguish between primary and secondary adrenocortical insufficiency. In primary adrenocortical insufficiency, the levels exceed 250 pg per milliliter and usually are greater than 400 pg per milliliter. By contrast, plasma ACTH levels in secondary adrenocortical insufficiency are inappropriately low, ranging from 0 to 50 pg per milliliter. The plasma aldosterone response to ACTH can also be used to differentiate primary from secondary adrenocortical insufficiency, but there is less extensive experience with this procedure.

Further diagnostic procedures are needed only in exceptional cases, for example, in suspected secondary adrenocortical insufficiency with a normal response to ACTH or in cases in which plasma ACTH levels are unavailable. In these cases the metyrapone or insulin hypoglycemia tests can be helpful. The latter test is usually performed in suspected hypopituitarism, since simultaneous assessment of both growth hormone and ACTH can be performed (Ch. 225). The metyrapone test is performed in patients in whom hypoglycemia is contraindicated or those with prior glucocorticoid therapy, since it provides essentially the same information and is of less potential risk to the patient. An abnormal response to metyrapone establishes the diagnosis of secondary adrenocortical insufficiency, since the primary form would have been excluded by the ACTH stimulation test. The presence of low normal or low ACTH levels further confirms this diagnosis.

In spontaneous adrenocortical insufficiency of any type, the laboratory evaluation should include a blood glucose, serum calcium and phosphorus, and thyroid function tests, including TSH and thyroid antibody determinations. If there is oligo-

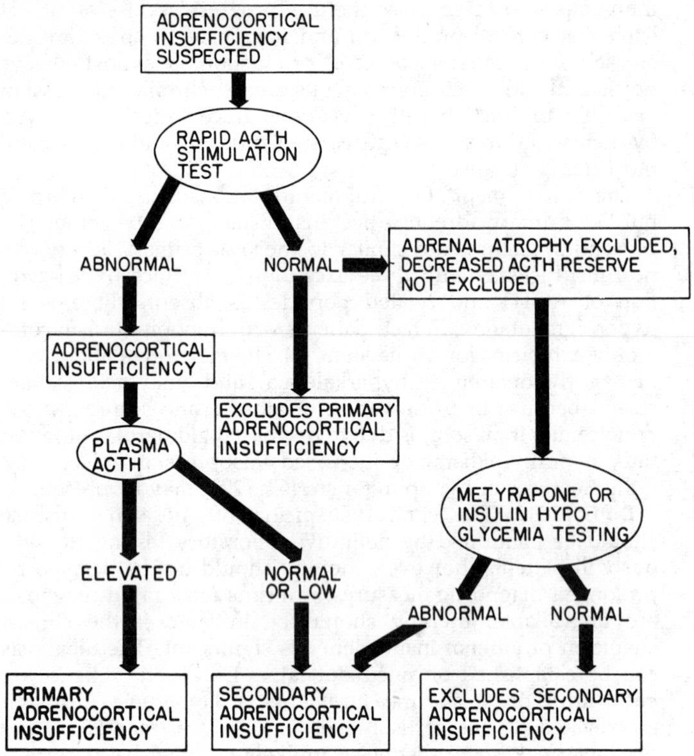

Figure 229–5. Evaluation of suspected primary or secondary adrenocortical insufficiency. Boxes enclose clinical decisions and circles enclose diagnostic tests. (Reprinted from Baxter JD, Tyrrell JB: *In* Felig P, Baxter JD, Broadus AE, Frohman LA (eds.): Endocrinology and Metabolism. New York, McGraw-Hill Book Company 1981, p 458.)

menorrhea or amenorrhea, FSH and LH levels should be determined. Finally, first- and second-degree relatives should be screened for endocrine deficiency syndromes because of the increased risk in these individuals. In secondary adrenocortical insufficiency, patients should be examined for other pituitary dysfunction, pituitary or hypothalamic tumors, and prior glucocorticoid therapy (Ch. 225). In acute adrenocortical insufficiency, the precipitating cause should be determined, since this is often infectious.

TREATMENT. *Acute Adrenocortical Insufficiency.* In an acute crisis, therapy should be instituted as soon as possible after the diagnosis is suspected (Table 229–5). A soluble glucocorticoid, such as cortisol hemisuccinate or phosphate, should be given intravenously. Volume depletion, electrolyte abnormalities, and hypoglycemia should be corrected and general supportive measures instituted. Precipitating factors should be assessed and corrected. If recovery is satisfactory, the glucocorticoid dose can then be reduced on the second day and then tapered to oral maintenance doses by the fourth to fifth days. Mineralocorticoid replacement is unnecessary when high doses of cortisol are given, but should be given if a synthetic glucocorticoid such as prednisolone or dexamethasone is used and when the cortisol dose has been tapered to near-maintenance levels.

TABLE 229–5. THERAPY OF ADRENAL INSUFFICIENCY

Acute Crisis

1. Hydrocortisone, 100 mg IV, every 6 hr for 24 hr. If stable, reduce to 50 mg every 6 hr and then taper to oral maintenance in 4 to 5 days. Maintain or increase dose to 200 to 400 mg per 24 hr if complications persist or occur.
2. Correct volume depletion, dehydration, hypotension, and hypoglycemia with intravenous saline and glucose.
3. Correct precipitating factors, especially infection.

Maintenance

1. Hydrocortisone 15 to 20 mg p.o. q A.M.; 5 to 10 mg at 4 to 6 P.M.
2. 9α-Fluorocortisol 0.05 to 0.1 mg q A.M. (primary).
3. Follow weight, blood pressure, and electrolytes.
4. Educate patient and increase cortisol dosage during stress.

Chronic Adrenocortical Insufficiency. The treatment of the primary form of this condition requires both glucocorticoid and mineralocorticoid replacement, whereas the secondary form usually requires only glucocorticoid replacement (Table 229–5). Patients must be made aware that a lifetime of replacement is necessary and of the need to increase glucocorticoid replacement in times of stress. Each patient should carry an identification bracelet or card. Cortisol at levels similar to physiologic production is given in a way that crudely approximates the circadian rhythm. Thus, for ordinary maintenance, 15 to 20 mg of cortisol are given in the early morning and 5 to 10 mg in the late afternoon. An equivalent amount of prednisolone or prednisone (about 5 mg per day) or cortisone acetate (37.5 mg per day) is also acceptable; however, the potency of dexamethasone has probably been underestimated, and this steroid is not recommended. For mineralocorticoid replacement, 9α-fluorocortisol 0.05 to 0.1 mg orally per day is recommended. Follow-up is mainly by clinical assessment of a feeling of well-being, examination of signs of glucocorticoid or mineralocorticoid excess or deficiency, and measurements of serum electrolytes. Measurements of plasma cortisol, ACTH, and renin are usually not helpful. The doses may need to be adjusted somewhat. Many of the subjective complaints of Addison's disease can be reversed within a few days; a somewhat longer time is required before strength returns to normal and hyperpigmentation subsides.

In times of stress, it is sometimes difficult to predict the need for increased glucocorticoid administration. It is best to err on the side of overreplacement rather than underreplacement. For minor illnesses such as significant upper respiratory infections, the cortisol dose should be doubled or tripled and then tapered as soon as possible. It is not usually necessary to change the 9α-fluorocortisol dose. Patients with vomiting and substantial diarrhea should seek medical attention and receive parenteral cortisol. Patients who may not have early access to medical attention should keep injectable cortisol available and be instructed in its use.

In the event of major trauma, treatment should be similar to that for adrenal crisis discussed above. In the case of elective

TABLE 229–6. STEROID COVERAGE FOR SURGERY

1. Correct electrolytes, blood pressure, and hydration if necessary.
2. Hydrocortisone phosphate or hemisuccinate, 100 mg IM, on call to operating room.
3. Hydrocortisone phosphate or hemisuccinate, 50 mg IM or IV, in recovery room and every 6 hr for the first 24 hr.
4. If progress is satisfactory, reduce dosage to 25 mg every 6 hr for 24 hr; then taper to maintenance dosage over 3 to 5 days. Resume previous 9α-fluorocortisol dose when patient is taking oral medications.
5. Maintain or increase cortisol dosage to 200 to 400 mg per 24 hr if fever, hypotension, or other complications occur.

From Baxter JD, Tyrrell JB: The adrenal cortex. *In* Felig P, Baxter JD, Broadus AH, Froham LA (eds.): Endocrinology and Metabolism. New York, McGraw-Hill Book Company, 1981, p 462.

major surgery the protocol described in Table 229–6 has been shown to be effective.

PROGNOSIS. Survival of patients in whom adrenocortical insufficiency was adequately diagnosed and treated now approximates that of the normal population. This is in sharp contrast to the period before steroids were available or when only mineralocorticoid replacement was available, at which time the survival rate was usually two years or less.

HYPOALDOSTERONISM

PATHOGENESIS. Hypoaldosteronism can occur in association with hypocortisolism or as an isolated defect. The major cause of isolated hypoaldosteronism is defective renal renin secretion (hyporeninemic hypoaldosteronism) (Ch. 76). Other rarer causes include isolated adrenal biosynthetic defects (18-hydroxylase syndrome), transient deficiency following removal of an aldosterone-producing tumor, unresponsiveness to aldosterone (pseudohypoaldosteronism) with normal or increased aldosterone production, marked potassium depletion, and heparin administration.

HYPORENINEMIC HYPOALDOSTERONISM. This is seen in patients with renal disease due to a variety of causes such as interstitial nephritis, diabetes mellitus, or multiple myeloma. It has also been observed following removal of an aldosterone-producing tumor or rarely without any apparent cause in association with hypertension. The hyporeninemia leads to decreased aldosterone production and impaired ability of the zona glomerulosa to respond to stimuli. However, the gland usually retains some capacity to secrete aldosterone through stimulation by potassium. Hypoaldosteronism results secondarily in hyperkalemia, which is disproportionate to the extent of renal disease. Chronic renal disease per se ordinarily does not lead to hyperkalemia unless the glomerular filtration rate is severely impaired (e.g., less than 15 ml per minute). In fact, hyporeninemic hypoaldosteronism is probably a common cause of hyperkalemia in patients with renal disease and creatinine clearance rates greater than 15 ml per minute. Although these patients can develop hyponatremia, in adults this is less common, probably because of the fact that the primary disease tends to favor sodium retention. These patients also tend to develop a metabolic acidosis due to the lack of H^+-secreting actions of aldosterone; this can be accentuated by a decreased glomerular filtration rate. This form of acidosis has been classified as type IV renal tubular acidosis (Ch. 83.2).

TREATMENT. The treatment of hypoaldosteronism involves therapy for the primary condition plus mineralocorticoid replacement as described above for primary adrenocortical insufficiency. However, in some patients with hypertension, treatment with 9α-fluorocortisol is not indicated and diuretics are used instead. Conversely, some patients require higher doses of mineralocorticoids, probably because the renal disease renders them more refractory to the steroid.

Cushing's Syndrome

J. Blake Tyrrell

Cushing's syndrome results from chronic glucocorticoid excess. It is seen most commonly in patients receiving long-term therapy with supraphysiologic doses of glucocorticoids. Spontaneously occurring Cushing's syndrome is a rare disorder, the precise incidence of which is unknown. It occurs as a result of either primary tumors of the adrenal gland that hypersecrete cortisol or from excess ACTH secretion that may be of pituitary or nonpituitary (ectopic ACTH syndrome) sources.

Cushing's disease, the subtype of spontaneous hypercortisolism due to excessive pituitary ACTH secretion, accounts for two thirds of reported cases. This disorder is most common in women, with a female to male ratio of at least 5:1, and usually begins clinically between the ages of 20 and 40 years.

Secretion of ACTH from ectopic tumors is found in about 15 per cent of cases with documented Cushing's syndrome. The true incidence of this disorder is probably much higher, since many patients lack the typical clinical features of cortisol excess because of the dominance of the manifestations of cancer and the rapidity of progression and thus the disorder may go undiagnosed. Because of the current predominance of oat cell carcinoma of the lung in males, the ectopic ACTH syndrome has a female to male ratio of 1:3 and an age onset most frequently between 40 and 60 years.

Primary adrenal tumors secreting cortisol account for approximately 15 per cent of cases of Cushing's syndrome. In adults there is an equal frequency of adenoma and carcinoma. In childhood prior to the age of ten years, adrenal carcinoma is the most frequent cause of Cushing's syndrome. Both adenomas and carcinomas secreting cortisol are more prevalent in women than in men. The average age at diagnosis is approximately 40 years, and 70 per cent of cases occur in adults.

PATHOLOGY. Pituitary adenomas (Ch. 225) are present in over 90 per cent of patients with Cushing's disease. These tumors are usually small; 50 per cent are 5 mm or less in diameter. They are typically basophilic and unencapsulated and contain ACTH, β-LPH, and β-endorphin. The few patients with Cushing's disease who do not have pituitary adenomas have (1) diffuse hyperplasia; (2) hyperplasia with multiple nests of adenomatous cells; (3) an adenoma or adenomatous hyperplasia of the intermediate lobe of the pituitary, or (4) no obvious pituitary disorder.

Adrenocortical hyperplasia in Cushing's disease results in modest increases in combined adrenal weight due to hyperplasia of the zonae reticularis and fasciculata. In the ectopic ACTH syndrome, adrenal enlargement and hyperplasia of the zona reticularis are usually more marked with a concomitant reduction in the number of zona fasciculata cells. Bilateral nodular hyperplasia occurs in approximately 20 per cent of cases of ACTH excess and may be due to more prolonged stimulation of the adrenal cortex by ACTH. In this case, in addition to diffuse hyperplasia of the zonae reticularis and fasciculata, there are multiple nodules that vary from microscopic to several centimeters in diameter and that contain clear cells similar to those of the zona fasciculata.

Cortisol-secreting adenomas are usually encapsulated, range from 2 to 6 cm in diameter, typically secrete cortisol alone, and are usually composed of zona fasciculata–like cells. Adrenal carcinomas that secrete cortisol are usually large at the time of diagnosis, may be palpable as abdominal masses, and may secrete a number of steroids. Histologically these tumors may appear benign or exhibit considerable pleomorphism, and the histologic appearance does not predict benign or malignant behavior. Therefore the diagnosis of adrenal carcinoma is dependent on the demonstration of either local tumor invasiveness or metastatic spread. Extension of these tumors occurs locally, and common sites of metastases are the liver and lung.

ETIOLOGY AND PATHOGENESIS. The etiology of Cushing's disease is unknown. It is possible that primary pituitary tumors arise spontaneously. In cases in which diffuse or adenomatous hyperplasia is present, it is possible that excessive secretion of CRF or some other factor stimulates the pituitary. The ectopic

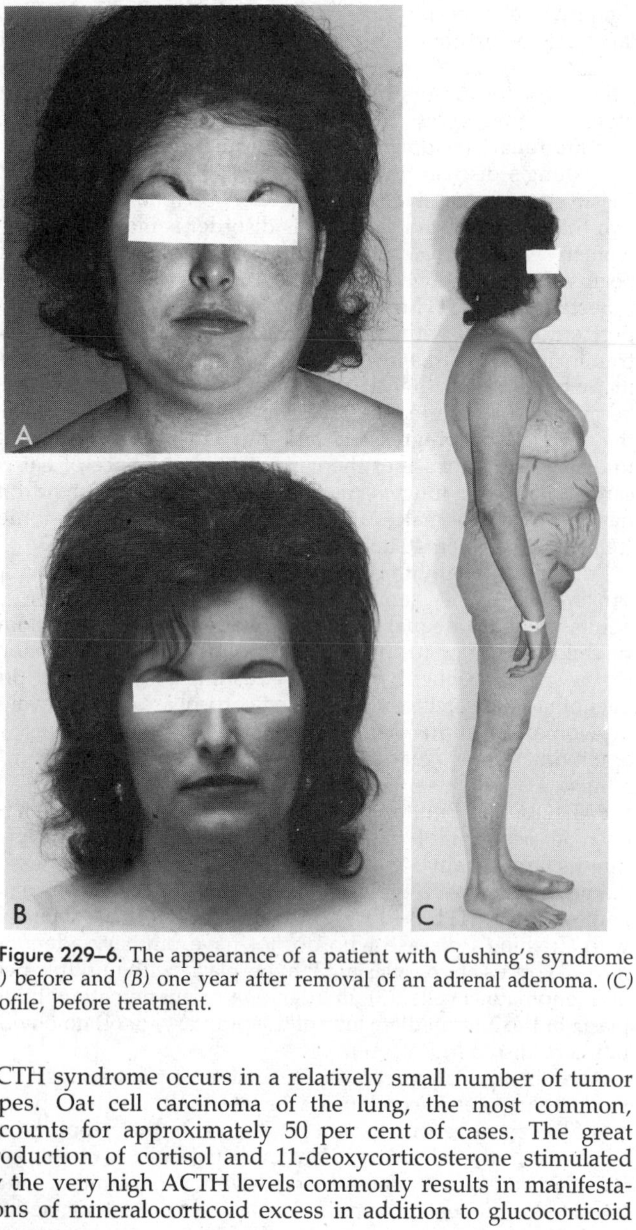

Figure 229–6. The appearance of a patient with Cushing's syndrome *(A)* before and *(B)* one year after removal of an adrenal adenoma. *(C)* Profile, before treatment.

ACTH syndrome occurs in a relatively small number of tumor types. Oat cell carcinoma of the lung, the most common, accounts for approximately 50 per cent of cases. The great production of cortisol and 11-deoxycorticosterone stimulated by the very high ACTH levels commonly results in manifestations of mineralocorticoid excess in addition to glucocorticoid excess.

Other ACTH-secreting tumors include thymomas, islet cell tumors of the pancreas, carcinoid tumors, medullary carcinomas of the thyroid, and pheochromocytomas. Many other tumors have been found to secrete ACTH, but occur very rarely. Cortisol–producing adrenal tumors arise spontaneously and are not under normal control by the hypothalamic-pituitary axis; their secretion of cortisol and the other steroids is autonomous, episodic, and random.

CLINICAL FEATURES. The classic features, most typically seen in Cushing's disease (Fig. 229–6, Table 229–7) usually develop insidiously over several years. The most common manifestation is central obesity with rounding of the face and fat accumulation around the trunk, supraclavicular areas, and dorsocervical spine. Serial photographs are sometimes helpful in recognizing these gradual changes. Whereas classically this pattern of obesity spares the extremities, generalized obesity including the extremities occurs in about 50 per cent of patients. Atrophy of the skin and underlying connective tissue is frequent. This leads to facial plethora, easy bruisability, and red to purple depressed striae. The last occur most commonly over the lower abdomen, but can also be more generalized on the trunk and upper legs. Patients also have poor healing of minor or major injuries and abrasions and an increased incidence of superficial

TABLE 229–7. INCIDENCE OF CLINICAL FEATURES OF CUSHING'S SYNDROME

Feature	%
Obesity	94
Facial plethora	84
Hirsutism	82
Menstrual disorders	76
Hypertension	72
Muscular weakness	58
Back pain	58
Striae	52
Acne	40
Psychologic symptoms	40
Bruising	36
Congestive heart failure	22
Edema	18
Renal calculi	16
Headache	14
Polyuria/polydipsia	10
Hyperpigmentation	6

Modified from Plotz CM, et al.: Am J Med 13:597, 1952, and Ross EJ, et al: Q J Med 35:149, 1966, and reprinted from Baxter JD, Tyrrell JB: The adrenal cortex. *In* Felig P, Baxter JD, Broadus AE, Frohman LA (eds.): Endocrinology and Metabolism. New York, McGraw-Hill Book Company, 1981, p 472.

fungal infections. Hirsutism is present in approximately 80 per cent of female patients as a result of excessive adrenal androgen secretion. Hypertension is present in the majority of patients; it is rarely accompanied by hypokalemia in Cushing's disease, although this is more common in the ectopic ACTH syndrome or adrenal carcinoma. Hypertension appears to contribute greatly to the mortality of untreated Cushing's syndrome.

Additional common manifestations include hypogonadism in both male and female patients, psychologic disturbances (usually depression), which occur in the majority, and proximal muscle weakness. Osteopenia is present in virtually all patients and involves primarily the ribs and vertebral bodies. With more longstanding disease, frank osteoporosis is common (Ch. 249). Back pain is common, and compression fractures of the spine occur in approximately 20 per cent. Renal stones, secondary to hypercalciuria, and thirst and polyuria, which may be due to hyperglycemia or to hypercalciuria, can also occur. Routine

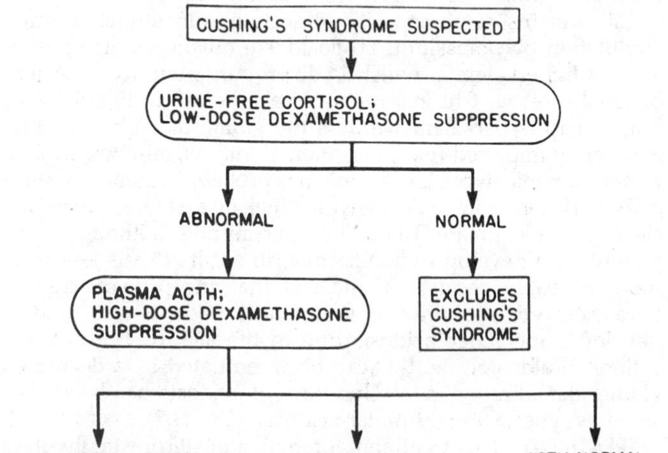

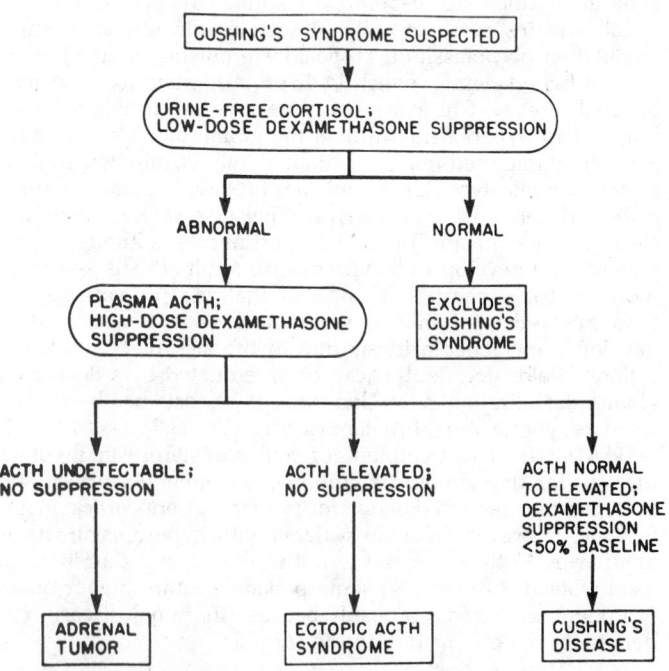

Figure 229–7. Evaluation of Cushing's syndrome. Boxes enclose clinical decisions and circles enclose diagnostic tests. See the text for details and the potential for false-positive and false-negative results. (Reprinted from Baxter JD, Tyrrell JB: *In* Felig P, Baxter JD, Broadus AE, Frohman LA (eds.): Endocrinology and Metabolism. New York, McGraw-Hill Book Company, 1981, p 475.)

laboratory tests may suggest the diagnosis but are nonspecific. These include high normal or modestly elevated values for the hematocrit, slightly elevated white cell counts, and a depressed percentage of lymphocytes and eosinophils. Electrolyte abnormalities occur only rarely in Cushing's disease, and the presence of hypokalemia should suggest the ectopic ACTH syndrome or adrenal carcinoma.

DIAGNOSIS. A suggested plan for the evaluation of suspected Cushing's syndrome is shown in Figure 229–7. If the syndrome is suspected the 24-hour urine free cortisol should be measured and the overnight 1 mg dexamethasone suppression test performed.

If results of both of these tests are normal, the diagnosis of Cushing's syndrome is excluded, with two exceptions: (1) Rare patients whose disease activity is episodic can have normal tests during periods of inactivity. In these cases, repeated evaluation during periods of disease activity will estabish the diagnosis. (2) Rare patients with Cushing's disease will have delayed clearance of dexamethasone, presumably on a genetic basis, and therefore will have a normal response to a low dose of dexamethasone. However, these patients will have elevated urine free cortisol levels.

If the 24-hour urine free cortisol level is elevated and the 1 mg overnight dexamethasone suppression test is abnormal, then spontaneous Cushing's syndrome is present provided that several abnormalities that lead to false-positive responses can be excluded. In obesity, estrogen therapy, drug therapy that increases dexamethasone metabolism (listed in Ch. 29), and chronic renal failure, results of the dexamethasone suppression test can be abnormal, although the 24-hour urine free cortisol is almost always in the normal range. In the case of obesity and estrogen therapy, the two-day low-dose dexamethasone test should be performed; the results are almost always normal in the absence of Cushing's syndrome. Response to both the 24-hour urine free cortisol and the 1 mg dexamethasone suppression tests can be abnormal in alcoholism, acute and chronic illness, depression and other states of substantial emotional stress, and anorexia nervosa. In these cases, in the absence of spontaneous Cushing's syndrome the abnormalities will subside following cessation of the condition. In any event, caution must be exercised before the diagnosis of spontaneous Cushing's syndrome is made in the presence of these conditions.

ETIOLOGIC DIAGNOSIS. Once the diagnosis of Cushing's syndrome has been established, it is essential to determine its specific cause. The two most useful procedures are the measurement of basal plasma ACTH levels and the high-dose dexamethasone suppression test. In Cushing's disease, ACTH levels are normal to modestly elevated (50 to 200 pg per milliliter) and in 90 per cent of these patients, plasma or urinary steroid levels are suppressed to less than 50 per cent of baseline values in response to the high-dose dexamethasone test. In the ectopic ACTH syndrome, plasma ACTH values are often markedly elevated and are more than 200 pg per milliliter in two thirds of patients. In about 95 per cent of these patients, hypothalamic-pituitary control of ACTH and cortisol secretion is absent, and there is no response to high-dose dexamethasone suppression. Exceptions occur in patients with relatively benign carcinoids or thymomas in whom ACTH levels may be only modestly elevated and in whom the high dose of dexamethasone may suppress ACTH release. With glucocorticoid–secreting adrenal tumors, plasma ACTH levels are suppressed to either low normal or undetectable levels, and dexamethasone suppression testing produces no reduction in cortisol levels.

Two major problems are encountered in determining the cause: (1) In approximately 10 per cent of patients with Cushing's disease the cortisol levels are not suppressed adequately in response to dexamethasone, and (2) approximately 5 per cent of patients with ectopic tumors have suppression in response to high-dose dexamethasone and thus may appear to have Cushing's disease. Testing with CRF will certainly aid in the differentiation of these two causes, since, in general,

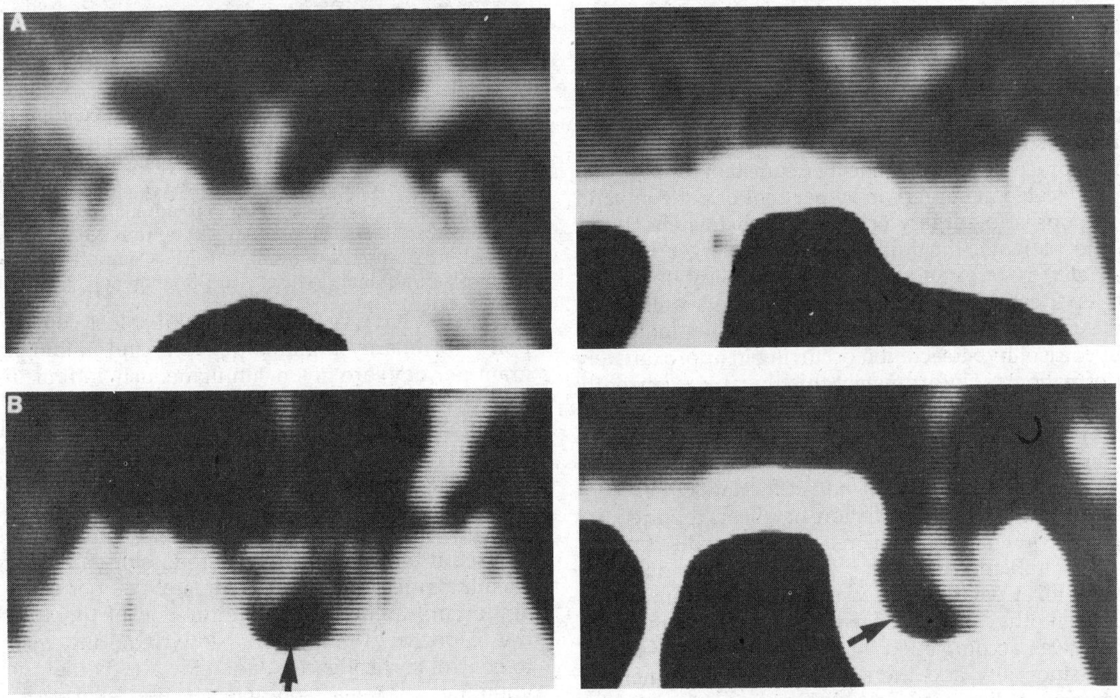

Figure 229–8. CT scans of normal and abnormal pituitary glands. The sections shown are computer re-formations derived from 1.5-mm axial sections through the sella turcica. Coronal re-formations are shown on the left and sagittal ones on the right. *A*, Normal pituitary gland. The upper border is flat; the pituitary stalk (seen on the coronal section) is midline; and the gland is relatively homogeneous in density. The lateral margins of the sella turcica (see coronal section) are formed by the contrast-enhancing cavernous sinuses. *B*, In a patient with Cushing's disease, a 3- to 4-mm pituitary adenoma is visualized as a low-density lesion in the anterior inferior portion of the anterior lobe (arrows). (Reprinted from Findling JW, Tyrrell JB: *In* Greenspan FS, Forsham PH (eds.): Basic and Clinical Endocrinology. Los Altos, Lange Medical Publications, 1983, p 59.)

responsiveness is observed in Cushing's disease but not in the ectopic ACTH syndrome. In some cases, lack of suppression with pituitary adenomas occurs with larger tumors that will be apparent when computed tomography (CT) is performed. Also, this problem is more frequent when there is nodular adrenal hyperplasia. With these cases it is necessary to use additional procedures to establish the diagnosis. These include extensive tumor screening such as the use of head and body CT, selective venous sampling of the petrosal sinuses that drain the anterior pituitary and of other suspected regions, and utilization of higher doses of dexamethasone.

Tumor Localization. In Cushing's disease high-resolution contrast-enhanced CT of the pituitary is the procedure of choice (Fig. 229–8). Because of the small size of these tumors, however, such scans allow definite tumor localization in only approximately 60 per cent of cases. Other radiologic procedures including plain sellar radiographs, polytomography, arteriography, and pneumoencephalography are of little additional utility. In the absence of a radiologically evident lesion consistent with an adenoma it is recommended that selective venous sampling for ACTH be performed prior to surgical interventions. This technique has been useful in establishing a pituitary cause of Cushing's syndrome, including in those patients with dexamethasone–nonsuppressible Cushing's disease, and in excluding a pituitary cause when an occult ectopic ACTH-secreting tumor is present. The technique requires an experienced radiologist, since sampling from the inferior petrosal sinuses is required to assess pituitary ACTH secretion adequately. A gradient of 2:1 of central to peripheral ACTH levels establishes the presence of Cushing's disease.

CT and ultrasonography of the adrenal (Fig. 229–9) should be used in patients with suspected adrenal tumors or in whom the cause is in doubt. Adrenal tumors are usually larger than 2 cm in diameter when diagnosed and thus are readily visible with those procedures. Adrenal scanning should also be performed when ACTH levels or dexamethasone studies are inconclusive. In this case they will help differentiate hyperplasia from primary adrenal tumors and may help to establish the diagnosis of nodular adrenal hyperplasia.

TREATMENT. Pituitary microsurgery with a transsphenoidal approach is the current method of choice for the initial therapy of Cushing's disease. It is critical that it be performed by a surgeon with substantial experience with the technique as it is not a common procedure. Under ideal circumstances, pituitary tumors can be located at surgery in 90 per cent of patients, and successful responses to surgery occur in approximately 80 per cent of all the patients, including those with larger tumors. Surgical mortality is rare, and significant complications occur in less than 2 per cent of patients. Heavy-particle irradiation is also effective therapy for Cushing's disease, with long-term correction of cortisol hypersecretion occurring in approximately 80 per cent of patients. Unfortunately this therapy is currently available in only one center in the United States. Conventional radiotherapy is successful in only 15 to 25 per cent of adults and should not be used as initial therapy because it precludes any further radiation therapy. In contrast, an 80 per cent response rate to conventional radiation has been reported for Cushing's disease in childhood; the reason for this discrepancy is unclear. Bilateral adrenalectomy, previously an accepted initial therapy for Cushing's disease, should be limited to patients in whom other therapies are unsuccessful. In the past, this procedure was accompanied by a high degree of surgical morbidity and mortality and the subsequent development of Nelson's syndrome (discussed below). Reserpine, bromocriptine, cyproheptadine, and sodium valproate have been used to suppress ACTH and treat Cushing's syndrome, but only a minority of patients respond. In general their use is recommended for adjunctive therapy in patients who have had unsuccessful responses to other therapy.

Drugs that inhibit adrenal cortisol secretion can also be used as adjunctive therapy or in patients in whom more definitive

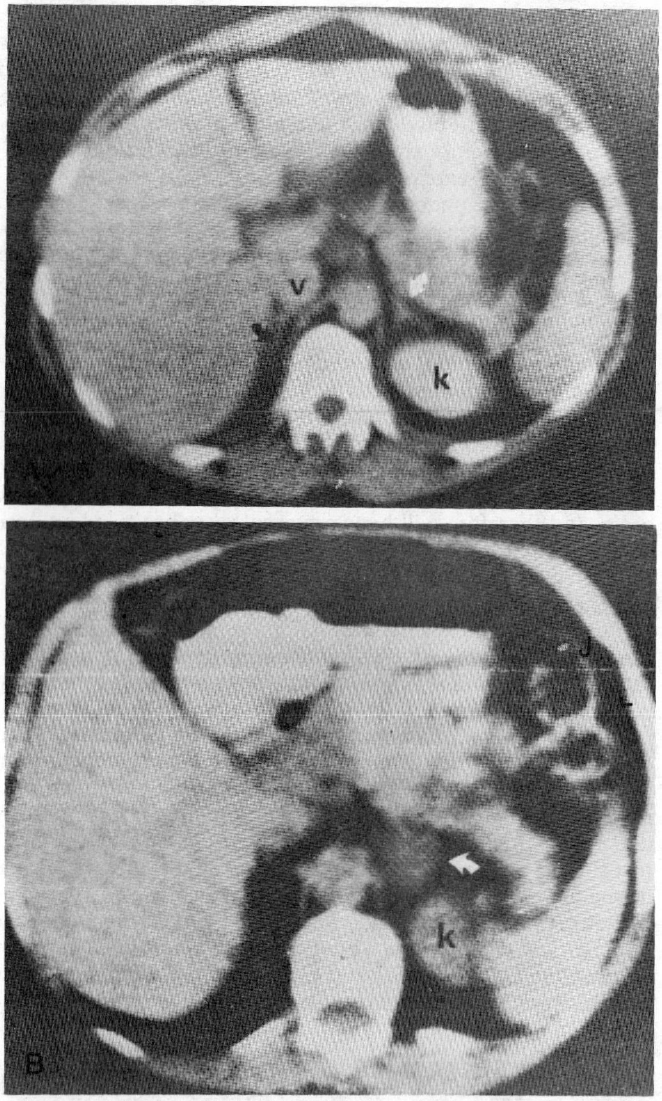

Figure 229–9. CT scans in Cushing's syndrome. *A*, Patient with ACTH-dependent Cushing's syndrome. The adrenal glands are not detectably abnormal by this procedure. The curvilinear right adrenal (black arrow) is shown posterior to the inferior vena cava (v) between the right lobe of the liver and the right crus of the diaphragm. The left adrenal (white arrow) has an inverted Y appearance anteromedial to the left kidney (k). *B*, A 3-cm left adrenal adenoma (white arrow) anteromedial to the left kidney (k). (From Korobkin M, White EA, Kressel HY, Moss AA, Montagne J-P: Computed tomographs in the diagnosis of adrenal disease. Am J Roentgenol 132:231, 1979.)

treatments have been unsuccessful. Most commonly, metyrapone* (ordinarily 2 grams per day) and aminoglutethimide (1 gram per day) are given simultaneously in four divided doses. These drugs are expensive, have frequent side effects that are predominantly gastrointestinal upsets, and result in secondary increases in ACTH levels that sometimes are sufficient to overcome the enzyme inhibition. They have not been used successfully for long-term therapy of Cushing's disease. Alternatively, mitotane, 3 to 6 grams per day in divided doses, can be used if tolerated. Although remission rates with the drug in Cushing's disease are approximately 80 per cent, relapse usually occurs following discontinuation of therapy. In addition, the response to mitotane is slow, requiring weeks to months to control cortisol excess, and side effects that include nausea, vomiting, diarrhea, somnolence, and skin rash occur in the majority of patients. Since the use of these drugs may produce hypoadrenalism, careful monitoring of steroid levels and glucocorticoid replacement may be required.

In the ectopic ACTH syndrome the tumor hypersecreting ACTH should be removed. This may be possible in the minority

*This use is not listed in the manufacturer's directive.

of patients with the more benign tumors such as thymoma, bronchial carcinoid, or pheochromocytoma. Unfortunately in the majority of patients the tumors are malignant and metastasize prior to the diagnosis of cortisol excess. In such patients, drug therapy as discussed above is used to control cortisol excess. Metyrapone and aminoglutethimide are preferred to mitotane because of their more rapid onset of action. Also hypokalemia should be corrected as required, and in some patients spironolactone therapy may be useful in blocking the mineralocorticoid effects of cortisol and 11-deoxycorticosterone. Bilateral adrenalectomy might be considered in a rare patient in whom drug therapy is inadequate and the cortisol excess rather than the tumor is life threatening.

The treatment of adrenal tumors is primarily surgical. Patients with unilateral adrenal adenoma should undergo resection of the affected adrenal. Since ACTH secretion and the contralateral adrenal are suppressed in these patients, glucocorticoid replacement therapy is required pending recovery of the normal adrenal, which frequently requires 9 to 12 months. Although surgical cure of adrenocortical carcinoma is unusual, surgical removal of the primary tumor is indicated to reduce cortisol secretion even when metastases are present. Mitotane 6 to 12 grams per day in divided doses, if tolerated, is recommended for patients with residual or nonresectable carcinoma, and approximately 75 per cent of patients achieve reduced steroid secretion. Only about one third of patients undergo reduction in tumor bulk, however, and it is not clear whether the drug prolongs survival. Metyrapone and aminoglutethimide can be used in patients who do not respond to or tolerate mitotane. The prognosis is poor with adrenal carcinoma; most patients survive less than five years following the onset of symptoms.

NELSON'S SYNDROME. Defined as the clinical progression of an ACTH–secreting pituitary adenoma following bilateral adrenalectomy for Cushing's disease, this syndrome appears to occur in at least one third of such patients. Fortunately the incidence of this disorder has dropped dramatically because of the decreased use of bilateral adrenalectomy for treatment of Cushing's disease.

The syndrome most likely results from enhanced progression of the pre-existing pituitary adenoma due to reduction of cortisol feedback inhibition of the tumor. Nelson's syndrome is seen with increasing hyperpigmentation usually within 1 to 2 years following adrenalectomy. In addition, these patients frequently exhibit local manifestations, including hypopituitarism, visual loss, headache, cavernous sinus invasion with extraocular muscle palsies, and rarely malignant changes with metastatic spread. Plasma ACTH levels are dramatically elevated and usually range from 1000 to 10,000 pg per milliliter. The majority of these tumors are greater than 1 cm in diameter and are readily localized by CT of the sella turcica.

The treatment of Nelson's syndrome is considerably less successful than that of Cushing's disease because of the large size and aggressive nature of these tumors. Although pituitary microsurgery is the preferred initial therapy, complete tumor resection is usually not possible. Heavy-particle irradiation may be utilized either as primary therapy or after surgery in patients with intrasellar tumors; however, in those with extrasellar extension, conventional postoperative radiation therapy should be undertaken. Although pharmacologic inhibition of ACTH secretion has been attempted with cyproheptadine, bromocriptine, and valproic acid, it appears that only a minority of patients respond. Nevertheless, trials of these medications are indicated if surgical and radiotherapeutic treatments are unsuccessful.

Mineralocorticoid Excess States

John D. Baxter

PRIMARY ALDOSTERONISM

Increased inappropriate production of aldosterone from the adrenal is known as primary aldosteronism, and leads to sodium retention with hypertension, suppression of plasma renin and to hypokalemia and its manifestations. It is due mainly to an adrenocortical adenoma, bilateral adrenocortical hyperplasia, or rarely to an adrenal carcinoma. The disease occurs in all age groups, with a peak incidence during the third and fourth decades. About 70 per cent of the adenomas occur in women. Although primary aldosteronism almost always results in hypertension (normotensive primary hyperaldosteronism is extremely rare), the syndrome is present in only a very small proportion (less than 2 per cent) of patients with hypertension. Nevertheless, this largely reversible form of hypertension should be considered in all hypertensive patients.

ALDOSTERONE-PRODUCING ADENOMAS. With an aldosterone-producing adenoma (Conn's syndrome), aldosterone excess leads to sodium retention and to potassium and hydrogen loss. Other steroids that are normally synthesized in the zona glomerulosa (i.e., deoxycorticosterone, corticosterone, and 18-hydroxycorticosterone) are also produced in excess, although they are probably not important in the overall pathophysiology. Sodium retention results in expansion of the extracellular fluid volume, increase in total body sodium content, and elevation of serum sodium concentration. Ultimately there is a major redistribution of fluid with an increased intracellular sodium content in tissues; this may contribute to increased vascular reactivity. Although it is clear that prolonged sodium retention is a major contributor to the associated hypertension, it has been proposed that aldosterone may have other hypertensive actions as well. The electrolyte abnormalities of hyperaldosteronism result in muscular weakness, a tendency to cardiac irritability and arrhythmia, carbohydrate intolerance, resistance to vasopressin (nephrogenic diabetes insipidus), and abnormalities in baroreceptor function. The last results in more volume-dependent hypertension. The expansion of the extracellular fluid and plasma volume is registered by the stretch receptors at the juxtaglomerular apparatus and by sodium chloride flux at the macula densa with suppression of renin release, low plasma renin levels, and unresponsiveness of renin release to the provocative stimuli that usually effect release. Thus, increased aldosterone production with a suppressed renin system defines the disorder.

Long term, the sustained hypertension leads to a bodily compensation by decreasing somewhat the plasma volume, although the hypertension continues to be aldosterone dependent. The hypertension can also lead to many of the complications of hypertension such as renal damage, stroke, and myocardial infarction.

BILATERAL ADRENAL HYPERPLASIA. Bilateral adrenal hyperplasia can be diffuse or nodular, and selectively involves the glomerulosa cells. In most series it accounts for perhaps 20 per cent of the patients in whom primary aldosteronism is diagnosed; however, its precise incidence is not known, since there is a gradient between what is termed low-renin essential hypertension without frank aldosterone excess and this syndrome. Adrenal hyperplasia is not known to precede development of an adenoma.

The pathophysiology of hyperplasia shows at least four differences from that of adenoma; (1) Even though the plasma renin is suppressed, unlike the case with an aldosterone-producing adenoma, it responds to postural and other stimuli. (2) The adrenal appears to be hypersensitive to angiotensin II, exhibiting a marked increase in aldosterone production rather than insensitivity. (3) The aldosterone hypersecretion tends to be less than with the adenoma, a feature that is useful in the differential diagnosis. By contrast the blood pressure in the two groups tends to be similar. (4) The hypertension tends not to respond to adrenalectomy, implying that common factors produce both hypertension and enhanced adrenal sensitivity to angiotensin II. Whereas the mechanism for the development of hyperplasia is unknown, it is attractive to hypothesize that there is abnormal production (or loss) of a factor that enhances adrenal and vascular sensitivity to angiotensin II.

CLINICAL PRESENTATION. Patients usually appear for treatment because of elevated blood pressure detected on routine screening or, less commonly, because of symptoms of hypokalemia. The blood pressure elevations range from mild to severe, with mean presenting pressures in the range of 200 mm Hg systolic and 120 mm Hg diastolic. Malignant hypertension is rare. A history of hypertension in pregnancy is common with female patients who develop the disorder. When present, symptoms of hypokalemia include the nonspecific complaints of tiredness, loss of stamina, weakness, nocturia, and lassitude. Symptoms of more severe depletion include alkalosis, rarely with a positive Trousseau or Chvostek sign; increased thirst and polyuria with low urine specific gravity and unresponsiveness to vasopressin; paresthesias; cardiac arrhythmias such as ventricular tachycardia; and postural hypotension with dizziness. The serum sodium is rarely less than 139 mEq per liter in the absence of diuretic therapy. In spite of fluid overload, edema is only rarely present. The heart is usually only mildly enlarged, if at all, and electrocardiographic changes are usually those of moderate left ventricular hypertrophy and potassium depletion. There tend to be fewer funduscopic changes relative to the hypertension than in other forms of hypertension.

DIAGNOSIS. The hallmarks of the disorder are hypertension with hypokalemia, suppression of the renin-angiotensin system, and increased aldosterone production. A suggested evaluation plan is shown in Figure 229–10. The initial step in diagnosis is to determine whether hypokalemia is present, since this is the hallmark of mineralocorticoid excess. All patients with hypertension should be screened, especially those with spontaneous hypokalemia, after diuretics have been withheld for at least three weeks.

The evaluation of hypokalemia requires control of the sodium balance, since sodium depletion from decreased intake or diuretics can decrease urinary potassium excretion and thus mask hypokalemia. Random serum potassium levels may be normal in up to 20 per cent of patients with primary aldosteronism, but salt loading will unmask hypokalemia in virtually all patients. If according to the dietary history the patient's usual sodium intake is 120 mEq per 24 hours or greater, measurement of normal potassium levels on three occasions obviates the need for further evaluation. If dietary intake is inadequate or unclear, the patient is instructed to consume a normal diet supplemented with 1 gram of NaCl with each meal for four days, and the serum potassium is then measured.

If the plasma potassium value is low, other causes of hypokalemia should be ruled out: diuretic therapy, gastrointestinal loss due to vomiting or diarrhea, other mineralocorticoid excess syndromes (discussed below), starvation, insulin and glucose therapy, metabolic acidosis, renal disease, and renovascular and accelerated hypertension. The tests described below should allow these to be ruled out.

Random unstimulated plasma renin activity (PRA) or plasma renin concentration (PRC) should be determined as the next step in diagnosis. In primary aldosteronism this will be suppressed even after short-term diuretic therapy, salt restriction, assumption of erect posture, or exercise, although other causes of low renin must be excluded. If PRA is normal or high, primary aldosteronism is unlikely.

If the plasma renin value is low or marginally low, 24-hour urinary aldosterone and the plasma aldosterone should be measured. Urinary measurement is superior to plasma measurement for detecting mild primary aldosteronism. Plasma measurements are elevated in most cases of primary aldosteronism, however, and are more useful in the differential diagnosis of the various forms of primary aldosteronism. It is critical to monitor the salt intake and posture, as discussed earlier, because patients with essential hypertension and a low salt intake will have increased aldosterone levels. The urinary aldosterone is increased to over 17 μg per 24 hours in most cases of primary aldosteronism regardless of the cause. With an adenoma the overnight recumbent plasma aldosterone levels will almost always exceed 20 ng per deciliter. In hyperplasia the plasma aldosterone levels are ordinarily less than 20 ng per deciliter and frequently are in the normal range. The effect of hypokalemia that decreases aldosterone secretion must also be

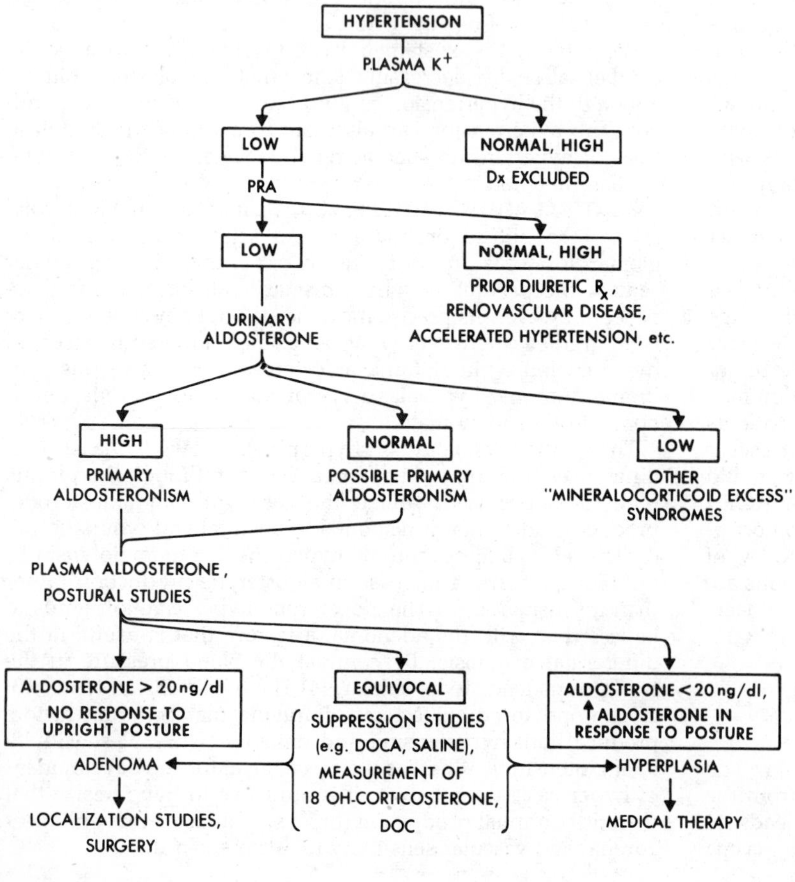

Figure 229–10. Flow diagram for the evaluation of primary aldosteronism. PRA = plasma renin activity. Dx = diagnosis. Rx = therapy. (Reprinted from Biglieri EG, Baxter JD: *In* Felig P, Baxter JD, Broadus AE, Frohman LA (eds.): Endocrinology and Metabolism. New York, McGraw-Hill Book Company, 1981, p 569.)

considered. Thus, in the presence of hypokalemia and suppressed PRA, aldosterone levels in the normal range are inappropriately high and thus abnormal.

In the presence of marginally suppressed PRC and mild elevation of plasma or urinary aldosterone, one of the stimulation tests (discussed earlier) may be necessary to diagnose primary aldosteronism. In general they are unnecessary if accurate plasma and urine aldosterone measurements can be obtained. Marginal cases are usually due to primary aldosteronism with hyperplasia, in which case antimineralocorticoid therapy is indicated. In many cases such therapy can be initiated and the case re-evaluated at a later time.

If the diagnosis of primary aldosteronism is made, it is important for therapy to distinguish between adenoma and hyperplasia. The levels of plasma aldosterone provide an initial indication; if these are substantially elevated, e.g., above 30 ng per deciliter, postural studies are unnecessary. 18-Hydroxycorticosterone measurements may even be better for discrimination, but these are not generally available. Since plasma aldosterone levels in hyperplasia but not adenoma are still under control by the renin-angiotensin system, the plasma aldosterone response to posture can be discriminatory. Patients with an adenoma will not show an increase in plasma aldosterone concentration and PRA (or at most a slight increase), whereas patients with hyperplasia will show such increases. These procedures will allow a diagnosis to be made in most instances. If uncertainty still exists, the response to DOCA, 9α-fluorocortisol, or saline can be measured and will almost always allow a distinction. More recent studies indicate that the converting-enzyme inhibitor captopril can be used alternatively. The inhibitor causes a drop in plasma aldosterone concentration in patients with hyperplasia but not adenoma.

Once an adenoma is suspected, CT of the adrenals should be performed. In most cases this will permit localization of the tumor. In the less than 20 per cent of patients in whom an adenoma is not found, selective venous sampling with measurements of aldosterone-cortisol ratios is usually helpful, can determine whether adenoma or hyperplasia is present, and can lateralize an adenoma.

TREATMENT. Unilateral adrenalectomy is indicated for aldosterone-producing adenomas. Prior to surgery the blood pressure and serum potassium should be normalized by treatment with the mineralocorticoid antagonist spironolactone (200 to 400 mg per day) or the potassium–sparing diuretic amiloride (20 to 40 mg per day). Medical therapy can be continued in the rare patient in whom surgery is contraindicated. This form of treatment also tends to reactivate the suppressed renin-angiotensin system so that the incidence of postoperative hypoaldosteronism is reduced. Also the response of the blood pressure to this therapy provides an excellent indication of the anticipated response to surgery.

Following surgery the blood pressure returns to normal in around 50 per cent of patients with reduction of hypertension in another 25 per cent. However, hypertension, but not hyperaldosteronism, returns in about 40 per cent by ten years postoperatively.

Most patients with bilateral hyperplasia will not respond to surgery; therefore medical therapy is recommended. These patients should be given spironolactone or amiloride in doses described above; this will correct the hypokalemia, but will not correct the hypertension in most cases. Additional antihypertensive medications are usually necessary. There is also a rare subgroup of patients with hyperplasia whose hyperaldosteronism is responsive to glucocorticoids; treatment of these patients with a glucocorticoid in normal replacement amounts or slightly above such amounts is recommended. Whether all patients with hyperplasia should be screened for this responsiveness is controversial.

OTHER FORMS OF HYPERTENSION ASSOCIATED WITH MINERALOCORTICOID EXCESS

There are several other mineralocorticoid-excess conditions. DOC excess can occur in the 11β- and 17α-hydroxylase syndromes (Ch. 233) and in occasional patients with Cushing's syndrome. This is particularly true when the latter is due to an ectopic ACTH-producing carcinoma. It can also be seen in certain adrenal carcinomas. In all these cases the PRC is suppressed as it is in primary aldosteronism; however, plasma aldosterone levels are usually suppressed as well in these conditions. Rarely iatrogenic causes of mineralocorticoid-excess hypertension result from excessive ingestion of licorice, carbenoxolone (for ulcer treatment), 9α-fluorocortisol for postural hypotension, or mineralocorticoid-containing nasal sprays (not available in the United States). It can be present in rare cases of relative generalized insensitivity to glucocorticoids when elevated cortisol levels have mineralocorticoid actions. There are some rare syndromes in which there are hypertension, hypokalemia, and suppressed PRC with no detectable elevations of known mineralocorticoids (e.g., Liddle's syndrome, Ch. 83.5). Some of these syndromes could represent primary hypersensitivity to mineralocorticoids. In all of these conditions there are hypertension, hypokalemia, and suppression of PRC without an associated increase of aldosterone.

SECONDARY HYPERALDOSTERONISM

Secondary hyperaldosteronism results from stimulation of the adrenal glomerulosa by extra-adrenal factors, usually the renin-angiotensin system. It can be physiologic or contribute to the pathology of disease states. A physiologic increase occurs during excessive potassium intake as part of the body's defense against hyperkalemia. Secondary hyperaldosteronism can occur during the luteal phase of the menstrual cycle and occasionally during oral contraceptive use. Aldosterone secretion increases progessively during normal pregnancy; levels are elevated by the fifteenth week of gestation and are ten times those of nonpregnant women in the third trimester. This is presumably due to an increase in renin and angiotensin, possibly due to the decrease in blood pressure that occurs in pregnancy. Interestingly, renin levels are more elevated during the first trimester, whereas plasma aldosterone levels are highest during the third trimester. This may be due to a progessive increase in sensitivity of the adrenal glomerulosa to angiotensin II. Aldosterone secretion increases when there is excessive sodium loss and when there is dietary restriction of sodium. Aldosterone increases in some patients with congestive heart failure and with significant hypoalbuminemia. Renin and aldosterone levels are commonly elevated in cirrhosis when ascites is present; this is accentuated by decreased clearance of aldosterone. The increased aldosterone further promotes sodium retention and potassium loss; this explains the rationale of using mineralocorticoid antagonists in the treatment of ascites. Elevated aldosterone levels are found in Bartter's syndrome (Ch. 83.5). Finally, secondary hyperaldosteronism and hypertension can occur with renal artery stenosis, unilateral renal ischemia, accelerated hypertension, and renin-secreting tumors.

Aron DC, Tyrrell JB, Fitzgerald PA, Findling JW, Forsham PH: Cushing's syndrome: Problems in diagnosis. Medicine 60:25, 1981. *An analysis of the problems and approaches when results do not conform to the usual norms.*

Baxter JD, Tyrrell JB: The adrenal cortex. *In* Felig P, Baxter JD, Broadus AE, Frohman LA (eds.): Endocrinology and Metabolism. New York, McGraw-Hill Book Company, 1981, pp 385–510. *An extensive review of the physiology and pathology of the adrenal cortex.*

Biglieri EG, Baxter JD: The endocrinology of hypertension. *In* Felig P, Baxter JD, Broadus AE, Frohman LA (eds.): Endocrinology and Metabolism. New York, McGraw-Hill Book Company, 1981, pp 551–598. *An analysis of the pathophysiology and approaches to diagnosis and treatment of not only primary aldosteronism but also of other types of endocrine hypertension.*

Chrousos GP, Schulte HM, Oldfield EH, Gold PW, Cutler GB Jr, Loriaux DL: The corticotropin-releasing factor stimulation test. An aid in the evaluation of patients with Cushing's syndrome. N Engl J Med 310:622, 1984. Orth ON: The old and the new in Cushing's syndrome. N Engl J Med 310:649, 1984. *These papers establish the utility of CRF in the differential diagnosis of Cushing's syndrome and are accompanied by a thoughtful editorial overview of the procedures in the differential diagnosis of cortisol excess.*

Crapo L: Cushing's syndrome: A review of diagnostic tests. Metabolism 28:955,

1979. *A detailed evaluation of the many diagnostic approaches to Cushing's syndrome. Required reading for a background in this area.*

Finkelstein M, Shaefer JM: Inborn errors of steroid biosynthesis. Physiol Rev 59:353, 1979. *This article examines the enzymology and metabolic derangements that occur in association with steroid hormone biosynthetic defects.*

Irvine WJ, Toft AD, Feek CM: Addison's disease. *In* James VHT (ed.): The Adrenal Gland. New York, Raven Press, 1979, pp 131–164. *An extensive analysis of the pathophysiology of Addison's disease and the associated disorders.*

Keeton TK, Campbell WB: The pharmacologic alteration of renin release. Pharmacol Rev 31:81, 1980. *An overview of renin release with emphasis on pharmacological factors that alter it.*

Keller-Wood ME, Dallman M: Corticosteroid inhibition of ACTH secretion. Endocr Rev 5:1, 1984. *A review of the kinetics and mechanisms whereby glucocorticoids block both CRF and ACTH release.*

Krieger DT: Physiopathology of Cushing's disease. Endocr Rev 4:22, 1983. *This analysis of Cushing's disease emphasizes its possible causes.*

Lieberman S, Greenfield NJ, Wolfson A: A heuristic proposal for understanding steroidogenic processes. Endocr Rev 5:128, 1984. *A review of the enzymology and the pathways in steroid biosynthesis.*

Munck A, Guyre P, Holbrook NJ: Physiological functions of glucocorticoids in stress and their relation to pharmacological actions. Endocr Rev 5:25, 1984. *A new proposal that explains how glucocorticoids are useful in the body's response to stress.*

Parker LN, Odell WD: Control of adrenal androgen secretion. Endocr Rev 1:392, 1980. *An excellent examination of the factors that regulate adrenal androgen production.*

230. DIABETES MELLITUS

Jerrold M. Olefsky

DEFINITION. Diabetes mellitus is a heterogeneous primary disorder of carbohydrate metabolism with multiple etiologic factors that generally involve absolute or relative insulin deficiency or insulin resistance or both. All causes of diabetes ultimately lead to hyperglycemia, which is the hallmark of this disease syndrome.

CLASSIFICATION AND DIAGNOSIS

The currently accepted classification and criteria for the diagnosis of diabetes mellitus are based on the 1979 report of the National Diabetes Data Group and are comparable to the standards set forth by the World Health Organization (Table 230–1). Diabetes can be separated into two general disease syndromes: (1) *Type I,* or *insulin-dependent diabetes mellitus* (IDDM), is present in patients with little or no endogenous insulin secretory capacity. These patients develop extreme hyperglycemia, ketosis, and the associated symptomatology unless treated with insulin, and they are therefore entirely dependent on exogenous insulin therapy for immediate survival. This form of the disease usually, but not always, develops prior to early adulthood. Older terms for this syndrome are juvenile onset, ketosis prone, or brittle diabetes. (2) *Type II,* or *noninsulin-dependent diabetes mellitus* (NIDDM), occurs in patients who retain significant endogenous insulin secretory capacity. Although treatment with insulin may be necessary for control of hyperglycemia, these patients do not develop ketosis in the absence of insulin therapy and are not dependent on exogenous insulin for immediate survival. Previous terms for this form of the disease are maturity or adult onset, nonketotic, and stable diabetes. The diagnosis of diabetes in patients with the insulin-dependent form of the disease is usually unequivocal, and the distinction between type I and type II diabetes can usually be made on clinical grounds. However, there are occasional patients with minimal, but clearly detectable, endogenous insulin secretion in whom the disease is difficult to categorize initially; when these patients are followed over longer periods, however, the necessary distinction can usually be made.

TABLE 230–1. CLASSIFICATION OF DIABETES

1. Insulin-dependent, or type I diabetes (IDDM). Formerly called juvenile-onset or ketosis-prone diabetes.
2. Noninsulin-dependent, or type II diabetes (NIDDM). Formerly called adult-onset, maturity-onset, or nonketotic diabetes.
   A. Obese (~80%)
   B. Nonobese (~20%)
3. Secondary diabetes
   A. Pancreatic disease (e.g., pancreatectomy, pancreatic insufficiency, hemochromatosis)
   B. Hormonal (excess counterinsulin hormones, e.g., Cushing's syndrome, acromegaly, pheochromocytoma)
   C. Drug-induced (e.g., thiazide diuretics, steroids, phenytoin)
   D. Associated with specific genetic syndromes (e.g., lipodystrophy, myotonic dystrophy, ataxia telangiectasia)
4. Impaired glucose tolerance (IGT). Formerly called chemical, latent, borderline, or subclinical diabetes.
5. Gestational diabetes: glucose intolerance with onset during pregnancy.

The diagnosis of NIDDM is based on a distinction between normal and abnormal levels of glycemia and therefore is less precise. Prior to the report of the National Diabetes Data Group, oral glucose tolerance tests were commonly used to establish this diagnosis. This approach is fraught with difficulties because oral glucose tolerance is affected by numerous other variables that can cause mild abnormalities of glucose metabolism independent of diabetes. Concomitant illness, stress, physical inactivity, hypocaloric or low carbohydrate intake, various drugs, and aging are among those factor that can adversely influence glucose tolerance. Therefore, when employed, glucose tolerance testing must be rigorously controlled by administering a standard oral glucose load (75 grams), insuring an appropriate antecedent diet (eucaloric with at least 200 grams carbohydrate per day), adequate physical activity, and the absence of drugs affecting carbohydrate metabolism. Even with these precautions, only a minority (15 to 25 per cent) of individuals who have normal fasting plasma glucose levels with abnormal glucose tolerance tests go on to develop overt diabetes. In recognition of the above facts, the National Diabetes Data Group recommended relatively stringent criteria for establishing the diagnosis of NIDDM: (1) fasting venous plasma glucose concentration > 140 mg per deciliter on at least two separate occasions, or (2) in the absence of fasting hyperglycemia, a diagnosis of NIDDM can be made following ingestion of the standard 75-gram oral glucose tolerance test if the 2-hour venous plasma glucose and one other sample (the 30-, 60-, or 90-minute sample) exceed 200 mg per deciliter.

Impaired glucose tolerance exists if the fasting plasma glucose level is less than 140 mg per deciliter and if the 30-, 60-, or 90-minute plasma glucose concentration exceeds 200 mg per deciliter along with a 2-hour plasma glucose level between 140 and 200 mg per deciliter. Microvascular complications of diabetes rarely occur in individuals with impaired glucose tolerance, and the great majority of these cases do not deteriorate to overt diabetes in long-term follow up. Most instances of impaired glucose tolerance, therefore, are probably unrelated to the disease syndrome of NIDDM. Almost all patients who meet the criteria for NIDDM during oral glucose tolerance testing show fasting hyperglycemia (greater than 140 mg per deciliter) when they are repeatedly evaluated. Furthermore, in those few patients who meet the criteria for NIDDM in the absence of fasting hyperglycemia, most do not develop fasting hyperglycemia during prolonged follow-up, and clinical symptoms of diabetes are unusual. Thus the clinical significance of impaired glucose tolerance is unclear. As previously mentioned, only a minority (2 to 35 per cent, depending on the population examined) of these patients go on to develop overt NIDDM when followed for up to 20 years. In evaluating the meaning of impaired glucose tolerance, the real challenge is to develop markers to detect which patients with impaired glucose tolerance have a benign nonprogressive abnormality of glucose intolerance and which have a prediabetic state. Patients with impaired glucose tolerance who secrete low amounts of insulin, compared to normal individuals, have a much higher risk of developing overt diabetes (perhaps up to 40 per cent), whereas those who secrete high amounts of insulin seldom (about 5 per cent) progress to frank diabetes. In view of the above, it would seem that glucose tolerance testing is unnecessary for patient management in the absence of clinical signs and symptoms of diabetes, although this is still a highly useful procedure for epidemiologic or research purposes. An exception to this would be in a pregnant subject suspected of having gestational diabetes, since criteria for this diagnosis are less stringent and vigorous management of minimal degrees of hyperglycemia are deemed important.

Serum and plasma glucose concentrations are identical and run 10 to 15 per cent higher than whole blood determinations (the latter are infrequently performed nowadays). The glucose concentration in capillary blood is essentially identical to that in venous blood during the fasting state, but under postprandial conditions, tissues readily take up glucose and capillary blood glucose concentrations can be 10 to 30 mg per deciliter greater than concomitant venous blood glucose levels.

There is an age-related decline in glucose tolerance that has been extensively studied. Insulin secretion is not decreased in aging, whereas insulin resistance is a common finding in aged populations. This insulin resistance is due to a post-receptor binding defect in insulin action. Age-related variables such as inadequate diet, increasing adiposity with decreased lean body mass, and physical inactivity can contribute to this insulin-resistant state, but the aging process itself also plays a significant role. The glucose intolerance of aging tends to be mild and is most easily detected following an oral glucose challenge. When mild abnormalities of oral glucose tolerance tests were used to diagnose diabetes, age adjusted criteria for these tests had to be employed. However, with the current more stringent criteria noted above, this problem is largely obviated since the glucose intolerance of aging does not cause significant fasting hyperglycemia (more than 140 mg per deciliter) and only rarely would cause glucose intolerance severe enough to meet the new criteria in the absence of fasting hyperglycemia.

EPIDEMIOLOGY AND CLINICAL PRESENTATION

The prevalence of diabetes has been difficult to quantitate accurately because the criteria for the diagnosis of NIDDM have varied from survey to survey over the years; the less stringent the criteria the greater the prevalence and vice versa. It is hoped that the widely accepted, uniform, WHO and National Diabetes Data Group standards will successfully address this problem. Furthermore, the prevalence of diabetes differs widely among different populations, depending on ethnic group constituents, age, economic conditions, and probably other environmental factors. For example, the prevalence of diabetes is extremely high among Pima Indians (about 35 per cent) and certain Micronesian cultures (about 35 per cent). Indians, particularly after emigrating from their country, have a higher rate of diabetes than other ethnic groups. Thus, Indians living in South Africa, Trinidad, Singapore, Malayasia, and Fiji exhibit a higher prevalence of diabetes than the local population and than those living on the Indian subcontinent. A low prevalence of diabetes has been noted in Eskimos, Athabascan Indians (Alaska), and Chinese (although prevalence increases in Chinese populations living in Western countries). The proportion of IDDM to NIDDM also differs widely among different populations; IDDM is extremely rare in Pima Indians, Micronesians, and Eskimos, but is more common in Caucasian populations. *Overall, in the United States the prevalence of diabetes is probably between 2 and 4 per cent, with IDDM comprising 7 to 10 per cent of all cases.* The prevalence of IDDM (0.2 to 0.3 per cent) is probably more accurate than the estimates for NIDDM, because of the relative ease of ascertainment and the fact that many patients with NIDDM are asymptomatic and the disease is undiagnosed.

A few facts concerning the prevalence of major diabetes-related complications serve to underscore the enormous impact of this disease. Approximately 25 per cent of all new cases of end-stage renal failure occur in patients with diabetes. About 20,000 amputations (primarily of toes, feet, and legs) are carried out in patients with diabetes, representing approximately half of the nontraumatic amputations performed in the United States. Furthermore, diabetes is the leading cause of new cases of blindness, with approximately 5000 new cases occurring each year.

INSULIN-DEPENDENT DIABETES MELLITUS (IDDM, TYPE I). These patients have little or no endogenous insulin and usually present with relatively abrupt clinical symptoms of *polyuria, polydipsia,* and *polyphagia. Weight loss,* fatigue, and infection can often accompany the initial presentation. Because of the extreme hypoinsulinemia and hyperglucagonemia these patients readily develop *ketosis,* and the initial onset of this disease may be clinically evident as full-blown ketoacidosis. At the time of the first clinical presentations, symptoms can usually be traced back for several days to a few weeks. However, B cell destruction may have started months, or maybe even years, prior to the onset of clinical symptoms. Unfortunately, detection of this preclinical state of disease is seldom possible, so that methods to delay or prevent the full-blown clinical disease, even if such methods existed, will have limited feasibility and have not been systematically attempted. The peak age of onset of IDDM is 11 to 13 years, coinciding with early adolescence and puberty. A secondary peak is noted at age 6 to 8 years, and by the third decade of life the incidence falls to a steady, but still substantial level. It is unusual for IDDM to begin past age 40. Once IDDM is diagnosed, insulin therapy is required to achieve initial metabolic control. In many patients a "honeymoon" period follows initial treatment in which the disease remits and little or no insulin is required. This remission is due to a partial return of endogenous insulin secretion, which may last for several weeks or months and occasionally 1 to 2 years; ultimately, however, the disease recurs, and insulin therapy is required permanently.

NON-INSULIN DEPENDENT DIABETES MELLITUS (NIDDM, TYPE II). Patients with NIDDM typically present with polyuria and polydipsia of several weeks' to months' duration. Polyphagia can occur but is less common, whereas weight loss, weakness, and fatigue are frequent. Dizziness, headaches, and blurry vision are common accompanying complaints. In many patients no symptoms are apparent and the disease is diagnosed by routine blood or urine testing. In others, diabetes is advanced, and the presenting complaints are related to neuropathic, retinopathic, or vascular complications. NIDDM patients are usually but not always older than 40 at presentation and 70 to 90 per cent are overweight. Endogenous insulin secretion is relatively preserved and may even be excessive; thus, ketosis is rare, explaining why NIDDM is categorized as nonketotic or ketosis resistant.

SECONDARY DIABETIC STATES. In addition to the major categories of diabetes (IDDM and NIDDM), a large number of secondary forms of diabetes have been described. Secondary diabetes exists when some other readily identifiable primary disease entity or pathophysiologic state causes or is strongly associated with the diabetic state (Table 230–2). In general, these cases are unusual and comprise only a small proportion of the total cases of diabetes. Any disease process that limits insulin secretion or impairs insulin action can cause secondary diabetes, and numerous syndromes exist. Disorders that lead to pancreatic destruction such as chronic pancreatitis, cystic fibrosis, or hemochromatosis can reduce insulin secretion enough to cause diabetes. Conditions in which excess amounts of counterinsulin hormones are secreted, such as Cushing's disease, acromegaly, pheochromocytoma, and glucagonoma, can also produce diabetes. A number of drugs such as thiazide diuretics, glucocorticoids, and adrenergic agents can lead to, or at least exacerbate, diabetes. Many unusual genetic diseases are associated with a higher than normal incidence of diabetes through unknown mechanisms; these include muscular dystrophy, myotonic dystrophy, Friedreich's ataxia, Turner's syndrome, and others.

Finally, several rare syndromes have been recently identified, whose biochemical mechanisms are well described and which

TABLE 230–2. SOME FEATURES DISTINGUISHING BETWEEN INSULIN-DEPENDENT AND NONINSULIN-DEPENDENT DIABETES

	IDDM	NIDDM
Synonym	Type I	Type II
Age of onset	Usually <30	Usually >40
Ketosis	Common	Rare
Body weight	Nonobese	Obese (80%)
Prevalence	0.2%–0.3%	2%–4%
Genetics		
HLA association	Yes	No
Monozygotic twin studies	40%–50% concordance rate	Concordance rate near 100%
Circulating islet cell antibodies	Yes	No
Associated with other autoimmune phenomena	Occasional	No
Treatment with insulin	Always necessary	Usually not required
Complications	Frequent	Frequent
Insulin secretion	Severe deficiency	Variable: moderate deficiency to hyperinsulinemia
Insulin resistance	Occasional: with poor control or excessive insulin antibodies	Usual: due to receptor and postreceptor defects

primarily involve abnormalities of insulin-glucose physiology. Certain patients with extreme insulin resistance, acanthosis nigricans, and diabetes have been identified with circulating anti-insulin receptor antibodies. These antibodies are part of a more generalized autoimmune process, since proteinuria, leukopenia, and antinuclear and anti-DNA antibodies also exist. Other patients with the triad of acanthosis nigricans, insulin resistance, and diabetes do not have antireceptor antibodies but instead have a profound decrease in cellular insulin receptors. Typically these are young females with hirsutism and polycystic ovaries. In one such patient, several family members were also found to have decreased insulin receptors and insulin resistance, suggesting that this disorder is due to a genetically mediated decrease in insulin receptors. Patients have been reported in whom abnormal insulin products are synthesized and secreted and the specific molecular lesions identified. Familial hyperproinsulinemia involves a defect in the proinsulin molecule that prevents normal cleavage of proinsulin to insulin in the pancreatic B cell. This leads to the secretion of large amounts of proinsulin (which is biologically less active than insulin) instead of insulin. This disorder can lead to impaired glucose tolerance but has not yet been associated with overt fasting hyperglycemia. Rarely patients carry mutations in the insulin structural gene itself that lead to the secretion of insulin species with single amino acid substitutions resulting in markedly reduced biologic activity. These patients have a clinical picture of typical NIDDM. These mutant insulins are immunologically reactive and are secreted in large quantities in response to the hyperglycemic state. The clinical hallmark of this condition is the presence of hyperglycemia and marked hyperinsulinemia in a patient with normal sensitivity to exogenous insulin.

GENETICS

Diabetes has long been termed a geneticist's nightmare. The disease clearly aggregates in families and has a strong familial component. However, the precise genetic contribution to diabetes has been difficult to ascertain for at least four reasons: (1) no specific genetic marker has been identified. Glucose tolerance is the currently used method of diagnosis, but because of differences in the way tests are performed and the criteria used, it is difficult to compare one study to another; (2) There is a great deal of etiologic heterogeneity between IDDM and NIDDM and within these categories. This indicates genetic heterogeneity even though the phenotype (hyperglycemia) is comparable. It is also possible that, depending on environmental factors, there can be variable phenotypic expression of a common genotype; (3) It is likely that a "diabetogenic gene" interacts with external factors as well as with other genetic components, making the specific genetic influences underlying the final phenotypic expression of the diabetes hard to detect; (4) Actual transmission rates of diabetes from generation to generation are low.

Genetic factors are clearly important in the etiology of diabetes. This is demonstrated by classical twin studies. When twins below the age of 40 years are studied, if one twin has diabetes (mostly IDDM based on age) then the other twin develops diabetes only 50 per cent of the time. If the two pairs are concordant, the second twin usually develops diabetes within a couple of years of the first. For a purely genetic disease, concordance should be 100 per cent. This suggests that while genetic factors are important in IDDM, they are only predisposing and must interact with environmental influences if diabetes is to develop. This does not exclude the possibility that in some patients IDDM occurs entirely because of genetic or environmental factors. In twins over 40 years the concordance rate for diabetes (almost all NIDDM based on age) approaches 100 per cent. This suggests that genetic factors are more important in this form of diabetes and may be causal, or closely associated with causal mechanisms.

Despite the contribution of genetic factors, direct transmission of diabetes from parent to offspring is surprisingly low. If one parent has IDDM the risk to the offspring of developing IDDM is on the order of 2 to 5 per cent. If one child has IDDM the average risk for another sibling is 5 to 10 per cent. However, the risk is much greater if the second sibling is HLA (human leukocyte antigen) identical to the first, intermediate if HLA haploidentical, and very low if HLA nonidentical. The type of diabetes tends to run true in families, and the incidence of NIDDM in the offspring of an IDDM parent is probably not greater than normal. If one parent has NIDDM the risk is 10 to 15 per cent for offspring developing the disease. When both parents have NIDDM, the transmission risk increases but adequate data are not available to quantitate the increase in risk. If one sibling has NIDDM, the risk for another sibling is 10 to 15 per cent. These low rates of transmission make it difficult to trace models of inheritance in family studies, but the facts are clinically important in counseling and reassuring diabetic patients who wish to have children.

Strong associations have been identified between IDDM and specific HLAs coded by the major histocompatibility complex region located on the short arm of the sixth chromosome (Ch. 436). Four loci, designated A, B, C, and D, are now recognized in this region. Loci A, B, and C are defined serologically while the D locus is detected by the mixed lymphocyte (MLC) reaction. A DR locus can also be identified and typed using a serologic test. Although not proven, antigens at the D locus detected by MLC may be identical to the antigens at the DR locus identified serologically. At each of these loci numerous alleles (genes) exist, some of which confer increased risk for the development of IDDM. These high risk alleles include: HLA-DR3, HLA-Dw3, HLA-DR4, HLA-Dw4, HLA-B8, and HLA-B15 (the small w means that the antigen identified at the D locus by MLC has been provisionally accepted by the International Histocompatability Workshop; the w is deleted when identification is considered definite). The HLA-A, B, and C antigens are present on virtually all nucleated cell types, whereas the HLA-D or DR antigens or both show tissue restriction and are predominantly expressed on B lymphocytes and macrophages. It is possible that D/DR antigens are also expressed on islet cells, but this is unproven at the current time.

An HLA haplotype refers to a particular set of alleles at the four closely linked HLA loci, A, B, C, and D on one of the sixth chromosomes (each person inherits two haplotypes, one from each parent). In this system, some of the alleles are in linkage disequilibrium. This means that certain HLA antigens encoded by alleles at the different HLA loci occur together more frequently within the same haplotype than would be predicted by random statistical chance taking gene (allele) frequency into account. The antigens encoded by the HLA alleles associated with higher risk for IDDM do not directly cause or predispose to the disease. Rather, these alleles are felt to be in linkage disequilibrium with genes in the HLA region (possibly certain immune response genes) that are directly related to the etiology of IDDM. In other words, through linkage disequilibrium one "looks" at the "diabetogenic gene" via the more easily measured HLA antigens.

Current evidence indicates that the D locus is more important than the B locus because it is more closely linked to the etiologically important genes. In this event, the predictive value of the HLA-B antigen is through its linkage disequilibrium to the D locus. The relative risk for IDDM conferred by HLA-B8 or HLA-B15 is two to four times normal and is four to ten times normal for DR3/Dw3 or DR4/Dw4. Interestingly, homozygosity at any of these alleles (i.e., DR3/DR3) does not lead to greater risk than when the allele occurs on only one haplotype. However, if both sixth chromosomes bear two different diabetes-associated alleles at a particular locus (i.e., DR3/DR4) the increase in risk is more than additive. It should be kept in mind that the diabetes-associated HLA antigens are quite frequent in the nondiabetic population (although, clearly less frequent than in IDDM). For example, 30 to 35 per cent of normal persons are positive for DR3 or DR4. Thus, far more people who are positive for these antigens are normal than have IDDM (e.g., if the average risk for IDDM in a population is 0.2 per cent, and if a particular HLA haplotype confers a ten-fold increase in risk, then the risk would still be only 2 per cent for those with this haplotype). This is an important point to realize in thinking about HLA typing for screening or predictive value in a practical or clinical sense.

Despite all this information, the model of inheritance for IDDM is obscure, although it is clearly not autosomal dominant. The low penetrance of the diabetes-associated genes combined with the relative degrees of HLA associations suggests that the genetic predisposition must interact with specific environmental factors for IDDM to occur. Additionally, the disease could be multigenic, with at least two genes necessary (allelic or nonallelic) for IDDM to develop (with this model environmental factors would still be necessary).

In NIDDM no HLA associations have been identified, demonstrating the differences in etiology between the two major forms of diabetes. Although the location of the genetic component for NIDDM is not known, potentially important changes have been noted on the eleventh chromosome, which contains the insulin gene. A 1.5 to 3.4 kilobase insertion of extra DNA, about 500 base pairs upstream from the 5′ flanking end of the insulin gene, has been described as a polymorphism more frequent in patients with NIDDM compared to normal persons or patients with IDDM. If this insertion (or some more specific aspect of this polymorphism) proves to be an accurate marker for NIDDM, then this will be of great value in predicting subjects at risk and in tracing inheritance patterns. Furthermore, if this insertion influences gene regulation then it might have causal significance in terms of insulin biosynthesis. However, since NIDDM patients usually have adequate amounts of insulin within B cells, it is not readily apparent how this potential gene abnormality could influence functional dynamics of insulin secretion.

PATHOGENESIS

Before discussion of the pathogenetic aspects of diabetes it is important to review briefly some of the essential features of insulin and glucose physiology. Insulin is produced in the pancreatic B cell as the primary biosynthetic product preproinsulin containing 109 amino acid residues (MW ~ 11,500). This peptide is rapidly converted to proinsulin (86 amino acid residues, MW ~ 9000) by cleavage of the amino terminal 23 amino acid "pre" sequence. Within the B cell secretory granules, proinsulin is converted by proteolytic cleavage to insulin (51 amino acids, MW ~ 6000) and C peptide (31 amino acids, MW ~ 3000). Thus, the final B cell secretory product is 95 per cent insulin and C peptide in equimolar amounts and 5 per cent unconverted proinsulin. In familial hyperproinsulinemia, mutations in the proinsulin sequence prevent proteolytic conversion within the secretory granule, leading to release of large amounts of proinsulin having only 7 to 10 per cent of insulin's biologic activity. The regulation of insulin release is extremely complex, being influenced by glucose, amino acids, gut insulinogenic hormones, glucagon, neural influences, and other factors. However, glucose is the most important stimulus for insulin secretion.

After a brief circulating time ($t\frac{1}{2}$ 4 to 8 minutes) insulin interacts with target tissues to exert its biologic effects. At the target cell, insulin action is initiated by binding of the hormone to specific cell surface insulin receptors. Following formation of the insulin receptor complex one or more signals are propagated (second messengers) that interact with a variety of cellular effector systems such as enzymes and glucose transport proteins to produce insulin's ultimate biologic effects. Insulin exerts its major effects on carbohydrate homeostasis by stimulating peripheral glucose disposal and inhibiting hepatic glucose production. A variety of abnormalities in insulin biosynthesis, secretion, and action can lead to diabetes.

There are a number of other hormones that affect carbohydrate homeostasis termed anti-insulin or counteregulatory hormones (glucagon, growth hormone, cortisol, and catecholamines). Among these, glucagon is probably most important in terms of the pathophysiology of diabetes. Glucagon is 29 amino acids (MW ~ 3000) in length and is synthesized in the pancreatic alpha cells as proglucagon (MW ~ 9000 to 11,000). Its release is stimulated by hypoglycemia, amino acids, neural influences, and stress. Its major effect on glucose metabolism is exerted at the liver where it binds to surface receptors, stimulates cyclic AMP generation, and promotes glycogenolysis, gluconeogenesis, and ketogenesis. Its lipolytic effects are minimal in man, and glucagon has little if any effect on peripheral glucose uptake. Thus, glucagon affects glucose metabolism by influencing hepatic glucose production, and glucagon levels are absolutely or relatively increased in both IDDM and NIDDM.

NIDDM. Abnormalities of insulin and, to a lesser extent, glucagon secretion and action are central to the pathogenesis of NIDDM. Syndromes involving abnormalities of insulin biosynthesis have already been discussed. These include familial hyperproinsulinemia and mutations in the structural gene for insulin leading to secretion of a biologically defective insulin molecule. These rare syndromes lead to mild degrees of glucose intolerance or a clinical picture indistinguishable from NIDDM. Beyond these unusual syndromes, however, insulin biosynthesis is qualitatively normal in NIDDM.

Secretion of insulin is not normal in NIDDM. In some patients with impaired glucose tolerance, substantially reduced amounts of insulin are secreted in response to a glucose load. These subjects are not insulin resistant and the defect in insulin secretion appears adequately to account for their abnormal glucose metabolism. These patients have a relatively high propensity to develop overt NIDDM (up to 50 per cent) and should be followed for progression. Other patients with impaired glucose tolerance secrete normal or increased amounts of insulin, although in some cases the dynamics of secretion may be altered with a delay in release of insulin following a glucose stimulus. These patients are insulin resistant primarily because of decreased insulin receptors. This is true in both the obese and nonobese categories of this classification. In relatively few (about 5 per cent) of the hyperinsulinemic insulin-resistant patients with impaired glucose tolerance is there progression to fasting hyperglycemia.

The great majority of patients with NIDDM are both insulin deficient and insulin resistant. The decrease in insulin action exists whether they are obese or nonobese (although approximately 80 per cent are obese). Patients with NIDDM may have normal or elevated fasting insulin levels, but they almost always secrete decreased amounts of insulin following oral glucose or meals. Other functional abnormalities that have been identified include a marked decrease in early release of insulin (first phase) after intravenous administration of glucose, and much greater blunting of the insulin response to glucose compared to other insulin stimuli (amino acids, sulfonylureas, glucagon, or B agonists). These latter findings have given rise to the idea that B cell dysfunction in NIDDM may be characterized by a defect in glucose recognition by islet cells.

In addition to these abnormalities of insulin secretion, patients with NIDDM are also insulin resistant. Insulin action is a complex sequence of events beginning with binding to surface receptors; insulin resistance can be due to any abnormality at any step along the insulin action pathway. For convenience, the cellular causes of insulin resistance can be broadly divided into receptor and postreceptor defects (Fig. 230–1). A receptor defect involves a decrease in insulin binding due to a decrease in either receptor number or affinity or to both. A postreceptor defect refers to any biologically significant abnormality in the activity of effector proteins (such as insulin-sensitive enzymes or transport proteins) or an impairment in the coupling or transducing mechanisms between insulin receptor complexes and effector units. In a pure sense, a postreceptor defect is really a postbinding defect since insulin receptor function could be abnormal independent of its binding properties. In subjects with impaired glucose tolerance who are insulin resistant, receptor defects exist (decreased receptor number), but postreceptor function is normal. In NIDDM, insulin resistance exists in the great majority of patients. Although a receptor defect (decreased number) is present in most insulin-resistant NIDDM patients, this does not appear to be the major abnormality. Postreceptor defects also exist, and these appear to play the predominant role in causing the insulin-resistant state. As far as glucose homeostasis is concerned, at least one type of postreceptor defect has been biochemically defined in NIDDM; that is, these patients exhibit a decrease in the intrinsic activity of the glucose transport effector system.

Insulin deficiency and insulin resistance both contribute to the hyperglycemia of NIDDM. In addition, another abnormality also contributes to the hyperglycemia; hepatic glucose production rates are increased in NIDDM, and the magnitude of this increase is proportional to the level of fasting hyperglycemia. This hepatic abnormality is, at least partially, due to resistance to insulin's normal restraining effect on liver glucose production. Additionally, glucagon levels are often elevated, either absolutely or relatively, in NIDDM, and it is possible that excess glucagon stimulation also contributes to the increase in glucose production.

Thus, insulin deficiency, insulin resistance, and accelerated hepatic glucose production all exist in NIDDM, and all contribute to the hyperglycemia (Fig. 230–2). It is tempting to suggest a unifying pathogenetic hypothesis in which one metabolic lesion is primary and the others secondary. Unfortunately it is not possible to choose any particular sequence at this time. All three abnormalities can be generated in animal models by inducing hyperglycemia and hypoinsulinemia, and all three are at least partially reversible with weight loss, oral sulfonylureas, or insulin therapy.

IDDM. A strong genetic component is involved in the etiology of IDDM, but extragenetic factors must also contribute, at least in most patients. Several lines of evidence suggest a role for *viruses* in IDDM: (1) Autopsies of IDDM patients dying within a few months of the disease's onset have revealed an "insulitis" consisting of round cell infiltration of islet tissue. (2) A modest seasonal variation to the incidence of IDDM has been noted in some studies. (3) A clinical history of preceding viral-type illness, particularly Coxsackie B and mumps, is often reported at the onset of IDDM. (4) Increased viral titers, including coxsackievirus B4, have been reported in IDDM patients at or near the time of the disease's onset. (5) Certain diabetogenic viruses (encephalomyocarditis M, coxsackievirus B, and rheovirus) can cause diabetes when inoculated into rodents. Further, the susceptibility of different rodent strains to develop viral-induced diabetes appears to be under genetic control. (6) Diabetogenic viruses can also directly infect B cells in culture, causing cell lysis and death. (7) Finally, direct support for virus-induced diabetes has been obtained in humans. Coxsackievirus B4 was isolated from the pancreas of a boy with new-onset IDDM who died of severe ketoacidosis closely following a

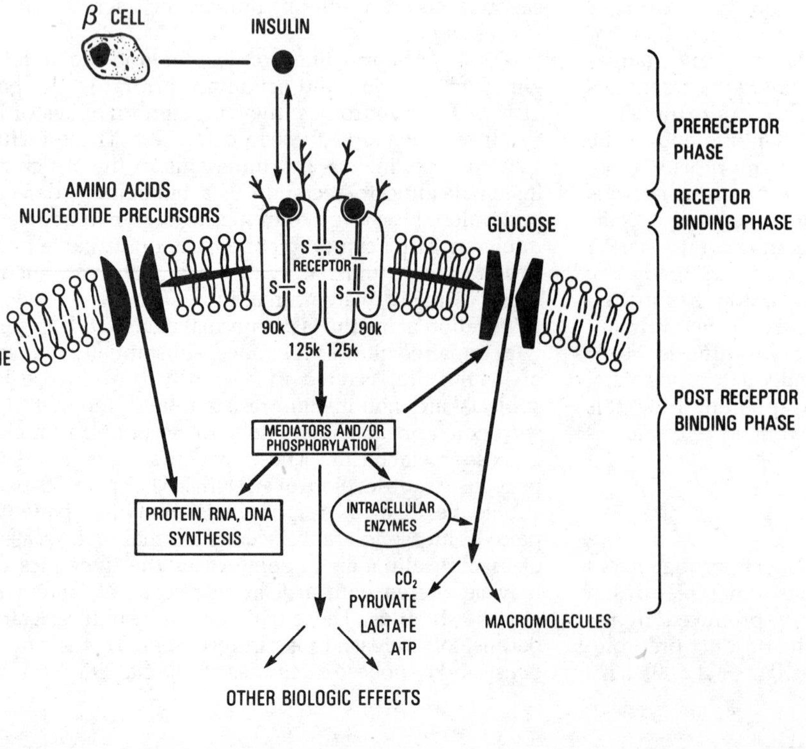

Figure 230–1. Model of insulin action and categories of insulin resistance. Abnormalities can occur at the prereceptor phase, involving biosynthesis and secretion of abnormal beta cell products; at the receptor binding phase, involving decreased insulin binding to receptors due to decreased receptor number or affinity; or at the postreceptor binding phase, involving any defect in the insulin action cascade distal to the initial binding event.

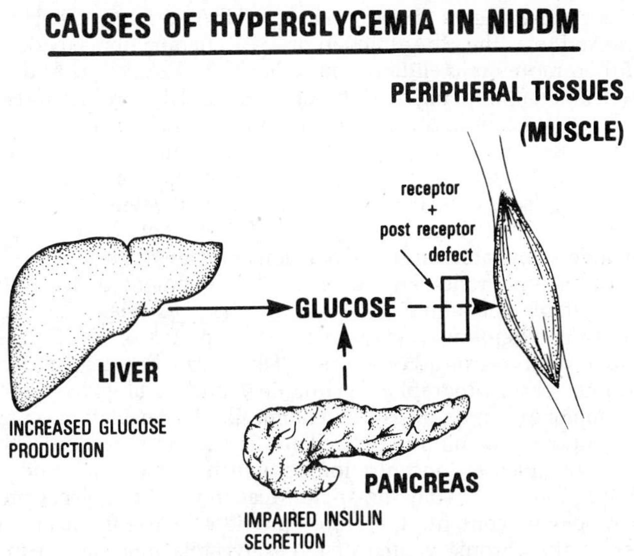

Figure 230–2. Summary of the metabolic abnormalities in NIDDM which contribute to the hyperglycemia. Increased hepatic glucose production, impaired insulin secretion, and insulin resistance due to receptor and postreceptor defects all combine to generate the hyperglycemic state.

flulike illness associated with rising serum titers of neutralizing antibody to the virus. The viral isolate was inoculated into experimental animals, producing diabetes, and viral antigens could be demonstrated in the B cells from the infected animals.

Autoimmunity may also play a role in the etiology of IDDM. Circulating antibodies to thyroid, gastric mucosa, and the adrenal are far more common in patients with IDDM than in normal persons. More importantly, up to 90 per cent of patients with new-onset IDDM have demonstrable titers of plasma islet cell antibodies. These antibodies are heterogeneous, some binding to cytoplasmic antigens common to all islet cells and others directed against the B cell surface. The latter lyse B cells in culture in the presence of complement, consistent with a pathophysiologic role in vivo. These islet cell antibodies are also observed in BB rats, an animal model that spontaneously develops an IDDM-like syndrome. In humans, titers of islet cell antibodies fall after the onset of clinical disease; by five years only 20 per cent of patients have demonstrable titers, and by 10 to 20 years the prevalence falls to 5 to 10 per cent. Patients who continue to demonstrate antibodies after several years may be examples of heterogeneity within IDDM. In these patients IDDM may represent a primary autoimmune disease, since they are largely female, show a great prevalence of other organ-specific antibodies, and have a strong family history of autoimmune disease. Patients with onset of IDDM at an older age tend to fall in this group. Genetically, they may also be different, since they have a greater prevalence of HLA-B8 and DR3. In cases of IDDM in which islet cell antibodies are cleared within one year of the disease's onset, patients are more often male, do not typically show signs of other autoimmune phenomena, experience onset of disease at a younger age, and have a higher association with HLA-B15 and HLA-DR4. Circulating antibodies may not be the only component of the immune response associated with IDDM; a cell-mediated immune response may also be involved. Increased K cells (killer lymphocytes) have been reported in IDDM along with alterations in T-lymphocyte subpopulations. Both antibody-induced and cell-mediated immune phenomena may be involved in the pathogenesis of IDDM.

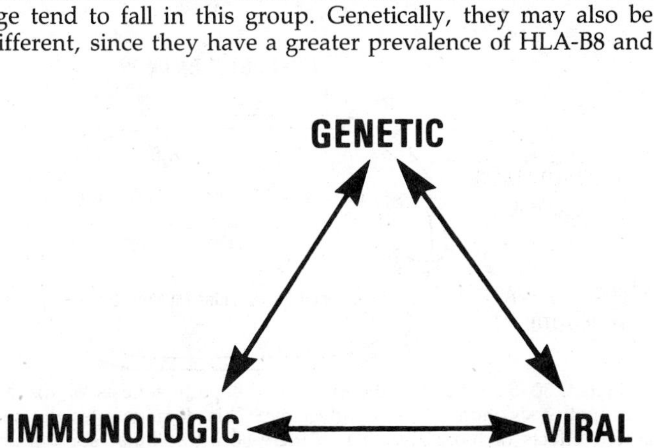

Figure 230–3. An interplay of genetic, immunologic, and viral etiologies contributes to the pathogenesis of NIDDM. The importance of each factor probably differs in subpopulations of IDDM, demonstrating the heterogeneity of this disease.

Strong arguments can be made for the role of genetic susceptibility, viruses, and altered immunity in the etiology of IDDM (Fig. 230–3). However, the contribution of these factors and the sequential relationship among them cannot be stated at this time. Clearly, immune responses could provide the causal link between the HLA associations and clinical IDDM, since the HLA alleles are thought to be associated through linkage disequilibrium to immune response genes. One way to integrate these factors would be to postulate that susceptibility to IDDM is inherited through genes closely associated with the HLA loci. Given this proper genetic background, environmental agents such as certain viruses exhibiting B cell tropism and possibly chemical agents can injure and in some cases destroy B cells. Following B cell injury, an immune response (possibly antibody and cell mediated) directed against B cells occurs owing to release of B cell antigens into the circulation, alteration of B cell antigens, cross-reactivity with viral antigens, or primary modulation of the immune response. In any event, the immune response would then exacerbate or complete the initial viral or chemical B cell injury. Of course this is only one of several sequences that can be proposed, but it is consistent with most of the available data. IDDM is probably heterogeneous, and no single sequence of pathogenetic events will necessarily explain all cases. For example, IDDM patients who are HLA-B8/DR3 display other organ-specific autoantibodies and probably have a primary autoimmune disease and do not need an environmental factor to develop the disease. Based on the intertwining of genetic, viral, and immune influences, it also follows that B cell destruction in IDDM does not usually occur acutely. It is likely that this process is gradual over months to years, even though the clinical onset of metabolic decompensation is usually abrupt when destruction of B cell mass reaches a critical point or an intercurrent illness occurs. This raises the possibility of intervention therapies (immune or other) following the onset of B cell injury but prior to clinical manifestations of IDDM, since by the time IDDM appears B cell destruction may be too far advanced for effective therapy. Such an approach would require a method to detect preclinical IDDM. Such methods are currently under intense study.

C peptide is secreted in equimolar amounts compared to insulin. Since C peptide has a much longer half-life than insulin, it provides an excellent measure of insulin secretory capacity, especially in those patients with circulating anti-insulin antibodies that interfere with usual insulin radioimmunoassays. In patients with type I diabetes who have been treated with insulin for longer than five years, C peptide levels are usually undetectable. However, C peptide may be measured in many of these patients during the first years of their disease. This suggests that the loss of beta cell secretion in IDDM is not abrupt, but continues for several years after the diabetes becomes clinically apparent. For the most part, ease of diabetic management and stability of metabolic control in IDDM are correlated with the degree of the residual insulin secretion. Those patients with the highest levels of circulating C peptide are easier to treat, and those with undetectable levels are more unstable. Some of the major clinical and pathophysiologic distinctions between IDDM and NIDDM are listed in Table 230–2.

TREATMENT

In this section, details concerning the various methods of diabetic management will be discussed. However, since the severity and clinical picture of diabetes are quite variable, therapeutic methods are also varied. In particular, major differences exist in the approach to NIDDM versus IDDM, and whenever possible therapeutic distinctions for these two forms of diabetes will be made.

RELATIONSHIP BETWEEN HYPERGLYCEMIA AND COMPLICATIONS. It is important to start with more general principles and to identify overall therapeutic goals. A consideration of therapeutic goals involves one of the most important questions in the field; that is, what is the relationship between hyperglycemia and the development of diabetic complications? Simply put, are complications due to hyperglycemia or are they due to genetic factors independent of hyperglycemia? This is the central clinical question in diabetes concerning which a voluminous literature exists.

Hyperglycemia is the most obvious metabolic abnormality in diabetes. It is therefore reasonable to suspect that elevated glucose levels play a role in diabetic complications. Consistent with this is a large body of retrospective evidence showing that better control is usually associated with fewer complications. Unfortunately, in the absence of randomized, prospective studies in which significant differences in glycemic control are achieved between matched experimental and control groups over an extended period, current clinical studies can provide only nonconclusive evidence. Classical diabetic complications can occur in secondary diabetes (in which genetic aspects of diabetes are presumably missing) and in normal kidneys following transplantation into diabetic patients. Furthermore, in twin studies the degree of retinopathy is comparable in twins concordant for IDDM, whereas in discordant pairs the nondiabetic twin does not have retinopathy. Certain abnormalities seen in diabetes, such as retinal capillary leakage (as demonstrated by fluorescein angiography), slowed motor nerve conductive velocity, and microalbuminuria, can be reversed by intensive insulin therapy, but the relationship between these physiologic abnormalities and clinically significant complications has not been demonstrated. In animal experiments a number of studies have shown good correlation between the level of hyperglycemia and microvascular complications similar (but perhaps not identical) to those seen in human diabetes. In animals, these complications can also be prevented or reversed with insulin therapy.

Several biochemical mechanisms have been proposed that may link hyperglycemia to complications. Proteins can be nonenzymatically glycosylated in vivo, and the degree of this glycosylation is directly related to the degree of hyperglycemia. Chromatography of red blood cell hemolysates shows four minor components (HbA_{1a1}, HbA_{1a2}, HbA_{1b1}, HbA_{1c}) of HbA, referred to as the HbA_1 fraction or "fast" hemoglobins (because of their more rapid elution from columns). HbA_1 is due to post-translational, nonenzymatic modification of HbA and comprises about 6 per cent of total hemoglobin in normal persons. HbA_{1c} comprises approximately two thirds of these minor components and is increased in the presence of hyperglycemia. To form HBA_{1c}, glucose combines with the N terminal valine of β chains to form a Schiff base aldimine (Fig. 230–4). This compound is relatively unstable, and the reaction is readily reversible. The aldimine undergoes an Amadori rearrangement to form the more stable ketoamine. HbA can also be glycosylated through the same chemical reaction at the N terminus of the α chain and ε amino groups of lysines. HbA_{1c} can be measured by various chromatographic techniques, and total glycosylated hemoglobin can be measured chemically. Glycosylation occurs continuously within the red cell and is a direct reflection of the average glucose concentration to which the cell is exposed throughout its 120-day life span. Measurement of glycosylated hemoglobin content, therefore, provides a useful means to assess the chronic degree of hyperglycemia that existed in a given patient over the preceding several weeks and is not affected by acute changes in plasma glucose level. Additionally, the nonspecific and nonenzymatic nature of hemoglobin glycosylation raises the possibility that glycosylation of other body proteins can occur, leading to structural or functional changes that may be related to chronic diabetic complications. Increased amounts of glycosylated low-density lipoprotein (LDL) molecules, for example, circulate in hyperglycemic diabetic patients and do not bind normally to LDL receptors. Since abnormal glycosylation may affect all tissues, this mechanism could be related to a variety of diabetic complications.

Additional biochemical lesions related to hyperglycemia have been proposed for nervous tissue. *Sorbitol* is a polyhydroxyl alcohol (polyol) produced from glucose by aldose reductase in nerve tissue; once formed, sorbitol can be converted to fructose (Fig. 230–5). It is theorized that this polyol pathway is particularly active in diabetes because of the hyperglycemia. This could lead to increased intracellular osmolarity (due to accumulation of sorbitol and fructose) with water influx, swelling

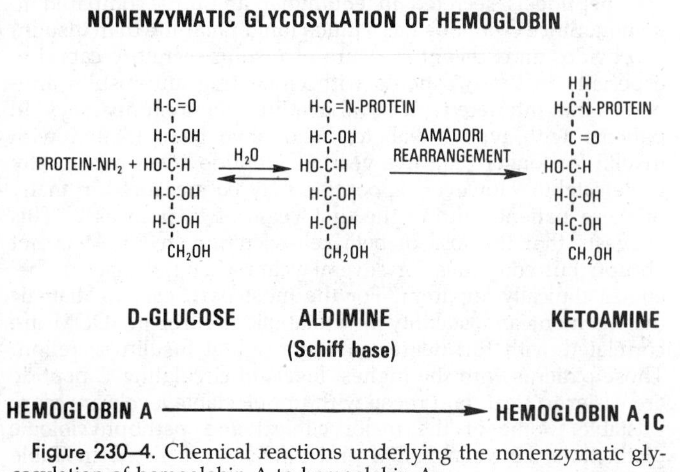

Figure 230–4. Chemical reactions underlying the nonenzymatic glycosylation of hemoglobin A to hemoglobin A_{1C}.

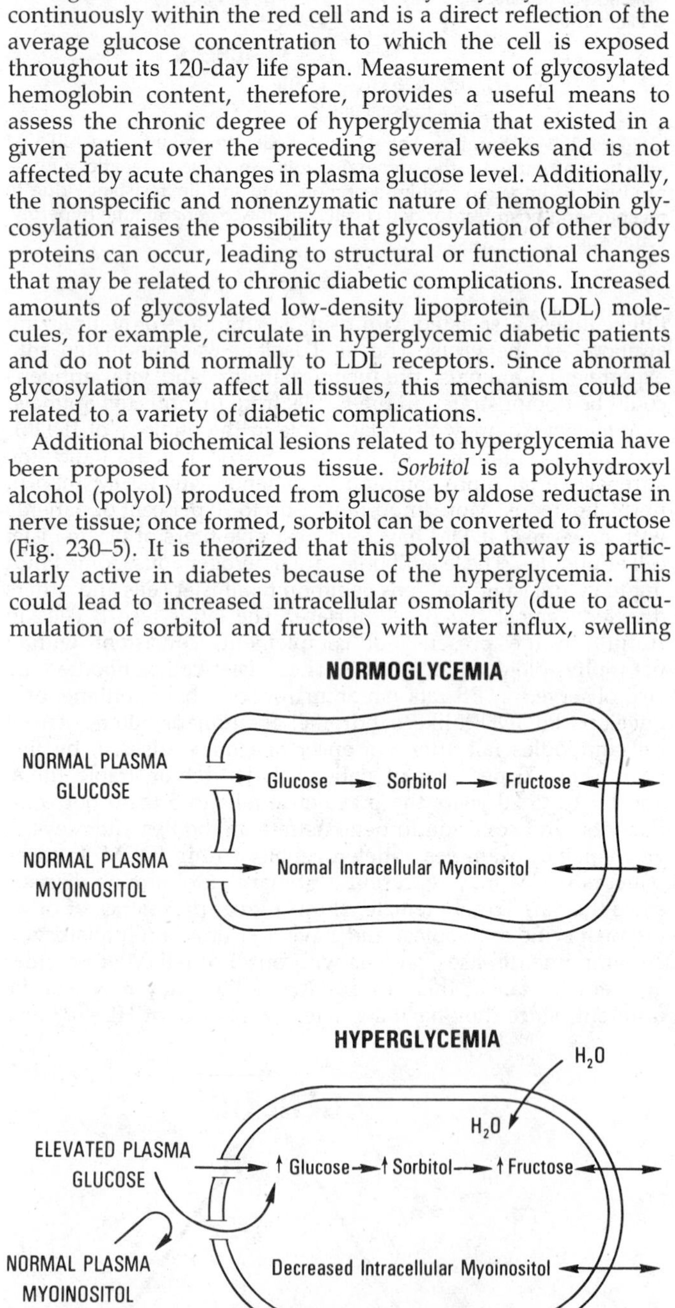

Figure 230–5. Metabolic theories for the pathogenesis of diabetic neuropathy secondary to hyperglycemia. This demonstrates the suggested effects of hyperglycemia to increase intracellular sorbitol and fructose concentrations leading to an osmotic increase in intracellular water content. In addition, it has been suggested that hyperglycemia depletes intracellular myoinositol content by competitively inhibiting the uptake of myoinositol from the extracellular space.

of Schwann cells, anoxia, and demyelination. Consistent with this, an increase in sorbitol content has been found in nerve tissue of diabetic rats, and it is reversible with insulin therapy. However, Schwann cell swelling and increased water content have not yet been demonstrated, and further testing of the polyol pathway hypothesis is necessary. Another hyperglycemia-related metabolic lesion in nervous tissue has been proposed involving *myoinositol*. Concentrations of this compound are decreased in peripheral nerves of diabetic rats, and this is associated with a decrease in nerve conduction velocity. These abnormalities can be prevented by insulin or oral myoinositol supplements. It is possible that uptake of myoinositol by nerves is inhibited by hyperglycemia, leading to depletion and pathologic sequelae. A link may exist between polyol and myoinositol metabolism in that increased activity of the polyol pathway contributes to the reduction in nerve myoinositol content.

The above discussion cites clinical and biochemical evidence supporting the relationship between hyperglycemia and complications. On the other hand, there is evidence against this relationship. For example, patients have been reported with diabetic complications at the time of onset of IDDM, when hyperglycemia should not have preexisted for a significant time. Additionally, some patients with very poor glycemic control never develop complications. Ultimately, however, the main argument against the relationship is simply that it has not been proven with certainty by well-controlled, prospective studies in man.

Taking all factors into account, it seems reasonable to me to conclude that although a definitive relationship between hyperglycemia and complications has been neither established nor disproved at present, the bulk of evidence weighs in favor of such a relationship. With this in mind it seems prudent to establish as a therapeutic goal the maintenance of plasma glucose levels as close to normal as possible in diabetic patients. The major complication of aggressive antidiabetic therapy is hypoglycemia, which, if severe enough, can unequivocally produce immediate and irreversible CNS damage. Therefore, diabetic management should be pushed until glucose levels are normal or near normal, unless recurrent, overt episodes of hypoglycemia develop. If this occurs, then compromises are necessary in the degree of glycemic control achieved. Other therapeutic goals include (1) normal growth and development in children, (2) normal pregnancy and childbirth in females, (3) reduction of diabetes-related atherosclerosis risk factors, especially in adult diabetic patients, and (4) minimal interference with normal life style in all diabetics.

DIETARY TREATMENT. Dietary treatment is an integral part of the overall therapeutic plan in all diabetic patients. In many NIDDM patients dietary therapy can be the predominant method of treatment. Dietary therapy is concerned with the total number of calories ingested, the distribution of calories throughout the day, the individual food sources that make up these calories, and maintenance of proper nutrition. Dietary therapy is much different in NIDDM and IDDM, because patients in the former are usually obese, whereas in the latter they are not, and NIDDM patients retain endogenous insulin secretion while IDDM patients do not.

Total Caloric Intake. Since most NIDDM patients are overweight, caloric restriction is advisable and can be of great benefit. The essential tenet of weight reduction is straightforward: if caloric expenditure exceeds intake, weight will be lost. There are many ways to calculate daily caloric expenditure, but on the average this amounts to 30 to 35 kcal per kilogram in normal man; 25 kcal per kilogram is attributed to the basal metabolic rate and the rest to physical activity. Daily caloric requirements are about 30 kcal per kilogram in sedentary individuals and approximately 35 kcal per kilogram in moderately active subjects. For those who engage in brisk physical exertion for prolonged intervals throughout the day caloric expenditure can exceed 35 kcal per kilogram. Another factor affecting caloric requirements (at least on a per kilogram basis) is the degree of adiposity. Adipose tissue is predominantly storage triglyceride, which is relatively inert metabolically with a decreased caloric need per unit weight. Thus, the greater the degree of adiposity, the lower the caloric requirement per kilogram. In very obese, sedentary individuals, daily caloric requirements can be as low as 25 kcal per kilogram of body weight.

A number of approaches to weight reduction exist that vary in the degree of caloric restriction and rate of weight loss, dietary constituents, as well as behaviorial and psychological support measures. These include nutritionally sound and modestly restricted diets that achieve slow gradual weight loss over several months, nutritionally balanced and very low calorie diets for rapid weight loss, and behavior modification, pharmacologic aids, and even surgical procedures (i.e., gastric plication) in the massively obese patient in whom medical therapy fails. These approaches are discussed in detail in Chapter 216.

For all these methods, inducing the initial period of weight loss is not the major problem in weight reduction, but, rather, the major problem is weight regain or recidivism. Motivated patients can usually successfully lose weight over the initial dietary period, but it is the unusual patient who successfully keeps the pounds off. The major challenge in weight reduction therapy is to develop a proper supportive environment and patient motivation to maintain weight loss after it has been achieved. In the NIDDM patient, significant caloric restriction is usually successful in lowering plasma glucose levels even before significant weight loss is achieved. Depending on the degree of obesity that was present initially and the amount of weight loss, continued beneficial effects on glycemic control can be maintained after the goal weight is achieved and a eucaloric diet is initiated. In general, the more recent the onset of NIDDM, the more responsive the patient will be to the beneficial effects of weight reduction. In patients with pronounced fasting hyperglycemia, very low calorie diets (300 to 600 kcal per day) are often useful in achieving rapid glycemic control as well as an initial rapid rate of weight loss (which can often be of important psychological and motivational benefit). Very low calorie diets usually consist of liquid formula meals and should not be utilized unless they contain adequate amounts (a minimum 30 to 40 grams per day) of high quality protein and are supplemented with vitamins and micronutrients. NIDDM patients on such diets should be supervised by a physician.

The mechanisms whereby weight reduction ameliorates hyperglycemia in NIDDM are not completely clear. Weight loss leads to a reduction in the accelerated rates of hepatic glucose production, ameliorates the degree of insulin resistance by increasing insulin receptors and reducing the magnitude of the post-receptor defect in insulin action, and possibly improves beta cell secretion. However, the precise cellular mechanisms leading to these effects are not known. Patients with IDDM are seldom obese, and an important nutritional goal is maintenance of adequate nutrition, particularly to assure normal growth and development in children and pregnant women.

Distribution of Calories. In addition to total caloric consumption, attention should also be paid to the distribution of calories throughout the day in any dietary prescription. Two principles should be kept in mind: (1) calories should be spread as evenly as possible throughout the major daily meals to avoid a large concentration of calories at any one meal and not to overwhelm the diabetic patient's impaired capacity to metabolize food; and (2) in those patients receiving exogenous insulin, caloric intake should be temporally adjusted to coincide with the time course of action of the administered insulin. The latter point highlights a major difference in dietary consideration between patients with IDDM and NIDDM. In NIDDM, endogenous insulin secretion is still present and the beta cell can respond at the appropriate times (albeit to a limited degree) to food ingestion, regardless of when it occurs throughout the day. This is even true, although to a lesser extent, in NIDDM subjects who are treated with insulin. Thus, in these patients it is sufficient to balance calories throughout the day, but the patient has a good deal of leeway to determine the timing of specific meals as long as calories are ingested at times of peak exogenous insulin action. For practical purposes, the only insulin present in patients with IDDM is that which is administered exogenously. Therefore, patients must pay close attention to the timing of meals and must be certain that there is reasonable concordance between meal ingestion and the time course of action of the insulin they have taken. To a certain extent the patient can elect a temporal pattern suitable to his lifestyle and preference and the insulin therapy regimen can then be tailored appropriately. In this way greater flexibility is allowed that improves overall patient compliance and quality of life.

Nutrient Content of Diet. A great deal of attention is currently being paid to the individual components comprising the diabetic diet. When patients consume eucaloric diets, it is important that they be properly balanced and nutritionally sound. A generally accepted protein requirement is 0.8 grams per kilogram per day for adults, but larger amounts are usually consumed in Western diets. Thus, protein usually comprises about 15 per cent of total caloric consumption. With this as a base, the proportions of fat and carbohydrate (CHO) are inversely related. Previous attempts to restrict total CHO intake are no longer deemed advisable, and most authorities now advocate liberalization of CHO intake to 50 to 55 per cent of total calories. This means that total fat intake should not exceed 30 to 35 per cent, and because diabetic patients are predisposed to macrovascular disease, saturated fat (primarily animal fat) intake should be reduced so that the polyunsaturated-saturated fat ratio is equivalent to 1:0. Ideally, cholesterol intake should not exceed 450 mg per day. The makeup of the CHO portion of the diet also requires attention. In the past it was felt that diabetics should rigorously avoid sucrose because it is rapidly absorbed and raises the blood glucose level inordinately. While this may be true when sucrose is consumed as the sole nutritive component, as in soft drinks or certain candies, it is less of a problem when modest amounts of sucrose are eaten in a mixed meal setting. Because of this, up to 5 per cent of total CHO can be consumed as sucrose, as long as it is taken in the context of a mixed meal and spaced out through the day. This allows the diabetic a wider variety of food choices, making the diet more palatable; a side benefit of this approach is that it improves patient adherence to the dietary prescription and to the other elements of the overall therapeutic plan. The remainder of the CHO predominantly consists of starches. All complex CHO cannot be lumped together as a single food group because the glycemic response to different starches differs widely, being lowest for lentils and pasta and highest for wheat and potatoes. More work needs to be done to determine the glycemic potency of a large number of foods, singly and together, in diabetic patients before the precise composition of the CHO in the diet can be recommended with certainty. At this stage it is advisable for the diabetic to consume 50 to 55 per cent of calories as CHO with a modest restriction in sucrose intake and emphasis on ingestion of those complex CHOs with low glycemic potency.

Fructose is a nutritive sweetener that may also have a place in the diabetic diet. This simple CHO is somewhat sweeter than sucrose and has similar properties when prepared in foods. Thus, fructose can be substituted for sucrose in most foods with little change in taste or texture. The advantage is that fructose is absorbed from the gastrointestinal tract more slowly than sucrose and is predominantly taken up and metabolized by the liver through non-insulin–dependent mechanisms. Within the liver, fructose is phosphorylated and eventually converted to glycogen or triglyceride through the triose phosphate intermediates. Thus, little fructose escapes hepatic uptake to enter the peripheral circulation, and only a small amount of fructose is converted to glucose for release from the liver. Ingestion of fructose leads to a minimal postprandial rise in plasma glucose or insulin levels in normal persons and in diabetics when taken alone or as part of a mixed meal. For these reasons, fructose offers some advantage in the diabetic diet, and amounts up to 75 grams per day can be safely consumed. The major exception occurs in patients with severely uncontrolled NIDDM or in poorly insulinized IDDM patients. In these conditions glycogen production is inhibited and fructose enters the gluconeogenic pathway and is ultimately released as glucose, causing hyperglycemia.

Dietary fiber can also influence CHO absorption. Glycemic excursions are reduced and insulin secretion diminished when normal persons and subjects with NIDDM consume fiber-enriched diets. This effect is mediated through delayed gastric emptying and overall slowing of the rate of CHO digestion and absorption. Since large amounts of fiber (10 to 15 grams per meal) are needed to observe these effects, major changes in dietary patterns would be necessary to achieve beneficial results. Nevertheless, when fiber is consumed as natural foods, there do not seem to be any untoward effects of increased fiber ingestion, and some studies indicate that increased fiber intake can lower serum triglyceride levels. The only potential caveat to this statement involves growing children and pregnant women, since subtle undesirable changes in micronutrient absorption due to high fiber ingestion have not been ruled out.

A minority of diabetic patients adhere to the recommended dietary regimens. To a large extent this is due to inadequate understanding on the part of the patient as well as the physician regarding dietary goals and methods. An additional factor is that dietary therapy must be individualized, taking into account each patient's life style, economic status, food preferences, and social needs. This can be a time-consuming process, and few physicians have the time or training to participate with patients in this type of detailed dietary management. For this reason it is critical to incorporate a dietitian or nutritionist trained in the principles of dietary therapy of diabetes as part of the health care team. One cannot simply give pamphlets, instructional aids, and meal plans and expect even motivated patients to adhere to the necessary regimens. Detailed instruction by a nutrition counselor is necessary to tailor the diet to each patient's special needs. Dietary therapy is a chronic treatment modality and therefore the longer view is important. Occasional deviations from recommended meal plans for special occasions are acceptable, providing the patient has a clear understanding of how this should be managed. Often, this allows for better patient compliance with the overall diet plan. Periodic meetings with a nutrition counselor are necessary to implement and maintain individualized dietary regimens.

ORAL HYPOGLYCEMIC AGENTS. Oral hypoglycemic agents are often therapeutically effective in NIDDM patients. In 1970, serious questions were raised concerning the use of these agents: results of the University Group Diabetes Program (UGDP) indicated that these drugs increased the rate of sudden death from heart disease in patients with mild NIDDM. However, because of numerous questions concerning the design and interpretation of the UGDP study, concerns about the use of oral hypoglycemic agents have greatly diminished. In patients who do not respond satisfactorily to diet and do not have severe hyperglycemia (i.e., plasma glucose levels consistently greater than 250 mg per deciliter), oral agents are an appropriate therapeutic choice. In patients with severe hyperglycemia, insulin therapy is preferable, at least initially, to gain more rapid control of clinical symptoms and to prevent hyperosmolarity. While sulfonylureas are effective in patients with NIDDM, they are ineffective in IDDM. Some have suggested that combinations of oral agents with insulin can reduce insulin requirements in IDDM; however, this has not been proven, and would be of minor clinical importance anyway.

The mechanism of action of sulfonylureas is complex. In the short term, they augment B cell insulin secretion. However, after several months of therapy, insulin levels return to pretreatment values while glucose levels remain improved. These findings led to the demonstration that sulfonylureas exert extrapancreatic effects on glucose metabolism: (1) they reduce the accelerated rates of hepatic glucose production in NIDDM; (2) they partially reverse the postreceptor defect in insulin action; and (3) they increase the number of cellular insulin receptors. These all represent significant components of the insulin resistance of NIDDM, so sulfonylureas can improve glycemia by improving insulin's effectiveness at target cells. The relative importance of each of these actions in ameliorating hyperglycemia is unclear, but it is likely that the pancreatic and extrapancreatic effects of these agents combine to produce the hypoglycemic action of these drugs.

There are several different kinds of sulfonylureas, differing primarily in potency, pharmacokinetics, and modes of metabolism as outlined in Table 230–3. *Tolbutamide* is metabolized to inert products by the liver and has a relatively short half-life, necessitating administration two or three times a day. Although it is the least potent of the available sulfonylureas on a weight basis, it has not been clearly demonstrated that any sulfonylurea produces greater hypoglycemic potency at maximal doses in diabetic patients. Therefore, for practical purposes, the differences in relative potency of the different drugs simply mean that more or less of a given agent should be used. *Tolazamide* and especially *acetohexamide* are metabolized by the liver to biologically active products that are then excreted by the kidneys. These drugs have intermediate half-lives and are usually given twice (but sometimes once) a day. Contrary to earlier data, *chlorpropamide* also undergoes considerable hepatic degradation into less active metabolites excreted in the urine. This compound can cause significant water retention and hyponatremia by potentiating ADH action on the kidney. Chlorpropamide has the longest circulating half-life and duration of action (about 60 hours) and is given only once a day. Hypoglycemia is the major complication of sulfonylureas, and this can be particularly severe with chlorpropamide because of its long duration of action. Elderly NIDDM subjects are more susceptible to hypoglycemia, especially those prone to skip meals. The route of metabolism of the different compounds may influence the choice of agent. One should be cautious about the use of chlorpropamide, acetohexamide, and, to a lesser extent, tolazamide in patients with compromised renal function because of the route of excretion. Second-generation sulfonylureas, such as *glybenclamide,* have been extensively used in Europe, but as of this writing, have not yet been released for use in the United States. These agents are metabolized by the liver and have relatively long duration of action and can be given once a day. It is claimed, but not rigorously demonstrated, that the second-generation sulfonylureas are more effective than the first-generation drugs.

The other major category of oral hypoglycemic agents consists of the biguanides, such as *phenformin.* The exact mechanism of action of these drugs is not clear, although they may interfere with hepatic gluconeogenesis. However, these drugs were strongly implicated in the development of lactic acidosis and have been prohibited from clinical use in the United States by the Food and Drug Administration. When they were used, they were often given in combination with a sulfonylurea.

In NIDDM the usual practice is to begin with a low dose of a given sulfonyluria, advancing the dose until the therapeutic response is satisfactory or a maximal dose is reached. Occasionally patients who do not respond to one drug can be switched to another with beneficial effect. Certain drug interactions occur with sulfonylureas, that is, phenylbutazone and anticoagulants compete for hepatic removal mechanisms with sulfonylureas. A disulfiram (Antabuse)-like reaction can occasionally occur following alcohol consumption by patients taking sulfonylureas. This is most frequently reported with chlorpropamide, but has not yet been noted with the second-generation agents. Potential interactions of this sort should always be kept in mind in the appropriate clinical context.

Approximately 10 to 20 per cent of NIDDM patients do not respond to oral agents, and treatment is termed primary failure. Secondary failure occurs when a patient responds initially to an oral agent, but then ceases to respond in the next year or two. This occurs in 5 to 20 per cent of patients, but these proportions obviously depend on the particular NIDDM population studied. For example, patients with new-onset diabetes respond better than those with longstanding disease. In some cases, secondary failure is due to dietary noncompliance in a patient who previously successfully adhered to a dietary regimen. However, this is often not the case, and the mechanisms of secondary failure in many patients with NIDDM remain unknown.

Debate exists as to which patients with NIDDM are appropriate candidates for oral sulfonylurea therapy. In view of the evidence implicating hyperglycemia with diabetic complications, the therapeutic goal with oral agents should be the maintenance of glucose levels as near to normal as possible. In patients with mild to moderate fasting hyperglycemia (140 to 230 mg per deciliter), dietary therapy should be tried first; if the above therapeutic goals are not achieved with this approach, then a sulfonylurea can be added. The problem arises in patients with more severe fasting hyperglycemia (more than 230 mg per deciliter) who have pronounced clinical symptoms despite dietary treatment. In these patients, some would advise an initial period of sulfonylurea therapy, and if satisfactory control is not achieved then insulin treatment should be substituted. Others would suggest an initial period of insulin therapy following which the patient is switched to sulfonylureas: if satisfactory control is achieved, the drug is continued. Alternatively, insulin can be used indefinitely in these patients. Clearly this is a gray area, and the particular approach should be individualized to each patient, taking into account the total clinical context of the patient's disease, acceptance of the various therapeutic methods, level of diabetes education, and

TABLE 230–3. CHARACTERISTICS OF SULFONYLUREAS

Generic Name	Brand Name	Dosage Range (mg)	Duration of Action (hr)	Comments
Tolbutamide	Orinase	500–3000	6–12	Metabolized by liver to inert products, given 2–3 × /day
Chlorpropamide	Diabinase	100–500	60	Metabolized by liver (~70%) to less active metabolite, and excreted intact (~30%) by kidneys; can potentiate ADH action, given 1 × /day
Acetohexamide	Dymelor	250–1500	12–24	Metabolized by liver to active metabolite given 1–2 × /day
Tolazamide	Tolinase	100–1000	10–18	Metabolized by liver to active product, given 1–2 × /day
Glyburide	Micronase	2.5–30	10–30	Metabolized by liver to inert products, given 1 × /day
Glipizide	Glucotrol	5–40	18–30	Metabolized by liver to inert products, given 1 × /day

motivation. In a patient in whom severe fasting hyperglycemia is maintained, with marked clinical symptoms and incipient hyperosmolarity, oral agents are probably not appropriate, at least initially. In these patients insulin therapy should be the primary mode of treatment and can be continued indefinitely, or a therapeutic trial of sulfonylureas can be substituted once the hyperglycemia has been brought under control by the initial period of insulin treatment. In general, response to sulfonylurea therapy is best if the onset of diabetes is recent and the patient is over 40 years of age and not thin.

INSULIN TREATMENT. Insulin is the primary mode of therapy in all patients with IDDM and in many with NIDDM (see above). The goals of therapy include: (1) normal growth and development in children, (2) normal pregnancy, delivery, and conceptus in women, (3) minimal interference with psychosocial adjustment, (4) acceptable glycemic control, with minimal hypoglycemia, and (5) prevention of complications. Little disagreement exists concerning goals 1 to 3; however, different views exist of how best to achieve goals 4 and 5. There are many different methods of insulin therapy, and the method chosen is highly dependent on one's view of goals 4 and 5. If a physician holds closely to the important relationship between control and complications, then "acceptable control" will be much more rigorously defined and a method of insulin treatment that is designed to produce the desired response will be chosen. On the other hand, those who question the link between hyperglycemia and complications are advocates of looser control and will utilize a less intensive method of insulin delivery. In general, it is quite easy to eliminate overt symptoms of hyperglycemia with any method of insulin therapy, but it is extremely difficult, and probably impossible, to achieve euglycemia on a 24-hour basis. How close one comes to this ideal depends on the method of insulin delivery chosen, which in turn depends on one's philosophy of diabetic management.

Insulin Preparations. To begin a discussion of the methods of insulin treatment, let us first consider the many different kinds of insulin available. Commerical insulin comes in concentrations of 100 units per milliliter (U-100) and 500 units per milliliter (U-500). The various insulin preparations differ in their time course of action (rapid, intermediate, and long acting), degree of purity, and source (beef, pork, beef-pork, or human synthetic insulin); these properties are outlined in Table 230–4. By adjustment of pH during preparation, the size of the zinc-insulin crystal can be modified; the larger the crystals, the slower the release after subcutaneous injection, and this accounts for the differences in time of action between semilente (rapid-acting) and ultralente (long-acting) insulin. Lente (intermediate-acting) insulin is simply a 30:70 mixture of semilente and ultralente respectively. The other method to delay the onset of action of injected insulin is to mix it with a protein (protamine) and adjust the pH. This results in NPH (intermediate) and PZI (long-acting) preparations. It should be cautioned that the values for peak onset and duration of action

TABLE 230–4. PROPERTIES OF VARIOUS INSULIN PREPARATIONS

Class	Type	Peak Effect	Duration of Action (hr)
Rapid	Regular crystalline insulin (CZI)	2–4	6–8
	Semilente	2–6	10–12
Intermediate	Neutral protamine (NPH)	6–12	18–24
	Lente	6–12	18–24
Long Acting	Protamine zinc, (PZI)	14–24	36
	Ultralente	18–24	36

listed in Table 230–4 are simply estimates. There is a great deal of variability in these values from patient to patient as a result of circulating anti-insulin antibodies that alter the pharmacokinetics of insulin, variation in subcutaneous absorption, individual responses, and other factors. Additionally, absorption of insulin may be quite variable within a single patient from day to day, since absorption of subcutaneous insulin is markedly increased by vigorous exercise of the injected extremity or massage of the injection site. Differences in purity also exist. Conventional insulin preparations contain less than 10,000 parts per million (ppm) of impurities; improved single peak insulin, less than 50 ppm; and "purified" insulin, 1 to 10 ppm. The impurities mentioned are predominantly proinsulin, with smaller amounts of insulin dimers, proinsulin-like products, glucagon, pancreatic polypeptide, somatostatin, and vasoactive polypeptide. For practical purposes, commercially available insulin preparations are labeled as purified (1 to 10 ppm); if they are not specifically labeled they contain 20 to 50 ppm. The older less pure forms are no longer widely distributed. Essentially all preparations can be obtained as purified pork, beef, or beef-pork mixtures. Finally, highly purified human insulin is now available as a product of recombinant DNA biosynthesis or chemical conversion of pork to human insulin.

Methods of Treatment. The insulin regimen can be more or less intensive, depending on the number of injections per day, types of insulin used, and frequency and method of assessing control. Many NIDDM patients, and occasional IDDM patients, can achieve excellent glycemic control with a single daily (morning) injection of an intermediate-acting insulin. Occasionally, because of postbreakfast hyperglycemia, it is necessary to mix a short-acting preparation with this single dose. In most patients who realize excellent control with this regimen, endogenous insulin secretion is retained. A somewhat more intensive method to regulate glycemia involves a split-dosage regimen. This includes morning (before breakfast) and evening (before dinner) injection of mixtures of intermediate- and rapid-acting insulin. About two thirds of the total daily dose is usually given in the morning and about one third in the evening; the proportion of intermediate- to rapid-acting insulin at each injection is usually two thirds to one third. Patients receiving single-dose therapy who require more than 50 to 60 units per day should usually be tried on a split-dose regimen. In a 70-kg man, normal 24-hour insulin output has been estimated at 25 units per day. Therefore, in normal-sized diabetic subjects starting insulin therapy, it is reasonable to begin with a total daily dose of about 20 units per day with upward adjustments every several days based on the level of blood and urinary glucose. In mildly obese IDDM patients, starting doses can be 5 to 10 units per day higher. Because of insulin resistance, obese NIDDM patients requiring insulin will often need 60 to 90 units per day. With the above methods of insulin delivery, assessment of glycemic control can be carried out in several ways. Measurements of urinary glucose and ketones can be obtained before breakfast and once or twice throughout the day. Patients should be instructed to void 30 minutes before obtaining urine for glucose determination (double voiding), particularly for the morning sample, so that the urinary glucose is more representative of the corresponding blood glucose. Regardless of how carefully urinary glucose is determined, it provides only a rough approximation of blood glucose levels. Factors such as renal threshold, renal blood flow, and urine volume greatly affect the meaning of urine glucose measurements (i.e., a 4+ reaction in a concentrated urine sample is of little significance compared to a 4+ reaction in a dilute sample). For these reasons, urinary glucose is a poor way to monitor diabetic control and if at all possible should not be relied upon as the sole guide on which to base the insulin regimen. Twenty-four hour urinary glucose excretion can be periodically assessed to provide a better estimate of day-long control (less than 5 grams per day is excellent control) or glycosylated hemoglobin can be measured to assess the overall state of glycemic control during the preceding few weeks. The best current method to assess glycemic control is home-, or self-, monitoring of glucose (see below). This requires the patient to assess his own blood glucose level daily and to make appropriate adjustments in insulin dosage. This approach places a large part of the management responsibility in the hands of the patient and emphasizes the need for a continuous outpatient patient education program.

When patients with new-onset IDDM are started on insulin therapy, after an initial period of stabilization, insulin requirements frequently decrease dramatically over the ensuing few weeks. This is the so-called honeymoon phenomenon, and it is sometimes possible to maintain near-normal levels of glycemia without administering any insulin. This honeymoon phase may last for a few weeks and sometimes as long as one to two years. It is invariably followed by worsening of metabolic control with permanent recrudescence of the insulin-dependent state. Some experts have recommended that during this honeymoon period insulin administration should never be completely stopped, even if dosages have to be reduced to homeopathic levels. The reason for this is the fear that if there is a prolonged period in which insulin is not administered, once insulin therapy is reinstituted an anamnestic response with rising titers of anti-insulin antibodies might occur. However, with use of the highly purified insulin preparations now available, or with biosynthetic human insulin, this may be less of a problem.

If more intensive insulin management is required to achieve closer to normal glycemic control, then multiple daily injections of insulin or continuous subcutaneous insulin infusion (CSII) are used. At the current time these approaches are generally limited to patients with IDDM. However, if ideal control of glycemia is the therapeutic goal, there is no reason these methods could not be used in patients with NIDDM whose disease cannot be satisfactorily controlled by other means. Multiple injections involve administration of regular insulin before each meal, with the dose adjusted to the anticipated meal size. This is usually combined with either a long-acting insulin in the morning or an intermediate-acting preparation in the evening.

The most intensive method of insulin delivery is CSII. This consists of constant insulin delivery into a subcutaneous site in the abdominal wall via an open loop delivery device consisting of a small insulin pump that must be worn by the patient essentially 24 hours a day. The key to this method of therapy is the constant delivery of basal insulin. The basal insulin infusion is supplemented by a preprandial bolus of insulin given 15 minutes prior to meal ingestion. This gives the patient a fair degree of flexibility in the timing and content of meals, since the preprandial bolus is given at the patient's discretion in an amount picked to match meal size. In general, the basal insulin infusion accounts for about 50 per cent of the total daily insulin dose and usually averages 0.5 to 1 unit per hour. Typically, preprandial boluses are 5 to 10 units, depending on meal size, time of day, and proximity to time of exercise. To be successful, intensive insulin therapy regimens must be combined with home- (or self-) glucose monitoring. This requires the patient to obtain capillary blood by finger prick for glucose measurement, using a reflectance meter. There are numerous devices and algorithms for constant insulin delivery and various approaches to the frequency and method of self-glucose measurements. A detailed discussion of these issues is beyond the scope of this chapter, but suffice it to say that with properly motivated and educated patients and physicians, excellent control can be achieved in nearly all subjects. Patients generally accept this mode of therapy quite well and report an increased feeling of well-being. However, CSII should not be used indiscriminately, since pump dysfunction does occur, and hypoglycemia is a real problem, especially nocturnally. Additionally, a great deal is asked of patients when they participate in these programs in terms of dedication, education, and changes in life style.

Many other insulin treatment schedules have been proposed, all of which represent variations on the above common themes. Some of these are listed in Table 230–5. No single method is inherently superior to any other, and it is probably best for a physician to become accustomed to one or two methods and use them more or less exclusively so that he will be familiar with problems associated with insulin therapy and its individualization. All of these approaches are meant as guidelines rather than rigid algorithms, and considerable flexibility should be allowed to achieve optimal individualization.

TABLE 230–5. DIFFERENT INSULIN REGIMENS

Split dose intermediate (NPH or lente) + regular insulin		
	A.M. dose:	⅔ TDD*
		~ 70% intermediate
		~ 30% regular
	P.M. dose:	⅓ TDD
		50%–70% intermediate
		30%–50% regular
Intermediate + preprandial regular insulin		
	Breakfast:	Regular, 25%–40% TDD
	Lunch:	Regular, 25%–30% TDD
	Dinner:	Regular, 25%–30% TDD
	Night:	NPH or lente, 15%–25% TDD
Ultralente + preprandial regular insulin		
	Breakfast:	Regular, 15%–25% TDD
	Lunch:	Regular, 15%–25% TDD
	Dinner:	Regular, 15%–25% TDD
		Ultralente, 40%–60% TDD
Triple A.M. mixture: regular, lente + ultralente insulin		
Double A.M. mixture: regular + NPH (or lente) insulin		

*TDD, total daily dose

Regardless of the insulin regimen employed, an established daily dose in a given patient must not be considered to be fixed. Even long-established insulin dosages may need to be increased because of changes in growth status, subtle intercurrent illness or stress, or development of anti-insulin antibodies. Dosages may need to be decreased because of consistent increases in physical activity, dietary changes, or changes in concomitant drug therapy (e.g., stopping steroids). Additionally, absorption may vary from one anatomic site to another, and the rate of absorption of insulin can be augmented by exercise involving a particular injection site. This simply means that the physician and the patient must constantly review the treatment program and be prepared to make changes when indicated.

Complications of Insulin Therapy. Several complications are associated with insulin treatment, but the most significant of these is *hypoglycemia*. This is because even the best mode of insulin delivery is still an imperfect method to mimic the homeostatic mechanisms in normal subjects. Normal persons respond to food ingestion, exercise, and stress in such a way as to keep the blood glucose level within narrowly defined limits. One can hope to approach this, but not match it, with the methods used for delivery of exogenous insulin. For example, when normal individuals exercise, peripheral glucose uptake increases, and this is matched by a corresponding increase in hepatic glucose production. A decrease in insulin secretion allows the increase in hepatic glucose production to occur. Obviously this degree of fine tuning is difficult to achieve with exogenous insulin administration. Consequently hypoglycemia is a common complication of insulin therapy as the result of overzealous insulin administration or inappropriate timing. Most often this occurs in a situation in which tight control is attempted. Occasional mild episodes of hypoglycemia are probably acceptable if they appear in a patient in whom excellent control is generally achieved and who is fully aware of their occurrence and of methods to abort them. However, frequent and severe hypoglycemic reactions are unacceptable. These are serious and occasionally can be fatal. Furthermore, the long-term effects on the central nervous system of frequent hypoglycemic episodes have not been determined. If satisfactory control cannot be achieved without recurrence of such reactions, then compromises in the overall therapeutic plan must be made. It would seem imprudent to expose patients to known complications of hypoglycemia in the hope that superior control will prevent chronic diabetic complications in the future.

An interesting aspect of hypoglycemic episodes is the so-called *Somogyi phenomenon.* This involves rebound hyperglycemia due to excessive secretion of counterregulatory hormones following a previous episode of hypoglycemia. The classic situation involves nocturnal hypoglycemia followed by marked hyperglycemia prior to breakfast. This can induce a self-defeating cycle in which the insulin dose is progressively raised in response to the fasting hyperglycemia when a reduction in insulin dose, to prevent the nocturnal hypoglycemia, would be more appropriate.

A minority of patients beginning insulin therapy experience a variety of local allergic reactions at the injection site. Manifestations include local itching, erythematous indurated lesions, and occasional small, discrete subcutaneous nodules. These local reactions are usually self-limited and eventually disappear with continued insulin treatment. Antihistamines may be used for symptomatic relief if necessary. The frequency of these problems has decreased significantly with the use of the newer more highly purified insulins. Rare patients may develop systemic reactions, including generalized urticaria and even anaphylactic reactions. This usually occurs when insulin therapy has been stopped for a time and then reinstituted. If these symptoms cannot be controlled by antihistamines, and if insulin treatment is mandatory for the patient's well-being, then formal desensitization regimens are necessary. Other local reactions at the injection site include lipoatrophy and hypertrophy. Lipoatrophy at the injection site is a benign condition usually due to impurities in the insulin preparation. It can usually be corrected by changing to a highly purified pork insulin and injecting this into the lipoatrophic areas, which then fill in with subcutaneous fat in a normal fashion. Most likely the new highly purified human insulin preparations will also be suitable for this purpose. Insulin hypertrophy is attributed to the local lipogenic effects of the injected insulin. In advanced cases the underlying tissue can be fibrous and less vascular, making the overlying skin anesthetic. This explains why many patients prefer these areas as sites of injection. The problem can usually be corrected by carefully rotating injection sites.

FUTURE MODES OF THERAPY

Even with the most meticulous mode of insulin therapy in the most motivated patients, euglycemic control is difficult to achieve for prolonged periods. Thus the search for better, more effective, and, in some cases, curative forms of therapy continues. Transplantation of the pancreas or islet cells continues to receive extensive study. Numerous logistical, immunologic, and technical problems need to be overcome before such therapies become available for routine clinical purposes, but there are signs that some positive results might be seen in the next several years. This is the one mode of therapy that might actually be considered curative. Efforts continue to be expended in developing newer and better external or implantable insulin-delivery devices. Unquestionably the mechanical and engineering aspects of insulin-delivery devices will continue to improve dramatically over the next several years, and pumps that are smaller, safer, and more flexible will be produced. It also seems likely that reliable implantable devices are in the offing. However, unless such devices can be used to administer insulin via the portal route, the advantage of implantable pumps appears to be mostly esthetic. An additional hope for internal devices is that a closed loop system can be designed. This would require development of a reliable, fail-safe glucose sensor integrated into the appropriate algorithms for insulin delivery. If such artificial pancreases become readily available they would obviously have wide applicability. Finally, since hyperglucagonemia has been implicated in the pathogenesis of the hyperglycemia in diabetes, agents that specifically suppress glucagon secretion have been sought. Attempts to develop a glucagon-specific somatostatin derivative continue; such a compound might be a useful adjunctive therapy in the management of diabetes.

ACUTE COMPLICATIONS

A number of acute metabolic complications of diabetes exist, including diabetic ketoacidosis, hyperosmolar nonketotic coma, lactic acidosis, and hypoglycemia.

Diabetic Ketoacidosis (DKA)

DKA is due to insulin deficiency. Before consideration of the pathogenesis of this metabolic derangement, it is important to review the normal physiologic effects of insulin on carbohydrate, protein, and fat metabolism, since DKA simply represents a reversal of these normal insulin-stimulated processes.

PHYSIOLOGY OF FED AND FASTED STATE. When food is ingested, insulin functions as the major anabolic hormone facilitating the disposition of carbohydrate, protein, and fat and their synthesis into macromolecules for storage (Fig. 230–6*A*). Glucose is absorbed into the portal vein, and approximately 60 per cent of the ingested glucose-derived carbons end up in liver glycogen in the postprandial period. A significant portion of this is probably not a result of direct hepatic glucose uptake, but is due to peripheral metabolism of glucose to three-carbon fragments (lactate, pyruvate) that are then recycled to the liver where they enter the gluconeogenic pathway and are synthesized into glycogen. Glycogen then serves as the storage form of carbohydrate for later release. When glucose is metabolized via the glycolytic (anaerobic) pathway, 2 moles of ATP are generated per mole of glucose. Aerobic, or oxidative, metabolism (Krebs' cycle) is far more efficient as an energy-producing process and generates 12 moles of ATP per mole of glucose. Insulin exerts multiple anabolic effects on this process. It stimulates glucose uptake and glycogen synthesis by muscle and inhibits glycogenolysis. In liver, insulin does not directly stimulate glucose uptake, but it does actively promote glycogenesis and inhibit glycogenolysis. Although most of the ingested glucose, or glucose derived carbon, ends up in the liver in the postprandial period, the central nervous system (CNS) (primarily brain) is the predominant tissue of glucose consumption, accounting for about 70 per cent of total glucose utilization. Glucose is the primary source of energy for brain, and glucose uptake and metabolism in this tissue are independent of insulin. A major purpose of glucose homeostasis is to store glucose as liver glycogen postprandially when glucose and insulin levels are high, so that it can be released in the interprandial period for CNS consumption. Protein digestion and absorption lead to a postprandial rise in circulating amino acid levels. Insulin plays a dominant role in converting amino acids to protein by stimulating amino acid uptake in muscle and liver and by augmenting protein synthesis and inhibiting proteolysis. Fat is absorbed as chylomicrons that enter the circulation via the lymphatic system. Insulin affects fat assimilation in a number of ways. Lipoprotein lipase is an enzyme, synthesized primarily by fat and muscle tissue, that is secreted into the extracellular space and incorporated into the surface of nearby endothelial cells. In this location, lipoprotein lipase hydrolyzes fatty acids from triglyceride-rich lipoproteins (chylomicrons and very low density lipoproteins); these fatty acids are then taken up, predominantly by adipose tissue, where they are esterified into triglyceride for storage in the fat droplet of adipocytes. Insulin stimulates the synthesis and secretion of lipoprotein lipase and also strongly inhibits lipolysis of triglycerides stored in adipose tissue. Additionally, by promoting glucose uptake, insulin increases the supply of glycerol within adipocytes for esterification of fatty acids. Insulin is also lipogenic and stimulates the synthesis of fatty acids from glucose or other substrates that form pyruvate.

Many of these insulin effects are antagonized by the coun-

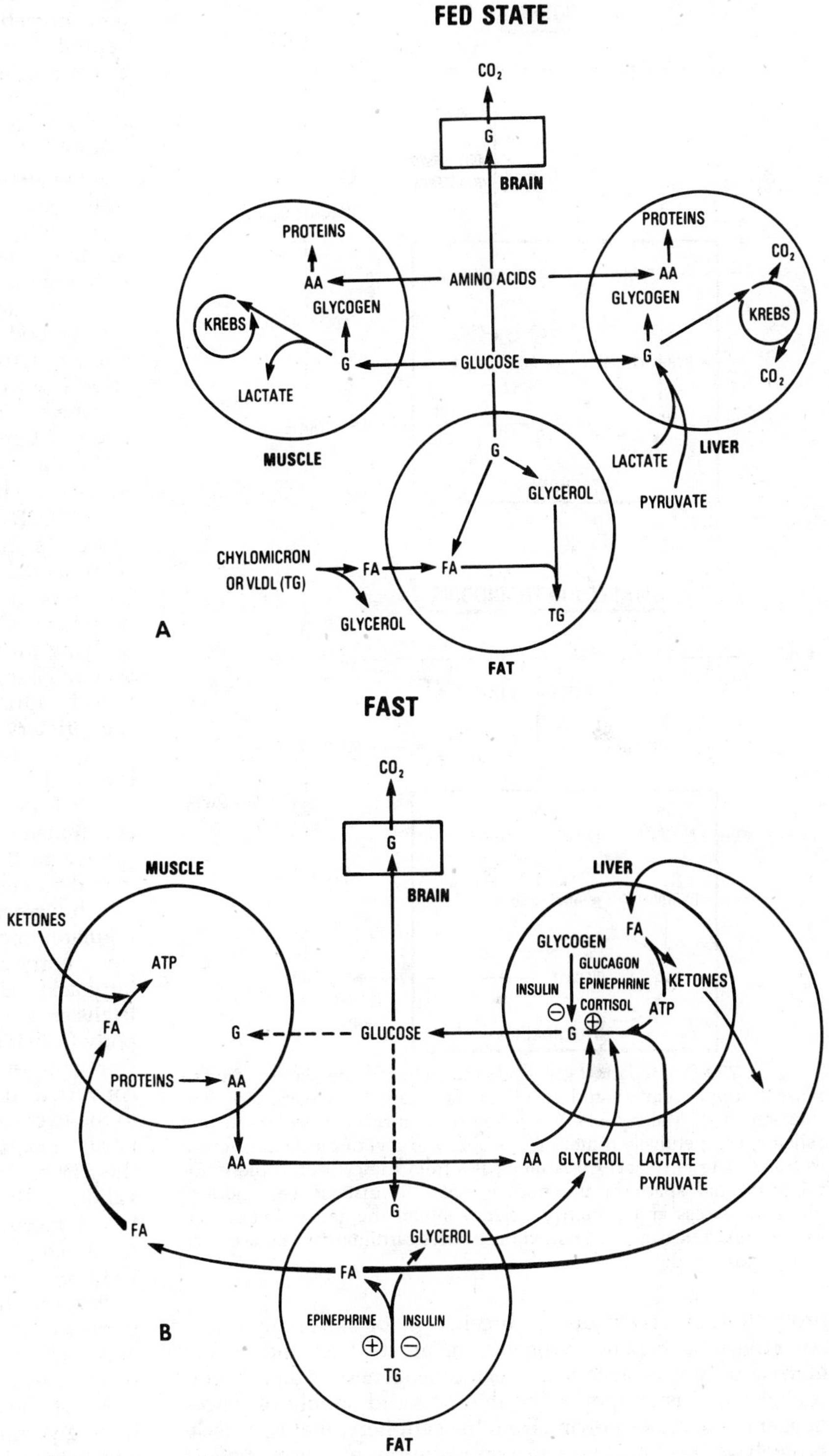

Figure 230–6. *A,* Fuel homeostasis during the immediate postprandial fed state. The key features of this diagram are the storage of glucose, amino acids, and fatty acids as the macromolecules glycogen, protein, and triglyceride in tissue depots; each of these processes is facilitated by the anabolic effects of insulin. *B,* Reversal of the anabolic effects of insulin during the insulinopenic fasting state. The major purpose of these homeostatic responses is to maintain a supply of glucose for obligate glucose uptake by the CNS while other tissues cease their consumption of glucose in favor of fatty acids from adipose tissue depots.

terregulatory hormones, glucagon, epinephrine, cortisol, and growth hormone. When mild (fasting) or severe (DKA) insulin deficiency exists, the processes outlined in Figure 230–6*A* are reversed, and characteristic metabolic derangements occur. This is illustrated in Figure 230–6*B*. A 24-hour fast causes mild insulin deficiency, and this results in a marked decrease in peripheral glucose uptake. This is accompanied by a decrease in synthesis of glycogen, protein, and triglyceride, along with increased breakdown of these storage macromolecules by accelerated glycogenolysis, proteolysis, and lipolysis. These catabolic processes increase as a result of the lack of insulin effect, but breakdown of macromolecules is also augmented by increased concentrations of counterregulatory hormones. Thus, glucagon stimulates glycogen breakdown and is also strongly ketogenic but has no in vivo effect on glucose uptake, lipolysis, or proteolysis. Epinephrine promotes glycogenolysis and lipolysis and also inhibits peripheral glucose uptake. Cortisol probably has effects that are additive or possibly synergistic with the other counterregulatory hormones and may independently stimulate proteolysis. Growth hormone probably plays a minor role in these events mediated through inhibition of glucose uptake. Taken together, insulin deficiency plus increased counterregulatory hormones lead to a marked decrease in glucose metabolism by insulin-sensitive tissues, "sparing" glucose for the obligate CNS utilization. The source of glucose in this setting is the liver. For the initial 12 to 24 hours, hepatic glucose

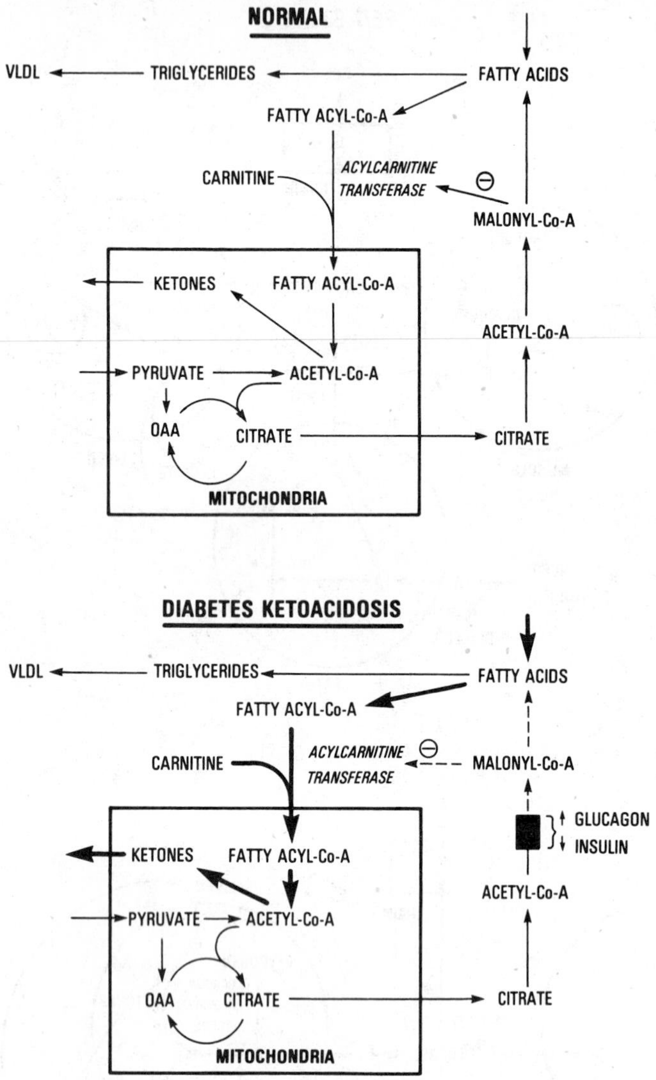

Figure 230–7. Hepatic fatty acid and ketoacid metabolism in the normal (upper panel) and insulinopenic diabetic ketoacidotic state (lower panel). Malonyl-Co-A is a key regulatory intermediate in this scheme, competitively inhibiting the ability of acyl carnitine transferase to translocate fatty acyl-Co-A molecules from the cytosol to the intramitochondrial space in the normal state. In diabetic ketoacidosis, glucagon excess and insulin deficiency inhibit the generation of malonyl-Co-A, releasing the inhibition of acyl carnitine transferase. See text for further details.

production is largely due to breakdown of stored glycogen. After this time, hepatic glycogen stores are depleted and hepatic glucose output is sustained by gluconeogenesis. Hepatic gluconeogenesis is supported by the increased supply of gluconeogenic substrates flowing from the periphery, that is, muscle proteolysis, leading to an increased supply of gluconeogenic amino acids (mainly alanine) and increased lipolysis resulting in enhanced glycerol release from adipose tissue. Some lactate and pyruvate are supplied from anaerobic metabolism of glucose in peripheral tissues (Cori cycle). Thus the liver is the central clearing house in this process by converting the breakdown products of stored fat and protein to supply glucose for the CNS in a setting (fasting) in which exogenous glucose is unavailable. In this situation the predominant energy source for non-CNS tissues is circulating free fatty acids (FFA) derived from breakdown of adipose tissue triglyceride (the CNS cannot utilize FFA as a metabolic fuel). Free fatty acids also supply the liver with the energy necessary to drive gluconeogenesis. Ketone bodies are produced in the liver from fatty acid oxidation under conditions of insulin deficiency and glucagon excess. In fasting this serves an important homeostatic purpose, since ketone bodies can be utilized by the CNS and muscle for energy, markedly reducing the need for protein breakdown to supply gluconeogenic precursors for liver glucose production. Ketone bodies provide a mechanism to convert adipose tissue energy stores into a substrate that can be metabolized in the CNS; this spares critical body proteins, allowing humans to survive relatively long-term fasts.

PATHOPHYSIOLOGY OF DKA. In DKA, all of these homeostatic processes are out of control, leading to pronounced hyperglycemia and ketonemia. The hyperglycemia is due to a combination of increased hepatic glucose production and decreased peripheral glucose uptake. The biochemical mechanisms underlying the hyperketonemia are somewhat more complex, as seen in Figure 230–7. Ketone bodies are produced in hepatocyte mitochondria by beta oxidation of fatty acids, and glucagon is the primary hormone responsible for inducing the hepatic ketogenic state. It does this by lowering malonyl coenzyme A levels, the first committed substrate in fatty acid synthesis, which leads to a marked increase in the activity of carnitine acyl transferase I. This enzyme translocates fatty acids from the cytosol to the intramitochondrial space where they are converted to ketones. Hepatic carnitine levels are also increased, which further drives this transfer step by mass action. The key regulatory point in understanding ketogenesis is that in the fed state, entry of fatty acids into the mitochondria is low, limiting fatty acid oxidation and ketogenesis in favor of fatty acid and triglyceride synthesis; thus the liver is rate limiting in ketone body formation. When insulin is low and glucagon high (as in starvation or DKA), fatty acids freely enter mitochondria to be converted to ketones, and therefore the supply of fatty acids to the liver is rate limiting for ketogenesis. Fatty acids are freely permeable across the hepatocyte plasma membrane, and thus the plasma concentration of FFA drives ketogenesis. In starvation, fatty acid levels are only moderately increased, leading to enhanced, but controlled, ketogenesis; in DKA, FFA levels are much higher, leading to uncontrolled ketogenesis. Another factor enhancing ketonemia in DKA is related to ketone body utilization. Insulin normally stimulates ketoacid uptake by peripheral tissues, and this is inhibited in DKA; additionally, very high levels of ketones may saturate the uptake mechanisms, further limiting utilization.

All of the pathophysiologic sequelae of DKA follow from hyperglycemia and hyperketonemia (Fig. 230–8). Thus, acidosis and ketonuria are directly due to the buildup of the ketoacids

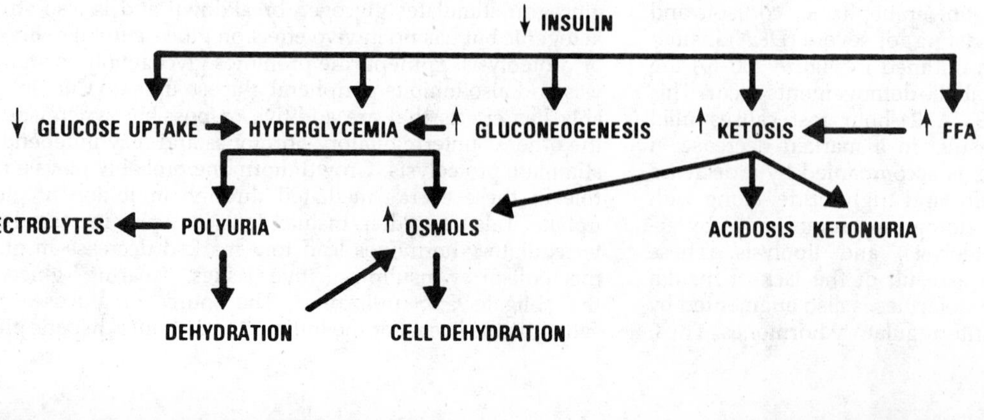

Figure 230–8. Pathophysiology of diabetic ketoacidosis. Severe insulin deficiency leads to hyperglycemia and ketonemia, and from this all of the other pathophysiologic sequelae result.

beta hydroxybutyrate and acetoacetate. The hyperglycemia and hyperketonemia produce an osmotic diuresis that causes intravascular volume depletion and dehydration and urinary electrolyte loss. The hyperosmolarity further exaggerates intracellular dehydration.

CLINICAL PICTURE. Diabetic ketoacidosis can be a life-threatening situation, and the clinical presentation is often dramatic. An antecedent history of polyuria and polydipsia for one to several days is typical, and nausea, vomiting, and anorexia are frequent accompanying symptoms. Occasionally abdominal pain is a predominant feature, sometimes mimicking an acute abdominal condition. Often this is due to gastric stasis and distention. In the obtunded patient with gastric distention, nasogastric suction should be considered to avoid vomiting with aspiration. Physical findings include tachypnea, dehydration, and disorientation, or even coma. If systemic acidosis is severe, Kussmaul respirations are present. Precipitating causes of DKA include failure of the patient to take insulin, infection, intercurrent illness, trauma, or emotional stress. When a known diabetic presents with signs and symptoms of DKA, the diagnosis is usually straightforward. However, DKA can also be the initial presenting episode of diabetes. DKA is a disease of IDDM, only rarely occurring in NIDDM, and only when precipitating causes are extreme.

Although the diagnosis of DKA can be strongly suspected on a clinical basis, confirmation is based on laboratory analyses. The diagnosis is made by demonstrating hyperglycemia and hyperketonemia in the presence of acidosis. However, the severity of these abnormalities can vary over a wide range. Occasionally the presenting episode may be severe ketonemia and acidosis and only mild hyperglycemia (200 to 400 mg per deciliter). Other patients may have severe hyperglycemia and only mild ketonemia and acidosis. Occasionally, alcoholic patients have ketonemia and hyperglycemia, and this condition, termed alcoholic ketoacidosis, must be differentiated from DKA (see next section). Direct quantitative measurements of acetoacetate and beta hydroxybutyrate are not usually readily available, and most physicians rely on reagent strips (Ketostix) or tablets (Acetest) for measurements. With this method, a nitroprusside reaction is the indicator; nitroprusside reacts mainly with acetoacetate, to a lesser extent with acetone, and not at all with beta hydroxybutyrate. Since beta hydroxybutyrate levels are much higher than acetoacetate levels in DKA, this method can sometimes be confusing. For example, when concomitant lactic acidosis exists, acetoacetate production may be inhibited in the presence of very high levels of beta hydroxybutyrate. In this setting the nitroprusside reaction may not be strongly positive. During the course of insulin therapy for DKA, beta hydroxybutyrate levels may fall out of proportion to acetoacetate levels, giving the impression that therapy is less effective than it actually is. Serum sodium levels are usually mildly decreased. This is due to the hyperglycemia- and hyperketonemia-induced hyperosmolarity, which attracts extracellular water from the intracellular space, leading to dilution of serum sodium. It should be kept in mind that the osmolar contribution of the hyperketonemia can often approach the contribution of the hyperglycemia. Serum bicarbonate levels are depressed, and the magnitude of decrease is in proportion to the degree of acidosis. BUN levels are usually modestly elevated as a result of dehydration and a component of prerenal azotemia. Serum potassium levels can be high, low, or normal, depending on the degree of dehydration and acidosis. In all cases, severe total body and intracellular potassium depletion exists. Because of cellular buffering mechanisms, which exchange intracellular potassium for extracellular hydrogen ion, extracellular potassium levels are often maintained in acidotic states. Nevertheless, greater than 95 per cent of total body potassium is intracellular, so in the presence of acidosis, extracellular potassium levels do not reflect total body potassium stores unless the potassium concentration is plotted on a nomogram related to serum pH (Fig. 230–9).

TREATMENT OF DKA. The treatment of DKA should be started as soon as it is diagnosed. The goals of therapy are to increase the rate of glucose utilization by insulin-dependent tissues, to reverse ketonemia and acidosis, and to correct the depletion of water and electrolytes. To accomplish this, treatment can be divided into four general areas: (1) insulin administration, (2) replacement of fluid and electrolytes, (3) treatment of any precipitating problems, and (4) avoidance of complications.

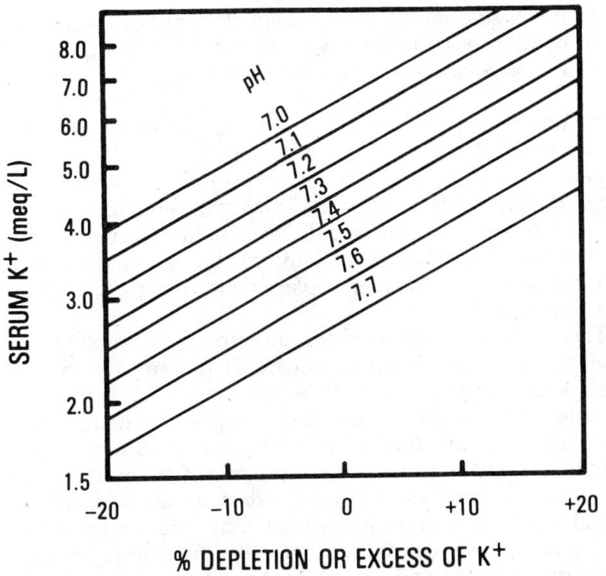

Figure 230–9. Nomogram depicting the relationship between total body potassium depletion, serum potassium, and serum pH. Per cent potassium depletion or excess is calculated by drawing a horizontal line from the ordinate intercept of the serum potassium concentration to the intersection of the diagonal line corresponding to the coexisting serum pH. From this intersection a vertical line is dropped to the abscissa and per cent potassium depletion or excess is read from the abscissal intercept. For example, at a serum potassium concentration of 4.0, at a concommitant serum pH of 7.2, an approximate 10 per cent depletion of total body potassium stores exists.

A variety of *insulin* regimens are possible, ranging from constant intravenous infusion to intermittent administration of intravenous, subcutaneous, or intramuscular boluses. The aim of all forms of insulin administration is to achieve a rapid and maximal insulin effect. In vivo insulin action is near maximal at an insulin concentration of about 200 μU per milliliter, and achieving higher levels has little further benefit. Since insulin is rapidly cleared from the circulation ($t\frac{1}{2}$ = 7 minutes), boluses must be given frequently (every 30 to 60 minutes) to maintain maximally effective insulin levels. With constant intravenous administration, serum insulin levels are maintained at a steady state throughout the infusion. In normal subjects, an infusion rate of 10 units per hour will result in an insulin level of approximately 200 μU per milliliter by 30 minutes, and if this mode of treatment is chosen a priming dose (10 to 20 units) should be given initially. Advocates of constant intravenous infusion maintain that the rate of metabolic improvement is smoother and more predictable and hypoglycemia is less common. Additionally, problems of variable or inadequate absorption from subcutaneous or intramuscular sites are avoided. One difficulty with this method occurs in the occasional patient with severe insulin resistance due to sepsis or high titers of insulin antibodies. If clear-cut metabolic improvement is not seen within the first few hours of constant insulin infusion, a bolus of insulin (20 to 30 units) should be given and the rate of insulin infusion increased.

Fluid replacement should also be started immediately. Patients with DKA are dehydrated and hypovolemic and usually have fluid deficits of 5 to 8 liters or more. Thus, rapid expansion of intravascular volume is essential, and this is achieved by an initial infusion of 1 to 2 liters of normal saline, or equivalent, over the first one to two hours. Of course, caution should be used in those patients with underlying cardiovascular or oliguric renal disease. Following initial rapid fluid administration, the rate of replacement can be slowed to restore estimated losses by 16 to 24 hours, depending on the patient's degree of dehydration and underlying cardiovascular-renal status. Much of the initial decline in plasma glucose level is due to volume expansion with reduction of hyperosmolarity, along with increased glomerular filtration and corresponding urinary glucose loss. In general, the aim should be to initiate metabolic correction rapidly, but once the patient has shown clear-cut substantial improvement, further replacement therapy can proceed more cautiously.

The electrolyte content of administered fluids must be closely monitored. Over the entire course of therapy the goal is to replace the electrolyte deficit, which averages 200 to 400 mEq each for sodium, potassium, and phosphate. Patients are usually ingesting some form of calories by 16 to 24 hours, and this provides the most physiologic replacement method. Potassium replacement requires the most attention. Regardless of the initial serum potassium level, total body reserves are depleted and serum levels will fall dramatically as acidosis and hyperglycemia are corrected. As glucose is taken up by cells under the influence of insulin, potassium is also transported intracellularly, and as acidosis is reversed the cellular buffering process exchanging intracellular potassium for extracellular hydrogen ion diminishes. To prevent hypokalemia, potassium should be included in the intravenous fluids once it is established that renal perfusion and urine flow are adequate following initial intravascular fluid expansion. To accomplish this, 40 mEq of potassium can be added to each liter of intravenous fluids as the phosphate salt. Phosphate depletion is also uniform in DKA, and some replacement is advisable, particularly if serum phosphate levels are low. This can be accomplished by administering 10 to 20 mmol per hour and can be combined with potassium replacement by giving potassium phosphate. Bicarbonate replacement should be initiated in patients with severe acidosis ($pH < 7.0$). This can be administered at the rate of 44 mEq per liter with appropriate monitoring of pH until it rises above 7.0. Three to four ampules of bicarbonate (44 mEq per ampule) will usually suffice to achieve this goal. Excessive bicarbonate replacement is contraindicated since this will exacerbate the tendency toward hypokalemia and may also result in rebound CNS acidosis. The latter occurs because carbon dioxide is more readily diffusible across the blood-brain barrier than is bicarbonate ion, causing CNS pH to fall at a time when peripheral pH is rising. This can lead to stupor and worsening of CNS status at a time when metabolic improvement is occurring.

Therapy should be monitored by frequent assessment of clinical status and laboratory measurements of urine and serum glucose and ketone levels. A fall in plasma glucose level is the earliest sign of effective therapy, and therefore plasma glucose should be frequently monitored. Once plasma glucose levels fall to approximately 250 mg per deciliter, 5 per cent glucose should be added to the intravenous fluids. Occasionally children or adolescents with DKA exhibit marked mental deterioration, including development of coma 4 to 6 hours after therapy has begun. Usually this is associated with a marked fall in hyperglycemia and serum osmolality, and cerebral edema has been noted in a few autopsy cases. Overall this is probably a rare complication of therapy. Because of the importance of plasma glucose monitoring in assessing the effectiveness of therapy, administration of glucose has no place in the initial stages of DKA treatment.

While insulin and fluid and electrolyte replacement therapy are being administered, a concomitant search for underlying precipitating factors should be undertaken. Leukocytosis often accompanies uncomplicated DKA and so should be viewed appropriately when one is searching for underlying infection. Hypothermia can be associated with DKA, and therefore fever should be a strong impetus to screen rigorously for a site of infection.

The major complications of DKA are mostly the result of treatment and include *hypokalemia, late hypoglycemia, rebound CNS acidosis,* and *CNS deterioration* (possibly due to cerebral edema). However, with proper attention to therapeutic details the former two can always be avoided, and the latter are fortunately rare. Recurrence of DKA can occur in the hospital if the vigorous phase of therapy is relaxed too soon. Maintenance of a flow chart with all therapies and laboratory tests recorded is an important means of coordination so that unexpected results do not go undetected and inappropriate therapies are not given.

Alcoholic Ketoacidosis

Alcoholic ketoacidosis can sometimes present a problem in the differential diagnosis of DKA when the patient is not a known diabetic or when a diabetic patient ingests large amounts of alcohol. This syndrome is characterized by hyperketonemia, acidosis, and dehydration. Serum glucose levels can be normal or sometimes elevated to the lower range of values seen in DKA. In the latter case a diagnostic problem can occur. The clinical picture of alcoholic ketoacidosis occurs in alcoholics following a recent, and sometimes prolonged alcoholic debauch; abstinence during the immediately preceding 12 to 24 hours is a common finding. The patient is usually anorexic, sometimes with nausea and vomiting, and some degree of starvation over the preceding one to three days is always present. The starvation, perhaps accompanied by stress-related hyperglucagonemia, creates a ketogenic state in the liver. This is accompanied by elevated FFA levels similar to those seen in starvation, which are perhaps augmented by adrenergic activation related to alcohol withdrawal, creating the metabolic environment for ketoacidosis. It is unusual for these patients to have hyperglycemia, but it can occur. When it does, the pathogenesis is unclear. In some patients, abnormalities of glucose tolerance exist after therapy, and thus the hyperglycemia may be stress related in previously glucose-intolerant patients. Alternatively, adrenergic mechanisms related to alcohol withdrawal could suppress residual endogenous insulin secretion, facilitating mild hyperglycemia. Regardless of the underlying mechanisms, the metabolic abnormalities are rapidly reversed by intravenous administration of fluids and glucose. Only occasionally is insulin needed in the early stages of treatment.

Nonketotic Hyperosmolar Syndrome

The term *nonketotic hyperosmolar coma* has frequently been applied to this syndrome, but by no means do all patients display coma or even mental obtundity. Rather, this syndrome comprises a spectrum ranging from mild degrees of hyperosmolarity with minimal CNS symptoms to severe hyperosmolarity with accompanying coma. The biochemical hallmarks are extreme hyperglycemia (mean 1000 mg per deciliter, range 600 to 2400 mg per deciliter) in the absence of overt ketoacidosis. Dehydration, hypovolemia, and disorientation are accompanying features. This syndrome usually develops over a much longer interval than DKA, with symptoms of polyuria antedating clinical presentation by several days and sometimes weeks. This syndrome usually occurs in elderly patients with NIDDM (often not previously diagnosed) who for some reason are unable to keep up with the osmotic diuresis by adequate water ingestion and this results in severe dehydration. The severe hyperglycemia is at least partly caused by decreased renal glucose excretion due either to intrinsic underlying renal disease or to decreased glomerular filtration and prerenal azotemia secondary to the marked hypovolemia and dehydration. Frequently this condition is associated with steroid, diuretic, or phenytoin therapy as a precipitating cause. Other precipitating factors include infections, cerebrovascular events, or therapeutic maneuvers such as hypertonic peritoneal dialysis or parenteral nutrition.

Serum sodium and potassium levels are usually normal while

serum bicarbonate levels are often somewhat depressed. This is usually not associated with significant ketonemia and probably reflects an underlying component of lactic acidosis due to hypovolemia. The BUN is uniformly elevated because of hypovolemia and prerenal azotemia. In these cases, though, acidosis is mild, and serum osmolality can be approximated by the formula:

$$\text{serum osmolality (mOsm per liter)} = 2 \times [Na^+ + K^+ \text{ (mEq/L)}] + \frac{\text{plasma glucose (mg/dl)}}{18} + \text{BUN (mg/dl)}/2.8.$$

However, since urea is freely diffusible across cell membranes it does not alter the effective serum osmolality, which is the clinically important factor to consider in this hyperosmolar condition. Most experts do not consider BUN levels in this calculation and prefer to estimate effective serum osmolarity as:

$$\text{Eosm} = 2 \times [Na^+ + K^+ \text{ (mEq/L)}] + \text{plasma glucose (mg/dl)}/18.$$

Values above 300 mOsm per liter are abnormal and above 320 mOsm per liter are indicative of clinically significant hyperosmolarity.

The reason ketosis is not a feature of this condition has not been satisfactorily explained. FFA levels are not as high in this syndrome as they are in DKA, and most investigators attribute the relatively lower FFA levels and decreased rates of ketogenesis to higher residual insulin levels in patients with hyperosmolar syndrome. This answer is not entirely satisfactory, however, since measured peripheral insulin levels overlap with those reported in DKA. On the other hand, peripheral insulin levels do not always reflect portal insulin concentrations, and significant differences in portal insulin levels may exist in DKA versus hyperosmolar syndrome, with the higher levels in hyperosmolar syndrome restraining hepatic ketogenesis.

In some series, the mortality has ranged up to 50 per cent. However, the relatively high mortality reflects selection criteria since mortality tends to be higher with greater severity of the hyperosmolality. The first priority of treatment should be intravascular volume expansion to restore circulatory integrity. This is accomplished by infusion of 1 to 2 liters of normal saline, or equivalent, over one to two hours, provided absolute cardiovascular contraindications do not exist. Even normal saline is hypotonic relative to serum in these patients, and therefore this therapy will initiate the correction of the hyperosmolality. As in DKA, insulin can be administered by constant intravenous infusions or bolus therapy. Since absorption of insulin administered subcutaneously or intramuscularly is variable because of dehydration and hypovolemia, and since late hypoglycemia is a more common complication of the hyperosmolar syndrome, constant intravenous administration of insulin can be very effective in this condition, leading to a predictable and fairly constant, smooth decline in plasma glucose levels. Once plasma glucose begins to decrease, and provided acceptable volume expansion and urine flow have been established, potassium phosphate salts should be added to the intravenous fluids. Subsequent to the initial volume expansion, intravenous fluids can consist of 0.5 normal saline with added potassium phosphate. Once plasma glucose levels decline to approximately 250 mg per deciliter, 5 per cent glucose should be added to the intravenous fluids. The above comments are meant more as guidelines than hard and fast rules, since, as in DKA, therapy must be individualized as far as replacement of fluids and electrolytes is concerned. This is best done by maintaining an organized flow chart with frequent measurements of plasma glucose, electrolytes, blood pressure, and urine volume. Despite even the best therapy, morbidity and mortality are high in this condition. Thrombosis and embolic events as well as infections, particularly pneumonia with accompanying adult respiratory distress syndrome, contribute significantly to adverse outcomes. In summary, rigorous but carefully monitored hydration and reestablishment of circulatory integrity are critical for successful therapy. These goals should be pursued while hyperosmolarity is corrected by administration of relatively hypotonic fluids with adequate free water along with insulin to reduce the hyperglycemia. Concomitantly a careful workup should be instituted to uncover precipitating factors with appropriate therapy when necessary.

CHRONIC OR LATE COMPLICATIONS OF DIABETES

Retinopathy

Eye disease is common in diabetes, and permanent loss of vision is one of the most striking and feared complications. Approximately 25 per cent of all newly reported cases of blindness are attributed to diabetes. When diabetics of all ages and types are considered together, the incidence of blindness from diabetic retinopathy is 0.2 per cent per year in all diabetics and 0.6 per cent per year in diabetics with retinopathy. This is 11 and 29 times greater, respectively, than the incidence of blindness from all other causes combined in the general population.

The major form of diabetic eye disease is diabetic retinopathy. Two general categories exist: nonproliferative or background retinopathy and proliferative retinopathy. Nonproliferative retinopathy can include venous abnormalities, microaneurysms, retinal hemorrhages, retinal edema, and exudates. This may progress to proliferative retinopathy, characterized by neovascularization, glial proliferation, and vitreoretinal traction. In general, diabetic retinopathy is progressive and tends to worsen with the duration of disease. However, most diabetics do not develop proliferative retinopathy. The incidence of this complication is substantially lower in NIDDM then in IDDM, even when corrected for duration of disease. However, since there are many more patients with NIDDM than IDDM, the absolute numbers of NIDDM and IDDM patients with proliferative retinopathy are roughly comparable.

NONPROLIFERATIVE RETINOPATHY. Probably the earliest retinal change is increased capillary permeability seen on fluorescein angiography. This abnormality can be readily reversed by effective glycemic control, but the relationship of this form of capillary permeability to retinopathy is unknown. Nonperfusion of retinal capillaries occurs early in diabetic retinopathy (so-called capillary dropout), and this leads to areas of retinal ischemia and infarction. Microaneurysms are small (15 to 50 μm diameter) excrescences along capillaries and are particularly prominent along the edges of areas of capillary nonperfusion. Fusiform aneurysms, or general dilatation of capillary loops, can also occur. Retinal veins are often tortuous and dilated; dilatation can be segmental, giving rise to a beaded or "sausage string" appearance. Exudates can be of two types: (1) *Hard, waxy exudates* are white to yellowish, shiny, with defined borders but without surrounding pigmentation. These exudates are due to lipid- and protein-containing fluid that has leaked from surrounding capillaries. (2) *Cotton-wool, or soft, exudates* are really areas of nonperfusion representing retinal microinfarcts and are often surrounded by microaneurysms. Clinically, an increase in cotton-wool areas indicates progressive capillary dropout and is a poor prognostic sign. Subretinal hemorrhages tend to be small and dot shaped and may resorb within a few weeks. Larger, flame-shaped hemorrhages occur in the superficial retinal layers and resorb more slowly. Preretinal hemorrhages are more serious and can impair vision if they are large or if they impinge on the macula. Following resorption, scarring and vitreous retraction or retinal detachment can occur. Edema of the retina is due to abnormal capillary permeability and ischemia. When persistent macular edema exists, vision is seriously impaired, and usual forms of therapy (photocoagulation) may not be effective. The primary pathogenetic events underlying these changes of nonproliferative background retinopathy are unclear, but loss of supporting capillary pericytes, endothelial proliferation, and hyperviscosity with red cell aggregation, together or alone, have all been proposed.

PROLIFERATIVE RETINOPATHY. The hallmark of proliferative retinopathy is new vessel formation or neovascularization. These capillary fronds or loops can grow on the surface of the retina or extend into the vitreous. Often this is accompanied by proliferation of glial elements in the region of the optic disc or along the new vessel arcades. Traction between the vitreous and the neovascular and glial elements can ultimately develop, leading to retinal detachment or large-scale hemorrhage into the vitreous. These events will lead to serious loss of vision or blindness. It has been suggested that the stimulus for neovascularization is retinal ischemia with local release of growth-promoting factors.

Photocoagulation is the therapy of choice for proliferative diabetic retinopathy. With this therapy, a light beam is focused on the retina to produce a burn or coagulum in a precisely defined area. By this means, one can selectively destroy microaneurysms, leaky vessels, neovascular elements, and areas of microinfarction or edema. Destruction of vessels prone to hemorrhage or causing traction directly prevents further deterioration. Destroying areas of retina that are poorly perfused and hypoxic may curtail the ischemic stimulus for neovascularization, preventing further proliferative changes. Regardless of the mechanism, the cooperative trial of the Diabetic Retinopathy Study Research Group clearly showed that photocoagulation decreases the incidence of retinal detachment, hemorrhage, and loss of vision. Thus, photocoagulation involves selective treatment of new vessels as well as panretinal treatment to destroy 20 to 30 per cent of the remaining retinal tissue. Whether photocoagulation therapy for preproliferative retinopathy should be undertaken is not yet clear; control studies are currently under way to resolve this question. All patients with significant diabetic retinopathy should be followed by an ophthalmologist and photocoagulation considered when new vessel formation or preretinal hemorrhage occurs. Photocoagulation early in the course of diabetic retinopathy may ultimately prove advisable. In the past, hypophysectomy was used as treatment for proliferative retinopathy. However, the therapeutic responses to this maneuver are quite variable, and significant complications exist. With the advent of photocoagulation, use of hypophysectomy has been largely abandoned. In patients with severe vitreal involvement, total vitrectomy may offer some possibility of improvement and preservation of vision.

Other Complications of Diabetes Affecting Vision

In addition to retinopathy, the eyes are affected in other ways by diabetes mellitus. Diabetics may experience temporary blurring of vision and *changes in refraction,* most likely due to osmotic changes in lens shape as a result of fluctuations in hyperglycemia. These changes can be disconcerting, but patients should be advised not to seek new refractions until a stable period of metabolic control is produced. It may take six to eight weeks before the hyperglycemia-induced changes in visual acuity subside. *Glaucoma* is also more frequent in diabetics. Rubeosis iridis is due to capillary neovascularization of the iris, which can produce closed-angle glaucoma. Usually occurring when diabetic retinopathy is advanced, this form of glaucoma is generally refractory to treatment. Open-angle glaucoma is also more frequent in diabetics, and this may relate to fibrosis or scarring of the canals of Schlemm, which drain the anterior chamber. Although *cataracts* are common in diabetes, it has not been rigorously demonstrated that the incidence of cataracts is increased in this condition. For the most part, cataracts in diabetics are indistinguishable from senile cataracts in nondiabetic patients, and the indications for surgery are the same as in nondiabetics. It is possible that the presence of diabetes accelerates the development of senile cataracts so that they occur at an earlier age than in nondiabetics. It has been postulated that hyperglycemia leads to increased sorbitol production in the lens, resulting in osmotic changes that accelerate cataract formation. While evidence in favor of this theory exists, it still remains to be proved. Opacities in the lens termed snowflake cataracts are occasionally noted in young patients whose diabetes is in poor control. This form of cataract is more specific for diabetes but can occur in other conditions and, unlike the senile cataract, can regress when glycemic control is achieved.

Nephropathy

Kidney disease is common in diabetes (See also Ch. 84 for an extensive discussion of the kidney in diabetes), and renal failure is one of the major causes of death.

PATHOLOGY. The dominant form of diabetic nephropathy is microvascular disease affecting the renal glomerulus. A number of distinct morphologic and functional abnormalities characterize diabetic glomerulopathy. Early in diabetes the kidney increases in size, and the associated glomerular hypertrophy leads to an increased glomerular filtration rate with hyperfiltration and microalbuminuria in up to 50 per cent of patients with new-onset IDDM. The hyperfiltration and increased kidney size revert to normal following effective insulin therapy and are unassociated with other glomerular lesions. Later in the disease, diffuse thickening of the glomerular basement membrane is noted along with increased mesangial volume. Patients with substantial histologic changes can exhibit normal renal function; however, impaired renal function probably does not occur in the absence of morphologic changes. Later in the disease, when decreased renal function is evident, the mesangium further expands and occupies a greater proportion of the glomerular volume while the thickness of the glomerular basement membrane is not necessarily increased. Glomerular occlusion accompanies this picture. Often characteristic nodular hyaline-like deposits, termed nodular glomerulocapillary sclerosis or Kimmelstiel-Wilson lesions, are evident in the center of peripheral glomerular capillary lobules.

CLINICAL AND FUNCTIONAL ASPECTS. The manifestations of diabetic nephropathy are quite heterogeneous. Asymptomatic, mild proteinuria can remain constant for many years. In other patients proteinuria may increase and be followed by progressive reduction in glomerular filtration and renal function. Persistent proteinuria (3 to 5 grams per day or greater) is a poor prognostic sign, usually heralding renal failure within five years. However, exceptions exist. The proteinuria may progress to include all of the classical features of the nephrotic syndrome. Once azotemia develops, progression to renal failure and uremia is inevitable within a few months to two to three years.

The diagnosis of diabetic nephropathy is usually made on clinical grounds, and renal biopsy is rarely indicated. Invasive diagnostic procedures should be aimed at detection of reversible features such as infection or obstruction. Contrast studies should not be conducted without clear indications, since rapid deterioration of renal function with acute renal failure sometimes follows intravenous pyelography or angiography in azotemic diabetic patients. When the study is performed, patients should be well hydrated before testing.

If renal failure develops in a diabetic, dialysis or transplantation must be considered. As recently as 10 to 15 years ago, uremic diabetics were thought to be extremely poor risks for dialysis with very low survival rates and high rates of complications, particularly infections and deterioration of vision. However, in recent years, results have been much better with a first-year survival of over 80 per cent and three-year survival of over 60 per cent. Additionally, far fewer cases of progressive visual impairment and blindness occur. Thus, in the absence of other negative factors, the presence of diabetes should not be considered a contraindication to dialysis, and decisions to initiate this form of therapy should generally proceed as in nondiabetic uremic patients. Chronic ambulatory peritoneal dialysis (CAPD) has been tried in some patients, but overall experience is still limited. Indications for CAPD vary widely among treatment centers, as does enthusiasm for this mode of therapy. Recent experience with renal transplantation has also been encouraging. Regardless of donor source (cadaver or related donor), survival rates after renal transplantion in diabetics approach that in nondiabetics. Interestingly, diabetic-type glomerular changes have been noted in biopsy specimens from the transplanted kidney from many of these patients.

Neuropathy

Diabetic neuropathy is perhaps the most common disabling chronic complication of diabetes. Although death seldom results from neuropathic changes alone, a great deal of morbidity and reduced quality of life can be attributed to diabetic neuropathy. The incidence and severity of neuropathy generally progress with duration of diabetes, and severe neuropathy can often exist in the absence of other chronic diabetic complications. A number of different classification schemes have been proposed, but none is entirely satisfactory, primarily because the causes of diabetic neuropathy are not known, and therefore classification must be descriptive in nature rather than based on pathogenetic mechanisms. Table 230–6 provides a simplified method of classification that may prove useful. Polyneuropathy is a diffuse symmetric disorder of peripheral nerve function. Asymmetric neuropathy implies a cluster of signs and symptoms that can be anatomically related to dysfunction of a single nerve trunk (mononeuropathy) or to more than one nerve trunk (mononeuropathy multiplex) either simultaneously or successively. It has been proposed that the symmetric or diffuse neuropathies are due to "metabolic" abnormalities of the neurons or the Schwann cells, whereas the asymmetric or focal neuropathies are due to vascular occlusion and ischemia. Diabetic neuropathy is very common in both IDDM and NIDDM, and mild to severe disease can exist in up to 50 per cent of patients. The incidence of symmetric neuropathy is comparable in IDDM and NIDDM when corrected for duration of disease, but focal neuropathies are more common in older NIDDM patients, suggesting a vascular contribution to the etiology.

SYMMETRIC DISTAL POLYNEUROPATHY. This form of diabetic neuropathy can be divided into two types: (1) relatively asymptomatic and (2) painful. The first form is diffuse, distal, usually in the lower extremities with a stocking type of distribution. It is characterized by numbness, tingling, or pins-and-needles sensation, often worse at night. Although the course may wax and wane, it is generally progressive and irreversible. Decreased sensory perception occurs and may result in neuropathic ulcers and Charcot joints. Symptoms of the painful form can range from burning or dull aching sensations to cramping or excruciating, lancinating pain. The pain is often worse at night and partially relieved by movement. Hyperesthesia can be so marked that even light touch is so painful that the patient cannot tolerate bed covers. Physical examination is similar in both types and is often rather unremarkable. The single most common finding is absence of deep tendon reflexes in the lower extremities (i.e., loss of knee and ankle jerks). Decreased perception of pain and light touch may be evident, and sometimes loss of vibratory sensation exists. The onset of pain may be abrupt or gradual and usually resolves by three months to one to two years. In some cases, institution of glycemic control coincides with resolution of pain; this may be causal. Paradoxically, insulin therapy with glycemic control can sometimes exacerbate or bring on painful neuropathic symptoms. In these cases, symptoms will subside in a few weeks if control is maintained. In some patients the decrease in pain reflects progression of the neuropathy with loss of pain sensation. A number of therapies have been tried, but these are usually unsatisfactory. Narcotic addiction may result when painful neuropathy is severe and long lasting. Combinations of B vitamins have been used, but success is unusual. Phenytoin or carbamazepine has also been used, and at least temporary or partial relief of pain and paresthesias has been reported in 25 to 50 per cent of patients. These agents should be tried at full anticonvulsant doses and discontinued if a response is not seen within two weeks. Combination therapy with amitriptyline and fluphenazine has also been advocated; there have been some reports of good results by one week. Treatment with any of these pharmacologic agents is only symptomatic and does not affect the course of the disease. Insofar as hyperglycemia causes neuropathy, maintenance of good control should be the primary emphasis. The possible role of sorbitol accumulation or myoinositol depletion in the pathogenesis of diabetic neuropathy was discussed earlier. Inhibitors of aldose reductase and oral myoinositol supplementation have been recently tried with some reports of success. Further studies will be necessary to determine the importance of these methods in the future treatment of diabetic neuropathy.

TABLE 230–6. CLASSIFICATION OF DIABETIC NEUROPATHY

1. Symmetric distal polyneuropathy
2. Asymmetric neuropathy
   A. Cranial mononeuropathy and mononeuropathy multiplex
   B. Peripheral mononeuropathy and mononeuropathy multiplex
   C. Neuromuscular syndromes
3. Autonomic neuropathy

NEUROPATHIC LESIONS AND THE DIABETIC FOOT. Loss of sensation can lead to the development of a Charcot joint as a result of repeated undetected trauma. More commonly, neuropathic ulcers develop, particularly on the plantar aspect of the foot. This can be due to weakness of the intrinsic muscles of the foot secondary to neuropathy, leading to abnormal pressure distribution. Weight bearing is then accentuated on the metatarsal heads, causing degeneration of the underlying fat pads and eventually leading to the typical open, draining neuropathic ulcer. Ulcers can also result from penetrating wounds caused by stepping on tacks or other sharp objects the patient does not feel. The best therapy is preventive. All diabetics should be trained to examine their feet daily for callous formation, blisters, or trauma. Shoes should be properly fitted; orthotic or other devices to aid in proper weight distribution are sometimes helpful. Patients should be advised never to walk barefoot. In all cases the feet should be kept clean and dry, and professional trimming of toenails and callosities is often advisable. Neuropathic foot ulcers can lead to gangrene and the requirement for amputation. Meticulous foot care substantially decreases the incidence of these ulcers and is a major form of preventive therapy that all diabetics should receive. Once open ulcers develop, healing can still occur if peripheral circulation is adequate. A high index of suspicion should be maintained for underlying osteomyelitis. Treatment is supportive with bed rest, elevation of the foot, warm (but not hot) foot soaks, debridement, and in some cases antibiotics. Protective plaster casts are sometimes advised. If these therapies fail and gangrene develops, amputation is the only recourse.

ASYMMETRIC NEUROPATHY. Diabetic mononeuropathies of the cranial nerves usually involve cranial nerve III, VI, or IV in order of frequency. This gives rise to extraocular muscle paralysis with diplopia. The most common syndrome is isolated third nerve palsy accompanied in 80 per cent of cases by sparing of the pupillary reflex. Pupillary sparing suggests that the underlying lesion is occlusion of a nutrient artery with ischemia of deep but not superficial oculomotor nerve fibers. Onset is usually abrupt and is frequently preceded by pain behind or above the eye. More than one cranial nerve is sometimes involved, and occasionally findings are bilateral. Spontaneous recovery is the rule within 3 to 12 months, but recurrences can occur. Mononeuropathies of peripheral nerves most frequently occur at sites of external pressure or entrapment (i.e., carpal tunnel). Manifestations include footdrop, wristdrop, or other symptoms related to the particular nerve involved. The clinical course is similar to that of the cranial mononeuropathies. Along with other forms of diabetic neuropathy these syndromes are usually associated with modestly increased protein content of the spinal fluid.

Another diabetic neuropathic syndrome involves *radiculopathy*. This syndrome is characterized by dysesthesias and painful hyperesthesia localized to the anatomic distribution of one or more spinal nerves. Symptoms can resemble herpes zoster, although skin lesions are seldom noted. On occasion, symptoms can be bilateral. Drug therapy similar to that used for painful symmetric polyneuropathy has been tried, but symptoms usually resolve spontaneously in weeks to months. Again, repeated episodes have been noted.

Neuromuscular syndromes related to diabetic retinopathy have been described. In the upper extremity, bilateral atrophy of the interosseous muscles as well as the thenar and hypothenar eminences of the hand can lead to profound loss of motor power with significant functional impairment. In the lower extremities, wasting and weakness of proximal leg muscles and pelvic girdle musculature have been termed diabetic amyotrophy. The clinical picture may be asymmetric, and elderly men are more commonly affected. Diabetic neuropathic cachexia is a syndrome of elderly male diabetics characterized by marked weight loss, painful peripheral polyneuropathy, and depression. The weight loss is so marked that patients appear cachectic, leading to a diagnosis of suspected underlying malignant disease. Other complications of diabetes are typically absent, and patients spontaneously recover in about one year.

AUTONOMIC NEUROPATHY. Autonomic diabetic neuropathies can be protean in their manifestations, leading to distressing clinical symptoms corresponding to the organ systems involved. Urinary bladder dysfunction is common, leading to urinary retention of large residual volumes. A definitive diagnosis can be made with a voiding cystometrogram, and therapy with cholinergic agents can sometimes be helpful. As the disease progresses, urinary tract infections become more frequent (possibly because of repeated catheterization), endangering the kidneys. In advanced cases, bladder neck resection to improve voiding may be necessary. Impotence with retrograde ejaculation is extremely common in men with longstanding diabetes. However, impotence in the diabetic male does not eliminate the need for exploration of possible psychogenic causes, which may be reversible. A variety of gastrointestinal tract syndromes can also occur. Gastroparesis diabeticorum involves delayed gastric emptying, retention, and hypotonicity. Symptoms include nausea, abdominal distention, belching, and general postprandial discomfort. Since this syndrome disrupts eating habits, control of the diabetes can be made more difficult. Treatment with metoclopramide has been useful in some but by no means all cases. Dysfunction of the small and large bowel can lead to malabsorption or diabetic diarrhea or both. Diabetic diarrhea often occurs at night, and fecal incontinence is a frequent feature. Autonomic involvement of sympathetic nervous system may lead to orthostatic hypotension and sometimes can be disabling. Attempts to expand intravascular volume with a high salt diet and sometimes mineralocorticoids are frequently effective but must be cautiously employed, since underlying cardiovascular disease is common in diabetic patients.

Cardiovascular Disease

Cardiovascular disease is the major cause of death in diabetic patients and is far more prevalent than in the nondiabetic population because of accelerated atherogenesis. Not only is cardiovascular disease more frequent, but onset is at an earlier age, and manifestations are more severe. The etiology of the accelerated atherosclerosis in diabetes is incompletely understood, but the causes are probably multifactorial. Most forms of hyperlipoproteinemia are more common in diabetic subjects, and high-density lipoprotein levels tend to be decreased in patients with uncontrolled diabetes. Furthermore, in patients with chronic hyperglycemia, circulating lipoproteins become glycosylated, adversely altering their turnover and sites of tissue deposition. This phenomenon might contribute to the increased risk of atherosclerosis in the absence of grossly elevated circulating lipid levels. Abnormalities of endothelial cell function have also been proposed that would enhance the susceptibility of arterial walls to injury. Increased platelet aggregation and hyperviscosity have also been proposed. Medical management of these risk factors is similar to that in nondiabetic subjects. Thus, specific diet and drug therapy for the various hyperlipoproteinemias should be used when indicated (Ch. 183). On occasion, lipid-lowering drugs such as nicotinic acid may accentuate glucose intolerance. Because of the high risk for atherogenesis, diabetics should be strongly encouraged to abstain from cigarette smoking. Arterial hypertension is a frequent concomitant of diabetes and should be treated promptly. Interestingly, epidemiologic studies have suggested that the existence of hypertension causes little in the way of additive risk for atherosclerosis in diabetics. The diabetic has a substantially greater risk for the development of all forms of cardiovascular disease even when hypertension and hyperlipoproteinemia are taken into account.

The pattern of coronary artery disease (CAD) has been reported to be different in diabetics and nondiabetics, exhibiting in diabetics a greater tendency toward diffuse distal lesions in addition to the usual proximal lesions. However, systematic studies have not uniformly confirmed this notion, suggesting that if this is a feature of CAD in diabetes, then only a minority of patients show diffuse distal occlusive disease. This is important, since one would expect coronary artery bypass surgery to be less successful in patients with distal disease and poor runoff. Overall the indications for myocardial revascularization are probably no different in diabetics and nondiabetics, although a greater incidence of postoperative complications is seen in diabetics. The presence of diabetes substantially eliminates the sex differences in CAD, since the incidence of CAD is roughly comparable in premenopausal diabetic women and age-matched diabetic men. Complications of myocardial infarction are more frequent in diabetics, and postinfarction survival is less. Although angina pectoris is common in diabetic patients, atypical anginal syndromes are seen more frequently than in nondiabetics. Various atypical pain patterns have been described. Painless myocardial infarction has been described in diabetes, probably due to disturbance of afferent nerve fibers. This diagnosis should be suspected in diabetic patients with the sudden onset of left ventricular failure. A syndrome of diabetic cardiomyopathy has been described and is characterized by congestive heart failure in the absence of proximal CAD. It is thought that this syndrome is due to small-vessel occlusive disease. Whether a distinct cardiomyopathy exists in diabetes in the absence of any CAD is still being debated.

Peripheral vascular disease is far more frequent in the diabetic than in the nondiabetic population, and this is particularly so for distal vascular insufficiency of the lower limbs. When combined with the neuropathic complications of diabetes, this unfortunately presents an ideal setting for the development of ischemia and gangrene, necessitating amputation. Because of the marked distal small-vessel disease, vascular bypass surgery is often unsatisfactory. Most forms of cerebrovascular disease and stroke are also seen more frequently in diabetes.

Dermatologic Lesions

Dermatologic abnormalities are common in diabetes. For example, these patients are more prone to various skin infections such as carbuncles and furuncles. These can often be extensive and difficult to treat. Vaginal candidiasis is frequent in hyperglycemic glycosuric women. Antifungal agents are effective in treating this disorder, but recurrences are common until glycosuria is effectively controlled. Necrobiosis lipoidica diabeticorum consists of round or oval, sharply defined, plaque-like lesions on the anterior surface of the lower legs. The borders of these lesions are frequently elevated, and the center may be depressed. The centers tend to be yellowish, while the borders are hyperpigmented. Although this lesion is uncommon in diabetics, when it does occur, the plaques can ulcerate upon minimal trauma. Diabetic dermopathy (shin spots) is the most frequent dermatologic lesion seen in diabetic patients, occurring in 60 per cent of males and 30 per cent of females. These lesions are common over the tibial area, but also can be observed on forearms and thighs. They begin as small reddish papules that gradually heal, leaving thin hyperpigmented atrophic areas behind. Typical xanthomatoses can occur secondary to hyperlipoproteinemia. In insulin-dependent diabetic subjects, tight waxy skin over the dorsum of the hands in conjunction with joint contractions has been observed. This may be an important clinical observation, since these patients appear to have accelerated development of other microangiopathic complications.

CONCLUSIONS

Diabetes mellitus is a chronic disease and therefore the approach to the patient and methods of management must encompass a long-term view. Patients with diabetes will be interacting with health care providers for the remainder of their lives. The patient must become well educated concerning the disease and eventually learn to individualize all the various components of therapy to his or her own personal circumstances. Ultimately many of the day-to-day therapy and management decisions rest in the hands of the patient. Since much of the treatment of diabetes involves intensive self-care, in a very real sense the patient may be his or her own most important physician. This requires education, motivation, and pychological adjustment.

Brand PW: The diabetic foot. *In* Ellenberg M, Rifkin H (eds.): Diabetes Mellitus. Theory and Practice. 3rd ed. New Hyde Park, NY, Medical Examination Publishing Co., 1983, pp 829–849. *An in-depth review of the clinical manifestations and management of diabetic foot problems.*

Bunn HF: Evaluation of glycosylated hemoglobin in diabetic patients. Diabetes 30:613, 1981. *A review of the biochemistry, clinical significance, and use of glycosylated hemoglobin in diabetes.*

Cahill GF, Jr: Starvation in man. N Engl J Med 282:668, 1970. *A classic article in which the available information on substrate and hormonal interrelationships in the fed and fasted state is synthesized into an organized homeostatic picture.*

Cudworth AG, Wolf E: The genetic susceptibility to type I (insulin-dependent) diabetes mellitus. Clin Endocrinol Metab 11:389, 1982. *A discussion of the HLA associations in type I diabetes mellitus.*

Diabetic Retinopathy Study Research Group: Preliminary report on the effects of photocoagulation. Am J Ophthalmol 81:383, 1976. *A report of the multicenter study demonstrating the utility of photocoagulation in diabetic retinopathy.*

Feig PU, McCurdy DK: The hypertonic state. N Engl J Med 297:1444, 1977. *A discussion of the pathophysiology and clinical treatment of the hyperosmolar syndrome.*

Feingold KR: Hypoglycemia: A pitfall of insulin therapy. West J Med 139:688, 1983. *An excellent clinical discussion of this important complication of the therapy of diabetes, with 56 references.*

Foster DW, McGarry JD: The metabolic derangements and treatment of diabetic ketoacidosis. N Engl J Med 309:159, 1983. *A thorough and current review of the pathogenesis and treatment of this disorder.*

Galloway JA: Insulin treatment for the early 80s: Facts and questions about old and new insulins and their usage. Diabetes Care 3:615, 1980. *A review of the biochemical and clinical features of the various insulin preparations available.*

Given BD, Mako ME, Tager H, Baldwin D, Markese J, Rubenstein AH, Olefsky J, Kobayashi M, Kolterman O, Poucher R: Circulating insulin with reduced biological activity in a patient with diabetes. N Engl J Med 302:129, 1980. *The first description of a patient producing a biologically defective insulin molecule.*

Goetz FC: Recent progress in the management of end-stage diabetic nephropathy. Clin Endocrinol Metab 11:579, 1982. *An up-to-date discussion on the relative success rates of dialysis and transplantation in end-stage diabetic nephropathy.*

Grogen CH, Lernmark A: Islet cell antibodies in diabetes. Clin Endocrinol Metab 11:409, 1982. *A literature review of islet cell antibodies in diabetes mellitus.*

Kreisberg RA: Diabetic ketoacidosis: New concepts and trends in pathogenesis and treatment. Ann Intern Med 88:681, 1978. *A discussion of pathogenetic mechanisms and a review of treatment methods in diabetic ketoacidosis.*

Lernmark A, Baekkeskov S: Islet cell antibodies—Theoretical and practical implications. Diabetologia 21:431, 1981. *A discussion of the potential role of autoantibodies directed against beta cells in the pathogenesis of diabetes.*

L'Esperance FA Jr, James SA Jr: The eye and diabetes mellitus. *In* Ellenberg M, Rifkin H (eds.): Diabetes Mellitus. Theory and Practice. 3rd ed. New Hyde Park, NY, Medical Examination Publishing Co., 1983, pp 727–757. *A general review of the ocular complications of diabetes mellitus with particular emphasis on retinopathy.*

McGarry JD, Foster DW: Regulation of hepatic fatty acid oxidation and ketone body production. Ann Rev Biochem 49:395, 1980. *Detailed review of the intermediary metabolism of ketogenesis and the pathogenesis of diabetic ketoacidosis.*

National Diabetes Data Group: Classification and diagnosis of diabetes mellitus and other categories of glucose intolerance. Diabetes 63:843, 1977. *A description of the unified classification system and methods and criteria for diagnosis of diabetes mellitus.*

Olefsky JM, Kolterman OG: Mechanisms of insulin resistance in obesity and non-insulin dependent (type II) diabetes. Am J Med 70:151, 1981. *A review of the pathogenesis and contribution of insulin resistance in NIDDM.*

Peacock I, Tattersall R: Methods of self monitoring of diabetic control. Clin Endocrinol Metab 11:485, 1982. *A review of the rationale and technique of self-monitoring of glucose in diabetes mellitus.*

Rimoin DL, Rotter JI: Genetic syndromes associated with diabetes mellitus and glucose intolerance. *In* Kobberling J, Tattersall R (eds.): Genetics of Diabetes Mellitus. New York, Academic Press, 1982, pp 149–181. *A detailed discussion of all of the genetic diseases that can be associated with diabetes mellitus.*

Rotter JI, Anderson CE, Rimoin DL: Genetics of diabetes mellitus. *In* Ellenberg M, Rifkin H (eds.): Diabetes Mellitus. Theory and Practice. 3rd ed. New Hyde Park, NY, Medical Examination Publishing Co., 1983, pp 481–503. *A review of the inheritance patterns and the genetic contributions to the etiology of type I and type II diabetes mellitus.*

Rotwein P, Chyn R, Chirgwin J, Cordell B, Goodman HM, Permutt MA: Polymorphism in the 5′-flanking region of the human insulin gene and its possible relation to type 2 diabetes. Science 213:1117, 1981. *Report of an increased frequency of a unique polymorphism of the insulin gene in NIDDM.*

Schade DS, Santiago JV, Skyler JS, Rizza RA: Intensive insulin therapy. Princeton, Excerpta Medica, 1983. *A recent monograph outlining the physiologic principles and methods of administering intensive therapy by multiple injections as well as CSII.*

Skyler JS: Complications of diabetes mellitus: Relationship to metabolic dysfunction. Diabetes Care 2:499, 1979. *A discussion of the value of glycemic control in the late complications of diabetes mellitus.*

Tattersall RB: Home blood glucose monitoring. Diabetologia 16:71, 1979. *An article dealing with measuring blood glucose instead of relying on urine values.*

Unger RH, Orci L: Glucagon and the A cell. Physiology and pathophysiology. N Engl J Med 304:1518, 1575, 1981. *A review of the physiology of glucagon secretion and action as well as its role in the pathophysiology of diabetes.*

Viberti GC, Pickup JC, Jarrett RJ, Keen H: Effect of control of blood glucose on urinary excretion of albumin and B_2 microglobulin in insulin-dependent diabetes. N Engl J Med 300:638, 1979. *A report showing the reversibility of microalbuminuria by insulin treatment in type I diabetes.*

Yoon J-W, Austin M, Onodera T, Notkins AL: Virus-induced diabetes mellitus. N Engl J Med 300:1173, 1979. *A report of a well-documented case of viral-induced diabetes.*

231. HYPOGLYCEMIC DISORDERS

F. John Service

Hypoglycemia is a pathophysiologic state and not a disease. Just as pain, fever, or vomiting requires identification of the underlying condition, hypoglycemia warrants diagnosis of the primary disorder causing the low plasma glucose level.

Hypoglycemia can be defined as a glucose concentration below the lower limit of normal. However, since hypoglycemic disorders are clinical syndromes almost invariably associated with symptoms from the low concentration of glucose, hypoglycemia is usually considered to be a glucose concentration in the range below the level at which symptoms could be expected to occur.

PHYSIOLOGY

Plasma glucose concentration is maintained within narrow bounds, in spite of intermittent food ingestion and periods of fasting, as the net balance between the rates of glucose production and utilization. Following food ingestion the increase in plasma glucose, in concert with an incretin effect from enteric factors, results in a increase in plasma insulin that accelerates glucose utilization and suppresses hepatic glucose production. As the plasma glucose concentration falls postprandially, plasma insulin decreases, which restores glucose utilization and production to the preprandial rates. There is then a transition from a state of glucose storage to one of carefully husbanded glucose production at rates designed to satisfy the obligatory needs of the body. In the postabsorptive period four to six hours after food ingestion, plasma glucose concentrations are generally 80 to 90 mg per deciliter with rates of glucose production and utilization of approximately 2 mg per kg^{-1} per min^{-1}. About half of the glucose produced is metabolized by the central nervous system. Glucose production at this time is primarily from hepatic glycogenolysis (70 to 80 per cent), with a small contribution from gluconeogenesis (20 to 25 per cent). Hepatic glycogen stores become exhausted after 24 to 36 hours of fasting.

Glycogenolysis is stimulated by epinephrine and glucagon and inhibited by insulin. Several enzymes are involved in the cleavage of glucose moieties from glycogen and the final appearance of free glucose in the circulation. Abnormalities of these enzymes may result in hypoglycemia. For example, deficient activity of glucose 6-phosphatase (von Gierke's disease) may cause severe hypoglycemia, whereas deficient activities of glycogen phosphorylase and debrancher enzyme cause milder degrees of hypoglycemia (Ch. 179). Deficiency of glycogen synthetase results in severe hypoglycemia in newborns.

Gluconeogenesis is the generation of new glucose from noncarbohydrate substrates. Defects in this process result in hypoglycemia after prolonged fasting when glycogen stores have been depleted. Lactate and pyruvate, glycerol, and amino acids account for approximately 58 per cent, 13 per cent, and 29 per cent of the glucose produced via gluconeogenesis. Defects in gluconeogenesis may arise from (1) diminished substrate availability, e.g., ketotic hypoglycemia in children; (2) altered redox state, which inhibits several important gluconeogenic enzymes, e.g., alcohol hypoglycemia; and (3) inhibition of fatty acid oxidation, which diminishes the energy source for gluconeogenesis, e.g., poisoning from the unripe ackee fruit.

Alanine and glutamine are the most important amino acids that act as glucose precursors. The carbon source of alanine is muscle-derived pyruvate, and the nitrogen source for the transamination of pyruvate to alanine is thought to be branched-chain amino acids. Impaired metabolism of leucine, a branched-chain amino acid, observed in maple syrup urine disease (see Ch. 193) is associated with reduced alanine production and sometimes with hypoglycemia.

After three days of fasting, glucose production is primarily derived from hepatic gluconeogenesis; after prolonged fasting, renal gluconeogenesis may account for approximately 50 per cent of glucose production. The effects of insulin, glucagon, catecholamines, cortisol, and growth hormone on glucose homeostasis and recovery from hypoglycemia are shown in Table 231–1. Insulin is the primary hypoglycemic hormone; the others act by a variety of mechanisms to elevate glucose concentrations. Although plasma glucagon, catecholamines, cortisol, and growth hormone increase in response to insulin-induced hypoglycemia, glucagon makes the major contribution to the acute recovery from hypoglycemia. Catecholamines can result in a modest elevation of glucose concentration in the presence of glucagon deficiency or severe hypoglycemia.

CLINICAL EVALUATION

Defects of many of the mechanisms that maintain plasma glucose in the normal range are associated with readily recognizable clinical syndromes. In some instances the symptoms and signs of the primary disorder predominate over those of hypoglycemia, or at least point to the existence of the primary disorder causing hypoglycemia. In some patients with multisystem disease, poor nutrition, or multiple-drug use, the basis for hypoglycemia may be uncertain and the patient too ill to undergo extensive evaluation. Common causes of hypoglycemia are listed in Table 231–2.

In the majority of patients with symptoms of hypoglycemia who appear healthy, screening laboratory tests should include plasma glucose, serum insulin, calcium, phosphate, uric acid, lipids, creatinine, liver function evaluation, insulin antibodies, and plasma and urine corticosteroids. Documentation of drug-induced hypoglycemia may be difficult. A detailed history must be obtained, and every medication, including nonprescription drugs, used by the patient must be examined.

TABLE 231–1. HORMONAL CONTROL OF GLUCOSE HOMEOSTASIS

Hormone	Hepatic Glucose Production	Extrahepatic Glucose Utilization	Basal Glucose Production	Relative Importance to Recovery from Insulin-Induced Hypoglycemia
Insulin	↓	↑	↓	
Glucagon	↑	–	↑	+ + +
Catecholamines*	↑	↓	–	+
Cortisol	↑	↓	↑	–
Growth hormone†	↑	↓	–	–

NOTE: ↑ = increase; ↓ = decrease; – = no effect.

*Epinephrine is approximately ten times more potent than norepinephrine. Its action is primarily through a beta-adrenergic mechanism. In the presence of glucagon deficiency, catecholamines make a modest contribution to the recovery from hypoglycemia.

†Has an acute and transient hypoglycemic effect.

When a patient is observed with symptoms of hypoglycemia, 10 to 20 ml of blood in addition to that for glucose determination should be withdrawn. The specific analyses can be determined by the clues generated from the history and physical examination. Such an opportunity may provide sufficient data to establish the cause of the hypoglycemic disorder or narrow the diagnostic possibilities. Glucose should be administered following blood withdrawal to any patient suspected of being hypoglycemic. Prompt treatment will shorten the duration of hypoglycemia, and if the patient is not hypoglycemic no harm will have been done.

In patients with asymptomatic hypoglycemia one must be alert to artifactual hypoglycemia. Whole blood glucose values may be spuriously low in polycythemia vera because of the unequal distribution of glucose between erythrocyte and plasma or excessive glycolysis by erythrocytes, or both, and in leukemia from excessive glycolysis by leukocytes. Prompt measurement of glucose in plasma in these conditions should provide accurate results.

An uncommon and challenging problem is the low plasma glucose concentration in an asymptomatic patient in whom laboratory error and spurious result have been ruled out. Such patients may have adapted to longstanding hypoglycemia or have mild symptoms that have been completely unrecognized.

A flow diagram of a clinical approach to the evaluation of a suspected hypoglycemic disorder is presented in Figure 231–1. Note that the evaluation is directed to patients who appear healthy. For those who do not appear healthy the results of the history and physical examination will determine the direction of the investigation.

Hypoglycemic disorders cause a constellation of symptoms that usually recur as discrete episodes at irregular intervals. A useful but not infallible historical aid is the timing of symptoms in relation to food intake: those occurring within six hours of food intake are the *food-stimulated hypoglycemias* and those occurring beyond six hours of food intake are the *food-deprived hypoglycemias*.

Considerable effort should be expended to obtain from the patient and family members a detailed description of symptoms and careful attention paid to their occurrence in relation to food intake. The food-stimulated hypoglycemias usually cause symptoms of catecholamine release—sweating, shakiness, anxiety, palpitations, and weakness—and rarely those of impairment of central nervous system function. The food-deprived

TABLE 231–2. COMMON CAUSES OF HYPOGLYCEMIA

Medications
Ethanol
Factitial
Insulinoma
Non–islet cell tumors
Multifactorial in sick patient
Islet dysplasia of infancy
Ketotic hypoglycemia

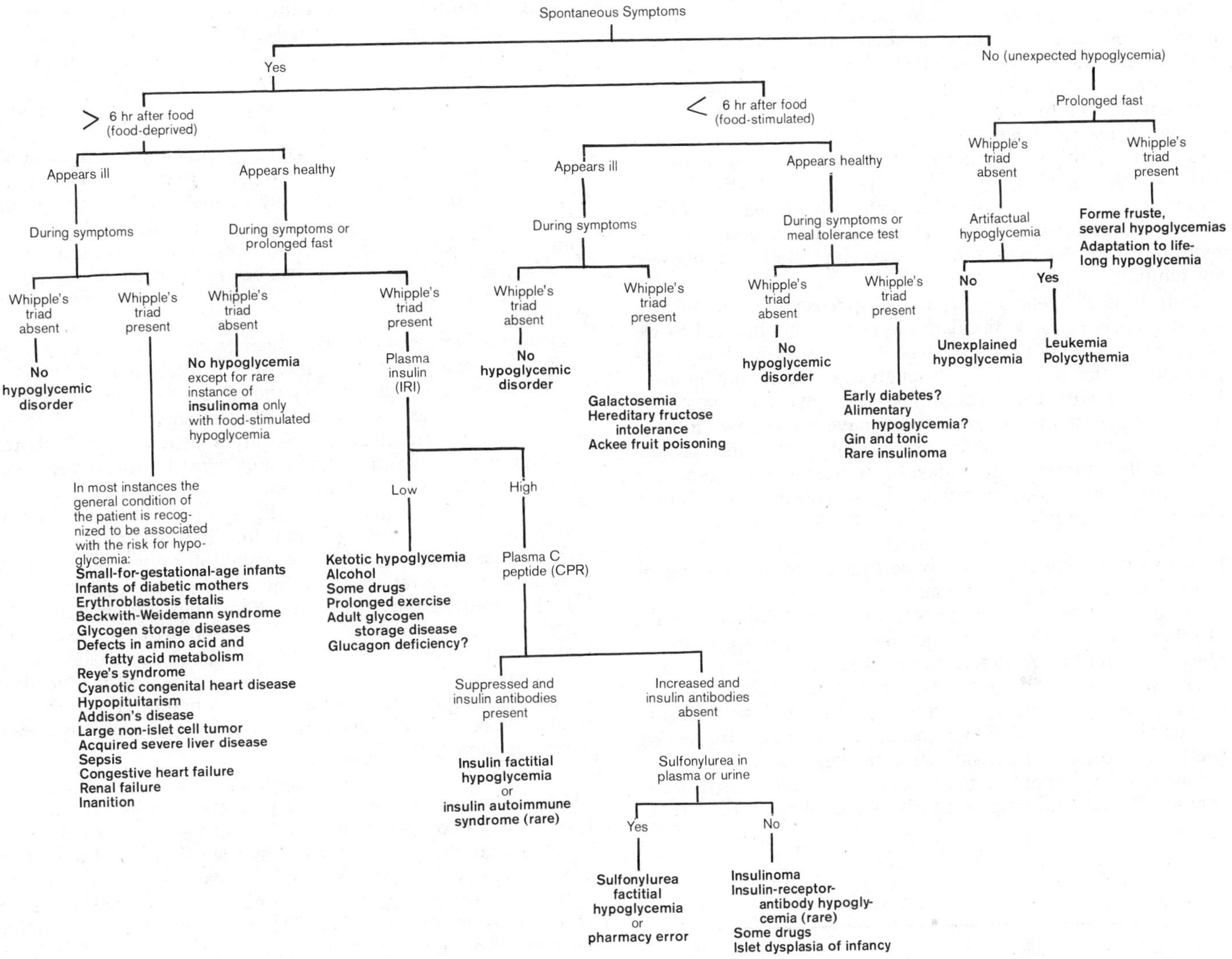

Figure 231–1. Evaluation of hypoglycemic disorders.

hypoglycemias, on the other hand, usually result in impairment of central nervous system function—reduced intellectual capacity, confusion, irritability, abnormal behavior, convulsions, and coma. Sometimes there is complicating hypothermia. Often the symptoms of catecholamine release that precede the central nervous system symptoms go unrecognized. Symptoms of hypoglycemia usually occur at plasma glucose concentrations of about 45 mg per deciliter or less (whole blood glucose of 40 mg per deciliter or less). Although some studies suggest that a rapid fall in glucose concentration results in symptoms even when plasma glucose does not decrease below 45 mg per deciliter, the weight of evidence does not support this relationship. The symptoms of hypoglycemia are nonspecific. For this reason it is necessary to demonstrate a low plasma glucose value concomitant with symptoms and subsequent relief of symptoms by correction of the hypoglycemia, i.e., *Whipple's triad*. This triad should be demonstrated before hypoglycemia can be considered to be the basis for a patient's symptoms. Although food, especially free carbohydrate, will relieve symptoms regardless of the cause of the hypoglycemia, persons without a hypoglycemic disorder may feel better after eating. It is therefore imperative to confirm that symptoms are due to hypoglycemia.

FOOD-STIMULATED HYPOGLYCEMIAS

Subsequent to the conceptualization of hyperinsulinism as a disease, after insulin became available for the treatment of diabetes, many patients with postprandial symptoms were found to have concomitant blood sugar concentrations within or even above the normal range. For such cases the term *functional hypoglycemia* was coined. Eventually reliance on a subnormal glucose concentration at the time of spontaneous symptoms came to be replaced by the oral glucose tolerance test. Reproduction of those symptoms experienced during ordinary daily activities and documentation of a plasma glucose nadir ≤50 mg per deciliter (or its equivalent) during the oral glucose tolerance test have been considered confirmation of the presence of a food-stimulated hypoglycemic disorder. Use of the oral glucose tolerance test is fraught with risk of misdiagnosis since (1) in at least 10 per cent of healthy persons the plasma glucose nadir is less than 50 mg per deciliter; (2) there is no correlation between the nadir of plasma glucose concentrations and the occurrence of symptoms of hypoglycemia in patients with symptoms suggestive of food-stimulated hypoglycemia; and (3) the results of oral glucose tolerance tests are variable upon repeated testing. Measurement of plasma cortisol responses, calculation of rates of glucose descent, and hypoglycemic indices have not improved the accuracy of the oral glucose tolerance test. Furthermore, many patients with symptoms typical of a food-stimulated hypoglycemic disorder experience symptoms after a "placebo" oral glucose tolerance test.

Recent studies have measured plasma glucose responses to mixed nutrient meals designed as more representative of the body's usual challenge to glucose homeostasis than large oral glucose loads. These results have been compared to those following standard glucose test meals (75 to 100 grams of glucose) (Fig. 231–2). Although patients had symptoms during both tests, none of the patients who had a hypoglycemic nadir after oral glucose intake evinced hypoglycemia after mixed nutrient intake. In addition, there was no EEG evidence of hypoglycemia in those who had symptoms during the test meal. Therefore the oral glucose tolerance test should not be used for the evaluation of hypoglycemia in patients with symptoms in the postprandial period. Instead, plasma glucose should be measured during the spontaneous occurrence of symptoms or after ingestion of a meal typical of that followed by symptoms.

Unfortunately, reliance on the oral glucose tolerance test for the diagnosis of food-stimulated hypoglycemia has led to extensive literature not on disorders of hypoglycemia but on the oral glucose tolerance test. Although there undoubtedly are a few patients with true postprandial hypoglycemia, most persons with symptoms following meals have been shown to have psychoneurosis. The use of low carbohydrate–high protein diets, sulfonylureas, biguanides, or anticholinergic agents for the treatment of food-stimulated hypoglycemias has limited experimental support.

Hypoglycemia following the ingestion of substances that are toxic to susceptible persons may be considered in the category of food-stimulated hypoglycemias.

The ingestion of large amounts (equivalent of three highballs) of ethanol and carbohydrate (gin and tonic) may cause hypoglycemia within three to four hours in some healthy persons.

The unripe ackee fruit may result in hypoglycemia in children or adults with chronic malnutrition by inhibiting the transport of long-chain fatty acids into mitochondria, thereby suppressing their oxidation and depressing gluconeogenesis.

Postprandial hypoglycemia occurs in children with galactosemia (Ch. 178) and hereditary fructose intolerance (Ch. 181).

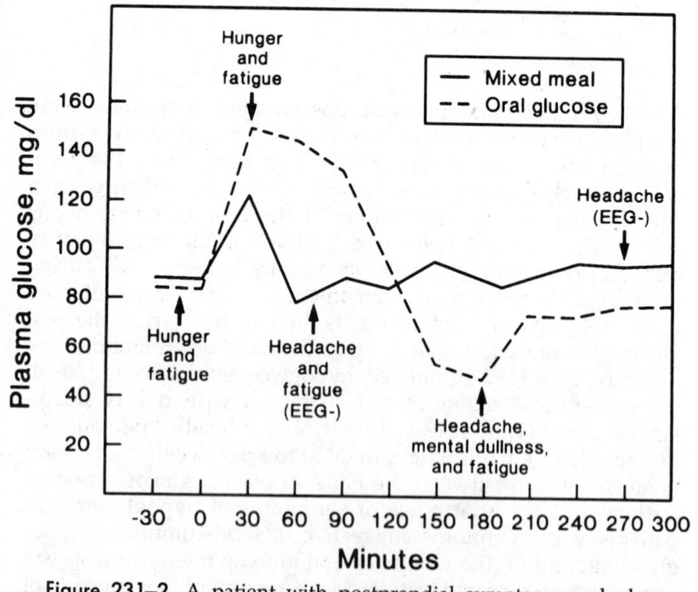

Figure 231–2. A patient with postprandial symptoms and plasma glucose responses to an oral glucose tolerance test consistent with a diagnosis of reactive hypoglycemia underwent a mixed meal study. Similar symptoms occurred in both studies; they bore no consistent relationship to the concomitant plasma glucose concentrations. Monitoring by EEG during occurrence of symptoms after the mixed meal showed no abnormalities. It was concluded that the symptoms could not be ascribed to a disorder of glucose homeostasis and that the OGTT should not be used for diagnosis of reactive hypoglycemia. (From Service FJ: *In* Hypoglycemic Disorders: Pathogenesis, Diagnosis, and Treatment. Boston, GK Hall, 1982. Reprinted with permission.)

FOOD-DEPRIVED (FASTING) HYPOGLYCEMIAS

Drug-Induced Hypoglycemias

Drugs constitute the most common cause of hypoglycemia if insulin and sulfonylureas used by diabetic persons are included. Factors increasing the risk of drug-induced hypoglycemia are extremes of age, antecedent food deprivation, and impaired renal and hepatic function. The drugs most commonly implicated as the cause for hypoglycemia in addition to insulin and sulfonylurea are salicylates, propranolol, and alcohol. Other drugs recently reported to cause hypoglycemia are disopyramide (Norpace), sulfamethoxazole, and trimethoprim (Bactrim, Septra) in the presence of renal failure and pentamidine (Lomidine)* and quinine when used for cerebral malaria. Since a wide variety of drugs has been implicated as the cause of hypoglycemia, the reader is referred to review articles on this subject.

Ethanol-induced hypoglycemia arises from inhibition of gluconeogenesis as a result of the increase in the NADH-NAD ratio in instances of depleted hepatic glycogen. The increased NADH-NAD ratio suppresses the conversions of lactate to pyruvate, α-glycerophosphate to dihydroxyacetone phosphate, and glutamate to α-ketoglutarate and several tricarboxylic cycle reactions. Infusion of ethanol into healthy subjects for four hours results in hypoglycemia, reduced rates of hepatic glucose production, suppressed plasma insulin concentrations, increased plasma lactate, β-hydroxybutyrate, glycerol, and free fatty acid concentrations, and increased lactate-pyruvate and β-hydroxybutyrate-acetoacetate ratios. Hypoglycemia usually develops within 6 to 36 hours of the ingesting of even moderate amounts of alcohol by persons chronically malnourished or by healthy persons who have missed one or two meals. Healthy children are especially susceptible to alcohol-induced hypoglycemia. Blood alcohol levels may not be elevated when the patient is hypoglycemic.

Insulinoma

Approximately 60 per cent of patients with insulinoma are female. Insulinomas are uncommon in persons less than 20 years of age and rare in those less than 5 years of age. The median age at diagnosis is about 50 years, except in patients with the multiple endocrine neoplasia (MEN) syndrome in which it is in the mid 20s. Ten per cent of patients with insulinoma are older than 70 years of age.

Of patients with insulinoma 80 per cent have single benign tumors, 11 per cent have multiple benign tumors, 6 per cent have single malignant tumors, and the remainder have multiple malignant tumors or islet hyperplasia. Ten per cent of insulinoma patients have MEN syndrome type 1 (Ch. 240), and 80 per cent of these patients have multiple insulinomas; however, only 60 per cent of patients with multiple insulinomas have the MEN syndrome.

Some tumors secrete hormones in addition to insulin: gastrin, 5-hydroxyindoles, ACTH, glucagon, and somatostatin. In rare instances, insulinomas have occurred in non–insulin-dependent diabetic persons but have never been documented in an insulin-dependent subject.

CLINICAL PICTURE. Symptoms may be present for many years prior to the diagnosis. In one series 85 per cent of patients had various combinations of diplopia, blurred vision, sweating, palpitations, or weakness; 80 per cent had confusion or abnormal behavior; 53 per cent had unconsciousness or amnesia; and 12 per cent had grand mal seizures. Twenty per cent of cases may be misdiagnosed, the belief being that the patient has a neurologic or psychiatric disorder.

Hypoglycemia usually occurs several hours after a meal, most commonly before the evening meal (Fig. 231–3). In rare instances, symptoms may occur solely in the postprandial period rather than during fasting. Symptoms may be aggravated by exercise, alcohol use, a high protein–low carbohydrate diet, treatment with sulfonylureas, and fasts. Less than 20 per cent of patients with insulinoma gain weight.

*Pentamidine (Lomidine) is an investigational drug available from the Centers for Disease Control, Atlanta, GA.

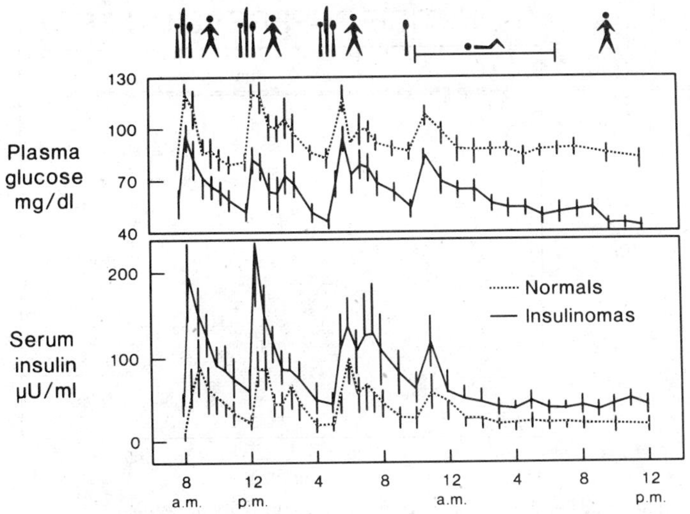

Figure 231–3. Serial measurements of plasma glucose and serum insulin in patients with insulinoma and healthy subjects under ordinary life conditions. Plasma glucose declined to hypoglycemic levels in the late postabsorptive and fasting states in those with insulinoma. Hyperinsulinemia was observed in response to meals and also in the postabsorptive and fasting states. (Fork, knife, spoon = meal; spoon = snack; standing figure = exercise; reclining figure = sleep.) (From Service FJ, Nelson RL: Insulinoma. Comp Ther 6:70, 1980. Reprinted with permission.)

DIAGNOSIS. The diagnosis of insulinoma is based on the demonstration of Whipple's triad and hyperinsulinemia or an inappropriately normal insulin level for a low glucose value. Insulin antibodies should be undetectable unless the patient has taken exogenous insulin. Useful screening tests are *daily fasting plasma glucose and insulin determinations* and the *intravenous tolbutamide test*. The latter (Fig. 231–4) has approximately a 90 per cent diagnostic accuracy. This test should be performed only in persons for whom the fasting plasma glucose is known to exceed 50 mg per deciliter on the day of the test and who have not been food deprived for several days preceding the test. Diagnostic criteria should be based on absolute values during the last hour of the test, i.e., plasma glucose <55 mg per deciliter, blood glucose <50 mg per deciliter, and serum insulin >20 μU per milliliter at the 120- to 180-minute period of the test. Diagnostic criteria will reflect local laboratory procedures and so should be generated at each institution. Diagnostic criteria based on percentage of recovery of basal plasma glucose at the end of the test are less accurate. If the plasma glucose responses to intravenous tolbutamide are normal, the insulin values give little additional information.

Prolonged supervised fasting is the single most reliable test for the diagnosis of insulinoma. During the fast the patient should be active during the day. Noncaloric beverages can be consumed. The frequency of blood sampling during the fast should be guided by the patient's history of tolerance to food withdrawal. The frequency of sampling should be increased as the plasma glucose approaches the hypoglycemic range. Whenever blood is withdrawn for glucose determination, a sample should also be drawn for determination of serum insulin and, if factitial hypoglycemia is suspected, of C peptide and sulfonylurea. During the fast the patient's intellectual status should be checked regularly by simple mathematic tasks such as serial sevens. During prolonged fasting healthy women experience lower plasma glucose concentrations than do healthy men: values as low as 42 mg per deciliter in men and 34 mg per deciliter in women may be unaccompanied by symptoms. Therefore it is essential to continue the fast to the point at which symptoms develop, or to 72 hours. Serum insulin concentrations may be in the "normal" range in about 50 per cent of determinations when the plasma glucose is in the hypoglycemic range (Fig. 231–5); 10 per cent of patients with insulinoma may have all insulin values in this normal range during hypoglycemia; however, this normal serum insulin concentration is probably excessive if it is above 6 μU per milliliter and certainly excessive if it is above 10 μU per milliliter during hypoglycemia. Various glucose-insulin ratios provide less diagnostic accuracy (Fig. 231–6).

In a large series, Whipple's triad was demonstrated within 12 hours of the last meal in 29 per cent of patients, within 24 hours in 71 per cent, within 36 hours in 79 per cent, within 48 hours in 92 per cent, within 60 hours in 97 per cent, and within 72 hours in 98 per cent. In rare instances, patients with insulinoma may not develop hypoglycemia during prolonged fasting of even up to 96 hours. At the time of hypoglycemic symptoms, plasma glucose concentrations were ≤46 mg per deciliter in 100 per cent of patients, ≤39 mg per deciliter in 75 per cent, ≤35 mg per deciliter in 50 per cent, and ≤28 mg per deciliter in 25 per cent.

The *intravenous glucagon test*, which is considered to be positive if the peak insulin response exceeds 130 μU per milliliter, has a diagnostic accuracy of 50 to 80 per cent. The C *peptide suppression test* is based on the observation that exogenous insulin-induced hypoglycemia suppresses C peptide concentration in normal persons but not in those with insulinomas (Fig. 231–7). The criteria for normal C peptide suppression will depend on the C peptide assay. The utility of other tests such as glycosylated hemoglobin, human pancreatic polypeptide, and infusions of alcohol, calcium, epinephrine and propranolol, diazoxide, and somatostatin-tolbutamide in the diagnosis of insulinoma is unproven or inadequate. Human chorionic gonadotropin or one of its subunits may be a marker for functioning

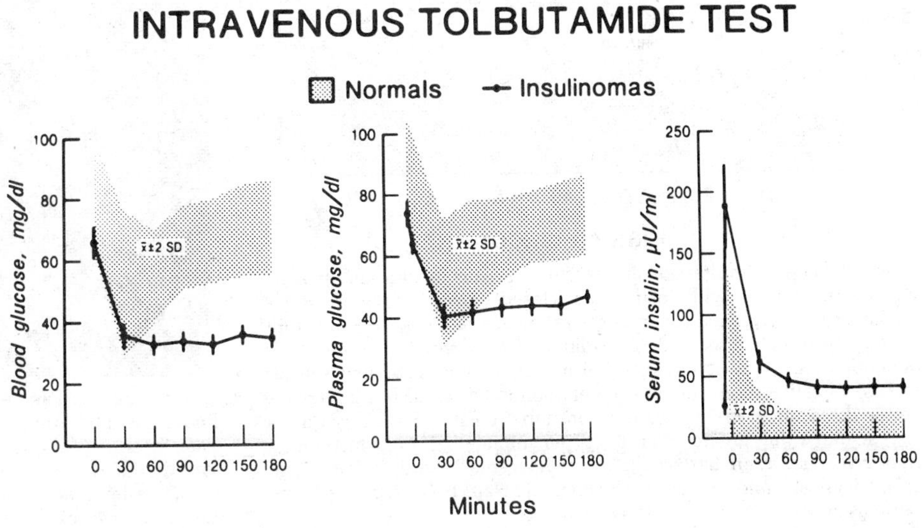

Figure 231–4. Intravenous tolbutamide test results in 34 patients with insulinoma (M ± SEM) and healthy subjects (shaded). Fourteen with insulinoma had glucose measured in whole blood; 20 had glucose measured in plasma. Criteria for diagnosis of insulinoma is a blood glucose level of 50 mg per deciliter or less, plasma glucose 55 mg per deciliter or less, and serum insulin greater than 20 μU per milliter at the 120 to 180 minute part of the test. (From Service FJ: *In* Hypoglycemic Disorders: Pathogenesis, Diagnosis, and Treatment. Boston, GK Hall, 1982. Reprinted with permission.)

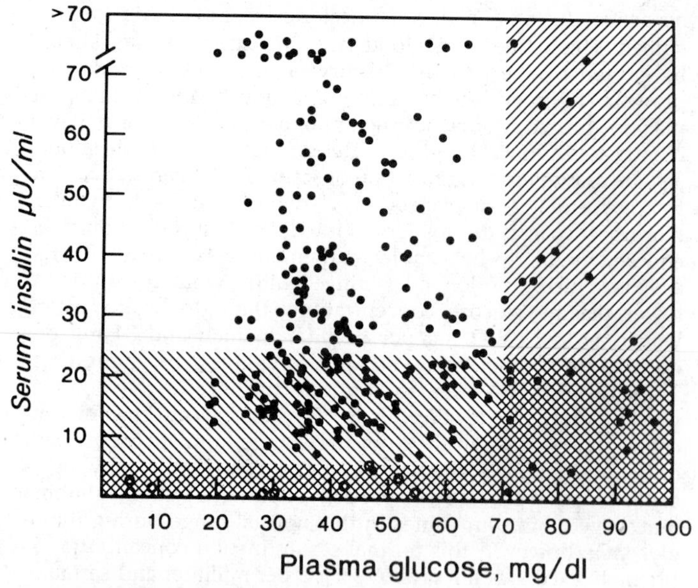

Figure 231–5. Simultaneously measured serum insulin and plasma glucose in 72 patients with insulinomas (closed circles) and six patients with noninsulin-mediated hypoglycemia (open circles). Ten per cent of those with insulinoma for whom multiple simultaneous insulin and glucose determinations were made all had insulin values in the normal range during concomitant hypoglycemia. (From Service FJ: *In* Hypoglycemic Disorders: Pathogenesis, Diagnosis, and Treatment. Boston, GK Hall, 1982. Reprinted with permission.)

malignant insulinomas. Eighty per cent of patients with insulinoma may have elevated proinsulin concentrations (>20 per cent of total immunoreactive insulin).

LOCALIZATION. Only after the diagnosis of insulinoma has been confirmed biochemically should a localization procedure be done. Pancreatic angiography has been reported to have a high rate of success if stereoscopy, magnification, and subtraction are used (Fig. 231–8). Insulinomas appear as homogeneous, intensely vascular, sharply circumscribed masses within the substance of the pancreas.

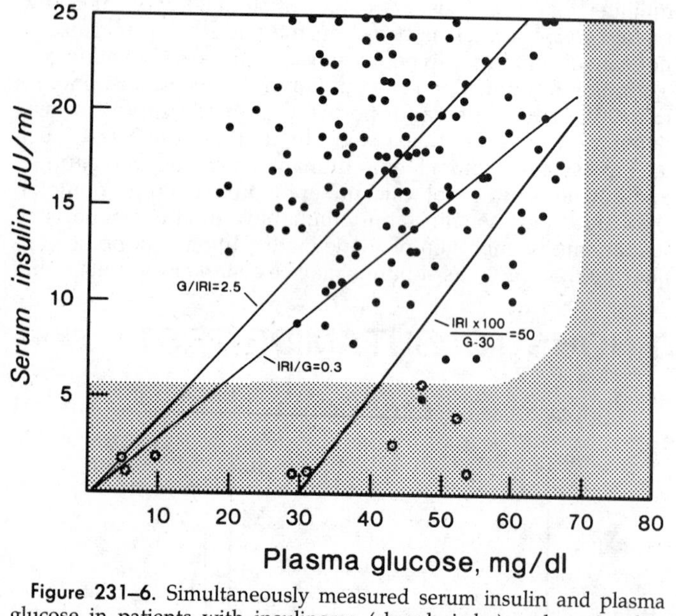

Figure 231–6. Simultaneously measured serum insulin and plasma glucose in patients with insulinoma (closed circles) and noninsulin-mediated hypoglycemia (open circles). Various ratios—glucose:insulin = 2.5, insulin:glucose = 0.3, insulin × 100 ÷ glucose − 30 = 50 (amended ratio)—designed to establish relative hyperinsulinemia result in false-negative interpretation of data points below each ratio line. A better discrimination to determine insulin-mediated hypoglycemia is any insulin value greater than 6 μU per milliliter during concomitant hypoglycemia. (From Service FJ: *In* Hypoglycemic Disorders: Pathogenesis, Diagnosis, and Treatment. Boston, GK Hall, 1982. Reprinted with permission.)

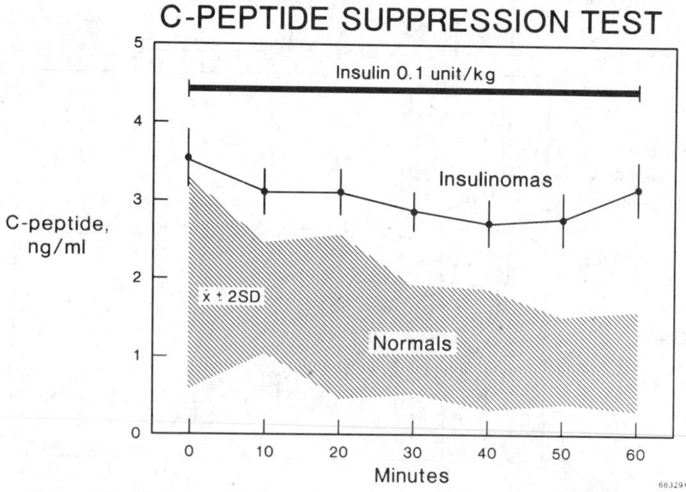

Figure 231–7. C-peptide suppression test in 17 insulinomas (M ± SEM) and controls (shaded). In response to insulin-induced hypoglycemia, insulinomas fail to suppress C-peptide. (From Service FJ, Nelson RL: Insulinoma. Comp Ther 6:70, 1980. Reprinted with permission.)

Computed tomography has had limited success in localization. Real-time high-resolution ultrasonography done both preoperatively and intraoperatively is currently demonstrating a high degree of accuracy. The indications for and value of selective venous sampling for insulin determinations done either by the percutaneous transhepatic route or directly at the time of surgery remain undetermined. Failure to localize an insulinoma by any of these techniques should not deter pancreatic exploration in a patient for whom the diagnosis has been firmly established. Surgeons experienced in insulinoma surgery are highly successful in finding the tumor even when it has not been localized preoperatively.

TREATMENT. Surgical removal is the preferred form of treatment for insulinoma. In a large series, 54 per cent of subjects underwent successful enucleation of the tumor; 38 per cent,

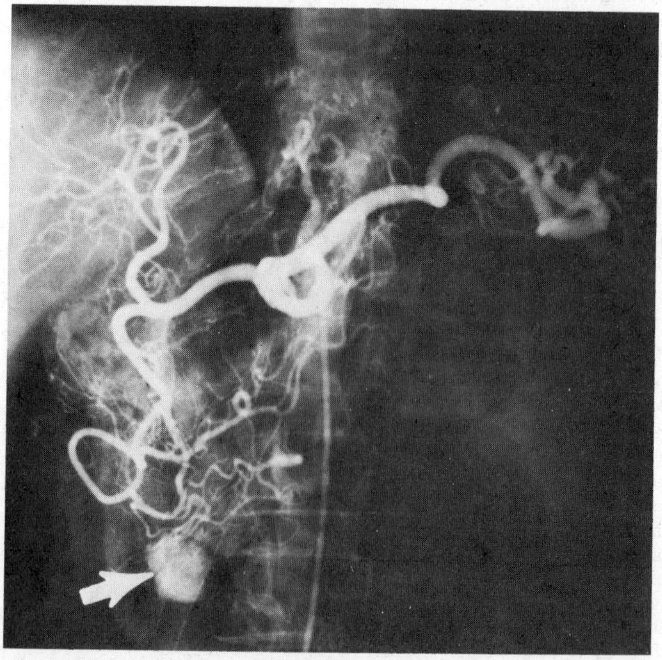

Figure 231–8. Pancreatic angiogram: intense vascular blush of insulinoma (white arrow) in the inferior portion of the head of the pancreas (late arterial phase of celiac artery injection). (From Stephens DH, Sheedy PF: Computed tomography. *In* Margulis AR, Burhenne HJ (eds.): Alimentary Tract Radiology. Vol 3. Abdominal imaging. St. Louis, CV Mosby, 1979. Reprinted with permission.)

partial pancreatectomy; and the remainder, a variety of other procedures. In the series, 84 per cent were cured, 7 per cent had diabetes, and the remainder required medical treatment to control persistent hypoglycemia from malignant insulinoma, islet hyperplasia, or a tumor missed during surgery. There was no operative mortality, and the postoperative complication rate was 10 per cent.

Intraoperative glucose monitoring should not be relied upon for surgical management, since there is a high (23 per cent) incidence of failure of plasma glucose to increase after successful insulinoma removal.

The median diameter of benign tumors has been reported to be 1.5 cm. Malignant tumors are usually large. Tumors are evenly distributed throughout the pancreas whether benign or malignant, single or multiple. Ectopically located insulinoma and islet hyperplasia are very rare. There is no correlation between the severity of symptoms and size of the insulinoma.

Treatment of persistent hypoglycemia in a patient with malignant insulinoma, in a patient in whom insulinoma cannot be found at pancreatic exploration, or in one who refuses surgery is best accomplished with diazoxide, which inhibits insulin release, although phenytoin and propranolol have been used successfully in some cases. Malignant insulinoma metastasizes primarily to local structures such as regional lymph nodes and liver; distant metastases are uncommon. The chemotherapeutic regimen of choice consists of streptozotocin and 5-fluorouracil. Survival exceeds that in adenocarcinoma of the pancreas.

Factitial and Autoimmune Hypoglycemia

Nondiabetic persons who secretly take insulin or sulfonylureas are predominantly women in the third and fourth decades of life who are employed in health-related occupations. Patients with factitial hypoglycemia have an erratic pattern in the occurrence of symptoms and may tolerate prolonged periods of fasting. With the exception of the rare instance of the insulin autoimmune syndrome, the presence of insulin antibodies is strong evidence of repeated injection of insulin. In addition, the presence of low plasma concentrations of C peptide concomitant with elevated insulin levels and hypoglycemia indicates an exogenous source of insulin. Insulin antibodies will result in spurious radioimmunoassayable plasma insulin concentrations: very high if the double-antibody assay is used and undetectable if the charcoal-coated–dextran assay is used. Results of tests for insulinoma (including the C peptide suppression test if the patient is taking a sulfonylurea) may be indistinguishable between an insulinoma patient and a patient who secretly took the hypoglycemic agent prior to the test. Concentrations of sulfonylurea should be measured in the plasma or urine if it is suspected of being the hypoglycemic agent. The clinical pattern in diabetic subjects consists of increased frequency of hypoglycemia during treatment and persistence of hypoglycemic episodes after complete cessation of use of the agent. The presence of insulin antibodies is of no help in the diagnosis in the insulin-treated patient. An inverse relation between C peptide and insulin levels during hypoglycemia is diagnostic of surreptitious insulin administration. Insulin has been used for suicide, homicide, and child abuse. Errors in filling prescriptions by substitution of a sulfonylurea for the intended medication have led to hypoglycemia.

In rare instances, patients may have hypoglycemia who apparently have never had an insulin injection but have insulin antibodies. These patients may range in age from a few days old to elderly. Hypoglycemia may be severe, occur during fasting or postprandially, and is often self-limited. Too few cases have been adequately described to ascertain whether free insulin concentrations are abnormal during episodes of hypoglycemia; free C peptide concentrations appear to be appropriately suppressed. Discrimination between autoimmune and factitial hypoglycemia rests on demonstrating differences in the characteristics of the insulin antibodies and the absence of bovine and porcine proinsulin and C peptide-specific antibodies. Neither the biochemical characteristics of this syndrome nor the mechanism of the hypoglycemia has been elucidated. Hypoglycemia has been observed in a few persons with insulin receptor antibodies that presumably act like insulin agonists. Most of the reported patients had pre-existing insulin-resistant diabetes and evidence for autoimmune disease prior to the development of hypoglycemia. This syndrome may respond to glucocorticoid therapy but not to immunosuppressive agents or plasmapheresis.

Non–Beta Cell Tumor Hypoglycemia

A wide variety of tumors of mesenchymal or epithelial origin and some malignant hematologic diseases have been associated with hypoglycemia.

Mesenchymal tumors account for 45 to 64 per cent of the reported cases. Approximately one third of the tumors are located in the chest and two thirds are in the abdomen, usually in the retroperitoneum. They usually are large and therefore readily detectable. Hepatomas account for 22 per cent of cases.

No single pathogenetic mechanism satisfactorily explains all cases of tumor-related hypoglycemia. In some, more than one mechanism may be involved. Metastatic destruction of the adrenals or pituitary and extensive metastatic involvement of the liver can impair glucoregulatory mechanisms. Some tumors evince a high rate of glucose utilization. In others, substances such as tryptophan metabolites may impair gluconeogenesis. The conflicting data regarding the presence or absence of elevated concentrations of insulin-like growth factors in the serum of these patients may be due to methodologic differences in measuring the substances. Total or partial surgical removal of the tumor usually results in amelioration of the hypoglycemia.

Hypoglycemia in Hepatic, Renal, and Endocrine Disorders

Symptomatic hypoglycemia is uncommon in liver disease because glucose homeostasis can be maintained with as little as 20 per cent of healthy parenchymal cells, but biochemical hypoglycemia has been reported in a wide variety of acquired hepatic diseases. The hypoglycemia of congestive heart failure, sepsis, and Reye's syndrome is considered to be due to hepatic mechanisms.

Hypoglycemia is uncommon in adrenocortical insufficiency. Hypoglycemia in hypopituitarism is common in children under six years of age but less so beyond that age. Asymptomatic hypoglycemia has been observed in isolated growth hormone deficiency after prolonged fasting. Spontaneous hypoglycemia has been reported to be a frequent finding in isolated ACTH deficiency. Adults surgically deprived of epinephrine are not subject to hypoglycemia.

Hypoglycemia in nondiabetic persons with renal failure may be due to inadequate gluconeogenic substrate availability. Glucagon deficiency is a theoretic mechanism for hypoglycemia, but the existence of this disorder has not been confirmed.

Froesch ER, Zopf J, Widmer U: Hypoglycemia associated with non-islet cell tumor and insulin-like growth factors (letter). Gorden P, Kahn CR, Roth J, Megyeshi K (response to letter). N Engl J Med 306:1178–1179, 1982. *The letter and response describe the controversy regarding the concentrations of insulin-like growth factors in non–beta cell tumor hypoglycemia.*

Garber AJ, Bier DM, Cryer PE, Pagliara AS: Hypoglycemia in compensated chronic renal insufficiency. Substrate limitation of gluconeogenesis. Diabetes 23:982–986, 1974. *Data are presented indicating that hypoglycemia in chronic renal failure may be due to inadequate availability of alanine.*

Hogan MJ, Service FJ, Sharbrough F, Gerich JE: Oral glucose tolerance test compared with a mixed meal in the diagnosis of reactive hypoglycemia. A caveat on stimulation. Mayo Clin Proc 58:491–496, 1983. *The authors demonstrate the inadequacy of the oral glucose tolerance test for the diagnosis of postprandial symptoms. Patients considered to have food-stimulated hypoglycemia after oral glucose tolerance testing had no hypoglycemia after a mixed meal despite the presence of postprandial symptoms. In addition, EEG monitoring during postprandial symptoms showed no changes.*

Le-Ran A, Anderson RW: The diagnosis of postprandial hypoglycemia. Diabetes 30:996–999, 1981. *The authors report the results of oral glucose tolerance testing in a large group of healthy persons, in 10 per cent of whom the glucose nadir was ≤47 mg per deciliter. In addition, the nonspecificity of the postoral glucose symptoms is underscored by the observation of symptoms following administration of a placebo.*

Marks V: Hypoglycemia. Oxford, Blackwell Scientific Publications, Ltd., 1981. *This is an authoritative reference work on hypoglycemic disorders.*

Scarlett JA, Mako ME, Rubenstein AH, Blix PM, Goldman J, Horwitz DL, Tager H, Jaspan JB, St Jernholm MR, Olefsky JM: Factitious hypoglycemia. Diagnosis and measurement of serum C-peptide immunoreactivity and insulin-binding antibodies. N Engl J Med 297:1029, 1977. *Seven cases of surreptitious injection of insulin are described. The authors emphasize the importance of the triad of low plasma glucose and high plasma insulin levels and suppression of plasma C peptide for diagnosis of this condition. In addition, there is a useful discussion of characteristics of antibodies to insulin, proinsulin, and C peptide of human, porcine, and bovine origin for the distinction between factitial and autoimmune hypoglycemia.*

Seltzer HS: Severe drug-induced hypoglycemia: A review. Comp Ther 5:21–29, 1979. *This review is an excellent reference source regarding the drugs implicated and the conditions conducive to drug-induced hypoglycemia.*

Service FJ: Hypoglycemic Disorders: Pathogenesis, Diagnosis, and Treatment. Boston, G. K. Hall, 1983. *This book is recommended for those desiring more detailed description of hypoglycemic disorders. For those interested in hypoglycemias in the pediatric age range the chapter, Hypoglycemia in infants and children, by E. Tsalikian and M. W. Haymond, is an excellent reference source.*

Taylor SI, Greenberger G, Marcus-Samuels B, Underhill LH, Dons RF, Ryan J, Roddam RF, Rupe CE, Gorden P: Hypoglycemia associated with antibodies to the insulin receptor. N Engl J Med 307:1422–1426, 1982. *The authors report a nondiabetic patient with fasting hypoglycemia ascribed to the action of autoantibodies to the insulin receptor. Although the few other patients with this syndrome had a history of prior diabetes, evidence for coexistent autoimmune disease is a clue to the presence of antireceptor antibodies.*

232. PANCREATIC ISLET CELL TUMORS

Carl Grunfeld

THE ISLETS OF LANGERHANS

Dispersed throughout the exocrine pancreas are nests of endocrine cells, the islets of Langerhans. The islet itself is a miniature organ with a distinctive organization of individualized cells, each of which produces a single hormone (Fig. 232–1). Insulin-containing B cells form the core of the islet and make up 60 per cent of the endocrine pancreas. They are surrounded by a rim of A cells that secrete glucagon and constitute 25 per cent of the islet. In the ventral portion of the head of the pancreas, glucagon-secreting cells are rare, and the rim is predominantly made up of cells containing pancreatic polypeptide. D cells containing somatostatin or gastrin are primarily found between the A and B cells. The location and function of cells containing other hormones, such as vasoactive intestinal polypeptide, have not yet been precisely defined.

The cells of the islets are capable of communication with each other through gap junctions. These transmembrane channels permit the exchange of small signal molecules as well as some polypeptides. Complete structural integrity of the islet is probably required for normal function.

Cells of the islets may become hyperplastic in response to prolonged stimulation of hormone secretion. Thus, A cells containing glucagon are often increased in diabetes mellitus. B cells increase after prolonged excessive caloric ingestion or in the presence of insulin resistance.

ISLET CELL TUMORS

Tumors can arise from any of the hormone-producing cells of the islets of Langerhans. Patients with islet cell tumors may seek help either because of distinct syndromes due to the hypersecretion of hormones by the tumors or because of mass effects of local or metastatic tumor spread. Nearly all benign islet cell tumors and more than 80 per cent of carcinomas secrete clinically significant amounts of hormone. Some tumors, particularly those arising from more than one cell type, have been shown to produce multiple hormones. Clinical presentation usually reflects the dominance of one hormone.

The tumor is named after the hormone responsible for the syndrome or, in asymptomatic patients, the hormone found in highest concentration in the circulation or in the tumor. For

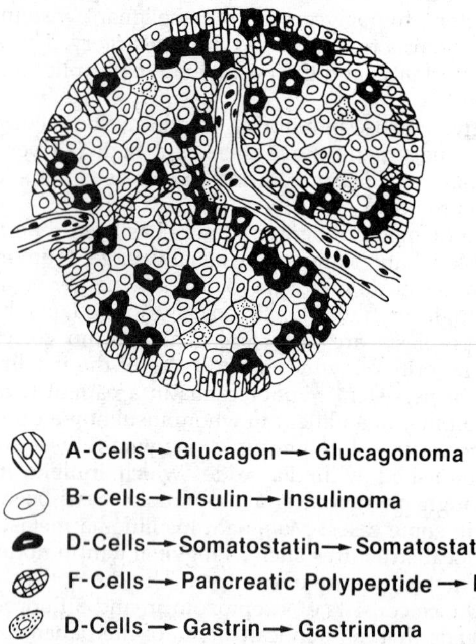

Figure 232–1. Morphology of the islets of Langerhans. This schematic representation of a typical islet demonstrates the distinctive distribution of hormone-secreting cells within the islet. Insulin-containing B cells, forming the core of the islet, are surrounded by glucagon-containing A cells. D cells are interspersed. In the posterior portion of the head of the pancreas, the proportion of cells containing pancreatic polypeptide is increased and the number of glucagon-secreting cells is strikingly decreased. Each cell type is capable of neoplastic transformation, yielding an adenoma or carcinoma that synthesizes the characteristic hormone. (Modified from Unger RH, Orci L: Glucagon and the A cell: Physiology and pathophysiology. N Engl J Med 304:1518, 1981. Reprinted with permission.)

example, a tumor producing insulin is known as an insulinoma, and one producing glucagon is a glucagonoma. The tumors also retain the morphologic characteristics of the cell of origin.

DIAGNOSIS. Diagnosis of islet cell tumors is usually made by detecting elevated basal or fasting levels of the suspected hormone in the presence of the characteristic syndrome. Provocative tests have also been developed that use pharmacologic agents to discriminate between secretion from a tumor and from a normal pancreas. In addition, tumors usually secrete a larger proportion of prohormone or other species of high molecular weight than do normal islet cells. Once the diagnosis is made, imaging techniques such as ultrasound, computed tomography, and angiography are helpful in localizing the tumor and in detecting hepatic and lymph node metastases (see Fig. 231–8). These techniques should not be relied upon to make the diagnosis of the islet cell tumor, as there are a significant number of false-negative and false-positive results of tests. When a tumor is not readily detectable, selective venous catheterization can be used to obtain samples for radioimmunoassay, thereby identifying the area of the pancreas responsible for hypersecretion of the excess hormone. Controversy exists as to whether or not extensive preoperative tumor localization is required.

PATHOLOGY. There is no distinctive pathologic finding that can distinguish between benign and malignant islet cell tumors, although vascular invasion is suggestive of malignancy. The diagnosis of carcinoma is made when metastases are found at presentation or subsequent to resection of a solitary tumor. Elevated levels of human chorionic gonadotropin are useful in helping to establish the preoperative diagnosis of malignancy.

ASSOCIATED SYNDROMES. Pancreatic islet cell tumors may also be part of the multiple endocrine neoplasia (MEN) syndromes (see Ch. 240). It is critical to identify patients with this syndrome as they may have multiple islet cell tumors. Identification of the tumor or area of the pancreas responsible for excess secretion is essential to allow limited pancreatic resection by the surgeon. Unfortunately in patients with a MEN syndrome, tumors may continue to recur, necessitating total pancreatectomy. The presence of hypercalcemia in patients with islet cell tumors is suggestive of the MEN 1 syndrome, as 85 per cent of all patients with MEN type 1 have hyperparathyroidism at some time.

THERAPY. The primary therapy of solitary islet cell tumors is surgical resection. When a patient has islet cell carcinoma with metastasis, therapy is directed toward ameliorating the symptoms of the presenting syndrome and may include pharmacologic inhibitors of hormone secretion and action, chemotherapeutic agents, or surgical debulking. The specific agents are discussed under each tumor.

Similar syndromes resulting from hypersecretion of pancreatic hormones can occur secondary to diffuse hyperplasia of islet cells. The architecture of the pancreas may be disordered, with nests of islet cells arising from exocrine ducts. The treatment of hyperplastic syndromes is partial or near-total pancreatectomy.

The characteristic syndromes associated with islet cell tumors are outlined in Table 232–1.

Insulinoma

The most common islet cell tumor is the insulinoma, which may produce life-threatening hypoglycemia. Insulinoma is reviewed in Ch. 231.

Gastrinoma

The second most common islet cell tumor is the gastrinoma associated with Zollinger-Ellison syndrome, producing recurrent peptic ulcers due to hypersecretion of gastric acid. This syndrome is discussed in Ch. 99.

VIPoma or the Diarrheogenic Syndrome

CLINICAL PRESENTATION. VIP (vasoactive intestinal polypeptide)-oma or the diarrheogenic syndrome, associated with islet cell tumors, severe watery diarrhea, and hypokalemia, is also called pancreatic cholera, Verner-Morrison syndrome, WDHA (watery diarrhea, hypokalemia, achlorhydria) syndrome, or WDHH (watery diarrhea, hypokalemia, hypochlorhydria) syndrome. Patients have profound but intermittent secretory diarrhea, with peak diarrhea output exceeding 3 liters per day in 80 per cent. A more general discussion of secretory diarrhea is contained in Ch. 102. Unlike the diarrheal discharge of chronic laxative abuse, in this diarrhea the discharge is rich in electrolytes; fecal potassium loss can reach 300 mEq per day. Serum potassium is usually less than 3 mEq per liter and is accompanied by acidosis due to severe losses of bicarbonate.

The severe hypokalemia may lead to profound weakness, to flaccid paralysis, and to renal failure due to hypokalemic nephropathy. More than half of the patients have frank diabetes or glucose intolerance, which is probably secondary to hypokalemia, a known inhibitor of insulin secretion (see Ch. 76 for a discussion of hypokalemia). Hypercalcemia is found in half of the patients during attacks and is not usually indicative of hyperparathyroidism (and the MEN 1 syndrome), as parathyroid hormone levels are suppressed and the hypercalcemia remits with resection of the primary islet cell tumor. Despite hypercalcemia, tetany due to hypomagnesemia has been described. Dilation of the gallbladder or small intestine may be seen during radiographic examination, and flushing of the skin has been reported.

DIFFERENTIAL DIAGNOSIS. Secretory diarrhea may result from three other endocrine tumors: gastrinoma, carcinoid, and somatostatinoma. However, peak volume of diarrhea rarely exceeds 3 liters per day in these syndromes. Further, the diarrhea in Zollinger-Ellison syndrome is caused by hypersecretion of gastric acid and can be reversed by gastric suction or with cimetidine. The diarrheogenic syndrome is almost always accompanied by achlorhydria or hypochlorhydria; decreased gastric acid secretion persists when the diarrhea is in remission and the serum potassium is normal.

PATHOLOGY. Eighty per cent of the patients with the diarrheogenic syndrome are found to have islet cell tumors. Nearly half are malignant. When the diarrhea is constant, the probability of malignancy is increased. Patients without islet cell tumors often have diffuse islet cell hyperplasia. The diarrheogenic syndrome has also been reported with bronchial tumor, pheochromocytoma, and ganglioneuroblastoma.

The diarrhea probably results from excess secretion of VIP. Infusion of VIP into laboratory animals and humans results in secretory diarrhea, hypokalemia, inhibition of gastric acid secretion, and hypercalcemia. Increased plasma VIP levels have been found in patients in whom islet cell tumor, islet cell hyperplasia, bronchogenic carcinoma, ganglioneuroblastoma, or pheochromocytoma was found to be the cause of the syndrome. VIP is difficult to detect in the circulation of normal man; therefore the absence of VIP does not rule out the diagnosis. An islet cell tumor producing only pancreatic polypeptide (another presumed hormone of unknown normal function) has also been reported to be associated with this syndrome. Rare tumors have been accompanied by elevated levels of prostaglandin E_2.

THERAPY. Treatment of the diarrheogenic syndrome is primarily by surgery. Because of the profound systemic effects of this tumor, resection is considered even in the presence of metastases. When no tumor is found, subtotal pancreatectomy is usually attempted. If hyperplasia is then identified on histopathology and symptoms persist, total pancreatectomy should be considered. Metastatic tumor has been successfully treated with streptozotocin. The tumors may be transiently

TABLE 232–1. SYNDROMES ASSOCIATED WITH ISLET CELL TUMORS

Tumor	Major Findings	Minor Findings	Other Hormones in Tumor or Plasma	% Malignancy	Hyperplasia	MEN Syndrome
Insulinoma	Adrenergic: palpitations, tremor, hunger, sweating Neuroglycopenic: confusion, seizures, transient focal deficit, coma	Ischemic cardiovascular disease, permanent neurologic deficits	Gastrin, glucagon, pancreatic polypeptide, somatostatin	10	Occasional	10%
Gastrinoma	Peptic ulcers, enhanced acid secretion	Diarrhea, malabsorption, weight loss, dumping	ACTH, insulin, glucagon, VIP, 5-HIAA, MSH, somatostatin, calcitonin, pancreatic polypeptide	40–60	10%	25%
VIPoma	Watery diarrhea, hypokalemia, hypochlorhydria	Hypercalcemia, hyperglycemia, weakness, hypomagnesemia	Pancreatic polypeptide (?), prostaglandins (?)	40	20%	Rare
Glucagonoma	Rash, diabetes, weight loss, anemia	Diarrhea, abdominal pain, thromboembolic disease	Pancreatic polypeptide, 5-HIAA	60	Occasional	Occasional
Somatostatinoma	Diabetes, cholelithiasis, steatorrhea, malabsorption, weight loss	Ingestion, abdominal pain, anemia, diarrhea, ductal obstruction, hypoglycemia (?)	ACTH, gastrin, calcitonin, PGE_2, glucagon, pancreatic polypeptide, VIP, 5-HIAA, substance P	66	None reported	One case (MEN 3)

responsive to steroids, indomethacin, somatostatin, or trifluoperazine, which may be useful in preparing patients for surgery or as a palliative for metastatic disease.

Glucagonoma

CLINICAL PRESENTATION. The glucagonoma syndrome is characterized by a waxing and waning skin rash (necrolytic migratory erythema), diabetes, hypoaminoacidemia, weight loss, and anemia. The classic cutaneous lesion begins as an erythematous base, becomes indurated, and develops superficial central blistering. The blisters then erode and crust over. Healing may be accompanied by hyperpigmentation. This process takes 7 to 14 days with lesions developing in one area while others are resolving. The rash is most prominent on the perineum, along intertriginous folds, and around the mouth and nose. Glossitis, stomatitis, and cheilitis often occur in association with facial lesions. Onycholysis and brittle nails may be present.

Although cutaneous lesions were the hallmark of the first reported cases, the rash is actually present in only two thirds of patients with glucagonoma. The remaining patients usually present because of widespread metastatic disease. Rarely, patients are found during the evaluation of diabetes mellitus or are detected in the course of evaluation for the MEN 1 syndrome.

Frank diabetes occurs in 60 per cent of patients with glucagonoma, and an additional 30 per cent have glucose intolerance. Even in patients with severe hyperglycemia, diabetic ketoacidosis is rarely observed in the glucagonoma syndrome, despite the known ability of glucagon to stimulate hepatic ketogenesis. It is thought that the presence of normal or elevated levels of insulin suppresses lipolysis, limiting the free fatty acid substrates for hepatic ketone production.

Weight loss and anemia are found at the time of diagnosis in half of the patients with glucagonoma. Gastrointestinal symptoms include diarrhea, abdominal pain, and nausea and vomiting. Thromboembolic disease has also been described.

Glucagonoma is infrequently found in the MEN 1 syndrome. However, rare MEN 1 kindreds have been reported in which some members have glucagonoma and others have hyperglucagonemia without clinically detectable tumors. In addition, a familial glucagonoma syndrome has been reported in the absence of other endocrine tumors.

DIAGNOSIS. The diagnosis of glucagonoma is made by detecting elevated levels of glucagon and excluding other conditions associated with hyperglucagonemia, including diabetic ketoacidosis and hyperosmolar syndrome, chronic renal failure, cardiovascular collapse, and cirrhosis of the liver. Normal circulating levels of glucagon are 50 to 150 pg per milliliter. Most patients with glucagonoma have levels in excess of 500 pg per milliliter (occasionally as high as 10,000 pg per milliliter), while glucagon levels in the previously mentioned syndromes average 200 to 500 pg per milliliter.

Once the diagnosis of glucagonoma is confirmed, computed tomography or angiography may be helpful in localizing the tumor and detecting the presence of metastases. At the time of presentation 60 per cent of glucagonomas have metastasized, most commonly to the liver and local lymph nodes.

THERAPY. Surgery is the treatment of choice for glucagonoma confined to the pancreas. Surgery may also be indicated with metastatic disease, as debulking of the tumor mass may ameliorate the glucagonoma syndrome. Streptozotocin, with or without 5-fluorouracil and dacarbazine (DTIC), may induce significant remission. Somatostatin and its long-acting analogues consistently decrease glucagon secretion from glucagonomas. Phenoxybenzamine may also inhibit glucagon secretion from tumors.

The skin rash resolves within a few days of successful surgery and may improve during tumor remission induced by chemotherapy. The immediate cause of the cutaneous lesions is thought to be hypoaminoacidemia, found in 90 per cent of patients with glucagonoma, secondary to enhanced hepatic catabolism of amino acids. An impressive improvement of the rash occurs with hyperalimentation of amino acids, indicating that amino acid deficiency rather than hyperglucagonemia per se may be the basis of the skin lesion.

Somatostatinoma

CLINICAL PRESENTATION. Less than 20 cases of somatostatinoma have been reported; most were found incidentally during laparotomy or during the workup of obstructive jaundice, with identification made retrospectively on the basis of elevated concentrations of somatostatin in the tumor or in the patient's plasma. The tumors contain granules characteristic of D cells.

A syndrome associated with hypersomatostatinemia has been proposed that includes diabetes mellitus, cholelithiasis, steatorrhea with malabsorption, dyspepsia, and significant weight loss. Patients may also have hypochlorhydria, watery diarrhea, anemia, and flushing. The diabetes is usually mild; ketosis has not been described.

The pathophysiology of the syndrome is consistent with the known physiologic and pharmacologic effects of somatostatin. Infusion of somatostatin in man inhibits the release of multiple hormones, including insulin, glucagon, secretin, gastrin, and motilin. Hyperglycemia results from suppression of insulin secretion, but ketosis has not been noted, presumably because of the concomitant inhibition of glucagon secretion. Suppression of secretin, motilin, and gastrin, which decreases hydrochloric acid secretion, gastric emptying, and duodenal motility, tends to cause indigestion and abdominal pain. Inhibition of gallbladder contraction is thought to predispose to cholelithiasis. Malabsorption is produced by inhibition of pancreatic exocrine function.

It is difficult to make the prospective diagnosis of somatostatinoma, as all of these symptoms are nonspecific and are found more commonly in other disorders. The incidence of cholelithiasis is increased in patients with any form of diabetes. Malabsorption may occur in diabetics with chronic pancreatitis. This diagnostic difficulty is further compounded by recent reports of patients with documented somatostatinoma but with none of the components of the proposed syndrome. Three of these patients had severe hypoglycemia and were suspected of having insulinomas. Their tumors also contained small amounts of insulin, and it was proposed that secretion of small amounts of insulin from the tumors with concomitant suppression of compensatory release of glucagon from the normal pancreas resulted in hypoglycemia. Other patients presented with obstructive jaundice; no symptoms of the syndrome were elicited in retrospect.

Somatostatinomas may secrete additional hormones that modify the clinical syndrome. Striking elevations of serum calcitonin can cause watery diarrhea due to the effects of calcitonin on water and electrolyte transport in the gut. Somatostatinomas can produce ACTH, causing Cushing's syndrome. A somatostatinoma accompanied by secretion of prostaglandin E_2 was found in a patient with prominent flushing. A patient with Zollinger-Ellison syndrome was found to have an endocrine tumor of the gut secreting both gastrin and somatostatin. Hyperplasia of cells containing pancreatic polypeptide (resulting in excess secretion of this hormone) has been reported in the presence of somatostatinoma.

DIAGNOSIS. The diagnosis of somatostatinoma is made by detecting elevated basal or stimulated levels of circulating somatostatin. Tolbutamide infusion results in marked elevation of somatostatin in patients with somatostatinoma but not in controls, and has been used to detect tumors in patients with normal basal somatostatin levels.

THERAPY. Two thirds of patients with somatostatinoma have metastases at the time of presentation; this may reflect the difficulty in the clinical diagnosis of this syndrome. Streptozotocin therapy produces regression in tumor size and reduction of plasma somatostatin level.

Other Hormones Produced by Islet Cell Tumors

PANCREATIC POLYPEPTIDE. Islet cell tumors producing pancreatic polypeptide have been associated with watery diarrhea, hypokalemia, and achlorhydria. One patient had normal serum levels of VIP, but pancreatic polypeptide concentration was a thousand times normal. Pancreatic polypeptide has been detected in many endocrine tumors of the pancreas and gut, but most of these tumors usually produce higher levels of another polypeptide hormone.

ACTH. Pancreatic islet cell tumors producing ACTH account for nearly 10 per cent of cases of Cushing's syndrome due to ectopic ACTH production. Such tumors are usually found to secrete multiple hormones, including insulin, gastrin, serotonin, or somatostatin. However, it is more common to find Cushing's *disease* due to a pituitary adenoma associated with other islet cell tumors in patients with MEN type 1.

GROWTH HORMONE–RELEASING FACTOR. Acromegaly has been reported in patients with islet cell tumors secreting growth hormone–releasing factor. Although these patients often have hyperplasia of the growth hormone–secreting cells of the pituitary, it is very difficult to distinguish them from patients with classic acromegaly due to a pituitary adenoma (see Ch. 225). In either case the sella may be normal or enlarged, and growth hormone levels may show paradoxic responses to provocative testing.

SEROTONIN. Production and secretion of serotonin by islet cell tumors has been reported as a cause of the diarrheogenic syndrome. Since VIP levels were not measured, this may represent synthesis of a second hormone by a mixed adenoma. Carcinoid syndrome has also been reported in association with carcinoma of exocrine pancreatic duct cells.

Moossa AR: Tumors of the Pancreas. Baltimore, Williams & Wilkins, 1980. *Includes detailed chapters on the pathology, pathophysiology, radiology, and surgical treatment of islet cell tumors.*

Morrison AB: Islet cell tumors and the diarrheogenic syndrome. Monogr Pathol 21:185, 1980. *A complete review of all definitive and probable cases of the diarrheogenic syndrome.*

Pipeleers D, Couturier E, Gepts W, Reynders J, Sommers G: Five cases of somatostatinoma: Clinical heterogeneity and diagnostic usefulness of basal and tolbutamide-induced hypersomatostatinemia. J Clin Endocrinol Metab 56:1236, 1983. *Four of these patients with documented somatostatinoma showed none of the symptoms of the proposed somatostatinoma syndrome.*

Stacpoole PW: The glucagonoma syndrome. Clinical features, diagnosis and treatment. Endocr Rev 2:347, 1981. *A recent comprehensive review of all cases reported to date.*

233. DISORDERS OF SEXUAL DIFFERENTIATION

Julianne Imperato-McGinley

NORMAL SEXUAL DIFFERENTIATION

The fetus is bipotential for sexual differentiation. The bipotentiality includes the gonad, the internal sex structures, and the external genitalia.

Development of the Bipotential Gonad

In fetuses of both sexes an undifferentiated gonad develops during the fifth week of fetal life. A thickened area of coelomic or germinal epithelium appears on the medial aspect of the mesonephros, and proliferation of germinal epithelium cells and underlying mesenchyme produces a prominence on the medial side of the mesonephros designated the gonadal ridge. Following this, cords of cells known as primary sex cords proliferate from the epithelium into the mesenchyme. The gonad at this stage consists primarily of mesodermal cells of coelomic epithelial origin. The primordial germ cells are visible early in the third week among the endodermal cells of the wall of the yolk sac near the origin of the allantois. They are spherical and larger than mesenchymal cells, with large vesicular nuclei and abundant cytoplasm. During folding of the embryo, part of the yolk sac is incorporated into the embryo, and the primordial germ cells migrate by a combination of ameboid movement and passive transfer along the dorsal mesentery to the gonadal ridges. During migration the germ cells multiply by mitosis. By the fifth week of fetal life they begin to migrate into the underlying mesenchyme, and by the end of the sixth week the undifferentiated or bipotential gonad is formed (Fig. 233–1). The primordial germ cells develop into spermatogonia in the male and ova in the female, the sex cords become either seminiferous tubules or primary ovarian follicles, and the mesenchymal cells form either the Leydig cells or the theca and stromal cells in the female.

Gonadal Differentiation—Development of the Testes and Ovaries

Testicular or seminiferous cords evolve from primary sex cords of the indifferent gonad at approximately the seventh week of gestation in a 15- to 20-mm male embryo (Fig. 233–1). The Sertoli cells differentiate within each cord, enlarge, aggregate, and engulf the germ cells. The distal ends of the seminiferous cords then interconnect to form a network of solid cords, the rete testes, which is in direct contact with the wolffian (mesonephric) ducts. By the sixth month, the ends of the rete testes develop a lumen continuous with the mesonephric tubules, which later develop into the ductuli efferentia. The fetal Leydig cells are apparent by eight weeks of fetal life, and at three months of gestation they completely fill the interstitial spaces.

Ovarian differentiation from the indifferent gonad begins at approximately 50 days of gestation (Fig. 233–1). The primary

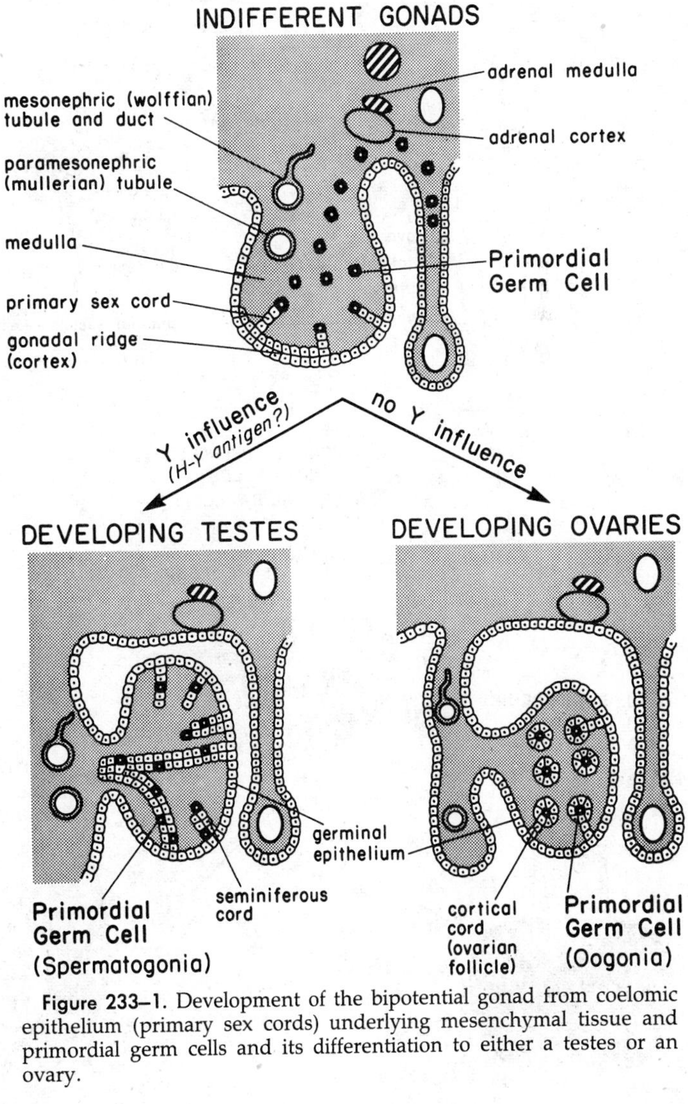

Figure 233–1. Development of the bipotential gonad from coelomic epithelium (primary sex cords) underlying mesenchymal tissue and primordial germ cells and its differentiation to either a testes or an ovary.

sex cords form irregular groups of cells called medullary cords containing primitive granulosa cells that engulf primordial oogonia. The oogonia are in the prophase of meiosis at day 50 to 55. The leptotene stage begins at day 60, the pachytene stage at approximately day 80, and by day 90 the oogonia enter the diplotene stage. As the oogonia differentiate, the primitive granulosa cells organize around them and form a single layer constituting the primordial follicle. Primary follicles are formed when the primordial follicle containing oocytes of the diplotene stage becomes separated by connective tissue. At 18 to 20 weeks of gestation, there are approximately 7 million oogonia and oocytes, whereas at birth the number decreases to approximately 2 million.

Phenotypic Differentiation

Ductal Development

In every fetus, both *wolffian (mesonephric) ducts,* which develop into epididymis, vas deferens, and seminal vesicles in the male, and *müllerian (paramesonephric) ducts,* which develop into fallopian tubes, uterus, and upper third of the vagina in the female, are present (Fig. 233–2). The wolffian ducts appear at 25 to 30 days of gestation, and the müllerian ducts at 44 to 48 days. In the male the initial event is regression of the müllerian ducts, completed at about seven and one half weeks of gestation, followed by stabilization and differentiation of the mesonephric wolffian ducts to form the epididymis, vas deferens, seminal vesicles, and ejaculatory ducts. In the female the wolffian ducts regress at approximately ten and one half weeks, and the müllerian ducts differentiate to form the fallopian tubes, uterus, and upper portion of the vagina.

Development of the External Genitalia

The external genitalia of both sexes (like the gonad) develop from common primordia, the urogenital tubercle, urogenital folds, and urogenital swellings schematically represented in Figure 233–2. In the male, external genital masculinization begins shortly after wolffian ductal differentiation. The urogenital tubercle elongates to become the glans penis, the urogenital folds fuse and become the shaft of the penis, and the urogenital

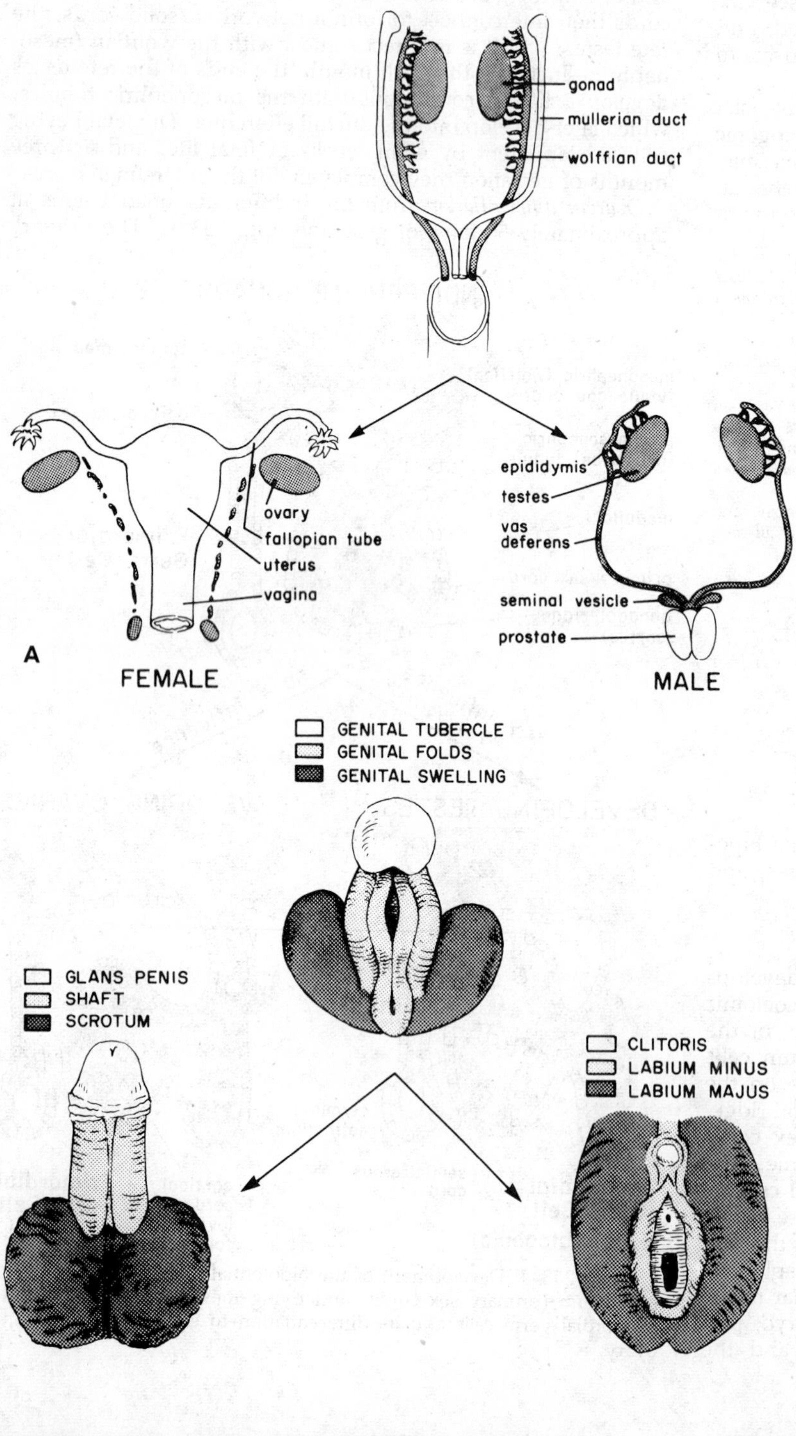

Figure 233–2. Summary of male and female sexual differentiation. *A,* Internal sexual differentiation from wolffian and müllerian ducts. *B,* Development of male and female external genitalia from common primordia.

swellings become the scrotum. The prostate arises from endodermal buds in the urethral lining at 10 weeks and grows into the mesenchyme, which forms the muscular and connective tissue components. Male external sexual differentiation is completed by 14 weeks of gestation. However, descent of the testes and growth of the penis occur between 20 weeks of gestation and term. In the female the urogenital tubercle becomes the clitoris, the urogenital swellings the labia majora, and the urogential folds the labia minora. Female differentiation occurs after the embryo has reached 10½ weeks.

Determinants of Phenotypic Differentiation

Since the fetus is bipotential, what are the determinants of the male or female phenotype?

Female Phenotypic Differentiation

Ovarian tissue containing primary follicles is found in human abortuses with a 45 XO complement. Thus, ovarian differentiation does not appear to require a 46 XX chromosomal complement. Adults, however, with a 45 XO complement no longer have ovarian follicles, and only streak gonads made of whorls of connective tissue remain. Deletion of either the long or short arm of the X chromosome will result in streak gonads. A complete 46 XX complement, therefore, although not necessary for ovarian differentiation, is essential for maintenance of normal ovarian follicular development. Deletion of the short arm of the X chromosome (XXp-) is associated with streaked gonads and the skeletal and somatic anomalies of subjects with 45 XO Turner's syndrome. In contrast, long arm deletions (XXq-) are usually associated with streak gonads and none of the stigmata of Turner's syndrome. See Ch. 236 for a complete discussion of XO and XX gonadal dysgenesis.

In the absence of gonads, either ovaries or testes, the wolffian anlagen regress and the müllerian ducts differentiate to form fallopian tubes, uterus, and upper portion of the vagina, and the external genital primordia differentiate as female (Fig. 233–2). Thus, femaleness appears to be the innate tendency of every fetus and does not require gonadal influence.

Male Phenotypic Differentiation

TESTICULAR DIFFERENTIATION. The development of the male phenotype is more complex; to initiate the process the testes must develop and function normally. Testicular influence is necessary to alter the tendency of the fetus to develop as female. In man, normal testicular differentiation is controlled by the Y chromosome. Analysis of Y chromosome structural abnormalities in man suggests that the short arm (Yp) of the chromosome near the centromere carries the gene(s) directing testicular formation. Simple absence of the (Yp) of the Y chromosome results in a female phenotype, with streak gonads.

What is the mechanism of Y chromosomal control of testicular differentiation? It has been postulated that a testicular organizing substance produced locally by cells within the gonad and under the control of the Y chromosome imposes testicular organogenesis on the gonadal primordium early in gestation, thereby preventing the undifferentiated gonad from developing as an ovary (Fig. 233–3). The inducer substance may be the H-Y histocompatibility antigen, present on the cell surface of individuals with a Y chromosome: (1) Males with two Y chromosomes have more circulating H-Y antigen than normal 46 XY males. (2) In most individuals with Y chromosome deletions the H-Y gene is found on the short arm of the Y chromosome near the centromere, a region known to be testis determining. (3) In general, whenever testicular tissue is found in patients with disorders of sexual development serologic H-Y antigen is detected. Exceptions to the associations have recently been demonstrated, raising the possibility that the H-Y antigen commonly measured in neutralization reactions may not be the only form of testicular organizing factor present.

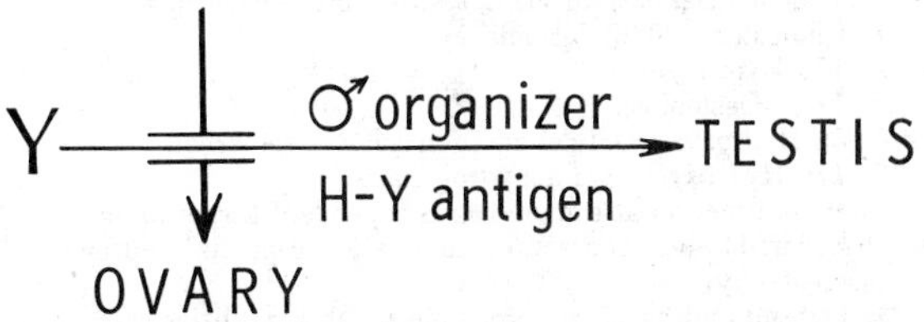

Figure 233–3. Testicular organizing substance under Y chromosome (?H-Y antigen) control imposing testicular organogenesis on the indifferent gonad.

A minimum of three genes may be responsible for H-Y antigen secretion with a fourth gene controlling the gonad-specific H-Y antigen receptor. The H-Y structural gene is hypothesized to be autosomal and under the regulating influence of genes located on both X and Y chromosomes. In the presence of the Y chromosome the H-Y structural gene becomes activated. A regulator gene on the X chromosome that represses the autosomal structural gene is postulated. The action of the X-linked controlling gene must require a 46 XX complement, since a uniplex dose is insufficient for complete repression (XO subjects have been found to be H-Y antigen positive but with an intermediate titer).

DIFFERENTIATION OF MALE GENITAL STRUCTURES. Two secretions from the developing fetal testes are essential for male phenotypic differentiation, testosterone and müllerian inhibiting factor. Responsiveness to both hormones is present only during the critical period of male sexual differentiation, from the eighth to the fourteenth weeks of gestation. In the male fetus at eight weeks of gestational age the histologic appearance of differentiated Leydig cells and the onset of testosterone formation are temporally related and appear to be under the stimulation of placental chorionic gonadotropin. The initiation of testicular testosterone formation from the Leydig cells coincides with wolffian differentiation and differentiation of the male external genitalia. However, for differentiation of the external genitalia, testosterone acts as a prohormone and is converted to 5α-dihydrotestosterone by the microsomal enzyme, steroid Δ^4 5α-reductase.

Thus, testosterone and its metabolite dihydrotestosterone are essential for sexual differentiation in the male fetus, with selective roles for each hormone during embryogenesis. Testosterone acting locally mediates differentiation of the wolffian ductal system to the vas deferens, epididymis, and seminal vesicles, while the local conversion of testosterone to dihydrotestosterone mediates development of male external genitalia and prostate (Fig. 233–4). Male pseudohermaphrodites with 5α-reductase deficiency and decreased dihydrotestosterone production (see Male Pseudohermaphroditism) have defined the necessity for dihydrotestosterone in the formation of male external genitalia and prostate and have delineated specific actions for the two androgens in utero.

Both testosterone and dihydrotestosterone bind to the same high-affinity androgen receptor protein within the cells of androgen-dependent target areas. Testosterone enters the target cell by a process of passive diffusion and either binds to a cytoplasmic receptor or is converted to dihydrotestosterone, which binds to the receptor. This androgen receptor complex then binds to acceptor sites in nuclear chromatin and ultimately initiates transcription of messenger ribonucleic acid (RNA), resulting in the complex metabolic processes of androgen action (Ch. 221).

The inhibition of the müllerian anlage is not under androgen control; müllerian inhibiting factor, a high molecular weight glycoprotein, is a product of the Sertoli cells of the seminiferous tubules. Its secretion begins shortly after the initiation of seminiferous tubular differentiation and continues through the perinatal period.

In summary, normal male phenotypic development requires that the testes differentiate and function normally, so that at a critically sensitive period in utero (8 to 14 weeks) müllerian

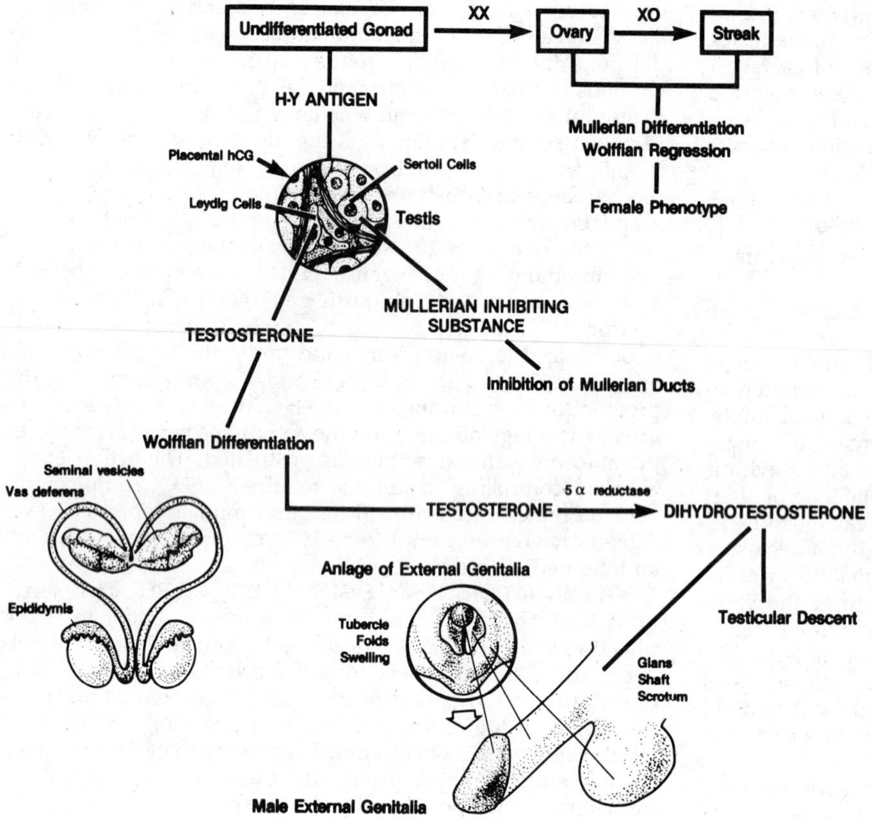

Figure 233–4. Schematic representation of the factors involved in male and female sexual differentiation.

inhibiting factor, secreted by the Sertoli cells, and testosterone, secreted by the Leydig cells, are produced in sufficient amounts. Müllerian inhibiting factor, acting locally, suppresses the müllerian anlage, and testosterone, also acting locally, causes differentiation of the wolffian anlage to epididymis, vas deferens, and seminal vesicles. Testosterone circulates and is converted by the enzyme 5α-reductase to dihydrotestosterone in the cells of the urogenital tubercle, urogenital sinus, and urogenital folds, resulting in differentiation of the male external genitalia (Fig. 233–4). Depending upon specific target tissue, either testosterone or dihydrotestosterone complexes with the cytoplasmic receptor, and this receptor-hormone complex is transferred to the nucleus to initiate androgen action.

Genetic Control of Male Sexual Differentiation

The multifactorial process of male sexual differentiation is under complex genetic control. Testicular differentiation requires the presence of gene(s) normally found on the Y chromosome. The enzymes involved in testosterone biosynthesis, as well as the the enzyme 5α-reductase converting testosterone to dihydrotestosterone, are known to be regulated by genes located on the autosomes. Genes located on the X chromosome control the cytoplasmic receptor at the androgen-dependent target areas. Inherited forms of müllerian inhibiting factor deficiency are transmitted as a recessive trait, either autosomal or X linked. Thus, normal male phenotypic development is regulated by multiple genes located on the autosomes as well as both X and Y chromosomes.

Austin CR, Edwards RG (eds.): Mechanisms of Sex Differentiation in Animals and Man. New York, Academic Press, 1981. *All aspects of sexual differentiation are covered. Chapters 4 and 5 are particularly informative.*

Wachtel S: H-Y Antigen and the Biology of Sex Determination. New York, Grune & Stratton, 1983. *The state of the art concerning H-Y antigen and sexual differentiation.*

ABNORMALITIES OF SEXUAL DIFFERENTIATION

Male Pseudohermaphroditism

The known etiologic factors in male pseudohermaphroditism or incomplete masculinization can be divided into three basic categories: (1) disorders of testicular differentiation and development; (2) disorders of testicular function; and (3) disorders of function at the androgen-dependent target areas. Table 233–1 lists the specific clinical entities within each category.

Disorders of Testicular Differentiation and Development

XY GONADAL DYSGENESIS. *Clinical Presentation.* Subjects with pure gonadal dysgenesis have a 46 XY chromosomal complement, but are phenotypic females with primary amenorrhea, tall stature, eunuchoidal proportions, and scant axillary and pubic hair. A uterus and fallopian tubes are present, and

TABLE 233–1. CLASSIFICATION OF THE CAUSES OF MALE PSEUDOHERMAPHRODITISM

I. Disorders of testicular differentiation and development
 A Testicular dysgenesis, affecting both Leydig cell and seminiferous tubule development
  1. Y chromosomal abnormalities
  2. XY gonadal dysgenesis
  3. XO/XY gonadal dysgenesis
  4. Testicular regression syndrome
 B. Leydig cell agenesis or dysgenesis—selective absence or decrease in Leydig cell differentiation and function—seminiferous tubule embryogenesis occurring normally
  1. Abnormality of the HCG-LH receptor: absence of precursor Leydig cell
II. Disorders of testicular function
 A. Abnormalities of müllerian inhibiting factor synthesis—persistent müllerian duct syndrome
 B. Enzyme deficiencies affecting testosterone biosynthesis
  1. Cholesterol 20,22-desmolase
  2. 17α-Hydroxylase
  3. 17,20-Desmolase
  4. 3β-Hydroxysteroid dehydrogenase:Δ^{5-4} isomerase
  5. 17β-Hydroxysteroid dehydrogenase
III. Disorders of function at the androgen-dependent target areas
 A. Disorders of androgen action (complete and partial androgen insensitivity)
  1. Cytosol androgen–receptor binding abnormalities
  2. Post cytosol androgen–receptor binding abnormalities
 B. Disorders of testosterone metabolism
  1. 5α-Reductase deficiency

streak gonads are found. In the incomplete forms of this condition, variable amounts of functional testicular tissue are found, and consequently at birth the subjects frequently have clitoromegaly, ambiguous genitalia, or, rarely, a penile urethra. Virilization at puberty is also variable. In pure gonadal dysgenesis, postpubertal gonadotropins are increased and in the castrate range with female levels of testosterone. However, when functioning testicular tissue is present, testosterone can be increased from slightly above the female level to a low normal male level. Additionally, if müllerian inhibiting factor is produced there may be partial or complete absence of müllerian structures (Fig. 233–5).

Pathophysiology. In pure gonadal dysgenesis the testes do not differentiate at all, and in the absence of a functional testis phenotypic development is female, with wolffian duct regression and müllerian differentiation. In the incomplete forms there is variable testicular development with varying degrees of fetal masculinization. The etiology of this condition is unknown, but it could be due to a number of theoretic causes involving testicular organizing substance (H-Y antigen). There could be a lack of, or decreased secretion of, testicular organizing substance, abnormalities in its structure, or lack or decrease in its gonadal specific receptor. Interestingly, serologic analyses of subjects with pure gonadal dysgenesis have revealed a negative H-Y antigen titer in some subjects, while others have a positive titer, suggesting genetic heterogeneity. Since H-Y antigen has been postulated to be the testicular organizing substance, the presence of streaked gonads in H-Y antigen-positive individuals has been explained by either postulating a defect in the gonadal receptor for testicular organizing H-Y antigen or by postulating the presence of a structurally inactive form of H-Y antigen.

Approximately 13 familial cases of pure gonadal dysgenesis have been described, and inheritance appears to be either X-linked recessive or autosomal dominant–sex limited. Within families there may be variable expressivity of the gene defect, with some sibs having the pure form and a female phenotype and others with ambiguous genitalia.

Management and Therapy. The streak gonads should be removed since approximately 20 to 30 per cent of subjects will develop gonadoblastomas or dysgerminomas within the streak gonads. Dysgerminomas may be malignant, and approximately 5 to 8 per cent of gonadoblastomas also contain malignant elements. In pure gonadal dysgenesis, infants are invariably reared as female and come to the attention of the physician at puberty because of lack of secondary sexual development. Estrogen and progesterone replacement therapy should be instituted after prophylactic removal of the streak gonads. In complete forms, the child should be reared in the sex that will be more functional, and appropriate surgical correction of the genitalia carried out. Intra-abdominal testicular tissue should always be removed because of the increased risk of malignancy.

MIXED GONADAL DYSGENESIS. ***Clinical Presentation.*** Classically, subjects with mixed gonadal dysgenesis have a streak gonad on one side and a testis on the contralateral side. Most demonstrate XO/XY mosaicism on chromosomal analysis. The phenotypic spectrum ranges from phenotypic females, with or without the clinical characteristics of Turner's syndrome, to subjects with ambiguous genitalia, to normal phenotypic males. The genitalia are sufficiently ambiguous in most affected subjects that approximately two thirds are raised as girls, with the stigmata of Turner's syndrome occurring in one third. Affected subjects have a uterus, and most have bilateral fallopian tubes. The vas deferens, if present, is on the side of the testis, and frequently a fallopian tube also exists adjacent to the vas deferens. Virilization generally occurs at puberty. The testes appear histologically normal before puberty. However, after puberty the seminiferous tubules demonstrate thickened walls and contain few if any germ cells. Consequently, affected subjects are infertile. If pubertal gynecomastia occurs, a gonadal tumor should be suspected.

Pathogenesis. XO/XY mosaicism in subjects with this condition can be best explained as resulting from mitotic nondisjunction or anaphase lag, resulting in loss of the Y chromosome. Perhaps the lack of testicular differentiation of the streak gonad is related to the preponderance of the XO cell line in that gonad. Despite good Leydig cell function with virilization at puberty, the testis must have been functionally dysgenetic (between the eighth to fourteenth weeks of gestation—the critically responsive period) as evidenced by absence of or incomplete virilization of the external genitalia. Theoretically a delay in testicular differentiation and function in utero could result in delayed secretion of testosterone and müllerian inhibiting factor, completely or partially missing the critically responsive period and resulting in the presence of female or ambiguous genitalia and müllerian structures.

There are subjects with an XO/XY chromosomal complement and bilaterally streaked gonads as well as XO/XY subjects with bilateral testes. Thus the classic clinical syndrome of mixed gonadal dysgenesis may be one clinical entity in a spectrum ranging from streaked gonads and a female phenotype to varied abnormalities of testicular development (symmetric or asym-

ABNORMALITIES OF TESTICULAR DIFFERENTIATION SECONDARY TO Y CHROMOSOME ABNORMALITIES

	Deletion of Y chromosome	Deletion of short arm of Y chromosome	Gene mutation(s) of short arm of Y chromosome (nonvisible damage)	Phenotype
Bilateral streaked gonads (gonadal dysgenesis)	XO	XY(p-)	XY	Female
↕	XY ⇅ XO	XY(p-) ⇅ XY	↕	
Asymmetric gonadal dysgenesis (MGD)	XO/XY	XY(p-)/XY	XY	Male
↕	XY ⇅ XO	XY(p-) ⇅ XY	↕	
Bilateral dysgenetic testes	XO/XY	XY(p-)/XY	XY	Pseudohermaphroditism
↕	XY ⇅ XO	XY(p-) ⇅ XY	↕	
Bilateral testes	XY	XY	XY	Normal male

Figure 233–5. Abnormalities of testicular differentiation secondary to Y chromosomal defects.

metric) and genital ambiguity, possibly depending upon the preponderance of a particular cell line, either XO or XY, within the gonad at the time of differentiation (Fig. 233–5).

Management and Therapy. Because of the increased incidence of tumor formation, an intra-abdominal testis that cannot be brought into the scrotum should be removed as well as the streak gonad. If the subject is being raised as male, a scrotal testis should be preserved. In instances in which the testes cannot be brought to the scrotum and must be removed, or the external genitalia are severely ambiguous, or both conditions exist, the sex of rearing should be female and appropriate genital surgery performed.

XY AGONADISM, TESTICULAR REGRESSION, OR VANISHING TESTES SYNDROME. *Clinical Presentation.* Typically these subjects are 46 XY phenotypic females presenting with a total absence of gonads and no müllerian or wolffian internal structures. The lack of müllerian structures, together with a total lack of gonadal remnants, separates this entity from pure XY gonadal dysgenesis. The condition appears to be secondary to regression of the differentiating testis before the onset of androgen secretion, resulting in lack of wolffian differentiation, but after the onset of secretion of müllerian inhibiting factor, resulting in inhibition of female internal structures. There is, however, a phenotypic spectrum of agonadal subjects perhaps related to testicular regression occurring at various times, during or after the critical period of male sexual differentiation. Affected subjects can therefore vary widely in phenotypes: from those with total absence of internal sex structures and female external genitalia, to subjects with ambiguous genitalia, to normal males with absent testes and a microphallus.

Pathophysiology. The etiology of the testicular regression is unknown. These subjects are unequivocally 46 XY, and chromosomal abnormalities have never been demonstrated. Familial cases of agonadism in XY subjects occur, however, suggesting that in some cases it may be an inherited condition. Variable phenotypic expression in agonadal siblings from the same kindred also occurs suggesting that this condition is a clinical, spectrum due to the time of regression of the embryonic testes.

LEYDIG CELL AGENESIS OR DYSGENESIS, GONADOTROPIN UNRESPONSIVENESS. *Clinical Characteristics.* Adult subjects with Leydig cell agenesis or dysgenesis have either normal female external genitalia or slight posterior fusion of the labia majora and have been raised as females. Two prepubertal cases have been described, one with totally female genitalia and the other with a bifid scrotum, a clitoral-like phallus, and a urogenital sinus. An epididymis and vas deferens are present in all affected subjects, indicating that little testosterone is needed at a critical period to initiate wolffian differentiation. No müllerian structures are found, confirming the fact that müllerian inhibiting factor is not secreted by the Leydig cells, but is secreted by the Sertoli cells of the seminiferous tubules. In the adults, normal appearing Sertoli cells with few spermatogonia and few or no Leydig cells are present in the testis.

Pathophysiology. In adult cases, plasma androgen levels are in the female range and do not significantly change with administration of human chorionic gonadotropin (HCG). Luteinizing hormone (LH) levels are significantly elevated, while follicle-stimulating hormone (FSH) levels are in the normal range. In the children, there is no demonstrable plasma androgen response to administration of HCG.

Theoretically the absence or decrease in Leydig cells can result from (1) an absence of or decrease in precursor cells destined to become functioning Leydig cells under HCG-LH stimulation or (2) a decrease in the HCG-LH receptor or receptor response of the precursor Leydig cells. It can also be theorized that the HCG-LH receptor mediates Leydig cell differentiation, and without these receptors, precursor Leydig cells are not formed. A complete phenotypic spectrum of subjects with this disorder can be anticipated, dependent upon the severity of the developmental defect.

Management and Therapy. Those subjects in whom the diagnosis is made in infancy or early childhood should be raised in the sex in which they will be more apt to function normally. In most instances this would be as female because of the severe genital ambiguity. Thus the testes should be removed and corrective genital surgery performed.

Those subjects in whom the diagnosis is made in adulthood who were raised as females and have a female gender identity should have the testes removed, and female sex hormone therapy should be instituted to induce and maintain breast development.

Disorders of Testicular Function

In disorders of testicular function, the testes have differentiated normally, but there is an abnormality in the secretion of either müllerian inhibiting factor or testosterone.

MÜLLERIAN INHIBITING FACTOR DEFICIENCY. *Clinical Presentation.* Males with this condition have a uterus and bilateral fallopian tubes. They have bilateral testes with normal male differentiation of wolffian structures and external genitalia and undergo normal male puberty. This entity most frequently occurs as unilateral cryptorchidism with a contralateral inguinal hernia containing müllerian structures, "uteri inguinale," and a testis. The presence of the inguinal hernia most often brings affected males to a physician's attention. Although fertility has been described, azoospermia is frequently noted. More than 70 cases of this entity have been reported, including at least 8 families with 2 affected sibs. The majority of pedigree studies suggest an X-linked or autosomal recessive inheritance. In one family study, however, inheritance was compatible with X-linked or autosomal dominant inheritance. In approximately 5 per cent of affected patients, either seminomas or other germ cell tumors occur.

Pathogenesis. This entity could be due to a number of abnormalities affecting the synthesis, structure, timing of secretion, or action of müllerian inhibiting factor. Documentation of the actual biochemical abnormality will have to await characterization of the factor or its receptor. The ultimate effect is lack of suppression of the müllerian anlage resulting in the presence of a uterus. Androgen secretion is adequate during the critical period of sexual differentiation, with normal sexual differentiation of the wolffian ducts and external genitalia.

Management and Therapy. In affected males the müllerian structures should be surgically removed if they are in the inguinal canal. Since malignant change in müllerian structures has never been reported, surgical removal is not necessary if they are located in the abdomen. The cryptorchid testes should be brought into the scrotal sac as early as possible and the patient examined frequently for the development of testicular tumors.

Imperato-McGinley J: Sexual differentiation–Normal and abnormal. Curr Top Exp Endocrinol 5:231–307, 1983. *Of particular interest in this review is the section on male pseudohermaphroditism, including an up-to-date bibliography for each clinical entity described.*

DEFICIENCIES OF TESTOSTERONE BIOSYNTHESIS. *Clinical Features.* Five enzymatic reactions convert cholesterol to testosterone; deficiencies of all have been described. These enzyme deficiencies constitute the nonvirilizing forms of the adrenogenital syndrome. The five enzymatic steps include (1) cholesterol 20,22-desmolase, (2) 3β-hydroxysteroid dehydrogenase:Δ^{5-4}isomerase, (3) 17α-hydroxylase, (4) 17,20-desmolase, and (5) 17β-hydroxysteroid dehydrogenase (Fig. 233–6). A deficiency of the enzymes cholesterol 20,22-desmolase and 3β-hydroxysteroid dehydrogenase:Δ^{5-4} isomerase also impairs production of aldosterone and cortisol. 17α-Hydroxylase deficiency impairs cortisol production, while 17,20-desmolase and 17β-hydroxysteroid dehydrogenase deficiencies affect only androgen biosynthesis. Since androgens are the precursors of estrogens, it follows that estrogen production is also low in all of the enzyme deficiencies except 17β-hydroxysteroid dehydrogenase (Table 233–2). These disorders appear to be inherited as autosomal recessive traits. Genotypic females are phenotypically normal at birth, with the exception of females with 3β-

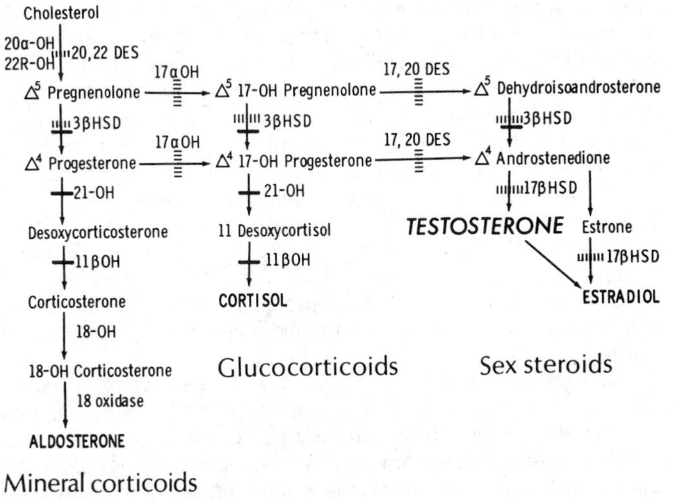

Figure 233–6. Congenital adrenal hyperplasia. *A,* Enzyme deficiencies resulting in male pseudohermaphroditism. Cholesterol 20,22-desmolase, 17α-hydroxylase, 3β-hydroxysteroid dehydrogenase:Δ^{5-4} isomerase, 17,20-desmolase, 17β-hydroxysteroid dehydrogenase. *B,* Enzyme deficiences resulting in female pseudohermaphroditism. 21-hydroxylase, 11β-hydroxylase, 3β-hydroxysteroid dehydrogenase:Δ^{5-4} isomerase. (DES = desmolase; OH = hydroxylase; HSD = hydroxysteroid dehydrogenase.)

hydroxysteroid dehydrogenase deficiency, who may be mildly virilized.

The testes differentiate normally, and normal amounts of müllerian inhibiting factor are secreted, so that no müllerian structures are present. However, the impaired secretion of testosterone by Leydig cells at the critical period of sexual differentiation in utero (8 to 14 weeks of gestation) causes ambiguity of the external genitalia. Wolffian differentiation is usually normal. In general, the severity of the enzyme defect is reflected in the degree of external genital ambiguity at birth and the amount of virilization at puberty. Each specific enzyme deficiency, however, may show considerable variation in clinical presentation, and affected males with the same enzyme deficiency may present with totally female external genitalia or as males with mild hypospadias and cryptorchidism.

The possible causes for the abnormalities of enzymatic function include mutant genes at structural loci coding for the amino acid sequences of the enzymes changing the enzyme structure and altering its catalytic efficiency, or mutations at sites other than the structural loci. These mutations can be classified as *regulatory,* altering the rate of synthesis or degradation of the enzyme; *architectural,* affecting incorporation of enzyme molecules into active sites in the cell; or *temporal,* affecting the development of the tissue or the time of activation of regulatory systems.

Congenital Lipoid Adrenal Hyperplasia (Cholesterol 20,22-Desmolase Deficiency). In 1957, a genetic male from a consanguineous marriage was described with wolffian differentiation but with female external genitalia. The infant died in adrenal crisis at 6 days of age, and at autopsy the adrenals showed enormous accumulation of lipids in the cortical cells. Consequently the disorder was labeled congenital lipoid adrenal hyperplasia. Subsequent autopsy reports of other affected genotypic male infants have confirmed that the large, yellowish adrenals contain cells with foamy, spongy cytoplasm and stain positively for lipids.

The affected genotypic males have abdominal or inguinal testes with wolffian differentiation. There are no müllerian structures. The external genitalia are either female or severely ambiguous. As would be expected, genotypic female infants have normal female internal and external accessory sex organs.

Approximately 20 cases have been described with equal numbers of both sexes affected. Most of the affected have died in adrenal crisis in infancy, because of severe deficiencies of glucocorticoid and mineralocorticoid production. Only two children have survived to early childhood, a six-year-old male pseudohermaphrodite and an eight-year-old phenotypic female but genetic and gonadal male. Both children had severe adrenal insufficiency in infancy, and congenital adrenal hypoplasia was diagnosed. It was only with reevaluation in childhood, when they were found to have testes, that the correct diagnosis was established.

PATHOGENESIS. A deficiency in the conversion of cholesterol to pregnenolone results in decreased glucocorticoid, mineralocorticoid, and sex steroid production (Fig. 233–6). All plasma steroid values are low to unmeasurable, and little or no urinary 17-ketosteroids, 17-hydroxysteroids, or aldosterone is found (Table 233–2). In the conversion of cholesterol to pregnenolone, at least three enzymes are involved: 20α-hydroxylase, 22α-hydroxylase and 20,22-desmolase. These reactions are mitochondrial mixed-function oxidase reactions requiring a flavoprotein and non-heme iron protein that function in the transport of electrons from NADPH to cytochrome P-450 as the terminal enzyme. A cytochrome P-450 enzyme of the adrenal cortex has been shown to catalyze the formation of pregnenolone from cholesterol, 20α-hydroxycholesterol, 22R- and 22S-hydroxycholesterol, or 20,22-dihydroxycholesterol.

TABLE 233–2. XY MALE PSEUDOHERMAPHRODITISM WITH AN ENZYMATIC DEFECT IN TESTOSTERONE BIOSYNTHESIS

	Genitalia		Secretion				
Enzyme Deficiency	*Female or urogenital sinus*	*Ambiguous*	*Cortisol*	*Aldosterone*	*Androgens*	**Puberty**	**Comments**
Cholesterol 20,22-desmolase	+ + + +	+	↓	↓	↓	↓	
3β-Hydroxysteroid dehydrogenase:Δ^{5-4} isomerase	+	+ + + +	↓	↓	↑ DHEA	Gynecomastia despite low estrogens	Intact peripheral 3βHSD with conversion of Δ^5 to Δ^4 steroids
17α-Hydroxylase	+ + + +	+ +	↓	B ↑ DOC ↑	↓	Gynecomastia despite low estrogens	Hypertension due to ↑ DOC with ↓ renin and aldosterone
17,20-Desmolase	+ + + +	+	—	—	↓		
17β-Hydroxysteroid dehydrogenase	+ + + +	+ +	—	—	↓ T ↑ Δ^4	Gynecomastia due to increased estrogen and decreased T	Peripheral conversion of androstenedione to E_1

↑ elevated; ↓ decreased; — normal; + relative frequency of occurrence; B = corticosterone; DOC = desoxycorticosterone; DHEA = dehydroepiandrosterone; T = testosterone; Δ^4 = androstenedione; 3βHSD = 3β-hydroxysteroid dehydrogenase; E_1 = estrone

In a study of adrenal tissue from a child who died with this condition, a deficiency of the enzyme 20α-hydroxylase was suggested as the cause. In another study of adrenal tissue from an affected infant, partial deficiency of cytochrome P-450, with decreased cholesterol 20,22-desmolase activity, was demonstrated. Thus there may be genetic heterogeneity in the expression of this disorder. Theoretically a deficiency of any of the three enzymes or cofactors could result in decreased conversion of cholesterol to pregnenolone.

MANAGEMENT AND THERAPY. In the newborn, signs of adrenal insufficiency with hyperkalemia and hyponatremia occur within the first two weeks, and this condition must be distinguished from 3β-hydroxysteroid dehydrogenase deficiency or congenital adrenal hypoplasia. In a phenotypic female infant, or an infant with ambiguous genitalia and adrenal insufficiency, demonstration of a 46 XY karyotype or demonstration of enlarged adrenals by a radiographic technique will help distinguish this condition from congenital adrenal hypoplasia. The finding of low urinary 17-ketosteroids and low plasma dehydroepiandrosterone levels will distinguish it from 3β-hydroxysteroid dehydrogenase deficiency. Once the diagnosis is established, glucocorticoid and mineralocorticoid therapy should be immediately instituted and is essential for survival. In genotypic males, sex hormone therapy should be instituted at puberty in accordance with the sex of rearing. In most instances, because of the severity of the genital defect, the sex of rearing would be female. Genotypic females will also require appropriate female sex hormone therapy at puberty.

3β-Hydroxysteroid Dehydrogenase:Δ^{5-4} Isomerase Deficiency. CLINICAL PRESENTATION. In 1961 the first three cases of 3β-hydroxysteroid dehydrogenase:Δ^{5-4} isomerase deficiency were described in both males and females. Affected 46 XY subjects had genital ambiguity, although mild to moderate hypospadias is more common than severe perineoscrotal hypospadias. Internal male sexual differentiation is normal, with wolffian differentiation and müllerian ductal inhibition. Curiously, genetic males who reach puberty develop gynecomastia, the etiology of which is not known. At birth affected females have normal or slightly virilized external genitalia, with clitoral hypertrophy and slight labial fusion.

Severely affected children have adrenal insufficiency and die in infancy as a result of salt-losing crisis if not adequately treated. In the milder cases sufficient cortisol and aldosterone are synthesized and consequently adrenal insufficiency is not present in infancy. A mild deficiency of the enzyme has recently been described in a genotypic female with primary amenorrhea, breast development, hirsutism, and clitoromegaly at puberty. Treatment of the adrenal defect by administration of glucocorticoids resulted in the onset of menstruation with ovulation, suggesting that the amenorrhea was secondary to the suppressive effect of excess circulating adrenal androgens on gonadotropins and that the enzymatic defect within the ovary was mild. A very subtle enzyme deficiency may be present in some women with hirsutism and menstrual irregularities.

PATHOGENESIS. In the adrenal the enzyme deficiency ultimately results in decreased cortisol production, which causes increased ACTH secretion and consequent increased production of Δ^5,3β-hydroxysteroids (Fig. 233–6). Plasma levels of pregnenolone, 17α-hydroxypregnenolone, and dehydroepiandrosterone and their sulfate conjugates are usually increased, with decreased levels of aldosterone and cortisol. The slight virilization of the external genitalia in the female is most probably due to the mild androgenic effect of the excess plasma dehydroepiandrosterone or its subsequent peripheral conversion to Δ^5-androstenediol and other androgens (Table 233–2). Surprisingly, plasma Δ^4 steroids, i.e., progesterone, 17α-hydroxyprogesterone, androstenedione, and occasionally testosterone, may be normal or even increased. These findings have been interpreted as reflecting intact hepatic and peripheral 3β-hydroxysteroid dehydrogenase:Δ^{5-4} isomerase enzyme activity. Also in some affected subjects, the gonadal defect is not as severe as the adrenal defect. Thus the same enzyme may be under different genetic control in different areas, or there may be different isoenzymes within the adrenal, gonad, and liver.

MANAGEMENT AND THERAPY. In infancy the diagnosis is suggested in a 46 XY male with ambiguous genitalia and adrenal insufficiency. In distinction to an infant with cholesterol 20,22-desmolase deficiency, urinary 17-ketosteroid values are normal to high with increased plasma dehydroepiandrosterone. Treatment involves mineralocorticoid and glucocorticoid replacement therapy, as in cholesterol 20,22-desmolase deficiency. If needed, sex steroid therapy should be instituted at puberty to induce sexual development in accordance with the sex of rearing.

17α-Hydroxylase Deficiency. CLINICAL PRESENTATION. The first case of 17α-hydroxylase deficiency, described in 1966, was in a 35-year-old genetic and phenotypic female with a lack of secondary sexual development, hypertension, and hypokalemic alkalosis. Since then, many cases have been reported in both genetic males and females. In 46 XY subjects the defect of the external genitalia is usually severe, resulting in completely female external genitalia at birth. Müllerian structures are absent, and wolffian structures are either developed or hypoplastic. Often gynecomastia develops at puberty with little or no virilization. Thus, males with this enzyme deficiency can have the same phenotype in adulthood as subjects with the complete androgen insensitivity syndrome. In 46 XX females with this condition secondary sexual development is absent at puberty and there is primary amenorrhea. Classically the affected subjects also have hypertension and hypokalemia.

PATHOGENESIS. The enzyme 17α-hydroxylase converts pregnenolone and progesterone to 17α-hydroxypregenolone and 17α-hydroxyprogesterone, respectively (Fig. 233–6). These enzymatic steps are necessary for the ultimate formation of cortisol and C19 androgens, including testosterone. Thus a deficiency results in decreased plasma cortisol, with an increase in ACTH and hypersecretion of the plasma precursor 17-deoxysteroids (pregnenolone, progesterone, desoxycorticosterone, corticosterone, 18-hydroxycorticosterone) and increased excretion of their urinary metabolites. Those steroids requiring 17α-hydroxylation are decreased, i.e., plasma 17α-hydroxypregnenolone, 17α-hydroxyprogesterone, 11-deoxycortisol, cortisol, androstenedione, dehydroepiandrosterone, testosterone, and estrogen. Consequently, urinary levels of 17-hydroxysteroids and 17-ketosteroids are low. Despite markedly impaired cortisol production, signs of glucocorticoid deficiency do not generally occur, because of the inherent glucocorticoid activity in the high levels of circulating corticosterone. Excess circulating desoxycorticosterone results in increased sodium retention with increased plasma volume, resulting in hypertension, hypokalemia, and suppression of plasma renin. The plasma aldosterone value is also low secondary to a low level of plasma renin (Table 233–2).

In affected adults, gonadotropin values are elevated, sex steroid levels are low, and in the male there is little or no testicular 17α-hydroxyprogesterone and testosterone response to HCG administration. Consanguinity has been documented in some cases, as has an occurrence of the disorder in siblings of both the same and opposite sex, supporting an autosomal recessive mode of inheritance.

MANAGEMENT AND THERAPY. Hypertension associated with hypokalemic alkalosis in an XY individual with female external genitalia or ambiguous genitalia should suggest the diagnosis. It should also be suspected in any XX female with the same symptom complex who has primary amenorrhea and lack of secondary sexual development. Glucocorticoid replacement therapy is administered to reverse the metabolic abnormality and lower the blood pressure. Appropriate sex steroid therapy concordant with the sex of rearing should be administered at puberty.

17β-Hydroxysteroid Dehydrogenase Deficiency. CLINICAL PRESENTATION. The first case of 17β-hydroxysteroid dehydrogenase deficiency was described in 1965. To date, this condition has been described only in 46 XY males. Affected subjects have either female external genitalia or mild ambiguity of the genitalia and, with few exceptions, were raised as girls. In subjects with totally female appearing external genitalia at birth, the abnormality is not noted until puberty, when virilization frequently occurs with clitoral enlargement. At puberty there are two distinct clinical presentations. Some subjects develop gynecomastia in addition to virilization, while others undergo strong virilization with a male pattern of body hair, deep voice, android build, and no gynecomastia. All subjects raised as females throughout childhood who were castrated prior to or during their teenage years have maintained a female gender identity. However 5 of 6 individuals, from four different kindreds, who were not castrated changed gender identity from female to male with virilization at puberty; also 7 of 25 affected subjects, from a large Arab kindred, with this condition changed gender role from female to male with the hormonal events of puberty.

PATHOGENESIS. 17β-Hydroxysteroid dehydrogenase is a microsomal enzyme catalyzing the conversion of androstenedione to testosterone, the final step in the synthesis of testosterone (Fig. 233–6). It also catalyzes the oxidation-reduction of estrone and estradiol, dehydroepiandrosterone, and Δ^5-androstenediol. The enzyme is not restricted to the adrenal and gonads, but is present in many tissues of the body. In affected 46 XY subjects, the enzyme deficiency results in increased circulating plasma levels of androstenedione, while plasma levels of testosterone are low to low normal (Table 233–2). Plasma luteinizing hormone is increased, while plasma follicle-stimulating hormone is normal to increased. Spermatic vein blood demonstrates an abnormally elevated ratio of androstenedione to testosterone. Approximately 90 per cent of circulating testosterone arises from the extragonadal conversion of androstenedione. Thus in the adult the defect appears to affect the testes while peripheral enzyme activity appears to be intact. However, for masculinization of the external genitalia to be minimal or absent in the fetus, peripheral conversion of androstenedione to testosterone and dihydrotestosterone in the anlage of the external genitalia must be insignificant or absent during early gestation. Thus, peripheral as well as testicular 17β-hydroxysteroid dehydrogenase activity appears deficient in utero, whereas peripheral enzyme activity appears to be intact in the adult. The elevated plasma levels of androstenedione result in increased peripheral conversion to estrone (Table 233–2). In some subjects the conversion of estrone to estradiol also appears to be as severely impaired as the conversion of androstenedione to testosterone, while in others it is impaired to a lesser degree or not at all suggesting that the 17β-hydroxysteroid dehydrogenase enzyme(s) converting estrone to estradiol and androstenedione to testosterone may be under different regulatory control. The lower the plasma testosterone-estradiol ratio, the greater the likelihood of gynecomastia developing in an affected subject at the time of puberty.

MANAGEMENT AND THERAPY. 46 XY affected subjects with female external genitalia should be raised as females and castration carried out either before or during early puberty to avoid significant virilization. Female sex hormone therapy should be instituted at puberty. In those subjects with ambiguous genitalia that can be surgically corrected, a male sex of rearing should be considered. If the diagnosis is made peripubertally or postpubertally, careful psychosexual evaluation should be performed to determine the gender identity before any therapy is instituted. If a gender change from female to male has occurred with puberty, corrective male genital surgery is needed.

17,20-Desmolase Deficiency. CLINICAL PRESENTATION. In 1972 a child with male ambiguous genitalia was described with a defect postulated to be secondary to 17,20-desmolase deficiency. A male pseudohermaphroditic cousin and maternal 46 XY "aunt" were included in the report. Since then nine cases of the enzyme deficiency in 46 XY males have been reported, all phenotypic females or subjects with severely ambiguous genitalia. Recently the first case of a genetic female with primary amenorrhea and lack of secondary sexual development has been reported.

PATHOGENESIS. Partial or complete lack of the enzyme 17,20-desmolase in the adrenal and gonads results in decreased cleavage of the two-carbon side chain from either 17α-hydroxyprogesterone or 17α-hydroxypregnenolone with a resultant decrease in androstenedione and dehydroepiandrosterone production, respectively (Fig. 233–6). This step is essential for the ultimate formation of testosterone and estrogens. Two types of 17,20-desmolase deficiency have been described, one affecting both the Δ^4 and Δ^5 pathways and one affecting the Δ^4 pathway alone, with normal plasma levels of dehydroepiandrosterone (Fig. 233–6). In prepubertal subjects with both Δ^4 and Δ^5 17,20-desmolase pathways affected, low plasma levels of dehydroepiandrosterone and androstenedione are present, which do not increase following administration of ACTH.

It is not known why the basal plasma levels of progesterone, pregnenolone, 17α-hydroxyprogesterone, and 17α-hydroxypregnenolone are elevated, particularly in prepubertal subjects with this enzyme deficiency. Since the enzyme 17,20-desmolase is not involved in cortisol biosynthesis, ACTH levels should be normal with subsequent normal amounts of the C21 precursor steroids mentioned above (Fig. 233–6).

MANAGEMENT AND THERAPY. In genotypic males the sex of rearing will depend upon the degree of ambiguity of the external genitalia. In the more severe cases, patients should be raised as females, with castration carried out in early childhood. Sex hormone therapy at puberty will invariably be necessary. In genotypic females, estrogen and progesterone supplementation will invariably be needed at the time of puberty.

Finkelstein M, and Shaeffer J: Inborn errors of steroid biosynthesis. Physiol Rev 59:353–406, 1979. *An all-encompassing review of the nonvirilizing and virilizing forms of congenital adrenal hyperplasia. A gem.*

Disorders of Function at Androgen-Dependent Target Areas

COMPLETE ANDROGEN INSENSITIVITY—TESTICULAR FEMINIZATION. ***Clinical Presentation.*** In this inherited form of male pseudohermaphroditism, genetic and gonadal males have a female phenotype and totally female psychosexual orientation. The testes differentiate normally with adequate secretion of müllerian inhibiting factor, resulting in the absence of fallopian tubes, uterus, and upper portion of the vagina. Despite normal to high-normal plasma levels of testosterone, wolffian structures are absent, and the external genitalia are totally female. Affected subjects are raised as girls, and the condition is rarely suspected prior to puberty. A prepubertal diagnosis is occasionally made when inguinal or labial masses are palpated in a phenotypic female child and are found to be testes.

Adequate breast development occurs at puberty, but pubic and axillary hair is scant to absent. Medical attention is usually sought at this time because of primary amenorrhea. A diagnosis of complete androgen insensitivity or testicular feminization should be considered in a phenotypic female with primary amenorrhea, good breast development, scantness or absence of pubic and axillary hair, a short vagina, and absence of the cervix and uterus. Rarely, patients with 17α-hydroxylase deficiency may have the same phenotypic presentation at puberty.

Pathogenesis. In patients with complete androgen insensitivity, absence of high-affinity dihydrotestosterone binding to the cytosol receptor (receptor-negative) has been demonstrated in cultured fibroblasts from genital skin. Qualitative abnormalities of the androgen receptor have also been described. Some subjects have partial cytosol receptor–binding under the usual assay conditions at 37° C, with normal binding at 26° C, demonstrating a structural alteration of the receptor at elevated temperatures that is reversible. Others show another qualitative defect demonstrated by failure of stabilization of the androgen receptor with sodium molybdate. Finally, postreceptor variants with normal cytosol receptor binding have also been demonstrated. In the latter individuals, the mutation may affect nuclear binding or the steps in the initiation of androgen action subsequent to nuclear binding, i.e., failure of RNA synthesis or an abnormality in its processing (Fig. 233–7).

It has been postulated that the X chromosomes of all mammals including man are homologous and genes X-linked in one species are X-linked in all. A defect in the receptor-negative form of complete androgen insensitivity has been found to be maternally transmitted with only males expressing the condition, suggesting inheritance as X-linked recessive or autosomal dominant–sex limited (males). Studies of genital skin fibroblasts from mothers of affected subjects demonstrate two clonal populations, one with normal dihydrotestosterone binding and one with absence of binding to the cytosol receptor, confirming X-linkage in this form of androgen insensitivity. Attempts to demonstrate linkage to known X-borne markers such as color blindness, hemophilia, XG immunoglobulin, and G6PD have been unsuccessful.

Plasma testosterone levels are normal to high with mild to moderately elevated plasma levels of luteinizing hormone (LH). A possible explanation for the elevated LH is the relative androgen insensitivity at the level of the hypothalamus resulting in partial negative feedback via conversion of testosterone to estradiol with no direct androgen inhibition. Follicle-stimulating hormone (FSH) levels are normal to elevated. Castration results in further elevation of LH and FSH levels, indicating prior partial feedback control. Urinary estrogens and plasma estradiol levels are generally in the low female range. An increased production rate has been shown for estrone and estradiol, which is mainly testicular in origin. The elevation of plasma estrogens together with the androgen unresponsiveness results in an unopposed estrogen effect that may be the cause of the breast development at puberty.

The histology of the testes cannot be distinguished from that of normal prepubertal males. Postpubertal histologic sections, however, reveal immature tubular development; they contain Sertoli cells and spermatogonia, but no evidence of spermatogenesis. Clumping of tubules with the formation of tubular adenomas is frequently found. The Leydig cells are hyperplastic with abundant smooth endoplasmic reticulum and mitochondria with tubular cristae, which correlate with the elevated plasma testosterone levels.

Management and Therapy. The frequency of testicular neoplasms in complete androgen insensitivity is approximately 2 to 5 per cent, tumors rarely occurring before the age of 25 to 30 years. For this reason the testes should be removed following puberty to allow complete breast development. Following castration, intermittent estrogen replacement therapy is necessary to maintain adequate breast turgor. In general, the vagina is adequate for normal coital function. Occasionally it is too shallow, but can frequently be enlarged with vaginal dilators, thereby bypassing the necessity for reconstructive surgery.

PARTIAL ANDROGEN INSENSITIVITY. ***Clinical Presentation.*** Partial forms of androgen insensitivity have been described. Affected subjects range from XY subjects with genital ambiguity and minimal to moderate pubertal virilization and gynecomastia, to those with a normal male phenotype, normal male secondary sexual development, and infertility. Within affected families the phenotype can vary, demonstrating that a single mutant gene can have variable phenotypic expression.

Pathogenesis. In general, the endocrine profile is similar to that demonstrated in subjects with complete androgen insensitivity. Plasma LH and testosterone levels are generally elevated. The total amount of 17β-estradiol produced and the quantity secreted by the testes can be greater than those found in patients with complete androgen insensitivity. However, despite increased estrogen production, the degree of feminization at puberty is not as marked as in complete androgen insensitivity, which may be a consequence of the incomplete androgen resistance with a less severe androgen and estrogen imbalance at the cellular level.

In many affected males with incomplete androgen insensitivity, the binding capacity and affinity of the androgen cytosol receptor for dihydrotestosterone is normal. Thus this condition may be a variant of complete androgen insensitivity with normal cytosol-binding activity. Other affected males, however, have a reduced number of cytosol-binding sites for dihydrotestosterone; this may represent a variant of complete androgen insensitivity with absence of androgen-binding activity. Qualitative defects in the receptor, i.e., thermolability and failure of

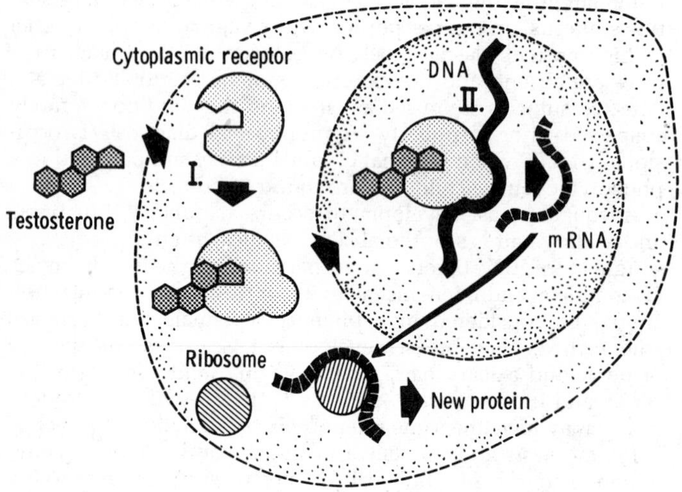

I. Abnormalities affecting binding to the cytosol receptor

A. Quantitative

1. Absent binding to cytosol receptor

B. Qualitative

1. Thermolability
2. Failure of stabilization with sodium molybdate

II. Nuclear or post nuclear receptor binding defect

Figure 233–7. Illustration of the abnormalities of androgen action resulting in androgen insensitivity.

stabilization with sodium molybdate as in complete androgen insensitivity, have also been shown.

The mildest form of incomplete androgen insensitivity may be infertility in phenotypically normal men with either azoospermia or severe oligospermia. The mean plasma levels of LH and testosterone can be either normal or elevated. The most frequent finding in cultured genital skin fibroblasts is a decrease in androgen binding capacity to the androgen cytosol receptor by over 50 per cent in comparison to that found in normal skin samples. Recently a qualitative defect affecting failure of receptor stabilization has also been identified. A major unknown in this form of androgen resistance is its frequency as a cause of infertility.

Management and Therapy. Incomplete forms of androgen insensitivity can be distinguished biochemically from male pseudohermaphroditism with defects in testosterone biosynthesis. All of these conditions can have the same phenotypic presentation prior to puberty. In the absence of a demonstrable cytosol receptor abnormality, a decrease in the anabolic response to androgen administration, i.e., decreased nitrogen retention, may help clarify the diagnosis. True hermaphrodites most commonly have an XX karyotype and can often be distinguished on that basis. Incomplete androgen insensitivity in puberty commonly results in gynecomastia and varying degrees of virilization. Following puberty, a normal to elevated plasma testosterone level with a normal androstenedione-testosterone ratio as well as normal plasma progesterone and dehydroepiandrosterone levels will distinguish subjects with this condition from subjects with 17β-hydroxysteroid dehydrogenase deficiency, 17α-hydroxylase deficiency, and 3β-hydroxysteroid dehydrogenase deficiency who can have the same appearance. Those subjects with moderate to severe defects in masculinization of the external genitalia should be raised as females and if possible castrated before puberty because of the possibility of virilization. Estrogen therapy should be added at puberty. Those with mild hypospadias can be raised as males but will require surgery for correction of both the hypospadias and the gynecomastia.

Griffin JE, Leshen M, Wilson, JD: Androgen resistance syndromes. Am J Physiol 243:E-81–87, 1982. *A comprehensive review, particularly of the biochemical abnormalities in complete and partial androgen insensitivity.*

5α-REDUCTASE DEFICIENCY. ***Clinical Presentation.*** In 1974, steroid 5α-reductase deficiency was first described as a cause of male pseudohermaphroditism in 38 subjects from a large Dominican kindred and two sibs from Dallas. This condition has subsequently been described in subjects throughout the world. Most subjects have perineal hypospadias with separate urethral and vaginal openings within a urogenital sinus. Rarely, a blind vaginal pouch opens into the urethra. The patients have an epididymis, vas deferens, and seminal vesicles. The incidence of cryptorchidism is significantly higher in childhood than adulthood, suggesting that it is not uncommon for the testes to descend during puberty in this condition.

The pubertal events include deepening of the voice, development of a muscular habitus, growth of the phallus, rugation and hyperpigmentation of the scrotum, and testicular descent. The prostate is small or absent, even in elderly subjects. Subjects have erections with ejaculation from the perineal urethra. Facial hair is decreased or absent and body hair is decreased. In only one subject has mild acne been reported, and none have temporal hairline recession.

Pathogenesis. The enzyme Δ^4,5α-reductase with NADPH as a cofactor catalyzes the reduction of the double bond at the 4–5 position of both C19 steroids, such as testosterone, and C21 steroids. It is present in high quantities in the liver and peripheral tissues, particularly the sebaceous glands, hair follicles, and skin of the external genitalia, where it actively converts testosterone to dihydrotestosterone, a more potent androgen. In subjects with 5α-reductase deficiency, the biochemical abnormality is characterized by normal to elevated levels of plasma testosterone with decreased levels of dihydrotestosterone resulting in an increased testosterone to dihydrotestosterone ratio. There is decreased production of the urinary 5α-reduced metabolites of testosterone, i.e., androsterone and androstanediol, causing elevated etiocholanolone-androsterone and etiocholanediol-androstanediol ratios. The urinary 5α-reduced metabolites of C21 and C19 steroids other than testosterone, i.e., cortisol, corticosterone, 11β-hydroxyandrostenedione, and androstenedione, are also decreased. Diminished 5α-reductase activity has been demonstrated both in skin slices and in fibroblasts cultured from genital skin. Based on consanguinity and biochemical data of parents, who demonstrate an intermediate defect in enzyme activity, an autosomal recessive inheritance has been demonstrated.

Male pseudohermaphrodites with 5α-reductase deficiency represent a unique clinical model, defining major actions for testosterone and dihydrotestosterone in male sexual differentiation and development. Since the developmental defect is limited to the external genitalia and prostate, the normal development of these structures appears to be effected through the actions of dihydrotestosterone. In contrast, wolffian differentiation develops normally and appears to be a testosterone-mediated function (Fig. 233–8). At puberty the affected males develop rugation and hyperpigmentation of the scrotum,

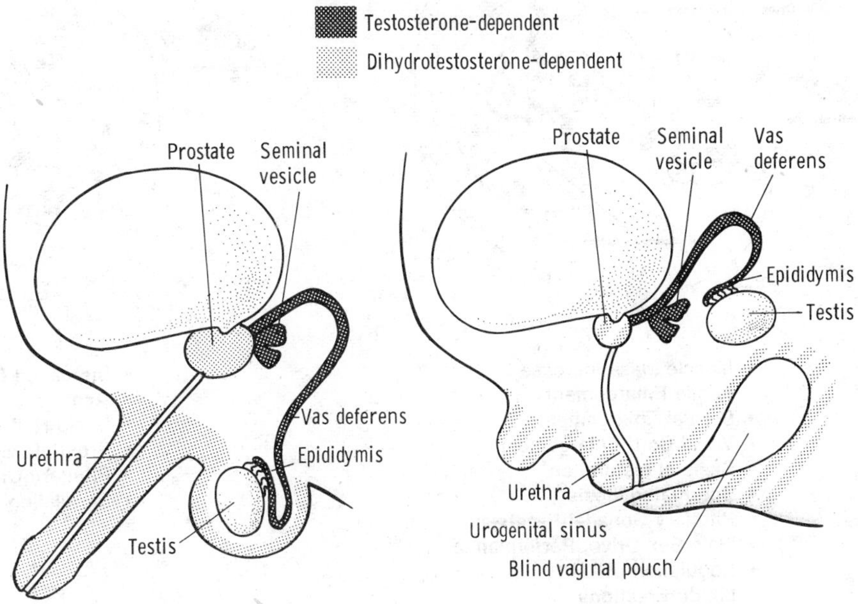

Figure 233–8. Illustration of the hypothesis for the specific actions of testosterone and dihydrotestosterone in male sexual differentiation in utero.

growth of the phallus, an increase in muscle mass, and deepening of the voice (Fig. 233–9). Their ultimate height is also similar to that of their fathers and normal male sibs. Thus the aforementioned pubertal events are mainly effected through the actions of testosterone. In contrast, prostatic development or enlargement, acne, normal male facial and body hair, and temporal recession of the hairline do not occur in affected males, and appear to be effected mainly through the actions of dihydrotestosterone.

Since both androgens share a common cytosol receptor, it is puzzling that the effects of dihydrotestosterone in dihydrotestosterone-dependent areas are not mimicked by testosterone. Two possible explanations can be submitted: (1) the cytosol receptor at certain target sites is modified so that it favors 5α-dihydrotestosterone over testosterone or (2) the 5α-dihydrotestosterone receptor complex has a higher affinity for the acceptor sites in chromatin.

In affected subjects with descended testes, testicular biopsy has demonstrated complete spermatogenesis; thus testosterone may be more important than dihydrotestosterone in the process of spermatogenesis. The question of fertility, however, remains unanswered. The cryptorchid testes of most subjects demonstrate seminiferous tubular damage with either Sertoli cells only or aberrant spermatogenesis. Plasma LH is increased despite normal to high plasma levels of testosterone, suggesting a role for dihydrotestosterone in the negative feedback control of LH. The elevated plasma LH levels correlate with the microscopic findings of Leydig cell hyperplasia. Plasma FSH levels are also elevated, which may be a consequence of the cryptorchidism with its damaging effect on spermatogenesis. Affected males have erections, with ejaculation from the perineal urethra, and thus these male sexual functions appear to be mediated through the actions of testosterone, either directly or via conversion to estradiol in the brain. Conversely, administration of pharmacologic amounts of dihydrotesterone causes a substantial decrease in plasma testosterone with subsequent loss of libido and impotence.

A documented gender change from female to male in untreated affected subjects from the Dominican kindred underscores the importance of testosterone exposure of the brain in utero, the early postnatal period, and at puberty in the determination of male gender identity. Theoretically, "masculinization" of the brain occurs under the influence of testosterone and, together with activation of testosterone-mediated puberty, a male gender identity develops, overriding the female sex of rearing. It has been proposed that gender identity becomes fixed by 18 months to 4 years of age, around the time of language development. However, from studies with these patients, it appears that the development of gender identity in man is continually evolving throughout childhood and adolescence, becoming fixed with puberty.

Imperato-McGinley J, Peterson RE, Gautier T: Male pseudohermaphroditism secondary to 5α-reductase deficiency: A review. *In* Resko J (ed.): Fetal Endocrinology. New York, Academic Press, 1981, pp 359–382. *A review of the cases reported, as well as the clinical and biochemical findings in this interesting experiment of nature.*

Imperto-McGinley J, Peterson RE, Gautier T, Sturla E: The impact of androgens on the evolution of male gender identity. *In* Kogan SJ, Hafez ESE (eds.): Clinics in Andrology: Pediatric Andrology. Vol. 7. The Hague, Matinus Nihoff, 1981, pp 99–105. *A study of gender change from female to male in a large kindred with 5α-reductase deficiency—a comprehensive theory concerning the aquisition of gender identity in males.*

XX Males and True Hermaphroditism

XX Males

Clinical Presentation. Since the first case report in 1962, reports of approximately 50 cases of XX males have been published, including members within the same family. A rare condition, the incidence in newborn males is estimated to be 1 in 20,000. Classically XX adult males have short stature, a normal-sized penis, small firm testes generally less than 2 cm, and infertility. One third have gynecomastia. The phenotypic appearance resembles that of males with Klinefelter's syndrome (XXY) with the notable exception that XX males are shorter in stature, even shorter than the average male. In general, the histologic features of the testes also resemble those of subjects with Klinefelter's syndrome. The seminiferous tubules of the testes are hyalinized and contain only Sertoli cells or occasionally a few immature spermatogonia, correlating clinically with azoospermia or oligospermia. The Leydig cells are hyperplastic. Levels of FSH and LH are elevated, with decreased plasma testosterone and increased plasma estradiol levels. More recently, XX children with bilateral testes have been reported with ambiguous genitalia, suggesting a phenotypic spectrum in this condition.

Pathogenesis. The etiologic factors for the expression of

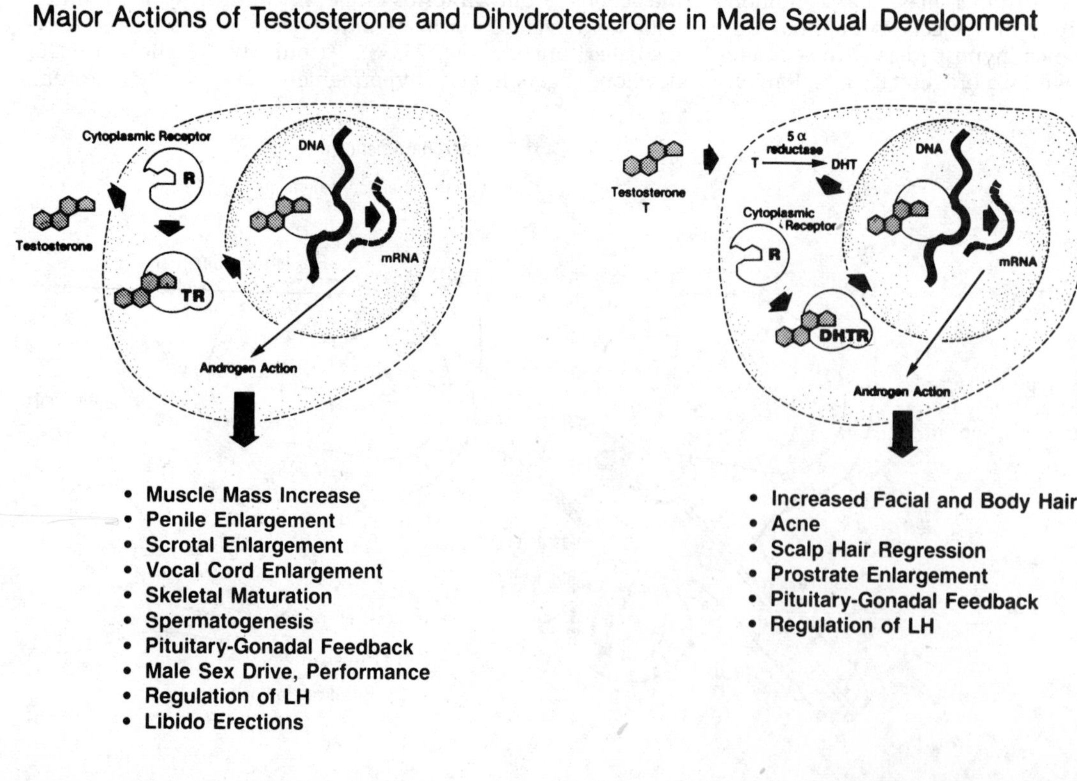

Figure 233–9. Illustration of the major actions of testosterone and dihydrotestosterone at puberty.

masculinity in XX individuals have been the subject of much speculation. Three possible mechanisms have been proposed—(1) translocation of part of the Y chromosome to the X chromosome or to an autosome, (2) undetected mosaicism XX/XY or XXY, or (3) a mutant autosomal gene determining maleness in an XX individual. Studies of H-Y antigen in subjects with this condition have revealed a positive titer. Recently, chromosome preparations from 8 of 12 46 XX males were clearly distinguishable from normal 46 XX female preparations secondary to alterations in shape, as well as an increase in the tip of the short arm of the X chromosome. DNA digests from the nuclei of cells from testes of an XX male have demonstrated Y-specific DNA fragments. Thus, the condition in a high percentage of 46 XX males appears to be a consequence of a paternal X-Y interchange affecting the testes-determining area of the Y chromosome.

True Hermaphroditism

Clinical Presentation. The morphologic expression of true hemaphroditism is the presence of both ovarian and testicular tissue, with each gonad containing its corresponding gamete. Most subjects have ambiguous genitalia, although approximately 7 per cent of true hermaphrodites have normal female external genitalia, and 12 per cent have a penile urethra; 75 per cent of affected subjects are raised as males. Although a rare form of intersex, it is relatively common among the Bantu of South Africa. The most common gonadal associations are an ovary and testis or an ovotestis and ovary, each occurring in 30 per cent of cases. Bilateral ovotestes occur in 20 per cent of the cases; an ovotestis and testis in only 10 per cent. The ovotestis frequently has ovarian and testicular tissue arranged in an end-to-end fashion. Although the ovarian portion is usually histologically normal, the testicular portion is clearly histologically abnormal, and spermatogenesis has never been observed. Gonadal tumors occur in approximately 2 per cent.

A fallopian tube is always found adjacent to an ovary. A fallopian tube is also most commonly found adjacent to an ovotestis; an epididymis is present in approximately one third of the cases. A uterus is present in approximately 90 per cent of affected subjects. In familial reports of true hermaphroditism, however, there is no uterus in the majority of those affected, and there are bilateral descended ovotestes.

With puberty, variable virilization and feminization occur. About half of affected subjects will menstruate; in those raised as males with mild or moderate hypospadias or a penile urethra, menstruation can present as cyclic hematuria. Gynecomastia will develop in 80 per cent of subjects. Pregnancy and childbirth have been reported in true hermaphrodites following removal of testicular tissue and correction of the external genitalia. A few subjects with functional testicular tissue are fertile.

Pathogenesis. A 46 XX complement is present in approximately two thirds of cases, XX/XY mosaicism in one third of cases, and 46 XY complement in one tenth of the cases. XX true hermaphrodites have been reported to be H-Y antigen positive, suggesting translocation of Y chromosomal material to either the X chromosome or an autosome, or undetected XX/XY chimerism. Although they are H-Y antigen positive, a reduced titer has been reported, suggesting random inactivation of an X chromosome that bears the translocated H-Y locus. When cells were cultured from the testicular portion of the ovotestis of an XX true hermaphrodite, they were H-Y antigen positive, whereas cells cultured from the ovarian portion were H-Y antigen negative. These observations suggest that the ovotestes arise from an H-Y+/H-Y− mosaic primordium. A reported case of true hermaphroditism in a subject whose brother and paternal uncle were XX males suggests that XX males and XX true hermaphrodites may be variants of the same condition.

Management and Therapy. The sex assignment in true hermaphroditism diagnosed in infancy and childhood is best determined by the appearance of the external genitalia, together with the gonadal tissue and internal structures. If an ovary-ovotestis and a uterus are present, the ovotestis and any male internal structures should be removed and feminizing surgery of the external genitalia performed. If bilateral ovotestes are present, and if a good line of demarcation is seen between ovarian and testicular tissue, the testicular portion should be removed, the genitalia surgically feminized, and the child raised as female. If a testis is present on one side and an ovotestis on the contralateral side, the testis should be brought into the scrotum and the child raised as male if the external genitalia can be surgically corrected. If an ovary is present on one side and a testis on the contralateral side, the sex of rearing should be decided by evaluation of the appearance of the external and internal sex structures, and appropriate surgical correction should be performed. Peripubertal or postpubertal surgical correction of the internal and external sex structures should depend exclusively upon the gender identity of the affected individual. Although testicular tumor formation is rare, if the individual is to be raised as male the testis should be brought into the scrotum, so that periodic examination can be carried out.

De La Chapelle A: The etiology of maleness in XX men. Hum Genet 58:105–116, 1981. *A review of clinical characteristics and hypotheses in the occurrence of this unique condition.*

Van Niekerk WA: True hermaphroditism—An analytic review with a report of 3 new cases. Am J Obstet Gynecol 126:890, 1976. *An extensive review of all reported cases to 1976, covering clinical presentation and etiology.*

Female Pseudohermaphroditism

Female pseudohermaphroditism can result from either fetal or maternal androgenic influences (Table 233–3). Cases of undetermined etiology have also been described.

Congenital Adrenal Hyperplasia—Virilizing Forms

Three adrenal enzyme defects, 21-hydroxylase deficiency, 11β-hydroxylase deficiency, and 3β-hydroxysteroid dehydrogenase deficiency, can result in increased androgen production in utero with virilization of the female fetus. They are the virilizing forms of congenital adrenal hyperplasia (Fig. 233–6). 21-Hydroxylase and 11β-hydroxylase deficiency can result in severe virilization of the female fetus, whereas the virilization reported with 3β-hydroxysteroid dehydrogenase deficiency is very mild. Since 3β-hydroxysteroid dehydrogenase deficiency is also a cause of male pseudohermaphroditism, it is discussed in the section Male Pseudohermaphroditism, as are the non-virilizing forms of congenital adrenal hyperplasia. The enzyme defects causing virilization of the female fetus result in decreased cortisol production, with increased pituitary ACTH and resultant adrenal androgen overproduction. In the genotypic female, since ovaries and not testes are present, müllerian inhibiting factor is not produced, and the internal structures are female, i.e., uterus and fallopian tubes. Despite the increase in androgen production severe enough to masculinize the external genitalia, wolffian differentiation has never been described. Affected 46 XY males with either 21-hydroxylase or 11β-hydroxylase deficiency appear phenotypically normal at birth.

21-HYDROXYLASE DEFICIENCY. ***Clinical Features.*** First de-

TABLE 233–3. CLASSIFICATION OF CAUSES OF FEMALE PSEUDOHERMAPHRODITISM

- I. Androgenic influences
  - A. Fetal
    - 1. Congenital adrenogenital syndrome:
      - a. 21-Hydroxylase deficiency;
      - b. 11β-Hydroxylase deficiency;
      - c. 3β-Hydroxysteroid dehydrogenase:Δ^{5-4} isomerase deficiency
  - B. Maternal
    - 1. Excess maternal androgen production
    - 2. Maternal ingestion of virilizing substances
- II. Idiopathic

scribed in 1950, 21-hydroxylase deficiency is the most common cause of ambiguous genitalia in 46 XX infants. Its incidence varies from approximately 1 in 300 births in Alaskan Eskimos to 1 in 15,000 births in Caucasians in Wisconsin. The spectrum of masculinization varies from female infants with minimal clitoromegaly and fusion of the labioscrotal folds to infants with a penile urethra and the appearance of a cryptorchid male. Classically, if affected XX children are untreated in infancy, there is rapid acceleration of growth, enlargement of the clitoris, increase in muscle mass, precocious development of pubic axillary and body hair, and advancement of bone age. Although they are tall in childhood, premature closure of the epiphyses eventually results in short stature in adulthood. At the time of expected puberty, there is absence of breast development and menstruation. Untreated males with this condition also show precocious maturation and are short in stature in adulthood. The excessive androgen production can inhibit gonadotropin secretion, so that untreated adult males, although strongly virilized, can have small soft testes and azoospermia. However, because of the adrenal androgen excess, they are capable of having erections. Frequently, however, true puberty occurs in untreated males with normal FSH and LH secretion, testicular enlargement, and spermatogenesis. ACTH-dependent testicular "tumors" have been described and can occur either unilaterally or bilaterally; most probably they are of adrenal origin.

Two forms of 21-hydroxylase deficiency have been described, a simple form and a salt-losing form. Infants with the salt-losing form usually have an adrenal crisis within the first two weeks of life. Infants with the simple form do not show signs of adrenal crisis; ambiguity of the external genitalia is the most prominent feature.

Pathogenesis. 21-Hydroxylase deficiency results in decreased synthesis of cortisol with consequent increase in ACTH and increase in plasma progesterone, 17α-hydroxyprogesterone, and C19 androgens (dehydroepiandrosterone, androstenedione, and testosterone; Fig. 233–6). In the newborn, determination of plasma 17α-hydroxyprogesterone is the test most diagnostic for this condition. The increased adrenal androgen production in the female fetus in utero results in virilization of the external genitalia. In the salt-losing form, there is a deficiency of aldosterone production. However, an additive factor in the salt loss may be due to increased production of progesterone and 17α-hydroxyprogesterone, which act as aldosterone antagonists.

The gene for 21-hydroxylase deficiency is closely linked to the HLA-B locus of chromosome 6. Obligate carrier parents and sibs predicted to be heterozygotes by HLA typing frequently demonstrate increased 17α-hydroxyprogesterone levels in response to a one-hour ACTH stimulation test. Although the tests are extremely helpful in heterozygote detection, they are not uniformly conclusive. Family members, both males and females, have also been identified who have biochemical evidence of 21-hydroxylase deficiency but are without signs of virilization, hirsutism, amenorrhea, or infertility. These individuals are designated as having a cryptic form of 21-hydroxylase deficiency. It is proposed that they are genetic compounds, the result of two recessive gene defects, a severe and a mild defect in 21-hydroxylation. Why they are clinically asymptomatic remains unanswered. A late-onset or attenuated variant of 21-hydroxylase deficiency has also recently been documented in adult women with hirsutism, or virilization and menstrual irregularities. HLA typing and ACTH testing of affected subjects' parents and sibs with this form also document linkage to the HLA-B locus of chromosome 6, as in the classic form of congenital adrenal hyperplasia.

Management and Therapy. Affected females with 21-hydroxylase deficiency have ovaries and normal internal female structures with potential for fertility. Therefore, diagnosis and treatment should be carried out early and the child appropriately treated and raised as a female. Surgical correction of the masculinized external genitalia should be performed early so that gender confusion does not occur later on in childhood and adolescence. Medical therapy involves adequate glucocorticoid replacement therapy to lower ACTH secretion and to suppress adrenal androgen excess. Overtreatment should be avoided to prevent the signs and symptoms of glucocorticoid excess, which can lead to growth retardation.

Overt salt losers must be given mineralocorticoid as well as glucocorticoid replacement therapy. Many affected subjects without overt signs of adrenal crisis have impaired mineralocorticoid production, characterized by decreased sodium content and plasma volume with resultant increase in plasma renin. The increased plasma renin has been postulated to increase release of ACTH, necessitating more glucocorticoid replacement therapy. Thus mineralocorticoid supplementation should be considered in any subject with increase of plasma renin, despite the absence of signs of adrenal insufficiency.

Assessment of adequate therapy in a child is made on the basis of maintaining normal growth velocity, without signs of excess of either androgen or exogenous glucocorticoid. Monitoring plasma 17α-hydroxyprogesterone and plasma androgens has been helpful in regulating the glucocorticoid dosage; normalization of plasma androstenedione is the most reliable predictor of optimal therapy.

11β-HYDROXYLASE DEFICIENCY. ***Clinical Features.*** In 1955 a deficiency of the enzyme 11β-hydroxylase was identified as a cause of congenital adrenal hyperplasia with hypertension. To date approximately 60 cases have been described. In females with 21-hydroxylase deficiency, the enzyme deficiency at birth results in normal female genitalia to varying degrees of masculinization of the external genitalia. Adolescence results in mild hirsutism, clitoral hypertrophy, and irregular menses to severe virilization. Males with this condition show precocious male sexual maturation but develop gynecomastia at puberty. The cause of the gynecomastia is not known, but it has been postulated to be secondary to elevated plasma desoxycorticosterone levels.

Pathogenesis. 11β-Hydroxylase deficiency results in decreased cortisol production, which causes an increase in ACTH, in C19 androgen secretion, and in desoxycorticosterone production (Fig. 233–6). Elevation of the plasma 11-desoxycortisol level is diagnostic of this enzyme deficiency and distinguishes it from 21-hydroxylase deficiency. Plasma cortisol as well as the urinary cortisol metabolites tetrahydrocortisone and tetrahydrocortisol can be normal to low. Urinary 17-ketosteroids, reflecting adrenal androgen overproduction, and urinary 17-hydroxysteroids, reflecting elevated levels of plasma 11-desoxycortisol, are increased. Excretion of pregnanetriol, a metabolite of 17α-hydroxyprogesterone, is usually normal or slightly increased. Plasma desoxycorticosterone is increased as is its urinary metabolite tetrahydrodesoxycorticosterone, while corticosterone and aldosterone are decreased. The increased production of desoxycorticosterone results in salt retention, increased plasma volume, hypertension, and decreased plasma renin. Some affected subjects are not hypertensive and have a deficiency of the enzyme that appears to be limited to the 17α-hydroxylated pathway, with normal levels of plasma desoxycorticosterone and its urinary metabolites. This has been explained by postulating the presence of either two 11β-hydroxylase enzyme systems or two different regulatory systems for 17α-hydroxylated steroids and for 17-desoxysteroids.

Management and Therapy. Glucocorticoid replacement therapy will effect biochemical normalization, decrease blood pressure, and arrest precocious development. In females, surgical correction of the external genitalia should be carried out, as in females with 21-hydroxylase deficiency.

Virilization of the Female Fetus Secondary to Excess Maternal Androgen Production or Exogenous Maternal Administration of Virilizing Hormones

Masculinization of the female infant has been demonstrated in mothers with ovarian luteomas, virilizing adrenal tumors, and untreated maternal congenital adrenal hyperplasia. Why virilization of the female fetus does not occur in all states of maternal hyperandrogenicity may be related to the onset and the degree of hyperandrogenicity and the potency of the androgens secreted. The placenta may also offer some protection for the fetus by aromatization of the maternal androgens to estrogens.

Administration of testosterone or its derivatives to pregnant women has been associated with virilization of the female fetus. These substances stimulate virilization of the external genitalia with no effect on differentiation of the wolffian ductal system. A causal relationship of the progestational agents progesterone, medroxyprogesterone, and 17α-hydroxyprogesterone has not been definitely proven. Paradoxic masculinization of the female fetus associated with maternal administration of diethylstilbestrol early in pregnancy has been reported rarely. The degree of genital masculinization is correlated with the time of initiation of treatment. The mechanism for the genital masculinization has been postulated to be secondary to inhibition of the enzyme 3β-hydroxysteroid dehydrogenase:Δ^{5-4} isomerase by diethylstilbestrol, with consequent elevation of the weak androgen dehydroepiandrosterone and possibly other Δ^5-androgenic steroids.

New M, Levine LS: Congenital adrenal hyperplasia and related conditions. *In* Stanbury JB, et al (eds.): Metabolic Basis of Inherited Disease. 5th ed. New York, McGraw Hill Book Company, 1983, Ch. 47. *Contains an excellent review of 21-hydroxylase deficiency with particular emphasis on genetics.*

234. THE TESTIS

Mortimer B. Lipsett

INTRODUCTION

Fetal Development

The primordial gonad arises in the urogenital ridge from intermediate mesoderm during the fifth week of gestation (Ch. 233). Early in its development, the bipotential primitive gonad (Fig. 234–1) is composed of two unipotential mesodermal primordia, each with a distinct physiologic as well as morphologic capacity: (1) a cortical component, consisting of the germinal epithelium; and (2) a medullary component, made up of the primary sex cords derived from the germinal epithelium, and mesonephric and blastemal elements. A third constituent, the primordial germ cell, which appears to be bipotential, arises in an extragonadal site and migrates to the gonads. Under the influence of the Y organizer, a surface protein of cells carrying the Y chromosome, the medullary component differentiates as a testis (Fig. 234–1). The cortical component can differentiate as an ovary only in the absence of Y organizer.

When the gonad destined to become a testis begins to differentiate in a male direction during the seventh to eighth week of embryonic life, the cortical component involutes. Within the medulla, seminiferous tubules form from the primary sex cords and anastomose with the rete testis and testicular ducts, and Leydig cells develop. Leydig cells proliferate predominantly during the first half of gestation, but then gradually decrease in number and involute after birth. Leydig cells acquire the capacity to synthesize testosterone, and this steroid hormone has been found in the fetal testis. At the time of pubescence morphologic differentiation of Leydig cells occurs, and testosterone production is greatly increased. Fetal development of the testis and the accessory sex structures is discussed more fully in Ch. 233.

Chemistry and Physiology of the Testicular Hormones

The testicular hormone *testosterone,* secreted from the Leydig cell, has the primary role in the development and maintenance of the male accessory sex organs, prostate, and seminal vesicles, in the elaboration of semen, and in the development of masculine secondary sexual characteristics. These properties define a class of substances, the androgens; the important androgen secreted by the testis is testosterone. The 5α-reduced derivative of testosterone, 5α-dihydrotestosterone, is the active form of the hormone at the nuclear receptor within the male accessory sex structures, and is responsible for inducing growth of these organs.

The adrenal cortex secretes little testosterone. The weak androgenic potency of adrenocortical steroids such as androstenedione and dehydroepiandrosterone can be attributed to their conversion to testosterone in small yield.

Healthy young men secrete about 7 mg of testosterone per day. Testosterone originates in the Leydig cells, although the seminiferous tubule has a weak capacity for testosterone synthesis. Clinical signs of androgen deficiency are absent and testosterone secretion is normal in certain testicular disorders in man associated with defective seminiferous tubules but with intact Leydig cells.

Pathways for the biosynthesis of testosterone by the Leydig cell resemble those in other steroid-synthesizing glands (see Fig. 233–6). Precursors such as acetate and low-density lipoprotein cholesterol are converted enzymatically to testosterone via 17-hydroxypregnenolone and 17-hydroxyprogesterone. The Leydig cell can also aromatize testosterone to estradiol. In adult men, 10 to 15 μg of estradiol is secreted daily; an additional 25 to 30 μg is produced peripherally by aromatization of testosterone and from estrone formed from adrenal androstenedione (Fig. 234–2). Blood estrogen in the male then depends on testicular secretion and rates of peripheral aromatization of adrenal and testicular precursors. Estrone, however, is predominantly a product of adrenal cortical secretions.

The liver is the main site of catabolism of testosterone and of the conjugation of its known metabolites with glucuronic or sulfuric acid; other tissues play a less important role in its metabolism. The major identifiable urinary metabolites are the 17-ketosteroids, androsterone and etiocholanolone, which are excreted principally as glucuronides and account for 20 to 40 per cent of the testosterone secreted. A small amount of testosterone (0.2 to 2 per cent) is excreted as testosterone glucuronide.

Spermatogenesis and the Sertoli Cell

SPERMATOGENESIS. About 90 per cent of the mass of the testis is due to the seminiferous tubules where spermatogenesis takes place. The seminiferous epithelium is composed of the germ cells and the nonproliferating Sertoli cells. In the human the duration of spermatogenesis is about 74 days and includes mitosis of the spermatogonia, meiosis in the subsequent generation of spermatocytes to reduce the diploid number of chromosomes to the haploid number, and finally transformation of the spermatocyte to the mature spermatozoon. These processes depend critically on normal Sertoli cell function. It has been difficult to discern clearly the effect of hormones at any specific level of spermatogenesis. The germ cell does not possess hormone receptors and thus cannot be a direct hormonal target.

SERTOLI CELL. In the human the Sertoli cell does not undergo mitosis after birth. There are inter-Sertoli cell tight junctions so that the Sertoli cells constitute a barrier between the germ cells and the external environment. Macromolecules can thus enter the Sertoli cell compartment only with difficulty. The various stages of spermatogenesis are arranged within the Sertoli cells so that the final release of the spermatogonium occurs at the apical end of the Sertoli cell into the lumen.

The Sertoli cell is a biosynthetically active tissue. It is responsible for secretion of the luminal fluid of the testis. It synthesizes a variety of proteins: androgen-binding protein, closely similar to that synthesized by the liver; plasminogen activator; ceruloplasmin; transferrin; and others of unknown function. In effect, the Sertoli cell maintains a culture medium for the germ cell, synthesizing those same proteins that have been found necessary to maintain many cells in plasma-free tissue culture.

The Sertoli cell is a target for two hormones, follicle-stimulating hormone (FSH) and androgen. FSH is apparently active

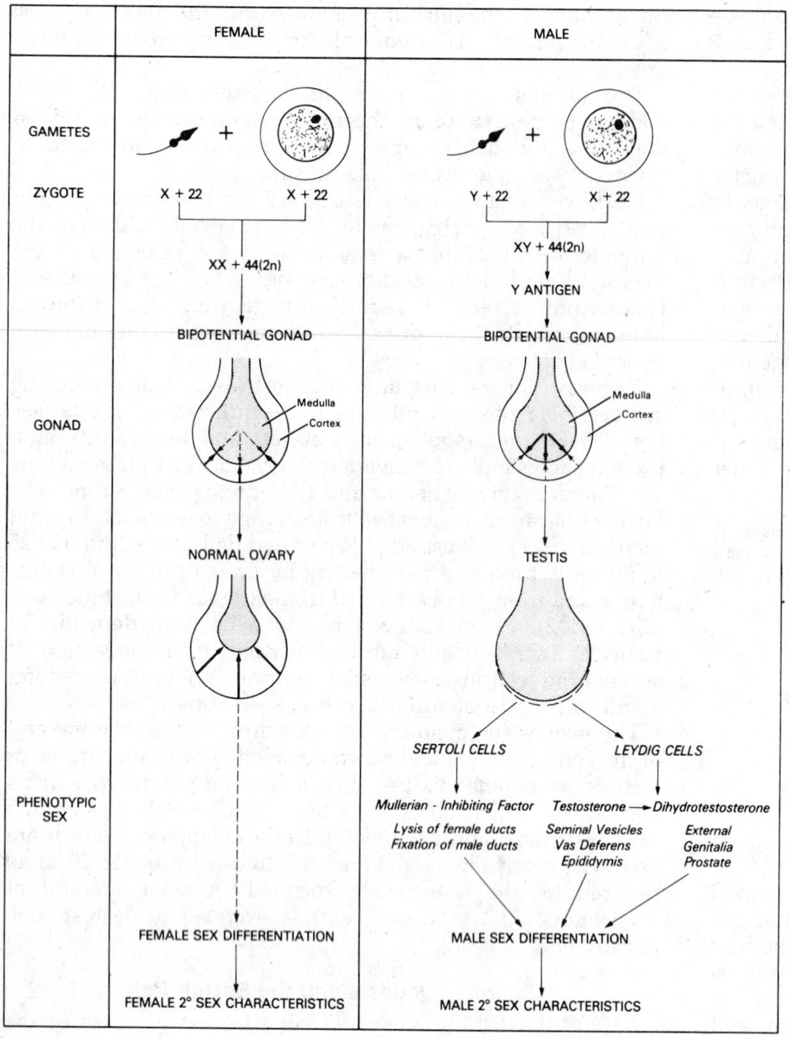

Figure 234–1. Diagrammatic scheme of human sex determination and differentiation.

only at initiation of spermatogenesis when it demonstrates the same features of other peptide hormones: surface receptors, generation of cAMP, and phosphorylation of intracellular proteins. The maintenance of Sertoli cell function and thus of spermatogenesis is dependent on high levels of androgen and the classic androgen receptor has been found in the Sertoli cell. In hypophysectomized men, spermatogenesis can be maintained by administration of human chorionic gonadotropin (HCG), intratesticular implants of androgen, or high doses of androgen, resulting in each case in a high intratesticular concentration of androgen. For optimal spermatogenesis, FSH may be needed.

There are multiple interactions between the compartments of the testis and between these compartments and the hypothalamic-pituitary unit (Fig. 234–3). The roles of the estrogen and androgen receptors in the Leydig cell during normal physiologic circumstances have not been clarified, although a high dose of estrogen can directly decrease several Leydig cell enzymes necessary for testosterone synthesis. In spite of these many new data, the relationship between luteinizing hormone (LH) and the Leydig cell remains the critical factor, and consideration of plasma levels of LH and testosterone will clarify most clinical situations.

Testosterone exerts a negative feedback on LH secretion, and it seems likely that both androgen and estrogen receptors modulate LH secretion. The hypothalamus and the pituitary have the capacity to metabolize testosterone to dihydrotestosterone and estradiol. Plasma FSH also is suppressed by testosterone, but an additional factor, inhibin, a polypeptide of about 20,000 daltons derived from the Sertoli cell, also modulates

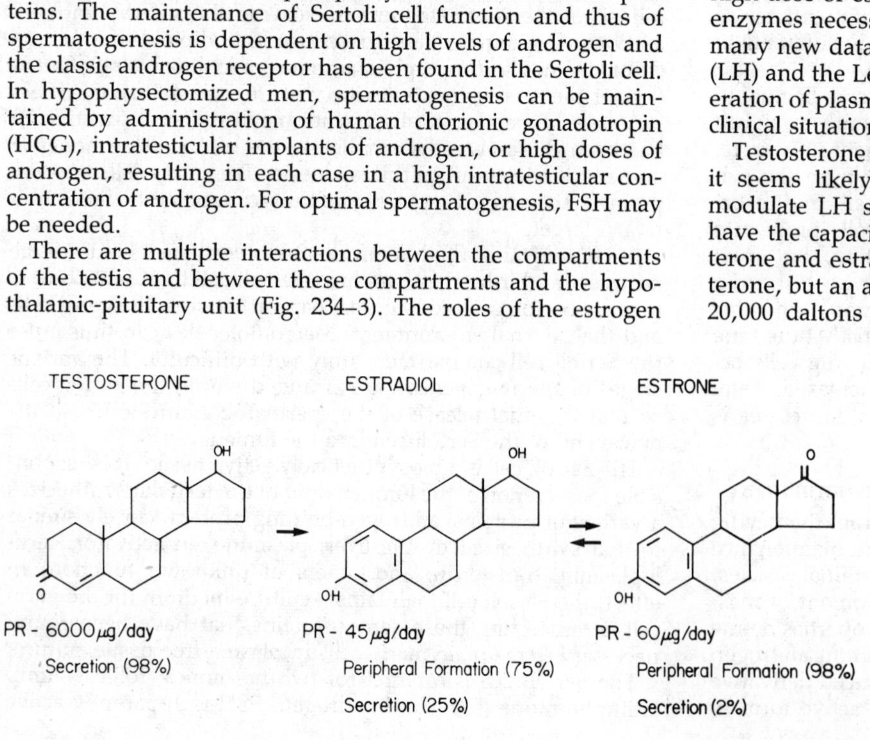

Figure 234–2. Production rates (PR) and origins of estradiol and estrone in men.

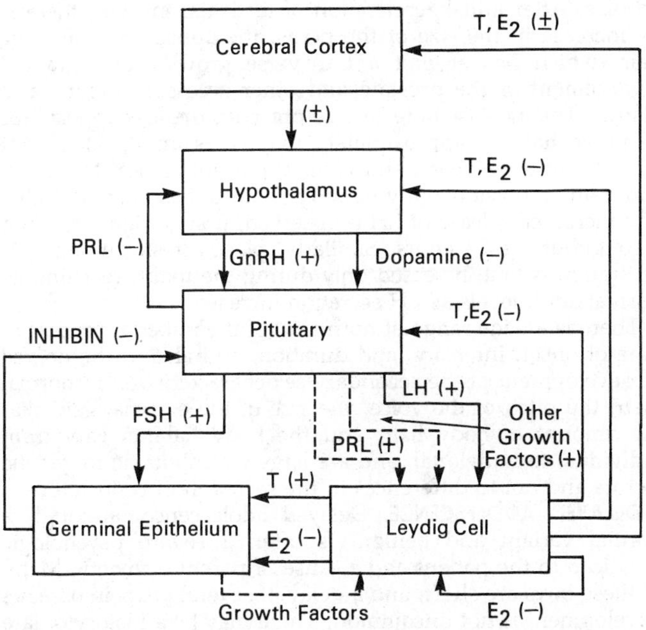

Figure 234–3. Diagram of interrelations between hypothalamus, pituitary and testis. Dotted lines indicate those actions that remain somewhat equivocal. GnRH = gonadotropin-releasing hormone; PRL = prolactin; T = testosterone; E_2 = estradiol.

FSH secretion at the pituitary level. Thus plasma FSH and LH levels are high in the absence of Leydig cell secretions, but FSH alone is increased when there is severe seminiferous tubule disease. Whether this is an important normal regulatory mechanism is not clear, but pulsatile injections of testosterone and estradiol at physiologic levels will also maintain normal plasma FSH in the castrated experimental animal. Prolactin at high levels directly inhibits the secretion of FSH and LH and may modulate Leydig cell secretions. The brain, as well, can alter hypothalamic-pituitary function.

Evaluation of Testicular Function

CLINICAL ASSESSMENT. Adequacy of androgen production can be estimated from the degree of development of the penis and scrotum, size of the prostate, general maturity and status of male secondary sex characteristics, habitus and skeletal proportions, muscular development, and sexual potency. This assessment has limitations in the mature adult, however, because regression of secondary sexual characteristics is slow even after complete loss of Leydig cell function. Furthermore, facial and body hair can be highly variable owing to genetic differences in the distribution of the pilosebaceous apparatus and differences in responsiveness of these skin appendages to hormonal stimulation. In the American Indian, the black African, and some Orientals facial and body hair is sparse or absent despite normal testicular function and plasma testosterone concentration.

URINARY 17-KETOSTEROIDS. About 80 per cent of the urinary 17-ketosteroids (17-KS) is derived from adrenocortical steroids that have little intrinsic androgenic activity. Less than 3 mg daily is derived from Leydig cell secretions. Androsterone and etiocholanolone, the principal urinary metabolites of testosterone, are also metabolites of adrenocortical 11-deoxysteroids. Thus, since urinary 17-KS are an index chiefly of adrenal cortical function, they cannot be used to assess testicular function. Testosterone, which has a hydroxyl group at carbon atom 17, is not a 17-ketosteroid.

The normal range of 17-KS excretion in men is 8 to 20 mg per day (mean, 15 mg). Before puberty only small amounts are detectable in urine. In adult men and women after the third decade, urinary 17-KS decreases gradually owing to lessening adrenal secretion of dehydroepiandrosterone. The excretion of 17-KS may be reduced in eunuchoidism, although the values obtained in such patients are often within the normal range. In panhypopituitarism the function of both the testis and the adrenal cortex is impaired, and the excretion of urinary 17-KS is greatly decreased. Low values are also frequently found in chronic debilitating disease and renal insufficiency. Measurement of urinary 17-KS has little clinical value in diseases of the testis or adrenal cortex except as a screening test for congenital adrenal hyperplasia and adrenal tumors (see Ch. 229).

PLASMA AND URINARY TESTOSTERONE. Measurement of plasma, salivary or urinary testosterone, the last as the glucuronide conjugate, provides reliable indices of Leydig cell function. The production rate of testosterone can be estimated, but the method is too cumbersome for routine use. Young adult males excrete 40 to 100 μg per day of testosterone glucuronide; women excrete less than 6 μg, and boys before puberty less than 0.5 μg. The concentration of testosterone in plasma of young adult men ranges from 0.3 to 1.2 μg per deciliter (mean 0.65 μg per deciliter), and the concentration in women varies from 0.034 to 0.06 μg per deciliter (mean, 0.054 μg per deciliter). More than 98 per cent of testosterone in plasma is bound to a specific β-globulin, sex-steroid binding globulin, and thus only 1 to 2 per cent is available for diffusion into cells. The administration of HCG to adult men induces a rise in plasma and urinary testosterone; this procedure has been used to assess the responsiveness of the Leydig cell and to distinguish between primary and secondary testicular disease.

PLASMA AND URINARY GONADOTROPINS. Gonadotropin releasing hormone (GnRH) is secreted in pulsatile fashion, and this results in marked fluctuations of plasma LH and only small changes in FSH. In normal men, there may be 8 to 15 LH secreting episodes per 24 hours, and LH levels may vary from 40 to 250 per cent of the mean level. In practice, this means that at least three measurements are necessary to estimate mean LH levels. Mean plasma FSH concentration is 12 mIU per milliliter (range, 4 to 27 mIU per milliliter). The mean LH concentration is 9 mIU per milliliter (range, 4 to 19 mIU per milliliter). Increased excretion or plasma concentrations of these hormones suggest primary testicular disease; isolated increases of FSH point to severe disease of the germinal epithelium. The lower level of sensitivity of most of the immunoassays is such that a gonadotropin concentration in the lower part of the normal range cannot be distinguished from decreased levels. Plasma LH can now be bioassayed as well, and the ratio of bioassayable LH and radioimmunologic LH will vary according to hormonal status. A case of apparently biologically inactive but fully immunoperative LH has been reported.

ASSESSMENT OF HYPOTHALAMIC-PITUITARY GONADOTROPIN RELEASE. Clomiphene citrate, an analogue of the nonsteroidal estrogen chlorotrianisene, is an estrogen antagonist and competes with estrogen at pituitary and/or hypothalamic receptors. When administered to normal men by mouth, 100 to 200 mg per day for five to seven days, it evokes a mean increase in the concentration of plasma FSH of 130 per cent and of plasma LH of 160 per cent. It also induces a rise in urinary FSH and LH and of plasma testosterone. Little or no increase in FSH or LH secretion is elicited in men with pituitary disease.

The identification and synthesis of the hypothalamic decapeptide GnRH have enabled the physician to establish pituitary responsiveness directly (see Ch. 225). It has been valuable in distinguishing between pituitary and hypothalamic disease. In general, a heightened response to GnRH indicates that there is a somewhat increased secretion of the gonadotropins and, by implication, decreased secretion of the testicular regulatory substance.

TESTICULAR BIOPSY. This procedure can be of great value in the diagnosis and prognosis of testicular disorders. It provides information concerning the gametogenic function of the testis—the status of the seminiferous tubules and the stages of spermatogenesis. Biopsy of the testis is of use in diagnosis of tubular disease, in assessing processes of sperm maturation, and in distinguishing azoospermia resulting from obstruction to the passage of sperm from azoospermia of other causes.

EXAMINATION OF SEMEN. Specimens of semen for analysis should be obtained two to three days after the last ejaculation. The volume of the specimen, the total number of sperm, and the motility and morphology of the sperm are determined. The minimal number of sperm necessary for normal fertility is unknown, but a total sperm count of 60 million may be considered normal. Less than this in general means decreased fertility. Because of the wide variations in sperm count among several specimens from the same patient, evaluation of therapy requires long control periods. Assessment of motility and morphology may require examination of many specimens to establish an accurate baseline. The quality of the sperm is only roughly quantified by these crude indices. When spermatogenesis is induced in men with hypogonadotropic hypogonadism, only a few million sperm are necessary for impregnation. The fertilizing capacity of sperm is now being assessed by penetration of the zona pellucida–free hamster ovum.

SEX CHROMATIN PATTERN. The number of X chromosomes in the sex chromosome complex can be assessed indirectly by cytologic methods because of sexual dimorphism in the nuclear structure of somatic cells. Preparations suitable for examination can be obtained from smears of buccal mucosa, skin biopsy specimens, or blood (see Ch. 35). This test is widely used in the investigation of abnormalities of sex differentiation, particularly of males with defective testes and azoospermia or severe oligospermia. When a chromatin-positive (female-type) nuclear sex chromatin pattern is detected in a phenotypic male with bilateral testes, it suggests that an associated congenital primary testicular disorder may be present.

Catt KJ, Harwood JP, Clayton RN, et al: Regulation of peptide hormone receptors and gonadal steroidogenesis. Recent Prog Horm Res 36:557, 1980. *The authors give a comprehensive review of testicular gonadotropin receptors and the events of steroid biosynthesis.*

Clermont Y: Kinetics of spermatogenesis in mammals: Seminiferous epithelium cycle and spermatogonial renewal. Physiol Rev 52:198, 1972. *This is a description of the mechanisms of spermatogenesis and provides a good framework for understanding the dynamics of the process.*

Lipsett MB: Regulation of testicular functions. Andrologia 8:43, 1976. *This article describes the interactions between steroids and gonadotropins in men.*

Lipsett MB: Physiology and pathophysiology of the Leydig cell. N Engl J Med 303:682, 1980. *The Leydig cell and its physiologic aberrations are described.*

Mainwaring WIP: The Mechanism of Androgen Action. New York, Springer-Verlag, 1977. *This monograph discusses the basic biochemistry of androgen at the cellular level.*

Parvinen M: Regulation of the seminiferous epithelium. Endocr Rev 3:404, 1982. *This is a comprehensive review of spermatogenesis in the human and the effects of hormones on the process.*

PUBERTAL DEVELOPMENT IN THE MALE

There are wide variations in the age of onset, duration, and sequence of events that characterize the biologic pattern of male puberty. In normal boys signs of puberty may appear at any age between 10 and 17 years; the average age of onset is 12 to 13 years. Once initiated, the major changes are usually completed or well advanced in three to four years; in a small percentage of normal persons, maturity is not attained until the age of 21, and rarely thereafter.

The stimulus for release of pituitary gonadotropin at puberty originates in the hypothalamus and is mediated by a neurohormonal secretion, GnRH. A certain level of physiologic maturation, presumably including the central nervous system, is necessary before this complex and incompletely understood mechanism is activated. This level of development can be best correlated with the degree of osseous and epiphyseal development (bone age) rather than with the chronologic age. Small amounts of FSH and LH are secreted by prepubertal children. The hypothalamic-pituitary-testicular negative feedback mechanism is operative and set at a low level before pubescence.

The sequence of events that marks the pubertal period starts with an acceleration in the growth of the testes and scrotum. The initial increase in testicular size, occurring between 11 and 12 years, is largely attributable to changes in the seminiferous tubules. After initial acceleration of testicular growth, there is an increase in the size of the penis, the appearance of pubic hair, which has at first a transverse growth, and gradual enlargement of the prostate and other accessory organs and glands. The increase in testis size precedes the first appearance of pubic hair by approximately two years and peak height velocity by three years, and is an important clinical feature in ascertaining onset of early puberty. With pubescence, pulsatile and increased release of LH is observed, first at night and then throughout the 24 hours. Similarly, plasma testosterone concentration is first increased only during the night, reaching its normal adult levels as LH secretion increases.

There is a wide range of normality of the pubertal process in time of onset, intensity, and duration, and also in the degree of development of the secondary sex characteristics. In normal men, the pitch of the voice, the size of the external genitalia, the amount of body hair, and the body habitus vary from individual to individual, and are largely attributable to genetic factors and not to differences in the secretion of testosterone.

DELAYED ADOLESCENCE. Delayed adolescence, although a normal variant and benign, is often a severe psychologic handicap to the patient and a cause of parental anxiety. Many of these boys are short, and a delay of several years in osseous development is not uncommon. There may be a history of late onset of puberty in other members of the family. Retardation of puberty can be due to inadequate dietary intake or to chronic illness, because these may be associated with either diminished secretion of pituitary gonadotropin or Leydig cell dysfunction.

Pubertal failure or arrest in pubertal development secondary to pituitary-hypothalamic dysfunction or gonadal disease must be excluded in cases of delayed puberty. To exclude pituitary tumor, roentgenographic examination of the skull and careful examination of the fundi and visual fields are required, as well as search for other signs of neurologic involvement in boys who are significantly delayed in their sexual development, particularly when this is accompanied by stunting of growth. It is advisable to assess other pituitary functions, especially if the delayed maturation is accompanied by short stature or a decreased rate of growth. A buccal smear for sex chromatin and determination of plasma gonadotropins may clarify the clinical situation. The response to clomiphene or to GnRH will not differentiate between delayed puberty and hypogonadotropic hypogonadism, because both groups are unresponsive to clomiphene, and GnRH causes a similar pattern of LH and FSH release in both groups.

Treatment. Treatment should be directed toward correction of the basic disturbance, e.g., measures to improve nutrition or treatment of a pituitary neoplasm. Substitution therapy with male sex hormone should be started at about 13 or 14 years of age so that the onset of the patient's maturation coincides with that of his contemporaries. The use of this regimen does not preclude subsequent induction of spermatogenesis with FSH and HCG in those individuals with hypogonadotropic hypogonadism.

Less well defined is the treatment of boys in whom no apparent etiologic factor is found. Many will mature spontaneously before 17 years of age and merely represent an extreme of the normal range. Although indiscriminate use of hormonal treatment in this group is unwise, sociopsychologic considerations may make it expedient to treat such boys. A therapeutic trial with human chorionic gonadotropin, 500 to 1000 IU three times weekly injected intramuscularly, or with a long-acting testosterone preparation 200 mg every two to three weeks for three to six months will cause virilization, and often maturation will progress after treatment is discontinued.

Marshal WA, Tanner JM: Variations in the pattern of pubertal changes in boys. Arch Dis Child 45:13, 1970. *This paper provides a detailed description of the stages in male pubertal development and variations from the normal patterns. Physicians interested in these clinical problems should read this paper.*

SEXUAL PRECOCITY

Isosexual precocity in boys is defined as the occurrence of signs of masculinization before the age of ten years. Skeletal maturation is accelerated and the epiphyses fuse at a premature age, leading to a short stature in adult life. On the other hand, mental and dental development are not precocious. Sexual precocity occurs about three times more frequently in girls than in boys. There are four main causes of isosexual precocity in boys: *cerebral, adrenocortical, testicular,* and *tumors secreting HCG.*

CEREBRAL CAUSES. *Cerebral causes of sexual precocity* are associated with premature activation of the hypothalamic-pituitary mechanism and the release of pituitary gonadotropins. This form, designated true precocious puberty or complete isosexual precocity, is manifested by maturation of the Leydig cells, enlargement of the testis, and spermatogenesis.

True precocious puberty may be caused by organic lesions of the brain either directly or indirectly involving the posterior hypothalamus, such as hypothalamic and pineal tumors, hamartoma of the tuber cinereum, craniopharyngioma, hydrocephalus, postencephalitic lesions, congenital defects, tuberous sclerosis, and neurofibromatosis. The *McCune-Albright syndrome* of sexual precocity, polyostotic fibrous dysplasia, and pigmented areas of skin is rare in boys. The mechanism whereby such lesions activate the hypothalamic-pituitary secretion of gonadotropins is unknown. Cerebral lesions, particularly tumors, accompanied by precocious puberty may affect other hypothalamic functions, causing diabetes insipidus, bulimia, obesity, somnolence, emotional lability, or disturbances in temperature regulation. The syndrome of diabetes insipidus and precocious puberty suggests *aberrant pinealoma.* Signs of puberty may precede the onset of detectable neurologic involvement, and prolonged observation with repeated careful neurologic examinations, roentgenograms of the skull, and determinations of the visual fields is necessary before it is possible to exclude cerebral neoplasm. When no organic cause is found, the condition is described as *idiopathic precocious puberty;* in some instances, it is transmitted as a sex-limited autosomal dominant trait. In the idiopathic cases, seizure disorders and abnormal electroencephalographic patterns are appreciably more frequent than in normal children.

In all varieties of precocious puberty, plasma and urinary testosterone values are increased, because either Leydig cell secretion is stimulated or testosterone is produced elsewhere. In true precocious puberty, pituitary gonadotropin is secreted in the pulsatile manner that normally occurs with pubescence. Analogues of GnRH have been shown to suppress pituitary and testicular function and are of use in true isosexual precocious puberty. Rarely secretion of HCG by extrapituitary neoplasms, such as hepatoblastoma, causes isosexual precocity.

In forms of isosexual precocity not related to intracranial causes, in contrast to the enlarged phallus the testes remain immature and true puberty does not occur. Accordingly, this type has been called *incomplete sexual precocity or precocious pseudopuberty.*

ADRENOCORTICAL CAUSES. *Adrenocortical hyperfunction* resulting from congenital virilizing adrenal hyperplasia or a virilizing adrenocortical tumor is the most common cause of precocious pseudopuberty in boys. With few exceptions the testes remain prepubertal in size despite enlargement of the penis and scrotum and development of other secondary sexual characteristics. In congenital adrenal hyperplasia ectopic nodules of hyperplastic adrenal tissue are occasionally palpable in the testis, and may be confused with Leydig cell tumor, especially in rare instances in which striking enlargement of the testis is found. The excretion of 17-KS is increased in relation to chronologic age, and plasma levels of 17-hydroxyprogesterone and its metabolite, urinary pregnanetriol, are high in congenital adrenal hyperplasia.

TESTICULAR CAUSES. *Interstitial cell tumor of the testis* is a rare cause of isosexual precocity. In almost all reported cases the tumor has been unilateral, and the contralateral testis is immature. Gynecomastia is occasionally present. The excretion of 17-KS is usually normal, although occasional high values have been reported. Plasma testosterone concentration has generally been in the low normal adult male range. Spermatogenesis has been observed in the tubules surrounding the tumor only, thereby confirming the importance of high intratesticular androgen concentrations for spermatogenesis. There are now well-documented cases of apparently autonomous Leydig cell function that had previously been attributed to hypothalamic-pituitary activation.

SECONDARY TO HCG. *Iatrogenic sexual precocity* has been produced by the administration of male sex hormone, but is seen most frequently in boys who have been treated with large doses of HCG for cryptorchidism. Ectopic production of HCG by tumors may rarely lead to precocious puberty.

HYPOGONADISM

Hypogonadism may refer to a decrease in either the endocrine or the gametogenic function of the testis or to both. Primary hypogonadism is due to testicular disease, whereas secondary hypogonadism is a result of hypothalamic-pituitary disease. The excretion or blood level of gonadotropins is normal or high in primary hypogonadism, and is decreased in secondary hypogonadism. Primary lesions of the testis involving only spermatogenesis, resulting in infertility without hypoandrogenism, occur commonly. On the other hand, whenever testosterone secretion is deficient, spermatogenesis is impaired.

ANDROGEN DEFICIENCY. The clinical signs of androgen deficiency depend upon the age of onset and upon severity and duration of the deficiency. Total loss of testicular androgenic function, usually secondary to surgical castration or congenital defects of the testes, before or during early puberty results in eunuchoidism in adulthood. Eunuchoidism causes disproportionate growth of the long bones owing to delay in epiphyseal closure. The span exceeds the height by several inches, and the distance between the symphysis pubis and the sole (lower segment) measures more than 55 per cent of the height. Tall stature is common but not invariable. (The characteristic skeletal proportions of the eunuch are not pathognomonic and may be found in otherwise normal men.) The shoulders tend to be narrow and, although the habitus may be lean or obese, excessive fat deposition often occurs about the pectoral region, hips, thighs, and lower abdomen. Muscular development is poor. Except for the appearance of sparse pubic hair, secondary sex characteristics fail to appear, and the voice remains juvenile. Gynecomastia occurs in association with Klinefelter's syndrome and with male pseudohermaphroditism. Acne and baldness do not occur. Sex drive and potency are absent or greatly reduced. The hematocrit and hemoglobin levels are characteristic of those for women and increase with administration of androgen.

The effects on somatic and sexual development of partial loss of testicular androgenic function are less striking and vary greatly in degree. Characteristic of the milder forms of eunuchoidism are the scant growth of facial hair and a female distribution of pubic hair. In men who have attained sexual maturity, castration does not result in complete regression of secondary sexual characteristics, and the signs of androgen deficiency are less conspicuous. The most common signs are reduction in prostatic size, diminished rate of growth of the beard and body hair, the appearance of fine wrinkles around the eyes, and a pasty, sallow complexion. Semen volume is reduced. Potency and libido, although usually diminished, occasionally persist. There may be vasomotor phenomena, including hot flushes.

Androgen deficiency is best treated by preparations of testosterone for intramuscular, oral, and buccal or sublingual administration. The mode of administration depends, for the most part, on the preference of the patient and the cost.

Esterification of testosterone with organic acids potentiates its activity when injected as an oily solution. Testosterone propionate in doses of 25 to 50 mg by intramuscular injection two or three times weekly is adequate for replacement therapy. However, longer-acting esters are available that can be administered less frequently. One dose of 300 mg of testosterone cyclopentylpropionate or testosterone enanthate is highly effective when injected at two- to three-week intervals.

Methyltestosterone is an effective preparation for oral and buccal or sublingual use. It is usually administered in doses of 50 mg (30 to 75 mg) orally or about 25 mg per day sublingually. It is not metabolized to 17-KS as is testosterone. Fluoxymesterone (Halotestin) in doses of 10 mg daily has also been used for substitution therapy. None of the oral androgens is as effective as the testosterone esters given by injection. No potent protein anabolic steroid lacking androgenic properties is available at present, although intensive efforts have been made to obtain one.

Undesirable effects of androgens include edema caused by retention of extracellular electrolyte (a rare effect except with use of large doses or in elderly persons with diminished cardiac reserve), polycythemia, acne, gynecomastia, and premature closure of the epiphyses. Rarely, methyltestosterone and other oral androgens cause reversible intrahepatic cholestatic jaundice. Androgen therapy may be contraindicated in patients with carcinoma of the prostate. The use of androgens by normal men to increase athletic performance remains controversial; it is certain, though, that the androgens will markedly decrease spermatogenesis.

Primary Hypogonadism (Primary Failure of the Testis)

The problem of classification of primary hypogonadism has not been entirely resolved, because the etiology of many of the disorders in this group is uncertain. Primary hypogonadism may result from genetic and developmental defects, such as seminiferous tubule dysgenesis and Laurence-Moon-Biedl syndrome, or from other causes: trauma, destruction of spermatogonia after orchitis, exposure to ionizing radiation, chemotherapy, and surgical castration. Disorders in this group may or may not be accompanied by androgen deficiency, although in some eunuchoidism is a constant or frequent feature. Disorders of spermatogenesis characterized only by oligospermia and infertility are likewise examples of primary hypogonadism. Plasma LH is increased with hypofunction of the Leydig cells as in old age or myotonic dystrophy. Plasma FSH is increased whenever tubular damage is severe enough to compromise Sertoli cell function. A high plasma FSH concentration almost always signifies irreversible infertility.

Klinefelter's Syndrome; Seminiferous Tubule Dysgenesis

This syndrome is characterized classically by small, firm testes, azoospermia, gynecomastia, and elevated urinary gonadotropins. The features become apparent during early puberty, and may include eunuchoidism. Histologically there is atrophy and hyalinization of the seminiferous tubules; Leydig cells tend to occur in large clumps and are apparently increased in number, but total Leydig cell volume is probably normal. The few remaining tubules are lined by Sertoli cells; rarely, germ cells are present. Elastic fibers in the tunica propria are absent, indicating failure of pubertal maturation. The cause of the syndrome is a developmental defect of the gonad associated with and probably resulting from a sex chromosome abnormality. Klinefelter's syndrome and its variants are now defined by the single constant finding of an increase in the number of X chromosomes in at least one cell line.

The discovery that most persons with the classic features of Klinefelter's syndrome are chromatin positive, followed by the detection of sex chromosome abnormalities, served to identify an especially well-defined disorder caused by a nonfamilial, genetically determined gonadal defect, sometimes called "seminiferous tubule dysgenesis." This disorder, which occurs sporadically, is an important cause of male infertility and a common type of sexual anomaly which occurs with a frequency in the order of 1 in 500 newborn males.

The most frequent clinical feature of Klinefelter's syndrome is the small size of the testes, the long diameter usually being less than 2 cm. The testes are firmer than normal owing to hyalinization of the tubules. Patients with this disorder are often tall, and the skeletal proportions frequently are eunuchoid as a consequence of the disproportionately long lower extremities, even though epiphyseal fusion is not delayed and skeletal maturation usually follows the normal male pattern (Fig. 234–4). Cryptorchidism and hypospadias are infrequent, and gynecomastia is present in fewer than 50 per cent of the cases. Mental retardation and psychopathic behavior are not uncommon, and there is often evidence of poor social adaptation. This disorder has been reported in association with mongolism and with leukemia. It has been suggested that chronic pulmonary disease and varicose veins are more prevalent in affected adults. The frequency of impaired glucose tolerance and of mild diabetes is increased.

In the classic form of the disease plasma FSH is increased as a result of the extensive tubular destruction. Plasma LH is usually high but may be normal in those few men with normal Leydig cell function. The plasma concentration of testosterone is often low, and may increase only slowly with the daily administration of human chorionic gonadotropin for four to five days.

The common abnormality of the sex chromosomes in Klinefelter's syndrome is a 47,XXY karyotype. Less common types of sex chromosome abnormalities in this disorder include phenotypic males with the genotypes 48,XXYY, 48,XXXY, or 49,XXXXY that have been found so far only in mentally retarded persons. Unusually tall stature has been found in the XXYY group, along with a tendency to more aggressive and delinquent behavior. The 48,XXXY sex chromosome complex is associated with two sex chromatin bodies in a proportion of diploid somatic nuclei, and the 49,XXXXY constitution with three sex chromatin bodies. In addition to mental retardation, the XXXXY men have had severe congenital malformations, including very small, usually undescended testes; hypoplastic external genitalia; minor skeletal deformities, including radioulnar synostosis; and other congenital anomalies. It seems that with increasing numbers of X chromosomes, the severity of the abnormalities increases.

Instances of sex chromosome mosaicism have also been described in which at least two populations of cells with different cell chromosome complexes were found in the same individual, e.g., XY/XXY (one cell line with an XY sex chromosome complex and another with an XXY sex chromosome complex), XY/XXXY, XX/XXY, and XXXY/XXXXY. Sex chromosome mosaics arise from a mitotic error in an early division after fertilization in a zygote that originally had either a normal or an abnormal sex chromosome constitution. The detection of a chromatin-positive sex chromatin pattern on buccal smear should not by itself be used as incontrovertible evidence of sterility. Active spermatogenesis was found in the testes of an XY/XXXXY mosaic, and additional examples of potential fertility may be found in chromatin-positive males with other forms of sex chromosome mosaicism, especially XY/XXY. In several carefully studied men with Klinefelter's syndrome, only an XX sex chromosome constitution was found. The maternal origin of the two X chromosomes suggests that a Y chromosome was present early in ontogeny and was lost or more likely translocated to an X chromosome or autosome, or that these men were mosaics and the Y-bearing cell line has escaped detection.

The typical XXY sex chromosome constitution of seminiferous tubule dysgenesis may arise from an abnormality of meiosis during gametogenesis or from a mitotic error in the fertilized zygote (see Ch. 35). The positive association of this disorder with advanced maternal age and the results of surveys of color blindness (a sex-linked recessive trait) and of the Xg blood group suggest a maternal origin with nondisjunction occurring during oogenesis. Using X-linked markers, a paternal origin of one X has been established in several informative pedigrees, nondisjunction during spermatogenesis giving rise to an XY-

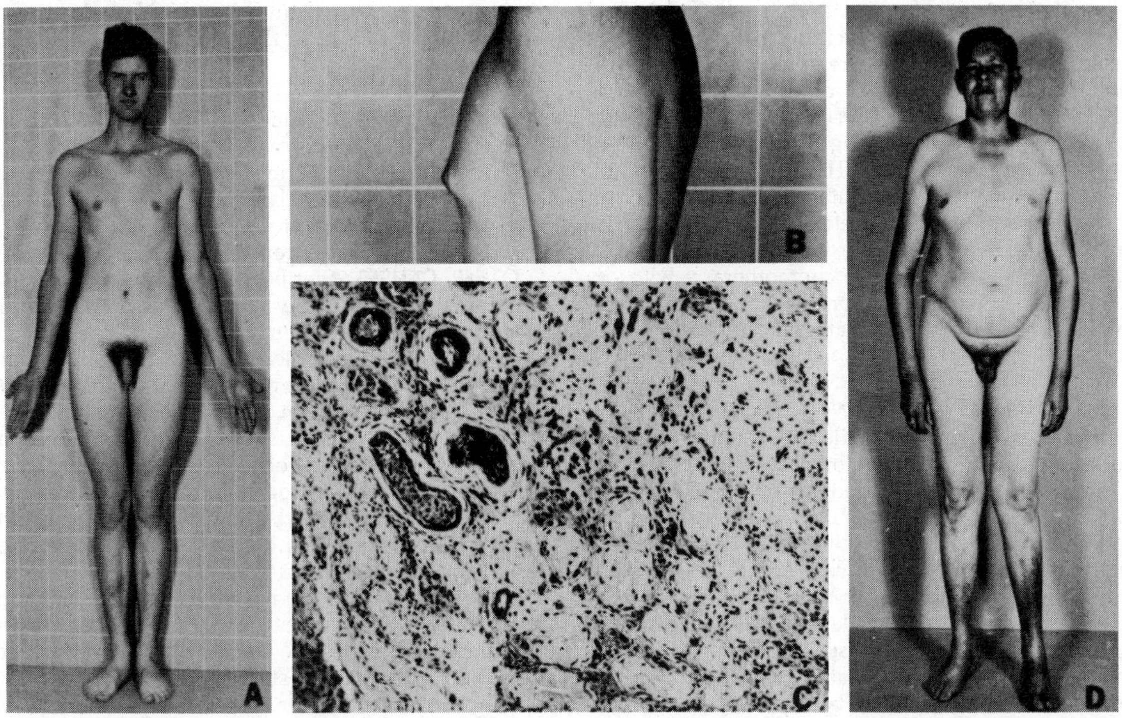

Figure 234–4. *A* and *B*, Typical 19-year-old phenotypic male with chromatin-positive seminiferous tubule dysgenesis (Klinefelter's syndrome). This patient had a positive sex chromatin pattern and an XXY karyotype. His 17-ketosteroid excretion was 11.2 mg per 24 hours, and his urinary gonadotropin excretion was more than 100 mu. These patients vary widely in their habitus and degree of virilization. This patient is well virilized, but had long extremities with eunuchoidal proportions and exhibited gynecomastia. The testes measured 1.8 × 0.9 cm and were small and firm. Testicular biopsy, *C*, revealed a severe degree of hyalinization of his seminiferous tubules and Leydig cell hyperplasia. *D*, Forty-eight-year-old man with chromatin-positive Klinefelter's syndrome who came to medical attention only because his severe leg varicosities were thought to reveal a "female trait." (From Van Wyk JJ, Grumbach MM: *In* Williams RH [ed.]: Textbook of Endocrinology. 4th ed. Philadelphia, W. B. Saunders Company, 1968.)

bearing sperm and fertilization yielding an XXY zygote. More complex sex chromosome anomalies may arise from meiotic or mitotic errors, or from a combination of both.

The gonadal defect is a consequence of the abnormal sex chromosome constitution. The single Y chromosome is a sufficiently powerful male determiner to suppress the cortical component (ovarian anlage) of the primordial gonad despite the presence of two (or even four) X chromosomes. The fetal testes that develop may have either an adequate number or a deficiency of germ cells, but bring about normal male differentiation of the genital tract. At puberty, if the function of the Leydig cells is adequate as occurs rarely, male secondary sexual characteristics develop, but the seminiferous tubules lack or are severely deficient in germ cells. Tubular hyalinization usually does not begin until the later prepubertal period. It seems likely that the characteristic appearance of the testes in adolescent and adult cases depends on the direct or indirect action of pituitary gonadotropins from the onset of puberty on an inherently defective testis, which, before this time, shows only subtle signs of an abnormal histologic structure.

TREATMENT. If there is evidence of androgen deficiency, testosterone replacement is indicated. Testosterone treatment may produce transient increase in gynecomastia and nipple tenderness. Mastectomy may be necessary in some patients, primarily for cosmetic reasons.

Chromatin-Negative Klinefelter's Syndrome

This term, a misnomer, was bestowed before the fundamental distinction was made on the basis of karyotype. The small testes and azoospermia suggest the Klinefelter phenotype. The testicular lesion resembles that of Klinefelter's syndrome, but the testis can react to injury in only a limited number of ways. The patients have none of the associated anomalies seen in Klinefelter's syndrome, but hypogonadism is sometimes present. It is probable that so-called chromatin-negative Klinefelter's syndrome is the end-stage of several different disease processes, the final result being hyalinization of the tubules with loss of spermatogonia. Some of these patients may be unrecognized mosaics with one cell line bearing an XXY karyotype and would thus be classified as having Klinefelter's syndrome. Plasma testosterone levels have varied from normal to low.

XYY Syndrome

Although the XXY syndrome is discussed under the topic of primary hypogonadism, in fact primary hypogonadism is unusual in XYY subjects. The XYY syndrome is characterized by a chromosome complement of 47 with an extra Y chromosome and a sex chromatin–negative buccal smear that contains nuclei with two small fluorescent Y chromatin masses, and is estimated to occur in 1 per 500 to 1 per 1000 male births. Newborn males and young boys with this syndrome have a normal phenotype. A number of associated characteristics have been reported in the adolescent and adult XYY male. These include tall stature (often over 6 feet), severe acne, and skeletal abnormalities, e.g., radioulnar synostosis. In studies of criminals with a history of aggressive crimes, an increased frequency of the XYY genotype has been noted. On the other hand, most adult XYY males are physically and mentally normal, and the genotype is present with greater frequency in tall men.

Although the extra Y apparently confers the potential for increased stature, Leydig cell function and plasma and urinary testosterone concentrations have been normal.

Germinal Aplasia (Sertoli-Cell-Only Syndrome)

This condition is characterized by seminiferous tubules lined with Sertoli cells, little or no tubular fibrosis, and absent germinal cells. The patients are first seen by the physician because of sterility. Leydig cell function is normal. Azoospermia is an invariable finding. The testes are somewhat reduced in size. Plasma FSH levels are increased four- to five-fold, whereas LH levels are within normal limits. There is an exaggerated response of LH to GnRH, indicating some abnormality of Leydig cell control or LH secretion. The karyotype is 46,XY. Germinal aplasia is probably a congenital disease of the Sertoli cell, and these cells are abnormal by electron microscopy. The lesion has also been described after exposure of the testes to ionizing radiation and after extensive chemotherapy with cytotoxic agents. There is no treatment for the spontaneous form, but even severe damage to the spermatogenic epithelium may be reversible.

Myotonic Muscular Dystrophy

Testicular atrophy, occurring in middle age, is found in about 80 per cent of affected men with myotonic dystrophy (see Ch. 538.1). This syndrome is characterized by myotonia, muscle wasting, frontal baldness, and lenticular opacities. Signs of androgen deficiency occur in 18 per cent of the patients and gynecomastia in 12 per cent. As the disease progresses, increasing tubular fibrosis results in high plasma FSH levels and Leydig cell failure leads to high LH levels. The testis shows tubular fibrosis, hyalinization, and disordered spermatogenesis. There are other metabolic abnormalities which, in association with the testicular findings, have been described as accelerated aging.

Anorchia

Absence of both testes in phenotypic males has been described but is exceedingly rare. Careful surgical exploration is required to establish the diagnosis. In a few cases, catheterization of the spermatic vein revealed a testosterone gradient, suggesting that a nidus of Leydig cells in the expected position of the testis remained functional. Unilateral anorchia is more common, and may result from testicular atrophy after herniorrhaphy, from attempted orchiopexy, or from a developmental disturbance, in which case there may be associated anomalies of the genitourinary tract.

Infertility

In many testicular lesions, the defect involves only spermatogenic function and results in infertility. Endocrine manifestations are absent. Either the semen lacks sperm or the number or quality of sperm is diminished. Testicular biopsy has a major role in differentiating the various disturbances in spermatogenic activity and in determining prognosis. Azoospermia is usually associated with severe tubular fibrosis, germinal aplasia, or spermatogenic arrest, and oligospermia with germinal cell desquamation, hypospermatogenesis, incomplete spermatogenic arrest, and less severe forms of tubular fibrosis. In general, only azoospermia or severe oligospermia is associated with increased plasma FSH concentrations. In most cases the cause is unknown. Azoospermia may also result from obstruction in the afferent ducts secondary to gonorrhea, tuberculosis, or a nonspecific infection. Absence or atresia of the vas deferens and a rudimentary epididymis are common bilateral lesions in boys with cystic fibrosis, but may occur spontaneously. Azoospermia in the presence of a normal FSH suggests obstructive disease and warrants biopsy and urologic consultation.

OLIGOSPERMIA. This condition is composed of many variants. There may be partial arrest of spermatogenesis at the primary or secondary spermatocyte stage or at the spermatid stage. Abnormalities of the meiotic chromosomes and reduction in chiasma formation have been noted in men with oligospermia. Sperm morphology may be abnormal. Of interest are the nonmotile sperm seen in *Kartagener's syndrome* (sinusitis, bronchiectasis, and situs inversus). The cause of immotility is the absence of the dynein arms of the microtubular elements of the sperm tail, and this defect is related to the immobility of the cilia in the bronchi. In some men with severe oligospermia the fibroblasts have only one half the normal number of androgen receptors. Thus the effect of decreased androgen action at the tubule is the putative cause of the associated infertility.

VARICOCELE. This condition is associated with decreased sperm count and infertility in 25 to 65 per cent of men, and there are varying abnormalities of sperm morphology. In general, measures of endocrine function have been normal. Results of varicocelectomy have been uneven, the incidence of restored fertility varying from 25 to 75 per cent. The role of the varicocele in producing infertility remains obscure.

OTHER CAUSES. Sterility is a common sequel of bilateral cryptorchidism and may occur in association with unilateral cryptorchidism. Sterility may follow orchitis caused by mumps, gonorrhea, brucellosis, leprosy, or occasionally other systemic infection; it may be of developmental origin, as in seminiferous tubule dysgenesis. Even relatively minor illnesses may cause profound depression in sperm count. Starvation and chronic debilitating diseases associated with inanition adversely affect spermatic function. Estrogen and androgen administration also inhibit spermatogenesis by suppression of gonadotropins with concomitant decrease in intratesticular testosterone concentration. The increasing survival and cure rates of men with lymphomas treated with multiple chemotherapeutic agents has led to assessment of testicular function after treatment. The seminiferous tubules are sensitive to alkylating agents in particular, and permanent sterility may follow therapy. Recovery of function, which occurs rarely, may be monitored by measurement of plasma FSH. If fertility is an objective after therapy, sperm banking is an option.

TREATMENT OF INFERTILITY IN THE MALE. Although important advances have been made in the evaluation of spermatogenic function, treatment of infertility caused by primary testicular disease is unsatisfactory. The results of therapy of hormonally normal men with oligospermia by the use of large doses of androgenic steroids, gonadotropins, pregnenolone, thyroid hormone, clomiphene, and vitamin preparations have been generally unsuccessful. The intermittent use of large doses of testosterone to take advantage of the "rebound effect" on spermatogenesis has not been established as efficacious, although occasional men seem to benefit. The use of testololactone, which inhibits aromatization, has been shown to increase the sperm count in some men with oligospermia. This suggests a role for intratubular estrogen in the etiology of some types of oligospermia.

Secondary Hypogonadism

Secondary hypogonadism is due to decreased secretion of gonadotropins, and may result from neoplastic, inflammatory, traumatic, vascular, or degenerative lesions involving the pituitary or hypothalamus. These lesions include such entities as pituitary adenoma, craniopharyngioma, astrocytoma, infarction, carotid aneurysm, granulomas such as tuberculosis, histiocytosis X, and hemochromatosis. In many instances, the nature of the underlying lesion is not known. A functional and reversible depression of gonadotropin secretion occurs in malnutrition, in chronic disease states associated with inanition and nutritional deficiencies, and in some patients with myxedema. High concentrations of androgen and estrogen, as in the adrenogenital syndrome, may cause secondary hypogonadism by suppression of gonadotropin secretion. Excessive estrogen, either from ingestion or an endogenous source, as from a feminizing adrenal tumor, depresses the secretion of pituitary gonadotropin. The testicular atrophy that occurs in some patients with severe liver disease is due in part to increased levels of estrogen. Decreased gonadotropin secretion may also result from the nutritional and metabolic disturbances accompanying hepatic cirrhosis. Alcohol, or its metabolite acetaldehyde, has direct toxic effects on the Leydig cell.

Decreased secretion of pituitary gonadotropins occurs either as an isolated defect, *hypogonadotropic hypogonadism*, or, more commonly, in association with a deficiency of growth hormone and other anterior pituitary hormones. On the other hand, hypoadrenocorticism or hypothyroidism secondary to pituitary failure is rarely found without concurrent involvement of gonadotropic function and secondary hypogonadism. Secondary hypogonadism is usually characterized by both inadequate androgenic function and, with rare exceptions (see below), absent or deficient spermatogenesis.

The clinical manifestations vary with age of onset, degree of the deficiency, and whether there is coexistent deficiency of other anterior pituitary hormones. Hypopituitarism occurring during childhood, commonly designated "pituitary dwarfism," results in proportionate dwarfism and complete sexual infantilism. The characteristic features of prepubertal or pubertal gonadotropic failure are eunuchoid habitus, small testes, lack of development of secondary sexual characteristics, an increased frequency of anosmia or hyposmia, low or absent gonadotropins, and low plasma testosterone concentration. The absence of gynecomastia, regarded by some as a salient feature, is of no clinical value in differentiating primary from secondary hypogonadism. It is important to detect organic disease of the pituitary region. Such evaluation should include study of the visual fields, roentgenography of the sella turcica, and, when indicated, such procedures as tomography of the sella, computed tomography, and carotid and venous angiography.

A familial form of isolated hypogonadotropic hypogonadism limited to males occurs in association with anosmia or hyposmia *(Kallmann's syndrome)* and is transmitted as either an X-linked or a sex-linked dominant trait. Aplasia of the olfactory lobes has been found in autopsied cases. Leydig cell responsiveness to HCG in some of these patients may be decreased. Both familial and sporadic forms of isolated FSH and LH deficiency are known, and these may be associated with a variety of somatic anomalies and neurologic defects. Although the initial response to GnRH has been variable, with continued administration the response becomes normal. These data suggest that hypothalamic synthesis or release of GnRH is impaired in these patients and in most patients with hypogonadotropic hypogonadism.

The testis in patients with hypogonadotropic hypogonadism remains infantile, the tubular diameter being the same as that of the fetal testis. When pituitary function is decreased in adult life, tubular collapse, fibrosis, and hyalinization occur at variable times after the onset of gonadotropic failure.

Isolated LH Deficiency. There is a group of eunuchoidal men with relatively normal-sized testes and some spermatogenic function to whom the term "fertile eunuch" has been applied. The patients are not fertile, however, because spermatogenesis is decreased, and libido and potency are absent. Leydig cells are absent or few in number, and androgen deficiency is always present. The concentration of plasma LH and the excretion of urinary LH are low or undetectable, whereas the secretion of FSH is normal. Chorionic gonadotropin stimulates Leydig cell function, ameliorates the androgen deficiency, and increases spermatogenesis. These patients have a relative deficiency of LH, which may arise from an abnormality in the hypothalamus (and the synthesis or release of GnRH) or in the pituitary gland. A kindred with two affected brothers has been reported. Rarely, a pituitary tumor or idiopathic delayed adolescence may manifest itself as isolated LH deficiency.

Treatment. A physiologic approach to the treatment of secondary hypogonadism characterized by decreased spermatogenesis requires the use of gonadotropins or GnRH. FSH preparations derived from animal sources are not consistently effective and, when injected repeatedly, stimulate antibody formation that reduces the effect of the hormones. However, gonadotropins prepared from menopausal urine have been used successfully in combination with HCG to induce spermatogenesis in patients with hypogonadotropic hypogonadism. As little as 25 IU of FSH three times a week in combination with 1000 IU of HCG three times a week has induced spermatogenesis. Impregnation often occurs with total sperm counts below 20 million. This suggests that the infertility seen in men with oligospermia whose sperm counts may be higher is due to factors other than sperm number. Spermatogenesis has been induced in hypogonadotropic hypogonadism with pulsatile injection of GnRH. Testosterone cannot be used in place of HCG, because intratesticular testosterone concentrations do not reach the levels attained when the Leydig cells are stimulated by HCG. HCG does not have a direct effect on the seminiferous tubules, although in a few instances of partial gonadotropic failure in which some FSH secretion remained, spermatogenic as well as Leydig cell function improved after its use. HCG has been effective in maintaining spermatogenesis after hypophysectomy for diabetic retinopathy, or after initiation of spermatogenesis with FSH. When only androgen substitution therapy is needed, one of the long-acting testosterone preparations is preferred.

Boyden TW, Pamenter RW: Effects of ethanol on the male hypothalamic-pituitary-gonadal axis. Endocr Rev 4:389, 1983. *A comprehensive discussion of the effects of alcohol.*

Brasel JA, Wright JC, Wilkins L, Blizzard RM: An evaluation of seventy-five patients with hypopituitarism beginning in childhood. Am J Med 38:484, 1965. *This is a comprehensive review of the clinical syndrome of hypopituitarism with many data about hypogonadism.*

Paulsen CA, Gordon DL, Carpenter RW, Gandy HM, Drucker WD: Klinefelter's syndrome and its variants: A hormonal and chromosomal study. Recent Prog Horm Res 24:321, 1968. *This is a comprehensive review of the clinical manifestations and laboratory findings of a large group of men with Klinefelter's syndrome.*

CRYPTORCHIDISM

The terms "cryptorchidism" and "undescended testes" are used synonymously to designate testes that have never descended into the scrotum. Unilateral cryptorchidism is approximately four times as common as bilaterally undescended testes. A cryptorchid testis may be situated in the abdomen, within the inguinal canal, or in an ectopic position outside the scrotum and the normal pathway of descent. The majority of undescended testes are inguinal. To avoid needless treatment, it is essential to distinguish this condition from retractile testes, which lie in the lower or upper scrotum and are withdrawn into the inguinal region and occasionally into the abdomen by slight stimulus.

The testes usually descend into the scrotum about the eighth fetal month; but occasionally descent is delayed until shortly after birth. Incomplete descent is common in premature male infants. Undescended testes are found at birth in 3 to 4 per cent of full-term male infants. During the first month of life 50 per cent of undescended testes reached the scrotum. Spontaneous descent occurs frequently during the first year of life and is less common after this age. Only 0.5 per cent of male infants have undescended testes at 12 months of age. The prevalence of unilateral and bilateral cryptorchidism in large series of adult males has been variously estimated at 0.2 to 0.4 per cent.

The etiology is not understood. Not infrequently a normal testis resides in the superficial inguinal pouch, its descent arrested by Scarpa's fascia. However, the cryptorchid testis is often dysgenetic. In rare instances, unilateral or bilateral cryptorchidism is the only overt anatomic abnormality of the external genitalia in individuals with fetal testicular dysfunction.

DIAGNOSIS. The most difficult aspect of diagnosis is distinguishing the true undescended testis from the more common retractile testis of childhood; repeated examinations may be necessary, especially in obese boys. It is important to ascertain by careful inquiry whether the testes have at any time been observed in the scrotum. In cryptorchidism the ipsilateral side of the scrotum is empty and poorly developed. The patient should be carefully examined while standing, squatting, and in a recumbent position, in a warm room and with warm hands. Bimanual examination and palpation while the patient performs a Valsalva maneuver or while the examiner applies pressure to the lower abdomen are also useful procedures. In boys with retractile testes, elicitation of the cremasteric reflex often results in a localized puckering of the scrotal skin. If the testis is palpated in the normal pathway of descent, gentle manipulation should be used in an attempt to displace it into the scrotum. Such mobile testes do not require therapy and will remain in the scrotum with the advent of puberty. Failure to palpate a testis on multiple occasions suggests that the testis is intra-abdominal, atrophic, or absent. An increase in plasma FSH and an augmented response to GnRH indicates severe Sertoli cell dysfunction.

TREATMENT. The treatment of undescended testes is a vexing and controversial subject; experienced observers differ in their approach to the problem. Major considerations are (1) the potential fertility of the undescended testis, (2) the likelihood of spontaneous descent, and (3) the propensity of the undescended testis to undergo malignant change.

During or after puberty the undescended testis shows degenerative changes that eventually proceed to atrophy. These changes have been ascribed to the deleterious effect of the higher temperature of an extrascrotal environment on the testes, especially on the germinal epithelium. The tubules gradually undergo progressive fibrosis and loss of germinal elements, although androgenic function may persist for many years. These degenerative changes may also be manifestations of a dysgenetic testis. This distinction is important, because the risk of cancer in the dysgenetic gonad is considerably greater than in the normal gonad.

Men with bilateral undescended testes are sterile. However, general agreement is lacking as to the age at which the fertility potential of the cryptorchid testis is impaired. A lag in development of the seminiferous tubules and, in some instances, a mild degree of fibrosis in undescended testes after the age of six to ten years have been observed. The significance of these changes is uncertain, but after puberty irreversible degenerative changes frequently occur.

The incidence of cancer in undescended testes is considerably greater than in scrotal testes, and more so in abdominal than in inguinal testes. The probability of cancer occurring in a cryptorchid testis is 30 to 50 times greater than in the normal testis.

The most important problem in the treatment of patients with cryptorchidism is the age at which it is advisable to attempt correction. Treatment consists of orchiopexy or of the administration of HCG followed by orchiopexy when necessary. Therapy must be started before pubescence and probably by age 6 if irreparable testicular damage is to be prevented. In the more common unilateral cryptorchidism, the scrotal testis, if normal, is adequate for fertility. Treatment is recommended for cosmetic reasons, to facilitate examination for neoplasm, and as additional insurance against infertility in the event that the scrotal testis is defective or impaired at a later age.

In bilateral cryptorchidism preservation of fertility is the major consideration, but the results of treatment are disappointing. Bilateral orchiopexy is generally followed by tubular fibrosis and atrophy. Since many undescended testes descend before puberty, it is justifiable to delay treatment until nine years of age unless the testis is ectopic or associated with a hernia.

When hormonal therapy is effective, it is probable that the testis would have descended spontaneously at puberty under the stimulus of endogenous gonadotropin. To minimize a theoretical risk of damage to the tubule, short intensive courses of 1000 units of HCG administered intramuscularly daily for three days or 1000 units three times a week for three weeks may be used. Hormonal treatment is contraindicated when the testis lies outside the normal pathway of descent.

If the undescended testis is atrophic and biopsy at the time of surgery shows irreversible changes, it is generally advisable to perform orchiectomy, provided that the contralateral testis is in the scrotum. This also applies to a testis that, despite all attempts at mobilization, cannot be brought into the scrotum.

Batata MA, Whitmore WF Jr, Chu FCH, et al: Cryptorchidism and testicular cancer. J Urol 124:382, 1980. *A review of the incidence of cancer and of the results of treatment.*

Raifer J, Walsh PC: Testicular descent: Normal and abnormal. Urol Clin N Amer 5:223, 1978. *A discussion of embryology, mechanisms and treatment.*

IMPOTENCE

Impotence is a complicated problem that may be either relative or complete and may involve any phase of the sexual act. Although it is a symptom of androgen deficiency and of genitourinary or neurologic disease, in many instances it is psychic in origin. Multiple sclerosis, tabes dorsalis, and diabetic neuropathy are commonly associated with impotence. Impotence without apparent impairment of libido has been described in patients with temporal lobe lesions. Many drugs used in the therapy of hypertension can cause impotence. When impotence is the principal complaint of a patient, it is often the result of an emotional disturbance, and in this case androgen therapy is valueless. Stress can decrease gonadotropin secretion and thereby affect androgen secretion and spermatogenesis (see Ch. 236). Increased prolactin, resulting from tumor or drugs, may produce impotence by directly suppressing LH via a "short-loop" feedback, and, consequently, testosterone secretion. Rarely primary hyperprolactinemia may cause impotence. With tests now available, specific causes of impotence can be identified more often. In one recent series, only 14 per cent of impotent men were identified as having psychogenic impotence; in an additional 7 per cent the cause was not known.

Slag MF, Morley JE, Elgon MK, et al: Impotence in medical clinic outpatients. JAMA 249:1736, 1983. *A large study of men in an outpatient clinic who were carefully studied for causes of impotence.*

"MALE CLIMACTERIC"

The male climacteric, as an analogue of the menopause, does not exist. Although during the fifth or sixth decade ovarian failure with a consequent rise in gonadotropin excretion is an anticipated physiologic accompaniment of the aging process, spontaneous testicular deficiency of sufficient degree to produce symptoms is rare. Many of the symptoms ascribed to this syndrome are common in psychoneurotic middle-aged and elderly men. The diagnosis of testicular failure should be documented by finding an increased plasma level of gonadotropin and a low level of plasma testosterone, and should be confirmed by obtaining a therapeutic response to androgen therapy but not to placebos. In healthy men there are only minor decreases in plasma testosterone concentrations with increasing age. A progressive increase in plasma LH levels after age 60 has been described, indicating mild compensated Leydig cell failure. Plasma estradiol increases with age as a result of increased conversion of testosterone to estradiol in peripheral tissues. The frequency of alterations in tubular histology increases progressively after age 30, prominent changes being thickening of the basement membrane, intratubular fibrosis, and loss of germ cells. Plasma FSH increases after age 70 in response to this seminiferous tubule damage.

ORCHITIS

Acute orchitis, a common complication of mumps, is a rare occurrence in the course of other specific infectious diseases (see Ch. 335).

Chronic orchitis is associated with painless, hard, sometimes nodular enlargement of the testis. *Syphilis*, the most common cause, may produce an interstitial orchitis in which the testis is characteristically smooth and wooden in consistency ("billiard ball" testis); involvement is frequently bilateral. Other causes include *tuberculosis, leprosy, brucellosis, glanders,* and certain parasitic infections such as *filariasis* and *bilharziasis*. In these diseases, Leydig cell function almost always remains intact, but severe tubular destruction may result.

TABLE 234–1. TUMORS OF TESTIS: CLASSIFICATION*

I. Primary tumors
  A. Germinal
    1. Seminoma
    2. Embryonal tumors
      a. Embryoma
      b. Choriocarcinoma
      c. Embryonal carcinoma
      d. Teratocarcinoma
      e. Adult teratoma
    3. Combinations of seminoma and embryonal tumor and of the various types of embryonal tumors
    4. Gonadal tumors in intersexes (gonadoblastomas)
  B. Nongerminal tumors
    1. Interstitial cell tumor
    2. Sertoli cell tumor
    3. Tumors of testicular stroma: fibroma, lipoma, etc.
II. Secondary tumors
  A. Lymphoma, plasmacytoma, leukemia, etc.
  B. Metastatic carcinoma

*From Melicow MM: Classification of Tumors of the Testis. J Urol 73:547, 1955.

TUMORS OF THE TESTIS

Tumors of the testis are uncommon, constituting about 0.7 per cent of all forms of cancer in the male. They occur in about 0.002 per cent of men, and frequently are malignant. The greatest incidence occurs in the third and fourth decades. Testicular tumors may arise from any of the cellular components of the testis or their embryonal precursors.

Considerable uncertainty applies to classification, especially of those neoplasms whose origin has been ascribed to the totipotent germ cell. A classification of testicular tumors is shown in Table 234–1.

Germinal Tumors

Most common are germinal tumors, and, of these, seminoma exceeds in frequency all other testicular tumors. *Seminoma,* although usually fairly uniform in cellular architecture, may contain embryonal elements such as chorionic syncytium in the primary growth or in metastatic lesions. In contrast to the embryonal tumors, which tend to invade the spermatic cord and to metastasize early, especially to lung, seminomas in general are relatively slow growing and commonly invade the iliac and periaortic lymph nodes before generalized dissemination is demonstrable. In addition, seminomas are frequently highly radiosensitive, whereas embryonal tumors are usually resistant to radiotherapy. The significantly increased incidence of germinal tumors, particularly seminoma, in undescended testes and in the dysgenetic gonads of intersexes has been discussed above.

Many patients with germinal tumors excrete increased amounts of chorionic gonadotropin. This may almost always be attributed to the presence of trophoblastic elements in the tumor. Response to therapy or evidence of recurrence may be monitored by measurement of plasma HCG levels. Other fetal protein markers such as carcinoembryonic antigens may also be secreted by these cancers.

The germ cell tumors of the testis are responsive to therapy. Removal or radiation of regional and paraortic lymph nodes has produced survival rates of 80 to 95 per cent in men with seminoma. Choriocarcinoma and embryonal cell carcinoma have responded to multiagent chemotherapeutic regimens. With the addition of cisdiamminedichloroplatinum to combinations of methotrexate, dactinomycin, and chlorambucil, response rates of 40 to 70 per cent have been achieved in men with metastatic disease. About 40 per cent of these patients are apparently in long-term remission.

Interstitial Cell Tumors

Tumors of this type are rare, occur at any age, and are usually but not invariably benign. The tumors are small and often difficult to palpate. In boys interstitial cell tumors cause sexual precocity but not true puberty, because spermatogenesis is absent in the contralateral testis. The only recognizable endocrine manifestation in the adult is gynecomastia, which has been observed in about 10 per cent of cases. Malignant interstitial cell tumors that retain their steroid-synthesizing capacities have been reported.

Fraley EE, Lange PH, Kennedy BJ: Germ-cell testicular cancer in adults. N Engl J Med 301:1370, 1979. *A review of embryology, endocrinology, and therapy of germ-cell tumors of the testis.*

Hainsworth JD, Greco FA: Testicular germ cell neoplasms. Am J Med: 75:817, 1983. *The diagnosis and treatment of these tumors is well described in this excellent review (121 references).*

235. DISEASES OF THE PROSTATE

Patrick C. Walsh

The adult prostate weighs approximately 20 grams and lies immediately below the base of the bladder surrounding the proximal portion of the urethra. This tubuloalveolar gland secretes a colorless, slightly acidic fluid that contains fibrinolysin, citric acid, acid phosphatase, spermine, potassium, calcium, and zinc. The differentiation, growth, and function of the prostate are under the regulation of testicular androgens. Testosterone, which is secreted by the testes under the control of pituitary luteinizing hormone, is the principal circulating androgen. Testosterone enters the prostatic cell by passive diffusion where it is converted to dihydrotestosterone, the principal intracellular androgen. Dihydrotestosterone then binds to a specific cytosolic receptor protein, translocates to the nucleus, and influences in a complex fashion the expression of genetic information (see Ch. 221 for details).

Unlike most other organ systems, patients with diseases of the prostate do not present with complaints referable to disorders of prostatic function. Indeed, the exact role of prostatic secretion in normal reproduction is unclear. Rather, patients present with inflammatory, congestive, or neoplastic disturbances that most often give rise to difficulties with micturition. For this reason, men are often unaware of the existence of the prostate until one of these disorders develops. Starting at puberty, the prostate increases from approximately 4 grams to 20 grams in weight by age 20. Thereafter, for the next several decades prostatitis is the most common prostatic disorder. Beyond the fifth decade, benign prostatic hyperplasia and prostatic carcinoma predominate.

PROSTATITIS

Prostatitis, which refers to any condition associated with prostatic inflammation, is the most imprecise diagnosis in all of medicine. The disease can be acute or chronic and can have either bacterial or nonbacterial causes.

ETIOLOGY AND PATHOGENESIS. Bacterial prostatitis is most commonly caused by gram-negative organisms (predominantly *Escherichia coli*) and more rarely by enterococcus. Possible routes of infection include ascending urethral infection, reflux of infected urine into the prostatic ducts that empty into the posterior urethra, invasion by rectal bacteria via direct extension or lymphogenous spread, and hematogenous infection. Whether infectious prostatitis is a sexually transmitted disease is uncertain. The etiology of nonbacterial prostatitis is unknown. Except in rare instances, the disease does not appear to be caused by fungi, obligate anaerobic bacteria, trichomonads, viral agents, T-mycoplasma, or *Chlamydia.*

CLINICAL MANIFESTATIONS, DIAGNOSIS, AND DIFFERENTIAL DIAGNOSIS. Much of the confusion concerning prostatitis is attributable to imprecise methods of diagnosis. Many male patients have multiple genitourinary complaints centered on the prostate. Often the medical history and physical findings are not helpful in the differential diagnosis. Furthermore, when done as isolated procedures, midstream urinalysis and culture offer little diagnostic assistance. The two most useful tools in forming a differential diagnosis are examination of the expressed prostatic secretions (EPS) and quantitative bacterial localization cultures. Although microscopic examination of the EPS is important, it can be misleading. The clinician should always compare the microscopic appearance of the EPS to smears of the spun sediment of the first voided 10 ml of urine (the urethral specimen) and the midstream urine (bladder specimen) to localize the site of the inflammatory response. The presence of >20 white blood cells per high power field in the EPS is abnormal. During prostatic inflammation EPS typically contain leukocytosis and abnormal numbers of lipid-laden macrophages (oval fat bodies). The most accurate and useful method of establishing the diagnosis of bacterial prostatitis is the performance of simultaneous quantitative bacterial cultures of the urethral urine, bladder urine, and EPS. Four specimens are collected: the first voided 10 ml (VB1), the midstream aliquot (VB2), the EPS, and the first voided 10 ml immediately after prostatic massage (VB3). All specimens are cultured quantitatively by surface streaking onto blood and MacConkey agar. The diagnosis of bacterial prostatitis is confirmed when the quantitative bacterial colony counts of the prostatic specimens (EPS and VB3) significantly exceed those of the urethral (VB1) and bladder (VB2) specimens by at least 1 logarithm. Based on these diagnostic maneuvers, the inflammatory diseases of the prostate have been subdivided into four categories: (1) acute bacterial prostatitis, (2) chronic bacterial prostatitis, (3) nonbacterial prostatitis, and (4) prostatodynia.

Acute bacterial prostatitis is a fulminating bacterial infection characterized by fever, chills, low back and perineal pain, and intense irritative voiding symptoms. Rectal examination usually discloses a markedly tender prostate that is swollen, firm, and warm. Prostatic discomfort and the risk of bacteremia generally make prostatic massage unwise. Because bacterial cystitis usually accompanies the disease, the pathogen can be identified by culture of a voided specimen of urine. The disease often responds dramatically to therapy with antibacterial agents.

Chronic bacterial prostatitis is one of the most common causes of relapsing urinary tract infection in men. The majority of patients complain of irritative voiding symptoms (dysuria, urgency, frequency, and nocturia) and pain in various sites (suprapubic, perineal, low back, scrotal, and penile). However, patients are usually asymptomatic until significant bacteriuria develops. Rectal palpation discloses no specific or characteristic finding. The diagnosis is based upon quantitative bacterial localization cultures. Characteristically, these patients have relapsing urinary tract infections caused by the same pathogen. Although the urine may be sterilized and symptoms may disappear during treatment with antimicrobial agents, the organism often persists unaltered in the prostatic fluid; when therapy is discontinued, reinfection of the urine and reappearance of symptoms occur.

Nonbacterial prostatitis, a disease of uncertain cause, is the most common type of prostatitis seen today. The symptoms, physical findings, and microscopic appearance of the EPS in nonbacterial prostatitis and chronic bacterial prostatitis are indistinguishable. However, the patient with nonbacterial prostatitis has no history of documented urinary tract infection, and localization cultures exclude an infectious etiology. The etiology of this disorder is unknown. Finally, some male patients complain of symptoms that mimic prostatitis, especially a painful prostate, but they have negative cultures and no history of documented urinary tract infections. Contrary to the findings in the other categories, the EPS is normal. Since these men do not actually have prostatitis, the diagnostic term *prostatodynia* has been suggested.

All patients with lower urinary tract complaints require a full evaluation. The differential diagnosis of patients with lower urinary tract irritative symptoms should include carcinoma of the bladder, urethral stricture, prostatic obstruction, pericolic abscess, neurogenic bladder, diabetes mellitus, bladder calculus, and detrusor-sphincter dyssynergia. Because the symptoms in men with nonbacterial prostatitis are identical to those of patients with flat in situ carcinoma of the bladder, urinary cytologic studies and cystoscopy should be performed in these patients to exclude the presence of a malignancy.

TREATMENT. In patients with bacterial prostatitis, the use of antibacterial agents is complicated by the fact that most of the agents that are useful against gram-negative bacteria diffuse poorly into prostatic fluid. The factors that limit diffusion include lipid solubility, pKa, protein binding, and molecular size and shape. Although trimethoprim fulfills all theoretical criteria, and experimentally high levels can be demonstrated in canine prostatic fluid, only one third of patients with chronic prostatitis are cured by treatment with trimethoprim.

In patients with acute bacterial prostatitis, hospitalization may be required. Rest in bed, sexual abstention, increased hydration, analgesics, antipyretics, stool softeners, and suprapubic bladder drainage (the latter for the rare patient who has urinary retention) have been recommended. The diffuse and intense inflammation of acute prostatitis allows many drugs to diffuse readily into the prostatic fluid. Therapy should be begun with trimethoprim-sulfamethoxazole (160 mg of trimethoprim and 800 mg of sulfamethoxazole), administered twice daily until the results of culture and sensitivity are known. Therapy with the appropriate antibiotic should then be continued for at least 30 days in an effort to prevent the evolution of chronic prostatitis. In patients with chronic bacterial prostatitis, trimethoprim-sulfamethoxazole has the best cure rate that has been documented. Among patients who receive therapy continuously for four to six weeks, the cure rate has been 32 to 71 per cent. If patients fail to respond to this treatment, therapy with erythromycin, minocycline, or oral carbenicillin indanyl sodium may be attempted. In those patients who are not cured by medical therapy, continuous suppressive treatment with low dose medication can be attempted. The most suitable choices are trimethoprim-sulfamethoxazole, 1 regular tablet daily, or nitrofurantoin, 100 mg by mouth daily. Even though the pathogen persists in the prostatic ducts, suppressive therapy usually prevents bacteriuria and controls the symptoms.

In patients with nonbacterial prostatitis, because the cause of the disease is unknown, definitive therapy is difficult. In these patients treatment is usually directed toward controlling the symptoms. A trial of clinical treatment with a tetracycline preparation or erythromycin in maximal doses is a reasonable approach to initial treatment. Most patients benefit from a frank discussion of the nature of their condition, short-term use of anticholinergic or anti-inflammatory agents, and hot sitz baths. Although prostatic massage is advocated by many, its benefits are questioned by others. The proper management of men with prostatodynia is unclear.

Feit RM, Fair WR: Prostatitis. Sex Trans Dis 5:78, 1978. *A concise article describing the diagnosis and management of the common forms of prostatitis.*

Meares EM Jr: Prostatitis syndromes: New perspectives about old woes. J Urol 123:141, 1980. *The author has provided an extensive review of the syndromes classified under the term prostatitis. The diagnosis, pathogenesis, and management of each disorder are clearly outlined. It is the most authoritative article published on this subject.*

Mears EM Jr, Barbalias GA: Prostatitis: Bacterial, nonbacterial, prostatodynia. Semin Urol 1:146, 1983. *The most up-to-date review of the subject.*

BENIGN PROSTATIC HYPERPLASIA

INCIDENCE AND PREVALENCE. Benign prostatic hyperplasia (BPH) is probably the most common neoplastic growth in men. The disease characteristically occurs in men older than age 40; few if any patients with true nodular hyperplasia have been observed before this age. In men over the age of 50, the frequency of symptomatic BPH varies from 50 to 75 per cent. The mean age of detection by race is about 65 years for whites and approximately five years earlier for blacks. The probability of a 40-year-old man's requiring an operation for BPH if he lives to 80 years of age is approximately 10 per cent.

ETIOLOGY AND PATHOGENESIS. Although the development of BPH is almost a universal phenomenon in aging men, the cause and pathogenesis of this disorder are not well understood. The two major factors necessary for the onset of BPH are the presence of the testes and aging. Consequently, much interest has been directed at identifying a hormonal etiology. There are several factors that strongly support the possibility that BPH in men is under endocrine control: (1) BPH does not occur in men who are castrated prior to puberty; (2) regression of established BPH has been reported to occur following castration; and (3) in a canine model, BPH can be produced by treatment with hormones. The prostate appears to become more sensitive to androgens as the gland enlarges and as plasma levels of testosterone decline. These observations suggest that other factors, such as estrogen induction of increased androgen receptor levels, may sensitize the prostate to adequate levels of dihydrotestosterone and accelerate growth. Medical approaches to the management of BPH must await further elucidation of these factors.

CLINICAL MANIFESTATIONS. Enlargement of the prostate causes no obvious physiologic manifestations. The disturbances that result are entirely secondary to effects on the urethra, the bladder, and the kidneys. In early cases the patient usually has minimal symptoms because the detrusor musculature is capable of compensating for the increased outlet resistance to urine flow. With increasing obstruction, however, the patient develops a constellation of symptoms called "prostatism": diminution in the caliber and force of the urinary stream, hesitancy in initiating voiding, inability to terminate micturition abruptly with postvoid dribbling, a sensation of incomplete emptying of the bladder, and occasionally urinary retention. These are *obstructive symptoms* and they must be carefully distinguished from *irritative* lower urinary tract symptoms such as dysuria, frequency, and urgency. Disastrous results can follow a prostatectomy performed on a patient whose symptoms stemmed from irritation, such as an inflammatory or infectious process, rather than from obstruction. As the amount of residual urine increases, the patient may note nocturia, diurnal frequency, a mass in the lower abdomen, and overflow urinary incontinence. In patients with slowly progressive obstruction, the patient may gradually adjust to the symptoms and present with "silent prostatism." On examination these patients may show the secondary anemia of renal insufficiency, a lower abdominal midline mass representing a distended bladder, and other findings associated with renal insufficiency (see Ch. 82).

DIAGNOSIS AND DIFFERENTIAL DIAGNOSIS. Usually there is no difficulty in establishing the diagnosis of BPH. The patient usually presents with lower urinary tract obstructive symptoms. Prior to examination the physician should observe the patient voiding to completion to document the decrease in size and force of the urinary stream. The prostate is palpated with attention to size, consistency, and shape. Hyperplasia usually produces a smooth, firm, and elastic enlargement of the prostate. However, the size of the prostate on rectal examination does not permit one to estimate the degree of bladder neck obstruction. Patients with marked enlargement of the prostate may have no urinary tract obstruction, and others with a large intravesical median lobe may have marked outflow obstructive symptoms without palpable enlargement of the gland. In addition to revealing the individual characteristics of the prostate, the rectal examination also affords the physician an opportunity to evaluate the intactness of the rectal sphincter, which indirectly reflects the state of vesical innervation.

A urinalysis and urine culture are performed to evaluate the presence of infection; a serum creatinine is obtained to evaluate renal function; and a serum acid phosphatase sample is drawn (preferably prior to prostatic examination). In patients whose disease is in an early stage and who have only mild symptoms, no further studies are necessary. However, in men with marked outlet obstructive symptoms, intravenous urography and cystourethroscopy should be performed. The intravenous urogram with a postvoiding film will document the degree of upper tract obstruction, identify the presence of bladder calculi, and estimate the degree of bladder emptying. Cystourethroscopy is valuable in confirming the presence of vesical neck obstruction, in evaluating the degree of detrusor hypertrophy (presence of trabeculation, cellules, and diverticula), and in excluding the presence of a bladder tumor.

Several other conditions produce bladder neck obstruction: carcinoma of the prostate, bladder neck contracture, urethral stricture, bladder calculus, carcinoma of the bladder, chronic prostatitis, and neurogenic bladder. The presence of irritative lower urinary tract symptoms, such as dysuria, urgency, and frequency, should alert the physician to consider conditions other than obstruction as the cause for the patient's symptoms. In the absence of a large amount of residual urine, frequency and nocturia are not caused by BPH. Bladder neck contracture, urethral stricture, bladder calculi, and bladder neoplasms are best evaluated with endoscopy.

TREATMENT AND PROGNOSIS. At present, there is no effective medical management for the treatment of BPH; surgery is the only effective form of therapy. The vast majority of men over the age of 60 have some evidence of BPH, so the mere presence of this disorder is not an indication for its treatment. The general indications for the relief of prostatic obstruction are (1) acute urinary retention, (2) hydronephrosis, (3) recurrent urinary tract infection aggravated by residual urine, (4) severe hematuria from a congestive prostate, and (5) outflow obstructive symptoms that are of sufficient concern to the patient to cause him to desire treatment. When the patient is seen early in the course of the disease, when his symptoms are mild, and before any of these relative indications are present, he is often curious about the natural history of the disease. This question is difficult to answer, because many patients who receive no treatment whatsoever will have no change in their symptoms over many years. Consequently in the group of patients that lack definitive indications for prostatectomy, it appears advisable to examine the patient periodically to observe the natural history of the disease rather than to anticipate its development by advising prophylactic prostatectomy. Simple prostatectomy can be performed in a variety of ways. However, transurethral resection of the prostate is the procedure with the least morbidity.

Walsh PC: Benign prostatic hyperplasia. *In* Harrison JH, Gittes RF, Perlmutter AD, Stamey TA, Walsh PC (eds.): Campbell's Urology. 4th ed. Philadelphia, W. B. Saunders Company, 1979, pp 949–964. *A comprehensive review of all aspects relative to the diagnosis and treatment of benign prostatic hyperplasia.*

Walsh PC, Hutchins GM, Ewing LL: The tissue content of dihydrotestosterone in human prostatic hyperplasia is not supranormal. J Clin Invest 72:1772, 1983. *Recognition that human BPH occurs in the presence of normal levels of dihydrotestosterone should focus research efforts to identify other factors that may sensitize this tissue and accelerate growth.*

Wilson JD: The pathogenesis of benign prostatic hyperplasia. Am J Med 68:745, 1980. *A concise and lucid discussion of the endocrine factors that may be responsible for the development of benign prostatic hyperplasia. Experimental studies are integrated with clinical findings to formulate a sound understanding of the pathogenesis of this common disease.*

CARCINOMA OF THE PROSTATE

INCIDENCE, PREVALENCE, EPIDEMIOLOGY. The prostate is the third leading site of cancer in males, accounting for about 17 per cent of all male cancers. The only female cancers that account for more new cancer cases per year are cancers of the breast and uterus. Approximately 5 per cent of white males and 6 per cent of nonwhite males will develop cancer of the prostate. Furthermore, it is calculated that 1.7 per cent of newborn white males and 2.3 per cent of newborn nonwhite males will eventually die of the disease. Although carcinoma of the prostate does not develop in eunuchs, there is no other evidence to suggest that a direct relationship exists between hormone levels and the development of prostatic cancer. Similarly, no relationship between the development of benign prostatic hyperplasia and prostatic cancer has been demonstrated. Furthermore, there is little relationship between prostatic cancer and industrial carcinogens, cigarette smoking, use of alcohol, disease patterns, circumcision, weight, height, blood group, or hair distribution.

PATHOLOGY. More than 95 per cent of all prostatic carcinomas are adenocarcinomas. The tumor is multifocal in 85 per cent of the cases, suggesting a multifocal rather than a single site of origin. Prostatic carcinoma can spread by local extension or by lymphatic or hematogenous dissemination. As carcinoma of the prostate progresses, the tumor extends to the urethra, the bladder neck, the seminal vesicles, and the trigone. The most common sites of lymph node metastases, in descending order of frequency, are the obturator, hypogastric, iliac, presacral, and periaortic nodes. Osseous metastases constitute the most common form of hematogenous spread. The most frequent sites of involvement are, in decreasing order, the pelvis, the lumbar spine, the femora, the thoracic spine, and the ribs. The most common sites for visceral metastases include the lung and liver. Pulmonary metastases are detected clinically or radiographically in less than 6 per cent of patients.

The prognosis of patients with prostatic cancer correlates well with the grade and stage of the tumor, although grading is somewhat difficult because most tumors exhibit a heterogeneous histologic pattern: (Table 235–1): *Stage A* disease is not palpable clinically but is found histopathologically following prostatectomy. It is subdivided into two biologically meaningful subclasses: Stage A1, focal or well differentiated carcinoma, and Stage A2, diffuse or poorly differentiated carcinoma. *Stage B* tumors are limited to the prostate and on rectal examination can be subdivided into Stage B1, a solitary nodule involving less than one lobe of the prostate, and Stage B2, cancer in which one lobe or more is involved. *Stage C* tumors extend beyond the prostatic capsule but have not metastasized. *Stage D* represents metastatic carcinoma of the prostate and includes any patient with an elevated serum acid phosphatase level. Stage D can be subdivided into Stage D1, the presence of metastatic disease in lymph nodes, and Stage D2, patients with clinical metastatic carcinoma.

CLINICAL MANIFESTATIONS AND DIAGNOSIS. Early in the clinical evolution of prostatic cancer symptoms may be entirely absent. Later, patients develop symptoms of urinary outflow obstruction or bone pain. Hematuria, lymphadenopathy, and lower extremity edema are uncommon presenting symptoms of prostatic cancer. A careful routine rectal examination is the only means of detecting prostatic cancer at an early stage. Carcinoma of the prostate characteristically has a hard consistency, felt as a region of dense induration within the substance of the prostate. With tumor penetration of the capsule, the margins of the prostate may become obscured and tumor may be palpated extending to the seminal vesicles and regions of the bladder neck. Other causes of prostatic induration include focal regions of benign hyperplasia, prostatic calculi, granulomatous prostatitis, prostatic infarction, and postoperative changes. Approximately 50 per cent of prostatic nodules are malignant.

A clinical suspicion of prostatic cancer requires histologic verification by needle biopsy. If the biopsy is positive, the patient should have a serum acid phosphatase determination, an intravenous urogram and a bone scan. Because of the lack of specificity of bone scans, skeletal radiographs should be performed of any suspicious areas. Routine lymphangiography or staging pelvic lymphadenectomy is generally unnecessary in the management of patients with prostatic cancer.

TABLE 235–1. CARCINOMA OF PROSTATE

Stage (Whitmore)	Definition of Stage	Usual Treatment
A	Not palpable; found by histopathology	
A_1	Focal, well differentiated	Observation
A_2	Diffuse, poorly differentiated	Radical prostatectomy
B	Palpable, but limited to prostate	
B_1	Solitary nodule < one lobe	Radical prostatectomy
B_2	One lobe or more involved	Megavolt radiation
C	Extension beyond capsule	Megavolt radiation
D	Metastatic disease; acid phosphatase ↑	Hormonal therapy
D_1	Pelvic lymph nodes only	Rarely chemotherapy
D_2	More widespread metastases	

Serum acid phosphatase is elevated in most patients with bony metastases and, more rarely, with localized carcinoma. It is not sufficiently sensitive or specific for screening, so is used mainly to follow the progress of the disease. Acid phosphatase, not inhibited by l-tartrate, is characteristically elevated in the serum of patients with Gaucher's disease (Ch. 185).

TREATMENT. There is considerable debate concerning the best mode of therapy for each particular stage of carcinoma of the prostate. In selecting treatment there is often the dilemma of attempting both to maintain the quality of life and to increase the duration of survival. Men with carcinoma of the prostate are often old and suffer from other illnesses that may pose a greater threat than the cancer itself. Furthermore, although there are a variety of relatively effective therapeutic modalities from which to choose, there is little information that accurately compares their relative efficacy. Each form of treatment is associated with undesirable side effects. In selecting therapy the physician must determine the long-term threat that the tumor poses to the quality and duration of survival in each individual patient and must select a form of treatment that provides the proper balance between efficacy and morbidity.

In patients with Stage A1 prostatic cancer, observation but no further treatment is necessary. Patients with Stage A2 and B1 prostatic cancer who are less than 70 years old are ideal candidates for radical prostatectomy. In these patients, the tumor will be confined to the pathologic specimen in 84 to 95 per cent of the cases, and the long-term survival of these patients is excellent. Although the complications of radical prostatectomy are often emphasized, in the hands of the experienced surgeon the incidence of urinary incontinence should be less than 2 per cent. Previously, most patients were impotent postoperatively. However, with use of a new surgical technique this undesirable side effect can be avoided. In patients with Stage B2 prostatic cancer, 50 to 60 per cent will have involvement of the seminal vesicles. Because only 5 per cent of patients with involvement of the seminal vesicles survive 15 years free of tumor, patients with Stage B2 disease are not ideal candidates for radical surgery. For the treatment of Stage B2 and C disease, megavoltage radiation provides excellent palliation and the possibility of cure. For the treatment of Stage D disease, hormonal therapy is the preferred modality for initial treatment, but there are two major areas of controversy: (1) What are the relative merits of estrogen therapy versus therapy with bilateral orchiectomy or the combination of estrogen plus castration? (2) What is the preferred timing of endocrine treatment?

The physiologic effects of estrogen therapy and orchiectomy are similar, i.e., they produce regression of cancer of the prostate by suppressing plasma testosterone levels. Orchiectomy alone, estrogen therapy, or the combination of the two appears to be equally effective in the treatment of metastatic carcinoma of the prostate.

The second point of controversy surrounds the proper timing of endocrine therapy: Should it be instituted as soon as the diagnosis is made, or should treatment be delayed until the patient becomes symptomatic? In one study, patients with Stage A and B carcinoma of the prostate who were treated with estrogen had a higher death rate than did patients who were not receiving estrogen. The increase in death rate was caused by cardiovascular complications, suggesting that early treatment with estrogens can be harmful under some circumstances. The survival rate of patients with Stage C and D carcinoma treated with initial hormonal therapy was identical to the survival rate in those patients in whom hormonal therapy was delayed until symptoms appeared. Therefore, delaying hormonal therapy until symptoms occur has no adverse effect on the survival rate in patients with established metastatic disease. Estrogen therapy or orchiectomy should probably be delayed until symptoms appear. At that time, treatment with estrogen (diethylstilbestrol, 1 mg per day) or orchiectomy may be utilized. Reactivation of symptoms following an initial response to hormonal therapy, usually indicates a tumor no longer under hormonal control. Attempts at further endocrine therapy (adrenalectomy, hypophysectomy, or antiandrogen therapy) are usually disappointing. At present the only hope for treatment of these patients is chemotherapy. Several large scale clinical studies are currently in progress to evaluate different cytotoxic agents for the treatment of metastatic carcinoma of the prostate.

Catalona WJ, Scott WW: Carcinoma of the prostate. *In* Harrison JH, Gittes RF, Perlmutter AD, Stamey TA, Walsh PC (eds.): Campbell's Urology. 4th ed. Philadelphia, W. B. Saunders Company, 1979, pp 1085–1124. *This article provides a comprehensive review of all aspects relative to the diagnosis and treatment of carcinoma of the prostate.*

Scott WW, Menon M, Walsh PC: Hormonal therapy of prostatic cancer. Cancer 45:1929, 1980. *The hormonal therapy of prostatic cancer is approached from a physiologic standpoint. These findings are integrated with clinical studies to provide a sound basis for recommending timing and forms of treatment.*

Walsh PC, Jewett HJ: Radical surgery for prostatic cancer. Cancer 45:1906, 1980. *Radical prostatectomy for the treatment of prostatic cancer is somewhat controversial. This article provides a sound rationale for this form of treatment and identifies those patients most likely to benefit from surgical treatment.*

Walsh PC, Lepor H, Eggleston JC: Radical prostatectomy with preservation of sexual function: Anatomical and pathological considerations. Prostate 4:473, 1983. *By eliminating the fear of impotence associated with radical prostatectomy, patients and their physicians may be encouraged to diagnose prostatic cancer at an earlier stage when it is still curable.*

236. THE OVARIES

Griff T. Ross

Throughout postnatal life, normally functioning ovaries secrete sex steroid hormones and, from menarche to menopause, produce oocytes which differentiate into ova, the definitive female gametes. Since sex steroid hormones participate in the growth, differentiation, and function of a variety of extragonadal and extragenital tissues, ovarian function is not the exclusive concern of the gynecologist or the endocrinologist but of all physicians. When signs and symptoms consistent with inappropriate sex steroid hormone activity are encountered in any female patient, the physician should consider ovarian dysfunction in the differential diagnosis and proceed to determine its pathophysiologic origin.

A rational approach to the diagnosis and treatment of disorders of ovarian function depends upon knowledge of (1) the relationships of follicle growth, gametogenesis, and sex steroid hormone production; (2) regulation of these functions in health; (3) extraovarian actions of sex steroid hormones on target tissues; and (4) methods for the clinical and laboratory evaluation of these factors in health and disease. In this chapter this information will be briefly summarized and applied to the diagnosis and treatment of specific disorders of ovarian function in girls before and after puberty and in women before and after menopause.

Gross and Microscopic Anatomy

The mature ovaries are oval structures approximately $4 \times 3 \times 1$ cm in diameter with an average combined weight of about 14 grams. Each of these structures is attached to the lateral pelvic wall by the infundibulopelvic ligament, to the posterior surface of the broad ligament by the mesovarium, and to the uterus by the ovarian ligament. Nerves, blood vessels, and lymphatics traverse the mesovarium of each ovary to enter an inner hilum, which is contiguous with a central medulla. The medulla is surrounded by an outer cortex, bounded in turn by a derivative of coelomic epithelium called the germinal epithelium (Fig. 236–1). The hilum of each ovary also contains steroid hormone–secreting cells, called hilar cells. In addition to blood vessels, the medulla of each ovary contains the cellular debris remaining after follicle maturation and regression, and the cortex contains follicle complexes in all stages of maturation.

The *follicle complex* is the indispensable structural and functional component of the human ovary; neither steroidogenesis nor gametogenesis occurs in the absence of follicles. Its cellular

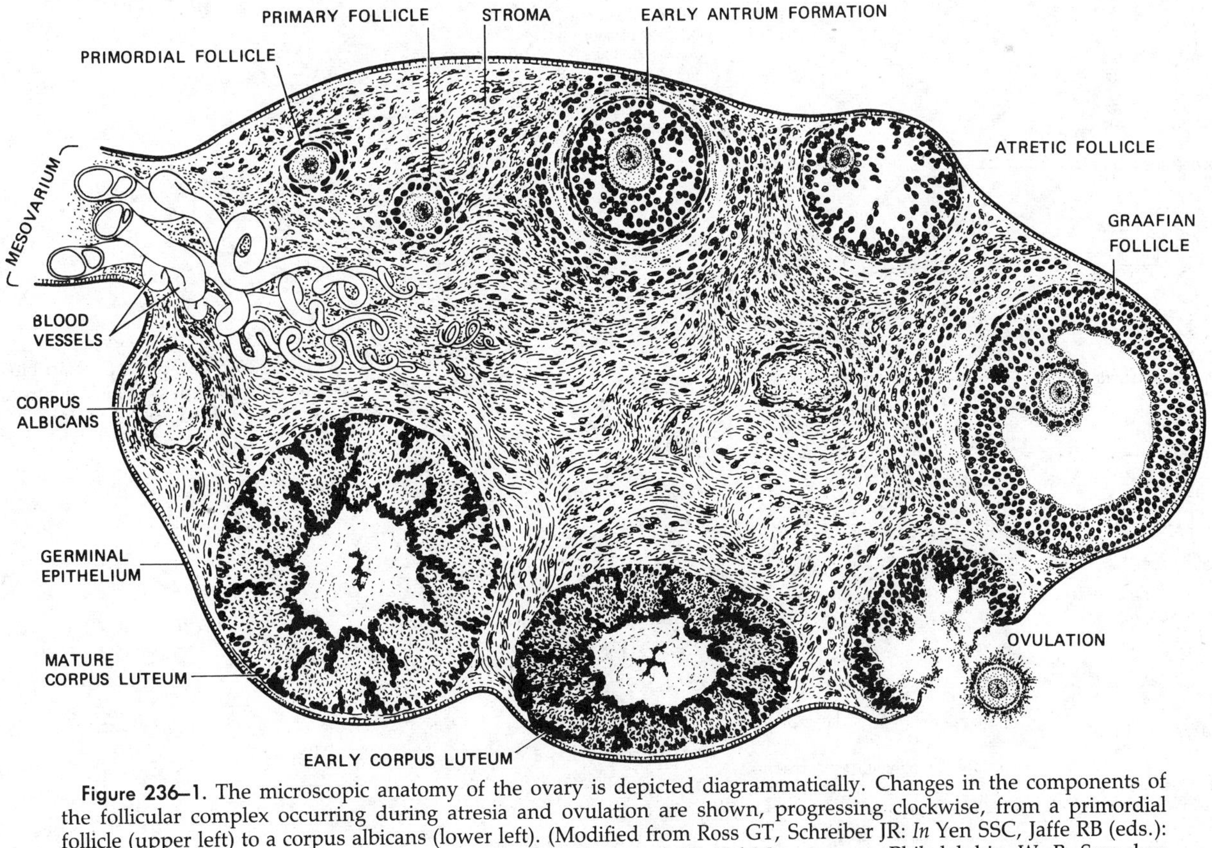

Figure 236–1. The microscopic anatomy of the ovary is depicted diagrammatically. Changes in the components of the follicular complex occurring during atresia and ovulation are shown, progressing clockwise, from a primordial follicle (upper left) to a corpus albicans (lower left). (Modified from Ross GT, Schreiber JR: *In* Yen SSC, Jaffe RB (eds.): Reproductive Endocrinology—Physiology, Pathophysiology and Clinical Management. Philadelphia, W. B. Saunders Company, 1978, pp 63–79.)

components consist of an *oocyte, granulosa cells,* and some interstitial cells called *theca cells*. Characteristic changes in the morphology of each component occur during follicle growth and differentiation. Interactions among these components give rise to the gamete (ovum) and to sex steroid hormones essential for establishing and maintaining early pregnancy should the ovum be fertilized.

The primordial follicle is bounded by a membrane, the basal lamina, which excludes blood and lymph vessels and is selectively permeable to solutes in plasma. Inside the basal lamina, less than a dozen spindle-shaped granulosa cells surround a primary oocyte, the nucleus of which is in prophase of the first meiotic division. This collection of cells is surrounded in turn by stroma, which consists of supporting connective tissue cells, contractile cells, and some steroid hormone–secreting interstitial cells, all intermingled with blood and lymph vessels (Fig. 236–1). Interstitial cells surrounding an individual follicle are called theca cells.

Morphologic Correlates of Normal Ovarian Function

From the time of their appearance in the fetal ovary until their disappearance from ovaries of postmenopausal women, selected primordial follicles begin to grow while others remain inactive. The normal progression of growth of follicles depends upon adequate stimulation by pituitary gonadotropins.

Growth and differentiation of the primordial follicle terminate in either *ovulation*, with extrusion of a secondary oocyte, or *atresia*, with retention and degeneration of the oocyte in situ. Pari passu, with either ovulation or atresia, developing follicles produce sex steroid hormones: estrogens, androgens, and progestogens. The steps in biosynthesis of sex steroid hormones are summarized diagrammatically in Figure 236–2. Two alternative pathways exist for synthesizing progestogens, androgens, and estrogens: the so-called Δ^5 pathway, in which 17α-hydroxypregnenolone and dehydroisoandrosterone are intermediates, and the Δ^4 pathway, in which pregnenolone is converted to progesterone and 17α-hydroxyprogesterone and androstenedione are the alternative intermediates. The "preferred" pathway in the human ovary is unknown.

Prior to the menarche, all developing follicles undergo atresia. After the menarche, while atresia continues, one follicle begins to grow more rapidly than its peers and moves to the surface of the cortex in preparation for ovulation. Steroid hormones secreted by this "dominant" follicle act on the hypothalamus and pituitary to stimulate a "surge" in luteinizing hormone (LH) secretion that anticipates its rupture (ovulation) by 35 to 40 hours (see Ch. 225).

This LH surge is indispensable for ovulation, but the mechanism by which it induces ovulation remains obscure. Hypotheses include an LH-induced increase in intrafollicular pressure, stimulation of contractile elements in the stroma, or proteolytic digestion of the basal lamina. Of these, the last is currently favored.

After the follicle has ruptured and the oocyte has been extruded, blood vessels and fibroblasts from the surrounding theca penetrate the basal lamina and permeate the residual granulosa cells, which rapidly differentiate into luteal cells with steroid hormone–secreting organelles. Fibroblasts, luteal cells, related thecal cells, and blood vessels together form the definitive *corpus luteum* (Fig. 236–1), which secretes increasing amounts of estrogens and progestogens for a period of about eight days. Then, unless fertilization occurs, steroid hormone production declines progressively over the last six to eight days of the cycle and menstruation begins. The corpus luteum is replaced by an avascular scar called a *corpus albicans*. If pregnancy occurs, (human) chorionic gonadotropin (hCG) produced by the conceptus stimulates continued production of estrogens

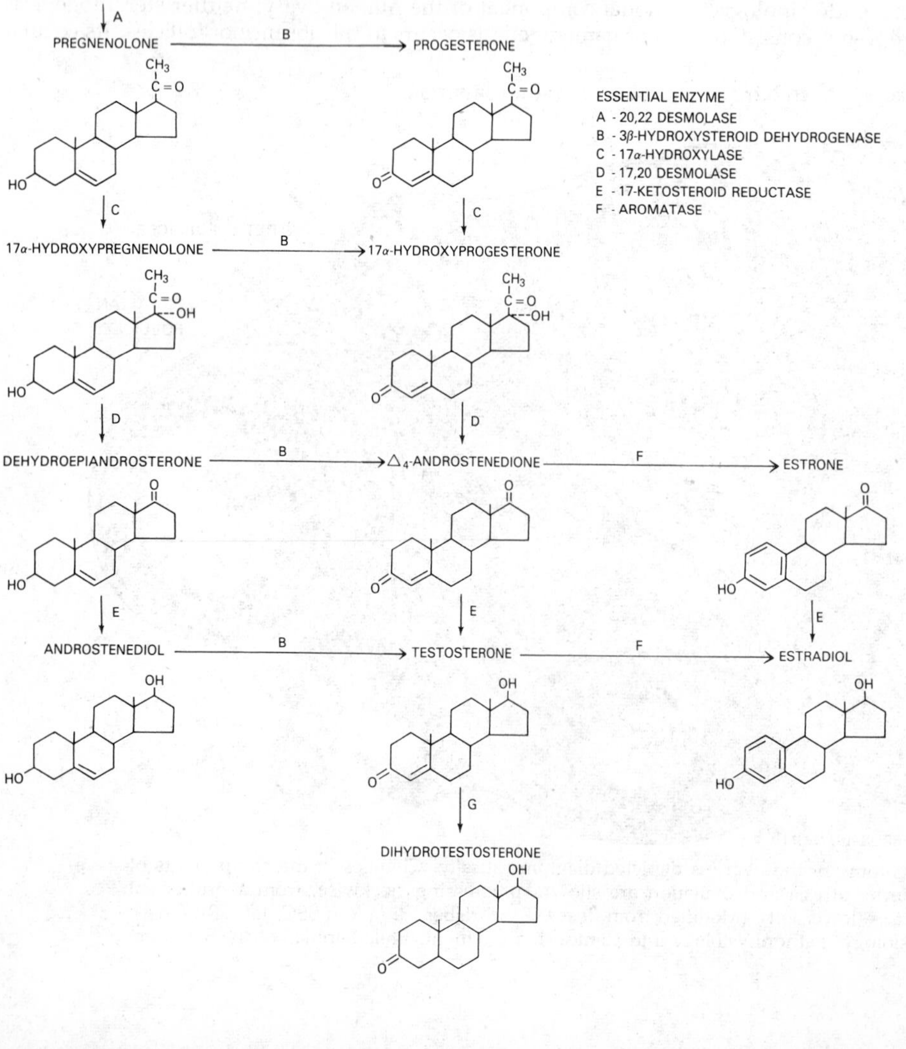

Figure 236–2. Steps in ovarian biosynthesis of steroid hormones. (Modified from data of Ross GT: *In* Rudolph AM (ed.): Pediatrics 16:1726, 1977.)

and progestogens by the corpus luteum. This persists throughout pregnancy. In addition to progesterone, hCG stimulates the corpus luteum of pregnancy to secrete relaxin, a peptide, the function of which remains obscure.

Since no oocytes are produced and no primordial follicles are formed after six months postnatally, successive cycles of atresia and ovulation deplete the supply of primordial follicles. As the number of follicles declines, the intermenstrual interval becomes irregular, anovulatory cycles occur, menses finally cease, and the *menopause* is established despite the presence of a few primordial follicles and increased pituitary gonadotropin secretion. Why these remaining follicles fail to grow or secrete steroid hormones remains unknown.

As a result of both depletion of follicles and failure of the remaining ones to mature, the ovaries shrink and ovarian weight markedly declines after the menopause. Four or five years after the last menstrual period, the last follicles disappear and only stroma persists. Ovarian estrogen synthesis ceases, but variable quantities of estrogen (mostly estrone) continue to be produced by aromatization of androgens, principally androstenedione, produced by both ovaries and adrenals, chiefly the latter. The quantity of estrone produced through this pathway is greater in obese than nonobese postmenopausal women and greater in postmenopausal than premenopausal obese women.

Hormonal Correlates of Normal Ovarian Function

The normal progression of these morphologic and functional changes requires gonadotropin secretion:

1. Once initiated, normal progression of follicle growth, steroid hormone production, ovulation, and atresia are gonadotropin dependent.

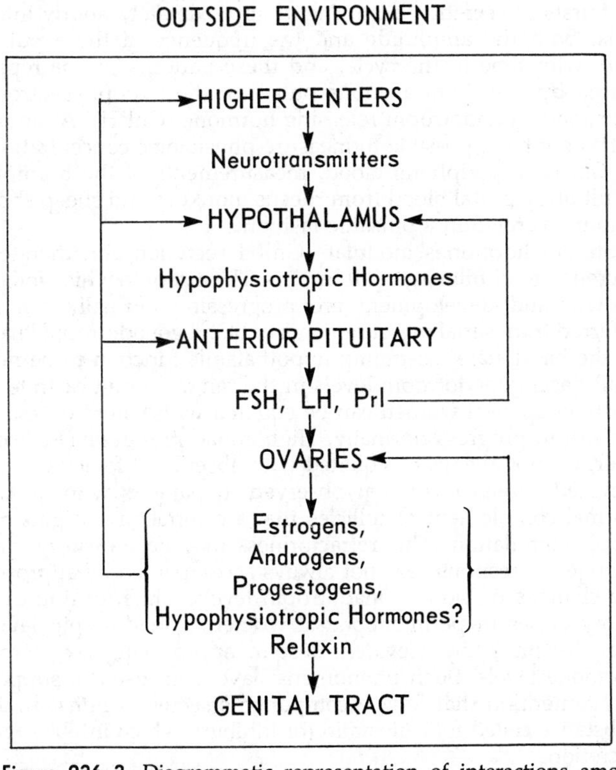

Figure 236–3. Diagrammatic representation of interactions among components of the hypothalamic-pituitary-ovarian axis. "Feedback loops," some negative and some positive (see text), of ovarian steroid and peptide hormones on anterior pituitary, hypothalamus, and higher centers are indicated by lines and appropriate arrows on the left-hand side of the figure. "Short loop feedback" of pituitary peptide hormones on hypothalamic sites, and of ovarian hormones acting locally to regulate follicular growth and development within the ovary, are indicated by lines and appropriate arrows on the right-hand side. Substances designated in lower case letters are the mediators of effects on various loci indicated in capital letters. Relevant details concerning these complex interactions will be found in the text of this chapter and in Ch. 225.

2. Sex steroid hormones produced in response to gonadotropins act locally to modulate these gonadotropin-dependent phenomena.

3. After the menarche, ovarian sex steroid hormones produced by the dominant preovulatory follicle and its successor, the corpus luteum, act systemically to coordinate functions of the hypothalamic-pituitary unit, the ovary, and the endometrium essential for maintaining ovulatory menstrual cycles and initiating pregnancy. These interactions are summarized diagrammatically in Figure 236–3.

4. The structural and functional status of follicular development (and thus of the ovaries) can be inferred from the status of sex steroid hormone production at any age throughout life. Moreover, since measures of sex steroid hormone secretion reflect the developmental status of the follicle chosen to ovulate during each cycle after the menarche, evaluation of sex steroid hormone production provides an appraisal of both steroidogenesis and gametogenesis in ovaries of women in any age group.

Sex Steroid Hormones and Clinical Evaluation of Ovarian Function

MEASUREMENTS OF SEX STEROID HORMONES. There are three major sex hormones produced by the mature human ovary: 17β-estradiol, progesterone, and testosterone. The pathways for the synthesis of these compounds and the relationship of estrogens and progesterone to follicle-stimulating hormone (FSH) and LH in the normal menstrual cycle have been shown in Figure 236–2. Table 236–1 shows the normal plasma concentrations of estrogens and progesterone during the menstrual cycle, together with their production rates.

For evaluating sex steroid hormone production, sensitive methods are available for measuring their concentrations in practical volumes of blood or aliquots of 24-hour urine specimens. These "chemical" or immunologic assays are expensive and not always easily accessible. Moreover, in a given patient, results may not be as reliable as evaluating the biologic activity of sex steroids in suitable target tissues of the hormones.

RESPONSES IN SEX STEROID HORMONE–DEPENDENT TISSUES. The sex steroid hormone target tissues include breasts, pubic and axillary hair, bone, vaginal epithelium, endocervical glands, endometrium, hypothalamus, and pituitary gland, and such metabolic processes as linear growth, basal body temperature regulation, and hepatic synthesis of some serum proteins. Responses of the target tissues to sex steroid hormones will often enable the physician to accurately assess ovarian function.

Target tissues dependent upon sex steroid hormones are responsive throughout life, but changing quantities of sex hormones produced at different times in life, coupled with limited accessibility of some of these tissues, render some end-organ responses more useful than others in the evaluation of ovarian function.

The Vaginal Epithelium. Estrogens and progestogens regulate rates of proliferation and differentiation of the stratified squamous epithelial cells which form the mucosa of the vagina. These cells exfoliate into the vagina and can be studied in smears of suitably stained vaginal secretions. The proportions of morphologically distinctive cells are altered by the prevailing sex steroid hormone milieu. Superficial cells predominate when estrogenization is adequate or excessive, whereas basal and parabasal cells predominate when estrogenization is low. Under the influence of progestogens, numbers of both superficial and basal cells decline and numbers of polymorphonuclear cells increase. This examination provides a rapid and inexpensive screen for the adequacy of estrogenic activity in the absence of vaginal infection.

The Endocervical Glands. Estrogens and progestogens regulate the amount and composition of endocervical mucus, an aqueous solution of proteins and electrolytes. Estrogens increase the quantity, the viscosity, and the elasticity or "spinnbarkeit" of the cervical mucus, as well as the tendency of

TABLE 236–1. PLASMA CONCENTRATIONS, METABOLIC CLEARANCE RATES (MCR) AND PRODUCTION RATES, AND OVARIAN SECRETION RATES OF SEX STEROID HORMONES AS A FUNCTION OF TIME IN CYCLE

Steroid	Time in Cycle	Plasma Concentration (ng/dl)	Plasma MCR (Liters/Day)	Plasma Production Rate (μg/Day)	Ovarian Secretion Rate (μg/Day)
Estradiol	Early	6	1350	81	70
	Mid-cycle	33–70		445–945	400–800
	Luteal	20		270	250
Estrone	Early	5	2210	110	80
	Mid-cycle	15–30		331–662	250–500
	Luteal	11		243	160
Estriol	Early	0.7	2100	14	18
	Luteal	1.0		23	
Progesterone	Follicular	3–10	2510	750–2500	1500
	Luteal	6–20		15,000–50,0000	24,000

electrolytes to crystallize in a "ferning" pattern (after water evaporates from smears of mucus on a glass slide). In contrast, progesterone not only inhibits endocervical mucus secretion but also reduces its viscosity, its elasticity, and its tendency to "fern." Simultaneous evaluation of endocervical mucus and vaginal epithelium enhances the value of each test.

The Endometrium. The cavity of the uterus is lined by mucosa, which consists of a superficial avascular layer of columnar epithelial cells overlying spindle-shaped stromal cells, penetrated by crypts of the surface epithelial cells and richly vascularized. Estrogens stimulate proliferation of both epithelial and stromal cells so that the mucosa thickens. In contrast, progestogens inhibit mitosis in estrogen-primed epithelial and stromal cells, stimulate secretory activity and glycogen storage in epithelial cells, increase vascularity of the stromal layer, and initiate "decidual" changes in stromal cells.

As the corpus luteum secretes less estrogen and progestogen, necrosis of stromal blood vessels is followed by multifocal necrosis and exfoliation of the epithelium which denudes the mucosa of all epithelial cells (except those lining glandular crypts). This initiates menstrual bleeding. It has been proposed that the reduction in steroids mobilizes lysosomal enzymes, which hydrolyze phospholipids. This would stimulate synthesis of prostaglandin $F_2\alpha$ which in turn is thought to stimulate endometrial necrosis and bleeding. After menses, mucosal continuity is restored by estrogen-stimulated proliferation of epithelial cells in the crypts.

Endometrial response to estrogens is sufficiently reliable to enable a pathologist to recognize the early, mid, or late proliferative (or preovulatory) phase of normal cycles. Morphologic changes in response to progesterone are sufficiently reproducible to enable a skilled observer to date the specimens in relation to an idealized 28-day cycle in which ovulation is assumed to have occurred on the fourteenth day. When the time of specimen collection is related to the onset of next menses, a discrepancy of more than two days in the actual and expected dates has been equated with inadequate corpus luteum function. For making these assessments of sex steroid hormone activity in sexually mature women, suitable specimens of endometrium can be obtained during an office visit, with minimal discomfort to the patient.

After the menarche, the appropriateness of ovarian estrogen secretion and endometrial response to the hormone can be inferred from a *progestogen withdrawal test*, performed by giving a single intramuscular injection of 100 mg of progesterone in oil, or alternatively by giving 10 mg of medroxyprogesterone acetate by mouth each day for five days. Vaginal bleeding within one week after the injection or after completing the five-day course of medroxyprogesterone has been equated with ovarian estrogen production equivalent to a mean serum estradiol level of 60 ng per deciliter, whereas failure to bleed indicates much lower serum estradiol levels of the order of 15 ng per deciliter.

The Hypothalamic Thermoregulatory Center. Estrogens reduce and progestogens increase basal body temperatures so that a progressive "thermogenic shift" of more than 0.3° C occurring after a nadir in serial basal body temperatures is a presumptive sign of ovulation, corpus luteum formation, and progesterone secretion. Although useful, this sign is not an entirely reliable test of the adequacy of corpus luteum function, since elevation of basal body temperature requires less progesterone than does adequate secretory transformation of the endometrium. Furthermore, taking body temperatures daily for five minutes before arising and recording these for 18 to 35 days is tedious, and patients often fail to comply fully.

The Hypothalamic-Pituitary Unit. The hormone concentrations in blood during a normal menstrual cycle in relation to the preovulatory LH surge or "peak" during spontaneous ovulatory cycles have been related to "feedback" effects (inhibitory or stimulatory) on pituitary cells by simultaneous changes in blood estrogen and progestogen concentrations. The smooth curves shown for FSH and LH are actually generated by pulses or bursts of secretion occurring at approximately hourly intervals. Both the amplitude and the frequency of these pulses vary with time in the cycle, and these patterns can be reproduced by giving intravenous pulses of the hypophyseotropic hormone, gonadotropin releasing hormone (GnRH). Although it has not been possible to measure physiologic concentrations of GnRH in peripheral blood, measurements of the hormone in pituitary portal blood from rhesus monkeys and sheep show it to be secreted in a pulsatile fashion.

Steroid hormones modulate GnRH secretion and therefore secretion of pituitary gonadotropins. The extent to which follicle growth and development are progressing normally can be inferred from serial measurements of blood gonadotropin levels in the basal state, assuming hypothalamic function to be normal. Basal gonadotropin levels in the range seen in castrate or postmenopausal women can be equated with failure of follicle growth to progress normally. High gonadotropin levels, however, cannot always be equated with absence of follicles, since elevated levels have been observed in patients who have a normal complement of follicles that are refractory to gonadotropic stimulation. This refractoriness may be transitory, and changes in response are not always accompanied by appropriate changes in blood gonadotropin levels. Thus, during ovulatory cycles in perimenopausal women, gonadotropin levels may be markedly elevated despite appropriate sex steroid hormone levels. Such phenomena have been used to support the contention that follicle components secrete a nonsteroidal substance called folliculostatin (or inhibin), which inhibits FSH secretion.

When basal gonadotropin levels are low in the face of signs and symptoms of estrogen deficiency in sexually mature women, hypothalamic-pituitary dysfunction or failure can be inferred. Pulsatile variations in gonadotropin levels may alter the validity of a single sample for evaluating basal secretion of the hormones. A sample taken from pooled specimens collected consecutively over the course of two to three hours will minimize this source of variation.

Bones, Breasts, and Pubic Hair. Vaginal epithelium, endocervical glands, and endometrium will respond to estrogen prior to puberty, but sampling these is not practical. Instead, response in such target tissues as bone, breasts, and pubic hair is more easily appraised. Estrogens stimulate ductular and stromal proliferation, and progestogens stimulate alveolobular development in breasts.

Estrogens stimulate growth of pubic hair, but the mechanism of hormone action is obscure.

Although the exact mechanism of action is unknown, estrogens are required for the normal formation, mineralization, and maturation of bones. Standards have been established for determining radiographically whether "bone age" is advancing appropriately in relation to chronologic age from infancy to adulthood. These standards are based on radiographs of left-sided extremities (hands, wrists, elbows, shoulders, hips, and knees) in normal children of different ages. Estrogen deficiencies retard and excesses advance bone age in relation to chronologic age, but the changes are slow to appear.

During childhood, deficiencies of estradiol are manifest by delayed or inadequate maturation and excesses by premature maturation in these steroid hormone–sensitive target tissues. During the postpubertal years, regression of breast development and osteopenia are signs of deficient, and breast engorgement and tenderness are signs of excess sex steroid hormone secretion.

Benirschke K: The endometrium. *In* Yen SSC, Jaffe RB (eds.): Reproductive Endocrinology. Philadelphia, W. B. Saunders Company, 1978, pp 241–260. *A pathologist provides a well illustrated discourse on endometrial morphology in health and disease.*

Espey LL: Ovarian contractility and its relationship to ovulation: A review. Biol Reprod 19:540, 1978. *Contains references to processes that may be involved in mechanics of ovulation.*

Knobil E: Neuroendocrine control of the menstrual cycle. Recent Prog Horm Res 36:53, 1980. *A literate treatment of results of a decade of intensive studies of hormonal events pacing the primate menstrual cycle; required reading for serious students of reproductive biology.*

Rebar RW: Practical evaluation of hormonal status. *In* Yen SSC, Jaffe RB (eds.): Reproductive Endocrinology. Philadelphia, W. B. Saunders Company, 1978, pp 469–518. *A clinician describes a systematic approach to assessing ovarian function and clinical diagnosis. Bibliography is exhaustive.*

Ross GT, Lipsett MB (eds.): Reproductive endocrinology. Clin Endocrinol Metab 7:467, 1978. *A collection of reviews on the "state of the art" of information about human ovarian function throughout life.*

Ross GT, Schreiber JR: The ovary. *In* Yen SSC, Jaffe RB (eds.): Reproductive Endocrinology. Philadelphia, W. B. Saunders Company, 1978, pp 63–79. *A treatise on ovarian morphology, physiology, and function, written by physicians for physicians.*

SEX STEROID HORMONES AND OVARIAN FUNCTION DURING INFANCY AND EARLY CHILDHOOD

Normal

Ovaries of infant and prepubertal girls respond in the same fashion as ovaries of postmenarchal women to the same gonadotropic stimulus. Ovarian follicles of prepubertal girls are smaller and secrete less steroid hormones prior to undergoing atresia because pituitary gonadotropin secretion is insufficient. The low blood estrogen levels characteristic of prepubertal girls do not elicit pituitary gonadotropin secretion comparable to that which occurs in adults following oophorectomy or primary ovarian failure. Indeed, failure of gonadotropins to rise in response to such blood estrogen levels in adults would be consistent with hypothalamic-pituitary dysfunction or failure. Ovulatory cycles are induced during chronic pulsatile administration of GnRH to prepubertal female rhesus monkeys and cease when GnRH is discontinued. In postpubertal girls, rising blood estrogens elicit an inhibition of FSH and a stimulation of LH secretion. In contrast, both FSH and LH secretion are inhibited following administration of extremely small doses of estradiol to prepubertal girls. The hypothalamic-pituitary unit during childhood is extremely sensitive to the inhibitory effects of estrogens. As puberty progresses, this sensitivity to inhibitory effects declines and gives way to a positive feedback effect of estrogens on LH secretion. Differences in hypothalamic-pituitary function therefore appear to account for differences in ovarian function before and after puberty.

Two additional observations provide circumstantial evidence for changes in steroid hormone regulation of hypothalamic-pituitary function after puberty in girls. First, pulsatile changes in blood LH levels, reflecting pulsatile secretion of LH and consistent with pulsatile secretion of GnRH, have been observed in specimens collected from pubescent girls during sleeping but not waking hours, and no such changes have been noted in clearly prepubertal girls. Second, ovulatory menstrual cycles have been induced during chronic pulsatile GnRH therapy in girls with hypogonadotropic hypogonadism, delayed puberty, and primary amenorrhea resulting from hypothalamic failure.

Abnormal

WITH NORMAL SEX STEROID HORMONE PRODUCTION. Ovarian diseases associated with normal sex steroid hormone production are uncommonly recognized during infancy and childhood. Instead, these become apparent at the expected age of puberty and will be discussed later.

WITH DECREASED SEX STEROID HORMONE PRODUCTION. Since ovarian steroid hormone production is normally low during infancy and prepubertal childhood, signs and symptoms associated with, but not resulting from, inadequate ovarian function are more useful clues for the presence of ovarian disease. These include failure to grow (the most common basis for seeking medical advice), musculoskeletal deformities, café-au-lait spots, pigmented nevi, a variety of congenital malformations, and cranial nerve deficits.

Although sex steroid hormone deficiencies produce few signs or symptoms during infancy and childhood, identification of the disorder at this time permits the physician to plan therapeutic strategies to deal with such problems as pubertal delay, primary amenorrhea, virilization at puberty, and the propensity of dysgenetic gonads to undergo malignant degeneration. All ovarian diseases associated with sex steroid hormone deficiency in infancy and childhood will be associated with sex steroid hormone deficiency later in life. Details related to specific syndromes are discussed in the next section under Delayed Puberty and Primary Amenorrhea.

WITH INCREASED SEX STEROID HORMONE PRODUCTION: PRECOCIOUS PUBERTY AND PSEUDOPUBERTY. The signs and symptoms of ovarian diseases associated with sex steroid hormone deficiency are unimpressive in infants and prepubertal girls. In contrast, the signs and symptoms of sex steroid hormone excess are dramatic, since all of the target tissues respond to stimulation in infants and children. Thus, accelerated linear growth and advanced bone age, breast growth and maturation, appearance of pubic and axillary hair, maturation of the external genitalia, and even cyclic vaginal bleeding may occur during the first year of life. The last-named event represents the syndrome of *isosexual precocious puberty,* in which premature maturation of the hypothalamic-pituitary axis results in ovulatory menstrual cycles indistinguishable from those that occur physiologically after puberty.

Similar signs may occur when the sex steroid hormone excess derives from ovarian or adrenal tumors or from normal ovaries responding to gonadotropins secreted by nonovarian tumors (so-called ectopic gonadotropin secretion). This is referred to as *isosexual precocious pseudopuberty.* In some instances pubertal changes may proceed along heterosexual, virilizing lines. The premature maturation of secondary sexual characteristics in these patients is referred to as *heterosexual precocious pseudopuberty.*

Target tissue responses to androgen excess in virilizing syndromes of heterosexual precocious pseudopuberty may be dramatic. Oily skin, severe acne, pubic and axillary hair growth, excessive facial and body hair, temporal hair recession, clitoral enlargement, and even episodic vaginal bleeding may occur in these girls. These syndromes rarely result from ovarian diseases but more commonly from adrenal cortical hyperplasia secondary to genetically determined deficiencies in enzymes required for the biosynthesis of cortisol (see Ch. 229). Ordinarily these are diagnosed during the neonatal period, but mild allelic variants associated with milder deficits occasionally escape detection until later.

Isosexual precocious puberty is rarely associated with life-threatening disease. Iso- and heterosexual precocious pseudopuberty may be associated with either life-threatening or reversible benign diseases. Thus, making the distinction promptly has important implications for treatment. Distinguishing the syndromes, however, may be difficult for at least two reasons.

First, the sequence of maturational events in the syndromes of both precocious puberty and precocious pseudopuberty is similar to that occurring during spontaneous puberty. In these syndromes, as in spontaneous puberty, breast and pubic hair development are the first changes to appear. Premature development of breasts (premature thelarche) or pubic hair (premature pubarche or adrenarche) may occur as isolated self-limited events with no further progression of pubertal maturation. Distinguishing among these alternatives early in the clinical course of any of them is often difficult.

Second, periodic vaginal bleeding may occur in isosexual precocious puberty and in both iso- and heterosexual precocious pseudopuberty. In these instances, only clear-cut presumptive indicators of ovulation which develop late in the clinical course will distinguish between these two syndromes.

CLINICAL EVALUATION OF PATIENTS WITH PRECOCIOUS PUBERTY AND PSEUDOPUBERTY. Fortunately, in some instances the history and physical examination will provide information useful for distinguishing isosexual precocious puberty from isosexual and heterosexual precocious pseudopuberty.

The History. The first element to explore carefully in eliciting the history is the temporal sequence in which signs and symptoms of sex steroid hormone excess appeared. Breast budding usually appears before or very shortly after pubic hair growth begins during normal pubescence. If pubic hair growth is not followed shortly by breast budding, the sequence suggests a diagnosis of premature adrenarche. Conversely, breast hypertrophy persisting for months without appearance of pubic hair suggests premature thelarche.

Careful questioning of the mother and other women with whom an infant or child has intimate contact may reveal a source of either inadvertent oral ingestion (oral contraceptive pills, for example) or percutaneous absorption (cosmetics or powders containing steroids) of estrogens or androgens. A diagnosis of *factitious pseudopuberty* on this basis eliminates the need for more complicated and expensive diagnostic tests.

A history of seizures or seizure equivalents provides presumptive evidence for an intracerebral tumor that may be associated with precocious puberty if the tumor stimulates pituitary gonadotropin secretion.

The Physical Examination. The physician should look very carefully for evidences of virilization. When present, virilizing signs exclude the diagnosis of isosexual precocious puberty. In their absence, however, a diagnosis of pseudopuberty cannot be excluded, since virilizing signs take a finite period of time to develop. Moreover, isosexual changes may result from estrogens produced by peripheral aromatization of androgens secreted by adrenal or ovarian tumors.

Physical examination of organ systems that are not estrogen targets may provide valuable clues for distinguishing among the etiologic variants of precocious puberty and pseudopuberty. The constellation of cutaneous café-au-lait spots, facial asymmetry, polyostotic fibrous dysplasia, and other skeletal abnormalities such as sclerotic changes in the base of the skull and cranial nerve deficits suggests a diagnosis of the *McCune-Albright syndrome* in a girl with signs of precocious puberty (see Ch. 251). Other neurologic deficits may be associated with central nervous system tumors such as phakomas, hamartomas, and neoplasms of the floor of the third ventricle which initiate isosexual precocious puberty. As noted, neurologic deficits are more likely to be associated with precocious puberty.

Signs and symptoms of thyroid hormone deficiency have been observed in girls with precocious puberty associated with thyroid-stimulating hormone (TSH)-deficient hypothyroidism. Thyroid hormone replacement therapy halts progression of the pubertal changes in these girls, and they will subsequently undergo puberty at the usual time.

Careful abdominal and rectal examination is helpful in distinguishing true precocious puberty from pseudopuberty, since most adrenal and ovarian tumors associated with iso- or heterosexual precocious pseudopuberty are palpable. Benign adrenal adenomas secreting androgens or estrogens may not be large enough to be palpated, but functioning adrenal carcinomas are almost always palpable. Ovarian cysts may also secrete sufficient estrogen to initiate isosexual pseudopuberty. Ovarian cysts may occur prior to development of ovulatory cycles in true isosexual precocity. Hence, the presence of these cysts does not exclude a diagnosis of true isosexual precocious puberty, and laparotomy is indicated to assure that the lesion is not an ovarian tumor.

When vaginal bleeding is the only sign or symptom of precocity, vaginal inspection is essential to rule out bleeding secondary to local irritation from infection or foreign bodies and to eliminate bleeding vaginal or cervical neoplasms. This examination should be done prior to embarking on more complex diagnostic studies, since vaginal bleeding as the first sign of precocious puberty is exceedingly uncommon.

TABLE 236–2. SIGNS USEFUL IN DIAGNOSING SYNDROMES OF PRECOCIOUS PUBERTY AND PSEUDOPUBERTY*

	Breast Enlargement	Pubic Hair	Vaginal Bleeding	Virilizing Signs	Advanced Bone Age	Neurologic Deficits	Abdominopelvic Masses
Premature thelarche	+	–	–	–	–	–	–
Premature adrenarche	–	+	–	–	±	–	–
Precocious puberty							
Idiopathic	+	+	+	–	+	–	Rarely
Due to CNS tumor	+	+	+	–	+	+	–
McCune-Albright syndrome†	+	+	+	–	+	+	–
Primary hypothyroidism‡	+	Rarely	+	–	–	–	Rarely
Isosexual precocious pseudopuberty							
Ovarian tumors	+	+	+	–	+	–	+
Adrenal tumors§	+	+	+	–	+	–	+
Ovarian cysts	+	+	+	–	+	–	+
Factitious¶	+	+	+	–	+	–	–
Heterosexual precocious pseudopuberty							
Ovarian tumors	+	+	+	+	+	–	Rarely
Adrenal tumors§	+	+	+	+	+	–	+
Congenital adrenal hyperplasia	+	+	+	+	+	–	–

*Modified from data of Ross GT, Vande Wiele RL: *In* Williams, RH (ed.): Textbook of Endocrinology. 5th ed. Philadelphia, W. B. Saunders Company, 1974, pp 368–422.

†Facial asymmetry and other musculoskeletal abnormalities are diagnostic.

‡Retarded bone age is diagnostic.

§Mass in upper abdomen is suggestive.

¶History of exposure is essential.

A summary of physical findings and tests useful for distinguishing entities associated with precocious puberty and precocious pseudopuberty is summarized in Table 236–2. Table 236–3 provides a scheme for further evaluating patients with and without physical signs of virilization.

Diagnostic Tests. In addition to the history and physical examination, useful maneuvers include ultrasonic scanning of adrenals and ovaries and computed tomographic (CT) scans of adrenals for confirming impressions obtained by palpation. CT scans of the head are indicated when a history of seizures is elicited or neurologic deficits are discovered in a patient with signs of precocious puberty or pseudopuberty.

Radiographic determination of bone age should be made. Plain skull films are useful in screening for pituitary and parapituitary tumors.

On occasion, measurement of steroid and peptide hormone concentrations in blood will provide diagnostically useful information. High blood levels of 17-OH-progesterone or 11-deoxycortisol which decline following oral administration of suppressive doses of dexamethasone (see Ch. 229 and 237) are useful for distinguishing adrenal cortical hyperplasia from adrenal cortical adenomas and carcinomas or from ovarian tumors secreting androgens. High levels of serum testosterone suggest an ovarian source of excess androgen, whereas high levels of dehydroisoandrosterone (DHA) or its sulfate ester (DHAS), the principal precursors of urinary 17-ketosteroids, are more consistent with adrenal sources of excess androgen.

Blood immunoreactive LH levels in excess of those encountered in any physiologic state in women and girls are diagnostic of ovarian dysgerminomas and teratomas which secrete hCG that is antigenically and biologically similar to LH and stimulates ovarian steroid hormone secretion and pseudopubertal changes in prepubertal girls. Blood FSH:LH ratios compatible with those in sexually mature women are helpful for diagnosing precocious puberty. If obtaining blood specimens is impractical, determining gonadotropin concentrations in timed urine collections serves the same purpose.

TABLE 236–3. SCHEMA FOR DIAGNOSTIC EVALUATION OF PATIENTS WITH PRECOCIOUS PUBERTY AND PSEUDOPUBERTY

I. Virilizing signs present
  A. With palpable abdominal or pelvic masses
    1. If location suggests adrenal tumor:
      a. Do CT scan to rule out bilateral tumors
      b. Look for metastases in chest, liver
    2. If location suggests ovarian tumor
      a. Confirm mass with ultrasonic scanning
      b. Examine under anesthesia and explore surgically
  B. Without palpable abdominal or pelvic masses: measure serum androgens and androgen precursors: DHA, DHAS, T
    1. If all elevated, do Decadron suppression test
      a. If suppressible, suspect congenital adrenal hyperplasia due to 11- or 21-hydroxylase deficiency; measure 17-OHP, 11-DOC to distinguish
      b. If not suppressible, suspect adrenal carcinoma or rare ovarian tumor; use scans appropriately, measure hormones in venous effluent to lateralize before surgery
    2. If testosterone is disproportionately elevated, suspect ovarian tumor, and use ultrasonic scan to lateralize before surgery
II. Virilizing signs absent
  A. With palpable abdominal or pelvic masses
    1. If location suggests adrenal tumor, proceed as in 1.A.1
    2. If location suggests ovarian tumor, proceed as in 1.A.2
  B. Without palpable abdominal or pelvic masses
    1. If vaginal bleeding has occurred, inspect vagina for infection, foreign body, tumor
    2. If vaginal bleeding has not occurred, do complete neuroophthalmologic exam
      a. If abnormal, involve neurosurgeon in choice of further studies for intracerebral tumors likely to produce precocious puberty
      b. If normal, determine bone age by x-ray
        (1) If retarded, diagnostic of precocious puberty due to primary hypothyroidism
        (2) If normal or advanced, measure serum DHA, DHAS
          (a) If values consistent with age, consider premature thelarche, early precocious puberty, factitious pseudopuberty, forme fruste of McCune-Albright syndrome
          (b) If values increased for age, consider premature adrenarche, early precocious puberty, pseudopuberty due to occult ovarian or adrenal tumor

TABLE 236–4. CRITERIA FOR DISTINGUISHING TANNER STAGES 1 THROUGH 5 IN BREASTS AND PUBIC HAIR MATURATION*

For Breasts	Stage	For Pubic Hair
No palpable glandular tissue; areola not pigmented; except for nipple, breast does not project from anterior chest wall	1	None
Glandular tissue is palpable at least coextensively with the diameter of the areola; nipple and breast project as a single mound from anterior chest wall	2	Occasional wispy strands, usually along the labia
Increased glandular tissue to palpation; breasts enlarged; areola increasing in diameter and becoming more darkly pigmented, but contours of breast and areola remain in a single plane	3	More, darker, coarser hair extending superiorly over the pubis
Further enlargement; increased areolar pigmentation; areola and nipple form a secondary mound above level of the breast	4	Dark, coarse, curly hair, covering the mons pubis in the adult pattern, but not extending to medial aspects of thighs
Areola and nipple no longer project but have receded to make a smooth contour in profile view	5	Mature; extends to thighs but otherwise remains in female pattern

*Modified from data of Ross GT, Vande Wiele, RL: *In* Williams, RH (ed.): Textbook of Endocrinology. 5th ed. Philadelphia, W. B. Saunders Company, 1974, pp 368–422.

SEX STEROID HORMONES AND OVARIAN FUNCTION DURING LATE CHILDHOOD

Normal

NORMAL PUBERTY. To determine if the extent of pubertal development is normal for a girl's chronologic peer group, it is necessary to know the mean age and range of ages associated with the onset of breast and pubic hair development and the rates of progression in maturation, as well as the mean age and age ranges of the normal pubertal growth spurt and of normal menarche. To give the assessment an objective, quantitative dimension, degrees of breast and pubic hair development have been assigned numbers ranging from 1 (least mature) to 5 (adults). Criteria for these states are listed in Table 236–4.

The pubertal growth spurt, manifested by acceleration in the rate of linear growth, is an important landmark. It usually begins after breast development has been initiated and is often completed by the time maturation has progressed to Stage 3.

Menarche marks the completion of pubertal change. It appears at a mean age of 12.6 years, with a standard deviation of 1.2 years. The age range of menarche is 9 to 16 years in the United States population. Thus, *the occurrence of menarche before the age of 9 or failure to occur after the age of 16 merits evaluation.* Since the beginning of breast maturation anticipates the menarche by one to two years, failure to initiate changes in sexual characteristics by age 12 merits study.

DELAYED PUBERTY. In some girls who will undergo puberty spontaneously, delays in both the age at onset and rates of progression of pubertal changes exceed three standard deviations from the means for normal girls. These delays may create psychologic problems, generate parental anxiety, and pose problems in diagnosis and management. Unfortunately, the diagnosis is confirmed only by spontaneous onset and completion of puberty, and a decision to temporize can be justified only after excluding other diagnosable entities.

As an alternative to temporizing, sex steroid hormones can be used to induce pubertal changes in secondary sexual characteristics when the psychologic burden of delay is intolerable. Although no apparent permanent damage to fertility results from giving sex steroid hormones, the extent of linear growth may be compromised if treatment is too aggressive.

Abnormal

DYSFUNCTIONAL UTERINE BLEEDING. Prolonged and severe vaginal bleeding associated with endometrial hyperplasia and anovulation may occur after the menarche. In these girls no response in plasma LH is seen following 1 mg injections of estradiol benzoate, a manipulation which elicits an increase in blood LH levels in normal postpubertal girls. Progestogens will sometimes induce a "medical curettage" and stop bleeding. If this fails, a gynecologist should be consulted.

PRIMARY AMENORRHEA. During later childhood, when pubescence normally begins, the majority of ovarian diseases present with signs and symptoms suggestive of decreased ovarian sex steroid hormone production. In addition to short stature, these include retarded development of secondary sexual characteristics (delayed puberty) or primary amenorrhea or both. The relationships between sex steroid hormone production and primary amenorrhea are shown in Table 236–5.

WITH NORMAL SEX STEROID HORMONE PRODUCTION. When pubertal changes have begun at an appropriate age and secondary sexual characteristics have matured fully and in proper sequence but menses have not appeared, primary attention should be directed to the genital tract. Müllerian dysgenesis and amenorrhea traumatica are major considerations.

Müllerian Dysgenesis. Müllerian ducts normally give rise to fallopian tubes, the uterus, the cervix, and the upper vagina in genetic females (Fig. 233–2). For unknown reasons, one or more of the derivatives may not develop, and the failure may go unrecognized until the age of puberty. The anomalies vary in severity from an imperforate hymen to complete aplasia of all müllerian duct derivatives with vaginal atresia. Although aplasia usually involves all of the derivatives, single component defects have been described. Thus, vaginal aplasia associated with absence of the uterus and cervix is the most common defect, with an estimated frequency of 1 per 4000 female infants. In about 10 per cent of cases, vaginal aplasia is associated with a functionally normal uterus and cervix. Congenital absence of the cervix associated with a functionally normal uterus and patent vagina is extremely rare, less than 20 cases having been reported.

TABLE 236–5. SEX STEROID HORMONE PRODUCTION AND PRIMARY AMENORRHEA

- I. With normal sex steroid hormone production
  - A. Müllerian dysgenesis
  - B. Amenorrhea traumatica
- II. With decreased sex steroid hormone production
  - A. Disorders of fetal development and differentiation
    - 1. Of the genitalia
      - a. Male pseudohermaphroditism due to deficient testosterone synthesis
        - (1) 20,22-Desmolase
        - (2) 3β-Hydroxysteroid dehydrogenase
        - (3) 17α-Hydroxylase
        - (4) 17,20-Desmolase
        - (5) 17-Ketosteroid reductase
      - b. Male pseudohermaphroditism due to 5α-reductase deficiency
      - c. Male pseudohermaphroditism due to androgen resistance
        - (1) Complete testicular feminization
        - (2) Incomplete testicular feminization
        - (3) Familial incomplete male pseudohermaphroditism
      - d. Female pseudohermaphroditism with fetal and postnatal androgen excess
    - 2. Of the gonads
      - a. Gonadal dysgenesis with stigmata of Turner's syndrome
      - b. Mixed gonadal dysgenesis
      - c. Pure gonadal dysgenesis
      - d. True hermaphroditism
  - B. Congenital and acquired disorders
    - 1. Follicular insensitivity to gonadotropins
      - a. 17-hydroxylase deficiency
      - b. "Resistant ovaries"
    - 2. Hypothalamic pituitary diseases
      - a. Familial hypogonadotropic hypogonadism
      - b. Pituitary and parapituitary tumors
      - c. Idiopathic panhypopituitarism
      - d. Anorexia nervosa
    - 3. Miscellaneous systemic diseases
- III. With increased sex steroid hormone production
  - A. Androgen secreting ovarian and adrenal tumors
  - B. Male pseudohermaphroditism due to 5α-reductase deficiency
  - C. Polycystic ovarian disease

Normal ovarian sex steroid hormone secretion induces cyclic endometrial growth and shedding after menarche. In girls with a normal uterus but cervical aplasia, vaginal aplasia, or an imperforate hymen, the menstrual effluent is retained, producing endometriosis and cyclic abdominal pain without external evidence of menses. Examination under anesthesia is essential for determining the extent of the defect and should be done by a surgeon experienced in creating vaginas for these patients. When the defect consists of an imperforate hymen only, restoration of normal function is accomplished by incising the hymenal membrane. Attempts at plastic reconstruction of a functional vagina and a patent outflow tract have met with variable success, and successful pregnancy has been reported only rarely.

Amenorrhea Traumatica. In addition to müllerian dysgenesis, endometrial synechiae associated with endometrial resistance to estrogenic and progestational steroid hormone stimulation and withdrawal may result in primary amenorrhea. Endometritis, usually tuberculous, is the predisposing etiology.

WITH DECREASED SEX STEROID HORMONE PRODUCTION FETALLY AND POSTNATALLY. ***Errors in Genital Differentiation.*** Errors in gender assignment to genetic males during the neonatal period account for about 50 per cent of cases of primary amenorrhea. These errors are usually based on gross abnormalities in genital differentiation.

Virilization of gonaductal and genital anlagen in genetic males is dependent upon two secretory products of fetal testes: (1) testosterone, which stimulates development of wolffian duct derivatives and virilization of derivatives of the urogenital sinus and genital tubercle (following its conversion to dihydrotestosterone in the target tissues); and (2) müllerian regression factor, which results in degeneration of müllerian ducts. Abnormalities are discussed in Ch. 233.

Errors in Gonadal Development. GONADAL DYSGENESIS. The term "gonadal dysgenesis" is used to designate the most common error in fetal gonadal differentiation, occurring with an estimated frequency of 1 per 5000 to 7000 newborns or 1 per 2700 newborn phenotypic females. The gonads are streaks composed of fibrous stroma and devoid of gametogenic components. In most instances sex chromosomal aberrations are found in karyotypes prepared from cultures of somatic cells and presumably predispose to reduction in the number of germ cells available at the time of follicle formation during fetal life. The limited number of follicles formed is depleted by atresia prior to puberty in most instances. Occasionally, a few will persist postnatally, mature, and produce sufficient estrogen to initiate pubertal changes. Rarely, these will be sufficient for completing puberty, and there are case reports of ovulation followed by pregnancy and delivery of normal infants at term.

Streak gonads also occur in persons in whom there are no detectable morphologic abnormalities of the sex chromosomes, suggesting that other factors may result in depletion of germ cells and reduction in number of follicles formed. Thus, there are two familial varieties of gonadal dysgenesis caused by gene mutations, both of which occur sporadically as well. A paucity of follicles has been seen in ovaries of fetuses and infants with trisomy 13 or 18 syndromes (see Ch. 35). A paucity of primordial follicles and failure of maturation of these have been described in ovaries of girls with ataxia telangiectasia (see Ch. 492). Whether chromosomal breakage and immunoglobulin deficiencies, both characteristic manifestations of the latter syndrome, predispose to a reduction in oocytes and follicles remains to be determined.

The syndrome of sexual infantilism, short stature, musculoskeletal abnormalities, and streak gonads, referred to as *Turner's syndrome,* is associated with abnormalities of sex chromosome number or morphology. Among these patients, one of virtually every variety of chromosomal breakage, with or without reunion, has been described (see Ch. 35). However, the most common karyotype is 45,X, in which the second sex chromosome is totally deleted. Short stature and other somatic stigmata associated with chromatin-negative nuclear sex without "F" bodies (see Ch. 35) in a patient with female external genitalia and failure to achieve puberty are diagnostic of the 45,X syndrome. Many of the somatic stigmata of Turner's syndrome occur in Noonan's syndrome, in arthrogryposis, in the Klippel-Feil syndrome (see Ch. 523), and in a variety of other syndromes in which sex chromosomes are normal. Girls with these latter disorders have chromatin-positive nuclear sex (Barr bodies) and 46,XX karyotypes.

MIXED GONADAL DYSGENESIS. The term "mixed gonadal dysgenesis" has been used to designate asymmetrical gonadal development with a germ cell tumor or a testis on one side and an undifferentiated streak, a rudimentary gonad, or no gonad on the other side. Gonaductal differentiation is usually concordant with gonadal differentiation, but the extent of genital virilization is variable. In patients with germ cell tumors, 90 per cent of whom are reared as females, virilization is mild, and some breast development occurs at puberty. In contrast, among patients with a testis and a streak, only 70 per cent are raised as females, virilization at puberty is marked, and no breast development occurs. Short stature and other stigmata associated with a 45,X karyotype in Turner's syndrome are less commonly observed among patients with tumors than among patients with testes.

Nuclear sex is usually chromatin negative. "F" bodies should be sought, but failure to demonstrate an "F" body is not a definitive test for the Y chromosomes, since Y chromosomes that do not fluoresce have been identified among patients with 45,X/46,XY sex chromosomal mosaicism and mixed gonadal dysgenesis. Thus, to rule out the presence of cell lines containing "Y" chromosomes in patients with anomalous external genitalia and chromatin-negative nuclear sex but no "F" bodies, the karyotype should be determined.

No endocrine tests are diagnostic of either tumor or testis. Visualization, biopsy, and removal of all gonadal tissue seem indicated to remove sources of androgen in girls with X/XY karyotypes in whom virilization occurs at puberty and to eliminate the neoplastic potential of dysgenetic gonads. Suitable sex steroid hormone replacement therapy should be undertaken at the appropriate time.

PURE GONADAL DYSGENESIS. The term "pure gonadal dysgenesis" has been used to distinguish sexually immature taller girls (>150 cm) with bilateral streak gonads and minimal extragenital extragonadal somatic stigmata from sexually immature shorter girls (<150 cm) with streak gonads associated with the musculoskeletal defects usually regarded as manifestations of Turner's syndrome. This distinction is clinically useful in view of the high incidence of gonadal tumors in patients with pure gonadal dysgenesis and an XY karyotype.

Pure gonadal dysgenesis is a genetic disorder occurring in siblings, whereas Turner's syndrome is rarely observed in siblings. Heredofamilial gonadal dysgenesis can be associated with either an XY or XX karyotype, and the disorder is sometimes referred to as familial XX or XY gonadal dysgenesis. The two karyotypes are transmitted differently, and there are some other distinguishing clinical features. The 45,XY syndrome, transmitted as an X-linked recessive trait (see Ch. 35), is associated with gonadal tumors in about 25 per cent of cases and clitoral hypertrophy in 10 to 15 per cent of cases. These changes are found in less than 5 per cent of patients with the XX syndrome. The high incidence of tumors of germ cell origin among persons with an XY genotype mandates gonadectomy in these patients.

Sex chromosomal aneuploidy is less common among patients with pure gonadal dysgenesis. Mosaic karyotypes such as 45,X/46,XX have been described in sporadic cases of pure gonadal dysgenesis.

TRUE HERMAPHRODITISM. Gonadal differentiation may proceed differently on the two sides, giving rise to a unilateral testis or ovary or ovotestis, with an ovary or a testis or an ovotestis on the other side. When both sperm and oocytes are found in these gonads, true hermaphroditism is diagnosed. Hermaphroditism is further discussed in Ch. 233.

Disorders Due to Follicular Insensitivity to Gonadotropins. 17-HYDROXYLASE DEFICIENCY (see also Ch. 229). Failure of follicle growth to progress normally results in primary amenorrhea in women congenitally unable to synthesize estrogen because of deficiency of 17-hydroxylase. In these women steroid hormone synthesis does not progress beyond progesterone (Fig. 236–2), and estrogen deficiency gives rise to sexual infantilism and primary amenorrhea associated with increased serum and urinary gonadotropins. Furthermore, excessive synthesis of an adrenal cortical salt-retaining steroid hormone, desoxycorticosterone, predisposes to hypertension with hypokalemic alkalosis. Ovarian biopsies show numerous large cysts and numerous primordial follicles with complete failure of orderly follicular maturation despite high serum gonadotropin levels. The association of sexual infantilism and primary amenorrhea with hypertension suggests the diagnosis. When present, high serum levels of progesterone and desoxycorticosterone (DOC) are diagnostic. The hypertension may respond to glucocorticoid replacement therapy.

RESISTANT OVARIES. Some sexually immature normotensive girls with high serum and urinary gonadotropins have ovaries that contain primordial follicles that neither mature nor secrete estrogens despite stimulation with massive doses of exogenous gonadotropins. Since ovulation may follow administration of estrogens, the defect possibly lies in the inability to initiate estrogen synthesis prior to antrum formation.

Disorders Due to Hypothalamic-Pituitary Dysfunction or Failure. The pituitary must secrete sufficient quantities of gonadotropins to stimulate ovarian follicular maturation and sex steroid hormone secretion. If it does not, secondary sexual characteristics do not mature and no menses occur. Failure may result from inadequate hypothalamic stimulation or from primary pituitary diseases (such as neoplasms or granulomas) that adversely affect pituitary function. All varieties of sexual immaturity resulting from inadequate pituitary gonadotropin secretion are referred to as syndromes of *hypogonadotropic hypogonadism.* It is important to distinguish among them in order that treatment be directed toward the specific underlying disease (see Ch. 225).

FAMILIAL HYPOGONADOTROPIC HYPOGONADISM (see also Ch. 234). Kallmann's syndrome is a familial disorder characterized by anosmia or hyposmia secondary to dysplasia of the rhinencephalon, sexual immaturity, and variable expression of midline defects. The trait is transmitted as an X-linked recessive or male-limited autosomal dominant trait, although genetic heterogeneity may occur. Ovaries of these women contain numerous primordial follicles, but follicular maturation is severely retarded even when compared to that in ovaries of neonates. Successful pregnancies after induction of ovulation with gonadotropins support the contention that the hypogonadism results from inadequate gonadotropin secretion. Successful induction of ovulation after chronic pulsatile administration of gonadotropin-releasing hormone to persons with this syndrome suggests that the disease is of hypothalamic rather than pituitary origin.

ANOREXIA NERVOSA. Primary amenorrhea resulting from hypothalamic dysfunction occurs as a complication of anorexia nervosa. Anorexia nervosa is discussed extensively in Ch. 215.

SECONDARY TO PITUITARY AND PARAPITUITARY TUMORS. Disorders of hypothalamic control of pituitary hormone secretion, including gonadotropins, are associated with third ventricle tumors and parapituitary tumors. Destruction of anterior pituitary tissue by primary pituitary neoplasms or by metastatic infiltration of other neoplasms may result in hypogonadism and primary amenorrhea associated with signs and symptoms of deficiencies of other pituitary hormones (see Ch. 225 and 511). Neurologic and neuroradiologic examinations are essential for proper evaluation. Surgical ablation is indicated when feasible.

SECONDARY TO SYSTEMIC DISEASE. The hypothalamic-pituitary unit may fail to function appropriately in a number of debilitating, stressful, systemic diseases that interfere with somatic growth and development. Chronic renal failure is perhaps the most common of these. It would be rare indeed for such a disease process to be discovered during the course of an evaluation for primary amenorrhea.

WITH INCREASED SEX STEROID HORMONE PRODUCTION. The quantities of testosterone and of dihydrotestosterone produced normally in female fetuses are inadequate to effect virilization of the primordia of the urogenital sinus and external genitalia. Excessive androgen arising endogenously from the adrenals or exogenously from hormonal therapy of pregnant women will produce virilization of the external genitalia and result in female pseudohermaphroditism. The extent of anomalous genital differentiation varies from an enlarged clitoris to ambiguity sufficient to make gender assignment by inspection hazardous.

Excessive maternal ovarian androgen production during gestation sometimes results in virilization of the urogenital sinus and genital tubercle derivatives in genetic females with normal ovaries.

Excessive fetal adrenal androgen secretion is usually associated with defective cortisol synthesis, and failure to suppress pituitary adrenocorticotropin secretion results in congenital adrenal hyperplasia and excessive adrenal androgen secretion (see Ch. 229). In female fetuses with deficiencies of either the 11β-hydroxylase or 21-hydroxylase enzyme system, excessive adrenocortical androgen secretion not only results in virilization of the external genitalia, and occasionally the urogenital sinus as well, during fetal life but also stimulates development of heterosexual precocious pseudopuberty and suppresses pituitary gonadotropin secretion postnatally.

Ordinarily, signs and symptoms of adrenal cortical insufficiency in these girls during the neonatal period lead to recognition and appropriate treatment at that time. Allelic variants associated with milder enzyme deficits may not be recognized until signs and symptoms of heterosexual precocious pseudopuberty, primary amenorrhea, or severe acne and hirsutism lead to recognition of the pathophysiologic basis of the disorder. Chromatin-positive nuclear sex eliminates the diagnosis of male pseudohermaphroditism. Other diagnostic tests are discussed in Ch. 229 and 237.

Male Pseudohermaphroditism Due to 5α-Reductase Deficiency. Male pseudohermaphrodites with 5α-reductase deficiency are usually raised as girls. However, at puberty breasts fail to develop, pubic hair and beard develop, no menses occur, virilization of the external genitalia takes place, and these persons assume male gender roles. By standards for girls at puberty, testosterone production is increased (see Ch. 233).

Polycystic Ovarian Disease. A syndrome of primary amenorrhea with hirsutism, other virilizing signs, insulin-resistant diabetes, acanthosis nigricans, and obesity has been shown to be associated with enlarged polycystic ovaries secreting excessive androgen. The diabetes seems to result from circulating antibodies directed toward plasma membrane receptors for insulin, suggesting an autoimmune component in the etiology of the disorder. The disease must be distinguished from androgen-secreting ovarian and adrenal tumors which are associated with primary amenorrhea and sometimes with diabetes.

Jaffe RB: Disorders of sexual development. *In* Yen SSC, Jaffe RB (eds.): Reproductive Endocrinology. Philadelphia, W. B. Saunders Company, 1978, pp 271–296. *A concise but comprehensive summary of the literature relevant to errors in fetal genital differentiation and neonatal gender assignment.*

Kulin HE: The maturation of ovulatory potential in man. Horm Res 12:46, 1980. *Applications of timed urine collections to the study of disorders of puberty are discussed in detail.*

Marshall WA, Tanner JM: Variations in pattern of pubertal changes in girls. Arch Dis Child 44:291, 1969. *A classic paper, required reading for all serious students.*

Rosenfield RL: The ovary and female sexual maturation. *In* Kaplan SA (ed.): Clinical Pediatric and Adolescent Endocrinology. Philadelphia, W. B. Saunders Company, 1982, pp 217–268. *A scholarly treatment of prepubertal, peripubertal, and early postpubertal ovarian function in health and disease.*

Styne DM, Grumbach MM: Puberty in the male and female: Its physiology and disorders. *In* Yen SSC, Jaffe RB (eds.): Reproductive Endocrinology. Philadelphia, W. B. Saunders Company, 1978, pp 189–240. *A well-organized discussion with excellent bibliography relevant to normal or abnormal sex steroid hormone production before and after puberty in boys and girls.*

SEX STEROID HORMONES AND OVARIAN FUNCTION AFTER THE MENARCHE

Normal

Regular ovulatory menstrual cycles and fertility provide the best evidence that ovarian function is normal after the menarche; and since ovulatory menstrual cycles require normal hypothalamic, pituitary, and uterine interactions as well, one can infer that all components of the system are functioning normally. Conversely, menstrual disorders and infertility are the most common signs that ovarian function is abnormal in women after the menarche. In women with cyclic menses and infertility and in women with secondary amenorrhea, abnormal ovarian function may result in normal, decreased, or increased sex steroid hormone production. Table 236–6 provides a systematic framework for evaluating ovarian function in these women. In this table, as before, causes are stratified on the basis of sex steroid hormone production. Although measurements of plasma sex steroid hormone concentrations are not always necessary, the range of normal values which takes cyclic changes into account is summarized in Table 236–1.

Abnormal

INFERTILITY (WITH CYCLIC VAGINAL BLEEDING). ***With Normal Sex Steroid Hormone Production.*** Prior to undertaking diagnostic evaluation of women with infertility, ejaculates obtained from their husbands should be examined for abnormalities of sperm number, morphology, and motility. When sex steroid hormone production is normal and menses are regular, infertility is not due to any known ovarian disease. Since determining the cause of infertility in these women involves invasive procedures, a gynecologist with experience in evaluating such patients should be consulted. This referral is particularly appropriate now that in vitro fertilization and embryo transfer are regarded as acceptable methods for treating infertility due to tubal factors in women who ovulate. Moreover, recently in women in whom oocytes are not produced, pregnancies have been established by transferring embryos recovered from donor women artificially inseminated with sperm provided by the husband of the infertile woman.

With Decreased Sex Steroid Hormone Production. Infertility may result from anovulation or luteal insufficiency, both of which occur in women with cyclic bleeding.

LUTEAL INSUFFICIENCY. Corpus luteum function inadequate for establishing and maintaining early pregnancy has been shown to be the cause of infertility or repeated early abortions in some women with regular menstrual cycles. Mean luteal phase blood progesterone concentrations in these women are reduced when compared with those in fertile women who carry pregnancies to term. When rigid criteria based on endometrial morphology have been used for diagnosis, replacement therapy with progesterone has resulted in term pregnancies with delivery of normal infants, suggesting that inadequate luteal phase progesterone is the basis for the problem in some of them.

Inadequate (short) luteal phases occur frequently in women

who continue to ovulate and menstruate despite elevated blood prolactin levels, so that pituitary adenomas should be considered among the diagnostic possibilities in women with luteal insufficiency.

ANOVULATION. Anovulation can be associated with cyclic vaginal bleeding. Monophasic basal body temperature charts, serum progesterone consistent with follicular phase levels, and endometrial biopsies showing proliferative endometrium after the onset of bleeding are diagnostic. Anovulation may also be associated with excessive vaginal bleeding secondary to persistent proliferative endometrium resulting from estrogenic stimulation uninterrupted by progesterone. The syndrome is referred to as anovulatory *dysfunctional uterine bleeding,* and as in prepubertal girls with this disorder, giving estradiol benzoate fails to elicit an appropriate increase in LH secretion in these women. Endometrium should be sampled; if bleeding does not stop after giving progesterone, curettage may be necessary.

With Increased Sex Steroid Hormone Production. Although rare, persistent cyclic vaginal bleeding, ovulation, and fertility are consistent with ovarian and adrenal sources of excess androgen sufficient to cause virilization in a woman. More commonly, however, this constellation is associated with secondary amenorrhea (see below).

SECONDARY AMENORRHEA. Abnormalities at any level of the hypothalamic-pituitary-ovarian-uterine axis can interrupt ovulatory menstrual cycles. When menses fail to recur for six to twelve months in nonpregnant or parturient women who are not breast-feeding, a diagnosis of secondary amenorrhea is established. Secondary amenorrhea is not a disease entity but a sign that function has been compromised in one or more components of the hypothalamic-pituitary-ovarian-uterine axis. In all cases, sufficient diagnostic tests should be done to exclude pregnancy or life-threatening disease from the list of possible causes. Subsequent evaluation should be directed toward longitudinal monitoring to assure that the problem is not secondary to a serious disease, or to restore fertility if the patient wishes to become pregnant.

As in women with cyclic vaginal bleeding and infertility, sex steroid hormone production may be classified as normal, decreased, or increased (see Table 236–6). In these women, an objective test of estrogen production, based on endometrial response to progesterone administration and withdrawal, and, when indicated, determinations of blood FSH, LH, and prolactin can be used to assist in identifying the possible etiologic factors.

With Normal Sex Steroid Hormone Production. Amenorrhea in the face of cyclic changes in ovarian steroid hormone levels and activities consistent with those occurring during ovulatory cycles, or failure to bleed after receiving estrogens and progestogens, indicates failure of endometrial response to steroid hormone stimulation and withdrawal, obstruction of the outflow tract, or total absence of endometrium. When outflow tract obstruction and hysterectomy have been eliminated, endometrial refractoriness must be the cause. Cervical stenosis and intrauterine synechiae resulting from postpartum, postabortal, or tuberculous endometritis or following myomectomy or cesarean section must be considered. Surgical correction of these lesions is followed by resumption of menses in most cases.

With Decreased Sex Steroid Hormone Production. In women with secondary amenorrhea, decreased sex steroid hormone production results from either primary or secondary ovarian failure. In primary ovarian failure, decreased steroid hormone production results from physiologic or pathologic depletion of follicles, from transitory failure of follicles to respond to gonadotropic stimulation in young women, or from combinations of the two phenomena during the perimenopausal period. Low estrogen activity and high blood gonadotropins are characteristically seen.

In secondary ovarian failure, reduced ovarian sex steroid hormone production results from inadequate gonadotropic stimulation of follicles. Reduced blood FSH and LH levels and sometimes increased blood prolactin levels are indicative of dysfunction or failure of the hypothalamic-pituitary unit. Measurements of blood FSH and LH, high in primary failure but normal to low in secondary ovarian failure, distinguish the two categories.

When secondary ovarian failure is diagnosed, the cause of the hypothalamic-pituitary dysfunction must be determined. The process may be intrinsic to the hypothalamus or the pituitary or extrinsic to these organs, and other diagnostic measures are required to differentiate the two types (see Ch. 225).

"Postpill" amenorrhea persisting for more than a year after a woman discontinues oral contraceptives requires an evaluation to exclude other causes of secondary amenorrhea. These include pregnancy, premature ovarian failure, polycystic ovarian disease, and pituitary tumors. Ovulatory cycles will be resumed spontaneously in most women in whom these other causes have been excluded. Moreover, in women in whom amenorrhea persists without other demonstrable causes, normal pregnancies have followed ovulation induction, and postpartum, spontaneous, ovulatory menstrual cycles have resumed.

With Increased Sex Steroid Hormone Production. Ovarian tumors autonomously secreting estrogens or androgens or both may cause amenorrhea during the reproductive years. Ovarian secretion of androstenedione provides substrate for estrogen production by peripheral aromatization. The quantities of androgen derived from the androstenedione may be insufficient to produce signs of virilization but sufficient to stimulate estrogen production. The pathophysiologic basis of the amen-

TABLE 236–6. SEX STEROID HORMONE PRODUCTION AND OVARIAN DYSFUNCTION AFTER THE MENARCHE

I. Sex steroid hormone production and infertility
  A. With normal sex steroid hormone production
  B. With decreased sex steroid hormone production
    1. Luteal insufficiency
    2. Anovulation
  C. With increased sex steroid hormone production
II. Sex steroid hormone production and secondary amenorrhea
  A. With normal sex steroid hormone production
    1. Amenorrhea traumatica
      a. Postinfectious
      b. Postoperative
    2. Hysterectomy
  B. With decreased sex steroid hormone production
    1. Primary ovarian failure (gonadotropins elevated)
      a. Due to depletion of follicles
        (1) In gonadal dysgenesis
        (2) In autoimmune diseases
        (3) After chemotherapy
        (4) After irradiation
        (5) After surgery
        (6) After toxic exposure (smoking)
      b. Due to follicle resistance to gonadotropins
    2. Secondary ovarian failure (gonadotropins normal or low)
      a. Hypothalamic-pituitary dysfunction or failure with hyperprolactinemia
      b. Hypothalamic-pituitary dysfunction or failure with euprolactinemia
        (1) Due to primary hypothalamic or pituitary disorders
          (a) Tumors
          (b) Postoperative
          (c) Postirradiative
          (d) Posttraumatic
          (e) Postinfectious
          (f) Postinfarctional
          (g) The "empty sella"
        (2) Due to secondary hypothalamic or pituitary disorders
          (a) Psychogenic amenorrhea
          (b) Anorexia nervosa and excessive weight reduction
          (c) "Postpill" amenorrhea
          (d) Nonovarian endocrinopathies; thyroid diseases, adrenal diseases, diabetes
          (e) Systemic diseases
  C. With increased sex steroid hormone production
    1. Ovarian tumors secreting androgens or estrogens
    2. Adrenal tumors secreting androgens
    3. Increased peripheral aromatization of androgens
    4. Polycystic ovarian disease

orrhea is similar to that seen when ovarian estrogen or androgen production is excessive, and results from the integrated effect of sustained peripheral estrogen production on the hypothalamic-pituitary unit and the steroid hormone–dependent target organs.

POLYCYSTIC OVARIES (STEIN-LEVENTHAL SYNDROME). Grossly, the ovaries are sometimes enlarged with a glistening surface and a cortex thickened by excessive collagen deposition. Microscopically, these ovaries contain numerous follicular cysts with thecal hyperplasia and hypertrophy (sometimes called hyperthecosis). "Lutein cells" are sometimes seen in the stroma. The microscopic appearance of these follicles is consistent with that of follicles undergoing atresia in response to excessive stimulation by interstitial cell–stimulating hormone (LH or hCG).

High concentrations of androstenedione have been found in venous effluent from these ovaries, and antral fluid from the follicular cysts contains more androgens and less estrogens and progestogens than antral fluid from follicles destined for ovulation.

The constellation of thecal hypertrophy, stromal lutein cells, and elevated antral fluid androgen levels are consistent with the observation that peripheral blood LH levels are higher and FSH levels lower than those seen in samples collected during the follicular phase of ovulatory cycles in normal women.

Despite levels of androgens in ovarian venous and peripheral blood that are frequently sufficient to produce hirsutism, or rarely, virilization, there is considerable evidence of estrogenic activity in target tissues from these women. The endometrium is hyperplastic and sometimes undergoes neoplastic changes (atypical for young women); pituitary FSH secretion is decreased and LH secretion is increased, both consistent with normal hypothalamic-pituitary response to estrogenic stimulation. Production of estrogens results from peripheral aromatization of androstenedione so that daily estrone production rates are increased two- to four-fold over those seen in the follicular phase of women with ovulatory menstrual cycles.

The following pathogenetic sequence is consistent with the clinical observations: (1) Estrone acts on the hypothalamic-pituitary unit to suppress FSH secretion and stimulate LH secretion. (2) Inhibition of FSH secretion reduces FSH-dependent aromatase induction so that less estradiol is produced. (3) Increased LH secretion stimulates thecal and stromal hyperplasia, hypertrophy, and androstenedione secretion. (4) Increased ovarian androstenedione production stimulates atresia, inhibits follicle growth and estradiol production in the ovaries, and produces signs of androgen excess in the extraovarian tissues. (5) Increased peripheral aromatization of androstenedione leads to increased estrone production. (6) Estrone acts upon target tissues to produce chronic anovulation and "continuous estrus," with signs of androgen excess.

How the cycle of events originates remains speculative. Among others, increased adrenal androstenedione production prior to the menarche, leading to increased estrone production in the periphery, remains a viable possibility.

Ovarian enlargement and continuously increased androstenedione and estrone production also occur in women with ovarian tumors, adrenal tumors, Cushing's syndrome, and virilizing congenital adrenal hyperplasia. Discussion of how the distinction can be made will be deferred until diagnosis and treatment of hirsutism are discussed (see Ch. 237). The clinical features of polycystic ovarian disease with hirsutism are similar to those for idiopathic hirsutism. In both syndromes, ovarian function may be deranged. To minimize repetition in relation to diagnosis and treatment of these disorders, the reader is referred to Ch. 237.

Evaluating the Patient with Secondary Amenorrhea. THE HISTORY. In eliciting the medical history of a woman with secondary amenorrhea, the physician should make a candid appraisal of coital habits, including contraceptive methods used and, if parous, a detailed review of events during prepartum, intrapartum, and postpartum periods of all pregnancies. These data are essential for correctly interpreting results of assays for chorionic gonadotropin in blood or urine, and in deciding about the need for further tests to distinguish pregnancy from gestational trophoblastic neoplasms, or tumors of ovaries or other tissues which secrete chorionic gonadotropins and threaten the woman's life.

Intra- or postpartum hemorrhages requiring blood transfusions, coupled with failure to lactate or to resume menses, are consistent with presumptive diagnosis of Sheehan's syndrome (postpartum pituitary necrosis), whereas persistent galactorrhea and amenorrhea after weaning are suggestive of a pituitary tumor secreting prolactin. Galactorrhea and amenorrhea unrelated to parturition have similar implications. Postpartum endometritis or vigorous dilatation and curettage predisposes to intrauterine synechiae and amenorrhea traumatica (Asherman's syndrome).

Probing dietary habits may provide presumptive evidence for hypothalamic dysfunction secondary to precipitous weight reduction or the syndrome of anorexia nervosa (see Ch. 215). Drugs, including psychotropic agents, antihypertensives, and oral contraceptives, predispose to amenorrhea with or without galactorrhea in some women, and careful questioning about medications is relevant. Secondary amenorrhea is more common among women who participate in marathon running and other strenuous forms of exercise than among their sedentary peers. Along with inquiry about nonovarian endocrinopathies, evidence should be sought for hypothalamic-pituitary dysfunction or failure from postoperative, postirradiative, post-traumatic, postinfectious, and postinfarctive insults. Signs and symptoms of estrogen deficiency, including vasomotor instability, reduction of vaginal secretions, vaginitis, and dyspareunia, suggest a diagnosis of primary ovarian failure resulting from premature or physiologic menopause.

THE PHYSICAL EXAMINATION. Some diagnostically useful signs which should be kept in mind during physical examination include (1) general nutritional status; (2) amount, type, and distribution of hair; (3) cutaneous manifestations of thyroid, ovarian, and adrenal cortical disease, including oiliness, acne, excessive dryness, cutis marmorata, melanotic pigmentation, telangiectasia, bruising, and striae; (4) volume of breasts and presence of galactorrhea; (5) neurologic deficits, including visual field defects and other evidence for pituitary, parapituitary, or other intracerebral tumors; (6) abdominal masses suggestive of adrenal tumors; and (7) quality of vaginal mucosa, cervical mucus, size of uterus, and ovarian and parametrial masses.

DIAGNOSTIC TESTS. No diagnostic tests should be performed until pregnancy has been eliminated as a cause of secondary amenorrhea. Sensitive methods for measuring chorionic gonadotropin in blood or urine are indispensable.

Prevailing levels of estrogen significantly influence endometrial responses to exogenous progestogens so that presence or absence of withdrawal bleeding following progestogens provides a useful screening test of ovarian sex steroid hormone production and thus of ovarian function in women with secondary amenorrhea. Moreover, when coupled with measurements of blood FSH, LH, and prolactin concentrations, the test provides a rational basis for categorizing the etiologic varieties of secondary amenorrhea.

To minimize the effects of exogenous sex steroid hormones on basal gonadotropin concentrations, specimens of blood (see above) should be collected on the first visit and retained until results of the progestogen withdrawal test are known. If bleeding occurs, five conclusions are valid: (1) the hypothalamic-pituitary unit responds to changes in the sex steroid hormone milieu, (2) the pituitary secretes FSH and LH, (3) ovarian follicles respond to the gonadotropins, (4) the endometrium responds to both stimulation and withdrawal of estrogens and progesterone, and (5) the outflow tract is patent. Measurements of sex steroid hormone or gonadotropin levels are not useful in women who bleed following progesterone. However, since about 15 per cent of patients with prolactin-secreting tumors will bleed following progesterone, measuring prolactin is indicated.

If bleeding does not occur, 50 μg of ethinyl estradiol or equivalent amounts of other estrogens should be administered for 21 days and the progesterone withdrawal test repeated. Failure to bleed can be equated with a refractory endometrium, and measuring blood hormone concentrations is not necessary. Instead, the patient should be referred to a gynecologist for further evaluation and treatment.

In every patient in whom bleeding fails to occur following progesterone alone but does occur after giving estrogen and progestogen, blood FSH, LH, and prolactin concentrations should be measured. High levels of FSH and LH are consistent with primary ovarian disease, whereas low or normal levels suggest secondary ovarian failure resulting from hypothalamic-pituitary dysfunction or failure.

Increased levels of prolactin are suggestive of hypothalamic-pituitary dysfunction associated with prolactin-secreting pituitary adenomas, and the higher the prolactin levels, the greater the likelihood that a tumor is present. Plain skull films should be obtained in all cases and complemented with computed tomography as indicated. Skull x-rays should be examined for signs of an "empty sella" resulting from a congenitally abnormal diaphragma sella which permits the subarachnoid space to extend into the sella turcica, forming a cavity around which pituitary tissue is molded (see Ch. 225). The empty sella may also be associated with euprolactinemic amenorrhea (see below).

When blood prolactin is normal in a patient with signs of decreased sex steroid hormone production and low blood FSH and LH concentrations, primary hypothalamic or pituitary disorders that result in tissue destruction must be distinguished from secondary hypothalamic-pituitary disorders, nonovarian endocrinopathies, and systemic diseases. To choose tests which will assist in distinguishing hypothalamic and pituitary tumors from an empty sella and other causes of hypothalamic-pituitary dysfunction or failure, consultation should be obtained with colleagues in neurology, neurosurgery, and radiology (see Ch. 225).

Davajan V, Israel R: Infertility: Causes, evaluation, and treatment. *In* DeGroot LJ, et al. (eds.): Endocrinology, Vol 3. New York, Grune & Stratton, 1979, pp 1459–1472. *A lucid, logical approach to evaluating infertile couples.*

DiZerega GS, Ross GT: Luteal phase dysfunction. Clin Obstet Gynaecol 8:733, 1981. *A clinically oriented review of an important cause of infertility.*

Ross GT, Hillier SG: Luteal maturation and luteal phase defect. Clin Obstet Gynaecol 5:391, 1978. *A review of hormonal control of corpus luteum function in mammals, including humans.*

Ross GT, Vande Wiele RL: The ovaries. *In* Williams RH (ed.): Textbook of Endocrinology. 5th ed. Philadelphia, W. B. Saunders Company, 1974, pp 368–422. *An extensive discussion of the physiology and pathophysiology of ovarian function to facilitate clinical diagnosis and treatment of disorders in these throughout life.*

Toaff R, Balla S: Traumatic hypomenorrhea-amenorrhea (Asherman's syndrome). Fertil Steril 30:379, 1978. *An informative discussion of these phenomena for clinicians.*

Yen SSC: Chronic anovulation. *In* Yen SSC, Jaffe RB (eds.): Reproductive Endocrinology. Philadelphia, W. B. Saunders Company, 1978, pp 297–323. *An interpretation of the pathophysiologic bases for anovulation, amenorrhea, and dysfunctional uterine bleeding in the light of disorders of "feedback" mechanisms which the author's research has illuminated.*

SEX STEROID HORMONES AND OVARIAN FUNCTION AFTER THE MENOPAUSE

Normal

When the primordial follicles remaining in the ovary cease to mature in response to gonadotropins, ovarian estrogen secretion declines markedly. However, some estrogen continues to be produced by extraovarian conversion (aromatization) of androstenedione to estrone, and estrone becomes the major circulating estrogen after the menopause. The adrenals contribute more androstenedione than do the ovaries in postmenopausal women.

As a result of decreased estrogen production, estrogenic effects are reduced at the target tissues. Thus, the vaginal epithelium thins, cervical mucus declines, vaginal secretions decrease, endometrium atrophies, the breasts atrophy, hypothalamic thermoregulatory function alters, pituitary gonadotropin secretion rises, and osteoporotic changes in bone accelerate. These changes, however, become sufficiently severe to warrant estrogen replacement therapy in no more than 25 per cent of postmenopausal women. Except for the thermoregulatory dysfunction which results in "hot flushes," the changes are insidious and may never reach symptomatic levels.

Abnormal

WITH NORMAL OR DECREASED SEX STEROID HORMONE PRODUCTION. Since decreased ovarian estrogen secretion is normal after the menopause, it is difficult to know where to draw the line between "normal" and "decreased" ovarian steroid hormone production in postmenopausal women.

Intolerable symptoms of "decreased" ovarian steroid hormone production include hot flushes and vaginitis. Subjective sensations of hot flushes are associated with average maximal increments of about 2.5° C in peripheral skin temperatures. These may recur at hourly intervals, persist for about half an hour, are usually preceded by pulsatile increments in blood LH concentrations, and usually subside spontaneously after a year or two. Vaginitis and dyspareunia, related to thinning and reduction in glycogen content of vaginal epithelium, are unlikely to subside spontaneously.

WITH INCREASED SEX STEROID HORMONE PRODUCTION. Syndromes associated with increased steroid hormone production are easily recognized in postmenopausal women. If the steroid is estrogen, breast engorgement and tenderness, increased vaginal secretions, and vaginal bleeding are common signs and symptoms. On the other hand, if increased androgen production occurs, virilizing signs such as male pattern balding, oily skin, acne, increased libido, clitoral enlargement, changes in the larynx and voice, and hirsutism may occur singly or in combination. These excess steroids are almost invariably produced by adrenal cortical or ovarian tumors, and most of these are palpable. Endometrial carcinomas give rise to vaginal bleeding, and these occur more commonly in women with increased estrogen production, whether secreted by ovarian tumors or resulting from excessive aromatization of androstenedione secreted by normal or neoplastic adrenal tissue. Obesity, age, and liver disease all enhance aromatization in postmenopausal women.

Korenman SG, Sherman BM, Korenman JC: Reproductive hormone function: The perimenopausal period and beyond. Clin Endocrinol Metab 7:625, 1978. *A clinician who has studied hormonal events during and following the menopause examines the clinical relevance of these studies.*

MacDonald PC, Edman CD, Hemsell DL, Porter JC, Siiteri PK: Effect of obesity on conversion of plasma androstenedione to estrone in postmenopausal women with and without endometrial cancer. Am J Obstet Gynecol 130:448, 1978. *Contains references to the pioneering observations by MacDonald and Siiteri et al. on the phenomenon of extraglandular aromatization as a source of estrogens after the menopause.*

OVARIAN TUMORS

Ovarian tumors may give rise to signs and symptoms of ovarian dysfunction in any age group. They will be discussed as a group to minimize repetition.

Ovarian tumors include the following major types: (1) common "epithelial" tumors derived from coelomic epithelial cells; (2) sex cord stromal tumors consisting of theca cells, granulosa cells, stromal cells, Sertoli cells, Leydig cells, or their progenitors; (3) lipid cell tumors composed of cells similar but not identical to Leydig cells, lutein cells, and adrenal cortical cells; (4) germ cell tumors, which include dysgerminomas; and (5) gonadoblastomas composed of cells resembling germ cells, granulosa cells, and Sertoli cells. Each of these major classes includes a number of different histologic variants, too numerous to mention here. Cells of the common epithelial tumors, the most frequently occurring ovarian tumors, rarely secrete hormones, but some cells in each of the other varieties may produce hormones in quantities sufficient to stimulate target tissue responses suggestive of excess ovarian steroid hormone secretion.

Although only 5 per cent of ovarian tumors secrete sufficient hormone to produce overt signs and symptoms of response in the appropriate target tissues, a larger proportion of them secrete small amounts of hormones, which may include estrogens, androgens, progesterone (rarely), chorionic gonadotropin (which stimulates steroid hormone production by the nontumorous portion of the ovaries), thyroxine, serotonin, or, more rarely, other peptide hormones (see Ch. 172). In addition to hormone secretion by tumor cells per se, both primary and metastatic ovarian tumors appear to stimulate surrounding normal ovarian stroma to "luteinize" and secrete sex steroid hormones, particularly androgens.

Some tumors are associated with clinical manifestations of decreased hormone production. The prolonged periods of amenorrhea caused by steroid hormone suppression of gonadotropins may alternate with periods of excessive vaginal bleeding secondary to endometrial hyperplasia.

Ovarian tumors occur in all age groups, but most of them are less common in younger persons, especially infants and children. Steroid hormone–secreting ovarian tumors produce overt manifestations of pseudopuberty in a small proportion of girls with the syndrome. Amenorrhea and erratic bleeding may occur in association with tumors during the reproductive years. In postmenopausal women increased estrogens, either secreted by the tumor or produced by aromatization of androgens secreted by the tumor, stimulate endometrial proliferation and are often accompanied by bleeding and occasionally by changes suggestive of endometrial neoplasia.

Some clinical features of ovarian tumors producing hormones are summarized in Table 236–7. Fortunately most of them are palpable, and scanning with ultrasound makes it possible to identify some too small to palpate. Whenever a pelvic mass is discovered during evaluation of ovarian dysfunction in any girl or woman, it is the physician's responsibility to determine the nature of the mass and treat it appropriately.

In addition to frank neoplasms, there are some "tumor-like" conditions characterized by ovarian enlargement and sex steroid hormone secretion similar to that seen with bona fide tumors (from which they must be differentiated). These include the following: (1) pregnancy luteomas (nodular theca–lutein hyperplasia) that result in virilization of the mother (and occasionally her female fetus as well) and regress spontaneously post partum; (2) ovarian stromal hyperplasia and hyperthecosis, sometimes associated with virilizing syndromes; (3) multiple luteinized follicle cysts or corpora lutea which result from excessive gonadotropic stimulation by hCG, secreted by gestational trophoblastic neoplasms, or by mixtures of menopausal gonadotropins and hCG used in ovulation induction; (4) inclusion cysts, containing surface epithelium (germinal epithelium); (5) simple cysts without lining cells; and (6) paraovarian cysts.

Ovarian enlargement resulting from multiple follicle cysts, excessive ovarian androgen secretion, and ovarian enlargement are seen in patients with polycystic ovaries or the Stein-Leventhal syndrome. Since coincidental ovarian tumors occur in patients with the Stein-Leventhal syndrome, diagnostic evaluation should include visualization of the ovaries.

Sometimes ovarian enlargement, caused by endometrial cysts, occurs in women with endometriomas. Around the menarche and around the menopause, cysts may increase and decrease in size in relation to the menstrual cycle; they require close surveillance and repeated examination to exclude the possibility of neoplasms.

Babaknia A, Calfopoulos P, Jones HW Jr: The Stein-Leventhal syndrome and coincidental ovarian tumors. Obstet Gynecol 47:233, 1976. *Coincidental neoplasma were found in 28 of 181 patients with surgically proven Stein-Leventhal syndrome.*

Scully RE: Ovarian tumors with endocrine manifestations. *In* DeGroot LJ, et al. (ed.): Endocrinology, Vol 3. New York, Grune & Stratton, 1979, pp 1473–1488. *An excellent discussion of the clinical manifestations of ovarian tumors for any physician who undertakes the medical care of women.*

TREATMENT OF OVARIAN DYSFUNCTION

Sex steroid hormone replacement therapy is virtually the only treatment of primary ovarian failure; other alternatives are available for restoration of ovarian function in persons with secondary ovarian failure. None of the available regimens is without hazard. The physician and the patient should have a candid discussion of the risks, benefits, and alternatives prior to electing the modality to be used.

Complications of Sex Steroid Hormone Therapy

WITH ORAL CONTRACEPTIVES IN PREMENOPAUSAL WOMEN. Oral contraceptive preparations containing a combination of estrogens and progestogens produce a hormonal milieu similar to that found during the luteal phase of an ovulatory menstrual cycle, or during early pregnancy. The term "pseudopregnancy" is used sometimes to describe the condition, since the metabolic effects of this hormonal mixture of estrogens and progestogens mimic those seen during pregnancy. For example, blood levels

TABLE 236–7. CLINICAL FEATURES OF HORMONE-PRODUCING OVARIAN TUMORS*

Tumor	Hormones Produced†	Incidence: Age in Years: Peak	Incidence: Age in Years: Range	Incidence: Malignancy	Incidence: Bilaterality	Size Range in cm (per cent Palpable)	Miscellaneous
Androblastoma (arrhenoblastomas)	*Androgens*, estrogens	20–40	4–69	20%	Rare	< 5– > 25 (85)	Most common virilizing ovarian neoplasm
Dysgerminoma	Androgens, *chorionic gonadotropin*	10–30	6–76	100%	15%	3–50 (60)	May be "mixed" with other tumors originating from germ cells
Gonadoblastoma	*Androgens*, estrogens	10–30	6–38	50%	40%	< 1– > 30 (?)	Usually occur in genetic males with female external genitalia
Granulosa-theca cell	*Estrogens*, androgens, progestogens	30–70	< 1–92	5–20%	10–15%	< 1– > 30 (80–90)	Most common functioning ovarian neoplasm
Hilar cell	*Androgens*, estrogens	45–75	4–86	Rare	Rare	1–9 (50)	Hypertension in 50%, diabetes in 50%
Lipoid cell (adrenal-like)	*Androgens*, estrogens	20–50	6–78	20%	Rare	0.5–30	Diabetes associated with lesion in 50%
Teratomas, benign	Serotonin, thyroxine	10–40	< 1–78	Rare	10%	2–45 (90)	Carcinoid syndrome only in patients with large carcinoid tumors
Teratomas, malignant	Chorionic gonadotropin	6–15	6–42	100%	Rare	> 5 (100)	Not all secrete chorionic gonadotropin

*Modified from data of Rose GT, Vande Wiele, RL: *In* Williams RH (ed.): Textbook of Endocrinology, 5th ed. Philadelphia, W. B. Saunders Company, 1974, pp 368–422.

†When more than one hormone is secreted, the major one is *italicized*.

of carrier proteins such as cortisol-binding globulin, thyroid hormone–binding proteins, transferrin, and ceruloplasmin are elevated as they are in pregnancy. This results in increased "total" blood levels of the ligands but seems to have little pathophysiologic significance.

The contraceptive steroid preparations may reproduce the syndrome of *idiopathic recurrent jaundice,* related to disorders in bile conjugation and excretion, and therefore are contraindicated in patients with a history of recurrent jaundice of pregnancy. There is a two-fold increase in the incidence of *gallstones* associated with alterations in the composition of bile, particularly increased cholesterol content of bile (see Ch. 129).

Benign hepatic adenomas and *focal nodular hyperplasia of the liver* have an increased incidence in women taking oral contraceptive preparations. The tumors are rare but are prone to rupture with exsanguinating hemorrhage.

There is no convincing evidence that oral contraceptives increase the incidence of breast cancers. In contrast, an association of increased incidence in *endometrial cancers* with estrogens (endogenous and exogenous) seems to be established for women receiving estrogens after menopause (see below). Close surveillance is therefore indicated. Oral contraceptives may stimulate rapid growth of uterine leiomyomas, requiring surgical intervention. If these agents are given to a woman who has these tumors, the uterine size should be assessed frequently.

The most serious complication of using oral contraceptives is an increased incidence of *thromboembolic phenomena,* originally thought to be due exclusively to the estrogen component but now known to involve the progestogens as well. The incidences of *cerebrovascular thrombosis* and *hemorrhage* are increased ninefold and twofold, respectively, among women using oral contraceptives. Spontaneous incidence of these cerebrovascular accidents is extremely low in a control population of the same age. Other cerebrovascular effects include induction or *intensification of migraine* headaches among women with this diathesis. *Thrombophlebitis, pulmonary embolism,* and also *hepatic vein thrombosis* have been reported to be increased in frequency. Alternative methods of contraception should be prescribed for women with a history of thromboembolic disorders.

Hypertension associated with the use of oral contraceptives may now be the most frequent form of endocrine hypertension and seems to be related to activation of the renin-angiotensin system. The incidence of induced hypertension rises with duration of use to levels of 5 per cent of users after five years. Hypertension usually regresses after discontinuation of the drugs in women who were normotensive prior to taking the agents. The blood pressure should therefore be followed closely. Conversely, in any woman found to be hypertensive, an inquiry must be made about the use of such hormonal preparations.

The incidence of *abnormal glucose tolerance tests* rises with duration of use. In women with diabetes severe enough to require insulin, dosage must be adjusted upward after taking the agents. Fasting blood glucose concentrations and urine tests for glucose should be done at least annually in women receiving oral contraceptives, particularly women at increased risk for developing diabetes.

Estrogens *increase serum triglyceride levels,* and the pathologic consequences of this action appear to be amplified by smoking, obesity, hypertension, and diabetes. These effects are particularly evident among older women. Serum lipids should be measured prior to instituting this form of therapy, which is contraindicated in those having pre-existing hyperlipidemia.

There is no evidence that using oral contraceptives affects subsequent fertility adversely; 85 per cent of nulliparous and 93 per cent of parous women in one large series conceived during the two years immediately after discontinuation of oral contraceptive use. "Postpill" amenorrhea has been discussed earlier.

A potpourri of other side effects includes salt and water retention, increased nitrogen retention and weight gain, nausea, vomiting, bloating, depression, and sleep disturbances. These all contribute to the unwillingness of some women to use oral contraceptives and compel consideration of alternative methods.

Although the incidence of certain complications is increased, the absolute risk is still low and may be tolerable if the benefit is likely to be significant. An agreement on the need for close surveillance, adhered to scrupulously by physician and patient alike, will reduce the likelihood of serious morbidity if complications occur.

WITH ESTROGENS IN POSTMENOPAUSAL WOMEN. The therapeutic use of estrogens in postmenopausal women can be summarized as follows: (1) The minimal effective dose of estrogens should be given for as short a time as required for symptomatic relief of hot flushes if the severity of symptoms and the patient's assessment of the need for symptomatic relief are sufficient. (2) Estrogens can be used successfully in relieving vaginitis and dyspareunia, but establishing relative merits of topical and systemic administration requires further study. (3) If given around the time of the menopause, estrogens may retard bone loss, but it has not been shown that this will prevent subsequent development of fractures related to osteoporosis (see Ch. 249). (4) There is no convincing evidence for usefulness of estrogens in treating primary psychologic problems in this age group.

With regard to risks, the following summary represents a reasonable current consensus: (1) There are no persuasive data that customary doses of estrogens alter the incidence of thromboembolic phenomena, stroke, or heart disease in women undergoing a natural menopause. (2) Estrogens stimulate cystic hyperplasia of the endometrium, a premalignant condition. (3) The spontaneous incidence rate of endometrial cancer (1 per 1000 women not receiving estrogens) is increased several-fold after using conjugated estrogens (estrone sulfate) in doses of 0.625 to 1.25 mg per day for two to four years. These cancers tend to be low grade and in early stages when detected, and are associated with a high cure rate. Progestogens given for several days during treatment cycles decrease the incidence of cystic hyperplasia, but this regimen has not been shown to reduce the incidence of endometrial cancer. The endometrium should be sampled prior to beginning treatment and whenever bleeding supervenes. The effectiveness of endometrial sampling in the absence of bleeding is questionable. (4) In postmenopausal as in premenopausal women, estrogens increase cholesterol content of the bile and double the incidence of gallstones. (5) There is no convincing evidence that giving estrogens increases the incidence of carcinoma of the breast in postmenopausal women.

In postmenopausal women, then, it appears that the risk of giving estrogens is tolerable, particularly if therapy is deemed necessary by doctor and patient alike. The recommendations and assessments cited above were arrived at by a national Consensus Development Conference in 1979.

Consensus: Estrogen Use and Postmenopausal Women. National Institutes of Health Consensus Development Conference Summary, Vol 2, No 8, September 13–14, 1979. *A consensus on the state of the art as relates to risks and benefits.*

Mishell DR Jr: Contraception. *In* DeGroot LJ, et al. (eds.): Endocrinology, Vol 3. New York, Grune & Stratton, 1979, pp 1435–1450. *An authoritative discussion of the risks and benefits of contraceptive modalities.*

Schenker JG, Weinstein D: Ovarian hyperstimulation syndrome: A current survey. Fertil Steril 30:255, 1978. *A comprehensive review, sufficient in itself for the needs of many clinicians, but with references for those interested in pursuing the subject further.*

Weinstein M: Estrogen use in postmenopausal women: Costs, risks, and benefits. N Engl J Med 303:308, 1980. *A critical evaluation of risks and benefits of the use of estrogens in postmenopausal women.*

Regimens of Treatment

Once the physician has determined whether steroid hormone production is normal, decreased, or increased, and has ascertained the locus of the problem, treatment is generally directed toward restoring manifestations of ovarian function to normal for the peer group. Accordingly, therapy will be considered in relation to the age group of a patient.

PRIOR TO THE MENARCHE. ***With Normal Sex Steroid Hormone Production.*** In those instances in which attention is drawn to müllerian dysgenesis by signs or symptoms unrelated to ovarian function (e.g., in girls with Klippel-Feil syndrome), a route of egress of menstrual fluids is established, but reconstruction of a vagina is usually delayed until the patient contemplates marriage.

With Decreased Sex Steroid Hormone Production. When delayed pubertal changes are due to primary ovarian failure, sex steroid hormone replacement therapy must be used judiciously to assure a girl some parity with her peers in development of secondary sexual characteristics such as breasts and pubic hair. The girl and her parents should be prepared to cope with problems of irregular vaginal bleeding which complicate initiation of replacement therapy with estrogens. Ethinyl estradiol (30 to 50 μg per day), or a biologically equivalent dose of some other oral estrogen, is given continuously for periods of 90 days, coupled with a progestogen such as medroxyprogesterone acetate for the last seven days of this period. This is followed by a week to ten days of no treatment, during which vaginal bleeding should occur. The use of GnRH to induce pituitary gonadotropin secretion is under study and promises to be effective when delayed pubertal changes are due to ovarian failure secondary to hypothalamic-pituitary dysfunction or failure. As noted, it is sometimes wise to temporize rather than use sex steroid hormones for initiating pubertal changes in girls with idiopathic delayed puberty.

With Increased Sex Steroid Hormone Production. When the source of sex steroid hormone excess is an ovarian or adrenal tumor, surgical removal of the tumor must be attempted. When congenital adrenal hyperplasia is the cause, suppression of ACTH secretion with exogenous glucocorticoids will slow advancing pubertal changes (see Ch. 229).

Regimens available for inhibiting progression of isosexual precocious puberty, preventing premature closure of epiphyses and thus preventing short stature, are unsatisfactory. Although menses can be suppressed effectively with progestogens in children with precocious puberty, other stigmata such as advancing bone age with premature closure of epiphyses and short stature progress. Moreover, this therapy is often complicated by signs and symptoms of glucocorticoid excess. Giving long-acting analogues of GnRH inhibits the effects of endogenous pulses of this hypophysiotropic hormone with the result that signs of precocious puberty, including advancing bone age, regress. To date, there are no untoward results of this treatment. Furthermore, pubertal changes are resumed when the drug is discontinued.

AFTER THE MENARCHE. ***With Normal or Decreased Sex Steroid Hormone Production.*** If sex steroid hormone production is normal, then therapy must be directed toward whatever problem gives rise to the patient's concerns. As long as ovarian sex steroid hormone production and ovulatory menstrual cycles persist, a woman engaging in sexual intercourse is at risk for pregnancy, desired or undesired, and prevention of pregnancy may be the reason for consulting a physician.

The oral contraceptives that suppress ovulation by suppressing gonadotropin secretion provide the most effective protection against unwanted or unplanned pregnancies. However, side effects such as nausea (sometimes with vomiting), weight gain, fluid retention, hypertension, hyperglycemia and glycosuria, gallstones, hepatic adenomas, and thrombophlebitis complicate use of these substances. Moreover, ethical constraints limit their usefulness in some women, and inability to follow the prescribed regimen limits their effectiveness in others.

In some of these latter women, intramuscular injections of large doses of long-acting progestogens are effective, but, again, side effects such as "breakthrough" vaginal bleeding have limited their acceptability. In others, intrauterine devices, which permit ovulation and menstruation to continue but prevent implantation, provide a satisfactory alternative. However, pregnancies occurring with the device in situ and increased infections complicate use of intrauterine devices.

If sex steroid hormone is decreased as a consequence of primary ovarian failure, sex steroid hormone replacement may be indicated. On the other hand, if the cause of decreased sex steroid production is secondary ovarian failure, a series of options exist, and choices depend upon the patient's concerns. The first option is to do nothing if reassurance is all the patient requires. However, if cyclic vaginal bleeding is important to the woman's self-image and there are no contraindications, cyclic administration of sex steroid hormones, preferably a combination of estrogens and progestogens, will result in cyclic bleeding. Finally, if a woman wishes to become pregnant, her husband is fertile, and her ovaries contain responsive follicles, a number of other choices are available.

Infertility and early abortions secondary to euprolactinemic luteal insufficiency have been reversed successfully with vaginal suppositories of progesterone. In women with hyperprolactinemic luteal insufficiency or anovulation, suppression of prolactin secretion with ergolines, such as bromocriptine, has been used effectively to induce ovulation followed by pregnancy with delivery of normal infants at term (see Ch. 238). If there is a prolactin-secreting pituitary tumor, surgical removal of the tumor results in resumption of ovulatory menstrual cycles in 60 to 90 per cent of young women, depending on its nature and size.

In euprolactinemic women with decreased sex steroid hormone production and low to normal gonadotropins who bleed following progesterone withdrawal, stimulating pituitary gonadotropin secretion will result in ovulation followed by normal pregnancies. The use of clomiphene citrate, an estrogen antagonist which blocks the feedback inhibition of gonadal steroids on the hypothalamus, has induced ovulations followed by pregnancies. In recent clinical investigations, pulsatile injections of GnRH around the clock for 20 days or more have also induced ovulation in such patients. Pregnancy rates appear to be lower than those associated with spontaneous ovulations.

If attempts at inducing ovulation by stimulating pituitary gonadotropin secretion fail, follicle growth can be stimulated by daily injections of menopausal gonadotropins containing FSH and LH in ratios around 1:1 until serum estradiol levels, determined daily, rise to levels consistent with those seen in late follicular phase of spontaneous cycles (400 to 600 pg per milliliter). Then follicle rupture and corpus luteum function are stimulated by one or more injections of hCG, a surrogate for LH. Morbidity may result from multiple ovulations with multiple fetuses or from a syndrome of massive ovarian enlargement, ascites, hydrothorax, hemorrhage resulting from intravascular coagulation and fibrinolysis, and hypovolemia and shock following administration of hCG, particularly in women who conceive. Monitoring estrogen levels in blood or urine daily during ovulation induction and withholding hCG when these become excessive reduce the incidence to acceptable levels but do not eliminate these complications.

With Increased Sex Steroid Hormone Production. Methods for distinguishing ovarian from adrenal tumors secreting excess androgens are discussed in relation to treatment of hirsutism (see Ch. 237). In these women, signs and symptoms of excess steroid hormone production will disappear slowly following complete removal of the tumor. When excess steroid hormone secretion is gonadotropin dependent, oral contraceptives containing mixtures of estrogens and progestogens will suppress pituitary gonadotropin secretion, reduce steroid hormone production, and ameliorate signs and symptoms. The usefulness of potent, long-acting GnRH antagonists for this purpose is under study.

When excess steroid hormone production is ACTH dependent, glucocorticoids given orally will suppress pituitary ACTH secretion. However, chronic suppression renders the pituitary–

adrenal cortical axis incapable of responding to stress with increased glucocorticoid production so that the patient is vulnerable to the hazards of acute adrenal cortical insufficiency (see Ch. 237). Treatment of women with polycystic ovarian disease is sufficiently complex to merit separate consideration. If restoration of fertility is the primary goal, clomiphene or exogenous gonadotropins may be used to induce ovulation. In some instances in which clomiphene has not been effective, surgical resection of a significant amount of ovarian tissue has resulted in resumption of spontaneous ovulatory menstrual cycles and restoration of fertility. Since these salutary results of surgery do not always persist for the remainder of the patient's reproductive life, surgical intervention is not the treatment of choice when alternative therapies are effective.

When the objectives of treatment relate to control of hirsutism, the principles outlined in Ch. 237 are applicable to patients with polycystic ovarian disease.

AFTER THE MENOPAUSE. ***With Normal or Decreased Sex Steroid Hormone Production.*** Except for occasional neoplasms not affecting sex steroid hormone production, there are no ovarian disorders associated with normal sex steroid hormone production in postmenopausal women.

Few well-designed prospective studies have been done to establish either the safety or the efficacy of giving sex steroid hormones to all postmenopausal women in order to prevent signs and symptoms of reduced sex steroid hormone production in some of them. As noted, the existence of a "syndrome" to which all women are equally susceptible is questionable.

Complications of osteoporosis occurring after the menopause are major medical problems of aging in women. Although the hormonal milieu is contributory, the pathophysiologic basis of osteoporosis after the menopause is multifactorial (see Ch. 249). Other factors contributing to the risk include smoking, low body weight, decreased dietary calcium, inadequate vitamin D intake, and inadequate exercise, and these should be corrected in any event.

In the face of the multiplicity of factors contributing to osteoporosis after the menopause, it is not surprising that it would be difficult to establish either prophylactic or therapeutic benefit from giving estrogens. However, the consensus is that daily low doses (0.625 to 1.25 mg of conjugated estrogen) or equivalent doses of others should be used. Alternatives to oral routes of administration are under study.

In contrast to osteoporosis, the efficacy of estrogens for relief of intolerable hot flashes, dyspareunia, and vaginal infections is easily demonstrated. The dose of estrogens should be the minimal amount required for relief, and the need for continuing treatment indefinitely once the symptoms have been ameliorated is questionable. Attempts should be made to progressively reduce and finally stop treatment altogether.

With Increased Sex Steroid Hormone Production. Treatment of disorders resulting in excess steroid hormone secretion after the menopause is identical to that recommended for use prior to the menopause.

Consensus: Estrogen Use and Postmenopausal Women. National Institutes of Health Consensus Development Conference Summary, Vol 2, No 8, Sept. 13–14, 1979. *A consensus on the state of the art as it relates to risks and benefits.*

Mishell DR, Jr: Contraception. *In* DeGroot LJ, et al. (eds.): Endocrinology, Vol 3. New York, Grune & Stratton, 1979, pp 1435–1450. *An authoritative discussion of the risks and benefits of contraceptive methods.*

Research on the menopause. Technical report series 670. World Health Organization, Geneva, 1981. *A summary of the world literature on the menopause.*

Schenker JG, Weinstein D: Ovarian hyperstimulation syndrome: A current survey. Fertil Steril 30:255, 1978. *A comprehensive review, sufficient in itself for the needs of many clinicians, but with references for those interested in pursuing the subject further.*

Weinstein M: Estrogen use in postmenopausal women. Costs, risks, and benefits. N Engl J Med 303:308, 1980. *A critical evaluation of risks and benefits of the use of estrogens in postmenopausal women.*

ACKNOWLEDGMENT

The skillful assistance given by Mrs. Ollie S. Monger in preparing the original and by Mary Gilliland and A.M. Ross in preparing the revised manuscript is gratefully acknowledged.

237. HIRSUTISM

D. Lynn Loriaux

DEFINITIONS. ***Normal Hair Growth.*** Except for the palms of the hands and the soles of the feet, the bodies of men and women are covered with hair follicles. The hairs growing from these follicles are of two types, *vellous* and *terminal.* Vellous hair is the soft, downy hair that is characteristic of the faces of children. Terminal hair (the hairs of the scalp and eyebrows being examples) is usually more deeply pigmented, of greater diameter, and stiffer. Androgens induce follicles to change the nature of the hair produced from vellous to terminal (or vice versa, as in male pattern baldness) in certain areas of the body, including the mons pubis, axillae, chest, and face (mustache and beard). There is a spectrum of androgen-dependent hair follicle response, the mons pubis being the most sensitive and the beard hairs usually being the least sensitive. In other areas, notably the arms and legs, increased androgen stimulation is not obligatory for the change from vellous to terminal hair. These follicles are considered to be partially androgen dependent.

Hirsutism. In women, excessive growth of body hair is called hirsutism. This is not a disease per se, but it may be a sign of disease. Certain patterns of hair growth can be said to be clearly abnormal in women, e.g., terminal hair on the upper abdomen or shoulders and upper back. Only 3 per cent of women have terminal hair over the sternum. Thus, terminal hair in these locations suggests an underlying disorder. More often, however, women complaining of hirsutism come to the physician not with hair in these abnormal locations, but with the subjective impression that either the rate of hair growth or the distribution of hair, or both seems to be changing. This can be an early indication of serious illness. In the majority of patients, however, no underlying disease can be found.

ETIOLOGY. Etiologically, hirsutism can be divided into two categories: androgen-independent hirsutism and androgen-dependent hirsutism. Ordinarily, the distinction between the two varieties can be made on clinical grounds.

In *androgen-independent hirsutism* the hair is usually vellous and evenly distributed over both androgen-independent areas, such as the forehead, and androgen-dependent areas, such as the chin and upper lip (Fig. 237–1). The more common causes of androgen-independent hirsutism are listed in Table 237–1.

In *androgen-dependent hirsutism,* the hair is of the terminal type and the distribution is restricted to androgen-responsive areas such as the chin, upper lip, and chest. Androgen-dependent hirsutism, caused by androgen excess, may be found in association with other signs of androgen effects, as noted below. The causes of androgen-dependent hirsutism are listed in Table 237–2. Since androgens in women are secreted only by the adrenal glands and by the ovaries, one or the other of these two glands must be the source of the excess androgen, except in cases of factitious hirsutism caused by exogenous androgen administration.

PATHOGENESIS OF ANDROGEN-DEPENDENT HIRSUTISM. Androgen-dependent hirsutism is the result of an elevated plasma protein unbound testosterone concentration. The pathophysiologic mechanism underlying the increased plasma testosterone concentrations found in the adrenal causes of hirsutism, such as adrenal cancer and virilizing adrenal adenomas, and the ovarian causes of hirsutism, including ovarian neoplasms, polycystic ovarian disease, and idiopathic hirsutism, is the excessive secretion of testosterone and/or its immediate precursor, androstenedione. Androstenedione contributes to plasma testosterone by being converted to testosterone in the liver and other peripheral tissues.

The syndromes of congenital adrenal hyperplasia (CAH) also cause hirsutism through increased androgen secretion, but the mechanism is more complex (see Ch. 229). The more common of these virilizing syndromes, 21-hydroxylase deficiency, results

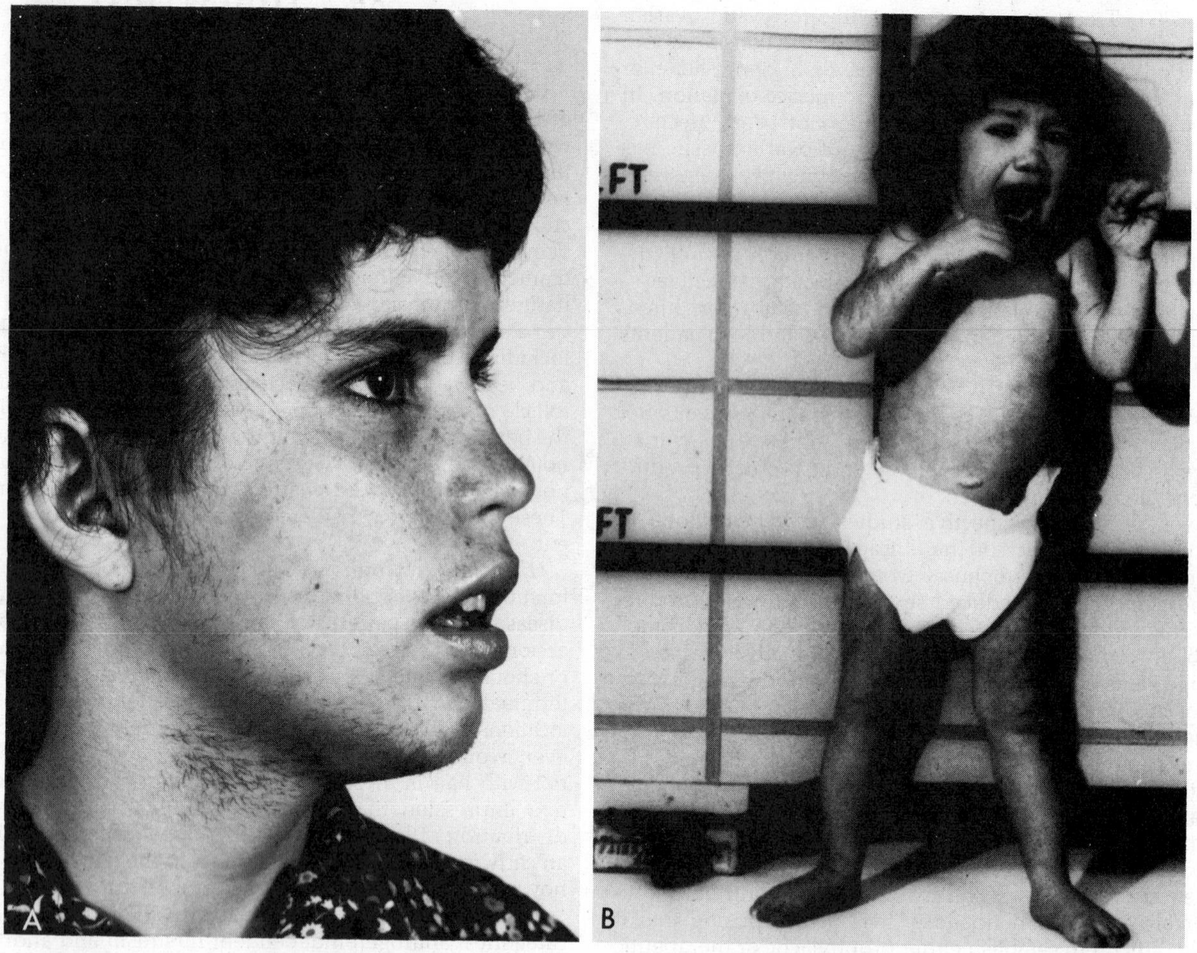

Figure 237–1. Examples of androgen-dependent and androgen-independent hirsutism. *A*, Androgen-dependent hirsutism in a woman with the polycystic ovarian syndrome. The terminal hairs are confined to the beard and mustache areas. *B*, A child with androgen-independent hirsutism induced by diazoxide. Note the even distribution of the hair over arms, legs, abdomen, chest, and face.

in the impaired ability of the adrenal gland to synthesize cortisol. Impaired cortisol production causes increased ACTH stimulation of the adrenal gland with resultant overproduction of 17-hydroxyprogesterone, the substrate for 21-hydroxylase activity, and its metabolic product androstenedione (see Fig. 233–6). Androstenedione is partially converted to testosterone, the hormone responsible for hirsutism and virilization. A second and less common form of CAH, 11-hydroxylase deficiency, is also associated with excessive testosterone production. This presumably results from the conversion of 11-deoxycortisol, the cortisol biosynthetic intermediate just before the 11-hydroxylase block, to androstenedione and thence to testosterone (see Fig. 233–6).

CLINICAL MANIFESTATIONS. The consequences of elevated plasma testosterone concentrations include hirsutism, acne, temporal balding, increased muscle strength, altered libido, and, in virilized patients, clitoral enlargement and deepening of the voice. There is usually also defeminization with amenorrhea, decrease in the size of the breasts, and change from the female body habitus. The various disorders leading to androgen excess vary primarily in the time of onset of the symptoms and the degree to which they progress.

TABLE 237–1. CAUSES OF ANDROGEN-INDEPENDENT HIRSUTISM

1. Medications:
   - Phenytoin
   - Diazoxide
   - Glucocorticoids
   - Minoxidil
2. Metabolic disorders:
   - Starvation (anorexia nervosa)
   - Porphyria cutanea tarda
   - Hypertrichosis lanuginosa
3. Genetic disorders
   - Cornelia de Lange syndrome
   - Seckel's dwarfism
   - Congenital hypertrichosis

TABLE 237–2. CAUSES OF ANDROGEN-DEPENDENT HIRSUTISM

1. Ovarian causes:
   - Neoplastic
     - Sertoli-Leydig cell tumors (arrhenoblastoma)
     - Granulosa-stromal cell tumors
     - Gynandroblastoma
     - Lipoid cell tumor
     - Gonadoblastoma
   - Non-neoplastic
     - Polycystic ovarian disease
     - Hyperthecosis
     - Idiopathic hirsutism
2. Adrenal abnormalities:
   - Neoplastic
     - Adrenocortical carcinoma
     - Virilizing adrenal adenoma
   - Non-neoplastic
     - Congenital adrenal hyperplasia
       - 21-Hydroxylase deficiency
       - 11-Hydroxylase deficiency
     - Cushing's disease
3. Medications:
   - Androgens (such as Danazol, Halotestin)
   - "19-Nor" progestins

Idiopathic hirsutism and polycystic ovarian disease tend to present a similar clinical picture, and in fact there may be a continuous spectrum between them. Patients with these disorders rarely become virilized and as such do not have clitoral enlargement or masculinization of the larynx. The hirsutism is usually first noticed in the peripubertal period and tends to stabilize after one to two years of progressive worsening. Menses are often irregular in polycystic ovarian disease and may cease altogether with time. On physical examination hirsutism and the frequent occurrence of enlarged ovaries are usually the only abnormal findings.

Hirsutism that has its onset before or after the pubertal period is suggestive of more serious disease. Adrenal carcinoma can appear at any time in life. These tumors are generally inefficient in producing steroid hormone and hence are large at the time of presentation. Forty per cent are palpable, 90 per cent are detectable by intravenous pyelography, and perhaps all are detectable with computed tomography. The rare virilizing adrenal adenomas, on the other hand, are quite efficient in the synthesis of steroid hormones and are usually only a few centimeters in diameter at the time that symptoms first appear.

Congenital adrenal hyperplasia usually becomes clinically apparent at birth or during childhood. It is characterized, in girls, by rapid growth, by heterosexual precocious puberty, and by hypertension in those having the 11-hydroxylase–deficient variety. Rarely, congenital adrenal hyperplasia may first become clinically apparent at the time of puberty or thereafter. When this occurs, the major clinical manifestations are hirsutism, acne, and menstrual irregularity.

Ovarian neoplasms with manifestations of excessive androgen secretion usually occur in adults (Table 237–2). Most will lead to overt virilization with time, and the majority are palpable on pelvic examination.

DIAGNOSIS. Important historical points include age at onset of hirsutism, rate of progression of hirsutism, the body areas involved, the menstrual history, libidinal changes, changes in appetite and weight, and the family history regarding hirsutism. Important physical findings include the nature of the hair (vellous versus terminal), the hair distribution, and the presence or absence of the signs of virilization noted above. Additionally, a careful examination for abdominal and pelvic masses must be made.

The laboratory evaluation of the hirsute woman relies on the measurement of plasma testosterone and plasma 17-hydroxyprogesterone, and on the imaging of the adrenal glands with computed tomography and the ovaries with ultrasonography.

In normal women, the upper limit of plasma testosterone concentrations is about 80 ng per deciliter. Values in excess of 200 ng per deciliter are rarely associated with idiopathic hirsutism or polycystic ovarian disease but are frequently associated with adrenal and ovarian tumors. Hence, values in this range make the diagnosis of an adrenal or ovarian neoplasm much more likely. Additionally, testosterone values in this range will ultimately lead to virilization, making definitive diagnosis and treatment imperative. Plasma testosterone values of less than 200 ng per deciliter are more likely to be associated with a benign process, but periodic re-evaluation (i.e., at three- to six-month intervals) is necessary to ensure that those patients with a progressive disorder will be identified as early as possible.

The measurement of plasma 17-hydroxyprogesterone is the single best test for the diagnosis of congenital adrenal hyperplasia resulting from 21-hydroxylase deficiency. Plasma 17-hydroxyprogesterone values are less than 200 ng per deciliter in normal women. Most patients with 21-hydroxylase deficiency have values at least five times this level. The most reliable diagnostic test for this disorder is determination of the plasma level of 17-hydroxyprogesterone 30 minutes after an intravenous injection of 250 μg synthetic ACTH. In normal subjects the value rarely exceeds 400 ng per deciliter. Patients with 21-hydroxylase deficiency achieve levels of 3000 ng per deciliter or greater. Since 17-hydroxyprogesterone can also be secreted by certain ovarian and adrenal neoplasms, it is essential that plasma 17-hydroxyprogesterone levels be shown to normalize after three days of adrenal suppressive therapy, using 0.5 mg of dexamethasone four times daily to document the adrenal origin of the abnormality.

The diagnosis of 11-hydroxylase deficiency depends, similarly, upon the measurement of plasma 11-deoxycortisol. Because this steroid is also secreted by adrenal neoplasms, distinguishing the 11-hydroxylase type of congenital adrenal hyperplasia from adrenal neoplasms again requires the demonstration that adrenal suppression with dexamethasone lowers the plasma 11-deoxycortisol into the normal range.

Adrenal neoplasms should be sought with computed tomography or ultrasonography, but pelvic ultrasonography is sufficient for diagnosing most virilizing ovarian tumors and does not expose the ovaries to ionizing radiation. If an adrenal or ovarian mass is found and congenital adrenal hyperplasia has been excluded, surgical exploration should be undertaken for definitive diagnosis and initial treatment.

TREATMENT. The treatments of Cushing's disease, adrenal neoplasms, and congenital adrenal hyperplasia are discussed in Ch. 229. Patients with congenital adrenal hyperplasia should be treated with 12 to 15 mg of hydrocortisone per square meter per day, or its equivalent, given preferably at bedtime, to suppress ACTH secretion and thus adrenal androgen production.

The treatment of idiopathic hirsutism and polycystic ovarian disease is less well defined. Many treatment regimens have been proposed. These include hypothalamic-pituitary-ovarian suppression with oral contraceptives, adrenal suppression with exogenous glucocorticoids, electrolysis, wax and chemical depilatories, and simple shaving. Antiandrogens such as cyproterone acetate have been employed in European countries.

Since the extent of hirsutism in women with idiopathic hirsutism and polycystic ovarian disease is usually stable and rarely progresses to virilization, the problem is primarily a cosmetic one with its attendant psychologic ramifications. Although the psychologic discomfort associated with these disorders may be great, it is difficult to justify potentially dangerous hormonal therapies for the treatment of these patients. Thus, the potential complications of treatment with oral contraceptives, glucocorticoids, and antiandrogens should be carefully considered before treatment with these agents is initiated.

The disadvantages of electrolysis include expense, potential scarring, and the need to continue the treatment on a regular basis for an indefinite period. Using wax or chemical depilatories can be painful and untidy. Shaving, on the other hand is safe, effective, and inexpensive. Although shaving is alleged to exacerbate hirsutism, this is not borne out by clinical study. Many women will reject shaving on the basis that it is unfeminine. They will often relent, however, when it is pointed out that they have no such misgivings about shaving their legs and underarms. On balance then, shaving is the cheapest, safest, and most effective form of treatment for idiopathic hirsutism and should be employed whenever possible.

PROGNOSIS. Since hirsutism is a symptom of many different disorders, prognosis for remission is linked to the efficacy of treatment for these maladies. It should be emphasized again that most patients complaining of hirsutism have no serious underlying disorder. Complete extirpation of an androgen-producing neoplasm can be expected to result in the resolution of hirsutism. However, the recovery period may be as long as two years, and patients should be warned not to expect a dramatic decrease in hair growth immediately following therapeutic intervention.

Hirsutism tends to progress to a given level and to stabilize without treatment in idiopathic hirsutism and polycystic ovarian disease. Patients are often aware that the process does not seem to be progressing, but the assurance that it probably will not progress is often helpful in allaying anxiety.

Blankstein J, Faiman C, Reyes FI, et al.: Adult onset familial adrenal 21-hydroxylase deficiency. Am J Med 68:441, 1980. *The best documented cases of this rare cause of hirsutism.*

Chrousos GP, Loriaux DL, Mann DL, Cutler GB: Late-onset 21-hydroxylase deficiency mimicking idiopathic hirsutism or polycystic ovarian disease. Ann Intern Med 96:143, 1982. *Clinical and laboratory description of a rare genetic disorder associated with hirsutism with review of the literature and 80 references.*

Ferriman D, Gallway M: Clinical assessment of body hair in women. J Clin Endocrinol Metab 21:1440, 1961. *Delineates normal and abnormal hair growth patterns in women.*

Kirschner MA, Zucker IR, Jespersen D: Idiopathic hirsutism, an ovarian abnormality. N Engl J Med 294:637, 1976. *The best pathogenetic study of idiopathic hirsutism.*

Korobkin M, White EA, Kressel HY, et al.: Computed tomography in the diagnosis of adrenal disease. Am J Roentgenol 132:231, 1979, *An up-to-date discussion of the power of this technique for diagnosing adrenal mass lesions.*

Lipsett MB: Benign masculinizing adrenal adenomas. N Engl J Med 289:802, 1973. *A concise discussion of this rare disorder.*

238. NONMALIGNANT DISEASES OF THE BREAST

George Tolis

Diseases of the breast are important in medical practice. In this chapter some of the developmental aspects and the function (lactation) of the breast will be reviewed briefly as a background for more extensive discussions of two clinically important disorders, gynecomastia and galactorrhea. Carcinoma of the breast, by far the most important disease of that organ, will be discussed in Ch. 239.

DEVELOPMENTAL ASPECTS OF THE MAMMARY GLAND. The human breast has a tubuloalveolar structure and consists of 15 to 25 lobes radiating from the nipple. Each lobe is subdivided into lobules from which emerge lactiferous ducts. The mammary line is well developed in the five-week embryo, but it is not until the fifth gestational month that both the nipple and the secondary buds develop. Until puberty the human mammary gland does not develop unless a pathologic condition occurs (e.g., feminizing adrenal carcinoma). With the onset of puberty, the areola enlarges and becomes pigmented and a significant growth of the tubular duct of the female breast ensues. Estrogens primarily stimulate the development of the mammary duct; progesterone seems to play a major role in alveolar growth. The role of other factors (such as growth hormone, insulin, somatomedins, epidermal growth factor, glucocorticoids, and thyroxine) in the normal growth of the mammary gland is incompletely understood.

INITIATION AND MAINTENANCE OF LACTATION. The hormonal factor absolutely required for lactation is prolactin. In the absence of adequate circulating prolactin, lactation does not occur or ceases if previously established. Furthermore the experimental administration of a specific antiserum to prolactin inhibits galactopoiesis. For prolactin activity to be fully expressed, optimal concentrations of other hormones (such as estrogens, thyroxine, and insulin) are also required. The effects of prolactin upon the female breast are modulated by various factors such as age, hormones, and medications. The administration of estrogens in the postpartum period will suppress lactation in many women by a mechanism independent of serum prolactin levels. Since serum prolactin concentrations do not decrease, it appears that in this situation estrogens block the action of prolactin. In contrast, the suppression of lactation by bromocriptine, a dopamine analogue, is due to the inhibition of prolactin release from the pituitary gland. In the breast-feeding mother basal serum prolactin levels fall gradually, yet the amount of milk secreted increases. Although no association exists between the resting serum prolactin levels and the amount of milk produced, there may be a correlation between the amount of lactation and the degree of prolactin increment induced by vigorous suckling.

GALACTORRHEA

Nonpuerperal lactation or galactorrhea is an abnormal physical sign which occurs in both men and women. The amount of milk secreted forms the basis of the grading system used in quantitating the disorder. Grades I and II: Milk can be expressed manually but the patient may not necessarily be aware of it otherwise. Grades III and IV: Copious milk secretion occurs in an intermittent or continuous manner. The degree of galactorrhea so defined does not correlate with the pathologic significance of the underlying disorder (i.e., pituitary tumors may be associated with Grade II galactorrhea; the use of psychotropic drugs may lead to Grade IV galactorrhea). Galactorrhea usually is of benign significance. It becomes an important clinical sign especially when it is associated with disturbances of menstruation or impairment of fertility.

ETIOLOGY AND PATHOGENESIS. The classification of galactorrhea is more meaningful if it takes into account the serum prolactin (PRL) levels (Table 238–1). *Normoprolactinemic galactorrhea* is usually benign as far as hypothalamic-pituitary pathology is concerned. In acromegaly secondary to a growth hormone–secreting tumor, excess milk production may be due to the intrinsic lactogenic activity of growth hormone or to a circulating PRL of different molecular form than that measured by the standard radioimmunoassay. Even when serum PRL is in the normal range, the level may be inappropriately increased for a particular individual, since further lowering of the PRL with bromocriptine may be effective treatment. It has also been speculated that prior to the development of galactorrhea there may have been an increase in PRL which led to an increase in the number of lactogenic receptors and therefore to enhanced sensitivity.

Hyperprolactinemic galactorrhea should prompt a thorough investigation. Increased serum levels of PRL can result either from a decrease in its metabolic clearance (e.g., in liver failure or hypothyroidism) or from an increase in PRL production. The latter can result from conditions decreasing the inhibitory

TABLE 238–1. CAUSES OF NONPUERPERAL GALACTORRHEA

I. Central origin
- A. Organic
  - 1. Suprahypophyseal lesions
    - a. Hypothalamic disorders—infiltrative processes (histiocytosis, metastatic diseases); masses (craniopharyngioma, meningioma); infarction; embolism
    - b. Pituitary stalk lesions—section; impingement by tumors (all types with suprasellar extension); vascular insult
  - 2. Hypophyseal tumors
    - a. Prolactin secreting* (solitary; part of multiple endocrine adenomatosis syndrome mixed with GH, TSH, ACTH)
- B. Functional
  - 1. Drug related
    - a. Psychotropic (butyrophenones, phenothiazines)*
    - b. Antihypertensive (reserpine, alpha-methyldopa)
    - c. Cannabinoids (morphine, heroin)
    - d. Contraceptives
    - e. Antigastroplegics (metoclopramide)*
  - 2. Unclassified (idiopathic, stress, empty sella syndrome)

II. Peripheral origin
- A. Due to pituitary prolactin
  - 1. Due to primary failure of target endocrine gland
    - a. Hypothyroidism
    - b. Addison's disease
  - 2. Due to excess estrogen formation from target endocrine glands
    - a. Feminizing adrenal carcinoma
    - b. Polycystic ovarian syndrome
  - 3. Due to decreased metabolic clearance of PRL
    - a. Renal failure
    - b. Liver failure
    - c. Hypothyroidism
  - 4. Due to local breast conditions
    - a. Mechanical stimulation or suckling
    - b. Thoracic and/or breast trauma, burn
    - c. Inflammation, i.e., mastitis, herpes zoster
- B. Due to ectopic prolactin production
  - 1. Renal neoplasia
  - 2. Bronchogenic neoplasia

*Most common causes of highest serum PRL levels.

hypothalamic (dopaminergic) control of the pituitary or from the presence of a prolactin-secreting pituitary tumor. A decrease in the hypothalamic suppression of the secretion of PRL by the pituitary can be due either to lesions in the hypothalamus (e.g., gliomas, craniopharyngioma, histiocytosis, infarction) or to disruption of the hypothalamic-pituitary neurovascular connections (e.g., pituitary stalk section, tumoral impingement on the stalk such as by suprasellar extension of pituitary tumor). Functional causes of decreased dopaminergic control are mainly due to the intake of drugs which may (1) inhibit dopamine synthesis (e.g., alpha-methyl paratyrosine); (2) deplete the pool of catecholamine (e.g., reserpine); (3) dilute the catecholamine content in the presynaptic neurons (e.g., the false neurotransmitter methyldopa); or (4) occupy the postsynaptic receptor sites (e.g., haloperidol). Other drugs which stimulate the pituitary lactotrope are exogenous opiates and contraceptive steroids, especially those with high estrogen content. In susceptible animals, administration of a large dose of estrogen may induce pituitary prolactin-secreting tumors and result in hyperprolactinemia.

Galactorrhea and hyperprolactinemia may occur in primary myxedema or in Addison's disease. The mechanism whereby hypothyroidism leads to hyperprolactinemia is unknown, but it is believed to be mediated via excessive thyrotropin-releasing hormone (TRH) secretion. Whether excess corticotropin releasing factor (CRF) accounts for the hyperprolactinemic galactorrhea of Addison's disease or Cushing's syndrome is unknown. Other conditions leading to excess PRL secretion include the polycystic ovary syndrome and adrenal carcinoma, presumably because of the excess estrogen production found in these syndromes.

Excess production of PRL has been reported in patients with bronchogenic or renal neoplasms. Ectopic sources of PRL should be considered in the differential diagnosis.

CLINICAL PRESENTATION AND DIFFERENTIAL DIAGNOSIS. The clinical presentation of galactorrhea is highly variable, with milk production anywhere on the scale of I to IV (see above). There may be no other symptoms, or the patient may present the signs or symptoms of any of the disorders listed in Table 238–1. It is particularly important to determine carefully any drugs the patient may be taking.

In humans, the incidence of prolactin-secreting tumors (prolactinomas) is far higher in women then in men. A more general discussion of pituitary tumors has been presented in Ch. 225. Galactorrhea associated with amenorrhea is the most common presentation of a prolactinoma in women. Galactorrhea alone is found in less than one third of patients with prolactinoma. Prolactinomas in men produce galactorrhea much more rarely and, partly because of this, tend to present later as larger, space-occupying tumors.

One should measure serum PRL in every patient with galactorrhea. If the level is elevated and there is no evidence of psychotropic drug intake or primary hypothyroidism, one should exclude the presence of a pituitary tumor. If the tumor is non-prolactin-secreting and impinges upon the stalk, then the administration of TRH (500 μg intravenously) will provoke an increase of at least two-fold in serum PRL in the majority of patients (see Ch. 224 for normal response of PRL to TRH). If the tumor is composed of prolactin-secreting cells, then the diagnosis can be established with a combination of radiologic techniques and hormonal assays. If serum PRL levels exceed 500 ng per milliliter, a macroadenoma of the pituitary will generally be demonstrable by a plain skull film of the sella turcica by both the anteroposterior and lateral views. If the levels are between 100 and 500 ng per milliliter, the plain skull film may be normal but complex motion tomography will demonstrate a microadenoma in 85 per cent of the patients. In as many as 20 per cent of such patients TRH may elicit a doubling of serum PRL levels. If the levels of PRL are less than 100 ng per milliliter, no sella pathology may be detected even when high resolution computed tomography is utilized. In these cases a larger proportion of patients may respond to TRH. If PRL is not released by TRH in patients with hyperprolactinemia, the diagnosis of an autonomously secreting adenoma is strongly suspected. In our series surgical exploration successfully identified a tumor in 14 out of 16 patients who had equivocal radiologic examination of the sella but who did not respond to TRH with an increase in serum PRL.

TREATMENT. The treatment of the patient with galactorrhea depends on the primary disease. Discontinuation of medications or treatment of conditions such as hypothyroidism should lessen milk secretion. In persistent hyperprolactinemia without radiologic evidence for prolactinoma, bromocriptine will often be sufficient therapy (see below for treatment schedule). In such patients annual evaluation by sella radiology may be necessary if, upon discontinuation of the medication, hyperprolactinemia again supervenes. If a microadenoma is strongly suspected, the same strategy can be followed even for the woman who desires pregnancy. Small (10 mm or less) noninvasive microadenomas do not seem to grow rapidly during the gestational period. If there are signs of tumor growth despite bromocriptine treatment, transsphenoidal tumor resection is the preferred treatment. If during bromocriptine treatment there is no radiographic evidence of growth of the tumor, if the serum PRL is maintained within normal limits, and if the clinical abnormality is corrected, the patient can be kept on this regimen indefinitely. Reasons for discontinuation of medical therapy are (1) patient noncompliance, (2) cost of the medication, (3) development of side effects, and (4) failure of the medication to control the clinical and hormonal disorder (e.g., continuation of galactorrhea-amenorrhea and nonsuppression of serum PRL). In these instances, which are not uncommon, transsphenoidal resection of the pituitary adenoma could be undertaken in specialized centers. Pituitary tumor irradiation is the alternative to surgery. For those patients with galactorrhea and large adenomas, with or without parasellar and suprasellar extension, a combination of surgery, radiotherapy, and bromocriptine offers the best results. There have been reports of rapid decrease in tumor size with the use of bromocriptine alone, but there have been other reports to the contrary. Bromocriptine should not be the sole treatment of prolactin-secreting macroadenomas.

The management of patients with idiopathic normoprolactinemic galactorrhea is very difficult. Reports of the efficacy of pyridoxine and cyproheptadine in the treatment of these patients are not convincing and may represent only a placebo effect. Bromocriptine has been used to treat normoprolactinemic galactorrhea, but the number of "responders" not unexpectedly is smaller than in hyperprolactinemic patients. A trial of bromocriptine in normoprolactinemic galactorrhea may be warranted, based on the reasoning that (1) the levels of PRL, although within the normal range, may be inappropriately high for a given patient, and (2) there may be a discrepancy between the biologically active versus the immunologically detectable PRL molecule.

Bromocriptine should be administered carefully in the treatment of galactorrhea. Our custom is to begin with 1.25 mg (occasionally even with half that dose) every night for one week, and then to increase it by 1.25 mg every week until a dose of 2.5 mg twice daily is reached. A total daily dose of 10 mg is rarely exceeded, although the dose can be increased to 20 mg per day. Bromocriptine is taken with a meal, and the patient is asked to avoid abrupt postural change in order to prevent orthostatic hypotensive episodes. Nausea and behavioral changes (of the manic type) are other side effects. Currently there is no evidence for teratogenicity or other defects in the offspring of mothers who conceived while receiving bromocriptine. The drug passes the placental barrier, however, and exposed children have been followed for less than ten years. It is probably prudent, therefore, for women to discontinue the medication on the days of planned insemination and during pregnancy.

GYNECOMASTIA

Gynecomastia is defined as a palpable, firm mass, measuring at least 2 cm in diameter in the subareolar region. It represents excessive development of the male breast with a feminine appearance, and is the most common disorder of the male breast; about 85 per cent of male breast masses are due to gynecomastia. Pathologically it may be florid with proliferation of glandular or fibrous elements, characterized by increase of stromal tissue. The florid type may regress or progress to the fibrous type; the fibrous type is typically irreversible.

Gynecomastia usually begins at puberty when it may be unilateral or bilateral. When gynecomastia is unilateral it is more commonly on the left side for reasons unknown. Approximately 40 per cent of pubescent boys may develop some transient gynecomastia, with the highest incidence being between 14 and 15.5 years of age. Autopsy studies of elderly men have revealed true gynecomastia in as many as 40 per cent of subjects. The development of gynecomastia from late puberty to male senescence may signal a serious underlying disorder, such as adrenal or testicular tumor, and in such cases early diagnosis and treatment may be lifesaving.

ETIOLOGY AND PATHOPHYSIOLOGY. A classification of gynecomastia is contained in Table 238–2. The pathophysiology of gynecomastia has been partly clarified. For the majority of patients it seems to be associated with a disturbance in the balance of estrogenic-androgenic effects on the mammary epithelium. The pathogenesis of gynecomastia may be complex. For example, both increased estrogen production and aromatization of secreted androgens to estrogens may occur in adrenal tumors and congenital adrenal hyperplasia. In nonadrenal neoplasms associated with human chorionic gonadotropin (HCG) production, the excess estrogen levels are due to increased secretion of estrogens by the testes. Finally, the estrogen level may be only relatively increased in comparison to the testosterone level, as in Klinefelter's syndrome or in testicular failure, with an increased estrogen-androgen ratio. An increased extraglandular formation of estrogens from androgens is believed to play a significant role in the gynecomastia seen in patients with chronic liver disease, starvation, and thyrotoxicosis. In these conditions, as a result of decreased hepatic extraction, there is increased androgen available for peripheral conversion to estrogens. The latter mechanism seems to be operative in some patients with idiopathic gynecomastia but its significance in that syndrome has not been fully elucidated.

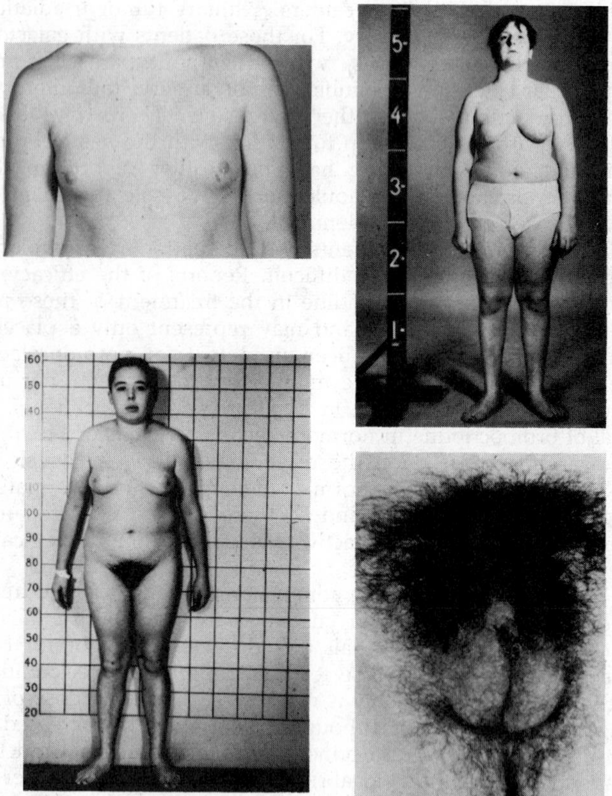

Figure 238–1. *Upper left,* Pubertal gynecomastia (physical examination: normal). *Upper right,* Gynecomastia associated with obesity (physical examination: normal except for increased adiposity). *Lower left and right,* Phenotypic appearance of body habitus and external genitalia in a genetically male patient with the syndrome of incomplete testicular feminization (physical examination: female escutcheon, hypospadias, bifid scrotum, normal-sized testes). (Courtesy of Dr. H. Guyda.)

TABLE 238–2. CLASSIFICATION OF THE CAUSES OF GYNECOMASTIA

All true gynecomastia is caused by an estrogenic effect on the male breast. This may result from excessive estrogen or from deficient androgen.

I. Physiologic—newborn, puberty, senescence
II. Pathologic
  A. Increased estrogen secretion
    1. Hermaphroditism
    2. Klinefelter's syndrome
    3. Congenital adrenal hyperplasia
    4. Neoplastic
      a. Adrenal carcinoma
      b. Testicular tumor (Sertoli cell, Leydig cell, choriocarcinoma)
      c. Paraneoplasms secreting human chorionic gonadotropin (lung, liver, kidney, stomach, lymphopoietic system)
  B. Increased conversion of androgens to estrogens
    1. Adrenal carcinoma
    2. Liver disorders (failure secondary to infectious or nutritional causes, carcinoma)
    3. Nutritional (refeeding after starvation)
    4. Thyrotoxicosis
  C. Decreased androgen secretion
    1. Primary testicular failure (anorchia, Klinefelter's syndrome, enzymatic defects in testosterone synthesis)
    2. Secondary testicular failure (castration; infectious orchitis; mumps and other viruses, lepromatous, tuberculous; neurologic disorders: paraplegia, muscular dystrophy; renal failure; panhypopituitarism; prolactin-secreting tumors)
  D. Decreased androgen activity due to receptor protein abnormalities
    1. Complete testicular feminization
    2. Incomplete testicular feminization
    3. Reifenstein's syndrome
III. Pharmacologic—a combination of mechanisms
  A. Cannabinoid—methadone and marijuana
  B. Psychotropics—phenothiazine, butyrophenone, reserpine
  C. Antihypertensives—reserpine, alpha-methyldopa, spironolactone
  D. Cardiac—digitalis
  E. Gastrointestinal—cimetidine, metoclopramide, domperidone
  F. Antituberculous—isoniazid
  G. Hormonal
    1. Sex steroids—estrogens, androgens
    2. Gonadotropins—human chorionic gonadotropin
    3. Antiandrogens
  H. Cytotoxic—cyclophosphamide, mustine, vincristine, mitotane
  I. Miscellaneous—penicillamine
IV. Idiopathic

Peptide hormones may contribute to the genesis of gynecomastia directly or indirectly. Human placental lactogen (HPL) is secreted by some testicular tumors, but its role in the proliferation of mammary epithelium is not clear. Some patients with hyperprolactinemia associated with prolactin-secreting pituitary tumor have gynecomastia. This is probably secondary to a decrease in androgen secretion (suppression of gonadotropins), possibly to a decrease in the peripheral conversion of testosterone to its active metabolite dihydrotestosterone.

In the syndrome of complete testicular feminization, androgen production by the testes is normal but pituitary luteinizing hormone (LH) output is enhanced (because the absence of cytoplasmic androgen receptors in the pituitary impairs feedback control) and leads to testicular estrogen production. The increased estrogen, coupled with a defect in the action of androgen owing to the lack of the receptor in the mammary gland, leads to excessive estrogenic expression and gynecomastia. A similar mechanism has been invoked in incomplete testicular feminization and in Reifenstein's syndrome. Perhaps variations in hormone receptor levels may account for other cases of gynecomastia associated with normal circulating levels of estrogens and androgens.

Gynecomastia occurs in patients receiving various drugs, in particular estrogens (orally, parenterally, or as ointments). Other drugs, however, can also lead to gynecomastia by altering the effective estrogenic-androgenic ratio of activity in the breast. Some lead to decreased testosterone synthesis (e.g., chemotherapeutic agents, high doses of spironolactone) or interfere with testosterone action (e.g., cyproterone, low doses of spironolactone). They may cause increased estrogen production (e.g., HCG) or may themselves have an estrogen-like effect (digitalis, tetrahydrocannabinol).

DIAGNOSIS AND DIFFERENTIAL DIAGNOSIS. It is obviously important to be sure that true gynecomastia is present. The most common error is to confuse the "false gynecomastia" of obesity with true gynecomastia. The obese breast lacks glandular elements on palpation. Palpation will also differentiate gynecomastia from such disorders as carcinoma or neurofibroma. It should be evident that even the presence of true gynecomastia with onset at the time of puberty does not call for a major medical investigation in view of its high incidence (see above) and benign prognosis.

The differential diagnosis of gynecomastia may be accomplished on the basis of history and physical examination. In most instances laboratory studies will be important as well. For example, examination of the head and neck may reveal the presence of signs of compression of the anterior visual pathways consistent with suprasellar extension of a pituitary tumor, or diplopia, lid lag, or goiter consistent with Graves' disease. Examination of the breasts may reveal the presence of galactorrhea, in which case measurement of serum prolactin (PRL) is mandatory. The skin and abdomen may reveal signs of liver failure and examination of the testes may establish microrchidia, in which case a chromosomal disorder should be suspected (e.g., Klinefelter's syndrome). Alternatively, asymmetrical enlargement of a testis raises suspicion of a malignant process.

Laboratory studies will be selected in part based on the clinical circumstances revealed by the history, physical examination, and the age of the patient. A study of liver function is usually indicated. Useful hormone assays include the determination of serum estrogens (estrone and estradiol), androgens (androstenedione and testosterone), and luteinizing hormone (LH), and of urinary 17-ketosteroids. Excess serum estrogens are found in patients with Leydig cell tumors and adrenal carcinoma; in such patients serum LH and testosterone levels are low. Elevated serum LH is found in primary testicular failure (in which case testosterone levels are low) and in HCG-secreting tumors (due to cross-reaction of HCG in the assay for LH if a specific HCG assay is not done). If HCG is elevated, serum testosterone may be normal but serum estrogens tend to be elevated. Abnormally high LH occurs in the syndrome of peripheral androgen resistance and is accompanied by normal or elevated testosterone levels. Finally, excessive excretion of 17-ketosteroids almost invariably reflects disease of the adrenal cortex. Inability to demonstrate abnormal values in any of the aforementioned measurements does not exclude a metabolic cause of gynecomastia. More elaborate methods are required to facilitate in vivo study of the binding or the biologic action of sex steroids in order to elucidate further the cases of idiopathic gynecomastia.

Radiologic studies can be of significant help in selected cases. Four radiographic patterns have been identified: (1) the presence of ductlike structures (54 per cent incidence in one series); (2) marked proliferation of the ducts occupying almost the entire breast; (3) homogeneous density occupying either or both subareolar breast areas; and (4) nonhomogeneous density in subareolar or most breast regions. The last appearance was found more often in adults, whereas homogeneity was more prevalent in pubertal gynecomastia. Xeromammography in a patient with a breast mass raises strong suspicions for cancer when the mass is solid, spiculated, and located eccentrically in relation to the nipple; benign gynecomastia, by contrast, is symmetrical in relation to the nipple.

TREATMENT. Regression of gynecomastia can occur in the majority of patients. It is spontaneous in the pubertal cases (up to 90 per cent regress within one to three years). In the rest of the patients, removal of the offending agent or appropriate drug treatment will result in significant improvement when utilized not too late in the course of the abnormality. Thus, impressive improvement occurs with the removal of a sex steroid–producing tumor or treatment of thyrotoxicosis, whereas poor results are obtained in longstanding cases of Klinefelter's or fibrous gynecomastia. In cases of androgen deficiency, androgen administration certainly leads to improvement; however, the active biotransformation of aromatizable androgens to estrogens sustains gynecomastic changes. Attempts to use nonaromatizable androgens or dihydrotestosterone may have promise. As well, independent or combined administration of antiestrogens could theoretically protect the breast tissue from the estrogenic side effects; well-documented series are not as yet reported. If gynecomastia is long lasting, the ensuing fibrotic changes are irreversible, so that even the removal of the causative agent (e.g., drug withdrawal) may not lead to a return of the breasts to normal size. Cosmetic mastectomy may be the preferred mode of "treatment," depending upon the wishes of the patient.

Galactorrhea

Friesen HG, Tolis G: The use of bromocriptine in the galactorrhea-amenorrhea syndromes. Clin Endocrinol 6S:91, 1977. *An important document in the North American literature. It is based on the Canadian Cooperative Study and should be a standard reference.*

Kleinberg DL, Noel GH, Frantz AG: Galactorrhea: A study of 235 cases, including 48 with pituitary tumors. N Engl J Med 296:589, 1977. *This study confirms and extends previous observations. It is among the most comprehensive reports on etiologic entities associated with galactorrhea.*

Koppelman MCS, Jaffe MJ, Rieth KG, Caruso RC, Loriaux DL: Hyperprolactinemia, amenorrhea and galactorrhea. Ann Intern Med 100:115, 1984. *The authors report on their experiences with 25 patients with this syndrome and emphasize its benign clinical course. Because of this they advocate conservative treatment.*

Tolis G: Galactorrhea. *In* Krieger DT, Bordin WC (eds.): Current Therapy in Endocrinology 1983–1984. Toronto and St. Louis, B.C. Decker and C.V. Mosby Companies, 1983, pp 427–428. *Report based on author's data and literature review of normoprolactinemic and hyperprolactinemic galactorrhea.*

Tolis G, Franks S: Prolactin pathophysiology. *In* Clinical Neuroendocrinology: A Pathophysiological Approach. New York, Raven Press, 1979, pp 291-318. *This paper is based primarily on numerous studies reported by the authors during the last decade. It contains an extensive review of work that has been amply confirmed.*

Tucker A: Control of lactation. Semin Perinatol 3:199, 1979. *A scholarly analysis of the current concepts of lactogenesis.*

Yen SSC: Lactogenesis and lactation. *In* Yen SSC, Jaffe RB (eds.): Reproductive Endocrinology. Philadelphia, W. B. Saunders Company, 1978, pp 165-167. *Lucid description of current knowledge with regard to control of lactation in humans. The whole chapter on prolactin must be read even by the advanced reader.*

Gynecomastia

Chandrakant CK, Parekh NJ: The male breast. Radiol Clin North Am 21:137, 1983. *A thorough review and presentation of the authors' own series of radiologic issues in the evaluation of gynecomastia.*

Large DM, Anderson DC: Twenty-four hour profiles of circulating androgens and estrogens in male puberty with and without gynecomastia. Clin Endocrinol 11:505, 1979. *A significant contribution. It documents the long-held view that there is an estrogen-androgen imbalance associated with pubertal gynecomastia.*

Large DM, Jones JM, Shalet SM, Scarffe JH, Gibbs AC: Gynaecomastia complicating the treatment of myeloma. Br J Cancer 48:69, 1983. *A detailed hormonal study of patients with gynecomastia receiving cytotoxic agents.*

Wilson JD, Aiman J, MacDonald P: The pathogenesis of gynecomastia. Adv Intern Med 25:1, 1980. *This review is based on the authors' longstanding experience in the steroid field and presents a "state of the art" contribution with regard to the pathophysiology of gynecomastia.*

239. CARCINOMA OF THE BREAST

George P. Canellos

Carcinoma of the breast is the most common malignant tumor of women, accounting for approximately 35,000 annual deaths. It is estimated that 1 of every 13 women in the United States will develop breast cancer at some time in her life—approximately a 7 per cent chance. Greater public awareness and increased application of self-examination and mammographic screening are now identifying about 105,000 new cases annually in the United States.

ETIOLOGY. Hormonal and genetic factors predispose to the development of this tumor. A maternal history of breast cancer increases the risk three-fold; the tumor tends to occur at an earlier age in descendants of patients who have had breast cancer. Ovarian function and estrogenic hormones have been implicated as causative factors. Elevated blood levels of estradiol plus estrone and prolactin have been found in the daughters of breast cancer patients. In some experimental animals the estrogens estradiol and estrone are carcinogenic. A generally increased risk for breast cancer has been associated with nulliparity, late first pregnancy, and premenstrual symptoms of breast swelling. A decreased risk has been associated with castration before the age of 40. Multiparity, especially beginning before 20 years of age, and prolonged lactation with long-term nursing exert a protective effect probably related to suppression of ovulation.

The incidence of breast cancer rises progressively from age 30 to 90, although the greater number of cases occur between 45 and 59. Mortality from the disease is much higher in Western and/or developed countries. It is rare in Japan, and when it occurs the course tends to be more benign than that seen in the United States. There is no clear explanation for the different incidence between Japanese and American women, although the Western high fat diet and obesity are thought to affect storage and metabolism of estrogens. Certain defined ethnic groups, such as the Parsis of India, have a higher than expected incidence of breast cancer.

The same etiologic factors which contribute to the development of breast cancer may participate in the genesis of benign breast disorders such as fibroadenoma and fibrocystic disease, since patients with breast cancer tend to have had a higher frequency of benign breast disease. The hazards of radiation exposure have been debated in light of the use of mammography. A direct linear relationship seems to exist between the amount of radiation exposure and the risk of breast cancer and amounts to less than 1 per cent increased risk per rad. These estimates were derived from studies of atomic bomb survivors, women treated with radiation for acute postpartum mastitis, and those who received repeated fluoroscopic examinations of the chest.

PATHOLOGY. Carcinoma of the breast is a neoplasm of the ductal epithelium in over 90 per cent of cases. The presence of fibrosis confers its scirrhous character. Neoplastic degeneration can occur in the lobules (lobular carcinoma), usually as low grade tumor or carcinoma in situ, and can often be bilateral. This form of breast carcinoma and noninfiltrating (intraductal) carcinoma constitute 5 to 10 per cent of all breast cancer and rarely ever disseminate. Another relatively benign variant of ductal epithelium is medullary carcinoma, which occurs in about 20 to 25 per cent of cases. This tumor has a significantly higher ten-year survival (84 per cent). There is an equal frequency of nodal metastases but a better prognosis when nodes are positive when compared to other infiltrating ductal cancers.

Paget's disease of the breast (nipple) is a crusted, eczematoid lesion caused by subareolar intraductal carcinoma which begins in the minute ducts of the nipple and grows up toward the skin. Large, clear vacuolated tumor cells (Paget's cells) occur in the deeper layers of the epidermis.

Inflammatory carcinoma represents a particularly malignant variant. It is characterized by erythema, pain, and fullness of the breast owing to dermal lymphatic invasion of anaplastic tumor cells. The median survival of such patients is usually less than 18 months.

The biologic behavior of human breast cancer is highly variable, as reflected in measured mean tumor volume doubling times of 105 to 212 days with a wide range of 15 to 1869 days.

CLINICAL MANIFESTATIONS. ***Primary Disease.*** The majority of patients present with a painless breast mass which was self-detected. Unfavorable prognostic signs include skin involvement, inflammatory signs, fixation to the chest wall, tumor size in excess of 5 cm, palpable axillary nodes, and nipple involvement. The prognosis for development of subsequent metastases can be determined from the extent of axillary node involvement. Patients with negative nodes have a 20 to 30 per cent chance of relapse over ten years. The frequency of relapse rises 66 per cent when one to three nodes are involved and to 85 per cent when more than three nodes are involved. A number of histologic findings have been reported to increase the likelihood of axillary metastases. These include poor differentiation, blood vessel invasion, and lack of lymphoid infiltration of the tumor.

The present clinical staging system incorporates the features described above:

Stage I—tumor <2 cm without skin involvement and with no clinically suspicious axillary nodes.

Stage II—tumor <2 cm with clinically suspicious nodes; any tumor 2 to 5 cm with or without clinically suspicious nodes.

Stage III—any tumor >5 cm; skin involvement or chest wall attachment; any sized tumor with clinically fixed axillary nodes; edema of arm; infraclavicular nodes.

Stage IV—metastatic disease.

The accuracy of clinical diagnosis for isolated breast masses is about 70 per cent. The use of low dose mammography has an accuracy of about 90 per cent. The currently recommended guidelines for screening mammography restrict its use to women 50 years old or older. Women aged 40 to 49 years should have the technique used for annual screening only if they have a prior history of breast cancer or if their mother or sister(s) has breast cancer. In the 35 to 39 age group, women should have annual mammography only if there is prior history of breast cancer, since these patients have a 10 per cent chance of developing cancer in the contralateral breast.

Metastatic Disease. There is a risk of metastatic disease at any time up to at least 20 years postmastectomy, although the majority of metastases are clinically evident by five to seven years. The most common sites of metastases in patients who have positive axillary nodes include the locoregional area, the bones, and the viscera. Routine bone scans at the time of surgery have not been useful in identifying metastatic disease, since only about 6 per cent are abnormal in Stage I or Stage II patients. The incidence of positive scans rises to 25 per cent in Stage III patients. The use of brain scans as a survey technique for metastases is equally inefficient, since about 98 per cent are normal even in the presence of recurrent disease. Biochemical markers have rarely been useful in the detection of clinically undetectable metastatic disease. The serial measurement of alkaline phosphatase, carcinoembryonic antigen, and gamma glutamyl transpeptidase has been proposed as useful in the early detection of metastatic disease, since abnormalities in at least one of these three tests may precede clinical detection by three months. Preoperative measurement of carcinoembryonic antigen (CEA) is not of diagnostic value in early breast cancer, since the incidence of minimal elevation (30 per cent) is approximately the same as for normal women. Persistent postoperative elevation, however, has correlated with the likelihood of relapse. Sixty-eight per cent of patients with metastatic disease have an elevated CEA, with the highest frequency in those with hepatic metastases (93 per cent).

ESTROGEN RECEPTOR PROTEIN (ERP) (Table 239–1). It is possible to measure cytoplasmic proteins which function as receptors to bind and transfer estrogens to the nuclei of cells. These can be measured as femtomoles of ^{3}(H) estradiol bound per milligram of cytosol protein. Approximately 60 per cent of

TABLE 239–1. SOME FEATURES OF THE ESTROGEN RECEPTOR PROTEIN (ERP)

Occurs in breast cancer (male and female), but also in some other tumors, e.g., melanoma
Cytoplasmic protein with 4S, 8S peaks (8S peak correlates with response), expressed as femtomoles of ^{3}H estradiol bound per milligram of protein
Fifty to 60 per cent of tumors will have levels >3 femtomoles per milligram of protein; 50 to 60 per cent ERP-positive tumors respond to endocrine ablation, hormone therapy, or antiestrogen
Breast tumors are positive in 30 per cent of premenopausal patients and 70 per cent of postmenopausal patients
ERP status of metastatic lesion usually reflects value of primary tumor—unchanged by chemotherapy
ERP-negative tumors tend to have higher kinetic (labeling) indices and to recur sooner than ERP-positive tumors

primary breast tumors have measurable ERP, usually >10 femtomoles per milligram. The presence and the quantity of ERP tend to vary with the menstrual status. Approximately 30 per cent of breast carcinomas in premenopausal women and >60 per cent of such tumors in postmenopausal women contain measurable ERP. The concordance for the presence or absence of ERP between primary and metastatic tumor is high (80 per cent), as it is between multiple metastatic sites. The level is unaffected by chemotherapeutic agents. There is a positive correlation between the presence of the ERP and response to hormonal manipulation: approximately 50 to 60 per cent ERP-positive patients experience objective tumor regression; less than 5 per cent of ERP-negative patients benefit from hormonal treatment. ERP-positive tumors tend to be more differentiated, have lower mitotic activity, and are associated with a longer time interval between primary treatment and metastases in those who subsequently relapse.

The ERP is heterogeneously distributed in the cells of a breast tumor. ERP-positive tumors which recur following endocrine treatment tend to have low or absent ERP. The subsequent response to chemotherapy does not appear to be affected by ERP status or response to previous hormonal treatment. In addition to receptors for estrogen, the cytosol of breast tumors contains receptor proteins for progesterone (PRP) in about 50 per cent of cases. The presence of both ERP and PRP is associated with the highest response rate to hormonal treatment. Tumors lacking both receptors (30 per cent of all cases) rarely respond.

TREATMENT (Table 239–2). ***Primary Therapy.*** There has been a gradual departure from the classic Halsted radical mastectomy to more conservative surgery for primary breast tumors. The modified radical mastectomy with preservation of the pectoralis major muscle and removal of axillary nodes has been the standard approach to Stage I and II tumors. An increasing body of evidence suggests that simple mastectomy alone may suffice in patients with small primary tumors and clinically uninvolved axillary nodes. The routine use of postoperative radiation therapy following either modified radical mastectomy or simple (total) mastectomy does not improve survival but does decrease local recurrence. Exploration (or sampling) of ipsilateral axillary nodes for evidence of microscopic involvement remains an important procedure to identify patients at higher risk of developing distant metastases. An alternative to mastectomy has been the use of primary radiation therapy following excision of the tumor ("lumpectomy"). External beam radiation and iridium needle implants are capable of delivering 8000 to 10,000 rads to the tumor. The local control rate for small primary tumors appears comparable to mastectomy.

Stage III tumors have a high potential for local recurrence and distant metastases with a five-year survival between 20 and 30 per cent. Such tumors are treated primarily by radiation therapy preceded or followed by some form of systemic therapy. In some instances mastectomy can be performed after radiation, but extensive skin infiltration, ulceration, attachment to chest wall, or inflammatory changes require radiation and/or chemotherapy as the initial form of therapy.

In some instances reconstructive surgery with insertion of a prosthesis can be accomplished following radical surgery.

Hormonal Treatment. In all instances a measurement of ERP should be made on all primary tumors, since subsequent metastases would be expected to have a similar ERP constitution. Lacking an ERP measurement, certain clinical features predict response to hormonal treatment: (1) a disease-free interval in excess of two years; (2) a small tumor; (3) metastatic disease confined to bone, skin, lung, and nodes; and (4) the patient's being more than five years postmenopausal.

The likelihood of response to hormonal treatment can be predicted from the height of the ERP value as well as the presence of progesterone receptors. The preferred initial approach to hormonal treatment of premenopausal patients is oophorectomy. Without knowledge of the ERP status, about 33 per cent of patients will respond for a mean duration of 12 to 16 months and are likely to survive almost two years longer than nonresponders. In the past, response to oophorectomy could be used to predict subsequent benefit from further endocrine ablation such as adrenalectomy or hypophysectomy. Although criteria for response are variable, response to adrenalectomy is likely in 40 to 60 per cent of those who have responded to oophorectomy and in <30 per cent of nonresponders. Metastases to the central nervous system and liver rarely respond to either oophorectomy or adrenalectomy.

Transsphenoidal hypophysectomy is about as effective as adrenalectomy in patients who have responded to previous hormonal treatment. The mean duration of response to either mode of therapy is about 18 months, although responses up to five years have been noted in a minority of patients. Measurement of pituitary hormones suggests that transfrontal hypophysectomy is superior to the transsphenoidal approach. Antitumor response may be seen without complete ablation of pituitary endocrine function as measured by radioimmunoassay of serum levels of pituitary hormones in basal or stimulated states. Endocrine ablation in postmenopausal patients has been gradually replaced by antiestrogen therapy with tamoxifen or "medical adrenalectomy" with aminoglutethimide.

Medical Adrenalectomy. Aminoglutethimide will inhibit adrenal estrogen synthesis in castrated or postmenopausal women by inhibiting adrenal conversion of cholesterol to pregnenolone. This results in a marked but not complete inhibition of the synthesis of progesterone, testosterone, androstenedione, and other Δ^4 class steroids. An additional action of the drug is inhibition of the conversion, in peripheral extra-adrenal tissues, of androstenedione to estrone (aromatization), which is a precursor to estradiol. The extra-adrenal sources normally account for almost all of the estrogen produced in postmenopausal women. The adrenal production of cortisol is also suppressed, resulting in a compensatory rise of ACTH, which can overcome the blockade by aminoglutethimide. Effective suppression of estrogen production by aminoglutethimide must therefore in-

TABLE 239–2. THERAPEUTIC APPROACH TO BREAST CANCER

Stage I—Optimal local treatment	
ERP +	No further therapy (in pre- and postmenopausal); hormone therapy is investigational
ERP −	Adjuvant chemotherapy (optional in premenopausal)
Stage II—Optimal local treatment	
ERP +	Premenopausal: adjuvant chemotherapy; addition of hormonal therapy is investigational
ERP +	Postmenopausal: adjuvant chemotherapy and/or hormone therapy is recommended but remains investigational
ERP −	Adjuvant chemotherapy recommended for premenopausal and most postmenopausal patients
Stage III—Locally advanced	
	Optimal local treatment with radiation and surgery if possible. This may be preceded and followed by chemotherapy.
Stage IV	
ERP +	Skin, soft tissue, bone, lymph nodes, pleura: hormonal therapy
ERP +	Liver, lymphangitic spread to lung, multiple metastatic sites (three): chemotherapy plus hormonal therapy
ERP −	Chemotherapy

clude the addition of glucocorticoid, preferably hydrocortisone rather than dexamethasone. Metabolism of the latter steroid can be accelerated by aminoglutethimide. Clinical trials of aminoglutethimide, employing 250 mg four times a day with 40 mg of hydrocortisone daily, have demonstrated a 30 to 40 per cent objective response rate of breast carcinoma in postmenopausal women. The response rate is somewhat higher in women with ERP-positive tumors. Comparative trials show a response rate equivalent to that obtained by surgical adrenalectomy or hypophysectomy. Toxic side effects, which occur in about 20 per cent of cases, include dizziness, somnolence, rash, or a combination, which generally improve over a few days but may not wane for one or two weeks.

Additive Hormone Therapy. Estrogens, androgens, and progestational agents have been used to treat advanced breast cancer in postmenopausal women. Prior to the introduction of antiestrogens the most commonly used hormonal agents were the estrogens, and among these the usual preparation was diethylstilbestrol, 5 mg three times a day.

Response is usually slow, occurring over several weeks and lasting about 12 to 14 months. A positive response is more likely to occcur in women ten years beyond the menopause. The general response rate is about 30 per cent, but this rises to about 50 per cent in ERP-positive patients. Carcinoma in the skin, lymph nodes, and breast is more likely to respond than osseous metastases. Anorexia, nausea, and vomiting may occur at the initiation of therapy, but these symptoms can be relieved by changing to other estrogenic preparations. The chronic toxicity of estrogens includes fluid retention, softening of skin, and breast engorgement. The most troublesome side effect, usually seen at the beginning of treatment, is increased bone pain and/or hypercalcemia, which can be controlled by hydration, diuresis, and/or mithramycin. If the hormone is continued, the flare reaction can actually herald an antitumor response. Patients whose disease progresses while they are receiving estrogens may respond to the sudden cessation of treatment. This rebound regression can occur in up to 30 per cent of treated patients and usually predicts response to other forms of endocrine therapy.

Androgenic hormones are usually less effective than estrogens in postmenopausal patients with soft tissue metastases. They are equal to or superior to estrogens in the treatment of osseous metastases. The usual preparations are testosterone propionate, 100 mg intramuscularly three times a week, or fluoxymesterone, 10 mg by mouth twice a day. The side effects are mainly virilization, erythrocytosis, and increased libido. The mechanism of the therapeutic action of estrogens and androgens in breast carcinoma is unknown, although suppression of pituitary function as well as a direct toxic effect on the cancer cell has been proposed.

Progestational agents in high dosage have also been used successfully, especially in patients who have previously responded to estrogens or androgens. Progestational hormones are less toxic than sex steroids, but they have not been as extensively studied as primary hormonal treatment. The tumor response rate varies from 5 to 25 per cent, but response rarely occurs in patients refractory to other hormones. The use of sex steroid hormones as first line endocrine treatment must be weighed against the fact that safe and effective antiestrogen therapy, with tamoxifen, can achieve comparable responses. Corticosteroids offer the potential of transient antitumor benefit by virtue of their suppression of pituitary ACTH and secondary decrease of adrenocortical function. The toxicity of long-term corticosteroids reduces the usefulness of this form of hormonal therapy.

Antiestrogen Therapy. A number of antiestrogen compounds, such as nafoxidine, clomiphene, and tamoxifen, have the ability to interfere with the effect of estrogen on certain target tissues. The most commonly used and safest antiestrogenic drug is tamoxifen, which competes with estradiol for the high affinity cytoplasmic receptor, binds to it, and makes it refractory to subsequent estrogenic stimuli. In a dosage of 20 to 40 mg per day the drug is capable of inducing remissions of metastatic breast carcinoma, with a duration of response equal to or exceeding that seen with androgens, estrogens, and hypophysectomy. Eventual refractoriness to tamoxifen or other hormonal therapy does not preclude a subsequent hormonal response if that patient is crossed-over to the alternative therapy.

Antitumor response in premenopausal women with advanced cancer has been noted with tamoxifen, although it has not replaced oophorectomy as primary treatment of the ERP-positive patient. The drug is primarily indicated for ERP-positive postmenopausal women. As with other forms of hormonal treatment, responses are most frequent for lesions of soft tissue, lymph nodes, and bone. A tumor which is positive for ERP and which has responded to prior endocrine therapy can be predicted to have a 60 to 80 per cent response rate to tamoxifen, lasting 12 to 18 months on the average. The side effects of tamoxifen are minimal. There is transient nausea or vomiting in about 10 per cent of cases. If a "flare" consisting of increased bone pain and hypercalcemia occurs, it is usually short lived and, as with estrogen treatment, usually heralds an antitumor response.

The primary hormonal therapy for premenopausal women with ERP-positive metastatic disease is oophorectomy followed by antiestrogen therapy or endocrine ablation. Postmenopausal patients with ERP-positive tumors are usually treated with antiestrogens, followed by medical or surgical adrenalectomy for previous hormonal responders. The combination of medical adrenalectomy and antiestrogen therapy is still investigational.

Cytotoxic Chemotherapy. A variety of cytotoxic agents of differing biochemical mechanism of action have demonstrated antitumor activity in advanced breast cancer.

The most commonly used agents include cyclophosphamide, L-phenylalanine mustard (L-PAM), methotrexate, 5-fluorouracil, and doxorubicin (Adriamycin). Each drug used as a single agent can induce a partial regression in about 20 to 30 per cent of cases, but complete responses are rarely seen. When active agents are used in combination chemotherapy programs, the results are superior to the single agents in overall responses, as well as in the achievement of complete remissions. Combination chemotherapy is particularly effective in patients with extensive metastatic disease in the liver and lymphangitic pulmonary metastases, two sites which rarely respond to hormonal therapy. All metastatic sites are capable of responding to combination chemotherapy regimens, including osseous lesions. Neither the previous response to endocrine therapy nor the ERP status influences the response to cytotoxic chemotherapy, and, conversely, prior administration of chemotherapy does not negate a subsequent hormonal response. About 20 per cent of patients achieve a complete remission with combination chemotherapy, which is rarely seen with hormonal therapy or single agent cytotoxic drugs. The more commonly used combination chemotherapy regimens include cyclophosphamide or L-PAM, methotrexate, and 5-fluorouracil (CMF or PMF). An alternative regimen substitutes doxorubicin for methotrexate (CAF). Among the variety of programs available, no one of them has clearly emerged as superior. Cytotoxic chemotherapy in advanced disease can induce remissions lasting in excess of 12 months but rarely exceeding 24 months. It is rare also that all drug therapy can be discontinued in patients with complete remission.

As with hormonal therapy, bone films in patients treated with drugs can often show an increase in osteoblastic reaction as part of the healing process, and this may be falsely interpreted as disease progression. The simultaneous addition of cytotoxic chemotherapy to hormonal therapy, either endocrine ablation or tamoxifen, has shown no clear improvement in survival over the sequential use of these methods. Marked osteolytic destruction of the femur or humerus may necessitate insertion of a prosthesis to prevent pathologic fracture.

Radiation therapy has an important palliative role in metastatic cancer. Metastatic lesions to the brain or meninges can often be effectively treated with complete disappearance of radiographic abnormalities. Intrathecal chemotherapy may also be required when meningeal infiltration is the predominant abnormality. Pain resulting from metastatic bone lesions can be relieved, as well as impending spinal cord compression by tumor.

Adjuvant Therapy. Patients can be identified as being at high risk for developing metastatic disease according to the presence of microscopic involvement of axillary lymph nodes by tumor. Two categories of risk include those with one to three positive nodes (moderate risk) and those with more than three nodes (high risk). Chemotherapy given as an adjuvant to primary treatment is intended to eradicate or significantly retard the growth of microscopic metastases. The current information suggests a definite role for adjuvant combination chemotherapy of premenopausal women in the moderate and high risk groups. Disease-free survival has been significantly prolonged in premenopausal women by the use of combination chemotherapy. The latter is superior to single-agent treatment. More recent trials have shown similar advantages of adjuvant chemotherapy for postmenopausal patients. The addition of hormonal agents to cytotoxic drugs will enhance the disease-free survival of patients with ERP-positive tumors, but overall survival may not be superior to the sequential use of these methods. Some postmenopausal patients in similar risk categories may also benefit, but further controlled trials are required to establish the definite value of adjuvant chemotherapy in postmenopausal patients.

MALE BREAST CANCER. Carcinoma of the male breast is rare, accounting for 0.9 per cent of all breast cancer. The epidemiology, clinical presentation, and primary therapy are very similar to those of female breast cancer. The etiology is unknown, although abnormalities of estrogen metabolism have been reported. Carcinoma of the breast occurs in higher frequency in patients with Klinefelter's syndrome. The management of metastatic disease includes castration as the primary approach, which will yield a response rate in excess of that seen following oophorectomy in premenopausal women (40 to 60 per cent). Similarly, adrenalectomy and hypophysectomy can effectively palliate metastatic disease. ERP has been noted in male breast cancer, but the results of additive hormonal therapy are considerably less than in female breast cancer.

Casebeer K, et al.: Recommendations of the consensus development panel on breast cancer screening. Cancer Res 38:476, 1978. *The proceedings of the NCI-sponsored meeting on the medications for mammography screening.*

Crichlow RW: Breast cancer in man. Semin Oncol 1:145, 1974. *A concise review of the literature on this rare form of breast cancer.*

Henderson IC, Canellos GP: Cancer of the breast. The past decade. N Engl J Med 302:17, 78, 1980. *Comprehensive review of the literature concerning primary and metastatic disease treatment.*

Legha SS, Davis HL, Muggia FM: Hormonal therapy of breast cancer: New approaches and concepts. Ann Intern Med 88:69, 1978. *A review of the approaches to hormonal treatment.*

Legha SS, et al.: Complete remissions in metastatic breast cancer treated with combination drug therapy. Ann Intern Med 91:847, 1979. *The natural history of a series of patients who achieved complete remission with combination chemotherapy.*

McCarthy KS Jr, Silva JS, Cox EB, Leight GS Jr, Wells SA Jr, McCarthy KS Sr: Relationship of age and menopausal status to estrogen receptor content in primary carcinoma of the breast. Ann Surg 197:2, 1983. *Up-to-date study of ERP and age.*

Rosen PP, Saigo PE, Braun DW, Weathers E, Kinne DW: Prognosis in stage II ($T_1N_1M_0$) breast cancer. Ann Surg 194:5, 1981. *The Memorial Hospital experience with this common stage.*

Rossi A, Bonadonna G, Valagussa P, Veronesi U: Multimodal treatment in operable breast cancer: Five-year results of the CMF programme. Br Med J 282, 1981. *The most recent review of the Milan data.*

Senn HJ: Current status and indications for adjuvant therapy in breast cancer. Cancer Chemother Pharmacol 8:139, 1982. *A comprehensive and critical statement on adjuvant therapy.*

Wolmark N, Fisher B: Surgery in the primary treatment of breast cancer. Breast Cancer Res Treat 1:339, 1982. *The NSABP experience with primary treatment.*

Wynder EL, MacCormack FA, Stellman SD: The epidemiology of breast cancer in 785 United States caucasian women. Cancer 41:2341, 1978. *A review of demographic and hormone-related risk factors with a good review of the literature.*

240. POLYGLANDULAR DISORDERS

John N. Loeb

A number of different syndromes are characterized by autonomous hyperfunction or hypofunction of more than one endocrine gland. Although the majority of these syndromes are clearly of genetic origin, the fundamental mechanisms leading to hyperfunction or hypofunction thus far remain unknown in any instance. The syndromes to be considered in this chapter are those in which dysfunction appears to be autonomous within the affected endocrine glands themselves; multiple glandular abnormalities resulting from primary abnormalities in the hypothalamic-pituitary axis or to various locally infiltrative processes are discussed elsewhere.

SYNDROMES CHARACTERIZED BY MULTIPLE ENDOCRINE GLAND HYPERFUNCTION OR NEOPLASIA

The major syndromes characterized by multiple endocrine hyperfunction are those of multiple endocrine adenomatosis (MEA) or multiple endocrine neoplasia (MEN). A number of these syndromes are clearly inherited as autosomal dominant traits and are clinically distinct. The term MEN is now generally preferred because it is more inclusive, comprising both hyperplastic and carcinomatous as well as adenomatous abnormalities. Table 240–1 compares the clinical features of some of these syndromes.

MULTIPLE ENDOCRINE NEOPLASIA, TYPE 1 (WERMER'S SYNDROME). In 1954 Wermer reported the familial occurrence of *multiple tumors of the anterior pituitary, parathyroid glands, and pancreatic islet cells* in association with a high incidence of peptic ulcer. This complex of abnormalities is now most commonly referred to as multiple endocrine neoplasia, type 1 (MEN 1). The syndrome may also include tumor or hyperfunction of the adrenal and thyroid glands, but the relation of these latter endocrinopathies to the underlying genetic abnormality is less well defined. Although it has been proposed that the fundamental defect in MEN 1 is an abnormal differentiation of neural crest tissue, current evidence in support of this hypothesis is by no means conclusive (see also below, under MEN 2).

More than half of patients with MEN 1 have adenomas of two or more different endocrine glands, and involvement of three or more different glands is seen in up to 20 per cent of affected individuals. The approximate frequencies of glandular involvement in patients exhibiting any manifestation of endocrine hyperfunction are, in descending order, parathyroids (90 to 95 per cent), pancreatic islet cells (30 to 35 per cent), and anterior pituitary (15 to 20 per cent). Less commonly there may be hyperfunction (adenomas) of the adrenal cortex and thyroid gland; carcinoid tumors have been reported occasionally. Initial manifestations are most commonly detected in middle age, and many years may elapse between the manifestation of the first endocrine abnormality and ensuing ones. The clinical course is highly variable, depending in part upon which glands are affected and whether the neoplasm results in hypersecretion or instead in compression of surrounding normal glandular tissue with concomitant loss of function. By far the greatest majority of patients (over 90 per cent) have problems related to hypercalcemia, peptic ulcer, hypoglycemia, or pituitary dysfunction. In patients with pituitary neoplasms symptoms are most commonly attributable to pituitary enlargement, with headache or visual-field abnormalities, or to hypopituitarism. Acromegaly, the galactorrhea-amenorrhea syndrome with hyperprolactinemia, and, considerably more rarely, Cushing's syndrome, may also be seen.

Parathyroid gland involvement is by far the most common manifestation of MEN 1 but may be clinically "silent" for many years. Patients may have a history of kidney stones or progressive renal failure as the first manifestation of hyperparathyroidism, or, much more commonly, hypercalcemia may be detected incidentally upon routine screening. All four parathyroid glands are frequently abnormal, and pathologic study may reveal either hyperplasia or multiple adenomas. Parathyroid carcinoma is rare.

Islet cell tumors of the pancreas can be either adenomas (generally multiple) or carcinomas; they may be preceded by diffuse hyperplasia of islet tissue and most typically secrete excess gastrin. Hypersecretion of gastrin may give rise to the *Zollinger-Ellison syndrome* (see Ch. 99) characterized by marked hypersecretion of hydrochloric acid, peptic ulceration (sometimes involving esophageal, distal duodenal, or jejunal sites), and, often, diarrhea. Abdominal pain, bleeding, and perforation are more common than in ordinary instances of peptic ulcer, and radiographic signs consistent with hypersecretion of gastric acid (e.g., hypertrophied gastric rugae) are frequently seen. Many patients in whom the Zollinger-Ellison syndrome initially appears in isolation represent a subset of individuals with MEN 1; approximately half of such patients ultimately develop manifestations of additional endocrine neoplasms.

Hypersecretion of insulin by islet cell neoplasms may produce hypoglycemia as an initial manifestation, whereas the elaboration of other substances may, considerably more rarely, result in a variety of other syndromes. Vasoactive intestinal peptide and prostaglandins have been proposed as agents possibly responsible for the intractable watery diarrhea that can be seen even in the absence of hypersecretion of gastrin and the Zollinger-Ellison syndrome, and hypersecretion of glucagon with hyperglycemia, weight loss, and a characteristic skin rash ("necrotizing migratory erythema") has been reported. Islet cell tumors may also secrete pancreatic polypeptide or, rarely, ACTH or serotonin.

Symptoms caused by *pituitary adenomas* in MEN 1 are most commonly due to local encroachment of tumor on other structures, with headache or visual-field abnormalities, or to deficiency of one or more of the tropic hormones. Many of these tumors secrete prolactin and may give rise to the galactorrhea-amenorrhea syndrome. More rarely there is hypersecretion of growth hormone with resulting acromegaly. Hypersecretion of ACTH in MEN 1 is almost always attributable to an ectopic (pancreatic) site.

Adrenocortical hyperfunction may be due to ectopic production of ACTH or to independently functioning adrenal adenomas or carcinomas. Functioning adenomas most commonly elaborate hydrocortisone, giving rise to signs of glucocorticoid excess, but predominant secretion of aldosterone has been reported in rare instances. Hyperfunction of the *thyroid* gland has been reported least frequently of all, and, in part owing to the high incidence of thyroid abnormalities in the population at large, it is possible that sporadic instances of thyroid hyperfunction in MEN 1 represent incidental occurrences unrelated to the underlying genetic abnormality. Adenomas, thyroiditis, and rarely papillary and follicular cell carcinomas have all been reported in association with MEN 1; medullary carcinomas are *not* a part of this syndrome (cf. MEN 2, below). *Other tumors* that can form a part of the clinical picture of MEN 1 include schwannomas, multiple cutaneous lipomas, thymomas, and both bronchial and small intestinal carcinoids.

Management of the various manifestations of MEN 1 is, for the most part, similar to management of the identical manifestations when they occur in sporadic form and hence is considered elsewhere in this textbook. As indicated above, parathyroid involvement, when it occurs, frequently involves more than one gland, and histopathology far more commonly reveals diffuse hyperplasia than a single adenoma. In such instances a number of surgeons now advocate total parathyroidectomy with reimplantation of a glandular fragment in a location conveniently accessible to subsequent exploration if necessary (e.g., the muscle of the forearm). Management of severe peptic ulceration in MEN 1 requires either long-term cimetidine therapy or near-total gastrectomy—rather than an attempt to eliminate the source of excess gastrin—since hypersecretion of gastrin by islet-cell tissue in this syndrome is almost always attributable to either multiple tumors or diffuse hyperplasia.

Because of the sporadic nature of the sequential manifestations of this syndrome, it is important to follow affected individuals with particular attention to the development of new abnormalities. Once the diagnosis has been established in a given patient and baseline films of the sella turcica and prolactin levels have proved to be normal, the major requisite is a careful interval history and a periodic (e.g., yearly) determination of the serum calcium and phosphorus. Because of the high incidence of affected first-degree relatives, such family members should be carefully evaluated for evidence of the syndrome.

MULTIPLE ENDOCRINE NEOPLASIA, TYPE 2 (SIPPLE'S SYNDROME). A second and entirely distinct syndrome, multiple endocrine neoplasia, type 2 (MEN 2 or MEN 2A), is characterized by *medullary carcinoma of the thyroid, pheochromocytoma, and parathyroid hyperplasia.* First partially described by Sipple in 1961, this syndrome, like MEN 1, is inherited as an autosomal dominant trait. The pheochromocytomas are frequently multi-

TABLE 240–1. COMPARISON OF THE CLINICAL FEATURES OF THE MAJOR SYNDROMES CHARACTERIZED BY MULTIPLE ENDOCRINE GLAND HYPERFUNCTION

Endocrine Abnormality	MEN 1*	MEN 2 ("2A")*	MEN 3 ("2B")*
Hyperparathyroidism [Hyperplasia or multiple adenomas]	90–95%, with high incidence of hypercalcemia and nephrolithiasis	25–30%, but only 10% with frank hypercalcemia or nephrolithiasis	Rare
Pancreatic islet cell hyperfunction [Hyperplasia, adenomas, or carcinoma, with hypersecretion (*e.g.*, of gastrin or insulin)]	30–35%	—†	—
Pituitary adenomas ["Nonfunctioning" or with hypersecretion of prolactin (common) or growth hormone (rare)]	15–20%	—	—
Multiple cutaneous lipomas	20%	—	—
Thyroid adenomas, adrenal cortical adenomas, carcinoid tumors	Rare	—	—
Thyroid C-cell hyperplasia with hypersecretion of calcitonin ± medullary carcinoma	—	"100%"‡	"100%"‡
Pheochromocytoma	—	Probably > 20%	Probably > 20%
Multiple mucosal neuromas; marfanoid habitus	—	—	Characteristic
Inheritance	Autosomal dominant	Autosomal dominant	Autosomal dominant, but frequently "sporadic"

*Percentages indicate approximate frequencies among affected individuals manifesting hyperfunction of at least one endocrine gland.
†— = *not* part of the syndrome.
‡Generally taken to be an essential component of the syndrome.

ple, involving both adrenal glands as well as extra-adrenal sites, and the medullary carcinoma of the thyroid generally appears to be multifocal in origin. A particularly convenient and virtually constant feature of the medullary thyroid carcinomas is the hypersecretion of calcitonin, which serves as a useful marker for the presence of this neoplasm. Elevated levels of calcitonin, either under basal conditions or in response to the provocative stimuli of calcium and pentagastrin infusions, are an indication of parafollicular C-cell hyperplasia in the thyroid gland and may herald the presence of the genetic abnormality well before pathologic changes appear that are unequivocally malignant. As in the instance of the pancreatic adenomas in MEN 1, the medullary carcinomas of the thyroid in MEN 2 may secrete a variety of hormones that are not secreted by the corresponding normal tissues: ACTH, prolactin, histaminase, vasoactive intestinal peptide, serotonin, and a number of prostaglandins. Only rarely does medullary carcinoma of the thyroid present as a palpable mass. Pheochromocytoma is observed in only about one half of affected individuals, and hyperparathyroidism in about one quarter. Only about 10 per cent of individuals with MEN 2 exhibit hypercalcemia or nephrolithiasis (cf. the much higher incidence of overt hyperparathyroidism in MEN 1). Glial tumors and meningiomas may also be seen in MEN 2, but occur far less frequently.

It has been suggested that MEN 2 represents a form of neuroectodermal dysplasia in which so-called APUD cells (cells capable of *a*mine *p*recursor *u*ptake and *d*ecarboxylation and possessing rather characteristic histologic staining properties)—following their normal embryonic migration to the foregut and subsequent localization in a variety of endocrine tissues—later become neoplastic and secrete excessive amounts of hormone in response to a specific genetic defect. Although the evidence for a common APUD cell origin is somewhat better for MEN 2 than it is for MEN 1, it is still by no means wholly convincing. In particular, the high incidence of parathyroid involvement is difficult to reconcile with this theory, since the bulk of present evidence suggests an epithelial rather than a neural crest origin for this tissue.

The pheochromocytomas of MEN 2 are generally benign and are treated surgically. Because they are frequently bilateral, an anterior surgical approach is often recommended; CT scan, multiple-site venous sampling for catecholamines, and angiography can all be helpful in planning surgery. Medullary carcinoma of the thyroid, on the other hand, runs a typically malignant course, and, because of its multifocal nature, requires total thyroidectomy. Elevated levels of calcitonin per se constitute a sufficient indication for total thyroidectomy, even when the tumor is otherwise clinically silent. The tumor is frequently slowly growing, and limited node dissection is thus justified; completeness of tumor removal and the possibility of subsequent recurrence are both conveniently monitored by serum calcitonin levels. The isolated finding of medullary carcinoma of the thyroid should prompt a particularly careful inquiry into the family history since it is likely that at least 10 per cent of such tumors are familial.

MULTIPLE ENDOCRINE NEOPLASIA, TYPE 3 (MUCOSAL NEUROMA SYNDROME). This syndrome (MEN 3 or MEN 2B) resembles MEN 2 but differs in four important respects: (1) The medullary carcinoma of the thyroid and the pheochromocytomas may be accompanied by striking and often disfiguring neuromas of the lips, buccal mucosa, and tongue, as well as by ganglioneuromas of the gastrointestinal tract, thickened corneal nerves visible upon slit-lamp examination, and cafe-áu-lait spots, neuromas, or neurofibromas of the skin; (2) the body habitus may somewhat resemble that seen in patients with Marfan's syndrome; (3) parathyroid hyperplasia sufficient to result in frank hyperalcemia is rare; and (4) mean survival time in MEN 3 is considerably shorter than that in MEN 2 (30 versus 60 years). In contrast to MEN 1 and MEN 2, MEN 3 is frequently sporadic, a history of affected family members being obtainable in not more than half of the cases.

McCUNE-ALBRIGHT SYNDROME. In 1937, McCune and Albright and their associates both described a syndrome characterized by a triad of *polyostotic fibrous dysplasia, cafe-áu-lait pigmentation of the skin* (typically over the forehead, nuchal or sacral areas, or buttocks), and *precocious puberty of the female.* The precocious puberty, although predominantly seen in the female, may occur in males as well. This syndrome may be accompanied by a variety of other endocrine abnormalities, including pituitary hyperfunction (with Cushing's syndrome, acromegaly, or gigantism), bilateral pheochromocytomas, hyperthyroidism, and hypercorticism resulting from adrenal adenoma. Frank malignant disease has not been described. Although the sexual precocity appears to be hypothalamic in origin, patients with adrenal adenomas and hyperthyroidism have been found to have low plasma levels of ACTH and TSH, respectively. The cause of the bone lesions is unknown. The disease appears to be sporadic.

SYNDROMES CHARACTERIZED BY MULTIPLE ENDOCRINE GLAND HYPOFUNCTION

Syndromes characterized by hypofunction of multiple endocrine organs will be discussed under the separate headings of Schmidt's syndrome and the syndrome of polyglandular deficiency associated with mucocutaneous candidiasis. As noted below, however, evidence that the two syndromes actually represent different entities is incomplete. Table 240–2 compares the clinical features of these syndromes.

MULTIPLE ENDOCRINE DEFICIENCY SYNDROME (SCHMIDT'S SYNDROME). In 1926, Schmidt described two patients with biglandular failure characterized by *idiopathic Addison's disease and lymphocytic thyroiditis.* This syndrome has subsequently been expanded to include "primary" failure of other endocrine glands, including the gonads, parathyroids, and endocrine pancreas, as well as a number of nonendocrine abnormalities of presumed autoimmune origin (see below). Virtually any

TABLE 240–2. COMPARISON OF THE CLINICAL FEATURES OF THE MAJOR SYNDROMES CHARACTERIZED BY MULTIPLE ENDOCRINE GLAND HYPOFUNCTION

	Multiple Endocrine Deficiency Syndrome (Schmidt's Syndrome)	Polyglandular Deficiency with Mucocutaneous Candidiasis
Hypoadrenalism	Common	Common
Hypothyroidism	Common	Less common
Hypoparathyroidism	Less common	Common
Gonadal failure	Less common	Less common
Diabetes mellitus	Less common	Rare
Pituitary insufficiency	Rare	Rare
Autoantibodies to endocrine tissues and gastric parietal cells	Often present	Often present
Sex distribution	Strong female predominance	Female preponderance about 4 : 1
Inheritance	Usually "sporadic"; relatively high frequency of certain HLA alleles	Generally inherited as autosomal recessive; no apparent HLA association
Time of onset	Usually becomes evident during adult life	Typically becomes evident during childhood preceded by chronic mucocutaneous moniliasis
Other associated "autoimmune" diseases and characteristics	Pernicious anemia; celiac disease; alopecia; vitiligo; antibody-mediated IgA deficiency; myasthenia gravis; isolated red-cell aplasia	Pernicious anemia; celiac disease; alopecia; vitiligo; IgA deficiency; hypergammaglobulinemia; chronic active hepatitis; proliferative glomerulonephritis

combination of the foregoing endocrine deficiencies may appear in a single individual. The order of appearance is extremely variable; a lag of as much as 17 years has been observed in the manifestation of sequential deficiencies. Hypothyroidism and hypoadrenalism are particularly common; diabetes mellitus, hypoparathyroidism, and gonadal failure are somewhat less so. The frequencies of the different glandular failures probably vary greatly with ascertainment; if one considers juvenile-onset diabetes mellitus as part of the syndrome, the association of this with autoimmune thyroid disease may be the most commonly encountered combination.

Characteristic of this syndrome is the presence of autoantibodies to endocrine tissue and at times to gastric parietal cells as well. Such antibodies are often detectable before the appearance of clinical glandular insufficiency and are a hallmark of syndromes of "idiopathic" endocrine failure. Their presence has been implicated in the pathogenesis of the glandular destruction itself rather than merely as reflecting an immune response to tissue antigens released during antecedent glandular degeneration. Thus, for example, approximately two thirds of patients with idiopathic Addison's disease are reported to have autoantibodies to adrenal tissue, whereas such antibodies are generally absent in patients whose adrenal insufficiency is secondary to tuberculous destruction. About twice as many females are affected with idiopathic adrenal insufficiency as males. Although most cases of multiple deficiency syndromes are sporadic, their occasional appearance in kindreds, as well as the relatively high gene frequency of the HLA-B8 and HLA-Dw3 alleles in affected persons, provides strong evidence for a genetic component contributing to the pathogenesis of polyglandular failure. Other "autoimmune" diseases that may accompany the aforementioned endocrine deficiencies include pernicious anemia, celiac disease, myasthenia gravis, alopecia, vitiligo, isolated red-cell aplasia, and antibody-mediated IgA deficiency. Because it occurs in the same families and has the same HLA associations, Graves' disease is considered by many to be another facet of the syndrome.

Although the constellation of adrenal, thyroid, and gonadal failure in a single patient can easily be confused with primary pituitary insufficiency, measurement of the appropriate tropic hormones now permits a ready differentiation of the two syndromes. Occasionally the simultaneous presence of hyperpigmentation in such an individual suggests a diagnosis of primary adrenal failure on "clinical" grounds alone. Because of the sporadic appearance and variable sequence of subsequent endocrine deficiencies, patients with a proven idiopathic endocrine deficiency should be periodically screened for evidence of additional endocrine involvement.

POLYGLANDULAR DEFICIENCY ASSOCIATED WITH MUCOCUTANEOUS CANDIDIASIS. A clinical picture somewhat different from that of Schmidt's syndrome is presented by patients with the so-called candidiasis-endocrinopathy syndrome. Characteristically this syndrome is dominated by the presence of extensive mucocutaneous candidiasis that appears in early childhood and is followed by the development of idiopathic adrenal insufficiency or hypoparathyroidism or both. Most typically, but not invariably, the appearance of these endocrinopathies postdates the acquisition of chronic monilial infection (mean age of onset, 13 versus 3 years, respectively). As in Schmidt's syndrome, antibodies against endocrine tissues are frequently demonstrable, and pernicious anemia with antibodies against gastric parietal cells may also be present. Diabetes mellitus, in contrast, is relatively rare. Also contrasting with Schmidt's syndrome, which most typically becomes evident in adult life, is the fact that there is no apparent association with the presence of specific HLA alleles, and the apparent inheritance of the syndrome as an autosomal recessive trait. Chronic active hepatitis and proliferative glomerulonephritis have also been reported. The mucocutaneous candidiasis is associated with hypergammaglobulinemia, IgA deficiency, and anergy to *Candida albicans*, and typically is relatively resistant to therapy. No evidence for disseminated candidiasis has been found in autopsied individuals, nor has *Candida* yet been cultured from an affected endocrine gland.

Albright F, Butler AM, Hampton AO, Smith P: Syndrome characterized by osteitis fibrosa disseminata, areas of pigmentation and endocrine dysfunction, with precocious puberty in females. N Engl J Med 216:727, 1937. *One of the two classic descriptions of the McCune-Albright syndrome. Excellent figures.*

Eisenbarth GS, Wilson PW, Ward F, Buckley C, Lebovitz H: The polyglandular failure syndrome: Disease inheritance, HLA type, and immune function. Ann Intern Med 91:528, 1979. *Excellent review summarizing evidence for association of the syndrome of familial polyglandular failure with the HLA-B8 allele.*

Irvine WJ, Barnes EW: Adrenocortical insufficiency. Clin Endocrinol Metab 1:549, 1972. *Exhaustive review contrasting the characteristics of idiopathic and other types of primary adrenal insufficiency. Contains a wealth of material on the association between idiopathic Addison's disease and other examples of idiopathic end-organ failure.*

Marx SJ, Spiegel AM, Levine MA, Rizzoli RE, Lasker RD, Santora AC, Downs RW Jr, Aurbach GD: Familial hypocalciuric hypercalcemia: The relation to primary parathyroid hyperplasia. N Engl J Med 307:416, 1982. *Excellent review of hereditary causes of primary parathyroid hyperplasia, including explicit discussion of the different MEN syndromes.*

Prosser PR, Karam JH, Townsend JJ, Forsham PH: Prolactin-secreting pituitary adenomas in multiple endocrine adenomatosis, type I. Ann Intern Med 91:41, 1979. *Evidence for a high incidence of prolactin-secreting pituitary tumors in MEN I.*

Schimke RN: Syndromes with multiple endocrine gland involvement. Prog Med Genet (ns) 3:143, 1979. *Concise review providing a rationale for the current classification of polyglandular disorders. Useful bibliography.*

Schimke RN: Genetic aspects of multiple endocrine neoplasia. Annu Rev Med 35:25, 1984. *A useful recent review.*

Trence DL, Morley JE, Handwerger BS: Polyglandular autoimmune syndromes. Am J Med 77:107, 1984. *An up-to-date recent review of these interesting disorders supplemented by 110 references.*

241. THE ADRENAL MEDULLA AND THE SYMPATHETIC NERVOUS SYSTEM

Philip E. Cryer

The sympathochromaffin system consists of two components: (1) the sympathetic nervous system and (2) the chromaffin tissues, including the adrenal medulla. The primary endocrine, neurotransmitter and perhaps paracrine products of the sympathochromaffin system are the catecholamines—epinephrine (Adrenaline), norepinephrine (noradrenaline), and dopamine. Cells of the sympathochromaffin system also contain, and in some instances are known to synthesize and release, a variety of peptides of potential biologic importance, including enkephalins. Their pathophysiologic roles, if any, are unknown.

Catecholamine excess commonly results in hypertension along with typical symptoms. It has long been suspected, but is still not proven, that increased sympathetic nervous system activity is the cause of primary (essential) hypertension. Catecholamine overproduction from chromaffin cell tumors—pheochromocytomas—is an uncommon, but curable, cause of hypertension. Deficient sympathetic neuronal norepinephrine release results in postural (orthostatic) hypotension, a sharp decrease in blood pressure when a person stands. Under certain conditions, deficient adrenomedullary epinephrine secretion results in hypoglycemia. These three prominent examples of sympathochromaffin pathophysiology are discussed in the paragraphs that follow. Possible roles of the sympathochromaffin system in the pathophysiology of a variety of human disorders—such as cardiac, hepatic, and renal failure, diabetes, asthma, thyroid disease, myocardial infarction, and cardiac arrhythmias, among others—are emerging but will not be discussed here.

PHYSIOLOGY OF THE SYMPATHOCHROMAFFIN SYSTEM

CATECHOLAMINE BIOSYNTHESIS. The term *catecholamines* is often used to refer to epinephrine and norepinephrine, although dopamine is also a catecholamine, i.e., has the dihydroxyphenyl ("catechol") ring structure and an amine side chain (Fig. 241–1). The catecholamines are synthesized from the amino acid tyrosine, which is derived from the diet or formed by hydroxylation of the essential amino acid phenylalanine. Tyrosine hydroxylase, the enzyme that converts tyrosine to dihydroxyphenylalanine (dopa), is the rate-limiting enzyme in catecholamine biosynthesis. In the presence of a nonspecific decarboxylase, dopa is converted to dopamine, which is the final product in some systems (e.g., interneurons in the sympathetic ganglia). After transport into cytoplasmic vesicles (storage granules), dopamine can be converted to norepinephrine in the presence of dopamine β-hydroxylase. Norepinephrine is the final product in sympathetic postganglionic neurons. Other tissues, such as the adrenal medulla, have cells that also contain phenylethanolamine-N-methyltransferase, the enzyme that converts norepinephrine to epinephrine, which is the final product of those cells.

Catecholamines are stored in cytoplasmic granules and released from the cell by exocytosis in response to neural stimulation. The major determinants of tyrosine hydroxylase activity and synthesis, and thus of catecholamine biosynthesis, are product inhibition and the frequency of transsynaptic neural stimulation of catecholamine-releasing cells. Product inhibition decreases the activity of tyrosine hydroxylase; repetitive stimulation increases synthesis of the enzyme.

CATECHOLAMINE DEGRADATION AND ELIMINATION. Catecholamines are degraded by two principal enzyme systems, catechol-O-methyltransferase (COMT) and monoamine oxidase (MAO) (Fig. 241–1). COMT converts norepinephrine and epinephrine to their respective O-methyl derivatives, the metanephrines (normetanephrine and metanephrine). MAO converts norepinephrine and epinephrine to dihydroxymandelic acid. These intermediates, the metanephrines and dihydroxymandelic acid, can then serve as substrates for MAO and COMT respectively, resulting in their conversion to the major end product of extra-CNS catecholamine metabolism, vanillylmandelic acid (VMA). Dopamine metabolism (not shown in Figure 241–1) by MAO and COMT leads to the formation of

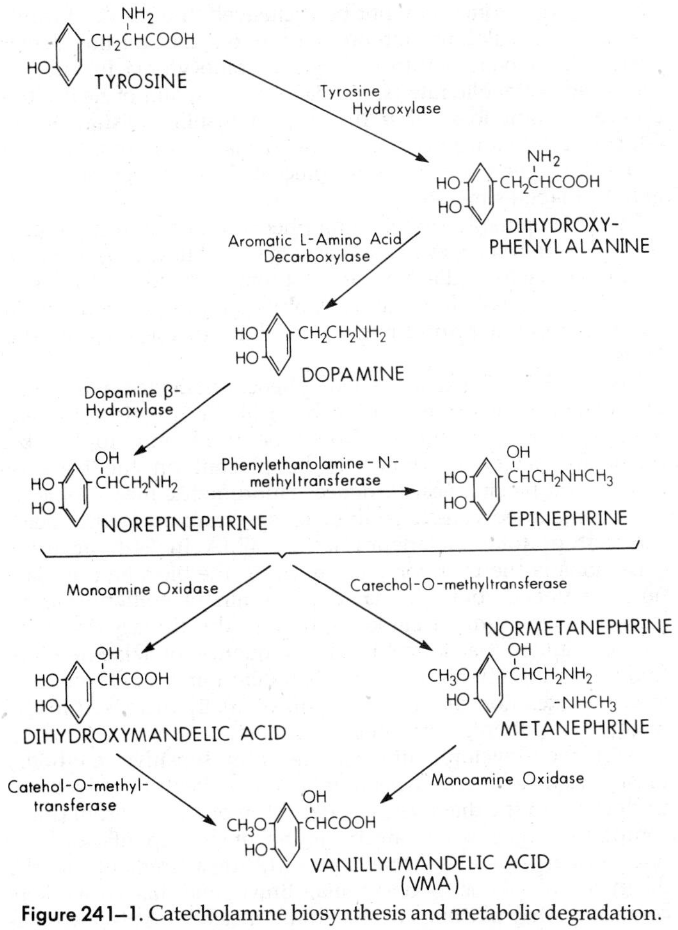

Figure 241–1. Catecholamine biosynthesis and metabolic degradation.

homovanillic acid (HVA), which is identical to VMA except that it lacks a hydroxyl group on the β carbon of the side chain.

In general, catecholamine degradation within the sympathochromaffin cells is via MAO, whereas that of released catecholamines is via COMT. Released catecholamines are also conjugated, largely to sulfate in humans, and this may be another important route of inactivation. The relative importance of conjugation in relation to cellular uptake and degradation by MAO and COMT remains to be established. Nonetheless, 60 to 80 per cent of plasma epinephrine and norepinephrine and roughly half of the catecholamines excreted in the urine are conjugated.

Catecholamines are cleared rapidly from the circulation. Plasma half-times are 1 to 2 minutes. Clearance is largely extrarenal; less than 5 per cent appears in the urine unaltered.

BIOLOGIC ROLES OF THE CATECHOLAMINES. Epinephrine, norepinephrine, and dopamine are neurotransmitters in the CNS. Outside of the CNS, epinephrine is a hormone of the adrenal medulla, and norepinephrine is primarily the neurotransmitter of sympathetic postganglionic neurons. Dopamine is probably also a neurotransmitter, although its physiologic role has not been defined clearly.

Neurally regulated secretion of epinephrine from extra-adrenal chromaffin tissue (not sympathetic neurons) occurs, but in the absence of the adrenal medulla even stimulated plasma epinephrine levels in adults are not high enough to produce measurable biologic effects. Biologic actions of extra-adrenal epinephrine, if any, must be paracrine/neurotransmitter, not hormonal, in nature, at least in adults. Thus, epinephrine functions primarily as a hormone of the adrenal medulla and its plasma concentration is a valid index of its secretion.

Norepinephrine is released from axon terminals of sympathetic postganglionic neurons in direct relation to adrenergic receptors on innervated target cells. Most released norepinephrine is dissipated locally by reuptake into an axon terminal ($uptake_1$), where it is either stored in vesicles or metabolized, or by uptake into other cells adjacent to the synaptic cleft ($uptake_2$), where it is metabolized. Only a small fraction escapes into the circulation. The plasma norepinephrine concentration is a reasonable index of sympathetic neural activity under common physiologic conditions, at least in the basal state and during upright activity in humans. However, under some conditions, such as hypoglycemia, substantial amounts of norepinephrine (along with large amounts of epinephrine), are released from chromaffin tissues, specifically the adrenal medulla. Under such conditions the plasma norepinephrine concentration is clearly not an index of sympathetic neural activity. During vigorous physical activity and in a variety of pathologic states such as surgery, acute myocardial infarction, and diabetic ketoacidosis, circulating norepinephrine is probably derived from both the sympathetic nerves and the adrenal medulla, and its concentrations can be high enough to produce measurable effects. Under these conditions norepinephrine may function as a hormone as well as a neurotransmitter.

This physiology is relevant to the clinical use of plasma catecholamine measurements. Norepinephrine release from sympathetic neurons in amounts sufficient to produce biologically active norepinephrine concentrations in the synaptic cleft can be associated with very small, even undetectable, increments in its plasma concentration. On the other hand, if norepinephrine is released directly into the circulation (as from a pheochromocytoma) substantial increments in its plasma concentration are required to produce biologically active synaptic cleft concentrations.

BIOLOGIC ACTIONS OF THE CATECHOLAMINES. Catecholamines produce a variety of hemodynamic and metabolic effects. These are the result of catecholamine occupancy of adrenergic receptors (adrenoceptors) on the surface of target cells and a consequent series of intra-membrane and intracellular biochemical events. Adrenergic receptors are divided into

α- and β-adrenergic receptors, which are subdivided into α_1- and α_2-adrenergic receptors and β_1- and β_2-adrenergic receptors on the basis of measurements of the responses to various agonists and antagonists and the binding of a variety of ligands (generally antagonists) and competition for binding of these ligands by agonists and antagonists in vitro. In general, β-adrenergic receptors are linked through a stimulatory guanine nucleotide regulatory protein to adenylate cyclase, and α_2- (but not α_1-) adrenergic receptors are linked through an inhibitory protein to adenylate cyclase. A discussion of adrenergic receptors is beyond the scope of this chapter although selected examples are given.

Catecholamines increase the rate and force of myocardial contraction (β_1) and produce vasoconstriction (α) in most vascular beds, although vasodilatation (β_2) occurs in some vascular beds, e.g., those of skeletal muscle. Norepinephrine produces increased vascular resistance and blood pressure (systolic and diastolic); the increased blood pressure reflexively limits the increase in heart rate. Probably because it has a higher affinity than norepinephrine for β_2-adrenergic receptors, epinephrine normally produces a somewhat different pattern: increased systolic, but not diastolic, blood pressure and increased heart rate.

Catecholamines increase the plasma glucose concentration through complex actions. These involve both stimulation of hepatic glucose production and limitation of glucose utilization and are mediated by both direct and indirect mechanisms. Foremost among the indirect mechanisms is limitation of insulin secretion (α). The direct actions are largely β mediated. Catecholamines also stimulate lipolysis, ketogenesis, glycolysis, and mobilization of amino acids such as alanine. They also increase thermogenesis.

Symptoms that occur when the sympathochromaffin system is activated include palpitations, anxiety, headache, and diaphoresis. All but the last are attributable to released catecholamines; diaphoresis has been attributed to a sympathetic cholinergic mechanism.

PHEOCHROMOCYTOMA

Pheochromocytomas are catecholamine-releasing tumors that typically produce hypertension. They are an uncommon cause of hypertension; fewer than 1 in 200 hypertensive patients harbors a pheochromocytoma. Yet it is important to detect a pheochromocytoma for several reasons: (1) Hypertension due to a pheochromocytoma is usually curable by surgical removal of the tumor. (2) Patients with a pheochromocytoma are at risk for a lethal hypertensive paroxysm. (3) Some pheochromocytomas (probably less than 5 per cent) are malignant; early detection and removal would be expected to reduce the frequency of metastatic disease. Parenthetically, malignancy is established convincingly only by proven metastases; histologic criteria in the primary tumor are not reliable. (4) The presence of pheochromocytomas can be a clue to the presence of associated endocrine and nonendocrine familial disorders (Ch. 240). Pheochromocytomas are components of the multiple endocrine neoplasia type 2 (MEN 2) and type 3 (MEN 3) syndromes. These familial disorders are inherited as autosomal dominant traits. MEN 2 includes medullary carcinoma of the thyroid, primary hyperparathyroidism, and pheochromocytoma. MEN 3 includes medullary carcinoma of the thyroid, multiple mucosal neuromas, and pheochromocytoma. Pheochromocytomas are not a component of the MEN 1 syndrome (pituitary and pancreatic adenomas and hyperparathyroidism). Familial pheochromocytomas also occur as an isolated disorder, in neurofibromatosis, and in the von Hippel-Lindau syndrome.

PATHOLOGY. Pheochromocytomas arise from chromaffin cells. Chromaffin cells are widespread and associated with sympathetic ganglia during fetal life. Postnatally most chromaffin cells degenerate; the major residual clusters of chromaffin cells comprise the adrenal medulla. Thus, it is not surprising that approximately 90 per cent of pheochromocytomas arise from the adrenal medulla. Extra-adrenal pheochromocytomas (paragangliomas) have been found in sites ranging from the carotid body to the pelvic floor. However, the majority are associated with sympathetic ganglia in the abdomen and most of the others with ganglia in the posterior mediastinum. Multiple pheochromocytomas, including bilateral adrenomedullary tumors, occur in up to 10 per cent of apparently sporadic cases. Bilateral adrenomedullary pheochromocytomas, with or without extra-adrenal tumors, are the rule in familial pheochromocytoma. Bilateral adrenomedullary hyperplasia, thought to be a precursor to pheochromocytoma, has been found in members of affected families.

The vast majority of pheochromocytomas release norepinephrine, and most also release some epinephrine. Rarely, a pheochromocytoma releases epinephrine predominantly or even exclusively.

CLINICAL MANIFESTATIONS. The clinical manifestations of pheochromocytomas are commonly due to the effects of released catecholamines and only rarely to the mass effect of the tumor. Common symptoms are *headache, palpitations,* and *diaphoresis.* Less common symptoms include abdominal or chest pain, gastrointestinal symptoms, weakness, or visual symptoms. Symptoms are typically paroxysmal and associated with increments in blood pressure. Hypertension is sometimes truly intermittent. In many cases, hypertension is sustained, but exhibits marked fluctuations with peak values occurring during symptomatic episodes. In general, these paroxysmal clinical expressions can be explained by episodic catecholamine release. Plasma catecholamine levels are higher during symptomatic, hypertensive episodes than during asymptomatic, less hypertensive, or even normotensive intervals. The event(s) that precipitates episodic catecholamine release is usually not identifiable. However, the relationship between plasma catecholamine concentrations and blood pressure is not tight. This may reflect contrasting effects of norepinephrine and epinephrine but raises the possibility that hypertension in a patient with a pheochromocytoma may not be exclusively the result of direct effects of circulating norepinephrine on the cardiovascular system. Metabolic features of pheochromocytoma include an increased metabolic rate (some patients complain of heat intolerance, weight loss, or both) and an insulin-resistant state. Glucose intolerance occurs, but overt diabetes is unusual and probably reflects a coexistent defect in insulin secretion, i.e., genetic diabetes mellitus.

The rare epinephrine-releasing pheochromocytomas can produce different paroxysms. These may include hypotension, prominent tachycardia, noncardiac pulmonary edema, and cardiac arrhythmias. It is conceivable that tumor products in addition to epinephrine might contribute to these manifestations.

DIAGNOSIS. The diagnosis of pheochromocytoma is based upon clinical suspicion and biochemical confirmation. In general, radiographic studies should be used only to localize pheochromocytomas known to be present on the basis of clinical and biochemical evidence. Fluorometric measurements of unconjugated catecholamines or spectrophotometric measurement of total metanephrines or VMA in 24-hour urine collections is the traditional approach to the biochemical diagnosis of pheochromocytoma. If predominant epinephrine release is suspected on clinical grounds, the urinary catecholamines can be fractionated. The frequency of false-negative findings is slightly higher with VMA determinations. Nonetheless, the excretion of all three is substantially increased in the majority of patients with pheochromocytomas.

With the development of sufficiently sensitive methods, plasma catecholamine measurements have been effectively introduced into the diagnosis of pheochromocytoma. From direct comparison of plasma catecholamine measurements and 24-hour urinary metanephrine and VMA measurements in the diagnosis of pheochromocytoma, Bravo and his co-workers concluded that plasma catecholamine measurements were superior because there was less overlap in the data between affected and unaffected hypertensive patients (Fig. 241–2). However, the two approaches yield somewhat different information. Urinary measurements provide an index of catecholamine release integrated over time. Thus they might reflect intermittent plasma catecholamine elevations that could be missed by plasma measurements that provide information relevant only to a time frame of a few minutes. Conceptually similar is the measurement of catecholamines in platelets.

Most patients with a pheochromocytoma have markedly elevated plasma catecholamine values. Three points warrant emphasis, however. First, occasional patients with pheochromocytomas and typical histories of paroxysms have normal plasma catecholamine concentrations during an asymptomatic, normotensive interval. Second, some patients, commonly those investigated because of family history of pheochromocytoma, have no symptoms or signs and have normal plasma catecholamine concentrations, but are found to have pheochromocytomas. These are not innocent tumors; lethal hypertensive paroxysms have occurred in such patients. Third, patients thought to have predominant epinephrine-secreting pheochromocytomas on clinical grounds can also have substantial overproduction of norepinephrine.

Strict attention to the details of sample collection, handling and storage, the sources of possible biologic variation, and the effects of drugs is critical if diagnostic error is to be avoided in the biochemical assessment of patients with suspected pheochromocytomas. Patients should be studied in the drug-free state if at all possible. Elevated plasma catecholamine concentrations are to be expected during physical or mental stress and in any acute illness. Elevations, at times marked, have been well documented in patients with acute myocardial infarction, shock, burns, diabetic ketoacidosis, and cerebrovascular accidents, as well as during and immediately after surgery. Stable plasma catecholamine elevations also occur in patients with chronic disorders—for example, hypothyroidism, congestive heart failure, chronic obstructive pulmonary disease, anemia, duodenal ulcer, and depression. Lastly, elevated plasma catecholamine concentrations have been found in some, but certainly not all, patients thought to have essential hypertension.

It is my practice to obtain samples for determination of plasma norepinephrine and epinephrine in the basal state, with the patient supine, when pheochromocytoma is suspected. Substantial elevations over reference values provide strong support for the diagnosis of pheochromocytoma and are commonly found in affected patients. Samples are also obtained during symptomatic paroxysms. However, the interpretation of such values is more judgmental since reference values cannot be defined precisely. Patients without pheochromocytoma might be expected to have somewhat elevated plasma norepinephrine and epinephrine levels during such symptomatic episodes. Thus the biochemical diagnosis of pheochromocytoma is more convincingly supported if plasma catecholamine levels are elevated in the basal state and rise further during symptomatic episodes.

It is useful to record the blood pressure and whether or not symptoms are present when plasma samples for catecholamine measurements are drawn from a patient suspected of having a pheochromocytoma. Clearly, normal plasma (or urinary) catecholamine values obtained when the patient is normotensive and free of symptoms do not exclude the presence of a pheochromocytoma. Theoretically, 24-hour urinary catecholamine or metabolite measurements might detect intermittent catecholamine release missed by plasma sampling, so these measurements as well as plasma norepinephrine and epinephrine measurements should be obtained unless the diagnosis is obvious.

Substantial plasma norepinephrine elevations are required to produce hypertension in normal humans (e.g., venous plasma norepinephrine elevations to approximately 1000 pg per milliliter are required to raise the diastolic pressure, and elevations to approximately 2000 pg per milliliter are required to produce diastolic hypertension). Plasma epinephrine elevations within the physiologic range do not raise the diastolic blood pressure. It is reasonable, therefore, to consider normal or even moderately elevated plasma catecholamine levels obtained when the patient is hypertensive to be strong evidence against the diagnosis of pheochromocytoma.

Most patients ultimately found to have pheochromocytomas have distinctly elevated plasma and urinary catecholamine levels. The considerations raised in the preceding paragraphs also apply to patients in whom the diagnosis is less clear cut and to the always difficult problem of the degree of certainty of a negative conclusion. Obviously one can never be absolutely certain during life that a given patient does not have a pheochromocytoma. As in many other areas of medicine, clinical judgment must be based upon probability.

Recently, oral clonidine (0.3 mg) has been found to suppress plasma catecholamine levels in hypertensive patients without pheochromocytoma but not in patients with pheochromocytoma. Thus the clonidine suppression test has been suggested to distinguish patients with primary hypertension with elevated basal plasma norepinephrine levels from those with hyperten-

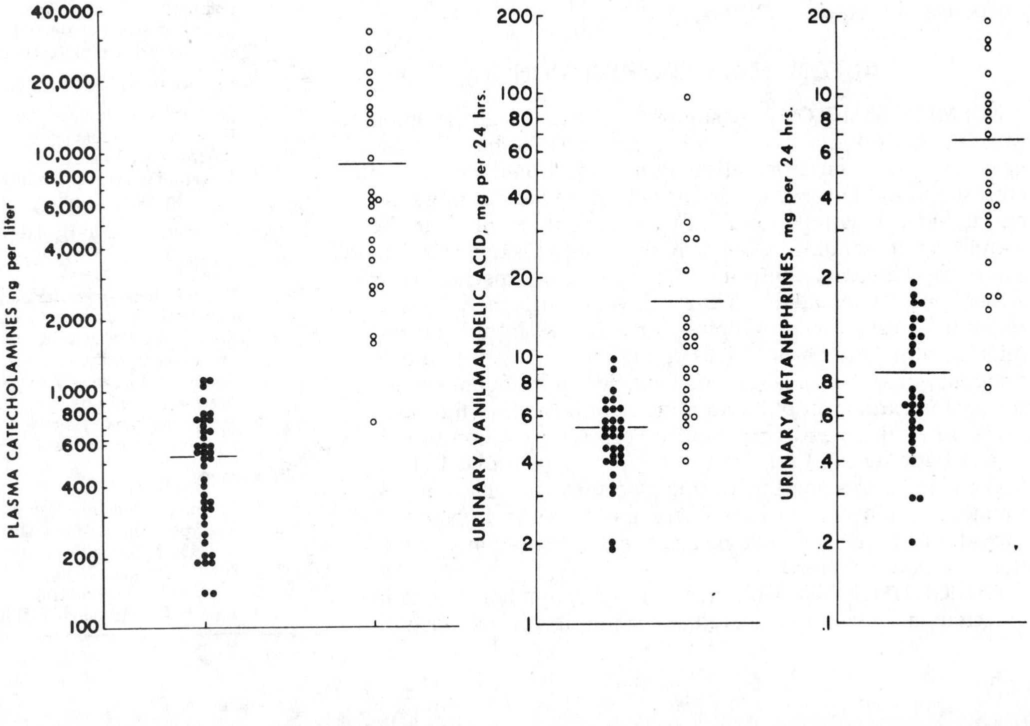

Figure 241–2. Plasma total catecholamine concentrations and urinary vanillylmandelic acid and metanephrine excretions in patients with pheochromocytomas (open symbols) and in hypertensive controls (closed symbols). Note the semi-logarithmic scales. (From Bravo EL, Tarazi RC, Gifford RW, Stewart BH: Circulating and urinary catecholamines in pheochromocytoma. N Engl J Med 301:682, 1979, with permission.)

sion due to a pheochromocytoma. Definition of the utility of this test awaits further experience. False negatives have already been reported. Further, hypotension can follow administration of 0.3 mg clonidine.

LOCALIZATION. Given biochemical confirmation of pheochromocytoma, anatomic localization is desirable. Normal adrenal glands can usually be imaged with modern computed tomography (CT) and the majority of adrenomedullary pheochromocytomas can be seen with this technique. CT is the recommended initial localizing procedure. It is conceivable that ultrasonography of the adrenals might be positive despite negative CT scans in an unusually thin patient. External scanning after the injection of radioactive agents that localize in pheochromocytomas has the conceptual advantage of measuring function rather than anatomy and the practical advantage of permitting scanning of the entire trunk of the body and might, therefore, be expected to localize extra-adrenal pheochromocytomas better than CT scans. The initial experience with [^{131}I]-m-iodobenzylguanidine (MIBG) scans has been encouraging in this regard.

TREATMENT. Treatment is surgical removal of the pheochromocytoma. Patients are usually prepared for surgery by administration of an α-adrenergic antagonist, such as phenoxybenzamine or prazosin, in doses sufficient to produce normal blood pressure and to prevent paroxysms. These drugs can also be used to treat chronic catecholamine excess in patients with metastatic tumor, although they do not influence the growth of a malignant pheochromocytoma. A β-adrenergic antagonist, such as propranolol, can be added to the preoperative regimen if arrhythmias are, or become, a problem.

Most patients are cured by surgery. The differential diagnosis of persistent hypertension includes a missed pheochromocytoma, a surgical complication resulting in renal ischemia, and underlying primary hypertension.

OTHER NEURAL CREST TUMORS. Pheochromocytomas are tumors of differentiated neural crest cells, the chromaffin cells. Tumors of more primitive cells also occur. These include neuroblastoma, a rather common malignant tumor of infancy and early childhood, usually arising in the adrenal medulla, and ganglioneuroma, a generally benign tumor often arising in sympathetic ganglia. These tumors commonly synthesize catecholamines, but usually do not release catecholamines in sufficient quantities to produce clinical manifestations. Presumably the catecholamines are largely inactivated within the tumor. Nonetheless, measurements of catecholamine metabolites such as HVA and VMA are useful, particularly in assessing the response to therapy.

AUTONOMIC HYPOFUNCTION

NORMAL PHYSIOLOGY. Assumption of the upright position causes a sharp reduction in venous return to the heart. In the absence of compensatory mechanisms this would result in a corresponding decrease in cardiac output, in arterial pressure, and in blood flow to the brain. Syncope would result from the simple act of standing. Obviously there are effective compensatory mechanisms. The primary compensatory mechanism is a baroreceptor-initiated, CNS-mediated, sympathetic neural reflex that results in a norepinephrine release from axon terminals within the tissues. This results in a sharp increase in systemic vascular resistance (and limitation of the fall in venous return and cardiac output) and, thus, maintenance of the blood pressure in the standing position. Postural activation of this sympathetic reflex is reflected in a rapid, approximately twofold rise in plasma norepinephrine concentrations. Thus, measurement of the plasma norepinephrine response to standing provides a relatively simple means of assessing the integrity of this sympathetic reflex.

PATHOPHYSIOLOGY. Defective postural adaptation results in a decrement in blood pressure upon standing, termed postural (orthostatic) hypotension. Conceptually, postural hypotension can be caused by one or more of three general mechanisms: (1) absolute or relative intravascular volume contraction; (2) resistance to the cardiovascular actions of norepinephrine; and (3) an afferent, central or efferent defect in the sympathetic neural reflex arc. Patients with postural hypotension due to intravascular volume contraction or resistance to the action of norepinephrine exhibit an exaggerated plasma norepinephrine response to standing. They have *hyper*adrenergic postural hypotension. In contrast, patients with postural hypotension due to a defect in the sympathetic reflex arc have a blunted plasma norepinephrine response to standing. They have *hypo*adrenergic postural hypotension.

HYPERADRENERGIC POSTURAL HYPOTENSION. The causes of hyperadrenergic postural hypotension are listed in Table 241–1. These should be considered in all patients with postural hypotension, including those with overt autonomic disease, because they are commonly treatable. A given patient can have multiple hypotensive mechanisms; correction of one can result in clinical improvement. For example, in a patient with relatively mild autonomic hypofunction, otherwise trivial sodium depletion may result in symptomatic postural hypotension that can be treated by sodium repletion.

HYPOADRENERGIC POSTURAL HYPOTENSION. Hypoadrenergic postural hypotension can result from afferent, central or efferent lesions in the sympathetic neural arc. Diseases recognized to cause secondary hypoadrenergic postural hypotension produce lesions in the brain, spinal cord, or peripheral nerves (Table 241–1). Diabetes is a common cause. In the absence of such diseases, autonomic hypofunction is considered to be idiopathic or primary. Undoubtedly a heterogenous group of disorders of unknown etiology, primary autonomic dysfunction can be divided into two clinical and pathophysiologic syndromes. *Primary autonomic dysfunction type 1,* most commonly referred to as idiopathic orthostatic hypotension, is characterized by autonomic hypofunction in the absence of central nervous system disease. In addition to a blunted plasma norepinephrine response to standing, common to both the type 1 and type 2 disorders, as a group patients with the type 1 disorder have low basal plasma norepinephrine concentrations. They are thought to have lesions of the peripheral autonomic nerves.

TABLE 241–1. DIFFERENTIAL DIAGNOSIS OF POSTURAL HYPOTENSION

I. Hyperadrenergic postural hypotension
  A. Intravascular volume contraction
    1. Hemorrhage
    2. Severe chronic anemia
    3. Sodium (and water) depletion—aldosterone deficiency, diuretics, gastrointestinal or renal diseases
    4. Relative volume contraction—pregnancy
  B. Resistance to released norepinephrine
    1. Sodium depletion (see above)
    2. Glucocorticoid deficiency
    3. Bartter's syndrome
    4. Vasodilator drugs—nitroglycerin; hydralazine and minoxidil; prazosin, bromocriptine, and other α-adrenergic antagonists

II. Hypoadrenergic Postural Hypotension
  A. Secondary
    1. Brain lesions—vascular accidents involving the brainstem, toxic/nutritional encephalopathies, demyelinating and degenerative disorders, neoplasms, trauma, infections, tricyclic antidepressants, and phenothiazines
    2. Spinal cord lesions—cervical transection, mass lesions (tumor, abscess), syringomyelia, combined systems disease, tabes dorsalis
    3. Peripheral nerve lesions—diabetic adrenergic neuropathy, alcoholism, amyloidosis, porphyria, vincristine
  B. Primary
    1. Primary autonomic dysfunction
      a. Type 1: Idiopathic orthostatic hypotension
      b. Type 2: Idiopathic orthostatic hypotension with somatic neurologic deficit (Shy-Drager syndrome, multiple system atrophy)
    2. Familial dysautonomia (Riley-Day syndrome)

Primary autonomic dysfunction type 2 is perhaps best known as the Shy-Drager syndrome; it has also been referred to as multiple system atrophy or idiopathic orthostatic hypotension with somatic neurologic deficit. In addition to autonomic hypofunction, patients with the type 2 disorder have degenerative central nervous system disease most commonly manifested as parkinsonism. Such patients have normal basal plasma norepinephrine concentrations and their autonomic lesions are thought to be in the central nervous system.

Impairment of both sympathetic and parasympathetic neural functions is the rule in primary autonomic dysfunction. Thus a variety of symptoms, such as diminished sweating and heat intolerance, difficulty in focusing, gastrointestinal symptoms, urinary and fecal incontinence and impotence, in addition to postural symptoms, occur commonly.

Treatment involves correction of the underlying cause of postural hypotension (Table 241–1) when possible. Symptomatic treatment approaches include sodium loading (NaCl) tablets plus fludrocortisone, (0.1 to 0.3 mg daily), which can produce hypokalemia and might precipitate cardiac failure in a patient with heart disease. Although not approved by the FDA at this writing, the agonist midodrine (which constricts veins as well as arterioles) appears to be an effective drug.

EPINEPHRINE DEFICIENCY

Glucagon normally plays a primary role in promoting glucose recovery from *hypoglycemia*. Epinephrine is not critical when glucagon secretion is intact but compensates largely, and becomes critical, when glucagon secretion is deficient. Glucose recovery from hypoglycemia fails to occur only in the absence of both glucagon and epinephrine.

In patients with insulin-dependent diabetes mellitus (IDDM), glucagon secretory responses to hypoglycemia are commonly blunted or absent. This defect occurs relatively early in the course of the disease and is selective for the response to plasma glucose decrements. Its mechanism is unknown. To the extent that they have deficient glucagon secretory responses, patients with IDDM are dependent upon epinephrine to promote recovery from hypoglycemia. If deficient epinephrine secretory responses also develop, as they sometimes do late in the course of the disease (or if the hyperglycemic actions of epinephrine are blocked as with propranolol administration), patients can become defenseless against hypoglycemia. Studies have shown that patients judged to have inadequate glucose counterregulation on the basis of an insulin infusion test and subsequently found to have recurrent, severe hypoglycemia during intensive treatment of their diabetes, have combined deficiencies of glucagon and epinephrine secretion in response to glucose decrements. In contrast, patients judged to have adequate glucose counterregulation, and subsequently found to have few severe hypoglycemic episodes during intensive treatment, have comparably deficient glucagon secretion but normal epinephrine secretion. Thus, inadequate glucose counterregulation due to combined deficiencies of glucagon and epinephrine secretion results in a 25-fold increase in the risk of severe hypoglycemia during intensive therapy of IDDM.

Bravo EL, Tarazi RC, Fouad FM, Vidt DG, Gifford RW Jr: Clonidine suppression test: A useful aid in the diagnosis of pheochromocytoma. N Engl J Med 305:623, 1981. *A suppression test for the diagnosis of pheochromocytoma.*

Cryer PE: Physiology and pathophysiology of the human sympathoadrenal neuroendocrine system. N Engl J Med 303:436, 1980. *A review from the perspective of plasma norepinephrine and epinephrine measurements.*

Cryer PE: Diseases of the adrenal medullae and sympathetic nervous system. *In* Felig P, Baxter JD, Broadus AE, Frohman LE (eds.): Endocrinology and Metabolism. New York, McGraw-Hill Book Company, 1981, pp 511–550. *A more detailed discussion of sympathochromaffin physiology and pathophysiology.*

Cryer PE, Gerich JE: The relevance of glucose counterregulatory systems to patients with diabetes: Critical roles of glucagon and epinephrine. Diabetes Care 6:95, 1983. *Review of hypoglycemic glucose counterregulation in normal and diabetic persons.*

Manger WM, Gifford RW Jr: Hypertension secondary to pheochromocytoma. Bull NY Acad Med 58:139, 1982. *An extensive clinical experience.*

Schirger A, Sheps SG, Thomas JE, Fealey RD: Midodrine. A new agent in the management of idiopathic orthostatic hypotension and Shy-Drager syndrome. Mayo Clin Proc 56:429, 1981. *A promising drug for the treatment of hypoadrenergic postural hypotension.*

Thomas JE, Schirger A, Fealey RD, Sheps SG: Orthostatic hypotension. Mayo Clin Proc 56:17, 1981. *An extensive clinical experience.*

White NH, Skor D, Cryer PE, Bier DM, Levandoski L, Santiago JV: Identification of type 1 diabetic patients at increased risk for hypoglycemia during intensive therapy. N Engl J Med 308:485, 1983. *Demonstration that combined glucagon and epinephrine deficiencies result in a 25-fold increased risk of severe hypoglycemia during intensive treatment of insulin-dependent diabetes mellitus.*

Zweiffler AJ, Julius S: Increased platelet catecholamine content in pheochromocytoma. N Engl J Med 306:890, 1982. *An alternative to plasma catecholamine measurements in the diagnosis of pheochromocytoma, although seldom necessary.*

242. THE CARCINOID SYNDROME

Philip E. Cryer

Carcinoid tumors arise from enterochromaffin (Kulchitsky) cells that are located predominantly in the gastrointestinal mucosa. Enterochromaffin cells have the potential to produce a variety of biologically active amines and peptides, including serotonin, bradykinin, and histamine, as well as prostaglandins. Carcinoid tumors are relatively common. Those that release sufficient quantities of mediators into the systemic circulation to produce the clinical carcinoid syndrome—flushing often with diarrhea and sometimes with wheezing or cardiac failure—are rare. Carcinoid tumors are most commonly found in the appendix or rectum, but these rarely produce the carcinoid syndrome. The tumors that produce the syndrome typically arise in the ileum, although the carcinoid syndrome can also result from tumors of the stomach, bile duct, duodenum, pancreas, lung, or even the ovary. Despite the release of a variety of mediators, the biochemical common denominator of the carcinoid syndrome is the overproduction of serotonin and the excretion of its major metabolite, 5-hydroxyindoleacetic acid (5-HIAA).

A variety of ectopic humoral syndromes have been associated with histologic carcinoid tumors. These include Cushing's syndrome (ACTH) and dilutional hyponatremia (vasopressin) with bronchial carcinoids, gynecomastia (chorionic gonadotropin) with gastric carcinoids, and hypoglycemia (insulin) with pancreatic carcinoids. Typically, such patients do not have the carcinoid syndrome.

BIOSYNTHESIS AND DEGRADATION OF SEROTONIN. Serotonin is synthesized from dietary tryptophan (Fig. 242–1). In the

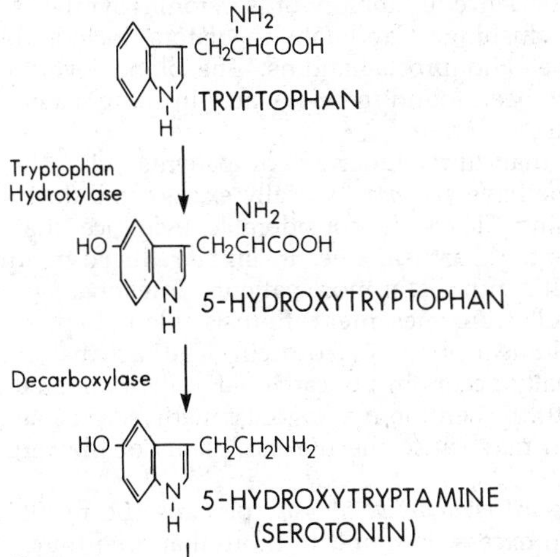

Figure 242–1. Synthesis and degradation of serotonin.

presence of tryptophan hydroxylase, tryptophan is converted to 5-hydroxytryptophan, which, in the presence of aromatic L-amino acid decarboxylase, is converted to 5-hydroxytryptamine (serotonin). Through a series of reactions, including that involving the enzyme monamine oxidase, 5-hydroxytryptamine is converted to 5-hydroxyindoleacetic acid.

Approximately 90 per cent of serotonin in the body is normally found in the gut. Serotonin synthesis accounts for only 1 per cent of the metabolism of tryptophan in normal individuals. This may be as high as 60 per cent in patients with the carcinoid syndrome. Indeed, a pellagra-like skin rash has been attributed to diversion of tryptophan from nicotinic acid synthesis in such patients. Normal individuals excrete less than 10 mg of 5-HIAA per 24 hours. Patients with the carcinoid syndrome commonly excrete 50 to 100 mg per 24 hours.

CLINICAL MANIFESTATIONS. Clinical carcinoid syndrome is usually associated with an ileal carcinoid tumor that has metastasized to the liver. Although carcinoids in sites, such as the lung or ovary, that do not drain into the portal circulation can rarely produce the carcinoid syndrome without evident hepatic metastases, carcinoid syndrome due to an ileal carcinoid is almost invariably associated with overt hepatic metastases. Presumably the liver clears mediators released from the tumor, and this clearance is impaired by metastatic tumor, resulting in the clinical syndrome.

More than 90 per cent of patients with the carcinoid syndrome have episodes of *cutaneous flushing*. The flush usually begins in the face and may spread to the trunk or even the extremities. It is red initially and then becomes purple; it commonly lasts only a few minutes, but may continue for hours. *Telangiectasias* of the face can result from frequent flushing. The heart rate increases and the blood pressure tends to decrease during a flush. This is in contrast to patients with pheochromocytomas who typically have episodes of pallor with hypertension. Bronchial carcinoids may be associated with more intense and long-lasting flushing episodes. In patients with gastric carcinoids, flushing tends to be patchy initially and may be anywhere on the body. Headache commonly follows the flush.

Flushing can be precipitated by alcohol, food, stress, or palpation of the liver, or it may follow the administration of catecholamines, pentagastrin, or reserpine. A single mediator that causes the carcinoid flush has not been identified. It is not serotonin, since inhibition of serotonin synthesis does not prevent flushing. Candidate mediators include bradykinin, histamine, and prostaglandins. The blood levels of each of these has been found to be elevated in some patients with the carcinoid syndrome.

More than three quarters of patients with the carcinoid syndrome have *diarrhea*, typically exacerbated during episodes of flushing. There is considerable evidence that serotonin mediates the diarrhea, since it can be reduced by inhibition of serotonin synthesis in most patients. Intestinal symptoms can also result from mesenteric fibrosis. Pleural, peritoneal, and retroperitoneal fibroses also occur. The fact that such fibrosis occasionally occurs in noncarcinoid patients treated for a long term with the serotonin antagonist methysergide suggests that serotonin may cause the fibrotic lesions of the carcinoid syndrome.

Right-sided endocardial fibrosis, perhaps the result of chronic serotonin excess, is found in more than one third of patients with the carcinoid syndrome. Cardiac failure, due to pulmonic stenosis or tricuspid insufficiency or both, is less common but implies a poor prognosis. Involvement of the left side of the heart is uncommon. It does occur in patients with bronchial carcinoids, which implies that the responsible mediator(s) is ordinarily cleared during passage through pulmonary capillaries.

Bronchoconstriction with wheezing during an episode of flushing is less common, occurring in about 20 per cent of patients. Like flushing, but unlike diarrhea, bronchoconstriction is not prevented by inhibition of serotonin synthesis.

Somatostatin has been reported to decrease flushing, diarrhea, and bronchoconstriction in patients with the carcinoid syndrome. The mechanism(s) of this effect is not known.

DIAGNOSIS. Diagnosis is based upon clinical suspicion—usually a history of flushing and diarrhea—associated with markedly increased urinary 5-hydroxyindoleacetic acid excretion. Metastatic hepatomegaly is common. Since carcinoid tumors produce the carcinoid syndrome rarely, the histologic diagnosis of a carcinoid tumor does not establish the presence of the carcinoid syndrome. Platelet serotonin levels are elevated in most patients with the carcinoid syndrome. Gastric carcinoids appear to have low decarboxylase activity since 5-hydroxytryptophan, rather than serotonin, is the major product of indole metabolism in some such patients.

Provocative tests, such as the precipitation of episodes with intravenous administration of epinephrine, are seldom necessary and potentially dangerous, since severe hypotension and bronchoconstriction can occur.

False-positive urinary 5-HIAA determinations are common and should be suspected particularly when the values are minimally elevated, e.g., 10 to 20 mg per 24 hours. Increased 5-HIAA excretion can follow the ingestion of chocolate, bananas, tomatoes, pineapples, walnuts, and avocados and the use of drugs, including mephenesin, methocarbamol, reserpine, acetaminophen, and glyceryl guaiacolate (the last in some cough syrups). Increased values have also been reported in Whipple's disease and nontropical sprue.

Computed tomography, radionuclide scans, ultrasonography, and conventional barium contrast x-ray studies can be used to define tumor anatomy. Despite widespread metastases, the primary tumor can be small and difficult to demonstrate.

TREATMENT. In the presence of documented metastases, resection of a primary ileal carcinoid tumor is not indicated. It may become necessary because of intestinal obstruction or because of intussusception. Rarely, surgical removal of an isolated tumor (e.g., a bronchial or ovarian carcinoid) is curative. Devascularization of metastatic tumor by percutaneous arterial embolization has been reported to produce symptomatic relief in some patients.

Survival of less than five years after the onset of the carcinoid syndrome is the rule, but survival for more than 20 years is well documented. Thus, high-risk attempts at curative therapy are generally not indicated. Carcinoid tumors are not radiosensitive. Low-risk chemotherapy has not been very effective.

Symptomatic therapy includes nutritional support plus the provision of nicotinamide to prevent pellagra. Diarrhea has been treated with serotonin antagonists such as methysergide or cyproheptadine as well as with opiates. The drug parachlorophenylalanine, a tryptophan hydroxylase inhibitor, reduces diarrhea. However, allergic reactions and CNS side effects have occurred, and the drug remains experimental. No drug is consistently effective in preventing flushing; H_1 and H_2 histamine antagonists, including cimetidine, are often tried. Phenothiazines and the α-adrenergic antagonist phenoxybenzamine have also been used, as have glucocorticoids. Recently, treatment with leukocyte interferon was reported to decrease flushing and diarrhea in six of nine patients with the carcinoid syndrome. Symptomatic improvement, reduction of 5-HIAA excretion, and reduction in tumor size was reported in a patient treated with tamoxifen.

Frolich JC, Margolius HS: Prostaglandins, the kallikrein-kinin system, Bartter's syndrome and the carcinoid syndrome. *In* Felig P, Baxter JD, Broadus AE, Frohman LE, (eds.): Endocrinology and Metabolism. New York, McGraw-Hill Book Company, 1981, pp 1247–1274. *A more detailed discussion of the carcinoid syndrome.*

Melia WM, Nunnerly HB, Johnson PJ, Williams R: Use of arterial devascularization and cytotoxic drugs in 30 patients with the carcinoid syndrome. Br J Cancer 46:331, 1982. *Promising symptomatic responses to tumor devascularization but not to cytotoxic drugs.*

Oberg K, Funa K, Alm G: Effects of leukocyte interferon on clinical symptoms and hormone levels in patients with mid-gut carcinoid tumors and carcinoid syndrome. N Engl J Med 309:129, 1983. *Unanticipated clinical and biochemical responses with demonstrable reductions in tumor size.*

Part XVIII
DISEASES OF BONE AND BONE MINERAL METABOLISM

243. MINERAL AND BONE HOMEOSTASIS

Claude D. Arnaud

THE INTEGRATED CALCIOTROPIC HORMONE SYSTEM

A highly integrated and complex endocrine system maintains calcium, phosphate, and magnesium homeostasis in all vertebrates. It involves an interplay between two polypeptide hormones, parathyroid hormone (PTH) and calcitonin, and a sterol hormone, 1,25-dihydroxycholecalciferol [1,25$(OH)_2$D]. Biosynthesis and secretion of the polypeptide hormones are regulated by a negative feedback mechanism that involves calcium ion activity in the extracellular fluids (Fig. 243–1). Biosynthesis of 1,25$(OH)_2$D from the major circulating metabolite of vitamin D, 25-hydroxycholecalciferol (25OHD), takes place in the kidney and is regulated by PTH and calcitonin as well as by the extracellular fluid concentrations of calcium and phosphate. Other hormones, such as insulin, growth hormone, somatomedin, cortisol, thyroxine, epinephrine, estrogen, testosterone, and inorganic phosphate, together with some compounds not yet identified and certain physical factors, undoubtedly play roles in the modification and regulation of organ responses to PTH, calcitonin, and 1,25$(OH)_2$D.

Parathyroid hormone, calcitonin, and 1,25$(OH)_2$D regulate the flow of minerals into and out of the extracellular fluid compartment through their actions on intestine, kidney, and bone (Fig. 243–1, Table 243–1). The target cells of these organs function as a barrier between the extracellular fluid compartment and the intestinal lumen, the renal tubular lumen, and the bone fluid compartment (Fig. 243–2). These target cells are highly specialized for solute transport against a concentration gradient and thus are often described as being polarized.

PARATHYROID HORMONE. Under normal circumstances, PTH prevents serum calcium from falling below physiologic concentrations by stimulating calcium movement from the bone fluid compartment and the intestinal and renal tubular lumina into the blood. Whereas its effects on bone and kidney are direct, PTH acts indirectly on the intestine, through the mediation of vitamin D. The hormone stimulates the conversion of 25OHD to 1,25$(OH)_2$D via a 1α-hydroxylase in the mitochondria of the renal tubule (this stimulation works directly and indirectly through a decrease in serum phosphate levels). The 1,25$(OH)_2$D thus formed stimulates intestinal absorption of calcium via a vitamin D–dependent calcium pump.

Parathyroid hormone also prevents serum phosphate levels from rising above normal physiologic concentrations by increasing renal tubular excretion of phosphate. This regulatory action is important because phosphate, like calcium, is also released into the blood by PTH-induced bone resorption. This function can be particularly appreciated in patients with end-stage renal failure and associated severe hyperparathyroidism. These patients develop hyperphosphatemia because large quantities of phosphate are released from bone and the kidney can no longer excrete it.

CALCITONIN. Calcitonin prevents abnormal increases in both serum calcium and serum phosphate. It decreases the translocation of calcium from the renal tubule and bone fluid compartment into the blood and thus can be considered as a counterregulator of PTH in this regard. The effects of calcitonin on the intestinal absorption of calcium and vitamin D metabolism are uncertain.

VITAMIN D. Vitamin D, as 1,25$(OH)_2$D, acts primarily to maintain the cellular calcium transport system in the intestine, which causes the active extrusion of calcium against a concentration gradient from the interior of the cell (ionized calcium concentration = 10^{-7} to 10^{-6} M), across the antiluminal membrane, and into the extracellular fluid (ionized calcium concentration = 10^{-3} M) (Fig. 243–3). Thus, PTH and 1,25$(OH)_2$D are interdependent. The renal production of 1,25$(OH)_2$D depends upon the prevailing concentration of PTH in the blood, and the ability of PTH to increase plasma calcium depends upon a calcium transport system maintained by 1,25$(OH)_2$D.

CONTROL MECHANISMS. Figure 243–1 shows the relationships among the different components involved in maintaining a normal level of plasma calcium. Each of the three overlapping feedback loops involves one of the target organs of the calciotropic hormones and the four controlling elements—i.e., plasma calcium, PTH, calcitonin, and 1,25$(OH)_2$D. The left limbs of the loops depict physiologic events that increase plasma calcium, and the right limbs events that decrease plasma calcium. Under physiologic conditions, there are small fluctuations in plasma calcium. Decreases in plasma calcium increase

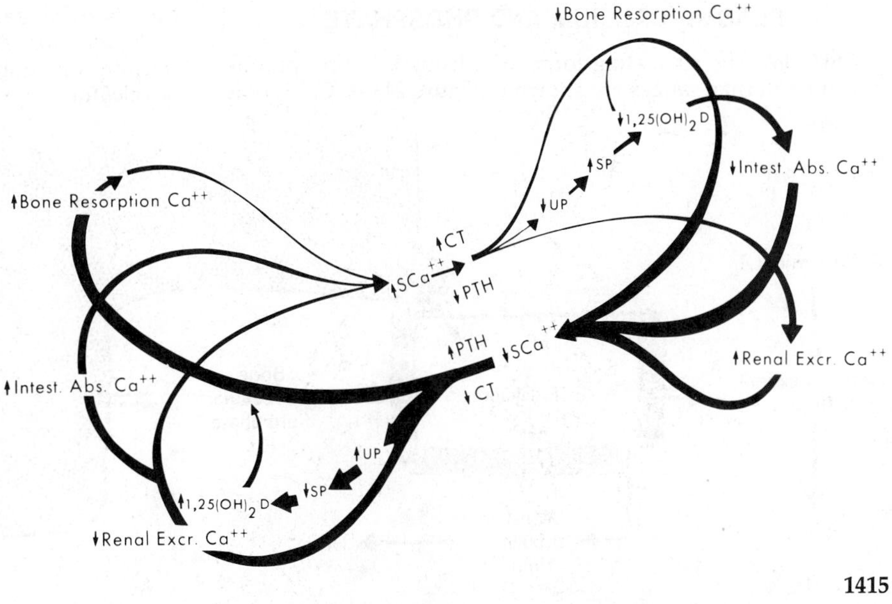

Figure 243–1. Schema of calcium homeostasis, consisting of three overlapping control loops that interlock and relate to one another through the level of blood concentrations of ionic calcium, parathyroid hormone, and calcitonin. Each loop involves a calciotropic hormone target organ (bone, intestine, kidney). The limbs on the left depict physiologic events that increase the blood concentration of calcium, and the limbs on the right, events that decrease this concentration. See text for detailed descriptions. (From Arnaud CD: Calcium homeostasis: Regulatory elements and their integrity. Fed Proc 37:2558, 1978.)

TABLE 243–1. ACTIONS OF MAJOR CALCIUM-REGULATING HORMONES

	Bone	Kidney	Intestine
PTH	Increases resorption of calcium and phosphate.	Increases resorption of calcium; conversion of 25OHD to $1,25(OH)_2D$. Decreases resorption of phosphate; resorption of bicarbonate.	No direct effects.
Calcitonin	Decreases resorption of calcium and phosphate.	Decreases resorption of calcium and phosphate. Questionable effect on vitamin D metabolism.	No direct effects.
Vitamin D	Maintains Ca^{2+} transport system.	Decreases resorption of calcium.	Increases absorption of calcium and phosphate.

Adapted from Arnaud CD, Kolb FO: The calciotropic hormones and metabolic bone disease. *In* Greenspan FS, Forsham PH (eds.): Basic and Clinical Endocrinology. Los Altos, Lange Medical Publications, 1983, p 188.

PTH secretion and decrease calcitonin secretion. These changes in hormone secretion lead to increased bone resporption, decreased renal excretion of calcium, and increased intestinal calcium absorption (via PTH stimulation of $1,25(OH)_2D$ production; left side of Fig. 243–1). As a consequence of these events, plasma calcium rises slightly above physiologic levels, inhibiting PTH secretion and stimulating calcitonin secretion. These changes in plasma hormone concentrations decrease bone resorption, increase renal excretion of calcium, and decrease intestinal absorption of calcium (right side of Fig. 243–1), causing plasma calcium to fall below the physiologic level. This sequence of events probably occurs within milliseconds, so that plasma calcium is maintained at physiologic levels with minimal oscillation. The "butterfly" scheme in Figure 243–1 not only shows the relationships among elements that control mineral homeostasis under physiologic conditions but also suggests how potential pathogenetic mechanisms and adaptive responses elicited by disease or treatment would operate in this system.

PLASMA CALCIUM AND PHOSPHATE

CALCIUM. The circulating forms of calcium and phosphorus and their normal ranges are shown in Figure 243–4. Calcium is distributed in three major fractions: ionized, protein-bound, and complexed. The ionized form (Ca^{2+}), the only biologically active species, constitutes 46 to 50 per cent of total calcium. The protein-bound fraction, roughly equivalent to the ionized fraction in amount, is biologically inert. However, the calcium bound to albumin (80 per cent) and globulin (20 per cent) is important because it provides a readily available reservoir of this important cation. Since the binding of calcium to these proteins obeys the mass-law equation, calcium can dissociate from its binding sites to provide a first-line defense against hypocalcemia. Moreover, hyperproteinemia (e.g., hyperglobulinemia in myelomatosis) can increase and hypoproteinemia (e.g., hypoalbuminemia in cirrhosis of the liver or nephrosis) can decrease total plasma calcium without changing the concentration of ionized calcium. Formulas have been developed to estimate the percentage of calcium bound to the plasma proteins based on the differential binding affinities of albumin and globulin; for example,

$$\text{Per cent protein-bound Ca} = 8 \times \text{albumin (grams per deciliter)} + 2 \times \text{globulin (grams per deciliter)} + 3.$$

Such formulas permit the calculation of diffusible calcium (see below) by subtracting protein-bound from total calcium. Such estimates can be notoriously inaccurate, however, especially in patients with low plasma protein concentrations. The only accurate means of determining the plasma concentration of ionized calcium in hypo- or hyperproteinemic states is to measure it directly by an ion-selective electrode procedure. The fraction of plasma calcium that is complexed to organic (e.g., citrate) and inorganic (e.g., phosphate or sulfate) acids is small (approximately 8 per cent), and, like the ionized fraction, it is ultrafilterable (diffusible). Complexed calcium probably has little importance as a reservoir for ionized calcium, but in states of hyperphosphatemia, such as chronic renal failure, excessive complexing of calcium with phosphate may contribute to the decrease in plasma ionized calcium observed in this condition.

The normal range for serum calcium (Fig. 243–4) is small (1.2 mg per deciliter) compared to the total concentration of serum calcium (8.9 to 10.1 mg per deciliter), and the same is true for the ionized fraction. Thus, values for total calcium below 8.9 mg per deciliter, assuming that plasma protein concentrations are normal, reflect clinically significant hypocalcemia, and values above 10.1 mg per deciliter reflect hypercalcemia. In recent years, serum calcium has been measured with reasonable accuracy in most clinical laboratories. However, stored plasma samples may yield artifactual decreases in circulating calcium concentrations, and contaminated serum samples may yield artifactual increases. The latter problem is most frequently caused by inadvertent contamination of the blood-drawing tubes with calcium when they are manufactured or contamination of laboratory equipment by airborne calcium carbonate dust from laboratory chalk boards. Thus, it is important to use *fresh serum* for calcium measurements and eliminate sources of calcium contamination in order to obtain reliable measurements of calcium.

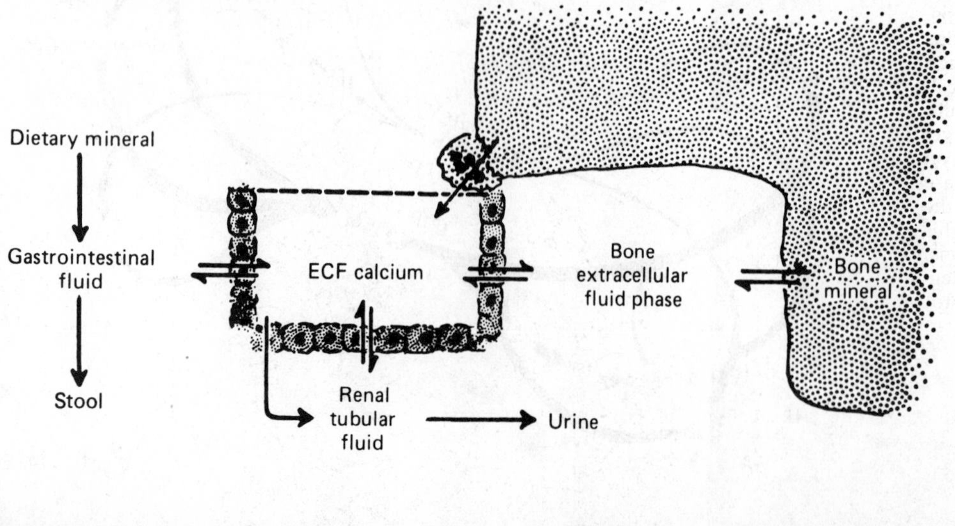

Figure 243–2. Cellular barrier separating the extracellular fluid compartment from the intestinal lumen, the renal tubular lumen, and the bone fluid compartment. PTH, calcitonin, and $1,25(OH)_2D$ act on these cells (directly or indirectly) to regulate the flow of calcium into and out of the extracellular fluid. (From Rasmussen H, et al.: Effect of ions upon bone cell function. Fed Proc 29:1191, 1970.)

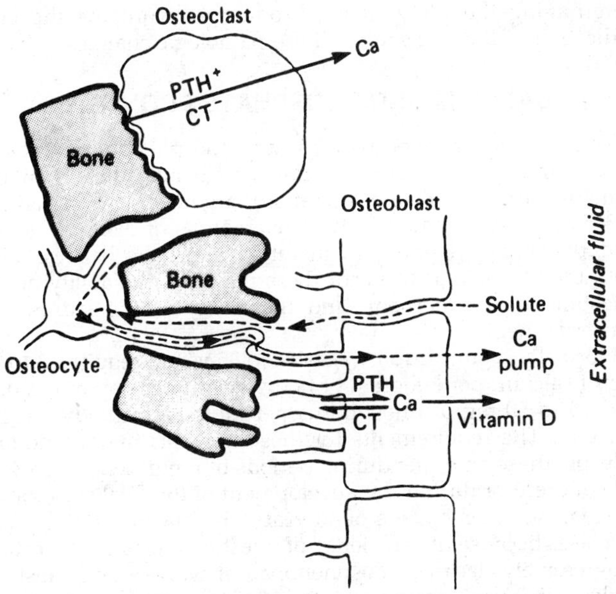

Figure 243–3. Relationships between calciotropic hormones, bone cells, and calcium transport. Bone crystal is represented by the shaded areas. The osteoclast, with an active "ruffled border," is shown resorbing bone—a process stimulated by PTH^+ and inhibited by calcitonin (CT^-). The osteoblasts are actively extruding calcium (Ca) from the bone fluid (between cells and crystals) under the influence of hormones. Processes connecting deep osteocytes are shown participating in calcium transport (dotted arrows). (From Arnaud CD, Kolb FO: The calciotropic hormones and metabolic bone disease. *In* Greenspan FS, Forsham PH (eds.): Basic and Clinical Endocrinology. Los Altos, Lange Medical Publications, 1983, p 189.)

The plasma calcium concentration varies little in spite of large changes in dietary calcium because of the adaptive alterations in the endocrine system regulating this mineral. Minor diurnal changes (decreases in the afternoon) have been recorded. In addition, plasma calcium decreases with age in men but not in women, probably due to a decrease in the serum albumin concentration in men. Total (but not ionized) serum calcium also decreases during pregnancy, and this change may also be due to the well-documented decrease in the serum albumin concentration in this condition.

Hypocalcemia produces a myriad of symptoms, and when severe can result in tetany and possibly convulsions (see Ch. 510). *Hypercalcemia* can produce functional changes in most organ systems, and these changes may lead to a confusing variety of symptoms and objective findings (see Ch. 246).

PHOSPHORUS. Only 15 per cent of plasma phosphate is bound to proteins in the blood (Fig. 243–4). The rest is ultrafilterable and consists mainly of free HPO_4^{2-} and $NaHPO_4^-$ (85 per cent), with free $H_2PO_4^-$ making up the remainder (15 per cent). By convention, plasma phosphate is expressed in terms of the amount of elemental phosphorus involved.

In comparison to calcium, phosphate has a wider range of normal plasma values (2.5 to 4.5 mg per deciliter) (Fig. 243–4). Moreover, increases or decreases in dietary phosphate are promptly reflected in changes in the same direction in serum phosphorus and urinary phosphorus excretion. There are also marked diurnal variations in serum phosphorus and urinary phosphorus excretion, even during a fast, which are caused in part by diurnal changes in plasma cortisol. Serum phosphorus concentrations in young children are almost double those in adults, and they increase slightly with age in women.

Serum phosphorus can be measured accurately and precisely in most laboratories. However, spuriously high values may be obtained if (1) serum extracts or dialysates are exposed to acid longer than is prescribed (resulting in hydrolysis of organic compounds containing phosphorus) or (2) hemolyzed serum is used (red blood cells contain phosphorus).

Hyperphosphatemia. Acute, severe hyperphosphatemia, as might be induced by intravenous phosphate infusion, can cause hypocalcemia sufficiently severe to result in tetany and even death. The less severe hyperphosphatemia induced by phosphate ingestion rarely causes symptoms; however, if the patient has an associated disorder in which there is a tendency toward hypocalcemia (e.g., mild hypoparathyroidism or chronic renal failure), frank hypocalcemia may develop.

Hypophosphatemia (see also Ch. 207). Acute respiratory alkalosis, the administration of a large quantity of carbohydrate, and insulin administration all cause a rapid decrease in serum phosphorus. Severe hypophosphatemia may occur during the treatment of diabetic ketoacidosis or forced nutrition of undernourished patients and can cause both skeletal myopathy and cardiomyopathy. These conditions may lead to rhabdomyolysis, as evidenced by increases in serum creatine phosphokinase (Ch. 76). The levels of 2,3-diphosphoglyceric acid and

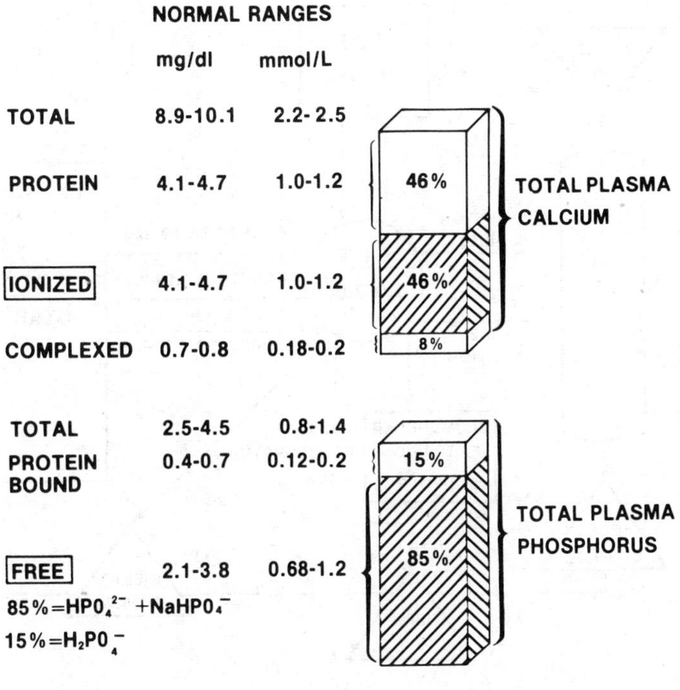

Figure 243–4. Distribution and normal ranges of calcium and phosphorus in the plasma.

adenosine triphosphate (ATP) in erythrocytes may also decrease; the decrease in 2,3-diphosphoglyceric acid in turn may decrease oxygen delivery to tissues, and the decrease in ATP may cause hemolytic anemia. Chronic, moderate hypophosphatemia frequently results in osteomalacia or rickets, as in the genetic disorder X-linked hypophosphatemia (Ch. 207). Generally, restoration of serum phosphate concentrations to normal corrects abnormal organ function in hypophosphatemic conditions, except in X-linked hypophosphatemic rickets, which requires regimens specially tailored for individual patients.

INTERRELATION OF PLASMA CALCIUM AND PHOSPHATE

The physiologic importance of the relationship between the circulating concentrations of ionized calcium and diffusible (free) phosphate is poorly understood, especially with regard to the formation and dissolution of amorphous calcium phosphate ($Ca_3(PO_4)_2$) and hydroxyapatite ($Ca_{10}(PO_4)_6(OH)_2$) in bone. However, available evidence indicates that the ion product of normal plasma concentrations of calcium and phosphate (the Ca × P ion product) is considerably higher than that necessary to form these two compounds. Thus, in comparison to bone, plasma is saturated with calcium and phosphate, and this can be considered an important driving force in bone mineralization. The positive effect of vitamin D on bone mineralization is probably indirect and resides in its ability to maintain the Ca × P ion product in the normal range by increasing calcium and phosphate absorption by the gut and their resorption by bone (Fig. 243–1).

The biologic significance of the Ca × P ion product has been questioned in recent years, but it is important to recognize that products below 20 mg per deciliter (0.7 mmol per liter) usually reflect a mineralization defect in bone, and products above 70 mg per deciliter (2.2 mmol per liter) a propensity toward soft tissue calcification. There are exceptions to these numerical guidelines that will become apparent in future chapters, but, short of directly measuring changes in bone formation in bone biopsy specimens or changes in calcium content in soft tissues, determining the Ca × P ion product may provide the best indication of the presence of these pathologic changes.

CALCIUM AND PHOSPHATE ECONOMY

The quantitative aspects of calcium and phosphorus metabolism, under conditions of metabolic balance (dietary intake equal to urinary and fecal excretion), are illustrated in Figures 243–5 and 243–6, respectively. The amounts of dietary calcium and phosphate required to maintain metabolic balance vary with the physiologic need for these minerals, the ability of the intestine to absorb them, and the ability of the kidneys to conserve them.

Normally, young adults (ages 21 to 35 years) require 12 to 15 mg of calcium per kilogram of body weight per day in the diet and 15 to 20 mg of phosphorus per kilogram of body weight per day. The requirements for these minerals may be double or triple these amounts during periods of rapid skeletal growth (in children) or during the development of the fetal skeleton in pregnancy. After the age of 40 years, the calcium requirement increases because the efficiency of intestinal calcium absorption progressively declines. Postmenopausal women and most elderly men must ingest approximately 50 per cent more calcium than young adults to avoid negative balance.

Dietary deprivation of calcium or phosphorus induces adaptive changes in the production and secretion of the calciotropic hormones that minimize the development of negative balance. In the case of calcium, only 30 to 50 per cent of ingested calcium is normally absorbed (Fig. 243–5). With decreased intake, serum calcium decreases slightly, and the sequence of events depicted in the left limbs of the feedback loops in Figure 243–1 is activated. In severe, chronic dietary deficiency of calcium in normal subjects, PTH stimulates an increase in plasma $1,25(OH)_2D$ levels, which can increase fractional calcium absorption up to 75 per cent; hence, the total body calcium is minimally perturbed. However, this adaptive response requires a chronic increase in plasma concentrations of PTH. The destructive effects of such hyperparathyroidism on bone (see Ch. 246) may be of little consequence to the young adult, in whom the net loss of total body calcium is minimal, but they may be devastating to individuals with high calcium requirements (e.g., young children and pregnant women) or to patients who cannot

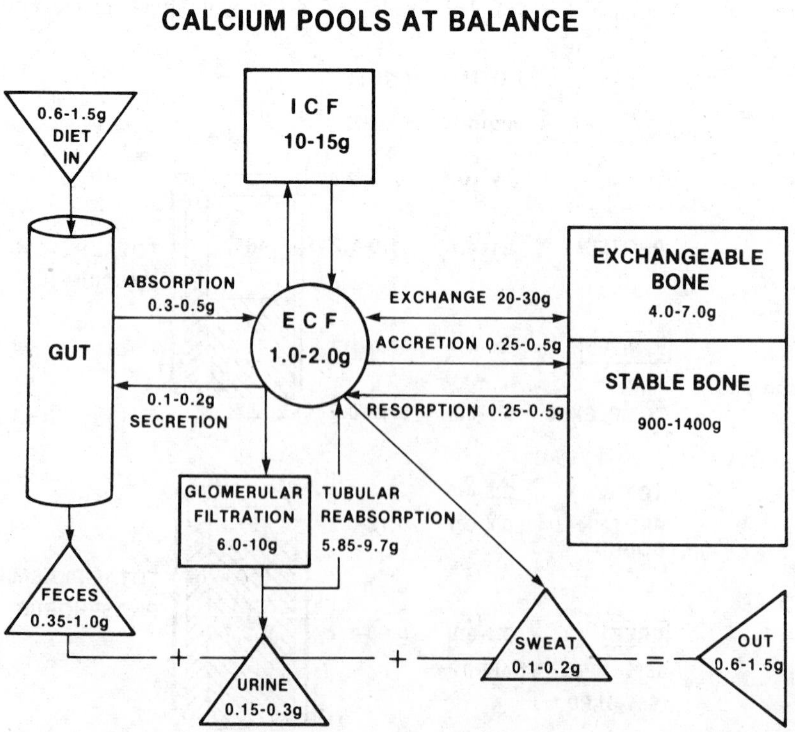

Figure 243–5. Normal distribution of calcium in the body. ICF denotes intracellular fluid, and ECF extracellular fluid.

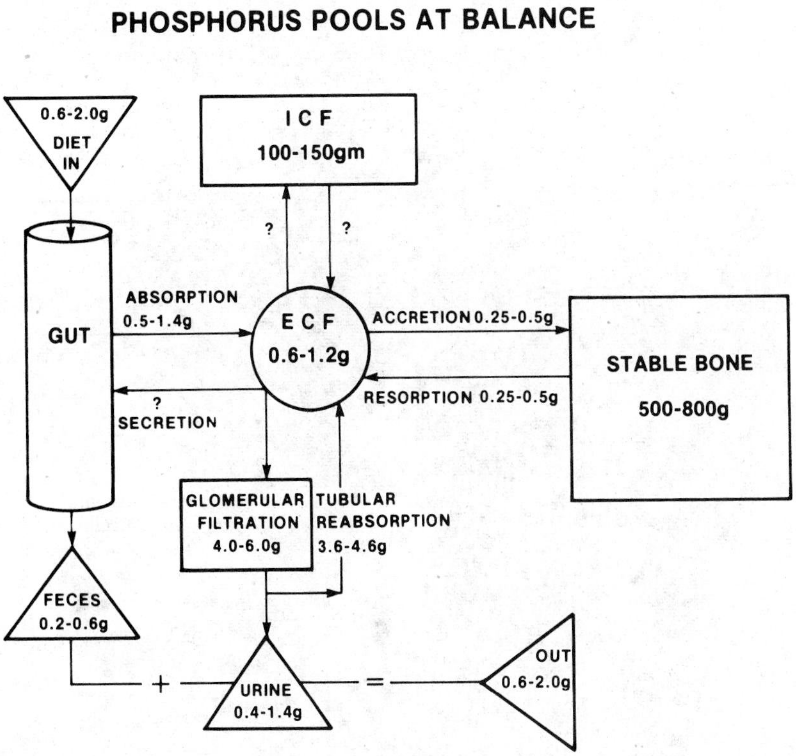

Figure 243–6. Normal distribution of phosphorus in the body. ICF denotes intracellular fluid, and ECF extracellular fluid.

adapt adequately to calcium deprivation by increasing intestinal absorption of calcium (e.g., the elderly).

Whereas the intestine plays the major role in the body's adaptation to a dietary deficiency of calcium, the kidney, with its ability to rapidly reduce urinary phosphate excretion, plays the major role in maintaining phosphate balance during a dietary deficiency of this mineral. Normally, 70 to 80 per cent of dietary phosphorus is absorbed, and therefore any increase in its fractional absorption during deprivation would have little influence in preventing the development of negative balance. However, 80 per cent or more of absorbed phosphorus is normally excreted in the urine; thus, decreasing excretion by 50 per cent, for example, would have an effect comparable to that of almost tripling dietary intake.

The mechanism(s) involved in the decrease in urinary excretion of phosphorus in response to dietary deprivation is not entirely understood. Hypophosphatemia in this condition is associated with increased production of $1,25(OH)_2D$, increased intestinal absorption of calcium, mild hypercalcemia, and decreased PTH secretion (Fig. 243–1, left middle limb). Any one or a combination of these changes could account for part or all of the decrease in urinary excretion of phosphorus. However, it is also possible that other, as yet undescribed, factors may also play a role.

BONE

Function of Bone

Bone has four major functions: (1) Bones provide rigid support to extremities and to the body cavities that contain vital organs. When bone is weak or defective, erect posture may be impossible and vital organ function may be compromised. (An example is the cardiopulmonary dysfunction that occurs in patients with severe kyphosis due to vertebral collapse.) (2) Bones are crucial to locomotion in that they provide efficient levers and sites of attachment for muscles. With bony deformities, these levers become defective, and severe abnormalities of gait develop. (3) Bone provides a hospitable environment for the dispersed hematopoietic system. (4) Bone provides a large reservoir of ions, such as calcium, phosphorus, magnesium, and sodium, that are crucial for life and can be mobilized when the external environment fails to provide them.

Structure of Bone

Two thirds of the weight of bone is mineral; the remainder is water and collagen. Minor organic components, such as proteoglycans, lipids, noncollagenous proteins, and acidic proteins that contain γ-carboxyglutamic acid, are probably important, but their functions are poorly understood.

There are two types of bone mineral. The major form consists of hydroxyapatite in crystals of varying maturity. The remainder is amorphous calcium phosphate, which lacks a coherent x-ray diffraction pattern, has a lower calcium-to-phosphate ratio than pure hydroxyapatite, occurs in regions of active bone formation, and is present in larger quantities in young bone.

As a living tissue, bone is unique in that it is not only rigid and resists forces that would ordinarily break brittle materials but is also light enough to be moved by coordinated muscle contractions. These characteristics are a function of the strategic location of two major types of bone (Fig. 243–7). Cortical bone, composed of densely packed, mineralized collagen laid down in layers, provides rigidity and is the major component of tubular bones. Trabecular (cancellous) bone is spongy in appearance, provides strength and elasticity, and constitutes the major portion of the axial skeleton. Defective or scanty cortical bone leads to fractures of the long bones, whereas defective or scanty trabecular bone leads to vertebral fractures. Fractures of long bones may also occur because normal reinforcement by trabecular bone is lacking.

Microscopically, there are two types of bone structure: woven and lamellar. Both may be found in either cortical or trabecular bone. Woven bone is a normal constituent of embryonic bone but in adult bone usually reflects the presence of disease. Lamellar bone is stronger than woven bone and is formed more slowly. It progressively replaces woven bone as the skeleton develops from birth. Whereas woven bone has nonparallel collagen fibers, many osteocytes per unit area of matrix, and mineral that is poorly incorporated into collagen fibrils, lamellar bone has a parallel arrangement of collagen fibers, few osteocytes per unit area of matrix, and mineral that is well incorporated into collagen fibrils. Cortical lamellar bone is present in

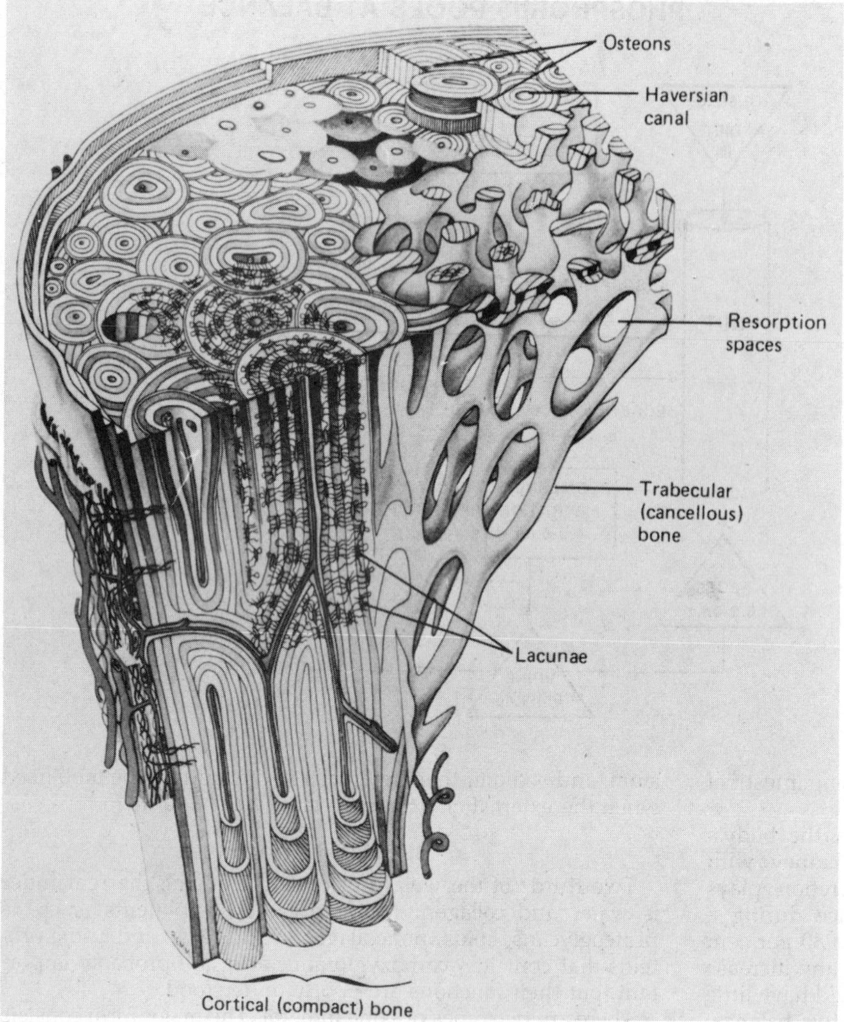

Figure 243–7. Diagram of some of the main features of the microstructure of mature bone seen in both transverse (top) and longitudinal sections. Areas of cortical (compact) and trabecular (cancellous) bone are included. The central area in the transverse section simulates a microradiograph, with the differences in density reflecting variations in mineralization. Note the general construction of the osteons, the distribution of the osteocyte lacunae, the haversian systems, resorption spaces, and the different views of the structural basis of bone lamellation. (Adapted from Warwick R, Williams PL [eds.]: Gray's Anatomy. 35th ed. Edinburgh, Churchill Livingstone, 1973, p 217.)

concentric layers surrounding the vascular channels that compose the haversian systems of cortical bone (osteons) (Fig. 243–7). In contrast, the lamellar bone of trabeculae is present in layers and is laid down in long sheaves and sheets (Fig. 243–8).

Formation and Resorption of Bone

Bone is formed and resorbed continuously throughout life. These important processes depend upon three major types of bone cells, each with different functions.

OSTEOBLASTS. Osteoblasts are thought to be derived from a

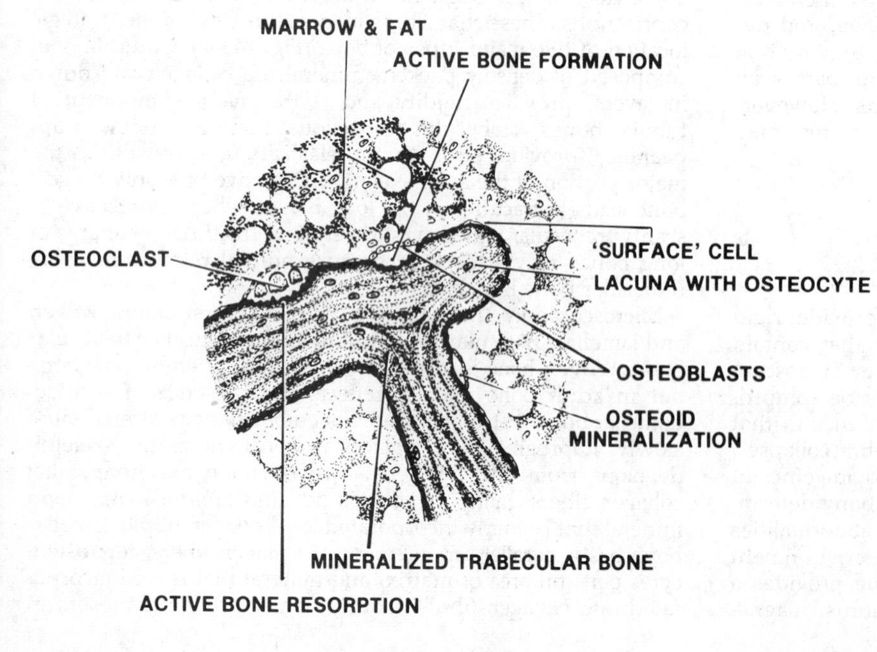

Figure 243–8. Schema of typical microscopic appearance of a section of undemineralized trabecular bone showing active bone resorption and formation.

population of dividing cells, present on bone surfaces, that arise from mesenchymal cells in the connective tissue in bone. These specialized cells form new bone on bone surfaces previously resorbed by osteoclasts and have alkaline phosphatase activity. The exact role of alkaline phosphatase in osteoblast function remains uncertain. Osteoblasts are actively involved in the synthesis of the components of bone matrix (primarily collagen) and probably facilitate the movement of mineral ions between extracellular fluid and the bone surface (Fig. 243–3). The evidence supporting such ion transport by osteoblasts is sparse, but there is widespread agreement that osteoblast-mediated transport of calcium and phosphate is involved in the mineralization of collagen, which in turn is crucial for the formation of bone. In the process of bone formation, osteoblasts gradually become encased in the bone matrix they have produced.

OSTEOCYTES. Once trapped in the mineralized matrix, the functional and morphologic characteristics of osteoblasts change, and they are then called osteocytes. Protein synthesis decreases markedly, and the cells develop multiple processes that reach out through lacunae (Figs. 243–3, 243–7, and 243–8) in bone tissue to "communicate" with processes of other osteocytes within a unit of bone (osteon) and with the processes of surface osteoblasts (Fig. 243–3). The physiologic importance of osteocytes is controversial, but it is believed that they permit mineral movement in and out of regions of bone that are removed from surfaces.

OSTEOCLASTS. Osteoclasts are multinucleated giant cells that are responsible for the resorption of bone (Figs. 243–3 and 243–8). They are probably derived from circulating mononucleated macrophages, which differentiate into the mature osteoclasts by fusion in the bone environment. These cells contain all of the enzymatic components that, when secreted into their environs, solubilize matrix and release calcium and phosphate. Once released, mineral is transported through the osteoclasts into the extracellular fluid and ultimately into blood. Opinion has varied over the years concerning the relative importance to extracellular homeostasis of osteoclastic resorption of bone and the translocation of mineral from the surface of bone into the extracellular space by surface osteoblasts. It is likely that the major role of osteoclastic bone resorption is in bone remodeling (see below).

Dynamics of Bone

The term "modeling," as applied to bone, denotes processes involved in the formation of the macroscopic skeleton. Thus, modeling ceases at maturity (age 18 to 20). The term "remodeling" denotes those processes, occurring at bone surfaces before and after adult development, that are required to maintain the structural integrity of bone.

Abnormalities of remodeling are responsible for metabolic bone diseases. These abnormalities involve alterations in the balance between bone formation and resorption, which lead to diminished structural integrity of bone and ultimately compromise its functions. Normally, in spite of continuous bone remodeling, there is no net gain or loss of skeletal mass after longitudinal growth has ceased (Figs. 243–5 and 243–6). This has led to the view that bone resorption and formation are closely coupled and that this coupling is the result of the coordinated activity of "packets" of interacting osteoblasts and osteoclasts. These packets have been termed "basic multicellular units." The activity of such a unit is characterized by osteoclastic resorption of a defined quantity of bone (on the surface in trabecular bone and by actual excavation in cortical bone), followed by repair of the defect by osteoblasts. During the repair process, collagen (osteoid) is laid down and subsequently mineralized.

Using timed, sequential labeling of bone with orally administered tetracycline (which binds to recently mineralized collagen) and histomorphometric analysis of transiliac bone biopsies from normal adult humans, it has been possible to time the activities of a basic multicellular unit. Estimates indicate that osteoclastic resorption proceeds for about one month in a normal 30-year-old adult, and osteoblastic repair for about three months. The term "sigma" is used to denote the total duration of activity of a typical basic multicellular unit. The concept of sigma has added a new dimension to the understanding of the pathogenesis of metabolic bone disease. Thus, an imbalance between bone formation and resorption could be due not only to alterations in the relative numbers and activities of osteoblasts and osteoclasts but also to abnormalities in the relative duration of the activities of these two cell types.

General Evaluation of Patients with Metabolic Bone Disease

The early detection and treatment of metabolic bone disease is important because it may be difficult or impossible to restore skeletal mass after bone has been lost. This is particularly true of the bone loss that occurs in postmenopausal women and the elderly. It is insidious but causes symptoms only when skeletal mass has decreased to the point that fractures occur with minimal trauma. Establishing bone loss can be difficult because available techniques cannot always detect a decrease in skeletal mass in individual patients. It is necessary, therefore, to have a high index of suspicion for the presence of metabolic bone disease in patients at risk for its development, so that treatment can be instituted early. Since specific metabolic bone diseases are discussed in other chapters, this section will provide only a broad overview of the evaluation of patients with these disorders.

Any one or a combination of the risk factors listed in Table 243–2, especially if accompanied by symptoms such as back pain and muscular weakness or a history of bone fracture with minimal trauma, should raise the question of whether a patient has metabolic bone disease. The extent and type of investigation done should be determined by the specific metabolic bone disease suspected. More than one pathologic process may be involved in producing skeletal disease in an individual patient. Thus, once metabolic bone disease is discovered, the clinician should evaluate the patient for the presence of all of the diseases and risk factors that could alter skeletal metabolism and aggravate the bone disease.

In postmenopausal or elderly patients who have sustained a

TABLE 243–2. MAJOR RISK FACTORS FOR THE DEVELOPMENT OF METABOLIC BONE DISEASE

A. Physiologic Factors
  1. Non-black race
  2. Postmenopausal
  3. Aging
B. Dietary, Environmental, and Physical Factors
  1. Decreased calcium intake
  2. Decreased phosphate intake
  3. Decreased vitamin D intake
  4. Sunlight deprivation
  5. Immobilization
C. Drugs
  1. Corticosteroids
  2. Thyroid hormone
  3. Anticonvulsants
  4. Alcohol
  5. Antacids containing aluminum
  6. Heparin
  7. Cancer chemotherapy
D. Diseases
  1. Endocrinologic
    a. Hyperparathyroidism
    b. Hyperthyroidism
    c. Hyperadrenocorticism
    d. Sex hormone deficiency
  2. Gastrointestinal
    a. Intestinal malabsorption
    b. Malabsorption due to gastric or intestinal resection
    c. Chronic obstructive biliary disease
  3. Renal
    a. Functional impairment of any cause
    b. All tubular disorders resulting in calcium or phosphate loss
    c. ? Nephrosis

recent fracture with minimal trauma, the cause of the osseous demineralization underlying the fracture should be investigated. Although a generalized decrease in skeletal mass due to the osteoporosis associated with menopause or aging is the most likely cause, the first diagnostic consideration should be osseous malignancy, and such patients should be investigated for multiple myeloma (using immunoelectrophoresis of serum and urine protein, Ch. 163) and metastatic malignancy (using radionuclide bone scans). The clinician should also assess vitamin D nutritional status and parathyroid function (serum measurements of calcium, phosphorus, magnesium, alkaline phosphatase, 25OHD, and immunoreactive PTH). Hypercalcemia, if found, should be investigated as described in Chapter 246. Hypocalcemia, especially if it is accompanied by hypophosphatemia, suggests the presence of vitamin D deficiency and osteomalacia. Such a diagnosis is confirmed if serum concentrations of 25OHD are low and serum concentrations of immunoreactive PTH and alkaline phosphatase are increased. These findings should prompt an investigation of possible causes of vitamin D deficiency, such as intestinal malabsorption (e.g., a 72-hour stool fat measurement).

If the noted serum measurements are normal and no evidence for malignancy can be found, the next major objective is to establish the extent and location of bone demineralization so that the effects of treatment can be assessed over time. The only clinical measurement of value is patient height. Decreased height usually reflects the progression of spinal crush fractures and is probably the best indication of disease activity. Although lateral x-rays of the spine, done serially, show only gross decreases in bone mineral, they are the only means of directly assessing new vertebral crush fractures. They should be performed initially and repeated routinely every two years or if there is significant recurrence of back pain. Roentgenograms of the proximal femur yield information about the integrity of the femoral neck and trochanter, which are major sites of osteoporotic fractures that can result in permanent incapacitation and even death (10 to 20 per cent) in the elderly. Disappearance of the superior trabecular pattern that traverses the greater trochanter (arrow in Grade 3 sketch, Fig. 243–9) signals that osteoporosis is sufficiently severe to place the patient at increased risk for hip fracture. It is probably wise to obtain x-rays of these areas at the initial evaluation of postmenopausal or elderly patients for two reasons. First, if grade 2 or 3 trabecular patterns are present, patients should be cautioned to eliminate hazards that may cause falls in their home environments. Second, they provide a basis for comparison with similar x-rays obtained during long-term follow-up and treatment.

There are several clinically applicable techniques for measuring bone mass. The first involves careful x-rays of the hands and measurement of the endosteal and periosteal diameters of the second to fourth metacarpal bones with a precision caliper. The combined cortical thickness of bones is then determined by subtracting the internal from the external diameter. The precision of this measurement is about ± 2 per cent, and values obtained are reasonable reflections of appendicular skeletal mass. The second technique, single photon absorptiometry, measures the attenuation by bone (usually the radius) of a gamma ray beam generated by a ^{125}I or ^{247}Am source. The precision of this measurement is also about ± 2 per cent, and values obtained reflect predominantly appendicular skeletal mass.

Two recently developed techniques can directly measure the mineral content in almost any bone in the body, although both have been used mainly to assess the axial skeleton. The first technique, dual photon absorptiometry, measures the combined mineral content of several vertebrae in both cortical and trabecular bone, as well as that present in overlying structures (e.g., in calcified abdominal aorta). It uses equipment that can be modified from equipment available in most nuclear medicine units. The second technique, which uses computer-assisted tomography, is much more selective than the first, measuring the mineral content of only vertebral trabecular bone. Both techniques are amazingly precise. Although these techniques are currently available only at larger centers, recent advances should make them generally available soon.

The clinical usefulness of techniques that measure bone mineral content is unclear. Unfortunately, they cannot definitely exclude the presence of osteoporosis because there is a large overlap in measurements between patients with proved osteoporotic fractures and age-matched subjects without fractures. However, it may be possible to use single measurements to estimate the fracture risk in individual patients, once data concerning the incidence of fracture are available from long-term, prospective follow-up of such patients.

Presently, histomorphometric analysis of transiliac bone biopsies has achieved almost the status of a fine art. The procedure is most useful in establishing a diagnosis of osteomalacia (Ch. 245) and in determining if, in a given patient, diminished bone density is associated with significant changes in the duration of bone formation or resorption.

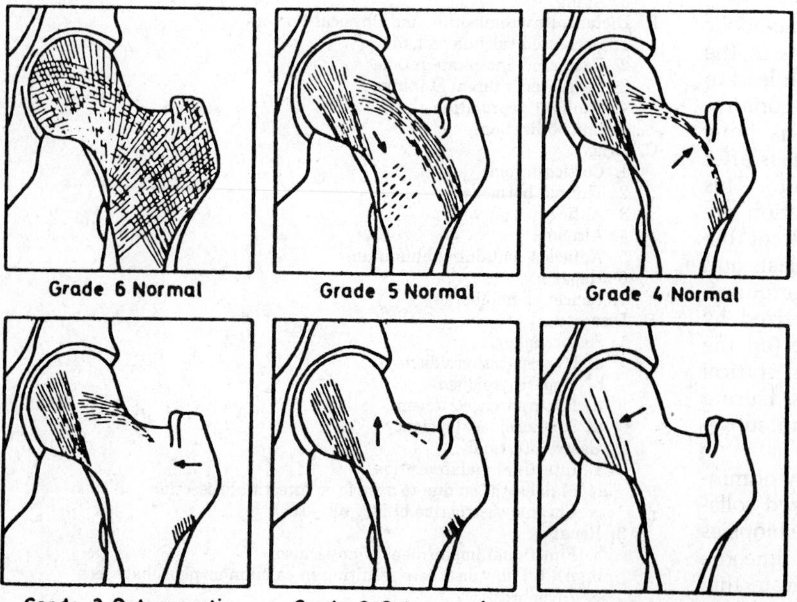

Figure 243–9. The effects of increasingly severe osteoporosis on the pattern of trabecular bone in the upper end of the femur. Arrows show progressive radiologic disappearance of trabecular groups. (Adapted from Singh M, et al.: Femoral trabecular-pattern index for evaluation of spinal osteoporosis. Ann Intern Med 77:64, 1972.)

Arnaud CD: Calcium homeostasis: Regulatory elements and their integration. Fed Proc 37:2557,1978. *Original description of "butterfly" diagram of calcium homeostasis and its usefulness in understanding pathogenic schemes and predicting effects of treatment.*

Aurbach GD, Marx S, Spiegel AM: Parathyroid hormone, calcitonin and the calciferols. *In* Williams RH (ed.): Textbook of Endocrinology. Philadelphia, W. B. Saunders Company, 1981, pp 922–1031. *Focuses on the calciotropic hormones and diseases associated with their abnormal production, secretion, and metabolism.*

Avioli L, Raisz L: Bone metabolism and disease. *In* Bondy PK, Rosenberg LE (eds.): Metabolic Control and Disease. Philadelphia, W. B. Saunders Company, 1980, pp 1709–1786. *Provides an excellent, in-depth description of bone metabolism and disease.*

DeGroot LJ (ed.): Endocrinology. Vol 2. New York, Grune & Stratton, 1979, pp 551–692. *Comprehensive review of the basic science of the mineral-regulating hormones, arranged in 13 chapters written by internationally renowned experts. Topics include parathyroid hormone, calcitonin, and vitamin D chemistry, biosynthesis, secretion, metabolism, and action.*

244. VITAMIN D

Daniel D. Bikle

Vitamin D is a steroid hormone with two molecular forms: vitamin D_3 (cholecalciferol) and vitamin D_2 (ergocalciferol). Vitamin D_3 is produced in the skin of animals, including humans. Vitamin D_2 is derived from the plant sterol ergosterol. It differs from vitamin D_3 in that the side chain has a double bond at C22–23 and a methyl group attached to C24. Vitamin D_2 is the usual form of vitamin D available for pharmaceutical use, although both vitamin D_2 and D_3 are used as food supplements. Despite subtle differences in physiology and biochemistry, vitamin D_2 and D_3 have equivalent potency and mechanisms of action in humans. Therefore, in the ensuing discussion, lack of a subscript after the D indicates that both forms of vitamin D are implied.

To achieve biologic potency, vitamin D must be metabolized further. Two of these metabolites, 25-hydroxyvitamin D (25OHD) and 1,25-dihydroxyvitamin D (1,25$(OH)_2$D), are produced by successive hydroxylations; the hepatic enzyme vitamin D 25-hydroxylase acts at the C25 position to form 25OHD, and the renal enzyme 25OHD 1-hydroxylase acts at the C1 position to form 1,25$(OH)_2$D. Both 25OHD (calcifediol) and 1,25$(OH)_2$D (calcitriol) are available in drug form to treat disorders of calcium homeostasis. A third metabolite, 24,25-dihydroxyvitamin D (24,25$(OH)_2$D), also shows promise as a therapeutic agent but as yet is available only for investigational purposes. 24,25$(OH)_2$D, like 1,25$(OH)_2$D, is produced from 25OHD principally in the kidney.

VITAMIN D ENDOCRINE SYSTEM

The vitamin D endocrine system can be divided into three levels (Fig. 244–1): bioavailability of vitamin D from skin and gut, metabolism of vitamin D to its active forms principally by the liver and kidney, and the action of these metabolites on target tissues.

BIOAVAILABILITY. Vitamin D_3 production in the skin is a multistep process. Irradiation of 7-dehydrocholesterol by ultraviolet (UV) light converts it to previtamin D_3, which then undergoes thermal isomerization to vitamin D_3. No clear regulation of vitamin D_3 production, other than the amount of UV irradiation that reaches the 7-dehydrocholesterol in the epidermis, has been observed.

Vitamin D is also available from the diet, as it is commonly used as a food supplement in dairy products. Vitamin D is absorbed principally in the jejunum by a process (chylomicron formation) that is facilitated by bile salts, fatty acids, and monoglycerides. Most of the vitamin D absorbed passes through the lymphatic system before entering the bloodstream. The hydroxylated metabolites of vitamin D (i.e., 25OHD and 1,25$(OH)_2$D) depend less on chylomicron formation for their absorption.

Vitamin D and its metabolites are transported in blood bound mainly to an alpha globulin (molecular weight, 58,000) called vitamin D binding protein (DBP). This protein has a higher affinity for 25OHD and 24,25$(OH)_2$D than for vitamin D and 1,25$(OH)_2$D. Since the amount of DBP in blood (5×10^{-6}M) far exceeds that of vitamin D and its metabolites (see accompanying table), 1 per cent or less of the total amount of these metabolites is actually free to diffuse into cells. It is unclear whether DBP serves principally as a circulating reservoir for the vitamin D metabolites in blood or whether it facilitates the transport of these metabolites into target tissues. Changes in DBP levels

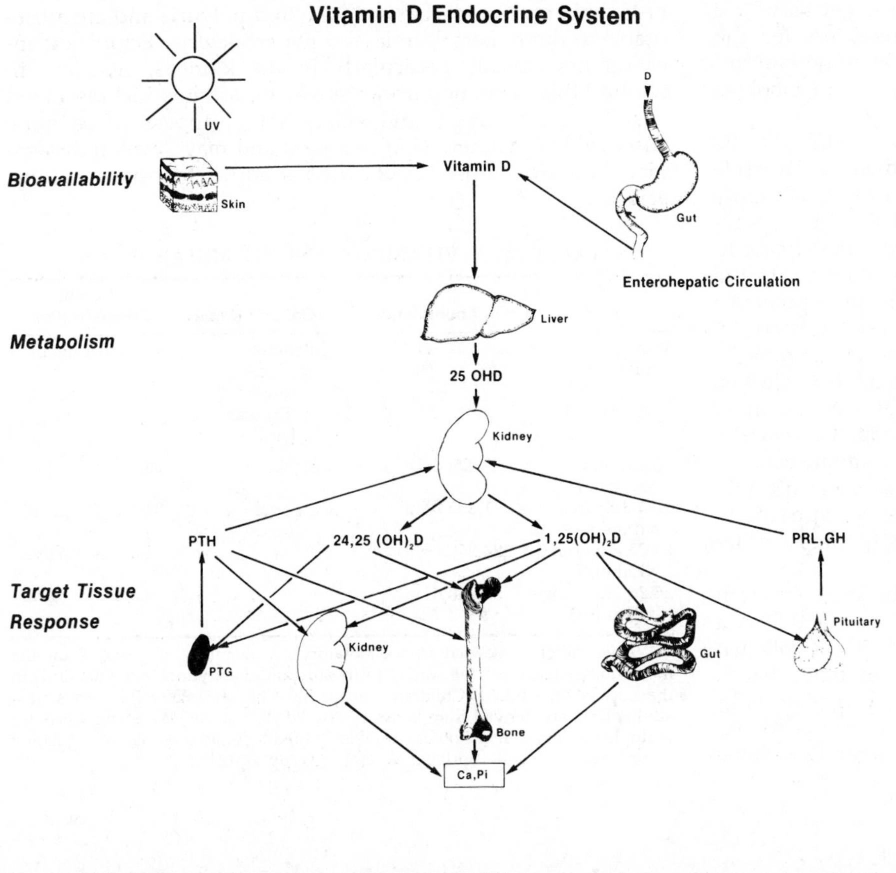

Figure 244–1. The vitamin D endocrine system. Vitamin D is made available to the body by photogenesis in the skin and absorption from the intestine. Vitamin D is then hydroxylated in the liver to 25OHD, then in the kidney to 1,25$(OH)_2$D and 24,25$(OH)_2$D. The active vitamin D metabolites act on different tissues to produce a variety of responses. The three target tissues principally responsible for calcium (Ca) and phosphate (Pi) homeostasis are kidney, bone, and intestine. Endocrine tissues such as the parathyroid gland (PTG) and anterior pituitary are also target tissues. Their hormones, parathyroid hormone (PTH), prolactin (PRL), and growth hormone (GH), help regulate vitamin D metabolism in the kidney; in addition, PTH has a direct effect on bone and kidney regulation of calcium and phosphate homeostasis. (Reproduced with permission from Bikle DD: The vitamin D endocrine system. *In* Stollerman GH, et al. (eds.): Advances in Internal Medicine, Volume 27. Copyright © 1982 by Year Book Medical Publishers, Inc., Chicago.)

(pregnancy and estrogen increase DBP, and liver disease and proteinuria decrease DBP) affect total concentrations of vitamin D metabolites without necessarily affecting the free concentrations. The relative importance of free and total concentrations of the vitamin D metabolites has not been established.

METABOLISM. ***Liver.*** The first step in the bioactivation of vitamin D occurs in the liver, where vitamin D 25-hydroxylase converts vitamin D to 25OHD. This cytochrome P450 mixed function oxidase is found in both microsomes and mitochondria. Since 25OHD production is governed principally by the supply of substrate (i.e., vitamin D), circulating 25OHD levels are a good indicator of vitamin D bioavailability. Hepatic production of 25OHD appears to be well preserved in all but the most severe cases of liver disease unless the vitamin D stores are depleted. However, compounds such as phenytoin and phenobarbital, which induce drug-metabolizing enzymes in the liver, alter the hepatic metabolism of vitamin D in such a manner as to lead to clinical bone disease.

Kidney. The 25OHD produced by the liver is further metabolized to $1,25(OH)_2D$ and $24,25(OH)_2D$, principally in the kidney, by 25OHD 1-hydroxylase and 24-hydroxylase, respectively. Little if any $1,25(OH)_2D$ is produced outside the kidney (except by the placenta) under normal circumstances, although other tissues, such as bone, cartilage, skin, and intestine, may produce $25(OH)_2D$ under some circumstances. Lymphomatous or sarcoid tissue may also contain 1-hydroxylase activity. Both 1-hydroxylase and 24-hydroxylase are cytochrome P450 mixed function oxidases located exclusively in the mitochondria of the proximal renal tubule. Their activities are closely regulated by a variety of ions and hormones, the most important of which are calcium, phosphate, $1,25(OH)_2D$ itself, and parathyroid hormone (PTH). Low serum calcium and phosphate levels and elevated PTH levels stimulate $1,25(OH)_2D$ production. High $1,25(OH)_2D$ levels inhibit $1,25(OH)_2D$ production but increase $24,25(OH)_2D$ production.

TARGET TISSUE RESPONSE. Although bone, gut, and kidney are the primary target tissues for vitamin D, many other tissues, including the pituitary, parathyroid glands, pancreas, brain, and skin, contain a specific receptor for $1,25(OH)_2D$ and respond to it by a change in function. Muscle contains no receptors for $1,25(OH)_2D$ but appears to be a target tissue for 25OHD. Whether all tissues that contain receptors for the vitamin D metabolites have a physiologically important response to normal circulating concentrations of the metabolites has not been established.

Intestine. Of the various tissues affected by $1,25(OH)_2D$, the intestine has been the most extensively studied. $1,25(OH)_2D$ regulates calcium transport across the intestine in a highly integrated sequence of events. First of all, $1,25(OH)_2D$ appears to increase the permeability of the brush border membrane to calcium, permitting calcium to enter from the lumen into the intestinal epithelial cell down a steep electrochemical gradient. The calcium that enters the cell must be accumulated by subcellular organelles, such as the mitochondria, to prevent cytosolic calcium concentrations from reaching toxic levels; $1,25(OH)_2D$ stimulates this accumulation. The calcium must then be transported through the cell and pumped across the basolateral membrane into the bloodstream. A unique calcium binding protein (CaBP), induced by $1,25(OH)_2D$ in the intestine as well as in a number of other target tissues, appears to modulate intracellular calcium concentrations, perhaps by facilitating the removal of calcium from the cell.

Bone. The role of the vitamin D metabolites in calcium movement in and out of bone is less clear. $1,25(OH)_2D$ is a potent stimulator of bone resorption and inhibitor of collagen production (bone formation) in vitro. On the other hand, $24,25(OH)_2D$ may stimulate bone and cartilage formation without stimulating bone resorption. These results have engendered a controversy as to whether all the effects of vitamin D on bone are mediated by $1,25(OH)_2D$ or whether other metabolites, $24,25(OH)_2D$ in particular, have a unique biologic role.

Although the vitamin D metabolites may play a role, independent of PTH, in regulating renal calcium and phosphate excretion, this role has not been well defined.

MEASUREMENT IN SERUM

Most assays for the vitamin D metabolites use naturally occurring binding proteins. Radioimmunoassays employing poly- or monoclonal antibodies and a bioassay evaluating bone resorption from cultured bone in vitro have also been developed. The principal difficulty in measuring vitamin D metabolites is that chromatographic separation of the metabolites from each other and from other interfering substances is required. Nevertheless, most laboratories generally agree on the measurements of 25OHD and $1,25(OH)_2D$ (Table 244–1). Measurement of vitamin D itself remains difficult because of its poor solubility in aqueous solutions and modest affinity to the binding proteins used in the assays.

HYPOVITAMINOSIS D

Vitamin D deficiency results from insufficient vitamin D in the diet, insufficient production of vitamin D in the skin, inadequate absorption of vitamin D from the diet, or abnormal conversion of vitamin D to its bioactive metabolites. Vitamin D deficiency appears clinically as rickets in children and osteomalacia in adults. This subject is discussed in detail in the chapter on Osteomalacia (Ch. 245).

HYPERVITAMINOSIS D

Hypervitaminosis D may occur in three general settings: (1) excessive consumption, usually for therapeutic purposes, of vitamin D, vitamin D analogues (such as dihydrotachysterol), or vitamin D metabolites; (2) the abnormal conversion of vitamin D to its biologically active metabolites, as occurs in sarcoidosis and possibly other granulomatous diseases; or (3) a change in the sensitivity of the target tissue to vitamin D, as can occur with the remission of a variety of gastrointestinal diseases associated with calcium malabsorption. The initial signs and symptoms of vitamin D intoxication include weakness, lethargy, headaches, nausea, and polyuria and are attributable to the hypercalcemia and hypercalciuria. Ectopic calcification may occur, particularly in the kidneys, resulting in nephrolithiasis or nephrocalcinosis; other sites include blood vessels, heart, lungs, and skin. Infants appear to be quite susceptible to vitamin D intoxication and may develop disseminated arteriosclerosis, supravalvular aortic stenosis, and renal acidosis.

TABLE 244–1. VITAMIN D AND ITS METABOLITES

Name	Abbreviation	Generic Name	Serum Concentration*
Vitamin D	D	Calciferol	1.6 ± 0.4 ng/ml
Vitamin D_3	D_3	a) Cholecalciferol	
Vitamin D_2	D_2	b) Ergocalciferol	
25 hydroxyvitamin D	25OHD	Calcifediol	26.5 ± 5.3 ng/ml
1,25 dihydroxyvitamin D	$1,25(OH)_2D$	Calcitriol	34.1 ± 9.8 pg/ml
24,25 dihydroxyvitamin D	$24,25(OH)_2D$		1.3 ± 0.4 ng/ml
25,26 dihydroxyvitamin D	$25,26(OH)_2D$		0.5 ± 0.1 ng/ml

*Values differ somewhat from laboratory to laboratory, depending on the methodology used and the sunlight exposure and dietary intake of vitamin D in the population studied. Children tend to have higher $1,25(OH)_2D$ levels than adults. Data are derived from Lambert PW, Fu IY, Kaetzel DM, et al.: Assay for multiple vitamin D metabolites. *In* Bikle DD (ed.): Assay of Calcium Regulating Hormones. New York, Springer-Verlag, 1983, pp 99–124.

The dose of vitamin D required to produce toxicity varies among patients, reflecting differences in absorption, storage, and subsequent metabolism of the vitamin as well as in target tissue response to the active metabolites. For example, an elderly patient with senile osteoporosis and a low turnover rate for bone also tends to have a reduced ability to absorb calcium in the intestine and a reduced ability to produce $1,25(OH)_2D$ in the kidney. Such a patient can usually ingest 50,000 to 100,000 IU of vitamin D per day without developing hypercalcemia or hypercalciuria. In contrast, a patient of similar age with a similar degree of osteoporosis but in whom the osteoporosis develops as a result of primary hyperparathyroidism would almost certainly be harmed by this amount of vitamin D. In the latter patient the ability of vitamin D to stimulate bone resorption and intestinal calcium absorption is enhanced in part because of the greater rates of $1,25(OH)_2D$ production and bone turnover observed in primary hyperparathyroidism. Patients with sarcoidosis appear to develop vitamin D intoxication because $1,25(OH)_2D$ production in the abnormal tissue apparently is not subject to the normal feedback mechanisms that regulate renal production of $1,25(OH)_2D$. Analogues of vitamin D, such as dihydrotachysterol, or the renal metabolite of vitamin D, $1,25(OH)_2D$, which bypass the normal rate-limiting step of vitamin D bioactivation (the renal 1α-hydroxylase), are more likely than vitamin D or 25OHD to result in hypercalcemia if used in excess.

Hypervitaminosis D is treated by stopping the administration of vitamin D or its analogues or metabolites. If the hypercalcemia is severe, the patient should be placed on a low calcium diet and given glucocorticoids (e.g., 60 mg of prednisone every day) and generous amounts of fluids. Acute hypercalcemia, when symptomatic, can be treated with saline and furosemide diuresis, as described under the general management of hypercalcemia. Hypercalcemia lasts only for a few days when caused by $1,25(OH)_2D$ excess, but it may persist for weeks or months when caused by vitamin D excess. The hypercalcemia of sarcoidosis tends to respond within days to glucocorticoid therapy.

Barbour GL, Coburn JW, Slatopolsky E, Norman AW, Horst RL: Hypercalcemia in an anephric patient with sarcoidosis: Evidence for extrarenal generation of 1,25-dihydroxyvitamin D. N Engl J Med 305:440, 1981. *An instructive case of an anephric patient with sarcoidosis in whom hypercalcemia and elevated $1,25(OH)_2D$ levels developed in parallel and then decreased in parallel following prednisone therapy.*

Bikle DD: The vitamin D endocrine system. Adv Intern Med 27:45, 1982. *A review of the physiology and pathophysiology of the vitamin D endocrine system.*

Bikle DD (ed.): Assay of Calcium Regulating Hormones. New York, Springer-Verlag, 1983.

Bikle DD, Morrissey RL, Zolock DT, Rasmussen H: The intestinal response to vitamin D. Rev Physiol Biochem Pharmacol 89:63, 1981. *A comprehensive discussion of intestinal calcium and phosphate transport and the role of $1,25(OH)_2D$ in this process.*

Fraser DR: Regulation of the metabolism of vitamin D. Physiol Rev 60:551, 1980. *A thorough, well-balanced review of vitamin D metabolism in the liver and kidney.*

Haddad JG Jr: Transport of vitamin D metabolites. Clin Orthop 142:249, 1979. *A good review of the vitamin D binding protein in blood.*

Lee DBN, Zawada ET, Kleeman CR: The pathophysiology and clinical aspects of hypercalcemic disorders. West J Med 129:278, 1978. *This article discusses all the major hypercalcemic disorders, including the diagnosis and treatment of hypervitaminosis D.*

Mason RS, Frankel T, Chan Y-L, Lissner D, Posen S: Vitamin D conversion by sarcoid lymph node homogenate. Ann Intern Med 100:59, 1984. *Provides direct evidence that sarcoid tissue in a lymph node may be capable of metabolizing 25OHD to $1,25(OH)_2D$ and $25,26(OH)_2D$.*

245. OSTEOMALACIA AND RICKETS

Daniel D. Bikle

DEFINITIONS

Osteomalacia and rickets are caused by the abnormal mineralization of bone. Osteomalacia refers to the defect that occurs in bone in which the epiphyseal plates have closed (i.e., in adults), whereas rickets refers to the defect that occurs in growing bone (i.e., in children). Abnormal mineralization in growing bone affects the transformation of cartilage into bone at the zone of provisional calcification. As a result, an enormous profusion of disorganized, nonmineralized, degenerating cartilage appears in this region, leading to widening of the epiphyseal plate (observed radiologically as a widened radiolucent zone) with flaring or cupping and irregularity of the epiphyseal-metaphyseal junctions. This latter problem gives rise to the clinically obvious beaded swellings along the costochondral junctions (rachitic rosary) and the swelling at the ends of the long bones. Growth is retarded by the failure to make new bone. Once bone growth has ceased (i.e., after closure of the epiphyseal plates), the clinical evidence for defective mineralization becomes more subtle, and special diagnostic procedures may be required for its detection.

PATHOGENESIS

The best known cause of abnormal bone mineralization is vitamin D deficiency. Vitamin D, through its biologically active metabolites, insures that the calcium and phosphate concentrations in the extracellular milieu are adequate for mineralization to occur. Vitamin D also may permit osteoblasts to produce a bone matrix that can be mineralized, and then allows them to mineralize that matrix in a normal fashion. Phosphate deficiency is another condition that can cause defective mineralization. It may act independently or in conjunction with other predisposing abnormalities since most hypophosphatemic disorders associated with osteomalacia or rickets also affect the vitamin D endocrine system. Dietary calcium deficiency has been implicated recently as a cause of rickets and may contribute to the osteomalacia and osteoporosis found in elderly patients. Osteomalacia or rickets may develop despite adequate levels of calcium, phosphate, and vitamin D if the bone matrix cannot undergo normal mineralization. For example, the deficiency in alkaline phosphatase in patients with hypophosphatasia can cause a defect in mineralization. This enzyme cleaves pyrophosphate, an inhibitor of bone mineralization, and a deficiency results in reduced removal of this inhibitor. Finally, drugs such as etidronate and heavy metals such as aluminum can interfere with mineralization and lead to osteomalacia or rickets.

Table 245–1 lists diseases associated with osteomalacia and rickets according to the presumed mechanism responsible for the mineralization defect. Diseases that appear under multiple headings affect bone mineralization via multiple mechanisms. It is important to understand the mechanism by which a particular disease interferes with bone mineralization in order to choose appropriate diagnostic procedures and therapy.

Disorders in the Vitamin D Endocrine System

The exact mechanism or mechanisms by which vitamin D maintains normal bone development is unknown, but disorders in the vitamin D endocrine system are the leading cause of rickets and osteomalacia through decreased bioavailability of vitamin D, abnormal metabolism of vitamin D, and abnormal response of target tissues to the biologically active vitamin D metabolites.

Decreased Bioavailability

REDUCED SUNLIGHT EXPOSURE. The human skin can generate adequate amounts of vitamin D if exposed to sufficient ultraviolet irradiation. However, in countries with limited sunlight or where the population dresses in a fashion that reduces sunlight exposure, circulating levels of vitamin D metabolites are often low. These low levels may help explain why the incidence of osteomalacia is higher in Great Britain, the Scandinavian countries, the Middle East, and India than in the United States.

NUTRITIONAL VITAMIN D DEFICIENCY. The fortification of dairy products with vitamin D has made nutritional vitamin D-

TABLE 245–1. THE OSTEOMALACIC SYNDROMES*

A. Disorders in the vitamin D endocrine system
   1. Decreased bioavailability
      - Insufficient sunlight exposure
      - Nutritional vitamin D deficiency
      - Nephrotic syndrome (urinary loss)
      - Malabsorption (fecal loss)
         - Billroth type II gastrectomy
         - Sprue
         - Regional enteritis
         - Jejunoileal bypass
         - Pancreatic insufficiency
         - Cholestatic disorders
         - Cholestyramine
   2. Abnormal metabolism
      - Liver disease
      - Chronic renal failure
      - Vitamin D dependent rickets type I
      - Tumoral hypophosphatemic osteomalacia
      - X-linked hypophosphatemia
      - Hypoparathyroidism (?)
      - Chronic acidosis (?)
      - Anticonvulsants
   3. Abnormal target tissue response
      - Vitamin D dependent rickets type II
      - Gastrointestinal disorders

B. Disorders of phosphate homeostasis
   1. Decreased intestinal absorption
      - Malnutrition
      - Malabsorption
      - Antacids containing aluminum hydroxide
   2. Increased renal loss
      - X-linked hypophosphatemic rickets
      - Tumoral hypophosphatemic osteomalacia
      - De Toni-Debré-Fanconi (phosphaturia, aminoaciduria, glycosuria, bicarbonaturia)
      - Cystinosis
      - Oculocerebralrenal syndrome (Lowe's syndrome)
      - Paraproteinemias
      - Wilson's disease
      - Glycogen storage diseases
      - Galactosemia
      - Tyrosinemia
      - Cadmium poisoning
      - Neurofibromatosis

C. Calcium deficiency
   1. Dietary insufficiency
   2. Excessive renal loss (?)
   3. Malabsorption of calcium (?)

D. Primary disorders of bone matrix
   1. Hypophosphatasia
   2. Fibrogenesis imperfecta ossium
   3. Axial osteomalacia

E. Inhibitors of mineralization
   1. Aluminum
      - Chronic renal failure
      - Total parenteral nutrition
   2. Etidronate
   3. Phenytoin (?)
   4. Fluoride (?)

*This table categorizes diseases that produce osteomalacia according to the presumed mechanism(s) by which bone mineralization is inhibited. A question mark indicates that the association of the disease to osteomalacia or the mechanism by which it produces osteomalacia is not established.

deficient rickets uncommon in the United States, although it is still prevalent in other parts of the world. Even in the United States vitamin D deficiency may occur in children of vegetarian mothers who avoid milk products (and presumably have reduced vitamin D stores) and in children who are not weaned to vitamin D-supplemented milk by age 2. The contribution of nutritional vitamin D deficiency to osteomalacia in elderly people is unknown. Osteomalacia has been observed in 25 to 30 per cent of bone biopsies from elderly patients who have suffered hip fractures in Scandinavia and Great Britain. Most likely, both reduced vitamin D intake and reduced sunlight exposure contribute to the development of osteomalacia in the elderly.

NEPHROTIC SYNDROME. Even when vitamin D intake is adequate, vitamin D and its metabolites can be lost in the urine. The vitamin D metabolites in serum are tightly bound to an alpha globulin called vitamin D binding protein (DBP), which has a molecular weight of 58,000. Patients with the nephrotic syndrome may lose substantial amounts of DBP into their urine and consequently have very low circulating levels of the vitamin D metabolites. The incidence of osteomalacia in patients with the nephrotic syndrome is unknown; osteomalacia has only recently been recognized as a complication of this renal disease.

MALABSORPTION. Fecal loss of vitamin D and its metabolites occurs in patients with malabsorption for several reasons. Ingested vitamin D is absorbed primarily in chylomicrons; disorders that involve the biliary tract, pancreas, or mid to distal portions of the small intestine reduce the efficiency of this process. Endogenous vitamin D and its metabolites undergo enterohepatic circulation; disorders of the distal small bowel disrupt this circulation. In cholestatic disorders, urinary excretion of vitamin D metabolites is increased and intestinal absorption is decreased. Drugs, such as cholestyramine, that are used in the treatment of cholestatic disorders may compound the problem by binding to the vitamin D metabolites and enhancing their fecal excretion. The resulting bone disease is often a combination of osteomalacia and osteoporosis. The extent of osteomalacia in patients with cholestatic and gastrointestinal disorders varies from country to country. It appears to be higher in Great Britain and Northern Europe than in the United States. Fully 25 to 50 per cent of British and European patients who have undergone Billroth type II gastrectomy or jejunoileal bypass or who have cholestatic liver disease or inflammatory bowel disease have osteomalacia when evaluated by bone biopsy. Pancreatic insufficiency appears to be associated with a lower incidence of osteomalacia than these other forms of gastrointestinal disease.

Abnormal Metabolism

LIVER DISEASE. The hepatic production of 25-hydroxyvitamin D (25OHD) is not tightly controlled. Neither cholestatic nor parenchymal liver disease has much effect on 25OHD production. The low levels of circulating 25OHD found in patients with liver disease can usually be attributed to reduced hepatic synthesis of DBP, poor nutrition, or malabsorption rather than to failure by the liver to metabolize vitamin D. Regardless of the mechanism, patients with chronic liver disease are predisposed to developing osteomalacia.

CHRONIC RENAL FAILURE (also see Ch. 78). Metabolism of 25OHD to 1,25-dihydroxyvitamin D ($1,25(OH)_2D$) and 24,25-dihydroxyvitamin D ($24,25(OH)_2D$) in the kidney is tightly regulated. Renal disease results in reduced circulating levels of both these metabolites. With the reduction in $1,25(OH)_2D$ levels, intestinal calcium absorption falls and bone resorption appears to become less sensitive to parathyroid hormone (PTH)—a result that leads to hypocalcemia. Phosphate excretion by the diseased kidney is decreased, resulting in hyperphosphatemia and aggravation of the hypocalcemia. As a consequence, hyperparathyroidism develops, possibly facilitated by the fact that the levels of the vitamin D metabolites are too low to inhibit parathyroid hormone (PTH) secretion. The net effect of deficient $1,25(OH)_2D$ and $24,25(OH)_2D$ and excessive PTH on bone is complex. Patients may have osteitis fibrosa (reflecting excessive PTH), osteomalacia (in part reflecting vitamin D deficiency), or a combination of the two. One particularly debilitating form of renal osteodystrophy is found in a small percentage of patients in whom only osteomalacia occurs. These patients have normal or only modestly elevated levels of PTH and alkaline phosphatase; hypercalcemia, especially after small doses of $1,25(OH)_2D$, and refractoriness to $1,25(OH)_2D$ therapy are often found. Such patients appear to have increased aluminum content in their bones, particularly in the zone where mineralization is occurring (calcification front).

VITAMIN D-DEPENDENT RICKETS TYPE I. Vitamin D-dependent rickets type I, or pseudo-vitamin D deficiency, is a rare, autosomal recessive disease in which there is a low level of $1,25(OH)_2D$ resulting from a selective deficiency in the renal production of $1,25(OH)_2D$. Although affected patients do not respond to doses of vitamin D that are adequate to treat vitamin D deficiency (i.e., 400 to 4000 IU per day), they do respond to moderate doses (4000 to 40,000 IU per day) of vitamin D or physiologic doses (0.5 to 1.0 μg per day) of $1,25(OH)_2D$.

TUMOR-INDUCED HYPOPHOSPHATEMIC OSTEOMALACIA. Certain unusual tumors (usually mesenchymal) produce osteomalacia associated with low serum levels of phosphorus and $1,25(OH)_2D$ and increased phosphaturia. The cause of this syndrome is unknown, but it is presumed that a humoral product of the tumor suppresses both $1,25(OH)_2D$ production and phosphate reabsorption in the kidney. Removal of the tumor reverses the abnormalities.

X-LINKED HYPOPHOSPHATEMIA. X-linked hypophosphatemia (vitamin D-resistant rickets, or VDRR) is characterized by renal phosphate wasting, hypophosphatemia, and a subtle decrease in $1,25(OH)_2D$ production. Although most cases are diagnosed in childhood and have an X-linked dominant form of inheritance, sporadic adult cases and autosomal transmission occur. Most patients have $1,25(OH)_2D$ levels that are inappropriately low for the degree of hypophosphatemia, which ordinarily increases $1,25(OH)_2D$ production. Treatment with oral phosphate and vitamin D suppresses $1,25(OH)_2D$ to even lower levels. The primary abnormality in these patients is thought to be a defect in renal tubular phosphate transport, resulting in renal phosphate wasting. This defect may secondarily alter vitamin D metabolism. X-linked hypophosphatemia is a fairly common form of metabolic bone disease that should be suspected in all individuals who have low levels of serum phosphate and evidence of bone disease.

HYPOPARATHYROIDISM. Parathyroid hormone is a major stimulator of $1,25(OH)_2D$ production. One would expect osteomalacia to develop when the hormone is absent, because of the reduction in $1,25(OH)_2D$ production. However, osteomalacia appears to be a rare complication of hypoparathyroidism.

CHRONIC METABOLIC ACIDOSIS. Acute metabolic acidosis results in reduced $1,25(OH)_2D$ production. Although chronic metabolic acidosis is associated wih osteomalacia, especially when accompanied by renal loss of phosphate and bicarbonate (as in proximal renal tubular acidosis), it is unclear whether chronic metabolic acidosis has a direct effect on the renal metabolism of vitamin D. Distal renal tubular acidosis and chronic respiratory acidosis are not associated with osteomalacia.

ANTICONVULSANTS. Phenytoin and phenobarbital induce drug-metabolizing enzymes in the liver that alter the hepatic metabolism of vitamin D. This effect may account for the lower circulating levels of 25OHD found in patients treated with anticonvulsants. Surprisingly, these drugs do not lead to a reduction in $1,25(OH)_2D$ levels. Institutionalized children and adults treated with anticonvulsants have a high incidence of rickets or osteomalacia. Outpatient studies of adults treated with anticonvulsants suggest a lower but still substantial incidence of osteomalacia by biochemical criteria, although large studies that incorporate bone biopsy evaluations have not been performed. Clinically debilitating osteomalacia is unusual in outpatient populations treated with anticonvulsants.

Abnormal Target Tissue Response

VITAMIN D-DEPENDENT RICKETS TYPE II. Vitamin D-dependent rickets type II is a rare condition that occurs in childhood and is not responsive to even huge doses of vitamin D. Unlike patients with vitamin D-dependent rickets type I (see Abnormal Metabolism, above), children with type II disease have high circulating levels of $1,25(OH)_2D$. Their problem appears to be a deficiency of normal intracellular receptors for $1,25(OH)_2D$.

GASTROINTESTINAL DISORDERS. Less exotic examples of abnormal target tissue response include a variety of gastrointestinal diseases, such as sprue, short bowel, and regional enteritis, in which calcium and phosphate malabsorption occur not only because of vitamin D deficiency but also because of decreased absorptive surface, steatorrhea, and rapid transit time.

Disorders of Phosphate Homeostasis (also see Ch. 207)

Chronic hypophosphatemia may lead to rickets or osteomalacia independently of other predisposing abnormalities. However, the principal diseases in which hypophosphatemia is associated with osteomalacia or rickets also include other abnormalities that can interfere with bone mineralization. Chronic phosphate depletion is caused by decreased intestinal absorption or increased renal clearance. Acute hypophosphatemia can result from movement of phosphate into cells (e.g., after infusion of insulin and glucose), but this condition is transient and does not result in bone disease (see Ch. 207).

Decreased Intestinal Absorption

MALNUTRITION. Seventy to 90 per cent of dietary phosphate is absorbed, primarily in the jejunum. This process is not tightly regulated, although vitamin D, at least in animal models, stimulates phosphate absorption. Meat and dairy products are the principal dietary sources of phosphate, and vegetarian diets that exclude them can result in phosphate deficiency. The incidence of osteomalacia in vegetarians who avoid all meat and dairy products is unknown. However, since these dietary practices also lead to decreased vitamin D intake, such individuals may be predisposed to bone disease.

MALABSORPTION. Intrinsic small bowel disease and surgical rearrangement of the small bowel interfere with phosphate absorption and, if coupled with diarrhea or steatorrhea, can result in phosphate depletion. The hypophosphatemia may contribute to the osteomalacia seen in such patients, especially when vitamin D levels are reduced (see Decreased Bioavailability of Vitamin D, above).

ALUMINUM HYDROXIDE ANTACIDS. A number of widely used antacids (for example, Mylanta, Maalox, Basaljel, and Amphojel) contain aluminum hydroxide, which binds phosphate and prevents its absorption. Patients who ingest large amounts of these antacids may become depleted in phosphate. This mechanism may contribute to the severity of the osteomalacia observed in patients with chronic renal failure, and in patients who have undergone partial gastrectomy but who continue to ingest large quantities of antacids (see Ch. 248).

Increased Renal Loss

Eighty-five to 90 per cent of the phosphate filtered by the glomerulus is reabsorbed, primarily in the proximal tubule. This process is regulated by PTH, which reduces renal tubular phosphate reabsorption, and probably also by vitamin D, which appears to increase renal tubular phosphate reabsorption. Many diseases that affect renal handling of phosphate are associated with osteomalacia. X-linked hypophosphatemia and tumoral hypophosphatemic osteomalacia have been described above. The De Toni-Debré-Fanconi syndromes are also associated with osteomalacia (Ch. 83.5). They include a heterogeneous group of unusual disorders that are characterized by phosphaturia, aminoaciduria, glycosuria, and bicarbonaturia, and frequently by mild acidosis and hypercalciuria. In general, the osteomalacia or rickets associated with these proximal tubular disorders responds only to large doses of vitamin D. The associated bone disease is most likely the result of a combination of systemic acidosis, hypophosphatemia, and abnormal vitamin D metabolism.

Calcium Deficiency

Calcium deficiency may contribute to the mineralization defect that complicates gastrointestinal disease and proximal tubular disorders, but it is less well established as a cause of osteomalacia than is vitamin D or phosphate deficiency. However, in one carefully performed study of children who ingested a low-calcium diet, there was clinical, biochemical, and histologic evidence of osteomalacia. The serum phosphate and 25OHD levels were normal but the serum calcium levels were low. Since intestinal absorption of calcium decreases with age, the daily requirement for calcium increases from approximately 800 mg in young adults to 1400 mg in the elderly. Calcium deficiency can result not only from inadequate dietary intake but also from excessive fecal and urinary losses.

Primary Disorders of the Bone Matrix

Intrinsic disorders of bone in which matrix is produced but not mineralized are rare. Three diseases appear to fit this category, but none are well understood.

Hypophosphatasia

Hypophosphatasia is a familial disease that is transmitted in an autosomal recessive pattern. Children with this disease usually present with a severe form of rickets, whereas adults may present merely with a predisposition to fractures. The biochemical hallmarks are low serum (and tissue) levels of alkaline phosphatase and increased urinary levels of phosphoethanolamine. The reason why these patients develop osteomalacia or rickets is unclear, but the following mechanism has been suggested. Skeletal alkaline phosphatase cleaves pyrophosphate, an inhibitor of bone mineralization; patients deficient in alkaline phosphatase may be unable to hydrolyze this inhibitor and so develop a mineralization defect.

Fibrogenesis Imperfecta Ossium

Fibrogenesis imperfecta ossium is a rare, painful disorder that affects middle-aged males in what appears to be a sporadic fashion. Serum alkaline phosphatase is increased. The bones have a dense, amorphous, mottled appearance radiologically and a disorganized arrangement of collagen with decreased birefringence, histologically. Presumably, the disorganized collagen matrix retards normal bone mineralization.

Axial Osteomalacia

Unlike fibrogenesis imperfecta ossium, axial osteomalacia is not painful, involves only the axial skeleton, shows no disorganization of collagen on bone biospy, and is not associated with increased serum alkaline phosphatase. The reason for the mineralization disorder in this rare disease is uncertain.

Inhibitors of Mineralization

Several drugs are known to cause osteomalacia or rickets by inhibiting mineralization, but in no case is the mechanism fully understood.

Aluminum

Patients on hemodialysis are exposed to aluminum in the dialysate if tap water is used and through the antacid preparations used to control serum phosphate. Most develop bone disease. Bone biopsies show a correlation between the extent of osteomalacia in these patients and the amount of aluminum deposited in bone. It is likely that the aluminum blocks normal mineralization. Severely affected patients respond to a reduction in their exposure to or body stores of the metal.

Many patients who are treated by total parenteral nutrition for extended periods of time develop bone disease characterized by osteomalacia. In some cases the aluminum content of the casein hydrolysate used to provide amino acids is high. Replacement of casein hydrolysate with purified amino acids may correct or prevent this complication.

Etidronate

Etidronate, the only diphosphonate available for clinical use in the United States, produces osteomalacia at doses greater than 5 to 10 mg per kilogram of body weight. Therefore, the dose must be limited. Etidronate affects osteoblast function and inhibits calcium phosphate crystallization. It is unclear why this drug and not other diphosphonates results in osteomalacia.

Phenytoin

As discussed previously (see Anticonvulsants), phenytoin therapy may cause osteomalacia by inducing enzymes that alter the hepatic metabolism of vitamin D. In addition, phenytoin directly and adversely affects bone mineral metabolism in animals. This effect may also contribute to bone disease.

Fluoride

Fluoride stimulates bone formation, but if it is administered in high doses without adequate calcium supplementation, the bone is poorly mineralized. The mechanism or mechanisms by which fluoride alters osteoblast function and bone mineralization is unknown.

DIAGNOSIS

In children the presentation of rickets is generally obvious from a combination of clinical and radiologic evidence. The diagnostic challenge is to determine the etiology. The most common causes—malabsorption, liver disease, chronic renal failure, X-linked hypophosphatemic rickets, and vitamin D deficiency—are readily distinguished on the basis of history, clinical findings, and routine analyses of blood and urine. In adults the clinical, radiologic, and biochemical evidence for osteomalacia is often subtle. In situations in which osteomalacia should be suspected (malnutrition, liver disease, malabsorption, renal failure, and unexplained osteopenia), the clinician must decide whether to biopsy the bone for histomorphometric examination. When bone biopsy is performed, the information obtained is valuable both for planning and for following therapy. However, this definitive procedure is not yet widely available. When bone biopsy is not used, diagnosis is less certain, but the radiologic and biochemical tests discussed in the paragraphs that follow are still useful in selecting patients for a therapeutic trial of vitamin D, calcium, or phosphate, or all three.

Clinical Features

The clinical presentation of rickets depends on the age of the patient and, to some extent, the etiology of the syndrome (Fig. 245–1). The affected infant or young child may be apathetic, listless, weak, hypotonic, and growing poorly. A soft somewhat misshapen head with widened sutures and frontal bossing may be observed. Eruption of teeth may be delayed, and teeth that do appear may be pitted and poorly mineralized. The enlargement and cupping of the costochondral junctions produce the "rachitic rosary" on the thorax. The tug of the diaphragm against the softened lower ribs may produce an indentation at the point of insertion of the diaphragm—Harrison's groove. Muscle hypotonia can result in a pronounced pot belly and a waddling gait. The limbs may become bowed, and joints may swell because of flaring at the ends of the long bones (including phalanges and metacarpals). Pathologic fractures may occur in patients with florid rickets.

Adult patients with osteomalacia may complain of poorly localized bone pain that is characterized as a constant, dull ache. Muscle weakness, usually of the proximal muscles, may be present, and severely affected patients may be unable to walk. A fracture, often of the hip, may be the initial presentation. In general, however, it is difficult to diagnose osteomalacia on clinical grounds alone.

Radiologic Features

The radiologic features of rickets, like the clinical manifestations, can be quite striking, especially in the young child. In growing bone, the radiolucent epiphyses are wide and flared, with irregular epiphyseal-metaphyseal junctions. Long bones

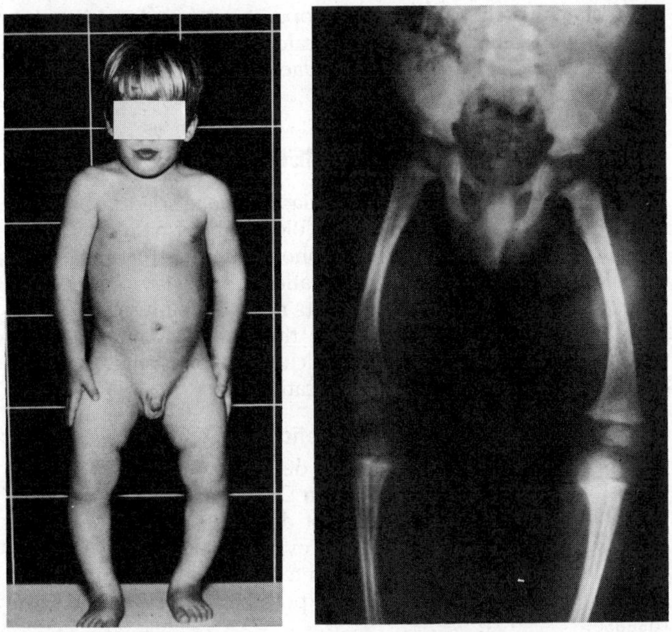

A B

Figure 245–1. The clinical (*A*) and radiologic (*B*) appearance of a young boy with X-linked hypophosphatemic rickets. The most striking abnormalities are the bowing of the legs, apparent in both femora and tibiae, with flaring of the ends of these bones at the knee. (Photographs courtesy of Dr. Sara B. Arnaud.)

may be bowed. The cortices of the long bones are often indistinct. Occasionally, evidence of secondary hyperparathyroidism—subperiosteal resorption in the phalanges and metacarpals and erosion of the distal ends of the clavicles—is observed. Pseudofractures (also known as Looser's zones or Milkman's fractures) are an uncommon but nearly pathognomonic feature of rickets and osteomalacia (Fig. 245–2). These radiolucent lines are most often found along the concave side of the femoral neck, the pubic rami, the ribs, the clavicles, and the lateral aspect of the scapulae. Pseudofractures may result from unhealed microfractures at points of stress or at the entry point of blood vessels into bone. They may progress to complete fractures that go unrecognized and thereby lead to substantial deformity and disability. Bone density is not a reliable indicator of osteomalacia, since bone density can be decreased in patients with vitamin D deficiency or increased in patients with chronic renal failure. In adults with normal renal function, radiologic evidence of a mineralization defect is often subtle and not readily distinguishable from osteoporosis.

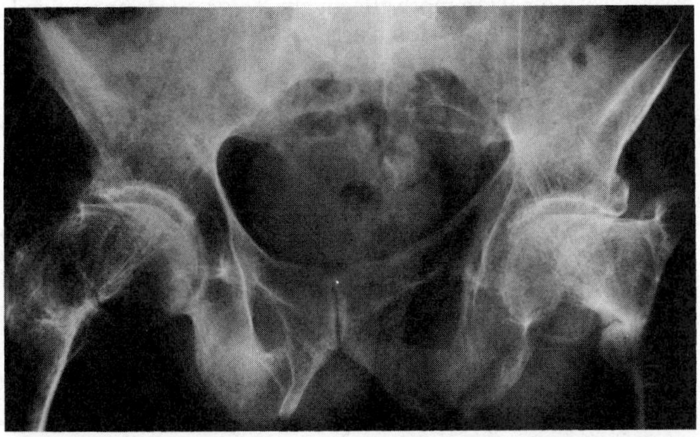

Figure 245–2. Roentgenogram of the pelvis of an elderly female with severe osteomalacia. This film reveals marked bowing (varus deformity) of both femoral necks, with pseudofractures of the medial aspect of the femoral necks and the superior aspect of the left pubic ramus. (Photograph courtesy of Dr. Harry K. Genant.)

Biochemical Features

The multiple etiologies of rickets and osteomalacia do not produce a single pattern of biochemical abnormalities. Furthermore, osteomalacia may be found on bone biopsy with no abnormality in serum or urinary levels of minerals and electrolytes. However, certain general patterns can be recognized.

Vitamin D Deficiency

Vitamin D deficiency, whether it is caused by nutritional deficiency, malabsorption, or abnormal metabolism, results in decreased intestinal absorption of calcium and phosphate. In conjunction with the resulting secondary hyperparathyroidism, vitamin D deficiency leads to increase in bone resorption, urinary phosphate excretion, and urinary calcium reabsorption. The net result tends to be a low normal serum calcium level, low serum phosphate level (unless chronic renal failure prevents phosphaturia), elevated serum alkaline phosphatase level, increased PTH level, decreased urinary calcium level, and increased urinary phosphate level. Finding a low 25OHD level in combination with these other biochemical alterations confirms the diagnosis of vitamin D deficiency. Caution is necessary in interpreting such biochemical data, however. Other factors, such as age and diet, must also be considered. For example, serum phosphate values are normally lower in adults than in children, and alkaline phosphatase levels are lower and are less reliable indicators of vitamin D deficiency in adults than in children. Dietary history is important, since urinary phosphate excretion and, to a lesser degree, urinary calcium excretion reflect dietary phosphate and calcium content. Since phosphate excretion depends on the filtered load (the product of the glomerular filtration rate [GFR] and serum phosphate), urinary phosphate levels may be normal if either the GFR or serum phosphate levels are reduced, despite the presence of hyperparathyroidism. Expressions of renal phosphate clearance that account for these variables (e.g., renal threshold for phosphate, or TmP/GFR) are a better indicator of renal phosphate handling than is total phosphate excretion.

Chronic Renal Failure (Ch. 78)

Most patients with chronic renal failure and renal osteodystrophy have osteitis fibrosa alone or in combination with osteomalacia. If not well controlled, these patients will have a low serum level of calcium and high serum levels of phosphate, alkaline phosphatase, and PTH. A few patients develop severe secondary hyperparathyroidism in which the PTH level increases dramatically, with restoration of the serum calcium to normal or even elevated levels (sometimes called tertiary hyperparathyroidism). Another small subset of patients with renal osteodystrophy present with normal or low serum levels of PTH and alkaline phosphatase. Their serum calcium levels are often elevated after treatment with small doses of $1,25(OH)_2D$. These patients have pure osteomalacia on bone biopsy and are thought to suffer from aluminum intoxication (see Ch. 248). Regardless of the type of bone disease, most patients with chronic renal disease have low $1,25(OH)_2D$ and $24,25(OH)_2D$ levels and, unless treated with vitamin D, tend to have low 25OHD levels as well.

Vitamin D–Dependent Rickets Types I and II

In these rare diseases, serum and urinary levels of calcium and phosphate resemble those in vitamin D–deficient rickets. However, serum 25OHD levels are normal or high. In type I patients, serum $1,25(OH)_2D$ levels are low in comparison to serum 25OHD levels, whereas in type II patients, serum $1,25(OH)_2D$ levels may be extraordinarily high.

Anticonvulsants

Patients on long-term anticonvulsant therapy tend to have the biochemical findings of mild vitamin D deficiency, including a low serum 25OHD level. Since these patients have normal serum $1,25(OH)_2D$ levels, some investigators have suggested that anticonvulsants may directly inhibit calcium transport in intestine and bone.

Hypophosphatemic Disorders

A low serum phosphate level and high renal clearance of phosphate are characteristic of diseases such as X-linked hypophosphatemic rickets, tumoral hypophosphatemic osteomalacia, and the variety of proximal renal tubular disorders that are associated with osteomalacia. Serum calcium is generally normal. In both X-linked hypophosphatemic rickets and tumoral hypophosphatemic osteomalacia, serum $1,25(OH)_2D$ is inappropriately low for the serum phosphate, although it is often in the low normal range. The proximal tubular diseases that present with the full De Toni-Debré-Fanconi syndrome also result in increased urinary levels of bicarbonate, amino acids, and glucose, as well as metabolic acidosis. Levels of the vitamin D metabolites have not been reported in large series of such patients.

Calcium Deficiency

In one study children suspected of having rickets on the basis of calcium-deficient diets had normal serum levels of 25OHD and phosphate, elevated serum levels of alkaline phosphatase, and low serum and urinary levels of calcium. Additional studies of calcium deficiency are necessary to confirm these observations.

Mineralization Disorders

Disorders attributed to an intrinsic defect in mineralization of the bone matrix do not produce the biochemical abnormalities observed in vitamin D deficiency. For example, patients who have developed osteomalacia as a result of long-term hemodialysis or total parenteral nutrition frequently are found to have hypercalcemia and hyperphosphatemia with low or normal levels of PTH. It is possible that the skeleton in these patients is unable to adequately buffer calcium and phosphate from the intestine, total parenteral nutrition solutions, or dialysate, resulting in marked oscillations of serum calcium and phosphate.

Histologic Features

Because of the difficulty in diagnosing osteomalacia in adults by clinical and radiologic means, transcortical bone biopsy is becoming increasingly popular. The rib and iliac crest are the sites generally biopsied. To assess osteoid content and appositional rate, the bone biopsy specimen is processed without decalcification. This requires special equipment.

In osteomalacia, bone is mineralized poorly and slowly, resulting in wide osteoid seams ($\sim 12\mu$) and a large fraction of bone covered by unmineralized osteoid. States of high bone turnover (increased bone formation and resorption), such as hyperparathyroidism, can also cause wide osteoid seams and increased osteoid surface, producing a superficial resemblance to osteomalacia. Therefore, the rate of bone turnover should be determined by labeling bone with tetracycline which provides a fluorescent marker of the calcification front. When two doses of tetracycline are given at different times, the distance between the two labels divided by the time interval between the two doses equals the appositional rate of bone formation. Normal appositional rate is approximately 0.74 μ per day. Mineralization lag time, the time required for newly formed osteoid to be mineralized, can be calculated by dividing osteoid seam width by the appositional rate. It is normally about 20 to 25 days. Because tetracycline labels the calcification front, the fraction of the osteoid surface undergoing active mineralization (normally about 60 per cent) can also be determined. Depressed appositional rate, increased mineralization lag time, and reduced calcification front clearly distinguish osteomalacia from high turnover states such as hyperparathyroidism. Low turnover states such as senile osteoporosis can also have low appositional rates and reduced calcification fronts, but these are distinguished from osteomalacia by normal or reduced osteoid seam width.

TREATMENT

The goal in treating osteomalacia and rickets is to normalize the clinical, biochemical, and radiologic abnormalities without producing hypercalcemia, hyperphosphatemia, hypercalciuria, nephrolithiasis, or ectopic calcification (especially nephrocalcinosis). To realize this goal, patients must be followed carefully, and as the bone lesions heal or the underlying disease improves, the dose of vitamin D, calcium, or phosphate needs to be adjusted to avoid such complications.

Vitamin D Deficiency

Simple nutritional vitamin D deficiency responds to oral doses of 2000 to 4000 IU of vitamin D per day, taken for several months, followed by replacement doses of 200 to 400 IU per day. Radiologic and biochemical evidence of healing requires several months. If the patient fails to respond to treatment, the physician should consider other possible causes of the bone disease.

Intestinal Malabsorption and Liver Disease

Patients with intestinal malabsorption or liver disease may respond to large doses of oral vitamin D (25,000 to 100,000 IU per day), or they may require parenteral administration of the vitamin. Since patients with steatorrhea absorb 25OHD (calcifediol) better than they do vitamin D, 50 to 100 μg of calcifediol per day or every other day should be tried if large doses of vitamin D fail to raise circulating levels of 25OHD into the high normal range. Vitamin D therapy should be supplemented with 1 to 3 grams of calcium per day. Only the osteomalacic component of the bone disease associated with these conditions responds to vitamin D; the osteoporotic component does not. Consequently, patients must be carefully selected for vitamin D treatment and carefully followed. Histomorphometric evaluation of bone biopsies is particular useful in this regard.

Chronic Renal Failure

Most patients with renal osteodystrophy respond to $1,25(OH)_2D$ (calcitriol, 0.5 to 1.0 μg per day) or dihydrotachysterol (DHT, 0.25 to 0.5 mg per day), calcium supplementation (1 to 3 grams per day), and phosphate restriction (dietary restriction supplemented with phosphate binders such as aluminum hydroxide). The goal is to achieve and maintain normal serum levels of calcium, phosphate, PTH, and alkaline phosphatase. This regimen treats osteitis fibrosa more effectively than the osteomalacia. Some authorities recommend the use of calcifediol rather than calcitriol or DHT since calcifediol may treat the osteomalacia more effectively. This issue is unresolved. Patients with only osteomalacia usually fail to respond to $1,25(OH)_2D$ alone, but they have responded to $1,25(OH)_2D$ in combination with $24,25(OH)_2D$, a metabolite not yet available for clinical use. The osteomalacia in renal osteodystrophy also appears to respond to the removal of aluminum with deferoxamine, a drug approved for the treatment of iron overload. Neither $24,25(OH)_2D$ nor deferoxamine has been approved by the United States Food and Drug Administration for the treatment of renal osteodystrophy, and both must currently be considered investigational drugs for this purpose.

Hypophosphatemia

The bone disease in patients with X-linked hypophosphatemia responds to the combination of phosphate (1 to 3 grams per day) and either large doses (25,000 to 100,000 IU) of vitamin D or more physiologic doses (0.25 to 1.0 μg per day) of $1,25(OH)_2D$. Neither phosphate nor vitamin D alone is as effective. Unfortunately, oral phosphate preparations also act as laxatives, and tolerance of full doses is therefore sometimes difficult to achieve. Less information is available regarding the efficacy of vitamin D and phosphate in other hypophosphatemic syndromes. When hypophosphatemia is associated with metabolic acidosis, as it often is in the De Toni-Debré-Fanconi syndrome, correction of the acidosis with bicarbonate may improve the associated metabolic bone disease.

Calcium Deficiency

Calcium supplements (1 to 3 grams per day) are useful in the treatment of calcium deficiency resulting from deficient diets, intestinal malabsorption, and aging. The amount of calcium should be adjusted to achieve adequate intestinal absorption, as monitored by urinary calcium excretion and serum levels of calcium and PTH.

Inhibitors of Mineralization

Restricting the use of aluminum-containing antacids in patients with chronic renal failure or peptic ulcer, removing aluminum and other impurities from the water used in hemodialysis, and substituting purified amino acids for the aluminum-containing casein hydrolysate in total parenteral nutrition solutions should reduce the incidence of aluminum intoxication. Chelation and removal of aluminum from the body with deferoxamine shows promise as a remedy of the future.

Patients on long-term anticonvulsant therapy may benefit from the prophylactic use of 2000 to 4000 IU of vitamin D per day and 500 and 1000 mg of calcium per day, especially if their serum 25OHD levels are low.

Etidronate, which is used in the treatment of Paget's disease, should be limited to a dose of 5 mg per kilogram and restricted to therapeutic periods of six months with at least six months between treatment periods.

Fluoride, which is currently under investigation for the treatment of osteoporosis, must be accompanied by 1 to 2 grams of calcium per day.

Bikle DD: Calcium absorption and vitamin D metabolism. Clin Gastroenterol 12:379, 1983. *An up-to-date review of the effect of vitamin D on the intestine and the gastrointestinal diseases that lead to osteomalacia.*

Contrib Nephrol 18, 1980. *This entire issue is devoted to renal oseodystrophy and the role of the vitamin D metabolites in its treatment.*

Frame B, Parfitt AM: Osteomalacia: Current concepts. Ann Intern Med 89:966, 1978. *An excellent review of osteomalacia, with a complete list of the diseases that produce it and a full description of the mineralization defect.*

Fukumoto Y, Tarui S, Tsukiyama K, et al: Tumor-induced vitamin D-resistant hypophosphatemic osteomalacia associated with proximal renal tubular dysfunction and 1,25-dihydroxyvitamin D deficiency. J Clin Endocrinol Metab 49:873, 1979. *A good description of a case of tumoral hypophosphatemic osteomalacia.*

Glorieux FH, Marie PJ, Pettifor JM, Delvin EE: Bone response to phosphate salts, ergocalciferol, and calcitriol in hypophosphatemic vitamin D-resistant rickets. N Engl J Med 303:1023, 1980. *This article describes modern therapy for this disorder.*

Goldstein DA, Haldimann B, Sherman D, Norman AW, Massry SG: Vitamin D metabolites and calcium metabolism in patients with nephrotic syndrome and normal renal function. J Clin Endocrinol Metab 52:116, 1981. *This article describes the pathogenesis of osteomalacia in the nephrotic syndrome.*

Hahn TJ, Halstead LR: Anticonvulsant drug-induced osteomalacia: Alterations in mineral metabolism and response to vitamin D_3 administration. Calcif Tissue Int 27:13, 1979. *This review describes the mechanisms by which anticonvulsants produce osteomalacia.*

Klein GL, Targoff CM, Ament ME, et al.: Bone disease associated with total parenteral nutrition. Lancet 2:1041, 1980. *This article describes the development of osteomalacia in patients on long-term total parenteral nutrition.*

Long RG, Sherlock S: Vitamin D in chronic liver disease. Prog Liver Dis 6:539, 1979. *This review of hepatic osteodystrophy emphasizes the abnormalities of the vitamin D endocrine system observed in and the recommended treatment for patients with liver disease.*

Mankin HJ: Rickets, osteomalacia, and renal osteodystrophy. Parts I and II. J Bone Joint Surg Am 56A:101, 352, 1974. A thorough review with an excellent accounting of the history of the subject, an excellent description of the clinical presentation of rickets, and a complete list of the etiologies of bone mineralization disorders.

Marie PJ, Pettifor JM, Ross FP, Glorieux FH: Histological osteomalacia due to dietary calcium deficiency in children. N Engl J Med 307:584, 1982. *This study indicates that calcium deficiency alone may be sufficient to cause osteomalacia.*

Parfitt AM, Gallagher JC, Heaney RP, Johnston CC, Neer R, Whedon GD: Vitamin D and bone health in the elderly. Am J Clin Nutr 36:1014, 1982. *A review of the importance of adequate vitamin D intake in adults, discussing among other issues the high incidence of osteomalacia found in patients with hip fractures.*

Rasmussen H, Bordier P: Vitamin D and bone. Metab Bone Dis Relat Res 1:7, 1978. *A mechanistic discussion of the effect of vitamin D and its metabolites on bone, emphasizing the concept that different vitamin D metabolites have different biologic effects.*

Scriver CR, Reade TM, DeLuca HF, Hamstra AJ: Serum 1,25-dihydroxyvitamin D levels in normal subjects and in patients with hereditary rickets or bone disease. N Engl J Med 299:976, 1978. *This report contains a good description of vitamin D-resistant rickets (X-linked) and vitamin D-dependent rickets type I.*

246. THE PARATHYROID GLANDS, HYPERCALCEMIA, AND HYPOCALCEMIA

Claude D. Arnaud

PARATHYROID HORMONE

STRUCTURE AND SYNTHESIS. *Parathyroid hormone (PTH)*, an 84 amino acid, linear polypeptide with a molecular weight of 9500, is the principal regulator of the concentration of ionic calcium in extracellular fluid. The biosynthesis and intracellular processing of the hormone are complex (Fig. 246–1). The original hormonal gene product of the parathyroid cell is a 115 amino acid precursor termed pre-proparathyroid hormone. Like other exportable proteins, it is synthesized on ribosomes bound to the membrane of the endoplasmic reticulum and discharged vectorially into its cisternal space. When the growing polypeptide chain attains a length of 20 to 30 amino acids, the first two amino-terminal methionine residues of the "pre" sequence are removed by a putative methionyl amino peptidase. With further growth of the chain, the hydrophobic 23 amino acid "pre" sequence acts to bind the polyribosome-precursor complex to the reticular membrane. This process provides the precursor access to the cisternal space of the endoplasmic reticulum and, presumably, to the enzyme ("clipase") that removes the presequence, leaving the 90 amino acid proparathyroid hormone structure. Proparathyroid hormone is converted to parathyroid hormone in the Golgi apparatus by proteolytic removal ("tryptic clipase") of the remaining 6 amino acids at the amino terminus. Here, the 84 amino acid polypeptide is readied for secretion either in a secretory granule or in its free form. There is no evidence that either of the parathyroid hormone precursor molecules or the "pre" or "pro" peptide sequence normally finds its way into the circulation.

In contrast to the rapid regulation of secretion, hormone biosynthesis is only slowly influenced by changes in concentrations of extracellular ionic calcium. Intracellular stores of parathyroid hormone may be regulated by a degradative pathway that is stimulated by high and inhibited by low extracellular calcium. This degradative pathway is of considerable current interest. Not only may it provide an important mechanism for regulating parathyroid hormone economy, as noted later, but the fragments of the hormone produced during its intracellular degradation may also provide a major source for the multiple immunoreactive forms of the hormone known to circulate in the blood (see below).

The amino acid sequences of bovine, porcine, and human parathyroid hormone have been determined (Fig. 246–2). The differences among them prevent complete immunologic cross-reactivity. This probably accounts for the difficulties that have been encountered in developing radioimmunoassays for the measurement of human parathyroid hormone, using antisera directed against bovine or porcine peptides, which previously were more readily available than the human peptide. All of the structural information required for full biologic activity of native, 84 amino acid parathyroid hormone lies within the 34 amino acids at the amino terminus. The active fragments of the bovine and human hormones, multiple fragments of the mid and carboxyl regions of the bovine and human hormones, and recently the full sequence of human parathyroid hormone have been synthesized and are commercially available for investigational use. Limited studies of the mid- and carboxyl-region fragments have shown them to be biologically inert.

CONTROL OF SECRETION. Parathyroid hormone is rapidly

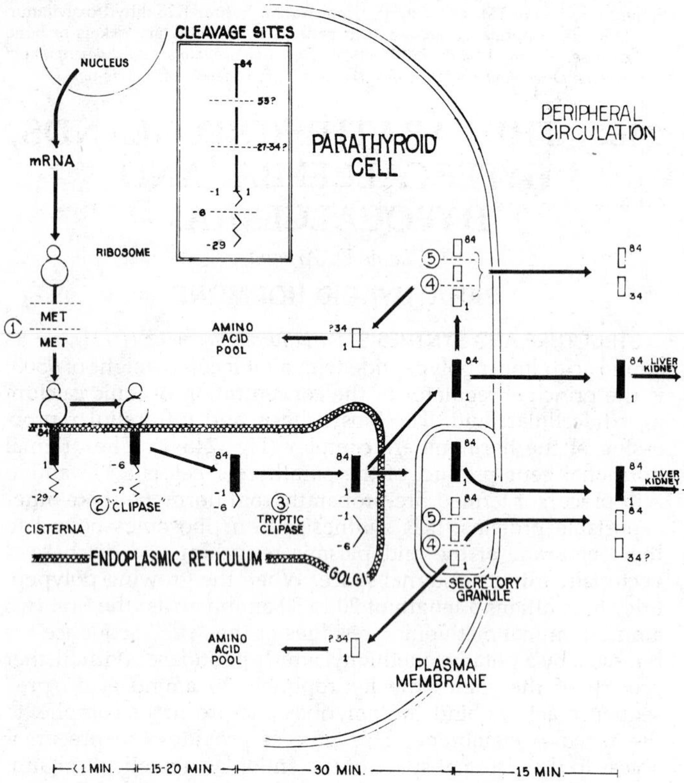

Figure 246–1. Proposed intracellular pathway for the biosynthesis of parathyroid hormone. Pre-proparathyroid hormone (Pre-ProPTH), the initial product of synthesis on the ribosomes, is converted into proparathyroid hormone (ProPTH) by removal of (1) the NH_2-terminal methionyl residues and (2) the NH_2-terminal sequence (-29 through -7) of 23 amino acids during synthesis and within seconds afterwards, respectively. The conversion of Pre-ProPTH probably occurs during transport of the polypeptide into the cisterna of the rough endoplasmic reticulum. By 20 minutes after synthesis, ProPTH reaches the Golgi region and is converted into PTH by (3) removal of the NH_2-terminal hexapeptide. PTH is either stored in a secretory granule or released into the cell cytoplasm, where it remains until it is released into the circulation in response to a fall in the blood concentration of calcium. Intact PTH [PTH(1-84)] undergoes at least two cleavages while in the secretory granule (and possibly in the cytoplasm) (4,5). These cleavages generate amino-, mid-, and carboxyl-region fragments. The mid- and carboxyl-region fragments are secreted into the circulation along with PTH(1-84), whereas the amino-region fragments are further degraded by the cell. The PTH(1-84) released into the circulation undergoes metabolic degradation in the liver and kidney (6), and this adds to the pool of circulating fragments. The time needed for these events is given below the schema. (Adapted from Habener JF, et al.: Biosynthesis of parathyroid hormone. Rec Prog Hormone Res 33:287, 1977.)

released from the parathyroid glands in response to a fall in plasma ionic calcium. It acts on kidney, intestine (indirectly, see below), and bone to restore the concentration of this cation to just above a normal set point, which, in turn, inhibits the secretion of the hormone. This negative feedback cycle is depicted in the "butterfly" diagram shown in Figure 243–1, in which the cycle is dissected into three loops, each involving one of the major target organs of parathyroid hormone. The concentration of extracellular ionic calcium is the major regulator of parathyroid hormone secretion. A more general discussion of calcium metabolism and its homeostasis is provided in Ch. 243. Other factors influence secretion only indirectly. For

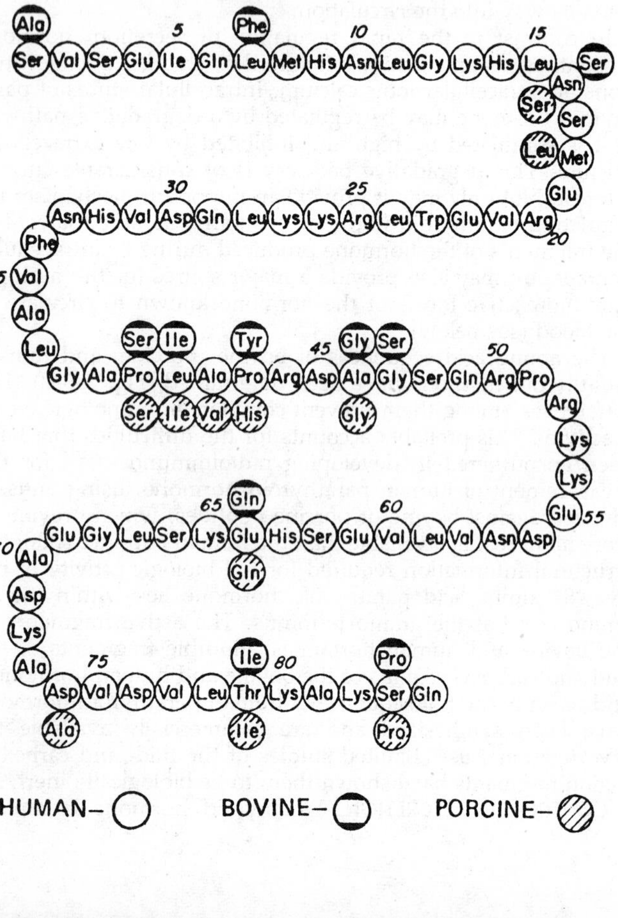

Figure 246–2. Parathyroid hormone. The figure shows the structure of human PTH and indicates at which positions the amino acid residues differ for bovine and porcine PTH. (Reprinted with permission from Keutmann HT, et al.: Complete amino acid sequence of human parathyroid hormone. Biochemistry 17:5728, 1978. Copyright 1978 American Chemical Society.)

example, plasma phosphate alters the degree to which calcium is complexed, and blood pH, the degree to which it binds to albumin. The effects of extracellular magnesium concentrations on secretion are qualitatively similar to those of ionic calcium but are physiologically less important. Paradoxically, severe, prolonged hypomagnesemia markedly inhibits secretion of parathyroid hormone and may be associated with hypocalcemia (see below). Known, direct parathyroid hormone secretagogues of questionable physiologic importance include β-adrenergic agonists, prostaglandins, and histamine. These agents, as well as decreased ionic calcium, stimulate the production of cyclic 3′5′-adenosine monophosphate (cyclic AMP) in parathyroid cells in vitro, and it is presumed that this compound mediates their actions on hormone secretion.

THE CIRCULATING HORMONE. Circulating parathyroid hormone is heterogeneous. It consists of the intact 84 amino acid polypeptide and multiple fragments of the hormone. These fragments are derived from the mid and carboxyl regions of the hormone molecule and therefore are likely to be biologically inactive. There is no evidence that biologically active fragments are secreted by the parathyroid gland or that they are present in the circulation. It is not possible at present to determine precisely the relative quantities of intact parathyroid hormone and of its fragments in serum, but grossly there are more circulating fragments than intact hormone. This difference is due primarily to the fact that the fragments survive longer in the circulation. The fragments are derived both from the degradative metabolism of intact parathyroid hormone (Fig. 246–1) and from glandular secretion, but the quantitative importance of these sources is uncertain.

Biologically active parathyroid hormone normally circulates in the blood at extremely low concentrations (<50 pg per milliliter). It is likely that there are individual, constitutionally derived "set point" values for the plasma ionic calcium above which glandular secretion rates are decreased and below which they are increased. However, steady state levels of parathyroid hormone are probably determined primarily by the degree to which the parathyroid glands must adapt to individual, chronic, environmentally induced changes in the level of plasma ionic calcium (e.g., dietary calcium and phosphate). There is an inverse relationship between fasting levels of serum calcium and serum immunoreactive parathyroid hormone (iPTH) in normal subjects (Fig. 246–3). Serum iPTH also increases with age (Fig. 246–4).

ACTION OF PARATHYROID HORMONE. The major function of PTH is to defend against hypocalcemia. It carries out this function by promoting virtually all of the actions that could be teleologically postulated: (1) release of calcium from bone, (2) conservation of calcium by the kidney, (3) enhanced absorption of calcium from the gut (indirectly via vitamin D), and (4) reduction in plasma phosphate. These physiologic effects of parathyroid hormone will be described after a brief summary of what is known concerning its mechanism of action.

MECHANISM OF ACTION OF PTH. Parathyroid hormone binds to specific plasma membrane receptors of target cells. These occupied receptors interact with a membrane-bound protein that is regulated by guanyl nucleotides; this protein in turn activates membrane-bound adenylate cyclase to convert ATP to cyclic AMP (Fig. 246–5). Cyclic AMP, by virtue of its ability to initiate a cascade of enzyme-activating intracellular phosphorylations, is considered to be one of possibly several intracellular "second messengers" responsible for mediating the final expression of the action of the hormone. The details of these enzyme activations and the manner in which they relate to discrete effects of the hormone are unknown. Other potential second messengers of parathyroid hormone (e.g., calcium itself) that might act in concert with or modulate the actions of cyclic AMP are under investigation. A more general description of the mechanisms by which polypeptide hormones act on target cells is contained in Ch. 221.

Information concerning the structural requirements for the action of parathyroid hormone at the site of its receptor is rapidly becoming available. The region of the molecule essential

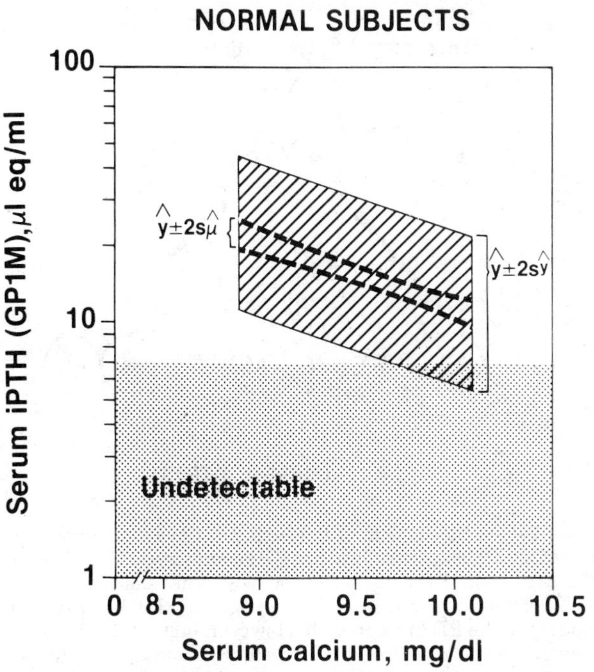

Figure 246–3. Serum immunoreactive parathyroid hormone (iPTH) (log scale) as a function of serum total calcium in 150 normal subjects (r = −0.424; p <0.001). (From Purnell D, et al.: Treatment of primary hyperparathyroidism. Am J Med 56:801, 1974.)

for receptor binding is the amino acid sequence 25-30, and for receptor activation, the 1-7 sequence. Recently, two analogues of bovine PTH that are truncated at the amino terminus have been developed. One of these, [8]Nle,[18]Nle,[34]Tyr bovine PTH(3-

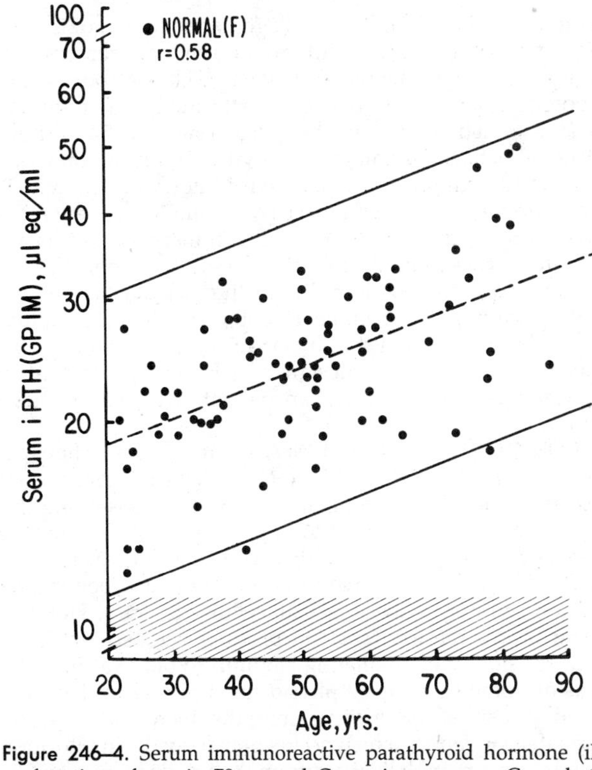

Figure 246–4. Serum immunoreactive parathyroid hormone (iPTH) as a function of age in 78 normal Caucasian women. Cross-hatched area at bottom represents limit of assay detectability. Mean increase in serum iPTH between age 20 and 90 is 80 per cent and is significant (p <0.001). (From Gallagher JC, et al.: The effect of age on serum immunoreactive parathyroid hormone in normal and osteoporotic women. J Lab Clin Med 95:376, 1980.)

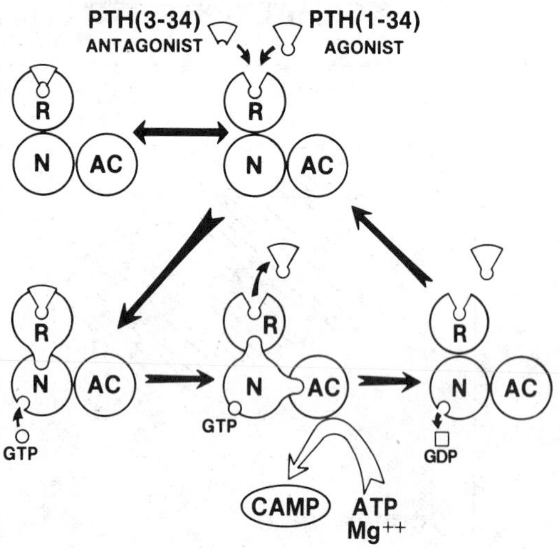

Figure 246–5. Mechanism of PTH action on membrane-bound adenylate cyclase. The biologically active PTH agonist ^{8}Nle,^{18}Nle,^{34}Tyr bovine PTH(1-34) amide [PTH(1-34)] and the biologically inactive PTH antagonist ^{8}Nle,^{18}Nle,^{34}Tyr bovine PTH(3-34) amide [PTH(3-34)] are capable of binding to the PTH receptor (R). However, only PTH(1-34) is capable of converting the receptor to a high-affinity state, so that the guanyl nucleotide regulatory protein (N) can be stimulated to bind guanosine triphosphate (GTP). The binding of GTP to N converts R to a low-affinity state, inducing dissociation of PTH(1-34) *and* the formation of an N-adenylate cyclase (AC) complex, leading to the activation of this enzyme and the increased production of intracellular cAMP. In contrast, the binding of PTH antagonist to R does not change the affinity of R; consequently, R cannot interact with N or induce activation of AC. (From Arnaud CD, Kolb FO: The calciotropic hormones and metabolic bone disease. *In* Greenspan FS, Forsham PH (eds.): Basic and Clinical Endocrinology. Los Altos, Lange Medical Publications, 1983, p 193.)

34) amide [bPTH(3-34)], has both agonist and antagonist properties in vitro. It binds to parathyroid hormone receptors in the kidney to the same degree as bovine PTH(1-34) but is much less potent in converting the receptor to the high-affinity state necessary to activate adenylate cyclase (Fig. 246–5). Although bPTH(3-34) acts as an antagonist in vitro, it fails to antagonize concomitantly administered parathyroid hormone in vivo. The other analogue, ^{34}Tyr bovine PTH(7-34) amide, has antagonist but no agonist properties in vitro. Preliminary studies indicate that it antagonizes parathyroid hormone in vivo but that large doses are required, possibly due to the fact that its ability to bind to parathyroid hormone receptors is weak. In spite of this, the development of this analogue represents an important advance in the effort to design a PTH antagonist that can rapidly reverse hypercalcemia in patients with severe hyperparathyroidism.

ACTION OF PTH ON THE KIDNEY. Parathyroid hormone acts most immediately on the kidney (1) to increase renal tubular reabsorption of calcium and magnesium, thus conserving these two divalent cations, and (2) to increase phosphate and bicarbonate excretion by inhibiting their proximal tubular reabsorption. These latter effects have several important, albeit indirect, effects on the homeostasis of extracellular calcium. Hormone-induced bicarbonaturia tends to produce acidosis, which decreases the ability of circulating albumin to bind calcium, thus increasing ionic calcium by physiochemical means. Hormone-induced phosphaturia assures that the increased release of phosphate from bone, which occurs obligately during hormone-induced calcium mobilization from bone, does not produce hyperphosphatemia. Increased serum phosphate would tend to complex calcium and thereby counteract the physiologic effect of parathyroid hormone to increase plasma ionic calcium.

The most important indirect effect of the phosphaturic action of the hormone is illustrated in the intestinal feedback loop in Figure 243–1. Parathyroid hormone, either directly or by its hypophosphatemic action, stimulates renal tubular 25OH 1α-hydroxylase to convert the major circulating metabolite of vitamin D, 25-hydroxycholecalciferol (25OHD), to its major, biologically active metabolite, 1α,25-dihydroxycholecalciferol [1,25$(OH)_2$D]. This latter metabolite acts directly on the intestinal mucosal cell to increase calcium absorption and on bone to increase resorption (see arrow between the intestinal and bone loops in Fig. 243–1). The metabolism of vitamin D is discussed in detail in Ch. 244.

In the process of stimulating adenylate cyclase in renal tubular cells, parathyroid hormone increases the urinary excretion of cyclic AMP. Presumably, cyclic AMP is simply released into the tubular fluid following its intracellular synthesis, since it has no known extracellular function. Urinary cyclic AMP is increased by the administration of other hormones active in the kidney, including epinephrine and glucagon, but its renal production and excretion are almost entirely due to parathyroid hormone. It can therefore be used as an indirect measure of the action of parathyroid hormone on the kidney, as noted below.

ACTION OF PTH ON BONE. Parathyroid hormone increases the net release of calcium and phosphate from bone into extracellular fluid. In this defense of calcium homeostasis the hormone influences the differentiation and activities of bone cells. These cellular events appear to depend upon a permissive effect of biologically active vitamin D metabolites (e.g., 1,25$(OH)_2$D), but the precise mechanism involved in this important relationship between parathyroid hormone and vitamin D is poorly understood. The physiology and pathophysiology of mineral metabolism demonstrate a wide range of interactions between parathyroid hormone (tropic) and vitamin D (permissive), as will be noted here and in the chapters on metabolic bone diseases.

ASSAY IN BIOLOGIC FLUIDS. The major tool for measuring parathyroid hormone in biologic fluids is radioimmunoassay. Values for serum iPTH vary from laboratory to laboratory, however, because of the differences in the source (bovine or human) and purity of the parathyroid hormone preparations used as standards and in the specificity of the antisera. Therefore, interpretation of serum iPTH values requires knowledge of the normal range for each assay system. Until recently, most radioimmunoassays of human PTH have used ^{125}I-labeled bovine PTH as the radioligand and cross-reacting antisera directed against porcine or bovine PTH. Use of synthetic human PTH or its fragments, which have recently become commercially available, may help to minimize some of the inconsistencies in the future. However, variations in the specificities of antisera used in different assays will continue to result in different iPTH values for the same serum sample. Such differences reflect true differences in the concentrations of the various forms of circulating parathyroid hormone.

At present, all available antisera that have a sufficiently high affinity for parathyroid hormone to be useful in radioimmunoassays are multivalent and contain antibodies directed at multiple regions of the PTH molecule. Antisera directed against the mid or carboxyl region of the PTH molecule recognize inactive mid- or carboxyl-region fragments and intact, biologically active PTH, and antisera directed against the amino region recognize amino-region fragments and intact PTH. Because the quantities of mid- and carboxyl-region fragments in the circulation are greater than those of amino-region fragments or intact PTH, values for serum iPTH are higher in mid- and carboxyl-region assays than in amino-region assays.

Mid- and carboxyl-region assays have provided surprisingly good diagnostic tools in the evaluation of patients suspected of having parathyroid disease, even though the resulting values for serum iPTH primarily reflect circulating, biologically inactive hormone (i.e., mid- and carboxyl-region fragments) (see below). This is fortunate because the concentrations of intact PTH in the circulation are so low that, with rare exception, they are beyond the sensitivity limits of all the amino-region assays yet developed.

Ideally, radioimmunoassays for parathyroid hormone should do the following: (1) be able to measure serum iPTH in over 95 per cent of normal subjects, (2) demonstrate an inverse relationship between serum iPTH and total serum calcium over the normal range of serum calcium (Fig. 246–3), (3) show consistently low or undetectable serum iPTH values in all patients with hypoparathyroidism as well as in all patients with hypercalcemia of nonparathyroid origin, other than cancer, and (4) demonstrate iPTH values greater than the upper limits of normal in 90 per cent of patients with surgically proved primary hyperparathyroidism.

Until recently, bioassays for parathyroid hormone lacked sufficient sensitivity for the study of circulating parathyroid hormone. This obstacle has now been overcome by two novel approaches. One is a cytochemical bioassay that is based on the PTH-specific stimulation of glucose-6-phosphate dehydrogenase in guinea pig renal slices. This assay is extremely sensitive, measuring femtogram amounts of parathyroid hormone. Its disadvantage is its technical complexity. The other assay, which is more convenient, uses a nonhydrolyzable analogue of guanosine triphosphate, 5′guanyl-imidodiphosphate [Gpp(NH)p], to greatly augment the sensitivity of adenylate cyclase to parathyroid hormone in canine kidneys in vitro. In the presence of Gpp(NH)p, as little as 10 pg per milliliter of intact PTH elicits significant stimulation. However, even with this sensitivity, the measurement of parathyroid hormone in normal serum requires the immunoextraction of 3 ml of serum. This assay is accurate, precise, and simple and can be performed rapidly.

DeGroot LJ (ed.): Endocrinology. Vol 2. New York, Grune & Stratton, 1979, pp 587–636, 713–716. *Comprehensive review of PTH chemistry and physiology.*

Goltzman D, Henderson B, Loveridge N: Cytochemical bioassay of parathyroid hormone: Characteristics of the assay and analysis of circulating hormonal forms. J Clin Invest 65:1309,1980. *Describes the clinical application of the cytochemical bioassay of serum PTH for the evaluation of patients with parathyroid dysfunction.*

Nissenson RA, Abbott SR, Teitelbaum AP, Clark OH, Arnaud CD: Endogenous biologically active human parathyroid hormone: Measurement by a guanyl nucleotide-amplified renal adenylate cyclase assay. J Clin Endocrinol Metab 52:840,1981. *Describes the guanyl nucleotide-amplified adenylate cyclase bioassay of serum PTH.*

Nissenson RA, Teitelbaum AP, Abbott SR, Pliam N, Silve C, Zitzner L, Nyiredy K, Arnaud CD: Parathyroid hormone receptors in kidney and bone: Relation to adenylate cyclase activation. *In* Cohn DV, Talmage RV, Mathews JL (eds.): Hormonal Control of Calcium Metabolism. Amsterdam, Excerpta Medica, 1981, pp 44–54. *Review of the current knowledge about the interaction between PTH receptors and adenylate cyclase.*

PRIMARY HYPERPARATHYROIDISM

DEFINITION. Primary hyperparathyroidism describes a disorder or group of disorders resulting from excessive, relatively uncontrolled secretion of parathyroid hormone by a single or multiple parathyroid glands. The actions of parathyroid hormone on bone and kidney usually result in hypercalcemia, the biochemical hallmark of the disorder, but this fails to inhibit PTH secretion normally. Most patients are now detected by routine measurement of the serum calcium while relatively asymptomatic and without other readily demonstrable manifestations of the disease. When present, symptoms can be remarkably varied and vague and are related to hypercalcemia, hypercalciuria (nephrolithiasis), or osteitis fibrosa cystica (bone pain).

ETIOLOGY. The etiology of primary hyperparathyroidism is unknown. In several families the disease has been inherited as an autosomal dominant trait. Patients studied for the detection of thyroid carcinoma following previous neck x-irradiation have incidentally shown a greater than expected number of cases of primary hyperparathyroidism. It is difficult to interpret such studies, however, because information about the general incidence and natural history of primary hyperparathyroidism is incomplete.

Calcium infusions in the hyperparathyroid patients with mild hypercalcemia incompletely suppress serum immunoreactive parathyroid hormone levels. This strongly suggests that increased hormone secretion in these patients is due, at least in part, to a set point error in the level of ionic calcium at which abnormal tissue is suppressed. This defect can be demonstrated in vitro. Higher concentrations of calcium are required in the medium to decrease parathyroid hormone secretion from parathyroid cells isolated from abnormal glands than are required for cells isolated from normal glands.

INCIDENCE. Routine, automated measurement of serum calcium has vastly increased the detection of primary hyperparathyroidism. The incidence of primary hyperparathyroidism increases in both men and women after age 50, but it is two to four times more common in women. The disease is rare in children. In a careful epidemiologic study of cases detected in Rochester, Minnesota, over a ten-year period, the age-adjusted incidence rate was estimated to be 42 per 100,000. Studies of selected populations (mostly older than 40 years of age) have revealed prevalence rates of primary hyperparathyroidism as high as 1 in 1000 to 1 in 200 of those surveyed.

PATHOLOGY. Histologically, abnormal parathyroid glands from patients with primary hyperparathyroidism have been characterized as being hyperplastic, adenomatous, or malignant. Unfortunately, it is often difficult, if not impossible, to distinguish between an adenoma and chief cell hyperplasia in a given gland, and, occasionally, abnormal parathyroid tissue that is benign has many of the histologic features of malignant tissue. Thus, it has generally been necessary to revert to the gross pathology observed at surgery to classify parathyroid lesions. The surgeon determines the number of abnormal glands present on the basis of their size and gross appearance, and the pathologist determines whether the biopsy specimens are parathyroid tissue. Single gland involvement ("adenoma") is observed in about 80 per cent of patients and multiple gland involvement ("hyperplasia") in about 20 per cent. Less than 2 per cent of hyperfunctioning glands are carcinomatous as judged by a combination of gross appearance, histology, and the ultimate biologic behavior of the abnormal tissue. Multiple glands are almost always involved in familial primary hyperparathyroidism and the hyperparathyroidism associated with multiple endocrine neoplasia (MEN) syndromes. Abnormal parathyroid glands usually weigh between 0.2 and 2.0 grams (25 to 75 mg is normal) and have a characteristic yellow-red color and "bulging" appearance in situ. Occasionally, very large glands (e.g., >10 grams) are observed. The severity of the clinical manifestations, especially the degree of hypercalcemia, is generally proportional to the quantity of hyperfunctioning tissue present and the level of serum immunoreactive PTH (iPTH). The predominant cell type in most abnormal glands is the chief cell, although so-called "water-clear cells" and oxyphilic cells may be admixed, and very occasionally either of these cells may predominate. The secretory capabilities of the "water-clear" and oxyphilic cells are unknown.

Virtually all patients with primary hyperparathyroidism have histomorphometric evidence of excess parathyroid hormone action in bone biopsies from the iliac crest, although most of these patients do not have radiographic evidence of bone disease. An increase in the amount of bone surface undergoing resorption, increased numbers of osteoclasts, osteocytic osteolysis, and, in moderate to severe cases, marrow fibrosis are characteristic of this lesion, which is termed osteitis fibrosa cystica. Only far advanced disease is associated with classic bone cysts and fractures. It is not uncommon to observe extensive evidence of a mineralization defect characterized by large quantities of unmineralized osteoid and disorganized (woven versus lamellar) bone.

Between 20 and 30 per cent of patients have nephrolithiasis, not infrequently complicated by pyelonephritis. Gross nephrocalcinosis or calcification of the renal papillae is unusual, but careful microscopic examinations of kidneys with special calcium stains occasionally reveal peritubular and tubular calcifications at autopsy. The incidence of such soft tissue calcification in patients with mild to moderate disease is unknown; however, it may be relatively frequent because chondrocalcinosis and calcific tendinitis can be demonstrated on x-ray in approximately 7.5 to 18 per cent of cases. Calcification of other organs such as stomach, lung, and heart has been observed in patients with hyperparathyroid crisis (serum calcium >15.0 mg per deciliter).

Myopathy is relatively common in primary hyperparathyroidism, and muscle biopsy may show neuropathic atrophy of both Type I and Type II muscle fibers. These histologic changes parallel clinical, neurologic, and electromyographic dysfunction.

PATHOPHYSIOLOGY. The excessive release of parathyroid hormone from hyperfunctioning parathyroid tissue causes exaggerated physiologic responses of target organs (see Fig. 243–1) and inappropriately raises the concentration of ionized calcium in extracellular fluid. In contrast to other hypercalcemic states, in primary hyperparathyroidism the first lines of defense against hypercalcemia (increased renal and intestinal loss of calcium) are not fully operative, since the kidney and intestine are target organs for PTH and are themselves contributing to the pathogenesis of the hypercalcemia. Early in the course of the disease, when serum calcium values are <11.5 mg per deciliter (normal range, 8.9 to 10.1 mg per deciliter), urinary calcium is often relatively low for the degree of hypercalcemia and may be normal. When serum calcium values exceed 12.0 mg per deciliter, the increased filtered load of calcium overwhelms renal tubular reabsorption and hypercalciuria develops. This assists in limiting the further rise of plasma calcium but at the cost of producing kidney stone diathesis secondary to continued hypercalciuria, along with other changes in urine composition (e.g., increased pH resulting from bicarbonaturia).

Factors other than urinary loss may tend to limit the degree of hypercalcemia in primary hyperparathyroidism. First, calcium may be "lost" from the extracellular fluid by being deposited in soft tissues. This metastatic calcification may cause symptoms (e.g., joint pain owing to calcific tendinitis and chondrocalcinosis) or compromise function (e.g., nephrocalcinosis leading to renal failure). Secondly, the permissive effect of vitamin D is necessary for the action of parathyroid hormone; in its absence patients with even severe hyperparathyroidism become either eucalcemic or nearly so. In fact, stores of vitamin D may become depleted in a patient who previously was marginally replete because of the increased renal conversion of 25OHD to 1,25$(OH)_2$D, which is caused by excessive parathyroid hormone. As a result, such patients may have severe osteomalacia in addition to osteitis fibrosa cystica. Finally, hypercalcemia per se may increase the degradation of biologically active forms of parathyroid hormone peripherally (i.e., in the liver and possibly the kidney) and in the parathyroid tissue itself. In this way plasma calcium not only may regulate parathyroid hormone secretion but also may be an important factor in determining the relative quantities of circulating, biologically active parathyroid hormone and inactive hormone fragments. Increased secretion of calcitonin might be expected to play an important role in correcting the hypercalcemia of primary hyperparathyroidism (see Fig. 243–1), but this seems not to occur in the majority of patients. In fact, the secretory reserve of calcitonin often appears to be depleted.

Parathyroid hormone decreases renal tubular reabsorption of phosphate, and in excess tends to cause hyperphosphaturia and hypophosphatemia. Normally, these effects both support mineral homeostasis (by stimulating 1,25$(OH)_2$D production) and protect it (by clearing from the blood phosphate that is removed from bone during resorption of calcium). In patients with primary hyperparathyroidism, however, hypophosphatemia tends to worsen hypercalcemia by causing increased production of the hypercalcemic compound 1,25$(OH)_2$D and decreased complexing of blood ionic calcium by phosphate.

Patients with primary hyperparathyroidism generally have mild to moderate hyperchloremic acidosis, primarily because excess hormone decreases urinary hydrogen ion excretion and increases urinary bicarbonate excretion. These effects also tend to aggravate existing hypercalcemia by decreasing the ability of blood albumin to bind ionic calcium, and by increasing the dissolution of bone mineral.

Urinary cyclic AMP is increased in as many as 80 per cent of patients with primary hyperparathyroidism. Presumably, increased hormonal occupancy of renal receptors stimulates adenylate cyclase to produce an increase in this intracellular second messenger. Interestingly, the phosphaturic and cyclic AMP responses to exogenously administered parathyroid hormone are blunted in patients with primary hyperparathyroidism, suggesting refractoriness or "desensitization" of one or more of the cellular components responsible for these effects. This desensitization, as well as the increased excretion of nephrogenous cyclic AMP, has been used as a diagnostic test for the presence of hyperparathyroidism.

Patients with radiologic evidence of osteitis fibrosa cystica (a bone lesion caused by excess PTH), almost always have increased serum concentrations of the bone isoenzyme of alkaline phosphatase. This enzyme is produced by osteoblasts and probably constitutes one of several enzymes involved in osseous mineralization. These patients also excrete in their urine greater than normal quantities of small peptides that contain hydroxyproline. This amino acid is unique to collagen, which is the major structural protein in bone. Combined increases in serum alkaline phosphatase and urinary excretion of hydroxyproline reflect grossly increased bone turnover, which can be documented further by studies of the dynamics of intravenously administered, isotopically labeled calcium (^{47}Ca, ^{45}Ca).

SYMPTOMS. Most patients with primary hyperparathyroidism are relatively asymptomatic when the diagnosis is made, or else they have nonspecific symptoms, especially those of weakness and easy fatigability. When symptoms do occur, they can generally be attributed to either hypercalcemia with associated hypercalciuria or to osteitis fibrosa cystica.

Hypercalcemia. The symptoms attributable to hypercalcemia involve a number of systems: (1) Central nervous system—impaired mentation, loss of memory for recent events, emotional lability, depression, anosmia, somnolence, and even coma. (2) Neuromuscular—weakness (especially of the proximal musculature), arthralgias, severe pruritus (which may be due to metastatic calcification in the skin), and the restless leg syndrome (no comfortable position for legs when attempting to sleep). The joint pains may be due to associated gout, intra-articular deposition of calcium pyrophosphate crystals (pseudogout), calcific tendinitis, or chondrocalcinosis. (3) Gastrointestinal—anorexia, nausea, vomiting, dyspepsia, constipation, and possibly an increased incidence of peptic ulcer and acute pancreatitis. (4) Renal—polyuria, nocturia, and susceptibility to calcium oxalate or calcium phosphate stones, which sometimes leads to renal failure from calcium nephropathy, with associated symptoms of uremia. (5) Cardiovascular—increased frequency of hypertension. In general, all of these abnormalities are related to the degree of increase in ionized calcium in extracellular fluid, but the correlation is a crude one. One patient may be severely incapacitated at a level of serum calcium that produces only moderate symptoms in another.

Osteitis Fibrosa Cystica. Bony abnormalities can be demonstrated by special techniques in biopsy specimens from the iliac crest in most patients with primary hyperparathyroidism. However, symptomatic bone disease is now rare in this disorder. Patients may infrequently complain of diffuse or localized (e.g., to the back) bone pain. Very rarely patients may have a pathologic fracture through a bone cyst. The radiographic changes in osteitis fibrosa cystica are described later.

PHYSICAL SIGNS. Most patients with primary hyperparathyroidism have no abnormal physical signs of the disorder. When present, such signs are usually confined to the neuromuscular system or to organ systems in which soft tissue calcification can be noted. Neurologic abnormalities are nonspecific and include impaired mentation, hyperactive deep tendon reflexes, sensory loss for pain and vibration, proximal muscle weakness (particularly the thighs), abnormal tongue movements (resembling fasciculations), glossal atrophy, and ataxic gait.

Soft tissue calcification can result in arthritis (chondrocalcinosis or calcific tendinitis), conjunctivitis (conjunctival calcium phosphate crystals), and "band keratopathy," which is characterized by deposition of opaque calcium phosphate in vertical lines parallel to and within the ocular limbus, usually laterally (3 o'clock) in the cornea. These ocular signs, which can be best seen with slit lamp examination, are rare in hyperparathyroidism unless the serum phosphate is elevated, as occurs after the onset of renal failure.

Primary hyperparathyroidism is a prominent component of the rare multiple endocrine neoplasia syndromes (MEN I or IIa), which are described in Ch. 240. The clinician should look for evidence of these abnormalities—e.g., acromegaly, hypopituitarism, pheochromocytoma, and medullary carcinoma of the thyroid—during the physical examination.

Enlarged parathyroid glands are only rarely demonstrable on physical examination. In fact, even in the presence of primary hyperparathyroidism, a nodule felt in the neck is almost certainly one of the thyroid rather than the parathyroid.

Rarely, patients may exhibit bone tenderness on examination, and even more rarely bone deformities, fractures through an osteoclastic cyst, or the presence of an epulis (brown tumor of the jaw).

RADIOGRAPHIC MANIFESTATIONS. The most specific and frequent radiographic sign of osteitis fibrosa cystica is that of subperiosteal bone resorption. This sign is best demonstrated in magnified, fine grain, industrial radiographs of the fingers (particularly the index finger) (Fig. 246–6*A*). Particular attention should be paid to the radial surface of the phalanx, where the cortex is almost completely resorbed, leaving only a lacey edge. Other radiographic manifestations of the disease range from generalized osteopenia to bone cysts ("brown tumors") and erosion of distal phalangeal tufts or the distal ends of the clavicles. Figure 246–6*B* provides an example of severe osteitis fibrosa cystica involving the skull.

Soft tissue calcifications (e.g., calcific tendinitis, chondrocalcinosis, nephrocalcinosis, and pulmonary calcifications) may be detected on routine films incidentally. The latter two are demonstrated best with bone scanning techniques, using radioactively labeled diphosphate compounds.

Nephrocalcinosis is rarely seen radiographically, but lithiasis is common. Since the stones are usually radiopaque (i.e., calcium oxalate and calcium phosphate stones), nephrotomograms are helpful in identifying, localizing, and measuring them. This procedure is important in determining the "activity" of the stone disease (see Ch. 89). An increase in stone diameter with time can be taken as objective evidence of "active" stone disease and is probably an additional indication for treatment of hyperparathyroidism (see below). Primary hyperparathyroidism may also be associated, although less commonly, with uric acid stones (not radiopaque). Thus, x-ray examination of the urinary tract with contrast material is also important.

DIFFERENTIAL DIAGNOSIS. In general, the major problem in the differential diagnosis of primary hyperparathyroidism is distinguishing this disease from other conditions associated with hypercalcemia. Hypercalcemia associated with thiazide

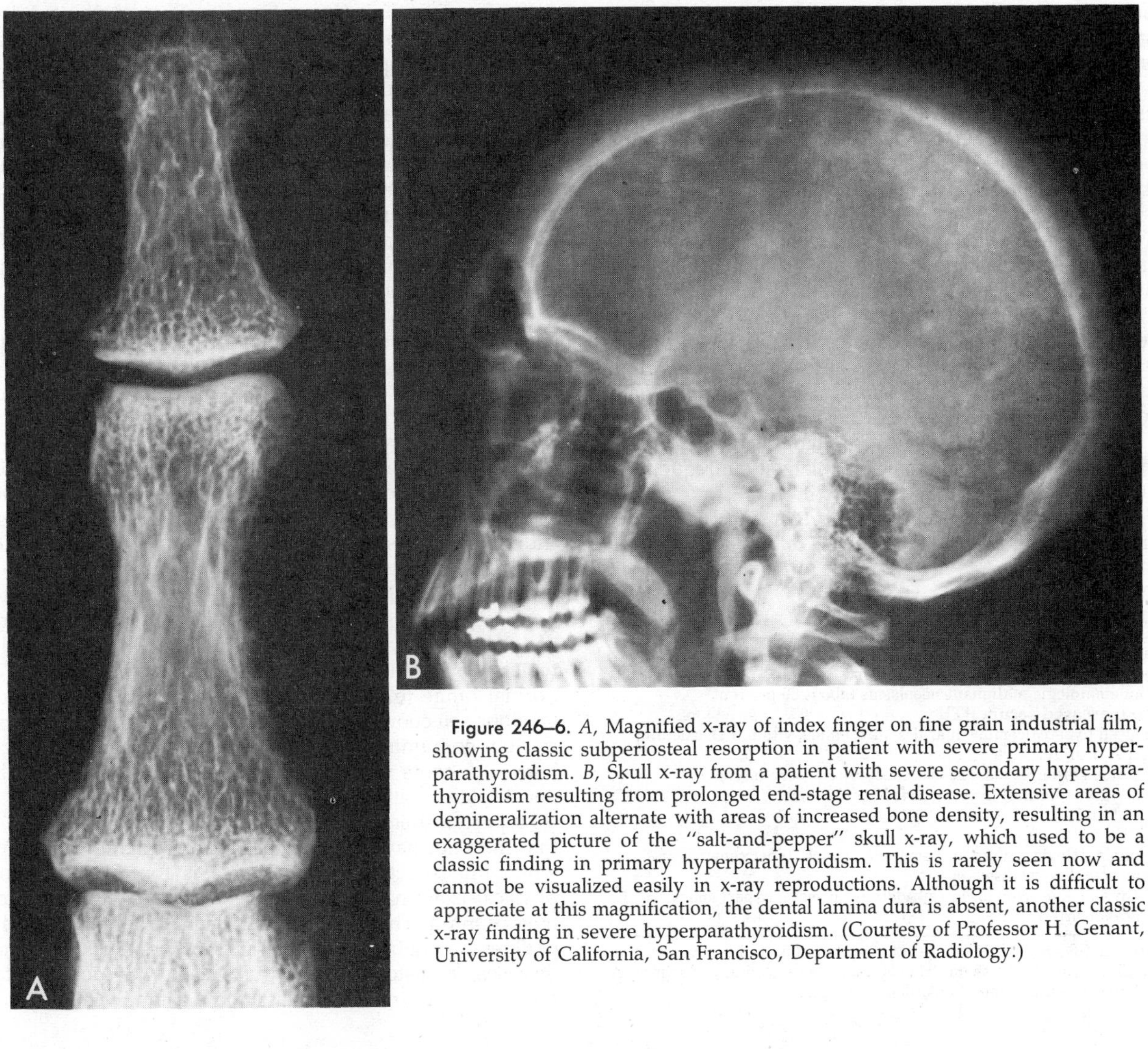

Figure 246–6. *A*, Magnified x-ray of index finger on fine grain industrial film, showing classic subperiosteal resorption in patient with severe primary hyperparathyroidism. *B*, Skull x-ray from a patient with severe secondary hyperparathyroidism resulting from prolonged end-stage renal disease. Extensive areas of demineralization alternate with areas of increased bone density, resulting in an exaggerated picture of the "salt-and-pepper" skull x-ray, which used to be a classic finding in primary hyperparathyroidism. This is rarely seen now and cannot be visualized easily in x-ray reproductions. Although it is difficult to appreciate at this magnification, the dental lamina dura is absent, another classic x-ray finding in severe hyperparathyroidism. (Courtesy of Professor H. Genant, University of California, San Francisco, Department of Radiology.)

diuretic therapy and with nonhematologic malignancy are the most frequently encountered among these. Other important causes of hypercalcemia are (1) hematologic malignancies involving bone (myeloma, lymphoma, and leukemia); (2) granulomatous diseases (sarcoidosis, tuberculosis, and berylliosis); (3) endocrine disorders, including thyrotoxicosis and acute adrenal insufficiency; (4) familial hypocalciuric hypercalcemia (a genetic disorder formerly called benign familial hypercalcemia); (5) excessive ingestion of calcium, vitamin D, or vitamin A; (6) extensive skeletal immobilization (e.g., spica body cast) in normal young people and prolonged bed rest in patients with osteolytic metabolic bone disease; and (7) idiopathic hypercalcemia of infancy.

Pathophysiologically, hypercalcemic disorders can be segregated into those caused by excess parathyroid hormone and those caused by factors other than parathyroid hormone (Table 246–1). Only patients with primary hyperparathyroidism and certain patients with malignant diseases have both hypercalcemia and elevated levels of circulating parathyroid hormone. In all other patients with hypercalcemia the secretion of parathyroid hormone is suppressed.

The underlying causes of the hypercalcemia in conditions without increased secretion of parathyroid hormone are varied and for the most part uncertain. They are discussed below under "Nonparathyroid Causes of Hypercalcemia." The most important among these, in terms of the differential diagnosis of primary hyperparathyroidism, are the hypercalcemia of malignancy and familial hypocalciuric hypercalcemia.

Hypercalcemia of Malignancy. It is unlikely that metastases to bone produce chronic hypercalcemia simply by physical displacement of bone. Rather, malignant tumors probably produce osteolytic humoral factors that act either systemically or locally in the immediate vicinity of a metastasis. These factors include parathyroid hormone–like substances, prostaglandins, osteoclast-activating factor (OAF), and probably other factors yet to be discovered. Any one or a combination of these factors might be secreted systemically by a tumor or released locally by its bony metastases in sufficient quantities to stimulate osteolysis and produce hypercalcemia. Osteoclast-activating factor is largely responsible for the production of hypercalcemia in patients with hematologic malignancies, especially multiple myeloma. Ectopic secretion of prostaglandins of the E_2 series may be associated with hypercalcemia, as documented by the presence of prostaglandin metabolites in urine, and more specifically by the response of the hypercalcemia to treatment with inhibitors of prostaglandin synthesis, such as indomethacin (see Ch. 223). Extensive experience now shows, however, that the primary involvement of prostaglandins in the production of hypercalcemia of malignancy is relatively infrequent, so that other humoral factors must be sought.

More than 35 years ago, Fuller Albright postulated that parathyroid hormone was the major cause of the hypercalcemia of malignancy. In the absence of renal failure, a large proportion of patients with this disease have the same degree of hypophosphatemia as do patients with moderate to severe primary hyperparathyroidism. In my experience, as many as 70 to 80 per cent of hypercalcemic patients with nonhematologic malignancies exhibit normal (80 per cent) to increased (20 per cent) values for serum immunoreactive parathyroid hormone (iPTH). The presence of immunoreactive parathyroid hormone in the serum of a hypercalcemic patient is considered to be abnormal. Other laboratories using different assays have reported lower frequencies for measurable levels of iPTH in the hypercalcemia of malignancy. Serum values for iPTH tend to be much higher in patients with primary hyperparathyroidism than in patients with malignancy with equal degrees of hypercalcemia. These results suggest (1) that the iPTH measured in the sera of patients with malignancy-associated hypercalcemia is an incidental finding and not pathogenetically related to the hypercalcemia, or (2) that the iPTH is quantitatively misrepresented by assays used to detect it and that, in fact, sufficient quantities of a biologically active parathyroid hormone–like compound with low PTH immunoreactivity circulates in the plasma of these patients to explain the hypercalcemia. I favor the latter alternative, based on studies concerning the heterogeneity of circulating PTH in patients with ectopic hyperparathyroidism and on the fact that such patients usually excrete increased nephrogenous cyclic AMP in amounts comparable to that found in patients with primary hyperparathyroidism. Patients with the ectopic syndrome have not only greater hypercalciuria but also much lower values for serum $1,25(OH)_2D$ than do patients with primary hyperparathyroidism. This suggests that the range of biologic actions of the parathyroid hormone–like substance in patients with ectopic disease may be different from that of native parathyroid hormone.

Benign Familial Hypercalcemia. Benign familial hypercalcemia (or familial hypocalciuric hypercalcemia) is probably the second most important consideration in the differential diagnosis of primary hyperparathyroidism. This recently described condition is rare and is inherited as an autosomal dominant trait. It is characterized by asymptomatic hypercalcemia, hypocalciuria, a tendency toward mild hypermagnesemia, and normal to low levels of serum iPTH. Histologically, the parathyroid glands either are normal or show equivocal "hyperplasia," and subtotal parathyroidectomy has consistently failed to restore eucalcemia. The response of nephrogenous cyclic AMP to exogenous and endogenous parathyroid hormone is greater in patients with familial hypocalciuric hypercalcemia than in normal subjects or in patients with primary hyperparathyroidism. The hypercalcemia in this familial syndrome may be due, at least in part, to renal hypersensitivity to the hypocalciuric effects of parathyroid hormone. In this sense then, familial hypocalciuric hypercalcemia could be considered to be a form of hyperparathyroidism. However, the notable absence of the characteristic sequelae of primary hyperparathyroidism (e.g., renal stones and osteitis fibrosa cystica) in these patients clearly indicates that tissue hypersensitivity to parathyroid hormone is probably not generalized.

DIAGNOSTIC INVESTIGATIONS. *General.* The presence of hypercalcemia is established when at least three measurements of total serum calcium are increased above the normal range, which is 8.9 to 10.1 mg per deciliter. If laboratories use a wider normal range (e.g., 9.0 to 11.0 mg per deciliter), based either on poor selection of normal control subjects or problems with calcium contamination in the laboratory (Ch. 243), large numbers of patients with mild hypercalcemia (i.e., 10.2 to 11.0 mg per deciliter) will go undetected.

Hypercalcemia generally reflects serious underlying disease that may not have been suspected on initial evaluation. Thus, when unsuspected hypercalcemia is found, the history and physical examination should be repeated with specific objectives in mind. These include detailed evaluation of the duration of illness, drug intake, the possible presence of other endocrine diseases, a history of nephrolithiasis with documentation if possible, symptoms of malignancy, a family history of endo-

TABLE 246–1. DIFFERENTIAL DIAGNOSIS OF HYPERCALCEMIA

Due to increased serum PTH
Primary and "tertiary" hyperparathyroidism
Some nonhematologic malignant neoplasms (about 80 per cent)
Not due to increased serum PTH
Drug-induced hypercalcemia (thiazides, furosemide, vitamin D, calcium, vitamin A, lithium)
Granulomatous diseases (sarcoidosis, tuberculosis, berylliosis)
Genetic diseases (familial hypocalciuric hypercalcemia)
Immobilization
"Idiopathic"
Some nonhematologic malignant neoplasms (about 20 per cent)
Malignant hematologic diseases
Nonparathyroid endocrine diseases (Addison's disease, hyper- and hypothyroidism)

From Arnaud CD, Kolb FO: The calciotropic hormones and metabolic bone disease. *In* Greenspan FS, Forsham PH (eds.): Basic and Clinical Endocrinology. Los Altos, Lange Medical Publications, 1983, p 208.

crine and mineral disorders, and the possible presence of palpable lymph nodes or masses, unusual skin pigmentation or lesions, and an enlarged thyroid, liver, or spleen.

Illness of long duration associated with kidney stones but no weight loss favors primary hyperparathyroidism; illness of short duration associated with weight loss without nephrolithiasis favors a nonparathyroid cause for hypercalcemia, particularly malignancy. A history of thiazide intake might explain an increase in serum calcium to 11.0 mg per deciliter, but higher values usually indicate that the effects of this drug have augmented the hypercalcemia of another condition (e.g., mild hyperparathyroidism). Patients who are taking thiazides and are hypercalcemic should be re-evaluated one month after discontinuing the drug. Vitamin D in doses exceeding 50,000 units per day can cause hypercalcemia in adults, and its ingestion may not have been elicited in the initial history. Hypercalcemic patients may be abnormally sensitive to vitamin D. Thus, intake of less than 50,000 units per day may aggravate existing hypercalcemia in sarcoidosis or primary hyperparathyroidism. What may appear initially to be a severe form of the primary disorder may prove to be relatively mild when vitamin D intake is curtailed. Excess calcium ingested in the form of antacids containing calcium carbonate (>5 grams per day) can cause severe hypercalcemia in susceptible individuals, especially when coupled with additional intake of alkali (bicarbonate) as in the "milk-alkali syndrome." This condition is rare in the absence of other abnormalities. Many patients actually have underlying primary hyperparathyroidism and are taking calcium carbonate and alkali for associated gastric hyperacidity.

The family history may hold the key to both the correct diagnosis and the correct treatment of a hypercalcemic patient. Systematic inquiry regarding a history of neck exploration and the presence of hypercalcemia, nephrolithiasis, metabolic bone disease, intractable peptic ulcer disease, and endocrine tumors in family members is essential. There is no specific family history in the syndrome of familial hypocalciuric hypercalcemia, although a history of unsuccessful parathyroid surgery in more than one hypercalcemic relative is characteristic of this condition. The diagnosis can be made definitive only by documenting hypercalcemia in the immediate relatives of the patient. If a multiple endocrine neoplasia syndrome or familial hyperparathyroidism is present, the patient will almost certainly have enlargement ("hyperplasia") of all four glands, and subtotal parathyroidectomy (removal of three and one half glands), as opposed to single gland removal, would be indicated.

Radioimmunoassay of Parathyroid Hormone. The availability of sensitive and specific radioimmunoassays of parathyroid hormone in serum has revolutionized the approach to the diagnosis of primary hyperparathyroidism during the past few years. Previously, patients were first extensively evaluated for nonparathyroid disorders that could cause hypercalcemia, and the diagnosis of hyperparathyroidism was one of exclusion. Now measurements of serum iPTH and calcium allow the assignment of patients either to a group that is very likely to have a surgically resectable parathyroid lesion(s) or to groups that require further diagnostic evaluation for the cause of hypercalcemia (Fig. 246–7).

The author's experience in the diagnosis of primary hyperparathyroidism, using a radioimmunoassay of serum parathy-

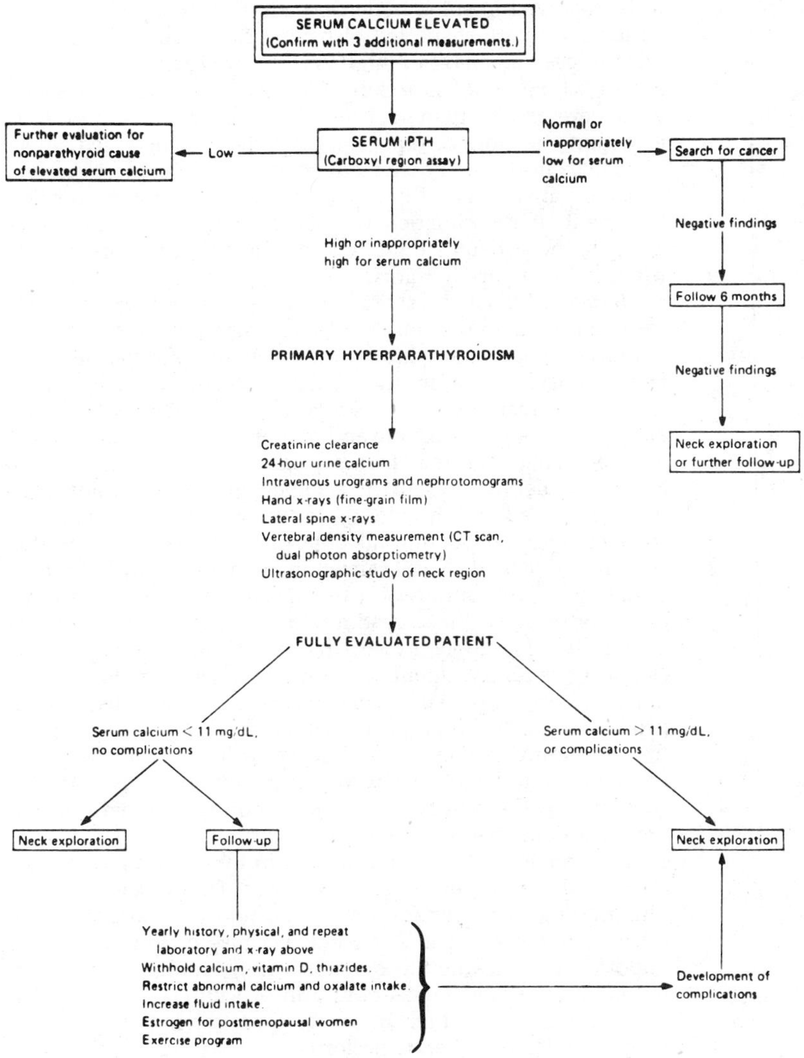

Figure 246–7. Use of PTH radioimmunoassay in the diagnosis and management of patients with hypercalcemia. (From Arnaud CD, Kolb FO: The calciotropic hormones and metabolic bone disease. *In* Greenspan FS, Forsham PH (eds.): Basic and Clinical Endocrinology. Los Altos, Lange Medical Publications, 1983, p 211.)

roid hormone that is specific for the mid region of the molecule, is illustrated in Figure 246–8. Ninety per cent of patients with surgically proved disease had values of serum iPTH that exceeded the upper limit of normal, and 10 per cent had values that were in the upper range of normal but inappropriately high for the total calcium concentration. Not shown are serum iPTH values in patients with nonparathyroid hypercalcemia (e.g., sarcoidosis and vitamin D intoxication). These are low or undetectable except in ectopic hyperparathyroidism caused by nonparathyroid cancer (see below). Thus, it is possible, by measuring calcium and iPTH in a single morning fasting serum sample, to categorize correctly 80 to 90 per cent of the hypercalcemic patients who have a potentially resectable hyperfunctioning parathyroid gland(s) and to categorize a similar percentage of the patients who have nonparathyroid hypercalcemia and who therefore require further study to discover the underlying cause of this derangement (see below). The advantages of using the serum iPTH as the principal laboratory probe to "triage" the hypercalcemic patient are clear. In the majority of patients with primary hyperparathyroidism, a correct diagnosis can be made in an outpatient setting, eliminating the costs and inconveniences of hospitalization and the multiple indirect tests required for a similar, less definitive diagnosis by exclusion.

Values of serum iPTH, measured with an assay specific for the mid or carboxyl region, are much lower for a given serum calcium in malignancy-associated hypercalcemia than in primary hyperparathyroidism (Fig. 246–9). This interesting phenomenon is probably due to the fact that patients with the hypercalcemia of malignancy have relatively low serum quantities of carboxyl- and mid-region fragments in comparison to

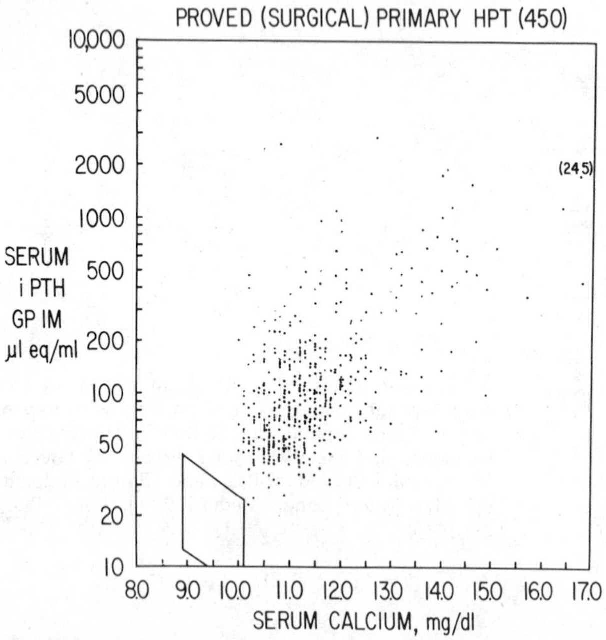

Figure 246–8. Serum iPTH values as a function of serum calcium concentration in 450 patients with surgically proved primary hyperparathyroidism. The area enclosed by the solid lines represents the normal range ± 2 SD for serum iPTH and serum calcium. Note that there is a 10 per cent overlap of serum iPTH with the normal range. Greater than 95 per cent of normal sera and all hyperparathyroid sera have measurable iPTH. Formal discriminative analysis of serum iPTH and serum calcium separates 100 per cent of hyperparathyroid patients from normal subjects. (From Arnaud CD, et al.: Human parathyroid hormone: Biologic and immunologic activities of its synthetic (1-34) tetratriacontapeptide and the utility of a carboxyl-terminal-specific radioimmunoassay in assessment of hyperparathyroid syndromes. Excerpta Medica International Congress Series No. 346, Calcium-Regulating Hormones, 1975, p 19.)

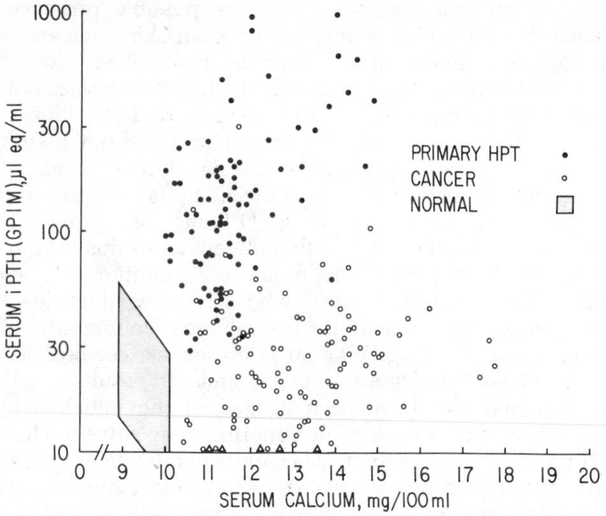

Figure 246–9. Relationship between serum iPTH and serum calcium in primary hyperparathyroid patients (●) and hypercalcemic patients with cancer(○). Note that for a given serum calcium value, serum iPTH is lower in patients with cancer. Of 105 patients with cancer, 5 had undetectable serum iPTH (Δ). Area enclosed with solid lines indicates normal range ± 2 SD for serum iPTH and serum calcium. (From Benson RC, Jr, et al.: Radioimmunoassay of parathyroid hormone in hypercalcemic patients with malignant disease. Am J Med 56:823, 1974.)

patients with primary hyperparathyroidism, but essentially equivalent quantities of intact parathyroid hormone. Irrespective of the pathophysiology involved, the relationships shown in Figure 246–9 help greatly in determining the course of action to be followed in some hypercalcemic and hypophosphatemic patients who are suspected of having cancer (e.g., those with weight loss, anemia, or a high erythrocyte sedimentation rate) but in whom proof is lacking (Fig. 246–7). If serum calcium values are greater than 12.5 mg per deciliter and serum iPTH is within the normal range or only slightly increased, more intensive efforts should be made to identify a neoplastic lesion, and the patient should be followed with temporizing medical treatment. If the situation is not clarified after six to twelve months, the patient should be re-evaluated for the presence of primary hyperparathyroidism.

Clinical Chemistry. Several serum and urine measurements may be helpful in the course of assigning patients to either the parathyroid or the nonparathyroid categories of hypercalcemia. Hyperphosphatemia in the absence of severe renal failure favors a nonparathyroid cause. Hypophosphatemia, when dietary phosphate is adequate and oral phosphate binding agents are not being ingested, favors primary hyperparathyroidism but is frequently present in ectopic hyperparathyroidism as well. Increased serum chloride favors primary hyperparathyroidism. Increased serum alkaline phosphatase is more often present in patients with cancer than in those with primary hyperparathyroidism and, in the absence of radiographic evidence of osteitis fibrosa cystica, should alert one to the likely possibility of ectopic hyperparathyroidism. Although polyclonal hypergammaglobulinemia might suggest multiple myeloma or sarcoidosis, this abnormality has been observed in primary hyperparathyroidism with disappearance after parathyroidectomy. Anemia and increases in the erythrocyte sedimentation rate have been recorded in primary hyperparathyroidism, but these findings suggest a nonparathyroid cause of hypercalcemia, particularly malignancy.

Measurement of the urine calcium in hypercalcemic patients is generally not useful unless it is low (<100 mg per 24 hours). This finding may give the only indication that familial hypocalciuric hypercalcemia is present. Because of the therapeutic importance of making this diagnosis (i.e., avoiding neck exploration), measurement of 24-hour urine calcium is recommended in the routine evaluation of any hypercalcemic patient before parathyroid exploration is performed.

Nephrogenous Cyclic AMP. Approximately 40 to 50 per cent of the cyclic AMP excreted in the urine is derived from the renal tubular cell. Its production and cellular release into the urine are almost entirely under the control of parathyroid hormone (see above). This component of urinary cyclic AMP can be accurately estimated and is termed nephrogenous cyclic AMP. It is increased above normal in 80 per cent of patients with primary hyperparathyroidism and in a large proportion of patients with the syndrome of ectopic hyperparathyroidism. Thus, it is not helpful in distinguishing between these two common disorders. Because low levels of nephrogenous cyclic AMP are present in patients with nonparathyroid hypercalcemia (excluding ectopic hyperparathyroidism), the test is useful in those patients whose serum iPTH is equivocally increased. In such patients, a low level of nephrogenous cyclic AMP would suggest that the serum iPTH value was artifactual and would argue against primary hyperparathyroidism, whereas a normal or increased level would confirm the validity of the serum iPTH value and favor this condition.

Other Diagnostic Tests. The glucocorticoid suppression test may be used in the rare event that the results of all the diagnostic tests already discussed are equivocal. It is based on the empirical observation that the hypercalcemia of conditions such as vitamin D intoxication, sarcoidosis, lymphoproliferative syndromes, and myeloma generally responds to the administration of 300 mg of cortisone or 60 mg of prednisone given daily in divided doses for ten days, whereas the same treatment only rarely results in a decrease in serum calcium in primary or ectopic hyperparathyroidism. The mechanisms involved in steroid-induced suppression of hypercalcemia are poorly understood, and variables other than steroids (e.g., hydration) may influence the level of serum calcium during the ten days of the test. A positive test (i.e., a significant decrease in serum calcium) should argue against neck exploration and for intensive investigation for another cause of hypercalcemia. A negative test would be consistent with primary or ectopic hyperparathyroidism.

Other diagnostic tests used less frequently include measurement of phosphate clearance (which is increased in primary hyperparathyroidism) and measurement of nephrogenous cyclic AMP after PTH administration (which is decreased in primary hyperparathyroidism, most likely because of a desensitization mechanism).

Finally, radiographs of the hands on fine grain industrial film should be obtained whenever hypercalcemia presents a diagnostic problem. Although the finding of definitive subperiosteal bone resorption is relatively unusual (approximately 8 to 10 per cent of patients with primary hyperparathyroidism), it is diagnostic of hyperparathyroidism and is probably the most reliable and readily available evidence supporting the need for neck exploration in patients with severe, life-threatening hypercalcemia.

PREOPERATIVE LOCALIZATION OF ABNORMAL PARATHYROID TISSUE. The abnormal parathyroid tissue causing primary hyperparathyroidism will be discovered and excised in greater than 90 per cent of initial neck explorations performed by an experienced parathyroid surgeon. Thus, there is no need for preoperative localization prior to first surgery except under unusual circumstances. In general, localization procedures are reserved for those patients in whom the first neck exploration was unsuccessful or for those who suffer recurrent disease. Noninvasive procedures include esophagography, ultrasonography, computed tomography, and isotopic scanning with thallium. Invasive procedures include arteriography, differential venous catheterization with measurement of iPTH in the serum samples obtained, and needle aspiration of a tumor with ultrasonic guidance.

Esophagography may occasionally identify a relatively large parathyroid gland, deep in the tracheoesophageal groove, which was inadvertently missed on first exploration because of its aberrant shape. Generally, however, the procedure is unrewarding. It is now possible to identify parathyroid lesions that are less than 1 cm in diameter by ultrasound examination of the neck or by thallium scanning. Further technological development in these areas is expected, and, because of the simplicity of the procedures, evaluation prior to initial neck exploration may become routinely advisable. Ultrasonography has not proved useful in identifying mediastinal parathyroid lesions, but computed tomography has. These noninvasive procedures may also have diagnostic value in the patient with severe hypercalcemia who has not undergone previous neck exploration. When a mass lesion(s) is identified in a location(s) consistent with normal or aberrant parathyroid tissue, the patient probably has primary hyperparathyroidism, and neck exploration should be performed early, before values for serum iPTH are available (usually requires several days) if the patient's condition is sufficiently serious.

Of the invasive procedures, thyroid arteriography is the most useful to the surgeon when a lesion is identified. As with the noninvasive procedures, the results are specific only in the sense that the location of an identified lesion is consistent with that of a normal or aberrant parathyroid gland. This procedure is not without risk, since neurologic complications such as transient occipital blindness and hemiplegia have been recorded.

Differential catheterization of the thyroidal and mediastinal veins for the purpose of obtaining serum for iPTH analysis can be performed after the veins have been identified during arteriography. The procedure is simple if a lesion has been identified by arteriography, since all that is required of iPTH analysis of the blood draining the lesion is confirmation that it is parathyroid in origin. If arteriography has not identified a lesion, all of the small veins should be entered and sampled. It is frequently difficult to obtain proper blood samples from small veins because the lumen may be obstructed by the catheter tip and because the sample may be diluted with blood from larger veins. It is important that a bioassay for PTH or a radioimmunoassay of PTH that recognizes only intact PTH (assays specific for the amino region or intact PTH) be used for measurements of iPTH in sera obtained during differential venous catheterization. Step-up differences in iPTH concentrations between peripheral sera and sera from veins draining parathyroid lesions are greater using such assays because of the relatively low concentrations of intact PTH in the peripheral circulation. By contrast, mid- and carboxyl-region specific assays measure the high concentrations of mid- and carboxyl-region fragments in the peripheral circulation and provide smaller step-up increases.

TREATMENT. The medical treatment of hypercalcemia is described in detail below ("Nonparathyroid Causes of Hypercalcemia"). The discussion here will be confined to the definitive treatment of hyperparathyroidism per se. The surgical removal of abnormal parathyroid tissue should be considered in all patients in whom the diagnosis of primary hyperparathyroidism has been established. Although patients with only biochemical abnormalities do not always develop clinically significant sequelae, they often do. Furthermore, the majority of these patients have histologic evidence of hyperparathyroidism in bone biopsies. This should be kept in mind before a long-term medical follow-up program is embarked upon, especially in older women who may have already suffered considerable bone loss as a result of age-related factors. Age per se should not be a contraindication to neck exploration. In fact, it is better to perform elective parathyroidectomy in an older person than to face hypercalcemia later as a complication of another age-related, serious illness (e.g., myocardial infarction).

If surgery is withheld and one embarks on following a patient who has hyperparathyroidism with only biochemical abnormalities, there remains a group of compelling indications for neck exploration: (1) radiographic evidence of metabolic bone disease, (2) demonstration of decreasing renal function, (3) active nephrolithiasis, (4) serum calcium concentrations greater than 11.0 mg per deciliter, and (5) the development of one or more "complications" of hyperparathyroidism, such as serious psychiatric disease, peptic ulcer that is resistant to treatment, pancreatitis, or severe hypertension. In any patient proposed for long-term follow-up, certain follow-up studies should be done systematically (Fig. 246–7). At a minimum, these should include a yearly history and physical examination, determinations of serum calcium and creatinine clearance, x-rays of the hand on fine grain industrial film to detect subperiosteal bone resorption, and a plain film of the abdomen to detect renal calcifications. If inactive nephrolithiasis has been detected on initial examination, nephrotomograms should be done to determine if new stones have developed or old stones have increased in size. By definition, either of these would be interpreted as the recrudescence of active stone disease, which would in turn be an indication for surgery.

The most critical consideration in the surgical treatment of patients with primary hyperparathyroidism is the selection of the surgeon. He should not only have extensive experience in parathyroid surgery but also be able to recognize an abnormal, enlarged parathyroid gland—a difficult skill to attain. The surgeon usually attempts to identify all four parathyroid glands (using biopsy if absolutely necessary), with the plan of removing a single enlarged parathyroid gland or three and one half parathyroid glands if multiple glands are involved. Less commonly, one side of the neck is explored first and any single enlarged parathyroid gland is removed. If the second parathyroid gland on the same side is normal, the other side of the neck is not explored. If the second parathyroid gland is abnormal, it is removed and the other side of the neck is explored and all the parathyroid tissue removed except for one half of a gland. The second approach has the advantage of leaving the unoperated side without scar tissue and easier to explore at a future time for recurrent hyperparathyroidism, but has the disadvantage of not firmly establishing whether multiple glands are enlarged.

Autotransplantation of parathyroid tissue to the muscles of the forearm may be of considerable value in special circumstances, such as when the last known parathyroid gland is removed because of recurrent primary hyperparathyroidism. Such patients are likely to be rendered hypoparathyroid without successful transplantation. The functioning of such transplants can be easily assessed by determining if there is a step-up in the concentration of parathyroid hormone in venous blood from the ipsilateral forearm in comparison with the other forearm.

Approximately 20 per cent of abnormal parathyroid glands are in the mediastinum, but the great majority of these (approximately 95 per cent) are high enough that they can be readily identified and removed during routine neck exploration. In the remaining cases abnormal parathyroid tissue is located elsewhere in the mediastinum and can be approached for excision only by splitting the sternum. Before the advent of localization procedures (see above), the success rate in removing abnormal parathyroid tissue from the mediastinum was only 50 per cent. The decision to carry out mediastinal exploration depends to a large extent on the accuracy and completeness of the information obtained during initial neck exploration. If the exploration was inadequate or the records are incomplete, neck surgery probably should be repeated.

Postoperatively, serum calcium concentrations decrease to within the normal range or below within 24 to 48 hours. It is possible to determine if all of the abnormal parathyroid tissue has been removed by measuring urinary cyclic AMP (which should be decreased) within two hours of parathyroidectomy. Patients who have significant bony demineralization may develop significant hypocalcemia postoperatively, presumably owing to the avidity of demineralized bone for extracellular fluid calcium. This "hungry bone syndrome" can be distinguished from hypoparathyroidism by the absence of hyperphosphatemia and the presence of increased concentrations of serum iPTH. Treatment of this syndrome, which may be difficult, requires very large quantities of intravenous calcium given continuously by infusion and administration of calcium carbonate by mouth in doses of 1 to 5 grams per day, depending upon the serum calcium response. Administration of vitamin D (usually 50,000 to 100,000 units daily) is of equivocal value but should be given. The biologically active metabolite of vitamin D 1,25$(OH)_2$D may prove to be an effective therapeutic agent in the future.

Most patients who develop hypocalcemia and mild hyperphosphatemia have temporary hypoparathyroidism, as evidenced by low normal values for serum iPTH. A small percentage of these patients will develop permanent hypoparathyroidism requiring treatment (see below).

Worsening of renal function (either temporary or permanent), metabolic acidosis, hypomagnesemia, pancreatitis, and gout or pseudogout are other complications that may occur in the postoperative period. Deterioration in renal function should be anticipated in patients who have abnormal renal function preoperatively, and prophylactic mannitol infusions should be given early in the postoperative period to initiate an osmotic diuresis. Likewise, a flaring of gout or pseudogout should be anticipated in patients with intra-articular calcification or a history of prior arthritic attacks.

PROGNOSIS. The natural history of primary hyperparathyroidism is not known. This is because the majority of patients, once the diagnosis is established, are subjected to neck exploration and removal of the abnormal parathyroid glands and are cured.

A large proportion of patients have "biochemical" hyperparathyroidism—i.e., only a slightly increased serum calcium (10.1 to 11.0 mg per deciliter) and no clinical manifestations of the disease. In a large prospective study (150 patients), relatively few (10 to 30 per cent) progressed to a more severe form of the disease within five years. In this study, no clinical or biochemical abnormality was found to be predictive of such a progression.

It is presumed that patients with mild to moderately severe manifestations of primary hyperparathyroidism represent progression from a previously "biochemical" form of the disease. A relatively small portion of this group of patients also attains some degree of disease stability; some patients have been observed for as long as 10 to 15 years without apparent progression. Except for a very small number who progress to severe disease, the remaining patients in this group probably progress slowly in the signs and symptoms of the disease and suffer a gradual deterioration of renal function. Patients with severe primary hyperparathyroidism (serum calcium $>$15 mg per deciliter) will almost certainly die of their disease unless it is detected and appropriately treated.

Surgical resection of benign parathyroid lesions is generally curative in primary hyperparathyroidism. Recurrences are rare in patients who have single gland disease, but relatively common when multiple glands are involved. The calcium nephropathy of hyperparathyroidism may be irreversible; whether improvement in hypertension occurs after successful treatment of hyperparathyroidism has not been estabished. Active nephrolithiasis generally becomes inactive unless factors other than primary hyperparathyroidism are present to perpetuate this problem. There have been anecdotal reports that severe psychiatric symptoms may disappear after the removal of abnormal parathyroid glands. All but the more severe forms of osteitis fibrosa cystica demonstrate improvement within months of parathyroidectomy and essentially complete resolution within a year. At present it is not known if the surgical treatment of hyperparathyroidism in patients who also have postmenopausal or senile osteoporosis results in improvement of the osteopenic disease. However, this will be important to determine because as many as 8 to 10 per cent of patients with age-related osteopenia have increased circulating levels of immunoreactive parathyroid hormone and may suffer from some form of curable hyperparathyroidism.

Arnaud CD, Clark OH: Primary hyperparathyroidism. *In* Krieger DT, Bardin CW: Current Therapy in Endocrinology 1983–1984. Philadelphia and St. Louis, B. C. Decker, Inc., and C. V. Mosby Company, 1983, pp 277–282. *Review of the medical and surgical treatment of primary hyperparathyroidism.*

Benson RC Jr, Riggs BL, Pickard BM, Arnaud CD: Radioimmunoassay of parathyroid hormone in hypercalcemic patients with malignant disease. Am J Med 56:821,1974. *Prospective study of serum calcium and serum PTH in 108 unselected patients with the hypercalcemia of cancer and 87 patients with primary hyperparathyroidism. Cancer patients had a lower serum PTH for a given degree of hypercalcemia than did patients with primary hyperparathyroidism.*

Christensson T, Hellström K, Wengle B, Alveryd A, Wikland B: Prevalence of hypercalcemia in health screening in Stockholm. Acta Med Scand 200:131, 1976. *In this study at least 3 per cent of 15,903 residents of Stockholm (predominantly middle-aged) had "asymptomatic hypercalcemia" and, most probably, primary hyperparathyroidism.*

DeGroot LJ (ed.): Endocrinology. Vol 2. New York, Grune & Stratton, 1979, pp 693–737. *Extensive and inclusive review of primary hyperparathyroidism by internationally renowned experts. The subjects discussed include clinical features, differential diagnosis, parathyroid hormone radioimmunoassay, localizing techniques, medical management, and surgical management.*

Foley TP Jr, Harrison HC, Arnaud CD, Harrison HE: Familial benign hypercalcemia. J Pediatr 81:1060, 1972. *First description of the syndrome of familial benign hypercalcemia, or familial hypocalciuric hypercalcemia.*

Heath H III, Hodgson SF, Kennedy MA: Primary hyperparathyroidism: Incidence, morbidity and potential economic impact in a community. N Engl J Med 302:189, 1980. *Only available systematic, epidemiologic study of the incidence of primary hyperparathyroidism in a well-characterized general population.*

Reading CC, Carboneau JW, James EM, Karsell PR, Purnell DC, Grant CS, van Heerden JA: High-resolution parathyroid sonography. Am J Roentgenol 139:539,1982. *An evaluation of high-resolution ultrasonography in the localization of pathologic parathyroid tissue.*

Stark DD, Moss AW, Gooding GAW, Clark OH: Parathyroid scanning by computed tomography. Radiology 148:297,1983. *An evaluation of computed tomography in the localization of pathologic parathyroid tissue.*

HYPOPARATHYROIDISM

DEFINITION. Hypoparathyroidism, or deficient secretion of parathyroid hormone, is characterized clinically by symptoms of neuromuscular hyperactivity and biochemically by hypocalcemia, hyperphosphatemia, and diminished to absent levels of circulating immunoreactive parathyroid hormone.

ETIOLOGY. There are three types of hypoparathyroidism: surgically induced, idiopathic, and functional. *Surgically induced hypoparathyroidism,* the most common of these, may occur after any surgical procedure in which the anterior neck is explored, including thyroidectomy, removal of abnormal parathyroid glands, and excision of various malignant lesions in the neck. Parathyroid glands need not actually be removed for hypoparathyroidism to ensue. In such cases it is presumed that the blood supply to the parathyroid glands has been compromised.

Idiopathic hypoparathyroidism occurs spontaneously and can be categorized according to whether it appears early or late in life. Aside from congenital absence of the glands, as in DiGeorge's syndrome (see Ch. 429), the syndromes occurring at an early age are genetic and are transmitted most frequently as an autosomal recessive trait. This type of hypoparathyroidism is called multiple endocrine deficiency–autoimmune–candidiasis (MEDAC) syndrome or juvenile familial endocrinopathy–hypoparathyroidism–Addison's disease–moniliasis (HAM) syndrome. Hypoparathyroidism, Addison's disease, and mucocutaneous candidiasis characterize the disorder. Circulating antibodies specific for parathyroid and adrenal tissues are frequently present, but they correlate poorly with clinical manifestations. Sporadic cases of MEDAC syndrome have been reported, as well as cases that have an autosomal recessive mode of inheritance. The majority of these are generally seen at a later age, and some have hypoparathyroidism only. This syndrome is described in Ch. 240. The late onset form of idiopathic hypoparathyroidism occurs sporadically and circulating glandular antibodies are absent. The cause of parathyroid gland destruction in these cases is unknown.

Functional hypoparathyroidism occurs in patients with severe and prolonged hypomagnesemia of whatever cause (see Ch. 208). Since magnesium is required for release of parathyroid hormone from the glands, serum iPTH is characteristically low or undetectable in this syndrome. Infusion of magnesium increases serum iPTH rapidly (within minutes), and restoration of magnesium to normal levels ultimately restores eucalcemia. Magnesium is probably also required for the peripheral action of parathyroid hormone; the hypocalcemia in patients with functional hypoparathyroidism may be due, in part, to the failure of PTH to act normally on its target tissues.

Neonatal hypoparathyroidism occurs in infants of mothers who have primary hyperparathyroidism. It is presumed that in utero exposure to maternal hypercalcemia results in prolonged suppression of fetal parathyroid glands and failure of the parathyroid glands to respond to hypocalcemic stimuli after birth.

PATHOLOGY. Patients with MEDAC syndrome may have lymphocytic infiltration and fibrosis of glands. In the few patients with late onset idiopathic hypoparathyroidism who have been examined, fatty infiltration, fibrosis, and atrophy have been found. Longstanding cases of hypoparathyroidism have characteristic soft tissue calcifications in the lens and basal ganglia of the brain. All types of bone cells are diminished, and both formation and resorption surfaces in bone are decreased.

PATHOPHYSIOLOGY AND CLINICAL CHEMISTRY. The pathophysiology and biochemical consequences of parathyroid gland removal can be appreciated by referring to the "butterfly" diagram (Fig. 243–1). In hypoparathyroidism the right limbs of the three feedback loops predominate. There is (1) decreased bone resorption; (2) decreased renal phosphate excretion, increased serum phosphate, decreased $1,25(OH)_2D$, and decreased intestinal absorption of calcium; and (3) increased excretion of calcium for the prevailing serum concentration of calcium. Patients have hypocalcemia and generally hyperphosphatemia, provided that dietary phosphate has been normal. Urinary calcium is usually low unless eucalcemia has been restored with treatment. In that case, urinary calcium is generally inappropriately high for the level of serum calcium and occasionally reaches hypercalciuric levels. Nephrogenous cyclic AMP is decreased but increases briskly with the administration of parathyroid hormone.

Hypocalcemia and mild alkalosis (resulting from decreased bicarbonate excretion), if sufficiently severe, cause increased neuromuscular excitability with consequent tetany and, rarely, convulsions.

CLINICAL MANIFESTATIONS. The clinical manifestations of hypoparathyroidism depend upon the severity of the disease (degree of hypocalcemia) and its chronicity. The rate of decrease in the serum calcium appears to be a major determinant in the development of the neuromuscular complications (see below) of hypocalcemia. Thus, these symptoms are more likely to occur within one to two days after parathyroidectomy, when serum calcium decreases acutely, and at serum calcium values that may be considerably higher (e.g., 8.0 mg per deciliter) than might be found in patients who have had more severe hypocalcemia (e.g., 6.0 mg per deciliter) for a longer time. It is therefore important to observe patients carefully for the development of the clinical signs heralding tetany, immediately and for several days after neck surgery, in the region of the parathyroid glands, rather than relying entirely on the absolute concentration of the serum calcium.

Hypocalcemia causes a decreased threshold of excitation, repetitive responses to a single stimulus, reduced accommodation, and, at the extreme, continuous activity of nervous tissues. Such neural activity occurs spontaneously in both sensory and motor fibers in hypocalcemic states and gives rise to neuromuscular symptoms and signs. Symptoms include numbness and tingling around the mouth, in the tips of the fingers, and sometimes in the feet. An attack of tetany usually begins with this prodrome and is followed by muscle spasms in the extremities and face. The hands, forearms, and, less commonly, feet become contorted in a characteristic way (Fig. 246–10). First, the thumb is strongly adducted, followed by flexion of the metacarpophalangeal joints, extension of the

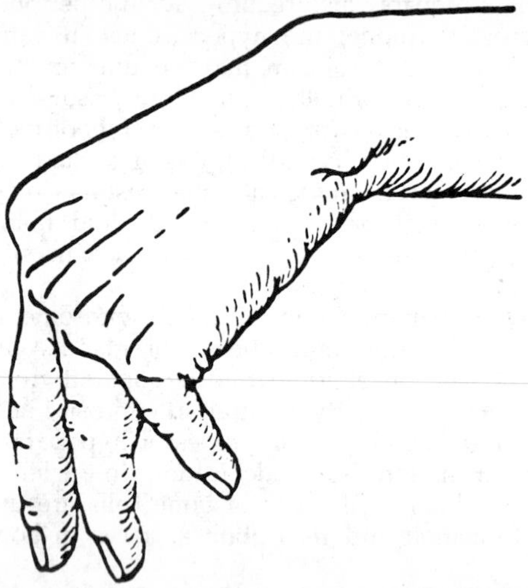

Figure 246–10. Position of hand in hypocalcemic tetany (Trousseau's sign). (From Ganong WF: Review of Medical Physiology. 11th ed. Los Altos, Lange Medical Publications, 1983, p 319.)

interphalangeal joints (with fingers together), and flexion of the wrist and elbow joints. This somewhat grotesque spastic condition may be quite painful but is more alarming than dangerous. Because of its alarming quality, patients may hyperventilate and secrete more epinephrine. Hyperventilation causes hypocapnia and alkalosis and worsens hypocalcemia by increasing the binding of ionic calcium to plasma proteins. Increased epinephrine secretion produces further anxiety, tachycardia, sweating, and peripheral and circumoral pallor. Prolonged hyperventilation in normal subjects can lower serum ionic calcium and produce tetany, but great care should be exercised in attributing such findings to hyperventilation alone.

Patients with hypoparathyroidism may have convulsions, especially during childhood. A more generalized form of tetany may be followed by prolonged tonic spasms, or the patient may have a typical epileptiform seizure (grand mal, jacksonian, focal, or petit mal), with characteristic associated electroencephalographic (EEG) findings. Because restoration of eucalcemia results in a decrease in the number of seizures without improvement in the EEG findings associated with seizures, it is thought that hypocalcemia lowers the excitation threshold of pre-existing epilepsy in such patients. The characteristic EEG changes associated with hypocalcemia per se do disappear after restoration of eucalcemia. Laryngeal spasm and stridor may occur during tetany and may precipitate seizures because of hypoxia. The relatively unusual finding of papilledema and increased intracranial pressure resulting from hypocalcemia in association with convulsions may suggest the diagnosis of brain tumor.

Latent tetany can be detected by several relatively specific physical signs. *Chvostek's sign* is elicited by tapping the facial nerve just anterior to the ear lobe, just below the zygomatic arch, or between the zygomatic arch and the corner of the mouth. The response ranges from twitching of the lip at the corner of the mouth to twitching of all of the facial muscles on the stimulated side. Simple twitching at the corner of the mouth occurs in 25 per cent of normal subjects, but more extensive muscle contraction (ala nasi and orbital muscles) is a reliable sign of latent tetany.

Trousseau's sign is demonstrated with a sphygmomanometer cuff inflated about the arm to above the systolic blood pressure for at least two minutes. A positive response consists of the development of typical ipsilateral carpal spasm (Fig. 246–10), with relaxation only occurring five to ten seconds after the cuff is deflated. Apparent spasm disappearing instantly should be regarded with suspicion. Trousseau's sign is the most reliable physical finding of latent tetany, and serial tests for this sign should be done and the results recorded in the immediate postoperative period after anterior neck surgery.

Beyond the neurologic manifestations described above, there are a number of other possible manifestations of hypocalcemia: (1) basal ganglia calcification and occasional extrapyramidal neurologic syndromes; (2) papilledema and increased intracranial pressure; (3) psychiatric disorders; (4) skin, hair, and fingernail abnormalities; (5) susceptibility to *Candida* infections; (6) inhibition of normal dental development; (7) lenticular cataracts; (8) intestinal malabsorption; (9) prolongation of the $Q\text{-}T_c$ and S-T intervals of the electrocardiogram, in rare cases 2:1 heart block, and even more rarely heart failure requiring digitalis and diuretics; and (10) increased serum concentrations of creatine phosphokinase and lactic dehydrogenase.

Extrapyramidal neurologic syndromes, including classic parkinsonism, may occur in patients with chronic hypoparathyroidism. Such manifestations are presumably caused by the basal ganglia calcification observed in the majority of such patients. Many untreated patients without extrapyramidal syndromes are unduly sensitive to the dystonic side effects of phenothiazine drugs, suggesting that calcification of the ganglia may have more general pathologic importance than was once believed. Treatment of hypocalcemia usually improves the neurologic disorder, and decreases in basal ganglia calcification have been documented radiologically.

Psychiatric disorders occur but are unusual in defined populations of hypoparathyroid patients. Mental retardation occurs in about 20 per cent of children with the disease, but this condition improves with restoration of eucalcemia in some. Tooth development is impaired in many children with the disease; hypoplasia of enamel, increased susceptibility to caries, delayed eruption, gaps between the teeth, and dysplastic dentin have been observed.

Lenticular cataracts are the most common sequelae of hypoparathyroidism. Visual impairment is observed only after five to ten years of cataract development. Fully mature cataracts in hypoparathyroidism are confluent and produce total opacity of the lens. Such cataracts are different from senile cataracts, which are frequently confined to one segment of the lens. Successful treatment of hypocalcemia generally halts the progress of cataracts, and, rarely, opacities may diminish in size.

The skin of patients with longstanding hypoparathyroidism may be dry and scaling, the nails ridged longitudinally, and the hair coarse, dry, friable, and falling. An occasional patient will suffer exfoliative dermatitis or atopic eczema, and existing psoriasis may be made worse. All of these lesions tend to improve and disappear with restoration of eucalcemia. *Candida* infections can complicate skin, nail, and hair abnormalities. They also improve with treatment of hypocalcemia but may require specific antifungal therapy as well.

Intestinal malabsorption with steatorrhea occurs in rare cases of longstanding untreated hypoparathyroidism. The disorder is presumed to be due to decreased serum calcium because it is reversed by successful treatment of hypocalcemia but not by a gluten-free diet. The problem is particularly difficult to manage because the treatment of hypoparathyroidism largely depends upon the ability to increase calcium transport across a normal gastrointestinal tract with drugs. Conversely, malabsorption may cause functional hypoparathyroidism by producing magnesium deficiency.

Hypocalcemia causes prolongation of the $Q\text{-}T_c$ interval in the electrocardiogram, but clinical cardiac abnormalities are rare in hypoparathyroidism. Congestive heart failure, requiring digitalis and diuretics, has been reported, but this condition usually reverses following successful treatment of hypocalcemia.

DIAGNOSIS. The detection of hypoparathyroidism depends upon maintaining a high index of suspicion in certain clinical situations. Serum calcium should be measured yearly in patients who have had anterior neck surgery or who are suspected of having the MEDAC syndrome. Cutaneous candidiasis, cataracts, incidental discovery of basal ganglia calcification, convulsions, numbness and tingling of the fingers, facial muscle spasm (spontaneous or self-induced), delayed dentition, and developmental retardation should all prompt serum calcium measurement.

In the absence of renal failure, the diagnosis of hypoparathyroidism is virtually certain if hypocalcemia and hyperphosphatemia are found. However, some patients may be actually relatively depleted in phosphate because of dietary restriction or the ingestion of aluminum hydroxide gels. In addition, in patients who have undergone parathyroidectomy for primary hyperparathyroidism, bone uptake of minerals may be so great as to produce hypophosphatemia (the "hungry bone syndrome"). The measurement of serum iPTH is crucial for diagnosis. Increased values in a range appropriate to the degree of hypocalcemia would essentially exclude the presence of hypoparathyroidism and suggest the possibility of end-organ resistance to parathyroid hormone (i.e., pseudohypoparathyroidism [see below], vitamin D deficiency, and vitamin D dependency) or secondary hypoparathyroidism resulting from such disorders as dietary deficiency of calcium, intestinal malabsorption of calcium, or excessive intake of drugs containing absorbable phosphate.

Undetectable serum iPTH confirms the diagnosis of hypoparathyroidism, provided that the assay used is sufficiently sensitive to measure serum iPTH in the large majority of normal subjects. Serum iPTH may be barely detectable in some patients with hypoparathyroidism if the assay employed is very sensitive, but such low values may be due to nonspecific effects of serum per se in radioimmunoassays that do not adequately control for this factor.

Patients with functional hypoparathyroidism resulting from hypomagnesemia also have low to undetectable levels of serum iPTH. Detection of this condition depends upon the measurement of serum magnesium and its diagnosis upon the demonstration that successful treatment with magnesium salts restores eucalcemia and increases serum iPTH (see Ch. 208).

TREATMENT. Theoretically, the most appropriate therapy for hypoparathyroidism would be the physiologic replacement of parathyroid hormone. This approach is impractical at present because the hormone must be administered parenterally and because synthetic human parathyroid hormone is too expensive. Such treatment might become practical in the future for some patients who are poorly controlled on conventional regimens.

Because of the absence of parathyroid hormone and the consequent hyperphosphatemia, the renal enzyme that converts 25OHD to $1,25(OH)_2D$, 1α-hydroxylase, is relatively inactive in patients with hypoparathyroidism. Conversion of circulating 25OHD to $1,25(OH)_2D$ is poor, and serum levels of this most active vitamin D metabolite are low or undetectable. In fact, hypoparathyroid patients are resistant to pharmacologic quantities of vitamin D for this reason.

The lowering of serum phosphate levels, using diets low in phosphate (i.e., restricting dairy products and meat) and oral aluminum hydroxide gels to bind intestinal phosphate, might be expected to increase the conversion of 25OHD to $1,25(OH)_2D$, but such treatment has received little attention. Rather, treatment with pharmacologic doses of vitamin D_2 or its more potent analogue, dihydrotachysterol, in combination with oral calcium, has been the mainstay regimen for many years. Unfortunately, unpredictable hypercalcemic episodes sometimes occur with this therapeutic regimen unless serum calcium is monitored at least once per month. A single episode of vitamin D intoxication can irreversibly impair renal function and can last from weeks to months because the body stores vitamin D and its metabolite 25OHD. The treatment of the vitamin D intoxication is similar to that described for severe hypercalcemia (see below), but with the additional use of corticosteroids (60 mg of prednisone or 300 mg of cortisone in four divided doses per day), which appear to antagonize vitamin D action.

Tetany caused by hypoparathyroidism requires emergency treatment with intravenous calcium to prevent laryngeal stridor and convulsions, the occurrence of which cannot be predicted. A 10 per cent solution of calcium gluconate (10 to 20 ml) should be given slowly (not more than 10 ml per minute) intravenously until symptoms are relieved or until serum calcium rises above 7 mg per deciliter. Hypercalcemia should be avoided; maintaining calcium levels between 7.5 and 9.0 mg per deciliter is adequate. Caution should be exercised in patients taking digitalis because calcium potentiates the action of this drug on the heart. Electrocardiographic monitoring during intravenous administration of calcium is prudent. It may be necessary to maintain serum calcium at levels that prevent tetany for several days before treatment with vitamin D or its metabolites or analogues (see below) becomes effective. This is accomplished by combining oral with intravenous calcium administration. Oral calcium is begun as soon as possible, starting with 200 mg of elemental calcium (as the gluconate or chloride salt) every two hours, increasing to 500 mg with each dose. If serum calcium falls below 7.5 mg per deciliter after six hours of the combined intravenous and oral regimen, continuous calcium infusion should be started. Five hundred ml of 5 per cent glucose and water containing 10 ml of 10 per cent calcium gluconate (1 gram) is given over six hours initially, with the quantity of calcium increased in increments of 5 ml (0.5 grams) every six hours until satisfactory control is achieved. In patients with hyperparathyroidism and bone disease who have undergone successful excision of a hyperfunctioning parathyroid gland(s), hypocalcemia may be profound and extremely resistant to treatment. As much as 10 grams of elemental calcium administered intravenously by infusion over 24 hours may be required to increase serum calcium above 7.5 mg per deciliter. Such patients are notoriously resistant to vitamin D.

Most patients with severe hypoparathyroidism require some form of long-term treatment with vitamin D. An effective regimen is as follows: dihydrotachysterol, 4 mg per day for two days, then 2 mg per day for two days, then 1 mg per day until dose adjustment is required, as judged by serum calcium values. Ideally, serum calcium should be maintained between 8.5 and 9.0 mg per deciliter, leaving a margin for the calcium to fluctuate upward to levels that are still not dangerous. The major advantage of dihydrotachysterol is its relatively rapid onset of action and short half-life. With regard to the latter, hypercalcemia caused by inadvertent overdosage is relieved within one to three weeks after the drug is discontinued; in comparison, the hypercalcemic effects of overdoses of vitamin D persist for 6 to 18 weeks. Dihydrotachysterol offers another advantage in that parathyroid function can be tested fairly soon after withdrawal of the drug. Hypocalcemia occurring within two weeks of withdrawal proves the persistence of hypoparathyroidism. The disadvantage of dihydrotachysterol is its cost.

The only natural vitamin D preparation currently available for general clinical use is ergocalciferol, or vitamin D_2, which is derived from plant sources (vitamin D_3 is the naturally produced compound in humans). In initiating vitamin D_2 therapy, the development of hypercalcemia can best be avoided by giving small doses initially (0.2 mg [8,000 units] to 0.5 mg [20,000 units]), with gradual increases only after steady state levels of serum calcium are achieved at each dose level. Most patients can be managed successfully with 1.0 mg (40,000 units) to 3.0 mg (120,000 units) of vitamin D_2 daily. The occasional patient who requires more than 3.0 mg per day is a candidate for the shorter acting analogues or metabolites of vitamin D.

Relatively little information is now available concerning the long-term management of hypoparathyroidism with the vitamin D_3 metabolites 25-OH-D_3 (calcifediol) or $1,25(OH)_2D_3$ (calcitriol). Both appear to be biologically effective and superior to vitamin D_2 with respect to the rapidity of onset and termination of action. Neither seems to have major advantages over dihydrotachysterol, except in patients who are particularly difficult to manage. The initiation and termination of action appears to be faster for $1,25(OH)_2D_3$ than for dihydrotachysterol. Both metabolites are even more expensive than dihydrotachysterol.

Since vitamin D acts primarily to increase intestinal calcium absorption, dietary calcium must be adequate: an approximate total (dietary and supplemented) intake of 1.0 gram daily in patients under 40 and 2 grams in patients over 40. Supplements can be provided by administering calcium as the gluconate, chloride, or carbonate salt. There are disadvantages to each. Calcium gluconate tablets contain relatively small quantities of calcium (9 per cent by weight), so that a large number of tablets must be given. Calcium chloride tablets contain larger quantities of calcium (27 per cent) but tend to produce gastric irritation. Calcium carbonate tablets also contain large quantities of calcium (40 per cent) but tend to produce alkalosis, which may aggravate hypocalcemia.

Patients with milder hypoparathyroidism may require only calcium supplementation (1 to 5 grams daily) and moderate degrees of phosphate restriction (including aluminum hydroxide gels) to maintain serum calcium in a therapeutic range. This treatment should be tried whenever a successful outcome is thought to be possible in order to avoid vitamin D intoxication entirely.

Long-term restoration of serum calcium to normal or nearly normal levels usually results in improvement in most manifestations of surgical and idiopathic hypoparathyroidism, including the skin disorders and associated candidiasis. Unfortunately, the latter appears to persist in the MEDAC syndrome, and resolution usually can be achieved only with iodoquinol or with systemic amphotericin (alone or combined with transfer factor) therapy.

Hypercalciuria can complicate successful restoration of a normal plasma calcium owing to the absence of the influence of parathyroid hormone to maintain normal renal tubular reabsorption of calcium. Accurate measurement of 24-hour urine calcium is therefore mandatory as serum calcium approaches the normal range during calcium and vitamin D treatment in order to avert possible renal stone formation. Thiazide diuretics, which cause increased renal tubular reabsorption of calcium, may be useful in such patients and may have the added advantage of partially restoring eucalcemia as a result of this action.

Anast CS, Mohs JM, Kaplan SL, Burns TW: Evidence for parathyroid failure in magnesium deficiency. Science 177:606, 1972. *First definitive demonstration of functional hypoparathyroidism in a magnesium-deficient patient with a selective intestinal defect in the absorption of magnesium.*

Attie JM, Kafif RA: Preservation of parathyroid glands during total thyroidectomy. Improved techniques utilizing microsurgery. Am J Surg 130:399, 1975. *Describes techniques in thyroid surgery that should help prevent destruction of the parathyroid glands and consequent hypoparathyroidism.*

Avioli LV: The therapeutic approach to hypoparathyroidism. Am J Med 57:34, 1974. *An important review of the problems encountered in the treatment of hypoparathyroidism.*

Harrison HE, Lifshitz F, Blizzard RM: Comparison between crystalline dihydrotachysterol and calciferol in patients requiring pharmacologic vitamin D therapy. N Engl J Med 276:894, 1967. *A classic review of the relative merits of vitamin D and dihydrotachysterol in the treatment of vitamin D resistant states, including hypoparathyroidism.*

Hunt G, Morgan DB: The early effects of dihydrotachysterol on calcium and phosphorus metabolism in patients with hypoparathyroidism. Clin Sci 38:713, 1970. *A careful evaluation of the effects of dihydrotachysterol in patients with hypoparathyroidism.*

Neer RM, Holick MF, DeLuca HF, Potts JT Jr: Effects of 1α-hydroxyvitamin D_3 and $1,25(OH)_2D_3$ on calcium and phosphorus metabolism in hypoparathyroidism. Metabolism 24:1403, 1975. *These authors investigated the acute effects of $1\alpha OHD_3$ and $1,25(OH)_2D_3$ in five patients with surgical hypoparathyroidism and found that these compounds are rapid acting. Since urinary hydroxyproline levels did not increase, they concluded that these compounds act on the intestine rather than on bone to increase serum calcium.*

Nusynowitz ML, Frame B, Kolb FO: The spectrum of the hypoparathyroid states: A classification based on physiologic principles. Medicine 55:105, 1976. *Broad and in-depth evaluation of all forms of hypoparathyroidism.*

Parfitt AM: The incidence of hypoparathyroid tetany after thyroid operations. Relationship to age, extent of resection and surgical experience. Med J Aust 1:1103, 1971. *Detailed compilation of the factors involved in the production of hypoparathyroidism resulting from thyroidectomy.*

Parfitt AM: The spectrum of hypoparathyroidism. J Clin Endocrinol Metab 34:152, 1972. *This detailed analysis of serum calcium values in hypoparathyroid patients formed the basis for the author's classification of the severity of the disease.*

Parfitt AM: Adult hypoparathyroidism. Treatment with calcifediol. Arch Intern Med 138:874, 1978. *A systematic study of the therapeutic efficacy of 25OHD in hypoparathyroid patients for a total of 19 patient-years.*

Parfitt AM: Surgical, idiopathic, and other varieties of parathyroid hormone–deficient hypoparathyroidism. *In* DeGroot LJ (ed.): Endocrinology. Vol 2. New York, Grune & Stratton, 1979, pp 755–768. *Comprehensive review of parathyroid hormone–deficient hypoparathyroidism.*

PSEUDOHYPOPARATHYROIDISM AND PSEUDOPSEUDOHYPOPARATHYROIDISM

DEFINITIONS. *Pseudohypoparathyroidism* describes a rare clinical state of hypoparathyroidism that results from target tissue resistance to parathyroid hormone, associated with a secondary, hypocalcemia–induced increase in parathyroid gland function. Patients with pseudohypoparathyroidism classically have a variety of congenital defects in growth and skeletal development, including short stature and foreshortened metacarpal and metatarsal bones (Fig. 246–11). Patients with *pseudopseudohypoparathyroidism* have analogous developmental defects without clinical hypoparathyroidism. Some patients with pseudohypoparathyroidism have target tissue resistance to the hormone but no developmental abnormalities, and others with developmental abnormalities have spontaneous remission of clinical hypoparathyroidism. Very rarely, patients have developmental abnormalities and clinical hypoparathyroidism with typical osteitis fibrosa cystica, a syndrome described by the barbarism "pseudohyperhypoparathyroidism."

ETIOLOGY AND GENETICS. It is difficult to conceive that all these combinations of manifestations could be ascribed to a single underlying biochemical defect. Although abnormal target tissue responses to parathyroid hormone may be the underlying theme, it is likely that an array of separate, rate-limiting steps, from receptor binding of parathyroid hormone to final expression of the cellular actions of the hormone (see Fig. 246–5) could be involved.

In some patients with pseudohypoparathyroidism, the guanyl nucleotide–sensitive regulatory protein (N protein), which couples parathyroid hormone–occupied receptors to adenylate cyclase, is decreased by 50 per cent in the red blood cells (see Fig. 246–5). In such patients this defect appears to produce resistance to several other hormones that apparently exert their actions by stimulating the increased production of cellular cyclic AMP (e.g., vasopressin and glucagon). Other possible mechanisms, as yet largely untested, include the secretion of a biologically inert form of parathyroid hormone, an intrinsic abnormality of parathyroid hormone receptors, autoantibodies to the parathyroid hormone receptor, a defect in adenylate cyclase, a disturbance in the process by which parathyroid hormone alters the distribution of ions across membranes, abnormalities of cellular protein kinases or other hormone-dependent enzymes, or gross cellular abnormalities that permit all of the actions of the hormone except the actual transfer of minerals from the cell to the blood.

Patients with pseudohypoparathyroidism generally fail to respond normally to the administration of large doses of parathyroid hormone with an increase in urinary phosphate excretion and nephrogenous cyclic AMP. A few have normal cyclic AMP responses but diminished phosphate responses, whereas others may have the reverse. The implication is that cyclic AMP may not be involved in the biologic actions of PTH. However, these results can be explained by several alternative explanations, including the possibility that urinary excretion of cyclic AMP does not accurately reflect all of the cyclic AMP–related cellular events critical to parathyroid hormone action and that only small changes in intracellular cyclic AMP are required for parathyroid hormone action.

Levels of $1,25(OH)_2D$ have been reported to be low in pseudohypoparathyroidism, and, because of this, defective conversion of 25OHD to $1,25(OH)_2D$ has been suggested as the mechanism involved in the abnormal mineral homeostasis in these patients. Support for this argument is derived from the success achieved in restoring serum calcium and urinary phosphate excretion to normal levels with $1,25(OH)_2D$ administration in patients with pseudohypoparathyroidism. Again, alter-

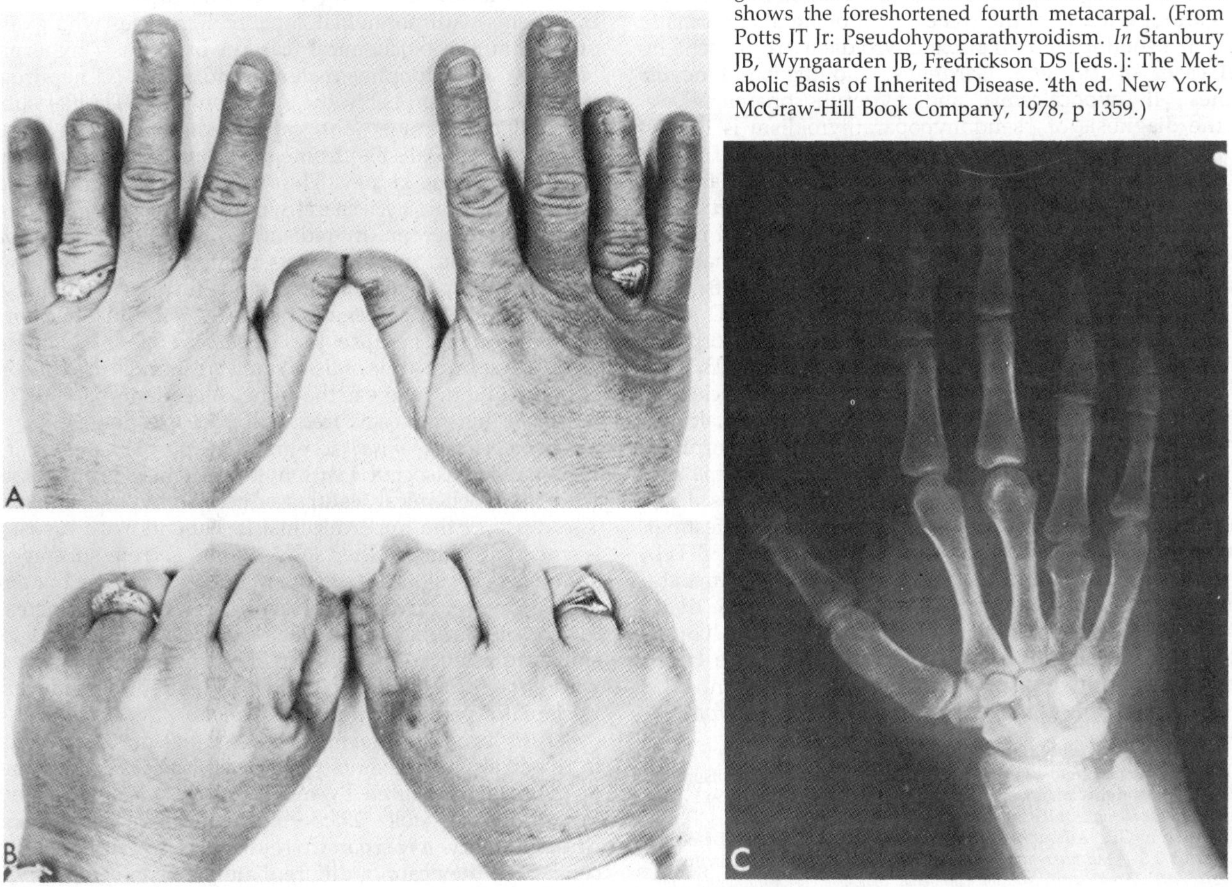

Figure 246–11. Hands of patient with pseudohypoparathyroidism. *A,* Note the shortened fourth finger. *B,* Note the "absent" fourth knuckle. *C,* Film shows the foreshortened fourth metacarpal. (From Potts JT Jr: Pseudohypoparathyroidism. *In* Stanbury JB, Wyngaarden JB, Fredrickson DS [eds.]: The Metabolic Basis of Inherited Disease. 4th ed. New York, McGraw-Hill Book Company, 1978, p 1359.)

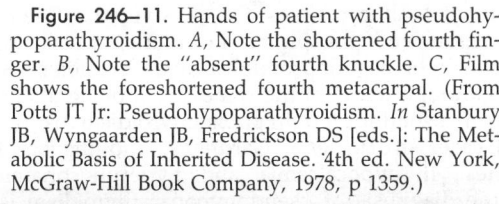

native explanations for these observations are not only possible but likely. Increased renal tubular cyclic AMP may be involved in the stimulation of 1-α hydroxylation of 25OHD. If this is true, normal tissue responsiveness to parathyroid hormone may be necessary for the production of $1,25(OH)_2D$. This would account for the low levels of serum $1,25(OH)_2D$ found in pseudohypoparathyroidism. Likewise, $1,25(OH)_2D$ might be expected to improve the responsiveness of bone to parathyroid hormone in patients with deficient production of $1,25(OH)_2D$ simply because the hypercalcemic action of parathyroid hormone depends upon the presence of biologically active metabolites of vitamin D. Finally, the phosphaturia induced in pseudohypoparathyroidism by $1,25(OH)_2D$ administration could be due to the restoration of eucalcemia; it is well known that phosphaturia occurs when the serum calcium is restored to normal in patients with surgical hypoparathyroidism.

Although pseudohypoparathyroidism is inherited, the mode of its transmission is unclear. A sex-linked dominant mechanism is possible, since there is a female-to-male ratio of 2:1 for the disease. It is difficult to explain how the developmental defects of pseudohypoparathyroidism can be inherited without abnormalities occurring in the adenylate cyclase system. Furthermore, four cases of male-to-male transmission of the developmental defects have been recorded.

PATHOPHYSIOLOGY AND CLINICAL CHEMISTRY. The biochemical findings in patients with pseudohypoparathyroidism are identical to those observed in patients with surgical or idiopathic hypoparathyroidism, except that serum iPTH is increased appropriately for the degree of hypocalcemia. The pathophysiology of the disease can be visualized best by referring to Figure 246–1. Parathyroid hormone action is blocked in all three of the left limbs of the feedback loops. The result in the right limbs is (1) decreased bone resorption caused by decreased bone cell responsiveness to parathyroid hormone; (2) increased serum phosphate caused by decreased renal tubular responsiveness to the phosphaturic action of PTH, which in turn decreases production of $1,25(OH)_2D$ and intestinal calcium absorption; and (3) increased renal excretion of calcium for the degree of hypocalcemia, which is caused again by decreased renal tubular responsiveness to the hypocalciuric effects of parathyroid hormone. The consequent hypocalcemia stimulates parathyroid hormone secretion.

PATHOLOGY. In patients who are hypocalcemic, the parathyroid glands are hyperplastic. Aside from the unique developmental abnormalities noted under Clinical Manifestations, below, the findings are the same as in surgical hypoparathyroidism.

CLINICAL MANIFESTATIONS. Most of the symptoms and signs of pseudohypoparathyroidism are the same as those of surgical and idiopathic hypoparathyroidism, and are due almost entirely to hypocalcemia. However, there are certain unique developmental features. Many patients are mentally retarded, have short stocky builds, are obese, have rounded faces, and display one or more short metacarpal or metatarsal bones. A classic sign of the brachymetacarpia, usually most marked in the fourth and fifth metacarpals, is the formation of a dimple over the head of the involved metacarpals when the patient makes a fist (Fig. 246–11). The fingers may be foreshortened. The calvarium is thickened in one third of patients, and there may be delayed dentition, defective enamel, and absence of teeth. There also may be exostoses, coxa vara, coxa valga, and bowing of the radius, tibia, and fibula.

DIAGNOSIS. The diagnosis of pseudohypoparathyroidism or pseudopseudohypoparathyroidism is likely when the described developmental abnormalities are discovered. When normal serum calcium and phosphorus are found in such a patient, the diagnosis of pseudopseudohypoparathyroidism is almost certain, although many of the same developmental abnormalities seen in pseudopseudohypoparathyroidism are present in unusual cases of Turner's, Gardner's, and the basal nevus syndromes. If hypocalcemia and hyperphosphatemia are found, the diagnosis of pseudohypoparathyroidism is highly likely. Increased serum iPTH and markedly diminished phosphaturic and nephrogenous cyclic AMP responses to parathyroid hormone distinguish pseudohypoparathyroidism from surgical, idiopathic, and functional hypoparathyroidism in patients with equivocal signs of the developmental abnormalities. If serum phosphorus is normal or low in such patients, secondary hyperparathyroidism resulting from vitamin D deficiency, dietary calcium deficiency, or intestinal malabsorption of calcium must be excluded. Measurement of serum 25OHD should help determine the presence of vitamin D deficiency, and dietary history or analysis, the presence of dietary calcium deficiency. The third underlying cause, intestinal malabsorption of calcium, may present difficulties because hypocalcemia per se may produce malabsorption (see above), and, unless magnesium deficiency is present, patients with intrinsic intestinal malabsorption usually have increased levels of serum iPTH. Therapeutic tests may be needed. When treatment of malabsorption with a gluten-free diet restores eucalcemia, the diagnosis is probably gluten-sensitive enteropathy (see Ch. 103). If correction of hypocalcemia with a regimen used in the treatment of hypoparathyroidism cures the malabsorption syndrome, the underlying diagnosis is probably pseudohypoparathyroidism.

Albright F, Burnett CH, Smith PH, Parson W: Pseudohypoparathyroidism—an example of "Seabright-Bantam syndrome." Endocrinology 30:922, 1942. *First description of pseudohypoparathyroidism.*

Chase LR, Melson GL, Aurbach GD: Pseudohypoparathyroidism: Defective excretion of 3'5'-AMP in response to parathyroid hormone. J Clin Invest 48:1832, 1969. *First demonstration of renal blockade of parathyroid hormone–stimulated cyclic AMP excretion in pseudohypoparathyroidism.*

Drezner MK, Burch WM: Altered activity of the nucleotide regulatory site in the parathyroid hormone-sensitive adenylate cyclase from the renal cortex of a patient with pseudohypoparathyroidism. J Clin Invest 62:1222, 1978. *Demonstration that the addition of GTP to renal cortical membranes from a patient with pseudohypoparathyroidism restores their sensitivity to parathyroid hormone stimultion of adenylate cyclase in vitro. These results suggest that the molecular defect in some patients with this disease may be an abnormality of the regulatory protein that couples parathyroid hormone to adenylate cyclase.*

Farfel Z, Brickman AS, Kaslow HR, Brothers VM, Bourne HR: Defect of receptor-cyclase coupling protein in pseudohypoparathyroidism. N Engl J Med 303:237, 1980. Levine MA, Downs RW Jr, Singer M, Marx SJ, Aurbach GD, Speigel AM: Deficient activity of guanine nucleotide regulatory protein in erythrocytes from patients with pseudohypoparathyroidism. Biochem Biophys Res Commun 94:1319, 1980. *The work described in these two papers was done simultaneously and independently by two different groups. The results are essentially the same: the activity of the guanyl nucleotide regulatory protein in the red blood cell membranes of some patients with pseudohypoparathyroidism was significantly reduced. Taken with the results of the study by Drezner and Burch (see above), they support the hypothesis that deficient activity of this protein is the molecular basis for hormone resistance in some patients with this inherited disorder.*

Potts JT Jr.: Pseudohypoparathyroidism. *In* DeGroot LJ (ed.): Endocrinology. Vol 2. New York, Grune & Stratton, 1979, pp 769–776. *Comprehensive review of pseudohypoparathyroidism.*

HYPERCALCEMIA AND ITS TREATMENT

Many diseases and conditions of nonparathyroid origin are associated with hypercalcemia (Table 246–1). Malignancy-associated hypercalcemia and familial hypocalciuric hypercalcemia are discussed extensively in relation to the differential diagnosis of primary hyperparathyroidism (see above), because these disorders frequently resemble primary hyperparathyroidism in their clinical presentation and biochemical characteristics. This section will describe the spectrum of disorders that can produce hypercalcemia by mechanisms unrelated to parathyroid hormone (these are listed in Table 246–1 under the category of hypercalcemia "not due to increased serum PTH"). This section will also discuss the medical treatment of hypercalcemia, whether of parathyroid or nonparathyroid origin.

Nonparathyroid Causes of Hypercalcemia

Malignancy

As discussed above, the underlying cause of hypercalcemia in patients with nonhematologic malignancies who exhibit the other common biochemical features of primary hyperparathyroidism (i.e., hypophosphatemia and increased nephrogenous cyclic AMP) is probably the secretion of a PTH-like substance by malignant tissue. The cancers that are most commonly associated with this syndrome are bronchogenic carcinoma and carcinoma of the kidney. Thus, although not strictly accurate, the term "ectopic hyperparathyroidism" has been used (as well as pseudohyperparathyroidism) to segregate these patients from those with malignancy-associated hypercalcemia who do not have hypophosphatemia and increased nephrogenous cyclic AMP. This segregation appears to be justified on therapeutic grounds because the hypercalcemia in patients with ectopic hyperparathyroidism rarely responds to corticosteroid administration, whereas the hypercalcemia in patients who do not have this syndrome frequently does respond.

Carcinoma of the breast accounts for approximately half of the malignancies associated with hypercalcemia. It is not associated with the biochemical features of ectopic hyperparathyroidism. The cause of the hypercalcemia in patients with breast cancer is uncertain. Many other solid tumors secrete substances that stimulate the cellular elements in bone to increase bone resorption. However, cultured breast cancer cells can increase the release of calcium from devitalized bone in vitro in a manner similar to osteoclasts. Thus, the direct interaction of tumor cells with bone (i.e., metastasis) may be required to produce hypercalcemia in patients with breast cancer.

Serum levels of phosphate are normal or slightly increased in hypercalcemic patients with breast cancer, and serum levels of iPTH (as measured by mid- or carboxyl-region assays) are low or undetectable. These biochemical findings usually exclude primary hyperparathyroidism as a cause of hypercalcemia, but they cannot differentiate between ectopic hyperparathyroidism and breast cancer associated with hypercalcemia. The measurement of nephrogenous cyclic AMP may be helpful in this regard. It is almost always increased in patients with the syndrome of ectopic hyperparathyroidism and normal or decreased in patients with breast cancer. The hypercalcemia of patients with breast cancer usually responds to corticosteroids.

The finding of increased serum levels of iPTH and hypophosphatemia in hypercalcemic patients with a history of successfully treated breast cancer or with active disease almost certainly reflects associated primary hyperparathyroidism. Successful treatment of the latter (see above) may completely resolve the hypercalcemia. Frankly increased levels of serum iPTH in hypercalcemic patients with nonhematologic malignancies other than breast cancer should be interpreted similarly. As described in Figure 246–9, serum iPTH (as measured by mid- or carboxyl-region assays) is either normal or slightly increased in most patients with the syndrome of ectopic hyperparathyroidism. Thus, values of serum iPTH that are greater than two times the upper limit of normal in such patients indicate the coexistence of malignancy and primary hyperparathyroidism.

Multiple myeloma is the most common of the hematologic malignancies causing hypercalcemia. Approximately 20 to 30 per cent of patients with this disease have increased calcium levels. As in breast cancer, serum phosphate is normal or slightly increased, and corticosteroid administration frequently resolves the hypercalcemia. Patients with multiple myeloma often present with vertebral compression fractures and can be mistakenly diagnosed as having idiopathic osteoporosis. Roentgenograms of the spine may not distinguish between these two diseases. Interestingly, radionuclide bone scans often do not identify the bony lesions of multiple myeloma; a "positive scan" is more consistent with metastatic malignancy. A definitive diagnosis of multiple myeloma can usually be made if immunoelectrophoresis of serum or urine protein shows immunoglobulin abnormalities or if bone marrow biopsies show increased plasma cells.

The underlying cause of the hypercalcemia in patients with multiple myeloma is probably increased osteoclastic osteolysis induced by the local elaboration by myeloma cells of a small, as yet uncharacterized, peptide, osteoclast-activating factor (OAF) (Fig. 163–2). However, in some patients with this disease, the hypercalcemia may not be due to osteolysis but to extensive binding of calcium by the high circulating concentrations of myeloma proteins, which results in an increase in the protein-bound, biologically inert fraction of the plasma calcium (Ch. 243).

Hypercalcemia is unusual in other hematologic or lymphoproliferative malignancies, but it can occur in acute lymphocytic leukemia and more rarely in Hodgkin's disease, lymphosarcoma, and reticulum cell sarcoma. Although it has not been proved, the cause of hypercalcemia in these conditions is thought to be osteolysis induced by osteoclast-activating factor (or a similar substance) that is elaborated by tumor deposits (accumulations of malignant cells) in bone. Such lesions are common in patients with acute leukemia (50 to 90 per cent), but the incidence of hypercalcemia is quite low (5 per cent), suggesting that leukemic cells only rarely develop the capacity to produce significant quantities of osteolytic substances. High serum levels of 1,25-dihydroxyvitamin D have been reported in three patients with non-Hodgkin's lymphoma and hypercalcemia; it was speculated that the increased 1,25 dihydroxyvitamin D was synthesized in the neoplastic tissue.

Drugs

Thiazide diuretics regularly cause small increases in the plasma levels of total and ionized calcium in normal subjects by increasing serum protein concentrations (hemoconcentration due to volume depletion) and increasing renal tubular reabsorption of calcium. The widespread use of these agents for hypertension and as diuretics has complicated the diagnosis of hypercalcemia. Two simple rules are valuable in the evaluation of such patients. First, thiazide diuretics rarely increase serum calcium levels above 11.0 mg per deciliter, and therefore patients with higher values probably have a hypercalcemic disorder that is not related to thiazide administration. Secondly, serum calcium should be restored to the normal range (8.9 to 10.1 mg per deciliter) in normal patients within three weeks of discontinuing thiazides. There is no evidence that the mild hypercalcemia caused by thiazide diuretics causes adverse effects.

Furosemide, a diuretic commonly used in the treatment of severe hypercalcemia (see below), has been reported to cause mild hypercalcemia when administered chronically. There is no explanation for this apparent paradox.

Vitamin D was once used in large doses (>50,000 units per day) to treat rheumatologic conditions; not surprisingly, vitamin D intoxication (see Ch. 244) and consequent hypercalcemia were common complications of that type of therapy. It is relatively rare now but should be considered in the differential diagnosis of hypercalcemia, particularly in those patients treated with large doses of vitamin D or its metabolites (e.g., for hypoparathyroidism and renal osteodystrophy) and in individuals who are prone to self-medication with large doses of vitamins and minerals. The hypercalcemia associated with vitamin D intoxication usually is accompanied by slight to moderate increases in serum phosphate unless there is some independent reason for phosphate depletion. As with other nonparathyroid disorders, this biochemical feature helps distinguish vitamin D intoxication from primary hyperparathyroidism, but the diagnosis can be confirmed by demonstrating decreased or undetectable serum levels of iPTH and serum levels of 25OHD that are greater than 300 ng per milliliter. Corticosteroids characteristically reverse the hypercalcemia of vitamin D intoxication, as they do the hypercalcemia of breast cancer and hematologic malignancies.

Vitamin A, when ingested in doses of 50,000 to 100,000 units daily (10 to 20 times the minimum daily requirement), may result in hypercalcemia and diffuse bone pain. It is presumed that increased bone resorption underlies these abnormalities, even though skeletal x-rays are generally normal. In some cases these films may show multiple calcifications of the periosteum along the shafts of the phalanges and metacarpals. The diagnosis is confirmed by demonstrating that serum vitamin A levels are two to three times higher than normal. Symptoms, skeletal lesions, and hypercalcemia resolve rapidly after discontinuation of the vitamin.

Lithium, used in doses typical for manic-depressive illness, can cause mild hypercalcemia, which resolves after the drug is discontinued. The mechanism by which lithium induces hypercalcemia is unclear, although increased serum iPTH levels have been demonstrated recently in patients taking this drug. Further investigation is needed to determine whether increased secretion of PTH plays an important role in the hypercalcemia associated with lithium treatment.

Milk-Alkali Syndrome (Burnett's Syndrome). Ingestion of antacids that contain large amounts of calcium (i.e., >5 grams per day) can produce hypercalcemia in susceptible individuals and should be suspected, particularly in neurotic or psychiatrically ill patients who may be medicating themselves surreptitiously. If excessive calcium intake and the resulting hypercalcemia continue for a long time, the kidney may be damaged and renal failure may occur. This course of events was more frequent many years ago when the treatment of peptic ulcer included the use of large quantities of calcium in the form of milk or calcium carbonate and soluble alkali.

Granulomatous Diseases

Hypercalcemia occurs in 10 to 20 per cent of patients with *sarcoidosis* but is rare in other granulomatous diseases. When hypercalcemia is present, serum levels of phosphate and alkaline phosphatase are generally increased and hypercalciuria is common. Other manifestations of the sarcoidosis, such as hilar lymphadenopathy, enlarged liver or spleen, peripheral lymphadenopathy, skin lesions, and hyperglobulinemia, are usually present. An increased serum level of angiotensin-converting enzyme in a hypercalcemic patient is highly suggestive of sarcoidosis (see Ch. 67), and the demonstration of noncaseating granulomatous lesions in a biopsied lymph node (e.g., the scalene) is confirmatory.

The presence of low serum levels of phosphate and increased serum levels of PTH in a hypercalcemic patient with sarcoidosis indicates primary hyperparathyroidism. Diagnosis may be difficult in such patients when sarcoidosis involves the kidneys and compromises renal function.

Patients with sarcoidosis are very sensitive to the hypercalcemic effects of vitamin D. They have an increased ability to convert vitamin D to its biologically active form, $1,25(OH)_2D$. The site of this increased conversion may be the abnormal granulomatous tissue that these patients harbor. This tissue appears capable of hydroxylating 25OHD to form a compound that has chromatographic properties similar to those of $1,25(OH)_2D$. Although proof is lacking at present, it is presumed that the mechanism underlying the hypercalcemia in other granulomatous diseases is similar to that responsible for the hypercalcemia in sarcoidosis. Treatment with corticosteroids lowers serum calcium levels in hypercalcemic patients with sarcoidosis in the same way as in vitamin D intoxication.

Nonparathyroid Endocrine Diseases

Hyperthyroidism frequently (in 20 per cent of patients) causes mild hypercalcemia, which resolves soon after treatment for the hyperthyroidism is instituted. The hypercalcemia is accompanied by normal or slightly increased concentrations of serum phosphate, decreased concentrations of serum iPTH, and increased excretion of hydroxyproline. As might be expected, bone biopsies from patients with hyperthyroidism are hypercellular and show increases in both formation and resorption surfaces of bone. It is presumed that the hypercalcemia in these patients is due to the uncoupling of bone formation and resorption so that resorption predominates. Serum levels of calcium above 11.5 mg per deciliter are rare in patients with hyperthyroidism; when they occur, they suggest the presence of another hypercalcemic disorder.

Acute adrenal insufficiency may be associated with hypercalcemia. Although the mechanism is poorly understood, increases in serum protein concentrations associated with severe hemoconcentration may be involved. Glucocorticoid replacement restores serum calcium concentrations to normal.

Familial Hypocalciuric Hypercalcemia

(See above, p. 1438.)

Immobilization

Immobilization of patients in body casts or by quadraplegia frequently causes hypercalcemia as a result of increased dissolution of bone. Hypercalcemia is generally mild in adults but can be severe in children (e.g., >15.0 mg per deciliter). This difference in severity is probably due to the higher turnover rate of bone in children. The mechanism responsible for enhanced dissolution of bone in immobilized patients is unclear, but available evidence from histomorphometric examination of bone biopsies from these patients suggests that bone formation surfaces are decreased and bone resorption surfaces are increased. The hypercalcemia associated with immobilization usually resolves rapidly when patients can bear weight with their lower extremities (as little as one or more hours per day). Treatment of hypercalcemia in adults is rarely needed because it is mild. However, the severe hypercalcemia seen in immobilized children requires prompt treatment using the measures detailed below (i.e., increased fluids, sodium chloride, phosphate, and possibly calcitonin).

Idiopathic Hypercalcemia of Infancy

Idiopathic hypercalcemia of infancy is rare. It is associated with several congenital cardiovascular and facial defects. Hypersensitivity to vitamin D is suspected as the cause of the hypercalcemia because corticosteroids can lower the serum calcium concentrations in these patients. Moreover, there may be increased conversion of vitamin D to $1,25(OH)_2D$ in affected infants.

Neonatal primary hyperparathyroidism, also a rare disease, is easily confused with idiopathic hypercalcemia of infancy. The treatments for these two diseases are different and depend completely upon the correct diagnosis. Measurement of serum iPTH is key in this latter regard; levels are increased in primary hyperparathyroidism and decreased or undetectable in idiopathic hypercalcemia.

Renal Failure and Renal Transplantation

Hypercalcemia may occur during the development of severe secondary hyperparathyroidism caused by chronic renal failure or after renal transplantation. The pathogenesis and treatment of the hypercalcemia associated with these conditions is described in Ch. 248. Hypercalcemia is a frequent complication of acute renal failure, but its cause is poorly understood. It is usually managed successfully by hemodialysis with dialysis baths that contain low concentrations of calcium.

Medical Treatment of Hypercalcemia

Acute Severe Hypercalcemia

The medical treatment of acute severe hypercalcemia (>13.0 mg per deciliter) should be started immediately, because the condition is life-threatening. Serum levels of calcium, magnesium, sodium, and potassium must be monitored every two to four hours. If possible, patients should remain ambulatory, since immobilization may increase serum calcium in some patients. In patients with heart disease who are in danger of developing heart failure due to volume overload from fluid administration, central venous pressure should be monitored so that appropriate measures can be taken if the pressure increases.

The diagnostic approach to determining the underlying cause of hypercalcemia outlined here should be instituted early so that the cause of hypercalcemia can be specifically identified and treated.

In addition to these measures, dietary calcium should be restricted, and all drugs that might cause hypercalcemia (e.g., thiazides or vitamin D) discontinued. If the patient is taking digitalis, it may be wise to reduce the dose because the hypercalcemic patient may be more sensitive to the toxic effects of this drug. Ideally, the patient should be admitted to an intensive care unit for electrocardiographic monitoring while antihypercalcemic measures are instituted. Beta-adrenergic blockade is useful in protecting the heart against the adverse effects of severe hypercalcemia, especially serious arrhythmias.

The mainstay of therapy is a regimen of hydration, initially with normal saline, plus forced diuresis using furosemide or ethacrynic acid. The objective is to increase the urinary excretion of calcium rapidly, thus decreasing the exchangeable calcium pool and the serum calcium concentration. Saline is given to increase sodium excretion because sodium clearance parallels calcium clearance during water or osmotic diuresis. Furosemide and ethacrynic acid inhibit the tubular reabsorption of calcium and aid in maintaining diuresis. Approximately 4 to 6 liters of isotonic saline (sometimes as much as 12 liters are needed) should be given intravenously each day, along with 20 to 100 mg of furosemide or 10 to 40 mg of ethacrynic acid every 1 to 2 hours (intravenously or orally). Such a regimen usually increases urinary calcium excretion to 500 to 1000 mg per day and lowers serum calcium by 2 to 6 mg per deciliter after 24 to 48 hours. Potassium and magnesium depletion are complications of therapy, and appropriate replacement should be instituted early.

After serum calcium has decreased to a reasonably safe level (<13 mg per deciliter), a chronic regimen may be instituted. At the minimum, this should consist of a daily oral regimen of 40 to 160 mg of furosemide or 50 to 200 mg of ethacrynic acid, 400 to 600 mEq of sodium chloride (in tablet form), and 3 liters of fluid. Serum calcium, magnesium, and potassium should be monitored daily at first, and then weekly when serum calcium has stabilized. Magnesium and potassium should be replaced as necessary. Patient compliance with this regimen can be monitored by measuring 24 hour urinary excretion of sodium (which should exceed 300 mEq per day) and 24 hour urinary volume (minimum required is 2500 ml per day).

Chronic Treatment of Moderately Severe Hypercalcemia

Whereas the acute treatment of severe hypercalcemia (>13.0 mg per deciliter) is nonspecific and relatively straightforward, requiring primarily hydration and saline diuresis (see below), the chronic treatment of moderately severe hypercalcemia (<13.0 mg per deciliter) requires knowledge of the underlying disease and involves trial and error in formulating an effective drug regimen. The problem is less difficult in diseases of nonparathyroid origin because treatment of the underlying disease (e.g., hyperthyroidism), discontinuation of drugs (e.g., thiazide diuretics), or treatment with corticosteroids (e.g., 300 mg of cortisone or 60 mg of prednisone given daily in divided doses for sarcoidosis, multiple myeloma, or vitamin D intoxication) usually results in satisfactory resolution of hypercalcemia. However, the medical treatment of hypercalcemia in those diseases associated with excess circulating levels of PTH or PTH-like substances is considerably more difficult. The drugs that are available may not be completely effective and may have serious side effects.

All patients with moderately severe hypercalcemia should maintain a high fluid intake (3 to 5 liters per day) and, unless contraindicated because of associated diseases, a sodium chloride intake of at least 300 to 400 mEq per day. These measures increase the renal excretion of calcium while maintaining the concentration of urinary calcium below that conducive to renal stone formation. Periodic measurements of serum electrolytes should be made because this regimen can cause magnesium and potassium depletion. These ions should be replaced if their serum concentrations decrease. Except in patients with breast cancer, in whom the administration of estrogens or androgens may induce hypercalcemia for unknown reasons, hypercalcemic postmenopausal women with either primary hyperparathyroidism or the syndrome of ectopic hyperparathyroidism should be given cyclic estrogen-progestin therapy (as described in Ch. 249). Estrogens suppress bone resorption and have been used successfully in the long-term management of mild hypercalcemia in women with primary hyperparathyroidism.

If hypercalcemia is not controlled (10.0 to 11.0 mg per deciliter) using these simple measures, other agents may be tried. Oral phosphate, either as neutral or potassium phosphate, may be given in doses as high as 2 to 4 grams of elemental phosphorus per day. Initial doses should be relatively low (1 to 2 grams per day in divided doses every 6 hours) because gastrointestinal side effects (e.g., nausea and diarrhea) may occur; these should disappear, however, with time. During treatment with phosphate, serum levels of calcium, phosphate, and creatinine should be monitored to determine whether the serum calcium level has decreased and whether hyperphosphatemia or impaired renal function has developed. Increases in serum phosphorus above 5 mg per deciliter should be avoided because extraskeletal calcifications (e.g., in the kidney) may be induced. Phosphate should be discontinued if the serum creatinine level increases significantly.

If phosphate therapy fails, the only effective approach to the treatment of hypercalcemia is to use mithramycin. This cytotoxic antibiotic has been used to treat testicular tumors but also ameliorates hypercalcemia by dramatically inhibiting bone resorption, presumably by killing osteoclasts. However, the drug is associated with renal and hepatic toxicity, thrombocytopenia, nausea, vomiting, stomatitis, and facial swelling. Therefore, it is usually reserved for hypercalcemic patients with malignancy. The intravenous administration of 15 to 25 μg of mithramycin per kilogram of body weight generally restores serum calcium to nearly normal levels within a few days. The duration of this effect varies, but it can last as long as a month. When hypercalcemia recurs, mithramycin can be administered again, provided that thrombocytopenia has not occurred and renal and hepatic function have not been impaired. Lower doses (10 to 15 μg per kilogram of body weight) can be tried, with the expectation that there will be fewer side effects. In general, the toxic effects of mithramycin can be reversed by discontinuing the drug.

The treatment of hypercalcemia with calcitonin, although rational, has been disappointing, and there is no convincing evidence that it is effective in the chronic management of hypercalcemia in these patients.

Indomethacin, given orally in doses of 25 mg every 6 hours, may be tried, but it is rarely effective. The rationale for its use is that the hypercalcemia may be due to increased bone resorption caused by excess prostaglandin released by the cancer.

Bilezikian JP: Hypercalcemia. *In* Krieger DT, Bardin CW: Current Therapy in Endocrinology 1983–1984. Philadelphia and St. Louis, B. C. Decker, Inc., and C. V. Mosby Company, 1983, pp 272–277. *Brief but incisive review of the treatment of hypercalcemia.*

Rodman JS, Sherwood LM: Disorders of mineral metabolism in malignancy. *In* Avioli LV, Krane SM (eds.): Metabolic Bone Disease. Vol 2. New York, Academic Press, 1978, pp 577–631. *A systematic assessment of the diagnosis, etiology, and management of patients with malignancy-associated hypercalcemia.*

Suki WN, Yium JJ, Von Minden M, Saller-Herbert C, Eknoyan G, Martinez-Maldonado M: Acute treatment of hypercalcemia with furosemide. N Engl J Med 283:836,1970. *Classic paper outlining the acute treatment of hypercalcemia.*

Symposium on the etiology and medical management of hypercalcemia. Metab Bone Dis 2:143,1980. *A series of review articles describing recent advances in understanding the causes and medical treatment of hypercalcemia.*

247. THE ULTIMOBRANCHIAL CELLS AND CALCITONIN

Claude D. Arnaud

INTRODUCTION. The ultimobranchial cells develop from neural crest tissue in the ultimobranchial cleft during embryonic life. They form a discrete organ in submammalian vertebrates called the ultimobranchial gland. In the mammal, the anlage of the cells merges with the embryonic thyroid gland, ultimately becoming dispersed in the central region of each lobe (of the thyroid gland), adjacent to the follicular cells.

Calcitonin, a 32 amino acid, 3700 molecular weight polypeptide with a 1-7 disulfide bridge, is biosynthesized and secreted by the ultimobranchial (parafollicular or "C") cells. It is synthesized as a large molecular weight precursor.

Calcitonin is rapidly released by the "C" cells in response to small increases in plasma ionic calcium. It acts on kidney and bone to restore the level of this cation to just below a normal set point, which in turn inhibits the secretion of the hormone. Calcitonin is a physiologic antagonist to parathyroid hormone, and these agents presumably act in concert to maintain the normal concentration of ionic calcium in the extracellular fluid. These relationships are illustrated in Figure 243–1.

The actual importance of calcitonin in the calcium homeostasis of adult humans is not established. An excess or deficiency of parathyroid hormone or vitamin D produces dramatic clinical disorders. In contrast, an excess (medullary carcinoma of the thyroid) or deficiency (post-thyroidectomy) of calcitonin produces few discernible and no serious abnormalities in mineral metabolism. The basal plasma levels of calcitonin and its responsiveness to induced hypercalcemia or pentagastrin injection are lower in women than in men and decrease with age. In adult humans, calcitonin may function primarily to restrain the bone resorptive effects of parathyroid hormone. If so, the long-term combination of a progressive decrease in calcitonin secretion and reserve and an increase in parathyroid hormone secretion may contribute to the osteoporosis of aging.

Calcitonin exists in multiple molecular forms in ultimobranchial tissue and plasma. In contrast to parathyroid hormone, however, the major circulating species are not hormone fragments but immunoreactive forms with molecular weights larger than 32 amino acid calcitonin. It is likely that some of these forms represent polymers of calcitonin with disulfide molecular links. The different antisera used in radioimmunoassays recognize these forms differently, and therefore the normal range for plasma calcitonin must be established for each assay. The concentrations of calcitonin are extremely low (<100 pg per milliliter). Induced hypercalcemia and pentagastrin injection cause an increase in plasma calcitonin in approximately 40 to 50 per cent of normal women and 70 to 80 per cent of normal men. However, it is unlikely that gastrin is a physiologic calcitonin secretagogue. Other calcitonin secretagogues of unproved physiologic significance include glucagon, β-adrenergic agonists, and alcohol.

When bone turnover rates are high, calcitonin administration produces rapid and profound hypocalcemia and hypophosphatemia. This is largely due to the fact that the hormone decreases bone resorption. Calcitonin also increases urinary excretion of calcium and phosphate, but its action on the kidney is transient and variable. Calcitonin stimulates adenylate cyclase in bone and kidney, but whether cyclic AMP is the major intracellular mediator of calcitonin action has not been established. It is also unclear whether calcitonin influences intestinal calcium absorption.

HYPOCALCITONINEMIA

No clinical condition has been reported to date in which hypocalcitoninemia plays a definitive role, except possibly the osteoporosis of aging (see above).

MEDULLARY CARCINOMA

DEFINITION. Medullary carcinoma, a malignancy of the parafollicular cells of the thyroid gland, is the only recognized disorder in which calcitonin is inappropriately secreted in excess. It occurs sporadically but also may be inherited as an autosomal dominant trait as part of the multiple endocrine neoplasia (MEN) syndromes, Types II and III. These syndromes include medullary carcinoma of the thyroid gland and pheochromocytoma. Patients with MEN II have a normal appearance but a high incidence of hyperparathyroidism, most frequently resulting from enlargement of multiple parathyroid glands. Patients with MEN III have a striking appearance owing to ganglioneuromas of the labia and mucosae, a marfanoid habitus, and other somatic abnormalities. Hyperparathyroidism is unusual.

INCIDENCE. Medullary carcinoma constitutes between 3.5 and 10 per cent of all thyroid malignancies. The incidence in males and females is almost equal, there being a male-to-female ratio of 1.3:1 in sporadic cases and 1:1 in familial cases. In general, familial cases present at a younger age than do sporadic cases.

PATHOLOGY. Medullary carcinoma manifests as a solid, often hard mass confined to but not encapsulated in the substance of the thyroid gland. In sporadic cases, it is often unilateral, but in familial cases it is frequently bilateral. It is composed of sheets of cells with granular cytoplasms, and usually contains irregular masses of amyloid and fibrous tissue. Most patients who present with a thyroid mass have metastases to cervical lymph nodes. Some lesions spread to the upper mediastinum. Spread beyond the mediastinum, usually delayed until late in the natural history of the disease, is most commonly to lungs, liver, bones, and the adrenal glands.

PATHOPHYSIOLOGY. Medullary carcinomas secrete large quantities of calcitonin and respond to provocative stimuli such as increased serum calcium or intravenous pentagastrin. Although calcitonin produces hypocalcemia and hypophosphatemia in experimental animals, these biochemical findings are unusual in patients with medullary carcinoma in spite of extremely high levels of immunoreactive calcitonin. This paradox is probably due to a combination of factors, including homologous desensitization of tissues that normally respond to calcitonin.

Medullary carcinoma may secrete many other bioactive substances in addition to calcitonin, each with the potential of causing clinical symptoms. These substances include biogenic amines, ACTH and corticotropin-releasing hormone, prostaglandins, nerve growth factor, and possibly a prolactin-releasing hormone. Diarrhea is present in 20 per cent of patients. It relents after surgical excision of the tumor and is therefore thought to be humorally mediated. Cushing's syndrome is present in about 5 per cent of cases and is secondary to secretion of excessive ACTH.

CLINICAL MANIFESTATIONS AND DETECTION. The majority of patients with sporadic medullary carcinoma present with an asymptomatic thyroid mass. Patients with MEN III may complain of the neuromas they harbor and their marfanoid habitus. Hypercalcemia may be detected on routine blood screening in patients with MEN II and primary hyperparathyroidism. Most important, hypertension in patients with MEN II and III may lead to the diagnosis of pheochromocytoma, which is more life threatening than is medullary carcinoma.

Paraneoplastic syndromes, such as Cushing's syndrome or intractable diarrhea, should alert the physician to the possible existence of medullary carcinoma. Certainly, a history of more than one family member with thyroid cancer should raise suspicion in a patient with bizarre symptoms.

Other neural manifestations in MEN III include medullated nerves on slit lamp examination of the eye and ganglioneuromas of the gastrointestinal tract. The latter can cause gastrointestinal obstruction as well as megacolon.

Medullary cancers occasionally calcify. The discovery of a calcified thyroidal mass does not indicate that it is benign; rather, it is probably an indication for the measurement of serum immunoreactive calcitonin (see below).

DIAGNOSIS. The cornerstone for the investigation of patients suspected of having medullary carcinoma is the radioimmunoassay of calcitonin in plasma. Although not specific for this tumor, increased levels of immunoreactive calcitonin in patients with a thyroid mass, pheochromocytoma, or a family history of medullary carcinoma virtually assure the diagnosis. Serum immunoreactive calcitonin may be increased in many other conditions, however, including other malignancies that secrete calcitonin ectopically (especially small cell carcinoma of the lung), chronic renal failure, gastrointestinal disorders such as tumors of the pancreas and pernicious anemia, subacute Hashimoto's thyroiditis, and pregnancy. These conditions should be considered in the interpretation of a high value.

The diagnostic power of the calcitonin radioimmunoassay is greatly enhanced when combined with provocative tests. For example, as many as 30 per cent of members of a family with MEN II who actually harbor small medullary carcinomas will have normal unstimulated plasma levels of immunoreactive calcitonin. They can only be detected by intravenous administration of 0.5 μg of pentagastrin* per kilogram of body weight over five to ten seconds, or 150 mg of calcium chloride over ten minutes. Plasma levels of immunoreactive calcitonin increase abnormally in the majority of these patients, thus establishing the diagnosis; surgery can then be performed before metastatic spread occurs. The calcitonin radioimmunoassay should be able to measure normal plasma levels of immunoreactive calcitonin (males, <100 pg per milliliter; females, <70 pg per milliliter). Without such sensitivity it is unlikely that the assay will be able to detect relatively small increases above the stimulated normal range, thus making the test impossible to interpret.

To rule out familial medullary carcinoma, immunoreactive calcitonin should be measured during a provocative test in all primary relatives of all patients with medullary carcinoma, regardless of family history. In a few affected patients with minimal parafollicular cell disease, false-negative results will be obtained with any of the tests outlined. Provocative testing should therefore be performed yearly in primary relatives with previous negative tests, since approximately 50 per cent of the members of a given family with MEN II should eventually develop medullary cancer. Its timely detection will permit definitive surgical treatment.

TREATMENT. After exclusion or treatment of pheochromocytoma, total thyroidectomy is mandatory. This is especially true in patients with MEN II because medullary carcinoma is almost always bilateral and polycentric. Lymph nodes in the midline compartment should be removed and those in both internal jugular chains sampled. If jugular lymph nodes are involved, a modified neck dissection should be performed. Postoperatively, all patients should be studied with a provocative test(s) to determine if residual tumor is present and should be given thyroid hormone replacement. The overall prevalence of residual medullary cancer after such surgery is about 35 per cent. The majority of these patients are older and have had regional metastases at surgery. Long-term follow-up with provocative tests every year is advised for all patients. Although it is usually difficult to determine the location of metastases responsible for a positive result in a provocative test, local recurrences are likely and can be dealt with surgically. There is no known effective chemotherapeutic, isotopic, or radiologic treatment for medullary carcinoma.

PROGNOSIS. Patients with sporadic medullary carcinoma have the least favorable prognosis. Metastases are usually present, and only 46 per cent of these patients survive for ten years. Patients with MEN II appear to fare better, with few having been recorded as dying from their disease. Conversely, in the Mayo Clinic series of patients with MEN III, 67 per cent have had residual disease after surgery, and 18 per cent have died of medullary cancer. The reasons for the apparent difference in the prognosis of MEN II and MEN III are unknown.

*This use is not listed in the manufacturer's directive.

THERAPEUTIC USE OF CALCITONIN

Calcitonin is used to treat Paget's disease of bone and hypercalcemia of all causes (see Ch. 250). The preparation most frequently employed is synthetic salmon calcitonin because this species is about 30 times more potent in lowering serum calcium than are mammalian calcitonins (porcine, human). The rationale for its use in both Paget's disease and hypercalcemia is its inhibitory effect on bone resorption. In unusual cases, high titers of circulating antibodies are formed against salmon calcitonin. These antibodies may block the action of the hormone and its beneficial effects. In such cases, synthetic human calcitonin may be successfully substituted, but this species of the hormone is not readily available commercially at present.

Austin L, Heath H III: Calcitonin: Physiology and pathophysiology. N Engl J Med 304:269, 1981. *Lively review of recent advances in calcitonin research in health and disease.*

Gagel RF, Melvin KEW, Tashjian AH Jr, Miller HH, Feldman ZT, Wolfe HJ, DeLellis RA, Cervi-Skinner S, Reichlin S: Natural history of the familial medullary thyroid carcinoma–pheochromocytoma syndrome and the identification of preneoplastic stages by screening studies: A five-year report. Trans Assoc Am Physicians 88:177, 1975. *The first description of the diagnostic power of the calcitonin radioimmunoassay in the diagnosis of familial medullary carcinoma.*

Sizemore GW, Carney JA, Heath H III: Epidemiology of medullary carcinoma of the thyroid gland: A five year experience (1971–1976). Surg Clin North Am 57:633, 1977. *Describes this group's extensive experience with both the familial and sporadic forms of medullary carcinoma of the thyroid gland.*

Williams ED: Medullary carcinoma of the thyroid. *In* DeGroot LJ (ed.): Endocrinology. Vol 2. New York, Grune & Stratton, 1979, pp 777–792. *Comprehensive review of medullary cancer of the thyroid gland.*

248. RENAL OSTEODYSTROPHY

Eduardo Slatopolsky

Renal osteodystrophy is a generic term that describes the complex lesions of bone that are present in the majority of patients with advanced renal failure. The main components of renal osteodystrophy are osteitis fibrosa and osteomalacia. A lesser role is played by osteosclerosis and osteoporosis. Osteitis fibrosa, a consequence of increased parathyroid hormone activity, is characterized by an increase in the number of osteoclasts, an increase in bone resorption, and marrow fibrosis. Osteomalacia, a condition secondary in part to alterations in vitamin D metabolism, is characterized by a decreased mineralization rate of osteoid tissue shown histologically by an abnormal calcification front in bone. Osteosclerosis is caused by localized areas of mineralized woven bone, which appears as increased bone density on radiographic studies. Osteoporosis is defined as a decrease in the mass of normally mineralized bone and represents only an infrequent and minor component of renal osteodystrophy.

OSTEITIS FIBROSA (also see Chapter 246)

Secondary hyperparathyroidism is a universal complication of chronic renal disease. Chief cell hyperplasia of the parathyroid glands and high levels of immunoreactive parathyroid hormone (i-PTH) are among the earliest findings affecting mineral metabolism in patients with chronic renal failure. The factors that contribute to the development of secondary hyperparathyroidism in renal insufficiency include (1) phosphate retention, (2) altered vitamin D metabolism, (3) skeletal resistance to the calcemic action of PTH, (4) impaired degradation of parathyroid hormone, and (5) altered feedback regulation between ionized calcium and the secretion of PTH.

PHOSPHATE RETENTION. Considerable evidence supports an important role of phosphate retention in producing secondary hyperparathyroidism. Long-term feeding of a diet high in phosphate to animals with normal renal function can produce secondary hyperparathyroidism. Conversely, restriction of dietary phosphate can prevent the development of secondary hyperparathyroidism in chronic renal failure. The effect of phosphate retention is mediated via lowering ionized calcium concentration. This effect probably is caused by a combination of factors, such as complexing ionized calcium, decreasing the production of 1,25-dihydroxycholecalciferol ($1,25(OH)_2D_3$), the active metabolite of vitamin D, and decreasing bone calcium mobilization from the skeleton. In patients with far advanced renal failure (glomerular filtration rate [GFR] less than 20 ml per minute), correction of hyperphosphatemia alone does not completely reverse secondary hyperparathyroidism, since many other factors also contribute to the increased PTH levels in blood.

ALTERATIONS IN VITAMIN D METABOLISM (see Ch. 244). Renal osteodystrophy may arise in part because of defective renal production of the active form of vitamin D in advanced renal failure. The liver hydroxylates vitamin D_3 to 25-hydroxycholecalciferol ($25(OH)D_3$), the predominant form of vitamin D_3 present in plasma. $25(OH)D_3$ is further hydroxylated to $1,25(OH)_2D_3$ by the enzyme 25-hydroxycholecalciferol-1α-hydroxylase, which is localized in the mitochondrial fraction of the proximal tubular cells (Fig. 244–1). Parathyroid hormone and low-phosphate diets play a key role in the stimulation of 1α-hydroxylase. On the other hand, lack of parathyroid hormone or hyperphosphatemia decreases the activity of 1α-hydroxylase. The evidence that alterated vitamin D metabolism contributes to abnormal calcium metabolism in advanced renal failure is considerable. Metabolic balance studies and radioisotopic techniques have shown reduced intestinal absorption of calcium in patients with far advanced renal insufficiency. Low levels of $1,25(OH)_2D_3$ in serum and calcium malabsorption are usually present in patients with a GFR of less than 40 per minute.

SKELETAL RESISTANCE TO THE ACTION OF PARATHYROID HORMONE. Skeletal resistance to the calcemic action of PTH may also play a role in the development of hypocalcemia seen in patients with renal insufficiency. Higher circulating levels of PTH may be needed for the maintenance of a normal plasma calcium in patients with renal failure.

IMPAIRED DEGRADATION OF PTH SECONDARY TO REDUCED RENAL FUNCTION. The liver and the kidney play key roles in the metabolism of parathyroid hormone. The uptake of i-PTH by the liver is selective for the intact hormone. The liver does not remove either amino terminal or carboxy terminal PTH fragments from the circulation. The kidney, on the other hand, removes both intact PTH and amino and carboxy terminal fragments from the circulation. Thus, in patients with chronic renal insufficiency, the high levels of circulating i-PTH result in part from increased PTH secretion, caused by chief cell hyperplasia, and in part from a decreased catabolism secondary to a decreased number of nephrons and decreased hepatic metabolism of intact PTH.

ALTERED FEEDBACK REGULATION BETWEEN IONIZED CALCIUM AND THE SECRETION OF PARATHYROID HORMONE. The control of the secretion of PTH by ionized calcium levels in plasma may be blunted in patients with chronic renal insufficiency. Hyperplastic parathyroid glands display less sensitivity to calcium than do normal tissues. This suggests that the mechanism for increased PTH levels may be caused by a shift in the set-point for calcium as well as the increased tissue mass. The set-point is defined as the amount of calcium necessary to suppress the secretion of parathyroid hormone by 50 per cent. Thus, a normal concentration of plasma calcium may not be sufficient to suppress hyperplastic glands, and plasma calcium may have to be increased to or even above the upper limits of normal to control the release of PTH in patients with secondary hyperparathyroidism.

OSTEOMALACIA (see Ch. 245)

Osteomalacia is defined as an increase in the osteoid seam width accompanied by a decrease in the mineralization front. The presence of excess osteoid per se does not necessarily indicate osteomalacia. An increase in osteoid tissue may be secondary to abnormalities in mineralization (osteomalacia) or caused by an increased rate of bone collagen synthesis, which is normally mineralized. The use of double tetracycline labelling of the calcification front in vivo can differentiate between these two possibilities. Therefore, the use of this technique and quantitative bone histology are critical for the diagnosis of osteomalacia. The mechanisms whereby altered vitamin D metabolism leads to impaired mineralization of bone are poorly understood. Whether vitamin D or $1,25(OH)_2D_3$ can directly stimulate bone mineralization or whether they lead to mineralization by increasing the levels of calcium and phosphate in the extracellular fluid surrounding bone remains a matter of controversy. Although the plasma levels of $1,25(OH)_2D_3$ are reduced in patients with far-advanced renal insufficiency, overt osteomalacia is found in only a small fraction of patients with end-stage uremia and may be absent even in anephric patients. Thus other factors, such as the plasma level of phosphorus, could also participate in the pathogenesis of osteomalacia in uremic patients. Hypophosphatemia per se can produce severe osteomalacia even in patients with normal renal function. Additional factors include alterations in collagen synthesis and maturation, defective bone crystal maturation, increased bone magnesium, elevated levels of pyrophosphate, and diminished calcium carbonate. The combination of these factors may play a role in the maturation of the bone and potentially contribute to the development of osteomalacia. Acidosis also contributes to the skeletal disease. In chronic renal insufficiency the skeleton plays an important role in buffering the hydrogen entering the body. Administration of bicarbonate and correction of the acidosis in azotemic patients can reduce fecal calcium excretion.

There is another type of osteomalacia that usually does not respond to any metabolite of vitamin D. Patients with this type of osteomalacia have pathologic fractures and complain of severe bone pain, and characteristically they have low levels of parathyroid hormone. When biopsies have been performed in these patients and the tissue stained appropriately, deposition of aluminum in the interface between the osteoid tissue and the calcification front has been found. Aluminum has a toxic effect on the osteoblast. The source of the aluminum may be a high aluminum content in the water or the ingestion of phosphate-binders containing aluminum or both. Finally, the lack of parathyroid hormone in patients who have had total parathyroidectomy leads to low bone turnover and rarely may precipitate the development of osteomalacia.

CLINICAL MANIFESTATIONS

Most of the symptoms related to renal osteodystrophy appear only when renal failure is advanced. On the other hand, certain biochemical alterations may appear early in the course of renal insufficiency. Knowledge of the presence of these alterations may help the physician to introduce treatment early in the course of renal failure and aid in the prevention of severe complications in bone and mineral metabolism.

Bone pain can develop and progress slowly to a point at which the patient becomes bedridden. Moreover, this can occur whether the skeletal pathology is osteitis fibrosa or osteomalacia. The bone pain is generally vague and commonly located in the lower back, hips, knees, and legs. Low-back pain may arise from the collapse of the vertebral body, and sharp chest pain may indicate spontaneous rib fracture. Physical findings are frequently lacking.

Muscular weakness when present is usually proximal, appears slowly, and progresses with time. Plasma levels of the muscle enzymes, creatinine phosphokinase and transaminase, are usually normal, and the electron micrographic changes are nonspecific. The pathogenesis of such muscular weakness is uncertain. In patients with myopathy, electron micrography has revealed localized disorganization of the myofibrils and dispersion of the Z-band material, which reverts to normal following treatment with $25(OH)D_3$.

Pruritus due to calcium deposition in skin is a common symptom in uremic patients, particularly with severe secondary hyperparathyroidism. Peripheral ischemic necrosis and vascular calcification also have been reported in these patients. The lesions may involve the tips of the toes and fingers, and the skin becomes violaceous. Ulcerations and scar formation may occur with clear demarcation of the lesions from the surrounding skin.

Calcific periarthritis, which is associated with acute pain and swelling around one or more joints, may be caused by deposition of hydroxy apatite crystals and is accompanied by marked hyperphosphatemia. *Skeletal deformities* are common in azotemic children who are growing. Bowing of the tibia and femur and deformities from slipped epiphyses are not uncommon. Children with renal rickets sometimes exhibit typical radiographic findings of viamin D deficiency. In adults with renal failure, particularly those with osteomalacia, marked skeletal deformities with lumbar scoliosis, thoracic kyphosis, and deformity of the thoracic cage may be observed. *Growth retardation* is usually seen in young children before and during maintenance hemodialysis.

BIOCHEMICAL FEATURES

One of the early changes in patients with renal insufficiency (GFR 60 to 80 ml per minute) is the presence of elevated levels of circulating i-PTH. As the disease progresses (GFR less than 40 ml per minute), hypocalcemia and low levels of $1,25(OH)_2D_3$ are present in these patients. In patients with advanced renal insufficiency the serum calcium may remain close to normal and values below 7.5 mg per deciliter are infrequent. Usually hypocalcemia is more marked in those patients who have severe osteomalacia and in those with profound metabolic acidosis. Occasionally, hypercalcemia may be observed in uremic patients, particularly those undergoing long-term dialysis. This can arise from severe hyperparathyroidism, from the ingestion of large amounts of calcium and vitamin D, from unrelated diseases such as sarcoidosis or malignancies, or from a "pure" mineralizing defect. This has been described in patients who have osteomalacia secondary to aluminum retention.

Hyperphosphatemia is usually common in patients with a GFR of less than 25 ml per minute. The degree of hyperphosphatemia depends on the amount of phosphate ingested in the diet, the fraction absorbed in the intestine, and the amount excreted in the urine. Obviously, if the patient ingests phosphate binders, the serum phosphate level may remain normal despite advanced renal insufficiency. Patients with severe hyperparathyroidism and advanced renal insufficiency usually have higher concentrations of serum phosphate in plasma.

Hypermagnesemia occurs in patients when renal insufficiency is very advanced, usually with a GFR of less than 15 ml per minute. The increase in serum magnesium levels is usually associated with an increased content of magnesium in bone, a factor that may affect crystal formation.

Total serum alkaline phosphatase levels are commonly higher in uremic patients with osteitis fibrosa than in those with osteomalacia. Coexistent liver disease should be excluded as a cause of elevated alkaline phosphatase levels.

RADIOGRAPHIC FEATURES

The main radiographic feature of secondary hyperparathyroidism is *osteitis fibrosa,* manifested as an increase in bone resorption, more commonly seen on the subperiosteal surfaces of bone (Fig. 246–6). Erosions that occur in conjunction with formation of new bone may appear as cysts or osteoclastomas (brown tumors). The presence of subperiosteal erosion correlates with serum i-PTH and histomorphometric features of osteitis fibrosa on bone biopsy. Subperiosteal resorption of the phalanges may be the most sensitive radiographic sign of secondary hyperparathyroidism. The tuft of the terminal phalanx or the second or third digit commonly shows resorption. With severe tuft erosion there may be a collapse of the soft tissue and a change in the contour of the tuft so that the finger appears to show clubbing. Bone erosions may also occur at the upper end of the tibia, the neck of the femur or the humerus, and the lower surface of the medial end of the clavicle. In the skull, resorption leads to the mottled and granular appearance commonly associated with altering areas of osteosclerosis.

Osteosclerosis is thought to be another feature of osteitis fibrosa arising from an increase in the thickness and number of trabecula in spongy bone. Osteosclerosis can lead to a typical "rugger jersey" appearance of the spine.

The x-ray features of *osteomalacia* are far less distinctive than those of secondary hyperparathyroidism. The Looser zone or pseudofracture are the only pathognomonic findings of osteomalacia in the adult (Fig. 245–2). A typical x-ray feature of rickets, that is, widening of the epiphyseal growth plate, cannot develop after epiphyseal closure and, hence, is limited to children. With mechanical stress and severe prolonged vitamin deficiency, a Looser zone may extend across the full width of the bone and produce a true fracture with displacement of fragments. Uremic patients with osteomalacia commonly have secondary hyperparathyroidism with concomitant x-ray features of the latter. Thus, a diagnosis of osteomalacia rests on histologic examinations, and one can only be certain of this diagnosis from bone therapy.

EXTRASKELETAL CALCIFICATIONS. The factors that predispose to the appearance of soft tissue calcification include an increase in the calcium phosphate product in plasma, the degree of secondary hyperparathyroidism, the magnitude of alkalosis, and the degree of local tissue injury. Three major varieties include (1) calcification of the medium sized arteries, (2) articular or tumoral calcifications, and (3) visceral calcifications affecting the heart, lung, and kidney.

TREATMENT

The objectives of the treatment of patients with renal osteodystrophy are (1) to return the blood levels of calcium and phosphorus to normal, (2) to suppress secondary hyperparathyroidism, (3) to reverse the histologic abnormalities in the skeleton, and (4) to prevent and reverse extraskeletal deposits of calcium and phosphate. It is very important to begin measures for the control of the abnormal mineral metabolism of renal disease early in the course, when the GFR is 30 to 40 ml per minute. Guidelines for the management of renal osteodystrophy are summarized in Table 248–1.

TABLE 248–1. GUIDELINES FOR MANAGEMENT OF RENAL OSTEODYSTROPHY

A. *Control of serum phosphate* (P) (3.5–5.0 mg/dl)

- Restrict phosphorus intake in diet to 600 to 800 mg per day
- Phosphate-binding antacids: aluminum carbonate or hydroxide; individualize dosage: Basalgel, Dialume, Alucap, Amphogel, 1 to 4 capsules with each meal
- Hypophosphatemia should be avoided
- Predialysis phosphorus: 4.5–5.5 mg/dl

B. *Adequate calcium intake*

- Oral calcium supplements, providing 1 to 2 gm per day when serum P is controlled: Os-Cal, Titralac
- Dialysate Ca, 6.5 to 7.0 mg per dl (3.25 to 3.5 mEq per liter)

C. *Use of vitamin D sterols*

- Vitamin D_2 or D_3: 50,000 to 250,000 IU (1.25 to 6.25 mg)
- Dihydrotachysterol: 0.25 to 2.0 mg per day
- 25-hydroxyvitamin D_3 (calcifediol): 20 to 100 μg per day (Calderol)
- 1,25-dihydroxyvitamin D_3 (calcitriol): 0.5 to 1.0 μg per day (Rocaltrol)

D. *Parathyroidectomy:*

- Severe secondary hyperparathyroidism (bone erosions and increased i-PTH) plus any of the following:
  - Persistent hypercalcemia (serum Ca > 11.5 to 12.0 mg per dl)
  - Progressive or symptomatic extraskeletal calcification
  - Persistently elevated serum calcium × phosphorus product
  - Pruritus not responsive to medical treatment
  - Calciphylaxis (ischemic ulcers and necrosis)
  - Symptomatic hypercalcemia after renal transplantation

CONTROL OF PHOSPHORUS. To control phosphorus, dietary phosphate intake should be reduced to 700 to 800 mg per day by restricting the ingestion of dairy products and by decreasing the amount of protein in the diet. In addition to dietary control of phosphorus, patients with advanced renal failure very likely need phosphate-binders to reduce the intestinal absorption of phosphate. Phosphate-binders should be ingested with the meal in order to increase their efficiency in binding phosphate. One of the obstacles to the use of aluminum-containing gels is the potential development of aluminum accumulation. Therefore, they should be used with caution and if the patient develops symptoms and signs suggesting aluminum-induced osteomalacia, aluminum-containing gels should be discontinued. If the phosphorus level is not controlled, the patient will develop severe secondary hyperparathyroidism and extraskeletal calcification. The addition of calcium carbonate in a dose of 1 to 2 grams with each meal helps to bind phosphate and to reduce the amount of aluminum binders necessary for the treatment of hyperphosphatemia. Calcium carbonate also provides dietary calcium and thereby helps to correct the negative calcium balance characteristic of far advanced renal insufficiency. The goal when using phosphate binders is to reduce the serum phosphorus to near normal. If the patient is not yet receiving dialysis treatment, the serum phosphorus should be maintained between 3.5 and 4.5 mg per deciliter.

CONTROL OF CALCIUM. The plasma calcium level should be maintained at the upper limits of normal. If a patient has severe hyperphosphatemia, the administration of large amounts of calcium can aggravate the deposition of calcium phosphate salts and metastatic calcification; thus the hyperphosphatemia should be corrected before calcium administration. Supplemental calcium administration should be discontinued if the serum calcium increases above 11.5 mg per deciliter. The concentration of calcium in dialysate can clearly affect serum calcium levels in patients treated with maintenance hemodialysis. The ideal calcium concentration in the dialysate is between 6.5 and 7.0 mg per deciliter. Despite dietary control of phosphate, the use of phosphate binders, the adequate intake of calcium in the diet, and appropriate levels of calcium in the dialysate, a significant number of uremic patients still develop skeletal disease. Thus, vitamin D and its metabolites are important and effective agents in the treatment of renal osteodystrophy.

VITAMIN D. $1,25(OH)_2D_3$, the most active metabolite of vitamin D, has a short half-life, approximately 10 to 15 hours. This is the drug of choice in the treatment of hypocalcemia and secondary hyperparathyroidism. The usual dose is 0.5 to 1 microgram per day. If the main histologic lesion is osteomalacia, excellent results have been obtained with the use of $25(OH)D_3$ (20 to 100 μg per day), in addition to $1,25(OH)_2D_3$. The most common and important side effect of vitamin D and its metabolites is hypercalcemia; less frequently hyperphospatemia develops.

PARATHYROIDECTOMY. The treatment modalities outlined in the previous paragraphs can improve the homeostasis of calcium and phosphorus, reverse the symptoms of bone disease, and suppress PTH secretion. However, such measures may not be entirely successful, and parathyroidectomy may be required in some cases. Indications for parathyroid surgery include severe secondary hyperparathyroidism (bone erosions and high levels of i-PTH) plus any of the following: (1) persistent hypercalcemia, particularly when symptomatic; (2) intractible pruritus that does not respond to dialysis or other medical treatment; (3) progressive extra-skeletal calcification in conjunction with a high calcium-phosphorus product that is consistently about 75 to 80 mg per deciliter despite appropriate phosphate restriction; and (4) the appearance of calciphylaxis with ischemic lesions of the soft tissues. Because of lack of compliance, many patients are unable to control their serum phosphorus levels. In these cases, neither calcium supplements nor vitamin D or its metabolites can be recommended safely.

Moreover, this type of patient usually develops severe secondary hyperparathyroidism and surgical parathyroidectomy may be the treatment of choice.

Post-operative hypocalcemia may pose a problem if the remaining parathyroid tissue is inadequate. The chances for developing hypocalcemia are enhanced if severe osteitis fibrosa is present preoperatively. Pre-operative treatment of such patients with $1,25(OH)_2D_3$ in the dose of 1 to 2 μg per day may obviate such problems. Serum levels of phosphorus and magnesium sometimes decrease after parathyroid surgery, and aluminum-containing phosphate binders should be withheld if the serum phosphorus falls below 3.0 mg per deciliter. Rapid remineralization of the skeleton occurs during this period, and once the "hungry bones" have been mineralized, serum calcium rises. A fall in elevated plasma alkaline phosphatase level towards normal may be a clue that rapid skeletal remineralization is nearly complete and indicates that calcium supplements and vitamin D dosage may be reduced or discontinued. In the past, the removal of three and a half parathyroid glands was the procedure of choice; more recently, surgeons have gained experience with total parathyroidectomy followed by autotransplantation of parathyroid tissue into the patient's forearm. The tissue that is transplanted to the forearm is more accessible for subsequent surgical removal if necessary. Total parathyroidectomy without autotransplantation has little place in the management of renal bone disease, and this may predispose to the development of isolated mineralization defects or osteomalacia in uremic patients. Cryopreservation of removed parathyroid tissue is a useful precaution so that hypoparathyroidism may be treated by reimplantation of parathyroid tissue.

ALUMINUM-INDUCED OSTEOMALACIA. If the patient has aluminum-induced osteomalacia, phosphate binders containing aluminum should be discontinued at once. Phosphate should be controlled by using a more restrictive phosphate diet, and the serum phosphorus level may be allowed to increase to 6 mg per deciliter. Although still experimental and not approved for general use, deferoxamine, a drug known to chelate iron, also has an effect on aluminum. Preliminary reports have shown that use of this substance produced a significant improvement in patients with aluminum-induced osteomalacia.

Coburn JW, Slatopolsky E: Vitamin D, parathyroid hormone and renal osteodystrophy. *In* Brenner BM, Rector FC (eds.): The Kidney. 2nd ed. Philadelphia, W. B. Saunders Company, 1981, pp 2213–2305.

Massry SG: Divalent ion metabolism and renal osteodystrophy. *In* Massry SG, Glassock RJ (eds.): Textbook of Nephrology. Baltimore, Williams and Wilkins, 1983, pp 7.104–7.148. *These two references offer comprehensive, up-to-date reviews of the pathogenesis, diagnosis, prevention, and treatment of renal osteodystrophy. They also review the alterations in calcium and phosphate metabolism found in renal disease. Both contain extensive reference lists.*

249. OSTEOPOROSIS

B. Lawrence Riggs

GENERAL CONSIDERATIONS

DEFINITION. Osteoporosis is defined as an absolute decrease in the amount of bone to a level below that required for mechanical support or, as Fuller Albright succinctly put it many years ago, "There is too little bone." The bone that is present is normal chemically and histologically.

PATHOPHYSIOLOGY. For bone to be lost, there must be an absolute or relative increase in bone resorption over bone formation. Bone remodeling occurs at discrete foci in the skeleton, termed "bone remodeling units." A team of osteoclasts appears, constructs a resorption tunnel in cortical bone or a resorption groove on the surface of trabecular bone and then, several weeks later, is replaced by osteoblasts, which fill in the resorption space to form a new bone structural unit. The time required for completion of this sequence normally is about three months but may be longer in osteoporotic patients. Osteoporosis could be caused by an increase in the activity or duration of action of osteoclasts (leading to the excavation of a larger resorption space), by a decrease in the activity or duration of action of osteoblasts (leading to an incompletely refilled resorption space), or by a combination of both. All three mechanisms have been observed in the various types of osteoporosis. Thus, osteoporosis may be associated with low, normal, or high bone turnover.

EPIDEMIOLOGY. Osteoporosis is an enormous public health problem. About one million fractures in the United States each year are attributable to osteoporosis. Among women over age 65, 25 per cent will have one or more vertebral fractures caused by osteoporosis. By extreme old age, one woman in three and one man in six will have had a hip fracture. These fractures are associated with a mortality of 15 per cent, result in long-term domicilliary care in 50 per cent of the cases, and cost over $1 billion each year for only the short-term medical and surgical care. Indeed, falls are the leading cause of accidental death in the elderly, primarily because of hip fractures.

RISK FACTORS FOR OSTEOPOROSIS. Risk factors for bone loss are cumulative and, in any given patient, may be multiple. These can be categorized into five groups and are described in the following paragraphs.

(1) The phenomenon of age-related bone loss is perhaps most important. Beginning in early middle age, all individuals lose bone with aging. Over a lifetime, women lose about 45 per cent of the bone from their vertebrae and about 55 per cent from their proximal femur; men lose about half of this amount. The major cause of age-related bone loss appears to be insufficient bone formation in individual bone remodeling units.

(2) Insufficient accumulation of skeletal mass in young adulthood predisposes to fractures later in life as age-related bone loss ensues. Differences in bone density at skeletal maturity explain in part racial and sexual differences in the incidence of osteoporosis. White women have the lightest skeleton and black men have the heaviest; white men and black women have skeletons of intermediate density. This rank order corresponds to the rank order for occurrence of fractures. Women of short stature and of northern European extraction tend toward a more gracile skeleton and also have an increased incidence of osteoporosis later in life. Moreover, if the rate of bone loss with age is constant, those white women with the lowest bone density values at skeletal maturity are at the greatest risk for fracture in later life. The amount of bone in young adulthood has been shown to have significant genetic determinants, and osteoporotic patients often have affected relatives.

(3) Bioavailability of calcium is a third important factor. In contrast to the requirements for other mineral nutrients, the basal requirement for calcium is relatively high because of obligatory fecal and urinary losses—about 150 to 250 mg per day. When the amount of absorbed dietary calcium is insufficient to offset these losses, calcium must be withdrawn from bone, which contains 99 per cent of total body stores. Both menopause and aging increase the requirement for dietary calcium mainly by decreasing the efficiency of intestinal calcium absorption. Estimates based on metabolic balance suggest that premenopausal women require 1,000 mg of calcium per day to maintain calcium balance and postmenopausal women require 1,400 mg per day. Yet the dietary calcium intake of American women from middle life onward is only about 550 mg per day.

(4) The menopause and other abnormalities in endocrine function contribute to osteoporosis. Longitudinal studies of appendicular, mainly cortical, bone after oophorectomy have shown accelerated loss (total, about 8 per cent more than predicted) for about seven years. The extent of axial, mainly trabecular, bone loss due to estrogen deficiency is controversial but probably is somewhat more than appendicular bone loss. The negative calcium balance induced by menopause is associated with increased bone turnover—bone resorption increases more than does bone formation. It has been suggested that estrogen deficiency might increase the responsiveness of bone to circulating endogenous parathyroid hormone. Because

women have lower serum levels of immunoreactive calcitonin than men and because the menopause may further decrease calcitonin secretion, calcitonin deficiency may contribute to bone loss. Both intestinal calcium absorption and serum levels of 1,25-dihydroxyvitamin D are decreased in osteoporosis.

(5) Various risk factors for bone loss in the environment have been identified. These include high protein intake, high alcohol consumption, smoking, and decreased physical activity. Obesity is protective, possibly because of increased loading stress to the spine and, in postmenopausal women, because of increased conversion (in fat tissue) of adrenal androgens to estrogens.

SPECIFIC OSTEOPOROSIS SYNDROMES

Osteoporosis can be associated secondarily with a large number of disorders (Table 249–1). In 60 per cent of cases in men and 80 per cent in women, the disease occurs in middle-aged and older persons without any secondary abnormality. This common, primary form of the disease has been termed "involutional osteoporosis."

JUVENILE OSTEOPOROSIS. A rare syndrome of osteoporosis occurs in prepubertal children, usually between ages 8 and 14 years. The radiographic features of the syndrome are indistinguishable from those of involutional osteoporosis. Histologically, bone formation is normal or decreased but bone resorption is strikingly increased. Onset is acute, and multiple vertebral fractures occur over a period of two to four years. Then there is spontaneous remission and resumption of normal bone growth. Thus, treatment consists of protection of the spine until the remission occurs. There is no evidence that drug therapy is beneficial. Sex steroids are contraindicated because they may result in early closure of the epiphyseal growth plates. The syndrome is distinguished from osteogenesis imperfecta by lack of blue sclera and other characteristic stigmata, by the lack of a history of fractures of long bones, and by the absence of family history for bone disease. Cushing's syndrome should be excluded by adrenal function tests. Although the etiology is unknown, the temporal relationship to puberty suggests that hormonal factors may be important.

IDIOPATHIC OSTEOPOROSIS IN YOUNG ADULTS. This term is used to describe the relatively uncommon occurrence of osteoporosis in younger men or premenopausal women in whom no etiologic factor can be found. Undoubtedly, it is etiologically heterogeneous. In some patients, it runs a clinical course similar to that of involutional osteoporosis; in others, it is rapidly progressive and may lead to severe disability or even death (from respiratory failure) several years after onset. Except when the characteristic clinical features are present, it may be difficult to exclude a variant form of osteogenesis imperfecta tarda. Bone biopsy may help because patients with osteogenesis imperfecta invariably have very low bone turnover whereas patients with idiopathic osteoporosis often have high bone turnover.

TABLE 249–1. CLASSIFICATION OF CAUSES OF OSTEOPOROSIS

Primary osteoporosis	Bone marrow disorders
Juvenile	Multiple myeloma and related disorders
Idiopathic (young adults)	Systemic mastocytosis
Involutional osteoporosis	Disseminated carcinoma
Endocrine diseases	Connective tissue diseases
Hypogonadism	Osteogenesis imperfecta
Ovarian agenesis	Homocystinuria
Hyperadrenocorticism	Ehlers-Danlos syndrome
Hyperthyroidism	Marfan's syndrome
Hyperparathyroidism	
Diabetes mellitus (?)	
Gastrointestinal diseases	Miscellaneous causes
Subtotal gastrectomy	Immobilization
Malabsorption syndromes	Chronic obstructive pulmonary disease
Chronic obstructive jaundice	Chronic alcoholism
Primary biliary cirrhosis	Chronic heparin administration
Severe malnutrition	Rheumatoid arthritis (?)
Alactasia	

TABLE 249–2. INVOLUTIONAL OSTEOPOROSIS

	Type I	Type II
Age	51–65 yrs*	> 75 yrs*
Sex ratio (F:M)	6:1	2:1
Bone loss: Type	Mainly trabecular	Trabecular and cortical
Rate	Accelerated	Not accelerated
Fracture type	Mainly vertebral	Both vertebral and hip
Parathyroid function	Decreased	Increased
Calcium absorption	Decreased	Decreased
Metabolism of 25(OH)D to $1,25(OH)_2D$	Secondary decrease	Primary decrease
Major etiologic factors	Menopause	Decreased bone formation; Secondary hyperparathyroidism

*Both types occur in the decade from 66 to 75 years.

INVOLUTIONAL OSTEOPOROSIS. It is becoming increasingly clear that the common variety of osteoporosis occurring in men and women with increasing frequency after middle life may consist of two distinct syndromes. Type I osteoporosis ("postmenopausal" osteoporosis) occurs in a relatively small subset of postmenopausal women who are 51 to 65 years of age. Less frequently, a similar syndrome occurs in men of comparable age. Type II osteoporosis ("senile" osteoporosis) occurs in a large proportion of women or men who are more than 75 years of age. Osteoporosis occurring in the decade from 66 to 75 years may represent a combination of both types. These two syndromes can be shown to differ with respect to epidemiology, patterns of trabecular and cortical bone loss, parathyroid function, and cause (Table 249–2).

Type I osteoporosis is the classic form of the disease described in 1940 by Fuller Albright and his associates and characteristically occurs in women within 15 years of menopause. Less commonly, men are affected with a form of osteoporosis that is otherwise indistinguishable from that occurring in postmenopausal women. Vertebral fracture is its main clinical manifestation but Colles' fracture of the distal radius occurs frequently. Both of these fracture sites contain large amounts of trabecular bone. Recent measurements of bone density have clearly established that patients with type I osteoporosis have accelerated loss of trabecular bone but their rate of loss of cortical bone is similar to or only slightly less than that for age-matched normal subjects. The accelerated bone loss leads to decreased parathyroid hormone secretion which, in turn, leads to decreased production of 1,25-dihydroxyvitamin D [$1,25(OH)_2D_3$]. The decreased circulating levels of serum $1,25(OH)_2D_3$ results in impaired calcium absorption, which may further increase bone loss. The predilection for women and the temporal proximity to menopause implicate estrogen deficiency as an etiologic agent. Yet only a relatively small subset of postmenopausal women have this form of osteoporosis, but all are deficient in estrogen. In postmenopausal women, most investigators have found no differences between those with and those without osteoporosis. Thus, some factor or factors in addition to menopause must determine individual susceptibility.

Type II osteoporosis occurs in persons 75 years of age or older and is manifested mainly by hip fracture and vertebral fracture, but fractures of the proximal humerus, proximal tibia, and pelvis may also occur. In patients with type II osteoporosis, individual bone densitometric values for the proximal femur, vertebrae, and bones of the appendicular skeleton are in the lower part of the age- and sex-adjusted normal range. Thus, type II osteoporosis is characterized by proportionate loss of both cortical and trabecular bone and a rate of loss similar to that in the general population. There may be two major causes for type II osteoporosis—impaired bone formation and secondary hyperparathyroidism. First, from the fourth decade of life onward, less bone is formed than is resorbed at individual remodeling foci, and this imbalance increases with aging. Second, the age-related increase in parathyroid function occurs concomitantly with and probably results from the age-related decrease in calcium absorption. Although serum levels of 25(OH)D are generally normal, serum levels of $1,25(OH)_2D$ decrease in the elderly and may be even lower in patients with hip fracture. These decreases may be caused by impaired metabolism of 25(OH)D to $1,25(OH)_2D$, an abnormality that has been documented in aging rats. The recent observation that overall bone turnover among women may increase with aging (as assessed by measurement of serum bone gla-protein and other biochemical markers) suggests that secondary hyperparathyroidism may increase the number of individual bone remodeling units and thus increases bone turnover at the tissue level. Because bone formation remains decreased at the level of individual remodeling units, increased bone turnover would result in increased bone loss.

ENDOCRINE DISEASES. Osteoporosis may be associated with a number of syndromes of endocrine dysfunction. *Hypogonadism* in either sex leads to an increased incidence of osteoporosis. Hypogonadism is probably the main cause of osteoporosis associated with ovarian agenesis *(Turner's syndrome)* although a genetic abnormality of bone maturation probably also is present. Endogenous or exogenous *hyperadrenocorticism* is associated with both decreased bone formation and increased bone resorption that lead to rapid bone loss. The decrease in bone formation results from inhibition of collagen biosynthesis. The increase in bone resorption may be indirectly mediated, possibly by an increased sensitivity of bone to parathyroid hormone. Patients with glucocorticoid excess also have impaired calcium absorption, and this can be reversed by administering vitamin D or its active metabolite. An effect of corticosteroids on vitamin D metabolism, however, has not been conclusively established.

Although *hyperthyroidism* consistently increases bone turnover, in most patients formation and resorption remain coupled. Symptomatic osteoporosis associated with hyperthyroidism therefore is relatively unusual and, when present, generally occurs in postmenopausal women. Although osteitis fibrosa is the characteristic skeletal abnormality associated with *hyperparathyroidism*, about 5 per cent of patients, mostly postmenopausal women, present with osteopenia and vertebral compression fractures. It has been suggested that patients with either juvenile- or adult-onset *diabetes mellitus* have an increased risk for osteoporosis, but others have challenged this view. Osteoporosis associated with *acromegaly* is believed to be rare and, when present, is the result of concomitant hypogonadism. In fact, because of the anabolic effect of growth hormone excess on the skeleton, most patients with acromegaly have an increase in both trabecular and cortical bone mass.

GASTROINTESTINAL DISEASES. These conditions can cause either osteoporosis or osteomalacia, and they generally produce a mixture of both. About 5 per cent of patients with *subtotal gastrectomy*, particularly in those with the Billroth II type, subsequently develop bone disease. *Malabsorption syndromes* impair absorption of calcium and vitamin D; usually this results in osteomalacia but, if mild, the predominant lesion may be osteoporosis. Chronic obstructive jaundice may be associated with bone disease because the enterohepatic circulation of active vitamin D metabolites is impaired. This mechanism may play a role in the osteomalacia associated with *primary biliary cirrhosis*. In the United States, however, osteoporosis associated with a profound depression in bone formation is the typical finding. Its etiology is unknown. *Severe malnutrition* involving both protein and calcium deficiency—as has been observed in prisoners of war and in patients with anorexia nervosa—may cause osteoporosis. Finally, *alactasia* has been reported in up to 30 per cent of osteoporotic subjects. This disorder may be a risk factor for osteoporosis because it produces intolerance to milk and, thus, is associated with a low calcium intake.

BONE MARROW DISORDERS. *Multiple myeloma* is associated with diffuse osteoporosis in about 10 per cent of patients and in a lesser proportion of other myeloproliferative disorders. It is mediated by an increased local production of osteoclast activating factor (a lymphokine with potent bone-resorbing properties) by bone marrow cells. Diffuse osteoporosis also may occur when *disseminated carcinoma* involves the bone marrow.

CONNECTIVE TISSUE DISEASES. An unusually severe form of osteoporosis may occur in *osteogenesis imperfecta*. This disease is usually inherited as an autosomal dominant trait and is associated with blue sclera, deafness, thin skin, and impaired biosynthesis of type I collagen. Although onset usually is in childhood, some patients present with premature spinal osteoporosis in the absence of a history of limb bone fracture. The *Marfan* and *Ehlers-Danlos syndromes* also may be associated with spinal osteopenia but less frequently include vertebral fractures. Osteoporosis commonly occurs in patients with *homocystinuria*, an autosomal recessive disorder caused by deficient cystathionine synthase activity. The resultant increase in homocysteine and other metabolites in the circulation interferes with cross-linking of collagen.

MISCELLANEOUS CAUSES. Total *immobilization*, such as occurs in traumatic quadriplegia, results in a loss of up to 1 per cent of bone per month, especially in the trabecular bone of the axial skeleton. After loss of 40 to 50 per cent of bone from the spinal column, a new steady state is reached and bone mass is maintained. Bone loss is associated with both depressed bone formation and enhanced bone resorption. Significant bone loss also occurs during total bed rest among nonparalyzed individuals. If immobilization is transient, replacement of bone mass occurs on remobilization, provided that there has been only thinning of bone trabeculae rather than loss of trabeculae and other structural elements.

Not infrequently, osteoporosis is associated with *chronic obstructive pulmonary disease*. Whether this is related to the consumption of tobacco, which is believed to be a bone toxin, or to the pulmonary disease itself is unknown. Young alcoholics also have been shown to have thinner bones than other subjects of similar age. Long-term therapy with *heparin* has been reported to cause severe loss of bone and spontaneous fractures. Heparin decreases the stability of lysosomes, and release of collagenase and other lysosomal enzymes may be responsible for the bone loss. Finally, although it has been suggested that osteoporosis may be a complication of rheumatoid arthritis, most of the bone loss in these patients can probably be accounted for by corticosteroid use and by immobilization.

CLINICAL CONSIDERATIONS

CLINICAL PRESENTATION. Osteoporosis is manifested by *back pain, loss of height* and *spinal deformity*, especially kyphosis, and *fractures of the hips, wrist*, and, less frequently, other bones. The most characteristic symptom of osteoporosis is back pain caused by vertebral compression. Typically, a woman within 20 years after menopause develops acute lumbar or thoracic back pain after some ordinary activity such as raising a window or lifting a sack of groceries. The pain may be mild or severe, and it may be localized or exhibit flank radiation. It remits in days or weeks but then recurs. After several episodes of acute intermittent pain, the patient may develop a chronic mechanical backache resulting from spinal deformity. Untreated or unsuccessfully treated patients may develop *severe kyphosis* and a loss of 4 to 8 inches of height. In severe cases, the rib cage comes to rest on the pelvic brim. The frequency of occurrence of vertebral fractures and the number of fractures that eventually occur vary widely between patients, but the average is one per year. In general, elderly women progress more slowly and commonly develop substantial dorsal kyphosis and cervical lordosis—the so-called dowager's hump—in the absence of significant pain. Half of the hip fractures in elderly men and women are spontaneous and half are associated with falls.

RADIOLOGIC FINDINGS. Roentgenograms of the spinal column show accentuation of the vertebral end-plates, prominence of the weight-bearing, vertical trabeculae (due to disappearance of the horizontal trabeculae), and loss of contrast in radiodensity between the interior of the vertebral body and adjacent soft tissue (Fig. 249–1). Vertebral deformity may take the form of collapse (reduction of anterior and posterior height), anterior wedging (reduction in anterior height, usually occurring in the thoracic spinal column), or "ballooning" (biconcave compression of the end-plates by pressure of the intervertebral discs, usually occurring in the lumbar spinal column). Also, localized herniation of the nucleus pulposus into the vertebral body (Schmorl's nodes) may occur. Osteoporosis due to glucocorticoid excess should be considered when there is associated osteoporosis of the skull, fractures of the ribs and pelvic rami, and prominent partially mineralized callus at the sites of fracture. In the absence of pseudofractures, osteomalacia may be difficult to distinguish from osteoporosis, but it often has a "ground glass" appearance rather than the characteristic "clear glass" appearance of osteoporosis. Posterior wedging of a vertebra suggests a destructive lesion rather than osteoporosis.

DIAGNOSTIC EVALUATION. All newly discovered patients with osteoporosis should have a general medical evaluation to exclude secondary diseases that may cause osteoporosis and to assess severity. Systemic symptoms or abnormal physical findings suggest the presence of an underlying disease. Serum calcium and phosphorus levels are normal in primary osteoporosis. Serum alkaline phosphatase level also is normal except for transient elevations during healing of vertebral fractures. Sustained elevation of alkaline phosphatase level, in the absence of liver disease, suggests osteomalacia or a destructive skeletal process.

Multiple myeloma may be present in the absence of symptoms and with a normal hematogram and erythrocyte sedimentation rate. Although most cases can be diagnosed by serum and urine protein electrophoresis, bone marrow examination occasionally is required (see Ch. 163). Sometimes this is necessary to diagnose some cases of disseminated carcinoma. Transiliac bone biopsy may be needed to exclude osteomalacia or to stage the abnormality in bone remodeling.

Severity of osteoporosis can be assessed most easily by determining the amount of height loss and the number of vertebral fractures, but it can be assessed more precisely by measuring vertebral density directly with either dual photon absorptiometry or quantitative computed tomography. Although currently confined to only a few research centers, these procedures should soon be widely available.

TREATMENT

GENERAL THERAPEUTIC MEASURES. Acute back pain responds to analgesics, heat, and gentle massage to alleviate muscle spasm. Sometimes a brief period of bed rest is required. Chronic back pain often is caused by spinal deformity and thus is

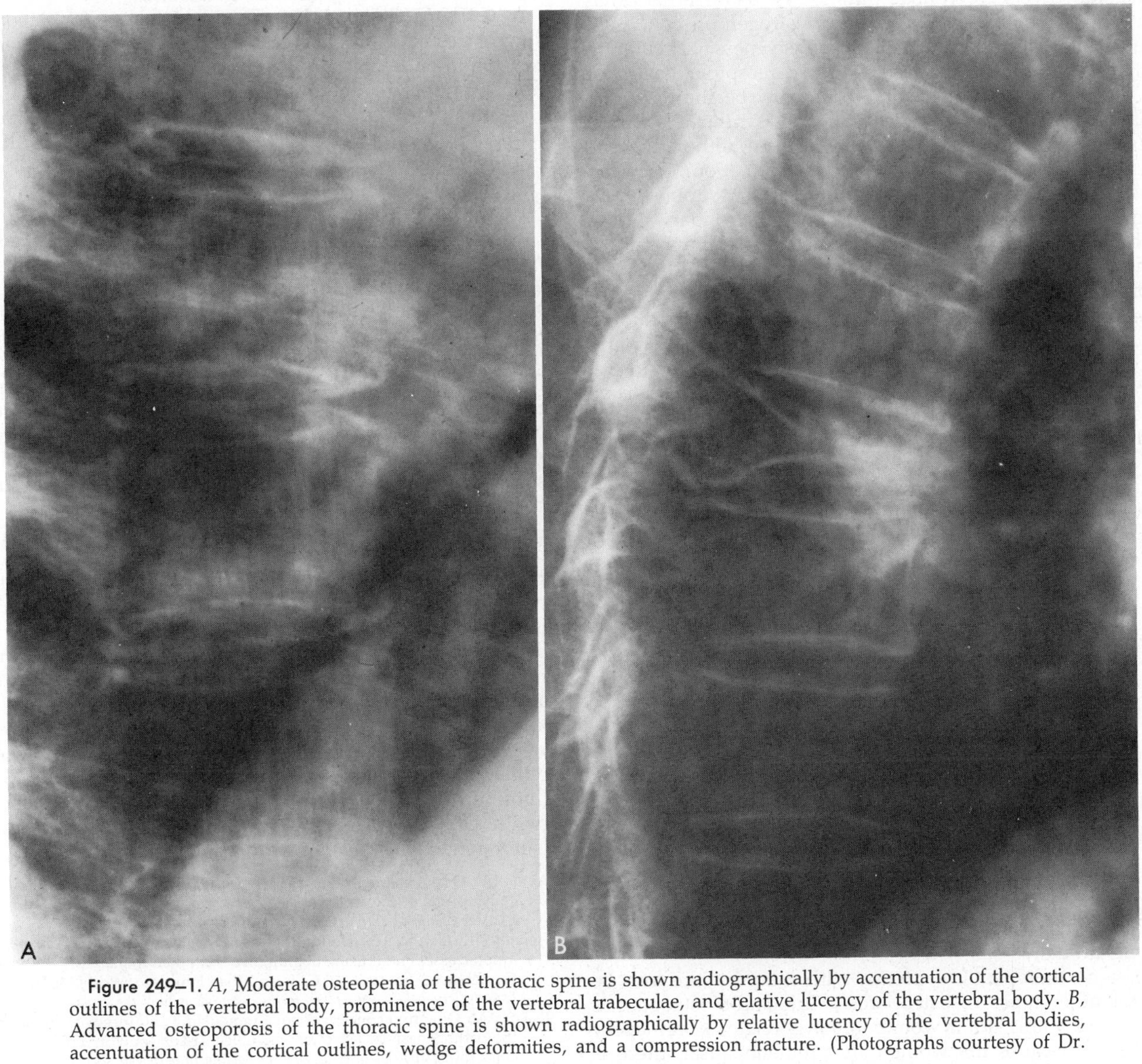

Figure 249–1. *A*, Moderate osteopenia of the thoracic spine is shown radiographically by accentuation of the cortical outlines of the vertebral body, prominence of the vertebral trabeculae, and relative lucency of the vertebral body. *B*, Advanced osteoporosis of the thoracic spine is shown radiographically by relative lucency of the vertebral bodies, accentuation of the cortical outlines, wedge deformities, and a compression fracture. (Photographs courtesy of Dr. Harry K. Genant.)

difficult to relieve completely. Instruction in posture and gait training and institution of regular back extension exercises to strengthen the flabby paravertebral muscles usually are beneficial. Occasionally, an orthopedic back brace is required. All patients with osteoporosis should have a diet adequate in calcium, proteins, and vitamins, should be reasonably active physically, and should take precautions to prevent falls.

DRUG THERAPY. Calcium, vitamin D, estrogen, anabolic steroids, and calcitonin inhibit bone resorption. When a new steady state is attained after three to six months of treatment, there is a coupled reduction in bone formation that approximates the reduction in bone resorption. Thus, the best result that can be obtained with this class of therapeutic agents is maintenance of the existing skeletal mass or slowing of its rate of loss.

Calcium, which is prescribed to offset the impaired calcium absorption that is often present in osteoporosis and to decrease parathyroid hormone secretion, is safe, well-tolerated, and inexpensive. *Vitamin D* and its active metabolites have a similar function but must be used judiciously, because the dose that increases calcium absorption is not much smaller than the dose that increases bone resorption.

Estrogen is more effective than calcium but has significant side effects. These commonly include induction of menstruation, mastodynia, and fluid retention; less common but more serious side effects are venous thrombosis, endometrial carcinoma, and cholelithiasis. The effect of estrogen on bone may be mediated by decreasing skeletal responsiveness to circulating parathyroid hormone. Because estrogen receptors have not been demonstrated in bone, its action may be indirect. The mechanism of action of androgens and synthetic anabolic agents probably is similar to that of estrogen, although some data suggest a weak stimulation of bone formation. *Calcitonin* is an effective antiresorption agent, but calcium supplementation must be given concurrently to prevent secondary hyperparathyroidism. Disadvantages include the requirement for parenteral administration, a relatively high cost, and the development of neutralizing antibodies in some patients.

Therapy for patients with involutional osteoporosis should be individualized. For patients with mild disease, particularly in those older than 75 years, only calcium supplementation (1.0 to 1.5 grams per day) need be employed. For more extensive disease, especially in women within 15 years of menopause, low-dose estrogen therapy (such as cyclic doses of 0.625 mg daily of conjugated estrogen or 0.025 mg daily of ethynyl estradiol) may be used. Because the risk of endometrial hyperplasia (and, therefore, carcinoma) is reduced or eliminated by concomitant progestin therapy, 5 mg daily of medroxyprogesterone acetate is given during the last ten days of the cycle. Even a hysterectomized woman should receive cyclic therapy. If fractures continue on this regimen, the dosage of both the estrogen and progestin should be doubled. Elderly women may prefer synthetic anabolic steroids to estrogens.

Vitamin D and its active metabolites probably should be reserved for patients with a documented or suspected impairment in calcium absorption. This can be inferred from a relatively low urinary calcium excretion rate (<75 mg per day), especially if this does not increase significantly with calcium supplementation. Calcitonin is most likely to be effective in patients with osteoporosis associated with a high bone turnover. In the absence of a bone biopsy, this can be inferred from values in the upper portion of the normal range for serum phosphorus and urinary calcium. The recommended dose is 100 units daily accompanied by at least 1.0 gram of supplementary calcium daily.

The same therapeutic approach with modifications can be used for other types of osteoporosis. Idiopathic osteoporosis occurring in young adult women often is relatively refractory to therapy. Because the women are premenopausal, there is no reason to prescribe sex steroids. Some of these patients have impaired calcium absorption, which is correctable with vitamin D therapy. The mainstay of treatment, therefore, is calcium supplementation with or without pharmacologic doses of vitamin D. Calcitonin can be added to reduce the increased level of bone resorption that may be present.

Men with osteoporosis usually do not have a deficiency of sex steroids and thus have no need for hormonal treatment. But 10 to 20 per cent have partial or complete hypogonadism from various causes. Patients with documented low plasma testosterone levels should receive replacement therapy with, for example, testosterone enanthate (Delatestryl) in a dose of 200 to 400 mg intramuscularly every four weeks. Calcium supplementation with or without pharmacologic doses of vitamin D should also be given.

The most common cause of secondary osteoporosis is chronic use of pharmacologic dosages of glucocorticoids. The single most effective measure is reduction of dosage or, if possible, complete discontinuation of the glucocorticoids. Administering the glucocorticoids once daily or on alternate days may maintain a more favorable balance between anti-inflammatory and immunosuppressive effects and the osteopenic effect. All patients should be given calcium supplements, and postmenopausal women should be given estrogens. Although glucocorticoids inhibit calcium absorption, the use of pharmacologic dosages of vitamin D or its metabolites in this circumstance is controversial and may abet the calciuric effects of glucocorticoids. There is increasing evidence that glucocorticoids do not induce major alterations in vitamin D metabolism.

INVESTIGATIONAL DRUGS. The ideal therapy for osteoporosis should result in an increase in bone formation over bone resorption and consequently an increase in bone mass. Three investigational regimens have been described that may have this effect: low-dose therapy with the synthetic 1-34 fragment of parathyroid hormone, combined oral therapy with phosphate and calcitonin, and combined therapy with fluoride and calcium. Only the last has been studied in detail and has given reproducible results.

Sodium fluoride is a potent stimulator of osteoblasts, and recent studies on bone cells *in vitro* have shown that this effect is direct. Sodium fluoride can induce a substantial increase in trabecular bone of the axial skeleton. But concurrent administration of supplementary calcium is required to prevent or minimize the incomplete mineralization that may occur when fluoride is given alone. Bone biopsy studies suggest that fluoride therapy may bypass the normal remodeling sequence and induce osteoblast formation *de novo* on previously quiescent surfaces. Although fluoridic bone may be structurally less sound than an equivalent amount of normal bone, the substantial increase in bone mass increases net bone strength.

Patients treated with fluoride at the Mayo Clinic had fewer new fractures. Unfortunately, a significant subset (25 to 40 per cent) responded to sodium fluoride therapy incompletely or not at all, possibly because they had an intrinsic abnormality in osteoblast function. At least one third of treated patients develop gastric or rheumatic side effects: the former consist of nausea or epigastric burning distress caused by gastric irritation and the latter consist of periarticular pain, particularly in the knees, ankles, and feet. Both types of symptoms disappear when treatment is discontinued and usually do not recur after reinstitution of sodium fluoride at a lower dosage. Sodium fluoride has not been approved for treatment of osteoporosis by the United States Food and Drug Administration, and so it is not generally available in a high-dose form.

Avioli LV: Osteoporosis. *In* Peck WA (ed.): Bone and Mineral Research. Annual 1. Amsterdam, Excerpta Medica, 1983, pp 280–318. *Comprehensive survey of new developments with detailed literature review.*

Genant HK, Gordan GS, Hoffman PG Jr: Osteoporosis: part I. Advanced radiographic assessment using quantitative computed tomography—Medical Staff Conference, University of California, San Francisco. West J Med 139:75, 1983. *Description of this new method for assessing density of the spine.*

Parfitt AM: Quantum concept of bone remodeling and turnover: Implications for the pathogenesis of osteoporosis. Calcif Tissue Int 28:1, 1979. *A lucid review of the role of abnormalities of bone remodeling in pathogenesis of osteoporosis.*

Parfitt AM: Morphologic basis of bone mineral measurements: Transient and steady state effects of treatment in osteoporosis. Min Electrolyte Metab 4:273, 1980. *The theoretical basis for differences in early and late effects of therapeutic agents on bone remodeling and bone density in osteoporosis.*

Riggs BL, Seeman E, Hodgson SF, et al.: Effect of the fluoride/calcium regimen on vertebral fracture occurrence in postmenopausal osteoporosis. N Engl J Med 306:446, 1982. *Effect of calcium, estrogen, and sodium fluoride, alone and in combination, on fracture occurrence.*

Riggs BL, Melton LJ III: Evidence for two distinct syndromes of involutional osteoporosis. Am J Med 75:899, 1983. *Summary of evidence that supports this concept.*

Riggs, BL, Wahner HW, Seeman E, et al.: Changes in bone mineral density of the proximal femur and spine with aging. J Clin Invest 70:716, 1982. *Bone density measurements in normal and osteoporotic subjects using dual photon absorptiometry.*

Steinbach HL: The roentgen appearance of osteoporosis. Radiol Clin North Am 2:191, 1964. *Classic article on the radiologic appearance of osteoporosis.*

250. PAGET'S DISEASE OF BONE (OSTEITIS DEFORMANS)

Frederick R. Singer

INCIDENCE AND EPIDEMIOLOGY

Paget's disease is a common bone disorder second in incidence to osteoporosis. In areas of prevalence it affects approximately 3 per cent of the population over age 40. The disease is commonly diagnosed in the United Kingdom and in the countries to which its inhabitants have migrated, including the United States, Canada, South Africa, Australia, and New Zealand. The disease also is common in France, Germany, and Italy. Patients are rarely found in China, Japan, India, or Scandinavia. There is no major predilection for either sex.

There is evidence of an autosomal dominant transmission that is linked to histocompatibility leukocyte antigens. As high as 50 per cent of patients have been reported to have at least one relative with the disease.

PATHOLOGY

Paget's disease may affect one or many bones but in the majority of patients most of the skeleton is uninvolved. The earliest phase is characterized by a localized osteolytic process in which proliferation of multinucleated osteoclasts is the dominant lesion. The osteoclasts of Paget's disease are occasionally quite large and may exhibit more than 100 nuclei in a cross-section of one cell. Adjacent to the advancing osteolytic front, the pathology is characterized by a mixed osteolytic and osteoblastic process of great intensity. Numerous plump osteoblasts line bony trabeculae that have previously been partially resorbed by osteoclasts. The marrow spaces may be devoid of hematopoietic cells and instead are filled with fibroblasts, connective tissue, and blood vessels. The resultant architecture of the bone takes on a "mosaic" pattern in which the cement lines are arranged in a haphazard pattern instead of the normal symmetry of parallel collagen fibers in both cortical and trabecular bone. Occasionally this abnormal mosaic pattern is present with little or no cellular activity. Osteolytic, mixed osteolytic and osteoblastic, and "burned out" Paget's disease may be present in a single bone. Paget's disease can usually be readily distinguished from primary hyperparathyroidism, osteomyelitis, and osteomalacia by light microscopy, but electron microscopy studies have provided evidence of a characteristic lesion. The nuclei, and at times the cytoplasm, of the osteoclasts frequently contain abnormal inclusions that resemble the nucleocapsids of viruses of the Paramyxoviridae family. Further evidence of a viral presence in these cells has been obtained by the use of immunohistologic staining. Antisera to respiratory syncytial virus and measles virus have produced positive results in the osteoclasts of Paget's disease but in no other disorder.

ETIOLOGY

Sir James Paget, in his original description of the disease, proposed that the entity was inflammatory in nature. The recent ultrastructural and immunohistologic studies support the concept of a "slow" virus infection, although definitive proof is still to be obtained. Other hypotheses for which there are insignificant supporting data include an abnormality of hormone secretion, a neoplastic state, a vascular anomaly, an autoimmune state, and an inborn error of connective tissue biosynthesis.

CLINICAL FEATURES

In many patients Paget's disease is not appreciated until an abnormal radiograph or laboratory test is encountered either in the course of a routine evaluation or during assessment of an unrelated complaint. The most common complaints of symptomatic patients are *skeletal deformity* and *musculoskeletal pain.* The bones most likely to be abnormal on physical examination are the cranium, the clavicles, and the long bones, particularly of the lower extremities. The complications associated with skull lesions include hearing loss, vertigo, tinnitus and, less commonly, headaches. Severe enlargement of the base of the skull may lead to basilar impression and compression of the spinal cord, the brain stem, the cerebellum, and the basilar and vertebral arteries. Slurred speech, impaired swallowing, diplopia, and urinary incontinence may result. Deformity of the facial bones (leontiasis ossea) is much less common in patients with Paget's disease than in patients with fibrous dysplasia, a disease which usually is diagnosed several decades earlier in life. The spine may be involved at any level, but lumbar and thoracic vertebrae are most commonly affected. One or more vertebrae, consecutive or not, can manifest the disease. Back pain may be severe and of complex origin since degenerative arthritis is common in this age group, and impingement of skeletal tissue on nerve roots or the spinal cord can occur. The sudden onset of intolerable pain suggests that a compression fracture has occurred. Disease affecting the pelvis and proximal femur produces a common severe pain syndrome, weight-bearing pain from degenerative arthritis of the hip. Ambulation may also be impaired when significant lateral or anterior bowing of the femur or tibia develops. These bones are also prone to pathologic fracture. Evidence of disease activity in long bones is manifested by increased skin temperature over the affected bone. This results from the increased cutaneous blood flow associated with the hypervascular bone beneath.

Defects in Bruch's membrane of the retina, termed angioid streaks, may be observed in about 10 per cent of patients and seldom are associated with impaired vision. Cardiac enlargement and frank congestive heart failure may be a manifestation of prior increased cardiac output, which is thought to be a consequence of increased vascularity of affected bones. This usually occurs in patients with more than 30 per cent of the skeleton affected by Paget's disease or when the skull is severely involved. Bone tumors such as osteosarcoma and giant cell tumor may develop in lesions of Paget's disease (Ch. 252). A rapid worsening of bone pain or the relatively sudden development of a mass or both are the common modes of presentation.

RADIOLOGY. The radiologic features of Paget's disease are so characteristic that it is seldom necessary to obtain a bone biopsy for diagnosis. The earliest manifestation is a localized osteolytic lesion most readily detected in the skull and at either end of a long bone. In the skull, the circumscribed radiolucent area has been termed osteoporosis circumscripta (Fig. 250–1). The osteolytic lesion in an extremity bone usually progresses with a sharply defined V-shape at an average rate of progression of 1 cm per year. Linear cortical radiolucencies may develop in the femur or tibia on the convex surface of a curved bone and may be precursors of fractures. An uncommon variant of the osteolytic lesion may occur at the distal end of the tibia in which a cystic-like expansion of the bone is seen. Osteolytic disease of the vertebral bodies is often associated with sclerotic margins

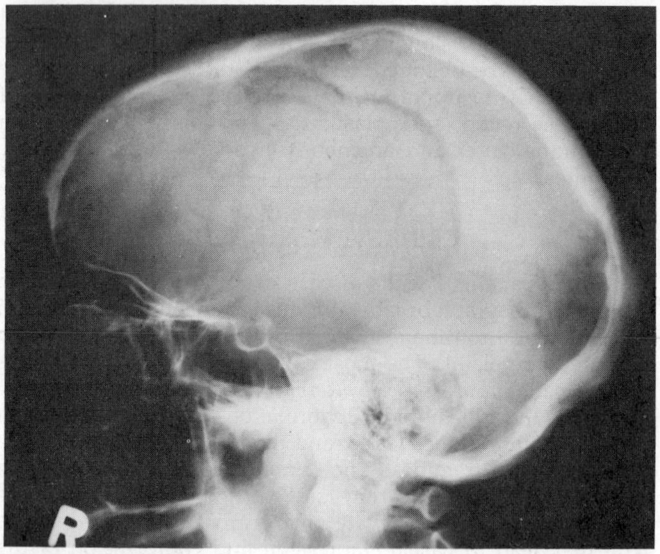

Figure 250–1. Osteoporosis circumscripta of the skull involving the frontal, parietal, and temporal bones.

giving a "picture frame" appearance. These vertebrae are prone to compression fractures.

The radiographic manifestations of osteoblastic activity generally appear years or even decades after the onset of osteolysis. In the skull a "honeycomb" appearance of patchy new bone may fill in the underlying osteoporosis circumscripta, and subsequently the classic "cotton-wool" lesions of exuberant chaotic bone formation appear with a strikingly thickened calvarium (Fig. 250–2). In the long bones, the osteolytic lesions evolve into thickened bone with irregular trabeculation. In the pelvis, thickening of the iliopectineal line, the "brim sign," is nearly pathognomonic of Paget's disease. It is also found in patients with osteopetrosis but rarely in patients with osteoblastic metastases. Enlargement of the ischial and pubic bones is also typical of Paget's disease. Sclerosis of the pagetic vertebral body may be difficult to distinguish from malignant bone involvement, but if the vertebral body is clearly larger than adjacent vertebral bodies, Paget's disease is likely. Computerized tomography of the spine is a useful means of evaluating the detailed anatomy of the spine and is particularly helpful in defining arthritic and neurologic complications in the patient with back pain.

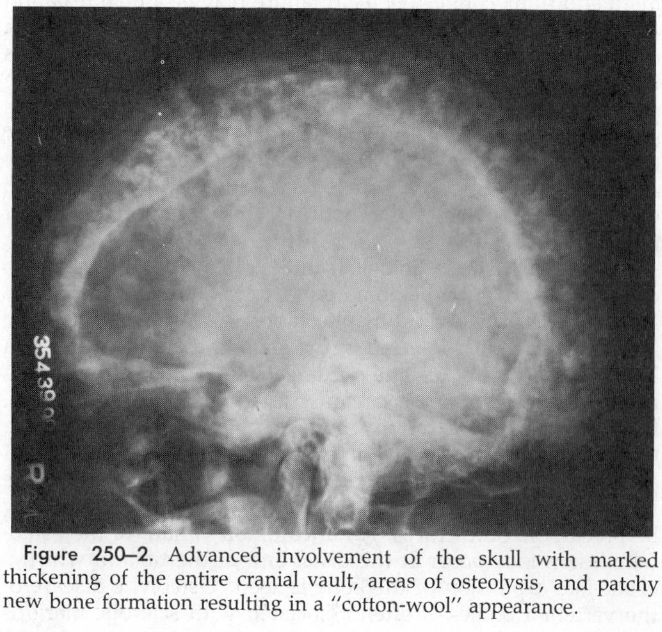

Figure 250–2. Advanced involvement of the skull with marked thickening of the entire cranial vault, areas of osteolysis, and patchy new bone formation resulting in a "cotton-wool" appearance.

The bone scan is the most sensitive means to detect active lesions of Paget's disease, although it is not a specific diagnostic test. The earliest lesions may not be discernible roentgenographically at the same time an area of increased uptake of the radiolabeled scanning agent is obvious.

BIOCHEMICAL FEATURES

The extent and activity of Paget's disease has been found to correlate reasonably well with serum alkaline phosphatase activity (an index of osteoblastic activity) and urinary hydroxyproline excretion (an index of bone matrix resorption). Patients with very limited active disease have normal biochemical parameters, whereas increases of 50-fold greater than normal sometimes occur in patients with polyostotic disease of greatest extent. The serum calcium concentration is normal except in patients who are immobilized or in whom malignancy or primary hyperparathyroidism develops. Hypercalciuria precedes hypercalcemia in these patients. Hyperuricemia, with or without clinical gout, is sometimes found and may reflect increased turnover of purines.

MEDICAL AND SURGICAL THERAPY

CALCITONIN. Most patients with Paget's disease do not require any therapy or may only require analgesic agents such as aspirin or indomethacin. Effective and safe therapy of Paget's disease only became possible in 1975 with the availability of salmon calcitonin. Subcutaneous injections of 50 to 100 MRC units daily or on alternate days produce an average decrease of 50 per cent in biochemical parameters and improve many of the manifestations of the disease. Relief of bone pain, healing of osteolytic lesions, reduction of increased cardiac output and elevated skin temperature, stabilization of auditory acuity, and reversal of various neurologic deficits have all been convincingly documented during chronic therapy. Treatment may be necessary for years in patients with active osteolytic lesions. Side effects include nausea, facial flushing, and polyuria, but they seldom require interruption of therapy. Salmon calcitonin elicits an antibody response in more than 50 per cent of patients, since its amino acid sequence differs considerably from human calcitonin. Approximately 25 per cent of patients acquire high enough antibody titers to become resistant to hormone action. These patients respond to human calcitonin (still experimental in the United States) or to other forms of therapy.

DIPHOSPHONATES. An alternate form of therapy is disodium etidronate, whose main advantage is its oral mode of administration. At a dose of 5 mg per kilogram of body weight daily for an initial treatment period of six months this drug produces benefits similar to calcitonin. However, healing of osteolytic lesions has seldom been documented. Long-term use of higher doses should be avoided because of impairment of bone mineralization and resulting susceptibility to fracture.

CYTOTOXIC AGENTS. Mithramycin is a cytotoxic antibiotic which has not been approved for therapy of Paget's disease by the FDA but has been used in selected patients because of its great potency. Dosage has not been standardized but intravenous infusions of 10 to 15 μg per kilogram daily for 10 days or once weekly have been reported to suppress many of the manifestations of the disease. The platelet, renal, and hepatic toxicity of this agent warrants great caution in its use. It should be reserved for patients with marked symptomatology who fail with other agents.

The effectiveness of medical therapy can usually be assessed by measurement of serum alkaline phosphatase activity alone at intervals of two to four months. The appropriate duration of therapy varies in respect to the type of lesions encountered in the patient and the specific drug administred.

Surgery is an important adjunct to medical therapy in selected patients. Occipital craniectomy may be necessary in patients with basilar impression, and decompression of neurologic structures affected by vertebral lesions is another procedure of critical importance. More commonly orthopedic procedures are required to enable more normal ambulation in patients with pelvic and lower extremity disease. Degenerative arthritis of the hip is a common complication that can produce severe pain and limit ambulation. Results of total hip replacement are excellent. Deformity of the tibia may also limit ambulation because of knee and ankle pain. Tibial osteotomy leading to restoration of a more normal knee-ankle alignment can also markedly alleviate joint pain and restore a near normal gait. If possible 1 to 3 months of medical therapy should be administered prior to surgery in order to reduce the amount of intra- and postoperative bleeding and to prevent immobilization hypercalcemia postoperatively.

Altman RD, Singer FR: Proceedings of the Kroc foundation conference on Paget's disease of bone. Arthritis Rheum 23:1073, 1980. *A comprehensive coverage of etiologic, metabolic, and therapeutic aspects of the disease.*

Barry H: Paget's Disease of Bone. Baltimore, Williams & Wilkins Company, 1969. *A general review of Paget's disease written by an orthopedic surgeon and emphasizing surgical and neoplastic aspects of the disease.*

Mills BG, Singer FR, Weiner LP, Suffin SC, Stabile E, Holst P: Evidence for both respiratory syncytial virus and measles virus antigens in the osteoclasts of patients with Paget's disease of bone. Clin Orth Rel Res 183:303, 1984. *A study documenting antigens of two paramyxoviridae viruses in osteoclasts of Paget's disease.*

Nagant De Deuxchaisnes C, Krane SM: Paget's disease of bone; clinical and metabolic observations. Medicine 43:233, 1964. *Excellent review of clinical and metabolic features of Paget's disease.*

Singer FR: Paget's Disease of Bone. New York, Plenum Press, 1977. *A monograph written for the practitioner that emphasizes clinical manifestations of the disease and the approach to therapy.*

251. OSTEONECROSIS, OSTEOSCLEROSIS, AND OTHER DISORDERS OF BONE

Gordon J. Strewler

OSTEONECROSIS

Osteonecrosis is synonymous with aseptic or avascular necrosis of bone; these terms describe infarction of bone, presumably resulting from ischemia. Such infarcts may be asymptomatic or associated with self-limited pain if they occur in the shaft, as in sickle cell disease or hyperbaric injury (caisson disease). Syndromes with greater morbidity occur with infarcts of subarticular bone, especially in the femoral head.

ETIOLOGY. The most common cause of osteonecrosis is fracture or dislocation of the femoral neck. Other bones susceptible to post-traumatic osteonecrosis are the proximal pole of the carpal scaphoid and the body of the talus. Nontraumatic vascular compromise, usually of the femoral head, is the likely cause of osteonecrosis in sickle cell disease (sludging of sickled erythrocytes), caisson disease (gas bubble emboli), Gaucher's disease (obstruction by histiocytes), hemophilia, and polycythemia vera. Other important etiologies are glucocorticoid therapy, cytotoxic chemotherapy, radiation injury, and renal transplantation. The prevalence of osteonecrosis after renal transplantation ranges from 3 to 41 per cent in various reports. In addition to corticosteroid therapy, precedent renal osteodystrophy and persistent secondary hyperparathyroidism may be etiologic factors. Osteonecrosis is associated with alcoholism, chronic pancreatitis, hyperuricemia, and diabetes mellitus, but diabetics seem to be relatively protected against its development after renal transplantation. The epiphyseal regions of growing bone in children are susceptible to osteonecrosis; here the relative roles of constitutional factors and trauma are poorly defined. Over 50 eponymic syndromes, collectively called osteochondroses, are associated with osteonecrosis at various epiphyseal sites. The commonest, once again, is the femoral head (Perthes' disease).

PATHOGENESIS. While in some disorders (e.g., sickle cell disease), osteonecrosis can readily be ascribed to vascular obstruction, in others, such as glucocorticoid excess, its cause is unknown. There is little support for such proposed mechanisms of steroid-induced osteonecrosis as increased intramedullary pressure with obstruction of venous outflow, fat embol-

ization, or osteopenia with nonhealing microfractures. Also poorly understood are the mechanisms by which infarction of bone leads to its eventual collapse. Dead bone does not lose mechanical stability; bone resorption occurring as part of the reparative process may weaken the infarcted area, predisposing the infarcted bone to fractures and fragmentation.

CLINICAL MANIFESTATIONS. Besides the femoral head, common sites of nontraumatic osteonecrosis include the femoral condyles, distal tibia, humeral head, and talus. The presenting symptom is pain, often of acute onset. Radiologic diagnosis may be delayed for weeks or months because dead and living bone are radiologically indistinguishable. It is mostly slow reparative processes that are visualized radiographically. Patchy lucencies reflect resorption, whereas linear subchondral lucencies reflect collapse of bone; patchy sclerosis indicates growth of new bone over the scaffolding of dead trabeculae. These reparative processes may lead to healing if fragmentation or collapse of weakened bone does not supervene. Initial therapy consists of avoidance of weight bearing, but surgery, such as transpositional osteotomy, arthrotomy with removal of fragments, or arthroplasty, may be required.

Davidson JK (ed.): Aseptic Necrosis of Bone. New York, American Elsevier, 1976. *Review of the radiology and pathology of osteonecrosis, with chapters on traumatic, dysbaric, and hemoglobinopathy-related syndromes.*

Glimcher MJ, Kenzora JE: The biology of osteonecrosis of the human femoral head and its clinical implications. III. Discussion of the etiology and genesis of the pathological sequelae; comments on treatment. Clin Orthop 140:273, 1979. *A thoughtful review of the pathogenesis of osteonecrosis and its clinical implications.*

DISORDERS OF INCREASED BONE DENSITY

Radiographic evidence of increased bone density usually reflects increased bone mass per unit volume, rather than increased mineral per unit of bone mass. This increase can result from accelerated synthesis and mineralization of the bone matrix or from decreased bone resorption. The pathogenesis of such disorders is rarely known, and their histologic characteristics are often indistinguishable; hence, they are classified in the accompanying table on the basis of their radiographic appearance. In the table the term osteosclerosis refers

TABLE 251–1. CAUSES OF OSTEOSCLEROSIS*

A. Osteosclerosis found predominantly in spongy trabecular bone
- Neoplastic causes (prostatic carcinoma, breast carcinoma, gastrointestinal adenocarcinoma, carcinoid tumors, transitional cell carcinoma, myeloma, lymphoma, leukemia)
- Hematologic causes (sickle cell disorders, systemic mastocytosis, myelofibrosis, polycythemia vera)
- Metabolic causes (renal osteodystrophy, Paget's disease, primary hyperparathyroidism, fluorosis, vitamin D-resistant rickets)

B. Osteosclerosis involving cortical and trabecular bone
- Osteopetrosis
  - Malignant (congenita)
  - Benign (tarda)
- Pyknodysostosis
- Sclerosteosis

C. Osteosclerosis found predominantly in compact cortical bone
- Hypertrophic osteoarthropathy
- Pachydermoperiostosis
- Vitamin A intoxication
- Progressive diaphyseal dysplasia (Camurati-Engelmann disease)
- Hereditary hyperphosphatasia
- Endosteal hyperostosis
  - Van Buchem's disease (hyperostosis corticalis generalisata)
  - Autosomal dominant (Worth's disease)

D. Focal osteosclerosis
- Osteopoikilosis
- Osteopathia striata
- Melorheostosis

*Adapted from Genant HK: Review of the osteoscleroses. *In* Margulis AR, Gooding CA (eds.): Diagnostic Radiology. San Francisco, University of California, 1981, pp 109–122.

to increased bone density; as indicated, sclerosis can involve predominantly cortical or trabecular (cancellous) bone or both. Sclerosis of the cortex can produce increased width as the result of new bone formation, and this is sometimes referred to as hyperostosis. Bone shape can also be altered by disorders of modeling, the process by which bones assume their adult shape during development.

Trabecular Osteosclerosis

This form of osteosclerosis is the most frequently encountered. Its causes can be categorized as neoplastic, hematologic, or metabolic.

Neoplastic. Prostatic and breast carcinoma, as well as other neoplasms with osteoblastic metastases, can present on occasion as diffuse osteosclerosis; however, localized blastic or lytic areas are generally also present and permit radiologic diagnosis of malignancy. Generalized osteosclerosis is a rare presentation of myeloma and other hematologic malignancies.

Hematologic. In 40 per cent of cases of agnogenic myeloid metaplasia with myelofibrosis, diffuse skeletal sclerosis is seen. Osteosclerosis is also preceded by myelofibrosis when it occurs in mastocytosis and polycythemia vera. Sickle cell disease is manifested in bone by sclerosis, medullary bone infarcts, and subchondral osteonecrosis.

Metabolic. Renal osteodystrophy characteristically gives rise to sclerosis of the vertebral end-plates—the "rugger-jersey" spine—and to trabecular sclerosis in the metaphyses of long bones and the skull (Ch. 248). Cortical erosions of secondary hyperparathyroidism are also typically present. Diffuse osteosclerosis is an unusual presentation of Paget's disease and is rare in primary hyperparathyroidism. Fluorosis occurs endemically in areas of India and Africa where the fluoride content of water is high, following industrial exposure in aluminum and fertilizer plants, and, increasingly, in individuals treated for osteoporosis (see Ch. 249). Uniform sclerosis of bone is accompanied by exostoses and roughened cortical calcifications at muscle and ligamentous insertions, which suggest the diagnosis. Periarticular pain and limitation of motion are common. Histologically, thick trabeculae are covered by wide osteoid seams, which indicate the presence of osteomalacia.

Cortical and Trabecular Osteosclerosis

Osteopetrosis

Osteopetrosis (Albers-Schönberg disease or marble bone disease), a rare disorder of greatly increased bone density, occurs in several distinct forms. The malignant, autosomal recessive form (osteopetrosis congenita) results in replacement of the marrow space with bone, which causes anemia, infection, and early death. The benign, autosomal dominant form (osteopetrosis tarda) may be asymptomatic and rarely limits survival. A mild form with autosomal recessive rather than dominant inheritance is characterized by renal tubular acidosis and absence of the isozyme carbonic anhydrase II in erythrocytes. In obligate heterozygotes for this disorder, carbonic anhydrase II activity is half of normal. This is undoubtedly an important clue to the nature of osteoclast dysfunction in these individuals.

PATHOLOGY. Osteosclerosis results from defective osteoclast function with a failure of normal bone resorption. The medullary cavity is occupied by thickened bone trabeculae with central zones of entrapped calcified cartilage, which indicate a failure to resorb the primary spongiosa. Osteoclasts are abundant. In some cases defective osteoclast function is suggested by the absence of a ruffled border, the redundantly invaginated membrane structure normally adjacent to bone in actively resorbing osteoclasts.

MALIGNANT OSTEOPETROSIS. The malignant, autosomal recessive form of osteopetrosis presents in infancy with failure to thrive and delayed development. Proptosis, blindness, and frequently deafness and hydrocephalus ensue before age two,

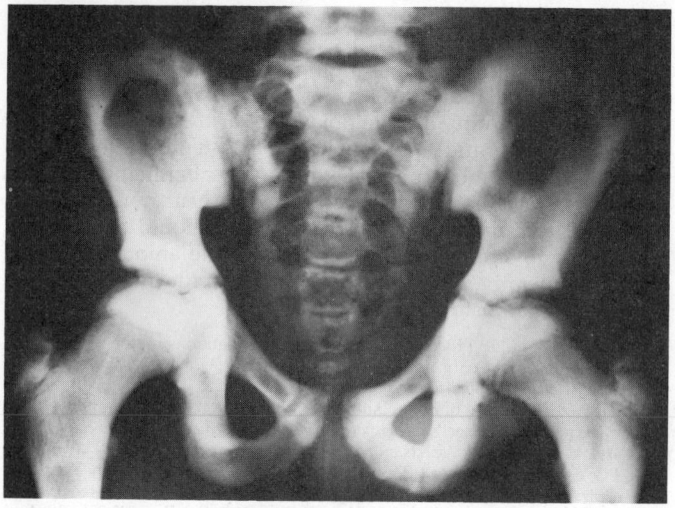

Figure 251–1. Roentgenogram of the pelvis of a teenager with the benign, autosomal recessive form of osteopetrosis.

as bone encroaches upon the cranial foramina. Despite its solid appearance, osteopetrotic bone is fragile, and fractures are frequent. Osteomyelitis is common. Obliteration of the marrow space causes extramedullary hematopoiesis, with hepatosplenomegaly and hypersplenism. Leukoerythroblastic anemia and thrombocytopenia are accompanied by elevated acid and alkaline phosphatase levels and, on occasion, hypocalcemia. Radiologically, the bone is everywhere sclerotic, often with metaphyseal bands of increased density. The long bones are poorly modeled and clublike; ragged metaphyseal-epiphyseal junctions may suggest rickets. Untreated, malignant osteopetrosis results in death from infection, bleeding, or anemia.

BENIGN OSTEOPETROSIS. This autosomal dominant variant is asymptomatic in about half of cases and is usually detected in family studies or as an incidental radiologic finding. The remainder of patients present with fractures of brittle osteopetrotic bone (about 40 per cent) or with osteomyelitis, usually of the mandible. Radiographically, the picture resembles that in the malignant form, but bones are well-modeled (Fig. 251–1). The only laboratory abnormality is an increased acid phosphatase level in some patients.

TREATMENT. Several animal models of osteopetrosis are available. The observation that the disease in mice and rats could be cured by transplantation of marrow or spleen cells has led to the successful use of bone marrow transplantation from HLA-identical sibs for treatment of malignant, autosomal recessive osteopetrosis. Establishment of a chimeric state is accompanied by remarkable regression of osteosclerosis and the reversal of anemia and incomplete nerve deficits. Defective function of killer T cells, which may predispose to infectious complications, may also be reversed by marrow transplantation. A conceptual by-product of these experiments has been the demonstration that the osteoclast originates from hematopoietic elements, thus ending a long debate about its ancestry.

Pyknodysostosis

This disease has only recently been distinguished from osteopetrosis. Inherited as an autosomal recessive trait, it is characterized by short stature and generalized osteosclerosis and is distinguished from osteopetrosis by several additional features: an obtuse mandibular angle with receding chin, multiple wormian bones with persistently open cranial fontanelles, and hypoplasia of terminal phalanges and clavicles. Fractures are common. Toulouse-Lautrec is thought to have suffered from pyknodysostosis.

Cortical Osteosclerosis

Hypertrophic Osteoarthropathy

This term describes subperiosteal formation of new bone in the long bones, secondary to some other condition. It usually occurs in conjunction with digital clubbing and arthritis (see

Ch. 461). The etiologies include pulmonary, hepatic, and intestinal disease. Bronchogenic carcinoma (except small cell carcinoma) is the commonest cause of hypertrophic osteoarthropathy and of clubbing; other causes of hypertrophic pulmonary osteoarthropathy are pleural tumors, lung abscesses, and empyema. Hypertrophic osteoarthropathy occurs in as many as 30 per cent of patients with chronic liver disease, often without clubbing. It is occasionally seen in ulcerative colitis and regional enteritis. Hypertrophic osteoarthropathy is unusual in cyanotic congenital heart disease, although clubbing is typically observed.

Hypertrophic osteoarthropathy is usually confined to the distal tibia and fibula and the distal radius and ulna. When advanced, it may involve other bones. However, it rarely involves the distal phalanges, even in the presence of clubbing. Bone pain, tenderness, and soft tissue swelling may be present, but the condition is sometimes asymptomatic. The periosteum is thickened, and subperiosteal formation of new bone is radiographically evident. Initially present as a separate stripe, new bone may eventually fuse with the cortex. The differential diagnosis includes pachydermoperiostosis, hypervitaminosis A, syphilis, and polyarteritis nodosa. The pathogenesis is unknown. However, blood flow to affected extremities is increased, and the condition sometimes responds to vagotomy; these findings suggest that central reflex changes may be operative.

Pachydermoperiostosis

Pachydermoperiostosis is an autosomal dominant condition in which periosteal formation of new bone occurs from puberty in the same distribution as in secondary hypertrophic osteoarthropathy. Also classically present are marked clubbing and thickened, oily skin. Facial features are coarse, and the thickened forehead and scalp are often marked by transverse folds (cutis verticis gyrata). The appearance may superficially resemble acromegaly. Pachydermoperiostosis is differentiated from secondary hypertrophic osteoarthropathy by the family history and lack of an antecedent cause.

Vitamin A Intoxication (Ch. 217)

Previously witnessed mostly in abusers of vitamins, this disorder is being seen more often, sometimes with hypercalcemia, in those treated with 13-cis-retinoic acid for cystic acne, ichthyosis, or malignancy. The characteristic periosteal new bone is often seen as a fusiform excrescence on the midshaft.

Progressive Diaphyseal Dysplasia

This rare disorder, also known as Camurati-Engelmann disease, is inherited as an autosomal trait. Classically, it is manifest in childhood by a thin body habitus, muscle wasting and weakness with a waddling gait, and bone pain. Serum biochemistry is usually normal, but the alkaline phosphatase level may be increased; the erythrocyte sedimentation rate is also elevated. X-rays show characteristic hyperostosis of the diaphyseal cortices with symmetrical fusiform enlargement of the long bones. The skull is sometimes involved. These changes progress with time, at a pace that slows in adulthood. Bone pain and muscle weakness sometimes respond to corticosteroids, but the bony changes do not. Like other autosomal dominant traits, progressive diaphyseal dysplasia exhibits considerable phenotypic variation; asymptomatic individuals and a mild adult variant (Ribbing disease) are common.

Hereditary Hyperphosphatasia

Hereditary hyperphosphatasia has also been called congenital hyperphosphatasia, osteoectasia with hyperphosphatasia, and juvenile Paget's disease; the last, however, is a poor term since Paget's disease is probably not heritable. Children affected by this rare, crippling, autosomal recessive condition present before age two with an enlarging skull, bowing of the extremities, bone pain, and fractures. Alkaline and acid phosphatase levels and the urinary hydroxyproline level are greatly increased. The calvaria is thickened, with focal densities that resemble cotton-wool balls. Elsewhere, bones are thickened symmetrically and may be demineralized, sometimes with loss of the normal cortex. Several patients have responded dramatically to calcitonin.

Endosteal Hyperostosis

This disease occurs in autosomal recessive (van Buchem's disease, hyperostosis corticalis generalisata) and dominant forms. The distinguishing feature is asymptomatic enlargement of the mandible from childhood, with sclerosis of the skull and thickening of the diaphyseal cortices of long bones.

Focal Osteosclerosis

Osteopoikilosis is an asymptomatic, autosomal dominant trait. Pea-sized sclerotic spots, prominent in the metaphyseal area, are accompanied in some kindreds by unique cutaneous lesions (dermatofibrosis lenticularis disseminata). These are yellowish papules or plaques with increased elastin. The combination is known as the Buschke-Ollendorff syndrome. *Osteopathia striata,* another autosomal dominant disorder of the sclerosing type, is usually asymptomatic and is characterized by symmetrical, parallel arrays of fine streaks in the long bones and pelvis. *Melorheostosis* is a progressive, painful disorder in which discrete hyperostotic areas appear to flow down the long bones like dripping wax. No hereditary predisposition is evident.

Beighton P, Cremin BJ: Sclerosing Bone Dysplasias. New York, Springer-Verlag, 1980. *A radiographic atlas with useful comments on nosology and a good bibliography.*

Coccia PF, Krivit W, Cervenka J, Clawson C, Kersey JH, Kim TH, Nesbit ME, Ramsay NCK, Warkentin PI, Teitelbaum SL, Kahn AJ, Brown DM: Successful bone-marrow transplantation for infantile malignant osteopetrosis. N Engl J Med 302:701, 1980. *The first successful treatment of this disorder.*

Murray RO, Jacobson HG: The Radiology of Skeletal Disorders: Exercises in Diagnosis. 2nd ed. Vol. 4. Edinburgh, Churchill Livingstone, 1977. *The question-answer format and a charming prose style make this an eminently readable book.*

Schneerson JM: Digital clubbing and hypertrophic osteoarthropathy: The underlying mechanisms. Br J Dis Chest 75:113, 1981. *A review of clubbing and hypertrophic osteoarthropathy, with 180 references.*

Sly WS, Hewett-Emmett D, Whyte MP, Yu Y-SL, Tashian RE: Carbonic anhydrase II deficiency identified as the primary defect in the autosomal recessive syndrome of osteopetrosis with renal tubular acidosis and cerebral calcification. Proc Natl Acad Sci USA 80:2752, 1983. *Elucidation of the probable pathogenesis of one variant of osteopetrosis.*

OTHER DISORDERS OF BONE

Fibrous Dysplasia

Fibrous dysplasia occurs in both monostotic and polyostotic forms. The latter is often associated with cutaneous café au lait spots and precocious pseudopuberty in females, and this triad is called Albright's syndrome (also the McCune-Albright syndrome).

The etiology of fibrous dysplasia is unknown. It is not heritable. Individual lesions are composed of dense fibrous tissue in medullary bone, interspersed with thin bone trabeculae (often covered by wide osteoid seams) and sometimes islands of cartilage. Radiographically, the lesions have a multilocular appearance beneath a thinned cortex (Fig. 251–2). Within, they have the appearance of ground glass, owing to their fine trabeculation. Although monostotic and polyostotic forms are histologically indistinguishable, monostotic lesions are not associated with an endocrinopathy. They commonly involve the proximal femur, tibia, or ribs, may occur at any age, and can cause bone pain, fractures, or deformity. Malignant transformation occurs in about 1 per cent of lesions.

Polyostotic fibrous dysplasia usually presents between the ages of 3 and 10. It may involve over 50 per cent of the skeleton and frequently produces "shepherd's-crook" deformity of the femur and discrepancies in leg length; skull involvement may cause gross facial disfigurement (leontiasis ossea). Fractures are common. Serum biochemistry is frequently normal except for elevation of the alkaline phosphatase level. The café au lait spots sometimes seen in polyostotic fibrous dysplasia have

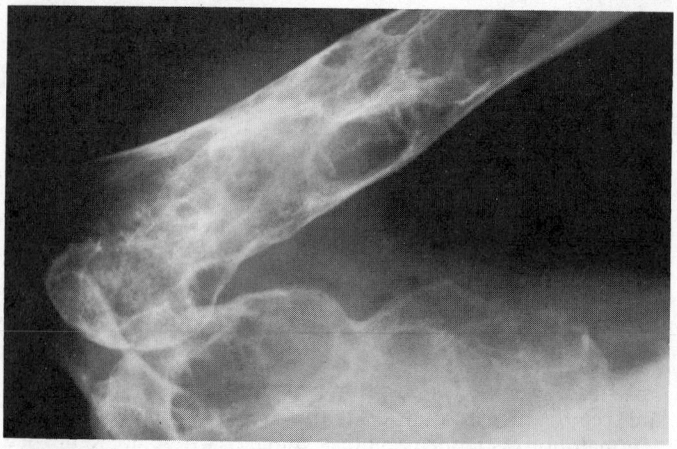

Figure 251–2. Roentgenogram of the humerus and scapula of a patient with extensive polyostotic fibrous dysplasia. Both bones are extensively involved with typical lesions.

jagged borders that Albright likened to the coast of Maine, to distinguish them from those in neurofibromatosis, which have smooth borders like the coast of California.

About half of girls with polyostotic fibrous dysplasia undergo precocious pseudopuberty, which may precede detection of the bony abnormality. Precocious pseudopuberty has also been reported in a few boys with this syndrome. Sexual maturation in both sexes is associated with low gonadotropin levels, and fertility does not occur (hence, it is termed *pseudo*puberty). Histologically, the ovaries display multiple follicle cysts. Several other endocrinopathies have been described in Albright's syndrome; these include hyperthyroidism (in about 20 per cent), gigantism with acromegaly, and Cushing's syndrome. Levels of thyroid-stimulating hormone (TSH) are suppressed in hyperthyroidism associated with Albright's syndrome, and adrenocorticotropic hormone (ACTH) is likewise suppressed when adrenal hyperfunction occurs in Albright's syndrome. In all these glands, which thus function autonomously, receptors for the respective tropic hormones—luteinizing hormone (LH), follicle-stimulating hormone (FSH), TSH, and ACTH—are coupled to adenylate cyclase. However, the nature of the regulatory defect remains to be defined and may be unrelated to the receptor-adenylate cyclase system.

In addition to these disorders of endocrine hyperfunction, hypophosphatemic osteomalacia has been described in association with Albright's syndrome.

Hereditary Multiple Exostoses

This relatively common disorder (also called diaphyseal aclasis) is inherited as an autosomal dominant trait with high penetrance. Irregular bony excrescences protrude from the expanded metaphyses of the long bones. These osteocartilaginous exostoses arise from the growth plate and grow as the bone does. They may subsequently become isolated from the epiphysis or remain in continuity, but they reproduce normal structure, with an outer cortex and an inner spongiosa continuous with that of the bone of origin. Growth ceases in adulthood. Disability results principally from limb-length discrepancies: linear bone growth decreases as the bone grows transversely. Less common are syndromes of nerve, spinal cord, and vascular compression. The exostoses undergo sarcomatous degeneration in 3 to 10 per cent of affected individuals, and this must be suspected when a lesion enlarges rapidly, especially during adulthood.

Enchondromatosis (Dyschondroplasia, Ollier's Disease)

A sporadic condition, enchondromatosis becomes symptomatic in childhood as multiple, growing, cartilaginous masses within the trabecular bone, which produce swelling and interfere with linear bone growth. As with cartilaginous exostoses, these arise from the growth plate, growth ceases at puberty, and replacement of cartilage by mature bone may follow. Enchondromas appear radiologically as radiolucent defects in the metaphyseal area of the tubular and flat bones, often with central calcific stippling. The affected area may be expanded, with thinning of the cortex. Enchondromatosis must be distinguished from hereditary exostoses and from fibrous dysplasia. Malignant degeneration is uncommon. When enchondromatosis is associated with multiple hemangiomas (Maffucci's syndrome), the enchondromas or hemangiomas undergo malignant transformation in 15 per cent of cases.

Achondroplasia

Chondrodystrophies are disorders of cartilaginous growth that typically eventuate in disproportionate short stature. The commonest of them is achondroplasia. Affected individuals are easily recognizable: the limbs are short; the trunk is of relatively normal length; and the head is large, with a bulging forehead and scooped-out nose. Achondroplasia is inherited as an autosomal dominant trait. About 80 per cent of cases represent new mutations; the mutation rate increases with paternal age. To account for short bones and a shortened cranial base but a normal cranial vault, the mutation must affect endochondral ossification, as in the limbs and chondrocranium, but not membranous ossification, as in the vault. Surprisingly, the growth plate is not grossly disorganized histologically and chondrocytes are normal ultrastructurally—the pathogenesis of achondroplasia remains an enigma. Radiographically, the cranial base and foramen magnum are small, lumbar lordosis is greatly exaggerated, and the lumbar spinal canal narrows from the upper to lower lumbar spine, as indicated by a decreasing interpeduncular distance. The long bones appear massive, owing to their disproportionately normal width. Complications can include hydrocephalus, presumably related to the small size of the foramen magnum, and spinal cord and root compression, a potential consequence of even minimal impingement by a disk or osteophyte upon the small spinal canal. Reproductive potential is limited by social factors as well as cephalopelvic disproportion. Despite its problems, achondroplasia is compatible with good health and a normal lifespan.

Grabias SL, Campbell CJ: Fibrous dysplasia. Orthop Clin North Am 8:771, 1977. *A review of clinical, radiologic, and orthopedic aspects of monostotic and polyostotic forms of fibrous dysplasia.*

McKusick VA: Heritable Disorders of Connective Tissue. 4th ed. St. Louis, CV Mosby, 1972. *This scholarly, profusely illustrated book remains an excellent source for the inherited diseases of bone.*

Rimoin DL: The chondrodystrophies. Adv Hum Genet 5:1, 1975. *Achondroplasia and a host of less common causes of disproportionate short stature are discussed.*

252. BONE TUMORS

Henry J. Mankin

PRIMARY TUMORS OF BONE

Primary bone tumors are uncommon but they are important since they are most frequent in the young (the second to the fourth decades) and they tend to be extraordinarily malignant. Beyond their random occurrence, bone tumors have been associated with (1) genetic disorders of preosseous cartilage (hereditary multiple osteocartilaginous exostoses and enchondromatosis), (2) radiation injury, (3) Paget's disease, (4) bone infarcts, and (5) chronic osteomyelitis.

CLASSIFICATION AND STAGING

Any connective tissue element that exists in the osseous or preosseous skeleton can be the cell of origin of a neoplastic process; both benign and malignant tumors may be classified according to cell type as osseous, cartilaginous, fibrous, and "other" (including vascular, neural, marrow, lipid, and tumors of unspecified origin). Furthermore, within each broad category, several radiologically, histologically, and biologically distinct types of tumors exist, providing a sometimes puzzling array of diagnoses from which to choose for a patient who presents with an obvious radiographic lesion.

Prior to treatment, all primary bone tumors must be "staged" in order to assess the local extent of the lesion (T), the grade of the tumor (G), and the presence or absence of distant metastases (M). The determination of T is best done by physical examination, radiographs, and special imaging studies, including angiography, computerized and planar tomography, and ^{99m}Tc bone scanning. The grade of the tumor can only be determined by study of biopsy material using both standard and specialized techniques. Since most bone tumors metastasize to the lungs and occasionally other bones, full lung tomograms or computerized tomography of the chest and a bone scan are required to establish "M."

BENIGN BONE TUMORS

Most benign tumors of bone present as a mass or deformity detectable on physical examination, as an incidental finding on a radiograph, or occasionally as a result of a pathologic fracture through a weakened area of the bone. With few exceptions, benign lesions are small and painless. For some, the radiographic features are so characteristic as to be easily recognizable. Benign bone tumors show well-defined cortical margins, absence of a soft tissue mass, and sclerotic bony margination separating the lesion from the normal tissues. Some lesions may require biopsy for definition, and some, particularly those that threaten the integrity of the skeleton, require treatment, which for most of these lesions is "intralesional" (such as simple excision or curettage and packing of the defect with auto- or allograft bone), resulting in a "cure" in a high percentage of the cases.

MALIGNANT PRIMARY TUMORS OF BONE

Multiple myeloma, the most common primary malignancy of bone, is discussed in Ch. 163. Other primary malignant tumors of bone are rare. The majority of these are osteosarcoma and (depending on the age group studied) chondrosarcoma; round cell tumors (Ewing's sarcoma and primary lymphoma of bone), giant cell tumors, and malignant fibrous tumors follow in order of diminishing frequency.

OSTEOSARCOMA. The peak age of incidence for osteosarcoma is in the second decade with a second lesser peak occurring in later years (in association with Paget's disease). The tumor has a predilection for the distal femur or proximal tibia of the rapidly growing child and occurs more frequently in males. Osteosarcoma in later life usually occurs as a complication of Paget's disease, irradiation injury of bone, or a bone infarct.

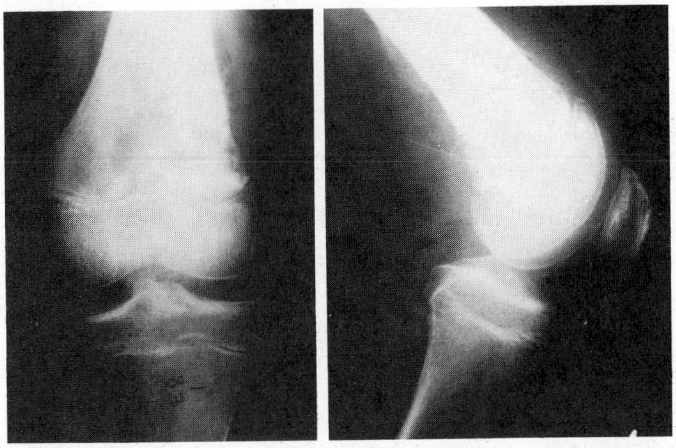

Figure 252–1. Anteroposterior lateral radiographs of the distal femur of a 10-year-old girl, showing the classic picture of an osteosarcoma. Note the destruction and blastic productive changes both within the bone and in the adjacent soft tissue mass, which is seen best extending posteriorly on the lateral film.

Pain, limitation of movement, and swelling are the principal complaints, and even at earliest observation, the radiographic findings show obvious destruction and a soft tissue mass outside the bone (Fig. 252–1). Productive changes within and without the bone suggest the presence of the osteosarcoma. Typically, the serum alkaline phosphatase level is markedly elevated. Fully one fourth of patients have metastases to the lungs at the time of the initial examination or shortly after. If left untreated, the course is fulminant with a rapid progression of the tumor, widespread metastases, and death in less than a year.

Treatment consists of wide excision of the primary tumor, which in many cases will require amputation of the extremity, but in selected instances includes a local resection and limb reconstruction with auto- or allograft or metallic implants. Chemotherapeutic agents such as doxorubicin, high dose methotrexate with citrovorum rescue or cis-platinum or both may improve the prognosis of patients with pulmonary micrometastases, with reported survival figures ranging from 50 to 80 per cent, at three years. Resection of pulmonary nodules in conjunction with aggressive chemotherapy appears to be successful in effecting cure in over 20 per cent of the patients so treated.

ROUND CELL SARCOMA. *Ewing's sarcoma* is a highly malignant tumor of unknown cytogenesis, which primarily affects teenage children and produces a very destructive, lytic tumor often of the pelvis, shaft of the femur, or other long bones. Symptoms and signs include not only local pain, swelling, and a palpable mass, but at times systemic findings such as fever, malaise, chills, and a rapid sedimentation rate. The prognosis for this tumor is particularly poor without treatment, but the lesions, like the lymphomas of bone, are remarkably radiosensitive. The combination of local radiation and chemotherapy provide a long survival rate exceeding 60 per cent. *Non-Hodgkin's lymphoma* and less frequently *Hodgkin's lymphoma* may make their appearance as a bony focus difficult to distinguish radiographically and sometimes histologically from Ewing's sarcoma. Staging of these individuals is essential to be certain that the bony tumor is solitary rather than an osseous focus of diffuse disease. The treatment is similar to that of lymphoma of other sites, depending principally on the radiosensitivity of the primary site and the response of the tumor to chemotherapeutic drugs.

CHONDROSARCOMA. The chondrosarcomas are extraordinarily variable in clinical presentation, degree of malignancy, and biological behavior. Central chondrosarcomas, most prevalent in middle age, occur most frequently in the pelvis and proximal portions of the appendicular skeleton. Both radiation and chemotherapy are relatively ineffective, particularly for large tumors. With accurate staging, however, surgery may produce a cure in up to 85 per cent of patients, depending on the stage of the disease.

METASTATIC TUMORS OF BONE

Certain of the malignant neoplasms and tumors of the hematopoietic system have a propensity for metastasis to the skeleton. At times, the presenting complaint for a patient with a primary breast, lung, prostatic, renal, or thyroid carcinoma may be pain in the spine, ribs, or long bones or a pathologic fracture through a metastatic focus. In males, the most frequent source of metastastic carcinoma is carcinoma of the prostate, followed closely by carcinoma of the lung and gastrointestinal tract; in women, carcinoma of the breast is by far the most frequent cause of metastatic bone disease. The frequency of metastatic carcinoma far exceeds that of primary tumors of bone, especially in later life, so that staging of any individual with a bone tumor should include a careful clinical, imaging, and laboratory evaluation of the more frequent sites of origin.

Conversely, patients who are under treatment for primary tumors of the organs just cited should have frequent bone scans, which are far more sensitive than radiographs in revealing the presence of distant metastases.

Radiographic findings in metastatic bone disease vary with the type of primary tumor and the bony site involved, but almost always the tumorous deposits are in the axial and proximal appendicular skeleton, are centrally placed within the bone, and are quite destructive in appearance. About 90 per cent of prostatic, 50 per cent of breast, and 25 per cent of lung carcinomatous metastases evoke a sclerotic response in the affected bone producing a mottled increase in osseous density on the radiograph. The treatment of skeletal metastases from a primary carcinoma depends on the patient's general condition, the radiosensitivity of the lesion, the site and extent of involvement, and the proximity of the tumor to vital structures such as the spinal cord. Regression and long-term remission can be achieved in some patients with carcinoma of the prostate and breast simply with the use of hormones and radiation (see Ch. 235 and 239). When the integrity of the skeletal system is threatened or a pathologic fracture of a long bone has occured, prophylactic or therapeutic open reduction and internal fixation is clearly indicated and frequently provides the patient with considerable relief of pain and restoration of function.

Enneking WF: Musculoskeletal Tumor Society. New York, Churchill Livingston, 1983. *A comprehensive text detailing the principles and technical aspects of surgical management of bone tumors.*

Huvos AG: Bone Tumors, Diagnosis, Treatment and Progress. Philadelphia, W.B. Saunders Company, 1979. *A detailed text describing the classification system, radiologic characteristics, and pathologic patterns for a variety of benign and malignant bone tumors.*

Mankin HJ: Current concept in cancer: Advances in diagnosis and treatment of bone tumors. N Engl J Med 300:543, 1979. *A review article on recent trends in diagnosis and management of bone tumors.*

Part XIX
INFECTIOUS DISEASES
Section One INTRODUCTION

253. INTRODUCTION TO MICROBIAL DISEASES

Charles C. J. Carpenter

Those diseases for which specific cures are possible and for which immunoprophylaxis is available are caused primarily by infectious agents. Throughout the developing world, acute infections, predominantly acute diarrheal illnesses and acute respiratory disease, are by far the leading causes of mortality. In more circumscribed areas of Asia, Africa, and South America, protozoal diseases (especially malaria) and helminthic infections (notably schistosomiasis and onchocerciasis) continue to affect millions of individuals and to cause hundreds of thousands of deaths annually. In the developed world, microbial disease processes remain the most common curable causes of both morbidity and mortality. Pneumococcal pneumonia, although curable by timely antimicrobial therapy, and in large part preventable by immunization of susceptible population groups, remains among the ten leading causes of death in North America. New problems associated with infectious diseases continue to make their appearance in patients immunocompromised by treatment with cytotoxic or immunosuppressive drugs, or both. Such patients are susceptible to life-threatening infections caused by a wide range of opportunistic, normally commensal, microorganisms. The great variety of unusual infections occurring in immunosuppressed patients presents a continuing diagnostic and therapeutic challenge.

Rapid progress has continued in the development and application of vaccines effective against major life-threatening viral illnesses, and the utilization of recombinant deoxyribonucleic acid (DNA) technology and hybridoma-derived antibodies give promise of yielding effective means of preventing additional bacterial, protozoal, and helminthic infections. The eradication of smallpox has been a reality for several years, and more widespread immunization against poliomyelitis has led to further decline in the incidence of this frightening disease. An effective vaccine against hepatitis B became commercially available in 1982 in quantities adequate to immunize the populations at greatest risk in North America. The preparation of the hepatitis B vaccine is unique in that it consists of an antigen derived from the serum of humans with hepatitis B antigenemia, and the lengthy purification process has made the vaccine so expensive as to limit its use to high-risk populations. Concomitant with this development, however, has been the recognition that non-A, non-B hepatitis (presumably caused by two or more viruses, for which there are no specific diagnostic tests) is now the leading cause of post-transfusion hepatitis. The availability of the remarkably effective human diploid cell rabies vaccine has greatly decreased the cost and discomfort of immunization against this uniformly fatal illness; the development of this vaccine has fortuitously occurred concomitantly with an increase in endemic sylvatic rabies in many parts of the United States. Recent in vitro studies give promise, at long last, that the development of an effective antimalarial vaccine, using recombinant DNA technology, is near fruition.

However, despite heartening progress in the prevention and treatment of a number of major microbial illnesses, new infectious diseases continue to appear, and additional previously recognized disease syndromes have been shown to be caused by microbial agents. During the past four years, two additional previously recognized illnesses, Lyme disease and adult T cell leukemia, have been shown to result from infectious processes. Furthermore, the acquired immune deficiency syndrome (AIDS) was first recognized in 1979, and its incidence has increased exponentially since that time. This illness has recently extended beyond the initially recognized susceptible population of male homosexuals, intravenous-drug users, and hemophiliacs. Recently, both children and female sexual partners of male patients with AIDS, as well as occasional transfusion recipients, have, albeit in small numbers, developed this disease. Epidemiologic data suggest that AIDS, which results in virtually complete destruction of cellular immune mechanisms, may result from an infectious agent that resembles hepatitis B in its mode of transmission. Recently, both viral isolation and serologic studies have strongly supported an etiologic role for a retrovirus in AIDS. Human T cell lymphotropic virus type III (HTLV-III) and lymphadenopathy-associated virus (LAV) have been implicated by American and French investigators, respectively, as etiologic agents. Published data do not permit a definite conclusion as to whether or not HTLV-III and LAV are identical, or closely related, retroviruses. Susceptibility to infection and the development of clinical illness following exposure to the putative etiologic virus may, however, be influenced by subclinical immunodeficiency in the groups at greatest risk. For example, male homosexuals are repeatedly exposed to a variety of agents (e.g., cytomegalovirus) that may cause transient impairment of the cellular immune response.

Once the clinical syndrome of AIDS develops, the management of this group of patients poses unique challenges from the standpoint of infectious diseases, since the patients invariably develop multiple serious infections, often with microorganisms that are resistant to available therapeutic agents (e.g., cryptosporidia, *Mycobacterium avium–intracellularis*, disseminated cytomegalovirus). Patients with fully developed AIDS have generally succumbed to the illness within two years after the diagnosis has been established. Although one or more opportunistic infections (e.g., *Pneumocystis carinii*) may respond to appropriate antimicrobial therapy, no therapeutic approach has been effective yet in correcting the defect in cellular immunity. Several trials with potentially helpful agents, including immune interferon and interleukin II, are underway. AIDS represents the most devastating of the health problems that plague the homosexual community, and the ultimate extent of this disease cannot be estimated. The frequent development of an unusually aggressive form of Kaposi's sarcoma in patients with AIDS may provide an important clue as to the relationship between altered immune function and neoplasia.

Microbial diseases have provided original models for critical studies of immune processes; recently, another newly recognized illness, Lyme disease, has been shown to be of infectious etiology and has provided a unique look at the immune interaction between host and parasite. Lyme disease is now known to be caused by a borrelia-like spirochete, which is transmitted by the tick *Ixodes dammini*. Many of the features of Lyme disease mimic those of Reiter's syndrome, another post-infectious, immunologically mediated rheumatologic illness; clinical similarities between certain cases of Lyme disease and rheumatoid arthritis have provided added impetus to the search for an infectious, and therefore potentially eradicable, etiologic agent in rheumatoid arthritis.

Because of the clear-cut etiologic role between certain retroviruses and neoplasia in experimental animals, a search for viral etiologic agents in human cancer has been under way for several decades. The first clear-cut link between a specific virus and human neoplasia has recently been established, with the demonstration of a strong epidemiologic relationship between a unique retrovirus, human T cell leukemia virus, and adult T cell leukemia in three distinct geographic locations (Southern Japan, the Caribbean, and the Southeastern United States). This demonstration provides great impetus to search for chemotherapeutic agents effective against retroviruses. It also encourages a more intensive search for viral etiologic agents in other human neoplastic processes.

In the face of rapid and sometimes bewildering changes,

both in the nature of the infectious diseases with which the clinician is confronted and the therapeutic armamentarium at his disposal, two basic principles continue to guide the physician's approach to patient management. When faced with a sick patient, a physician's primary responsibility is to determine whether or not the illness does indeed represent an acute infectious process—a decision made more complex by such factors as frequent lack of fever in elderly patients with pneumonia, lack of leukocytosis in many patients on cytotoxic drug therapy, and so forth. There is probably no situation in clinical medicine in which the thoughtful attention to all relevant details of the patient's medical history and a meticulous physical examination remain more important to the welfare of the patient. Once a physician has made the decision that a patient has an infectious process, his next responsibility must be to determine whether or not the patient has a potentially fulminant, life-threatening illness, which could cause death within the next few hours in the absence of prompt and appropriate therapy. Such illnesses obviously include such life-threatening diseases as acute bacterial meningitis, falciparum malaria, and gram-negative bacteremia but may also include such generally nonlethal illnesses as acute bacterial pneumonia. Because of the difficulty in determining which infectious processes are potentially death-dealing, it is incumbent on the physician, when faced with a patient with an acute infectious process, to establish a tentative diagnosis as rapidly as possible (e.g., with the use of Gram stained preparation in the case of acute bacterial pneumonia or purulent meningitis) and to initiate specific therapy for the presumed pathogen as rapidly as possible. In no other major group of illnesses is the rapid initiation of appropriate therapy so important as in acute infectious diseases.

Despite the prophylactic and therapeutic advances that have resulted from the rapid evolution of cellular and molecular biology, the microbial world continues to present the thoughtful physician with some of the most perplexing, and potentially rewarding, problems in the practice of medicine.

254. THE FEBRILE PATIENT

Sheldon M. Wolff

Fever is one of the most common symptoms that physicians encounter. In the vast majority of patients the fever is secondary to an infectious process, often viral in origin. In such patients, the febrile state is self-limited and relatively little is needed in terms of diagnostic workup or therapy. However, when the fever persists for more than a few days or is excessively high, a more thorough evaluation is indicated. Certain aspects of the febrile patient are worth emphasizing. For example, fever is *never* the sole manifestation of an illness. Constitutional symptoms such as headache, myalgias, or malaise almost always accompany fever. In addition, except in rare instances, the type or pattern of fever is of no diagnostic value. When a quotidian fever pattern occurs in the proper setting, then malaria should be considered. Furthermore, a Pel-Ebstein pattern should suggest Hodgkin's disease, but is not diagnostic. In fact, viral diseases can cause hectic fevers accompanied by chills and be indistinguishable from the response of patients with bacteremia or fungemia. Thus, when approaching a patient with fever, careful history taking, thorough physical examination, and close observation are all indicated.

Some patients with febrile illnesses will have persistent symptoms (and fever) for more than two weeks despite a thorough evaluation by history, physical examination, and laboratory tests, including appropriate cultures of blood, sputum, urine, and, if indicated, stools. Such patients can be considered to have a fever of unknown origin (FUO), and they require extensive evaluation.

When attempting to determine the cause of a prolonged fever, the wide spectrum of diseases that cause fever must be considered. Factors such as age, social and economic factors, geography, and recent exposure are all important determinants of the causes of prolonged fevers. In the overwhelming majority of FUO patients, an underlying cause is discovered or the patient recovers spontaneously.

CAUSES OF FEVER OF UNKNOWN ORIGIN. ***Infections.*** Approximately one third of all FUO patients will have an infectious etiology to explain their illness. Any infectious agent can be the cause of an FUO, although it is rare for a virus to be the cause of such a condition. Although most will be obvious, self-limited, or responsive to therapy, other infectious diseases may still present as an FUO. In particular, certain sites such as bone, sinuses, heart valves, subphrenic area, biliary tract and the urinary tract may be infected and not provide localizing signs.

Neoplasias. Some tumors are likely to be associated with fever and may present as an FUO. At least 20 per cent of FUO patients will have an underlying tumor as a cause of the FUO. The percentage of such patients is increasing. Examples of such neoplasms include Hodgkin's and other lymphomas, hypernephroma, preleukemia, and atrial myxoma. However, tumors of almost any origin may present as an FUO, and this may occur in the absence of metastases. In addition, the fever may precede the clinical appearance of the underlying disease by weeks or months.

Hypersensitivity Diseases. Although most collagen vascular diseases can present as an FUO, systemic lupus erythematosus, Still's disease (in children and adults), and certain of the systemic necrotizing vasculitides such as temporal arteritis are more likely than others. Certain drug reactions may present as an FUO. Scleroderma is one of the collagen vascular diseases that rarely or never presents as an FUO.

Granulomatous Diseases. There are three major granulomatous diseases of unknown etiology that may present as fevers of unknown origin. The most common of these is sarcoidosis. Most, but not all, sarcoid patients who present with an FUO have extrapulmonary disease often involving the liver. In regional enteritis, fever can sometimes be much more prominent than any gastrointestinal signs or symptoms. Many of the well-known causes of granulomatous hepatitis, such as tuberculosis, sarcoidosis, or systemic fungal infections, can present as an FUO. In addition, there is a separate group of patients with granulomatous hepatitis of unknown cause and FUO. Thus, any FUO patient whose symptoms persist despite thorough noninvasive workup should have a liver biospy.

Inherited Diseases. There are at least four inherited diseases that present as an FUO. The most common of these is familial Mediterranean fever (FMF). Although FMF is most common in Armenians, Sephardic Jews, and Arabs, it can occur in almost any ethnic group. It is in the latter situation that the diagnosis is most often missed and the patient is considered to have an FUO. Patients with an inherited hyperlipidemia (Type 1) may have fever as a presenting complaint. In patients with Fabry's disease, an X-linked inherited error of glycosphingolipid metabolism characterized by telangiectases and lancinating pain, fever may be a prominent sign. Cyclic neutropenia often presents as an FUO, and a small percentage of patients with this disease seem to have a familial form.

Factitious Diseases. A small number of patients who present with an FUO turn out to have a factitious or self-induced illness. In general, these patients are young female adults who are in the health-related professions. Such patients can be roughly separated into two groups. The first consists of patients who feign illness by manipulating thermometers and often have a bona fide febrile illness prior to the onset of their so-called FUO. The second group is predominantly in the third or fourth decade of life, and these patients have more profound psychiatric problems. They will often induce disease and in fact can do themselves considerable harm.

EVALUATION OF THE PATIENT WITH AN FUO. The approach to the patient with an FUO requires an awareness of the myriad etiologies and a willingness to demonstrate a thoroughness in the workup that few other situations in medicine demand. Careful attention to the history is required. Has there been any exposure to infectious agents? Any unusual travel? These and many other questions must be asked. If the answers are positive, then follow-up laboratory procedures will be required. A thorough and complete physical examination is mandatory. Furthermore, repeated attention must be paid to any changes, such as the appearance of septic phenomena in the skin, fundi, nailbeds, or other areas.

Approximately 10 per cent of FUO patients will defy extensive evaluation and continue to have fevers without a diagnosis forthcoming. Such patients require close observation and follow-up, and workups may have to be repeated. A patient with an ongoing active debilitating illness requires earlier re-evaluation than the patient with a chronic, slowly progressive course. The longer a patient has an FUO, the less likely he is to have an infectious or neoplastic cause for the fever.

The laboratory evaluation of the patient with an FUO should be logical and complete. Knowledge of the causes of fever directs the physician toward appropriate laboratory tests. Certain examinations are mandatory such as skin tests, liver function tests, and complete blood counts. However, tests should not be performed just for the sake of completeness if they have little or no chance of providing useful information. Appropriate cultures must be made, but again reason should prevail regarding the number and sites.

Radiographic studies must include the chest, sinuses (if headache or pain is present), the entire gastrointestinal and biliary tracts, and the urinary tract. Radionuclide scanning should be employed after the appropriate x-rays have been obtained. Finally, CT scans and ultrasonography should be obtained when indicated.

If all of these noninvasive procedures have been performed and a diagnosis still has not been made, then invasive procedures must be employed. Bone marrow and liver biopsies should be done. When indicated, other biopsies will prove of value. For example, biopsy of a skin lesion, biopsy of an enlarged node, or temporal artery biopsy may prove useful in selected patients. The availability of needle biopsy techniques and the use of scanning methods and, when indicated, peritoneoscopy make exploratory laparotomy no longer indicated in the evaluation of FUO patients.

Aduan RP, Fauci AS, Dale DC, Herzberg JH, Wolff SM: Factitious fever and self-induced infections. Ann Intern Med 90:230, 1979. *A comprehensive review of a large group of patients with factitious and self-induced diseases.*

Dinarello CA, Wolff SM: Approach to the patient with fever of unknown origin. *In* Mandell G, Bennett JE, Douglas RG (eds.): Principles and Practices of Infectious Diseases, Vol 1. New York, John Wiley & Sons, 1979, pp 421-428. *A detailed discussion of the evaluation and diagnostic procedures to be followed in patients with fevers of unknown origin.*

Dinarello CA, Wolff SM: Fever of unknown origin. *In* Mandell G, Bennett JE, Douglas RG (eds.): Principles and Practices of Infectious Diseases, Vol 1. New York, John Wiley & Sons, 1979, pp 407–421. *A categorization of the types of diseases that can present in patients with fevers of unknown origin.*

Larson EB, Featherstone HJ, Petersdorf RG: Fever of undetermined origin: Diagnosis and follow-up of 105 cases, 1970–1980. Medicine 61:269, 1982. *A comparison by Dr. Petersdorf's group of their recent experience and the data they published in 1961.*

Petersdorf RG, Beeson PB: Fever of unexplained origin. Medicine 40:1, 1961. *The classic paper on fever of unknown origin.*

Wolff SM, Fauci AS, Dale DC: Unusual etiologies of fever and their evaluation. Ann Rev Med 26:277, 1975. *A summary of a 15-year study of a large group of patients with chronic or recurring fevers.*

255. PATHOGENESIS OF FEVER

Charles A. Dinarello

DEFINITION. Fever is an elevation of temperature above the normal amplitude of daily variation. Infections are most commonly associated with fever, but several noninfectious diseases may also have fever as their primary clinical presentation. Although the vast majority of patients with elevated body temperature are experiencing fever, there are a few instances in which elevated temperature is not fever but rather hyperthermia. These include heat stroke syndromes, certain metabolic diseases, and the effects of pharmacologic agents that interfere with thermoregulation.

Fever is best understood at the hypothalamic level, and the home thermostat can be used as an analogy for hypothalamic control of body temperature. The thermoregulatory center located in the anterior hypothalamus regulates internal temperature at about 37° C (98.6° F) primarily by its ability to balance heat production and peripheral heat loss. During fever, the thermostat setting in the hypothalamic center shifts upward, e.g., from 37 to 39° C. This results in signals to increase heat production and decrease peripheral heat loss. Heat production from shivering muscles and heat conservation from peripheral vasoconstriction continue until the temperature of the blood supplying the hypothalamus matches the higher thermostat setting. In contradistinction to fever, the setting of the thermoregulatory center during hyperthermia remains unchanged at normothermic levels, while, in an uncontrolled fashion, body temperature increases and overrides the ability to lose heat. Exogenous heat exposure and endogenous heat production are two mechanisms by which hyperthermia can result in dangerously high internal temperatures. In comparison to fever, hyperthermia is a much rarer cause for elevated body temperature, but it is nevertheless important to make the distinction. Hyperthermia can be rapidly fatal, and its treatment differs from that of fever.

PATHOGENESIS. Several substances in addition to infectious agents have been recognized to cause fever. The most widespread and potent of these is the lipopolysaccharide of gram-negative bacteria, also called *endotoxin.* Endotoxin will produce fever in humans when as little as 2 ng per kilogram is injected intravenously. Other substances that produce fever include toxins from gram-positive bacteria, drugs in sensitized individuals, and incompatible blood products. It has become a custom to refer to endotoxin and other substances that produce fever as *exogenous pyrogens.* Exogenous pyrogens share no common physicochemical structure, are derived from varied sources of microbial and nonmicrobial origin, and, in general, do not directly affect the hypothalamus but rather produce fever through the action of a mediator molecule, *endogenous pyrogen.*

ENDOGENOUS PYROGEN. Endogenous pyrogen, a small molecular weight protein, was first described by Beeson in 1948. Subsequent animal and human studies established the importance of endogenous pyrogen in mediating fever and as being responsible for the upward resetting of the hypothalamic thermostat. This substance is produced in response to infections, toxic substances, or immunologic reactions. It is not species specific, and endogenous pyrogen produced from human cells causes fever in animals. Endogenous pyrogen is a product of phagocytic leukocytes but, unlike other substances released by phagocytes, it is not preformed. Following stimulation by exogenous pyrogens, phagocytes synthesize endogenous pyrogen de novo and release the substance into the circulation. Monocytes, fixed mononuclear phagocytes such as Kupffer cells of the liver, alveolar macrophages, and splenic sinusoidal cells are capable of releasing the pyrogen, but lymphocytes and neutrophils are not. In patients with severe bone marrow depression and no circulating phagocytic cells, the tissue macrophages are a potential source of endogenous pyrogen and may account for the fever observed in these individuals. Studies also suggest that certain tumors produce endogenous pyrogen in vitro. These include human lymphoma cell lines, circulating monocytic leukemia cells, and renal carcinomas. Pyrogen production by certain tumor cells may be one mechanism by which fever is produced in patients with these tumors.

Human subjects injected with endogenous pyrogen made by their blood leukocytes respond with chills and fever. The pyrogen has been demonstrated in sterile pleural, peritoneal, and joint effusions and is readily produced in vitro when human phagocytes are stimulated. The induction of endogenous pyrogen from human phagocytic cells in vitro by a variety of exogenous pyrogens is one of the methods used to study the pathogenesis of fever in humans. Most substances that produce fever when injected into humans induce the release of endogenous pyrogen in vitro.

Animal studies have shown that the preoptic area of the anterior hypothalamus is the primary site of action for the induction of fever by endogenous pyrogen. Thermosensitive cells in the preoptic anterior hypothalamus increase their rate of discharge when endogenous pyrogen is injected. In addition, there is a concomitant rise in the concentration of monoamines and prostaglandins in the third and fourth cerebral ventricles and in the vicinity of the thermoregulatory center. Synthesis of prostaglandins, particularly of the E series, is an important result of the action of endogenous pyrogen on the hypothalamus. Like endogenous pyrogen, prostaglandin E_2 produces fever when injected into the anterior hypothalamus. See Figure 255–1.

ACTION OF ANTIPYRETICS. Aspirin and other antipyretics have no effect on the synthesis and release of endogenous pyrogen from phagocytic leukocytes. Therefore, their role in reducing fever is not directly related to their peripheral anti-inflammatory properties. The potency of an antipyretic in reducing fever is proportionately related to its ability to inhibit the synthesis of brain prostaglandins, and thus the primary mechanism of antipyretics is the prevention of prostaglandin synthesis in the hypothalamus. The ability of endogenous pyrogen to raise the hypothalamic thermostat setting is due to its ability to increase the concentration of hypothalamic prostaglandin, and hence antipyretics lower fever by preventing pyrogen-induced prostaglandin synthesis. This is corroborated by the clinical observation that antipyretics do not lower normal body temperature but only the elevated temperature of fever. Corticosteroids prevent fever by reducing the amount of endogenous pyrogen released from phagocytes. Therefore, the ability of corticosteroids to reduce fever is related to their peripheral anti-inflammatory properties.

DIAGNOSIS. Individuals maintain body temperature at about 37° C despite wide variations in environmental temperatures. For some individuals, normal body temperature can be below or above 37° C without constituting a pathologic process. During a 24-hour period, body temperature varies from a low point in the early morning to the highest levels at 4 to 6 P.M. The amplitude of this daily variation, also called circadian temperature rhythm, is about 0.6° C (1° F), and individuals retain their circadian rhythm throughout life despite intervening bouts of prolonged illness. An elevation above the normal amplitude of daily temperature for an individual is considered fever. During fever, the morning low and evening high temperature pattern can still be observed. In the occasional situation in which elevated temperature is really hyperthermia, this rhythm is absent. A diagnosis of hyperthermia is often made because of a preceding history of heat exposure or use of certain drugs that interfere with normal thermoregulation. In some patients the hypothalamic set-point is elevated owing to local trauma, hemorrhage, tumor invasion, or intrinsic hypothalamic malfunction. The term "hypothalamic fever" is sometimes used to describe elevated temperature caused by abnormal hypothalamic function. However, the majority of patients with hypothalamic damage have hypothermia or do not thermoregulate properly to mild environmental termperature changes. In those patients in whom hypothalamic fever is suspected, diagnosis depends on demonstrating other abnormal hypothalamic functions, such as production of hypothalamic-releasing factors, abnormal response to cold, and absence of circadian rhythm.

MANIFESTATIONS OF FEVER. The subjective symptoms of fever include sensations of feeling cold or warm, headache, myalgias, arthralgias, and general malaise. The objective signs besides elevated temperature include increased respiratory rate, widened pulse pressure, and rapid heart rate. There are exceptions, however. Patients with typhoid fever and certain hypothalamic tumors have lower pulse rates than expected during fever. Laboratory findings are altered in fever. The most notable of these is elevated erythrocyte sedimentation rate resulting from increased haptoglobin, fibrinogen, ceruloplasmin, and C-reactive protein levels. These are often called "acute phase reactants" and account for the elevation in globulins seen on serum protein electrophoresis. In some patients the neutrophil count is elevated and young marrow forms appear in the peripheral blood, but these leukocyte changes may reflect the disease causing the infection rather than the fever itself. Serum iron and zinc levels are decreased during fever, and the low iron may play a role in the anemia that frequently accompanies chronic fever.

Metabolic rate is increased during fever (13 to 15 per cent per degree above 37° C), thus requiring more calories and increased oxygen. The metabolic consequences of fever can be detrimental. For example, muscle breakdown occurs in which the amino acids are inefficiently consumed for energy. Muscle protein breakdown appears to be triggered by endogenous pyrogen-induced PGE_2 production. Also, fever is accompanied by an increase in urinary calcium, which reflects progressive

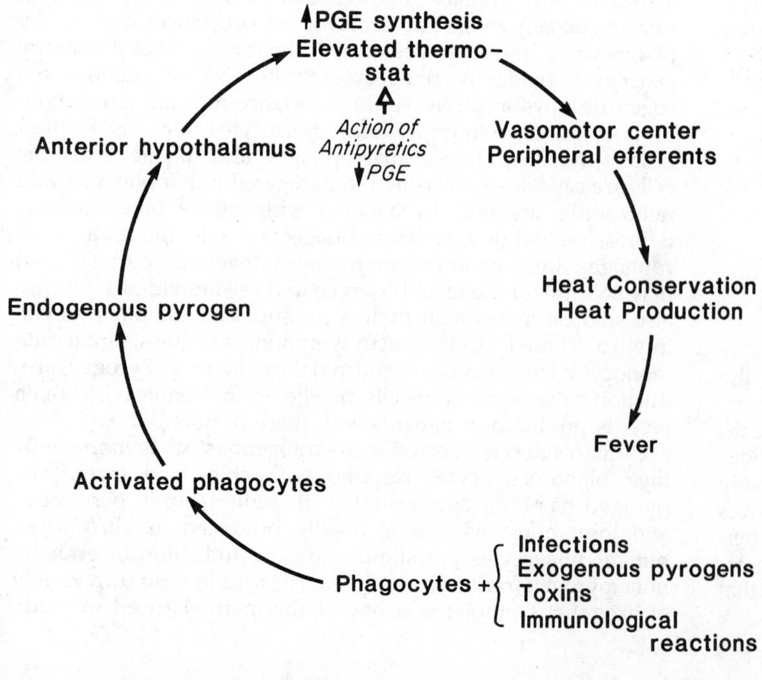

Figure 255–1. Mechanisms for the production of fever.

breakdown of bone. Aminoaciduria and proteinuria reflect the generalized breakdown of tissue during fever.

Fever caused by infectious, toxic, or immunologic diseases rarely exceeds 41.1° C (106° F), and there is clinical as well as animal evidence that the hypothalamic set-point for pyrogen response has a thermal ceiling. Extremely high fever (hyperpyrexia), however, can occur in any patient with significant disease, but it is most frequently observed in patients with central nervous system hemorrhage. In general, there are only a few clinical conditions in which moderately elevated temperature is detrimental. These are in patients with central nervous system disease, decreased cardiovascular function, and prior history of febrile seizure, and in pregnant women. The increased oxygen demand, cardiac output, and pulse rate associated with fever are particularly dangerous to patients with a compromised myocardium. Fever may also be teratogenic for the developing fetus.

TREATMENT. Most individuals with fever caused by infectious diseases, such as upper respiratory tract infections or flu syndromes, experience unpleasant symptoms and treat their fever with antipyretics. There is no evidence that moderately elevated temperature is harmful to patients who are not in one of the risk groups noted above. It is often desirable to withhold antipyretic therapy so that fever can be used as an index of improvement or worsening of a disease. On the other hand, there are no data on humans to suggest that fever is beneficial, although in some animal models survival from certain bacteremias is increased in febrile as compared with normothermic animals. Presently, there is renewed interest in the use of hyperthermia in treating disease, particularly disseminated cancers. In these situations, there may be beneficial aspects of elevated temperature for certain host defense mechanisms as well as the injurious effects of high temperature on some neoplastic cells. In most clinical settings, the use of oral antipyretics suffices to reduce fever. In febrile adults, a single oral dose (600 to 900 mg) of acetaminophen or aspirin reduces body temperature to normal levels in three to six hours. Peak plasma levels of the drugs vary and the times of peak drug concentration also vary considerably between one and five hours following oral administration.

Acetaminophen and aspirin in comparable oral doses have approximately equal ability to lower body temperature. The need to repeat the dose of antipyretics may be related to continued synthesis and release of endogenous pyrogen and the short duration of action of antipyretics. In adults, the total daily dose of acetaminophen should not exceed 3 grams under ordinary circumstances and should be lower in patients with impaired hepatic function. The dose limits in children are adjusted on the basis of body surface or weight.

Acetaminophen should be used as an antipyretic in patients who are allergic to salicylates or who have gastrointestinal intolerance to aspirin. In addition, acetaminophen is preferable to aspirin in patients with hemophilia, von Willebrand's disease, or other diseases of blood coagulation or who are being treated with oral anticoagulants. Aspirin is contraindicated in patients with peptic ulcer or asthma. However, with the exceptions cited above, there is no advantage to using acetaminophen rather than aspirin for the reduction of fever.

Several physical methods can also be used to reduce body temperature. The most common is water or alcohol sponging. The use of air-conditioned rooms, fans, and cooling blankets will also reduce core temperature by facilitating air and surface heat conduction from the skin. If physical methods are used to reduce core temperature at a time when the hypothalamic set-point remains elevated, shivering and vasoconstriction will occur as the hypothalamic drive to raise core temperature competes with the peripheral removal of heat. Thus, the ideal circumstance for reducing body temperature during fever combines the use of an antipyretic that lowers the hypothalamic set-point with physical methods that promote heat dissipation. In some circumstances, overzealous methods to reduce fever can lead to hypothermia. This is often the case when phenobarbital, chlorpromazine, or large doses of corticosteroids are administered in conjunction with antipyretics and sponging.

Any patient with fever of 41.1° C (106° F) (hyperpyrexia) requires urgent medical care. For some patients with preexisting cardiovascular, pulmonary, or central nervous system diseases, or in children who have had a febrile seizure, the temperature at which the individual is at risk may be considerably lower. Efforts to reduce hyperpyrexia should be instituted with rapidity before physiologic changes secondary to prolonged high temperature produce significant morbidity. These may include acidosis, hypovolemia, cardiac arrhythmias, respiratory and contraction alkalosis, and electrolyte abnormalities. It is helpful to use physical methods to reduce body temperature during hyperpyrexia, but core temperature should be carefully monitored.

Dinarello CA: Interleukin-1. Rev Inf Dis 6:54, 1984. *A comprehensive review of the interrelationship between fever and the acute phase response.*

Dinarello CA, Wolff SM: Molecular basis of fever in humans. Am J Med 72:799, 1982. *A detailed review of the pathogenesis of fever with discussion of the production and action of human endogenous pyrogen.*

Atkins E: Fever: Its history, cause and function. Yale J Biol Med 55:283, 1982. *A concise review of the history and function of fever.*

Milton AS (ed.): Pyretics and Antipyretics. Berlin, Springer Verlag, 1982. *A monograph (600 pages) with over 25 recognized contributors updating the mechanisms of fever production and antipyresis.*

256. SHOCK SYNDROMES RELATED TO SEPSIS

John N. Sheagren

Sepsis is defined as the presence of various pus-forming and other pathogenic organisms or their toxins in the blood or tissues. The presumptive diagnosis of sepsis is often made on the basic of historical, physical, and laboratory data even in the absence of proof. The most serious complications are produced when infection spreads from the original focus to the bloodstream. Bacteremia can produce two very different types of complications: microbiologic and inflammatory. The microbiologic complications result from the local and systemic proliferation and seeding of the causative organism, which cause direct tissue or organ damage. The inflammatory complications are produced locally and can result in tissue or organ destruction independent of toxic factors produced by the causative organism. Bacteremia triggers intravascular activation of the same inflammatory systems that are protective within tissues. These combine with stress-generated endocrine responses to produce a sequence of metabolic events. The end stage of these events is the systemic vascular collapse traditionally termed *septic shock.*

Morbidity and mortality associated with septic shock are quite high: approximately two thirds of such patients die. Therefore, prevention of septic shock should be the primary goal. It is possible to recognize clinically the changes that occur in patients in the early stages of the septic shock syndrome. Intervention at early stages of the syndrome can reduce morbidity and mortality.

INCIDENCE AND EPIDEMIOLOGY. Infections most commonly occur in the hospital setting. Many infected patients become bacteremic. It is estimated that of 100 randomly chosen patients who appear to be infected (septic) in a hospital setting, approximately 90 per cent will actually be infected. Of those in whom infection is ultimately documented, about 20 per cent will develop some evidence of hemodynamic instability and appear, at least temporarily, "shocky." About half of that group of shocky patients (or about 10 per cent of all septic-appearing patients) will go on to frank septic shock and/or manifest serious end organ malfunction related to the septic episode such as adult respiratory distress syndrome (ARDS), renal failure, or disseminated intravascular coagulation (DIC). Since about 5 per cent of all hospital patients either are admitted with or develop an infection during hospitalization, the number of patients at risk of developing septic shock is large. The clinician must be familiar with the manifestations and differential diagnosis of the septic-appearing patient and have in mind rapid comprehensive diagnostic and therapeutic plans of action.

Shock Related to Gram-Negative as Opposed to Gram-Positive Organisms. Many authors state that septic shock more commonly follows gram-negative than gram-positive septic episodes, and many textbooks still refer to generic septic shock as gram-negative sepsis or endotoxic shock because endotoxin is found only in gram-negative bacterial cell walls. Recent studies suggest that in a theoretical group of 100 patients who are bacteremic with gram-negative microbes, the incidence of metabolic complications and shock is high (about 25 per cent). However, about 10 per cent of patients with gram-positive bacteremia, especially those infected with *Staphylococcus aureus*, develop shock. The incidence of suppurative complications (metastatic seeding to bones, joints, viscera, and so on), on the other hand, is much higher with gram-positive microorganisms. Gram-positive bacteria have the capability of adhering to endothelial cells to a much greater degree than do gram-negative organisms, so that seeding to heart valves and other organs is much more common.

PATHOGENESIS. Sepsis can cause shock in many ways, either related to the primary focus of infection or to the systemic effects of bacteremia. These mechanisms of shock are listed in Table 256–1.

The classic *septic shock syndrome* results primarily from the sequence of events triggered by bacteremia during which cell wall bacterial substances (endotoxin in gram-negative organisms and the peptidoglycan/teichoic acid complex in gram-positive organisms) activate the complement, coagulation, kinin, and ACTH/endorphin systems. This activation results in a series of metabolic events that ultimately progress to a state of shock (see Table 256–1, inflammatory-system–mediated shock). This type of shock traditionally has been erroneously referred to as gram-negative or endotoxic shock. Clinically, severe sepsis produces hemodynamic changes in two phases. Septic patients initially have hemodynamic changes primarily reflecting vasodilation. The patient is hyperdynamic with increased cardiac output and decreased systemic vascular resistance. As this hyperdynamic state develops, the peripheral processes of complement-mediated leukoagglutination and capillary damage cause a severe capillary leak syndrome. Intravascular volume begins to decrease, resulting in the "unloaded patient" in full-blown septic shock. This second phase of septic shock occurs when blood pressure falls dramatically as intravascular volume decreases, and as cardiac output, previously elevated, declines. Several factors contribute to the decline in cardiac output: peripheral resistance in late septic shock begins to increase, and several cardiodepressants are demonstrable, namely vasopressin and encephalin (one of the products of the endorphin system activation). Individual organs may be damaged independently of the hypotensive events; for example, direct pulmonary damage by the activated leukocytes may result in ARDS, or the patient may develop renal malfunction whether or not frank hypotension has occurred. Presumably these end organ manifestations are related to localized direct inflammatory damage caused by the events previously described. It is in this stage that disseminated intravascular coagulation associated with severe hypoperfusion may occur with extremely high morbidity and mortality.

TABLE 256–1. MECHANISMS OF SHOCK CAUSED BY SEPSIS

1. Shock related to a localized primary focus of infection
   Hypovolemic shock: severe local infection may
   —cause sufficient local fluid accumulation to produce systemic hypovolemia.
   —produce severe diarrhea with gastrointestinal fluid loss.
   —erode into a local vessel with mycotic aneurysm formation and rupture.
   Cardiogenic shock: extension of a pericardiac infection (usually pneumonia) into the pericardium may cause purulent pericarditis and tamponade.
   Toxigenic shock (the toxic shock syndrome): a toxin is produced locally, causing
   —endothelial cell damage with capillary leakage.
   —cardiodepression.
2. Shock related to bacteremic infections
   Cardiogenic shock: seeding of the organism through the bloodstream may cause
   —valvular malfunction (endocarditis).
   —myocarditis secondary to multiple metastatic myocardial abscesses.
   —purulent pericarditis (metastatic).
   Inflammatory-system–mediated shock: bacterial cell wall substances activate the complement, coagulation, kinin, and ACTH/endorphin systems and thus cause
   —vasodilation (roles of endorphins, kinins, and complement).
   —capillary leakage (primarily due to the intracapillary adherence and aggregation of activated polymorphonuclear leukocytes).
   —disseminated intravascular coagulation.
   —cardiodepression (encephalins, vasopressin, possibly other substances).

Figure 256–1 outlines the sequence of early events initiated from the localized focus of infection. From these events are derived the various complications of bacteremia, which include metastatic abscess formation and the metabolic complications described earlier. Antibiotics limit metastatic abscess formation (the microbiologic complications of bacteremia). However, a number of other metabolic events, when activated and independent of bacterial proliferation, still produce substantial morbidity and mortality. Therefore, anti-inflammatory therapy is recommended.

The ACTH/Endorphin System. During systemic stress, increased ACTH release occurs. For each molecule of ACTH produced, a molecule of one of the endorphins or encephalins is also produced. The endorphins are very powerful opiate-like substances that have a variety of other metabolic effects. The endorphins provide pain relief during severe stress, and high levels of circulating endorphins may have the same side effects as opiates, resulting in hypotension, changes in vascular permeability, and alterations in mentation.

Coagulation/Kinin System Activation. Bacterial endotoxins and other cell wall materials directly activate the coagulation system both by initiating platelet aggregation and by activating Hageman factor. These coagulation events are triggered simultaneously by intravascular bacterial cell wall products. Subsequently, kinin system activation (see Ch. 442) results in the production of bradykinin, a powerful vasodilator.

Complement System Activation. The complement system is also directly activated by high molecular weight bacterial and fungal polysaccharides primarily by means of the alternative pathway. A sequence of intravascular events ensues, resulting in microvascular instability as well as massive chaotic activation of circulating polymorphonuclear leukocytes (PMNs). The activated PMN has enhanced bactericidal capabilities but also an

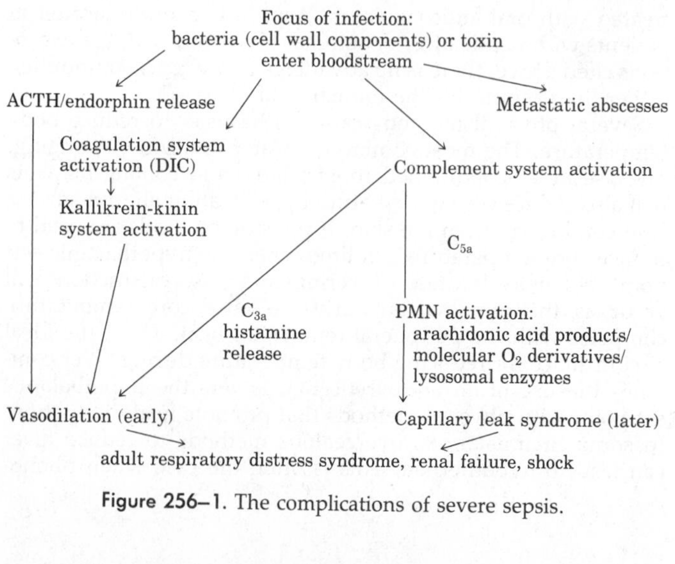

Figure 256–1. The complications of severe sepsis.

enhanced capability of damaging host tissues. The activated PMN possesses increased amounts of lysosomal enzymes and produces a variety of toxic metabolites of molecular oxygen, all of which are both bactericidal and cytocidal. Furthermore, the activated PMN produces both inflammatory prostaglandins and several products of the lipoxygenase system, many of which enhance inflammation by also producing vasodilation, capillary leakage, chemotaxis, and PMN activation. The activated PMNs adhere to each other (the *leukopenic phase* of sepsis during which PMN aggregates form in capillaries) and to endothelial cells to cause severe endothelial cell damage and capillary leakage.

CLINICAL MANIFESTATIONS. ***The Septic Patient.*** The clinical situation in which a patient is considered septic (highly likely to be infected) is common. Patients in this setting usually have fever. High fever and the presence of a chill strongly indicate that bacterial sepsis is occurring. Starting with the clinical recognition of fever, the managing physician must be constantly on the alert for signs that the patient's condition is deteriorating in a manner suggestive of septic shock. Thus, clinically it is useful to try to identify subgroups of patients who are not only likely to be infected but have additional systemic signs of toxicity that suggest that they may be toxemic or bacteremic and in danger of developing full-bown shock. When a clinical diagnosis of septic shock can be made, the mortality rate is exceedingly high. It is important to develop the concept of the "preshock phase of septic shock" predicated on identifying a subgroup of infected patients more likely than others to develop shock. Treatment before shock develops may prevent some of the morbidity and mortality associated with sepsis.

Table 256–2 lists several systemic signs and a variety of physical findings likely to be predictive of the development of septic shock. Extremes of body temperature are often associated with shock. Specifically, fever in excess of 40.6° C and hypothermia associated with sepsis should be alerting signs that hypotension may soon follow. Also, in the febrile patient with a distinct change in mentation the mortality rate is higher. In association with such a finding, primary central nervous system infection may be present, and lumbar puncture is often indicated. Febrile patients who have hemodynamic instability (who are orthostatic with a blood pressure decrease of 30 mm Hg or greater) should be considered on the verge of developing septic shock.

While it is not possible to distinguish between simple dehydration and early septic shock solely on the basis of orthostatic blood pressure changes, hemodynamic monitoring will show an increase in peripheral vascular resistance in the former case and a reduction in the latter. Also, fluid challenge alone will rapidly stabilize the condition of the purely hypovolemic patient. Sepsis is associated in the early stages with a state of "warm shock" in which there is a decrease in orthostatic blood pressure but good perfusion in the extremities (they are warm and pink rather than cool and cyanotic). Since the lung is such an important organ in systemic septic shock, tachypnea with hypoxemia or the development of a metabolic acidosis or both may be predictive of impending ARDS. The development of peripheral edema, often with a suddenly decreased serum albumin concentration, just as in toxigenic shock (see section on the Toxic Shock Syndrome in Ch. 270), is often caused by an unrecognized bacteremic event.

Laboratory Data Suggesting Bacteremia or Toxemia. Several laboratory tests are often helpful in the evaluation of a potentially septic patient (Table 256–2). The blood may show hypoxemia and a metabolic acidosis. Serum lactate elevation is highly predictive of deterioration leading to septic shock. Decreasing urine output, often associated with rising blood urea nitrogen and creatinine, may be seen early in sepsis as renal failure occurs. Serum albumin measurements may show decreases in excess of that calculated by catabolism alone. Often such patients show signs of progressive peripheral edema. In early sepsis, the total white count may be low, with most of the decrease in the PMN count, owing to complement-induced leukoaggregation. As white cells aggregate, platelets become caught up in the process. Thrombocytopenia is predictive of high risk of septic shock and ARDS.

TABLE 256–2. PHYSICAL SIGNS AND LABORATORY DATA LIKELY TO BE PREDICTIVE OF THE DEVELOPMENT OF SEPTIC SHOCK

1. Extremes of body temperature (fever >40.6° C or hypothermia)
2. Altered mental status
3. Orthostatic blood pressure decrease (>30 mm Hg)
4. Decreasing urine output
5. Unexplained edema, usually associated with a falling serum albumin concentration
6. Tachypnea with hypoxemia and/or the development of a metabolic acidosis
7. Elevated serum lactate concentration
8. Development of leukopenia (predominantly neutropenia)
9. Development of thrombocytopenia with or without petechial skin rash

In the future, assistance in clinical decision making will be provided by rapid laboratory measurements of the activation of many of the systems shown in Figure 256–1. For example, the rapid identification of a falling total complement level and elevated levels of C5a, prostaglandins, or endorphins might predict subgroups of septic patients at risk of developing shock.

DIAGNOSIS. The presumptive diagnosis of sepsis must be made when the setting and attendant clinical signs are suggestive. In general, patients with fever should be considered septic until proved otherwise. Therapy should always be initiated for high-risk febrile patients in advance of microbiologic confirmation of sepsis.

Evaluation of the Septic Patient. The setting in which the episode is occurring should be evaluated promptly. Crucial to appropriate initial decision making are the background history, which may help to define the type of host defense defect present, and prior cultural data, which might be predictive of the infecting organism. The physical examination should be directed at quickly but thoroughly searching for the septic source as well as signs of end organ failure that might indicate progression to shock such as altered mental status, progressive edema, hypotension, and so on (Table 256–2). All potentially infected foci should be appropriately sampled, and the material obtained should be Gram-stained and cultured.

Differential Diagnosis of Severe Sepsis. Having done a thorough preliminary evaluation, one can reassess the clinical situation on subsequent days and stop antibiotic therapy if the episode later seems not to be infectious. Many nonseptic events can cause high fever with or without vascular instability. For example, a variety of hypersensitivity reactions (often caused by drugs) may mimic sepsis. Vasculitic diseases may present with high fever, unstable blood pressure, and altered mentation. Pulmonary emboli occur frequently in the hospital setting, and especially if the patient develops fever the embolic event initially may be confused with sepsis. Myocardial infarction may result in hemodynamic instability, and in the subset of patients who develop higher than average fever, may lead to initial confusion with sepsis.

There are infectious syndromes against which antimicrobials are of no use in which bacterial sepsis may be suspected. For example, viral syndromes such as those caused by influenza viruses, enteroviruses, adenoviruses, cytomegalovirus, and hepatitis viruses may all have very high fever and be quite difficult to diagnosis. Malaria, common in other parts of the world, can be extremely hard to identify when it is afflicting patients in the United States. It is sometimes difficult initially to differentiate malaria from severe sepsis unless the parasite is detected on the peripheral blood smear.

TREATMENT. ***Antibacterial Therapy.*** Extremely broad coverage is required in patients with the syndrome of severe sepsis. It is best to initiate therapy with a combination of antibiotics when the infecting organism is unknown. An aminoglycoside should always be used, and gentamicin remains the aminoglycoside of choice unless other considerations (such as abnormal renal function and known microbial resistance) dictate the use of tobramycin or amikacin. In the granulocytopenic patient, the aminoglycoside should be combined with high doses of carbenicillin, ticarcillin, or mezlocillin. In the patient likely to have an anaerobic focus of infection in which *Bacteriodes fragilis* is likely to be present, such as an intra-abdominal or gynecologic infection, or decubitus and lower extremity vascular and neuropathic ulcers, clindamycin is combined with gentamicin. For all other patients, gentamicin plus cefazolin, the best first-generation cephalosporin, is the combination of choice. When cultures define the causative microbe(s) or other data point to a specific organism, therapy can be tailored to the most appropriate, most specific, least toxic, and least expensive single antibiotic.

Antishock Therapy. The most important component of the therapy of shock associated with sepsis is volume replacement. Sufficient quantities of an appropriate solute (or, where indicated, albumin or whole blood) should be administered to the septic patient in an attempt to provide adequate volume support. Hemodynamic monitoring of the patient's clinically deteriorating septic condition is mandatory and is preferably carried out in the intensive care unit (see Ch. 71 on Critical Care Medicine). For example, while fluid administration should be vigorous from the beginning, adequate volume support means administering just enough fluid to bring the patient's pulmonary capillary wedge pressure to the high normal range. As outlined in Figure 256–2, an attempt can be made to counter the adverse inflammatory sequelae of bacteremia with appropriate anti-inflammatory drug therapy. Used most commonly in severely septic patients are massive doses of methylprednisolone sodium succinate, a dose of 30 mg per kilogram being appropriate. One should not use longer acting glucocorticoids such as dexamethasone that extend the period of immunosuppression. This controversial topic has recently been extensively reviewed (see Sande and Root, chapter on "Glucocorticoid Therapy in the Management of Severe Sepsis").

The use of other anti-inflammatory drugs such as the antiprostaglandins is under active investigation. These agents may selectively suppress inflammatory damage caused by the activated PMN without interfering with the antibacterial capabilities of these important host defense cells.

Some clinicians are beginning to use naloxone in severe sepsis on the basis of the documented contribution of the endorphin system to hemodynamic instability in experimental models of septic shock. However, in primate models naloxone, like alpha agonists (aramine and levophed) appears to increase blood pressure without leading to improved tissue perfusion. Therefore, naloxone as routine therapy for patients with severe sepsis is premature. Further investigation of the use of naloxone in severe sepsis and septic shock is indicated.

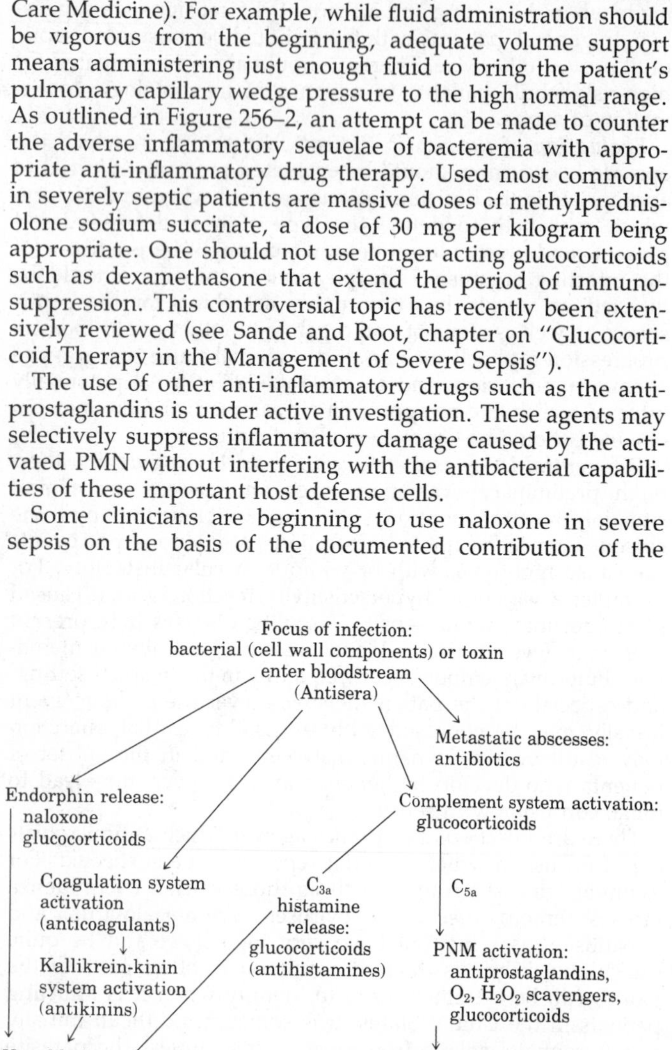

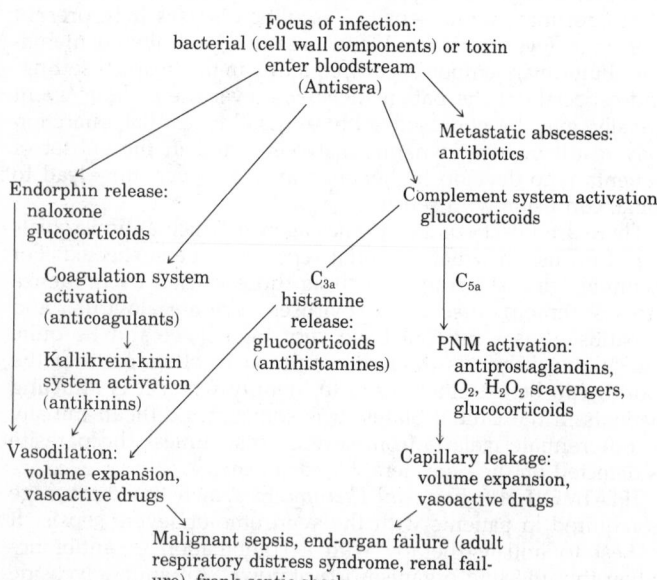

Figure 256–2. Therapy for the complications of severe sepsis.

In DIC, one should not use anticoagulant therapy when the cause is thought to be sepsis. Many other modalities of therapy are being evaluated in septic shock.

The Role of Surgery and Hyperbaric Oxygen. Surgical debridement and drainage of septic foci is especially important. All severe localized infections, especially with gas formation, should be widely debrided and drained. Hyperbaric oxygen has been used in patients with the gangrene syndromes and clostridial myonecrosis. Whether or not it stabilizes patients' conditions or influences the ultimate outcome is unknown.

Antiendotoxin Antiserum. Recently, it has been demonstrated that an antiserum against endotoxin enhances survival in patients bacteremic with gram-negative organisms. In a recent prospective randomized study, an antiserum directed against the "core" (common) lipopolysaccharide moiety of an *Escherichia coli* mutant significantly reduced mortality in severely septic patients (Ziegler, 1982). Thus, ultimately the infusion of a monoclonal antiendotoxin antiserum may be beneficial in patients showing signs of the early stages of septic shock.

PROGNOSIS. Most febrile patients lacking other signs of severe sepsis (as described in Table 256–2) will usually do well even when bacteremic. Such patients usually respond quickly to volume administration, antibacterial therapy, and drainage of the primary focus of infection. However, the presence of shock dramatically increases morbidity and mortality. Even when the inciting infection is localized, the presence of shock (with the exception of the toxic shock syndrome) is associated with a 50 per cent mortality. As noted earlier, full-blown, bacteremia-associated septic shock has greater than 70 per cent mortality. A favorable outcome in a patient in frank shock depends on the skill of management in the intensive care unit. Early diagnosis and therapy of severely septic patients will decrease the morbidity and mortality.

PREVENTION. Prevention of infection, especially in the hospital, is the key to reducing morbidity and mortality associated with septic shock. Strict adherence to the hospital infection control program with avoidance of Foley catheters and meticulous attention to the placement and maintenance of intravascular lines dramatically reduces the incidence of bacteremic infections. The concept of the preshock approach to the therapy of septic shock is useful; in all such patients fluids should be administered and broad antibiotic coverage started early. In addition, in some overtly bacteremic patients anti-inflammatory therapy will probably reduce morbidity and mortality. Controlled studies of anti-inflammatory therapy in severe sepsis are under way and better guidelines soon should be forthcoming.

Abraham E, Shoemaker WC, Bland RD, Cobo JC: Sequential cardiorespiratory patterns in septic shock. Crit Care Med 11:799, 1983. *Describes the hemodynamic patterns occurring in patients as they develop septic shock.*

Hoffman SL, Punjabi NH, Kumala S, et al.: Reduction in mortality in chloramphenicol-treated severe typhoid fever by high-dose dexamethasone. N Engl J Med 310:82, 1984. *A prospective controlled study showing significant reduction in mortality in patients in the "preshock" stage of typhoid fever who were given 6 mg per kilogram of dexamethasone along with antibiotic and volume support.*

Jacob HS, Craddock PR, Hammerschmidt DE, Moldow CF: Complement-induced granulocyte aggregation: An unsuspected mechanism of disease. N Engl J Med 302:789, 1980. *Describes how complement-induced granulocyte aggregation leads to capillary and organ damge.*

Sande M, Root RR: Septic Shock: Newer Concepts in Pathophysiology and Treatment. New York, Churchill Livingstone, Inc. (in press). *Complete up-to-date review of all aspects of septic shock including papers on the roles of endorphins, complement, prostaglandins, the PMN, and glucocorticoid therapy.*

Sheagren JN: Septic shock and corticosteroids. N Engl J Med 305:456, 1981. *A brief review of the rationale and potential problems of corticosteroid administration to patients in septic shock.*

Sprung CL, Civetta J, Rackow EC, et al.: The Pulmonary Artery Catheter—Methodology and Clinical Applications. Baltimore, University Park Press, 1983. *A complete review of the use of the Swan-Ganz catheter.*

Weissman G, Smolen JE, Dorchak HM: Release of inflammatory mediators from stimulated neutrophils. N Engl J Med 303:27, 1980. *An excellent description of the events leading to and occurring in the activated PMN.*

Zeigler EJ, McCutchan JA, Fierer J, et al.: Treatment of gram-negative bacteremia and shock with human antiserum to a mutant *Escherichia coli.* N Engl J Med 307:1225, 1982. *Describes therapy of bacteremic patients with human antiserum to endotoxin core resulting in a significant reduction in mortality.*

257. THE COMPROMISED HOST

John I. Gallin

COMPONENTS OF THE HOST DEFENSES. The host defenses comprise complex and interrelated systems, which are outlined in Table 257–1. Familiarity with these systems provides a basis for the diagnosis and management of patients with compromised defenses.

Physical Barriers. Intact skin and mucous membranes prevent microbial invasion. The skin is a complex organ, consisting of several cell types which, in addition to providing a physical barrier, produce numerous antimicrobial agents such as lactic acid, ammonia, urea, and free fatty acids. These protect the host from superficial challenges. The mucous membrane secretions, which trap inhaled microorganisms, contain soluble factors such as immunoglobulin A, lactoferrin, lysozyme, and α_1-antitrypsin, which have antibacterial activity. Proper function of the nasal and respiratory passage cilia facilitates microbial clearance. In addition, host defenses require normal anatomy of the respiratory, genitourinary, and gastrointestinal systems.

Inflammatory Response. The circulating phagocytes (neutrophils, monocytes, eosinophils, and basophils) are the central components of the inflammatory response. The phagocytes are manufactured and undergo maturation in the bone marrow, and upon appropriate stimulation are delivered to the bloodstream where they circulate and are distributed to local tissue sites. Recruitment of phagocytic leukocytes from the bloodstream involves a complex process called diapedesis or emigration. The initial step of this process is not completely understood but seems to require phagocyte aggregation and adherence to the endothelium. The phagocytic cells pass between the endothelial cells as they migrate to tissue sites. The availability of the potential space between endothelial cells through which phagocytes migrate is modulated by local tissue products of the complement cascade (the anaphylatoxins, or small molecular weight cleavage products of the third and fifth complement components, C3a and C5a) and the potent vasodilator bradykinin produced by activation of the fibrinolytic and kinin generating systems. The complement cascade and the fibrinolytic and kinin generating systems are activated by microbial products, such as endotoxin, and a variety of substances secreted by leukocytes, platelets, and fibroblasts. Locomotion of phagocytes requires cell adherence to their substratum, deformability, machinery for random locomotion, and the ability to sense a gradient of a chemical signal (chemotactic factor) and convert random locomotion (kinesis) to directed locomotion (chemotaxis). The locomotory apparatus includes an intact actin and myosin system for movement and an intact microtubule system to stabilize the cell during locomotion and organize the intracellular granules, which are secreted extracellularly during locomotion and appear to be important modulators of the inflammatory process.

The chemotactic factors are humoral mediators and include products from activation of the complement system (C5a) and the arachidonic acid cascade (leukotriene B_4). Other chemoattractants result from activation of the kinin generating system, products from neutrophils, macrophages, lymphocytes (lymphokines), and fibroblasts (collagen and other peptides), some bacterial products, as well as oxidation products of certain fatty acids. Some chemotactic factors are highly preferential for particular cell types (i.e., histamine and other mast cell products are preferential for eosinophils, whereas an alveolar macrophage product is preferential for neutrophils). After recruitment, microorganisms that have been opsonized by complement products and immunoglobulins to facilitate adherence to the phagocyte membrane are then ingested, killed, and digested. These events require complex biochemical and biophysical events with specific mechanisms for elimination of different classes of microorganisms (see Ch. 148).

Reticuloendothelial System. The reticuloendothelial system is the major system for the clearance of circulating microorganisms from the bloodstream. The main components of the system are the tissue, or "fixed," phagocytes, consisting of splenic macrophages, alveolar macrophages, Kupffer cells, lymph node macrophages, and microglial cells in the brain. Many or perhaps all of these macrophages are derived from circulating monocytes that migrate from the bloodstream into the extravascular space where they differentiate into the tissue macrophages.

The Immune Response. The T and B lymphocytes are the main components of the immune response. T lymphocytes are the functional cells of cell-mediated immunity or delayed hypersensitivity. Mature B cells, or plasma cells, produce antibodies and are the cells of humoral immunity. The functions of T and B lymphocytes are closely related. For example, helper T cells facilitate B cell function, whereas suppressor T cells are important regulators of B cell function. The thymus gland controls the maturation of the T lymphocytes; factors controlling B cell maturation in humans are not known.

Upon appropriate signal, lymphocytes are released from the bone marrow into the circulation, where they are distributed throughout the body. The mechanism of mobilizing lymphocytes to tissue sites from the circulation is poorly understood but may involve chemotaxis. At tissue sites lymphocytes perform their specific tasks. The T lymphocytes are believed to be critical in eliminating such pathogens as *Mycobacterium tuberculosis, Histoplasma capsulatum, Candida albicans,* and certain viruses. The B cells respond to antigens (which may first have to be processed by macrophages) by synthesis of the immunoglobulins (antibodies), which have important roles in complement activation, virus neutralization, and opsonization. (For a detailed review of the various components of the immune response, see Ch. 427.)

ETIOLOGY. Infection is a major cause of morbidity and mortality in patients undergoing treatment for neoplasia or collagen vascular diseases, or therapy to prevent organ rejection following organ transplantation. In each of these clinical settings there may be an inherent defect of host defenses. However, the most common cause for the recurrent infections in each of these settings is the use of drugs which suppress the cellular and/or humoral components of the inflammatory and immune responses. Thus drugs which cause neutropenia, such as Cytoxan or myelosuppressive agents; drugs which suppress phagocytic cell function, such as corticosteroids or aspirin; drugs which suppress the T or B cell systems, such as Cytoxan (presumably inhibits T suppressor cells) or methotrexate (presumably inhibits antigen-specific lymphocyte transformation); and drugs used to prevent graft versus host disease, such as cyclosporin A (presumably inhibits antigenic triggering of immunocompetent cells), all have the potential to compromise

TABLE 257–1. THE HOST DEFENSES

Physical barriers
Skin
Mucocus membranes
Inflammatory response
Circulating phagocytes
Humoral mediators
Reticuloendothelial system
Fixed phagocytes
Immune response
T cells (cell-mediated immunity, delayed hypersensitivity)
B cells (antibody responses)
Other mediators (i.e., lymphotoxin)

the host defenses and predispose the patient to infection. These drug-related effects are probably the most common cause for the compromised host seen in the hospital.

A host may also be compromised as a consequence of environmental factors, such as protein-calorie malnutrition, thermal injury, alcoholism, and irradiation. Host defense defects can also result from a number of inherited and congenital disorders, as well as from acquired defects associated with numerous diseases. The particular type of infection will depend on the nature of the fundamental defect.

PATHOGENESIS AND PATHOLOGY. Pathologic models in support of predicted abnormalities of host defenses are well described for certain components of the defense system. Other examples are emerging as we understand what parameters are important to assess. Examples related to infection from penetration of the skin are obvious and include penetrating trauma and severe burns.

Mucous membrane secretions are abnormally viscid in cystic fibrosis, and mucous plug formation with obstruction and subsequent pneumonia can result. Mucociliary movement is abnormal in Kartagener's syndrome (situs inversus, chronic sinusitis, and bronchiectasis), and this is related to absence of a particuar cilial subunit (dynein arms). Mucus secretion and cilial integrity may also be damaged by decreases in temperature and humidity, exposure to inhalants such as cigarette smoke and atmospheric pollutants, supplemental oxygen, endotracheal tubes, and thermal injury. Infection by certain respiratory viruses (i.e., influenza) and *Mycoplasma pneumoniae* can damage the mucociliary system, resulting in increased susceptibility to bronchitis and pneumonia. Recurrent bacterial pneumonias result from anatomic derangement of bronchi by obstruction from neoplasm, foreign objects, mucous plugs, or local collapse secondary to bronchiectasis and from chronic aspiration.

Gastrointestinal "blind loops" following certain surgical procedures result in overgrowth with coliform bacteria which consume vitamin B_{12} or folic acid and thereby contribute to neutropenic states. Genitourinary tract infections with gram-negative bacteria are associated with congenital and acquired abnormalities such as congenital ureteral abnormalities, urethral stricture, urethral changes following pregnancy, and urethral obstruction from stones, prostatic hypertrophy, and prostatic carcinoma.

Other anatomic defects increasing susceptibility to infection include damaged heart valves following endocarditis or rheumatic fever. Aortic aneurysms can be infected with salmonellae (particularly *Salmonella choleraesuis*), staphylococci, and streptococci. Peripheral vascular disease of diabetes mellitus is associated with infection of the distal phalanges of the toes. Foreign objects, including prosthetic devices, sutures, gauze, and intravenous or Foley catheters, interfere with normal anatomic integrity and are subject to microbial colonization and subsequent microbial dissemination.

Patients who have had splenectomy are at increased risk for *Streptococcus pneumoniae* infection, especially infants and young children. The precise basis for this is not known, but decreased clearance of bacteria by the reticuloendothelial system is thought to be important. Children with sickle cell hemoglobinopathies, as well as patients with hemoglobinopathies from a variety of causes, are susceptible to *Salmonella*, *Streptococcus pneumoniae*, and *Bartonella* infection. The host defect in the hemoglobinopathies may relate to splenic dysfunction, but abnormal alternative complement pathway function and impaired phagocytosis and killing of the indicated organisms by leukocytes have been described. Splenic dysfunction is also seen in splenomegaly from a variety of causes, including passive congestion, certain collagen-vascular diseases (systemic lupus erythematosus and Felty's syndrome), and lymphomas. These examples of splenic dysfunction are associated with neutropenia from neutrophil trapping and destruction in the spleen.

A number of other conditions predispose to compromised defenses. During viral influenza there is increased susceptibility to pneumococcal and staphylococcal pneumonia. The mechanism for this is poorly understood, but impaired mucociliary function, neutropenia, and adverse effects of the virus on phagocytic cell function have been implicated. Neoplasms, malnutrition, diabetes mellitus, and effects of a variety of pharmacologic agents, especially corticosteroids and myelosuppressive agents, compromise host defenses by affecting the production, distribution, and function of leukocytes. Prolonged use of antimicrobial drugs predisposes toward colonization with microorganisms resistant to the antibiotics, particularly *Staphylococcus aureus*, resistant gram-negative bacilli such as *Pseudomonas*, *Serratia*, and the gram-negative coccobacilli *Acinetobacter* species, as well as fungi *(Candida)*, and the compromised host is more likely to become infected with these organisms.

Leukopenias. Perhaps the best evidence for a role of leukocytes in host defenses is the severe infections associated with leukopenias. Leukopenia exists when the peripheral white blood count is below 4000 per cubic millimeter. Although all leukocytes can be depressed, most frequently neutrophils are the cell type affected. In general, when the granulocyte count is below 500 to 1000 cells per cubic millimeter, patients are at increased risk of infection, and when there are fewer than 200 cells per cubic millimeter, the inflammatory response is essentially absent and severe infection is the rule. Both the degree of granulocyte depression and its duration are important variables relating to the severity and rate of infection. Lymphopenia exists when the number of lymphocytes is below 1400 per cubic millimeter in children and 1000 per cubic millimeter in adults. The complete absence of leukocytes is not compatible with life in a normal environment. The particular type of infection associated with leukopenia depends upon which leukocyte population is depressed. Absence of thymus-dependent lymphocytes or T cells, as in thymus aplasia (DiGeorge's syndrome) or thymus hypoplasia (Nezelof's syndrome), is associated with severe defects of cell-mediated immunity (see Ch. 429). Absent B lymphocytes (Bruton's X-linked agammaglobulinemia) is associated with a severe abnormality of humoral mediated immunity (see Ch. 429). Combined T and B cell lymphopenia (see Ch. 429) has a particularly poor prognosis.

The causes of leukopenias are multiple and are related to depressed marrow production (idiopathic, drug-induced, leukemias, tumor invasion of the bone marrow, and nutritional deficiencies), peripheral destruction (immune mechanisms, splenic trapping), or peripheral pooling with overwhelming bacterial infection. Leukopenia is seen following infection with bacteria (typhoid, paratyphoid fever, tuberculosis, brucellosis), viruses (influenza, measles, infectious mononucleosis, rubella), rickettsiae, and protozoa (malaria, kala-azar). (For a complete review of the leukopenias, see Ch. 150.)

Leukocyte Dysfunction. The leukocyte dysfunction syndromes also demonstrate the primary importance of leukocytes in host defenses. Patients with T cell dysfunction include those with acquired immune deficiency syndrome, mucocutaneous candidiasis, and nucleoside phosphorylase deficiency. Combined T and B cell dysfunction is seen in adenosine deaminase deficiency and the Wiskott-Aldrich syndrome (see Ch. 429). Neutrophil dysfunctions attributable to abnormal adherence, chemotaxis, degranulation, and bactericidal activity are reviewed in Ch. 149. Defects of the humoral components of the inflammatory response include abnormalities of mediators. These include deficiencies of certain complement components (C3 and C5) with abnormal anaphylatoxin, opsonin, and chemotactic factor production. Inhibitors acting on the chemotactic factors have been described in patients with Hodgkin's disease, sarcoidosis, alcoholism, and cirrhosis. Patients deficient in the late complement components (C6 and C7) have increased susceptibility to *Neisseria* infections.

CLINICAL MANIFESTATIONS. The clinical history can be very important when evaluating a patient suspected of having a host defense defect. The type, frequency, duration, and location of infections, the intensity of the inflammatory reaction, and associated illnesses or clinical problems, such as allergies or atopic dermatitis, as well as the family history, are important and are summarized in Table 257–2.

Leukopenias. The clinical manifestations of leukopenia without infection are minimal, or those of the underlying disease. With acute drug-induced leukopenia, chills, fever, and prostration may be the initial manifestations and may be attributed to invasion by bacteria. However, these symptoms may occur within an hour of administering a drug which results in a hapten-antibody type reaction, such as with aminopyrine, and may relate to release of endogenous pyrogens from immune lysis of leukocytes. The initial symptoms may transiently disappear, to be followed by recurrent fever, chills, headaches, and frequently ulceration of the oropharynx and sometimes the rectum and vagina. These ulcerations are called aphthous ulcers and may be the initial clinical manifestation of neutropenia. The ulcers often have a gray membrane, but frank pus is absent. Patients receiving cytotoxic drug therapy get similar ulcers, independent of neutropenia, which may be difficult to distinguish from aphthous ulcers. Following or concomitant with this stage there are usually symptoms of local bacterial invasion. Frequently bacterial invasion is overwhelming without impressive clinical manifestations because of lack of an inflammatory reaction. Minimal skin lesions characterized by local erythema and tenderness or minimal roentgenographic findings often are the only indications of overwhelming infection with gram-negative bacilli. Careful and frequent inspection of the patient is thus required. With agranulocytosis, regional lymph nodes become enlarged. In the absence of aggressive therapy or spontaneous remission, death from overwhelming infection (usually gram-negative bacilli) ensues. If remission of the agranulocytosis occurs, immature granulocytes appear in the circulation before mature cells.

Patients with severe leukopenia also have an increased incidence of *Pneumocystis carinii* and cytomegalovirus infection as well as infection with the systemic mycoses, including candidiasis, invasive aspergillosis, and mucormycosis. Systemic candidiasis, defined as tissue invasion with or without colonization of superficial surfaces, is the most common mycosis in the neutropenic patient. Prolonged drug therapy for a bacterial infection predisposes to candidiasis and especially *C. albicans* because of normally occurring local colonization. The presence of thrush in the mouth, vagina, or skin indicates candidiasis in these patients, and indwelling catheters may serve as portals of entry. In systemic candidiasis symptoms are usually confined to the distal esophagus or the bladder, with rare local symptoms in the lung, liver, spleen, or kidney. Symptomatic lesions in the distal esophagus in compromised hosts are usually indicative of candidiasis and are characterized by dysphagia, odynophagia, pyrosis, retrosternal pain, and gastrointestinal bleeding. On x-ray irregular scalloping of the esophageal lining is manifest. Aspergillosis (penetration of hyphae into tissues) is an infection seen in neutropenic patients who are also on corticosteroid therapy; mucormycosis is also seen in this setting, especially in patients with diabetes mellitus. Aspergillosis almost invariably involves the lung, causing symptoms suggesting pneumonia or pulmonary emboli. Pulmonary mucormycosis is almost indistinguishable from aspergillosis.

Disorders of the Inflammatory Response. Patients with defective phagocyte chemotaxis present with minimal physical findings or findings characteristic of their underlying disease. The signs and symptoms of the infection are delayed because too few phagocytes arrive too late. Patients with defective leukocyte chemotaxis frequently have severe periodontal disease and dermatologic abnormalities, and these patients have frequent sinopulmonary infections with recurrent otitis media, bronchitis, and pneumonia. *Staphylococcus aureus* is the most frequent infectious agent, but *Streptococcus pneumoniae* and *Hemophilus influenzae* are also common.

A syndrome in which defective neutrophil and monocyte chemotaxis has been an associated host defense defect is found in patients with eczematous and pustular dermatitis, markedly elevated IgE (especially against *Staphylococcus aureus* and *Candida albicans*), low grade eosinophilia, "cold" staphylococcal skin infections, and recurrent bronchitis and pneumonias with subsequent bronchiectasis (Job's syndrome and its variants). About 50 per cent of patients with this disease have mucocutaneous candidiasis. The chemotactic defect in these patients, however, is variable, and it is not clear whether this is the primary host defense defect. Many of the patients appear to have a T cell defect, although how the T cell abnormality relates to the neutrophil and monocyte chemotactic defect is presently not known. It is possible that the primary problem is related to the lymphocyte and not the phagocyte. These patients frequently have subcutaneous and lymph node abscesses requiring surgical drainage, and their facies have a characteristic broad nasal bridge. Many patients are teenagers at the time of evaluation for host defense defects, and few patients over 30 years of age have been noted. Usually these patients have had recurrent pneumonias since early childhood, and many have thoracotomy scars from lobectomy for the severe bronchiectasis, bronchopleural fistulas, and cyst formation. The syndrome appears to be familial in some cases. Similar clinical spectrums with high IgE and a chemotactic defect are seen in patients with incontinentia pigmenti and an unusual type of ichthyosis.

Defective neutrophil and monocyte chemotaxis, delayed degranulation of neutrophils, and abnormal microbial killing are also noted in patients with the Chédiak-Higashi syndrome, a rare disease with autosomal recessive inheritance characterized by partial oculocutaneous albinism, nystagmus, neutropenia, recurrent cutaneous infections (particularly with *Staphylococcus aureus*), and giant lysosomes in all cells containing lysosomes. Patients with either congenital or acquired (from thermal injury) deficiency of specific granules also have defective neutrophil chemotaxis. All of these patients usually have multiple subcutaneous scars from their recurrent infections.

An impressive list of diseases with chemotactic defects and recurrent infections has emerged in recent years and includes the following: diabetes mellitus, leukemias, malignancies (melanoma and breast carcinoma), rheumatoid arthritis, Felty's syndrome, systemic lupus erythematosus in some patients, thermal injury, bone marrow transplantation (associated with graft versus host disease and administration of antithymocyte globulin), congenital ichthyosis with *Trichophyton rubrum* infection, hypogammaglobulinemia, α-mannosidase deficiency, chronic renal failure (especially if the patient is on chronic hemodialysis), severe protein-calorie malnutrition, severe bacterial infections, and viral influenza. The mechanism for the chemotactic defect has not been delineated in most of these diseases, and it is not clear whether the chemotactic defect is a cause or effect of the recurrent infections. However, a few well documented case reports of patients with severe pyogenic infections and defective leukocyte locomotion attributable to actin dysfunction or abnormal microtubule assembly clearly illustrate the importance of leukocyte chemotaxis in the host defense system.

Other phagocyte disorders include deficient phagocytosis which can be related to abnormal opsonization as in sickle cell disease or to possible dysfunction of the fifth complement component, Leiner's syndrome, and congenital deficiency of certain complement components (C3 and C5) or immunoglobulins. Clinical manifestations of these deficiencies are recurrent otitis media, bronchitis, pneumonia, and sepsis with encapsulated bacteria. These deficiencies, as well as those with abnormal killing of bacteria, as in chronic granulomatous disease in which there is defective superoxide and hydrogen peroxide generation, are reviewed in Ch. 149.

Immune Dysfunctions. Patients with T cell abnormalities have

TABLE 257–2. INFECTIONS IN PATIENTS WITH HOST DEFENSE DEFECTS

Host Defect	Clinical Examples	Clinical Manifestation of Infections	Infectious Agents
Inflammatory response			
Neutropenia	Aplastic anemia Agranulocytosis Leukemias	Pneumonia; ulcers of skin, oral cavity, rectum, and vagina; fever; depressed inflammatory response	Gram-negative bacilli (especially *E. coli, Pseudomonas* sp., *Klebsiella, Staph. aureus)* fungi *(Candida, Aspergillus), Pneumocystis carinii*
Chemotaxis	Chédiak-Higashi syndrome Specific granule deficiency Deficiency of 110,000 dalton glycoprotein	Subcutaneous abscesses	*Staph. aureus, Strep. pyogenes*
	Job's syndrome and variants (variable chemotactic defect)	"Cold" abscesses, bronchitis, otitis, pneumonia, bronchiectasis	*Staph. aureus, C. albicans, H. influenzae*
	Newborns	Bacteremia	Gram-negative bacilli
	Protein-calorie malnutrition; others (see text)	Bacteremia	Gram-negative bacilli
Phagocytosis			
Cellular defect	Systemic lupus erythematosus, megaloblastic anemia, chronic myelocytic leukemia	Otitis, bacteremia, pneumonias, meningitis	Encapsulated bacteria
Opsonin deficiency			
C3 deficiency	Inherited or acquired (i.e., systemic lupus erythematosus)	Otitis, bacteremia, pneumonia, meningitis	*Pseudomonas, Proteus, Staph. aureus, Strep. pneumoniae*
C5 dysfunction (possible)	Leiner's syndrome of newborn infants	Generalized seborrheic dermatitis, severe diarrhea, local and systemic infections	Gram-negative bacilli
Alternative complement pathway	Sickle cell disease	Pneumonia, osteomyelitis	Salmonella, *Strep. pneumoniae*
Bactericidal activity	Chronic granulomatous disease	Recurrent infection of lymph nodes, skin, lung, liver, bone, and other tissues	Catalase (+) microorganisms *(Staphylococcus, Klebsiella, E. coli, Serratin marcescens, Pseudomonas, Proteus, Salmonella, Candida, Aspergillus, Nocardia)*
Immune response			
T cells			
Deficiency	Thymic aplasia (DiGeorge's syndrome) and thymic hypoplasia (Nezelof's syndrome)	Otitis, pneumonia	Tuberculosis, *Listeria,* BCGosis, leprosy, *Candida,* cryptococci, aspergillosis, *Pneumocystis,* toxoplasmosis, *Strongyloides,* herpes simplex, herpes zoster, cytomegalovirus, measles
	Acquired immune deficiency syndrome	Pneumonia, oral thrush, esophagitis, meningitis, disseminated infection	*Pneumocystis, Candida, Cryptococcus,* herpes simplex, cytomegalovirus, Epstein-Barr virus, *Mycobacterium tuberculosis, Toxoplasma gondii, Cryptosporidiosus*

Dysfunction	Mucocutaneous candidiasis	Candida of mucous membranes or oral cavity, esophagus, vagina, nailbeds	*Candida albicans*
	Purine nucleoside phosphorylase deficiency	Chronic pneumonias, diarrhea, candidiasis	Fungal and viral infections
B cells	Bruton's X-linked agammaglobulinemia	Bacteremia, pneumonias, sinusitis	Fulminant hepatitis, poliomyelitis, measles, chickenpox
	Dysgammaglobulinemias, agammaglobulinemia, multiple myeloma, chronic lymphocytic leukemias		
	IgA deficiency and nodular lymphoid hyperplasia of the intestine	Diarrhea, malabsorption	*Giardia lamblia*
Mixed T and B cells	Common variable hypogammaglobulinemia (may be due to excess T suppressor cells inhibiting B cells)	Sinusitis, bronchitis, pneumonia, bacteremia	High and low grade bacterial pathogens, *Pneumocystis,* cytomegalovirus
	Ataxia telangiectasia (decreased IgA and IgE)	Sinusitis, bronchitis, pneumonia	*Strep. pneumoniae, H. influenzae,* rubella, *Giardia lamblia*
	Wiskott-Aldrich syndrome (defective antibody response to polysaccharides, decreased IgE, IgM, abnormal monocyte chemotaxis)	Otitis, pneumonia	Infections seen in T and B cell dysfunction
	Severe combined immunodeficiency, adenosine deaminase deficiency	Severe infection involving multiple sites	Infections seen in T and B cell dysfunction
Mixed defects	Hodgkin's disease and lymphoma (lymphocytopenia, delayed hypersensitivity, abnormal monocyte chemotaxis)	Pneumonia, bacteremia, hepatitis	Tuberculosis, histoplasmosis, *Salmonella, Listeria, Brucella abortis, Pneumocystis,* cytomegalovirus, herpes zoster, herpes simplex, *Cryptococcus, Candida, Aspergillosis*
	Diabetes mellitus (abnormal chemotaxis, phagocytosis, compromised neurovascular supply)	Cellulitis, urinary tract infections	*Staphylococcus aureus,* gram-negative bacilli, *Candida,* mucormycosis
	Uremia (chemotactic defect, depressed, delayed hypersensitivity, lymphopenia)	Bacteremia, pneumonia, urinary tract infection	*Staph. aureus, E. coli, Klebsiella, Pseudomonas*
	Burns (chemotactic defect, necrosis)	Cellulitis, bacteremia, pneumonia	*Staphylococcus, Strep. pyogenes, Pseudomonas* sp., *Candida,* herpes simplex
	Cystic fibrosis (mucociliary dysfunction)	Bronchitis, pneumonia	*Staph. aureus, Pseudomonas*
	Splenectomy	Pneumonia and osteomyelitis	*Streptococcus pneumoniae, Salmonella*
Iatrogenic	Foreign body (intravenous catheters, prosthetic devices)	Bacteremia, local abscesses	*Staph. aureus,* gram-negative bacilli, *Candida*
	Antibiotics	Bacteremia	*Staph. aureus,* gram-negative bacilli *(Serratia, Pseudomonas, Mima-Herellea), Candida*
	Corticosteroid therapy (depressed delayed hypersensitivity, neutrophil margination and adherence)	Bacteremia, pneumonia	*Candida, Pneumocystis, Staph. aureus,* gram-negative bacilli, others

recurrent infections from intracellular bacteria such as *M. tuberculosis*, leprosy, BCGosis, *Listeria*, and *Legionella*. These patients also become infected with other fungi (cryptococcosis, *Candida* and aspergillosis), protozoa (*Pneumocystis carinii*, toxoplasmosis, and *Strongyloides*), and viruses (herpes simplex, varicella/zoster virus, cytomegalovirus, and measles). The clinical presentation of these patients is discussed in Ch. 429.

In other patients the number of T cells is normal, but there is abnormal effector cell response to antigenic stimulation. Delayed skin responses to *Candida* and other naturally occurring antigens is absent, and lymphocytes from many of the patients do not respond to in vitro stimulation with antigens, especially *Candida*, by producing lymphokines or by replication. A well defined group of patients with T cell dysfunction have mucocutaneous candidiasis with *Candida albicans* infection restricted to the skin, nails, and mucous membranes. Another small group of patients deficient in purine nucleoside phosphorylase have T cell dysfunction with recurrent viral and fungal infections.

A dramatic form of an acquired defect of cell mediated immunity is the acquired immune deficiency syndrome (AIDS) (Ch. 430). AIDS is characterized by a remarkably selective deficiency of the number and function of the T helper cells. As a consequence, these patients are susceptible to infection with *Pneumocystis carinii*, *Candida albicans* (oral thrush and esophagitis), *Cryptococcus neoformans* meningitis or disseminated disease, cytomegalovirus, herpes simplex virus, toxoplasmosis, and mycobacterial infections, especially disseminated *Mycobacterium avium-intracellulare*. The latter infection is common in AIDS patients but rare in other immunosuppressed patients.

The prototype disease for B cell deficiency is Bruton's X-linked agammaglobulinemia with absent fully developed B cells and grossly deficient synthesis and secretion of antibody. These patients are subject to infection with encapsulated virulent pathogens such as *Streptococcus pneumoniae*, *Hemophilus influenzae*, and *Pseudomonas aeruginosa*. Untreated, these infections spread rapidly, and patients have sinorespiratory infections with recurrent pneumonias and otitis media, as well as osteomyelitis, dermatitis, and meningitis. The patients usually respond to appropriate antimicrobial drugs, probably because of normal phagocyte and T cell function. Infections caused by intracellular microorganisms such as *M. tuberculosis*, *Histoplasma*, and fungi are relatively infrequent.

Diseases with combined deficiencies of T and B cells are associated with severe infections. Such patients usually succumb early in life to many different forms of infection, including *Pneumocystis carinii*, cytomegalovirus, other viruses, and bacterial pathogens of high and low grade virulence.

DIAGNOSIS. Initial evaluation of patients with recurrent infections requires a thorough history. For example, a history of contact dermatitis (poison ivy) helps eliminate T cell dysfunction, whereas a history of mucocutaneous candidiasis suggests a T cell abnormality. Aphthous ulcers may be early signs of severe neutropenia. Staphylococcal skin infections and recurrent pneumonias suggest a chemotactic defect, and a history of recurrent infections with catalase positive microorganisms suggests chronic granulomatous disease.

Tests useful in the laboratory evaluation of compromised hosts are summarized in Table 257–3. Initial laboratory screening studies can be very informative. A white blood count and differential count will serve as a screen for the leukopenias. In occasional patients in whom the clinical course suggests cyclic neutropenia, daily white blood cell counts for several months are necessary. The morphology of the white cell can be particularly helpful. For example, multilobed nuclei are seen in polymorphonuclear leukocytes in vitamin B_{12} or folate deficiency, and when considering the Chédiak-Higashi syndrome the characteristic giant lysosomes can be seen. An excellent screening test used to diagnose chronic granulomatous disease is the ability of granulocytes to reduce nitroblue tetrazolium dye. This test, which is available in most medical centers, reflects leukocyte oxidative metabolism and is markedly abnormal in chronic granulomatous disease and a few related disorders of phagocyte function (see Ch. 149). Other tests capable of detecting chronic granulomatous disease include the chemiluminescence assay as well as a new spectrofluorometric assay employing lipophilic fluorescent probes of membrane potential. The latter assay is simple and fast. An abnormality of the latter assay may reflect a fundamental defect of ion transport in leukocytes obtained from patients with chronic granulomatous disease.

TABLE 257–3. DIAGNOSTIC TESTS USED IN THE EVALUATION OF HOST DEFENSE DEFECTS

Host Defense	Test
Bone marrow production	Peripheral white blood count*
	Marrow aspirate*
	Bone marrow reserve test†
Inflammatory response	Rebuck skin window*†
	Leukocyte function
	Adherence*†
	Chemotactic response*†
	Phagocytosis‡
	Degranulation‡
	Bactericidal activity*†
	Oxidative metabolism
	Nitroblue tetrazolium dye reduction (NBT test)*†
	Hexosemonophosphate shunt activity‡
	Leukocyte glucose-6-phosphate dehydrogenase and myeloperoxidase‡
	Cytochrome b‡
	Chemotactic and opsonic activity of serum*†
	Complement levels (CH50,* C3*, C4†)
Immune response	
T cell system (cellular immunity)	Delayed hypersensitivity skin tests to common antigens*
	Sensitization to dinitrochlorobenzene‡
	Chest x-ray to assess thymus gland*
	Quantitation of T cells†
	T cell rosettes
	Specific membrane markers
	Lymphocyte transformation studies†
	Nonspecific mitogens (pokeweed, concanavalin A)
	Specific antigens (PPD, mumps, streptokinase-streptodornase, *Candida albicans*)
	Lymphokine and monokine production‡
	Chemotactic lymphokines
	Interleukins
	Macrophage migration-inhibitory factor
B cell system (humoral immunity)	Quantitative immunoglobulins*
	Immunoglobulin subclasses‡
	Kinetics of antibody synthesis following primary and secondary immunization‡
	Antibodies to common viruses†
	Specific antibody response after immunization* (typhoid H and O agglutinins)

*Screening tests.
†Generally available at major medical centers.
‡Available only in specialized laboratories.

Qualitative immunoglobulin tests assess B cell function, and in the presence of borderline hypogammaglobulinemia the capacity of patients to produce specific antibodies after immunization is important. Most hospital laboratories can measure typhoid H and O agglutinins before and after immunization with standard vaccines, and antibodies to common viruses are also usually available. In addition, antibody titers to some antigens used for childhood immunization (e.g., tetanus, diphtheria) can often be obtained through referral laboratories. T cell function can be screened by delayed hypersensitivity skin testing to common antigens (PPD, *Candida*, mumps, streptokinase, and streptodornase). A chest x-ray will help in evaluation of the thymus gland and may reveal evidence for recurrent pneumonias or bronchiectasis. Total hemolytic complement (CH50), C3, and C4 levels are available in many laboratories, although studies of individual complement components can be obtained only in a few research centers.

More specific studies are often necessary to define host defense defects. Marrow reserves can be evaluated by a bone marrow aspirate and with an etiocholanolone administration test. The inflammatory response can be estimated in vivo with a Rebuck skin window, which assesses the ability of leukocytes to accumulate at a superficial abrasion. More precise characterization of the cellular and humoral components of the inflammatory response require studies in vitro. Leukocyte adherence is measured by the ability of cells to stick to nylon wool. Locomotion can be qualitatively evaluated by looking at cells moving on glass slides and by measuring cell migration into different kinds of filter paper. Chemotactic factors are assessed by their ability to attract normal leukocytes. These studies of the inflammatory response are generally available in medical centers, as are studies for the quantitation of leukocyte phagocytosis and killing of bacteria. Studies of leukocyte hexose monophosphate shunt activity, leukocyte actin and myosin, or microtubule function are presently restricted to a few clinical research laboratories.

In-depth studies of the immune system include quantitation of T and B cells (and their subpopulations), using specific membrane markers. B cell function can be evaluated by the kinetics of antibody synthesis following primary and secondary immunization. Measurement of immunoglobulin G subclasses is also available. T cell function can be further characterized in vivo by monitoring the delayed hypersensitivity response after contact sensitization with dinitrochlorobenzene. T cell functional correlates of delayed hypersensitivity can be assessed in vitro by measuring proliferative responses (tritium incorporation) to nonspecific stimuli such as mitogens (phytohemagglutinin, pokeweed mitogen, and concanavalin A) or specific stimuli such as antigens (PPD, mumps, streptokinase-streptodornase, or *Candida albicans*). Quantitation of the release of lymphokines and monokines (i.e., migration inhibitory factor, interleukins, or chemotactic lymphokines) is generally available in medical centers. Other specific tests of T cell function are available only in highly specialized laboratories.

Particularly puzzling patients with no demonstrable defect of host defenses should raise one's suspicion of the possibility of a psychologic disorder with self-inflicted lesions. Psychologic problems can be very serious, with patients or parents of children inoculating foreign material subcutaneously or performing other manipulations that can manifest as severe abscesses or unexplained fevers; many of these patients are medical or paramedical professionals. Continual culture of fecal flora from wounds and localization of infections to conveniently reached areas (such as the left side of the body in right-handed individuals) should lead one to suspect psychologic problems.

MANAGEMENT. ***General Considerations.*** Management of the compromised host is based in part on the specific problems. Risk from environmental factors such as crowded living conditions, contaminated hospital respirators, or intravenous lines must be rigidly controlled. Intravenous lines should be used only when necessary; metal (scalp vein) devices should be used whenever possible, as microbial colonization with these is less than with plastic catheters. Similarly, all catheters, especially Foley catheters, should be used as little as possible, and they should be changed regularly. Antimicrobial agents should be carefully selected and used with as much microbial specificity as possible.

Certain procedures are associated with bacteremia or local spread of infection, and compromised hosts undergoing these procedures may be at increased risk. In particular, dental manipulation, bronchoscopy, certain gastrointestinal studies (gastroscopy, jejunal biopsy, liver biopsy, sigmoidoscopy, barium enema, retrograde cholangiograms), urinary tract manipulations (catheterization, cystoscopy, retrograde pyelogram), angiograms (cardiac catheterization), orthopedic surgery, and, on rare occasions, bone marrow aspiration have all been associated with bacteremia.

Prophylactic Antibiotics. In severely compromised hosts, administration of appropriate antimicrobials (depending on the expected bacteremia) prior to and for several hours after the procedure may prevent development of disseminated foci of infection. Oxacillin (2 grams intravenously for adults or 200 mg per kilogram intravenously for children) plus gentamicin (1.5 mg per kilogram intramuscularly or intravenously for adults or 3 to 5 mg per kilogram intramuscularly or intravenously for children) 30 to 60 minutes before and 8 and 16 hours after procedure is one regimen useful for dental or surgical patients. There is increasing evidence that oral nonabsorbable "prophylactic" antibiotics such as gentamicin, vancomycin, and neomycin may be appropriate for decreasing sepsis and pulmonary and anal-rectal infections in patients receiving induction chemotherapy for tumors. This is particularly true if the white blood cell count is less than 1000 cells per cubic millimeter for more than two weeks. However, such oral antibiotics are associated with malabsorption as well as poor patient compliance because of bad taste, often made worse by the nausea and vomiting from induction chemotherapy. Therefore, unless good patient compliance is anticipated, oral nonabsorbable antibiotics should not be used.

Considerable controversy exists regarding the necessity for isolating patients with compromised defenses. Obviously judgment is required as to which patients require isolation. Patients with severely compromised defenses (such as patients with agranulocytosis plus corticosteroid therapy) may benefit by isolation from hospital personnel, as may those with draining staphylococcal wounds or herpes zoster. However, isolation is disruptive to hospital routine and should not be continued any longer than required. Hospital personnel with minor infections, such as active oral herpetic lesions, should avoid contact with severely compromised patients such as neonates or adult patients in laminar flow facilities. Since malnourished patients have major problems with inflammatory and immune responses, adequate diet and correction of a malnourished state is often critical to the care of a compromised host.

Leukopenias. The compromised host with leukopenia, and in particular granulocytopenia, poses a particularly difficult management problem. Usually the faster the granulocytopenia evolves, the more severe the consequences. This is especially true if immunosuppressive drugs such as corticosteroids are being used concurrently. If there is any possibility of an environmental or drug-induced leukopenia, the etiologic agent should be eliminated. When infections occur, inflammatory manifestations are markedly diminished or absent, and careful and frequent examination of the patient for subtle findings of infection is required. Surveillance cultures of the oral cavity, stool, and open wounds, as well as culture of withdrawn catheter tips, can be very helpful in the selection of initial antimicrobials when these patients become infected.

A particularly difficult management problem is the granulocytopenic patient with fever. In most series, about one third of these patients will have positive cultures, one third will have sepsis, and one third will have no evidence of infection. In general, combination antibiotics such as an aminoglycoside (i.e., tobramycin), a broad-spectrum antipseudomonal penicillin (i.e., ticarcillin), and gentamicin are recommended as initial therapy. The duration of therapy is governed by the clinical response and culture results. If there is a good clinical response with a rise in granulocyte count, antibiotics can be discontinued when the patient has been afebrile for 48 hours. If a pathogen is isolated, appropriate antibiotics are selected and serum antibiotic levels are monitored; signs of local infection must be searched for repetitively. If the patient becomes afebrile but remains neutropenic, combination antibiotics are continued, although increased problems with fungal infection may result. In the setting of persistent neutropenia and positive blood cultures, white blood cell transfusions may be appropriate. If there is no clinical response and no pathogen is isolated, it is appropriate to add a cephalosporin antibiotic. If still no response is seen over an additional 48 hours, strong consideration of disseminated fungal infection should be entertained, and initiation of empiric therapy with amphotericin B is appropriate; white blood cell transfusions may then be considered.

Neutropenic patients with documented mycotic infections

require special attention. Heavy colonization with *Candida* (thrush of the mouth, esophagus, or vagina) should be treated with a topical antifungal agent such as nystatin (Mycostatin, Miconazole, or Ketoconazole). Patients with *Candida* urinary tract colonization, as judged by pseudohyphae in the urine, who have no fever or other evidence of infection and in whom a Foley catheter is required, may benefit from bladder irrigation for several days with amphotericin B (50 μg per milliliter). If a bladder catheter is not in place, oral 5-fluorocytosine should be considered, especially if the clinical situation is not urgent and renal function is normal. With severe candidiasis, intravenous amphotericin B should be used. Patients with compromised defenses who demonstrate transient candidemia that is thought to be related to contaminated intravenous lines may benefit from a short course of intravenous amphotericin B to try to prevent the establishment of disseminated foci. Fungemia in patients with malignancies and compromised defenses, especially lymphoreticular or hematopoietic malignancies, is frequently associated with disseminated fungal infection, and in these patients early use of amphotericin, sometimes prior to microbiologic confirmation, should be considered. Ketoconazole is particularly useful in the management of chronic *Candida* infection of the nails and oral cavity in patients with Job's syndrome.

Use of agents such as lithium and androgens to stimulate the bone marrow has been of use in some patients. Bone marrow transplantation to reconstitute patients with agranulocytosis and other immunodeficiencies is attractive but still under investigation and at present is restricted to only a few medical centers. Use of leukocyte transfusions to transiently correct leukopenias may prove to be beneficial. Initial studies using leukocyte transfusions are encouraging, but methods for collection and storage of leukocytes and techniques for the prevention of antileukocyte antibody formation in recipients remain particular problems.

Disorders of the Inflammatory Response. Management of patients with neutrophil dysfunction syndromes requires aggressive therapy of particular infections with careful selection of antimicrobial drugs. Aggressive use of antimicrobials and early surgical drainage of abscesses in some patients (i.e., with chronic granulomatous disease) is appropriate. Long-term chemoprophylaxis has not been established as beneficial, although it may help in selected situations; chemoprophylaxis prior to procedures commonly associated with bacteremia is appropriate. Trimethoprim-sulfamethoxazole may be useful as a prophylactic agent in selected patients with chronic granulomatous disease because it significantly prolongs infection-free intervals. Patients allergic to sulfamethoxazole appear to benefit from prophylactic trimethoprim-dicloxacillin. There is increasing evidence that leukocyte transfusions are important adjunct therapy for life-threatening infections in chronic granulomatous disease. Leukocytes used for transfusion in chronic granulomatous disease should not be irradiated since graft versus host disease is no problem in these patients and irradiation damages phagocyte function. Although bone marrow transplantation may have a role in the future, currently the severe complication of bone marrow transplantation excludes its use in patients with phagocyte defects.

Manipulation of leukocyte function with pharmacologic agents may be an important future approach to management of patients with leukocyte dysfunction. Ascorbic acid has improved granulocyte function in a few patients with the Chédiak-Higashi syndrome. Levamisole,* which previously was thought to be of use in patients with hyper IgE-recurrent infection (Job's) syndrome, has been shown to be nonefficacious and is no longer indicated. Vitamin E, which is thought to protect phagocytes from auto-oxidative damage, is under investigation for treating certain patients with phagocyte defects.

*Investigational drug.

Aside from the infectious complications of the inherited phagocyte defect syndromes, a number of other problems often appear with specific syndromes. Abnormal, chronically inflamed gingivae and a predisposition to periodontal disease are common findings in all the inherited syndromes of phagocyte dysfunction. Special attention to routine oral hygiene procedures seems to be the most reasonable approach to this chronic problem. Twice-daily tooth brushing with 3 per cent H_2O_2 and baking soda brings about dramatic improvement in the dental health of some patients.

Patients with chronic granulomatous disease can develop granulomatous inflammation, which is not obviously infectious, at any anatomic site. With time and repeated episodes, the physical size of such granulomatous masses can cause disease by mass effect; esophageal, gastric antrum, and duodenal obstruction due to such granulomatous masses have all been described. Although such obstructions usually resolve with empiric antibiotic therapy, surgical resection of involved areas has been used to clear obstruction that did not respond to antimicrobials.

Several skin conditions are commonly seen in patients with defective phagocyte function. Patients with chronic granulomatous disease often have seborrheic dermatitis involving the scalp, axillary, and pubic hair. This dermatitis tends to wax and wane in severity, and often becomes secondarily infected with common skin flora, especially *Staphylococcus aureus*. Dramatic improvement is usually seen during periods of intravenous antibiotic therapy for other infections. For chronic management of this dermatitis, daily local scrubs with hexachlorophene or iodine-containing soaps and application of hydrocortisone cream locally can be helpful. Of course, with continued use of these soaps, possible side effects from absorption of hexachlorophene or iodine must be monitored. Patients with chronic granulomatous disease also have chronic inflammation of the nares that can be severe, painful, and cause denuding of skin around the tip of the nose. When this nasal inflammation is mild, it needs no specific therapy other than good local hygiene. However, if it becomes severe, it should be treated with 7- to 10-day courses of antibiotics. Penicillinase-resistant penicillin, given orally, usually proves effective, with courses of therapy repeated as inflammation flares.

Disorders of the Immune Response. Patients with IgG immunoglobulin deficiency with recurrent bacterial infections usually benefit from replacement therapy with human gamma globulin. Maintenance of plasma IgG around 200 mg per milliliter is reported to decrease severe infections, although sinusitis, bronchitis, and otitis may persist. Intramuscular injection of IgG (100 mg per kilogram) at monthly intervals is usually adequate. Immunoglobulin also may be administered by slow subcutaneous infusion, although replacement immunoglobulin preparations that can be administered intravenously recently have become available. Globulin injection is beneficial only in patients deficient in immunoglobulin G. An alternative therapy is infusion of fresh plasma, 10 to 20 ml per kilogram, at intervals of three to four weeks. The advantage is that, in addition to replacing IgG, it replaces IgM and IgA, although the IgA never enters the secretory pools. The disadvantage is the risk of transmitting hepatitis and the volumes required. Despite gamma globulin, repeated infections and progression of pulmonary fibrosis and bronchiectasis may persist.

Attempts at immune reconstitution have also included bone marrow transplantation, infusion of histocompatible lymphocytes, and administration of alpha interferon, gamma interferon, and interleukin. Despite transient signs of improvement of several deficiencies, no impressive long-lasting cures have consistently been seen with these approaches.

Treatment of patients with T cell deficiencies is largely a research procedure. Attempts to reconstitute cell-mediated immune responses with BCG, killed *C. parvum*, cimetidine, muramyl dipeptide, lithium compounds, and interferon have had mixed success. Some patients have responded to fetal thymus graft with increased numbers of T cells and improved T cell function, especially those with the fungal infections, candidiasis, or coccidioidomycosis. Other patients have responded to immune reconstitution with transfer factor therapy. However, efficacy with transfer factor only seems to be long-lasting when it is used in combination with antifungal therapy and when the transfer factor is obtained from donors sensitive to the fungus. At present, therapeutic use of transfer factor should be considered investigational and its use restricted to investigators actively evaluating its therapeutic potential.

Dale D, Guetry D, Wewerka JR, Bull JM, Chusid MJ: Chronic neutropenia. Medicine 58:128, 1979. *A nice survey of chronic neutropenias, particularly with regard to diagnosis and natural history. Good for medical students and house officers.*

Donabedian H, Gallin JI: The hyperimmunoglobulin E-recurrent infection (Job's) syndrome. A review of the NIH experience and the literature. Medicine 62:195, 1983. *A comprehensive review of the pathogenesis and management of this complex disease.*

Easmon CSF, Gaya H: Second International Symposium on Infections in the Immunocompromised Host. London, Academic Press, 1983. *A comprehensive overview of host defenses, ranging from pathophysiology of parasitic and viral infection to therapeutic use of antiviral agents and immunopotentiators. Excellent book for fellows and established clinicians in infectious diseases with selected fine chapters for students.*

Gallin JI: Abnormal phagocyte chemotaxis: Pathophysiology, clinical manifestations and patient management. Rev Infect Dis 3:1196, 1981. *A comprehensive review of the presentation and management of these unusual patients.*

Gallin JI, Buescher ES, Seligmann BE, Gaither T, Nath J, Katz P: Recent advances in chronic granulomatous disease. Ann Intern Med 99:657, 1983. *Detailed updated review and discussion of the recent advances in the pathogenesis and management of chronic granulomatous disease.*

Gallin JI, Fauci AS: Advances in Host Defense Mechanisms. Vol. 1. Phagocytic Cells. Vol. 2. Lymphoid Cells. Vol. 3. Chronic Granulomatous Disease. New York, Raven Press, 1982–1983. *A new series designed to integrate highly sophisticated science with applicability to clinically relevant host defense mechanisms. Geared for broad readership, including students, fellows, and specialists in infectious diseases.*

Good RA (ed.): Proceedings of a workshop on intravenous immune globulin: Its use and potential. J Clin Immunol 2 (Suppl) 4S–48S, 1982. *A clearly written collection of papers analyzing the use of intravenous immune globulin. Good for fellows and specialists who need a review of this emerging therapy.*

Grieco MH (ed.): Infections in the Abnormal Host. New York, Yorke Medical Books, 1980. *A collection of chapters by leading investigators. Very complete approach. Ideal for fellows and residents.*

Lichtenstein LM, Fauci AS: Current Therapy in Allergy and Immunology, 1983–1984. New York, B.C. Decker, Inc., 1983. *Contains clearly written chapters on the management of the immunocompromised host. A practical guide for those managing these difficult patients.*

Klebanoff SJ, Clark RA: The Neutrophil: Function and Clinical Disorders. Amsterdam, North Holland Publishing Company, 1978. *An "encyclopedia" of neutrophil function and disorders. Excellent references through 1977. Ideal for fellows; selected chapters are superb for students.*

258. PREVENTION AND TREATMENT OF HOSPITAL-ACQUIRED INFECTIONS

*Richard P. Wenzel**

HISTORY. The father of infection control is Ignaz Semmelweis (1818–1865), whose observations in Vienna—prior to formulation of the germ theory—laid the foundations for hospital epidemiology. At the Allgemeines Krankenhaus, Semmelweis compiled mortality data on two obstetrics wards: on one ward (I), in which all women were attended by obstetricians and medical students, the mortality was over 8 per cent; on the other ward (II), in which all women were attended by midwives, the mortality was 2 per cent. In retrospect the cause of death with puerperal sepsis was the Group A β-hemolytic streptococcus, *S. pyogenes*. Semmelweis made two very important observations: (1) there was a lower mortality on ward I when medical students were on vacation, and (2) the odor of the autopsy room was noted on ward I whenever students were present. Furthermore, a colleague and pathologist, Professor Kolletschka, accidentally cut his own finger while performing a postmortem examination on one of the women who died of puerperal sepsis. Professor Kolletschka developed a syndrome very similar to that of the obstetric patients and died. Semmelweis reasoned that some element was carried on the hands of students and physicians from the autopsy room (where they performed postmortem examinations) to the obstetrics ward (where they examined patients). Eventually Semmelweis introduced the practice of handwashing with an antiseptic (chloride of lime) between the autopsy room and the delivery room and before the examination of each patient. Thereafter, the mortality in ward I fell to less than 2 per cent.

INTRODUCTION. Each year approximately 40 million people are hospitalized in the United States. Between 5 and 10 per cent, or 2 to 4 million patients, will develop an infection that was not present or incubating upon admission. Such infections are referred to as hospital acquired or nosocomial.† Nosocomial infections are directly responsible for an estimated 75,000 to 150,000 deaths, and lead to excess hospitalization (Table 258–1) with an economic burden of approximately 5 billion dollars per year. Several features distinguish nosocomial infections from community-acquired infections: the former are often (50 to 70 per cent) caused by aerobic gram-negative rods; they frequently occur in patients with altered host immune defenses; and they require therapy with more toxic antibiotics. Staphylococcal disease accounts for 10 to 20 per cent of hospital-acquired infections, and in some hospitals an increasing proportion of these are resistant to methicillin and other penicillinase-resistant antibiotics. The distribution of infections by anatomic site in acute care hospitals (Table 258–1) indicates that infections of the urinary tract account for 35 to 40 per cent of all nosocomial infections; postoperative wounds, 20 per cent; bloodstream, 5 to 10 per cent; lung, 15 per cent; and others, 15 to 20 per cent. Although the data on infections acquired in nursing homes are limited, estimates are that they may total 7 million or more each year.

No matter how effective an infection control program may be, it is impossible to eliminate all infections, in part because many arise endogenously in patients whose immune defense mechanisms are impaired, such as patients with leukemia and those who have received organ transplants. In addition, many patients have indwelling catheters, which provide organisms access to the body. Interspersed among such endemic infections, epidemics occur. An epidemic implies an unusual and significant increase in the incidence of a particular disease. It is estimated that 4 per cent of infected patients acquire their infections as part of a major epidemic; another 4 to 6 per cent are thought to acquire their infection as part of a cluster of epidemiologically linked infections. Both epidemic and endemic infections may result from a transient breakdown in proper technique or another common source event. Recognition of endemic infection may allow for correction of the problem before epidemic rates occur. The major point is that infection control efforts should focus on preventable infections.

Infection or colonization results when a sufficient number of organisms with ability to attach to skin or mucosal surfaces reaches a susceptible host. Colonization implies a peaceful coexistence between organism and host, whereas infection results from an altered balance of power in favor of the organism. Three major routes are recognized by which organisms are transmitted to hospitalized patients: direct contact, the air (via droplet nuclei less than 5 μ in diameter), and common source vehicles such as contaminated nebulizers. The most

TABLE 258–1. IMPACT OF HOSPITAL-ACQUIRED INFECTIONS IN ACUTE CARE INSTITUTIONS

Anatomic Site	Number of Infections per 100 Admissions	Proportion of All Hospital-Acquired Infections	Estimated Direct Mortality	Mean Number of Excess Hospital Days per Infection
Urinary tract	2.5	35–40%	<1%	2
Postoperative wound	1.5	20%	<1%	7
Pulmonary	1	15%	?*	?
Bloodstream	0.5–1	5–10%	25%	30
Others	1	15–20%	Varies with site	Varies with site

*Gross mortality was 35 per cent in an uncontrolled study at a university hospital.

*The author gratefully acknowledges the assistance of Bruce F. Farber, M.D., Division of Infectious Diseases, University of Pittsburgh Hospital, Pittsburgh, Pennsylvania.

†Nosocomial is derived from the Greek word for hospital.

likely mode of transmission of infection in the hospital is direct contact via the hands of medical personnel. Furthermore, the rate of transmission by all mechanisms is highest in patients in close proximity to the reservoir. Simple handwashing is effective in preventing direct contact transmission and remains the most important infection control measure. Additionally, infections can be minimized by elimination of the reservoir. If the reservoir is an inanimate object (e.g., a pressure monitor transducer head), infection control is readily accomplished. Unfortunately the reservoirs for most nosocomial infections are patients themselves. Thus, isolation techniques (see below) are utilized to contain certain organisms that cannot be readily eliminated.

HIGH RISK LOCATIONS. Certain areas of any hospital are likely to be the locale of high rates of endemic infections as well as of outbreaks or epidemics. The high risk areas include the critical care areas, burn units, and dialysis units. Critical care areas are usually the birthplace and area of highest prevalence of antibiotic resistance in the hospital, including methicillin-resistant *S. aureus* and aminoglycoside-resistant gram-negative rods. Recently the importance of *S. epidermidis* bloodstream infections in patients in intensive care units has been stressed.

Critical Care Areas. Medical, surgical, and neonatal critical care areas provide a concentration of patients at high risk for developing nosocomial infections. This is a reflection of patients' underlying diseases, the frequent use of invasive monitoring, and alteration of normal flora by antibiotics. Often patients are in close proximity to each other, promoting transmission by busy medical personnel who fail to wash their hands between contacts. Cross-infection has been reported to be particularly common among thermally injured patients. Furthermore, the widespread use of topical antibiotics may select for colonization and infection with multiply resistant organisms. The major pathogens include *Pseudomonas aeruginosa, Providencia stuartii,* other gram-negative rods, and, in some burn units, methicillin-resistant *S. aureus.*

Proper design of critical care units with regard to separation of patients by partitions and placement of sinks at the entranceway to individual patient cubicles, as well as optimal nursing-to-patient ratios, may minimize the risks of cross-infection. Other suggested infection control measures include (1) the notification of the infection control team by the unit of all new procedures or products and (2) use of a clinical flow sheet listing all catheters, dates of insertion, and rationale for continued use.

Dialysis Units. Both bacterial and viral infections occur with increased frequency in patients with chronic renal failure. Bacterial infections often affect fistulas and arteriovenous access shunts. With infected fistulas, up to one third of patients may have no objective signs of infection, and may complain only of intense pain. With *S. aureus* infections of fistulas or shunts, up to 20 per cent may develop secondary endocarditis. Evidence of viral infection (including both non-A non-B and type B viral hepatitis) is found in virtually all units. Often the virus is introduced by one of the blood products used. Once introduced, transmission to other patients and staff can occur by accidental needle stick exposure, contaminated dialysis equipment, and possibly other contact. Renal patients are more likely to become chronic carriers of hepatitis B surface antigen (HB_sAg) than are patients in the community who become infected with hepatitis B. Staff members working in these units are also at increased risk of infection. Recent data from the Centers for Disease Control indicate that in 1982 only 0.4 per cent of dialysis personnel and 0.5 per cent of patients acquired hepatitis B. The annual incidence of non-A non-B hepatitis in patients was 1.6 per cent. Thus, there would appear to be a dramatic reduction in hepatitis B relative to the late 1970's and a 3 to 1 ratio of non-A non-B to type B infection in dialysis patients. The infections may result in chronic liver disease, including a susceptibility to delta infection in chronic carriers of HB_sAg, and may expose offspring of pregnant workers to the risk of neonatal hepatitis. With the recent introduction of an effective vaccine for hepatitis B, susceptible hospital personnel who are exposed to blood products are advised to receive it. The vaccine is given in three 1 ml doses administered intramuscularly at times zero, one month, and six months. In addition, the risk to the staff can be minimized and epidemics identified early or prevented with proper control practices: (1) Strict handwashing procedures should be observed. (2) Serologic surveillance of patients and dialysis staff for hepatitis at three- to six-month intervals is recommended unless anti-HB_S antibody is present. (3) Protective clothing should be worn in the area. (4) Eating, drinking, smoking, and mouth pipetting should be prohibited in the unit. (5) Contaminated materials should be autoclaved or incinerated. (6) Contaminated surfaces should be washed with 0.5 to 1.0 per cent sodium hypochlorite prior to routine cleanup. (7) Needles used to draw blood should be discarded in boxes, and not recapped. (8) Pregnant staff members might consider transferring to another area of the hospital in order to avoid acquiring viral hepatitis and transmitting the infection to the baby.

SURVEILLANCE. Surveillance refers to the routine and orderly collection of information regarding the occurrence of a disease. In the hospital it is primarily used to define endemic rates and to identify high and low risk areas. Data from surveillance identify clusters and epidemics when certain threshold rates are exceeded. Thus, surveillance is the basis for alteration of existing procedures and practices. The impact of various methods of surveillance in reducing infections is currently under study. A minimal data base is necessary in order to establish priorities for a proper infection control program and to satisfy the requirements of the Joint Commission for Accreditation of Hospitals (JCAH). In general, surveillance is performed by infection control practitioners, most of whom are nurses. In addition, the practitioners gathering data often reinforce isolation procedures and identify new problems by their visibility on the wards and by communication with staff nurses and physicians. The starting point for data collection varies; review of nursing care plans, antibiotic use, bacteriology reports, and fever curves have all been used to identify patients at high risk. Once high risk patients are identified, trained practitioners can then review their charts, seeking any evidence for infection. Practitioners who wish to compare infection rates among similar categories of hospitals should use identical definitions for infection (Table 258–2). Infection rates for a defined period are later compiled by identifying the number of infections (numerator) and the total number of patients at risk (denominator). By convention, the number of patients admitted or discharged is often substituted for the number of patients at risk. Infection rates by site, service, organism, and procedure are tallied. In hospitals with sophisticated surveillance, infection rates by underlying diagnosis are also reported. In addition, a summary of antibiotic sensitivity patterns for hospital pathogens may help clinicians select proper initial antimicrobial therapy of nosocomial infections.

Analysis of data collected by surveillance requires knowledge of basic epidemiologic measurements. These include the following: (1) Incidence—the number of new cases of a disease in a population at risk over a specified unit of time. An example is the number of new cases of wound infection per 100 patients

TABLE 258–2. DEFINITIONS OF NOSOCOMIAL INFECTION* USED IN SURVEILLANCE

Anatomic Site	Criteria
Urine	≥100,000 colonies of bacteria per milliliter of urine
Postoperative wound	Pus at the incision site
Blood	Positive culture (exclude contaminant)
Pulmonary	New infiltrate on chest film associated with purulent sputum (exclude atelectasis and pulmonary embolus with infarction)
Burns	$\geq 10^6$ organisms per gram of biopsy tissue

*Infections which are not incubating or present upon admission.

at risk per month. (2) Prevalence—the number of persons with a disease (newly acquired or not) at a given time. An example is the number of patients on January 1 with an obvious wound infection per 100 patients on the ward. (3) Attack rate—the number of new cases of a disease in a particular population exposed to a particular risk. No defined unit of time is implied, although the period of risk is assumed to be limited. An example is the number of patients with a wound infection per 100 undergoing appendectomies.

Surveillance data should be summarized in a report for distribution throughout the hospital. This enables the various services to review their performance routinely and to become aware of potential problems. If a change in the infection rate appears to be significant, it is necessary to use statistical testing to be sure.

URINARY TRACT INFECTIONS. The upper and lower urinary tracts are the source of 35 to 40 per cent of all nosocomial infections. About 80 per cent of infections occur in patients who have undergone some form of instrumentation, usually catheterization.

A simple in-and-out catheterization is frequently used to obtain urine samples from patients who cannot give a clean voided sample. Although this procedure carries a relatively low risk of significant bacteriuria in healthy ambulatory men and women (2 to 3 per cent), the risk is 6 per cent in hospitalized women, 9 per cent in postpartum women, and 23 per cent in postpartum women who have had complicated labors. Although the risk may be justified in postoperative patients with transient retention, routine catheterization should be discouraged in healthy obstetric patients at the time of delivery.

Indwelling Foley catheters are used in 10 to 20 per cent of hospitalized patients. They are the major predisposing agents of nosocomially induced urinary tract infection. The risk associated with these catheters is dependent upon the length of time they remain in place: bacteriuria occurs at a rate of 5 per cent per day that the indwelling catheter is left in place. Evidence of upper tract involvement by antibody coating tests and the presence of circulating endotoxins are not infrequent in patients with catheter-related infection. In addition, urinary infections serve as the most common predisposing source for secondary gram-negative rod bacteremia. Secondary bacteremia occurs in 3 per cent of bacteriuric patients. However, recent data suggest that the rate of secondary bacteremia with *Serratia marcescens* bacteriuria is very high (16/100) and that all bacteriuric patients with the organism should be given appropriate therapy regardless of symptoms.

The principal organisms involved in nosocomial urinary tract infections are as follows: *E. coli* (33 per cent), enterococci (15 per cent), *Proteus* (15 per cent), *Klebsiella* (10 per cent), and *Pseudomonas* (10 per cent). Unlike community-acquired urinary tract infections, these organisms are usually resistant to sulfonamides and ampicillin. Newer β-lactam antibiotics and aminoglycosides are effective in most cases, but outbreaks of multiply resistant organisms have occurred.

Hematogenous spread of bacteria to the urinary tract is uncommon. In most catheter-related infections, organisms gain entrance to the system and ascend into the bladder. There are several areas where contamination is likely to occur: the junction of the catheter and urethral meatus, the internal aspect of the collection vessel tubing with retrograde flow to the bladder, and the urethra at the time of catheterization resulting from inadequate preparation or improper technique. Bacteria can migrate from the perineum along the outside of the catheter into the bladder. This is probably the major route of infection occurring within the first week of catheterization. In one well-described outbreak, the risk of acquiring a Foley catheter–related urinary tract infection was significantly greater in patients who had a catheterized roommate with a similar infection. Cross-infections seemed to occur by the hands of medical personnel, with contamination of the collection system and subsequent migration around the catheter into the bladder.

All patients requiring indwelling catheters should have closed drainage systems in an effort to maintain the sterility of the system and help prevent cross-infections among patients. Proper care of the closed system is important in minimizing the risk of infection. Basic practices include the following: (1) Aseptic insertion by trained personnel. In one study patients catheterized by specially instructed physicians had significantly less bacteriuria at 48 hours than did those catheterized by licensed practical nurses. Catheter care teams have not been shown to be cost effective or efficacious. (2) Drainage bags should be hung and kept upright below the level of the patient's bladder to prevent retrograde flow. They should never be allowed to rest on the floor or to be inverted. (3) Drainage bags should be emptied frequently to avoid distention and contamination. All vessels used to measure urine output should be disinfected between patients to avoid cross-infection. (4) The system should not be irrigated unless absolutely necessary. Small specimens of urine can be aspirated from the proximal lumen of the catheter with a sterile syringe after proper disinfection. (5) Routine changing of the catheters is probably unnecessary unless they become obstructed or encrusted.

Perineal care and use of antimicrobial lubricants either around the catheter or impregnated within the catheter are not of proven efficacy. Similarly, the use of disinfectants in the drainage bag has not reduced infections in patients catheterized one week or less. Furthermore, the practice of culturing the tip of catheters at the time of removal has been shown not to be a valuable monitor of infection.

Several authors have suggested the use of prophylactic irrigation of closed drainage systems with acetic acid or polymyxin-neomycin solutions. Their use should probably be reserved for those who require irrigation to relieve obstruction by clots. The efficacy of prophylactic antibiotics appears to be limited to the first four days of catheterization. Although this may be of value in selected patients such as those undergoing prostate surgery, prolonged or widespread use should be discouraged, since it will most likely select for resistant organisms. In addition, the efficacy of prophylactic antibiotics has not been critically evaluated in closed drainage systems.

NOSOCOMIAL PNEUMONIAS. Approximately 1 per cent of hospitalized patients will develop a nosocomial pneumonia. Hospital-acquired pneumonias tend to be more common in university than community hospitals owing to differences in patient populations. Although crude mortality for nosocomial pneumonias in university patients has been reported to be 35 per cent, prospective studies of the direct morbidity and mortality of hospital-acquired pneumonias (apart from the influence of underlying diseases) are lacking. *Pseudomonas* pneumonia appears to carry a particularly high mortality (70 per cent), as do pneumonias in the compromised hosts and those which are superinfections. A recent survey by the Centers for Disease Control's National Nosocomial Infectious Study suggested that 7 per cent of nosocomial pneumonias led to secondary bacteremias.

The most common cause of nosocomial pneumonias is the gram-negative bacilli, accounting for over 50 per cent of all cases. No study has employed transtracheal aspirates or lung aspirates to confirm the etiology of nosocomial pneumonias in a large series of patients. *Klebsiella, S. aureus, Pseudomonas aeruginosa,* and *E. coli* are frequently isolated from sputum. These organisms colonize the upper airways of up to 50 per cent of critically ill hospitalized patients, usually within four to five days of admission. Once colonized, a patient is at higher risk for the development of pneumonia; in one study of intensive care unit patients, pneumonia occurred in 23 per cent of colonized, in contrast to 3 per cent of noncolonized, patients. Factors influencing colonization are multiple and poorly understood. Organisms appear to come from exogenous sources (especially *Pseudomonas*) via respiratory care equipment or the hands of medical personnel; organisms (especially Enterobacteriaceae) may also come from the patient's own gastrointestinal tract. One measure to reduce pharyngeal colonization rates is proper handwashing to prevent cross-contamination.

Aspiration of gastric contents with subsequent pneumonitis is common in the patient with cerebrovascular disease, seizures, drug overdose, cardiopulmonary arrests, and any condition which alters the patient's respiratory clearing mechanisms. Similarly, postoperative patients are at higher risk of developing pneumonia. Chemical pneumonitis from aspiration of gastric contents generally develops immediately and may be associated with respiratory failure. The pneumonia may result in death or resolve over a five-day period. Chemical pneumonitis does not require antimicrobial therapy, and studies have demonstrated the lack of efficacy of steroid therapy. Bacterial pneumonia, however, may develop as a complication of aspiration. Bacterial infection is characterized by deterioration after a transient period of recovery.

Frequently, postoperative and seriously ill patients have endotracheal or nasotracheal tubes or tracheostomies. Although these protect the patient from aspiration, they also bypass normal defense mechanisms and predispose to tracheal injury from suctioning. Uncommonly, secretions and gastric contents may be aspirated around the tube. There are occasionally serious problems associated with respiratory therapy. Outbreaks of pharyngeal colonization and pneumonia have been associated with the use of contaminated anesthesia equipment, ventilators, and IPPB machines with medication nebulizers. Usually, the gases from oxygen and air compressors, and internal parts of the machines, do not become contaminated or promote bacterial growth. The changeable tubing and masks can become contaminated if not disinfected or sterilized between patients. The greatest source of contamination is large volume Venturi nebulizers. Nebulizers produce liquid in aerosol (droplet) form by either ultrasonic or centrifugal means. These droplets can emit aerosols containing large numbers of gram-negative rods that may be delivered to terminal bronchi, resulting in pneumonia. Contamination of the large volume cascade humidifier may occur during cleaning or replenishing water. Organisms capable of growing under these conditions include *P. aeruginosa, P. cepacia, Serratia marcescens, Acinetobacter calcoaceticus,* and *Flavobacterium meningosepticum.* Pneumonia caused by any of these suggests the possibility of exogenous contamination. The risk of contamination appears to be minimal with small volume medication nebulizers as long as the medications used are sterile. Humidifiers usually do not serve as a potential risk to patients, because bacteria are not transported by molecules of water in vapor form.

The immune compromised host with pulmonary infiltrates represents a particularly difficult diagnostic and therapeutic problem. These are generally patients whose diseases are being treated with steroids or cytotoxic agents or both. Although the most common cause for their pneumonias are aerobic gram-negative rods, up to 25 per cent may become infected with fungi, herpesviruses, *Legionella pneumophila, Legionella (tatlockia) micdadei, Nocardia,* acid-fast bacilli, and combinations of these. Optimal therapy generally requires a tissue diagnosis, often an open lung biopsy of diffuse infiltrates, or needle aspirate of solitary nodules. Hospitals with clusters of patients with *Legionella pneumophila* have usually identified water as the significant vehicle, and control of contamination has been followed by a reduction in number of cases.

A great deal of attention has been focused on the infection control practices necessary to minimize the risk of pneumonias from respiratory care equipment. Although the data are incomplete, important points include the following: (1) Large volume reservoir nebulizers should be replaced by humidifiers if possible. Water used for humidification should be sterile. (2) All medication used for respiratory therapy should be sterile and preferably administered as a single unit dose. (3) Equipment such as tubing that comes into direct contact with patients should be changed between patients and every 24 to 48 hours when in continuous use.

BLOODSTREAM INFECTIONS. Hospital-acquired bloodstream infections may be primary (without an apparent source) or secondary to infection at a distal site. The distinction is important for both epidemiologic and clinical reasons. Secondary bloodstream infections complicate 3 per cent of urinary tract infections, 5 to 7 per cent of postoperative wound and pulmonary infections, and 7 per cent of cutaneous infections. *E. coli, S. aureus, K. pneumoniae, S. marcescens,* and *P. aeruginosa* are the usual pathogens. Identification of the source allows one to treat both the underlying condition and the complicating bacteremia. For example, bacteremia developing in patients with a urinary tract infection should suggest the possibility of obstruction, which may require surgery as well as antibiotics.

When true primary bacteremias occur, even in the compromised host, one must always consider the possibility of an infusion- or instrument-related infection. Twenty-five per cent of all patients hospitalized receive intravenous infusions, and the use of hyperalimentation and arterial and Swan-Ganz catheters has increased greatly in recent years.

Infections related to intravenous fluids or intravascular devices may occur from either intrinsic or extrinsic contamination of the system (see Fig. 258–1). Contamination of the infusion or administration set at the site of manufacture (intrinsic) may be extremely difficult to detect. In the early 1970's, at least 400 cases of *Enterobacter* sepsis occurred secondary to contaminated dextrose infusions. Because only a small proportion (0.7 to 0.9 per cent) of all manufactured bottles were contaminated and because these were shipped to many different hospitals, the association of contaminated fluids and septicemia was difficult to detect. Certain clues, however, should serve as a flag for such a possibility: (1) sepsis occurring in an otherwise low risk patient receiving an intravenous solution, or (2) a cluster of primary bloodstream infections with an unusual pathogen. Only certain organisms are capable of growing well in intravenous solutions (pH as low as 4.5). *Klebsiella, Enterobacter,* and *Serratia* can readily grow in 5 per cent dextrose in water, exceeding 10^5 colonies per milliliter within 24 hours at room temperature. Thus, careful examination of intravenous infusion bags or bottles may be useful, but even when the infusion contains 10^6 organisms per milliliter, cloudiness may be difficult to detect with the unaided eye. *Pseudomonas cepacia, Citrobacter freundii,* and *Flavobacterium* species are also likely to contaminate intravenous infusions. In contrast, *Proteus* species, *Pseudomonas aeruginosa, S. aureus, E. coli, Acinetobacter* species, and *Candida* species are all unable to survive in significant numbers under these conditions.

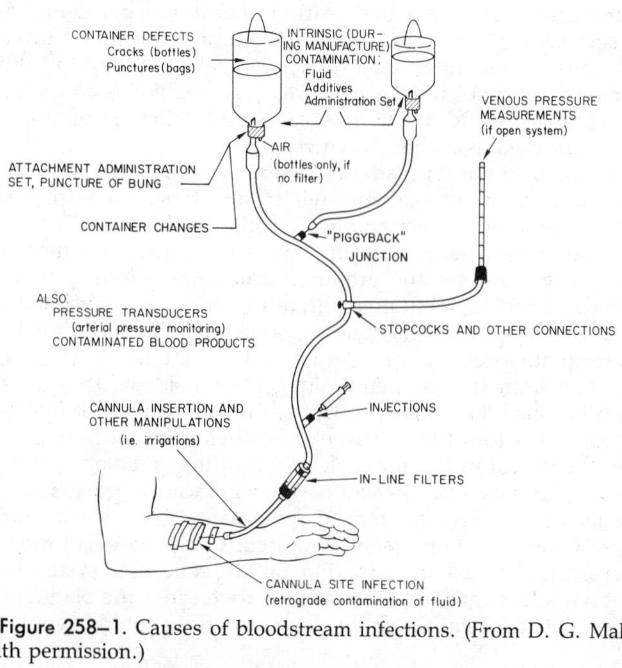

Figure 258–1. Causes of bloodstream infections. (From D. G. Maki, with permission.)

Extrinsic contamination, usually at the catheter site, is the most likely source of infusion-related infections. Steel needles carry a lower risk than plastic catheters. The incidence of a catheter-related infection rises with the length of time the catheter is left in place. Inflammation at the catheter site (a "cord," redness, swelling, pain), when present, strongly suggests catheter-associated sepsis. Catheters introduced via surgical cutdowns, femoral catheters, and devices left in place for more than 48 hours are particularly at risk. In contrast to contamination of the infusion, cannula-related sepsis is likely to be caused by gram-positive organisms, predominantly by *S. aureus* (50 per cent), *S. epidermidis*, and enterococci, although some are caused by gram-negative rods. Preliminary data suggest that intra-arterial catheters should not remain in place longer than four days. A semiquantitative technique of culturing the catheter tip when it is removed has been described by Maki et al. to aid in the diagnosis of catheter-related sepsis. The technique requires that the indwelling catheter be removed after a thorough antiseptic preparation of the insertion site. The distal section of the catheter is then cut off with a sterile scissors, beginning several millimeters inside the former skin surface–catheter interface, and placed into a sterile screw-capped container. The tip is then rolled four times back and forth on an agar plate in the microbiology laboratory. Colony counts of greater than 15 suggest the presence of a concordant catheter-related sepsis.

An unusual complication of catheters is suppurative thrombophlebitis, a purulent infection involving the entire vein, often occurring in the burn patient. Although local evidence of infection may be absent, the patients have unremitting sepsis. Therapy requires surgical excision of the vein, beginning proximal to the involved section, as well as antimicrobial therapy.

In recent years, the use of Hickman-Broviac intravenous catheters has become popular, both for infusing fluids and for withdrawing blood from selected patients. The catheters are tunneled under the skin of the chest wall midway between the nipple and sternum and enter the subclavian vein superiorly. The tip of the catheter is placed in the right atrium; the origin of the catheter on the outside of the chest wall has a Luer lock and contains heparinized saline solution when not in use. Several studies have shown an association between the use of these catheters and subsequent bloodstream infection. Although the attack rate is as high as 20 to 40 per cent of patients, the incidence of bloodstream infection is low, approximately 3 per 1000 days of use. The most frequent isolates are *S. epidermidis* (20 per cent), *S. aureus* (20 per cent), *Candida* sp. (15 per cent), and gram-negative rods. Although it is not always necessary to remove the catheter in the face of sepsis, generally it is wise to do so if the etiologic agent is *Corynebacterium*, *Nocardia*, or a fungus.

Parenteral hyperalimentation presents some unique problems regarding infection control. The hypertonic solutions require the use of central venous catheters which are left in place for prolonged periods of time. Although the high concentrations of glucose do not support bacterial growth, *Candida* species grow well in this milieu. *Candida* and other bacteria can colonize the occlusive dressings used to cover the catheter insertion site. Preparation of the solution under strict sterile technique is required. In addition, supervision of therapy by hyperalimentation teams, including surgeon, nurse, and pharmacist, seems to reduce the attack rate of fungemia from 10 to 20 per cent to 1 to 2 per cent.

The use of topical antibacterial ointments around intravenous catheter sites does not reduce the risk of infection. Their use may increase the risk of colonization by *Candida* around hyperalimentation lines. Similarly, bacterial filters have not yet been demonstrated to be efficacious in reducing fungemia. Recently the use of transparent plastic dressings for intravenous catheters has been popularized. Their efficacy in reducing catheter-related sepsis has not been established.

Recommended measures to reduce the incidence of catheter-related sepsis include strict aseptic technique in inserting a cannula after preparation of the skin, the use of steel needles for intravenous infusions whenever possible, changing arterial lines at least every four days, and changing intravenous catheter and administration sets at least every 48 hours. The use of flow sheets to keep track of the multiple monitoring devices used in intensive care areas should be encouraged.

Despite the use of control measures, bloodstream infections related to infusion therapy will occur. The following is offered as a general guide in the approach to the hospitalized patient with sepsis:

1. Determine the most likely source of infection (is it primary or secondary?). If secondary, where is the other infection site: urinary tract, lung, wound, or elsewhere?

2. What intravenous and intra-arterial devices are in place? How long have they been there? Is there any evidence of local inflammation? If the bacteremia is primary or caused by an unusual pathogen, or occurs while the patient is receiving appropriate antimicrobial therapy, the following measures should be undertaken: (a) Discontinue the intravenous device immediately. (b) After iodine prep of the latex injection port at the distal end of the intravenous tubing (allow iodine to remain at least two minutes and then remove with 70 per cent isopropyl alcohol), aspirate 10 ml of the intravenous contents. Place 5 ml into each of two blood culture bottles (one set), and send to the bacteriology laboratory. (c) Remove the indwelling catheter aseptically, and send it to the laboratory for semiquantitative culture. (d) Record the lot number of all intravenous products the patient was receiving.

3. Draw blood cultures and obtain appropriate cultures at distal sites.

4. Initiate intravenous antimicrobial therapy. Until sensitivities are available, initial antibiotic selection should be based on the surveillance data for the hospital ward(s) in which the patient has resided. This suggestion is prompted by the fact that the probability of specific aminoglycoside-resistant gram-negative rods and the probability of methicillin-resistant *S. aureus* may be different in intensive care unit areas and in the general wards.

5. Treat the underlying sources of infection. In the setting of breakthrough bacteremia (occurring while the patient is on appropriate therapy), special attention should be given to the possibility of an undrained abscess, a vascular focus of infection, or inadequate levels of antibiotic. Polymicrobial sepsis suggests the presence of a gastrointestinal, hepatobiliary, or genitourinary source, often with obstruction.

POSTOPERATIVE WOUND INFECTIONS. The rate of infection at the incision site following surgery depends on the skill of the surgeon and the degree of contamination at the time of operation. Contamination of a postoperative wound with subsequent infection can occur from either an endogenous or an exogenous source. The risk of endogenous contamination is dependent upon the type of operation being performed. Surgical fields involving the colon or other nonsterile structures are more likely to get infected than those involving clean areas such as with hip replacement. Another likely source of endogenous contamination is an active site of infection at a peripheral location. For example, an untreated urinary tract infection or infected ulcer is associated with a two to three times increased rate of postoperative wound infection and should be treated prior to elective surgery.

In contrast to endogenous contamination, exogenous contamination usually occurs from a break in technique at the time of surgery. A wide variety of sources have been described, including operating room personnel and surgical materials. In addition, certain practices appear to be associated with a higher infection rate, e.g., failure of the patient to use an antiseptic soap during the preoperative shower, and shaving of the operative site.

Prophylactic antibiotics given just prior to surgery have been shown to reduce the incidence of infection following certain procedures. Effective chemoprophylaxis requires that the antimicrobial cover only the most likely pathogens, be initiated just prior to surgery, and be given for brief periods of time (no more than 48 hours after surgery). There must be high tissue and blood levels of drug at the time of surgery. When wound infections do occur, they are generally caused by *S. aureus* or gram-negative rods. Patients with *S. aureus* infections should be placed on "contact" or "drainage/secretion" precautions to minimize the risk of cross-contamination. Treatment usually requires drainage followed by antibiotic therapy for approximately seven days.

If pus is found after surgery and no organisms are recovered from routine cultures, then a possibility exists that infection is caused by anaerobic bacteria, rapid-growing atypical mycobacteria, or a saprophytic fungus. The latter two situations are distinctly unusual and should be considered only if there are clinical or laboratory features suggesting nonvegetative bacterial infection.

Wound infections occurring unusually early (within 24 to 48 hours of surgery) should suggest the possibility of infection with β-hemolytic Group A streptococci *(S. pyogenes), Clostridium* species (gas gangrene) or organs causing necrotizing fasciitis. These are especially serious and life-threatening infections requiring immediate evaluation and therapy. Their management is discussed elsewhere in this text.

OTHER INFECTION SITES. A wide variety of infections occur in hospitalized patients in addition to those previously discussed. Nosocomial meningitis usually occurs following neurosurgical shunting procedures and is usually caused by *S. aureus, S. epidermidis,* or gram-negative rods, rarely by *Candida* as a late infection. In the compromised host, nosocomial meningitis may occur without prior surgery. *Listeria, Cryptococcus,* and gram-negative rods are the likely pathogens. Group B streptococci are a common cause of meningitis in the neonate, and there have been recent reports of *Citrobacter* bloodstream infection and meningitis in a few neonatal units.

Infections following the insertion of artificial joints are particularly difficult to treat. Those occurring in the hospitalized patient usually are "early onset" infections. *S. epidermidis, S. aureus,* and gram-negative rods are involved. In a large study of infections following total knee arthroplasty at the Mayo Clinic, the significance of anaerobes was stressed. Unless the infection is of a superficial wound, salvage of the prosthesis is infrequent. Infections with a late onset (beyond eight weeks) account for at least 50 per cent of infections involving prosthetic joints.

In the last ten years, the percentage of infants delivered by cesarean section has risen. Currently, up to 25 per cent of all deliveries are performed in this manner. In contrast to the incidence of endometritis following vaginal deliveries (1 per cent or less), that following cesarean section ranges from 20 to 30 per cent. The specific contribution to the increased infection risk by the cesarean section, underlying disease, or use of fetal monitoring is unclear.

INFECTION CONTROL COMMITTEE. In order to be accredited by the Joint Commission for Accreditation of Hospitals (JCAH), all hospitals in the United States are required to have an infection control committee that meets at least six times a year. The committee formulates and reviews hospital policies with regard to infection control practices. Usually, its members are diverse, representing the medicine, surgery, microbiology laboratory, nursing, and pharmacy departments. One member of the committee serves as the hospital epidemiologist, usually someone with training in infectious diseases or clinical microbiology who has a strong interest in infection control.

An important task of the committee is to adopt and enforce proper isolation practices to prevent the transmission of communicable diseases within the hospital. Most hospitals utilize a limited number of types of isolation based upon the route of transmission of the disease. The Centers for Disease Control (CDC) released a new set of isolation guidelines in 1983 (Table 258–3). Of note is that their earlier recommendation for "protective" isolation was deleted because efficacy has not been demonstrated. Hospitals may want to utilize the CDC guidelines verbatim or modify them for local use. An isolation manual listing the precautions and the type of isolation a specific disease requires should be distributed to each ward. Infection control practitioners then review on-ward practices to assure compliance and to prevent unnecessary isolation, which is costly and inefficient. "Isolation" is used to imply that a private room is necessary, and "precaution" is used when a private room is optional or not indicated.

INANIMATE OBJECTS. The inanimate environment of a hospital may serve as a potential reservoir for microorganisms. Water in flower vases may contain up to 10^9 organisms per milliliter (usually *Pseudomonas*), and stethoscopes are capable of being colonized. The risks associated with toilets and laundry chutes appear minimal. In one cancer hospital, fireproofing

TABLE 258–3. NEW ISOLATION PROCEDURES RECOMMENDED BY THE CENTERS FOR DISEASE CONTROL IN 1983

Isolation Category	Private Room Necessary	Masks	Gowns	Gloves	Hand-washing	Examples of Diseases for Which It Is Recommended
Strict	+	+	+	+	+	Pharyngeal diphtheria; varicella; zoster (localized in immunocompromised patient or disseminated)
Contact	+	For those in close contact	If soiling likely	If contact with infective material	+	Staphylococcal furunculosis in newborns; Herpes simplex disseminated, severe primary, or neonatal; methicillin-resistant *S. aureus*
Respiratory	+	For those in close contact	—	—	+	Measles; meningococcal pneumonia, meningitis, or meningococcemia; *H. influenzae,* pneumonia, or meningitis
Tuberculosis (AFB)	+	If patient is coughing	Only to prevent gross contamination	—	+	Tuberculosis
Enteric precautions	Only if patient's hygiene is poor	—	If soiling likely	If contact with infective material	+	Viral hepatitis A; *Salmonella, Shigella,* or *C. difficile* enterocolitis
Drainage/secretion precautions	—	—	If soiling likely	If contact with infective material	+	Minor or limited skin infections including those caused by *S. aureus*
Blood/body fluid precautions	Only if patient's hygiene is poor	—	If soiling with blood or body fluids likely	If contact with blood or body fluid	+	AIDS; Creutzfeldt-Jakob disease; viral hepatitis B

materials were shown to be a reservoir for *Aspergillus*, which caused deep tissue infections in patients, some of whom are only briefly immunosuppressed. In all outbreaks of nosocomial *Aspergillus* pulmonary infections, the mode of transmission was airborne.

Based on the limited amount of information available, several recommendations can be made: (1) Flower vases probably do not belong in burn units or intensive care areas. (2) Patients on isolation should be issued a single stethoscope to be used by all physicians entering the room. In addition, alcohol swabs will kill most bacteria on the stethoscope to be used on high risk patients (those with severe dermatitis or burns). (3) Prior to construction or installation of waste disposal chutes, fire-proofing material, or other environment changes, an infection control specialist should be consulted. (4) In general, routine culturing of the inanimate environment should be discouraged. Only in working up an outbreak might this be essential.

STERILIZATION AND DISINFECTION. In order to reduce the number of organisms that come in contact with patients, sterilization, disinfection, and antiseptics are employed. Sterilization refers to the killing of all forms of microbiologic life, including spores. The term disinfection implies that there is a marked reduction of the number of microorganisms but that spores are not killed. Antiseptics are degerming agents which can be used on the skin.

Sterilization. Two types of sterilization are generally employed in hospitals: autoclaving and gas. The former, use of moist heat under pressure, is the more effective and less expensive method. Boiling at normal atmospheric pressure is not sufficient to sterilize (kill spores). Gaseous sterilization, using ethylene oxide, is an acceptable alternative for use on items that cannot withstand heat. The gas is effective at lower temperatures and can penetrate plastics and other materials. However, ethylene oxide is an explosive and a skin irritant, and is potentially mutagenic and carcinogenic. The Occupational Safety and Health Administration has proposed to reduce the current permissible exposure limit for ethylene oxide from 50 parts per million to 1 part per million as an eight-hour time-weighted average. Regardless of the method of sterilization used, biologic sterility testing with spore strips must be used to document adequacy of the sterilization process. *Bacillus stearothermophilus* spores are very heat resistant and are used to monitor sterilization processes using moist heat. *Bacillus subtilis* spores are used to monitor the efficacy of gas sterilization processes.

Disinfection. Several different classes of chemical disinfectants exist. Commonly used agents include chlorine, iodine, phenols, hexachlorophenes, alcohols, and second generation quaternary ammonium compounds. They vary in their ability to kill microorganisms, and the type of agent utilized depends upon the likely pathogens and the properties of the object to be disinfected. Two epidemics of idiopathic neonatal hyperbilirubinemia have been linked to excessive use of a phenolic disinfectant plus detergent. Thus, alternatives are recommended for use in the newborn area. Particular care must be taken with hepatitis B virus and the Jakob-Creutzfeldt agent. Both are resistant to killing by most disinfectants, but they are thought to be susceptible to high concentrations of hypochlorite. For the Jakob-Creutzfeldt agent, the preferred method is autoclave sterilization for unusually long times (one hour at 121° C). It has recently been suggested that if autoclave sterilization is not possible, a one-hour exposure to 1 N sodium hydroxide inactivates Jakob-Creutzfeldt agent. Furthermore, it is less corrosive than hypochlorite for all materials except aluminum.

Recently there have been reports of bloodstream infections and pseudoinfections and peritonitis traced to contaminated povidone iodine and polyximer iodine antiseptic compounds. The organisms were *Ps. cepacia* and *Ps. aeruginosa*, respectively, species that are naturally resistant to many antibiotics, have minimal growth requirements, and are ubiquitous. Their ability to survive in an iodine-containing product has stimulated research into the chemistry of these agents and an increased awareness of infectious complications with antiseptics.

With the recent isolation of *Legionella pneumophila* from cooling towers, the question of decontamination arises. The Centers for Disease Control recommend that cooling towers undergo periodic maintenance to ensure low levels of slime bacteria and algae in accordance with the American Society of Heating, Refrigeration and Air Conditioning Engineers and the Environmental Protection Agency. Field trials are being planned to evaluate the efficacy of various water additives to eliminate *L. pneumophila*.

With respect to the acquired immune deficiency syndrome (AIDS), the Centers for Disease Control (CDC) have recommended that the same precautions be used when caring for patients with viral hepatitis B, in whom blood and body fluids likely to have become contaminated with blood are considered infective. The same guidelines also hold for reusable instruments. Specifically, the CDC stated that lensed instruments should be sterilized after use on AIDS patients. A similar statement regarding endoscopes was made by the American Hospital Association's Advisory Committee on Infections Within Hospitals.

HANDWASHING. Proper and frequent handwashing is the most important control measure available in preventing the transmission of infectious diseases in hospitalized patients. The role of antiseptics is secondary in importance to standard handwashing with plain soap and water before and after routine patient contact.

The normal flora of the skin consists of a transient and permanent group of organisms. Transiently present organisms are more often the gram-negative rods and at times *S. aureus*. Permanent flora include the micrococci *S. epidermidis* and *Propionibacterium acnes*. Recent data suggest that certain gram-negative rods appear to be persistent after standard handwashing efforts and thus may be part of the permanent flora. *S. aureus* can also become part of the permanent flora of the anterior nares and thereby repeatedly colonize the hands. Soap and water appear to be generally effective in removing the transient flora. Various antiseptics, including isopropyl and ethyl alcohol, are more effective in reducing, but not eliminating, the permanent flora. Hexachlorophene is highly effective against *S. aureus*, but has little or no activity against gram-negative rods and fungi. In addition, absorption of hexachlorophene through the skin has been shown to cause vacuolization of brain tissue in some infants and experimental laboratory animals, and therefore its routine use for washing babies in the newborn and premature units is discouraged. Aqueous benzalkonium chloride (Aqueous Zephiran) is relatively ineffective and will sustain the growth of gram-negative rods. Its use as an antiseptic should be discouraged. Iodine remains an excellent antiseptic with a wide range of action, but causes local irritation. Chlorhexidine is also an effective antiseptic, but may cause dermatitis with excessive use.

EMPLOYEE HEALTH. The employee health division should be concerned with protecting both patients and employees from the transmission of infectious diseases. Problems most frequently arise regarding the transmission of tuberculosis, viral hepatitis, herpesvirus infections, and meningococcal infections.

Tuberculosis. The risk of tuberculosis is related to exposure to unsuspected cases among patients. After patients have been placed upon respiratory isolation, the risk becomes minimal. Unfortunately, routine chest x-rays are not specific or sensitive enough to screen for suspected cases. The addition of a tuberculin skin test for all patients who have respiratory symptoms or radiographic abnormalities may lead to earlier diagnosis and may prevent early transmission.

All employees should receive a tuberculin skin test (intermediate strength or 5 tuberculin units PPD-S) prior to beginning work. These are repeated yearly or three months after exposure to an initially unsuspected case. Employees who convert their PPD skin test result from negative to positive (10 mm induration or greater) should be considered for therapy with isoniazid (INH), 300 mg per day for one year.

Viral Hepatitis. Transmission of hepatitis A to employees or other patients is very unusual. Unlike hepatitis B and non-A non-B viral hepatitis, hepatitis A is transmitted almost exclusively by the oral-fecal route. In addition, peak viral excretion maximally occurs prior to the development of symptoms. Enteric precautions are probably effective in protecting medical personnel from acquiring hepatitis A from hospitalized patients with the disease.

Hepatitis B is transmitted by parenteral or mucous membrane exposure to infected blood or body fluids. Because of their frequent exposure to blood from accidental needle sticks and blood spills, medical personnel are at increased risk. The prevalence of both HB_sAg and anti-HB_s has been shown to be higher in medical personnel than in control populations: approximately 15 per cent of physicians are positive for anti-HB_s, and 1 per cent carry HB_sAg. Dentists and oral surgeons appear to be at even higher risk.

The infection control committee in conjunction with the employee health division should set up a standardized procedure with regard to the prevention of hepatitis. Despite the institution of proper isolation of infected patients, needle stick accidents will occur. Data on the best way to manage these exposures are incomplete. Currently it seems reasonable to draw blood from both the donor (source) and the recipient in order to clarify the risk of transmitting hepatitis B to a susceptible hospital employee. If the donor shows evidence of infection with hepatitis B and the recipient is susceptible, then both high titered anti-hepatitis B immunoglobulin (HBIG) and the first dose of vaccine should be offered to the hospital worker. At one month and six months, the second and third doses of vaccine should be given. A second dose of high titered globulin is *not* necessary. If there is concern about the transmission of either hepatitis A or non-A non-B hepatitis, standard immune serum globulin could be given, although its efficacy in preventing non-A non-B disease is uncertain. This virus has replaced hepatitis B as the most common cause of post-transfusion–related hepatitis, and non-A non-B is responsible for at least 80 per cent of post-transfusion hepatitis. Its exact role in needle stick associated disease, however, is unknown.

Herpes Infections. Nonimmune personnel having direct contact with the oral secretions of patients are at risk for developing herpes skin infections. Usually a nurse involved in suctioning a tracheostomy comes in contact with virus-contaminated secretions at the site of a locally traumatized or minimally lacerated finger. This exposure is followed by the development of a localized, painful, herpes simplex infection referred to as "whitlow." These infections are often misdiagnosed as bacterial infections and may get secondarily infected if incised and drained. The use of gloves will probably prevent the transmission of herpes, although personnel with vesicles should avoid contact with immunosuppressed patients.

Meningococcal Disease. Few events produce more panic among hospital employees than exposure to a patient suspected of having meningococcal disease. Nevertheless, cases among exposed medical personnel are very rare. Secondary attack rates are significantly higher in household contacts. Close contact with the index case appears to be required. Guidelines recommended by the Centers for Disease Control include the following: (1) Suspected cases of meningococcal disease should be placed on respiratory isolation immediately. (2) A contact list of those who have had *close* (possible secretion) contact with the case should be compiled. The Public Health Department should be notified immediately to supervise the identification of contact exposures made in the community prior to admission. (3) Personnel who have known close contact should be given antimicrobial prophylaxis as soon as possible, and should not await cultural confirmation of the diagnosis or susceptibility testing. Recommended prophylaxis for adults is rifampin, 600 mg orally twice daily for two days. If rifampin is not tolerated, minocycline, 100 to 200 mg orally every 12 hours, can be given for three days. Sulfonamides may be used only if the organism has been shown to be sensitive. Penicillin is not effective for prophylaxis for elimination of the carrier state. (4) Routine nasopharyngeal cultures of employees are not useful. (5) Indiscriminate use of prophylactic therapy should be discouraged (in those who have had fleeting or casual contact). (6) In the setting of an epidemic, the use of vaccines as an adjuvant to antimicrobial prophylaxis should be considered if the offending organism is in the serogroup A or C.

American Hospital Association: A hospitalized approach to AIDS. Recommendations of the Advisory Committee on Infections Within Hospitals. Infect Control 5:242, 1984.

Bennett J, Brachman S: Hospital Infections. Boston, Little, Brown & Company, 1979. Wenzel, R: Handbook of Hospital Acquired Infections. Boca Raton, Fla., CRC Press, 1981. *Two comprehensive texts devoted solely to the problem of hospital-acquired infections.*

Centers for Disease Control: Acquired immune deficiency syndrome (AIDS): Precautions for clinical and laboratory staffs. Morbid Mortal Wkly Rep 31:577, 1982.

Cundy K, Ball W: Infection Control in Health Care Facilities. Microbiologic Surveillance. Baltimore, University Park Press, 1976. *A review of the limited amount of data available regarding potential risks of inanimate objects in promoting infection.*

Garner JS, Simmons BP: CDC guidelines for isolation precautions in hospitals. Infect Control 4 (Special Suppl):245, 1983.

Kunin CM: Detection, Prevention and Management of Urinary Tract Infections. Philadelphia, Lea & Febiger, 1979. *A readable reference that provides both basic and advanced knowledge regarding all aspects of urinary tract infections.*

Maki DG, Weise EC, Sarafin HW: A semiquantitative culture method for identifying intravenous catheter related infection. N Engl J Med 296:1305, 1977. *Description of the microbiologic technique to help determine the likelihood of catheter-induced sepsis.*

Proceedings of the Second International Conference on Nosocomial Infections, Centers for Disease Control, Atlanta, August 5–8, 1980. Am J Med 70:379, 631, 899, 1981. Proceedings of the International Symposium and Workshop on Nosocomial Infection, Jerusalem, Israel, April 27 to May 2, 1980. Rev Infect Dis 3:635, 1981. Proceedings of the First International Symposium on Hospital Acquired Infections, Vienna, Austria, April 24–28, 1983. Infect Control 4:363, 440, 1983; 5:18, 1984. *Three recent conferences updating information on hospital-acquired infections.*

Russell AD, Hugo WB, Ayliffe GAJ: Principles and Practice of Disinfection, Preservation and Sterilization. Boston, Blackwell Scientific Publications, 1982. *Provides detailed discussion of the chemical agents and modes of action, as well as tests of sterility. Two chapters are devoted specifically to issues in the hospital.*

Simmons RL, Howard RJ: Surgical Infectious Diseases. New York, Appleton-Century-Crofts, 1982. *Comprehensive review of infections in surgical patients.*

259. ADVICE TO TRAVELERS

Jeffrey A. Gelfand

Travelers frequently make precise arrangements for connecting flights, hotels, theater tickets, and tours, but give little or no advance consideration to their health while traveling. This can result in disrupted plans, physical misery, serious illness, and considerable expense. Vaccination requirements for entering different countries vary and depend on where the traveler has stopped en route. There are several publications that address these issues. The Centers for Disease Control (CDC) publishes an annually updated guide, *Health Information for International Travel.* It contains a compendium of the vaccination requirements for entry into other countries, epidemiologic information, current CDC recommendations for vaccinations, chemoprophylaxis, and other helpful information. It can be obtained by writing the Superintendent of Documents, United States Government Printing Office, Washington, D.C. 20402. The publication number is the year followed by 8280 (i.e., 84–8280). Finally, local health departments and "Traveler's Clinics" (now available in a number of teaching hospitals) can provide up-to-the-minute information about changing epidemiologic and vaccination requirements.

Travel to such areas as Europe, Australia, and New Zealand poses no greater health hazard than travel in the United States and Canada. The risks of travel to other areas vary greatly from country to country and depend on the traveler's local living conditions and length of stay. In general, brief visits to large cities, with accommodations in good tourist hotels and meals in reputable restaurants, carry little risk of exotic infection. Travel to rural areas may greatly increase such risks.

GENERAL MEASURES. Gastronomic curiosity and gourmet tastes should be restrained by prudence. Meat and fish should be well cooked. Smoking, salting, and drying are not sufficient to kill tapeworm cysts. Peelable raw fruits and vegetables with unbroken skin are safe if peeled by the diner; the skin should be discarded. Lettuce is especially to be avoided because it is virtually impossible to cleanse it of protozoal cysts. In general, dairy foods, including local cheeses, should be avoided. Milk can be safely consumed after boiling. Untreated water should be avoided, as should ice. Alcohol does not confer "sterility" to local water, and many pathogens can tolerate alcohol better than can the traveler. Very hot tap water is safer but not risk-free. Bottled water is not necessarily safe, although carbonated bottled water and beverages usually are. Tea and coffee made with boiled water are safe. Beer and wine present few hazards (save for the next morning).

While recent evidence suggests that following such rules will not help the traveler evade the ever-present threat of uncomplicated traveler's diarrhea, these measures are likely to reduce the probability of developing more serious food-bourne bacterial and parasitic diseases. Swimming in fresh water in tropical areas where schistosomiasis is found should be avoided; salt water and chlorinated pools are safe. Measures to prevent insect bites (clothing, netting, repellents) should be considered where appropriate. Patients should be cautioned against taking over-the-counter medications proferred by pharmacists and physicians abroad. These medications, as well as prescription drugs, may contain agents of dubious efficacy and significant toxicity. For example, chloramphenicol may be present in cold remedies. Finally, lists of English-speaking physicians can be supplied by United States and other consulates general. Practical advice on securing such information after hours can be found in *Traveling Health—A Complete Guide to Medical Services in 23 Countries,* a traveler's guide to foreign health services.

IMMUNIZATIONS. The two immunizations occasionally required for entry into other countries are for yellow fever and cholera. In general, these vaccinations are not required for travel from the United States to Canada, Mexico, Europe, or Caribbean countries, nor for re-entry to the United States. All travelers should receive a tetanus–diphtheria toxoid booster if the tetanus immunization status is uncertain or if ten or more years have passed since the last vaccination. Poliomyelitis is a real threat in developing nations, and all travelers to such areas should receive a booster dose of trivalent oral polio vaccine (TOPV). Persons not previously immunized should receive the primary series of TOPV. Those with depressed immune function should receive inactivated polio vaccine.

Cholera. The risk of cholera to most tourists is low, and cholera vaccines are of limited effectiveness in protecting against clinical cholera. Vaccination is not recommended unless the traveler will be visiting an area experiencing an outbreak or will be living in an endemic area with poor sanitation. Travel to other countries from such areas may require vaccination as a condition of entry.

Hepatitis A. Immune serum globulin is effective in reducing the risk of hepatitis A. A dose of 5 ml is recommended for adults traveling to the developing world for periods of over three months and is repeated every four to six months. For those staying in endemic areas for a briefer period, a dose of 2 ml can be used.

Measles. For those born after 1956 without prior physician-documented history of the disease or immunization, vaccination is advised.

Plague. Plague vaccine is recommended only for those traveling to enzootic rural areas of Asia, South America, and Africa.

Rabies. Prudence would dictate that anyone anticipating exposure to animals in an enzootic or epizootic area ought to receive pre-exposure prophylaxis. Simple residence for several months in such an area is sufficient for some to advocate vaccination. A new human diploid cell vaccine is now available in the United States.

Smallpox. Smallpox vaccine should not be given for international travel.

Typhoid. Typhoid vaccination is only partially effective, and the protective effect may be overcome by large inocula. It is recommended for travelers to endemic areas experiencing an outbreak. Highly susceptible travelers (patients with achlorhydria, immunosuppression, or sickle cell disease) should be immunized.

Typhus. This vaccine should be considered only for those traveling to the highland areas of Africa, the Andes, and the Himalayas.

Yellow Fever. Yellow fever vaccination is recommended for travel to endemic areas of South America and Africa. Vaccination is also required for travel to and between such areas. It can only be given at designated yellow fever vaccination centers (travelers should check with the local board of health).

MALARIA CHEMOPROPHYLAXIS. Falciparum malaria can kill within 48 hours. Travelers to areas where malaria is endemic should receive chloroquine prophylaxis. A weekly dose of 500 mg (300 mg base) of chloroquine phosphate should be taken by adults (50 kg body weight) beginning two weeks before arrival in an endemic area and continuing while there and for six weeks after leaving. Travelers returning from prolonged, heavy exposure in areas where *P. vivax* and *P. ovale* are endemic can be given a course of primaquine phosphate during the last two weeks of postexposure chloroquine prophylaxis to prevent relapse from extraerythrocytic infection, although such therapy is not recommended for the average traveler. Glucose-6-phosphate dehydrogenase deficiency should be ruled out prior to primaquine therapy.

Travelers to areas with chloroquine-resistant falciparum malaria are advised to take a weekly dose of a fixed ratio tablet containing sulfadoxine (500 mg) and pyrimethamine (25 mg), marketed under the name Fansidar (Hoffman-LaRoche) and recently licensed for sale in the United States. This should be taken in addition to the weekly dose of chloroquine, the preferred prophylaxis for *P. vivax.* Even for countries listed as having chloroquine-resistant *P. falciparum,* the occurrence of these strains may be limited to certain areas only. More detailed references should be consulted for information about Fansidar-resistant *P. falciparum,* prophylaxis in pregnancy, and other selected topics.

TRAVELER'S DIARRHEA. Diarrhea, sufficiently severe to disrupt plans, strikes one quarter to one half of travelers to certain areas. Enterotoxigenic *E. coli* (ETEC) are associated with from 40 to 70 per cent of cases of diarrhea in travelers, depending on location and culture techniques. Other agents, notably shigellae, salmonellae, campylobacter, vibrios, *Entamoeba histolytica, Giardia,* reovirus, and Norwalk virus, may be causes. In the tropics, traveler's diarrhea usually begins in the first week and lasts on the average about three and a half days. In addition to the general measures previously recommended—which may not prevent simple traveler's diarrhea—prophylactic measures have been investigated. One agent widely used abroad, iodochlorhydroxyquin (Entero-Vioform), has been associated with severe neurotoxicity and is of dubious efficacy. Both doxycycline and trimethoprim/sulfamethoxazole (TMP/SMX) have been used and are effective prophylaxis for traveler's diarrhea. However, allergic reactions, photosensitivity reactions, and the demonstrated emergence of resistance to these drugs by ETEC lead most authorities to advise against such prophylaxis for routine travel. Bismuth subsalicylate (Pepto-Bismol), 60 ml taken four times a day during the trip, is effective and safe prophylaxis for those not already taking salicylates in high doses but is impractical for most.

Many authorities advise travelers to wait until diarrhea begins and then to institute therapy. Pepto-Bismol, 30 to 60 ml taken every half hour for eight doses, reduces the number of loose stools by about 50 per cent and increases the rate of recovery within 24 hours. A recent double-blind, controlled study demonstrated that either TMP/SMX (160 mg TMP; 800 mg SMX) or TMP alone (200 mg), taken twice daily for five days, substantially reduced the severity of traveler's diarrhea. The opiate drugs may actually intensify dysentery with shigellae and therefore should be used sparingly and only for mild disease. A reasonable approach, therefore, would be to treat mild disease with Pepto-Bismol and with judicious use of opiates to reduce periods of great inconvenience. More serious illness could be treated with either TMP/SMX or TMP alone, with the understanding that drug reactions could be a hazard with antimicrobial therapy. Finally, replacement of fluid losses is critical for therapy of severe disease. Several commercial preparations of World Health Organization rehydration salts are now commercially available.

ADVICE ON RETURNING HOME. The most important single bit of advice is to remind the traveler to include the history of travel when seeking medical attention. The clinical onset of certain diseases may be months or even years after the traveler returns home, and the traveler should be reminded of this possibility.

Centers for Disease Control: Health information for international travel, 1983. Morbid Mortal Weekly Rep 28 (Suppl), 1983. Available from the Superintendent of Documents, United States Government Printing Office, Washington, D.C. 20402, HEW Publication No. (CDC) 83–8280. *This is a thorough and very helpful guide to the medical aspects of international travel, from vaccination requirements to the importation of pets.*

DuPont HL, Galindo E, Evans DG, Cabada FJ, Sullivan P, Evans DJ: Prevention of traveler's diarrhea with trimethoprim-sulfamethoxazole and with trimethoprim alone. Gastroenterology 84:75, 1983. *A placebo-controlled, double-blind trial of TMP/SMX or TMP alone in United States students studying in Mexico. Prophylaxis was very effective.*

DuPont HL, Hornick RB: Adverse effect of Lomotil therapy in shigellosis. JAMA 226:1525, 1973. *Although the frequency of stools was diminished by this commonly used antidiarrheal agent, fever and toxemia were increased in patients with this infection by an invasive pathogen.*

DuPont HL, Reves RR, Galindo E, Sullivan PS, Wood LV, Mendiola JG: Treatment of travelers' diarrhea with trimethoprim/sulfamethoxazole and with trimethoprim alone. N Engl J Med 307:841, 1982. *This critical paper is the basis for recommending therapy with these drugs.*

DuPont HL, Sullivan P, Pickering LK, Haynes C, Ackerman PB: Symptomatic treatment of diarrhea with bismuth subsalicylate among students attending a Mexican university. Gastroenterology 73:715, 1977. *Treatment of traveler's diarrhea with Pepto-Bismol reduced loose movements and speeded recovery.*

Gorbach SL: Traveler's diarrhea. N Engl J Med 307:881, 1982. *A clear, practical, concise, and thoughtful view of the subject by an authority.*

Hillman SM, Hillman RS: Traveling Healthy—A Complete Guide to Medical Services in 23 Countries. New York, Penguin Books, 1980. *This paperback guide is a highly useful compendium. Included are practical advice, first aid, sensible suggestions for patients with pacemakers and numerous other disorders, glossaries of emergency medical terms in languages from Danish to Serbo-Croatian, and a pharmacopeia listing commonly used drugs and their equivalents abroad. An outstandingly valuable little book for travelers.*

Immunization and chemoprophylaxis for travelers. Med Lett 25:37, 1983. *Reviews current immunization requirements and recommendations and also contains a complete list of all countries with malaria risk, the nature of those risks, and malaria chemoprophylaxis recommendations.*

Portnoy BJ, DuPont HL, Pruitt D, Abdo JA, Rodriguez JT: Antidiarrheal agents in the treatment of acute diarrhea in children. JAMA 236:844, 1976. *An evaluation of two of the most commonly used agents for treating diarrhea. Neither was effective in a controlled study.*

Steffen R, Van der Linde F, Gyr K, Schär M: Epidemiology of diarrhea in travelers. JAMA 249:1176, 1983. *A retrospective analysis of 16,568 European travelers' experiences. The data suggest that dirty fingers reach the best of hotels and restaurants and that four stars do not protect a guest from diarrhea.*

Wyler DJ: Malaria-resurgence, resistance, and research. N Engl J Med 308:875;934, 1983. *A comprehensive review. Includes such problems as Fansidar-resistant P. falciparum and other topics beyond the scope of this chapter.*

Section Two BACTERIAL DISEASES

Pneumonia

260. INTRODUCTION TO PNEUMONIA

Herbert Y. Reynolds

Pneumonia is a general term denoting a group of clinical diseases that result from microbial infection of lung parenchyma. It is a commonly encountered disease and, in one form or another, continues to be a leading cause of death in the United States. Histologically, pneumonitis represents an inflammatory reaction in the interstitium of alveoli and an accumulation of exudate in alveolar lumina. Consolidation and a degree of impaired gas-exchange may occur in affected lung tissue. With successful inactivation of the infecting agent, resolution occurs and normal lung structure is usually restored. Exceptions to the complete healing phase occur in certain necrotizing pneumonias, those caused by staphylococcal or gram-negative bacteria, after which lung scars or fibrosis may develop. Bronchopneumonia denotes multiple patchy and diffuse areas of involvement and often implies that a less severe form of disease exists because signs and radiographic evidence of consolidation are absent.

Mycoplasmal, pneumococcal, certain other primary bacterial pneumonias, and the necrotizing (frequently nosocomial) pneumonias are considered in Ch. 261 to 266. Because staphylococcal pneumonia is so closely related to influenza, it is discussed under influenza (see Ch. 78), as well as under staphylococcal disease (see Ch. 270). The pneumonias caused by viruses, rickettsiae, certain fungal species, i.e., *Histoplasma*, coccidioidomycosis, *Aspergillus*, *Legionella* and other taxonomically less well defined species, such as *Pneumocystis carinii*, are considered in the individual chapters dealing with those infections.

PATHOGENESIS. Microorganisms reach lung tissue in several ways: (1) by direct inhalation of infectious particles from ambient air or by aspiration of secretions from the mouth and nasopharynx, (2) by deposition in lung vasculature following hematogenous spread from another site, and (3) by exogenous penetration of lung tissue. The last-named route includes trauma as well as iatrogenic inoculation of lung tissue with bacteria during chest surgery or from other kinds of diagnostic or therapeutic procedures, e.g., bronchoscopy. The inhalation-aspiration route is by far the most significant. Also important are the size and configuration of inhaled particles and droplets, which determine the site or level of deposition in the respiratory tract. For example, approximately 90 per cent of particles between 5 and 10 μ in diameter impact at some point along the trachea or in major bronchi, whereas those between 0.5 and 3 μ in size may escape filtration and be deposited in terminal air spaces. Particles <0.5 μ in diameter remain suspended in air and may leave the body via expired air. Because many bacteria are in this small size range, they frequently plumb the airways to the alveoli.

Of importance in developing pneumonia are the forces that can keep microorganisms in the lung. The mucosal surfaces of the nose and mouth and the gingival border possess numerous microorganisms that are considered to be normal flora; yet surprisingly few species of aerobic gram-negative bacilli routinely colonize these areas, especially the potentially pathologic gram-negative rod bacteria. With almost any alteration in health status of the host, there is a substantial increase in the recovery of Enterobacteriaceae and *Pseudomonas* bacteria in cultures or swabs taken from the naso-oropharynx. Poor nutrition, debilitation, and hospitalization itself seem to enhance colonization. An assay in vitro that allows these bacteria to react with buccal cells or nasal and tracheal ciliated epithelial cells from such patients will show increased attachment of bacteria. Common to both viruses and mycoplasmas is their injury of the ciliary epithelium lining the trachea and conducting airways. After viral infections in particular, bacteria may not be cleared normally from the lower airways owing to damage in the ciliary clearing action of the respiratory epithelium. Subsequent stasis of mucus and secretions allows for bacterial multiplication, or breaks in the cellular junctions of the lining surface may permit submucosal penetration of bacteria. Viruses shed from infected respiratory epithelium in proximal airways can be aspirated into alveoli and ingested by macrophages, thereby infecting these cells and impairing their phagocytic and bactericidal capacity. This is a well-recognized sequence predisposing to bacterial superinfection, frequently with staphylococci, with pneumonia as a common aftermath. Finally, special features of invading microorganisms can be important in establishing the beachhead of infection—a large inoculum, unusual virulence, or secretion of exo- or endotoxins and other enzymes that directly affect the function of host cells or structurally damage lung tissue. Some common bacteria (*Hemophilus spp.*, pneumococci, and *Neisseria spp.*) that colonize the airways of those with chronic bronchitis can produce an IgA protease that cleaves secretory IgA_1 and that may favor attachment to the mucosa.

LUNG HOST DEFENSES. Many microbial agents can infect the lungs and cause pneumonia, but bacteria do so most frequently. Although a common disease, bacterial pneumonia is a relatively rare occurrence in normal people, considering the burden of microorganisms in the ambient air and our frequent exposure to infectious respiratory droplets and secretions from the sneezing and coughing of fellow humans. This attests to the effectiveness of the lung host defense system. This defense system consists of a complex interrelationship between anatomic barriers and cleansing mechanisms present in the nasopharynx and upper airways and with local cellular and humoral factors operant in the terminal air-exchange units (alveoli). This might be described as the "natural defense system" of the respiratory tract. With respect to infectious agents, normal lungs are generally kept sterile beyond the first bronchial divisions.

In the upper respiratory tract and large airways, a combination of mechanisms excludes particulate material: (1) anatomic barriers such as the epiglottis and tight apical cellular junctions between epithelial lining cells, (2) frequent branching of the pulmonary tree (to effect aerodynamic filtration of inspired air), (3) mucociliary clearance of particulates that impact on the mucosa, and (4) the cough response. When infectious agents, bacteria in particular, elude the physical or mechanical defenses described above and are deposited in the alveoli, another group of host factors takes over. This switch occurs because lung structure changes at the level of respiratory bronchioles, and in the terminal units (alveolar ducts and alveoli) ciliated epithelium and mucus-secreting cells (goblet cells and mucous glands) are no longer present. Therefore, mucociliary clearance does not occur in the terminal units; nor does coughing effectively clear material from the alveoli. Thus microbial clearance and removal of other antigenic material from alveoli are dependent entirely on cellular and humoral factors.

If a bacterium of critical size reaches an alveolus (in the absence of edema fluid of either circulatory or inflammatory origin), the microbe may encounter at least three substances that conceivably might inactivate it, exclusive of its eventual inactivation by phagocytosis. First, surfactant, secreted by Type II pneumocytes, may have some antibacterial activity against staphylococci and rough colony strains of some gram-negative rod bacteria. Second, immunoglobulins, principally of the IgG class and, in lesser concentration, monomeric and secretory forms of IgA, may have specific opsonic antibody activity for the bacterium. Third, complement components, especially properdin factor B, might interact with the bacterium and trigger the alternative complement pathway. One or all of these substances can prepare the bacterium for ingestion by an alveolar macrophage, or the activated complement sequence can lyse it directly. Although alveolar macrophages avidly phagocytose some inert particles, they ingest viable bacteria with considerably less enthusiasm. Coating or opsonizing the organisms will enhance phagocytosis approximately ten-fold. Immunoglobulin G appears to be the principal substance capable of increasing alveolar macrophage phagocytosis, although complement (C3b) can function to enhance or amplify the process. Some particulates that activate the alternate complement pathway can interact with fragments of fibronectin found in the alveoli lining fluid, which in turn bind to a specific receptor on alveolar macrophages. Thus, nonimmune opsonins may aid phagocytosis. Once phagocytosis has occurred, the alveolar macrophage can inactivate susceptible organisms. Intracellular killing proceeds but often at a slower rate than that measured in PMNs and along less well studied metabolic pathways. Whereas PMNs may kill ingested bacteria with one or a combination of four antimicrobial systems (H_2O_2, superoxide anion [O_2^-], myeloperoxidase, or halide anion), the process is less certain in alveolar macrophages.

Following ingestion of bacteria, the fate of alveolar macrophages is not certain. They are long-lived tissue cells that can survive months to years and presumably are capable of handling repeated bacterial and other microbial challenges. Because they are mobile cells, they can migrate to other alveoli through the pores of Kohn or move to more proximal areas of the respiratory tract and get aboard the mucociliary escalator for elimination from the lungs. In addition, macrophages gain entry into lung lymphatics and can be carried to regional lymph nodes, which can be sites for initiating humoral and cellular immune responses for the lung. Undoubtedly, macrophages are instrumental in degrading antigenic material and presenting it to appropriate lymphocytes in these nodes. This exit also gives potential access to systemic lymphoid tissue.

Alveolar macrophages are the most numerous resident phagocytes present in the alveoli. They are the bona fide first line of cellular defense on the airside of the lower respiratory tract. A few PMNs, about one per 100 alveoli, are present, but primarily they are reserve phagocytic cells close by in the intravascular compartment. A plentiful supply of PMNs resides in the blood of lung capillaries as part of the body's pool of marginated PMNs. Even though PMNs are in close proximity to alveolar spaces, they are nonetheless separated by several planes of tissue-capillary endothelium, interstitial space, and alveolar epithelium. Depending upon the species of bacteria that is inhaled into the lungs, alveolar macrophages and/or PMNs are selected to respond to the inoculum. Experimentally in mice, a small dose of aerosolized *Staphylococcus aureus* is contained solely by macrophages, whereas *Klebsiella* and *Pseudomonas* evoke a PMN exudate in alveoli. Or, if a sufficiently large bacterial inoculum or particularly virulent microorganisms reach the lower respiratory tract, the lung parenchyma mounts an extensive inflammatory response, which is a potent mechanism to augment host defense. The development of the inflammatory response and hence pneumonia is a deliberate and controlled reaction in the lungs. The ingredients of initiation, amplification, and, finally, suppression are present. When the lung parenchyma mounts an extensive inflammatory response it may be perceived as clinical illness, and a chest roentgenogram usually reveals an infiltrate.

Granulocyte movement into the alveoli is an orderly reaction initiated from the alveolar side. This is termed directed migration or chemotaxis. At least two mechanisms for chemotactic activity exist that can set in motion the inflammatory response in the alveoli and amplify the PMN response. *The first* is best illustrated with the example of gram-negative rod bacteria known to contain lipopolysaccharide substances termed endotoxins. Some complement components, particularly factor B, are present in small amounts in bronchoalveolar fluids. Bacterial endotoxin can directly activate the alternative complement pathway, leading to the formation of fragments such as C5a that are known to be potent stimulators of PMN chemotaxis. In addition, the inflammatory response may include activation of the kinin system. This could result in generation of kallikrein, which has chemotactic activity, and bradykinin, which is capable of increasing vascular permeability and could account for the accumulation of fluid and other humoral substances in alveoli that accompany pneumonia. *The second mechanism* may emanate from the alveolar macrophage itself. Following phagocytosis of opsonized bacteria, chemotactic factors are synthesized and secreted that will selectively attract PMNs. These small molecular weight, noncomplement factors include some leukotriene substances (LTB_4) derived from arachadonic acid along its lipoxygenase pathway.

Once PMNs and other components of edema fluid have filled alveolar spaces, an exudative inflammatory reaction exists in lung parenchyma and pathologically pneumonitis is present. Ultimately lung tissues become consolidated. Proteolytic enzymes (PMN-derived elastase) are released but largely neutralized by several inhibitor proteins, $alpha_1$ proteinase and bronchial mucosal inhibitor, which minimize autodestruction of lung tissue. Pending successful containment of the infection, resolution and healing phases eventually occur. At present, however, little is known about the processes that turn off or limit the acute inflammatory reaction of pneumonia and initiate recovery. Serum-derived chemotactic factor inactivator can inhibit immune-complex deposition in animal lung tissue and modify the ensuing inflammatory response. The identification of such inhibitors and the potential for manipulating them is a part of lung immunophysiology that is still in its infancy.

CLINICAL PRESENTATION. For the physician to discover that a pneumonia, i.e., an intrapulmonary process of some sort, is present in an adult patient is not a difficult feat, but two more things are necessary—to assemble evidence that the disease is indeed microbial in origin and not an infarct or neoplasm and to identify the specific microbe that is involved. Every aspect of management—the choice of treatment, the complications to be watched for, and the hour-by-hour prognosis—depends on the nature of this information. To obtain it accurately *and in proper time* requires the physician to be wholly familiar with the various ways in which each one of the microbial pneumonias expresses itself. Some forms of pneumonia encountered relatively rarely arise as complications of familiar microbial diseases such as measles or tuberculosis or streptococcal disease. Occasionally, well-known viruses such as influenza or chickenpox cause pneumonia, or the physician may be asked to see a patient with psittacosis. In the compromised host, necrotizing pneumonias caused by *Pseudomonas* and other gram-negative bacilli are commonplace. Most of the time, in an adult patient the physician is dealing with *mycoplasmal pneumonia* or with *one of three bacterial pneumonias*, pneumococcal, staphylococcal, or some other form of necrotizing pneumonia in an obviously altered host. This narrowing of the probabilities does not really lighten the seriousness of making the correct choice, for the most effective treatment for pneumococcal pneumonia is without much value in *Klebsiella* pneumonia. A choice of therapy based on a diagnosis of mycoplasmal pneumonia when the patient actually has staphylococcal pneumonia could result in a fatality. Recently recognized bacteria (*Legionella spp.*), unexpected combinations of microbes in immunocompromised hosts (viral and lethal *Pneumocystis carinii* in homosexuals and illicit-drug users) or antibiotic-resistant strains are part of a changing spectrum of pneumonia that can be encountered in community-acquired disease or as complications in hospitalized patients. Unusual microbial etiologies are to be expected.

As indicated above, in most persons with pneumonia, the physician's opportunity for error comes not from overlooking altogether that respiratory disease is present, but from minimizing its importance ("a little bronchitis") or from lightheartedly mislabeling a quite serious *nonmicrobial* condition, such as pulmonary infarction, as "a viral pneumonia." Therefore, to establish that a pneumonic process is present and to amass evidence that it is most probably microbial in origin, two things are of importance: obtaining a relevant clinical history and using some readily available and simple laboratory techniques. Young adults often have the classic symptoms that can be readily pinpointed to the lower respiratory tract, whereas infants and the elderly may have so few respiratory symptoms as to cause concern that infection may be arising from another organ system. Elderly or severely ill patients may have an unimpressive amount of cough, scant sputum production, little evidence of respiratory symptoms, and a deceptive absence of fever. Only after excluding infection systematically in other organ systems does the respiratory tract receive greater consideration. The onset of fever and agitation or altered mentation frequently ushers in an acquired or nosocomial lung infection in a hospitalized or immunocompromised patient (see Ch. 264). Obviously, a high index of suspicion is needed, plus confirming evidence from the physical examination and other laboratory aids.

A conscientious medical history and physical examination are essential. The oral account from an ambulatory patient may be straightforward and describe a prodromal upper respiratory infection, sudden and precise onset of chills followed by fever, painful cough, fatigue and apprehension, and failure of antipyretic medication to provide relief. With a chronically ill hospitalized patient, the search for a source of a temperature spike always includes a chest radiograph, which may happen to show a new infiltrate; an extensive history is less necessary. Answers to a few specific queries are always needed; e.g., has there been prior illness, hemoptysis, use of antibiotics, chills, or pleuritic chest pain? Once the nature of respiratory illness has been determined, other problems invariably come to mind, which should be weighed appropriately. Does the patient have any obvious risk factors or underlying illnesses that make him or her susceptible to a specific bacterial infection? Are there any special epidemiologic considerations, and—of special importance—are any other members of the immediate family ill? Is this a recurrent pneumonia? What other peculiar problems of the patient may complicate medical management, such as drug allergies, compromised renal or hepatic function, poor superficial arm veins that prevent easy intravenous access, and so on? Will the patient require hospitalization or outpatient management? Some of the considerations are not relevant for every case. The point for emphasis, however, is the use of a mental checklist to organize and cover most facets of the patient's presentation. This leads to initiation of an orderly plan for the management of the particular respiratory infection.

Auscultation and percussion of the chest may reveal typical signs of lung consolidation that affirm the existence and location of infection. If the pneumonic process has been viewed on chest radiograph prior to examination of the patient, as may occur in a busy emergency room or in an intensive care unit where routine chest films are obtained, the physician may not always follow through with a detailed physical examination. This is a mistake because valuable contributory information may be missed. Appearance of the skin and mucous membranes can help assess fluid status, indicate jaundice or cyanosis, which can accompany serious pneumonia, reveal needle tracks in illicit drug users, and disclose lesions suggesting peripheral emboli. Assessment of oral hygiene, condition of the teeth and gingiva, and adequacy of the gag reflex could all point to a likely aspiration syndrome and anaerobic infection. Fingernail beds roughly reflect oxygenation, or the presence of clubbing may give a clue to underlying lung disease. Acute endocarditis can complicate pneumonia; hence auscultation of the heart and a search for signs of emboli are important. Just watching the patient breathe or observing his position in bed as he attempts to splint his chest or to minimize pleuritic pain can help one gauge the discomfort the patient is experiencing. Upper abdominal tenderness may reflect diaphragmatic irritation resulting from inflamed pleural surfaces, but the association can be confusing in the patient. High fever can cause changes in mental status, but meningitis can occasionally complicate pneumonias as well, especially those caused by gram-negative bacilli; thus a neurologic examination should also be part of the evaluation.

DIAGNOSIS AND MANAGEMENT. The physician in possession of the patient's history, the results of the physical examination, and the chest radiograph knows a lot about the setting of the illness, the likely cause, and the probable extent of involvement. A good sputum specimen, well Gram stained, may suggest a causative agent, and an elevated white blood cell count with a left shift of the differential reinforces the impression of acute disease. With this data base a good diagnosis is possible, but the final decision on the causative agent may have to await culture results. Thus, an element of uncertainty is present and antibiotic therapy is somewhat empiric. At this point in formulating a plan of action, three principles of patient management bear repeating and deserve emphasis: (1) obtain all the necessary specimens for appropriate bacteriologic cultures before antimicrobial therapy is begun so that there is a reasonable chance for laboratory recovery of the organism; (2) ensure that the drug therapy is as specific as one's certainty of the etiologic agent allows, yet sufficiently broad—temporarily at least—to cover the common yet unsuspected microorganisms as well; and (3) tailor or change the antimicrobial coverage in several days when the results of the cultures are available. A few days of a broad-spectrum antimicrobial coverage will usually not cause superinfections or selection of the drug-resistant bacteria so long as the physician discontinues unnecessary drugs and appropriately narrows the antimicrobial spectrum as soon as possible.

Since appropriate examination and culture of respiratory secretions are so necessary for the rational treatment of pneumonia, the physician should be vigorous in his attempt to get adequate specimens. If the patient is not producing sputum, an attempt to induce secretions by nebulization of ultrasonic water particles is reasonable. Such particles (which may vary in size between 0.8 and 10 μ in diameter) serve as an irritant and stimulate most subjects to cough. Attempts to obtain lung secretions by passing a small rubber catheter through the nose or mouth rarely get beyond the vocal cords of an alert patient and accomplish little more than further distressing an already sick patient in order to obtain a sample of oropharyngeal fluids.

In addition to sputum cultures, the desirability of having blood and pleural fluid (if evidence of pleural effusion is present) specimens for culture must be weighed. Several blood cultures are recommended because the causative bacterium can be obtained in a reasonable percentage of patients, especially with lobar pneumococcal pneumonia, in which the recovery rate may be 10 to 25 per cent. A parapneumonic effusion is a common occurrence, and one may be evident on initial presentation or develop in the course of the illness, despite appropriate antibiotic treatment. Indications for use of a diagnostic thoracentesis vary. On *initial* evaluation if the patient has clinical evidence of pleural space fluid, substantiated by decubitus chest radiographs or ultrasonography, a thoracentesis is indicated to determine whether the fluid is exudative or whether empyema exists. Empyema is usually associated with pneumonitis or lung abscess in adjacent lung tissue, and the fluid is exudative and like pus; microorganisms may be seen on stained smear and usually grow from cultures, especially anaerobic ones. Aside from culturing the pleural material, cellular analysis (total cell count and differential count) and certain chemical tests (pH, LDH, glucose, total protein, and on occasion lactic acid, amylase, lipids, and cytology) will identify pleural fluid to be a transudate or exudate (see Ch. 58). If an empyema exists or analysis of an exudate meets certain criteria (e.g., pH <7.2, or purulent material with high white cell count), repeated thoracenteses to drain the fluid or use of an indwelling chest tube to promote continuous drainage is usually deemed necessary to hasten healing and to prevent or minimize future pleural adhesions. *Later* in the disease course, if a parapneumonic effusion develops, thoracentesis is indicated if (1) fever persists for 72 hours after beginning treatment with appropriate antibiotics; (2) a large effusion develops that is contributing to discomfort and difficult breathing or is perceived to be increasing in size; and (3) there is evidence that once freely movable fluid has become loculated. In contrast, if a small effusion develops but the patient continues to improve and remains afebrile, it is acceptable to watch the condition, because the fluid will likely diminish and be absorbed. Needle pleural biopsy should be included with a thoracentesis procedure if the etiology of the lung infection is not definite or prior cellular analysis of pleural fluid suggests that an unsuspected primary pleural process is present. Histology and culture of pleural tissue are often invaluable in the diagnosis of carcinomatosis or mycobacterial infection.

In the patient who has a new lung infiltrate, fever, and the clinical setting of pneumonia but who is unable to provide an adequate expectorated sputum sample, the question of how vigorous to be in obtaining respiratory secretions is always difficult to resolve. The situation arises most often in the debilitated, chronically ill patient or the immunosuppressed host, and many factors such as patient tolerance, hematologic parameters, and probability of opportunistic infection dictate the decision on how invasive to be. Each of the procedures noted below carries with it some risk of producing a potentially serious complication in a patient who may be already quite sick. The use of any of these procedures should be carefully limited to those necessary situations in which the additional knowledge to be obtained could be of significant benefit to the patient. The confidence and skill with which certain procedures are performed reflect the experience of the physician involved, so that preference of one technique over another may reflect community availability of an appropriate operator.

Percutaneous transtracheal aspiration is a direct approach that eliminates much of the contaminating oral microbial flora. Aspiration is performed through a plastic angiocatheter (No. 14 or 16 needle size) and needle inserted through the cricothyroid membrane into the airway lumen, and material is aspirated after a small injection of saline solution which makes the patient cough. Transtracheal specimens can become contaminated with mouth flora and yield confusing results if shortcomings in the procedure are not recognized. However, bacteriologic data obtained are more reliable than those gotten from routine sputum samples. Both anaerobic and aerobic cultures should be planted when a tracheal aspirate is obtained. Although this procedure is generally safe, occasionally some hazard accompanies it, such as air leak, leading to subcutaneous or mediastinal emphysema, or tracheal bleeding. A review of over 1200 such aspirations found the mean incidence of complications from subcutaneous emphysema and hemorrhage (not just blood-tinged sputum) to be less than 0.5 per cent (range reported, 0 to 1.6 per cent).

The availability of *fiberoptic bronchoscopy* with bronchial lavage and brushing provides another approach to lower respiratory secretions. The risk of bronchoscopy is small even in patients with extensive pneumonia; correction of thrombocytopenia, if present, with platelet transfusions and the administration of supplemental oxygen during the procedure are indicated. Often a direct view of the affected lung anatomy, particularly if a loss of volume in the lung lobe accompanies the infection, may provide evidence of an endobronchial obstruction. Removal of secretions or a mucous plug could make the procedure therapeutic as well as diagnostic.

Usually, the lavage fluid or brush culture will contain the offending pathogen; however, microbial cultures from the bronchoscopy specimens also contain contaminating flora from the nasopharynx. Interpretation of culture results is often confusing, and identifying the predominant organism may be difficult. To date, no one has perfected a completely reliable way of collecting bronchoscopy lavage specimens that avoids this contamination, although a variety of new telescoping, protected catheters are available. Transbronchial biopsy can be added to the procedure to provide lung tissue for culture and histology. Biopsies of pieces 2 to 3 mm in size are usually obtained. Upon reviewing the diagnostic accuracy of about 230 fiberoptic bronchoscopy procedures, which included bronchial brushing and transbronchial biopsy specimens and were performed in immunocompromised hosts with lung infection, the yield of a specific etiologic diagnosis was about 50 per cent. Brushing gave the correct diagnosis in about 27 per cent and biopsy in about 40 per cent; the combination was about 50 per cent. Complications arising from bronchoscopy include hemorrhage in about 7 per cent and pneumothorax in 5 to 7 per cent. Occasionally, a chest tube is needed to treat the pneumothorax. In about 15 to 25 per cent of patients having bronchoscopy, a postbronchoscopy fever (38.3 to 38.9° C) will develop four to eight hours after the procedure. This usually lasts less than 24 hours. Fever does not seem to reflect a complicating pneumonia, although bacteria are introduced from the nose and throat into the lung with the procedure. The episode can usually be managed with antipyretic therapy alone and without an antibiotic.

Direct examination and culture of affected lung tissue is often indicated. Physicians who care for adult patients with pneumonia generally do not think in terms of needle aspiration of lung tissue. Pediatricians, on the other hand, confronted with undiagnosed pneumonias in infants, feel more comfortable with the procedure and use it frequently. Precise indications for a needle aspirate lung biopsy in an adult cannot be formulated unequivocally; however, a localized, peripheral infiltrate which is "well situated" may lend itself to a needle approach with relatively small risk of complication. Spreading microorganisms along the needle track or soiling the pleural surface is always a consideration, but in actual practice it seems to occur rarely. A small pneumothorax may complicate a needle aspiration in about 25 per cent of cases, but the frequency of this occurrence depends somewhat on the type and size of the needle used. Self-limited hemoptysis occurs in about 5 per cent of patients. Often the factor of most significance is the skill and experience of the physician doing the procedure; this usually dictates the frequency and success with which needle aspiration is used within a particular hospital or medical community. The need to do a *small open thoracotomy* to obtain lung tissue is often easier to agree upon. This approach gives the best piece of tissue and is tolerated surprisingly well by even the sickest patient. Generally thoracic surgeons are extremely skillful in managing this situation. Open lung biopsy is often necessary in the immunocompromised patient with an advancing, undiagnosed pulmonary infiltrate and pneumonia. However, two failings often are observed with the procedure. Medical personnel wait too long to get the biopsy, thus delaying appropriate antimicrobial therapy, or they do not coordinate the handling of the tissue with the microbiologist and pathologist to ensure optimal analysis. A brief presurgical consultation with all the principals is most helpful. The pathologist can often suggest the best area of lung to biopsy, and having the microbiology laboratory prepared can ensure that the most appropriate cultures are quickly planted.

Invariably the initial therapy must be chosen on the basis of the skillful interpretation of essentially *clinical* phenomena and must be heavily weighted toward protecting the patient against the most dangerous of the conceivable diagnoses in that particular set of circumstances. Antimicrobial therapy—plus appropriate support with fluids, antipyretic drugs, oxygen, suction or postural drainage, and the other modalities employed to treat serious lung infection—remains the cornerstone of medical management. Intelligent use of antimicrobial drugs is not easy, and frequent reappraisal of their choice and patient response must be practiced. Once the patient's therapy is underway, the physician can not relax but must remain alert for complications that can develop. A resurgence of fever after an initial period of defervescence is a frequent clue. One of a number of problems could be the cause. Poor coughing and an accumulation of secretions or a mucous plug can obstruct an airway, leading to partial collapse of a lung lobe or segment. Vigorous postural drainage and endotracheal suctions may remove secretions and help re-expand the lung portion and should be tried if possible for 24 hours before resorting to bronchoscopy. The development of loculated pleural fluid has been addressed already and usually requires thoracentesis and possible chest tube drainage. Secondary bacterial infection following a viral pneumonia or superinfection occurring after broad-spectrum antimicrobial therapy may cause fever and worsening of the patient's condition; thus reculturing sputum and blood is necessary. Drug allergy causing mild blood eosinophilia and lingering fever is a frequent and often unsuspected complication that requires discontinuation or substitution in the antibiotic regimen. Finally, complete resolution of the pneumonic process or closure of a lung abscess must be observed, for failure of this part of the healing phase may require additional attention. Sputum cytologies and bronchoscopy might be indicated to rule out a partially obstructing airway lesion or endobronchial tumor.

Bordelon JY, Legrand P, Gewin WC, Sanders CV: The telescoping plugged catheter in suspected anerobic infections. Am Rev Respir Dis 128:465, 1982. *Equipment not yet perfected.*

Czop JK, McGowan SE, Center DM: Opsonin-independent phagocytosis by human alveolar macrophages: Augmentation by human plasma fibronectin. Am Rev Respir Dis 125:607, 1982. *Existence of nonimmune opsonins adds another mechanism for increasing phagocytosis, a process that is becoming increasingly complex to understand.*

Fick RB, Reynolds HY: Changing spectrum of pneumonia: News media creation or clinical reality? Am J Med 74:1, 1983. *An overview of a troublesome situation. Antibiotic therapy also is discussed.*

Kilian M, Mestecky J, Kulhavy R, Tomana M, Butter WT: IgA_1 proteases from *Hemophilus influenzae, Streptococcus pneumoniae, Neisseria meningitides* and *Streptococcus sanguis:* Comparative immunochemical studies. J Immunol 124:2596, 1980. *A fascinating adaptative feature of bacteria to thwart host defenses.*

Marini JJ, Pierson DJ, Hudson LD: Acute lobar atelectasis. A prospective comparison of fiberoptic bronchoscopy and respiratory therapy. Am Rev Respir Dis 119: 971, 1979. *A pertinent clinical trial demonstrating that vigorous respiratory therapy is important.*

Matthay RA, Mortiz ED: Invasive procedures for diagnosing pulmonary infection—a critical review. Clin Chest Med 2:3, 1981. *Summarizes the literature on the diagnostic yield of bronchoscopic, transtracheal, and lung biopsy techniques to obtain lung diagnoses and bacteriologic cultures.*

Niederman MS, Rafferty TD, Sasaki CT, Merrill WW, Matthay RA, Reynolds HY: Comparison of bacterial adherence to ciliated and squamous epithelial cells obtained from human respiratory tract. Am Rev Respir Dis 127:85, 1983. *The kinetics of Pseudomonas aeruginosa binding to cells are explored. Provides good background references.*

Palmer DL, Davidson M, Lusk R: Needle aspiration of the lung in complex pneumonias. Chest 78:16, 1980. *A procedure whose time is arriving.*

Rehm SR, Gross GN, Pierce AK: Early bacterial clearance from murine lungs. Species dependent phagocyte response. J Clin Invest 66:194, 1980. *An interesting research model showing that various bacteria may be cleared in the lungs by different types of phagocytes—alveolar macrophages or polymorphonuclear granulocytes.*

Reynolds HY: Lung host defenses—status report. Chest 75:239(Suppl.), 1979. *An appraisal stressing control of the lung inflammatory response and assessing ways that immune responses are initiated in the airways.*

Reynolds HY: Lung inflammation: Role of endogenous chemotactic factors in attracting polymorphonuclear granulocytes. Am Rev Respir Dis 127:16(Suppl.), 1983. *Summarizes macrophage- and complement-derived chemotactic substances.*

261. PNEUMOCOCCAL PNEUMONIA

David T. Durack

DEFINITION. Pneumococcal pneumonia is a common bacterial infection of the lungs caused by *Streptococcus pneumoniae.* This illness is usually characterized by sudden onset, high fever, shaking chills, pleuritic chest pain, and a racking cough which raises thick, blood-stained sputum.

HISTORICAL NOTE. The pneumococcus was described simultaneously by Pasteur in France and by Sternberg in the United States in 1881. Pasteur isolated the organism from frothy saliva on the lips of a child who had died with rabies, whereas Sternberg found it in the throats of healthy people. Thus, both original isolations correctly indicated that this species could be a constituent of the normal flora of the upper airways. Weichselbaum showed that the organism caused pneumonia. The crucial discovery by Avery, MacLeod, and McCarty that DNA was the genetic material which transformed a rough, avirulent strain of pneumococcus into the smooth, virulent form led directly to the development of the science of molecular biology as we know it today. MacLeod and his colleagues demonstrated in the 1940's that a vaccine derived from pneumococcal polysaccharide provided some immunity to pneumonia. Austrian's work led to recognition of the continuing need for a vaccine in the antibiotic era, and to reintroduction of a useful vaccine in the 1970's.

MICROBIOLOGY. Pneumococci are gram-positive streptococci, each organism measuring about 0.8 μ in diameter. They associate in pairs much more often than in chains. They are not quite spherical, so that on a Gram-stained slide these diplococci look like two short, fat bullets pointing away from each other, with bases touching.

Pneumococci are facultative anaerobes. They flourish in nutrient media containing 5 to 10 per cent blood or serum, and their growth is encouraged by carbon dioxide. On blood agar plates they form circular colonies 0.5 to 1.5 mm in diameter. These are dome shaped at first, but often become umbilicated as time passes owing to autolysis of the cocci in the older, central part of the colony. Autolysis is a characteristic attribute of pneumococci; for example, a broth culture full of living pneumococci sometimes spontaneously becomes sterile, containing nothing but bacterial debris, within a day. This self-destruction is caused by the pneumococcal enzyme L-alanine muramyl amidase. Pneumococci also elaborate a hyaluronidase, but unlike other common pathogens such as staphylococci, clostridia, and pseudomonas they produce no known toxins. Colonies of pneumococci growing on blood agar are surrounded by a zone of green (alpha) hemolysis caused by a hemolysin, which under anaerobic conditions causes clear (beta) hemolysis. Pneumococci undergo rapid autolysis when exposed to bile or sodium deoxycholate, and are highly sensitive to optochin. These characteristics are exploited in the laboratory to distinguish pneumococci from other alpha-hemolytic streptococci.

Possession of a capsule is an important attribute of pneumococci. These capsules consist of a high molecular weight polysaccharide polymer that forms a glutinous coat around each bacterium. Variations in the composition of these capsular carbohydrates allow serologic differentiation of at least 83 antigenically distinct types of pneumococci. The capsule is also a crucial virulence factor. It confers resistance to ingestion by phagocytes; this can be partially or completely overcome if type-specific antibody and complement are available to opsonize the pneumococci. Encapsulated, virulent strains form smooth, glistening, mucoid colonies, whereas noncapsulated, nonvirulent strains form rough, dry, granular colonies. The Type 3 pneumococcus is a particularly virulent strain that is noted for producing an abundance of capsular polysaccharide; its colonies are therefore unusually large and mucoid. Incubation of pneumococci with specific antiserum to the capsule causes it to swell and become visible under the microscope. This is the quellung reaction, which can be used for rapid confirmation of presence of pneumococci in clinical specimens as well as for typing.

Pneumococci are ordinarily highly sensitive to a broad range of antibiotics, including the penicillins, cephalosporins, chloramphenicol, erythromycin, tetracyclines, clindamycin, and vancomycin. They are relatively resistant to aminoglycosides. For penicillin, the minimal inhibitory concentration (MIC) is usually 0.01 μg per milliliter or less, but intermediate (MIC 0.2 to 1.0 μg per milliliter) or high-level resistance (MIC 1.0 μg per milliliter or more) can occur. Penicillin resistance in pneumococci, in contrast to gonococci, is mediated by chromosomal mutations, not by plasmids. High-level resistance was extremely rare until 1977, when many resistant strains appeared among pneumococci isolated from children in Durban and Johannesburg, South Africa. Subsequently, a large number of strains that were resistant to many other antibiotics as well as to penicillin were isolated from patients and carriers in these cities. Currently intermediate resistance can be expected in 2 to 5 per cent of clinical isolates in the United States, and high-level resistance in 0.5 to 1 per cent. Therefore, sensitivity tests should be performed on isolates from blood or cerebrospinal fluid when practicable. The necessity for *routine* sensitivity testing of isolates from sputum is debatable. Because the prevalence of resistance seems to be increasing gradually, clinicians should be alert to the possibility of antibiotic treatment failures in future.

EPIDEMIOLOGY. Pneumococci are commonly present in the upper respiratory tract as part of the normal microbial flora. Various studies have found that 10 to 60 per cent of healthy people carry one or more types of pneumococci at any one time. These are most often the higher-numbered, less pathogenic types, with the exception that Type 3 is carried quite commonly by normal people. Lower-numbered, more pathogenic types are found less frequently in the oropharynx, but presumably must have been acquired transiently by patients who develop pneumococcal pneumonia.

Pneumococci cause about 50 per cent of *all* bacterial pneumonias and 90 per cent of all cases of *lobar* pneumonia. In children, Types 6, 14, 18, 19, and 23 predominate. In adults, Types, 1, 3, 4, 6, 7, 8, 12, 14, 18, 19, and 23 cause about four fifths of pneumococcal infections. Typing is not merely of academic interest, because polyvalent vaccines must include antigens from the predominant types.

The ratio of males to females among patients with pneumococcal pneumonia is about 3:2. Most cases occur during winter and early spring, when viral respiratory infections are prevalent. Pneumococcal pneumonia is generally a sporadic rather than epidemic disease; it should not be regarded as contagious. Rarely, epidemics of pneumonia have occurred in closed communities when the carriage rate of a pathogenic pneumococcus has become unusually high and a viral respiratory infection passes through the group. This observation demonstrates that pneumococci carried in the nasopharyngeal flora of normal persons can cause infection under suitable circumstances. When bacterial pneumonia complicates influenza, the pneumococcus is the most common etiologic agent, followed in frequency by staphylococci. Therefore, epidemiologists are able to monitor the advent and progress of influenza epidemics by watching the monthly death rate from pneumonia.

PATHOGENESIS. Microorganisms enter the lower airways every day in everyone. The likelihood that pneumonia will result is directly proportional to the *inoculum size* and *virulence* of the organisms, and inversely related to the adequacy of pulmonary *host defenses.* These include the epiglottal and cough reflexes, the carpet of mucus lining the large airways (which is kept moving away from the alveoli at a rate of 1 to 3 cm per hour by the cilia of the respiratory epithelium), lymphatic drainage of alveoli, alveolar macrophages, opsonins, antibodies, and neutrophil leukocytes. Partial or complete obstruction of a bronchus interferes with local defenses and strongly predisposes to infection.

Pneumonia occurs when one or more of these defenses is impaired and pneumococci are aspirated (Table 261–1). The central importance of aspiration in pathogenesis is supported by experiments in laboratory animals. Other experiments have shown that fluid-containing alveoli are far more susceptible to infection than are dry alveoli, hence the increased risk of pneumonia in patients with heart failure. Like any aspiration pneumonia, pneumococcal pneumonia shows a predilection for dependent portions of the lung: the lower lobes and the

TABLE 261–1. CONDITIONS THAT PREDISPOSE TO PNEUMOCOCCAL PNEUMONIA AND OTHER LOWER RESPIRATORY TRACT INFECTIONS BY INTERFERING WITH THE NORMAL DEFENSE MECHANISMS

Impairment of Defenses	Causes
Depressed epiglottal and cough reflexes	Unconsciousness, seizures, alcohol, anesthesia, CNS depressants, neuromuscular diseases
Decreased activity of cilia	Smoking, inhaled pollutants and toxic gases, upper respiratory infections, pertussis, chronic bronchitis, intubation, Kartagener's syndrome
Increased secretions	Common cold, other viral respiratory infections, anesthesia, bronchiectasis
Decreased lymphatic flow	Congestive heart failure, tumor
Atelectasis	Tumor or foreign body in bronchi, anesthesia, trauma
Fluid in the alveoli	Congestive heart failure, aspiration, hypoproteinemia, trauma
Abnormality of phagocytes	Neutropenia, sickle cell disease, influenza, asplenia
Abnormality of humoral immunity	Hypogammaglobulinemia, congenital or acquired, e.g., multiple myeloma; starvation, sickle cell disease, hypocomplementemia

posterior segments of the upper lobes. However, the right middle lobe is involved more often than in other forms of aspiration pneumonia.

The mouse provides a useful model for study of the pathogenicity of pneumococci. Most encapsulated strains are "mouse virulent," i.e., injection of only one to ten pneumococci into the peritoneal cavity of a mouse will result in its death from overwhelming pneumococcal bacteremia. If the capsule is removed by treatment with a polysaccharidase before inoculation, more than 1 million of the same pneumococci are needed to kill a mouse. Similarly, a rough (unencapsulated) mutant is far less virulent than its smooth parent. These observations indicate the crucial importance of the capsule as a virulence factor.

Opsonizing antibodies to the capsule are vitally important in host defense against pneumococci. This is evident from the clinical observation that patients with immunoglobulin deficiency are at increased risk for pneumococcal infections. For example, pneumococcal pneumonia occasionally provides the presenting evidence of multiple myeloma. During the first few days of an infection, only nonspecific antibodies possessing relatively weak opsonizing capacity are present in serum. If the patient survives, monospecific anticapsular antibody usually appears after five to ten days, promoting efficient phagocytosis and thus assisting in recovery. Because the issue of death or recovery is often decided before this, great efforts have been made to provide a patient with specific antibodies early enough to influence the course of illness. In the preantibiotic era, passive immunity was provided by administration of specific horse or rabbit antisera, resulting in significant improvement in outcome. Today, a degree of active humoral immunity can be provided by administering polyvalent pneumococcal vaccine to selected high-risk patients.

PATHOLOGY. Once a sufficient inoculum of sufficiently virulent pneumococci has reached the alveoli, pneumonia develops and evolves in a stereotyped fashion. First, fluid pours out from capillaries to fill the alveoli, spreading concentrically outward via the pores of Kohn and the smallest airways to fill adjacent alveoli and acini. This infected tide carries pneumococci into contiguous areas until its flow is stopped by an anatomic barrier, usually the visceral pleura investing a segment or lobe of the lung. Edema fluid containing pneumococci also enters the bronchi, by way of which it can bypass segmental anatomic divisions to involve nearby segments or other lobes. The normal smooth, slippery surface of the pleura overlying an affected segment or lobe becomes roughened as dilated vessels leak plasma and inflammatory cells, forming a patch of fibrinous pleurisy. The movements of breathing then give rise to pleuritic chest pain and a friction rub at the site. Often there is an associated exudative effusion.

Next, the interaction of pneumococci with serum opsonins and complement in the alveolar exudate generates chemotactic factors, which stimulate an outpouring of neutrophils into the alveoli. These phagocytes, together with many red cells that spill out from damaged capillaries, pack the alveoli to cause *consolidation.* Although neutrophils do not phagocytose bacteria efficiently when suspended in fluid, they can ingest pneumococci that are trapped against cell surfaces such as the alveolar wall (surface phagocytosis) or immobilized in consolidated exudate. Thus a finely balanced contest develops between the spreading pneumococcal infection and pursuing phagocytes brought to the site by the host's inflammatory reaction. Even without treatment, polymorphonuclear phagocytes will eventually contain the acute infection in a majority of patients. Therefore, antibiotic treatment should be regarded as only one of many antibacterial mechanisms working together to overcome pneumococcal infection. Antibiotics need not *kill* pneumococci to be effective; bacteriostatic agents work as well as bactericidal drugs because in this infection treatment need only tip the balance slightly in favor of the host, whose phagocytes will then effect cure. Unfavorable factors for the host include a high inoculum, a virulent infecting strain, a wide area of involved lung, lack of specific opsonizing antibody, and anatomic abnormalities such as bronchial obstruction, especially when the patient is elderly and debilitated by other diseases.

Finally, macrophages migrate into the consolidated alveoli and ingest the debris left behind as the acute infection resolves. This, together with expectoration of alveolar contents by coughing, results in ultimate resolution of the exudate. Because the alveolar wall is not destroyed when consolidation occurs, recovery is complete in most cases, with restoration of normal pulmonary anatomy.

In a fully developed case of pneumonia, all of the three main stages of the inflammatory reaction described above may be present at once. At the periphery is a spreading zone of serous edema fluid containing bacteria but few cells. Within is a zone of early consolidation, marked by hemorrhage and migration of neutrophils into alveoli, causing the pathologic appearance graphically described as "red hepatization." In the oldest part of the lesion is found a zone of advanced consolidation in which leukocytes predominate; this is termed "gray hepatization." Here the process of resolution begins.

Pneumococcal pneumonia can develop in a patchy, multifocal, and peribronchial rather than segmental or lobar distribution. This form of the disease may be termed *bronchopneumonia.* It is more common in elderly, immobile, or debilitated patients, especially those with cardiac failure, and is often a preterminal complication contributing to, or causing, death.

Spread of Infection. Pneumococci can infect contiguous pleural or pericardial spaces by direct spread from the lung. The organisms may travel via lymphatics, spread across anatomic barriers breached by inflammation, or pass through new communications such as bronchopleural fistulas. The thoracic duct, fed by lymphatic drainage from infected lung, can carry pneumococci to the bloodstream, causing *bacteremia.* Hematogenous seeding of distant susceptible sites can lead to pneumococcal meningitis, endocarditis, pericarditis, arthritis, or ophthalmitis. All these metastatic infections have become uncommon in the antibiotic era.

CLINICAL FINDINGS. The bedside examiner finds a patient suffering from a serious febrile illness, intermittently sweating, breathing fast, distressed by frequent bouts of coughing, and preoccupied with pleuritic pain. The patient may be too ill to cooperate fully with history or examination until these symptoms improve.

Many patients have had an upper respiratory infection for several days before the onset of pneumonia. This may be as mild as a common cold or as severe as influenza. Then they experience an abrupt chill, followed quickly by fever, cough, and chest pain, often with rapid progression over 12 to 24 hours. Patients may vomit once or twice early in the course. The *chill* is often severe, being accompanied by a teeth-chattering, bed-rattling rigor lasting from 10 to 30 minutes. Chills may continue intermittently, but frequently only a single episode of true rigor occurs; repeated rigors over several days are unusual unless a complication has developed. The *fever* is usually high and continuous, ranging between 39.5 and 41° C. This contributes to the patient's striking malaise, weakness, myalgia, and prostration. Temperature should be measured rectally, because the patient is usually breathing rapidly through his mouth. Anxiety, restlessness, and delirium are common.

Cough occurs in more than 90 per cent of patients; it may be dry at first, but soon the patient begins to raise sputum. This is blood tinged or bloody in about three fourths of cases. The blood is usually well mixed through the sputum rather than streaked on the surface, because bleeding occurs directly into the exudate in the alveoli. This gives the sputum a characteristic "rusty" or "prune-juice" appearance. The pneumococcal capsular polysaccharide itself may be present in the sputum in such abundance as to lend it a sticky, tenacious mucoid character, especially in Type 3 infections. In some cases the sputum is simply mucopurulent.

Chest pain is common and frequently severe. It is stabbing in nature, localized over the involved lobe, and sharply exacerbated by deep breathing or coughing. The patient often carefully adjusts his position in bed in order to "splint" the ribs, reducing chest wall movement over the area of pleurisy. Diaphragmatic pleurisy may cause upper abdominal pain or pain referred to the shoulder.

On examination, the patient's brow is usually beaded with sweat and his skin is hot. The "fever blisters" of reactivated herpes simplex virus infection are commonly present around the lips. Rapid pulse and wide pulse pressure accompany the fever. Respiratory distress is evident, with tachypnea, dyspnea, and use of the accessory muscles. Breathing may be so restricted by pleuritic pain that each shallow breath is followed by an audible, grunting expiration. Mild central cyanosis may be present owing to alveolar hypoventilation as a consequence of shallow breathing, and to shunting of venous blood through consolidated lung. Shock may supervene.

On inspection, chest wall movements may be diminished on the affected side owing to the combined effect of consolidation of the underlying lung and splinting of voluntary muscles. Palpation confirms decreased respiratory movement and will occasionally reveal a palpable pleural rib. The trachea is usually central but occasionally deviates toward the affected side if there is associated atelectasis or away from it if there is a large pleural effusion. Vocal fremitus is increased owing to conduction of vibrations from patent bronchi through solid lung.

Percussion reveals dullness over the affected lung, unless the area of consolidation is too small or too deep to be detectable. Even light percussion may cause local pain at the site of underlying pleurisy.

Auscultation over consolidated lung reveals bronchial breath sounds, increased vocal resonance, whispered pectoriloquy, egophony ("*e to a* change"), and crackling rales. A localized pleural friction rub is often present.

Other findings that may be present include *jaundice,* which occurs in a few severe cases and indicates a worse prognosis, and *abdominal distention,* which can be due to gastrectasia (acute gastric dilatation) or generalized ileus. *Neck stiffness* could be due to concomitant meningitis, and the neurologic examination should be complete enough to exclude this complication and to detect any focal neurologic signs. Signs of shock or heart failure can be present in severe cases. *Systolic murmurs* in the aortic area are common, most often signifying no more than a high cardiac output. Murmurs caused by aortic or mitral regurgitation should raise the possibility of pneumococcal endocarditis.

Many patients with pneumococcal pneumonia have milder symptoms and less striking physical signs. Not all need admission to hospital.

LABORATORY FINDINGS. The leukocyte count is usually elevated to 15,000 to 30,000 cells per cubic millimeter, with an increased percentage of mature and immature neutrophils. These often show toxic granulation. Painstaking examination of a Gram-stained smear of the buffy coat (if time is available) will show intraleukocytic pneumococci in a few cases, especially in patients who are asplenic. Leukopenia occurs in some severe cases, and is associated with a worse prognosis. The infection is usually too short lived to cause anemia; if present, anemia probably reflects a pre-existing condition. Moderate free-water depletion caused by fever and sweating is reflected by raised serum sodium concentration in most patients. Hypovolemia may occur owing to the combined effects of vomiting, vasodilatation, and ileus. The erythrocyte sedimentation rate may be elevated, but is of little value in diagnosis.

Examination of *Gram-stained sputum* is an important step in evaluation of a patient with pneumonia. Smears containing many epithelial cells associated with normal flora should be discarded, because they are heavily contaminated with saliva and can only be misleading. Presence of many polymorphonuclear leukocytes indicates that the specimen is sputum. A smear showing predominant gram-positive bullet-shaped diplococci associated with pus cells together with a positive *sputum culture* for pneumococci provides good evidence (but not proof) of pneumococcal infection in a patient with pneumonia. Interpretation of the sputum Gram stain should be tempered by the knowledge that false positives are common (because pneumococci are part of the normal flora), and that the Gram stain may not correlate with the results of sputum culture. Sputum from many patients with pneumococcal pneumonia shows only mixed flora. In practice, the sputum Gram stain is sometimes more useful by helping to rule out staphylococcal or gram-negative pneumonia than by helping to rule in pneumococcal disease.

In seriously ill patients with pneumonia, further measures to identify the causative organism may be considered necessary. Transtracheal aspiration provides a more reliable specimen for Gram stain and culture than sputum, but about one third of transtracheal specimens will yield one or more contaminating organisms from the upper airways. Direct needle aspiration of the lung will not yield contaminants, but a false-negative result is obtained in about one third of cases. Bronchoscopy is of limited value in diagnosis of acute pneumonia, except when endobronchial obstruction must be excluded. Fortunately, these techniques are not necessary for diagnosis and management of most cases of pneumococcal pneumonia.

Two *blood cultures* should be taken prior to treatment from all patients with pneumonia who are ill enough to be hospitalized. Fifteen to 25 per cent of patients with pneumococcal pneumonia have positive blood cultures. Unlike a positive sputum culture, a positive blood culture proves the diagnosis, and also indicates that the patient has a higher risk of complications and death than patients with negative blood cultures.

Counterimmunoelectrophoresis (CIE) and co-agglutination are modern techniques that can identify pneumococcal polysaccharide in clinical specimens such as cerebrospinal fluid, urine, and blood within one to three hours by utilizing specific antigen-antibody reactions. Since the lungs in pneumococcal pneumonia can contain as much as 1 to 2 grams of polysaccharide, it is not surprising that this substance can be found in patients' blood and urine. CIE will be positive on blood from half or more of patients with bacteremia. High levels indicate severe disease and a worse prognosis. Although more valuable in evaluation of meningitis than of pneumonia, CIE occasionally confirms a diagnosis missed by blood and sputum cultures and provides another means to type the pneumococcus. Polysaccharide can sometimes be detected in the urine of a patient with pneumococcal infection for days or even weeks after eradication of living pneumococci.

ROENTGENOGRAPHY. The chest x-ray usually shows a homogeneous opacity in one or more segments or lobes of the lung (Fig. 261–1). An air bronchogram is almost always present, and volume loss is slight or nonexistent. Patients with bronchopneumonia have diffuse, patchy infiltrates on x-ray rather than consolidation. In a patient with emphysema, pneumonia causes poorly defined opacities that are honeycombed with small holes, presumably emphysematous spaces that escape consolidation (Fig. 261–2). Rarely, pneumococcal pneumonia may produce a spherical opacity on the chest film.

Resolution after treatment may be rapid, progressing to completion in two weeks or less, but in some cases the radiologic appearance of consolidation persists for several weeks despite successful treatment. This may cause unjustified alarm and despondency on the part of the physician; therefore, frequent follow-up x-rays should be avoided in patients who are clinically cured. On the other hand, follow-up x-rays are mandatory for patients who do not recover promptly. They may reveal various causes of treatment failure, including tumor, lung abscess, empyema, or bronchopleural fistula.

DIFFERENTIAL DIAGNOSIS. Many other infections can simulate pneumococcal pneumonia. *Klebsiella pneumoniae* causes a form of lobar pneumonia that may be radiologically indistinguishable. Some cases show a bulging interlobar fissure on x-ray, but this sign is not specific. *Klebsiella* pneumonia shows some predilection for the upper lobes, and frequently causes necrosis

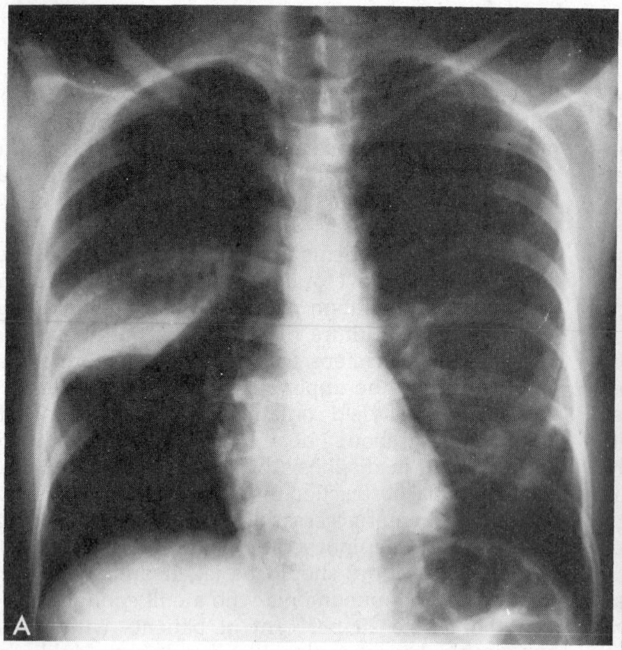

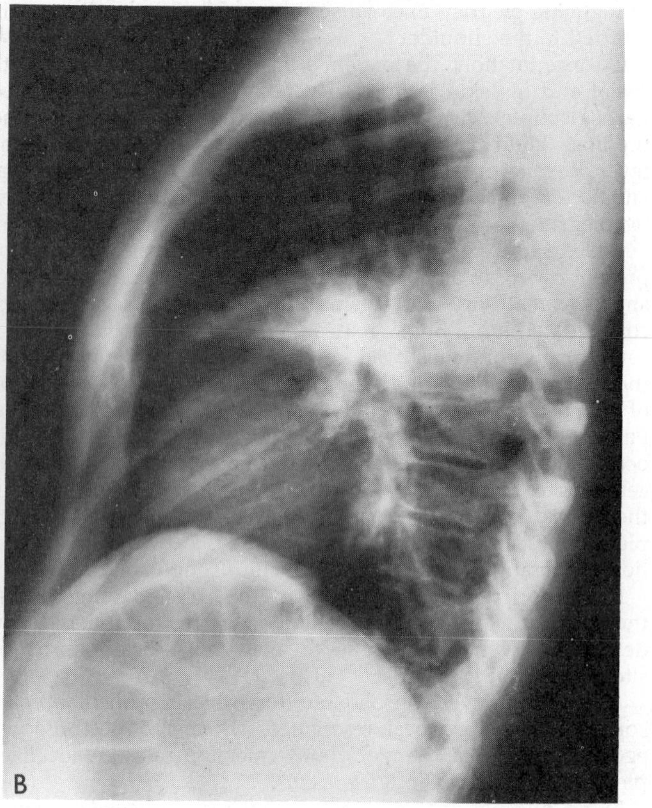

Figure 261–1. Chest x-ray from a typical case of pneumococcal pneumonia showing segmental consolidation in the anterior and posterior segments of the right upper lobe, bounded by pleural surfaces. *A*, Posteroanterior view. *B*, Lateral view.

of pulmonary parenchyma so that patients produce sputum likened to red currant jelly. Staphylococcal pneumonia occurs as a complication of influenza or as part of disseminated staphylococcal infections; it often causes multiple patchy infiltrates that may progress to form pneumatoceles or abscesses. *Hemophilus influenzae* type b pneumonia may be clinically indistinguishable from pneumococcal infection, but is much more common in children under five years of age than in adults. *Streptococcus pyogenes* and *Neisseria meningitidis* (usually group Y) are other rare causes of pneumonia that can be distinguished with certainty only by the results of culture.

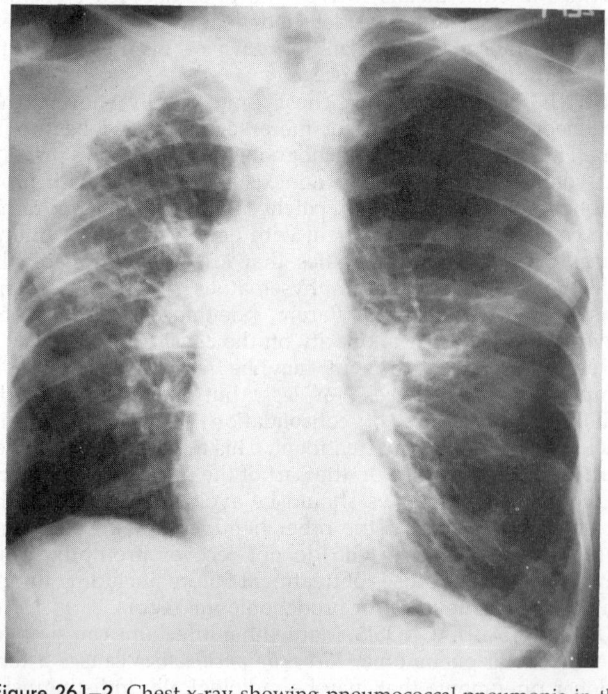

Figure 261–2. Chest x-ray showing pneumococcal pneumonia in the right upper lobe of a patient with severe emphysema. Instead of homogeneous consolidation there is diffuse, patchy ("Swiss-cheese") opacification.

Mycoplasma and chlamydial pneumonias are usually less acute in onset and less likely to cause lobar consolidation. Patients with tuberculous pneumonia show less acute prostration and are less likely to have neutrophil leukocytosis. Legionnaires' disease usually does not evolve as rapidly as pneumococcal pneumonia and is more likely to be associated with gastrointestinal upset.

The differential diagnosis between pulmonary infarction and pneumonia is frequently difficult, but must be made in order to treat these conditions correctly. Misdirected treatment of pulmonary embolus as pneumonia (or vice versa) can have serious consequences. Careful consideration of the differential features (Table 261–2) may be sufficient to clarify the diagnosis, but in some cases only pulmonary angiography can resolve the issue.

Infections below the diaphragm such as subphrenic or hepatic abscesses can cause fever, cough, low chest pain, referred pain to the shoulder, atelectasis, and pleural effusion, thus closely simulating lower lobe pneumonia. Gonococcal perihepatitis can mimic right lower lobe pneumonia.

TREATMENT. *Supportive measures* are important for the comfort and safety of patients with pneumococcal pneumonia. They should be put at bed rest, without undue disturbances except for regular checks of respiratory rate, blood pressure, and urine output until there is clearly no danger that shock will develop.

Adequate *analgesia* is needed, both to relieve distress and to allow deeper breathing and coughing to help raise secretions. Codeine tablets may suffice, but will not be adequate for some patients with severe pleurisy or those not absorbing oral drugs because of ileus. These patients should receive parenteral meperidine, 50 to 100 mg every three to six hours until relief is provided, unless there is *real* danger of harming the patient by depressing the respiratory center. In many patients with pneumonia, the benefits of parenteral narcotic treatment for

TABLE 261–2. COMPARATIVE FEATURES OF PNEUMOCOCCAL PNEUMONIA AND PULMONARY INFARCTION (IN PRACTICE, EXCEPTIONS TO THESE GUIDELINES ARE COMMON, MAKING THIS A DIFFICULT DIFFERENTIAL DIAGNOSIS)

	Pneumococcal Pneumonia	Pulmonary Infarction
Predisposing factors	Alcoholism, measles, debility	Recent trauma or operation; immobility
Previous upper respiratory infection	Yes	No
Fever, sweating	Yes, usually >39.5°C	Yes, usually <39.5°C
Rigors	Yes	No
Cough	Severe, in paroxysms	Slight or none
Purulent sputum	Yes	No
Hemoptysis	Yes; rusty color, well mixed with sputum	Yes; bright red blood
Pleuritic chest pain, pleural rub	Yes	Yes
Dyspnea, cyanosis	Yes	Yes
Sputum Grain stain	Gram-positive diplococci or mixed flora; leukocytes present	Mixed flora from saliva; few leukocytes
Leukocytosis	Yes; often >15,000/mm^3	Yes; often <15,000/mm^3
Shift to the left, toxic granulations	Yes	No
Bilirubin	May be elevated	May be elevated
Arterial oxygen	Moderate reduction	Moderate reduction
Chest roentgenogram	Lobar or segmental opacity	Pleural-based, segmental, wedge-shaped opacity
Radionuclide scan	Matched ventilation and perfusion defect	Matched ventilation and perfusion defect
Pulmonary angiogram	Normal	Obstruction of pulmonary arteries

pleuritic pain far outweigh any risks, so they should not be allowed to suffer because of excessive reluctance to use a respiratory depressant. Aspirin should be avoided because it interferes with evaluation of progress by means of the temperature chart. Moreover, haphazard use of antipyretics can actually increase the patient's discomfort by subjecting him to intermittent swings in temperature with associated heavy sweats. If antipyretic therapy seems truly necessary, it should be given on a round-the-clock dosage schedule.

Because pneumococcal pneumonia is common in alcoholics, delirium tremens often develops during treatment, requiring additional nursing care, sedation, and fluid replacement. Its manifestations must be distinguished from those of unsuspected meningitis.

Oxygen should be administered to moderately or severely ill patients until improvement begins, preferably by a mask with humidification to avoid desiccation of the mucosae of the upper airways. Intubation and mechanical ventilation may be necessary if respiratory failure develops.

Intravenous fluids should not be given automatically, because some patients with mild disease have no disturbance of fluid balance. Significant fluid and electrolyte depletion should be treated, with the aim of keeping up a good urine flow with specific gravity less than 1.020, and maintaining the serum sodium below 145 mEq per liter. Because the degree of free water depletion caused by fever is usually greater than the degree of salt depletion, half-normal saline or quarter-normal saline plus 5 per cent dextrose will usually provide correct replacement therapy.

If the patient has significant distention and discomfort from ileus or gastrectasia, oral treatment should be avoided and nasogastric suction should be instituted until peristalsis returns. Otherwise, patients may be given clear liquids until improvement begins, after which a light diet can be given when the patient requests it. Because the illness is usually brief, tube feeding or hyperalimentation should not be necessary.

Even though many patients would recover completely without treatment, *antibiotics* reduce mortality, shorten the duration of illness, and prevent development of complications, especially bacteremia and metastatic infections. Therefore all patients should be treated as soon as a clinical diagnosis of pneumococcal pneumonia is made, without waiting for results of cultures.

Penicillin is the drug of choice. The selection of one of several well-tried regimens employing one of the various forms of penicillin (Table 261–3) should be based upon the severity of the illness and the convenience of the patient. Neither oral nor intramuscular therapy should be used for patients in shock. For most patients the course of penicillin need not be prolonged beyond five to seven days.

For patients allergic to the penicillins, a cephalosporin can usually be substituted, because the cross-reaction rate is very low. Care should be taken, however, to administer the first dose in a setting in which an immediate allergic reaction can be treated adequately. For added safety a simple scratch test through a drop of the cephalosporin solution placed on the skin, to look for wheal and flare reaction, may be performed. Patients who cannot tolerate either penicillins or cephalosporins may be treated with erythromycin. This antibiotic is also active against *Mycoplasma pneumoniae.* Therefore, it is particularly useful for patients with mild symptoms who could have either mycoplasmal or pneumococcal pneumonia, and who could be treated as outpatients.

Response to treatment is usually rapid, gratifying both patient and physician. Temperature often falls to normal by crisis within 24 hours, but persistence of fever with resolution by lysis over several days is *not* uncommon and need not be interpreted as treatment failure. Fever recurring or persisting after three days may be due to a focus of extrapulmonary pneumococcal infection that is more resistant to treatment, such as empyema, pericarditis, or arthritis. Other causes of fever during treatment include polymicrobial infection, drug fever, or another underlying disease that was overlooked or misdiagnosed. Failure of the pneumonia to resolve may be due to obstruction of a bronchus by tumor or foreign body, or to infection with more than one organism.

COMPLICATIONS. At least 10 to 20 per cent of patients with pneumococcal pneumonia develop a concomitant *pleural effusion.* The true incidence is considerably higher, but the effusions pass unnoticed because patients are not routinely x-rayed in the lateral decubitus position. Small effusions usually resolve spontaneously after successful treatment, and pleural aspiration is not mandatory. Pleural fluid should be obtained, cultured, and tested for pH, cell count, protein, and lactic dehydrogenase concentration in severely ill patients, in those with large effusions, in those who do not recover smoothly, and whenever empyema is suspected.

Most parapneumonic effusions resolve after treatment, but a few progress to *empyema.* This complication is more likely to

TABLE 261–3. STANDARD ANTIBIOTIC REGIMENS FOR TREATMENT OF PNEUMOCOCCAL PNEUMONIA

For patients with mild symptoms, treated outside hospital	Penicillin V, 500 mg PO four times daily for seven days *or* Erythromycin, 250 mg PO four times daily for seven days*
For inpatients with uncomplicated pneumonia	Crystalline penicillin G, 1.0 million units (600 mg) IV every six hours for five to seven days *or* Procaine penicillin G, 300,000–600,000 units IM every twelve hours for five to seven days
If the patient is allergic to penicillin	Cefazolin, 0.5 gram IM or IV every eight hours for five to seven days
If the patient is allergic to penicillin and cephalosporin	Erythromycin, 250 mg IV every eight hours for five to seven days
For inpatients with pneumonia plus meningitis, pericarditis, arthritis, or endocarditis	Crystalline penicillin G, 3.0–4.0 million units IV every four hours for ten days (meningitis) or two to four weeks (pericarditis, endocarditis)

*If etiology is uncertain, erythromycin is a good first choice because it also treats mycoplasma pneumonia.

develop in untreated cases, or in patients whose treatment was delayed or inadequate. Empyema occurs in less than 5 per cent of adequately treated patients. The clinical distinction between simple effusion and empyema is important, because most empyemas require drainage. Small or moderate effusions noted early in the course of treatment often do not require drainage, even though the fluid has the biochemical characteristics of an exudate and occasionally is infected with pneumococci. Later, if the fluid turns to thick pus composed of fibrin, serum, organisms, and disintegrating leukocytes releasing enzymes and nucleic acids, spontaneous resolution is unlikely to occur. By this time the effusion has evolved into a true empyema; loculations that cannot be drained by simple needle aspiration have usually formed, and secondary bacterial infection with anaerobes or other denizens of the oropharynx may have occurred. Drainage via a chest tube should be instituted. Because a thick, infected exudate often cannot move freely with changes in position, radiographic diagnosis of empyemas can be difficult. Loculated empyemas can be misinterpreted on x-ray as unresolved pneumonia, or tumor. Ultrasonography and needle aspiration can help to make the diagnosis.

The possibility that pneumococcal *meningitis* is present in a patient with pneumonia must be carefully considered (even though this complication is uncommon), because meningitis requires a much higher dosage of penicillin than pneumonia for cure (Table 261–3). If there is any doubt about this issue, a spinal tap should be performed. A small subgroup of patients, usually alcoholics, develop the triad of pneumonia, meningitis, and endocarditis (Austrian's syndrome). These patients are always bacteremic, and their prognosis is very grave; about 80 per cent will die despite treatment. First- or second-generation cephalosporins or erythromycin must not be used in a patient with pneumococcal meningitis; if a patient with this complication is allergic to penicillin, chloramphenicol, 1.0 gram intravenously every six hours, should be added to the treatment regimen. Alternatively, a third-generation cephalosporin that provides good concentrations in cerebrospinal fluid (such as cefotaxime 2.0 gram intravenously every four hours) could be used.

Pneumococcal pericarditis, peritonitis, endocarditis, and arthritis all may occur in association with pneumonia. These conditions are discussed in Ch. 53, 269, and 446, respectively.

PROGNOSIS. The overall case fatality rate for untreated pneumococcal pneumonia is about 25 per cent. This varies widely among subgroups: in young people without pre-existing diseases and without bacteremia, mortality would be only 1 in 20 even without treatment, whereas in bacteremic, elderly patients with chronic heart or lung disease, mortality would be about ten times higher.

Recognized adverse prognostic factors include pneumonia occurring in old age or in infancy; chronic heart, lung, or liver disease; malnutrition; debilitation; bacteremia; positive CIE for polysaccharide in blood; shock, meningitis, endocarditis, or pericarditis; alcoholism or delirium tremens; advanced pregnancy; involvement of more than one lobe; infection with virulent serotypes, e.g., Type 3; leukopenia; jaundice; and delayed treatment.

In the pre-penicillin era, both serotherapy and sulfonamide treatment improved the prognosis significantly. Penicillin further improved these figures, so that overall mortality is now about 5 per cent. However, for those patients with several major adverse prognostic factors, mortality remains higher than 20 to 30 per cent, even with penicillin treatment and modern intensive care.

PREVENTION. Even though the sputum of a patient with pneumococcal pneumonia contains the etiologic organism, there is negligible risk that medical staff and other patients who come in contact with him will "catch pneumonia." Isolation during treatment is therefore not necessary.

Antibiotic treatment given empirically for viral upper respiratory infections undoubtedly prevents or aborts some cases of pneumococcal pneumonia. However, because upper respiratory infections are hundreds of times more common than pneumonia, the cost and risks of treating all of them with antibiotics outweigh the benefit of preventing an occasional case of pneumonia. In young children with absent or hypofunctioning spleens, long-term, low-dose penicillin prophylaxis may be appropriate, but in this setting the primary aim is to prevent fulminant pneumococcal *bacteremia* rather than pneumonia.

The presently available polyvalent pneumococcal vaccine (Pneumovax 23) contains purified polysaccharide antigens derived from the 23 types most commonly recovered from infected patients. These 23 types cause about 90 per cent of pneumococcal infections, and the vaccine is estimated to be about 80 per cent effective. This means that theoretically the vaccine could prevent about two thirds of pneumococcal pneumonias, and possibly some other pneumococcal infections. Not all vaccinated persons will produce protective levels of antibody, and infections caused by types contained in the vaccine have occurred after vaccination. It does not seem to be effective in prevention of pneumococcal otitis. Children less than two years of age should not receive this vaccine, because their antibody response is inadequate. This is unfortunate because among asplenic patients, very young children are at the greatest risk for severe pneumococcal infection.

Present recommendations call for vaccination of high-risk patients over two years old, including those with sickle cell disease; patients with splenic hypofunction or asplenia; the elderly; and patients with chronic cardiac or respiratory disease. Apart from children with asplenia, this is essentially the same population that should receive influenza vaccine.

Because the vaccine consists of purified polysaccharide, there is no risk of inadvertently causing infection if an immunosuppressed patient is vaccinated. Even though such patients' antibody responses are unpredictable, it is reasonable to vaccinate them in the hope that partial protection will result. Side effects are limited to local tenderness. Immunity appears to be long lasting; patients should not be revaccinated in less than five years, lest a more severe local reaction occur.

Austrian R: Random gleanings from a life with the pneumococcus. J Infect Dis 131:474, 484, 1975. *A potpourri of interesting observations on pneumococci, by a true authority.*

Austrian R, Douglas RM, Schiffman G, Coetzee AM, Koornhof HJ, Hayden-Smith, Reid RDW: Prevention of pneumococcal pneumonia by vaccination. Trans Assoc Am Physicians 89:184, 1976. *This paper summarizes the rationale for vaccination against pneumococcal infection and gives the results of initial clinical studies proving efficacy of the currently available vaccine.*

Coonrod JD, Kunz LJ, Ferraro MJ (eds.): Direct Detection of Microorganisms in Clinical Samples. New York, Academic Press, 1983. *The title of this comprehensive volume is self-explanatory. It provides numerous references to detection of pneumococci in body fluids, including notes on counterimmunoelectrophoresis (CIE) and coagglutination.*

Fraser RG, Paré JAP: Diagnosis of Diseases of the Chest. 2nd ed. Philadelphia, W.B. Saunders Company, 1978, pp 689–695. *A standard, authoritative text that sets down the salient radiographic features of pneumococcal pneumonia.*

Heffron R: Pneumonia, with Special Reference to Pneumococcus Lobar Pneumonia. New York, Commonwealth Fund, 1939. *This is a classic description of large numbers of patients studied in the preantibiotic era. Valuable today for its superb detail on clinical findings and the natural history of pneumonia.*

Hook EW, Horton CA, Schaberg DR: Failure of intensive care unit support to influence mortality from pneumococcal bacteremia. JAMA 249:1055, 1983. *This clinical brief shows that even the most intensive modern medical care cannot save 30 to 76 per cent of patients with pneumococcal bacteremia and thus emphasizes the need for vaccines.*

Istre GR, Humphreys JT, Albrecht KD, et al.: Chloramphenicol and penicillin resistance in pneumococci isolated from blood and cerebrospinal fluid: A prevalence study in metropolitan Denver. J Clin Microbiol 17:472, 1983. *A short recent paper with current information on the prevalence of antibiotic resistance among clinical isolates of pneumococci in the United States.*

Jacobs MR, Koornhof HJ, Robins-Browne RM, et al.: Emergence of multiply resistant pneumococci. N Engl J Med 299:735, 1978. *An important report describing the emergence of a large number of strains of antibiotic-resistant pneumococci in South Africa. Emphasizes the potential for worldwide spread of resistant strains, and supports the need for an effective vaccine.*

Jay SJ, Johanson WG Jr, Pierce AK: The radiographic resolution of *Streptococcus pneumoniae* pneumonia. N Engl J Med 293:798, 1975. *This study demonstrates that radiographic changes may persist for several weeks after successful treatment of bacteremic pneumococcal pneumonia. The authors recommend follow-up x-ray not earlier than six weeks after onset for patients who are doing well.*

Lerner AM, Jankauskas K: The classic bacterial pneumonias. Disease-a-Month, February 1975, pp 1–46. *A general description of pneumococcal pneumonia, with additional comments on other bacterial pneumonias.*
Robbins JB, Austrian R, Lee C-J, et al.: Considerations for formulating the second-generation pneumococcal capsular polysaccharide vaccine with emphasis on the cross-reactive types within groups. J Infect Dis 148:1136, 1983. *An extensive review of pneumococcal serotypes, related specifically to human infection and vaccines.*

262. MYCOPLASMAL INFECTIONS

Stephen G. Baum

INTRODUCTION

The most significant human infections caused by mycoplasmas are diseases of the respiratory tract, including pharyngitis, tracheobronchitis, and pneumonia. Recently one species of mycoplasmas, *Mycoplasma hominis*, and a closely related organism, *Ureaplasma*, have been etiologically implicated in some diseases of the human urogenital tract.

The high incidence of mycoplasmal infection is not generally appreciated. Factors responsible for this include lack of familiarity with mycoplasmal syndromes; the absence of specific, rapid tests for diagnosis in the early phases of these diseases; and the relative difficulty of growing the organisms in the diagnostic laboratory.

Accurate etiologic diagnosis of mycoplasmal diseases, however, is of considerable clinical importance. Mycoplasmal infections do not respond to the antimicrobial therapies usually used for respiratory or genital infections but treatment with erythromycins or tetracyclines leads to amelioration of symptoms, decrease in the likelihood of spread, and eventually, true microbiologic cure.

HISTORY. In the late 1930's, a group of pneumonias was delineated that did not resemble typical bacterial lobar pneumonia. Because the cause of the pneumonias was unknown, and because the radiographic appearance and low mortality distinguished these cases from pneumococcal and other bacterial respiratory infections, these were called *primary atypical pneumonias*. A decade later, when sulfa drugs were in use and penicillin was hailed as a cure for all bacterial infections, it was recognized that this group of pneumonias was also atypical in its lack of response to penicillin and sulfa drugs.

In the intervening years, recognition of many new viral, bacterial, rickettsial, and chlamydial organisms has revealed the cause of some of these atypical pneumonias. In the 1950's, the organism responsible for many cases of so-called atypical pneumonia was isolated by Eaton and was shown to be similar to one causing pleuropneumonia in cattle; hence the names Eaton agent and pleuropneumonia-like organisms (PPLO). In 1962, Chanock and co-workers showed that this agent belongs to the family of mycoplasmatacea (then newly described), and so it was reclassified as *Mycoplasma pneumoniae*.

Mycoplasmas are ubiquitous in the animal kingdom. There are about ten species that colonize the respiratory or genital tract of humans. In addition, a related organism, *Ureaplasma urealyticum*, is frequently cultured from the human genital tract. Because of the ubiquity of these agents and the fact that related members of the order Mycoplasmatales infect various animals, the etiologies of a large variety of contagious, neoplastic, and inflammatory syndromes have been ascribed to infection by these organisms. However, only one species of *Mycoplasma*, *M. pneumoniae*, has been unquestionably proved to cause disease in humans.

DESCRIPTION OF THE ORGANISM AND RELATIONSHIP TO PATHOGENESIS. The mycoplasmas, members of the class Mollicutes, represent the smallest free-living forms, i.e., they do not require host cells for replication. For many years the question of whether these organisms were viruses or bacteria was debated. However, it appears that they are neither, and there is no significant deoxyribonucleic acid similarity between mycoplasmas and any known bacterium or virus.

The average diameter of mycoplasmas (125 to 150 nm) is in the size range of large viruses. They have no cell wall but are bounded by a limiting membrane containing lipid. Absence of a cell wall renders them susceptible to lysis by hypotonic solutions but insensitive to cell-wall active antibiotics such as the penicillins. Mycoplasmas and *Ureaplasma* can be grown on agar supplemented with serum proteins and sterols. Most *Mycoplasma* species form 200- to 300-μm colonies, which look much like a fried egg. They have a peripheral halo and a thicker central portion lying just below the surface of the agar. *M. pneumoniae* colonies, however, lack the halo and resemble a mulberry. *Ureaplasma* was previously called "T-strain" *Mycoplasma* because it formed tiny colonies on agar. When *M. pneumoniae* is grown on agar containing mammalian erythrocytes, it rapidly produces a clear zone of hemolysis similar to β-hemolysis of some bacteria. *M. pneumoniae* also differs from many other mycoplasmas in that it grows more slowly, ferments glucose to produce acid, adsorbs red cells to growing colonies, and reduces the dye tetrazolium under aerobic conditions. All of these characteristics have been exploited to establish a rapid microbiologic diagnosis.

When mycoplasmas contaminate tissue culture systems, as they often do, they are found intracellularly. This fact has led to speculation as to the mechanisms of persistence of these organisms in vivo. However, electron microscopic studies using tracheal organ culture systems have demonstrated most of the infecting organisms extracellularly at the base of the cilia of epithelial cells.

Two properties of *M. pneumoniae* seem to correlate extremely well with its pathogenicity in humans. *M. pneumoniae* has a selective affinity for respiratory epithelial cells and produces hydrogen peroxide. The H_2O_2 is thought to be responsible for much of the initial cell disruption in the respiratory tract. H_2O_2 also causes damage to erythrocyte membranes. In the laboratory, this damage results in hemolysis, and, in the patient, may alter erythrocyte antigens, thereby stimulating cold agglutinins. These agglutinins appear in the serum of over 50 per cent of patients who develop mycoplasmal pneumonia and are capable of clumping red blood cells in vitro at 4° C. They are different from cold precipitins or cryoglobulins occurring in other diseases. Cold agglutinins are IgM antibodies directed at the I antigen on the surface of normal erythrocytes. There is increasing evidence that cold agglutinins are antibodies to a glycolipid in the membrane of *M. pneumoniae*, which happens to cross-react with a similar erythrocyte antigen. Cold agglutinins occur rarely in other diseases, including influenza and adenoviral pneumonia.

RESPIRATORY DISEASES CAUSED BY *M. pneumoniae*

DEFINITION. Respiratory infection by *M. pneumoniae* may be asymptomatic or may lead to inflammation of the upper airways (pharyngitis or tracheitis) or lower respiratory tract (bronchitis or pneumonia). In the vast majority of cases, disease is self-limited, but proper antibiotic therapy can shorten the duration of symptoms.

EPIDEMIOLOGY. The monitoring of large populations over prolonged periods has disclosed that each year about one out of every thousand people in the United States will experience mycoplasmal pneumonia. The incidence of all other mycoplasmal upper and lower respiratory infections is probably ten times that of mycoplasmal pneumonia. Studies of selected "closed" populations such as exist in military recruit camps, boarding schools, and colleges have shown that from one quarter to three quarters of all pneumonias occurring in these groups are caused by *M. pneumoniae*.

Mycoplasmal respiratory infection is most common in children and young adults, with a peak incidence in the age range of 5 to 20 years; however, infants and elderly patients are also infected. Distribution is worldwide. Although documented epidemics have occurred primarily in the fall months, this disease does not have the marked seasonal predominance that is found with influenza.

Infection is spread from person to person by respiratory secretions expelled during bouts of coughing. The organism is present in these secretions for several days prior to the onset of symptoms and peaks in titer in the sputum during the first week of clinical illness. Of significance to the spread of this disease is the fact that *M. pneumoniae* organisms persist in the sputum, albeit in reduced numbers, for weeks after the cessation of appropriate antimicrobial therapy.

In open populations under nonepidemic conditions, the infection seems to be spread most easily between playmates and within the household. The index case is usually a child. The majority of households having an index case will experience secondary infections, and the majority of susceptible family members will become infected, with resultant symptomatic disease or asymptomatic seroconversion.

In comparison with viral respiratory disease, the incubation period for mycoplasmal infection is relatively long, averaging two to three weeks. Therefore, unless two or more people from a household are simultaneously infected from an index case, it is unusual for several family members to be ill at the same time, and the disease may take several months to run its course through a household.

CLINICAL PRESENTATIONS. Mycoplasmal infection of the upper airways is impossible to distinguish clinically from infection by other agents. On the other hand, mycoplasmal pneumonia has several characteristics that may help the physician to diagnose this disease (see Fig. 262–1). The onset of mycoplasmal pneumonia is usually insidious in contrast to the abrupt onset of adenoviral or influenzal pneumonia. Mild fever is usually the first sign of infection. The hallmark of the disease is severe, disabling, paroxysmal cough, which usually becomes prominent two or three days after the onset of fever and often requires narcotic medication for suppression. Although usually nonproductive, the cough may yield small amounts of whitish sputum. Occasionally the sputum may contain flecks of blood, but grossly purulent sputum and marked hemoptysis are rare. Production of purulent or bloody sputum is actually more prevalent in tracheobronchitis than in pneumonia.

Headache occurs commonly in conjunction with the cough. During the first week of illness, many patients complain of burning soreness in the chest, though true pleuritic pain is uncommon. Fever rarely exceeds 39.5° C (102 to 103° F), and mild myalgias and malaise occur early in the disease. A history of shaking chills, severe myalgias, or gastrointestinal complaints is unusual.

On physical examination, the pharynx may be slightly injected or inflamed. Much diagnostic emphasis has been placed on the presence of bullous myringitis in patients with mycoplasmal respiratory disease. This finding was noted in less than 25 per cent of volunteers experimentally infected with *M. pneumoniae*, and is very rare in naturally occurring mycoplasmal infection. Bacteria are much more commonly cultured than *M. pneumoniae* from patients with bullous myringitis, and the relationship between *M. pneumoniae* infection and bullous myringitis or otitis remains tenuous.

Examination of the chest usually fails to show signs of dense consolidation or fluid accumulation. Auscultation reveals fine rales either unilaterally or bilaterally, which are often not very impressive. Findings from the remainder of the physical examination are usually normal.

In this regard, the radiographic appearance of the lungs frequently presents a surprise. There is marked patchy infiltration of the lungs consistent with extensive interstitial pneumonia; bilateral involvement is evident in about one quarter of the patients. Infiltration is most prominent at the base of the lungs, although mycoplasmal pneumonia can be seen in any pulmonary segment. There may be slight blunting of the costovertebral angle on the affected side(s) in 10 to 20 per cent of patients, but large pleural effusions are rare. If thoracentesis is performed, it yields a serous or serosanguinous transudative fluid.

COMPLICATIONS. Spread of infection within the lung and pleural effusions are the most common pulmonary complications. Involvement of a number of extrapulmonary sites has been attributed to infection with *M. pneumoniae*, usually occurring as complications of pulmonary disease. Occasionally, they have been seen without pneumonia, and mycoplasmal causation has been substantiated on the basis of culture of the organism from involved organs, four-fold or greater rises in mycoplasma-specific antibodies, or demonstration (described later) of less specific cold hemagglutinins.

Three extrapulmonary complications are relatively common (occurring in 2 to 10 per cent of patients). These deserve comment because, when present, they help to confirm the diagnosis of mycoplasmal pneumonia.

Erythema Multiforme Major (Stevens-Johnson Syndrome). Some patients with mycoplasmal pneumonia develop blistering lesions involving the mouth, eyes, and skin. Usually, although the lesions look quite severe, they heal with minimal scarring. However, when the cornea is involved, blindness may ensue, and local and systemic steroid therapy is often recommended in these instances. This dermatologic syndrome has many causes, including adverse reaction to drugs. When, however, it occurs in conjunction with interstitial pneumonia in a child or young adult, its presence helps confirm the clinical diagnosis of mycoplasmal pneumonia.

The pathogenesis of this syndrome is unknown. There is one report of isolation of *M. pneumoniae* from skin lesions, but most authorities consider Stevens-Johnson syndrome an allergic reaction. A great variety of other skin rashes in mycoplasmal pneumonia has been described, but these are not diagnostically helpful.

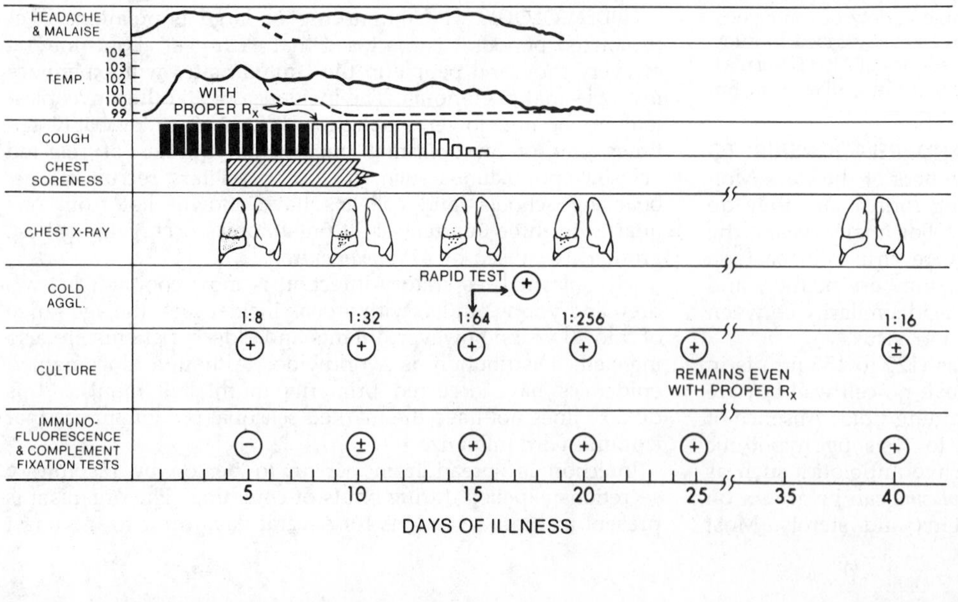

Figure 262–1. Major clinical manifestations of mycoplasmal pneumonia.

Raynaud's Phenomenon. A second syndrome, manifesting itself in the skin of fewer than 5 per cent of mycoplasmal pneumonia patients, is Raynaud's phenomenon. This consists of a painful blanching of the distal parts of fingers and toes that occurs upon exposure to a cold environment. Blanching may occur whether or not the patient has a history of Raynaud's phenomenon unrelated to mycoplasmal infection. There is no experimental evidence on the pathogenesis of this complication in *M. pneumoniae* infection. However, it is tempting to hypothesize that high titers of cold hemagglutinins could play a role by creating minute thrombi in the microcirculation of the distal extremities when exposed to cold. Patients with sickle cell disease may have particularly severe symptoms when they contract mycoplasmal pneumonia. In the presence of extremely high titers of cold agglutinins (1:20,000), gangrene of the distal parts of fingers and toes in these patients has been reported.

Hemolysis. Patients with cold agglutinin titers of greater than 1:500 may experience rapid and severe hemolysis with decreases of 50 per cent in hematocrit. This complication occurs in less than 5 per cent of patients in the second or third week of illness.

LESS COMMON COMPLICATIONS. Among the organ systems reported to be rarely involved in mycoplasmal infection are the cardiovascular, skeletal, and central nervous systems. In a very few cases involving each of these systems, the organism has been cultured directly from the affected organ. However, since mycoplasmal respiratory infection is very common (one per 100 people per year), it is quite possible that in those cases in which *Mycoplasma* was not cultured from the site, the extrapulmonary syndrome was due to a second agent and that two diseases, such as viral aseptic meningitis and mycoplasmal upper respiratory infection, occurred concurrently.

NEUROLOGIC COMPLICATIONS. Aseptic meningitis, meningoencephalitis, cranial nerve neuritis, peripheral neuritis, Guillain-Barré syndrome, transverse myelitis, and psychosis all have been reported as complications of *M. pneumoniae* infection. Most often, etiologic diagnosis is made on the basis of exclusion of other agents and antibody response to *M. pneumoniae*. Spinal fluid cell counts and glucose and protein levels are extremely variable in these cases, ranging from normal to patterns consistent with aseptic meningitis. In some cases, elevated cerebrospinal fluid proteins were found to contain antibodies to *M. pneumoniae*, but these often paralleled serum antibody levels, and it was unclear whether or not cerebrospinal fluid antibody represented diffusion from the serum. There are only two or three reports of isolation of *M. pneumoniae* from cerebrospinal fluid or neural tissue, and the prevailing hypothesis is that mycoplasmal central nervous system disease occurs on the basis of allergic reaction.

Patients with neurologic complications seem to have greater mortality than is commonly associated with mycoplasmal disease. This could signify either a group of patients at markedly increased risk of death from mycoplasmal infection or alternatively, support the hypothesis that these patients had a second (concurrent) undiagnosed disease with greater inherent mortality.

CARDIOVASCULAR COMPLICATIONS. Pericarditis and myocarditis are the most commonly reported cardiovascular complications of mycoplasmal infection. In general, the major criteria of heart disease have been congestive failure and abnormal electrocardiographic results. Large pericardial effusions have not occurred. There have been a few deaths during the acute phase of the disease, but recovery without sequellae is the rule. In most cases documentation of *M. pneumoniae* infection has been made by noting seroconversion. In one retrospective study based on seroconversion, 8 per cent of patients with *M. pneumoniae* infection had evidence of pericarditis or myocarditis. The average age of these patients was 46 years, considerably older than the mean for patients with *M. pneumoniae* infection.

MUSCULOSKELETAL COMPLICATIONS. Arthralgias are common in association with mycoplasmal pneumonia, but frank arthritis is rare. When it does occur, arthritis may continue long after the other manifestations of mycoplasmal infection are gone. Large joints seem to be preferentially affected, and the arthritis may be migratory. *Mycoplasma* has not been cultured from joint fluid of immunocompetent patients.

M. pneumoniae and other mycoplasmas have been implicated as the causative agents of a number of other connective tissue diseases, including rheumatoid arthritis, juvenile rheumatoid arthritis, and Reiter's syndrome. Nonhuman mycoplasmas have been shown to cause arthritis in the animals they infect, and *M. pneumoniae* has been cultured on sevaral occasions from the joints of immunocompromised patients. To date, however, there is no evidence that human mycoplasmas cause joint disease, except perhaps as an acute manifestation of pneumonia.

CLINICAL COURSE. Mycoplasmal respiratory disease is almost invariably self-limited and very rarely results in death. In the absence of treatment, upper respiratory infection usually lasts one to three weeks, and pneumonia may persist from four to six weeks. Recovery is gradual, with clinical improvement preceding roentgenographic clearing. Development of any of the severe cardiovascular, dermatologic, hematologic, or neurologic complications described earlier may prolong resolution. Proper treatment, which is often not begun until other antibiotics have failed, would appear to shorten the duration of symptoms by about half. Results might be even better than this if treatment were begun earlier. Relapse occurs in 5 to 10 per cent of patients. In most cases these patients receive courses of therapy less than two weeks in duration.

Two groups of patients commonly appear to develop severe disease. The first group consists of infants who, until recently, were thought not to be particularly susceptible to *M. pneumoniae* infection. Many infants develop severe respiratory distress requiring intubation and supported respiration. Fortunately, despite severe illness the prognosis for these children is excellent. The second group contains patients with sickle cell disease. In addition to digital gangrene, these patients are prone to develop large multilobar pneumonias and pleural effusions. The possibility of mycoplasmal infection should be considered in a patient with sickle cell crisis and interstitial pneumonia.

PATHOLOGY. Since death is rare in patients with mycoplasmal pneumonia, descriptions of pathologic changes in this disease rest on a very small number of specimens. The tracheobronchial tree and lungs are generally hyperemic. There is evidence of interstitial pneumonia with engorged lungs consistent with the findings on x-ray. Cellular infiltrate, usually minimal, consists mostly of mononuclear elements. Tracheal organ culture systems have been used to demonstrate that infection with *M. pneumoniae* causes a marked decrease of ciliary action, followed by complete loss of cilia and sloughing of epithelial cells.

IMMUNITY. There is a variety of antibody responses to infection with *M. pneumoniae*. It is unclear what role these immune responses play in the pathogenesis of, and recovery from, infection. Secretory IgA antibody is thought to be the most protective immunoglobulin in this disease. Individual immunity may be relatively short-lived, and there are well-documented instances of recurrent disease within two to ten years following primary infection.

DIAGNOSIS. A clinical diagnosis of mycoplasmal pneumonia should be seriously entertained whenever interstitial pneumonia occurs in a young adult. Examination of the Gram-stained sputum is helpful in that it reveals inflammation but no bacterial organisms. The peripheral leukocyte count may be normal or slightly elevated. There is minimal shift toward immature forms, and mild lymphopenia may exist. The diagnosis is substantiated by finding a cold agglutinin titer greater than 1:32 in the serum.

Hospital bacteriology or serology laboratories titrate cold agglutinins in patients' serum using Rh-positive, type O erythrocytes to avoid reactions due to major blood-group isoantibodies present in the patient's serum. However, a simple, rapid bedside procedure for finding cold agglutinins can be performed using only the patient's blood. One milliliter of freshly drawn blood is placed in a tube containing anticoagulant. The tube used for prothrombin determinations is suitable. The tube is chilled on ice for two or three minutes and then gently rotated in a horizontal position. Development of small clumps of erythrocytes, similar to those seen when typing blood, which disappear on warming the tube between the hands, indicates the presence of cold agglutinins. The agglutination-dissociation cycle can be repeated many times with the same blood sample. This differentiates the reaction from direct hemagglutination by viruses—a process that generally cannot be recycled. A positive test result correlates with a cold agglutinin titer of 1:64 or greater. When the cold agglutinin titer is extremely high, an easily dissociable clot may form in the tube. Blood from a patient with an unrelated disease should be used as a control. Cold agglutinins are usually found during the second and third weeks of illness and may peak one month or more after the onset of symptoms.

Diagnosis of mycoplasmal pneumonia should be further supported by finding rising titers of specific antibodies to the *Mycoplasma* organism. These can be measured by complement fixation, inhibition of hemadsorption, or immunofluorescence techniques. In addition, patients with mycoplasmal pneumonia may develop a false-positive test result for syphilis.

Definitive diagnosis of mycoplasmal pneumonia rests, however, on coupling an antibody rise with culturing *M. pneumoniae* from sputum. Although growth on agar may take two to three weeks, rendering results useless for initiating drug therapy, a more rapid (three to four days) presumptive diagnosis can be based on the use of a diphasic medium available in some diagnostic laboratories.

DIFFERENTIAL DIAGNOSIS. The most common respiratory infections mimicking mycoplasmal pneumonia are influenza and adenoviral and legionnaires' disease. These tend to be more fulminant in onset and are associated with more severe systemic symptoms and greater respiratory insufficiency. Patients with legionnaires' disease are likely to be older males with histories of smoking. Often one cannot definitively distinguish between these diseases, and a therapeutic trial with erythromycin (which will also treat *Legionella pneumophila*) may be warranted. Psittacosis and ornithosis (chlamydial diseases) and Q fever (a rickettsial disease) should also be considered in the diagnosis. In such cases, exposure to birds on the one hand and to cattle on the other may prove diagnostically helpful.

THERAPY. Treatment with appropriate antibiotics can terminate symptoms abruptly and usually must be begun on the basis of clinical diagnosis. Penicillins, cephalosporins, and aminoglycosides, such as streptomycin, kanamycin, and gentamicin, have little or no effect against these organisms.

M. pneumoniae is sensitive in vitro and in vivo to erythromycin and to the tetracyclines. These agents appear to be equally effective in diminishing the symptoms of the disease. Because there are fewer adverse effects, especially in children under age ten years, erythromycin is preferred. The dosage for either drug is 250 to 500 mg four times daily for two weeks. Although erythromycin and the tetracyclines are effective in ending symptoms, *M. pneumoniae* can be isolated from the sputum of patients for several weeks after the onset of therapy. The mechanism of persistence is unknown but does not depend on the emergence of drug-resistant organisms.

PREVENTION. The frequency of mycoplasmal infection makes the development of a vaccine an attractive objective. Inactivated vaccines, while producing rises in serum antibody levels, give little protection. This observation has aroused the suspicion that IgA antibodies in nasopharyngeal secretions may have more significance than serum antibodies in preventing the disease.

The possible roles of IgA antibodies and delayed hypersensitivity in combating disease have prompted the trial of intranasally administered vaccines using temperature-sensitive (ts) mutants of *M. pneumoniae*. The rationale was that these mutants would induce a localized nasopharyngeal immune response but would not replicate in the warmer lower respiratory tree and cause disease. The results of initial trials of these vaccines have been variable.

GENITAL INFECTION BY MYCOPLASMA AND UREAPLASMA

INTRODUCTION. One strain of human mycoplasmas, *M. hominis*, and a closely related organism, *Ureaplasma urealyticum*, frequently colonize the male and female genital tracts. During the past decade, there has been increasing interest in discovering the role these organisms might play in causing disease of the genitourinary system.

EPIDEMIOLOGY. *M. hominis* and ureaplasmas can be included in the group of venereally transmitted infectious agents. Infants are colonized during birth, but carriage of the organism is lost during the first year of life. After this, the prevalence of colonization increases with age and sexual experience as it does for other sexually transmitted organisms. At all ages, females seem to be more readily colonized than males, and colonization is found most frequently in patients from lower socioeconomic groups.

CLINICAL PRESENTATIONS. *M. hominis*, *U. urealyticum*, or both organisms have been implicated in nongonococcal urethritis and inflammatory disease of the prostate, vagina, cervix, upper urinary tract, and female pelvic organs. In addition, colonization by one or both of these organisms has been associated with male and female infertility, habitual abortion, and recurrent production of premature and underweight infants.

INFECTION OF THE LOWER URINARY TRACT. Chlamydia are responsible for a large percentage of cases of nongonococcal urethritis (NGU). *U. urealyticum* is probably the cause of many of the remaining cases of NGU. Evidence for this stems from the many patients with NGU from whom ureaplasmas are cultured and from these patients' poor clinical response to treatment with sulfa drugs, to which chlamydia are susceptible and to which *Ureaplasma* is not. *M. hominis* probably does not cause urethritis. This organism has been cultured from men with prostatitis, but its causative role is unclear.

INFECTION OF THE UPPER URINARY TRACT. *M. hominis* has been isolated from the kidneys and ureters of patients with clinical pyelonephritis. Antibody to the organism was detected in serum and urine from some of these patients, providing moderately strong evidence that *M. hominis* causes some cases of pyelonephritis. *U. urealyticum* infection has not been detected in patients with pyelonephritis, but the agent may infrequently play a role in urinary calculus formation. This relationship might be expected from the organism's ability to metabolize urea to ammonia, producing alkaline urine in which calcium is poorly soluble, a trait it shares with some *Proteus* bacteria that are also associated with urinary stone formation.

INFECTION OF THE FEMALE GENITAL TRACT. *M. hominis* probably causes a small proportion of the cases of vaginitis and cervicitis. Infection of the uterus and fallopian tubes with this organism has also been documented. *Ureaplasma* rarely, if ever, causes infection in the female pelvis.

MYCOPLASMAS AND REPRODUCTIVE ABNORMALITIES. *U. urealyticum* has been cultured from the sperm of males with fertility disorders. Treatment to eradicate *Ureaplasma* has resulted in increased motility and number of sperm as well as improved morphology. No evidence has been collected as to improvement in fertility after therapy.

Ureaplasma has also been isolated from internal organs of the products of conception of patients with repeated spontaneous abortions. In addition, in some studies *U. urealyticum* was more often isolated from the genital tracts of women with this syndrome than from control populations. Finally, treatment with tetracycline prior to conception in women with histories of habitual abortion has been reported to increase fetal salvage rate. Unfortunately, few if any of these studies took into account the presence of chlamydia, which might have been responsible for the reproductive disorders.

LOW BIRTH WEIGHT. Prior to the realization that tetracycline is contraindicated in pregnancy, it was shown that tetracycline treatment of mothers who habitually gave birth to underweight fetuses would increase birth weight. In addition, vaginal colonization by ureaplasmas was correlated with decreased birth weight. However, these studies did not take into account the presence or absence of chlamydia.

PUERPERAL INFECTION. *M. hominis* infection and septicemia have been associated with some cases of postpartum fever. This organism has been found in the blood of up to 10 per cent of women with fever after delivery, and antibody response indicating true infection has been noted in many cases.

THERAPY. Mycoplasmas and *Ureaplasma* are all susceptible to the tetracyclines. *U. urealyticum* is sensitive to erythromycin, but *M. hominis* is not. Spectinomycin, an antimicrobial agent used in cases of penicillin-resistant gonococcal disease, appears to be effective against both *M. hominis* and *U. urealyticum*. Since both *U. urealyticum* and *C. trachomatis* are sensitive to tetracycline, it is recommended that patients with NGU be treated with a tetracycline at a dose of 1 to 2 grams daily for one to two weeks. The patient should abstain from sexual intercourse during this period, and sexual partners should be evaluated for therapy.

In addition, tetracycline therapy prior to conception and erythromycin therapy during pregnancy should be considered for couples with recurrent infertility or gestational problems who are shown to harbor *U. urealyticum* in the genitourinary tract.

Episodes of postabortal and puerperal fever are usually self-limited and do not require antimicrobial therapy directed at mycoplasmas. Should such therapy be deemed necessary, tetracycline is the drug of choice.

Couch RB: Mycoplasma disease. *In* Mandell G, Douglas RG, Bennet JE (eds.): Principles and Practice of Infectious Diseases. 2nd ed. New York, John Wiley & Sons, 1984. *An up-to-date chapter dealing with both clinical and microbiologic aspects.*

Roberts DB: The etiology of bullous myringitis and the role of mycoplasmas in ear disease: A review. Pediatrics 65:761, 1980. *A definitive review of several studies indicating no significant relationship between this organism and ear disease.*

Taylor-Robinson D, McCormack WM: The genital mycoplasmas. N Engl J Med 302:1003, 1980; 302:1063, 1980. *A comprehensive two-part article on epidemiology, microbiology, clinical presentation, and therapy.*

263. PNEUMONIA DUE TO KLEBSIELLA

(Friedländer's Pneumonia)

Herbert Y. Reynolds

Within the family of Enterobacteriaceae, three related bacteria—*Klebsiella, Enterobacter,* and *Serratia*—constitute a tribe designated as Klebsielleae. The genus *Klebsiella* consists of four species: *K. pneumoniae,* which accounts for about 95 per cent of the clinical isolates; *K. ozaenae,* which occurs infrequently and is associated with a form of chronic atrophic rhinitis (ozena) and purulent infection of the mucous membrane; *K. rhinoscleromatis,* which is the cause of scleroma, a granulomatous process rarely encountered in the United States, which can involve the respiratory mucosa of the nose, paranasal sinuses, middle ear, and oropharynx; and a close variant of *K. pneumoniae, K. oxytoca.* All of the species are nonmotile lactose fermenters with cellular capsules. On solid culture media, klebsiellae produce large, mucoid colonies reflecting polysaccharide capsular material. Capsular antigens, termed K antigens rather than somatic O antigens, provide one serologic basis for distinguishing *Klebsiella* strains. Bacteriocin production by *Klebsiella* strains is another typing method that seems useful.

Klebsiella pneumoniae may be present in the oropharynx of normal persons, although the prevalence is low (1 to 6 per cent). There is no tendency for contacts to acquire the organism from a carrier, and it is difficult to implant organisms in the pharynx of healthy volunteers. As with a number of other pathogenic bacteria, the prevalence of *Klebsiella* in pharyngeal cultures increases (up to 20 per cent) in hospitalized subjects. The organism is an important cause of nosocomial infection in infants in nurseries and intensive care units. Pulmonary infections most likely arise from inhalation or aspiration of organisms from the oropharynx during circumstances in which the major pulmonary antibacterial defense mechanisms are compromised. For example, classic primary *Klebsiella* pneumonia usually occurs in patients with underlying conditions such as alcoholism, chronic obstructive airways disease (emphysema-bronchitis), or diabetes mellitus. Operationally, infections may be considered as primary if *Klebsiella* organisms are isolated from specimens obtained when the patient first seeks medical aid. The designation "secondary" is then applied to those infections that either represent superinfection of an underlying infection or are opportunistic in origin. The present chapter is concerned with the primary pneumonia. The management of the so-called "secondary" *Klebsiella* bronchopulmonary infections is essentially the same as for any nosocomial pneumonia (see Ch. 264). There are no clinical features that readily distinguish nosocomial *Klebsiella* lung infection from that caused by other aerobic gram-negative bacilli.

In patients with primary pneumonia, males predominate heavily (80 to 90 per cent) and most infections occur in middle-aged and older patients. A common coexisting disease is alcoholism (66 per cent). Both chronic bronchopulmonary disease and, to a lesser extent, diabetes mellitus appear to predispose to *Klebsiella* pneumonia.

PATHOLOGY. The outstanding characteristic of *Klebsiella* pneumonia is its destructiveness; it is a necrotizing pneumonia, leading in many instances to cavitation. In fatal cases lobar involvement most often occurs, but infection may be lobular or may be a combination of both; an upper lobe is most frequently involved. The pleural surface is covered by a fibrinous exudate, and adhesions form early. Empyema is appreciably more frequent than in pneumococcal pneumonia and probably occurs in about one fifth of cases. Microscopically, in the acute stage the alveolar walls are congested. Usually the alveoli are filled with an exudate composed of a mixture of predominantly polymorphonuclear cells. There is abscess formation in association with necrosis of the alveolar walls. Other findings at autopsy may include extrapulmonary sites of dissemination, e.g., pericarditis or meningitis. Evidence of alcoholic hepatitis and alcoholic cirrhosis is common.

CLINICAL MANIFESTATIONS. The onset is usually sudden, associated with cough productive of sputum (90 per cent), pleuritic chest pain (80 per cent), and true rigors (60 per cent). Early prostration is a usual feature. Occasionally the acute onset is preceded by a nondescript upper respiratory infection and cough. Rarely, epigastric pain and vomiting are the initial symptoms. A gray-green, blood-tinged sputum is usual, but it can be a nonputrid, homogeneous, thick mixture of blood and mucus, brick red in color, resembling currant jelly. On examination, the patient appears acutely ill, febrile, dyspneic, and often cyanotic. Tachycardia is present in proportion to the fever. Chest examination usually reveals signs of pulmonary consolidation. There may be loss of lung volume as manifested by decreased size and expansion of the involved hemithorax and diaphragmatic elevation. Auscultation may reveal suppressed breath sounds with few rales, despite evidence of considerable consolidation. Involvement of more than one lobe is frequent (in two thirds of patients), with a predilection for upper lobes.

LABORATORY AND ROENTGENOGRAPHIC FINDINGS. Peripheral leukocyte counts vary from marked leukopenia to leukocytosis, but leukopenia (and neutropenia) is a poor prognostic sign. In one quarter of patients the total leukocyte count may be in the normal range. On sputum culture, other gram-negative bacilli may be isolated in addition to *Klebsiella*. A mixed sputum flora containing other gram-negative bacilli such as *Pseudomonas spp.* is especially common in secondary infections. A pulmonary source is often incriminated in patients with *Klebsiella* bacteremia. This is an unusual association, because in other types of gram-negative bacillary bacteremia the urinary tract usually represents the major primary source, followed by the gastrointestinal tract.

The roentgenographic features are variable and include massive lobar consolidation, lobular involvement, lung abscess formation with either multiple small thin-walled or large abscess cavities, and residual parenchymal fibrosis. Bulging of a fissure, sharp advancing borders of the infiltrates, and abscess formation occur with greater frequency than in other types of pneumonia. The pneumonic infiltrate is relatively dense, but shadows of similar density can be seen with other types of bacterial pneumonia. Bronchopneumonic distribution is less characteristic but can occur, and even bilateral perihilar infiltrates are reported.

COMPLICATIONS. Rapid destruction of pulmonary tissue with suppuration or residual fibrosis occurs in as many as half of the surviving patients. Necrosis may occur within 24 to 48 hours, and abscess formation may be recognized within four days. Less common pulmonary complications include pleural effusion and pneumothorax. Rarely, massive pulmonary gangrene complicates lobar *Klebsiella* pneumonia; surgical removal of the lung tissue may be required to ensure patient survival. In the past, activation of quiescent pulmonary tuberculosis has been reported. It is believed that some of these cases actually represent a slough of localized tuberculous disease by the necrotizing *Klebsiella* pneumonia.

The course of illness is not marked by frequent extrapulmonary manifestations, but they can occur and include pericarditis, meningitis, gastroenteritis, erythematous skin rashes, and nonsuppurative polyarthritis.

PROGNOSIS AND TREATMENT. In the preantimicrobial era, the case mortality of *Klebsiella* pneumonia ranged from 51 to 97 per cent. The use of antimicrobials has markedly decreased mortality, but in some series the mortality remains nearly 50 per cent. In these series there has been a predominance of severely ill, alcoholic patients, although good results have been reported even in this group. Analysis of the mode of death frequently reveals that inadequate removal of tenacious pulmonary secretions was a significant factor. The correlation of bloodstream invasion and fatality is frequently close.

The majority of strains of *Klebsiella* are susceptible in vitro to chloramphenicol, the cephalosporins, and the aminoglycosides. Some of the "second and third generation" cephalosporins (cefoxitin and cefotaxime) and new penicillin antibiotics (piperacillin and mezlocillin) have good activity against *Klebsiella* also; however, clinical experience is still limited for some of these antibiotics in serious infections. The antimicrobial regimen of choice varies according to the gravity of the acute clinical situation and the extent of the underlying problem. Because necrosis of lung tissue can occur so rapidly, it is essential that maximally effective antimicrobial therapy be started immediately. In patients with life-threatening infection, which is at least potentially always the case, a two-drug regimen of intravenous cephalothin and an aminoglycoside (gentamicin) is recommended. After several days of such therapy, if the infection is well under control, the cephalothin may be discontinued. Meticulous measures directed at supportive care—maintenance of clear airways, adequate but not excessive ventilation and oxygenation, adequate fluid and electrolyte replacement, and often control of delirium tremens—are essential.

An emerging problem is the developing resistance of *Klebsiella* to multiple antibiotics, including gentamicin. In such a situation another aminoglycoside should be chosen, and, if possible, drug susceptibility studies should be done. Streptomycin, amikacin, and tobramycin are the principal drugs from among which a choice must be made.

CHRONIC CAVITARY KLEBSIELLA DISEASE

Occasionally chronic cavitary disease of the lung will result from infection with *Klebsiella*. In some cases this chronic disease is a known sequel to a primary pneumonia. In other cases, there is no convincing history of such an acute process and the disease appears to have persisted in subacute or chronic form for many months. Because of the rarity of this form of *Klebsiella* disease, its natural history has not been well characterized. It should be treated initially with the drug-pairing regimen of cephalothin and gentamicin, which can be appropriately modified as improvement occurs. The general treatment should be that for any other lung abscess, including surgical excision in rare cases (see Ch. 63).

Bauernfeind A, Petermuller C, Schneider R: Bacteriocins as tools in analysis of nosocomial *Klebsiella* pneumoniae infections. J Clin Microbiol 14:15, 1981. *Perhaps a simpler method of typing and good for epidemiologic studies.*

Bloomfield AL: The fate of bacteria introduced into the upper air passages. V. The Friedländer bacilli. Bull Johns Hopkins Hosp 31:203, 1920. *A historical account but still pertinent.*

Knight L, Fraser RG, Robson HG: Massive pulmonary gangrene: A severe complication of *Klebsiella* pneumonia. Can Med Assoc J 112:196, 1975. *A rare complication that requires surgical resection.*

Lerner AM: The gram-negative bacillary pneumonias. Disease-a-Month, November 1980, pp 1–56. *Excellent review.*

O'Callaghan RJ, Rousset KM, Harkness NK, Murray ML, Lewis AC, Williams WL: Analysis of increasing antibiotic resistance of *Klebsiella pneumoniae* relative to changes in chemotherapy. J Infect Dis 138:293, 1978. *An all too common problem with many bacteria.*

264. PNEUMONIA CAUSED BY OTHER AEROBIC GRAM-NEGATIVE BACILLI (Pseudomonas, Escherichia coli, and Serratia)

Herbert Y. Reynolds

Bacterial species that belong to the families Enterobacteriaceae and Pseudomonadaceae are considered together because of (1) similarities in the pulmonary infection they produce and (2) common circumstances in which they cause disease. Only a few of the bacteria that are frequently encountered as respiratory pathogens will be discussed individually. Others may be important in special instances, but statistically are less of a problem. Specialized texts on microbial diseases and the periodical literature can supply more detailed information about rare or unusual infections.

The family Enterobacteriaceae is composed of numerous interrelated bacilli, all of which are gram-negative, are nonsporulating, grow on ordinary media, and rapidly ferment glucose. The following genera are included in the family: *Shigella, Escherichia, Salmonella, Arizona, Citrobacter, Edwardsiella, Klebsiella, Enterobacter, Serratia, Proteus, Providencia,* and *Erwinia.* The nonfermenting aerobic gram-negative bacilli are recognized with almost equal frequency. Organisms in this category include *Pseudomonas aeruginosa, P. maltophilia, P. pseudomallei, P. cepacia, P. stutzeri, Acinetobacter lwoffi* (previously *Mima polymorpha*), *Acinetobacter anitratus* (previously *Herellea vaginicola* and *Achromobacter anitratus*), *Alcaligenes spp., Achromobacter spp., Flavobacterium spp., Moraxella spp.,* and *Aeromonas hydrophila.* Infections caused by *Pseudomonas pseudomallei* (melioidosis) are presented in Ch. 290.

Pulmonary infections associated with the small aerobic gram-negative bacilli belonging to the genera *Bordetella, Brucella, Hemophilus,* and *Yersinia,* as well as nonsporulating anaerobic gram-negative bacilli, e.g., *Bacteroides* and *Fusobacterium,* are discussed in the individual chapters dealing with each of these infections. Pneumonia caused by *Klebsiella* is the subject of Ch. 263.

Aerobic gram-negative bacilli are frequently the cause of respiratory infection in two groups of patients: those who develop a superinfection or acquire an infection in the hospital (nosocomial), and those who are immunocompromised. These topics are discussed in detail in Ch. 257 and 258.

NOSOCOMIAL PNEUMONIA—PREDISPOSING FACTORS

Many common aerobic gram-negative bacteria normally inhabit the human gastrointestinal tract, and a significant number of healthy, normal people have oropharyngeal colonization with a small number of these bacteria. Certain species such as *Pseudomonas aeruginosa* can be isolated from various skin sites (hands and axillae) in some instances. Since these bacteria are part of the normal microbial flora, they rarely cause primary infection. However, they are a menace for superinfection or secondary hospital-acquired infections. The magnitude of this infectious disease problem is large in terms of patient morbidity and mortality and financial burden to the health care system. Hospital-acquired infections develop in approximately 5 to 7 per cent of all hospitalized patients, with infections of the urinary tract and surgical wounds still causing most of them. However, lower respiratory tract infections account for 15 to 20 per cent of these infections in medical and surgical patients. Perhaps more disturbing than the frequency of respiratory infections is the poor success generally cited for treatment and control. Serious underlying disease is usually present, and, despite antimicrobial therapy, the case mortality from nosocomial pneumonia may approach 50 per cent, depending somewhat on the specific causative bacterium and the clinical setting of the patient. Because *Klebsiella pneumoniae, Pseudomonas aeruginosa, Serratia spp.*, and, less frequently, other gram-negative rods are the cause of severe, nosocomial respiratory infections in hospitalized and/or immunocompromised patients, some general comments about the enviromental setting and alterations in lung host defenses will be offered before focusing on individual disease entities.

Conditions which lead to nosocomial pneumonia are usually obvious. Susceptible patients invariably have one or a combination of the following: (1) chronic debilitating illness, often requiring prolonged hospitalization; (2) prior therapy with antimicrobial drugs having a broad spectrum; (3) a breach of the airway by tracheostomy or endotracheal tube; and (4) impaired host immunity (cellular and/or humoral) owing to a primary disease or as a consequence of immunosuppressive therapy.

The hospital environment itself is a prime source of opportunistic microorganisms and a good repository for some hardy drug-resistant strains. However, the term "nosocomial," strictly defined as an infection originating in a hospital or as one that is not clinically evident or incubating at the time of hospital admission, may not include all the circumstances inducing it. Other descriptions, such as iatrogenic or autogenic infection and superinfection, are often more appropriate.

Chronic illness and hospitalization per se are associated with some striking changes in patterns of bacterial colonization of the respiratory tract which seem significant. Generally the oropharynx of a normal person is not a very suitable environment for growth of aerobic gram-negative bacteria. Yet colonization develops rapidly in patients admitted to a medical intensive care unit, for example, and occurs in about half of them within a few days of admission. Patients with diabetes mellitus or alcoholism also have an increased carriage of gram-negative bacilli in their oropharynx. Such colonization of the respiratory tract apparently plays a major role in the pathogenesis of nosocomial respiratory infections through aspiration of oropharyngeal secretions which inoculate the airways. Thus, a change in nutritional milieu of the oronasopharynx induced by chronic disease, prior antibiotics, gingival disease, metabolic disease, and many other causes promotes sticking and adherence of certain bacteria to buccal mucosal cells, which may lead to colonization. Moreover, altered mentation, which depresses control of swallowing mechanisms or coughing, compounds the aspiration problem. When pharyngeal and sputum cultures become positive for Enterobacteriaceae or Pseudomonadaceae and other pathogenic bacteria, it is likely that the respiratory tract is also colonized with these microorganisms. Such a finding should alert one to impending respiratory infection. New techniques to assess adherence of bacteria to the patient's buccal mucosa cells or respiratory ciliated cells cultured in vitro may prove important in selecting patients who are susceptible to bacterial colonization. Such susceptible persons might profit from enhanced surveillance or prophylactic use of a topical antimicrobial drug in the oropharynx to prevent colonization with potential pathogens. The future will decide the usefulness of this approach.

The importance of prior antimicrobial therapy as a determinant of oropharyngeal colonization with gram-negative bacilli is not as obvious as might be expected. Some studies which recorded development of colonization in hospitalized patients have failed to find strong evidence that prior or concomitant antimicrobial use was a requisite factor, although such therapy usually increases the occurrence of colonization. On the contrary, in principle, broad-spectrum antimicrobial therapy that reduces a proportion of the normal bacterial flora of the gastrointestinal tract and naso-oropharyngeal area should improve the opportunity for more drug-resistant strains to emerge. Perhaps of greater significance is the emergence of fungal strains in the wake of a bacterial void so that colonization with these opportunistic organisms presages respiratory infection.

An interruption in the continuity of the airway with an endotracheal tube, for example, is often associated with bacterial colonization of the tracheobronchial tree and with recurrent respiratory infections. Important mechanical barriers that guard entry into the lungs are bypassed and microorganisms have direct access. Some aspiration of upper airway secretions often continues despite the inflated cuff around the tube, and the situation can be compounded if ventilatory equipment is attached that may itself contain a source of bacteria and, in fact, forcefully aerosolize them into the airway. In the time since it was demonstrated that contaminated inhalation respiratory equipment could be the source of nosocomial pneumonia, significant improvement has occurred in the general care and handling of this equipment, with the pleasing result that this form of iatrogenic infection is less frequent.

The immunocompromised patient presents a complex array of disordered host defenses, and the lungs are but one organ system at risk for infection. Predisposition to pneumonia with gram-negative bacilli occurs because a number of cellular components in the respiratory tract are vulnerable to the direct effects of various antineoplastic chemotherapy drugs and anti-inflammatory agents, or they may have been depleted because renewal from the bone marrow, for example, is inadequate. (See Lung Host Defenses in Ch. 257.)

Granulocytopenia is the most common abnormality in patients who have ineffective granulocytopoiesis or are receiving cytotoxic chemotherapy. With an inadequate systemic supply of circulating phagocytic cells, a lack of reserve or marginated granulocytes develops in capillary storage areas, such as the lung capillary vasculature. As a result the lower respiratory tract lacks secondary phagocytes that can be attracted to alveolar areas to attack bacteria, and the inflammatory response is diminished.

Although alveolar macrophages do not appear to be as easily depleted as the short-lived polymorphonuclear granulocytes in the immunosuppressed subject, subtle metabolic effects from cytotoxic drugs probably do impair their phagocytic and bactericidal capacity, thereby accounting for the greater susceptibility of the host to respiratory infections. Available evidence indicates that bone marrow–derived circulating monocytes are the precursors of tissue macrophages in the lungs. After the monocyte enters the pulmonary lymphoreticular system, it undergoes further development into a mature phagocytic macrophage which has a life span of months or years. Alveolar macrophages obtained by lung lavage from leukemia patients who have been leukopenic (monocytopenic) for several months are functionally and morphologically normal, despite intensive chemotherapy. Moreover, some human pulmonary macrophages are capable of a slow rate of replication, which suggests that the number of lung macrophages can be maintained in part by local cell proliferation when the usual influx of cells from peripheral blood and from bone marrow is absent.

Lymphoid tissue is extensive along the airways, and its alteration could directly affect the lung's handling of antigenic substances contained in respired air. Certain populations of lymphocytes are sensitive to radiotherapy (T cells) and may be eliminated when various forms of irradiation therapy are given. Cytotoxic drugs such as cyclophosphamide have various effects on both major subpopulations of lymphocytes (B and T cells). Cytotoxic agents, therefore, have the potential for blunting cell-mediated immune responses as well as for impeding the development of immunoglobulin-producing lymphocytes and plasma cells that secrete local secretory antibodies onto respiratory mucosal surfaces. Deficiencies in circulating humoral antibodies also occur in persons who are heavily immunosuppressed.

The consequence of injury to other cell types in the lung, such as surfactant-secreting Type II alveolar epithelial cells, various mucus-producing cells, and ciliated epithelial cells, is largely conjectural, because the deleterious effects of immunosuppressive agents on these cell types have not been established. Yet it seems plausible that drastic regimens of immunosuppressive therapy may impair the function of these cells. The cumulative effects of diminished surfactant production promoting lung atelectasis, altered mucus secretion, and reduced ciliary clearance all could contribute to stasis and accumulation of lung secretions which promote local bacterial growth and subsequent pneumonia.

PNEUMONIA CAUSED BY PSEUDOMONAS

Pseudomonas, which is a distinct genus of bacteria and is not included in the family Enterobacteriaceae, is widespread in the environment and is generally part of the usual bacterial flora of hospitals and intensive care units. *Pseudomonas* organisms are frequently carried on the skin (axillary and anogenital areas) of normal people and transiently may be part of the intestinal flora in a significant number (up to 20 per cent). Almost any alteration in normal health status, such as hospitalization or antimicrobial or immunosuppressive therapy, is associated with increased carriage of *Pseudomonas* organisms.

For this discussion, *Pseudomonas* respiratory infection refers to infection caused by *Pseudomonas aeruginosa*, which is the most important pathogen of the genus. The reader should remember, however, that other *Pseudomonas* species can cause serious infections (*P. pseudomallei* [melioidosis] and P. *mallei* [glanders]). Moreover, other less frequently encountered species are being implicated in human infection. *P. cepacia* has the distinction of being at least one in this group of clinical pathogens that is generally not susceptible to gentamicin, hence making drug susceptibility testing necessary for proper drug selection. Increasingly, this species is becoming a problem for those with cystic fibrosis.

PREDISPOSING FACTORS. *Pseudomonas* rarely produces infection in a normal person but is a frequent cause of sepsis and pneumonia in the abnormal host. It continues, along with *Klebsiella*, to be among the organisms most frequently isolated from patients with nosocomial pneumonia. In the past, chronic lung or heart disease apparently increased susceptibility to *Pseudomonas* pneumonia; now leukopenia (granulocytopenia) and other evidence of immunosuppressive disease or treatment is more common. *Pseudomonas* infection is likely to be an acquired or secondary pneumonia following any one of the predisposing causes already outlined. As a form of primary pneumonia, it is essentially limited to patients who are receiving inhalation therapy that incorporates reservoir nebulization. Following *Pseudomonas* bacteremia, pulmonary complications are well described, consisting of nodular areas of lung infarction with massive bacterial infiltration of arterial and venous walls. Such bacteremia produces a form of necrotizing pneumonia. This presentation may occur in illicit intravenous-drug users who develop *Pseudomonas* tricuspid endocarditis. People with cystic fibrosis (CF) have a special problem with *Pseudomonas*. This organism may not initiate lung infection and tissue destruction in CF, for staphylococci are usually the culprit, but *Pseudomonas* eventually becomes the long-term nemesis. Sputum and lungs of CF subjects are persistently colonized with the organism, which causes frequent episodes of bronchitis and pneumonia. Infection-free intervals become shorter, and multiple courses of parenteral antibiotic therapy are required to control *Pseudomonas* in the lungs. A mucoid, slime-producing strain of *P. aeruginosa* has a peculiar affinity for the CF lung.

PATHOGENESIS AND PATHOLOGY. The ubiquitous *Pseudomonas* organisms seem benign and harmless when they encounter a normal person. For the altered or compromised host, they are invasive and virulent. The bacterium is well equipped with an arsenal of extracellular toxins (exotoxin A), proteolytic enzymes (elastase and collagenase), hemolytic factors (phospholipases), leukocidin, pigments (pyocyanin and fluorescein), and cell wall endotoxin, which variously affect host tissues and inflammatory cells. Also, *Pseudomonas* has a capsular slime coat which may provide added protection. An adequate supply of granulocytes seems to be an important determinant in host resistance to infection. Once pseudomonads become enmeshed in lung tissue, they are difficult to eradicate completely, and colonization or chronic infection may persist.

On microscopic section, the intra-alveolar inflammatory exudate is a mixture of polymorphonuclear leukocytic and mononuclear cells, or the cellular infiltrates may consist predominantly of mononuclear cells admixed with fragmented pyknotic nuclei of necrotic neutrophils. At a later stage, alveolar spaces are filled with a deeply basophilic granular material containing large macrophage-like cells and dense colonies of gram-negative bacilli. In an abscess there is often focal hemorrhage. The dominant microscopic lesion is that of alveolar septal necrosis. In association with these necrotizing lesions, necrosis of arterial walls and secondary thrombosis of vessels have been encountered when the *Pseudomonas* pneumonia is of bacteremic origin or associated with nebulizing therapy equipment. In primary *Pseudomonas* pneumonia, as reported by Tillotson and Lerner (1968), vascular involvement is not a feature. *Pseudomonas cepacia* is also associated with a necrotizing granulomatous pneumonia.

CLINICAL FEATURES. In patients with *Pseudomonas* pneumonia, apprehension, toxicity, confusion, and progressive cyanosis are characteristic; hemoptysis is unusual. Relative bradycardia may occur. Alteration in diurnal temperature patterns, with the peak temperature in early morning, was noted by Tillotson and Lerner. The physical signs over the thorax are those found with any pneumonic process. The development of empyema is common and may occur in 30 to 50 per cent of patients. In CF patients with chronic and recurrent episodes of *Pseudomonas* pneumonia, cough and sputum and chest signs are evident, but they may have only low grade fever and little elevation in white blood cell count. Infection is confined to the respiratory tract, and septicemia or peripheral sites of infection virtually never occur. Roentgenograms reveal bilateral pneumonic infiltrates, usually in the lower lobe, that are often nodular and may undergo necrosis, with abscesses that may be small but are often greater than 1 cm in diameter. A pattern of interstitial infiltration may be seen. With resolution of pneumonia, areas of lung with poor expansion and residual "scarring" may be noted on follow-up chest films.

LABORATORY FINDINGS. The usual laboratory tests such as leukocyte counts are of little help, their results being either normal or moderately increased but most often reflecting the bone marrow status of an underlying disease. Cultures of sputum are of only moderate help, because *Pseudomonas* organisms are frequently present as commensals in patients who are receiving antimicrobial therapy or in those who are critically ill. Distinguishing tissue infection from colonization may be facilitated by a serum antibody response to *Pseudomonas* exotoxin A. Infection and invasive disease may elicit an antibody titer of 1:1000 in patients who are not immunosuppressed. If the situation necessitates establishing with certainty the organism involved, specimens could be collected by transtracheal aspiration or by other methods already suggested. With empyema, thoracentesis with staining and culture of the fluid will help confirm the diagnosis and facilitate the selection of optimal therapy.

PROGNOSIS AND TREATMENT. Prognosis varies with the underlying condition of the patient. Patients with CF often have chronic *Pseudomonas* infection punctuated by acute episodes of pneumonia. Although the infections can be suppressed and controlled for a variable period of time, up to many years, eventually recurrent *Pseudomonas* infections cause considerable morbidity and the demise of the patient. Case mortality rates in the range of 80 per cent are not uncommon in the immunocompromised patient with nosocomial *Pseudomonas* pneumonia, especially if bacteremia develops. However, in recent years, the mortality seems distinctly less and appears to be about 50 per cent. Several important advances have occurred. First, better antimicrobial drugs are available. The use of an aminoglycoside (gentamicin, tobramycin, or netilmicin) and carbenicillin (or ticarcillin) in combination for *Pseudomonas aeruginosa* infections has had a dramatic impact. Tobramycin seems to be the drug of choice for nonresistance strains, and amikacin is best reserved for use when resistance to another aminoglycoside develops. Several new penicillins are available as alternatives to carbenicillin and tricarcillin, if *Pseudomonas* drug resistance is a problem. These are piperacillin, mezlocillin, and azlocillin. They are active against many gram-negative bacilli but are ineffective against beta-lactamase-producing bacteria. Because *Pseudomonas* resistance can develop if one of the penicillin antibiotics is used alone, they are given in combination with an aminoglycoside. One advantage of these new penicillins is their lower sodium content. Several newer "third generation" cephalosporins have activity against *Pseudomonas* strains (cefoperazone, ceftazidin*, and cefulodin*) and may offer additional options for antibiotic selection. However, clinical use of these drugs for serious *Pseudomonas* infections is still rather limited. Undoubtedly, it will be necessary to search for additional antimicrobials in the future to keep ahead of the adaptable *Pseudomonas* strains. Second, medical personnel are much more aware of their role in the transmission of this ubiquitous microorganism, and appropriate changes in patient care techniques have been made. Third, meticulous cleanliness of respiratory ventilation equipment and use of disposable endotracheal or tracheostomy suctioning devices are routine.

Other forms of supportive care are also essential. Because *Pseudomonas* organisms are difficult to clear from infected lung tissue, patients will frequently relapse after drug therapy is discontinued, despite what is considered an adequate course of therapy. Re-treatment is usually necessary and should be done in conjunction with drug susceptibility testing. With successful treatment, *Pseudomonas* may still reappear in the sputum, making it necessary to distinguish between relapse and persistent colonization of the respiratory tract. Changing lung infiltrates and clinical signs help separate the two. Passive antibody administration of anti-*Pseudomonas* gamma globulin or prophylactic immunization of high-risk patients with *Pseudomonas* lipopolysaccharide antigens may become practical in the future. Granulocyte transfusion therapy in appropriate patients is a reasonable possibility.

PNEUMONIA DUE TO OTHER AEROBIC GRAM-NEGATIVE BACILLI (E. coli, Serratia Marcescens, and Proteus spp.)

Many bacterial species other than *Klebsiella pneumoniae* that belong to the families Enterobacteriaceae and Achromobacteraceae may produce pulmonary infection. In addition, in many hospitals other gram-negative organisms such as *Serratia marcescens* are being encountered, especially in hospital-associated secondary pneumonia.

Primary *E. coli* pneumonia tends to be present as a scattered pneumonic process in the lower lobes. Empyema formation is less common than with *Klebsiella* or *Pseudomonas*. *E. coli* bacteremia from a urinary or gastrointestinal source results in lung infection more commonly than does bacteremia from other gram-negative bacilli.

Proteus species also produce a clinical picture similar to that of *Klebsiella* (see Ch. 263), with fever, chills, dyspnea, pleuritic chest pain, and cough productive of purulent sputum. Signs of consolidation are usual. Roentgenograms reveal dense infiltrates in the posterior segment of an upper lobe or superior segment of the right lower lobe. Progression to lung abscess or empyema is common.

Serratia infections, which are always secondary, have been associated with "pseudohemoptysis" resulting from a red pigment produced by some strains of *Serratia marcescens*. Other features may include abscess formation, empyema, or both.

Clinical experience with the other bacterial genera such as *Flavobacterium* and *Acinetobacter* is limited, but suggests that their clinical manifestations are similar to those of secondary *Klebsiella* infections.

The antimicrobial regimen of choice may be selected according to the physician's knowledge of the epidemiologic pattern of drug resistance to be anticipated in a given community, but should be confirmed, when possible, by tests on an individual patient's organism.

Doggett RG (ed.): *Pseudomonas aeruginosa*—Clinical Manifestations of Infection and Current Therapy. New York, Academic Press, 1979. *A fine book with experienced authors covering all important features of* Pseudomonas *disease.*

Fick RB, Reynolds HY: *Pseudomonas* respiratory infection in cystic fibrosis: A possible defect in opsonic IgG antibody. Bull Eur Physiopathol Resp 19:151, 1983. *More details about mechanisms of infection in these patients.*

Gilardi GL: Infrequently encountered *Pseudomonas* species causing infection in humans. Ann Intern Med 77:211, 1972. *Emphasizes that other* Pseudomonas *organisms can be pathogenic.*

Higushi JH, Johanson WG: Colonization and bronchopulmonary infection. Clin Chest Med January 1982, p 133. *By authors who have spearheaded this clinical association.*

Jonas M, Cunha BA: Bacteremic *Escherichia coli* pneumonia. Arch Intern Med 142:2157, 1982. *Still a virulent infection and perhaps overlooked among the other gram-negative pneumonias.*

LaForce FM: Hospital-acquired gram negative rod pneumonias: An overview. Am J Med 70:664, 1981. *A good update.*

Pierce AK, Sanford JP: Aerobic gram-negative bacillary pneumonias: State of the art. Am Rev Respir Dis 110:647, 1974. *Still a good review.*

Pollack M, Longfield RN, Karney WW: Clinical significance of serum antibody responses to exotoxin A and type-specific lipopolysaccharides in patients with *Pseudomonas aeruginosa* infections. Am J Med 74:980, 1983. *A new laboratory parameter that seems helpful.*

Reynolds HY, Fick RB Jr.: *Pseudomonas aeruginosa* pulmonary infections (emphasizing nosocomial pneumonia and respiratory infections in cystic fibrosis). In Sabath LD (ed.): *Pseudomonas aeruginosa*—the Organism, Diseases It Causes and Their Treatment. Bern, Hans Humber, 1980, pp 71–88. *This reference complements the present chapter. Of more importance is the book itself, which is another excellent volume on most facets of the bacterium.*

Reynolds HY, Levine AS, Wood RE, Zierdt CH, Dale DC, Pennington JE: *Pseudomonas aeruginosa* infections: Persisting problems and current research to find new therapies. Ann Intern Med 82:819, 1975. *Most helpful on the immunocompromised patient. Reviews approaches to immunotherapy.*

Tillotson JR, Lerner AM: Characteristics of pneumonias caused by *Escherichia coli*. N Engl J Med 277:115, 1967. *Best description of this infection.*

Tillotson JR, Lerner AM: Characteristics of nonbacteremia *Pseudomonas* pneumonia. Ann Intern Med 68:295, 1968. *The classic clinical description.*

265. ASPIRATION PNEUMONIA

Herbert Y. Reynolds

Pneumonitis is an important host response of the respiratory tract to a variety of substances, liquid and particulate, that can be inhaled into the airways. The nature of the inciting material dictates the degree of inflammation and the extent of its effect on the lungs. These materials can be divided for convenience

*Investigational drugs in U.S.A.

into (1) inert, nontoxic substances; (2) acid gastric contents; (3) fluid admixed with food particles, which can cause mechanical obstruction to airways; and (4) oropharyngeal secretions laden with bacteria. A variety of liquids, if breathed into the lungs, cause acute pulmonary edema, including fresh and sea water (near-drowning), acid gastric juice, and halogenated aromatic hydrocarbons. Also, innumerable chemical agents inhaled as fumes or vapors cause irritation, edema, bronchorrhea, and varying degrees of alveolitis or bronchitis (see Ch. 560). Aspiration of solid foreign bodies, which usually occurs in children or in those suffering maxillofacial trauma, may be suspected if acute coughing or wheezing develops. Often the only residual clue is radiographic evidence of a persisting infiltrate or a localized area of lung collapse or of overinflation, suggesting endobronchial obstruction. Thus, there are many causes and kinds of inocula that produce a pulmonary inhalation syndrome of dyspnea, cough, airway irritation, alveolitis, pulmonary edema, and, frequently, infection. Lung infection and abscess are such frequent concomitants that their control is an important part of therapy and management (see Ch. 281).

PATHOGENESIS. With normal swallowing the tongue rises against the hard palate to propel a bolus into the pharynx, and aspiration is prevented by closure of the soft palate, glottis, and epiglottis. However, aspiration of small amounts of pharyngeal fluid is a normal occurrence, especially during deep sleep. Yet the saliva and nasal drainage, admixed with normal bacterial flora of the nose and mouth, which trickle into the trachea and bronchi incite no reaction or symptoms; presumably normal mucociliary clearance removes the secretions and microorganisms. In the absence of gastric regurgitation, which might add acid to the oral secretions, the pH of oropharyngeal fluid is neutral, and this fact may minimize irritation.

The normal microbial flora of the oral cavity is complex, and each anatomic site—mucous membranes, tooth surfaces, and gingival crevices—has elements of an individual flora. Anaerobic bacteria predominate over aerobic ones in a ten-fold ratio and the microbiota is diverse. Anaerobes isolated from the gingiva include *Bacteroides oralis, B. melaninogenicus, Fusobacterium,* and other spirochetal forms. *Streptococcus mutans* and *S. sanguis* are found on tooth surfaces and in dental plaque, whereas the tongue and buccal surfaces contain many forms of aerobic gram-positive and gram-negative bacteria such as *Streptococcus viridans, Neisseria catarrhalis,* enterococci, *S. pneumoniae, Staphylococcus aureus,* and *Hemophilus spp.* Furthermore, *Candida spp.* and certain known pathogens, such as *S. pyogenes* and *N. meningitidis,* presumably as part of a carrier state, can be recovered in asymptomatic people. Enterobacteriaceae are rare, but their carriage increases tremendously with hospitalization and serious illness. Why aspiration syndromes are particularly associated with indigenous, saprophytic, noninvasive anaerobic strains of bacteria is not completely understood. Concomitant lung tissue necrosis, presence of poorly vascularized lung or malignant tissue, plentiful facultative bacterial growth in existing bronchiectatic airways, or poor dental hygiene with an unusually large number of anaerobic bacteria in the gum tissue, coupled with malnutrition, immunosuppressive therapy, diabetes, or alcoholism, all may variously combine to make the host more susceptible to local lung growth of these organisms. Mixed infections with a variety of anaerobic and aerobic bacteria are common.

The aspiration of gastric acid secretions with low pH (<2.5) is usually thought to be an important cause of aspiration injury. Originally this entity defined the aspiration syndrome. Mendelson noted that obstetric patients who aspirated liquid gastric contents (40 of the 66 patients were so classified) developed an asthma-like syndrome which also included cyanosis, rales, rhonchi, and occasionally pulmonary edema. This developed acutely but resolved quickly (in 36 hours) with an uncomplicated recovery in 75 per cent and no mortality. This clinical sequence is less severe than the fulminant, life-threatening disease that acid aspiration produces in animal models and in nonobstetric patients, which is characterized by widespread, rapid damage from a chemical burn of the airways and alveoli. Acute pulmonary edema, hemorrhage, and degeneration of the alveolar epithelial surface occur, accompanied by necrosis of Type I pneumocytes; a few hours later, the pulmonary transudate has been replaced by an infiltration of polymorphonuclear granulocytes and deposition of fibrin in alveoli. Alveolar epithelial permeability for albumin and larger-sized molecules ($>170{,}000$ MW) is increased, so that many plasma components cross the blood-air barrier. Affected lung tissue evolves through an edematous, hemorrhagic, consolidated phase in which hyaline membranes are present if the patient or animal survives. Resolution features regeneration of bronchial epithelium, fibroblast proliferation, and resorbing inflammation. The clinical parallel of these changes is the adult respiratory distress syndrome, in which treatment is directed toward improving oxygenation in noncompliant, atelectatic lungs with poor ventilation and perfusion match-up.

What has been described is a catastrophic disease of extreme seriousness, yet the presentation usually encountered is far less severe. The animal model results from instillation of 1 to 5 ml per kilogram of dilute acid into the experimental lung. In most clinical situations, less toxic fluids or secretions are aspirated and usually in smaller quantities.

Blood may accumulate in the lung if aspiration follows hematemesis or hemoptysis; chest trauma with lung contusion is also a common source of blood in the airways. Blood may cause acute local airway obstruction and may result in areas of atelectasis and lung infiltration. The residual blood itself is eventually well handled in the lungs. Although it may cause consolidation, it incites only a moderate inflammatory response and no necrosis of lung tissue. Alveolar macrophages ingest red blood cells and degrade them within a few days; hemosiderin-laden macrophages eventually can be found in sputum. However, repeated bleeding in an area of the lung can result in chronic inflammatory changes and interstitial fibrosis.

Of more pertinence to injury mechanisms that result from aspiration are the effects of nonacid (pH >2.5) liquid containing small, nonobstructing particles of food. This combination may be the most prevalent in hospitalized patients who are being fed through nasogastric tubes, or who have endotracheal tubes or tracheostomies. Similar circumstances may pertain to patients with neurologic disabilities, esophageal motor dysfunction, or a tracheoesophageal fistula. Repeated aspirations of small quantities of regurgitated liquid and foodstuff plus inhalation of oronasopharyngeal secretions during sleep may result in frequent and chronic insults to the airways. Although periodic bouts of fever and pneumonitis occur and chest radiographs often show infiltrates or residual scarring, it is often surprising how well this type of repeated aspiration is tolerated. Neutral, nonacid, clear, inert liquids incite little inflammatory response in the lungs; however, formula feeding, dairy products, and creamy liquids or soups cause more reaction. The size of the particles, their chemical composition, and the ease with which they disintegrate or undergo phagocytosis and biodegradation determine the degree of local inflammatory response. Hemorrhagic pneumonia and a parenchymal granulomatous response can occur from these kinds of insult. Concomitant bacterial infection does not seem to be a uniform complication, but excluding it can be difficult. A chemical alveolitis can produce the same physical and roentgenographic signs as bacterial pneumonitis. Infectious complications and lung abscess are more frequent in inebriated patients and those with depressed consciousness.

CLINICAL PRESENTATION. Aspiration syndromes constitute a spectrum ranging from tracheal obstruction from a bolus of meat to bronchial obstruction from a peanut or tooth, to inhalation of vomitus or blood during an emergency intubation procedure, to aspiration of fluids leaking around an endotracheal tube with development of a localized lung infiltrate. The overt and acute situations present no problem in diagnosis, but do require prompt action to remove an obstruction or suction out the airways, to control dyspnea and cough, and to correct hypoxia. Following apparent aspiration of acid gastric contents containing partially digested food particles, a brief latent period (up to one or two hours) may occur before clinical signs of respiratory distress develop. Often the patient has a disturbance of consciousness resulting from a sedative drug or general anesthesia. Tachypnea, fever (up to 39° C), diffuse rales, and hypoxemia develop in 70 to 90 per cent of patients, whereas cough, wheezing, cyanosis, and apnea occur in about one third. In the setting of aspirated gastric contents, lung infection develops in about 25 per cent of patients and becomes evident in three to five days. Apnea and shock are ominous signs that are likely to be associated with a fatal outcome. The adult respiratory distress syndrome frequently develops.

Inapparent or subtle forms of aspiration are often difficult to detect and troublesome to manage because of uncertainty about the diagnosis or because the condition cannot be easily remedied. The process may be recurrent and chronic. Persons who have lost consciousness from drug overdoses, inebriation, generalized seizures, or neurovascular injury are often assumed to have aspirated stomach or oropharyngeal fluid, although actual evidence of foreign material in the throat or trachea may be lacking. If pneumonia develops and an infiltrate is visible on radiograph, aspiration is a reasonable assumption, provided that a specific primary infection can be excluded. Following cardiopulmonary resuscitation or emergency intubation, patients may inhale fluid or blood, and subsequent pneumonitis is reasonably ascribed to aspiration. Once a patient is intubated or has a tracheostomy in place, the danger of aspiration is not over. A bit of red-colored gelatin appearing in the endotracheal suctioning catheter is a vivid indication that the patient is aspirating around an endotracheal tube. If a few drops of Evans blue dye are placed on the tongue of an intubated patient and dye is obtained by suctioning through the endotracheal tube, aspiration is proved. Such leakage of dye into the trachea will occur in about 20 per cent of patients who are intubated with a high volume, low pressure cuffed tube. Such a balloon cuff marks a technologic improvement over the low volume, high pressure cuffed tubes in standard use until a few years ago. With the stiffer, smaller balloon tube, the incidence of pericuff aspiration of blue dye was about 56 per cent. The incidence of aspiration in patients with tracheostomies has been reduced from about 80 per cent to 15 per cent by use of large volume, low pressure cuffs.

Other factors that contribute to potential aspiration in the hospitalized patient are presence of a nasogastric tube, supine position in bed, cloudy mental status, and inadequacy of cough reflex. Nasogastric tubes have been associated with aspiration. Imprecise gastric placement and poor mechanical suction or drainage may allow fluid to accumulate; the nasogastric tube passes through both upper and lower esophageal sphincters, making them incompetent and thus providing an easy route for liquid to travel. A greater risk may be posed by a small bore "pediatric" tube inserted through the nose and esophagus for intragastric feeding with liquid formula and hypertonic fluids. With this small tube it is impossible to evacuate the stomach of residual liquid prior to the next feeding. If gastric emptying is delayed and feeding is overly zealous, gastric overflow and regurgitation may occur. Careful regulation of the amount of feeding can obviate this complication. Other factors listed can be controlled by conscientious nursing care, which protects the patient until normal reflexes to cough and to swallow return.

Problems of chronic aspiration usually have a well-defined cause related to failure of mechanical closure of the airway during swallowing or to esophageal dysphagia. Neurologic sequelae affecting striated muscles of the pharynx (bulbar palsy), laryngectomy for cancer, and a variety of esophageal diseases are common causes. Overflow regurgitation of accumulated food and fluid occur with hypopharyngeal (Zenker's) diverticulum and functional esophageal obstruction (achalasia), so that aspiration pneumonia is a common complication. The esophagus is often affected in progressive systemic sclerosis, and difficult swallowing enhances the risk of aspiration. Occasionally, tumor, chest trauma, or irradiation therapy may create a complicating tracheoesophageal fistula through which swallowed fluid and small pieces of food are directly inhaled into the airways; persistent pneumonia and lung abscess usually develop.

LABORATORY AND RADIOGRAPHIC FINDINGS. Normal oropharyngeal fluids, including saliva and tracheobronchial secretions, have a neutral pH and a low glucose content (<5 mg per deciliter). With overt aspiration of acid stomach fluid, it may be possible transiently to record a low pH in fluid recovered from the airways, but the fluid is quickly buffered by plasma components and may be neutral. Recovery of food particles in suctioned airway fluid is prima facie evidence of aspiration. Because the glucose content is normally low in airway fluid, aspiration of oral feeding formulas can significantly elevate the glucose level (>25 to 90 mg per deciliter) in tracheobronchial secretions. As with most pneumonias, the peripheral white blood cell count is usually elevated.

Sputum analysis is essential, but microbial cultures can be confusing. The patient may complain of a foul taste to the sputum; it may smell putrid and contain some blood as well. A sputum Gram stain may not show a predominant organism but rather may contain a mixture of gram-positive and gram-negative flora and inflammatory cells. Failure to isolate an aerobic bacterial pathogen on culture should make one consider anaerobic organisms. Pending the patient's initial response to empiric antibiotic therapy, suitable culture specimens obtained by transtracheal aspirate or direct needle puncture must be considered. Expectorated sputum is of no value for anaerobic cultures because of contamination by normal mouth flora. If pleural fluid is present, a thoracentesis is indicated. If an abscess is present and bronchoscopy has been performed, anaerobic cultures should be made from the irrigation fluid, but the results can be confusing owing to contamination with mouth flora.

The bacteriology from 70 prospective cases of suspected aspiration in 38 community-acquired and 32 hospital-acquired infections (cultures obtained from blood, pleural fluid, or transtracheal aspiration) has provided some important information: Mixed bacteriologic infections (anaerobic and aerobic) were found in 26 per cent of the former compared with almost 60 per cent of the latter. Aerobic infections only were highest in the hospitalized patients (19 per cent versus 8 per cent). The high incidence of aerobic organisms probably reflects the frequency of aerobic gram-negative bacilli in the oropharynx of many chronically ill, hospitalized patients. Infection with anaerobes alone occurred in 66 per cent of the community-acquired aspirations but in only 22 per cent of hospital cases. The most frequent anaerobic isolates were *Bacteroides melaninogenicus*, peptostreptococcus, *Fusobacterium nucleatum*, peptococcus, and *B. fragilis;* of aerobic bacteria the most frequent were *Streptococcus pneumoniae*, *Staphylococcus aureus*, *Klebsiella spp.*, *Pseudomonas aeruginosa*, and *E. coli.*

On the chest radiograph, certain locations of a lung infiltrate have special importance in confirming or alerting the physician to the diagnosis of aspiration pneumonitis. In a recumbent, supine position, posterior segments of the upper lobes or the superior segments of the lower lobes may be dependent; in the upright position, basal segments of the lower lobes are susceptible. With acid aspiration, multiple lobes can be involved and the entire lung fields can show evidence of infiltration and alveolar filling if widespread pulmonary edema and the adult respiratory distress syndrome ensue.

If aspiration is complicated by an anaerobic lung infection, the initial localized pneumonitis may be subpleural and may spread to adjacent segments of lung or into the pleural space. As liquefaction and necrosis occur, the center of the pneumonia becomes a thin wall abscess, resulting in a cavity; if bronchial drainage develops, there will be an air-fluid level. Radiographically, one to two weeks is required for this sequence to occur. The picture of the abscess is not specific, and similar findings can occur with fungal and tuberculous infections, with aerobic bacterial infections, and occasionally from cavitating carcinoma. In these instances, the abscess tends to have a thicker, irregular, or shaggy wall.

THERAPY AND MANAGEMENT. Because pulmonary aspiration of gastric contents poses a hazard in emergency surgical patients and obstetric patients, attempts have been made to decrease gastric acidity with an H_2-receptor histamine antagonist, such as cimetidine or ranitidine. Such prophylactic therapy will increase pH signficantly and reduce gastric fluid volume in many (80 per cent) but not all patients, so its effects must be monitored.

Massive aspiration of blood or vomitus, especially with acid liquid, is an emergency. Debris must be cleared from the throat and airways, a patent airway established with an endotracheal tube, and adequate oxygenation provided. The situation may not stabilize, and intravenous fluid therapy for shock, plus assisted mechanical ventilation with use of end-expiratory pressure and high inspired concentrations of oxygen, may be needed. The use of corticosteroid therapy in this acute situation to minimize the chemical inflammatory reaction in lung parenchyma remains controversial. With experimental acid instillation into the lung, corticosteroid action lessens the impact of injury, provided that the drug is given prior to the injury. Delayed treatment is less helpful. In the clinical situation the drug can only be given after the initiating insult. However, administration of a high dose of intravenous corticosteroid as part of the immediate therapy will not likely cause complications and might contribute positively. Such therapy should not be continued for more than 24 hours after the insult was perceived to have occurred. Use of antibiotic therapy is likewise confusing. Bacterial pneumonia may follow acid aspiration in 25 to 45 per cent of cases, typically during the first week when the patient may be recovering from chemical pneumonitis. With the initial aspirating insult, oral bacteria undoubtedly inoculate the airways, so it might seem logical to eliminate them straightaway with early antibiotic therapy. Unfortunately, prophylactic antibiotic therapy does not seem to prevent pneumonia or favorably influence mortality. Thus, the prudent course may be to withhold antibiotic therapy but *carefully* observe the patient for evidence that bacterial infection has supervened. A new fever spike, progressive chest infiltrates, purulent sputum, or cultures showing pathogenic bacteria would dictate the addition of antibiotics. Similarly, with aspiration of inert, nontoxic fluids, bacterial infection may not invariably follow, so withholding antibiotics is recommended unless a clear indication for their use develops. This approach may suffice as well for patients who regurgitate liquid food feedings or who are noted to aspirate around cuffed endotracheal tubes. Nursing care directed toward evacuating residual gastric contents before refeeding, maintaining an upright position during eating, encouraging progressive ambulation, and improving pulmonary status to hasten extubation is the preferred course.

Aspiration of oropharyngeal secretions in patients with depressed levels of consciousness in whom dental and gingival hygiene are poor may lead to a necrotizing pneumonia, lung abscess, or empyema. Infection with a variety of anaerobic bacteria is a certainty; if the patient has been hospitalized or is chronically ill, concomitant infection with aerobic bacteria is likely. Antibiotic therapy is directed initially at the anaerobes, for which intermittent, high dose parenteral penicillin G is usually sufficient. An alternative choice is clindamycin, particularly if penicillin allergy is of concern. If aerobic bacterial coverage is deemed reasonable, inclusion of an aminoglycoside and an antistaphylococcal antibiotic is indicated. In this situation a combination such as gentamicin and clindamycin or the equivalent is good. In addition, vigorous maneuvers to promote pulmonary drainage of secretions (chest wall clapping and postural drainage) are advocated. Drainage of pleural fluid is often necessary.

Usually, a pulmonary abscess will eventually close with appropriate therapy, although some weeks may be required for this to happen. Antibiotic therapy is indicated until healing occurs, and a course of three to four weeks, or possibly several months, is often needed, rather than the customary ten to fourteen days of treatment suggested for routine pneumonias. Closure of the abscess cavity should be followed radiographically; if resolution does not occur, additional diagnostic evaluation is indicated, including sputum for cytology and fiberoptic bronchoscopy. Pulmonary carcinoma can be present in such an abscess area.

With chronic aspiration syndromes often not much can be offered, and in some instances radical procedures must be contemplated. For those with esophageal disorders care with eating and mechanical dilation of obstruction to promote better emptying and flow-through of ingested food may suffice. Occasionally to remedy defects in laryngeal closure, an arytenoid-epiglottic flap is reconstructed; oversewing the larynx necessitates a tracheostomy, prevents speech, and is a drastic solution. Such patients may have persistent areas of lung infiltration on chest radiograph which change or wax and wane in appearance. Continuous low grade fever may occur. The response is a low grade reactive pneumonitis which is not attended by many systemic symptoms or overwhelming infection. Antibiotic therapy is not indicated continuously and should be reserved for well-defined episodes.

Andrews AD, Brock JG, Downing JW: Protection against pulmonary acid aspiration with ranitidine. A new histamine H_2 antagonist. Anaesthesia 37:22, 1982. *Other similar articles, including those on the use of cimetidine, should be reviewed for timing of doses and expected results.*

Bartlett JG: The triple threat of aspiration pneumonia. Chest 68:560, 1975. *A nice review with helpful classification of aspiration syndromes.*

Bartlett JG: Aspiration pneumonia. Clin Notes Respir Dis 18:3, 1980. *Update of the preceding entry with pertinent references.*

Bynum LJ, Pierce AK: Pulmonary aspiration of gastric contents. Am Rev Respir Dis 111:1129, 1976. *Good clinical review focusing only on the problem of aspirating gastric contents.*

Huxley EJ, Viroslav J, Gray WR, Pierce AK: Pharyngeal aspiration in normal adults and patients with depressed consciousness. Am J Med 65:564, 1978. *Evidence seems conclusive that normal people can aspirate during sleep.*

Lorber B, Swenson RM: Bacteriology of aspiration pneumonia. A prospective study of community and hospitalized cases. Ann Intern Med 81:329, 1974. *Complements the Bartlett references and adds details about the etiology of infection in this disease.*

Mendelson CL: The aspiration of stomach contents into the lungs during obstetric anesthesia. Am J Obstet Gynecol 52:191, 1946. *The classic description, yet this disease in pregnant patients differs in severity from that in other patients who aspirate stomach acid secretions.*

Spray SB, Zuidema GD, Cameron JL: Aspiration pneumonia—incidence of aspiration with endotracheal tubes. Am J Surg 131:701, 1976. *A common problem that has been alleviated somewhat with the new endotracheal design of a high volume, low pressure cuff.*

Winterbauer R, Durning R Jr., Baron E, McFadden M: Aspirated nasogastric feeding solution detected by glucose strips. Ann Intern Med 95:67, 1981. *Interesting approach to diagnosis.*

Wynne JW, Modell JH: Respiratory aspiration of stomach contents. Ann Intern Med 87:466, 1977. *A thorough review with detailed discussion of therapy.*

266. LEGIONELLOSIS

David W. Fraser

DEFINITION. Legionellosis refers to acute bacterial infections of humans caused by *Legionella pneumophila, L. micdadei, L. bozemanii, L. dumoffii, L. gormanii, L. longbeachae, L. jordanis, L. oakridgensis, L. wadsworthii, L. feeleii,* or *L. morrisii.* As several additional species have been identified but not yet named, the list can be expected to lengthen. Infections caused by *Legionella spp.* have occurred in two distinct forms: legionnaires' disease, which is characterized by pneumonia, involvement of other organ systems, and (at least for *L. pneumophila*) a two- to ten-day incubation period; and Pontiac fever, which is characterized by fever without pneumonia or involvement of other organ systems and an incubation period of 5 to 66 hours.

ETIOLOGY. Members of the genus *Legionella* are aerobic, weakly staining, gram-negative bacilli that will not grow on most commonly used bacteriologic media but will grow on media containing supplementary L-cysteine, ferric salts, and activated charcoal. Growth is best at 35° C, but colonies may take up to 12 days to appear on primary culture, especially if the inocula are small. They do not form spores but contain vacuoles that stain with Sudan black B. Many strains are flagellated. In tissue, *L. micdadei* is partially acid fast if the Kinyoun modification is used. In all species, 60 per cent or more of cellular fatty acids have branched chains. They are catalase-positive but do not ferment sugars. *Legionella* species can be distinguished most readily by direct immunofluorescence but phenotypic differences are seen in regard to the presence and color of colonial autofluorescence in ultraviolet light, the pattern of fatty acids in gas liquid chromatography, browning of yeast extract agar medium supplemented with L-tyrosine, ability to hydrolyze hippurate, and gelatinase and oxidase activity. Nine serogroups of *L. pneumophila* and two of *L. longbeachae* have been identified that can be distinguished by direct immunofluorescence or slide agglutination. In addition, antigens are shared among the six serogroups of *L. pneumophila,* the species of Legionellae, and other genera of gram-negative bacilli. Legionellae are found in a wide variety of watery environments. *L. pneumophila* can survive more than one year in tap water. The means by which these fastidious bacteria survive so well in water has not been established, but the presence of algae, amebae, and other bacteria may be important. Apparent variations in the virulence of strains of *L. pneumophila* have been related to the presence or absence of plasmids and particular surface antigens.

EPIDEMIOLOGY. Although only recently recognized to cause human disease, three species of *Legionella* were first isolated decades ago (*L. micdadei,* 1943; *L. pneumophila,* 1947; *L. bozemanii,* 1959). Legionellae cause outbreaks of both pneumonic and nonpneumonic disease, as well as sporadic cases of pneumonia. The incidence of sporadic *L. pneumophila* pneumonia caused by serogroups 1 or 2 has been estimated from a prospective serologic study to be 12 cases per 100,000 population per year. The incidence of pneumonia caused by the other Legionellae is unknown but is probably much lower. Five per cent of recognized pneumonia cases caused by *L. pneumophila* and most so far recognized as being caused by *L. micdadei* are nosocomial. Cases of *Legionella* pneumonia have been documented in six continents. Cases occur throughout the year but primarily in the summer. Epidemiologic factors associated with increased risk of *L. pneumophila* pneumonia include male sex, middle or old age, cigarette smoking, excessive consumption of alcohol, travel, work in construction, residence near excavation or construction, and underlying medical conditions or therapy commonly associated with immunosuppression. Immunosuppression is also common in those with *L. micdadei* pneumonia.

The only proven mode of spread of *Legionella* is the airborne route. Outbreaks have been traced to airborne spread of bacteria released in aerosols by air-conditioning cooling towers, evaporative condensers, and industrial grinding machinery and inhaled by people downwind. *L. pneumophila* infections have been traced to contamination of the hot water in potable water systems, but whether spread in these cases is by aerosolization, drinking, or mucous membrane contact is unknown. Person-to-person spread has not been documented.

Clusters of *Legionella* infections have occurred in one or two epidemiologic patterns. Outbreaks of legionnaires' disease (named for the group most affected in the 1976 Philadelphia outbreak) are characterized by attack rates of 0.1 to 5.0 per cent for people presumed to be exposed. All documented point-source outbreaks have been caused by *L. pneumophila,* and the usual incubation period has been two to ten days (mean = 5.5 days). More than 30 outbreaks have been recognized. Pontiac fever outbreaks (named for the city in which an outbreak occurred in 1968) are characterized by attack rates of 95 to 100 per cent for people intensively exposed and by incubation periods of 5 to 66 hours (mean = 36 hours). Five such outbreaks have been documented, caused by *L. pneumophila* in four and *L. feeleii* in one. No differences in the source or mode of spread of the organism appear to explain the epidemiologic (or clinical—see later discussion) differences between legionnaires' disease and Pontiac fever.

PATHOGENESIS. Legionnaires' disease appears to occur two to ten days after inhalation of *L. pneumophila.* About half of those infected develop clinical illness. The only consistent pathologic condition found is in the lung and includes areas of acute fibrinopurulent pneumonia bounded by lobular septa. The infiltrate comprises polymorphonuclear leukocytes and macrophages, many of which are necrotic, mixed with proliferating Type II pneumocytes and fibrin. Large numbers of bacteria can be demonstrated by Dieterle silver stain or direct immunofluorescence in areas of pneumonia and commonly clustered in macrophages. Bacteria can also be seen in areas of pleuritis. The lung architecture is usually intact, although focal septal necrosis is sometimes seen, and frank lung abscess may occur in immunosuppressed people. Respiratory bronchioles are affected, but larger bronchioles and bronchi (and their cilia) are spared, perhaps explaining in part the usual paucity of sputum and rarity of person-to-person spread. Healing is commonly complete, but in some patients residual fibrosis can be detected by diminished capacity to diffuse carbon monoxide.

The degree to which involvement of organs other than the lungs is due to direct invasion by *L. pneumophila* or to remote effects of the organism in lung tissue is uncertain. Rarely, *L. pneumophila* has been visualized in mediastinal lymph nodes, blood vessels, liver, spleen, bone marrow, and kidneys and has been recovered from blood. *L. pneumophila* has some of the properties of endotoxins and produces a soluble hemolysin and lymphocytotoxin, but the role of these or other toxins in the pathogenesis of disease is unclear.

L. pneumophila organisms are ingested by monocytes, including human alveolar macrophages. In unactivated macrophages, the bacteria multiply freely—apparently helped by their ability to inhibit phagosome-lysozyme fusion. In macrophages that are activated, as by incubation with lymphocytes stimulated by concanavilin A, *L. pneumophila* multiply more slowly and may indeed be killed. The intracellular location of *Legionella* may help explain the poor agreement between antibiotic sensitivities observed in vitro and in vivo. Although complement-mediated killing of *L. pneumophila,* apparently by the classic pathway, is accelerated by specific antibody in vitro, a protective effect of antibody has not been shown in humans. The possibility that opsonic activity of serogroup-specific antibody is more protective of bacterium than host has been suggested.

Little is known about the pathophysiology of the Pontiac fever syndrome of *L. pneumophila* or *L. feeleii* infection or of the cases of pneumonia caused by Legionellae other than *L. pneumophila.* Pathologically, the latter cases resemble *L. pneumophila* pneumonia. No differences have been found in *L. pneumophila* strains that cause legionnaires' disease and Pontiac fever.

CLINICAL MANIFESTATIONS. *Legionella* infections occur in at least two distinct syndromes: legionnaires' disease and Pontiac fever. Pontiac fever is an acute influenza-like illness characterized by fever, headache, and myalgia. Cough, sore throat, diarrhea, confusion, and chest pain occur but are not usually prominent. Pneumonia does not occur, although one patient had a pleural friction rub during convalescence. The illness is debilitating for two to seven days, but all patients recover completely.

Legionnaires' disease varies in severity from a mild grippe to a severe multisystem disease affecting lungs, liver, kidney, gastrointestinal tract, and central nervous system. Typically, patients have the subacute onset of malaise, weakness, anorexia, dry cough, and fever, without accompanying upper respiratory symptoms. Illness progresses over the next day or two, commonly with repeated rigors, pleuritic chest pain, headache, watery diarrhea, generalized abdominal pain, and confusion. Sputum may be expectorated but is often scant and nonpurulent and may be streaked with blood. Patients appear acutely ill, usually with temperatures of 38.9 to 40.4° C. The degree of tachypnea reflects the severity of the pneumonia, but the pulse rate is often slower than would be expected from the temperature. Pulmonary rales are common early, and signs of consolidation may appear later. Nonfocal neurologic disturbances (confusion, clumsiness, ataxia, slurred speech, and apparent hallucinations) occur and often are of a severity disproportionate to the degree of fever or metabolic derangements.

Laboratory testing shows normal or moderately elevated leukocyte counts with an excess of juvenile neutrophils. Erythrocyte sedimentation rate is greatly elevated. Modest elevations of serum concentrations of transaminases are common. Microscopic hematuria is seen in one third of patients and is often accompanied by cylindruria and proteinuria. Azotemia is found at some time during the illness in about 15 per cent of patients and occasionally necessitates dialysis. Chest radiographs may show patchy infiltrates early in the disease, which later progress to dense consolidation, often in a lobar or segmental pattern and commonly bilaterally. Cavitation is sometimes seen in the immunocompromised host. Pleural effusions are seen in up to one third of patients but are small except in occasional immunosuppressed patients. Gram staining of transtracheally aspirated material usually shows moderate numbers of neutrophils, but large numbers of bacilli are rarely seen. The protein and cellular composition of pleural fluid suggests an exudate in half and a transudate in the other half of the cases in which it is examined. Cerebrospinal fluid is usually normal, although small numbers of lymphocytes have been seen. Without specific therapy fever, pneumonia, and accompanying hypoxemia may progress for five to seven days and be complicated by the syndrome of inappropriate secretion of antidiuretic hormone. Death occurs in 15 to 20 per cent of patients and is usually the result of progressive pneumonia; however, in a few cases a syndrome resembling septic shock precedes death. With specific therapy temperature generally begins to decrease within 24 hours and may be normal within two days, although radiographically the pneumonia may continue to progress for two to five days. Radiographic resolution of *L. pneumophila* pneumonia may take many weeks, longer than for pneumococcal or *Mycoplasma* pneumonia. Residual scarring can be seen histologically and radiographically. In rare cases patients with severe neurologic involvement show mild residual aphasia and impaired memory. Amnesia for the acute illness is common.

Rare cases of *Legionella* infection localized outside the lungs have involved perirectal abscess, focal myocarditis, hemodialysis fistula infection, or pyelonephritis. Coinfection with other bacteria may occur in such sites.

DIAGNOSIS. *Legionella* pneumonia must be distinguished from pneumonia caused by other bacteria or infections caused by *Mycoplasma pneumoniae, Chlamydia psittaci, Coxiella burnetii,* influenza virus, or several other respiratory viruses. Clinical clues that are of differential value for *L. pneumophila* pneumonia include very high fever with repeated rigors, lack of preceding upper respiratory symptoms, diarrhea, unexplained impairment of mental function, hematuria, abnormal liver function, negative routine bacteriologic cultures, and failure to respond to therapy with penicillins, cephalosporins, or aminoglycosides. Epidemiologic clues (see above) may also be helpful in suggesting the diagnosis. With *Legionella* pneumonia, staining well-collected lower respiratory secretions by the Gram method reveals neutrophils accompanied by no bacteria or by weakly staining gram-negative bacilli.

Specific diagnosis is made by isolation of *Legionella* from lung tissue, respiratory secretions, pleural fluid, or blood; detection of specific antigens in lung tissue, respiratory secretions, extrapulmonary tissue, or urine; or demonstration of a significant rise in serum antibody titer during convalescence. Charcoal yeast extract (CYE) agar or buffered CYE agar supports growth of all species, but isolation of *L. pneumophila* from sputum is aided by the incorporation of cefamandole (or vancomycin), polymyxin B, and anisomycin in the agar to inhibit other organisms. A biphasic medium with CYE agar as the solid phase has been successful for culture of *L. pneumophila* from blood. Direct immunofluorescence using species- and serogroup-specific conjugated antisera is useful in detecting *Legionella* in tissue and secretions. For *L. pneumophila,* about two thirds of infected patients have organisms detectable in lower respiratory tract secretions, and they remain detectable for an average of four days after specific therapy is started. *L. pneumophila* serogroup 1 antigen can be detected in the urine of most infected patients by latex agglutination, enzyme-linked immunoassay, or radioimmunoassay and may persist for many weeks. The procedure used for serologic detection of infection is usually indirect immunofluorescence, but this procedure is not well standardized for strains other than *L. pneumophila* serogroup 1. About 80 per cent of patients with *L. pneumophila* pneumonia have a four-fold or greater rise in antibody titer to 1:128 or greater within two to six weeks after onset of symptoms. Rises in titer are not always serogroup specific and may involve IgM, IgG, or IgA. Because rises in titers to *L. pneumophila* have been found in patients with culture-confirmed plague, tularemia, or *Bacteroides fragilis* bacteremia and in patients with simultaneous rises in antibody titers to *M. pneumoniae* or *Leptospira interrogans,* it is likely that serologic diagnosis is not always specific.

THERAPY. Patients with severe *Legionella* pneumonia require supportive respiratory therapy, including supplemental oxygen and mechanical ventilation with or without positive end-expiratory pressure. Careful management of fluid and electrolytes may be necessary in cases of renal insufficiency and inappropriate secretion of antidiuretic hormone. Dialysis may be needed as a temporary measure in frank renal failure. Vasoactive amines, such as dopamine, may be helpful in managing septic shock.

Experimental studies have provided conflicting information as to antimicrobials that may be effective as specific therapy. However, assay systems suggest that erythromycin and rifampin are effective against all *Legionella* species. Retrospective studies of epidemic cases suggest that therapy of *L. pneumophila* pneumonia with erythromycin is associated with a decrease in case-fatality ratio from 24 to 5 per cent.

Recommended initial therapy for pneumonia suspected to be caused by any of the *Legionella* species is erythromycin, 2 grams per day (50 mg per kilogram per day for children) given in four divided doses orally, or in seriously ill patients, intravenously. The dose for adults can be doubled if clinical response is not prompt. Patients with confirmed disease who do not respond to high-dose erythromycin given intravenously may be given rifampin, 600 mg daily, in addition. Because of concern about development of resistance to the drug, rifampin should not be given alone. Therapy should continue for 14 days, although pulmonary cavitation may require therapy to be prolonged. The possibility of relapse after specific therapy is stopped should be remembered. In cases of relapse, erythromycin therapy should be resumed promptly. The potential value of sulfamethoxazole-trimethoprim, tetracyclines, and cefoxitin in treating *Legionella* pneumonia deserves further study.

Initial treatment of adults with pneumonias of uncertain cause but suspected to be of bacterial origin can usefully include erythromcyin—with or without an aminoglycoside—because of the relative safety of erythromycin and its broad spectrum of activity against the most common bacterial agents of pneumonia in this group. Doses are as recommended for *Legionella* pneumonia.

No specific therapy is needed for Pontiac fever.

PREVENTION. Outbreaks caused by organisms from contaminated cooling towers, evaporative condensers, or industrial grinding coolants can be stopped by turning off this equipment or perhaps by treating it with chemicals effective against *L. pneumophila,* such as calcium hypochlorite, quaternary ammonium compounds, and dibromonitrilopropionamide. Whether these chemicals would be helpful in preventive maintenance of these units is unknown. Outbreaks traced to potable water have been controlled by raising the temperature of the hot water to ≥55° C or by hyperchlorination (to ≥2 mg free residual chlorine per liter). Secretion precautions in hospitalized cases may be helpful in decreasing the theoretical possibility of person-to-person spread. In the laboratory caution should be exercised to prevent generation of aerosols of live organisms or to contain them in a biologic safety cabinet.

Edelstein PH, Meyer RD, Finegold SM: Laboratory diagnosis of legionnaires' disease. Am Rev Respir Dis 121:317, 1980. *Detailed paper from the clinical laboratory most experienced in diagnosis of legionnaires' disease; covers culturing, direct immunofluorescence staining, and serology. Complete set of references.*

Fraser DW, Tsai TR (sic), Orenstein W, Parkin WE, Beecham HJ, Sharrar RG, Harris J, Mallison GF, Martin SM, McDade JE, Shepard CC, Brachman PS, Field Investigation Team: Legionnaires' disease. Description of an epidemic of pneumonia. N Engl J Med 297:1189, 1977. *The 1976 Philadelphia outbreak.*

Horowitz MA, Silverstein SC: Intracellular multiplication of Legionnaires' disease bacteria (*Legionella pneumophila*) in human monocytes is reversibly inhibited by erythromycin and rifampin. J Clin Invest 71:15, 1983. *One of a series of papers that emphasize the role of cell-mediated immunity in legionellosis.*

Kirby BD, Snyder KM, Meyer RD, Finegold SM: Legionnaires' disease: Report of 65 nosocomially-acquired cases and review of the literature. Medicine 59:188, 1980. *The largest series of cases seen by one group of clinicians.*

Muder RR, Yu VL, Zuravleff JJ: Pneumonia due to the Pittsburgh pneumonia agent: New clinical perspective with a review of the literature. Medicine 62:120, 1983. *Clinical summary of* L. micdadei *pneumonia.*

Sathapatayavonas B, Kohler RB, Wheat LJ, White A, Winn WC Jr: Rapid diagnosis of legionnaires' disease by latex agglutination. Am Rev Respir Dis 127:559, 1983. *Utility of urinary antigen detection in diagnosis of legionellosis.*

Thornsberry C, Feeley JC, Jakubowski W, Balows A (eds.): Proceedings of Second International Symposium on *Legionella*. Washington, D.C.: American Society of Microbiology (in press). *State of the art as of June 1983. Concise reviews and helpful original papers on bacteriology, epidemiology, ecology, pathogenesis, and diagnosis.*

Wilkinson HW, Reingold AL, Brake BJ, McGibboney DL, Gorman GW, Broome CV: Reactivity of serum from patients with suspected legionellosis against 20 antigens of *Legionellaceae* and *Legionella*-like organisms by direct immunofluorescence assay. J Infect Dis 147:23, 1983. *Useful caution about interpretation of serologic tests in suspected legionellosis.*

Winn WC, Myerowitz R: The pathology of *Legionella* pneumonias: A review of 74 cases and the literature. Hum Pathol 12:401, 1981. *Documents the similarity of pneumonias caused by the various Legionellae.*

Streptococcal Diseases

267. STREPTOCOCCAL DISEASES

Richard M. Krause

Streptococci are ubiquitous, gram-positive globular bacteria that grow in chains. They were first described by Billroth in 1874 in purulent exudates from erysipelas lesions and infected wounds. Subsequently they were shown to cause different forms of streptococcal disease, including streptococcal sore throat, scarlet fever, streptococcal skin infections (impetigo or pyoderma), suppurative infections including abscesses and pneumonia, food poisoning, septicemia, bacterial endocarditis, and urinary tract infections. A single streptococcal species may be responsible for a variety of diseases, and many different kinds of streptococci may be cultured from humans and animals.

The first classification of these organisms was based on their capacity to lyse red blood cells. When streptococci are cultured on blood agar plates, three types of hemolytic reactions are observed. Streptococcal colonies surrounded by a clear zone of hemolysis are termed beta, colonies surrounded by green partial hemolysis are termed alpha, and the nonhemolytic colonies are termed gamma.

Primarily through the efforts of Lancefield, the beta-hemolytic streptococci were further differentiated into a number of immunologic categories, designated groups A to H and K to T, on the basis of specific polysaccharide antigens. Most streptococci causing pharyngitis and impetigo belong to group A. Rheumatic fever occurs only after group A pharyngitis. Streptococci belonging to certain other Lancefield groups are now recognized as important causes of infection. Alpha-hemolytic and gamma streptococci can cause sepsis with systemic illness.

Group A streptococcal pharyngitis has been intensely studied over the years because it may give rise to the delayed, nonsuppurative sequelae acute rheumatic fever (ARF) and acute glomerulonephritis (AGN). While ARF is less common in the United States today than 30 years ago, it still persists as a common cause of heart disease in much of the developing world.

CLASSIFICATION OF STREPTOCOCCI OF CLINICAL IMPORTANCE

The classification of streptococci on the basis of hemolysis patterns on blood agar plates and antigenic composition was a major advance. Nevertheless, it is frequently necessary to employ a combination of features, including growth characteristics and biochemical reactions, to fully characterize these organisms because they are such a heterogeneous group. A classification of streptococci with a clinical orientation for the most important streptococcal infections is presented in Table 267–1. While group A streptococci remain important human pathogens, beta-hemolytic non-group A, alpha hemolytic, and nonhemolytic streptococci are of increasing importance as the cause of suppurative infections in all regions of the body.

GROUP A INFECTIONS. Group A streptococci are the most common cause of streptococcal pharyngitis. They are recognized by the characteristic group A carbohydrate cell wall antigen, which is identified by serologic reactions to specific rabbit antiserum. In this way they can be distinguished from other beta-hemolytic streptococci that are also frequently isolated from the human pharynx, vagina, or skin.

GROUP B INFECTIONS. Group B streptococci are identified serologically by their characteristic cell wall polysaccharide. Group B streptococci were first recognized as a cause of bovine mastitis, but since the 1960's they have emerged as a major cause of neonatal sepsis with or without meningitis. Carriage of group B streptococci in the female genital tract is a major source of these infections.

GROUP D INFECTIONS. Group D streptococci consist of two major categories: enterococci (such as *S. faecalis*) and nonenterococci (such as *S. bovis*). Strains isolated from clinical cultures are usually nonhemolytic or alpha hemolytic, but beta-hemolytic strains are seen.

Enterococci are present in the normal intestinal flora and are a significant cause of community-acquired and hospital-acquired sepsis, as demonstrated by the cultivation of these organisms from the blood. Enterococci are a frequent cause of urinary tract infections, particularly in patients with structural abnormalities of the urinary tract. They are also a frequent cause of endocarditis. Enterococci are frequently resistant to many antibiotics, which complicates treatment. For the treatment of enterococcal endocarditis, combined therapy should be employed, including intravenously administered penicillin in high doses plus an aminoglycoside antibiotic. In combination, these drugs have a synergistic killing effect on enterococci.

In contrast to enterococci, nonenterococcal group D streptococci isolated from patients with endocarditis are extremely sensitive to penicillin. Because of these differences in antibiotic sensitivity, it may be necessary to perform additional biochemical tests to differentiate enterococci from nonenterococcal group D organisms. One simple procedure that may be useful is to attempt growth in a broth containing 6.5 per cent sodium chloride. Enterococci will usually grow under these conditions, whereas other streptococci will not.

OTHER STREPTOCOCCAL INFECTIONS. Not infrequently, the beta-hemolytic streptococci cultured from the throat or other

TABLE 267–1. CLINICAL CLASSES OF STREPTOCOCCAL INFECTIONS

Lancefield Groups	Hemolysis on Blood Agar	Representative Species	Major Clinical Syndromes	Colonization (Carriage)
A	Beta	*S. pyogenes*	Pharyngitis (scarlet fever), pyoderma, wound infection, sepsis, rheumatic fever, acute glomerulonephritis	Pharynx
B	Beta	*S. agalactiae*	Perinatal sepsis, newborn meningitis, subacute bacterial endocarditis, urinary tract infection, adult sepsis	Adult urogenital tract, gastrointestinal tract, throat, rectum, pharynx
C and G	Beta	—	Mild pharyngitis	Pharynx
D	Variable (usually nonhemolytic)	Enterococci *(S. faecalis)*	Subacute bacterial endocarditis, urinary tract infection	Bowel
		Nonenterococci *(S. bovis)*	Subacute bacterial endocarditis	
Nongroupable: viridans streptococci	Alpha (green)	*S. salivarius, S. sanguis, S. mutans*	Subacute bacterial endocarditis, caries	Oropharynx, saliva
Anaerobic (microaerophilic streptococci)	Gamma (nonhemolytic) or variable	*Peptostreptococcus*	Abscesses, gangrene, necrotizing fascitis, peritonsillar abscess	Mouth, intestine, vagina

sites are identified as group C or G organisms. Most commonly when they infect the pharynx, these organisms produce no symptoms or illness. But on occasion a low grade pharyngitis occurs, which may be exudative. A rise in the convalescent antistreptolysin O titer indicates that these groups actually can cause an infection of the pharynx and other sites and are not just passively carried. An unexpected event was the occurrence of ten cases of group C streptococcal sepsis, including meningitis, in New Mexico in the summer of 1983. In addition to group C and G, case reports indicate that under diverse circumstances streptococci belonging to most of the other groups can cause sporadic infections, including meningitis, infected heart valves, visceral abscesses, and soft tissue infections following surgical procedures. Furthermore, these less common organisms are now known to cause opportunistic infections in individuals whose resistance has been compromised by other diseases or treatments.

The predominant aerobic flora of the oral pharynx normally consists of a large variety of streptococci. These are classified as *viridans*, alpha hemolytic, or green streptococci. It is probable that they play some useful role by maintaining a favorable ecologic balance. However, they can produce disease in abnormal circumstances. They are a common cause of subacute bacterial endocarditis and enter the bloodstream most often from diseased teeth and gums.

Special interest has now centered on a species of these organisms identified as *S. mutans*. These bacteria colonize the oral cavity and have been implicated in the development of dental caries. They produce a mucoid substance that becomes part of the plaque adhering to the tooth enamel. The bacteria remain embedded in the plaque and excrete metabolic products that are a factor in the production of caries. Currently there is evidence that dental caries can be prevented by decreasing sugar in the diet to diminish the growth of these bacteria as well as by practicing proper oral hygiene to remove the plaque containing the *S. mutans* organisms. Work is also in progress on a possible vaccine.

Anaerobic streptococci are also a prominent part of the normal flora in the mouth, intestine, and vagina. It is suspected that they maintain an ecologic balance on the surface of these tissues, but the mechanism is unknown. The presence of this normal flora appears to be important, however, because when the ecologic balance is disturbed by the use of antibiotics, pathogens such as *Candida albicans* may cause infections of these sites.

Anaerobic streptococci may cause abscesses in many different regions of the body, including retropharyngeal spaces, paranasal sinuses, dental structures, and the brain. Visceral infections include lung abscesses and empyema fluids, abscesses of the liver and other intra-abdominal viscera, and perirectal and pelvic abscesses. Anaerobic streptococci are especially prone to thrive in dead or devitalized muscle, skin, or subcutaneous tissue. A rapidly progressing necrotizing fasciitis or *progressive synergistic gangrene* is usually produced by these anaerobic streptococci along with *Staphylococcus aureus*. While these anaerobic organisms are usually sensitive to penicillin, debridement and drainage of abscesses is an important aspect of treatment.

GROUP A STREPTOCOCCAL INFECTIONS

BACKGROUND AND PATHOGENESIS. Although streptococci were identified as the cause of scarlet fever and tonsillitis in 1895, determination of the origin and epidemiology of streptococcal infections stems from the serologic classification of the organisms into groups by Lancefield and into types by Lancefield and Griffith. With these developments it was possible to identify group A streptococci as the most common cause of streptococcal pharyngitis. The ability to measure serologic responses was another important advance. Most widely used has been the antistreptolysin O (ASO) test developed by Todd in 1932. This was a major achievement because a rise in an ASO titer or a markedly elevated titer was indicative of a prior streptococcal infection. These immunologic and bacteriologic developments led to the firm conclusion that ARF and AGN were nonsuppurative sequelae to group A streptococcal infections and that infections by *none* of the other streptococcal groups resulted in such sequelae. The rare exception to this rule is that on occasion group C streptococcal infections appear to cause AGN. ARF is only observed after group A pharyngitis, whereas AGN is seen after pharyngitis and other streptococcal infections such as pyoderma.

Epidemics of streptococcal disease in the armed forces have been known since the Civil War. The epidemics in World War I, World War II, and the Korean War were studied in detail, and much of the current knowledge concerning the epidemiology of group A streptococcal disease rests on this research. A major advance was the prevention of rheumatic fever by penicillin treatment of streptococcal pharyngitis and the use of penicillin prophylaxis to prevent recurrences of ARF in patients who had had prior ARF. Epidemics have not been confined to the armed forces, however. Epidemics of streptococcal sore throat and scarlet fever were once commonly observed among school children, and this resulted in extensive programs for the early detection and treatment of pharyngitis for the prevention of rheumatic fever. While epidemics of streptococcal pharyngitis are now less common, sporadic outbreaks in school or other closed populations still occur as minor epidemics. As a result occasional cases of ARF and AGN are still seen in civilian populations.

In the United States, England, and much of Europe, the incidence of streptococcal disease has declined dramatically in the last two decades. There is a belief in some quarters that this decrease is due in part to those properties of the group A streptococci that account for their ability to spread widely in a community and to produce acute disease. While such changes in streptococcal characteristics may have occurred, it is also possible that extensive use of antibiotics has decreased the reservoir of virulent streptococci and therefore their spread. It should be remembered that the untreated patient is the source of secondary spread to susceptible individuals.

Group A streptococci are subdivided into M types on the basis of an antigen known as *M protein*. More than 70 antigenically distinct M types have been identified. This substance plays a very important role in the pathogenesis of group A streptococcal infections. The M protein is a surface component of the streptococcus and is correlated with its ability to resist phagocytosis. Streptococci that have large amounts of M protein are highly resistant to phagocytosis, whereas those with no or small amounts of M protein are susceptible to phagocytosis. Following an infection with streptococci of a particular M type, homologous type-specific immunity develops, so that the individual is resistant to infection by organisms of the same M type. Because this type-specific antibody can persist for many years, reinfection with the same M type is rare. Penicillin or other antibiotic therapy can suppress the type-specific immune response, however; for this reason reinfection with the same M type has been seen in recent years. Because immunity is M-type–specific and because there are numerous M types of streptococci, repeated streptococcal infections caused by different M types are common, particularly in childhood and early adult life.

Because of the importance of M-type–specific immunity in resistance to group A streptococcal infections, intensive research has centered on the immunochemistry of the M protein and the immune response to it. The complete chemical structure of several different M proteins is now known, and with the use of recombinant deoxyribonucleic acid technology, pure type 6 M protein has been produced by *Escherichia coli*. It should now be possible to examine at the molecular level the chemical basis for the antiphagocytic properties of M protein and to explore the molecular interactions that occur when specific antibody promotes phagocytosis of group A streptococci. While these recent developments on the chemistry of M protein again have raised the possibility of a multivalent streptococcal vaccine for use in regions where streptococcal disease still flourishes, a number of theoretical and practical impediments have to be overcome before the development of such a vaccine.

The T antigen is another streptococcal surface protein that has assisted in the classification of streptococci isolated from clinical material. As with M proteins, there are multiple serotypes of T antigens. While T antigens (unlike M proteins) play no part in virulence, they have become very useful antigenic markers, particularly in the recognition of less virulent strains that have lost their M protein. The T antigen classification also has been useful in identifying strains isolated from patients with pyoderma for which an M protein has not yet been identified.

In addition to the M and T proteins, two other major elements of the streptococcal cell wall are the group-specific C carbohydrate and the backbone matrix, a peptidoglycan similar to that in many other gram-positive bacteria. When injected into animals, the backbone matrix produces many of the same biologic reactions as do the endotoxins of gram-negative bacteria. Derivatives of it are known to function as an adjuvant.

Because group A streptococcal infections have been such an important health problem in the past, the organisms and their products have been intensely studied in an effort to determine the cause of ARF and AGN, but the precise nature of the pathogenesis of these complications is unknown. (See Ch. 268 and 80.) Group A streptococci grown in vivo and in vitro produce a great variety of antigenic extracellular products such as the two hemolysins streptolysin O and streptolysin S, streptokinase, hyaluronidase, nicotinamide adenine dinucleotidase (NADase), several deoxyribonucleases (DNAses), and proteinases. The antibody responses to several of these substances are useful in diagnosis. Hemolysis surrounding colonies on the surface of blood agar plates is due primarily to the action of streptolysin S. It is not antigenic. Streptolysin O is reversibly inhibited by oxygen. Because anaerobic conditions prevail beneath the surface of the blood agar, hemolysis in this region is due to streptolysin O. Streptolysin O is produced by almost all group A strains as well as by many group C and G organisms. Since streptolysin O is a good antigen, titration of ASO antibodies in human sera is the most widely used serologic procedure in clinical practice to detect a prior group A streptococcal infection. In recent years, a test to measure anti-DNAse B antibodies has been used in the evaluation of streptococcal pyoderma.

It is assumed that extracellular products play a role in the pathogenesis of streptococcal infections, but the exact relationship is conjectural. Nevertheless, it is probable that the breakdown of fibrin and nucleic acids by streptokinase and the DNAses, respectively, produces the characteristic thin pus of streptococcal infections. It is also possible that hyaluronidase contributes to the rapid spread of the organisms through the tissues, as is seen in streptococcal cellulitis. None of these substances has been implicated in the pathogenesis of ARF or AGN. The erythrogenic toxins cause the typical erythema of scarlet fever. There are three serologically distinct toxins, each neutralized by its respective antibody. For this reason scarlet fever may occur more than once. All strains of streptococci do not produce an erythrogenic toxin. These toxins are induced by lysogeny of group A streptococci with a temperate bacteriophage.

Group A streptococci most commonly infect the tonsils, nasopharynx, and skin. A number of features of streptococcal skin infections set them apart from streptococcal tonsillitis. For this reason, the clinical features of skin infections will be considered separately.

EPIDEMIOLOGY. Streptococcal pharyngitis and tonsillitis are the most common group A streptococcal infections. Their most frequent occurrence is in children between 5 and 15 years of age, but both younger and older persons are still highly susceptible to infection. This is particularly true when special environmental circumstances enhance transmission. For example, mobilization of troops during wartime results in an increased incidence of streptococcal infections in individuals 18 to 25 years of age. The high attack rate in children and military recruits is related to the mode of transmission of group A streptococcal infections. Transmission occurs as a result of close contact between susceptible individuals and either infected persons or healthy individuals who carry contagious streptococci in the pharynx. Organisms are transmitted from one person to another on saliva droplets produced by sneezing or coughing. For this reason, transmission of this disease requires close association with an individual who harbors infectious streptococci in the pharynx. The streptococci that contaminate the fomites and dust in the environment are not the cause of pharyngeal infection even though the organisms are viable and can be cultivated on blood agar from these environmental sources.

Untreated patients are the primary source of the spread of streptococcal disease, especially during the period of acute pharyngitis and for the first several weeks of convalescence. Studies of kindergarten and school-age children indicate that an untreated child is often the source of the disease in the classroom as well as in the home. It is therefore important to identify and treat patients as soon as possible to prevent secondary spread of the disease.

Patients not treated with antibiotics may carry group A streptococci in the nasopharynx for several weeks or months. Furthermore, many individuals will acquire the organism and carry it for similar periods of time without any signs or symptoms of acute pharyngitis. Epidemiologic studies have revealed that untreated patients and asymptomatic carriers are highly infectious during the first one to three weeks after acquisition of pharyngeal group A streptococci. Throat cultures from such individuals frequently reveal large numbers of group A streptococcal colonies; these people have been labeled "dangerous" carriers. Long-term carriage for many weeks or months is seen frequently, but usually the throat culture yields only a small number of group A streptococcal colonies. Furthermore, the streptococci isolated after three weeks frequently have a diminished amount of M protein. The small number of streptococci in the throat and the loss of M protein are probably responsible for the lack of transmission of streptococci from individuals during convalescence and from those who remain persistent carriers for weeks or months.

Nasal or throat carriage (or both) of virulent streptococci is also a source of infection of open wounds and skin abrasions as well as of puerperal sepsis. Secondary infection of the lungs may occur, particularly after a respiratory infection such as influenza. Indeed, streptococcal pneumonia may be seen with greater frequency during an influenza epidemic.

A confusing aspect of streptococcal pharyngitis is that a significant number of individuals have "silent" infections that are detected by positive throat cultures *and* a rise in the ASO titer. In early studies it was learned that at least 25 to 30 per cent of all patients who developed ARF had had a preceding silent throat infection. Such silent infections complicate the control of spread of streptococcal disease in a family or community. Epidemiologic studies have shown that patients with subclinical or silent infection are capable of disseminating the streptococci to other individuals who then may develop overt disease.

Currently there is debate concerning reasons for the declining frequency of severe acute pharyngitis with exudate. Certainly the number of such patients with severe disease is much smaller than it was 30 years ago, while the mild form appears more common. It is unknown whether this change in the clinical picture is due to a decline in the virulence of the streptococci, to host factors, or to the widespread use of antibiotics to treat patients who had been infected with the more virulent forms of streptococci, thus eliminating these organisms from the reservoir of potential pathogens.

A number of epidemiologic factors influence the spread of streptococcal disease. Clearly, socioeconomic factors that promote crowding will result in close contact between individuals and therefore in the spread of streptococci. Climate, season, and geography also can enhance the spread of streptococci because of their influence in bringing people into close contact. It has already been mentioned that military recruits are susceptible because they are clustered in large camps under crowded conditions. Similarly, streptococcal disease is common in civilian populations where poverty and poor housing promote crowded living conditions and therefore the spread from one individual to another. It is probable that these factors continue to influence the widespread occurrence of streptococcal disease in developing countries. For this reason ARF and rheumatic heart disease are common in these regions.

Scarlet fever is now uncommon in the United States. The reasons for this are not clear because the decline began before the widespread use of antibiotics. Streptococcal strains that produce scarlet fever are the same as those that produce group A infections except that they are lysogenized by a bacteriophage that induces the production of erythrogenic toxin.

Whereas streptococcal pharyngitis is most common in the winter months when close contact between individuals is greatest, streptococcal pyoderma occurs in the late summer and early fall. Presumably this is due to exposure of uncovered skin during the warmer months to minor trauma and insect bites, which favor skin infections. Although streptococcal pharyngitis and streptococcal pyoderma occur worldwide, geography clearly influences the occurrence of these two diseases. Pharyngitis is more common in temperate and cold climates, and pyoderma is more frequent in hot or tropical climates.

The attack rate of ARF after streptococcal infections may vary widely. During the major epidemics of World War II and the Korean War, the attack rate was 3 per cent or more in military recruits with untreated group A streptococcal infections. Since that time, studies of children and other civilian populations, particularly those experiencing the sporadic infections that occur today, have suggested that the attack rate may be as low as 0.3 per cent or less. Two features were associated with the large military epidemics of pharyngitis in which the ARF attack rates were high: (1) the magnitude of the immune response associated with infection and (2) the long duration of convalescent carriage of strains after untreated infection. For example, patients who had very high ASO responses were more likely to have attacks of ARF than those who had low or moderate responses. The mild acute streptococcal pharyngitis seen in recent years is followed by a small increase in the ASO titer and a brief period of pharyngeal carriage. This changing pattern in the severity of pharyngitis, in combination with antibiotic therapy, may be responsible for the decreased incidence of ARF. Whatever the reasons for the decrease, this event has implications concerning methods of medical management, including the use of penicillin prophylaxis, which is a matter that will be discussed later.

The epidemiology and the bacteriology of the streptococcal infections that precede ARF differ in important respects from those of the streptococcal infections that precede AGN. In the early years of streptococcal bacteriology, ARF was seen as a complication of epidemic pharyngitis due to nearly all of the different types of group A streptococci. For example, certain M types such as 1, 3, 5, 6, 14, 18, 19, and 24 have all produced epidemics of pharyngitis in the United States that have resulted in ARF. In contrast, AGN was not a constant complication of these epidemics. The occurrence of AGN has been associated with epidemics of pharyngitis due to a limited number of M types, such as type 12. Such differences in the bacteriology of ARF and AGN have raised speculation concerning "rheumatogenic" and "nephritogenic" strains of streptococci. However, such designations become blurred on the basis of epidemiologic information. Sporadic outbreaks of AGN due to types 1, 3, and 6 have been seen, all of which have been associated with ARF. There is no doubt that certain outbreaks of type 12 pharyngitis have resulted in an unusually high incidence of AGN, but type 12 strains in the general population have not consistently resulted in outbreaks of AGN. Therefore, no single M type can be arbitrarily designated nephritogenic. Clearly the *antecedent* streptococcal infection that results in AGN must be due to an organism that has acquired some special characteristic other than a particular M protein. Despite intensive study, there is no certainty as to the nature of this special characteristic. Efforts are under way to identify streptococcal antigens in the immune complexes of patients with AGN that are associated with "nephritogenic" streptococci. It is tempting to speculate that strains acquire the "nephritogenic" property by some form of gene transfer from those streptococci that already possess the capacity to produce AGN.

As attention was focused on the epidemiology of streptococcal infections and AGN, additional M serotypes that had not been associated with pharyngitis were identified, primarily from skin infections. Nearly 20 new M serotypes have been identified from skin cultures as the cause of impetigo. AGN has been associated with skin infections due to several of these types, such as M type 49.

STREPTOCOCCAL SORE THROAT. The usual incubation period

of streptococcal pharyngitis is between two and four days. Typically in both children and adults there is a rather abrupt onset of sore throat. A particular characteristic is pain on swallowing. Hoarseness is rare. Other symptoms include headache, malaise, feverishness, and anorexia. Chilliness is common, but not rigor. Nausea, vomiting, and abdominal pain are common in children. The patient appears mildly to moderately ill, but signs and symptoms depend upon the severity of the illness. Temperature frequently exceeds 38.5° C. In the moderately severe case, examination of the throat reveals diffuse erythema, edema, and lymphoid hyperplasia of the posterior pharynx. The uvula may be edematous. The tonsils are enlarged and reddened, with either a punctate or a confluent yellow-gray exudate. There may be discrete areas of exudate about 1 to 2 mm in diameter on the posterior pharynx. The anterior cervical nodes are usually enlarged. The white blood cell count is usually greater than 12,000 per cu mm. When properly taken, the throat culture usually reveals large numbers of group A beta-hemolytic streptococci. Not uncommonly, group A streptococci are the predominant organisms observed on the culture plate. The course of streptococcal pharyngitis is usually self-limited and the fever abates within a week. The constitutional symptoms and sore throat disappear during this time.

A pharyngitis of the severity just described is typical of the infections seen in earlier years in civilian populations and during military epidemics, but such infections occur less commonly today. Most patients do not have all of the signs and symptoms just described. For example, in mild pharyngitis, there may be no exudate and the throat culture may reveal modest numbers of group A streptococci.

If antimicrobial therapy has not been used, group A streptococci persist in the pharynx for weeks or months following acute pharyngitis. A small number of patients who are treated with penicillin will carry the streptococci for several weeks. If the course of antibiotics has been adequate, these patients need not be retreated. They are unlikely to be a source of spread to other individuals.

The diagnosis of streptococcal pharyngitis in infants and small children presents a special challenge. The disease lacks a well-defined onset. Often there is rhinorrhea as a dominant manifestation. Fever is low grade. Usually the physical signs in the throat are not helpful in the differential diagnosis. A throat culture is positive when properly taken. Despite the mildness of the pharyngitis in infants, suppurative complications such as otitis media can occur.

SCARLET FEVER. Scarlet fever occurs in those patients with streptococcal pharyngitis in whom the infected organism produces an erythrogenic toxin and who are not immune to the toxin because of prior exposure. The enanthem of scarlet fever includes a tongue that may be bright red with large papillae (raspberry tongue) or coated with the red papillae protruding (strawberry tongue). These manifestations of the disease are rarely seen in adults. The rash appears shortly after the onset of the sore throat, usually within two days, and involves the neck, upper chest, and back and then spreads to the remainder of the trunk and the extremities. The palms and the soles are spared. The rash consists of a diffuse erythema that blanches on pressure, with numerous 1-mm punctate elevations that give a sandpaper texture to the skin. There is a generalized facial flush with a pale area often seen around the mouth, the *circumoral pallor.* The distribution of the rash is variable. The trunk and inner aspects of the arms and thighs are most often affected, but in milder cases the rash is seen only in the axilla or groin. Linear striations of confluent petechiae are known as *Pastia's lines.* A tourniquet applied to the arm for five minutes results in large numbers of petechiae distal to the obstruction in nearly all cases (the *Rumpel-Leede sign*). The erythema usually disappears by the sixth to ninth day after the onset of infection. Desquamation of the skin is a characteristic of scarlet fever. It begins with a fine scaling of the face and body and is usually completed during the second week. There then occurs an extensive and characteristic desquamation of the palms and soles. Eosinophilia has been observed, particularly during the period of desquamation.

SUPPURATIVE COMPLICATIONS. The most frequent suppurative complications of streptococcal pharyngitis are perinasal sinusitis, otitis media, and mastoiditis. Suppurative cervical adenitis may occur, as well as impetigo. Bacteremia was seen more commonly in earlier times prior to the use of antibiotics; this resulted in metastatic lesions in joints, bones, and other sites. Group A streptococcal meningitis is now uncommon.

An unusual and infrequent complication of streptococcal tonsillitis is *peritonsillar abscess,* or *quinsy.* While it is probable that the streptococcal infection leads to the formation of the abscess, the abscesses themselves do not contain group A streptococci but a variety of oropharyngeal flora, including anaerobic bacteria. This complication should be suspected if there is an abrupt increase in (1) soreness in the throat, (2) swelling in the neck, and (3) fever during or shortly after streptococcal pharyngitis. Inspection of the throat will reveal the displacement of the tonsil on the affected side toward the midline. A fluctuant mass may be felt in the affected area with a gloved finger; it should be treated promptly because complications arise when the infection extends further into the neck and surrounding tissues.

NONSUPPURATIVE COMPLICATIONS. The nonsuppurative complications of streptococcal disease are ARF and AGN. These are discussed in Ch. 268 and 80.

DIAGNOSIS. Group A streptococcal pharyngitis must be differentiated from pharyngitis due to other bacterial and viral agents. Gonococcal tonsillopharyngitis should be suspected if there is a history of homosexuality or fellatio. *Vincent's angina* usually has an insidious onset without the constitutional symptoms characteristic of a streptococcal sore throat. Signs of this infection, including an exudate, are commonly unilateral, whereas streptococcal pharyngitis is not. *Diphtheria* is now rare, although it should be recognized by the presence of the characteristic diphtheritic membrane as well as the other signs and symptoms of the disease.

The major confusion in the differential diagnosis will stem from viral respiratory infections, which not only occur more frequently than do streptococcal infections but which also may cause pharyngeal and tonsillar exudate. While many upper respiratory infections have a "common cold–like" quality, the symptoms may overlap considerably with those of streptococcal disease. It should be remembered that adenoviruses can cause an exudative pharyngitis that clinically is indistinguishable from that due to group A streptococci. A severe exudative pharyngitis with fever and toxicity is seen in infectious mononucleosis. The generalized symptoms and signs associated with infectious mononucleosis, however, should assist in the differential diagnosis. Pharyngitis due to group A coxsackieviruses (herpangina) or to herpes simplex will result in formation of vesicles. When these rupture they may leave shallow ulcers that can often be differentiated by inspection from streptococcal disease. Because it is frequently not possible to distinguish streptococcal from nonstreptococcal sore throat on clinical grounds, precise diagnosis requires a throat culture.

Before any antimicrobial therapy is administered, swabs should be passed through the mouth under direct vision and a good light and rubbed over the tonsils and posterior pharynx. The swab should be streaked directly, with a minimum of delay, on a sheep blood agar plate of low dextrose content. After incubation overnight, the number of hemolytic streptococci present should be recorded in a roughly quantitative manner. These organisms will be very numerous in nearly all cases if they are the cause of the infection. The presence of a few colonies does not provide convincing evidence that they are responsible for the illness, because 5 to 10 per cent of the general population may be nasopharyngeal carriers of these organisms. Serologic grouping and typing of the isolated organisms are usually not necessary for routine clinical diagnosis. Because the growth of group A streptococci is inhibited in vitro by paper discs containing less than 0.02 unit of bacitracin, some laboratories routinely determine the bacitracin susceptibility of hemolytic streptococci. Hemolytic bacteria resistant to such low concentrations of bacitracin are unlikely to be group A streptococci. On the other hand, approximately 5 per cent of non-group A hemolytic streptococci are also susceptible to this low concentration.

If the pharyngitis persists with adequate penicillin therapy, it is unlikely to be due to group A streptococci. It should be remembered, however, that viral pharyngitis is often of brief duration, and if such patients are treated with penicillin, it may appear that there has been a therapeutic response when in fact the disease has abated spontaneously.

The ASO test is not useful in the diagnosis of streptococcal pharyngitis. An elevation in titer is evidence of a recent infection and is employed in the diagnosis of patients with rheumatic fever and rheumatic heart disease.

TREATMENT. There are three reasons for treating streptococcal pharyngitis: (1) the prevention of suppurative complications, (2) the prevention of the nonsuppurative complications ARF and AGN, and (3) the prevention of spread of the disease through family contacts or to persons in small social units such as school rooms and army barracks. Prevention of ARF depends upon the eradication of the organism from the pharynx, and this requires treatment for at least ten days. Because signs and symptoms frequently subside in a few days, there is a tendency to shorten the time antibiotics are given. Brief periods of antibiotic therapy do not eliminate the streptococci from the pharynx. Patients treated briefly have a greater risk of developing ARF than do those who are adequately treated for at least ten days.

Penicillin is the drug of choice. Group A streptococci are highly susceptible to the action of penicillin. Despite its use for the last 40 years, no penicillin-resistant strains have developed. A single intramuscular injection of 1.2 million units of benzathine penicillin G provides a sufficiently prolonged level of penicillin in the blood to eradicate the organism. For children weighing less than 60 pounds, the dose is 600,000 units. If oral therapy is used, 250,000 units of penicillin G or 250 mg of penicillin V, three or four times daily, is the treatment of choice. If penicillin allergy is suspected or known to exist, erythromycin is the drug of choice, 20 mg per pound per day (not to exceed 1 gram per day) for a period of ten days. Erythromycin resistance is not yet a serious problem in the United States. Many group A streptococci have developed resistance to tetracycline, and it is no longer recommended for treatment of group A infections. Sulfonamides, when used to treat streptococcal pharyngitis, are ineffective in preventing rheumatic fever. They do not suppress the immune response, do not terminate pharyngeal carriage of streptococci, and thus do not reduce the attack rate of subsequent rheumatic fever. They may be used, however, as continuous prophylaxis to prevent new infections.

Treatment of streptococcal sore throat should be started as soon as a definite diagnosis of streptococcal infection is made. It has been shown, however, that a short delay (even for several days) in initiating antimicrobial therapy while awaiting throat culture results does not significantly interfere with rheumatic fever prevention. One exception to this statement involves the patient with a history of rheumatic fever. In such a patient, the prevention of rheumatic recurrence is not always possible unless treatment is instituted at the first clinical sign of streptococcal infection. For such a patient, any delay of therapy entails the risk of reactivation of the disease.

If severe suppurative streptococcal infections such as mastoiditis, pneumonia, wound infections, or other forms of sepsis are present, patients should receive 600,000 units of procaine penicillin G twice a day intramuscularly for several days until the illness is under control. Then a shift can be made to benzathine penicillin or oral penicillin. It may be necessary to prolong therapy for several weeks whenever pus or necrosis is present, particularly when adequate debridement is not possible, and mixed infection with anaerobes should be excluded.

STREPTOCOCCAL PNEUMONIA

Streptococcal pneumonia is now uncommon. It can be seen, however, as a complication of influenza, measles, pertussis, or varicella. It is characterized by abrupt onset of fever, chills, myalgia, dyspnea, cough, pleuritic chest pain, and hemoptysis. Patients are severely ill. Radiologically, there is usually bronchopneumonia. Lobar consolidation is less common. One characteristic feature of streptococcal pneumonia is the early and rapid accumulation of a large volume of thin empyema fluid. The pneumonic infection can extend to the mediastinum and pericardium. Bacteremia occurs in 10 to 15 per cent of the cases. Bacteriologic diagnosis depends on recovering group A streptococci from the sputum, empyema fluid, and blood. Because the patient is very ill, treatment should be started promptly. Therapy consists of 4 to 6 million units of parenteral procaine penicillin G given daily; this total daily dose is given in two to four intramuscular injections. There must also be adequate drainage of the empyema fluid. This may require insertion of a chest tube.

STREPTOCOCCAL SKIN INFECTIONS

PYODERMA. Group A streptococci can produce localized purulent skin infections known as pyoderma. While some of the lesions represent secondary infections of wounds or burns, most commonly the infection is primary and is usually referred to as *streptococcal impetigo* or *impetigo contagiosa*. Intensive studies over the past 20 years have revealed a number of important bacteriologic and epidemiologic differences between streptococcal impetigo and streptococcal pharyngitis (Table 267–2). Impetigo occurs in the summer and fall, whereas pharyngitis is seen in the winter and spring. Children between the ages of

TABLE 267–2. COMPARISON OF THE FEATURES OF STREPTOCOCCAL PHARYNGITIS AND PYODERMA*

Features	Pharyngitis	Pyoderma
Clinical Illness	Acute	Indolent
Laboratory		
Leukocytosis	Usually present	Often absent
Antistreptolysin O response	Common	Uncommon
Epidemiology		
Seasonal occurrence	Winter and spring	Late summer and early fall
Geographic distribution	More common in temperate or cold climates	Common in hot or tropical climates
Age	School-age children	Children of preschool age
Transmission	Direct spread from human reservoirs	Unknown; insects may be mechanical vectors
Carrier state	Common in pharynx of many populations	Unusual on skin
Preceding trauma	Not present	May predispose to infection
Complications		
Acute nephritis	Occurs; partially preventable (50%)	Occurs; preventability unknown
Acute rheumatic fever	Occurs; preventable	Does not occur
Treatment		
Local	Not important	Removal of crusts and scrubbing with hexachlorophene soap
Systemic	Single intramuscular injection of benzathine penicillin or oral penicillin for 10 days	May not be necessary; extensive lesions may require intramuscular benzathine penicillin

*Modified from Wannamaker LW: N Engl J Med 282:23, 78, 1970.

two and five years are more commonly infected. They are usually from underprivileged families residing in the southern United States or the tropics. Nevertheless, outbreaks can be seen among children of similar circumstances in other areas of the United States, such as those in American Indian reservations.

Epidemiologic studies have not clarified the mode of spread of streptococcal pyoderma, but it is reasonable to assume that personal contact with infected patients and perhaps insect vectors may be important. Despite the uncertainty about the mode of spread, a number of important epidemiologic and clinical facts have emerged from recent studies. In general, the streptococci that cause pyoderma are the higher numbered M types, whereas pharyngitis is usually due to M types 1 through 40. Children who develop streptococcal impetigo and who carry the higher types on the skin may then develop pharyngeal carriage of these skin strains, which are unlikely to cause pharyngitis. Such pharyngeal carriage must be taken into consideration in the diagnosis of respiratory disease in these children, because carriage of these strains alone is not indicative of streptococcal pharyngitis.

Differences have been seen also in the immune response, depending on the site of the streptococcal infection. While the ASO response is usually brisk following streptococcal pharyngitis, it is weak or absent in patients with impetigo. It has been suggested that inactivation of streptolysin O by the lipids present in the skin accounts for this feeble antibody response. Brisk antibody responses do occur, however, to DNAse B in patients with impetigo. M type-specific protective antibodies are almost always produced after streptococcal pharyngitis, but the response to the M type-specific antigens is variable in the case of impetigo. It is not surprising, therefore, that lesions due to the same serotype may persist for months if untreated.

The lesions of streptococcal impetigo occur over the exposed areas of the body. They are more common on the lower extremities, undoubtedly because abrasions of the skin are more common in these areas. The lesions begin as papules but rapidly evolve into vesicles surrounded by erythema. They may be localized but are often multiple. As the papules enlarge, they break down over five or six days to form a thick crust. The lesions heal slowly, leaving a depigmented area. While there may be some regional lymphadenitis, systemic symptoms are not usually present.

While streptococcal impetigo can be suspected from the history as well as the examination, definite diagnosis requires bacteriologic culture. The crust must be removed to obtain specimens from the base of the lesion after washing the infected area of the skin with sterile water. Soap or other detergents can kill or reduce the number of group A streptococci. Culturing the surface of the lesion itself will usually give a negative result. Culture results may show both group A streptococci and *Staphylococcus aureus,* but it is generally believed that the streptococcus is the primary pathogen. In many instances mild impetigo responds to local treatment. The crusts should be removed and the skin washed with soap and water. Topical antibiotics and other antiseptics have little or no value in treatment or prevention. When the lesions are more extensive, parenteral use of benzathine penicillin is indicated. The lesions respond well to penicillin therapy. The antibiotic regimen is the same as used for the treatment of pharyngitis. Even though the *S. aureus* present may produce penicillinase, this does not interfere with penicillin treatment. Prevention of impetigo is achieved with good personal hygiene and liberal use of soap and water.

The importance of streptococcal impetigo beyond the inconvenience and some disfiguration of the skin relates to its association with AGN. Not all strains of group A streptococci that cause impetigo and other forms of pyoderma result in AGN; nevertheless, certain M types such as 49, 55, and 57 have been associated with sporadic cases as well as large epidemics of pyoderma-associated AGN. These have occurred in many different geographic regions. Although there is evidence to suggest that treatment of streptococcal pharyngitis will prevent AGN 50 per cent of the time, there is no conclusive evidence that treatment of an individual case of pyoderma will prevent subsequent occurrence of AGN. Nevertheless, treatment of the individual is important, particularly in a setting in which AGN is occurring or has occurred in the past, because this eradicates the streptococcus from the environment. The individual is therefore not a risk to siblings and other school children.

A more severe ulcerated form of pyoderma is known as *ecthyma.* During the Vietnam conflict, this was seen in combat troops serving in the jungle. The ulcers, located on the ankle or dorsum of the foot, are circular, have a punched-out appearance and are 0.5 to 3 cm in diameter. They contain purulent material and may be covered with a yellow-gray crust. They are surrounded by a zone of erythema, and in more severe cases there may be cellulitis and lymphadenitis.

ERYSIPELAS. Erysipelas (St. Anthony's fire) is an acute infection of the skin and subcutaneous tissues caused by group A streptococci. The disease is more common in infants, young children, and elderly people. It is most commonly seen on the face and has a "butterfly" distribution when the bridge of the nose and the cheeks are involved. Eyelids are edematous and often swollen shut. The source of the infection is the patient's nasopharynx. Erysipelas may also develop from streptococcal infections elsewhere on the body, including surgical incisions and wounds. In some cases the disease has been seen in association with dermatophytosis.

As with streptococcal pharyngitis, the onset is usually abrupt, and similar systemic symptoms are frequently present. The lesion initially begins with an area of mild discomfort at the site of infection. Erythema follows and enlarges rapidly, reaching a maximum in three to six days. The lesion, pink to deep red in color, has an advancing irregular margin. It is warm to the touch. Vesicles and bullae may appear, which then rupture and become crusted. As the margin advances, the central area begins to clear and the skin returns to a normal appearance, usually with some residual pigmentation.

While recovery is usually seen in a week or ten days, this varies with the severity of the infection. High fever and bacteremia were often present before antibiotics were available, and mortality was not uncommon, particularly in patients who had bacteremia. Death is rare when the disease is adequately treated with penicillin or another appropriate antibiotic. Early diagnosis and treatment are important in infants and in elderly, debilitated, or immunosuppressed individuals. Death can occur in these cases if treatment is not prompt. Not uncommonly the disease will recur in the same site, particularly if there are areas of lymphatic obstruction.

Large numbers of group A streptococci can usually be cultured from the nasopharynx of patients with early erysipelas. Efforts to culture the streptococci from the edema fluid of the lesion are not always successful. Diagnosis is primarily made on the basis of clinical findings.

PREVENTION AND PROPHYLAXIS OF GROUP A STREPTOCOCCAL DISEASES AND THEIR NONSUPPURATIVE SEQUELAE

Views on the antibiotic treatment of streptococcal pharyngitis to prevent ARF and AGN are undergoing re-evaluation because of the decrease in the severity of streptococcal pharyngitis in recent years and the dramatic decline in the occurrence of ARF. Do the low attack rates of ARF (1 to 2 per 100,000 people per year for the age group 5 to 17 years) justify intensive efforts to detect streptococcal infections by bacteriologic cultures? Do they justify a prolonged course of antibiotic therapy for all patients in whom streptococcal infection is suspected, however mild it may be? Views are currently changing on these matters, and there is now discussion of some relaxation of the vigorous efforts used in the past to diagnose and treat streptococcal pharyngitis.

From this debate several principles are emerging. While direct proof is lacking, it is probable that the decline in the incidence of both ARF and streptococcal pharyngitis is due at least in part to the widespread use of penicillin to treat this infection during the past 25 years. It is difficult to believe that this decline in disease has occurred as a result of genetic changes in the streptococci. This would have required the simultaneous occurrence of similar genetic events in a large number of different streptococci during this interval, which seems unlikely. Certainly the decline in both diseases has been too precipitous to have been the result of changes in the genetic background of the population that would have enhanced natural immunity. These considerations suggest that the treatment of pharyngitis with penicillin has been a major factor in reducing the incidence of this infection; it follows that penicillin treatment has also influenced the decline in ARF. It seems likely that continuation of treatment in the future will maintain this low incidence. It is known that virulent group A streptococci lurk in the shadows and are the cause of occasional outbreaks of streptococcal pharyngitis. It is certainly conceivable that such outbreaks would become more common if penicillin treatment were no longer used. Therefore, arguments to discontinue the use of penicillin to treat streptococcal pharyngitis, even though the disease is less virulent today than in previous times, are reminiscent of the arguments to discontinue the use of pertussis or poliomyelitis vaccines now that these diseases are rare. We know that failure to vaccinate will result in the re-emergence of these diseases.

Until there is more evidence concerning the benign nature of the streptococcal diseases that are occurring today, it will be prudent to maintain vigilance concerning streptococcal infections. Nevertheless, a consensus is emerging that the milder forms of pharyngitis need not be treated until the diagnosis is confirmed by throat culture. Furthermore, many specialists question the value of a throat culture in all cases of upper respiratory disease. These authors would reserve the throat culture for laboratory confirmation of streptococcal disease that is suspected on clinical grounds. Current recommendations call for a second throat culture at the end of ten days of treatment to be certain that the streptococcus has been eliminated. This is probably no longer necessary in the routine case. Furthermore, throat cultures of family members in contact with the usual case of streptococcal pharyngitis seem unnecessary.

Despite the decrease in the severity of streptococcal diseases and the decrease in incidence of ARF and AGN, small outbreaks of streptococcal infection still occur that result in sporadic cases of ARF and AGN. Certainly the occurrence of an index case of either ARF or AGN should alert the physician to the possibility that an outbreak of streptococcal disease is occurring in a family or school.

It is apparent from this dicussion concerning the infrequency of ARF and the milder nature of streptococcal disease that there is probably much less risk today of the recurrence of rheumatic fever in patients with prior history of the disease following an untreated streptococcal infection. Continuous antibiotic prophylaxis has been employed in the past to prevent recurrences of rheumatic fever in such patients, and while discussions are under way concerning modification of the recommendations, the three regimens listed below are still recommended at this time.

1. Benzathine penicillin G in a single injection of 1.2 million units will provide protection for about 30 days. The disadvantages and discomfort of this regimen have to be weighed against the individual patient's susceptibility to rheumatic recurrences. Those with rheumatic heart disease, those who have had a recent attack of rheumatic fever, and those exposed to an environment in which the incidence of streptococcal infection is frequent deserve the most effective protection. For such patients, benzathine penicillin by monthly injection is recommended.

2. Sulfonamide given daily by mouth in the form of 1.0 gram of sulfadiazine or one of the other sulfapyrimidines provides satisfactory prophylaxis, but failures will occur. Toxic reactions may be observed during the first 60 days of continuous treatment. These have been rare, however, with the small doses of sulfadiazine that have been employed extensively.

3. Penicillin in oral doses of 200,000 units (125 mg) of penicillin G twice daily has been employed widely for prevention of streptococcal infections. This regimen has not been any more effective, however, than the daily dose of 1.0 gram of sulfadiazine. Indeed, 200,000 units of penicillin twice daily has not proved as yet to be clearly superior to the single dose. It is possible that the oral dose of penicillin may have to be increased to nearly therapeutic proportions to be more effective than sulfonamides, and this would increase further its expense and impracticability.

GROUP B STREPTOCOCCAL INFECTIONS

In the past, group B streptococci were primarily of interest to veterinarians because they were the cause of bovine mastitis. However, in recent years human strains of group B streptococci that appear to be distinct from the bovine strains have received considerable attention because they frequently produce neonatal sepsis. Group B streptococci are subdivided by means of surface polysaccharides into five serotypes: Ia, Ib, Ic, II, and III. Recent evidence suggests that group B streptococci normally colonize the intestine, and it is speculated that there is then secondary spread from the rectum to the vagina. This raises the possibility of sexual transmission of these organisms. Vaginal carriage is asymptomatic in postpubertal women. The incidence of carriage and of neonatal infection varies widely depending on socioeconomic status and geographic residence.

Infections due to group B streptococci are associated with perinatal events. Maternal infections include chorioamnionitis, septic abortion, and puerperal sepsis. Group B streptococci are now recognized as one of the most frequent causes of neonatal sepsis and meningitis. Extensive clinical and epidemiologic studies have delineated two forms of the disease. "Early onset disease" primarily involves infection of the lungs. The disease usually occurs within the first ten days of life, but cases after this period have been reported. The organisms are usually acquired from the maternal genital tract. This may be secondary to aspiration of infected amniotic fluid. Septicemia may be present. Early onset disease occurs as frequently as in 5 of every 1000 live births, although this varies depending upon the regions of the country and the specific hospital reporting. Early onset disease tends to occur in infants of certain high-risk pregnancies, such as those involving prematurity, prolonged rupture of membranes, and maternal infection. The other form of group B streptococcal neonatal infection has been referred to as "late onset disease." Affected infants develop meningitis and bacteremia. The infant is usually over ten days old, but cases have occurred at four or five days of age. Infection is due to nosocomial transmission. The disease has a much lower mortality rate than early onset disease. Type III organisms predominate as the cause of early and late onset disease.

Because all the evidence suggests that early onset disease in the newborn infant is acquired by vertical transmission from the mother who has vaginal colonization by group B streptococci, intravenous administration of ampicillin sodium has been used to treat such women during labor in an effort to prevent transmission. While several reports clearly indicate that transmission of group B streptococci carriage to the newborn infant has been prevented, the number of deliveries has not been sufficiently large to determine whether early onset disease has also been prevented. All newborns who acquire group B carriage in the ear, nose, umbilicus, and rectum do not develop early onset disease. Nevertheless, prevention of vertical transmission of carriage is a promising development, particularly if current studies also show the prevention of early onset disease.

Another strategy to prevent early onset disease has been penicillin treatment of all newborn infants immediately after birth. Several controlled studies involving the treatment of thousands of infants have shown a decrease in the number of cases of early onset disease due to group B streptococci, but there is also an indication that disease due to penicillin-resistant pathogens increased during this neonatal period of observation. Additional studies now in progress may clarify this matter. At this time, routine use of penicillin at birth to prevent group B streptococcal infections cannot be recommended.

While group B streptococci frequently may be cultured from the throat, they rarely if ever cause pharyngitis. Group B streptococcal infection can, however, cause urinary tract infections in both sexes. Infected men are likely to be elderly. Group B streptococci may produce suppurative gangrenous lesions in adults with insulin-dependent diabetes mellitus who have peripheral vascular insufficiency. Any large series of infectious diseases will reveal group B streptococci as a cause of endocarditis, pneumonia, empyema, meningitis, peritonitis, and terminal bacteremia in patients with malignancy.

All group B streptococci are susceptible to penicillin. It is the drug of choice for these infections. Thus far, most strains are susceptible to erythromycin. Tetracycline should not be used because the organisms have developed resistance to this antibiotic.

Baker CJ: Group B streptococcal infections. Adv Intern Med 25:475, 1980. *A brief but comprehensive review of the clinical features, epidemiology, and clinical microbiology of this most important cause of sepsis and meningitis in the newborn. Approximately 100 references are annotated.*

Holm SE, Christensen P: Basic Concepts of Streptococci and Streptococcal Diseases. Surrey, England, Readbooks Ltd., 1982. *Over 100 short papers on many aspects of the bacteriology, epidemiology, and pathogenesis of streptococcal diseases. An excellent source of recent articles in journals.*

McCarty M: Streptococci. *In* Davis BD, Dulbecco R, Eisen HN, Ginsberg HS (eds.): Microbiology. New York, Harper & Row, 1980, pp 607–622. *A good brief review of all aspects of streptococcal bacteriology and streptococcal disease.*

Read SE, Zabriskie JB (eds.): Streptococcal Diseases and the Immune Response. New York, Academic Press, 1980. *An exhaustive symposium of immunology in general and streptococcal diseases in particular by leading American and British investigators.*

Rheumatic Fever Committee, American Heart Association: Prevention of rheumatic fever. Circulation 55:s1, 1977. *Standard recommendations for the prevention of rheumatic fever, which should be basic knowledge for all physicians.*

Shulman ST (ed.): Management of Pharyngitis in an Era of Declining Rheumatic Fever. Columbus, Ohio, Ross Laboratories, 1984. *A collection of papers that thoroughly reviews the changing patterns of streptococcal diseases and the implications of these changes for treatment and management.*

Wannamaker LW: Infections of the throat and skin. N Engl J Med 282:23, 78, 1970. *A critical review of the clinical microbiology and epidemiology of "skin strains" of group A streptococci.*

Wannamaker LW: Immunology of streptococci. *In* Nahmias AJ, O'Reilly RJ (eds.): Immunology of Human Infection. Part I: Bacteria, Mycoplasmae, Chlamydiae, and Fungi. New York, Plenum Medical Book Company, 1981, pp 47–92. *An excellent review of the humoral and cellular immune responses to many different streptococcal products and antigens. Includes 400 references.*

Wood HF, Feinstein AR, Taranta A, Epstein JA, Simpson R: Rheumatic fever in children and adolescents. III. Comparative effectiveness of three prophylaxis regimens in preventing streptococcal infections and rheumatic recurrences. Ann Intern Med 60 (S5):31, 1964. *A classic controlled long-term study of the prevention of rheumatic recurrences and the relative effectiveness of the three regimens commonly in use for secondary prophylaxis.*

Yow MD, Mason EO, Leeds LJ, Thompson PK, Clark DJ, Gardner SE: Ampicillin prevents intrapartum transmission of group B streptococcus. JAMA 241:1245, 1979. *One of the first papers to demonstrate that women who are colonized with group B streptococci and are treated with intravenous ampicillin sodium during labor do not vertically transmit group B streptococci to their newborn infant.*

268. RHEUMATIC FEVER

Alan L. Bisno

DEFINITION. Rheumatic fever is a delayed, nonsuppurative sequel of upper respiratory infection with group A streptococci. The disease is characterized by inflammatory lesions involving primarily the joints, heart, and subcutaneous tissues; its pathogenesis remains obscure. The clinical manifestations include polyarthritis, carditis, subcutaneous nodules, erythema marginatum, and chorea in varying combinations. In its classic form, the disorder is acute, febrile, and largely self-limited. However, damage to heart valves may be chronic and progressive, causing cardiac disability or death many years after the initial episode. Persons who have had rheumatic fever are inordinately susceptible to recurrent episodes following group A streptococcal upper respiratory infections. Both initial and recurrent attacks of acute rheumatic fever are largely preventable by treatment or prophylaxis of the antecedent streptococcal infection.

ETIOLOGY. The development of acute rheumatic fever (ARF) requires antecedent infection with a specific organism, the group A *Streptococcus*, at a specific body site, the upper respiratory tract. Cutaneous streptococcal infection, a frequent precursor of poststreptococcal acute glomerulonephritis, has never been shown to cause rheumatic fever. The explanation for this phenomenon remains obscure. It may indicate a requirement for a site with a rich endowment of lymphoid tissue, such as the pharynx, for initiation of the disease process. It may relate to the blunted immunologic response to certain streptococcal antigens observed following skin infection. Still another possible explanation is that so-called "pyoderma" strains of group A streptococci lack rheumatogenic potential.

Strains representing a number of the more than 70 M protein serotypes of group A streptococci are capable of eliciting ARF. Whether *all* clinically virulent strains of *S. pyogenes* are equally "rheumatogenic" remains a matter of controversy. There is evidence to suggest, however, that group A streptococci may vary in their rheumatogenic potential. Analysis of epidemics of ARF caused by a variety of serotypes shows a striking absence of certain highly prevalent types (e.g., type 12) and an overrepresentation of others, particularly type 5. Reports from the preantibiotic era document epidemics of streptococcal tonsillitis, even among rheumatic subjects, in which ARF failed to appear. Prospective studies from Trinidad, where poststreptococcal acute glomerulonephritis and ARF occur simultaneously in the same indigent population, indicate that the streptococcal strains responsible for each sequel are serotypically distinct.

PATHOGENESIS. The mechanism by which group A streptococci elicit the connective tissue inflammatory response which constitutes ARF remains unknown. Various theories have been advanced: (1) direct tissue invasion by streptococci themselves or by variants of the organism with incomplete cell walls; (2) toxic effects of streptococcal products, particularly streptolysins S or O, both of which are capable of initiating tissue injury; (3) a serum sickness–like reaction mediated by antigen-antibody complexes, perhaps localized to sites of tissue injury; and (4) "autoimmune" phenomena induced by the similarity of certain streptococcal and human tissue antigens.

Efforts to discriminate among these potential pathogenetic mechanisms have been hampered by the lack of an animal model of rheumatic fever. Many authorities currently favor the theory that ARF is an "autoimmune" disorder, in which tissue damage is mediated by the host's own immunologic responses to the antecedent streptococcal infection. This theory is made more credible by the relatively long latent period between the onset of pharyngitis and ARF and by the demonstration of numerous examples of antigenic similarity between somatic constituents of the group A *Streptococcus* and human tissues. The most intensively studied of these antigenic cross-reactions has been that between streptococci and human heart. Many patients with ARF or rheumatic heart disease demonstrate in their sera antibodies that cross-react with heart tissue in a variety of test systems. These "heart reactive antibodies" (HRA) are also present, although in lower titer, in sera of some patients with uncomplicated streptococcal infection. HRA are also present in the sera of patients with postcardiotomy and postmyocardial infarction syndromes and in endomyocardial fibrosis, and it is possible that they represent a secondary response to myocardial antigenic determinants exposed or modified by tissue damage.

Two pieces of evidence suggest, however, that the presence of HRA in ARF patients is not secondary but rather is based upon cross-reactions between streptococcal and host antigens. Rabbits immunized with group A streptococcal cell walls develop antibodies that bind to sarcolemma and subsarcolemmal sarcoplasm in cardiac myofibers and skeletal muscle, as well as to smooth muscle of vessel walls and of endocardium. HRA in rheumatic patients but not in those with nonstreptococcal-related illness may be absorbed by streptococcal constituents. Antigens of the group A *Streptococcus* that share antigenic determinants with heart tissue have been localized both to the cell wall (including the M protein molecule) and to the cell membrane.

Another intriguing cross-reaction is that described between the group A carbohydrate in cell walls of *S. pyogenes* and a glycoprotein in human and bovine heart valves. The cross-reactive substance appears to be N-acetyl glucosamine, the terminal residue in rhamnose side chains of group A carbohydrate. This cross-reaction is of special interest because serum levels of antibodies to group A carbohydrate remain elevated for years in patients with rheumatic valvulitis (but not in rheumatic patients without valvulitis) and decline remarkably if valve resection is performed.

Patients with ARF have, on the average, higher titers of serum antibodies to virtually all streptococcal extracellular and somatic antigens than do patients with uncomplicated streptococcal infections. Perhaps for this reason, much of the immunologic investigation of rheumatic fever has focused upon humoral antibodies (e.g., HRA, anticarbohydrate antibodies, and anti–brain-cell antibodies) that cross-react with human and streptococcal antigens. Data relating to cellular immunity are more limited. ARF patients exhibit an exaggerated cellular reactivity to streptococcal constituents, particularly streptococcal cell membrane antigens, as demonstrated by inhibition in vitro of migration of peripheral blood lymphocytes.

Chronic remittent nodular lesions have been produced in dermal connective tissue following injection into experimental animals of a streptococcal mucopeptide-polysaccharide cell wall complex. Taken together, these and other reported antigenic cross-reactions and toxic phenomena could theoretically account for most of the manifestations of ARF. As yet, however, there is no direct evidence that any of them is of pathogenetic significance.

Several observations suggest that development of rheumatic fever may be modulated, at least in part, by the specific genetic constitution of the host. These include (1) the tendency of rheumatic fever to affect more than one member of a given family; (2) the fact that only a small percentage of all individuals experiencing an immunologically significant streptococcal infection develop ARF; (3) the tendency of rheumatic individuals to experience recurrent attacks; and (4) the propensity of rheumatic subjects to exhibit exaggerated immunologic responses to streptococcal antigens. Analyses of the relative frequencies of histocompatibility antigens in rheumatic subjects and controls have been inconclusive. A preliminary report, however, suggests that a particular B cell alloantigen is present in three quarters of rheumatic subjects but in less than 20 per cent of controls.

EPIDEMIOLOGY. The epidemiology of ARF mirrors that of streptococcal pharyngitis. The peak age incidence is 5 to 15 years, but both primary and recurrent cases are frequently seen in adults. ARF is rare in children less than 4 years of age, a fact that has led some observers to speculate that repetitive streptococcal infections are necessary to "prime" the host for the disease. There is no clear-cut sex predilection, although females are more likely to develop certain manifestations such as Sydenham's chorea and mitral stenosis.

Rheumatic fever occurs in all parts of the world; there is no known racial predisposition. In temperate climates, ARF peaks in the cooler months of the year, in the winter and early spring or shortly after schools open in the fall. The major environmental factor favoring occurrence appears to be crowding, as in military barracks or similar closed institutions and in large households. Crowding favors interpersonal spread of group A streptococci and perhaps enhances streptococcal virulence by frequent human passage. At present, ARF is primarily a disease of lower socioeconomic classes, particularly those massed in the densely populated core areas of major urban metropolitan centers. The disease remains rampant in developing areas such as the Middle East, the Indian subcontinent, and many nations of Africa and South America. It has been estimated that rheumatic heart disease causes 25 to 40 per cent of all cardiovascular disease in the third world.

The precise incidence of ARF in the United States is difficult to ascertain. In many localities the disease is not reportable. Cases manifested by carditis alone may not come to medical attention during the acute phase, and instances of polyarthritis or cardiac disease of other etiologies are frequently confused with ARF. All observers agree, however, that the incidence of ARF and the prevalence of rheumatic heart disease have declined dramatically both in America and in Western Europe over the past four to five decades. Studies of the incidence of ARF (hospitalized and nonhospitalized cases) among children aged 5 to 19 years in Baltimore and Nashville during the 1960's indicated rates in the range of approximately 24 to 34 per 100,000 population. The rate for blacks was about twice that for whites, a fact thought to be related to socioeconomic rather than to genetic factors. During roughly the same time period, the ARF attack rate among school-aged children in the most congested of Manhattan's Spanish-American neighborhoods was estimated to be 78 per 100,000. At present, however, rates of less than 2 per 100,000 school children have been reported from several centers. In the affluent suburbs of many United States cities, ARF is becoming extremely rare.

The frequency with which ARF develops following untreated group A streptococcal upper respiratory infection differs with the epidemiologic circumstances. In the years following World War II, careful prospective studies were conducted among personnel in military recruit camps suffering from exudative tonsillitis or pharyngitis caused by M typable group A streptococci. Under such circumstances, in which cases of streptococcal pharyngitis tend to be clinically severe and to appear in discrete epidemics, approximately 3 per cent of untreated patients developed ARF. Studies of endemically occurring streptococcal infection among open populations of children are complicated by the difficulties of differentiating cases of mild, nonexudative streptococcal pharyngitis from viral pharyngitis occurring in streptococcal carriers; nevertheless, the ARF attack rate in such circumstances is clearly lower than in the military experience, with an overall attack rate of less than 1 per cent.

Certain features of the antecedent streptococcal infection are associated with an increased risk of ARF. Among these are the magnitude of the ASO titer rise and the persistence of the infecting organism in the pharynx. Prospective civilian studies indicate that ARF is more likely to occur following clinically severe exudative pharyngitis than following mild, nonexudative illness. On the other hand, one third or more of cases of ARF occur after streptococcal infections which are asymptomatic or so mild as to have been forgotten by the patient.

Patients with a history of ARF are at greatly increased risk of recurrent disease following an immunologically significant streptococcal infection. In long-term prospective studies of rheumatic subjects carried out at Irvington House, a rheumatic fever sanatorium outside New York City, one of every five documented streptococcal infections gave rise to a recurrence of ARF. The risk of recurrence is greater in patients with preexisting rheumatic heart disease and in those experiencing symptomatic throat infections; the risk declines with advancing age and with increasing interval since the most recent rheumatic attack. Nevertheless, rheumatic patients remain at increased risk well into adult life, perhaps indefinitely.

PATHOLOGY. ARF is characterized by exudative and proliferative inflammatory lesions in the connective tissues, especially those of heart, joints, and subcutaneous tissues. The early lesions consist of edema of the ground substance, fragmentation of collagen fibers, cellular infiltration, and fibrinoid degeneration. In the heart, diffuse degeneration and even necrosis of muscle cells may be observed. At a slightly later stage, focal perivascular inflammatory lesions develop. These so-called *Aschoff nodules* (Fig. 268–1), considered pathognomonic of rheumatic fever, consist of a central area of fibrinoid surrounded by lymphocytes, plasma cells, and large basophilic cells, some of them multinucleate. Many of these cells have elongated nuclei with a distinctive chromatin pattern, sometimes called "caterpillar" or "owl-eye" nuclei, depending on their orientation in microscopic cross-section. Cells containing these nuclei are called "Anitschkow myocytes," despite the fact that most authorities believe them to be of mesenchymal origin.

Cardiac findings may include pericarditis, myocarditis, and endocarditis. Foci of coronary arteritis may also be observed. A thickened and roughened area ("MacCallum's patch") is frequently present in the left atrium above the posterior leaflet of the mitral valve. Valvular lesions appear early as small verrucae along the line of closure. Later, as healing occurs, the valves may become thickened and deformed, the chordae shortened, and the commissures fused. These changes result in valvular stenosis or insufficiency. The mitral valve is most commonly involved, followed by the aortic, the tricuspid, and, rarely, the pulmonic.

Pathologically, the *arthritis* of ARF is characterized by a fibrinous exudate and sterile effusion without erosion of the joint surfaces or pannus formation. *Subcutaneous nodules* have many histologic features in common with the Aschoff nodules. They consist of central zones of fibrinoid necrosis surrounded by histiocytes, fibroblasts, occasional lymphocytes, and rare polymorphonuclear cells. Inflammation of the smaller arteries and arterioles may occur throughout the body. Despite pathologic evidence of diffuse vasculitis, aneurysms and thrombosis are not typical features of ARF.

CLINICAL MANIFESTATIONS. Rheumatic fever may involve a number of different organ systems, most notably the heart, joints, skin, and central nervous system. The clinical picture of the disease may thus be quite variable, depending upon which systems are attacked, whether they are involved singly or in combination, the order in which they are affected, and the severity of the involvement. Five clinical features of the disease are so characteristic of it that they are recognized as "major manifestations" according to the revised Jones criteria (see below) for diagnosis of ARF: carditis, polyarthritis, chorea, subcutaneous nodules, and erythema marginatum. Certain other findings, frequently present but nonspecific, have been designated "minor manifestations." These include arthralgia, fever, history of previous rheumatic fever or evidence of preexisting rheumatic heart disease, and certain laboratory findings (see below).

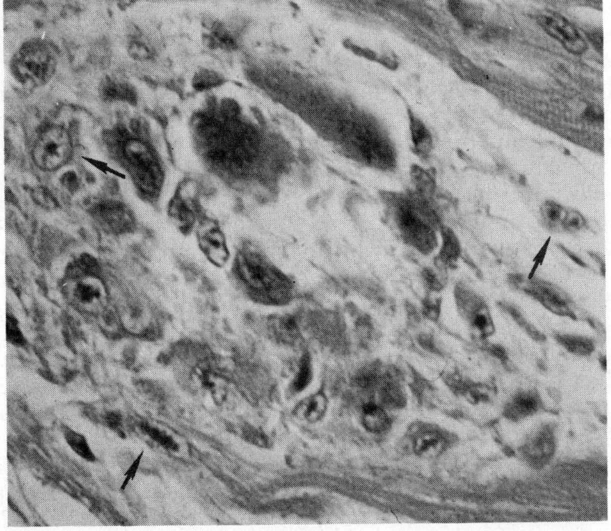

Figure 268–1. Myocardial Aschoff nodule demonstrates areas of fibrinoid degeneration and numerous large cells with polymorphous nuclei; several of the nuclei have "owl eye" or "caterpillar" configurations (arrows). (× 630.) (Courtesy of Robert Peace, M.D.)

In cases in which it can be determined, the *latent period* between the antecedent streptococcal infection and the onset of symptoms of ARF ranges between one and five weeks. The average latent period is 19 days for both primary and recurrent attacks. When acute polyarthritis is the presenting complaint, the onset is often rather abrupt and may be marked by high fever and toxicity. If isolated carditis is the initial manifestation, the onset may be insidious or even subclinical. Between these two extremes, a wide variety of gradations exists in the initial presentation of ARF. In most attacks, fever and joint involvement are the earliest clinical manifestations, although they may occasionally be preceded by abdominal pain localized to the periumbilical or infraumbilical areas. At times the location and severity of the pain, as well as fleeting signs of peritoneal inflammation, may lead to a misdiagnosis of acute appendicitis. Carditis, if it is to appear, usually does so within the first three weeks of the illness. In contrast, chorea tends to occur later in the course of the disease, sometimes after all other manifestations have subsided. Fortunately, chorea and polyarthritis almost never occur simultaneously. Epistaxis may be a feature of ARF, occurring both at the onset and throughout the acute phase of the illness; it may be quite severe.

Overall, arthritis occurs in approximately 75 per cent of first attacks of ARF, carditis in 40 to 50 per cent, chorea in 15 per cent, and subcutaneous nodules and erythema marginatum in fewer than 10 per cent. The incidence of individual manifestations, however, varies with age. Carditis is more frequent in the youngest age groups and is relatively rare in first attacks occurring in adults. Chorea occurs primarily in persons between age five years and puberty. It is seen more frequently in females and virtually never occurs in adult males. Thus, most attacks of ARF occurring in adults are manifested primarily by arthritis.

Arthritis. Joint involvement ranges from arthralgia alone to acute, disabling arthritis characterized by swelling, warmth, erythema, severe limitation of motion, and exquisite tenderness to pressure. The larger joints of the extremities are usually involved—most frequently the knees and ankles, but also the wrists and elbows. The hips and small joints of the hands and feet are affected occasionally. Involvement of shoulders and lumbosacral, cervical, sternoclavicular, and temporomandibular joints occurs in a relatively small percentage of cases. The synovial fluid contains thousands of white blood cells with a marked preponderance of polymorphonuclear leukocytes; bacterial cultures are sterile.

Characteristically, the articular involvement in ARF assumes a pattern of *migratory polyarthritis*. This does not mean that inflammation in one joint disappears before the next is attacked. Rather, a number of joints are affected in succession and the periods of involvement overlap. Inflammation in one joint may subside while another is becoming symptomatic, so that the process seems to migrate from joint to joint. In untreated cases, as many as 16 joints may be affected, and about half the patients develop arthritis in more than six joints. When effective anti-inflammatory therapy is administered early in the course of the disease, the involvement not infrequently remains monoarticular or pauciarticular.

In most instances, inflammation in any one joint begins to subside spontaneously within a week and the total duration of involvement is no more than two or three weeks. The entire bout of polyarthritis rarely lasts more than four weeks and resolves completely, leaving no residual joint damage. Some authors have described the rare occurrence of *Jaccoud's arthritis*, so-called chronic post–rheumatic fever arthropathy of the metacarpophalangeal joints, following repetitive bouts of rheumatic polyarthritis. This entity is not a true arthritis but a form of periarticular fibrosis; its relationship to rheumatic fever remains unresolved.

Carditis. Rheumatic fever may involve the endocardium, myocardium, and pericardium, and thus the disease is capable of inducing a true *pancarditis*. Carditis is the most important manifestation of ARF because it is the only one capable of causing significant permanent organ damage or death. Although the clinical picture may at times be fulminant, it is more frequently mild or even asymptomatic and may escape notice in the absence of more obvious associated findings such as arthritis or chorea. The diagnosis of carditis requires the presence of one of the following four manifestations: (1) organic cardiac murmurs not previously present, (2) cardiomegaly, (3) pericarditis, or (4) congestive heart failure. In practice, the characteristic murmurs of ARF are almost always present in cases of rheumatic carditis, unless the ability to hear them is obscured (e.g., loud pericardial friction rub, large pericardial effusion, low cardiac output, severe tachycardia). The diagnosis of carditis should be made with caution in the absence of one of the following three murmurs: apical systolic, apical mid-diastolic, and basal diastolic. Such murmurs, if they are destined to develop, do so usually within the first week and almost always within the first three weeks of illness. (An exception to this rule may occur in the patient with "pure" chorea; see later discussion.) The *apical systolic murmur* of relative or actual mitral regurgitation encompasses most of systole. It is blowing, relatively high pitched, and heard best at the apex; it radiates to the axilla and at times to the base of the heart or the back. It must be distinguished carefully by quality, location, and radiation from a variety of functional precordial systolic murmurs heard in normal individuals, especially in children. The *apical mid-diastolic* (Carey-Coombs) murmur is a low-pitched sound replacing or immediately following the third heart sound and ending distinctly before the first heart sound. It may be heard in a variety of conditions associated with increased flow across the mitral valve and is thus not pathognomonic of ARF. It may be differentiated from the diastolic rumble of mitral stenosis by the absence of an opening snap, presystolic accentuation, or accentuated first sound at the mitral area. The high-pitched, decrescendo *basal diastolic murmur* of aortic regurgitation is best heard along the upper left sternal border or over the aortic area. It may be brief and faint, best heard after expiration with the patient leaning forward.

Other prominent auscultatory findings in patients with active rheumatic carditis include tachycardia, which persists during sleep; protodiastolic, presystolic, or summation gallops; an indistinct or "mushy" quality to the first heart sound (resulting in some cases from first degree heart block); pericardial friction rub; or muffling of heart tones caused by pericardial effusion. In the early stages of congestive heart failure, rapid distention of the hepatic capsule may lead to right upper quadrant aching and tenderness over the liver. All the usual clinical findings of pericarditis or congestive failure may be observed.

A number of different rhythm disturbances may occur during the course of ARF. By far the most common is first degree atrioventricular block. Second and third degree heart block, nodal rhythm, and premature contractions may also be observed; atrial fibrillation, on the other hand, is usually a feature of chronic rather than acute rheumatic involvement. Conduction disturbances do not in themselves indicate acute carditis, and their presence or absence is unrelated to the subsequent development of rheumatic heart disease.

In cases of ARF with severe carditis, areas of patchy pneumonitis are sometimes seen. Many observers feel that these pulmonary infiltrates represent a specific *rheumatic pneumonia*. The case is difficult to prove, however, because of the confusion induced by such confounding clinical entities as pulmonary edema, pulmonary embolization, superimposed bacterial pneumonia, and the acute respiratory distress syndrome in these severely ill and toxic patients.

Sydenham's Chorea (Chorea Minor, "St. Vitus' Dance"). This neurologic syndrome occurs after a latent period which is variable but on the average longer than that associated with the other manifestations of ARF. It frequently occurs in "pure" form, either unaccompanied by other major manifestations or, after a latent period of several months, at a time when all other evidences of acute rheumatic activity have subsided. Chorea is characterized by rapid, purposeless, involuntary movements, most noticeable in the extremities and face. The arms and legs flail about in erratic, jerky, incoordinated movements which may sometimes be unilateral (hemichorea). Facial tics, grimaces, grins, and contortions are evident. The speech is usually slurred or jerky. The tongue, when protruded, retracts involuntarily, while asynchronous contractions of lingual muscles produce a "bag of worms" appearance. The involuntary motions disappear during sleep and may be partially suppressed by rest, sedation, or volition.

Patients with chorea display generalized muscle weakness and an inability to maintain a tetanic muscle contraction. Thus, when the patient is asked to squeeze the examiner's fingers, a squeezing and relaxing motion occurs which has been described as "milkmaid's grip." The knee jerk may have a pendular quality. There is no cranial nerve or pyramidal involvement, and sensory modalities are unaffected. The electroencephalogram may display abnormal slow wave activity.

Emotional lability is characteristic of Sydenham's chorea and often may precede other neurologic manifestations, leaving teachers and parents puzzled over apparently inexplicable personality changes.

Subcutaneous Nodules. These are firm, painless subcutaneous lesions which vary in size from a few millimeters to approximately 2 cm. The skin overlying them is freely movable and is not inflamed. The lesions tend to occur in crops over bony surfaces or prominences and over tendons. Sites of predilection include the extensor surfaces of elbows, knees, and wrists; the occiput; and spinous processes of the thoracic and lumbar vertebrae. Nodules are virtually never seen as the sole major manifestation of ARF; they almost always appear in association with carditis, and the cardiac involvement in such cases tends to be clinically severe. Nodules ordinarily do not appear until at least three weeks after the onset of an attack, usually lasting one to two weeks. They may appear in repeated crops in patients with protracted carditis. Similar nodules may be seen in systemic lupus erythematosus and in rheumatoid arthritis. Subcutaneous nodules in the latter disease are larger and more persistent than those in rheumatic fever.

Erythema Marginatum. The rash begins as an erythematous macule or papule, which then extends outward, while the skin in the center returns to normal. Adjacent lesions coalesce, forming circinate or serpiginous patterns (see Color plate 9). The lesions are neither pruritic nor indurated, and they blanch on pressure. They vary greatly in size, and appear mostly upon the trunk and proximal extremities, sparing the face. Erythema marginatum may be raised or flat; the latter was termed *erythema annulare* in the older literature. The lesions are evanescent, migrating from place to place, at times changing before the observer's eyes, and leaving no residual scarring. The erythema may be brought out by the application of heat. Individual lesions may come and go in minutes to hours, but the process may go on intermittently for weeks to months uninfluenced by anti-inflammatory therapy; its persistence is not necessarily an adverse prognostic sign. In the great majority of cases, erythema marginatum is accompanied by carditis; it also tends to be associated with subcutaneous nodules.

LABORATORY FINDINGS. No specific laboratory test is diagnostic of ARF. Usually there is a leukocytosis with an increase in the proportion of polymorphonuclear leukocytes. A mild to moderate normocytic normochromic anemia is the rule. In some patients the serum glutamic oxaloacetic transaminase level is elevated. Evidences of acute inflammation are prominent, including readily detectable quantities of C-reactive protein in the blood and elevation of the erythrocyte sedimentation rate. An exception is "pure" chorea, which may appear long after indices of inflammation have returned to normal. The urine may contain protein, white cells, and red cells. Biopsy studies have revealed a variety of renal abnormalities, but the classic proliferative glomerular abnormalities which characterize post-streptococcal acute glomerulonephritis occur quite rarely, if at all, in ARF. Electrocardiographic and radiographic studies may reveal evidence of rhythm disturbances, pericarditis, pericardial effusion, or congestive heart failure.

The major laboratory contribution to the workup of ARF is the documentation of recent group A streptococcal infection. Throat culture should always be performed but is positive in only a minority of cases. This is perhaps due to the time lapse of several weeks between the onset of the pharyngeal infection and the throat culture. The serum titer of antistreptolysin O (ASO) is elevated in 80 per cent or more of ARF patients. If two streptococcal antibody tests, e.g., ASO plus either anti–DNAse B or antihyaluronidase, are performed, an elevated titer of at least one will be found in 90 per cent of ARF patients. A battery of three tests will establish the presence of recent, immunologically significant streptococcal infection in more than 95 per cent of individuals experiencing an acute rheumatic attack. The definition of an "elevated" titer varies, depending upon the test employed, age of the patient, and geographic locale. In practice ASO titers greater than 200 to 250 Todd units per milliliter are generally considered elevated. At times, serial sampling may detect a rising titer of streptococcal antibodies in patients seen early in the course of a rheumatic attack.

A simple slide agglutination test (Streptozyme) is positive in high titer in over 90 per cent of ARF patients. However, the test must be performed by a technician skilled in interpreting hemagglutination reactions, and values of 1:100 to 1:200 should be considered equivocal. Care should be taken to test simultaneously controls of known titer.

COURSE AND PROGNOSIS. The average duration of an untreated attack of ARF is approximately three months. The duration tends to be longer, up to six months, in patients with severe carditis. Less than 5 per cent of patients have continuing rheumatic activity for longer than six months. In a few of these the disease is limited to chorea and is otherwise benign. Other patients exhibit evidence of persistent inflammatory activity, including arthritis, carditis, and subcutaneous nodules. "Chronic rheumatic fever" occurs more frequently in patients who have had one or more previous attacks; cardiac involvement in chronic rheumatic fever tends to be frequent and severe.

Death from intractable myocarditis during the acute phase of ARF is now very rare. Once the acute attack has subsided, the only long-term sequel is that of rheumatic heart disease, manifested primarily by insufficiency and/or stenosis of the mitral and aortic valves. The prognosis from a cardiac standpoint is very much dependent upon the clinical findings at the time the patient is first seen. In one large study, for example, 347 patients were examined during an acute rheumatic attack and again ten years later. Among patients who had been free of carditis during their acute attack, only 6 per cent had residual heart disease on follow-up. Patients with no pre-existing heart disease and with mild carditis during their acute attack (i.e., apical systolic murmur without pericarditis or heart failure) had a relatively good prognosis in that only approximately 30 per cent had heart murmurs ten years later. About 40 per cent of subjects with apical or basal diastolic murmurs and 70 per cent of subjects with failure and/or pericarditis during their acute attacks had residual rheumatic heart disease. The prognosis was worse in patients with pre-existing heart disease and in those who had experienced recurrent attacks of ARF in the ten-year interval.

The data cited above indicate that patients who do not develop carditis during an acute attack and are protected from ARF recurrences are most unlikely to suffer from rheumatic heart disease. The patient with "pure" chorea represents an exception to this rule. A significant proportion of such patients who have no evidence of carditis when first examined may develop rheumatic valvular disease on prolonged follow-up. Although the explanation for this phenomenon is unknown, it is conceivable that, in view of the long latent period associated with chorea, signs of carditis might have been present earlier but subsided by the time the neurologic abnormality became evident.

DIAGNOSIS. Although ARF is readily recognized in the individual who presents with multiple major manifestations or in epidemic circumstances, at other times the disease may be extraordinarily difficult to diagnose with confidence. This is because of the variability of its clinical presentation, the frequency with which only a single major manifestation is detected, and the fact that there is no definitive diagnostic laboratory test. Nevertheless, precise diagnosis is especially important in this disease because of the necessity to advise the patient regarding prolonged antimicrobial prophylaxis (see below).

The diagnostic criteria of T. Duckett Jones, as subsequently modified by a committee of the American Heart Association, attempt to minimize over- and underdiagnosis (Table 268–1). Two major manifestations, or one major and two minor manifestations, indicate a high probability of ARF, *provided that there is supporting evidence of recent streptococcal infection.* Although a positive throat culture for group A streptococci technically satisfies this requirement, it is important to realize that streptococcal carriage rates of 15 per cent are not uncommon among school-aged children during the fall and winter. Elevated titers of antibodies to streptococcal extracellular products, although not diagnostic of ARF, do indicate a recent, *immunologically significant* streptococcal infection. Conversely, if a battery of streptococcal antibody tests fails to reveal any evidence of recent infection, the diagnosis of ARF must be considered unlikely. This statement does *not* necessarily hold true in patients whose only rheumatic manifestation is Sydenham's chorea. Because of the long latent period associated with chorea, previously elevated antibody titers may have declined to normal.

The modified Jones criteria are of course only guidelines. They are most difficult to apply confidently when polyarthritis is the single major manifestation present. Under such circumstances, serious consideration must be given to various other entities, including rheumatoid arthritis, Still's disease, viral arthritides (e.g., rubella, hepatitis B), the early prepurpuric phase of Henoch-Schönlein purpura, and septic arthritis. The last-named entity has come to the fore with the resurgence of

TABLE 268–1. JONES CRITERIA (REVISED) FOR GUIDANCE IN THE DIAGNOSIS OF RHEUMATIC FEVER*

Major Manifestations	Minor Manifestations
Carditis	*Clinical*
Polyarthritis	Previous rheumatic fever or rheumatic heart disease
Chorea	Arthralgia
Erythema marginatum	Fever
Subcutaneous nodules	*Laboratory*
	Acute phase reactions
	Erythrocyte sedimentation rate, C-reactive protein, leukocytosis
	Prolonged P-R interval

Plus

Supporting evidence of preceding streptococcal infection (increased ASO or other streptococcal antibodies; positive throat culture for group A *Streptococcus;* recent scarlet fever).

The presence of two major criteria, or of one major and two minor criteria, indicates a high probability of the presence of rheumatic fever if supported by evidence of a preceding streptococcal infection. The absence of such evidence should make the diagnosis doubtful, except in situations in which rheumatic fever is first discovered after a long latent period from the antecedent infection (e.g., Sydenham's chorea or low-grade carditis).

*From Circulation 32:64, 1965, with permission.

gonococcal arthritis as a relatively common cause of febrile polyarthralgia and polyarthritis in adolescent females in certain population groups.

Serum sickness is frequently a serious consideration, particularly if the patient has received penicillin or other antibiotics for a preceding respiratory infection. Systemic lupus erythematosus, sickle cell hemoglobinopathies, and infective endocarditis may involve the joints and the heart. Other differential diagnostic considerations include congenital heart lesions, viral and idiopathic forms of myocarditis and pericarditis, and functional heart murmurs. Nonfamilial forms of chorea have been described in systemic lupus erythematosus, and rarely in association with the use of birth control pills. It remains uncertain how often episodes of chorea occurring during pregnancy ("chorea gravidarum") represent attacks of rheumatic fever. Other disorders that may at times be confused with ARF are gout, sarcoidosis, Hodgkin's disease, and acute leukemia.

Following an episode of acute streptococcal pharyngitis, a small proportion of patients may experience persistent symptoms of malaise, arthralgia, low grade fever, and lymphadenopathy plus laboratory evidences of mild inflammation. It is difficult to classify such cases, but the affected individuals do not meet the criteria for diagnosis of ARF and, moreover, do not appear to be at risk for the delayed cardiac sequelae of ARF.

TREATMENT. Antibiotics neither modify the course of a rheumatic attack nor influence the subsequent development of carditis. Nevertheless, it is conventional to give a course of antibiotics designed to eradicate any group A streptococci remaining in the tonsils and pharynx, at least in part to prevent spread of the organism to close contacts. The recommended regimens are as follows: intramuscular benzathine penicillin G, 600,000 units for children less than 60 pounds and 1,200,000 units for heavier individuals; or penicillin V orally, 125 to 250 mg four times daily for ten days. Penicillin-allergic individuals may receive erythromycin. The specific dosage varies somewhat with the preparation selected but is in the range of 20 to 40 mg per kilogram of body weight per day divided in two to four equal doses. The maximum dose is one gram per day. Following completion of this therapy, continuous antistreptococcal prophylaxis should commence (see below).

Treatment with anti-inflammatory agents is effective in suppressing many of the signs and symptoms of ARF. These agents do not "cure" the disease, nor do they prevent the subsequent evolution of rheumatic heart disease. They should be avoided in very mild or equivocal cases, because, by suppressing the clinical manifestations, they may obscure the diagnosis. The two drugs most widely used are aspirin and corticosteroids. The former is used in patients with acute polyarthritis, provided that carditis is either absent or mild and there is no evidence of congestive heart failure. Aspirin is very effective in decreasing fever, toxicity, and joint inflammation. It should be given in a dosage of 90 to 100 mg per kilogram per day. This is administered in equally divided doses, every four hours for the first 24 to 36 hours; thereafter it may be given in four doses during waking hours. A salicylate level of 25 mg per deciliter is usually satisfactory. The incidence of nausea and vomiting may be minimized by starting somewhat below the optimal dosage level and gradually increasing over a few days. The patient should be observed for evidence of significant gastrointestinal bleeding and for signs and symptoms of salicylism. After two weeks, the dosage is reduced to 60 to 70 mg per kilogram per day for an additional six weeks. These dosage schedules represent general guidelines only. The precise aspirin dose must be determined by the patient's clinical response, blood salicylate levels, and tolerance of the drug.

Corticosteroids are generally reserved for patients who have severe carditis manifested by congestive heart failure, who are unable to tolerate large doses of salicylates, or whose signs and symptoms are inadequately suppressed by aspirin. As with aspirin, the dosage must be individualized. Prednisone, 40 to 60 mg per day in divided doses, may be used initially; after two to three weeks it should be withdrawn slowly over an additional three-week period. In cases of fulminating carditis with profound heart failure, intravenous corticosteroids may be employed. Aspirin should be administered for a month after discontinuation of prednisone. As is the case for other patients receiving corticosteroids, the physician should be alert to problems such as gastrointestinal bleeding, sodium and water retention, potassium depletion, and impairment of glucose tolerance. Suppression of the pituitary-adrenal axis or of the host immune system is a potential problem but not ordinarily a major one during this relatively short course of treatment. The role of nonsteroidal anti-inflammatory agents in management of ARF remains to be defined.

Following cessation of anti-inflammatory therapy, clinical or laboratory evidence of ARF may reappear. Such therapeutic "rebounds" occur more frequently after corticosteroid therapy than after treatment with aspirin. They may be minimized by prolonging salicylate therapy for 9 to 12 weeks and, when corticosteroids have been required, by continuing aspirin use for a month after corticosteroids have been discontinued.

Congestive heart failure is managed by the usual measures of bed rest, sodium restriction, diuretics, and, if necessary, oxygen and digitalis. The potential risk of digitalis-induced arrhythmias in the patient with active myocarditis must be borne in mind.

All patients should be kept at bed rest for the first three weeks of illness, during which time carditis will usually manifest itself if it is destined to appear. Bathroom privileges and an occasional period in a chair may be allowed unless arthritis or chorea make this infeasible or unless incipient or frank heart failure supervenes. Subsequently the level of physical activity should be guided by the patient's clinical status, primarily by the presence and activity of rheumatic carditis. Patients with congestive heart failure should be kept at bed rest as long as failure is present. Patients with Sydenham's chorea require a quiet environment, and sedatives such as phenobarbital may be helpful.

Once the acute attack has subsided completely, the patient's subsequent level of physical activity is dependent upon his cardiac status. Patients without residual heart disease may resume full and unrestricted activity. It is important that the patient not be subjected to unwarranted invalidism, either because of his own inaccurate perceptions of the nature of the rheumatic process or because of those of his parents, teachers, or employers.

PREVENTION. "Primary prevention" of ARF consists of accurate diagnosis and appropriate treatment of streptococcal sore throat (Ch. 267). Although straightforward in theory, primary prevention is often frustratingly difficult to achieve. In many of the densely populated, indigent communities in which the risk of ARF is greatest, children with self-limited illnesses such as sore throats may never come to medical attention, and throat culture services are usually unavailable to aid in diagnosis. Moreover, in one third or more of cases, ARF may arise after a clinically inapparent streptococcal infection.

Perhaps the most effective strategy for avoiding the mortality and chronic cardiac disability associated with ARF is that of "secondary prevention." This strategy focuses upon the group of persons who have already suffered a rheumatic attack and who are inordinately susceptible to a recurrence following an immunologically significant streptococcal upper respiratory infection. Recurrent attacks tend to be mimetic in nature so that patients who have suffered carditis with their previous attack are likely to have repetitive cardiac involvement and progressive cardiac damage. Because even patients who experienced only arthritis or chorea may develop carditis with recurrent attacks of ARF, *all* patients who have experienced a documented attack of ARF should receive continuous antimicrobial prophylaxis to prevent either symptomatic or asymptomatic streptococcal infections. The specific regimens to be used are indicated in Ch. 267. By far the most effective of these is monthly benzathine penicillin G. Rheumatic recurrences are very unusual in patients faithfully adhering to this regimen.

The total duration of rheumatic prophylaxis remains unresolved. Some authorities recommend lifelong prophylaxis. On the other hand, the risk of rheumatic recurrence is known to diminish with increasing age and increasing interval since the most recent rheumatic attack. Patients who escape carditis during their initial attack are less likely to experience rheumatic recurrences and less likely to develop carditis if a recurrence does ensue. These facts, coupled with the relative rarity of ARF itself in most parts of the United States at present, suggest that prophylaxis need not be perpetual for all rheumatic subjects. Continuous prophylaxis should be maintained indefinitely for all those with clinically significant rheumatic heart disease. Other rheumatic subjects should be protected until reaching adulthood, for at least five years after their most recent attack, and if they are in an epidemiologic circumstance which places them at high risk of streptococcal acquisition (e.g., parents of small children, school teachers, military recruits, pediatricians). The decision to remove a rheumatic subject from continuous prophylaxis should be an individualized one, based upon the physician's assessment of the risk and likely consequences of recurrence, and taken with the patient's informed consent. Patients taken off prophylaxis must be instructed to return immediately for medical follow-up whenever symptoms of pharyngitis occur.

Patients with rheumatic valvular heart disease must receive prophylaxis designed to avoid bacterial endocarditis whenever they undergo dental or surgical procedures likely to evoke bacteremia. This is not necessary in the rheumatic subject who is free of residual heart disease. The regimens for prevention of endocarditis (see Ch. 269) are entirely different from those prescribed for prevention of ARF, and the fact that a patient is receiving rheumatic fever prophylaxis in no way exempts him from endocarditis prophylaxis. This is a frequent point of confusion not only among patients but among physicians and dentists as well.

Bisno AL: The concept of rheumatogenic and non-rheumatogenic group A streptococci. *In* Read SE, Zabriskie JB (eds.): Streptococcal Diseases and the Immune Response. New York, Academic Press, 1980, pp 789–803. *Summarizes data supporting the hypothesis that group A streptococci vary in rheumutogenic potential.*

Bisno AL, Pearce IA, Wall HP, Moody MD, Stollerman GH: Contrasting epidemiology of acute rheumatic fever and acute glomerulonephritis: Nature of the antecedent streptococcal infection. N Engl J Med 283:561, 1970. *The epidemiology and bacteriology of endemically occurring streptococcal infections and their nonsuppurative sequels in an indigent, urban southern United States population.*

Committee on Rheumatic Fever and Bacterial Endocarditis, American Heart Association: Prevention of rheumatic fever. Circulation 55:1A, 1977. *Official recommendations of the American Heart Association for primary and secondary prevention of rheumatic fever. Includes specific antibiotic regimens.*

Feinstein AR, Spagnuola M: The clinical pattern of acute rheumatic fever: A reappraisal. Medicine 41:279, 1962. *An extremely careful and comprehensive analysis of the clinical patterns observed in 374 episodes of ARF admitted to the Irvington House rheumatic fever sanatorium.*

Land MA, Bisno AL: Acute rheumatic fever: A vanishing disease in suburbia. JAMA 249:895, 1983. *Up-to-date data on the occurrence of ARF in a middle-sized United States community. Discussion of recent trends in rheumatic fever incidence in the United States.*

Markowitz M, Gordis L: Rheumatic Fever. 2nd ed. Philadelphia, W. B. Saunders Company, 1972. *An excellent general textbook with authoritative coverage of areas of public health interest: epidemiology, primary prevention, and community health services.*

Sanyal SK, Thapar MK, Ahmed SH, et al.: The initial attack of acute rheumatic fever during childhood in north India: A prospective study of the clinical profile. Circulation 49:7, 1974. *The frequency of occurrence of the major clinical manifestations of ARF is carefully documented in patients admitted to a general hospital in north India, and the findings are compared with those from large series in the United States.*

Stollerman GH: Rheumatic Fever and Streptococcal Infection. New York, Grune & Stratton, 1975. *A comprehensive, extremely readable summary of all aspects of rheumatic fever. The bibliography is excellent.*

United Kingdom and United States Joint Report: The natural history of rheumatic fever and rheumatic heart disease: Ten year report of a cooperative clinical trial of ACTH, cortisone and aspirin. Circulation 32:457, 1965. *This definitive international study of the natural history of rheumatic fever relates the risk of developing rheumatic heart disease to the cardiac status during the acute attack. Long-term prognosis was not improved by the use of corticosteroids or ACTH.*

Wood HF, Feinstein AR, Taranta A, et al.: Rheumatic fever in children and adolescents. III. Comparative effectiveness of three prophylaxis regimens in preventing streptococcal infections and rheumatic recurrences. Ann Intern Med 60(Suppl 5):31, 1964. *This beautifully designed and executed Irvington House study provides definitive data on the efficacy of secondary prophylaxis.*

Endocarditis

269. INFECTIVE ENDOCARDITIS

David T. Durack

When microbes colonize the endocardium, they cause the disease termed *infective endocarditis.* The organism is usually a common bacterium, the site affected is usually one of the heart valves, and the characteristic lesion is a vegetation. For general use, the term infective endocarditis is more appropriate than *bacterial endocarditis,* because this disease also can be caused by fungi and chlamydia. Serviceable terms in general use include *subacute* and *acute bacterial endocarditis* (SBE and ABE), *native valve endocarditis* (NVE), *prosthetic valve endocarditis* (PVE), and *nonbacterial thrombotic endocarditis* (NBTE).

HISTORY. Throughout the last hundred years, infective endocarditis has fascinated students of internal medicine. Although the disease is not particularly common, it has traditionally been given prominence in textbooks and in teaching. Many notable scholars have studied and written on endocarditis, including Virchow, Osler, Thayer, Libman, Friedberg, and Beeson. Contrary to popular belief, the first systemic dose of penicillin was administered at Columbia University in 1940 to a patient with endocarditis, not in Oxford in 1941. The first demonstration that infective endocarditis (previously always fatal) could be cured in a large number of cases by administering penicillin came from Loewe and his colleagues in New York in 1944.

MICROBIOLOGY. Most of the species of bacteria that have been isolated from humans have been reported to cause endocarditis. However, a few common species account for the great majority of infections. Gram-positive streptococci and staphylococci dominate the list: together these organisms cause more than 80 per cent of infections on native valves. Table 269–1 shows representative figures for the reported frequency of the main etiologic microbes on native valves, on prosthetic valves, and in drug addicts. Individual and local experience may differ widely.

The Gram-Positive Cocci. The various alpha-hemolytic (viridans) streptococci together cause more cases of endocarditis than any other bacteria. These relatively avirulent streptococci are found in large numbers in the oropharyngeal and gastrointestinal flora. The species that cause SBE most often (in order of frequency) are *Streptococcus sanguis, S. mutans, S. intermedius,* and *S. mitis.* Next in frequency among the streptococci causing endocarditis are the Group D streptococci, *S. bovis* and *S. faecalis. S. bovis* bacteremia and endocarditis are strongly associated with the presence of lower gastrointestinal lesions, including polyps and colonic cancer. Therefore, recovery of this species from blood cultures should be followed up by investigation for colonic lesions, whether or not the patient has symptoms. *S. faecalis* (enterococcus) causes endocarditis in association with infections of the genital and urinary tract in women of childbearing age and of the urinary tract in elderly men with prostatic disease.

S. pneumoniae occasionally causes acute endocarditis. The triad of coexisting pneumococcal pneumonia, meningitis, and endocarditis is known as *Austrian's syndrome.* It is found in debilitated alcoholics and carries a very poor prognosis.

A few cases of endocarditis are caused by nutritionally dependent streptococci that require media supplemented with

TABLE 269–1. APPROXIMATE FREQUENCY OF VARIOUS ORGANISMS CAUSING INFECTIVE ENDOCARDITIS ON NATIVE VALVES, IN DRUG ABUSERS, AND ON PROSTHETIC VALVES*

	NVE (%)	Intravenous Drug Abusers (%)	Early PVE (%)	Late PVE (%)
Streptococci	65	15	10	35
Viridans, alpha-hemolytic	35	5	<5	25
S. bovis (group D)	15	<5	<5	<5
S. fecalis (group D)	10	8	<5	<5
Other streptococci	<5	<5	<5	<5
Staphylococci	25	50	50	30
Coagulase-positive	23	50	20	10
Coagulase-negative	<5	<5	30	20
Gram-negative aerobic bacilli	<5	15	20	15
Fungi	<5	5	10	5
Miscellaneous bacteria	<5	5	5	5
Diphtheroids, propionibacteria	<1	<5	5	<5
Other anaerobes	<1	<1	<1	<1
Rickettsia	<1	<1	<1	<1
Chlamydia	<1	<1	<1	<1
Polymicrobial infection	<1	5	5	5
Culture-negative endocarditis	5–10	5	<5	<5

*These are representative figures collated from the literature; wide local variations in frequency are to be expected.

Adapted from Durack DT: Infective and non-infective endocarditis. *In* Hurst JW (ed.): The Heart. Chap. 54. New York, McGraw-Hill Book Company, 1982, pp 1250–1277.

L-cysteine or pyridoxine for growth. These fastidious organisms can be difficult to isolate from blood cultures, and the infections they cause are more difficult to cure than infections caused by other streptococci.

Staphylococcus aureus is the leading cause of acute bacterial endocarditis, the predominant species in narcotic addicts with endocarditis, and an important cause of PVE (Table 269–1). *Staphylococcus epidermidis* rarely causes NVE. In contrast, it is a leading cause of PVE.

Other Etiologic Organisms. Gram-negative and fungal infections are described later. Endocarditis caused by *Hemophilus* species is usually associated with *H. aphrophilus, H. paraphrophilus,* or *H. parainfluenzae,* rarely with *H. influenzae. Neisseria gonorrhoeae* endocarditis, an acute disease that often involves the right side of the heart, has become rare since the introduction of penicillin. Endocarditis caused by anaerobic bacteria is also rare, accounting for less than 1 per cent of cases.

PATHOGENESIS AND PATHOLOGY. Figure 269–1 illustrates the sequence of events in pathogenesis of SBE, which usually develops on abnormal heart valves. Previously, the underlying cardiac condition was most often chronic rheumatic valvular heart disease. Today, the leading pre-existing condition for SBE in the United States is congenital heart disease in its various forms, including mitral valve prolapse. Next in frequency is rheumatic disease, but the number of such cases will decline further in the United States and other developed countries as the prevalence of chronic rheumatic heart disease in the general population continues to fall. Other important predisposing conditions are cardiac surgery (especially if a prosthetic valve has been implanted) and previous episodes of infective endocarditis. ABE can attack previously normal as well as damaged

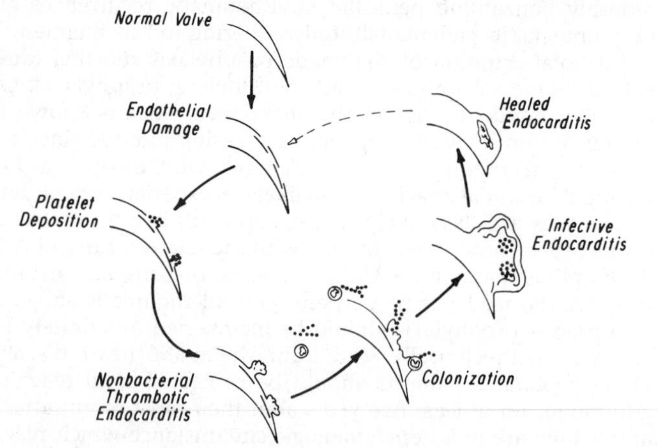

Figure 269–1. A diagram to illustrate the main events in pathogenesis of subacute bacterial endocarditis. Adapted from Durack DT: Infective and non-infective endocarditis. *In* Hurst JW (ed.): The Heart. Chap. 54. New York, McGraw-Hill Book Company, 1982.

valves. Estimates of the frequency of the main underlying heart conditions for patients of various ages with acute or subacute endocarditis are shown in Table 269–2. Table 269–3 lists estimates of the relative risks for endocarditis posed by various cardiac lesions.

The pathogenetic sequence leading to SBE begins with endothelial damage. When subendothelial connective tissue containing collagen fibers is denuded of endothelium, platelets aggregate at the site. These aggregates have been found occasionally on normal valves, but they occur more frequently on the surfaces of valves damaged by congenital or rheumatic disease or by a previous episode of infective endocarditis. These microscopic platelet thrombi may form and resolve harmlessly, but sometimes they are stabilized by deposition of fibrin and grow to form nodular sterile vegetations that are referred to as NBTE. Microscopic examination shows bundles of degenerating platelets held together by strands of fibrin, with few other cells present. This process can be induced in experimental animals by passing a catheter into the heart; NBTE forms at sites where the catheter damages the endothelium. Intracardiac pressure-monitoring catheters produce NBTE in humans in the same way. For unknown reasons, patients with cachexia caused by advanced malignancy or other wasting diseases are prone to form NBTE, which in this setting is usually termed *marantic endocarditis.* The sterile vegetations found in a few patients with systemic lupus erythematosus (Libman-Sacks endocarditis) are another form of NBTE.

The vegetations of NBTE are irregular friable white or tan masses of variable size that are usually found along the lines where valves touch upon closing. They may be so small as to be easily missed on inspection but are frequently rather large. Because there is no inflammatory reaction at the site of attachment, the vegetations of NBTE can often be picked off easily with forceps at necropsy to leave a normal-looking valve surface. These easily dislodged vegetations embolize frequently, often blocking peripheral arteries and causing infarction in myocardium, spleen, kidney, brain, gut, or extremities.

When NBTE is colonized by circulating bacteria, infective endocarditis results. Two important factors that determine

TABLE 269–2. APPROXIMATE FREQUENCY OF THE MAJOR CATEGORIES OF PRE-EXISTING CARDIAC LESIONS IN PATIENTS WITH INFECTIVE ENDOCARDITIS

	Children under 2 Years Old (%)	Children 2 to 15 Years Old (%)	Adults 15 to 50 Years Old (%)	Adults > 50 Years Old (%)	Adults, Intravenous Drug Abusers
No known heart disease	50–70	10–15	10–20	10	50–60
Congenital heart disease	30–50	70–80	20–30	10–20	10
Rheumatic heart disease	Rare	10–20	30–40	20–30	10
Degenerative heart disease	0	0	Rare	10–20	Rare
Previous cardiac surgery	5	10–15	10–20	10–20	10–20
Previous endocarditis	Rare	5	5	5–10	10–20

Adapted from Durack DT: Infective and non-infective endocarditis. *In* Hurst JW (ed.): The Heart. Chap. 54. New York, McGraw-Hill Book Company, 1982, pp 1250–1277.

TABLE 269–3. ESTIMATED RELATIVE RISK FOR INFECTIVE ENDOCARDITIS POSED BY VARIOUS CARDIAC LESIONS

Relatively High Risk	Intermediate Risk	Very Low or Negligible Risk
Prosthetic heart valves	Mitral valve prolapse	Atrial septal defects
Aortic valve disease	Pure mitral stenosis	Arteriosclerotic plaques
Mitral insufficiency	Tricuspid valve disease	Coronary artery disease
Patent ductus arteriosus	Pulmonary valve disease	Syphilitic aortitis
Ventricular septal defect	Previous infective endocarditis	Cardiac pacemakers
Coarctation of the aorta	Asymmetric septal hypertrophy	Surgically corrected cardiac lesions (without prosthetic implants, more than 6 months after operation)
Marfan's syndrome	Calcific aortic sclerosis	
	Hyperalimentation or pressure-monitoring lines that reach the right atrium	
	Nonvalvular intracardiac prosthetic implants	

Adapted from Durack DT: Infective and non-infective endocarditis. *In* Hurst JW (ed.): The Heart. Chap. 54. New York, McGraw-Hill Book Company, 1982, pp 1250–1277.

which organisms will be most likely to cause endocarditis are the frequency with which they are found in the blood and their ability to adhere to fibrin and platelet thrombi. Viridans streptococci enter the blood from the oral cavity frequently (probably daily) and adhere well. They are the leading cause of SBE (Table 269–1). In contrast, *Escherichia coli* adheres poorly and rarely causes endocarditis even though it very frequently causes bacteremia.

Once lodged upon the surface of NBTE, bacteria multiply rapidly and attain high numbers within the vegetation, after which many enter the stationary or resting phase. The presence of bacteria is a powerful stimulus for further localized thrombosis, which causes vegetations to enlarge by accretion of new layers of fibrin. Because these layers protect bacteria from phagocytes, the vegetation provides a sanctuary in which even avirulent bacteria can flourish.

Approximate figures for the frequency with which vegetations are found at various locations in the heart are given in Table 269–4. The frequency with which a cardiac valve is involved by endocarditis is related to the mean blood pressure acting upon it. Accordingly, the aortic and mitral valves are infected far more often than the tricuspid and pulmonary valves. This rule holds for SBE but not for acute endocarditis in intravenous drug abusers, in whom tricuspid valve infection is common (Table 269–4).

Endocarditis usually develops at sites where blood flows from a high-pressure source (e.g., the left ventricle) through an orifice (e.g., a ventricular septal defect) into a low-pressure sink (e.g., the right ventricle). Examples of cardiovascular conditions subject to infection that fit these criteria include mitral regurgitation, aortic stenosis, ventricular septal defect, patent ductus arteriosus, and coarctation of the aorta. Vegetations are usually located on the "downstream" side of these anatomic abnormalities, where pressure effects and turbulence favor deposition of bacteria from the swift stream of blood.

TABLE 269–4. FREQUENCY WITH WHICH ANATOMIC SITES ARE INVOLVED IN SUBACUTE ENDOCARDITIS, ACUTE ENDOCARDITIS, AND ENDOCARDITIS IN DRUG ADDICTS

	SBE (%)	ABE (%)	Endocarditis in Intravenous Drug Abusers (%)
Left-sided valves	85	65	40
Aortic	15–26	18–25	25–30
Mitral	38–45	30–35	15–20
Aortic and Mitral	23–30	15–20	13–20
Right-sided valves	5	20	50
Tricuspid	1–5	15	45–55
Pulmonary	1	Rare	2
Tricuspid and pulmonary	Rare	Rare	3
Left- and right-sided sites	Rare	5–10	5–10
Other sites (patent ductus, VSD, coarctation, jet lesions	10	5	5

Adapted from Durack DT: Infective and non-infective endocarditis. *In* Hurst JW (ed.): The Heart. Chap. 54. New York, McGraw-Hill Book Company, 1982, pp 1250–1277.

Vegetations also may develop at sites where a turbulent regurgitant jet of blood strikes the wall of a cardiac chamber, causing endothelial roughening and reactive endocardial fibrosis. These are called *jet lesions*.

The vegetations of infective endocarditis are variable in appearance. Some are small wartlike nodules, while others have the cauliflower-like polypoid appearance that gave rise to the descriptive term *vegetation*. Some are less than 1 sq mm in size, while others are so large as to block the valve orifice and cause functional stenosis. They may be white, red, tan, or gray. Vegetations in patients with ABE or fungal endocarditis are often larger than those of SBE. Microscopic examination shows colonies of bacteria or masses of fungal hyphae embedded in fibrin and platelets. Infected vegetations usually contain surprisingly few leukocytes. Inflammatory cells may accumulate at the base of the vegetation, where it attaches to the valve. This distorts the valve, superimposing new damage on any pre-existing pathology. If this reaction is severe, the valve may perforate, or an abscess may develop in adjacent tissues. Abscess formation is common in ABE and PVE but not in SBE.

Antibodies to many of the commensal organisms that cause SBE are present in low titer before infection occurs, increase in number during the course of SBE, and decrease after successful treatment. These antibodies do not arrest the progress of SBE and do not provide immunity to future endocardial infection.

The healing process begins even in untreated endocarditis but only reaches completion if antibiotic treatment kills the bacteria. Host cells move in to organize the vegetation; macrophages ingest bacterial and cellular debris; and fibroblasts lay down new collagen. The vegetations gradually shrink over a period of weeks or months and become endothelialized. Recognizable but nonviable bacteria can sometimes be found in sections of valves resected at operation or necropsy, months after infection has been eradicated. The healed valve is often scarred, thickened by fibrosis, and calcified. It may be perforated, and the supporting structures may be damaged. Residual hemodynamic dysfunction, mild or severe, is therefore likely. This condition may worsen over time, although bacteria have been eradicated by treatment long before. The scarred valve remains susceptible to reinfection for life.

CLINICAL FEATURES. All the clinical and laboratory manifestations of infective endocarditis reflect the effects of a systemic intravascular infection and the patient's physiologic and immunologic reaction to it.

History. The onset of subacute endocarditis is usually insidious, with nonspecific complaints, general malaise, anorexia, weakness, and fatigue. This nonspecific syndrome is often described as a "flu-like illness." Low grade intermittent fevers with chills and night sweats are usual. Headaches, myalgias, arthralgias, and back pain are common. A history of heart murmur, congenital heart disease, rheumatic fever, or cardiac surgery may help identify the underlying lesion. The patient may conceal intravenous drug abuse, which should be kept in mind during both interview and examination as a possible mode of infection.

Symptoms of heart failure must be carefully sought because their presence is of great prognostic significance. Embolization and infarction can cause sudden onset of neurologic symptoms such as hemiparesis or abdominal pain due to splenic, renal, or gut infarction. Embolization of a coronary artery can cause silent or symptomatic myocardial infarction. Perforation of a valve or rupture of chordae tendineae can cause sudden onset of severe heart failure.

Physical Examination. Patients with subacute endocarditis may have nonspecific symptoms of subacute systemic infection including pallor, asthenia, and sweating. A variety of interesting peripheral signs may be found on further examination, including petechiae, splinter hemorrhages, Roth's spots, Osler's nodes, Janeway's lesions, and clubbing of the fingers. Some of the characteristics of these signs are summarized in Table 269–5.

Examination of the spleen often shows moderate enlargement but no notable tenderness unless there is a splenic abscess or recent embolic infarction.

On examination of the cardiovascular system, the peripheral pulse is usually rapid because of fever, heart failure, or both. A "collapsing" pulse may be present, indicating aortic incompetence associated with pre-existing aortic valve disease or new aortic insufficiency associated with endocarditis. Individual peripheral arteries may be occluded by emboli, or they may be the site of a mycotic aneurysm.

One or more cardiac murmurs is present in virtually all patients with endocarditis. Murmurs may be caused by pre-existing heart disease, by endocarditis itself, or by both. Up to 15 per cent of patients do not have a heart murmur when first examined, but nearly all develop a murmur before the disease has run its course. New murmurs and changing murmurs are more likely to occur in acute endocarditis than in subacute disease. Development of a new murmur of aortic insufficiency during a febrile illness of unknown origin strongly suggests the diagnosis of endocarditis.

COMPLICATIONS. Heart failure is by far the most important complication of infective endocarditis because it exerts more influence on prognosis and treatment than any other complication. In one representative series, some degree of heart failure was present in 75 per cent of patients with aortic valve disease and endocarditis, in 50 per cent with mitral valve involvement, and in 19 per cent with tricuspid disease.

Arterial embolization is diagnosed in about one third of patients with subacute endocarditis and in up to two thirds of patients with acute endocarditis. Many small or large arterial emboli go undetected. Any artery may be affected. In order of frequency, arteries supplying the brain, lung, myocardium, spleen, and extremities are involved.

Neurologic manifestations of endocarditis are common and clinically important. These include toxic confusional states, stroke, meningoencephalitis, cranial or peripheral nerve lesions, and psychiatric symptoms. About 10 per cent of patients with endocarditis have complaints involving the central nervous system, while 30 to 50 per cent have nervous system involvement at some point during the course of the disease. Cerebral infarction is usually caused by embolism, while cerebral hemorrhage, which is less common than infarction, may be associated with emboli or rupture of a mycotic aneurysm. Heparin therapy increases the risk that an intracranial hemorrhage will occur during the course of infective endocarditis.

Cerebritis secondary to impaction of infected emboli or hematogenous spread of bacteria is quite common, especially in acute bacterial endocarditis caused by *S. aureus*. Cerebritis may progress to form a frank cerebral abscess, which is found in 1 to 5 per cent of cases of acute endocarditis. However, brain abscesses rarely complicate subacute endocarditis.

In up to 15 per cent of patients, examination of the cerebrospinal fluid may show reactive changes consisting of the presence of polymorphonuclear leukocytes and moderately elevated protein concentration. Such reactions are particularly common in acute staphylococcal endocarditis. In most cases cerebrospinal glucose concentrations do not decrease, cultures are negative, and true bacterial meningitis does not develop, except in a few patients with acute pneumococcal or staphylococcal endocarditis.

Mycotic aneurysm is an unusual but important complication that is diagnosed in 3 to 5 per cent of patients. The true incidence is probably higher, but a number pass undetected, especially small aneurysms in the brain. Mycotic aneurysms are caused by an inflammatory reaction in the arterial wall associated with septic microemboli to vasa vasorum or impaction of an infected embolus in the arterial lumen. The site most often involved is the proximal aorta, including the sinuses of Valsalva, followed by arteries to the viscera, extremities, and brain. Living organisms are seldom found in the wall of these aneurysms, even when the underlying endocardial infection is still active. Presumably, the damage that weakens the arterial wall was done by an earlier inflammatory reaction to infected emboli. If an aneurysm enlarges to a certain critical size (prob-

TABLE 269–5. CHARACTERISTICS OF PERIPHERAL SIGNS OF INFECTIVE ENDOCARDITIS

	Petechiae	Splinter Hemorrhages	Roth's Spots	Osler's Nodes	Janeway's Lesions	Clubbing
Appearance	Tiny red hemorrhagic spots	"Splinters" under nails; red when fresh, then brown or black	Small bright red patches with white centers	Pea-sized red or purplish nodules	Red macules	Curvature of the nails in two planes, with swelling of the terminal phalanges
Distribution	Anywhere, especially above clavicles, in mouth and in conjunctivae	Distal third of nails	Retinae	Fingers and toes; occasionally hands and feet	Palms and soles; occasionally on flanks, forearms, ankles, feet, ears	Fingers and/or toes
Incidence	Common, in both SBE and ABE	Common, in both SBE and ABE	Infrequent; usually in SBE	Infrequent; usually in SBE	Infrequent; usually in ABE	Rare; in SBE only
Pathology	Increased capillary permeability; microemboli	Blood in avascular squamous epithelium under nail; due to microemboli or increased capillary fragility	Inflammation and hemorrhage	Intracutaneous local vasculitis; bacteria rarely found; occasional abscess formation; probably embolic in origin	Origin uncertain; possibly embolic or allergic in origin	Soft tissue proliferation, occasionally periosteal new bone formation
Pain	None	None	None	Mild to moderately severe	None	Usually none; sometimes painful
Duration	Days	Weeks	Days	Days	Several hours to days	Weeks to months
Diagnostic significance	Nonspecific; also found in septicemia, after cardiac surgery, and in many other disorders	Nonspecific; found in up to 10% of normal people, and up to 40% of patients with mitral stenosis	Strongly suggestive of endocarditis but not diagnostic	Almost pathognomonic for endocarditis	Unusual in bacteremia without endocarditis	Nonspecific; found in many cardiopulmonary disorders; can be congenital

Adapted from Durack DT: Infective and non-infective endocarditis. *In* Hurst JW (ed.): The Heart. Chap. 54. New York, McGraw-Hill Book Company, 1982, pp 1250–1277.

ably about 1 cm in diameter), it is likely to continue to enlarge and eventually rupture as a result of the physical force of the arterial pressure, despite eradication of the infecting organisms by antimicrobial therapy.

Most patients with subacute endocarditis have some abnormalities in the urinary sediment. In some cases this is due to glomerulonephritis, a relatively common complication that is usually not severe enough to cause significant renal failure. Glomerulonephritis is caused by deposition of immune complexes on the glomerular basement membrane. Other inflammatory manifestations of subacute infective endocarditis that may be mediated by immune complexes include arthritis, tenosynovitis, and possibly pericarditis, Osler's nodes, and Roth's spots. In a few patients with long-term SBE, glomerulonephritis is severe enough to make dialysis necessary. Renal function usually recovers steadily within a few weeks after the start of effective treatment.

SPECIAL FORMS OF INFECTIVE ENDOCARDITIS

ACUTE BACTERIAL ENDOCARDITIS. Several important features distinguish acute from subacute bacterial endocarditis. The diagnosis is usually made within seven days from onset of symptoms. The clinical course is usually measured in days rather than in weeks or months. The associated systemic illness is more severe, and early mortality is higher.

Acute endocardial infection is usually caused by primary pathogens capable of producing invasive infection at other sites. *S. aureus* is the most common cause of acute endocarditis. This species alone accounts for 50 to 70 per cent of cases. The patient is more likely to suffer rapid destruction of the valve, including perforation, so the likelihood that valve replacement will be required is greater. Patients with acute bacterial endocarditis are also more likely to have one or more focal infections outside the heart—in brain, bone, lungs, or other sites. Such foci could be either primary (that is, the portal of entry for endocarditis) or secondary hematogenous infections. In contrast, the organisms that cause subacute bacterial endocarditis rarely cause localized hematogenous infection elsewhere in the body.

Abscesses in the fibrous cardiac skeleton or myocardium are much more likely to form in acute than in subacute endocarditis. If such abscesses are adjacent to the fibers of the conduction system, they may cause conduction defects. Abscesses may be responsible for antibiotic treatment failure.

Because acute bacterial endocarditis is caused by invasive organisms and progresses rapidly, treatment should not be delayed until blood culture results are available. It is important to clear the bloodstream of circulating organisms as soon as possible, both to reduce the risk of death from septicemia and to lessen the chances that metastatic infection will develop elsewhere. When acute endocarditis is strongly suspected, empiric antibiotic therapy should be started immediately after three blood culture samples have been drawn.

ENDOCARDITIS IN DRUG ADDICTS. Endocarditis is the most important of the many infective complications experienced by intravenous drug abusers. Salient features that distinguish endocarditis in this subgroup from the disease in general include: a younger age of onset, a higher proportion of acute cases, a correspondingly higher proportion of cases involving normal cardiac valves, and a high frequency of tricuspid valve infection. The etiologic organisms can gain entry into the bloodstream in various ways: directly, by injection of contaminated materials; or indirectly, from the patient's skin flora, from cellulitis caused by subcutaneous injection of drugs, or from suppurative thrombophlebitis or drug-related infections in other sites such as the lungs. *S. aureus* is the leading etiologic organism. Addicts also have an increased incidence of endocardial infection with gram-negative bacilli, especially *Pseudomonas* species, and fungi.

Drug addicts with acute endocarditis usually experience a brief severe illness, with heavily positive blood cultures. Because the etiologic organisms are often primary pathogens, hematogenous infection elsewhere in the body is common. A common finding on admission is multiple patches of pneumonitis visible on chest x-ray. These are caused by multiple small septic pulmonary emboli arising from vegetations on the tricuspid or occasionally the pulmonary valve. Although acute disease is typical, subacute endocarditis in addicts is not rare, especially in those who have had previous episodes of endocarditis.

The prognosis for young drug addicts with right-sided *S. aureus* infection is good, with mortality rates of less than 5 per cent. Factors that worsen the prognosis include left-sided involvement, particularly aortic, and infection with gram-negative bacilli or fungi. Recurrent episodes of endocarditis are common in addicts who continue to use drugs after their first episode of endocarditis, especially if a prosthetic valve has been inserted.

PROSTHETIC VALVE INFECTION. Prosthetic valve endocarditis should be regarded as a special category, because it differs in many ways from other forms of endocarditis. By definition, early PVE occurs within 60 days of valve placement and late PVE more than 60 days postoperatively. Early PVE occurs at a rate of about 1 per cent, although this figure varies between hospitals. Late PVE is estimated to occur at an overall rate of about 1 per cent per year. The rate for an aortic valve prosthesis is four to five times higher than for a mitral prosthesis.

The progress of PVE may be either acute or subacute, but this cannot be predicted reliably from the infecting organism. For example, even *S. epidermidis*, a nonpathogen that causes indolent chronic disease on native valves, can cause an acute syndrome in early PVE.

The spectrum of organisms causing PVE is quite distinct. *S. epidermidis*, which rarely infects native valves, is a leading cause of both early and late prosthetic valve infection. Gram-negative bacilli and fungi infect prosthetic valves notably more often than they do native valves, especially in early onset cases. The later the onset of PVE after operation, the more nearly the spectrum of etiologic organisms resembles that of native valve endocarditis.

In addition to forming vegetations, infection may spread around the circumference of the sewing ring of the prosthesis, often causing partial dehiscence and paravalvular leaks. Abscess formation in fibrous tissue or myocardium adjacent to the sewing ring is common. Despite these adverse factors, when a prosthetic valve is replaced for infection, early reinfection with the same organism is uncommon.

In general, PVE is harder to cure than most other forms of endocarditis (Table 269–6). This is due partly to the increased frequency of antibiotic-resistant organisms in PVE, and partly to the fact that a foreign body is present at the site of infection. Not surprisingly, the risk of relapse after antibiotic therapy is much higher for PVE than for native valve infection. Valve replacement is often necessary to achieve cure. Antibiotic treatment usually must be continued for a minimum of four to six weeks, sometimes for many months. In some cases in which repeated valve replacement is contraindicated, cure cannot be achieved but suppressive antibiotic therapy is continued indefinitely.

GRAM-NEGATIVE BACTERIAL ENDOCARDITIS. This term usually refers to infection with enteric or environmental gram-negative aerobic bacilli such as *Klebsiella*, *Pseudomonas*, *Serratia*, *Enterobacter*, and *E. coli*. (*Hemophilus* species usually cause subacute endocarditis and are not considered in this group.) Gram-negative endocarditis is a rare disease except in two settings: early prosthetic valve infection and intravenous drug addiction. In these two groups, gram-negative bacilli can account for up to 15 to 20 per cent of cases.

Gram-negative endocarditis often but not always progresses acutely. Patients may develop septic shock. The mortality rate is higher than for gram-positive infections, approaching that of fungal endocarditis. Antibiotic treatment alone is often unsuc-

TABLE 269–6. ESTIMATED BACTERIOLOGIC CURE RATES FOR ETIOLOGIC ORGANISMS TREATED WITH ANTIMICROBIAL THERAPY ALONE OR ANTIMICROBIALS PLUS SURGERY*

Native Valve Endocarditis	Antimicrobial Therapy Alone	Antimicrobial Therapy Plus Surgery
Viridans streptococci, group A streptococci, *S. bovis*, pneumococci, gonococci	98	98
S. fecalis	90	>90
S. aureus (in young drug addicts)	90	>90
S. aureus (in elderly patients with chronic underlying diseases)	50	70
Gram-negative aerobic bacilli†	40	65
Fungi	<5	50

Prosthetic Valve Endocarditis	Early PVE	Late PVE	Early PVE	Late PVE
Viridans streptococci, group A streptococci, *S. bovis*, pneumococci, gonococci	‡	80	‡	90
S. fecalis	‡	60	‡	75
S. aureus	25	40	50	60
S. epidermidis	20	40	60	70
Gram-negative aerobic bacilli†	<10	20	40	50
Fungi	<1	<1	30	40

*Morbidity and mortality will be significantly greater than these figures for bacteriologic cure indicate.

†Excluding *Hemophilus* species.

‡Insufficient data to estimate rate.

Adapted from Durack DT: Infective and non-infective endocarditis. *In* Hurst JW (ed.): The Heart. Chap. 54. New York, McGraw-Hill Book Company, 1982, pp 1250–1277.

cessful, so valve replacement is frequently necessary. Treatment with combinations of two or more antibiotics for six weeks or more is often necessary. Relapse after antibiotic treatment is much more common than for gram-positive infection.

FUNGAL ENDOCARDITIS. Like gram-negative endocarditis, fungal infection of the endocardium is rare except in two groups of patients: those with prosthetic valves and intravenous drug addicts. Although a wide variety of fungal species have been recovered from patients with endocarditis over the years, only two predominate, *Candida* and *Aspergillus spp. C. albicans* endocarditis occurs in patients with central intravascular lines, especially hyperalimentation lines that are allowed to reach the level of the tricuspid valve. Therefore, these infections often involve the right side. *C. parapsilosis* and *C. tropicalis* are more likely to occur in drug addicts and can infect valves on both sides of the heart. Fungal vegetations tend to be bulky and often cause infarctions as a result of embolization of peripheral arteries. Because blood cultures are commonly negative in fungal endocarditis (see earlier discussion), surgical removal of a large embolus from an artery to one of the limbs may be diagnostic as well as therapeutic. Histologic section examination may show hyphae of the infecting fungus.

Few drugs are available for treatment of fungal endocarditis. Amphotericin B is generally used, but the chances of achieving cure with drug therapy alone is extremely low. Cure rates can be greatly increased by surgical removal of vegetations and valve replacement, but mortality remains relatively high compared with that for other forms of endocarditis (Table 269–6).

ENDOCARDITIS IN INFANTS AND CHILDREN. Infective endocarditis is an unusual occurrence in infants. When it does occur, it is most often only one component of systemic bacterial infection caused by an invasive organism such as *S. aureus*. The endocardial infection is likely to follow an acute course and is not uncommonly discovered as an unexpected finding at necropsy in an infant who has died with bacterial infection. Often a normal cardiac valve is involved, as in other forms of acute endocarditis. The remainder of cases are associated with congenital cardiac defects. Because the diagnosis is often delayed or missed, endocarditis in infants has a higher mortality than in other age groups.

In children more than one year old, infective endocarditis is not rare. Most affected children have subacute disease involving congenital cardiac defects. The spectrum of etiologic organisms and the approach to diagnosis and treatment are similar to those in adult infective endocarditis. However, the age and physical size of children must be carefully considered when choosing the best time for cardiac surgery, especially when prostheses must be implanted.

ENDOCARDITIS IN OBSTETRIC AND GYNECOLOGIC PRACTICE. Pregnancy itself poses little increased risk for infective endocarditis, but a few cases develop during delivery or in the puerperium. If the mother has pre-existing valvular disease, bacteremias associated with perinatal infective complications such as amnionitis, endometritis, parametritis, septic thrombophlebitis, or urinary tract infection can seed the endocardium. Septic abortion or pelvic infection related to intrauterine contraceptive devices can also lead to endocarditis in susceptible patients. The leading etiologic organisms in this setting are *S. faecalis*, *S. agalactiae* (Group B), *S. aureus*, and occasionally *Bacteroides* or gram-negative enteric bacilli.

NOSOCOMIAL ENDOCARDITIS. Intensive medical care can predispose to endocarditis in many ways. Endothelial damage can be caused by intracardiac surgery, pressure-monitoring catheters, ventriculoatrial shunts, and hyperalimentation lines if they reach into the right atrium. Portals of entry for microorganisms are provided by wounds, burns, biopsy sites, intravenous and arterial catheters and pacemakers, hemodialysis access sites, urinary catheters, and intratracheal airways. Nosocomial bacteremias are common in seriously ill patients. Therefore, it is not surprising that hospital-acquired infective endocarditis has become increasingly common in the past two decades as intensive care units have proliferated. Perhaps the highest risk is found in severely burned patients, who may sustain repeated episodes of bacteremia while pressure-monitoring catheters are kept in the right side of the heart for long periods. In contrast, diagnostic right heart catheterization for brief periods in patients in a coronary care unit, who seldom develop bacteremia, presents a very low risk for infective endocarditis.

The microbes likely to cause nosocomial endocarditis are staphylococci, *Candida* species, and gram-negative bacilli. The prognosis is worse than for most other forms of infective endocarditis. This is because the patients have serious pre-existing diseases that may obscure the symptoms and signs, thus delaying diagnosis. Also, nosocomially acquired organisms are more likely than streptococci to be resistant to antibiotics.

CULTURE-NEGATIVE ENDOCARDITIS. This term refers to the situation in which the endocardium is infected, but blood cultures remain persistently negative. Possible causes include antibiotic therapy or infection by slow-growing or fastidious microorganisms that are missed because of suboptimal blood culture technique. Culture-negative endocarditis is an uncommon disease. Therefore, when blood cultures from a patient not receiving antibiotics remain persistently negative, that patient probably does not have endocarditis. Fungal endocarditis is an exception. Blood cultures are positive in only about half of patients with *Candida* endocarditis and in less than one fifth of those with *Aspergillus* infection. When culture-negative disease does occur, it is much more likely to follow a subacute than an acute course.

If the clinical findings strongly support the diagnosis of culture-negative endocarditis, a therapeutic trial of antibiotic therapy may be given. This usually consists of a penicillin plus an aminoglycoside for subacute infection, a combination which would cover viridans streptococci, enterococci, *Hemophilus* species, and diphtheroids. If the disease is acute, treatment for *Staphylococcus aureus* must be included. To be of diagnostic value, a proper therapeutic trial must be continued for at least two weeks unless new information changes the situation.

INFECTIVE ENDARTERITIS. An infection located within an artery can mimic infective endocarditis. Possible sites of vegetations include patent ductus arteriosus, coarctation of the aorta, arteriovenous fistulas, and prosthetic vascular grafts. In the past, about one quarter of all patients with an uncorrected patent ductus arteriosus eventually developed bacterial endarteritis. Because many of the underlying lesions are surgically correctable, infective endarteritis is now uncommon in developed countries, with the exception of infections in arteriovenous shunts constructed for the purpose of hemodialysis. When bacterial endarteritis occurs in an aneurysm, the etiologic organisms are usually found within a multilayered thrombus in the lumen of the aneurysm rather than in vegetations.

RECURRENT ENDOCARDITIS. The term *recurrent endocarditis* includes both *relapses* and *reinfections.* Recurent endocarditis has been reported in from 2 to 30 per cent of cases. This wide variation is partly explained by variable duration of follow-up. Intravenous drug abusers are at higher risk than any other group for recurrent endocarditis. A few patients with more than three separate episodes of infective endocarditis have been reported.

The likelihood of relapse after treatment of different forms of infective endocarditis can be predicted from published experience (Table 269–6). Because occasional relapses occur even after optimal treatment, careful follow-up for several months after treatment is mandatory. Most relapses occur within a few days or weeks of ending treatment, but occasional late relapses occur as a result of a few organisms surviving in a metabolically inactive state deep within vegetations.

Reinfection means a new episode of endocarditis has developed after cure of a previous episode. Usually a different species or strain of etiologic organism is involved, but if the second organism is a common viridans streptococcus that appears identical to the first, one cannot be certain whether an episode of recurrent endocarditis represents reinfection or relapse.

DIFFERENTIAL DIAGNOSIS. The differential diagnosis of endocarditis is very wide because its manifestations are numerous and often nonspecific. SBE must be considered in the evaluation of every patient with fever of unknown origin. It can be confused with rheumatic fever, osteomyelitis, tuberculosis, meningitis, intra-abdominal infections, salmonellosis, brucellosis, glomerulonephritis, myocardial infarction, stroke, endocardial thrombi, atrial myxoma, connective tissue diseases, vasculitis, occult malignancy (especially lymphomas), congestive heart failure, pericarditis, and even psychoneurosis. ABE shares many manifestations with septicemias caused by *S. aureus, Neisseria,* pneumococci, and gram-negative bacilli in patients who do not have endocarditis. It may mimic pneumonia, meningitis, brain abscess, stroke, malaria, acute pericarditis, vasculitis, and disseminated intravascular coagulation.

INVESTIGATIONS. ***Routine Tests.*** Results of urinalysis are abnormal in about 50 per cent of cases, showing microscopic hematuria or slight proteinuria or both. Gross hematuria suggests that renal infarction may have occurred. Red cell casts and heavy proteinuria indicate that immune complex glomerulonephritis may be present.

The automated blood count shows only nonspecific abnormalities. Anemia is usual in SBE and fairly common in ABE. Anemia is most often of the hypoproliferative type, with a normochromic normocytic smear. ABE may cause acute hemolysis. A prosthetic valve may cause chronic low grade hemolysis in the absence of infection.

A moderate leukocytosis with some immature forms apparent on smear is often found in SBE, but in many cases the leukocyte count is normal. Patients with ABE usually show a striking neutrophilia with band forms, vacuoles, Döhle bodies, and toxic granulation. In a few cases, careful examination of a Gram-stained smear of the buffy coat will reveal organisms within neutrophils.

The erythrocyte sedimentation rate is almost always elevated, except in a few acute cases of very brief duration.

Blood Culture. This is the single most important investigation in diagnosis of endocarditis. Blood cultures should be drawn from all patients with fever and heart murmur unless their illness is clearly due to another diagnosed disease or the fever resolves quickly without recurrence. Blood cultures should also be taken if a patient with a heart lesion susceptible to endocarditis has other symptoms or signs consistent with infection.

The bacteremia of infective endocarditis is usually continuous, with between 1 and 100 organisms per milliliter of blood in subacute cases. Therefore, it is seldom necessary to draw a large number of blood cultures. The causative organism can be recovered from culture samples taken on the first day of admission in over 90 per cent of patients with culture-positive endocarditis. No more than three separate venous blood cultures should be drawn on the first day. If these show no growth by the second day, two or three further culture samples may be drawn. If the patient has received prior antibiotic therapy, further blood samples may be taken over the following week in a search for recrudescence of bacteremia after antibiotic effect has passed. Otherwise, repeated blood cultures are likely to be uninformative and wasteful.

Ten to 20 ml of blood should be drawn for each culture after careful skin preparation. Skin preparation is especially important because common skin flora (*S. epidermidis* and diphtheroids) can cause endocarditis, and their isolation from blood cultures can cause diagnostic confusion. Pour plates can help to distinguish contaminants from true positive cultures. The culture medium should be adequately supplemented to allow growth of fastidious, nutritionally variant bacteria. When endocarditis is suspected, cultures should be incubated for three weeks and stains made at intervals even if no growth is apparent on inspection.

Subacute endocarditis stimulates the humoral immune system to produce both nonspecific and specific antibodies. A positive test for rheumatoid factor is found in 40 to 50 per cent of subacute cases but rarely in ABE. It can provide a useful diagnostic clue in culture-negative cases. A polyclonal increase in gamma globulins is characteristic. Occasional false-positive serologic test results for syphilis occur.

Hemolytic complement levels may be moderately elevated, normal, or low. The lowest levels are found in patients with immune complex glomerulonephritis. Circulating immune complexes are present in more than 80 per cent of patients with either ABE or SBE but are not diagnostically important in practice. All these immunologic findings revert to normal after eradication of the organisms.

Electrocardiography. Electrocardiography may reveal evidence of otherwise silent myocardial infarction due to embolization of a vegetation to a coronary artery. When a disturbance of conduction develops during the course of endocarditis, extension of infection into the myocardium may have occurred. This could be focal myocarditis or an abscess located close to the conduction system.

Echocardiography. Echocardiography may detect valvular vegetations or help in evaluation of underlying heart disease and cardiac function. This tool can be very helpful, but its sensitivity and specificity for diagnosis of endocarditis are limited. Negative echocardiographic study results do not rule out endocarditis. Very small vegetations cannot be detected, and all the leaflets of the valves cannot be visualized in every patient. Occasionally false-positive readings for vegetations occur, particularly in patients with myxomatous degeneration of a valve.

The larger vegetations typical of acute infection in narcotic addicts and of fungal endocarditis are easier to demonstrate than the smaller lesions found in some patients with SBE. Vegetations on prosthetic valves are difficult to visualize. Sequential echocardiographic studies of vegetations during and after treatment are unreliable as a criterion for success or failure of antibiotic therapy.

Radiography. The chest x-ray is most useful in endocarditis to provide evidence of congestive heart failure. Multiple small patchy infiltrates in the lungs of an intravenous drug abuser with fever strongly suggest the diagnosis of septic emboli arising from right-sided infective endocarditis. Valvular calcification may identify a valve affected by chronic rheumatic or congenital disease. A mycotic aneurysm could cause widening of the aorta.

Abnormal motion of a prosthetic valve can be detected by fluoroscopy, indicating presence of a vegetation or partial dehiscence of the valve from the aortic root. This information can indicate that valve replacement is needed during management of PVE.

Computerized axial tomography can be very useful to define the cause of focal neurologic lesions in patients with endocarditis. Such lesions could be caused by various complications, including cerebritis, infarction, hemorrhage from a mycotic aneurysm, or brain abscess. Angiography is occasionally necessary to demonstrate mycotic aneurysms in the brain or elsewhere.

Cardiac catheterization and cineangiography are not necessary for most patients who respond well to antimicrobial therapy without developing cardiac failure. When treatment seems to be failing and/or operation is considered, cardiac catheterization can provide vital information. In one study of 35 patients who underwent cardiac catheterization during active endocarditis, the precatheterization assessment was significantly modified for 23, the diagnosis of site of valve involvement was altered for 14, and six valve ring abscesses were revealed. Surgery was postponed or cancelled for six patients when catheterization indicated only mild hemodynamic abnormalities. There were no serious complications. This study suggests that catheterization is so useful for selected patients with endocarditis that it should not be avoided for fear of dislodging emboli.

TREATMENT. *General Measures.* The patient should be informed of the diagnosis and treatment plan and comforted. Heart failure, if present, should be managed with bed rest, salt restriction, and drug treatment as necessary. High temperatures and headaches can be treated symptomatically.

Antibiotic Therapy. For optimal antibiotic therapy, certain microbiologic information on the infecting organism is necessary. For most bacteria, both the minimal inhibitory concentration (MIC) and minimal bactericidal concentration (MBC) of the antibiotics likely to be used should be determined. This will form the basis for choice of definitive therapy.

The serum bactericidal titer (SBT or Schlichter test) is frequently used and sometimes useful in the management of endocarditis. The infecting organism is exposed in vitro to the patient's serum, which is drawn while antibiotic therapy is being administered, to determine the maximum dilutions of serum that will inhibit and kill the organism. Clinical experience indicates that the SBT should be 1:8 or higher at intervals during each day of treatment. The SBT provides assurance that the antibiotic(s) present in the patient's serum is actually capable of killing the infecting organism. For gram-positive organisms the serum usually can kill the organism without difficulty, and SBTs are often very high (1:128 to 1:1024). In such cases, SBTs need not be measured repeatedly. The SBT is most likely to be clinically helpful when the physician is treating an unusual organism, using unusual antibiotics, using an unusual regimen (such as oral treatment), or encountering treatment failure. If treatment with unusual combinations of antibiotics is needed, further laboratory tests should be performed to find out whether they are synergistic, indifferent, or antagonistic in combination.

Bactericidal antibiotics should be used for treatment of endocarditis whenever possible. Some patients have been cured with bacteriostatic drugs, but results of treatment with these agents are usually poor, presumably because host defense mechanisms are inadequate in the vegetation. With respect to treatment, the vegetations of infective endocarditis provide a contrast to bacterial pneumonia, in which phagocytes are plentiful and bacteriostatic antibiotics are usually effective. Curative antibiotic therapy for endocarditis must eradicate organisms completely, without the help of phagocytes to eliminate microbes that are relatively resistant to antibiotics because they are in the resting phase.

Clinical experience with treatment of the common forms of bacterial endocarditis caused by gram-positive cocci is so extensive that specific therapeutic regimens can be recommended with confidence. Standard regimens for streptococcal and staphylococcal endocarditis are listed in Table 269–7. Regimens for treatment of endocarditis caused by less common organisms are not listed. For these, treatment must be chosen on the basis of more limited published experience, together with the results of tests performed upon the infecting organism in the microbiology laboratory. One of the beta-lactam antibiotics should be included in the regimen whenever possible.

Empiric Therapy. When the causative organism is unknown, the choice of empiric therapy depends upon whether the patient has acute or subacute disease. For ABE, broad-spectrum therapy that will cover *S. aureus* as well as many species of streptococci and gram-negative bacilli is required. For SBE, a regimen that will treat most streptococci including *S. faecalis* is appropriate. To meet these requirements, the following regimens are suggested (see opposite page):

TABLE 269–7. TREATMENT REGIMENS FOR INFECTIVE ENDOCARDITIS CAUSED BY GRAM-POSITIVE COCCI

Organism	Antibiotic Regimen	Duration, weeks	Comments
Alpha-hemolytic (viridans) streptococci, *S. bovis*	1. Penicillin G 2 million units every 6 hours IV plus streptomycin 10 mg per kilogram every 12 hours IM, *or*	2	For patients <65 years old without renal failure, eighth-nerve defects, or serious complications
	2. Penicillin G 2 million units every 6 hours IV *plus* streptomycin 10 mg per kilogram every 12 hours IM (for first 2 weeks only), *or*	4	For patients with complicated disease, e.g., CNS involvement, shock, moderately penicillin-resistant organism, failed previous treatment
	3. Penicillin G 4 million units every 6 hours IV, *or*	4	For patients >65 years old, with renal failure or eighth-nerve defect
	4. Cefazolin 2 grams every 8 hours IV, *or*	4	For patients allergic to penicillin
	5. Vancomycin 15 mg per kilogram every 12 hours IV	4	For patients allergic to penicillin
Group A streptococci, *S. pneumoniae*	1. Penicillin G 2 million units every 6 hours IV, *or*	2–4	These organisms are usually highly sensitive to pencillin; 2 weeks will be adequate for most cases
	2. Cefazolin 2 grams every 8 hours IV	2–4	
S. fecalis, other penicillin-resistant streptococci	1. Ampicillin 2 grams every 4 hours IV *plus* gentamicin 1.0 mg per kilogram every 8 hours IV, *or*	4–6	Four weeks will be adequate for most cases
	2. Vancomycin 15 mg per kilogram every 12 hours IV *plus* streptomycin 15 mg per kilogram every 12 hours IM	4–6	Four weeks will be adequate for most cases
S. aureus	1. Nafcillin 2 grams every 4 hours IV, *or*	4 or longer	Standard regimen
	2. Nafcillin as above *plus* gentamicin 1.5 mg per kilogram every 8 hours IV for the first 3–5 days, *or*	4 or longer	For patients with severe disseminated staphylococcal disease, gentamicin synergy may be advantageous during early stages of treatment
	3. Cephalothin 2 grams every 4 hours IV, *or*	4 or longer	For patients allergic to penicillin
	4. Vancomycin 15 mg per kilogram every 12 hours IV	4 or longer	For patients allergic to penicillin and cephalosporin; for resistant organisms

1. For ABE, a combination of nafcillin, 2 grams intravenously every four hours plus ampicillin, 2 grams intravenously every four hours plus gentamicin, 1.5 mg per kilogram intravenously every eight hours.

2. For SBE, a combination of ampicillin, 2 grams intravenously every four hours plus gentamicin, 1.5 mg per kilogram intravenously every eight hours.

These regimens should be adjusted if and when the causative organism is identified.

Duration of Therapy. Because infective endocarditis carries significant mortality even when well managed, it is important that treatment be continued long enough to ensure that relapse will not occur. On the other hand, patients with the most easily treated forms of endocarditis should not be subjected to unnecessarily long and expensive treatment in hospital. Extensive experience with treatment of the streptococci provides sufficient grounds for firm recommendations on duration of therapy for these organisms (Table 269–7).

In contrast, the natural history of *S. aureus* endocarditis is highly variable. Some patients recover swiftly without complications, but others remain febrile for several weeks, often with manifestations of disseminated staphylococcal disease such as osteomyelitis. While four weeks of therapy will be adequate for most cases, this must not be regarded as a rigid rule because some patients require treatment for six to eight weeks or longer to achieve cure. In general, the less extensive the published experience with a particular infective agent, the more one should lean toward prolonging treatment in order to provide a reasonable margin of safety. Guidelines on duration of treatment for other organisms are not listed in Table 269–7 because the duration required varies greatly according to individual circumstances.

Anticoagulants. Although the infected vegetation is essentially a thrombotic lesion, there is no evidence that anticoagulants provide a useful therapeutic effect in endocarditis. In fact, simultaneous treatment with antibiotics plus heparin carries a higher risk of serious or fatal intracerebral hemorrhage from mycotic aneurysm or infarction than treatment with penicillin alone. However, coumadin can be given to most patients with endocarditis without excessive risk.

It is therefore best to avoid use of heparin entirely in endocarditis and to discontinue or avoid anticoagulation therapy if possible. However, coumadin may be given if there is a clear-cut indication, taking care not to allow the prothrombin time to rise above 1.5 times normal values. An antibiotic treatment regimen that does not require intramuscular injections should be used if the patient is receiving anticoagulants.

Surgical Treatment. Modern operative treatment constitutes the greatest advance in management of endocarditis since the advent of antibiotics. Because surgery may be needed for any patient during the course of endocarditis, they should be managed close to a thoracic surgical unit. Consultation should be obtained early, so that immediate operation can be performed if necessary.

Aortic or mitral valvular incompetence with consequent acute left ventricular failure can occur without warning, even in the most favorable forms of endocarditis. These patients need valve replacement in order to reverse cardiac failure resulting from new or worsening valvular dysfunction. Replacement of an infected prosthesis is often necessary for cure because prosthetic valve infection is more difficult to eradicate with antibiotics than is native valve infection. Repeated major emboli constitute a relative indication for valve replacement. Occasionally, a patient remains septic despite antibiotic therapy. Operation may then be required for infection control rather than for the hemodynamic consequences of infection. Operation to close a patent ductus arteriosus or septal defect, to excise a coarctation of the aorta, or to relieve asymmetric septal hypertrophy may be required as part of treatment of endocarditis engrafted upon these lesions.

Good surgical management for endocarditis depends on correct timing for valve replacement. If operation is undertaken too soon, unnecessary operative mortality and early and late morbidity of valve replacement may result. Some patients will respond quickly to medical therapy, so that operation can be postponed indefinitely. If time is available for treatment of septicemia, renal failure, pneumonia, myocarditis, conduction defects, or other complications before valve replacement, ventricular function will improve and operative risk will be correspondingly lower. Given a few days, antibiotic therapy should eradicate or at least greatly reduce the population of organisms on the valve, thus increasing the chance that an artificial valve can be inserted without itself becoming infected. However, if surgery is delayed too long patients may die suddenly, or their hemodynamic status may deteriorate so that operation is no longer feasible. This is a tragic error, because some of these patients could have been saved by earlier operation.

Frequent re-examination of the patient, together with echocardiography and/or cardiac catheterization to extend the clinical findings, is indicated in every case in which operation may be needed. The natural history of the type of endocarditis being treated should be taken into account. Penicillin-sensitive streptococcal endocarditis can almost always be bacteriologically cured (Table 269–6), and the prognosis is good if cardiac failure does not occur. Thus, operation should usually be considered only for patients with cardiac failure who do not respond to medical treatment. Similarly, narcotic addicts with acute staphylococcal endocarditis have a relatively good prognosis, so operation should be reserved for those who develop serious heart failure. At the other end of the spectrum, the likelihood that fungal prosthetic valve endocarditis can be eradicated with antifungal drugs alone is negligible, even in the absence of heart failure (Table 269–6). Such patients usually should undergo valve replacement early, without waiting to test the remote possibility that antifungal treatment could eradicate the infection. Aortic valve involvement, staphylococcal infection in patients other than drug addicts, gram-negative infection, prosthetic valve infection, and extension of infection into the myocardium should be regarded as other relative indications favoring early valve replacement.

PROGNOSIS. Infective endocarditis is unusual among infectious diseases in that it is always fatal if untreated. Most of the rare cases of apparent recovery reported in the preantibiotic era probably did not have infective endocarditis, which can be diagnosed with absolute certainty only at operation or necropsy. The median interval between onset of symptoms and death in patients with untreated subacute endocarditis was about six months, with wide individual variation. Almost all patients with acute infective endocarditis died in less than four weeks.

Favorable prognostic factors include infection with penicillin-sensitive streptococci, a youthful patient, absence of serious pre-existing diseases, and early diagnosis and treatment. The rate of recovery for many young drug addicts with *S. aureus* infection of the tricuspid valve is excellent—greater than 95 per cent.

Heart failure is by far the most important adverse prognostic factor. Other adverse factors include aortic valve involvement, renal failure, culture-negative disease, gram-negative or fungal infection, prosthetic valve infection, and presence of an abscess in the valve ring or myocardium.

Today, bacteriologic cure can be achieved in most patients with bacterial endocarditis (Table 269–6). This is not true for infection with resistant gram-negative bacilli and fungi, but fortunately these are uncommon. Despite the ability to eradicate most organisms, both early and long-term mortality and morbidity of infective endocarditis remain significant because of damage already done before treatment. Follow-up of patients cured of infective endocarditis shows a five-year survival of only 60 to 70 per cent.

PREVENTION. Because endocarditis is a serious disease, antibiotics are usually given to susceptible patients during medical and dental procedures known to cause bacteremia, in an

TABLE 269–8. AUTHOR'S RECOMMENDATIONS FOR PROPHYLAXIS OF ENDOCARDITIS*

Types of Regimen	Indications	Drug and Dosage
Standard	For dental procedures and oral or upper respiratory tract surgery	Penicillin V 2 grams orally 1 hour before, then 1 gram 6 hours later†
Special	Parenteral regimen for high-risk patients; also for gastrointestinal or genitourinary tract procedures	Ampicillin 1 to 2 grams IM or IV *plus* gentamicin 1.5 mg per kilogram IM or IV, 0.5 hours before†
	Parenteral regimen for penicillin-allergic patients	Vancomycin 1 gram IV *slowly* over 1 hour, starting 1 hour before; *add* gentamicin 1.5 mg per kilogram IM or IV if gastrointestinal or genitourinary tract is involved†
	Oral regimen for penicillin-allergic patients (oral and respiratory tract procedures)	Erythromycin 1 gram orally 1 hour before, then 0.5 gram 6 hours later†
	Oral regimen for minor gastrointestinal or genitourinary tract procedures	Amoxicillin 3 grams orally 1 hour before, then 1.5 grams 6 hours later†
	Parenteral regimen for cardiac surgery including prosthetic valve placement	Cefazolin 2 grams IV on induction of anesthesia, repeated 8 and 16 hours later,‡ *or* Vancomycin 1 gram IV *slowly* over 1 hour, starting on induction of anesthesia, then 0.5 gram IV 8 and 16 hours later‡

*These are empiric suggestions. No regimen has been proven effective, and prevention failures may occur with any regimen. These recommendations are not intended to cover all clinical situations; practitioners should use their own judgment on safety and cost-benefit issues in each individual case. Several additional doses may be given if the period of risk for bacteremia is prolonged, but prophylaxis should not be extended for days.

†Pediatric dosages: ampicillin 50 mg per kilogram; erythromycin 20 mg per kilogram for first dose, then 10 mg per kilogram; gentamicin 2 mg per kilogram; vancomycin 20 mg per kilogram; penicillin V, cefazolin, and amoxicillin for children weighing more than 60 pounds, use same dose as for adults; for children weighing less than 60 pounds, use half the adult dose.

‡Gentamicin 1.5 mg per kilogram IV may be given with each dose only if postoperative gram-negative infections have occurred with significant frequency.

Adapted from Durack DT: Nine controversies in the management of endocarditis. *In* Petersdorf RG, et al. (eds.): Update V. Harrison's Principles of Internal Medicine. New York, McGraw-Hill Book Company, 1984, pp 35–46.

attempt to prevent this infection. Unfortunately, there is no proof that this practice is effective. Meaningful cost-benefit ratios cannot be calculated, and any recommendations are therefore necessarily empiric.

One approach is to consider two factors in each situation: (1) the relative risk for endocarditis posed by the patient's heart condition and (2) the relative risk for endocarditis posed by the procedure. If both risks are judged to be significant, prophylactic antibiotics should be given. If one or both of these risk factors is judged to be negligible, prophylaxis should be omitted. The first of these two questions can be approached by using a ranking like that shown in Table 269–3. The second can be approached by knowing something of the frequency of bacteremia after the procedure in question and the number of cases of endocarditis attributed to it. For example, if a patient with aortic stenosis were to have dental extraction or urologic surgery, attempted prevention with antibiotics would be appropriate. If the same patient were to undergo gastroscopy, antibiotics would not be indicated because that procedure poses very little risk for endocarditis.

Prophylaxis for endocarditis is probably not required to cover most gastrointestinal diagnostic procedures such as endoscopy or radiocontrast studies, nor for normal delivery, therapeutic abortion, dilation and curettage, insertion or removal of intrauterine contraceptive devices in the absence of local infection, cardiac catheterization, insertion of pacemakers, endotracheal intubation, or bronchoscopy. However, some physicians choose to cover even these low-risk procedures in patients with prosthetic valves because they are at higher risk for endocarditis.

The indication for prophylactic antibiotics in patients with mitral valve prolapse remains controversial. MVP increases an individual's risk for endocarditis by five to eight times and underlies a significant proportion of cases of subacute bacterial endocarditis. However, mitral valve prolapse is very common in the general population, while endocarditis is relatively uncommon, so prolapse should be regarded as a low-risk lesion for endocarditis. Many authorities currently recommend prophylaxis for patients with prolapse, especially those with mitral regurgitation, but an estimate of benefits in relation to costs has indicated that prophylaxis for prolapse is probably not cost-effective. In the author's opinion, it is reasonable to give prophylaxis to MVP patients undergoing procedures that cause significant bacteremia because the costs and risks of oral penicillin therapy for an individual are very low, and a serious disease may occasionally be prevented. However, use of antibiotics in this setting should be considered optional rather than mandatory. Parenteral prophylaxis for MVP patients probably should be avoided to reduce the risk of anaphylaxis.

Specific recommendations for prophylaxis of endocarditis are listed in Table 269–8.

AHA Committee Report: Treatment of infective endocarditis due to viridans streptococci. Circulation 63:730A, 1981. *A brief, authoritative statement on treatment options for endocarditis caused by streptococci.*

Bisno AL: Treatment of Infective Endocarditis. New York, Grune & Stratton, 1982. *This book deals with many aspects of endocarditis besides treatment. It provides a good source for references.*

Durack DT: Infective and non-infective endocarditis. *In* Hurst JW (ed.): The Heart. Chap. 54. New York, McGraw Hill Book Company, 1982, pp 1250–1277. *A general review of infective and noninfective endocarditis in a leading cardiology textbook (181 references).*

Durack DT: Prophylaxis of endocarditis. *In* Mandell GL, Douglas RG, Bennett JE (eds.): Principles and Practice of Infectious Diseases. New York, John Wiley & Sons (in press), 1984. *This chapter analyzes the problems of endocarditis prophylaxis in detail and reviews current recommendations (52 references).*

Karchmer AW, Dismukes WE, Buckley MJ, Austen WG: Late prosthetic valve endocarditis: Clinical features influencing therapy. Am J Med 64:199, 1978. *This paper reports on patients with late prosthetic valve endocarditis, comparing survival according to etiologic organisms and medical as opposed to surgical treatment. Various features that carry a poor prognosis are identified, and relative indications for surgery are discussed.*

Rahimtoola SH: Infective Endocarditis. New York, Grune & Stratton, 1978. *A heavily referenced book, with good material on pathogenesis, pathology, and endocarditis in addicts and fungal endocarditis.*

Reisberg BE: Infective endocarditis in the narcotic. Prog Cardiovasc Dis 22:193, 1979. *A useful review of infective endocarditis in narcotic addicts. The importance of tricuspid valve infection and the effect of different infecting organisms and the sites involved on prognosis are analyzed.*

Weinstein L: Infective endocarditis. *In* Braunwald E (ed.): Heart Disease. A Textbook of Cardiovascular Medicine. Philadelphia, W. B. Saunders Company, 1984, pp 1136–1182. *A long, detailed chapter in a major cardiology textbook (382 references).*

Staphylococcal Infections

270. STAPHYLOCOCCAL INFECTIONS

John N. Sheagren

Staphylococci are ubiquitous in nature. All humans are colonized by "nonpathogenic" staphylococci. In addition the "pathogenic" coagulase-producing *Staphylococcus aureus* is present transiently in a high percentage of people and is chronically carried by about 15 per cent of the normal population. As would be expected, staphylococci, whether causative of infection or as contaminants, are frequently isolated from cultures.

S. aureus itself is one of the most important bacterial pathogens of man. It can be aggressively invasive, spreading rapidly through soft tissues, directly invading bones and other support structures and ultimately, under conducive circumstances, seeding the bloodstream to produce a fulminant picture of septic shock and disseminated intravascular coagulation. Conversely, *S. aureus* can lie dormant deep within tissues for years without causing disease. The balance between host and parasite that results in infection with a given strain of staphylococci is not known and continues to be the subject of active research.

Staphylococci are the most important hospital-associated gram-positive organisms and rank only behind *Escherichia coli* in overall incidence of infections in the hospital setting. In the community, staphylococci, particularly *S. aureus*, are the leading cause of acute, serious, and progressive skin, soft tissue, and posttraumatic infections. A thorough understanding of the pathogenetic mechanisms and clinical manifestations of staphylococcal infections is crucial to the care of septic patients in every medical environment.

BACTERIOLOGY. Staphylococci are members of the family micrococcaceae of which there are two genera of major clinical importance, the micrococci and the staphylococci. These two genera are both catalase positive, but only staphylococci can anaerobically ferment glucose to produce acid. The staphylococci in turn have three clinically important species: *S. aureus*, *S. epidermidis*, and *S. saprophyticus*. *S. aureus* alone has the capacity to produce coagulase, which is detected by timed incubation of a sample of a broth culture with citrated rabbit plasma. This test results in the production of a clot and permits the relatively rapid separation of *S. aureus* from the coagulase-negative species (*S. epidermidis* and *S. saprophyticus*). Almost all laboratories label all coagulase-negative organisms as "*S. epidermidis*," which results in the failure to differentiate at least one clinically important subspecies, *S. saprophyticus*. *S. saprophyticus* is coagulase negative but ferments mannitol and can also be identified by resistance to novobiocin. *S. saprophyticus* is a frequent cause of urinary tract infections, almost always in young women; these organisms are sensitive to all generally prescribed urinary tract antibiotics.

As regards *S. aureus*, the word *aureus* comes from the Latin word meaning gold and refers to the fact that most *S. aureus* colonies develop a bright golden-yellow color on blood agar media. However, *S. aureus* speciation is now assigned to all strains producing coagulase, whether or not they are golden in color. In addition to the production of coagulase by *S. aureus*, almost all strains ferment mannitol and contain deoxyribonuclease (DNAase). Staphylococci grow well both anaerobically and aerobically: thus, both aerobic and anaerobic bottles in a blood culture set from a truly bacteremic patient are usually positive.

The name staphylococcus comes from the fact that these organisms grow in clusters in liquid or semisolid media or within tissues when causing infection. However, in material obtained from abscesses, the organisms can sometimes be confusing in morphology, being quite variable in size, shape, and tendency toward clustering. Occasionally the organisms may grow in pairs or even chains, and confusion with streptococci is possible. Nonetheless, to the trained eye the size and general characteristics of the organism usually permit an accurate diagnosis of a pure staphylococcal lesion when the stained smear is carefully examined.

No reproducible serologic typing schemes are available to classify staphylococci. However, bacteriophage typing has been extremely useful in identifying strain characteristics of *S. aureus* and in providing epidemiologic data. Recently, bacteriophage typing has begun to be applied to *S. epidermidis*, and over 50 per cent of recovered strains can now be typed by this system. Bacteriophages are viruses that attach to the mucopeptide-teichoic acid complex of the cell wall. Over 100 different phages are now available for use in typing *S. aureus*, and five major groups of organisms having generally similar characteristics have been designated (phage groups I through V). For example, some phage groups of staphylococci are more likely to produce certain toxins than are others. Coagulase-negative *S. epidermidis* has also been divided into subgroups, known as biotypes, based on biochemical testing.

EPIDEMIOLOGY. Staphylococci may colonize almost all animal species and, as noted earlier, *S. epidermidis* is universally present on the human skin. The carrier state of *S. aureus* is clinically important. Humans carry *S. aureus* predominantly in the nasopharynx, although some individuals can be heavily colonized in the axillae, groin, and perirectal region. The heavily colonized individual may become a source of recurrent infections both to himself and to surrounding contacts. Most humans probably carry a few *S. aureus* organisms among the normal flora of every body site but at such a low level that routine cultures rarely reveal the organism. As stated earlier, about 15 per cent of normal, non-hospital-associated persons more or less chronically carry a heavy growth of *S. aureus* in their noses.

The definition of the carrier state is a simple one: from swab culture of the anterior nares of a carrier, multiple colonies of *S. aureus* are visually identified on a blood agar culture plate. Clearly this definition is imprecise, because the more intensely one focuses attention on the organism the higher will be the percentage of normal individuals found to carry it. Nonetheless, colony counts of the nasopharyngeal flora consistently indicate a small group of persons who harbor relatively large numbers of the organism.

The factors that result in high growth rates and numbers of *S. aureus* in the nares of certain individuals and not in others are unknown. There is no evidence that the immune response to the organism (for example, secretory immunoglobulins or other inhibitory substances) plays a major role in the acquisition and loss of the organism from the nose and throat, as is the case for the meningococcus. Data indicate that the teichoic acid moiety in the cell wall of *S. aureus* mediates the adherence of the organism to nasal mucosal cells, a phenomenon of major import in mucous membrane colonization. Also, it is highly probable that the carrier state is influenced by the ability of other members of the normal bacterial flora of the nose, throat, and skin to suppress growth of a given strain of staphylococcus. Most probably, other staphylococci or micrococci (or both) will turn out to be instrumental in controlling the growth of a newly introduced staphylococcal strain. In fact, clinical use of this concept has already been attempted via the process termed *bacterial interference*. Bacterial interference is the concept that a nonpathogenic strain of staphylococcus, once established, seems to reduce the likelihood of acquisition of another, more pathogenic strain (see later section).

There is an interesting association between the nasal carriage of *S. aureus* and any condition associated with small breaks in the skin and mucous membranes. It has been known for a long time that patients with a variety of dermatoses, especially atopic dermatitis, are very likely to be heavily colonized with *S. aureus.* In fact, patients with eczematous skin diseases may be heavily colonized in the lesions but have few organisms on the intervening normal skin. Possibly related to these observations is the fact that patients who regularly use needles have an increased rate of carriage of *S. aureus.* Drug addicts, diabetics injecting insulin, patients on hemodialysis, and even patients receiving brief courses of allergy shots all have an increased rate of nasal carriage of *S. aureus.* This phenomenon is clinically important, because the organism carried in the nose and throat is often identical to that in the bloodstream of drug-abusing patients with endocarditis. Similarly, studies done years ago demonstrated that patients who entered hospitals for surgical procedures and who were carriers of *S. aureus* had increased rates of wound infections with the carried organism. Thus, the sequence of events leading to infection with *S. aureus* seems to be the following: persons who for whatever reason begin to carry the organism in the nose are at risk of seeding the organism to other bodily sites and to breaks in the skin (for example, wounds or points of insertion of intravascular catheters). From such colonized peripheral sites, the organism may invade and cause destructive and rapidly progressive local and systemic septic complications.

Carriage of staphylococci within the gastrointestinal tract has not been extensively studied. However, normally a few staphylococci can usually be isolated. *S. epidermidis* is not uncommonly isolated from the stool but probably represents contamination from the perianal skin. Staphylococci, especially *S. aureus,* may grow to very high titers in the gastrointestinal tract in the presence of antibiotic therapy and cause gastrointestinal symptoms; the presumption is that antibiotics suppress the more sensitive normal floral components that are responsible for inhibiting the growth of *S. aureus.* This rationale is similar to that for the emergence of *C. difficile* in the syndrome of antibiotic-associated colitis (see Ch. 278).

Newborn infants rapidly experience an increasing rate of colonization following birth. It is not uncommon within nurseries to note infant colonization rates of 25 to 30 per cent. Most infants remain asymptomatic; on occasion, however, outbreaks of disease within nurseries may occur, sometimes traceable to a common carrier. Adult patients become increasingly colonized with *S. aureus* the longer they remain in the hospital. Once a hospitalized individual becomes a carrier (expecially individuals with open, actively infected lesions), the nasally carried organisms may spread to other anatomic sites, to clothing and other items within the room, and to individuals with whom the patient has contact. The most effective technique for stopping transmission of staphylococci from person to person, especially in a hospital setting, is to wash one's hands meticulously immediately before and immediately after examining each patient. This process is particularly important when examining a patient with a gross, obviously staphylococcal lesion or with a chronic exudative dermatosis. Such patients should always be managed by appropriate isolation procedures while they are hospitalized.

PATHOGENESIS. Whether or not an infection develops with any microorganism depends on the balance between the aggressiveness of the organism and the level of defense provided by the host. Thus, organisms that are highly virulent may regularly infect normal hosts and, conversely, nonpathogenic (saprophytic) organisms usually only cause infection in the face of a significant impairment of host defense. The following paragraphs will first describe those microbial characteristics that lead to the presence or absence of virulence and then the primary mechanisms by which the host attempts containment.

Microbial Virulence. The factor that makes certain strains of staphylococci virulent and others nonpathogenic is unknown. A variety of extracellular enzymes is produced by *S. aureus,* many probably participating in the pathogenic capabilities of the organism. For example, in the case of streptococci, hyaluronidase probably assists the organism in its rapid spread through tissues. A variety of other enzymes may also degrade other tissue elements, may lyse inflammation-associated coagulation (coagulase), and may be directly toxic to either white cells (leukocidins) or platelets. A variety of studies in experimental models has shown a high correlation between coagulase production and organism virulence.

Numerous toxins are produced by *S. aureus.* Some have endotoxic capabilities when injected into tissues (for example, the alpha and beta toxins). *S. aureus* frequently produces an enterotoxin, and at present six enterotoxins (A through F) have been described. Enterotoxin F is identical to pyrogenic exotoxin C, the toxin involved in the toxic shock syndrome. Another well described toxin is the exfoliative toxin responsible for the staphylococcal scalded skin syndrome.

The capsular and cell wall components of *S. aureus* clearly participate in the pathogenesis of certain clinical syndromes produced by the organism. Many *S. aureus* strains have a polysaccharide capsule covering the complex rigid cell wall matrix that consists of peptidoglycan and teichoic acid (ribitol in *S. aureus* and predominantly glycerol in *S. epidermidis*). In most strains of *S. aureus* a unique substance, *protein A,* is also part of the cell wall. Protein A is an immunologically active substance having high affinity for the FC fragment of immunoglobulins, particularly subgroups of IgG. Thus, protein A binds to and aggregates IgG molecules and, interestingly, fixes complement in the process. Protein A has emerged as an extremely useful immunochemical substance for extraction or quantitation (or both) of IgG molecules from biologic specimens. Whether protein A plays some role in any of the clinical syndromes produced by *S. aureus* is unknown. However, it is intriguing to speculate that protein A interacting nonspecifically with plasma immunoglobulins and fixing complement in the process might contribute both to the pathogenesis of septic shock and to the rapid onset of glomerular damage often present in patients with staphylococcal bacteremia or endocarditis.

The presence of a capsule varies greatly from strain to strain and may explain some of the biologic differences between organisms as they invade tissues or the bloodstream. The capsule inhibits phagocytosis by interfering with the interaction between the underlying teichoic acid–peptidoglycan complex and complement, which is activated primarily via the alternative pathway. Thus, encapsulated strains are protected in tissues from the complement-mediated attack by polymorphonuclear leukocytes (PMNs). Along with the enzymes described above, the capsule undoubtedly increases the ability of *S. aureus* to protect itself as it spreads through tissues and therefore is an important virulence factor for tissue infections. Paradoxically, while unencapsulated organisms are more likely to be contained in tissues, should the bloodstream be reached (for example in a narcotics addict directly injecting carried organisms into the blood stream), the syndrome of septic shock and disseminated intravascular coagulation (DIC) may result. The syndrome of septic shock follows massive intravascular complement, coagulation system, and kinin system activation (see Ch. 256). In such a situation, unencapsulated strains of *S. aureus* produce septic shock exactly like gram-negative bacteria wherein the cell wall lipopolysaccharide (endotoxin) activates the responsible inflammatory systems.

Host Defense Aspects. The primary mechanism by which the host defends against staphylococci, expecially *S. aureus,* is via the nonspecific defense system. The specific, antibody and T cell-mediated, host defenses appear to participate very little, if at all, in defense against *S. aureus.* Thus, while antibodies are of theoretical value against encapsulated strains of *S. aureus,* no data exist to show that antibody (commonly present in the sera of most individuals against a variety of cell wall antigens and toxins of *S. aureus*) is of any clinical value. Previous attempts to develop vaccines against the organism have not yielded documented clinical benefits.

The nonspecific host defense system consists of the barrier

systems (skin and mucous membranes) plus the complement-mediated polymorphonuclear (PMN) leukocyte assault on invading organisms. Patients with defects in intracellular killing of bacteria by the PMN (for example, as in the chronic granulomatous disease of childhood or the Chediak-Higashi syndrome) are particularly prone to develop serious infections with *S. aureus*.

Certain pathologic states with highly elevated levels of IgE predispose the patient to recurrent, chronic infections with *S. aureus*. Job's syndrome is a condition wherein an elevated IgE level associated with eczematous skin changes somehow predisposes the patient to recurrent soft tissue infections. No one knows how or why staphylococcal infections are enhanced by highly elevated levels of IgE. The theory is that mast cell activation in the neighborhood of a focus of *S. aureus* infection somehow impairs normal PMN-mediated defense mechanisms. Some recent studies have shown that antihistamines may at least partially correct the defect demonstrated in these patients.

The presence of a foreign body has a dramatic effect on the development of staphylococcal infections. For example, infections with *S. epidermidis* strains are particularly common in patients harboring foreign bodies such as prosthetic heart valves, cerebrospinal fluid shunts, and artificial joints. As for *S. aureus*, the inoculum required experimentally to produce a skin infection in a healthy individual is very large (10^6 to 10^7 organisms); however, the presence of even a small foreign body such as a suture reduces the dose required to produce an infection to less than 100 organisms. Thus, foreign bodies must provide a nidus of chronic inflammation in which leukocyte accumulation is impaired. An area ripe for productive clinical investigation is how a foreign body impairs host defenses.

CLINICAL MANIFESTATIONS

This section will review two broad categories of types of human disease produced by staphylococci: first discussed will be diseases related to the production of toxins by staphylococci (exclusively *S. aureus*) and then diseases related to direct organism invasion.

TOXIN-PRODUCED DISEASES. As noted above, *S. aureus* produces a variety of toxins. Clinically, the most important toxins are the enterotoxins and exfoliative toxin. The distinction between the different types of toxins is becoming less clear: for example, the toxin involved in the toxic shock syndrome (pyrogenic exotoxin C) has recently been shown to be identical to enterotoxin F; furthermore, that toxin clearly has exfoliative properties.

Staphylococcal Gastroenteritis. While gastrointestinal disease may be caused by massive, physical overgrowth of *S. aureus* within the gastrointestinal tract, most cases of gastroenteritis follow the ingestion of foods containing a preformed toxin. The toxin itself is not produced within the gastrointestinal tract. A number of extracellular toxins are produced in large amounts when the culture media contains high amounts of carbohydrate (as in sugary and starchy foods contaminated by *S. aureus*) and when such a mixture is incubated at appropriate conditions of temperature and acidity. Toxin ingestion results in increased intestinal peristalsis, profuse nausea, vomiting, diarrhea, and in some cases fever. The organism and its preformed toxin can usually be identified in point source outbreaks from the epidemiologically implicated foodstuff. Toxin-mediated staphylococcal gastroenteritis is usually self-limited, lasting anywhere from 12 to 24 hours; however, supportive therapy (fluid and electrolyte maintenance) may on occasion be required. Antibiotics are not useful.

The Toxic Shock Syndrome (TSS). TSS is almost certainly caused by the production of a toxin at the site of a localized, often relatively asymptomatic or unnoticed infection with any strain of *S. aureus* capable of toxin production. The most common site of infection is the vagina, almost invariably in association with tampon usage. The few (less than 10 per cent) TSS cases that have not been associated with infection of the female genital tract have usually been associated with infected foreign bodies (such as sutures) in surgical wounds. As noted earlier, both enterotoxin F and pyrogenic exotoxin C were described by independent investigators as putative toxins responsible for the syndrome. Recent studies have confirmed the two substances to be identical. Toxin production by strains of *S. aureus* isolated from cases of TSS have been shown to be related to lysogeny, the presence of a temperate bacteriophage. Presumably, the clinical manifestations of the syndrome are produced when the toxin is absorbed either through mucous membranes or from a subcutaneous tissue site of colonization or infection. The toxin probably produces its systemic effects by directly damaging peripheral tissues.

The clinical syndrome that results is dramatic. The patient, almost always unaware of the focus of toxin production, experiences the abrupt onset of high fever, myalgias, and profuse nausea, vomiting and watery diarrhea. Within the first several days, a sunburn-like rash appears, and the conjunctivae become injected. On biopsy of the skin lesions, the epidermis exhibits cleavage in the basilar layers, differentiating it from the staphylococcal scalded skin syndrome (discussed later) and from viral and drug eruptions. The patient often becomes progressively more ill and is frequently in frank shock when presenting for care. A diffuse capillary leak syndrome rapidly develops, and the serum albumin concentration often plummets to less than 2 grams per 100 ml. Hypotension and frank shock are common and are often associated with the adult respiratory distress syndrome (ARDS), acute renal failure, and abnormalities in literally every organ system evaluated. For example, almost all patients exhibit an altered state of mentation, hepatocellular malfunction, elevated levels of muscle enzymes, thrombocytopenia, and a low serum calcium concentration (far out of proportion to the hypoalbuminemia). Highly elevated levels of calcitonin are present for which no explanation presently exists.

Therapy is both supportive and specific. Identification of the site of infection, drainage thereof (most frequently consisting of removal of contaminated tampons), and antibiotic therapy with beta-lactamase-resistant antistaphylococcal agents are all indicated. Antibiotics do not change the course of the initial illness but seem to prevent relapse, at least in tampon-associated cases. It is important to realize that patients with TSS are rarely bacteremic, and therefore this type of shock syndrome is different from bacteremic, inflammatory system-mediated shock (see Ch. 256), wherein complement, coagulation, and kinin system activation seem to be primary events.

The prognosis in TSS is favorable despite the fact that most patients are critically ill for a period of time in the hospital. However, between 5 and 10 per cent of patients studied so far succumb to the illness. Since recurrences, generally milder, are relatively common following tampon-associated TSS (up to 10 per cent over the subsequent three menstrual cycles), women who have recovered from TSS should avoid tampon use for at least six months following the illness.

The Staphylococcal Scalded Skin Syndrome (SSSS). SSSS is another toxin-mediated disease produced by certain strains of *S. aureus*, usually of phage group II. These organisms produce an exfoliative toxin that when injected experimentally into infant mice produces dramatic skin desquamation and mimics in every way the clinical syndrome seen in human infants. This disease is also produced by a toxin originating in a distant focus of infection: a toxin-producing organism produces and releases the exfoliative toxin that after absorption and systemic dissemination causes cleavage of the middle layers of the epidermis, bulla formation, and ultimately slippage of the superficial layer of the epithelium on gentle pressure (a positive *Nikolsky's sign*). The skin is often tender and very erythematous, producing a sunburn-like rash during the initial phase. Infants are most commonly involved, and outbreaks of this syndrome have occurred in nurseries after introduction of a toxin-producing strain. Often mild or asymptomatic omphalitis is the source.

In older children, the portal of infection can be any minor skin abrasion, furuncle, or some other infected local site. The conjunctival sac may be the source as a result of mild conjunctivitis, and this source often goes undetected. The syndrome has occasionally been reported to involve adults. The rash proceeds rapidly to desquamation, but healing is rapid and is related to how promptly the peripheral site has been treated. Mortality of SSSS is very low.

Differentiation of SSSS from viral exanthems and drug allergies is very important. The most important disease with which SSSS can be confused is *toxic epidermal necrolysis (TEN)*, an often fatal variant of erythema multiforme usually caused by a drug allergy (see Ch. 557). The two illnesses can be differentiated on skin biopsy, and therapy is very different for each: local care and antibiotics suffice to cure SSSS, whereas high dose systemic glucocorticoids are indicated in TEN, with mortality still remaining high.

DISEASES RELATED TO DIRECT INVASION AND SYSTEMIC SPREAD OF STAPHYLOCOCCI. In the following subsections, the classic clinical manifestations of invasive staphylococcal infection, bacteremia, and endocarditis are described. Under each section will be addressed not only the classic clinical manifestations but diagnostic, therapeutic, and prognostic aspects of each illness.

Dermal Infections. Most minor skin infections in man are caused either by *S. aureus* or group A beta-hemolytic streptococci. There is no way clinically to differentiate between diseases produced by the penicillin-sensitive streptococci and *S. aureus;* obviously, this is an important point, for all skin infections in which antibiotic therapy seems indicated therefore require the use of a beta-lactamase-resistant antibiotic (see Ch. 27). Direct invasion through minor breaks in skin and mucous membranes is the hallmark of disease produced by *S. aureus.* A wide variety of dermal and soft tissue infections may result, including cellulitis, local abscess formation (furuncles and carbuncles), lymphangiitis, and lymphadenitis. Direct extension then can occur to deep support structures such as bones and joints and result in primary osteomyelitis and septic arthritis. Even dermal staphylococcal infections that appear minor are important to recognize because they may become a source of bacteremia. When a patient with a localized *S. aureus* skin infection manifests fever and chills, bacteremia must be assumed to be present, and prompt diagnostic and therapeutic intervention should be initiated.

Diagnosis of dermal infections is usually relatively easy. The aspirate of a large, well developed abscess (furuncle or carbuncle) almost always reveals typical creamy pus, and on Gram stain the clustered organisms are mixed with inflammatory debris. One should not neglect performing Gram stains of materials from every dermal infection because occasionally gram-negative organisms may cause a clinical picture similar to that of gram-positive infections, especially in immunocompromised hosts, and obviously the initial therapeutic approach will be very different.

Therapy must always be initiated with a beta-lactamase-resistant antibiotic if antimicrobial therapy is indicated at all. In fact, the backbone of therapy of dermal staphylococcal infections continues to be debridement and drainage. Only large lesions associated with signs of surrounding cutaneous spread or systemic clinical symptoms need be treated with antibiotics. It is usually wise, however, before incising a large staphylococcal abscess (even when localized) to treat the patient with an oral dose of a penicillinase-resistant antibiotic (250 mg of dicloxicillin). Such a dose should be administered 30 minutes to one hour before incision and drainage is carried out.

The prognosis for most localized infections is excellent, but infections due to *S. aureus* often recur. Population surveys have found that each year most persons develop one to several isolated local lesions, most probably caused by *S. aureus.* However, not infrequently, an individual may suffer from recurrent crops of extremely debilitating local skin lesions. In this situation the patient is usually found to be carrying the causative organism in the anterior nares, the axilla or groin and/or perirectal region. Most such individuals are nasal carriers, and an attempt to eradicate nasal carriage is worth making (see later section on Treatment of Chronic Carriers).

Bone and Joint Infections. Through a variety of mechanisms, *S. aureus* commonly involves bone (osteomyelitis, see Ch. 274) and joints (see Ch. 446 on Septic Arthritis). Direct inoculation by *S. aureus* can occur in trauma or penetrating wounds. Bone and joint infections can also result from bacteremia. In children and young adults it is assumed that bacteremia originates from a minor dermal source (such as folliculitis) or somehow directly enters the bloodstream from heavily colonized mucous membranes. Seeding of *S. aureus* from the blood tends to occur to areas previously traumatized or harboring foreign bodies. In young children, the organism tends to seed into the diaphyseal plates of the long bone, areas of greatest vascularity. The affected area (usually on the ankle, knee, or shin) becomes acutely warm and swollen and may appear at first to be a primary cellulitis. Fever and shaking chills are common. Blood cultures are usually positive. In adults, the syndrome of hematogenous osteomyelitis is usually less acute, often involving the lumbar vertebrae. The individual will begin to develop low grade fever, night sweats, and back pain that gradually becomes localized to an area of point tenderness. In such cases, *S. aureus* may grow from the blood, but more commonly the organism is isolated from an aspirate of the bone or intervertebral space obtained by an orthopedic surgical consultant.

Staphylococcal septic arthritis usually involves a joint afflicted by pre-existing chronic arthritis (such as rheumatoid arthritis or osteoarthritis). Again, an episode of bacteremia causes seeding to a previously inflamed joint. The only indication in some patients is the development of increasing symptoms in one joint, usually accompanied by fever. Joint aspiration reveals a purulent effusion; Gram stains may be negative, but the organism is usually culturable. *S. epidermidis* increasingly is being described as a cause of chronic osteomyelitis, especially in debilitated patients such as those on hemodialysis or with underlying neoplastic diseases.

The diagnosis of staphylococcal bone and joint infections depends on recovering the organism from an aspirate of the involved site; every effort should be made, with the assistance of orthopedic surgeons, to aspirate or biopsy the involved area *before* antibiotics are started. Newer techniques permit core biopsies to be obtained from deep tissues and may in future permit more frequent definitive bacteriologic diagnosis of low grade, chronic bone and joint infections. The diagnosis becomes especially difficult if patients have been treated with antibiotics before appropriate culture material has been obtained. In such cases a rising or significantly elevated teichoic acid antibody titer may assist in diagnosing deep infections due to *S. aureus* (see later section on The Teichoic Acid Antibody Assay).

Treatment of osteomyelitis in adults must be prolonged. While it is becoming customary to treat children with a brief course of parenteral antibiotics, adults on oral antibiotics tend to relapse if a prolonged parenteral course of antibiotics is not administered. Four weeks of parenteral therapy is the minimun acceptable course, and most clinicians prefer to treat for six weeks. An oral antistaphylococcal agent (for example, dicloxacillin 2 grams daily) should be continued for several weeks following discharge. Gradual reduction of the dose of oral antibiotic over a three- to six-month period may leave the patient symptom-free for an extended period of time. Some clinicians treat isolated septic arthritis for only two weeks. However, it is extremely difficult to differentiate septic arthritis *without* bone involvement from that with osteomyelitis. Therefore, a four-week course of therapy with appropriate parenteral antibiotics is recommended. Staphylococcal osteomyelitis tends to relapse even after years of quiescence, and one can never be sure of complete eradication of the disease. Once a relapse has occurred, chronic recurrence will be the rule. In such situations carefully planned surgical debridement and drainage under the cover of a prolonged parenteral and oral course of antibiotics may result in extended quiescence or even apparent cure.

Staphylococcal Pneumonia and Empyema. Although most cases of *S. aureus* pneumonia follow acute viral infections of the lower respiratory tract (especially influenza), the disease occasionally occurs de novo in elderly and debilitated individuals. *S. aureus* pneumonia is most often acquired in the hospital. Primary staphylococcal pneumonia is most common in children and usually evolves radiologically from patchy pulmonary infiltrates into harder nodules and then pneumatoceles. Rapid development of pleural effusions and empyema often accompanied by pneumothorax may occur. Staphylococcal bronchitis and recurrent pneumonias are also seen in children and young adults with cystic fibrosis, and a young adult suffering from recurrent bronchitis from which *S. aureus* and/or *Pseudomonas aeruginosa* (usually with mucoid colonial morphology) are isolated should have a sweat test evaluation.

Adult patients with influenza have an increased incidence of *S. aureus* pneumonia. The patient is usually recovering from typical symptoms of influenza when the rapid onset of fever, chills, and chest pain supervenes. Gram stain of the sputum in such cases reveals large clumps of gram-positive cocci. Therapy must be intense with appropriate antibiotics. Nonetheless, such patients often do poorly and frequently develop secondary infections with gram-negative organisms, chronic respiratory failure, and progressive debility. Mortality rates remain high. Even in young people, morbidity is substantial, related to serious, rapidly progressive pulmonary disease often with empyema as well as the sequelae of the accompanying bacteremia.

In particular, pleural effusions accompanying *S. aureus* pneumonia require early drainage to prevent empyema formation. If thorough drainage cannot be accomplished by needle aspiration, a chest tube must be inserted. Every effort should be made to avoid the debilitating, prolonged sequelae that result from an extensive, multiloculated *S. aureus* infection of the pleural space.

Staphylococcal Meningitis, Cerebritis, and Brain Abscess. Meningitis due to *S. aureus* most commonly develops as a complication of a central nervous system diagnostic or neurosurgical procedure. Occasionally, however, meningitis may develop during an episode of bacteremia from a peripheral site. Many patients with staphylococcal bacteremia, with or without endocarditis, develop transient but sometimes focal central nervous system symptoms. On lumbar puncture, such patients commonly have a PMN pleocytosis with elevated protein but a normal to low normal glucose concentration and a *negative* Gram stain. These individuals probably have begun to develop multiple perimeningeal foci or areas of cerebritis (or both) and not yet frank meningitis. Almost certainly, if left untreated such patients would develop frank brain abscesses or fulminant staphylococcal meningitis. On occasion, such a patient may also exhibit purpura, disseminated intravascular coagulation, and shock in which the differentiation from *meningococcal meningitis* (see Ch. 272) is difficult. Treatment of such patients is particularly difficult, for the initial inclination is to use penicillin, an inappropriate antibiotic choice. Thus, for any patient whose Gram stain of the spinal fluid does not reveal identifiable organisms (such as meningococci or penumococci), a beta-lactamase resistant antibiotic must be included in the initial antibiotic coverage.

Brain abscesses in general are usually caused by anaerobes, but not infrequently *S. aureus* is found to accompany them. Therefore, antistaphylococcal drugs should be included with antianaerobic antibiotics in the initial coverage of such individuals. For example, nafcillin plus chloramphenicol is a combination frequently used for the patient who has a brain abscess with the source and causative organisms not yet defined. Surgical drainage is required only if the abscess is large and encapsulated.

Therapy of staphylococcal meningitis and cerebritis is usually that of the underlying syndrome (for example, endocarditis). However, even in the rare patient with an uncomplicated case of pure meningitis, therapy should be prolonged, at least four weeks parenterally, in contrast to the customary 10 to 14 days of therapy for patients with uncomplicated meningitis caused by *S. pneumoniae* or *N. meningitides*.

Staphylococcus epidermidis may cause meningeal signs and symptoms, almost always in a patient with a central nervous system shunt in place. In such instances, the infection has originated in the shunt, and the organism has proliferated and seeded back into the spinal fluid. In many such cases, the individual known to have a shunt in place simply has fever with few if any central nervous system signs. Only an aspirate of the shunt itself will reveal the organism. Therapy may result in quiescence of symptoms, but removal of the infected shunt is almost always required before cure can be accomplished.

Staphylococcal Urinary Tract Infections. Here the species spectrum changes, and coagulase-negative staphylococci become the more common infecting organisms. *S. epidermidis* may occasionally cause urinary tract infections, especially in elderly hospitalized men with obstructive urinary tract pathology or indwelling Foley catheters.

Staphylococcus saprophyticus accounts for between 5 and 10 per cent of urinary tract infections in otherwise healthy young women. Presumably the organism colonizes the genitalia and for reasons not yet ascertained may ascend the urethra to involve the bladder and cause symptomatic cystitis. *S. saprophyticus* is easily treated, being sensitive to essentially all commonly used antibiotics, including penicillin, ampicillin, sulfonamides, and cephalosporins.

S. aureus may involve the urinary tract by either of two mechanisms: first, the organism may seed to the renal cortex during an episode of staphylococcal bacteremia; second, usually in patients with lower urinary tract pathology or indwelling Foley catheters, the organism may ascend to cause a primary lower urinary tract infection. Approximately 10 per cent of patients with staphylococcal bacteremia eventually excrete the organism in the urine; other studies have found that about 25 per cent of patients with a defined urinary tract infection caused by *S. aureus* had had a preceding bacteremic episode. Thus, small cortical abscesses must occur frequently during bacteremia and ultimately rupture in some patients into the tubules and the urine. Most such patients respond promptly to therapy for the underlying disease, and renal carbuncles are now rare.

Conversely, some patients with a primary staphylococcal urinary tract infection may develop secondary bacteremia, that occurrence being reported in about 5 per cent of such patients. In some patients, the renal infection may seed to the perinephric and retroperitoneal structures, with resultant chronic infection and fibrosis. Frank perinephric abscess is a complication associated with high morbidity and mortality. This condition occurs most frequently in patients with chronic underlying renal diseases who are also often diabetic. Aggressive drainage along with prolonged antibiotic therapy is required for cure.

Staphylococcal Endocarditis. This condition follows staphylococcal bacteremia during which a nidus of infection becomes established on one or more heart valves. Endocarditis consists of two clinical syndromes (see Ch. 269): the first is "subacute" bacterial endocarditis, and the second is "acute" bacterial endocarditis.

SUBACUTE BACTERIAL ENDOCARDITIS. The patient presents with a history of days to weeks of low grade fever with or without chills, myalgias, night sweats, and weight loss. The word subacute refers to the clinical manifestations: the clinical course is one of a chronic, febrile illness. The patient almost always has a history of pre-existing organic valvular heart disease, and the species of staphylococcus involved is usually *S. epidermidis*. *S. epidermidis* accounts for approximately 5 per cent of all cases of subacute endocarditis, the vast majority being caused by streptococcal species. *S. epidermidis* is the most common cause, however, of endocarditis occurring in association with prosthetic heart valves (see Ch. 269). The organism, being a contaminant from the patient's or surgeon's skin flora, is inoculated at the time of the surgical valve replacement. Most such infections occur within the initial two months after surgery. In such instances, the outlook for therapy with antibiotics alone is poor, and reoperation with removal of the infected valve or valve ring is often required. More than half of such patients die.

ACUTE BACTERIAL ENDOCARDITIS. The word acute refers to the clinical presentation of the patient who experiences the rapid onset of fever, chills, and myalgias, often with back pain or some gastrointestinal symptoms. The fever is often quite high (103 to 105° F), and the individual at first has the feeling of developing a very bad case of the flu. In the majority of cases, the individual has not had a history of pre-existing valvular heart disease, although it is assumed that many of these individuals have had asymptomatic organic valvular lesions (such as a fenestrated or bicuspid aortic valve, mitral valve prolapse, and so forth). Frequently, therapy for such individuals, who previously had been well, is delayed because the patient and the physician do not realize the gravity of the situation.

S. aureus is almost always the cause of the syndrome of acute endocarditis. At the time of presentation, the patient may not have an obvious heart murmur or show evidence of embolic phenomenon. Thus, the differentiation between primary staphylococcal bacteremia, which may remain uncomplicated, and acute staphylococcal bacterial endocarditis is clinically difficult. The physician must closely follow every patient whose blood samples grow *S. aureus* and must examine carefully each day for the presence of a new murmur, the signs of embolic phenomena, or the observable development of vegetation(s) by echocardiography. Valve destruction, especially of the aortic valve, may progress quite rapidly (see Ch. 269 on Acute Aortic Insufficiency), and surgery may be necessary even within the first few days of presentation of a patient with an acutely insufficient aortic valve. The physician should not hesitate to operate on such a patient, because the possibility of infection of the prosthetic valve is high; over half of such patients will survive the surgical procedure and do well.

The diagnosis of staphylococcal endocarditis depends on the finding of the causative organism in the blood of a patient with one of the clinical syndromes described earlier. It is almost unheard of for a patient to have culture-negative endocarditis caused by staphylococci without having had *intensive* antibiotic therapy during the few days immediately prior to obtaining blood cultures. However, such may be the case in the postsurgical patient for whom prophylactic antibiotics may have been administered or in the drug addict who may surreptitiously have taken antibiotics.

The syndrome of *S. aureus* endocarditis in the drug addict is somewhat different from the acute bacterial endocarditis syndrome already described. In the drug abuser, the vegetation is almost always on one of the right sided heart valves, usually the tricuspid valve. Therefore, pleuritic chest pain and pulmonary infiltrates are common occurrences due to embolization. In drug-abusing patients who have surreptitiously taken antibiotics, the syndrome may be of a much lower grade and may mimic that of subacute bacterial endocarditis. In fact, it is so hard at the time of presentation to make the diagnosis of endocarditis in the drug addict that any person with a history (recent or distant) of parenteral drug abuse who presents with a fever should be considered to have bacterial endocarditis (usually with *S. aureus*) until proven otherwise.

The treatment of bacterial endocarditis must be prolonged (see Ch. 269). Four weeks of parenteral therapy is the minimum for staphylococcal endocarditis, although some authors have reported that two weeks may suffice for the drug addict, usually a young, otherwise healthy individual with right-sided endocarditis. All staphylococcal infections should be treated with a "cidal" antibiotic, and serum bactericidal levels must be monitored to guide effective therapy. For infections caused by beta-lactam antibiotic-resistant staphylococci, whether *aureus* or *epidermidis* species, a cephalosporin is not adequate therapy (see later discussion of treatment) although data may indicate sensitivity to the cephalosporins in vitro. As noted earlier, patients with prosthetic valve endocarditis often require surgery to eradicate the infection. Even those patients with prosthetic valve infections who respond to antibiotics alone probably should be treated with a prolonged course of oral therapy following the six-week course of parenteral therapy in the hospital. In patients with prosthetic valve endocarditis, usually due to *S. epidermidis*, treatment for six weeks parenterally in the hospital followed by an appropriate oral antistaphylococcal drug for a period of several months is recommended.

The prognosis for patients with staphylococcal endocarditis is guarded. Patients with prosthetic valve endocarditis have about a 50 per cent mortality rate, depending on the organism involved, how long after surgery the endocarditis develops, whether or not additional surgery is required for therapy, and the status of underlying left ventricular function. Patients with acute bacterial endocarditis caused by *S. aureus* will do well if they are young and otherwise healthy and especially if the vegetations are on the right-sided valves. The older the patient with left-sided valvular involvement, the higher the mortality (approaching 60 to 80 per cent). Pre-existing symptomatic heart disease is a particularly ominous prognostic sign. The patients who have the subacute syndrome due to *S. epidermidis* not on prosthetic valves, in which the organism is susceptible to the usual antibiotics, usually do quite well: survival rates are comparable with those of patients with streptococcal endocarditis (in the range of 80 to 90 per cent).

Staphylococcal Bacteremia. Sustained bacteremia due to *S. epidermidis* is uncommon. Although blood cultures frequently yield the organism, 80 to 90 per cent of the time it is a contaminant. The occasional case of true, sustained *S. epidermidis* bacteremia is usually caused by infection of an intravascular line or a prosthetic valve. The commonest species causing true bacteremia, especially in the hospital, is *S. aureus*.

There are two varieties of *S. aureus* bacteremia: primary and secondary. Primary bacteremia exists when a patient presenting with fever and chills grows *S. aureus* out of multiple blood cultures but does *not* have an identifiable seeding focus of infection. In this situation, the patient may have unrecognized endocarditis and should be treated accordingly. Secondary bacteremia is that associated with an obvious, peripheral focus of infection, for example, an intravascular line. Many such patients have a benign clinical course after line removal and a brief course of antibiotic treatment. The problem is to select from the overall group of such patients those that have not developed metastatic septic complications. Patients without metastatic sequelae require only a short (14-day) course of therapy. The typical patient who develops *S. aureus* bacteremia has usually been hospitalized for some other medical problem and has had a neglected peripheral or central venous or arterial access line in place. The patient suddenly develops fever and chills with or without signs of local infection at the site of the line. Other common sources are hemodialysis access shunts, postsurgical or traumatic wounds, and decubitus ulcers. The diagnosis of staphylococcal bacteremia is made when *S. aureus* grows from several blood cultures obtained before an empiric course of antibiotics is begun. Some patients already will have an obvious metastatic complication of the bacteremic episode when first examined.

The complications of an episode of *S. aureus* bacteremia are of two varieties: the first type is nonsuppurative, involving patients who develop the septic shock syndrome, including, in some, disseminated intravascular coagulation; the second type is suppurative, involving the metastatic spread of the organism via the bloodstream to heart valves or other organs. The development of endocarditis in this setting turns out to be distinctly uncommon; most suppurative spread occurs to bones, joints, and kidneys, occasionally to other deep viscera, and rarely to the meninges. Following the episode of bacteremia, the patient is placed first on broad, empiric and later on specific antistaphylococcal antibiotic therapy. Throughout this period, the patient must be examined carefully each day for metastatic suppurative sites. Laboratory evaluation may also be helpful, yielding pyuria and the organism from the urine, abnormalities of liver function, and other data. Vegetations may become demonstrable by echocardiography. Radionuclide scans may reveal infectious foci within bones, joints, or soft tissues.

Those patients who develop a clinically evident metastatic focus are treated as dictated by the type of complication that has evolved. Approximately 20 per cent of previously healthy persons who acquire *S. aureus* bacteremia develop some type of complication. In the absence of clinical findings after two weeks of observation, some experts now recommend discontinuation of antibiotics. At this point the results of a teichoic acid antibody (TA-AB) analysis reassure the clinician that no metastatic seeding had occurred. While most positive TA-AB titers will be from patients who already have developed obvious metastatic sequelae, a small subgroup of clinically well patients will also develop a positive TA-AB test. These persons probably have had subclinical suppuration and could be at risk of relapse in the days and weeks to follow. In this subgroup of patients continued parenteral therapy may be advisable with noninvasive search, despite the absence of clinical signs, for deep collections using such tests as echocardiograms, sonography, and bone, gallium, and computed tomography scans. Administration of an oral antistaphylococcal drug (dicloxacillin) should be continued for several weeks if there is any doubt about the possibility of residual metastatic abscesses.

If the following criteria are present, patients qualify for a short course (14 days) of antibiotic therapy following an episode of *S. aureus* bacteremia:

1. Host defenses are normal.
2. The patient should have no seedable sites (pre-existing valvular heart lesions, implanted prostheses, chronic arthritis).
3. The primary focus of infection should be obvious and easily managed.
4. There should be a prompt, complete response to the initial course of antimicrobial therapy.
5. The *S. aureus* recovered should be fully sensitive to the antibiotics initially chosen.
6. No clinical evidence of a metastatic, suppurative complication should be found.
7. No rise in the titer of teichoic acid antibodies should occur over a 14-day period of observation.

Septic Shock Syndromes Due to Staphylococci. Staphylococci can produce shock by five mechanisms:

1. The local infection can generate a massive inflammatory reaction resulting in sufficient "third spacing" (i.e., fluid accumulation into the area of infection) to lead to hypovolemic shock.
2. Enterotoxin producing *S. aureus* occasionally causes diarrhea severe enough to cause hypovolemia and shock.
3. Cardiogenic shock can be produced by staphylococci by causing either valve malfunction (usually aortic), multiple myocardial abscesses, or purulent pericarditis.
4. Endotoxic-like shock can be produced via intravascular complement activation (see Ch. 256 on Shock Syndromes Related to Sepsis).
5. Toxigenic shock—the toxic shock syndrome—can produce shock probably by direct capillary endothelial and end-organ damage.

Massive local infection due to staphylococci is uncommon, and such infections usually involve several organisms, usually anaerobes coinfecting with *S. aureus. S. epidermidis* may be a part of the flora in these infections but is probably not pathogenic. Specifically, patients with one of the gangrene syndromes (for example, necrotizing fasciitis or synergistic gangrene) may develop shock not caused by bacteremia but by fluid accumulation in the infected area. Such individuals require massive fluid and albumin .replacement, extensive local debridement, and broad antibiotic coverage.

Diarrhea, nausea, and vomiting may be so severe in some patients with staphylococcal food poisoning that shock may develop from hypovolemia secondary to gastrointestinal fluid loss. Hospitalization with fluid replacement may be required and will usually suffice because the disease is self-limiting.

Cardiogenic shock is self-explanatory (see Ch. 43).

During acute sepsis *S. aureus* may produce shock that in every way mimics that produced by endotoxin during gram-negative organism septicemia (See Ch. 256). Briefly, the primary event in endotoxic shock is the following: on entering the bloodstream, endotoxin activates a sequence of endocrine and inflammatory events leading first to vasodilation and subsequently to a primarily complement and PMN-mediated capillary leak syndrome resulting in full-blown septic shock. The coagulation and kinin systems also become activated, and such patients may suffer frank DIC. The presence or absence of a capsule seems to be a major factor determining whether or not a particular strain of *S. aureus* in the bloodstream will cause an endotoxic shock-like syndrome. Encapsulated organisms are virulent in tissues and are *more* likely to reach the bloodstream in the course of a peripheral infection. However, once there they are *less* likely to produce the septic shock syndrome. Unencapsulated strains activate complement readily in tissues and therefore are *more* likely to be contained and are least likely to reach the bloodstream and to cause bacteremia. Yet, these are the organisms that can cause shock when directly inoculated into the bloodstream, as by a parenteral drug user or when having colonized an intravascular line.

For a discussion of the toxigenic shock caused by *S. aureus*, refer to the earlier section on the toxic shock syndrome.

Miscellaneous Staphylococcal Infections. This section focuses on several relatively unusual infections that require special diagnostic and therapeutic considerations.

STAPHYLOCOCCAL PYOMYOSITIS. This malady is primarily a tropical disease, rare enough to be reportable in the United States. The patient develops pain, warmth, and swelling over a muscle region usually of the lower extremities and buttocks. The overlying skin may appear quite normal or may look like a mild cellulitis; however, when drainage is attempted, the surgeon discovers that the infection extends into muscle, often with extensive destruction. In the tropics, the disease afflicts malnourished individuals.

S. AUREUS EPIDURAL ABSCESS. This infection is often related to the presence of vertebral osteomyelitis wherein periosseus inflammation extends into the epidural space. The inflammation causes localized tenderness over the spine at point of infection followed by weakness and progressive neurologic signs of paraplegia. Effective therapy depends on early diagnosis and *prompt* surgical intervention and drainage.

DIAGNOSIS. The diagnosis of staphylococcal infections continues to be made clinically. Knowledgeable interpretation of the Gram stain of an adequately obtained specimen will usually suggest the presence of staphylococci. Culture of such a specimen almost always will yield the responsible staphylococcus, and absolute confirmation is provided by the presence of positive blood cultures. Some judgment is required in deciding whether *S. epidermidis* in blood cultures is a contaminant or a true infection. The presence of the organism *in more than two* consecutive blood cultures and associated with proper clinical circumstances (the presence of an indwelling intravascular catheter or a prosthetic device) strongly suggests true bacteremia. The vast majority (80 to 85 per cent) of *S. epidermidis* isolated from blood culture bottles are single organisms, usually in only one of the two bottles in a set, and are contaminants. While *S. aureus* may on occasion contaminate blood cultures, the clinician must determine the significance of the isolation of *S. aureus* from the blood under any condition. In most cases multiple blood cultures will be positive, and there is no question about the diagnosis of the true bacteremic state. If there is any doubt as to the origin of *S. aureus* either in blood, urine, or other fluid specimens, appropriate therapy should be continued.

The Teichoic Acid Antibody (TA-AB) Assay. This assay measures the presence (and titer) or absence of antibodies to staphylococcal cell wall teichoic acids. It is of no use in diagnosing infections with *S. epidermidis* because it only identifies antibodies to the ribotol teichoic acid moiety in the wall of *S. aureus.* Approximately 90 per cent of patients with *S. aureus* endocarditis develop a significant titer of teichoic acid antibodies. The test is fairly sensitive but only modestly specific for other types of serious, deep-seated *S. aureus* infections. The major role of the TA-AB assay is not primarily to diagnose *S. aureus* infections, most of which are diagnosed on clinical grounds, but to assist the clinician in deciding how long to treat bacteremic patients. Patients with *S. aureus* bacteremia who develop disseminated or metastatic abscesses will usually develop an increase in the titer of TA-AB acid antibodies as opposed to those with benign, self-limited bacteremias. The predictive value of a negative assay in someone who has experienced an episode of *S. aureus* bacteremia is high; therefore, the test is useful in *ruling out* metastatic infections in such patients. Other situations in which the teichoic acid antibody may be of some use in clinical decision making are the following:

1. For patients with endocarditis and negative blood cultures, usually because of prior antibiotic therapy (in a drug addict). A rise in TA-AB titers to a positive level confirms the diagnosis.
2. For deep tissue infections thought likely to be due to *S. aureus* but inaccessible to culturing (osteomyelitis or visceral abscesses). Again, a rising TA-AB titer is confirmatory, but a negative test does *not* rule out the involvement of *S. aureus.*
3. To determine the response to therapy of patients with endocarditis. Patients responding to therapy will have a prompt (two- to four-weeks) decrease in the titer of antibodies. A titer that remains elevated suggests an undrained focus of residual infection.
4. To detect relapse. Relapse is associated with a rapidly rising antibody titer; thus, sequential titers may help the clinician analyze febrile episodes occurring late in the course of treatment of an episode of endocarditis.

TREATMENT. Effective therapy of staphylococcal infections depends on early, effective debridement and drainage of the primary focus of infection along with the selection of antibiotics to which the organisms are susceptible. At present, 90 per cent of all organisms, whether nosocomial or community-acquired, are resistant to penicillin. Therefore, no patient suspected of having an infection with *S. aureus* should be started on a penicillinase-susceptible penicillin. Most staphylococci are still susceptible to nafcillin and oxacillin; methicillin is an antiquated drug, more toxic than either of the aforementioned parenteral alternatives. Usual doses of nafcillin and oxacillin are in the range of from 6 to 12 grams daily, and patients with endocarditis should receive between 9 and 12 grams daily. In the penicillin-allergic individual, the cephalosporins can be used in the absence of a history of an anaphylactic type of penicillin hypersensitivity; however, the most effective alternative continues to be vancomycin. Vancomycin is used in a dose of 2 to 4 grams per day parenterally and should be equal to the penicillins and cephalosporins in terms of therapeutic outcome.

Beta-Lactam Antibiotic–Resistant Staphylococci (BLARS). These organisms are usually referred to as "methicillin-resistant staphylococci." However, methicillin is simply the disc used to determine resistance of these organisms and many such organisms remain sensitive by disk and other in vitro methods to the cephalosporins. However, the clinical responses to the cephalosporins of cephalosporin-sensitive but methicillin-resistant organisms have not been good. Thus, when any species of staphylococcus has been identified as being methicillin-resistant (or, therefore, nafcillin- or oxacillin-resistant) it should be considered resistant to all beta-lactam antibiotics regardless of contrary in vitro data. The drug of choice in the treatment of BLARS is vancomycin. Alternative drugs include rifampin and trimethoprim/sulfamethoxazole (TMS). Some BLARS remain sensitive to the aminoglycosides, and aminoglycosides may provide a synergistic effect with whatever other antibiotic is used. These recommendations hold true both for *S. aureus* and *S. epidermidis.*

Treatment of Chronic Carriers. Certain individuals may suffer recurrent staphylococcal infections of the skin (furunculosis), and eradication of the nasal carrier state may be required to terminate the series of infections. Nasal carriage termination may be difficult by local means. Traditionally, individuals so afflicted have been advised to observe meticulous personal hygienic measures such as frequent bathing or showering, using pHisoHex or other bactericidal soap preparations, and the application of an antibacterial ointment such as bacitracin to the anterior nares. While such a treatment program will clear a portion of chronic carriers, many will relapse and develop recurrent crops of boils. The drug most helpful in this situation is rifampin, known to be excreted in bactericidal concentrations in external secretions. Rifampin should always be used with another oral antistaphylococcal drug that, even though present in low concentrations, will delay the emergence of rifampin resistance. Thus, a seven- to ten-day course of rifampin* (300 mg twice daily) plus, for example, dicloxacillin (125 mg four times a day) or in the penicillin-allergic patient cephalexin or TMS is very effective in eliminating nasal carriage of *S. aureus* and the associated dermal infections. A percentage of individuals will reacquire the organism and the course of therapy may have to be repeated; the physician should be sure to ascertain that the carried organism is still sensitive to rifampin. In the future, recolonization of such individuals with nonpathogenic staphylococci may play an important adjunctive role in preventing recrudescence of carriage by an aggressive organism.

Bacterial Interference. Bacterial interference is the process of recolonizing an individual with an organism in order to displace a more pathogenic microbe. Initially, investigators found that patients heavily colonized with an aggressive strain of *S. aureus* that was associated with recurrent infections (boils, omphalitis, or conjunctivitis) could be helped by being recolonized with a nonpathogenic strain (designated strain 502A) of the organism. Multiple reports in 1960's and 1970's attested to the efficacy of bacterial interference. However, from time to time, there were reports of a serious infection caused by the 502A strain of *S. aureus.* The use of bacterial interference to treat recurrent infections due to a carried strain of *S. aureus* therefore has declined. The potential usefulness of this process should be kept in mind as one considers therapeutic approaches to patients with recurrent furunculosis recalcitrant to repeated courses of therapy. It is probable that other species of truly nonpathogenic staphylococci or micrococci will also be found to interfere with *S. aureus* colonization and that clinical application of this technique will be common in the future.

PREVENTION. Prevention of nosocomial staphylococcal infections depends on breaking the chain of transmission between a carrier and a susceptible noncarrier. Transmission from person to person is interrupted by thorough handwashing before and after examination of each patient. Certain other hospital infection control recommendations and procedures apply in particular to staphylococcal infections. For example, hospitals are required to have specific recommendations about the placement and maintenance of intravascular catheters; such instructions should be followed *meticulously.* Staphylococci are among the leading causes of infection of indwelling intravascular catheters, and proper catheter maintenance substantially reduces the incidence of nosocomial infections with these organisms.

While in theory vaccines containing capsular polysaccharides

*This use of rifampin is not listed in the manufacturer's directive.

might enhance host defenses against the encapsulated strains of staphylococci, vaccines developed in the past were not shown to be of major clinical benefit. It is probable that some acquired immunity does develop against staphylococci, since the incidence of *S. aureus* infections decreases with increasing age. However, firm evidence is lacking that enhancement of humoral or cellular immunity against staphylococci significantly assists the host in its struggle with the organism.

Kaplan MH, Tenenbaum MJ: *Staphylococcus aureus*: Cellular biology and clinical application. Am J Med 72:248–57, 1982. *Reviews the clinically relevant molecular biologic aspects of S. aureus.*

Musher DM, McKenzie SO: Infections due to *Staphylococcus aureus*. Medicine 56:383–409, 1977. *A nice review of most clinical aspects of S. aureus infections.*

Sheagren JN: Endocarditis complicating drug abuse. *In* Remington JN, Swartz MN (eds.): Current Clinical Topics in Infectious Diseases. New York, McGraw-Hill Book Company, 1981, pp 211–33. *Describes the syndrome of endocarditis in the drug-abuser and highlights the role of S. aureus therein.*

Sheagren JN: Guidelines for the use of the teichoic acid antibody assay. Arch Int Med 144:250–252, 1984. *A brief summary of indications for the use of the teichoic acid antibody assay.*

Sheagren JN: *Staphylococcus aureus*—the persistent pathogen. N. Engl J Med (in press). *A complete, up-to-date review of all newer aspects of infections with S. aureus.*

Bacterial Meningitis

Morton N. Swartz

271. BACTERIAL MENINGITIS

Meningitis is an inflammation of the arachnoid, the pia mater, and the intervening cerebrospinal fluid. The inflammatory process extends throughout the subarachnoid space about the brain and spinal cord and regularly involves the ventricles. Pyogenic meningitis, considered in this chapter, is usually an acute infection due to bacteria which evoke a polymorphonuclear response in the cerebrospinal fluid (CSF). One of its major forms, that caused by meningococci, is considered in Ch. 272; less acute forms of bacterial meningitis, characterized by a mononuclear cell response in the CSF, are discussed in Ch. 298 and 497.

ETIOLOGY AND INCIDENCE. Approximately 17,500 cases of bacterial meningitis are estimated to occur annually in the United States. If all cases are included irregardless of the age of patients, data from the Centers for Disease Control in 1978 indicated that *Hemophilus influenzae* type b is the most frequent bacterial cause (46 per cent), followed by *Neisseria meningitidis* (27 per cent) and *Streptococcus pneumoniae* (11 per cent). About 70 per cent of all cases occur in children under 5 years of age.The relative frequencies with which the different bacterial species cause meningitis are age related. In the newborn, gram-negative bacilli (most frequently *E. coli,* but also other enteric bacilli and *Pseudomonas*) and group B streptococci are the principal causes. In the past 15 years the group B (type III principally) *Streptococcus* has increased in importance in neonatal meningitis; in some hospitals it is the single most frequent etiology, surpassing *E. coli.* Beyond the first month of life and extending through childhood, *H. influenzae* and *N. meningitidis* are the most frequent causes of bacterial meningitis. In adults *S. pneumoniae* and *N. meningitidis* are responsible for most cases. Meningococcal meningitis is the only type that occurs in outbreaks; its relative frequency among the meningitides will depend on whether statistics have been gathered during an epidemic period. In about 10 per cent of patients with pyogenic meningitis the bacterial cause cannot be defined. Simultaneous mixed meningitis is rare, occurring in the setting of neurosurgical procedures, penetrating head injury, or intraventricular rupture of a cerebral abscess; the isolation of anaerobes should strongly suggest the last of these.

TABLE 271–1. BACTERIAL CAUSES OF MENINGITIS

	Neonates (≤ 1 month) (%)	Children (1 month–15 years) (%)	Adults (> 15 years) (%)
S. pneumoniae	0–5	10–20	30–50
N. meningitidis	0–1	25–40	10–35
H. influenzae	0–3	40–60	1–3
Streptococci	20–40 *	2–4	5
Staphylococci	5	1–2	5–15
Listeria	2–10	1–2	5
Gram-negative bacilli	50–60 †	1–2	1–10

*Almost all isolates from neonatal meningitis are group B streptococci.
†Of all cases of neonatal meningitis, *E. coli* accounts for about 40 per cent and *Klebsiella-Enterobacter* for about 8 per cent.

Important changes have occurred in the frequencies of several types of bacterial meningitis over the past 10 to 20 years. Gram-negative bacillary meningitis has almost doubled in frequency, probably reflecting more frequent and extensive neurosurgical procedures as well as other nosocomial factors. *Listeria monocytogenes* has increased eight- to tenfold as a cause of bacterial meningitis in urban general hospitals, reflecting the enlarging immunosuppressed population at particular risk.

CLINICAL SETTINGS. The clinical setting in which meningitis develops may provide a clue to the specific bacterial cause. Meningococcal disease, including meningitis, may occur sporadically and in cyclic outbreaks; military recruits are particularly susceptible, but large urban outbreaks also occur, as in Brazil in 1971 (see Ch. 272).

Certain predisposing factors are frequently associated with the development of *pneumococcal meningitis. Acute otitis media* (± *mastoiditis*) occurs in about 30 per cent of patients. *Pneumonia* is present in about 25 per cent of patients with pneumococcal meningitis, a much higher frequency than in meningitis caused by *H. influenzae* or *N. meningitidis. Acute pneumococcal sinusitis* is occasionally the initial focus from which infection spreads to the meninges. A significant head injury (recent or remote) has occurred in about 10 per cent of patients with pneumococcal meningitis. CSF rhinorrhea (usually caused by a defect or fracture in the cribriform plate) is present in about 5 per cent of patients with pneumococcal meningitis. Meningitis occurring in young children with sickle cell anemia is most likely to be due to *S. pneumoniae.* A variety of defects in host defenses (primary or acquired immunoglobulin deficiencies, the asplenic state) may predispose to pneumococcal disease, particularly meningitis. Alcoholism is an underlying problem in 10 to 25 per cent of adults with pneumococcal meningitis in urban hospitals.

S. aureus meningitis is seen most commonly as a complication of a neurosurgical procedure, following penetrating skull trauma, or secondary to staphylococcal bacteremia and endocarditis. Meningitis caused by *gram-negative bacilli* takes one of three forms: neonatal meningitis, meningitis following trauma or surgery involving the central nervous system, or spontaneous meningitis in adults (e.g., bacteremic *Klebsiella* meningitis in a patient with diabetes mellitus). The most common causes of gram-negative bacillary meningitis in the adult are *E. coli* (about 30 per cent) and *Klebsiella-Enterobacter* (about 40 per cent). The most frequent causes of bacterial meningitis in patients with neoplastic disease are gram-negative bacilli (particularly *Pseudomonas aeruginosa* and *E. coli), Listeria monocytogenes, S. pneumoniae,* and *S. aureus.* Meningitis caused by *group A streptococci* is uncommon, but occasionally occurs following acute otitis media, mastoiditis, or sinusitis. *Clostridium perfringens* is a rare cause of meningitis usually secondary to a penetrating injury.

The age-related incidence (children under five years) of *H. influenzae* type b meningitis is so striking that the occurrence of this disease in an adult should raise the question of the presence of an underlying anatomic or immunologic defect, circumventing the usual barrier interposed by serum bactericidal mechanisms.

Neonatal Meningitis. The incidence of meningitis is higher in the first month of life than in any other single month. The principal cause, *E. coli* strains containing the K1 capsular antigen, is usually acquired by the neonates from their mothers who carry the organism in their stool. In the newborn the group B *Streptococcus* can produce either an "early onset" (occurring within eight days of delivery and characterized by a fulminant illness with septicemia, severe respiratory distress, and sometimes meningitis) or a "late onset" (occurring ten days to two months after delivery and presenting a more insidious, slowly progressive illness which usually includes meningitis) infection. Type III strains predominate in the latter, but in the "early onset" form the serotypes are variable. Group B streptococci are acquired by the neonate either in passage through the birth canal or through nosocomial spread in the nursery.

The clinical signs in neonatal meningitis suggest sepsis but not necessarily central nervous system involvement: fever (in only 60 per cent), jaundice, diarrhea, lethargy, poor feeding or vomiting, respiratory distress (including apnea), seizures, irritability, bulging fontanel (in only 30 per cent), and nuchal rigidity (15 per cent). Frequently, only by examination of the CSF can the presence of meningitis be ruled in or out.

PATHOLOGY. The purulent exudate is distributed widely in the subarachnoid space, most abundant in the basal cisterns and about the cerebellum initially, but also extending into the sulci over the cerebrum. The exudate in pneumococcal meningitis tends to be more evident over the convexities of the brain than in the basilar region. There is no direct invasion of cerebral tissue by the infecting organism or the inflammatory exudate, but the subjacent brain becomes congested and edematous. The effectiveness of the pial barrier accounts for the fact that cerebral abscess does not complicate bacterial meningitis. Indeed, when these two processes coexist, the sequence usually has been that of an initial abscess subsequently leaking its contents into the ventricular system, producing meningitis. Structures adjacent to the meninges may show a variety of pathologic changes secondary to bacterial meningitis. *Cortical thrombophlebitis* results from venous stasis and adjacent meningeal inflammation. Infarction of cerebral tissue may follow. *Involvement of small pial arteries* with peripheral aneurysm formation and vascular occlusion occurs occasionally in bacterial meningitis. In fulminating cases (particularly meningococcal meningitis), *cerebral edema* may be marked even though the CSF pleocytosis is only moderate. Rarely such patients develop temporal lobe and cerebellar herniation, resulting in compression of the midbrain and medulla. *Damage to cranial nerves* occurs in areas where dense exudate accumulates; the third and sixth cranial nerves are also vulnerable to damage by increased intracranial pressure. *Ventriculitis* probably occurs in most cases of bacterial meningitis; rarely this progresses to the accumulation of pus, *ventricular empyema*. *Hydrocephalus* can develop during meningitis from obstruction to CSF flow within the ventricular system (obstructive hydrocephalus) or extraventricularly (communicating hydrocephalus). *Subdural effusions* are sterile transudates which develop over the cerebral cortex in about 15 per cent of infants with bacterial meningitis. Rarely such effusions become infected, producing a subdural empyema. In the past the diagnosis has been made almost exclusively in infants, in whom abnormal transillumination or increasing head size can be detected. Now, sterile or infected (showing peripheral contrast enhancement) subdural collections can be demonstrated readily by CT scan as low density areas about the cerebrum.

PATHOGENESIS. Bacteria may reach the meninges by several routes: (1) systemic bacteremia, (2) direct ingress from the upper respiratory tract or skin through an anatomic defect (e.g., skull fracture, eroding sequestrum, meningocele), (3) passage intracranially via venules in the nasopharynx, or (4) spread from a contiguous focus of infection (infection of the paranasal sinuses, leakage of a brain abscess). Bacteremic spread to the meninges is probably the most frequent path of infection. However, not all bacteremic organisms have the same likelihood of causing meningitis. Most bacterial species causing meningitis (*H. influenzae b, N. meningitidis, S. pneumoniae, E. coli* K1, group B III *Streptococcus*) have definable capsules which are antiphagocytic. Whether the capsular polysaccharide, in addition, confers some special meningeal tropism, possibly through surface receptors, is not known. The primary focus initiating the bacteremia is usually in the upper respiratory tract or lung (pneumonia) but may be in the heart (endocarditis) or the gastrointestinal or urinary tracts. Once established in any part of the meninges, infection quickly extends throughout the subarachnoid space. In addition, evidence from animal models of bacterial meningitis suggests that a secondary bacteremia may follow meningeal infection and itself contribute to continuing further inoculation of the cerebrospinal fluid.

CLINICAL MANIFESTATIONS. ***History.*** An acute onset of fever, generalized headache, vomiting, and stiff neck are common to many types of meningitis. Although some patients develop bacterial meningitis in the absence of respiratory symptoms, the majority of patients with pyogenic meningitis of the three common causes have had an antecedent or accompanying upper respiratory tract infection, acute otitis (or mastoiditis), or pneumonia. Myalgias (particularly in meningococcal disease), backache, and generalized weakness are common symptoms. The illness usually progresses rapidly with development of confusion, obtundation, and loss of consciousness. Occasionally the onset may be less acute, with meningeal signs present for several days to a week prior to hospitalization.

General Physical Findings. Evidences of meningeal irritation (drowsiness and decreased mentation, stiff neck, positive Kernig's and Brudzinski's signs) are usually present. In certain patients the findings of meningitis may be easily overlooked; infants, obtunded patients, or elderly patients with congestive failure or pneumonia may develop meningitis without prominent meningeal signs. Their lethargy should be investigated carefully and meningeal signs should be sought; if any doubt exists, examination of the CSF is indicated.

The presence of a petechial, purpuric, or ecchymotic rash in a patient with meningeal findings almost always indicates meningococcal infection and requires prompt treatment because of the rapidity with which this infection can progress (see Ch. 272). Rarely, extensive petechial and purpuric lesions occur in meningitis caused by *S. pneumoniae* or *H. influenzae*. Very rarely skin lesions almost indistinguishable from those of meningococcal bacteremia occur in patients with acute *S. aureus* endocarditis who also have meningeal signs and a CSF pleocytosis (secondary either to staphylococcal meningitis or to embolic cerebral infarction). Usually one or two of the lesions in such a patient are those of purulent purpura; aspiration of material reveals staphylococci on Gram stain. In the summer months viral aseptic meningitis (particularly caused by echovirus 9) may produce meningeal signs, macular and petechial skin lesions, and a CSF pleocytosis of several hundred to 1000 cells, with neutrophils predominating initially.

Neurologic Findings and Complications. *Cranial nerve abnormalities,* involving principally the third, fourth, sixth, or seventh nerves, occur in 10 to 20 per cent of patients with bacterial meningitis. These usually disappear shortly after recovery. Hearing loss occurs in 20 to 25 per cent of children with bacterial meningitis. In about half of those it is a conductive loss, frequently associated with otitis media, and transient. In the other half a persistent sensorineural hearing loss (unilateral or bilateral) occurs; the most likely sites of involvement appear to be the inner ear (infection possibly spreading from the subarachnoid space along the cochlear aqueduct) and the acoustic nerve. In children permanent hearing impairment is more common following meningitis due to *S. pneumoniae* than to *H. influenzae* or *N. meningitidis*.

Seizures (focal or generalized) occur during the acute phase of bacterial meningitis in 20 to 30 per cent of patients and may be due to readily reversible causes (high fever in infants; penicillin neurotoxicity when large doses are administered intravenously in the presence of renal failure) or to focal cerebral injury. Seizures can occur during the first few days, or can appear with associated focal neurologic deficits caused by cortical vein phlebitis seven to ten days after the onset of the meningitis.

Brain swelling and increased CSF pressure are associated with seizures, third nerve dysfunction, abnormal reflexes, coma, hypertension, and bradycardia. Papilledema is rare in bacterial meningitis even with high CSF pressures. Its presence should indicate the possibility of some other associated or independent suppurative intracranial process (subdural empyema, brain abscess). Marked central hyperpnea sometimes occurs in patients with severe bacterial meningitis; CSF acidosis (principally caused by increased lactic acid levels) provides much of the respiratory stimulus.

Focal cerebral signs (hemiparesis, dysphasia, visual field defects) occur in about 15 per cent of patients with bacterial meningitis. They may develop during early meningitis secondary to occlusive vascular processes or some days later. It is important to distinguish lateralizing findings resulting from postictal changes (Todd's paralysis), which usually persist for no more than several hours.

Prompt treatment of bacterial meningitis usually results in rapid recovery of neurologic function. Persistent or late onset of obtundation and coma without focal findings suggests the development of brain swelling, subdural effusions (in the infant), hydrocephalus, loculated ventriculitis, cortical thrombophlebitis, or sagittal sinus thrombosis. The last three are commonly associated with fever and a continuing CSF pleocytosis.

Residual neurologic damage remains in 10 to 20 per cent of patients who recover from bacterial meningitis. In infants surviving neonatal meningitis, significant sequelae are much more frequent (30 to 50 per cent).

LABORATORY DIAGNOSIS. ***Cerebrospinal Fluid Examination.*** Initial CSF pressure is usually moderately elevated (200 to 300 mm H_2O). Striking elevations (over 400 mm) occur in occasional patients with acute brain swelling complicating meningitis in the absence of an associated mass lesion.

GRAM-STAINED SMEAR. By the time of hospitalization, most patients with pyogenic meningitis have large numbers (at least 10^5 per milliliter) of bacteria in the cerebrospinal fluid. Careful examination of the Gram-stained smear of the spun sediment of CSF reveals the etiologic agent in 70 to 80 per cent of cases. In most instances when gram-positive diplococci (or short chaining cocci) are observed on stained CSF smear they are pneumococci. In certain clinical settings it is important to distinguish this organism from the relatively pencillin-resistant enterococcus, which would require the addition of an aminoglycoside to penicillin in treatment. If sufficient organisms are present in the CSF, prompt identification of a pneumococcus can be made by the quellung reaction, employing pooled pneumococcal antisera. Culture of the cerebrospinal fluid reveals the etiologic agent in 80 to 90 per cent of patients with bacterial meningitis.

SPECIAL IMMUNOLOGIC AND SEROLOGIC PROCEDURES. In patients in whom the etiologic agent is not identified on Gram-stained smear of the CSF, rapid diagnosis may often be made by detection of specific bacterial antigens by latex agglutination (LA) or countercurrent immunoelectrophoresis (CIE). These techniques have been employed most extensively in the rapid diagnosis of meningitis caused by *H. influenzae* type b, but have also been used in the diagnosis of meningococcal (groups A,B,C, and Y) and pneumococcal meningitis. Antigen detection by LA is more sensitive and provides results more rapidly than CIE. Since *E. coli* K1 and *N. meningitidis* serogroup B share a common antigenic determinant, immunologic cross-reactivity may cause a false-positive reaction with the group B meningococcal reagent. Since the bacterial cause can be found on Gram-stained smear in most cases of bacterial meningitis, the role of latex agglutination appears to be as an adjunct in rapid diagnosis when no organisms are observed or in providing a specific rather than a morphologic (Gram stain) diagnosis.

The limulus gelation assay for endotoxin is positive in the CSF of patients with meningitis caused by gram-negative bacteria but not in the case of meningitis caused by gram-positive organisms.

CELL COUNT. The cell count in untreated meningitis usually ranges between 100 and 10,000 per cubic millimeter, with polymorphonuclear leukocytes predominating initially (80 per cent or more) and lymphocytes appearing subsequently. Extremely high cell counts (>50,000 per cubic millimeter) may occur rarely in primary bacterial meningitis, but should also raise the possibility of intraventricular rupture of a cerebral abscess. Cell counts as low as 10 to 20 may be observed early in bacterial meningitis (particularly that caused by *N. meningitidis* and *H. influenzae*). Occasionally, in granulocytopenic patients or in the elderly with overwhelming pneumococcal meningitis, the CSF may contain very few leukocytes and yet may appear grossly turbid because of the presence of myriads of organisms. Meningitis caused by several bacterial species (*M. tuberculosis, T. pallidum*) characteristically produces a lymphocytic pleocytosis. *Listeria monocytogenes* meningitis in infants may produce a primarily lymphocytic response in the CSF; in the adult there is usually a polymorphonuclear response, but rarely lymphocytes predominate.

GLUCOSE. The CSF glucose is reduced to values of 40 mg per deciliter or below (or less than 50 to 60 per cent of the simultaneous blood level) in over 50 per cent of patients with bacterial meningitis; this finding can be very valuable in distinguishing bacterial meningitis from most viral meningitides or parameningeal infections. A normal CSF glucose does not exclude the diagnosis of bacterial meningitis. The simultaneous blood glucose level should be determined, because patients with diabetes mellitus (or who are receiving intravenous glucose infusions) will have an elevated level of glucose in the CSF, and its significance can be appreciated only on comparison with the simultaneous blood level. However, it may take 90 to 120 minutes for equilibration to occur after major shifts in the level of glucose in the circulation. The hypoglycorrhachia characteristic of pyogenic meningitis appears to be due to interference with normal carrier-facilitated diffusion of glucose.

PROTEIN. The level of protein in the CSF is usually elevated above 100 mg per deciliter, and the higher values are more commonly observed in pneumococcal meningitis. Extreme elevations, up to 1000 mg per deciliter or more, indicate impending or actual subarachnoid block secondary to the meningitis.

OTHER ABNORMALITIES IN THE CSF. Elevated levels of lactic acid occur in pyogenic meningitis. Lactic dehydrogenase levels (particularly isozymes 4 and 5 derived from granulocytes) are commonly elevated in patients with bacterial meningitis. Although the levels of lactic dehydrogenase are higher in patients with bacterial meningitis than in those with viral infections of the central nervous system, these alterations are not of help in determining the specific etiologic agent involved.

Other Laboratory Tests. BLOOD and RESPIRATORY TRACT CULTURES. Bacteremia is demonstrable in about 80 per cent of patients with *H. influenzae* meningitis, 50 per cent of those with pneumococcal meningitis, and 30 to 40 per cent of those with meningococcal meningitis. Cultures of the upper respiratory tract have not proved helpful in establishing an etiologic diagnosis. Determination of serum creatinine and electrolytes is important in view of the gravity of the illness, the occurrence of specific abnormalities secondary to the meningitis (syndrome of inappropriate secretion of antidiuretic hormone), and problems in therapy in the presence of renal dysfunction (seizures and hyperkalemia with high-dose penicillin therapy). In patients with extensive petechial and purpuric skin lesions, evaluation for coagulopathy is indicated.

Radiologic Studies. In view of the frequency with which pyogenic meningitis is associated with primary foci of infection in the chest, nasal sinuses, or mastoid, roentgenograms of these areas should be taken at the appropriate time after institution of antimicrobial therapy. Computerized tomography (CT) scans are not indicated in most patients with bacterial meningitis. If a mass lesion (cerebral abscess, subdural empyema) is suspected by history, clinical setting, or physical findings (papilledema), then radionuclide or CT scans should be performed. *Bacterial meningitis is a medical emergency requiring immediate diagnosis and rapid institution of antimicrobial therapy.* Delay in performing a diagnostic lumbar puncture in order to obtain a CT scan should be avoided except on the basis of findings indicative of a parameningeal collection or other intracranial mass lesion. Changes may be observed on CT scan during meningitis itself: enlargement of the subarachnoid spaces, including the interhemispheric area; generalized contrast enhancement of the leptomeninges and the ependyma; or areas of diminished density in a patchy pattern owing to associated cerebritis and necrosis. In the patient with meningitis whose clinical status deteriorates or fails to improve, the CT scan may be helpful in demonstrating suspected complications: sterile subdural collections or empyema; ventricular enlargement secondary to communicating obstructive hydrocephalus; prominent persisting basilar meningitis; extensive areas of cerebral infarction resulting from occlusion of major cerebral arteries or veins; or marked ventricular wall enhancement, suggesting ventriculitis or ventricular empyema.

DIAGNOSIS. The diagnosis of bacterial meningitis is not difficult in a febrile patient with meningeal symptoms and signs developing in the setting of a predisposing illness. The diagnosis may be less obvious in the elderly, obtunded patient with pneumonia or the confused alcoholic patient in impending delirium tremens. Examination of the CSF should be carried out promptly under these circumstances or whenever there is any question of meningitis.

Headache, fever, vomiting, stiff neck, and CSF pleocytosis are features of meningeal inflammation and are common to many types of meningitis (e.g., bacterial, fungal, viral) and also to some parameningeal processes. The CSF findings are most helpful in distinguishing among these processes (see Ch. 496). In the patient with meningitis whose CSF does not reveal the etiologic agent on examination of Gram-stained smear, particularly when the CSF glucose is normal and the polymorphonuclear pleocytosis is atypical, certain treatable processes which can mimic bacterial meningitis should be considered in differential diagnosis: (1) *Parameningeal infections.* The presence of infections (chronic ear or nasal accessory sinus infections, lung abscess) predisposing to brain abscess, epidural (cerebral or spinal) abscess, subdural empyema, or pyogenic venous sinus phlebitis should be sought. Neurologic findings may appear in the course of primary bacterial meningitis, but their presence should alert the physician to the need for close scrutiny for the presence of a space-occupying infectious process in the central nervous system. Neurologic symptoms or findings antedating the onset of meningeal symptoms should suggest the possibility of a parameningeal infection. The isolation of an anaerobic organism should suggest the possibility of intraventricular leakage of a cerebral abscess. (2) *Bacterial endocarditis.* Bacterial meningitis may occur during bacterial endocarditis caused by pyogenic organisms such as *S. aureus* and enterococci. In subacute bacterial endocarditis sterile embolic infarctions of the brain may occur and produce meningeal signs and a CSF pleocytosis containing several hundred cells, including polymorphonuclear leukocytes. A history of dental manipulation, fever, and anorexia antedating the meningitis should be sought; careful examination for heart murmurs and peripheral stigmata of endocarditis is indicated. (3) *"Chemical" meningitis.* The clinical and CSF findings (polymorphonuclear pleocytosis and even reduced glucose level) of bacterial meningitis may be produced by chemically induced inflammation. Acute meningitis following a diagnostic lumbar puncture or spinal anesthesia may be due to bacterial (usually *Pseudomonas* species or coliform organisms) or chemical contamination of equipment or anesthetic agent. Endogenous chemical meningitis resulting from leakage into the subarachnoid space of material from an epidermoid tumor or a craniopharyngioma can produce a polymorphonuclear pleocytosis and hypoglycorrhachia. Birefringent material may be seen on polarizing microscopy of the CSF sediment.

NON-NEUROLOGIC COMPLICATIONS. ***Shock.*** When shock occurs in pyogenic meningitis it is usually a manifestation of an accompanying intense bacteremia, as in fulminant meningococcemia, rather than of the meningitis itself. Management is guided by the principles of septic shock therapy with appropriate modifications for myocardial failure (see Ch. 272).

Coagulation Disorders. Coagulopathies are frequently associated with the intense bacteremias (usually meningococcal, occasionally pneumococcal) and hypotension which can accompany meningitis. The changes may be mild such as thrombocytopenia (with or without prolongation of prothrombin and partial thromboplastin times) or more marked with clinical evidences of disseminated intravascular coagulation (see Ch. 272).

Septic Complications. Endocarditis. Previously, 5 to 10 per cent of patients with pneumococcal meningitis, particularly those with bacteremia and pneumonia as well, developed acute endocarditis, most commonly on the aortic valve. The incidence is currently much lower, as a result of earlier treatment of the initiating infection. In such patients, febrile relapse and a new murmur may appear shortly after completion of antimicrobial therapy for meningitis.

Pyogenic Arthritis. Septic arthritis may result from the bacteremia associated with meningitis caused by *S. pneumoniae*, *N. meningitidis*, or *H. influenzae*.

Prolonged Fever. With appropriate antimicrobial treatment of meningitis of the three most common bacterial causes, patients become afebrile within two to five days. Sometimes fever persists beyond this or recurs after an afebrile period. In the patient with persisting headache, obtundation, and cerebral findings, inadequate drug therapy or neurologic sequelae (cortical venous thrombophlebitis, ventriculitis, subdural collections) are important considerations. Re-evaluation of the CSF, particularly Gram-stained smear and culture, is essential under these circumstances. Drug fever may be responsible in the patient who continues to show clinical improvement in all other respects. Metastatic infection (septic arthritis, purulent pericarditis, thoracic empyema, endocarditis) may be the cause of continuing or recurrent fever.

A syndrome consisting of fever, arthritis, and pericarditis three to six days after initiation of effective antimicrobial therapy of meningococcal meningitis occurs in about 10 per cent of patients (see Ch. 272).

RECURRENT MENINGITIS. Repeated episodes of bacterial meningitis generally indicate a host defect, either in local anatomy or in antibacterial and immunologic defenses (e.g., recurrent *N. meningitidis* infections in patients with congenital or acquired deficiencies of complement, particularly late-acting components). *S. pneumoniae* is by far the most frequent cause of recurrent meningitis. Eleven per cent of patients with pneumococcal meningitis have had more than one episode, whereas 0.5 per cent of patients with meningitis caused by other organisms have had recurrent attacks. A history of head trauma is much more frequent in patients with recurrent meningitis. Organisms may directly enter the subarachnoid space, through a defect in the cribriform plate (the most common site), in association with the empty sella syndrome, via a basilar skull fracture, through an erosive sequestrum of the mastoid, through congenital dermal defects along the craniospinal axis (usually evident before adult life), or as a consequence of penetrating cranial trauma or neurosurgical procedures. The anatomic defect may produce a frank CSF leak (rhinorrhea or, less commonly, otorrhea) or may entrap a vascular cuff of meninges which might subsequently serve as a direct route for organisms to reach the meninges. CSF rhinorrhea may be intermittent, and meningitis may occur months or years after head injury.

Any patient with bacterial meningitis, particularly if meningitis is recurrent, should be evaluated carefully for any congenital or post-traumatic defects. The presence of CSF rhinorrhea should be sought at admission and subsequently (rhinorrhea may clear during active meningitis only to recur when inflammation has resolved). Clinical clues suggesting the presence of a CSF fistula through the cribriform plate, pericranial air sinuses, or temporal bone include (1) salty taste in the throat, (2) positionally dependent rhinorrhea (rhinorrhea only in the lateral recumbent or prone position suggests an otic or sphenoid origin), (3) anosmia (cribriform plate leak), (4) hearing loss or full feeling in the ear, often with a finding of fluid or bubbles behind the tympanic membrane (leakage into the middle ear). Demonstration of glucose in nasal secretions with glucose oxidase "sticks" (Dextrostix) suggests the presence of CSF. Quantitative determination of glucose and chloride content of nasal secretions can definitively establish the presence of CSF rhinorrhea.

Recurrent pneumococcal meningitis may occur without apparent predisposing circumstances, and cryptic CSF leaks should be sought actively in such patients by polytomography of the frontal and mastoid regions and by radioisotope techniques. (Radioiodine-labeled albumin is introduced intrathecally, and pledgets of cotton placed in the nares are subsequently examined for the radionuclide. Radioisotopic cisternography has been used successfully recently.) Intrathecal introduction of fluorescein as a visual tracer (under ultraviolet light) can be employed similarly in detecting active leaks. Surgical closure of CSF fistulas should be carried out to prevent further episodes of meningitis. Newer extracranial approaches via the ethmoid sinuses for repair of cribriform plate or sphenoid sinus dural defects are successful and avoid the higher morbidity associated with craniotomy.

In most patients with CSF otorrhea and rhinorrhea following an acute head injury, the leak ceases in one or two weeks. *Persistent rhinorrhea for more than four to six weeks is an indication for surgical repair.* Prolonged administration of penicillin will not prevent pneumococcal meningitis and may encourage infection with more drug-resistant species.

Rarely, recurrent meningitis of nonbacterial etiology may mimic bacterial meningitis. *Mollaret's meningitis* consists of repeated febrile episodes of mild meningeal symptomatology, usually without neurologic abnormalities. Initially, large "endothelial" cells may be seen in the CSF along with polymorphonuclear leukocytes, which subsequently are replaced by lymphocytes. *Behçet's syndrome,* characterized by relapsing oral and genital ulcers and ocular lesions (hypopyon), may exhibit a variety of neurologic abnormalities, including recurrent meningitis.

PROGNOSIS. The introduction of antimicrobial agents has converted bacterial meningitis from a disease that was almost always fatal to one in which the majority of patients survive without significant neurologic residua. The mortality rate for bacterial meningitis varies with the etiologic agent and the clinical circumstances. With current antimicrobial therapy the mortality rate for *H. influenzae* meningitis is below 5 per cent and that for meningococcal meningitis is about 10 per cent. The highest mortality is with pneumococcal meningitis, in which the rate is about 25 per cent. Poor prognostic factors include advanced age, presence of other foci of infection, underlying diseases (leukemia, alcoholism), coma, and delay in instituting appropriate therapy.

TREATMENT. ***Antimicrobial Agents.*** *Antimicrobial therapy should be begun promptly in this life-threatening emergency.* Treatment should be aimed at the most likely causes based on available clinical clues (age of the patient, presence of a purpuric rash, a recent neurosurgical procedure, CSF rhinorrhea). If the infecting organism is observed on examination of the Gram-stained smear of the CSF sediment, specific therapy is initiated. If the etiologic agent is not seen on smear (or not detected by CIE), treatment for bacterial meningitis of unknown etiology should be carried out (see below).

With the exception of chloramphenicol, the commonly employed antimicrobial agents do not readily penetrate the normal blood-brain barrier; but the passage of penicillin and other antimicrobials is enhanced in the presence of meningeal inflammation. Antimicrobial drugs should be administered intravenously throughout the treatment period; reduction in dosage as the patient improves should be avoided, because normalization of the blood-brain barrier during recovery reduces the CSF levels of drug that are achievable. Bactericidal drugs (penicillin, ampicillin) are preferred whenever possible in the treatment of meningitis caused by susceptible bacteria. Several antimicrobial drugs (first or second generation cephalosporins, clindamycin) which do not provide effective levels in the cerebrospinal fluid should not be used.

Meningitis of Specific Bacterial Cause. The treatment of choice for pneumococcal meningitis in the adult is penicillin (24 million units daily in divided doses every two hours) or ampicillin (12 grams daily in divided doses every two to three hours). In the patient with a major penicillin allergy, chloramphenicol (4 to 6 grams intravenously daily in the adult) is a reasonable alternative. Penicillin (ampicillin) is the most extensively studied and effective agent in the treatment of pneumococcal meningitis, but limited studies of chloramphenicol indicate that it can produce comparable therapeutic results. However, several points of caution should be made: (1) resistance to chloramphenicol has been reported from Spain in 45 per cent of pneumococcal strains, (2) the response to chloramphenicol of granulocytopenic patients may be suboptimal. Recently, isolates of *S. pneumoniae* that are relatively resistant (minimum inhibitory concentration (MIC) of 0.1 to 1.0 μg per milliliter) or highly resistant (South African strains with MIC of 4 to 8 μg per milliliter) to penicillin have been identified. In the United States, relative pneumococcal resistance to penicillin occurs in approximately 2 per cent of clinical isolates (in a few geographic areas the figures are as high as 8 or 16 per cent). In addition to cases of meningitis due to highly penicillin-resistant *S. pneumoniae* that occurred during the outbreak in South Africa in the late 1970's, seven cases of meningitis due to moderately penicillin-resistant strains (including two that were multiply-resistant) have been described in the United States and abroad. Thus, antimicrobial susceptibilities should be determined for all pneumococcal isolates from cerebrospinal fluid and blood. Chloramphenicol is a reasonable alternative to penicillin G in treatment of pneumococcal meningitis due to strains that are penicillin-resistant, provided they are not multiply-resistant. The multiply and highly penicillin-resistant strains in South Africa were susceptible only to vancomycin among the commonly employed antimicrobials. Of the currently available third-generation cephalosporins, cefotaxime has the greatest in vitro activity (MIC of 0.06 to 0.5 μg per milliliter) against moderately penicillin-resistant *S. pneumoniae,* but its effectiveness in meningitis due to such strains requires clinical evaluation.

The treatment of meningococcal meningitis is the same as for pneumococcal meningitis (see Ch. 272).

At present 25 per cent of isolates of *H. influenzae* b in the United States are ampicillin resistant. This has dictated a change in initial management of *H. influenzae* meningitis. Chloramphenicol (100 mg per kilogram intravenously daily for a child; 4 grams intravenously daily for an adult), either alone or in combination with ampicillin (300 to 400 mg per kilogram intravenously per day for a child; 12 grams intravenously per day for an adult), is the preferred treatment until drug susceptibilities are determined. If the organism proves susceptible to ampicillin, then this drug can be used alone in treatment. In the rare instance of *H. influenzae* meningitis due to a strain resistant to both ampicillin and chloramphenicol or occurring in a patient who cannot tolerate chloramphenicol, cefotaxime (180 mg per kilogram intravenously daily in divided doses every 4 to 6 hours for children) or moxalactam (100 mg per kilogram intravenously as a loading dose followed by 50 mg per kilogram every 6 hours for children) are alternatives.

Adult meningitis caused by methicillin-sensitive *S. aureus* should be treated with a penicillinase-resistant penicillin (nafcillin 10 to 12 grams intravenously per day). In the penicillin-allergic patient, vancomycin (2.0 grams intravenously in divided doses every 6 hours) is the alternative of choice. Since penetration of vancomycin into the CSF is limited, adjunctive intrathecal therapy (5,000 to 10,000 units of bacitracin slowly in 10 ml of CSF in the adult; or 5 to 20 mg of vancomycin in 10 ml of 5 per cent dextrose–0.85 per cent NaCl slowly in the adult)* has been used when CSF cultures have remained positive after 48 hours of intravenous therapy alone. For adult meningitis due to methicillin-resistant *S. aureus*, intravenous vancomycin (with adjunctive intrathecal bacitracin or vancomycin) is the treatment of choice. In refractory cases the addition of another drug for systemic therapy (rifampin or gentamicin) may be warranted.

Treatment of enterococcal meningitis in the adult involves the use of intravenous penicillin (24 million units daily) or ampicillin (12 grams daily), supplemented with parenterally administered gentamicin (3 to 5 mg per kilogram daily in divided doses every eight hours). In the patient who fails to respond promptly to parenteral therapy, adjunctive intrathecal therapy with gentamicin* (3 to 5 mg) should be considered.

The third generation cephalosporins (cefotaxime 12 grams daily intravenously in divided doses every 4 hours in adults; moxalactam 12 grams daily intravenously in divided doses every 6 hours in adults) are now being used extensively in the treatment of meningitis known to be due to susceptible gram-negative bacilli (*E. coli, Klebsiella, Proteus,* etc.). They should not be used in the treatment of meningitis due to less susceptible species such as *Pseudomonas aeruginosa* and *Acinetobacter*. Initial treatment (on the basis only of findings on Gram-stained smear of CSF) of adults with gram-negative bacillary meningitis involves either the combination of cefotaxime (or moxalactam) with an aminoglycoside (e.g., gentamicin 5 mg per kilogram daily intravenously in divided doses every 8 hours) or, alternatively, the combination of chloramphenicol (4 grams intravenously daily) with an aminoglycoside. Adjunctive intrathecal therapy with gentamicin* (3 to 5 mg administered at intervals of 24 hours for the first few days) may be indicated as well. Following identification of the specific pathogen and determination of its drug susceptibilities, alterations in antimicrobial therapy may be indicated. If the organism is *Pseudomonas aeruginosa*, parenteral and intrathecal gentamicin (or tobramycin) would be employed in combination with carbenicillin (30 to 40 grams intravenously daily).

Bacterial Meningitis of Unknown Etiology. Initial treatment of meningitis when the etiologic agent cannot be identified on Gram-stained smear of cerebrospinal fluid is based on available clinical clues. *In the neonate,* a wide range of gram-positive (group B streptococci, *Listeria*) and gram-negative organisms *(E. coli, Klebsiella, H. influenzae)* may be the cause, indicating the intravenous use of combined therapy with drugs such as ampicillin with gentamicin (or amikacin), or ampicillin with moxalactam, until results of cultures become available. *In children,* therapy is directed at the three most frequent pathogens: *H. influenzae, S. pneumoniae,* and *N. meningitidis.* The appearance of ampicillin resistance among strains of *H. influenzae* has necessitated the shift from single drug therapy (ampicillin) to a two-drug approach (ampicillin-chloramphenicol) in the treatment of meningitis of unknown cause in this age group, pending results of culture. *In adults,* therapy with ampicillin or penicillin is directed at the most common community-acquired pathogens (*S. pneumoniae* and *N. meningitidis*). However, because *H. influenzae* type b infections appear to be increasing in adults, and because of the increased incidence of gram-negative bacillary and staphylococcal meningitis in certain clinical settings, broader initial therapy may be indicated if clinical features suggest unusual organisms.

Duration of Therapy. The frequency of cerebrospinal fluid examinations depends on the clinical course, but a repeat examination should be done in 24 to 48 hours if there has not been satisfactory improvement. Routine "end-of-treatment" CSF examination is unnecessary in most patients with the common types of community-acquired bacterial meningitis. Meningococci are rapidly eliminated from the circulation and CSF with appropriate antimicrobial therapy, which should be continued for at least five to seven days after the patient becomes afebrile. If the patient has responded well, a follow-up lumbar puncture is not necesssary. *H. influenzae* meningitis should be treated for a minimum of ten days (at least for seven days after the patient becomes afebrile); re-examination of the CSF at that time usually shows cell counts of less than 60 (over 90 per cent mononuclear). Follow-up CSF examination may be omitted in those patients who have responded with very rapid and complete clinical resolution of the meningitis. Since pneumococcal meningitis produces a more intense inflammatory response, antimicrobial treatment should be continued for 10 to 14 days and follow-up examination of the CSF should be done and show resolution before discontinuing treatment. More prolonged therapy is indicated with concomitant parameningeal infection or mastoiditis. Treatment of gram-negative bacillary meningitis with parenteral antimicrobials is prolonged, usually for a minimum of three weeks (particularly in patients with a recent neurosurgical procedure) in order to prevent relapse. Repeated examinations of the CSF (particularly for cell count, Gram-stained smear, and culture) are necessary both during and at the conclusion of treatment to determine whether bacteriologic cure has been achieved.

Other Aspects of Treatment. Occasional patients with acute bacterial meningitis develop marked brain swelling (CSF pressure exceeding 400 mm H_2O), which may lead to temporal lobe or cerebellar herniation following lumbar puncture. To reduce this increased pressure, an intravenous infusion of 20 per cent mannitol solution (1.5 to 2.0 grams per kilogram) is administered over 20 to 60 minutes. Continued control of increased intracranial pressure, if needed thereafter, may be effected with mannitol, dexamethasone (10 mg intravenously, followed by 4 mg every six hours), or both. Brain swelling is about the only indication for the use of corticosteroids in the treatment of pyogenic meningitis; they should be employed only when the appropriate antimicrobial drugs are administered. Fluid restriction (1200 to 1500 ml daily in adults) is advisable during the first 24 to 48 hours to minimize brain swelling.

Patients with acute bacterial meningitis should receive constant nursing attention to ensure prompt recognition of seizures and to prevent aspiration. If seizures occur, they should be treated acutely with diazepam (Valium) administered slowly intravenously in a dose of 5 to 10 mg in the adult. Maintenance anticonvulsant therapy can be continued thereafter with intravenous phenytoin (Dilantin) until the medication can be administered orally. Sedation should be avoided because of the danger of respiratory depression and aspiration.

Surgical treatment of an accompanying pyogenic focus such as mastoiditis should be carried out when complete recovery from the meningitis has occurred, but under continuing antibiotic administration. Rarely, the mastoid infection (e.g., Bezold abscess) is so hyperacute that early drainage may be required after 48 hours or so of antibiotic therapy when the acute meningeal process will have subsided somewhat.

*Intrathecal use is not mentioned in the manufacturer's package insert approved by the U.S. Food and Drug Administration. Therefore its use in these circumstances must be considered investigational.

Berk SL, McCabe WR: Meningitis caused by gram-negative bacilli. Ann Intern Med 93:253, 1980. *Good descriptions of gram-negative bacillary meningitis occurring spontaneously and after neurosurgery.*

Carpenter RR, Petersdorf RG: The clinical spectrum of bacterial meningitis. Am J Med 33:262, 1962. *Clear description of clinical settings and findings in the common meningitides.*

Cherubin CE, Corrado ML, Nair SR, Gombert ME, Landesman S, Humbert G: Treatment of gram-negative bacillary meningitis: Role of the new cephalosporin antibiotics. Rev Infect Dis 4:S453, 1982. *Summary of results of cefotaxime treatment of 137 patients with various types of bacterial meningitis.*

Durack DT, Spanos A: End-of-treatment spinal tap in bacterial meningitis. Is it worthwhile? JAMA 248:75, 1982. *Places in perspective the role of end-of-treatment CSF examination.*

Geiseler PJ, Nelson KE, Levin S, Reddi KT, Moses VK: Community-acquired purulent meningitis: A review of 1316 cases during the antibiotic era, 1954–1976. Rev Infect Dis 2:725, 1980. *Extensive experience at one of the last contagious disease hospitals in the United States is recounted. Effects of prior antibiotic therapy on culture results are particularly well studied.*

Hand WL, Sanford JP: Posttraumatic bacterial meningitis. Ann Intern Med 72:869, 1970. *Provides a helpful approach to the problem of post-traumatic CSF rhinorrhea and meningitis.*

Hyslop NE Jr, Montgomery WW: Diagnosis and management of meningitis associated with cerebrospinal leaks. *In* Remington JS, Swartz MN (eds.): Current Clinical Topics in Infectious Diseases, Vol 3. New York, McGraw-Hill Book Company, 1982, pp 254–285. *Most complete review of the bacteriology, anatomy, diagnostic approach, and surgical repair of CSF leaks associated with meningitis.*

Mangi RJ, Holstein LL, Andriole VT: Treatment of gram-negative bacillary meningitis with intrathecal gentamicin. Yale J Biol Med 50:31, 1977. *Helpful guidance for management of this difficult-to-treat form of bacterial meningitis.*

New PFJ, Davis KR: The role of CT scanning in diagnosis of infections of the central nervous system. *In* Remington JS, Swartz MN (eds.): Current Clinical Topics in Infectious Diseases, Vol 1. New York, McGraw-Hill Book Company, 1980, pp 1–33. *Comprehensive review of the changes on CT scan in a wide variety of CNS infections. Large number of illustrative scans with good descriptions.*

Overturf GD: Treatment of the child with bacterial meningitis. *In* Remington JS, Swartz MN (eds.): Current Clinical Topics in Infectious Diseases, Vol 3. New York, McGraw-Hill Book Company, 1982, pp 218–253. *Excellent review of management of childhood meningitis.*

Rahal JJ Jr: Moxalactam therapy for gram-negative bacillary meningitis. Rev Infect Dis 4:S606, 1982. *Experience with moxalactam treatment of 20 patients with gram-negative bacillary meningitis.*

Swartz MN: Intracranial infections. *In* Rosenberg RN (ed.): The Science and Practice of Clinical Medicine, Vol 5. New York, Grune and Stratton, 1980, pp 1–40. *Comprehensive clinical review of purulent meningitis, aseptic meningitis, encephalitis, and parameningeal infections.*

Swartz MN, Dodge PR: Bacterial meningitis—a review of selected aspects. N Engl J Med 272:725, 779, 842, 898, 954, 1003, 1965. *Detailed account of experience at the Massachusetts General Hospital. Particularly good on clinical aspects, neurologic complications, and differential diagnosis.*

272. MENINGOCOCCAL DISEASE

DEFINITION. Meningococcal infections are due to *Neisseria meningitidis*. The best known syndromes are *meningococcal meningitis* ("epidemic cerebrospinal meningitis") and *fulminant meningococcemia*. Infections also occur in the upper and lower respiratory tracts, joints, pericardium, eyes, and genitourinary tract.

ETIOLOGY. *N. meningitidis* is a gram-negative coccus which appears on smears of infected fluids as biscuit-shaped diplococci, located either extracellularly or within polymorphonuclear leukocytes. Colonies are best isolated on blood, "chocolate," or enriched Mueller-Hinton agar in an atmosphere of 3 to 10 per cent CO_2. Modified Thayer-Martin selective medium is useful in detection of meningococcal carriers or in initial isolation of *N. meningitidis* from areas with an extensive indigenous flora. The organism is susceptible to drying or chilling, and specimens should be inoculated and incubated promptly.

Since other *Neisseria* species and related organisms *(Branhamella catarrhalis)*, as well as morphologically similar gram-negative coccobacilli (e.g., *Moraxella*), may be isolated from clinical specimens, biochemical and immunologic methods are needed for identification. *Neisseria* species are oxidase positive. Whereas *N. gonorrhoeae* metabolizes only glucose (but not maltose or lactose), *N. meningitidis* metabolizes both glucose and maltose (but not lactose). *N. lactamica*, a species sometimes present in throat cultures, may be mistaken for the meningococcus, since it too metabolizes both glucose and maltose; however, it also utilizes lactose. Occasional maltose-negative strains of *N. meningitidis* have been noted; fluorescent antibody or coagglutination tests or electrophoretic analysis of hexokinase isoenzymes may be helpful in distinguishing such strains from *N. gonorrhoeae*, particularly when isolated from atypical locations.

Nine serogroups of *N. meningitidis*—A, B, C, D, X, Y, Z, Z′ (also known as 29E), W135—have been defined. They differ in the structures of their capsular polysaccharides and can be identified by agglutination reactions with specific antisera. Most meningococcal disease is due to strains belonging to groups A, B, C, and Y. Twenty to 50 per cent of isolates from carriers are nongroupable (unencapsulated). Subcapsular protein antigens located in the outer bacterial membrane have been used to identify at least 15 serotypes among the various serogroups, providing a classification useful in epidemiologic studies. Serotype 2 strains are responsible for most cases of meningococcal disease due to group B (50 per cent) and group C (80 per cent) organisms (and also are associated with groups Y and W135), but they are rarely isolated from carriers not in direct contact with clinical cases. In contrast, other serotypes are commonly isolated, but primarily from carriers. Group A meningococcal strains show no variation in their outer membrane proteins and are unrelated serologically to the serotypes of other groups.

Strains of *N. meningitidis* produce extracellular proteases which cleave the IgA1 heavy chain in the hinge region. Although the role of this protease in infection is unknown, its elaboration also by the other principal causes of bacterial meningitis *(H. influenzae, S. pneumoniae)* and the importance of IgA in mucosal immunity at the pharyngeal portal for these organisms suggests a possible role in pathogenicity.

Fresh isolates of *N. meningitidis* from the pharynx of carriers and from patients with meningococcal disease contain pili, which appear to have an important role in attachment to human nasopharyngeal cells. The colonial morphology of fresh isolates of *N. meningitidis* from patients with invasive infection (transparent colonies) differs from that of isolates from asymptomatic carriers (opaque colonies). Meningococci from transparent colonies are more resistant to killing by normal serum than are meningococci from opaque colonies, suggesting that this property may be a marker for virulence.

Meningococci contain endotoxins, and these lipopolysaccharides may play a role in the purpura and other clinical features of meningococcemia.

INCIDENCE. *N. meningitidis* is second only to *H. influenzae* as a cause of bacterial meningitis reported in this country. It is estimated that 3000 to 6000 cases of meningococcal meningitis occur annually.

EPIDEMIOLOGY. The natural reservoir of *N. meningitidis* is the human nasopharynx, and transmission occurs principally through airborne droplets or close contact. Infection may occur as the asymptomatic carrier state (the most common form) or as sporadic cases, limited outbreaks, or widespread epidemics.

Carrier State. Nasopharyngeal carrier rates may fluctuate widely. In a nonepidemic period it is 3 to 10 per cent in a civilian population. The rate varies with age: 0.5 to 1.0 per cent in children 3 to 48 months of age and about 5 per cent in those 14 to 17 years of age. In the nonepidemic setting carriage usually lasts weeks to months. The carrier rate in close family contacts of a case of meningococcal disease is increased and may reach 40 per cent. In crowded populations (e.g., military training camps) the carrier rate ranges between 20 and 60 per cent and may reach 90 per cent during epidemics. Although it has often been stated that meningococcal outbreaks occur when the rate of nasopharyngeal carriage exceeds 20 per cent in a military camp, there is in reality no clear relation between the overall carriage rate in a community and the occurrence of meningococcal disease. The strain(serotype)-specific acquisition rate appears to be a more reliable indicator of an outbreak than the group-specific carriage rate.

Spread of disease appears to be mediated by carriers rather than by direct case-to-case transmission. An adult family member generally is the one who brings *N. meningitidis* into a household, where it spreads to others and often colonizes younger children and infants last. As yet unknown host and environmental factors are of decisive importance in determining whether the organism will be confined to the nasopharynx or whether dissemination will take place.

Meningococcal Disease. The annual attack rate for meningococcal disease in the United States in recent years has ranged between 0.7 and 1.3 year per 100,000 population. The highest incidence is in the first year of life (14.4 per 100,000), declining in the one- to four-year age group (4.6 per 100,000), and ultimately reaching the level of 0.3 per 100,000 in adults. During epidemics of meningococcal disease, overall annual attack rates of 5 to 24 cases per 100,000 are observed (as high as 370 per 100,000 in Sao Paulo, Brazil, in 1974). The peak incidence is in the winter and early spring.

During a nonepidemic period the risk of meningococcal illness for household contacts of an initial case is about 3 per 1000 (500- to 1000-fold higher than the overall endemic rate for meningococcal disease) and stems from the higher carriage rate in this setting. The secondary attack rate appears to be age related, with most cases occurring in younger children.

Major meningococcal epidemics, caused primarily by group A strains, tend to recur at 20- to 30-year intervals. More circumscribed outbreaks have taken place in interepidemic periods, as in Detroit in 1929, when about 750 cases occurred over an eight-month period. Aside from several minor urban outbreaks, particularly among alcoholics, in the Pacific Northwest and a small outbreak in Canada, group A strains have only rarely been implicated in meningococcal disease in North America during the past decade. However, serious epidemics caused by group A meningococci have occurred in Finland in 1973, in Brazil in 1974, and in northern Nigeria in 1977. The outbreak in Nigeria is but one of many that have occurred about once every ten years in the "meningitis belt" in sub-Saharan Africa. In the 1948–49 epidemic, about 93,000 cases were reported, with over 14,000 deaths. Although group A meningococci had been susceptible to sulfonamides in the past, resistant strains first appeared in the epidemics in Africa in the late 1960's and subsequently in Brazil and Finland.

Although group A meningococci have been involved in the most extensive epidemics of meningococcal disease, groups B and C have been responsible for more limited outbreaks and for numerous sporadic cases both in this country and abroad. In the United States in 1963 and 1964, outbreaks caused by group B meningococci (noteworthy for their frequent resistance to sulfonamides) occurred in military camps. By 1967 serogroup B was responsible for the majority of infections occurring in military and civilian populations. By the early 1970's serogroup C strains were those most frequently isolated, only to be supplanted by group B in the mid 1970's. In the period 1975–1980 the serogroups found among disease-related strains were as follows: B (56 per cent), C (19 per cent), Y (11 per cent), W135 (10 per cent), A (3 per cent), and ungroupable (1 per cent). Serogroup W135 has recently appeared as an important cause of meningococcal disease in this country (21 per cent in 1980), displacing group C as the second most frequent cause.

Just as serogrouping of meningococcal strains has been invaluable in the study of major epidemics and in the development and use of polysaccharide vaccines, serotyping can be helpful in evaluating changes in ambient strains. Between epidemics sporadic cases are caused by heterogeneous strains belonging to many serogroups and a variety of serotypes. In military recruit populations, the serogroup carried is not a valid indicator of epidemic potential. At intervals of about ten years a single serotype (e.g., serotype 2, present in most disease-related strains of groups B and C and in some strains of groups Y and W135 during this past decade) becomes pre-eminent, producing a higher endemic rate of disease, sometimes accompanied by scattered small outbreaks.

Nosocomial transmission of infection occasionally occurs. Meningococcal meningitis has developed in several physicians who gave mouth-to-mouth resuscitation to infected patients. Group Y meningococci particularly have been implicated in meningococcal pneumonia, and such patients, if not isolated, may be responsible for nosocomial spread of infection.

Immunity. The age-specific incidence of meningococcal disease is inversely proportional to the prevalence of antimeningococcal bactericidal antibodies (against serogroups A, B, C). At birth, over 50 per cent of infants have bactericidal antibody. From 6 to 24 months of age, the prevalence of antibodies is lowest, and thereafter it increases to early adulthood, when over 70 per cent of individuals have bactericidal activity. The protective role of bactericidal antibodies against *N. meningitidis* was demonstrated during an outbreak of group C meningitis among army recruits in 1968. Eleven per cent of recruits lacked serum antibody against the outbreak-associated strain, and one quarter of these susceptibles acquired this strain during their training period. Of the susceptibles exposed, 38 per cent developed systemic meningococcal disease; in contrast, only 1 per cent of the entire trainee group developed disease.

IgA antibody to meningococcal polysaccharide may have a paradoxic effect. When a large part of an individual's antibodies to a meningococcal serogroup is of this class, serum bactericidal activity of IgM and IgG is blocked, enhancing susceptibility to meningococcal disease. This odd phenomenon is observed for a short time following the induction of IgA by asymptomatic carriage of *N. meningitidis* or an immunologically related organism.

Following meningococcal meningitis serum bactericidal antibody develops, and the patient is immune to clinical reinfection with the same serogroup. However, this is not the usual means of acquiring immunity. Nasopharyngeal carriage of *N. meningitidis* is an effective immunizing process, producing rises in bactericidal antibody within five to twelve days of acquisition of the organism. About 90 per cent of carriers of group B, C, or Y meningococci develop increased serum bactericidal titers, primarily to the colonizing strain but also to heterologous strains. Similarly, nasopharyngeal carriage of nongroupable meningococci, strains rarely causing human disease, can induce antibodies against various groupable pathogenic isolates.

The group-specific capsular polysaccharides of group A and group C meningococci are good immunogens and have been used in successful vaccines. The capsular polysaccharide of group B meningococci is a polymer of α2-8–linked sialic acid and is a very poor immunogen. Human brain glycoproteins contain polysialosyl chains that cross-react immunologically with the group B capsular polysaccharide (but not with group A polysaccharide), perhaps accounting for the failure to develop an effective group B vaccine.

In young children, colonization with *N. lactamica* may induce cross-reactive antibodies to *N. meningitidis* and thus contribute to natural immunity. *N. lactamica* is relatively avirulent and has only rarely been involved in systemic infections. During the first eight years of life the age-related prevalence of meningococcal carriage is between 0.5 and 2 per cent, whereas that of *N. lactamica* is considerably higher (4 to 20 per cent).

In addition to antibody, complement is an important component of serum bactericidal activity. Isolated congenital deficiency of one of the late complement components (C5, C6, C7, or C8) is rare and has been associated with recurrent or chronic (chronic meningococcemia) infections with *N. meningitidis* or *N. gonorrhoeae*. Repeated episodes of meningococcal meningitis have occurred in patients with late complement component deficiencies in the absence of enhanced susceptibility to organisms other than *N. meningitidis*. Measurement of total hemolytic complement is helpful for screening purposes in a patient with recurrent systemic *Neisseria* infections. The course of infection, whether meningitis or meningococcemia, is not unusual, and the response to antimicrobial treatment is satisfactory. Complement deficiency, either congenital (late-acting components) or due to a complement-depleting (C1, C3, C4) underlying disease, also may be an important risk factor for the occurrence of first episodes of nonepidemic meningococcal disease: among 20 patients presenting with invasive infection 30 per cent had decreased complement function.

PATHOGENESIS AND PATHOLOGY. The factors that determine whether initial exposure to *N. meningitidis* will result in benign nasopharyngeal carriage or serious invasive infection are unclear. About one third of patients with invasive infection have had antecedent symptoms referable to the upper respiratory tract. Whether these prodromal symptoms are produced by *N. meningitidis* or a predisposing viral respiratory infection is difficult to determine, particularly since many cases of meningococcal disease occur in the winter when viral respiratory infections are frequent. A simultaneous outbreak of systemic meningococcal disease and influenza A2 infection has occurred in a closed institutional setting. The predisposing role of influenza for meningococcal lower respiratory infections may be clearer (e.g., the occurrence of numerous cases of meningococcal pneumonia complicating influenza during the 1918–19 pandemic).

The incubation period from the initiation of nasopharyngeal infection to bloodstream dissemination is difficult to determine but is probably under ten days. The incubation period may be quite short, judging by the fact that the interval between primary and secondary cases in the same household is often only one to four days. Also, among prospectively studied military recruits cultured within seven days preceding hospitalization for meningococcal disease, only about 20 per cent were carriers of the implicated strain. Once the organism has entered the circulation, the predominant (over 90 per cent) clinical expression is as meningitis or meningococcemia.

The pathologic findings in acute meningococcemia involve the microvasculature and are observed when shock and disseminated intravascular coagulation have occurred. The skin lesions show evidence of fibrin thrombi and vasculitis in small blood vessels. *N. meningitidis* can be seen in endothelial cells and in neutrophils surrounding damaged vessels. The prominent purpura has been attributed to the enhanced capacity to elicit the dermal Shwartzman reaction of its endotoxin compared to endotoxin from enteric gram-negative bacilli. Hemorrhagic adrenal infarction is often observed in patients with fulminant meningococcemia (Waterhouse-Friderichsen syndrome). Shock in this disease is a consequence of bacteremia and not of adrenal failure, since (1) fulminant meningococcemia can occur without adrenal hemorrhage, (2) serum cortisol levels are normal or elevated, and (3) patients who have recovered have not developed Addison's disease. It has been suggested that the shock, purpura, and widespread microvascular thrombi are consequences of an endotoxin-initiated generalized Shwartzman-like reaction or endotoxin-activated disseminated intravascular coagulation. Depressed levels of complement components are found in some patients with acute meningococcemia and may reflect complement activation by circulating endotoxin. Interstitial myocarditis is observed in about 70 per cent of cases of fatal meningococcal disease.

CLINICAL MANIFESTATIONS. Overt illness develops when the initial, often minimally symptomatic nasopharyngeal infection has progressed to bloodstream invasion. The subsequent clinical picture may be mild, or sudden in onset and fulminant, and may reflect principally the bacteremia or features referable to metastatic localization of infection. The most common clinical syndromes are acute meningococcemia, acute purulent meningitis, and a combination of the two (meningococcemia-meningitis).

Meningitis. Most cases occur in children between three months of age and adolescence. Isolated meningitis is less common than meningococcemia-meningitis. The clinical picture may be dominated by manifestations of either meningococcemia or meningitis. In the latter instance the findings are similar to those of meningitis caused by any of the common pyogens (see Ch. 271). Predisposing acute otitis media or pneumonia is unusual in contrast to *H. influenzae* or pneumococcal meningitis. The onset of meningeal symptomatology (1) may be rapid (less than 24 hours) without premonitory symptomatology, (2) may follow an upper respiratory infection of one or two weeks' duration, or (3) may evolve gradually over several days of upper respiratory or nonlocalizing symptoms. In the last-named instance CSF examination during this period may reveal minimal or no increase in cell count and no organisms on Gram-stained smear, but *N. meningitidis* may be isolated, indicating early meningeal involvement. A "clear" CSF in this setting should *not* preclude careful culture. The rapid onset of delirium is seen occasionally in bacterial meningitis (more frequently meningococcal), but it also may occur with a temporal lobe abscess or encephalitis. The neurologic features and complications of meningococcal meningitis are generally the same as for other bacterial meningitides.

The course of meningococcal meningitis may differ from that of other pyogenic meningitides in the occasional occurrence during convalescence of a nonseptic arthritis-pericarditis syndrome.

Meningococcemia. About 20 per cent of patients with meningococcal disease have meningococcemia without meningitis. The clinical expression of meningococcemia varies from an acute process (mild systemic illness or rapidly lethal course) to a chronic, indolent, relapsing disease that may go on for months.

Mild Acute Meningococcemia. This is the most common form of meningococcemia, characterized by the rapid development of malaise, fever, chills, myalgias, and arthralgias, often following a minor upper respiratory infection. In a few patients diarrhea has been an early symptom. The subsequent course may follow one of several paths: (1) Symptoms may abate in two or three days, and the diagnosis is made in retrospect when *N. meningitidis* is isolated from a blood culture. (2) Initial symptomatology is followed over 24 to 48 hours by recurrent chills and the appearance of erythematous macular lesions, particularly on the extremities, often accompanied by petechiae. In more severe infections, purpura and ecchymotic areas with gunmetal gray necrotic centers appear. Tachycardia and tachypnea are prominent. Mild hypotension may be present, and shock is a feature if fulminant meningococcemia ensues. In some patients headache may appear and confusion and stiff neck develop; the syndrome then becomes one of combined *meningococcemia-meningitis.* A meningoencephalopathic picture has been described in up to 15 per cent of patients. This probably represents a heterogeneous group (some with meningitis and others with fulminant meningococcemia and central nervous system changes secondary to shock), in whom confusion, delirium, or coma is striking. (3) Occasionally, initial malaise, fever, and arthralgias (accompanied by a few macular and petechial skin lesions) may persist for about a week, during which one or more joint effusions may develop. Blood cultures reveal *N. meningitidis,* and all manifestations promptly subside on treatment with penicillin.

Fulminant Meningococcemia. This is the most dramatic form of infection, with an abrupt onset and extraordinarily rapid progression (occasionally less than 10 hours from onset to fatal termination). It occurs in about 10 per cent of patients with meningococcal disease. Violent chills, high fever, dizziness, headache, and profound weakness develop over a few hours. Petechiae appear initially on the extremities; they rapidly increase in number and coalesce as new ones appear in the conjunctivae and buccal mucosa. Hypotension with peripheral vasoconstriction quickly appears. Purpura soon develops (Fig. 272–1). At this point the patient may still be febrile or may have become hypothermic. As shock supervenes, restlessness, mental obtundation, and coma may follow in rapid succession. Disseminated intravascular coagulation (DIC) is commonly present, with enlarging hemorrhagic areas in the skin and sometimes mucosal and gastrointestinal bleeding. Cardiac (my-

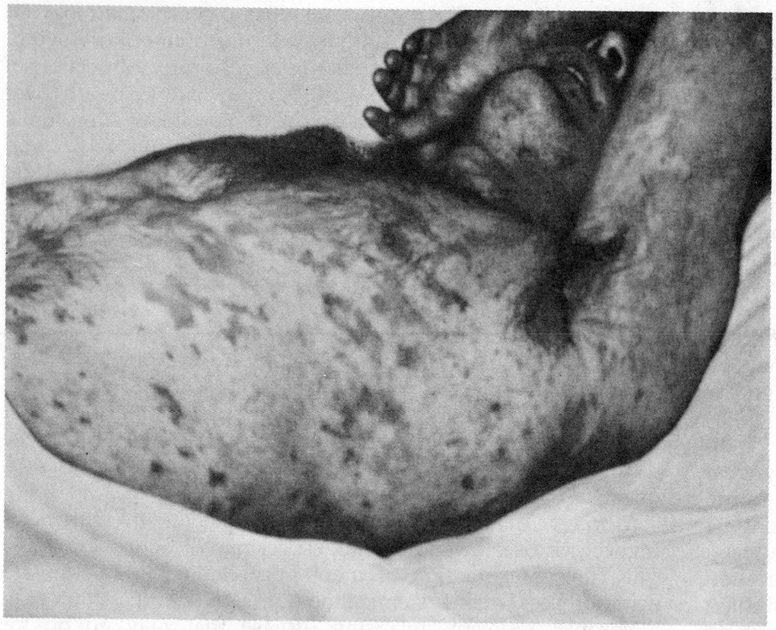

Figure 272–1. Skin lesions in fulminating meningococcemia. (Courtesy of Dr. Worth B. Daniels.)

ocarditis) and respiratory ("shock lung") failure may be terminal events. *The relentless course, once shock develops, makes mandatory early diagnosis and immediate institution of antibiotic treatment even while parts of the initial examination are being performed.*

CHRONIC MENINGOCOCCEMIA. This uncommon form of meningococcemia is characterized by intermittent febrile episodes lasting one to six days, or, rarely, by sustained fevers for several weeks. It begins with chills, migratory arthralgias (or occasionally mild arthritis), and headache, but minimal toxicity. A transient polymorphous (erythematous macules and papules, rare petechiae, and purpuric nodules) nonpruritic rash appears with each febrile episode. The total number of skin lesions is small, and Gram stain and culture only rarely reveal the etiologic agent. Biopsy reveals a leukocytoclastic angiitis, which may be mistaken for a collagen disease or allergic vasculitis. Splenomegaly is observed in 20 per cent of patients. Blood cultures are not positive during apyrexial periods and may not yield the organism until the second or third febrile episode.

Untreated, about 20 per cent of patients ultimately develop meningitis. Rarer complications include endocarditis and epididymitis.

Where the organism resides between episodes is unclear. Throat cultures frequently have not revealed meningococci. The occurrence of chronic meningococcemia in several patients with congenital late complement component deficiencies suggests a possible factor in pathogenesis.

Upper Respiratory Tract Infection. How frequently nasopharyngeal infection is symptomatic is unclear. Nasopharyngeal symptoms preceding some systemic meningococcal infections may be due to this organism or to ambient viral respiratory infections.

Pneumonia. Meningococcal pneumonia is much more often of bronchogenic than of hematogenous origin. Other than during the 1918 influenza pandemic, it has been reported only rarely until this past decade. Primary meningococcal pneumonia is most often due to group Y; in recent years among recruits pneumonia caused by group Y has become the most common form of meningococcal disease. Primary meningococcal pneumonia may be segmental, lobar, or bronchopneumonic in pattern. It sometimes follows antecedent influenza or adenoviral infection. Clinical features are similar to those of community-acquired pneumonias. The onset may be gradual or abrupt. Lower lobes are usually involved. Bacteremia occurs in about 15 per cent of cases. In some patients purulent sputum is produced, containing numerous gram-negative diplococci; in others sputum is scanty, and diagnosis is made on a transtracheal aspirate or by blood culture. Response to treatment with penicillin is prompt.

Meningococcal pneumonia occasionally develops in the course of clinical meningococcemia or meningitis, but the clinical picture is dominated by the extrapulmonary aspects.

To be distinguished from meningococcal pneumonia are occasional exacerbations of chronic bronchopulmonary infection in which the sputum may show numerous gram-negative, biscuit-shaped diplococci (usually noninvasive *Neisseria* species or *Branhamella catarrhalis*). Beta-lactamase–producing strains of *Branhamella catarrhalis* have been isolated with increasing frequency in such pulmonary infections, and they may not respond to treatment with penicillin or ampicillin.

Arthritis. Arthritis complicates 2 to 16 per cent of acute meningococcal illness and may take several forms: (1) *Isolated, acute suppurative meningococcal arthritis,* a rare type occurring in the absence of meningitis or clinical meningococcemia. The joint fluid has the characteristics of septic arthritis. (2) *Early onset (first two to three days) arthritis* during meningococcal meningitis or meningococcemia, the most common form. It is a polyarthritis with acutely inflamed joints; effusions are small or absent. It responds promptly to penicillin. (3) *Late onset (fourth to tenth day, when meningitis is subsiding) arthritis.* This is commonly a subacute mono- or oligoarthritis accompanied by joint effusions. It is associated with recrudescence of fever, pleuropericarditis, and, occasionally, new papulobullous skin lesions. Synovial and pericardial fluids are characteristically serosanguineous (but sometimes purulent) and sterile. Immunopathologic study of synovial lesions implicates immune complex formation in their genesis. Treatment involves joint aspiration and the use of anti-inflammatory agents.

Pericarditis. Pericarditis complicates 2 to 20 per cent of meningococcal disease. It may take several forms: (1) *Early onset pericarditis,* appearing in the first several days of clinical meningococcemia or meningitis, may be purulent and may be due to invasion by *N. meningitidis.* (2) *Late onset pericarditis,* developing four to ten days after onset of meningitis, may cause large sterile, serosanguineous effusions. The favorable response to anti-inflammatory agents and adrenal corticosteroids supports the proposed role of hypersensitivity in pathogenesis. (3) *Isolated purulent pericarditis,* occurring in the absence of meningitis or clinical meningococcemia, is the least common form of meningococcal pericarditis and usually presents with a purulent effusion and tamponade requiring surgical intervention.

Other Meningococcal Infections. Ocular involvement (panophthalmitis, conjunctivitis) occurs in less than 1 per cent of patients with meningococcal disease. Primary conjunctivitis, an acute purulent process, is even less common. Since dissemination develops in 10 per cent of children with primary meningococcal conjunctivitis, systemic therapy with penicillin should be employed along with topical antimicrobials.

Genital tract and anal infections with *N. meningitidis* occasionally occur, the latter in homosexual males. In the female symptomatic or asymptomatic infections of the cervix and vagina may be associated with salpingitis or subsequent clinical meningococcemia. Urethral infection is less common than anal infection but is usually symptomatic. Treatment, as for gonococcal infection, is warranted to eliminate symptomatic disease and to prevent the rare instance of disseminated infection.

COURSE AND COMPLICATIONS. Acute meningococcemia may run a varied course, from that of mild disease to that of fulminant illness with death in a day or less. Certain features (particularly if present simultaneously) indicate a poor prognosis: (1) petechiae for less than 12 hours prior to hospitalization (rapid development of crops of new petechiae and purpura from one hour to the next is ominous); (2) shock; (3) fever above 40° C; (4) absence of meningitis; (5) leukopenia; (6) thrombocytopenia or evidence of DIC; and (7) extremes of age.

Extensive purpura, acral cyanosis, hemorrhagic bullae, and peripheral gangrene are features of fulminant meningococcemia, usually occurring in the presence of shock and DIC. DIC may be evident on hospitalization or may develop precipitously in some patients who are stable initially. In acute DIC platelets, fibrinogen and factors II, V, VIII, and XIII are reduced. Abnormalities in three screening tests (prothrombin time prolongation, platelet count reduction, hypofibrinogenemia) aid in detection of DIC, which occurs to some extent in about one quarter of patients with meningococcemia. The partial thromboplastin time may also be prolonged. Confirmation is provided by demonstration of circulating fibrin degradation products in concentrations greater than 40 μg per milliliter. These coagulation defects can result in upper gastrointestinal bleeding, hematuria, and bleeding from the respiratory tract. Despite all therapeutic interventions, some patients show progressive deterioration with marked tachycardia, hyperventilation, refractory shock, metabolic acidosis, deepening coma, and "shock lung." Myocardial involvement may be manifest as either transient electrocardiographic changes or left ventricular failure.

In those who recover, resolution of the hemorrhagic or gangrenous lesions is slow and may require skin grafting. Areas of the hands and feet may remain edematous, cold, and cyanotic and may show demarcation after some weeks.

DIAGNOSIS. ***Laboratory Findings.*** Bacteriologic diagnosis is established by the finding of organisms on stained smears from an infected area (in an appropriate clinical setting), by isolation of *N. meningitidis* from blood or infected body fluids, or by demonstration by latex agglutination or counterimmunoelectrophoresis of group A, B, C, or Y polysaccharide antigen in blood or CSF. Blood cultures reveal *N. meningitidis* in about one third of patients with meningococcal meningitis and in 50 to 75 per cent with clinical meningococcemia or meningococcemia-meningitis. In rare patients with fulminant meningococcemia, diplococci can be seen on Gram-stained smears of blood or buffy coat. Demonstration of organisms on scrapings from skin lesions in acute meningococcemia has been variable: 70 per cent in one study, but much lower in more recent experience.

Since *N. gonorrhoeae* can be isolated from the pharynx and *N. meningitidis* can occasionally be found in the anogenital area, since both species may invade the bloodstream, and since gonococci and *N. lactamica* have on rare occasions been implicated in meningitis, accurate bacteriologic identification is important. However, 0.5 to 5 per cent of meningococci are maltose negative and may thus resemble gonococci and cause confusion.

Meningococcal polysaccharide antigen is demonstrated in the CSF of about 70 per cent of patients with meningococcal meningitis. Antigen is detected in the blood of 10 to 25 per cent of patients with meningococcemia, and its presence is associated with a poorer prognosis and higher incidence of late onset arthritis.

The CSF findings in meningococcal meningitis are those of pyogenic meningitis.

Differential Diagnosis. The differential diagnosis of meningococcal meningitis in the absence of clinical meningococcemia is that of acute meningitis with a purulent CSF formula. With the meningococcemia-meningitis syndrome it should be remembered that very rare instances of meningitis caused by *H. influenzae* and *S. pneumoniae* may be accompanied by petechial skin lesions. Occasional patients with enteroviral meningitis may have a brisk CSF pleocytosis (up to several thousand cells, with as many as 50 to 80 per cent neutrophils and a maculopetechial rash). Rarely, acute bacterial endocarditis caused by *Staphylococcus aureus* can produce a clinical picture almost indistinguishable from that of meningococcemia-meningitis, with a polymorphonuclear CSF pleocytosis and petechial and purpuric skin lesions. In *S. aureus* endocarditis there are a few skin lesions of purulent purpura which show the etiologic agent on Gram-stained smear. Occasionally measles or other viral exanthems may resemble early meningococcemia. Rocky Mountain spotted fever may mimic meningococcemia, but the absence of meningitis in the former, epidemiologic considerations, and demonstration of the etiologic agent aid in distinguishing between these processes.

Chronic meningococcemia, because of its protean manifestations, may be mistaken for Henoch-Schönlein purpura, acute vasculitis, gonococcemia, rheumatic fever, and subacute bacterial endocarditis.

TREATMENT. ***Antibiotic Management.*** As soon as the diagnosis is made, the patient should be put on respiratory isolation to minimize nosocomial spread of infection. Whereas practically all meningococci isolated prior to 1963 were susceptible to sulfadiazine (formerly the treatment of choice), since that time isolates resistant to sulfonamides have become common. Sulfonamide resistance in this country peaked in 1970, when 67 per cent of strains were resistant, and has since decreased (1980) to 12 per cent (8 per cent of group B, 30 per cent of group C, 4 per cent of group W135; all group Y strains susceptible). Should resistance to sulfonamides decline to less than 10 per cent, sulfonamides may again become appropriate drugs for prophylaxis.

Antimicrobial therapy should be initiated *immediately* in patients with suspected meningococcal meningitis or clinical meningococcemia because of the rapidity with which the illness may progress. Clinical isolates have been uniformly susceptible to penicillin and ampicillin (one penicillin-resistant genitourinary tract isolate, a strain with an R-factor mediated β-lactamase, has recently been described). Intravenous penicillin G is the drug of choice (24 million units daily in the adult in divided doses every two hours) for meningococcal meningitis. Alternatively, intravenous ampicillin can be employed in the adult (12 grams daily in divided doses every two to three hours). In patients allergic to penicillin, intravenous chloramphenicol (4 to 6 grams daily in the adult) is the recommended alternative, with appropriate monitoring of the hematopoietic system. The duration of treatment of meningococcal meningitis and the management of complications are considered in Ch. 271.

Intravenous penicillin G is the treatment of acute clinical meningococcemia without meningitis. Although 8 to 10 million units daily is usually adequate to sterilize the blood and most areas of metastatic infection, it may not provide therapeutic CSF levels in the patient with incipient meningitis. For this reason, initial therapy with "meningitis" doses is often employed. Treatment is continued until the patient has been afebrile for five days. Penicillin (5 to 8 million units daily intravenously in the adult) is effective treatment for chronic meningococcemia.

Other Aspects of Treatment. Treatment of severe meningococcemia requires supportive measures to deal with shock and other complications (DIC, congestive failure, metabolic acidosis, "shock lung"). These include cardiovascular monitoring in an intensive care setting, initial volume expansion, use of vasoactive agents, attention to fluid balances, maintenance of adequate oxygenation, and possible use of digitalis. A central venous pressure (CVP) catheter is placed (a flow-directed pulmonary catheter for evaluation of left atrial and ventricular filling pressures may be necessary if cardiac decompensation develops). Volume expansion (dextrose-saline infused rapidly) is necessary initially to assure that intravascular volume is optimal. If there is no sudden or progressive rise in CVP, then volume expansion (utilizing both crystalloid and colloid) is continued until shock is corrected or fluid overload (increased CVP, rales) develops. Urine output should be monitored and maintained at 40 to 50 ml per hour.

If rapid improvement does not follow volume expansion or if the CVP exceeds appropriate limits, a catecholamine should be added to enhance cardiac output and raise arterial pressure to the range of 90 to 100 mm Hg. Dopamine has been widely used because of its ability to increase renal blood flow (at dosage below 6 μg per kilogram per minute) while increasing cardiac contractility. It is administered by continuous intravenous (initial rate of 2 to 5 μg per kilogram per minute) infusion at a rate sufficient to maintain an adequate arterial pressure and urine volume.

Evidence as to whether adrenal corticosteroids have a beneficial effect in bacteremic shock is still conflicting. One or two pharmacologic doses (3 mg per kilogram of dexamethasone or 30 mg per kilogram of methylprednisolone intravenously) have been used in patients not responding to the aforementioned initial measures. Smaller maintenance doses do not appear beneficial, and continued administration predisposes to superinfection.

Adequate oxygenation is essential in a patient with shock, particularly if meningitis is also a feature (in which hypoxia can aggravate cerebral edema). Oxygen administration, and intubation with ventilatory assistance if needed, should be an integral part of therapy aiming at restoring the arterial P_{O_2} to appropriate levels (80 to 120 mm Hg). Acidosis should be corrected by intravenous administration of sodium bicarbonate (45 mEq) as needed. Digitalis is not of value in meningococcemic shock, but may have a possible role if fluid overload complicates volume expansion or secondary myocarditis. Generally, diuretics such as furosemide have been of more value in this acute situation.

The initial enthusiasm for heparin treatment of DIC in meningococcemia and septic shock has waned, since evidence of efficacy in reducing mortality has been conflicting despite improvement in coagulation factors. Heparin treatment on the basis of laboratory abnormalities alone is inadvisable. Reversal of hypotension is often associated with improvement in laboratory evidences of DIC and a halt in further clinical progression of the coagulopathy. Only if bleeding into deep tissues or from mucosal surfaces develops or thrombotic manifestations occur in the presence of DIC might heparinization be considered. After initiation of heparin therapy coagulation factor deficiencies can be repaired by administration of fresh frozen plasma. Once heparin is started, prothrombin time and partial thromboplastin time determinations are no longer helpful in following laboratory evidences of DIC; levels of fibrin degradation products, fibrinogen, and platelets are of greatest assistance.

PREVENTION. ***Chemoprophylaxis.*** Close contacts (e.g., same household or daycare center, medical personnel exposed by intimate contact such as mouth-to-mouth resuscitation) of a patient with meningococcal disease are at increased risk of developing systemic disease, and should receive chemoprophylaxis. Since secondary (or coprimary) cases usually occur within four days of the initial case, prophylactic treatment should begin as soon as the initial case is identified. Rifampin has been shown to be 80 to 90 per cent effective in eliminating meningococci from the nasopharynx of asymptomatic carriers, and minocycline has been almost as effective. Because of reports of vestibular side effects with minocycline, rifampin is the recommended drug for chemoprophylaxis. It is administered for two days: to adults at a dosage of 600 mg orally twice daily; to children (five to twelve years of age) at a dosage of 10 mg per kilogram twice daily; and to children three to twelve months of age, at a dosage of 5 mg per kilogram twice daily. Since even the high doses of penicillin used to treat meningococcal meningitis or meningococcemia may not eradicate nasopharyngeal carriage, rifampin should be administered also to the index patient prior to discharge from hospital. Rifampin-resistant strains appear readily and would be selected if use of the drug for prophylaxis were widespread.

Meningococcal Vaccine. Monovalent (group A or C), bivalent (groups A and C), and polyvalent (groups A, C, Y, and W135) meningococcal polysaccharide vaccines are commercially available. The vaccines are effective in adults, but they demonstrate less immunogenicity in children below two years of age. Vaccines containing group C polysaccharide have been administered routinely to all recruits in the armed forces, essentially eliminating serogroup C disease in this population. Group A vaccine has been used successfully to control epidemics in Africa, Brazil, and Finland.

The principal indication for use of meningococcal vaccines is the presence of outbreaks of meningococcal disease caused by *N. meningitidis* belonging to serogroup A or C (or more recently, Y and W135).

The routine immunization of individuals against meningococcal disease is not recommended because of the low risk of disease in the absence of outbreaks. However, vaccination should be considered for travelers to countries in which there is epidemic meningococcal disease. Since about 50 per cent of secondary cases among close contacts occur more than five days following the primary case, consideration should be given to the use of immunization as an adjunct to chemoprophylaxis to extend protection if the latter has been unsuccessful.

PROGNOSIS. The mortality from meningococcal meningitis before any treatment was available was about 75 per cent, and residual neurologic damage in the survivors was extensive. The advent of the sulfonamides brought a dramatic reduction in mortality to 5 to 15 per cent. Despite the emergence of sulfonamide-resistant *N. meningitidis,* mortality has been kept at the same low level through the use of high doses of penicillin G or ampicillin. The case-fatality ratio for patients with meningococcemia without accompanying meningitis is higher (25 per cent) than for meningococcal meningitis and reflects the fulminant course in some patients. The case-fatality ratio is highest in children under two years of age and in adults over 50.

Benoit FL: Chronic meningococcemia. Case report and review of the literature. Am J Med 35:103, 1963. *The best review of the clinical features of this fascinating entity.*

Band JD, Chamberland ME, Platt T, Weaver RE, Thornsberry C, Fraser DW: Trends in meningococcal disease in the United States, 1975–1980. J Infect Dis 148:754, 1983. *Most current review of incidence of meningococcal disease in the United States, with emphasis on the role of various serogroups and the prevalence of sulfonamide resistance.*

DeVoe IW: The meningococcus and mechanisms of pathogenicity. Microbiol Rev 46:162, 1982. *Comprehensive review of the biologic properties of* N. meningitidis *and of the epidemiologic and immunologic aspects of meningococcal disease.*

Feldman HA: Meningococcal infections. Adv Intern Med 18:117, 1972. *The best overview of the major aspects of meningococcal disease, including epidemiology, clinical aspects, treatment, and prevention. Authoritative; very well referenced.*

Greenfield S, Sheehe PR, Feldman HA: Meningococcal carriage in a population of "normal" families. J Infect Dis 123:67, 1971. *A most thorough description of the epidemiology of meningococcal carriage in a civilian urban population during a nonepidemic period.*

Goldschneider I, Gotschlich EC, Artenstein MS: Human immunity to the meningococcus. I. The role of humoral antibodies. J Exper Med 129:1307, 1969. *A most important paper, relating susceptibility to meningococcal infection to the lack of serum bactericidal activity against* N. meningitidis. *A lucid presentation of the basic facts necessary to understand the epidemiology of meningococcal disease.*

Goldschneider I, Gotschlich EC, Artenstein MS: Human immunity to the meningococcus. II. Development of natural immunity. J Exper Med 129:1327, 1969. *A second landmark paper by these authors on immunity to meningococcal infection. The role of the carrier state as an immunizing process is clearly demonstrated.*

Koppes GM, Ellenbogen C, Gebhart RJ: Group Y meningococcal disease in United States Air Force recruits. Am J Med 62:661, 1977. *A very good description of the spectrum of disease produced by group Y meningococci. The importance of pneumonia in a recruit population is emphasized.*
Peltola H: Meningococcal disease: Still with us. Rev Infect Dis 5:71, 1983. *Authoritative evaluation of the current status of meningococcal disease around the world.*
Peltola H, Makela PH, Kayhty H, et al.: Clinical efficacy of meningococcus group A capsular polysaccharide vaccine in children three months to five years of age. N Engl J Med 297:686, 1977. *A noteworthy study of a successful large-scale immunization program during a meningococcal epidemic.*

273. INFECTIONS CAUSED BY HEMOPHILUS SPECIES

DEFINITION. *Hemophilus* infections involve primarily the upper respiratory tract and the bronchopulmonary system. Invasive infections (bacteremia, meningitis, pericarditis, septic arthritis, cellulitis) may sometimes ensue; they occur predominantly in young children and are almost always due to one species, *Hemophilus influenzae* type b. Endocarditis is occasionally caused by *Hemophilus* species other than *H. influenzae* b. One *Hemophilus* species *(H. ducreyi)* is the cause of chancroid (see Ch. 305), and another (*H. vaginalis*—more recently designated *Gardnerella vaginalis*) is implicated in "nonspecific vaginitis." With the exception of these last two species, the normal habitat of the *Hemophilus* species is the upper respiratory tract.

GENERAL MICROBIOLOGIC FEATURES. The various *Hemophilus* species (Table 273–1) are similar in morphology (small, pleomorphic, gram-negative bacilli) and growth requirements (facultatively aerobic, media supplemented with blood). *H. influenzae* requires for aerobic growth both the X factor (hematin) and the V factor (NAD, NADP, or nicotinamide nucleoside) present in erythrocytes. Since some strains of *H. influenzae* grow best in 5 to 10 per cent carbon dioxide and other *Hemophilus* species have a CO_2 dependence, clinical specimens should be incubated in a CO_2 incubator. Media for isolation of *Hemophilus* species include chocolate agar, agar containing horse (but not sheep) blood, or enrichment agar (Levinthal).

H. hemolyticus rarely is isolated from sites outside the upper respiratory tract and is of dubious pathogenicity.

INFECTIONS DUE TO HEMOPHILUS INFLUENZAE. ***Etiology.*** *H. influenzae* strains are either encapsulated (typable) or unencapsulated (nontypable). The former consist of six distinguishable types, designated a to f. Nearly all strains causing invasive infection belong to type b, and the capsular polysaccharide contains both ribose and ribitol phosphate (PRP). However, encapsulated strains make up only a small percentage of clinical isolates of *H. influenzae.* Nontypable strains are more likely to be implicated in localized infections and rarely are associated with bacteremia. Encapsulated strains can be identified by a variety of methods employing antisera to their capsular antigens (immunofluorescence; production of immunoprecipitin halos ringing colonies on agar plates containing antiserum; demonstration by counterimmunoelectrophoresis of capsular antigen in culture supernatants). The outer membrane of *H. influenzae* strains contains a lipopolysaccharide with the properties of endotoxin. A classification of *H. influenzae* b into subtypes based on differences in outer membrane proteins has been developed and may be of potential use in epidemiologic studies.

Smears of clinical specimens usually show pleomorphic gram-negative coccobacilli. Occasionally, in underdecolorized gram-stained smears of spinal fluid, bipolar concentration of stain may incorrectly suggest gram-positive diplococci.

TABLE 273–1. DIFFERENTIAL PROPERTIES OF *HEMOPHILUS* SPECIES

Species	Growth Factor Requirement X	V	CO_2 Dependence	Hemolysis
H. influenzae	+	+	–	–
H. parainfluenzae	–	+	–	–
H. aphrophilus	–, +	–	+	–
H. paraphrophilus	–	+	+	–
H. hemolyticus	+	+	–	+
H. ducreyi	+	–	–	–

Incidence and Prevalence. Nontypable *H. influenzae* are commonly carried in the nasopharynx of asymptomatic individuals. Rates of carriage for encapsulated strains (usually type b) are much lower (less than 5 per cent of children and less than 1 per cent of adults). Nasopharyngeal carriage of *H. influenzae* b may develop in some persons in the presence of circulating antibody to PRP, and successful antibiotic treatment of *H. influenzae* meningitis may not eliminate it from the upper respiratory tract. The carrier state may persist for weeks to months.

H. influenzae b is the principal (estimated 8000 to 11,000 cases annually) cause of reported cases of bacterial meningitis in the United States. The frequency of invasive infections is inversely related to age; only a small percentage of cases occur in older children or adults. In the past decade many clinicians have had the impression that systemic disease caused by *H. influenzae* b has become more frequent in adults. Systemic infection with *H. influenzae* probably should be considered in the adult in the proper setting more frequently than was formerly the case.

Epidemiology. Infections in the first two months of life are rare, probably because of transplacental transfer of maternal antibody. Most cases of meningitis, septic arthritis, and cellulitis occur in children under two years of age. The mean age of children with epiglottitis is three to five years. Host factors appearing to contribute to increased susceptibility include immune globulin deficiencies, sickle cell disease, CSF fistulas, splenectomized states, and chronic pulmonary infections. Alcoholism appears to be a risk factor in adults.

Unlike *Neisseria meningitidis, H. influenzae* b does not cause epidemics in the community, but it is responsible for an increased incidence of secondary cases among susceptibles in families or in day-care centers exposed to an index case. The risk of serious *H. influenzae* illness among exposed household contacts of a child with *H. influenzae* meningitis is age dependent, with an incidence of 3.8 per cent among children under two years of age, 1.5 per cent among children two to three years of age, and 0.1 per cent among children four to five years of age. The rate of infection in household contacts without regard to age represents a 600-fold increase in risk over that in the population at large.

Pathogenesis and Immunity. Most nasopharyngeal infections with *H. influenzae* are unrecognized and occur by age five years. Type b strains may occasionally invade locally, producing epiglottitis, pneumonia, or buccal cellulitis, or may be disseminated via the bloodstream, producing meningitis. Pathogenicity of type b strains is due principally to the antiphagocytic activity of its PRP capsule. Nonencapsulated strains rarely produce bacteremic infection but can produce disease involving the upper (otitis media, sinusitis) and lower (pneumonia, exacerbations of chronic bronchitis) respiratory tracts.

Since the study of Fothergill and Wright, the conventional dogma has been that susceptibility to *H. influenzae* meningitis is inversely related to the presence of serum bactericidal activity (equated with anti-PRP antibody), which in turn correlates with age. In Finland, preliminary studies of anti-PRP antibodies by radioimmunoassay indicate an inverse correlation between age-related antibody levels and incidence of bacteremic *H. influenzae* disease; 90 per cent of children (3 to 12 months of age) had antibody levels less than 150 ng per milliliter, whereas all adults had higher levels. Antibodies to outer membrane proteins also play a role in immunity, but they appear to be protective primarily against strains of the same subtype.

The antibody response to *H. influenzae* b meningitis is age related (infants responding poorly and older children and adults developing high titers) and related to PRP load and clearance rate. Antigenemia may persist for as long as several weeks in younger children; an antibody response may be delayed until antigenemia has cleared. Anti-PRP antibody responses are observed within about three months in about 80 per cent of children with meningitis.

Anti-PRP antibodies can be generated by intestinal colonization or infection with bacteria (e.g., *E. coli* 075:K100:H5) exhibiting cross-reacting surface antigens. It has been suggested that the age-related acquisition of anti-PRP antibodies is too rapid and extensive to be accounted for by the low incidence of *H. influenzae* b carriage or disease, and that cross-reacting *E. coli* strains in the intestine may serve as the primary immunogen.

Clinical Manifestations. In one survey of children with serious *H. influenzae* infections, meningitis was the most common manifestation (about 50 per cent), followed by pneumonia (15 per cent), bacteremia without definable portal (10 per cent), cellulitis (10 per cent), epiglottitis (10 per cent), and pericarditis (4 per cent). Among adults with *H. influenzae* bacteremia, pneumonia is the commonest cause. About half the isolates are nontypable, and most of the typable strains belong to type b. Other sources of *H. influenzae* bacteremia in adults include obstetric infections (nontypable strains), meningitis, occult bacteremias, cellulitis, acute sinusitis, and epiglottitis. Metastatic *H. influenzae* infections in the adult include septic arthritis and purulent pericarditis.

MENINGITIS. (See Ch. 271). *H. influenzae* type b is the preeminent cause of bacterial meningitis in childhood, most cases occurring between ages four months and two years. The clinical features are not distinctive except as they relate to pyogenic meningitis occurring at that age. The manifestations may be nonspecific (fever, irritability, listlessness, poor feeding, vomiting) initially, especially in the younger child, and there may be only minimal nuchal rigidity. If the fontanel is still open, it may not be tense, particularly if the infant is dehydrated. Subdural effusions occur more frequently (20 to 30 per cent) with *H. influenzae* meningitis, but this is related to age and ease of detection by transillumination.

EPIGLOTTITIS. This pediatric otolaryngologic emergency begins abruptly with a severe sore throat, fever, and dysphagia; progression is swift, usually requiring hospitalization (and intubation) within 12 hours of onset. In the adult the onset of epiglottitis may be more prolonged and respiratory difficulty less pronounced initially despite severe pharyngitis and dysphagia; occasionally, the clinical picture may be mistaken for that of asthma. Airway obstruction in the child develops early with a sensation of choking, inspiratory (but not expiratory) distress, drooling, and anxiety. Speech is muffled, but the barking cough observed in croup is uncommon. The patient sits leaning forward with arms, back, and neck hyperextended to provide maximal airway. Pneumonia occurs in 15 to 25 per cent of patients, but simultaneous meningitis is uncommon. *Intraoral examination of the child (particularly in the supine position) may precipitate a cardiorespiratory arrest and should be performed only with the means of establishing an airway immediately at hand.* The pharynx is reddened; the epiglottis is bright red and markedly swollen. Lateral radiographs of the neck can demonstrate swelling of the epiglottis, but are of less value in acute cases (the procedure may delay establishment of an adequate airway) than in subacute ones.

Viral croup may resemble epiglottitis but occurs in younger children (3 to 36 months), has a more gradual onset, and frequently is preceded by an upper respiratory infection; the airway obstruction is subglottic.

PNEUMONIA. Most cases occur in children, are due to type b, and are accompanied by bacteremia. Lobar consolidation occurs more commonly than bronchopneumonia, and pleural effusions (or empyema) are present in 75 per cent of cases. Lung abscess is rare. Meningitis occurs in about 15 per cent of patients.

In the adult *H. influenzae* pneumonia occurs more frequently in the setting of chronic lung disease, alcoholism, immunologic deficiency, or preceding viral respiratory tract infection, but it may develop in previously healthy individuals. The majority of sputum isolates are nontypable, as are most blood isolates from the approximately 20 per cent of patients in whom bacteremia occurs. The radiologic pattern is more often that of bronchopneumonia. Small sterile parapneumonic effusions are common. The diagnosis can be suspected on the basis of findings on Gram-stained smears of sputum, but confirmation is provided by isolation of the organism from blood, pleural fluid, or lower respiratory tract.

BRONCHITIS. *H. influenzae* (nontypable) has been associated with purulent sputum and clinical exacerbations (dyspnea, wheezing, low grade fever) of chronic bronchitis. A direct etiologic role is difficult to establish because of the frequent (20 to 80 per cent) carriage of these organisms in the upper respiratory tract of normal adults.

CELLULITIS. *H. influenzae* b causes cellulitis in children below two years of age, but recently has also been observed to cause cellulitis on rare occasions in older adults. The cheek, periorbital area, head, and neck are the most common sites. An associated ipsilateral otitis media or upper respiratory infection is a frequent precursor. It begins with fever, local pain, and increasing toxicity. The lesion develops within a few hours and progresses rapidly; it is poorly demarcated, tender, and edematous. Although usually described as having a distinctive bluish purple color, the lesion is commonly erythematous like other types of cellulitis or may occasionally resemble angioedema. Bacteremia occurs in 80 per cent of cases and can result in metastatic infection. Diagnosis is made on the basis of the appearance and location of the lesion, the patient's age, Gram-stained smears and culture of an aspirate, and blood cultures.

BACTEREMIA WITHOUT OBVIOUS PORTAL. *H. influenzae* b is responsible for about 20 per cent of cryptogenic bacteremias occurring in febrile children with mild nonspecific illnesses managed on an ambulatory basis. Such patients are at considerable risk for subsequent serious localized infection (meningitis, pneumonia, epiglottitis). Unsuspected *H. influenzae* bacteremia also occurs in patients with neoplastic disease undergoing chemotherapy. Fulminant *H. influenzae* bacteremia with fatal shock and disseminated intravascular coagulation can develop in splenectomized patients.

SKELETAL INFECTIONS. Septic arthritis accounts for 1 to 8 per cent of cases of invasive *H. influenzae* b infection in children. It is the cause of pyogenic arthritis in about half the cases in children under two years of age. Weight-bearing joints are most often involved. Most commonly pyarthrosis is secondary to bacteremic spread from an upper respiratory tract infection or otitis media, but joint involvement may result from direct spread of adjacent osteomyelitis in the first year of life.

H. influenzae is a rare cause of osteomyelitis in children, usually occurring in the first year of life.

PERICARDITIS. *H. influenzae* b is the cause of 10 to 15 per cent of cases of purulent pericarditis in children. It is a rare cause of pericarditis in adults. Pericarditis may result from either bacteremic seeding of the pericardium or contiguous spread from infected lung or pleura. Over half of the cases in children have an associated pneumonia. High fever, tachycardia, tachypnea, and the hemodynamic manifestations of cardiac tamponade are commonly present. Treatment involves pericardiocentesis for diagnosis followed by surgical drainage (closed catheter drainage or anterior pericardectomy), along with antimicrobial therapy. With treatment 85 to 95 per cent of patients recover.

OTITIS MEDIA AND SINUSITIS. *H. influenzae* is second in frequency to *Streptococcus pneumoniae* as the cause of acute otitis media in children. In most instances the *H. influenzae* strains are not typable, but type b strains can be isolated in 10 per cent of cases. Serous middle ear fluid in children with chronic low grade otitis media with effusion may be colonized by *H. influenzae*, which may contribute to its persistence. *H. influenzae* also appears to be a significant cause of otitis media in older children and adults. The manifestations of acute otitis media caused by *H. influenzae* are indistinguishable from those caused by other pyogens: otalgia, fever, hyperemia of the tympanic membrane, and middle ear fluid. Tinnitus, vertigo, and nystagmus may develop.

Acute sinusitis is more common in adults than in children. In about 25 per cent of cases *H. influenzae* (nontypable) is the cause. Acute sinusitis is often preceded by a viral upper respiratory infection. Facial pain, frontal headache, purulent nasal discharge or nasal obstruction, anosmia, and nasal speech are common features. Sinus tenderness and opacity on transillumination are helpful findings.

CONJUNCTIVITIS. Most strains of *Hemophilus* isolated from conjunctivae are unencapsulated and formerly were designated as *H. aegyptius* (Koch-Weeks bacillus) on the basis of their hemagglutinating property. Currently these strains are considered as biotypes of *H. influenzae*. *H. influenzae* mucopurulent conjunctivitis occurs principally in children, particularly in the summer. The findings of acute catarrhal conjunctivitis are present, but petechial hemorrhages on the tarsal and epibulbar conjunctivae are suggestive of *H. influenzae* or a pneumococcal cause. Transient marginal corneal infiltrates are more common with this type of infection than with those resulting from pneumococci. Diagnosis is made on the basis of Gram-stained smears of conjunctival scrapings and culture of the outer eye.

H. influenzae conjunctivitis is often self-limited, clearing in 7 to 14 days. Treatment consists of moist soaks to keep the eyelids clean and topical antimicrobials (e.g., 10 to 30 per cent sulfacetamide eyedrops).

OTHER INFECTIONS. *H. influenzae* is a very rare cause of endocarditis and brain abscess. *H. influenzae* may occasionally be the cause of nonexudative pharyngitis (with prominent pain and dysphagia), but its presence in the pharynx often merely represents colonization. Rare cases of genital tract infections (salpingitis, endometritis, puerperal sepsis) and urinary infections have occurred.

Diagnosis. Certain serious infections (purulent meningitis, epiglottitis, facial and orbital cellulitis) in young children should suggest the possibility of *H. influenzae* b as the cause. In meningitis the presence of gram-negative pleomorphic coccobacillary forms in smears of CSF is highly suggestive of *H. influenzae*, but other organisms (*Pasteurella multocida, Acinetobacter*) which only rarely cause meningitis may have a similar appearance. Rapid and sensitive methods of antigen (PRP) detection such as counterimmunoelectrophoresis (CIE), latex particle agglutination, and enzyme-linked immunosorbent assay (ELISA) have detected *H. influenzae* b antigen in initial CSF specimens of 70 to 90 per cent of cases of *H. influenzae* meningitis; they are particularly helpful in early diagnosis and in the diagnosis of patients whose cultures may be negative because of prior antibiotic therapy. Antigenemia can be demonstrated in 60 to 100 per cent of patients with *H. influenzae* b meningitis but much less frequently in children with epiglottitis and cellulitis. False-positive reactions may occur owing to cross-reactive antigens in other bacteria such as *E. coli*, but these are infrequent.

Bacteremia is commonly demonstrable in patients with invasive infections (at least 80 per cent of children with meningitis, epiglottitis, or cellulitis) caused by *H. influenzae* b. *H. influenzae* is generally isolated on cultures of the epiglottis, joint fluid, and empyema fluid when it is the cause of infection in those areas.

Treatment. Currently, about 24 per cent of strains of *H. influenzae* b isolated in this country from systemic infections are ampicillin resistant (β-lactamase producing), with some variation (13 to 36 per cent) between geographic areas. About 15 per cent of strains (usually nontypable) associated with childhood otitis media are ampicillin resistant, as are 2 to 8 per cent of strains (mostly nontypable) isolated from adults with invasive infections or chronic bronchitis. Because of this prevalence of ampicillin resistance, systemic illnesses caused by *H. influenzae* (or when this organism is suspected) should be treated with chloramphenicol alone or in combination with ampicillin (see Ch. 271) until it is determined whether the organism produces β-lactamase; if it does not, then only the ampicillin need be continued. Rare strains of *H. influenzae* resistant to chloramphenicol have been isolated from children with meningitis. Very rare cases of meningitis caused by *H. influenzae* b resistant to both ampicillin and chloramphenicol have occurred. As yet there is no reason to change the initial therapy (chloramphenicol alone or with ampicillin) for invasive disease caused by this organism. For systemic infection associated with such a doubly resistant strain, or when the presence of such an organism is suspected on the basis of clinical response to conventional therapy, treatment should involve a third generation cephalosporin such as moxalactam or cefotaxime (see Ch. 271). Antimicrobial susceptibilities of *H. influenzae* isolates from systemic diseases should be determined if possible, particularly if the response to chloramphenicol is unsatisfactory. Chloramphenicol is bactericidal against *H. influenzae* at concentrations readily achieved in humans. Although antagonism has been demonstrated in vitro and in vivo between penicillin and chloramphenicol against *S. pneumoniae*, there appears to be no antagonism between these two drugs against *H. influenzae.*

Ampicillin (50 to 100 mg per kilogram per day in four divided doses) or amoxicillin (50 mg per kilogram per day in four divided doses), because each is active against *S. pneumoniae* and most strains of *H. influenzae*, is still the drug of choice for initial treatment of otitis media in children. Alternatives include trimethoprim (TMP)–sulfamethoxazole (SMX) (40 mg TMP–200 mg SMX twice daily per 20 pounds), the combination of penicillin (or erythromycin) with a sulfonamide, or cefaclor. Treatment should be continued for 10 to 14 days. Initial treatment of *H. influenzae* pneumonia in the adult should be with ampicillin, since these infections are infrequently caused by ampicillin-resistant strains, and there is sufficient time to shift therapy (chloramphenicol, cefamandole) if the response is unsatisfactory. Based on the bacteriology (*S. pneumoniae* and *H. influenzae* are frequently identified) of acute sinusitis, ampicillin is a reasonable initial antibiotic choice. (In the patient with rapidly progressive frontal sinusitis, *S. aureus* must be considered as a cause as well, and a penicillinase-resistant penicillin should be included in the initial therapeutic program.)

Prevention. An experimental vaccine consisting of purified capsular PRP has been tested on over 50,000 children in Finland and has been found to be well tolerated, immunogenic, and capable of preventing invasive *H. influenzae* b disease above the age of 18 months. Unfortunately, for children below 18 months of age, when the incidence of *H. influenzae* meningitis is greatest, it was a poor immunogen and was not protective. This vaccine is not yet approved for use in the United States. In view of what appears to be an age-specific defect in the response of infants to thymus-independent polysaccharide antigens, promising preliminary attempts have been made to overcome this limitation by linking the PRP antigen to a protein (tetanus toxoid), thus involving T cell participation and establishing immunologic memory.

The rate of secondary cases among young children who are close contacts of a patient with invasive *H. influenzae* b infection indicates the need for an effective prophylactic antibiotic program. Since rifampin has efficacy in eliminating nasopharyngeal carriage of *H. influenzae* b, the following management of household contacts has been recommended: (1) if another child less than four years of age resides in the household of an index case, all household members (including adults) should receive rifampin (20 mg per kilogram orally once daily for four days, with a maximal daily dose of 600 mg); (2) rifampin in the same dosage should also be administered to the index patient prior to discharge from the hospital, since nasopharyngeal carriage may reappear after discontinuation of ampicillin or chloramphenicol therapy for systemic infection; (3) rifampin prophylaxis is probably not indicated if over two weeks have elapsed since illness began in the index patient or if the youngest child in the household is four years of age or older.

INFECTIONS CAUSED BY OTHER HEMOPHILUS SPECIES. ***Hemophilus Parainfluenzae.*** This *Hemophilus* species is part of the normal flora of the nasopharynx and is found in dental plaque. It is very uncommonly responsible for human disease. It has been a rare cause of meningitis, epiglottitis, otitis media, puerperal bacteremia, brain abscess, and pneumonia in adults. Ampicillin is the drug of choice, except when ampicillin resistance is present (6 per cent of isolates), in which case chloramphenicol should be used. The most common association of *H. parainfluenzae* with disease has been with infective endocarditis. It may take as long as 14 to 18 days to grow out of blood cultures. The only distinctive clinical feature (also observed with *H. aphrophilus* endocarditis) appears to be the frequent occurrence of embolic occlusion of large arteries. For endocarditis in the adult, treatment with ampicillin (12 grams daily intravenously) alone or in combination with gentamicin (4 mg per kilogram per day in divided doses every eight hours intravenously) for four to six weeks has been employed successfully.

Hemophilus Aphrophilus. This organism is part of the normal gingival flora and is a rare cause of disease, generally acting as an "opportunist." The infections it produces, often following oropharyngeal foci of infection or trauma, include abscesses (particularly brain abscess), bacteremia, and endocarditis. Most strains are susceptible to penicillin, ampicillin, cephalothin, chloramphenicol, and gentamicin. Successful treatment of endocarditis has involved the use of ampicillin or penicillin, alone or in combination with streptomycin for four to six weeks.

H. Ducreyi. See Ch. 305.

Hemophilus Vaginalis. *Hemophilus vaginalis* is now designated as a new species, *Gardnerella vaginalis. G. vaginalis* is found in the vaginal flora of 40 per cent of normal women but in large numbers in the vaginal fluid of over 95 per cent of patients with nonspecific vaginitis. It appears that this organism, acting in concert with certain anaerobes, causes this type of vaginal infection. Oral metronidazole, which is active against both anaerobes and *G. vaginalis,* suppresses both organisms and produces clinical improvement. Such improvement does not occur on treatment with oral ampicillin or doxycycline. Findings suggesting the diagnosis of nonspecific vaginitis include the presence of "clue" cells (vaginal epithelial cells with numerous adherent small gram-negative bacilli) in a vaginal discharge with pH 5.0 (exhibiting a "fishy" amine-like odor upon addition of potassium hydroxide). Treatment with metronidazole is effective, but its possible toxicity must be considered in view of the mildness of the disease and the possibility of reinfection. *G. vaginalis* has also been a cause of puerperal fever with bacteremia, septic abortion, and neonatal bacteremia.

Hemophilus influenzae

Cherry JD: Acute epiglottitis, laryngitis, and croup. In Remington JS, Swartz MN (eds.): Current Clinical Topics in Infectious Disease, 2. New York, McGraw-Hill Book Company, 1981, pp 1–30. *Provides a particularly vivid clinical picture of acute* H. influenzae *epiglottitis. Valuable points on differential diagnosis and treatment are emphasized. A very well organized and thoroughly referenced presentation.*

Dajani AS, Asmar BI, Thirumoorthi MC: Systemic *Haemophilus influenzae* disease. J Pediatr 94:355, 1979. *This is a thorough review of an extensive pediatric experience with systemic* H. influenzae *b infections. It provides helpful data on the relative frequencies of the various clinical syndromes and an extensive bibliography.*

Feigen RD, Stechenberg BW, Chang MJ, Dunkle LM, Wong ML, Pelkes H, Dodge PR, Davis H: Prospective evaluation of treatment of *Hemophilus influenzae* meningitis. J Pediatr 88:542, 1976. *This report on 50 well-studied children with* H. influenzae *meningitis provides helpful information concerning the value of counterimmunoelectrophoresis in rapid diagnosis, the spectrum of neurologic complications, and the response to antibiotic treatment.*

Fothergill LD, Wright J: Influenzal meningitis: Relation of age incidence to bactericidal power of blood against causal organism. J Immunol 24:273, 1933. *This is the original and "classic" study demonstrating an inverse relationship between the presence of serum bactericidal antibody and the incidence of* H. influenzae *meningitis at various ages.*

Granoff DM, Ward JI: Current status of prophylaxis for *Haemophilus influenzae* infections. *In* Remington JS, Swartz MN (eds.): Current Clinical Topics in Infectious Disease, 5th ed. New York, McGraw-Hill Book Company, 1984. *Provides excellent background regarding secondary spread of* H. influenzae *infections and concrete recommendations for chemoprophylaxis of close family and day-care center contacts.*

Hirschmann JV, Everett ED: *Haemophilus influenzae* infections in adults: Report of nine cases and a review of the literature. Medicine 58:80, 1979. *This is a thorough review of the various clinical syndromes produced by* H. influenzae *in the adult. Extensively referenced.*

O'Reilly RJ, Anderson P, Ingram DL, Peter G, Smith DH: Circulating polyribosephosphate in *Hemophilus influenzae* type b meningitis. J Clin Invest 56:1012, 1975. *This is an important study showing that certain patients with impaired capacity to clear capsular polysaccharide from the blood following* H. influenzae *meningitis fail to develop the expected antibody response to PRP. Stimulating discussion.*

Peltola H, Käyhty H, Sivonen A, Mäkelä PH: *Haemophilus influenzae* type b capsular polysaccharide vaccine in children: A double-blind field study of 100,000 vaccinees three months to five years of age in Finland. Pediatrics 60:730, 1977. *This article describes a very well conducted, large scale trial of the type b capsular polysaccharide vaccine, which protected against bacteremic* H. influenzae *b disease in children older than 18 months of age but not in younger children. The data are extensive and well presented.*

Robbins JB, Schneerson R, Argaman M, Handzel ZT: *Haemophilus influenzae* type b: Disease and immunity in humans. Ann Intern Med 78:259, 1973. *This is a broad informative review of immunity to* H. influenzae *in the population and of the possible role of enteric bacteria (with cross-reacting antigens) in "natural" immunity to* H. influenzae *b.*

Spagnuolo PJ, Ellner JJ, Lerner PI, McHenry MC, Flatauer F, Rosenberg P, Rosenthal MS: *Haemophilus influenzae* meningitis: The spectrum of disease in adults. Medicine 61:74, 1982. *These 15 cases represent the largest series of cases of* H. influenzae *meningitis reported in the past 20 years. Particular emphasis is on predisposing factors in this unusual form of meningitis in adults.*

Syriopoulou V, Scheifele D, Smith AL, Perry PM, Howie V: Increasing incidence of ampicillin resistance in *Hemophilus influenzae.* J Pediatr 92:889, 1978. *Brief and to the point; ampicillin-resistance is increasing in both type b and non-b isolates of* H. influenzae *in various parts of the United States. Evidence presented is unequivocal.*

Wallace RJ Jr, Musher DM, Septimus EJ, McGowan JE, Quinones FJ, Wiss K, Vance PH, Trier PA: *Haemophilus influenzae* infections in adults: Characterization of strains by serotypes, biotypes, and β-lactamase production. J Infect Dis 144:101, 1981. *This is a detailed review of 103 cases of* H. influenzae *bacteremia or meningitis. Noteworthy is the frequency of nontypable strains among blood isolates in adults and the infrequency of ampicillin resistance in the same group.*

Hemophilus parainfluenzae and Hemophilus aphrophilus

Bieger RC, Brewer NS, Washington JA II: *Haemophilus aphrophilus:* A microbiologic and clinical review and report of 42 cases. Medicine 57:345, 1978. *A comprehensive review of the bacteriologic features, ecologic niche, and clinical impact of this uncommon cause of human disease.*

Chunn CJ, Jones SR, McCutchan JA, Young EJ, Gilbert DN: *Haemophilus parainfluenzae* infective endocarditis. Medicine 56:99, 1977. *This report from five medical centers represents the largest series described to date of* Hemophilus parainfluenzae *endocarditis. Helpful points on bacteriologic identification, distinctive clinical aspects (e.g., frequent emboli to major arteries), and antibiotic recommendations are presented.*

Oill PA, Chow AW, Guze LB: Adult bacteremic *Haemophilus parainfluenzae* infections: Seven reports of cases and a review of the literature. Arch Intern Med 139:985, 1979. *The type of infection (exclusive of endocarditis) caused by* H. parainfluenzae *and the antibiotic susceptibilities of this organism are summarized concisely.*

Gardnerella vaginalis (Hemophilus vaginalis)

Spiegel CA, Amsel R, Eschenbach D, Schoenknecht F, Holmes KK: Anaerobic bacteria in nonspecific vaginitis. N Engl J Med 303:601, 1980. *Strong circumstantial evidence implicating both anaerobic bacteria and* Gardnerella vaginalis (Hemophilus vaginalis) *in the production of "nonspecific vaginitis" is presented. Good references for those uninformed about this entity.*

Osteomyelitis

274. OSTEOMYELITIS

Francis A. Waldvogel

DEFINITIONS. Osteomyelitis is an infection of bacterial, sometimes of fungal, and exceptionally of viral origin that invades and destroys bone. Osteomyelitis is a well known, albeit rare, consequence of bacteremia (hematogenous osteomyelitis). In other situations, such as open fractures, wounds, and orthopedic procedures, the microorganism gains access to bone from a contaminated or infected contiguous structure (osteomyelitis secondary to contiguous infection). Finally, peripheral bones can also be invaded by contiguity in case of severe vascular insufficiency (osteomyelitis secondary to vascular insufficiency). In the latter case, other metabolic and neurologic factors play an important contributory role.

ETIOLOGY. Most cases of osteomyelitis are of bacterial origin, and *S. aureus* is still the most common etiologic agent, being responsible for more than 50 per cent of cases. Other etiologic agents include (1) gram-negative enteric organisms, which are often responsible for hematogenous vertebral osteomyelitis in the elderly; (2) certain *Salmonella* species, which cause osteomyelitis in patients with sickle cell disease; (3) *Pseudomonas aeruginosa,* often responsible for vertebral osteomyelitis in heroin addicts; (4) anaerobic organisms, which are sometimes isolated in pure or mixed cultures from infected bone in the vicinity of an anaerobic reservoir (maxilla, sinuses, sacrum); and (5) *Mycobacterium tuberculosis,* still a major cause of osteomyelitis of the spine in developing countries. In addition, various fungi can occasionally cause osteomyelitis after bacteremic spread, mostly in patients with intravenous access devices. Finally, rare cases of viral osteomyelitides have been described after chickenpox and smallpox.

INCIDENCE, PREVALENCE, AND EPIDEMIOLOGY. Hematogenous osteomyelitis has a biphasic incidence, occurring mainly in children, in whom it shows a predilection for the metaphysis of long bones, and in adults beyond the age of 50 years, in whom it most often involves the spine. Blunt trauma is considered by many to be a favoring factor in children. In adults, any factor favoring bacteremia (urinary tract infection, prostatitis, various skin infections, prolonged intravenous therapy, or repeated injections) can occasionally lead to hematogenous osteomyelitis of the spine. The prevalence of osteomyelitis secondary to a contiguous infection is difficult to determine and reflects the frequency of major trauma and of orthopedic procedures in a given population. It can be as high as 15 per cent in patients with multiple comminuted fractures or less than 1 per cent after total hip replacement performed under strictly aseptic conditions.

PATHOGENESIS AND PATHOLOGY. The various pathogenic mechanisms leading to bone destruction are as yet largely unknown. Since microorganisms per se are unable to destroy bone tissue, one has to postulate that the inflammatory reaction, the metabolic alterations, and the vascular changes triggered by the bacterial invasion play a preponderant role in the development of an osteomyelitic focus, i.e., in bone destruction and regeneration. From a strictly pathologic point of view, the following major changes can be identified: (1) bone necrosis, with death of the cellular constituents and disappearance of bone mass. Sometimes devitalized bone persists as a dead fragment called a sequestrum; (2) a heavy inflammatory reaction, in which granulocytes predominate initially but are replaced over time by a mononuclear infiltrate; (3) new bone apposition, originating from periosteal activation; this periosteal reaction is indeed often the first sign of osteomyelitis identified on x-rays. In some cases, this bone apposition can be exuberant and lead to bridging of two adjacent bone structures, as in vertebral osteomyelitis. In other cases, bone apposition is very modest, and x-ray examination may show only an intraosseous, punched-out radiolucent lesion, as in subacute hematogenous osteomyelitis (Brodie's abscess).

CLINICAL MANIFESTATIONS. Hematogenous osteomyelitis involving long bones starts as an acute episode with chills and fever. The young patient usually complains of an excruciating pain in the affected bone, most often the tibia or femur and more rarely the humerus or radius. Clinical examination shows normal skin over the affected limb, but the bone metaphysis is exceedingly painful on palpation. The adjacent joint is usually unaffected by the disease.

The clinical presentation is usually more progressive in hematogenous vertebral osteomyelitis: following an episode of fever, the middle-aged or elderly patient complains within the next few days or weeks of an ill-defined pain in the spine, most often in the lower dorsal or lumbar segments. On physical examination, the patient is moderately or sometimes highly febrile. There is paravertebral tenderness and spasm on palpation of the affected segment, but the overlying skin is normal. A careful neurologic examination should be carried out to exclude the possibility of a paraspinal abscess, a dreaded complication of vertebral osteomyelitis leading to paraplegia (see Ch. 496).

Osteomyelitis secondary to a contiguous focus of infection after open trauma or secondary to orthopedic reconstructive surgery is a real diagnostic challenge, since pain, low grade fever, local signs of inflammation, and x-ray findings are compatible with both postoperative changes and infection. Persistent fever and increasing signs of inflammation one week after trauma or surgery, persistent inflammation of the surgical incision with oozing of serosanguineous material, and increasing pain on weight-bearing are all helpful clinical signs in favor of infection.

DIFFERENTIAL DIAGNOSIS AND DIAGNOSIS. Whenever osteomyelitis is suspected, blood cultures should be immediately obtained. In hematogenous disease, they will yield the offending organism in 50 per cent of cases. In suspected osteomyelitis of the spine, direct aspiration or bone biopsy is often necessary for a full microbiologic diagnosis if blood cultures remain negative. In osteomyelitis secondary to a contiguous focus, careful probing of the wound with aspiration of the material under aseptic conditions for Gram stain and culture will often yield the necessary microbiologic information. Other laboratory tests are noncontributory: erythrocyte sedimentation rate is usually increased; the white blood cell count is normal or high; and blood chemical values, including alkaline phosphatases, are normal.

Radiologic changes are delayed, appearing several weeks after the onset of the disease. In hematogenous osteomyelitis

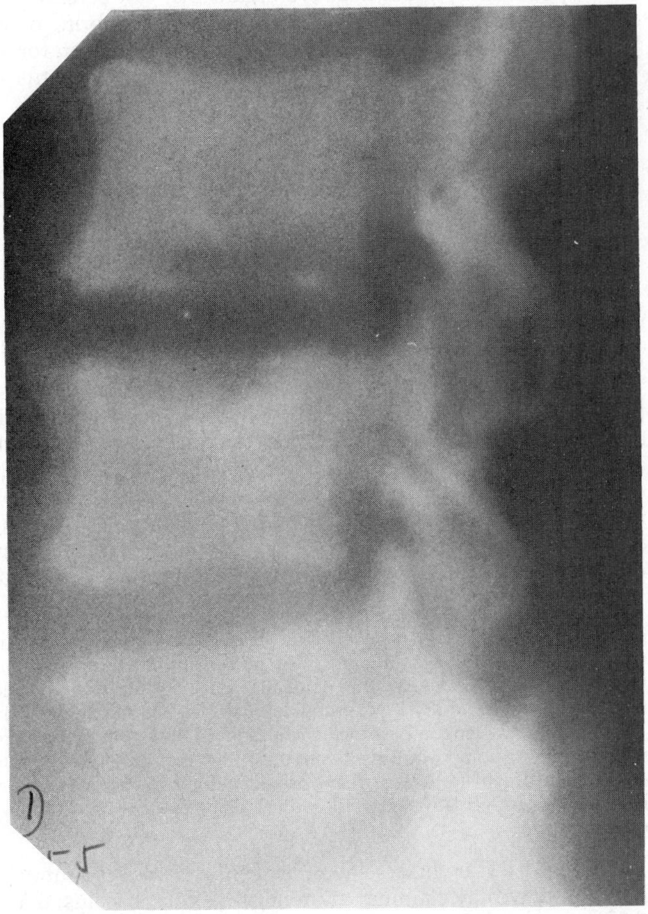

Figure 274–1. Tomogram showing vertebral osteomyelitis. Note the piecemeal necrosis of the two adjacent vertebral plateaus and the anterior bone apposition.

of long bones, periosteal elevation and subsequent bone destruction are the first changes to be observed. In vertebral osteomyelitis, progressive piecemeal destruction of two adjacent vertebral plateaus, narrowing of the intervertebral space, and progressive anterior periosteal bridging are the hallmarks of the disease, bone sclerosis being a late event (see Fig. 274–1). In tuberculous osteomyelitis of the spine, the changes just mentioned are delayed and occur over several months, periosteal reaction usually being absent.

In most cases of hematogenous osteomyelitis, ^{99m}Tc-polyphosphate uptake, although nonspecific, can be of great diagnostic help by identifying the suspected areas of infection for appropriate tomograms at a stage when conventional x-ray results are still normal. In osteomyelitis secondary to a contiguous focus of infection, radiologic techniques and bone scanning are less helpful, since they cannot distinguish between normal bone reaction and infection. Direct aspiration or biopsy for microscopical examination and culture is therefore the procedure of choice to establish the diagnosis.

Acute hematogenous osteomyelitis of long bones has to be differentiated clinically from septic arthritis, bursitis, and cellulitis. These more superficial infections are accompanied by local skin changes, and x-ray results remain normal. Osteomyelitis of the spine is a diagnostic challenge and has to be differentiated from bone tumors such as myeloma and metastases, which usually do not involve two adjacent vertebral plateaus. In case of doubt, bone biopsy may be indicated.

TREATMENT. Medical treatment of osteomyelitis includes the parenteral administration of an appropriate antibiotic, such as cloxacillin 8 grams per day* for *S. aureus* infections. As a general rule, those parenteral antibiotics used for septicemias are also effective in osteomyelitis due to the same organism if the drug is given for six weeks. Thus, osteomyelitis of the spine, which is often caused by gram-negative organisms, can be cured by ampicillin, a first or second generation cephalosporin, or an aminoglycoside (depending on sensitivity testing) given for six weeks. Bed rest is usually recommended until all signs of inflammation have abated, pain has subsided, and x-rays show signs of improvement. This is particularly true for osteomyelitis of the spine. Surgery is rarely indicated in hematogenous infection, except for drainage of intramedullary abscesses, removal of sequestra, and decompression if neurologic signs supervene in vertebral osteomyelitis. In osteomyelitis secondary to a contiguous focus of infection, careful evaluation of the situation by a skilled orthopedic surgeon is mandatory. In case of infected fractures or prostheses, stable union is a prerequisite for bacteriologic cure. Union should be achieved first despite sepsis, and infection is controlled subsequently by antibiotic therapy after removal of the foreign material. In case of nonunion of a fracture or loosening of the prosthesis, the foreign material should be removed, and if possible replaced by an external fixation device. Infected prostheses should also be removed and the infected focus cleaned out, with reinsertion of new material in a one-step or two-step procedure.

PREVENTION. At present, there is no preventive treatment available for hematogenous osteomyelitis, since the occurrence of the disease after bacteremia is unpredictable. Infection rates after insertion of hip prostheses have been shown to be markedly decreased by short-term coverage (two to three days) with parenteral antistaphylococcal antibiotics. Such coverage should also be considered in high-risk operations, such as reduction of comminuted fractures, open fractures, and insertion of joint prostheses.

*May exceed manufacturer's recommended dosage.

Kido D, Bryan D, Halpern M: Hematogenous osteomyelitis in drug addicts. Ther Nucl Med 118:356, 1973. *A concise study of 32 cases, most of them due to* Pseudomonas *species. Discusses their clinical and radiologic manifestations.*

Norden C: Experimental osteomyelitis II: Therapeutic trials and measurement of antibiotic levels in bone. J Infect Dis 124:565, 1971. *An interesting animal model allowing the study of the various pathogenic factors of osteomyelitis and the efficacy of various antibiotic regimens.*

Waldvogel FA, Medoff G, Swartz MN: Osteomyelitis: A review of clinical features, therapeutic considerations and unusual aspects I. II. III. N Engl J Med 282:198, 260, 316, 1970. *A retrospective review of 247 cases of osteomyelitis, their clinical and radiologic presentations, and their treatment.*

Waldvogel FA, Vasey H: Osteomyelitis: The past decade. N Engl J Med 303:360, 1980. *A review update of newer approaches in diagnosis and treatment of osteomyelitis, with emphasis on a combined surgical and medical approach.*

Wedge JH, Oryschak AF, Robertson DE, Kirkaldy-Willis WH: Atypical manifestations of spinal infections. Clin Orthop Rel Res 123:155, 1977. *Unusual presentations of vertebral osteomyelitis that underline its diagnostic challenge.*

Whooping Cough

275. WHOOPING COUGH (Pertussis)

Samuel L. Katz

DEFINITION. Whooping cough is an acute respiratory illness that classically affects infants and young children. The etiologic agent is usually *Bordetella pertussis;* occasionally *B. parapertussis* and rarely *B. bronchiseptica* produce a similar syndrome. The descriptive name derives from a distressing, prolonged inspiratory effort that follows paroxysmal coughing. Whooping cough is still responsible for a significant number of deaths in infants in areas where pertussis immunization is not practiced.

HISTORY. The disease was first recorded in the middle of the sixteenth century by Moulton and by DeBaillou. Sydenham applied the name "pertussis" to any illness accompanied by violent coughing, but the term became restricted to the epidemic disease that was a well-recognized clinical entity by the middle of the eighteenth century. In 1900 Bordet and Gengou observed coccobacilli in the sputum of a child with whooping cough, but it was not until 1906 that they were able to culture the organism. Many years passed before the Bordet-Gengou bacillus was universally accepted as the etiologic agent of whooping cough.

ETIOLOGY. When first isolated, *Bordetella pertussis* is a minute, nonmotile, weakly staining, gram-negative coccobacillus, 0.5 to 1.0 μ in length. Capsules can be demonstrated by special procedures, and bipolar metachromatic granules are present. The complex medium containing blood originally employed by Bordet and Gengou is still often used for cultivation. *Primary isolates, phase I organisms, will not grow on conventional laboratory media,* but will do so after prolonged passage. At the same time colonial morphology changes, marked pleomorphism of individual cells is evident, and there is an alteration in antigenic composition. This occurs in a series of phases, and the change from phase I to phase IV has been likened to the smooth to rough transition of other bacteria. Only phase I organisms are virulent, and *only phase I organisms* provide effective immunizing material.

The addition of blood to Bordet-Gengou medium is required for the growth of phase I organisms, but the blood acts to neutralize inhibitory substances, probably fatty acids, rather than to provide nutrients. Charcoal, starch, or ion exchange resins can be substituted for blood.

A single protein toxin purified from the organism's envelope is antigenic and responsible for the induction of histamine sensitization (HSF), activation of pancreatic islet cells (IAP), and lymphocytosis (LPF). Other toxins of *B. pertussis* include a heat-labile toxin and a heat-stable toxin (lipopolysaccharide). There are an extracytoplasmic adenylate cyclase, two hemagglutinins (the filamentous protein from fimbria, FHA, and the HSF-LPF-IAP hemagglutinin) as well as O and K surface and capsular antigens. The roles of these constituents in disease production and in the development of protective immunity are under investigation. The fimbrial hemagglutinin is apparently responsible for attachment of *B. pertussis* to ciliated respiratory epithelial cells. The systemic disease manifestations are likely caused by circulating HSF-IAP-LPF exotoxin secreted by bacterial cells.

Approximately 5 to 10 per cent of clinical whooping cough may be caused by *B. parapertussis*. The animal pathogen *B. bronchiseptica* is responsible for a very minor percentage of cases. These organisms can be differentiated from *B. pertussis* by growth requirements, enzyme production, and presence of species-specific antigens. It has been suggested that adenoviruses, alone or in concert with *B. pertussis*, may play an etiologic role in some cases of whooping cough.

EPIDEMIOLOGY. In communities of susceptibles the family attack rate is 80 to 90 per cent, which is extremely high for a bacterial disease, approaching that seen in varicella or measles. Transmission is by droplet infection. Carriers of *B. pertussis* are found infrequently, but persons previously immunized have been shown during outbreaks of disease to excrete the organism in the absence of clinical illness.

The mortality rate from whooping cough has fallen since the turn of this century owing to improved supportive therapy. The incidence of whooping cough, however, did not change until after the 1940's, when immunization of young children became standard practice. In the 1940's, approximately 200,000 cases of pertussis were reported annually in the United States; in 1983, 2258 cases were reported. At the same time, the fatality rate has dropped from 20 per 1000 patients to 3. The majority of deaths, over 70 per cent, occur in children under one year of age, with the preponderance in infants under the age of six months.

Neither immunization against pertussis nor natural disease provides lifelong protection. In the case of artificial immunization, an attack rate greater than 50 per cent has been reported when the interval after immunization exceeds 12 years. Thus in the face of routine immunization, it is possible that pertussis will become primarily a disease of older children and adults.

PATHOLOGY. Interpretation of pathologic material obtained at autopsy is difficult because of the common presence of complicating respiratory infections. Lesions caused by *B. pertussis* are found principally in the bronchi and bronchioles, but changes are also seen in the nasopharynx, larynx, and trachea. Masses of bacteria are intertwined with the cilia of the columnar epithelium together with mucopurulent exudate. Adherence of organisms to ciliated respiratory epithelial cells is the crucial element in pathogenesis of disease. There is also necrosis of the midzonal and basilar epithelium with infiltration of polymorphonuclear leukocytes and macrophages. Peribronchial accumulation of lymphocytes and granulocytes produces the picture of interstitial pneumonitis. Secondary atelectasis and localized emphysema are common.

CLINICAL MANIFESTATIONS. After an incubation period of 7 to 16 days, symptoms appear. It is customary to divide the clinical course into three stages, each of two weeks' duration, but variation is frequent.

Catarrhal Stage. Whooping cough begins with symptoms indistinguishable from those of a mild viral upper respiratory infection or common cold. Sneezing is frequent, the conjunctivae are injected, and a nocturnal cough appears. The temperature may be slightly elevated at this time. Infectivity is greatest at this stage.

Paroxysmal Stage. Seven to 14 days after onset, the cough becomes more frequent, diurnal, and then paroxysmal. In a typical paroxysm there is a series of 15 to 20 short coughs of increasing intensity, and then with a deep inspiration the air is drawn into the lungs, making the "whoop." A tenacious mucus plug is usually expelled, and vomiting frequently follows. Paroxysms may occur as often as every half hour, and are accompanied by signs of increased venous pressure. The conjunctivae are deeply engorged; there is periorbital edema; and petechial hemorrhages, particularly about the forehead, as well as epistaxis are common. During the attack the infant may be cyanotic until the crowing whoop occurs. In between paroxysms the child usually feels well though justifiably apprehensive.

Physical examination of the chest is usually unremarkable, although scattered rhonchi may be heard. The chest roentgenogram sometimes reveals hilar and mediastinal nodal enlargement. The presence of fever immediately suggests the development of a secondary infectious process.

Convalescent Stage. Gradually the paroxysms become less frequent and less intense; vomiting ceases, and slow recovery ensues. Often for many months even a mild, unrelated respiratory infection will induce a return of paroxysmal cough and whoop.

In very young infants the paroxysms and the whoop are often absent; instead, choking spells and apneic episodes may be the major manifestations. Second attacks of whooping cough as well as disease occurring in previously immunized individuals often present simply as an upper respiratory illness or bronchitis.

Complications. Complications may be related to the primary disease or to secondary events. Alterations in acid-base balance occur as a result of metabolic alkalosis when vomiting is severe. Recurrent vomiting can also lead to malnutrition. Anoxemic manifestations are seen when ventilation is markedly impaired. Central nervous system changes can result from cerebral anoxia or hemorrhages consequent to the elevated venous pressure. Rarely, cortical degeneration occurs, but the exact pathogenesis of the encephalopathy is unknown. A serous meningitis with lymphocytosis of the cerebrospinal fluid has been described. Localized areas of emphysema and atelectasis generally return to normal after the disease has run its course, and pneumothorax and interstitial emphysema are infrequently seen.

The major cause of death in whooping cough is complicating pneumonia or bronchopneumonia caused by other bacteria or viruses. In addition, secondary bacterial otitis media occurs frequently.

DIAGNOSIS. There is little difficulty in making the clinical diagnosis of whooping cough in a patient who, after a variable period of coryzal symptoms, develops paroxysmal coughing with a terminal inspiratory whoop. Toward the end of the catarrhal stage, or early in the spasmodic phase, leukocytosis often occurs. In contrast to the leukocytosis found in most bacterial diseases, the predominating cell type is the mature small lymphocyte. Characteristically the leukocyte count ranges from 15,000 to 30,000 per cubic millimeter, and 80 per cent of the cells are small lymphocytes. However, the leukocyte count either may be normal or may reach a level greater than 100,000 per cubic millimeter. Polymorphonuclear leukocytosis suggests a secondary bacterial complication.

Difficulty in recognizing whooping cough occurs in the catarrhal stage, in abortive or mild cases, and in young infants. Epidemiologic awareness may suggest the possibility, but microbiologic identification of the organisms is required. Physicians whose residency training was in the 1970's and 1980's may never have encountered a case of whooping cough. During the early stages *B. pertussis* can be isolated from approximately 90 per cent of patients. By the third or fourth week the organism can be recovered in only 50 per cent of cases, and in the convalescent stage it is unusual to obtain a positive culture.

Adequate specimens and appropriate media are essential if bacteriologic diagnosis is to be efficient. *Specimens are best obtained by pernasal swab rather than by the cough plate method.* A sterile cotton swab wrapped about a flexible copper wire is passed through the nares, and mucus is obtained from the posterior pharynx. The swab must not be allowed to dry out because *B. pertussis* is readily killed by desiccation. As quickly as possible the specimen is plated onto fresh Bordet-Gengou medium, to which penicillin has been added to prevent overgrowth of adventitious organisms. Incubation is at 35° C, and although the trained observer can recognize the small, bisected pearl colonies of *B. pertussis* within 48 hours, at least 72 hours of growth is usually required. Presumptive identification can be made by agglutination tests with appropriate antisera. It is virtually impossible to distinguish between *Bordetella* species on primary isolation except by serologic means.

A fluorescent antibody staining procedure that can be applied directly to clinical specimens as well as to organisms grown in culture has been utilized by many state diagnostic laboratories and the Centers for Disease Control. It greatly accelerates the identification of organisms after isolation, but is unreliable in its direct application to nasopharyngeal swabs or other clinical material.

Serologic procedures are of little help in the diagnosis of whooping cough because a rise in titer of most antibodies does not occur until at least the third week of illness. Tests are not well standardized, and few laboratories perform them.

It is difficult to distinguish abortive or mild cases of pertussis from tracheobronchitis caused by other agents except by bacteriologic means.

TREATMENT. Mild cases of pertussis require only supportive treatment. Specific therapy of severe whooping cough has been disappointing despite the in vitro susceptibility of *B. pertussis* to various antimicrobial agents and the protective effect of passively administered antibody in experimental disease.

Antimicrobials. A number of antimicrobial drugs have significant activity against *B. pertussis* in vitro. Agents that readily eradicate the organisms may shorten the course of the illness if given in the catarrhal or early paroxysmal stages. In the established paroxysmal stage the organisms can also be readily eliminated by antimicrobials, but the course of the illness is unaltered. Even in the paroxysmal stage the use of drugs may be justified in order to render the patient noninfectious.

Erythromycin, oxytetracycline, and several other drugs are effective in eliminating organisms. Erythromycin is the drug of choice. The daily dose is 50 mg per kilogram of body weight given in four divided doses. The organism is eliminated after a few days of therapy, but because bacteriologic relapse may occur, treatment should be continued for 14 to 21 days.

Immunotherapy. Hyperimmune human gamma globulin has previously been used in therapy of unimmunized patients, particularly small infants, with no efficacy demonstrated in controlled trials.

Supportive Therapy. Particularly in the young infant, supportive measures combined with careful nursing care are of paramount importance. Specific attention must be devoted to the maintenance of proper water and electrolyte balance, adequate nutrition, and sufficient oxygenation. Constant alertness for the presence of secondary infectious complications such as pneumonia is required.

PREVENTION. Unfortunately, the diagnosis is usually not made until the end of the catarrhal stage, and by then spread of the disease has already occurred. Exposed susceptibles should receive erythromycin prophylaxis, and contacts under four years of age who have been previously immunized should receive a booster dose of vaccine in addition to erythromycin. Booster doses of vaccine have been used to protect adults, such as hospital staff, but side effects tend to be frequent, and erythromycin chemoprophylaxis may be preferable.

Active Immunization. The fall in incidence of whooping cough in the very young is directly related to widespread immunization with suitable, killed suspensions of *B. pertussis.* The highest risk of serious morbidity and mortality is in the young infant. Women of childbearing age generally do not have significant levels of protective antibody in their sera, and these antibodies may be of a type (IgM) that does not cross the placenta. Consequently, newborns are not protected by maternal antibodies. Therefore active immunization is begun as early as is commensurate with the production of a satisfactory immune response. At present, it is recommended that the infant receive three injections of pertussis vaccine at eight-week intervals commencing at age two months. Each injection provides four NIH* units. The NIH unitage is based upon the ability of a vaccine to protect mice against a standard intracerebral infection. The pertussis suspension is incorporated into a triple vaccine with alum-precipitated diphtheria and tetanus toxoids (DTP). Booster injections are given one and five years after completion of the initial course. Administration of pertussis vaccine to those over six years of age is not generally recommended because of an apparent increased incidence of untoward reactions and the diminished risk of the illness itself in the older child. However, low doses have been administered to adults without incident. There is no protection against parapertussis.

As previously noted, immunization does not confer lifelong protection. Approximately 80 per cent of those vaccinated within four years of exposure will be protected, whereas 80 to 90 per cent of a matched unimmunized group with similar exposure will contact pertussis. The prophylactic efficacy of pertussis vaccine was clearly demonstrated when epidemics occurred in the United Kingdom in 1977–1979 and 1982 following a three- to five-year period during which vaccine acceptance had declined to very low levels. More than 170,000 cases of whooping cough were reported, including 42 deaths, principally among children under five years of age. Similar outbreaks have followed diminished vaccine utilization in Japan and Sweden.

Local reactions as well as fever, hyperirritability, or seizures may occur after injection of pertussis vaccine. The exact incidence of the more severe complication of encephalopathy is uncertain. A current British study suggests a risk of 1 in 300,000 immunizations for previously normal infants, with residual neurologic damage in 30 per cent of those affected. The occurrence of neurotoxicity appears to be decreasing as more refined immunizing suspensions are used, and certain components of *B. pertussis* may prove to be effective without engendering serious side effects. Despite the small, but real, incidence of neurologic complications of pertussis immunization, the risk is far less than the hazards of whooping cough in the young child. Nevertheless, in infants with a personal history of convulsions or other neurologic disorders, pertussis immunization should be deferred until the condition has stabilized and is under medical control. A Japanese vaccine containing only the two *B. pertussis* hemagglutinins, extracted, purified, and formalin-treated, is far less reactogenic than the whole bacterial cell vaccine that has been used for more than 40 years. If tests of its immunogenicity and prophylactic efficacy are convincing in field use, it may replace the killed whole cell vaccine.

Keller MA, Aftandelians R, Connor JD: Etiology of pertussis syndrome. Pediatrics 66:50, 1980. *A clarification of the interrelationships of* B. pertussis *and adenoviruses in whooping cough.*

Manclark CR, Hill JC: International Symposium on Pertussis. Washington, D.C., US Dept HEW NIH, 1979. *This 387-page volume contains informative papers on research dealing with the organism, its components, infection, disease control, and vaccine development.*

Mertsola J, Ruuskanen O, Eerola E, Viljanen MK: Intrafamilial spread of pertussis. J Pediatr 103:359, 1983. *Longitudinal household epidemiology of pertussis as influenced by prior vaccination.*

Miller DL, Alderslade R, Ross EM: Whooping cough and whooping cough vaccine: The risks and benefits debate. Epidem Rev 4:1, 1982. *Particularly cogent at this time when public confidence in pertussis vaccine has been eroded by media presentations.*

Olson LC: Pertussis. Medicine 54:427, 1975. *A time-tested review including all the "classics" among its more than 400 references.*

Sato Y, Kimura M, Fukumi H: Development of a pertussis component vaccine in Japan. Lancet 1:122, 1984. *The great hope for an improved less reactive vaccine in the 1980's.*

*National Institutes of Health.

276. DIPHTHERIA

Richard V. McCloskey

Diphtheria is an acute infectious disease caused by a bacillus, *Corynebacterium diphtheriae*. The infection usually localizes in the pharynx, larynx, nostrils, and occasionally the skin and gives rise to both local and systemic signs. The latter are related to the production of a potent, soluble exotoxin elaborated by the microorganisms multiplying at the site of infection.

HISTORY. *Corynebacterium diphtheriae* was observed in diphtheritic membrane by Klebs in 1883. Loeffler in 1884 cultivated *C. diphtheriae* and described its characteristics. The Greek name of the type species—from *Korynee,* club; *bakterion,* staff; and *diphtheria,* leather hide—describes the club-shaped bacillus that causes a leathery membrane in the pharynx. In 1888 Roux and Yersin discovered that bacillus-free filtrates from diphtheria bacillus cultures would kill guinea pigs and thus demonstrated the potent exotoxin fundamental to the pathogenesis of diphtheria. The test that first enabled physicians to distinguish between susceptible and resistant patients was described by Schick in 1913. In the same year, von Behring successfully immunized children with a toxin-antitoxin mixture. From 1923 to 1928, Glenny and Ramon treated toxin to develop toxoid. Immunization with toxoid remains the primary method for suppression of diphtheria. Between 1960 and 1970, Collier, Gill, and Pappenheimer and their colleagues described the means by which toxin disrupts protein synthesis.

ETIOLOGY. *C. diphtheriae* is a pleomorphic, unencapsulated, nonmotile gram-positive bacillus. Smears prepared with differential stains (Albert's stain) may reveal metachromatic granules. The organisms may be arranged in palisades, L or V forms, or in groups resembling "Chinese characters" when examined in stained preparations. Growth is aerobic, and potassium tellurite or coagulated serum (Loeffler's medium) promotes growth. Colonies of *Corynebacterium* species (as well as streptococci and staphylococci) growing on tellurite-containing media develop a grayish black color. *C. diphtheriae* characteristically produces both a brown-gray halo and a garlic odor when growing on Tinsdale's agar. *C. diphtheriae* cohabitates the mucous membranes of humans together with other morphologically similar saprophytic diphtheroids from which it must be distinguished, usually by differential fermentation of glycogen, starch, glucose, maltose, and sucrose. The characteristics of the three stable types of diphtheria bacillus are as follows: *gravis,* a short uniformly staining rod forming low circular coherent colonies on tellurite agar, which becomes a "daisyhead" when well developed; this type may cause slight hemolysis; *intermedius,* long pleomorphic clubbed rods forming small discrete delicate colonies on tellurite agar; *mitis,* long pleomorphic rods with prominent metachromatic granules forming "poached egg" colonies on tellurite agar.

EPIDEMIOLOGY. Intimate contact with other infected persons is required for the spread of diphtheria. Transmission is usually by way of infected droplets or nasopharyngeal secretions. Infective skin exudate is also involved in person-to-person spread. Carriers are persons harboring a toxinogenic strain of *C. diphtheriae* in the nasopharynx or on the skin. An asymptomatic carrier can only be detected by culture of the nasopharynx or skin. Attention is often directed toward carriers when close associates, siblings, or marital partners develop diphtheria. A carrier state may exist for several days before the onset of symptoms. A convalescent carrier state occurs after symptoms subside. The duration of a convalescent carrier state is greatly shortened by appropriate antibiotic treatment. Carriers constitute the reservoir from which the disease spreads to susceptible patients.

Recent surveys of diphtheria carriers show that 88 per cent have completed or partially completed a course of diphtheria immunization. In the past decade, diphtheria in the United States has been a disease of urban rather than rural populations. Diphtheria affects mainly poor persons living in crowded conditions with poor access to health care facilities. Morbidity and mortality are highest in children less than 14 years of age. In the United States, attack rates are highest among blacks and Mexican Americans between 5 and 14 years of age.

In tropical and subtropical areas, the disease is more often manifest as a skin disease than as a respiratory tract infection. Skin infections are important in maintaining endemism of *C. diphtheriae* infections in tropical and subtropical areas. Skin infections, because of greater contagiousness, result in higher environmental carrier levels of *C. diphtheriae* than does respiratory tract diphtheria. As the incidence of skin infections increases, so does the reservoir, acquisition, and transmission of *C. diphtheriae.* Such mechanisms have been thought to be important in spreading respiratory tract diphtheria in tropical and, more recently, in temperate climates.

Epidemiologists use several techniques to classify toxin-producing *C. diphtheriae* and to disrupt its method of spread. The three types—mitis, intermedius, and gravis—are identified by colonial morphologic characteristics and a number of biochemical properties. The classification does not necessarily imply that disease caused by an intermedius strain is invariably less severe than that produced by a gravis strain. Mitis strains, however, have produced less severe disease than that caused by the other two biotypes. Gravis types have produced epidemics in populations of unimmunized persons previously experiencing disease due to mitis or intermedius strains. Well-immunized populations more often experience disease caused by mitis types. Each type can cause epidemic diphtheria.

C. diphtheriae strains can be classified by patterns of bacteriophage lysis into at least 35 types. Each bacteriophage type is stable and specific. A lysotype may persist in the throats of healthy carriers for years. In a given geographic area a single lysotype may be obtained from both patients and asymptomatic carriers. Some bacteriophage types are confined to or more frequently found in certain countries, which suggests that the lysotyping scheme may reflect the adaptability of *C. diphtheriae* to selected populations. The ease with which a strain of *C. diphtheriae* can be induced to liberate the identifying bacteriophage into the surrounding medium may be directly correlated with high toxin production and high capacity to spread among a population.

Recent urban epidemics of diphtheria in the United States have been difficult to control, even though hundreds of thousands of persons completed diphtheria immunization through intensive efforts by medical personnel. Immunization with diphtheria toxoid of susceptible persons must be combined with a program that identifies carriers of diphtheria and terminates the carrier state by antibiotic treatment. Quarantine is not effective in an open urban society.

PATHOGENESIS. Myocarditis and neuritis are caused by the toxin elaborated by *C. diphtheriae* and absorbed by the infected patient. A great deal is known about the molecular mechanisms by which this toxin causes disease. The toxin is an acidic globular protein with a molecular weight of 62,000 to 63,000. It is characterized by extreme potency, a cellular site of activity, and a latent period before inhibition of cellular protein synthesis is manifest. Strains of *C. diphtheriae* infected by a lysogenic bacteriophage produce the toxin when iron is present in a critical concentration range in the medium. A fragment of toxin bypasses normal cellular digestive mechanisms and enters the cytoplasm. After crossing the cell membrane, toxin inactivates a factor *(elongation factor)* that is one of several soluble proteins needed for the translocation step of protein synthesis. The toxin catalyzes the reaction nicotine adeninedinucleotide + elongation factor = adenosine diphosphoribose–elongation factor complex + nicotinamide + hydrogen. When the elongation factor is linked with adenosine diphosphoribose, it is inactive. Translocation of peptidyl transfer ribonucleic acid (tRNA) from acceptor to donor sites on the ribosome is disrupted, and protein synthesis stops. The whole toxin is actually a proenzyme. The reaction with adenosine diphosphoribose (ribosylation reaction) is caused by a proteolytic fragment of the whole toxin (fragment A). Nontoxinogen *C. diphtheriae* elaborate a physicochemically similar but immunochemically dissimilar and biologically innocuous protein. Therefore, identification of toxin production in vitro by *C. diphtheriae* (toxinogenicity) is of paramount importance. This is usually accomplished by demonstrating immunoprecipitation lines produced by a strain of *C. diphtheriae* growing on agar on which is placed a filter paper strip containing a diluted, highly purified diphtheria antitoxin *(Elek's test)*. Other biologically active extracellular products of *C. diphtheriae* play some role in the production of diphtheria, since nontoxinogenic *C. diphtheriae* may cause clinical diphtheria although of a milder variety than that produced by toxinogenic organisms.

CLINICAL MANIFESTATIONS. Diphtheria may be a symptomless state or a rapidly fatal hypertoxic disease that devastates the heart and lungs. The primary determinants of diphtheria are the patient's immunity to diphtheria toxin, the virulence and toxinogenicity of the infecting strain of *C. diphtheriae*, and the anatomic location of the infection. Additional characteristics that may influence the symptoms elicited are age, coexisting systemic disease, and pre-existing local nasopharyngeal disease. The incubation period is usually two to six days. Most patients, excluding those with the mildest of nasal or skin infections, seek medical attention after several days of systemic illness. The speed of onset is variable. Younger patients may be desperately ill in the face of deceptively modest malaise and fatigue. The temperature gradually rises, seldom exceeding 102° F except in those most severely ill. Children are less likely than adults to complain of sore throat, which is not usually the initial complaint at any age. Other signs and symptoms depend on the extent of the local diphtheritic lesion. Further discussion may be divided on this basis.

Anterior Nasal Diphtheria. Patients with anterior nasal diphtheria may be minimally inconvenienced while producing a thick mucopurulent nasal discharge, which may irritate the external nares and upper lips. A creamy yellowish membrane, with or without crusting, may be seen in the nose. Severe intoxication from nasal diphtheria is not common.

Tonsillar (Faucial) Diphtheria. In tonsillar diphtheria the membrane begins as a thin mucilaginous structure involving one or both tonsils. It is not confined to tonsillar crypts. By the time medical advice is sought, usually there is a characteristic grayish-green color to some area of the membrane. The membrane, which is several millimeters thick, may be difficult to dislodge with a swab and when torn off often leaves a bleeding surface on the tonsil. Sometimes the membrane crosses anatomic borders and may extend beyond the anterior pillar of the tonsils, which are often enlarged. The four most common complaints during an outbreak in Texas were sore throat (85 per cent), pain on swallowing (23 per cent), nausea and vomiting (25 per cent), and headache (18 per cent). The most common sign was fever (85 per cent). Moderately tender lymph nodes, 1 to 2 cm in diameter, can usually be palpated in the anterior triangle of the neck.

Pharyngeal Diphtheria. Outside the palatine tonsil the membrane spreads to the uvula, the soft palate, and the pharyngeal wall. The marked swelling of the tonsils at this point often obscures large areas of membrane on the posterior aspect of the tonsil. The nasal mucosa may be involved and may bleed profusely. The greenish character of the membrane is more prominent. There may be necrotic black patches in those areas where the membrane first appeared. The so-called *diphtheritic fetor* is of little diagnostic value, occurring also during the course of infectious mononucleosis and Vincent's infection. A hot tender edema (bull neck) involving the anterior part of the neck may obscure the angle of the jaw, the border of the sternocleidomastoid muscle, the clavicle, and the enlarged lymph nodes, which become more prominent as the edema subsides. The child with pharyngeal diphtheria is pathetically weak, limp, unresisting, pale, and exhausted. Bleeding from the upper airway is a grave prognostic sign.

Laryngeal and Bronchial Diphtheria. The membrane may extend downward or may involve the larynx exclusively. The voice will become hoarse, inspiratory and expiratory stridor may appear, dyspnea and cyanosis occur, and accessory muscles of respiration are used. Casts of the major bronchi can be formed by the membrane. If not removed by bronchoscopy, this membrane may cause death by hypoxia.

Myocarditis. In diphtheritic myocarditis most of the electrocardiographic abnormalities appear during the first week of illness. There is a correlation between delayed conduction velocity of the median, ulnar, and common peroneal nerves and myocardial conduction system disturbances. Moreover, the delayed peripheral nerve conduction velocity precedes clinical evidence of myocarditis and myocardial conduction system abnormalities. The determination of peripheral nerve conduction delay may be used to predict the appearance of myocarditis and cardiac arrhythmias. ST-T wave changes that are destined to improve usually do so within ten days of appearance of the abnormalities.

The severity of the illness and the toxemia are roughly related to the incidence of electrocardiographic (ECG) abnormalities and acute circulatory failure. Acute circulatory failure is practically never seen with nasal diphtheria but may occur in 9 per cent with pharyngeal-laryngeal infection, largely as a consequence of the amount of toxin produced by the more extensive deeper respiratory infections. Acute circulatory failure appears as the sudden onset of pallor, hypotension, collapsed peripheral pulses, and profuse perspiration. Diphtheria with ST-T wave changes is associated with a significantly higher mortality (28 per cent) than diphtheria without ECG changes (6 to 10 per cent). Serial determinations of serum glutamic oxalacetic transaminase concentration will identify most patients with myocarditis.

Early identification of diphtheritic myocarditis is important in reducing morbidity and mortality. Patients with ECG abnormalities during diphtheria should undergo continuous monitoring in specialized cardiac units with supportive ancillary facilities. Treatment is aimed at the more serious arrhythmias and conduction disturbances. Atrioventricular (AV) block and left bundle branch block (LBBB) are ominous signs, associated with mortality of 60 to 100 per cent. Electric pacing with temporary transvenous pacing electrodes or myocardial demand pacemakers can resolve AV block and LBBB produced by diphtheritic myocarditis. Treatment regimens usually include salt restriction, careful fluid balance, and short-acting digitalis preparations if congestive heart failure is marked. Antiarrhythmic agents such as procainamide, lidocaine, and isoproterenol are used when indicated to suppress or control specific arrhythmias. High dose steroid therapy is often used in anticipation of reducing edema and fibrosis of the myocardium or conducting system, although there is no firm evidence that steroids actually accomplish these objectives.

Since patients who develop myocarditis are severely intoxicated, the physician should anticipate other toxic manifestations. Intensive nursing care may be needed to support respiration and to prevent permanent complications of peripheral neuritis. Thrombocytopenia due to platelet destruction may complicate the myocarditis, and platelet transfusions may be necessary.

DIAGNOSIS. The diagnosis of diphtheria must rest on clinical grounds alone, since treatment cannot await bacteriologic confirmation. Diphtheria must be considered whenever a membrane is present in the throat, especially if the uvula is involved. Infectious mononucleosis membrane is confined to the tonsils and remains creamy-white without necrotic patches for a longer time than diphtheritic membrane. Streptococcal pharyngitis is associated with fiery redness of the throat and white exudate. Severe throat pain and faucial distortion are not seen in uncomplicated diphtheria. The foul necrotic exudate complicating leukemia may be impossible to distinguish from diphtheria by examination alone. Vincent's angina may involve the gums and is identified by Gram stain of the exudate. Simultaneous infection with streptococci (32 per cent in a recent outbreak) does not alter the physical findings suggestive of diphtheria. The laboratory findings in diphtheria are nonspecific and include moderate leukocytosis and transient albuminuria.

TREATMENT AND PREVENTION. A patient with tonsillar or nasopharyngeal diphtheria requires isolation in the hospital with bed rest for 10 to 14 days. The early use of adequate amounts of diphtheria antitoxin (DAT) remains the most important specific mode of treatment. Every patient with diphtheria merits DAT therapy, even though a week or so may have passed since the onset of illness. Since DAT is horse serum, intradermal and conjunctival tests (or both) should be performed before administration. If either is positive, desensitization is time-consuming and hazardous but is justifiable because DAT is the only specific treatment available. The required dose of DAT may be simplified as follows: if membrane does not extend beyond the tonsil and there is no thrombocytopenia, the patient may be treated by intramuscular administration of 20,000 units. Patients with more extensive membrane require 80,000 to 100,000 units, preferably by the intravenous route. The minimum amount of DAT necessary to prevent complications is not known. Antibiotics are used to eliminate the organism from the upper respiratory tract and to terminate the carrier state. Penicillin and erythromycin are both effective. If the patient is unable to swallow, initial treatment with parenteral administration of penicillin produces less vomiting and pain at the site of administration than does parenteral erythromycin therapy. Tetracycline, rifampin, clindamycin, and ampicillin are effective in vitro against *C. diphtheriae*, but cephalexin, oxacillin, and lincomycin are not. Both benzathine penicillin and erythromycin therapy can be used to terminate the carrier state. Bed rest is strictly enforced. Airway obstruction requires tracheostomy. Bronchoscopy may be performed to remove membranes from larger bronchi. Expert nursing care is necessary to prevent pneumonia caused by gram-negative bacilli acquired in the hospital. Therapy is always expensive and not always successful.

The complications of diphtheria can be prevented by active immunization beginning in childhood, with booster immunization every ten years thereafter. Active immunization and early treatment of carriers are both necessary for control of the disease. Immunization should be begun with diphtheria-tetanus-pertussis vaccine (DTP) in infants at six weeks of age. Three 0.5-ml injections of DTP are given at monthly intervals, with a booster dose of 0.5 ml at one year. Children who have received this primary series should receive a booster dose before entry into school. For older children, primary immunization may be accomplished by two doses of pediatric diphtheria-tetanus (DT), 0.5 ml each, six weeks apart with a booster six months to one year later. Persons over 12 years of age should be primarily immunized with the same schedule, but adult-type diphtheria-tetanus vaccine (dT) should be used. Schick test are unnecessary before adult immunizations. Those heavily exposed (physicians, nurses, hospital workers) to diphtheria should receive a 0.5-ml booster dose of dT every five years. All others should receive 0.5 ml of dT at ten-year intervals. Patients exposed to a suspected case should receive a 0.5-ml dT booster dose if they have been immunized previously but have not had a booster immunization within ten years.

Barksdale L: Immunology of diphtheria. *In* Nahmias AJ, O'Reilly RJ (eds.): Immunology of Human Infection. New York, Plenum Publishing Corp. 1981, pp 171–199. *Recent and comprehensive review.*

Diphtheria, Tetanus, and Pertussis. Guidelines for vaccine prophylaxis and other preventive measures. Immunization Practices Advisory Committee. Centers for Disease Control. Ann Intern Med 95:723–728, 1981.

Dobie RA, Tobey DN: Clinical features of diptheria in the respiratory tract. JAMA 242:2197, 1979. *A description of the signs and symptoms of diphtheritic rhinitis, pharyngitis, and laryngotracheitis.*

Koopman JS, Campbell J: The role of cutaneous diphtheria infections in a diphtheria epidemic. J Infect Dis 131:239, 1975. *An analysis of how skin infections may spread* C. diphtheriae *infections.*

McCloskey RV, Eller JJ, Green M, Smilack J: The 1970 epidemic of diphtheria in San Antonio. Ann Intern Med 75:495, 1971. *A description of clinical and epidemiologic features of an epidemic of diphtheria in a community in the United States.*

Clostridial Diseases

277. CLOSTRIDIAL MYONECROSIS AND OTHER CLOSTRIDIAL DISEASES

John G. Bartlett

Clostridia are gram-positive, spore-forming anaerobic bacteria that are widely distributed in soil and in the normal intestinal microflora of animals. Sporulation permits survival in adverse conditions so that these organisms can be isolated with ease from almost any environmental source. Concentrations vary considerably, but any fertile loam is expected to contain at least 10^3 clostridia per gram. Clostridia have been found in the intestinal tract of almost all animals examined. Most humans harbor 10^9 to 10^{10} clostridia per gram of stool; these organisms are less commonly found in the normal flora of the skin, oral cavity, and female genital tract. *C. perfringens*, the most frequent clinical isolate, is found in virtually all soil samples and, along with *C. ramosum*, is the most frequent clostridial species found in the intestinal flora of humans. Nevertheless, there are over 60 recognized species, and about 30 species have been found in human infections. Many clinical laboratories do not perform the extensive biochemical testing necessary to speciate clostridial isolates, and even when this is done, many organisms do not fit current taxonomic schema.

Clostridia cause diverse disease processes including bacteremia, localized infections at various anatomic sites, and the histotoxic clostridial syndromes. The latter refers to well-characterized syndromes caused by toxins elaborated under appropriate cultural conditions by various clostridial species (Table 277–1). The most commonly encountered histotoxic species is *C. perfringens*, which is divided into five types designated A to E on the basis of the production of the four major lethal toxins designated alpha, beta, epsilon, and iota. All *C. perfringens*, and many other species of clostridia (Table 277–1), produce alpha toxin, a phospholipase that splits lecithin to phosphoryl choline and a diglyceride. Intravenous administration of alpha toxin in experimental animals causes massive hemolysis, platelet destruction, and widespread capillary damage. Other clostridial toxins cause diseases of the intestine (enteric toxins) or

TABLE 277–1. HISTOTOXIC CLOSTRIDIAL SYNDROMES

Disease	Agent	Toxin
Enteric diseases		
Food poisoning	*C. perfringens*, type A	Enterotoxin
Antibiotic-induced diarrhea or colitis	*C. difficile*	Toxins A and B
Enteritis necroticans	*C. perfringens*, type C	Beta toxin
Neurologic syndromes		
Botulism	*C. botulinum*	Botulinal toxins A, B, E, and F
Tetanus	*C. tetanus*	Tetanospasmin
Myonecrosis (gas gangrene)	*C. perfringens, C. novyi, C. septicum, C. histolyticum, C. bifermentans, C. fallax*	Multiple toxins, especially alpha toxin

of the nervous system (neurotoxins). The toxins of *C. botulinum* and *C. tetanus* are lethal to mice in doses of 1 ng. By extrapolation, the lethal dose in the bloodstream of humans is approximately 10^{-9} mg per kilogram body weight, making these toxins the most potent poisons known. The toxins of *C. difficile* and the alpha toxin of *C. perfringens* are about 100 to 1,000 times less potent in mouse lethality testing.

Smith LDS: The Pathogenic Anaerobic Bacteria. 2nd ed. Springfield, Charles C Thomas, 1975, pp 109–324. *The author, a noted authority in the field, provides a scholarly review of clostridia, including a description of the species, their natural habitat, their toxins, and their role in disease.*

CLOSTRIDIAL MYONECROSIS

DEFINITION. Clostridial myonecrosis, or gas gangrene, is a life-threatening infection involving muscle caused by toxins produced by clostridia, usually *C. perfringens*.

ETIOLOGY. Clostridial myonecrosis usually follows wounding from trauma or surgery, contamination with histotoxic clostridia, and toxin elaboration. It is estimated that 30 to 80 per cent of serious traumatic open wounds are contaminated by clostridia, although gas gangrene remains a relatively rare infection. This experience emphasizes the decisive role of local conditions that promote toxin production primarily by decreasing the oxidation-reduction potential. Contributing factors to tissue hypoxia include vascular insufficiency, the presence of foreign bodies, tissue necrosis, and concurrent infection involving other microbes.

The most frequent pathogen, *C. perfringens*, is found in approximately 80 per cent of cases with positive cultures. Other clostridial species implicated include *C. novyi, C. septicum, C. histolyticum, C. bifermentans*, and *C. fallax*. In many instances, there are several clostridial species isolated from the infected site. Species causing gas gangrene produce over 20 exotoxins, including seven that are lethal to experimental animals. Perhaps the most important toxin is *alpha toxin*, a lecithinase that destroys cell membranes, alters capillary permeability, destroys platelets, and causes severe hemolysis. In appropriate environmental conditions, the histotoxic clostridia replicate and elaborate toxins that diffuse out to adjacent soft tissue and thus promote local spread as well as extensive systemic effects.

CLINICAL MANIFESTATIONS. Gas gangrene is a devastating infection characterized by prominent findings at the site of injury and profound systemic toxicity. Most cases occur in association with wounding from trauma or surgery. The usual clinical settings are: (1) traumatic injury or penetrating wound; (2) surgery, especially intestinal or biliary tract operations; (3) uterine gas gangrene, which most frequently follows septic abortions; (4) soft tissue lesions associated with vascular insufficiency; (5) intestinal gas gangrene, which is most commonly found in compromised hosts, especially patients with leukemia or colonic carcinoma; and (6) "spontaneous gas gangrene," a rare form of the disease in which there is no readily identifiable predisposing condition. The experience during peacetime among civilians in the United States is that approximately 50 per cent of cases follow severe traumatic injury and 40 per cent follow surgery. The most frequent traumatic injuries are car accidents, crush injuries, industrial accidents, and gunshot wounds. The most frequent antecedent surgical procedures are elective colon resection, nonelective colonic surgery, and biliary tract surgery. About two thirds of cases involve extremities, and one third involve the abdominal wall.

The usual incubation period from the time of wounding to the onset of symptoms is one to four days with a range of eight hours to several weeks. The first symptom is usually sudden and severe pain at the site of injury. Observations at this time typically show tense edema and tenderness. Gas may be noted in the soft tissues by palpation, x-ray, computerized tomography, or ultrasound studies. The skin is initially pale and then progresses to a magenta or bronze discoloration, and there is often cutaneous necrosis with hemorrhagic bullae. As the lesion evolves, there may be a thin, serosanguinous discharge with characteristic sweet odor. The systemic findings that accompany the evolving changes at the wound are profound. These include diaphoresis, low grade fever, and tachycardia that is disproportionate to the temperature elevation. Common complications include hemolytic anemia, hypotension, and renal failure. The patient is typically anxious throughout the disease but remains alert despite profound systemic toxicity.

DIAGNOSIS. The diagnosis of clostridial myonecrosis is based on a constellation of clinical findings, observations at the site of injury, and supporting microbiologic data. X-rays or computerized tomography studies often show gas bubbles distributed in and around muscle, and Gram stains of discharge typically show large, gram-positive bacilli with blunt ends and a paucity of polymorphonuclear leukocytes. Approximately 15 per cent of patients have clostridial bacteremia. Nevertheless, the findings on Gram stain and the detection of gas in the soft tissue cannot be considered specific. Moreover, most patients with clostridial bacteremia do not have myonecrosis. The definitive diagnostic procedure is surgical incision to expose muscle that may appear pale and edematous, beefy-red or, in the most advanced stages, black and friable. The muscle is nonviable, it fails to contract with stimulation, and the cut surface does not bleed.

The differential diagnosis includes a number of soft tissue infections that may also involve clostridia, are associated with tissue necrosis, are characterized by a fulminant course, or are associated with gas formation. Important findings in the differential diagnosis are summarized in Table 277–2.

TREATMENT. The most important facet of treatment is extensive surgical debridement with wide excision of involved muscle, amputation when an extremity is involved, or hysterectomy with uterine gas gangrene. The preferred antibiotic is aqueous penicillin G in doses of 10 to 20 million units daily for adults. Chloramphenicol in doses of 1 gram intravenously every six hours is the preferred regimen for patients with penicillin hypersensitivity. Cephalosporins and clindamycin are less active against clostridia and cannot be considered suitable substitutes for penicillin. The therapeutic value of hyperbaric oxygen is controversial. Advocates claim that this will clearly demarcate the necrotic tissue to simplify surgery and improve survival rates. Nevertheless, controlled studies to document efficacy are not available, and there may be major problems in transferring critically ill patients to centers with this type of facility. Surgery should not be delayed. Supportive measures include fluid and electrolyte replacement, control of acidosis, transfusions for severe anemia, and appropriate measures for renal failure.

PROGNOSIS. Clostridial myonecrosis is a devastating infection that often requires mutilating surgery and prolonged hospital courses. The overall mortality rate in 116 reports summarizing over 1200 cases is 25 per cent.

PREVENTION. The inoculum of *C. perfringens* required to produce gas gangrene is reduced by 10^6 organisms in experimental animals if the organism is delivered into devitalized muscle containing dirt instead of normal tissue. As noted earlier, contamination of wounds by clostridia from either soil sources or from the endogenous fecal flora is common with both traumatic injuries and surgical incisions. The incidence of clostridial myonecrosis following battlefield injury was 10 per cent in World War I, 1 per cent in World War II, and 0.01 per cent (22 cases in 139,000 battle injuries) in the Vietnam War. These figures reflect improvements in the management of battlefield injuries with major emphasis on prompt and thorough debridement. There should also be care in preserving the vascular supply, particularly with the use of tourniquets and casts. Judicious decisions regarding closure of traumatic wounds and the prophylactic use of antibiotics are also important. There is no effective means of active immunization.

TABLE 277–2. DEEP AND SERIOUS SOFT TISSUE INFECTIONS

	Gas-Forming Cellulitis	Synergistic Necrotizing Cellulitis	Gas Gangrene	"Streptococcal" Myonecrosis	Necrotizing Fasciitis	Infected Vascular Gangrene	Streptococcal Gangrene
Predisposing conditions	Traumatic	Diabetes, prior local lesion, perirectal lesion	Traumatic or surgical wound	Trauma, surgery	Diabetes, trauma, surgery, perineal infection	Arterial insufficiency	Traumatic or surgical wound
Incubation period	>3 days	3–14 days	1–4 days	3–4 days	1–4 days	>5 days	6 hours–2 days
Etiologic organism(s)	Clostridia, others	Mixed aerobic-anaerobic flora	Clostridia, esp. *C. perfringens*	Anaerobic streptococci	Mixed aerobic-anaerobic flora	Mixed aerobic-anaerobic flora	*S. pyogenes*
Systemic toxicity	Minimal	Moderate to severe	Severe	Minimal until late in course	Moderate to severe	Minimal	Severe
Course	Gradual	Acute	Acute	Subacute	Acute or subacute	Subacute	Acute
Wound findings							
Local pain	Minimal	Moderate to severe	Severe	Late only	Minimal to moderate	Variable	Severe
Skin appearance	Swollen, minimal discoloration	Erythematous or gangrene	Tense and blanched, yellow-bronze, necrosis with hemorrhagic bullae	Erythema or yellow bronze	Blanched, erythema, necrosis with hemorrhagic bullae	Erythema or necrosis	Erythema, necrosis
Gas	Abundant	Variable	Usually present	Variable	Variable	Variable	No
Muscle involvement	No	Variable	Myonecrosis	Myonecrosis	No	Myonecrosis limited to area of vascular insufficiency	No
Discharge	Thin, dark, sweetish or foul odor	Dark pus or "dishwater," putrid	Serosanguinous, sweet or foul odor	Seropurulent	Seropurulent or "dishwater," putrid	Minimal	None or serosanguinous, no odor
Gram stain	PMNs and gram-positive bacilli	PMNs, mixed flora	Sparse PMNs; gram-positive bacilli	PMNs, gram-positive cocci	PMNs, mixed flora	PMNs, mixed flora	PMNs, gram-positive cocci in chains
Surgical therapy	Debridement	Wide filleting incisions	Extensive excision, amputation	Excision of necrotic muscle	Wide filleting incisions	Amputation	Debridement of necrotic tissue

Baxter CR: Surgical management of soft tissue infections. Surg Clin North Am 52:1483, 1972. *Soft tissue infections are reviewed using three categories: infections requiring incision and drainage, infections requiring excision of tissue, and infections not requiring extensive surgery.*

Dellinger EP: Severe necrotizing soft tissue infections. JAMA 246:1717–1721, 1981. *The author reviews management principles for severe soft tissue infections and emphasizes the differential diagnosis based on clinical presentation, Gram stain, and operative inspection.*

Heimbach RD: Gas gangrene: Review and update. HBO Review 1:41, 1980. *The author reviews gas gangrene and presents an endorsement for hyperbaric oxygen treatment that may be overly enthusiastic.*

MacLennan JD: The histotoxic clostridial infections of man. Bacteriol Rev 26:117, 1962. *This is a classic monograph that summarizes the clinical, pathologic, microbiologic, and epidemiologic features of serious soft tissue infections.*

Weinstein L, Barza M: Gas gangrene. New Engl J Med 289:1129, 1972. *A review of clinical features and management recommendations for gas gangrene.*

OTHER CLOSTRIDIAL DISEASES

SEPTICEMIA. Clostridia account for up to 3 per cent of all positive blood cultures in most clinical microbiologic laboratories. The most frequent species is *C. perfringens*, which accounts for 50 to 60 per cent. On rare occasions these patients have associated findings compatible with gas gangrene. More frequently they have associated infections involving a mixed aerobic-anaerobic flora that may include clostridia at the infected site, but most often they have other conditions in which neither the source nor the significance of the clostridia is apparent. Perhaps the most important point to emphasize is that the vast majority of patients with positive blood cultures for clostridia do not have devastating soft tissue infections that require emergent surgical intervention. Special notation must be made for bacteremia with *C. septicum*. Many of these patients have a hematologic malignancy, neutropenia, or colonic carcinoma. The usual portal of entry in these cases is the distal ileum or cecum, most patients are acutely ill, and aggressive antibiotic therapy with penicillin is indicated.

MISCELLANEOUS INFECTIONS. Clostridia are frequently isolated from infections involving the host's normal flora. This situation especially applies to cases in which the infecting flora originates in the colon, such as in intra-abdominal sepsis, wound infections after intestinal surgery, and wounds or decubitus ulcers located on the lower trunk or lower extremities. These organisms are also found in 5 to 10 per cent of anaerobic pulmonary infections and with similar frequency in nonvenereal infections of the female genital tract. Such infections usually involve a mixture of aerobic and anaerobic bacteria so that the role of clostridia is uncertain. The major concern is often gas gangrene and, as already emphasized, this diagnosis is best established by supporting clinical findings. Other considerations in the differential diagnosis include soft tissue infections associated with gas formation, such as gas-forming cellulitis, necrotizing fasciitis, infected vascular gangrene, and synergistic necrotizing cellulitis. All of these may involve clostridia as well as other microbes, but they are quite different in terms of prognosis, clinical findings, and type of surgery required (Table 277–2). Penicillin G is regarded as the preferred antibiotic for clostridial infections, and chloramphenicol is appropriate for patients who have a contraindication to penicillin; clindamycin and cephalosporins are regarded as somewhat inferior.

CLOSTRIDIA ENTEROTOXEMIAS. Clostridia cause three different types of enteric disease, each of which is ascribed to a unique toxin (Table 277–1). *C. difficile*, the major cause of antibiotic-associated colitis, is discussed in Ch. 278.

C. perfringens is commonly responsible for foodborne outbreaks of a self-limited enteric disease. The cause is an enterotoxin produced by some type A strains during sporulation. The pathophysiologic mechanism is: (1) ingestion of at least 10^8 viable vegetative cells; (2) enterotoxigenic potential of the ingested strain; (3) sporulation with toxin production in the alkaline medium of the small bowel; (4) diarrhea and cramps due to fluid secretion, morphologic damage to the intestinal mucosa, and altered motility in the small bowel. The usual vehicle is meat or food made with meat, such as stews, meat pies, gravies, or casseroles. The attack rate among exposed persons is usually 30 to 60 per cent and the incubation period ranges from 7 to 15 hours. Common symptoms are diarrhea (90 per cent), abdominal cramps (80 per cent), nausea (25 per cent), fever (25 per cent), and vomiting (10 per cent). The diagnosis is suspected in any outbreak of gastrointestinal disease associated with typical symptoms and incubation period among persons sharing a common and likely food source. Confirmation requires the recovery of *C. perfringens* in concentrations of at least 10^5 per gram of epidemiologically implicated food and recovery of at least 10^6 spores per gram of stool obtained within 48 hours after onset of symptoms from victims. Nearly all patients have spontaneous resolution of symptoms within 6 to 24 hours and do not require any specific form of therapy.

Enteritis necroticans is a serious gastrointestinal disease caused by the beta toxin of *C. perfringens*, type C. This disease, once called "darmbrand," occurred in epidemic form in malnourished individuals from Norway and Germany at the end of World War II. More recently, the same condition, known locally as "pigbel," has been found to be endemic in the highlands of New Guinea. Most victims are children who have participated in pig feasts that are believed to provide the source of the organism as well as a complex set of circumstances believed necessary for pathogenesis. The toxin is susceptible to proteolytic enzymes including trypsin. However, toxin inactivation in the small bowel fails because of enzyme deficiency ascribed to protein malnutrition, excessive consumption of sweet potatoes, which contain trypsin inhibitors, or colonization with *Ascaris lumbricoides*, which secrete trypsin inhibitors. The predilection for children presumably reflects antigenic naiveté. Pathologically, enteritis necroticans is a segmental disease of the small bowel that is characterized by mucosal infarction, edema, hemorrhage, and infiltration with polymorphonuclear cells. In advanced stages the bowel is thinned, friable, and subject to perforation. Medical therapy consists of intestinal decompression, penicillin or chloramphenicol, and intravenous fluid support. About half of the patients require resectional surgery, and the overall mortality rate is 15 to 40 per cent. Prevention in the endemic area is achieved with a beta-toxoid vaccine that is currently recommended for children in the endemic area.

Alpern RJ, Dowell VR Jr.: Nonhistotoxic clostridial bacteremia. Am J Clin Pathol 33:717–722, 1971. *A review of 86 patients with clostridia bacteremia, of whom none had gas gangrene, most had self-limited disease, and 84 had no identifiable portal of entry.*

Gorbach SL, Thadepalli H: Isolation of *Clostridia* in human infections: Evaluation of 114 cases. J Infect Dis 131:S81–S85, 1975. *The authors review their experience with 152 strains of clostridia recovered from 144 patients at Cook County Hospital. Sixty-five patients had soft tissue infections, or intra-abdominal sepsis, and 84 per cent of these had polymicrobial infections. Clostridia bacteremia in 49 patients usually occurred with no apparent relation to the clinical setting.*

Lawrence G, Walker PD: Pathogenesis of enteritis necroticans in Papua New Guinea. Lancet 1:125–126, 1976. *The authors, noted authorities in the field, provide a postulate for the pathophysiology of pigbel.*

Lawrence G, Shann F, Freestone DS, Walker PD: Prevention of necrotising enteritis in Papua New Guinea by active immunization. Lancet 1:227–230, 1979. *The authors provide data from a controlled trial showing success of vaccination with beta toxin toxoid.*

Koransky JR, Stargel MD, Dowell VR Jr.: Clostridium septicum bacteremia. Am J Med 66:63–66, 1979. *A review of 59 patients with* C. septicum *bacteremia that showed 71 per cent had malignancy, most presented with a fulminant clinical course, and most died unless appropriate antibiotics were given soon after admission.*

Ramsay AM: The significance of *Clostridium welchii* in the cervical swab and blood stream in postpartum and postabortum sepsis. J Obstet Gynecol Br Commonwealth 56:247–258, 1949. *The author refers to* C. perfringens (welchii) *as a "harmless saprophyte" in a discussion of 28 women with bacteremia, since most had minimal clinical disturbance despite the fact that the majority were studied before antibiotics were available.*

Shaudera WX, Tacket CO, Blake PA: Food poisoning due to *Clostridium perfringens* in the US. J Infect Dis 147:167–170, 1983. *The authors review the Centers for Disease Control's experience with* C. perfringens *food poisoning.*

278. PSEUDOMEMBRANOUS COLITIS

John G. Bartlett

DESCRIPTION. Pseudomembranous enterocolitis is a severe gastrointestinal disease characterized by exudative plaques on the intestinal mucosa. The most commonly involved site is the colon, in which case the preferred appellation is pseudomembranous colitis rather than "enterocolitis."

ETIOLOGY. Pseudomembranous enterocolitis is usually found in association with other conditions, although occasional cases occur in healthy persons with no identifiable risk factors. This condition was initially described in the preantibiotic era when it most frequently followed intestinal surgery. Additional recognized risk factors include intestinal obstruction, uremia, the hemolytic-uremic syndrome, Hirschsprung's disease, inflammatory bowel disease, shigellosis, intestinal ischemia, and neonatal necrotizing enterocolitis. During the past three decades, the disease has been recognized most frequently as a complication of antimicrobial use.

Studies of "antibiotic-associated pseudomembranous colitis" are divided into two periods with quite different observations. Reports from the 1950's and 1960's indicated that the small intestine usually was involved ("enterocolitis"), mortality rates were high, and the most frequently implicated drugs were chloramphenicol, tetracycline, and oral neomycin. *Staphylococcus aureus* was the suspected pathogen in most cases reported at that time. More recent studies of antibiotic-associated pseudomembranous colitis show that the lesions are generally confined to the colon, different antimicrobials are usually implicated (see later discussion), and the prognosis is considerably better than previously reported. The more recent work also indicates that *Clostridium difficile* is the responsible pathogen in the majority of cases.

INCIDENCE. Most patients with pseudomembranous colitis have recent antibiotic exposure, and the other risk factors noted appear to account for less than 10 per cent of all cases. The incidence of antibiotic-associated pseudomembranous colitis depends on the frequency with which endoscopy is performed to establish the diagnosis, antimicrobial use patterns, and epidemiologic patterns. Nearly all antimicrobials with an antibacterial spectrum of activity have been implicated. The most frequent are ampicillin, clindamycin, and cephalosporins. Less frequent are penicillins other than ampicillin, erythromycin, and sulfamethoxazole-trimethoprim. Drugs rarely implicated include tetracyclines, chloramphenicol, sulfonamides, and parenterally administered aminoglycosides. *C. difficile*–induced diarrhea or colitis may occur sporadically or in clusters within institutions. Epidemiologic studies indicate that *C. difficile* may be found in the colonic flora of about 3 per cent of healthy adults, is widely distributed in the environment, and is especially common in areas subject to fecal contamination from patients who have *C. difficile*–induced diarrheal complications. This last observation provides an explanation for focal outbreaks of the disease and emphasizes the importance of appropriate precautionary measures to limit spread.

MECHANISM. *C. difficile*–induced colitis is a toxin-mediated enteric disease in which there is no microbial invasion of the intestinal mucosa.

CLINICAL MANIFESTATIONS. Virtually all patients are at risk for antibiotic-associated pseudomembranous colitis, although there appears to be an increased risk with increasing age. The most common symptom is diarrhea consisting of watery or semiliquid stools without visible blood. Stool examination may show fecal leukocytes, but this is inconsistent and nonspecific. Many patients also have fever, which is usually moderate but may reach 40° C. Other common findings are abdominal cramps, lower quadrant tenderness, leukocytosis, and hypoalbuminemia. Systemic symptoms and abdominal findings are not invariably present, and some patients simply have annoying diarrhea. Complications in severe cases include dehydration, hypoalbuminemia with anasarca, electrolyte disturbances, toxic megacolon, and colonic perforation. Symptoms may begin at any time during the course of antimicrobial treatment or up to six weeks after antimicrobials have been discontinued. The differential diagnosis includes acute and chronic diarrhea caused by enteric pathogens other than *C. difficile*, intra-abdominal sepsis, and idiopathic inflammatory bowel disease.

DIAGNOSIS. The preferred method to establish the anatomic diagnosis is endoscopy. Gross inspection of the colon typically reveals punctate, raised, yellowish-white plaques with "skip areas" of a normal mucosa or a mucosa showing erythema or edema. The plaques are usually 2 to 10 mm wide but may enlarge and coalesce over extensive segments of the colon in the late stages. Pseudomembranes are often located throughout the colon, but up to 20 per cent of patients have segmental involvement of the right side of the colon, necessitating colonoscopy rather than sigmoidoscopy. Recognition of typical lesions on gross inspection often requires an experienced endoscopist using care to wipe away mucus to detect adherent plaques. Some cases are recognized only with histologic studies of biopsy specimens. Microscopic examination shows epithelial necrosis, goblet cells distended with mucus, and infiltration of the lamina propria with polymorphonuclear cells and eosinophilic exudate. The pseudomembrane is attached to the surface epithelium and is composed of fibrin, mucin, and polymorphonuclear cells.

The preferred diagnostic test to implicate *C. difficile* is a tissue culture assay of stool to demonstrate a cytopathic toxin that is neutralized by antitoxin to *C. difficile* or *C. sordellii.* Antitoxin neutralization with antisera to *C. sordellii* reflects antigenic cross-reactivity. Toxin titers may also be performed using serial dilutions of stool specimens, although there is little correlation between the toxin titer and the severity of the disease. Nearly all patients who have this toxin in the stool will also have *C. difficile* recovered using appropriate culture techniques. However, most clinical laboratories do not have the necessary expertise to recover and identify *C. difficile,* and occasional asymptomatic patients harbor the organism without the toxin. The best clinical correlation has been with the toxin assay.

Anatomic changes in the colonic mucosa noted in patients with the diarrheal complications of antibiotic use include an entirely normal colonic mucosa, erythema or edema, and colitis with friability, ulceration, or hemorrhage. Pseudomembranous colitis is regarded as the most severe and characteristic form of this complication. The toxin of *C. difficile* has been implicated in the entire spectrum of anatomic changes, but the frequency of this toxin correlates to a large extent with the severity of the disease process. Tissue culture assays for *C. difficile* toxin are positive in over 90 per cent of patients with pseudomembranous colitis and in approximately 20 per cent of those with antibiotic-associated diarrhea and an entirely normal colonic mucosa. Thus, the tissue culture assay described reflects a mechanism and does not establish the anatomic diagnosis. There is no identifiable pathogen in most patients with antibiotic-associated diarrhea or colitis in whom the assay for *C. difficile* toxin is negative, except for occasional cases that may involve *S. aureus.*

TREATMENT. The most important therapeutic decision is discontinuation of the implicated antimicrobial agent. This approach often results in resolution of symptoms with no necessity for further diagnostic tests or therapy. Patients with severe or persistent symptoms should undergo endoscopy to define anatomic changes and stool examination to detect *C. difficile* cytotoxin. Patients with severe fluid, albumin, or electrolyte depletion often require intravenous replacement and may require hyperalimentation. The role of corticosteroids and attempts to manipulate the flora, as with oral lactobacilli or fecal enemas, is uncertain. Antiperistaltic drugs are contraindicated.

Specific therapy is available for diarrhea caused by *C. difficile,* using cholestyramine to bind the toxin or vancomycin to inhibit the pathogen. The preferred agent for seriously ill patients is orally administered vancomycin, 125 to 500 mg four times daily for 7 to 14 days. Vancomycin is active against virtually all strains of *C. difficile,* the levels in the colon with oral administration are extremely high, and systemic toxicity is nil owing to poor absorption with oral administration even in the presence of an inflamed bowel. The major problems with vancomycin are high cost, noxious taste, and relapses in about 20 per cent of patients when vancomycin is discontinued. Relapses are characterized by the recurrence of typical symptoms, positive tissue culture assays for *C. difficile* cytotoxin, and stool cultures that yield vancomycin-sensitive strains of *C. difficile.* The mechanism of relapse is presumed to be reacquisition of the organism from an environmental source or failure to eradicate the pathogen from the gastrointestinal tract because of persistence of spores.

An alternative form of treatment is cholestyramine, one 4-gram packet three times daily for five days. The mechanism of activity is binding of the toxin by the anion exchange resin. This drug is not so predictably effective for initial treatment as vancomycin and should be reserved for less seriously ill patients or those who have suffered a relapse with vancomycin therapy. Alternative antibiotics include bacitracin or metronidazole, both in doses of 500 mg orally four times daily.

PROGNOSIS. Most patients with pseudomembranous colitis eventually recover even without specific forms of therapy. However, symptoms may be prolonged and debilitating, with persistent diarrhea for several weeks or months. Reports that focus on more seriously ill patients indicate mortality rates of 10 to 30 per cent. With early institution of vancomycin therapy there is a prompt symptomatic response, and virtually all patients recover. Following recovery, there are no recurrences except with the previously noted relapses following oral vancomycin therapy or re-exposure to another antimicrobial that has been associated with this complication.

PREVENTION. The most important preventive measure is judicious use of antimicrobial agents. Patients with *C. difficile*–induced diarrhea or colitis should be isolated and placed on enteric precautions to limit spread to susceptible hosts within institutions.

Bartlett JG: Antibiotic-associated pseudomembranous colitis. Rev Infect Dis 1:123, 1979. *Summary of evidence implicating* C. difficile *and experience with assays for the toxin of this microbe.*

Bartlett JG, Gorbach SL: Pseudomembranous colitis. Adv Intern Med 22:455, 1977. *Review of the topic with extensive reference list for publications prior to evidence implicating* C. difficile.

Bartlett JG, Tedesco FJ, Shull S, Lowe B: Relapse following oral vancomycin therapy of antibiotic-associated pseudomembranous colitis. Gastroenterology 78:431, 1980. *Review of experience with vancomycin therapy for 90 patients.*

Price AB, Davis DR: Pseudomembranous colitis. J Clin Pathol 30:1, 1977. *A review of histopathologic changes.*

Fekety R, Kim K-H, Brown D, Batts DH, Cudmore M, Silva J Jr.: Epidemiology of antibiotic-associated colitis. Am J Med 70:906, 1981. *A survey of the epidemiology of* C. difficile.

279. BOTULISM

John G. Bartlett

DEFINITION. Botulism is a severe neuroparalytic disease caused by toxins of *Clostridium botulinum.* There are four recognized disease categories: (1) foodborne botulism, (2) infant botulism, (3) wound botulism, and (4) unclassified cases.

ETIOLOGY. *C. botulinum* is a gram-positive, spore-forming obligate anaerobe that is widely distributed in nature and frequently found in soil, marine environments, and agricultural products. Adults regularly ingest *C. botulinum* spores from fresh agricultural products without deleterious consequences, and this organism is not recognized as a component of the normal fecal flora. Each strain produces one of seven antigenically distinct toxins of approximately 150,000 daltons, designated A through G. Human disease is caused by types A, B, E, and rarely F. These toxins are hematogenously disseminated to peripheral cholinergic synapses where they bind irreversibly and block acetylcholine release. The result is hypotonia with a descending symmetric flaccid paralysis. Botulinal toxin is the most potent poison of man; it has an estimated lethal dose in the bloodstream of 10^{-9} mg per kilogram.

FOOD POISONING. Foodborne botulism results from the ingestion of preformed toxin in inadequately prepared food. There are an average of 15 "outbreaks" annually in the United States, most of which involve a single case. The most frequently implicated vehicle in the United States is home-canned foods, which usually have a putrefactive odor. Meat and meat products are more commonly responsible in Europe, and preserved fish is most frequent in Japan, Scandinavia, and Russia. Type

A and B organisms predominate in the United States. Type E organisms are usually, but not exclusively, associated with an aquatic source in northern latitudes, where they are found in coastal waters, lakes, and intestines of fish that inhabit these areas.

CLINICAL MANIFESTATIONS. The incubation period is usually 18 to 36 hours but may be as short as two hours or as long as eight days. Persons with the shortest incubation period usually have the most severe disease. The bulbar musculature is affected first, with resultant diplopia, difficulty in focusing to a near point, dry mouth, and dysphagia. Common gastrointestinal symptoms include nausea, vomiting, and abdominal pain. Neurologic examination shows lateral rectus muscle weakness (cranial nerve VI), ptosis, dilated pupils with sluggish reaction, decreased gag reflex, or medial rectus paresis. This is followed by descending involvement of the motor neurons to peripheral muscles, including the muscles of respiration. Some patients have only mild illness, whereas others have severe paralysis that may continue, requiring intensive supportive care for weeks. Mentation remains clear, there is no fever, and neurologic dysfunction is bilateral but not necessarily symmetric. The principle causes of death are respiratory or bulbar paralysis and infectious complications during the period of supportive care.

DIAGNOSIS. The usual laboratory test in suspected cases is analysis of serum, stool, and food suspected of harboring botulinum toxin. This is done in a mouse assay in which specimens are injected intraperitoneally to demonstrate a lethal toxin that is neutralized by type-specific antitoxin. Possibly contaminated foods and patient stool may also be cultured for *C. botulinum.* Among patients with clinical evidence of botulism, the toxin is detected in sera from one third, the toxin is found in the stool from one third, and the organism is recovered in stool from 60 per cent of patients.

Botulism should be suspected in patients with acute flaccid paralysis, especially when there is bilateral sixth cranial nerve dysfunction, associated gastrointestinal symptoms, prior ingestion of possibly contaminated food, and typical symptoms in other persons who shared this food. The differential diagnosis includes myasthenia gravis, Guillain-Barré syndrome, tick paralysis, cerebrovascular accident involving branches of the basilar artery, trichinosis, the Eaton-Lambert syndrome, hypocalcemia, hypermagnesemia, organophosphate poisoning, atropine poisoning, paralytic poisoning caused by shellfish or puffer fish, and psychiatric syndromes. Electromyography is useful in differentiating botulism from other neurologic syndromes. This shows a diminished amplitude of muscle action potentials with a single supramaximal stimulus and facilitation of action potentials using paired or repetitive stimuli. These findings do not appear until the patient develops peripheral muscle weakness and are most likely to be positive in an affected limb.

TREATMENT. Ventilatory support is most important. Elimination of the toxin from the gastrointestinal tract may be facilitated using gastric lavage, cathartics, and enemas early in the course. Antitoxin is usually given irrespective of the duration of illness, since the toxin may persist in the blood for extended periods. Treatment is initiated using two vials of the trivalent antitoxin, each containing 7500 IU type A, 5500 IU type B, and 8,500 IU type E antitoxin; this is given intravenously and repeated at two to four hours. The antitoxin is horse serum and is associated with a 20 per cent incidence of hypersensitivity reactions, the most serious being anaphylaxis in 3 to 5 per cent. Efficacy of the antitoxin is most clearly established with type E botulism. Other therapeutic considerations include guanidine hydrochloride (15 to 50 mg per kilogram daily) to enhance acetylcholine release, but efficacy has not been established. Antimicrobial agents are advocated only for infectious complications.

PROGNOSIS. The case fatality rate for foodborne botulism was formerly 60 to 70 per cent. Improved methods of management, especially support of respiratory function, have reduced the fatality rate to less than 10 per cent in recent years. Patients who survive generally have complete recovery.

PREVENTION. Foodborne botulism is caused by germination of spores in food with toxin produced by vegetative forms, although the toxin may also be produced in vivo by simultaneous ingestion of spores. The disease may be prevented by destruction of spores in the original food source, inhibition of germination, or destruction of preformed toxin. Specific measures are as follows:

1. Destruction of spores with heat or irradiation. Spores of types A and B may survive boiling for several hours, especially at high altitudes (such as in Colorado) where the boiling point may be substantially lower. These spores may be destroyed if kept at 120° C for 30 minutes using pressure cookers. Spores of type E are most heat-labile and are killed with heating at 80° C for 30 minutes.
2. Germination may be inhibited by a reduction in pH, refrigeration, freezing, drying, or addition of salt, sugar, or other inhibitory substances such as sodium nitrite.
3. Inactivation of preformed toxin is accomplished by terminal heating for 20 minutes at 80° C or for 10 minutes at 90° C.

INFANT BOTULISM. Infant botulism results from production of *C. botulinum* toxin in vivo following colonization of the gastrointestinal tract in children ages one to nine months. This is the most common form of botulism in the United States, where 30 to 80 cases are documented annually. Spores of *C. botulinum* (but not the toxin) have been found in about 10 per cent of honey supplies, which presumably account for one third of cases. The disease spectrum varies considerably, ranging from "failure to thrive" or mild changes in bowel habits to the sudden infant death syndrome or "crib death." The most commonly recognized form of the disease is the "floppy baby syndrome." Initial symptoms are lethargy, diminished suck, weakness, feeble cry, and diminished spontaneous activity with loss of head control. This is followed by extensive flaccid paralysis. The diagnosis is established with the recovery of *C. botulinum* or its toxin in stool. The toxin has rarely been detected in the serum. Fecal carriage of the organism and the toxin may persist for weeks to months following clinical improvement and hospital discharge. The major therapeutic need is supportive care with special attention to nutrition and maintenance of respiratory function. The role of antitoxin, guanidine, and antibiotics in this form of botulism has not been established, and generally their use is not advised. The mortality rate for hospitalized patients given supportive care is only 2 per cent.

WOUND BOTULISM. This is a rare form of botulism in which a traumatic wound is infected by *C. botulinum* with toxin production in vivo. Clinical features are identical to those of foodborne botulism except that the incubation period is 4 to 14 days and there is a paucity of gastrointestinal symptoms. The diagnosis is established by recovering *C. botulinum* from the wound or by detection of the toxin in serum.

UNCLASSIFIED BOTULISM. This category includes persons over the age of 12 months who have typical symptoms and signs of botulism with no identifiable vehicle. It is possible that some cases result from production of toxin in vivo by organisms colonizing the intestine in a fashion comparable to the mechanism described for infant botulism.

SPECIAL NOTE. Physicians who suspect foodborne botulism should alert their state health department and the Communicable Diseases Center (telephone 404–329–3311 on weekdays; 404–329–3644 on nights, holidays, and weekends).

Dowell VR Jr., McCroskey LM, Hathaway CL, Lombard GL, Hughes JM, Merson MH: Coproexamination for botulinal toxin and *Clostridium botulinum.* JAMA 238:1829, 1977. *Reviews methods to establish the diagnosis in foodborne botulism.*

Merson MH, Hughes JM, Dowell VR, Taylor A, Barker WH, Gangarosa EJ: Current trends in botulism in the United States. JAMA 229:1305, 1974. *Summary of the CDC experience with foodborne botulism.*

Arnon SS: Infant botulism. Ann Rev Med 31:541, 1980. *A review of infant botulism.*

280. TETANUS

John H. Kerr

Tetanus, often called "lockjaw," is a disease of the nervous system characterized by intense activity of motor neurons resulting in severe muscle spasms. It is caused by an exotoxin of *Clostridium tetani.*

ETIOLOGY. *Clostridium tetani* is an actively mobile gram-positive bacillus which, in its spore-bearing form, has a characteristic "drumstick" appearance. It is a strict anaerobe, and spores will germinate only if the oxidation-reduction potential in the environment is +0.01 volt or less at pH 7. At 37° C, *Clostridium* grows well in a cooked meat medium and on blood agar plates, where slight hemolysis is often observed. Vegetative bacilli are readily killed by antiseptics and by heat, but the spores are highly resistant to antiseptics and variably resistant to heat. To kill all spores, boiling for at least four hours or autoclaving for 12 minutes at 121° C is required.

Clostridium tetani produces two exotoxins, tetanospasmin and tetanolysin. Tetanospasmin, a protein of molecular weight 150,000, is one of the most potent neurotoxins that have been isolated. Tetanolysin can cause hemolysis on blood agar plates, but does not seem to play any significant part in the pathogenesis of the disease.

EPIDEMIOLOGY. *Clostridium tetani* is commonly found in soil and in the feces of domestic animals and humans. Spores can be recovered from dust and clothing and, in suitably dry surroundings, may survive in a viable form for many years.

Tetanus is most common in warm climates and in highly cultivated rural areas. It remains a major public health problem in economically underdeveloped countries, where it causes several hundred thousand, mostly neonatal, deaths each year. Unhygienic practices such as dressing the umbilical stump with dung and neonatal circumcision in primitive conditions tend to maintain the high incidence of neonatal tetanus, which has a fatality rate exceeding 60 per cent except in a few outstanding centers. In more temperate and economically developed areas such as Europe and North America, the disease has become extremely rare because of better hygiene, improved wound care, and high immunization rates. In these countries, neonatal tetanus is almost unknown, and tetanus has increasingly become a disease of the elderly, probably because of impaired local responses to infection and of poorly maintained immunity.

PATHOGENESIS. For tetanus to occur, *Clostridium tetani* must be introduced into and multiply within the body. Spores may be carried in through large or small wounds but will germinate only if anaerobic conditions develop. This is most likely in wounds which contain necrotic tissue or foreign bodies, or in those which are heavily contaminated with soil or manure. If these conditions persist for more than a few hours, the clostridia multiply and may produce toxins. Tetanospasmin is released by autolysis of clostridial cells and diffuses into the local tissues, from where it may be spread throughout the body in the bloodstream. Most is taken up by the peripheral endings of motor neurons, although some enters sensory and autonomic nerve fibers. The toxin then travels along nerve fibers toward the central nervous system and, after a period of time related directly to the length of the nerve and inversely to the electrical activity in the axon, reaches and is concentrated within the cell body. At this stage, the electrical and functional characteristics of the cells are unaffected by the toxin within them. The symptoms of tetanus appear only after the toxin has passed across the synaptic cleft into the presynaptic terminals of spinal inhibitory interneurons where it combines with a ganglioside and interferes with the release of the inhibitory transmitter substance. Disinhibition of both alpha and gamma motor neurons occurs, leading to the increase in muscle tone, loss of coordination, and spontaneous simultaneous contractions of both agonist and antagonist muscles that constitute tetanic spasms.

An analogous process whereby tetanospasmin migrates centripetally along the sympathetic chain to produce disinhibition in the lateral horns of the spinal cord has been demonstrated in animals and probably explains the autonomic disturbances that complicate many of the severe cases in humans. In man, pathologic lesions caused directly by tetanospasmin have not been demonstrated unequivocally, and the toxin appears to kill by disrupting neurologic coordination. Even after the most severe form of the disease, recovery, if it takes place, is complete.

CLINICAL FEATURES AND CRITERIA OF SEVERITY IN TETANUS. The criteria of severity may be established in two ways: from the history, and from the symptoms and signs.

From the History. The severity of an attack of tetanus is related to the incubation period (the period from injury to the first sign of tetanus) and the onset period (the period from the first sign to the first generalized spasm). If the former is less than nine days and the latter less than 48 hours, the attack of tetanus may be expected to be severe. The length of the onset period is, in general, the more reliable guide.

From the Symptoms and Signs. In the mild case, tetanus usually presents with rigidity of muscles, which may be generalized or affect only one limb (local tetanus). Stiffness of the jaw muscles causes trismus, and stiffness of the facial muscles may cause a change of expression. Stiffness of the muscles of the neck and back may cause discomfort or even pain on attempted flexion of the spine.

In the moderate case, the patient has more severe generalized rigidity. Trismus is pronounced, the mouth can hardly be opened, and rigidity of the muscles of the face may cause the sneering "risus sardonicus." Opisthotonos may be pronounced, but more typically the stiffness of the antagonist muscles makes the patient lie "at attention" in bed, and the muscles of the back and abdomen are hard to the touch. Muscle spasms may appear as mild exacerbations of this generalized rigidity and may arise spontaneously or more commonly as a result of stimuli. The diagnostic characteristic of the moderate case, however, is the presence of dysphagia due to involvement of the pharyngeal muscles.

The patient with severe tetanus is distinguished from the patient with moderate tetanus by the presence of reflex spasms that may be of appalling intensity. If the spasms are untreated, opisthotonos becomes extreme and the intense muscle spasm may fracture vertebrae. Spasm of the laryngeal muscles, the diaphragm, and the intercostals prevents ventilation, and cyanosis occurs. Reflex spasms that cause cyanosis and cannot be controlled except by powerful relaxants such as curare are the characteristic features of the severe case of tetanus.

Autonomic Disturbances. Disturbances of the autonomic nervous system occur frequently in severely affected tetanus patients and may prove fatal, particularly when the disease occurs in drug addicts. Younger patients often develop a fluctuating hypertension and increasing tachycardia after a few days of treatment, and cardiovascular responses to stimuli such as the aspiration of secretions from the respiratory tract become exaggerated so that systolic blood pressures of over 300 mm Hg are not uncommon. Patients sweat profusely and may become extremely vasoconstricted peripherally with a sharp line of demarcation between warm and cold skin. Hyperpyrexia occurs in the absence of significant secondary infection and probably reflects the inability of the vasoconstricted patient to lose heat. High metabolic rates have been measured in spite of muscular paralysis, and the cardiac output is often disproportionately high in relation to tissue oxygen utilization, suggesting increased neurogenic drive to the heart. Raised plasma and urine catecholamine levels occur in association with these disturbances, and it seems likely that the sympathetic nervous system is grossly overactive and incoordinate. Prolonged overactivity has been followed by supraventricular tachycardia and multifocal ventricular ectopic beats, unresponsive hypotension, sudden bradycardia, and cardiac arrest.

Perhaps fortunately, patients with severe tetanus often remember little of their illness, but may recall weird and sometimes frightening dreams. Electroencephalography usually shows a sleep pattern with activation during stimulation such as tracheal aspiration.

DIAGNOSIS. The diagnosis of the established case of tetanus is all too easy, and strychnine poisoning is the only condition which is truly similar to established tetanus. Trismus may occur from dental infections, and the author has seen one case of hysterical tetanus. Overdose with or sensitivity to the phenothiazine group of drugs can be confused with tetanus, but the movements in these conditions usually include grimacing and jaw movements in which the jaw is opened widely.

TREATMENT. Treatment in tetanus is essentially symptomatic, but all patients with the disease should receive antimicrobial drugs, active and passive immunization, and should undergo wound excision. To allow the earliest possible detection of possibly lethal manifestations of the disease, such as severe muscular or laryngeal spasms, the treatment of tetanus should be conducted in a well-lighted intensive care unit rather than in isolation in a darkened side room.

Antibiotics. Treatment with penicillin (1 million units every six hours intramuscularly) or erythromycin (500 mg every six hours intravenously) should be commenced to ensure that all clostridia are killed.

Antitoxin. Human tetanus immunoglobulin (1000 units intravenously and 2000 units intramuscularly) should be administered as early as possible to produce a high blood level. Only toxin circulating in the bloodstream and that in the tissues near the wound will be accessible to this antitoxin, since that in transit up nerve fibers and that which has entered spinal interneurons and produced symptoms cannot be neutralized by blood-borne antitoxin. In animals, intrathecal antitoxin has been shown to combine with tetanospasmin in the synaptic clefts between motor neuron and interneuron and thus prevent the development of tetanic spasms. The administration of antitoxin by this route is currently being investigated, particularly in parts of the world where tetanus is common and medical facilities are scarce. The results to date do not match those that can be expected in a fully equipped intensive care unit.

Surgical Intervention. If a focus of infection or wound is found, surgical debridement should be carried out shortly after the administration of the intravenous antitoxin so that any toxin released into the circulation at surgery will be neutralized. In about 20 per cent of tetanus cases, no source of infection is ever identified.

Active Immunization. Because an attack of tetanus does not confer immunity to tetanus, active immunization with adsorbed toxoid should be started and a full course of three injections given during the recovery period.

Symptomatic Measures. MUSCULAR HYPERTONICITY. The trismus and increased muscle tone of the mild case of tetanus can usually be controlled adequately with small doses of diazepam (10 mg every three to four hours orally or parenterally). Barbiturates and chlorpromazine have also been widely and effectively employed against these symptoms.

DYSPHAGIA AND AIRWAY MANAGEMENT. Trismus is a common early symptom in tetanus and is frequently accompanied by incoordination of the swallowing and laryngeal protective reflexes. Correct management of the airway is of vital importance, because laryngeal spasm may occur spontaneously or may be induced by attempts to swallow saliva or to pass a nasogastric tube. In addition, dysphagia may allow inhalation of infected material and saliva from the mouth so that atelectasis and pneumonia can follow; the latter remains a common cause of death in tetanus.

To minimize pulmonary complications, protection of the airway by intubation with a cuffed tube is advocated as soon as dysphagia is suspected. The symptom may be demonstrated as a tendency to cough and clear the throat after swallowing a mouthful of water, and, in more advanced form, as an inability to swallow saliva so that the patient drools or spits it out. Orotracheal intubation should be performed under general anesthesia and after muscle paralysis, allowing an elective tracheostomy with a cuffed tube. Meticulous pulmonary care should be instituted and maintained until normal pharyngolaryngeal function returns.

MUSCLE SPASMS. Muscle spasms in tetanus can be either localized or generalized and of varying severity. Sustained contraction of the muscles is exhausting, painful, and, if the respiratory muscles become involved, dangerous. When large doses of diazepam or chlorpromazine are employed in attempts to control severe spasms, oversedation may lead to hypoventilation between spasms. In this situation, and when muscle spasms themselves interfere with ventilation, therapeutic paralysis should be induced with curariform drugs and the resultant ventilatory failure treated with intermittent positive pressure ventilation (IPPV). Curare or pancuronium is given intramuscularly or intravenously and with sufficient frequency to allow IPPV to proceed freely and to keep the patient comfortable. This method of treatment has proved most satisfactory when used early in the disease rather than after prolonged attempts to manage the patient with sedative agents. Smythe et al. (1974) have reported remarkable success in neonates with similar techniques.

Once curarization and IPPV have commenced, anxiety in the conscious but paretic patient should be minimized by frequent reassurance from the nursing staff and by mild hypnosis from diazepam or a barbiturate. Some of the most severely affected patients, however, become unresponsive and appear comatose for periods of one to three weeks during the critical phase of their illness, and in this situation sedative agents and muscle relaxants should be administered only if clearly indicated. Such patients usually regain consciousness during the recovery phase and appear normal apart from amnesia. After one to four weeks of treatment, curare requirements decrease and diazepam may be reinstituted to reduce muscle stiffness during weaning from IPPV.

Nutrition. Patients with mild tetanus may be fed orally, but once dysphagia develops a nasogastric tube should be inserted while the patient is anesthetized for tracheostomy. The considerable caloric (2500 calories per day) and fluid requirements of the tetanus patient can be satisfied effectively over the two- to four-week period of dysphagia by nasogastric feeding. Paralytic ileus occurs fairly frequently in severe tetanus, but usually responds to intermittent gastric drainage followed by the instillation of antacids and gut stimulants (e.g., metoclopramide).

Fluid Balance. The maintenance of a balanced fluid status in the severely ill tetanus patient is complicated by the considerable insensible fluid losses produced by profuse sweating and by unswallowed saliva. If reliance is placed entirely upon measured fluid input and output, fluid losses may be seriously underestimated and dehydration may result.

Underhydration in an immobilized patient increases the possibility of deep venous thrombosis and of pulmonary embolism, and the latter remains a common cause of death in tetanus. Although anticoagulation, started 24 hours after tracheostomy and continued until remobilization, has been practiced without significant complication in several centers, protection against pulmonary embolism has not been complete, and avoidance of dehydration is equally important.

Insensible fluid losses are best monitored by weighing the patient each day, and dehydration is avoided by measuring the specific gravity (or osmolality) of the urine regularly. Enough fluid should be given parenterally or by nasogastric tube to produce a daily urine flow of 1.5 to 2 liters and to maintain the urine specific gravity below 1.015. Particular care must be taken to react promptly to the severe hypovolemia which may develop rapidly when overactivity of the sympathetic nervous system causes excessive sweating in association with gastrointestinal stasis.

Cardiovascular Disturbances. In some tetanus patients who show severe muscular symptoms, cardiovascular changes in the form of tachycardia, hypertension, and increased responses to therapeutic maneuvers, such as tracheal aspiration, may appear after two to five days of treatment by curarization and artificial ventilation. These changes have been controlled successfully with adrenergic blocking agents. To reduce the tachycardia resulting from the intense sympathetic stimulation of the heart, a beta-adrenergic blocking agent such as propranolol (10 mg every three to six hours via nasogastric tube) should be administered until the heart rate averages less than 100; if hypertension persists, an antihypertensive (e.g., labetalol,* 50 to 100 mg every two to six hours) should be added.

*Investigational drug in the United States.

Although other combinations of antiadrenergic agents might be more effective, short-acting drugs are preferred, because, particularly in drug addicts and in elderly patients, the pattern of autonomic disturbance may change very rapidly. In these groups of patients, episodes of profound hypotension and bradycardia may suddenly occur and, on occasion, lead to cardiac arrest. Provided that resuscitation is prompt, the cardiovascular status may be restored rapidly and repeatedly by measures such as tracheal aspiration and mildly painful stimuli

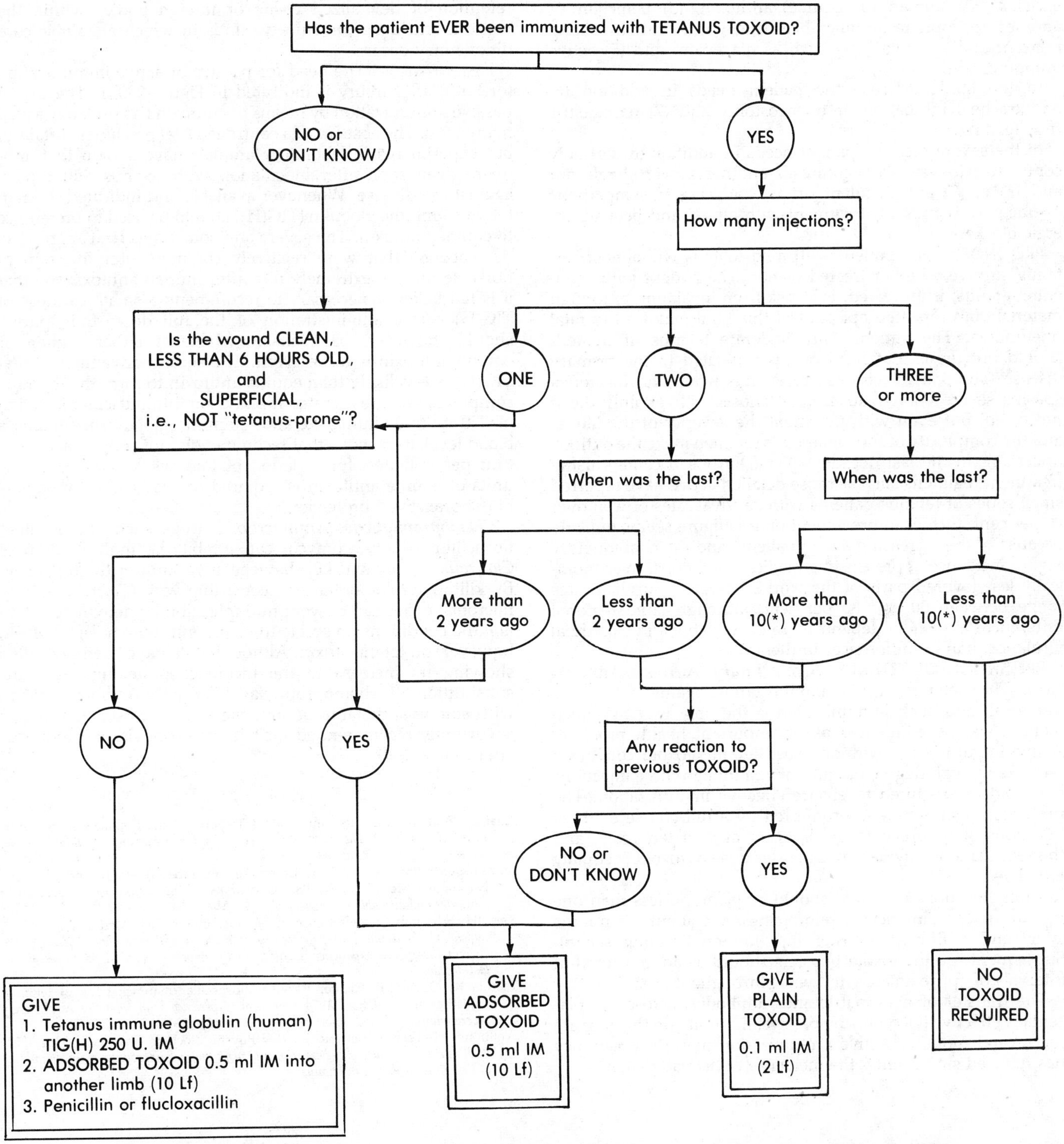

Figure 280–1. Tetanus prophylaxis for the injured patient. In addition, patients who have not received at least three previous injections of toxoid should be given further doses of adsorbed toxoid (0.5 ml IM) after six weeks and six months. The volumetric doses assume a toxoid concentration of 20 Lf per ml. (*) Five years if wound is "tetanus prone" or if patient is aged over 60 years.

which result in the release of endogenous catecholamines. These sudden and readily reversible episodes, during which the circulation appears unstimulated and dilated, must be contrasted with the unresponsive preterminal hypotension accompanied by tachycardia, vasoconstriction, and hyperpyrexia which has followed prolonged and unrelieved sympathetic overactivity. In view of the varying patterns of cardiovascular disturbance, continuous direct monitoring of heart rate and of arterial and central venous blood pressures has proved of much benefit in guiding therapy.

In summary, in a mild case the patient needs (1) wound excision, (2) human (or equine) antitoxin, (3) penicillin or another appropriate antimicrobial drug, (4) a centrally acting relaxant and sedative drug such as diazepam, and (5) active immunization.

In the moderate case the patient needs in addition (6) endotracheal intubation or tracheostomy and (7) nasogastric tube feeding.

In the severe case the patient needs in addition (8) virtually complete paralysis with curare or another powerful relaxant and IPPV, (9) anticoagulant drugs, and (10), if sympathetic overactivity is present, treatment with alpha- and beta-adrenergic blockers.

PROGNOSIS. The patient with mild tetanus will almost certainly survive whether treated or not. The patient with moderate tetanus, if untreated, is at risk from inhalation of foreign material, and repeated episodes of this kind may lead to fatal pneumonia. The patient with moderate tetanus, if treated, should not die except from causes unrelated to the primary disease. The patient with severe tetanus who is having reflex spasms severe enough to cause cyanosis will certainly die if untreated, but even with treatment the severity of the illness and the complexity of the therapeutic regimen make the outlook uncertain. In the last decade, several European centers using treatment regimens such as those detailed above have reported small series of tetanus patients with survival rates of well over 90 per cent; further improvement on this figure seems unlikely because of the increasing age of patients and the consequently higher incidence of pre-existing medical conditions. In economically less favored parts of the world, however, survival rates range between 30 and 80 per cent, although large regional differences appear to depend more on variations in clostridial virulence than on differences in therapy.

PREVENTION OF TETANUS. ***Before Injury.*** ACTIVE IMMUNIZATION. The need for active immunization against tetanus is universal, and such immunization is the only way by which tetanus will be eliminated as an important health problem. Active immunization with adsorbed tetanus toxoid conveys a remarkably high degree of immunity, although three injections of toxoid are required to ensure effective immunization. The protection against tetanus conferred by a full course of three injections of adsorbed toxoid lasts for at least ten years, and the reactivation provided by a booster dose of toxoid is equally long lived.

Three injections of toxoid should be given no less than one month apart in infancy, a reinforcing dose about 12 months later, and a fifth or booster injection on entering school. Subsequent routine toxoid boosters should be administered at intervals of approximately ten years throughout life.

The transfer of maternal tetanus antibodies across the placenta is effective in conferring passive immunity on the neonate for several months. Active immunization in early pregnancy has reduced significantly the incidence of neonatal tetanus.

After Injury. PREVENTION OF CONTAMINATION. Simple measures that prevent wound contamination can contribute significantly to the prevention of tetanus, as is shown by the effect of attention to treatment of the umbilical stump on the incidence of neonatal tetanus. The aim of surgery in prophylaxis is to remove all dead tissue and foreign bodies from a wound. This not only removes spore-bearing material but also denies the spores the anaerobic conditions necessary for their growth. Tetanus often occurs in patients in whom no wound is found, so that a precise definition of a "tetanus-prone" wound is difficult, although it is generally agreed that certain features increase the likelihood of tetanus. These features include an interval of more than six hours between injury and treatment, heavy contamination of the wound with soil or manure, the retention of devitalized tissue or foreign bodies within the wound, and deep puncture wounds in which anaerobic conditions may occur.

IMMUNIZATION. The need for passive or active immunization (or both) after injury is indicated in Figure 280–1. The use of passive immunization by means of antitoxin has probably saved many lives. The absence of a controlled trial precludes certainty, but experiments in laboratory animals have shown that antitoxin given soon after inoculation with tetanus will protect against the disease. Whenever available and indicated, human tetanus immune globulin (TIG(H)) should be used in preference to equine antitoxin. The severe and sometimes fatal anaphylactic reactions that were relatively common after injection of horse serum are extremely rare after human antitoxin, so that it is not believed necessary to recommend a small test dose of TIG(H) before administration of the full dose. Epinephrine should, however, be available whenever either human or equine antitoxin is to be given. The second advantage is that TIG(H) is less likely than equine antitoxin to form the immune complexes that are excreted rapidly. An intramuscular injection of 250 units of human tetanus immune globulin maintains a blood level at or above that recommended for prophylaxis (0.01 unit per milliliter) for a period of four weeks, whereas 1500 units of equine antitoxin is required to produce a comparable but shorter-lived protection.

Chemoprophylaxis. Antimicrobial drugs such as penicillin, floxacillin, or erythromycin can inhibit the multiplication of *Clostridium tetani* and kill the vegetative form of the organism. By killing aerobic organisms coexisting with *Clostridium,* antimicrobial drugs can prevent multiplication by denying *Clostridium* the conditions favorable to its growth; they have no effect, however, on tetanus toxin. Although data have been presented showing no increase in the incidence of tetanus after the substitution of chemoprophylaxis for passive immunization with equine antitetanus serum, the less toxic human antitoxin is currently recommended for tetanus prophylaxis if indicated after injury.

Adams EB, Laurence DR, Smith JWG: Tetanus. Oxford, Blackwell Scientific Publications, 1969. *The standard clinical text on the disease with a full bibliography up to the time of publication.*

Immunization Practices Advisory Committee: Diphtheria, tetanus and pertussis. NY State J Med 82:1563, 1982. *Current recommendations about immunization schedules and available materials.*

Kerr JH: Editorial: Current topics in tetanus. Intens Care Med 5:105, 1979. *A review which attempts to pull together the recent pathophysiologic findings and current therapeutic experience; includes all the important clinical references for the last decade.*

Tseuda K, Oliver PB, Richter RW: Cardiovascular manifestations of tetanus. Anesthesiology 40:588, 1974. *American experience with intensive care of very severe tetanus. Includes information about management in drug addiction.*

Wellhöner H: Tetanus neurotoxin. Rev Physiol Biochem Pharmacol 93:1, 1982. *Well-referenced review of the experimental work that has improved our understanding of the clinical changes in tetanus.*

281. DISEASES CAUSED BY NON-SPORE-FORMING ANAEROBIC BACTERIA

Sherwood L. Gorbach

DEFINITIONS. Anaerobic bacteria are the major constituents of the microflora that colonizes the gastrointestinal tract, upper respiratory tract, skin, and vagina. Under normal circumstances these organisms exist in a *commensal* (literal meaning "dining at the same table") relationship with their host. Anaerobic bacteria require reduced oxygen tension for growth; the more fastidious strains cannot survive exposure to atmospheric oxygen for more than five minutes. As a general rule, anaerobes associated with infectious processes are relatively aerotolerant. Teleologically, aerotolerance provides anaerobic bacteria with a survival advantage in mammalian tissues, since the extremely oxygen-sensitive forms perish almost immediately upon escape from their natural ecologic niche, while aerotolerant forms can establish a septic focus.

Regardless of the organ site, anaerobic infections have three characteristics in common. First, such infections are truly endogenous, since the pathogens originate from the normal flora of the host. Second, certain pathogenic conditions predispose to anaerobic infections by initiating spread of the normal flora beyond the confines of mucosal barriers. These inciting events also produce a low *oxidation-reduction potential* (Eh) in the tissues, thereby favoring the growth of anaerobic organisms. Compromised vascular supply, trauma, tissue destruction, and antecedent infections caused by aerobic bacteria or viruses that result in necrosis are among the situations that precede anaerobic infection. Third, the infecting flora is highly complex. Abdominal infections, for example, harbor an average of five different bacterial species, usually three anaerobes and two aerobic or facultative strains.

ANAEROBIC GRAM-NEGATIVE BACILLI. ***Bacteroides.*** *B. fragilis* is the preeminent anaerobic pathogen in humans. This distinction is based on its virulence, its ubiquity in various organ sites, and its resistance to many conventional antimicrobial drugs. The organism frequently produces abscesses and causes tissue destruction. The *B. fragilis* group has been divided into five distinct species, based on biochemical differences and DNA homology: *B. fragilis, B. distasonis, B. vulgatus, B. ovatus,* and *B. thetaiotaomicron.* Although these organisms are recognized pathogens, they all lack one of the prime virulence factors of other gram-negative organisms, endotoxin. While *Bacteroides* strains do possess a surface *lipopolysaccharide (LPS),* this substance differs in chemical composition from LPS of other gram-negative organisms. In addition, the *B. fragilis* LPS lacks the biologic activities of classic endotoxin, such as production of septic shock and vascular collapse in experimental animals. On the other hand, *B. fragilis* contains on its outer cell membrane a specific, large molecular weight capsule composed of polysaccharide. In a purified form the capsular material is highly antigenic, and it can produce abscesses when it is injected into experimental animals.

B. fragilis causes infections in the abdominal cavity that are associated with contamination by the intestinal flora. These organisms also are found in female pelvic infections and in mixed infections of skin and soft tissue such as decubitus ulcer, diabetic foot ulcer, and gangrene of the perineum.

The *Bacteroides melaninogenicus-asaccharolyticus* group is found in the normal flora and in association with various infections. The group has seven distinct species. The major distinguishing feature of *B. melaninogenicus* is the production of a brown-black pigment, formed in the colony after five to seven days of growth on blood agar. Many strains require blood and vitamin K or its analogues for growth. Young colonies of *B. melaninogenicus* show an intense red fluorescence under ultraviolet light even before the black pigment appears. This fluorescence can also be demonstrated in wounds infected by these organisms. Infections caused by *B. melaninogenicus* are most commonly found in the respiratory tract, head and neck region, and female pelvic area.

Fusobacterium. Several species comprise the genus, of which the major ones found in clinical specimens are *F. nucleatum* and *F. necrophorum.* In Gram-stained preparations, these organisms take up the strain poorly and appear as slender spear-shaped bacilli with parallel sides and tapered ends. The LPS of *F. nucleatum* causes septic shock and vascular collapse when injected intravenously into rabbits, in contrast to the material found in *B. fragilis,* which is biologically inactive in this model. *Fusobacterium spp.* are regular constituents of the normal flora of the oral cavity, gastrointestinal tract, and female genital tract. Among the infectious processes, these organisms are major causes of pleuropulmonary infections and various abscesses of the head and neck region. They are also responsible for bacteremia. The most common sites of origin are the female genital tract, orofacial region, and lower respiratory tract.

ANAEROBIC GRAM-POSITIVE COCCI. This diverse group of organisms ranks second in importance to *Bacteroides* in frequency of isolation from infected sites. The two genera are *Peptostreptococcus* and *Peptococcus.* (There are also gram-negative cocci known as *Veillonella,* which are only rarely involved as pathogens.) Peptostreptococci form long chains of cocci in culture. They produce gas and a foul odor in the test tube and in infected sites as well. Peptococci occur as irregular clumps of gram-positive cocci that resemble *Staphylococcus aureus* in morphologic appearance. These organisms are catalase positive and produce no odor.

Anaerobic gram-positive cocci are important components of the normal flora of humans. Within the oral cavity peptostreptococci represent a significant percentage of the anaerobic isolates in saliva and dental plaque. They are also among the leading components of the fecal flora and the vaginal flora. As pathogenic organisms these anaerobic cocci are found in virtually all sites where anaerobes have been identified. Approximately 50 per cent of such isolates in a clinical bacteriology laboratory are from surgical wounds, mostly associated with abdominal operations and hysterectomies. The gram-positive cocci are also found in skin and soft tissue infections and in blood cultures. About one third of anaerobic pleuropulmonary infections are associated with these gram-positive cocci. In the female genital tract they are probably the most important cause of salpingitis and are frequently isolated in cases of pelvic abscess.

GRAM-POSITIVE NON-SPORE-FORMING BACILLI. The two leading isolates are *Propionibacterium acnes* and various species of *Eubacterium. P. acnes* is the most frequent anaerobe found on normal skin. Many laboratories incorrectly identify it as a diphtheroid. This organism is commonly recovered from blood cultures, most often as a contaminant. It is also isolated from wound infections as part of a mixed flora. Although these organisms have little intrinsic pathogenicity, they are important causes of infection in patients with artificial heart valves, vascular grafts, orthopedic prostheses, or ventricular shunts. *Eubacterium* is isolated from wound infections, particularly in association with *Bacteroides.* As far as can be determined, *Eubacterium* plays no pathogenic role in the infective process. The basis for this statement is that eubacteria are virtually never isolated in pure culture from an abscess; they are rarely associated with bacteremia; and they have not been isolated, as a rule, after patients have failed to respond to antibiotic treatment.

PATHOGENESIS OF ANAEROBIC INFECTIONS. ***Unitarian Compared with Synergistic Infections.*** Our theoretical models of infections are based on concepts of microbial monoetiology. Pasteur established that certain microorganisms are responsible for a specific disease state. His theory was formalized by Robert

Koch in his famous postulates. Finally, Erhlich created the concept of a single drug, the "magic bullet," designed for a specific infection. Thus, the principal states: one microbe, one disease, one drug. This concept applies to classic infections such as typhoid fever, diphtheria, and cholera. However, the classic design does not fit most infections associated with anaerobic bacteria, since these processes harbor multiple strains of organisms with varying oxygen sensitivities and undefined pathogenic potentials. Anaerobic infections follow the model of bacterial synergy, in which several bacteria behave in a cooperative fashion to produce infection. In experimental model systems of mixed infection, various microbial components contribute virulence factors or growth substances that permit other more pathogenic forms to invade the tissues. A diphtheroid, for example, adds vitamin K to a septic process, which enables *B. melaninogenicus* to cause tissue necrosis. The growth of *B. melaninogenicus* is dependent on vitamin K supplied, in this instance, by a nonpathogenic partner. Most clinical anaerobic infections are mixed, containing several species of bacteria. Since it is not clear which are the primary pathogens and which are the symbionts and commensals, it is often necessary to treat all of the potential pathogens.

Virulence Factors. The microenvironment of an anaerobic abscess has features that insure its own survival. An abscess has an Eh of −250 mv, with an extremely low concentration of oxygen. Anaerobiosis is a hostile condition for host-defense mechanisms. Within this oxygen-free zone, neutrophils are unable to kill bacteria by their oxidative metabolic pathway. Low oxygen tension also inhibits the activity of aminoglycoside antibiotics, since they require an oxidative transport system to cross the bacterial cell envelope. The abscess itself contains a large concentration of microorganisms, approximately 10^8 to 10^9 per milliliter. A high inoculum and a relatively low growth rate are adverse conditions for the activity of beta-lactam antibiotics. Thus, host defenses and antibiotic interventions are hindered in an anaerobic abscess.

Individual anaerobic microorganisms possess virulence factors that promote their survival in the host's tissues. *B. fragilis* elaborates a polysaccharide capsule that provides protection against phagocytosis by neutrophils. These organisms also elaborate extracellular enzymes, such as lipases, proteases, nucleases, and heparinases, that contribute to the formation of abscess and necrosis. Membrane-associated enzymes are found in many virulent anaerobes, including beta-lactamases and superoxide dismutase (SOD). The beta-lactamases destroy antibiotics such as penicillin and cephalosporin. SOD, an enzyme present in virtually all pathogenic anaerobes studied thus far, seems to protect the organism in its initial exposure to oxygenated tissues.

Immunologic factors are affected by anaerobic bacteria. Several species of anaerobes are more resistant to phagocytosis than coliforms and other facultative organisms. Anaerobic bacteria can also interfere with phagocytosis of aerobes when both organisms are present in a mixed infection. For example, *B. fragilis* inhibits phagocytosis and killing of *Proteus mirabilis* in vitro, but the coliforms have no effect on phagocytosis of the anaerobes. *B. fragilis* appears to influence the alternate pathway of serum complement. Cell-mediated immunity also plays a role in anaerobic infections, at least in abscess formation by *B. fragilis*.

Role of Facultative Organisms. Facultative or aerobic organisms are frequent partners in anaerobic infections. In some settings these organisms seem to initiate the infective process, perhaps by promoting early tissue necrosis or by consuming oxygen in the tissues. In abdominal infections coliforms and *Bacteroides* are often isolated together.

An animal model of intra-abdominal infection has delineated the role of these pathogens in the septic process. Following intestinal perforation, the initial phase consists of peritonitis, bacteremia, and septic shock. This phase is caused, at least in the animal model, by coliforms such as *E. coli* and *Proteus*. The later occurrence of abscess formation, however, is associated with anaerobes, particularly *Bacteroides*. Antimicrobial drugs active only against coliforms suppress the initial septicemic and shock phase but have no effect on abscess formation. Similarly, antianaerobic drugs do not protect against coliform bacteremia, but they do suppress formation of abscess. The clinical picture is complex, with overlapping of the septic shock stage and the abscess stage. However, the therapeutic implications are clear: both components of abdominal sepsis should receive appropriate antimicrobial attention.

ANAEROBIC BACTERIA IN VARIOUS INFECTIONS. Aerobic and facultative microorganisms have been traditionally considered the major pathogens in infectious diseases. Recent improvements in laboratory techniques have facilitated the identification of anaerobic bacteria, and it has become clear that these oxygen-sensitive organisms share responsibility for a significant number of infections seen in clinical practice. Certain types of infection, such as those appearing in the abdomen, chest, female genital tract, and head and neck, characteristically are caused by anaerobes. Other infections such as lobar pneumonia, acute pharyngitis, and pyogenic meningitis are rarely associated with anaerobic bacteria.

Intra-abdominal Infections. Infections within the peritoneal cavity usually are related to contamination by the intestinal flora. The microflora of the upper intestine, from the stomach to the upper ileum, consists of sparse numbers of facultative gram-positive organisms derived from the oropharynx. Relatively few coliforms and obligate anaerobes are encountered. The lower bowel, on the other hand, harbors a luxuriant flora in which anaerobes outnumber facultative organisms such as coliforms by a factor of 1000 to 1. Hence, injuries to the upper intestinal tract, such as perforated ulcer or trauma, result in a small inoculum of microorganisms and a low risk of infection. But colonic perforations release a large inoculum of bacteria, causing a high rate of infection.

Peritonitis and intra-abdominal abscess are associated with anaerobic bacteria in 95 per cent of cases. The most frequent finding is a mixture of aerobes and anaerobes. (Infection by a single facultative organism such as *E. coli* is uncommon and usually is seen in *primary peritonitis* associated with cirrhosis of the liver.) In a large series of intra-abdominal infections, an average of five different organisms were isolated from each patient, including three types of anaerobes and two aerobes. Of the anaerobes, *Bacteroides*, *Clostridium*, anaerobic cocci, and *Fusobacterium* are the major pathogens. The specific site of infection does not determine the flora, since the same pathogens are found in peritonitis, appendicitis, subphrenic abscess, and diverticular abscess.

Anaerobic Pleuropulmonary Infections. Anaerobic infections of the lower respiratory tract produce four clinical conditions: *aspiration pneumonia, lung abscess, necrotizing pneumonia,* and *empyema*. The pathogenesis of these conditions is aspiration of oropharyngeal contents, a situation associated with compromised state of consciousness, obstruction of the esophagus, and neurologic deficits. The oral flora is permitted admission to normally sterile regions of the lower respiratory tract. Approximately 90 per cent of patients with aspiration pneumonia have anaerobes as the major infecting flora. The situation applies to patients who have aspirated outside the hospital or shortly after admission, since they harbor normal oral flora. When the aspiration event occurs after hospitalization or after treatment with antibiotics, at which time the oral flora becomes colonized by gram-negative facultative organisms, the aspirated flora assumes a different character. Coliforms and *Pseudomonas* account for most cases of hospital-acquired aspiration pneumonia. Lung abscess is associated with anaerobic bacteria in over 90 per cent of cases. The aerobes that occasionally cause a solitary lung abscess include *Klebsiella* and *S. aureus*. Necrotizing pneumonia is actually an earlier stage of lung abscess in which a specific segment or lobe of the lung is extensively damaged with multiple small abscesses. In the more advanced stage these abscesses coalesce to form a single large cavity, leaving in its wake a large area of destroyed lung. Necrotizing pneumonia is a more aggressive condition than lung abscess, with higher mortality. Anaerobes are responsible for the vast majority of cases. Empyema is an infection usually associated with underlying pneumonitis or lung abscess. Nearly 75 per cent of the cases of empyema are associated with anaerobes, most frequently in patients with chronic infection. The remaining cases are caused by the classic aerobic pathogens such as staphylococci, group A streptococci, and pneumococci; these organisms produce an acute onset and a more virulent course. Formerly, most cases of empyema were caused by these aerobic gram-positive organisms, but the situation has been reversed with the advent of antimicrobial agents.

Anaerobic pleuropulmonary infections involve multiple bacterial species including *B. melaninogenicus*, *F. nucleatum*, and anaerobic gram-positive cocci. *B. fragilis* is found in 15 per cent of cases. The fact that these organisms are found in the same relative concentrations in the various clinical cases suggests that the inoculum of oral contents is similar in each setting. Corroboration for this hypothesis is provided by animal studies in which a spectrum of pulmonary infection is produced by the same inoculum of mixed bacteria derived from gingival scrapings.

Obstetric and Gynecologic Infections. The source of infections of the female upper genital tract is the vaginal flora, which has aerobic and anaerobic bacteria as normal constituents. The clinical conditions in which anaerobes are frequently encountered include tubo-ovarian abscess, pelvic abscess, septic abortion, endomyometritis, and postoperative wound infection (following hysterectomy). Polymicrobic bacteremia is a frequent occurrence in patients with severe pelvic infections. One important difference between pelvic abscesses derived from the female genital tract and those in the abdomen is that pure anaerobic infections—those without coliforms or other facultative forms—occur with a higher frequency in the pelvic location. The major anaerobic pathogens are *Bacteroides* (*B. fragilis*, as well as *B. bivius* and *B. disiens*), gram-positive cocci (especially *Peptostreptococcus*), *Fusobacterium*, and *Clostridium*. Pelvic inflammatory disease, also known as salpingitis, is a milder condition that is caused by an array of organisms, including gonococci, *Chlamydia*, and anaerobes, particularly *Peptostreptococcus*.

Head and Neck Infections. Since the anaerobic bacteria in the normal flora of the upper airways have limited invasive properties, they require an antecedent event that permits their movement into deeper structures. Dental manipulation, trauma, prior bacterial or viral infections, and operative interventions can provide the initiating circumstance. Necrotizing infections of the gingiva are usually associated with *B. melaninogenicus*, as well as other anaerobes. This organism is also present in endodontal infections. Spirochetes have been found at the advancing border of inflammation in histologic sections of acute ulcerative gingivitis, noma, and lung abscess. Since these organisms cannot be grown in subculture, their role in pathogenesis cannot be assessed. In patients with *sinusitis*, anaerobes are recovered from 50 per cent of patients with chronic processes. However, acute or subacute sinusitis, lasting three months or less, is rarely associated with anaerobes. *Otitis media* may be either acute or chronic. As in sinusitis, anaerobes may be present in the chronic forms but are rarely present in the more acute cases. *Space infections*, occurring in the potential spaces formed by fascial planes of the head and neck, are usually associated with three types of organisms: either *S. aureus*, *Streptococcus pyogenes*, or anaerobic bacteria. The first two organisms occur in space infections related to overlying skin processes such as boils or impetigo. Anaerobes are associated with space infections that arise from diseases of the mucous membrane, dental manipulations, or in those cases that occur spontaneously. *Ludwig's angina* is an example of a space infection associated with anaerobes.

Of the central nervous system infections, *brain abscess* is the one most frequently associated with anaerobic bacteria. These organisms are isolated from 85 per cent of suppurative brain abscesses unrelated to trauma or operative procedures. Gram-positive cocci, followed in frequency by *Fusobacterium* and *Bacteroides*, are the most common strains, often in association with facultative streptococci and coliforms. *Subdural empyema* may also be caused by anaerobes, particularly when it occurs in association with a parameningeal focus in an ear or nasal sinus. Classic pyogenic meningitis, however, is rarely caused by anaerobes.

Skin, Bone, and Soft Tissue Infections. The predisposing factors in anaerobic skin and soft tissue infections are trauma, ischemia, and surgery. The organisms often derive from the fecal or oral flora, particularly in wounds associated with intestinal surgery, decubitus ulcer, and human bites. The clinical presentations are *crepitant cellulitis*, *synergistic gangrene* or *cellulitis*, and *necrotizing fasciitis*. Anaerobes are also regularly encountered in *diabetic foot ulcers;* 75 per cent of such lesions are associated with *Bacteroides*, anaerobic cocci, and *Clostridium*, usually in mixed culture. Anaerobic *osteomyelitis* is associated with trauma or prior surgery, although some cases arise from hematogenous spread.

CLUES TO PRESUMPTIVE DIAGNOSIS OF ANAEROBIC INFECTION. Clinicians should be able to suspect the diagnosis of an anaerobic infection before the bacteriologic results are available. Such decisions are based on certain features that should suggest the presence of anaerobes in an infectious process. (1) Any infection that is contiguous or in proximity to a mucosal surface normally harboring an anaerobic flora—the gastrointestinal tract, female genital tract, and oropharynx—could potentially include anaerobes as part of the infecting flora. (2) A foul-smelling discharge is pathognomonic evidence of anaerobic infection, since the odor is caused by metabolism of these organisms. The absence of odor, however, is not helpful, because 50 per cent of anaerobic infections lack the characteristic odor. (3) The presence of severe tissue necrosis, abscess formation, fasciitis, or gangrene raises the possibility of the presence of anaerobes. (4) Gas in the tissue is highly suggestive, although not absolutely diagnostic, of anaerobic organisms. (5) A mixed infection, indicated by a Gram stain of exudate showing a polymorphic array of organisms, strongly suggests anaerobic involvement. Certain anaerobes have a characteristic appearance under the microscope, especially *Clostridium*, *Fusobacterium*, *Actinomyces*, and certain strains of *Bacteroides*. (6) The failure to recover organisms by conventional aerobic culture in the presence of clinical infection suggests that more fastidious bacteria, such as anaerobes, are present. (7) Failure to respond to antibiotics that have poor anaerobic activity, such as aminoglycosides and certain penicillins and cephalosporins, provides another clue that anaerobes may be part of the infecting flora.

TREATMENT STRATEGIES FOR ANAEROBIC INFECTIONS. Successful therapy for anaerobic infections involves rational antibiotic selection in conjunction with judicious surgical resection and drainage. The operative approach may be ultimately decisive, but it should be emphasized that surgical intervention alone may be inadequate. Anaerobic infection can continue to simmer with intermittent sepsis and insidious extension of the process unless appropriate antimicrobial agents are employed. Selection of initial antibiotic therapy should be based on knowledge of the pathogens likely to be present in a specific clinical setting. Because many anaerobic infections tend to be mixed with coliforms and other facultative organisms, it is advisable to use antimicrobial drugs active against both components. With regard to the anaerobic components, important differences are seen in infections above and below the diaphragm. Anaerobic infections above the diaphragm, including those in the central nervous system, head and neck region, and pleuropulmonary area, tend to involve organisms sensitive to penicillin. This observation is not invariably true, since certain organisms, especially *B. melaninogenicus*, can elaborate beta-lactamases, which inactivate penicillins and cephalosporins. Anaerobic infections below the diaphragm, such as those in the abdominal cavity and female genital tract, commonly involve *B. fragilis* as a major pathogen. Since this organism is commonly resistant to several antimicrobial agents, infections in these sites require special consideration for choice of antimicrobial drugs.

TREATMENT. The range of choice among antimicrobial drugs is somewhat limited with regard to anaerobic bacteria in general and even more so with *B. fragilis.* A United States survey of antibiotic susceptibility among strains of *B. fragilis* from nine medical centers was conducted during 1981. Among the 750 isolates, cefoxitin was the most active beta-lactam antibiotic with resistance rates running from 3 to 17 per cent in various centers. Piperacillin and moxalactam were the next most active beta-lactam antibiotics. Since high blood levels can be achieved with these drugs, they can be used to treat clinical infections caused by this organism. Piperacillin showed the best activity, second only to cefoxitin. Disappointing results were seen with penicillin, carbenicillin, ticarcillin, cephalothin, cefamandole, and certain third generation cephalosporins such as cefotaxime and cefoperazone. The drugs in this grouping are not considered good choices for infections associated with *B. fragilis.* Clostridia, fusobacteria, and gram-positive cocci are usually sensitive to several drugs, including penicillins, cephalosporins, clindamycin, and metronidazole.

The explanation for variations in activity of the beta-lactam drugs against anaerobes is the presence in certain strains of constitutive beta-lactamases. This enzyme is found in most strains of *B. fragilis* isolated from clinical sources. It is also found in 20 to 40 per cent of strains of *B. melaninogenicus* and in occasional strains of *Fusobacterium.* The increased activity of cefoxitin and moxalactam against *B. fragilis* is based on their apparent resistance to hydrolysis by beta-lactamase elaborated by anaerobic organisms.

Metronidazole, a bacteriocidal drug, has excellent activity against *Bacteroides, Fusobacterium, Clostridium,* and most strains of anaerobic cocci. Resistance to metronidazole among *Bacteroides* is extremely rare. Since the drug has a spectrum limited almost exclusively to anaerobes, another agent such as an aminoglycoside should be included for facultative organisms. In clinical trials metronidazole has produced excellent results in intra-abdominal infections, female pelvic infections, brain abscess, and anaerobic osteomyelitis. Many failures, however, have been noted in anaerobic pleuropulmonary infections. Such failures are probably related to the relatively poor activity against microaerophilic organisms that may accompany this infectious process.

Clindamycin is highly active against most anaerobic isolates with resistance rates among *Bacteroides* running at about 5 per cent. Some resistant isolates of *Clostridium* and *Fusobacterium* have been encountered, but they have been relatively uncommon in clinical practice. The drug is also active against streptococci, both aerobic and anaerobic, and most strains of *S. aureus.* It has very little activity against coliforms and other facultative gram-negative organisms, so a second drug is used in mixed anaerobic infections. Clindamycin has produced excellent results in intra-abdominal infections, female pelvic infections, and skin and soft tissue infections. Some authorities consider it the drug of choice for anaerobic pleuropulmonary infections, preferring it to penicillin because of apparent failures associated with penicillin treatment; however, this issue remains controversial. Erythromycin is less active than clindamycin, although resistance patterns commonly overlap. The problem with erythromycin is the difficulty in administering it parenterally. By the oral route only low serum levels of erythromycin are obtained, often below the amount needed to inhibit many anaerobic bacteria.

Tetracyclines were once touted as drugs of choice for anaerobic infections, but recently their performance against *Bacteroides* and many gram-negative cocci has considerably altered this view. Widespread tetracycline resistance has been noted in recent surveys. As a result, this class of compounds is not recommended for treatment of anaerobic infections. Chloramphenicol shows excellent activity in vitro against *Bacteroides* and most other anaerobic pathogens. It also has activity against coliforms, staphylococci, and streptococci. While some clinical trials have shown good results with chloramphenicol, others have encountered therapeutic failures. In addition, animal models of anaerobic infection have shown poor results with chloramphenicol treatment. Anaerobic organisms can inactivate chloramphenicol by at least two mechanisms, acetylation and nitroreduction. It is possible that one or both of these mechanisms is responsible for the occasional clinical failures with this drug.

Aminoglycoside antibiotics are uniformly inactive against nearly all anaerobic bacteria. These drugs are included in antimicrobial regimens for therapy of mixed infections, although their role is clearly to suppress the facultative gram-negative components.

PROGNOSIS. Prognosis of anaerobic infections is related to the site of infection, the type of pathogen, the underlying condition of the patient, and the choice of antimicrobial therapy. In general, anaerobic pleuropulmonary infections have a good outcome, especially when adequate drainage can be achieved. Penicillin G has been successful in treating these infections in the past, curing up to 95 per cent of patients with aspiration pneumonia or lung abscess, for example. Recently, some failures have been noted with penicillin, and in such instances clindamycin has been used to advantage. Metronidazole treatment has been associated with failures in lung abscess. In certain series poor outcomes are noted in 25 to 50 per cent of treated patients.

Severe intra-abdominal infections have a failure rate of 10 to 20 per cent even with optimal surgery and antimicrobial therapy. Higher failure rates in controlled clinical trials have been associated with treatment regimens using antimicrobial agents with poor activity against *B. fragilis* such as cephalothin, doxycycline, cefamandole, and cefoperazone. Infections of the female genital tract generally have a good prognosis since most patients tend to be rather healthy prior to the onset of the septic process. Good results have been reported with cefoxitin, clindamycin, and metronidazole, usually in association with another antibiotic. In one clinical trial penicillin combined with gentamicin produced a poor result in endomyometritis when compared with the alternative regimen of clindamycin and gentamicin.

In general, clinical trials with new antimicrobial agents have corroborated the findings in animal models and susceptibility testing in vitro. Because of the vast array of anaerobic organisms and their varying patterns of susceptibility, it is best to base empiric therapy on known sensitivity patterns and performance of the specific drugs in controlled clinical trials.

Bartlett JG, Finegold SM: Anaerobic infections of the lung and pleural space. Am Rev Respir Dis 110:56, 1974. *A comprehensive review of anaerobic pleuropulmonary infections, based on the authors' extensive personal experience.*

Bartlett JG, Louie TJ, Gorbach SL, Onderdonk AB: Therapeutic efficacy of 29 antimicrobial regimens in experimental intra-abdominal sepsis. Rev Infect Dis 3:535, 1981. *An experimental model of intra-abdominal infections that explains the pathophysiologic events and the rationale for antimicrobial treatments.*

Finegold SM: Anaerobic Bacteria in Human Disease. New York, Academic Press, 1977. *A compendium of information on various anaerobic bacteria and their disease manifestations.*

Gorbach SL, Bartlett JG: Medical progress: Anaerobic infections. N Engl J Med 290:1177, 1974. *The clinical and microbiologic features of anaerobic infections in many organ sites.*

Kasper DL, Weintraub A, Lindberg AA, Lonngren J: Capsular polysaccharides and lipopolysaccharides from two *Bacteroides fragilis* reference strains: Chemical and immunochemical characterization. J Bacteriol 153:991, 1983. *The chemical structure of the capsular polysaccharide, an important virulence factor of the preeminent pathogen,* Bacteroides fragilis. *This is not an article for the casual reader.*

Sweet RL: Anaerobic infections in the female genital tract. Am J Obstet Gynecol 122:891, 1975. *Good bacteriology and careful collection techniques provide the basis for this important study.*

Tally FP, Cuchural G, Jacobus NV, Gorbach SL, Aldridge KE, Cleary TJ, Finegold SM, Hill GB, Iannini PB, McCloskey RV, O'Keefe JP, Pierson CL: Susceptibility of the *Bacteroides fragilis* group in the United States in 1981. Antimicrob Agents Chemother 23:536, 1983. *A nationwide survey of antimicrobial sensitivities in this important pathogen.*

Typhoid Fever and Salmonellosis

282. TYPHOID FEVER

Sherwood L. Gorbach

Typhoid ("cloudy") fever is a febrile illness of prolonged duration marked by hectic fever, delirium, enlargement of the spleen, abdominal pain, and a variety of systemic manifestations. Although caused primarily by *Salmonella typhi*, typhoidal disease occasionally is produced by other types of salmonellae. The portal of entry is the gastrointestinal tract, but typhoid fever is not truly an intestinal disease, having more systemic symptoms than those related to the bowel. There is a mortality of 1 to 5 per cent in drug-treated patients; the causes of death are intestinal perforation, hemorrhage, and severe toxemia.

EPIDEMIOLOGY. Improvements in environmental sanitation have reduced the incidence of typhoid fever in the industrialized nations. Approximately 500 cases occur each year in the United States, chiefly in young people. Most cases are sporadic, but are invariably related to a human carrier. The organism is essentially confined to humans, either in a disease state or as a carrier. Large-scale epidemics of typhoid occur on a regular basis, usually traced to contaminated food, which may be imported from an endemic area, or to contaminated water supplies. Another source of infection is the clinical bacteriology laboratory. Laboratory workers account for 2 to 5 per cent of typhoid cases each year.

Typhoid bacillus is a classic food- and waterborne pathogen. The major routes of passage are by the five F's: flies, fingers, food, feces, and fomites. *S. typhi* is extremely hardy and can survive for extended periods in polluted waters, contaminated foods, and soiled bedclothes.

Since *S. typhi* cohabits exclusively with man, the occurrence of a single case means the presence of a carrier. An investigation by public health authorities should be instituted to determine the source and the presence of other cases. Chronic carriers, as they are discovered, are registered with the health authorities. However, registered carriers represent only a minority of the potential reservoir and do not take account of the "imported" cases of typhoid, which include nearly half of the acute infections in the United States.

PATHOGENESIS AND PATHOLOGY. The pathologic events of typhoid fever are initiated in the intestinal tract following oral ingestion of typhoid bacilli. The organism penetrates the small bowel mucosa, sparing the stomach, and makes its way rapidly to the lymphatics, the mesenteric nodes, and, within minutes, to the bloodstream. There is a paucity of local inflammatory findings, which explains the lack of intestinal symptoms at this stage. This sequence of events is in marked contrast to that of other forms of salmonellosis and to shigellosis in which the intestinal findings are prominent at the onset.

The organism must survive passage through the stomach, warding off the destructive action of gastric acid. Food and beverages, the classic vehicles of typhoid fever, also serve as an excellent buffer to acid. The number of bacilli ingested is a critical determinant of infection. An inoculum of 10^9 bacilli produces disease in 95 per cent of apparently healthy people, whereas 10^3 organisms rarely cause symptoms. The higher the inoculum size, the shorter the incubation period.

Following the initial bacteremia, the organism is sequestered in macrophages and monocytic cells of the reticuloendothelial system. It undergoes multiplication, and re-emerges several days later in recurrent waves of bacteremia, an event which initiates the symptomatic phase of infection. Now in great numbers, the organism is spread throughout the host, infecting many organ sites. The intestinal tract may be seeded by direct bacteremic spread, as, for example, to Peyer's patches in the terminal ileum. Alternatively, the gallbladder contains a large number of bacilli, and contaminated bile is another method of infecting the gut.

Hyperplasia of the reticuloendothelial system, including lymph nodes, liver, and spleen, is characteristic of typhoid fever. The liver contains discrete, micronodular areas of necrosis, surrounded by macrophages and lymphocytes. Inflammation of the gallbladder is common, and may lead to acute cholecystitis. Patients with pre-existing gallbladder disease have a penchant for becoming carriers, because the bacillus becomes intimately associated with the chronic infection and may be incorporated within the gallstones themselves. Lymphoid follicles in the gut, such as Peyer's patches, become hyperplastic, with infiltration of macrophages, lymphocytes, and red blood cells. Subsequently, a follicle may ulcerate and penetrate through the submucosa to the intestinal lumen, discharging in its wake large numbers of typhoid bacilli. As the bowel wall is progressively involved, it becomes paper-thin, and is susceptible to transmural perforation into the peritoneal cavity. This occurs most commonly in the distal ileum, 25 cm from the ileocecal sphincter. Erosion into blood vessels produces severe intestinal hemorrhage.

An analogy has been drawn between the biologic effects of endotoxin and typhoid fever. Both cause chills, fever, headache, nausea, and vomiting, as well as the laboratory findings of leukopenia and thrombocytopenia. With endotoxin, however, increasing doses produce a state of tolerance in which further administration has no effect. By contrast, typhoid fever is a relentless and sustained state of illness. Administration of viable typhoid organisms to volunteers rendered tolerant to endotoxin still produces symptoms. Thus typhoid fever cannot be explained merely as a reaction to endotoxin, although this material may play some role in the disease state.

CLINICAL MANIFESTATIONS. Typhoid fever lasts about four weeks, evolving in a manner consistent with the pathophysiologic events. Classically, the illness is described as a series of one-week stages. Although in general the illness follows such a pattern, individual cases may deviate significantly, and the illness may persist (with accompanying bacteremia) with only slight improvement for four weeks or more. The *incubation period* is generally 7 to 14 days, with wide variations on either extreme. During the *first week,* the triad of fever, headache, and abdominal pain is commonly encountered. The onset usually is insidious with a stepladder rise of fever which later becomes persistent. It is accompanied by a dull headache. The pulse is often slower than would be expected for the degree of temperature elevation. Abdominal pain is localized to the right lower quadrant in most instances, although it can be diffuse. In approximately 50 per cent of patients, there is no change in bowel habits; in fact, constipation is more common than diarrhea in children. Near the end of the first week, enlargement of the spleen is noticeable. An evanescent and classic rash, "rose spots," becomes manifest at this time. It is observed in approximately 70 per cent of whites, but considerably less frequently in dark-skinned persons. Rose spots are deeply red, 2- to 4-mm macules, often present in clusters, blanching on pressure; they occur most often on the upper anterior abdominal wall and lower thorax. During the *second week,* the fever becomes more continuous. The patient looks sick and withdrawn, although he may be fully responsive. In some, marked deterioration in the mental condition, lassitude, delirium, and even coma may develop. Cough is commonly present and epistaxis is not infrequent. During the *third week,* the patient's illness continues in the "typhoidal state." There may be disoriented mentation and, in some cases, extreme toxemia. In this period there may be intestinal involvement, manifested clinically by greenish "pea-soup" diarrhea and the dire complications of intestinal perforation and hemorrhage. The *fourth week* usually but not invariably brings slackening of the fever and improvement in clinical status. The patient becomes more interested in the surroundings. There is significant weight loss, anemia, and profound fatigue. Typhoid fever is among the longest and most debilitating of microbial diseases.

Typhoid fever is a less severe illness in previously healthy persons who seek medical attention for the earliest symptoms of fever, lassitude, and headache. Prompt diagnosis and appropriate therapy interrupt the classic four-week scenario, producing an aborted illness consisting of little more than a few days of fever and malaise. Such patients should receive 14 days of antimicrobial therapy, but early discharge from the hospital can be considered, with the completion of drug treatment accomplished on an outpatient basis.

COMPLICATIONS. Since the typhoid bacillus is widely disseminated through recurrent waves of bacteremia, many organ sites are involved. Pneumonia occurs in 10 per cent of patients, although cough, without radiographic findings, is encountered in approximately two thirds. Rarely there is a small pleural effusion. During the severe toxemic phase, patients may aspirate gastric contents and develop a suppurative pneumonia. Severe headache, delirium, and even coma are often noted, but suppurative disease of the brain and meninges is quite uncommon, being seen in less than 1 per cent of patients. Typhoid pyelonephritis associated with renal pain, hematuria, and pyuria is occasionally encountered. The gallbladder and liver are often involved with inflammatory changes. Acute cholecystitis can occur during the initial period of typhoid fever. Jaundice, on the basis of diffuse hepatic inflammation, has been observed in some patients. The microorganism may spread to bone, especially ribs and spine, and to the large joints. Nerve deafness, conjunctivitis, keratitis, and optic neuritis have all been seen on rare occasions.

Although the litany of organ site involvement is long, the pre-eminent complications are intestinal hemorrhage and perforation. These events are most apt to occur in the third week and during convalescence and are not closely related to the severity of the disease. However, they tend to occur in the same patient, with the bleeding serving as a warning of a possible perforation to come. Bleeding may be sudden and severe, or a slow ooze. Prior to chemotherapy, the incidence of hemorrhage was 7 to 20 per cent in various series; it is somewhat less frequent since specific treatment has been available. The ileum is the main site of bowel perforation. The onset may be sudden with signs of acute abdominal distress. Or there may be a leak of intraluminal contents to form an abscess in the lower quadrant or pelvis, producing a more chronic, insidious course. Approximately 3 per cent of patients with typhoid fever will experience intestinal perforation.

RELAPSE. After defervescence has occurred and the patient has apparently "ridden through the storm," there remains a potential for recurrence. The relapse generally occurs eight to ten days after cessation of drug therapy and consists of a reenactment of the major manifestations such as fever, chills, skin rash, and bacteremia. Early chemotherapy of the initial infection may increase the potential for relapse because it prevents the development of natural immunity, an important feature in eventually controlling the organism within the host.

CARRIERS. After six weeks, approximately 50 per cent of typhoid victims are still shedding the organism in their feces. This figure progressively declines so that after three months only 5 to 10 per cent are excreters. A chronic carrier is defined as a person with stool cultures positive for *S. typhi* at least one year following an episode of typhoid or, in some cases, positive stool cultures without a documented history of disease. The possibility of spontaneously aborting the carrier state is very unlikely after this time. Chronic carriers are more common in older age groups, in women (a 3:1 ratio of women to men), and in people with gallbladder disease. The organism usually is harbored in the gallbladder, often forming part of gallstones, and persists in a noninflammatory symbiotic relationship with the host, causing neither local inflammation nor systemic symptoms. Occasionally, the gallbladder is free of the organism, and it is apparently carried in the large bowel. In the usual case, the bile contains enormous numbers of bacilli, up to 10^9 per milliliter, and they are discharged in the feces in varying concentrations. The organisms are viable and fully infective, so the carrier may be a source of new infection.

LABORATORY FINDINGS AND DIAGNOSIS. Many laboratory features of typhoid fever are consistent with prolonged sepsis. A normochromic, normocytic anemia persists throughout the infection; it may be made worse by intestinal blood loss or a reaction of the bone marrow to agents such as chloramphenicol. Thrombocytopenia occurs during the initial hectic period of the disease. Leukopenia is characteristic of the first week of illness, with the major depression in polymorphonuclear leukocytes.

The definitive diagnosis of typhoid fever is established by isolating the organism. During the first week, blood cultures are positive in 90 per cent of patients. If the clinical illness persists essentially unimproved, the bacteremia likewise persists, and the blood culture may be positive for several weeks or more. The blood culture thus is the primary diagnostic test. Stool cultures usually become positive in the second and third weeks when the organisms are shed from the lymphoid follicles of the intestinal wall. During the third week, urine culture yields typhoid bacilli in approximately 30 per cent of patients. Rose spots harbor the organism, and they can be sampled by small skin snips of the lesion that are cultured in nutrient broth. These are positive in two thirds of patients. A most useful source is the bone marrow, which is positive for *S. typhi* in 90 per cent of patients, even when they have received some antimicrobial therapy.

The titer of agglutinins (Widal test) against somatic (O) and flagellar (H) antigens rises during the third week of illness. An O titer of 1:80 or more in nonimmunized individuals is suggestive of typhoid fever. Higher initial titers or a four-fold rise provides stronger evidence. The H antigen is more nonspecific, and is likely to be elevated from prior immunization or infection by other enteric bacteria. There are many false-positive and occasional false-negative Widal reactions so that a diagnosis based on titer rises alone is tenuous.

DIFFERENTIAL DIAGNOSIS. In endemic regions the most perplexing diagnosis is between typhoid fever and malaria, because both diseases can cause fever, chills, splenomegaly, and neutropenia. Travelers to such areas may acquire either disease so that they present with the same diagnostic dilemma. Blood smears usually are positive in malaria, and typhoid is identified by isolating the organism in culture or, as an early clue, a positive Widal reaction. In certain parts of the world, Lassa fever or dengue is a diagnostic alternative. Other salmonellae can mimic typhoid fever. Among bacterial infections which may be confused with typhoid, tuberculosis, shigellosis, leptospirosis, and bacteremias associated with cholecystitis and pyelonephritis should be given consideration. Viral agents such as infectious mononucleosis and infectious hepatitis can present similar symptoms. Patients having delirium or coma with normal cerebrospinal fluid may be thought to have viral encephalitis rather than typhoid fever. Rickettsial diseases may be considered, but the absence of a characteristic rash would militate against this diagnosis.

TREATMENT. Drug resistance, mediated by plasmids, can occur among typhoid bacilli. Most strains are susceptible to chloramphenicol and ampicillin, although notable epidemics with strains resistant to either of these drugs have been reported in recent years. Hence, a great effort should be made in each case to isolate the organism and to perform drug susceptibility tests. Chloramphenicol remains the standard therapy because of its proved efficacy and its high activity against most clinical isolates of typhoid bacilli. The response to therapy is remarkably constant, as defervescence regularly occurs three to five days after initiating treatment. The clinical condition improves within one to two days, with decreased toxemia and slowly declining fever. In adults, chloramphenicol should be given in a total daily dose of 2 to 4 grams, administered in four equally divided doses. Occasionally in very sick patients it may be necessary to give the drug by the intravenous route, and the total daily dose of 2 to 4 grams should be used. Oral medication can then be given after improvement in the clinical status. Chloramphenicol is well absorbed from the intestinal tract, but is rather poorly absorbed from intramuscular sites. Thus the intramuscular route is to be avoided. The duration of treatment is two weeks; prolongation of this treatment does not reduce the incidence of complications or carriers. Intestinal perforation and hemorrhage can occur during what is apparently successful treatment. Relapse may follow an otherwise uneventful course and should be treated with the same drug.

Ampicillin has been recommended as alternative therapy, but it has been somewhat disappointing in comparison with chloramphenicol. The dose is 6 grams per day, intravenously, in four to six divided doses. Amoxicillin, a closely related drug, provides better absorption and increased efficacy. Several studies have shown that amoxicillin, in doses of 4 grams per day in four divided doses, has good activity, but is somewhat less effective than chloramphenicol. Sulfamethoxazole-trimethoprim has also been used effectively in the therapy of typhoid fever in a dose of 800 mg (sulfamethoxazole) and 160 mg (trimethoprim) twice daily for 14 days.

Corticosteroids are administered for severe toxemia and fever, and may produce a dramatic response in the patient with profound sepsis. The treatment should be given in high doses, 60 mg per day of prednisone divided in four doses, and rapidly tapered over the next three days. The wide experience with steroid treatment has failed to show any adverse effects, although the potentiality for masking intestinal perforation is still present. Thus steroids are best reserved for patients with severe toxicity.

Intestinal perforation is managed by standard surgical practices. All patients should be treated with nasogastric suction. Indications for operation are progressive peritoneal signs or localization of an abscess. Simple closure of the perforation is the treatment of choice. However, the ileum may be riddled with multiple perforations, and resection or exteriorization of the intestinal loop may be required.

Good nursing care plays a major role in the recovery from typhoid fever. The pyrexia can be managed with tepid baths and sponging. Salicylates and antipyretics should be used judiciously as they cause severe sweating and may lower the blood pressure.

A chronic carrier, who has been discharging *S. typhi* for longer than one year, can be treated with antimicrobials in an attempt to eliminate the infection. One regimen that works in approximately two thirds of patients is 6 grams of ampicillin per day in four divided doses for six weeks. Alternative drugs are amoxicillin and sulfamethoxazole-trimethoprim. Reappearance of the carrier state following such treatment is generally associated with gallbladder disease. In persons with gallstones or chronic cholecystitis, cholecystectomy eliminates the carrier state in 85 per cent. This procedure, however, is recommended only for those whose profession is not compatible with the typhoid carrier state, i.e., food handlers and health care providers.

PROGNOSIS. Prior to antimicrobial therapy, the case mortality of typhoid fever was around 10 to 15 per cent. The introduction of chloramphenicol has reduced this to 1 per cent, and most patients now succumb to either perforation or hemorrhage. However, in areas of the world with poor nutrition and limited medical facilities, the mortality rate may be higher. Factors that influence a lethal outcome are severity of the disease at time of admission (coma is a poor prognostic sign); age, with the very young and the very old being at greatest risk; and first infection, because a second attack, although uncommon, is less severe than the primary episode.

PROPHYLAXIS. For control of intrahospital spread, enteric precautions should be initiated; fecal, urine, and blood specimens should be disposed of by double-bag techniques and always handled with gloves. Additional precautions are unwarranted.

The currently available typhoid vaccine affords only 70 per cent protection and is associated with a high incidence of side effects, mostly at the site of injection. It is only recommended for high-risk situations and should not be given for short-term travel. Since the major forces of immunity act at the intestinal mucosal surface, an oral vaccine would offer theoretical advantages. A double mutant typhoid strain, Ty21a, lacking UDP-galactose-4-epimerase, has been developed by Professor Rene Germanier. This avirulent oral vaccine has undergone extensive field trials in Egypt and Chile. Not only has the vaccine been proven safe, it has shown a remarkable efficacy, 96 per cent, in preventing natural disease in an endemic area. A commercial product should be available sometime in the future.

Hoffman SL, Punjabi NH, Kumala S, Moechtar A, Pulungsih SP, Rivai AR, Rockhill RC, Woodward TE, Loedin AA: Reduction of mortality in chloramphenicol-treated typhoid fever by high dose dexamethasone. N Engl J Med 310:82, 1984. *In typhoid patients with delerium, obtundation, stupor, coma, or shock, dexamethasone therapy was highly efficacious.*

Hoffman TA, Ruiz CJ, Counts GW, Sachs JM, Nitskiu JL: Waterborne typhoid fever in Dade County, Florida: Clinical and therapeutic evaluation in 105 bacteremic patients. Am J Med 59:481, 1975. *Good account of an epidemic. The illness was generally mild. Chloramphenicol seemed to be superior to ampicillin for therapy.*

Hornick RB, Greisman SE, Woodward TE, DuPont HL, Dawkins AT, Snyder MJ: Typhoid fever: Pathogenesis and immunologic control. N Engl J Med 283:686, 739, 1970. *A good account of pathophysiology, including a discussion of the role of endotoxin. Human volunteer studies are reviewed.*

Johnson WD Jr, Hook EW, Lindsey E, Kaye D: Treatment of chronic typhoid carriers with ampicillin. Antimicrob Agents Chemother 3:439, 1973. *Using large doses of ampicillin orally, these authors cured ten chronic typhoid carriers.*

Kim J-P, Oh S-K, Jarret F: Management of ileal perforation due to typhoid fever. Ann Surg 181:88, 1975. *A life-threatening complication can be managed successfully by judicious surgical intervention.*

Pillay N, Adams EB, North-Coombes D: Comparative trial of amoxycillin and chloramphenicol in treatment of typhoid fever in adults. Lancet 2:333, 1975. *In a randomized clinical trial with 124 typhoid patients, chloramphenicol and amoxicillin performed equally well.*

Snyder MJ, Gonzalez O, Palomino C, Music SI, Hornick RB, Perroni J, Woodward WE, Gonzales C, Dupont HL, Woodward TE: Comparative efficacy of chloramphenicol, ampicillin, and co-trimoxazole in the treatment of typhoid fever. Lancet 2:1155, 1976. *Chloramphenicol was the superior agent for reduction of fever. Intravenous administration appears to be better than oral.*

Wahdan MH, Serie C, Cerisier Y, Sallam S, Germanier R: A controlled field trial of live *Salmonella typhi* strain Ty21a oral vaccine against typhoid: Three-year results. J Infect Dis 145:292, 1982. *An important vaccine, not only for excellent activity against an ancient enemy, typhoid fever, but also because this is the first oral bacterial vaccine.*

Wicks CB, Holmes GS, Davidson L: Endemic typhoid fever. Quart J Med 159:341, 1971. *Excellent compilation of clinical and laboratory findings in 265 patients with typhoid fever in Rhodesia.*

283. SALMONELLA INFECTIONS OTHER THAN TYPHOID FEVER

Richard B. Hornick

DEFINITION. Salmonellae comprise a large group of gram-negative bacilli that can cause a broad spectrum of disease in man and animals. The most common disorder in humans is gastroenteritis or salmonellosis, usually a mild, self-limited diarrheal illness. Systemic spread from the gut is unusual. Other patients may develop septicemia, a stubborn infection for the host to eradicate, even with antimicrobial therapy. Localized infections may present in the form of osteomyelitis, mycotic aneurysms, or abscesses. The unique human pathogen *S. typhi* produces enteric fever, an illness also caused by several other select *Salmonella* species. A prolonged carrier state which mimics that seen following infection with *S. typhi*, may result from *Salmonella* infections.

Many animals suffer fatal diarrheal disease caused by species of salmonellae that infect only animals. Some animals have an asymptomatic infection caused by strains that infect both humans and animals. Meat and eggs and other animal-derived food products serve as the most important source of infections in humans.

ETIOLOGY. Salmonellae are motile, gram-negative bacilli that do not ferment lactose or sucrose but metabolize glucose, maltose, and mannitol. They grow readily on many media.

Enrichment and transport media are useful for obtaining an increased yield from stool cultures, especially those collected as part of an epidemiologic survey.

Salmonellae contain a thick and complex lipopolysaccharide cell wall. This cell wall is the O antigen, made up of several specific O antigen types. The specificity of each of the O antigens is determined by the arrangement of the repeating sequence of sugars that constitute the outer layer of the cell wall. Strains lacking the outer layer are characterized as "rough" because of the wrinkled surface of the colonies. Such strains appear to be nonpathogenic. Antibodies directed at the R core protect against infections caused by many gram-negative bacilli. The inner or basal layer is the lipid moiety, a bridging structure between the outer two layers and the foundation of the cell wall. This whole substance is the endotoxin, the ubiquitous lipopolysaccharide material of all gram-negative bacilli that causes fever plus other severe host reactions during active disease.

There are at least 60 specific O-antigen complexes. Group-specific antibodies can be used to classify salmonellae into many serotypes. The H antigens are the flagellae of the organisms. Serotyping, using O and H antisera plus biochemical tests, has established the presence of at least 1700 species. A simplified characterization has been suggested based on host preferences and adaptations: (1) *Salmonella* serotypes highly adapted to man. These include *S. typhi, S. paratyphi A, S. schottmülleri* (paratyphi B), *S. hirschfeldii* (paratyphi C), and *S. sendai*. There is no animal reservoir for these strains, animal infection is rare, and accidental and human-to-human transmission is critical in the epidemiology of the disease they produce. (2) *Salmonella* serotypes highly adapted to specific nonhuman hosts. Most strains cause only illness in animals. *S. dublin* from cattle and *S. choleraesuis* from swine are two exceptions that often cause human disease. (3) *Salmonella* serotypes unadapted to specific hosts. This is a large group (>1400 strains), ubiquitous in nature, that usually causes gastroenteritis, rarely invades the bloodstream, and is responsible for about 85 per cent of all *Salmonella* infections in the United States. It is the strains within this last group that will be mainly discussed in this chapter. The most common serotypes involved in human disease are *S. typhimurium* (accounts for about 25 to 30 per cent of all cases), *S. enteritidis, S. heidelberg, S. newport, S. infantis, S. agona, S. montevideo, S. saint-paul,* and *S. javiana*. *Salmonella* infections are reportable diseases, and the ranking listed comes from the annual compilation published by the Centers for Disease Control.

EPIDEMIOLOGY. Humans ingest salmonellae primarily in contaminated food, less frequently in water, and in rare instances from exotic sources. Salmonellae can infect many species of animals. Those of greatest potential as a human health hazard are meat-producing animals and poultry. Eggs and egg products have been a consistent source of salmonellae. The organisms can be incorporated into the egg before the shell is completely calcified in the chicken, or the egg becomes contaminated during its expulsion from the chicken. Cracked or dirty eggs should raise a suspicion regarding contamination with salmonellae. An egg containing salmonellae requires at least three minutes of boiling to ensure complete bacterial killing. Poultry may become infected, have no significant disease, and yet be fecal shedders. During the processing of poultry, the carcasses may become surface contaminated from water baths or conveyer belts that were colonized by previously processed birds. Consumers handling such poultry products are at risk of infection. The organisms persist on the fingers for several hours and can be transferred to foods that can serve as culture media for further multiplication. The meat of animals usually does not contain abscesses, nor are the salmonellae isolated from mesenteric lymph nodes of meat-producing animals. Thus, most salmonellae are found on the surface of the meats and represent skin colonization from the contaminated surfaces of the processing plant. Raw milk is a persistent source of *S. dublin* for consumers. Up to 10 per cent of healthy cattle may carry this species.

Pet turtles have been an important source of salmonella infections in this country. Chickens and cattle can deposit ample salmonellae into the soil upon which the turtles feed. The legs of the common housefly can carry salmonellae, which they apparently acquire while feeding on feces. Transmission to human food is a possible but not a likely event. Carmine red dye, derived from female scale insects and larvae, has caused hospital epidemics of salmonellosis. The tainted dye was given to patients to determine intestinal transit time. Such dye has been used to color food, cosmetics, and drugs. Recently, an outbreak of salmonellosis occurred among teenagers and young adults using marijuana contaminated with *S. muenchen*, an organism isolated from poultry, swine, and cattle.

Human-to-human spread via contaminated food or water is the second most common means of transmitting salmonellae. Transient or convalescent carriers have frequently been the source of large foodborne outbreaks of gastroenteritis. Improper hand washing, inadequate refrigeration of prepared foods prior to serving, and insufficient cooking of poultry products have been common epidemiologic features of outbreaks occurring after large public feasts.

Most cases of salmonellosis occurring in healthy adults are of little medical significance. However, outbreaks in nursing homes or nurseries cause severe morbidity and unnecessary mortality. Epidemics may arise owing to contaminated hospital food; cross-infections have been documented in pediatric wards resulting from contaminated fingers or clothes of attending personnel or via aerosols from sick infants. A rare source of infection by *S. kottbus* has been infected breast milk. This unusual strain was being excreted by the donor of the milk. Faulty refrigeration allowed for multiplication of this species in the milk.

The most common form of illness produced is salmonellosis, a diarrheal disease. Children have the greatest incidence (median age, ten years), and the highest rate is in infants. In the United States, this disease occurs most frequently in the summer and early fall.

The epidemiologic characteristics of other strains causing systemic infection are also varied. *S. choleraesuis*, which is associated with swine and pork products, is an unusual isolate in the United States but is the predominant cause of localized or enteric fever syndromes. Children with this strain may develop a moderately severe form of enteric fever. Infected adults are more likely to present with bacteremia or localized infectious conditions such as abscesses in deep muscle groups, osteomyelitis, or mycotic aneurysms. This difference may be due to partial immunity developed in the adults and resulting from previous subclinical infections.

Enteric fever may be produced by *S. paratyphi A and B*. These are unusual infections in this country but are common in late-developing countries where typhoid fever is also prevalent. Patients with enteric fever induced by *S. paratyphi B* frequently respond less promptly to antibiotic treatment than do patients with typhoid fever.

PATHOLOGY. *Salmonella*-induced gastroenteritis causes death rarely. Infants and the aged are at the greatest risk. Death usually occurs as a result of the secondary effects of dehydration caused by the diarrhea. Intestinal mucosa is red and swollen and often shows petechial hemorrhages. Salmonellae induce a polymorphonuclear leukocyte infiltration in the lamina propria region. The organisms reach that area by penetrating through the epithelial cell layer. Those patients suffering from bacteremia or localized disease have collections of neutrophils in the areas of bacterial localizations. In contrast, *S. typhi* induces mononuclear cell responses in the liver or in the lamina propria and at sites of intestinal perforation. These differences in cellular responses may be due to small concentrations of endotoxin present at the sites of *S. typhi* multiplication.

PATHOGENESIS. Ingested salmonellae must penetrate through the epithelial cell layer in order to produce disease.

Stomach acid is an effective barrier to large inocula reaching the small and large intestine, where disease is initiated. Persons who are taking antacids, or who have achlorhydria because of drugs, marijuana use, surgery, or age, are at increased risk of acquiring salmonellae or other enteric pathogens. Passage through the stomach appears to be facilitated by ingestion of the bacilli in a small volume of fluid (50 ml or less). This small volume is not retained in the stomach. Nonspecific defense mechanisms in the small and large bowel such as rapid transit time, inactivation by enzymes or lysozymes, and nosocomial bacteria may decrease the number of bacteria able to penetrate through the epithelial cells.

Once the bacteria reach the lamina propria area, further penetration into the lymphatics or capillaries is impeded by the involved inflammatory response. Presumably the polymorphonuclear leukocytes effectively phagocytize and eliminate these salmonellae. Rarely does bacteremia occur in patients manifesting a diarrheal disease. Bacteremia is a more frequent event in children than in adults and may be due to a relatively incompetent immune system in the lamina propria.

The watery stools elicited by the ingestion of salmonellae probably originate in the upper small intestine, a section which has a great secretory capacity. An enterotoxin stimulates the secretion of electrolytes and fluid into the lumen. This process is similar to that associated with diarrhea induced by enterotoxigenic *E. coli.* No penetration occurs; the toxin is released on the surface of the cells and activates adenylate cyclase; secretion of chloride and sodium ions results. The inflammatory process associated with penetration in the ileum may cause diarrheal disease characterized by stools of smaller volume. These presumably result from the lesser capacity of the ileum to secrete fluid and perhaps from failure to absorb all the fluid presented to the inflamed ileum. The secretion in the ileum may be stimulated by the enterotoxins, by prostaglandins released from the inflammatory exudate, or by both. This latter mediator also activates the adenylate cyclase energy system. A smear of a small specimen of stool stained with methylene blue will reveal large numbers of neutrophils. These are indicative of involvement of the large bowel in the inflammatory process initiated by salmonellae.

The number of organisms necessary to induce gastroenteritis in man is largely unknown. Limited studies in volunteers have suggested that large doses of *S. typhimurium,* e.g., 10 million to 1 billion cells, are required to cause disease. Whether such large doses are involved in naturally occurring outbreaks is unknown. The incubation period falls within a relatively narrow range—12 to 24 hours. An inverse relationship between the size of the inoculum and the length of the incubation period probably exists, but evidence for this is lacking. The other members of the *Salmonella* genus that cause enteric fever or localized disease are ingested in the same fashion and presumably penetrate within a similar time frame, but symptoms and signs of disease do not appear for many days. During the incubation period, systemic spread is occurring and multiplication of the pathogens in the reticuloendothelial system and other organs proceeds until the spreading infection exceeds the defense mechanisms and disease is apparent. The short incubation period of salmonellosis suggests that this infection is superficial in the gut and causes disease through quick-acting substances such as enterotoxins. The self-limiting nature is consistent with rapid clearing mechanisms, e.g., short life span of the epithelial cells and efficient cellular clearing systems in the lamina propria.

Certain patients with chronic diseases are prone to *Salmonella* infections. There is a predilection for patients with sickle cell disease to develop septicemia or localized *Salmonella* infection. Osteomyelitis caused by one of the *Salmonella* strains is especially common. These patients are deficient in opsonizing capabilities, have reduced numbers of phagocytes in the spleen and elsewhere, and sustain bone and gut infarcts. Taken together, these changes can permit an easy access of salmonellae through the gut, an ability to survive in the circulation and to establish an infection in the bone. Patients with acute hemolytic processes caused by bartonellosis and malaria have an increased incidence of salmonellosis. Diseases that impair cellular immune mechanisms, e.g., leukemias and lymphomas, are associated with a high incidence of salmonellal septicemic infections. *S. typhimurium* has been one of the most frequently isolated strains from such patients. Patients with chronic *Schistosoma haematobium* infections of the genitourinary tract are prone to have chronic bacteriuria and bacteremia caused by *S. typhi* and *S. paratyphi* strains. Such patients may be chronic carriers, but also the associated obstruction of a ureter or calcification in the bladder contributes to the persistent *Salmonella* infection. Treatment of the schistosomiasis as well as the bacterial infection can be curative.

The pathogenesis of the chronic asymptomatic carrier state caused by salmonellae other than *S. typhi* is not clearly understood. A few persons will have chronic low grade infection in a diseased gallbladder identical to the typhoid carrier state. The paratyphi strains are involved in this manner. However, for those strains causing salmonellosis, carriage may persist for many months without evidence of biliary tract dysfunction. Some of those patients have received unnecessary antibiotic therapy for their diarrhea, and this can prolong the carrier state. In mice, the antibiotic eliminates part of the nosocomial flora that normally inhibits the colonization and multiplication of salmonellae. The mechanism involves the acid environment associated with the production of short chain fatty acids by the normal flora. This explanation, if applicable to the human situation, suggests that chronic carriage occurs primarily in the intestinal tract. Rarely will these patients shed salmonellae beyond eight months.

CLINICAL MANIFESTATIONS. ***Gastroenteritis.*** Gastroenteritis begins abruptly with nausea and crampy abdominal pain followed by the onset of diarrhea. The stools are watery, initially in large volume, and occasionally will contain mucus and a trace of blood. A smaller number of patients will have pastelike or semisolid stools that are associated with cramps in the lower quadrants. These stools are likely to contain mucus and blood, and white cells are seen on a methylene blue–stained specimen. Vomiting is not frequent and, if present, does not persist throughout the period of the diarrhea. Fever of 38.5 to 39° C is seen in 50 to 70 per cent of patients. Chills are noted in about 30 per cent of patients. Physical findings are few and relate to the inflammatory process in the gastrointestinal tract. Palpation tenderness resulting from contraction of loops of bowel is present but in variable locations of the abdominal cavity. Duration of symptoms in otherwise healthy adults is about two to five days. The disease persists for a longer period in patients debilitated by extremes of age, malignancy, or antibiotic or steroid therapy.

The symptoms and signs of enteric fever have been described for typhoid fever. An identical presentation is associated with disease produced by paratyphi strains.

Bacteremia. Patients with this form of salmonellal disease have a history of fever, chills, sweats, malaise, anorexia, and weight loss for several days to a week or more. Stool cultures may not reveal salmonellae, but blood cultures will be positive. A search for the source of bacteremia is mandatory but often unrewarding. Osteomyelitis, mycotic aneurysm or infection of a pre-existing aneurysm (abdominal aorta or femoral artery are common sites), pericarditis (minimal amount of exudate present), abscesses, arthritis, meningitis, pneumonia, and hepatitis are all representative of localized infections with bacteremia. Patients with solid tumors may have abscesses in these lesions that serve as a source of *Salmonella* bacteremia. Pheochromocytoma, ovarian cyst, renal cell carcinoma, uterine myomas and metastatic tumors to bone or skin are common examples of such tumors.

The isolation of *S. choleraesuis* from the blood of an adult is usually indicative of an abscess.

DIAGNOSIS. The diagnosis of any form of *Salmonella* infection is confirmed by isolation of the organism from blood or stool or both. Other isolations can be made from liver, abscesses, or localized infections when systemic disease is present. Fresh diarrheal stool specimens should be cultured. Serologic information is not helpful for salmonellosis but is useful for the systemic infections, especially enteric fever. About 65 to 70 per cent of patients with enteric fever will have a four-fold or greater increase in O and/or H antibody titers over a two- to three-week span.

Patients with gastroenteritis will have a normal white blood cell count. Hemoconcentration may occur with significant fluid loss. A smear of the diarrheal stool stained with methylene blue will often reveal numerous leukocytes, indicating colitis. Similar findings are noted with other bacteria that invade epithelial cells, e.g., *Shigella, Campylobacter, Yersinia.*

The differential diagnosis of *Salmonella* gastroenteritis includes a broad spectrum of enteric pathogens: enterotoxigenic *E. coli* (heat-stable and heat-labile toxins), *Campylobacter fetus subspecies jejuni, Vibrio parahaemolyticus, Shigella* species, *Yersinia enterocolitica,* and other bacteria associated with food-induced diarrhea. The diarrheal syndromes produced by these organisms can mimic that caused by salmonellae. Causation can be speculated on the basis of historical facts (seafood—*Vibrio parahaemolyticus;* refried rice—*B. cereus*), but confirmation requires cultural proof. Viral agents such as the parvoviruses and rotovirus can also cause the same illness; however, the highest attack rate is in infants and children. Isolation techniques for these viruses are not readily available. Unfortunately, most patients with infectious diarrhea have almost recovered from their illness when culture results are available. In certain patients, e.g., those with persistent diarrhea or those debilitated by other illness, specific cultural information is necessary to prescribe appropriate therapy. More rapid culture techniques are needed.

TREATMENT. Fluid replacement is the uniform approach to treatment of any patient with a diarrheal illness. It is especially critical in the management of patients who cannot readily tolerate a reduction in plasma volume. In most adults with salmonellosis, self-treatment with tolerated liquids is usually satisfactory. Fruit juices, broths, tea, and water are useful. Milk should be used with caution. In children an acquired lactase deficiency during the diarrhea is common, and milk can therefore prolong the diarrheal state because of the osmotic effect of undigested lactose. Intravenous fluids are necessary only for severely dehydrated patients unable to take oral replacement fluid because of nausea and vomiting.

Antibiotic treatment is not required to treat salmonellosis. Selected patients may benefit. Infants and elderly nursing-home patients who are known to be at greatest risk of mortality from this infection should be treated. A short course (three to five days) of ampicillin (4 to 6 grams per day) or amoxicillin (2 to 4 grams per day) may be used in adults. Sensitivity of the isolate to various antibiotics should be ascertained, since ampicillin-resistant strains are becoming increasingly common. Trimethoprim-sulfamethoxazole or chloramphenicol is an effective alternative. Antibiotic treatment will prolong the excretion of salmonellae in the stools and may not shorten the clinical course of the patient's illness. Adults usually recover without antibiotic therapy in two to five days.

The uncomfortable abdominal cramps may be relieved with atropine or drugs with a similar smooth muscle relaxing effect. However, such drugs have an antiperistaltic effect which can prolong the diarrhea. Thus, these drugs should be used intermittently for relief of pain only.

The treatment of the systemic forms of *Salmonella* infection requires appropriate antibiotic therapy. The approach is similar to that for typhoid fever. Three drugs have been generally effective: chloramphenicol, trimethoprim-sulfamethoxazole, and ampicillin or amoxicillin. Drainage of abscesses is mandatory. Resection of infected aneurysms is indicated, but the surgical results have been poor. Antibiotic coverage is required before, during, and after surgery.

PROGNOSIS. Gastroenteritis is a mild self-limiting infection, and recovery is complete in several days. Complications are mainly related to consequences of dehydration, e.g., azotemia, stroke, or myocardial infarction, occurring in those patients with significant arteriosclerosis or tenuous fluid balance. Mortality occurs in infants and the elderly. In some epidemics in nurseries or nursing homes, the rate has been 3 to 5 per cent. Immunity to reinfection is incomplete and repeated episodes of salmonellosis will occur following re-exposure.

The prognosis for patients with bacteremic forms of salmonellae may be poor, since many of these patients have underlying diseases. The mortality with *S. choleraesuis* infections has been reported to be as high as 20 per cent. Infants with meningitis have a mortality of 40 per cent, and residual neurologic defects are common.

PREVENTION. There is no vaccine to prevent gastroenteritis or the systemic forms of *Salmonella* infection. Typhoid fever prevention is possible with a new oral attenuated vaccine strain. Careful attention to handwashing, refrigeration of prepared foods, and proper cooking of poultry and their products can help reduce the opportunities to acquire salmonellosis.

Aserhoff B, Bennett JV: Effect of antibiotic therapy in acute salmonellosis on the fecal excretion of salmonellae. N Engl J Med 281:636, 1969. *This paper presents evidence that suggested antibiotic treatment prolongs the fecal secretion of salmonellae in patients with salmonellosis.*

Black PH, King LJ, Swartz MN: Salmonellosis: A review of some unusual aspects. N Engl J Med 262:811, 1960. *A classic paper that highlights many of the epidemiologic and clinical curiosities of* Salmonella*-induced disease.*

Giannella RA, Broitman SA, Zamcheck N: Influence of gastric acidity on bacterial and parasitic enteric infections: A perspective. Ann Intern Med 78:271, 1973. *A good review of the topic dealing with the gastric acid barrier.*

Huang CT, Lo CB: Human infection with *Salmonella choleraesuis* in Hong Kong. J Hyg 65:149, 1967. *The authors present a complete summary of the clinical manifestations of infection with this important* Salmonella *strain.*

Riley LW, DiFerdinando GT Jr, DeMelfi TM, Cohen ML: Evaluation of isolated cases of salmonellosis by plasmid profile analysis: Introduction and transmission of a bacterial clone by precooked roast beef. J Infect Dis 148:12, 1983. *A new epidemiologic tool for identifying* Salmonella *isolated from patients in scattered locations as coming from a common source.*

Other Bacterial Infections

284. EXTRAINTESTINAL INFECTIONS CAUSED BY ENTERIC BACTERIA

Charles C. J. Carpenter

Microorganisms indigenous to the gastrointestinal tract, the enteric bacteria, have become increasingly important causes of human disease over the past three decades. Bacterial infections caused by these organisms share an origin in the gut and similar epidemiologic and pathogenic characteristics and require a common approach to diagnosis, treatment, and prevention.

The enteric bacteria are the principle organisms found in infections of the abdominal viscera, peritoneum, and urinary tract, as well as frequent secondary invaders of the respiratory tract, burns, or other sites of disruption of cutaneous and mucous membrane barriers. Currently, the enteric bacteria constitute the most frequent cause of life-threatening septicemia. The majority of serious infections caused by enteric organisms may be regarded as the result of medical progress, because they have developed directly from increased use of broad-spectrum antimicrobial agents, more aggressive surgery, larger numbers of patients receiving immunosuppressive therapy, and greater use of invasive management techniques (tracheal intubation and intravenous cannulas). Antimicrobial therapy has a strong selective effect on the gastrointestinal flora and is the most important reason for the increasing role of normal colonic flora in systemic infection.

The normal human intestinal flora is extraordinarily complex and consists of over 100 bacterial species. Only a small proportion of these species is commonly involved in extraintestinal infections. The human colon contains 10^{10} to 10^{11} organisms per gram of content, and roughly 60 per cent of the bulk of the normal stool is contributed by bacteria. Ninety to 98 per cent of the normal colonic flora are obligate anaerobes. Most common among these are the gram-negative bacilli, *Bacteroides* and *Fusobacterium*, followed by gram-positive bacilli, including *Bifidobacterium*, *Eubacterium*, and *Corynebacterium* species, and a wide variety of anaerobic streptococci. Less common anaerobes in the colonic flora include the gram-positive spore-forming rods of the *Clostridium* species and the gram-negative cocci *Veillonella*. The aerobic gram-negative rods, most of which belong to the family Enterobacteriaceae, account for only 2 to 10 per cent of the normal colonic flora but cause the majority of life-threatening extraintestinal infections. Of these the most common are *Escherichia coli*, followed by the *Klebsiella-Enterobacter* group, *Proteus*, *Providencia*, *Edwardsiella*, and *Serratia*. *Salmonella*, *Shigella*, *Yersinia*, *Campylobacter*, and pathogenic *Vibrio* species occur only under pathologic conditions and are not constituents of the normal intestinal flora. *Pseudomonas* is an entirely unrelated species, usually found in small numbers in the colon under normal circumstances; *Pseudomonas* may, however, become far more prominent in the gut flora after antimicrobial therapy, especially in immunocompromised hosts. The same considerations apply to yeasts, especially *Candida*, which reside in small numbers in the normal large intestine but are increasingly prominent after antimicrobial therapy.

Although the upper gastrointestinal tract, from duodenum through ileum, under normal circumstances is also colonized with lesser numbers of bacteria (predominantly lactobacilli and gram-negative anaerobes), bacteria derived from the normal upper gastrointestinal tract seldom cause serious extraintestinal bacterial infections.

SPECIFIC LOCAL INFECTIONS CAUSED BY ENTERIC BACTERIA

The mixed intestinal flora participate in infections that originate from lesions of the bowel, including appendicitis, cholangitis, diverticulitis, and perforation (from diverticulitis, ileitis, colitis, or carcinoma). These lesions may lead to localized subdiaphragmatic, hepatic, and pelvic abscesses, which are frequent causes of occult fever in patients recovering from abdominal surgery or trauma; the same intestinal flora may also result in generalized peritonitis. Current data indicate that both aerobic and anaerobic bacteria play major roles in infection of the abdominal cavity. The relative importance of aerobic bacteria has been exaggerated in the past because such microorganisms as *E. coli* grow luxuriantly in both aerobic and anaerobic media and usually predominate in routine cultures. There is now compelling evidence that the anaerobic bacteria, especially *Bacteroides* species, play major roles in infection of the abdominal cavity and are largely responsible for the fecal odor of pus often obtained from such infected sites. Previous dicta have emphasized the need to suspect anaerobic bacteria when foul-smelling pus is present and when organisms can be visualized microscopically but fail to grow under routine conditions. Current data, however, indicate that anaerobes should be presumed to be present in any infection of the abdominal cavity caused by intestinal microorganisms, with the obvious implication that therapy effective against anaerobes (metronidazole or clindamycin) should be employed.

MENINGITIS AND BRAIN ABSCESS. During the first four weeks of life, purulent meningitis is frequently caused by enteric bacteria. Such cases may occur sporadically in nurseries and may be associated with septicemia and infection of any other tissue of the body. Infants with meningoceles are particularly susceptible to enteric bacterial meningitis. Meningitis caused by enteric bacteria occurs rarely in adults. Generally it develops as a complication of gram-negative bacteremia or of a neurosurgical procedure or when host immune response is impaired. Nontraumatic brain abscesses are usually caused by infection by multiple bacteria, including anaerobic bacteria similar to those found in the intestinal tract. The primary sites of infection, however, are usually chronically infected mastoid and paranasal sinuses or lung and less commonly abdominal and pelvic sites.

PERITONITIS AND BACTEREMIA ASSOCIATED WITH HEPATIC CIRRHOSIS. Occasionally individuals with cirrhosis of the liver and ascites develop *spontaneous peritonitis* without evidence of localized sepsis elsewhere. Similarly, patients with cirrhosis with or without ascites occasionally develop bacteremia that is generally caused by one of the enteric organisms, most frequently *E. coli*. The illnesses may be self-limited but should always be treated with antimicrobials active against the most likely pathogens. A definitive explanation for such spontaneous infections is lacking; possibilities include shunting of bacteria away from the liver and impairment of host humoral and cellular defense mechanisms.

PERIRECTAL ABSCESS. Perirectal abscess, in which multiple enteric bacteria are generally involved, is most often a localized infection that responds well to appropriate surgical drainage. However, perirectal abscess is a life-threatening complication in patients with marked granulocytopenia, especially leukemic patients receiving cytotoxic chemotherapy. Rectal examination should be performed gently in such patients, since bacteremia is a frequent complication, presumably because of inadequate localization of infection in the absence of adequate circulating granulocytes.

ABSCESSES AT SITES OF SUBCUTANEOUS INJECTIONS. Enteric bacilli occasionally cause abscesses in subcutaneous tissue at sites of hypodermic injections. This complication commonly affects insulin-dependent diabetic individuals. The abscesses are characterized by gas formation, which may lead to more serious clostridial infection. However, the subcutaneous infections caused by aerobic enteric bacilli usually respond well to appropriate antimicrobial therapy. Rarely *nonclostridial crepitant cellulitis*, a synergistic infection caused by intestinal aerobic and anaerobic bacteria, progresses rapidly, requiring urgent and extensive debridement as well as antimicrobial therapy.

SUPERFICIAL INFECTION. Enteric bacteria, especially *Proteus*, and environmental gram-negative bacilli, predominantly *Pseudomonas*, are commonly recovered from the surfaces of burns, varicose ulcers, decubitus ulcers, tracheostomy sites, and other unprotected surface areas. These organisms are of doubtful pathogenic significance, and satisfactory healing of surface wounds may proceed regardless of their presence. They may, however, occasionally cause fulminant gram-negative bacteremia, especially in patients with severe burns. The sinus exudate from chronic osteomyelitis or chronic otitis media often contains *Proteus* as the dominant organism, but again its pathogenic significance is doubtful.

SUPERINFECTION AND PNEUMONIA. Enteric bacteria frequently predominate in the oropharynx and bronchial secretions of patients who are elderly, chronically ill, or immunosuppressed, as well as in individuals who have been treated with antimicrobial agents. Generally, the presence of enteric bacteria in such patients simply represents superficial colonization with resistant bacterial strains after suppression of the primary flora. If tissue invasion is suspected on clinical grounds, transtracheal aspiration followed by Gram stain and culture of aspirated secretions is a useful method to distinguish between colonization of the oropharynx and true infection of the lower respiratory tract. The demonstration of elastin fibers in bronchial secretion is a reliable means of distinguishing necrotizing infections from simple colonization. Pneumonia caused by enteric bacteria is always a potentially life-threatening infection and is especially serious in patients who have difficulty clearing their secetions or require ventilator therapy. A single agent is generally responsible for the pneumonia, and successful therapy depends upon the isolation of and specific therapy for the microorganism.

URINARY TRACT INFECTIONS. Enteric bacteria are the organisms most frequently associated with urinary tract infections. *E. coli* is by far the most common microorganism in uncomplicated infections of the urinary tract. When other organisms, especially the enteric *Klebsiella-Enterobacter* group or environmental *Pseudomonas,* are involved in the absence of an indwelling urinary catheter, they usually point to structural or neurologic problems of the voiding system or to repeated instrumentation.

PROSTATIC INFECTIONS. Enteric bacilli predominate as etiologic agents in the chronic prostatitis that often accompanies prostatic hypertrophy in older men. The pathogenesis of prostatitis in such individuals is poorly understood and presents a particularly difficult therapeutic problem, since many of the agents most effective against the aerobic enteric bacilli (aminoglycosides) do not reach adequate concentrations in the prostate.

METASTATIC INFECTIONS. Despite the frequency with which enteric bacteria invade the blood and the fact that gram-negative enteric bacilli now account for the vast majority of recognized bacteremias, metastatic intravascular infection and localization of enteric bacilli on normal human heart valves remain rare. Less than 3 per cent of cases of endocarditis are caused by enteric bacilli in the absence of intravenous drug abuse. However, occasional cases of suppurative lesions such as arthritis, osteomyelitis, and panophthalmitis do occur after enteric bacteremia. Vertebral osteomyelitis occurs with increased frequency in men with prostatic disease; presumably the method of spread is by way of septic emboli through the vertebral venous plexus to the spine.

UNIQUE FEATURES OF PSEUDOMONAS INFECTIONS. *Pseudomonas,* although often responsible for infections similar to those caused by enteric gram-negative bacteria, are not truly enteric bacteria. Under certain circumstances, especially in patients on broad-spectrum antimicrobial therapy, patients with severe leukopenia with or without acute leukemia, or intravenous drug users, severe sepsis may be produced by *Pseudomonas.* In addition to the endotoxin that is in the cell wall of most gram-negative bacteria, *Pseudomonas aeruginosa* produces several enzymes, including collagenase, proteases, elastase, and an exotoxin (PA toxin) whose mode of action is similar to that of diphtheria toxin. *Pseudomonas* commonly occurs in tap water, may be resistant to antiseptics used in sterilizing instruments, and therefore frequently is introduced by cystoscopy or ventilator-associated aerosols. *Pseudomonas* is notoriously resistant to standard antimicrobial therapy and often emerges as a dominant microorganism on mucosal surfaces after eradication of the normal microbial flora by drugs. It may then become responsible for the phenomenon of superinfection, as in the bronchopulmonary infections that often complicate prophylactic antimicrobial therapy of chronic lung disease or in the urinary tract infections associated with chronic indwelling catheters.

Tissue invasion by *Pseudomonas,* most frequently recognized in patients with leukopenia or relapsing leukemia, is often characterized by a necrotizing vasculitis with bacterial invasion of the walls of arteries and veins. This may lead to the distinctive necrotic skin lesion (ecthyma gangrenosum) that may develop on any part of the body. This lesion may begin as a vesicle that later becomes necrotic; the typical lesion of ecthyma gangrenosum is a round indurated ulcer with a black center that varies from a few millimeters to 10 or more centimeters in diameter. Although not specific for *Pseudomonas* infection, the presence of ecthyma gangrenosum should make the physician suspect this microorganism.

GRAM-NEGATIVE BACTEREMIA

Bacteremia caused by gram-negative bacilli has been a problem of major importance only since the advent of antimicrobial therapy. Urinary tract infections are the source of about half of all cases of bloodstream invasion by enteric bacilli. Other causes include infections developing at the site of intravenous catheters, postoperative complications of gastrointestinal tract surgery, postpartum or postabortal sepsis, and infections of wounds, ulcers, burns, and internal prosthetic devices. Sometimes there is a clear-cut precipitating factor such as an invasive diagnostic procedure (endoscopy) or manipulation of an infected wound.

These bacteremias have clinical characteristics that closely resemble the known biologic effects of gram-negative bacterial endotoxins. The onset of symptoms often occurs with a shaking chill followed by a sharp rise in temperature. The onset is accompanied by leukopenia, but leukocytosis usually ensues within 12 hours. An important concomitant reaction may be a decrease in blood pressure with inadequate tissue perfusion. At least two factors, peripheral vasodilatation and decreased myocardial contractile force, may contribute to the circulatory dysfunction. In patients with inadequate tissue perfusion the cardiac output may be elevated or normal, associated with peripheral arterial dilatation, or it may be very low, associated with poor myocardial contractility. An initial manifestation is often hyperventilation with a consequent respiratory alkalosis, but with persistence of poor tissue perfusion metabolic acidosis ensues. The inadequate tissue perfusion may be manifested only by a modest alteration in the patient's intellectual status. Occasionally patients, especially the elderly, develop bacteremic shock without detectable elevation of temperature. For these reasons, bacteremia must always be considered in the evaluation of unexplained hypotension. Some patients with gram-negative bacteremia develop disseminated intravascular coagulation. This phenomenon is not unique to enteric bacteremia, since it also may occur with fungal, viral, rickettsial, and gram-positive bacterial infections. Although the mortality rate is high in patients with circulatory impairment associated with gram-negative bacteremia, the outcome is clearly related to a number of factors, including age, underlying disease, and antecedent cardiopulmonary status. However, with prompt diagnosis, appropriate antimicrobial therapy, hemodynamic monitoring, and correction of circulatory abnormalities, the majority of patients without major underlying disease should survive.

Generalized sepsis with enteric bacteria is one of several causes of the *adult respiratory distress syndrome (ARDS).* This syndrome is produced by widespread damage to capillary endothelium of the lung rather than direct pulmonary infection and requires adequate oxygenation, generally including positive end-expiratory pressure.

ENDOTOXIN. Endotoxins from a wide variety of unrelated bacterial species behave similarly, regardless of the pathogenicity of the microorganisms from which they are derived. In the intact microorganism, endotoxins exist as complexes of lipid, polysaccharide, and protein. The biologic activity appears to be a property of a lipid portion. The cell wall of gram-negative bacilli may be roughly divided into three areas. The outermost region contains the chains of specific sugars that characterize the O-specific antigens that determine individual serotypes within a bacterial species. This outer region is linked to a core polysaccharide that is similar in structure among related groups of bacteria. The core polysaccharide is in turn linked through trisaccharides to the major lipid component, termed *lipid A.* The major biologic properties of endotoxin may be accounted for by the complex lipid substance. Lipid A is immunogenic, producing antibodies that cross-react among the gram-negative bacilli. Antibody prepared against lipid A protects against challenge by heterologous gram-negative bacteria in certain animal models. Better protection, however, is obtained by immunization with specific O antigens that induce opsonizing antibodies. Current data suggest that the mortality rate of patients with gram-negative bacteremia is lower in individuals with initially high titers of antibody to the lipid A component. Recent controlled studies have demonstrated that adjunctive treatment of gram-negative infections with antiserum against core lipopolysaccharide significantly increases the survival of patients with bacteremic shock.

When injected intravenously into the experimental animal, the endotoxins cause fever, leukopenia, circulatory collapse, and capillary hemorrhages. Tolerance develops after repeated injections of endotoxin. The clinical features of enteric gram-negative bacteremia may resemble the reaction of laboratory animals or humans to intravenous injection of purified endotoxic preparations. The exact role of endotoxins in the manifestation of gram-negative bacteremia remains uncertain, because chills, fever, leukocytosis, and leukopenia may also result from infection by microorganisms containing little or no biologically active endotoxin in the cell wall (*Candida, Bacteroides spp.*).

Endotoxin is believed to be pyrogenic by virtue of its ability to induce macrophages to release endogenous pyrogen. This protein is carried by the circulation to hypothalamic temperature-regulating nuclei, producing alteration in thermoregulation. In the experimental animal, frequent repeated doses of endotoxin appear to exhaust the capability of macrophages to release endogenous pyrogen. More prolonged exposure of the experimental animal to endotoxin appears to produce antibodies that block endotoxin action.

ANTIBODIES. Antibodies reacting with most Enterobacteriaceae are demonstrable in the sera of normal humans, probably because of continual absorption of small quantities of antigen by the gastrointestinal tract. Gram-negative bacteria contain a wide variety of antigenic determinants. These antigens vary in pathogenetic significance in different species. Certain enteric bacilli contain *K* or *capsular polysaccharides*. The capsular polysaccharides constitute the Vi antigens of *S. typhi*, are prominent in *Klebsiella*, and appear to contribute to the virulence of *E. coli* associated with neonatal meningitis; capsular antigens may also be related to the invasiveness of *E. coli* in pyelonephritis. Capsular polysaccharides interfere with phagocytosis and are probably responsible for the increased virulence of encapsulated bacterial strains. Antibodies to the O or somatic antigens have been most extensively studied in *E. coli*. These antibodies may provide cross-protection against a variety of other enteric microorganisms. Most enteric bacilli are susceptible to immune lysis by the combined effects of antibody and complement, both in vivo and in vitro. Presumably immune lysis is of major importance in preventing the enteric bacilli from invading the bloodstream of normal humans.

MANAGEMENT OF EXTRAINTESTINAL ENTERIC BACTERIAL INFECTIONS

GENERAL PRINCIPLES. Intestinal gram-negative enteric infections are largely iatrogenic; therefore, many of these infections are preventable, especially those arising from indwelling intravenous catheters, instrumentation of the urinary tract, and contaminated suction and ventilation equipment. Elimination of such sources of contamination is the physician's compelling responsibility. The major clinical considerations are (1) early recognition of infection and bacteremia, (2) early recognition and prompt drainage of abscesses, (3) recognition that anaerobic bacteria, not readily cultured, are almost invariably involved in certain infected sites, and (4) differentiation of true infections from superficial contamination that often requires no treatment.

GRAM-NEGATIVE BACTEREMIA. Either the clinical presumption or the documented presence of gram-negative organisms in the blood should alert the physician to initiate a meticulous search for the site of infection, including intravenous or urinary catheters and renal, pelvic, or perirectal abscesses. The successful eradication of infection can seldom be achieved without removal of infected foreign objects and drainage of abscesses. Because of the rapid downhill course of many patients with gram-negative bacteremia, treatment must be begun on the basis of the presumptive diagnosis prior to isolation of the specific causative microorganism.

In settings in which bacteremia is apt to be most rapidly fatal (severe leukopenia, acute leukemia, immunosuppressed patients), the bacteremia often occurs in hospitals where multiple drug-resistant organisms such as *Serratia, Klebsiella,* and *Pseudomonas* play prominent roles. In the febrile immunosuppressed patient, after cultures have been obtained from the blood and other suspected sites of infection, therapy should be begun with an aminoglycoside and either carbenicillin or ticarcillin. The choice of a specific aminoglycoside depends on the frequency, in a given hospital, with which endemic strains are resistant to gentamicin or tobramycin. Once the specific organism has been isolated, therapy should be altered to include the most appropriate and least toxic agents.

Modification of drug therapy is dependent on the site of infection. Gram-negative meningitis in adults often requires a third generation cephalosporin, moxalactam, or intraventricular injection of aminoglycosides via reservoir. When *Klebsiella* is strongly suspected in a pulmonary infection, a cephalosporin should generally be added to an aminoglycoside.

When anaerobes are presumed to be present in abdominal, pelvic, or anogenital infections, an agent such as metronidazole, cefoxitin, clindamycin, chloramphenicol, or moxalactam should be included, the choice being based largely on susceptibility of the patient to the toxic effects peculiar to the chosen antimicrobial agent (for example, chloramphenicol should not be used in a leukopenic individual).

Acute, nonbacteremic urinary infections are likely to respond to oral agents such as sulfamethoxazole-trimethoprim, ampicillin, or tetracycline. The selection of specific drugs should be based on in vitro sensitivity testing. Oral carbenicillin should be reserved for treatment of *Pseudomonas* urinary tract infections outside the hospital because of the danger of selecting resistant organisms in the hospital environment. In patients with indwelling urinary catheters, antimicrobial therapy is ineffective in eradicating chronic urinary infections and should be reserved for acute episodes of sepsis.

Management of bacteremic shock is complex and requires monitoring by a properly placed Swan-Ganz catheter and therapy as outlined in Ch. 43. With optimal corrective measures designed to improve tissue perfusion, survival becomes dependent on removal of any infected foreign material, drainage of abscess cavities, appropriate antimicrobial therapy, and underlying host defenses.

Kreger BE, Craven DE, McCabe WR: Gram-negative bacteremia. IV. Re-evaluation of clinical features and treatment in 612 patients. Am J Med 68:344, 1980. *A large, up-to-date, authoritative analysis of the clinical manifestations of bacteremia caused by enteric bacteria.*

McCabe WR, Treadwell TL, DeMaria A: Pathophysiology of bacteremia. Am J Med 75(1B):7, 1983. *A thoughtful and authoritative discussion of the pathogenesis, clinical manifestations, and pathophysiology of bacteremia.*

Mangi RJ, Quintiliani R, Andriole VT: Gram-negative bacillary meningitis. Am J Med 59:829, 1975. *A comprehensive review of the experience at Yale New Haven Medical Center with gram-negative bacillary meningitis over a five-year period. It demonstrates the contribution of these organisms to the overall experience with bacterial meningitis (4.2 per cent of the cases) and the frequent association with neurosurgery (69 per cent) and neonatal cases (42 per cent). It documents the importance of the nosocomial origin of these cases.*

Young LS, Martin WJ, Meyer RD, Weinstein RJ, Anderson ET: Gram-negative rod bacteremia: Microbiologic, immunologic and therapeutic considerations. Ann Intern Med 86:456, 1977. *An excellent symposium on the laboratory, epidemiologic, and biologic features of gram-negative rod bacteremia. It has an extensive (134-item) bibliography.*

Zeigler EJ, McCutchan JA, Frerer J, Glauser MP, Sadoff JC, Douglas H, Braude AI: Treatment of gram-negative bacteremia and shock with human antiserum to a mutant *Escherichia coli*. New Engl J Med 306:1225, 1982. *This careful clinical study clearly demonstrates that therapy with human antiserum against core lipopolysaccharide of gram-negative enteric bacilli greatly reduces mortality in gram-negative bacteremia.*

285. SHIGELLOSIS

Charles C. J. Carpenter

DEFINITION. Shigellosis is a specific acute bacterial infection of the human intestinal tract caused by bacteria of the genus *Shigella*, with predominant involvement of the distal colon, sigmoid, and rectum. It most commonly is manifested as a clinically nonspecific diarrhea. In the more severe cases, the initial mild diarrhea is accompanied by fever and followed by true dysentery, with cramping abdominal pain, tenesmus, and frequent stools in which mucus, leukocytes, and erythrocytes are abundant.

ETIOLOGY. Shigellae (dysentery bacilli) are nonmotile gram-negative bacilli belonging to the family Enterobacteriaceae. Four species of shigellae are recognized on the basis of antigenic and biochemical properties: *S. dysenteriae* (Group A), *S. flexneri* (Group B), *S. boydii* (Group C), and *S. sonnei* (Group D). Among these species there are over 40 types, each of which is designated by the species name followed by a specific Arabic number. With the exception of *S. flexneri* 6, they do not ferment lactose. The most common species in the United States until 1965 was *S. flexneri*; this species has largely been replaced by *S. sonnei*. *S. sonnei* is now also the most commonly isolated shigella in Western Europe and Japan. *S. boydii* is so rarely encountered in the United States that its isolation suggests exposure during foreign travel. *S. dysenteriae* is now unusual in the more developed countries.

EPIDEMIOLOGY. ***Incidence and Prevalence.*** Despite generally high standards of hygiene, there were over 14,000 cases of shigellosis reported in the United States in 1980. *S. sonnei* has been the predominant etiologic species in North America, Western Europe, and Japan for the past two decades, and the great majority of patients have been children. The true incidence is undoubtedly several times higher than the number of reported cases.

In much of Eastern Europe and in the developing areas of the world, *S. flexneri* has continued to be the predominant causative agent. *S. dysenteriae* 1 (Shiga bacillus) has nearly disappeared as a major endemic cause of dysentery but re-emerged as a major epidemic problem in Central America from 1969 to 1972. Microepidemics caused by the Shiga bacillus recur sporadically throughout the developing world.

Spread of Infection. Shigellosis is found throughout the world. Seasonal patterns vary in different regions; shigellosis characteristically peaks in the late summer and early autumn in North America. Humans and the higher primates are the only known reservoirs of *Shigella* infection. During clinical illness and for a variable period (up to six weeks) following recovery, fecal excretion of shigellae continues. Although the organisms are quite sensitive to desiccation, they may survive for several months in foods and water. Transmission most often occurs by close person-to-person contact. Children in the one- to four-year age group are at highest risk of developing shigellosis; young males are affected more often than young females. In young adults the incidence is higher in women than in men, which probably reflects closer contact of women with ill children. Intrafamilial spread is especially likely to occur when the initial case has occurred in a preschool child. Attack rates in affected families range from 10 to 80 per cent.

Custodial institutions, especially those caring for the retarded, are frequent settings for large epidemics because of difficulty in maintaining adequate hygiene in these settings. Up to 30 per cent of individuals admitted to certain custodial institutions experience an episode of shigellosis within a year of arrival. Nursery schools and day care centers have especially high attack rates whenever shigellae are introduced.

Since shigellae are transmitted by the fecal-oral route, crowded living conditions, poor water supply, and inadequate sewage facilities all correlate significantly with increased risk of infection. Within the United States, shigellosis is excessively high in urban ghettos and Indian reservations. The male homosexual population is also at great risk for shigellosis, which is one of the more common causes of the "gay bowel syndrome."

The recent pandemic spread of *S. dysenteriae* 1 (Shiga bacillus) in Central America and Mexico subsided without major extension to either North or South America. As has been true of pandemics in the past, the reasons for the development of the 1969 to 1972 Central American Shiga bacillus pandemic remain obscure.

PATHOGENESIS AND PATHOPHYSIOLOGY. Since the microorganisms are relatively resistant to acid, shigellae have less difficulty than other enteric pathogens in passing the gastric barrier. In volunteer studies, as few as 200 ingested bacilli regularly initiate disease in 25 per cent of healthy adults. This contrasts strikingly with the much larger numbers of typhoid or cholera bacilli required to produce disease in normal individuals. During the incubation period, usually 36 to 72 hours, the organisms traverse the small bowel and proliferate in the distal jejunum, ileum, and colon. In the colon shigellae reach concentrations of 10^6 to 10^{10} organisms per gram of stool. Unlike the case with certain other enteric pathogens (*V. cholerae* and enterotoxigenic *E. coli*), epithelial cell penetration is essential to the pathogenesis of shigellosis. Multiplication of bacteria occurs within epithelial cells of the colon, predominantly in the villi; this is followed by an acute inflammatory response in the subjacent lamina propria. Destruction of the villous tips, distortion of the mucosal architecture, and formation of superficial microabscesses ensue. In the more severe cases, long segments of colon may be affected with a diffuse inflammatory process that remains confined to the lamina propria. The altered mucosa is friable and is covered with an exudate of polymorphonuclear leukocytes. Stool therefore contains large numbers of erythrocytes and leukocytes. Since the inflammation is superficial, bacteremia is rare, and colonic perforation seldom occurs.

S. dysenteriae and certain strains of *S. flexneri* and *S. sonnei* produce an enterotoxin that causes secretion of isotonic fluid by the small bowel. The role of this enterotoxin in clinical shigellosis is not certain; the enterotoxin may be responsible for the watery diarrhea that often precedes full-blown bacillary dysentery. It is possible that the enterotoxin is entirely responsible for the clinical manifestations in mild cases characterized by only short-term watery nonbloody diarrhea.

CLINICAL MANIFESTATIONS. Shigellosis is often a biphasic disease, beginning with cramping abdominal pain and watery diarrhea, sometimes accompanied by fever (up to 40° C) and generalized myalgias. Fluid and electrolyte losses are greatest during the initial phase of the illness. Such losses are rarely voluminous enough to be life-threatening except in very young children and the elderly. This first phase usually lasts for one to three days; in more severely ill patients, it is followed by a second phase that in the absence of treatment may last for weeks. The second phase is that of true dysentery; the character of the stool changes, with a decrease in the volume and the appearance of bright red blood and mucus in the feces. During this phase, tenesmus may become a complicating feature, and anorexia and weight loss are common. Fever is not prominent during the second phase of the illness.

Many patients infected with shigellae are entirely asymptomatic, and a large number simply have mild cramping abdominal pain and watery diarrhea that clinically cannot be differentiated from illnesses caused by several other microorganisms. Only the more severe cases, with classic bacillary dysentery, can readily be diagnosed clinically as shigellosis. Of the *Shigella* strains now encountered in the United States, *S. dysenteriae* is the most virulent and by far the least common. *S. flexneri* is intermediate in both virulence and frequency, and *S. sonnei*, which accounts for 80 per cent of cases in the United States, presents the mildest clinical picture.

The onset of shigellosis is often more fulminant in children, who may present with unexplained high fever with or without convulsions. Neurologic symptoms and signs, including delirium, headache, nuchal rigidity, and lethargy, rarely occur in adults but are common in young children. Roughly 25 per cent of children hospitalized for shigellosis experience convulsions. The cause of the convulsions is unknown. A small proportion of children infected by *S. dysenteriae* 1 develop a severe, often fatal hemolytic-uremic syndrome; this syndrome is associated with endotoxemia and circulating immune complexes.

DIAGNOSIS. Shigellosis should be considered in any patient with acute onset of fever and diarrhea. Diagnosis is more likely in the high-risk groups just described. Examination of the stool is quite useful in the diagnosis. Blood and pus are grossly apparent in severe bacillary dysentery; even in milder forms of the disease, microscopic examination of the stool often reveals numerous leukocytes and erythrocytes. The fecal leukocyte examination should be performed with a portion of liquid stool, preferably containing mucus. A drop of stool is placed on a microscopic slide and mixed thoroughly with two drops of methylene blue. A coverslip is placed over the mixture for microscopic examination. The presence of abundant polymorphonuclear leukocytes helps in distinguishing shigellosis from diarrheal syndromes caused by enterotoxigenic *E. coli* and *Vibrio cholerae* (in which fecal leukocytes are characteristically absent). The fecal leukocyte examination is not helpful in distinguishing shigellosis from diarrheal illnesses caused by other invasive enteric pathogens (nontyphoidal *Salmonella, Campylobacter, Yersinia, Entamoeba*). The peripheral white cell count is of little diagnostic value, since it may range from less than 3000 to more than 30,000. Sigmoidoscopic examination reveals diffuse erythema and a friable mucosa, with shallow ulcers 3 to 7 mm in diameter.

Definitive diagnosis depends upon isolating shigellae by selective media. A rectal swab, a swab of a colonic ulcer obtained by sigmoidoscopic examination, or a freshly passed stool specimen should be inoculated immediately on culture plates or into carrying media. Since isolation rates of shigellae from freshly passed stools of patients with shigellosis may be as low as 67 per cent, culturing for three successive days is recommended. Stool cultures are generally positive within 24 hours after onset of symptoms and may remain positive for several weeks in the absence of antimicrobial therapy. Blood cultures are so rarely positive as to be of no diagnostic value.

Appropriate culture media include blood, desoxycholate, and salmonella-shigella (S-S) agars. Selected colonies suggestive of shigellae should be placed on triple sugar–iron agar and lysine-iron agar. Colonies showing an alkaline slant and acid butt, without gas or hydrogen sulfide in either agar, should be definitively diagnosed by agglutination with polyvalent *Shigella* antisera. S-S agar is inhibitory for the most virulent of the *Shigella* species, *S. dysenteriae* 1.

Definitive bacteriologic diagnosis becomes of critical importance in distinguishing the more severe and prolonged cases of shigellosis from ulcerative colitis, with which it may be confused both clinically and on sigmoidoscopic examination. Occasionally patients with shigellosis have been subjected to colectomy because of a mistaken diagnosis of ulcerative colitis; a positive culture should clearly prevent such a misadventure.

TREATMENT. The three steps in the treatment of shigellosis include correction of fluid and electrolyte balance, antimicrobial therapy, and symptomatic relief. Although voluminous production of diarrhea is unusual in shigellosis, fluid loss may be lethal in the very young and the very old. Fluid losses in shigellosis are qualitatively similar to those in other infectious diarrheal diseases, and the patient should be treated with appropriate intravenous or oral electrolyte repletion fluids (see Ch. 286) in quantities adequate to correct clinical signs of saline depletion. The requirement for fluids is generally small, but fluid repletion will be lifesaving in exceptional cases.

The effectiveness of antimicrobial agents in treating shigellosis has been well established. Although infections with *S. sonnei, S. flexneri*, and *S. boydii* are generally self-limited except in the very young and very old, appropriate antimicrobial therapy may decrease the duration of symptoms by 50 per cent and decrease the duration of excretion of shigellae (an important epidemiologic factor) by a far greater percentage. Infection by *S. dysenteriae* 1 may result in a 10 to 30 per cent mortality rate in the absence of antimicrobial therapy, and appropriate antimicrobials are mandatory with this pathogen. Ampicillin is currently the drug of choice for sensitive strains of shigellosis in the United States. It should be administered orally in four divided doses for a total of 2 grams a day to adults and 100 mg per kilogram per day to children for a five-day period. Because of the increasing frequency of plasmid-mediated antimicrobial resistance to *Shigella* infections, drug susceptibility testing is important. For adults with ampicillin-resistant isolates, tetracycline in a single oral dose of 2.5 grams is usually effective. Sulfamethoxazole-trimethoprim administered in standard doses twice daily for five days is now the treatment of choice for *Shigella* strains of unknown antibiotic sensitivity in both adults and children.* Certain drugs that appear effective in vitro, including amoxicillin and nonabsorbable antimicrobials such as neomycin or kanamycin, are not effective in vivo. Sulfonamide resistance is so widespread as to nullify the value of these agents.

Agents that decrease intestinal motility should not be used. Such preparations as diphenoxylate and paregoric may exacerbate symptoms, presumably by retarding intestinal clearance of the microorganisms. There is no convincing evidence that pectin- or bismuth-containing preparations are helpful.

PROGNOSIS. The mortality rate in untreated shigellosis is dependent upon the infectious strain and ranges from 30 per cent in certain outbreaks caused by *S. dysenteriae* 1 to less than 1 per cent in most *S. sonnei* infections. Even with infection caused by *S. dysenteriae* 1, mortality rates should approach zero if appropriate fluid replacement and antimicrobial therapy are initiated early. A small number of patients, especially those with histocompatibility antigen B27, develop *Reiter's syndrome* weeks or months after recovery from shigellosis.

PREVENTION. Individuals excreting shigellae should be excluded from all phases of food handling until negative cultures have been obtained from three successive stool specimens collected after completion of antimicrobial therapy. In institutional outbreaks, strict and early isolation of infected individuals is mandatory. Targeted antimicrobial chemoprophylaxis has been disappointing. The most important control measure is scrupulous handwashing by all individuals involved in handling of food. Reporting of shigellosis cases to health authorities should be mandatory.

For the traveler to countries with major *Shigella* problems, no chemoprophylactic agent is an adequate substitute for good personal hygiene and the avoidance of contaminated food and water. Although an oral attenuated vaccine has provided significant protection in volunteer studies, no effective vaccine is now commercially available.

Dupont HL, Hornick RB: Adverse effect of Lomotil therapy in shigellosis. JAMA 226:1525, 1973. *A concise discussion of clearly defined untoward effects of diphenoxylate with atropine in shigellosis.*

DuPont HL, Hornick RB, Dawkins AT, Snyder MJ, Formal SB: The response of man to virulent *Shigella flexneri* 2a. J Infect Dis 119:296, 1969. *A precise description of the clinical course and antibody response in shigellosis induced by oral administration of* Shigella flexneri, *in varying doses, to informed young adult volunteers.*

Haltalin KC, Kusmiesz, HT, Hinton LV, Nelson JD: Treatment of acute diarrhea in outpatients. Am J Dis Child 124:554, 1972. *An unequivocal demonstration of the value of appropriate antimicrobial therapy in the management of shigellosis.*

Koster F, Levin J, Walker L, Tung KSK, Gilman RH, Rahaman MM, Majid MA, Islam S, Williams RC: Hemolytic-uremic syndrome after shigellosis. Relation to endotoxemia and circulating immune complexes. N Engl J Med 298:927, 1978. *New light on the pathogenesis of this frequently lethal complication of shigellosis in children.*

Pickering LK, DuPont HL, Olarte J: Single-dose tetracycline therapy for shigellosis in adults. JAMA 239:853, 1978. *This concise, provocative study clearly demonstrates the effectiveness of single-dose tetracycline in adults infected with antibiotic-sensitive* Shigella *and strongly suggests that this therapy is also effective in adults infected by* Shigella *that demonstrate resistance to tetracycline in vitro.*

*Not recommended for children under age two months.

Stoll BJ, Glass RI, Hug MI, Khan MU, Banu H, Holt J: Epidemiologic and clinical features of patients infected with *Shigella* who attended a diarrheal hospital in Bangladesh. J Infect Dis 146:177, 1982. *Emphasizes the broad range of clinical manifestation of this disease and the continuing importance of* Shigella *as a major enteric pathogen in developed countries.*

286. CHOLERA (Asiatic Cholera)

Nathaniel F. Pierce

DEFINITION. Cholera is an acute, sometimes fulminant, diarrheal disease during which *Vibrio cholerae,* serogroup 1, are abundant in liquid stool. It occurs only in humans and varies in severity from a mild diarrheal illness to a dramatically severe disease that causes death from hypovolemic shock in a few hours owing to the passage of voluminous, watery, electrolyte-rich stools. Cholera usually occurs in epidemic form; it has caused seven pandemics in the past two centuries.

ETIOLOGY. *Vibrio cholerae* are short, slightly curved, motile gram-negative rods that grow aerobically at 37° C. There are more than 60 O serogroups of *Vibrio cholerae,* but only serogroup 1 causes epidemic cholera. Some of the others sporadically cause acute diarrhea, which is occasionally severe. *Vibrio cholerae,* serogroup 1, occurs as two serotypes, *Ogawa* and *Inaba,* which reflect differences in the somatic antigen; there are also two biotypes: the *classic* and the *eltor.* The eltor biotype is recognized by its resistance to polymyxin B and by characteristic patterns of susceptibility to vibriophage. Distinction between the two biotypes has epidemiologic importance; the eltor biotype causes a higher proportion of mild or asymptomatic infections and survives better outside the human host.

EPIDEMIOLOGY. ***The Seventh Pandemic.*** The traditional "home" of cholera is the delta region of the Ganges and Brahmaputra rivers, where thousands of cases occur during annual epidemics. During pandemics the disease has spread in Asia, Africa, Europe, and North America. The current pandemic is due to the eltor biotype; it involves Southeast Asia, the Indian subcontinent, the Middle East, Africa, and the Gulf Coast of the United States. The world total of reported cases reached its peak in 1971, and cholera now appears to be endemic in many of these recently involved areas. Cholera has also been imported to Japan, Israel, Spain, Italy, and Portugal, where it has caused isolated outbreaks. Individual cases have also occurred among travelers returning from affected areas. In the United States, cholera has occurred sporadically along the Gulf Coast since 1973. All cases were caused by the same unusual strain of *Vibrio cholerae,* which suggests that Gulf Coast waters may have been contaminated since 1973.

Mode of Spread. Cholera is largely waterborne, usually by means of fecal contamination of drinking water. However, food exposed to contaminated water may also be the vehicle for infection. Examples of the latter include fresh vegetables washed in contaminated water and shellfish harvested from contaminated water. Evidence that *Vibrio cholerae* adhere to shellfish suggests that these may prove an especially important means of spread.

Secondary cases of cholera in affected households are common because of direct contamination of water or food with infected excreta. Persons with self-limited, mild, or asymptomatic infections outnumber those with serious illness and are probably the major means by which cholera is spread from affected to nearby nonaffected communities. Prolonged gallbladder carriage also occurs in about 3 per cent of older adults convalescent from cholera; however, their role in transmission of cholera is uncertain.

Susceptibility to Cholera. The age distribution of cholera cases reflects the level of naturally acquired immunity in the population. In endemic areas, adults ingest the organism many times and develop substantial immunity; in such areas, cholera is largely a disease of children. In Bangladesh, for example, attack rates among children under five years old are ten times those of adults. In contrast, attack rates in newly affected areas, where there is no naturally acquired immunity, are nearly equal among adults and children.

Vibrio cholerae are quickly killed by pH levels below 5.5. Thus, normal gastric acidity is an important barrier to infection. Impairment of gastric acidity by mucosal atrophy, the use of antacids, or subtotal gastrectomy increases susceptibility to cholera.

PATHOGENESIS. The incubation period for cholera is usually one to two days but may vary from 12 hours to six days. Cholera occurs when *Vibrio cholerae* are ingested, survive passage through the stomach, colonize and multiply in the small bowel, and release the cholera enterotoxin. Colonization is promoted by adherence of the vibrios to the small bowel mucosa. The enterotoxin is a protein (molecular weight 84,000) composed of A and B subunits. The B subunit binds irreversibly to its receptor, GM_1 ganglioside, on the brush border of small bowel epithelial cells. This assists entry of the A subunit into epithelial cells, which causes activation of adenylate cyclase, an increase in intracellular content of 3′,5′-cyclic adenosine monophosphate, and the secretion of electrolytes into the bowel lumen. Cholera enterotoxin does not cause morphologic damage to the bowel mucosa, does not alter its permeability to serum proteins, and does not affect the active absorption of monosaccharides (e.g., glucose) or amino acids. The secreted electrolyte solution passes through the gut and emerges as watery stool, which rapidly becomes free of fecal material. Flecks of mucus give the stool its characteristic "rice-water" appearance. The stool is isotonic with plasma but has concentrations of bicarbonate and potassium greater than plasma (see Table 286–1). All of the signs, symptoms, and metabolic disorders of cholera are related to the rapid loss of this electrolyte-rich liquid stool. This loss causes hypvolemia, base-deficit acidosis, and potassium depletion.

CLINICAL MANIFESTATIONS. Cholera begins with the abrupt onset of watery diarrhea. Many cases are mild, cause little morbidity, and cannot be distinguished clinically from other types of gastroenteritis. In severe cases, however, stool loss is dramatic, sometimes exceeding 1 liter per hour. Collapse resulting from hypovolemic shock occurs when unreplaced fluid losses equal about 10 per cent of body weight. This may happen within 6 hours but usually requires 18 to 24 hours. Greater fluid losses are rapidly lethal. Vomiting, painful cramps of the gastrocnemius muscles, and severe thirst are other prominent features of severe cholera.

The outstanding physical findings in severe untreated cholera are the results of marked isotonic fluid deficit. These include collapse, poor skin turgor, weak or absent peripheral pulses, hypotension, tachycardia, and cyanosis. Eyes are sunken, the voice is faint and high-pitched, heart sounds are faint, and bowel sounds are hypoactive. Adults are usually normally oriented but apathetic. Features that occur only in children under seven years are fever and occasionally coma or convulsions.

Initial laboratory findings reflect the loss of isotonic bicarbonate-rich stool (see Table 286–1). These include increased plasma protein concentration, increased plasma-specific gravity, low arterial pH, and low plasma bicarbonate concentration.

TABLE 286–1. TYPICAL CHEMICAL VALUES IN STOOL AND PLASMA FROM PATIENTS WITH SEVERE CHOLERA

		Plasma	
	Stool	*Untreated*	*Treated*†
Sodium*	138 (105)	141	142
Chloride*	102 (90)	107	106
Potassium*	18 (25)	4.5	3.6
Bicarbonate*	45 (30)	9	21
Arterial pH	—	7.21	7.43
Plasma specific gravity	—	1.040	1.026

*Milliequivalents per liter. Stool values in parentheses are for children less than 10 years old.

†Four hours after water and electrolyte replacement.

Plasma sodium concentration is normal. Small children occasionally have severe hypoglycemia.

DIAGNOSIS. Cholera should be suspected in any acute case of watery, shock-producing diarrhea, especially in an adult. Travel to or residence in a cholera-affected area makes the diagnosis more likely. A diagnosis of cholera should also be considered in exposed persons with acute attacks of mild, painless, nonbloody diarrhea.

After treatment has begun, a direct stool examination should be performed. A fecal smear stained with methylene blue usually reveals neither erythrocytes nor leukocytes, which is a feature also characteristic of infections with enterotoxigenic *Escherichia coli* and rotavirus. Dark-field microscopy of dilute feces reveals numerous bacilli with the rapid, darting movement characteristic of vibrios. Immobilization of these organisms by addition of group-specific antisera confirms that they are *Vibrio cholerae,* serogroup 1.

Stool should also be obtained for diagnostic culture. The simplest method involves direct plating of feces on thiosulfate-citrate-bile salt-sucrose (TCBS) agar, a medium highly selective for vibrios. Opaque flat yellow colonies form on TCBS agar within 18 hours at 37° C. Confirmation of serogroup and serotype is made by direct bacterial agglutination in specific antisera. The eltor biotype is identified by its resistance to polymyxin B.

The diagnosis can be confirmed by showing significant rises during convalescence in the serum titers of *Vibrio cholerae* agglutinating antibody or of complement-dependent vibriocidal antibodies. Serodiagnostic techniques are used mostly for epidemiologic studies.

TREATMENT. The mainstay of cholera therapy is prompt, complete replacement of lost water and electrolytes. In severe cases, this should be done immediately, before diagnostic studies. Fluid replacement therapy for cholera is fully effective for cholera-like diseases sometimes caused by other bacterial or viral agents.

Water and electrolytes can be replaced intravenously or in many cases orally. The choice depends upon the patient's condition and the treatment materials available. Intravenous rehydration is required for severely hypovolemic patients and is acceptable for those less seriously ill. Oral replacement of water and electrolytes can be used throughout the course of mild cases and in severe cases after hypovolemia has been corrected by rapid intravenous replacement. Oral therapy is especially useful in rural or underdeveloped areas where intravenous fluids are in short supply.

Lactated Ringer's solution is satisfactory for intravenous rehydration. Initial treatment should aim to restore an effective blood volume as rapidly as possible. Fluid should be given through a large bore needle at 50 to 100 ml per minute until a strong radial pulse is restored. The remainder of the initial deficit is then replaced within two hours. For example, a 50-kg patient with severe dehydration has a fluid deficit of about 5 liters (10 per cent of body weight); 1 to 2 liters is replaced within 20 minutes, and the remainder (3 to 4 liters) by the end of two hours. The response to rapid rehydration is usually dramatic, patients becoming alert, comfortable, and fully cooperative within an hour. After initial rehydration, if administration of intravenous fluids is continued, the infusion should be given at a rate equal to the rate of ongoing measured stool loss until diarrhea subsides. If stool loss cannot be measured, the rate should be sufficient to maintain a strong pulse and normal skin turgor. In severe cases, stool losses may average 10 to 25 ml per kilogram per hour for the first 24 hours. Overhydration can be detected by frequent examination of the neck veins and auscultation of the lungs.

Oral therapy is effective because enteric glucose absorption and glucose-facilitated sodium absorption are intact in patients with cholera. A suitable glucose-electrolyte solution is made by adding the following (in grams per liter) to drinking water: sodium chloride, 3.5; sodium bicarbonate, 2.5; potassium chloride, 1.5; and glucose, 20. If glucose is unavailable, sucrose (40 grams per liter) is nearly as effective. Oral rehydration requires 50 to 100 ml per kilogram, depending upon the degree of dehydration. Replacement of ongoing stool losses requires 5 to 15 ml per kilogram per hour. Thirst is a valuable guide to oral fluid requirements; however, patients may need encouragement to drink the large amounts required for rehydration (up to 1000 ml per hour for adults). Vomiting may occur but does not affect the success of oral therapy unless it is severe.

The treatment of small children with cholera resembles that of adults. The same solutions may be used for oral or intravenous replacement. If lactated Ringer's solution is given, oral supplementation with glucose and potassium is needed to prevent symptomatic hypoglycemia and hypokalemia. The rate of intravenous rehydration should be slower to minimize the risk of coma or seizures caused by cerebral edema. After rapid restoration of a strong radial pulse, by infusing up to 30 ml per kilogram in 30 minutes, the remainder of the initial deficit is replaced in about six hours. Thereafter, ongoing stool losses are replaced as they occur.

Adjunctive therapy with oral antibiotics markedly reduces the duration and volume of stool loss and shortens the period of vibrio excretion. Oral tetracycline (50 mg per kilogram per day in six-hourly doses for two days, maximum daily dose 2 grams) is usually most effective. Recently, *Vibrio cholerae* resistant to tetracycline have been encountered. Furazolidone or chloramphenicol are alternative choices in such instances. A normal diet should be given as soon as appetite returns. Drinking water should be freely available and frequently offered to small children.

The complications of cholera depend largely upon the adequacy of treatment. Uncorrected hypovolemia is the major cause of death. Transient oliguria occurs in many patients, but renal failure with acute tubular necrosis occurs only when hypovolemia is poorly corrected. Inadequate potassium replacement causes cardiac arrhythmias in adults and serious paralytic ileus in children. Water and electrolyte replacement without correction of acidosis can cause pulmonary edema. Uncorrected hypoglycemia can contribute to coma or seizures in children. Severe cholera during the third trimester of pregnancy carries a high risk of fetal death.

PROGNOSIS. Mortality from serious cholera, if untreated, reaches 50 per cent. With adequate replacement therapy, however, mortality approaches zero. Despite adequate therapy, a mortality of about 1 per cent persists among small children, owing largely to complicating coma and seizures.

PREVENTION. Immunization with killed cholera vaccine (containing 10 billion bacteria per milliliter) enhances protection for about six months for adults in endemic areas but is less effective for children or persons from nonendemic areas. Cholera vaccine does not alter fecal shedding of *Vibrio cholerae* and thus does not reduce disease transmission. Tetracycline taken prophylactically by household contacts of proven cases prevents secondary cases. Safe sewage disposal and pure water supplies are the only certain means of preventing cholera.

Barua D, Burrows W: Cholera. Philadelphia, W. B. Saunders Company, 1974. *A broad review of bacteriologic, epidemiologic, immunologic, and clinical aspects of cholera written by a variety of experts.*

Blake PA, Allegra DT, Snyder JD, Barrett TJ, McFarland L, Caraway CT, Feeley JC, Craig JP, Lee JV, Puhr ND, Feldman RA: Cholera—possible endemic focus in the United States. N Engl J Med 302:305, 1980. *This article describes the recent cholera outbreak in Louisiana. It is a valuable example of how an outbreak can occur in a developed nation.*

Carpenter CCJ, Mitra PP, Sack RB: Clinical studies in Asiatic cholera. Parts I–VI. Bull Johns Hopkins Hosp 118:165, 1966. *This is an excellent series of reports concerning the pathophysiology of cholera, rational fluid replacement, and the value of antibiotic therapy.*

Hirschhorn N: The treatment of acute diarrhea in children. An historical and physiologic perspective. Am J Clin Nutr 33:637, 1980. *A thorough review of the special concerns that surround treatment of acute diarrhea, including cholera, in children. The review serves to "bridge" the traditional pediatric literature and the recent literature on cholera and related diarrheal diseases.*

Moss J, Vaughan M: Activation of adenylate cyclase by choleragen. Ann Rev Biochem 48:581, 1979. *A complete review of the cellular basis of action of cholera toxin.*

Pierce NF, Hirschhorn N: Oral fluid—a simple weapon against dehydration in diarrhea. How it works and how to use it. WHO Chron 31:87, 1977. *This is a how-to-do-it article on the use of oral glucose-electrolyte solutions for replacement therapy of acute watery diarrhea. The article was designed especially to aid workers in developing nations where medical care facilities are limited.*
Wallace CK, Anderson PN, Brown TC, Khanra SR, Lewis GW, Pierce NF, Sanyal SN, Segre GV, Waldman RH: Optimal antibiotic therapy in cholera. Bull WHO 39:236, 1966. *This article describes studies on the efficacy of several antibiotics as adjuncts in cholera therapy.*

287. YERSINIA INFECTIONS

Thomas Butler

Plague

DEFINITION. Plague is a bacterial infection of animals and humans caused by *Yersinia pestis*. The most common clinical form is *acute regional lymphadenitis*, called *bubonic plague*. Less common forms include *septicemic*, *pneumonic*, and *meningeal plague*. Mortality is high in untreated cases, but antibiotic treatment administered early in the course of the disease markedly reduces fatalities. Plague has a widespread distribution in the world with significant foci in the Americas, Africa, and Asia. The natural reservoirs of *Y. pestis* are predominantly urban and sylvatic rodents, and it is transmitted among animals and occasionally to humans by bites of infected fleas.

HISTORY. *Y. pestis* has caused devastating pandemics with high mortality rates throughout history. The fourth great pandemic in the world is presently under way. The first three are believed to have occurred in the following times: the first originated in Egypt in 542 A.D. and spread to Turkey and Europe. The second pandemic started in the 14th century in Asia Minor and Africa; after spreading to Europe the black death killed about a fourth of the continent's people. The third occurred in Europe during the 15th to 18th centuries. The present fourth pandemic began around 1860 in the Chinese province of Yunnan. It spread to the southern coast of China, reaching Hong Kong in 1894. Subsequently plague was carried by ship to India, other countries of Asia, Brazil, and California. An estimated 10 million deaths were caused by this disease in India during this century. The plague bacillus was discovered by Alexandre Yersin in 1894 in Hong Kong. It was called *Pasteurella pestis* until 1970.

ETIOLOGY. The causative agent, *Y. pestis*, belongs to the family of bacteria Enterobacteriaceae. It is an aerobic gram-negative bacillus that is readily cultured in broth or agar media with an optimal growth rate at 28° C. The plague bacillus possesses a large number of antigens and toxins that have important roles in virulence and pathogenicity. In the capsular envelope there is a protein called Fraction 1 antigen, which confers antiphagocytic activity and can activate complement proteins of the host. Fraction 1 is produced well at 37° C but not at 28° C and below, indicating that this virulence factor develops while bacteria are in their mammalian hosts but is absent while bacteria are in fleas. Another antiphagocytic antigen of *Y. pestis* is the VW antigen. In the cell walls of *Y. pestis* there is a potent lipopolysaccharide endotoxin, which like endotoxins of other gram-negative bacteria produces fever, leukopenia followed by leukocytosis, disseminated intravascular coagulation, complement activation, and many kinds of tissue damage. In experimental systems, plague endotoxin causes local and generalized Shwartzman reactions, is mitogenic for B lymphocytes, and stimulates gelation of limulus lysate. Additionally, *Y. pestis* elaborates exotoxins that may play pathogenic roles. One of these is a protein called the *murine toxin*, which is cardiotoxic in animals and produces beta-adrenergic blockade, but the role of this exotoxin in human disease is unclear.

Another important protein secreted by *Y. pestis* is a coagulase, which causes blood that is ingested by the flea to clot in the proventriculus, thus blocking the transit into the stomach of the flea. These "blocked" fleas are efficient vectors for plague infection because they regurgitate *Y. pestis* into the bite wound when they attempt to feed. The coagulase of *Y. pestis* is active at 28° C and at lower temperatures but is inactive at higher temperatures such as 35° C. This explains the cessation of plague transmission during the very hot seasons in tropical countries.

DISTRIBUTION AND EPIDEMIOLOGY. Plague is currently endemic in several countries of Africa, the Americas, and Asia. The widespread distribution of plague in the world during the last decade indicates that the infection is firmly entrenched in the world's rodent populations. Vietnam reported more cases than other countries during the 1970's, with a high of 4056 cases in 1970. After Vietnam, which reported a total of 13,786 cases during the decade, other countries with high incidences of human plague were Burma with 2795 cases, Brazil with 1464 cases, Kenya with 393 cases, Peru with 316 cases, Sudan with 226 cases, Bolivia with 219 cases, the United States with 105 cases, and Zaire with 95 cases. In the United States, plague occurs naturally in sylvatic rodents, such as ground squirrels and rock squirrels, and is geographically limited almost entirely to the Southwestern states of New Mexico, Arizona, Colorado, Nevada, and California.

Plague is primarily a zoonotic infection. It is transmitted among the natural animal reservoirs by flea bites or by ingestion of contaminated animal tissues. Throughout the world the domestic and urban rats, *Rattus rattus* and *R. norvegicus*, are the most important reservoirs of the plague bacillus. In sylvatic foci of plague, however, as occur in the United States, the important reservoirs are the ground squirrel, rock squirrel, and prairie dog. Humans are an accidental host in the natural cycle of plague and appear to play no role in the maintenance of plague in nature. Only rarely, during epidemics of pneumonic plague, is the infection passed directly from person to person. Also rarely does the infection develop in humans by the direct handling of contaminated animal tissues.

The occurrence of human plague is always linked to the transmission of plague among the natural animal reservoirs. The incidence of plague in humans for any particular locality is therefore a function of both the frequency of infection in local rodent populations and the intimacy with which the people live with the infected rodents and their fleas. Although humans develop acquired immunity after plague infection, the role of immunity in determining host susceptibility to infection of individuals in a population appears to be small.

Two other epidemiologic features of plague infection are its focal range and seasonality. Foci of active plague infection are typically limited to single villages and even to single city blocks, with the adjacent villages and blocks being entirely plague free. This striking local concentration of plague has been related to the parochial behavior of rats, which stay near one food supply for extended periods. Only during the transport of rodents by man, as on ships or trains, are infected rodents and thus epidemics of plague likely to spread to distant geographic areas.

Plague occurs predominantly in warm tropical climates. Epizootics tend to occur during humid warm seasons and are sharply curtailed during very hot seasons when average daily temperatures exceed 30° C and during very dry seasons. These seasonal fluctuations have been related to flea behavior and physiology. Humid conditions permit fleas to wait longer periods between blood meals so they can survive off the bodies of their rodent hosts during the search for new hosts. Furthermore, during the best seasons for plague transmission, fleas proliferate on their hosts, and when the flea index (ratio of fleas to rodents) exceeds 1, the conditions are usually optimal for a plague epidemic.

PATHOGENESIS AND CLINICAL FEATURES. Although plague infection of man can assume many varied clinical forms, the most common is bubonic plague, which presents a distinctive clinical picture. During an incubation period of two to eight days following a bite by an infected flea, bacteria proliferate in the regional lymph nodes. Patients are typically affected by the sudden onset of fever, chills, weakness, and headache. Usually at the same time, or after a few hours or the next day, patients notice the *bubo,* which is signaled by intense pain in one anatomic region of lymph nodes, usually the groin, axilla, or neck. A swelling evolves that is so tender that the patient typically avoids any motion that would provoke tenderness of the affected nodes.

The buboes of patients with plague are oval swellings varying from about 1 to 10 cm in length and elevating the overlying skin, which may appear stretched or erythematous. They may appear either as a smooth uniform egg-shaped mass or an irregular cluster of several nodes with intervening and surrounding edema. Palpation will typically elicit extreme tenderness. There is warmth of the overlying skin and an underlying, firm nonfluctuant mass. Usually around the lymph nodes there is considerable edema, which can be gelatinous or pitting in nature. Occasionally edema extends into the skin region drained by the affected lymph nodes. Although infections other than plague can produce acute lymphadenitis, plague is unique for the suddenness of onset of the fever and the bubo, the rapid development of intense inflammation in the bubo, and the fulminant clinical course that can produce death as quickly as two to four days after the onset of symptoms. The bubo of plague is also distinctive for the usual absence of a detectable skin lesion and likewise for the absence of an ascending lymphangitis nearby.

In uncomplicated *bubonic plague,* the patients are typically prostrate and lethargic and often exhibit restlessness or agitation. Occasionally they are delirious with high fever, and seizures are common in children. Temperature is usually in the range of 38.5 to 40.0° C, and the pulse rate is increased to 110 to 140 beats per minute. Blood pressure is characteristically low, in the range of 100/60 mm Hg, due to extreme vasodilation. Pressure determinations may be unobtainable if shock ensues. The liver and spleen are often palpable and tender.

The pathology of bubonic plague is unmistakable and characterized by hemorrhage and necrosis. The capsules of the lymph nodes are obliterated by the destructive inflammatory process that involves the periglandular tissues as much as the lymph nodes themselves. The normal architecture that separates cortex from medulla is destroyed. The lymphoid cells of the medulla are necrotic. There are large phagocytic cells, polymorphonuclear leukocytes, red cells, and a granular material that is a pure culture of plague bacilli. Blood vessels are thrombosed.

The majority of patients with bubonic plague do not have skin lesions. About a fourth of patients in Vietnam, however, did show varied skin findings. The most common were pustules, vesicles, eschars, or papules near the bubo or in the anatomic region of skin that is lymphatically drained by the affected lymph nodes. These presumably represent sites of flea bite inoculations. When these lesions are opened, they usually contain white cells and plague bacilli. These skin lesions rarely progress to extensive cellulitis or abscesses. Ulceration may lead, however, to a larger plague carbuncle.

Another kind of skin lesion in plague is purpura, which is a result of the systemic disease. The purpura may become necrotic, resulting in gangrene of distal extremities that is the probable basis of the term black death. These purpuric lesions result from vasculitis and occlusion by fibrin thrombi, resulting in hemorrhage and necrosis.

A distinctive feature of plague, in addition to the bubo, is the propensity for massive growth of bacteria in the blood. In the early acute stages of bubonic plague, all patients probably have intermittent bacteremia. Single blood cultures obtained at the time of hospital admission from Vietnamese patients were positive in 27 per cent of cases. A hallmark of moribund patients with plague is high-density bacteremia, so that a blood smear revealing characteristic bacilli has been used as a prognostic indicator in this disease. Occasionally in the pathogenesis of plague infection bacteria are inoculated and proliferate in the body without producing a bubo. Patients may actually die with bacteremia but without detectable lymphadenitis. This syndrome has been termed septicemic plague to denote plague without a bubo. Some authors have called bubonic plague with high-density bacteremia *bubonic-septicemic.*

One of the feared complications of bubonic plague is secondary pneumonia. The infection reaches the lungs by hematogenous spread of bacteria from the bubo. In addition to the high mortality, plague pneumonia is highly contagious by airborne transmission. It is characterized by fever and lymphadenopathy with cough, chest pain, and often hemoptysis. Radiographically there is patchy bronchopneumonia or confluent consolidation. The sputum is usually purulent and contains plague bacilli.

Primary inhalation pneumonia is rare now but is a potential threat to the individual exposed to a patient with plague who has a cough. The disease can be so rapidly fatal that persons reportedly have been exposed, become ill, and died on the same day. Plague pneumonia is invariably fatal when antibiotic therapy is delayed more than 20 hours after the onset of illness.

Plague meningitis is a rarer complication and typically occurs more than a week after inadequately treated bubonic plague. It results from hematogenous spread from a bubo and carries a high mortality rate when compared with uncomplicated bubonic plague. There appears to be a strong association between buboes located in the axilla and the development of meningitis. Less commonly, plague meningitis appears as a primary infection without antecedent lymphadenitis. Plague meningitis is characterized by fever, headache, meningismus, and pleocytosis with a predominance of polymorphonuclear leukocytes. Bacteria are frequently demonstrable with a Gram stain of spinal fluid sediment, and endotoxin has been demonstrated in spinal fluid by the limulus gelation assay.

Plague can produce *pharyngitis* that may resemble acute tonsillitis. The anterior cervical lymph nodes are usually inflamed, and *Y. pestis* may be recovered from a throat culture or aspiration of a cervical bubo. This is a rare clinical form of plague that is presumed to follow the inhalation or ingestion of plague bacilli. In some societies, plague pharyngitis occurs predominantly in women and has been related to their practice of searching the hair for lice or fleas and killing them by crushing between the teeth.

LABORATORY FEATURES. The white blood cell count is typically elevated in the range of 10,000 to 20,000 cells per cubic millimeter, with a predominance of immature and mature neutrophils. Patients who are most severely ill tend to have higher counts. Occasionally some patients, especially children, may develop myelocytic leukemoid reactions with white cell counts as high as 100,000 per cubic millimeter. The white blood cells in the peripheral blood typically show cytoplasmic vacuolations, toxic granulations, and Dohle bodies that are characteristic of acute bacterial infections. Blood platelet counts may be normal or low in the early stages of bubonic plague. Although a generalized bleeding tendency from profound thrombocytopenia is rare, disseminated intravascular coagulation (DIC) is common. Fibrinogen-fibrin degradation products in the serum that are indicative of DIC were detected in elevated titers in most patients tested in Vietnam.

DIAGNOSIS. Plague should be suspected in febrile patients who have been exposed to rodents or other mammals in the known endemic areas of the world. A bacteriologic diagnosis is readily made in most patients by smear and culture of a bubo aspirate. The aspirate is obtained by inserting a 20-gauge needle on a 10-ml syringe containing 1 ml of sterile saline solution into the bubo and aspirating several times until the saline solution has become blood-tinged. Because the bubo does not contain liquid pus, it may be necessary to inject some of the saline solution and to immediately reaspirate it. Drops of the aspirate should be placed on microscope slides and air-dried for both Gram and Wayson's stains. The Gram stain will reveal polymorphonuclear leukocytes and gram-negative coccobacilli and bacilli ranging from 1 to 2 μm in length. With Wayson's stain *Y. pestis* appear as light blue bacilli with dark blue polar bodies, and the remainder of the slide has a contrasting pink counterstain. Smears of blood, sputum, or spinal fluid can be handled similarly.

The aspirate, blood, and other appropriate fluids should be inoculated onto blood and MacConkey's agar plates and into infusion broth. The organism is identified in triple sugar–iron agar by an alkaline slant and acid butt without gas or H_2S, by negative urease and indole reactions, by failure to utilize citrate, and by nonmotility. For definitive identification, cultures can be mailed in double containers to the Centers for Disease Control, Plague Branch, P.O. Box 2087, Fort Collins, Colorado 80422 (telephone no.: 303-482-0213). At this same laboratory, a serologic test, the passive hemagglutination test utilizing Fraction 1 of *Y. pestis*, can be performed on acute- and convalescent-phase serum. For patients with negative cultures, a four-fold or greater increase in titer or a single titer of greater than or equal to 1:16 is presumptive evidence for plague infection.

The differential diagnosis of bubonic plague includes tularemia, streptococcal and staphylococcal lymphadenitis, secondary syphilis, and lymphogranuloma venereum. For pneumonia, the physician also should consider common forms of bacterial and viral pneumonia. For meningitis and septicemia, the common bacterial causes need to be assessed by age groups.

TREATMENT AND PROGNOSIS. Untreated plague has an estimated mortality of greater than 50 per cent and can evolve into a fulminant illness complicated by septic shock. Therefore the early institution of effective antibiotic therapy is mandatory. In 1948, streptomycin was identified as the drug of choice for the treatment of plague by reducing mortality to less than 5 per cent. No other drug has been demonstrated to be more efficacious or less toxic. Streptomycin should be administered intramuscularly in two divided doses daily, totaling 30 mg per kilogram of body weight per day for ten days. Most patients improve rapidly and become afebrile in about three days. The ten-day course is recommended to prevent relapses because viable bacteria have been isolated from buboes of patients with plague during convalescence. The risk of vestibular damage and hearing loss caused by streptomycin is minimal during a ten-day course. This antibiotic should be used cautiously, however, during pregnancy, in older patients who would have trouble adapting to vestibular damage, and in patients with previous hearing difficulty. In such patients, the course of streptomycin can be shortened to three days after the patient becomes afebrile. Renal injury as a result of streptomycin therapy is rare with this regimen; however, renal function should be monitored. If the serum creatinine concentration rises significantly, the dose of streptomycin should be reduced. In mild renal failure the recommended dose is about 20 mg per kilogram per day and in advanced renal failure 8 mg per kilogram every three days. Most preparations of streptomycin available in the United States are in an oil base and can be administered only intramuscularly.

For patients allergic to streptomycin or for whom an oral drug is strongly preferred, tetracycline is a satisfactory alternative. It is administered orally in a dose of 2 to 4 grams per day in four divided doses for ten days. Tetracycline is contraindicated in children under seven years of age and in pregnant women in order to avoid staining of developing teeth. It is also contraindicated in patients with renal failure.

For patients with meningitis who will require a drug that penetrates well into the cerebrospinal fluid and for patients with profound hypotension in whom an intramuscular injection may not be well absorbed, chloramphenicol should be administered intravenously with a loading dose of 25 mg per kilogram of body weight followed by 60 mg per kilogram per day in four divided doses. After clinical improvement oral chloramphenicol administration should be continued to complete a total course of ten days; the dosage may be reduced to 30 mg per kilogram per day to reduce the magnitude of bone marrow suppression, which is reversible after completion of therapy.

Antibiotic resistance in human isolates of *Y. pestis* has never been reported, nor has resistance emerged during antibiotic therapy. The three antibiotics streptomycin, tetracycline, and chloramphenicol given alone are clinically very effective and relapses are exceedingly rare. Therefore, there is no rationale for using multiple antibiotics to treat plague.

Because patients are febrile and often have nausea or vomiting, hypotension, and dehydration, intravenous 0.9 per cent saline solution should be given to most patients for the first few days of the illness or until improvement occurs. Patients in shock will require additional quantities of fluid with hemodynamic monitoring and the judicious use of epinephrine or dopamine. There is no evidence that corticosteroids are beneficial in plague. Although disseminated intravascular coagulation is commonly present and purpura occasionally develops in severely ill patients, therapy with heparin has no proven benefit in plague infections.

The buboes usually recede without need of local therapy. Occasionally, however, they may enlarge or become fluctuant during the first week of treatment and require incision and drainage. The aspirated fluid should be cultured for evidence of superinfection, but this material is usually sterile.

PREVENTION. All patients with suspected plague should be reported to a health department and to the World Health Organization. Patients with uncomplicated infections who are promptly treated present no health hazards to other persons. Those with cough or other signs of pneumonia must be placed in strict respiratory isolation for at least 48 hours after the start of antibiotic therapy or until the sputum culture is negative. The bubo aspirate and blood must be handled with gloves. Standard bacteriologic techniques that safeguard against skin contact with and aerosolization of infected fluids and cultures should be adequate to protect laboratory personnel.

A formalin-killed vaccine, plague vaccine U.S.P. (Cutter Laboratories, Berkeley, California 94710) is available for travelers to epidemic or hyperendemic areas, for individuals who must live and work in close contact with wild rodents, and for laboratory workers who must handle live *Y. pestis* cultures. A primary series of two injections is recommended with a one- to three-month interval between them. Booster injections are given every six months for as long as exposure continues. In addition, persons living in endemic areas should protect themselves against rodents and fleas. Measures include living in rat-proof houses, wearing shoes and garments to cover the legs, and application of insecticide dusts to houses.

The control of plague by health departments requires knowledge of the epidemiology of infected animals, vectors, and the contact of humans with these animals in any particular area. In the United States the Plague Branch of the Centers for Disease Control in Fort Collins, Colorado, has a field team of entomologists, mammalogists, and epidemiologists to investigate cases of plague. A specific approach to each case should be chosen and usually consists of insecticide use around homes, trapping of animals, and education of people to avoid contact with certain animals. Urban plague has been successfully controlled in many cities around the world by quarantine, rat control, and insecticide use.

Brubaker RR: The genus *Yersinia:* Biochemistry and genetics of virulence. Curr Top Microbiol Immunol 57:111, 1972. *A review of features of the plague bacillus that render it virulent.*

Butler T: A clinical study of bubonic plague. Observations of the 1970 Vietnam epidemic with emphasis on coagulation studies, skin histology, and electrocardiograms. Am J Med 53:268, 1972. *This paper describes clinical features of serious cases in Vietnam.*

Butler T: Plague and other *Yersinia* infections. New York, Plenum Publishing Corp., 1983. *This recent monograph gives full clinical description and contemporary literature citations.*

Pollitzer R: Plague. Mongraph Series. Geneva, World Health Organization, 1954. *This is a classic monograph covering older literature.*

Reed WP, Palmer DL, Williams RC, Kisch AL: Bubonic plague in the Southwestern United States: A review of recent experience. Medicine 49:465, 1970. *This is a good review of cases in the United States.*

Other Yersinia Infections

DEFINITION. The non-plague yersinioses are caused by *Yersinia enterocolitica* and *Y. pseudotuberculosis*. These gram-negative rod bacteria produce fever, diarrhea, and abdominal pain that can mimic acute appendicitis. The common pathologic lesions in yersiniosis are acute enteritis and mesenteric lymphadenitis. Extraintestinal disease may result from septicemia or appear as arthritis and erythema nodosum.

ETIOLOGY. The *Yersiniae* are members of the bacterial order Enterobacteriaceae. Accordingly, they are gram-negative rods that are oxidase negative and grow on agars containing bile salts. They do not ferment lactose and grow faster at 25° C than at 37° C. Of the 34 different O serotypes of *Y. enterocolitica* that have been identified, the ones most commonly associated with human disease are types 3 and 9 in Canada and Europe and type 8 in the United States. Like other gram-negative bacteria, the *Yersiniae* contain a lipopolysaccharide endotoxin in the cell wall that may be responsible, in part, for the fever and inflammation. *Y. enterocolitica* elaborates an enterotoxin that is plasmid mediated, resembles the heat-stable enterotoxin of *Escherichia coli*, and may cause the diarrhea associated with this infection.

EPIDEMIOLOGY. The yersinioses are distributed worldwide. Large numbers of confirmed cases have been reported in Europe, Canada, the United States, and Japan. This infection has also been reported from Africa and Asia, but little information is available on the incidence of infection in tropical areas. In the United States, infection with *Y. enterocolitica* appears to be rare when compared with infection with *Salmonella* and *Shigella* species, but in other countries such as Finland and Sweden the incidence of infection is higher. Both adults and children are susceptible to infection. Males acquire the infection more commonly than females. The natural reservoirs of *Y. enterocolitica* are farm animals, especially pigs and goats, and other domestic animals, including dogs and cats. The natural reservoirs of *Y. pseudotuberculosis* include birds and other diverse domestic and farm animals. These animals harbor the bacteria in their intestines and excrete them in feces. Humans become infected by ingesting food or water contaminated by animal feces or directly by the ingestion of certain fomites. Person-to-person transmission seems to be rare. In the United States, well-defined outbreaks of *Y. enterocolitica* infection have occurred in a North Carolina family with a sick dog, in a New York school at which chocolate milk was the source of infection, in members of a Brownie scout troop in Pennsylvania who ate infected bean sprouts, and in persons who drank milk from a dairy in Tennessee. There are no clear seasonal patterns of infection.

PATHOGENESIS OF CLINICAL SYNDROMES. An inoculum with as many as 10^9 organisms may be required to produce infection. During the incubation period, estimated at four to ten days, bacteria proliferate in the small bowel; invade the mucosa, especially that of the ileum; and elicit an acute inflammatory response. Ulcerations may occur and polymorphonuclear leukocytes appear in the stool. Some bacteria migrate via the lymphatics to the mesenteric lymph nodes, where inflammation occurs. The initial symptoms incude fever and either diarrhea or abdominal pain. In these instances, the corresponding pathologic finding is terminal ileitis or mesenteric lymphadenitis or both. The colon is less frequently affected, but aphthoid ulcers and hemorrhagic colitis have been described in yersiniosis. The tissues are affected by acute inflammation, thrombosis of blood vessels, hemorrhage, and necrosis. The diarrhea results from the mucosal invasion by bacteria or the action of an enterotoxin. Diarrhea varies from semisolid or watery to grossly bloody. In some patients the abdominal pain is severe and located in the right lower quadrant and may be mistaken for appendicitis; the appendix is usually normal. A few days later, some patients may develop extraintestinal complications of arthralgias, arthritis, and erythema nodosum. Since the synovial and cutaneous tissues in these syndromes are sterile, an immunologic reaction has been postulated to explain their pathogenesis. Arthritis is more likely to occur in individuals of haplotype HLA-B27, and erythema nodosum occurs more commonly in women. Septicemia is a rare complication that occurs in the setting of prior liver disease, malignancies, or immunosuppressive therapy. Rarer clinical forms of yersiniosis include pneumonia, pharyngitis, and meningitis. Antibodies appear in the blood against the O and other antigens of *Y. enterocolitica*, and nearly all infections are self-limited. However, fatalities have occurred from extensive ulceration and necrosis of the intestine and septicemia.

DIAGNOSIS. The diagnosis requires the isolation of *Yersiniae* from stool, blood, or surgical specimens. The number of bacteria in stool may be small, and a cold-enrichment technique may be required. A rectal swab or piece of stool is placed into 0.067 M phosphate-buffered saline solution at a pH of 7.6 and incubated at 4° C for four weeks. Most other stool bacteria die, whereas *Y. enterocolitica* will grow. At weekly intervals, subcultures should be made on MacConkey agar. Identification is made by finding non-lactose-fermenting colonies that on triple sugar–iron agar give an acid-acid reaction (*Y. enterocolitica*) or alkaline-acid reaction (*Y. pseudotuberculosis*) without gas or hydrogen sulfide, are positive for urease, and are motile at 25° C but nonmotile at 37° C. *Y. enterocolitica* gives a positive reaction for ornithine decarboxylase, whereas *Y. pseudotuberculosis* does not. A diagnosis can be made from serologic test results by showing a rise in agglutinin titer in paired serum specimens. The existence of cross-reacting antigens in the genera *Brucella*, *Vibrio*, and *Salmonella* indicates that false-positive serologic results sometimes occur.

TREATMENT AND PROGNOSIS. Yersiniosis is usually self-limited and so rarely diagnosed that it is impossible to assess the possible benefits of antibiotic treatment. Most isolates of *Y. enterocolitica* are susceptible to streptomycin, gentamicin, tetracycline, chloramphenicol, and sulfamethoxazole-trimethoprim and resistant to the penicillins and cephalosporin antibiotics. *Y. pseudotuberculosis* isolates usually have been susceptible to penicillin. It is important to suspect the diagnosis in patients with severe abdominal pain to avoid unnecessary surgery for appendicitis. The recognition that early fever accompanies yersiniosis may be helpful, as is epidemiologic information pertaining to outbreaks in the community.

PREVENTION AND CONTROL. The presumed origin of *Y. enterocolitica* infection in farm and domestic animals suggests that transmission may be similar to that of *Salmonella*. Meat and dairy products and other farm produce should periodically be examined for *Y. enterocolitica* content. During outbreaks, public health authorities should identify sources of infection in food (especially milk), water, or persons.

Bottone EJ: *Yersinia enterocolitica:* A panoramic view of a charismatic organism. CRC Crit Rev Microbiol 5:211, 1977. *A useful review of microbiologic aspects of these infections.*

Carter PB, Lafleur L, Toma S: *Yersinia enterocolitica:* Biology, epidemiology, and pathology. Contrib Microbiol Immunol 5, 1979. *This volume contains research papers given at a symposium and is excellent for the serious student of these diseases.*

Kohl S: *Yersinia enterocolitica* infections. Pediatr Clin North Am 26:433, 1979. *This clinical discussion emphasizes disease syndromes in children.*

Vantrappen G, Agg HO, Geboes K, Ponette E: *Yersinia enteritis.* Med Clin North Am 66:639, 1982. *This article contains a good clinical description of gastroenterologic features of the disease.*

288. TULAREMIA

Richard B. Hornick

DEFINITION. Tularemia is a rare infectious disease in the United States caused by a small gram-negative pleomorphic rod, *Francisella tularensis*. This organism is acquired from an animal reservoir, frequently cottontail rabbits, by direct contact with diseased animal tissues, the bite of an infected tick or deer fly, ingestion of contaminated food or water, and inhalation of aerosolized bacteria. Clinical manifestations usually include a cutaneous ulcer with enlargement of regional lymph nodes. Rarely, a pneumonitis will result from inhalation of *F. tularensis* or secondary spread from the skin ulcer and lymph nodes. Confirmation of the diagnosis by cultural technique is not advocated because of the high contagion risk to personnel handling this organism. The therapeutic response to effective antibiotic therapy is rapid.

HISTORICAL FEATURES. The typhoidal form of tularemia was first described in Japan in 1818. The disease was thought to be due to ingestion of "poisonous hare meat." In 1890 in Norway, the tularemia bacillus was isolated from ill lemmings. A clear description of the organism occurred in 1906 when McCoy uncovered a "plague-like" disease among ground squirrels in Tulare County, California. Francis coined the name tularemia to honor the American geographic site of identification and also to stress that the disease was frequently bacteremic in animals. In Japan, tularemia may be referred to as Ohara's disease, or Yato-byo (wild hare disease).

ETIOLOGY, SPECIFIC LABORATORY DIAGNOSIS, AND EPIDEMIOLOGY. *F. tularensis* is a small gram-negative pleomorphic rod-shaped bacterium. Organisms are not seen in smears of infected tissue unless special staining techniques are used. Fluorescent antibody conjugate staining and modified Dieterle staining are the best methods for demonstrating them. All tularemia strains are serologically identical, but there are biochemical and virulence differences for mammals that have allowed differentiation of two strains. These are called Jellison A and B; the former, found only in North America, is lethal for domestic rabbits *(Oryctolagus)* and causes severe disease in man. The unique biochemical capabilities of this strain—e.g., it ferments glycerol and contains citrulline ureidase—do not explain its increased virulence. Strain B lacks these biochemical features, is not lethal for cottontails, causes milder disease in man, usually is isolated from rodents or from water, and is distributed over Europe, Asia, and North America. Reasons for the differences in virulence are unknown.

Culture Methods. The direct isolation of *F. tularensis* from blood (rarely), pus from ulcers or buboes, sputum, or pharyngeal or gastric aspirations in a patient with pneumonitis can be achieved by two methods. This is a class 4 organism requiring an effective hood or an adequate isolation laboratory to prevent human disease or epizootics. The two methods for isolation are intraperitoneal inoculation of guinea pigs and direct plating of a specimen onto glucose cysteine blood agar, cystine heart agar, or eugon agar. As few as one to five viable organisms will cause death of guinea pigs in five to ten days. Appropriate facilities are needed to prevent spread of the disease to other animals. The media employed to isolate the organism usually contain drugs to suppress other flora and allow the tularemia colonies to be visible. Useful additions are 0.1 mg of cycloheximide and 20 units of penicillin per milliliter of media. The colonies are small on these media; they appear in 48 to 72 hours of incubation at 37° C.

Serologic Diagnosis. The measurement of serum agglutinating antibodies is a useful and safer method of diagnosing tularemia. Titers begin to rise in about seven to ten days and peak in three to four weeks. Paired serum specimens obtained two weeks apart and demonstrating a four-fold or greater rise are diagnostic of tularemia. However, a single specimen with a titer of 1:160 or greater in a patient thought to have tularemia on clinical grounds is diagnostic. Antibiotic therapy does not appear to dampen the antibody response. Titers remain elevated for six to eight months and then decline in the subsequent one to one and a half years to low or undetectable levels. There is a cross-reaction with brucella antigen during the early phase of the antibody response. The brucella titer falls off faster than and is never so high as the tularemia titer.

Skin Testing. A skin test antigen has proved to be reliable for diagnostic and epidemiologic purposes. A positive test result, similar in appearance to a tuberculin test response, is present during the first week of illness, frequently before the agglutinins are detectable, and remains positive for years. There is no known cross-reacting skin test antigen. The antigen is derived from *F. tularensis* by ether extraction; however, it is not commonly available. It can be obtained from the Centers for Disease Control, Atlanta. In 10 per cent of patients, the skin test antigen may boost pre-existing agglutinating antibody titers. Skin test reactivity can be shown to be associated with sensitized lymphocytes.

Epidemiology. Tularemia is a sporadic disease; man acquires it when he is bitten by an infected tick or deer fly or when he handles an infected animal. In the process of field dressing a rabbit or skinning a muskrat, the hands may become contaminated with infected blood, subcutaneous abscesses, or liver and spleen that contain millions of organisms. The act of eviscerating the animal can create an aerosol that can be inhaled. The ingestion of contaminated water or food is the least likely method of acquiring tularemia. Many carnivores such as dogs, cats, bull snakes, and others may feed on diseased rabbits. This results in contamination of the teeth and saliva. These animals are relatively resistant to tularemia. Contact with the teeth of a pet dog or cat has resulted in ulceroglandular tularemia. Studies in volunteers have quantitated the susceptibility of man to infection and disease and the virulence of *F. tularensis* for man. As few as 50 type A organisms injected subcutaneously will cause ulceroglandular disease. Pneumonic tularemia can be induced by a similar inoculum size if the aerosolized and inhaled particles are small (less than 5 microns). Type B organisms require an inoculum about 1000 times larger to induce ulceroglandular or respiratory disease in man.

The incidence of tularemia is low, fewer than 200 cases a year having been reported in each of the past ten years. The peak incidence was in 1939, when almost 2300 cases were reported. Laws passed at that time prohibited the sale of wild rabbits, especially cottontails, and this legislation plus increased public awareness of the danger of handling sick or dying wild animals has contributed to the decline. Most cases occur in the Midwest, but the disease is not restricted to any one geographic location in the United States. Cottontail rabbits in urban and suburban areas throughout the country provide the reservoir from which tularemia can occur. Epizootics among these or other animals can cause epidemics in man. Tularemia has been reported only north of the thirtieth parallel. The cottontail rabbit is not found in Europe; various rodents such as voles, muskrats, and hares carry *F. tularensis* (Jellison B type) in that part of the world. Diseased jack rabbits, found west of the Mississippi River, may be an important source of contamination of ticks and deer flies.

In the summer months, most cases of tularemia are caused by tick or deer fly bites. Ulceroglandular disease begins with an ulcer at the site of the bite, e.g., groin, axilla, or scalp. In the fall, during hunting season, sporadic cases, usually ulceroglandular, occur among hunters and trappers. In the Scandinavian countries, epidemics have occurred in the winter months when farmers handling stored hay contaminated by diseased voles inhaled *F. tularensis* and developed pneumonic tularemia.

MECHANISMS OF INFECTION AND PATHOLOGY. The most common form of tularemia results from the penetration of *F. tularensis* into the skin. This penetration may be through hair follicles or minute areas of trauma. The development of the subsequent disease takes two to six days, depending upon the number of bacteria and their virulence. The organisms multiply in the dermis and induce a marked inflammatory process consisting primarily of mononuclear cells with a perivascular distribution. This process produces an erythematous tender papule. The inflamed area continues to swell until the induced ischemia causes the skin to ulcerate. The base of the ulcer becomes black and depressed. The edges are sharply demarcated. At the time of penetration some organisms may be phagocytized and transported in the lymph to regional nodes. There is no clinically apparent lymphangitis. The nodes enlarge and become painful when caseation occurs. Histologic sections reveal geographic necrosis and disruption of the capsule. Fluctuation of the node is a late and rare event. It may then rupture.

The necrotic, purulent, painful lymph node is termed a bubo. Healing of a bubo takes months even with appropriate antibiotic treatment. Aspiration of an unruptured node may lead to an indolent draining sinus tract. *F. tularensis* may remain in the necrotic tissue and purulent drainage for many weeks. The ulcer heals slowly and usually leaves a depigmented, rounded area in the skin.

Oculoglandular tularemia may occur when the conjunctival sac is infected from an ulcer or contaminated finger. Small yellowish granulomatous lesions develop on the palpebral conjunctivae, accompanied by enlargement of the preauricular lymph nodes. In untreated patients the cornea may perforate.

Inhaled small particle aerosols (<5 microns in diameter) containing *F. tularensis* (usually type A) are ultimately deposited in the terminal bronchioles and alveoli, although infection of the trachea and large bronchi also occurs. A peribronchial inflammation develops with infiltration by neutrophils and mononuclear cells. This produces necrosis of alveolar walls and results in localized pneumonitis. In man, small areas of pneumonitis represent the most common findings on chest roentgenograms. Often these are ill defined and difficult to interpret. Lobar consolidation or lung abscesses represent extensive spread and necrosis. These are infrequent in man. Mediastinal and peritracheal lymph nodes enlarge and may be apparent on chest x-ray films. They may be partially responsible, along with the bronchitis, for the substernal burning that is common in patients with tularemic pneumonia. The incubation period for this form of tularemia varies inversely with the size and virulence of the inhaled inoculum. Following an inoculum of 10 to 50 organisms, disease appears in about four to seven days in volunteers.

Typhoidal tularemia follows systemic spread of *F. tularensis* from the oropharynx and probably the gastrointestinal tract when a huge inoculum is swallowed. Enlargement of cervical lymph nodes, and presumably nodes in the mesentery, occurs. This latter process causes abdominal pain and is associated with an ileus. This is the most unusual form of tularemia in this country.

CLINICAL MANIFESTATIONS. Disease initiated by a tick bite is manifested by an ulcer at the site or adjacent to it. The tick defecates after feeding, and the infected feces may be scratched into the epidermis. Usually the lesion will be in the inguinal, axillary, or scalp skin. If contact with tularemia organisms results from the handling of an infected animal, an ulcerative lesion evolves in the skin of the hands, frequently around a fingernail. This lesion may be so trivial that it is ignored by the patient. The ulcer is depressed into the dermis, has sharply demarcated edges, and gradually develops a black base. In the initial stage of development the lesion produces a thick, yellowish exudate. Regional lymph nodes enlarge and are tender to palpation. Fever and chills are common. The temperature curve is usually remittent or continuous in character. Without antibiotic therapy, most patients remain febrile for several weeks, the ulcer heals slowly over weeks to months, and the enlarged lymph nodes persist for months. Untreated patients may occasionally develop a secondary necrotizing pneumonia as a consequence of bacteremia. These patients may be acutely ill.

Primary tularemia pneumonia presents with the sudden development of substernal burning and a nonproductive paroxysmal cough associated with fever and chills. Headache, myalgia, photophobia, malaise, and prostration are common findings. The temperature elevates quickly to 39.4 to 40° C and remains at that level (continuous fever curve) until antibiotic treatment is given. Sixty to 70 per cent of patients will survive without specific therapy, and in these a slow defervescence occurs over several months. X-ray of the lungs may reveal ill-defined, scattered oval areas of infiltration, with enlarged peritracheal lymph nodes. Pleural effusions, lobar consolidation, and lung abscess are other manifestations of this form of tularemia. Cervical lymph nodes are palpable and tender.

DIAGNOSIS AND DIFFERENTIAL DIAGNOSIS. The diagnosis of ulceroglandular tularemia is made by the clinical manifestations and serologic studies. Paired serum specimens collected over a two- to three-week period are required to demonstrate a fourfold rise in titer. A baseline agglutinin titer of 1:160 in a patient with a history of an indolent ulcer for two or more weeks is diagnostic of tularemia. Culture of an ulcer and blood should be performed only if the hospital laboratory has appropriate protective isolation hoods. Patients with sporotrichosis or *Mycobacterium marinum* infections may have ulcers suggestive of tularemia but are usually afebrile. Enlarged lymph nodes extending centripetally as a beaded chain are a characteristic finding in sporotrichosis. Lesions of the fingers infected with staphylococci or beta streptococci usually produce more pus and may be associated with lymphangitis. *B. anthracis* can produce an ulcer (anthrax) with black-based, sharply demarcated edges similar to that initiated by *F. tularensis*. A careful history and serologic data will help in the differential diagnosis. In patients in whom any form of tularemia is suspected, the use of the skin test antigen will be helpful. The test result is usually positive prior to the development of agglutinating antibodies.

Tularemia pneumonia must be differentiated from the more common bacterial, viral, and mycoplasmal pneumonias. The history and the presence of ulceroglandular disease are helpful. Skin testing and serologic studies are diagnostic. The chest x-ray may yield suggestive findings consisting of ill-defined, small, oval, multiple infiltrates but is not diagnostic.

Patients infected with *F. tularensis* usually have a normal leukocyte count with an elevation of the sedimentation rate and a positive C-reactive protein (CRP) determination. The white count is elevated when a bubo or a lung abscess is present.

COMPLICATIONS. Pericarditis and meningitis are rare events that usually occur in patients who have been misdiagnosed and have received inappropriate treatment. Pericarditis results from direct extension of the infection from the purulent, necrotic mediastinal lymph nodes or the involved lung. Constrictive pericarditis has been reported. Meningitis develops rarely, represents a seeding of the meninges during bacteremia, and is characterized by a lymphocytic pleocytosis in the cerebrospinal fluid.

TREATMENT. Patients with all forms of tularemia respond to the following antibiotics: streptomycin, gentamicin, tetracycline, and chloramphenicol. The aminoglycoside antibiotics are recommended, since they produce a prompt cure of patients with the most severe form of tularemia. Patients with pneumonitis are afebrile within 24 to 48 hours and do not relapse. Ulcers and tender lymph nodes heal over a period of seven to ten days. Gentamicin, 5 mg per kilogram per day in divided doses, is given for ten days. Streptomycin was the principal drug for treating tularemia before gentamicin; 1 gram is given every 12 hours for ten days. Treatment with tetracycline or chloramphenicol may produce an equally rapid response, but relapses occur in 15 to 20 per cent of the patients. These drugs are not recommended unless gentamicin or streptomycin is contraindicated. Doses of 3 to 4 grams of tetracycline or 3 grams of chloramphenicol daily for ten days can be employed. Naturally acquired resistance to any of these antibiotics has not been found.

Patients with ulceroglandular tularemia respond well to these antibiotics. Fluctuant lymph nodes should not be aspirated until the patient has finished the course of the antibiotic treatment. Isolation of patients with any form of tularemia is not required; there is no evidence of person-to-person spread.

PROGNOSIS. The mortality rate for untreated ulceroglandular disease is about 5 per cent. Patients infected with type B strains and untreated probably have a mortality rate less than 1 per cent. Many of these patients probably go undiagnosed, as the disease is mild and self-limiting. Treatment with antibiotics prevents death and promotes healing in a week to ten days.

The mortality rate for pneumonic tularemia in the preantibiotic period was 30 to 60 per cent. Treatment with streptomycin or tetracycline has lowered this figure to less than 1 per cent. Healing occurs without residual lung damage or deficits in pulmonary function.

PREVENTION. Patients who recover from tularemia have a high degree of resistance to reinfection. If *F. tularensis* is reintroduced into the skin, a positive skin test reaction ensues without ulceration. Resistance to pulmonary disease may be associated with sensitized lymphocytes and alveolar macrophages.

A live attenuated strain of *F. tularensis* has been prepared as a vaccine. This can be administered by the acupuncture route, and it produces excellent immunity. The vaccine can be obtained from the Commander, U.S. Army Medical Research Institute of Infectious Diseases, Frederick, Maryland 21701. Its use is limited to persons considered at high risk such as selected laboratory workers, forest rangers, game wardens, and perhaps others known to be exposed during an outbreak. The vaccine exerts its effect through the stimulation of cellular immune mechanisms. Circulating agglutinins are not associated with resistance to disease.

Buchanan TM, Brooks GF, Brachman PS: The tularemia skin test; 325 skin tests in 210 persons: Serologic correlation and review of the literature. Ann Intern Med 74:336, 1971. *This study is an extension of the study reported by Young et al. (see below). It clearly presents proof of the efficacy of the skin test as a diagnostic test for tularemia. In addition it shows the amount of antigen stimulation needed to cause a conversion to a positive reactor.*

Francis E: The occurrence of tularemia in nature as a disease of man. Public Health Rep 36:1731, 1921. *A classic paper demonstrating the transmission experiments documenting the role of the deer fly and lice in spreading tularemia from infected animals to uninfected rabbits, also showing that nasal washings of rabbits could be a source of virulent organisms. The author cites the chronicity of tularemia in man untreated with antibiotics and reports one of the first fatal cases of ulceroglandular disease in man.*

Saslaw S, Carlisle HN: Studies with tularemia vaccine in volunteers. IV. Brucella agglutinins in vaccinated and unvaccinated volunteers challenged with *Pasteurella tularensis.* Am J Med Sci 242:70, 1961. *This was the fourth paper in the series dealing with volunteers infected with tularemia. Earlier studies documented the minimal infective dose for man, and this study differentiated serologic responses to tularemia and brucella antigens.*

Tärnvik A, Sandström G, Löfgren S: Time of lymphocyte response after onset of tularemia and after tularemia vaccination. J Clin Microbiol 10:854, 1979. *Presents evidence on the development of cellular immunity in patients with tularemia or who have received the attenuated vaccine.*

Teutsch SM, Marone WJ, Brink EW, Potter ME, Eliot G, Hoxsie R, Craven RB, Kaufman AF: Pneumonic tularemia on Martha's Vineyard. N Engl J Med 301:826, 1979. *This study illustrates the suddenness with which tularemia may appear in a geographic area. Furthermore it indicates a unique mechanism by which man can acquire pneumonic tularemia.*

Young LS, Bicknell DS, Archer BG, Clinton JM, Leavens LJ, Feeley JC, Brachman PS: Tularemia epidemic: Vermont, 1968. Forty-seven cases linked to contact with muskrats. N Engl J Med 280:1253, 1969. *This represents one of the largest outbreaks occurring in the United States in the past 20 years. It is one of the best described epidemiologic studies of infection caused by the Jellison type B organism.*

289. ANTHRAX

Philip S. Brachman

DEFINITION. Anthrax is a zoonotic disease transmitted to humans through contact with animals or animal products. Its primary forms are cutaneous, inhalational, and gastrointestinal. Occasionally, meningitis and septicemia occur, almost always secondary to one of the primary forms. In the United States, the most common form of the disease is the cutaneous lesion; inhalation anthrax occurs rarely; gastrointestinal anthrax has never been reported in the United States. Synonyms for anthrax include charbon, malignant pustule, Siberian ulcer, malignant edema, splenic fever, milzbrand, woolsorter's disease, and ragpicker's disease.

ETIOLOGY. *Bacillus anthracis* is a gram-positive, nonmotile, spore-forming bacillus (1 to 1.3 $m\mu \times 3$ to 10 $m\mu$) that on ordinary laboratory media at 35 to 37° C produces round, grayish white, ground-glass–appearing, convex, tenacious colonies 2 to 5 mm in diameter with comma-shaped projections. Microscopic examination of artificial media growth shows long parallel chains of organisms, referred to as "boxcars." Material from a fresh lesion reveals shorter chains with individual organisms having slightly rounded ends. Fluorescent antibody staining and a specific gamma bacteriophage can be used to identify *B. anthracis.* Parenteral inoculation of mice, guinea pigs, or rabbits with agar-grown cells or washed liquid growth will result in death in 24 to 72 hours.

B. anthracis spores may persist for years in the industrial or agricultural environment.

INCIDENCE AND PREVALENCE. In 1975–1976 the worldwide incidence of anthrax was 1651 cases, undoubtedly an underestimate. Reports to the World Health Organization (WHO) concerning anthrax in countries throughout the world are inaccurate and sporadic. Cutaneous anthrax is reported to be endemic in Haiti, South Africa, and several Asiatic countries. Occasionally, inhalation anthrax is reported from some industrialized countries, primarily in Europe, and is directly related to processing hair or wool. Gastrointestinal anthrax is occasionally reported from some African and Asiatic countries and from Russia.

In the United States, the average annual occurrence in 1916–1925 was 127 cases, and in 1974–1983, 1.3 cases. Ninety-five per cent of the cases in the United States are cutaneous; the other five per cent are inhalational. Twenty of the 231 cases reported from 1955 through 1983 were fatal, for a case-fatality rate (CFR) of 8.7 per cent. Two hundred and twenty cases with 11 deaths were cutaneous (CFR, 5 per cent); 11 cases with 9 deaths were inhalational (CFR, 82 per cent). Anthrax meningitis occurs in less than 5 per cent of the cases.

EPIDEMIOLOGY. Cases are classified as either industrial (80 per cent) or agricultural (20 per cent). Industrial anthrax results from contact with animal products, usually from Asia or Africa, including goat hair, wool, hides and skin, and animal bones. Transmission is by direct contact with contaminated animal products, or by indirect contact with a contaminated environment or with airborne particles created during the processing of animal products. In some cases classified as industrial, the source of infection was clothing, yarn, insulation material, saddle pads, or fertilizer. Occasional laboratory-acquired infections are reported.

Agricultural anthrax results from contact with infected animals (cattle, horses, sheep, goats, or swine) or their discharges. Animal vaccine inadvertently injected into the injector's hand has also caused disease.

In the United States, the majority of cases are sporadic, although there are occasional epidemics. The largest epidemic occurred during ten weeks in 1957, when nine of 600 employees in a processing plant acquired anthrax; four cutaneous and five inhalation (four fatalities) cases were associated with one batch of contaminated goat hair imported from Asia.

Human-to-human transmission has not been reported.

PATHOGENESIS. Cutaneous anthrax results from the introduction of *B. anthracis* through a wound or by means of an infected animal fiber penetrating the skin. Organisms in the subcutaneous tissue germinate, multiply, and produce toxin with tissue necrosis. Organisms and toxin may be distributed by the vascular or lymphatic system, resulting in involvement of regional lymph nodes, septicemia, and toxemia.

Inhalation anthrax results from the inhalation of airborne droplet nuclei less than 5 μ in size, with subsequent deposition on the terminal alveoli, where they are phagocytized by macrophages, carried through the alveolar membranes, and deposited in the regional lymph nodes; there they germinate, multiply, and produce toxin. The resulting reaction causes necrosis of the mediastinal tissue, leading to hemorrhagic, edematous mediastinitis, a unique pathologic finding. There may be a direct toxic effect on the pulmonary capillary endothelium, causing pulmonary capillary thrombosis and respiratory failure. Primary anthrax pneumonia is not seen, although there may be secondary pneumonic involvement.

Gastrointestinal anthrax results from ingestion of contaminated meat and deposition of spores in the submucosa of the intestinal tract (commonly ileum or cecum), where they germinate, multiply, and produce toxin, with resultant edema, hemorrhage, and necrosis. A mucosal lesion may develop with hemorrhage; there may be regional lymph node involvement. Occasionally organisms are introduced through the oral mucosa (oropharyngeal anthrax) and deposited in the regional lymph nodes, where they germinate, multiply, and produce toxin.

Anthrax meningitis results from hematogenous spread of bacteria from a primary focus.

Bacillus anthracis produces a toxin consisting of three components: edema factor, lethal factor, and protective antigen. In human disease antibiotic therapy may sterilize the tissue (usually within 24 hours of initiation), but the persistence of the toxin results in continued development of clinical disease until it is metabolized.

Clinical disease probably imparts permanent immunity; purported second cases have not been confirmed.

CLINICAL MANIFESTATIONS. Cutaneous anthrax usually occurs on the upper extremities or face. There may be mild fever, malaise, and headache. After an incubation period of three to ten days (usually five to seven days), a small pruritic, painless papule (approximately 1.0 cm) develops at the site of inoculation. Several days later a small vesicle or ring of vesicles is noted; this may be surrounded by erythema and slight nonpitting edema. The lesion may enlarge to approximately 4 cm. Within several days a dark hemorrhagic area develops beneath the center of the vesicular tissue. Disruption of the tissue releases a clear or slightly serous liquid teeming with organisms. Beneath this tissue will be a well-demarcated depressed ulcer crater in the center of which a black eschar is developing. The eschar dries and separates from the tissue within one to three weeks, leaving a scar. There may be lymphangitis and regional lymphadenopathy. The lesion is not painful except when secondarily infected. Rarely the lesion is large and irregularly shaped. Significant edema may develop, particularly with lesions near the eye. Malignant edema refers to an especially serious form with spreading edema, induration, formation of bullae, high fever, and severe toxemia. Rarely, multiple simultaneous lesions have been reported, probably resulting from simultaneous coprimary infections.

Antibiotic therapy will not alter the progression of the lesion, although it may influence the development of secondary infection and of septicemia.

Inhalation anthrax has an incubation period of one to five days (commonly three to four days). This form of the disease is biphasic, with an initial phase similar to a mild upper respiratory tract infection, with mild fever, malaise, fatigue, myalgia, nonproductive cough, and occasionally a sensation of precordial oppression. The only physical finding may be rhonchi on auscultation of the chest. Within several days there may be clinical improvement, but then the second or acute phase develops with severe respiratory distress as manifested by dyspnea, cyanosis, respiratory stridor, and profuse diaphoresis. Subcutaneous edema of the chest and neck may develop. The vital signs are elevated; moist, crepitant rales may be heard; minimal pleural effusion may be evident; shock may develop. On chest x-ray, the typical finding is that of an enlarged mediastinum and possible pleural effusion. The patient usually dies within 24 hours.

Gastrointestinal anthrax has an incubation period of two to five days. In the abdominal form of the disease, the initial symptoms are nausea, vomiting, anorexia, and fever. With progression of the disease, significant abdominal pain, hematemesis, and bloody diarrhea may develop. In some instances the findings simulate an acute surgical abdomen. Ascites may be present. Further progression leads to toxemia, cyanosis, shock, and death. In the oropharyngeal form, patients develop fever, anorexia, cervical or submandibular lymphadenopathy, and edema. A primary anthrax lesion of the pharynx has also been reported.

Anthrax meningitis resembles typical hemorrhagic meningitis.

DIAGNOSIS. In cutaneous anthrax, the typical lesion is a painless, pruritic papule which progresses into a vesicle, beneath which a depressed black eschar develops. Microscopic and bacteriologic examination of fluid from a vesicle or exudate from beneath the eschar should reveal organisms. The differential diagnosis includes staphylococcal skin infections, tularemia, plague, contagious pustular dermatitis (ecthyma contagiosum or orf), and milker's nodule.

The classic physical finding of inhalation anthrax is widening of the mediastinum. The initial phase of inhalation anthrax is indistinguishable from a mild upper respiratory tract infection, and the acute phase of severe respiratory distress will resemble other diseases that cause respiratory insufficiency. Sputum cultures are not generally positive for *B. anthracis*.

Gastrointestinal anthrax has no characteristic signs and symptoms, but organisms may be demonstrable in feces or vomitus. The clinical course may resemble shigellosis or *Yersinia* gastroenteritis. Severe involvement may lead to surgery of the abdomen. Involvement of the upper gastrointestinal tract is not distinctive of infection with *B. anthracis*.

Anthrax meningitis resembles hemorrhagic meningitis or possibly a cerebrovascular accident, but there should be evidence of a primary site of infection. The organism should be demonstrable in the cerebrospinal fluid. In any of these forms of the disease, appropriate serum specimens may demonstrate a four-fold rise in indirect hemagglutination titer.

TREATMENT. The drug of choice in anthrax is penicillin; *B. anthracis* organisms resistant to penicillin have not been identified from clinical specimens. In mild cutaneous anthrax, oral potassium penicillin, 2 grams per day for five to seven days, is recommended. With extensive lesions or with significant systemic illness, intramuscular procaine penicillin, 4 to 6 million units per day for five to seven days, should be given. Tetracycline or erythromycin may also be used in oral doses of 2 grams per day for five to seven days. In malignant edema, additional therapy with intravenous hydrocortisone, 100 to 200 mg per day, has been reported to be effective.

The lesion in cutaneous anthrax should be covered with a clean dressing. Hospitalized patients should be on secretion precautions. No ointments have been shown to be effective; excision of the lesion has been reported to increase the severity of symptoms.

Therapy of inhalation anthrax is based primarily on empirical knowledge and extrapolation from animal experiments. Penicillin G should be administered intravenously in doses of 18 to 24 million units per day. Streptomycin, 1 to 2 grams per day intravenously, may also be used. Supportive therapy such as volume expanders and vasopressor agents should be used as necessary. There may be a need to ensure an adequate airway if edema results in compression of the trachea.

For gastrointestinal anthrax, the therapeutic regimen for inhalation anthrax should be initiated. Tetracycline, 1 gram per day intravenously, has also been reported to be effective.

Anthrax meningitis should be treated in the same way as inhalation anthrax.

PROGNOSIS. The case-fatality ratio for cutaneous anthrax is 20 per cent without treatment and less than 5 per cent with appropriate treatment. Inhalation anthrax is almost always fatal. Gastrointestinal anthrax has a case fatality rate of 25 to 75 per cent.

PREVENTION. Formaldehyde has been successfully used to decontaminate raw hair and wool; gamma irradiation, steam under pressure, and ethylene oxide sterilization have been used with less effectiveness. Currently, prevention is directed toward protecting the employee by use of an effective, cell-free vaccine, education, good personal hygiene, and use of protective clothing, including respirators if aerosols are created. Gastrointestinal anthrax can be prevented by education concerning the ingestion of potentially contaminated meat. Prophylactic antibiotics or hyperimmune serum have not been shown to be effective.

Agricultural cases can be prevented by practicing good animal husbandry, including annual immunization of animals.

Albrink WS, Brooks SM, Biron RE, Kopel M: Human inhalation anthrax, a report of three fatal cases. Am J Pathol 36:457, 1960. *A good review of the pathology of inhalation anthrax from personal observations.*

Brachman PS: Anthrax. *In* Evans A, Feldman H (eds.): Bacterial Infections of Humans: Epidemiology and Control. New York, Ms. Hilary Evans Publishing Company, 1982, pp 63–74. *Comprehensive summary of all aspects of anthrax, with emphasis on the epidemiology.*

Brachman PS: Inhalation anthrax, New York Academy of Science, Conference on Airborne Contagion, November 8, 1979. Ann NY Acad Sci 353:83, 1980. *An up-to-date review of all aspects of inhalation anthrax.*

Brachman PS, Plotkin SA, Bumford FH, Atchison MM: An epidemic of inhalation anthrax. II. Epidemiologic investigations. Am J Hyg 72:6, 1960. *A report on the epidemiologic investigation of an epidemic of inhalation anthrax in the United States.*

Feeley JC, Brachman PS: *Bacillus anthracis. In* Lenette EH, Spaulding EH, Traunt JP (eds.): Manual of Clinical Microbiology. 2nd ed. Washington, D.C., American Society for Microbiology, 1974, pp 143-147. *A thorough review of the laboratory identification of anthrax.*

Plotkin SA, Brachman PS, Utell M, Bumford FH, Atchison MM: An epidemic of inhalation anthrax. The first in the twentieth century. I. Clinical features. Am J Med 29:992, 1960. *Summarizes the clinical features of an epidemic of inhalation anthrax in the United States.*

Sirisanthana T, Navachareon N, Tharavichitkul P, Sirisanthana V, Brown AE: Outbreak of oral-oropharyngeal anthrax: An unusual manifestation of human infection with *Bacillus anthracis.* Am J Trop Med 33:144, 1984.

290. DISEASES CAUSED BY PSEUDOMONADS

Michael Barza

Melioidosis and glanders are due to closely related bacteria of the genus *Pseudomonas.* Like other pseudomonads, these are strictly aerobic, nonfermentative, gram-negative bacilli. Both species show distinctive bipolar staining with various dyes.

MELIOIDOSIS

DEFINITION. Melioidosis, caused by *P. pseudomallei,* is a rare disease which is acquired in equatorial areas. It may produce fulminant septicemia with widespread suppurative lesions or a chronic, tuberculosis-like illness with lung cavitation. Infection occurs through contact with contaminated soil or water.

ETIOLOGY. In 1912, Whitmore and Krishnaswami, while performing autopsies on derelicts in Rangoon who had died of a glanders-like illness, recovered a unique bacillus. Because of the resemblance to glanders, this bacterium came to be called *P. pseudomallei* and the disease, melioidosis.

EPIDEMIOLOGY. *P. pseudomallei* is found in a narrow belt ranging 20 degrees on either side of the equator. Most cases have been acquired in Southeast Asia, but some have been reported from the Philippines, Guam, Australia, and, rarely, Central or South America. Over 300 cases of melioidosis with 36 deaths were recorded among United States troops stationed in Vietnam.

The organism is widespread in soil and stagnant water, particularly in paddy fields. Epizootic disease occurs among sheep, goats, swine, and horses, but, in contrast to glanders, these animals do not seem to be a reservoir of human disease. Most human infections are believed to arise by contamination of skin abrasions by soil or water. This may explain the marked predilection for males. Ingestion and inhalation are occasional routes of entry. Rarely, laboratory workers have been infected in the course of working with this organism. Only one instance of human-to-human transmission has been reported.

Inapparent infection in the form of seroreactivity is common in endemic areas. Significant titers have been found in as many as 20 per cent of Vietnamese and in 1 to 2 per cent of United States soldiers who spent at least six months in Vietnam. Even higher rates were reported in soldiers wounded in Vietnam. This is of importance because of the remarkable ability of melioidosis, like tuberculosis, to become clinically manifest for the first time many years after exposure. A population of veterans in the United States is now at risk of this disease.

PATHOGENESIS AND PATHOLOGY. In acute septicemic melioidosis, organisms are disseminated widely throughout the body, particularly the lungs, liver, spleen, and lymph nodes. Lung lesions are usually due to hematogenous spread, but sometimes result from inhalation. Multiple small abscesses are formed, containing necrotic material, neutrophils, and abundant bacteria. With time, the lesions coalesce and may cavitate. A rim of hemorrhage may be evident in pulmonary abscesses.

In chronic melioidosis, the lungs and lymph nodes are most commonly affected. The lesions show a combination of central necrosis containing polymorphonuclear leukocytes, and peripheral granulomas. Giant cells may be seen. Organisms are sparse in these lesions.

CLINICAL MANIFESTATIONS. The incubation period is usually a few days, but may be as long as 20 years or more. In late-onset cases, the illness often seems to be triggered by intercurrent trauma or other disease such as diabetes mellitus, alcoholism, or cancer or by malnutrition. The most common manifestation of infection with *P. pseudomallei* is simply a positive serologic test result. Clinical disease ranges from an acute septicemic form to a subacute or chronic localized form. At both extremes, the lung is commonly involved.

Acute septicemic melioidosis causes fever, chills, tachypnea, and muscle pain, as well as signs and symptoms attributable to local abscess formation. Macroscopic abscesses are common in the liver, spleen, and lymph nodes. They are especially prominent in the lungs, chiefly in the upper lobes. Radiographic changes range from bronchopneumonia through lobar consolidation to nodular lesions which coalesce and may cavitate. There may be pleuritic chest pain and a pleural rub. Rales and rhonchi are often heard. Pustular skin lesions are sometimes seen. Routine laboratory tests show anemia and a variable polymorphonuclear leukocytosis.

Subacute or chronic melioidosis may occur in the wake of the acute infection or may arise indolently. The typical presentation is cavitary disease of the upper lobes of the lungs, resembling tuberculosis. The liver, skin, bones, and soft tissues may be affected, and sinus tracts may be formed. The general picture is of a chronic, wasting, usually febrile illness with occasional periods of remission.

Variations upon these themes may be encountered. A nodular abscess with regional lymphadenitis may occur at the site of the original infection, usually the skin. Focal and diffuse encephalitis, as well as pleural mass and effusion, have been described.

DIAGNOSIS. Melioidosis should be suspected in those who have resided in an endemic area and who manifest either an acute, febrile illness with widespread suppurative lesions, especially in the lungs and skin, or who exhibit progressive cavitary lung disease without a clear cause. Gram stain of infected material may show the organisms poorly, but Wright's, Giemsa, and other techniques usually demonstrate the bacteria and reveal the bipolar accentuation.

The laboratory should be alerted to the suspected diagnosis. The organisms usually grow well in ordinary media, although they may be sparse in chronic infections and may be overgrown by normal flora. Selective media may increase the yield. After several days of incubation, the colonies usually assume a typical "wrinkled" appearance on agar media. *P. pseudomallei* can be differentiated from other pseudomonads by a variety of biologic features. Fluorescent-antibody staining, one of the most definitive tests, cross-reacts with *P. mallei,* but the two organisms can be distinguished by the lack of motility of the latter.

Serologic studies may be helpful. The complement fixation test is suggestive at titers above 1:8 and the hemagglutination test at titers above 1:80. A four-fold rise in titer is essentially diagnostic. Serologic tests are occasionally negative in patients with active disease. Elevated titers may persist despite successful treatment of melioidosis.

TREATMENT. There is no general agreement upon an optimal regimen for the treatment of melioidosis. The choice of drugs must, to some extent, be based upon sensitivity tests. Most active in vitro are the tetracyclines, chloramphenicol, novobiocin, kanamycin, sulfonamides, and trimethoprim-sulfamethoxazole. For *acute septicemic illness,* high doses of tetracycline (80 mg per kilogram per day) *and* chloramphenicol (80 mg per kilogram per day) are recommended, together with one of the following: trimethoprim-sulfamethoxazole (9 and 45 mg per kilogram per day), sulfisoxazole (140 mg per kilogram per day), or kanamycin (30 mg per kilogram per day). Drug toxicity has been a problem at these high doses, so they should be reduced when this is feasible.

For *chronic melioidosis,* tetracycline, chloramphenicol, sulfisoxazole, or trimethoprim-sulfamethoxazole should be given in about half the dosage recommended for acute disease. One drug to which the organism is sensitive usually suffices. Because the bacteria are very difficult to eradicate, treatment for acute or chronic disease generally should be given for at least 3 months and as long as 6 to 12 months. Abscesses should be drained according to usual principles; however, surgical intervention without adequate antibiotic coverage can be dangerous. The indications for operation on patients with active lung disease are not settled.

PROGNOSIS. The mortality rate of untreated septicemic melioidosis exceeds 90 per cent, but with treatment this is reduced to about 50 per cent. Subacute or chronic infection carries a lower mortality which, with treatment, may be diminished to 10 per cent or less.

PREVENTION. No vaccine is available. It seems reasonable to recommend thorough cleansing of abrasions sustained in endemic areas. Despite the rarity of person-to-person transmission, patients with active infection, especially pulmonary infection, should probably be isolated.

Everett ED, Nelson RA: Pulmonary melioidosis. Observations in thirty-nine cases. Am Rev Respir Dis 112:331, 1975. *A thorough account of the clinical presentation of a large group of United States soldiers, most of whom had subacute or chronic pulmonary infection. Therapeutic recommendations, including the role of surgery, are discussed at length.*

Howe C, Sampath A, Spotnitz M: The pseudomallei group: A review. J Infect Dis 124:598, 1971. *An excellent review of the bacteriology and epidemiology of the disease, and of what little is known about the pathogenetic factors involved.*

John JF Jr: Trimethoprim-sulfamethoxazole therapy of pulmonary melioidosis. Am Rev Respir Dis 114:1021, 1976. *Presentation of a case and brief review of the limited information available regarding therapy of cavitary lung disease.*

Piggott JA, Hochholzer L: Human melioidosis. A histopathologic study of acute and chronic melioidosis. Arch Pathol 90:101, 1970. *A clear description of the pathologic features of this disease, based on autopsy study of ten patients with acute and six with chronic melioidosis.*

Whitmore A, Krishnaswami CS: An account of the discovery of a hitherto undescribed infective disease occurring among the population of Rangoon. Indian Med Gazette 47:262, 1912. *A fascinating account of the discovery of melioidosis among the beggars and drug addicts of Rangoon. The authors humbly describe how their simple experiments led to the gradual realization that they had stumbled onto a new disease.*

GLANDERS

DEFINITION. Glanders is primarily an infection of horses, mules, or donkeys. It is very rarely transmitted to humans but can produce an acute septicemic illness or a more chronic one involving principally the skin and lungs.

ETIOLOGY. The causative organism, *Pseudomonas mallei,* derives its species name from the Latin *malleus* (Greek *melis*), connoting "severe disease." It is a strictly aerobic, nonfermentative, gram-negative rod which closely resembles *Pseudomonas pseudomallei,* the agent of melioidosis, but is nonmotile.

EPIDEMIOLOGY. Glanders occurs almost exclusively in people handling horses, mules, or donkeys. In horses, there may be pulmonary involvement or subcutaneous nodules, especially about the head and neck ("farcy"). It is occasionally transmitted to domestic animals. In the rare instances of human infection, transmission appears to be via broken skin or possibly aerosol inhalation. Glanders has been eradicated from the United States, but cases still occur in Asia and South America. Laboratory personnel working with the organism may become infected. In contrast to melioidosis, glanders can be transmitted from person to person fairly readily.

PATHOLOGY AND PATHOGENESIS. The lesions of glanders range from acute cellulitis with necrosis and abscess formation to a chronic necrotizing process with granuloma formation.

CLINICAL MANIFESTATIONS. Within a few days of cutaneous inoculation, subcutaneous nodules appear with regional lymphadenitis. When the portal of entry is the upper respiratory tract, draining mucosal ulcers occur. Lower respiratory infection following inhalation may have a longer incubation period, 10 to 14 days, and results in a necrotizing lobar or bronchopneumonia, nodular infiltrates, or lung abscess; accompanying features include chills, myalgias, headache, and pleuritic chest pain. Systemic spread may complicate infection in any of these sites, producing a rapidly fatal illness with a generalized pustular rash.

Aside from fever and local suppuration, physical findings may include generalized adenopathy and splenomegaly. The white blood cell count may be mildly elevated. Occasionally there is severe leukopenia.

In some patients, a chronic form of disease occurs with subcutaneous or intramuscular abscesses. There may be lymphadenitis and ulceration of the nasal mucosa. Involvement of the liver, spleen, lung, eye, and central nervous system has been reported.

DIAGNOSIS. Glanders should be considered when persons handling potentially infected animals or laboratory material develop nodular, suppurative infections of the skin and upper respiratory tract or an acute, septicemic illness. Bacteria are sparse even in abscesses and may not be well seen with Gram stain. Giemsa, Wright's, or methylene blue stain, however, may reveal organisms with typical bipolar staining ("safety pin" appearance). *P. mallei* grows slowly on various standard laboratory media. The bacteria can be identified presumptively by their biochemical characteristics and lack of motility, as well as by fluorescent-antibody staining. Serologic tests (agglutination, complement fixation) may be useful.

TREATMENT. The mortality of untreated glanders is high. Experience with therapy is limited. Sulfadiazine appears to be effective. It should be administered in a dosage of 100 mg per kilogram per day for three weeks or more. By analogy with melioidosis, other drugs such as tetracycline, chloramphenicol, or an aminoglycoside might be administered concomitantly.

Infected animals should be destroyed, and infected humans should be isolated to prevent spread of the disease.

Howe C, Miller WR: Human glanders: Report of six cases. Ann Intern Med 26:93, 1947. *A review of cases which occurred among workers in a single laboratory. The diagnoses were made serologically, and all patients survived.*

291. LISTERIOSIS

Michael Barza

DEFINITION. Infection caused by *Listeria monocytogenes,* a distinctive gram-positive bacillus, occurs worldwide. The organism has a propensity to afflict people with underlying diseases but also affects previously healthy individuals. Meningitis, bacteremia, and focal infections, as well as devastating neonatal sepsis, can occur.

ETIOLOGY. In 1926, Murray, Webb, and Swann isolated a new bacterium from sick rabbits and guinea pigs. Because it produced a monocytosis in these animals, they suggested the species name *monocytogenes.* The first human isolation, in 1929, was from a patient with an illness resembling infectious mononucleosis.

EPIDEMIOLOGY. *L. monocytogenes* is widespread in soil, water, and sewage, and can survive in moist environments for months. A large variety of healthy mammals, fowl, and fish are sporadically colonized. Listeriosis is a well-recognized cause of abortion, septicemia, and encephalitis in various animal species.

Despite these observations, most infections in humans are of uncertain origin. Patients are usually urban dwellers with no evident contact with animals, unpasteurized milk, or contaminated food or water. This has led to the suspicion that asymptomatic human carriers may be important sources of infection. Indeed, colonization of the nose, throat, or genitalia of healthy individuals occasionally occurs. Moreover, the organism can be recovered from the feces of at least 1 per cent of well people and a higher proportion of household contacts of infected persons.

The frequency of listeriosis appears to be increasing. This may be due in part to heightened awareness, but probably also reflects the increasing population of patients with immunosuppressive disorders who now constitute the majority of patients with *Listeria* infection. Males are more often affected than females. In Europe two thirds of cases occur in neonates, whereas in the United States most occur in later life. The reasons for these differences in sex and geographic distribution are not known.

L. monocytogenes can be grouped into 11 serotypes, of which type 1 (usually 1b) and type 4 are the most common in the United States. Clusters of cases caused by a single serotype have occasionally been described in the community and in the hospital, suggesting that person-to-person and/or common-source spread may occur. Nursery outbreaks are well recognized.

PATHOLOGY AND PATHOGENESIS. *L. monocytogenes* shares with mycobacteria, fungi, *Salmonella* and *Brucella* the property of surviving within phagocytes, especially macrophages. Resistance to infection appears to depend mainly on the acquisition of cell-mediated immunity. Humoral immunity plays a lesser role. Accordingly, patients who have diseases which depress cellular immunity or who are taking immunosuppressive drugs are especially susceptible.

The portal of entry is not known but may be the intestine. In animals, *Listeria* multiply within epithelial cells of the gut. Presumably, bacteremia may ensue with seeding of various sites. The usual histologic response in humans is a polymorphonuclear leukocytosis with microabscess formation. However, there may occasionally be a monocytic reaction. In perinatal infection, miliary necrotizing granulomas are found in the liver, spleen, lungs, and central nervous system.

L. monocytogenes shows striking tropism for the fetus and placenta of most animals and for the central nervous system of monkeys and humans. Meningitis results in a dense, purulent reaction especially over the base of the brain. The infection sometimes extends more deeply to produce "cerebritis" or bacterial encephalitis. Brain abscess may supervene.

CLINICAL MANIFESTATIONS. After the neonatal period, listeriosis most commonly affects elderly patients, especially males. The major presentations are meningitis (55 per cent), bacteremia (25 per cent), endocarditis (7 per cent), and nonmeningitic infection of the central nervous system (6 per cent). More than one half of patients have an underlying disorder such as malignancy, cirrhosis, alcoholism, diabetes, or vasculitis, or are receiving immunosuppressive drugs such as corticosteroids. Gastrointestinal symptoms sometimes occur at the onset of the systemic illness, suggesting that the intestinal tract may be the portal of entry.

L. monocytogenes is a leading cause of bacterial *meningitis* among people with cancer, especially lymphoma and leukemia, and among recipients of renal transplants. About 30 per cent of patients have no preceding disease; however, *Listeria* accounts for fewer than 1 per cent of cases of meningitis in the population at large. The onset of illness is usually fairly sudden with headache and fever. Nuchal rigidity is present in 85 per cent of patients. Although the signs and symptoms generally resemble those of other pyogenic meningitides, coarse tremors or cerebellar ataxia may be striking. The cerebrospinal fluid in most patients (70 per cent) shows a polymorphonuclear leukocytosis and increased protein concentration; in fewer than half is the glucose decreased below 40 mg per deciliter. Occasionally, the course of *Listeria* meningitis is indolent and the spinal fluid contains a predominance of lymphocytes, leading to suspicion of tuberculous or cryptococcal infection.

Focal cerebritis or *brain abscess* may complicate the course of *Listeria* meningitis, especially in renal transplant recipients. In some patients, these focal lesions may appear without other evidence of meningitis. They usually affect the cerebral hemispheres or brainstem, causing hemiplegia or cranial nerve palsies. Aphasia, nystagmus, and dysconjugate gaze may occur as well. In the absence of meningitis, there is no nuchal rigidity and the spinal fluid abnormalities are relatively mild. Radionuclide scan and possibly computed tomographic (CT) scan may be helpful in delineating the lesions.

Bacteremia caused by *L. monocytogenes* usually affects patients under 50 years of age. About 90 per cent of patients have an underlying illness or are pregnant. There are no specific features to distinguish this from other forms of bacteremia. Fever, chills, and tachycardia are usual; hypotension and confusion may occur. Peripheral leukocytosis is the rule, but monocytosis has been reported. The major complications are meningitis and endocarditis.

Endocarditis caused by *L. monocytogenes* is rare. In contrast to other forms of listeriosis in adults, most patients have not had an immunosuppressive illness, but pre-existing valvular disease was noted in over half the cases. In several instances, infection occurred on a prosthetic valve.

Other *localized infections* include pneumonia, hepatitis, pericarditis, infected aortic aneurysm, osteomyelitis, conjunctivitis, intraocular infection, and primary skin infection. All of these are rare.

L. monocytogenes has occasionally been recovered from lymph nodes, blood, or spinal fluid of patients with a syndrome resembling infectious mononucleosis. However, this presentation is rare and is unrelated to EB-virus disease.

Perinatal infection, the most distinctive syndrome of listeriosis, may take one of two forms. In the first, the infant becomes infected in utero. The woman may be asymptomatic, or may sustain a mild influenza-like illness with fever, myalgias, diarrhea, sore throat, or urinary symptoms. Shortly thereafter, premature birth or stillbirth may occur. If the infant is born alive, signs of septicemia develop within hours. Fetal distress, pneumonia, diarrhea, seizures, and rash are common manifestations. Microabscesses, sometimes with a granulomatous component, are found in various organs. This disease, also known as "granulomatosis infantiseptica," has a very high mortality rate.

The second form of neonatal disease occurs after the first five to seven days of life. Meningitis is the usual presentation, but progressive hydrocephalus may occur. Infection is believed to be acquired during passage through the birth canal. Overall, about 10 to 20 per cent of neonatal meningitis is due to *L. monocytogenes.*

The role of listeriosis in spontaneous abortion is controversial. In one study, the organism was cultured from the cervix of 25 of 34 women who had had repeated abortions, but in none of 87 control patients. In another study, antibiotic treatment of three couples in which the wives had suffered repeated abortions resulted in successful pregnancies. However, a large body of data suggests that this sequence of events is unusual and that *Listeria* is not implicated in most instances of spontaneous abortion.

DIAGNOSIS. Beyond the neonatal period, there is little that is specific about the syndrome of listeriosis. Clearly, this organism must be suspected when meningitis occurs in a setting of diminished host defenses. However, the diagnosis rests upon bacteriologic grounds, and the key to diagnosis is awareness. Laboratories frequently misinterpret *L. monocytogenes* as diphtheroids, which are discarded as "contaminants." Gram stain of infected material may reveal the typical, pleomorphic, palisading, gram-positive bacilli. However, organisms are not seen in Gram stain of the spinal fluid in 60 to 75 per cent of patients with *Listeria* meningitis. Moreover, the organisms sometimes resemble streptococci, or in other instances, stain irregularly so that they are mistaken for *Hemophilus influenzae*. If the clinical setting is suggestive, the physician should alert the laboratory to the possibility of listeriosis. Cultures can then be examined for β-hemolysis, catalase positivity, and tumbling motility of organisms at room temperature, which distinguish *L. monocytogenes* from other agents.

Listeria is generally not difficult to grow from infected material unless the patient has received antibiotics. Selective media may be helpful with samples such as sputum and vaginal secretions that contain other bacteria. In addition to blood cultures, spinal fluid should be obtained if there is any suggestion of meningitis, for nuchal rigidity may be absent. In the newborn, material from the eye, ear, nose, throat, amniotic fluid, and meconium should be examined in addition to blood cultures.

TREATMENT. Ampicillin or penicillin G is the mainstay of therapy for listeriosis. The organisms are generally susceptible to these antibiotics as well as to trimethoprim-sulfamethoxazole, chloramphenicol, clindamycin, erythromycin, gentamicin, vancomycin, and tetracyclines, but individual strains may depart from the usual pattern. Cephalosporins should be avoided because of their limited meningeal penetration and generally poor activity against the organisms. In one retrospective study, ampicillin appeared somewhat better than penicillin G. There is some evidence that chloramphenicol, especially as a single agent, is less effective than ampicillin or penicillin G.

For initial therapy in adults, pending the results of sensitivity tests, ampicillin is recommended in a dosage of 200 mg per kilogram per day in six divided doses; alternatively, penicillin G, 300,000 units per kilogram per day in six or eight divided doses, may be used. Higher dosages may occasionally be required. There is synergy between these drugs and gentamicin or streptomycin in vitro. Thus, concomitant administration of an aminoglycoside, intrathecally for meningitis, might be considered in seriously ill patients or those who relapse. Therapy may have to be given for several weeks to prevent relapse. On the basis of activity in vitro, trimethoprim-sulfamethoxazole could be a useful alternative in the penicillin-allergic patient.

PROGNOSIS. The overall mortality of untreated listeriosis exceeds 70 per cent for meningitis or bacteremia. The outcome with treatment is influenced by coexisting diseases. In adults with meningitis, the mortality rate was 13 per cent in those without other disorders, 28 per cent in immunosuppressed patients without malignancy, and 60 per cent in those with malignancy. A low glucose concentration and high protein concentration in the cerebrospinal fluid appear to herald an unfavorable outcome of meningitis. Brain abscess or cerebritis carries a mortality rate of about 50 per cent, and residual defects are common.

Among patients treated appropriately for bacteremia with ampicillin or penicillin G, 90 per cent survive. Fatalities occur primarily among those with immunosuppressive illnesses in whom there is undiagnosed central nervous system infection. About one third of patients with endocarditis die, primarily of myocardial infarction, congestive heart failure, or subarachnoid hemorrhage.

Antibiotics have reduced the mortality rate of perinatal infection to about 50 per cent from almost 100 per cent. Patients being treated for bacteremia should be carefully watched for signs of meningitis, especially if they are being given antibiotics which penetrate the meninges poorly. Well demarcated brain abscesses require surgical drainage.

PREVENTION. There is no vaccine available to prevent listeriosis. On occasion, clusters of cases have occurred in hospitalized patients, suggesting possible cross-infection. Although such events are rare, it seems prudent to use isolation precautions for patients with listeriosis, especially if there are transplant recipients or patients with immunosuppressive disorders nearby.

It may be worthwhile to culture the cervix of women who have repeated abortions or whose infants die early in life and the blood of women who are febrile during pregnancy for the possibility of treatable *Listeria* infection.

Bottone EJ, Sierra MF: Listeria monocytogenes: Another look at the "Cinderella among pathogenic bacteria." Mt Sinai J Med 44:42, 1977. *A comprehensive review with emphasis on the bacteriologic properties and pathogenetic mechanisms of the organism.*

Green HT, Macaulay MB: Hospital outbreak of *Listeria monocytogenes* septicemia: A problem of cross-infection? Lancet 2:1039, 1978. *Just what the title says. Addresses the problem of whom, if anyone, to isolate in these circumstances.*

Lavetter A, Leedom JM, Mathies AW, Ivler D, Wehrle PF: Meningitis due to *Listeria monocytogenes*. N Engl J Med 285:598, 1971. *A retrospective comparison of the outcome of disease in 25 patients treated mainly with ampicillin or penicillin G. Although concomitant antibiotics may have skewed the results somewhat, the data suggest some advantage for ampicillin.*

Nieman RE, Lorber B: Listeriosis in adults: A changing pattern. Report of eight cases and review of the literature, 1968–1978. Rev Infect Dis 2:207, 1980. *A thorough review of the clinical aspects of listeriosis in the postnatal period, with a detailed analysis of risk factors and prognostic features.*

Perinatal listeriosis. Lancet 1:911, 1980. *A concise account of the current status of the diagnosis, treatment, and prevention of this highly fatal disease.*

Stamm AM, Dismukes WE, Simmons BP, Cobbs CG, Elliott A, Budrich P, Harmon J: Listeriosis in renal transplant recipients: Report of an outbreak and review of 102 cases. Rev Infect Dis 4:665, 1982. *An excellent review of this continuing problem. Has 110 references.*

Tuazon CU, Shamsuddin D, Miller H: Antibiotic susceptibility and synergy of clinical isolates of *Listeria monocytogenes*. Antimicrob Agents Chemother 21:525, 1982. *Stresses the lack of bactericidal activity of the penicillins (the drugs of choice) and of chloramphenicol and the excellent activity of trimethoprim-sulfamethoxazole in vitro.*

292. ERYSIPELOID

Michael Barza

DEFINITION. *Erysipelothrix rhusiopathiae* is an important cause of disease in animals. In humans, it produces a characteristic violaceous erythema of the fingers and hands known as erysipeloid (of Rosenbach). Disseminated infection and endocarditis rarely occur.

ETIOLOGY. *E. rhusiopathiae* is a slender, pleomorphic, non-spore-forming gram-positive rod which grows well on ordinary laboratory media. Its lack of motility or catalase production and its ability to form hydrogen sulfide on TSI slants help distinguish it from *Listeria monocytogenes* and *Corynebacteria* (diphtheroids).

EPIDEMIOLOGY. Erysipeloid is an occupational disease of persons exposed to infected animals or animal products. *E. rhusiopathiae* is found in various *animals*, including sheep, lamb, cattle, horses, dogs, and mice; *fish* and *shellfish*; and *fowl*, including turkeys, chickens, and ducks. It is carried by as many as 50 per cent of healthy swine and is an economically significant cause of disease in those animals and in turkeys. Swine develop septicemia, chronic arthritis with or without endocarditis, and a rhomboid urticarial skin reaction ("diamond skin"). *E. rhusiopathiae* appears to colonize the slime of fish. It survives in decaying organic matter. Although resistant to salting, pickling, and smoking, the bacteria are killed by heating at 55° C for 15 minutes.

Humans are quite resistant to infection by ingestion, but are readily infected through superficial abrasions in contact with contaminated material. Thus, the disease is most common in abattoir workers, butchers, fish-handlers, and the like. However, there is often no definite recollection of trauma.

CLINICAL MANIFESTATIONS. Within a few days of inoculation, rarely longer than a week, there is the onset of a purplish erythema, usually on the finger or hand. Pain or itching, tingling, and throbbing usually accompany and may antedate the skin lesions. The rash slowly spreads to involve other fingers, but rarely the fingertips or above the wrist. It is sharply demarcated, and there is central clearing. Vesicles and even bullae are sometimes seen. Lymphangitis or regional lymphadenitis occur in about 20 per cent of patients and constitutional symptoms such as fever in about 10 per cent. The joints in the affected extremity may be stiff and somewhat swollen. Untreated, the lesions usually resolve spontaneously over a period of weeks, but persistent sterile arthritis has been reported in up to 10 per cent of patients. In very rare instances, a generalized skin eruption occurs.

Occasionally, *E. rhusiopathiae* causes septicemia. This almost always signifies endocarditis. About half of these patients have no antecedent history of valvular disease; some have evidence of recent erysipeloid. The endocarditis may be very destructive, with a high mortality rate.

DIAGNOSIS. The characteristic skin lesion and history of animal contact point to the diagnosis. The violaceous hue, burning or painful sensation, and absence of suppuration or constitutional symptoms distinguish this from ordinary pyogenic infections. The organisms can rarely be grown from aspirates of infected material but can often (7 of 20 cases in one series) be cultured from full-thickness skin biopsy of the advancing edge. The septicemic disease is diagnosed by blood culture.

TREATMENT. The organisms are sensitive to penicillins, cephalosporins, erythromycin, clindamycin, tetracyclines, and chloramphenicol, but not to vancomycin or aminoglycosides. Uncomplicated cutaneous lesions generally respond well to oral penicillin G, although parenteral therapy is occasionally necessary. Surgical incision offers no benefit and may lead to secondary infection. A suggested regimen for endocarditis is intravenous penicillin G, 12 to 20 million units daily for four to six weeks. Valve excision may be required. With early and aggressive therapy, the survival rate is about 85 per cent.

There is no vaccine available to prevent the disease. Highly exposed persons should be advised to wear gloves and wash their hands frequently at work.

Grieco MH, Sheldon C: *Erysipelothrix rhusiopathiae*. Ann NY Acad Sci 174:523, 1970. *A concise and detailed review of the bacteriology, epidemiology, and clinical features of this disease. Many references.*

Klauder JV: Erysipeloid as an occupational disease. JAMA 111:1345, 1938. *An account of the epidemiology of the infection in 100 patients, together with a vivid, illustrated, clinical description.*

Klauder JV: *Erysipelothrix rhusiopathiae* infection in animals and in human beings. Ann NY Acad Sci 48:535, 1946. *A comparison of the disease in animals and humans, and detailed review of some unusual presentations in humans.*

Kramer MR, Gombert ME, Corrado ML, Ergin MA, Burnett V, Ganguly J: *Erysipelothrix rhusiopathiae* endocarditis. South Med J 75:892, 1982. *The first reported case in a drug addict. Points out the improved survival with current treatment, including valve replacement.*

Price JEL, Bennett WEJ: The erysipeloid of Rosenbach. Br Med J 2:1060, 1951. *A good clinical and epidemiologic description, with emphasis on the difficulties of bacteriologic diagnosis.*

293. ACTINOMYCOSIS

David J. Drutz

DEFINITION. Actinomycosis is a chronic suppurative and granulomatous bacterial infection characterized by contiguous spread, abscess formation, and sinuses that discharge grains ("sulfur granules"). There are four clinical forms: cervicofacial ("lumpy jaw"), thoracic, abdominal, and disseminated.

ETIOLOGY. Etiologic agents include *Actinomyces israelii, A. naeslundii, A. viscosus, A. odontolyticus, A. meyeri,* and *Arachnia propionica. Actinomyces bovis* produces lumpy jaw in cattle, but is virtually never a human pathogen. These filamentous bacteria are anaerobic or facultative, capnophilic, gram-positive, and non-acid-fast. Filaments may break up into coccobacilli. All are normal oral flora; none is recoverable from the environment. Sulfur granules may be found in normal tonsillar crypts in the absence of an inflammatory reaction.

Actinomycosis is characterized by "associate" bacteria (e.g., *Actinobacillus actinomycetemcomitans* or various streptococci in cervicofacial actinomycosis; *E. coli* and diverse enteric organisms in abdominal actinomycosis). Given the disruption of mucous membranes necessary for initiation of actinomycosis, their presence is not surprising. These aerobes may play a synergistic role by helping maintain the low oxygen tension necessary for growth of the actinomycetes.

EPIDEMIOLOGY. Actinomycosis occurs worldwide, and is unrelated to climate, occupation, race, or age. It may be more common in men than in women. Accurate data on incidence and prevalence are not available, but the disease is not rare. Actinomycosis occurs in many animal species, but is not transmissible to man.

PATHOGENESIS AND PATHOLOGY. The etiologic agents are poorly invasive, generally requiring a break in the mucous membrane and the presence of devitalized tissue suitable to their anaerobic growth requirements. Unlike *Nocardia* species, they are not usually opportunistic in a setting of depressed cell-mediated immunity.

In animal studies mycelia and grains are more difficult to eliminate than coccobacilli. When the suppurative response fails to eradicate the bacteria, a granulomatous reaction ensues, accompanied by intense fibrosis. Contiguous spread of infection characteristically ignores tissue boundaries, and ultimately produces draining sinus tracts and invasion of surrounding tissues.

The histopathologic picture is characterized by a mixed suppurative, granulomatous, and fibrotic process in which grains are a major distinguishing feature. When stained with hematoxylin-eosin, grains are centrally basophilic with eosinophilic rays (*Actinomyces* = "ray fungus"), terminating in pear-shaped "clubs." The clubs consist of an immune complex–derived sheath enclosing a single central filament that represents the organism itself. The grains stain well with methenamine silver, but Gram stain is needed to identify the actinomycetes.

CLINICAL MANIFESTATIONS. Cervicofacial actinomycosis accounts for 60 per cent of infections and generally occurs in a setting of tooth decay, gingival disease, dental extraction, or serious injury sufficient to disrupt mucosal integrity. Manifestations include pain (some are painless); woody-hard swelling, often in the parotid or mandibular region (attributable to fibrosis); discoloration; trismus; and multiple sinuses that discharge odorless pus containing yellow-white granules. Fever and leukocytosis may occur. The disease spreads by direct extension, and may involve tongue, salivary glands, pharynx, and larynx. Periostitis is followed by osteomyelitis. Cervical spine or cranial bone disease may lead to subdural empyema and central nervous system invasion. Cervicofacial actinomycosis may be confused with tuberculosis, nocardiosis, mycotic infections, osteomyelitis caused by other microorganisms, or neoplasm.

Thoracic actinomycosis accounts for 15 per cent of cases and may result from the aspiration of pharyngeal contents, dental plaque, or tonsillar grains; from organisms carried to the lung by a foreign body; by direct extension from cervicofacial or abdominal (especially hepatic) infection; or by hematogenous spread. There is often a history of underlying lung disease. Thoracic actinomycosis resembles other chronic inflammatory processes and malignancies. The tendency for the infection to cross pulmonary fissures and to form draining chest wall sinuses suggests the correct diagnosis. The pericardium and mediastinum may be invaded. Sulfur granules are rarely present in the sputum.

Abdominal actinomycosis accounts for about 20 per cent of cases and usually arises weeks to months following a perforation of the gastrointestinal tract. Most cases present in the right iliac fossa, reflecting a frequent association with appendicitis. Abdominal actinomycosis may spread by contiguity to other intra-abdominal structures (especially the liver), the lung, pelvis, spine, or abdominal wall. The eventual development of draining fistulas offers an important clue, and the diagnosis should be considered even in cases of perirectal abscess or fistula in ano. Abdominal actinomycosis may be confused with Crohn's disease, ulcerative colitis, tuberculosis, or malignancy. Colonization of the uterine cervix with *A. israelii* and other actinomycetes has become common with the use of intrauterine contraceptive devices (IUD's). Cases of pelvic actinomycosis have originated in this fashion.

Disseminated actinomycosis may result from the hematogenous spread of bacteria from any of the sites mentioned above, but most frequently follows thoracic disease. Hematogenous dissemination is rare. Tissues most commonly involved include the skin and subcutaneous tissues, bone, brain, liver, and kidneys.

DIAGNOSIS. The diagnosis of actinomycosis should be made by direct isolation of the infecting organism from clinical specimens, or from washed, crushed sulfur granules. Bacteriologic confirmation is achieved in less than 50 per cent of cases because of failure to obtain anaerobic cultures, or overgrowth by the "associate" bacteria. Examination of Gram-stained tissue for filamentous, branching, non-acid-fast, gram-positive organisms often provides the clue to diagnosis. The organisms can also be seen in Gram stains of crushed granules, but must be differentiated from those seen in the grains of botryomycosis, eumycetomas, or actinomycetomas (see Ch. 375). The diagnosis of pelvic actinomycosis is usually first suspected when organisms are seen on cytologic preparations from the cervix.

Transtracheal aspiration has been complicated by formation of actinomycotic neck abscess at the site of needle introduction.

There are no reliable serologic tests for actinomycosis and no skin tests. Fluorescent antibody staining techniques have been used to identify actinomycetes in tissue sections, to identify their presence in mixed cultures, and to verify their final identity after isolation. However, these tests are not generally available.

TREATMENT. Actinomycosis has a strong tendency to recur, at least partially because of inaccessibility of the disease process to antibiotic penetration. Therefore, prolonged treatment courses may be necessary. There is no generally agreed upon formula for antibiotic dose or duration, and treatment should be tailored to disease severity. Cervicofacial actinomycosis may be easier to cure than the other forms. Penicillin is the drug of choice. In severe cases, 10 to 20 million units are given intravenously daily for four to six weeks, followed by 2 to 5 million units of oral phenoxymethyl penicillin (or its equivalent) for a total of 12 to 18 months of treatment. Alternative antibiotics (given in full dosage) include tetracycline, erythromycin, lincomycin, or clindamycin. *A. israelii* is exquisitely sensitive to rifampin, but no data are available on therapy with this drug. Although *Actinobacillus actinomycetemcomitans* is not particularly susceptible to penicillin or ampicillin, patients with actinomycosis improve on these regimens. Therefore, it is not necessary to tailor therapy to the drug susceptibilities of "associate" bacteria. Adjunctive therapeutic measures for actinomycosis include surgery.

PROGNOSIS. The advent of antibiotics has greatly improved the prognosis for all forms of actinomycosis, and neither deformity nor death is common.

Berardi RS: Abdominal actinomycosis. Surg Gynecol Obstet 149:257, 1979. *A thorough and up-to-date review of all aspects of actinomycosis, with particular emphasis on the abdominal form.*

Bhagavan BS, Gupta PK: Genital actinomycosis and intrauterine contraceptive devices. Cytopathologic diagnosis and clinical significance. Hum Pathol 9:567, 1978. *An estimated 6 million women in the United States use intrauterine devices for contraception. This article discusses the role that actinomycosis may play in pelvic inflammatory disease.*

Flynn MW, Felson B: The roentgen manifestations of thoracic actinomycosis. Am J Roentgenol Radium Ther Nucl Med 110:707, 1970. *An outstanding guide to the roentgenographic diagnosis of pulmonary actinomycosis.*

Richtsmeier WJ, Johns ME: Actinomycosis of the head and neck. CRC Crit Rev Clin Lab Sci 11:175, 1979. *An excellent review, with an emphasis on infection of the head and neck.*

294. NOCARDIOSIS

David J. Drutz

DEFINITION. Nocardiosis is a subacute or chronic suppurative bacterial infection characterized by pneumonia and hematogenous dissemination, especially to the central nervous system. In immunosuppressed patients, the disease pursues a more acute, aggressive course.

ETIOLOGY. The etiologic agent is *Nocardia asteroides*, a gram-positive, aerobic actinomycete that is partially, and weakly, acid fast. Filamentous branching cells occur during logarithmic phase growth, but later fragment to small coccobacillary forms. There appear to be three subtypes of *N. asteroides*, occasionally manifesting divergent antimicrobial sensitivity patterns. There are also numerous other *Nocardia* species, and some aspects of classification are unsettled. All nocardiae contain mycolic acid and are similar to mycobacteria in this regard. All are commonly found in soil and on straw, grasses, and rotting vegetation. Nocardiae are resistant to rifampin, a useful point in taxonomy. *N. caviae*, *N. farcinica*, and *N. brasiliensis* can produce pulmonary and disseminated infection in man, but only rarely. *N. brasiliensis* is, however, a common cause of actinomycetoma (see Ch. 375).

INCIDENCE AND PREVALENCE. Nocardiosis occurs worldwide, in all ages, races, and climates. It is two to three times as common in men as in women, but there is no occupation-related susceptibility. Five hundred to 1000 clinical cases occur yearly in the United States, but because of underreporting the true incidence and prevalence of nocardiosis are unknown.

EPIDEMIOLOGY. Nocardiosis is presumed to result from inhalation of airborne bacteria. At least one common-source outbreak in immunocompromised patients has been reported. *N. asteroides* has been recovered from the sputum and other body sites in patients without apparent clinical disease.

Nocardiosis can occur in apparently normal persons or in those with chronic obstructive pulmonary disease, but is encountered more commonly in immunosuppressed patients. Associated clinical conditions include systemic lupus erythematosus, sarcoidosis, silicosis, alveolar proteinosis, chronic granulomatous disease, dysglobulinemias, solid or hematologic malignancies, and corticosteroid therapy. The recovery of *N. asteroides* from any immunocompromised person must be considered evidence of infection, not colonization, and must be appropriately treated.

Nocardiosis can occur as a primary cutaneous infection, usually following a local injury. Dissemination may occur.

PATHOGENESIS AND PATHOLOGY. In congenitally athymic nude mice, *N. asteroides* produces a fatal disseminated infection, but in their syngeneic thymus-bearing littermates, the disease is limited in extent and animals survive. *N. asteroides* growing in log phase prevents the phagolysosomal fusion necessary for alveolar macrophages to kill the ingested bacteria. These observations suggest that macrophages, T lymphocytes, and cell-mediated immunity play a crucial role in host defense against nocardiosis. The roles that serum factors and polymorphonuclear leukoyctes fulfill are poorly defined.

In humans, nocardiosis is characterized by suppuration and abscess formation. The intense fibrosis, extension by contiguous spread, sinus formation, grains, and granulomatous response that characterize actinomycosis and nocardial actinomycetoma are absent. Nocardiosis disseminates hematogenously, with a tendency to involve the central nervous system, kidneys, and skin. However, no organ is exempt. The histologic picture is dominated by suppuration, mimicking pyogenic bacterial infection. *N. asteroides* is usually overlooked in hematoxylin-eosin–stained tissue, but is seen with tissue Gram stain or Gomori methenamine silver (if staining time is extended). Acid-fast stains (appropriately modified to prevent overdecolorization) will demonstrate the organism, but its tendency to fragment into coccobacillary forms may cause it to be confused with *Mycobacterium tuberculosis* or atypical mycobacteria.

CLINICAL MANIFESTATIONS. Nocardiosis presents as a pneumonic process in about 75 per cent of cases; in others, the pulmonary involvement may be transient or inapparent. Fever and cough are common. The radiographic picture is characterized by segmental or lobar infiltrates, often with rapidly developing thick-walled cavities. Masses, nodules, empyema, bulging fissures, and even chest wall extension reminiscent of actinomycosis may be encountered. Other radiographic presentations include chronic solitary lung abscess or indolent progressive fibrosis. Hilar involvement and calcification are uncommon. The radiographic picture has no pathognomonic features, and is often complicated by pre-existing lung disease.

In 25 to 40 per cent of patients there is dissemination to the central nervous system. Occasionally, there is meningitis, but more frequently there are one or more space-occupying lesions, with headache and focal neurologic findings. Other common sites of dissemination include the skin and subcutaneous tissues, pleura and chest wall, kidney, eyes, liver, and lymph nodes. Fifty-five per cent of patients have no identifiable foci of secondary infection. However, dissemination is more common in the immunosuppressed, and must be aggressively sought. A negative chest film does not exclude disseminated nocardiosis.

DIAGNOSIS. In a patient with a generally intact immune system and a chronic disease course, nocardiosis may be confused with tuberculosis, mycoses, a variety of bacterial infections, or a malignancy. Repeated sputum cultures or more invasive diagnostic procedures may be required to reach the diagnosis. In the immunosuppressed patient, the disease may be confused or may coexist with any of the disorders named above, or with pneumocystosis *(P. carinii)*, Legionnaires' disease, cytomegalovirus infection, bleomycin lung, and others. In such patients, an aggressive diagnostic evaluation is indicated. Diagnostic flexibility is limited by the unavailability of reliable skin or serologic tests. Specimens of sputum, pleural fluid, tracheostomy secretions, transtracheal aspirates, bronchial washings and brushings, and transbronchial biopsy specimens should be stained and cultured. With failure of these methods, percutaneous lung aspiration or open lung biopsy should be carried out. Skin abscesses should be aspirated and smears examined for organisms. In addition, skin lesions should be biopsied, with portions submitted for histology and for culture. Computed tomographic (CT) scans of the brain should be obtained as otherwise silent cerebral abscesses or foci of cerebritis have been identified in this manner.

Nocardia asteroides will grow on most standard media. However, unless the organism is suspected, its recognition poses a practical problem because culture plates tend to be overgrown by microbial contaminants (especially in sputum) and are often discarded after 48 hours, whereas *N. asteroides* may require three to seven days for growth. As a result, the organism is more likely to be identified on media used for mycobacteria or fungi, which are observed for longer periods of time. Although chances for recovery of *N. asteroides* from the blood, urine, bone marrow, and spinal fluid are slim, cultures should nevertheless be obtained in difficult diagnostic situations.

TREATMENT. Most *N. asteroides* strains are sensitive to sulfonamides in vitro, and sulfonamides are the treatment of choice. Therapy should be initiated with 6 to 10 grams of sulfadiazine or sulfisoxazole daily. These regimens produce peak serum levels of 12 to 15 mg per deciliter. Subsequent dosage can be modified according to measured serum concentrations and clinical response. The duration of therapy is poorly standardized, but should be prolonged since relapse is common. In patients with intact host defenses, treatment should be continued for at least six weeks following clinical recovery. In the immunosuppressed, therapy should be given for at least one year. In patients with cerebral involvement, the progress of treatment should be monitored with serial CT scans. Surgery is usually required for brain abscesses and may also be necessary for subcutaneous abscesses or empyema.

Not all patients respond to sulfonamide therapy, especially those who are profoundly immunosuppressed. In these patients it may be necessary to reduce dosage of immunosuppressive drugs. It has also been common to employ supplemental drugs (cycloserine, ampicillin, tetracycline, erythromycin, streptomycin, and other aminoglycosides), but proof of efficacy of combined drug regimens is lacking. This statement also applies to co-trimoxazole, a fixed combination of one part trimethoprim to five parts sulfamethoxazole. Nevertheless, trimethoprim-sulfamethoxazole has come to be widely used, especially in immunocompromised patients or those with central nervous system involvement.

In patients unable to tolerate or not responding to sulfonamides, therapeutic alternatives include amikacin, minocycline, and chloramphenicol.

PROGNOSIS. Nocardiosis is not restricted to the immunosuppressed. However, those who are immunosuppressed have the most acute process, the greatest propensity to hematogenous dissemination, and the poorest prognosis. Prior to the sulfonamide era, only 25 per cent of patients recovered; in patients treated with a sulfonamide, the recovery rate is 54 per cent. However, Palmer et al. have recorded 75 per cent survival, even in immunosuppressed patients, when the diagnosis was established promptly and sulfonamide therapy begun. Thus, the chances for cure are directly related to the aggressiveness of management. Patients with cerebral involvement generally have a poorer prognosis.

Curry WA: Human nocardiosis. A clinical review with selected case reports. Arch Intern Med 140:818, 1980. *A current review, with valuable information concerning chemotherapy.*

Palmer DL, Harvey RL, Wheeler JK: Diagnostic and therapeutic considerations in *Nocardia asteroides* infection. Medicine 53:391, 1974. *A comprehensive literature review of 243 cases of nocardiosis (including 13 patients in their own experience) occurring between 1961 and 1972. Still the best single review on the subject.*

Simpson GL, Stinson EB, Egger MJ, Remington JS: Nocardial infections in the immunocompromised host: A detailed study in a defined population. Rev Infect Dis 3:492, 1981. *Twenty-one of 160 patients undergoing cardiac transplantation at Stanford developed nocardiosis. Percutaneous lung aspiration was of particular value in reaching the diagnosis; sputum survey cultures were rarely positive. Patients responded surprisingly well to sulfisoxazole, despite the fact that immunosuppressive therapy was not altered.*

Smego RA Jr, Moeller MB, Gallis HA: Trimethoprim-sulfamethoxazole therapy for Nocardia infections. Arch Intern Med 143:711, 1983. *This article provides an extensive literature review and argues that trimethoprim-sulfamethoxazole is likely to be superior to sulfonamides alone for patients with all forms of nocardiosis. The authors acknowledge that no direct comparative data exist but offer pharmacokinetic evidence and discussion of synergy in vitro to support the use of the combination.*

Stevens DA, Pier AC, Beaman BL, Morozumi PA, Lovett IS, Houang ET: Laboratory evaluation of an outbreak of nocardiosis in immunocompromised hosts. Am J Med 71:928, 1981. *Description of an apparent common-source outbreak of nocardiosis in a renal unit and/or possible person-to-person spread of infection.*

295. BRUCELLOSIS

*John E. Bennett**

DEFINITION. Brucellosis is an infectious disease characterized by fever, sweats, weakness, malaise, and weight loss. Infection is transmitted to man from animals or animal products containing bacteria of the genus *Brucella*.

ETIOLOGY. *Brucella suis, Brucella abortus, Brucella melitensis,* and *Brucella canis* may all cause human brucellosis. Brucellae are small, nonmotile, non-spore-forming, gram-negative rods. The four species are differentiated by biochemical and serologic reactions. Hogs are generally infected with *Br. suis,* cattle with *Br. abortus,* sheep and goats with *Br. melitensis,* and dogs with *Br. canis.* However, infections of swine with *Br. abortus* or of cattle with *Br. suis* may occur, and *Brucella* infection of caribou, deer, horses, moose, cats, and chickens has been reported. Animal-to-animal transmission is usually venereal or via ingestion of infected tissue or milk. Human infection most commonly results from ingestion of infected animal tissue or milk products, or through skin wounds directly bathed in freshly killed infected animal tissues, as in abattoir workers. Human infection via inoculation of the conjunctival sac has also been documented, and there is epidemiologic evidence to suggest rare infection via inhalation of aerosols containing *Brucella* organisms.

EPIDEMIOLOGY. Brucellosis is common in many countries of the world, with 500,000 cases per year being reported to the World Health Organization. Within the United States the number of cases reported to the Centers for Disease Control each year has gradually declined, with only 154 cases being reported in 1982. The actual number of cases in the United States is probably larger, but there is no doubt that the rigorous efforts to control brucellosis in this country have been effective.

Brucellosis most frequently occurs in persons with high rates

*This chapter is a revision of the chapter written by Thomas M. Buchanan, which appears in the 16th edition.

of exposure to *Brucella*-infected tissues, milk, or milk products. This includes slaughterhouse workers, livestock producers, veterinarians, and persons who ingest unpasteurized milk or milk products. During the ten-year period 1969–1978, 1171 (57 per cent) of the 2063 reported cases were in slaughterhouse employees.

Brucellae may remain viable in unpasteurized milk or cheese for approximately 10 or 90 days, respectively. Among the 3316 cases of brucellosis reported to the Centers for Disease Control in the 14-year period 1965–1978, ingestion of unpasteurized dairy products accounted for 8 per cent. The source of the dairy product was Mexico in 47 per cent, other foreign countries in 19 per cent, and the United States in 34 per cent. *Br. melitensis* in Mexican goat's milk cheese has been responsible for several outbreaks, including 29 cases from Texas in 1983. Isolation of *Brucella* from infected meat markedly decreases over a few days with refrigeration, and particularly with the curing and smoking processes used for ham and bacon. In the abattoir setting, persons with a combination of both high accidental cut rates and considerable exposure to the blood and lymph of freshly killed animals are most likely to develop *Brucella* infections. *Brucella* infections are often controlled by the patient's immune response, and asymptomatic infections are up to ten times more common than symptomatic disease and the clinical syndrome of brucellosis. Approximately 90 per cent of patients are immune to developing subsequent clinical brucellosis following recovery from their first infection. Therefore in populations with high exposures to potentially infected tissues (e.g., abattoir workers), most cases are seen in younger persons who have been exposed for shorter periods and are less likely to have developed immunity. Brucellosis affects men more commonly than women.

PATHOGENESIS AND PATHOLOGY. *Brucella* organisms penetrate the epithelial cells of the human skin (i.e., hands), oropharynx, conjunctivae, or lung. In the submucosa they interact with polymorphonuclear leukocytes (PMN) and/or tissue macrophages. Many are phagocytized, and, if the inoculum is sufficient, some spread via the lymphatics to regional lymph nodes. The most common sites of lymphadenitis in brucellosis are in the axillary, cervical, and supraclavicular locations, perhaps reflecting the high frequency of the hand-wound or oropharyngeal routes of infections. If the inoculum is sufficient to overcome host immune attempts at localization of *Brucella* organisms within the lymph nodes, bacteremia follows. The usual incubation period between infection and bacteremia with associated symptoms is 10 to 11 days with a heavy inoculum, and two to three weeks with a smaller inoculum. Incubation periods as short as seven days or as long as three months have been reported. Bacteremia is usually accompanied by phagocytosis of nearly all free *Brucella* organisms within a few hours by circulating PMN. These phagocytized brucellae are further localized most commonly to the spleen, liver, and bone marrow. Brucellae are located inside phagocytic vacuoles within PMN, and transient intracellular survival and even multiplication of *Brucella* organisms within phagocytes have been reported. In most instances, the inoculum is not large, the human host defenses prevail, granuloma formation does not occur, and the patient recovers. Similarly, even with a large inoculum, prompt treatment (within three to four weeks of onset of symptoms) of sufficient duration (four to eight weeks) results in rapid healing of the small granulomas and complete recovery. However, if the inoculum is large and the patient is not treated, small granulomas may fuse to form large granulomas that may eventually suppurate and serve as a source for recurrent bacteremia. Granulomas in the liver are common with infections caused by *Br. abortus* and *Br. suis*, but uncommon with hepatic involvement caused by *Br. melitensis*. Persistent bacteremia may lead to multiple system involvement, including most commonly infections and abscesses of the skeletal system (spine and joints), genitourinary tract (kidneys, bladder, epididymis, testes, urethra), optic nerve, lung, liver (abnormal liver function tests, jaundice), and cardiovascular system (endocarditis, myocarditis, pericarditis). *Br. suis* and *Br. melitensis* are more virulent than *Br. abortus*, and *Br. canis* usually causes a mild and easily treatable disease.

CLINICAL MANIFESTATIONS. Over 90 per cent of patients experience chilly sensations, sweats, and fever, accompanied by weakness and general malaise. The fever ranges from 38.3 to 40° C, and approximately 70 per cent of patients experience body aches. Over half of patients with brucellosis complain of anorexia and experience weight loss, averaging 15 to 20 pounds. Nearly 45 per cent of patients complain of headaches. Cough and/or arthralgias are present in approximately 20 to 25 per cent of patients. Diarrhea, constipation, visual disturbance, eye pain, dizziness, tinnitus, or genitourinary disturbance may occur, although less frequently. The most common signs of brucellosis in addition to fever are lymphadenopathy (up to 40 per cent), splenomegaly (up to 40 per cent), hepatomegaly (up to 8 per cent), and tenderness over the spine (up to 6 per cent), with the prevalence of each sign reflecting the chronicity of infection in the patient population studied. The average number of work days lost for an abattoir worker with brucellosis varies from 30 to 50 days. One third to one half of patients experience a sudden onset of symptoms; in the remainder the onset is gradual, over several days to weeks.

Observed complications in patients with untreated and longstanding brucellosis have included pleurisy, pleural effusion, lung abscess, millet-seed pulmonary calcification, empyema, pneumonia, chronic pulmonary granuloma, spondylitis, suppurative arthritis, osteomyelitis, hydrarthrosis, epididymitis, orchitis, cystitis, pyelitis, nephritis, optic neuritis, keratitis, uveitis, retinopathy, meningitis, encephalitis, neuritis, hemolytic anemia, thrombocytopenia or pancytopenia associated with hypersplenism, cholecystitis, pericholecystic or subdiaphragmatic abscesses, chronic cutaneous ulcers, endocarditis, myocarditis, thrombophlebitis, pulmonary embolization, and cardiac rupture. Patients suspected of central nervous system involvement with *Brucella* organisms should have cerebrospinal fluid (CSF) examined. *Brucella* meningoencephalitis or brain abscesses frequently produce increased CSF pressure and increased CSF protein levels. The CSF usually has increased gamma globulin levels and frequently contains *Brucella*-agglutinating antibodies. Many diseases more common than brucellosis have signs and symptoms that partially or almost totally mimic brucellosis. It is therefore important to exclude other more common illnesses and to obtain objective evidence of *Brucella* infection before making a diagnosis of brucellosis. Diseases that may resemble brucellosis include influenza; infectious mononucleosis; toxoplasmosis; viral hepatitis; acute pyelonephritis; ankylosing spondylitis; thyrotoxicosis; disseminated gonococcal infection; rheumatic fever; systemic lupus erythematosus; malaria; tuberculosis; sarcoidosis; leptospirosis; typhoid fever; Hodgkin's disease; lymphoblastic and lymphocytic leukemia; myeloblastic and myelocytic leukemia; metastatic carcinoma of the lung, colon, prostate, pancreas, stomach, or liver; and thiamin deficiency. If the patient has had recent exposure to animal tissue or products potentially infected with *Brucella* organisms, the clinical suspicion of brucellosis should be increased.

Objective findings useful for evaluation of possible brucellosis in a patient include physical signs, cultures, serologic data, and x-rays. The absence of at least intermittent fever of 38.3° C or higher makes a diagnosis of brucellosis extremely unlikely (less than 5 per cent of patients). Weight loss is present in approximately half of the patients; lymphadenopathy and splenomegaly are other common signs.

The definitive evidence of *Brucella* infection is the isolation of *Brucella* organisms from the patient. *However, culturing* Brucella *organisms may be dangerous to laboratory personnel. All cultures should be clearly marked "possible brucellosis." A laboratory should not undertake isolation and identification of* Brucella *unless Biosafety Level 3 facilities are available.* Early in the course of illness, particularly in association with fever and chills, the patient is likely to have *Brucella* bacteremia. Approximately 50 to 75 per cent of these patients who have not received antimicrobial drugs will yield *Brucella* organisms from their blood when one or two samples are cultured in standard blood culture bottles (containing trypticase soy broth) for one to three weeks in the presence of 5 to 10 per cent CO_2. Later in the course of the illness, bacteremia is less frequent and organisms are more likely to be isolated from infected lymph nodes, or from granulomas involving the spleen, liver, or skeletal system (most frequently, spine). During the past ten years only 15 to 20 per cent of brucellosis cases in the United States have been confirmed by culture. Most cases were diagnosed serologically.

The most reliable and standardized *serologic screening test* for brucellosis is the standard tube *Brucella* agglutination test, which measures antibodies directed predominantly at *Brucella* lipopolysaccharide antigens. A four-fold or greater rise in titer for sera drawn one to four weeks apart is indicative of recent exposure to *Brucella* or *Brucella*-like antigens. Separate sera should be tested on the same day, in the same laboratory, and under identical conditions to examine for seroconversion. Significant seroconversion is defined as four-fold or greater rise in titer from an initial titer of at least 40 or higher to an eventual titer of 160 or higher. The titer is the reciprocal of the maximal serum dilution that produces 50 per cent or more agglutination of the *Brucella* organisms under the test conditions. Most patients develop rising agglutination titers to *Brucella* antigens within one to two weeks of illness, and approximately 80 per cent of persons have an eight-fold or higher rise in their agglutinins during the acute illness. Within three weeks of illness, approximately 97 per cent of patients with brucellosis will have serologic evidence of their infection if a single serum sample is tested. With repeat testing, less than 0.7 per cent of all patients will remain seronegative (titer <160). Serum from patients infected with *Br. canis* usually fails to agglutinate the standard antigen but will react with antigen prepared from *Br. canis* or *Br. ovis*. Another cause of false negative agglutination test results is failure of the laboratory to test dilutions up to at least 1:320. The prozone phenomenon may cause lower dilutions to be negative. The maximal *Brucella* agglutination titers in sera from persons with asymptomatic *Brucella* infections may reach as high as titers in patients with clinical brucellosis. The *Brucella* skin test, cholera vaccination, or infection with *Vibrio cholerae, Pasteurella tularensis,* or *Yersinia enterocolitica* may cause seroconversion to elevated *Brucella* agglutination titers and not represent *Brucella* infection. Provided that these "cross-reactive" causes of seroconversion are ruled out, a four-fold rise in titer of *Brucella* agglutinating antibodies is indicative of current *Brucella* infection.

Significance of Elevated Antibody Titer. During the first one to two weeks of illness, the primary agglutinating antibody response to *Brucella* is of the IgM immunoglobulin class. Thereafter, IgG antibodies are formed in addition to IgM antibodies. Both IgG and IgM agglutinating antibodies are detected in the standard *Brucella* agglutination test. However, with early diagnosis and prompt treatment of sufficient duration, IgG agglutinating antibodies rarely persist beyond 6 to 12 months following onset of the disease. However, if the diagnosis is delayed for many months to years and no treatment is received, some patients (fewer than 15 per cent) will develop continuing *Brucella* infection with potentially serious complications. These patients will maintain elevated IgG *Brucella* agglutinins until diagnosed and treated. This information is useful to the clinician, because the *Brucella* agglutination performed in the presence of 0.05 M 2-mercaptoethanol (2-ME) recognizes only IgG agglutinating antibodies to Brucella. Thus in the absence of a rising agglutination titer, a single elevated 2-ME *Brucella* agglutination test titer is the most objective evidence that the patient has a current or recent infection. A titer of 160 or higher in the 2-ME test suggests either a current or recent asymptomatic infection or, if the patient is symptomatic, active infection with disease and the need for treatment. Titers of 40 to 80 in the 2-ME *Brucella* agglutination test are rarely associated with significant recent infections. In a patient with symptoms of three or more weeks' duration, a 2-ME *Brucella* agglutination titer of 20 or lower essentially eliminates the possibility that the patient's symptoms are due to brucellosis. A significant proportion of patients maintain elevated IgM agglutinating antibodies and consequently have elevated standard *Brucella* agglutination titers for many years, even after presumed complete cure of their brucellosis. In fact, standard *Brucella* agglutination titers of ≥160 are very common in completely asymptomatic abattoir workers. For this reason, the 2-ME *Brucella* agglutination test that measures only IgG agglutinating antibodies is the most useful indicator of whether the patient was cured (negative test). Of 92 patients with brucellosis followed recently by Buchanan and Faber for ≥18 months, 44 (48 per cent) retained positive standard *Brucella* agglutination test titers (≥160) after 18 months despite adequate treatment in nearly all cases. In contrast, only eight of these same patients retained positive titers (≥160) in the 2-ME *Brucella* agglutination test 12 months after treatment was initiated. None of the 84 patients with negative 2-ME titers after 12 months had significant signs or symptoms of brucellosis, and none developed chronic brucellosis. In contrast, four of the eight patients with persistent positive 2-ME titers still had signs and symptoms of brucellosis and required further treatment. Thus, the 2-ME *Brucella* agglutination test is the most useful objective indicator of whether a patient has responded to chemotherapy.

The Brucella skin test is not recommended for diagnostic purposes, because it may remain positive for many years following symptomatic or asymptomatic *Brucella* infection and it may interfere with interpretation of serologic tests by causing a rise in titer of the standard tube agglutination test.

TREATMENT. The drug of choice for brucellosis is tetracycline, given to adults as 500 mg orally four times a day and continued for four or preferably six weeks. The addition of streptomycin 1 gram intramuscularly each day for the first two weeks decreases the relapse rate and improves response in severely ill patients. Substitution of gentamicin or other aminoglycosides for streptomycin has been reported, as has usage of doxycycline instead of tetracycline. The merits of such exchanges are as yet unclear. The combination trimethoprim-sulfamethoxazole has been reasonably effective in a number of cases, particularly when the adult dose was two 80-400 mg tablets three or four times each day. Rifampin, 600 mg daily, has been a useful addition to other regimens and should be considered for cases refractory to tetracycline plus streptomycin or for patients with meningoencephalitis. Although penicillins and cephalosporins have not proven efficacious in brucellosis, moxalactam plus rifampin was reported to have cured a patient with chronic *Brucella* meningitis. With any effective treatment of brucellosis, fever may increase markedly for the first 24 hours, sometimes accompanied by delerium or shock. In severe brucellosis, concomitant administration of adrenal corticosteroids has been used for the first days of therapy to blunt this reaction. All antimicrobial regimens should be continued for four or preferably six weeks.

Relapses occur in less than 5 per cent of cases when the patient receives treatment early in the course of illness and for six weeks' duration. Relapse is more frequent when treatment is delayed or of insufficient duration. Most relapses occur within three months, and nearly all develop within ten months of completing initial therapy. Nearly all relapses rapidly respond to a repeat course of therapy.

PROGNOSIS. Brucellosis diagnosed within one month of onset of illness and treated with appropriate antimicrobial therapy for a sufficient period is a completely curable illness. Even before antimicrobial therapy was available, 85 per cent of patients recovered within three months. With chemotherapy, chronic brucellosis (illness lasting more than one year) or severe complications have become extremely rare. When either of these situations is found, it is almost invariably associated with a prolonged delay before diagnosis and/or failure to take prescribed medications. Acute brucellosis produces substantial malaise, weakness, fever, and weight loss and is frequently associated with an inability to work for one to two months, even with antimicrobial therapy. Without therapy, complications such as *Brucella* abscesses of the liver, spleen, vertebral column, heart valve, skin, meninges, lung, or bone marrow may occur, but with therapy, these complications are rare (less than 1 per cent). They almost invariably occur only in patients with continuous or intermittent fever of 38.3° C or higher and positive standard and 2-ME *Brucella* agglutination test results (titer greater than 160). When complications of brucellosis are demonstrated, they usually respond to a combination of surgical removal of the localized lesion and antimicrobial therapy. Hypersensitivity to *Brucella* antigens may occur, but in recent years it has been very unusual even among abattoir workers who are maximally exposed to potentially infected animal tissue. Therefore patients should be allowed to return to their former work, even if it means re-exposure to *Brucella* antigens, as development of hypersensitivity is unlikely. Also, immunity to reinfection follows the first *Brucella* infection in most (92 per cent) cases, and thus patients returning to work following treatment are less likely to acquire brucellosis than are previously uninfected employees. If these previously infected employees replace seronegative workers in areas of maximal exposure to freshly slaughtered animal tissues, fewer cases of brucellosis may result.

PREVENTION. Effective prevention of brucellosis in cattle results from a live attenuated *Brucella* vaccine. No vaccine is presently available for humans in the United States. The risk of acquiring brucellosis may be reduced by decreasing one's exposure to freshly killed animal tissue from potentially infected animals and by drinking only pasteurized milk and milk products. Slaughterhouse workers, meat inspectors, and veterinarians who occupationally examine large numbers of cattle and hogs may reduce their risk of infection by wearing protective gloves and goggles or eyeglasses and by avoiding hand or arm cuts that might provide a route of entry for *Brucella* organisms. Complete elimination of brucellosis in humans will first require elimination of *Brucella* infection in animals.

Buchanan TM, Faber LC: 2-Mercaptoethanol *Brucella* agglutination test: Usefulness for predicting recovery from brucellosis. J Clin Microbiol 11:691, 1980. *The most complete analysis of the standard and 2-ME* Brucella *agglutination tests, utilizing 15 to 29 sera from each of 92 patients with brucellosis who were followed closely for ≥18 months after initiation of treatment.*

Buchanan TM, et al.: Brucellosis in the United States, 1960–1972: An abattoir-associated disease. I. Clinical features and therapy. II. Diagnostic aspects. III. Epidemiology and evidence for acquired immunity. Medicine 53:403, 415, 427, 1974. *A detailed analysis of all aspects of brucellosis in 160 patients in a large Iowa abattoir.*

Cervantes F, Carbonell J, Bruguera M, Force L, Webb S: Liver disease in brucellosis. A clinical and pathological study of 40 cases. Postgrad Med J 58:346, 1982. *Biopsies and clinical features of 40 cases, mostly proved by serology, are analyzed.*

Gotuzzo E, Alarcon GS, Bocanegra TS, Carrillo C, Guerra JC, Rolands I, Espinoza LR: Articular involvement in human brucellosis: A retrospective analysis of 304 cases. Semin Arthritis Rheum 12:245, 1982. *An instructive analysis of sacroiliitis, arthritis, and spondylitis in 304 Peruvian cases, largely caused by* Br. melitensis.

Larbrisseau A, Maravi E, Aguilera F, Martinez-Lage JM: The neurological complications of brucellosis. Can J Neurol Sci 5:369, 1978. *A recent review of the neurologic complications of brucellosis, including meningoencephalitis, extradural* Brucella *granuloma, and neuritis.*

Marx A, Sandulache R, Pop A, Cerbu A: Biochemical basis of the serological cross-reactions between *Brucella abortus* and *Yersinia enterocolitica* serotype 0:9. Ann Microbiol 126B:435, 1975. *A biochemical study indicating cross-antigenicity in the lipopolysaccharide molecules of* Brucella abortus *and* Yersinia enterocolitica *serotype 0:9.*

Spink WW: The Nature of Brucellosis. Minneapolis, University of Minnesota Press, 1956. *A classic reference book detailing many aspects of brucellosis, and including an appendix of case histories of 139 bacteriologically proven cases.*

Young EJ: Human brucellosis. Rev Infect Dis 5:821, 1983. *Nine instructive cases of brucellosis are presented and the relevant literature reviewed.*

296. BARTONELLOSIS

Theodore C. Eickhoff

SYNONYMS. Synonyms for bartonellosis include Carrión's disease, Oroya fever, and verruga peruana.

DEFINITION. Bartonellosis is an insect-borne bacterial disease found only in South America, and characterized by two distinct stages. The first, Oroya fever, is an acute febrile hemolytic anemia with an appreciable mortality; the second, verruga peruana, is a benign cutaneous eruption of hemangiomatous papules and nodules.

ETIOLOGY. The disease is caused by *Bartonella bacilliformis,* a small gram-negative pleomorphic bacillus that may be cultivated readily in enriched bacteriologic media. The disease is transmitted to man by the bite of sandflies of the genus *Phlebotomus;* characteristic symptoms of Oroya fever follow an incubation period of two to six weeks.

EPIDEMIOLOGY. Although a number of epidemics have been reported, Oroya fever is more commonly seen as sporadic cases among populations of Peru, Colombia, and Ecuador, where occurrence of the disease is restricted to those who live or visit altitudes of 1500 to 9000 feet on both slopes of the Andes. This coincides in general with the ecologic zones supporting populations of the *Phlebotomus* vector.

The disease is transmitted by *Phlebotomus verrucarum,* a night-biting sandfly, and possibly by other unidentified species of sandfly. The principal reservoir of the disease appears to be man; no additional animal reservoirs have been implicated. Reports of cultivation of the agent from apparently healthy persons suggest that as much as 10 per cent of infection may be subclinical.

PATHOLOGY. In Oroya fever, the causative organism may be found in peripheral blood smears stained with Giemsa or Wright's stain, as well as in the reticuloendothelial cells. In the blood the parasite is found both free in the plasma and adherent to erythrocytes. Parasitization of the erythrocytes causes increased mechanical fragility and also increased sequestration of the cells in the spleen and liver. Because as many as 90 per cent of erythrocytes may be parasitized, a severe hemolytic anemia develops rapidly during the febrile period, erythrocyte counts decreasing within only a few days to levels of 1 to 2 million cells per cubic millimeter. Coombs' tests and tests for red cell agglutinins and hemolysins give negative results, and the mechanism of hemolysis remains poorly understood.

CLINICAL MANIFESTATIONS. The presenting symptoms of patients with Oroya fever are intermittent high fever, painful muscles and joints, tender enlarged lymph nodes, and the systemic symptoms and prostration of a severe anemia. The patient's skin color may reflect the presence of both jaundice caused by hemolysis and marked pallor caused by profound anemia. Peripheral blood films show macrocytosis, hypochromasia, poikilocytosis, Howell-Jolly bodies, and nucleated erythrocytes. Muscle and joint pain and headache may be severe. After three to six weeks, survivors begin a slow convalescence marked by disappearance of *bartonellae* from the blood and gradual normalization of temperature and red cell mass.

After a variable length of time, survivors may develop the second (verruga peruana) stage of the disease, characterized by cutaneous nodules that develop over one to two months. The "verrugas" are nodular hemangiomatous lesions, 0.5 to 2 cm in diameter, that most frequently involve exposed skin but occasionally may appear on mucous membranes or in viscera. The verrugas may persist for several months to several years in untreated persons, but mortality is infrequent. Occasional patients may experience only the fever and anemia without the skin manifestations or only the cutaneous lesions without the initial fever. Although these two aspects of the infection were once thought to be different diseases, there is ample evidence that both syndromes are manifestations of infection with the same organism. The skin lesions are believed to be an expression of developing immunity in the patient.

DIAGNOSIS. In the acute stage of Oroya fever both blood smears and blood culture usually reveal the presence of the agent. As the patient progresses toward the verruga stage of infection, the organism becomes more difficult to demonstrate in blood, but can be cultured from the cutaneous lesions.

TREATMENT AND PROGNOSIS. Mortality in the Oroya fever phase of the disease may approach 50 per cent, particularly when the infection is complicated by concurrent attacks of malaria, amebiasis, tuberculosis, or salmonellosis. The disease responds well to treatment with penicillin, tetracyclines, streptomycin, or chloramphenicol. Because of the high frequency of intercurrent *Salmonella* infections, chloramphenicol is widely used for seven or more days in a dose of 2.0 to 3.0 grams daily. Patients become afebrile in 24 to 48 hours, and, if they receive transfusions, recover strength rapidly. The mortality of the verruga stage of infection is less than 5 per cent, and the lesions respond variably to chemotherapy.

PREVENTION. Prevention requires control of the sandfly vector. Spraying of interior and exterior dwellings with residual insecticide has been helpful. Personal protection may be augmented by insect repellents and bed nets.

Archer GL, Coleman PH, Cole RM, Duma RJ, Johnston CL Jr: Human infection from an unidentified erythrocyte-associated bacterium. N Engl J Med 301:897, 1979. *Although bartonellae are the only well-characterized hemotropic bacteria known, this case report suggests the possibility that there may be others. See also the accompanying editorial by Ristic M, Kreier JP: Hemotropic bacteria, pp 937–939.*

Dooley JR: Haemotropic bacteria in man. Lancet 2:1237, 1980. Kreier JP, Ristic M: The biology of hemotrophic bacteria. Ann Rev Microbiol 35:325, 1981. *These two reviews are an excellent introduction to the broad topic of hemotrophic bacteria.*

Schultz MG: Daniel Carrión's experiment. N Engl J Med 278:1323, 1968. *A fascinating account of the young Peruvian medical student, Daniel Carrión, who demonstrated by his death that verruga peruana and Oroya fever were caused by the same etiologic agent.*

Presumptive Bacterial Disease

297. CAT SCRATCH DISEASE

Andrew M. Margileth

DEFINITION. Cat scratch disease (CSD) is usually a benign, self-limited disease characterized by tender regional chronic (≥ three weeks) lymphadenopathy and frequently preceded by a primary skin lesion following cat contact or scratches. Persistence of the adenopathy for several months in a generally healthy patient with gradual spontaneous resolution of the enlarged bubo is its natural course.

ETIOLOGY. Recently studies at the Armed Forces Institute of Pathology have implicated a small gram-negative bacillus as the causative agent of CSD. In 34 of 39 lymph nodes from patients with clinical and histopathologic criteria of CSD, pleomorphic rod-shaped bacilli were observed within the walls of capillaries, in or near areas of follicular hyperplasia, and within microabscesses. They were clearly seen with the Warthin-Starry silver impregnation stain and with immunoperoxidase stains using convalescent patient sera. Similar-appearing organisms were seen with light microscopy in the biopsied tissue of a primary inoculation cat scratch lesion on the finger of a patient with typical CSD.

EPIDEMIOLOGY. Since the initial description by Debré (1950), about 2000 patients with cat scratch disease have been reported in over 750 articles. An estimated 2000 unreported cases occur annually in the United States, primarily in children, but the true incidence is unknown. The disease is worldwide, occurring in all races with a predominance in males (61 per cent). In temperate zones, most cases have occurred during fall and winter. Seasonal variation is minimal in warmer climates. Several epidemics in the same house or geographic locality have been recorded.

TRANSMISSION AND COMMUNICABILITY. The mode of transmission is presumably by direct contact, since the bubo usually follows a scratch, bite, or lick from a young cat. Cat contact occurs in 90 per cent of patients. The disease has also developed after a dog bite or scratch and rarely after a scratch from a thorn, wood splinter, or fish bone. Person-to-person transmission has not been reported. Regional lymphadenopathy was produced experimentally in humans, monkeys, baboons, and Hartley guinea pigs after an intradermal injection of material aspirated from suppurative lymph nodes of human patients. Attempts to isolate an infectious agent from cat saliva or claws have been unsuccessful. The healthy cat—often a kitten—apparently acts as a mechanical vector for the infective agent, for skin tests with CS antigen on the implicated cats have been nonreactive. The writer's studies in family outbreaks have shown that the family cat usually transmits the causative agent no longer than two to three weeks.

PATHOGENESIS AND PATHOLOGY. No serologic test is available to measure antibodies to the causative agent. Fortunately, the cat scratch skin test is reliable and has a high degree of specificity; the reaction is a delayed hypersensitivity type. A positive reaction is usually detected at the time the clinical diagnosis is suspected; however, conversion may be delayed up to four weeks thereafter. Cutaneous reactivity lasts up to ten years. Second attacks have not been reported.

Biopsied lymph nodes may show distinct yet nonspecific stages, depending upon the interval between onset and biopsy. The early lesions reveal a reticulum cell hyperplasia followed by necrotizing granulomas, occasionally with giant cells, then multiple microabscesses, and, weeks to months later, frank abscess formation. Consequently, a presumptive histopathologic diagnosis of tularemia, brucellosis, tuberculosis, or sarcoidosis may be considered. Rarely a biopsy made before suppuration has appeared has shown histologic changes, including reticulum cell hyperplasia and granulomas, suggestive of Hodgkin's disease.

CLINICAL MANIFESTATIONS. The patient usually is not ill in spite of impressive lymphadenopathy; however, malaise, fever, sore throat, headache, and anorexia may be present. Three to ten days elapse from the time of the scratch or contact until a primary skin papule or pustule forms. It may exhibit one or more erythematous papules. Unilateral conjunctival granuloma or conjunctivitis occurred in 7 per cent of the author's 364 patients. An inoculation site (a scratch or a primary lesion, or both) may be detected in 54 to 96 per cent of patients, depending on the thoroughness of the examination and the duration of the bubo. Most primary lesions persist for one to three weeks, rarely for seven weeks. The primary lesion heals without scar formation. Regional lymphadenopathy usually develops about two weeks after the scratch (range, 3 to 50 days). Lymphangitis has not been observed. Tender nodes, present in 80 per cent of patients for the first one or two weeks, are commonly found in the head, neck, or axilla. Epitrochlear, inguinal, femoral, or popliteal areas are involved less frequently. Multiple site involvement occurred in 38 per cent of the author's cases. Node size varies from 1 to 8 cm. Enlargement persists for two to four months, rarely for 6 to 24 months. Suppuration occurs in about one tenth of patients seen in office practice and in about one quarter of those admitted to hospitals.

No clinical signs other than lymphadenopathy occurred in approximately half of the author's 707 patients observed throughout a 25-year period. In about one third of reported cases, patients had fever (38.3 to 41.2° C) lasting for 5 to 9 (1 to 30) days; 25 per cent of our 364 patients had malaise or an influenza-like syndrome lasting about 4 (1 to 21) days. Splenomegaly occurred in 16 per cent of the last 364 patients. Exanthems—maculopapular, petechial, or erythema nodosum or multiforme types—occurred in 4 per cent of the author's patients. The rash usually lasted 4 to 9 days. See Tables 297–1 and 297–2.

Unusual clinical manifestations include the oculoglandular syndrome of Parinaud (6 per cent, 42 of 707 of the author's cases), appearing as an ocular granuloma or conjunctivitis with parotid area swelling caused by preauricular lymphadenopathy;

TABLE 297–1. CLINICAL FEATURES IN 364 PATIENTS WITH CAT SCRATCH ADENOPATHY AND A POSITIVE SKIN TEST
(April 1975 to January 1983)

Category	Percentage of Patients
Animal contact	
Cat	89
Dog	9
None	2
Animal scratch	
Cat	71
Dog	2
None	27
Primary lesion	
Skin papule or pustule	45
Eye granuloma	7
Mucous membrane	2
Symptoms and signs	
None except adenopathy	52
Fever (38.3–42.1° C)	33
Malaise/fatigue	25
Splenomegaly	16
Sore throat	12
Headache	11
Anorexia/emesis/weight loss	10
Exanthem	4.4
Parotid swelling	3

encephalitis (45); thrombocytopenic purpura (8); osteomyelitis (5); and primary atypical pneumonia (4).

Children with central nervous system involvement may develop encephalopathy, meningitis, radiculitis, polyneuritis, or myelitis with paraplegia. Onset of neurologic symptoms is sudden, usually with fever, and occurs within one to six weeks of the onset of adenopathy. Major symptoms and signs in 41 cases of neurologic involvement were as follows: coma or convulsions in two thirds, neurologic abnormalities, noted above, in one fourth, and lethargy and/or confusion in one sixth. In 12 of 22 patients with neurologic involvement, cerebrospinal fluid pleocytosis, elevated protein, or both were detected. Electroencephalograms were abnormal in most patients. Severe manifestations have lasted for one to two weeks, with gradual recovery to normal status in one to six months in most patients.

DIAGNOSIS. Regional lymphadenopathy developing two weeks after cat contact, and especially if a primary inoculation papule or pustule followed a scratch, suggests cat scratch disease. Three of the four following manifestations would confirm the diagnosis in a typical case, whereas all four would be necessary in an atypical case: (1) a history of animal (usually cat) contact with presence of a scratch or a primary dermal or eye lesion; (2) aspiration of sterile pus from the node (a presumptive diagnostic test) or laboratory results excluding other etiologic possibilities; (3) a positive skin test result to cat scratch antigen (5 per cent false positives occur; use of only one antigen may give a false negative result in 10 to 20 per cent of patients); (4) node biopsy revealing histopathology consistent with CSD, especially if pleomorphic rod-shaped bacilli can be demonstrated with the Warthin-Starry silver stain.

If a negative skin test result is found to one or two different cat scratch antigens applied simultaneously and again four weeks later, and if results of other studies are negative, a biopsy must be considered to rule out a benign tumor or lymphoma. The presence of tenderness favors cat scratch or a pyogenic or mycobacterial adenopathy rather than a neoplasm. Ultrasonography has been very useful in deciding whether or not to aspirate nontender or nonfluctuant cervical masses. It may also aid needle placement for cyst or abscess aspiration.

Skin Tests. A skin test using cat scratch antigen is positive in 90 per cent of patients who are clinically suspected of CSD. A negative result often occurs if the duration of illness is less than three or four weeks, and about 5 per cent of patients with typical cat scratch disease will have negative test results with one or two different antigens. The positive reaction consists of a wheal or papule with 5 mm or more of induration, with or without erythema, occurring 48 to 72 hours after intradermal inoculation of 0.1 ml of antigen. Induration may persist for five to six days or longer. A positive test result may be obtained for years (10 to 28) after the initial episode.

False-positive reactions have been reported in veterinarians (12 to 29 per cent), healthy persons (4 to 5 per cent), and family contacts; the overall incidence is 5 per cent. Thus the limit of confidence for a positive reaction is about 95 per cent. If the reaction is negative at four-week intervals, the disease can be excluded with reasonable certainty, especially if two different antigens are used. Repeated skin testing with CS antigen in the same patients has not produced positive reactions. Skin tests with PPD-T and atypical PPD mycobacterium antigens have been rarely positive in patients with cat scratch disease.

Since CS antigen is not available commercially, all aspirated pus from affected nodes should be saved to prepare test antigen (Margileth, 1968, 1971). CS antigen for medical diagnosis is usually available from the author upon written request.

Laboratory Data. Laboratory tests are not diagnostic. Eosinophilia has been reported. At the onset the number of polymorphonuclear cells may be increased with a mild leukocytosis. A sedimentation rate, usually elevated during the first few

TABLE 297–2. CAT SCRATCH LYMPHADENOPATHY IN 364 PATIENTS—
CLINICAL CHARACTERISTICS OF INVOLVED NODES AND DURATION OF ADENOPATHY
(April 1975 to January 1983)

Adenopathy (N = 364)	Per Cent	Size (cm) (N = 364)	Per cent
Single node	41	1.0 to < 3.0	43
Multiple nodes	21	3.0 to < 5.0	38
Multiple sites	38	≥ 5.0	19
Tender nodes	79		
Suppuration	13		
Location (N = 470)	**Per Cent**	**Duration (N = 364)**	**Per Cent**
Head: total (N = 93*)	20	Prior to diagnosis**	
Submandibular	13	2 to < 4 weeks	51
Preauricular	19	1 to < 2 months	28
Neck: total (N = 193)	41	2 to < 4 months	14
Posterior	17	4 to < 6 months	3
Anterior	21	6 to < 12 months	3
Supraclavicular	3	Regression (months, < 1.0 cm)	
Extremities: total (N = 184)	39	1 to < 2	23
Axillary	22	2 to < 6	56
Epitrochlear	5	6 to < 12	14
Inguinal	7	12 to < 24	6
Femoral	5	≥ 24	1

*Occipital = 5 (1%).
**Duration ≥ 12 months = 4 (1%).

weeks of adenopathy, suggests an inflammatory lymphadenitis.

DIFFERENTIAL DIAGNOSIS. Cat scratch disease should be considered in all patients with persistent lymphadenopathy (over three weeks), because it is the most common cause of chronic regional lymphadenitis in children or adolescents. The presence of an inoculation (dermal or ocular) lesion strongly suggests CSD. Other less common causes are sporotrichosis, primary syphilis, lymphogranuloma venereum, typical or atypical tuberculosis, other bacterial adenitis, tularemia, brucellosis, histoplasmosis, coccidioidomycosis, sarcoidosis, toxoplasmosis, infectious mononucleosis, and benign or malignant tumors. In atypical forms of cat scratch disease, one may observe benign recurrent parotid lymphosialadenopathy, Parinaud's oculoglandular disease, encephalitis, pneumonia, thrombocytopenic purpura, erythema nodosum, and osteomyelitis, as well as fluctuant lymphadenopathy simulating cystic hygroma or a thyroglossal duct cyst. If CS skin test reactions are negative, as well as appropriate cultures and serologic and PPD-T and PPD Battery skin tests, a node biopsy will usually determine the cause.

TREATMENT. The best therapy is reassurance that the adenopathy is benign and in most cases will subside spontaneously within two or three months. Management consists of appropriate follow-up examination, analgesics for pain, and aspiration if suppuration ocurs. Lack of response to antimicrobials is the rule; if cat scratch disease is suspected, antimicrobial drugs are not recommended. In the child whose node suppurates, needle aspiration on an ambulatory basis is preferred to incision and drainage. After washing with Betadine cleanser, a needle (18 or 20 gauge) is inserted through normal unanesthetized skin at the base of the mass in order to avoid a chronic sinus tract in the event that a tuberculous lesion is present. Aspiration provides material for skin test antigen, relieves painful adenopathy, and usually allows the patient to become symptom free within 24 to 48 hours. If fluid recurs, reaspiration may be necessary. Application of moist soaks to the primary lesion may facilitate drainage and shorten the duration of lymphadenopathy. The efficacy of steroid therapy in CSD is questionable, and it is not recommended. Excisional biopsy of the node may be necessary in selected patients because of persistent pain or for diagnostic purposes. Spontaneous drainage occurred in 6 per cent of our last 364 patients.

PROGNOSIS. The prognosis is excellent; lymphadenopathy usually regresses spontaneously in two to three months. One attack appears to confer lifelong immunity. Complications and sequelae are almost nonexistent. Rare patients have been reported to have had chronic adenopathy for two years.

PREVENTION. Because of the number of household pets (50 million cats in the United States), cat scratch disease will be difficult to prevent. Disposal of the suspect cat is not recommended, because the cat involved is invariably well. Four to 9 per cent of family members scratched by the same cat may develop cat scratch disease. The patient with the disease does not require isolation or quarantine. Active or passive protection is not available.

Carithers HA: Cat scratch disease associated with an osteolytic lesion. Am J Dis Child 137:968, 1983, *A case report of a child with lytic bone involvement accompanying cat scratch disease and a review of three previously reported cases.*

Carithers HA: Oculoglandular disease of Parinaud. A manifestation of cat scratch disease. Am J Dis Child 132:1195, 1978. *The diagnostic criteria compiled from 14 patients with oculoglandular cat scratch disease are presented.*

Knight PJ, Mulne AF, Vassy LE: When is lymph node biopsy indicated in children with enlarged nodes? Pediatrics 69:391, 1982. *Based on examination of 239 children who underwent peripheral lymph node biopsy, the differential diagnosis and indications for biopsy are reviewed.*

Luddy RE, Sutherland JC, Levy BE, Schwartz AD: Cat-scratch disease simulating malignant lymphoma. Cancer 50:584, 1982. *A case report of a child with oculoglandular CSD with discussion of histopathology of infectious lymphadenopathy that clinically and histologically may simulate a malignant neoplasm.*

Margileth AM, Wear DJ, Hadfield TL, et al. Cat scratch disease: Bacteria in skin at the primary inoculation site. JAMA (in press), 1984. *Five patients with CSD had biopsy or aspiration of adenopathy and biopsy of the primary inoculation skin lesion. In three patients gram-negative pleomorphic bacilli were demonstrated in the skin lesion by the Warthin-Starry silver stain, and identical bacteria were also seen in the regional lymph nodes of two of these patients.*

Wear DJ, Margileth AM, Hadfield TL, Fischer GW, Schlagel CJ, King FM: Cat scratch disease: A bacterial infection. Science 221:1403, 1983. *In a series of 39 lymph nodes studied from patients with CSD, pleomorphic rod-shaped bacilli were observed in 34 by means of special stains.*

Diseases Due to Mycobacteria

298. TUBERCULOSIS

Emanuel Wolinsky

DEFINITION. Tuberculosis is a chronic infectious disease caused by mycobacteria of the "tuberculosis complex," mainly *Mycobacterium tuberculosis.*

HISTORY. During the Industrial Revolution of the 18th and 19th centuries the disease was known as the *white plague.* It was the leading cause of death in young people all over the world. Today, despite great progress in its treatment and control, it is still an important medical problem in many developing countries. A report from the World Health Organization in 1982 indicated that there were still 7 to 10 million new cases and about 3 million deaths each year from tuberculosis. In the United States the tuberculosis mortality has decreased from a rate of 202 per 100,000 in 1900 to less than 1 in 1982. The new case rate has also declined from about 60 per 100,000 in 1950 to 11 in 1982, but the rate has tended to level off during the past few years, resulting in a decline of approximately 5 per cent per year.

The rate of infection as determined by skin test surveys remains high in many developing countries. In the United States the rate has become increasingly difficult to estimate because of the abandonment of large-scale testing in cities. Information obtained in 1977 from selected urban areas of the country indicated that the rate of infection varied from less than 3 per cent in young children to 14 to 40 per cent in adults over the age of 65. Tuberculosis is becoming more and more a disease of middle-aged and older nonwhite men in residual urban pockets of disease associated with poverty and overcrowding.

The great physicians and scientists who were associated with landmark discoveries in tuberulosis include Laennec, who early in the nineteenth century disclosed the physical signs and morbid anatomy and who suggested the concept of one disease with involvement of many organ systems; Villemin, who in 1868 showed that the infection was caused by a transmissible agent; Koch, who demonstrated the tubercle bacillus in 1882; Roentgen, whose discovery of x-rays in 1895 was the begining of diagnostic radiology and allowed recognition of cavity formation; and Waksman, whose discovery of streptomycin in 1944 provided the first agent that could be used successfully in the chemotherapy of the disease.

ETIOLOGY. The microorganism that causes tuberculosis belongs to the genus *Mycobacterium,* which is classified in the family Mycobacteriaceae of the order Actinomycetales. Other families in this order are the Actinomycetaceae, with genera *Actinomyces* and *Nocardia,* and the Streptomycetaceae, which includes the genus *Streptomyces.* Taxonomists do not agree on the further classification of the genus *Mycobacterium,* but a useful concept is that of the tuberculosis complex to include *M. tuberculosis, M. bovis,* and probably *M. africanum.* Some taxonomists would subdivide *M. bovis* into European, Afro-Asian, and African variants. A few suggest that there should be just one species, *M. tuberculosis,* with subclassifications of bovine type, African type, and so forth.

M. tuberculosis is an obligate intracellular parasite that shares with other mycobacteria a characteristic staining quality. The popular abbreviation *AFB* for *acid-fast bacilli* is based on this quality. Acid-fastness is the result of retention of carbol fuchsin (or certain fluorochrome dyes) after washing with acid, alcohol, or both. It is not unique to mycobacteria, since *Nocardia* and certain *Corynebacterium* strains may also be acid fast. Mycobacterial cell walls are rich in lipids, existing mainly as complexes with peptides and polysaccharides. Certain stains can form a stable complex with one of these lipid compounds, mycolic acid, provided the latter is contained within an intact cell wall structure.

In addition to the members of the tuberculosis complex, the genus *Mycobacterium* may be divided into about 30 species. Again, there is disagreement among the taxonomists on the definition of many of these species (see Ch. 299).

PATHOLOGY AND PATHOGENESIS. Tuberculosis is derived from the word tubercle, meaning a small lump or nodule. Histopathologically, the tubercle is a more or less discrete focus of granulomatous inflammation consisting of lymphocytes, epithelioid cells, macrophages, and giant cells. The granulomas seen in tuberculosis are characterized by a form of tissue necrosis known as *caseation,* so called because the caseum has the consistency of soft cheese. Prior to the time of necrosis the lesion may heal completely by resolution, but once necrosis and caseation have occurred it heals by fibrosis, encapsulation, calcification, and scar formation. Breakdown of the lesion occurs when the caseum softens and liquefies and is expelled through the bronchial system. This process results in the formation of a cavity in the lung. Spread of disease may occur by local extension, by an intrabronchial route, or through the lymphohematogenous pathway. Early in the primary infection the organisms are transported to the draining lymph nodes and may be widely disseminated throughout the body. In the apical posterior areas of the upper lobes the seeded organisms may remain dormant in inactive lesions for many years only to reactivate during a period of lowered host immunity. The processes of healing and breakdown may occur sequentially and repeatedly so that various stages of the inflammatory reaction are seen in different areas.

The primary lesion in a nonsensitized individual consists of an area of nonspecific pneumonitis in a middle or lower lung zone at the site of deposition of the inhaled droplet nuclei. The initial inflammatory response is the same as that seen in any bacterial pneumonia and consists mainly of fibrin, edema, and polymorphonuclear leukocytes. The extent of this primary exudative response varies with the number and virulence of the bacilli inhaled, the native resistance of the host, and the effectiveness of the immune response. The change to a granulomatous type of reaction occurs coincidentally with the development of delayed hypersensitivity after two or three weeks. The mechanisms of cellular immunity may allow the host to wall off the lesion and to halt the lymphohematogenous spread. It is the softening and liquefaction of the caseous focus that leads to further trouble and the provision of a favorable environment for the rapid multiplication of the mycobacteria. In the encapsulated lesion that does not soften, the bacilli slowly lose their viability.

Stages in the natural history of untreated pulmonary tuberculosis may be described as follows:

1. During the primary phase and throughout the development of the lesions there are usually no symptoms. Even in the so-called manifest primary stage, symptoms may be mild or absent despite parenchymal lesions and enlarged hilar or mediastinal lymph nodes. Pleurisy with effusion may occur. Life-threatening complications at this stage are meningitis and miliary disease.
2. The primary disease usually heals, leaving evidence of its presence in the form of a calcified pulmonary scar along with calcifications in the draining lymph nodes, which together are known as a *Ghon complex.*
3. The third stage is one of latency, during which the bacilli remain dormant but still viable within inactive lesions. This situation may exist for the remainder of the patient's life.
4. Reactivation may occur in a relatively small proportion of infected individuals. This is the mechanism by which tuberculosis in the adult usually develops, either in the lung or in an extrapulmonary site.
5. Exogenous reinfection occasionally may be documented by the demonstration of bacilli with a different phage type or drug sensitivity pattern from those of the primary infection.

EPIDEMIOLOGY. Infection is usually transmitted from person to person by the inhalation of infective droplet nuclei that result from the aerosolization of respiratory secretions. The source of the infected material usually is an adult with cavitary pulmonary tuberculosis. The most important determinants of infectivity are the concentration of organisms in the sputum and the closeness and duration of contact with the index case. Other factors of importance are the cough frequency and the personal habits of the index case, the efficiency with which aerosols are produced by such activities as singing, loud talking, and laughing, and the air circulation and ventilation in the area of contact. A situation favorable to acquisition of infection would be an overcrowded and poorly ventilated house in which there were several young children and an adult with highly positive sputum.

Ingestion is no longer a common pathway for infection, although in the days of unpasteurized milk and widespread tuberculosis in cattle this was a common route of infection for *M. bovis,* especially for the production of tuberculosis of the tonsils and subsequent involvement of the submandibular lymph nodes. Another route of infection that still may be observed, however, is primary inoculation through the skin. Laboratory workers may inoculate themselves with actively growing cultures via needle puncture or broken glass, and pathologists may sustain a penetrating injury while doing a postmortem examination.

Many localized outbreaks or mini-epidemics have been reported in the past and continue to be observed today (Lincoln, 1967; Stead, 1979). The pattern of airborne transmission in a closed environment is well described in these accounts of infections aboard ships, in day care centers, nursing homes, prisons, industrial school dormitories, and school buses, and among members of a choir.

Tuberculosis Control. Tuberculosis is perpetuated by the repeated cycle of new infections that result from the inhalation of infected droplet nuclei coughed into the air by adults with cavitary pulmonary disease. This cycle may be attacked at several points. Case finding efforts are needed to recognize individuals with active disease so that they may be placed under treatment to terminate the infectivity. Large-scale roentgenographic surveys have been abandoned in favor of contact investigation, recognition of symptomatic cases at entry points to the medical care system, and surveillance of high-risk groups such as hospital personnel, prisoners, and nursing home patients.

Protection from the complications of primary disease may be afforded by vaccination with bacille Calmette-Guérin (BCG). This was a strain of *M. bovis* attenuated by many passages on artificial media. There are now many different strains, each unique, maintained in laboratories across the world. Vaccination has been utilized mainly in areas of the world that have a high rate of tuberculosis infection. Although vaccination may protect the individual, it does not reduce the overall rate of infection in the community, since it does not prevent the transmission of infection. Its effectiveness depends on an enhancement of the immune response, which enables the host to eliminate most of the bacilli before tissue destruction and dissemination occur. The efficacy of BCG is controversial. It has not been used extensively in the United States because it interferes with the subsequent use of the tuberculin test in recognizing tuberculosis infection and because the major source of morbidity is people already infected. Nevertheless, a case could be made for BCG in certain special circumstances such as to protect the infant whose mother has active disease and to prevent infection in close contacts of an index case with drug-resistant bacilli.

Chemoprophylaxis may be used to prevent infection in close contacts with negative skin tests, to prevent disease in those already infected, and to prevent subsequent recurrences in individuals with inactive pulmonary disease. The recommended drug for prophylaxis is isoniazid, once daily, in dosage of 300 mg for adults and 10 mg per kilogram (not to exceed 300 mg) for children. When taken for one year, such treatment results in a reduction of at least 70 per cent in the appearance of primary disease in household contacts. Protection is about 90 per cent in those who actually take the drug as prescribed. The effectiveness of shorter courses of therapy has not been adequately investigated. Six months of chemoprophylaxis, while not completely ineffective, protects less well than 12 months. The two principal drawbacks to this method of control are isoniazid hepatitis and the lack of compliance of about 30 per cent of patients to take the prescribed medication.

It has been estimated that the risk of developing active disease in recent tuberculin converters of any age is about 3.3 per cent in the first year after infection. From 5 to 15 per cent may progress to active disease within five years. The risk is greater in infants. Chemoprophylaxis is recommended for close contacts of patients with recently diagnosed active disease; for persons with recent infection documented by skin test conversion within the past two years; for individuals with positive skin test results, radiographic findings consistent with inactive tuberculous disease, and neither positive bacteriologic findings nor a history of adequate chemotherapy; and for individuals with positive skin test results who have additional risk factors (such as malignancy or severe diabetes) or who are undergoing prolonged immunosuppressive or corticosteroid therapy. Although chemoprophylaxis is utilized in this country as one of the important methods of tuberculosis control, it has not been accepted in many other parts of the world. Isoniazid will not prevent disease resulting from infection with isoniazid-resistant bacilli. Rifampin has been suggested as a substitute, although no good studies of its efficacy have been published.

IMMUNOLOGY. Tuberculosis is the classic example of disease caused by an intracellular parasite. Protection is afforded by the mechanisms of cell-mediated immunity rather than by those associated with antibodies. Immunity may be natural or acquired, but in either case it is the macrophage that assumes the major burden of protection. Polymorphonuclear leukocytes have the ability to phagocytize but not to destroy mycobacteria. Although the results of some experiments are contradictory, most researchers have been able to demonstrate that macrophages from an immunized animal kill the bacilli more efficiently and at a more rapid rate than do control cells. Macrophages may be activated by immunologically specific mechanisms as well as by nonspecific stimulation. Specific stimulation occurs when sensitized T lymphocytes contact mycobacterial antigens that have been properly processed by macrophages. The lymphocytes then release a number of active chemical substances known as *lymphokines,* one variety of which activates macrophages.

Native immunity certainly has played a role in the global aspects of tuberculosis. Good examples exist in the animal kingdom; the rat and the cat are quite resistant to infection with *M. tuberculosis,* in contrast to the guinea pig and the monkey, which are highly susceptible. Lurie was able to breed two races of rabbits, one susceptible and one resistant to infection. Although it is difficult to separate the factors of social and economic conditions from those of race, the Eskimo peoples and blacks are considered by some researchers to be more susceptible. The forces of natural selection probably contributed to the decline of tuberculosis prior to the introduction of chemotherapy, although improved socioeconomic conditions played an important role. Acquired immunity may occur as a result of natural infection or by vaccination. Recovery from tuberculosis confers protection against reinfection with a new inoculum, even though the original bacilli may remain latent for many years and be capable of producing recrudescent disease. Whether acquired by natural infection or vaccination, the protection is only relative and may be overwhelmed by a sufficiently large infecting dose.

The relationship between delayed hypersensitivity and immunity is still controversial. The two functions appear at about the same time after infection and are intimately related thereafter. Nevertheless, it has been shown in experimental animals that immunity may remain despite abolition of a positive skin test result by densensitization and that immunity may be induced by ribosome preparations that do not induce a positive skin test result.

The balance between the reactions of delayed hypersensitivity and those of the humoral antibody response is very important in determining the clinical presentation and prognosis in leprosy. A similar but less dramatic situation exists in tuberculosis. A more favorable prognosis may be expected for patients who have strong reactivity in their cell-mediated immune functions than for those who are hypoergic and have abundant antibody production. Patients with nonreactive tuberculosis tend to have disseminated disease with almost unopposed multiplication of the organisms in reticuloendothelial cells and a lack of granulomatous response. The question of whether the anergic state is the cause or the result of severe tuberculosis is moot. Recovery of the compromised cell-mediated immune functions, including delayed hypersensitivity, usually accompanies clinical improvement. A patient's location in the immune spectrum usually is dynamic and changeable rather than fixed.

The Tuberculin Skin Test. The biologically active material in the liquid medium after growth of *M. tuberculosis* was named *tuberculin* by Robert Koch. This crude material was later called *Old Tuberculin (OT).* A purified protein derivative of tuberculin *(PPD)* was made by Siebert in 1924 by precipitation with saturated ammonium sulfate. The World Health Organization adopted a large batch, designated *PPD-S,* as the international standard tuberculin. Five tuberculin units *(TU)* was defined as the biologic activity contained in a specified weight of PPD-S. Solutions with much greater stability were achieved by the addition of a wetting agent. All preparations of PPD commercially available in this country must be bioequivalent to 5 TU of PPD-S as demonstrated by comparative testing in humans.

The intracutaneous, or Mantoux, test is performed by injecting 5 TU contained in 0.1 ml of solution intracutaneously with needle and syringe. This is known as the intermediate strength test. It corresponds to 0.1 μg of the standard preparation. A more dilute solution containing 1 TU is available to test those who may be expected to have a very strong reaction, especially children. This preparation is known as first strength PPD and is essentially a five-fold dilution of the 5 TU material. Second strength PPD contains what is calculated to be 250 TU.

In the sensitized individual a reaction of redness, swelling, and induration will begin at about 6 hours, reach a maximum intensity at 36 to 60 hours, and then fade over the next several days. A positive result usually is defined as 10 mm or more of induration at 48 hours. This arbitrary definition is based on results of large-scale testing that showed that a reaction of 10 mm best separated those with from those without tuberculosis. The reading of the test is a subjective evaluation, with wide observer variation. It is only by averaging multiple readings made blindly by at least two expert readers that an accuracy within less than 3 mm may be approached.

It is unwise to have an arbitrary definition of a positive test result in the diagnostic evaluation of a sick patient. Many factors may diminish the response in a nonspecific manner. They include virus infections or live virus vaccination; immunosuppression by disease, drugs, or steroids; malnutrition; overwhelming infection of any kind; and old age. It is best to measure the induration as accurately as possible and, in addition, to describe the intensity of both the erythema and the induration. Erythema that persists for 48 hours is usually indicative of a positive test result. In case of doubt, it is often useful to repeat the test using 250 TU. If there is no reaction to the second strength material, the odds against the diagnosis of nondisseminated tuberculosis are approximately 50 to 1. It is helpful to determine the reaction to other antigens utilizing the so-called *anergy panel.* The most useful are mumps, *Candida,* trichophyton, tetanus toxoid, and a streptococcal antigen such as streptokinase. Failure to react to the panel indicates a generalized state of cutaneous anergy, which may be expected to include tuberculin. Several multiple puncture devices are available for performing a tuberculin test. Some are more reliable than others, but they should all be regarded as screening tests, and any doubtful or positive reactions should be tested with the Mantoux technique.

Intradermal administration of tuberculin in the recommended dosage does not induce an immunologic response even after repeated injections. However, a second injection from 2 weeks to 12 months after an original negative reaction may produce a booster response from recall of waning delayed hypersensitivity. To avoid the assumption that the positive reaction represents a new infection, it has been suggested that negative reactors be retested up to a week later in surveillance programs such as those for hospital personnel. Infection with any mycobacterium and probably with organisms of related genera, such as *Nocardia* and *Corynebacterium*, may give cross-reactions with the tuberculin test materials available today. Tuberculin reactivity is a quantitative function that may vary in intensity from time to time in a given person.

Factors Modifying the Course of Tuberculosis. Before chemotherapy, tuberculosis patients were considered to be at risk for recrudescent disease for the rest of their lives. Mitchell was able to follow over 2000 patients for 15 to 25 years after their moderately or far advanced disease had become inactive. He found a relapse rate of 28 per cent. Even with modern drug therapy relapse occasionally may occur, depending mainly on whether or not the patient was cooperative in taking medication. A study of 20,000 cases reported to the Centers for Disease Control in 1980 revealed that 7 to 8 per cent represented recurrent disease.

Many conditions are known to increase the risk for the recurrence of tuberculosis. Among these are emotional stress, malnutrition, drug addiction, alcoholism, immunosuppression by diseases that interfere with cell-mediated immunity, and the use of drugs such as corticosteroids. Gastric resection is a risk factor, presumably in relation to malnutrition. A risk over ten times that of suitable controls has been documented for patients with chronic renal failure on maintenance dialysis or for those with renal transplants. Influenza, pneumonia, and cancer of the lung may cause local reactivation of dormant lesions. Another local factor is the presence of pneumoconiosis, especially silicosis and coal worker's pneumoconiosis.

CLINICAL DESCRIPTION. ***Pulmonary Tuberculosis.*** Tuberculosis may involve any organ system, but the lung is the usual site of the primary lesion and the principal organ involved. In roughly one half of patients with extrapulmonary disease, however, the original pulmonary lesions may not be discernible clinically or radiographically.

PRIMARY TUBERCULOSIS. Primary tuberculosis refers to disease in a person not previously infected with a virulent mycobacterium of the tuberculosis complex. This definition excludes persons who have had BCG vaccination or infection with other mycobacteria. Primary tuberculosis formerly was seen almost exclusively in children and was known as the childhood type. At present it is not uncommon in adults of all ages. Most primary infections are subclinical and not detectable by ordinary radiographic procedures. They may be recognized, however, by a documented tuberculin skin test conversion. When accompanied by symptoms or radiographic evidence, or both, the disease is called manifest or overt primary tuberculosis. Complications of the primary infection include pleurisy with effusion, miliary disease, meningitis, bone and joint disease, and progressive primary infection. In progressive primary disease the lesions enlarge, caseate, liquefy, and cavitate. Primary disease in adults is especially prone to progression and cavity formation.

The morbidity and mortality associated with primary infection is related to age. Although usually benign in older children and adults, it is life-threatening when it occurs in infants. In a New York City study before the development of chemotherapy, tuberculosis in children less than six months of age had a mortality rate of 50 per cent. Congenital tuberculosis, often fatal, may be acquired from a mother with active disease by the hematogenous route or by the aspiration or ingestion of contaminated amniotic fluid. One of the unique findings in primary tuberculosis of young children is the development of consolidated and collapsed segmental lesions resulting from a combination of bronchial compression from enlarged hilar lymph nodes and extrusion of their caseous contents into the bronchial lumen. This situation usually is clinically benign despite the alarmingly unhealthy appearance of the chest roentgenogram. The spectrum of primary tuberculosis in adults was documented by Stead et al. in 1968. In almost half of 37 adults the disease progressed without interruption into chronic pulmonary tuberculosis.

REACTIVATION TUBERCULOSIS. This term refers to the pattern of disease in adults. It usually results from the reactivation of dormant foci in the posterior portions of the upper lobes, which had been seeded by the bloodstream during the early primary infection. Occasionally adult disease is the result of a new inoculum of tubercle bacilli in a person already sensitized by a previous infection. This condition is known as *exogenous reinfection*. Adult disease is characterized by chronicity, caseation, sloughing of liquefied caseous material, cavity formation, and the simultaneous occurrence of healing and progression in different areas of the lung. Lymph node involvement is usually minimal or absent, at least in those nodes that directly drain the pulmonary foci. Phage typing of strains recovered from different areas of the body and correlation between antimicrobial susceptibility patterns and the history of drug intake have been used to document both recrudescence of an old infection and exogenous reinfection.

The onset of disease may be *insidious, catarrhal, hemoptoic, or acute.* With insidious onset there is gradual development of fatigue, anorexia, weight loss, and other vague complaints. Later, a low grade intermittent fever may develop that is commonly associated with excessive sweating at night. The temperature elevation tends to occur in the late afternoon. The catarrhal onset is characterized by an increasingly productive cough and occasional blood streaking of the sputum. Fever and night sweats may also be noted. In the hemoptoic variety, the presenting symptom is hemoptysis either with or without some of the other symptoms already mentioned. Occasionally, the onset is acute and influenza-like with high fever, chills, myalgia, and productive cough. Pleuritic pain may be the presenting complaint, often without pleural fluid but sometimes ushering in the appearance of an effusion. Many cases of adult-type pulmonary tuberculosis in the past were discovered by routine chest films in asymptomatic persons. Some individuals might recall minor symptoms, such as slight pleurisy, night sweats, or tiredness, but others would deny all warning signs despite the presence of advanced disease. Before the advent of chemotherapy, it was not unusual for the patient to have hoarseness or perirectal abscess—both conditions being secondary to the long-term presence of highly positive sputum.

DIAGNOSIS. A careful history and physical examination often suggest the diagnosis of pulmonary tuberculosis before any laboratory test is ordered. The most characteristic physical findings of adult-type disease are rales heard posteriorly near the apex of one or both lungs. The chest radiographs will then confirm the presence of disease in the posterior portion of the upper lobes. Visualization of one or more cavities strengthens the diagnosis. In primary tuberculosis the initial pneumonic area may be anywhere in the lung, especially in the middle or lower lobes, with enlargement of the draining lymph nodes in the mediastinum. These characteristic patterns are not always seen, however. In a recent report from a large teaching hospital it was found that the diagnosis of tuberculosis was not suggested by the radiologist in 26 per cent of 100 consecutive cases. A wide variety of unusual patterns may be encountered, from mass lesions resembling malignancy to widespread interstitial disease of a nonspecific nature. Diabetics are more likely than nondiabetics to have lower lobe disease, which may also be noted as a bronchogenic spread from apical cavities.

Confirmation of the diagnosis should be sought by bacteriologic examination of the sputum. It may be necessary to obtain specimens by the inhalation of nebulized distilled water or saline solution or by gastric lavage. In addition to properly stained smears and cultures for acid-fast bacilli, it is useful to search for elastic fibers by unstained potassium hydroxide wet mounts. The presence of these fibers indicates destruction of lung tissue and should be accompanied by smears positive for AFB. Occasionally, it may be necessary to resort to bronchoscopy and even to lung biopsy to establish the diagnosis.

The tuberculin skin test is very useful in diagnosis, despite the fact that 5 to 20 per cent of those with newly diagnosed cases may have a negative response to the initial test. Transient depression of cell-mediated immune reactions may be either specific for tuberculin or a generalized anergy to all skin test antigens. For immediate diagnostic purposes in such cases, it is useful to apply a second strength PPD containing 250 TU, which will give a false negative reaction in no more than 1 to 2 per cent of patients without disseminated disease or severe debility.

Other laboratory tests are not particularly helpful. The blood count occasionally shows a leukemoid reaction, but more often there is a mild leukocytosis with a relative monocytosis. Many different serologic tests have been proposed, but none has proven useful enough at this time to be included as a diagnostic test.

Differential Diagnosis. Many subacute and chronic pulmonary conditions, both infectious and noninfectious, may be confused with tuberculosis. Some pulmonary mycoses, especially histoplasmosis, may present with a similar clinical and radiologic picture. Pyogenic lung abscess as well as pneumonia with a delayed resolution may be confused with tuberculosis. A pyogenic lung abscess is likely to have more fluid within it, hence a higher air-fluid level, and more dense consolidation around it. When repeated examinations of the sputum are negative for AFB, one should increase efforts at establishing another diagnosis. Tuberculomas may be confused with similar lesions arising from several different fungal infections and with pulmonary neoplasms. Sarcoidosis and tuberculosis may have similar manifestations. One third of cases of fever of unknown origin are due to infection, and extrapulmonary tuberculosis is still prominent among these cases.

TREATMENT. ***Historical Perspective.*** For many decades the physician relied upon nonspecific measures to treat tuberculosis. These measures included fresh air, good food, bed rest, and graded exercise, among others. The idea of the cottage sanatorium was started in this country in 1884 to accommodate these feeble attempts at treatment. Measures designated to collapse cavities and to put diseased portions of the lungs "at rest" included artificial pneumothorax, pneumoperitoneum, phrenic nerve crush, and various forms of thoracoplasty. Resectional surgery became popular after the introduction of effective drug therapy.

The era of chemotherapy began in 1945 with Waksman's discovery of streptomycin. In 1949 it was shown that treatment with the combination of streptomycin and para-aminosalicylic acid (PAS) delayed the emergence of streptomycin-resistant tubercle bacilli. With the introduction of isoniazid in 1952 it became possible to treat the disease with two drugs given by mouth. A course of 18 to 24 months was recommended by studies of relapse rates and the bacteriology of lesions removed at lung resection as related to duration of treatment. Ethambutol, marketed in 1961, replaced PAS because of its relative lack of annoying side effects. These drugs rendered all previous modes of therapy obsolete, and most sanatoriums in this country were closed by 1960. A study done in India in 1960 demonstrated that home treatment was not risky for the patient or his family. It was documented in 1973 that supervised intermittent treatment twice a week was just as beneficial as daily treatment, especially for the ambulatory continuation phase after a period of daily drug therapy. Such intermittent treatment is especially suited for uncooperative patients. The introduction of rifampin in 1966 provided not only another very powerful antituberculosis agent, but also the opportunity to shorten the duration of therapy by at least half. Published reports on short-course chemotherapy began to appear in 1972. It soon became obvious that the lessons learned from combination drug therapy prior to the use of rifampin did not apply to regimens containing isoniazid and rifampin. With proper combinations and rhythm of administration it is now possible to achieve excellent results with six months of treatment, provided that all doses are consumed as prescribed.

The Antituberculosis Drugs. *Isoniazid (INH)* is the most important drug in original treatment regimens. It is easily synthesized, highly stable, inexpensive, and well tolerated. The drug is well absorbed when given by mouth and may be administered parenterally. It is widely distributed throughout the body, including the central nervous system, and it reaches bacilli within cells. The drug exerts a bactericidal effect on actively multiplying bacilli. Adverse reactions may occur in approximately 5 per cent of cases with a daily dose of 5 mg per kilogram per day, usually given as 300 mg once daily for adults. A common toxicity is peripheral neuropathy, based on interference with the metabolism of pyridoxine. It is directly related to the dose and blood level and is more likely to be seen in genetically constituted slow acetylators and in malnourished individuals. Neuropathy can be prevented by the administration of 25 mg of pyridoxine daily and is not likely to occur when ordinary doses of INH are used in nonalcoholic, nondiabetic, well nourished, and relatively young patients. The most important adverse reaction is hepatitis of the hepatocellular variety. Although approximately 10 per cent of healthy individuals may have asymptomatic elevations of aminotransferases within the first two months of treatment, the enzyme levels usually return to normal despite the continued administration of the drug. The risk of hepatitis is related to age, being less than 1 per cent in those under 35 and increasing with age to 2.3 per cent at age 60. Hepatitis usually occurs within the first few months of treatment but occasionally appears in later stages. Heavy alcohol intake is associated with a greater risk of hepatitis. Several fatalities from INH hepatitis have been reported, mainly in patients whose reaction occurred late and in those who continued to take the drug despite progressive symptoms.

Some rare untoward effects include encephalopathy, loss of memory, optic atrophy, convulsions, hemolytic anemia, and purpura. The usual hypersensitivity reactions such as drug fever and skin rash occasionally may be seen. Isoniazid is one of several drugs that can produce a lupus-like syndrome. Although INH is excreted promptly and mainly by the kidneys, the half-life is prolonged only slightly in patients with renal failure.

Rifampin (RMP) is comparable to INH in its bactericidal effect on metabolically active bacilli. It is an antibiotic of the rifamycin family and is much more expensive than INH. Well absorbed when taken orally in a fasting state, the drug is widely distributed and penetrates well into cells and into the central nervous system. It differs from most of the antituberculosis drugs in that it has good activity against a variety of gram-positive and gram-negative bacteria. Its activity depends upon inhibition of DNA-dependent RNA polymerase activity. Rifampin is well tolerated by most patients in a dosage of 10 mg per kilogram per day, usually given to adults as 600 mg once daily by mouth. A parenteral preparation is not yet generally available, although it may be obtained from the manufacturer in emergency situations. Hepatitis is the most important adverse effect, occurring in about 1 per cent of patients. There are conflicting reports on the risk of hepatitis when INH and RMP are given together. Most studies now indicate no excessive risk. An exception occurs in the treatment of children, for whom a dosage of greater than 10 mg per kilogram per day of INH given with RMP is associated with a high risk of hepatitis.

Allergic reactions occasionally occur, especially in those individuals who take the drug irregularly or in those who are given intermittent treatment twice weekly in a dosage greater than 600 mg. These reactions include chills and fever and more rarely acute renal failure, thrombocytopenia, and massive hemolysis. Rifampin may induce enzymes in the liver that increase metabolic degradation of several other drugs, such as oral contraceptive agents and anticoagulants. The drug is excreted mainly by the liver and biliary tract and therefore must be given with caution to patients with liver failure.

Ethambutol (EMB) is a synthetic chemical compound of the ethylenediamine series discovered in 1961. It is well absorbed when given by mouth and is excreted mainly in the urine. Thus, the drug should be given with great care to patients with poor renal function, for whom dosage must be reduced and blood levels followed carefully. Aside from its principal toxicity, optic neuritis, there are very few adverse effects. Optic nerve toxicity is directly related to dosage and blood levels. At the recommended dosage of 15 mg per kilogram per day, optic neuritis is very rare, but some physicians administer 25 mg per kilogram per day for the first two or three months, at which dosage approximately 3 per cent of patients may have impaired visual acuity. When the higher dose is used, periodic examinations for visual acuity are indicated. The toxicity usually is reversible if administration of the drug is discontinued promptly.

Pyrazinamide (PZA) is a synthetic compound discovered in 1952 but originally rejected for general use in the United States because of excessive hepatoxicity when given in a dosage of 40 mg per kilogram per day. It has now become an important drug because of its excellent tissue sterilizing ability when used in combination with other bactericidal drugs. Toleration is acceptable at a lower dose than that originally used. It is well absorbed from the gastrointestinal tract, widely distributed throughout the body water, and penetrates well into the central nervous system. The drug is active against only one species of *Mycobacterium*, *M. tuberculosis*, and then only at the low pH of 5.0 to 5.5. It is especially useful to kill tubercle bacilli within macrophages, into whose acidic environment it penetrates well. It is excreted mainly by way of the kidneys. Allergic reactions are rare, but joint pains and occasionally gout may occur as the result of a hyperuricemic effect. Hepatitis may occur in about 1 per cent of patients receiving the recommended daily dose of 20 to 30 mg per kilogram, usually 1.5 grams for small and 2.0 grams for large adults, given by mouth once daily.

Streptomycin (SM) is an aminoglycoside antibiotic that has been chemically defined and synthesized. It is not absorbed when given by mouth. The principal method of elimination is through the kidneys, so that dosage adjustment is necessary when renal function is reduced. It is distributed largely in the extracellular fluid and does not enter appreciably into the central nervous system or into macrophages. The dosage is 10 to 15 mg per kilogram per day, given intramuscularly, usually as 0.75 to 1.0 gram once daily in adults with normal renal function. As with other aminoglycosides, damage to the renal tubules is common, as manifested by cylindruria, but renal function is not compromised unless blood levels of the drug are excessive. The major toxicity is exerted against the eighth nerve, of which the vestibular division is more likely to be affected, although deafness may also be produced. The seriousness of these reactions makes periodic testing of renal and eighth nerve function advisable, especially in the elderly. Measurements of blood levels should be obtained whenever renal function is in question. Allergic reactions are fairly common, as are paresthesias of the lips and extremities immediately after injection. The drug is bactericidal against tubercle bacilli. The maximum effect is exerted at a pH of 7.7.

Kanamycin and *capreomycin* are used as substitutes for SM when the organisms are resistant to that drug or on the rare occasions when the patient cannot tolerate SM. Dosages, methods of administration, and adverse reactions are similar to those of SM. More care is needed with kanamycin since it is slightly more ototoxic and nephrotoxic than SM, especially on the cochlear division of the eighth nerve.

Ethionamide and *cycloserine* are not used for initial therapy but are reserved for retreatment cases and for special situations of drug intolerance and bacillary resistance. Both drugs are given by mouth in dosages of 10 to 15 mg per kilogram per day. The administration of ethionamide is accompanied by rather severe gastrointestinal upset and occasionally by hepatitis, and allergic reactions are common. Allergic reactions with cycloserine are rare, but aberrations of mental function and seizures are quite common.

Drug Regimens. Until the landmark short-course chemotherapy studies of the British Medical Research Council and its cooperative investigators, the conventional drug regimens for initial treatment consisted mainly of INH and EMB for one and one half to two years, supplemented by RMP or SM for the first month or two in patients with far advanced disease. An intermittent regimen consisting of supervised twice-weekly drug administration can be used after the initial two or three months of daily treatment. Dosages in mg per kilogram recommended for intermittent treatment are as follows: INH 15, SM 25 to 30, EMB 50, and RMP 10 to 15 (usually no more than 600 mg total). With a fully compliant patient and drug-sensitive bacilli, the success rate is well over 95 per cent with long-term treatment. The main problems are related to the long-term administration of a drug regimen and include insuring compliance with recommended treatment and the cost of supervision and follow-up to the local health department.

SHORT-COURSE TREATMENT. The first report of successful short-course treatment was published in 1968 and involved experience in East Africa. From the results of many other trials conducted since then, it appears that the minimum requirements include therapy with INH and RMP for at least nine months. The addition of a third drug—EMB, SM, or PZA—for the first one to three months of intensive treatment guards against the eventuality of infection with INH- or RMP-resistant bacilli. To shorten the course to six months, a third drug is necessary. That drug should be PZA for the initial two months. Treatment may then be continued with daily INH plus RMP for the remaining four months. When the patient is in a high-risk group for infection with INH-resistant or RMP-resistant organisms, use of a four-drug regimen has been suggested for the first two months (INH/RMP/PZA/SM), followed by administration of two or three drugs, depending on drug susceptibility, for four months. A modification of the six-month treatment involving only 62 doses, fully supervised, is as follows: INH/RMP/PZA/SM daily for two weeks, then twice weekly for six weeks, then INH/RMP twice weekly for 18 weeks. These intensive regimens should be considered for patients who are likely to resist treatment, such as prisoners and urban homeless alcoholics. Preliminary reports have documented the effectiveness of these regimens.

Short-course treatment has the obvious advantages of smaller amounts of drugs used and less time needed at the ambulatory health facility for supervision of treatment. Another benefit of the INH/RMP combination is more rapid sputum conversion (by approximately two to three weeks) when compared with regimens without INH/RMP, although the conversion curves usually even out by the fourth month. In addition, if relapse occurs following short-course treatment, it is usually caused by drug-susceptible organisms.

The main disadvantage of intensive three- and four-drug regimens, drug toxicity, has proved to be less troublesome than was predicted. The number of patients removed from the study because of drug intolerance has been acceptable.

Results of Treatment. The success of treatment may be judged by clinical assessment, decreased bacillary count of the sputum, and clearing of the lungs as shown on radiographs. The temperature usually returns to normal within a week or two, but in some patients who are highly febrile defervescence may not occur for many weeks. The speed of radiographic improvement depends upon the nature and extent of pulmonary disease and the age of the patient. Chronic, cavitary, and fibrotic lesions do not clear rapidly. The sputum should be examined at frequent intervals during the first few months of treatment, since a decreasing number of acid-fast bacilli is the surest indication of successful treatment. With the best of regimens, it will take four to six weeks to convert sputum cultures to negative in 50 per cent of cases; to convert 75 per cent of cases usually requires about ten weeks. The rate of conversion depends on the same factors that determine the rate of radiographic clearing. Failure of the sputum to convert to negative or a rise in the bacillary count after an initial decrease represents a treatment failure. Such failures are usually the result of poor compliance on the part of the patient but occasionally are related to bacillary drug resistance or an inappropriate drug regimen. The aim of chemotherapy is an initial success rate of 100 per cent without relapses. When relapse occurs, it is usually within a year of the completion of therapy. Rarely, relapses may occur with decreasing frequency up to five to ten years after completion of therapy. This is so infrequent after adequate drug therapy that it is no longer necessary for the local health department to carry out periodic follow-up examinations.

Corticosteroids. Corticosteroids may be a useful adjunct to chemotherapy for selected patients. They usually produce a dramatic reversal of overwhelming sepsis. Absorption of the fluid may be hastened in tuberculous pleurisy and pericarditis, although there is no evidence that late complications in the pleural and pericardial spaces are prevented. In tuberculous meningitis it was often the custom to give steroids routinely, but there is no good evidence that this is necessary. Steroids should be given for as short a time as possible, preferably for no longer than three or four weeks. A more controversial issue is whether or not to use INH prophylaxis to cover the administration of steroids in the patient with a history of tuberculosis or with a positive tuberculin skin test result. This situation is most likely to occur in patients receiving steroids to prevent rejection of transplanted organs, to help control lymphoma or leukemia, or to control severe asthma. One year of INH preventive therapy is recommended when steroids will be used on a long-term basis.

Reversal of Infectiousness. Some experts believe that it takes only about two weeks of effective chemotherapy to render patients noninfectious to others, even when large numbers of viable acid-fast bacilli are still present in the sputum. The evidence for this is inconclusive, and it is more reasonable to consider a patient with smear-positive sputum to represent a gradually diminishing risk until the smears are negative.

Drug Resistance. The phenomenon of clinical bacillary resistance was recognized soon after SM was tried as single drug therapy. The emergence of drug-resistant strains was at least delayed, if not prevented, by the use of two or more drugs in combination. Resistant populations emerge by a selective process in which resistant cells are favored that have arisen by spontaneous random mutation at the rate of about 1×10^{-8} to 1×10^{-10} per bacterium per generation.

Modern drug regimens are designed to prevent the emergence of drug resistance unless the patient is noncompliant or if infection occurs with strains already resistant to one or more drugs—a situation known as *primary drug resistance.* The rate of primary drug resistance in a community will influence the choice of drug regimens for initial treatment. Accurate figures for this country were provided by a recent study from the Centers for Disease Control, which showed that the overall rate was 7 per cent and varied in different locations from 3 to 15 per cent, depending mainly on the relative numbers of Asian and Hispanic individuals in the population. Age was another important factor; the highest rate was seen in young children. The highest single drug rate was for INH, with SM second. The study also showed that the rate diminished slightly between 1965 and 1982. The importance of the overall drug resistance problem, both primary and acquired, was highlighted by another study from the Centers for Disease Control. Forty-one per cent of unsuccessfully treated patients harbored strains resistant to at least one drug. The known contacts of an index case excreting INH-resistant tubercle bacilli should receive careful follow-up, and appropriate treatment should be given if active disease develops. Alternatively, RMP either alone or with another drug such as EMB or PZA may be used, although it has not yet been proved that RMP is effective in prophylaxis.

Retreatment. Proper therapy for initial treatment failures and disease that relapses after apparently successful treatment requires special expertise. Accurate drug susceptibility testing is a prerequisite for devising the best drug regimen, but while awaiting test results the following guidelines may be followed: A single new drug should not be added to a regimen that has failed, since this may lead to rapid emergence of resistance to the new drug. Instead, a regimen should be chosen that contains at least two drugs that the patient has never received previously. In selecting the proper drugs, all available information should be gathered from the patient, the patient's family and former physicians, and health departments. Calls should be made to whatever laboratories have been involved in testing of organisms obtained from the patient to get firsthand bacteriologic data including drug sensitivity test results. The chosen regimen should be adjusted according to any newly available information. It may be necessary to use combinations of four or more drugs, some of which have high rates of adverse reactions. After two or three relapses, especially when the infecting strain is resistant to INH, RMP, and SM, the chances of success are slim. The best way to control the problem of retreatment of patients with multiply resistant strains is to prevent this unfortunate turn of events by proper supervision of the initial course of drug therapy.

Patients with Impaired Renal and Hepatic Function. Isoniazid is excreted mainly in the urine, and it has been reported that the drug will accumulate in patients with markedly impaired renal function. However, the drug is dialyzable, and others have reported that the half-life is prolonged only slightly in patients with renal failure. It is probably not necessary to reduce the dosage, but pyridoxine supplementation should be given and patients should be monitored for hepatitis and peripheral neuropathy. It may also be advisable to assay INH serum concentrations from time to time. Rifampin is metabolized in the liver and excreted mainly in the bile. When hepatic function is impaired, the drug may accumulate to toxic levels. Thus blood levels should be monitored. Both EMB and SM are cleared by dialysis and are excreted mainly through the urine. The dosage of SM must be reduced in proportion to the renal function; serum levels should be checked frequently, and the patient should be monitored for signs of eighth nerve toxicity. In a similar fashion, the dosage of EMB must be reduced, serum levels checked, and the visual acuity monitored. Since about 20 per cent of EMB is metabolized in the liver, it would be wise to check serum levels when there is hepatic failure. There is insufficient information upon which to base recommendations for use of PZA, ethionamide, and cycloserine in patients with impaired renal or hepatic function. Since PZA and cycloserine are excreted mainly by the kidneys, the dosage should be reduced and blood levels monitored when these drugs are used in patients with poor kidney function. It is not known how ethionamide is metabolized; only a very small amount may be found unchanged in the urine. Drug levels should be monitored to avoid accumulation.

Treatment of Pregnant Women. Ethionamide and SM should be avoided, the first because of teratogenic potential, and the second because eighth nerve damage has been reported in the fetus. Cycloserine and PZA should also be avoided because of a lack of information on possible adverse effects. Rifampin crosses the placental barrier readily and inhibits RNA polymerase. It should be used with caution and only with a very strong indication, perhaps only for the first few weeks of treatment. The combination of INH and EMB is the most suitable drug therapy for pregnant women.

Treatment of Children. There are conflicting recommendations for drug regimens and dosages of individual drugs for treatment of children with tuberculosis. The most suitable combination is INH 10 mg per kilogram daily (maximum of 300 mg daily) and RMP 15 mg per kilogram daily (maximum of 600 mg daily). A third drug should be added if there is risk of infection with drug-resistant organisms. The third drug, given for the first two or three months of therapy, may be SM, EMB, or PAS. All three drugs have drawbacks: SM has a high rate of adverse effects and must be given by injection; PAS is difficult to administer to children because of stomach irritation, and the drug is no longer available in the liquid form; young children cannot be monitored for the major toxicity of EMB, optic neuritis. Ethambutol is probably the best choice of therapy. It has been used successfully in other countries in a dosage of 15 mg per kilogram daily. The duration of treatment should be one year, although preliminary reports indicate that nine months may be sufficient.

Surgical and Collapse Procedures. The need for collapse procedures such as pneumothorax, penumoperitoneum, and phrenic nerve crush and for excisional surgery with or without thoracoplasty has been virtually eliminated by the success of chemotherapy. The surgeon may still be called upon to correct late complications of previous attempts at treatment such as bronchopleural fistula or persistent empyema.

EXTRAPULMONARY DISEASE. ***Thoracic Cavity and Chest Wall.*** Tuberculosis of the pleura is almost always associated with disease of the lung, arising by contiguous spread or rupture of a subpleural tubercle. It usually begins as a localized fibrinous inflammation, which produces pleuritic chest pain. Pleurisy with effusion is often associated with primary infection. When this occurs in young adults who are untreated, approximately 75 per cent may be expected to develop overt pulmonary tuberculosis within five years. The onset may be either abrupt or insidious, with cough and fever accompanying the chest pain. Pain and friction rub often disappear as pleural fluid accumulates. Most primary tuberculous pleural effusions will resorb spontaneously, sometimes within a week or two, but the diagnosis can be made on the basis of a positive tuberculin skin test result, the exudative characteristics of the fluid, and the preponderance of lymphocytes. Tubercle bacilli are usually very scarce in the fluid so that stained smears may be negative and cultures only weakly positive. Imprints and cultures made from pleural tissue removed by closed needle biopsy are more likely than the fluid to be positive. Histologic examination also may be helpful. Pleural effusions in young adults who have positive tuberculin skin test results are best treated as tuberculosis unless some other cause can be identified. The fluid should be aspirated for diagnosis and perhaps once or twice more if it accumulates rapidly. Chest tube drainage should be avoided. Corticosteroids should not be used routinely but may be given in selected cases to hasten symptomatic improvement and absorption of the fluid. Pleural effusion may also occur in disseminated tuberculosis with multiple organ and serous membrane involvement. Tuberculous empyema may be secondary to involvement of the vertebral column or result from a bronchopleural fistula.

Endobronchial tuberculosis commonly accompanies pulmonary disease but now rarely results in identifiable symptoms and signs. In primary tuberculosis of children it is the pressure of enlarged lymph nodes together with ulceration and rupture through the bronchial wall that produce endobronchial disease. Endobronchial disease in adults usually starts as inflammatory lesions from repeated implantations of tubercle bacilli originating in lung parenchyma. These lesions may progress to ulceration and narrowing of the bronchi and eventually to cicatricial stenosis. Secondary changes include atelectasis and obstructive pneumonitis, tension cavity from involvement of the distal small bronchi or bronchioles, and accumulation of fluid within cavities. The symptoms of endobronchial disease are spasmodic coughing and a localized wheeze. Bronchial ulceration or erosion of a caseating lymph node may cause positive sputum in the absence of recognizable pulmonary disease. Bronchoscopy usually serves to identify the lesions.

Although tuberculosis of the endocardium and myocardium has been described, the most common involvement of the heart is *pericarditis.* Rupture into the pericardium of nearby caseous lymph nodes is the common route of infection, although lymphohematogenous dissemination may occur. The serofibrinous pericardial effusion usually is associated with substernal pain, fever, pericardial friction rub, and left-sided pleural effusion. Cardiac tamponade occasionally develops in the acute stage. A search for tuberculosis elsewhere and a tuberculin skin test should be performed. A thorough examination of the pericardial fluid obtained by needle aspiration or surgical drainage also may be helpful. Obtaining a pericardial biopsy sample in the operating room may be justified in obscure cases because of the importance of early drug treatment. The differential diagnosis includes benign or viral pericarditis, pyogenic infection, other granulomatous inflammations, and malignant effusion. The diagnosis is made more difficult by the facts that the skin test reaction is negative in a sizable minority; the fluid rarely contains enough organisms to be positive by smear and often not even by culture; the characteristics of the fluid are nonspecific; and about half of the individuals have no other obvious sites of tuberculosis. The administration of corticosteroids may be beneficial, but antituberculosis drugs should be used in addition even when tuberculosis is only suspected.

The most important sequela is constrictive pericarditis, which usually occurs two to four years after the acute disease. At this stage the heart is small and relatively immobile and there is a paradoxical pulse and obstruction of venous return to the heart, with congestion of the liver, peripheral edema, and later ascites. Calcification of the pericardium may be seen on x-ray films. Treatment consists of removal of the pericardium, although it is preferable to perform the operation at an earlier stage.

The chest wall may be the site of one or more subcutaneous abscesses as a result of hematogenous dissemination or sometimes as the peripheral manifestation of an empyema necessitatis as it burrows through the chest wall. Chest wall abscesses may also result from drainage of underlying caseous lymph nodes along the intercostal lymphatics.

Extrathoracic. LYMPHATIC. Tuberculous lymphadenitis is the most common manifestation of extrathoracic disease throughout the world, and the most frequently involved nodes are cervical. The disease in this location was known as *scrofula,* or the *King's Evil.* The latter name was used because the condition was supposedly amenable to cure by the royal touch. Although it was once thought that infection with *M. bovis* was responsible for most cases of scrofula, a recent study from England emphasized that *M. tuberculosis* accounted for more cases than did the bovine organism, although the latter is relatively more common in lymphatic tuberculosis than in other forms of the disease. Infection of the tonsils through the ingestion of contaminated milk was the usual route of infection for the tonsillar node high in the neck, near the angle of the jaw. At present, scrofula in young children is mainly due to infection with mycobacteria other than *M. tuberculosis* and *M. bovis* (see Ch. 299). Supraclavicular node involvement usually arises by lymphatic spread from mediastinal disease. Nodes elsewhere in the neck, as well as those in the axilla and inguinal area, the other common sites of involvement, may be the result of drainage from a primary site or from hematogenous spread.

The infected nodes are usually detectable by sight and palpation. Although the nodes usually are not painful, they may be tender during the phase of rapid enlargement early in the infection. Later they become matted together and eventually soften, slough, and drain. Draining sinuses may persist for many months, sometimes for years, with intermittent healing and breakdown. The diagnosis may be made by bacteriologic study of the pus from draining sinuses or by biopsy together with bacteriologic studies. The presence of calcific densities in the neck and axilla as seen in the chest radiograph may provide evidence of healed tuberculous adenitis.

Lymphatic tuberculosis tends to heal but often not completely, so that relapse is common even many years after the primary infection. Treatment with antituberculosis drugs is usually successful, although the tendency to late relapse may still be seen, especially with two-drug regimens that do not include RMP. Excision of large caseous nodes in accessible sites sometimes is advisable.

GENITOURINARY. The second most common site of infection is the genitourinary tract. Disease is usually centered in the kidney, which becomes seeded either during the primary infection or later. These foci may remain dormant for many years. When reactivation occurs, one or more renal abscesses are produced, followed by spread to the remainder of the urinary tract. Extensive scarring of the ureters eventually occurs. This scarring produces obstructive hydronephrosis, which together with renal caseation may destroy the kidney completely. Specific symptoms may be lacking until the hydronephrotic kidney becomes secondarily infected or until the development of tuberculous cystitis manifested by frequency and dysuria. Long before the onset of symptoms, the examination of the urine may show hematuria, pyuria, and albuminuria, along with cultures negative for pyogens. The diagnosis is made by radiographic examination of the urinary tract, cystoscopy, and demonstration of tubercle bacilli by cultures of first morning voided urines. It was found that approximately 10 per cent of a general tuberculosis patient population had positive urine cultures, and in 7 per cent of these patients the urinary tract disease was completely unanticipated. Renal tuberculosis responds well to drug treatment. According to recent recommendations, conventional long-term regimens may be replaced by six- to nine-month courses of INH, RMP, and a third drug (either EMB or PZA). The role of surgery remains controversial. Some urologists would remove destroyed kidneys and repair strictures of the ureter, while others claim that surgery is almost never indicated.

Genital tuberculosis in the male may involve the prostate, seminal vesicles, and epididymis. The acute inflammation is later replaced by induration and hard nodules, sometimes followed by obstruction, calcification, and chronic draining sinuses of the scrotum. The diagnosis is made by finding tubercle bacilli in the urine, sinus drainage, or biopsied tissues. In the female, tuberculous salpingitis is the common manifestation, followed by disease of the uterus and ovaries. Sterility almost always results, and peritonitis may occur secondarily. The symptoms are those of chronic pelvic inflammatory disease. Diagnosis should be based on examination of tissue from the endometrium and from lesions visible through the laparoscope and cultures of the menstrual fluid or vaginal discharge. As with renal tuberculosis, drug therapy usually is successful, but excisional surgery may be indicated for residual lesions or persistently draining sinuses.

SKELETAL TUBERCULOSIS. The presence of a gibbus or hunchback deformity of the thoracic spine (Pott's disease) has served as a marker of tuberculosis since prehistoric times. *Tuberculous spondylitis* is still the most common manifestation of bone and joint infection. At present, it is mainly a disease of adults that arises by reactivation of dormant foci. The common areas of involvement are thoracic and lumbar; the cervical spine may be involved in 2 to 3 per cent of cases. The destructive process usually begins in the intervertebral discs, where it first produces narrowing of the disc space, then destruction of the two adjacent vertebral bodies through the bony end plates. Sometimes, however, the anterior portion of the vertebral body is destroyed first. Inflammation often extends into the soft tissues surrounding the spine, either in the form of a spreading, phlegmonous reaction or as a cold abscess that may be paravertebral, in and around the psoas muscle, or retropharyngeal, depending upon the site of disease. The symptoms are usually dominated by back pain, sometimes followed by the neurologic manifestations of compression of the spinal cord and nerve roots. There may be fever. Active tuberculosis of the lungs may be absent, although some evidence of past disease usually is seen.

Radiographic examination of the spine shows destructive lesions in the commonly involved sites. The paraspinal involvement appears as widening of the mediastinum or an oval-shaped density behind the heart. It may be manifested as a psoas abscess, a retropharyngeal abscess, or a mass in the groin or in the supraclavicular area. A similar radiographic appearance may occur in pyogenic infection of the spine. A needle biopsy sample usually is necessary to establish the proper diagnosis. Even when a pyogenic organism such as *Staphylococcus aureus* is isolated, caseating granulomas and a culture positive for *M. tuberculosis* sometimes can be found by biopsy. Occasionally open biopsy of the vertebral body may be necessary.

The disease has a natural tendency to heal by spontaneous fusion of the vertebral bodies. Treatment consists of antituberculosis chemotherapy according to the modern regimens described under Treatment. Preliminary results with short-course treatment are encouraging, but they cannot be recommended for routine use until further experience has accumulated. Published studies of the British Medical Research Council Working Party on Tuberculosis of the Spine have suggested that prolonged bed rest, immobilization of the spine, and spinal fusion operations are no longer necessary, although some indications still exist for surgical procedures: decompression of the spinal cord if there has been no neurologic improvement after several weeks of drug treatment and debridement and anterior spinal fusion for dangerous instability of the spine. The inflammatory reaction with or without pus around the spine often improves with drug treatment so that drainage is not always necessary.

Tuberculous arthritis occurs mainly in hips and knees but also may involve many other joints including elbows, shoulders, and the joints of the hands and feet. The patient usually has chronic monoarticular arthritis. Diagnosis is made by synovial biopsy and bacteriologic study of tissues and pus. The process usually responds to antituberculosis chemotherapy without the necessity for operative procedures, but occasionally excision of extensively destroyed synovium and temporary immobilization may be beneficial.

Tuberculous tenosynovitis is usually secondary to involvement of adjacent bone. At least two distinctive processes may result from involvement of the hand: carpal tunnel syndrome, and compound palmar ganglion, a distinctive bilobed swelling on either side of the volar carpal ligament. Chemotherapy often needs to be supplemented by debridement and evacuation of fibrinous material.

ABDOMINAL TUBERCULOSIS. *Intestinal tuberculosis* secondary to chronic pulmonary disease once was so common that patients were routinely screened by radiography of the small bowel upon admission to the sanatorium. This situation continued long after the ingestion of *M. bovis* was brought under control by the pasteurization of milk. Lately, the emphasis has been on primary intestinal disease in the absence of recognizable pulmonary lesions. The route of infection in these cases remains unknown. Tuberculosis may involve all parts of the alimentary canal from top to bottom, but by far the most common location is in the ileocecal area. The predominant tissue reaction may be either ulcerative or hyperplastic, with accompanying bleeding, perforation, fistula formation, obstruction, or combinations of two or more of these processes. The early symptoms are nonspecific, consisting mainly of anorexia, loss of weight, abdominal pain, and alternating periods of diarrhea and constipation. The clinical picture is not unlike that of Crohn's disease. Indeed, the differential diagnosis of these two conditions may not be possible, even on the basis of intestinal radiography. Tuberculosis of the colon also may occur and needs to be distinguished from carcinoma, diverticulitis, and inflammatory bowel disease of nonspecific nature. Perirectal abscess and fistula formation may result from lower colon lesions. The disease usually responds well to antituberculosis chemotherapy, but surgical correction may be necessary for the complications described earlier. The diagnosis often is made unexpectedly at surgery or autopsy.

Tuberculous peritonitis may result from bloodborne infection or by extension of disease from the intestine, mesenteric lymph nodes, or fallopian tubes. The classic form is that of a chronic adhesive peritonitis that produces a doughy, tender abdomen, abdominal masses, low grade fever, anorexia, and weight loss. A much more common manifestation is painless ascites. When this occurs in adults with alcoholic cirrhosis and ascites, it makes for a difficult differential diagnosis. Tuberculosis should be suspected when the combination of fever, ascites, and a positive tuberculin skin test reaction are found. Examination of the fluid is helpful. A high total protein concentration with a moderate number of leukocytes, mostly lymphocytes, is suggestive of tuberculosis. A more definitive diagnosis may be obtained by laparoscopy or laparotomy. Usually the entire peritoneal surface is studded with tubercles that are easily differentiated from carcinomatosis histologically. The fluid is rarely positive for AFB by stained smear and even by culture test is positive in somewhat less than 50 per cent of cases. Response to antituberculosis chemotherapy is good.

Isolated tuberculosis of the liver or spleen occasionally has been described. These organs are usually involved in disseminated or miliary tuberculosis, but occasionally a liver biopsy done in an attempt to explain enlargement of the liver, jaundice, or abnormal liver function studies leads to a diagnosis of tuberculosis when there is apparently no disease elsewhere.

CENTRAL NERVOUS SYSTEM. In the past, *tuberculous meningitis* was one of the most dreaded complications of primary tuberculosis in young children, appearing in about one in a thousand cases and almost always resulting in fatality. It usually occurred two to six months after the primary infection in infants and was commonly associated with miliary tuberculosis. In this country it is now more likely to be seen in adults than in children. Invasion of the meninges occurs by direct extension from subjacent caseous foci in the cerebral cortex, cerebellum, choroid plexus, middle ear, or spine. Brain infarcts secondary to tuberculous arteritis sometimes occur. The syndrome of inappropriate secretion of antidiuretic hormone may accompany the meningitis.

The inflammatory reaction is concentrated around the base of the brain where the thick exudate may eventually obstruct the basal foramina to produce hydrocephalus. Examination of the spinal fluid reveals a characteristic pattern of high protein, low sugar, and a moderate number (up to a few hundred) of leukocytes, most of which are lymphocytes. However, early in the course of the disease neutrophils may predominate; the shift to a lymphocytic exudate rarely does not occur; the sugar level may be normal or only slightly decreased; and the number of leukocytes may reach several thousand. Occasionally the protein content is high enough that a thin web or pellicle appears in undisturbed refrigerated fluid. Acid-fast bacilli may be seen in this web, although they are not visible in the sedimented fluid. Stained smears of the fluid are usually positive in no more than 25 per cent of samples, but there are a few colonies of tubercle bacilli in cultures in about 75 per cent of cases. The larger the sample of spinal fluid submitted, the greater the chance of finding the organism. The tuberculin skin test should be positive in approximately 75 per cent of cases, provided that those nonrective to 5 TU are retested immediately with 250 TU. A careful search reveals evidence of tuberculosis elsewhere in the majority of cases, although the disease in the lungs may appear to be inactive.

The onset is usually insidious, extending over a period of many weeks. Occasionally, however, there is a much more acute onset that resembles pyogenic or aseptic meningitis. The most common symptoms are headache, fever, lethargy, and confusion. Later, focal neurologic signs appear in the form of ocular palsies, other cranial nerve palsies, and increasing stupor progressing to coma. Stiffness of the neck is common. The outcome of therapy depends mainly on the stage of disease at the time treatment is instituted. Treatment should start immediately when tuberculous meningitis is suspected, without waiting for confirmation of diagnosis. A triple-drug regimen including INH and RMP is recommended. Ethionamide and PZA achieve therapeutic concentrations in spinal fluid even in the absence of an inflammatory reaction. Ethambutol penetrates reasonably well through inflamed meninges. It should be remembered that SM does not appear in therapeutic concentrations and that infections with INH-resistant organisms occur more often in children than in adults. It has been recommended that the third drug should be either ethionamide or PZA. Treatment should be continued for at least one year, although administration of the third drug may be discontinued after two or three months once it has been determined that drug resistance is not a problem. The use of corticosteroids is controversial. Intrathecal treatment is usually not necessary.

Tuberculomas of the brain may be seen at any age. Cases involving children still predominate in the developing countries, while in the United States they occur mainly in adults. The clinical presentation is that of a brain tumor with signs and symptoms of increased intracranial pressure, focal seizures, and focal neurologic defects. Indications of infection, such as fever, often are absent. Lesions may be single or multiple and must be differentiated from tumor and abscess of the brain. The spinal fluid may show slight lymphocytosis and elevated protein concentration, but often it is normal. The correct diagnosis may be suggested by radiographic scanning techniques, a positive tuberculin skin test reaction, and the presence of tuberculosis elsewhere, but the definitive procedures are needle aspiration through a burr hole and craniotomy for open biopsy. Drug treatment similar to that used for tuberculous meningitis should be used.

MISCELLANEOUS. Almost every organ and tissue of the body can be involved in tuberculosis. In the upper respiratory tract and oral cavity, the larynx and the middle ear are most prone to infection. *Tuberculous laryngitis* used to be a rather common complication that was considered to be secondary to longstanding highly positive sputum associated with chronic cavitary disease. It was extremely painful and resulted in such difficulty in swallowing that severe inanition resulted. Response to drug treatment, even to administration of SM alone, was rapid and dramatic. The new face of tuberculous laryngitis is that of a primary laryngeal lesion that must be distinguished from carcinoma. Tuberculous middle ear disease, formerly common, is now rare. It was usually associated with advanced pulmonary or disseminated disease. Involvement of the eye is in the form of chronic uveitis, such as chorioretinitis, iridocyclitis, or iritis. Phlyctenular conjunctivitis produces small yellowish vesicles. Direct inoculation into the eye may produce conjunctivitis or keratitis. The specific origin of eye disease is difficult to prove. Cutaneous tuberculosis has all but disappeared, except for lesions associated with direct inoculation in laboratory workers and pathologists. Other manifestations include lesions like lupus vulgaris in which tubercle bacilli may be located and the tuberculids that are considered to be hypersensitivity reactions in which the organisms usually are not found. The larger blood vessels may harbor infections in their walls. Tuberculosis is a rare cause of aortic aneurysm. At one time tuberculosis of the adrenal gland was a common cause of adrenal insufficiency. Occasional cases of tuberculosis of the thyroid, breast, and soft tissues elsewhere than in the chest wall are still being reported.

DISSEMINATED AND MILIARY TUBERCULOSIS. These terms are used synonymously, although miliary tuberculosis is but one form of disseminated tuberculosis in which the widely dispersed small tubercles resemble millet seeds. During life these lesions usually are first recognized in the chest roentgenogram as very small nodules of uniform size that are evenly distributed throughout both lungs. The acute form was predominately an early complication of untreated primary tuberculosis, occurring mainly in young children and often associated with meningitis. During the past three decades the predominant age group has changed to the elderly, and the disease has become more subacute in its progression.

The diagnosis often is missed because it is difficult to distinguish the tuberculosis symptoms from those of the many underlying conditions that could be responsible for the weight loss, increasing fatigue, and low grade fever. Skin test anergy and frequent absence of chronic pulmonary tuberculosis may compound the difficulty. This sort of subacute disseminated tuberculosis has been called *cryptic* or *nonreactive tuberculosis*. The situation was admirably presented and analyzed by Slavin et al. in 1980. In their series of autopsied cases, only 15 per cent of patients admitted during the antibiotic era had the correct diagnosis made antemortem. A composite of such a case would be an elderly anergic patient without previously recognized tuberculosis who presented to the hospital with malignancy, renal failure, a renal transplant, or chronic alcoholism. Constitutional symptoms would be nonspecific, mainly fever, loss of weight, and increasing fatigue. Examinations would reveal no obvious tuberculosis in lungs or other organs, no hepatosplenomegaly, and no enlarged peripheral lymph nodes. There would be moderate anemia, a slight elevation of alkaline phosphatase, and a negative initial bacteriologic workup. The correct diagnosis depends upon a high index of suspicion and the demonstration of characteristic microscopic lesions and mycobacteria by biopsy. The most productive tissue is the liver, usually sampled by needle biopsy, with bone marrow next in line. Blood cultures should be obtained since they are sometimes positive at this stage of disease. At a later stage choroidal tubercles may be seen and radiographs of the lungs may show the typical miliary pattern.

Miliary tuberculosis almost always results from the discharge of infected caseous material into the bloodstream, usually from a well hidden lymph node in the mediastinum or the abdomen. When multiple bacteremic episodes occur, the process may be protracted. The patient may have serositis manifested by pleural effusion, pericardial effusion, or ascites. Hematologic abnormalities may be so prominent that a primary blood disease is suspected. The most common abnormality is a leukemoid reaction, although leukopenia, thrombocytopenia, and hemolytic anemia may occur. More commonly the primary disease is hematologic, complicated by a secondary tuberculosis dissemination, especially when large doses of corticosteroids have been given.

Treatment should consist of an intensive antituberculosis drug regimen using three drugs, including INH and RMP, plus EMB or PZA. After a few months, when a good response has occurred and after the drug susceptibility pattern of the infecting strain is known, the third drug can be discontinued. The total duration of therapy utilizing the suggested regimen has not been established, but it probably should be at least one year. Disseminated mycobacteriosis has been recognized as one of the common opportunistic infections in immunosuppressed and debilitated patients, including those with acquired immunodeficiency syndrome. Nontuberculous mycobacteria cause these infections even more often than does *M. tuberculosis*—a fact that should be considered in the choice of proper treatment.

Andrew OT, Schoenfeld PY, Hopewell PC, Humphreys MH: Tuberculosis in patients with end-stage renal disease. Am J Med 68:59, 1980. *A study of 10 patients with tuberculosis from a group of 172 undergoing dialysis in San Francisco gave a risk ratio of 12. The problems of diagnosis and treatment are admirably discussed.*

Anonymous: Is BCG vaccination effective? Tubercle 62:219, 1981. *The failure of the most recent large-scale trial in South India to demonstrate protection is brought into focus by this concise article.*

Canetti G: The Tubercle Bacillus in the Pulmonary Lesion of Man. New York, Springer Publishing Company, Inc., 1955. *A classic monograph detailing and integrating the pathogenesis of the disease in relation to histopathology, bacteriology, and immunology, as well as the influence of chemotherapy on the lesions.*

Centers for Disease Control: Primary resistance to antituberculosis drugs—United States. Morbid Mortal Wkly Rep 32:521, 1983. *The final report of a seven-year study in which 20 selected laboratories throughout the country submitted over 12,000 cultures to the CDC laboratory to be tested for drug susceptibility in a uniform manner.*

Clemens JD, Chuong JJH, Feinstein AR: The BCG controversy; a methodological and statistical reappraisal. JAMA 249:2362, 1983. *The authors reanalyzed the major BCG trial reports and concluded that vaccination was highly protective. Their appraisal was based on the superior study design and statistical precision of the more favorable trials.*

Costello HD, Caras GJ, Snider DE Jr: Drug resistance among previously treated tuberculosis patients: A brief report. Am Rev Respir Dis 121:313, 1980. *Among 4000 unsuccessfully treated patients in the United States, 41 per cent harbored drug-resistant strains.*

Daniel TM: The immunology of tuberculosis. Clin Chest Med 1:189, 1980. *A good summary of the immune spectrum exhibited by tuberculosis patients, the importance of further purification of mycobacterial antigens, and the mechanisms of immunoregulation.*

Daniel TM, Balestrino EA, Balestrino OC, Davidson PT, Debanne SM, Kataria S, Kataria YP, Scocozza JB: The tuberculin specificity in humans of *Mycobacterium tuberculosis* antigen 5. Am Rev Respir Dis 126:600, 1982. *Despite the fact that antigen 5 appeared to be limited to* M. tuberculosis *and* M. bovis, *it proved to be no more specific than tuberculin PPD when tested in the field. A good review of the previous attempts to produce specific skin test antigens to differentiate various mycobacterioses.*

Dannenberg AM Jr: Macrophages in inflammation and infection. N Engl J Med 293:489, 1975. *This study utilizing skin lesions in rabbits demonstrates the dynamic nature of mycobacterial lesions. Macrophages enter the arena as novices, become activated locally by interaction with immune lymphocytes, ingest bacilli, die, and are replaced by fresh cells recruited from the circulation.*

Farer LS, Lowell AM, Meador MP: Extrapulmonary tuberculosis in the United States. Am J Epidemiol 109:205, 1979. *An analysis of tuberculosis cases reported to the Centers for Disease Control reveals but little change in the number or rate of extrapulmonary disease from 1964 to 1976. Cases are analyzed according to age, anatomic site, sex, and race.*

Fox W: The chemotherapy of tuberculosis: A review. Chest 76S:785, 1979. *An excellent review of antituberculosis drug treatment up to 1979.*

Goodwin RA, Des Prez RM: Apical localization of pulmonary tuberculosis, chronic pulmonary histoplasmosis, and progressive massive fibrosis of the lung. Chest 83:801, 1983. *The higher oxygen tension at the apices of the lungs has been used as an explanation for the localization of adult-type tuberculosis. A more satisfactory theory based on diminished tissue clearance of antigens and lymph stasis is promulgated in this paper.*

Lichtenstein IH, MacGregor RR: Mycobacterial infections in renal transplant recipients: Report of 5 cases and review of the literature. Rev Infec Dis 5:216, 1983. *Among the cases were two that probably represented reactivation tuberculosis in the transplanted kidney. A survey of 26 transplantation centers revealed a tuberculosis rate of 480 cases per 100,000.*

Lincoln EM: Epidemics of tuberculosis. Arch Environ Health 14:473, 1967. *A review of 109 epidemics in 12 countries, the majority of them occurring in schools.*

Lorin MI, Hsu KHK, Jacob SC: Treatment of tuberculosis in children. Pediatr Clin North Am 30:333, 1983. *The latest recommendations for treatment of children, from a Houston group with long-standing interest in pediatric tuberculosis.*

Lurie MB: Resistance to Tuberculosis: Experimental Studies in Native and Acquired Defensive Mechanisms. Cambridge, Harvard University Press, 1964. *The role of native immunity in tuberculosis is well illustrated in this book, which summarizes the author's experiments using inbred rabbits.*

Sahn SA, Lakshminarayan S: Tuberculosis after corticosteroid therapy. Br J Dis Chest 70:195, 1976. *A recent review that emphasizes the usefulness of preventive therapy with isoniazid in patients already infected with* M. tuberculosis.

Slavin RE, Walsh TJ, Pollack AD: Late generalized tuberculosis: A clinical pathologic analysis and comparison of 100 cases in the preantibiotic and antibiotic eras. Medicine 59:352, 1980. *This study, from the Department of Pathology at Johns Hopkins University, consisted of an analysis of 200 autopsied cases. It contains a wealth of useful information on one form of disseminated tuberculosis.*

Snider DE Jr, Layde PM, Johnson NW, Lyle MA: Treatment of tuberculosis during pregnancy. Am Rev Respir Dis 122:65, 1980. *Presented are guidelines for the use of antituberculosis drugs in pregnant women.*

Stead WW: Control of tuberculosis in institutions. Chest 76 (Suppl):797, 1979. *Reviews recent outbreaks in nursing homes, prisons, schools, and hospitals, and suggests common-sense methods of control.*

Stead WW, Kerby GR, Schlueter DP, Jordahl CW: The clinical spectrum of primary tuberculosis in adults. Ann Intern Med 68:333, 1968. *Primary pulmonary disease was documented in 37 adults, of whom 9 had only minor symptoms, 11 developed pleural effusion, and 16 showed progression to adult-type chronic pulmonary disease.*

Youmans GP: Mechanisms of immunity in tuberculosis. Pathobiol Annu 9:137, 1979. *In this review article a former Department of Microbiology Chairman who published extensively in this field explains why he believes that "tuberculin sensitivity is an immune phenomenon that is quite distinct from the specific acquired immune response."*

299. OTHER MYCOBACTERIOSES

Emanuel Wolinsky

Organisms of the tuberculosis complex are not the only mycobacteria associated with human disease. The most popular label at present for these other mycobacteria is "nontuberculous." They have become more prominent in the total picture of mycobacterial disease because of the declining incidence of tuberculosis and a greater awareness and recognition of the other mycobacterioses. Indeed, there is evidence that the frequency of nontuberculous pulmonary disease may be increasing in certain areas of the country. In addition, disseminated mycobacterial infection is now recognized much more frequently as an opportunistic infection in immunosuppressed individuals, especially in those with the acquired immune deficiency syndrome (AIDS). Infection with other mycobacteria has been blamed, perhaps unfairly, for the apparent failure of bacille Calmette-Guérin (BCG) vaccination to protect adults in South India from subsequent tuberculosis. Leprosy, also a mycobacterial disease, is discussed in Ch. 300.

HISTORICAL PERSPECTIVE. The presence of many other species of *Mycobacterium* in the environment and in cold-blooded animals was recognized within a few years after the discovery of the tubercle bacillus. Scattered reports of the isolation of other mycobacteria from human secretions or pus date back to 1885. Several perceptive studies were published in the 1930's and the 1940's, but the realization that human disease surely was associated with nontuberculous mycobacteria did not occur until the mid 1950's. Since then, knowledge has been increasing at a rapid pace, although there are still many unanswered questions regarding the epidemiology, pathogenesis, and treatment of the other mycobacterioses.

MYCOBACTERIA. ***Mycobacterium avium-intracellulare (MAI).*** Mycobacteria of this species or complex constitute the most important agents of nontuberculous mycobacteriosis throughout the world. The organism known as the avian tubercle bacillus was described in 1890, although tuberculosis of chickens had been recognized for 22 years before that time. Supposedly quite resistant to infection with *M. avium,* people with documented *M. avium* disease were the subject of occasional literature reports. Recognition of the expanded role of these mycobacteria in pulmonary and disseminated disease occurred in the 1950's, when the organism was misnamed *Nocardia intracellularis* and given the common name of Battey bacillus. The official name of *Mycobacterium intracellulare* was assigned in the 1960's. The realization that *M. intracellulare* could not be distinguished from *M. avium* in most laboratories dictated another change to the presently used term MAI or *M. avium complex.* In this complex one can recognize 28 types by seroagglutination, of which types 1 to 3 represent the classic *M. avium* strains. Strains of MAI grow slowly; usually are nonpigmented or slightly yellow, becoming more highly pigmented with age but independently of light; are resistant to most antituberculosis drugs; and often produce colony variants of two or three types, including smooth translucent, smooth domed, and rough opaque. Of the three variants, the translucent colonies are usually most drug resistant and most virulent for experimental animals. Strains of MAI may be associated with all varieties of mycobacterial disease, especially pulmonary disease, childhood lymphadenitis, and opportunistic infection in patients who have AIDS.

Mycobacterium scrofulaceum. This is a scotochromogenic mycobacterium similar in many ways to MAI. The pigmentation varies from light yellow to dark orange. In some publications these organisms are lumped together with MAI, and the combination is called the *MAIS complex.* The name derives from the fact that the organism was recognized as the cause of scrofula in young children. Rarely, *M. scrofulaceum* may be associated with pulmonary disease in adults. Most of the disease-associated strains belong to one of three seroagglutination types, but it is not uncommon to see a strain of *M. scrofulaceum* agglutinate in one of the MAI serotypes.

Mycobacterium kansasii. The "yellow bacillus" was described in 1953 in Kansas City and was later given the official name of *M. kansasii.* It is responsible for a large number of pulmonary mycobacteriosis cases in some areas of the world. The organisms may be recognized in the initial sputum smears as large cross-barred acid-fast bacilli. Positive cultures may be identified by their distinctive photochromogenicity. The yellow color is light-dependent, developing within hours after the colonies have been exposed to light. Most strains are fully susceptible to rifampin and only slightly resistant to isoniazid, ethambutol, and streptomycin. *M. kansasii* is not found in nature except occasionally in samples of water.

Mycobacterium fortuitum-chelonei. Strains of this group grow rapidly, even on ordinary laboratory media. They are sometimes spoken of as the *M. fortuitum complex,* but it is better to retain at least two separate species because they can be distinguished from each other readily in the laboratory, and *M. chelonei* tends to be much more drug resistant than *M. fortuitum.* Both species are pathogenic for mice and resistant to the usual antituberculosis drugs. Long known for their ability to produce injection site abscesses and severe infections of traumatic wounds, strains of this group recently have become prominent as the cause of sternal osteomyelitis after cardiac surgery, of wound infection after implantation of silicone breast prostheses, of disseminated and localized infection in dialysis patients, of prosthetic valve endocarditis, and of disseminated infections with skin lesions in the immunosuppressed host.

Mycobacterium marinum. This organism is distinctive by virtue of its photochromogenicity and an optimal growth temperature of 30 to 33° C. It was named and recognized as a pathogen of fish in 1926. It is a common contaminant in fresh and salt water, accounting for the frequent occurrence of skin infection in individuals who work or play in a marine environment. Deep infections of the hand may also occur. Almost all strains are resistant to isoniazid but susceptible to rifampin and ethambutol. The organisms are also susceptible to tetracycline and sulfonamides.

Other Slow-Growing Species. *Mycobacterium xenopi* has an optimal growth temperature of 43° C and has been found as a contaminant in hot water generators and storage tanks. From these sites several outbreaks have occurred of respiratory tract colonization and pulmonary disease in the hospital environment. Other species that may cause disease are *M. simiae, M. szulgai,* and *M. malmoense.* Two species that may be associated with superficial soft tissue disease but not with pulmonary disease are *M. ulcerans* and *M. hemophilum.*

Species of Low Pathogenic Potential. A few cases have been reported in which strains of the *M. terrae* complex (including *M. triviale*) were the cause of pulmonary disease, arthritis, or tenosynovitis. Strains of this complex may be found in the soil. An organism long associated with water and considered to be saprophytic is *M. gordonae.* Documented infections with this organism now range from bursitis to widely disseminated disease. Cases of pulmonary disease and synovitis also have been ascribed to *M. flavescens,* an organism with an intermediate growth rate that was previously considered to be nonpathogenic for humans.

EPIDEMIOLOGY. In contrast to tuberculosis, the other mycobacterioses are not transmitted from person to person but are acquired from the environment by mechanisms that are not well understood. For *M. xenopi* and *M. kansasii* the evidence points to aerosols of infected water. Strains of MAI may be found in domestic animals, soil, dust, and water. There is evidence that infected droplet nuclei may be produced along coastlines. Still largely unexplained is the geographic variability in the incidence of other mycobacterioses and the relative proportion of these infections attributable to each of the two most important agents of disease, MAI and *M. kansasii.* In this country the highest rates of *M. kansasii* disease have been reported from New Orleans, Dallas, Houston, Kansas City, and Chicago, while Milwaukee and the states of Georgia and Florida have reported a predominance of MAI disease. From one institution in St. Louis, 27 per cent of newly diagnosed cases of mycobacterial pulmonary disease were associated with an equal proportion of MAI and *M. kansasii.* Australia, Israel, and Japan have reported an overwhelming predominance of MAI infections over those caused by *M. kansasii.* These figures refer to pulmonary disease; they do not reflect the distribution of disseminated infections. A recent increase in MAI and a concomitant decrease in *M. kansasii* disease has been reported from Virginia (Kim et al., 1984).

PATHOGENESIS. The localization of disease in the lungs suggests that the inhalation of infectious aerosols represents the primary route of infection. In many cases infection occurs by inoculation as a result of puncture wounds, lacerations, and foreign bodies. The question of whether the disease in adults usually represents primary infection or recrudescence of dormant foci cannot be answered at this time.

CLINICAL DESCRIPTION. ***Pulmonary Disease.*** The classic description is that of chronic cavitary disease resembling tuberculosis that occurs in a middle-aged rural man who has one or more of the following predisposing conditions: pneumoconiosis, healed tuberculosis, chronic bronchitis and emphysema, bullous disease, bronchiectasis, and malignant disease. However, there are many exceptions: the disease may be seen in all age groups except in children, in either sex, and in some individuals without any apparent predisposing factor. It sometimes appears as an acute condition in which there is an infected bulla or cyst or in a case resembling pneumonia. Solitary pulmonary nodules also have been described. The common etiologic agent is MAI, with *M. kansasii* second and *M. xenopi* a distant third.

The diagnosis may be suspected from the clinical appearance and the x-ray film, but it is the laboratory that must supply the correct identification of the mycobacterial agent. Skin tests are not helpful owing to a lack of adequately standardized antigens and the poor specificity of the presently available reagents. Pulmonary changes are characterized by one or more thin-walled cavities with little or no pleural disease or spread to the basal segments of the lungs. The sputum usually contains many acid-fast bacilli visible on smear and yields a heavy growth of the infecting agent. It may be possible to recognize the large banded forms of *M. kansasii* in the direct smear. A single positive culture test result in which there are only a few colonies usually represents environmental contamination. Repeatedly positive specimens may be indicative of transient or long-term colonization of the respiratory tract when they are not associated with new or enlarging cavities and a compatible clinical picture.

Treatment for *M. kansasii* disease usually is highly successful, provided that rifampin is included in the regimen. It is recommended that isoniazid, rifampin, and ethambutol be given for one year after the sputum becomes negative for the organism. Results of preliminary trials of short-course treatment have not been encouraging.

Therapy for MAI disease, on the other hand, has proved to be difficult. Most strains are resistant to the available antituberculosis drugs as well as the other anti-infectives, and the drug regimens recommended up to now have been chosen empirically. The necessity for treatment must first be established by an observation period to determine the stability of disease and the rate of progression if it is advancing. During this period the sputum should be examined at frequent intervals, and the patient should receive a comprehensive course of bronchial hygiene, including cessation of smoking, bronchodilator therapy, chest physiotherapy, and antibiotics if there are purulent secretions. These maneuvers have served to eliminate the organism from the secretions of some patients with chronic pulmonary disease. It may be necessary to initiate therapy immediately in certain cases of severe acute disease with a new cavitary lesion and no other apparent cause. Drug treatment may be considered at three levels. Level 1 is a triple-drug regimen consisting of isoniazid, rifampin, and ethambutol for a duration of at least two years provided there is some response within the first few months. This level would be suitable for a patient who had chronic stable disease with consistently positive sputum test results and in whom the mycobacterial infection was adding to the burden of pulmonary disease. Level 2 treatment consists of the same three drugs plus daily streptomycin administration for at least two years. Administration of streptomycin may be reduced to two or three times a week after an initial response has been demonstrated. This treatment level would be suitable for a patient who had slowly progressive disease, who had a poor response to level 1 treatment, or who had a relapse after discontinuation of level 1 drug therapy. Drug treatment at level 3 may be empiric combinations of five or six drugs or more reasonably, a regimen consisting of isoniazid, ethambutol, streptomycin, and ansamycin LM 427. The latter drug is an investigational rifamycin derivative that may be obtained at present from the tuberculosis control unit of the Centers for Disease Control. Most strains of MAI are susceptible to this ansamycin in vitro.

The response to drug treatment depends to a large extent on the underlying chronic lung disease and on the rate of progression of the mycobacterial infection. For those patients who have rapidly progressive infection in lungs that are already severely damaged, the prognosis is poor even with level 3 treatment. Some of these individuals have defects in cellular immune functions, especially those associated with T cells. Resectional surgery should be considered after a few months of treatment for those patients who have adequate pulmonary function and sufficiently localized mycobacterial disease. Treatment is not necessary for solitary pulmonary nodules that result from MAI infection, usually recognized after resection.

Disease caused by *M. xenopi* and *M. szulgai* usually is amenable to drug therapy. The exact combinations of drugs to be used depend on the drug susceptibility patterns in vitro. Suggested for *M. xenopi* disease is a regimen consisting of isoniazid, rifampin, and streptomycin and for *M. szulgai*, rifampin, ethambutol, and either ethionamide or streptomycin.

Infections associated with *M. scrofulaceum*, *M. simiae*, and *M. fortuitum-chelonei* are more difficult to control because of natural drug resistance. Strains of *M. simiae* usually are resistant to all of the antituberculosis drugs except cycloserine and ethionamide. Limited information on susceptibility of *M. scrofulaceum* suggests that ethionamide, rifampin, and ethambutol are most likely to be active in vitro. The same considerations as those described for MAI infection are applicable to these resistant infections. Although pulmonary infections with *M. fortuitum-chelonei* are quite rare, there is some information about the response to drug treatment from cases of extrapulmonary disease. Before sensitivity test results are available, full doses of amikacin should be given intramuscularly, together with one or more of the following drugs: doxycycline, erythromycin, cefoxitin, and a sulfonamide.

Lymphadenitis. Mycobacterial lymphadenitis is almost exclusively a disease of children of preschool age. Data from British Columbia published in 1974 indicated that the case rate for this new kind of scrofula was 0.37 per 100,000 persons per year, about ten times higher than for that caused by *M. tuberculosis.* Involved nodes may be found in the femoral, inguinal, epitrochlear, and axillary areas, although the most common location is around the angle of the jaw. The route of infection to the groin area is obvious after a penetrating injury or splinter entry into an extremity. The cervical nodes probably become infected by mucous membrane penetration in the mouth or pharynx. Examination shows a child who has had a painless localized swelling for several weeks and who is otherwise healthy. An unknown number of cases go on to suppuration and breakdown. Draining sinuses, whether spontaneous or following incision and drainage, may persist for many months. *M. scrofulaceum* was the most common cause of this infection, with MAI the second. However, there has been a recent reversal of this ratio so that strains of MAI now are the most common isolates from these infected nodes. Rare cases caused by several other species have been reported.

Correct diagnosis depends on the physician's familiarity with the disease, a positive tuberculin skin test result (sometimes requiring the use of second strength purified protein derivative), the absence of a history of contact with tuberculosis, absence of thoracic disease, and the location as well as the appearance of the involved nodes. Other conditions that need to be differentiated are tuberculosis, pyogenic lymphadenitis, cat scratch disease, congenital cyst, and lymphoma. The treatment of choice is excision of the involved nodes. In about 10 per cent of cases there is a recurrence of the infection in another group of nodes near the original site, occasionally on the other side. Rarely, there may be a third episode. Recurrences should be treated in the same manner as the original infection. There is no convincing evidence that drug treatment is beneficial. It should be remembered that as a result of this infection a child may have a positive tuberculin skin test reaction for many years.

Skin and Soft Tissue Infections. CUTANEOUS GRANULOMAS. Localized groups of papules have been called swimming pool granuloma or fish tank granuloma, depending on the source of infection. In another form of the disease there is a local abscess at the inoculation site, usually on the hand, followed by a series of secondary nodules that progress centrally along the lymphatics in a manner not unlike that seen in sporotrichosis. A few deep hand infections have also been described. The infection is not uncommon as an occupational or recreational illness in people who work or play in a marine environment. With few exceptions, the etiologic agent is *M. marinum*. Most superficial infections are self limited. When treatment is deemed necessary, the physician may use a combination of rifampin and ethambutol, rifampin alone, one of the tetracyclines, or trimethoprim-sulfamethoxazole. All of these regimens have been reported to be successful.

LOCAL ABSCESS. Many cases of local abscess following subcutaneous or intramuscular injection have been reported, some in outbreaks. The trouble usually is traced to a contaminated multiple injection vial, and the etiologic agent usually is *M. fortuitum-chelonei*. Incision and drainage usually will suffice to control the infection.

LOCAL TRAUMA. Most of these infections caused by *M. fortuitum-chelonei* occur as a result of penetrating or lacerating wounds contaminated with soil. Expert surgical handling is necessary, along with appropriate drug therapy as outlined under Pulmonary Disease.

DISSEMINATED NODULES. Multiple nodules and abscesses may be associated with widely disseminated mycobacterial disease, almost always in an immunocompromised host. The species most often isolated is *M. fortuitum-chelonei*. In addition, such nodules have been described in renal transplant patients as a result of infection with *M. hemophilum*.

BURULI ULCER. This deeply penetrating ulcer caused by *M. ulcerans* is confined mainly to Africa, Papua New Guinea, Malaysia, and Australia. The treatment is difficult and controversial.

Skeletal Infections. The synovia, tendon sheaths, and bursae are involved more often than other parts of the skeletal system in nontuberculous mycobacterial infections. A wide variety of species may be associated, including environmental strains with little pathogenicity for man, such as *M. terrae*, *M. gordonae*, and *M. flavescens*. Leading the list of etiologic agents is *M. kansasii*, with *M. fortuitum-chelonei* and MAI following in that order. Many of these infections follow trauma in which the wound is contaminated with soil or water. Others have occurred after injections of corticosteroids into arthritic joints; in these cases it is difficult to determine which condition was primary. The most common site is the hand, where the infection produces an indolent but persistent tenosynovitis, including the carpal tunnel syndrome. Osteomyelitis may occur in the form of multifocal lesions from hematogenous dissemination, often as a slowly progressive rather than a fulminant infection. The principal etiologic agent in these cases is MAI.

Treatment for skeletal infection usually demands close cooperation between a skilled surgeon and a physician specializing in infectious disease. Drug therapy depends on the etiologic agent (refer to earlier discussion).

Postsurgical Infections. Infections following surgery mainly are caused by *M. fortuitum-chelonei*. They include prosthetic valve endocarditis, sternal wound infection and osteomyelitis after open heart surgery, wound infection after augmentation mammoplasty, and infections associated with hemodialysis and peritoneal dialysis.

Disseminated Disease. Patients who acquire disseminated disease usually are severely immunocompromised from the standpoint of cellular immune functions. The recently recognized acquired immune deficiency syndrome has been associated with a dramatic increase in disseminated mycobacterial infections, since up to 50 per cent of such patients coming to autopsy in several cities have been found to have disseminated MAI infections. Prior to 1980 there were relatively few cases of disseminated mycobacterial disease reported throughout the world. Such cases usually involved patients who had underlying hematologic malignancies or who were under treatment with corticosteroids, or both. Both children and adults were affected, and the most common etiologic agents were *M. kansasii* and MAI. The case fatality rate was very high, even with the most intensive multiple-drug treatment. Diagnosis is most commonly made by biopsy and culture of liver, bone marrow, or lymph nodes. Cultures of the blood are often positive. Skin lesions or subcutaneous nodules or abscesses should be biopsied and examined for acid-fast bacilli. Strains of *M. fortuitum-chelonei* often are associated with these superficial lesions. The tissues may show a nonspecific necrotizing reaction in which macrophages are loaded with acid-fast bacilli, rather than a granulomatous reaction.

Treatment for disseminated disease is based on the same principles as those outlined for pulmonary disease. Infections caused by drug-sensitive organisms such as *M. kansasii* can usually be brought under at least temporary control provided that the human host is able to provide an adequate immune response. For infections related to MAI a multiple-drug regimen is usually chosen empirically, with a core of ansamycin* LM 427 and clofazimine.* Attempts to modify the host response by the use of transfer factor or prostaglandin inhibitors such as indomethacin have not yet been fully evaluated.

*Investigational drugs available from Centers for Disease Control, Atlanta, GA.

Bailey WC: Treatment of atypical mycobacterial disease. Chest 84:625, 1983. *In addition to a review of therapeutic regimens, the author proposes a new mycobacterial classification system based on responsiveness of associated diseases to treatment.*

Chapman JS: The Atypical Mycobacteria and Human Mycobacteriosis. New York, Plenum Medical Book Company, 1977. *A very informative monograph from one of the leaders in the field.*

Dixon JH: Nontuberculous mycobacterial infection of the tendon sheaths in the hand. J Bone Joint Surg 63B:543, 1981. *A report from a hospital in London of six cases caused by* M. kansasii. *The long delay in establishing the correct diagnosis is emphasized.*

Gribetz AR, Damsker B, Bottone EJ, Kirschner PA, Teirstein AS: Solitary pulmonary nodules due to nontuberculous mycobacterial infection. Am J Med 70:39, 1981. *This paper from New York's Mt. Sinai Medical Center describes the findings in 20 resected nodules positive for AFB during the period from 1969 to 1979. Twelve yielded* M. avium-intracellulare *on culture;* M. tuberculosis *was found in only one.*

Kim TC, Arora NS, Aldrich TK, Rochester DF: Atypical mycobacterial infections: A clinical study of 92 patients. South Med J 74:1304, 1981. *This is a study of pulmonary disease as seen in Charlottesville, Virginia, from 1970 to 1979. The majority of cases were attributed to* M. avium-intracellulare, *with a pronounced decrease of* M. kansasii *disease during the second five-year period.*

Macher AM, Kovacs JA, Gill V, Roberts GD, Ames J, Park CH, Straus S, Lane HC, Parillo JE, Fauci AS, Masur H: Bacteremia due to *Mycobacterium avium-intracellulare* in the acquired immunodeficiency syndrome. Ann Intern Med 99:782, 1983. *Eight patients had positive blood culture results on 1 to 14 occasions, requiring only 7 to 14 days with an automated radiometric technique.*

Marchevsky A, Damsker B, Gribetz A, Tepper S, Geller SA: The spectrum of pathology of nontuberculous mycobacterial infections in open-lung biopsy specimens. Am J Clin Pathol 78:695, 1982. *From 1969 to 1980 at New York's*

Mt. Sinai Medical Center, biopsy material from 40 patients revealed AFB. M. avium-intracellulare *accounted for 24 cases and* M. tuberculosis *for 6. A variety of histopathologic reactions are described in addition to the classic granulomas.*

Mason UG, Greenberg LE, Yen SS, Kirkpatrick CH: Indomethacin-responsive mononuclear cell dysfunction in "atypical" mycobacteriosis. Cell Immunol 71:54, 1982. *Cells from nine patients were studied. Seven had MAI infection. Evidence was found in favor of abnormal immunoregulation mediated by an imbalance of arachidonic acid metabolic products.*

Moran JF, Alexander LG, Staub EW, Young WG, Sealy WC: Long-term results of pulmonary resection for atypical mycobacterial disease. Ann Thorac Surg 35:597, 1983. *This report documents the good results of resectional surgery in 37 patients seen by the surgical group at Duke University from 1967 to 1981. All disease was attributed to* M. avium-intracellulare.

Sutker WL, Lankford LL, Tompsett R: Granulomatous synovitis: The role of atypical mycobacteria. Rev Infect Dis 1:729, 1979. *Presented are data from 25 adult patients observed from 1970 through 1977. Positive culture results were obtained in 15 cases: 4* M. tuberculosis, *6* M. kansasii, *2 MAI, and 1 each* M. marinum, M. gordonae, *and* M. chelonei. *There is also a good literature review.*

Wolinsky E: Nontuberculous mycobacteria and associated diseases. Am Rev Respir Dis 119:107, 1979. *A "state of the art" review of the entire subject.*

Woodley CL, Kilburn JO: In vitro susceptibility of *Mycobacterium avium* complex and *Mycobacterium tuberculosis* strains to a spiropiperidyl rifamycin. Am Rev Respir Dis 126:588, 1982. *Information from the laboratories of the Centers for Disease Control form the basis for the investigation of the use of ansamycin LM 427 in the treatment of MAI disease.*

300. LEPROSY (Hansen's Disease)

Ward E. Bullock

DEFINITION. Leprosy is a chronic granulomatous disease of man that is caused by *Mycobacterium leprae.* It is a disease of great chronicity, and the spectrum of its clinical manifestations is broad. At one end of the spectrum is tuberculoid (TT) leprosy, in which the clinical manifestations are localized to a single area of skin and the associated nerve supply. At the opposite end of the spectrum is lepromatous (LL) leprosy, in which there is massive infection of the dermis by *M. leprae* as well as involvement of the nerves, nasopharynx, testes, and lymphoreticular system. The intermediate forms of leprosy display mixtures of the clinical, histopathologic, and immunologic features typical of TT or LL disease. The intermediate forms are less stable clinically and often progress toward the lepromatous end of the spectrum; spontaneous improvement with a shift toward the tuberculoid spectrum occurs less frequently unless antimicrobial therapy has been instituted. These "upward" or "downward" shifts, as defined by gain or loss of host resistance, may be marked by inflammatory reactions within infected tissues, the immunologic mechanisms of which are poorly understood. Such reactions produce considerable functional impairment when they involve the peripheral nerve trunks. Reactions of this type occur in individuals with intermediate forms of leprosy but not in those with TT or LL disease. LL leprosy is associated with a different type of tissue reaction, erythema nodosum leprosum (ENL), that likewise may precipitate acute nerve dysfunction, presumably as a result of the humoral response to antigens of *M. leprae.*

EPIDEMIOLOGY. ***Incidence and Prevalence.*** The World Health Organization has estimated the total number of leprosy cases in the world to be approximately 11 million. However, valid statistics are not available from several countries with a high prevalence of leprosy including China. The actual number of cases probably exceeds 15 million. The highest prevalence rates are in Asia and Africa, followed by Central and South America and Oceania. Overall, the prevalence rate does not exceed 25 to 55 per 1000 in these areas, although it may be greater than 200 per 1000 within particular villages and surrounding areas.

The proportion of cases with lepromatous leprosy varies considerably from region to region; in Asia and the Americas it ranges from 25 to 65 per cent. In Africa the lepromatous forms of disease are distinctly less common, constituting from 6 to 20 per cent of the leprosy population. Roughly 20 per cent of the known cases of leprosy in India are of the lepromatous type. Although most cases of leprosy are found in the tropics, leprosy can flourish in colder climates, as for example in Korea, northern China, and Siberia. Within the United States, leprosy is endemic in Hawaii and in small areas of Texas, Louisiana, and Florida. Nevertheless, of the 1480 new cases reported to the U.S. Public Health Service from 1978 through 1982, 89 per cent occurred in foreign-born patients. This percentage represents a significant shift since the period from 1947 to 1966 when only 55 per cent of patients were foreign born. The largest number of patients with leprosy from 1978 through 1982 have come from Vietnam.

TRANSMISSION. The incubation period of leprosy is generally three to five years but may range from six months to decades. The precise modes of transmission have not been established. Traditionally, it had been thought that transmission involved prolonged close exposure of susceptible persons to the skin of an index case, especially one with lepromatous infection. In an endemic area, the risk of acquiring leprosy among household contacts of lepromatous cases is about eight times that in normal households; the risk of acquisition in households with tuberculoid leprosy is approximately four times normal (Doull et al., 1962). In fact, very few leprosy bacilli are shed from the intact skin of lepromatous patients; large numbers of organisms may be shed from skin ulcers, but these are relatively uncommon. By contrast, the nasal secretions of those with lepromatous disease contain up to 2×10^8 *M. leprae* in a single nose blow. Thus, a major portal of entry may be the respiratory tract. To date, however, there is little evidence to document primary respiratory tract infection *prior* to the onset of skin lesions. The granulomatous inflammation of leprosy does not caseate except occasionally within nerves. Since lesions heal without calcification, there are no residual tissue markers of primary infection equivalent to the Ghon complex of tuberculosis that might suggest the initial site of infection.

The gastrointestinal tract is a possible route for primary infection, since breast milk contains large numbers of *M. leprae,* but primary lesions have not been recognized within the gastrointestinal tract. Biting insects may provide still another means of transmission, since viable *M. leprae* can be isolated from the midguts of laboratory-bred arthropods for at least 48 hours after they have fed on lepromatous cases.

Although man has been thought to be the only natural host of *M. leprae,* a disease resembling lepromatous leprosy has been recognized in up to 10 per cent of feral armadillos from certain regions of Louisiana. The organism recovered from these animals is indistinguishable from *M. leprae* by available techniques. Leprosy has also been discovered in the sooty mangabey, a New World monkey. Thus, there may exist reservoirs of *M. leprae* other than man.

Susceptibility to Leprosy. The host factors that determine susceptibility to disease once an individual has been infected with *M. leprae* are poorly understood. The incidence of new cases usually is highest among older children and young adults. Although the cell-mediated immune responses of younger children may be relatively immature at the time of initial exposure to *M. leprae* and thereby predispose to increased disease incidence, environmental factors undoubtedly play a major role as well. The index case in childhood leprosy frequently is a parent with untreated disease with whom the child will have had prolonged and close contact.

Leprosy is diagnosed more frequently in males than in females, the ratio being 3:1 in some areas. The apparent predominance of leprosy in males probably is specious, since census figures in many regions are uncontrolled for sex selection.

Genetic factors long have been held to be important in determining susceptibility to leprosy, especially to the lepromatous type. Strong support for this concept is lacking. In a large study of monozygotic twins, it was found that 37 of 62 (60 per cent) of monozygotic twin pairs were concordant for leprosy of similar type, whereas in 25 pairs (40 per cent) only one member had leprosy. Others have failed to detect differences from normal in the segregation patterns of multiple genetic polymorphic systems among leprosy cases. Likewise, no consistent associations have been found between leprosy and HLA-A, B, or C antigens, although one group has found a statistically significant preferential inheritance of HLA-DR2 by siblings with tuberculoid leprosy but not by healthy siblings or by siblings afflicted with lepromatous disease. No associations between DR2 and nonfamilial cases of tuberculoid leprosy were detected.

ETIOLOGY. The causative agent of leprosy is a bacillus measuring 0.3 to 0.4 μm × 4 to 7 μm that is acid-alcohol fast when stained by the Ziehl-Neelsen method. Although the lepra bacillus was the first to be identified as the cause of human disease by Hansen in 1874, successful cultivation of this organism in vitro has not yet been achieved conclusively, and hence relatively little is known of its biology. A significant advance was made in 1960, when Shephard observed that a small inoculum (10^4) of *M. leprae* prepared from infected human tissues will multiply in the footpads of mice to a plateau level of 10^6. During multiplication, the doubling time of *M. leprae* is extraordinarily long, ranging from 10 to 13 days. The mouse footpad model has also made it possible to study the efficacy of many compounds against *M. leprae* in vivo.

Systemic infections with *M. leprae* can be achieved in mice and rats that are congenitally athymic or have been neonatally thymectomized. It is difficult to maintain immunodeficient animals for prolonged periods, and thus the utility of these models has been limited. Nine-banded armadillos and some species of monkeys are susceptible to infection with *M. leprae.* The former tend to develop an overwhelming infection that is analogous to lepromatous leprosy. The armadillo model will be more useful when these animals can be bred to produce pathogen-free animals. The need for specific pathogen-free animals is critical because wild armadillos may be infected with other noncultivatable mycobacteria.

PATHOGENESIS AND HISTOPATHOLOGY. Whatever the portal of entry for *M. leprae* may be, the first clinical manifestations of leprosy appear in the skin. The histopathology of an early lesion may be indeterminate and reveal only nonspecific inflammation composed of a scanty lymphocytic infiltrate around the dermal appendages and neurovascular bundles. Rarely, an acid-fast bacillus can be seen within small nerves of the dermis. In untreated cases, indeterminate lesions may resolve spontaneously or evolve until the histopathology becomes more characteristic of leprosy. It is then possible to classify a lesion within the leprosy spectrum based on the cell types and the number of bacilli observed within the areas of granulomatous inflammation. The best standardized classification of leprosy is that developed by Ridley and Jopling, in which the leprosy spectrum is divided into five groups as outlined in Table 300–1.

Tuberculoid (TT) Leprosy. The lesion of TT leprosy is characterized by well-developed granulomas composed of epithelioid cells with a uniform appearance and giant cells of the Langhans or foreign body type. Lymphocytes are abundant at the periphery of the granuloma, and acid-fast bacilli usually cannot be identified. Dermal nerves involved by the granulomatous inflammation are destroyed.

Borderline Tuberculoid (BT) Leprosy. The pathology of TT and BT leprosy is similar except that acid-fast bacilli are more readily seen in the latter, especially in dermal nerves, although the number is small.

TABLE 300–1. IMMUNOLOGIC MANIFESTATIONS WITHIN THE LEPROSY SPECTRUM*

Manifestation	TT	BT	BB	BL	LL
Lepromin reaction	3+	1+	±	–	–
ENL	–	–	–	±	2+
Bacilli in nose	–	–	–	1+	2+
Bacilli in granuloma	0	1–3+	3–4+	4–5+	5–6+
Epithelioid cells	1+	1+	1+	–	–
Langhans giant cells	1+	2+	–	–	–
Foam cells	–	–	–	1+	3+
Lymphocytes	3+	2+	1+	1+	±
Nerve destruction (skin)	2+	2+	1+	±	–

*Modified from Ridley DS: Int J Leprosy 40:102, 1972.

Borderline (BB) Leprosy. In BB leprosy, the histologic picture may vary considerably from lesion to lesion or even within the same lesion. Typically, the granuloma formation is less well developed. Epithelioid cells are spread more diffusely throughout the granuloma, giant cells are not present, and there are fewer lymphocytes within the infiltrate. The dermal nerves are less damaged, and therefore more easily visible. Acid-fast bacilli are numerous.

Borderline Lepromatous (BL) Leprosy. In this form, histiocytes are the predominant cell type with relatively few lymphocytes scattered among them, sometimes in aggregates. Epithelioid cells are absent. The damage within dermal nerves is less than that observed in BB disease, but there is increased perineural inflammation. This produces lamination of the perineurium that imparts an "onion skin" appearance to the nerve. Large numbers of acid-fast bacilli are present.

Lepromatous Leprosy (LL). The inflammatory infiltrate is composed almost exclusively of histiocytic cells that have a foamy appearance. Masses of bacilli are present intracellularly, many in large clumps called globi. Lymphocytes are very sparse. Characteristically, there is a "clear zone" beneath the epidermal basement membrane in which there is no inflammatory infiltrate, as contrasted with the tuberculoid forms of leprosy in which the granulomas extend to the dermal-epidermal junction.

Granulomas can be identified in the lymphoreticular organs of persons with tuberculoid leprosy. However, granulomatous pathology is far more extensive in BL and LL disease. For example, the paracortical regions of lymph nodes are heavily infiltrated by masses of histiocytes and literally are "choked" with acid-fast bacilli; T lymphocytes, normally abundant in this area, are largely displaced. The germinal centers, containing a predominance of B lymphocytes, are spared; they tend to be increased in both size and number. In the spleen, the white pulp is especially prone to invasion by histiocytic cells, although the red pulp also may be infiltrated. Aggregates of foamy histiocytes are present in the liver, most frequently around the portal tracts and scattered within the lobules. Patients suffering from LL disease manifest a continuous bacteremia with up to 1×10^5 bacilli per milliliter of blood, and the total body burden of *M. leprae* may approach 10^{12}.

IMMUNOPATHOLOGIC CONSIDERATIONS. Intracutaneous injection of healthy individuals and of patients with TT or BT leprosy with a heat-killed suspension of *M. leprae* (integral lepromin) prepared from skin lepromas will induce local granuloma formation within a three- to four-week period. Conversely, patients with LL disease are completely anergic to lepromin. Thus, the lepromin test provides a crude indication of an individual's capacity to mount a cell-mediated immune response against infection in *M. leprae.* If more purified preparations of *M. leprae* are employed to skin test for delayed-type hypersensitivity or to measure the proliferative responses of lymphocytes in vitro, the response to these antigens decreases progressively across the leprosy spectrum, i.e., they are greatest in TT leprosy and least in LL cases. Moreover, in a high percentage of the latter group, there is a generalized impairment of the delayed-type hypersensitivity response to a variety of "recall" antigens as measured by skin testing and lymphocyte proliferative responses. The anergy to antigens of *M. leprae* is very persistent despite long-term treatment, whereas the anergy to other antigens tends to be reversible.

Serum levels of the immunoglobulins generally are within the normal range in tuberculoid patients, whereas polyclonal hypergammaglobulinemia is a common feature of lepromatous leprosy. More than 90 per cent of lepromatous sera contain antibodies to *M. leprae* that cross-react with other mycobacteria; as antimicrobial therapy is continued, titers of these antibodies decline over a period of years. Ten per cent or more of patients with LL disease will have biologic false-positive reactions in tests for syphilis employing cardiolipin-type antigens, and more than 30 per cent will have cryoglobulinemia. Circulating immune complexes are present in a substantial but variable percentage of lepromatous cases, and in more than 50 per cent the serum contains elevated levels of amyloid-related serum protein component (SAA), an acute phase reactant. Although the relationship of SAA to tissue amyloid is unclear, secondary amyloidosis is not an uncommon complication of longstanding lepromatous leprosy. At least 50 per cent of cases have greatly elevated serum levels of C-reactive protein. Less frequently, antinuclear antibodies and rheumatoid factor are present, as well as low titers of antibody to thyroglobulin. In tuberculoid forms of leprosy, the prevalence of these serologic abnormalities is very low, presumably because the host immunoregulatory control mechanisms are less disordered.

CLINICAL MANIFESTATIONS. The variations of histopathology within the skin and peripheral nerves are reflected clinically by a wide range of skin lesions and peripheral neuropathies. The typical indeterminate lesion is usually, but not always, seen in children. It is a hypopigmented macule, of which there are rarely more than three or four. The macule measures 2 to 5 cm in diameter, and sensation may be impaired slightly within the macular area. In many cases the macules resolve spontaneously, whereas in others they evolve to become lesions more typical of tuberculoid or lepromatous disease.

TT leprosy generally presents as a single large plaque or macule that is very well defined. Occasionally, up to two or three lesions are present. Plaques are erythematous with sharply elevated outer borders that slope toward a flattened center, which is rough, dry, hairless, and anesthetic. Macules may be either erythematous or hypopigmented in the center. Enlarged dermal nerve twigs and related peripheral nerve trunks may be palpable or visible within the involved skin area. The most frequently enlarged nerves are the greater auricular, the ulnar above the elbow, the peroneal as it curves around the head of the fibula, and the posterior tibial. As with skin lesions, nerve damage is localized. Any area of the body may be affected, although the axillae, inguinal region, and perineal areas are spared, presumably because of the proclivity of *M. leprae* to grow in cooler areas of the body.

BT leprosy closely resembles TT disease; however, the plaques or macules tend to be more numerous, and satellite lesions sometimes are present near the larger lesions. The peripheral nerve trunks frequently are enlarged by granulomatous infiltrates. Some of the more common complications are (1) traumatic plantar ulcerations of the feet, (2) foot drop, (3) loss of hand function as a result of flexion contracture and repeated trauma to anesthetic digits, and (4) corneal abrasions if there is corneal nerve dysfunction.

The lesions of BB leprosy are polymorphic in appearance. Generally they are numerous and vary considerably in size. Unlike the tuberculoid forms of disease, in which lesions are localized to one side of the body, the lesions of BB leprosy are more symmetrical. In some cases they appear as large, erythematous bands with sharply demarcated centers and outer edges. Others appear as irregular erythematous plaques with poorly defined outer margins and hypopigmented centers that have a characteristic "punched-out" appearance. Not infrequently, both types are present simultaneously, and satellite lesions are common. The lesions tend not to be as anesthetic as those in TT or BT disease.

Skin manifestations of BL leprosy are perhaps the most heterogeneous of all. They are numerous, are distributed bilaterally, and can present as macules, plaques, papules, or nodules. BL skin lesions tend to include some nodules with a "dimpled" appearance in the center, and some plaques have centers that appear hypopigmented and "punched out." As a rule, the nasal structures are not involved, although the ear lobes may be thickened. Nerve thickening can be quite prominent near the site of cutaneous lesions, but anesthesia is less evident than in the forms described above.

During early stages of LL leprosy, the extensive inflammatory response within the dermis gives rise to widely distributed erythematous macules or papules. In dark-skinned individuals these are difficult to see unless viewed obliquely in good light. With progression, plaques and nodules become evident. In later stages they are the predominant types of lesions. The skin becomes progressively thickened with infiltrate to produce the classic leonine facies in association with thinning and loss of eyebrows. Occasionally, cases of LL leprosy can present without obvious localized lesions but instead have diffuse lepromatous infiltrates in the skin. This type of disease is observed most frequently in Central America. Those who suffer from it are prone to develop a distinctive vasculitis (the so-called "Lucio's phenomenon") involving the dermal vessels that results in ischemic necrosis of the epidermis. The lesions are stellate in appearance and heal with atrophic scar formation.

In LL leprosy, the eyes frequently are involved by keratitis and iritis; there is progressive destruction of the nasal cartilage and anterior maxillary spinous process, resulting in saddle nose deformity. Incisor teeth may be lost, and chronic inflammation of the larynx can lead to life-threatening stenosis. Extensive infection of the testes is common, leading to fibrosis and hyalinization of the seminiferous tubules and azoospermia; the testicular damage is reflected by elevated gonadotropin levels, reduced plasma testosterone levels, and gynecomastia. The ovaries are infected only rarely. Nerve involvement is more extensive in LL leprosy than in other forms, although functional deficits are less severe because the intensity of the intraneuronal inflammation is reduced consequent to poor cell-mediated immunity to *M. leprae*. The neurologic damage usually manifests as mononeuritis multiplex, i.e., an asymmetrical sensory polyneuropathy.

Reactional States. Although leprosy itself is an extremely torpid infection, the clinical course all too frequently is punctuated by acute and subacute reactional states that produce serious morbidity and even death. The most common of these reactional states is erythema nodosum leprosum (ENL), which occurs only in patients with high bacterial loads—namely, those with BL or LL disease. Occasionally, untreated patients experience ENL. Much more frequently, effective antileprosy treatment triggers the onset of ENL, which occurs in more than 50 per cent of patients within the first year. The onset of ENL is sudden over a 24- to 48-hour period with eruption of painful red papules or nodules over the face, trunk, arms, and thighs. Nodules may proceed to frank suppuration, requiring several weeks to heal, generally without scarring. Occasionally, ENL is chronic, lasting for several months. Histologically, early ENL nodules reveal polymorphonuclear infiltration within the lepromatous granulomas, and frequently there is panniculitis; a panvasculitis may involve both arteries and veins in the dermis. It is widely believed that ENL activated by antimycobacterial therapy is precipitated by degradation of *M. leprae* with release of antigenic material. Antibodies to *M. leprae* are presumed to complex with these antigens, thereby inducing a number of serious constitutional disturbances, including severe pyrexia, iridocyclitis, neuritis, orchitis, lymphadenitis, and polyarthritis. In addition, there is a high prevalence of glomerulonephritis in ENL. Acute proliferative glomerulonephritis and focal mesangial hypercellularity with thickening of the glomerular capillary loops are the most consistent findings. Deposits of subendothelial or subepithelial electron-dense material are seen by electron microscopy, and discontinuous linear deposits of IgG, IgM, and C3 have been demonstrated along the capillary membranes by fluorescence microscopy. To date, it has not been established that antigenic material derived from *M. leprae* is actually present within the glomeruli. Notwithstanding the severity of the inflammatory response in many cases of ENL, hypocomplementemia is unusual.

Reversal Reactions. Patients with BT, BB, or BL disease may experience a quite different type of tissue reaction after they have been treated for several months. As the clinical status of these patients improves, typically from a BL to a BB classification, some will develop induration and erythema within infected areas of the skin. Histologic examination reveals an influx of lymphocytes into areas of granulomatous inflammation, with concomitant reduction in the number of bacilli. Reversal reactions generally develop over days or weeks and last for weeks or months. Although these reactions are regarded as an "upgrading" of the host's cellular immune responses, the clinical consequences can be serious. For example, augmentation of the inflammatory response within peripheral nerves can irreversibly damage the already compromised fascicles. Reactions quite similar in appearance to reversal reactions but that signal a deterioration in the immune response may be experienced by patients whose compliance with therapy is poor or in whom the *M. leprae* has become drug resistant. These so-called "downgrading" reactions are associated with worsening of the clinical condition and an increased bacillary index within tissues.

DIAGNOSIS AND DIFFERENTIAL DIAGNOSIS. Isolation of a phenolic glycolipid I that appears unique to *M. leprae* (Brennan and Barrow, 1980) offers promise that serologic tests may be developed that will aid in the early diagnosis of leprosy. At present, however, the diagnosis must be established by clinical examination and histopathologic study. An anesthetic or hypoesthetic skin lesion immediately suggests the diagnosis of leprosy; associated nerve thickening further supports the diagnosis. A skin biopsy is essential for confirmation and accurate classification of the disease. An adequate biopsy specimen must include both central and peripheral areas of a lesion and should be deep enough to remove subcutaneous fatty tissue en bloc. Elliptical excision biopsy 12 to 15 mm long is preferred to punch biopsy. When lesions of varying types are present, it is advisable to obtain biopsies from two different sites.

M. leprae in paraffinized tissues is poorly stained by the Ziehl-Neelsen method. A much better stain is obtained by the Wade-Fite method, or its equivalent, which restores the acid-fast property of *M. leprae* by impregnating the tissue section with an oily substance such as turpentine or peanut oil. Control sections known to contain acid-fast staining organisms should be prepared simultaneously. In patients with paucibacillary disease (i.e., TT or BT), serial histologic sections may have to be searched for hours to identify one or two bacilli; these most frequently will be located within dermal nerve twigs. The Ziehl-Neelsen stain is adequate for smear preparations as from nasal scrapings and the buffy coat of blood. Acid-fast staining bacilli are readily visualized in both types of smears in BL or LL disease. In buffy coat smears, mononuclear cells contain bacilli, as do occasional polymorphonuclear leukocytes.

Some clinical signs and symptoms that may be helpful in establishing the diagnosis of lepromatous leprosy include the following: (1) The ear lobes are thickened and have a "succulent" appearance. (2) The patient complains of a chronically stuffy nose with discharge that sometimes is bloody; frequently the examiner will note a fetid odor. (3) There may be ENL lesions scattered widely over the body, including the face. Erythema nodosum that is associated with other conditions usually is localized to the pretibial regions of the lower extremities. ENL is not seen in tuberculoid leprosy. (4) Not infrequently there is a brawny type of edema involving the lower extremities and the hands. Fusiform swelling of the digits that extends to the dorsum of the hands is seen, mimicking scleroderma.

Certain types of nerve deficits or deformities should suggest the possibility of leprosy in any form. These include (1) plantar ulcerations in a person who is neither diabetic nor tabetic; (2) footdrop without a history of poliomyelitis or heavy metal exposure; and (3) a characteristic claw deformity of the hands, with digital damage resulting from motor and sensory dysfunction of the ulnar nerve and other nerve supply to the hand. Occasionally, leprosy will be misdiagnosed as lupus erythematosus; fluorescent antibody staining of a skin biopsy may reveal immunoglobulin deposits resembling those of lupus within the epidermal basement membrane. A Wade-Fite stain is most helpful in such situations.

TREATMENT—PRINCIPAL DRUGS. ***Dapsone.*** The standard drug for leprosy continues to be 4,4′-diaminodiphenylsulfone (dapsone, DDS). DDS is thought to block the p-aminobenzoic acid condensation reaction necessary for folate synthesis. The minimal inhibitory concentration (MIC) of DDS for *M. leprae* that are susceptible to the drug ranges between 0.01 and 0.001 μg per milliliter as determined by the mouse footpad assay. DDS is inexpensive, a factor of great economic significance in countries with high prevalence rates of leprosy. Its toxicity is low; however, adverse reactions to DDS occasionally occur. The most serious are hemolysis, agranulocytosis, hepatitis, exfoliative dermatitis, and, very rarely, severe hypoalbuminemia. A devastating combination of exfoliative dermatitis and hepatitis, known as the "DDS syndrome," has been observed in perhaps 1 per 1000 cases in the early stages of treatment (less than seven weeks). Immediate cessation of DDS, intensive care, and massive corticosteroid therapy (in excess of 100 mg per day of prednisone or its equivalent) may be lifesaving.

Twenty-four hours after ingestion of DDS, 100 mg, the plasma concentration in a 60-kg person ranges from approximately 0.12 to 0.4 μg per milliliter. This rather wide range is explained by large individual differences in rates of clearance from the body, resulting in part from genetic polymorphism in acetylation of the drug. Thus, the half-life in plasma varies from 10 to 50 hours, with an average of 28 hours. Regardless of an individual's acetylation status, however, the plasma levels of DDS under daily therapy with 50 to 100 mg will remain well in excess of the MIC for susceptible *M. leprae*.

Rifampin.* The MIC of rifampin against *M. leprae* is less than 1 μg per ml, and it provides a rapid bactericidal effect against organisms in tissues and nasal secretions. As little as 4 weeks of therapy with rifampin prevents multiplication in the mouse footpad of acid-fast bacilli harvested from tissue specimens or nasal secretions of patients with lepromatous leprosy. A comparable loss of infectivity cannot be achieved with DDS until 10 to 12 weeks of treatment. Rifampin therapy also rapidly reduces the morphologic index (MI) of *M. leprae*. The MI expresses a ratio of the number of bacilli, within tissues or secretions, that stain uniformly by acid-fast methods and that therefore are considered viable over the number of bacilli that strain irregularly and therefore are considered to be nonviable. The MI of *M. leprae* in lepromatous patients falls to nearly zero within four weeks after the start of rifampin therapy. By contrast, three to six months of DDS therapy may be required for comparable reduction of the MI.

Clofazimine. Clofazimine (B663) is a phenazine iminoquinone derivative that is effective in the treatment of leprosy, although its mechanism of action is not well understood. There is some evidence that it may act by inhibiting template formation of deoxyribonucleic acid. The compound is highly lipophilic and is deposited within fatty tissues, the skin, and the reticuloendothelial system, where it is taken up by macrophages. Clofazimine is a dye and therefore causes skin pigmentation over time, with a coloration varying from a reddish hue to a deep purple with prolonged high dosage therapy. After discontinuation of clofazimine therapy, the pigmentation clears gradually over a period of months to years. Clofazimine is eliminated very slowly with a half-life following oral administration of 70 days or more. Urinary excretion is negligible, whereas approximately 50 per cent of an administered dose may be recovered unchanged from the feces, possibly as a result of incomplete absorption from the gut and excretion via the bile, in which high concentrations have been found. Given in high concentrations (200 to 300 mg per day) for extended periods of time, the drug is deposited in the small intestinal wall and thereby causes segmental thickening that may be associated with mid-abdominal burning or cramping pain, diarrhea, and rarely partial small bowel obstruction. Clofazimine has not been approved by the Food and Drug Administration. It may be obtained under protocol from the National Hansen's Disease Center, Carville, Louisiana.

*This use is not listed in the manufacturer's directive.

TREATMENT—CURRENT RECOMMENDATIONS. Of great concern has been the emergence of both primary and secondary resistance to DDS as a consequence of its long-term use as the single therapeutic agent to treat leprosy. Worldwide, the prevalence of secondary resistance currently ranges from 20 to 190 per 1000, depending on locale. Primary resistance to DDS of varying prevalence and degree also has been reported worldwide. In view of these findings, it is essential that a variety of antibiotics be administered to all patients with leprosy.

The principal aims of multidrug therapy are to stem the increase in prevalence of primary and secondary resistance to DDS by *M. leprae* and to reduce the duration of treatment. For treatment of multibacillary forms of leprosy (BB, BL, and LL types), the following triple drug combination is suggested by the World Health Organization (WHO): (1) a self-administered oral dose of DDS, 50 to 100 mg daily; (2) a self-administered oral dose of clofazimine, 50 mg daily plus a 300-mg dose given once monthly under supervision; and (3) an oral dose of rifampin, 600 mg once monthly under supervision. When clofazimine is totally unacceptable, ethionamide* or prothionamide† should be considered in a self-administered oral dose of 250 to 375 mg daily. The case for use of the latter antibiotics is more compelling in patients harboring *M. leprae* that is resistant to DDS. Proof of resistance requires special procedures that are available at centers for the treatment of leprosy.

Combined therapy should be given for a minimum of two years. If possible, such therapy should be continued until all skin scrapings and biopsies become negative for acid-fast bacilli, a process that may require several years.

The WHO recommendation for intermittent rifampin treatment is made in part because of the heavy economic burden that the drug places upon nations with a high prevalence of leprosy. The scientific rationale is based on preliminary clinical trials and studies of intermittent chemotherapy in the mouse footpad infection model. Despite the early promise of intermittent rifampin therapy and the low incidence of reactions to the drug when it is given in this manner (influenza-like syndrome, thrombocytopenic purpura, and shock), the WHO recommendation is based on incomplete data. Some experienced physicians prefer to give 450 or 600 mg of rifampin* daily for two to three years when possible.

For treatment of paucibacillary disease (indeterminant, TT, and BT types), the WHO recommends administration of rifampin,* 600 mg orally once per month under supervision for a six-month period plus DDS, 100 mg orally daily for six months, self-administered. If relapse occurs, the treatment regimen should be repeated. The number of *M. leprae* in patients with paucibacillary disease rarely exceeds 10^6. Therefore, the risk of selecting drug-resistant mutants by treatment appears to be quite low. Moreover, the cell-mediated immune defense mechanisms of these patients are better able to deal with the leprosy bacillus than are those of patients with multibacillary disease. However, the long-term efficacy of intermittent rifampin therapy for paucibacillary disease has not been established. Thus some leprologists elect to treat such cases with DDS, 50 to 100 mg daily plus rifampin, 450 to 600 mg daily for six months with DDS therapy continued for two to five years.

In patients with multibacillary disease who are treated appropriately, clinical improvement generally can be detected after the third month of treatment and clearly is evident by the sixth month. Disappearance of recognizable bacillary forms usually requires three to five years even though viable bacilli rapidly become undetectable by currently available assay methods. Thus patients with lepromatous leprosy have difficulty not only in disposing of viable *M. leprae* but also in clearing nonviable organisms.

Patients with lepromatous leprosy who are under treatment with a drug regimen that includes rifampin can be regarded as noncontagious after a two- to three-week period. However, even the untreated patient represents only a very low risk of contagion and can be admitted to any general hospital in which ordinary procedures of barrier nursing are observed. Tuberculoid leprosy should be viewed as noncontagious.

*This use is not listed in the manufacturer's directive.
†Investigational drug.

Treatment of Reactions. ENL is by far the most common reaction in lepromatous leprosy. When mild, it can be managed with aspirin. Severe episodes are controlled rapidly by high dosages of prednisone (60 to 80 mg per day). However, as the dosage is tapered, a flare-up of ENL is encountered frequently. Thalidomide* is very effective in treating severe ENL. The initial dosage is usually 200 mg given twice daily with gradual tapering over several weeks to maintenance levels of 50 to 100 mg per day. This dosage can be continued for several months. Administration of both prednisone and thalidomide to patients with severe ENL brings about very prompt improvement by means of the steroid action and yet permits rapid steroid withdrawal within a few days as the thalidomide takes full effect. The use of thalidomide in women of childbearing age is hazardous because of its teratogenicity. Clofazimine is also effective in the management of ENL, although it requires from four to six weeks to exert its effect. ENL reactions in patients with BL leprosy are poorly controlled by thalidomide and are best managed by judicious use of steroids and/or clofazimine.

Reversal reactions associated with severe neuritis or in which there is a risk of skin ulceration should be treated with steroids in high dosage, followed by very gradual tapering. Alternatively, steroids plus clofazimine can be employed to attempt more rapid withdrawal of the steroid. Reversal reactions are far more chronic than the usual episodes of ENL and may require anti-inflammatory therapy for several months. Thalidomide is ineffective in treating these reactions.

Treatment of Other Complications. A cold abscess within a peripheral nerve requires surgical drainage. A sudden increase in the intensity of nerve pain and/or increase in the functional deficit of a nerve under full medical therapy may be helped in some cases by surgical decompression to relieve the intraneural edema. Excellent corrective surgical procedures are available for deformity of the hands secondary to permanent loss of motor innervation. The common problem of footdrop can be greatly improved by transfer of the tibialis posterior muscle so that it becomes a dorsiflexor. Plantar ulceration secondary to sensory loss responds well to appropriate medical and surgical management. Subsequently the patient should be fitted carefully with special footwear that will increase the area of load-bearing and reduce pressure at the ulcer-prone site. Madarosis (complete loss of eyebrows) can be corrected by swinging scalp flaps to the eyebrow area after infection has been arrested. This cosmetic procedure can make the difference between social acceptance or nonacceptance, since laymen in regions endemic for leprosy are well aware of the cause of eyebrow loss. Leprotic iridocyclitis is an insidious complication in lepromatous patients that may progress without pain. Treatment with mydriatrics and steroids is essential to prevent destruction of the ciliary body. Lagophthalmos secondary to involvement of the seventh cranial nerve also must be corrected to prevent exposure keratitis.

PROGNOSIS. Most cases of TT leprosy are self-curing, as are many of those with indeterminate disease. Some individuals with BT leprosy may self-cure with or without permanent nerve damage; however, there is a tendency for others to lose cell-mediated immune responsiveness to *M. leprae* and to drift toward the lepromatous end of the disease spectrum. Notwithstanding the more favorable prognosis in tuberculoid leprosy, all patients should be treated as detailed above.

Most cases of lepromatous leprosy can be brought to a state of arrest if not cure, provided that compliance is good and that appropriate therapy is continued for a prolonged period. Death caused by amyloidosis or inadequately treated ENL is relatively infrequent.

PREVENTION AND PROPHYLAXIS. The household contacts of leprosy patients, especially children, should be examined care-

*Investigational drug in leprosy.

fully for signs of leprosy, and suspicious skin lesions must be biopsied. Generally, household contacts of TT and BT patients should not be given prophylaxis, although it is advisable that they be examined annually. Children who have had extensive household contact with BL or LL patients who have been untreated should be considered for DDS prophylaxis; DDS has been shown to be of prophylactic value in children under the age of 16 when given according to recommended dosage schedules (Filice and Fraser). Adults appear to be less susceptible to leprosy; since the efficacy of DDS prophylaxis in this group has not been established, preventive treatment of older age groups usually is not recommended.

Three major trials to determine the preventive role of BCG vaccine against leprosy have yielded different results. At this time BCG is not recommended for prevention of leprosy.

Bullock WE: Immunology of leprosy. *In* Nahmias A, O'Reilly R (eds.): Immunology of Human Infection, Part I. New York, Plenum Publishing Corporation, 1981, p 369. *A thorough discussion of the immunologic disturbances associated with leprosy.*

Filice GA, Fraser DW: Management of household contacts of leprosy patients. Ann Intern Med 88:538, 1978. *Detailed recommendations.*

Ridley DS, Jopling WH: Classification of leprosy according to immunity. A five-group system. Int J Leprosy 34:255, 1966. *Most helpful for comprehending the spectrum of leprosy. Good illustrations.*

Serjeantson SW: HLA and susceptibility to leprosy. Immunol Rev 70:89, 1983. *A good review of the genetic aspects of leprosy.*

WHO Study Group Report: Chemotherapy of leprosy for control programmes. WHO Technical Report Series No. 675. Geneva, WHO, 1982. *A new report containing important recommendations for changes in the treatment of leprosy.*

Yawalkar SJ, Vischer W: Lamprene (Clofazimine) in Leprosy. Basel, Ciba-Geigy Limited, 1978, pp 1–15. *A concise summary of what is known about this important drug.*

Sexually Transmitted Diseases

P. Frederick Sparling

301. INTRODUCTION AND COMMON SYNDROMES

Sexually transmitted diseases (STDs) are a diverse group of infections, caused by biologically dissimilar microbial agents, which are grouped together because of certain common clinical and epidemiologic features. In recent years there has been a surge of interest by physicians, researchers, and the public in STDs. This interest in part is due to the prior lack of knowledge about these common diseases, to relaxation of former taboos about sexuality, and to recognition of the medical and economic importance of STD. This has resulted in a remarkable accumulation of information about "classic" venereal infections such as gonorrhea, as well as "new" sexually transmitted diseases such as hepatitis A and B, shigellosis, giardiasis, acquired immune deficiency syndrome (AIDS), and others. This chapter will discuss certain common features of some of these infections, as well as the differential diagnosis and management of several of the common syndromes of genital infections.

DEFINITIONS. Those infectious agents which are frequently transmitted by sexual contact, and for which sexual transmission is epidemiologically important, are considered sexually transmitted diseases. In some cases, such as gonorrhea and genital herpes simplex virus infection, sexual transmission is the only important mode of transmission, at least between adults. In others, such as the hepatitis viruses, giardiasis, shigellosis, and amebiasis, there are also important nonsexual means of acquiring infection. Table 301–1 lists the important infectious agents that are commonly transmitted sexually, as well as their known or probable disease syndromes. Other diseases, such as cervical carcinoma, for which there is strong epidemiologic evidence of association with sexual transmission but for which there still is not a known cause, will not be considered here. Diverse infections such as blastomycosis, histoplasmosis, and others for which sexual transmission has been documented generally will be considered. "Sexual" includes the full range of heterosexual or homosexual behavior, including genital, oral-genital, oral-anal, and genital-anal contact.

EPIDEMIOLOGIC CONSIDERATIONS. Sexually transmitted infections are prevalent in many segments of society, but, for obvious reasons, are most prevalent in the groups with the most promiscuous sexual activity. It is not sexual activity per se, but the number of different sexual partners that determines the risk of acquiring STD. The highest rates of gonorrhea are found in the young (15 to 30) and unmarried, and in groups of low educational and socioeconomic status. Rates of gonococcal infection may be 50-fold higher in young single inner-city persons than in married middle to upper-middle class persons. Decisions regarding the cost-effectiveness of screening for STD should be governed by these considerations; screening is most effective in high-risk groups.

Multiple infections are frequent in patients with sexually transmitted infection. In venereal disease clinics, about 20 per cent of men with gonorrhea also have urethral chlamydial infection, and 30 to 50 per cent of women with gonorrhea also have cervical chlamydial infection. In women with vaginitis, one study showed that 16 per cent of cases were caused by mixed infection with various combinations of *Candida, Trichomonas,* and *G. vaginalis.* However, there is no convincing evidence that one sexually transmitted infection directly increases the risk of acquiring others. Rather, the frequent coexistence of multiple sexually acquired infections probably reflects the frequency of these organisms and the multiplicity of sexual partners among patients who were the subjects of these studies.

Control of sexually transmitted infections is complicated by the frequent lack of significant symptoms. The majority of gonococcal and chlamydial infections in women probably are associated with few symptoms. From 10 to 50 per cent of urethral gonococcal infections in men are oligo- or asymptomatic. Urethral chlamydial infections of men are more common than gonococcal infections and frequently are asymptomatic. The importance of the asymptomatic male is underscored by the repeated observation that women with gonococcal pelvic inflammatory disease have male partners whose infection is asymptomatic. Thus, one of the crucial issues in management is proper diagnosis and treatment of the asymptomatically infected partner.

STD IN HOMOSEXUAL MALES. Homosexual males are recognized as a group at particularly high risk of acquiring sexually transmitted disease. The current epidemic of AIDS in homosexual men is a major concern. This subject is discussed in Ch. 430. AIDS is but one of many STD-related problems in homosexual males, however. Currently, approximately 50 per cent of all male patients in the United States with infectious (primary and secondary) syphilis name other males as their contacts. Some homosexual males are exceptionally promiscuous and are at high risk of acquiring not only syphilis but also gonococcal urethritis, proctitis, and pharyngitis; herpes genitalis and proctitis; hepatitis A and B; and a variety of enteric infections that are rarely transmitted in heterosexual sex, including giardiasis, amebiasis, and shigellosis. These enteric infections are probably transmitted by oral-anal or anal-penile-oral contact. Several cities in the United States with relatively large populations of homosexual males have had major increases in prevalence of giardiasis, amebiasis, and shigellosis. In some studies, the incidence of acute shigellosis and hepatitis A and B in men aged 20 to 39 was six to ten times that of any other age group of men or women. A study of a population of homosexual men

TABLE 301–1. SEXUALLY TRANSMITTED AGENTS AND THEIR SYNDROMES*

Microorganism	Syndromes
Bacteria	
Neisseria gonorrhoeae	Urethritis, cervicitis, bartholinitis, proctitis, pharyngitis, salpingitis, epididymitis, conjunctivitis, perihepatitis, arthritis, dermatitis, endocarditis, meningitis, amniotic infection syndrome
Gardnerella vaginalis	"Nonspecific" vaginosis (in association with anaerobic bacteria)
Treponema pallidum	Syphilis (multiple clinical syndromes)
Hemophilus ducreyi	Chancroid
Calymmatobacterium granulomatis	Granuloma inguinale
Shigella species	Enteritis in homosexual men
Campylobacter species	Enteritis in homosexual men
Group B *Streptococcus*	Neonatal sepsis and meningitis
Chlamydiae	
Chlamydia trachomatis	Nongonococcal urethritis, purulent hypertrophic cervicitis, epididymitis, salpingitis, conjunctivitis, trachoma, pneumonia, perihepatitis, lymphogranuloma venereum, ? Reiter's syndrome
Mycoplasmas	
Ureaplasma urealyticum	Nongonococcal urethritis, ? premature rupture of membranes and abortion
Mycoplasma hominis	Postpartum fever, ? pelvic inflammatory disease
Viruses	
Herpes simplex virus	Genital herpes, proctitis, meningitis, disseminated infection in neonates
Hepatitis A virus	Hepatitis in homosexual men
Hepatitis B virus	Hepatitis, ? periarteritis nodosa, hepatoma; especially prevalent in homosexual men
Cytomegalovirus	Congenital infection (birth defects, infant mortality, mental deficiency, hearing loss); mononucleosis syndrome
Genital wart virus	Condyloma acuminatum
Molluscum contagiosum virus	Molluscum contagiosum
Protozoa	
Trichomonas vaginalis	Trichomonal vaginitis, occasional urethritis
Entamoeba histolytica	Enteritis in homosexual men
Giardia lamblia	Enteritis in homosexual men
Fungi	
Candida albicans	Vaginitis, balanitis
Ectoparasites	
Phthirus pubis	Pubic lice infestation
Sarcoptes scabei	Scabies

*The relative importance of sexual transmission in the epidemiology of several of these agents remains to be defined; these include Group B streptococci, hepatitis A virus, cytomegalovirus, *Candida albicans*, and others.

in New York City showed that nearly 40 per cent had *E. histolytica*, *G. lamblia*, or both in their stool. It is not clear whether the apparent increase in STD in homosexual men is due to increased recognition and reporting of these diseases or to changing patterns of sexual behavior among certain groups of homosexual men. Homosexual women apparently do not have increased rates of STD.

INCIDENCE OF STDs. The true incidence of the STDs is not known in the United States because of serious problems of underreporting. Nevertheless, some estimates are available (Table 301–2). Gonorrhea is the most common of the reported infectious diseases in the United States, and infections by genital chlamydiae (which are not reportable at present) are probably of similar or greater magnitude. The relative incidence of STD is quite variable in different areas of the world. For instance, chancroid is presently quite uncommon in the United States, but is about as common as gonorrhea in certain areas of the Far East.

COMMON SYNDROMES. ***Urethritis in Males.*** Urethritis in males is a very common syndrome. It is ordinarily classified as either gonococcal or nongonococcal urethritis (NGU), depending on whether the presence of gonococci can be demonstrated by Gram stain or culture. In venereal disease clinics, the prevalence of gonococcal and nongonococcal urethritis is similar, but NGU is considerably more common in private practice and in college infirmaries. A recent study of asymptomatic sexually active military men found a 1 per cent prevalence of urethral gonorrhea but a 12 per cent prevalence of urethral chlamydial infection.

A large number of studies have established *Chlamydia trachomatis* as a cause of approximately 40 per cent of cases of NGU. Case-control studies have provided suggestive evidence that *Ureaplasma urealyticum* (formerly "T-strain" mycoplasma) is a significant factor in chlamydia-negative NGU. In addition, urethral inoculation of volunteers with pure cultures of *U. urealyticum* produced rather typical NGU. In practice, however, it is difficult to define the importance of *Ureaplasma* infection in patients with urethritis, because up to 50 per cent of asymptomatic sexually active persons are colonized by these organisms. A very small proportion of cases of male NGU is due to *Trichomonas vaginalis* or herpes simplex virus infection.

Diagnosis of urethritis requires demonstration of an inflammatory urethral exudate. A discharge may not be evident if the patient has recently voided, and patients preferably should be examined several hours after their last urination. The discharge may be present only in the morning, prior to urination. Demonstration of discharge often requires urethral "milking," and may require insertion of a small calcium-alginate or similar swab into the anterior urethra, with examination of a direct Gram-stained smear of the swab for leukocytes. Presence of an average of at least five polymorphonuclear leukocytes per high power (100×) field suggests the diagnosis of urethritis.

The patient should be questioned for past history of urethritis, and for symptoms suggestive of systemic diseases such as Reiter's syndrome or disseminated gonococcal infection. Examination should be made for signs of conjunctivitis, arthritis, dermatitis, and epididymitis. Prostatitis is rarely present unless there are symptoms of perineal, suprapubic, or rectal discomfort, and rectal examination is not routinely indicated. Rectal examination and urine culture are indicated in men with dysuria but without signs of anterior urethral discharge.

Laboratory studies are ordinarily limited to a Gram stain of urethral exudate. Demonstration of typical gram-negative diplococci, many of which are inside neutrophils, establishes the diagnosis of gonococcal urethritis. At least 90 per cent of men with symptomatic culture-proven urethral gonorrhea have a positive Gram stain. In occasional patients, especially those with equivocal Gram stain, it may be necessary to culture the anterior urethra or freshly voided urine sediment for gonococci. This is particularly important in asymptomatic male contacts of patients with disseminated gonococcal infection or gonococcal salpingitis, since Gram stain of urethral contents is positive in only about 60 per cent of men with asymptomatic urethral gonorrhea.

Diagnosis of NGU is made by exclusion of gonorrhea. Dem-

TABLE 301–2. INCIDENCE OF CERTAIN SEXUALLY TRANSMITTED DISEASES IN THE UNITED STATES, 1977*

Disease	Estimated Annual Incidence
Gonorrhea	2,000,000
Nongonococcal urethritis in men	1,000,000
Trichomoniasis	800,000
Condyloma acuminatum	300,000
Pelvic inflammatory disease	250,000
Genital herpes simplex virus	200,000
Pediculosis pubis	150,000
Syphilis (primary and secondary)	75,000

*Source: STD Fact Sheet, HEW Publication (CDC) 79–8195.

onstration of genital chlamydiae or ureaplasmas requires cultural methods that are not routinely available at present. Monoclonal antibodies recently were made available for diagnosis of chlamydiae in secretions; early results indicate a sensitivity of over 90 per cent compared with culture, with nearly 100 per cent specificity. There is no serologic test that is clinically useful to diagnose infection by either of these agents. Examination of a saline suspension of urethral exudate for motile trichomonads occasionally may be revealing in patients with recurrent urethritis who fail to respond to appropriate therapy. A serologic test for syphilis should be obtained, but the diagnostic yield is low.

Management is outlined in Figure 301–1 and is discussed further in Ch. 302. Sexual partners of men with gonococcal or nongonococcal urethritis should be treated both to prevent reinfection of the patient and to prevent development of complications in the partners.

The syndrome of *postgonococcal urethritis* (persistence or recrudescence of urethritis after administration of therapy that has eradicated gonococcal infection) is usually due to concomitant urethral chlamydial infection that was not eradicated by the original treatment. This syndrome is more common after therapy with intramuscular procaine penicillin or a single oral dose of ampicillin than after a five-day regimen of tetracycline, undoubtedly because of the greater efficacy of tetracycline for treating chlamydial infections. Accordingly, there is considerable merit to use of oral tetracycline for treatment of gonococcal urethritis, either as the sole therapy or to follow up penicillin or ampicillin therapy.

Genital Ulcer Syndrome. Genital skin lesions may be either ulcerative or nonulcerative. In patients seen in a venereal disease clinic, the most common sexually transmitted nonulcerative genital lesions are due to scabies, genital warts, molluscum contagiosum, or *Candida* species, but differential diagnosis includes a long list of dermatologic conditions.

The most common cause of ulcerative genital lesions in patients in the United States is herpes simplex virus, but differential diagnosis includes syphilis, chancroid, lymphogranuloma venereum (LGV), granuloma inguinale (GI), and trauma. Chancroid is uncommon in Western nations, and LGV and GI are rare. The most important distinction is between syphilis and genital herpes. Sometimes, the appearance is virtually diagnostic: grouped painful superficial vesicles are nearly diagnostic of herpes, whereas a single clean-based nonpainful ulcer with indurated margins suggests primary syphilis. In recent studies, only about 60 per cent of penile syphilitic chancres had this classic appearance. Painful ulcers suggest herpes, or possibly chancroid. Genital herpes may present as a single ulcer, particularly in patients with recurrent herpes, and syphilis may present with multiple ulcers. Secondarily infected lesions of primary syphilis may be painful.

It is a useful rule to obtain a serologic test for syphilis on all patients with genital ulcers, and, if the initial serology is negative and if the diagnosis remains uncertain, to obtain a second serology about two weeks later. A dark-field examination for syphilis should also be done, and it should be repeated twice on successive days if syphilis is seriously suspected and the initial examination is negative.

Infection by herpes simplex virus may be efficiently diagnosed by viral culture or by immunofluorescent methods, but these are frequently unavailable in practice. Papanicolaou smear is suggestive of herpes in about two thirds of culture-positive cases. Giemsa or Wright's stain of cells scraped from the base of a vesicle may reveal multinucleate giant cells (Tzanck test), but this test is particularly insensitive in herpetic lesions which have become ulcerated. Serologic tests for herpesvirus are not helpful. Referral of patients to centers with capability of viral culture may be indicated in diagnostically difficult patients.

In addition to herpesvirus infection, chancroid should be suspected in patients with painful genital ulcers. Chancroid is more likely if there has been recent sexual contact in Africa or the Far East. Attempts should be made to isolate the causative agent, *Hemophilus ducreyi;* selective culture media are an improvement over previously available methods. No serologic tests are available.

Therapy clearly depends on the correct diagnosis. Topical antibiotics are never indicated. Initial genital herpes (first infection) is best treated with topical or oral administration of acyclovir or intravenous administration for severe infections (see Ch. 28). Therapy of chancroid is with co-trimoxazole or erythromycin. Occasional empirical trials of oral co-trimoxazole or erythromycin are warranted in patients with persistent genital ulcers not readily attributable to herpesvirus or syphilis, but repeated attempts to isolate *H. ducreyi* should be made in such instances. It is not possible to arrive at an unequivocal diagnosis of the cause of genital ulcers in all patients.

Lower Genital Tract Infections in Women. Infections of the female genitourinary tract produce a variety of syndromes, often with overlapping symptoms (dysuria, vaginal discharge, vulvar irritation). These infections are very common, relatively poorly understood by most physicians, sometimes difficult to treat, and often frustrating for both doctor and patient. However, the various syndromes usually can be distinguished on relatively simple clinical and laboratory grounds, and a precise microbial etiology often can be established.

It is most helpful first to determine the primary anatomic site of infection: urethra or bladder, endocervix, or vagina. This can sometimes be accomplished by history; women with urinary tract infection (UTI) usually experience "internal" dysuria, whereas women with dysuria associated with vaginitis usually experience "external" dysuria owing to passage of urine over

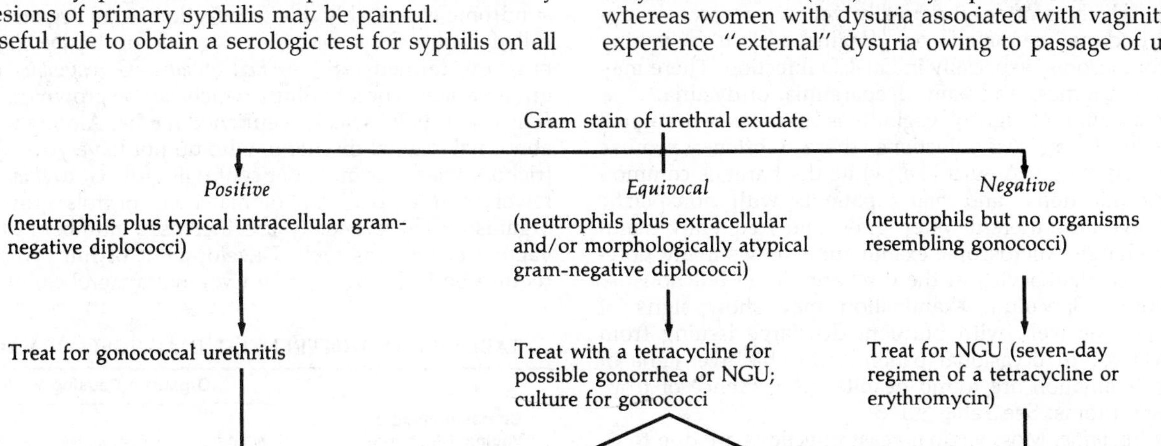

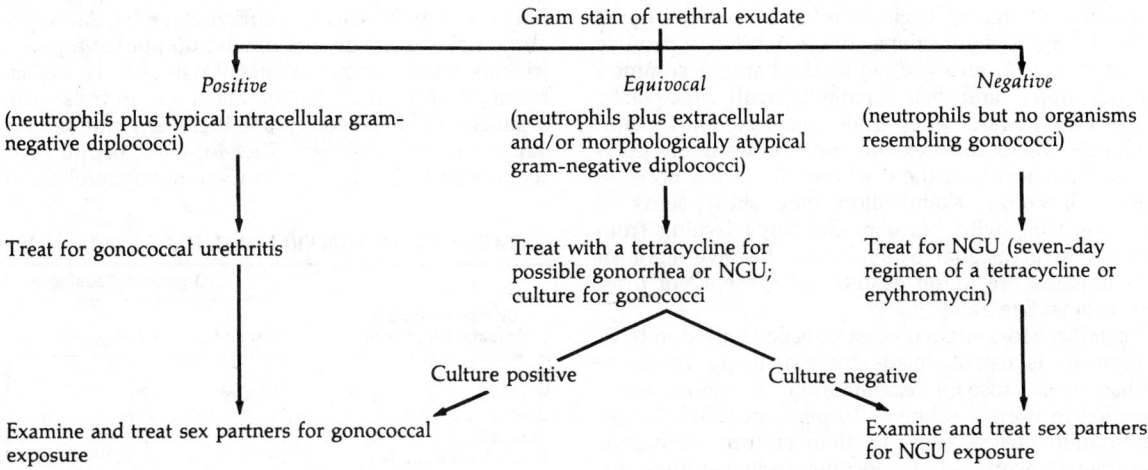

Figure 301–1. Management of male patients with urethritis.

inflamed labia. Cervicitis is diagnosed by physical examination; there are mucopurulent secretions emanating from the endocervical canal, and there is often a hypertrophic, mucoid, reddened "cobblestone" appearance to the cervical mucosa. Patients with cervicitis may also have urethritis or vaginitis. Vaginitis is associated with increased vaginal discharge of several types, as discussed below, and frequently there are associated signs and symptoms of vaginal, vulvar, and perineal irritation (dyspareunia, external dysuria, itching, pain). In patients with lower genitourinary infection, it is important to determine whether there is involvement of the upper genitourinary tract (pyelonephritis, salpingitis).

THE URETHRAL SYNDROME. Bacterial cystitis with or without pyelonephritis is usually diagnosed in women with dysuria, urinary frequency, and pyuria if they have colony counts of at least 10^5 bacteria per milliliter of urine. If similar symptoms are present but routine cultures grow less than 10^4 bacteria per milliliter of voided urine, the "urethral syndrome" is likely.

In a study of sexually active young women who presented to walk-in clinics with dysuria and urinary frequency, and who did not have vaginitis or active herpes simplex infection, 43 per cent had the urethral syndrome (urethritis). Among women with urethritis, 25 per cent had positive urethral cultures for *Chlamydia trachomatis.* Isolation of chlamydiae from the urethra was uncommon in women without urethritis. In other studies, gonococci also were shown to cause this syndrome. Thus, women as well as men may present with urethritis caused by gonococci and chlamydiae.

Management of patients with the urethral syndrome has not been carefully evaluated. Patients with symptoms of urinary tract infection who do not have bacteriuria should have urethral and cervical cultures for *N. gonorrhoeae.* If these cultures are also negative, a therapeutic trial may be made with a tetracycline or a sulfonamide for approximately seven days. There are no controlled trials of such therapy or of the management of sexual partners of women with the urethral syndrome.

VAGINITIS. In a large study of women in a primary care clinic who presented with lower genitourinary complaints, vaginitis was more than five times as common as urinary tract infections. In this and similar studies, there were three predominant types of vaginitis: yeast infection *(Candida albicans),* trichomonas *(T. vaginalis)* infection, and "nonspecific" vaginitis caused by organisms other than *Candida* and *T. vaginalis.* The incidence of these types of vaginitis varies in different patient populations, but in general *Candida* and nonspecific vaginitis are more common than *T. vaginalis* vaginitis.

Symptoms of vaginitis include increased volume of vaginal discharge, which is often abnormally yellow or green in appearance, and may be malodorous. Vaginal and vulvar itching may be troublesome, especially in *Candida* infection. There may be vaginal tenderness and pain, dyspareunia, or dysuria.

The most common sign of vaginitis is an increased vaginal discharge. In *T. vaginalis* infections, there is often a profuse and frothy discharge. A curd-like, white discharge is common in *Candida* infections, and many patients with nonspecific vaginitis have an adherent, often gray, and frequently malodorous discharge. Microscopic examination shows many polymorphonuclear leukocytes in the discharge in all but nonspecific vaginitis. Speculum examination may show signs of endocervicitis as well, with purulent discharge issuing from the cervical os. In occasional patients, no objective signs of vaginal inflammation are found despite the presence of troublesome symptoms. See Table 301–3.

Candida Vaginitis. Most vaginal yeast infections are due to *C. albicans.* Diagnosis is usually made by visualizing yeasts or pseudohyphae by microscopic examination of vaginal secretions suspended in normal saline or 10 per cent KOH. Microscopic examination is less sensitive than culture. However, many asymptomatic women have positive vaginal cultures for *C. albicans,* and therefore some authorities advocate using microscopy in preference to culture. The discharge in *Candida* vaginitis is not malodorous and has a pH of less than 4.5 when a drop is applied to pH paper with a range of 4.0 to 5.5.

Therapy of *Candida* vaginitis is with intravaginal nystatin twice daily for seven days, or with one of the imidazole compounds (clotrimazole or miconazole) once each night for seven days. Several studies suggest that therapy with the imidazoles is more effective than with nystatin. There is no convincing evidence that attempts to eradicate yeast from the gastrointestinal tract by administration of oral nystatin have a significant effect on rates of cure or relapse of *Candida* vaginitis. There is no evidence to warrant therapy of sexual partners. Attempts should be made to correct ancillary conditions which increase susceptibility to vaginal candidiasis: antibiotic therapy, diabetes, or oral anovulatory steroids. Relapse is a significant problem in some patients. No therapy is indicated for asymptomatic vaginal carriers of *C. albicans.*

T. Vaginale Vaginitis. Diagnosis is made ordinarily by visualizing motile trichomonads in a normal saline suspension of vaginal secretions. The organisms are easily seen at high-dry (100×) magnification, and may usually be seen under low power magnification. The saline suspension should be examined promptly. Culture is more sensitive, but about 80 to 90 per cent of culture-positive cases are detected by microscopy. Addition of a drop of 10 per cent KOH to vaginal secretions usually results in liberation of a detectable fish-like odor, attributed to release of volatile amines. The pH of vaginal secretions is usually greater than 5.0. In these latter two respects, *T. vaginale* vaginitis is similar to nonspecific vaginitis.

Therapy of trichomoniasis is with one of the nitroimidazoles, either metronidazole or newer compounds such as tinidazole. The latter is extensively used in Europe but is not approved in the United States. A single 2.0-gram oral dose of metronidazole is as effective as multiple-day regimens. Metronidazole is mutagenic, and there is evidence that it is a weak carcinogen in certain animal systems (but, so far, not in humans). Accordingly, it should be used with caution; it has been advocated for women with asymptomatic trichomoniasis, but others would reserve its use for women with symptomatic infections because of possible adverse effects. Metronidazole should not be used in the first trimester of pregnancy. Since over one third of male sexual partners of women with trichomoniasis are asymptomatic urethral carriers of *T. vaginale,* the male partners should also be treated with a single 2.0-gram dose of metronidazole.

Although *T. vaginale* can be transmitted sexually, it probably is transmitted by other means as well. This conclusion is based on prevalence studies which show one peak in young, sexually active women and a second peak in older women who have no other evidence for sexually transmitted infection.

Nonspecific Vaginosis. Recent work has confirmed that this syndrome is probably due to infection by an organism formerly called either *Corynebacterium vaginale* or *Hemophilus vaginalis,* but now termed *Gardnerella vaginalis. G. vaginalis* is a small, gram-variable coccobacillus, which can be grown quite successfully on partially selective enriched media. Among women with abnormal vaginal discharge who do not have yeast infection or trichomoniasis, over 90 per cent will grow *G. vaginalis,* whereas fewer than 10 per cent of matched controls grow the same organism. There usually are increased numbers of anaerobic vaginal bacteria as well. Development of full symptoms may require both *G. vaginalis* and vaginal anaerobes, although the

TABLE 301–3. DIFFERENTIAL DIAGNOSIS OF VAGINITIS

Characteristics of Vaginal Discharge	Organism Causing Vaginitis		
	C. albicans	*T. vaginalis*	*G. vaginalis*
pH	4.5	>5.0	>5.0
White curd	Usually	No	No
Odor with KOH	No	Yes	Yes
Clue cells	No	No	Usually
Motile trichomonads	No	Usually	No
Yeast cells	Yes	No	No

precise pathophysiology of this syndrome is still under investigation.

Diagnosis of nonspecific vaginosis is by exclusion of trichomoniasis, candidiasis, and purulent cervicitis. Abnormal cells termed "clue cells" are often seen in a wet mount of vaginal secretions in normal saline; these are stippled, granular-appearing vaginal epithelial cells that contain large numbers of adherent *G. vaginalis.* Few polymorphonuclear leukocytes are present. Addition of a drop of 10 per cent KOH usually results in production of an unpleasant fishy odor. The pH of the vaginal secretions is nearly always greater than 5.0.

Optimal therapy is being investigated. Some but not all studies show that oral ampicillin (500 mg four times daily for seven days) is effective. Metronidazole has only borderline activity in vitro against *G. vaginalis,* but in a dose of 500 mg by mouth twice daily for seven days it was effective in eradicating both *G. vaginalis* and the symptoms of vaginitis from 80 of 81 patients in one trial; similar results have been obtained in other trials. This suggests that the principal cause of this syndrome is an anaerobe, since metronidazole is principally effective against anaerobes. Interest is now focused on curved gram-negative anaerobic rods that are often found in women with nonspecific vaginosis. Oral tetracycline and topical vaginal creams containing sulfonamides are usually ineffective. Over 90 per cent of male partners are urethral carriers of *G. vaginalis,* and therefore probably should be treated with the same regimen as the patient.

Mixed Vaginitis. In 2 to 16 per cent of patients, vaginitis may be due to polymicrobial infection with two or three of the organisms *C. albicans, T. vaginalis,* or *G. vaginalis.* Such mixed infection may account for some instances of treatment failure. Particular care should be given to identification of all causative organisms in patients who have recurrent or relapsing vaginitis.

CERVICITIS. Two organisms are recognized as probable causes of mucopurulent endocervicitis: *N. gonorrhoeae* and *C. trachomatis.* Women who are sexual partners of men with chlamydia-positive NGU have a much higher rate of isolation of chlamydiae from the cervix than do women who are partners of men with chlamydia-negative NGU, and they also have significantly higher rates of mucopurulent cervicitis. Herpes simplex virus can also cause cervicitis, especially in primary infection. However, the clinical appearance in herpetic cervicitis is different, with cervical vesicles and ulcers rather than mucopurulent cervicitis.

True cervicitis should not be confused with cervical ectopy, which is merely the appearance of endocervical columnar epithelium on the exposed, visible exocervix. This results in a red-appearing cervix and may result in increased production of a mucoid vaginal discharge, but does not require therapy.

Diagnosis of mucopurulent endocervicitis requires visualization of purulent discharge from the cervical os. There often is a roughened "cobblestone" appearance to the cervix. Gram stain is about 60 per cent sensitive and over 90 per cent specific for gonorrhea if typical intracellular gonococci are seen, but cultures for *N. gonorrhoeae* should be taken. Tissue culture methods for isolation of *C. trachomatis* are not widely available. Cytology is not sufficiently sensitive to warrant widespread use. New monoclonal antibodies against *C. trachomatis* may allow rapid, sensitive, specific immunofluorescent diagnosis from patient secretions.

Antibiotic therapy appears to result in clinical improvement in mucopurulent cervicitis. Patients with negative cultures for the gonococcus probably should be treated with tetracycline or erythromycin in a dose of 500 mg four times daily for at least seven days; their sexual partners probably should be treated similarly. One should recognize that only modest data support these recommendations. No other form of cervicitis has been shown to respond to antimicrobial therapy.

Upper Genital Tract Disease in Women: Salpingitis. Full coverage of this important topic is precluded by space considerations. This is a very important clinical problem, resulting in considerable morbidity in the estimated 250,000 to 500,000 women who are affected yearly in the United States.

ETIOLOGY. The gonococcus may account for as much as 50 per cent of cases in the United States. About 15 to 20 per cent of women with gonococcal cervicitis probably subsequently develop salpingitis. Increasingly strong evidence now implicates genital chlamydial infections as another significant cause of salpingitis; in Sweden, more cases of salpingitis are due to *C. trachomatis* than to *N. gonorrhoeae.* There is less convincing evidence that *Mycoplasma hominis* may occasionally cause a similar syndrome. Many cases of salpingitis are caused by mixed infection with microaerophilic streptococci and enteric bacilli, often including *Bacteroides* species. These polymicrobial infections appear to be more common in recurrent attacks of salpingitis.

DIAGNOSIS. Clinical diagnosis of salpingitis is inexact. Perhaps only 20 per cent of patients have the classic syndrome of lower abdominal pain and tenderness, cervical tenderness, fever, leukocytosis, and elevated sedimentation rate. The most common findings are lower abdominal tenderness, which is usually bilateral, and adnexal and cervical tenderness. Patients with gonococcal salpingitis are more likely to present with fever, and more commonly have onset near the menses, whereas patients with nongonococcal salpingitis more commonly present with adnexal masses. Laparoscopy is commonly used to diagnose salpingitis in certain countries, but is invasive and requires general anesthesia. In the United States, laparoscopy is usually used only in selected patients whose differential diagnosis includes ectopic pregnancy, appendicitis, ruptured abscess, or other potential emergencies.

COMPLICATIONS. Complications are primarily infertility and ectopic pregnancies. Rates of involuntary infertility are about 15 per cent after one attack of salpingitis and about 75 per cent after three or more attacks. Total hysterectomy may eventually be necessitated by symptoms of chronic salpingitis.

THERAPY. A controlled trial of outpatient therapy showed that ten-day regimens of either oral tetracycline or ampicillin were equally effective in both gonococcal and nongonococcal salpingitis. Recent recommendations from the Centers for Disease Control suggest initial therapy with cefoxitin 2.0 grams intramuscularly, or ampicillin 3.5 grams orally, or aqueous procaine penicillin G 4.8 mU intramuscularly, each along with probenecid 1.0 gram orally, followed by doxycycline 100 mg orally twice daily for 10 to 14 days. There are no controlled data on efficacy of various regimens used for hospitalized patients. Current recommendations call for doxycycline 100 mg intravenously twice daily plus cefoxitin 2.0 grams intravenously four times daily; or clindamycin 600 mg intravenously four times daily plus gentamicin or tobramycin 1.5 mg per kilogram intravenously three times daily; or doxycycline 100 mg intravenously twice daily plus metronidazole 1.0 gram intravenously twice daily in patients with normal renal function. Patients should usually be hospitalized if they are very ill, are pregnant, have significant adnexal masses, or have failed previous therapy, or if the differential diagnosis includes surgical emergencies such as appendicitis or ectopic pregnancy.

PREVENTION. Sexual partners of women with gonococcal salpingitis must be identified, examined, and treated to prevent subsequent reinfection of the patient. About one half of the infected male partners of women with gonococcal salpingitis are asymptomatic. Treatment of women with tetracycline (as compared with penicillin) to eradicate chlamydiae from the cervix reduced the incidence of posttherapy salpingitis in one recent study (Rees, 1980), which suggests that increased emphasis on treatment of chlamydiae in the male and female genital tract might reduce the incidence of salpingitis.

Baldson MJ, Pead L, Taylor GE, Maskell R: *Corynebacterium vaginale* and vaginitis: A controlled trial of treatment. Lancet 1:501, 1980. *A randomized trial of the therapy of nonspecific vaginitis. Tetracycline was ineffective, but metronidazole was effective.*

Bowie WR, Wang S-P, Alexander ER, Floyd J, Forsyth PS, Pollock HM, Lin J-SL, Buchanan TM, Holmes KK: Etiology of nongonococcal urethritis: Evidence for *Chlamydia trachomatis* and *Ureaplasma urealyticum*. J Clin Invest 59:735, 1977. *An excellent epidemiologic and clinical study of the etiology and therapy of nongonococcal urethritis in males.*

Centers for Disease Control: Sexually transmitted diseases treatment guidelines 1982. Morbid Mortal Wkly Rep (Suppl) 31(2S):33S, 1982. *The current United States Public Health Service treatment guidelines for all STDs.*

Chapel TA, Brown WJ, Jeffries C, Stewart JA: How reliable is the morphologic diagnosis of penile ulcerations? Sex Trans Dis 4:150, 1977. *Difficulties in clinical distinction among lesions caused by* T. pallidum, *herpesvirus hominis,* and Hemophilus ducreyi *are clearly elucidated.*

Cunningham FG, Hauth JC, Strong JD, Herbert WNP, Gilstrap LC, Wilson RH, Kappus SS: Evaluation of tetracycline or penicillin and ampicillin for treatment of acute pelvic inflammatory disease. N Engl J Med 296:1380, 1977. *The best available study of antibiotic therapy of mild to moderate pelvic inflammatory disease.*

Jacobs NF Jr, Kraus SJ: Gonococcal and nongonococcal urethritis in men: Clinical and laboratory differentiation. Ann Intern Med 82:7, 1975. *A study of clinical and laboratory features which allow distinction between gonococcal and nongonococcal urethritis.*

Mårdh P-A, Møller BR, Paavonen J: Chlamydial infection of the female genital tract with emphasis on pelvic inflammatory disease. A review of Scandinavian studies. Sex Transm Dis 8 (Suppl):140, 1981. *Review of the role of chlamydiae in pelvic inflammatory disease.*

McCue JD, Komaroff AL, Pass TM, Cohen AB, Friedland G: Strategies for diagnosing vaginitis. J Family Pract 9:395, 1979. *A study in a primary care clinic of simple methods for diagnosing the etiology of genitourinary symptoms in women.*

Pheifer TA, Forsyth PS, Durfee MA, Pollock HM, Holmes KK: Nonspecific vaginitis: Role of *Haemophilus vaginalis* and treatment with metronidazole. N Engl J Med 298:1429, 1978. *A clinical and therapeutic study of nonspecific vaginitis, showing that both* G. vaginalis *and vaginal anaerobes are probably important in causation of the syndrome, and also that metronidazole is effective therapy.*

Rees E: The treatment of pelvic inflammatory disease. Am J Obstet Gynecol 138:1042, 1980. *Treatment of women with chlamydial infection of the cervix with tetracycline as compared with penicillin reduced the incidence of subsequent salpingitis.*

Sohn N, Robilotti JG Jr: The gay bowel syndrome: A review of colonic and rectal conditions in 200 male homosexuals. Am J Gastroenterol 67:478, 1977. *A brief clinical review of the numerous kinds of venereal infections acquired by male homosexuals.*

Stamm WE, Koutsky LA, Benedetti JK, Jourden JL, Brunham RC, Holmes KK: *Chlamydia trachomatis* urethral infections in men: Prevalence, risk factors, and clinical manifestations. Ann Intern Med 100:47, 1984. *Asymptomatic male urethral carriers of chlamydiae are very common.*

Stamm WE, Wagner KF, Amsel R, Alexander ER, Turck M, Counts GW, Holmes KK: Causes of the acute urethral syndrome in women. N Engl J Med 303:409, 1980. *Females may also develop a form of nongonococcal urethritis resulting from infection with* Chlamydia trachomatis.

Tait IA, Rees E, Hobson D, Byng RE, Tweedie MCK: Chlamydial infection of the cervix in contacts of men with nongonococcal urethritis. Br J Vener Dis 56:37, 1980. Chlamydia trachomatis *is shown to cause mucopurulent cervicitis, and appropriate antibiotic therapy to result in clinical improvement.*

Taylor-Robinson D, Csonka GW, Prentice MJ: Human intraurethral inoculation of ureaplasmas. Q J Med 46:309, 1977. *Inoculation of the investigator's urethra with ureaplasmas resulted in nonspecific urethritis.*

302. GONOCOCCAL INFECTIONS

INTRODUCTION. *Neisseria gonorrhoeae* is a common sexually transmitted organism which causes anterior urethritis in males and endocervicitis and urethritis in females. Other types of primary infection include pharyngitis, proctitis, conjunctivitis, and vulvovaginitis; the last-named disorder occurs principally in prepubescent females. Complications may occur by direct extension of infection, including epididymitis, prostatitis, Bartholin gland abscess, salpingitis, and perihepatitis. Bacteremia may occur, with production of characteristic cutaneous lesions, arthritis, and tenosynovitis; rare complications include endocarditis and meningitis. Conjunctival infection formerly was a common cause of blindness in neonates.

Gonorrhea is the most common reportable infectious disease in the United States, with about 1 million reported cases annually. The true incidence is probably at least 2 million cases annually.

EPIDEMIOLOGY. The only natural hosts for *N. gonorrhoeae* are humans. The organism normally resides on the columnar epithelium of mucosal surfaces and is usually transmitted by intimate sexual contact.

The prevalence of gonorrhea varies greatly in different groups. As many as 5 per cent of persons in high-risk populations may be infected at any time. Surveys of private practices in the United States in the 1970's showed that about 2 per cent of sexually active young women had positive endocervical cultures for the gonococcus. Highest prevalence was found in young (15 to 30) single persons of low socioeconomic and educational status, probably because these factors correlate positively with sexual promiscuity.

The risk of acquiring infection depends on the type of contact with an infected person. About 60 to 80 per cent of females in contact with a male with urethral gonorrhea will develop gonococcal cervicitis. In contrast, it is estimated that only 20 to 30 per cent of males having sex with an infected female will develop gonorrhea. This difference may be due to exposure of females to a larger inoculum of gonococci. A person having oral sex with a male with gonococcal urethritis has considerable risk of acquiring pharyngeal gonorrhea. Transmission of infection by oral contact with the genitals of an infected female is rare. Infection is apparently efficiently spread by penile-rectal contact.

Gonococci die rapidly upon drying, and transmission by fomites is rare. Epidemics were reported in prepubertal females living in close proximity in orphanages, but such episodes are now very uncommon.

Control of gonorrhea is difficult because of the frequency of asymptomatic infection. Perhaps 50 per cent of infections in females are asymptomatic or only minimally symptomatic, and at least 10 per cent of infected males are asymptomatic.

In past years there was considerable emphasis on case finding by endocervical culture of young, sexually active females. The merit of this strategy depends on the prevalence of infection in the community and the life style of the patient. A more cost-effective method for finding infected patients is to culture patients about six weeks after treatment for gonorrhea; as many as 15 to 20 per cent of such persons will be culture positive, usually because of reinfection.

THE ORGANISM. *N. gonorrhoeae* is a gram-negative, aerobic diplococcus. Many strains require 3 to 10 per cent CO_2 for optimal growth. They are highly autolytic and die rapidly when outside their normal human environment. They are sensitive to fatty acids and grow best on media with added starch to inhibit fatty acids present in agar. Iron required for growth is usually provided by addition of hemoglobin (chocolate agar). Several partially selective media are available; most employ antibiotics such as trimethoprim, vancomycin, colistin, and nystatin to inhibit growth of other microorganisms. Replacement of vancomycin with lincomycin seems to improve the rate of isolation of gonococci.

Presumptive identification in vitro is made by colonial morphology, Gram stain, and a positive oxidase test. Differentiation from the closely related meningococcus and the various nonpathogenic *Neisseria* is ordinarily by patterns of utilization of various simple carbohydrates; gonococci use glucose but not maltose or sucrose.

Gonococci are highly variable and occur in a number of different colonial forms. Small colonial types are piliated and more virulent in humans than the larger, nonpiliated variants. Variation is also found in certain outer membrane proteins which affect colony opacity. Opaque colonies may attach to certain mucosal surfaces better than transparent colonies, whereas transparent colonies are more likely to invade and cause salpingitis or bacteremia and arthritis. All gonococci and meningococci are able to use transferrin as a source of iron, whereas nonpathogenic *Neisseria* organisms are rarely able to do so. The importance of other surface components of the gonococcus in pathogenesis of infection is under intense investigation. A surface capsule has been reported, but its composition and biologic importance, if any, are unknown.

Gonococci can be serotyped on the basis of antigenic differences in pili, outer membrane proteins, and other antigens. They also can be reliably biotyped by definition of their nutritional requirements on defined agar media ("auxotypes"). These tests are not routinely available at present.

PATHOGENESIS. The minimal infective dose of gonococci for establishment of urethritis in male volunteers is between 100 and 1000 colony-forming units. Surface pili undoubtedly help to attach the bacteria to the mucosal surface, and they also help prevent ingestion and killing by polymorphonuclear leukocytes. Typical urethral infections result in a moderately severe inflammatory response, which is probably due to release of toxic lipopolysaccharide from gonococci, and possibly to production of chemotactic factors which attract neutrophilic leukocytes. Certain strains, particularly those requiring arginine, hypoxanthine, and uracil for growth (Arg^- Hyx^- Ura^- auxotype) are likely to cause asymptomatic urethral infection for reasons not completely understood. These strains are usually penicillin sensitive, resistant to the bactericidal effects of normal human serum, and particularly likely to cause bacteremia and septic arthritis.

In the preantibiotic era, symptoms usually persisted for two to three months before host defenses finally succeeded in eradicating the infection. Host defenses include serum opsonic and bactericidal antibodies, as well as local (mucosal) antibodies of the IgG and IgA classes. All gonococci produce an enzyme, IgA protease, which cleaves the major class of secretory IgA, perhaps accounting in part for persistence of local gonococcal infections.

Serum bactericidal antibodies are undoubtedly important in prevention of bacteremic infection. The best evidence for this has been provided by patients who suffer from homozygous deficiency of one of the complement components C6, C7, or C8. This results in deficiency of serum bactericidal activity but no alteration of serum opsonic activity. Such individuals are particularly prone to recurrent bacteremic gonococcal infection, or to recurrent meningococcal meningitis or meningococcemia.

CLINICAL PATTERNS OF DISEASE. ***Gonorrhea in Males.*** Gonococcal urethritis in males ("the clap," or "the strain") is characterized by a yellowish purulent urethral discharge and dysuria. The usual incubation period is two to six days. The discharge of gonorrhea is slightly more copious and purulent than in nongonococcal urethritis (NGU). Symptoms are probably produced by 90 per cent of infections, although asymptomatic infections do occur and may persist for many months. Males with asymptomatic infection do not seek treatment, whereas those with symptomatic infection are usually promptly treated and cured. This is the probable explanation for prevalence studies which show that up to 50 per cent of infected males are asymptomatic. Asymptomatic infection in males and females is of great epidemiologic importance, since such carriers may continue to spread infection to new sexual partners for months if they are not properly diagnosed and treated.

Complications of gonococcal urethritis in males are now rare. Urethral stricture was formerly a common complication, but was probably due in part to the use of caustic treatment regimens. Epididymitis and prostatitis, relatively common complications in the past, are seen only occasionally today. The principal complication is disseminated gonococcal infection, which is estimated to affect about 1 per cent of men with gonorrhea. This entity is discussed below.

The differential diagnosis of gonococcal urethritis is discussed in Ch. 301.

Gonococcal infections of the pharynx and rectum are common problems in homosexual males. Most patients with pharyngeal infection are asymptomatic, but occasional patients have exudative pharyngitis with cervical adenopathy. Gonococcal infection of the rectum causes a wide spectrum of symptoms, ranging from asymptomatic carriers to severe proctitis with tenesmus and bloody mucopurulent discharge. Although approximately 40 per cent of females with cervical gonorrhea also have positive rectal cultures, symptoms of proctitis in females are unusual. This has suggested that the trauma of rectal intercourse may contribute to the proctitis observed in males. Sigmoidoscopy may be indicated to exclude ulcerative colitis, Crohn's colitis, rectal lacerations, or other infections such as shigellosis, amebiasis, or syphilis, all of which are common in male homosexuals.

Gonococcal epididymitis is usually unilateral. Both *Chlamydia trachomatis* and the gonococcus are significant causes of epididymitis in men under 35 years, whereas coliform bacteria are the usual cause in older males. The differential diagnosis includes trauma, tumor, and torsion of the testicle, the last of which is suggested by sudden onset and elevation of the testicle. If there is question of testicular torsion, consultation with a urologist is necessary. In epididymitis there is often a urethral exudate, which should be cultured for gonococci and other bacteria. Treatment of gonococcal epididymitis includes scrotal elevation and seven to ten days of appropriate antibiotics, as indicated in Table 302–1.

Gonorrhea in Females. In prevalence studies, approximately one half of women infected with the gonococcus are asymptomatic or have so few symptoms that they do not seek medical care. The most commonly involved site is the endocervix (80 to 90 per cent), followed by the urethra (80 per cent), rectum (40 per cent), and pharynx (10 to 20 per cent). Most pharyngeal, urethral, and rectal infections cause few or no symptoms. Cervical infection may result in vaginal discharge or abnormal menstrual bleeding. Neither of these symptoms is specific for gonococcal infection. Gonococcal urethritis may mimic cystitis caused by enteric bacilli, although standard urine cultures are negative because gonococci do not grow on culture media ordinarily used to diagnose urinary tract infection. Gonorrhea should be suspected in sexually active young women with urethral symptoms. A pelvic examination should be done, and cultures should be taken for the gonococcus from the endocervix and from the urethra if symptoms of urethritis are present. Culture methods are discussed below under Laboratory Diagnosis. The differential diagnosis of cervicitis, vaginitis, and the urethral syndrome is discussed in Ch. 301.

The most important complication of gonorrhea is salpingitis. The less precise term "pelvic inflammatory disease" (PID) is often used synonymously. Although many other organisms can cause a similar syndrome, the gonococcus accounts for about half of the estimated 500,000 annual cases of PID in the United States. About 15 per cent of women with gonococcal cervicitis develop PID, often in close proximity to a menstrual period. Symptoms usually include abdominal pain, and often there is fever. Physical examination usually discloses cervical motion tenderness and bilateral adnexal tenderness; in a small proportion of cases the disease may be unilateral, causing confusion with appendicitis or ectopic pregnancy. There may be signs of generalized peritonitis. Laboratory studies often show an elevation of the white blood cell count and sedimentation rate. The diagnosis of PID is inexact, as shown by laparoscopic examination; many patients with PID will be missed if undue reliance is placed on presence of fever or elevation of white blood cell count or sedimentation rate.

Although PID is uncommon in pregnancy, it may be particularly severe, and pregnant patients with PID should probably be hospitalized. The incidence of gonococcal PID is increased about three-fold in women using an intrauterine device (IUD) for contraception.

A single attack of gonococcal PID seems to increase two-fold the risk of developing another bout of PID with subsequent gonococcal cervicitis. About half of the male sexual partners of women with gonococcal PID are infected, and half of these infections are asymptomatic. Failure to diagnose and treat properly the male partners exposes the patient to the risk of further attacks of PID. After the patient has been effectively treated, it often is wise to refer her and her sexual partners to a public health clinic for follow-up.

The major complication of gonococcal PID is tubal scarring and infertility. The incidence of involuntary infertility is estimated as 15 per cent after one attack of PID and about 50 per cent after three attacks. The incidence of ectopic pregnancy is increased from seven- to ten-fold in women with previous salpingitis, with resultant increased fetal and maternal mortality. Treatment is indicated in Table 302–1.

Gonococci may spread upward to the liver, causing perihepatitis (Fitz-Hugh–Curtis syndrome). Gonococcal perihepatitis causes tenderness and pain in the region of the liver which mimics acute cholecystitis. However, it resolves promptly with appropriate antibiotic therapy. Peritoneoscopy may be indicated rarely for diagnostic purposes; "violin-string" adhesions between the liver capsule and the peritoneum are seen.

Gonorrhea in Children. Infants born to a mother with cervicovaginal gonorrhea may develop gonococcal conjunctivitis, although routine use of prophylactic 1 per cent silver nitrate eye drops (or, in some hospitals, topical erythromycin or tetracycline) has markedly reduced the incidence of this problem. Neonates may also acquire pharyngeal, respiratory, or rectal infection, and may develop gonococcal sepsis. Older children up to one year of age usually acquire conjunctival or vaginal infection by accidental contamination from an adult, whereas from one year to puberty most childhood gonorrhea is the result of purposeful sexual abuse by an adult.

TABLE 302–1. ANTIBIOTIC REGIMENS RECOMMENDED FOR GONOCOCCAL INFECTIONS

Diagnosis	Treatment
Uncomplicated genital infection, men and women	Aqueous procaine penicillin G (APPG), 4.8 million units IM in two divided doses, plus 1.0 gram of probenecid PO *or* Tetracycline, 0.5 gram PO four times daily for seven days *or* Ampicillin, 3.5 grams (or amoxicillin, 3.0 grams), in a single PO dose, plus 1.0 gram of probenecid PO *or* Spectinomycin, 2.0 grams IM
Anorectal infections in men	APPG, 4.8 million units IM, plus 1.0 gram of probenecid PO *or* Spectinomycin, 2.0 grams IM
Pharyngeal infection	APPG, 4.8 million units IM, plus 1.0 gram of probenecid PO *or* Tetracycline, 0.5 gram PO four times daily for seven days
Treatment failure (patients should be recultured and isolates tested for production of β-lactamase)	Spectinomycin, 2.0 grams IM
Penicillinase-producing *N. gonorrhoeae* or infection acquired in Africa or the Far East where PPNG are common	Spectinomycin, 2.0 grams IM *or* Ceftriaxone, 125 mg IM
Gonorrhea in pregnancy	APPG, 4.8 million units IM, plus 1.0 gram of probenecid *or* Spectinomycin, 2.0 grams IM
Salpingitis—outpatient	APPG, 4.8 million units IM, plus 1.0 gram of probenecid, or cefoxitin, 2.0 grams IM, followed by doxycycline, 100 mg PO two times daily for ten days *or* Doxycycline, 100 mg PO two times daily for ten days
Salpingitis—inpatient	Doxycycline, 100 mg IV twice daily plus cefoxitin, 2.0 grams IV four times daily until improved, followed by doxycycline, 100 mg PO twice daily to complete 14 days of therapy; alternative regimens include clindamycin plus an aminoglycoside, cefoxitin, or doxycycline, 100 mg IV twice daily plus metronidazole, 1.0 gram IV twice daily until improved, followed by same drugs, same dose PO to complete 14 days of therapy
Disseminated gonococcal infection	Penicillin G, 10 million units IV daily until improvement, followed by ampicillin, 0.5 gram PO four times daily to complete a minimum of seven days of therapy *or* Ampicillin, 3.5 grams PO, plus 1.0 gram of probenecid, followed by ampicillin, 0.5 gram PO four times daily for seven days *or* Tetracycline, 0.5 gram PO four times daily for seven days

Gonococcal Bacteremia. Approximately 1 per cent of adults with gonorrhea develop the syndrome of gonococcal bacteremia, dermatitis, and arthritis, or disseminated gonococcal infection (DGI). In most series, the majority of patients with DGI are women. The regional incidence of DGI probably varies because of geographic differences in prevalence of the antibiotic-sensitive, serum-bactericidal–resistant strains of *N. gonorrhoeae* which cause this syndrome. The severity of the syndrome is variable, from a slowly evolving mild illness with little or no fever, mild arthralgias, and few skin lesions to a fulminant illness with high fever and prostration. Most episodes of DGI are relatively mild in comparison with meningococcemia.

Many patients with DGI have no local symptoms of gonococcal infection. Initial manifestations are usually migratory asymmetrical polyarthralgias and skin lesions which are often accompanied by fever. Many patients have tenosynovitis, typically involving the flexor tendon sheaths of the wrist or the Achilles tendon (colloquially known as "lover's heels"). Skin lesions are few in number (less than 30 usually), are acral in distribution (fingers, toes, extremities), and may be painful before they are visible. The individual lesions may be papules, pustules, or bullae on an erythematous base; less commonly seen are petechiae or necrotic lesions. The rash is not pathognomonic, but is sufficiently typical that it should strongly suggest DGI when seen in young patients with polyarthralgias. Blood cultures are often positive at this stage, and circulating immune complexes may be present. Gram stain of the skin lesions is positive in only about 5 per cent of patients, but gonococcal antigens can be detected in these lesions in about two thirds of patients by use of immunofluorescent-labeled antigonococcal antibody.

The early stage of gonococcemia may subside spontaneously, or may merge indistinctly after about one week into a second stage of septic arthritis. Skin lesions have usually disappeared by this time, and blood cultures are nearly always negative. Septic arthritis may occur without preceding skin lesions or polyarthralgia. One large joint (elbow, wrist, hip, knee, ankle) is usually involved, although some series report involvement of two joints in a significant minority of patients. On infrequent occasions symmetrical involvement of the fingers may mimic acute rheumatoid arthritis. Physical examination typically discloses a swollen, warm joint with evident intra-articular fluid. Aspiration of the joint often reveals a marked neutrophilic leukocytosis (50,000 to 100,000 leukocytes per cubic millimeter), although early in the development of the septic joint the synovial leukocyte count may be much lower. Cultures of joint fluid are usually positive if the leukocyte count is 80,000 or greater, but are often negative when leukocyte counts are 20,000 or less.

Other complications of gonococcal bacteremia include mild hepatitis, myocarditis, the Fitz-Hugh–Curtis syndrome, meningitis, and endocarditis. In the preantibiotic era gonococcal infection accounted for up to 10 percent of all endocarditis, but it is now rare. Gonococcal endocarditis is often a rapidly progressive infection with severe valvular damage; it should be suspected in patients with a new murmur, severe prostrating illness, severe myocarditis, or evidence of renal failure, or in the presence of stigmata of peripheral embolization.

The differential diagnosis of the gonococcal bacteremia arthritis syndrome includes Reiter's syndrome, rheumatic fever, rheumatoid arthritis, systemic lupus erythematosus, other infectious or postinfectious arthritis, subacute bacterial endocarditis, meningococcemia, and viral hepatitis. In young males,

Reiter's syndrome is the principal consideration. Conjunctivitis is rarely seen in gonococcemia, but is common in Reiter's syndrome. In the absence of typical skin lesions, DGI may not be suspected until culture results are known.

Diagnosis of DGI is secure when gonococci are recovered from the blood, skin lesions, or synovial fluid. The diagnosis of DGI is probably correct in patients in whom the only positive cultures are from local mucosal surfaces, but in whom there are both typical skin lesions and a prompt response to antigonococcal therapy.

LABORATORY DIAGNOSIS. Gram's stain of urethral exudate in symptomatic males has a sensitivity of 90 to 98 per cent and a specificity of 95 to 98 per cent. Accordingly, urethral cultures are not ordinarily indicated in untreated symptomatic males. Since the sensitivity of the Gram stain is only about 60 per cent in asymptomatic male urethral infection, cultures of the anterior urethra or fresh urine sediment are recommended when epidemiologic evidence suggests possible asymptomatic urethral infection. Gram stain of the endocervix is about 50 to 60 per cent sensitive and about 82 to 97 per cent specific in women with positive cervical cultures for *N. gonorrhoeae.* Care must be taken to avoid mistaking normal endocervical flora and neutrophils for gonorrhea; only smears showing several neutrophils with multiple, typical intracellular gram-negative diplococci should be read as presumptively positive for gonorrhea. All women should be cultured for *N. gonorrhoeae,* even if the Gram stain appears positive.

Cultures should be plated immediately if possible onto chocolate agar or chocolate agar containing selective antibiotics (e.g., modified Thayer-Martin medium, MTM). Holding medium such as Amies' or Stuart's transport media may be used if necessary, but viability of gonococci drops after 12 to 24 hours in such media. In infected women, a single endocervical culture on MTM is about 80 to 90 per cent sensitive, as judged by yields obtained with multiple cultures from multiple sites. About 3 to 5 per cent of women will have their only positive culture at the pharyngeal, urethral, or rectal site. The yield from these sites is too low to warrant routine pharyngeal, urethral, or rectal cultures. Urethral cultures are indicated in women with the urethral syndrome. Both cervical and rectal cultures should be obtained as part of the test of cure in women after treatment, since inclusion of the rectal culture increases the diagnostic yield of treatment failures by as much as 50 per cent. Pharyngeal cultures should be obtained from patients with symptomatic pharyngitis, or from persons exposed by fellatio to infected males. Patients with possible disseminated gonococcal infection should have culture samples taken from all possible mucosal sites (pharynx, urethra, cervix, rectum), as well as blood and synovial fluid.

Cultures of the cervix should be taken under direct visualization during speculum examination, using a cotton-tipped swab. Lubricant jellies may be deleterious to gonococci and should be avoided. Cultures of tampons can be used if speculum examination is not possible. Cultures of the anterior urethra of males should be taken with calcium alginate swabs or a sterile wire loop.

Positive cultures from the pharynx or rectum should be carefully evaluated by the microbiology laboratory to avoid confusion between gonococci and meningococci. Meningococci are more common than gonococci in throat cultures. Male homosexuals apparently transmit meningococci sexually, and positive rectal cultures for meningococci are relatively common in this group.

A variety of inexpensive office kits is available for culturing gonococci. These offer the advantages of media with long shelf life. They are approximately equal to standard cultures when their use is limited to urethral or cervical samples; the presently available systems should not be used for pharyngeal or rectal cultures.

A variety of serologic tests for gonorrhea has been developed in the past, and more are being tested currently. No test available in 1984 is sufficiently sensitive and specific to merit use for screening purposes. Patients with complications of gonorrhea usually have detectable serum antibodies against crude or purified gonococcal antigens, but none of the tests is routinely available at present.

TREATMENT. Gonococci frequently have chromosomal mutations which result in relative resistance to penicillin, tetracycline, and other antibiotics. The resistance in these strains is usually low level and can be overcome by appropriate doses of penicillin or tetracycline.

Gonococci which carry a β-lactamase (penicillinase) plasmid recently emerged in the Far East and elsewhere, and have spread to much of the world. Penicillinase-producing gonococci (PPNG) account for about 30 per cent of all gonorrhea in certain cities in the Philippines, but are quite uncommon (less than 0.5 per cent) in the United States. The prevalence of PPNG is only about 1 per cent in northern Europe, but seems to be rising. There are two closely related gonococcal penicillinase plasmids of either 3.2 or 4.4×10^6 daltons; each encodes a typical enteric-type TEM β-lactamase. The gonococcal plasmids are similar to penicillinase plasmids found in *Hemophilus* species. PPNG are resistant to clinically attainable doses of penicillins, but are sensitive to spectinomycin, and to certain cephalosporins (cefuroxime, cefoxitin, ceftriaxone*). PPNG are known to cause DGI and salpingitis.

The antibiotic regimens recommended for gonorrhea in the United States are summarized in Table 302–1. Because gonococcal infections commonly are associated with genital chlamydial infection, most authorities now recommend a seven-day course of a tetracycline for all patients with gonorrhea, either as sole therapy or as follow-up to initial penicillin or ampicillin therapy.

Although the risk of anaphylaxis after penicillin is low (0.05 per cent if there is no history of penicillin allergy), up to 1 per cent of patients treated with 4.8 million units of procaine penicillin develop an acute neurotoxic syndrome caused by inadvertent intravenous administration of procaine, and up to 5 to 15 per cent develop rash caused by penicillin. The procaine penicillin regimen has the advantages of proven efficacy for incubating syphilis, and single-dose administration. The latter is of considerable theoretical advantage because of potential patient noncompliance with multidose oral regimens. The seven-day oral tetracycline regimen has little toxicity, but its principal merit is concomitant treatment of coexistent genital chlamydial or ureaplasmal infections. In men, this clearly results in reduced incidence of postgonococcal urethritis, which is usually due to chlamydial infection. Recent evidence suggests that generalized use of tetracyclines for gonorrhea in women would result in clinically significant benefits owing to simultaneous treatment of coexistent chlamydial infection.

In pharyngeal gonorrhea, the single-dose ampicillin and spectinomycin regimens result in about 50 per cent treatment failures. Consideration should be given to use of a pretreatment pharyngeal culture in patients treated with either of these regimens.

Each of the recommended regimens is highly effective for genital gonorrhea. If patients fail to respond to therapy, they should be cultured so that their isolates can be tested for production of penicillinase, and spectinomycin should be used for retreatment. However, most apparent failures are really reinfections. Some studies show that 15 per cent of patients are reinfected within six weeks of successful therapy. On this basis, many authorities recommend that patients should be recultured six weeks after treatment.

In the absence of an effective vaccine, control of this disease depends on proper diagnosis and treatment of patients' sexual contacts. If patients are given simple instructions, many will bring their contacts to the physician for examination. There are sound epidemiologic reasons for treating contacts immediately.

---

*Investigational drug.

Local health departments are not utilized sufficiently for help in examination and treatment of contacts.

Treatment of salpingitis (PID) has not been studied adequately. Two studies comparing ten-day oral ampicillin and tetracycline regimens found that they were equally effective in gonococcal and nongonococcal PID. Little is known about the relative merits of various regimens for hospitalized patients. Most authorities recommend removal of intrauterine devices in women with PID. It is crucial to examine and treat all sexual partners of women with gonococcal PID.

Therapy of gonococcal arthritis is ordinarily highly successful with each of the recommended regimens (Table 302–1). Failure to improve in three days suggests that the patient does not have DGI. Septic joints should be aspirated, both to make the initial diagnosis and to remove inflammatory exudate. Open drainage is rarely indicated, except in infection of the hip in childhood. Repeat closed aspiration may be necessary if joint fluid rapidly reaccumulates, but most patients require only one or a few joint aspirations. Antibiotics should not be injected into the joint space. Most patients with DGI should be hospitalized initially, but outpatient therapy may be used occasionally in carefully selected, compliant patients with a definite diagnosis and only mild infection.

Gonococcal conjunctivitis should be treated by immediate saline irrigation and intravenous penicillin G.

PREVENTION. Although vaccines are presently under intense study, an effective gonococcal vaccine is still only a hope. Condoms will prevent most infection, but those who need them most will often not use them. Certain contraceptive foams have antigonococcal activity but are of unproven efficacy clinically. Prophylaxis with a single dose of a tetracycline antibiotic was partially protective in a recent study, but failed in patients exposed to relatively resistant strains and therefore cannot be recommended. Prophylaxis with a five-day course of oral tetracycline has not been studied, but is undoubtedly effective and may be used in selected patients.

Barlow D, Phillips I: Gonorrhoea in women: Diagnostic, clinical, and laboratory aspects. Lancet 1:761, 1978. *A concise description of the clinical and laboratory findings in a large group of women.*

Brinton CC Jr, Wood SW, Brown A, Labik AM, Bryan JR, Lee SW, Polen SE, Tramont EC, Sadoff J, Zollinger W: The development of a neisserial pilus vaccine for gonorrhea and meningococcal meningitis. *In* Robbins JB, Hill JC, Sadoff JC (eds.): Seminars in Infectious Disease. Vol IV: Bacterial Vaccines. New York, Thieme-Stratton Inc., 1982, pp 140–159. *A gonococcal pilus vaccine protected human volunteers against experimental urethral infection. Unfortunately, this vaccine may not work for all strains.*

Brooks GF, Gotschlich EC, Holmes KK, Sawyer WD, Young FE (eds.): Immunobiology of *Neisseria gonorrhoeae.* Washington, D.C., American Society for Microbiology, 1978. *A comprehensive presentation of present research.*

Buchanan TM, Arko RJ: Immunity to gonococcal infection induced by vaccination with isolated outer membranes of *Neisseria gonorrhoeae* in guinea pigs. J Infect Dis 135:879, 1977. *This is one of several papers in the current literature which shows that it is possible to produce partial immunity to gonococcal infection with a vaccine. All studies to date show that the protection is only approximately 1000-fold, and there is little cross-protection against unrelated strains.*

Cunningham FG, Hauth JC, Strong JD, Herbert WNP, Gilstrap LC, Wilson RH, Kappus SS: Evaluation of tetracycline or penicillin and ampicillin for treatment of acute pelvic inflammatory disease. N Engl J Med 296:1380, 1977. *A prospective randomized comparison of outpatient therapy for pelvic inflammatory disease. Either tetracycline or ampicillin given for ten days is effective.*

Dans PE, Judson F: The establishment of a venereal disease clinic. II. An appraisal of current diagnostic methods in uncomplicated urogenital and rectal gonorrhea. J Am Vener Dis Assoc 1:107, 1975. *A critical examination of the utility of various diagnostic methods, including multiple cultures and Gram stains.*

Eisenstein BI, Sox T, Biswas G, Blackman E, Sparling PF: Conjugal transfer of the gonococcal penicillinase plasmid. Science 195:998, 1977. *Gonococci contain a conjugal plasmid which enables them to transfer sexually their penicillinase plasmid with efficiency.*

Handsfield HH, Hodson WA, Holmes KK: Neonatal gonococcal infection. I. Orogastric contamination with *Neisseria gonorrhoeae.* JAMA 225:697, 1973. *Maternal gonococcal infection is frequently associated with complications of delivery, and the neonate may develop systemic infection by gonococci.*

Handsfield HH, Lipman TO, Harnisch JP, Tronca E, Holmes KK: Asymptomatic gonorrhea in men: Diagnosis, natural course, prevalence and significance. N Engl J Med 290:117, 1974. *Asymptomatic infection of the male urethra by gonococci is carefully described, and is shown to be much more common than previously recognized.*

Handsfield HH, Murphy VL: Comparative study of ceftriaxone and spectinomycin for treatment of uncomplicated gonorrhoea in men. Lancet 2:67, 1983. *Among newer antibiotics, ceftriaxone appears most promising for single-dose therapy of penicillin-resistant gonorrhea.*

Handsfield HH, Wiesner PJ, Holmes KK: Treatment of the gonococcal arthritis-dermatitis syndrome. Ann Intern Med 84:661, 1976. *This is probably the best evaluation of the efficacy of various regimens for therapy of disseminated gonococcal infection.*

Kaufman RE, Johnson RE, Jaffe HW, Thornsberry C, Reynolds GH, Wiesner PJ, and The Cooperative Study Group: National gonorrhea therapy monitoring study: Treatment results. N Engl J Med 294:1, 1976. *The results of a large multiclinic evaluation of various regimens for outpatient therapy of gonorrhea.*

Lebedeff DA, Hochman EB: Rectal gonorrhea in men: Diagnosis and treatment. Ann Intern Med 92:463, 1980. *This paper briefly reviews the clinical findings, diagnostic methods, and efficacy of various methods of treatment for gonococcal proctitis in men.*

Luciano AA, Grubin L: Gonorrhea screening: Comparison of three techniques. JAMA 243:680, 1980. *Culture of the first voided urine in asymptomatic males is shown to be a highly reliable method for diagnosis.*

Mulks MH, Plaut AG: IgA protease production as a characteristic distinguishing pathogenic from harmless Neisseriaceae. N Engl J Med 299:973, 1978. *Gonococci and meningococci commonly produce an enzyme which cleaves immunoglobulin A1, and thereby probably increases the ability of the pathogenic* Neisseria *to escape local immune mechanisms.*

Peterson BH, Lee TJ, Snyderman R, Brooks GF: *Neisseria meningitidis* and *Neisseria gonorrhoeae* bacteremia associated with C6, C7, or C8 deficiency. Ann Intern Med 90:917, 1979. *A brief review of the clinical and laboratory findings in patients with homozygous complement deficiency and meningococcal or gonococcal bacteremia.*

Roberts RB (ed.): The Gonococcus. New York, John Wiley & Sons, 1977. *Contains comprehensive reviews of most clinical aspects of gonococcal infection.*

303. LYMPHOGRANULOMA VENEREUM

Lymphogranuloma venereum (LGV) is an acute to chronic sexually transmitted disease caused by strains of *Chlamydia trachomatis.* LGV typically produces transient genital lesions followed by significant regional lymphadenopathy, which may progress to late fibrosis and tissue destruction in untreated cases.

ETIOLOGY. The organisms causing LGV are closely related to the *C. trachomatis* strains which cause trachoma (serotypes A–C) or nongonococcal urethritis (serotypes D–K). By use of a microimmunofluorescent procedure the LGV strains have been grouped into three serotypes (L1, L2, and L3), of which L2 is apparently the most common. On one occasion the related organism *Chlamydia psittaci* caused a similar syndrome. All chlamydiae apparently contain a common group antigen, but recently an LGV-specific protein antigen has been partially characterized. As is the case with all chlamydiae, the LGV strains can be isolated only in tissue culture or in yolk sac culture.

EPIDEMIOLOGY. LGV is more common in tropical and subtropical climates but does occur in relatively low incidence throughout the western world. The true incidence is unknown. Screening of patients in venereal disease clinics with the LGV complement fixation test has sometimes shown 10 per cent with positive serologies; however, this may merely reflect cross-reactions between antibodies directed against the *Chlamydia trachomatis* serotypes D–K (the causes of nongonococcal urethritis and related syndromes) and the LGV serotypes L1, L2, and L3.

The disease is almost always transmitted by sexual contact. The site of primary infection is usually around the genitals but may be anal or oral, depending on the mode of sexual practice.

PATHOGENESIS AND PATHOLOGY. The incubation period is uncertain but has been estimated to be anywhere from a few days to several weeks. In approximately one fourth of patients a small evanescent primary vesicular or ulcerative lesion develops at the site of inoculation, but in the other three fourths of patients no primary lesion is clinically evident. Occasional patients may have symptoms of nonspecific urethritis, presumably owing to intraurethral infection. Approximately two to six weeks after sexual contact most patients develop significant regional lymphadenopathy. Primary infection of the anterior vulva or penis results in inguinal adenopathy, whereas primary infection of the vagina or posterior vulva or rectum results in primary perirectal or pelvic adenopathy. Most patients seen in venereal disease clinics are males with inguinal adenopathy. In about one third of patients the adenopathy is bilateral. Involvement of lymphatic tissue may result in significant lymphedema and, if untreated, may lead to elephantiasis of the external genitalia. Chronic infection of the perirectal tissues may lead to rectal strictures. The histologic appearance of involved tissues is nonspecific with acute and chronic inflammation.

CLINICAL MANIFESTATIONS. The transient primary lesion usually appears as an infiltrated papule or small erosion. It may mimic herpes but is frequently unnoticed or not present. In its earlier stages the adenopathy syndrome is manifested by discrete tender movable nodes. After several days the nodes become matted, with an ovoid firm lobulated swelling with adherent erythematous overlying skin. In about 10 to 20 per cent of patients, nodes are involved above and below the inguinal ligament, and fibrosis may result in the so-called "groove sign" (linear depressions parallel to the inguinal ligament). The nodes may undergo necrosis, and, if not aspirated, spontaneous fistula tracts may develop. Lymphatic obstruction may result in vulvar edema or polypoid masses around the anal orifice. In early stages anal masses may resemble hemorrhoids. There may be fever, chills, and headache, associated with other nonspecific systemic symptoms such as nausea and weight loss. Infrequently, there is generalized rash, polyarthralgia, splenomegaly, generalized lymphadenopathy, or meningismus. Cutaneous manifestations may include erythema nodosum, erythema multiforme, urticaria, or a scarlatiniform eruption.

Late complications are usually limited to strictures or scarring of the rectum. This complication is more common in women, but is now fortunately rare. There is often no preceding adenopathy syndrome. The strictures may be bandlike or may involve extensive areas of the lower large bowel.

DIAGNOSIS. LGV must be considered in patients with enlarged inguinal lymph nodes, draining inguinal fistulas, and rectal strictures. Differential diagnosis includes reactive nodes secondary to distal sites of pyogenic infection on the extremities (which may be small and not noticed unless careful examination is performed), chancroid, granuloma inguinale, syphilis, and a variety of other diseases associated with adenopathy or adenitis. Diagnosis is made by one of two methods: either by direct demonstration of LGV organisms in lesion material or by appropriate serologic tests. Material may be obtained for culture from affected lymph nodes by inserting a needle into the area of fluctuance, being careful to insert the needle through normal skin. The aspirated pus is characteristically extremely viscous. Organisms may sometimes be directly demonstrated in this material by immunofluorescence, although this test is not routinely available. Culture may be performed in yolk sacs or in tissue cell culture. A complement fixation test, using group-specific antigen, is widely available for serologic diagnosis. In the presence of a compatible clinical syndrome a titer of greater than or equal to 1:16 is strongly suggestive of LGV. Serial samples frequently show a four-fold or greater rise in titer in the acute stage of the disease. Most patients with LGV develop peak titers of at least 1:64. Other serologic tests are under development, including indirect immunofluorescence and counterimmunoelectrophoresis; each of these tests uses antigens specific for LGV, but neither is widely available at present. A recently developed direct immunofluorescence test employing monoclonal antibodies against *C. trachomatis* serotypes L1, L2, and L3 offers promise for rapid specific diagnosis, but it is not yet widely available.

Other laboratory tests are of little help. Many patients have a modest elevation in total leukocyte count with predominance of lymphocytes. There may be a reversal of the albumin globulin ratio, and some patients have elevated cryoglobulins or rheumatoid factor.

TREATMENT. Both tetracycline and sulfonamide drugs are effective. Usual therapy for adults is tetracycline, 500 mg four times daily for at least three weeks. When tetracycline is contraindicated as in pregnancy, sulfisoxazole may be given in a dose of 500 mg four times daily for at least three weeks. Tense nodes should be aspirated through normal skin to prevent formation of fistulous tracts. Patients with early stages of the disease respond well to therapy, but those with late complications, including chronic lymphatic obstruction and rectal stricture, respond poorly or not at all to antibiotic therapy. Surgery may be needed to correct rectal stricture. After an initial course of treatment, patients should be seen at least every three months for one year, and the titer of the LGV complement fixation test should be followed. Retreatment should be given if there is a four-fold increase in serologic titer or if there is clinical evidence of relapse. Sexual contacts should be treated similarly.

PREVENTION. There are no specific data regarding modes of prevention. Presumably, use of condoms would help to prevent transmission. An effective vaccine is not available.

Caldwell HD, Kuo CC: Serologic diagnosis of lymphogranuloma venereum by counterimmunoelectrophoresis with a *Chlamydia trachomatis* protein antigen. J Immunol 118:442, 1977. *A specific test for LGV is under development.*

Klotz SA, Drutz DJ, Tam MR, Reed KH: Hemorrhagic proctitis due to lymphogranuloma venereum serogroup L2: Diagnosis by fluorescent monoclonal antibody. N Engl J Med 308:1563, 1983. *LGV may cause hemorrhagic proctitis that mimics ulcerative colitis in homosexual males; monoclonal antibodies provide rapid diagnosis.*

Schachter J: Lymphogranuloma venereum and other nonocular *Chlamydia trachomatis* infections. *In* Hobson D, Holmes KK (eds.): Nongonococcal Urethritis and Related Infections. Washington, D.C., American Society for Microbiology, 1977, pp 91–97. *An excellent short review of the biology of the organism and the clinical manifestations of the disease.*

Sowmini CN, Gopalan KN, Chandrasekhara Rao G: Minocycline in the treatment of lymphogranuloma venereum. J Am Vener Dis Assoc 2:19, 1976. *Tetracyclines were effective in infected military personnel in Vietnam.*

304. GRANULOMA INGUINALE (Donovanosis)

Granuloma inguinale, also known as donovanosis, is a slowly progressive ulcerative disease involving principally the skin and subcutaneous tissues of the genital, inguinal, and anal regions. It is primarily transmitted sexually, but probably can be transmitted by nonsexual contact as well. Multiple sexual contacts with an infected partner seem necessary for transmission of infection. The disease is uncommon in the United States, with less than 100 recorded cases annually. It is quite common, however, in certain other areas of the world, especially Papua New Guinea.

ETIOLOGY. The causative organism is *Calymmatobacterium granulomatis*, a gram-negative bacterium which is immunologically related to certain *Klebsiella* strains. Current evidence suggests that *C. granulomatis* is not a member of the *Klebsiella-Enterobacter-Serratia* family; its exact taxonomic status is uncertain. The organism can be grown in yolk sacs, but only with great difficulty on artificial medium. It is apparently a facultative intracellular parasite, since in infected lesions it is found primarily in histiocytes or other mononuclear cells.

CLINICAL MANIFESTATIONS. The initial lesion usually appears as a subcutaneous nodule which erodes through the surface and develops into a beefy, elevated granulomatous lesion. This usually is painless and unassociated with systemic symptoms. Secondary bacterial infection may cause a necrotic painful ulcerative lesion which may be rapidly destructive. A cicatricial form may also occur with a depigmented elevated area of keloid-like scar containing scattered islands of granulomatous tissue. Lesions in the genital area are commonly associated with pseudobuboes in the inguinal region; these swellings are usually not due to involvement of the inguinal lymph nodes but rather to granulomatous involvement of the subcutaneous tissues. Metastatic infection of bones or other viscera is occasionally seen. Clinical experience suggests that secondary carcinomas may be a complication of granuloma inguinale.

DIFFERENTIAL DIAGNOSIS. The differential diagnosis includes tumor, lymphogranuloma venereum, chancroid, syphilis, and other ulcerative granulomatous diseases. Chancroid is usually differentiated by its irregular undermined borders, which are not seen in the usual cases of granuloma inguinale. Dark-field examination and serologic tests should help to distinguish syphilis. Biopsies may be necessary to distinguish granuloma inguinale from certain tumors.

DIAGNOSIS. Diagnosis is made by demonstrating intracellular "Donovan bodies" in histiocytes or other mononuclear cells from lesion scrapings or biopsies. Wright's stain or Giemsa stain of fresh impression smears or unfixed biopsies will usually demonstrate the bacilli relatively easily, although multiple biopsies may be necessary in chronic cases. Culture is not practical at present. A serologic test has been devised but is not clinically available. Histologic examination of biopsies shows mononuclear cells with some infiltration by polymorphonuclear leukocytes but no giant cells.

TREATMENT. Treatment consists of tetracycline or sulfisoxazole in a dose of 0.5 gram four times daily for at least three weeks. Other regimens which have proved effective include ampicillin, chloramphenicol, gentamicin, or co-trimoxazole. Limited experience suggests that lincomycin may be used successfully. Patients should be followed for at least several weeks after discontinuation of treatment because of the possibility of relapse. Although the risk of communicability appears to be low, sexual contacts should also be examined; at present, treatment of contacts is not indicated in the absence of clinically evident disease.

PREVENTION. No effective prevention is known.

Breschi LC, Goldman G, Shapiro SR: Granuloma inguinale in Vietnam: Successful therapy with ampicillin and lincomycin. J Am Vener Dis Assoc 1:118, 1975. *Ampicillin was frequently effective in patients previously unresponsive to tetracycline.*

Garg BR, Lal S, Sivamani S: Efficacy of co-trimoxazole in donovanosis. A preliminary report. Br J Vener Dis 54:348, 1978. *Trimethoprim and sulfamethoxazole were effective.*

Kuberski T: Granuloma inguinale (donovanosis). Sex Trans Dis 7:29, 1980. *An excellent short review.*

Maddocks I, Anders EM, Dennis E: Donovanosis in Papua New Guinea. Br J Vener Dis 52:190, 1976. *A description of the epidemiology and clinical manifestations in an endemic area of granuloma inguinale.*

305. CHANCROID

Chancroid is a sexually transmitted infection caused by the gram-negative bacillus *Hemophilus ducreyi.*

EPIDEMIOLOGY. On a worldwide basis chancroid is considerably more common than syphilis, and in parts of Africa and in Southeast Asia is nearly as great a problem as gonorrhea. In the United States it is an uncommon disease, but the incidence is rising. Epidemics have been documented in several cities in North America in recent years. About 90 per cent of reported cases occur in males. An outbreak in Greenland was exceptional in that about 40 per cent of cases were noted in women. It is quite likely that there has been significant underdiagnosis in women in the past.

CLINICAL MANIFESTATIONS. The usual incubation period is two to five days, but may be up to 14 days. In the Greenland outbreak the incubation period averaged nearly two weeks in women. The initial clinical manifestation is an inflammatory macule that then becomes a vesicle-pustule and finally a sharply circumscribed, somewhat ragged, and undermined painful ulcer. The base is moist and may be covered with a grayish necrotic exudate. Removal of the exudate reveals purulent granulation tissue. There is usually surrounding cutaneous erythema. Lesions typically are single but may be multiple, possibly owing to autoinoculation of nearby tissues. There are rarely systemic symptoms. Inguinal adenopathy is noted in half of patients, approximately two thirds of whom have unilateral adenopathy. Lesions are usually noted on the shaft or glans of the penis or around the anal orifice in males. In females lesions may occur on the cervix, vagina, vulva, or perianal area. Lesions may occasionally occur primarily on or spread to the abdomen, thigh, breast, fingers, or lips. Intraoral lesions are quite uncommon.

There are reports of a transient genital ulcer, followed by significant inguinal adenopathy. This may be difficult to distinguish from lymphogranuloma venereum. Other uncommon clinical variants include the *phagedenic type* of ulcer with secondary suprainfection and rapid tissue destruction; *giant chancroid,* which is characterized by a very large single ulcer; *serpiginous ulcer,* which is characterized by rapidly spreading indolent shallow ulcers on the groin or the thigh; and a *follicular* type with multiple small ulcers in a perifollicular distribution.

DIFFERENTIAL DIAGNOSIS. The differential diagnosis includes syphilis, herpes genitalis, lymphogranuloma venereum, traumatic ulcers, and granuloma inguinale. Of these the most commonly confused are syphilis and herpes genitalis. Multiple infections are relatively common. Outpatients with suspected chancroid should have a serologic test for syphilis and preferably a dark-field examination as well.

DIAGNOSIS. The diagnosis of chancroid is made on the basis of the clinical appearance of the lesions plus either morphologic demonstration of typical organisms in the lesions or recovery of *H. ducreyi* by culture. Culture is the preferred method. Positive cultures can be obtained in over 80 per cent of cases. Best culture results seem to be obtained with a chocolate agar medium containing 3 μg per milliliter of vancomycin. Necrotic debris should be removed from the ulcer with physiologic saline. The base and edges of the ulcer should be swabbed with a cotton-tipped swab and inoculated directly onto the culture plate if possible; swabs may be put into Amies transport medium if culture plates are not immediately available. Smears obtained from the undermined edges should be gently rolled onto a slide. *H. ducreyi* is a small gram-negative bacillus with rounded ends, which typically forms chains or parallel aggregates in lesions. Typical organisms are seen in 50 to 80 per cent of cases. Organisms may also be obtained by aspiration of inguinal nodes. Nodes should be aspirated by placing the needle through normal skin to avoid formation of fistulous tracts. Nodes should not be incised. There is no serologic test for chancroid.

TREATMENT. The drug of choice is probably erythromycin, in a dose of 500 mg orally four times daily for ten days. Combinations of trimethoprim and sulfamethoxazole (co-trimoxazole) are highly effective. Ampicillin should not be used, since some strains of *H. ducreyi* produce a typical TEM-type β-lactamase and are quite ampicillin resistant. Interestingly, the plasmid containing the gene for production of β-lactamase is very closely related to the penicillinase plasmids found recently in *H. influenzae* and *Neisseria gonorrhoeae.* All regular sexual partners should be examined and epidemiologically treated with a similar regimen.

PREVENTION. No vaccine is available. Use of a condom is presumably helpful. There are no data regarding efficacy of antibiotic prophylaxis.

Hammond GW, Lian CJ, Wilt JC, Ronald AR: Comparison of specimen collection and laboratory techniques for isolation of *Haemophilus ducreyi.* J Clin Microbiol 7:39, 1978. *Use of selective media improves rates of cultural isolation.*

Hammond GW, Slutchuk M, Scatliff J, Sherman E, Wilt JC, Ronald AR: Epidemiologic, clinical, laboratory, and therapeutic features of an urban outbreak of chancroid in North America. Rev Infect Dis 2:867, 1980. *An excellent summary of a recent epidemic in Winnipeg.*

Lykke-Olesen L, Larsen L, Pedersen TG, Gaarslev K: Epidemic of chancroid in Greenland 1977–78. Lancet 1:654, 1979. *A remarkable epidemic, affecting 3 per cent of the adult population. Tropical climates are not necessary to disease transmission or expression.*

Plummer FA, D'Costa LJ, Nsanze H, Maclean IW, Karasira P, Piot P, Fast MV, Ronald AR: Antimicrobial therapy of chancroid: Effectiveness of erythromycin. J Infect Dis 148:726, 1983. *Documents the efficacy of erythromycin.*

306. SYPHILIS

DEFINITION. Syphilis is a subacute to chronic infectious disease caused by the bacterium *Treponema pallidum.* It is usually acquired by sexual contact with another infected individual. Syphilis is remarkable among infectious diseases in its large variety of clinical presentations. It progresses, if untreated, through primary, secondary, and tertiary stages. The early stages (primary and secondary) are infectious. Spontaneous healing of early lesions occurs, followed by a long latent period. In about 30 per cent of untreated patients, late disease of the heart, central nervous system, or other organs ultimately develops. At one time this disease was termed "the great imitator." Although the disease is less common now than previously, it remains a great challenge to the clinician because of its protean manifestations, and is of great interest to biologists as well because of the long and tenuous balance between the host and the invading spirochete.

ETIOLOGY. The etiology of syphilis was discovered in 1905 by Schaudinn and Hoffman when they visualized spirochetal organisms in early infectious lesions. The causative agent of syphilis, *Treponema pallidum*, is closely related to other pathogenic spirochetes, including those causing yaws *(Treponema pertenue)* and pinta *(Treponema carateum)*. *T. pallidum* is also related in a more distant manner to other pathogenic spirochetes, including *Leptospira* (cause of leptospirosis) and *Borrelia* (cause of relapsing fever).

T. pallidum is a thin, helical cell approximately 0.15 μ wide and 6 to 50 μ long. Ordinarily there are approximately 6 to 14 spirals. The organism is tapered on either end. It is too thin to be seen by ordinary Gram stain but can be visualized in wet mounts by dark-field microscopy (see below), or by silver stains or fluorescent antibody methods.

The organism bears considerable structural resemblance to gram-negative bacteria. A superficial hyaluronic acid slime layer is formed around the organism, and may contribute to virulence. Beneath the slime layer is the outer membrane, or outer envelope, which is structurally similar to the outer membrane of gram-negative bacteria. Between the outer membrane and the peptidoglycan cell wall are six axial fibrils. The axial fibrils are attached three at each end and overlap in the center of the organism. They are structurally and biochemically similar to flagellae, and may be in part responsible for the motility of the organism.

It has not been possible to culture *T. pallidum* in vitro. Motility is prolonged under microaerophilic to anaerobic conditions. *T. pallidum* was formerly considered a strict anaerobe, but recent evidence shows that it is a microaerophilic to aerophilic organism. It can be maintained by serial passage in rabbits without loss of virulence. Only a few strains of *T. pallidum* have been isolated in rabbits and carefully studied, and little evidence is available regarding the genetic diversity of the organism. All studied isolates have been susceptible to penicillin and are similar antigenically. Immunity to the homologous strain develops after prolonged infection in rabbits. The only known natural hosts for *T. pallidum* are man and certain monkeys and higher apes.

HISTORY. A great epidemic of syphilis occurred throughout Europe in the late fifteenth century. Because of the severity of the infection it was termed the "great pox" in contrast to another prevalent infection, smallpox. The pandemic started soon after Columbus returned from the West Indies, and one school holds that the disease was imported into a nonimmune population by the returning sailors. However, there is evidence in the Old Testament and also in ancient Chinese writings of similar diseases, and there are other reasons for disbelieving the Columbian origin of syphilis. It seems more likely that syphilis was endemic in Europe, but rose to particular prominence in the late fifteenth century because of wartime conditions.

The disease was recognized to be sexually transmitted in the early sixteenth century. Its name is derived from the sixteenth century poem by Fracastorius about the mythical shepherd, Syphilis, who was afflicted with the disease. The major cardiovascular and neurologic complications were recognized in the eighteenth and nineteenth centuries. Many great figures of Western civilization had syphilis of the central nervous system, with untold effects on the course of history. The disease was confused with gonorrhea for some time. A clear distinction between syphilis and gonorrhea was finally made by Ricord in the mid 1800's.

Syphilis was treated for centuries with various heavy metal preparations. Until 1910, inunctions of mercury were the mainstay of therapy, which was apparently moderately effective, although extremely toxic. In 1910, Ehrlich introduced arsphenamine, the "magic bullet." This and subsequent arsenical compounds were more effective and less toxic than mercurial compounds and were revolutionary at the time. They had to be administered for periods of up to two years to be effective. Bismuth salts also were effective and were frequently used in combination with arsenicals between World War I and World War II. The final revolution occurred in 1943, when penicillin was introduced for therapy of syphilis. It was so effective and exhibited so little toxicity that many thought that this ancient disease would soon be eradicated. Although syphilis did decline rapidly in incidence after World War II, it has proved to be a resilient foe and continues to be a significant problem.

PATHOGENESIS AND HOST RESPONSE. *T. pallidum* may penetrate through normal mucosal membranes and also may penetrate through minor abrasions of epithelial surfaces. In experimental rabbit syphilis, spirochetes can be found in the lymphatic system within 30 minutes of inoculation and are found in blood shortly thereafter. There have been occasional instances in man of transfusion syphilis resulting from use of blood from a donor who was in the incubation stage of his disease. Therefore it seems clear that syphilis is a systemic disease from the onset in man as well. However, the first lesions appear at the site of primary inoculation, presumably because of the large numbers of treponemes implanted at this site. In laboratory animals, there is an inverse relationship between numbers of treponemes inoculated and time required for development of the primary cutaneous lesion. The minimal number of treponemes required to establish infection is not known, but may be as low as one treponeme. Multiplication of organisms is very slow, with a division time in rabbits of approximately 33 hours. Similarly slow growth of treponemes in man probably accounts in part for the protracted nature of the illness, and for the relatively long incubation period.

T. pallidum is not known to produce any toxins. Although the outer membrane structurally resembles those of gram-negative bacteria, there is no biologically active endotoxin in *T. pallidum*. Treponemes are capable of specific attachment to host cells, but it is not known whether attachment results in damage to host cells. Most treponemes are found in intercellular spaces, but occasional treponemes can be seen within phagocytic cells. However, there is no evidence for intracellular survival of treponemes.

The primary pathologic lesion of syphilis is a focal endarteritis. There is an increase in adventitial cells, endothelial proliferation, and presence of an inflammatory cuff around affected vessels. Lymphocytes, plasma cells, and monocytes predominate in the inflammatory lesion, and in some cases polymorphonuclear cells are seen as well. The vessel lumen is frequently obliterated. With healing there is considerable fibrosis. Treponemes may be seen in most early lesions of syphilis, and in some of the late lesions such as the meningoencephalitis of general paresis.

Granulomatous reaction is also frequent in secondary syphilis and in late syphilis. The granuloma is histologically nonspecific, and cases of syphilis have been incorrectly diagnosed as sarcoidosis or other granulomatous diseases. Human inoculation studies suggest that the pathogenesis of the gumma, which is a granulomatous lesion, involves hypersensitivity to small numbers of virulent treponemes introduced into a previously sensitized host.

Intracutaneous inoculation of patients with syphilis in various stages with partially purified antigens of *T. pallidum* showed that delayed cellular hypersensitivity developed only in late secondary syphilis but was uniformly present in latent syphilis. There may be temporary hyporesponsiveness of lymphocytes from patients with primary and secondary syphilis to treponemal antigens. It is possible but not yet proved that the unusual waxing and waning of lesions in early syphilis depend on the balance between development of effective cellular immunity and suppression of thymus-derived lymphocyte function.

The host also responds to infection with production of numerous antibodies, and in some instances circulating immune complexes may be formed. The nephrotic syndrome has been recognized occasionally in secondary syphilis, and renal biopsies from such cases have shown membranous glomerulonephritis characterized by focal subepithelial basement membrane deposits. The deposits contain both IgG and C3, and treponemal antibody.

Rarely patients may develop paroxysmal cold hemoglobinuria. This is due to production of an IgG antibody that binds to the red cell at 4° C and, upon rewarming of the blood in the presence of complement, results in hemolysis. Thus patients may develop massive hemolysis and hemoglobinuria after cold exposure. This was formerly usually due to congenital syphilis but is now almost always due to other infections. Treatment with penicillin usually stops the attacks.

Antibodies useful in diagnosis are discussed under Serologic Tests, below.

EPIDEMIOLOGY. Syphilis, with the exception of congenital syphilis, is acquired almost exclusively by intimate contact with the infectious lesions of primary or secondary syphilis (chancre, mucous patches, condylomata lata). This is usually through sexual intercourse, including anogenital and orogenital intercourse. Health workers have sometimes been infected during unsuspecting examination of patients with infectious lesions. Infection by contact with fomites is extremely uncommon.

Syphilis is most common in large cities, and in young sexually active individuals. The highest rate in both men and women occurs at ages 20 to 24, followed by ages 25 to 29 and 15 to 19 years. Among predominantly rural areas in the United States the disease is most prevalent in the southeast.

Syphilis spares no class, race, or group, but is more prevalent in the United States among the poorly educated and economically deprived than among more prosperous groups. Increased numbers of different sexual partners and perhaps indiscriminate choice of partner increase the risk of acquiring sexually transmitted disease. Patients with primary and secondary syphilis name on the average nearly three different sexual contacts within the previous 90 days. A cornerstone of syphilis control is epidemiologic investigation of sexual contacts of patients with primary or secondary lesions, and of patients with early latent disease.

In recent years male homosexuals have apparently accounted for an increasing proportion of the total cases of infectious syphilis. The ratio of male:female cases of primary and secondary syphilis in the United States rose from 1.6:1.0 in 1965 to 2.5:1.0 in 1975, and is now about 3:1. In many large cities over 50 per cent of all infectious syphilis occurs in male homosexuals. Currently, more than half of all white males with infectious syphilis name at least one male sexual partner during the recent past. In contrast only 2 per cent of primary and secondary syphilis in females occurs in women who name a female sexual contact. Similar trends have been noted in other countries.

Another important method of case detection is routine serologic testing. Of the approximately 38 million blood specimens examined annually in the United States, approximately 1 million are reactive. Approximately 35 per cent of primary and secondary syphilis and 75 per cent of early latent syphilis are detected annually by either serologic screening or contact treating.

The annual incidence of syphilis has generally declined worldwide for approximately 100 years with the exception of periods of extensive war. Reported cases of infectious primary and secondary syphilis in the United States peaked in 1947 at approximately 73 cases per 100,000 population. With introduction of penicillin there was a rapid decline in primary and secondary syphilis after World War II, to annual rates of approximately 4 cases per 100,000 in 1957. This resulted in declining federal expenditure for syphilis control, however, and there was a subsequent resurgence in infectious primary and secondary syphilis in the United States, reaching peaks of over 12 cases per 100,000 several times in the period 1965–1983. Total reported cases of primary and secondary syphilis in 1983 were 33,613. Since many cases of syphilis are not reported, the true incidence is much higher, perhaps 75,000 to 100,000 annually.

Reported deaths from syphilis declined from 2434 in 1965 to 200 in 1976. Infant deaths from syphilis and first admissions for syphilitic psychoses have fallen by 98 to 99 per cent since 1940. Patients with clinically manifest late syphilis, particularly gummas, are becoming less common, perhaps as a result of the effectiveness of penicillin therapy for early syphilis. However, surveys indicate that there still are significant numbers of patients with untreated cardiovascular and neurologic syphilis, especially among older age groups. There is suggestive evidence that neurosyphilis may be presenting with atypical clinical manifestations and therefore may not be easily recognized.

NATURAL COURSE OF UNTREATED SYPHILIS. The incubation period from time of exposure to development of the primary lesion at the place of initial inoculation of treponemes averages approximately 21 days, but ranges from 10 to 90 days. A painless papule develops, and gradually breaks down to form a clean-based ulcer with raised indurated margins. This persists for two to six weeks and then heals spontaneously. Several weeks later the patient characteristically develops a secondary stage characterized by low grade fever, headache, malaise, generalized lymphadenopathy, and a mucocutaneous rash. There may be involvement of visceral organs. The secondary eruption may occur while the primary chancre is still healing or several months after the disappearance of the chancre. The secondary lesions heal spontaneously within two to six weeks, and the infection then enters latency. Some patients may later develop relapsing lesions similar to those of the secondary stage; rarely the relapse will take the form of recurrence of the primary chancre. About one third of untreated patients eventually develop late destructive tertiary lesions involving one or more of the eyes, central nervous system, heart, or other organs, including skin. These may occur at any time from a few years to as late as 25 years following infection.

The course of untreated syphilis has been extensively studied in two large groups of patients. In the Oslo Study (1891–1951), over 2000 untreated patients diagnosed clinically (without serologic tests or lumbar punctures) were followed for the ultimate course of the disease. None of these patients received treatment with arsenicals or other compounds. A smaller prospective study was also done in the United States among black American males in rural Alabama (the Tuskegee Study, 1932–1972). This study, which was initiated in the arsenical era because of uncertainty that the beneficial effects of treatment outweighed the toxicity of prolonged exposure to arsenical compounds, extended into the penicillin era. It has been subjected to much criticism because curative penicillin therapy was not given when it became available in the mid 1940's, although antimicrobial drugs given for other purposes may have influenced the course of the disease in some patients.

In the Oslo Study, relapsing secondary lesions developed in the first four years after infection in nearly 25 per cent of patients. Twenty-eight per cent eventually developed tertiary syphilis. The most common late lesions were benign tertiary gummas of the skin, mucous membranes, and skeleton. Cardiovascular syphilis was diagnosed in slightly over 10 per cent and symptomatic neurosyphilis in 6.5 per cent of patients. Syphilis was the primary cause of death in 50 per cent of males and 8 per cent of females. Pregnancy had a beneficial effect on the disease. Among autopsied patients cardiovascular syphilis was proved in 35 per cent of men and 22 per cent of women. Serious late complications were more common in men than in women.

The Tuskegee Study showed that among men age 25 to 50 years, death rates were 75 per cent greater in syphilitics than in appropriately matched noninfected control subjects. Cardiovascular or central nervous system syphilis was the primary cause of death in 30 per cent of syphilitic men. Among autopsied patients aortitis was found in about 50 per cent of syphilitics with a persistently positive serologic test. Central nervous system syphilis was found in only 4 per cent. There was no definite anatomic basis for some of the excess mortality among syphilitics noted in the Tuskegee Study. Thus the incidence of cardiovascular syphilis was higher but the incidence of neurologic syphilis was lower in the Tuskegee Study than in the Oslo Study. On the basis of these data, plus other uncontrolled clinical observations, it has been suggested that black patients are particularly prone to development of cardiovascular syphilis, and white patients to central nervous system syphilis, but the evidence is not definitive. The reasons for the possible racial differences are unknown.

The incidence of late complications of untreated syphilis is presently unknown, but seems less than noted previously. Cases of gumma are presently so rare as to be reportable.

CLINICAL MANIFESTATIONS. ***Primary Syphilis.*** The typical lesion of primary syphilis is the chancre, a painless, clean-based, indurated ulcer. The chancre starts as a papule, but then superficial erosion occurs, resulting in the typical ulcer. The borders of the ulcer are raised, firm, and indurated. Occasionally, secondary infections change the appearance, resulting in a painful lesion. Most chancres are single, but multiple ulcers are sometimes seen, particularly when skin folds are opposed ("kissing chancres"). The untreated chancre heals in several weeks, leaving a faint scar. The chancre is usually associated with regional adenopathy, which may be either unilateral or bilateral. The regional nodes are movable, discrete, and rubbery. If the chancre occurs in the cervix or in the rectum, the affected regional iliac nodes are not palpable. See Figure 306–1.

It was formerly taught that 90 per cent of chancres occurred in the genital region. Presently a much higher proportion of nongenital chancres is observed, particularly among male homosexuals, in whom chancres in or near the rectum are common. Rectal chancres may have an atypical appearance mimicking rectal fissures or other more benign lesions, and are frequently overlooked. Conversely, they have also been mistaken for malignant disease. In general it is reasonable to assume that any ulcer occurring in the genital area or, in male homosexuals, around the rectum is syphilitic until proved otherwise. Chancres may also be seen in the pharynx, on the tongue, around the lips, on the fingers, on the nipples, or in diverse other areas. The morphology depends in part on the area of the body in which they occur and also on the host immune response. Chancres in previously infected individuals may be small and may remain papular. Chancres of the finger may appear more erosive and may be quite painful.

The *differential diagnosis* of a genital ulcer should include lesions caused by herpesvirus hominis type II. Herpetic ulcers can usually be distinguished because they are multiple, superficial, and, if seen early, vesicular. They are often painful. Herpetic ulcers, unlike syphilitic ulcers, may have a positive Tzanck test—multinucleated giant cells in the base of the ulcer. The ulcers of chancroid are usually painful, often multiple, and frequently exudative and nonindurated. Lymphogranuloma venereum may produce a small papular lesion associated with a regional adenopathy. Other conditions which must be distinguished include granuloma inguinale, drug eruptions, carcinoma, superficial fungal infections, traumatic lesions, and lichen planus. Final distinction in most cases is made on the basis of dark-field examination, which is positive only in syphilis.

Secondary Syphilis. Approximately four to eight weeks following the appearance of the primary chancre, patients typically develop lesions of secondary syphilis. They may complain of *malaise, fever, headache, sore throat,* and other systemic symptoms. Most patients have generalized lymphadenopathy, including the epitrochlear nodes. Approximately 30 per cent of patients will have evidence of the healing chancre, although

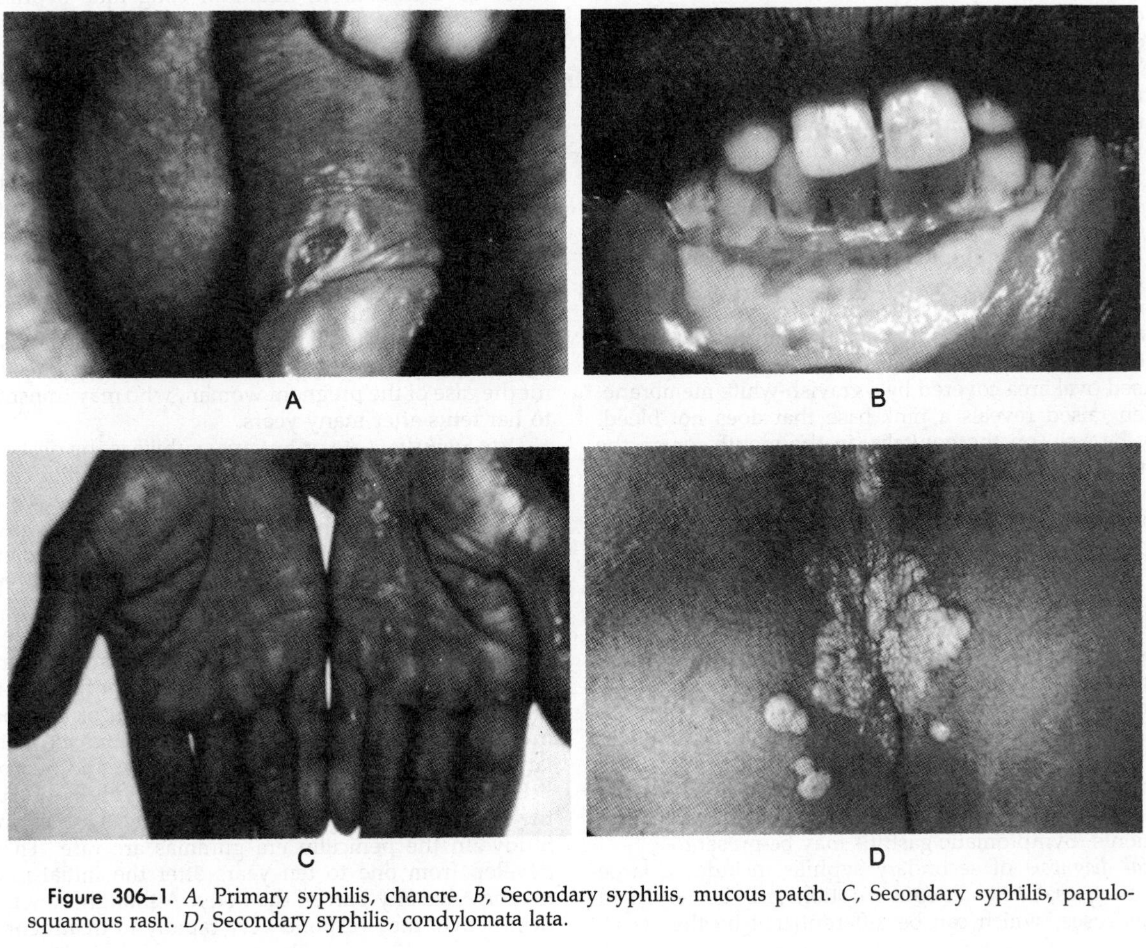

Figure 306–1. *A,* Primary syphilis, chancre. *B,* Secondary syphilis, mucous patch. *C,* Secondary syphilis, papulosquamous rash. *D,* Secondary syphilis, condylomata lata.

many patients, including male homosexuals and women, give no history of a primary lesion.

At least 80 per cent of patients with secondary syphilis have cutaneous lesions or lesions of the mucocutaneous junctions at some point in their illness. The diagnosis is usually first suspected on the basis of the cutaneous eruption. The rash is often minimally symptomatic, however, and many patients with late syphilis do not recall either primary or secondary lesions. The rashes are quite varied in their appearance, but have certain characteristic features. The lesions are usually widespread and are symmetrical in distribution. They often are pink, coppery, or dusky red, particularly the earliest macular lesions. They usually are nonpruritic, although occasional exceptions have been noted, and are almost never vesicular or bullous in adults. They are indurated except for the very earliest macular lesions and frequently have a superficial scale (papulosquamous lesions). They tend to be polymorphic and rounded, and on healing they may leave residual pigmentation or depigmentation. The lesions may be quite faint and difficult to visualize, particularly on dark-skinned individuals.

The earliest pink macular lesions are frequently seen on the margins of the ribs or the sides of the trunk with later spread to the rest of the body. The face is often spared except around the mouth. Subsequently a papular rash appears which is usually generalized but is *quite marked on the palms and soles.* These frequently are associated with a superficial scale and may be hyperpigmented. When the rash occurs on the face, it may be pustular, resembling acne vulgaris. On occasion the scale may be so great as to resemble psoriasis. Deep nodular lesions may cause confusion. Ulceration may occur, producing lesions resembling ecthyma. In malnourished or debilitated patients extensive destructive ulcerative lesions with a heaped-up crust may occur, the so-called rupial lesion. Lesions around the hair follicles may result in a patchy alopecia of the beard or of the scalp.

Ringed or annular lesions may occur, especially around the face, particularly on black individuals. Lesions at the angle of the mouth or the corner of the nose may have a central linear erosion (the so-called "split papule").

In warm, moist areas such as the perineum, large pale flat-topped papules may coalesce to form condylomata lata. These may also be seen in the axilla and rarely in a generalized form. They are extremely infectious. They are not to be confused with the common venereal warts (condylomata acuminata), which are small, often multiple, and more sharply raised than condylomata lata.

Other lesions of the mucous membranes are common. The palate and pharynx may be inflamed. Approximately 30 per cent of patients develop the so-called mucous patch. This is a slightly raised oval area covered by a grayish-white membrane, which when raised reveals a pink base that does not bleed. These may be seen on the genitalia, in the mouth, or on the tongue, and, like condylomata lata, are highly infectious.

Other manifestations of secondary syphilis include hepatitis, which has been reported in up to 10 per cent of patients in some series. Jaundice is rare, but an elevated alkaline phosphatase is common. Liver biopsy reveals small areas of focal necrosis and mononuclear infiltrate or periportal vasculitis. Spirochetes can often be visualized with silver stains. Periostitis with widespread lytic lesions of bone has been reported occasionally; use of bone scans appears to be a sensitive test for early syphilitic osteitis. An immune complex type of nephropathy with transient nephrotic syndrome has been rarely documented. There may be iritis or an anterior uveitis. From 10 to 30 per cent of patients have pleocytosis in the cerebrospinal fluid, but symptomatic meningitis is seen in less than 1 per cent of patients. Symptomatic gastritis may be present.

Differential diagnosis of secondary syphilis includes a large number of diseases. The cutaneous eruptions may be mimicked by pityriasis rosea, which can be differentiated by the occurrence of lesions along lines of skin cleavage and frequently by the presence of a herald patch in pityriasis rosea. Drug eruptions, acute febrile exanthems, psoriasis, lichen planus, scabies, and other diseases must also be considered in some cases. The mucous patch may superficially resemble oral candidiasis (thrush). Infectious mononucleosis may appear very similar to secondary syphilis, with sore throat, generalized adenopathy, hepatitis, and a generalized rash. Infectious hepatitis may also cause confusion. A high index of suspicion is required to make the diagnosis of syphilis in some cases. Unfortunately even classic cases with widespread, hyperpigmented, papulosquamous lesions involving the palms and the soles are not infrequently misdiagnosed in the current era. Fortunately, if the serologic tests for syphilis are obtained, they will be found to be positive in 99 per cent of patients. The condylomata lata and mucous patches contain large numbers of treponemes as seen on dark-field examination. Aspiration of lymph nodes may occasionally reveal motile *T. pallidum*.

Relapsing Syphilis. Condylomata lata are likely to recur. The skin manifestations tend to be unilateral, the eruptions more dense, marked, with fewer lesions, and sometimes solitary. They are also more infiltrated and of somewhat longer standing, and have some characteristics that resemble the skin lesions in late syphilis. This reflects the increasing immunity with the duration of the early disease. Neurorecurrences, as well as ophthalmic and other relapsing manifestations, may occur. If the patient has been inadequately treated, relapses may be delayed.

Latent Syphilis. By definition latent syphilis is that stage in which there are no clinical signs of syphilis and the cerebrospinal fluid is normal. Latency begins with the passing of the first attack of secondary syphilis and may last for a lifetime thereafter. It is usually detected by positive specific treponemal antibody tests for syphilis. The test must be shown to be reactive on more than one occasion to rule out technical errors. Diseases known to cause occasional false-positive treponemal reactions for syphilis, such as systemic lupus erythematosus, must be excluded. In addition, congenital syphilis must be excluded before the diagnosis of latent syphilis can be made. Patients may or may not have a history of earlier primary or secondary syphilis, although such history is obviously helpful in making a firm diagnosis of latent syphilis.

Latency has been divided into two stages: *early* and *late latency*. Early latency is ordinarily considered infection of less than four years' duration, based upon evidence in the Oslo Study that mucocutaneous relapse could occur at any time during the first four years. However, more recent evidence suggests that most relapses occur in the first year, and epidemiologic evidence shows that the most infectious spread of syphilis occurs during the first year of infection. *Therefore early latency in the United States is now defined as the first year after infection.* Late latent syphilis is ordinarily not infectious except for the case of the pregnant woman, who may transmit infection to her fetus after many years.

Late Syphilis. Late or tertiary syphilis is the destructive stage of the disease and can be crippling. Late syphilitic complications are still important medical problems, but newly recognized cases of late syphilis have been declining steadily in the United States since World War II. Although the incidence of late syphilis is unknown, the prevalence of various types of late syphilis has been approximated (Table 306–1).

Late syphilis is usually very slowly progressive, although certain neurologic syndromes may have sudden onset owing to endarteritis and thrombosis in the central nervous system. Late syphilis is noninfectious. Any organ of the body may be involved, but three main types of disease may be distinguished: late benign (gummatous), cardiovascular, and neurosyphilis.

LATE BENIGN SYPHILIS. Late benign syphilis or gumma was the most common complication of late syphilis in the Oslo Study. In the penicillin era gummas are rare. They typically develop from one to ten years after the initial infection and may involve any part of the body. Although they may be very destructive, they respond very rapidly to treatment and there-

TABLE 306–1. NEWLY DIAGNOSED TERTIARY SYPHILIS IN 105 PATIENTS IN DENMARK, 1961–1970

Type of Tertiary Syphilis	Number Observed*
Neurosyphilis	72
Asymptomatic	45
Tabes dorsalis	11
General paralysis	13
Meningovascular	1
Optic atrophy	2
Cardiovascular syphilis	44
Aortic insufficiency	16
Aortic aneurysm	13
Uncomplicated aortitis†	15
Late benign syphilis (gumma)	4

*Some patients had more than one form of late syphilis.
†Autopsy diagnoses only.

fore are relatively benign. Histologically the gumma is a granuloma. The histology is nonspecific and may be associated with central necrosis surrounded by epithelioid and fibroblastic cells and occasionally giant cells. There is sometimes vasculitis. *T. pallidum* is ordinarily not demonstrable by silver stains but can sometimes be recovered by inoculation of rabbits.

Gummas may be solitary or multiple. They are usually asymmetrical, and are often grouped. They may start as a superficial nodule or as a deeper lesion which breaks down to form punched-out ulcers. They are ordinarily indolent and slowly progressive with curving or polycyclic borders. They are indurated on palpation. There often is central healing with an atrophic scar surrounded by hyperpigmented borders. Cutaneous gummas may resemble other chronic granulomatous ulcerative lesions caused by tuberculosis, sarcoidosis, leprosy, and other deep fungal infections. Precise histologic diagnosis may not be possible. However, the syphilitic gumma is the only such lesion to heal dramatically with penicillin therapy. Another form of gumma is papulosquamous, and may mimic psoriasis.

Gummas may also involve deep visceral organs, of which the most common are the respiratory tract, the gastrointestinal tract, and bones. In earlier centuries gummas of the nose and palate commonly resulted in septal perforations and disfiguring facial lesions. Gummas may also involve the larynx or the pulmonary parenchyma. Gumma of the stomach may masquerade as carcinoma of the stomach or lymphoma. Gummas of the liver were once the most common form of visceral syphilis, presenting often with hepatosplenomegaly and anemia, occasionally with fever and jaundice. Skeletal gummas typically produce lesions in the long bones, skull, and clavicle. A characteristic symptom is nocturnal pain. Radiologic abnormalities when present include periostitis and either lytic or sclerotic destructive osteitis.

CARDIOVASCULAR SYPHILIS. The primary cardiovascular complications of syphilis are aortic insufficiency and aortic aneurysm, usually of the ascending aorta. Less commonly other large arteries may be involved, and rarely involvement of the coronary ostia results in coronary insufficiency. These complications in all cases are due to obliterative endarteritis of the vasa vasorum with resultant damage to the intima and media of the great vessels. This results in dilatation of the ascending aorta and eventually in stretching of the ring of the aortic valve, producing aortic insufficiency. The valve cusps remain normal. Death may eventually result from congestive heart failure. There has been some success with placing prosthetic heart valves in patients with syphilitic aortic insufficiency. Aneurysms occasionally present as a pulsating mass bulging through the anterior chest wall. Syphilitic aortitis may involve the descending aorta, but this is almost always proximal to the renal arteries, unlike atherosclerotic aneurysms, which typically involve the descending aorta below the renal arteries.

The disease usually begins within five to ten years after initial infection but may not become clinically manifest until 20 to 30 years after infection. Cardiovascular syphilis is thought to be more common in men than in women and possibly in blacks than in whites. The effects of genetic and nutritional factors on development of this and other complications of late syphilis are unclear. Cardiovascular syphilis does not occur after congenital infection—a phenomenon that remains unexplained.

Asymptomatic aortitis is best diagnosed by visualizing linear calcifications in the wall of the ascending aorta by x-ray. The signs of syphilitic aortic insufficiency are the same as for aortic insufficiency of other causes. In aortic insufficiency resulting from dilatation of the aortic ring, the decrescendo murmur is often loudest along the *right* sternal margin. Syphilitic aneurysms may be fusiform but are more typically saccular, and do not lead to aortic dissection. Approximately 10 to 25 per cent of patients with cardiovascular syphilis have coexistent neurosyphilis, and it is therefore mandatory to do a lumbar puncture in all patients with cardiovascular syphilis.

At present, syphilis is a relatively more common cause of aortic insufficiency among the elderly than among younger patients; this is due to the progressively decreasing incidence of new cases of late cardiovascular syphilis.

NEUROSYPHILIS. Neurosyphilis may be divided into four groups: asymptomatic, meningovascular, tabes dorsalis, and general paresis. Division is not absolute and there may be considerable overlap between syndromes. Current cases of neurosyphilis are more likely than heretofore to be variants of the classic syndromes, possibly as a result of use of antimicrobials for other diseases.

Asymptomatic Neurosyphilis. Asymptomatic neurosyphilis is diagnosed when there is a positive VDRL* in the cerebrospinal fluid (CSF) in the absence of signs and symptoms of neurologic disease. False-positive VDRL test results are very rare in CSF in the absence of a traumatic tap. The CSF usually shows an increased total protein and a lymphocytic pleocytosis, but these findings may be absent. If the CSF is normal two or more years after the initial infection, the patient is not likely to develop a positive CSF later. Athough up to 30 per cent of patients with untreated secondary syphilis have an abnormal CSF, penicillin therapy prevents progression to late symptomatic neurosyphilis. Because of this, routine lumbar punctures for examination of CSF are not indicated in early syphilis. Unfortunately, it has become common practice to avoid lumbar punctures in later stages of syphilis as well. Instead, patients are treated with doses of penicillin thought to be effective for neurosyphilis, if present. As a result, there are few data on the present frequency and course of asymptomatic neurosyphilis.

Some laboratories perform an FTA-ABS* test on spinal fluid. Interest in tests such as this has been prompted by good evidence that patients with untreated neurosyphilis may have a negative CSF-VDRL. There are published reports of positive FTA-ABS test results in the CSF of patients with otherwise normal spinal fluid, in whom there were clinical signs and symptoms compatible with neurosyphilis. However, the CSF FTA-ABS test has not been standardized, and there is some evidence that positive CSF test results are caused by passive transfer of serum antibody into spinal fluid. At present no diagnosis of asymptomatic (or symptomatic) neurosyphilis should be based solely on the CSF FTA-ABS* test.

Meningovascular Syphilis. An acute to subacute aseptic meningitis may occur at any time after the primary stage but usually within the first year of infection. It frequently involves the base of the brain and may result in unilateral or bilateral cranial nerve palsies. In about 10 per cent of cases, the onset of meningitis coincides with the rash of secondary syphilis. The spinal fluid shows a lymphocytic pleocytosis with increased protein and usually normal glucose concentration. The CSF-VDRL is nearly always positive. Rarely CSF glucose concentration is decreased. This syndrome can mimic tuberculous or fungal meningitis or nonpurulent meningitis of various causes.

*See Serologic Tests, below. Also refer to Table 306–2.

In other patients, the meningeal involvement may be less prominent but there is sufficient endarteritis and perivascular inflammation to result in cerebrovascular thrombosis and infarction, with signs and symptoms typical of those of cerebrovascular accidents of any cause. This usually occurs five to ten years after the initial infection and is more common in males. There often is an associated aseptic meningitis as well. Most cerebrovascular accidents are not due to syphilitic arteritis even in patients with a positive serologic test for syphilis. However, syphilis should be considered as the cause in young patients with a history of syphilis and without other causes for cerebrovascular accidents.

A variety of other meningeal syndromes may rarely be seen, including transverse myelitis and radiculitis. A rare syndrome of meningomyelitis may involve the lateral regions of the cord, resulting in anterior horn damage and paralysis of one or more extremities.

Tabes Dorsalis. Tabes dorsalis is a slowly progressive degenerative disease involving the posterior columns and posterior roots of the spinal cord, resulting in progressive loss of peripheral reflexes, impairment of vibration and position sense, and progressive ataxia. There may be chronic destructive changes in the large joints of the affected limbs in far advanced cases (Charcot's joints). Incontinence of the bladder and impotence are common. Sudden and severe painful crises of uncertain cause are a characteristic part of the syndrome. These may involve the larynx, vagina, rectum, or other organs. Not infrequently severe sharp abdominal pains lead to exploratory surgery. Lightning pains in the extremities may require opiates for relief. These may be triggered by exposure to cold or other stresses or may arise with no obvious precipitating cause.

The eyes are frequently involved as well. Optic atrophy is seen in 20 per cent of cases. The pupils are abnormal in 90 per cent of cases, with bilaterally small pupils which fail to constrict further in response to light but which do constrict normally to accommodation (Argyll Robertson pupils).

The cause of tabes dorsalis is unclear. Spirochetes cannot be demonstrated in the posterior column or dorsal root.

Onset of the disease is usually delayed, often 20 to 30 years after initial onset of infection. It is thought to be more common in whites and in males. Typical cases presenting with lightning pains, ataxia, Argyll Robertson pupils, absent deep tendon reflexes, and loss of posterior column function are easy to diagnose. Atypical cases may be more troublesome, particularly because the VDRL test result in the serum is normal in as many as 30 to 40 per cent of cases, and 10 to 20 per cent of cases (even before the advent of penicillin) have normal CSF-VDRL as well. The FTA-ABS test in serum is nearly always positive.

Treatment is unsatisfactory. Penicillin does not reverse the symptoms, although it does usually result in clearing of the abnormal spinal fluid. Carbamazepine in doses of 400 to 800 mg per day has been reported to be effective in treatment of the lightning pains.

Tabes dorsalis is now thought to be uncommon, although a survey of newly diagnosed late syphilis in Denmark in the decade 1961 to 1970 showed that in approximately 10 per cent of all persons with late syphilis and 40 per cent of all with clinical neurosyphilis there was evidence of tabes dorsalis.

General Paresis. This form of neurosyphilis is a chronic meningoencephalitis resulting in gradually progressive loss of cortical function. It typically occurs 10 to 20 years after the initial infection. Pathologically there is a perivascular and meningeal chronic inflammatory reaction with thickening of the meninges, a granular ependymitis, degeneration of the cortical parenchyma, and abundant spirochetes in the tissues.

The most devastating effect of general paresis is on the mind. With effective penicillin therapy this disease has become much less common; in the United States, first admissions to mental hospitals because of syphilitic psychosis have declined from 7694 in 1940 to 154 in 1968, the last year for which definite figures are available.

Symptomatically in its early stages general paresis results in nonspecific symptoms such as irritability, fatigability, headaches, forgetfulness, and personality changes. Later there is impaired memory, defective judgment, lack of insight, confusion, and often depression or marked elation. The patients may be delusional, and seizures are sometimes seen. There may also be loss of other cortical functions, including paralysis or aphasia.

Physical signs of the illness are primarily those of the altered mental status. Cranial nerve palsies are uncommon. Optic atrophy is rare. The complete Argyll Robertson pupil is also uncommon, but irregular or otherwise abnormal pupils are not infrequent. Peripheral reflexes are often somewhat increased.

The CSF is nearly always abnormal with lymphocytic pleocytosis and increased total protein. The VDRL is usually reactive in both spinal fluid and serum. The disease responds well to penicillin therapy if administered early, although as many as a third of treated patients may develop progressive neurologic decline in later years. Fever therapy induced with malaria was formerly an effective adjunct to treatment with arsenicals, but has now been abandoned.

Classic general paresis is now infrequently seen in the United States. However, it remains reasonable to suspect syphilis as the cause of undiagnosed neurologic illness. Since the VDRL may be negative in patients with late neurologic syphilis, the FTA-ABS test on serum must be performed before syphilis can be excluded.

Congenital Syphilis. Congenital syphilis results from transplacental hematogenous spread of syphilis from the mother to the fetus. The incidence of congenital syphilis among newborns or infants under one year of age in the United States rose from 180 cases in 1957 to 422 cases in 1972, but has since declined to about 100 cases annually. Each case of congenital syphilis represents a tragedy which possibly could have been prevented by better case reporting and by proper prenatal care. A VDRL should be obtained in all expectant mothers at the beginning and near the end of pregnancy.

It has generally been held that maternal syphilis cannot be transmitted to the fetus until the sixteenth to eighteenth week of pregnancy. However, spirochetes can be found in abortuses of as little as nine to ten weeks' gestation. The risk of fetal infection is greatest in the early stages of untreated maternal syphilis and declines slowly thereafter, but the mother may infect her fetus during at least the first five years of her infection. Adequate treatment of the mother prior to the sixteenth week will usually prevent manifest clinical illness in the neonate. Later treatment may not prevent late sequelae of the disease in the child. Untreated maternal infection may result in stillbirth, neonatal death, prematurity, or syndromes of early or late congenital syphilis among surviving infants.

Manifestations of early congenital syphilis are often seen in the perinatal period, but may not develop until the infant has been discharged from the hospital. The disease resembles secondary syphilis of the adult except that the rash may be vesicular or bullous, which is extremely rare in adults. There often is rhinitis, hepatosplenomegaly, hemolytic anemia, jaundice, and pseudoparalysis (immobility of one or more extremities) resulting from painful osteochondritis. There may be thrombocytopenia and leukocytosis. The early stages of congenital syphilis must be differentiated from rubella, cytomegalovirus infection, toxoplasmosis, bacterial sepsis, and other diseases.

Late congenital syphilis is defined as congenital syphilis of more than two years' duration. The disease may remain latent with no manifest late damage. Cardiovascular alterations have not been observed in congenital syphilis. Neurologic manifestations are common, and there may be eighth nerve deafness and interstitial keratitis. The latter occurs in over 10 per cent of patients but may not be manifest until the tenth year of life or later. Periostitis may result in prominent frontal bones, depression of the bridge of the nose ("saddle nose"), poor development of the maxilla, and anterior bowing of the tibias ("saber shins"). There may be late onset arthritis of the knees (Clutton's joints). The permanent dentition may show characteristic abnormalities known as Hutchinson's teeth; the upper central incisors are widely spaced, centrally notched, and tapered in the manner of a screwdriver. The molars may show multiple poorly developed cusps (mulberry molars). Some of the late manifestations such as interstitial keratitis and Clutton's joints may be due to hypersensitivity responses, and are benefited by corticosteroids in some cases.

DIAGNOSIS. ***Dark-Field Examination.*** The most definitive means of making a diagnosis is finding spirochetes of typical morphology and motility in lesions of early acquired or congenital syphilis. The dark-field examination is almost always positive in primary syphilis and in the moist mucosal lesions of secondary and congenital syphilis. It may occasionally be positive in aspirates of lymph nodes in secondary syphilis. Problems arise, however, because of false-negative results in primary syphilis owing to application by the patient of soaps or other toxic compounds to the lesions. A single negative result is therefore insufficient to exclude syphilis. Patients with suspicious lesions but with an initially negative dark-field examination should be instructed to avoid washing the lesion and to return daily for two successive examinations. Confusion may also arise because of presence of spirochetes which are morphologically indistinguishable from *T. pallidum* in the mouth, particularly around the gingival margins. For lesions in these areas, therefore, diagnosis often depends upon clinical appearance, history, and serologic testing.

To perform the dark-field examination, the surface of the suspected ulcerative lesion should be cleaned with saline solution and gauze without production of bleeding. Presence of red cells in the specimen makes it difficult to visualize small numbers of *T. pallidum*. Squeezing of the lesion (with gloves on) may help produce serous fluid, which is picked up on a glass slide, covered with a coverslip, and examined with the dark-field microscope. Living *T. pallidum* organisms demonstrate gradual motion to and fro, rotational movement around the long axis, and rather sudden 90 degree bending near the center of the organism. Since most physicians do not have the proper equipment and are not familiar with the techniques of dark-field microscopy, the state public health authorities can be called for assistance.

T. pallidum may also be demonstrated in biopsies or pathologic specimens by fluorescent antibody stains or by silver stains.

Serologic Tests. Two basic types of humoral antibody are stimulated by infection with *T. pallidum:* nonspecific antibody directed against diphosphatidyl glycerol (cardiolipin), which is a normal component of many tissues; and specific treponemal antibodies. Nonspecific antibodies against cardiolipin were formerly designated "reagin," a term which should be discarded to avoid confusion with another "reagin," IgE. The kinds of tests used in syphilis are summarized in Table 306–2.

TABLE 306–2. SEROLOGIC TESTS FOR SYPHILIS

Type	Use
Nonspecific (anticardiolipin) antibodies:	
VDRL (slide flocculation)	Screening, quantitation, following response to treatment
RPR (circle-card) (agglutination)	Screening
Kolmer (complement fixation)	Limited
Specific treponemal antibodies:	
FTA-ABS (immunofluorescence with absorbed serum)	Confirmatory, diagnostic, not for routine screening
MHA-TP (microhemagglutination)	Similar to FTA-ABS but can be quantitated and automated
TPI (immobilization)	Most specific but not generally available

VDRL = Venereal Disease Research Laboratories test.
RPR = Rapid plasma reagin test.
FTA-ABS = Fluorescent treponemal antibody absorption test.
TPI = *Treponema pallidum* immobilization test.
MHA-TP = Microhemagglutination assay for *T. pallidum*.

Nonspecific Tests. Anticardiolipin antibodies were first discovered by Wassermann in 1907, using extracts of congenitally syphilitic livers as the antigen for a complement fixation test. Subsequently it was shown that normal livers contained the same antigen as do many other tissues; the antigen for this class of test is now extracted from beef heart. As yet there is no convincing explanation for why patients infected with *T. pallidum* develop increasing titers of antibody against a normal tissue component.

The Wassermann test has now been replaced by related tests. The standard test in use today for detection of anticardiolipin antibody is the Venereal Disease Research Laboratories (VDRL) test, which is an easily quantitated slide flocculation test. Many similar tests, including the rapid plasma reagin (RPR) test and the unheated serum reagin (USR) test, are frequently used for screening for syphilis.

The VDRL and related tests are simple, well standardized, cheap, and easy to perform and are the screening tests of choice. The VDRL is the test of choice for following response of patients to treatment. Since the VDRL detects antibody against a normal tissue component, it may be falsely positive in a significant number of patients. The relative proportion of patients with a false-positive VDRL depends on the prevalence of syphilis in the community; the lower the prevalence of syphilis, the higher the proportion of positive VDRL tests which are due to nonsyphilitic causes.

The VDRL test begins to turn positive a week or two after the onset of the chancre. In large series of patients with primary syphilis, approximately two thirds have had a positive VDRL test. Obviously then a negative VDRL test does not exclude primary syphilis, particularly if the lesion is less than two weeks old. The VDRL is positive in 99 per cent of patients with secondary syphilis, the only exceptions being patients with such high titers of antibody that they are in antibody excess; dilution of the serum will then paradoxically result in conversion of a negative test to positive. VDRL reactivity tends to diminish in later stages of the disease, and only about 70 per cent of patients with cardiovascular or neurosyphilis have a positive VDRL test result.

The *quantitative titer* of the VDRL test is somewhat useful in diagnosis and quite useful in following therapeutic response. The titer is reported as the highest dilution which gives a positive response. Most patients with secondary syphilis have titers of at least 1:16. Most patients with false-positive VDRL tests have titers of less than 1:8. No single titer is in itself diagnostic. Significant rises (four-fold or greater) in paired sera, however, are strongly indicative of acute syphilis.

Treponemal Tests. There are many varieties of specific treponemal antibody tests. The first and still perhaps best test is the *Treponema pallidum* immobilization (TPI) test, which when properly performed is nearly completely specific for infection by *T. pallidum* or related pathogenic spirochetes. Unfortunately it is cumbersome and expensive and therefore is not routinely done in the United States at present. The most widely used treponemal antibody test is the fluorescent treponemal antibody absorption (FTA-ABS) test. Patient serum is absorbed with extracts of nonpathogenic cultivable treponemes to remove cross-reacting group treponemal antibody. The absorbed serum is reacted with dried *T. pallidum* on a glass slide, and specific antitreponemal antibodies are detected by subsequent addition of fluorescein-labeled anti-human gamma globulin. Other treponemal tests are based on agglutination of red cells to which *T. pallidum* antigens have been fixed, such as the microhemagglutination assay for *T. pallidum* (MHA-TP). Many other treponemal tests have been developed or are being investigated, but none is superior to the standard tests.

The precise nature of the antigens involved in these tests is not known. Characterization of the antigens of *T. pallidum* has been greatly hindered by inability to grow the organism in cell-free culture. Recent success in cloning *T. pallidum* antigens into

Escherichia coli may circumvent this problem. Antibodies reactive in the various tests are found in all major immunoglobulin classes (IgG, IgM, IgA). A modification of the FTA-ABS test has been developed using fluorescein-labeled anti-human IgM (IgM FTA-ABS). The IgM FTA-ABS test is of some use in diagnosis of early congenital syphilis but is of no use in distinguishing acute disease from old infections in adults.

The FTA-ABS test is best used as a confirmatory test. It is somewhat more difficult to perform than the VDRL test and cannot be easily quantitated. It is sensitive and has a high degree of specificity, being positive in only approximately 1 per cent of normal individuals. It is positive in 85 per cent of patients with primary syphilis, 99 per cent with secondary syphilis, and at least 95 per cent with late syphilis. It may therefore be the only test positive in patients with cardiovascular or neurologic syphilis. In late syphilis the FTA-ABS test usually remains positive for life despite adequate therapy. It (as well as the TPI and MHA-TP) is positive in other treponemal diseases such as pinta, yaws, and bejel.

The FTA-ABS test is reported in terms of relative brilliance of fluorescence, from borderline to 4+. Borderline reactivity has the same meaning as nonreactive for clinical purposes. Most laboratories report 1+ positive tests as reactive, but some studies have shown that such tests may be relatively difficult to reproduce. Occasional laboratories therefore only report as positive tests with 2+ or greater reactivity. In patients lacking historical or clinical evidence of syphilis but with a reactive FTA-ABS test, one should repeat the FTA-ABS test. Use of another treponemal test such as the MHA-TP may be helpful in certain problem cases.

The MHA-TP test is less sensitive than either the VDRL or the FTA-ABS test in primary syphilis. Its sensitivity and specificity otherwise are nearly identical to those of the FTA-ABS test, being positive in nearly all patients with secondary syphilis and in 95 per cent or more of patients with late syphilis. The reactivity of serologic tests for syphilis in various stages of disease is shown in Table 306–3.

False-Positive Serologic Test Results for Syphilis. The VDRL or RPR test may be positive in a variety of diseases other than syphilis. A false-positive result is defined as a reproducible positive test in a patient with no clinical or historical evidence of syphilis, and whose serum FTA-ABS or MHA-TP test is negative.

"Acute" (less than six months) false-positive VDRL test results occur with low frequency in atypical pneumonia, malaria, and other bacterial or viral infections, and may occur after smallpox or other vaccinations as well. *Chronic false-positive VDRL tests* (lasting longer than six months) are relatively common in autoimmune disorders such as systemic lupus erythematosus, in narcotic addicts, in leprosy, and in aged persons. From 8 to 20 per cent of patients with systemic lupus erythematosus have been reported as having a false-positive VDRL test, and the false-positive result may develop many years prior to the onset of other manifestations of the disease. A chronic false-positive VDRL test in females age 20 or younger carries a significant risk of future development of systemic lupus erythematosus, thyroiditis, or other autoimmune disorders, and such patients should be followed carefully for a considerable period of time. As many as one third of patients with narcotic addiction have a false-positive VDRL test. Over 1 per cent of patients aged 70 and 10 per cent of patients over age 80 have a low titer false-positive VDRL test. Most false-positive VDRL tests have a titer of 1:8 or less, although occasional patients with lymphoma and other diseases have been described with very high titer false-positive VDRL tests.

TABLE 306–3. FREQUENCY OF POSITIVE SEROLOGIC TESTS IN UNTREATED SYPHILIS

Stage	VDRL (%)	FTA-ABS (%)	MHA-TP (%)
Primary	70	85	50–60
Secondary	99	100	100
Latent or late	70	98	98

A positive FTA-ABS result is usually indicative of recent or past syphilis. However, there is an increased incidence of false-positive FTA-ABS results in systemic lupus erythematosus and in other chronic diseases associated with hyperglobulinemia, including rheumatoid arthritis, biliary cirrhosis, and others. False-positive results are of two kinds in systemic lupus erythematosus: the most common is one with a beaded pattern of fluorescence, which has been shown to be due to anti-DNA antibodies; there also may be homogeneous fluorescence of the treponeme indistinguishable from a true positive result in syphilis. Patients with systemic lupus who have a false-positive FTA-ABS result almost always have a negative VDRL result (and conversely, patients with SLE with a positive VDRL usually have a negative FTA-ABS).

Occasionally one encounters reproducible positive FTA-ABS results in patients with no clinical or historical evidence of syphilis and in whom there is no evidence of diseases associated with false-positive FTA-ABS results. It may be wise to obtain CSF for examination of total protein, cells, and VDRL reactivity in order to rule out neurosyphilis. If in doubt and if the patient is not allergic to penicillin, it is often wisest to treat such patients for possible syphilis.

IgM FTA-ABS Test for Congenital Syphilis. Mothers with a positive VDRL or FTA-ABS will deliver infants with a positive VDRL and FTA-ABS because of passive transfer of the IgG antibodies reactive in these tests. Since many infants with congenital syphilis are clinically normal at birth but develop serious symptomatic disease some weeks later, it is important to determine whether a newborn with a positive VDRL or FTA-ABS test has passively transferred maternal antibody or is actively infected. Since maternal IgM antibodies are not passively transferred to the fetus, an IgM FTA-ABS test has been developed to detect syphilis in the newborn. Unfortunately there is approximately a 35 per cent incidence of false-negative IgM FTA-ABS test results in delayed-onset congenital syphilis. There also is a false-positive rate of approximately 10 per cent. For these reasons the IgM FTA-ABS test is of limited use in diagnosis of neonatal syphilis.

If the mother has been adequately treated for syphilis during pregnancy and the infant is clinically normal at birth, one may elect to follow the infant carefully by serial examination and VDRL titers. If the positive VDRL in the infant is due to passively transferred maternal antibody, the titer of reactivity will fall markedly in the first two months of life. A rising titer indicates active disease and the need for treatment. Many physicians are unwilling to risk failure of proper follow-up of VDRL-positive but clinically normal neonates, and instead administer effective therapy immediately. The risk of penicillin allergy in neonates is very low.

TREATMENT. *T. pallidum* is highly susceptible to penicillin, being inhibited by less than 0.01 μg of penicillin G. Since treponemes divide slowly, and since penicillin acts only on dividing cells, it is necessary to maintain serum levels of penicillin for many days. Studies in animals and in man show that more therapy is required as the length of infection increases. Current recommendations for treatment of syphilis are summarized in Table 306–4.

Early (Less Than One Year) Infectious Syphilis. Early syphilis may be treated with a single injection of 2.4 million units of *benzathine penicillin G,* which provides low but effective serum levels for over two weeks. Extensive studies in the 1940's and 1950's with regimens which provided similar serum levels and duration of therapy showed that approximately 95 per cent of patients were cured by such treatment. Many of the remaining 5 per cent who had clinical or serologic evidence of relapse may actually have been reinfected. It is not necessary to examine the CSF at this stage, because penicillin prevents development of later neurosyphilis. Motile treponemes disappear from primary lesions in 24 hours.

TABLE 306-4. PENICILLIN TREATMENT PRACTICE IN SYPHILIS AS RECOMMENDED BY UNITED STATES PUBLIC HEALTH SERVICE

Indications for Syphilis Therapy†	Dosage and Administration*: Benzathine Penicillin G	Dosage and Administration*: Aqueous Benzyl Penicillin G or Procaine Penicillin G
Primary, secondary, and early latent syphilis (<1 year); epidemiologic treatment	Total of 2.4 million units; single IM dose of two injections of 1.2 million units in one session	Total of 4.8 million units IM in doses of 600,000 units daily for eight consecutive days
Late latent (>1 year) or when CSF was not examined in "latency"; asymptomatic neurosyphilis, symptomatic neurosyphilis, cardiovascular syphilis, late benign (cutaneous, osseous, visceral gumma)	Total of 7.2 million units IM in doses of 2.4 million units at seven-day intervals, over 21 days	Total of 9 million units IM in doses of 600,000 units daily over 15 days; in selected cases of symptomatic CNS syphilis, 2 to 4 million units of aqueous (crystalline) penicillin G intravenously every four hours for at least ten days
Congenital		
Early		
Up to two years of age	If CSF is normal: Total of 50,000 units per kilogram IM in a single or divided dose at one session	If CSF is abnormal: Total of 50,000 units per kilogram IM per day for ten consecutive days‡
Late		
Two to 12 years, weight 32 kg (71 lb) or less	Same as for early congenital syphilis	Same as for early congenital syphilis
Over 12 years, or over 32 kg	Same as for adult late latent syphilis	Same as for adult late latent syphilis

*Individual doses can be divided for injection in each buttock to minimize discomfort.

†In *pregnancy*, treatment is dependent on the stage of syphilis.

‡For aqueous penicillin, give in two divided doses per day; for procaine penicillin, give as one daily dose.

A single injection of 2.4 million units of *aqueous procaine penicillin*, which provides relatively high serum levels for a brief period, is ineffective in established early syphilis, but is curative if the disease is still in the incubating stage (e.g., in a patient who is being treated for gonorrhea and who happened to acquire syphilis simultaneously). Other regimens currently useful for gonorrhea have uncertain effects on incubating syphilis, and careful follow-up for syphilis is indicated in gonorrhea patients treated with regimens other than procaine penicillin. The incidence of incubating syphilis in gonorrhea patients is 2 per cent or more in several series.

For patients allergic to penicillin, tetracycline hydrochloride may be given in a total dose of 30 grams over 15 days, or erythromycin base may be given in a total dose of 30 grams over 15 days. Particularly careful follow-up is necessary in patients treated with drugs other than penicillin, because patients may not be fully compliant with these prolonged courses of oral therapy and these regimens have been less fully evaluated clinically. Cephaloridine or other cephalosporins may be effective but have not been well studied. Chloramphenicol is of equivocal efficacy and for this reason, as well as because of the risk of toxicity, should not be used. Spectinomycin has essentially no effect on syphilis.

Syphilis of More Than One Year's Duration. Larger doses of penicillin are needed for *neurosyphilis* (see Ch. 497) than for syphilis of less than one year's duration. In general, patients with general paresis respond better to treatment than do patients with tabes dorsalis, although patients with paresis should be expected to show residual effects of the infection. This is particularly true in advanced cases. Meningovascular syphilis usually responds well, except for residual damage to cranial nerves or cortical function resulting from ischemic infarcts. Published studies show that a total of 6.0 to 9.0 million units of penicillin G results in a satisfactory clinical response in approximately 90 per cent of patients with neurosyphilis.

Currently used benzathine penicillin regimens have received relatively little study in neurosyphilis. Benzathine penicillin G in a total dose of 7.2 million units given as 2.4 million units weekly for three successive weeks is effective in most patients. However, there are reports of patients who have failed standard penicillin therapy for neurosyphilis but who responded to intensive intravenous therapy which provided high serum levels of penicillin. Benzathine penicillin does not provide measurable levels of penicillin in the spinal fluid or aqueous humor of the eye. *Therefore in cases of symptomatic central nervous system syphilis, which is a serious disease, there is considerable rationale to treatment with intravenous penicillin G (20 million units per day for at least ten days in hospital).* Therapy of neurosyphilis not infrequently results in increased CSF pleocytosis for seven to ten days after starting treatment, and may transiently convert a normal CSF to abnormal.

Limited evidence suggests that treating *latent syphilis* with 7.2 million units total dose of benzathine penicillin is curative even if the patient has asymptomatic neurosyphilis. However, because of the possible lack of the efficacy of benzathine penicillin in some patients with central nervous system syphilis, it is desirable to examine CSF in all patients with latent syphilis to exclude asymptomatic neurosyphilis. Alternatively, one may reasonably elect to perform a lumbar puncture at the conclusion of the follow-up period (two years); if the CFS is normal, the patient can be reassured that neurosyphilis will not develop.

There is no evidence that therapy with antimicrobial drugs is clinically beneficial to patients with *cardiovascular syphilis*. Nevertheless, treatment of cardiovascular syphilis is recommended in order to prevent further progression of disease and because approximately 15 per cent of patients with cardiovascular syphilis have associated neurosyphilis.

There is no evidence as to the efficacy of other antimicrobials in treatment of later syphilis. Therefore if patients are allergic to penicillin, it is mandatory that the CSF be examined before therapy is undertaken. Either tetracycline, 2 grams daily for 30 days, or erythromycin, 2 grams daily for 30 days, is probably effective.

Syphilis in Pregnancy. All pregnant women should be examined with a VDRL or RPR test during pregnancy; if they are at high risk for syphilis, a second test should be obtained before delivery. Because of the risk to the fetus, evaluation and treatment of the VDRL-positive patient should be done as rapidly as possible, particularly for patients first seen in the later stages of pregnancy. If a confirmatory FTA-ABS is positive and the patient has not been treated, penicillin (or erythromycin for patients who are allergic to penicillin) should be administered in doses appropriate for early or late syphilis as outlined above. For patients who are VDRL positive but FTA-ABS negative and who have no clinical signs of syphilis, treatment may be withheld. In such patients a quantitative VDRL test and another FTA-ABS test should be repeated in four weeks. If the VDRL titer has risen by four-fold or more, or if clinical signs of syphilis have developed, the patient should be treated. If after repeat examination the diagnosis remains equivocal, the patient should be treated to prevent possible disease in the neonate. After treatment a quantitative VDRL titer should be followed monthly; if it rises four-fold, the patient should be treated a second time.

Congenital Syphilis. Proper treatment of the mother usually prevents active congenital syphilis in the neonate. However, infected infants may be clinically normal at birth, and the infant may be seronegative if the mother's infection was acquired late in pregnancy. The infant should be treated at birth if the mother has received no or inadequate treatment, or has been treated with drugs other than penicillin, or if the infant cannot be carefully followed up for several months after birth. CSF should be examined before treatment of the infant. If the CSF is normal, treatment may be with a single injection of 50,000 units per kilogram of benzathine penicillin G. If the CSF is abnormal, treatment should be with aqueous penicillin G, 50,000 units per kilogram intramuscularly or intravenously daily, given in two divided doses, for a minimum of ten days. Alternatively, a single daily intramuscular injection of procaine penicillin G, 50,000 units per kilogram, may be given for ten days. These recommendations are based upon the failure of benzathine penicillin to provide adequate treponemicidal levels in spinal fluid, and on evidence that aqueous or procaine penicillin does provide adequate CSF levels of penicillin.

Tetracycline should not be used to treat children of less than eight years of age. Antimicrobial agents other than penicillin are not recommended for treatment of congenital syphilis.

Follow-up Examinations. All patients with early syphilis or congenital syphilis should return for quantitative VDRL titers and clinical examination 3, 6, and 12 months after treatment. Patients with late latent syphilis should be examined also at 24 months after therapy; if CSF was not examined prior to therapy, a lumbar puncture should be done prior to discharge to rule out inadequately treated asymptomatic neurosyphilis.

The quantitative VDRL titer should return to normal within 12 months after therapy of primary syphilis or 24 months after therapy of secondary syphilis. In a small percentage of patients with early syphilis, the VDRL will remain reactive in low titer for long periods of time. Chronic low titer VDRL reactivity after therapy is much more common in late syphilis and should not be viewed with alarm. The FTA-ABS test usually remains positive for years, despite adequate therapy. The influence of therapy on serologic tests is shown in Table 306–5. A progressively rising VDRL titer after therapy (a four-fold or greater rise) is sufficient evidence for retreatment. Patients with treated early syphilis are fully susceptible to reinfection, and many clinical and serologic relapses after therapy are probably reinfections. As such they represent failures of proper epidemiologic case finding and preventive therapy of the patient's sexual contacts.

Patients with neurosyphilis should be followed with serologic tests for at least three years and with repeat examination of CSF at six-month intervals. The CSF pleocytosis is the first abnormality to disappear, but cell counts may not be normal for one to two years. The elevated CSF protein falls more slowly, followed by the positive CSF-VDRL test, which may take years to become negative. It is not known whether use of high-dose intravenous penicillin therapy will accelerate the return of CSF to normal. Rising CSF cell counts, protein, and VDRL titer obtained at follow-up are an indication for retreatment.

Epidemiologic Investigation and Treatment. All patients with syphilis should be reported to public health authorities. In the absence of an effective vaccine, control of syphilis depends on finding and treating persons with infectious lesions of primary and secondary syphilis before they can further transmit the disease, and on finding and treating persons with incubating syphilis before they have developed infectious lesions. All patients with early syphilis (less than one year) should be carefully interviewed by qualified persons to determine the nature of their recent sex contacts. Approximately 16 per cent of the named recent contacts of patients with early syphilis will be found to have active untreated syphilis on examination, and a similar proportion of individuals named as suspects or associates will also have active syphilis.

Most authorities, particularly in the United States, recommend treatment of sexual contacts of patients with early syphilis even if the contacts are clinically and serologically normal on examination. This is justifiable, because 30 per cent of clinically normal individuals named as contacts of persons with infectious lesions of syphilis within the previous 30 days will go on to develop syphilis if untreated. In general, preventive treatment is given to all sexual contacts of the past 90 days, although nearly all cases of syphilis in contacts will have developed within 60 days of exposure.

TABLE 306–5. EFFECT OF RECOMMENDED TREATMENT SCHEDULES ON SEROLOGIC TESTS FOR SYPHILIS

Stage of Disease When Treated	Time to Follow-up (Years)	Frequency of Positive Serologic Tests (%)	
		VDRL†	FTA-ABS
Primary (seropositive)*	2	0–3‡	>80
Secondary	2	0–24	>80
Late latent or tertiary	5–13	56–70	98

*Patients with primary syphilis and a positive VDRL test.
†Positive VDRL tests after treatment are almost always *low titer* unless reinfection or relapse has occurred.
‡The range of results reflects inclusion of data from several series, using different patient selection and treatment regimens.

Jarisch-Herxheimer Reaction. Up to 60 per cent of patients with early syphilis, and a significant proportion of patients with later stages of syphilis, experience a transient febrile reaction after therapy for syphilis. This usually occurs in the first few hours after therapy, peaks at six to eight hours, and disappears within 12 to 24 hours of therapy. Temperature elevation is usually low grade, and there is often associated myalgia, headache, and malaise. The skin lesions of secondary syphilis are often exacerbated during the Herxheimer reaction, and cutaneous lesions which were not visible may become visible. It is usually of no clinical significance and may be treated with salicylates in most cases. In patients with syphilis of the coronary ostia or of the optic nerve, there is a theoretical risk that local inflammation coincident with the Herxheimer reaction could precipitate serious damage. This is the subject of much discussion in the old literature, but there is little current evidence that "local Herxheimer reactions" constitute a significant risk to the patient. Corticosteroids have been used to prevent adverse effects of the Herxheimer reaction, but there is no evidence that they are clinically beneficial (other than reducing fever) or necessary. Institution of treatment with small doses of penicillin does not prevent the Herxheimer reaction.

The pathogenesis of the Herxheimer reaction is unclear. It may be due to liberation of antigens from the spirochetes. There is evidence of activation of the complement cascade, including transient consumption of C3, C4, C6, and C7, and of transient decrease in treponemal antibodies coincident with the Herxheimer reaction. There is also evidence for endotoxemia, obtained by positive limulus amebocyte gelation tests, at the time of the Herxheimer reaction, although *T. pallidum* does not contain biologically active endotoxin. These seemingly contradictory observations could be explained if the reaction resulted in release of endogenous endotoxin from the gut.

Persistence of Treponemes After Treatment. Studies in man and in rabbits have shown that spiral forms may be visualized by silver stains in lymph nodes after effective treatment. Living virulent treponemes have occasionally been recovered by rabbit inoculation from lymph nodes, CSF, or ocular fluids after effective treatment has been given. These documented cases of treponemal persistence are very rare, however. At present there is little reason to worry about persistence of virulent treponemes after therapy with penicillin, with the possible exception of central nervous system syphilis, which needs further evaluation. There is no evidence for selection of penicillin-resistant mutants of *T. pallidum* to date.

PROSPECTS FOR PREVENTION. Solid immunity develops in rabbits following prolonged infection with virulent *T. pallidum.* It has not yet been possible to transfer immunity passively in laboratory animals by either immune serum or immune lymphocytes alone, suggesting that both cellular and humoral systems are necessary for immunity. Rabbits have been effectively immunized with multiple injections of treponemes which have been rendered avirulent by irradiation or by exposure to cold. However, a very large number of injections and a large mass of treponemes are necessary to effect immunity in the laboratory animal. For this reason and since *T. pallidum* cannot yet be grown in a virulent state in cell-free medium, there is no immediate prospect for a vaccine. However, significant immunity does develop in man after prolonged infection. For the present, control depends entirely on clinical awareness on the part of physicians, adequate reporting to public health authorities, and vigorous application of epidemiologic investigation and preventive treatment of sexual contacts.

Drusin LM, Singer C, Valenti AJ, Armstrong D: Infectious syphilis mimicking neoplastic disease. Arch Intern Med 137:156, 1977. *A fascinating and frightening account of diagnostic problems caused by oral, rectal, or lymphatic syphilis, nearly leading to cancer surgery.*

Feher J, Somogyi T, Timmer M, Jozsa L: Early syphilitic hepatitis. Lancet 2:896, 1975. *A description of the frequency and histology of early syphilitic hepatitis.*

Fischer A, Kristensen JK, Husfelt V: Tertiary syphilis in Denmark 1961–1970. A description of 105 cases not previously diagnosed or specifically treated. Acta Dermatovener 56:485, 1976. *One of few studies of the prevalence of newly diagnosed late syphilis in the antibiotic era.*

Fulford KWM, Johnson N, Loveday C, Storey J, Tedder RS: Changes in intravascular complement and anti-treponemal antibody titres preceding the Jarisch-Herxheimer reaction in secondary syphilis. J Clin Exp Immunol 24:483, 1976. *A presentation of evidence that there may be an immunologic basis for the Jarisch-Herxheimer reaction.*

Gamble CN, Reardan JB: Immunopathogenesis of syphilitic glomerulonephritis: Elution of antitreponemal antibody from glomerular immune-complex deposits. N Engl J Med 292:449, 1975. *Clear evidence for an immune-complex etiology of syphilitic nephrosis.*

Gjestland T: The Oslo study of untreated syphilis: An epidemiologic investigation of the natural course of the syphilitic infection based upon a re-study of the Boeck-Bruusgaard material. Acta Derm Venereol 35:Suppl 34, 1955. *A medical classic, in which the long-term course of untreated syphilis is evaluated.*

Kaufman RE, Olansky DC, Wiesner PJ: The FTA-ABS (IgM) test for neonatal congenital syphilis: A critical review. J Am Vener Dis Assoc 1:79, 1974. *Unfortunately the initial hopes for the value of the FTA-ABS (IgM) test in congenital syphilis are dashed by experience.*

Lee TJ, Sparling PF: Syphilis. An algorithm. JAMA 242:1187, 1979. *An algorithm for management of patients who present with a positive VDRL or similar test.*

Lugar A, Schmidt B, Spendlingwimmer I, Horn F: Recent observations on the serology of syphilis. Br J Vener Dis 56:12, 1980. *A current evaluation of the merits of serologic tests for syphilis.*

Luxon L, Lees AJ, Greenwood RJ: Neurosyphilis today. Lancet 1:90, 1979. *A presentation of 17 cases, all of which were similar to types of neurosyphilis seen in the preantibiotic era.*

Magnuson HJ, Thomas EW, Olansky S, Kaplan BI, DeMello L, Cutler JC: Inoculation syphilis in human volunteers. Medicine 35:33, 1956. *A classic paper, in which prison volunteers were inoculated with virulent* T. pallidum. *Immunity to inoculation syphilis was observed only in individuals who had congenital or late syphilis.*

Musher DM, Schell RF, Jones RH, Jones AM: Lymphocyte transformation in syphilis: An in vitro correlate or immune suppression in vivo? Infect Immun 11:1261, 1975. *There is temporary T-lymphocyte hyporesponsiveness in secondary syphilis.*

Prewitt TA: Syphilitic aortic insufficiency. JAMA 211:637, 1970. *Observations on the epidemiology, serology, and clinical manifestations of syphilitic aortitis in the United States.*

Raskind MA, Eisdorfer C: Screening for syphilis in an aged psychiatrically impaired population. West J Med 125:361, 1976. *Syphilitic disease of the central nervous system may be more prevalent than hospital surveys suggest.*

Schroeter AL, Turner RH, Lucas JB, Brown WJ: Therapy for incubating syphilis: Effectiveness of gonorrhea treatment. JAMA 218:711, 1971. *A controlled study showing that single-dose procaine penicillin eradicates incubating syphilis.*

Sparling PF: Diagnosis and treatment of syphilis. N Engl J Med 284:642, 1971. *A critical review of syphilis serology.*

Syphilotherapy 1976: Position papers for the current USPHS recommendations. J Am Vener Dis Assoc 3:98, 1976. *Too many papers to be easily digested, but the definitive source for those who wish to have a summary of the available evidence.*

Tramont EC: Persistence of *Treponema pallidum* following penicillin G therapy: Report of two cases. JAMA 236:2206, 1976. *At least one of the cases of neurosyphilis probably was a true penicillin treatment failure.*

Turner TB: Syphilis and the treponematoses. *In* Mudd S (ed.): Infectious Agents and Host Reactions. Philadelphia, W. B. Saunders Company, 1970. *A scholarly review of the biology of the treponematoses.*

Wilner E, Brody JA: Prognosis of general paresis after treatment. Lancet 2:1370, 1968. *Neurosyphilis frequently shows clinical progression despite what is probably adequate therapy.*

Spirochetal Diseases Other Than Syphilis

307. NONSYPHILITIC TREPONEMATOSES*

Thomas Butler

DEFINITION. The nonsyphilitic treponematoses are the skin diseases called *yaws, bejel,* and *pinta.* They occur predominantly in tropical regions and are transmitted by skin contact with infected persons. Disfiguring ulcerations of the skin may be produced, and invasion of bone and other tissues has been described. Treatment with benzathine penicillin G is effective, and the World Health Organization has carried out extensive treatment campaigns in endemic areas.

ETIOLOGY. Yaws is caused by *Treponema pertenue;* pinta is caused by *T. carateum;* and bejel is caused by a treponeme that is indistinguishable from other species. Like *T. pallidum,* these treponemes are spirochetal bacteria with helical structures and measuring about 0.2 μ in diameter and 10 μ in length. They are visible by dark-field microscopy but cannot be cultivated in vitro.

DISTRIBUTION AND EPIDEMIOLOGY. Yaws is prevalent in rural areas of tropical Africa, the Americas, Southeast Asia, and Oceania. The highest incidence is in children between ages two and five years. Bejel occurs in Africa, in Eastern Mediterranean countries, on the Arabian peninsula, in Central Asia, and in Australia. It is most prevalent in arid regions. Pinta occurs in rural areas of tropical Central and South America. Pinta affects mostly older children and adolescents. Humans are the only known carriers of the nonsyphilitic treponematoses. The portal of entry is the skin, which must be broken, as by a scratch or insect bite, before the spirochete can enter. Transmission is believed to be by direct skin contact or indirectly by contaminated hands or fomites and is facilitated by conditions of poor personal hygiene and crowding.

CLINICAL FEATURES. *Yaws* produces a skin papule at the site of inoculation after an incubation period of three to four weeks. The most common sites are the legs and buttocks. The papule enlarges, ulcerates, and develops a serous crust from which treponemes can be recovered. Regional lymphadenitis may accompany the papule, which will heal spontaneously within six months. A generalized secondary rash will occur before or after healing of the initial lesion, and these rashes are also papular and often covered with brown crusts. Relapsing crops of lesions can occur. Papillomas may result, and the plantar surfaces of the feet are involved with hyperkeratotic lesions. Periostitis of long bones leads to tender bones, and fever may be present. Relapsing lesions may occur over several years, resulting in chronic ulcerations and destructive gummatous lesions affecting the skin and bones.

Bejel produces patches on the mucous membranes of the oral cavity and pharynx and can cause split papules at the mucocutaneous junction of the oral angles. Anal, genital, and other intertriginous skin areas can be affected by lesions that resemble secondary syphilis. Regional lymphadenitis is common, and generalized rashes are rare. Healing of these early lesions is followed by latency manifested by seropositivity or by late lesions that resemble tertiary syphilis. These include nodular ulcers of skin, deformities of bones, and gummatous lesions that can perforate the palate.

Pinta starts similarly as a cutaneous papule with regional lymphadenitis that is followed by a generalized maculopapular eruption. One to three years after healing of the initial lesion, large hyperpigmented macules that are brown or blue develop and subsequently lose their pigment and become white. The time required for lesions to pass through these stages varies, so that the same patient may have coexisting areas of increased pigment and loss of pigment.

DIAGNOSIS. By dark-field microscopy, the causative spirochetes from early skin lesions can be observed directly. Spirochetes have been demonstrated also in lymph node aspirates. Serologic tests for syphilis will detect cross-reacting antibodies in these diseases. The VDRL test, the serologic test for syphilis, and the fluorescent treponemal antibody absorption test will all give positive results if serum is taken at least two weeks after the appearance of initial lesions.

TREATMENT AND PROGNOSIS. Long-acting benzathine penicillin G given as 1.2 million units intramuscularly is the preferred treatment for patients with early lesions. For patients with late manifestations, this therapy should be repeated twice

*The author acknowledges the contribution of Dr. Thorstein Guthe on this subject in the 16th edition of *Cecil's Textbook of Medicine,* pages 1584–1589, and refers the interested reader to this more complete treatment of the subject, which includes photographs of skin lesions.

at approximately seven-day intervals. The early lesions will heal rapidly, and most seropositive patients will convert to seronegative status. Late destructive lesions take longer to show improvement.

PREVENTION. The prevalence of these diseases has been reduced in several areas of the world by mass treatment campaigns using penicillin. The World Health Organization has treated about 53 million cases of yaws and 350,000 cases of pinta in the field with good results. These campaigns, however, are not adequate to eradicate the disease. It has been suggested that reduction in transmission requires improvements in the sanitation and economic standards of people living in endemic areas.

Guthe T: Clinical serological and epidemiological features of framboesia tropica (yaws) and its control in rural communities. Acta Dermatovener 49:343, 1969.
Hackett CG, Guthe T: Some important aspects of yaws eradication. Bull WHO 15:869, 1956.
Hackett CJ, Lowenthal LJA: Differential Diagnosis of Yaws. WHO Monograph Series No. 45. Geneva, WHO, 1960.
Kantor I, Wilentz JM, Berger BB: Yaws. Arch Dermatol 103:546, 1971.

308. RELAPSING FEVER

Thomas Butler

DEFINITION. Relapsing fever is an acute febrile illness of humans that is caused by blood spirochetes belonging to *Borrelia* species. The two major kinds of relapsing fever are *louse-borne relapsing fever,* for which man is the reservoir and the body louse is the vector, and *tick-borne relapsing fever,* for which rodents and other animals are the predominant reservoirs and ticks are the vectors. The relapsing fevers are distributed worldwide in both tropical and temperate climates. The natural course of relapsing fever consists of one or more phases of fever and spirochetemia, which last for several days and are separated by afebrile intervals of several days without spirochetemia. Antiborrelial antibodies develop. Relapsing fever is usually a self-limited disease, but during epidemics of louse-borne relapsing fever high mortality rates have been recorded. The relapsing fevers are effectively treated with antibiotics, but after treatment patients will often experience a Jarisch-Herxheimer-like reaction that consists of a worsening of fever and signs of disease.

HISTORY. The term relapsing fever was coined by Craigie in Edinburgh in 1843. A year later in the same city, Henderson differentiated this disease from typhus fever. The etiologic agent of relapsing fever was first established in Berlin in 1873 by Obermeier, who used a microscope to observe spirochetes in the blood of patients. The transmission of *Borrelia* spirochetes by arthropod vectors was suggested in 1891 by Flugge, who postulated the body louse as a vector, and in 1905 by Dutton and Todd, who demonstrated the infection in the *Ornithodorus* ticks of Africa. The genus name *Borrelia* was proposed in 1907 in honor of the French bacteriologist A. Borrel.

Relapsing fever is certainly a disease of antiquity, and its known epidemic potential, particularly in times of war, migrations, and other conditions that favor human crowding and poor hygiene, suggests that relapsing fever has had a major impact on human history. Before the advent of microscopic diagnosis, however, it was not possible to distinguish relapsing fever from similar scourges of humankind such as malaria, typhoid fever, and typhus fever, and so the history of relapsing fever before 1873 is only speculative. Between 1910 and 1945, there have been at least seven epidemics of relapsing fever in North Africa, Sudan, Ethiopia, West Africa, Central Africa, Eastern Europe, and Russia. There were an estimated 15 million cases with over 5 million deaths and case fatality rates as high as 73 per cent.

ETIOLOGY. Relapsing fevers are caused by blood spirochetes of *Borrelia* species, which belong to the order of bacteria called Spirochaetales. *Borrelia* species differ from the other two genera of pathogenic spirochetes, *Leptospira* and *Treponema,* by structure, biochemical characteristics, and antigenic determinants. *Borrelia* spirochetes are spiral organisms that measure 5 to 40 μ in length and about 0.5 μ in diameter. They are too thin to be seen reliably by light microscopy of wet preparations, but they are easily visible when viewed by dark-field or phase contrast microscopy. They are stainable with aniline dyes, such as Wright or Giemsa stains, and can be visualized well in tissue by the application of silver stains, such as the Dieterle or Warthin-Starry stains. Like other bacteria, these spirochetes possess an outer cell wall (outer envelope) and an inner cytoplasmic membrane that contains muramic acid. Between the cell wall and the cytoplasmic membrane there are 15 to 20 flagella, which are anchored to the ends of the spirochete and wrap around its body until they meet at the middle region. In three dimensions the spirochetes have a helical configuration consisting of about four to ten coils with amplitudes of about 1 to 4 μ. Under dark-field or phase contrast microscopy, *Borrelia* spirochetes display an active corkscrew-like motility consisting of rotation and motion in helical waves to produce translational movement. *Borreliae* are microaerophilic and fermentative in their growth characteristics. They require long chain fatty acids for growth and are cultivable in Kelly's medium. *B. recurrentis,* the agent of louse-borne relapsing fever, is more fastidious than the tick-borne *Borreliae* and requires the further addition of asparagine and choline to Kelly's medium. The *Borreliae* grow slowly in Kelly's medium, with doubling times of 18 to 26 hours.

The species names of the tick-borne *Borrelia* are derived from the species names of *Ornithodorus* tick vectors that carry them. The more common ones in North America are *B. turicatae, B. hermsii,* and *B. parkeri* and in Africa *B. duttonii. Borrelia* spirochetes produce fever when injected into rabbits but do not possess endotoxin. In general, *Borrelia* spirochetes do not elicit acute inflammation, do not produce abscesses, and are confined predominantly to the plasma space of their mammalian hosts.

The relapsing feature of *Borrelia* infection has been attributed to antigenic variation in the infecting population of spirochetes. In experimental infections of rats with *B. hermsii,* three separate serotypes emerged sequentially during relapses, and specific antibody appeared in response to each of the antigenic variants.

DISTRIBUTION AND EPIDEMIOLOGY. The geographic distribution of the relapsing fevers is widespread, with occurrence in most continents of the world including the Americas, Europe, Africa, and Asia. Louse-borne relapsing fever has disappeared from the United States but still occurs in parts of South America, Europe, Africa, and Asia. From 1960 to 1979 louse-borne relapsing fever was documented in Ethiopia and Sudan. Although accurate statistics on the incidence of this disease are not available, Ethiopia appears to be the country with the highest incidence, estimated at approximately 10,000 or more cases a year. Tick-borne relapsing fever occurs in endemic foci in southern British Columbia, in the western United States, in the plateau regions of Mexico, and in Central and South America. This disease is present in all areas of Africa except for the Sahara Desert and the rain forest belt. It occurs also in Spain and Portugal. In Asia, tick-borne relapsing fever has been reported in Cyprus, Israel, Syria, Turkey, Iraq, Iran, southern Russia, China, Afghanistan, and India. Accurate statistics on tick-borne relapsing fever are not available, but the sporadic nature of human contact with rodent ticks and the small numbers of established diagnoses suggest that this form of relapsing fever occurs less frequently in humans than louse-borne relapsing fever.

The two types of relapsing fever, louse-borne and tick-borne, differ so much in their epidemiology that they must be considered separately. *Epidemic relapsing fever* refers to the louse-borne kind and *endemic* or *sporadic relapsing fever* to the tick-borne variety. The only species of *Borrelia* that causes louse-borne relapsing fever is *B. recurrentis.* Its vector is the human body louse, *Pediculus humanus humanus,* and the only known natural reservoir is humans. Thus, the cycle of infection is from person to person via the louse. Body lice acquire the infection by feeding on a spirochetemic person, and they remain infected for their entire life span, which is 10 to 61 days under laboratory conditions. The ingested spirochetes pass through the esophagus to the midgut, where they penetrate the gut epithelium to reach the hemolymph in which they will multiply. Spirochetes do not reach the salivary glands or ovaries of the lice. Therefore, infection is not transmitted to humans by bites of lice, and infection cannot be transmitted transovarially to offspring of infected lice. Infection is believed to be transmitted to humans by the crushing of lice on the skin, which allows liberated spirochetes to penetrate through a bite site or through intact skin. Body lice prefer the normal human body temperature of 37° C to higher temperatures; thus, lice are likely to leave the skin of a febrile patient to go to another person. This may explain, in part, the rapid transmission of infection during epidemics.

The persons at greatest risk for acquiring louse-borne relapsing fever are those living under crowded, unhygienic conditions that favor infestation with body lice. Migrant workers and soldiers in war are particularly prone to develop this infection. Males are at much greater risk than females, presumably because their lives more commonly expose them to infected lice. A strain-specific, short-lived acquired immunity develops following infection. This immunity helps to explain why migrant workers coming into an endemic area are more susceptible to infection than are the permanent inhabitants. In some endemic areas, such as Addis Ababa, Ethiopia, there is an increased incidence during the cool winter season when people wear heavier clothing that becomes louse-infested.

The species of *Borrelia* that cause tick-borne relapsing fever are numerous and include *B. duttoni* in East Africa, *B. hispanica* in Spain, *B. persica* in Asia, and *B. hermisii* and *B. turicatae* in North America. The vectors of these organisms are argasid ticks of the genus *Ornithodorus*. The major reservoirs of tick-borne relapsing fever are wild rodents, including squirrels, deer mice, rats, chipmunks, and rabbits, and occasionally lizards, toads, turtles, and owls. The infection is passed between the reservoir animals by tick bites, and humans are accidental hosts when they come into contact with infected animal ticks. The exception to the animal reservoirs may be *B. duttoni* in East Africa, which is carried by the domestic tick *Ornithodorus moubata*, for which humans appear to be the reservoir.

Ticks acquire the infection by biting and sucking blood from a spirochetemic animal. The spirochetes, after entering the hemocele, invade other tissues of the tick, including the salivary glands, the coxal glands on the legs, and the ovaries. Transmission of the infection to animals or to humans follows injection of infected saliva through the bite site or intact skin. Ticks are more durable vectors than body lice, being able to survive as long as 15 years between blood meals and to harbor viable spirochetes for years. In addition, female ticks can pass *Borrelia* spirochetes transovarially to their offspring, thus permitting ticks to be infective without having previously bitten an infected host.

Persons at greatest risk of infection are those who come in contact with infected ticks from wild rodents. In the United States the largest outbreak of tick-borne relapsing fever occurred in 62 campers and employees in the National Park at the Northern Rim of the Grand Canyon, Arizona, in 1973. They had all slept in log cabins that were inhabited by wild rodents. Another outbreak in Washington State affected 42 boy scouts who also camped in a log cabin. In tropical countries, people who live in dwellings that are not rodent proof are prone to infection.

PATHOGENESIS AND PATHOLOGY. After exposure to an infected louse or tick, spirochetes enter through the skin, and in the subcutaneous tissue they have access to the blood and lymphatic circulations. There are no symptoms during an incubation period estimated to last from 4 to 18 days after exposure while the spirochetes are dividing in the blood plasma. No local lesions develop at the skin site of entry, and there is no evidence for an intracellular phase of multiplication or sites of attachment of spirochetes to host cells. After the spirochetes have built up to a concentration of 10^6 to 10^8 per ml of blood, the symptoms of shaking chills, fever, headache, and fatigue begin suddenly. These symptoms may be continuous or intermittent and usually increase in intensity over several days. At this early stage of illness large numbers of spirochetes are regularly present in the plasma space and are easily visible on blood smears. A small number of the spirochetes are within circulating polymorphonuclear phagocytes, and some spirochetes have been phagocytosed by fixed macrophages of the reticuloendothelial system of the spleen, liver, and bone marrow. A decrease in blood platelets leads to diffuse petechial skin rashes. In some severely ill patients who have jaundice, liver function studies reveal intrahepatic obstruction of bile flow and hepatocellular inflammation.

There also is disseminated intravascular coagulation, which contributes to the decrease in platelets and produces prolonged prothrombin and partial thromboplastin times and elevated titers of fibrinogen-fibrin degradation products. During acute relapsing fever, there are decreased levels of serum complement, Hageman factor, and prekallikrein, suggesting that activation of certain plasma proteins contributes to the pathogenesis of features such as hypotension and disseminated intravascular coagulation.

In the hours after antibiotic treatment, most patients undergo a Jarisch-Herxheimer reaction characterized by rigor, rising temperature, and falling blood pressure. Disseminated intravascular coagulation is accelerated, and spirochetes are phagocytosed at increased rates while being cleared from the plasma. Some patients not receiving antibiotic treatment undergo a similar spontaneous crisis. It is during this crisis or Jarisch-Herxheimer reaction that patients are at the greatest risk of dying.

Autopsies performed in Ethiopia and Sudan in fatal cases of louse-borne relapsing fever showed characteristic disease most regularly in the spleen, liver, heart, and brain. The spleen is enlarged to as much as 900 grams, and the cut surface shows white microabscesses, which consist of necrosis and hemorrhage in the white pulp. Occasionally there are splenic infarcts and splenic rupture. The liver is also enlarged, often to over 2000 grams. The midzonal region shows scattered necrosis and hemorrhage, and Kupffer's cells are enlarged and numerous. The heart is normal in size but frequently shows evidence of myocarditis, consisting of interstitial edema and a cellular infiltrate of lymphocytes and plasma cells. Examination of the brain usually indicates cerebral edema, and in some cases there is hemorrhage into the subarachnoid space or cerebrum. Thus, the immediate causes of death in relapsing fever are varied and in any particular case may be liver failure, cerebral hemorrhage, or acute cardiac arrhythmia caused by myocarditis.

The majority of patients with relapsing fever recover from illness either with or without antibiotic treatment. Patients develop antiborrelial antibodies that can agglutinate, kill, or opsonize the spirochetes. In the absence of opsonizing antibody, spirochetes are rapidly phagocytosed and digested by polymorphonuclear leukocytes. These antibodies participate also in rendering patients immune to future infection with the same serotype of *Borrelia*.

CLINICAL SYNDROMES. The illness begins abruptly with shaking chills, fever, headache, and fatigue. Most patients have these symptoms almost continuously throughout the day, whereas some patients report the intermittent appearance of these symptoms several times a day. Patients complain frequently of myalgias, arthralgia, anorexia, dry cough, and abdominal pains. These symptoms are usually mild on the first day of illness and increase in intensity over a few days, until they result in prostration and a visit to a physician. The nonspecific nature of the symptoms leads the patient or the physician to believe the illness is flu-like.

The temperature is elevated in the range of 38.5° to 40° C, and the pulse rate is increased to about 115 beats per minute. The blood pressure is lowered to about 105/70 mm Hg. Patients appear lethargic or may be delirious. Common physicial signs are conjunctival injection, petechial skin rash that is more apparent on the trunk than on the extremities, and palpable liver and spleen. Jaundice is occasionally present. Generalized muscle weakness is common. Some patients have mental confusion or delirium or nuchal rigidity.

The laboratory results include a blood smear positive for spirochetes. The white blood cell count is usually normal, with increased band forms and decreased eosinophils. The platelet counts are often less than 50,000 per cubic millimeter, and there may be prolongation of prothrombin time and partial thromboplastin time. Liver function test results are frequently abnormal, with elevations in concentrations of serum alanine aminotransferase and bilirubin that are evenly divided between the conjugated and unconjugated fractions. Renal function studies often show mild abnormalities of the serum urea nitrogen and creatinine values, and patients may have proteinuria and microscopic hematuria.

DIAGNOSIS. The diagnosis of relapsing fever depends on the demonstration of spirochetemia. In most patients, this is readily accomplished by obtaining peripheral blood by either fingerstick or venipuncture methods and preparing a thin film on a microscope slide. *Borrelia* spirochetes are stained blue by aniline dyes. Thus a routine blood smear stained with Wright's or Giemsa stain is adequate. Blood smears, thin or thick, prepared for examination for malaria parasites, are also satisfactory. The spirochetes are 5 to 20 μ in length and lie in the plasma spaces between blood cells or may overlie the blood cells. Febrile patients with relapsing fever typically have large numbers of spirochetes in the blood, approximately 10^6 to 10^8 per ml, or several per high-power field. Patients who are afebrile in the interval between relapses will have smears negative for *Borrelia* and should be re-examined when the fever reappears. Spirochetemia also may be detected by dark-field or phase contrast microscopy. A drop of fresh blood is diluted with another drop of 0.9 per cent NaCl and overlaid with a coverslip. Spirochetes are readily identified by their characteristic rotational motility.

Serologic testing has been employed in endemic areas for seroepidemiology and examination of convalescent patients. Serum of convalescent patients contains antibodies that produce agglutination and immobilization of living spirochetes and that fix complement during reaction with spirochetal antigens. None of these tests, however, is standardized or commercially available for general use.

TREATMENT AND PROGNOSIS. The relapsing fevers are effectively treated with tetracycline and erythromycin. Tetracycline is the treatment of choice except in children less than seven years old and in pregnant women in whom tetracycline may stain developing fetal teeth. Recent studies in Ethiopia indicate that a single oral dose of tetracycline, 500 mg, is as effective in clearing spirochetemia and preventing relapse as a longer course of treatment. Erythromycin, 500 mg, given orally as a single dose, is equally effective and is a satisfactory alternative to tetracycline. For patients unable to take oral medication, intravenous injections of 250 mg of tetracycline or erythromycin are curative. For children weighing less than 30 kg, the dosage of tetracycline or erythromycin should be reduced to approximately 10 mg per kilogram. Penicillin G has been used to treat relapsing fever, but its use has been associated with slow clearance of spirochetes and relapses following treatment.

In most patients with louse-borne relapsing fever and in some with tick-borne relapsing fever, antibiotic treatment provokes a distressing Jarisch-Herxheimer-like reaction. During the reaction, the patient is extremely uncomfortable, feeling very cold with severe headache and myalgia. The blood leukocyte and platelet counts sharply decrease, and spirochetes disappear from the plasma. The patient may require intravenous infusions of 0.9 per cent NaCl to maintain adequate blood pressure. Over several hours, the temperature declines and the patient's condition improves. Attempts to ameliorate the severity of the reaction by giving antipyretic or anti-inflammatory drugs have not been entirely successful. The best approach is to anticipate reaction and to provide intensive nursing care and intravenous fluid support during the first day of treatment.

The prognosis is favorable for complete recovery in 95 per cent or more of treated cases of relapsing fever. Bad prognostic signs are the presence of jaundice, high spirochete counts in the blood, and hypotension. The prognosis of untreated disease is grave in the case of louse-borne relapsing fever, for which mortality rates of 40 per cent have been reported during recent epidemics. Untreated patients will also experience relapses. In louse-borne relapsing fever, the first attack lasts about six days and is followed by an afebrile period of about nine days. There usually is one relapse, which will last only about two days. In tick-borne relapsing fever, the first attack lasts about three days and is followed by an interval of about seven days, after which an average of three relapses occur, each lasting about two days. Relapses are usually milder in intensity than the first attacks.

PREVENTION. Available approaches for the control of relapsing fevers include the detection and treatment of human cases, vector control, rodent control, and public health education. Vaccines are not available for the prevention of relapsing fever. For louse-borne relapsing fever, the detection and treatment of cases has the effects of reducing the reservoir of infection and consequently of reducing transmission. More important is the control of louse infestation. Delousing of clothing and bodies with insecticides such as DDT can be employed, as can the application of insect repellents. In known epidemic situations, prophylactic antibiotics are a temporary measure to contain spread of infection to persons at high risk. The eventual control of this disease requires improvements in personal hygiene and housing conditions. For tick-borne relapsing fever, the treatment of human cases has no impact on the animal reservoirs. It is not possible to control this infection in wild rodents. Campers and hikers going into endemic areas should be advised to avoid cabins that are inhabited by rodents and ticks and to apply topical tick repellants to the skin.

Bryceson ADM, Parry EHO, Perine PL, Warrell DA, Vukotich D, Leithead CS: Louse-borne relapsing fever. A clinical and laboratory study of 62 cases in Ethiopia and a reconsideration of the literature. Q J Med 39:129, 1970.

Burgdorfer W: The epidemiology of the relapsing fevers. *In* Johnson RC (ed.): The Biology of Parasitic Spirochetes. New York, Academic Press, 1976, p 191.

Butler T, Hazen P, Wallace CK, Awoke S: *Borrelia recurrentis* infection: Pathogenesis of fever and petechiae. J Infect Dis 140:665, 1979.

Butler T, Jones PK, Wallace CK: *Borrelia recurrentis* infection: Single dose antibiotic regimens and management of Jarisch-Herxheimer reaction. J Infect Dis 137:573, 1978.

Warrell DA, Perine PL, Krause DW, Bing DH, MacDougal SJ: Pathophysiology and immunology of the Jarisch-Herxheimer–like reaction in louse-borne relapsing fever: Comparison of tetracycline and slow-release penicillin. J Infect Dis 147:898, 1983.

309. TROPICAL PHAGEDENIC ULCER

Anthony D. M. Bryceson

DEFINITION. Tropical phagedenic ulcer is an acute specific ulcer of skin and subcutaneous tissue, associated in its early stages with infection with *Borrelia vincentii* and anaerobic bacteria of the genus *Bacteroides*. The ulcer is usually situated below the knee, has certain typical characteristics, and commonly becomes chronic.

ETIOLOGY AND PATHOGENESIS. *B. vincentii* is a loosely coiled spirochete 5 to 10 μ long; it is a common oral commensal. *Bacteroides* is a curved, cigar-shaped rod 5 to 14 μ long, often beaded when stained; it, too, is an oral commensal and is common in moist soils. Either or both of these organisms are present in the acute stage of the ulcer. They gain entry through a tiny wound in the skin. Experimentally, they will cause ulcers only in malnourished subjects or animals. Other organisms, especially cocci, may also be found in established ulcers.

EPIDEMIOLOGY. The condition is common and widespread in the tropics and rare elsewhere. It may be found in all climates and at any altitude. In some countries hot wet areas are especially affected. In parts of some countries, active ulcers have a prevalence of 2 per cent and scars of 15 per cent. It is often the most common complaint of hospital outpatients, representing up to one third of new patients, and may be the most common cause of surgical admissions.

Tropical ulcer is typically a sporadic disease, especially affecting adolescent males. It is most common in the lower socioeconomic groups. Although the patient may not appear grossly malnourished, there is a clear clinical and experimental association with malnutrition. No specific nutritional deficiency has been identified, but tropical ulcer is rare in those who eat adequate animal protein and is especially common in labor gangs, ill-kept prisoners of war, and other physically deprived groups, among whom it can appear as an epidemic. This association with malnutrition and deprivation is also found in two other infections with the same organisms, cancrum oris (noma) and trench mouth (Vincent's angina).

PATHOGENESIS, CLINICAL MANIFESTATIONS, AND PROGNOSIS. The lesion starts at the site of a minor wound or insect bite, which the patient can usually recall. Often the site is neglected or treated with a native remedy, or sucked by mouth to clean it. A small blister appears, containing serosanguineous fluid, and ruptures, exposing an ash gray slough which has a characteristic foul smell. The ulcer spreads rapidly to involve subcutaneous tissue and often muscle and tendon down to bone. It reaches its final diameter of 1 to 40 cm in a few days. The central slough liquefies, exposing a gray-brown base. The ulcer is circular, with a raised edge and surrounding edema, and may encircle the limb. It is painful and bleeds easily. Regional lymph nodes may be enlarged and tender. The most common sites of tropical ulcers are over the bony parts of the leg at the level of, or just above, the ankle.

Histologic examination shows three layers: a superficial layer of coagulation necrosis in which organisms are abundant, a layer of granulation tissue, and a highly vascular base. The edge of the ulcer shows pseudoepitheliomatous hyperplasia.

Fifty per cent of ulcers heal spontaneously within three months, and 80 per cent within six months.

Chronic ulcers become less painful and lose their odor. They become irregular with a rigid base and edge and are filled with pink granulation tissue. Histologically there is much surrounding fibrosis. Squamous cell carcinoma develops in 9 per cent of chronic ulcers after a period of three months to 50 years. Tetanus and gangrene are rarer complications.

DIAGNOSIS. In the acute stage the appearances and smell are typical. The specific organisms can be demonstrated in a drop of fluid aspirated from the ulcer, either by dark-field microscopy or by Gram stain or staining with 1 per cent carbolfuchsin. Histologic examination is seldom needed. It is more difficult to identify the cause of chronic ulcers. The differential diagnosis includes yaws (serology and radiology), cutaneous diphtheria (climate, culture), Buruli ulcer (undermining, acid-fast bacilli), squamous cell carcinoma and melanoma (histology), and varicose ulcers (age group, venous abnormality).

TREATMENT. In the acute stage the patient is put to bed and the limb elevated. The ulcer is dressed with sterile saline or resorcinol monoacetate (Euresol). Hydrogen peroxide may be used for a few days to help slough out. Strong antiseptics are contraindicated. Penicillin is given by intramuscular injection for seven days; procaine penicillin, 600,000 units twice daily, or penicillin aluminium monostearate,* 1,200,000 units daily, is suitable. Metronidazole,† 200 mg thrice daily by mouth, is a suitable alternative to penicillin. The synergistic effect of the two drugs has not been tested.

This treatment controls the infection and cleans the ulcer. Ulcers under 5 cm in diameter should now heal satisfactorily. Ulcers over 5 cm should be grafted with split skin.

Chronic ulcers are treated initially in the same way and are then completely excised and grafted. A walking plaster may then be applied, and healing is complete within three weeks.

*No longer available in the United States.
†Investigational drug for this purpose.

PREVENTION. Good nutrition and physical health are the best preventives. Legs should be covered while walking in country where thorns or sharp grass may scratch them. Minor cuts and scratches should be washed and treated with local antiseptic.

Edington GM, Gillies HM: Tropical ulcers. *In* Pathology in the Tropics. London, Arnold, 1976, p 726. *Good pathologic account.*

Kuberski T, Koteka G: An epidemic of tropical ulcer in the Cook Islands. Am J Trop Med Hyg 29:291, 1980. *The little-known epidemic presentation.*

Lindler RR, Adeniyi-Jones C: The effect of metronidazole on tropical ulcers. Trans R Soc Trop Med Hyg 62:712, 1968. *One of the very few papers on chemotherapy.*

Lowenthal LJA: Tropical phagedenic ulcer: A review. *In* Lincicome DR (ed.): International Review of Tropical Medicine. New York, Academic Press, 1963, p 267. *Still the best major review.*

310. RAT BITE FEVERS

J. Bruce McClain

The term *rat-bite fevers* refers to illnesses caused by *Streptobacillus moniliformis* or *Spirillum minus.*

S. moniliformis previously has been called *Actinomyces muris, Streptothrix muris ratti,* or *Haverhilia multiformis.* It is an aerobic gram-negative branching rod in the same family as mycobacteria, 2 to 15 μ in length, and an inhabitant of the respiratory tracts of mice and rats.

Spirillum minus, sometimes called *Spirillum minor,* is a twisted gram-negative aerobic rod with bipolar tufts of flagella, which has not been grown on artificial media but which has been passed to animals. It is 2 to 5 μ in length and has been identified in the drainage from interstitial keratitis in rats.

EPIDEMIOLOGY. Neither streptobacillary nor spirillary rat-bite fevers are reportable diseases. The Centers for Disease Control receive two to three isolates annually. A survey from the 1940's of 400 rat bites reported 16 cases of clinical rat-bite fever, 8 of which had organisms identified. The highest reported rate of post–rat-bite fevers is 10 per cent. Many factors make the current prevalence in the United States difficult to determine: innate antibiotic responsiveness, the difficulty with which the causative organisms are isolated, and the lack of widely available serologic tests. The majority of recently reported cases are in laboratory workers with definite bite exposure, and these individuals constitute the population at highest risk. Other animals have been reported to transmit the disease, including weasels, dogs, cats, pigs, and mice. Streptobacillary fever may be transmitted by nonbite mechanisms, as demonstrated by an outbreak associated with consumption of unpasteurized milk in Haverhill, Massachusetts, and case reports of illness associated with trauma.

CLINICAL MANIFESTATIONS. ***Streptobacillary Fever (Haverhill Fever).*** The initial injury heals promptly in most cases. The incubation period from bite exposure is usually 3 to 4 days, with a range of 1 to 22 days. In the Haverhill outbreak most cases occurred within three days of exposure to contaminated milk. Ninety-five percent of patients will complain of fever, frequently in the 102° to 104° F range, usually with a sudden onset and a toxic effect on the patient. Bifrontal headache, nausea, vomiting, and myalgias usually accompany the fever initially. Occasionally there is a lessening of fever after a few days, with subsequent return of higher temperatures. A maculopapular rash develops within the first five days of illness in almost all patients. The rash is distributed distally and may involve the palms and soles of the feet. Occasionally the centers of the 0.3- to 1-cm lesions develop pustules. A fine desquamation occurs on healing in 20 per cent of patients. Arthritis occurs in 70 per cent of patients on the second through 14th days of illness and almost always involves more than one joint, especially the wrists and elbows. The arthritis is nondeforming, although in untreated cases it may persist for months and has been known to damage joints. Less frequently reported complications of streptobacillary fever are endocarditis, pericarditis, soft tissue abscesses, and amnionitis.

Spirillary Fever (Sodoku). The initial injury heals promptly in most cases, although induration, ulceration, or eschar may develop at the site of injury with the onset of illness. Regional adenopathy is frequently present. The incubation period is generally greater than 7 days, with a range of 1 to 36 days. The onset of sodoku is less abrupt than in streptobacillary fever, and temperatures are in the 102° F range. Fevers are recurrent with several days between episodes. Headaches, nausea, and vomiting are common, and a roseolar-urticarial rash is seen in half the patients. Arthritis is rare.

Spirilla are poorly characterized organisms. It seems that on occasion nonsodoku spirilla may cause illness in humans. These illnesses tend to be prolonged and to resemble endocarditis.

LABORATORY MANIFESTATIONS. Most patients with spirillary fever and less than 20 per cent with streptobacillary fever have false-positive results of serologic tests for syphilis. Leukocyte counts in both illnesses range from normal to 30,000 per cubic millimeter. Results of urinalysis usually are normal, although nephritic sediments have been seen in sodoku.

DIAGNOSIS. The diagnosis of streptobacillary rat-bite fever is made by culturing the organism from blood, joint fluid, or tissue or by demonstrating a four-fold rise in titer by an agglutination test that is available through the Centers for Disease Control. Titers may persist for two to four years. Streptobacilli from blood cultures will usually grow within a week. Their cultivation is complicated by requirements for animal serum in the medium and a CO_2 atmosphere as well as sensitivity to sodium polyanethol sulfonate (Liquoid, SPS), which is found in most automated blood culture systems at levels that are inhibitory (over 0.01 per cent). Specific measures to cultivate the organisms must be arranged with the laboratory.

Spirillary fever may be diagnosed by inoculation of mice with infected tissues or fluids and demonstration of morphologically compatible organisms in the peripheral blood by dark-field examination. Occasionally the diagnosis has been established by dark-field examination of peripheral blood or eschars in humans.

The differential diagnosis of rat-bite fever includes Still's disease, arthritis associated with hepatitis B, rubella, gonococcemia, meningococcemia, rickettsial disease, hypersensitivity vasculitis, and leptospirosis.

TREATMENT AND PROGNOSIS. Penicillin G, 1.2 million units per day in divided doses, is the treatment of choice for both types of rat-bite fever. Ampicillin or penicillin V, 2 grams per day is effective oral therapy. The duration of therapy should total ten days, and parenteral therapy may be followed with oral therapy. Higher doses have been used in endocarditis. The streptobacillary illness has responded to parenteral cephalosporin therapy. Oral cephalosporin therapy should not be substituted until more information is available. In the patient allergic to penicillin, both forms of the illness may be treated with tetracyclines, chloramphenicol, or streptomycin.

About 12 per cent of untreated patients with streptobacillary disease die, although in most cases the disease will run a course of 25 days with spontaneous resolution. Treatment with penicillin G will resolve most symptoms in one to four days, although patients who receive less than 400,000 units per day of penicillin have had illnesses persisting for several weeks. Penicillin resistance has been reported and should be kept in mind if treatment failure is suspected.

The mortality in untreated spirillary fever is 7 per cent. Without therapy the disease will last an average of 35 days. Spontaneous resolution is the rule. Penicillin therapy will cause resolution of symptoms in one or two days. A Herxheimer reaction is common.

Anderson LC, Leary SL, Manning PJ: Rat-bite fever in animal research laboratory personnel. Lab Anim Sci 33:292, 1983. *A case report and review of the clinical and epidemiologic characteristics of the group at risk for disease.*

Kowal J: Spirillum fever, report of a case and review of the literature. N Engl J Med 264:123, 1961. *An interesting review of nonsodoku spirillary illness.*

Roughgarden JW: Antimicrobial therapy of rat-bite fever. Arch Intern Med 116:39, 1965. *A comprehensive review of therapeutic results with various antimicrobials.*

Watkins CG: Ratbite fever. J Pediatr 28:429, 1946. *The best review of the clinical syndromes of rat-bite fever.*

311. LEPTOSPIROSIS

J. Bruce McClain

The term *leptospirosis* describes an infection with any serovar of *Leptospira interrogans*, regardless of the syndrome. Old names such as *canicola fever, Fort Bragg fever, Weil's disease,* or *peapicker's disease* are potentially confusing and should be avoided.

ETIOLOGY. *Leptospira* consists of two species: *interrogans*, which is pathogenic, and *biflexa*, which is saprophytic. Serotyping and serogrouping have established over 170 serovars in the species *L. interrogans*. The proper designation of a serovar is *L. interrogans* serovar pomona not *L.* pomona. The latter usage, although widespread, represents serovars as species and is incorrect.

The organism is a tightly coiled spirochete with one axial filament. With a diameter of about 0.15 μm, it is invisible on light microscopy and must be visualized by phase contrast or dark-field microscopy. It is easily cultured on Fletcher's medium and is an obligate aerobe.

EPIDEMIOLOGY. Leptospirosis is a ubiquitous enzootic disease. Reservoirs of infection include rodents, skunks, foxes, domestic livestock, and dogs. Many animals exhibit a prolonged urinary shedding of the organism without clinical illness. When humans contact infected tissues, fluids, or contaminated waters, they contract the illness. Transmission may occur through cuts, mucous membranes, and probably unabraded skin. In earlier series illness was reported associated with occupational exposure such as among sanitation, dairy, slaughter house, or fishing workers. The epidemiology has changed over the last 15 years, owing to the advent of multiuse land development with farmlands draining into recreational bodies of water. More recent reports indicate that at least half of cases result from nonvocational exposure. There has been a corresponding decrease in the age of persons infected, although males still comprise 80 per cent of cases. In the United States between 50 and 150 cases are reported annually. The national attack rate is 0.05 per 100,000, although rates as high as 1 per 100,000 occur in Hawaii. The disease is probably substantially underreported. Leptospirosis shows an annual peak in the summer months and has had a 4- to 5-year periodicity in attack rates over the last 25 years.

PATHOLOGY AND PATHOGENESIS. Gross anatomic findings in patients dying from leptospirosis are: (1) widespread hemorrhage in skin, mucosa, serosa, heart, lungs, spleen, liver, and kidneys; (2) hepatomegaly without prominent splenomegaly; (3) bile staining; and (4) enlargement of the heart and kidneys.

Histologic examination of the liver in autopsy material shows nonspecific inflammatory changes, bile stasis, and disruption of the limiting plate. Biopsy materials under light and electron microscopic examination show similar features with less destruction of architecture.

Kidneys in autopsy series show a spectrum of changes that reflect an initial tubular injury that is acellular. As the disease progresses and antibodies appear, inflammatory changes occur that result in an overt interstitial nephritis with disruption of the tubular architecture. Biopsy series show similar changes to a lesser degree. The glomeruli have foot-process fusion and mesangial hypertrophy but are otherwise spared. Leptospires are seen in most of the renal material.

Hemorrhagic manifestations are associated with areas of capillary wall damage and necrosis with perivascular round cell infiltration.

Striated muscle is frequently involved with degeneration of individual fibrils and loss of architecture associated with inflammation. This pattern is considered specific for leptospirosis. The myocardium is affected with similar changes. In one fourth of autopsy cases, myocarditis is listed as serious enough to be a contributing cause of death.

The mechanism by which *Leptospira* organisms cause damage to tissues is obscure. Toxic factors have been identified in culture supernatants, but organisms that do not produce some of these factors may cause serious disease. Early in the illness the evidence favors a direct leptospiral toxicity to certain tissues, while later in the illness damage secondary to inflammation is more pronounced.

CLINICAL FEATURES. Most natural infections appear 7 to 14 days after exposure, although the incubation period ranges from 2 to 20 days. The length of the incubation period has no prognostic significance. Clinical findings vary among reported series, but a general description includes: fever and headache, 95 per cent; myalgia and conjunctival suffusion, 80 per cent (in nonmilitary series suffusion is reported less often); gastrointestinal symptoms (nausea, vomiting, or abdominal pain), 60 per cent; cough or pharyngitis, 40 per cent; lymphadenopathy, 25 per cent; hepatomegaly, 15 per cent; rash, 10 per cent; and jaundice and gastrointestinal hemorrhage, 5 per cent each. Less commonly reported symptoms are splenomegaly, uveitis, and diarrhea. About one half of patients exhibit a "brutal beginning" with an abrupt onset of symptoms over a one- to two-hour period. The clinical picture that should bring leptospirosis to mind is a febrile patient with severe muscle aches and pain who is nauseated or vomiting. The presence of conjunctival suffusion may be very helpful in detecting the illness in military populations. It is not conjunctivitis as seen in allergic or viral conjunctivitis, but rather a *pericorneal reddening* or *hyperemia*.

The fever is high, usually above 102° C and frequently up to 104° C, and is accompanied by chills. Headache is severe and is characterized as retro-orbital or occipital. The presence of headache, high fever, and neck stiffness or pain due to profound myalgias suggests meningitis and may necessitate a lumbar puncture. Spinal fluid is usually acellular in the first five to seven days of illness, although leptospires may be seen. With the onset of antibody in the serum, an aseptic meningitis may occur in up to 90 per cent of patients, but only half will have meningeal symptoms. When a cutaneous hypesthesia is also present, patients may not tolerate the touch of a sheet. Other neurologic manifestations, such as changes in the level of consciousness, encephalitis, and cranial nerve palsies, have been reported less often. The muscle pains and tenderness are truly remarkable. The severity of myalgias may even prevent the patient from standing. The presence of nausea, vomiting, and anorexia with abdominal tenderness caused by muscle involvement can mimic pancreatitis. Acute dilatation of the gallbladder and cholecystitis can occur in leptospirosis and make the clinical evaluation of an ill patient very difficult, especially since there is already laboratory evidence of inflammation.

The illness usually lasts four to nine days. During that period all clinical findings resolve simultaneously, and both doctor and patients are surprised at how quickly the recovery has taken place and at how well the patient feels. In about 15 per cent of patients the illness persists beyond the ninth day. It rarely may last six to seven weeks.

Leptospirosis is generally a monophasic illness. In a minority of patients after an initial illness there will be a period of apparent recovery, after which symptoms worsen. This second phase is termed the *immune phase*. It lasts two to four days in most patients. It differs from initial illness in being more variable. Fever is not so high, myalgias and gastrointestinal symptoms are not so severe, but meningitis and abnormal spinal fluids and iridocyclitis are more common. The immune phase is so named because of its correlation with the onset of antibodies to leptospirosis in the blood, the disappearance of leptospiremia, and the onset of urine cultures positive for the germ.

The term *Weil's syndrome* is applied to one pole of a continuum of illness. It is not a specific subgroup of leptospirosis; it is simply severe leptospirosis. Any of the several manifestations of Weil's syndrome may occur alone. The clinical findings of intense jaundice, mental status changes, hemorrhage, purpura or petechiae, and renal insufficiency occurring in a previously normal patient are so memorable that it is not surprising that this was the syndrome that stimulated the search for leptospires. The first manifestation of severe illness is usually jaundice that develops between the fifth and ninth days. The intensity of jaundice has no prognostic significance. Renal insufficiency may develop concomitantly with jaundice. Oliguria is a grave prognostic sign. Hemorrhagic manifestations may develop: purpura and petechiae may appear on the oral, vaginal, or conjunctival mucosa. A biphasic pattern frequently may be seen, although the "stages" tend to merge into a single severe illness. Convalescence is rapid in most patients but may be delayed for up to ten weeks.

Childhood Disease. A recent report of nine pediatric cases reiterated the close contact of children to common reservoirs such as dogs. The pediatric syndrome shares many features of adult disease but is more intense, with several atypical features such as shock, hydrops of the gallbladder, skin desquamation, and chest x-ray abnormality.

LABORATORY FEATURES. Leukocyte counts are usually below 15,000 per cubic millimeter but may be as high as 50,000 per cubic millimeter. There is almost always neutrophilia. Hematocrit is normal in anicteric illness, but in prolonged illness anemia is common. The causes of anemia are many, with blood loss, microangiopathy, and leptospiral hemolysin all implicated in clinical cases. Thrombocytopenia is seen in severe cases. Coagulation studies occasionally demonstrate a vitamin K reversible prolongation of prothrombin time. However, this is not responsible for the hemorrhagic diathesis of severe leptospirosis. The sedimentation rate is elevated in half of cases.

Liver function tests reveal a mean SGOT/SGPT elevation of five times normal with occasional patients with elevations up to 20 times normal. The direct bilirubin concentration may rise as a manifestation of severe disease and may reach 64 mg per deciliter, but in most icteric cases it is below 20 mg per deciliter. The pattern is one of intrahepatic cholestasis.

Early in the illness 80 per cent of patients have abnormal urine findings. The most common abnormalities are microscopic hematuria, pyuria, and "2+" proteinuria. Gross hematuria rarely has been reported. One fourth of patients demonstrate elevations of the blood urea nitrogen between 20 and 100 mg per deciliter. The most common electrolyte abnormality is hyperkalemia, primarily in patients with renal failure.

The chest x-ray appears abnormal in one fourth of patients, including anicteric cases. The most common abnormality is patchy bronchopneumonia. A small pleural effusion is seen in 10 per cent of patients.

Electrocardiographic abnormalities occur in 10 to 40 per cent of patients, with bradycardia and low voltage accounting for one half of abnormalities. The remainder consists of nonspecific ST-T wave changes.

Cerebrospinal fluid may be abnormal in up to 90 per cent of patients. In 70 per cent of specimens the total cell count is below 500 per cubic millimeter, with frequent presence of neutrophils. Protein ranges from 50 to 110 mg per dl in 80 per cent of cases. The glucose concentration is usually normal.

IgM antibodies may be detected in blood by day four or five of illness in most patients.

DIAGNOSIS. A diagnosis of leptospirosis must be suspected in any patient with fever, myalgias, headache, and nausea or vomiting. The presence of conjunctival suffusion is an early and helpful sign. The most common misdiagnosis of a patient with leptospirosis is aseptic meningitis followed by viral hepatitis, viral syndrome, fever of unknown origin, bronchitis, influenza, nephritis, and rickettsiosis. The following differential points aid the clinician: (1) the myalgias of leptospirosis are not a prominent feature of viral hepatitis; (2) creatinine kinase is frequently elevated in leptospirosis, and this seldom occurs in viral hepatitis; (3) liver enzyme values in viral hepatitis may average 10 to 15 times higher than normal, but the average is five times higher in leptospirosis; (4) a conjunctival suffusion is very helpful in separating leptospirosis from other processes.

The diagnosis may be confirmed by culture (on Fletcher semisolid medium) of the blood in the first week of illness or of the urine thereafter. Cultures may take up to eight weeks to become positive. Since leptospires may be excreted in the urine for prolonged periods, the diagnosis may be established by urine culture in untreated patients even after clinical illness is over. Direct examination of the urine and blood are not sufficient to establish the diagnosis. There are many artifacts that may be mistaken for leptospires, especially by the inexperienced laboratory worker. When cultures are performed three to four times, organisms are recovered with regularity. The diagnosis may be established serologically by two methods. The macroagglutination is a screening test that uses pooled antigens from all of the serogroups of leptospirosis. Diagnosis is made by a four-fold rise in titer. This test is broadly available but will not detect infecting serovars that are not included in the pooled test antigens. The microagglutination requires a live pathogenic leptospiral culture and therefore is performed mainly in reference laboratories. Techniques for detecting genus-specific antibody or antigen using hemolytic assays and counterimmunoelectrophoresis have been published and are available as research tools. The most promising test for early diagnosis is a genus-specific antibody detection system.

PROGNOSIS. In most untreated cases this is a nonfatal, self-limited illness. The reported mortality of leptospirosis varies greatly among series. In military populations it is around 0.1 per cent. In civilian series it ranges from 5 to 10 per cent. In both military and civilian series mortality is related to age and presence of jaundice. Thirty per cent of patients over age 60 die. Jaundiced patients have a 15 per cent mortality. The differences in mortality may have to do with the underlying health of the host and the bias toward reporting of more serious cases. The military series involve large groups of well men in which high attack rates have been documented and physicians are sensitive to the diagnosis. If the patient lives, sequelae are uncommon even in severe cases. When sequelae occur, they consist of focal cerebral or peripheral nerve deficits or ocular problems caused by persistent uveitis. Several patients have been reported with persistent renal abnormalities.

THERAPY AND PREVENTION. Tetracycline or doxycycline (in controlled trials) are both effective in shortening the course of anicteric leptospirosis when they are given in the first two to four days of illness. Their efficacy in reducing symptoms if given later has not been established. Therapeutic trials were done in populations with no mortality in the placebo group, so the effect of these drugs on mortality is unknown. Doxycycline therapy prevents leptospiruria in infected patients. If leptospiruria is necessary for the mediation of renal damage, as some investigators have speculated, then doxycycline may affect the development of renal failure or Weil's syndrome. Although activities in vitro have been demonstrated for penicillins, aminoglycosides, and erythromycin, they have not been studied in a controlled trial. Uncontrolled experience suggests that penicillin is effective. The balance of therapy in leptospirosis consists of careful attention to the details of care in patients with renal, hepatic, hematologic, and central nervous system complications.

Doxycycline, 100 mg once a week, will prevent leptospirosis in high-risk groups for three weeks. Efficacy in longer periods of exposure has not been evaluated. There are no leptospiral vaccines for humans in use, although effective vaccines for animals are available.

Edwards GA, Domm BM: Human leptospirosis. Medicine 39:117, 1960. *An extensive analysis of the clinical and laboratory features of leptospirosis with a review of early papers.*

Feigin RD, Anderson DC: Human leptospirosis. CRC Crit Rev Clin Lab Sci 5:413, 1975. *The most comprehensive review of leptospirosis, including history, microbiology, pathogenesis, clinical findings, and therapy.*

McClain JBL, Ballou WR, Harrison SH, Steinweg DR: Doxycycline therapy of leptospirosis. Ann Intern Med 100:696, 1984. *A description of therapeutic effects of doxycycline in therapy of leptospirosis.*

Takafuji ET, Kirkpatrick JW, Miller RN, Karwacki JJ, Kelly PW, Gray MR, McNeil KM, Timboc HL, Kane RE, Sanchez JL: An efficacy trial of doxycycline chemoprophylaxis against leptospirosis. N Engl J Med 310:497, 1984. *Demonstrates efficacy in American soldiers with placebo controls.*

Diseases Caused by Chlamydiae

312. INTRODUCTION

Walter E. Stamm

Due to their obligate intracellular growth cycle, chlamydiae were originally considered large viruses and were variously called *Bedsonia* or *TRIC* (for *trachoma-inclusion conjunctivitis*) agents. These terms have been discarded, and chlamydiae now constitute a separate order (Chlamydiales), family (Chlamydiaceae), and genus *(Chlamydia)*. All members of the genus are obligate intracellular pathogens, but they more closely resemble bacteria than viruses in that they possess both deoxyribonucleic acid (DNA) and ribonucleic acid (RNA), divide by binary fission, have bacterial ribosomes and a cell wall not unlike that of Enterobacteriaceae, and can be inhibited by antibiotics. Compared with other bacteria, they have a small genome of 6 to 8 $\times$ 10^5 base pairs. They also lack adenosine triphosphate (ATP)–generating enzymes and hence depend entirely upon host cell metabolism for energy production.

The genus *Chlamydia* contains two species, *C. psittaci* and *C. trachomatis*. The former is a ubiquitous cause of infection in birds and lower mammals, with humans being occasional accidental hosts, while *C. trachomatis* infects humans and has no apparent natural animal hosts. Characteristically, *C. psittici* produces long lived, persistent infections of birds and mammals. Persistent infections caused by *C. trachomatis* in humans may also be common but have not been well documented. The two species can be readily differentiated in the laboratory in that *C. psittaci* forms diffuse intracytoplasmic inclusions that do not contain glycogen and thus do not stain with iodine, while *C. trachomatis* forms compact glycogen containing inclusions that readily stain with iodine. Sulfonamides inhibit growth of *C. psittaci* but not of *C. trachomatis*.

All chlamydiae possess a genus-specific, heat-stable lipopolysaccharide antigen that serves as the basis for the widely available complement fixation serologic test. Species- and immunotype-specific antigens have also been described and serve as the basis for subdividing *C. trachomatis* into 15 immunotypes using the microimmunofluorescence test of Wang and Grayston. Specific immunotypes tend to cause particular clinical syndromes. Types A, B, Ba, and C produce endemic trachoma (see Ch. 313). Types D, E, F, G, H, I, J, and K cause genital infections in adults (see Ch. 301) and ocular and respiratory infections in infants (see Ch. 63). Types L1 to L3 produce lymphogranuloma venereum (LGV) (see Ch. 303) and proctocolitis (see Ch. 104). LGV strains of *C. trachomatis* possess properties that distinguish them from non-LGV strains biologically, including more efficient cell entry and cell-to-cell infectivity in tissue culture, as well as mouse lethality upon intracerebral injection. A subtyping system for *C. psittaci* has not been developed.

Chlamydiae replicate by means of a unique life cycle unlike that of other bacteria. The 300-nM elementary body (the infective and extracellular form of a chlamydiae) initiates infection by attachment to specific receptors in the susceptible host cell's outer membrane. Subsequently, the elementary body enters the host cell by endocytosis. Within the resulting phagosome, the elementary body reorganizes within six hours into the larger 800- to 1000-nM and more metabolically active reticulate body. These reticulate bodies undergo repeated binary division until a large inclusion occupying much of the cell's cytoplasm and containing many reticulate bodies is formed. Reticulate bodies possess many ribosomes and synthesize DNA, RNA, proteins, and other molecules but cannot generate ATP. After 24 hours, some of the reticulate bodies condense to form compact elementary bodies in the mature inclusion, and the latter are released into the extracellular environment to begin the cycle anew.

C. trachomatis preferentially infects columnar epithelial cells, while *C. psittaci* has a broader host cell range, including macrophages. In most patients, *C. trachomatis* infections remain superficial, involving mucosal surfaces of the eye, nasopharynx, cervix, urethra, and rectum. Many of these infections produce few or no symptoms and tend to be subacute in nature and mild in terms of the signs they produce. Ascending infection of the endometrium, fallopian tube, liver capsule, epididymis, or lung produce more severe symptoms and signs and can be regarded as more extensive or invasive infections. LGV strains of *C. trachomatis* cause the most invasive disease, manifested either by proctocolitis or painful inguinal adenopathy and fever. *C. trachomatis* occasionally causes nongenital systemic infection, including culture-negative endocarditis, peritonitis, and pneumonia in adults.

Since many chlamydial infections produce either no symptoms or nonspecific symptoms and signs, laboratory confirmation of infection often must be sought. Available techniques include direct microscopic examination of tissue scrapings for typical inclusions or specific antigen, isolation of the organism, and assessment of antichlamydial antibody in serum or secretions. Cell culture techniques for cultivation of *C. trachomatis* have replaced the much more cumbersome isolation method using embryonated yolk sac. Widespread adoption of McCoy and HeLa 229 cell lines for isolation of *C. trachomatis* from patient secretions or biopsies has been a major factor contributing to recognition of the wide spectrum of infections caused by *C. trachomatis.* These cell lines require pretreatment with cyclohexamide and centrifugation of the inoculum onto the monolayer for efficient isolation of *C. trachomatis.* Inclusions formed in the cell culture monolayers can be visualized using iodine, Giemsa, or immunofluorescent staining procedures. Despite widespread use in research laboratories, cell culture procedures for isolation of *C. trachomatis* have not been generally available to clinicians because of the expense and technical difficulty. Lack of an available confirmatory diagnostic test has been a major factor contributing to the increasing incidence of genital and neonatal *C. trachomatis* infections in this country. Newer immunodiagnostic procedures that detect chlamydial antigen in patients' secretions are now being developed and many prove more useful than chlamydial culture for routine diagnostic purposes.

Chlamydial infection stimulates both a humoral and a cellular immune response, but neither appears to be completely protective against subsequent infection with either homologous or heterologous strains. Both local and systemic antibody can be demonstrated after acute infection, and immunoglobulin G (IgG) antibody neutralizes infective elementary bodies. In ocular infection, it has been advocated by some that the immune response actually participates in the disease process by producing continued inflammation. Serodiagnosis of chlamydial infections has limited applicability except in specific circumstances. The complement fixation test, available in most health department laboratories, should be used for confirmation of suspected psittacosis or LGV (see Ch. 20). The microimmunofluorescence test may be useful in the diagnosis of infant pneumonia (see Ch. 63), pelvic inflammatory disease, or Fitz-Hugh-Curtis syndrome but is available only in research laboratories. Uncomplicated genital infections evoke only low titer antibody responses, and acute infections cannot be easily distinguished from pre-existing antibody in many patients.

C. trachomatis infections can be treated with a variety of antimicrobial agents. Those agents with greatest demonstrated inhibitory activity in cell culture assays and in clinical studies include the tetracyclines (tetracycline HCl, doxycycline, and minocycline), erythromycin, sulfonamides, sulfamethoxazole-trimethoprim, chloramphenicol, and rifampin. The β-lactam antibiotics produce abnormal inclusions in cell culture and inhibit replication but have been largely ineffective in clinical treatment trials. The aminoglycosides, vancomycin, and spectinomycin have no activity against chlamydiae. In general, antibiotic therapy of chlamydial infections require 7 to 21 days of treatment; single-day regimens have been largely ineffective. Treatment failure usually indicates noncompliance, reinfection, or inadequate duration of drug therapy. Resistance to tetracycline or erythromycin has not been described.

313. TRACHOMA

Walter E. Stamm

C. trachomatis causes two epidemiologically distinct patterns of ocular infection. In endemic parts of the world, *C. trachomatis* immunotypes A, B, Ba, and C cause trachoma, a chronic eye disease that may lead to severe visual impairment or blindness. In nonendemic areas, immunotypes D through K produce a milder, self-limited conjunctivitis in infants born to mothers with cervical infection or in adults who acquire ocular infection after secondary spread from genital sites (see Ch. 63).

Since antiquity, trachomatous infection has been recognized in the Mediterranean basin and in the Orient, and it remains prevalent in Africa and Asia. Although the incidence has been decreasing over the last 30 years, more than 500 million persons have eye infections with chlamydiae, with millions blinded as a result. Trachoma flourishes in hot dry areas that have a shortage of available water and poor hygienic customs. Initial infection usually occurs in early childhood, and in certain parts of the world virtually the entire population is infected with chlamydiae before reaching adulthood. Repeated exposure to chlamydiae and the high prevalence of bacterial superinfection with *Hemophilus spp.*, pneumococci, staphylococci, and Enterobacteriaceae in these populations contribute to the severity of the resulting eye disease. In the United States, trachoma is occasionally seen on Indian reservations in the southwestern United States, in Mexican-Americans, and in immigrants from endemic areas, but such cases rarely result in major visual impairment, perhaps because bacterial superinfection is infrequent.

Persons with active trachoma shed chlamydiae in desquamated conjunctival cells, in conjunctival exudate, and in tears, which then may be transmitted by fingers, fomites, and perhaps flies. In endemic areas, transmission by these routes occurs through close personal contact, especially within family units and in groups of young children. Patients with early active infection shed more infective chlamydiae than those with chronic infection. However, even patients with long-term eye disease unaccompanied by signs of current activity may shed chlamydiae and thus serve as a source of infection.

Typical trachoma in children begins insidiously at about age two as a follicular conjunctivitis, most noticeable in the conjunctiva of the upper lid and the tarsal plate. Histologically, inclusion bodies appear within the conjunctival epithelial cells, polymorphonuclear leukocytes infiltrate the epithelium, and subepithelial lymphoid follicles develop. Reinfection is common during this period. Next the cornea becomes involved, with epithelial keratitis and subepithelial corneal infiltration resulting in opacities. Blood vessels from the limbus, accompanied by fibroblasts, invade the cornea to form a pannus. Progression of the inflammatory response leads to necrosis and scarring of the conjunctiva and gradual corneal vascularization from the upper limbus downward. Eventually a dense fibrovascular pannus extends over part or all of the cornea to grossly impair vision. Linear or stellate scars appear on the conjunctiva. Progressive scarring of the subepithelial tissues leads to deformation of the tarsal plate that results in entropion, trichiasis, and further corneal damage. Destruction of the conjunctival goblet cells and lacrimal ducts and gland produces xerosis. The latter changes often follow secondary bacterial infection, which may also produce corneal ulceration and accelerate loss of vision. Typically there are no systemic symptoms or signs of infection. The disease process evolves over about ten years in endemic areas but may be milder and more slowly progressive in other cases.

Adult inclusion conjunctivitis usually appears as an acute follicular conjunctivitis with preauricular lymphadenopathy. Untreated, it regresses slowly, but keratitis with marginal infiltrates, subepithelial opacities, and corneal neovascularization may develop in the conjunctiva. Unlike trachoma, adult inclusion conjunctivitis rarely impairs vision permanently.

The traditional diagnostic criteria for trachoma include lymphoid follicles on the upper tarsal plate, limbal follicles, typical conjunctival scars, and vascular pannus. Early in the disease the latter two can be detected only by slit lamp examination. The presence of any two of these features confirms the diagnosis. Laboratory confirmation of trachoma is based on (1) identification of typical inclusions in epithelial cells from a conjunctival swab or scraping (usually done by Giemsa or immunofluorescence staining); (2) cultivation of chlamydiae from a conjunctival specimen in cell culture; or (3) microimmunofluorescent antibody in high titer in tears. Approximately 20 to 60 per cent of children with early inflammatory trachoma have Giemsa-positive scrapings; higher yields result from cultures of chlamydiae.

In the differential diagnosis of ocular chlamydial infection, epidemic keratoconjunctivitis (usually caused by adenovirus type 8 or type 19), herpetic keratoconjunctivitis, Newcastle disease virus conjunctivitis, acute hemorrhagic conjunctivitis caused by enterovirus type 70 or coxsackievirus, reactions to allergens and irritating chemicals, and other bacterial causes of conjunctivitis must be considered. Some of these entities may coexist with chlamydial infections, and repeated ophthalmologic examinations and extensive laboratory evaluation may be required to establish a correct diagnosis.

Control of chronic trachoma in endemic areas has been attempted using tetracycline or erythromycin ointment in the eyes of all affected children in the community for 21 to 60 days. Oral administration of erythromycin has been used as an alternative. Antibiotic therapy usually suppresses clinical activity and chlamydial as well as bacterial growth but may not eradicate chlamydiae permanently. However, in endemic areas, repeated courses of drug treatment are beneficial because they reduce severity of eye disease and thus avoid progression toward blindness. Even one dose per month of doxycycline, 300 mg (2.5 to 4 mg per kilogram), can provide clinical benefit by converting severe to mild eye disease. Drug therapy has no influence on scars or pannus. Surgical correction is required in serious entropion or trichiasis. Topical corticosteroids and caustic substances have no place in therapy. For acute adult inclusion conjunctivitis, tetracycline HCl, 1.0 to 2.0 grams given orally daily in divided doses, or erythromycin, 1.0 to 2.0 grams given daily for two weeks, will successfully treat genital tract as well as ocular involvement. Sulfisoxazole, 4 grams daily, may also be effective. Sexual partners must be treated simultaneously in order to avoid reinfection.

The potential measures to prevent trachoma include efforts to increase the supply of water, practices to maintain cleanliness such as frequent handwashing and avoidance of use of common towels, and measures to reduce flies. It is also important to detect mild early infection in young children in endemic areas and to apply effective drug treatment repeatedly to prevent the blinding progression of the disease. Detection and treatment of adults who already have visual impairment probably can reduce the source of infection for children. Entire family groups or communities should be treated simultaneously. Efforts to prevent trachoma with a vaccine have been unsuccessful.

314. NEONATAL CHLAMYDIAL INFECTIONS

Walter E. Stamm

Between 5 and 22 per cent of pregnant women have *C. trachomatis* infection of the cervix, with neonatal infection occurring when the infant passes through the infected birth canal. Ascending intrauterine infection of the fetus has not been demonstrated. Shortly after birth, 30 to 50 per cent of infants born to infected mothers have cultural evidence of infection, 25 per cent manifest clinically apparent conjunctivitis, and 10 to 15 per cent acquire nasopharyngeal infection, which in some cases progresses to chlamydial neonatal pneumonitis. Otitis media and symptomatic nasopharyngitis may be caused by *C. trachomatis* in some infants.

Neonatal *C. trachomatis* inclusion conjunctivitis begins 5 to 14 days after birth. The infection must be differentiated from gonococcal ophthalmia (which has a shorter incubation period of 1 to 3 days) and from other common causes of neonatal conjunctivitis (*S. pneumoniae, H. influenzae, S. aureus,* and group D streptococci). Typical manifestations include lid and conjunctival swelling, mucopurulent ocular discharge, conjunctival hyperemia, and membrane formation. Untreated, the disease persists 3 to 12 months but usually heals without sequelae. Rarely, conjunctival scarring and corneal neovascularization occur. Neonates with inclusion conjunctivitis frequently have concomitant chlamydial infection of the nasopharynx, rectum, urethra, and vagina, usually without associated clinical manifestations at these sites.

The diagnosis can be rapidly established by demonstration of chlamydial inclusions in conjunctival scrapings stained by Giemsa or immunofluorescence. Cultures for *C. trachomatis* can also be used if available and will be positive in some smear-negative cases. Tear antibody to *C. trachomatis* can be demonstrated in most cases, but the test is not readily available.

Silver nitrate drops instilled at birth do not prevent chlamydial inclusion conjunctivitis and in some instances cause chemical conjunctivitis. For this reason, many health departments now recommend prophylactic use of erythromycin ointment at birth. However, topical erythromycin prophylaxis does not cure concomitant nasopharyngeal or rectal infection. Perhaps a better preventive approach would be screening and treatment of pregnant women for *C. trachomatis* infection before term. This approach essentially appears to eliminate *C. trachomatis* infections in neonates and should be the strategy of choice when cultures are available.

Since many infants with inclusion conjunctivitis have concomitant nasopharyngeal, rectal, and vaginal *C. trachomatis* infection, systemic rather than topical therapy should be used. In addition, relapses often follow topical therapy. Erythromycin, 40 to 50 mg per kilogram per day in four divided doses for 14 to 21 days, cures more than 80 per cent of cases. Both parents should be examined for *C. trachomatis* infection and should be treated with tetracycline or erythromycin (for nursing mothers) if cultures are not available.

Approximately 10 per cent of infants born to infected mothers develop a distinctive subacute chlamydial pneumonia between the first and fourth months of life. Typically, tachypnea, a stacatto cough, inspiratory rales, elevated serum globulin concentrations, and eosinophilia are seen but fever is absent. Hyperinflated lungs with scattered interstitial infiltrates are evident on chest x-ray examination. The disease lasts for weeks to months but is mild in most infants and will resolve without specific therapy. However, marked hypoxemia and apnea have been reported in some cases. Lung biopsies have demonstrated chlamydial inclusions, alveoli with inflammatory exudate, and a lymphocytic interstitial infiltration of the bronchial submucosa. In some cases, *C. trachomatis* have been recovered from lung tissue. Diagnosis in most instances can be suspected on clinical grounds and confirmed by the demonstration of chlamydial inclusions on Giemsa or immunofluorescent stained smears of the conjunctivae or nasopharynx. If available, *C. trachomatis* should be sought by cell culture of eye scrapings, nasopharyngeal swabs, or rectal swabs. Rising high titer immunoglobulin M (IgM) microimmunofluorescent antibody to *C. trachomatis* can be demonstrated in the majority of infants with pneumonia. Erythromycin, 50 mg per kilogram per day in four divided doses for 14 to 21 days, has been recommended for treatment of infant pneumonia, although there are no control trials demonstrating the benefits of this regimen.

Holmes KK: The chlamydia epidemic. JAMA 245:1718, 1981.
Mardh PA, Holmes KK, Oriel JD, Piot P, Schachter J (eds.): Chlamydial Infections. New York, Elsevier Science Publishing Company, Inc., 1982.
Schachter J, Caldwell HD: Chlamydiae. Ann Rev Microbiol 34:285, 1980.

315. PSITTACOSIS (Ornithosis, Parrot Fever)

William Schaffner

DEFINITION. Psittacosis is an infection of birds that is produced by *Chlamydia psittaci*. When transmitted to man, this agent can produce asymptomatic infection, a transient influenza-like illness, or serious pneumonic disease characterized by high fever, headache, cough, myalgia, and pulmonary infiltrates.

HISTORY. In 1879, Ritter, a Swiss physician, described seven cases of an unusual pneumonia that occurred after contact with tropical birds. Morange, in 1894, established the parrot as a vector and termed the disease *psittacosis* after the Greek *psittakos* (the parrot). Bedson demonstrated the filterable agent in 1930. Over 90 species of birds can harbor the agent, and it has a worldwide distribution.

ETIOLOGY. *C. psittaci* is an obligate intracellular bacterium morphologically and serologically related to the agents of lymphogranuloma venereum and trachoma. Parrots and parakeets are common carriers and until recently represented the major source of human infection. With better control of psittacine disease in aviaries, other birds now contribute more human infections. Cases have resulted from contact with turkeys, pigeons, ducks, and other fowl. Persons working with birds are at greatest risk, notably pet shop employees, pigeon handlers, and poultry workers, especially in turkey processing plants. There is no risk associated with eating poultry products.

The agent is present in the blood, tissue, feathers, and discharges of infected birds. Although the avian disease can be fatal, infected birds frequently show only minimal evidence of illness, such as ruffled feathers, lethargy, diarrhea, and failure to eat. Birds having active infections are most likely to transmit the disease, but asymptomatic carriers are common, and birds can shed transmissible agent for months.

Psittacosis is generally acquired by the respiratory route through inhalation of infected dried bird excreta or by handling of infected birds. Mouth-to-beak intimacies have led to infection in humans. Cases have been reported after only brief exposure to birds, and 20 per cent of patients can show no history of exposure to birds. Person-to-person transmission of psittacosis is rare. These cases of "human strain" psittacosis have been severe, with high mortality.

PATHOLOGY. In birds, the principal sites of disease are the liver, spleen, and pericardium. In man, the lung is most commonly involved. The psittacosis agent gains access to the human body via the respiratory route, rapidly enters the blood, and reaches the reticuloendothelial cells of the liver and spleen. After replication in these sites, invasion of the lung is by hematogenous spread. The mature pulmonary lesion is a lobular pneumonitis. The process is initiated by inflammation and progressive edema of the alveoli. Exudation is often accompanied by small hemorrhages, accounting for clinical hemoptysis. Thick, gelatinous plugs of mucus may fill major and minor bronchi and account for the severe cyanosis and progressive anoxia seen in fatal cases. Foci of necrosis may occur in more severely affected areas of the lung and are sometimes associated with capillary thrombi. The process is generally most severe in dependent bronchopulmonary segments. Large monocytes and macrophages containing cytoplasmic inclusion bodies, which represent the agent (LCL bodies), are characteristic. Hyperplasia and monocytic infiltration of pulmonary and hilar lymph nodes and splenic enlargement with occasional areas of focal necrosis occurs. Rarely the liver shows intralobular focal necrosis and swollen Kupffer cells containing the psittacosis elementary bodies. Changes in the myocardium, heart valves, pericardium, meninges, brain, adrenal glands, pancreas, and kidneys have been reported.

CLINICAL MANIFESTATIONS. Wide variations can occur in the clinical picture. The incubation period ranges from 7 to 15 days but may be longer. Asymptomatic or mild influenza-like infections probably are the rule. Moderate or severe infections, although less frequent, are more commonly diagnosed. The onset of illness may be insidious, but it often starts with chills and a fever that rises slowly to 39 to 40.5° C during the first week of illness. As with some other instances of intracellular infection, the pulse may be slow relative to the level of the fever. Headache is severe. Malaise, anorexia, nausea, vomiting, severe myalgias, particularly in the neck and back, and arthralgias are common. Cough is generally prominent but may be delayed until late in the first week. Small amounts of mucoid sputum with occasional blood streaking are the rule. Changes in mentation are often seen. Delirium or stupor may occur in severe cases toward the end of the first week, and usually are associated with severe pulmonary involvement, cyanosis, and other evidences of anoxia. Other neurologic manifestations are uncommon. A macular rash (Horder's spots) resembling that seen in typhoid has occasionally been described. Jaundice and progressive nitrogen retention have been reported in severe cases. Severe dyspnea, tachypnea, tachycardia, cyanosis, jaundice, delirium, and stupor are all poor prognostic signs.

The physical findings of pneumonia are usually sparse. Chest roentgenograms often reveal infiltrates not detected at the bedside. Examination may reveal only fever, painful muscle groups, an elevated respiratory rate, and a relative bradycardia. Fine, crepitant rales may be heard in localized areas over the lungs, but true consolidation is less common. Pleurisy with effusion can occur but is unusual. Mild hepatomegaly is frequent. A palpable spleen has been noted in a substantial number of patients. Splenomegaly in a patient with undiagnosed acute pneumonitis should raise the consideration of psittacosis. An erythematous pharynx may be noted. In rare instances there may be signs of pericarditis or myocarditis. In prolonged, severe illness, thrombophlebitis and pulmonary infarction have been reported as late complications.

Patients with mild cases may recover in seven days. More severe infections may last 12 to 21 days without specific treatment. Fever is ordinarily sustained or remittent and, when accompanied by bradycardia, resembles the fever of untreated typhoid infections. Defervescence is generally slow, and a prolonged convalescence is common. Relapses have been reported even after appropriate treatment. Reinfections have been described. Occasional cases of endocarditis caused by *C. psittaci* in patients with sterile blood cultures have been described.

LABORATORY FINDINGS. Simple laboratory studies are not helpful in establishing a diagnosis. The leukocyte count is usually normal or slightly elevated. The erythrocyte sedimentation rate is generally elevated. Chest roentgenograms generally show soft patchy infiltrates radiating outward from the hilum, which tend to be more prominent in dependent lobes or segments. Occasionally diffuse miliary, nodular, or frank lobar distribution of infiltrates is seen.

A specific diagnosis can be made only by isolation of the agent or by serologic studies. The agent is present in the blood and sputum during the first two to three weeks, but isolation is hazardous and should not be attempted except in special laboratories. Diagnosis is generally made by a four-fold rise in complement-fixing antibodies. A significant change in antibody titers is generally present by the twelfth to fourteenth day of disease; the titers are usually maximal by 30 days, then slowly wane. Treatment can delay or suppress antibody response. A serum complement-fixation titer of 1:32 during the acute illness is presumptive evidence of psittacosis. There is considerable cross-reaction between antigens prepared from psittacosis and lymphogranuloma venereum agents. False-positive complement-fixation tests may occur with Q fever, brucellosis, or legionnaires' disease.

DIFFERENTIAL DIAGNOSIS. Specific diagnosis of psittacosis is of extreme importance because of its potential severity, its response to antimicrobials, and the public health significance of psittacosis infection. All cases should be reported to the local health department. The syndrome of viral pneumonia accompanied by protracted high fever, unusually severe headache, and relative bradycardia should suggest psittacosis. Often a history of contact with birds is the only clue to diagnosis and may be elicited only by repeated questioning of the patient and family. When pneumonic symptoms are prominent, psittacosis must be differentiated from legionnaires' disease, viral pneumonias, mycoplasmal pneumonia, influenza, Q fever, tularemia, tuberculosis, fungal infection, and bacterial pneumonia distal to an obstructed bronchus. If pneumonic symptoms are not prominent, psittacosis can be confused with other systemic febrile illnesses such as typhoid fever, brucellosis, infectious mononucleosis, infectious hepatitis, miliary tuberculosis, or the viral meningoencephalitides.

TREATMENT. The tetracyclines are the drugs of choice, and early diagnosis and initiation of treatment may be lifesaving. After institution of therapy with 2 to 3 grams daily, both fever and symptoms are generally controlled within 48 to 72 hours, although the response may be indolent. Although the disease apparently responds to penicillin in doses above 2 million units daily and to erythromycin, tetracycline remains the drug of choice. Treatment should be continued for at least 10 days after defervescence to prevent relapse. With treatment, mortality rates as low as 1 to 5 per cent can be achieved.

Byrom NP, Walls J, Mair HJ: Fulminant psittacosis. Lancet 1:353, 1979. *The difficulty in differentiating psittacosis and legionnaires' disease at the bedside is emphasized.*

Jariwalla AG, Davies BH, White J: Infective endocarditis complicating psittacosis: Response to rifampicin. Br Med J 1:155, 1980. *Endocarditis caused by psittacosis is reviewed concisely.*

Macfarlane JT, Macrae AD: Psittacosis. Br Med Bull 39:163, 1983. *A well written review.*

Schaffner W, Drutz DJ, Duncan GW, Koenig MG: The clinical spectrum of endemic psittacosis. Arch Intern Med 119:433, 1967. *Good descriptions of clinical presentations.*

Rickettsial Diseases

316. INTRODUCTION

Charles L. Wisseman, Jr.

The diseases commonly referred to as the rickettsial diseases of man consist of several clinical entities, usually acute, self-limited fevers, caused by bacteria of the family Rickettsiaceae. They fall naturally into the typhus-like diseases (typhus groups, spotted fever group, and scrub typhus group), Q fever, and trench fever. The typhus-like diseases are caused by organisms of the genus *Rickettsia;* Q fever by *Coxiella burnetii;* and trench fever by *Rochalimaea quintana.*

Organisms of the *Rickettsia, Coxiella,* and *Rochalimaea* genera, although very different in many respects, are very small bacteria with a gram-negative bacterium-like cell wall, bacterial type internal structure (typical prokaryotic DNA arrangement with a genome size roughly equivalent to that of *Neisseria;* ribosomes), often a slime layer or microcapsule, and a substantial independent metabolic activity. Organisms of the genus *Rickettsia* and *Coxiella burnetii* are obligate intracellular parasites, i.e., they are known to grow only within eukaryotic host cells. *Rochalimaea quintana* can be grown on cell-free medium and grows extracellularly in the louse gut. All organisms of the genus *Rickettsia* have the capacity to penetrate through the host cell plasma membrane into the cytoplasm, can cause host cell lysis from without, and multiply by binary fission free in the host cell cytoplasm not surrounded by a vacuolar membrane. Different species vary in their capacity to interact with other host cell membranes. Thus members of the spotted fever group can penetrate into the host cell nucleus, and these, as well as *R. mooseri,* can escape through the plasma membrane without requiring complete host cell destruction as does *R. prowazekii. Coxiella burnetii* enters host cells passively by endocytosis and grows within a membrane-bound vacuole. These differences in action on host cell membranes are probably related to differences in disease patterns (host response) and immune mechanisms. Active penetration of host cells appears to be correlated with mouse lethal toxic action, hemolytic properties, and phospholipase action. Members of the genus *Rickettsia* that have been studied and *Coxiella burnetii* also have endotoxins similar in physiologic action to those of gram-negative bacilli.

All rickettsioses are transmitted by arthropod vectors, although Q fever is usually acquired from domestic animals (Table 316–1). With the exception of louse-borne typhus and trench fevers, in which man is the key vertebrate host and reservoir, all the rickettsioses are zoonoses, existing in a natural cycle involving arthropods (vectors and in some cases reservoirs) and vertebrate (usually mammalian) hosts. In these, man acquires the disease by accidentally intruding into the natural cycle and is a "dead-end" host not sustaining the infection cycle. The reservoir mechanism varies considerably among the rickettsioses. The nonsterile immunity in the vertebrate host, with persisting infection and potential or proved capacity for recrudescence, appears to be important in louse-borne typhus and trench fever, in which the main reservoir is man. In these infections, the vector (the human body louse) does not transmit the organism transovarially to the next generation, and, in the case of louse-borne typhus, the infection in the louse vector is almost invariably fatal to the louse in a week or two. On the other hand, in tick-, mite-, and chigger-borne rickettsioses, the organism is efficiently transmitted transovarially to succeeding generations, a process which probably constitutes the main reservoir mechanism, whereas the vertebrate infection serves only an amplifying role in some instances. *Coxiella burnetii,* possibly originally tick-borne, is sustained by vertical passage in its vertebrate host (e.g., sheep, cattle) by virtue of its capacity to multiply to phenomenal levels in placental tissues and to be excreted in milk.

Thus, although they are commonly lumped together under the "rickettsial diseases of man," and possess some points in common, there are major differences in the biologic properties of the organisms involved, in their interactions with host cells, and in their natural infection cycles and reservoir mechanisms. However, some similarities in cell tropism and the restricted ways in which man responds to injury have conspired to produce a group of clinical entities with many to few common features.

PATHOGENESIS, PATHOLOGY, IMMUNITY. Since the human diseases caused by members of the genus *Rickettsia* share many common features, it is convenient to consider here pathogenesis and immunity in a generalized framework.

The route of infection is frequently through the skin, injected through the vector mouth parts in tick-, mite-, and chigger-

TABLE 316–1. SUMMARY OF SOME EPIDEMIOLOGIC FEATURES OF SELECTED RICKETTSIAL DISEASES OF MAN

Disease	Organism	Natural Cycle: Arthropod Vector	Natural Cycle: Reservoir/ Mammalian Host	Usual Mode of Transmission to Man	Common Occupational or Environmental Association	Geographic Distribution
Typhus group						
Murine typhus	*Rickettsia mooseri* (*R. typhi*)	Flea	Rodents	Infected flea feces into broken skin or aerosol to mucous membranes	Rat-infected premises (shops, warehouses, grain elevators)	Scattered foci, worldwide
Epidemic typhus	*R. prowazekii*	Body louse	Man*	Infected crushed louse or feces into broken skin or aerosol to mucous membranes	Lousy human population with louse transfer	Worldwide
Brill-Zinsser disease	*R. prowazekii*	Recrudescence months to years after primary attack of louse-borne typhus			Unknown; ?stress	Worldwide
Spotted fever group (selected examples)						
Rocky Mountain spotted fever	*R. rickettsii*	Ixodid ticks	Ticks/small mammals	Tick bite, mechanical transfer to mucous membranes, ?airborne	Tick-infested terrain, houses, dogs	Western Hemisphere
Boutonneuse fever	*R. conorii*	Ixodid ticks	Ticks/rodents, dogs	Tick bite	Tick-infested terrain, houses, dogs	Mediterranean littoral, Africa, ?Indian subcontinent
Rickettsialpox	*R. akari*	Mouse mite	Mite/mice	Mouse mite bite	Unique mouse- and mite-infested premises (incinerators)	United States, U.S.S.R., Korea, ?Central Africa
Scrub typhus						
Tsutsugamushi disease	*R. tsutsugamushi* (multiple serotypes)	Chigger	Chigger/?rodents	Chigger bite	Chigger-infested terrain; secondary scrub, grass airfields, golf courses	Asia, Australia, New Guinea, Pacific islands
Q fever	*Coxiella burnetii*	?Ticks	Ticks/mammals	Inhalation of dried airborne infective material; ?tick bite	Domestic animals or products, dairies, lambing pens, slaughterhouses	Worldwide
Trench fever	*Rochalimaea quintana*	Body louse	Man	Infected crushed louse or feces into broken skin; ?aerosol to mucous membranes	Lousy human population with louse transfer	Africa, Mexico, ?South America, ?Eastern Europe

*Recent isolations of putative *R. prowazekii* from flying squirrels in the eastern United States have not been evaluated as reservoirs for human infection. Previous claims of involvement of domestic animals are now largely discounted.

borne rickettsioses and by contamination of broken skin by infected louse or flea feces in louse-borne typhus and murine typhus, respectively. Airborne rickettsiae in dried louse or flea feces may initiate airborne infection through the respiratory tract or conjunctiva. Aerosols of all rickettsiae are highly infectious via the respiratory tract.

Some local proliferation undoubtedly occurs at the inoculation site with all *Rickettsia* species. In some (e.g., scrub typhus, rickettsialpox, fièvre boutonneuse), a visible lesion (the *eschar*) develops at the inoculation site during the incubation period. Regional lymphadenopathy (as in scrub typhus) suggests lymphatic spread, whereas demonstration of rickettsiae in endothelial cells of small blood vessels at the inoculation site opens the possibility of early hematogenous dissemination. Patent rickettsemia probably appears only late in the incubation period, is regularly present at onset, and persists throughout the febrile period of disease despite the appearance of humoral antibodies by about the end of the first week of disease.

Disseminated focal infection of the small blood vessels (capillaries, arterioles, and venules) of the skin, and, to a lesser but significant extent, in other organs such as brain, lung, heart, and kidneys, is the single most important known pathophysiologic feature of these diseases. Thus, at focal points in the small blood vessels, rickettsiae infect, multiply in, and damage endothelial cells with cell necrosis, hypertrophy, and proliferation. Infection is limited to the endothelial cells in typhus and scrub typhus infections but may extend to all layers in Rocky Mountain spotted fever, causing necrosis of the media (Table 316–2). At the sites of endothelial damage, platelet-fibrin thrombi tend to form, which, along with endothelial hypertrophy and proliferation, partially or completely occlude vascular lumen. A typical perivascular inflammatory response develops, with polymorphonuclear and monocytic cells early and macrophages, lymphocytes, and occasional plasma cells later, coinciding approximately temporally with antibody response, suggesting the possibility of superimposition of a vascular immunopathologic component. This sequence suggests that a typical rickettsial infection evolves through an *early phase,* in which vascular damage is primarily the direct result of rickettsial infection, and a *late phase,* in which additional vascular damage is produced by immunologic mechanisms. The latter is unproved, but is consistent with the fact that in typhus and scrub typhus infections patients appear more "toxic" in this late phase and show greater vascular instability, and most deaths occur in the period *after* antibodies are demonstrable. On the other hand, the greater severity of vascular lesions and frequent deaths without detectable antibodies in early fatal cases of Rocky Mountain spotted fever suggest that direct rickettsia-induced vascular damage alone can initiate irreversible pathophysiologic changes.

The disseminated vascular lesions can account for many of the clinical and pathophysiologic abnormalities seen in these

TABLE 316–2. RICKETTSIA TARGET CELL RELATIONSHIPS, PATHOLOGIC LESIONS, AND CLINICAL MANIFESTATIONS OF HUMAN RICKETTSIOSES*

Disease	Target Cell	Host-Cell Association	Basic Lesion	Clinical Manifestations
Typhus-like fevers				
Typhus group	Endothelial	Free intracytoplasmic	Vasculitis	Acute self-limited fever
Scrub typhus	Endothelial	Free intracytoplasmic	Vasculitis	Acute self-limited fever
Spotted fever group	Endothelial, smooth muscle	Free intracytoplasmic and intranuclear	Vasculitis	Acute self-limited fever
Q fever	Reticuloendothelial	Intracytoplasmic vacuole	Granulomas	Acute self-limited fever, "atypical pneumonia," subacute hepatitis, subacute endocarditis
Trench fever	Unknown	Pericellular (in louse and cell culture)	Unknown	Recurring febrile episodes

*Adapted from Strickland (ed.): *Hunter's Tropical Medicine*. Philadelphia, W. B. Saunders Company, 1984.

infections, viz., rash, edema and increased extravascular fluid space, hypotension, and gangrene (in louse-borne typhus and Rocky Mountain spotted fever), as well as the clotting abnormalities (up to disseminated intravascular clotting), which have been recognized in several rickettsial diseases. The classic "typhus nodules" in the brain, most frequent in the midbrain and nuclear areas, are of the same vascular origin and help explain the mental changes and cranial nerve deficits. In Rocky Mountain spotted fever, discrete microinfarcts also may occur in the central nervous system with persisting electroencephalographic change. The heart often shows, in addition to the typical perivascular lesions, some edema, a diffuse mononuclear infiltrate of unknown origin, and a minor amount of muscle necrosis. Nonspecific electrocardiographic changes are common. Despite the dramatic histologic appearance of the heart, limited studies during World War II suggested that cardiac function was not impaired. This matter should be reinvestigated. Indeed, myocarditis has been suggested as a cause of death in Rocky Mountain spotted fever. Typical perivascular lesions occur in the portal areas of the liver, along with nonspecific focal areas of fatty degeneration in hepatocytes. However, the origin of abnormal blood transaminase levels remains unknown. The kidneys also show focal interstitial vascular lesions involving a few nephrons. The characteristic oliguria and azotemia of typhus have been attributed in the past to prerenal causes, e.g., hypotension, tissue catabolism, but evidence for transient immune complex disease should be sought by modern methods. The lungs show a variable degree of interstitial type pneumonitis on histologic examination and by x-ray regardless of route of infection. Cough is a common early clinical manifestation, but physical signs are scant.

Immunity to the infecting rickettsial strain following recovery from infection tends to be solid and longlasting but of a nonsterile type, i.e., the rickettsiae are not entirely eradicated and may remain "latent" for months to many years. The bases for immunity are not yet completely understood. An antibody response is detectable around the end of the first week of disease, but this does not cause an immediate control of rickettsemia. Cell-mediated immunity also develops, but the kinetics of its evolution in man have not yet been clearly documented. Laboratory studies suggest that both antibody-mediated and cell-mediated mechanisms contribute to immunity.

GENERAL CLINICAL DIAGNOSTIC CONSIDERATIONS. In classic form, the typhus-like rickettsial diseases (typhus group, spotted fever group, and scrub typhus group) display many common clinical features, which may vary in degree and in detail, e.g., fever, headache, cough, prostration, rash, altered mental state, hypotension, normal to low white blood count (Table 316–3). *Especially at the onset,* however, the signs and symptoms are those common to many acute infectious diseases, differential

TABLE 316–3. SOME CLINICAL FEATURES OF SELECTED RICKETTSIAL DISEASES

Disease	Usual Incubation Period (Days)	Eschar	Rash: Onset, Day of Disease	Rash: Distribution	Rash: Type	Usual Duration of Disease* (Days)	Usual Severity†	Fever After Chemotherapy (Hours)
Typhus group								
Murine typhus	12 (8–16)	None	5–7	Trunk → extremities	Macular, maculopapular	12 (8–16)	Moderate	48–72
Epidemic typhus	12 (10–14)	None	5–7	Trunk → extremities	Macular, maculopapular, petechial	14 (10–18)	Severe	48–72
Brill-Zinsser disease	—	None		Trunk → extremities	Macular	7–11	Relatively mild	48–72
Spotted fever group								
Rocky Mountain spotted fever	7 (3–12)	None	3–5	Extremities → trunk, face	Macular, maculopapular, petechial	16 (10–20)	Severe	72
Boutonneuse fever	5–7	Often present	3–4	Trunk, extremities, face, palms, soles	Macular, maculopapular, petechial	10 (7–14) 7	Moderate	—
Rickettsialpox	?9–17	Often present	1–3	Trunk → face, extremities	Papulovesicular	7 (3–11)	Relatively mild	—
Scrub typhus (tsutsugamushi disease)	1–12 (9–18)	Often present	4–6	Trunk → extremities	Macular, maculopapular	14 (10–20)	Mild to severe	24–36
Q fever	10–19	None		None		6 (2–21)	Relatively‡ mild	48 (occasionally slow)

*Untreated disease.
†Severity can vary greatly.
‡Occasional subacute infections occur (e.g., hepatitis, endocarditis).

clinical diagnosis is difficult, and specific laboratory diagnostic methods are limited. Sometimes an early sign, such as an eschar, which is variable even in the rickettsioses in which it occurs, is helpful. Later, rash, hypotension, changes in mental state, and the like may give clues. But rickettsioses vary in severity, and not all cases are classic. Moreover, in many areas, other infectious diseases exist which are confusing clinically, especially in that early period when the correct choice of chemotherapy may be lifesaving (as with Rocky Mountain spotted fever, meningococcemia, or cerebral malaria). Hence, one must be acutely sensitive to the different possibilities in one's area of practice and must devise a kind of strategy for the diagnosis and management, sometimes empirically on the basis of probabilities, of a rickettsia-like disease, using all available bits of epidemiologic, clinical, and laboratory information. Simple observation of the patient for the development of diagnostic clinical or laboratory features is a hazardous practice. In the United States, the single major factor contributory to the continuing 5 to 10 per cent mortality in Rocky Mountain spotted fever is delay in institution of specific chemotherapy. Listed below are some practical considerations that have emerged from analysis of experiences in several parts of the world.

The history of potential exposure (occupation, travel in endemic areas, recreational activities in wilderness areas), as well as of tick bite, is extremely important in alerting the physician to the possibility of a rickettsial disease. Modern air travel makes it possible to return from any part of the world within the incubation period of a rickettsial disease.

In a given area, certain diseases commonly cause difficult clinical differential diagnostic problems. For example, in the United States, the two diseases most commonly confused with Rocky Mountain spotted fever are measles and meningococcemia. In central and east Africa, two diseases which cause major differential diagnostic problems with louse-borne typhus are cerebral falciparum malaria and typhoid fever. Milder cases of typhus may be indistinguishable clinically from influenza. Patients with murine typhus fever commonly are found on enteric fever wards.

The most sophisticated modern laboratory diagnostic aids can sometimes help distinguish within hours between measles, meningococcemia, and Rocky Mountain spotted fever. Blood smears for malaria should be routine where malaria and rickettsial diseases coexist. Typhoid can be detected by cultures. Outside the United States and Europe, however, laboratory facilities may be unavailable, and an empirical therapeutic approach is often successful. For example, when it is not possible to distinguish between malaria, typhus, and typhoid, a combination of chloramphenicol and chloroquine, or other antimalarial appropriate for the resistance patterns of the area, often gives a satisfactory clinical response; or a "typhus suspect" not responding in 48 hours to a tetracycline drug can often be treated successfully with chloramphenicol.

Finally, outside the United States, a patient with a rickettsial infection may have another concurrent infection, e.g., typhus plus relapsing fever or trench fever; or typhus or scrub typhus plus malaria, bacterial pneumonia, or dysentery. These must also be diagnosed and treated specifically.

LABORATORY DIAGNOSIS. Methods for retrospective diagnoses (isolation of organism and serologic response) of rickettsial infections are reasonably well developed, although not universally available, but methods for specific diagnosis in the acute phase of disease, when crucial decisions about specific chemotherapy must be made, are generally unsatisfactory although improving. The following guidelines have been compiled especially for the practicing physician, beginning with methods applicable to the early, acute phase and proceeding to more specific methods, which sometimes tend to be only confirmatory or retrospective.

Exclusion of Diseases That Present Common Differential Diagnostic Problems in a Given Locality. Examples include malaria smear, skin lesion smear for meningococci, demonstration of measles antigen in respiratory epithelial cells by fluorescence microscopy, and cultures for typhoid and other enteric fevers.

Direct Demonstration of Rickettsiae in Tissues or Rickettsial Antigens in Urine in Acute Phase of Disease. Attempts to demonstrate rickettsiae directly in tissues or cells of patients and to demonstrate rickettsial antigens in body fluids, such as urine, have been explored for many years with variable degrees of success, although no method is yet available for routine diagnosis.

DIRECT MICROSCOPIC DEMONSTRATION OF RICKETTSIAE IN TISSUES. For diagnostic purposes, rickettsiae have been demonstrated in endothelial cells of skin biopsies, blood leukocytes (with or without a short period of incubation in vitro), and bone marrow smears in typhus and spotted fever infections of man or animals. The use of fluorescein-conjugated antisera permits identification of the organisms, specific at least to group. Refinement and standardization of these methods promise to yield practical routine methods for the early specific diagnosis of rickettsial infections and should be pursued vigorously.

DEMONSTRATION OF RICKETTSIAL ANTIGENS IN ACUTE PHASE URINE. Although theoretically feasible, reliable demonstration of rickettsial antigens in acute phase urine has been fraught with difficulty. Application of modern immunologic methods (radioimmunoassay, enzyme-linked immunosorbent assay [ELISA]) may improve sensitivity, specificity, and reliability and deserves concerted effort.

Isolation of Rickettsiae. The isolation of rickettsiae from the blood or tissues of a patient is hazardous, requires special laboratory facilities and trained personnel, usually does not yield results in time to influence patient management, and hence, was not encouraged as a routine procedure in the past. However, methods are improving, and moreover, it is now urgent to change this position because serologic retrospective diagnoses are ill equipped to identify new species or variants of rickettsiae. A growing diversity of rickettsial agents (e.g., the flying squirrel agent and *R. canada* in the typhus group, new members of the spotted fever group) is being recognized in the United States and elsewhere, whose importance as causes of human disease remains unknown; this is partly because conventional serologic tests for retrospective diagnosis are largely *group* specific, might not recognize variants at the species level, and would not detect infections with totally new agents. Isolation and characterization of the agent are the keystones of identification of new diseases.

Although isolation and identification of rickettsial agents are usually beyond the competence of the ordinary hospital laboratory, mechanisms do exist for accomplishing this. In the United States, properly collected and preserved specimens (frozen at −70° C or lower) can be sent through state health departments to the Centers for Disease Control in Atlanta, Georgia, where trained personnel and facilities exist to handle and characterize such agents. Also, the World Health Organization has established a series of reference laboratories that are capable of handling such agents.

Serologic Diagnosis. Serologic methods remain the mainstay of routine laboratory diagnosis of rickettsial infections and for epidemiologic purposes. However, since an antibody response rarely occurs with any of the rickettsioses before the end of the first week of disease, and since a rise in antibody titer is more or less essential to a solid diagnosis, convincing serologic diagnosis may become available only *after* the critical point has been passed with respect to lifesaving decisions about chemotherapy. At present, serologic tests consist of (1) nonspecific (Weil-Felix) tests generally available to hospital laboratories through commercially produced antigens (a part of the "febrile agglutinin" package) and (2) more specific tests, generally available at state health departments, the Centers for Disease Control, and the WHO reference laboratories.

In those rickettsioses studied, antibody response following

primary infection consists of an early transient IgM response and a slower more persistent IgG response. Recrudescent typhus (Brill-Zinsser disease) is characterized by a brisk IgG response with low to negligible IgM response. Antibodies persist for many years following louse-borne and murine typhus but fall to low or negligible levels two to three years after scrub typhus and uncomplicated Q fever. Persistent high titers with Phase I *C. burnetii* antigen suggest subacute infection, e.g., hepatitis or endocarditis.

WEIL-FELIX REACTION. Based upon unique sharing of polysaccharide antigens between certain *Proteus* strains and some rickettsiae, this agglutination test performed with suspensions of rough *Proteus* OX-2, OX-19, and OX-K strains has an historical aura and the advantage of simplicity, ready availability of antigens, and sensitivity to early antibody response.

Proteus agglutinins tend to appear early (toward the end of the first week), attain peak titers between three and four weeks after onset, and then rapidly decline. The Weil-Felix test is not positive in all rickettsial infections (rickettsialpox and Q fever) and is variable in recrudescent typhus (Brill-Zinsser disease). It will not distinguish between typhus and spotted fever group infections (*Proteus* OX-2 and OX-190). *Proteus* OX-K agglutination is not positive in all scrub typhus infections (about 70 per cent positive in primary infections and fewer in secondary infections) but may yield false positive results in relapsing fever and leptospirosis. Nevertheless, properly applied and interpreted, the test can be useful. Until more specific tests are generally available to physicians within a time frame useful for patient management, the Weil-Felix test, despite its deficiencies, will not die.

INDIRECT FLUORESCENT ANTIBODY TESTS (IFA). IFA tests are now generally used for diagnostic and epidemiologic purposes. They are sensitive and useful with anticomplementary sera or blood collected on filter paper. IFA tests may be positive when blocking factors interfere with CF or MA tests. They can be made group specific. Methods for improved species differentiation are under study. IgG, IgM, and IgA antibody titers can be determined directly. The IFA test is currently the most sensitive and reliable test available for the diagnosis of scrub typhus.

OTHER TESTS. Complement fixation and microliter agglutination tests, formerly the mainstay of rickettsial serodiagnosis and still useful, have been displaced by the IFA test. Toxin neutralization tests, passive hemagglutination tests, and radioimmune precipitation tests have special uses. New tests, such as the ELISA type test and latex agglutination tests, are under development and evaluation.

TREATMENT OF RICKETTSIAL DISEASES. The general principles of therapy are similar for all the common rickettsial diseases. Optimal management includes (1) specific antimicrobial therapy directed against the offending rickettsial agent; (2) supportive measures to correct physiologic abnormalities; (3) good nursing care to prevent serious complications; and (4) prompt, appropriate therapy of complications. In mild cases, patients treated early may require little more than the specific antimicrobial therapy. Vigorous supportive measures and good nursing may be lifesaving in severe cases.

Antirickettsial Therapy. *Prompt adequate antirickettsial therapy is the single most important factor in shortening the disease, reducing mortality, and speeding convalescence.* In cooperative uncomplicated patients this may be the only medication required.

Antimicrobial drugs of the tetracycline series are the drugs of choice for treatment of all rickettsial diseases. Although also highly effective, chloramphenicol is not recommended, unless tetracyclines cannot be used, because of the occasional complication of aplastic anemia. These drugs shorten the course of disease dramatically and reduce fatality rates virtually to zero except in neglected, complicated, or fulminating cases. The patient often begins to respond by 24 hours and is afebrile in one to four days, usually two to three days, depending on the specific rickettsia and the stage of disease at the time therapy is begun.

Penicillin, streptomycin, and sulfonamides are clinically ineffective. Practical concentrations of a wide range of aminoglycosides, semisynthetic penicillins, and cephalosporins do not inhibit *R. prowazekii* growth in vitro in cell cultures. *Note: Except for chloramphenicol,* none of the drugs (ampicillin, amoxicillin, co-trimoxazole) used for the treatment of typhoid fever, a serious differential diagnostic problem in some areas, gives clinical and/or in vitro evidence of effectiveness in typhus fever.

Tetracycline HCl is given orally in a total daily dose of 25 to 50 mg per kilogram of body weight. Two grams per day in divided doses at 4- to 6- or even 12-hour intervals usually suffices for adult patients. Chloramphenicol is given orally in amounts of 50 and 75 mg per kilogram of body weight per day for adults and children, respectively, usually in divided doses at 4- to 6- or even 12-hour intervals. (*Caution:* Doses larger than 25 mg per kilogram of body weight may be severely toxic for *newborn infants.*) Intravenous tetracycline is given in a dosage of 0.5 gram every 6 to 12 hours, to a maximum of 2 grams per day for adults. Chloramphenicol succinate, appropriately diluted, is given intravenously to adults in a dose of 1.0 gram every 8 to 12 hours. Parenteral therapy should be replaced with oral therapy as soon as the patient can swallow. When parenteral preparations are unavailable or intravenous drip therapy is impractical, oral preparations suspended in fluid may be administered by stomach tube.

Since neither tetracycline HCl nor chloramphenicol is rickettsicidal under ordinary circumstances, and since neither eradicates the organism from the body, ultimate freedom from clinical relapse (i.e., "cure") is probably dependent on an adequate immune response by the patient. Duration of therapy is dependent on the pharmacology of the particular drug employed; the susceptibility of the organism to, and rate of recovery from, the inhibitory effects of the drug employed, which may vary from one species of organism to another; and the stage of the disease at the time therapy is begun. Although not necessarily the minimal effective regimen, a practical conservative guide to duration of tetracycline or chloramphenicol therapy is to administer the drug until the patient has been afebrile for 48 hours and for an additional period until the total time elapsed from onset of disease is 12 to 14 days. Relapses respond to retreatment with the same drug. The usual precautions are observed for administering antimicrobials, e.g., adjustment of dosage to compensate for problems of immaturity in infants and of renal or hepatic dysfunction of rickettsial or other origin, staining of developing teeth, changes in microbial flora and superinfection, pregnancy, drug susceptibilities, or blood dyscrasias.

The introduction of new lipotropic tetracycline derivatives which produce prolonged high blood and tissue levels after a single dose (viz., doxycycline and minocycline) has literally revolutionized the management of louse-borne typhus. A *single* 100-mg dose of doxycycline will *cure* most adults, and a *single* 50-mg dose will cure most children, with only an occasional transient relapse which does not require additional therapy. A single 200-mg dose is rarely followed by relapse. Under extreme circumstances, single-dose doxycycline therapy, requiring only a single contact between patient and medical personnel, has been applied successfully on an outpatient basis. Unless in extremis from typhus or suffering from some unrelated disease, almost all patients will survive whether hospitalized, at home, or transiently disoriented in the bush. Single-dose doxycycline is currently the treatment of choice for louse-borne typhus. Comparable results have been obtained with minocycline, but because of its tendency to cause otitic complications, it is not recommended as a first choice drug.

Experience with single-dose doxycycline treatment of other rickettsioses indicates that a single 200-mg dose of doxycycline will cure some, but not all, cases of scrub typhus. On the other hand, very limited and uncontrolled observations suggest that a single dose will not suffice for the treatment of murine typhus or Rocky Mountain spotted fever, although a daily dose of 100 to 200 mg on a schedule described for tetracycline HCl is highly effective.

Antimicrobial resistance has not yet been encountered in naturally occurring rickettsial disease.

Steroids. Although not rigorously controlled, studies have shown that corticosteroids given in conjunction with antimicrobial drugs may cause rapid defervescence, dramatic reversal of neurologic impairment (coma, difficulty in swallowing), and an apparent improvement in the general well-being of the patient without adversely affecting the infectious process. A comatose typhus patient given steroid therapy in the evening may be sitting up on the side of the bed in the morning, conversing with his fellow patients and able to take medication and fluids by mouth. Similar effects may be seen in patients unable to swallow. More limited observations with scrub typhus and Rocky Mountain spotted fever have shown similar apparently beneficial effects, although reversal of intravascular clotting in Rocky Mountain spotted fever will not be effected. This has been accomplished by giving 100 mg of hydrocortisone intravenously and 200 to 300 mg of cortisone acetate intramuscularly in addition to tetracycline or doxycycline upon admission. *(Falciparum malaria must be excluded by blood smear in patients at risk to both diseases.)* Often within 24 hours a typhus patient is able to swallow the final dose of antibiotic (100 mg of doxycycline), to take oral fluids, to attend to elimination, and to move spontaneously to reduce the chances of developing pressure necroses or thrombophlebitis. Usually no more therapy of any kind, antimicrobial or steroid, is required, and nutrition presents no problem. This therapy is reserved for seriously ill or "uncooperative" patients.

Fluid and Electrolyte Balance. Oral fluids sufficient to ensure a daily urine output of at least 1500 ml suffice for the conscious, cooperative patient. The comatose patient will require parenteral fluids to maintain an adequate urine output. Fluids should be given slowly so as not to tax the potentially labile cardiovascular system. Excess electrolytes contribute to the general edema and to cardiac load when the fluid re-enters the vascular compartment. Urine output, the presence of oliguria, and laboratory determinations will serve as guides to the proper volume and proportion of electrolytes, glucose, and water.

Hepatic and Renal Systems. The cause of the disturbed liver (abnormal test results, rarely jaundice) and kidney (azotemia, albuminuria, oliguria) functions remains controversial, but these abnormalities are usually transient and disappear with convalescence.

Cardiovascular System, Including Blood. The most prominent manifestations of the typhus, scrub typhus, and spotted fever groups of rickettsial diseases can be attributed to abnormalities of the cardiovascular system. Hypotension is common, and peripheral vascular collapse, frequently in the second week of disease, is a leading cause of death and has been difficult to manage. Its cause is only incompletely understood. However, the widespread focal lesions of the small vessels are assumed to be contributory.

Albumin may be used to combat hypoproteinemia. Red cells are preferred to correct significant anemia. Heparin has been described as treatment for rickettsia-associated intravascular clotting, but other reports have failed to record benefit.

The management of peripheral vascular collapse is empirical and largely of unproved benefit: (1) oxygen; (2) judicious use of salt-poor concentrated albumin as a plasma expander and to reduce edema; (3) vasopressor drugs, e.g., levarterenol bitartrate (Levophed); and (4) corticosteroids such as hydrocortisone.

Pulmonary edema and congestive heart failure, resulting from excessive intake of salt and water or from rapid resorption of edema fluid with vascular healing, are treated with digitalis. No guidelines are available for the use of diuretics, but if their use is contemplated, consideration should be given to the state of renal function.

Massive intravascular hemolysis, described in glucose-6-phosphate dehydrogenase deficient subjects with murine or scrub typhus, has been managed with dialysis.

Other Complications. Bacterial pneumonia, still frequent in epidemic typhus, or other bacterial infections are treated with appropriate antimicrobial agents according to the causative organisms and their sensitivity patterns. Gangrene, decubitus ulcers, and thrombophlebitis are treated by the usual surgical and medical methods. Unless caused by a large destructive process (hemorrhage or thrombosis of a large vessel), neurologic abnormalities usually resolve with convalescence, although personality changes, electroencephalographic abnormalities, and deafness have been known to persist in some patients for months.

Nursing Care. Patients may be irrational or agitated and may injure themselves or even attempt self-destruction. Close observation and restraint may be required. Comatose patients should be turned frequently to prevent pressure necrosis, thrombophlebitis, and hypostatic pneumonia. Special skin care and protection of bony prominences may be desirable in view of the vascular damage associated with these diseases. Good oral hygiene reduces the chances of suppurative parotitis.

Special Considerations. Although classic Q fever often responds promptly to chemotherapy with tetracycline drugs or chloramphenicol as outlined above, the response in some cases is slower and less dramatic. Treatment of chronic infection is less satisfactory. Chemotherapy of *C. burnetii* endocarditis is especially unsatisfactory, probably because of the fact that most antirickettsial drugs are primarily rickettsiostatic. There has been very limited success with combined chemotherapy administered over a period of many months. Surgical replacement of the affected heart valve has been successful in some cases, but colonization of the artificial valve may occur.

Trench fever has been reported to respond to tetracycline drugs, but no information is available concerning the effects of brief chemotherapy on the persistence of the organism in the blood or on subsequent relapse rates.

General

Horsfall FL Jr, Tamm I (eds.): Viral and Rickettsial Infections of Man. 4th ed. Philadelphia, J. B. Lippincott Company, 1965. *Although dated in many respects, the chapters on rickettsial diseases present much basic information and background and constitute the most recent authoritative and comprehensive general coverage.*

Weiss E: Growth and physiology of rickettsiae. Bacteriol Rev 37:259, 1973. *This is a good review up to the date of its publication. Although much has transpired since, no more recent review is available.*

Laboratory Diagnosis

Elisberg BL, Bozeman FL: Serologic diagnosis of rickettsial diseases by indirect immunofluorescence. Arch Inst Pasteur Tunis 43:193, 1966. Fiset P, Ormsbe RA, Silberman R, Peacock M, Spielman SH: A microagglutination technique for detection and measurement of rickettsial antibodies. Acta Virol (Praha) 13:60, 1969. Murray ES, O'Connor JM, Gaon JA: Differentiation of 19S and 7S complement-fixing antibodies in primary versus recrudescent typhus by either ethanethiol or heat. Proc Soc Exp Biol Med 119:291, 1965. Philip RN, Casper EA, MacCormack JN, Sexton DJ, Thomas LA, Anacker RL, Burgdorfer W, Vick S: A comparison of serological methods for diagnosis of Rocky Mountain spotted fever. Am J Epidemiol 105:56, 1977. *These four papers provide some introduction into serologic diagnostic methods.*

Woodward TE, Pederson CE Jr, Oster CN, Bagley LR, Romberg J, Snyder MJ: Prompt confirmation of Rocky Mountain spotted fever: Identification of rickettsiae in skin tissues. J Infect Dis 134:297, 1976. *This method is currently under evaluation for rapid diagnosis in the acutely ill patient.*

Pathology

Pinkerton H, Strano AJ: Diseases caused by rickettsiae. *In* Binford CH, Connor DH (eds.): Pathology of Tropical and Extraordinary Diseases, Vol 1. Washington, D.C., Armed Forces Institute of Pathology, pp 87-100. *This publication presents a well-illustrated comparison of the pathologies of common rickettsial diseases, along with some additional references.*

Chemotherapy

Woodward TE: Therapy of the rickettsial diseases with a discussion of chemoprophylaxis. Arch Inst Pasteur Tunis 35:507, 1959. *This review presents briefly the evolution of chemotherapy of rickettsial diseases through the introduction of chloramphenicol and the early tetracyclines. More recent tetracyclines are not included; their use is described in many scattered publications and from the author's personal experience.*

317. THE TYPHUS GROUP

Charles L. Wisseman, Jr.

Three clinical and epidemiologic entities comprise the established diseases of the typhus group: (1) primary louse-borne epidemic typhus *(Rickettsia prowazekii);* (2) its recrudescent form, Brill-Zinsser disease *(R. prowazekii),* and (3) flea-borne murine typhus *(R. mooseri [R. typhi]).* These diseases are similar clinically and pathologically but differ in intensity of certain symptoms and signs, severity, and case fatality rate. Tables 316–1 to 316–3 summarize selected features of the organisms, the diseases, and their epidemiologies. This conventional listing of typhus group diseases has been complicated in the United States in recent years by (1) the isolation of a new species, *R. canada,* from ticks in Canada and its implication on serologic grounds as the possible cause of a Rocky Mountain spotted fever–like disease in Georgia; (2) the isolation of a rickettsia indistinguishable from *R. prowazekii* from flying squirrels in the eastern United States, and the recent recognition of sporadic human cases serologically identified as *R. prowazekii* infection in houses harboring flying squirrels; and (3) the strong one-way serologic cross-reactions between *R. canada* and *R. prowazekii.* Much more information, especially isolation and characterization of the agents from human cases, is needed for clarification.

EPIDEMIC LOUSE-BORNE TYPHUS FEVER

SYNONYMS. Synonyms include *classic, historic, and European typhus; jail, war, camp, and ship fever; Fleckfieber* (German); *typhus exanthématique* (French); *tifus exantemático* and *tabardillo* (Spanish); and *dermotypho* (Italian).

DEFINITION. Classic typhus fever is an acute infectious disease transmitted by the human body louse *(Pediculus humanus humanus)* and characterized clinically by sudden onset, sustained high fever of about two weeks' duration, a macular rash, and altered mental state. Brill-Zinsser disease is a recrudescence of typhus occurring months to years after primary infection, caused by organisms persisting in tissues since the primary infection, and clinically resembling a mild form of classic typhus.

ETIOLOGY (see Ch. 316). *Rickettsia prowazekii* is the etiologic agent of both classic typhus fever and Brill-Zinsser disease. No evidence has been obtained for significant variations in antigenic composition or virulence for man in strains from different areas, but attenuation has been observed as a laboratory phenomenon.

TRANSMISSION AND EPIDEMIOLOGY. The "classic" infection cycle is restricted to man and the human body louse *(Pediculus humanus humanus),* although the organism can also grow in the head louse *(Pediculus humanus capitis).* The louse acquires the rickettsia by feeding on the blood of a typhus patient during the rickettsemic phase. The organism multiplies in and destroys cells of the louse midgut. Large numbers of rickettsiae are excreted in the feces. The organism is not transmitted by bite. Instead, crushed infective lice or louse feces contaminate bite sites or other breaks in the skin, or airborne infective louse feces gain access through the respiratory tract.

The louse regularly dies of *R. prowazekii* infection, does not transmit the organism transovarially to the next generation, and is not a reservoir of typhus. Putative domestic animal reservoirs have largely been discounted as laboratory artifacts. The origin and extent of the flying squirrel typhus phenomenon is unknown, and, hence, the importance of its role as a reservoir of classic epidemic typhus or any manifestation other than the known sporadic cases in the eastern United States is not yet known. In most other areas, man, through the phenomenon of persisting infection and subsequent recrudescence (Brill-Zinsser disease), is the only known interepidemic reservoir and the mechanism by which the rickettsiae are made available again to lice. Neither the factors that precipitate recrudescence nor the precise rate of recrudescence are known, although one estimate suggests a rate less than 10 per 100,000 cases of primary infection. The efficiency with which lice become infected with *R. prowazekii* is apparently less during feeding upon Brill-Zinsser disease patients than upon primary typhus patients. Nevertheless, this phenomenon is known to have initiated typhus outbreaks and probably also contributes to sustaining endemicity.

Typhus can occur anywhere when living conditions and political, socioeconomic, environmental, and cultural factors predispose to lousiness and the transfer of lice among people. These are currently supplied in mountainous parts of the Northern and Southern Hemispheres, as well as equatorial regions, in deserts (Sahara, Arabian deserts) where heavy clothing is worn continuously, and in tropical regions.

Louse-borne typhus can occur as a truly epidemic disease, as a prolonged endemoepidemic disease (as in Ethiopia today), or as a highly endemic infection with sporadic, often unrecognized infections in young age groups but with occasional sharp village outbreaks involving all ages (as in Andean countries today).

PATHOLOGY. The general pathology and pathophysiologic features are described in Ch. 316.

CLINICAL MANIFESTATIONS AND COURSE. The following description applies to untreated full-blown classic typhus fever in adults. The incubation period usually is from 8 to 12 days but may be as short as 6 or as long as 15 days.

Prodromes of vague malaise and headache are not uncommon. The early phase is usually ushered in by the abrupt onset of fever, severe headache, myalgia of the back and legs, and chills or chilly sensations. The headache is intense and intractable and persists day and night. Over the first two or three days the temperature attains a level of 39 to 41° C, where it remains with only slight fluctuations until death or recovery. The skin is usually hot and dry. The face is flushed or dusky; the conjunctivae are suffused; photophobia is frequent. Deafness, tinnitus, and sometimes vertigo are prominent features. The mental state is dull. Weakness and prostration may be mild early, but after two or three days may become profound. Unproductive cough with sparse physical findings occurs in about two thirds of the cases. Nausea, vomiting, and diarrhea occur but are uncommon. Constipation is usually present.

The characteristic rash appears between the fourth and seventh days. The lesions first appear on the trunk and axillary folds and spread to the extremities, sparing the face, palms, and soles, except in very severely ill patients. At first the lesions are pinkish red macules that blanch on pressure. The evolution of the rash depends on the severity of the illness. In mild cases it may fade completely in one or two days; in cases of greater severity it may become maculopapular, then petechial, changing to reddish brown and lasting for one to two weeks before fading; in very severe cases the lesions may be exceedingly numerous, almost confluent, quickly becoming hemorrhagic or even purpuric. The rash may be absent in 5 to 10 per cent of cases. With experience and proper lighting, it may be seen without too much difficulty in dark-skinned persons.

At first the pulse rate is slow in relation to the temperature, but by the end of the first week it becomes rapid (110 to 140), weak, and frequently undulating or irregular. The blood pressure is usually low, sometimes with a systolic pressure below 80 mm Hg, and there may be brief episodes of severe hypotension. Cyanosis may be present.

The mental state progresses from dullness to stupor or occasionally to coma. The stupor may be interrupted by brief periods of delirium. Cranial nerves are selectively and variably involved (deafness, dysphagia, dysphonia). Coarse tremors may appear. Incontinence of urine and feces is encountered in severely ill patients.

Oliguria, proteinuria, and azotemia are common. Jaundice is rare, but elevations in serum transaminases may appear early. The white blood count may show a leukopenia early. In the second and third weeks of the disease it is normal or only slightly elevated unless complications ensue. Anemia may develop in the second or third week.

Death from typhus usually occurs between the ninth and eighteenth day of illness. The terminal period is usually characterized by a profound stupor, peripheral vascular collapse, and severe renal failure. When recovery is the outcome, the temperature begins to decline after 14 to 18 days and reaches a normal level by lysis in two to four days. The mental and physical state of the patient improve strikingly as the temperature falls, but strength returns more slowly (two to three months).

Secondary bacterial bronchopneumonia, otitis media, and parotitis are common in untreated patients. Thrombosis may affect the large arteries with serious results (e.g., hemiplegia). Thrombosis of small vessels may lead to gangrene, particularly of the toes, fingers, or ear lobes. Necrosis of the skin may occur over the bony prominences, especially over the sacrum or greater trochanter.

Severity of disease and case fatality rate increase with age, being less severe and often uncharacteristic in younger children and increasing rapidly with age over 40 years. In persons who contract typhus after having received killed typhus vaccine, the disease is greatly modified, with negligible mortality.

Brill-Zinsser disease is similar to primary typhus but milder. The fever, on the average, is lower and of shorter duration, the rash is less intense and often absent, and the case fatality rate is low.

PROGNOSIS. Depending on host factors, such as age, stress, nutritional state, and other concurrent diseases, case fatality rate in untreated typhus may range from 10 per cent or less to 60 per cent. Deep coma and severe hypotension and tachycardia associated with falling body temperature are signs of poor prognosis. Even such cases, however, often respond dramatically to appropriate chemotherapy and supportive measures. Appropriate treatment reduces the mortality rate in ordinary severe typhus fever virtually to zero.

TREATMENT. Treatment is described in Ch. 316. A single 200-mg oral dose of the long-acting tetracycline doxycycline is the treatment of choice under ordinary circumstances. The response of uncomplicated typhus to specific antirickettsial chemotherapy, whether begun early or late, is highly predictable. The temperature returns to normal limits in 48 to 72 hours, averaging about 60 hours, accompanied by progressive lessening of headache and improvement of mental status. Occasionally, some manifestations, such as deafness, may appear during response to early therapy but subsequently subside.

PREVENTION AND CONTROL. Infected lice and louse feces on a typhus patient present a special hazard to all nonimmune contacts, including physicians and attendants among whom infection is a common occupational hazard. Decontamination and delousing of the typhus patient and his clothing (including blankets and hats) are performed immediately upon hospitalization. Clothing and bedding are best decontaminated by heat, because this will kill the lice as well as the rickettsiae. After the patient is decontaminated and deloused, isolation and quarantine are not necessary.

Control of louse-borne typhus currently depends heavily upon control of the louse vector. Application of insecticide dusts (10 per cent DDT, 1 per cent malathion, 1 per cent lindane, or newer carbamates, depending upon local louse-resistance patterns) to fully clothed persons is very effective for reducing louse populations and controlling disease in acute outbreaks. Insecticides alone are less effective for long-term louse control in areas where conditions conducive to lousiness persist and where louse strains resistant to insecticides can be, and are, selected. The older methods of subjecting clothes and bedding to heat or fumigants (e.g., methylbromide) are effective but cumbersome. It is possible but unproved that repellent-treated clothing (e.g., M-1960, diethyltoluamide) would reduce the chances of louse acquisition.

Conventional typhus vaccines composed of killed organisms are no longer available in the United States, pending development of improved vaccines of proven protective potency. The attenuated E strain of *R. prowazekii,* when used as a living vaccine, is protective but may produce a mildly symptomatic, self-limited infection in 10 to 15 per cent of recipients. It is not generally available in the United States.

Under current circumstances, ordinary tourists or resident expatriates are not very likely to be exposed to louse-borne typhus, in contrast to murine typhus, even in endemic areas if they maintain the usual separate households, pay attention to personal hygiene, and do not mix intimately with the affected local population. On the other hand, anyone who comes in contact with members of the affected population (in crowds, markets, buses, schools, or churches) is at risk. Depending upon the circumstances, the wearing of insecticide- or repellent-treated clothing and the overnight exposure of clothing to a dichlorvos strip (No-Pest) in an airtight bag may reduce exposure to lice. Under very special *short-term* circumstances, chemoprophylaxis with 100 mg of doxycycline once or twice a week might be effective, but this has not been formally tested with louse-borne typhus, and the disease might develop after the drug is discontinued. Prompt chemotherapy on the first or second day of disease reduces typhus to a relatively minor inconvenience.

MURINE OR FLEA-BORNE TYPHUS FEVER

DEFINITION. Murine typhus fever is an acute infectious disease communicable from rodent hosts to man sporadically by means of the rat flea *(Xenopsylla cheopis).* The disease is similar clinically to classic epidemic typhus except that it is milder.

ETIOLOGY (see Ch. 316). *Rickettsia mooseri (R. typhi)* shares some common antigens with *R. prowazekii* and *R. canada* but differs in specific antigens, host range, and certain other biologic properties. Significant cross-immunity between *R. mooseri* and *R. prowazekii* is produced by infection but not by killed vaccines. DNA homology studies show a difference between *R. mooseri* and *R. prowazekii* sufficiently large to preclude easy transition from one to the other by simple variation or mutation, except on an evolutionary scale. Thus, *R. mooseri* is an unlikely source of some contemporary outbreaks of classic louse-borne epidemic typhus, as has been suggested, although limited outbreaks of louse-borne *R. mooseri* infection may have occurred.

TRANSMISSION AND EPIDEMIOLOGY. Murine typhus is not communicable from man to man. It is a zoonosis maintained in nature in a cycle involving rats and certain other small mammals as amplifying hosts and reservoirs and fleas and rat lice as vectors. In the rat flea and perhaps the other fleas infected by feeding upon rickettsemic rats, the organism grows in cells of the gut without killing the flea and is shed in the feces for the life of the flea. There is no transovarial transmission. It is transmitted to man, not by bite of the flea, but rather by contamination of broken skin with infective feces or by inhalation of dried infective feces.

Murine typhus is widely distributed over the world in the areas penetrated by *Rattus rattus* and *Rattus norvegicus* and where the vector fleas coexist. In some areas under appropriate conditions there may be spillover of *R. mooseri* from *Rattus* into other spatially closely associated small mammals and to man. Seasonal incidence of human infections appears to correlate with the periods of abundance of vector fleas, which in the United States is in the summer months. Rats are commensal animals closely associated with buildings or structures containing food (such as warehouses, markets, grain elevators, and dwellings).

PATHOLOGY. Although because of the low death rate few postmortem studies have been made, it is assumed that the lesions in man, as is the case in experimental infection of laboratory animals, are similar to those in louse-born typhus.

CLINICAL MANIFESTATIONS AND COURSE. The incubation period of murine typhus lasts from 6 to 14 days. The symptoms are similar to those of louse-borne typhus, the principal differences being that murine typhus is a milder and shorter disease, the rash is less extensive and persists for shorter periods, there are fewer complications, and the case fatality rate is lower.

Although murine typhus is often referred to as mild, and truly mild cases do occur, this is mildness *relative* to louse-borne typhus. On an absolute scale it can be severe and debilitating and may require two to three months for convalescence in untreated patients.

DIAGNOSIS. ***Clinical Diagnosis.*** The diagnosis of murine typhus may be suspected when a patient has sustained fever of several days' duration accompanied by headache, generalized aches and pains, and a macular or maculopapular rash appearing on the trunk on the fifth or sixth day after onset of fever. The patient with murine typhus may give a history of activities that have brought him into contact with places where rats are numerous. However, there is often no definite recollection of a flea bite. It is impossible on clinical evidence alone to distinguish an ordinary case of murine typhus from a case of Brill-Zinsser disease or a mild case of louse-borne typhus.

In many areas of the world where typhoid or other enteric fevers are common, where specific laboratory diagnostic tests are not readily available, and where chloramphenicol is routinely employed to treat enteric fevers, significant occurrence of murine typhus and sporadic louse-borne typhus may be unsuspected or unrecognized, being hidden among the enteric fevers by virtue of some clinical similarity and response to chloramphenicol. However, when ampicillin or trimethoprim-sulfamethoxazole is used for the treatment of suspected typhoid fevers, the typhus fevers do not respond and their presence may then be unveiled.

Laboratory Diagnosis. Diagnosis can often be made by specific rickettsial serologic tests or by isolation of the agent. (See Laboratory Diagnosis in Ch. 316.)

PROGNOSIS. The case fatality rate is usually less than 5 per cent in untreated patients and is virtually zero with rapid convalescence in uncomplicated murine typhus treated with appropriate antirickettsial drugs.

TREATMENT. Treatment follows the guidelines given in Ch. 316 with respect to the *multiple* dose antimicrobial regimen.

PREVENTION AND CONTROL. Individual preventive measures include avoiding endemic foci where rats and their fleas abound (e.g., warehouses, storage areas, grain elevators) or wearing repellent-treated clothing to prevent acquisition of fleas. A vaccine is not available.

General control measures are directed at reducing rat and flea populations. Among others, these include rat proof construction and prevention of access of rats to food materials; reduction of rat populations by poison baits (e.g., warfarin, alphanaphthylthiourea), trapping, or poison gases into burrows; and reduction of the flea population through application of appropriate insecticides (such as DDT) to rat runs. When contemplating a rodent control program, it is important to plan insecticide application for flea control prior to, or simultaneously with, the rodent control measures to prevent increased exposure of man to fleas seeking alternative hosts.

Gaon JA, Murray ES: The natural history of recrudescent typhus (Brill-Zinsser disease) in Bosnia. Bull WHO 35:133, 1966. *This paper summarizes the definitive work that validated Zinsser's hypothesis about the nature of the disease described by Brill.*

Miller ES, Beeson PB: Murine typhus fever. Medicine 25:1, 1946. Stuart BM, Pullen RL: Endemic (murine) typhus fever: Clinical observations of 180 cases. Ann Intern Med 23:520, 1945. *These two papers record a wealth of clinical observations on murine typhus fever.*

Proceedings of the International Symposium on the Control of Lice and Louse-Borne Diseases, Washington, D.C., December 4–6, 1972. Pan-American Health Organization Scientific Publication No 263, 1973. *This is the most comprehensive modern consideration of the problems of lice and louse-borne diseases available today.*

Traub R, Wisseman CL Jr, Farhang-Azad A: The ecology of murine typhus—a critical review. Trop Dis Bull 75:237, 1978. *Although current work is introducing some additional concepts, this publication comprehensively covers most of the published work up to the time of its preparation.*

Wohlbach SB, Todd JL, Palfrey FW: The Etiology and Pathology of Typhus. Cambridge, Mass., Harvard University Press, 1922. *This is the classic, definitive work on the etiology and pathology of louse-borne typhus fever.*

Zarafonetis CJD: The typhus fevers. *In* Coates JB, Havens WP (eds.): Medical Department, United States Army. Internal Medicine in World War II, Vol II. Infectious Diseases. Washington, D.C., Office of the Surgeon General, Department of the Army, 1963, pp 143-223. *Clinical aspects of louse-borne typhus seen by Army physicians during World War II are summarized in this publication.*

318. ROCKY MOUNTAIN SPOTTED FEVER

Charles L. Wisseman, Jr.

SYNONYMS. This disease is also known as *spotted fever* and *tick typhus* (England), *fiebre manchada* (Mexico), *fiebre petequial* (Colombia), and *febre maculosa* or *São Paulo typhus* (Brazil).

DEFINITION. Rocky Mountain spotted fever is a mild to severe, sometimes fatal, acute infectious disease of the Western Hemisphere caused by *Rickettsia rickettsii* and transmitted to man by several species of ticks. The disease is characterized by sudden onset with chills and headache, by fever of about two to three weeks' duration, and by a rash on the extremities and trunk beginning about the fourth day of disease.

ETIOLOGY. The disease is caused by *Rickettsia rickettsii*, the prototype species of the spotted fever group of rickettsiae with members of which it shares group antigens but from which it can be differentiated by more specific tests (see Ch. 316). Both mild and highly virulent strains exist in many parts of the United States. Although several other species of the spotted fever group of rickettsiae have been isolated from ticks, to date only typical *R. rickettsii* has been *isolated* from infections of man. More intensive efforts to isolate and characterize rickettsiae from patients are needed to clarify the role of other spotted fever group agents as possible causes of human disease.

DISTRIBUTION AND INCIDENCE. Although originally encountered in Rocky Mountain states (Montana and Idaho), Rocky Mountain spotted fever has been recognized in at least 46 states and is actually more prevalent in the south Atlantic states than in the West. In the eastern United States it extends from Cape Cod and some adjacent islands, through a focus on Long Island, to Florida, with almost half the cases in the United States occurring in Maryland, Virginia, North Carolina, and Georgia. The number of cases per year in the United States has risen steadily over the past several years to more than 1000 since 1979. The reasons for this increase are not fully understood, but may include abundance of ticks, extension of suburbs into tick-infested rural areas, and increased recreational activities in wilderness areas. Rocky Mountain spotted fever has also been recognized in several provinces of Canada, in Mexico, in Central America (Panama, Costa Rica) and in South America (Colombia, Brazil).

TRANSMISSION AND EPIDEMIOLOGY. Rocky Mountain spotted fever is a zoonosis maintained in a natural cycle between certain tick species and small (rodents, rabbits) and perhaps larger mammals. Man, a dead-end host for *R. rickettsii*, becomes infected when he intrudes into this zoonotic cycle (as for recreational or occupational reasons) and is bitten by an infected tick. Rocky Mountain spotted fever is not communicable from man to man by ordinary contact.

Although multiple tick species (both hard and soft varieties) are known to become naturally infected and may play a role in transmission among animals, the main tick vectors for man are hard (Ixodid) ticks: the wood tick *Dermacentor andersoni*, in the western United States; the dog tick, *Dermacentor variabilis*, in the eastern United States; *Amblyomma americanum* in Texas and Oklahoma; the brown dog tick, *Rhipicephalus sanguineus*, in northern Mexico (and introduced into the United States); and *Amblyomma cajennense* in Brazil and Colombia.

PATHOLOGY. The pathology of Rocky Mountain spotted fever conforms in general to the description of the rickettsial diseases in Ch. 316. Of special note is the fact that the vasculitis in Rocky Mountain spotted fever is not limited to the endothelium and is more severe than in typhus or scrub typhus, causing more pronounced thrombotic occlusion and necrosis of the muscular layers. Microinfarcts are seen with some frequency in the central nervous system.

CLINICAL MANIFESTATIONS AND COURSE. A history of tick bite can be elicited in many, but not all, patients. Variations in incubation period (2 to 14, average 7 days) and severity of disease are seen in Rocky Mountain spotted fever, with a tendency for an inverse relationship between the two. Very severe disease often is preceded by a short (two- to five-day) incubation period. Prodromes, when present, consist of anorexia, irritability, malaise, feverishness, and chilly sensations. Attacks may be so mild that the patient remains ambulatory, or so severe that death may occur within three to six days of onset. The more typical infections are sudden in onset, with severe headache, chills, fever, prostration, myalgia (especially of the back and legs) nausea with occasional vomiting, conjunctival injections, and photophobia. There may be abdominal muscular pain, tenderness of muscles on palpation, and arthralgia.

Body temperature reaches 39 to 40° C in the first two days, is sustained at elevated levels for about two weeks, and declines by slow lysis over three or four days. Hyperthermia in the range of 41° C is a serious sign. Body temperature falling to near or below normal levels in the face of severe hypotension and tachycardia carries a grave prognosis.

The characteristic rash appears on about the fourth day (two to six days), first about the wrists and ankles, and then extends rapidly over all or most of the body, including palms, soles, face, and, occasionally, the mucous membranes of the mouth and throat. At first, the lesions are pink macules, 2 to 5 mm in diameter, which blanch on pressure. In two or three days, they become fixed, darker red, or purplish, maculopapular, and, about the fourth day, petechial. Hemorrhagic lesions may coalesce. The rash begins to disappear as the fever subsides but often remains as pigmented spots for weeks.

Early in the disease the pulse is full, regular, and elevated in proportion to fever. Later, it becomes more rapid and feeble, and some degree of hypotension develops. The electrocardiogram may show minor S-T deflections and prolonged P-R intervals. In some cases, hypotension may attain shock levels, and gangrene of fingers, toes, ears, nose, or genitalia may develop. Thrombosis of larger vessels may lead to a loss of a portion of a limb or hemiplegia. The skin may become necrotic over body prominences. Hemorrhage from the nose, gastrointestinal tract, or kidney may occur. Platelet counts are frequently low. Varying degrees of disseminated intravascular coagulation have been observed.

Central nervous system involvement is manifest by restlessness, insomnia, delirium, stupor, and, in severe cases, coma. Convulsions, muscular rigidity, tremors, and athetoid movements may occur. Cranial nerve involvement is variable. Transient deafness is common, but peripheral neuritis is uncommon. Electroencephalographic changes may persist for many months. Incontinence of urine and feces may be present in severe cases.

The liver may be enlarged and serum albumin depressed, but jaundice is not common. Oliguria and some azotemia are common in severe cases. Anuria and marked azotemia may be seen in critically ill patients. Complicating secondary bacterial infections (bronchopneumonia, otitis media, parotitis) occur but are uncommon.

Convalescence may take weeks to months. Death, when it occurs in the nonfulminant variety, usually occurs late in the second week of disease (range about 9 to 18 days after onset).

DIAGNOSIS. An acute febrile illness with or without rash, in a person with a history of tick-bite, exposure to ticks (either in a tick-infested rural or suburban area or contact with a tick-infested dog), or, equally important, recreational or occupational activities that might have brought the patient into a tick-infested area, should alert the physician to the possibility of Rocky Mountain spotted fever. Although other diseases, especially those with rash, may present transient early differential diagnostic problems, the two diseases that have consistently caused the greatest confusion are measles and meningococcemia. The most promising laboratory diagnostic method for providing a specific diagnosis early enough in the disease to permit effective specific therapeutic intervention is the demonstration by the fluorescent antibody technique of spotted fever group rickettsiae in skin biopsies. Isolation attempts and serologic methods (see Laboratory Diagnosis in Ch. 316) are useful and important but rarely yield results in time for most efficient management.

PROGNOSIS. Although mild cases occur, the rapid, severe course in some patients makes it imperative to regard any suspected case of Rocky Mountain spotted fever as a medical emergency. In untreated cases, the overall case fatality rate is about 20 per cent, with areas of low (≤ 10 per cent) and high (≥ 60 per cent) rates. Prognosis depends on severity of infection, host factors (such as age, presence of other disease), and *the time after onset at which specific antirickettsial chemotherapy is started.* Even with effective antirickettsial drugs available, the case fatality rate has remained at 5 to 10 per cent. Analysis of fatal cases has shown that the single most important factor was *delay in institution of antirickettsial therapy,* whatever the reason. With the time between onset and death as short as three to six days, the critical period when antimicrobial therapy can influence the outcome may be very short indeed and does not leave much latitude for correcting errors in clinical diagnosis.

TREATMENT. *Prompt* administration of a tetracycline antibiotic, including doxycycline, or chloramphenicol daily for about six days, is the single most important specific therapeutic measure (see Treatment of Rickettsial Diseases in Ch. 316). Because specific etiologic diagnosis may be impossible in the first few days of disease, any patient seriously considered to have Rocky Mountain spotted fever should be treated as such while other diagnostic procedures continue. Other antimicrobial agents, such as the penicillins, cephalosporins, aminoglycosides, and trimethoprim-sulfamethoxazole, which are commonly employed for other proven or suspected bacterial infections, *are without effect* on Rocky Mountain spotted fever at clinically permissible doses. Reliance upon them to gain time for a laboratory-confirmed diagnosis may be devastating.

Specific treatment of uncomplicated Rocky Mountain spotted fever on the first or second day of disease usually results in rapid defervescence, sometimes by 24 to 48 hours, with few residua. In sharp contrast, in the untreated severe cases, tissue damage caused by progressive infection may be accompanied by increasingly serious physiologic derangements, as in the cardiovascular and blood clotting systems, which do not respond directly to antimicrobial therapy and which often are poorly responsive to therapies specifically directed at the physiologic derangements. A patient may progress to this dangerous state, associated with high mortality rate, in five to seven days after onset of disease, and occasionally even more rapidly. It is not uncommon for a patient with an unsuspected case of Rocky Mountain spotted fever to enter the hospital after two to four days of fever and to enter the critical phase while routine diagnostic tests are still in progress, perhaps even under the misguided security of some combination of beta lactam and aminoglycoside antibiotics.

PREVENTION AND CONTROL. Individual preventive measures are directed primarily at prevention of tick bite. The chances of ticks attaching should be minimized by (1) avoiding places especially likely to harbor ticks (e.g., brush where livestock and game take refuge); (2) wearing protective clothing designed to exclude ticks (preferably impregnated with a tick repellent, such as N-N-butylacetanilide or high concentrations of diethyltoluamide, or sprayed with the acaricide 0.5 per cent permethrin); and (3) carefully inspecting the *entire* body once or twice daily to remove all ticks. Ticks usually crawl about on the body or in the clothing for some time prior to attaching. Thus frequent inspection usually discloses ticks before they attach. Moreover, since the chance of transmission of Rocky Mountain spotted fever appears to be a function of the duration of attachment, early removal of an attached tick probably reduces the chances of infection. Ticks should be removed (from man or dogs) with a pair of forceps, exerting gentle steady traction so that the mouth parts are released intact from the skin. Most other commonly recommended methods of tick removal are less satisfactory. Contact between tick and fingers should be avoided, because rickettsiae in tick feces or body fluids may enter a break in the skin or be transferred to mucous membranes and initiate infection.

For families living in tick-infested areas, an especially effective preventive measure is for parents to establish the routine of examining themselves and their children for ticks every evening at bath time during the tick season, and to teach the children to examine themselves as soon as they are old enough.

Dogs frequently bring ticks into houses. Ticks should be removed with the same care to avoid possible infection as described above. Acquisition of Rocky Mountain spotted fever by inhalation of airborne dried infected tick feces from the dog's coat is suspected but not proven. Commercial repellent-impregnated plastic collars may reduce, but not necessarily eliminate, ticks on dogs. *Rhipicephalus sanguineus* ticks may become established indoors.

If an attached tick is found, even if it is positive for *R. rickettsii* by the "hemolymph" test, it is best practice today to place a person from whom such a tick has been removed under close observation, recording morning and evening temperatures for two weeks, and instituting full antirickettsial chemotherapy only, but promptly, when a significant rise in temperature first appears. Attempts at chemoprophylaxis are likely only to delay onset of disease.

R. rickettsii vaccines have been removed from the market because of limited effectiveness.

Area control of ticks is still very difficult and is usually considered impractical. Ticks are unusually resistant to most insecticides. Yet, some measure of control may be achieved in time on small plots of ground, such as suburban lots, by intensive acaricidal treatment, the clearing of underbrush, intensive gardening or cultivation, and a reduction of the wild animal population. Changes in land use may affect tick populations. Some progress is being made toward identifying the specific habitat alterations that affect tick populations.

Note: In the last few years there has been a flood of publications on many aspects of the problems of Rocky Mountain spotted fever. No unifying reviews have yet appeared. The following references are limited to clinical aspects of Rocky Mountain spotted fever, because they, especially through the references that each cites, give a broad access to the rapidly evolving newer knowledge of the pathophysiologic manifestation of this disease.

Bradford WD, Croker BP, Tisher CC: Kidney lesions in Rocky Mountain spotted fever. A light-, immunofluorescence-, and electron-microscopic study. Am J Pathol 97:381, 1979.
Bradford WD, Hackel DB: Myocardial involvement in Rocky Mountain spotted fever. Arch Pathol Lab Med 102:357, 1978.
Fine D, Mosher D, Yamada T, Burke D, Kenyon R: Coagulation and complement studies in Rocky Mountain spotted fever. Arch Intern Med 138:735, 1978.
Harrell GT: Rocky Mountain spotted fever. Medicine 28:333, 1949. *A classic.*
Hatwick MAW, O'Brien RJ, Hanson BF: Rocky Mountain spotted fever: Epidemiology of an increasing problem. Ann Intern Med 84:732, 1976.
Linnemann CC Jr, Janson PF: The clinical presentations of Rocky Mountain spotted fever. Clin Pediat 17:673, 1978.
Walker DH, Crawford CG, Cain BG: Rickettsial infection of the pulmonary microcirculation: The basis for interstitial pneumonitis in Rocky Mountain spotted fever. Hum Pathol 11:263, 1980.

319. TICK-BORNE RICKETTSIOSES OF THE EASTERN HEMISPHERE

Charles L. Wisseman, Jr.

DEFINITION. Three diseases, caused by three different members of the spotted fever group of rickettsiae, are currently the best recognized tick-borne rickettsioses of the Eastern Hemisphere and occur over distinct broad geographic areas: (1) African tick typhus *(R. conorii),* (2) North Asian tick-borne rickettsiosis *(R. sibirica),* and (3) Queensland tick typhus *(R. australis).* Each is a zoonosis, with man an accidental, dead-end host, and is transmitted by the bite of one or more species of ixodid ticks. The three diseases, mild to moderate in severity, closely resemble one another with a short (average five- to seven-day) incubation period, a primary lesion (eschar, tache noire), a fever of a few days' to two weeks' duration, and a maculopapular to almost nodular rash which appears three to five days after onset.

HISTORY, ETIOLOGY, DISTRIBUTION, AND EPIDEMIOLOGY. The problem of the identity of the etiologic agents of the tick-borne rickettsial diseases of man in the Eastern Hemisphere is complex and poorly resolved. In addition to the three well-described agents, *R. conorii, R. sibirica* and *R. australis,* which have been isolated from human infections, a number of new spotted fever group rickettsiae have been isolated from ticks in different areas—e.g., Switzerland, Czechoslovakia, Israel, Pakistan, Thailand—but their capacity to cause human disease is still unknown. In Malaysia infections of man and small mammals have been identified by spotted fever group specific serologic tests, but the causative rickettsia(e) has not yet been isolated and identified. Reports of *R. conorii* infection in Indochina, based on inadequate serology, are likely to be erroneous. In contrast, a new spotted fever group rickettsia, tentatively designated *R. israeli,* has been isolated from human cases. Much remains to be done to clarify the tick-borne causes of human rickettsial infections of the Eastern Hemisphere. Accordingly, the descriptions included here will be confined to the three established entities.

Following the recognition of *boutonneuse fever* in Tunisia, similar tick-borne diseases with local names (e.g., Marseille fever, Kenya tick typhus, South African tick typhus, Indian tick typhus) were described over a wide area, which encompassed parts of Africa, southern Europe, the Middle East, and the Indo-Pakistan subcontinent. Serologic studies and some strain comparison suggested that all are caused by strains of *R. conorii* and that the unifying term *African tick typhus* should be applied to all. This probably is correct to a large degree. However, serologic methods employed have limitations.

The recent findings of a multiplicity of established and probable new species of spotted fever group rickettsiae along with *R. conorii* in some of the areas of presumed African tick typhus *(R. conorii)* distribution (e.g., Europe, Israel, Pakistan) suggest that considerable work must yet be done to clarify the question of distribution and nature of "African tick typhus." In the Mediterranean littoral, the main vector of fièvre boutonneuse is the dog tick, *Rhipicephalus sanguineus,* and the disease is often acquired in and around human habitations, i.e., a domestic or urban pattern. In other areas, the causative agent of the local disease is transmitted by ticks which are parasitic on wild animals, and hence the disease is acquired in rural areas, e.g., certain stretches of the South African veldt.

North Asian tick-borne rickettsiosis (Siberian tick typhus), now known to be caused by *R. sibirica,* is distributed from European Russia through Siberia to the Soviet Far East and possibly to the Indo-Pakistan subcontinent. Several species of ixodid ticks have been implicated as vectors in different geographic regions. Its acquisition is characteristically in a sylvan or rural setting.

Queensland tick typhus is usually acquired in rural areas heavily infested with the tick *Ixodes holocyclus* and a history of tick bite and an eschar are common. The agent, *R. australis*, has only been isolated from the blood of patients. Antibodies have been detected in the blood of some small marsupials and a rat, suggesting a natural sylvan small animal–tick cycle.

The identity of the strains causing disease in Southeast Asia is unknown.

PATHOLOGY. The findings are similar to those in Rocky Mountain spotted fever except for the presence of the tache noire, the black button–like necrotic primary lesion that is generally found on the surface areas of the body ordinarily covered by clothing. The basic pathologic changes are found in the small blood vessels (see Ch. 316).

SYMPTOMS, LABORATORY FINDINGS, AND DIAGNOSIS. The three tick-borne rickettsioses that occur in different parts of the Eastern Hemisphere resemble one another closely. After an incubation period of about five to seven days, the disease begins with fever, headache, malaise, myalgia, and conjunctival injection. The primary lesion, which is present in most cases at the onset of fever, consists of a small ulcer 2 to 5 mm in diameter with a black center and a red areola; the regional lymph nodes are enlarged. The generalized erythematous maculopapular rash appears about the fourth day and quickly involves most of the body, including the palms and soles and often the face. In severe cases the rash becomes hemorrhagic. Fever abates during the second week. The prognosis is good except in the aged and debilitated. Complications and sequelae are unusual.

North Asian tick-borne rickettsiosis has been the subject of considerable laboratory and clinical observation by Soviet investigators. Mild hypotension, electrocardiographic changes, a reversal of the A/G ratio in serum (depressed albumin, early increased alpha globulins, followed by increase in gamma globulins), and abnormal liver function test results are noteworthy.

Agglutinins against *Proteus* OX-19 develop during the second week, and complement-fixing antibodies appear shortly thereafter. Diagnosis is established by the clinical picture, including the tache noire, the geographic location, and positive serologic reactions.

TREATMENT. The broad-spectrum antimicrobial drugs are as effective in patients with African tick typhus and North Asian tick-borne rickettsiosis as in those with other rickettsioses (see Ch. 316 for details of therapy). Presumably, these measures are also applicable to the other tick-borne rickettsioses of the Eastern Hemisphere. All the newly recognized strains display susceptibility in vitro to doxcycline of the same order as *R. rickettsii* and presumably would respond to similar therapeutic regimens.

PROPHYLAXIS. Prevention of human disease is based on avoiding the bites of infected ticks. In Ch. 318 details are set forth regarding personal prophylaxis, including the use of protective clothing, chemical repellents, and reduction of tick population by measures involved in terrain control. Vaccines for human use are not available.

Campbell RW, Abeywickrema P, Fenton C: Queensland tick typhus in Sydney: A new endemic focus. Med J Aust 1:350, 1979. *An introduction to Queensland tick typhus.*

Goldwasser RA, Klingberg MA, Klingberg W, Steiman Y, Swartz TA: Laboratory and epidemiological studies of rickettsial spotted fever in Israel. *In* Frontiers of Internal Medicine, Proceedings of 12th International Congress of Internal Medicine, Tel Aviv, 1974. Basel, Karger, 1975, pp 270-275. *Identification of a new tick-borne spotted fever group rickettsial infection of man in an area of established* R. conorii *endemicity.*

Hoogstraal, H: Ticks in relation to human disease caused by *Rickettsia* species. Ann Rev Entomol 12:377, 1967. *An excellent means of access to literature on tick-borne rickettsioses up to 1967.*

Lyskovtsev MM: Tickborne rickettsiosis. (Translation from the Russian.) Misc Publ Entomol Soc Am 6:41, 1968. *Access to tick-borne rickettsioses of the Soviet Union.*

320. RICKETTSIALPOX

Charles L. Wisseman, Jr.

DEFINITION. Rickettsialpox is a mite-borne rickettsial disease, mild and self-limited, which is characterized by an initial eschar-like lesion and a fever of a week's duration accompanied by headache, backache, and a generalized papulovesicular rash.

ETIOLOGY. Rickettsialpox is caused by *Rickettsia akari*, a member of the spotted fever group on the basis of shared group antigens but with unique specific antigens and biologic properties.

DISTRIBUTION AND INCIDENCE. The disease has been reported from cities in the United States (New York, Boston, West Haven, Ct., Philadelphia, Pittsburgh, and Cleveland) and from the U.S.S.R. In the first three years after the disease was described in 1946, about 500 cases were reported in the United States, mostly from New York, but the number reported has since decreased markedly. Although the reasons for the decrease are not established, it may be due to under-reporting of disease or to control measures.

TRANSMISSION AND EPIDEMIOLOGY. Although detailed information is sparse, it is clear that rickettsialpox is a zoonosis which can involve house mice *(Mus musculus)* and mouse mites *(Allodermanyssus sanguineus). R. akari* has also been isolated from rats in the U.S.S.R. and from voles (small field "mice") in Korea. It is unknown whether the basic natural cycle involves field rodents and their ectoparasites with occasional spillover into the mouse-mite cycle or whether the latter is in fact the basic sustaining cycle. Regardless, in the United States the mouse-mite cycle, greatly amplified and concentrated in discrete foci artificially created by, and frequented by, man himself (e.g., improperly fired apartment house incinerators), was responsible for bringing *R. akari* and man into effective contact with one another. The unusually large mite population, which infested the walls and floors of the incinerator rooms, had access to people entering the foci with a frequency not usually encountered under natural circumstances. Transmission is presumably by bite of the mite.

PATHOLOGY. As no fatal cases have been encountered, studies of the pathology of rickettsialpox have been limited to an examination of skin biopsies. Histologically, the eschar of rickettsialpox resembles the eschars of scrub typhus and boutonneuse fever. The skin lesions composing the rash show a typical perivascular infiltration by monouclear cells. Later, necrosis of the superficial epithelium leads to intraepidermal vesicle formation.

CLINICAL MANIFESTATIONS AND COURSE. The incubation period varies from about ten days to three weeks. An initial lesion (the eschar) appears at the site of the mite bite about a week before onset of fever in about 90 per cent of the cases, gradually enlarging and progressing from a papular lesion through vesicle formation, finally to form a dark encrusted lesion 0.5 to 1.5 cm in diameter. The onset of an intermittent fever is sudden and is accompanied by chills or chilly sensations, drenching sweats, headache, anorexia, and photophobia. The temperature ranges from about 38 to 40° C, lasts for about a week, is accompanied by headache, lassitude, and myalgia, and then gradually subsides. A sparse eruption appears on the trunk, extremities, and mucous membranes between the first and fourth days of fever, beginning as discrete maculopapular lesions and evolving into a vesiculopapular rash. The vesicles are firm, are sometimes surrounded by erythema, and, on drying, form a dark crust that falls off without leaving a scar.

DIAGNOSIS. ***Clinical Diagnosis.*** The clinical characteristics of the disease are so distinctive that in most patients a presumptive diagnosis may be made on clinical grounds. Chickenpox in adults poses the most difficult diagnostic problem. Important points in differentiation are as follows: the vesicles in rickettsialpox arise from the center of discrete papules; the lesions tend to appear at the same time instead of in crops; on the average, the number of lesions is fewer than in chickenpox; and there often is an initial lesion at the site of the mite bite.

Laboratory Diagnosis. Laboratory diagnosis depends on isolation of the agent and on serologic response measured by rickettsial group and specific antigens. The Weil-Felix result is negative (see Ch. 316).

PROGNOSIS. Even without specific therapy, the course of the disease is benign, and the prognosis excellent.

TREATMENT. Response to tetracycline drugs, given as outlined in Ch. 316, is rapid without relapse.

PREVENTION AND CONTROL. The transient emergence of rickettsialpox from a silent zoonosis to a human disease problem was an artifact of urban living, and its apparent disappearance is probably a result of minor changes in human behavior. The prevention and control of rickettsialpox depend on rodent and mite control by (1) the elimination of mice and mouse harborages, which should include proper care and firing of incinerators in dwellings, and (2) the application of residual acaricides to walls and other mite-infested areas. No vaccines have been developed.

Greenberg M, Pelliteri O, Klein IF, Huebner RJ: Rickettsialpox—a newly recognized rickettsial disease. II. Clinical observations. JAMA 133:901, 1947. *Original clinical description of a newly recognized spotted fever group infection.*

Lackman DH: A review of information on rickettsialpox in the United States. Clin Pediat 2:296, 1963. *A resource for information on rickettsialpox in the United States.*

321. SCRUB TYPHUS

Charles L. Wisseman, Jr.

SYNONYMS. Scrub typhus is also known as *chigger-borne rickettsiosis.* It has many local names, including *tsutsugamushi disease, Japanese river* or *flood fever, mite-borne typhus, rural typhus, Mossman fever,* and others.

DEFINITION. Scrub typhus is an acute, febrile, typhus-like disease of rural Asia transmitted by the bite of larval trombiculid mites (chiggers). The site of infection is often marked by an eschar accompanied by regional lymphadenitis.

ETIOLOGY. The disease is caused by infection with *Rickettsia tsutsugamushi (R. orientalis).* The organism differs somewhat from other members of the genus *Rickettsia.* It shares an antigen with *Proteus* OX-K. Multiple serotypes exist that produce substantial homologous immunity but only transient cross-immunity in man. Hence multiple attacks of scrub typhus are possible. Virulence of strains for mice and man varies from low to very high.

DISTRIBUTION AND INCIDENCE. Scrub typhus is widely distributed in eastern and southern Asia and the islands of the western and southern Pacific. It is known as far north as the island of Hokkaido in Japan and the Primorye region of asiatic U.S.S.R., as far south as the northern tip of Australia, and as far west as Pakistan and Tadzhikistan. Endemic infection is unknown in the New World, Europe, Africa, and Western Asia; but cases imported during the incubation period following infection in an endemic area have been recognized in the United States.

Scrub typhus is best known from its occurrence in substantial numbers when large groups of nonimmune persons enter an endemic area, such as in military operations, road building, land clearing, and certain agricultural settings such as rubber plantations. Application of modern epidemiologic and laboratory methods is currently revealing, as expected, that scrub typhus is a major cause of febrile disease in rural populations indigenous to endemic areas.

TRANSMISSION AND EPIDEMIOLOGY. Scrub typhus is acquired from the bite of infected larval trombiculid mites (chiggers). Humans acquire the infection when they intrude into an enzootic focus. Four main elements are constant features of such foci: (1) *R. tsutsugamushi;* (2) chiggers of the *Leptotrombidium deliense* group (*L. deliense, L. akamushi, L. fletcheri, L. arenicola, L. pallidum, L. pavlovskyi,* others); (3) wild rats, especially of the subgenus *Rattus;* and (4) transitional vegetation. The mites, whose larval "chiggers" are the only stage to feed on man and rats, efficiently transmit the rickettsia from one generation to the next through the egg (transovarial passage) and probably constitute the main reservoir of *R. tsutsugamushi* as well as serving as vectors. Rats, especially wild rats of the subgenus *Rattus,* and other small mammals (field mice, voles, shrews) serve as hosts for the parasitic larval mites. Some kind of transitional or secondary vegetation provides the habitat for the chigger-mammal association—e.g., in cleared forest areas; the fringe vegetation along roads, forest trails, or streams; abandoned agricultural areas. Within such habitats, infected chiggers may occur in very circumscribed foci or "mite islands," accounting for the marked focal distribution of scrub typhus cases and sudden outbreaks in field personnel. Suitable habitats are widely distributed from tropical to temperate zones and occur in such extreme settings as semideserts, alpine meadow in the Himalayas, disturbed rain forests, and seashores. In temperate zones, the chiggers are usually active at some time during the warm months, although *L. scutellare*–transmitted *winter* scrub typhus occurs in the Izu Islands of Japan. In tropical or subtropical regions, the disease may be more prevalent at one time of the year than another, depending on rainfall, flooding, and other factors.

PATHOLOGY. The pathologic features of scrub typhus conform generally to those described in Ch. 316. Of special note in scrub typhus is the primary local ulcer with regional and, later, generalized lymphadenopathy. Vascular thrombosis is less frequent than in epidemic typhus and Rocky Mountain spotted fever.

CLINICAL MANIFESTATIONS AND COURSE. The spectrum of clinical severity of untreated scrub typhus ranges from inapparent or mild to severe or fatal in different places and outbreaks. The following description pertains to a classic, relatively severe untreated case of scrub typhus.

The bite of the infecting chigger, which may be on any part of the body, is usually unnoticed; but in roughly 60 to 70 per cent of the primary infections and substantially fewer in second infections, a small painless papule develops during the 6- to 18-day (usually 9- to 12-day) incubation period. It enlarges, undergoes central necrosis, and crusts to form the eschar or primary lesion, which is well developed at the onset of disease. The regional lymph nodes are enlarged and tender. Prodromes of headache, malaise, anorexia, and weakness may occur. The onset is usually acute. The fever rises progressively during the first few days, sometimes accompanied by chills after about the third day, to 39.5 to 40.5° C, accompanied by severe headache, ocular pain, conjunctival injection, anorexia, generalized aches, malaise, apathy, and cough. Interstitial pneumonitis is common. The pulse remains relatively slow. Toward the end of the first week, a macular rash, later sometimes papular, often appears, first on the trunk and then on the extremities. About this time there is generalized lymphadenopathy, soft splenic enlargement, and sometimes hepatomegaly.

During the second week of disease, the temperature remains elevated and signs of complex multiple organ system involvement appear. Apathy may give way to more pronounced signs of meningoencephalitis: delirium and restlessness, stupor, coma, convulsions, muscular weakness, hyperesthesias, and coarse intention tremors. Cranial nerves are selectively involved: varying degrees of nerve deafness and papilledema and congestion of retinal vessels are common; dysarthria and dysphagia are less frequent. Signs of diffuse and focal myocarditis may appear: soft first heart sound, systolic murmurs, ectopic beats, occasional cardiac enlargement, transient gallop rhythm, and minor abnormalities of the electrocardiogram (prolonged P–R interval, inverted T waves). Classic congestive failure is rare, but varying degrees of circulatory failure may appear: increasing pulse rate, falling blood pressure (commonly below 100 mm Hg systolic), rapid shallow respirations, cyanosis, sweating, and cold clammy skin. Gangrene is rare, but edema may be overt in severe cases. Clinical evidence for renal insufficiency is often absent, but oliguria or anuria occurs in some. Spontaneous diuresis is fairly common late in the febrile course or in early convalescence.

In untreated cases, defervescence is by lysis usually after about 10 to 14 days (21 or more days in severe cases). Convalescence is prolonged. All abnormalities appear to be completely reversible, although some, such as cardiovascular instability, personality changes, and deafness, may occasionally persist for weeks to months. Long-term (ten years or more) follow-up of United States servicemen who survived scrub typhus in World War II failed to reveal any significant residua.

An early leukopenia (1000 to 5000 white blood cells per cubic millimeter) gives way to slightly depressed or normal total white blood counts, which may become somewhat elevated late in the disease. Total serum proteins are usually normal or low, but the albumin/globulin (A/G) ratio is often reversed. Occasional clotting disturbances have been reported recently, including disseminated intravascular clotting syndrome. Jaundice is rare, but serum transaminase enzyme levels may be elevated. Albuminuria is common. Isosthenuria, oliguria, and azotemia may occur.

Second and subsequent attacks may be atypical (milder, without eschar, and with sparse or no rash).

DIAGNOSIS. A typhus-like illness with a history of possible exposure in endemic areas and an eschar (in only about 60 to 70 per cent) with regional lymphadenitis should alert the physician to the possibility of scrub typhus. Differential diagnosis may be difficult in some endemic regions where the clinical picture may suggest other rickettsial infections (especially tick-borne typhus, which may also have an eschar) and other nonrickettsial infections (see General Clinical Diagnostic Considerations in Ch. 316). The Weil-Felix test with *Proteus* OX-K, not positive in all cases, is useful because of general availability. The indirect fluorescent antibody test is currently the serodiagnostic method of choice (see Laboratory Diagnosis in Ch. 316). Isolation can be accomplished by inoculating blood or tissue homogenates intraperitoneally into white mice.

PROGNOSIS. Untreated, the mortality ranges from essentially zero to over 30 per cent in different foci. Prompt antibiotic therapy reduces mortality virtually to zero.

TREATMENT. Tetracycline drugs, given as recommended in Ch. 316, and appropriate supportive measures are recommended treatment. Concurrent malaria should not be overlooked.

PREVENTION AND CONTROL. Effective killed vaccines have not yet been developed to prevent scrub typhus. Chemoprophylaxis with weekly doses of doxycycline is feasible. But practically, preventive measures against scrub typhus are directed primarily against the chigger vector. Mite-infested terrain should be avoided whenever possible. Individual prophylaxis against attack by larval mites consists of wearing protective clothing, impregnated with a mite repellent (benzyl benzoate, M-1960), and applying diethyltoluamide to exposed skin areas. The vector population in and around camp sites in endemic zones can be reduced (1) by treating the area intensively with acaricides, (2) possibly by reducing the rodent population through intensive poison bait campaigns, and (3) by destroying vegetation (using bulldozers, power oil burners, herbicides). However, appropriate and relevant environmental, medical, and ecologic considerations must temper decisions on the use of persisting acaricides and herbicides.

Brown GW, Robinson DM, Huxsoll DL: Scrub typhus: A common cause of illness in indigenous populations. Trans R Soc Trop Med Hyg 70:444, 1976. *Illustrates previously unrecognized burden of scrub typhus on human populations indigenous to endemic zones.*

Deller JJ Jr, Russell PK: An analysis of fevers of unknown origin in American soldiers in Vietnam. Ann Intern Med 66:1129, 1967. *Description of recent experience with scrub typhus in military operations.*

Olson JG, Bourgeois AL, Fang RCY, Coolbaugh JC, Dennis DT: Prevention of scrub typhus: Prophylactic administration of doxycycline in a randomized double blind trial. Am J Trop Med Hyg 29:989, 1980. *Suggests feasibility of simple chemoprophylaxis. Unfortunately, bibliography to previous work is incomplete.*

Traub R, Wisseman CL Jr: The ecology of chigger-borne rickettsioses (scrub typhus) (review article). J Med Entomol 11:237, 1974. *Comprehensive review and reference to literature on ecology of scrub typhus up to time of writing.*

322. TRENCH FEVER

Theodore C. Eickhoff

SYNONYMS. Trench fever is also called *five-day* or *quintan fever, shin-bone fever,* and *Volhynia fever.*

DEFINITION. Trench fever is a self-limited febrile disease transmitted by the body louse, *Pediculus humanus corporis,* and characterized by headache, fever, and severe pain in the bones, joints, and muscles. Fatalities are rare, but the disease is characterized in most patients by a relapsing course.

ETIOLOGY AND EPIDEMIOLOGY. The etiologic agent, *Rochalimaea quintana,* is a rickettsia-like agent that grows extracellularly in the louse gut, and is excreted in louse feces. Human infection follows accidental inoculation of contaminated feces into abraded skin or conjunctivae. The etiologic agent is differentiated from other rickettsiae by its ability to grow on artificial media, true rickettsiae being obligate intracellular parasites.

The disease was a major military problem during World Wars I and II in Europe and occurs in endemic form in Mexico, parts of North Africa, and eastern Europe and Asia. Humans are generally considered to be the principal reservoir, since the agent has been isolated from asymptomatic patients years after their initial infection. The louse then acquires its infection by ingesting the blood of an infected human. The recent finding that the so-called "vole agent" is in fact a strain of *Rochalimaea quintana* suggests that reservoirs may also exist in certain rodent populations.

PATHOLOGY AND CLINICAL MANIFESTATIONS. Histopathologic data are limited to skin biopsy studies that have revealed only nonspecific perivascular inflammation. Following an incubation period of 10 to 30 days, the presenting symptoms are fever, of either gradual or abrupt onset, severe weakness, headache, dizziness, and bone and body pain, frequently most dramatically severe in the shins. Physical and laboratory examination generally reveals only slight enlargement of the liver and spleen, pain and soreness in the muscles, and erythematous macules or papules which occur transiently in 70 to 80 per cent of patients. There may be a moderate leukocytosis. The initial febrile episode generally lasts three to five days but frequently recurs after a symptom-free interval of four to five days. Up to eight relapses of fever and symptoms similar to the initial episode have been described, but most patients fortunately experience only several such relapses. In some patients, the fever and symptoms are continuous for two to three weeks. In still others, the initial fever may decline, only to relapse without a true afebrile period, producing a typical "saddle-back" fever curve. Persistent rickettsemia is present during the initial attack, and continues during the relapses as well as the intervening asymptomatic periods; it may persist for months or sometimes years after apparent recovery.

DIAGNOSIS. A history of contact with lice within the appropriate incubation period is helpful. *R. quintana* can be cultivated on agar containing 10 per cent fresh defibrinated horse blood. Both a passive hemagglutination and an enzyme-linked immunosorbent assay test have proved useful in serologic diagnosis. During epidemics, typical cases may be diagnosed on clinical grounds alone. The differential diagnosis should include typhoid fever, typhus, dengue, relapsing fever, and leptospirosis.

TREATMENT AND PROGNOSIS. *Rochalimaea quintana* is highly sensitive in vitro to the tetracyclines and other broad-spectrum antimicrobials, and these may be expected to be as effective in the treatment of trench fever as in the treatment of other rickettsial diseases; there is, however, no direct information supporting their efficacy. Mortality is negligible, and the long-term prognosis is excellent. Approximately 85 per cent of patients recover fully within two months of onset; a few, however, continue to experience recurrences for months or years.

PREVENTION. Elimination of the louse vector by dusting clothing with residual insecticides should be as effective in controlling trench fever as in controlling epidemic typhus. Ten per cent DDT powders proved highly effective for louse control during World War II, but development of DDT resistance may require the use of lindane or malathion as a dusting powder.

Hurst A: Trench fever. Br Med J 2:318, 1942. *This is a lucid account of the clinical characteristics of trench fever in British troops in World War I.*

Vinson JW, Varela G, Molina-Pasquel C: Trench fever. III. Induction of clinical disease in volunteers inoculated with *Rickettsia quintana* propagated on blood agar. Am J Trop Med 18:713, 1969. *This study documents the isolation of the agent and induction of typical trench fever in volunteers.*

Weis E, Dasch GA, Woodman DR, Williams JC: Vole agent identified as a strain of the trench fever rickettsia, *Rochalimaea quintana*. Infect Immun 19:1013, 1978. *One of the few recent studies of trench fever, providing interesting, but speculative, epidemiologic insights.*

323. Q FEVER

Theodore C. Eickhoff

DEFINITION. Q fever is a self-limited rickettsial infection characterized by fever, chills, headache, and constitutional symptoms. In less than one half of patients, there may be an associated pneumonitis. It is unique among the rickettsial diseases of man in that infection is acquired by inhalation rather than by contact with an arthropod vector.

ETIOLOGY. The disease is caused by *Coxiella burnetii*, a rickettsial agent possessing a unique resistance to desiccation and to exposure in dusts and soils. The organism may be propagated in embryonated eggs and in mice, hamsters, and guinea pigs. Both patients and animals develop agglutinating and complement-fixing antibodies to the agents. *C. burnetii*, unlike other rickettsiae, does not stimulate the production of agglutinins to the X-strain of *Proteus vulgaris*.

EPIDEMIOLOGY. ***Incidence and Distribution.*** The true incidence of the disease in humans is impossible to determine because the majority of infections are undiagnosed. In the United States the disease, first found in Montana and California, is now recognized as prevalent in most of the states in which sheep and cattle are produced. Small numbers of cases have been reported from most of the remaining states. Serologic surveys have revealed that many persons exposed to infection in sheep and cattle ranches, abattoirs, meat packing plants or wool processing plants have serologic evidence of past infection. *C. burnetii* is now known to be distributed on a worldwide basis, except for Scandinavian countries.

TRANSMISSION. The epidemiology of Q fever is complex, involving two major patterns of transmission. The first pattern, described in Australia, is a disease cycle in wild animals with transmission of the agent from animal to animal by a tick vector. Such cycles involve up to 40 species of tick vectors. The agent can be transmitted indefinitely as an inapparent infection in the wild reservoir, such as kangaroos, by ticks, but it may also be transmitted laterally by arthropod vectors to a domestic animal in close contact with man. In these and similar cycles recognized in other parts of the world, *C. burnetii*, like the other rickettsial agents of human disease, is vector transmitted.

However, Q fever patients rarely give a history of tick bite. Human infection is now known to result almost exclusively from a second transmission cycle capable of sustaining itself independently of the wild animal cycle. The reservoirs of infection in the second pattern are domestic animals, principally cattle, sheep, and goats, in which *C. burnetii* produces an inapparent or at most mild infection. The organisms do, however, localize in placental tissue and mammary glands of pregnant animals. In sheep, *C. burnetii* is present in up to 10^{12} organisms per gram of placental tissue and to a lesser degree in amniotic fluid, milk, and feces. In the cow, and probably the goat, excretion occurs mainly through the placenta and milk. With all infected animals, the period of parturition is associated with the formation of a highly infectious aerosol. Such aerosols infect other cattle in the herd and also the human population in close contact with the animals. Further, because contaminated clothing, wool, hide, bedding, and soil may be the source of secondary aerosols, the infection may be transmitted by these vehicles at considerable distances from the infected cattle. The unique resistance of *C. burnetii* to prolonged exposure in nature contributes to the spread of the agent by such infectious microenvironments.

The domestic animal cycle has also resulted in several outbreaks of Q fever in personnel in United States medical schools carrying out research studies with pregnant ewes. In addition, Q fever is a recognized laboratory hazard; 50 cases were reported among personnel in one laboratory over a 15-year period. Only 21 of these personnel had been working directly with the organism. Rare reports of nosocomial transmission of Q fever suggest person-to-person transmission; this must be considered infrequent and unlikely.

C. burnetii is easily found in unpasteurized milk from infected cows. Several studies have reported serologic evidence of infection in raw milk drinkers, but there is no clear evidence of disease transmission via raw milk.

PATHOLOGY. Because the mortality rate is quite low, postmortem studies have been few. In patients with pneumonitis, the histopathology is similar to that seen in the viral pneumonias and psittacosis. During the acute phase of the disease, the systemic nature of Q fever is demonstrable both in biochemical abnormalities of liver function and in focal inflammation and noncaseating granulomas in hepatic biopsy specimens. Q fever endocarditis is the major serious complication of the disease, producing valvular vegetations from which rickettsiae may be isolated.

CLINICAL MANIFESTATIONS. After an incubation period of 10 to 28 days after exposure, most patients complain of an abrupt onset of high fever, rigors, headache, muscle pains, and severe malaise. The temperature may rise as high as 40° C and remain elevated, with considerable fluctuation, for one to two weeks. In contrast to all other rickettsial infections, there is no rash. In up to one half of patients there is roentgenographic evidence of pneumonitis, manifested clinically as a slight, nonproductive cough developing in the second week of fever.

Nevertheless, Q fever is more properly considered a severe systemic infection that infrequently causes significant pneumonitis. Hepatic involvement is common, manifested by hepatic enlargement, tenderness, or enzyme elevations; clinical jaundice is rare. Other complications of acute illness rarely reported include myocarditis, pericarditis, and encephalitis. The most serious late sequela, fortunately infrequent, is Q fever endocarditis, which may or may not be preceded by an illness compatible with the acute form of Q fever. Convalescence tends to be prolonged, lasting up to several months, even in uncomplicated cases.

DIAGNOSIS. Q fever should always be suspected in a patient having a severe febrile illness for which no obvious cause can be found. If the patient's vocation or avocation brings him into contact with sheep, cattle, or goats, or byproducts such as wool or hides, it should be particularly suspected.

The differential diagnosis of the acute systemic febrile illness includes influenza, infectious mononucleosis, brucellosis, typhoid fever, cytomegalovirus infection, leptospirosis, and toxoplasmosis. If pneumonitis is prominent, viral pneumonia, mycoplasma, psittacosis, and *Legionella pneumophila* must be considered as well. Evidence of hepatic involvement should suggest viral hepatitis or other intrahepatic processes in addition to those mentioned previously.

Diagnostic studies are usually limited to serologic studies. The complement-fixation test is the most generally available. Recent reports have emphasized the importance of phase variation in the selection of antigens for diagnostic use. Sixty-five per cent of patients will develop elevated titers against phase II antigen by the end of the second week of illness, and

90 per cent of patients will do so after four weeks. Elevated (≥1:200) antibody to phase I antigen is seen in patients with Q fever endocarditis, and the finding of such an elevated titer to phase I antigen during convalescence should raise the possibility of subacute or chronic infection.

TREATMENT AND PROGNOSIS. The tetracyclines and chloramphenicol are both effective in treatment of acute infections with *C. burnetii,* but owing to potential chloramphenicol toxicity, tetracycline is preferred, in a dose of 500 mg four times daily. The mortality is low (1 per cent or less) in untreated patients, and is lower still in those treated with antimicrobial drugs. Therapy should be continued for approximately one week, even though patients usually become afebrile within 48 to 72 hours. Patients occasionally may experience relapse after treatment, and when this occurs additional drug therapy should be administered.

Prognosis is less favorable for the rare patient in whom Q fever endocarditis develops. In some of these patients the disease has been reported to be unresponsive to antimicrobial therapy; long-term tetracycline therapy plus valve replacement as necessary is reported to reduce mortality in such patients to about 30 per cent.

PREVENTION. Experimental lots of yolk-sac vaccines have been effective in preventing clinical disease in volunteers experimentally infected via the respiratory route, and active immunization

is still under study. Control measures are presently limited to minimizing exposure to the agents. This is generally not feasible for those occupationally exposed, save for those working in research or diagnostic laboratories. Milk from cattle, sheep, and goats in endemic areas should be pasteurized or boiled before use.

Ascher MS, Berman MA, Ruppanner R: Initial clinical and immunologic evaluation of a new phase I Q fever vaccine and skin test in humans. J Infect Dis 148:214, 1983. *Description of a promising vaccine.*

Baca OG, Paretsky D: Q fever and *Coxiella burnetii*: A model for host-parasite interactions. Microbiol Rev 47:127, 1983. *A current comprehensive exposition of the basic biology of* C. burnetii.

Clark WH, Lenette EH, Railsback OC, et al.: Q fever in California. VII. Clinical features in one hundred eighty cases. Arch Intern Med 88:155, 1951. *Well over thirty years old, but still among the best clinical studies of Q fever to be found.*

Kimbrough RC, Ormsbee RA, Peacock M, et al.: Q fever endocarditis in the United States. Ann Intern Med 91:400, 1979. *Illustrates the current management of Q fever endocarditis, and the use of phase I and II antigens in serodiagnosis.*

Meiklejohn G, Reimer EG, Graves PS, Helmick C: Cryptic epidemic of Q fever in a medical school. J Infect Dis 144:107, 1981. *Provides an insight into the potential Q fever problem in research settings.*

Tigertt WD, Benenson AR, Gochenour WJ: Airborne Q fever. Bact Rev 25:285, 1961. *A thorough review of the epidemiology of Q fever, emphasizing the extreme infectivity of this agent.*

Tobin MJ, Cahill N, Gearty G, et al.: Q Fever endocarditis. Am J Med 72:396, 1982. *Good discussion of the management of Q fever endocarditis.*

Section Three VIRAL DISEASES

324. INTRODUCTION TO VIRAL DISEASES

Edwin D. Kilbourne

Viruses are the most pervasive of infectious agents, infecting not only animals and plants but also bacteria, which are themselves agents of disease. Indeed, the ultimate causes of diphtheria and scarlet fever are the lysogenic viruses which infect the responsible bacteria. Viruses are the simplest and smallest of microorganisms. They are essentially transmissible genomes—life reduced to minimal complexity. The simpler viruses are protein-wrapped packages of nucleic acid carrying the blueprints for their own replication. Although simple, a virus is highly specialized. It functions not as a random source of genes, but as an exquisitely specialized package of information narrowly adapted by evolution to a way of life which not only permits its replication in the proper environment (i.e., in the proper cells of the proper host) but somehow programs for its exit from this environment and its attachment to and penetration of cells of the next host. Thus, the influenza virus mutant, so avirulent that it does not damage respiratory tract epithelial cells and thus provoke a cough and thereby effect the expulsion of its progeny, will have small chance for survival.

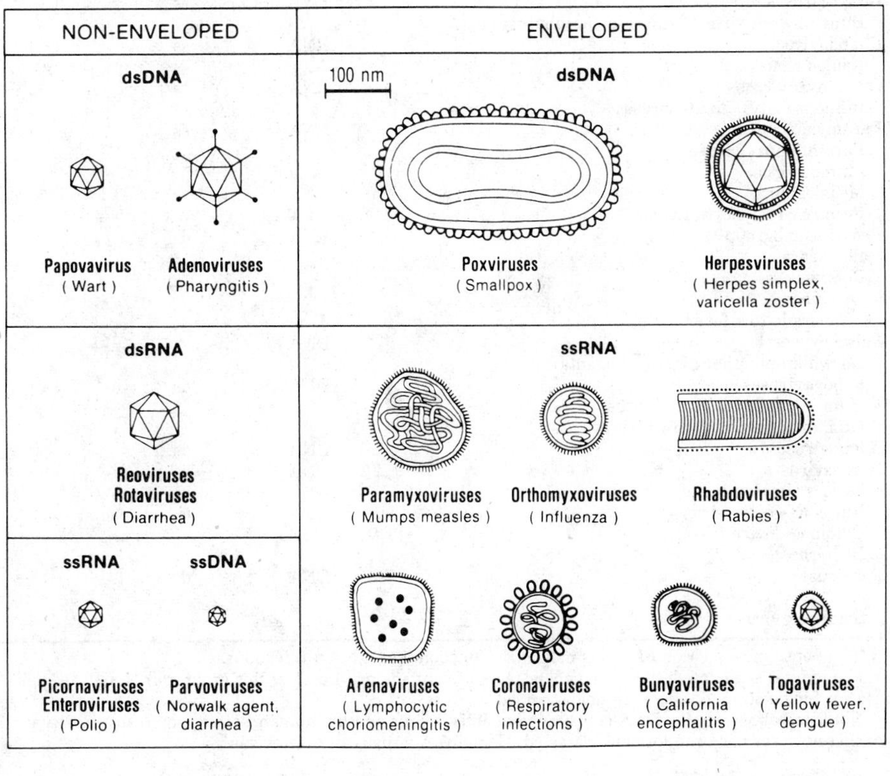

Figure 324–1. Families of known human viruses. (Modified from Matthews REF: Intervirology 12:158, 1979. By permission of S. Karger AG, Basel.)

Therefore, despite their utter dependence upon the cells of others and hence their formal lack of independence, viruses are most usefully considered as highly specialized organisms.

The dependence of viruses upon the host which they infect has favored the evolution of a temperate relationship for the most part of the viruses which are obligate and exclusive human parasites with man as their target and sustenance. Encountered early in life, sometimes damped by maternally transferred antibody, the obligate human viruses often cause asymptomatic infection and rarely kill. Paralysis in poliovirus infection is a rare event, measles encephalitis is uncommon, and fatal influenza usually occurs in previously damaged hosts.

But a large group of important and dangerous human viral infections are caused by viruses not specific for man. Such viruses as the agents of yellow fever and rabies cause primary infections of other hosts; they have not had to adapt to the human condition, and their ravages therefore are severe when human infection occurs as an accident of contact.

As shown in Figure 324–1, viruses come in a variety of shapes and sizes and vary widely in chemical composition (Table 324–1), from the simpler picornaviruses, which are composed only of RNA and protein, to the enveloped viruses, which contain glycoprotein spikes and lipid derived from the host cell membrane.

The relation of design and function of viruses is increasingly appreciated. Certain myxoviruses, including the influenza and parainfluenza viruses, possess a potent neuraminidase that probably abets their release from the mucin-coated cells of the respiratory tract. Most myxoviruses are fragile and unstable in the environment, whereas the enteroviruses, including poliovirus, can pass unscathed through the barrier of gastric acidity in their journey to the target cells of the small intestine.

Neither structural nor chemical similarity of viruses is any sure guide to the diseases that they may cause. Mumps and parainfluenza viruses are indistinguishable by electron microscopy and even share antigens in common, but one invades the salivary glands, pancreas, or meninges, whereas the other produces mild upper respiratory tract infection or infantile croup. Nor does viral dissimilarity predict dissimilar disease. The structurally variable, genetically plastic RNA virus of influenza and the geometrically precise DNA-containing adenovirus with its potential for latency both evoke similar clinical syndromes that may be difficult to differentiate.

BASIC CATEGORIES AND PROPERTIES OF HUMAN VIRUSES (VIRAL TAXONOMY). Is it important for the clinician to know that poliovirus is an enterovirus of the picornavirus family or that the agent of chickenpox is a herpesvirus? A physician who

TABLE 324–1. BASIC CATEGORIES AND PROPERTIES OF HUMAN VIRUSES

	Nucleic Acid			Virion		
Virus Families and Genera	*Type*	*Configuration*	*Sense**	*Size (nm)*	*Envelope*	**Obligate for Man**
Picornaviruses	RNA	ss	(+)	25	0	
Enteroviruses						
Poliovirus						Yes
Coxsackievirus						
Echovirus						
Rhinoviruses						
Togaviruses	RNA	ss	(+)			
Arbovirus A (alphavirus):				70	+	No
eastern, western, and Venezuelan encephalitis viruses						
Arbovirus B (flavivirus):				50	+	No
yellow fever, dengue viruses						
Rubella virus				60		Yes
Coronaviruses	RNA	ss	(+)	75–160	+	
Human coronavirus						Yes
Arenaviruses	RNA	ss	(−)†	50–300	+	No
Lymphocytic choriomeningitis virus; Lassa fever virus						
Bunyaviruses	RNA	ss	(−)†	90–100	+	No
Bunyamwera virus, California encephalitis virus						
Rhabdoviruses	RNA	ss	(−)	70 × 170	+	
Rabies virus						
Orthomyxoviruses	RNA	ss	(−)†	80–120	+	
Influenza A, B, and C viruses						†
Paramyxoviruses	RNA	ss	(−)	150 +	+	
Parainfluenza viruses						Yes (types 2 and 4)
Mumps virus						Yes
Measles virus						Yes
Respiratory syncytial virus						Yes
Reovirus subgroup	RNA	ds	(−)†	60–80	0	
Reoviruses						?
Rotaviruses						No
Orbiviruses:						No
Colorado tick fever						
Parvoviruses	DNA	ss		18–26	0	
Norwalk and other diarrheal agents						?
Papovaviruses	DNA	ds			0	
Human papilloma (wart) virus				52		Yes
Human polyoma JC, BK viruses				45		Yes
Adenoviruses	DNA	ds		70–90	0	Yes
Herpesviruses	DNA	ds		120–150	+	
Herpes simplex 1 and 2 viruses						Yes
Varicella-zoster virus						Yes
Cytomegalovirus						Yes
EB virus						Yes
Poxviruses	DNA	ds		170–260 × 300–450	+	
Smallpox virus						Yes

*(+) Sense means virion RNA has messenger function, i.e., RNA is infectious.
†Genome is segmented; therefore genetic reassortment among viruses of this group can occur.
ss = Single stranded. ds = Double stranded.
Not listed above are the DNA-containing hepatitis B virus and the human RNA retroviruses that have recently been associated with human T cell leukemia; neither of these viruses has been formally classified. Hepatitis A virus is an enterovirus.

possesses this information will not be surprised at the neurotropic potential of other enteroviruses, or at the reactivation of varicella virus as herpes zoster years after primary infection. If he appreciates the nuances of viral taxonomy he will know that it is a jungle of acronyms, sigla, neologisms, Greco-Latin hybrids, and morphologic descriptions. He will not be much aided by knowing that the togaviruses are cloaked (toga) with a host-derived envelope, because other enveloped viruses (Fig. 324–1, Table 324–1) are not so designated. However, the arbovirus designation of some members of the togavirus family will indicate to him that they are *ar*thropod *bo*rne. The term echovirus—*e*nteric *c*ytopathogenic *h*uman *o*rphan viruses—reminds him that these enteroviruses were recognized first as cytopathic agents in tissue culture and only later were associated with specific human diseases. In any case, it is the function of Table 324–1 to show where measles, mumps, and influenza viruses fit into the scheme of things and also to define the nature of their genomes as central to their replicative strategy and potential. Certain generalizations can be inferred on the basis of the nature of the viral nucleic acid. RNA viruses infrequently participate in true intrachromosomal genetic recombination with other viruses, and except for RNA tumor viruses (only recently found in humans) lack the capacity to integrate their genomes with that of the host—a capacity now proven for the DNA herpesviruses. On the other hand, certain of these viruses bear their RNA in pieces that can be readily reassorted during dual infection to create new viruses combining genes from both parents. Viruses as different as influenza and reoviruses share this property, which obviously enhances their adaptability and evolutionary potential. Viral nucleic acid may be double (ds) or single stranded (ss) in configuration, and RNA viruses contain either messenger RNA (mRNA) available for direct translation in the manufacture of viral proteins or RNA of nonmessage sense, which must be transcribed by a virion transcriptase to mRNA. Enveloped viruses (except for the poxviruses) emerge from infected cells by a budding process, incorporating host cell membrane lipids.

A CLASSIFICATION OF VIRUS INFECTIONS ACCORDING TO MECHANISM OF PATHOGENESIS. All viruses have in common the following replicative steps in the initial stage of pathogenesis: (1) *adsorption* through specific viral receptors to specific receptors on susceptible host cells; (2) *penetration* of the cell membrane; (3) *uncoating* of viral nucleic acid to permit expression of the viral genes (this step is usually carried out by host cell enzymes and coincides with the *eclipse period*, during which time infective virus cannot be found in the cell); (4) *macromolecular synthesis* of nucleic acid and protein; (5) *assembly* of virion components; and (6) *release* of infective virus from the cell. These events may occur in association with severe disruption of host cell function and rapid cytonecrosis, or host cell function may be virtually unaffected, depending on the nature of the invading virus. The damage to primary target cells may in itself directly cause the disease state, or characteristic symptoms may reflect involvement of secondary or even tertiary target cells in organs remote from the initial site of invasion (Fig. 324–2). Cellular damage may be the direct result of viral replication or may be indirectly mediated through the cellular immune response.

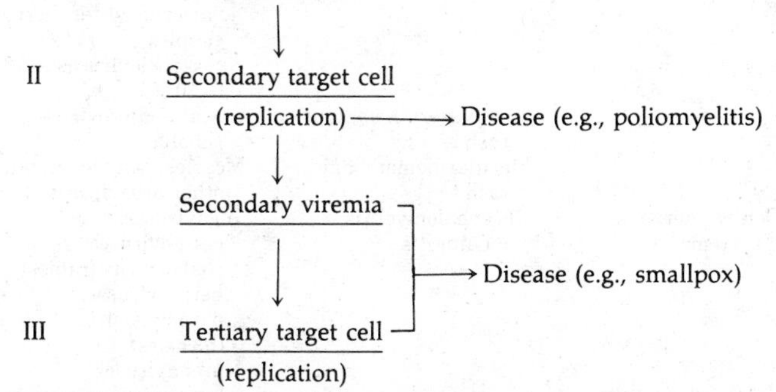

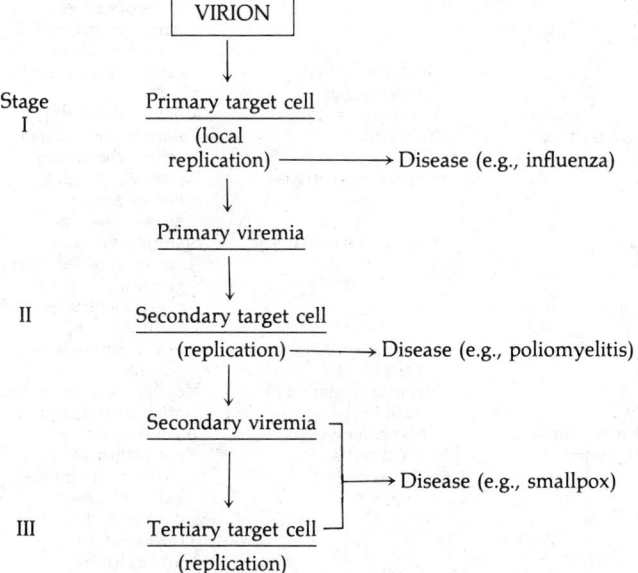

Figure 324–2. Stages of viral pathogenesis. Initial invasion may involve only primary target cells (influenza) or may lead to secondary or tertiary target cell invasion (poliomyelitis and smallpox), which results in the characteristic disease.

As illustrated in Table 324–2, initial and primary invasion of

TABLE 324–2. PATHOGENETIC CLASSIFICATION OF HUMAN VIRAL INFECTIONS

I. Primary and definitive infection of the respiratory tract
  A. Orthomyxoviruses (influenza A, B, and C viruses)—influenza
  B. Paramyxoviruses
    1. (Parainfluenza viruses 1–4)—rhinitis, laryngotracheitis "croup"
    2. Respiratory syncytial (RS) virus—croup, infantile pneumonia
  C. Rhinoviruses (1–89 +)—"common cold," rhinitis
  D. Coronaviruses—mild upper respiratory tract infection
II. Primary respiratory tract infection with secondary infection elsewhere
  A. Adenoviruses (types 1–28)—febrile pharyngitis, ocular involvement with some types (especially, type 8); viruses can multiply in the small intestine
  B. Paramyxoviruses
    1. Mumps virus—parotitis, orchitis, oophoritis, pancreatitis, meningoencephalitis, viremia
    2. Measles virus—conjunctivitis, rhinitis, pharyngitis, bronchitis, pneumonia, viremia, exanthem, encephalitis
  C. Rubella virus (German measles)—mild upper respiratory infection, viremia, exanthem, encephalitis
  D. Poxvirus (smallpox virus)—respiratory tract symptoms, exanthem (see Fig. 324–3)
  E. Herpesviruses
    1. (Varicella-zoster virus)—chickenpox; herpes zoster—extremely mild respiratory symptoms → pneumonia in adults, exanthem
    2. Cytomegalovirus (cytomegalic inclusion disease)—mild or absent respiratory symptoms, pneumonia, hepatitis, viremia (congenital transplacental infection may occur)
    3. EB virus—lymphoproliferative disease, infectious mononucleosis
III. Primary and definitive enteric infections
  Reoviruses, rotaviruses, and parvoviruses have recently been implicated in diarrheal disease of man on the basis of demonstration of their presence in high concentration by electron microscopy of fecal specimens and by specific immune response
  Although the enteroviruses and the hepatitis viruses multiply initially and principally in the gut, multiplication is not restricted to this site, and viremia and secondary manifestations occur
IV. Primary enteric infection with secondary infection elsewhere (all picornaviruses except rhinoviruses)
  A. Polioviruses (types 1–3)—pharyngitis, meningoencephalitis, poliomyelitis, viremia
  B. Coxsackievirus: group A (types 1–24); group B (types 1–6)—vesicular pharyngitis (herpangina), aseptic meningitis, exanthem (macular or vesicular), epidemic pleurodynia and myalgia, myocarditis, viremia
  C. Echoviruses (enteric cytopathogenic *h*uman *o*rphan viruses) (types 1–30 +)—upper respiratory infection, aseptic meningitis, gastroenteritis, exanthem (macular), viremia
  D. Herpesviruses (herpes simplex)—primary oral or genital infection
  E. Hepatitis virus A—virus not yet cultivable in cell culture systems, viremia
V. Percutaneous (parenteral) infections by viruses nonobligate for man
  A. Togaviruses (200 + viruses in 20 different antigenic groups)—all multiply in hematophagous (bloodsucking) vectors—mosquitoes, ticks, sandflies, or gnats—and in avian or nonhuman mammalian hosts; diverse systemic disease (see clinical classification, Table 324–3) and viremia
  B. Rhabdovirus—(rabies) encephalitis
  C. Arenaviruses—Lassa fever
  D. Bunyaviruses—California encephalitis
VI. Percutaneously acquired obligate human viruses
  A. Herpesvirus
    1. Herpes simplex type 2 virus—genital, venereal infection
    2. Hepatitis virus B (serum hepatitis) or hepatitis virus A (infectious hepatitis) when administered via hypodermic needle
VII. Transplacentally acquired (congenital or vertical) human viral infections (all characterized by maternal viremia)
  A. Rubella
  B. Cytomegalic inclusion disease
  C. Others on occasion

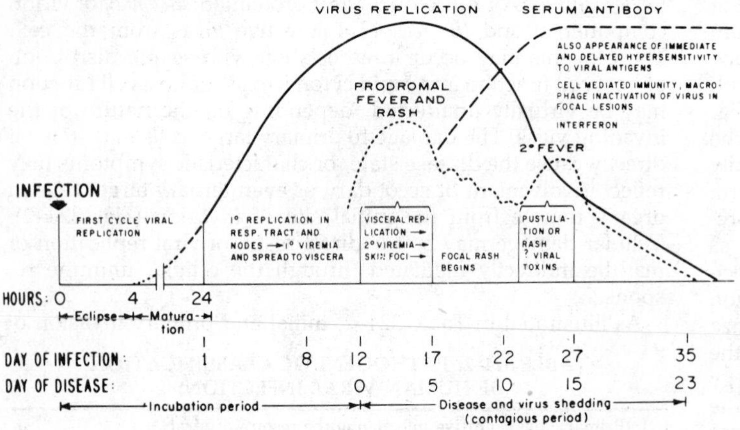

Figure 324–3. Pathogenesis of smallpox (based in part on inferences from animal models).

cells occurs with contagious viral infections (those spread from man to man) at respiratory or enteric portals. If replication is confined to these primary sites, as with rhinovirus and influenza virus infections in the respiratory tract, and rotavirus infection of the gut, then symptomatology similarly reflects this focal organ involvement. Viremia rarely occurs with these infections, and the malaise, myalgia, and other systemic signs of toxicity remain unexplained.

In other cases, the respiratory or intestinal tract, although the site of initial invasion, is not the definitive site of infection and disease. Measles and poliomyelitis viruses, although they first infect cells, respectively, of the respiratory tract or intestine, are spread through a viremic stage to other organs in which the characteristic disease is expressed. The transient involvement of the primary target cells may or may not be attended by minor or prodromal symptoms. It can be assumed that all virus diseases with rash, as well as those parenterally transmitted, must have a viremic stage. Furthermore, all viremic infections have the potential for congenital transplacental transmission. In fact, only rubella and cytomegaloviruses seem to be important causes of congenital disease.

The temporal aspects of viral pathogenesis are important to comprehend. A schematic profile of the pathogenic sequence in smallpox as a prototype is presented in Figure 324–3. Infection, probably initiated by one or very few viral particles, occurs in a cell or cells of the respiratory tract, in which the first cycle of viral replication takes place in a matter of hours. During the subsequent ten or eleven days of the *incubation period,* cell-to-cell spread locally in the respiratory tract and to regional nodes occurs by contiguity, associated with a transient primary viremia in which virus is disseminated to other viscera, including the liver and spleen. Symptoms of the disease begin about the twelfth day of infection in association with extensive visceral replication of virus, secondary viremia, and the establishment of skin foci. A prodromal fever and rash are associated with these events. On about the fifth day of disease (seventeenth day of infection) specific neutralizing antibody is first detectable in the serum. Thereafter it increases rapidly in titer coincidentally with the decline in fever, which occurs with appearance of the characteristic focal skin lesions.

Pustulation of the rash occurs between the ninth and fourteenth days as the result of cytonecrosis, from either viral toxins or perhaps immunopathologic reactions. This pustulation is associated with a secondary increase in fever and is not the result of secondary bacterial invasion.

Other events associated with the host's response which are difficult to indicate on a specific timetable are the appearance of both immediate and delayed hypersensitivity to viral antigens, the occurrence of cell-mediated immunity, and the inactivation of virus in focal lesions by macrophages. As with other viral infections, interferon probably plays a role in recovery, but the nature and extent of this role have not yet been defined.

A CLINICAL CLASSIFICATION OF VIRAL INFECTIONS. Finally, the physician must confront the end result of virus replication and the final stage of pathogenesis, which is clinical disease. Although certain viruses such as mumps, measles, and polioviruses are pathognomonic in their effects, clinical distinction among many virus infections is difficult. Indeed, fever and myalgia in the absence of obvious focal signs are generally regarded by physicians and laymen alike as manifestations of "a virus." Although the definitive diagnosis of viral infection

TABLE 324–3. CLINICAL CLASSIFICATION OF HUMAN VIRAL INFECTIONS (ACCORDING TO SITE OF CARDINAL SYMPTOMATOLOGY)

Site of Cardinal Symptoms	Presenting Disease	Causative Viruses
Upper respiratory tract	Rhinitis, pharyngitis, "common cold"	Rhinovirus, enterovirus, adenovirus, parainfluenza virus, coronavirus
Middle and lower respiratory tract	Tracheitis, bronchitis, pneumonia	Parainfluenza virus, RS virus, influenza viruses
Mouth	Gingivostomatitis, pharyngitis	Herpes simplex (type 1) virus
Genitalia	Vesicular or ulcerative lesions, orchitis, oophoritis	Herpes simplex (type 2) virus, mumps virus
Gastrointestinal	Gastroenteritis, hepatitis	Reoviruses, echoviruses, hepatitis viruses (A & B), rotaviruses, parvoviruses, yellow fever (arbovirus)
	Gastrointestinal hemorrhage	(Certain arboviruses)
	Pancreatitis	Mumps virus
Urinary tract	Nephritis	Yellow fever and some other arboviruses
Eye	Keratoconjunctivitis	Herpes simplex, herpes zoster, adenovirus type 8
Skin	Papular-vesicular rash	Smallpox virus, varicella-zoster, herpes simplex, coxsackieviruses A-16, 5, 10
	Macular-erythematous rash	Certain enteroviruses, rubella
	Macular-hemorrhagic rash	Measles, dengue, certain other arboviruses
Central nervous system	Encephalomyelitis, meningitis	Togaviruses, enteroviruses, rhabdovirus (rabies), herpesviruses, paramyxovirus (measles), arenaviruses, bunyaviruses, mumps
Peripheral lymph nodes	Lymphadenopathy	EB herpes virus
Salivary glands	Parotitis	Mumps virus

depends on isolation and identification of the virus and a study of specific immunologic response, consideration of the site of cardinal symptomatology is often helpful in reducing the range of etiologic possibilities (Table 324–3).

But as with other diseases, the clinical diagnosis of viral infections is aided by the context and circumstances in which infections occur. Acute pharyngitis in summer is usually caused by enteroviruses; in winter adenoviruses and rhinoviruses prevail. The individual case of influenza is easily confused with a number of other prostrating viral infections, but when the disease occurs in a sudden community-wide epidemic, it is readily diagnosed.

Viral infections are more frequent in childhood, at which time they are, in general, better tolerated. Except for the neonatal period, the severity of virus diseases increases with age *if such infection represents initial or primary contact with the virus.* On the other hand, reinfections of the adult (as with parainfluenza or adenoviruses) may be so modified by prior immune response that they are very mild or even asymptomatic. Needless to say, the severity of viral disease is often unfavorably influenced in chronically ill or immunologically compromised patients. In leukemic children with impaired cell-mediated immunity, varicella, among the mildest of viruses, can produce fatal illness; the rare paralytic complications of live poliovirus vaccines occur most commonly in children with immune deficiency states.

In summary, the clinical expression of disease in any given viral infection is a spectrum of response related to the virulence of the infecting virus (which tends to be relatively fixed), the infecting dose, the age and prior immunizing experience of the patient, and the integrity of his immune system and his general physiologic state, as well as host genetic factors which still remain to be defined.

These generalizations will gain substance in the separate consideration of individual virus infections in the chapters which follow.

Baltimore D: Expression of animal virus genomes. Bacteriol Rev 35:235, 1971. *Classic analysis of the differing replication strategies of viruses.*

Dulbecco R, Ginsberg HS: Virology. Harper & Row, 1980. *Excerpted from the classic* Microbiology *text. Good discussion of pathogenesis.*

Evans AS (ed.): Viral Infections of Humans—Epidemiology and Control. 2nd ed. New York, Plenum Medical Book Company, 1982. *Solid work with emphasis on viral epidemiology in general and particular.*

Fenner FJ, White DO: Medical Virology. 2nd ed. New York, Academic Press, 1976. *Dated but admirably succinct and well organized consideration of all aspects of human viral infections.*

Joklik WK: Principles of Animal Virology. New York, Appleton-Century-Crofts, 1980. *Strong basic text on virology and human virus diseases.*

Kilbourne ED: Segmented genome viruses and the evolutionary potential of asymmetrical sex. Perspect Biol Med 25:66, 1981. *Discussion of the potential evolutionary advantage of the several groups of viruses with segmented genomes, as well as practical applications of viral genetic reassortment.*

Luria SE, Darnell JE Jr, Baltimore D, Campbell A: General Virology. 3rd ed. New York, John Wiley & Sons, 1978. *Holistic consideration of general principles of virology, as well as a limited specific examination of prototype viruses of animals, plants, and bacteria.*

Reitz MS Jr, Kalyanaraman VS, Robert-Guroff M, Popovic M, Sarngadharan MG, Sarin PS, Gallo RC: Human T-cell leukemia/lymphoma virus: The retrovirus of adult T-cell leukemia/lymphoma. J Infect Dis 147:399, 1983. *Basic information about the first human leukemia virus to be isolated, written by the discoverer (R. C. Gallo) and his colleagues.*

Viral Infections of the Respiratory Tract

325/326. THE COMMON COLD*

Albert Z. Kapikian

DEFINITION. Although the term "common cold" does not denote a precisely defined disease, it has an almost universally comprehended meaning of an acute self-limited common illness of all age groups, in which the major clinical manifestations involve the upper respiratory tract, with nasal discharge (coryza) or nasal obstruction as the predominant symptom.

HISTORY. Although it was known since 1914 that bacteria-free filtrates of nasal secretions from patients with common cold could induce similar illnesses in volunteers inoculated intranasally, the discovery of etiologic agents from common colds eluded scientists for many years. Despite the isolation of numerous viruses that were associated etiologically with acute respiratory illnesses, such as influenza virus in 1933, and the adeno-, parainfluenza, and respiratory syncytial viruses in the 1950's, it soon became clear that the major etiologic agent(s) of the common cold had not yet been discovered. However, beginning gradually in the 1950's and escalating rapidly in the 1960's, largely because of the development of human diploid cell cultures (which were extremely sensitive for the propagation of certain viral agents), over 100 distinct common cold viruses were discovered and shown to be the major causative agents of the common cold. These heretofore fastidious agents were named rhinoviruses (rhin- is Greek for nose), since they caused predominantly nasal symptoms. Shortly thereafter, in the mid 1960's, another group of fastidious viruses, the coronaviruses, were discovered with the use of tissue and organ cultures and shown to be the second most important etiologic agents of the common cold and related diseases.

ETIOLOGY. Rhinoviruses have emerged as the major known causative agents of adult upper respiratory illnesses such as common colds. They have been isolated from approximately 15 to 40 per cent of adults with these illnesses (Table 325/326–1). The isolation rate is lower in children with upper respiratory tract illness, since only 4 to 5 per cent are rhinovirus positive. Rhinoviruses are classified as a subgroup of the picornavirus family and possess certain common characteristics, including small size (15 to 30 nm), ribonucleic acid (RNA) core, ether resistance, and complete or almost complete inactivation at pH 3. The latter property is a major characteristic distinguishing rhinoviruses from the other major subgroup of the picornaviruses, the enteroviruses (poliovirus, coxsackievirus, and echovirus), which are stable at pH 3. There are 89 officially designated rhinovirus serotypes, but the number will exceed 100 when the numbering system is extended further.

The second most important etiologic agents of common colds are the coronaviruses, which are associated with 10 to 20 per cent of common colds in adults. Their importance as etiologic agents of common colds in infants and young children has not been determined. These viruses possess certain common characteristics, including (a) a unique electron microscopic appearance characterized by pleomorphic 80 to 200 nm enveloped particles possessing relatively widely spaced club- or pear-shaped surface projections (reminiscent of the solar corona, from which the name coronavirus is derived); (b) an RNA genome; and (c) ether and acid lability. There are at least three distinct human coronavirus serotypes, designated B814, 229E, and OC43. Owing to difficulties in propagating these fastidious agents, fewer than 50 isolates have been recovered since their discovery; most epidemiologic studies have thus relied on serologic studies with the 229E and OC43 viruses for which suitable antigens could be prepared. As shown in Table 325/326–1, many other viruses such as influenza, parainfluenza, respiratory syncytial, adeno-, echo- and coxsackieviruses can also cause common-cold–like symptoms. These other agents are described in other sections of this text. A diagnosis of the etiology of a common cold cannot be made clinically, since the

*In the interests of an organized and coherent treatment of the topic, the originally planned chapters on The Common Cold and Rhinoviral Respiratory Disease have been combined into this single chapter.

TABLE 325/326–1. PERCENTAGE OF COMMON COLDS ASSOCIATED WITH SPECIFIC ETIOLOGIC AGENTS IN ADULTS*

Rhinoviruses (over 100 serotypes)	15–40%
Coronaviruses (at least 3 serotypes)	10–20%
Influenza viruses A, B, C, Parainfluenza viruses (4 serotypes) Respiratory syncytial virus (1 serotype) Adenoviruses (various serotypes)	5–10%
Coxsackieviruses (various serotypes) Echoviruses (various serotypes)	1–2%
Group A beta-hemolytic streptococci	2–10%
No specific agent known but presumed to be viral	30–50%

*Each of these agents can also cause common colds in the pediatric age group, but their relative roles are not clearly defined. Viruses associated with specific syndromes such as rubeola, rubella, and varicella have also been associated with common-cold–like symptoms in children.

agents causing the syndrome are so numerous. In addition, about one third to one half of common colds have yet to be associated with an etiologic agent.

INCIDENCE AND PREVALENCE. The common cold is probably the most frequently occurring illness in humans worldwide. The National Center for Health Statistics estimated that in the United States in 1981 the population experienced more than 93 million common colds for an incidence of 41.4 per 100 persons per year. Common colds represented 19.5 per cent of all acute conditions and were estimated to cause over 261 million days of restricted activity.

In the Cleveland Family Study, which spanned a period of about 10 years and included over 25,000 illnesses, common respiratory diseases accounted for 60 per cent of all illnesses. The overall incidence of common respiratory diseases (which included illnesses diagnosed as the common cold, rhinitis, laryngitis, bronchitis, and other undifferentiated acute respiratory illnesses) was 5.6 per person per year. Children under one year of age experienced about seven respiratory illnesses per year; the highest incidence occurred in the one-year age group (8.3 cases per year) and the incidence remained rather high through age five (7.4 cases per year). A progressive decrease was observed beginning at age six. As expected, adults had relatively fewer common respiratory illnesses than children (adults averaged over four per year). The average incidence was slightly greater in boys than in girls, whereas in adults, mothers experienced higher rates than fathers. In addition, the incidence of common respiratory diseases was greater in young children attending school than in those of the same age who were not in school; also, preschool siblings of school children had more respiratory illnesses than preschool siblings without brothers or sisters attending school. The incidence of common respiratory diseases increased progressively as family size increased from three to seven members. Such illnesses were introduced into the home most frequently by school children under six years of age, followed in order of decreasing frequency by preschool children, school children six years of age and over, mothers, and fathers. Analysis of secondary attack rates in families revealed that on the average 25 per cent of all exposures in the home were followed by illness; one- and two-year-olds experienced the highest secondary attack rates (about twice the average).

In a more recent survey of acute respiratory illnesses over a six-year period in Tecumseh, Michigan, the mean incidence of respiratory illnesses per person per year was 3. The highest incidence was in the one-year age group (6.1) and the next highest in the one- to two-year age group (5.7). A viral or potentially pathogenic bacterial agent was isolated from about 25 per cent of the specimens collected, with rhinoviruses accounting for 38.5 per cent of the total number of isolates, a figure representing more than twice the number of isolates of the next most frequently detected group, the parainfluenza viruses.

Studies of the prevalence of neutralizing antibodies in serum against various rhinovirus serotypes have revealed a gradual acquisition of antibody beginning early in childhood and reaching a maximum of at least 50 per cent in the fifth decade, thus providing further evidence that rhinovirus infections occur throughout early life and into adulthood. The prevalence of serum antibody to specific serotypes was not consistent. Although all individuals studied had neutralizing antibodies to each of the 55 serotypes tested, the prevalence of antibody to each serotype varied from about 10 to 80 per cent. Limited surveys of the prevalence of neutralizing antibody to rhinoviruses in various developed and developing countries including several tropical areas indicate a generally worldwide presence of rhinovirus antibody.

The prevalence of coronavirus serum antibody has been difficult to ascertain since only two serotypes, 229E and OC43, can be studied in cell cultures and, in addition, results have been variable in different locations with these two viruses. For example, in one study, 29 per cent of children and 69 per cent of adults had serum complement-fixing (CF) antibody to OC43 virus. Such antibody to 229E virus was present very infrequently in children, whereas about one third of adults were antibody positive. However, in the United Kingdom, about 25 per cent of children and 41 per cent of adults had neutralizing antibody to 229E virus. In United States marine recruits, over 80 per cent had serum hemagglutination inhibition antibody to OC43 virus and 12 per cent had CF antibody to 229E virus. A true evaluation of the prevalence of antibody to the coronavirus group must await the development of serologic assays for other members of this fastidious group of agents.

EPIDEMIOLOGY. In the temperate climates common colds occur most frequently in the colder months of the year. For example, in the Cleveland family study a consistent pattern of a low summer and high winter incidence of common respiratory diseases was documented. In September, a rise in respiratory illnesses to about six cases per person-year from a summer low of three cases per person-year was observed. After a slight dip in October an average rate of about seven cases per person-year was observed for each month from November through March. Some of the factors influencing the spread of common colds have already been described. However, with the discovery of rhinoviruses as the major etiologic agent of common colds, important questions relating to the epidemiology of these specific agents finally could be addressed.

Rhinoviruses are spread from person to person by direct contact, usually with transmission by infected droplets. In early volunteer studies, rhinoviruses induced common colds when administered in nasal drops or by swabbing the nasal mucosa or conjunctiva but not by swabbing the throat. More recent volunteer studies have highlighted a heretofore unrecognized mode of transmission that involves self-inoculation of the conjunctival or nasal mucosa with a rhinovirus-contaminated finger. Virus was recovered in 15 of 16 trials from fingers that were rubbed on plastic surfaces contaminated with rhinovirus one to three hours previously. In addition, rhinovirus was recovered from three of five subject pairs after exposures of uninfected skin to infected skin. The efficiency of transmission of infection from experimentally infected volunteers to susceptible volunteers by hand-to-hand contact followed by self-inoculation was compared with that of transmission by large- and small-particle aerosols. It was striking that 11 of 15 hand-to-hand exposures initiated infection, whereas only 1 of 12 large-particle exposures (donor and contact in social setting) and none of 10 small-particle exposures (donor and contact separated by double mesh barrier) induced such infection.

Rhinovirus communicability was evaluated in childless married couples in a study in which both lacked serum antibody. The overall transmission of a rhinovirus-related cold between partners was 38 per cent, which is similar to the secondary attack rate in the Cleveland Family Study or to those in epidemiologic studies of naturally occurring rhinovirus infections. Transmission rarely occurred unless (1) at least 1000 $TCID_{50}$ of virus was present in the donor's nasal washing, (2) the donor's hands and anterior nares were rhinovirus positive, (3) the donor had at least moderate symptoms, and (4) the partners spent many hours together (at least 122 hours during a seven-day period). Virus in saliva was not strongly associated with transmission.

The effect of exposure to cold temperatures on the course of common colds was evaluated in volunteers who were challenged with rhinovirus by small-particle aerosol or intranasal installation. Exposure to the cold environment did not have a significant effect on host resistance to rhinovirus infection and illness. Exposure to cold temperature did not induce a common cold in uninoculated volunteers. This finding is consistent with results of early studies on the epidemiology of common colds on the island of Spitzbergen. These early studies demonstrated that very few colds occurred during the bitter Arctic winter, but sharp outbreaks began shortly after the first ship arrived at the end of May. Thus, cold weather by itself did not induce common colds; the ingredient needed to initiate the outbreak was exposure to infected individuals. In early volunteer studies using common cold agents, fatigue and sleep deprivation caused an insignificant increase in the frequency with which colds occurred; however, in females, susceptibility was related to the menstrual cycle, with attempts to infect during menstruation being relatively unsuccessful.

The incubation period of rhinovirus-related common colds is quite short, ranging from one to five days with a mean of two days. Virus shedding generally begins with the onset of symptoms and continues for one week or even longer. Although there are over 100 distinct rhinovirus serotypes, no one serotype has assumed special importance because numerous serotypes usually circulate at the same time. Rhinoviruses can be detected during most months of the year but reach peak prevalence during the fall season. They are least prevalent during the cold winter months of December, January, and February when common colds still occur frequently. However, coronavirus infections have been found to be prevalent during the late fall, winter, and early spring, when rhinovirus infections occur infrequently. Thus, coronaviruses can be considered to be the major known etiologic agents of the common cold in the winter.

A cyclic pattern in infection rates of coronaviruses 229E and OC43 has been described. With the 229E virus, infections appear to occur in the same years in various locations, including Chicago, Maryland, Virginia, and Michigan; a two-year cycle of activity has been suggested. For OC43 virus, a two- to four-year cycle was found that did not coincide in all locations. The 229E virus was shed in nasal washings of volunteers for one to at least four days after challenge; the peak frequency of virus excretion generally coincided with the peak of clinical symptoms. Virus shedding was also detected in certain volunteers who did not develop colds after challenge. Reinfections have also been observed frequently with coronaviruses under natural conditions; recently, however, volunteers inoculated with the same coronavirus strain 8 to 12 months after initial challenge failed to develop illness on rechallenge. It appears that serum antibody to a specific rhinovirus serotype correlates with protection against natural or experimental challenge with that serotype. However, serum antibody may not in itself be responsible for protection but may be a reflection of the level of specific nasal secretory antibodies. In one volunteer study in which the protective effects of neutralizing antibody in serum and in nasal secretions were compared, it was found that only nasal secretory antibody was associated with resistance to rhinovirus infection and illness.

PATHOLOGY. The pathologic mechanisms whereby a common cold is induced by a virus are not known. However, the pathology of viral rhinitis in general has been described. In the initial acute period of viral rhinitis the nasal mucosa is thickened and edematous and depending on the degree of hyperemia is pale gray to red in color and covered by a thin watery mucoid discharge. The nasal cavities are narrowed by the enlargement of the turbinates. Histologically, there is extreme edema of the mucosal tissue, which is also infiltrated sparsely with neutrophils, lymphocytes, plasma cells, and eosinophils. Secretory hyperactivity of the mucus-secreting submucosal glands is also observed. The edematous nasal mucosa can cause obstruction of the orifices of the accessory air sinuses and lead to sinusitis. Bacterial superinfections can result in serious sequelae including osteomyelitis, cavernous sinus thrombophlebitis, epidural or subdural abscess, meningitis, or brain abscess. Nevertheless, such complications are exceedingly rare.

Information on the pathologic findings in acute rhinovirus infections is extremely limited. Biopsies of nasal epithelium were obtained from volunteers prior to and after rhinovirus inoculation and from volunteer controls who were not inoculated. Fixed smears prepared with Papanicolaou's stain demonstrated that most of the cells were ciliated columnar epithelial cells. Smaller numbers of nonciliated epithelial cells, goblet cells, and mononuclear and polymorphonuclear cells were also observed. However, consistent histologic changes were not observed in specimens obtained during infection or illness.

CLINICAL MANIFESTATIONS. The major clinical manifestation of common colds occurring under natural or experimental conditions is coryza or nasal congestion. The most common complaints in rhinovirus-positive respiratory illnesses in 139 civilian adults were rhinorrhea and sneezing, which were recorded in one half to two thirds of the cases. The next most frequent complaint was sore throat, which occurred in nearly one half, while hoarseness and cough were less common, being present in one quarter to one half of the cases. Temperature elevation was unusual. An oral temperature of 99.6° F (37.6° C) or greater at the time of study was documented in less than 1 per cent of the cases. Nonrespiratory complaints were not common except for headache, which occurred in approximately one quarter of the cases. The mean duration of symptoms was about 9 days with a median of 7.4 days and a mode of 4 days.

The clinical manifestations of coronavirus-229E–like infections under natural conditions in adults are quite similar. Of nine patients who shed this agent, all had coryza, eight had nasal congestion, seven had sneezing, and five had sore throat at the time of study. Less common manifestations were headache (in four), cough (in three), muscular or general aches (in three), and chills and fever (in two). Coryza or nasal congestion was the chief complaint in eight of the nine patients.

Administration of rhinoviruses or coronaviruses to volunteers has provided an opportunity to define the clinical manifestations associated with these agents under carefully controlled conditions (Table 325/326–2). The mean incubation period of colds induced by coronaviruses was significantly longer (about one day), the duration of the illness somewhat shorter, and the mean maximum number of paper tissues used per day (for nasal discharge) greater than in rhinovirus-induced illnesses. In later studies, each of six other coronavirus strains was also administered by the nasal route to volunteers: cumulatively, 35 of 49 volunteers developed common-cold–like illnesses. Thus, the ability to induce common colds in adults under experimental conditions is now as firmly established for the coronaviruses as for the rhinoviruses.

Rhinoviruses also cause common colds in children. The role of rhinoviruses as etiologic agents of bronchitis, bronchiolitis, bronchopneumonia, pneumonia, and croup is unclear. However, it appears certain that rhinoviruses are not important causes of these syndromes, even though administration of a rhinovirus by small-particle aerosol induces a tracheobronchitis in volunteers. Coronaviruses can also cause common-cold–like illnesses in children. In one study, coronavirus 229E was recovered from two infants with pneumonia, and serologic evidence of coronavirus infection was demonstrated in 8.2 per cent of pediatric patients hospitalized with lower respiratory tract disease. However, in other studies such an association was not found. Coronavirus OC43 infections also were observed in four military recruits with pneumonia with pleural

TABLE 325/326–2. COMPARISON OF THE CLINICAL FEATURES OF COLDS PRODUCED BY INTRANASAL ADMINISTRATION OF CORONAVIRUSES OR RHINOVIRUSES

	Coronaviruses		Rhinoviruses	
	229E	*B814*	*Type 2 (HGP or PK)*	*DC*
Number of volunteers inoculated	26	75	213	251
Number getting colds	13 (50%)	34 (45%)	78 (37%)	77 (31%)
Incubation period (days)				
Mean	3.3	3.2	2.1	2.1
Range	2–4	2–5	1–5	1–4
Duration (days)				
Mean	7	6	9	10
Range	3–18	2–17	3–19	2–26
Maximum number of tissues used daily				
Mean	23	21	14	18
Range	8–105	8–120	3–38	3–60
Malaise	46%	47%	28%	25%
Headache	85%	53%	56%	56%
Chill	31%	18%	28%	15%
Pyrexia	23%*	21%*	14%	18%
Mucopurulent nasal discharge	0	62%	83%	80%
Sore throat	54%	79%	87%	73%
Cough	31%	44%	68%	56%
Number of volunteers with colds of indicated severity				
Mild	10 (77%)	24 (71%)	63 (80%)	36 (47%)
Moderate	2 (15%)	7 (20%)	12 (15%)	28 (36%)
Severe	1 (8%)	3 (9%)	4 (5%)	13 (17%)

*Between 99.2° F (37.3° C) and 100.4° F (38° C). After Bradburne, Bynoe, Tyrrell: Br Med J 3:767, 1967.

reaction. The etiologic significance of such associations is not known. Rhinovirus and coronavirus infections have been associated with exacerbations of chronic bronchitis in adults. The association of rhinovirus infections with exacerbations of chronic lung disease has been reported in several studies; rhinoviruses have characteristically been the single most frequently detected agents (14 to 43 per cent). A transient decrease in pulmonary function has also been observed in volunteers infected with rhinovirus.

Complications of common colds include sinusitis, otitis media, acute infectious exacerbations in patients with chronic bronchitis, precipitation of asthma, and extensions of infections into the central nervous or cardiovascular systems, as noted in the pathology section. The role of bacteria acting in concert with the virus infection in certain of these complications must be kept in mind in establishing therapeutic regimens.

DIAGNOSIS. Since most respiratory viruses can induce common colds, an etiologic diagnosis cannot be made on clinical grounds. Specific viral diagnosis of the common cold is essentially a research procedure that requires tissue or organ cultures for virus isolation or antigens for certain serologic studies. Complement fixation (229E, OC43), hemagglutination-inhibition (OC43), enzyme-linked immunosorbent assay (229E), or radioimmunoassay (OC43) can be performed in order to demonstrate serologic evidence of infection with certain coronaviruses. However, antigens for such tests are not generally available. The most important test for a patient with a common-cold–like illness is a throat culture for group A beta-hemolytic streptococci because symptoms of illnesses associated with the common cold viruses and the streptoccoccus may overlap. Appropriate antibiotic therapy is available for treatment of this bacterial infection.

TREATMENT AND PREVENTION. There is no specific treatment for patients with the common cold. Only symptomatic treatment measures should be employed. The use of acetyl salicylic acid (aspirin) for children with colds should be approached with caution because of the epidemiologic association of this drug with Reye's syndrome when the drug is administered during a viral illness, usually influenza or varicella—both of which can cause symptoms resembling those of the common cold (Table 325/326–1). The Committee on Infectious Diseases of the American Academy of Pediatrics stated in a special report, "In balancing this probability (the risk) with the benefits of aspirin, it is the opinion of the Committee that aspirin should not be prescribed under usual circumstances for children with varicella or those suspected of having influenza on the basis of clinical or epidemiologic evidence."

Antibiotics have no value in the therapy of the uncomplicated common cold. Previous tonsillectomy did not significantly affect the number of common respiratory illnesses or the induction of experimental colds in volunteers in the Cleveland Family Study. The use of vitamin C for the treatment or prevention of common colds has aroused great interest and much controversy. Available evidence indicates that its use does not reduce the number of episodes of respiratory illness but does decrease somewhat the total number of days of disability. The routine use of large doses of vitamin C for preventive treatment of common colds does not appear to be warranted from evidence available at this time.

Although there was great enthusiasm for producing a vaccine against common colds in the 1960's, when the rhinoviruses were finally cultivated in tissue cultures with ease, this enthusiasm rapidly waned when the number of distinct serotypes gradually increased to 89. Currently over 100 serotypes are known to exist, and no one serotype or group of serotypes appears to be consistently more important than others. Experimental rhinovirus vaccines against single serotypes have been made and shown to be effective in preventing or modifying illnesses induced by the serotype present in the vaccine. Although some heterotypic antibody responses have been observed with decavalent rhinovirus vaccines, the production of a rhinovirus vaccine appears to be impractical because of the multiplicity of serotypes. Until the number of serotypes of coronaviruses can be elucidated and the role of antibody in preventing or modifying illnesses can be established, consideration of a coronavirus vaccine is premature. Antiviral drugs or compounds may hold promise as specific treatment measures. Interferon inducers or interferon itself applied topically in the nose have been shown to be effective in reducing symptomatic illness induced by a rhinovirus under experimental conditions.

One method available for preventing rhinovirus colds may

be the application of rigid personal hygienic measures when a family member has a common cold. This would entail hand washing and avoidance of finger-eye and finger-nose contact.

Committee on Infectious Diseases of the American Academy of Pediatrics (Fulginiti VA, Brunell PA, Cherry JD, Ector WL, Gershon AA, Gotoff SP, Hughes WT, Mortimer EA Jr, Peter G): Special report. Aspirin and Reye syndrome. Pediatrics 69:810, 1982. *After weighing the available evidence, this Committee has made a strong recommendation against the use of aspirin under usual circumstances in children with varicella or influenza (both of which can cause common-cold–like symptoms).*

D'Alessio DJ, Peterson JA, Dick CR, Dick EC: Transmission of experimental rhinovirus colds in volunteer married couples. J Infect Dis 133:28, 1976. *A carefully conducted study describing the communicability of rhinoviruses in married couples. Conditions for transmissibility of infection are elucidated.*

Dingle JH, Badger GF, Jordan WS: Illness in the home. A study of 25,000 illnesses in a group of Cleveland families. Cleveland, The Press of Western Reserve University, 1964. *A classic study of illnesses experienced by a group of families over an almost ten-year period. Detailed epidemiologic data are given on the patterns of illnesses, including common respiratory diseases.*

Douglas RG Jr, Lindgren KM, Couch RB: Exposure to cold environment and rhinovirus common cold. Failure to demonstrate effect. New Engl J Med 279:743, 1968. *This classic study examines the role of cold temperatures on host resistance to rhinovirus infection and illness.*

Dykes MHM, Meier P: Ascorbic acid and the common cold. JAMA 231:1073, 1975. *A thoughtful and careful analysis of numerous studies on the efficacy and safety of ascorbic acid in the prevention and treatment of the common cold. The authors conclude that "the unrestrictive use of ascorbic acid for these purposes cannot be advocated on the basis of the evidence currently available."*

Editorial: Cold comfort for hot children. Br. Med J 286:1163, 1983. *Reviews some of differential diagnoses when a child has a fever. Also examines the role of aspirin in Reye's syndrome and concludes that ". . . aspirin should be avoided in children with fever, especially during epidemics of influenza or chickenpox."*

Gwaltney JM Jr: Rhinoviruses. *In* Evans AS (ed.): Viral infections of humans. Epidemiology and control. New York, Plenum Medical Book Company, 1982, pp 491–517. *An up-to-date review of rhinoviruses from the epidemiologic perspective by a major contributor to this field (178 references).*

Gwaltney JM, Moskalski PB, Hendley JO: Hand-to-hand transmission of rhinovirus colds. Ann Intern Med 88:463, 1978. *An important paper by a pioneer group in rhinovirus research describing the efficient transmission of rhinovirus in common colds by hand exposure followed by self-inoculation. This route was more efficient for transmission than large- or small-particle aerosols.*

Jackson GG, Dowling HF, Anderson TO, Riff L, Saporta J, Turck M: Susceptibility and immunity to common upper respiratory viral infections—the common cold. Ann Intern Med 53:719, 1960. *The authors examine clinical aspects of experimentally induced common colds in volunteers. They also study environmental and physiologic factors in relation to susceptibility to common colds.*

Larson HE, Reed SE, Tyrrell DAJ: Isolation of rhinoviruses and coronaviruses from 38 colds in adults. J Med Virol 5:221, 1980. *This study demonstrates that the isolation rate of fastidious viruses from common colds can be enhanced substantially with the use of organ cultures and volunteers. This type of carefully executed study may also eventually lead to the discovery of new etiologic agents of common colds.*

Monto AS: Coronaviruses. *In* Evans AS (ed.): Viral infections of humans. Epidemiology and control. New York, Plenum Medical Book Company, 1982, pp 151–165. *An up-to-date review of the coronaviruses from the epidemiologic perspective (65 references).*

Reed SE: The behavior of recent isolates of human respiratory coronavirus in vitro and in volunteers: Evidence of heterogeneity among 299E related strains. J Med Virol 13:179, 1984. *Studies at the Common Cold Unit in Salisbury continue to expand our knowledge of the immunologic relationships among various strains of coronaviruses. Such studies may have an important bearing on vaccine approaches.*

Robbins SL, Cotran RS: Pathological Basis of Disease. 2nd ed. Philadelphia, W.B. Saunders Company, 1979, pp 881–882. *In a chapter on nasal cavities and accessory air sinuses, the authors describe the pathologic changes in viral rhinitis and also discuss bacterial complications.*

327. VIRAL PHARYNGITIS, LARYNGITIS, CROUP, AND BRONCHITIS

Maurice A. Mufson

DEFINITION. Viral infections that localize to the upper and middle respiratory passages produce an acute inflammatory response and depending upon the anatomic site involved, evoke the clinical manifestations of pharyngitis, laryngitis, croup (laryngotracheobronchitis), and bronchitis. These infections do not ordinarily involve the pulmonary alveoli. Pharyngitis, laryngitis, and bronchitis can occur in persons of any age. Croup occurs exclusively in children and mainly during the second year of life. The illnesses often begin abruptly with predominant upper respiratory tract signs and symptoms and limited systemic findings, and the uncomplicated illness abates after five to ten days. However, croup can be a life-threatening illness; the most common complications include respiratory failure and pneumonia.

ETIOLOGY. Many viruses that primarily infect the upper and middle respiratory passages can cause pharyngitis, laryngitis, croup, and bronchitis (see Table 327–1). The main viral pathogens of pharyngitis and laryngitis include rhinoviruses, coronaviruses, influenza A and B viruses, adenoviruses, parainfluenza viruses, enteroviruses, and respiratory syncytial virus. The principal viral pathogens of croup are the parainfluenza viruses types 1, 3, and 2 (in decreasing frequency). Influenza A and B viruses and respiratory syncytial virus are uncommon causes of croup. Acute viral bronchitis has been associated with influenza A and B virus, coronavirus, adenovirus, respiratory syncytial virus, and rhinovirus infections. In any individual case, the etiology of pharyngitis, laryngitis, croup, and bronchitis cannot be determined on the basis of the clinical characteristics of the illness. A definitive etiologic diagnosis can be made only by application of diagnostic virology tests.

Pharyngitis also can occur as part of systemic viral illnesses associated with *Epstein-Barr virus* (see Ch. 338) or *cytomegalovirus* (see Ch. 337) infection, and laryngitis and bronchitis occur in *measles* virus infection (see Ch. 332). When coryza represents the main feature of an upper respiratory infection, the term *common cold* (see Ch. 325) prevails. When the infecting virus is an influenza virus, the designation *influenza* describes an acute respiratory tract infection with fever and prostration (see Ch. 330). Since many viruses can cause either pharyngitis, laryngitis, croup, or bronchitis, and since the anatomic site of infection underlies the basis for the clinical manifestations, it seems preferable to retain these terms and modify them by adding the name of the infecting virus when it has been identified.

INCIDENCE AND PREVALENCE. Viral pharyngitis, laryngitis, and bronchitis occur commonly. Most children and adults experience three to five viral infections of the upper respiratory tract each year. Since croup is a serious illness of infants and children immediately recognizable by a distinctive complex of symptoms and signs (see later discussion), estimates of its incidence have been calculated among two populations studied during several years (Denny, 1983). The incidence of croup reached a peak during the second year of life, at 14.9 and 47.0 cases per 1000 children per year, and by age four to five it declined to 3.1 and 14.5 cases, respectively, in the two different populations.

EPIDEMIOLOGY. Viral pharyngitis, laryngitis, croup, and bronchitis occur during all months of the year, with peaks of occurrence paralleling epidemics of individual viruses. Respiratory syncytial virus, influenza A and B viruses, coronaviruses, parainfluenza virus type 1, and to a lesser extent type 2, occur in epidemics, mainly in the late fall, winter, and spring. The other viral pathogens occur endemically, although they may exhibit some seasonal variation from year to year. Virus infections of the respiratory tract spread by direct person-to-person contact, by infectious aerosols, or by fomites.

CLINICAL MANIFESTATIONS. ***Viral Pharyngitis.*** Acute viral pharyngitis is usually characterized by a scratchy and sore throat, but pain upon swallowing is not a prominent or constant feature. When dysphagia is present, it suggests a streptococcal infection. Cough is not a feature of acute viral pharyngitis. Fever and malaise accompany influenza and adenovirus infections, but these findings are infrequent with the other respiratory viral pathogens. Pharyngeal erythema and edema and enlarged and tender lymph nodes may be the only physical findings. Adenovirus pharyngitis may be associated with conjunctivitis. Exudative tonsillitis occurs in adenovirus infections, infectious mononucleosis associated with Epstein-Barr virus infection, herpetic pharyngitis (with or without vesicles or small ulcers), as well as streptococcal pharyngitis. Exudative tonsillitis alone does not serve to distinguish these infections. An attempt

TABLE 327–1. ETIOLOGY OF VIRAL PHARYNGITIS, LARYNGITIS, CROUP, AND BRONCHITIS

Virus	Serotype	Occurrence in Indicated Illness			
		Pharyngitis	*Laryngitis*	*Croup*	*Bronchitis*
Respiratory syncytial		+		+	+++
Parainfluenza	1	++	++	++++	++
	2	+	+	+++	+
	3	++	++	++++	++
Influenza	A	+++	+++	+	+++
	B	++	+		+
Adenovirus	1–7	++++	++	+	++
Coronavirus	Few	++	+		+++
Rhinovirus	Many	++++	+++		++
Enterovirus	Many	++			
Herpes simplex	1	++			

Frequency and importance of virus occurrence are graded from minimal importance (+) to major importance (++++). Blank = uncommon occurrence.

must be made to estabish the cause in these cases and should include appropriate diagnostic laboratory tests.

Viral Laryngitis. In acute viral laryngitis, hoarseness predominates, associated with difficulty in talking, pain on clearing respiratory secretions, and often fever, depending upon the infecting virus. Cough and pharyngitis may be present. The larynx is erythematous and edematous, and the regional lymph nodes are slightly enlarged and tender. Wheezes may be audible upon auscultation.

Viral Croup. The clinical picture of croup characteristically includes inspiratory stridor, hoarseness, and a brassy cough. This distinctive triad of symptoms reflects the acute and intense edema and mucoid exudative secretions of the larynx and associated obstruction of the subglottic portion of the upper airway. These symptoms develop acutely, accompanied by fever, cough, tachypnea, and wheezing. Retractions of the chest wall occur. Hemoptysis does not occur. Rhonchi, rales, or wheezes, alone or in combination, may be audible upon auscultation of the lungs. Radiographic examination of the neck can demonstrate subglottic narrowing, and a chest roentgenogram may show hyperinflation of the lungs. In the uncomplicated case, the findings resolve in several days, but some children develop respiratory failure and pneumonia. Children who previously experienced multiple episodes of croup manifest hyperreactive airways several years later.

Viral Bronchitis. In acute viral bronchitis, cough, with or without sputum production, and fever are the main features. The sputum is slightly mucoid or watery and white. Other common symptoms include hoarseness, nonpleuritic substernal chest pain, and malaise. Rhonchi or rales may be heard upon auscultation of the chest. The chest roentgenogram may show increased intensity of the vascular pattern, but pulmonary infiltrates do not occur. Acute bronchitis associated with influenza or coronavirus infection occurs often as an exacerbation of chronic bronchitis.

TREATMENT AND PROGNOSIS. The treatment of pharyngitis, laryngitis, and bronchitis associated with virus infections of the upper respiratory tract aims at the relief of distressing local and systemic symptoms. These illnesses are self-limited and not severe. Antibiotics are not indicated, except when secondary bacterial infection occurs. In pharyngitis, pharyngeal pain or dysphagia should be treated with analgesics and fluids. The treatment of laryngitis and bronchitis also requires analgesics, fluids, and rest. Cough in adults and older children that is relentless and causes fatigue should be treated with cough suppressant preparations.

The less serious cases of croup can be managed by having the child rest in bed at home. Vaporizers that produce a mist of moist air may be beneficial. Children with severe croup require hospitalization, supportive treatment, and constant monitoring for the development of respiratory distress. If hypoxemia develops, oxygen therapy is essential; hypoxemia requiring oxygen can develop even before cyanosis becomes evident. Subglottic edema may be reduced by the administration of racemic epinephrine. Administration of corticosteroids in the treatment of croup may have limited benefit.

Buscho RO, Saxtan D, Shultz PS, Finch E, Mufson MA: Viruses and *Mycoplasma pneumoniae* infections in exacerbations of chronic bronchitis. J Infect Dis 137:377, 1978. *A longitudinal study of acute viral exacerbations among a group of adult men with chronic bronchitis, employing virus isolation and serodiagnosis. Exacerbations were significantly associated with influenza and coronavirus infections compared with periods of remission.*

Denny FW, Murphy TF, Clyde WA Jr, Collier AM, Henderson FW: Croup: An 11-year study in a pediatric practice. Pediatrics 71:871, 1983. *A comprehensive investigation of the viral etiology and epidemiology of croup among a large population of ambulatory children. Viral infections were identified by virus isolation attempts on oropharyngeal cultures.*

Gwaltney JM Jr, Hendley JO: Transmission of experimental rhinovirus infection by contaminated surfaces. Am J Epidemiol 116:828, 1982. *The first demonstration that environmental surfaces contaminated with rhinovirus-containing secretions could serve as a reservoir for the spread of these viruses to susceptible persons.*

Koren G, Frand M, Barzilay Z, MacLeod SM: Corticosteroid treatment of laryngotracheitis *v* spasmodic croup in children. Am J Dis Child 137:941, 1983. *Recent re-evaluation of the effectiveness of corticosteroid therapy for croup. Double-blind random design was employed in the treatment of two categories of croup using a single high dose of dexamethasone. Six hours after the start of corticosteroid therapy, the respiratory rate of patients classified as having spasmodic croup had decreased significantly compared with the placebo group, but no change in respiratory rate was detected among patients classified as having laryngotracheitis.*

Sherter CB, Polnitsky CA: The relationship of viral infections to subsequent asthma. Clin Chest Med 2:67, 1981. *Review of the evidence for a causal relationship between virus infections of the respiratory tract during childhood and subsequent asthma.*

328. RESPIRATORY SYNCYTIAL VIRUS

Robert M. Chanock

DEFINITION. Respiratory syncytial virus (RSV) is the most important cause of viral lower respiratory tract disease in infants and children. This ubiquitous virus causes an extensive epidemic every year during fall, winter, or early spring. During these epidemics there is a dramatic increase in admission to hospitals of infants and young children with severe lower respiratory tract disease. Older children and adults commonly undergo reinfection, but disease is usually milder than that experienced during infancy and early childhood.

ETIOLOGY. The virus was first isolated in 1956 from a symptomatic laboratory chimpanzee during an outbreak of illness resembling the common cold. Shortly thereafter, a similar virus was recovered from children with pneumonia or croup, and its characteristic syncytial (giant cell) cytopathic effect in tissue culture was noted. RSV is an enveloped virus that belongs to the family Paramyxoviridae, genus *Pneumovirus*. It resembles the parainfluenza viruses of the genus *Paramyxovirus* but differs from them in morphology of its nucleocapsid, in failure to agglutinate erythrocytes (hemagglutination), and in absence of a neuraminidase enzyme. The viral genome consists of a single negative (−) strand of ribonucleic acid (RNA) approximately 15,000 bases in length. The genetic information of RSV is expressed as a series of viral messenger RNAs (mRNAs) transcribed from the viral genome that code for ten viral-specific proteins. One of these proteins, nucleocapsid protein, coats the viral RNA to form a helical nucleocapsid. This structure is enclosed within a bilayer lipid membrane that is studded with two different viral glycoproteins. One of these, the fusion protein, lyses the host cell membrane, permitting entry of virus into the cell. This protein is also responsible for fusion of infected cells to neighboring cells, a process that results in syncytium formation, a prominent feature of the virus during its growth in tissue culture.

Although antigenic variation among strains has been noted, it does not have epidemiologic significance. A related RSV is a common cause of respiratory disease in calves, but this virus does not appear to infect humans.

EPIDEMIOLOGY. RSV has a worldwide distribution. Whenever appropriate studies have been performed, RSV has been found to be the major pediatric respiratory tract pathogen. The highest incidence of severe lower respiratory tract disease is observed in infants between one and six months of age, with a peak incidence at two months. Serious lower respiratory tract disease occurs more commonly in males than in females and in nonblack than in black infants. Approximately 50 per cent of infants who live through a single RSV epidemic become infected. In certain settings, such as day care centers, the attack rate approaches 100 per cent during an outbreak.

Reinfection occurs with high frequency during childhood. Adults are also reinfected frequently, particularly when there is exposure to a large amount of virus. For example, during annual RSV epidemics, 25 to 50 per cent of the staff of pediatric wards undergo reinfection. In families into which virus is introduced, spread of RSV among older siblings also occurs with high frequency (40 per cent). In individuals of all ages, reinfection is usually symptomatic, and adults exposed to a large amount of virus may develop an influenza-like disease.

Most individuals infected with RSV have upper respiratory illness. However, a surprisingly large proportion of infants (25 to 40 per cent) also develop lower respiratory tract disease. Hospitalization of infants for RSV disease varies with environmental and socioeconomic conditions. Overall, 1 in 120 to 1 in 200 infants requires hospital care for RSV pneumonia or bronchiolitis during the first year of life. RSV is responsible for approximately 50 to 75 per cent of bronchiolitis and for 20 to 25 per cent of pneumonia that necessitate admission of infants and young children to hospital.

In developed countries, severe RSV lower respiratory tract disease is usually nonfatal (0.5 to 2.5 per cent). Fatal RSV disease occurs most often in infants with other underlying illnesses, particularly congenital heart disease (37 per cent), bronchopulmonary dysplasia, serious renal disease, and diseases such as cancer that are treated with immunosuppressive drugs. In a British study of 46 infants and children who died with lower respiratory tract disease, 13 were infected with RSV. In addition, a number of babies dying from sudden infant death syndrome are infected with RSV.

RSV has a clear seasonality in temperate zones of the world. In urban centers, epidemics occur yearly in the late fall, winter, or spring but not during the summer. In the northern hemisphere, the virus is rarely isolated during August or September. Each RSV epidemic lasts approximately five months, with 40 per cent of infections occurring during the peak month in the temporal center of the outbreak. In the northern hemisphere, most outbreaks peak in February or March, but the peak may occur as early as December or as late as June. RSV is spread

by infected respiratory secretions in the form of large droplets or through fomite contamination.

During epidemic intervals, RSV is one of the commonest causes of hospital-acquired infection on pediatric wards. The risk of infection increases as hospital stay is extended beyond one week. The mortality in such hospital-acquired infections is considerably higher than in community-acquired infetions because the patients involved are frequently at high risk because of other diseases, malnourishment, or immunosuppressive drugs.

Since reinfection with RSV is common and often associated with disease, it is clear that immunity is neither permanent nor complete. However, multiple reinfections induce temporary immunity to infection, and their cumulative effect prevents severe lower respiratory tract disease. Studies in adult volunteers indicate that immunity to induced infection correlates better with the level of nasal neutralizing immunoglobulin A (IgA) antibody than with serum antibody. On the other hand, there is some evidence that maternally transmitted antibody in small infants offers some protection from serious lower respiratory tract disease. Nonetheless, a considerable amount of severe RSV disease occurs in young infants who possess a moderate level of maternally derived serum neutralizing antibody.

CLINICAL MANIFESTATIONS. During infancy, RSV infection usually causes upper respiratory symptoms. In 25 to 40 per cent of infections the respiratory tract below the larynx is also involved. Lower respiratory tract signs are preceded by a prodromal phase of rhinorrhea that is sometimes accompanied by a decrease in appetite. Low grade fever is common. Cough is often accompanied by wheezing, and if disease is mild, symptoms may not progress beyond this stage. Examination usually reveals moderate tachypnea, diffuse rhonci, fine rales and wheezes, as well as profuse rhinorrhea and intermittent fever. Otitis media is also common. The chest x-ray usually appears normal. In most instances, uneventful recovery occurs after 7 to 12 days.

In more severe cases, coughing and wheezing progress and the child becomes dyspneic and refuses feedings. Hyperexpansion of the chest is evident, and there may be intercostal and subcostal retractions. Severe tachypnea is common even in the absence of visible cyanosis, and in advanced disease as the child tires and hypoxia becomes more extreme, listlessness and apnea occur. The chest may appear normal on x-ray examination, but often there is a combination of air trapping (hyperexpansion) and peribronchial thickening or interstitial pneumonia. Segmental or lobar consolidation is also occasionally seen, usually involving the right upper lobe. Pleural effusion is rare. In infants with underlying cardiac or respiratory disease, the progression of symptoms may be rapid. In these instances, respiratory failure requiring intubation and ventilation may appear on the second or third day of illness.

Almost all infants who require hospitalization are hypoxemic on admission and remain so for a prolonged period—up to several weeks—although recovery has ensued. The hypoxemia reflects an abnormally low ventilation-perfusion ratio. Hypercarbia may also be present.

In infants who were born prematurely, and sometimes in normal infants under six weeks of age, apneic spells may develop during RSV infection. This often occurs in the absence of significant respiratory signs and may be the predominant symptom bringing the infant to medical attention. Such apneic spells, while often recurrent during acute infection, are usually self-limited and rarely cause neurologic or systemic damage. However, exceptions to this pattern occur, and such episodes are an indication for hospitalization and careful medical supervision. Apnea at the peak of severe illness is a poor prognostic sign.

In the newborn infant, most RSV infections produce only

upper respiratory symptoms. Bronchiolitis is rare, and severe infection is more often characterized by lethargy, irritability, and fever or unstable body temperature than by specific respiratory signs.

Children who have apparently recovered completely from RSV bronchiolitis or pneumonia may still retain both measurable and symptomatic respiratory abnormalities for many years. A study of 23 children examined ten years after an episode of bronchiolitis found that although all were symptom free (a criterion for admission to the study), 20 had some measurable physiologic abnormality of lung function or arterial blood gases.

Acute RSV infections are common in adults, particularly in medical personnel or in those caring for small children. These infections are occasionally asymptomatic but usually are associated with rhinorrhea, pharyngitis, cough, constitutional symptoms of headache and fatigue, and fever. Disease usually lasts about five days but may be more prolonged, particularly in hospital staff. Alterations in pulmonary function, such as elevated total respiratory resistance and increased airway reactivity, often last for eight weeks. There is some evidence that RSV infection in the elderly is a cause of febrile bronchitis and severe or even fatal pneumonia.

DIAGNOSIS. Presumptive diagnosis of RSV infection can often be made on the basis of the clinical syndrome in relation to the time of year and other epidemiologic features. Definitive diagnosis depends upon the laboratory. In older children and adults, an increase in serum RSV antibody concentration, either complement fixing (CF) or neutralizing, is a fairly sensitive index of reinfection with RSV. Serologic tests in infants are less sensitive, particularly in patients under four months of age. In young infants, only 2 to 15 per cent of RSV infections are detectable by CF and 2 to 20 per cent by neutralization assay. Antibody measurement by solid-phase immunoassay (enzyme-linked immunosorbent assay; ELISA) recently has been shown to be a more sensitive indicator of infection in small infants than CF or neutralization. At all ages, however, isolation of virus or detection of antigen in respiratory secretions is the procedure of choice. Specimens are best obtained by aspiration or gentle washing out of nasopharyngeal secretions. These may be examined by inoculation of tissue culture, immunofluorescence, or ELISA. Infectivity of RSV in secretions is labile; hence samples should be placed on wet ice while being transported to a tissue culture laboratory.

TREATMENT AND PREVENTION. Treatment of RSV infections of the lower respiratory tract consists primarily of supportive care: mechanical removal of secretions, proper positioning of the infant, administration of humidified oxygen, and in severe cases respiratory assistance. When wheezing is an important symptom, some infants, particularly those over a year of age, will benefit from the use of theophylline or adrenergic drugs.

Ribavirin (1-b-D-ribofuranosyl-1,2,4-triazole-3-carboxamide), delivered by small-particle aerosol, shows some promise for treatment of severe RSV disease in young infants. In one study, the drug hastened recovery and diminished virus shedding.

Because immunity to RSV is neither permanent nor complete, the goal of immunoprophylaxis is prevention of severe lower respiratory tract disease. It should be possible to achieve this through the cumulative effect of repeated vaccination. Efforts to develop an effective vaccine have been frustrated by the ineffectiveness of formalin-inactivated virus and by the genetic instability of satisfactorily attenuated temperature-sensitive mutants that initially showed promise as live virus vaccine strains. Perhaps recent success in cloning complementary deoxyribonucleic acid (cDNA) copies of RSV genes in *E. coli* may open the way to the preparation of immunogenic viral surface glycoprotein antigens, or alternatively, recombinant DNA techniques may prove useful in constructing stable attenuated mutants that can be used in a live vaccine.

Chanock RM, Kim HW, Brandt CD, Parrott RH: Respiratory syncytial virus. *In* Evans AS (ed.): Viral Infections of Humans: Epidemiology and Control. New York, Plenum Publishing Corp., 1982, pp 471–489. *A summary of biologic properties of RSV as well as its epidemiology and the pathogenesis of the disease.*

Hall CBH, Geiman JM, Biggar R, Kotok DI, Hogan PM, Douglas RG Jr.: Respiratory syncytial virus infections within families. N Engl J Med 294:414, 1976. *Longitudinal surveillance of RSV infections in families. During an epidemic, infection occurred in 44 per cent of families; within these families the infection rate was 62 per cent in infants and 43 per cent in adults, the latter rate representing reinfection.*

Hall CBH, McBride JT, Walsh EE, Bell DM, Gala CL, Hildreth S, Ten Eyck LG, Hall WJ: Aerosolized ribavirin treatment of infants with respiratory syncytial viral infection. N Engl J Med 308:1443, 1983. *Administration of ribivirin by small-particle aerosol hastened recovery of infants with severe RSV lower respiratory tract disease.*

Henderson FW, Collier AM, Clyde WA Jr., Denny FW: Respiratory-syncytial-virus infections, reinfections and immunity. N Engl J Med 300:530, 1979. *Longitudinal surveillance of children in a day care center demonstrated high frequency of reinfection; also, after several reinfections partial immunity developed to RSV.*

Henderson FW, Collier AM, Sanyal MA, Watkins JM, Fairclough DL, Clyde WA Jr., Denny FW: A longitudinal study of respiratory viruses and bacteria in the etiology of acute otitis media with effusion. N Engl J Med 306:1377, 1982. *Important role of RSV infection in initiating acute otitis media with effusion.*

329. PARAINFLUENZA VIRAL DISEASES

Robert M. Chanock

DEFINITION. Infection with parainfluenza viruses occurs early in life and is an important cause of *pediatric respiratory tract disease*. The spectrum of illness varies from mild upper respiratory disease to severe croup, pneumonia, or bronchiolitis. Reinfection is common in later life and is associated with mild respiratory tract disease.

ETIOLOGY. The parainfluenza viruses are enveloped viruses that belong to the family Paramyxoviridae, genus *Paramyxovirus*. The single stranded ribonucleic acid (RNA) viral genome has negative polarity (antimessenger sense) and is approximately 15,000 bases in length. Its genetic information is expressed as a series of messenger RNAs (mRNAs) transcribed from the viral genome that code for seven viral-specific proteins. One of these proteins, nucleocapsid protein, coats the viral RNA to form a helical nucleocapsid. This structure is enclosed within a lipid bilayer envelope that is studded with the two viral glycoprotein surface antigens, the hemagglutinin-neuraminidase, and the fusion protein. Parainfluenza viruses share many properties with the influenza viruses, but they differ from these agents in their wider RNA nucleocapsid (18 nm as compared with 9 nm) and in the distribution of hemagglutination and neuraminidase functions on their surface glycoproteins. Both parainfluenza hemagglutinin and neuraminidase are located on the same surface glycoprotein, whereas these functions reside on separate surface glycoproteins of the influenza viruses. The parainfluenza viruses have common antigens that are not shared by the influenza viruses. Mumps virus shares the foregoing properties, as well as related antigens, with the parainfluenza viruses.

There are four antigenically distinct serotypes of human parainfluenza virus. These viruses were first recognized by cytopathic effects that developed in infected tissue cultures (type 2) or by the hemadsorption reaction in which guinea pig erythrocytes become adsorbed to an infected tissue culture monolayer (types 1, 3, and 4). Initially, these viruses were designated *hemadsorption viruses*, but later they were classified as parainfluenza viruses. Related parainfluenza viruses cause respiratory disease in mice (Sendai virus, a subtype of type 1), dogs (SV5, a subtype of type 2), calves (bovine shipping fever virus, a subtype of type 3), and birds (seven distinct serotypes not closely related to human parainfluenza viruses). Animal and avian parainfluenza viruses are distinct antigenically from human parainfluenza viruses and do not appear to infect humans.

EPIDEMIOLOGY. The four parainfluenza virus types have wide geographic distribution. The first three types have been identified in most areas where appropriate tissue culture and hemadsorption techniques have been applied to the study of childhood respiratory tract diseases. So far, type 4 viruses (subtypes 4A and 4B), which are more difficult to recover in tissue culture, have been isolated in fewer areas, but serologic studies suggest that they are also relatively ubiquitous. Each of the four parainfluenza virus types causes acute respiratory tract disease in humans.

The parainfluenza viruses are exceeded only by *respiratory syncytial virus (RSV)* as an important cause of lower respiratory tract disease in young children. These viruses, particularly type 3, commonly reinfect older children and adults to produce upper respiratory tract disease. Illness usually occurs less often and is less severe during reinfection than during primary infection.

There is considerable diversity in both epidemiologic and clinical manifestations of infections caused by the parainfluenza viruses. Parainfluenza virus type 1 is the principal cause of croup (laryngotracheobronchitis) in children, and parainfluenza virus type 3 is second only to RSV as a cause of pneumonia and bronchiolitis in infants less than six months of age. Parainfluenza virus type 2 resembles type 1 virus in clinical manifestations but causes serious illness less frequently. Infections with parainfluenza virus type 4 are detected infrequently, and associated illnesses are usually mild.

The parainfluenza viruses are most important as respiratory tract pathogens during infancy and childhood, when they (types 1 through 3) cause a spectrum of effects ranging from inapparent infection to life-threatening lower respiratory tract disease. Studies in different parts of the world indicate that types 1, 2, and 3 are associated with approximately 40 to 70 per cent of severe croup. In addition to croup, these three viruses are also responsible for a smaller but appreciable percentage of other acute respiratory tract diseases of infancy and early childhood. Eighty per cent of individuals undergoing primary infection with type 3 virus develop a febrile illness, and in one third there is involvement of the lower respiratory tract. Approximately one half of initial type 1 virus infections and two thirds of initial type 2 virus infections produce a febrile illness. Severe croup, although the most dramatic and serious manifestation of initial parainfluenza virus infection, is noted in only 2 to 3 per cent of primary type 1 or type 2 virus infections.

Primary parainfluenza virus infection generally occurs early in life. Type 3 virus often causes illness during the first months of life while infants still possess circulating neutralizing antibody derived from their mothers. In contrast, in young infants, maternally derived antibody appears to prevent both infection and severe disease caused by type 1 and type 2 viruses. After age four months, there is an increase in the number of cases of croup and other lower respiratory tract diseases caused by type 1 and type 2 viruses. This high incidence continues until approximately six years of age, after which age there is a much lower incidence. It is unusual for type 1 or type 2 virus to cause lower respiratory tract illness during adolescence or adult life, although this does occur on occasion.

At present, type 1 and type 2 virus epidemics are synchronous, occurring during the autumn of odd-numbered years. For many years, type 3 virus exhibited an endemic pattern, with infection occurring during all seasons of the year. Within this endemic pattern, small outbreaks occurred, but there was no predictable periodicity. Within the past five years, there has been a shift toward yearly spring epidemics of type 3 virus infection. Nosocomial infection with the parainfluenza viruses, particularly type 3 virus, is common and often leads to serious lower respiratory tract disease.

Transmission of parainfluenza viruses is by direct person-to-person contact or large droplet spread. The high rate of infection early in life, coupled with the high frequency of reinfection, suggests that these viruses spread readily from person to person. Reinfected individuals appear to be infectious, and a relatively small inoculum is able to initiate infection. Type 3 virus appears to be the most transmissible of the parainfluenza viruses.

In experimental infection of adult volunteers, the interval between administration of type 1, 2, or 3 virus and onset of upper respiratory tract symptoms ranged from three to six days. The incubation period in pediatric infections has not been defined; however, the interval between exposure to type 3 virus and the subsequent initial shedding of this virus is two to four days. Resistance to type 1 or type 2 parainfluenza virus infection and associated upper respiratory disease appears to be a function of local respiratory tract, secretory, immunoglobulin A (IgA)-neutralizing antibodies. Infants may also be partially protected from infection and disease by serum antibodies. This protective relationship is suggested by the relative sparing of young infants from type 1 and type 2 virus infection and associated disease at a time when they possess serum antibodies passively acquired from their mother. Also, the risk of infection with type 3 virus during the first four months of life is inversely related to the level of neutralizing antibody present in cord serum at birth. However, the protective effect of passive immunity is less than that observed for type 1 and type 2 viruses, since a significant number of infants with moderately high levels of maternally derived serum antibody become infected with type 3 virus and develop severe illness.

CLINICAL MANIFESTATIONS. In children, the most common type of illness consists of rhinitis, pharyngitis, and bronchitis, usually with fever. The most common initial symptoms are cough, hoarseness, and fever. The cough may be croupy, but respiratory distress is not present. Approximately three fourths of such ill children have temperatures above 37.8° C; fever usually lasts two to three days. Coarse breath sounds, rhonchi, erythema of the pharyngeal mucous membranes, and rhinitis are characteristic physical findings. Cervical adenopathy is uncommon.

When croup develops, the initial symptoms of rhinitis, pharyngitis, fever, and cough progress. After several days, the cough worsens and becomes brassy, seal-like, or barking and stridor ensues. At this stage, most children recover uneventfully after 24 to 48 hours, but in some air hunger develops, with cyanosis, sternal and intercostal retractions, and progressive airway obstruction. The lateral x-ray of the neck (which should be obtained only under carefully controlled medical supervision, if at all) shows glottic and subglottic narrowing (the "steeple sign") and differentiates this disease from epiglottitis.

When bronchiolitis or pneumonia develops, fever persists and the cough progresses and becomes somewhat productive. It is accompanied by wheezing, tachypnea, and retractions and in severe cases by cyanosis. The x-ray shows interstitial or perihilar infiltrates and air trapping. In some patients a combined bronchopneumonia-croup syndrome occurs.

DIAGNOSIS. Presumptive diagnosis of parainfluenza virus infection can be made on the basis of age, history, clinical findings, and relation to known or characteristic prevalence of virus in the community. Definitive diagnosis, however, requires recovery of the virus from appropriate specimens taken from the respiratory tract or identification of viral antigens in respiratory tract secretions by immunofluorescence or another form of immunoassay. Serodiagnosis by hemagglutination inhibition, complement fixation, or neutralization can establish that infection with a member of the parainfluenza virus group has occurred, but frequent heterotypic responses make type-specific diagnosis by serology extremely difficult.

TREATMENT. Symptomatic treatment of croup usually includes humidification of air by ultrasonic nebulizer and periodic inhalation of racemic epinephrine. Antibiotics are usually contraindicated. The use of corticosteroids is controversial, but many physicians prescribe high doses of dexamethasone if croup is severe. Specific antiviral treatment or effective vaccines for prevention of parainfluenza virus disease are not available.

Chanock RM, Parrott RH, Johnson KM, Kapikian AZ, Bell JA: Myxoviruses: Parainfluenza. Am Rev Respir Dis 88:152, 1963. *A discussion of the importance of parainfluenza viruses in pediatric respiratory tract disease and the first description of pattern of spread and reinfection.*

Denny FW, Murphy TF, Clyde WA, Jr, Collier AM, Henderson FW: Croup: An 11-year study in a pediatric practice. Pediatrics 71:871, 1983. *Eleven-year evaluation of the role of parainfluenza viruses in croup. These viruses accounted for 74 per cent of all virus isolates from croup patients.*

Fox JP, Hall CE: Infections with other respiratory pathogens: Influenza, mumps, and respiratory syncytial viruses; *Mycoplasma pneumoniae*. *In* Fox JP (ed.): Viruses in Families. Littleton, John Wright/PSG Inc, 1980, pp 335–381. *Longitudinal surveillance of families for parainfluenza virus infection and illness. Infection rate was 44 per 100 person years for all ages, while attack rate for illness associated with parainfluenza virus infection was 76 per cent for babies under age 2 years and 25 per cent for adults.*

Glezen WP, Denny FW: Epidemiology of acute lower respiratory disease in children. N Engl J Med 288:498, 1973. *Excellent summary of contribution of parainfluenza viruses to pediatric respiratory disease.*

Glezen WP, Loda FA, Denny FW: Parainfluenza viruses. *In* Evans AS (ed.): Viral Infections of Humans: Epidemiology and Control. New York, Plenum Publishing Company, Inc., 1982, pp 441–454. *Summary of natural history of parainfluenza virus infection and pathogenesis of disease.*

330. INFLUENZA

R. Gordon Douglas, Jr.

DEFINITION. Influenza is an acute, usually self-limited febrile illness that occurs in outbreaks of varying severity almost every winter. Although the causative virus is transmitted by the respiratory route, systemic symptoms are out of proportion to those in the respiratory tract. Infection with influenza virus can produce several other clinical syndromes common with infection with respiratory viruses, such as common colds, pharyngitis, croup, tracheobronchitis, bronchiolitis, or pneumonia. Conversely, infections with other respiratory viruses, such as respiratory syncytial virus, rhinovirus, or adenovirus, may produce sporadic cases indistinguishable from those of typical influenza. In addition to enormous morbidity and loss of time from school and work, influenza epidemics are associated with substantial mortality caused in large part by pulmonary complications.

HISTORY. Epidemics of respiratory disease similar to modern influenza have been recorded through the centuries. Since the year 1510, 31 pandemics have been described, 5 of which have occurred in the 20th century (1900, 1918, 1957, 1968, and 1977). Of these, the pandemic of 1918 was the most severe, accounting for at least 21 million deaths. Influenza A virus was first isolated in 1933 and influenza B virus in 1936. Effective inactivated viral vaccines were first produced in the 1940's, and antiviral chemotherapy became available in the late 1960's. Since 1968, over 200,000 deaths have occurred in the United States from epidemic influenza.

ETIOLOGY. Influenza viruses belong to the family Orthomyxoviridae. Influenza A virus constitutes one genus and influenza B virus another. The virion is a medium-sized (80 to 100 nm in diameter) enveloped sphericle or elongated particle covered with surface projections that are glycoproteins possessing either hemagglutinin (H) or neuraminidase (N) activity (Fig. 330–1). The envelope is composed of a lipid bilayer, on the inner surface of which is the matrix (M) protein. Within the envelope are eight segmented pieces of nucleocapsid, formed by a single species of protein, the nucleoprotein (NP), and by pieces of segmented single stranded ribonucleic acid (RNA). Three polymerase (P) proteins and two nonstructural (NS) proteins of unknown function are found within the envelope. The H is responsible for binding of the virus to the cell. Antibody to this protein neutralizes viral infectivity, and thus is the major determinant of immunity. The viral N is instrumental in release of virus from cells. Antineuraminidase antibody is not neutralizing but limits viral replication and therefore the severity of infection. The M protein plays a role in stability of the membrane and in organization of the virion during assembly. The three polymerases are important in viral replication. The internal M, NP, and P proteins are antigenically indistinguishable in all influenza A viruses but vary for influenza B and C viruses. Thus, type-specific (A, B, or C) distinction of influenza viruses depends on serologic reactions mediated by these internal antigens. However, the surface proteins (H and N) do vary, not only among influenza virus types but also among subtypes of influenza A.

The viral genome comprises eight segments of RNA, seven of which code for a single viral protein each. The eighth codes for the two nonstructural proteins. Reassortment of gene segments occurs frequently during infection to provide an unusually high frequency of genetic recombination. Influenza B and C viruses have been studied much less but appear to be structurally similar to influenza A virus. Antigenic variation is much less frequent with influenza B, and it may not occur with influenza C.

EPIDEMIOLOGY. ***Antigenic Variation.*** One of the unique and most remarkable features of influenza virus is the frequency with which changes in antigenicity occur. Such changes help

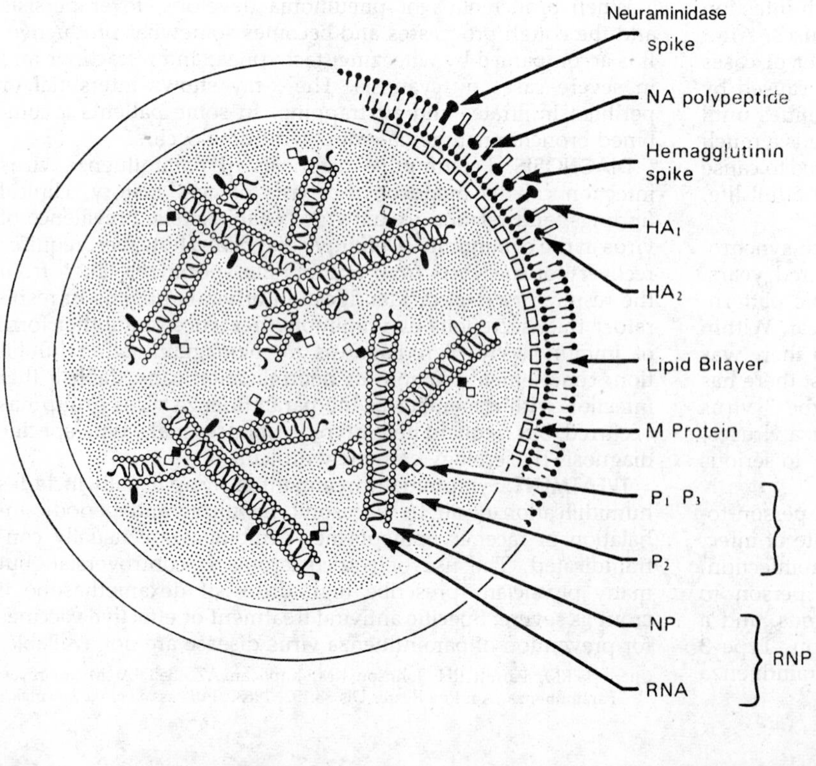

Figure 330–1. Schematic model for influenza virus virions. (Modified from Ginsberg HS: Orthomyxoviruses. *In* Davis BD, Dulbecco R, Eisen HN, Ginsburg HS (eds.): Microbiology, 3rd ed. Hagerstown, MD, Harper & Row, Publishers, 1980, p. 1119.)

explain why influenza continues to be a major epidemic disease in humans. As noted previously, antigenic variation involves only the H and N proteins among the proteins of influenza virus. The H is the most important since it is more frequently involved in antigenic variation than the N protein and since antibody to this protein neutralizes infection. Antigenic variation is referred to as *antigenic drift* or *antigenic shift,* depending on whether the variation is great or small.

Antigenic Drift. Antigenic drift refers to relatively minor changes that occur frequently (every year or every few years) within an influenza A subtype. Each subtype is named by its hemagglutinin and neuraminidase. To date, three hemagglutinins (H1, H2, and H3) and two neuraminidases (N1 and N2) have been recognized. The former designations, HO and HSW1, are now classified as variants of H1. Each strain within the subtype is identified by site and year of isolation. Thus, influenza A/Bangkok/79/H3N2 indicates an influenza virus of type A and subtype H3N2 that was isolated in 1979 in Bangkok. The original H3N2 variant, A/Aichi/68/H3N2, was isolated in Aichi, Japan, in 1968. All isolates worldwide for the next three years were serologically identical. Subsequent antigenic drifts resulted in recovery of variants possessing minor differences: A/England/72/H3N2, A/Port Chalmers/73/H3N2, A/Scotland/74/H3N2, A/Georgia/74/H3N2, A/Victoria/75/H3N2, A/Texas/77/H3N2, A/Bangkok/79/H3N2, A/Philippines/2/82/H3N2, and so on. Antigenic drift results from point mutations that usually affect the RNA segment coding for the hemagglutinin. Complete nucleotide sequencing of hemagglutinins of several H3 strains has been determined, in support of this hypothesis. As a result, there is an alteration in protein structure that involves one or a few amino acids and results in minor changes in antigenicity. There is immunologic selection in which a new virus is favored over the old for person-to-person transmission because of the less frequent presence of antibody in the population.

Antigenic Shift. Major antigenic shifts result from genetic reassortment when two influenza viruses simultaneously infect a single cell. Such an event results in a hemagglutinin or neuraminidase, or both, that is completely new in comparison with the previously circulating strain. Because of the high level of immunity to the old strain and lack of immunity to the new strain within the human population, the new strain, provided that it possesses intrinsic viral properties such as virulence and transmissibility, can readily cause a major outbreak of influenza.

Epidemic Influenza. An epidemic is an outbreak of influenza confined to one location such as a city, town, or country. In a given community, epidemics of influenza A virus infection have a characteristic pattern. A graphic description of an epidemic due to an A/Victoria/75/H3N2 like virus, which occurred in 1976 in Houston, Texas, is shown in Figure 330–2. Such localized epidemics begin rather abruptly, reach a sharp peak in two to three weeks, and last five to six weeks. Reports of increased numbers of children with febrile respiratory illness are often the first indication of influenza in a community. This is usually soon followed by the occurrence of influenza-like illnesses among adults. The next event is increased hospital admissions of patients with pneumonia, exacerbation of chronic obstructive pulmonary disease, croup, and congestive heart failure. There are increases in school and industrial absenteeism and in the number of deaths caused by pneumonia and influenza. Although the latter finding is a highly specific indicator of influenza, it invariably lags behind the others. Viral isolation studies show a peak that parallels that of acute febrile respiratory illness. Year-round studies indicate that almost all isolates are obtained during the epidemic period. It is rare to recover influenza virus during other periods of the year, although occasionally there is serologic evidence of infection during other months.

Epidemics occur almost exclusively during the winter months—October through April in the northern hemisphere and May through September in the southern hemisphere. When observed in large countries such as the United States or

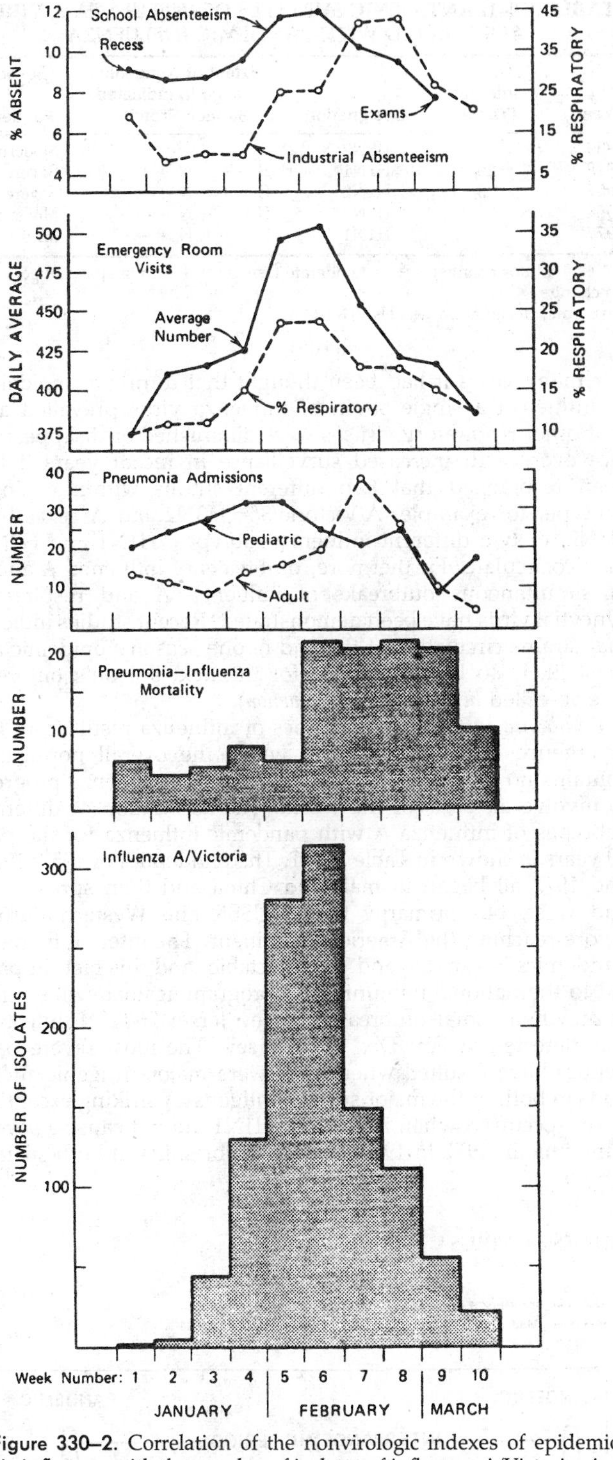

Figure 330–2. Correlation of the nonvirologic indexes of epidemiologic influenza with the number of isolates of influenza A/Victoria virus according to week, Houston, 1976 (industrial absenteeism is indicated by percentage with respiratory complaints). (From Glezen WP, Couch RB, Six HR: N Engl J Med 298:589, 1978.)

Australia, regional differences in the time of occurrence of influenza outbreaks are apparent. It is not uncommon to have major outbreaks occurring in some communities or regions while others are experiencing no activity whatsoever. Often those so spared will experience similar outbreaks at a later time, particularly if the prevalent virus demonstrates significant antigenic variation compared with previously prevalent viruses. During epidemics, the average overall attack rates are estimated to be 10 to 20 per cent; however, in selected populations or age groups, attack rates of 40 to 50 per cent are not uncommon.

TABLE 330–1. ANTIGENIC SUBTYPES OF INFLUENZA A VIRUS ASSOCIATED WITH PANDEMIC INFLUENZA

Year	Interval (Years)	Designation	Extent of Antigenic Change in Indicated Surface Protein*	Severity of Pandemic
1889	—	H3N2	?	Moderate
1918	29	H1N1†	H + + + N + + +	Severe
1957	39	H2N2	H + + + N + + +	Severe
1968	11	H3N2	H + + + N –	Moderate
1977	9	H1N1	H + + + N + + +	Mild

*+ = Minor change; + + = moderate change; + + + = major change; – = no change.
†Former designation was Hsw1N1 (35).

For many years it had been thought that during an epidemic of influenza a single strain of influenza virus prevailed and that other respiratory viruses were diminished or disappeared. However, with increased surveillance in recent years it has been recognized that two different strains within a single subtype, for example, A/Victoria/3/75/H3N2 and A/Texas/1/77/H3N2, or two different influenza subtypes, H1N1 and H3N2, may cocirculate. Furthermore, outbreaks of influenza A and B or simultaneous outbreaks of influenza A and respiratory syncytial virus have been demonstrated. Recent studies indicate that strains circulating at the end of one season's epidemic are most likely to be responsible for the next season's outbreak (the so-called *herald wave phenomenon*).

Pandemic Influenza. Pandemics of influenza result from the emergence of a new virus to which the overall population contains no immunity, so that epidemics of influenza progress to involve all parts of the world. The association of different subtypes of influenza A with pandemic influenza for the past 80 years is shown in Table 330–1. The pandemics of 1957, 1968, and 1977 all began in mainland China and then spread east and west, but primarily to the USSR and Western Europe before reaching the American continent. The interval between pandemics is variable and unpredictable, and this fact, in part, led to the national immunization program against swine influenza, when a small outbreak of A/New Jersey/76/H1N1 infection was detected at Fort Dix, New Jersey. The most severe pandemics have resulted when there were major antigenic alterations in both of the major surface antigens. A striking exception to this occurred when A/USSR/77/H1N1 did not cause a severe pandemic in 1977 to 1978, despite major shifts in both surface glycoproteins. This discrepancy may be due to the fact that much of the world's population of 1977 to 1978 had been alive during the previous H1N1 era, from 1947 to 1957, and thus possessed protective immunity. Furthermore, it appears that transmissibility from person to person and intrinsic virulence (severity of disease) are virus-coded functions that vary much as does antigenicity. Intrinsic virulence with H1N1 viruses appears to be milder than with H3N2 viruses.

Proposed Mechanism of Epidemic Behavior. The scheme shown in Figure 330–3 ties together the concepts of antigenic shifts and antigenic drifts in relation to population immunity. When a new virus, here called A HXNX, is introduced into a population lacking appropriate antibody, pandemic influenza results. After one or more waves of pandemic influenza, the level of immunity in the population increases. Such a chain of events provides a setting for emergence of a variant showing antigenic drift, since the level of immunity to it will be less than that to the original strain. Repeated epidemics caused by strains showing antigenic drift within the HXNX subtype occur in subsequent years. After 10 to 30 years of circulation of variants within this given subtype, the population's immunity to all variants within the subtype is very high, and the conditions for the spread of a new virus are favorable. Such a virus originates by genetic reassortment. Thus, it possesses an H or N protein, or both, that is markedly different with respect to the A HXNX subtype. When such a virus circulates, the next pandemic occurs. While the concepts of immunity of the population and antigenic variation are important in understanding the epidemiology of influenza, they do not provide the entire explanation. It is apparent that virus factors must contribute to virulence and transmissibility. Furthermore, it should be emphasized that other than the association of influenza outbreaks with colder seasons, the factors that allow an epidemic to develop remain unexplained. The factors responsible for the tapering off of an epidemic after five or six weeks, when only a portion of susceptible persons are infected, are also unknown. Finally, the host or medium where the virus has been between epidemics is not understood.

Mortality. In addition to the substantial morbidity associated with epidemic or pandemic influenza, mortality is also associated with such outbreaks. Pneumonia and influenza deaths fluctuate annually in predictable fashion, with peaks in the winter and troughs in the summer. When pneumonia and influenza deaths exceed the epidemic threshold, this is almost always due to influenza A virus activity or occasionally to influenza B virus activity.

PATHOLOGY AND PATHOGENESIS. Influenza virus infection

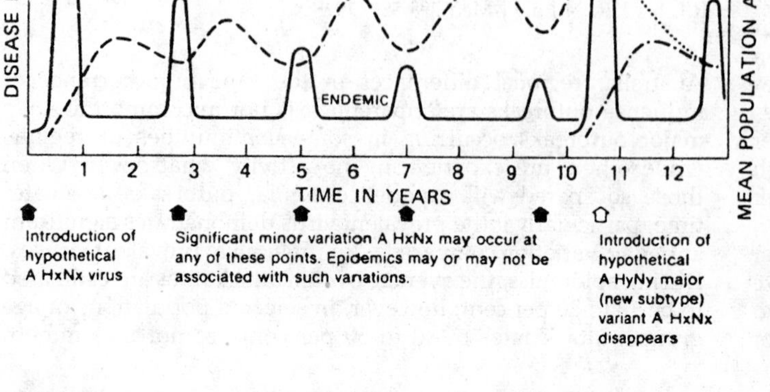

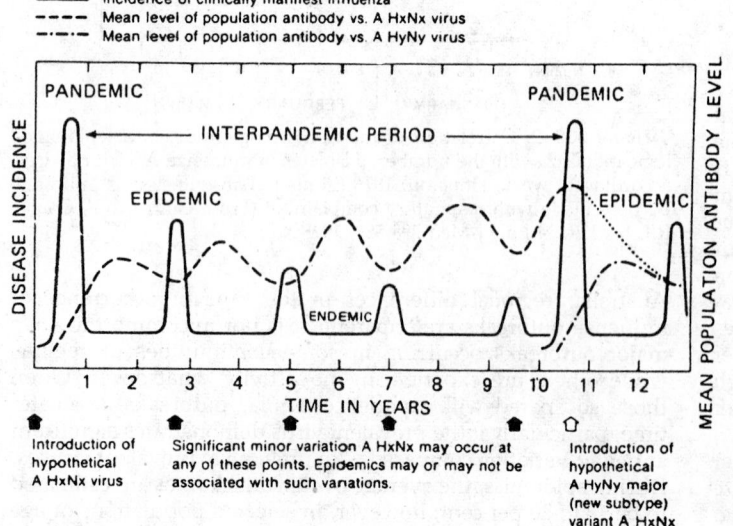

Figure 330–3. Schema of occurrence of influenza pandemics and epidemics in relation to the level of immunity in the population. AHxNx and AHyNy represent influenza viruses with completely different hemagglutinins and neuraminidases. (From Douglas RG Jr: *In* Galasso GJ, Merigan TC, Buchanan RA (eds.): Antiviral Agents and Viral Diseases of Man. New York, Raven Press, 1979.)

is acquired by transfer of virus-containing respiratory secretions from an infected to a susceptible person. Small-particle aerosols (less than 10 μ mass medium diameter) may be most significant in such person-to-person transmission. Once the virus has been deposited in the respiratory tract epithelium, unless it is prevented by specific secretory antibody, nonspecific mucoproteins, or mechanical actions of the mucociliary blanket, it attaches to and penetrates columnar epithelial cells. After absorption has taken place, the virion initiates its replication cycle. This cycle lasts four to six hours, and virus release continues for several hours before cell death ensues. Infection of adjacent and nearby cells follows, so that within a few replication cycles large numbers of cells in the respiratory tract are infected. The duration of the incubation period until onset of illness and virus shedding, which occur in close proximity, varies from 18 to 72 hours, depending in part on the inoculum size. Quantitation of virus in respiratory tract specimens reveals a characteristic pattern that correlates with severity of illness. This correlation suggests that a major mechanism in the production of illness is cell death resulting from viral replication. Serum or secretory antibody or cell-mediated immune mechanisms are not detectable at this time, indicating that immunologic mechanisms are probably not involved in production of illness. The occurrence of systemic illness and fever suggests hematogenous dissemination of virus or release of cellular products into the blood, but infectious virus only rarely has been detected in the blood.

Interferon is frequently detected in respiratory tract and serum specimens. Shedding of virus precedes by one to two days the appearance of interferon, which is correlated with improvements of signs and symptoms and decrease of virus titer and thus suggests that interferon is active in the recovery process. Nasal and bronchial biopsy specimens from persons with uncomplicated influenza reveal desquamation of the ciliated columnar epithelium. Individual cells show shrinkage, pyknotic nuclei, and loss of cilia. In addition, the lungs in fatal influenza show extensive hemorrhage, hyaline membrane formation, and paucity of polymorphonuclear cell infiltration. Patients with secondary bacterial pneumonia have the changes characteristic of bacterial pneumonia in addition to the tracheobronchial findings of influenza in the tracheobronchial tree.

Neutralizing, hemagglutination-inhibiting, antineuraminidase, complement-fixing, enzyme-linked immunosorbent assay (ELISA), and immunofluorescent antibodies begin to develop in the sera of persons with primary influenza virus infection during the second week after exposure to antigen and reach a peak by four weeks. Secretory antibodies develop in the respiratory tract after influenza infection and consist predominantly of immunoglobulin A (IgA) antibodies that reach peak titers in 14 days. Protection against infection is afforded by serum HAI titers of 1:40 or greater, serum-neutralizing titers of 1:8 or greater, or nasal-neutralizing antibody titers 1:4 or greater.

CLINICAL FINDINGS. Many patients can pinpoint the hour of onset. Initially, systemic systems predominate, and symptoms include feverishness, chilliness or frank shaking chills, headache, myalgias, malaise, and anorexia. In more severe cases, prostration is observed. Usually myalgias or headache are the most troublesome symptoms, and their severity is related to the level of the fever. Arthralgias are commonly observed. Ocular symptoms, although less commonly present, are helpful diagnostically and include photophobia, tearing, burning, and pain on moving the eyes. Respiratory symptoms, particularly dry cough and nasal discharge, are usually also present at the onset but are overshadowed by the systemic symptoms. Nasal obstruction, hoarseness, and dry sore throat may also be present.

Fever is the most important physical finding. The temperature usually rises rapidly to a peak of 38 to 40° C and occasionally to 41° C within 12 hours of onset, concurrently with the development of systemic symptoms. Fever is usually continuous but may be intermittent, especially if antipyretics are administered. On the second and third days of illness, the temperature elevation is usually less than on the first day. As fever subsides, the systemic symptoms diminish. Typically, the duration of fever is three days, but it may last from one to five or more days. In a few cases, a second fluctuation in fever occurs on the third or fourth day, resulting in a biphasic fever curve. Early in the course of illness, the patient appears toxic, the face is flushed, and the skin is hot and moist. The eyes are watery and reddened. Clear nasal discharge is common, but nasal obstruction is uncommon. The mucous membranes of the nose and throat are hyperemic, but exudate is not observed. Small tender cervical lymph nodes are often present, and transient scattered rhonchi or localized areas of rales are found in less than 20 per cent of cases.

As systemic signs and symptoms diminish, respiratory complaints and findings become more apparent. Cough is the most frequent and troublesome of these symptoms and may be accompanied by substernal discomfort or burning. Nasal obstruction, discharge, pharyngeal pain, and injection are also common. Such symptoms and signs usually persist three to four days after fever subsides; however, cough, lassitude, and malaise may persist for one, two, or more weeks before full recovery.

This pattern of illness just described occurs with any type or subtype of influenza A or B virus. Attack rates are higher in children than in adults, although the incidence of pulmonary complications is lower in children. Maximum temperatures are higher in children, cervical adenopathy may be more frequent, and croup occurs only among children.

PULMONARY COMPLICATIONS. Three kinds of pulmonary complications are well recognized: *primary influenza viral pneumonia, secondary bacterial pneumonia,* and *mixed viral and bacterial pneumonia.* In addition, during an outbreak of influenza, less distinct and milder pulmonic syndromes often occur that may represent viral tracheobronchitis, localized viral pneumonia, or possibly mixed viral and bacterial infection.

Primary Influenza Viral Pneumonia. This syndrome first became well documented in the pandemic of 1957 to 1958. However, it is clear that many of the deaths in the 1918 to 1919 outbreak were due to this syndrome in healthy young adults. Primary influenzal viral pneumonia has occurred predominantly among persons with cardiovascular disease, especially rheumatic heart disease with mitral stenosis. Although this syndrome occurs in healthy young adults in every large outbreak, other chronic disorders and pregnancy have been implicated as risk factors in some epidemics. Following a typical onset of influenza, there is rapid progression of fever, cough, dyspnea, and cyanosis. Physical examination and chest roentgenograms reveal bilateral findings consistent with the adult respiratory distress syndrome. Blood gas studies show marked hypoxia. Gram stain of the sputum fails to reveal significant bacteria, and bacterial culture yields sparse growth of normal flora. Viral cultures of sputum or tracheal aspirates yield high titers of influenza virus. Such patients do not respond to antibiotics, and mortality is high.

Secondary Bacterial Pneumonia. Bacterial superinfection is often clinically distinguishable from primary viral pneumonia. The patients are most often elderly or have chronic pulmonary, cardiac, metabolic, or other diseases. Following a typical influenza illness, a period of improvement lasting from one to four days may occur. Recrudescence of fever is associated with symptoms and signs of bacterial pneumonia, such as cough, sputum production, and a localized area of consolidation apparent on physical and chest roentgenogram examination. Gram stain and culture sputum reveal predominance of a bacterial pathogen, most often *S. pneumoniae, S. aureus,* or *H. influenzae.* Such patients will usually respond to specific antibiotic therapy.

Mixed Viral and Bacterial Pneumonia. During an outbreak of influenza, many cases are observed that do not clearly fit into either of the categories just described. The disease is not relentlessly progressive, and yet the fever pattern may be persistent and not biphasic. These patients may have a milder form of primary viral, secondary bacterial, or mixed viral and bacterial infection. Many will respond to antibiotics. Milder forms of primary viral pneumonia involving only one lobe or segment have been described that do not invariably lead to death. Such cases are more likely to be confused with a pneumonia due to *M. pneumoniae* than to that produced by bacterial infection. In children, pneumonia may occur but is less common than in adults. In addition, bronchiolitis and croup may be caused by influenza A or B virus infection.

Exacerbation of Chronic Obstructive Pulmonary Disease. In adults with chronic obstructive pulmonary disease, influenza A or B virus infection may lead not only to pneumonia but also to acute exacerbation of chronic bronchitis, a syndrome that is associated with other respiratory viruses and bacteria as well.

NONPULMONIC COMPLICATIONS. ***Reye's Syndrome.*** Reye's syndrome is a frequently recognized hepatic and central nervous system complication of influenza A and B infection as well as varicella-zoster virus infection. The syndrome occurs exclusively in children, most often between the ages of 2 and 16 years. Because of the epidemic nature of the occurrence of influenza A and B virus infections, Reye's syndrome also has an epidemic occurrence. Large outbreaks have occurred in the United States since 1967 in association with influenza A and B outbreaks. Reye's syndrome occurs several days after a typical upper respiratory, gastrointestinal, or chickenpox infection. The most significant manifestation is change in mental status, ranging from lethargy to delirium, obtundation, seizures, and respiratory arrest. In 75 per cent of the cases, central nervous system manifestations are preceded by nausea and vomiting, lasting one to two days. The children are usually afebrile and have hepatomegaly but are not jaundiced. Mortality is related to the stage of coma on admission and has decreased from approximately 40 per cent when the syndrome was first described to 10 per cent today. Lumbar puncture reveals normal protein values and cell counts confirming the presence of encephalopathy rather than encephalitis or meningoencephalitis. The most frequent laboratory abnormality is elevation of the blood ammonia value, which occurs in almost all patients. Hypoglycemia is present more often in patients with antecedent varicella-zoster or gastrointestinal illness, as compared with upper respiratory illness. Serum glutamic oxaloacetic transaminase (SGOT), serum glutamic pyruvic transaminase (SGPT), and bilirubin values are commonly elevated, as are creatine kinase (CK) and lactic dehydrogenase (LDH) levels. The prothrombin time is usually increased. Stage 4 or 5 coma on admission, evidence of increased intracranial pressure, and blood ammonia level greater than 300 μg per deciliter are all associated with mortality. Among survivors, 30 per cent of those who develop either decerebrate posturing or seizures during hospitalization have serious neurologic sequelae. Pathologically, the striking feature is absence of inflammatory changes. Liver biopsy specimens are usually pale yellow. Microscopic examination shows fatty infiltration of the hepatocytes with numerous small droplets of lipid uniformly distributed. The main ultrastructural finding is alteration of the hepatocyte mitochondria, including swelling and pleomorphism. Pathologic findings most often detected in the brain are cerebral edema, anoxia, and anoxic neuronal degeneration, but there is no inflammation. The pathophysiologic mechanism is unknown. Recently, an association with aspirin therapy during the antecedent illness has been indicated, but this finding has also been challenged.

Other Complications. Myositis and myoglobinuria with tender leg muscles and elevated serum CK levels have been reported, mostly occurring in children. Myocarditis, pericarditis, and myocardial infarction rarely have been associated with influenza A and B virus infection. Guillian-Barré syndrome has been reported to occur after influenza A, but no definite causal relationship has been established. Transverse myelitis and encephalitis have also been reported rarely.

DIAGNOSIS. In an individual case, influenza often cannot be distinguished from infection with a number of other viruses and bacteria that produce headache, muscle aches, fever, and cough. On occasion, other respiratory viruses can produce an influenza-like illness, as can streptococcal pharyngitis. In the summer months, enteroviruses produce a clinically indistinguishable picture, and the acute manifestations of many other infections, such as dengue, may mimic influenza. On the other hand, in the context of an epidemic, influenza may be readily distinguished from other acute infections. When the local, state, or national health authorities report the occurrence of an epidemic of influenza A or B virus infection in a given community, and a patient is seen with the acute onset of fever, headache, muscle aches, and cough, it is highly likely that these symptoms are caused by an influenza virus infection.

Definitive diagnosis depends on detection of infectious virus or viral antigen in secretions from patients or the detection of a serum antibody response. Influenza virus is readily isolated from throat or nasal swab specimens, sputum, or tracheal secretion specimens in the first two or three days of illness. Usually infectivity is detected within 48 to 72 hours in monkey kidney cell cultures. Viral antigen may be detected more rapidly in such specimens by use of immunofluorescence or ELISA, but these techniques are not widely available. Serologic methods are less useful clinically because they require a convalescent sera obtained 10 to 14 days after the onset of infection. However, they are of great use in epidemiologic studies and to document the occurrence of an outbreak. A four-fold increase in antibody titer comparing an acute to convalescent phase is diagnostic. The complement fixation antibody test is most useful for diagnosis because it is not dependent on strain or subtype variation, as is hemagglutination inhibition.

TREATMENT. Amantadine shortens the duration of fever and of systemic and respiratory symptoms by about 50 per cent. The dose is 100 to 200 mg per day orally for three to five days. Rimantadine, although not yet licensed, has a similar effect and reduces the likelihood of the mild transient central nervous system side effects that occur with amantadine. Other symptomatic measures include antipyretics and cough suppressants. Many authorities consider that aspirin should not be used, especially for persons under 16 years of age, because of its possible association with the occurrence of Reye's syndrome. There is no evidence that amantadine or rimantadine is effective in treatment of pulmonary complications of influenza.

Currently, primary influenza viral pneumonia in its severe stages is best managed in an intensive care unit with supportive measures such as respiratory therapy, supplemental oxygen, and fluids. Secondary bacterial pneumonia should be treated with appropriate antibiotics. When from studies of the sputum it is not clear which bacterium may be infecting the patient, coverage should include antibiotics that are effective against *S. aureus*, *S. pneumoniae*, and *H. influenzae*.

PREVENTION. The mainstay of prevention is the use of inactivated influenza virus vaccines. These vaccines provide about 80 per cent protective efficacy. The antigenic composition is reviewed annually so that the vaccine contains the most recently circulating strains. Usually the vaccine is a trivalent product containing one or more subtypes of influenza A and influenza B. The recent vaccines have been purified by density gradient centrifugation or chromatography and have very low reaction rates. One to two per cent of persons vaccinated will have fever and systemic symptoms peaking at 8 to 12 hours after vaccination, and up to 25 per cent may have mild local reactions at the site of vaccination. "Split" virus (subvirion) vaccines contain antigens with disrupted virus and may be less reactigenic than "whole" virus vaccines. The highest priority for vaccination should be given to persons with cardiac or pulmonary conditions requiring ongoing medical care and to residents of nursing homes and other chronic care facilities. Physicians, nurses and other personnel who have extensive contact with high-risk patients constitute the next priority for vaccination. Finally, persons over age 65 and persons with other chronic disease of any age should be vaccinated. Vaccine may also be given to well persons under age 65 who wish to reduce the likelihood of acquiring influenza.

Amantadine and rimantadine are also effective in preventing influenza A and should be used to supplement vaccine programs. Persons who are not vaccinated in the fall should be placed on amantadine when an outbreak occurs or throughout the influenza season for the highest risk group. If vaccine is available, persons may be vaccinated simultaneously, and amantadine therapy should be stopped after 14 days. Alternatively, if vaccine is not available, amantadine administration may be continued for the duration of the outbreak, the dose being 100 to 200 mg per day orally.

A Consensus Development Conference: Diagnosis and treatment of Reye's syndrome. JAMA 246:21, 1982. *Up-to-date summary of Reye's syndrome with description of staging.*

Barker WH, Mulloohy JP: Pneumonia and influenza deaths during epidemics: Implications for prevention. Arch Intern Med 142:85, 1982. *Rationale for influenza vaccination.*

Center for Disease Control: Prevention and Control of Influenza. Morbidity and Mortality Weekly Report 33:253–266, 1984. *Rationale and details of extensive revisions of recommendations for use of influenza vaccine.*

Dolin R, Reichman RC, Madore HP, Maynard R, Linton PN, Webber-Jones J: A controlled trial of amantadine and rimantadine in the prophylaxis of influenza A infection. N Engl J Med 307:580, 1982. *Definitive study comparing prophylactic efficacy of amantadine and rimantadine.*

Glezen WP, Couch RB, Six HR: The influenza herald wave. Am J Epidemiol 116:4, 1982. *Prediction of epidemic influenza from previous year's outbreak.*

Hauptmann R, Clarke LD, Mountford RC, Bachmayer H, Almond JW: Nucleotide sequence of the hemagglutinin gene of influenza virus A/England/321/77. J Gen Virol 64:215, 1983. *Studies on the molecular mechanism of antigenic drift.*

Younkin SW, Betts RF, Roth FK, Douglas RG: Reduction in fever and symptoms in young adults with aspirin or amantadine. Antimicrob Agents Chemother 23:577, 1983. *Recent study comparing therapeutic effects of amantadine and aspirin.*

331. ADENOVIRUS DISEASES

Stephen G. Baum

The clinically most significant diseases caused by adenoviruses are infections of the respiratory system and the eye. Recently, adenoviruses have been shown to play a major role in causing diarrheal disease in children and respiratory and urinary tract infections in immunocompromised patients. Adenoviruses are the object of intensive research efforts because they possess several fascinating and important biologic capabilities. Today they are perhaps the best characterized human virus group.

HISTORY. The term adenovirus derives from the fact that Rowe and colleagues first isolated these agents in 1953 from surgically removed adenoids that had been placed in tissue culture. The adenoidal cells underwent spontaneous cytopathic effects (CPE), and the virus could be passed serially in epithelial cells with reproducible characteristic CPE. In the past 30 years, 41 serotypes of human adenovirus have been identified (types 1 to 41). These have been isolated from adenoidal tissue, respiratory secretions, conjunctival exudate, urine, and stool samples. Many of the serotypes have been associated with specific syndromes, but over half the adenovirus types have not been shown to cause disease.

ETIOLOGIC AGENT. Adenoviruses are double-stranded DNA viruses that average 70 nm in diameter and have a unique outer structure, which permits their morphologic identification by electron microscopic examination. The virus is icosahedral with 20 equilateral triangular faces and 12 vertices. The faces are made up of hexon subunits, and the vertices each contain a penton subunit. From each vertex, an antenna-like structure, the fiber, projects with a knob at the end. Each class of these surface subunits differs antigenically from the others. The hexon contains group-specific and type-specific antigens. The 41 serotypes of adenovirus have been divided into four groups according to ability to agglutinate different erythrocytes. This artifactual grouping correlates well with the ability of different serotypes to cause specific syndromes and to induce tumors in animals.

In acute infections, adenoviruses cause cell death and lysis with release of new progeny virions. The mechanisms of latency and animal oncogenesis are not completely understood, although many of the functions of adenovirus have been accurately mapped on the deoxyribonucleic acid (DNA) genome. Adenoviruses can form a family of hybrid viruses with an unrelated DNA virus, SV40. Portions of the DNA of adenovirus and SV40 are covalently linked within an adenovirus outer coat. The hybrid virus has unique biologic and oncogenic capabilities in vitro and in animals in vivo. Neither adenovirus alone nor the hybrid viruses have been shown to cause cancer in humans.

A small defective DNA parvovirus has been isolated from some adenovirus preparations and from some patients with adenovirus infection. This *adeno-associated virus (AAV)* requires adenovirus for its replication. It is not known to cause disease by itself and does not appear to contribute to adenovirus pathogenesis.

EPIDEMIOLOGY. Most people experience an adenovirus infection during the first decade of life. The initial infecting serotype and the syndrome it causes are a function of the age of the patient and the route of infection. Studies of large populations show that adenoviruses cause 3 to 5 per cent of all clinically apparent infections in children. Adenoviruses are the most common viral isolates in this age group, and at least half of these isolations are associated with subclinical infections. Respiratory infection is transmitted by person-to-person contact or through contaminated swimming water.

Conjunctival infection may be transmitted directly, through water, or by fomites such as towels or ophthalmologic equipment and solutions. Pneumonia and urinary tract infection in immunocompromised patients may be acquired exogenously or may represent reactivation of latent infection. There are many adenoviruses that infect other animals and birds, but these play no known role in human disease.

CLINICAL PRESENTATIONS OCCURRING MOSTLY IN CHILDREN. ***Respiratory Infection.*** Infants most commonly manifest adenovirus infections as coryzal symptoms, but occasionally adenovirus type 7 causes fulminant bronchiolitis and pneumonia in this age group. In older children, pharyngitis and tracheobronchitis are most prevalent. Adenoviruses are the most common viral isolate from children with the whooping cough syndrome. It is not known whether this virus contributes to the pathogenesis of *Bordetella pertussis* infection or whether adenovirus alone can cause the syndrome.

Pharyngoconjunctival Fever. This syndrome occurs in small epidemics in summer camps where it is probably spread in swimming water. Adenovirus type 3 has been the most common isolate. The incubation period is three to five days, and symptoms, which are acute, include pharyngitis, rhinitis, conjunctivitis, cervical adenitis, and elevation in temperature to about 38° C. The bulbar and palpebral conjunctivae have a granular appearance. The symptoms last one to two weeks. Permanent sequelae are rare, and there is no specific therapy.

Intestinal Disease. Immunoelectron microscopy has revealed viruses in the stool in many cases of infantile diarrhea. The most common viruses visualized are rotaviruses and adenoviruses. These adenoviruses appear to be defective in their replication and require special cells for isolation in tissue culture. Two new serotypes, types 40 and 41, have been found most often in this situation. Intussusception in children has also been linked to adenovirus types 1, 2, 3, and 5, although a causal role is unproven. Many of the children with this syndrome have intercurrent adenoviral respiratory infection.

Hemorrhagic Cystitis. Adenovirus types 11 and 21 have been associated with hemorrhagic cystitis in American and Japanese children. Boys are affected more often than girls, in contrast to the situation with bacterial cystitis. Gross hematuria may persist for one to two weeks.

CLINICAL PRESENTATIONS OCCURRING MOSTLY IN ADULTS. ***Respiratory Infection.*** The first isolation of adenoviruses directly from sick patients occurred during an epidemic of acute respiratory disease in military recruits. This population seems extremely susceptible to infection with types 4 and 7, as it is to infection with *Mycoplasma pneumoniae* and the meningococci. In general, the manifestations are those of atypical pneumonia, of which up to 40 per cent of cases are caused by adenovirus. Fever to 39° C, cough, pharyngitis, rhinorrhea, and pulmonary rales are the most common signs and symptoms. Radiographic examination of the chest shows patchy interstitial infiltrates that are unilateral in most cases. Small pleural effusions can occur.

In nonepidemic situations, it is impossible to make a definitive clinical diagnosis of adenoviral pneumonia. Some factors useful in comparing adenoviral with mycoplasmal pneumonia are: lower incidence of cold agglutinins, shorter incubation period, and better correlation of x-ray and physical findings in the chest in adenovirus infection. Influenza and parainfluenza viruses produce similar syndromes. Adenoviral pneumonia usually lasts one to two weeks. There is no specific therapy, and bacterial superinfection and death are rare.

Adenoviruses have been isolated from the lungs of immunocompromised patients with pneumonia and from the urine of renal transplant recipients and patients with acquired immune deficiency syndrome (AIDS). Many of the higher serotypes were first isolated from such patients. In some of these instances, adenovirus operates as an opportunistic agent; in others it may play a primary role in causing disease.

Neurologic disease, most often appearing as meningoencephalitis, has been attributed to adenovirus. It sometimes occurs in minor epidemic form and is frequently associated with recent respiratory infection. The clinical presentation is that of encephalitis or aseptic meningitis. There are no pathognomonic findings.

Epidemic Keratoconjunctivitis. The initial epidemic of adenoviral keratoconjunctivitis involved shipyard workers who sustained minor eye trauma from paint and rust fragments. Adenovirus type 8 was isolated in this and many other epidemics. Serotypes 19 and 37 have caused keratoconjunctivitis that was spread by fomites such as roller towels. The incubation period is from 3 to 24 days. The onset is insidious, and both eyes often are affected. Eye irritation and exudation may last one to four weeks. Preauricular adenopathy often occurs early. Corneal involvement is a late complication and may persist for a month or more with blurring of vision. Residual blindness is unusual. There is no specific antiviral therapy as there is for herpes keratitis. Secondary spread to household contacts occurs in about 10 per cent of cases, varying with the duration of the index case.

TREATMENT AND PREVENTION. There is no effective antiviral chemotherapy for human adenoviral infections. Live, enteric coated oral adenovirus vaccines of types 4 and 7 have been effective in immunizing military populations. In epidemic situations, mass immunization with the live virus vaccine promptly interrupts the epidemic. The vaccine is not recommended or available for civilians because of the low incidence and sporadic occurrence of infection with adenovirus types 4 and 7.

Baum SG: Adenovirus. *In* Mandell A, Douglas RA, Bennet JE (eds.): Principles and Practice of Infectious Diseases. 2nd ed. New York, John Wiley & Sons, 1984. *An expanded version of the material in this chapter, containing correlative tables, fully referenced.*

Horwitz MS: Adenoviruses. *In* Fields BN, Melnick JL, Chanock R, Roizman B, Shope RE (eds.): Human Viral Diseases. New York, Raven Press (in press), 1984. *An encyclopedic chapter on the molecular biology of the adenoviruses.*

RNA Viral Infections Characterized by Cutaneous Lesions

332. MEASLES (Morbilli, Rubeola)

Samuel L. Katz

DEFINITION. Measles is an acute, highly contagious disease characterized by fever, coryza, cough, conjunctivitis, enanthem, and exanthem. Its morbidity and mortality vary greatly with host and environmental factors, and its epidemiology has been altered strikingly in the past 22 years in those nations where vaccine has been utilized widely.

ETIOLOGY. The virus is an enveloped, RNA paramyxovirus (genus morbillivirus) measuring 120 to 250 nm in diameter, similar to other members of the paramyxovirus family but lacking a neuraminidase. Its single antigenic serotype has been remarkably stable throughout the world for many years with no variation noted. Related animal morbilliviruses are canine distemper and bovine rinderpest, which show some cross-reactivity with measles. The virus contains six major polypeptides, which are responsible for a number of structural and functional properties, including hemagglutination (of primate erythrocytes), hemolysis, cell fusion, viral assembly, and virus penetration. Isolation of virus from clinical specimens is most successful with primary kidney cell cultures of human or simian origin. Laboratory passage has selected variants which grow well in other primary and continuous cell lines of mammalian and avian origin.

Certain simian species provide a reliable animal model of measles after respiratory tract or parenteral inoculation of human isolates. Some virus strains have been adapted to produce central nervous system infection in rodents.

EPIDEMIOLOGY. Classic descriptions of measles epidemiology are no longer applicable to those many areas of the world where measles vaccination is widely practiced. Instead of an inevitable childhood illness, the disease has become an unusual one. The age pattern has shifted to a greater proportion of cases among adolescents and young adults who remain susceptible because of lack of either childhood immunization or exposure to natural infection. In contrast, the epidemiology has been unaltered in developing nations where vaccine programs have been sporadic, incomplete, or totally lacking. Isolated communities such as the Faröe Islands (Panum) are infrequently attacked by measles, at which time manifest illness appears in virtually all persons not previously infected.

Throughout most of the world, measles was a disease of children; most adults acquired active immunity in childhood. Beyond the age of ten more than 90 per cent of the population had specific antibody. Although the peak attack rate coincided with the beginning of school (age six) in technologically advanced societies, it occurs much younger in most developing countries. Morbidity and mortality rates do not appear to be influenced by sex or race. Case fatality rates are highest in children less than five years of age, and are also relatively high in the aged. Congenital infection has occurred but intrauterine infection is more apt to produce a stillborn or premature infant.

There is no evidence that the virus may vary in virulence in nature. The excess morbidity and mortality of the disease in developing, isolated, or crowded populations may be explained as a corollary of (1) more prevalent infection of infants under one year of age, (2) poor environmental conditions, (3) inadequate medical care, and (4) secondary bacterial infections. A strikingly increased mortality rate is observed in areas where protein-calorie malnutrition is prevalent.

Communicability. Measles is one of the most highly contagious infections. Demonstration of virus in nasopharyngeal secretions during the prodromal, pre-eruptive phase and in the first days of rash is in accord with epidemiologic evidence that infection is disseminated and acquired by the respiratory tract. Close physical proximity or direct person-to-person contact is the usual requisite for infection.

Immunity. An unmodified attack of measles is usually followed by lifelong immunity. This observation is in accord with the observed enduring persistence of antibodies after infection. The mechanism of lifelong immunity after measles is undefined. Although persistence of infective virus seems not to occur, defective virus is demonstrable years after infection in the brain and peripheral lymph nodes of those rare individuals afflicted with subacute sclerosing panencephalitis (SSPE) (see Ch. 504).

Careful studies of isolated or closed populations after administration of live virus vaccine have demonstrated a lower level of antibody titer than in populations in which measles virus is circulating. Anamnestic antibody response in the absence of disease has been shown in immune contacts of patients with measles. However, studies of children in protected environments have demonstrated that re-exposure or reinfection is not necessary for maintenance of enduring immunity. Passively transferred maternal antibody protects the young infant for the first four to eight months of life.

PATHOLOGY AND PHYSIOLOGIC RESPONSES. Pathologic changes in fatal measles usually represent the compound effect of viral and secondary bacterial infection. Pneumonia is almost invariably present; it is most frequently interstitial. More representative are changes of the uncomplicated viral disease within the tonsillar, nasopharyngeal, and appendiceal tissue removed during the prodrome. These changes consist of round cell infiltration and the presence of multinucleated giant cells. Similar cells are commonly observed in tissue cultures infected with measles virus. Cytoplasmic and nuclear inclusions may be seen in epithelial cells. Koplik's spots show inflammatory mononuclear cell infiltration of buccal submucous glands and necrosis of focal vesicular lesions of the mucosa. Rash is the result of proliferation of capillary endothelial cells in the corium and the coincident exudation of serum, and occasionally erythrocytes, into the epidermis. Viral microtubular aggregates are found in the endothelium of dermal capillaries, but not in the epidermal layer. Simultaneous with the onset of rash, measles-specific antibodies are detectable in serum and, by immunofluorescence, in areas of rash. A marked leukopenia is frequently observed throughout the febrile period. Initially, the leukopenia is occasioned by a decline in lymphocytes on the first day of fever; subsequently, granulocytopenia ensues as well. Measles virus replicates in lymphoid tissues (spleen, thymus, lymph nodes), can multiply in vitro in peripheral blood T and B lymphocytes and monocytes, and can be isolated from blood leukocytes during the course of the disease. The virus is propagable in suspensions of leukocytes in vitro.

Immunosuppressive Effects of Measles. It has long been known that cell-mediated immunity is impaired during measles. There is transient suppression of the tuberculin reaction (observed also with measles vaccines), improvement in eczema and allergic asthma, delay in wound healing, and the induction of remissions in nephrosis. Actual infection of activated lymphocytes may explain the depression of cell-mediated immunity during the acute disease. In severe disease, the magnitude of depression of the total lymphocytes has been positively correlated with a lessened chance of recovery.

CLINICAL MANIFESTATIONS. After an incubation period that averages 11 days, measles becomes clinically manifest with symptoms of fever, malaise, myalgia, and headache. Within hours *ocular symptoms* of photophobia and burning pain are manifested by conjunctival injection, tearing, and exudate in the conjunctival sac. Concomitantly, or soon thereafter, *catarrhal inflammation of the respiratory tract* leads to sneezing, coughing, and nasal discharge. Less commonly, hoarseness and aphonia may reflect laryngeal involvement. In this prodromal stage of one to four days' duration, petechial lesions of the palate and pharynx or tiny white spots on the buccal mucosa *(Koplik's spots)* may herald the appearance of skin rash. The white lesions described by Koplik characteristically occur lateral to the molar teeth, and typically are mounted on red areolae of injected mucosa, which may coalesce to form a diffuse red background. They constitute a valuable, if not pathognomonic, diagnostic sign. The enanthem may involve other mucous membranes such as the palpebral conjunctiva and vaginal lining. It may "overlap" the subsequent appearance of the cutaneous rash by one to three days. See Figure 332–1.

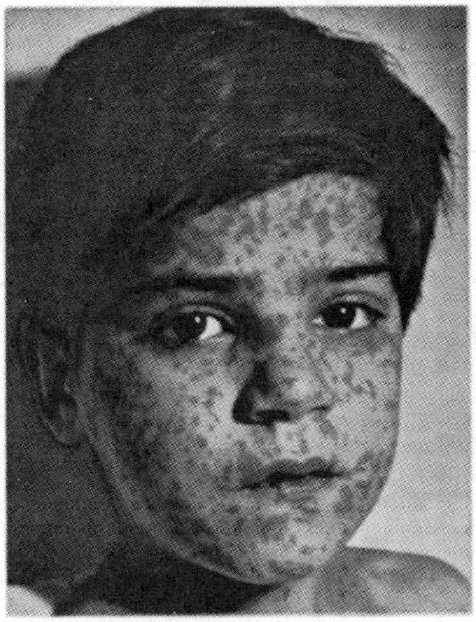

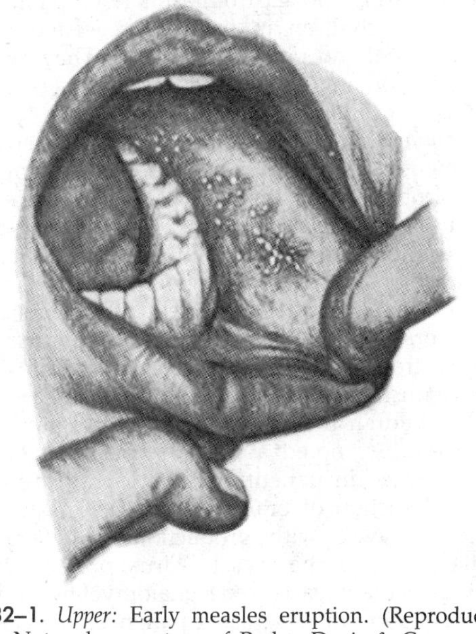

Figure 332–1. *Upper:* Early measles eruption. (Reproduction from Therapeutic Notes, by courtesy of Parke, Davis & Company.) *Lower:* Koplik's spots in measles (Hecker, Trumpp, and Abt).

The *rash* of measles follows the prodromal symptoms by two to four days, occasionally as late as seven days. It first appears behind the ears or on the face and neck as a blotchy erythema, spreads downward to cover the trunk, and finally is manifest on the extremities. The hands and feet may escape involvement. Initially, the eruption consists of discrete, reddish-brown macules that blanch with pressure. Subsequently, these lesions become papular, tend to coalesce, and may develop a hemorrhagic, nonblanching component. Rash is sometimes very extensive in children with protein-calorie malnutrition, and skin lesions associated with kwashiorkor may develop at the site of the exanthem. The rash fades in the order of its appearance; its disappearance about five days after onset is attended by a fine, powdery desquamation that spares the hands and feet. At its maximum the exanthem usually marks the termination of malaise and fever in the uncomplicated illness.

The *fever* of measles is commonly of the typhoidal, progressively rising type, and falls by lysis. It persists for about six days, and frequently reaches 40 or 41° C. Throughout the febrile period, productive *cough* and auscultatory evidence of bronchiolitis may be evident. These manifestations may persist after defervescence, and cough is often the last symptom to disappear. Bronchopulmonary symptomatology is an integral part of the primary viral infection; roentgenographic evidence of pulmonary involvement is frequently seen in the uncomplicated disease in the absence of leukocytosis and obvious bacterial infection. Generalized lymphadenopathy accompanies the acute febrile illness and may persist for several weeks thereafter.

COMPLICATIONS. It is difficult to distinguish between those complications directly attributable to the virus of measles and those resulting from secondary bacterial infections. The persistence or recurrence of fever and the development of leukocytosis are presumptive evidence of the usual bacterial sequelae of *otitis media* or *pneumonia.* Superimposed bacterial infection is common, and pneumonia accounts for most of the severe or fatal cases. Pneumococcus, *Streptococcus hemolyticus, Staphylococcus aureus,* and *Hemophilus influenzae* are the usual secondary invaders.

Serious complications directly related to the measles virus are rare. *Laryngitis* of sufficient severity to embarrass respiration has been observed, and may warrant tracheostomy. Keratoconjunctivitis is part of the acute phase but rarely progresses to actual corneal ulceration. *Electrocardiographic abnormalities* may be found in as many as 30 per cent of children, but clinical evidence of cardiac disease is absent. *Abdominal pain* or *diarrhea* may be related to invasion of lymphoid tissue of the appendix or Peyer's patches. These symptoms may lead to unnecessary surgery before the appearance of the typical rash. The frequency of stomatitis and gastrointestinal symptoms is greater in malnourished children in tropical areas and may reflect coincident bacterial and parasitic infection. They may result in severe dehydration and acidosis as fluid and electrolyte losses rise in the face of diminished oral intake.

Encephalomyelitis. A rare (0.1 per cent) but serious consequence of measles is a demyelinating encephalomyelitis that may appear from 1 to 14 days after the onset of infection. This complication is associated with a recurrence of fever, and headache, vomiting, and stiff neck. Stupor and convulsions usually follow. Localizing neurologic symptoms may be present. Death ensues in about 10 per cent of patients; more than half of survivors suffer permanent residuals of varying severity. Abnormal electroencephalograms were recorded in 51 per cent of children with measles *without clinical signs of encephalitis.* In some of the children the abnormal encephalographic findings were persistent. As noted above, the presence of virus has been demonstrated in patients with subacute sclerosing panencephalitis. Infection of brain cells results in an incomplete viral replicative cycle with production of defective virions lacking one ("M") of the measles-virus proteins. Studies of patients with acute measles encephalomyelitis and of those with late onset subacute sclerosing panencephalitis show high titers in serum and cerebrospinal fluid of antibodies to all the measles virus proteins except M. This protein is an internal membrane protein crucial to viral assembly.

Other late sequelae of measles are thrombocytopenic purpura and exacerbation or activation of pre-existing pulmonary tuberculosis. The late complication of subacute sclerosing panencephalitis (see Immunity, above) is discussed in Ch. 504.

Giant-Cell Pneumonia. In children with severe disease compromising normal cellular and humoral immune mechanisms, measles virus may induce an interstitial pneumonia characterized by giant cells and intracellular inclusion bodies. The disease is usually fatal; if the patient survives, persistence of virus and poor or absent antibody formation are evident in convalescence. The pneumonia may occur in the absence of rash so that its etiologic relation to measles may be unsuspected.

Measles Modified by Antibody Administration. Attenuation of the natural disease by antibody prophylaxis may result in an illness of lessened severity comparable with the milder infection of the maternally immunized newborn. Fever alone may be observed, but some degree of exanthem is usually apparent. Koplik's spots may not appear. In general, the course is truncated and relatively uncomplicated. Lasting immunity is uncertain and serologic studies should be obtained to check for measles-specific antibodies after modified illness.

Atypical Measles—A New Disease. From 1963 to 1967, two types of measles vaccine, one live attenuated, the other inactivated or "killed," were available in the United States. The live attenuated vaccine has since 1967 been the sole product licensed and utilized in this country. From 1965 to 1968 a series of reports was published describing a severe, atypical form of disease occurring after exposure to natural measles of children who had previously received the inactivated vaccine. These patients had high fever, pneumonia, pleural effusion, obtundation, and an unusual rash. The exanthem frequently was initially urticarial and rapidly progressive to maculopapular, petechial, and sometimes vesicular lesions. It was most striking, and often began, on the extremities and was sometimes accompanied by edema of hands and feet. Concomitantly these patients' sera revealed extraordinarily high titers of measles-specific antibodies (25,000 to 200,000 by hemagglutination-inhibition testing).

Subsequent investigations showed that patients who had received inactivated measles vaccines failed to develop antibodies to the "F" protein of the virus. This polypeptide is responsible for cell fusion, viral penetration, and hemolysis. Lack of antibodies to the cell fusion factor permitted these patients to support measles infection in superficial respiratory mucosal cells by cell-to-cell spread. The other measles virus antigens released by these infected cells stimulated a hyperimmune response to those polypeptides that had been present in the inactivated vaccines. Thus the atypical measles syndrome is an imbalance of immune response.

In addition to the rash and pulmonary findings, these patients may have elevated liver enzymes, disseminated intravascular coagulation, and marked myalgia. The pulmonary changes have persisted for longer than 18 months in patients followed with serial chest films. Initial diagnoses on presentation have included Rocky Mountain spotted fever and meningococcemia because of the similarities of rash and toxicity. Since inactivated vaccines were available only from 1963 through 1967, the past recipients are now in adolescence or young adulthood. This atypical measles syndrome is of increasing importance to the internist.

DIAGNOSIS. The experienced layman can diagnose typical measles. The querulous, bleary-eyed child, his face blotched and his nose crusted with exudate, presents a characteristic, if miserable, picture as he breathes open-mouthed between paroxysms of sneezing and coughing. The severity of the catarrhal symptoms distinguishes the disease from other eruptive fevers. In the prodromal period the diagnosis should be suggested by (1) fever higher than that of the usual respiratory virus infection, (2) known measles in the community, and (3) Koplik's spots on the buccal mucosa.

Differential diagnosis (see Table 332–1) includes consideration of rubella, scarlet fever, exanthem subitum, infectious mononucleosis, secondary syphilis, drug eruptions, and infection with certain coxsackie- and echoviruses. Of value in excluding these possibilities are the milder course, postauricular nodes, and pinker rash of rubella; the sore throat, eventual desquamation, strawberry tongue, and leukocytosis of scarlet fever; and serologic tests for infectious mononucleosis and syphilis. The rash of exanthem subitum does not appear until the termination of fever. Fever, enanthem, and catarrh are uncommon with the cutaneous manifestations of drug hypersensitivity. Erythema infectiosum is an afebrile illness with rash on the cheeks, arms, and legs. There is no prodrome or accompanying respiratory tract involvement.

Specific Diagnosis. Specific diagnosis depends on the isolation of measles virus from throat washings, blood, or urine by inoculation of tissue culture with materials obtained optimally during the prodrome or first days of rash. Increase in specific antibody may be detected as early as the first or second day of rash by the complement fixation test. Antibody is also demonstrated by neutralization and hemagglutination-inhibition

TABLE 332–1. A GUIDE TO THE DIFFERENTIAL DIAGNOSIS OF MEASLES

	Conjunctivitis	Rhinitis	Sore Throat	Enanthem	Leukocytosis	Specific Laboratory Tests Available
Measles	+ +	+ +	0	+	0	+
Rubella	±	±	±	±	0	+
Exanthem subitum	±	±	0	0	0	0
Enterovirus infection	0	±	±	0	0	+
Scarlet fever	±	±	+ +	0	+	+
Infectious mononucleosis	0	0	+ +	±	±	+
Drug rash	0	0	0	0	0	0

0 Not usually present; no test available.
± Variable in occurrence.
+ Present; test available (virus or bacterial culture, serology).
+ + Present and severe.

procedures. The latter is generally employed because of rapidity and reliability.

Presumptive diagnosis may be made if giant cells are detected in stained smears of nasal exudate in the pre-eruptive period.

PROGNOSIS. Uncomplicated measles is rarely fatal, and complete recovery is the rule. Fatalities are almost always the result of pneumonia, occurring principally in children below the age of two years. Mortality in economically underdeveloped countries may be 250 times that observed in the United States or northern Europe. Case fatality rates are also high in elderly and tuberculous patients. Congestive cardiac failure is a common cause of death in patients over 50 years old.

Antimicrobial drugs effective against the usual secondary invaders have reduced the case fatality rate of measles sharply. They have not proved effective in prophylaxis of bacterial complications, but in therapy.

Encephalitis occurs as frequently in mild as in severe measles (i.e., about one in a thousand cases). However, the incidence of neurologic sequelae after administration of attenuated live virus vaccine is only one in a million.

TREATMENT. There is no specific antiviral therapy for measles.

Symptomatic Therapy. In the absence of complications, bed rest is the essence of treatment in this usually benign, self-limited disease. Codeine sulfate may be useful in the amelioration of headache and myalgia and is effective in the management of cough. Aspirin may be employed for its analgesic and antipyretic actions. Fluids should be encouraged. Bright light is not an ocular hazard, but photophobia may require darkening of the patient's room.

Antimicrobial Prophylaxis. The course of uncomplicated measles is not influenced by antimicrobial drugs, and their use during the acute illness has resulted in no decrease of secondary bacterial complications (otitis, sinusitis, pneumonia). Instead, the same rates of complications (about 10 to 15 per cent) have been observed, but with organisms resistant to the antibiotics used during the viral illness. If careful observation of the patient is possible, rational therapy is based on the prompt recognition and etiologic definition of complications, followed by initiation of the appropriate antimicrobial drug in proper dosage.

PREVENTION. ***Vaccination.*** A highly effective vaccine available for the prevention of measles is derived from the Edmonston strain of virus isolated originally in the laboratory of Dr. John Enders. This live virus vaccine produces immunity by infection and therefore needs to be given only as a single injection. It induces antibody response of somewhat lesser magnitude than that following natural infection. In children over one year of age, seroconversion after vaccination is 90 to 97 per cent. Although a gradual fall in antibody titer occurs in the absence of exposure to wild type virus (see Epidemiology: Immunity), serum antibody is demonstrable in most individuals more than 15 years after a single administration of vaccine. The occasional failure of live virus vaccine to protect has recently been related to vaccination at less than 12 months of age, at which time maternal antibody may inhibit replication of the vaccine virus. It is now recommended that measles immunization be deferred until 15 months of age in technologically advanced countries in which infantile infection is uncommon. Reimmunization is not harmful and is recommended for those who have received vaccine before age one year. The current vaccine is fully effective and safe in susceptible adults also.

Contraindications to live virus vaccine include pregnancy, immunodeficiency, leukemia, and other systemic malignant diseases, active tuberculosis, and administration of resistance-depressing drugs such as corticosteroids and antimetabolites.

Eradication of measles through administration of live virus vaccines is a scientifically reasonable possibility. The introduction of immunization in the United States in 1963 has led to a decrease in incidence from about 500,000 cases annually to fewer than 1500 cases in 1983. Although it may be possible to eliminate indigenous measles in the United States, the problem of "imported infection" has arisen with the influx of susceptible children from Southeast Asia and certain Latin American nations.

Annunziato D, Kaplan MH, Hall WW, Ichinose H, Linn JH, Balsam D, Paladino VS: Atypical measles syndrome: Pathologic and serologic findings. Pediatrics 70:203, 1982. *Excellent clinical description and explanation of a syndrome now seen in young adults.*

Choppin PW, Richardson CD, Merz DC, Hall WW, Scheid A: The functions and inhibition of the membrane glycoproteins of paramyxoviruses and myxoviruses and the role of measles virus M protein in subacute sclerosing panencephalitis. J Infect Dis 143:352, 1981. *The ultimate correlation of molecular virology and clinical expression of measles and related viruses.*

Hinman AR, Brandling-Bennett AD, Bernier RH, Kirby CD, Eddins DL: Current features of measles in the United States: Feasibility of measles elimination. Epidem Rev 2:153, 1980. *A "state-of-the-art" review of measles surveillance, immunization, and plans for eradication of indigenous disease in the United States.*

Johnson RT, Griffin DE, Hirsch RL, Wolinsky JS, Roedenbeck S, deSoriano IL, Vaisberg A: Measles encephalomyelitis—clinical and immunologic studies. N Engl J Med 310:137, 1984. *Pathogenesis of central nervous system complications studied by modern immunologic approaches.*

Katz SL, Krugman S, Quinn TC (eds.): International symposium on measles immunization. Rev Infect Dis 5:389, 1983. *An all-inclusive presentation of measles and its prevention throughout the world.*

Panum PL: Observations Made During the Epidemic of Measles on the Faröe Islands. Delta Omega Society, 1940. *A classic clinical epidemiologic description of measles introduced into an isolated population with disease among all susceptibles born since the previous epidemic 65 years earlier.*

Sabin AB, Arechiga AF, deCastro JF, Sever JL, Madden DL, Shekarchi I, Albrecht P: Successful immunization of children with and without maternal antibody by aerosolized measles vaccine. JAMA 249:2651, 1983. *A new approach to vaccine administration, with promise of great benefit for developing nations.*

333. RUBELLA (German Measles)

Samuel L. Katz

DEFINITION. Rubella is an acute, usually benign infectious disease characterized by a three-day rash, generalized lymphadenopathy, and minimal or absent prodromal symptoms. Since 1941, it has been known to cause congenital malformations when infection occurs during the early months of pregnancy.

Rubella was recognized as a distinct clinical entity by German physicians in the mid-eighteenth century; it continued to be the subject of moderate interest through the next two centuries until 1941, when the Australian ophthalmologist Gregg called attention to its role as a teratogen. Over the next 20 years the association of rubella in early pregnancy with fetal defects (cataracts, heart disease, and deafness) was corroborated by a number of clinical epidemiologic studies. In 1962, techniques for viral culture and serologic confirmation became available.

ETIOLOGY. Rubella virus is a pleomorphic agent when viewed by electron microscopy, usually spherical, with a central nucleoid 30 nm in diameter contained within an outer envelope 60 to 70 nm wide. Its genome is RNA, and the virus is classified as a special member (genus rubivirus) of the togavirus group on the basis of its biochemical, biophysical, and ultrastructural properties. Unlike most of the togaviruses it does not utilize an arthropod vector in its natural cycle. In the human, its natural host, the virus behaves like a paramyxovirus, and many of its laboratory characteristics are like those of that group. It will multiply in a variety of primary cell culture systems and in some continuous cell lines, usually without detectable cytopathic effects. Hemagglutination of avian erythrocytes provides a convenient method for virus assay, and by inhibition of this hemagglutination the presence and titer of antibody are readily measured. By polyacrylamide-gel electrophoresis eight distinct viral polypeptides have been identified.

EPIDEMIOLOGY. Prior to the availability of rubella vaccines, the disease was worldwide in distribution, produced major epidemics at six- to nine-year intervals, and occurred mainly in school-age children, but also produced outbreaks in settings such as military recruit bases and college campuses where large numbers of susceptible young adults gathered in relatively crowded conditions. The use, since licensure in 1969, of more than 125 million doses of rubella vaccine in the United States has strikingly altered the epidemiology. There has been no major epidemic since 1964–1965, and the age-specific attack rate has altered with a significant increase in the proportion of cases reported in adolescents and young adults who failed to be immunized in childhood. In other nations, where rubella vaccine has not been widely utilized, the epidemiology has remained unchanged and epidemics were observed in 1971–1972 and in 1978–1979. Because the usual disease may be quite nonspecific clinically, with evidence that nearly one third of adults may undergo infection without rash, epidemiologic reporting has been variable. Since 1966, congenital rubella has been a reportable disease. It is probable that rubella is spread by the respiratory route by close and sustained personal contact. The usual infection is contagious during the period of prodromal symptoms and for as long as seven days after the appearance of rash. However, the infant with congenitally acquired infection may excrete virus in respiratory secretions and in urine for months after birth and is contagious during this time. In hospital environments, especially in nurseries, the congenital rubella baby has been a source of nosocomial infection of personnel involved in his care.

Immunity is lifelong in duration after initial infection. Authenticated second attacks are exceedingly rare, and require serologic documentation because of the nebulous nature of the clinical syndrome. *Subclinical* reinfection demonstrated by increase in IgG serum antibody has been documented with increasing frequency as better serologic methods and increased surveillance have become available. Reinfection occurs most commonly in crowded populations in which the density of infection and probability of spread are high. Such reinfections are not associated with viremia and thus pose little threat in pregnant women. IgM response serves to distinguish primary infection from reinfection. Immunity that follows artificial immunization with live virus vaccine is apparently of equal duration even though the antibody titers induced may be somewhat lower. (See Prevention, below.)

PATHOLOGY. Death from postnatal rubella is an almost unheard-of event, so the histology has not been studied. Since 1962, it has been possible to investigate the pathogenesis and to correlate clinical findings with virologic events. After initial invasion of the upper respiratory tract, virus spreads to local lymphoid tissue where it multiplies and starts a viremia of approximately seven days' duration. Respiratory tract shedding of virus and the viremia rise to peak levels until the onset of rash, at which time the latter becomes undetectable, whereas respiratory secretions contain diminishing quantities of virus over the succeeding 5 to 15 days. Specific antibodies can be demonstrated with the onset of rash, and circulating immune complexes are detectable soon thereafter.

Congenital Rubella. Necropsies of fetal and neonatal victims of intrauterine infection have shown a variety of embryonal defects related to developmental arrest involving all three germ layers.

The virus establishes chronic persistent infection of many tissues, with inhibition of mitosis and a resultant intrauterine growth retardation. Delayed and disordered organogenesis produces embryopathic structural defects (eye, brain, heart, large arteries), and continued viral infection in fetal and postnatal cells causes organ and tissue damage (hepatitis, nephritis, myocarditis, pneumonia, osteitis, meningitis, cochlear degeneration, pancreatitis).

CLINICAL MANIFESTATIONS. *Postnatally Acquired Rubella.* Fourteen to 21 days after exposure, the onset of rubella is manifested by the appearance of a rash with mild accompanying constitutional symptoms of malaise and occasional sore throat. Palpable, tender, and occasionally visible lymphadenopathy involves postauricular and suboccipital nodes. Moderate fever, coryza, and faint conjunctivitis may accompany the rash. Generalized peripheral lymphadenopathy and, more rarely, splenomegaly may occur.

The exanthem of rubella is usually apparent within 24 hours of the first symptoms as a faint macular erythema that first involves the face and neck. Characterized by its brevity and evanescence, it spreads rapidly to the trunk and extremities, sometimes leaving one site even as it appears at the next. The pink macules that constitute the rash blanch with pressure and rarely stain the skin. Rubella virus has been isolated from the skin lesions as well as from uninvolved sites. The truncal rash may coalesce, but the lesions on the extremities remain discrete. The eruption vanishes by the third day. Rubella may occur without rash. An enanthem has been described that is inconstant in form and occurrence. The lesions consist of red macules that usually involve the soft palate. Infections with adenoviruses, enteroviruses, and Epstein-Barr virus can mimic rubella with rash, fever, and lymphadenopathy. In the absence of an epidemic and of serologic (or virologic) confirmation, the clinical diagnosis of rubella is not reliable.

COMPLICATIONS. Recovery is almost always prompt and uneventful. In contrast to measles, secondary bacterial infections are not encountered in rubella. Arthritis is more common among adolescents and adults with rubella, particularly females. It appears three or more days after onset of rash and may last five to ten days. Large joints (knees, elbows, ankles) are most often involved, but small and medium-sized joints may also be affected. Surveys during urban epidemics have revealed rates of 5 to 15 per cent in males and 10 to 35 per cent in females. There appears to be no association with later rheumatoid arthritis or other joint disease.

Thrombocytopenia, when sought by serial platelet counts, is a common complication but rarely of clinical significance. The unusual patient who develops purpuric manifestations may also have evidence of increased capillary fragility and a prolonged bleeding time. A meningoencephalitis of short duration may occur one to six days after the appearance of rash. Its incidence is estimated at 1 in 6000 cases, and it is fatal in approximately 20 per cent of those afflicted. Rubella encephalopathy is not associated with demyelinization (in contrast to other postviral encephalitides). Survivors may have electroencephalographic abnormalities, but intellectual function seems to be preserved.

Congenital Rubella. Congenital transplacental infection of the fetus occurs as a consequence of maternal infection (which may or may not be clinically evident), usually in the first four months of pregnancy. Virus is demonstrable in placental and fetal tissues obtained by therapeutic abortion at that time. If pregnancy is not interrupted, fetal infection persists, and upon delivery of the infant, virus is recoverable from the throat, urine, conjunctivae, bone marrow, and cerebrospinal fluid of the living infant and from most organs at autopsy. From 20 to 80 per cent of infants born to mothers infected in the first trimester of pregnancy have stigmata of infection readily recognizable in the first year of life. These include *cardiac lesions* and *eye defects* (cataracts, glaucoma, retinitis, microphthalmia). Most infants in whom virus is detectable do not have evidence of disease at birth or may simply have intrauterine growth retardation. In others, disease of intermediate severity occurs. Most prominent of these manifestations is *thrombocytopenic purpura,* which disappears soon after birth. *Hepatosplenomegaly* with active hepatitis may persist for months. Other involvement includes *interstitial pneumonia, meningoencephalitis, hearing loss* of varying extent, and *lesions of the long bones.* A chronic recurrent erythematous rash associated with the presence of rubella virus in the skin has been reported in some patients. Recently, a progressive panencephalitis simulating subacute sclerosing panencephalitis has been observed in the second decade following congenital infection. The long-term sequelae for most congenital rubella infants include psychomotor retardation, hearing loss, and retinopathy.

A striking finding has been the persistence of virus in the pharynx, urine, and cerebrospinal fluid for as long as one year after birth (9 per cent). Infective virus was present in a congenital cataract after three years, and in the urine of a victim of congenital rubella 29 years after her birth. This evidence of continuing viral synthesis occurs coincidentally with circulating antibody (initially of maternal origin). The character of the antibody changes during the first months from IgG (presumably maternal) to IgM, indicating a primary response of the infant to the persisting viral antigen. Studies of older infants and children with stigmata of congenital rubella show them to be free of demonstrable virus and to possess the IgG immunoglobulins that characteristically persist after other viral infections. The defect in host response that is responsible for viral persistence has not yet been defined fully, but there is depressed T cell response to rubella virus antigens in some congenitally infected infants.

DIAGNOSIS. Rubella may be diagnosed clinically with assurance only during an epidemic. Distinction from measles may be made on the basis of fainter, nonstaining rash, the milder course, and the minimal or absent systemic complaints. Sore throat is a more prominent complaint in scarlet fever; the course of infectious mononucleosis is often more protracted, and splenomegaly is more frequent than in rubella. Specific diagnosis of rubella is made by isolation of the virus in any of several cell culture systems, or by demonstration of neutralizing, hemagglutination-inhibiting (HI), or complement-fixing antibody response during infection. HI antibodies are most rapidly and reproducibly available in diagnostic laboratories throughout the nation. A simple, ten-minute latex-agglutination card assay for antibodies enables the physician to determine rubella susceptibility or immunity within the time of an office or clinic visit.

PROGNOSIS. Complete recovery from postnatally acquired rubella is almost invariable. The rare deaths attributable to rubella follow the infrequent complication of meningoencephalitis. Infection in pregnancy constitutes a grave hazard to the fetus but not to the mother.

TREATMENT. There is no specific antiviral therapy. Few patients suffer discomfort severe enough to warrant symptomatic medication. Headache and myalgia may be controlled by aspirin.

PREVENTION. ***Passive Immunization.*** *Administration of gamma globulin to the pregnant woman may only mask her symptoms of infection yet not protect the fetus from viral invasion.* Its use may thus only obscure the picture and confound decision about the need for therapeutic abortion.

Active Immunization. Rubella may be prevented in children and adults by the parenteral administration of attenuated live virus vaccines produced in cell cultures. Seroconversion rates after immunization are at least 95 per cent. As with other live virus vaccines, serum antibody titers are somewhat lower than those that follow natural infection. However, antibody persists for at least 15 years after vaccination. Natural reinfection of individuals immunized with vaccine is not uncommon, although such infection is asymptomatic and without viremia. In children, vaccination is attended by little or no reaction; but in women, malaise, arthralgia, and mild, acute arthritis occur frequently, the incidence being directly related to age. It was initially recommended in the United States that immunization be carried out principally in childhood. The success of these efforts, with reduction of rubella cases to fewer than 1000 in 1983, has encouraged a more aggressive attempt to immunize susceptible women and adolescent girls. Current policy recommends vaccination of all such persons who have no history of previous rubella immunization. Of this population, only nonpregnant individuals should be immunized, and contraception (when appropriate) should be carried out for at least three months after vaccination. The inadvertent administration of vaccine to pregnant women has demonstrated that attenuated vaccine viruses can reach the products of conception; but in 143 such cases studied, no infant has been observed with congenital malformations as a result. The use of vaccine in the United States prevented a large epidemic of rubella expected in the early 1970's and has reduced the reported annual occurrence from more than 50,000 cases annually (with epidemic peaks of 200,000 to 500,000) to an all-time low of 953 in 1983, with only 20 cases of congenital rubella.

Centers for Disease Control: Rubella and congenital rubella—United States, 1980–83. Morbid Mortal Wkly Rep 32:505, 1983. *Fourteen years since licensure of rubella vaccine, a statement of achievements and the need for a focus on unimmunized adults and hospital personnel.*

Clarke M, Schild GC, Miller C, Seagroatt V, Pollock TM, Finlay S, Barbara JAJ: Surveys of rubella antibodies in young adults and children. Lancet 1:667, 1983. *The English approach to prevention of congenital rubella, very different from that in the United States and with persistence of congenital rubella 13 years after its initiation.*

Gregg NM: Congenital cataract following German measles in the mother. Trans Ophthal Soc Aust 3:35, 1941. *The original "classic" associating rubella in pregnancy with congenital malformations.*

Hanshaw JB, Dudgeon JA: Rubella. *In* Viral Diseases of the Fetus and Newborn. Philadelphia, W. B. Saunders Company, 1978. *For the interested scholar, an all-inclusive presentation with nine pages of references.*

Herrmann KL: Rubella virus. *In* Lennette EH, Schmidt NJ (eds.): Diagnostic Procedures for Viral, Rickettsial and Chlamydial Infections. 5th ed. Washington, D.C., American Public Health Association, 1979. *Excellent presentation of the laboratory support for confirmation of the clinical diagnosis.*

Hinman AR, Orenstein WA, Bart KJ, Preblud SR: Rational strategy for rubella vaccination. Lancet 1:39, 1983. *The architects of United States rubella eradication re-examine the problem.*

Tingle AJ, Yang T, Allen M, Kettyls GD, Larke RPB, Schulzer M: Prospective immunological assessment of arthritis induced by rubella vaccine. Infect Immunol 40:22, 1983. *The unresolved issue of rubella's relationship to rheumatoid arthritis and other disorders.*

334. FOOT AND MOUTH DISEASE (Aphthous Fever, Epizootic Stomatitis)

Catherine M. Wilfert

Foot and mouth disease (FMD) is a highly contagious illness of cloven-hoofed animals, especially cattle, sheep, goats, and pigs. The etiology was first ascribed to a filterable agent in 1898 by Loeffler and Frosch. The virus is now known to be a member of the picornavirus family. It belongs to the aphthovirus genus, which is composed of small (diameter of 25 to 30 nm) acid-labile RNA viruses containing naked icosahedral nucleocapsids. The disease in animals is characterized by fever and increased salivation, with the appearance of vesicular lesions on the mucous membranes of the mouth, tongue, and lips, between the paws, and on the teats and udder. Vesicular fluid is highly infectious. There are seven different serotypes of FMD which tend to be found in localized geographic areas. This virus is highly communicable among animals, and the epidemic spread of this agent among domestic animals can result in tremendous loss of livestock. The rigid quarantine regulations of the Bureau of Animal Diseases, U.S. Department of Agriculture, in the United States has freed this country of FMD. Indeed, public law prevents importation of the virus into the mainland of the United States even for experimental purposes. An inactivated vaccine for use in animals utilized polyvalent, cell culture–grown FMD virus. More recently, DNA recombinant technology and chemically synthesized peptides corresponding to specific regions of a capsid polypeptide have been successfully used as immunogens in animals.

FMD in its natural hosts is clinically indistinguishable from two other diseases which do occur in the United States. These are vesicular stomatitis virus of horses, cattle, and occasionally humans, and vesicular exanthema of swine. The rapid diagnosis of FMD in cattle is important to allow its differentiation from the other two diseases. This is accomplished by a qualified laboratory with the use of differential inoculations of infectious material into appropriate hosts.

Man is an extremely rare incidental host of FMD. The illness is usually self-limited, febrile, and characterized by excessive salivation and vesicular lesions on the buccal or lingual epithelium, and possibly the skin of the hands, feet, and other parts of the body. Humans apparently carry the virus for at least 24 hours in their nasopharynx and can transmit it to other humans or susceptible animals via infectious droplets. For diagnostic purposes vesicular fluid can be used as antigen in a serotype specific complement fixation test. Antibody assessment can be accomplished by hemagglutination inhibition assays and tissue culture neutralization assays. This illness has no relationship to hand-foot-and-mouth disease caused by coxsackieviruses.

Bittle JL, Houghten RA, Alexander H, Shinnick TM, Sutcliffe JG, Lerner RA, Rowlands DJ, Brown F: Protection against foot-and-mouth disease by immunization with a chemically synthesized peptide predicted from the viral nucleotide sequence. Nature 298:30, 1982.

Kleid DG, Yansura D, Small B, Dowbenk T, Moore DM, Grubman MJ, McKercher PD, Morgan DO, Robertson BH, Bachrach HL: Cloned viral protein vaccine for foot and mouth disease: Responses in cattle and swine. Science 214:1125, 1981. *Description of recombinant DNA technology applied to development of specific polypeptide antigen.*

335. MUMPS (Epidemic Parotitis)

Catherine M. Wilfert

DEFINITION. Mumps or epidemic parotitis is an acute communicable viral infection. The characteristic clinical manifestations were described in the fifth century B.C. by Hippocrates.

ETIOLOGY. Mumps virus is placed in the Paramyxovirus genus of the paramyxoviridiae family. The diameter of the virus particle is approximately 150 nm, and it has enveloped helical nucleocapsids. It is an RNA virus with a nonsegmented single stranded genome that apparently codes for six polypeptides, three of which are nucleocapsid proteins and three of which are envelope proteins. One of the surface glycoproteins is the spike containing the hemagglutinin and neuraminidase (HN). The hemagglutinin causes the agglutination of erythrocytes of several species. The second surface glycoprotein spike (F) is responsible for the cell fusing and hemolyzing activities of the virus. The remarkable feature of the two paramyxovirus glycoproteins F and HN is that they must be cleaved once by a cellular protease for the virus particles to become infectious. If the cells lack the protease, only noninfectious virus particles are produced. The paramyxoviruses enter cells by fusing with cell membranes and liberating their nucleocapsids into the cytoplasm of the host cell. Mumps virus replication occurs in a variety of cell cultures and is infective for monkeys and chick embryos. It is relatively heat labile, with loss of infectivity resulting from heating to 55 to 60° C for 20 minutes.

EPIDEMIOLOGY. Mumps virus infection is endemic in all areas of the world and occurs throughout the year. Mumps is predominantly a disease of childhood, and prior to the advent of vaccine the majority of clinically evident infections were seen in children between the ages of five and ten years. Serologic evidence suggested that approximately 85 per cent of mumps infections occurred in those under 15 years of age.

Infection is transmitted via respiratory droplets, but mumps virus is less communicable than measles or varicella. Epidemiologic evidence suggests that the period of infectivity is from several days before onset of symptoms until the subsidence of the salivary gland swelling. Prolonged or recurrent excretion of virus is unknown. As many as 25 to 40 per cent of mumps infections are entirely asymptomatic. For these reasons attempts to control the spread of mumps infection by isolation of a patient are usually futile. The asymptomatic patients excrete virus, may transmit infection, and have a self-limited infection. The resulting immunity is comparable to that following symptomatic infection. There are no known animal reservoirs for mumps.

PATHOGENESIS AND PATHOLOGY. The portal of entry of the virus is thought to be the upper respiratory tract. The time interval after exposure to virus before the appearance of the clinical symptoms ranges from 14 to 21 days, with the usual incubation period being 16 to 18 days. After entering the host, the virus replicates and viremia occurs, which may result in secondary invasion of several organ systems. Tissues such as the salivary glands (predominantly the parotids), meninges, testes, pancreas, ovaries, thyroid, and heart may show evidence of infection. Virus is also excreted in the urine, and transient abnormalities in renal function have been found.

Pathologic examination of involved tissues has been infrequent because of the usually benign nature of the illness. Available studies of salivary glands indicate that there is no disruption of the general architecture of the gland. The involved salivary ducts may demonstrate changes in the epithelial lining cells, ranging from edema to complete desquamation. The ducts are dilated, and the lumen may be filled with cellular debris and polymorphonuclear cells. There may be a moderate amount of periductal edema around the involved ducts. Mononuclear inflammatory cells predominate in the interstitium. The pathology of other involved tissues is similar, and no specific hallmarks allow the diagnosis of mumps infection to be made solely on the basis of the observed pathology.

CLINICAL MANIFESTATIONS. Salivary gland involvement usually precedes other clinical symptoms, lasts for two to seven days, and may be unilateral or bilateral. Infection of the salivary glands is manifested by pain, and the characteristic swelling of the parotid gland provides the diagnosis of mumps. The infection less frequently involves the submandibular or sublingual salivary glands. Although other manifestations of mumps most often coincide with the parotid swelling, they may precede or occur in the absence of salivary gland involvement.

Meningitis. Central nervous system involvement with mumps virus occurs frequently. Viral meningitis has been said to occur in 65 per cent of hospitalized persons with parotid swelling when lumbar puncture is done. The cerebrospinal fluid (CSF) shows a predominantly lymphocytic pleocytosis in affected individuals, although only one half of them will display clinical signs of meningitis. The signs of meningeal involvement are most often manifest two to ten days after the onset of parotitis and last three to five days. Illness is characterized by fever, headache, nausea, vomiting, nuchal rigidity, is self limited, and clears with minimal (if any) sequelae.

Encephalitis. A more serious and much less frequent central nervous system manifestation is encephalitis or encephalomyelitis. The onset is usually later than the transient meningitis and occurs 10 to 14 days after the clinical salivary gland involvement. The patient appears severely ill, is deeply obtunded, and may have seizures or die. Although occurring much less often than the encephalitis associated with measles or varicella, mumps encephalitis is clinically and pathologically indistinguishable from them.

In 1967 suckling hamsters inoculated intracerebrally with the virus developed hydrocephalus. Virus replication occurred within ependymal cells of the ventricles and choroid plexus. Two to six weeks after infection, as inflammation resolved, aqueductal stenosis and hydrocephalus developed at a time when viral antigens and infectious virus were no longer demonstrable. The clinical application of such observations remains to be established, but recognition that sequelae of a virus infection can occur when the virus is no longer detectable is a useful concept.

Epididymo-orchitis. The complication of mumps infection best known by nonmedical persons is the involvement of the testes. This manifestation occurs predominantly in postpubertal males with 20 to 30 per cent manifesting orchitis during the course of mumps infection. Bilateral testicular involvement occurs in 2 to 6 per cent of patients with orchitis. Orchitis usually begins abruptly with fever, chills, headache, and lower abdominal pain. The systemic reaction ordinarily parallels the extent of gonadal involvement. The testis swells rapidly and becomes very painful and tender. The pain and swelling disappear as fever subsides, usually within five days of onset. Testicular tenderness may persist for a longer period. There is no theoretical or factual basis for the fear of sexual impotence following mumps orchitis. In the vast majority of instances the disease is unilateral. At least one half of those patients who have unilateral disease have completely normal testes after the acute infection; the remainder may have some degree of unilateral testicular atrophy, which does not result in sterility.

Pancreatitis. Pancreatitis may occur in association with mumps infection, with typical symptoms of abdominal pain, fever, and vomiting. Symptoms gradually subside over a period of three to seven days, and the patient usually recovers completely. Studies in vitro have demonstrated that mumps virus can replicate in human pancreatic beta cells and pancreatic epithelial cells. There is no firm epidemiologic or clinical evidence linking mumps virus infection to subsequent development of diabetes mellitus.

Other Clinical Manifestations. Especially in adults, infection of other tissues may rarely occur. Oophoritis has been described in adult females. The characteristic lower quadrant or back pain suggests the clinical diagnosis, but involvement of the ovaries may occur in the absence of recognizable symptoms. Sterility is not a known consequence of mumps oophoritis. Extremely rare manifestations of infection include polyarthritis, mastitis, myocarditis, thyroiditis, dacryoadenitis, and bartholinitis.

HOST RESPONSE. In the normal individual a single infection with mumps virus confers permanent immunity against clinically evident infection. It is probable that reinfection, defined as an antibody rise after exposure to the virus, may occur, but neither virus shedding nor clinical illness has been demonstrated with such reinfection. Although second attacks of parotitis have been observed, there are other possible causes, including coxsackievirus or lymphocytic choriomeningitis virus infections, starch ingestion, sarcoidosis, iodine sensitivity, and thiazide therapy. At present there is no documentation by culture or serology of two clinical attacks of mumps virus infection in the same individual.

Mumps virus infection induces the formation of specific humoral antibodies. Initially antibody of the IgM class and subsequently antibody of the IgG class are formed. Neutralization of infectivity, inhibition of hemagglutination, and the inhibition of neuraminidase activity are functions attributable to antibody to the HN protein. Specific neutralizing antibodies can be detected during the first week of symptoms and ordinarily persist for a lifetime. Hemagglutinating inhibiting and complement-fixing antibodies become detectable from one to three weeks after onset and usually reach peak titers within three to six weeks.

In vitro, mumps virus replicates in human lymphoblastoid cell lines with T cell characteristics and in peripheral blood mononuclear cells. Pokeweed mitogen enhances replication that occurs primarily in T lymphocytes, suggesting that these cells might be infected during natural infection.

DIAGNOSIS. The clinical diagnosis is strongly suggested when a known exposure to mumps is followed in two to three weeks by an illness with compatible clinical findings such as parotitis. In the absence of parotitis or if parotitis has occurred previously, specific laboratory studies are necessary to confirm the diagnosis.

Johnson and Goodpasture established that mumps was caused by a filterable virus. Successful propagation of virus in chick embryos preceded the now generally employed standard tissue culture techniques. Virus has been isolated from such varied sources as blood, CSF, urine, saliva, salivary gland tissue, and human milk. Viral diagnostic laboratories are available in many academic and large hospital settings for unusual or complicated situations.

Many diagnostic laboratories are better able to offer serologic diagnosis than viral isolation. Evaluation of sera for antibodies to mumps virus is readily accomplished. With acute serum one can determine if a person has ever had mumps infection. An increase in antibody titer on convalescent serum is indicative of recent mumps virus infection. Complement-fixation (CF) tests are most commonly employed by diagnostic laboratories for this purpose. Occasionally it is useful to obtain additional information about the temporal relationship of an illness to the antibody response. Two complement-fixing antigens, the nucleoprotein or soluble (S) antigen and the viral surface antigen (V), have been recognized for years. CF antibodies against the S antigen are detectable within two to three days of onset, peak at about ten days, and disappear in eight to nine months. CF antibodies against the V antigen, which includes the HN and F proteins, are not detectable until approximately the tenth day of infection and persist for years. Comparison of the transient nature of the S antibodies with the delayed appearance of the V antibodies may assist in defining recent infection.

PROGNOSIS. In general the prognosis of infection with mumps virus is excellent. Fatalities have been associated with encephalitis, myocarditis, and nephritis but are extremely rare. An occasional sequel to mumps virus infection is deafness, which may occur even in the absence of other evidence of central nervous system involvement. The loss of hearing may be preceded by tinnitus and a sense of fullness of the ear. Deafness is relatively uncommon but occurs suddenly during the period of parotid swelling. It is usually unilateral, but an estimated 20 per cent of those affected may have bilateral disease. Once deafness has occurred, the damage is irreversible.

TREATMENT. Mumps is a self-limited infection, and there is no specific therapy available.

PREVENTIVE MEASURES. *Passive Protection.* A common question concerns what to do when a susceptible person is exposed to mumps infection. Administration of hyperimmune globulin or pooled serum IgG after such exposure has not decreased the number of patients acquiring illness nor has it lessened the severity of illness. There is a single controlled study reporting that administration of hyperimmune globulin after the appearance of parotitis can decrease the incidence and severity of orchitis. Other studies under epidemic conditions failed to demonstrate any alteration in the attack rate or in the subsequent development of orchitis or meningoencephalitis. Therefore, the use of hyperimmune globulin is of dubious value.

Immunization. Live attenuated mumps virus vaccine is available for prophylactic use. The attenuated virus vaccine is produced in tissue cultures of chick embryo fibroblasts and is administered parenterally. Virus is not shed by the vaccinee, and immunization does not cause any side effects. The vaccine produces 95 to 100 per cent serologic conversion from antibody negative to positive in vaccinated susceptibles. Although the antibody levels are considerably lower, they parallel those produced by natural infection and have persisted for the 14 to 16 years that the vaccine has been available for study. The presence of detectable mumps antibody correlates with protection against clinical illness. Immunized children in contact with naturally occurring mumps have been protected against clinical illness. It is recommended for administration to children more than one year of age and to adolescents and adults for induction of immunity. Live attenuated mumps vaccine has been combined with measles and rubella virus vaccines.

There is only a single serologic strain of mumps virus; hence a single infection with either natural or attenuated virus confers immunity. Approximately 40 million doses of mumps vaccine have been distributed since 1968, and this increasing use of mumps vaccination has resulted in a marked decline in the incidence of reported disease in the United States.

The vaccine will not offer protection against mumps if someone has already been exposed to natural infection and is in the incubation period of illness. On the other hand, no harmful effects have been noted after administration of vaccine to an exposed susceptible. If the original exposure is not followed by mumps infection, the vaccine would then induce protection against subsequent exposures.

Fleischer B, Kneth HW: Mumps virus replication in human lymphoid cell lines and in peripheral blood lymphocytes: Preference for T cells. Infect Immun 35:25, 1982. *In vitro studies suggesting that activated T lymphocytes are the major site of replication of mumps virus in peripheral white blood cells.*

Gordon JE, Kilham L: Ten years in the epidemiology of mumps. Am J Med Sci 218:358, 1949. *A general, thorough description of mumps prior to the advent of vaccine.*

Jensik SC, Silver S: Polypeptides of mumps virus. J Virol 17:363, 1976. *Viral glycoprotein containing neuraminidase and hemagglutinating activity corresponds to V antigen of mumps virus.*

Kilham L, Margolis G: Induction of congenital hydrocephalus in hamsters with attenuated and natural strains of mumps virus. J Infect Dis 132:462, 1975. *Experimental induction of intrauterine infection with attenuated and wild type mumps virus resulting in central nervous system infection.*

Koplan JP, Preblud SR: A benefit-cost analysis of mumps vaccine. Am J Dis Child 36:362, 1982. *Statistical demonstration of the reduction in morbidity, mortality, and costs associated with a mumps vaccination program.*

Orvel C: Structural polypeptides of mumps virus. J Gen Virol 41:527, 1978. *The experimental definition of mumps virus polypeptides is described.*

Prince GA, Jenson AB, Billups LC, Notkins AL: Infection of human pancreatic beta cell cultures with mumps virus. Nature 271:158, 1978. *The demonstration by immunofluorescence of mumps antigen in human beta cells.*

Westmore GA, Pickard BH, Stern H: Isolation of mumps virus from the inner ear after sudden deafness. Br Med J 1:14, 1979. *A case report documenting mumps virus in the inner ear in association with subsequent deafness.*

Diseases Caused by Herpes-Type Viruses

336. HERPES SIMPLEX VIRUS INFECTIONS

R. Gordon Douglas, Jr.

Herpes simplex virus produces diseases ranging from inapparent infections and fever blisters to fatal encephalitis. The word herpes is derived from the Greek word "herpein," meaning "to creep," in reference to the skin manifestations.

ETIOLOGY. Herpes simplex virus (herpesvirus hominis, HSV) is a member of the Herpetoviridae family, which consists of a group of large enveloped DNA-containing viruses, belonging to two genera: herpesvirus and cytomegalovirus. Members of the herpesvirus genus that infect man include herpes simplex virus types 1 and 2, varicella-zoster virus, and Epstein-Barr virus. Only a single member of the cytomegalovirus genus, human cytomegalovirus, causes disease in man. Herpes simplex virus has an internal core containing double-stranded DNA, which is surrounded by an electron dense capsid, an icosahedron of 162 hollow capsomeres surrounded by a lipid-containing laminated envelope studded with glycoprotein projections. Because of the variable size of the envelope, the overall diameter of the virus ranges from 150 to 200 nm.

Viral replication occurs primarily within the cell nucleus, and viral envelopes are derived, at least in part, from the nuclear membrane. Complete replication is associated with lysis of the infected cell.

Herpes simplex viruses differ in host range from other members of the Herpetoviridae family. For example, herpes simplex types 1 and 2 grow well in a variety of human and animal cell lines, in embryonated hens' eggs, and in laboratory animals. Varicella-zoster virus is more restricted, not replicating in embryonated hens' eggs or in experimental animals, and only replicating in a few cell lines. Human cytomegalovirus is further restricted in host range to human fibroblast cell lines, and Epstein-Barr virus will not yield productive infection in any animal, egg, or conventional cell culture system, but viral replication occurs in continuous human lymphoblastoid cell cultures.

HSV types 1 and 2 share common antigens so that cross-reacting antibodies are induced following infection with either virus. They can be differentiated by monoclonal antibody and restriction enzyme techniques. As shown in Table 336–1, they differ also by route of transmission, by usual site of disease, by type of complications, by differences in physical properties, and by biologic characteristics.

EPIDEMIOLOGY. Herpes simplex viruses are distributed worldwide. There are no known seasonal patterns of infection. Since infection with virus is followed by development of antibody that persists for life, incidence of infection can be determined by antibody studies. The prevalence of antibody is inversely related to socioeconomic status. In lower socioeconomic groups, almost 100 per cent of adults have antibody to HSV, whereas in higher socioeconomic groups, this proportion falls to 30 to 50 per cent. The time of maximal acquisition of infection varies with the two types. The prevalence of antibody to HSV type 1 rises during childhood, whereas the major period of infection with HSV type 2 follows puberty.

Transmission apparently occurs by direct contact from person to person, and there is no animal reservoir. HSV type 1 is transmitted primarily by contact with oral secretions, and HSV type 2 by contact with genital secretions. A small percentage of adults may be excreting HSV type 1 or type 2 at any time, and this may occur in the absence of active lesions. Apparently, transmission can occur both from overtly infected persons and from asymptomatic excretors. The portal of entry is most commonly the oral cavity for HSV type 1 and the genital tract for HSV type 2. However, either type of HSV may be intro-

TABLE 336–1. COMPARISON OF PREDOMINANT CHARACTERISTICS OF HSV TYPE 1 AND TYPE 2

Characteristics	HSV-1	HSV-2
Transmission	Oral route	Genital route
Usual site of lesions	Skin of face and mouth, upper trunk	Genitals, skin of thighs, buttocks
Complications		
Keratitis	+	−
Encephalitis (adults)	+	−
Neonatal infection	−	+
Physical characteristics		
Temperature sensitivity (40° C)	−	+
Heparin sensitivity	+	−
Biologic characteristics		
Pock size on chorioallantoic membranes	Small	Large
Plaques in cell cultures	Small	Large
Syncytial formation in human embryonic kidney cells	Small	Large
Experimental infection in mice	Less neurotropic	More neurotropic

duced directly into the eye, a skin site, or the oral cavity or genital area. Transmission of HSV type 2 to skin sites other than those in the genital area can occur to infants born to mothers with genital infections. Also, anal and perianal infections of HSV type 2 are common among homosexual populations. Autoinoculation from either oral or genital sites to hands, thighs, or buttocks is not unusual. Extraoral acquisition of HSV is a hazard in certain occupations, and persons such as dentists, respiratory care unit personnel, and wrestlers are at higher risk. Laboratory-acquired infection and nosocomial outbreaks in hospital personnel or in neonatal nurseries have been reported.

Recurrent infections are one of the hallmarks of the Herpetoviridae family, and they occur frequently with both HSV type 1 and type 2. Recurrent infections of the lips or perioral area with HSV type 1 occur in 20 to 40 per cent of the population, and some data suggest that this rate may be increased among persons with the major histocompatibility type, HLA-A1. Recurrences may occur as frequently as once every several weeks or as infrequently as once or twice per year. They usually occur at the same site and occur despite the presence of circulating or local antibodies. They may be triggered by sunlight, fever, local trauma, menstruation, emotional stress, or other factors. Recurrent HSV type 2 usually occurs as lesions on the external genitalia, and with either type recurrences may appear at other sites, e.g., the eye.

Genital recurrences occur in up to 60 per cent of those with initial episodes. This frequency depends on sex, HSV type, and presence and titer of neutralizing antibody. Although most recurrences are due to reactivation of latent virus, exogenous reinfection accounts for some cases.

PATHOGENESIS AND PATHOLOGY. Following spread of virus from one person to another, the virus replicates locally in peribasal and intermediate epithelial cells, resulting in lysis of cells and initiation of a local inflammatory response. This results in a characteristic thin-walled vesicle on an inflammatory base. Histologic study reveals multinucleated cells with ballooning degeneration, marked edema, and the characteristic Cowdry type A intranuclear inclusions which are indistinguishable from those caused by varicella-zoster virus. Lymphatics and regional lymph nodes may become infected, and in neonates or compromised hosts viremia and visceral dissemination may occur. In most persons, however, infection is controlled at the local site by host defense mechanisms. Although neutralizing antibody may contribute, cellular immune mechanisms, such as the production of interferon and induction of T cell reactivity and development of both natural killer cell and antibody-dependent lymphocyte cytotoxicity, are thought to have the major function in controlling HSV infections. Adults and children with depressed cell-mediated immune mechanisms appear to be more susceptible to severe disseminated HSV infections than those with depressed humoral immunity. Disease resulting from primary infection with HSV type 2 is more severe in those who have not experienced HSV type 1 infection previously than in those who have and who consequently possess immunity to HSV type 1. This suggests that heterotypic protective immunity is present.

Following primary infection, HSV becomes latent in the ganglia of the nerves supplying the infected areas; for HSV type 1 the trigeminal ganglion and for HSV type 2 the lumbosacral ganglia are most frequently involved. The virus does not remain latent at the skin or mucous membrane site. While the virus is latent, infectious virus is no longer detectable in specimens from patients and lesions do not occur. Viral DNA, but not intact virus, can be demonstrated in the ganglia. Methylation of viral DNA may play an important role in the maintenance of HSV latency. Productive infection in epithelial cells with cell lysis follows reactivation. In contrast, neurons do not undergo cell lysis during recurrences. Infectious virus appears to spread peripherally along sensory nerves to skin sites where productive infection leads to cell lysis, an inflammatory response, and development of the characteristic lesions.

CLINICAL MANIFESTATIONS. ***Primary Infection.*** Most commonly, primary infection with HSV type 1 is asymptomatic, but *gingivostomatitis* will occur in a small number, usually children one to three years of age. It can also occur in older children and adults. Following an incubation period of 2 to 12 days, prodromal symptoms of low grade fever and cervical adenopathy may occur. As the oral lesions appear, the temperature rises to 38.3 to 38.9° C, and there is intense oral pain, increased salivation, and foul breath. The oral lesions begin on the buccal and gingival mucosa and tongue and appear as multiple vesicles on an erythematous base. The vesicles coalesce and rupture, and ulcerative lesions appear with an erythematous margin covered with a yellowish, necrotic membrane. Leukocytosis is common. The disease varies considerably in severity and duration; however, it is self-limited and usually disappears by 14 days. The lesions heal without scar formation. In children, dehydration may occur because of poor fluid intake, drooling, and fever.

In adolescents, symptomatic primary infection with HSV type 1 more commonly takes the form of *pharyngitis* rather than gingivostomatitis, although the two may occur in combination. Pharyngitis alone also may be seen in younger children. Pharyngitis caused by HSV is characterized by sore throat, cervical adenopathy, exudate, fever, and headache in about two thirds of cases. It also may be associated with leukocytosis, dysphagia, chills, and myalgia. Submaxillary adenopathy is usually absent. Autoinoculation of other skin sites by the hands, with development of characteristic lesions, can occur in persons with either gingivostomatitis or pharyngitis.

Herpes simplex virus infections of the eye are usually caused by HSV type 1. Primary infection is an acute *keratoconjunctivitis* with or without skin involvement. If the lids are uninvolved, acute conjunctival follicular disease with nonsuppurative preauricular adenopathy is present. The presence of vesicles on the lid margins, which may require a magnifying lens or a slit lamp to see, is helpful in diagnosis. Overt involvement of the lids with multiple vesicles and lid edema may occur. Corneal involvement most characteristically takes the form of a branching (dendritic) ulcer. However, corneal manifestations may be atypical, especially early in illness, and consist of diffuse punctate lesions or wandering serpiginous ulcers without clear-cut branching. The disease is self-limited and resolves entirely without scarring in many cases. However, corneal involvement may lead to permanent scarring.

Primary *genital infection* is most common in adolescents and in young adults and is usually caused by HSV type 2. In the male, characteristic vesicular lesions on an erythematous base usually appear on the glans penis or the penile shaft. In the female, lesions may involve the vulva, perineum, buttocks, cervix, and vagina and are frequently accompanied by vaginal discharge. Primary infection in both sexes may be associated with fever, malaise, anorexia, and tender bilateral inguinal adenopathy. Although vesicular lesions may persist for several days, they usually ulcerate rapidly and become covered with a grayish-white exudate. These lesions are often exquisitely tender, and in the female urethral involvement may result in dysuria or urinary retention. Lesions of primary genital herpes may persist for several weeks before healing is complete. Herpetic sacral radiculomyelitis may rarely accompany genital infection.

Although manifestations of primary infection are generally oral or genital with either type of HSV, primary infection may involve other skin sites. When it involves the fingers, it is referred to as herpetic whitlow.

Primary perianal and rectal HSV infections are being recognized more frequently, particularly in male homosexuals. Pain, tenesmus, discharge, difficulty in urinating, and sacral paresthesias, as well as fever, chills, malaise, and headache occur commonly. Examination reveals vesicles and ulcerations. The disease is usually self-limited except in the setting of acquired immune deficiency syndrome (AIDS), in which proctitis may be progressive.

Recurrent Infections. The most common manifestation of recurrent infection with HSV type 1 is herpes labialis (fever blister, herpes simplex). The lesions of recurrent labial herpes are localized to the mucocutaneous junction of the lips or adjacent skin. The lower lip is more frequently involved than the upper lip, and in an individual patient lesions tend to occur at the same site. It is notable that although primary infections commonly occur within the mouth, recurrent oral herpes infections rarely involve mucous membranes. They are frequently heralded by prodromal symptoms, such as tingling or itching, which last for a few hours. Vesicles then appear and are often associated with considerable pain. The lesions progress from vesicle to ulcer to crust within 48 hours. Pain is most severe in the first 24 hours, and healing is complete within eight to ten days.

Recurrent ocular infection may take the form of epithelial infections or trophic ulcers, stromal disease (interstitial or disciform keratitis), iridocyclitis, or combinations of these. It is usually unilateral. Often the characteristic branching (dendritic) ulcers that stain with fluorescein are observed, and these are virtually diagnostic of HSV infection. Stromal disease is manifested by various forms of infiltrates underlying the ulcers, which result in opacification. Superficial keratitis usually heals, but recurrent infection with deep stromal involvement and uveitis may persist. Gradual diminution in visual acuity takes place with recurrent attacks, and permanent visual loss may result.

Recurrent genital lesions in both sexes are associated with less severe systemic symptoms and less extensive local involvement than primary attacks. They are often preceded by a prodrome of tenderness, itching, burning, or tingling. However, in occasional individuals, severe recurrent attacks may occur over a period of one or more years.

Other Manifestations. ENCEPHALITIS. Herpes simplex encephalitis is a rare complication of herpes virus infection. It is thought to be the most common sporadic viral encephalitis in the United States and is fully described in Ch. 499. The virus is believed to spread by neural routes into the brain, most often during recurrent infection, but also during primary infection. Almost all isolates from brain tissue of adults with encephalitis are HSV type 1. Encephalitis may also occur as part of disseminated neonatal infection with HSV type 2.

ASEPTIC MENINGITIS. Infrequently, in association with HSV type 2 genital infection, the clinical syndrome of aseptic meningitis, including fever, headache, stiff neck, and cerebrospinal fluid (CSF) pleocytosis, may occur. HSV type 2 has been isolated from the spinal fluid and blood in such cases. Isolation from the CSF, however, is rare.

CONGENITAL INFECTIONS. Congenital infection is very rare and probably results from retrograde spread of HSV type 2 from maternal genital infection to the placenta. Such infection may be recognized at birth by central nervous system manifestations such as microcephaly, intracranial calcifications, microphthalmia, seizures, and chorioretinitis, which are common to a number of chronic intrauterine infections.

NEONATAL INFECTIONS. Neonatal infections result from passage of the infant through an infected maternal genital tract or retrograde ascending infection if the membranes have ruptured. The overall risk of neonatal infection is low in women with primary or recurrent HSV type 2 infection after 32 weeks' gestation, but is higher if lesions are present at delivery. Infants born to mothers with primary infection during pregnancy are at greater risk of developing severe infection than are those whose mothers have recurrent genital herpes. Disease may range from mild self-limited skin infection to fatal disseminated infection with or without encephalitis. Localized skin disease occurs in 10 per cent of cases and is self-limited. Isolated involvement of the central nervous system (encephalitis) and eye (chorioretinitis) may lead to death or serious sequelae.

Disseminated neonatal infection usually appears a few days after birth, and vesicles may or may not be present. Vesicles eventually occur in 50 per cent of the infants, but may be absent early in infection. Patients may show constitutional signs and symptoms, irritability, seizures, respiratory distress, jaundice, petechiae, ecchymosis, and shock-like syndrome. Neurologic signs occur in 50 per cent of cases and include seizures, cranial nerve palsies, lethargy, and coma. CSF pleocytosis with increased protein and normal glucose also is commonly observed. Many of these patients will develop destructive encephalitis, disseminated intravascular coagulation, or hepatic and adrenal necrosis. About 75 per cent of patients die, and few recover without sequelae.

COMPROMISED HOSTS. Patients compromised by immunodeficiency or immunosuppression, by malnutrition, or by disorders of skin integrity such as burns or eczema are at greater risk of developing severe herpes simplex viral infections. Frequently the cardiac transplant recipient, and less so the renal transplant recipient, excretes HSV in throat washings for the first few months following grafting. Although some such patients may not have overt disease, some develop lesions which can be severe and persist for many weeks to months. Lesions may spread down the respiratory or gastrointestinal tracts and result in tracheobronchitis, pneumonia, or esophagitis. Patients with hematologic and lymphoreticular neoplasms and children with congenital thymic disorders may develop severe, chronic, progressive mucocutaneous HSV infection or disseminated disease. Disseminated disease has also been observed in pregnancy and in geriatric populations. Herpetic esophagitis may be related to nasogastric intubation and results in dysphasia and substernal pain. Burn wound infections with HSV are becoming increasingly well recognized, as are HSV infections in patients with a variety of other skin disorders.

Severe herpes infections, particularly progressive perianal ulcers, colitis, esophagitis, and pneumonia, are prominent features of AIDS.

ERYTHEMA MULTIFORME. About 5 to 15 per cent of all cases of erythema multiforme are regularly preceded by an attack of herpes simplex. Either HSV type 1 or HSV type 2 infections may be involved, and the cutaneous manifestations may range from mild to severe (Stevens-Johnson syndrome) and may be recurrent.

OTHER SYNDROMES. Attempts have been made to relate HSV infections to a variety of neurologic syndromes such as multiple sclerosis, Bell's palsy, some atypical pain syndromes, ascending myelitis, trigeminal neuralgia, temporal lobe epilepsy, and others, but there is no definitive proof of a causal relationship for any of these associations. However, there is evidence of infectious virus (HSV type 2), viral antigens, and viral DNA sequences in cervical carcinoma cells, but the exact role of HSV type 2 in the production of cervical cancer is not clear.

DIAGNOSIS. In most minor infections, diagnosis is dependent on clinical recognition. Gingivostomatitis must be differentiated from aphthous stomatitis, Stevens-Johnson syndrome, Vincent's infection, infectious mononucleosis, herpangina, and streptococcal or diphtheritic pharyngitis. Pharyngitis caused by HSV infection must be differentiated from that caused by streptococci, EB virus, and other viruses. Cervical adenopathy, exudate, and fever are more common in HSV than in other kinds of viral pharyngitis. If dendritic ulcers are present in patients with keratitis, they are virtually diagnostic of HSV infection; however, these ulcers have also been observed in varicella-zoster virus infections, and corneal abrasions are occasionally mistaken for HSV infection. The presence of multiple vesicular genital lesions or ulcerative lesions associated with pain helps differentiate herpes simplex genital infections from other forms of venereal disease such as syphilis and chancroid. Infections of other skin sites, particularly if they have a dermatomal distribution, must be distinguished from varicella-zoster virus infection. Severe anorectal pain, difficulty in urination, and sacral paresthesias are more common in HSV perianal and rectal disease than in other forms of proctitis. Recurrent herpes labialis is easily recognized clinically. Recurrent intraoral lesions are usually not herpes simplex but rather aphthous stomatitis or some other malady, but intraoral lesions may occur with HSV infections in the immunocompromised or immunosuppressed patient. Recurrent eye and genital infections commonly can be recognized by their characteristic clinical manifestations. Congenital infections may be difficult to distinguish from similar syndromes caused by rubella virus, cytomegalovirus, or *Toxoplasma gondii*. Neonatal infection with HSV may be mistaken for neonatal sepsis, erythema toxicum, streptococcal infection, and enteroviral infection. In more severe infections viral isolation attempts are helpful. Severe skin infection in older patients and disseminated infection in immunocompromised patients may also be diagnosed by recovery of virus. Burn wound infections, unless there are typical vesicular areas, usually must be diagnosed by viral isolation or biopsy for intranuclear inclusions.

Definitive diagnosis can be made by isolation of HSV from lesions. However, 1 to 15 per cent of asymptomatic normals will shed HSV in oral secretions and presumably a similar number in genital secretions. Therefore, isolation of virus from these sites may not be related to active disease. HSV types 1 and 2 replicate in a variety of cell lines, and cytopathic effects appear rapidly, usually within 24 to 48 hours. Specimens should be collected early by aspiration of vesicles or swabbing the open lesions, and promptly inoculated into cell cultures. If transportation to the laboratory must be delayed, specimens can be stored at 4° C for a few hours, or, if storage is longer than 24 hours, they should be stored at −70° C.

Histologic diagnosis is based on the presence of giant cells, intranuclear inclusions, or both in scrapings of lesions or biopsies of tissue. Scrapings may be smeared, fixed with ethanol or methanol, and stained with Giemsa, Wright, or Papanicolaou (preferred) stain. Usually only giant cells are seen on scrapings and smears, and intranuclear inclusions in HSV infection cannot be distinguished from those of varicella-zoster virus infection.

Development of serum antibodies when none existed previously is often helpful in recognizing primary infection but is of little value in recurrent infections. Measurement of IgM antibodies to HSV may be helpful in the diagnosis of neonatal infection. Such antibodies usually appear within the first four weeks of life in infected infants and persist for many months. Unfortunately, measurement of IgM antibodies in older persons has not proved useful in separating primary from recurrent infection.

TREATMENT. Specific antiviral chemotherapy is now available for some HSV infections. Vidarabine (adenine arabinoside, ara-A), has been shown to be effective and is licensed in the United States. Ophthalmic ointment (3 per cent) is administered as one half inch of ointment into the lower conjunctival sac five times a day at three-hour intervals. Intravenous vidarabine is effective in patients with HSV encephalitis. It is administered to patients with proven or suspected HSV encephalitis in a dose of 15 mg per kilogram per day for ten days. This drug is somewhat insoluble (maximum 0.75 mg per milliliter with warming) and thus requires substantial amounts of fluid, and patients may experience difficulties with fluid overload. Intravenous vidarabine has also been shown to be effective in neonatal disseminated herpes simplex infections. It is not effective topically against herpes labialis or other skin or genital infections.

Idoxuridine (IDU or 2′-deoxy-5-iodouridine) and trifluorothymidine have also been shown to be effective in the treatment of HSV keratitis, and are licensed for this purpose in the United States.

Acyclovir is effective for treatment of primary herpes genitalis, progressive mucocutaneous disease in immunosuppressed patients, and herpes keratitis. It is available as a topical 5 per cent ointment and as an intravenous form. An oral form is under study. Topical therapy is effective in primary but not in recurrent genital infections. Intravenous and oral acyclovir are more effective in recurrent and may be effective in primary genital infections. Topical acyclovir therapy is not recommended for recurrent herpes labialis.

As one might expect, immune serum globulin is not effective for treatment, since recurrent infections develop in the presence of high titers of circulating antibodies.

PROPHYLAXIS. Medical and dental personnel should be strongly encouraged to avoid direct contact with potential infectious lesions by wearing gloves. Patients with extensive herpetic lesions should be isolated. Either temporary abstinence or at least the use of condoms has been recommended to prevent genital spread when one sexual partner has active lesions. Continued use of condoms may be useful if there is a history of recurrent genital infections.

Prevention of neonatal disease in offspring of mothers with genital infection presents special problems in which considerable controversy exists. If there is clinically apparent cervical infection or genital virus excretion is detected at parturition before membranes rupture, a cesarean section is recommended. If rupture of the membranes has occurred, it is uncertain whether cesarean section will be effective in preventing infection, although rapid delivery by either route is clearly indicated to lessen exposure to the infant. If no lesions are obvious at delivery, only rarely is virus recoverable and vaginal delivery appears safe.

Corey L, Adams HG, Brown ZA, Holmes KK: Genital herpes simplex virus infections: Clinical manifestations, course and complications. Ann Intern Med 98:958, 1983. *Recent, well referenced review of genital HSV.*

Goodell SE, Quinn TC, Mkrtichian E, Schuffler MD, Holmes KK, Corey L: Herpes simplex virus proctitis in homosexual men. Clinical, sigmoidoscopic and histopathological features. N Engl J Med 308:868, 1983.

Hirsch MS, Schooley RT: Treatment of herpes virus infections. N Engl J Med 309:963, 1983. *An up-to-date, well referenced review of acyclovir, vidarabine, and other therapeutic agents in HSV infections.*

Whitley RH, Soong SJ, Hirsch MS, Karchmer AW, Dolin R, Galasso G, Dunnick JK, Alford CA, the NIAID Collaborative Antiviral Study Group: Herpes simplex encephalitis. Vidarabine therapy and diagnostic problems. N Engl J Med 304:313, 1981. *Follow-up of original controlled study with emphasis on diagnosis and prognosis.*

Wong KK, Hirsch MS: Herpes virus infections in patients with neoplastic disease. Ann Intern Med 76:464, 1984. *Well referenced summary of diagnosis and therapy with vidarabine, acyclovir, and alpha interferon.*

337. CYTOMEGALOVIRUS INFECTION

David J. Lang

DEFINITION. Infections caused by cytomegalovirus (CMV) may be asymptomatic or may cause disseminated and even fatal multisystem disease, depending upon the mode and timing of virus acquisition and the immune competence of the host. CMV infections occur commonly, although with variable severity, in the fetus and in immunocompromised individuals.

ETIOLOGY. CMV is a species-specific member of the herpesvirus group. Like other herpesviruses, CMV has the capacity to replicate persistently in the face of normal host immunity and to establish latent infections subject to reactivation. CMV cytopathology is focal in vitro, and replication of the virus is largely limited to cell cultures of species-specific fibroblasts. In vivo, however, CMV replicates in epithelial as well as fibroblastic elements. Subtypes of CMV can be distinguished, although the variants are without apparent clinical significance.

EPIDEMIOLOGY. CMV is worldwide in distribution, and the incidence of infection lacks consistent seasonality. Persistence, latency, and reactivation of CMV have made it difficult to interpret the etiologic significance of the recovery of the virus.

The age of acquisition of CMV is variable. In less developed parts of the world, CMV infection is acquired universally in infancy, probably at or shortly after parturition. Where interpersonal contact is reduced and sanitation is more universal, the acquisition of CMV infection is delayed and occurs gradually through infancy, childhood, and even adulthood. No specific genetic factors have as yet been identified that contribute to CMV colonization, infection, or persistence. Transmission of CMV is associated with close interpersonal (including sexual) contact or with direct introduction of cells or body fluids. CMV virus has been recovered from virtually all organs and tissues and can be found in urine, saliva, blood, semen, milk, secretions of the uterine cervix, and stool. This very prevalent virus is opportunistic; it reactivates in, is transmitted to, and spreads from hosts whose defenses are compromised. Since these patients are often found in hospital settings, this virus can provide a troublesome nosocomial problem, although spread occurs infrequently.

Prenatal CMV infection is the most common known congenital infection of humans. It occurs in about 1 per cent of infants born in the United States (0.5 to 8 per cent depending upon the population studied). Most of these infections reflect prenatal transmission of CMV reactivated during pregnancy in otherwise healthy immune women. As many as 30 per cent of pregnant women may shed CMV at some time and from some site during pregnancy. Active CMV shedding and perinatal transmission occur more frequently in young women.

PATHOGENESIS AND PATHOLOGY. CMV replicates slowly in vitro. Infected cells swell and develop characteristic intranuclear and paranuclear inclusions. In vitro CMV infections are accompanied by some changes associated with morphologic transformation. It has been possible to transform cells permanently by infecting with irradiated virus and in this way interfering selectively with the full cycle of virus replication and cytopathology. These CMV-transformed cells have malignant potential in certain animals. Whether CMV plays a role in the pathogenesis of malignancy in humans is unresolved.

CMV can and frequently does reactivate in immune hosts. When immune function is immature or compromised, reactivated virus can spread, causing significant injury and functional impairment. The pathogenesis of transplacental spread in the presence of intact maternal immunity remains unclear.

That CMV is carried in circulating cells of healthy individuals appears certain on the basis of epidemiologic observations. It is estimated that approximately 5 per cent of donor units of blood can transmit CMV. Nevertheless, it has been difficult to recover this virus from the circulating cells of healthy individuals.

Latent CMV may also be transmitted with transplanted organs. The superimposition of iatrogenic immunosuppression then further encourages CMV spread. Transmission of CMV with blood products has provided a particularly difficult problem for blood banks. The use of CMV antibody-negative units has been recommended for high-risk groups such as selected newborns or allograft recipients.

CLINICAL MANIFESTATIONS. ***Postnatal CMV Infection in Normal Hosts.*** In healthy individuals CMV infection is usually asymptomatic or unrecognized. Occasionally primary CMV infection is accompanied by a self-limited mononucleosis-like syndrome characterized by fever, splenomegaly, mild hepatocellular dysfunction, lymphoid hyperplasia including the presence of atypical lymphocytes, occasional thrombocytopenia, hemolysis, and inconsistent skin rash. Pharyngitis is not prominent. The fever may range from 39° to over 40° C (103 to 105° F) and in some instances is accompanied by night sweats and chills. Between febrile episodes the patient, although tired, does not feel very ill.

Some cases of mild to moderate hepatitis have been associated with CMV infection, and infrequently a normal host will experience an interstitial pneumonitis caused by this virus. There have been reports associating prior CMV infection with the Guillian-Barré syndrome. CMV infections have also been associated with isolated thrombocytopenia, hemolytic anemia, and ulcerative gastrointestinal disease.

Postnatal CMV Infection in Abnormal Hosts. Individuals undergoing open-heart surgery requiring perfusion and others receiving multiple units of blood may experience a mononucleosis-like illness about three to six weeks later. The illness can be mistaken for bacterial sepsis or endocarditis, a particularly important distinction in recipients of cardiac prostheses.

CMV infections have been a major problem for allograft recipients. Latent virus may be reactivated by immune suppression. Alternatively, the response to the allograft or, in the case of marrow transplantation, a graft versus host reaction, may stimulate virus reactivation. Immune suppression limits the ability of the host to restrict virus spread. Infection with this virus can be associated with significant and even fatal interstitial pneumonitis, hepatitis, encephalitis, and diffuse cytomegalic inclusion disease.

CMV infections have been found prominently in the acquired immune deficiency syndrome (AIDS). There has been speculation concerning the etiologic relevance of CMV to AIDS and to Kaposi's sarcoma. However, CMV (and other) infections associated with AIDS are more likely to be opportunistic, since immunologic impairment is prominent in this condition. Nevertheless, since CMV infections are often associated with some depression of the helper-suppressor T cell ratio, the differentiation between cause and effect, opportunism and pathogenesis, remains unclear.

Prenatal and Perinatal CMV Infection. Prenatal CMV infections were first appreciated through retrospective pathologic studies. Since the recognition of the infection depended on post-mortem examinations, it was initially concluded that prenatal CMV infection was rare and always fatal. The severe disseminated infection was termed *cytomegalic inclusion disease.* Subsequently, cytologic techniques identified CMV infection in living infants by the presence of large nuclear-inclusion–bearing cells in urinary sediment. The isolation of virus in vitro proved to be an even more sensitive technique. It became apparent that infants congenitally infected with CMV could survive and that manifestations of these infections resembled those associated with other prenatal infections. The CMV-infected infants were often small for gestational age and microcephalic. In some cases they exhibited intracerebral calcifications, hepatosplenomegaly, chorioretinitis, thrombocytopenia with purpura, macular rash, hemolytic anemia, and a variety of structural and functional organ impairments.

Prospective studies determined that congenital infections with CMV were not unusual or rare. Overall, about 1 per cent of babies were found to be prenatally infected with CMV. Prenatal CMV infection is particularly prevalent among infants of primiparous, young, unmarried, and promiscuous women. Most CMV-infected infants appear normal at birth, but as many as 10 to 20 per cent of such apparently symptomless congenital CMV infections are associated with learning disabilities, hearing impairment, or evidence of cognitive dysfunction.

Women who are immune prior to conception may give birth to CMV-infected infants. The birth to one woman of more than one CMV-infected infant with identical viral strains has been documented. It seems certain that at least some prenatal CMV infections are acquired from previously latent maternal virus reactivated during gestation.

Perinatal acquisition of CMV infection (from infected cervix, breast milk, or saliva) is usually asymptomatic. However, an infant born to a CMV-seronegative woman may develop significant postnatal pneumonia or hepatitis if infected with CMV via transfusions.

DIAGNOSIS. The laboratory isolation of CMV is accomplished in tissue culture and requires the prompt transportation of refrigerated specimens to a prepared virus laboratory. Up to five weeks can be required for recovery and identification of virus. Occasional prolonged shedding of virus and the intermittent reactivation of latent CMV may confuse the interpretation of virus recovery. The isolation of CMV at certain times (from urine taken during the first days of life) or from unusual sites (blood, spinal fluid, or tissues specifically involved in the disease process) makes the etiologic association of virus and clinical condition more likely. Demonstration of simultaneous seroconversion or significant (four-fold or greater) serologic change further strengthens the association. CMV serology may be assessed by complement-fixation, immunofluorescence, enzyme-linked immunosorbent assay (ELISA) procedures, and indirect hemagglutination. The use of CMV-specific IgM serology to identify recent infections may be rendered less useful by the presence of rheumatoid factor (false positives) and by the tendency of CMV IgM to persist in some instances and to reappear when latent virus is reactivated.

DIFFERENTIAL DIAGNOSIS. Congenital infections caused by toxoplasmosis, rubella, syphilis, and herpes simplex virus may be difficult to distinguish from those caused by CMV. All may be associated with intrauterine growth retardation, hepatic and splenic enlargement, purpura, thrombocytopenia, and hemolysis. Congenital toxoplasmosis can be associated as well with chorioretinitis and intracerebral calcifications.

Congenital rubella is associated with glaucoma, microphthalmia, cataracts, and cardiac malformations more frequently than is congenital CMV infection. The retinitis of congenital rubella, unlike that of CMV, is often marked by punctate retinal pigmentation.

Herpes simplex virus can be transmitted transplacentally, although usually neonatal herpes infection reflects the perinatal acquisition of the virus. Herpes infections are often associated with vesicular skin lesions, although systemic visceral and central nervous system infection may occur without rash.

In all of these instances the distinctions are made ultimately by laboratory studies. Specific IgM determinations are available for CMV, toxoplasmosis, rubella, and herpes simplex. The presence of a positive test for specific IgM to only one of these agents is usually diagnostic. The recovery of the specific agent in the case of CMV, rubella, or herpes simplex is also a rigorous means of identification. Differentiation of all of these conditions is important, since specific treatment is available for herpes simplex and for toxoplasmosis. The distinction of congenital syphilis or of bacterial sepsis, other potentially confusing entities in the neonate, is also important to facilitate specific therapy.

Postnatally acquired CMV infections may be difficult to distinguish from those caused by Epstein-Barr virus (EBV). EBV mononucleosis is often associated with a positive heterophil-agglutination reaction. CMV mononucleosis is always heterophil-negative. Hepatitis associated with CMV infection is generally milder than that associated with hepatitis A, B, or non-A, non-B viruses. The ultimate distinction between these conditions is dependent upon the results of virus-specific tests.

CMV interstitial pneumonitis cannot be identified on clinical grounds alone but requires the use of virologic studies applied to clinical samples, especially those from lung biopsies and needle aspirations.

PROGNOSIS. The outlook for normal development is poor in infants who are infected prenatally with CMV. Even among those with the apparently symptomless congenital CMV infections, as many as 20 per cent by school age may manifest significant sensorineural dysfunction.

Among individuals with acquired CMV infections, the prognosis is dependent upon the immune status of the host. In otherwise healthy persons, acquired CMV infections are self-limited and generally not associated with late complications. Among immunocompromised individuals, including transplant recipients, the outlook may vary from those who recover, maintain (allograft) function, and are without sequelae, to those who die with progressive interstitial pneumonitis. Disseminated CMV may predispose to significant life-threatening bacterial infections.

TREATMENT. A variety of nucleoside analogs, other antiviral drugs, transfer factor, antiserum, and steroids have been administered in an effort to treat CMV infections. None of these has been conclusively successful. Some drugs such as cytosine and adenine arabinoside have been associated with transient depression of virus titers. None has altered the clinical condition, nor has any of these agents curtailed the ultimate course of the virus infection. The intensive use of interferon in renal transplant recipients has reduced the shedding of virus and apparently improved the associated clinical conditions. Withdrawal of immunosuppression has been used as a means to control CMV infections in allograft recipients.

PREVENTION. "Attenuated" CMV vaccine strains have been produced in England and the United States. These candidate vaccine strains have been administered to volunteers, including health care workers, and to some individuals awaiting an allograft. The vaccines proved to be immunogenic and have not thus far been associated with detectable virus shedding or reactivation. Inoculated individuals who later received transplants and were immunosuppressed nevertheless did experience CMV reinfection and associated virus shedding.

Because of the questions associated with the production and use of attenuated CMV strains coupled with the evidence that immunity does ameliorate if not prevent prenatal and postnatal CMV infections, attention is also being directed to the development of subunit and peptide immunogens.

Adler SP: Transfusion-associated cytomegalovirus infections. Rev Infect Dis 5:977, 1983. *Comprehensive up-to-date review of transfusion-associated CMV infections with discussion of mechanisms as well as straightforward clinical issues.*

Betts RF: Cytomegalovirus infection in transplant patients. Prog Med Virol 23:44, 1982. *A very good discussion of the reciprocal impact of CMV upon all varieties of allograft. Contains an excellent summary of epidemiologic factors.*

Ho M: Cytomegalovirus, Biology and Infection. New York, Plenum Publishing Corp., 1982. *Treatise covering all aspects of CMV infection in humans. Small but thorough section pertinent to murine CMV. Very comprehensive bibliography.*

Mintz L, Drew WL, Miner RC, Braff EH: Cytomegalovirus infections in homosexual men. Ann Intern Med 99:326, 1983. *Prospective study covering aspects of sexual transmission of CMV in a homosexual population, with implications for AIDS.*

Zaia JA, Lang DJ: Cytomegalovirus infection of the fetus and neonate. Neurol Clin 2:387, 1984. *Recent review covering all aspects of pre- and perinatal CMV infection with discussion of some current hypotheses as well as comprehensive data review.*

338. INFECTIOUS MONONUCLEOSIS

*John A. Zaia**

DEFINITION. Infectious mononucleosis is an acute infection caused by Epstein-Barr virus (EBV). Symptomatic disease includes fever, sore throat, lymphadenopathy, and lymphocytosis with splenomegaly.

ETIOLOGY. EBV is a member of the herpesvirus group and was first isolated in tissue culture cell lines derived from Burkitt's lymphoma. Observation of EBV antibody seroconversion in a laboratory technician with infectious mononucleosis led to the etiologic connection of EBV with infectious mononucleosis. EBV has been isolated from cultures of peripheral blood, nasopharynx, and lymph nodes of persons with acute infectious mononucleosis.

Attempts to transmit infectious mononucleosis experimentally to volunteers by means of blood, throat washings, or stool suspensions from patients in the acute phase of infectious mononucleosis have been inconclusive or negative, probably because of the inclusion of seropositive nonsusceptible persons in the volunteer group. Infectious mononucleosis can be transmitted by blood transfusion. Seropositive college students with antibody to the viral capsid antigen (VCA) do not develop acute infectious mononucleosis. The disease is seen only in seronegative individuals.

INCIDENCE AND PREVALENCE. As in the other human herpesvirus infections, the incidence and prevalence of EBV infection are functions of socioeconomic factors that determine crowding and hygienic conditions. Infection occurs early in life in the less developed countries and is usually inapparent. In the more developed nations, EBV infection occurs later in life, usually in older children and adolescents. The ratio of asymptomatic to symptomatic disease in the middle class college population is approximately 2:1.

---

*With the assistance of David J. Lang.

EPIDEMIOLOGY. The source of EBV infection is contaminated body fluid(s), usually oropharyngeal secretions. EBV is readily demonstrated in the saliva of patients with infectious mononucleosis and also occurs late after infection in persons who have periodic reactivation of this virus. Antibody-positive individuals have been shown to be permanent carriers and to become intermittent excretors of EBV. Contact with infected saliva during intimate oral contact or from contaminated eating and drinking utensils provides the usual means of infection. Infections are transmitted by extracellular virus and occasionally by infected cells, as during blood transfusions. The incubation period is estimated to be between five and seven weeks when the disease occurs in young adults.

PATHOLOGY AND PATHOGENESIS. The pathology of EBV infection is confined to the lymphoid tissues. There is extensive hyperplasia of the lymph nodes, with partial obliteration and distention of lymphoid sinuses by macrophages, atypical lymphocytes, and plasma cells. Lymphoid follicular structure is maintained with occasional areas of focal necrosis and perivascular infiltration by atypical mononuclear cells. In the liver, patchy mononuclear cell infiltrates occur in the portal areas and in the lobular sinusoids. The bone marrow may contain granulomas.

The lymphoproliferative manifestations are related to two pathogenetic aspects of EBV infection: an initial virus infection with virus-induced proliferation of B lymphocytes and a secondary reaction of T lymphocytes to control the infection. The resultant immunopathologic events lead to the clinical syndrome of infectious mononucleosis. The peripheral blood contains large atypical lymphocytes (Downey cells), which consist of both transformed B cells and reactive T cells. Although these cells can be seen in other viral infections, they are most pronounced in infectious mononucleosis.

CLINICAL MANIFESTATIONS. Following a prodromal period lasting four to five days in which malaise, fatigue, and headache can occur, the principal clinical features of fever, sore throat, and cervical lymphadenopathy appear. Signs and symptoms can be quite variable and atypical, especially in children and the elderly. In the usual case of mononucleosis, fever persists for seven to ten days and may be greater than 39.5° C. Concomitantly, sore throat develops during the first week of disease, with inflammation and edema of the pharynx and exudative tonsillitis. A palatal enanthem can occur, consisting of petechiae on the palate, which cannot be distinguished from streptococcal pharyngitis. Lymph node enlargement is especially prominent in the anterior and posterior cervical nodes, but generalized adenopathy is often present. The lymph nodes are readily palpable and can be exquisitely tender. The lymphadenopathy persists for several weeks.

Splenomegaly occurs in approximately 50 per cent of patients and is greatest during the second and third weeks of illness. A rare complication of infectious mononucleosis is splenic rupture, which can be life-threatening. Although hepatosplenomegaly occurs in only 10 per cent of patients, liver function test results are frequently abnormal and clinical jaundice may develop during the first two weeks of illness. Elevated serum enzyme levels can persist for several weeks. During the first week as many as 10 per cent of patients develop a skin rash consisting of transient erythematous maculopapular eruptions on the trunk and proximal extremities. Although usually rubelliform in nature, the rash occasionally can be scarlatiniform, urticarial, or even hemorrhagic. Use of ampicillin and other antibiotics is frequently associated with skin rash. Bilateral supraorbital edema has been described as an early clinical finding.

Complications involving the central nervous system include Guillain-Barré syndrome, Bell's palsy, transverse myelitis, and meningoencephalitis. In addition, pneumonitis, myocarditis, pericarditis, nephritis, acquired hemolytic anemia, thrombocytopenic purpura, agranulocytosis, and aplastic anemia have been described during EBV infection.

The X-linked lymphoproliferative syndrome is a genetically inherited disease in which EBV infection can result in a lethal outcome. Susceptible individuals have been described with overwhelming EBV infection and fatal hepatitis, lymphoma, or agammaglobulinemia following EBV infection.

DIAGNOSIS. Infectious mononucleosis is diagnosed on the basis of clinical manifestations, characteristic blood abnormalities, and heterophile and EBV antibody titers. The white blood cell count may be normal or slightly low during the first week of infectious mononucleosis, but during the second and third weeks the white blood cell count is elevated to between 10,000 and 20,000 per square millimeter. The white blood cell differential count generally shows more than 50 per cent mononuclear cells, of which at least 10 per cent are atypical, with considerable pleomorphism. The atypical lymphocytosis may persist for several months. Occasionally, the total white blood cell count in the second and third weeks of illness is markedly elevated and can be as high as 50,000 per square millimeter. The Downey cells appear as large variably shaped cells with round, indented, or lobulated nuclei and with basophilic vacuolated cytoplasm.

Heterophile antibodies, mostly of the IgM class, develop transiently during the course of infectious mononucleosis and can be directed against sheep, horse, and bovine erythrocytes and also against such factors as I/i blood groups, immunoglobulin, nuclear factors, and Proteus OX19. The most frequent and useful heterophile antibodies in infectious mononucleosis are the agglutinins for sheep or horse erythrocytes and the hemolysins of bovine red blood cells. The development of antibody to sheep erythrocyte agglutinins in infectious mononucleosis was first described in 1932 by Paul and Bunnell. These antibodies were subsequently shown to be adsorbed by guinea pig kidney cell suspensions but not by bovine erythrocytes. The antibodies are referred to as the *heterophile agglutinins of Paul-Bunnell-Davidson (PBD).* The heterophile agglutinins are, with very rare exceptions, specific for infectious mononucleosis and form the basis for the currently available slide agglutination tests. These commercially available test kits give quick results and are generally specific for infectious mononucleosis, although false negative results can be observed when heterophile antibody titers are low, and false positive results occasionally can be seen. The PBD heterophile agglutinins are usually detectable during the first week of illness, but approximately 10 per cent of adolescent patients and a larger percentage of children fail to develop heterophile antibodies.

The EBV-specific serologic tests consist of the viral capsid antigen (VCA), the viral membrane antigen, the viral early antigens (EA), and the viral nuclear antigens (EBNA). Diagnostically significant increments in titer of antibody to VCA from acute to convalescent phases are observed in no more than 10 to 20 per cent of infectious mononucleosis patients. This is because VCA antibody is usually produced prior to clinical symptoms that are mediated by early immunopathologic events. IgM antibody to VCA is frequently present and is of proven value in the serodiagnosis of primary EBV infection. Antibody to EA is observed in 70 to 85 per cent of patients in the acute phase of infectious mononucleosis. This test is interpreted in two ways: diffuse staining of the nucleus and cytoplasm is seen during the acute phase of infectious mononucleosis, and a restricted staining of the cytoplasm is seen in prolonged cases of EBV infection. Antibody to EBNA appears only weeks or months after onset of illness and can be utilized to document EBV infection when early sera are not available. The EBV-specific antibody assays are not essential for the diagnosis of infectious mononucleosis when the heterophile antibody test result is positive. These tests should be reserved for heterophile-antibody–negative cases of mononucleosis-like illnesses and for evaluation of syndromes suggestive of EBV complications.

DIFFERENTIAL DIAGNOSIS. Infectious mononucleosis resembles several disorders associated with the nonspecific findings of fever, exudative tonsillitis, lymphadenopathy, and splenomegaly. Adenoviral pharyngitis and tonsillitis, streptococcal pharyngotonsillitis, diphtheria, and Vincent's angina can have oropharyngeal pathology similar to that associated with EBV infection. Mononucleosis syndromes are associated with cytomegalovirus infection, toxoplasmosis, hepatitis A, and hepatitis B and cannot be readily distinguished from infectious mononucleosis. Appropriate serologic tests should be used to exclude these entities. The heterophile agglutination tests specific for infectious mononucleosis are never positive in these conditions.

Blood dyscrasia, especially acute lymphocytic leukemia, can be similar to changes associated with infectious mononucleosis. Bone marrow examination should be performed in those individuals having a lymphoproliferative disease that lacks the diagnostic criteria of infectious mononucleosis.

TREATMENT. Infectious mononucleosis can be treated with corticosteroids when life-threatening complications are present. A ten-day course of prednisone is used starting with 60 mg per square meter on the first day and gradually decreasing this dosage by 5 mg per square meter per day. This is indicated for such complications as airway obstruction, neurologic complications, thrombocytopenia purpura, hemolytic anemia, and myocarditis.

The possible use of corticosteroid therapy for the treatment of uncomplicated infectious mononucleosis remains controversial. A well controlled study of steroid therapy demonstrated a decrease in the number of days of fever in the steroid-treated group. There is no clear evidence that this treatment increases the risk of other complications or the long-term potential risks of EBV infection such as lymphoproliferative disease and malignancy. At present, because of the known increased risks of lymphoproliferative neoplasm occurring in immunosuppressed allograft recipients with EBV infection, it would appear prudent to use steroid therapy only for severe complications of EBV infection.

PROGNOSIS. Infectious mononucleosis is generally a self-limited disease in which the acute symptoms subside within four to six weeks. Marked fatigue usually accompanies the convalescent period, and the patient should anticipate certain limitations to normal activity. Occasionally, these symptoms of fatigue persist for several months with or without abnormal liver function tests or other laboratory abnormalities. There is no explanation for the prolonged period of convalescence, which can last for many months in certain persons.

Andiman WA: The Epstein-Barr virus and EB virus infections in childhood. J Pediatr 95:171, 1979. *A review of EBV infection in the pediatric patient.*

Epstein MA, Achong BG: The Epstein-Barr Virus. New York, Springer-Verlag, 1979. *A complete review of laboratory and clinical aspects of EBV infection.*

Fleisher GR, Collins M, Fager S: Limitations of available tests for diagnosis of infectious mononucleosis. J Clin Microbiol 17:619, 1983. *Description of specificity and sensitivity of diagnostic tests for EBV.*

Hoagland RJ: The transmission of infectious mononucleosis. Am J Med Sci 229:262, 1955. *A classic description of EBV epidemiology.*

Horowitz CA, Henle W, Henle G, Schapiro R, Borken S, Bundtzen R: Infectious mononucleosis in patients aged 40 to 72 years: Report of 27 cases, including 3 without heterophil-antibody responses. Medicine 62:256, 1983. *A description of clinical EBV infection in older persons.*

Purtilo DT, Sakamoto K, Saemundsen AK, Sullivan JL, Synnerholm AC, Anvret M, Pritchard J, Sloper C, Sieff C, Pincott J, Pachman L, Rich K, Cruzi F, Cornet JA, Collins R, Barnes N, Knight J, Sandstedt B, Klein G: Documentation of Epstein-Barr virus infection in immunodeficient patients with life-threatening lymphoproliferative diseases by clinical, virological, and immunopathological studies. Cancer Res 41:4226, 1981. *Review of X-linked lymphoproliferative syndrome.*

339. VARICELLA AND HERPES ZOSTER

Sidney Kibrick

DEFINITION. Varicella (chickenpox) is an acute infectious disease, characterized by a generalized vesicular eruption which appears in crops over several days. It is most common in childhood.

Herpes zoster (shingles) is an acute infectious disease involving sensory ganglia and their cutaneous areas of innervation. It is characterized by pain along the distribution of the affected nerve and crops of clustered vesicles over the corresponding dermatome. It is usually unilateral and involves a single or adjacent dermatomes. The disease represents reactivation of a latent varicella virus in individuals with partial immunity to this agent.

ETIOLOGY. The agent responsible for these disorders is the varicella-zoster virus (V-Z virus), a member of the herpesvirus group. Weller isolated etiologic agents from both diseases in 1953 and subsequently established their similarity. Only one serotype is recognized. The virion, which is about 200 nm in diameter, has a DNA core, an icosahedral capsid, and a lipid containing envelope. Man is the only known natural host. The virus is quite labile and loses its infectivity quickly (probably within hours) in the external environment.

VARICELLA

EPIDEMIOLOGY. The disease is spread by airborne droplets and by direct contact with infected lesions. It may also be spread from person to person by a third individual (i.e., by indirect contact) within a limited time and distance, as on a hospital ward. Varicella is communicable from one to two days before onset of the rash until all the vesicles have crusted—five or six days after the rash appears in the average case, somewhat longer in more severe cases. The prodrome and early stages of eruption represent the periods of greatest communicability.

Although V-Z virus may be spread by respiratory secretions, it has rarely been possible to isolate this agent from nasal or pharyngeal secretions. By contrast, infectious virus is easily recovered from vesicle fluid.

Incidence and Prevalence. Varicella is primarily a disease of childhood. In temperate zones it is most common between two and eight years, with a peak on beginning school. Cases occur throughout the year but predominate in winter and spring. Inapparent infections are rare. Newborns of mothers who have had the disease are protected by maternal antibodies for up to about six months, but the degree of protection varies. Varicella is one of the most contagious of infectious diseases. Susceptible children exposed to cases in the same household had a secondary attack rate of 87 per cent. Histories of this disease in adults are often unreliable; in one study only 8 per cent of adults with supposedly negative histories acquired varicella from household contacts. Individuals with varicella usually develop lifelong immunity (but may subsequently develop zoster).

PATHOGENESIS AND PATHOLOGY. It is assumed that the virus enters and initially replicates in the respiratory tract. A viremia follows that disseminates virus throughout the body. Focal lesions then appear in the skin and occasionally in the viscera and enlarge by virus spread from infected to contiguous cells. The occurrence of the lesions in crops is consistent with an intermittent viremia. With appearance of circulating antibody (about one to four days after onset of the rash) the viremia ceases and symptoms begin to subside.

The histopathology of the skin lesions in varicella, herpes zoster, and herpes simplex is identical. Cells in the basal and prickle layers undergo ballooning degeneration, and edema fluid quickly accumulates, elevating the stratum corneum to form a clear vesicle containing large amounts of infective virus. The adjacent infected cells develop an eosinophilic inclusion in each nucleus. In addition, multinucleated giant cells containing such inclusions begin to form at the edges and base of the lesion. As the vesicles begin to dry, they become cloudy with accumulated inflammatory cells and desquamated epidermal cells, and the viral content declines. Finally the lesions crust, the epithelial cells at their base regenerate, and the crusts are shed. In fatal cases, areas of focal necrosis associated with cells showing characteristic intranuclear inclusions may be found throughout the respiratory tract, kidneys, adrenals, liver, and other organs.

The pathologic changes associated with varicella encephalitis are nonspecific and are similar to those seen in the other viral postinfectious encephalitides (see Ch. 506).

CLINICAL MANIFESTATIONS. After an incubation period of 14 to 16 days (range, 10 to 23 days), the disease is usually manifested in young children by low grade fever, malaise, and rash. In older patients, the eruption may be preceded by a one- or two-day prodrome consisting of fever and constitutional signs such as malaise, myalgia, and headache. The lesions, which first appear on the trunk and scalp, begin as small red macules and progress rapidly over 12 to 24 hours through stages to papules, vesicles, pustules, and crust formation. Pruritus is associated with the vesicular stage and may be quite marked. The vesicles are thin walled, superficial, and surrounded by prominent red areolae, which fade as the lesions dry. The crusts may fall off in a week or persist for several weeks, especially in lesions that become secondarily infected. Underlying areas generally heal completely over weeks to months; occasionally a pit or scar may persist.

The exanthem appears in successive crops over a one- to six-day period. Thus, as the disease progresses, a characteristic feature is the presence of lesions in various stages of development in the same anatomic area. Those in the final crop may regress after reaching the maculopapular stage.

The varicella rash has a centripetal distribution, being most abundant on the trunk and face and relatively sparse on the extremities, especially the distal extremities. It is usually increased, however, in areas of irritated, damaged, or inflamed skin.

Vesicles may also occur on the mucous membranes, especially in the mouth. Other sites which may be involved include the vaginal mucosa, conjunctiva, and pharynx. Lesions on mucous membranes break down to form shallow, generally painful white ulcers, which heal without crusting.

Fever parallels the severity of the rash and persists while new lesions continue to appear. Prolongation or recurrence of fever is associated either with bacterial superinfections, most commonly involving the skin lesions, or with some other complication of the disease. As with many other viral infections, varicella is usually more severe in adults than in children, with higher fever, more marked rash, and more frequent complications.

About 16 to 33 per cent of adults, and uncommonly children, develop clinical or radiologic evidence of pneumonitis during the disease. Chest films show diffuse nodular densities throughout both lung fields with a tendency to concentrate at the bases and hilum. The changes may persist for several months in severe cases. In some patients, fibrotic scars remain and gradually calcify, resembling the radiologic changes in healed miliary tuberculosis.

Encephalitis may occur with both mild and severe cases of varicella and is responsible for 90 per cent of the neurologic complications of this disease. Its incidence is estimated at less than one per 1000 cases. The manifestations are similar to those associated with measles or vaccinial encephalitis and may be quite severe with coma, seizures, appreciable mortality, and permanent sequelae. In about one third of patients with encephalitis, especially in children, cerebellar dysfunction with ataxia is the most prominent feature, and such patients generally do well, recovering completely within one to three weeks. Transverse myelitis, neuritis, and aseptic meningitis have also been observed.

Patients who are susceptible to varicella and who have leukemia, lymphoma, or congenital or acquired immunodeficiency or are on immunosuppressive medication represent a high-risk group for development of more severe disease, progressive varicella. Newborns of mothers who have onset of varicella less than five days before delivery or within 48 hours after delivery also fall into this category, presumably because they have received no maternal antibodies against this disease. This condition is characterized by continued eruption of lesions and high fever. In addition, pneumonia, disseminated visceral disease, secondary bacterial infection, central nervous system involvement, and hemorrhagic phenomena are more common, and mortality is significantly increased.

Additional manifestations that have been noted in varicella include *bullous rash, hepatitis, carditis, nephritis, orchitis, thrombocytopenia, and arthritis.* About 10 per cent of cases of Reye's syndrome (acute encephalopathy and fatty degeneration of the viscera) have been associated with an immediately preceding varicella (see Ch. 507).

Maternal infection with V-Z virus during the first four months of pregnancy has been reported to result occasionally in a syndrome of severe congenital malformation characterized by low birth weight for age, atrophy of a limb, scarring of the skin of that extremity, neurologic deficits, and eye abnormalities. The incidence of such cases appears to be quite low.

DIAGNOSIS. The typical case of varicella can be easily recognized on the basis of its characteristic clinical features. A history of exposure within the preceding several weeks is helpful. The demonstration of multinucleated giant cells in Wright- or Giemsa-stained scrapings of young vesicles (Tzanck smear) or in biopsies of affected tissues establishes the lesions as due to either V-Z or herpes simplex virus. Further differentiation among varicella, herpes zoster, and herpes simplex can then generally be made on the basis of associated clinical findings.

Viral isolation and/or serologic tests are generally necessary only to confirm unusual cases. Sera for testing should be collected within the first week after onset of illness and two to four weeks later. The virus can be readily isolated from vesicle fluid and identified in appropriate tissue cultures, or the presence of viral antigen can be confirmed by immunofluorescence. The demonstration of a rising titer of complement-fixing antibodies to V-Z antigen is also useful but must be interpreted with care, as this virus shares some antigenic components with herpes simplex virus. Complement-fixing antibodies decline rapidly and may not be detectable after six to twelve months. Neutralizing antibodies persist, but their determination is technically difficult. Immune status may be determined by an indirect fluorescent test with the patient's serum for antibody against V-Z virus-induced membrane antigen in infected cells (FAMA test). The presence of such antibody indicates immunity.

Other entities with a generalized vesicular eruption include smallpox (now extinct), eczema vaccinatum, eczema herpeticum, rickettsialpox, disease caused by certain coxsackieviruses, and some allergic rashes. None of these meet the criteria for diagnosis of varicella, and their differentiation from this disorder should present little difficulty.

TREATMENT. There is no specific therapy for varicella. Treatment is symptomatic and directed at relief of local discomfort and control of secondary infection. Supportive therapy includes acetaminophen (Tylenol) for high fever and constitutional symptoms and lukewarm starch baths, calamine lotion, and/or antihistamines for pruritus. The Centers for Disease Control recommend that salicylates not be used pending clarification of their possible causative role in Reye's syndrome. Nails should be kept clean and short to minimize skin infection from scratching. Patients with varicella pneumonia or encephalitis may need ventilatory support and attention to hydration, electrolyte balance, and nutrition. Bacterial or fungal superinfection may be important in the compromised host. Patients who develop varicella while on immunosuppressive doses of steroids should have the dose of such medication reduced to one to one and a half times physiologic levels (0.7 to 1.0 mg of cortisone per kilogram per day or its equivalent) as rapidly as is consistent with safety, and should be maintained at this level until the disease has subsided. Patients receiving other immunosuppressive therapy should also have the dose of their medication reduced.

Treatment with adenine arabinoside* (Ara-A, vidarabine), a DNA inhibitor, is of value for reducing the incidence of complications in immunocompromised patients with varicella. Early treatment is most effective. A dose of 10 mg per kilogram intravenously every 24 hours in a 12-hour infusion for five to seven days has been used. Acyclovir, another DNA inhibitor presently undergoing clinical trials, is less toxic and appears to be equally effective.

PREVENTION. Human immune serum globulin given to normal children within three days of exposure to varicella does not prevent but will attenuate the disease. V-Z immune globulin (VZIG), a more potent preparation, prepared from outdated normal blood with high antibody titers for V-Z virus, prevents varicella in normal hosts and reduces morbidity and mortality in susceptible high-risk hosts. VZIG is intended primarily for susceptible pediatric patients who meet high-risk criteria, for high-risk newborns, and on an individual basis for susceptible older compromised hosts. It is also available for prophylaxis for the patient with a history of chickenpox who has subsequently received a bone marrow transplant. Since such subjects are at high risk for severe disseminated disease, VZIG should be administered within 96 hours after exposure. It may be obtained by calling the local regional American Red Cross Office. Exposed patients on immunosuppressive therapy should not only receive VZIG but also have the dose of their medication reduced until the risk of varicella is past.

An attenuated live virus vaccine is currently being tested. It appears to be effective even in compromised hosts. Field trials in this country have been limited, however, by controversies regarding the long-term consequences and safety of a vaccine prepared with a virus that may establish a latent infection. It is presently being used in controlled studies on children with leukemia and other malignant diseases in whom the potential benefits outweigh the possible risks.

HERPES ZOSTER

EPIDEMIOLOGY. Herpes zoster represents a reactivation of a latent varicella infection; this disease may occur, therefore, in any subject who has had a prior infection with V-Z virus. Although shingles has been reported following contact with either varicella or herpes zoster, such cases most probably represent a coincidental reactivation of V-Z virus. The sporadic occurrence of herpes zoster as compared with the seasonal prevalence of varicella indicates that herpes zoster does not usually result from exogenous infection.

Susceptible persons may acquire varicella by close contact with patients with herpes zoster, but the estimated attack rate, 15 per cent or less, is considerably lower than that following similar exposure to varicella. This probably reflects the more limited skin and mucosal involvement, the presence of preexisting antibodies, and the decreased role of respiratory spread in patients with herpes zoster. Although the patient with herpes zoster does not disseminate virus so readily as the patient with varicella, vesicles yielding virus can persist longer than in varicella—for four to seven days after onset of the rash, longer in compromised hosts. As in varicella, the crusts in herpes zoster are not infectious.

Incidence and Prevalence. Herpes zoster may occur at any age but is uncommon in young hosts. The attack rate increases with age, with the peak incidence occurring in those over 50 years. In infancy or childhood the disease generally results from reactivation of an infection with V-Z virus acquired either in utero or in early infancy while protected by maternal antibodies. Although multiple episodes may occur, they are uncommon in the normal host. Data on age incidence suggest that 50 per cent of individuals will have had one episode by the age of 85 and 1 per cent will have had two attacks. The disease is more common in hosts with impaired cellular immunity, e.g., patients receiving immunosuppressive drugs and those with certain malignancies, especially Hodgkin's disease and lymphomas.

PATHOGENESIS AND PATHOLOGY. The exact pathogenesis of herpes zoster is not known. It is hypothesized that the V-Z virus enters the cutaneous endings of sensory nerves during varicella and travels centripetally along the nerve fibers to the sensory ganglia, where it becomes latent within the neurons. Although latency of V-Z virus in sensory ganglia remains to be proved, the virus has been demonstrated in ganglia of affected dermatomes obtained at autopsy from patients with active herpes zoster. Subsequently, in association with a variety of conditions, including development of malignancy, local x-irradiation, immunosuppressive therapy, tumor involvement of the dorsal root ganglion or adjacent structures, and treatment with certain drugs such as arsenicals, reactivation of the virus occurs. In many patients no obvious association or stimulus is apparent, and reactivation has been attributed to a decrease in host resistance with age. Virus replicates in the affected ganglia, producing an active ganglionitis causing pain along its sensory distribution. Virus is then believed to pass down the nerve and multiply again in the skin, where it produces the characteristic segmental, clustered, vesicular lesions of herpes zoster. A transitory viremia may also occur, as indicated by the appearance of a disseminated, generally sparse, varicella-like rash, usually several days after the dermatomal lesions, in up to one third of the patients. Rarely, spread to the viscera may also occur. The attack of herpes zoster is presumably terminated by the reactivated defense mechanisms of the host. Resolution and limitation of the rash correlate poorly with the antibody response. An impaired cellular immunity probably plays an important role in the pathogenesis of this disease.

Pathologic studies of involved sensory ganglia in herpes zoster reveal extensive lymphocytic infiltration, focal hemorrhage, and nerve cell destruction, followed in weeks to months by fibrosis. In addition, there is inflammation in the adjacent segments of the cord or brain stem. There may also be a localized leptomeningitis involving the affected segments; this process may occasionally spread to the anterior horn, resulting in motor paralysis, a rare complication of this disease.

The pathologic changes of zoster encephalitis are similar to those seen in varicella. The histopathology of the cutaneous lesions and the disseminated visceral lesions in herpes zoster is identical with that of varicella.

CLINICAL MANIFESTATIONS. Segmental or cutaneous paresthesias and pain of a burning or stabbing nature are characteristic of herpes zoster. These symptoms may be intermittent or constant and generally accompany the rash. Occasionally they may precede it by four or five days, presenting a prodromal picture easily confused with a variety of other illnesses characterized by localized pain. Malaise and fever may be present. The cutaneous lesions of zoster, like those of varicella, begin as erythematous maculopapules that progress over the next several days to form single or confluent clumps of vesicles, pustules, and crusts. Regional adenopathy generally accompanies the rash. New lesions continue to appear in crops for several days or longer, progressing to crusts which may persist for several weeks or more. Deep-seated lesions may result in scarring, and severe involvement may lead to gangrene. Typically, the rash appears in a unilateral, dermatomal distribution corresponding to the innervation of the affected sensory nerves. Occasionally the lesions may overlap onto adjacent dermatomes. Rarely, affected dermatomes may be separated or on opposite sides of the body.

The lesions of herpes zoster occur with the greatest frequency in those dermatomes in which the rash of varicella is most commonly found, i.e., the trunk in over 50 per cent of patients and, less often, the cervical and lumbar regions. The cranial nerve most commonly affected is the trigeminal, especially the ophthalmic branch. Ophthalmic zoster may be associated with a keratoconjunctivitis and impairment of oculomotor function

*Investigational drug for this purpose.

manifested by extraocular muscle weakness, ptosis, and mydriasis. Adjacent nerve roots may also be involved. Herpes zoster oticus (Ramsay Hunt syndrome) results from involvement of the facial and auditory nerves. Presenting features include vesicles in the external ear and ipsilateral facial paralysis, which is usually transitory. This localization of zoster may be accompanied by hearing loss, vertigo, loss of taste, tongue vesicles, and other signs consistent with involvement of additional cranial ganglia, especially those of the ninth and tenth cranial nerves.

Since the primary lesion of herpes zoster is in the nervous system, the cerebrospinal fluid may show a pleocytosis and elevation of protein. This is most frequent in patients with involvement of the cervical ganglia. Symptoms referable to meningeal involvement are minimal or absent. Although the cerebrospinal fluid changes may last for several weeks, recovery is usually complete.

Motor paralysis occasionally accompanies herpes zoster but is not common. It usually occurs within the first few weeks after onset of the rash, attains peak severity within days, and may persist for weeks or more. The paralysis almost always involves muscle groups innervated by nerves arising from the same spinal segment as that associated with the rash. About 75 per cent of such patients show complete or functional recovery. Major central nervous system infections with herpes zoster are rare, but cases of transverse myelitis, disseminated encephalitis, and acute cerebellar ataxia have been described.

The occurrence of segmental neuralgic pain without accompanying vesicles (zoster sine herpete) in serologically confirmed cases of V-Z infection has suggested that this virus may occasionally be activated in sensory ganglia without spread to the skin. Evidence in support of this hypothesis is limited.

Generalized herpes zoster occurs in 2 to 5 per cent of patients, most commonly in compromised hosts. It usually begins within a week or two of the localized rash, and is manifested as a varicella-like rash of varying severity, occasionally with widespread visceral involvement and fatal termination.

The neuralgia associated with herpes zoster generally subsides with recovery from the illness. It is rarely present in pediatric patients with this disease. In about 50 per cent of patients over 60 years it may persist for up to several months, and in a small percentage it may continue for a year or more.

Herpes zoster in pregnancy has not been shown to cause adverse effects in either the mother or the fetus.

DIAGNOSIS. Herpes zoster can generally be recognized by the characteristic development of pain and clustered vesicles in a unilateral, segmental distribution. Herpes simplex virus may occasionally produce a similar-appearing eruption, zosteriform simplex. Multiple recurrences are common with herpes simplex but uncommon in herpes zoster. Support for the diagnosis of herpes zoster may be obtained by the demonstration of multinucleated giant cells and intranuclear inclusions in stained scrapings of vesicular lesions (Tzanck smear) or in biopsies of affected tissues, but this does not differentiate between lesions of herpes zoster and herpes simplex. Such differentiation may be made by fluorescent antibody staining of cells in scrapings from vesicles. Specific diagnosis can also be made by isolation of the virus from vesicle fluid (and occasionally from cerebrospinal fluid with pleocytosis) in appropriate tissue culture systems. The virus may then be identified by standard serologic procedures, using specific antisera.

Methods for serologic diagnosis of herpes zoster are available but are not commonly employed. The complement fixation test, which is useful for confirmation of varicella, is less satisfactory for herpes zoster, since some patients show an elevated antibody titer in the acute phase serum with little subsequent rise. In addition, cross reactions occur with herpes simplex virus, so that simultaneous serologic tests must be carried out against both viruses before an antibody rise against V-Z virus may be considered as diagnostic.

TREATMENT. Uncomplicated herpes zoster requires only symptomatic and supportive therapy: analgesics such as aspirin or codeine for the neuralgia, and antihistamines and drying lotion for the pruritus. Ophthalmic zoster should be treated promptly by an ophthalmologist. Severe, prolonged postherpetic neuralgia presents a problem in management, since it is refractory to the usual analgesics and often leads to depression and occasionally to addiction in the search for relief. The combined use of analgesics, tranquilizers, and soporifics to break the pain cycle, followed by more limited use of such medication may be helpful. Treatment with prednisone is of questionable value.

Immunocompromised patients on immunosuppressive therapy who develop herpes zoster should have the medication dosage reduced as far as is practical. Treatment of such patients with adenine arabinoside early in the course of the infection (≤ 72 hours) has been shown to reduce systemic spread of virus as indicated by decreases in cutaneous spread of lesions and visceral disease. Controlled studies with acyclovir in such patients have given similar results.

Dissemination of herpes zoster lesions has been shown to occur in the presence of high levels of antibody. Administration of V-Z antibody preparations, therefore, would not be expected to affect the course of this illness.

PREVENTION. At present no effective means for prevention of herpes zoster is available.

Balfour HH Jr, Bean B, Laskin OL, Ambinder RF, Meyers JD, Wade JC, Zaia JA, Aeppli D, Kirk LE, Segreti AC, Keeney RE, the Burroughs Wellcome Collaborative Acyclovir Study Group: Acyclovir halts progression of herpes zoster in immunocompromised patients. N Engl J Med 308:1448, 1983. *Detailed double-blind collaborative evaluation of acyclovir.*

Herrmann KL: Congenital and perinatal varicella. Clin Obstet Gynecol 25:605, 1982. *A review with comments on management.*

Marcy SM, Kibrick S: Varicella and herpes zoster. *In* Hoeprich PD (ed.): Infectious Diseases. 3rd ed. New York, Harper & Row, 1982, pp 876–891. *Includes detailed accounts of less common complications of these disorders.*

Reichman RC, Mazur MH, Whitley RJ: *In* Dolin R (moderator): Herpes zoster–varicella infections in immunosuppressed patients. Ann Intern Med 89:375, 1978. *An edited transcription of a Combined Clinical Staff Conference at the Clinical Center, Bethesda, Md. (113 references).*

Weller TH: Varicella and herpes zoster. *In* Lennette EH, Schmidt NJ (eds.): Diagnostic Procedures for Viral, Rickettsial and Chlamydial Infections. Washington, D.C., American Public Health Association, 1979, pp 375-398. *A summary of procedures for isolation and study of varicella–herpes zoster virus in the laboratory. Includes data on interpretation of results.*

Weller TH: Varicella-herpes zoster virus. *In* Evans AS (ed.): Viral Infections of Humans, Epidemiology and Control. 2nd ed. New York, Plenum Publishing Corporation, 1982, pp 569–595. *The epidemiology and clinical features of varicella and herpes zoster are reviewed. Vaccine studies are summarized. Up-to-date, clearly written, and heavily referenced.*

Weller TH: Varicella and herpes zoster. Medical progress. N Engl J Med 309:1362, 1434, 1983. *A review of recent advances in knowledge about varicella and herpes zoster. Heavily referenced.*

Whitley RJ, Soong SJ, Dolin R, Betts R, Linneman C Jr, Alford CA Jr, the NIAID Collaborative Antiviral Study Group: Early vidarabine therapy to control the complications of herpes zoster in immunosuppressed patients. N Engl J Med 307:971, 1982. *Detailed double-blind collaborative evaluation of vidarabine.*

340. VARIOLA AND VACCINIA

Donald A. Henderson

The Thirty-third World Health Assembly "declares solemnly that the world and all its peoples have won freedom from smallpox . . . an unprecedented achievement in the history of public health. . . ." (Resolution 33.3, May 8, 1980, Geneva, Switzerland.)

This announcement was made some 30 months after the last known endemic case—a 23-year-old Somali cook who developed smallpox on October 26, 1977. In 1978, two additional cases of smallpox occurred in Birmingham, England, following a laboratory accident, but except for these cases no others have been found.

To confirm that eradication had been achieved, each country where smallpox had been endemic since 1967 and those at risk of importations conducted a search for cases for at least two years after the last known case. At the end of this period, World Health Organization (WHO)-appointed International Commissions reviewed the records of work and conducted extensive field visits to confirm the results. Between 1973 and 1979, 21 different commissions visited and certified eradication in 49 countries.

Finally, a Global Commission for the Certification of Smallpox Eradication reviewed the findings of each of the International Commissions and made special field visits. After satisfying itself that eradication had been achieved, the Commission reported its findings to the World Health Assembly. The Assembly members concurred and recommended that "smallpox vaccination be discontinued in every country except for investigators at special risk," and advised that "an international certificate of vaccination against smallpox should no longer be required of any traveller."

Thus concluded the first successful global program to eradicate a disease—one whose origins antedate written history and which over the centuries had proved to be one of the most devastating diseases known to man (McNeill).

HISTORY. Because of the need for variola virus to spread continually from person to person to survive, historians speculate that it emerged at some time after the first agricultural settlements, about 10,000 B.C. The presence of the distinctive smallpox rash on the mummy of Pharaoh Ramses V (1160 B.C.) documents its existence more than 3000 years ago (Dixon). In ancient times, only a few populated areas, probably in India, could have sustained its transmission. In the early Christian era descriptions suggestive of smallpox appear in historical accounts of western Asia, and by the eighth century it had established itself in Europe. Central and southern Africa were probably infected sometime later. In 1520, Spanish conquistadors brought the disease to the Americas.

Case-fatality rates of 20 per cent and greater were characteristic, and where population densities permitted the disease to become endemic virtually all persons eventually contracted smallpox. Deities to smallpox became a part of the culture in India, China, and a number of African countries. At the end of the eighteenth century, it was killing an estimated 400,000 Europeans each year and was responsible for one third of all cases of blindness.

VACCINATION. Edward Jenner's discovery in 1796 that smallpox could be prevented by "vaccination" with material from a cowpox lesion was widely acclaimed. Before his discovery, the only defense against smallpox was to deliberately inoculate (variolate) scabs or pustular material from smallpox patients into the skin of susceptibles. The resulting infection was usually less severe than infection acquired naturally by inhalation. Although case-fatality rates among those with induced infection were "only" 1 to 2 per cent, they readily transmitted infection to others. Within three years after Jenner first published his findings, more than 100,000 had been vaccinated in England. By 1803, the new vaccine had been transported to the Americas, Asia, and Africa, often by means of children who were vaccinated arm-to-arm in succession during the voyages.

During the nineteenth century, vaccination was increasingly widely practiced in temperate-climate countries, but the difficulties of sustaining the virus through arm-to-arm inoculation resulted in an uncertain supply. The discovery, late in the nineteenth century, that vaccinia virus could be propagated on the flank of a calf was an important advance. However, such vaccine remained viable for only a few days at ambient temperature. Finally, in the 1950's a commercially feasible technique was developed for producing a dried heat-resistant vaccine.

In the industrialized countries, smallpox incidence declined steadily, and Europe and North America succeeded in interrupting smallpox transmission after World War II. In these areas, the impetus for vaccination had diminished early in the century when a less virulent strain, variola minor, replaced variola major. Variola minor, with a case-fatality rate of about 1 per cent, was a less significant problem than variola major. In most of Africa, however, 5 to 15 per cent died of smallpox, and in Asia the virulent variola major prevailed. Neither in Africa nor in Asia was vaccination widely practiced.

ERADICATION OF SMALLPOX. Each year since 1948, the World Health Assembly had encouraged its member countries to take more vigorous control measures. It was a problem to all countries. Even those without disease feared importations and conducted vaccination programs to prevent epidemics should cases be imported. Although the global control of smallpox was in everyone's best interests, progress was slow. Finally, in 1959, the Assembly decided that a global eradication program should be undertaken. During the succeeding seven years, a number of countries undertook campaigns, but few succeeded in interrupting smallpox transmission. The few countries [illegible] were successful were plagued by importations from neighbors. Serious setbacks in WHO's other eradication program, the malaria program, caused the concept of eradication itself to be viewed with skepticism.

In 1966, the Assembly decided that one further effort should be made. It voted to allot $2.5 million annually for an intensified eradication program. A ten-year goal was proposed. The program commenced on January 1, 1967 (Henderson). In 1967, smallpox was endemic in 33 countries, and 14 additional countries reported importations. Although 131,000 cases were officially reported, later studies showed the true number to be about 10 to 15 million. Four geographic reservoirs of smallpox were identified: (1) Africa south of the Sahara; (2) a group of Southeast Asian countries, extending from Bangladesh through India, Nepal, Pakistan, and Afghanistan; (3) Indonesia; and (4) Brazil. The estimated population of these countries was more than 1.2 billion.

WHO's strategy called for each country to undertake a program of vaccination with the objective of reaching at least 80 per cent of the population during a two- to three-year period. During this time, a reliable reporting system was to be developed to identify foci of smallpox that would be eliminated by isolation of patients and vaccination of contacts. Extensive vaccination was believed necessary to increase population immunity and so reduce the number of cases to permit disease surveillance and containment activities to be effective.

Experience soon showed that the surveillance-containment strategy was more effective than had been thought, and, in fact, this proved to be the key to the program's success. In part, this was due to the unique characteristics of smallpox. An infected patient was able to transmit infection only from the time of first appearance of rash until the last scabs had separated. There were no chronic carriers or individuals with latent infection and no animal reservoir. The rash was sufficiently characteristic to be diagnosed with a high degree of accuracy by clinicians and villagers alike. The presence or absence of smallpox in an area could thus be reliably determined without laboratory studies. Moreover, approximately two thirds of recovered patients had characteristic residual facial scars. Thus, it was possible to determine both the present status of smallpox and its past history in an area.

To persist, smallpox virus had to be transmitted in a continuing chain of infection from patient to susceptible contact. By isolation of the patient and by vaccination of contacts, a barrier to transmission was created and a chain of infection interrupted. In small villages and in scattered populations, chains of transmission often terminated without intervention. Because smallpox did not spread rapidly, and then only to those in face-to-face contact, secondary cases usually were found among neighbors and relatives, and cases tended to cluster within parts of a town and in localized geographic regions. A patient rarely infected more than two or three others, and, even in infected households, three and sometimes four generations of cases occurred. Because of these factors, early detection of outbreaks and their containment proved effective in stopping transmission, even when there was a low level of population immunity (Foege et al.).

Smallpox vaccine that conferred excellent and durable immunity was an important factor in the program's success. Studies during the program revealed vaccine efficacy ratios of more than 90 per cent after 20 years. Because the lyophilized vaccine retained its potency after incubation at 37° C for at least one month, the logistics of vaccine storage and distribution were greatly simplified. The vaccination technique was greatly facilitated by the inexpensive newly developed bifurcated needle, a device best described as a large sewing needle with part of the eye ground off to leave two small prongs. Vaccine was held between the tines by capillarity. Fifteen rapid punc-

… with the needle held perpendicular to the …que was learned quickly and produced a high …ccessful vaccinations.

…THE PROGRAM. By 1969, eradication programs were in progress in all of the infected and immediately adjacent countries except for Ethiopia, whose program began in 1971. By 1970, the number of endemic countries had decreased from 33 to 18. Eleven of the 15 that became smallpox free were in western and central Africa. Brazil registered its last case in 1971 and Indonesia and Afghanistan in 1972. By 1973, all of Africa had become smallpox free except for Ethiopia and Botswana. In Asia, there remained only four smallpox-endemic countries: India, Pakistan, Nepal, and Bangladesh. However, the population of these four was over 700 million, and the techniques of surveillance and containment which had been applied in other areas had been less successful.

A new strategy in India began in the autumn of 1973 (Basu et al.). Far more rapid case detection and more effective containment of outbreaks were required. Accordingly, for one week each month more than 100,000 health workers were mobilized to search house by house, to detect cases. Hundreds of special surveillance-containment teams contained the outbreaks which were found. Between searches, the teams asked questions at markets and in schools to uncover rumors of cases. A similar strategy was adopted in the neighboring countries. By the summer of 1974, new cases began to decline, and a cash reward was offered to anyone who reported a case. In May 1975 the last case was detected in India, and on October 16, 1975, the last case in Asia.

The only remaining endemic country was Ethiopia. More than half of its population of 25 million lived more than a day's walk from any road, and its health structure was all but nonexistent. With the end of smallpox in Asia, resources were shifted to Ethiopia. In August 1976, the last case was isolated. Unfortunately, Somalian guerrilla forces had meanwhile introduced the disease into neighboring Somalia, and yet another year was to elapse before finally, on October 26, 1977, the last case occurred.

POSSIBLE SOURCES FOR A RETURN OF SMALLPOX. As of June, 1984, variola virus was known to exist in only two laboratories, each of which had been inspected by international teams. The risk of accidental escape is extremely small.

Extensive studies had been conducted since 1967 to discover a possible animal or other natural reservoir of the virus. None was found. The best evidence that such a reservoir does not exist is that all smallpox outbreaks detected in otherwise smallpox-free areas since 1967 were traced to known human cases.

Almost 200 cases of a newly recognized disease that is clinically indistinguishable from smallpox but caused by the related monkey pox virus occurred in six central and west African countries between 1970 and 1984. Almost all of the patients lived in small villages in the tropical rain forest. Person-to-person transmission occurred in several instances, but it is apparent that the virus is transmitted only with difficulty. Genome maps of this and other animal poxviruses reveal many differences between them and variola, suggesting that mutation to variola would be highly unlikely.

The recurrence of smallpox resulting from a deliberate release of variola virus cannot be ruled out. However, the potential damage of such an act should not be exaggerated. Smallpox does not spread rapidly as does influenza or measles, and an outbreak caused in this manner should be able to be contained within three to four weeks. Moreover, if someone were to decide to employ biologic weapons, there are other agents whose virulence and characteristics of spread are superior to those of variola virus.

As insurance against unforeseen events, WHO has established vaccine storage reserves of some 200 million doses of vaccine. Additional stocks are being retained by a number of governments.

Barring improbable circumstances, a human case of smallpox will never again be seen. However, the problem of mistaken diagnosis is a real one. For this reason, WHO medical officers with expertise in diagnosis remain on call to investigate rumors, and an expertise in laboratory diagnosis will be maintained by WHO Diagnostic Reference Laboratories (Centers for Disease Control, Atlanta, and the Institute for Virus Preparations, Moscow).

VARIOLA (Smallpox)

ETIOLOGY. Variola virus is one of a group of orthopoxviruses which includes vaccinia, monkey pox, rabbit pox, cowpox, camel pox, buffalo pox, and ectromelia (Nakano). The poxviruses are the largest viruses so recognized. The virions are brick-shaped structures with a diameter of about 200 mμ. The genome consists of a single molecule of a double-stranded DNA.

INCIDENCE AND PREVALENCE. The disease was declared to be eradicated on May 8, 1980.

PATHOLOGY AND PATHOGENESIS. The site of entry of the smallpox virus was probably the respiratory tract. In the 12-day incubation period the virus multiplied in the regional lymphoid tissues. Viremia occurred at the onset of fever and continued during the first two or three days of the pre-eruptive phase. During this time, the virus localized in mucous membranes, skin, and internal tissues. Antibodies appeared as early as the fourth day of disease. The virus multiplied in the epithelial cells of the skin and mucous membranes, causing pustulation. Patients became infectious at the time of onset of rash. Scabs separated during the third to fourth week of illness and, although virus could be detected in scabs, they were less infectious than vesicular or pustular secretions.

CLINICAL MANIFESTATIONS. The incubation period of smallpox was about 12 days with a range of 7 to 17 days. The illness began with severe malaise, prostration, head- and backache, and high fever lasting two to five days (Rao). Following the initial febrile period, a macular rash developed, which quickly became papular, and within two days the papules developed into vesicles and then pustules. On the eighth or ninth day of rash, crusting began. The scabs separated over the succeeding two to three weeks, leaving pigment-free skin. Subsequently, scarring or pitting developed. An important diagnostic feature of variola was the fact that lesions in any one area were all at the same stage of development, whereas in varicella they are in all stages. The eruption was characteristically more severe on the face and the distal parts of the arms and legs, and less severe over the trunk and abdomen. This centrifugal distribution was distinct from the rash of varicella, which tends to be centripetal. Lesions were often found on the palms of the hands and the soles of the feet, a finding uncommon in childhood varicella, although not unusual in the adult form. The characteristic pustular lesions of smallpox were round, raised, and tense, with a tendency to central depression as they began to dry. The majority of deaths occurred during the second week of rash.

VARIOLA MINOR AND INTERMEDIATE FORMS. In the early twentieth century, a milder clinical form of smallpox (variola minor, alastrim) became prevalent in the Americas, Europe, and parts of southern and eastern Africa. Case-fatality rates were 1 per cent or less. Variola major and minor were distinct although at times coexisting. Each of the two types gave rise to illnesses with a spectrum of severity ranging from fatal hemorrhagic cases to mild cases with only a few lesions. In outbreaks of variola major the severe cases predominated, whereas in variola minor most cases were mild. There was cross-protection between each of these forms and vaccinia.

DIFFERENTIAL DIAGNOSIS. Most cases of smallpox could readily be identified by the typical deep-seated rash, the centrifugal distribution of lesions, and the fact that in any area on the body all lesions were at the same stage of development. The infrequent severe hemorrhagic cases were frequently mistakenly diagnosed as meningococcemia, acute leukemia, or drug toxicity. Mild cases with few lesions were confused with varicella. Most problematic were severe cases of chickenpox in adults, which often were misdiagnosed as smallpox. Of help in diagnosis, however, was the fact that in any outbreak 80 per cent or more of the cases were clinically typical.

LABORATORY TESTS. Diagnosis of a poxvirus infection can be rapidly established by electron microscope identification of virus particles in vesicular or pustular fluid or scabs. Differentiation as to which poxvirus may be causing illness requires that the virus be isolated on chick chorioallantoic membrane and its properties characterized by specific biologic tests. WHO Reference Laboratories are prepared to undertake necessary diagnostic studies. For patients who have recovered, neutralizing antibody in serum specimens serves to identify which poxvirus was responsible for the illness.

TREATMENT. No specific treatment is available.

IDENTIFICATION OF A SUSPECT CASE OF SMALLPOX. Because smallpox has been eradicated, the occurrence of a single case has profound international implications. Should a suspect case be identified, *immediate notification of local, state, and national health officials is essential.* From time to time clinicians may suspect smallpox in a severely ill patient with fever and rash. Most suspected cases in recent years have been cases of varicella in adults. Visualization of varicella particles in vesicular, pustular, or scab material by electron microscopy will confirm the diagnosis. Under the electron microscope, orthopoxviruses such as vaccinia, monkey pox, and smallpox appear alike and must be further characterized by other biologic tests. Should a case prove to be smallpox, the source of virus must be assumed to be inadvertent or deliberate release from a laboratory.

A suspect patient should be placed under strict isolation and the diagnosis determined as an emergency measure. Additional measures will be dictated by epidemiologic circumstances.

VACCINIA (Vaccination)

No countries now require international certificates of vaccination and none conduct vaccination programs. Vaccination is recommended only for investigators who are working with poxviruses in the laboratory or who are engaged in field studies of monkey pox virus.

THE VACCINE. Vaccinia virus is believed to have derived from cowpox virus, although comparisons of contemporary strains of cowpox virus and vaccinia virus show them to have different biologic characteristics. Vaccinia virus is grown on the scarified flank of a calf or sheep. After purification and the addition of stabilizing agents, the suspension is freeze dried. Inoculated intradermally, vaccinia virus induces a mild infection and confers protection against all orthopoxviruses known to infect man—monkey pox, variola, and cowpox.

VACCINE PROTECTION. Following successful vaccination, protection against variola is virtually complete for five years, but effectiveness wanes over time. In poxvirus laboratories, vaccination at least every three years has been customary, and none so vaccinated has developed disease.

RISKS OF VACCINATION. Those who are candidates for vaccination are adults, a diminishing proportion of whom have received primary vaccinations as children. Although the risk of complications following revaccination is very low, primary vaccination of adults has been thought to be associated with a high incidence of serious complications, especially postvaccinial encephalitis. Most of the studies that document this are from Europe, where especially pathogenic strains had been used. Studies in the United States, where the New York Board of Health strain was used, reveal a much lower incidence of complications. A special study of vaccination complications among military recruits failed to document any cases of postvaccinial encephalitis among an estimated 2 million primary vaccinees.

FIRST VACCINATION (PRIMARY TAKE). Three days after vaccination a papule appears at the vaccination site. The papule is small, round, bright red, and hard but superficial. The papule changes to a vesicle, and by the seventh day is fully developed.

It is whitish, umbilicated, and multilocular and contains cl lymph. An erythematous areola expands to reach a maximal diameter about nine days after vaccination. Crusting begins at the center, and the dry brownish crust falls off about three weeks after vaccination, leaving a scar.

REVACCINATION. When vaccination is performed on persons who possess some immunity, a gradation of cutaneous responses is observed. Individuals who have not been vaccinated for several decades may develop what appears to be a primary take. In persons with an intermediate level of immunity, the course of development of the lesion is more rapid and the maximal diameter of erythema is reached in from three to seven days. In the highly immune person, virus multiplication may not occur. However, in such persons, a hypersensitivity response to vaccinial protein may occur. A papule and sometimes a vesicle with erythema may develop. The reaction reaches its peak in the first 48 hours, but by the sixth day, there is no evidence of an inflammatory process. This reaction was formerly termed a "reaction of immunity," implying that the individual was immune to smallpox. However, experiments have shown that vaccine that has been inactivated by heat may induce a similar response.

To distinguish the hypersensitivity type of reaction from one in which virus multiplication has taken place, the site of inoculation is examined between the sixth and eighth days. If there is evidence of induration or congestion, virus multiplication may be assumed. If there is no evidence of induration or congestion, virus multiplication may or may not have taken place, and repeat vaccination is advised.

CONTRAINDICATIONS. Four groups of persons are at special risk of complications: (1) persons with eczema or other forms of chronic dermatitis; (2) pregnant women; (3) patients with leukemia, lymphoma, and other reticuloendothelial malignancies; and (4) those receiving immunosuppressive drugs, especially glucocorticosteroids. Vaccinees in close contact with persons with eczema may infect them, sometimes with serious consequences. If vaccination is required for persons at special risk, vaccinia immune globulin (0.3 ml per kilogram intramuscularly) should be administered simultaneously.

COMPLICATIONS. ***Postvaccinal Encephalitis.*** Encephalitis following vaccination is a rare event and occurs between the eighth and fifteenth days. The disease may be associated with fever, headache, vomiting, drowsiness, and sometimes paralysis, meningitic signs, coma, and convulsions. The cerebrospinal fluid usually shows an increase in cells. Paralysis, when it occurs, is generally spastic in type. Recovery may be complete, or residual paralysis and other central nervous system symptoms may persist. There is no treatment. Studies conducted in the United States in 1963 and 1968 (Neff et al., Lane et al.) revealed 28 cases, 9 fatal, among 11.3 million primary vaccinees. No cases occurred among 16.3 million revaccinees.

Progressive Vaccinia (Vaccinia Gangrenosa). Progressive vaccinia is an exceedingly rare but often fatal complication among vaccinated persons who have deficient immune responses. The initial vaccinial lesion fails to heal and progresses to involve adjacent skin with necrosis of tissue. Dissemination of virus may result in metastatic vaccinial lesions in other parts of the skin, bones, or viscera. In the United States studies, 12 cases, including 2 deaths, occurred among 11.3 million primary vaccinees and 8 cases, including 2 deaths, among 16.3 million revaccinees. Treatment with vaccinia immune globulin and thiosemicarbazone* is beneficial.

Eczema Vaccinatum. Eczema vaccinatum is sometimes a serious complication, which may occur in persons with either active or healed eczema. It may occur among eczematous subjects who are in contact with recent vaccinees. The disease tends to localize at sites where eczematous lesions are or have been present.

---

*Available for experimental use only.

e globulin and the thiosemicarbazone* drugs apy.

cinia. Generalized vaccinia represents a sec- resulting from bloodborne dissemination of vaccinia virus. Almost all cases occur after primary vaccination. The lesions become evident between six and nine days after vaccination. The number of lesions may range from a few to a generalized involvement of the skin. It is a self-limited illness, and complete recovery occurs without specific therapy.

Fetal Vaccinia. Fetal vaccinia results from a bloodborne dissemination of vaccinia virus in the pregnant woman given primary vaccination. It may occur during any trimester of pregnancy and frequently results in death of the fetus.

Miscellaneous Complications. A great variety of rashes has been reported to be caused by vaccination. Most common are erythema multiforme and variously disturbed urticarial, maculopapular, blotchy erythematous eruptions.

Basu RN, Jerek Z, Ward NA: The Eradication of Smallpox from India. New Delhi, India, World Health Organization, 1979. *A well-written, detailed, profusely illustrated book describing the epidemiologic and operational aspects of the program in India.*

*Available for experimental use only.

Dixon CW: Smallpox. London, J & A Churchill, Ltd., 1962. *A 500-page, well-illustrated book, which presents a comprehensive historical account of smallpox and vaccination as well as the clinical features, pathogenesis, and epidemiology of the disease and laboratory characteristics of the virus.*

Foege WH, Miller JD, Lane JM: Selective epidemiologic control in smallpox eradication. Am J Epidemiol 94:311, 1971. *A description of the surveillance-containment methodology in West Africa and its implications for the global program.*

Henderson DA: Smallpox: Eradication of a killer. *In* Medical and Health Annual. Chicago, Encyclopaedia Britannica, 1979, pp 125–141. *An illustrated account of the global eradication program.*

Lane JM, Ruben FL, Neff JM, Miller JD: Complications of smallpox vaccination, 1968. N Engl J Med 281:138, 1969. *With the paper by Neff et al., one of the few detailed studies of the frequency of complications following smallpox vaccination.*

McNeill WH: Plagues and People. Garden City, N.Y., Anchor Press/Doubleday, 1976. *An historian's account of the impact on history of a number of pestilential diseases, among which smallpox is prominently featured. Although some of the interpretations are subject to dispute, the book provides an unusual perspective.*

Nakano JH: Poxviruses. *In* Lennette EH, Schmidt NJ (eds.): Diagnostic Procedures for Viral, Rickettsial and Chlamydial Infections. New York, Americn Public Health Association, 1979, pp 257–308. *An exhaustive description of the virologic characteristics and diagnostic methods for the poxviruses.*

Neff J, Lane JM, Pert JH, Moore R, Miller JD, Henderson DA: Complications of smallpox vaccination. N Engl J Med 276:1, 1967. *With the paper by Lane et al., one of the few detailed studies of the frequency of complications following smallpox vaccination.*

Rao AR: Smallpox. Bombay, India, Kothari Book Depot, 1972. *Written by a clinician who treated more than 3000 cases, this book is an excellent reference on the clinical aspects of variola major.*

World Health Organization, Final Report of the Global Commission for the Certification of Smallpox Eradication. Geneva, WHO, 1979. *A comprehensive report of the eradication program, the activities which were conducted to certify eradication, and much useful statistical data about the program and its progress.*

Enteroviral Diseases

Raphael Dolin

341. INTRODUCTION

Enteroviruses cause a wide variety of diseases in humans and other mammals. These viral agents comprise a separate genus (enterovirus) within the Picornavirus (*pico*, small; *rna*, ribonucleic acid) family, and share the following common properties: (1) size of 17 to 30 nm, (2) capsids with cubic symmetry, (3) RNA genome, and (4) four major and one minor structural polypeptides. The virion lacks a lipid envelope, which renders the viruses resistant to lipid solvents.

Enteroviruses have been historically subdivided into *polioviruses, groups A* and *B coxsackieviruses,* and *echoviruses.* These divisions were based on antigenic relationships and differences in host range. Sixty-seven distinct immunotypes (species) were originally identified, although these have been reduced to 63 because of reclassification and redundancy in numbering (Table 341–1). However, this classification is not entirely satisfactory, since several enteroviruses have properties which overlap groups defined by the criteria cited above. Therefore, newly recognized enteroviruses are no longer classified as echoviruses or coxsackieviruses, but are simply designated "enterovirus," and are numbered sequentially beginning with enterovirus 68. To avoid confusion within the older literature, the previous classification (coxsackievirus groups A and B, and echovirus) has been retained for the 63 original immunotypes (Table 341–1).

Since infections with polioviruses are presented in Ch. 502, this discussion will be limited to consideration of nonpolio enteroviruses.

CHARACTERISTICS OF NONPOLIO ENTEROVIRUSES

COXSACKIEVIRUSES. Coxsackieviruses were originally isolated from stools of children who were suffering from paralytic poliomyelitis in Coxsackie, New York. Unlike polioviruses, these viruses cause disease in suckling mice and were therefore presumed to be distinct from polioviruses (see Table 341–1). Subsequently, additional coxsackievirus immunotypes have been isolated from widespread geographic locations. These viruses are divided into two groups, A and B, depending on the histopathology of lesions induced in mice. Group A coxsackieviruses produce a generalized myositis of skeletal muscle, which results in flaccid paralysis. Group B coxsackieviruses produce a focal myositis and a generalized infection of brown fat, myocardium, pancreas, and central nervous system, which results in spastic paralysis. Group B coxsackieviruses can be readily cultivated in primate tissue culture, whereas group A coxsackieviruses grow inconsistently or not at all in tissue culture. Twenty-three immunotypes of group A and six of group B have been identified.

ECHOVIRUSES. Echoviruses were first isolated from the stools of healthy children, but were not pathogenic for primates or suckling mice. They were given the acronym echo (*e*nteric

TABLE 341–1. CHARACTERISTICS OF HUMAN ENTEROVIRUSES

Virus	Number of Immunotypes	Numerical Designation	Isolated in Tissue Culture	Pathogenic for Suckling Mice	Pathogenic for Primates
Polioviruses	3	1–3	Yes	No	Yes
Coxsackieviruses A	23	A1–A24*	Occasionally†	Yes	No‡
Coxsackieviruses B	6	B1–B6	Yes	Yes	No
Echoviruses	31	1–34§	Yes	No	No
Enteroviruses**	4	68–71	Yes	Variable	No¶

*A23 has been reclassified as echovirus 9.
†Primary isolation in tissue culture is difficult for most immunotypes except A7, 11, 13, 15, 16, 18, 20, and 21.
‡Coxsackie A7 is neuropathogenic for monkeys.
§Echovirus 10 is reovirus 1; echovirus 28 is rhinovirus 1A; echovirus 34 is a variant of coxsackievirus A24.
¶Enterovirus 70 is neuropathogenic for monkeys.
**Hepatitis A virus will likely be classified as an enterovirus in the future.

TABLE 341–2. ILLNESSES ASSOCIATED WITH NONPOLIO ENTEROVIRUSES*

Coxsackieviruses Group A	Coxsackieviruses Group B	Echoviruses	Enteroviruses
Asymptomatic infection Undifferentiated febrile illness with or without respiratory symptoms; common cold (21, 24); pneumonitis of infants (9, 16) Aseptic meningitis (1-14, 16, 17, 21, 22, 24); rare paralysis or encephalitis (4-7, 9, 10, 16) Mucocutaneous infection: herpangina (2-6, 8, 10, 22); lymphonodular pharyngitis (10); hand-foot-and-mouth disease (5, 9, 10, 16); exanthem (4, 5, 6, 9, 16) Acute hemorrhagic conjunctivitis (24)	Asymptomatic infection Undifferentiated febrile illness with or without respiratory symptoms; URI and pneumonia (4, 5) Aseptic meningitis (1-6); rare paralysis or encephalitis (2-5) Myocarditis (1-5)† Pericarditis (1-5)† Pleurodynia (1-6) Generalized disease of newborn (1-5) Exanthem (1-5)	Asymptomatic infection Undifferentiated febrile illness with or without respiratory symptoms (4, 9, 11, 20, 25) Aseptic meningitis (all); rare paralysis or encephalitis (all except 23, 26, 28, 29, 32) Exanthem (2, 4, 6, 9, 11, 16, 18) Neonatal diarrhea (18)	Asymptomatic infection Undifferentiated febrile illness with or without respiratory symptoms; pneumonia, bronchiolitis (68) Aseptic meningitis (70, 71); paralysis (70) Acute hemorrhagic conjunctivitis (70) Hand-foot-and-mouth disease (71) Exanthem (71)

*Immunotypes with strongest association are in parentheses.
†Myopericarditis has less frequently been associated with coxsackieviruses A1, 4, 9, and 16 and echoviruses 1, 3, 6 to 9, 11, 14, 19, 22, and 30.

*c*ytopathic *h*uman *o*rphan), indicating that they were not associated with disease. Subsequently, a variety of diseases have been associated with echoviruses, and 31 immunotypes have been recognized. Most echoviruses can be readily cultivated in tissue culture (see Table 341–1).

NEWLY RECOGNIZED ENTEROVIRUSES. Four newly recognized enteroviruses, immunotypes 68 to 71, have been reported since the adoption of the new classification schema. Illnesses produced by enteroviruses 68 and 71 are similar to those produced by coxsackieviruses and echoviruses (Table 341–2). Enterovirus 70 causes acute hemorrhagic conjunctivitis and is discussed in Ch. 94. Enterovirus 69 has not as yet been associated with illness. In addition, hepatitis A virus is now known to have the biophysical properties of enteroviruses and will likely be classified within the enterovirus genus in the future. Hepatitis A infections are discussed in Ch. 120.

GENERAL FEATURES OF NONPOLIO ENTEROVIRAL INFECTIONS

EPIDEMIOLOGY. Enteroviruses have a worldwide distribution. In temperate climates, the incidence of infection and illness is markedly increased in the summer and early fall, although enterovirus-associated disease has been reported at other times as well. In tropical climates, enterovirus infections occur throughout the year. The prevalence of individual immunotypes varies widely according to geographic locale and year. Generally, one or two immunotypes account for the bulk of enterovirus-induced disease during any given season, but occasionally multiple immunotypes may be equally prevalent. Because of the prolonged shedding of virus from the gastrointestinal tract (see below), the presence of enteroviruses in surface waters and in sewage is a good indicator of the prevalence of infection in the community.

Transmission of enteroviruses is primarily by the fecal-oral route, and the frequency of infection is increased by factors that promote such transmission, e.g., poor hygiene and low socioeconomic status. Young children have the highest attack rates and serve as the vehicles for spread within communities. Once infection occurs within a family, susceptible (nonimmune) family members are rapidly infected. Coxsackievirus infections appear to be somewhat more communicable than echovirus infections.

PATHOGENESIS AND CLINICAL MANIFESTATIONS. Models of the pathogenesis of enteroviral infection are based largely on studies with polioviruses. However, the pathogenesis of nonpolio enteroviral infection appears to be similar, except for the major organs that are affected. Initial replication of the virus takes place in the oropharynx or in the gastrointestinal tract. Viral infection may be limited to the mucosa, or may proceed deeper into lymphoid tissue. The latter may be followed by viremia and dissemination of virus to distant organs, such as the heart or the central nervous system. The marked variation in clinical manifestations associated with nonpolio enteroviral infections reflects the relative involvement of different target organs (Table 341–2).

The bulk of enteroviral infections (50 to 80 per cent) are asymptomatic, and many of the remainder consist of "undifferentiated febrile illnesses," often with respiratory symptoms. The latter illnesses are generally mild and last a few days. The enterovirus infections most frequently coming to the attention of a physician are those resulting in central nervous system, heart, or skin involvement. Enteroviruses have been associated with a wide variety of clinical syndromes referable to those organ systems (Table 341–2), the most important of which are discussed below. As with "undifferentiated febrile illnesses," these syndromes are rarely sufficiently distinctive to permit diagnosis of infection with a particular immunotype. Immunotypes from different groups can produce similar syndromes, and alternatively a single immunotype can produce clinically diverse illnesses. Thus, coxsackievirus B1 can induce aseptic meningitis in one patient and pericarditis in another, even during the same outbreak. The factors that determine which clinical manifestation will be expressed in any individual infection are poorly understood.

LABORATORY DIAGNOSIS. Laboratory diagnosis is based on virus isolation and/or immunotype-specific antibody rises in acute and convalescent serum specimens. Enteroviruses can frequently be isolated from throat secretions and stools obtained from patients with enteroviral infections. Such isolations are most frequent in younger children, particularly in lower socioeconomic groups. However, interpretation of the significance of such isolates in individual cases is difficult. Intercurrent subclinical infections or prolonged fecal shedding of virus (up to three months) may occur, so that an etiologic association between an isolate and a current disease episode cannot be made with certainty. A rising titer of immunotype-specific antibodies in acute and convalescent sera indicates that a recent infection has taken place, but similarly does not assign an etiologic role to the virus in question. The strongest evidence for enteroviruses as etiologic agents of a variety of diseases originates from two sources: (1) large scale studies in which isolation rates from cases are matched with controls and (2) isolation of virus from sites from which asymptomatic shedding of virus does not occur, e.g., cerebrospinal fluid, myocardium, or pericardial fluid. In this regard, virus culture of blood has been reported to be useful in infants with enterovirus-related illness.

Serologic diagnosis of enteroviral infections is particularly difficult because group specific tests, such as complement fixation, do not exist, and thus immunotype-specific neutralization tests must be carried out. Since there are 67 currently recognized immunotypes, neutralization tests against all potential agents cannot be performed. Of necessity, neutralization tests must be limited to those directed against the patient's isolate (if one is present), or perhaps against isolates prevalent in the community. A possible exception is the case in which only a few immunotypes are likely to be present (e.g., hand-foot-and-mouth disease—coxsackievirus A16; myocarditis—coxsackieviruses B1 to 6). In addition, patients may be seen late in the course of illness, at which time high, stable antibody titers are present, which further reduces the utility of serologic tests.

PREVENTION AND TREATMENT. Highly successful live and inactivated virus vaccines directed against poliovirus infections have been developed (see Ch. 502). Immunity to nonpolio enteroviruses has been less well studied, but appears to be similarly dependent on the presence of immunotype-specific local and humoral antibodies. Thus, the development of vaccines against these agents is theoretically possible. However, the large number of immunotypes among nonpolio enteroviruses (67), as compared to polioviruses (3), and the benign nature of most enteroviral-induced disease have precluded the development of such vaccines.

Specific antiviral chemotherapy or chemoprophylaxis directed at enteroviral infection is not currently available. Treatment consists of symptomatic or supportive therapy for severe illness, particularly that involving the central nervous system or the heart (see below). However, the vast majority of enteroviral illnesses are self-limited and require no therapy. Appropriate control measures include maintenance of good hygienic practices such as hand washing, and proper disposal of potentially infectious stools. Isolation of patients is impractical and rarely indicated.

Grist NR, Bell EJ, Assad F: Enteroviruses in human disease. Prog Med Virol 24:114, 1978. *An excellent review with a comprehensive bibliography. Emphasis is on recent developments in the field.*

Moore M: Enteroviral disease in the United States, 1970–1979. J Infect Dis 146:103, 1982. *A summary of the most recent ten-year experience of surveillance data from the Centers for Disease Control. Provides an excellent epidemiologic overview.*

Young NA: Picornaviridae. *In* Mandell GL, Douglas RG, Bennett JE (eds.): Principles and Practice of Infectious Diseases. New York, John Wiley & Sons, 1979, p 1083. *The best single work which covers the molecular biology, epidemiology, and clinical manifestations of enteroviral diseases. Contains an exhaustive bibliography.*

POLIOMYELITIS AND ASEPTIC MENINGITIS

The most important enteroviral infections are poliomyelitis, discussed in Ch. 502, and aseptic meningitis caused by coxsackieviruses and enteroviruses, discussed in Ch. 499.

342. PARALYSIS AND OTHER NEUROLOGIC COMPLICATIONS OF NONPOLIO ENTEROVIRUSES

Paralysis has been rarely associated with nonpolio enteroviral infections. The majority of reported cases have been diagnosed on the basis of isolation of echoviruses and coxsackieviruses from stool, with relatively few isolations from central nervous system tissue or cerebrospinal fluid. Generally, muscle weakness rather than paralysis has been observed in these patients. When present, paralysis and weakness are generally less extensive than in poliomyelitis, and tend to resolve over a variable period of time. Cranial nerve and severe bulbar involvement have also been reported. Coxsackievirus A7 has been the immunotype most commonly implicated in paralytic disease, and small outbreaks have been recognized in the USSR and Scotland. A poliomyelitis-like syndrome has also been reported to accompany acute hemorrhagic conjunctivitis caused by enterovirus 70 (see Ch. 94). Other neurologic complications include transverse myelitis and the Guillain-Barré syndrome, although the precise relationship of these illnesses to enteroviral infection is unclear.

Infants, children, and occasionally young adults infected with nonpolio enteroviruses have developed encephalitis as manifested by seizures, coma, cerebellar ataxia, hemiplegia, or extrapyramidal movements. Up to 10 per cent of children who acquired enteroviral meningitis during the first year of life have developed mild mental retardation and spasticity, suggesting that involvement of central nervous system parenchyma may be more frequent than has previously been suspected. Echovirus infection of the central nervous system in agammaglobulinemic patients has resulted in a chronic meningoencephalitis associated with a dermatomyositis-like syndrome.

Grist NR, Bell EJ: Enteroviral etiology of the paralytic poliomyelitis syndrome. Arch Environ Health 21:382, 1970. *A good review of the uncommon association of nonpolio enteroviruses with paralytic disease.*

Wilfert CM, Buckley RH, Mohanakumarz T, Griffith JF, Katz SL, Whisnant JK, Eggleston PA, Moore M, Treadwell E, Oxman MN, Rosen FS: Persistent and fatal central nervous system echovirus infections in patients with agammaglobulinemia. N Engl J Med 26:1485, 1977. *A description of the syndrome of chronic echovirus central nervous system infection and dermatomyositis in patients with abnormal B cell function.*

343. EPIDEMIC PLEURODYNIA (Bornholm Disease, Epidemic Myalgia, Devil's Grip, Sylvest's Disease)

DEFINITION. Epidemic pleurodynia (*pleura,* side; *odyne,* pain) is an acute febrile disease characterized by sudden, sharp chest (intercostal) or abdominal pain. Pain is paroxysmal in nature, and relapses frequently occur after periods of well-being.

ETIOLOGY. Group B coxsackieviruses (1 to 6) are the major causes of pleurodynia. Outbreaks have also been associated with echovirus 1, and sporadic cases with coxsackieviruses A4, A6, and A10 and echoviruses 1, 6, 9, and 19.

EPIDEMIOLOGY. Epidemic pleurodynia was first described in the mid-nineteenth century in Iceland and Norway. In 1933, Sylvest published a classic monograph describing the illness on the Danish island of Bornholm. Subsequently, outbreaks and sporadic cases have been described in many parts of the world. In contrast to the annual occurrence of aseptic meningitis, epidemics of pleurodynia occur much less frequently, often 10 to 20 years apart. As with other enteroviral infections, illness is most common in summer and early fall. Person-to-person transmission occurs, particularly within families, with incubation periods of two to five days. Attack rates are highest in children, but the peak incidence is at a somewhat older age (5 to 15 years) than with other enteroviral infections.

PATHOGENESIS. Although detailed studies of the histopathology of pleurodynia are not available, the infection appears to involve skeletal muscle rather than pleura or peritoneum. Often muscle tenderness and occasionally swelling can be noted at the site of pain. Hyperesthesia can be elicited over affected muscles as well. In contrast, pleural rubs have been infrequently and inconstantly noted, and peritonitis has not been present in cases that have come to laparotomy. However, coxsackievirus B has not been unequivocally isolated from affected muscle.

CLINICAL MANIFESTATIONS. Characteristically, pleurodynia begins as an abrupt paroxysm of pain, located over the lateral chest (ribs) or upper abdomen. The pain is of variable intensity, but can be severe, and is often described as "catching," "stabbing," "crushing," or "vise-like." Acute shortness of breath is also frequently present. Adults most commonly have chest pain, whereas children more frequently have abdominal pain, generally in the epigastrium and upper abdomen. Patients have been described with pain primarily in the lower abdomen, as well as in the extremities. Prodromal symptoms are not present in the majority of cases, although up to 25 per cent of individuals report headache, malaise, myalgia, and sore throat prior to the onset of pain. Fever of 37.8 to 40.0° C is present at the onset of pain, but resolves between paroxysms. Multiple paroxysms of pain occur and last from two to ten hours, during which time the patient may appear diaphoretic and acutely ill. The initial paroxysm of pain is most severe, and subsequent ones are generally milder. Splinting of the chest or guarding of the abdomen is usually observed, so that in one outbreak 9 of 49 patients underwent laparotomy before the disease was recognized. Tenderness or swelling of the affected muscles, or both, has been noted in up to 25 per cent of cases. During paroxysms, patients tend to lie quietly in bed and try to avoid any motion which may aggravate the pain. The patient may appear relatively well between bouts of pain.

Acute illness generally lasts one to six days, but a range of up to three weeks has been reported. Approximately 10 per cent of the patients experience at least one recurrence of pain within one or more months after the last paroxysm. Such recurrences often develop at the same site as the initial paroxysm of pain.

LABORATORY DIAGNOSIS. Specific diagnosis is made by isolation of coxsackie B virus from the throat or stools of acutely ill patients, along with rises in immunotype-specific neutralizing antibody titers in acute and convalescent sera. Detection of virus is most frequent in samples taken early in illness. Other laboratory tests are not helpful in making the diagnosis. White blood cell and differential counts are generally normal, although mild leukopenia has been reported in approximately 25 per cent of cases.

DIFFERENTIAL DIAGNOSIS. Because of the location of the pain, Bornholm disease can be confused with a variety of acute chest diseases, including pneumonia, pulmonary infarction, and myocardial ischemia. The absence of physical and roentgenographic signs of pulmonary infiltrates, the lack of sputum production, and a normal ECG help exclude these diagnoses. When the pain is primarily abdominal, differentiation from other causes of an acute abdominal pain can be difficult. The absence of signs of peritonitis and a normal white cell count may be helpful. The most useful distinguishing clinical feature of Bornholm disease is the paroxysmal nature of the pain. Epidemiologic information, such as the occurrence of a cluster of cases in the late summer, may also suggest the diagnosis.

PROGNOSIS AND TREATMENT. Patients with epidemic pleurodynia will eventually recover fully, although relapses are common (see above). Occasionally, malaise or asthenia may persist for months after the acute illness. Complications are uncommon, but may include aseptic meningitis (3 to 7 per cent of cases), orchitis (less than 5 per cent) and rarely pericarditis.

Treatment is entirely supportive and symptomatic. Episodes of acute pain can usually be controlled by salicylates or other mild analgesics. Occasionally, narcotic analgesics may be required for relief.

Finn JJ Jr, Weller TH, Morgan HR: Epidemic pleurodynia: Clinical and etiologic studies based on one hundred and fourteen cases. Arch Intern Med 83:305, 1949. *An excellent clinical review of the subject.*

Huebner RJ, Risser JA, Bell JA, Beeman EA, Biegelman PM, Strong JC: Epidemic pleurodynia in Texas: A study of 22 cases. N Engl J Med 248:267, 1953. *Demonstration of the viral etiology of an outbreak of pleurodynia.*

Pickles NW: Sylvest's disease (Bornholm disease). N Engl J Med 250:1033, 1954. *A vivid and dramatic discussion of the clinical presentation.*

Sylvest E: Epidemic Myalgia: Bornholm Disease. London, Oxford University Press, 1934, pp 1-155. *The classic monograph in the field.*

344. MYOCARDITIS AND PERICARDITIS CAUSED BY ENTEROVIRUSES

Enteroviruses are well recognized causes of myocarditis and pericarditis, with clinical manifestations that appear to be age dependent. Neonatal infection is a severe illness in which extensive involvement of the myocardium, widespread dissemination to other organs, and high fatality rates are seen. In older children and adults, pericarditis is most prominent, and the disease is generally self-limited.

ETIOLOGY. The group B coxsackieviruses, immunotypes 1 to 5, are the enteroviruses most frequently implicated in pericarditis and myocarditis. Depending on the study, group B coxsackieviruses have been reported to cause from 3 to 44 per cent of cases of acute pericarditis and approximately 33 per cent of cases of acute myocarditis. Group A coxsackieviruses (1, 4, 9, and 16) and echoviruses (1, 3, 6 to 9, 19, and 22) have also been implicated, but considerably less frequently. Since routine serologic testing is available for group B but not for group A coxsackieviruses or echoviruses, it is conceivable that the proportion of cases caused by the latter groups may be higher. The etiology of the majority of cases of "idiopathic" pericarditis and myocarditis remains unknown.

EPIDEMIOLOGY. Enteroviral myopericarditis occurs most frequently during the summer and early fall, and both epidemics and sporadic cases are seen. Neonatal myocarditis was first recognized in outbreaks in nurseries for the newborn in South Africa, Rhodesia, and the Netherlands in the mid-1950's. Subsequent reports have been largely confined to sporadic cases. Illness in nursery outbreaks appears to be postnatally acquired, presumably by the fecal-oral route. However, cases in which infection was acquired at birth and even in utero have been described. In the latter cases, infection of mothers appeared to take place within two weeks of delivery.

Among older children and adults, myopericardial involvement with enteroviral infection is sporadic, and even in the presence of outbreaks of enteroviral infection myopericardial involvement in this age group is uncommon. Despite the likely overreporting of serious infections, only 3 per cent of group B coxsackievirus infections reported to the World Health Organization involved the myocardium predominantly.

PATHOGENESIS. Infection of the heart by enteroviruses is most likely a result of viremia after initial replication of virus in the gastrointestinal tract. Histopathology of acute enteroviral myocarditis consists of a mixed polymorphonuclear leukocytic and lymphocytic infiltrate, which can be either diffuse or focal. Focal myocardial muscle degeneration and necrosis are also seen. The histopathology of enterovirus-induced pericarditis is similar, and is frequently accompanied by focal areas of subepicardial myocarditis. For this reason, some authors prefer the term "myopericarditis" rather than simply "pericarditis."

During acute illness, virus may be isolated from myocardium, pericardium, or pericardial fluid, and therefore the pathogenesis appears to be direct viral invasion of myopericardium. However, chronic inflammatory lesions from which infectious virus cannot be isolated have been described in humans and in experimental myocarditis. Chronic lesions, and perhaps clinically apparent relapses, may have an immunopathologic basis. Direct evidence is lacking in humans, but in weanling mice the severity of coxsackie B3 myocarditis is increased by intact T-lymphocyte functions.

CLINICAL MANIFESTATIONS. ***Neonatal Myocarditis.*** Myocarditis of the newborn presents from two days to three weeks after birth (mean of seven days) with the acute onset of fever and listlessness, often accompanied by coryza and/or diarrhea. When congestive heart failure is present, respiratory distress and tachycardia are prominent. In approximately one third of patients, a biphasic illness is seen. The first phase consists of a febrile prodrome followed by a period of well-being lasting one to seven days, after which the phase of clinically evident cardiac involvement appears. The latter is predominantly myocarditis with little or no pericarditis. Circulatory failure can develop rapidly and be profound, as manifested by cyanosis, abdominal distention, and edema. In addition, viral infection may be disseminated widely, with involvement of the central nervous system, lungs, liver, pancreas, spleen, and kidney. In cases of fulminant disease, death may ensue within 24 hours, although the majority of fatalities occur two to seven days after the onset of illness. Among survivors, cardiac function and general well-being improve rapidly once the fever and acute illness have resolved.

Myopericarditis of Older Children and Adults. In older children and adults, the clinical features of enteroviral infection of the heart are those of acute pericarditis. Sixty to 90 per cent of patients present with fever and chest pain, preceded by an upper respiratory tract illness in approximately two thirds of cases. The chest pain is most frequently precordial and dull, but can on occasion be sharp with pleuritic and positional components. Dyspnea, malaise, myalgias, and arthralgias are frequently seen. Physical examination reveals a pericardial friction rub, often transient, in 36 to 76 per cent of cases. Pericardial effusions have been reported in 0 to 45 per cent of cases, but acute cardiac tamponade is rare. Increased areas of cardiac dullness and gallop rhythms have been reported in up to 25 per cent of patients in some series, but are ordinarily not observed. Despite histopathologic evidence of subepicardial myocarditis accompanying pericarditis, clinically apparent congestive heart failure is unusual. When present, the latter indicates widespread myocardial involvement. Serologic evidence for enteroviral infection in cases clinically diagnosed as acute myocardial infarctions has been reported, but the etiologic role, if any, of viruses in that setting is unknown. Pleural effusions, particularly left-sided, have been reported in 20 to 50 per cent of cases of enterovirus-associated myopericarditis.

LABORATORY DIAGNOSIS. The etiology of illness is established by isolation of enterovirus from the myocardium, pericardium, or pericardial fluid. Specimens from these sites should be submitted for virus isolation whenever available. However, only throat and/or stool cultures are obtained in the majority of cases. Isolation of virus from these latter sites, along with rises in immunotype-specific serum antibodies, provides circumstantial evidence for the diagnosis of enteroviral myopericarditis. Diagnosis is made more difficult by the fact that many patients present late in the course of illness, when virus shedding has ceased, and when high, stable titers of antibodies are already present. In the latter case, detection of immunotype-specific IgM antibodies indicates recent infection.

The laboratory hallmark of myopericarditis is an abnormal ECG, seen in virtually all cases. Changes in pericarditis or mild myopericarditis are S-T segment elevation and T wave flattening or inversion. In severe myocarditis, Q waves, conduction disturbances, and arrhythmias can be seen. In the latter cases, elevations of myocardial enzymes have been noted. Chest x-ray reveals enlargement of the cardiac silhouette in 50 to 75 per cent of cases, which may reflect either cardiac dilatation or pericardial effusion. To determine the presence and location of effusions, echocardiograms can be very helpful. Analyses of pericardial fluid in documented viral myopericarditis have been infrequent, but the characteristics of the fluid are generally those of an exudate, with a predominantly polymorphonuclear leukocytic content. Considerable overlap exists between the cell counts, differentials, and protein content of pericardial fluid in cases of viral pericarditis and fluid from cases of pericarditis of other etiologies.

Other laboratory tests are generally not helpful in establishing the diagnosis. A moderate polymorphonuclear leukocytosis may be present, and elevated erythrocyte sedimentation rates have been reported in 70 to 90 per cent of patients.

DIFFERENTIAL DIAGNOSIS. Neonatal myocarditis can mimic pneumonia, bacterial sepsis, or other disseminated viral infections such as those caused by herpes simplex and cytomegalovirus. The prominent ECG changes, evidence of congestive heart failure, and absence of skin lesions may be helpful in suggesting the diagnosis of neonatal myocarditis. The differential diagnosis of myopericarditis in older patients is discussed in Ch. 51 and 52.

PROGNOSIS. Neonatal myocarditis was initially reported to have an extremely high case-fatality rate; however, recent experience suggests that with aggressive supportive therapy, mortality is less than 50 per cent. Long-term follow-up of survivors is not available.

The majority of older children and adults with enteroviral myopericarditis recover without clinically apparent sequelae. The duration of illness is highly variable (days to weeks), and up to 20 per cent of patients experience one or more episodes of recurrent myopericarditis within one year of the initial illness. Electrocardiographic abnormalities may persist in 10 to 20 per cent of patients, and long-term cardiomegaly has been described in 5 to 10 per cent. Constrictive pericarditis is an extremely rare complication. Chronic congestive heart failure also appears to be an unusual sequel of illness, although in one series 5 of 22 patients were reported to have this complication. The role of enterovirus-induced myocarditis in chronic cardiomyopathies of unknown etiology remains controversial.

TREATMENT. Specific antiviral chemotherapy for enteroviral infections is not available. Management of patients with enteroviral myopericarditis consists primarily of control of pain with analgesics and treatment of arrhythmias or congestive heart failure as they appear (see Ch. 42 and 50). In experimentally induced myocarditis in mice, vigorous exercise is deleterious, and therefore bed rest or restriction of activity is frequently recommended to patients. Corticosteroids also increase the severity of infection in the same animal model, but anecdotal reports of corticosteroid treatment of cases in humans have claimed either benefit or lack of harm. Controlled studies of corticosteroid therapy of enteroviral myopericarditis are not available.

PREVENTION. Specific preventive measures have not been developed. In neonatal myocarditis, patients and mothers should be isolated as a unit, and women at term should subsequently be admitted to a separate facility. Isolation of cases of myopericarditis in older children and adults is not indicated (see Ch. 89).

Grist NR, Bell EJ: A six-year study of coxsackievirus B infections in heart disease. J Hyg 73:165, 1974. *A solid, laboratory based investigation of the problem.*

Lansdown ABG: Viral infections and diseases of the heart. Prog Med Virol 24:70, 1978. *A comprehensive review of infections with all known virus groups, as well as with enteroviruses.*

Lerner MA: Myocarditis and pericarditis. *In* Mandell GL, Douglas RG, Bennett DE (eds.): Principles and Practice of Infectious Diseases. New York, John Wiley & Sons, 1979, p 711. *A thoughtful review of the subject, with a good presentation of the evidence for a viral etiology. Mechanisms of pathogenesis are also discussed.*

Sainani GS, Krompotic E, Slodki SJ: Adult heart disease due to coxsackievirus B infection. Medicine 47:133, 1968. *A study of 22 adult patients which illustrates the clinical presentations and difficulty in establishing an etiologic diagnosis.*

Woodruff J: Viral myocarditis: A review. Am J Pathol 101:425, 1980. *A good general review of the subject.*

345. MUCOCUTANEOUS INFECTIONS CAUSED BY ENTEROVIRUSES

ENANTHEMS

Herpangina (*herpes,* vesicular eruption; *angina,* inflammation of the throat) is a vesicular eruption of the posterior pharynx which is most frequently caused by coxsackievirus A (1 to 6, 8, 10, 16, and 22), although other enteroviruses have also been implicated. Lesions most commonly occur on the soft palate and anterior pillars of the tonsils, and less commonly on the posterior pharyngeal wall or buccal mucosa. Illness begins abruptly with fever ranging from 37.8 to 40.5° C, sore throat, and dysphagia. The pharynx appears mildly injected, with little or no tonsillar exudate. Discrete oropharyngeal lesions can be seen, which begin as macules, progress to gray papules, and eventually become erythematous-based vesicles, 2 to 5 mm in diameter. Lesions progress from macules to papules over a period of one to two days, and may evolve into ulcers that can last up to one week. The lesions are usually less than six in number, occasionally up to twelve, and are only moderately painful. Malaise, myalgia, and headache frequently accompany the fever at the onset of illness, but resolve over two to four days as the fever abates. Abdominal pain and vomiting have also been noted during acute illness.

Acute lymphonodular pharyngitis is a syndrome in which lesions occur with a distribution similar to that seen in herpangina. However, the lesions consist of small nodules of lymphocytes on an erythematous base, rather than vesicles or ulcers. Mild to moderate fever, headache, and sore throat are present as in herpangina, and symptoms last 4 to 14 days. Coxsackievirus A10 has been isolated from patients with this syndrome.

Hand-foot-and-mouth disease (vesicular stomatitis with exanthem) is a mucocutaneous infection with both an enanthem and an exanthem. The enanthem consists of vesicles and/or ulcers in the anterior pharynx, most commonly on the anterior buccal mucosa, tongue, lips, and hard palate. The oral lesions are accompanied in 75 per cent of cases by vesicular or papulovesicular lesions on the palms, soles, or extensor surfaces of the hands and feet. Occasionally, lesions are seen on the buttocks or genitalia. Lesions are surrounded by erythema and are usually tender. Initially, patients complain of sore throat or refuse to eat, and manifest a low grade fever (38 to 39° C) for 24 to 48 hours. Illness is generally mild and lasts less than one week. This syndrome is caused most frequently by coxsackievirus A16, less frequently by A5, A9, and A10, and occasionally by B2 or B5 or enterovirus 71.

EPIDEMIOLOGY. As with other enteroviral infections, the enanthems are seen most frequently during the summer and early fall. Attack rates are highest in younger children, but cases occur in adolescents and young adults as well. Both sporadic cases and outbreaks have been described. Several children within a family unit can become infected sequentially, with an incubation period of two to ten days. Less frequently, illness can spread to adults. Asymptomatic infection of contacts is common.

DIFFERENTIAL DIAGNOSIS. Herpangina and acute lymphonodular pharyngitis involve the posterior pharynx, whereas hand-foot-and-mouth disease involves the anterior pharynx. The latter is associated with cutaneous lesions which are absent in herpangina. Primary herpes simplex stomatitis is also an anterior stomatitis, but often has gingivitis and more prominent systemic signs and symptoms, including cervical lymphadenitis. Chickenpox occasionally has an enanthem, but cutaneous lesions are more numerous and widely distributed than in hand-foot-and-mouth disease. Bacterial pharyngitis or tonsillitis is generally manifested by more systemic signs of illness, as well as by the presence of more extensive pharyngeal exudate. However, individual cases of bacterial infection may be difficult to distinguish from those caused by enteroviruses. Bacterial pharyngitis, as well as pharyngitis caused by viruses other than enteroviruses, generally does not produce vesicular lesions.

LABORATORY DIAGNOSIS. The principles of diagnosis are the same as those discussed in Ch. 89. Virus is frequently isolated from throat, stool, or vesicular lesions.

TREATMENT. The enteroviral enanthems are benign, self-limited illnesses which ordinarily require only symptomatic therapy for sore throat and headache.

EXANTHEMS

Nonpolio enteroviruses cause a variety of exanthems that accompany "undifferentiated febrile illness" or specific disease syndromes such as aseptic meningitis, or that occur independently. The rate of exanthems associated with enteroviral infection is highest in young children, and the pathogenesis of the majority of these exanthems has not been clearly established. Virus has been isolated from the vesicular exanthem associated with hand-foot-and-mouth disease, and it is likely that these lesions are the result of viremia. Virus isolation has not been reported from enteroviral maculopapular exanthems, and some authors have suggested that an immunopathologic component may be present.

The characteristics of the enterovirus exanthems are not sufficiently distinctive for establishment of an etiologic diagnosis on clinical grounds alone. Multiple immunotypes of echoviruses, coxsackieviruses, and enterovirus 71 cause exanthems. The most common clinical presentation is that of a *morbilliform* exanthem which is caused most frequently by echovirus 9. The rash consists of fine, discrete macules and/or papules, and occurs primarily on the face, neck, and, to a lesser extent, chest and extremities. It is most commonly confused with rubella, although posterior cervical and auricular lymphadenopathy are generally not present. Occasionally, rashes may have petechial components and even frank purpura, which may lead to confusion with meningococcemia. Fever is generally low grade and is present at the time that the rash develops. The rash and fever last for three to seven days. Both outbreaks and sporadic cases have been described.

Roseoliform exanthems have been caused most commonly by echovirus 16 ("the Boston exanthem"). Typically, fever (38 to 39.5° C) appears first, and the rash develops as the fever subsides. The rash consists of salmon pink macules and papules on the face and chest, but may involve the extremities on occasion. Fever lasts for 24 to 36 hours, and the rash persists for one to five days. The rashes in roseoliform as well as rubelliform exanthems are usually not pruritic or painful, and complete resolution is the rule. As with other enteroviral-induced illnesses, exanthems are seen most frequently in the summer and early fall. Attack rates are highest in very young children, and both epidemic and sporadic cases are seen.

Diagnosis of enteroviral exanthems depends on laboratory demonstration of viral infection, as discussed in Ch. 89. In general, patients with enteroviral exanthems are only mildly ill, although occasionally infants may be more severely affected. Since little morbidity is associated with enteroviral exanthems, supportive or symptomatic therapy is rarely required. However, the presence of enteroviral exanthems should alert physicians to the potential development of other types of enteroviral illness in the community.

Adler JL, Mostow SR, Mellin H, Janney JH, Joseph JM: Epidemiologic investigation of hand-foot-and-mouth disease. Am J Dis Child 120:309, 1970. *A detailed investigation of an outbreak due to coxsackievirus A16.*

Horstmann DM: Viral exanthems and enanthems. Pediatrics 41:867, 1968. *A concise review of the subject.*

Huebner RJ, Cole RM, Beeman EA, Bell JA, Peers JH: Herpangina. Etiologic studies of a specific infectious disease. JAMA 145:628, 1951. *Demonstration of association of herpangina with coxsackievirus A infection.*

Neva FA, Feemster RF, Gorbach IJ: Clinical and epidemiological features of an unusual epidemic exanthem. JAMA 155:544, 1954. *The original description of the Boston exanthem.*

Sabin AB, Krumbiegel ER, Wigand R: ECHO type 9 virus disease. J Dis Child 96:197, 1958. *A detailed review of the spectrum of disease associated with an epidemic of this immunotype and the types of rashes which were present.*

346. ACUTE HEMORRHAGIC CONJUNCTIVITIS

DEFINITION. Acute hemorrhagic conjunctivitis (AHC) is an acute viral infection of the eye characterized by painful conjunctival inflammation, subconjunctival hemorrhages, and swelling of the eyelids. AHC has occurred in explosive epidemics in Africa, India, and Asia.

ETIOLOGY. Epidemic AHC has been caused primarily by enterovirus 70. A smaller number of cases have been caused by coxsackievirus A24 and by adenovirus 11.

EPIDEMIOLOGY. Epidemics of AHC caused by enterovirus 70 first appeared almost simultaneously in Ghana and Indonesia in 1969. Extensive outbreaks were subsequently observed in northern and southeastern Africa, as well as in India, Southeast Asia, and other areas of the Far East. Localized outbreaks have occurred in the United Kingdom, continental Europe, and the USSR. The USSR outbreaks have been most often related to index cases in travelers and subsequent spread at eye clinics. Cases in the United States had been reported only in Southeast Asian refugees until 1981, when cases originating in the Western hemisphere with subsequent spread to the southern United States were first noted.

Patterns of antibody prevalence to enterovirus 70 suggest

that AHC has emerged as a relatively new disease. In endemic areas, antibody studies of serum specimens obtained prior to 1969 revealed low or absent levels of neutralizing antibody to enterovirus 70 in the population. After the occurrence of epidemics in 1969–72, antibody prevalence rates of 40 to 50 per cent were noted, indicating that widespread subclinical as well as clinical infection had taken place. Attack rates for clinical illness are highest among young adults, but infection is most common in young children. It is estimated that tens of millions of cases of AHC caused by enterovirus 70 have occurred since 1969. Simultaneously, a variant of coxsackievirus A24 has been implicated in several hundred thousand cases of AHC, including cases in mixed outbreaks.

PATHOGENESIS. In contrast to other enteroviral infections, AHC is spread by fomites and by direct inoculation of conjunctiva from contaminated fingers. Incubation periods are relatively short (12 to 72 hours), and likely reflect the large inoculum transmitted by these means. Transmission rates are increased by crowding and by poor hygiene. Enterovirus 70 appears to replicate preferentially at 33 to 35° C, which may represent an adaptation to conjunctival temperatures, rather than to the higher temperatures of the gut.

CLINICAL MANIFESTATIONS. AHC begins abruptly with pain, photophobia, swelling of the eyelids, and serous or seromucous conjunctival discharge. Involvement is initially unilateral but rapidly spreads to the other eye. Subconjunctival hemorrhages are present in up to 90 per cent of patients with disease caused by enterovirus 70, but are less frequent in disease caused by coxsackievirus A24. Lesions vary in size from petechiae to hemorrhages that cover the entire bulbar conjunctiva. Conjunctival folliculitis and preauricular lymphadenopathy are also frequently present. Slit lamp examination often reveals corneal erosions or punctate epithelial keratitis. Low grade fever, headache, coryza, and malaise may be present in up to 20 per cent of cases.

LABORATORY DIAGNOSIS. Virus can be recovered from conjunctival scrapings in a high proportion of cases. Unlike other enteroviral infections, virus is rarely isolated from the throat or stool. The diagnosis is supported by immunotype-specific antibody rises in acute and convalescent sera.

PROGNOSIS. Signs and symptoms peak on the first day of illness, abate over the next 48 hours, and resolve within ten days. Permanent sequelae are rare, although discoloration from hemorrhages can persist for days. Keratitis rarely leads to permanent corneal damage. Occasionally, secondary bacterial infection may follow the acute viral conjunctivitis. In adults, a rare aseptic meningitis accompanied by a poliomyelitis-like motor paralysis has been reported usually in association with enterovirus 70 infection. Paralysis develops 5 to 42 days after acute illness and has been observed almost exclusively in adults with an increased prevalence in men. The pathogenesis of the neurologic syndrome is unclear, although enterovirus 70 has been reported to be neuropathogenic in monkeys.

TREATMENT AND PREVENTION. Treatment is entirely symptomatic. If bacterial conjunctivitis develops, topical application of antibacterial ophthalmic ointment is indicated. Prevention of spread of AHC depends on careful handwashing, avoidance of contaminated towels or clothing, and sterilization of ophthalmologic instruments.

Arnow JC, Hierholzer JC, Higbee J, Harris DH: Acute hemorrhagic conjunctivitis: A mixed virus outbreak among Vietnamese refugees on Guam. Am J Epidemiol 105:68, 1977. *Description of an outbreak caused by enterovirus 70 and adenovirus 11.*

Christopher S, Theogaraj S, Godbole S, John TS: An epidemic of acute hemorrhagic conjunctivitis due to coxsackievirus A24. J Infect Dis 146:16, 1982. *Report of a large outbreak of AHC in India with good clinical descriptions and virologic studies.*

Hierholzer JC, Hilliard KA, Esposito JJ: Serosurvey for "acute hemorrhagic conjunctivitis" virus (enterovirus 70) antibodies in the southeastern United States, with review of the literature and some epidemiologic implications. Am J Epidemiol 102:533, 1975. *A detailed review of the seroepidemiology and spread of this agent.*

347. RESPIRATORY TRACT ILLNESS ASSOCIATED WITH ENTEROVIRUSES

Enteroviruses have been associated with upper respiratory tract illness, primarily the "common cold syndrome," in both children and adults. Lower respiratory tract illness, including bronchitis, tracheitis, bronchiolitis, croup, and pneumonia, has been induced by enteroviruses in children, but infrequently in adults. The majority of respiratory tract symptoms have presented as part of the "undifferentiated febrile illness" or "summer grippe" associated with enteroviral infections (see Table 341–2). Coxsackievirus A21 has caused outbreaks of pharyngitis in military recruits and has induced respiratory tract disease in normal adult volunteers. Group B coxsackieviruses, enterovirus 68, and several echoviruses (chiefly echovirus 11) have also been implicated as causes of respiratory tract illness. Respiratory illness induced by enteroviruses cannot be differentiated on clinical grounds from that caused by respiratory tract viruses, such as rhinoviruses, parainfluenza viruses, respiratory syncytial virus, or adenoviruses. However, infection with the latter groups of viruses occurs most frequently during the winter months, whereas enterovirus infection is seen most frequently in the summer and early fall. Viral respiratory tract infections are discussed in Ch. 73 to 78.

Viral Disease of the Gastrointestinal Tract

348. VIRAL GASTROENTERITIS (Acute Infectious Nonbacterial Gastroenteritis, Epidemic Diarrhea, Winter Vomiting Disease)

Raphael Dolin

DEFINITION. The term "nonbacterial gastroenteritis," along with the descriptive phrases cited above, refers to a group of acute, common, self-limited illnesses characterized chiefly by vomiting and/or diarrhea. An infectious etiology for these diseases had been previously suspected, but it has only been recently that specific viral agents that cause at least a portion of such illnesses have been detected.

ETIOLOGY. Two groups of viral agents that induce acute gastroenteritis have been described. The first is the Norwalk-like agents, generally named after the location of the outbreak from which they have been derived (Norwalk, Hawaii, Montgomery County, Marin County, Snow Mountain, "W," Ditchling, Cockle, and Parramatta agents). These agents have not been cultivated in vitro and have been only partly characterized. They are small (approximately 25 to 32 nm in diameter), nonenveloped viral agents found in the stools of acutely ill patients. Since the Norwalk-like agents have been only partly characterized biochemically, definitive classification within virus families is not possible at this time. Preliminary analysis of the Norwalk-like agents has detected at least five antigenic types.

The second group is the rotaviruses, which have been classified within the family of Reoviridae. They are 66 to 70 nm in diameter, contain double-stranded RNA in 11 discrete segments, and have a characteristic double shell appearance. Although strain differences have not been fully analyzed, human rotaviruses appear to be of two subgroups and at least four neutralization serotypes. Human rotaviruses have recently been grown efficiently in vitro by employing rhesus monkey kidney cells in roller tubes to which trypsin has been added. Rotaviruses can be detected directly in stool by a variety of techniques (see later discussion).

In addition, other groups of viruses have been implicated in outbreaks of gastroenteritis. These include noncultivatable adenoviruses, astroviruses, caliciviruses, and coronaviruses. The etiologic association of these agents with human gastroenteritis is less well established than that for rotaviruses and Norwalk-like agents. Additional studies are required to determine the relative importance of those virus groups.

The enteroviruses (coxsackieviruses, echoviruses), discussed in Ch. 89 to 95, commonly infect the gastrointestinal tract but do not appear to be major causes of acute gastroenteritis. Echovirus 18 has been implicated in an outbreak of diarrhea in a nursery for newborns.

EPIDEMIOLOGY. Because of the lack of suitable detection methods, seroepidemiologic studies have been carried out only with the Norwalk and Snow Mountain agents within the Norwalk-like group. Naturally occurring illness with these agents appears to be exceedingly common and widespread, and to involve all age groups. In one study, evidence of infection with the Norwalk agent was found in 34 per cent of 70 outbreaks of acute nonbacterial gastroenteritis. Infection with the Norwalk or Snow Mountain agent generally occurs late in childhood, so that antibody prevalence rates rise from less than 20 per cent by age 5 to 50 per cent or greater by age 19. Illness occurs most frequently during the winter months, but outbreaks in other seasons have been reported. Both sporadic cases and explosive outbreaks have been noted, including several common source outbreaks, which have involved shellfish, drinking water, and swimming pools.

In contrast to the Norwalk-like agents, illness associated with rotaviruses has a striking predilection for the very young. Rotavirus-induced gastroenteritis occurs most frequently between 6 and 24 months of age, and occasionally up to four years of age. Widespread infection occurs, so that 52 to 90 per cent of individuals above two years of age have serum antibody against rotavirus. Illness in neonates, older children, and adults is infrequent but can occur. Asymptomatic reinfection in older age groups is common.

Rotavirus infections are worldwide in distribution, and are seen primarily during the winter months in both Northern and Southern Hemispheres. Cases occur both sporadically and in distinct outbreaks. Rotavirus infections have accounted for 42 to 55 per cent of infants and young children hospitalized with gastroenteritis in studies carried out throughout the world.

PATHOGENESIS. Acute infection with Norwalk and Hawaii agents results in reversible histopathologic lesions, which primarily involve the upper jejunum, with relative sparing of the stomach and rectum. The jejunal mucosa remains intact, but there is marked blunting of villi and shortening of microvilli. The lamina propria is infiltrated with both polymorphonuclear and mononuclear cells. Acute illness is also accompanied by malabsorption of d-xylose and fat. Rotavirus infections induce a similar pathology in the duodenum and jejunum, although inflammatory changes can on occasion be seen in the stomach and rectum.

In human volunteer studies, resistance to rotaviral infection correlated with the presence of circulating antibody, while the relationship to local antibody was less clear-cut. Resistance to infection with the Norwalk-like agents appears to be unrelated to serum antibody titers, but other determinants of immunity are not well understood.

CLINICAL MANIFESTATIONS. Illness induced by the Norwalk-like agents consists of nausea, abdominal cramps, vomiting and/or diarrhea, often accompanied by headache and myalgias. Onset of illness is often abrupt, and both vomiting and diarrhea usually occur, although either can be present alone. Low grade fever (38.9° C) can be found in approximately 50 to 60 per cent of patients. The incubation period for illness is generally from 18 to 48 hours, and disease manifestations last from 48 to 72 hours. Disease remits spontaneously and without known sequelae. Rotavirus infections have clinical features similar to those described for the Norwalk-like agents. Incubation periods range from 24 to 96 hours, and among hospitalized children illness lasts for five to eight days. Even in the latter cases, illness appears to be generally mild, although occasionally more severe and rarely fatal cases have been reported.

DIAGNOSIS. Infection with Norwalk-like agents currently can be detected only by immune electron microscopy or by radioimmunoassay, which are specialized techniques not widely available. Norwalk agent is found in stools during the first four to five days of illness, and serum antibody rises are noted two to six weeks later. Rotaviruses are easily detected in stools by a variety of techniques, including complement fixation (CF), immunofluorescence, conventional electron microscopy, and enzyme-linked immunosorbent assays (ELISA). Virus can be found in stools for up to eight days and occasionally longer after onset of illness, and serum antibody rises are seen by two weeks after illness.

Infection with Norwalk-like agents or rotaviruses can be suspected on the basis of epidemiologic information (age, time of year, secondary cases). Although illness is generally milder than that observed with several bacterial pathogens, individual cases cannot be differentiated from other causes of acute gastroenteritis on clinical grounds alone. Fecal leukocytes are absent in Norwalk-induced disease, and are usually absent in rotavirus infections, which may prove helpful for early differentiation from *Shigella* or *Salmonella* enteritis (see Ch. 173 and 179).

TREATMENT. Acute viral gastroenteritis is generally a benign, self-limited illness which requires no specific therapy. In some cases, particularly in the very young or debilitated, fluid replacement may be necessary; this can generally be provided in the form of clear liquids by mouth. With severe fluid loss, intravenous fluid and electrolyte replacement should be administered promptly. Occasionally, symptomatic treatment of headache or nausea may be required. Administration of bismuth subsalicylate has resulted in a mild reduction in symptoms in Norwalk-induced illness, but the effect of administration of inhibitors of intestinal motility in viral gastroenteritis has not been studied. Restriction of activity during acute illness according to the patient's own symptoms appears to be prudent.

PREVENTION. There are currently no available methods for prevention of viral gastroenteritis, which represents a major uncontrolled public health problem. Considerable interest exists in the development of live attenuated vaccines directed against rotaviruses. Candidate vaccines would have to be safe and effective in very young age groups.

Dolin R, Blacklow R, Chanock RM: Biological properties of Norwalk agent of acute infectious nonbacterial gastroenteritis. Proc Soc Exp Biol Med 140:578, 1972. *The initial description of experimentally induced illness associated with the Norwalk agent and the biologic properties of the infectious agent.*

Dolin R, Reichman RC, Roessner KD, Tralka TS, Schooley RT, Gary W, Morens D: Detection by immune electron microscopy of the Snow Mountain agent of acute viral gastroenteritis. J Infect Dis 146:184, 1982. *Description of the use of immune electron microscopy for detection of the Snow Mountain agent, as well as the humoral immune response to infection.*

Greenberg HB, Wyatt RG, Kalica AR, Yolken RH, Black R, Kapikian AZ, Chanock RM: New insights in viral gastroenteritis. *In* Perspectives in Virology. Vol XI. New York, John Wiley & Sons, 1981, p 163. *Current review of Norwalk and rotavirus infections, with an extensive bibliography.*

Kapikian AZ, Kim HW, Wyatt RG, Cline WL, Arrobio JO, Brandt CO, Rodriguez WJ, Sack DA, Chanock RM, Parrot RH: Human reovirus-like agent as the major pathogen associated with winter gastroenteritis in hospitalized infants and young children. N Engl J Med 294:965, 1976. *A prospective study demonstrating the importance of rotavirus infection in very young children.*

Sato K, Inaba Y, Shinozaki T, Fujii R, Matumoto M: Isolation of human rotavirus in cell cultures. Arch Virol 69:155, 1981. *Description of the technique employed to cultivate human rotavirus efficiently in vitro.*

Tyrrell DAJ, Kapikian AZ: Virus Infections of the Gastrointestinal Tract. New York, Marcel Dekker, Inc., 1982. *An entire volume devoted to viral infections of the gastrointestinal tract, with chapters on virology, pathophysiology, and immune response. An excellent reference source for in-depth reading.*

Arthropod-Borne Viral Fevers

349. INTRODUCTION

Karl M. Johnson

Arthropod-borne viruses (arboviruses) and the diseases they produce in man can be defined in a variety of ways. In biologic terms, any virus which multiplies in one or more arthropods and is therafter transmitted to a vertebrate such that this mechanism is significant in the natural maintenance of the agent is an arbovirus. More than 400 distinguishable viruses have been tentatively so classified, and about 100 of these are known to infect man. Arboviruses also can be organized into virologic families based on morphologic, biophysical, and biochemical properties. Most of those which cause human disease belong to one of two such families: the Togaviridae and the Bunyaviridae, which in turn have been subdivided into genera such as alphaviruses, flaviviruses, phleboviruses, bunyaviruses, and nairoviruses. Within these genera, in turn, agents have been clustered immunologically on the basis of shared antigens. For example, most mosquito-borne flaviviruses can be readily distinguished from tick-borne members of this genus by this means (see Table 349–1).

Finally, arboviruses can be separated by the clinical syndromes they produce in man. Although mild undifferentiated fever is the most common consequence of infection, more serious illness can sometimes be induced by certain of these viruses. These individual descriptions are placed in one of the following groups: (1) *fevers of undifferentiated type,* with or without rash; (2) *encephalitides,* often severe and with significant case-fatality rates; and (3) *hemorrhagic fevers,* also frequently severe and fatal. Some of the variables used to classify arboviruses and the diseases they produce are illustrated in the accompanying table. All of the agents contain RNA, and all except the reoviruses have lipid-containing envelopes.

The largest number of viruses has been associated exclusively with mild, undifferentiated disease, and most of these are encountered in tropical and semitropical countries (see Table 350–1). Those to be described represent but a small sample that has caused many human illnesses in either endemic or significant epidemic patterns.

All arboviruses conspicuously associated with encephalitis are included. Similarly, viruses causing hemorrhagic fever are described. All are zoonotic agents, but not all are vector-borne arboviruses. Except for the nairovirus *Congo-CHF* and the unclassified Bunyavirus, *Hantaan,* which causes hemorrhagic fever with renal syndrome, arboviruses causing hemorrhagic fever are flaviviruses. Other zoonotic viruses causing hemorrhagic fever include three Arenaviruses, *Junin, Machupo,* and *Lassa,* and the as yet unclassified agents, *Marburg* and *Ebola.*

Arenaviruses are fundamentally parasites of wild rodents and display a high order of host specificity, characterized by chronic infection with persistent viremia and shedding of virus in urine. Lymphocytic choriomeningitis virus (see Ch. 499) is the prototype of the family and is associated with the common house mouse, *Mus musculus.* Other Arenaviruses are usually restricted to a single rodent species in nature and are thus sharply circumscribed as geographic pathogens by the distribution and ecology of the specific rodent host.

All of the agents considered in these chapters are zoonotic viruses, and infection in man produced by them is determined by geographic and ecologic features peculiar to a given agent. All of these viruses most often produce clinically undifferentiated febrile disease in man. Thus, the most important elements in differential diagnosis of possible zoonotic viral disease are a *carefully taken history* emphasizing geography and exposure, and the use of *specific diagnostic tests.* In many parts of the world, malaria is the most likely cause of acute febrile disease in adults. The finding of malaria parasites in blood, however, may not solve the clinical problem; it should be remembered that either a simultaneous zoonotic viral infection or a drug-resistant parasite may account for the lack of response to supposed specific chemotherapy.

Virus isolation, together with an antibody rise to that agent in sequentially obtained sera from the patient, provides strong evidence for an etiologic association between virus and the observed illness. *Whole blood* is the best source of virus for nearly all of the disease here described, and it *should be obtained on the very first day the patient is seen,* because viremia often disappears rapidly during clinical illness, especially in the case

TABLE 349–1. CLASSIFICATION PARAMETERS FOR ARBOVIRUSES AND CERTAIN OTHER ZOONOTIC VIRUSES CAUSING ACUTE HUMAN DISEASE

Virus Family	Virus Properties	Vector	Human Disease	Examples
Togaviridae	Spherical, 50–70 nm (alpha), 40–50 nm (flavi); single-stranded infectious RNA			
Alphaviruses		Mosquitoes	Undifferentiated fever, encephalitis	Mayaro, Ross River, eastern equine encephalitis
Flaviviruses		Mosquitoes, ticks	Undifferentiated fever, encephalitis, hemorrhagic fever	Dengue, West Nile, St. Louis encephalitis, yellow fever
Bunyaviridae	Spherical, 90–100 nm; RNA segmented, circular, noninfectious			
Bunyaviruses		Mosquitoes	Undifferentiated fever, encephalitis	California encephalitis
Phleboviruses		Mosquitoes, phlebotomine flies	Undifferentiated fever	Sandfly, Rift Valley fevers
Nairoviruses		Ticks	Hemorrhagic fever	Congo-CHF
Hantaan virus		Rodents	Hemorrhagic fever	Hemorrhagic fever, renal syndrome
Arenaviridae	Spherical or pleomorphic, 50–300 nm; segmented, circular, noninfectious RNA	Rodents	Hemorrhagic fever	Junin, Machupo, Lassa
Reoviridae, arboviruses	Spherical, isometric, nonenveloped, 65-80 nm; RNA is 10 linear segments	Ticks	Undifferentiated fever	Colorado tick fever
Marburg-Ebola viruses	90 × 700-800 nm rods; single-stranded RNA	Unknown	Hemorrhagic fever	

of the encephalitides. An acute-phase serum sample for antibody studies should be collected at this same time, and a convalescent specimen gotten 7 to 30 days later usually discloses an increase in specific antibodies when measured by the complement-fixation (CF), hemagglutination-inhibition (HI), immunofluorescent (IF), or neutralization (N) method. Binding assays for antibodies, particularly of immunoglobulin M (IgM) subclass, may often provide specific diagnosis during the acute phase of illness.

Fenner F: Classification and nomenclature of viruses. Intervirology 7:1, 1976. *Definitive exposition of internationally accepted game rules by the chairman of the committee in charge.*

Shope RE, Sather GE: Arboviruses. *In* Lennette EH, Schmidt NJ (eds.): Diagnostic Procedures for Viral, Rickettsial and Chlamydia Infections. 5th ed. Washington, D.C. American Public Health Association, 1979, pp 767–814. *Carefully detailed explanation of current technology, with an excellent discussion of indications and limitations of various diagnostic procedures.*

Undifferentiated Fevers

350. DENGUE

Robert B. Tesh

DEFINITION. "Classic" dengue is an acute, self-limited illness characterized by fever, prostration, headache, myalgia, rash, lymphadenopathy, and leukopenia. It is caused by a mosquito-borne flavivirus. Typically the disease lasts five to seven days and is followed by one or more weeks of depression and weakness.

ETIOLOGY. Four antigenically related but distinct subtypes of dengue virus have been recovered from patients. Infection with each of these agents results in long-lasting immunity against the homologous virus and partial immunity, which persists only for about six months, against the other three heterologous subtypes.

EPIDEMIOLOGY. Dengue fever affects millions of people annually; in terms of human morbidity, it is by far the most important arthropod-transmitted viral illness. Dengue is mainly a disease of the tropics and subtropics, although it can also occur in temperate areas during warm weather. In fact, the first accurate clinical description of the disease was provided by Benjamin Rush during an epidemic in Philadelphia in the summer of 1780. However, the inability of *Aedes aegypti*, the principal mosquito vector, to survive prolonged winter weather has prevented the disease from becoming permanently established in temperate regions of the world.

The basic cycle of dengue virus involves man and certain *Aedes* mosquitoes. The character of dengue outbreaks often varies from one locality to another, depending on climatic conditions, the size and age of the susceptible human population, and the abundance and vector competence of the local mosquitoes. Thus dengue may appear as a nearly silent continuously endemic infection, as repeated seasonal epidemics, or as massive outbreaks affecting populations previously free of the disease for many years. Classic dengue is generally a much milder disease in children than in adults.

When a dengue-infected mosquito feeds or probes, it usually introduces virus-contaminated saliva into its host. If the person is susceptible (nonimmune), the virus multiplies, and within five to seven days viremia follows. This viremic period usually corresponds with the acute phase of the illness and lasts about six days. During this time, the patient is infectious to mosquitoes. After ingestion of infected human blood by a susceptible mosquito, eight to ten days is required at warm temperatures for the virus to multiply in the insect's body and to infect its salivary glands. The mosquito is then infectious for life.

Aedes aegypti is by far the most important vector. It breeds, rests, and feeds in or near human habitations. It is strongly attracted to man, biting in daylight or twilight. These attributes make it an ideal virus vector and explain why dengue is principally an urban disease. In rural areas other *Aedes* species such as *Ae. albopictus* transmit infection, but their habits and smaller human populations make explosive epidemics uncommon.

PATHOLOGY. Dengue virus infection occasionally produces hemorrhagic fever and shock. This syndrome is discussed in Ch. 359. Since classic dengue is rarely fatal, the only information available about its pathology is from biopsies of the skin rash. Such lesions consist of endothelial swelling, perivascular edema, and mononuclear infiltration of small vessels. Petechiae are characterized by extravasation of blood without significant inflammatory reaction.

CLINICAL MANIFESTATIONS. The incubation period of dengue fever is five to eight days. The onset in adults is sudden; during the first 12 to 24 hours the patient develops progressively severe malaise, fever, chills, headache, backache, and generalized myalgia. By the second day the patient is usually acutely ill and prostrate with fever up to 40° C, severe headache, retro-orbital pain, photophobia, generalized muscle aches, and joint stiffness. Other frequent symptoms include anorexia, altered taste sensations, nausea, vomiting, abdominal tenderness, sore throat, and depression. During this early phase, a flush or fleeting erythematous eruption may appear on the face, neck, and chest. The lymph nodes usually become enlarged and palpable, but the liver and spleen do not. The fever generally lasts five to seven days. Occasionally the temperature briefly falls on the third or fourth day, giving a "saddleback" fever curve.

About the third or fourth day of illness, a maculopapular or scarlatiniform rash appears, beginning on the trunk and spreading in centripetal fashion. This lasts several days, becomes itchy as it fades, but rarely desquamates. Initially, the leukocyte count may be normal; but by the third or fourth day of illness, a generalized leukopenia develops. Toward the end of the febrile period, small clusters of petechiae may appear, especially on the lower extremities, but the thrombocyte count and clotting time are normal in classic dengue. Convalescence begins on the sixth or seventh day when the fever ends, but full recovery often takes several weeks because of lingering weakness and depression.

DIAGNOSIS. During epidemics of dengue fever, when a large number of cases occurs within a short time, the diagnosis is relatively easy. Isolated cases of the disease are more difficult to recognize, because influenza, rubella, and a number of other arbovirus diseases may be mistaken for dengue. Thus laboratory confirmation of a *few* cases during an epidemic and of *every* case when the pattern is sporadic is important. Dengue is endemic in a number of countries in the Caribbean, South and Central America, Africa, and Southern Asia; thus a history of travel during the previous ten days is essential whenever dealing with a suspect case in areas where the disease is rare.

Isolation of the virus is the preferred method of diagnosis. Dengue virus can frequently be recovered from the blood or serum of patients during the febrile stage of their illness. Inoculation of specimens into live mosquitoes or mosquito cell cultures is the most sensitive culture technique. Serologic diagnosis, using acute and convalescent specimens drawn 14 to 21 days apart, is the alternative. However, interpretation of serologic results may be difficult if the patient has been infected before with another flavivirus. An anamnestic immune response generally develops after a second flavivirus infection, making identification of the specific infecting agent difficult or impossible.

TREATMENT AND PROGNOSIS. There is no specific therapy. Bed rest is indicated, as well as the usual supportive measures to maintain fluid and electrolyte balance, particularly if repeated vomiting occurs. Secondary bacterial infection is uncommon but should be anticipated and treated appropriately. Aspirin should be avoided in dengue patients to prevent exacerbation of the thrombocytopenia and hemorrhagic manifestations which occasionally develop. The prognosis in patients with classic dengue is excellent, although convalescence may be prolonged.

PREVENTION. No vaccines for dengue viruses are yet available. Individual protection is difficult, because the mosquito vectors bite during the day, and continuous use of repellents is not practical. Community protection is possible through effective control or eradication of the *Aedes* vectors. Dengue patients should be protected from mosquitoes during the first five or six days of their illness in order to prevent further virus transmission, and space-spraying of buildings frequented by patients should be done to eliminate mosquitoes possibly infected prior to the diagnosis of the disease.

Halstead SB: Dengue and dengue hemorrhagic fever. *In* Steele JH (ed.): CRC Handbook Series in Zoonoses, Sect. B: Viral Zoonoses. Vol. 1. Boca Raton, CRC Press, 1981, pp 421–435. *A good review of the disease and its epidemiology.*

Kuberski TT, Rosen L, Reed D, Mataika J: Clinical and laboratory observations on patients with primary and secondary dengue type 1 infections with hemorrhagic manifestations in Fiji. Am J Trop Med Hyg 26:775, 1977. *A comparison of symptoms in patients with primary and secondary dengue infections. Hematologic and serologic results as well as the level and duration of viremia are reported.*

Schlesinger RW: Dengue Viruses. Vol 16. New York, Springer-Verlag, 1977. *This monograph covers all aspects of dengue viruses. The clinical picture of classic and hemorrhagic dengue fever is described in detail.*

351. WEST NILE FEVER

Robert B. Tesh

DEFINITION. West Nile fever is an acute, febrile, mosquito-borne viral illness marked by headache, myalgia, lymphadenopathy, and rash. It is generally self-limited, although occasional deaths resulting from encephalitis occur in aged persons.

ETIOLOGY. The disease is caused by a small ribonucleic acid–containing virus (family Togaviridae, genus *Flavivirus*), which is closely related antigenically to Japanese B, Murray Valley, St. Louis, and Rocio encephalitis viruses. West Nile virus also is related to dengue and yellow fever viruses.

EPIDEMIOLOGY. Millions of people have been infected with West Nile virus, which occurs in many rural areas of Africa, the Middle East, southwest Asia, and southern Europe. The disease occurs in both endemic and epidemic forms. In areas where West Nile virus is highly endemic, infection occurs early in childhood and most of the adult population is immune. In regions where the virus is less active, sporadic epidemics of West Nile fever occur among persons of all ages. Epidemics usually occur during the summer months and are correlated with seasonal peaks in populations of culicine mosquitoes. The virus is thought to be maintained in nature by a cycle involving *Culex* mosquitoes and birds, with man serving as only an incidental host.

CLINICAL MANIFESTATIONS. The disease begins suddenly after an incubation period of three to six days. The character of clinical illness produced by West Nile virus infection is largely age dependent. Infants and young children generally experience a mild, nonspecific febrile illness. Adolescents and adults usually develop a dengue-like disease, characterized by fever, rash, severe frontal headache, orbital pain, backache, generalized myalgia, anorexia, lymphadenopathy, and leukopenia. The rash is nonpruritic and maculopapular in type, occurs mainly on the trunk, and clears without desquamation. Other, less frequent symptoms include sore throat, nausea, vomiting, and diarrhea. A few patients in this age group also develop signs of meningeal involvement (stiff neck, Kernig's sign) during the acute phase of their illness. The cerebrospinal fluid in these cases usually shows a slight increase in cells and protein. In elderly and debilitated patients, West Nile virus infection sometimes produces meningoencephalitis and occasionally causes death. Neurologic symptoms in the latter patients may include depressed sensorium, somnolence, involuntary twitches, and coma.

West Nile fever is generally a self-limited disease, lasting three to six days, although general weakness and fatigue may persist for one or two weeks after the illness. In patients who develop neurologic involvement, the encephalitic signs do not usually appear until the fourth or fifth day of illness, and after the temperature has returned to normal.

DIAGNOSIS. Clinically this disease is so similar to dengue and phlebotomus fever that laboratory diagnosis is essential in all cases. Virus isolation is by far the best method, and blood specimens obtained as late as the fourth symptomatic day yield a reasonably high percentage of strains when inoculated into newborn mice or a variety of cell cultures. Serologic diagnosis may also be attempted with acute and convalescent serum samples, but previous infection with related flaviviruses, such as the 17D yellow fever vaccine strain, may render interpretation of results extremely difficult owing to the heterologous immune response that develops after a second flavivirus infection.

TREATMENT AND PREVENTION. Management of patients is completely symptomatic. Complications are uncommon. Since there is no vaccine available, the only effective prevention of West Nile fever is to avoid mosquito bites. Mosquito control programs can reduce the vector population and thus the incidence of the disease. Visitors to areas where West Nile virus is endemic should use mosquito netting, screens, and insect repellent.

Goldblum N: West Nile fever in the Middle East. Proc 6th Int Congr Trop Med Malar 5:112, 1959. *A review of the clinical picture and epidemiology of West Nile fever in Israel.*

Southam CM, Moore AE: Induced virus infections in man by the Egypt isolates of West Nile virus. Am J Trop Med Hyg 3:19, 1954. *This paper reports in great detail the clinical course of terminal cancer patients inoculated with West Nile virus. Encephalitic symptoms were common in this group of patients.*

Taylor RM, Work TH, Hurlbut HS, Rizk F: A study of the ecology of West Nile virus in Egypt. Am J Trop Med Hyg 5:579, 1956. *This paper describes results of field and laboratory studies to identify the mosquito vectors and vertebrate reservoirs of West Nile virus. It is a classic work in arbovirology.*

352. PHLEBOTOMUS FEVER

Robert B. Tesh

DEFINITION. Phlebotomus fever, also referred to as sandfly or pappataci fever, is an acute, self-limited, flu-like illness of two to four days' duration, which is transmitted by the bite of infected phlebotomine sandflies. The disease occurs annually during the warm season in the Mediterranean littoral and central Asia. Sporadic cases have also been recognized in tropical America.

ETIOLOGY. The phlebotomus fever group of arboviruses (family Bunyaviridae, genus *Phlebovirus)* currently consists of 36 antigenically distinct and geographically dispersed virus serotypes. Although many of these agents are capable of producing "classic" phlebotomus fever, most cases of the disease are due to the Naples and Sicilian serotypes.

EPIDEMIOLOGY. Phlebotomus fever is a public health problem mainly in the Old World where it occurs in both endemic and epidemic forms. The occurrence of the disease in this region closely parallels the geographic distribution and abundance of *Phlebotomus papatasi,* its principal vector. In areas where the disease is endemic, most of the indigenous population is infected and thereby acquires immunity early in life. The disease in children is a relatively benign, nonspecific febrile illness. However, when nonimmune adults enter an endemic area and are bitten by infected sandflies, they develop "classic" phlebotomus fever. For this reason, historically the disease has been of some military importance.

The principal vector, *Phlebotomus papatasi,* is a tiny (2 to 3 mm) sand-colored midge. Because of their small size, they can readily pass through ordinary screens and mosquito netting. Sandflies usually move in short hops and rarely travel more than a few hundred meters from their resting and breeding sites. The larvae develop in loose soil and organic debris in stone walls, wells, gardens, animal shelters, and privies, usually near human dwellings. *P. papatasi* is active mainly at night and readily feeds on humans. Available evidence suggests that many viruses in the phlebotomus fever group are maintained in the sandfly population by transovarial (hereditary) transmission. This mechanism ensures survival of the viruses during winter months when the vector is inactive and during periods when susceptible vertebrate hosts are not available.

Phlebotomus fever also occurs in tropical America; however, in this region the important vectors are sylvan species belonging to the genus *Lutzomyia*. Therefore cases of the disease in the New World are sporadic in occurrence and found mainly in persons who enter the tropical forests for work and recreation.

PATHOGENESIS. Since there are no fatalities, the pathology of this disease in humans is unknown. Experimental studies in man, however, indicate that after intracutaneous inoculation the incubation period is three to six days. Viremia is brief and lasts only one or two days, usually being confined to the day prior to and that of the onset of symptoms. Postinfection immunity is type specific and probably lifelong.

CLINICAL MANIFESTATIONS. The disease is sudden in onset and is characterized by fever, headache, myalgia, photophobia, retro-orbital pain, and marked conjunctival injection. The face often has an erythematous flush, but a true rash is absent. Nausea and vomiting sometimes occur, but other gastrointestinal and respiratory symptoms are uncommon. Most patients with phlebotomus fever develop a marked leukopenia, consisting of an initial lymphopenia followed by a protracted neutropenia. The acute symptoms last only two to four days; however, a general feeling of weakness and depression often persists for a week or more.

DIAGNOSIS AND TREATMENT. Epidemiologic or travel history represents the best clue to diagnosis. Virus isolation is difficult. Serologic procedures may be carried out but serve principally to exclude other possible causes such as dengue, West Nile fever, and influenza. Management of patients is symptomatic. No vaccine is available, but insecticides are highly effective in controlling the peridomestic sandfly vectors.

Bartelloni PJ, Tesh RB: Clinical and serologic responses of volunteers infected with phlebotomus fever virus (Sicilian type). Am J Trop Med Hyg 25:456, 1976. *A description of the clinical, hematologic, and serologic responses of volunteers infected with sandfly fever. References are given to other similar studies.*

Sabin AB, Philip CB, Paul JR: Phlebotomus (pappataci or sandfly) fever. JAMA 125:693, 1944. *A report of research on sandfly fever among American troops during World War II. It presents a detailed clinical description of the disease.*

Tesh RB, Saidi S, Gajdamovic SJ, Rodhain F, Vesenjak-Hirjan J: Serological studies on the epidemiology of sandfly fever in the Old World. Bull WHO 54:663, 1976. *A review of the epidemiology of phlebotomus fever in the Old World. It includes a map showing the geographic distribution of the principal vector,* Phlebotomus papatasi.

353. RIFT VALLEY FEVER

Robert B. Tesh

DEFINITION. Rift Valley fever is an acute viral illness, usually of short duration, which is characterized by high fever, headache, retro-orbital pain, myalgia, prostration, photophobia, and conjunctival injection. A small percentage of patients with this disease develop hemorrhagic and encephalitic complications which are sometimes fatal. Humans generally acquire the disease by contact with infected domestic animals, although the virus may also be mosquito borne.

ETIOLOGY. The causative agent is a 90-nm, ribonucleic acid–containing virus that is antigenically related to a number of viruses in the phlebotomus fever group (family Bunyaviridae, genus *Phlebovirus*). However, because of the virulence of Rift Valley fever virus for animals and humans, the disease that it causes is considered separately.

EPIDEMIOLOGY. The known geographic distribution of the virus includes most of the eastern half of Africa. Rift Valley fever is primarily a disease of domestic ruminants. Epizootics produce heavy mortality among lambs and calves and cause increased rates of abortion among ewes and cows. Outbreaks of the disease in domestic animals are sporadic; the virus is presumed to be transmitted from animal to animal by infected mosquitoes. The maintenance mechanism of the virus between epizootics is unknown.

Humans usually acquire the virus by aerosol transmission or by direct contact with blood or tissues of infected animals. Veterinarians, ranchers, herdsmen, slaughterhouse employees, and persons working in animal disease diagnostic laboratories are all at special risk during epizootics. Rift Valley fever virus is highly infectious to humans; cases of the disease have occurred in persons who have only been present in a room where a sick animal has been slaughtered or autopsied. It is uncertain what role, if any, mosquitoes play in the transmission of Rift Valley fever to man. During an extensive Rift Valley fever epizootic in Egypt during 1977 and 1978, many thousands of people became ill with the disease and more than 600 deaths were recorded. Because of the value of domestic animals in many economically depressed regions of Africa, animals are often housed within family compounds. Furthermore, sick or dying animals are usually killed to salvage their meat. Both of these practices greatly increase the risk of virus transmission to humans.

CLINICAL MANIFESTATIONS. The incubation period is three to six days. Uncomplicated Rift Valley fever in man is similar to phlebotomus fever. The disease begins suddenly with fever up to 40° C, chills, severe headache, retro-orbital pain, photophobia, generalized myalgia, and prostration. Patients with this disease appear acutely ill, with flushed faces and marked conjunctival injection. Occasionally nausea, vomiting, and diarrhea occur. Physical examination early in the disease is unremarkable. The white blood count may be decreased, normal, or elevated. In most cases the illness lasts two to four days, although sometimes a brief recrudescence of fever occurs, giving a biphasic temperature curve. Recovery in uncomplicated cases is complete.

A few patients with Rift Valley fever develop serious complications. One is loss of central visual acuity and occasionally blindness. The eye symptoms do not usually become apparent until several days or weeks after the febrile illness has ended. Funduscopic examination in these cases shows white macular exudates and occasionally retinal hemorrhages. In some patients, vision gradually improves; in others, it does not.

A second complication is hemorrhagic manifestations. These usually appear between the second and fourth days of illness, about the time that the patient becomes afebrile. The patient becomes progressively jaundiced and drowsy and manifests petechiae, purpura, bleeding gums, hematemesis, and melena. Liver function test results, including bilirubin, serum transaminases, alkaline phosphatase, and prothrombin time, are abnormal. The prognosis in these cases is poor; death often occurs within a week and is due to shock and hepatic failure.

A third complication is meningoencephalitis. Neurologic symptoms appear several days after the febrile period ends and may include mental confusion, hallucinations, vertigo, meningismus, paresis, convulsions, and coma. The cerebrospinal fluid shows increased protein and pleocytosis. The outcome is gradual recovery or death.

PATHOGENESIS. At autopsy, patients with hemorrhagic complications have petechiae and hemorrhages throughout the gastrointestinal tract. The most characteristic lesion is in the liver and consists of diffuse central necrosis and hemorrhage. Affected hepatic cells show eosinophilic cytoplasmic degeneration similar to that seen in yellow fever. The brain in fatal cases of encephalitis shows focal necrosis and perivascular infiltration with macrophages and lymphocytes.

DIAGNOSIS. Rift Valley fever is primarily a disease of place and particular human activity. A history is more valuable than any other procedure. Blood obtained during the febrile period almost always contains virus. Serologic diagnosis is also fairly specific, although low level cross-reactions may occur with some heterologous antigens in the phlebotomus fever group.

TREATMENT AND PREVENTION. Management of patients with this disease is entirely symptomatic. Those with hemorrhage and shock obviously need blood replacement.

Live attenuated and formalin-killed vaccines are available in limited quantities for certain high-risk groups such as veterinarians and laboratory workers. These are protective for at least two years. Individual antimosquito measures would also seem prudent during epizootics.

Peters CJ, Meegan JM: Rift Valley fever. *In* Steele JH (ed.): CRC Handbook Series in Zoonoses, Section B: Viral Zoonoses. Vol. 1. Boca Raton, CRC Press, 1981, pp 403–420. *A complete review of all aspects of the disease.*

354. FEVERS CAUSED BY ALPHAVIRUSES: CHIKUNGUNYA, O'NYONG-NYONG, MAYARO, ROSS RIVER, AND OCKELBO

Robert B. Tesh

DEFINITION. Chikungunya, o'nyong-nyong, Mayaro, Ross River, and Ockelbo virus infections are acute nonfatal illnesses that usually include fever, arthralgia, and rash. They are caused by a group of antigenically related, geographically diverse, mosquito-borne viruses.

EPIDEMIOLOGY. These five diseases affect persons of all ages, although they are generally milder in children. Clinically, they are practically indistinguishable, but their epidemiology is quite different. Chikungunya is the most widely distributed of the five diseases and occurs in sub-Sahara Africa, India, Southeast Asia, and the Philippines. Epidemics are sporadic in occurrence and usually appear during warm rainy months. In rural Africa, the virus is maintained in a cycle involving wild primates and forest mosquitoes (*Aedes africanus* and *Ae. furcifer*). Urban outbreaks of chikungunya are usually associated with *Aedes aegypti*. In this situation the virus is probably transmitted from man to mosquito to man.

Little is known about the epidemiology of o'nyong-nyong fever. It has occurred in Uganda, Kenya, Tanzania, Malawi, and Senegal. Between 1959 and 1962, a major epidemic of this disease swept across East Africa, affecting millions of people. The suspected vectors are *Anopheles funestus* and *An. gambiae*.

Mayaro virus has been isolated in Trinidad, Surinam, Brazil, Colombia, and Bolivia. Cases of this disease have been associated mainly with persons who live or work in tropical forests, mostly males. Sylvan mosquitoes of the genus *Haemagogus* are thought to be the principal vectors. Wild animals probably serve as the virus reservoir.

Ross River fever, also known as "epidemic polyarthritis," has occurred in Australia, New Guinea, the Solomon islands, Fiji, American Samoa, and a number of other South Pacific islands. In southern Australia, sporadic cases of the disease usually occur during warm weather among vacationers traveling in rural areas. There the virus is thought to be maintained in a wild vertebrate-mosquito cycle, with *Culex annulirostris* and *Aedes vigilax* serving as principal vectors. However, explosive epidemics of this disease have also occurred on several South Pacific islands where the virus appeared to be transmitted from man to mosquito to man, analogous to urban outbreaks of chikungunya. In the latter epidemics, *Aedes polynesiensis* was the presumed vector.

Less is known about the epidemiology of Ockelbo fever. The disease was first recognized in Sweden. A similar illness has also been reported in Finland and adjacent regions of the Soviet Union, where it is referred to as "Pogasta disease" and "Karelian fever," respectively. In all three countries, the disease typically occurs in late summer among picnickers, berry collectors, and other persons entering wooded areas. A single recovery of the virus has been made from *Culiseta* mosquitoes.

CLINICAL MANIFESTATIONS. The usual incubation period for this group of illnesses is three to five days. Typically, the onset is abrupt with fever, headache, myalgia, and weakness. In Mayaro and chikungunya infections, the fever may reach 39 to 40° C. A saddleback or biphasic temperature curve sometimes occurs with chikungunya. In Ross River, Ockelbo, and o'nyong-nyong infections, the fever is generally lower and constitutional symptoms are milder. Arthralgia and rash may appear with the initial symptoms or develop several days later. Arthralgia is the most striking feature of these illnesses. It is usually bilateral and mainly affects joints in the extremities. Symptoms vary from excruciating pain to vague joint stiffness. Affected joints are often swollen and tender, but other signs of inflammation are absent. Previously injured joints are particularly susceptible. The rash is maculopapular in type and occurs mainly on the trunk and extremities, although the palms and soles may also be affected. The rash clears in four or five days without desquamation, leaving a brownish stain to the skin. Lymphadenopathy is also common. Many patients have a leukopenia with relative lymphocytosis during the first week of illness. One serious but rare complication of chikungunya virus infection is hemorrhagic manifestations. Epistaxis, hematemesis, melena, petechiae, and purpura have all been reported occasionally.

DIAGNOSIS. These viruses can usually be recovered from the blood or serum of patients during the first few days of illness by inoculation of newborn mice or various cell cultures. Standard serologic techniques are also highly reliable in making a specific diagnosis, provided that a first serum specimen is collected early in the disease and a second is obtained 10 to 14 days later. Diagnosis during epidemics is relatively easy; the occasional or isolated case is more difficult to recognize. The differential diagnosis includes other diseases producing fever, arthralgia, and rash.

TREATMENT AND PROGNOSIS. Treatment is symptomatic, and the prognosis is excellent. In general, these illnesses last only about one week, although the arthralgia sometimes persists for several weeks or months. In such a case, recurrent attacks of joint pain and swelling are common. The pathogenesis of the joint disease is unknown.

Skogh M, Espmark A: Ockelbo disease: Epidemic arthritis—exanthema syndrome in Sweden caused by Sindbis-virus like agent. Lancet 1:795, 1982. *Brief description of Ockelbo disease.*

Tesh RB: Arthritides caused by mosquito-borne viruses. Ann Rev Med 33:31, 1982. *A review of the clinical manifestations and epidemiology of diseases caused by five alphaviruses. Many references are given.*

355. COLORADO TICK FEVER

Theodore C. Eickhoff

DEFINITION. Colorado tick fever (CTF) is an acute, benign, tick-transmitted viral infection that occurs throughout the Rocky Mountain area, and is characterized by headache, back pain, a biphasic febrile course lasting about one week, and leukopenia.

ETIOLOGY. CTF virus is an arbovirus that is transmitted to humans by the bite of the hard-shelled wood tick, *Dermacentor andersoni*. Human cases appear to be limited to the combined geographic distribution of the vector, and the major mammalian reservoirs, ground squirrels and chipmunks. CTF virus is in the orbivirus genus of the reoviruses and is unrelated to other arbovirus groups.

EPIDEMIOLOGY. The disease occurs during the spring and summer months, when tick exposure in the mountains is common. Disease activity appears to follow springtime in the mountains, for cases occur at lower altitudes during April and May, and at higher altitudes during June and July, presumably reflecting the slower emergence of ticks at higher altitudes. Most patients give a history of having found attached ticks, but others will not be aware of the tick attachment and bite, even though they may have seen ticks on their body or clothing. Cases may occasionally be encountered in other areas of the country as a result of travel outside the endemic area during the incubation period, or accidental transportation of infected adult ticks in clothing or bedding.

The virus has been recovered from as many as 14 per cent of *Dermacentor andersoni* collected in endemic areas. Replication of the virus within these ticks has been documented. It is not clear whether the virus is passed transovarially within the vector species. The reservoir of the virus probably resides in numerous small mammals, particularly golden mantled ground squirrels and chipmunks, which have a prolonged viremia and infect nymphal ticks. Overwintering may thus occur in either nymphal ticks or hibernating small mammals. Adult ticks then transmit the virus to other small animals, with humans being accidental hosts.

INCIDENCE AND PREVALENCE. The disease has been reported from most states in the Rocky Mountain area and from western Canadian provinces, but the largest number of cases has generally been reported in Colorado. Several hundred cases are diagnosed annually in the endemic area, but it is likely that this represents only a fraction of the total. Mild or wholly subclinical infections do occur, but their frequency has not been systematically evaluated.

The virus has been isolated from other species of ticks and from numerous species of small mammals, suggesting that the disease may occur over a wider geographic area than is presently appreciated.

PATHOGENESIS. There is no unusual local reaction at the site of the tick bite inoculation, and the site of initial localization and replication of the virus is unknown. The onset of symptoms occurs three to seven days after tick exposure. Viremia can be demonstrated at the time of onset of fever, not only persisting during the febrile illness itself, but remarkably persisting in red blood cells long after the virus has disappeared from serum and neutralizing antibody has appeared. The virus can be demonstrated within erythrocytes by fluorescent antibody staining for up to 120 days, and has been grown from washed erythrocytes 100 days after the original infection.

Few pathologic data in man are available, since only one fatal case has been recorded. In experimental animals, the heart, lungs, spleen, bone marrow, and lymph nodes are important sites of viral replication. Occasional patients have clinical evidence of central nervous system or meningeal involvement, and CTF virus has been recovered from cerebrospinal fluid.

CLINICAL MANIFESTATIONS. The disease begins abruptly, with chilly sensations, fever of 38 to 40° C, myalgias most prominent in the back and legs, headache, retro-orbital pain, and photophobia. Malaise and nausea may occur, but vomiting is uncommon. Physical findings during the first two to three days of illness are nonspecific. The patient may be flushed, with conjunctival and pharyngeal erythema. Lymphadenopathy is not prominent, although mild splenomegaly is sometimes present. Rashes have been reported in up to 12 per cent of patients, commonly macular or maculopapular and distributed over the entire body, sometimes petechial and involving primarily the extremities. Tachycardia is in proportion to the temperature elevation.

In approximately half of the cases, a distinctly biphasic illness occurs, the so-called "saddleback" fever. Symptoms abate after two to three days, temperature becomes normal or nearly so, and the patient feels relatively well for one or two days, following which there is an abrupt return of fever, headache, and back pain, often more intense than in the first phase. The second phase lasts two to four days and then subsides, leaving the patient with weakness and lassitude that disappear entirely during the succeeding week or two. Some patients do not exhibit the typical biphasic course, and experience only one bout of fever, or have a typical illness but with a third phase of fever, or have a single prolonged febrile illness lasting five to eight days.

Central nervous system involvement has occurred in a few patients, invariably children. The presenting findings have been those of aseptic meningitis with nuchal rigidity and mononuclear pleocytosis, or encephalitis with a depressed sensorium or stupor. Hemorrhagic manifestations have been described in a few children with encephalitis.

Laboratory findings very early in the illness are generally not helpful, but leukopenia is usually present by the third day of illness, and becomes even more pronounced during the second phase, reaching levels as low as 2000 per cubic millimeter. The most striking decrease is in the granulocyte series, with a relative lymphocytosis, and there is frequently an accompanying thrombocytopenia. Atypical, vacuolated lymphocytes are frequently observed. Bone marrow examination reveals a maturation arrest in the granulocyte series. The white blood count returns to normal during convalescence.

DIAGNOSIS. The diagnosis should be suspected in any person with a history of tick exposure in the endemic area three to seven days prior to the onset of a febrile illness. Findings during the first phase, however, cannot be differentiated from many other acute febrile illnesses. A brief symptom-free interval followed by a second febrile illness should strongly suggest CTF. Profound leukopenia is usually present by that time, and lends support to the diagnosis.

The diagnosis is confirmed by isolation of the virus from serum or whole blood, via inoculation of suckling mice. More rapid diagnosis is possible by direct immunofluorescent staining of virus in the patient's erythrocytes. A diagnostic rise in both neutralizing and complement-fixing antibodies can generally be detected by examination of acute and convalescent sera.

The differential diagnosis can be troublesome, inasmuch as Rocky Mountain spotted fever is transmitted in the tick fever endemic area by the same vector, *Dermacentor andersoni.* Paradoxically, Rocky Mountain spotted fever has become an unusual disease in the state of Colorado and is outnumbered by CTF in Colorado by 20-fold. Nevertheless, differential diagnosis may be impossible early in the course of disease, before the characteristic rash of Rocky Mountain spotted fever appears. A relatively symptom-free interval after two or three days would be most unusual in Rocky Mountain spotted fever, and strongly favors the diagnosis of CTF.

TREATMENT. Therapy is entirely supportive, there being no specific therapy. Salicylates may be necessary to minimize headache and myalgias, but are neither required nor advisable in most patients.

PROGNOSIS. The disease is almost invariably benign, and the prognosis is excellent. Severe illness, complicated by central nervous system involvement, is seen infrequently and only in children.

PREVENTION. Both inactivated and live attenuated vaccines have been studied, but the modest number of cases and the benign nature of the disease suggest little need for active immunization.

The most effective means of preventing the disease is the use of protective clothing or repellents by people outdoors in endemic areas during the spring and summer months, together with frequent body inspection and prompt removal of ticks. Transfusion-associated disease can be prevented by exclusion of convalescent donors for a minimum of six months.

Goodpasture HC, Poland JD, Francy DB, Bowen GS, Horn KA: Colorado tick fever: Clinical, epidemiologic and laboratory aspects of 228 cases in Colorado in 1973–1974. Ann Intern Med 88:303, 1978. *A recent, thorough clinical study.*

Oshiro LS, Dondero DV, Emmons RW, Lennette EH: The development of Colorado tick fever virus within cells of the haematopoietic system. J Gen Virol 39:73, 1978. *Recommended for those interested in the unusual host-parasite relationship in CTF.*

356. ARTHROPOD-BORNE VIRAL ENCEPHALITIDES

Thomas P. Monath

Of the more than 450 arboviruses presently registered, 13 are important causes of encephalitis, some responsible for intermittent epidemics, and 14 are occasionally associated with encephalitis (see Table 356–1). Arboviral encephalitis is a significant health problem in Europe and the Soviet Union (tick-borne encephalitis), parts of Asia (Japanese encephalitis), and in the New World where the disease assumes great importance, owing to a proliferation of etiologic agents, widespread occurrence, potential for epidemic spread, and concurrent affliction of domestic animals and man. Only the African continent is spared from epidemiologically important arboviral encephalitides. The physician faced with a case should attempt to establish an early specific diagnosis, because it provides information about the occurrence of a potentially epidemic disease and directs investigative, preventive, and control measures by the responsible public health authority.

The viruses under consideration are transmitted between wild or domestic animals by the agency of blood-feeding mosquitoes or ticks (see Fig. 356–1). Vertebrate hosts circulate virus in their blood at titers sufficiently high to infect a specific arthropod vector(s). After ingestion of an infectious blood meal, a temperature-dependent delay (extrinsic incubation period) of a week or more is required for replication in salivary gland tissue before transmission by bite can occur; thereafter arthropods remain infective for life. Man is not an essential host in the transmission cycles of the arboviral encephalitides. Human infection is most often abortive or subclinical, and the severe manifestations of central nervous system inflammation occur in only a small fraction of persons infected. The ratio of inapparent to clinically overt infections is a distinctive, age-dependent quality of each disease.

CLINICAL FEATURES. In encephalitis, the brain parenchyma itself is affected, resulting in diffuse or localizing signs of cerebral dysfunction. Signs of meningeal irritation are also nearly always present *(meningoencephalitis),* but may be masked in the very young, the elderly, or the comatose patient. In some patients, inflammation of the leptomeninges may occur without evidence for disturbance of brain function (aseptic meningitis). A still milder form of arboviral central nervous system infection is manifested by fever and headache only; in such cases, however, cerebrospinal fluid pleocytosis may be present, indicating a forme fruste of meningitis.

The neurologic disease usually begins after a variable period of nonspecific, grippe-like symptoms. The clinical features and rate of evolution of encephalitis are quite variable. A degree of alteration of the state of consciousness is a universal finding in encephalitis. Convulsions, more often generalized than focal, may occur. Paresis, paralyses, hyperactive reflexes, and plantar extensor responses reflect damage to corticospinal tracts. A prominent feature of some infections (especially St. Louis and

TABLE 356–1. ARTHROPOD-BORNE VIRUSES WHICH CAUSE ACUTE CENTRAL NERVOUS SYSTEM INFECTION AND ENCEPHALITIS

Virus	Taxonomic Group	Mode of Transmission	Geographic Distribution	Disease in Domestic Livestock
I. Viruses Principally Associated with the Encephalitis Syndrome; Epidemic and Endemic				
Eastern equine encephalitis	Togaviridae, alphavirus	Mosquito	Eastern North America, Caribbean, South America	Equines, penned pheasants
Western equine encephalitis	Togaviridae, alphavirus	Mosquito	Western North America, South America	Equines
Venezuelan equine encephalitis	Togaviridae, alphavirus	Mosquito, possibly other modes (see text)	Florida, Central and South America	Equines
St. Louis encephalitis	Togaviridae, flavivirus	Mosquito	North America, Caribbean, Central and South America	None
Japanese encephalitis	Togaviridae, flavivirus	Mosquito	East, Southeast Asia; India	Equines, swine
Rocio encephalitis	Togaviridae, flavivirus	Mosquito	Brazil	None
Murray Valley encephalitis	Togaviridae, flavivirus	Mosquito	Australia	(Equines)*
California encephalitis and La Crosse	Bunyaviridae, California serogroup	Mosquito	North America	None
Tick-borne encephalitides: Russian spring-summer and Central European encephalitis	Togaviridae, flavivirus	Tick, ingestion of milk	Europe, USSR	None
Louping ill	Togaviridae, flavivirus	Tick	British Isles	Sheep, equines, cows
Powassan	Togaviridae, flavivirus	Tick	North America	None
II. Viruses Principally Associated with Other Syndromes, but Occasionally Causing Encephalitis; Epidemic and Endemic				
Sindbis (febrile illness with rash)	Togaviridae, alphavirus	Mosquito	Africa, Europe	None
West Nile (febrile illness with rash)	Togaviridae, flavivirus	Mosquito	Africa, Middle East	(Equines)*
Yellow fever (hemorrhagic fever)	Togaviridae, flavivirus	Mosquito	Africa, tropical America	None
Rift Valley fever (febrile illness, hemorrhagic fever)	Bunyaviridae, phlebotomus fever group	Mosquito, direct contact	Africa	Sheep, cows, goats
Colorado tick fever (febrile illness)	Reoviridae, orbivirus	Tick	Western North America	None
Tick-borne hemorrhagic fevers:				
Kyasanur Forest disease	Togaviridae, flavivirus	Tick	India	None
Omsk hemorrhagic fever	Togaviridae, flavivirus	Tick	Central Asia	None
Crimean hemorrhagic fever-Congo	Bunyaviridae, nairovirus	Tick	Eastern Europe, USSR, Africa	None
III. Rare and Sporadic Infections Associated with Encephalitis				
Semliki Forest†	Togaviridae, alphavirus	Mosquito	Africa, Southeast Asia	(Equines)*
Ilheus	Togaviridae, flavivirus	Mosquito	South America	None
Negishi	Togaviridae, flavivirus	Tick	Japan	None
Langat†	Togaviridae, flavivirus	Tick	Asia	None
Thogoto	Orthomyxovirus	Tick	Africa	None

*Disease suspected but not well documented.
†Encephalitis recorded in laboratory infections or experimental infections of cancer patients only; significance in naturally acquired infections unknown.

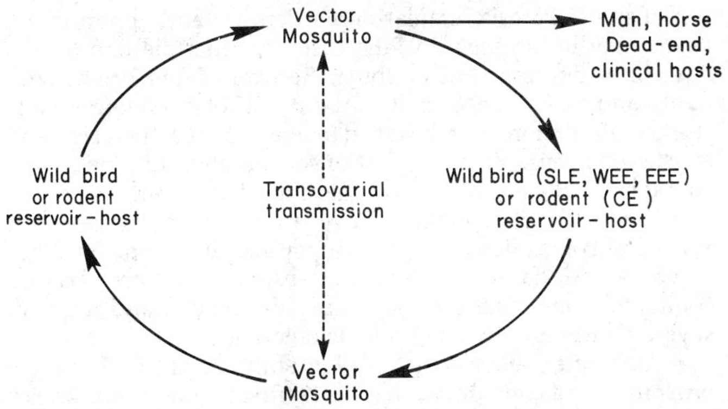

Figure 356–1. Generalized transmission cycle of the mosquito-borne encephalitides in North America.

Japanese encephalitis) is involvement of extrapyramidal structures, with tremor and muscular rigidity. Cerebellar dysfunction is manifested by muscular incoordination, dysmetria, and ataxic speech. Cranial nerve palsies are not uncommon and reflect damage to brainstem nuclei or supranuclear tracts. Autonomic disturbances (sialorrhea, cardiovascular irregularity, urinary retention) may be present. Infection of the cerebral cortex or hypothalamic–thalamic–temporal lobe regions produces confusion; defective memory; changes in speech, personality, and behavior; and the appearance of pathologic reflexes (e.g., suck, snout). Hyperthermia and the syndrome of inappropriate antidiuretic hormone secretion indicate disturbance of the pituitary-hypothalamic axis. Spinal cord involvement may be manifested by lower motor neuron and sensory deficits, hyperreflexia, and bladder paralysis. Interference with respiratory function, laryngeal paralysis, cardiac arrhythmia, and cerebral edema are potentially life-threatening complications. Surviving patients may be left with permanent neuropsychiatric sequelae. In the pregnant female, infection of the developing fetus may result in central nervous system damage or fetal death.

Clinical laboratory findings are relatively nonspecific. A modest peripheral leukocytosis is usual. The cerebrospinal fluid is under increased pressure and contains white blood cells (predominantly polymorphonuclear cells early and lymphocytes later). The cell count is generally less than 500 per cubic millimeter. Cerebrospinal fluid protein may be moderately elevated; glucose and lactate concentrations are normal. Changes in serum enzyme levels have been reported, reflecting myocarditis or damage to skeletal muscle or liver.

PATHOLOGY AND PATHOGENESIS. Two basic pathologic processes are common to the arboviral encephalitides; (1) neuronal and glial damage mediated by intracellular viral infection, and (2) an inflammatory response involving migration of immunologically active cells (lymphocytes, microglia, macrophages) into the perivascular space and brain parenchyma. Endothelial cell swelling and proliferation, vasculitic changes, and destruction of myelin sheaths in deep white matter areas are present in some of the arboviral encephalitides. Since the immune mechanism is responsible for the inflammatory response, an immunopathologic component has been postulated to occur in arboviral encephalitis. A balance apparently occurs between dual roles of the immune response in (1) viral clearance and recovery from infection and (2) enhancement of pathologic processes and acceleration of death.

After inoculation of virus by the bite of an infected arthropod, primary replication occurs in local tissues and in regional lymph nodes. Virus is carried by efferent lymphatics to the thoracic duct and into the bloodstream. This primary viremia seeds extraneural tissues, which in turn support further replication and release into the circulation. Viremia is modulated by replication in extraneural sites, by the rate of viral clearance by the reticuloendothelial system, and by the appearance of humoral antibodies. If viremia is prolonged and intense enough, the neural parenchyma is invaded, with or without ensuing clinical disease. The sites of extraneural infection vary from virus to virus. In the case of many alpha- and flaviviruses, experimental studies have shown that striated muscle and vascular endothelium are important sites of replication; in the case of Venezuelan encephalitis virus, myeloid and lymphoid tissue tropism has been emphasized. The mode of penetration of virus across the blood-brain junction is incompletely understood, but it is likely that passive movement of virus across cerebral capillaries plays a role. Factors that increase vascular permeability (heavy metal poisons, CO_2 inhalation, vasoactive amines) promote viral neuroinvasion. In experimental animals infected with flaviviruses, virus enters the central nervous system by way of the olfactory neuroepithelium. Olfactory neurons are infected by blood-borne virus, and the infection spreads by axonal transport to the brain.

The immature brain is more susceptible to damage by some arboviruses (e.g., western and Venezuelan equine and California encephalitis), accounting for the predominance of encephalitis in the younger age groups. But other central nervous system infections principally affect the elderly (e.g., St. Louis encephalitis), or have a bimodal incidence, striking both children and the very old. In endemic areas, accumulated immunity with increasing age may reduce the incidence of disease in the elderly. The reasons for the increased incidence and severity of some diseases in old persons are poorly understood; underlying hypertensive and arteriosclerotic cerebrovascular disease is suspected to play a role in viral neuroinvasion.

DIFFERENTIAL DIAGNOSIS. The primary task is to differentiate viral encephalitis from acute central nervous system infection by organisms which may respond to antibiotic therapy. Early clinical manifestations of bacterial meningitis (especially if partially treated), brain abscess, subdural empyema, and cerebral thrombophlebitis may mimic viral encephalitis, and cerebrospinal fluid changes are sometimes similar. Culture and repeated examination of the cerebrospinal fluid will help clarify the etiology in cases of bacterial meningitis. Diagnostic tests (computed tomography [CT], electroencephalography, brain scan) help define localized lesions, such as abscess. Subacute bacterial endocarditis may present with meningoencephalitis. Tuberculosis and fungal meningitis cause a mononuclear pleocytosis but reduced glucose values in the cerebrospinal fluid. Other infections that occasionally cause meningoencephalitis include Rocky Mountain spotted fever, leptospirosis, falciparum malaria, trichinosis, *Naegleria*, typhoid, and *Mycoplasma pneumoniae*.

Acute infection with viral agents other than arboviruses is associated with meningoencephalitis, including herpesviruses, mumps virus, enteroviruses, lymphocytic choriomeningitis virus, rabies, influenza, adenoviruses, respiratory syncytial virus, and encephalomyocarditis virus. Principal clues to an arboviral etiology are the history, presence of an outbreak of similar disease in the community, summer-fall occurrence, and the probable geographic locality in which infection was acquired. Echo- and coxsackieviruses cause summer-fall outbreaks in arbovirus epidemic areas, but the predominant syndrome produced is aseptic meningitis, and there may be clinical clues to the diagnosis (e.g., presence of rash, pleurodynia). In the individual case, herpes encephalitis presents the most important diagnostic challenge, since chemotherapy may be indicated. The presence of localizing neurologic signs, other clinical features (previous herpetic infection, subacute onset, predominant behavioral or confusional disturbance), and tests (e.g., CT scan) to detect a mass-like lesion are clues to the clinical diagnosis of herpes encephalitis. If brain biopsy is performed, fluorescent antibody tests and virus isolation attempts may be performed for both herpes and, if suspected, the arthropod-borne encephalitides.

Acute encephalitis may occur following exanthematous viral infections of childhood or administration of rabies or smallpox vaccines. The history of antecedent illness or vaccination and the prominence of myelitis in many cases are clues to the diagnosis.

Cerebrovascular accident may be confused with viral encephalitis. St. Louis encephalitis, a disease of the elderly, has been misdiagnosed as stroke. Subarachnoid hemorrhage produces meningismus, fever, headache, and neurologic signs that mimic an infectious etiology; CT scanning and lumbar puncture clearly distinguish these etiologies.

Metabolic (toxic) encephalopathies (caused by hypoxia, hypoglycemia, diabetic ketoacidosis, hepatic and renal failure, remote carcinoma, intoxications, and addisonian crisis) may present features suggesting infectious encephalitis. Careful history and physical, neurologic, and cerebrospinal fluid examination usually differentiate these conditions.

Neoplastic or *granulomatous diseases* involving the central nervous system and a variety of diseases of uncertain etiology (cat scratch disease, Behçet's disease, Reye's syndrome, acute multiple sclerosis, Lyme arthritis, and systemic lupus erythematosus) must occasionally be considered in the differential diagnosis.

Western Equine Encephalitis (WEE)

ETIOLOGIC AGENT. WEE virus, a member of the family Togaviridae, alphavirus genus, was first isolated in 1930 from a horse with encephalitis in California. A relative of WEE virus (Highlands J virus) present in the eastern United States is not associated with human (and rarely with equine) disease. WEE virus is pathogenic for a wide range of laboratory animals, embryonated eggs, and cell cultures. Isolation and viral assays are generally performed in infant mice inoculated intracranially or by plaque formation in primary avian cell cultures.

EPIDEMIOLOGY. ***Incidence and Prevalence.*** Between 1955 and 1981, 963 cases of WEE were reported in the United States. The annual incidence has varied from less than 10 cases to over 170 cases in epidemic years. Although classically an important disease on the west coast, the area most affected in recent years has been the central tier of states from the Mississippi River west to the Rocky Mountains, including adjacent parts of Canada. In Argentina and Uruguay, equine epizootics occur with little involvement of humans.

Epidemics generally occur in early or mid-summer, and may be precipitated by heavy snow melt or flooding, which produces conditions favorable for breeding of mosquito vectors. Cases of encephalitis in equines frequently precede the appearance of human disease by several weeks. The disease principally affects residents of rural agricultural communities. The incidence is higher in males than in females because of increased exposure to the vector during farming and recreational pursuits. WEE is most severe in infants and young children; these age groups also represent the immunologically most susceptible population in endemic areas. The case-fatality rate is between 3 and 7 per cent. In the western United States, mixed outbreaks of WEE and St. Louis encephalitis are the rule.

Transmission. The virus circulates between wild birds and *Culex tarsalis* mosquitoes. *Culex tarsalis,* an abundant breeder in irrigated areas and flooded pastures, is responsible for infection of man and equines, which develop low or undetectable viremias and do not perpetuate the chain of transmission. In temperate areas, transmission ceases during the winter months; the mechanism(s) whereby WEE virus persists in local winter reservoirs or is reintroduced in the spring is unknown.

CLINICAL FEATURES AND PATHOLOGY. The disease usually begins with generalized and nonspecific symptoms of fever, headache, malaise, and aches, lasting one to four days. Somnolence and lethargy, photophobia, vomiting, and neck stiffness signal the neurologic infection and progress, often quite rapidly, to stupor, coma, and, in a high proportion of children, convulsions. Paresis, cranial nerve deficits, and abnormal reflexes may be present. In fatal cases patients die one to two days after development of coma. Recovery often begins suddenly and progresses rapidly. About half of surviving infants suffer retardation, cerebellar damage, choreoathetosis, and spastic paralysis. Young age at onset, duration of illness, and convulsions during the acute phase are harbingers of permanent sequelae. Adults may have a prolonged convalescent syndrome of asthenia and neuropsychiatric complaints, but objective residua are rare and parkinsonism is extremely uncommon. Congenital infections are documented and result in severe and progressive neurologic deterioration.

A moderate leukocytosis and left shift are usual. The cerebrospinal fluid contains white cells (at first polymorphonuclear, then mononuclear), rarely in excess of 500 per cubic millimeter, and elevated protein concentration (usually 90 to 110 mg per deciliter).

Pathologic examination of the brains of infants reveals massive neuroparenchymal destruction; children dying months or years after the acute insult often have large cystic lesions in many areas of the brain. In older children and adults, acute WEE is characterized by focal necrosis and perivascular cuffing, predominantly in the basal ganglia and thalamic nuclei, but also in deep cerebral white matter. The highest titers of virus and interferon have also been found in basal ganglia and thalamus.

DIAGNOSIS. Viral isolation from blood or cerebrospinal fluid is almost never successful; a postmortem diagnosis may sometimes be achieved by isolation of the virus from brain tissue. Diagnosis is usually achieved by demonstration of a rise in hemagglutination-inhibiting (HI), fluorescent, complement-fixing (CF), or neutralizing (N) antibody titers in appropriately timed paired sera. An acute phase serum is obtained as early as possible in the illness, and a second serum a minimum of 10 to 14 days later.

TREATMENT. No specific chemotherapeutic agent is known. Supportive and good nursing care is essential and may reduce mortality. Control of high fever by sponging or ice packs and administration of antipyretics orally or rectally is recommended. Prompt administration of anticonvulsants (intravenous diazepam for acute control and phenytoin for more prolonged control) should be used to prevent protracted seizures and attendant hypoxia. Dehydration caused by fever, vomiting, and insufficient oral intake may be prominent, especially in children, and fluid and electrolyte balance must be restored and maintained by intravenous infusions. Management of airways in semicomatose and comatose patients is essential. Arterial blood gases should be monitored and respiratory assistance provided if hypoxia occurs. Prevention and treatment of secondary bacterial infections may be required; good pulmonary toilet and care of urinary catheters are essential. If clinical signs suggest cerebral edema or if the cerebrospinal fluid pressure is very high (>400 mm H_2O), measures to reduce brain swelling are indicated. Clinical signs that suggest progressive intracranial hypertension include deepening obtundation; prolonged delerium; respiratory, ocular, and motor signs of diencephalic deterioration; and loss of brainstem reflexes. Treatment consists of intracranial pressure monitoring, osmotic agents (mannitol), neuromuscular blocking agents, and/or hyperventilation.

PREVENTION AND CONTROL. An experimental formalin-inactivated vaccine grown in chick embryo cell cultures has been used exclusively for protection of laboratory workers. A commercial vaccine is available for horses; since equines are dead-end hosts, vaccination plays no role in preventing human disease. A high level of vaccine immunity in equines reduces their value as sentinels of WEE activity (see Epidemiology). In threatened or ongoing epidemics, residents should be advised to avoid mosquito bite by use of protective clothing, repellents, window screens, and restricted outdoor activity in the early morning, late afternoon, and evening. Public health measures include spray application of insecticides aimed at the adult *Culex tarsalis* vector.

EASTERN EQUINE ENCEPHALITIS (EEE)

ETIOLOGIC AGENT. EEE virus, first isolated in 1933, is an alphavirus. Two antigenic subtypes (North and South American) are distinguishable by special serologic tests. Methods for viral isolation and assay are as described for WEE.

EPIDEMIOLOGY. ***Incidence and Prevalence.*** The disease in man is relatively rare; 147 recognized cases were reported in the United States between 1955 and 1981. The largest outbreak occurred in 1959 in New Jersey (32 cases), but the usual pattern is one of a predominant equine epizootic involving 100 to 300 animals and associated with several human cases. The Atlantic and Gulf coastal areas are prone to recrudescent viral activity. Enzootic transmission and sporadic cases occur in inland freshwater swamp areas of the United States east of the Mississippi River. Outbreaks also occur in eastern Canada and in the Caribbean area (Jamaica, Hispaniola, Cuba) caused by the North American viral subtype. Equine epizootics have appeared in Panama, Brazil, Guyana, Venezuela, and Argentina, but human disease is rare or unrecognized.

Despite the small size of EEE epidemics, their cost in terms of severity is high. The case-fatality rate is 60 to 70 per cent. The incidence and mortality are highest in children under 15 and in persons over 55 years, with no sex predilection. A risk of human disease may be predicted by the occurrence of equine cases or outbreaks of fatal encephalitis in penned exotic birds (pheasants, chukar partridges), which precede the appearance of human cases by several weeks or more. Vaccination of horses and birds or inadequate surveillance may abrogate their usefulness as sentinels. Outbreaks occur during the late summer and early fall.

Transmission. In temperate areas, EEE virus circulates between wild birds and *Culiseta melanura* mosquitoes in fresh water swamp habitat. Transmission is favored by excessive rainfall during the autumn of the preceding year and the summer of the current year. Sporadic infections may be acquired in or near fresh water swamps by the bite of the primary enzootic vector, which is principally attracted to birds and rarely feeds on horses and man. Other species, in particular *Aedes sollicitans* and *Coquillettidia perturbans*, are implicated in epidemic-epizootic spread and extension of viral activity from swamp to salt marsh and woodland habitat. Transmission between penned pheasants and chukars is by contact, through pecking and cannibalism. The overwintering cycle is presently unknown.

CLINICAL FEATURES AND PATHOLOGY. The disease is more acute and rapidly progressive than the other arboviral encephalitides. The onset is abrupt, with high fever, vomiting, somnolence, stupor, coma, myoclonus, and generalized convulsions appearing within 24 to 48 hours. Autonomic disturbances (sialorrhea) may be prominent, and respiratory difficulty and cyanosis are frequent. A curious feature of the disease in children is facial, periorbital, or generalized edema. Death usually occurs during the first week after onset; in surviving patients, recovery begins during the second week and may progress rapidly. Residual damage, in 30 to 50 per cent of the patients, is often severe, especially in children, and is characterized by retardation, spastic paralyses, and atrophy of brain substance.

Examination of the cerebrospinal fluid provides a clue to the diagnosis. Early in infection, EEE is characterized by high cell counts (500 to 2000 per cubic millimeter) and a predominance of polymorphonuclear cells. The total cell count falls after day three or four, but polymorphonuclear cells persist as a significant fraction. Red blood cells may be present, the protein elevated, and glucose normal. A striking peripheral leukocytosis and left shift are frequent findings.

In contrast to St. Louis and western equine encephalitis, the brain is grossly edematous and congested, and the inflammatory response is predominantly polymorphonuclear rather than mononuclear. Focal vasculitic lesions, endothelial cell swelling, and intravenous and arteriolar thrombus formation are present. Demyelination, necrosis, neuronolysis, and neuronophagia are prominent. The areas most affected are basal ganglia, thalamus, hippocampus, and frontal and occipital cortex.

SPECIFIC DIAGNOSIS. Isolation of virus from blood and spinal fluid is rarely successful. A postmortem diagnosis can be achieved by virus isolation from brain in approximately 75 per cent of fatal cases. Serologic diagnosis is as described for WEE virus; because of the rapid course of the clinical disease, sera should be obtained at two- to three-day intervals during the acute phase of illness. An early serologic diagnosis can often be made by this means.

TREATMENT. Treatment is supportive (see previous discussion of WEE).

PREVENTION AND CONTROL. An experimental formalin-inactivated chick embryo cell culture vaccine is used to protect laboratory and field workers. Vaccination prevents disease in equines but does not interrupt transmission or prevent human infection. Reduction of mosquito populations by appropriate use of insecticides may be effective in threatened or established outbreaks.

VENEZUELAN EQUINE ENCEPHALITIS (VEE)

ETIOLOGY. The causative agent is an alphavirus first isolated in 1938 from a sick horse in Venezuela. Five antigenic subtypes (I to V) are separable by serologic tests; multiple antigenic variants of subtypes I and III are also recognized. Subtypes IAB and IC are responsible for epidemics involving man and equines. In Florida, subtype II is enzootic and produces sporadic human disease. Definition of the antigenic subtype and variant responsible for infection requires isolation of the virus and characterization by a specialty laboratory.

EPIDEMIOLOGY. ***Incidence and Prevalence.*** Large equine epizootics occur at five- to ten-year intervals in Venezuela, Colombia, Ecuador, and Peru. The capacity of VEE virus to invade new territory was demonstrated in 1969, when subtype IAB virus appeared in Guatemala and spread in waves throughout Central America, Mexico, and south Texas. Individual epizootics have involved many thousands (sometimes more than 100,000) of animals, with up to 40 per cent mortality rates. Associated human morbidity has also been great (up to 30,000 clinical cases). Truly subclinical infections are rare. The predominant syndrome is a self-limited grippe-like illness, and only about 4 per cent of infected persons, principally children under 15 years, develop encephalitis. The case-fatality rate in children up to five years old with encephalitis is approximately 35 per cent, but in older persons it is less than 10 per cent. Laboratory infections are common in unvaccinated persons working with the virus or infected animals.

Transmission. Transmission of subtypes IAB and IC viruses during epizootic-epidemics is effected by a large variety of mosquito vectors, including species of the genera *Aedes, Psorophora,* and *Mansonia;* equines are the principal viremic hosts. Viremia in man is of sufficient magnitude to infect mosquitoes, but man-mosquito-man transmission is of minor importance in the generation and maintenance of an outbreak. Virus may be present in pharyngeal excretions of human patients; contact or aerosol person-to-person spread, although possible, is not epidemiologically important. Aerosol transmission in the laboratory is nevertheless well documented. The interepidemic maintenance transmission cycle of these viral subtypes is unknown.

The other members of the VEE viral complex, including subtype II in Florida, have enzootic transmission cycles involving *Culex (Melanoconion)* species mosquitoes and small forest rodents and marsupials. Equines are not involved in transmission; human disease is sporadic and relatively uncommon, but may be clinically severe.

CLINICAL FEATURES AND PATHOLOGY. The incubation period is two to five days. Onset is sudden, with fever, chills, generalized malaise, and headache; these symptoms are followed by myalgia (especially in the lumbar region), nausea, vomiting, and occasionally diarrhea. Physical examination reveals fever, tachycardia, conjunctival injection, and, in some cases, nonexudative pharyngitis. Acute symptoms generally subside in four to six days; a convalescent fatigue syndrome may follow, lasting up to three weeks. A biphasic course has sometimes been noted; acute symptoms reappear after a brief remission, within a week after the initial onset.

Evidence of mild central nervous system involvement (photophobia, somnolence, confusion) may be present in cases of the typical, grippe-like illness described above. Severe encephalitis develops in a small proportion of those infected, principally children, and is characterized by meningeal signs, convulsions, tremor, stupor, coma, spastic paralysis, abnormal reflexes, cranial nerve palsies, and central respiratory failure. Residual neurologic damage occurs in severe cases. Congenital infections acquired during the first and second trimesters result in fetal encephalitis and death.

In the first few days of illness, the peripheral leukocyte count may be depressed, with decrease in both lymphocytes and neutrophils, or normal, with a relative lymphopenia. Eosinopenia and vacuolization of monocytes have been described. In cases with central nervous system signs, the cerebrospinal fluid contains up to 500 cells per cubic millimeter, predominantly lymphocytes. The serum lactic dehydrogenase and glutamic-oxaloacetic transaminase levels may be elevated. Impaired glucose tolerance and insulin release were found in experimental animals after VEE infection, but there are no reports of a diabetogenic effect in man.

The neuropathologic features of the disease in man have not been clearly documented. In the congenitally infected fetus there is massive and widespread necrosis of brain tissue, hemorrhages, and resorption of brain material, resulting in hydranencephaly.

DIAGNOSIS. Virus can be isolated from the blood during the first three or four days after onset, with peak titers on day two. Isolation from throat swabs or washings may also be successful. HI and N antibodies appear in the first week and CF antibodies in the second week after onset; serodiagnosis is achieved by testing appropriately timed paired sera.

TREATMENT. No specific therapy is available, and treatment of encephalitis cases is supportive (see earlier discussion of WEE).

PREVENTION AND CONTROL. An experimental live, attenuated vaccine (TC-83) is used in adult laboratory personnel and provides solid immunity to the immunizing subtype (IAB) and its closest relative (IC), but incomplete protection against infection with some heterologous VEE viruses. Epidemics and epizootics can be prevented by effective vaccination of equines (the principal viremic hosts), using live, attenuated, or inactivated TC-83 vaccines. In the face of an ongoing epidemic, spraying of insecticides to reduce the adult (infective) mosquito populations is the only means of immediate control; vaccination of equines at the periphery of the outbreak prevents spread.

ST. LOUIS ENCEPHALITIS (SLE)

ETIOLOGY. St. Louis encephalitis virus, a member of the flavivirus genus of the family Togaviridae, shares close antigenic relationships with Japanese encephalitis, Murray Valley encephalitis, and West Nile viruses. The virus is pathogenic for infant and adult mice inoculated intracerebrally and may also be assayed in a variety of avian and mammalian cell cultures. Strain differences in pathogenicity and genome composition are recognized and provide a geographic and epidemiologic classification. Strains associated with *Culex pipiens*-borne epidemics in the eastern United States are distinct from endemic strains transmitted by *Culex tarsalis* in the western states.

EPIDEMIOLOGY. ***Incidence and Prevalence.*** The virus is present in all parts of the Western Hemisphere, but causes epidemics only in North America and some Caribbean islands. During epidemic years, the virus has been responsible for up to 80 per cent of all reported cases of encephalitis of known etiology in the United States. A total of 4965 cases were reported between 1955 and 1981. In recent years, epidemics have occurred mainly in urban-suburban localities of the Ohio–Mississippi River basin, in eastern and central Texas, and in Florida. Small outbreaks have also occurred in rural areas of the western United States. Epidemics generally occur between July and September, with a peak in August, but may arise later in the year in warm areas such as Florida. No racial difference in disease susceptibility exists, but, owing to socioeconomic factors, attack rates have been higher in the black than in the white population of some cities. Prior exposure and immunity to dengue may provide a degree of cross-protection against clinical SLE.

The overall case-fatality rate is approximately 9 per cent; mortality is negligible in persons under 20 years, and it rises steeply after age 55 to approximately 30 per cent in patients over 65 years of age. The inapparent:apparent infection ratio is 800:1 in children up to nine years, 400:1 in persons 10 to 49 years, and 85:1 in persons over 60 years.

In tropical America, a high prevalence of antibody in many areas indicates widespread transmission; disease is sporadic and rarely recognized.

Transmission. In most of the eastern United States, SLE virus circulates between wild birds and *Culex pipiens* mosquitoes. *Culex pipiens* breeds in polluted water and achieves high densities in urban-suburban areas with poor sanitation. In Florida and in parts of the Caribbean, *Culex nigripalpus* is the principal vector. The cycle in the western United States also involves wild birds, but the vector is *Culex tarsalis*. The ecology of SLE and WEE viruses in the west is thus similar, and transmission occurs in rural, agricultural areas. Horses develop antibodies but not overt disease or significant viremia. The primary vectors (*C. pipiens, nigripalpus, tarsalis*) are responsible for transmission to man.

Above-average summer temperatures and deficient rainfall (which creates stagnant pools suitable for *Culex pipiens* breeding) are associated with epidemics in the eastern United States. *Culex tarsalis*–borne SLE in the western states is favored by warm spring temperatures, heavy winter-spring precipitation, high river runoff, and flood conditions.

During the winter, the virus is probably maintained locally in infected hibernating adult female *Culex*.

CLINICAL FEATURES AND PATHOLOGY. Three clinical syndromes are recognized: febrile headache, aseptic meningitis, and encephalitis. As discussed above, encephalitis is a more frequent presentation in the elderly and the milder syndromes in young patients. The incubation period is 4 to 21 days. Onset is characterized by a variable period of nonspecific symptoms, including fever, headache, generalized malaise, drowsiness, myalgias, and sore throat, followed by the acute or subacute onset of meningeal or encephalitic signs or both. Fever ranges from 38.3 to 41° C; poor prognosis is associated with persistent high temperatures of 40 to 41° C. Nausea and vomiting and photophobia are common. Neurologic abnormalities include altered sensorium, meningismus, cranial nerve deficits (principally lower motor neuron N. VII), abnormal reflexes, and tremors. Signs of thalamic, brainstem, and cerebellar dysfunction include myoclonic twitching, nystagmus, and ataxia in up to 25 per cent of patients. Motor abnormalities are infrequent and sensory changes extremely uncommon. Convulsions occur in 10 per cent of patients and are a poor prognostic sign. In general, extrapyramidal abnormalities (tremor of tongue, face, and limbs) and the altered state of consciousness are the most significant findings. Signs of markedly increased intracranial pressure are very unusual. Acute inflammatory polyradiculoneuropathy (Guillain-Barré syndrome) has occasionally been associated with SLE, both as an acute presentation and during the convalescent period. Approximately half of the patients with fatal outcome succumb during the first week and 80 per cent within two weeks after onset. Complications of the neurologic disease include pneumonia, bacterial septicemia, pulmonary embolism, and gastrointestinal hemorrhage. Underlying conditions, especially hypertensive and arteriosclerotic disease, chronic brain syndromes, diabetes mellitus, and chronic bronchopulmonary disease, appear to play a role in determining severity and outcome, and may relate to the virulence of the disease process in older persons.

In uncomplicated cases of SLE, there is a moderate peripheral neutrophilic leukocytosis and left shift. Cerebrospinal fluid is under increased pressure and contains up to 500 cells per cubic millimeter, with polymorphonuclear predominance early, changing to lymphocyte predominance within several days. Spinal fluid protein is mildly elevated and glucose usually normal; in one series, however, cerebrospinal fluid glucose was less than 50 per cent of the blood level in 5 of 23 adult patients. Elevations of serum enzymes (creatine phosphokinase and glutamic-oxaloacetic transaminase) are frequently found. Serum aldolase levels may be elevated, but muscle biopsies have shown no changes. The electroencephalogram typically shows amorphous delta wave activity and diffuse generalized slowing most prominent in the frontal and temporal regions. The brain scan is normal. Disproportionately high cerebral blood flow in relation to metabolic demands has been documented, indicating a disturbance in cerebrovascular autoregulation. Mild hyponatremia and fluid overload in about one third of patients with encephalitis are due to the syndrome of inappropriate secretion of antidiuretic hormone.

Genitourinary tract symptoms (urgency, frequency, incontinence, and retention), microscopic hematuria, pyuria, and proteinuria, and elevated blood urea nitrogen are frequent. SLE viral antigen in cells of the urinary sediment has been detected by fluorescent techniques and virus-like particles in urine by immunoelectronmicroscopy. The possibility that the kidney is a site of SLE replication and injury remains problematic.

A convalescent fatigue syndrome characterized by weakness, fatigue, nervousness, tremulousness, sleeplessness, irritability, depression, difficulty in concentrating, and headaches occurs in 30 to 50 per cent of older persons and clears in 80 per cent of these within three years.

Pathologic changes in fatal cases are limited to microscopic examination. Leptomeningitis is characterized by lymphocytic inflammation. Parenchymal changes consist of lymphocytic perivascular cuffing, cellular nodule formation, and neuronal degeneration. Changes are most pronounced in substantia nigra, thalamus and hypothalamus, cerebellar cortex, cerebral cortex, and basal ganglia.

DIAGNOSIS. In approximately half of the fatal cases, a diagnosis may be made by virus isolation from brain tissue or immunofluorescent staining of frozen sections of brain. The virus is rarely isolated from blood or spinal fluid obtained during the acute phase of illness. Serologic diagnosis is achieved by demonstration of changing antibody titers; the HI, immunoassay, and N tests demonstrate antibody within the first week after onset, and titers rise during the ensuing two weeks. CF antibodies appear 10 to 20 days after onset. Rapid early diagnosis is possible by measurement of IgM antibodies by enzyme-linked immunosorbent assay (ELISA) and serum and cerebrospinal fluid. Specific serologic diagnosis may be complicated by cross-reactions in persons with prior exposures to dengue and other related flaviviruses.

TREATMENT. Treatment is supportive (see earlier discussion of WEE). Hyponatremia and clinical signs of water intoxication are generally of mild to moderate severity and are managed by restricting fluid intake.

PREVENTION AND CONTROL. No vaccine is available. Surveillance of vectors, antibody prevalence in wild birds, or serologic conversions in sentinel fowl are used to detect viral transmission before the occurrence of human infections. The information may be used to initiate vector control efforts. Source reduction and larviciding of vector breeding sites are useful preventive measures. In the case of an established outbreak, avoidance of mosquito bites and spraying to reduce infected adult mosquitoes are the only effective means of control.

CALIFORNIA ENCEPHALITIS

ETIOLOGY. Four members of the California serogroup of the Bunyavirus genus, LaCrosse, California encephalitis, Jamestown Canyon, and snowshoe hare viruses, cause encephalitis. California encephalitis virus occurs in the western United States (California, New Mexico, Utah, Texas) and has been implicated in only three human cases. In contrast, LaCrosse virus, distributed more widely in the eastern half of the United States and southern Canada, is a major human pathogen. It was first isolated from the brain of a child who died of encephalitis in 1964 at LaCrosse, Wisconsin. Recently Jamestown Canyon and snowshoe hare viruses have been implicated in sporadic human encephalitis cases in the north central United States and in Canada. Mice and a variety of cell cultures are useful for virus isolation and assay.

EPIDEMIOLOGY. ***Incidence and Prevalence.*** Between its recognition as a nosologic entity in 1964 and 1981, a total of 1310 cases of LaCrosse viral encephalitis have been reported in the United States, with an annual incidence of 50 to 150 cases. Undoubtedly far underreported, it occurs as an endemic rather than an epidemic disease, with individual or small clusters of cases scattered across the affected areas. It is most prevalent in the north central states, where it is responsible for as many as 20 per cent of cases of acute central nervous system infection in children. It primarily affects persons less than 15 years of age living in rural and suburban areas characterized by deciduous hardwood forests. Focal "hot spots" (communities, even backyards) of recurrent summertime viral activity are recognized. Cases occur between July and September, with peak incidence in August. The case-fatality rate is low (less than 1 per cent).

TRANSMISSION. The vectors of LaCrosse virus are *Aedes* mosquitoes (principally *Ae. triseriatus*), which breed both in forest tree-holes and in peridomestic artificial containers. The vector serves as a reservoir of LaCrosse virus, which is efficiently passed transovarially from female mosquitoes to progeny. The virus survives the winter months in infected eggs of *Aedes triseriatus*. In the summer months, wild rodents (squirrels, chipmunks) contribute to a cycle of transmission as viremic hosts. Man becomes infected by the bite of an infected mosquito but does not play a role in transmission.

CLINICAL FEATURES. The true clinical spectrum of California virus infection is not known, but undoubtedly includes nonspecific febrile illness, aseptic meningitis, and meningoencephalitis. Encephalitis may be quite severe in the acute stage, but the disease is almost always self-limited and death is extremely uncommon. The disease begins with a nonspecific syndrome of fever, headache, sore throat, and gastrointestinal symptoms, with appearance of the neurotropic disorder within one to three days. In mild cases of encephalitis, central nervous system signs appear on the third day after onset and subside within seven to eight days. In the more severe form, neurologic signs appear earlier (within 24 to 48 hours of onset), usually in the form of generalized seizures and altered consciousness, and are more prolonged. Papilledema or abnormal optic disc margins have been noted, but signs of progressive intracranial hypertension are rare. Intensive care and respiratory support are frequently required in severe cases. The question of permanent sequelae is unsettled. Although there are conflicting reports, many workers believe LaCrosse virus infection is responsible for residual psychologic problems, emotional lability, hyperkinesis, infantilism, compulsive behavior, and auditory and visual perceptual problems. There are case reports of hemiparesis and persistent seizure disorders.

The peripheral white cell count is often moderately elevated, with a predominance of granulocytes and band forms. The cerebrospinal fluid shows up to 500 lymphocytes per cubic millimeter, normal or mildly elevated protein, and normal glucose concentrations. The abnormalities on the electroencephalogram include generalized slowing in the delta and theta range, indicating diffuse cortical dysfunction. Focal delta wave activity related to cortical destruction or focal seizures is also a common finding.

DIAGNOSIS. The virus has been recovered from the brain in fatal cases, but not from blood or spinal fluid obtained during the acute phase. Diagnosis is best achieved by tests for antibody in paired acute and convalescent sera. The counterimmunoelectrophoresis, HI, CF, FA, ELISA, and N tests are applicable. However, the most practical, sensitive, and reliable methods are the HI test using the LaCrosse viral antigen and the IgM antibody capture ELISA.

TREATMENT. Treatment is supportive.

PREVENTION AND CONTROL. There is no vaccine. Vector control methods are of uncertain usefulness in this disease because of the multifocal, endemic pattern of disease incidence and the inherited nature of infection in mosquito vectors. In defined "hot spots" of recurrent viral activity, efforts to eliminate breeding sites for *Aedes triseriatus* should be made. Avoidance of mosquito bites and protection of children by limiting exposure and use of repellents are reasonable suggestions to parents.

JAPANESE ENCEPHALITIS

ETIOLOGY. Japanese encephalitis is caused by a flavivirus first isolated in 1934 from the brain of a fatal human case in Japan. Unlike SLE, it causes epizootics of clinical encephalitis in equines. The virus also produces abortion and stillbirth in swine, an important economic problem in parts of Asia. Serologic cross-reactivity with other flaviviruses may lead to confusion in diagnostic tests.

EPIDEMIOLOGY. ***Prevalence and Incidence.*** The disease is endemic and epidemic in Asia, including Japan, Korea, Taiwan, China, Okinawa, Vietnam, the Philippines, Burma, Malaysia, Bangladesh, east and south India, Thailand, and Indonesia. Morbidity in some outbreaks is high (thousands of cases); case-fatality rates of 50 per cent or more have been reported but reflect underrecognition of nonfatal cases. In hyperendemic areas, over 70 per cent of adult populations surveyed have antibodies, and children under 15 years old are principally affected by the disease. In areas without a high prevalence of background immunity (e.g., northern India), however, all age groups are affected; and in Japan, where school children have been protected by vaccination campaigns targeted at this age group, occurrence of encephalitis in the elderly has become evident. The inapparent:apparent infection ratio is over 500:1 in children and decreases with age; in Korea, the ratio among American servicemen was estimated at 25:1. In temperate areas, JE is a summertime disease; in the tropics, it occurs year-round as a sporadic infection. Epidemics have been most frequent at the northern fringe of the tropical zone. JE is predominantly a rural disease, and the incidence in males is often higher than in females.

Transmission. The natural cycle involves *Culex* mosquito vectors and vertebrates susceptible to viremic infection, including wild birds and swine. Man and equines are incidental (dead-end) hosts. The vector species varies with geographic area; *Culex tritaeniorhyncus,* a rice-paddy breeder, is the most widespread and important. Overwinter survival and springtime recrudescence in temperate areas are unexplained, but evidence suggests that transovarial viral transmission in mosquitoes may play a role.

CLINICAL FEATURES AND PATHOLOGY. The spectrum of illness includes febrile headache, aseptic meningitis, and meningoencephalitis. The disease is more severe than St. Louis encephalitis. Onset is abrupt, with fever, headache, and gastrointestinal symptoms. Meningeal irritation develops within 24 hours and is followed on the second or third day by the appearance of irritability, impaired consciousness, convulsions (especially in children), muscular rigidity, mask-like facies, ataxia, coarse tremor, involuntary movements, cranial nerve deficits, paresis, hyperactive deep tendon reflexes, and pathologic reflexes. Weight loss and dehydration are often striking findings. In patients with mild involvement, fever subsides on the sixth or seventh day and neurologic signs resolve by the end of the second week after onset. In severe cases, hyperpyrexia and progressive neurologic dysfunction and coma result in death between the seventh and tenth days, or the patient undergoes a prolonged recovery, often leaving permanent sequelae. Cardiorespiratory complications are frequent during the acute stage in these patients. Atypical forms with predominance of bulbar or myelitic signs have been described. A poor prognosis is associated with prolonged high fever, frequent or prolonged seizures, high protein content in the cerebrospinal fluid, Babinski signs, and early appearance of respiratory depression.

The occurrence of sequelae correlates with severity of the acute stage of illness; young children are most susceptible, and sequelae, including mental impairment, emotional lability, choreoathetosis, tremor, parkinsonism, autonomic disturbances, motor paralysis, and pathopsychologic syndromes, including schizophrenia, have been reported in up to 75 per cent of patients.

Transplacental infection, resulting in fetal death and abortion, has been reported.

Clinical laboratory tests show a moderate peripheral leukocytosis early in the disease (usually characterized by neutrophilia) and cerebrospinal fluid pleocytosis, polymorphonuclear early but predominantly mononuclear later in the disease. Spinal fluid protein is mildly elevated and glucose concentration normal.

Neuropathologic changes and distribution of lesions are similar to those described for St. Louis encephalitis (see earlier discussion of SLE).

DIAGNOSIS. In many patients dying during the first week after onset, the virus may be isolated from brain or viral antigen demonstrated by immunofluorescence. Isolations from blood or spinal fluid are uncommon, and diagnosis is best achieved by serologic tests. HI and N antibodies appear during the first and CF antibodies during the second week after onset. In areas where other flaviviral infections are common, cross-reactions make serodiagnosis difficult; increased precision may be obtained by measuring early, specific IgM antibodies by immunoassays on serum or cerebrospinal fluid.

TREATMENT. Treatment is supportive (see earlier discussion of WEE).

PREVENTION AND CONTROL. Inactivated, partially purified mouse brain vaccines produced in Asia are used principally in preschool- and school-age children. Although not yet licensed for use in the United States, a vaccine produced in Japan is available on a limited scale to United States citizens traveling to high-risk areas. Information should be sought from state health departments or the Centers for Disease Control. Since three doses of the inactivated vaccine are used, and approximately one month is required to confer protection, vaccination is not a practical measure in the face of an ongoing epidemic. Reduction of vector mosquito populations by ultra-low volume application of insecticides may be used to abort outbreaks.

MURRAY VALLEY ENCEPHALITIS AND ROCIO ENCEPHALITIS

Murray Valley encephalitis and Rocio encephalitis are similar to Japanese encephalitis in pathogenesis and clinical features and are caused by closely related flaviviruses.

Murray Valley encephalitis has occurred in small epidemics in the Murray and Darling River valleys of Victoria and New South Wales, Australia. The virus is endemic in Northern Australia and New Guinea, where it is maintained in a bird-mosquito cycle. It has been postulated that the virus is intermittently brought south by migratory birds; in southern Australia, transmission involves water birds, domestic fowl, and *Culex annulirostris* mosquitoes. Diagnosis requires laboratory studies similar to those for other flaviviruses. No vaccine is available.

Rocio encephalitis was first described in 1975, when a new flavivirus by the same name was isolated from the brains of patients with fatal encephalitis during an epidemic in São Paulo State, Brazil. In several discrete outbreaks in 1975–1976, over 1000 cases occurred in this region, but the disease has not been recognized elsewhere. The transmission cycle is poorly understood, but probably involves wild birds and mosquitoes. An inactivated suckling mouse brain vaccine has been prepared but has been found to be of low potency.

TICK-BORNE ENCEPHALITIS

ETIOLOGIC AGENTS. A complex of six antigenically related tick-borne flaviviruses consists of Powassan, tick-borne encephalitis virus (TBE), louping ill, Kyasanur Forest disease (KFD), Omsk hemorrhagic fever (OHF), and Langat viruses. The predominant syndrome in KFD and OHF is hemorrhagic fever (see earlier discussion of VEE),but meningoencephalitis may be a component of the disease spectrum. Two subtypes of TBE virus (Central European encephalitis and Russian spring-summer encephalitis) are distinguished by special serologic tests, are ecologically distinct, and differ in virulence for man. Powassan and louping ill viruses are rare causes of encephalitis in North America and the British Isles, respectively. These viruses are serologically easily distinguished from mosquito-borne flaviviruses, but induce cross-reactions within the complex. The viruses may be isolated and assayed in infant mice and a variety of cell cultures.

EPIDEMIOLOGY. ***Incidence and Prevalence.*** TBE occurs in Europe (including European Russia), southern Scandinavia, and the far eastern USSR. Several hundred to 2000 cases are reported annually, with morbidity rates of up to 20 per 100,000 inhabitants. Inapparent infections are common. The disease is seasonal, corresponding to peak summertime tick vector populations. Adults over 20 years are principally affected, and persons frequenting tick-infested foci (e.g., forestry workers, shepherds, campers) are at highest risk. Family outbreaks are caused by drinking infected milk (see Transmission, below). In Europe, the disease is relatively mild (case-fatality rate 1 to 2 per cent); but in the Far East, it is severe (20 to 25 per cent). In the United States, the disease should be considered in persons with a history of travel to endemic areas.

Louping ill causes encephalitis in sheep and cattle in Scotland and in northern England and Ireland. Sporadic human cases have been recognized in veterinarians, butchers, and laboratory workers. Serologic surveys indicate that natural infections are uncommon. Powassan virus encephalitis has been documented in a total of 15 cases in the northeastern United States and eastern Canada. The case-fatality rate is 50 per cent. The virus is not associated with animal disease. Serosurveys indicate that human infections in the endemic area are rare (prevalence rates less than 1 per cent).

Transmission. In Europe, the vector of TBE is *Ixodes ricinus*, and in the Far East, *I. persulcatus*. The tick vector also serves as a reservoir of the virus, which is transmitted both transovarially and from one stage (instar) to the next. Larval ticks parasitize small rodents, which serve as amplifying viremic hosts during the spring and summer; hibernating rodents may also harbor the virus during the winter. Man is a dead-end host, incidental to the transmission cycle. Large vertebrates (goats, sheep, cattle) are hosts for nymphal and adult ticks and may become infected and shed virus in the milk. Outbreaks have occurred in families or groups of individuals ingesting unpasteurized goat or sheep milk or cheese.

Louping ill virus is maintained in nature by *Ixodes ricinus* ticks and a variety of hosts, including small mammals, ground-dwelling birds (grouse), and, probably, sheep. Humans become infected by direct contact with infected sheep, or by tick bite. The transmission cycle of Powassan virus involves *Ixodes cookei*, *I. marxi* (and possibly other tick species), and mammals, particularly rodents and carnivores. Human infection is acquired by tick bite; because of the small size of the vector, a history of bite is infrequently obtained.

CLINICAL FEATURES. TBE in Europe typically (but not invariably) has a diphasic course, beginning 7 to 14 days after exposure with an influenza-like syndrome lasting one week, followed by a period of clinical remission for several days, and then abrupt onset of aseptic meningitis or meningoencephalitis. The latter is usually benign, although severe paralytic illness, myelitis, myeloradiculitis, and bulbar forms may occur. Convalescence is often prolonged, and residual paralysis may follow in severe cases. In the Far East, TBE begins suddenly with fever, headache, and gastrointestinal symptoms, followed rapidly by appearance of depressed sensorium, coma, convulsions, and paralysis. Bulbar paralysis and cervical myelitis are frequent findings. In fatal cases, death occurs in the first week after onset. Survivors have a high incidence of residual paralyses, especially lower motor neuron paralysis of upper extremities or shoulder girdle. Aseptic meningitis and milder forms of encephalitis also occur. Chronic forms of TBE have been described, with active clinical and pathologic abnormalities a year or more after onset.

The clinical features of louping ill resemble the European form of TBE. Powassan encephalitis is characterized by a variable period of fever and nonspecific symptoms, followed by the development of encephalitic signs, which are frequently severe. Residual paralysis may occur.

Peripheral blood and cerebrospinal fluid changes are similar to those described in other forms of flaviviral encephalitis.

DIAGNOSIS. The virus may be isolated from brain tissue. In TBE, virus isolation from blood is also possible during the early phase of illness. Serologic diagnosis is achieved by the HI, CF, N, or ELISA techniques.

TREATMENT. Treatment is supportive (see earlier discussion of WEE).

CONTROL. In eastern Europe and the USSR, TBE vaccines are used in high-risk groups (forestry and agricultural workers, military personnel). Avoidance of tick exposure by use of protective clothing and repellents may be recommended to visitors in areas of high TBE activity. Surveillance of viral transmission and use of insecticides to control ticks have met with variable success. In years of high rodent population density, rodent control in natural foci has also been recommended.

Bennett NM: Murray Valley encephalitis, 1974. Clinical features. Med J Aust 2:446, 1976. *A useful guide to the clinical aspects of this rare infection.*

Blaškovič D, Nosek J: The ecological approach to the study of tick-borne encephalitis. Prog Med Virol 14:275, 1972. *Comprehensive review of the ecology, epidemiology, prevention, and control of tick-borne encephalitis; exhaustively referenced.*

Calisher CH, Thompson WH (eds.): California Serogroup Viruses. New York, Alan R. Liss, Inc., 1983. *Symposium covering all aspects of this virus group.*

Grabow JD, Matthews CG, Chun RWM, Thompson WH: The electroencephalogram and clinical sequelae of California arbovirus encephalitis. Neurology 19:394, 1969. *Clear descriptions of clinical course and residual damage in children with California encephalitis; should be consulted together with reference by Matthews et al.*

Hilty MD, Haynes RE, Azimi PH, Cramblett HG: California encephalitis in children. Am J Dis Child 124:530, 1972. *Useful clinical descriptions of this infection.*

Johnson KM, Martin DH: Venezuelan equine encephalitis. Adv Vet Sci Comp Med 18:79, 1974. *A superbly written, detailed, and well-referenced review of the clinical, virologic, and epidemiologic aspects of this disease.*

Leon CA, Jaramillo R, Martinez S, Fernandez F, Tellez H, Lasso B, Guzman R de: Sequelae of Venezuelan equine encephalitis in humans: A four-year follow-up. Int J Epidemiol 4:131, 1975. *The only well-documented study of neurologic residua of this infection.*

Lincoln AF, Sivertson SE: Acute phase of Japanese B encephalitis. Two hundred and one cases in American soldiers, Korea, 1950. JAMA 150:268, 1952. *The leading reference in English to the clinical features of Japanese encephalitis.*

Lopes O de S, Sachetta L de A, Coimbra TLM, Pinto GH, Glasser CM: Emergence

of a new arbovirus disease in Brazil [Rocio]. II. Epidemiologic studies on 1975 epidemic. Am J Epidemiol 108:394, 1978. *First description of this newly recognized disease; contains only epidemiologic information.*
Matthews CG, Chun RWM, Grabow JD, Thompson, WH: Psychological sequelae in children following California arbovirus encephalitis. Neurology 18:1023, 1968. *Useful to the physician facing questions from patients about sequelae in children recovering from this infection.*
Monath TP (ed.): Saint Louis Encephalitis. Washington, D.C., American Public Health Association, 1980. *Encyclopedic coverage of all aspects of St. Louis encephalitis, including clinical features and differential and definitive laboratory diagnosis. Contains references to all previously published studies.*
Venezuelan Encephalitis. Washington, D.C., Pan-American Health Organization Publication No. 243, 1972. *Proceedings of a symposium containing a wealth of published and unpublished information; all aspects of the disease are covered, but emphasis is on virology and ecology-epidemiology.*
Wallis RC: Recent advances in research on the eastern encephalitis virus. Yale J Biol Med 37:413, 1965. *A review; emphasizes epidemiologic and ecologic aspects.*

Viral Hemorrhagic Fevers

357. INTRODUCTION*

Karl M. Johnson

The viral hemorrhagic fevers form a group of acute diseases in which bleeding is a prominent clinical manifestation. These diseases occur in different parts of the world, are caused by ribonucleic acid (RNA)–containing viruses, and may be transmitted to man by mosquitoes, by ticks, or by direct contact with excreta of virus-infected rodents (see Table 358–1). Despite its longstanding fame as a cause of acute hepatocellular necrosis, *yellow fever* is included under this heading because of its recognized ability to induce gastrointestinal hemorrhage and a shock syndrome similar to that seen with other viruses of the group.

After a variable period of a few days to one to three weeks, during which the virus multiplies in lymphoid cells and produces a viremia, hemorrhagic fever patients experience fever, myalgia, and other nonspecific symptoms. Bleeding ensues, generally near the end of the febrile period, and although usually not sufficient per se to account for it, such hemorrhage is the harbinger of a clinical crisis dominated by hypovolemic shock. In at least two conditions, hemorrhagic fever with renal syndrome and dengue hemorrhagic fever, there is evidence that shock is caused by a widespread capillary vascular lesion in which plasma protein escapes the circulation much faster than erythrocytes. Thrombocytopenia and deficits in various circulating hemostatic factors are frequently present, but it is not clear whether they are etiologically related to this condition.

How the hemorrhagic syndrome is produced thus remains a mystery. No evidence for a direct virus-induced lesion of capillary endothelium has been obtained to date. Disseminated intravascular coagulation (DIC) has been shown in a few instances and postulated in others. Nevertheless, we have no clear idea about the important pathophysiologic events that induce hemorrhage and shock. Acute hepatocellular damage is present in many of these diseases and may play some role. Altered immunologic function also may be important; inflammatory reaction to tissue injury is notably absent in most hemorrhagic fevers, B cell lymphocyte suppression is suggested by high incidence of secondary bacterial infection and delay in antibody formation in Junin, Machupo, and Congo-CHF infections, and antigen-antibody complexes may prove to be important in dengue, Lassa, and Hantaan virus disease. Elucidation of the operative variables is important because case management and development of effective vaccines appear to offer more hope of averting fatal infection than interruption of nonhuman natural virus cycles.

358. YELLOW FEVER

Thomas P. Monath

DEFINITION. Yellow fever is an acute mosquito-borne viral infection characterized, in its severe form, by fever, jaundice, hemorrhage, and albuminuria. The disease is endemic-epidemic in tropical regions of the Americas and Africa (see Fig. 358–1), where it remains a major public health problem, but it does not occur in Asia.

*The views of the author in this and subsequent chapters do not purport to reflect the positions of the Department of the Army or the Department of Defense (Para. 4-3, AR 360-5).

ETIOLOGY. Yellow fever virus is the prototype of the flavivirus taxonomic group, which is composed of a variety of other medically important, antigenically related viruses, including several which also cause hemorrhagic fevers (see Table 358–1). Yellow fever virus and other flaviviruses are spherical, enveloped, RNA-containing particles of approximately 38 mμ in size; virions develop by budding from intracytoplasmic membranes of infected cells and accumulate in cisternae of the endoplasmic reticulum. Since the virus shares antigenic determinants with many other flaviviruses, serologic responses to infection are often nonspecific or difficult to interpret. Strains of yellow fever virus from Africa and South America are distinguishable in special serologic tests; strain variation in virulence markers for laboratory animals also occurs. However, no clear geographic differences have been shown in the clinical features of the human disease. Yellow fever virus is pathogenic for a variety of cell cultures, newborn mice, adult mice (when injected intracerebrally), and some monkey species. Rhesus monkeys have been used as an experimental model of the human disease.

EPIDEMIOLOGY. Two epidemiologic forms of yellow fever are classically distinguished on the basis of different mosquito vectors and vertebrate hosts involved in the cycle of virus transmission. These forms are clinically and pathoanatomically identical. In the *urban* form, yellow fever virus is passed from a viremic person to another, nonimmune individual by the peridomestic mosquito, *Aedes aegypti*. As with other arboviruses, a period of extrinsic incubation in the vector is required before virus can be transmitted. *Jungle* (or sylvan) yellow fever is a zoonotic infection, acquired through the bite of forest mosquito vector species, which maintain the virus in a monkey-mosquito-monkey cycle. The epidemiology of the disease in the Americas and in Africa differs and must be considered separately.

Between 50 and 300 cases of *jungle yellow fever* are recognized annually in South America. The virus is active primarily in Brazil, Peru, Bolivia, and Colombia in forested and sparsely populated areas under limited cultivation, drained by tributar-

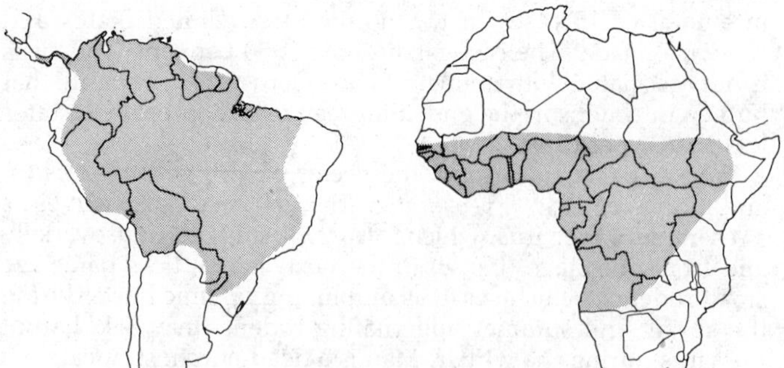

Figure 358–1. Shaded areas indicate zones of yellow fever endemicity. Some countries do not require certificate of yellow fever vaccination from travelers; nevertheless, vaccination is recommended for travel outside the urban areas of countries in the endemic zones. Yellow fever should be suspected in unvaccinated persons with fever and jaundice acquired in these areas.

TABLE 358–1. VIRAL HEMORRHAGIC FEVERS: ETIOLOGIC AND EPIDEMIOLOGIC CONSIDERATIONS

	Causative Agent	Vector(s)	Vertebrate Host(s)	Geographical Distribution	Epidemiologic Features of Involvement of Man	Control	Remarks
Yellow fever (urban)	YF virus—a flavivirus	*Aedes aegypti* in cities	Man	Human populations (usually urban) in tropics of South and Central America and Africa	Person-to-person passage by *Aedes aegypti*	*Aedes aegypti* control; vaccination	Sylvan YF can spread to cities
Yellow fever (sylvan)	YF virus—a flavivirus	*Haemagogus* mosquitoes in New World; *Aedes* species in Africa	Monkeys of several genera and species	Forests and jungles of South and Central America and West, Central, and East Africa	Man infected by exposure in jungle (e.g., woodcutters, hunters)	Vaccination	Human cases sporadic and unpredictable; disease often a "silent" epizootic in forests
Dengue hemorrhagic fever	Dengue viruses of four types; flaviviruses	*Aedes aegypti*	Man (involvement of other primates has been postulated)	Tropical and subtropical cities of Southeast Asia and Philippines; Caribbean	Small children usually involved in cities where *Aedes aegypti* densities ae high	*Aedes aegypti* control; mosquito repellent, screens, etc.	Disease may represent an immunologic over-response to a sequential infection with a different dengue strain
Omsk hemorrhagic fever	OHF virus—a flavivirus	Ticks of genus *Dermacentor*	Small rodents and muskrats	Omsk region of USSR; northern Rumania	People exposed in fields and wooded lands	Tick repellents and protective clothing	
Kyasanur Forest disease	KFD virus—a flavivirus	Ticks of several species in genus *Haemaphysalis*	Monkeys (rhesus and langur) and small rodents and birds	Mysore State, India	People exposed in fields and wooded lands	Tick control; tick repellents and protective clothing	Monkey mortality signals epidemic activity
Argentine hemorrhagic fever	Junin virus, an arenavirus	None recognized	Small rodents; *Akodon; Calomys laucha, musculinus*	Argentina: NW of Buenos Aires extending west to Province of Cordoba	Field workers at harvest time are particularly at risk	None practical	Infected rodents contaminate environment with urine
Bolivian hemorrhagic fever	Machupo virus—an arenavirus	None recognized	Small rodent, *Calomys callosus*	Beni Province of Bolivia	Residents of small rodent-infested villages and homes; 1971 nosocomial outbreak in Cochabamba, Bolivia	Rodent control in villages	High mortality in man
Lassa fever	Lassa virus, an arenavirus LCM-related	None required	Small rodent, *Mastomys natalensis*	West Africa; Nigeria, Liberia, Sierra Leone	Residents of small, rodent-infested villages; dramatic nosocomial outbreaks	None known; possibly rodent control	High mortality in man
Crimean hemorrhagic fever	Congo-CHF virus—a nairovirus	Ticks of several genera	Larger domestic animals implicated; also African hedgehog	Southern USSR, Bulgaria, East and West Africa	Cowhands and field workers in USSR; nosocomial outbreaks reported	Tick control relating to livestock; full isolation in patient care	Human disease important in USSR; importance to man in Africa not known
Korean hemorrhagic fever (hemor. nephrosonephritis)	Hantaan virus—a bunyavirus	None recognized	Small rodents: *Apodemus, Clethrionomys*	Korea; northern Eurasia to and including Scandinavia	Rural or sylvan exposure (military, forest occupations farmers, laboratory workers)		Urban rats may be reservoirs Related viruses present in North and South America, Africa, without recognized human disease

ies of the Amazon, Orinoco, and Magdalena rivers. Human cases reach a peak during the rainy months. Human cases are often sporadic, but small epidemics (involving 20 to 50 cases) are not uncommon. In the past, large outbreaks have been associated with monkey epizootics which appear at 5- to 40-year intervals and spread through natural corridors into forested areas, such as Central America, normally outside the enzootic zone. In the forest canopy, the virus circulates in a primary cycle involving monkeys and marmosets and mosquitoes of the genus *Haemagogus*. The exact location of virus activity in the vast tropical forests of South America is difficult or impossible to ascertain at any time, and indeed the virus is constantly moving, thus assuring a supply of susceptible hosts adequate for maintenance of the cycle. Presence of the virus is, however, sometimes evident on the basis of monkey deaths, because some New World species succumb to the infection. Humans may acquire the disease during activities, such as woodcutting, which bring them into contact with *Haemagogus* mosquitoes. Dramatic outbreaks have occurred when groups of unvaccinated laborers have penetrated jungle areas.

In the Americas, *urban yellow fever* has not occurred since 1954 (in Trinidad), largely because of the eradication of *Aedes aegypti* mosquitoes from population centers of South America. Nonetheless, some *aegypti*-infested areas of northern South America remain in juxtaposition to the jungle cycle, and the risk of a viremic individual traveling to receptive regions of the Caribbean and southern United States is recognized. The recent occurrence of dengue epidemics in the Caribbean is prima facie evidence that this region is receptive to yellow fever.

The situation in Africa is considerably more complex. Relatively few sporadic cases are recognized annually, but this reflects inadequate surveillance and diagnostic facilities. Large epidemics, which occur at irregular intervals in areas of West, Central, and East Africa between 0 and 15 degrees N, have involved as many as 100,000 cases, with 30,000 deaths. Epidemics sustained by the peridomestic *Ae. aegypti* vector have occurred in both the urban and rural environments of West Africa. Epidemic yellow fever in savannah and forest-savannah transition areas of West Africa has been transmitted by tree-hole breeding *Aedes*, including *furcifer-taylori, africanus,* and *luteocephalus,* with both monkeys and man as intermediate hosts. During the long dry season adult mosquitoes disappear, and the virus may survive in transovarially infected eggs of *Aedes* vectors.

In the more extensive forests of Central and East Africa, a jungle cycle analogous to that in the Americas operates, with *Aedes africanus* as the principal vector. Sporadic cases and epidemics in persons entering the forest or living at the forest fringe have resulted from exposure to this mosquito. In some areas, another vector, *Ae. simpsoni,* links the jungle cycle with human populations and has been responsible for intensive interhuman transmission.

All races are equally susceptible to yellow fever infection. The disease in native populations of Africa is thought to be milder than in whites, but this is probably a reflection of background immunity and cross-protection by related endemic flaviviruses; some outbreaks of yellow fever involving Africans have been severe, with high death rates. Nonimmune persons of all ages and both sexes are equally susceptible. The age and sex distribution is, however, determined by natural immunization and vaccination, and by occupational exposures. Adult males employed in woodcutting or agricultural pursuits are primarily affected by jungle yellow fever.

PATHOLOGY AND PATHOGENESIS. Gross pathologic lesions include icterus; hemorrhages or petechiae of the mucous membranes, stomach, duodenum, renal capsule, and urinary bladder; and small amounts of pleural and peritoneal fluid. Histopathologic changes of the liver may be characteristic, but even experienced pathologists may not be able to make an unequivocal diagnosis in atypical cases. Conditions with which yellow fever has been confused on the basis of liver pathology include Lassa fever, African (Marburg-Ebola virus) hemorrhagic fever, viral hepatitis, and leptospirosis. The typical yellow fever lesion is marked by cloudy swelling, then by coagulative necrosis of hepatocytes in the midzone of the liver lobule, sparing cells bordering the central vein. Eosinophilic degeneration of hepatocytes results in the formation of *Councilman bodies;* intranuclear eosinophilic granular inclusions (Torres bodies) have also been described. Multi- and microvacuolar fatty change is nearly always present, especially after the eighth day of illness. An inflammatory response is absent or mild. The reticulin framework is preserved. Characteristic changes have been seen in biopsy specimens taken as early as the third day of illness; interpretation of biopsy or necropsy material obtained after the tenth day is often difficult. Renal glomerular changes are relatively insignificant compared to acute tubular necrosis and fatty metamorphosis, which may be marked. The myocardial fibers show cloudy swelling, degeneration, and fatty infiltration. Lymphocytic elements in the spleen and nodes are depleted, and large mononuclear or histiocytic cells accumulate in the splenic follicles. The brain may show edema and petechial hemorrhages.

The *pathologic physiology* of yellow fever is poorly understood. Direct viral injury to the cells of major target organs such as the liver undoubtedly underlies the pathogenic process. Hepatic coma has not been clinically or electroencephalographically defined, and the role of hepatic failure in the disease is uncertain. Some patients have prominent signs of acute renal failure, and deaths have been attributed to uremia. It is not known whether acute tubular necrosis is due to direct viral injury or is secondary to hemodynamic causes or hepatocellular necrosis. Deaths (especially late in the disease) have occurred because of cardiac failure or arrhythmia, but are rare. Hemorrhage undoubtedly exacerbates hypotension and oliguria and may precipitate vascular collapse and death. Evidence for disseminated intravascular coagulation as the basis for the hemorrhagic diathesis is conflicting. Acidosis and hyperkalemia are probable terminal events. At present, the complex pathophysiologic interrelationships of yellow fever cannot be specified, and directions for specific therapeutic interventions are consequently undetermined.

CLINICAL MANIFESTATIONS. Yellow fever infection produces a clinical spectrum from very mild, nonspecific, febrile illness to a malignant, sometimes fatal form with pathognomonic features. The precise frequency with which the various clinical forms occur is uncertain; however, abortive infections are the rule, and the classic symptoms of severe yellow fever are found in only 10 to 20 per cent of cases. The incubation period (interval between bite of infected mosquito and onset of symptoms) is generally three to six days.

The mild case will not be suspected or clinically diagnosed except in the setting of an epidemic. In its mildest form it is characterized by sudden onset of fever and headache, without other symptoms, lasting 48 hours or less. In other patients, the fever is higher, the headache more distressing, and the illness accompanied by a grippe-like syndrome with nausea, myalgia, slight albuminuria, and bradycardia in relation to the presence of fever (Faget's sign). The illness lasts several days, with uneventful recovery.

The severe forms of yellow fever begin abruptly with fever to 40° C, chills or chilliness, severe headache, and generalized myalgia often most acute in the lower back. The patient appears distressed and anxious, the conjunctiva congested, the face and neck flushed, the tongue reddened at the tip and edges, the breath foul smelling. Anorexia, nausea, and vomiting are present, and minor gingival hemorrhages or epistaxis may occur. Despite a persistent or rising temperature, the pulse may fall. This syndrome, persisting for approximately three days, corresponds to the "period of infection," during which yellow fever virus is present in the blood. It may be followed by a "period of remission," with partial or complete defervescence and mitigation of symptoms, usually lasting several to 24 hours. The fever and systemic symptoms then reappear with more *frequent vomiting, epigastric pain, prostration,* and the *appearance of jaundice* ("period of intoxication"). Viremia is generally absent, and antibodies appear during this phase. Hematemesis, coffee grounds–appearing or black vomit (vomito negro), is a characteristic and frightening sign. Other hemorrhagic manifestations include melena, metrorrhagia, petechiae, ecchymoses, and diffuse oozing from the mucous membranes. Dehydration resulting from vomiting and increased insensible losses is frequent. Renal damage is marked by the sudden appearance of albuminuria, which may rapidly increase, and by diminishing urine output. The pulse remains dissociated from fever, but may weaken as the blood and pulse pressures decrease. The patient recovers either rapidly after a period of intoxication of three to four days or over a protracted course of up to two weeks. Fatalities (occurring in up to 50 per cent of severe yellow fever cases) generally occur on the seventh to tenth day of illness, and are preceded by increasing albuminuria, hemorrhages, rising pulse, hypotension, oliguria, and azotemia. Hypothermia, a severe agitated delirium, intractable hiccup, stupor, and coma are terminal signs.

In individual cases hepatic, renal, or myocardial involvement predominates, with clinical signs of relatively pure hepatitis, acute renal failure, or hypotension and hypokinetic heart failure. Pre-eminent central nervous system involvement, producing meningoencephalitic signs, has also been described. Atypical, fulminant cases occur, with death on the second or third day in the absence of hepatic or renal signs.

Physical findings during the period of intoxication include scleral and dermal icterus, hemorrhagic manifestations, epigastric (rarely hepatic) tenderness without organomegaly, and the changes already noted in vital signs.

The convalescent stage is sometimes prolonged, with profound asthenia lasting one to two weeks. Late death, occurring at the end of convalescence or even weeks after complete recovery from the acute illness, is a rare phenomenon attributed to yellow fever myocardial damage, cardiac arrhythmia, or failure. Suppurative parotitis (resulting from dehydration) and secondary bacterial pneumonia are recognized complications.

CLINICAL LABORATORY FINDINGS. Leukopenia (neutropenia) occurs most often during the early phase of illness; the white blood count is, however, often normal or elevated. Prolongation of the clotting, prothrombin, and partial thromboplastin times is marked in cases with jaundice. The platelet count may be decreased, and fibrin split products may be present in serum. The total and conjugated serum bilirubin rise together and may reach levels of 15 to 20 mg per deciliter in severe cases. Serum glutamic oxaloacetic transaminase and serum glutamic pyruvic transaminase levels are markedly elevated in all icteric (but inconstantly and to lower levels in anicteric) patients, with peak values between days five and ten of the illness, and return to normal by days ten to twenty. The alkaline phosphatase is generally normal. In patients with severe hepatic damage, hypoglycemia has been noted.

During the period of infection, the urine may contain a small amount of albumin, which then increases suddenly on the fourth or fifth day, reaching levels of 3 to 5 (rarely as high as 40) grams per liter. The urine contains bile; the cell sediment may be abnormal but is not diagnostically helpful. The cerebrospinal fluid is clear, without cells, but it is often under increased pressure, and contains a mildly raised concentration of protein. ST-T wave electrocardiographic abnormalities have been described.

DIAGNOSIS. In endemic areas, recognition and diagnosis of a case are of great importance because it may indicate the presence of an epidemic and stimulate preventive or control measures. Because the incubation period is sufficient to permit an infected person to travel a long distance, the diagnosis should be suspected in all patients with fever and jaundice coming from tropical America or Africa. Specific diagnosis depends upon histopathologic study, isolation of the virus, or demonstration of a specific antibody response. The hemorrhagic diathesis renders liver biopsy hazardous, and pathologic diagnosis is thus a postmortem procedure. The virus is most readily isolated (by inoculation of mice or cell cultures) from serum obtained during the first three or four days of illness (period of infection), but it may be recovered from serum up to the twelfth day and occasionally from liver at death. Rapid early diagnosis may be possible by direct detection of yellow fever antigen in serum by means of enzyme immunoassay.

Serologic methods useful in the diagnosis of yellow fever include hemagglutination-inhibition (HI), complement-fixation (CF), neutralization (N), fluorescence, and immunoassay tests. The HI and N antibodies appear within a week of onset; the CF antibodies appear later. Paired, acute, and convalescent phase specimens are usually required to establish the diagnosis by rise in antibody titer. Cross-reactions with other flaviviruses and the high prevalence of background immunity to flaviviruses in tropical populations make serodiagnosis difficult. Determination of immunoglobulin (IgM) antibody titers by fluorescent assay or immunoassay may provide a more precise diagnosis.

Virus isolation and serologic tests are applicable to the diagnosis of all clinical forms of yellow fever and are the only means available of establishing the cause of abortive and mild infections.

DIFFERENTIAL DIAGNOSIS. Mild yellow fever cannot be clinically distinguished from a wide array of other infections. In the presence of jaundice and the other signs of severe yellow fever, conditions that must be differentiated include viral hepatitis, falciparum malaria, spirochetal infections (tick-borne relapsing fever and Weil's disease), Rift Valley fever, typhoid, Q fever, typhus, and surgical, drug-induced, and toxic causes. Other diseases (usually without jaundice) that may be confused with yellow fever include Lassa, African (Marburg-Ebola virus), Bolivian, and Argentine hemorrhagic fevers.

PROGNOSIS. Up to 50 per cent of patients with severe forms of yellow fever die; unfortunately, patients in most reported series have been cared for under primitive conditions. The fatality rate of *all* patients with clinical illness is much lower (2 to 5 per cent). The prognosis should be guarded for the patient who, after a brief remission, enters a period of intoxication with rising fever, jaundice, and albuminuria. Features which correlate with a poor prognosis include early onset of bilirubinemia and albuminuria rising to high levels; prolongation of the prothrombin time below 25 per cent of normal; a rising and weakening pulse during the period of intoxication; severe hemorrhage; and the appearance of shock, coma, hypothermia, and intractable hiccup.

Relapses have not been described. The possibility of late death from myocardial or renal injury must be considered.

TREATMENT. No specific therapy exists. Complete bed rest, supportive care, and close monitoring of vital functions are essential. During the period of infection, mild sedatives, analgesics, and antiemetics may be indicated, and attention should be given to fluid and electrolyte balance. Aspirin is contraindicated because of the bleeding diathesis. Supportive measures are of critical importance during the period of intoxication if vomiting is severe, if hemorrhage appears, or if hypertension, hypokinetic heart failure, oliguria, azotemia, and electrolyte and acid-base imbalance become evident. In theory, these consequences of severe yellow fever might be lessened by intensive counter-regulation. In patients with evidence of acute tubular necrosis, dialysis may be indicated. Cautious consideration may be given to early heparin treatment of disseminated intravascular coagulation if laboratory tests indicate its occurrence.

Secondary bacterial infections or concurrent infections (in particular, malaria) should be treated by the usual appropriate means.

Return to activity should be gradual.

PREVENTION AND CONTROL. The patient with yellow fever should be isolated from possible contact with mosquitoes under netting or in a screened room. Yellow fever 17D is one of the safest live, attenuated vaccines available and provides effective, long-lasting immunity. For purposes of international certification, vaccination is considered valid for ten years, but immunity has been documented to last more than thirty years and may be lifelong. Since yellow fever exists as a silent enzoosis over wide areas of the tropics (see Fig. 358–1) and appears in epidemic form with little warning and without early recognition, vaccination of travelers is imperative. Immunity can be demonstrated within ten days after vaccination. Mild vaccine reactions occur rarely, and serious complications have been exceedingly uncommon. No untoward consequences for the fetus have been recorded, but on theoretical grounds, pregnant women should not be vaccinated unless the risk of acquiring yellow fever is considered great. The vaccine is prepared in chicken embryos and should not be used in persons hypersensitive to egg proteins. The French neurotropic viral vaccine produced in mouse brain is no longer manufactured; remaining stocks are used to a limited extent in parts of Africa.

In the event of an epidemic, the disease may be controlled by mass vaccination and the use of insecticides to reduce infected vector populations.

359. HEMORRHAGIC FEVER CAUSED BY DENGUE VIRUSES (DHF)

Karl M. Johnson

DEFINITION. Dengue hemorrhagic fever is an acute, infectious, urban mosquito-borne disease. Endoepidemic in pattern, it is clinically defined as a dengue disease that worsens two or more days after onset and is characterized by hypoproteinemia and one or more hemostatic abnormalities such as thrombocytopenia, prolonged bleeding time, or elevated prothrombin time. The *dengue shock syndrome* consists of hemorrhagic fever plus shock (hypotension or a pulse pressure of 20 mm Hg or less) and hemoconcentration (hematocrit at least 20 per cent greater than convalescent value).

ETIOLOGY. All evidence suggests that dengue hemorrhagic fever is caused by each of the four recognized dengue virus types. How they produce such disease is still not clear. A current hypothesis is that severe dengue disease is produced by an immunologic reaction that occurs in some individuals experiencing a second dengue infection. However, hemorrhagic fever has been unequivocally caused by primary dengue infection.

EPIDEMIOLOGY. Dengue hemorrhagic fever was first seen in epidemic proportions in Manila and Bangkok (1954) and in Singapore (1960). Other outbreaks have been reported from Malaysia, South Vietnam, India, Indonesia, Oceania, and recently in Cuba. In Bangkok age-specific rates in children have reached 7 to 8 per 1000. In most outbreaks cases occur only in children, principally below the age of eight years; otherwise, the epidemiology of infection leading to dengue hemorrhagic fever is basically similar to that associated with ordinary dengue fever.

PATHOLOGY. Autopsy data are scant. The chief abnormalities include generalized vascular congestion and dilatation with edema and multiple focal hemorrhages in most organs, mild to moderate pleural effusion and ascites, mononuclear cell infiltration of interstitial tissues and alveolar walls of lungs, focal myocardial congestion, and a decrease in mature lymphocytes with proliferation of mononuclear forms in the germinal centers of lymph follicles.

Tissue necrosis is unusual. Perivascular mononuclear cell infiltration is common, but there is no evidence for direct damage to vessels or intravascular thrombosis. Globulin deposition on endothelial surfaces of arterioles has been noted in some cases. The marrow may exhibit megakaryocyte maturation arrest and generalized transitory hypoplasia.

Focal necrosis, usually mild, is observed in the liver, and Councilman bodies similar to those seen in yellow fever may be present.

PATHOGENESIS OR MECHANISM OF DISEASE. Vascular congestion, dilatation, and increased permeability lead to the extensive edema and hemorrhage observed in the gastrointestinal tract, the skin, and other tissues. The cause of these vascular changes is unknown, but they result in loss of plasma volume and associated electrolyte disturbances. Platelet deficiency probably plays a role in the hemorrhages. Bleeding time is usually prolonged, prothrombin times are somewhat prolonged, clot retraction is poor, and the blood fibrinogen is slightly reduced. Depression of C3 and C4 proactivation levels indicates activation of both arms of the complement system. None of these changes is very profound. The circulatory collapse and shock observed appear to be far in excess of what might be expected from the extent of loss of edema fluid and blood. The adrenal changes suggest exhaustion of steroid reserve. Death in some cases has been accompanied by severe hyperkalemia.

CLINICAL MANIFESTATIONS. The onset is that of a dengue infection, usually abrupt, with fever. Nausea and vomiting are common. The throat appears injected, and there may be a dry cough. About the second or third day petechiae appear, usually first on the face or distal portions of the extremities but sparing the axillae and chest. The tourniquet test may be conspicuously positive before petechiae appear. Purpura and large ecchymoses as well as other manifestations of bleeding tendency are occasionally prominent. There may be severe abdominal pain and tenderness. About the third or fourth day, vomiting may produce copious coffee-ground-like material. Melena also is not uncommon, but gross bleeding from the intestines is rare. Shock is likely to occur in severe cases about the fourth day, and this critical state lasts about 12 to 24 hours. At this time the temperature falls to normal, the blood pressure and pulse pressure are low or unmeasurable, and the limbs are cool and present a purple or brownish mottled appearance. Perspiration is frequently profuse. The face and hands appear edematous. Restlessness and apprehension are conspicuous as the patient enters shock. Thrombocytopenia is noted during this period, and bleeding time is prolonged. Leukocytes remain at approximately normal levels, but are elevated in number in serious cases more frequently than they are depressed. The total and differential leukocyte counts are not those observed in dengue. Although the numbers of both immature and mature polymorphonuclear cells are decreased, there is an increase in lymphocytes and sometimes in monocytes.

DIAGNOSIS. Hemorrhagic fever begins as an extension of a classic dengue infection, and the early dengue syndrome intergrades into the milder and atypical manifestations of the later hemorrhagic syndrome. The diagnosis in a febrile child acutely ill for only two or three days is rendered highly probable by the presentation of petechiae, purpuric lesions, and unusual ecchymosis of the skin with most prominent distribution on the extremities and face, together with melena, thrombocytopenia, and a relatively normal leukocyte count. In a milder case or at an earlier stage, the tourniquet test may be of great assistance in detecting unusual capillary fragility. The rapid development of circulatory collapse and shock during the fourth to sixth day, associated with the aforementioned findings, differentiates this from most other exanthematous diseases. Meningococcemia and the Waterhouse-Friderichsen syndrome need careful consideration. Thrombocytopenic purpura can be expected to have an entirely different onset and is usually not associated with fever. Laboratory methods available for diagnosis are those described for dengue fever.

TREATMENT. There is no specific therapy, but case-fatality rates can be greatly reduced by skillful management directed toward combating shock. Close monitoring of pulse, respiration, and blood pressure during the course of treatment is essential for at least 48 hours, because shock can occur and recur. Oxygen should be administered if there is cyanosis or labored breathing. Hypovolemia should be treated by administration of lactated Ringer's solution or 5 per cent glucose in normal saline, on the basis of 20 ml per kilogram of body weight, administered rapidly. In profound or unresponsive shock, plasma or a plasma expander (dextran in normal saline) can be given at the rate of 20 ml per kilogram of body weight. When signs improve, 5 per cent glucose in normal saline or in lactate-supplemented Ringer's solution should be given at the rate of 10 ml per kilogram per hour, and continued until vital signs are normal. Acidosis should be corrected with sodium bicarbonate as necessary.

Whole blood should be given only if blood loss is known to be large. Administration of whole blood to a patient with elevated hematocrit may result in heart failure. Paraldehyde or chloral hydrate may be required for children who are markedly agitated. Salicylates administered during the febrile period may cause bleeding and acidosis, and they should not be given to febrile patients during a hemorrhagic fever outbreak. Pressor amines, alpha-adrenergic blocking agents, and steroids have not been demonstrated to be of value in treatment.

PROGNOSIS. Death is almost always associated with shock, and ranges from 5 to 50 per cent, depending to a large extent upon the condition of patients on admission and the facilities available for treatment. Residual effects have not been observed, and, in contrast to primary dengue, recovery is usually prompt and complete seven to ten days after onset.

PREVENTION. Prevention is similar to that for dengue fever.

360. TICK-BORNE FLAVIVIRUS DISEASES: KYASANUR FOREST DISEASE AND OMSK HEMORRHAGIC FEVER

Karl M. Johnson

DEFINITION. Kyasanur Forest disease (KFD) and Omsk hemorrhagic fever (OHF) produce acute febrile illness with hemorrhagic manifestations and/or mild encephalitis in India and western Siberia, respectively.

ETIOLOGY. These diseases are produced by antigenically related flaviviruses which also share antigens with other tick-borne flaviviruses causing encephalitis (see Ch. 358). Neutralizing antibody measurement is required to distinguish OHF infection from that of tick-borne encephalitis (RSSE), which also occurs in western Siberia. The OHF agent produces hemorrhagic pneumonia in inoculated muskrats, and KFD virus induces encephalitis and hemorrhage in langur and bonnet monkeys.

EPIDEMIOLOGY. These viruses are maintained in discrete geographic foci by circulation between wild and domestic vertebrates and ixodid ticks of the genera *Ixodes, Dermacentor,* and *Haemaphysalis.* Rodents, birds, bats, sheep, goats, and cattle experience clinically silent, viremic infection; in addition, these agents are transmitted transovarially in ticks, thus providing a mechanism for winter or dry season virus survival. Viremia with overt fatal infection occurs naturally in muskrats and monkeys, and major epizootics among these mammals often precede or accompany epidemics.

Residents of rural forested areas are at highest risk of infection, and seasonal patterns of disease transmission are determined by the influence of temperature or moisture on tick activity. Winter outbreaks of OHF occur among trappers and skinners of muskrats, and both viruses have induced aerosol-transmitted infection in laboratory workers.

CLINICAL MANIFESTATIONS AND PATHOLOGY. The incubation period ranges from 3 to 12 days and is terminated by the abrupt onset of fever, headache, myalgia, and gastrointestinal disturbances. There is leukopenia and, after four to five days, the onset of mildly hemorrhagic bronchopneumonia, petechiae, and mild bleeding from the intestines. Epistaxis may occur. Pneumonia and clinical shock are the most serious clinical signs, but occur in a minority of infections. KFD patients, in addition, frequently exhibit recurrent fever with signs of meningitis or encephalitis during the second week of illness.

Pathologic lesions noted at autopsy include scattered necrotic foci in liver and gastrointestinal mucosa, hemorrhagic bronchopneumonia, capillary hemorrhages without inflammation in many tissues, and, in the case of KFD, occasional inflammatory vascular lesions in the brain.

DIAGNOSIS AND TREATMENT. Isolation of virus from blood or brain tissue or serologic diagnosis by standard methods is possible. Treatment is symptomatic.

PROGNOSIS AND PREVENTION. Mortality ranges from 0.5 to 5 per cent. There are no definitive methods for prevention.

361. CRIMEAN HEMORRHAGIC FEVER

Karl M. Johnson

DEFINITION. Crimean hemorrhagic fever (CHF) is an acute febrile disease, often marked by severe hemorrhage, high mortality, and nosocomial transmission, occurring in the Soviet Union, Bulgaria, the Middle East, and Pakistan.

ETIOLOGY. The CHF agent is a nairovirus first isolated from human blood specimens in 1967. It is pathogenic for suckling mice and grows in several types of cultured cells. This virus is indistinguishable from Congo virus of Africa in complement fixation and neutralization tests. Strains from Eurasia and Africa are thus referred to as Congo-CHF virus.

EPIDEMIOLOGY. Congo-CHF virus is naturally transmitted by several species of hard ticks belonging to the genera *Hyalomma, Rhipicephalus, Amblyomma,* and *Boophilus.*

Active foci of infection exist in the lower Don and Volga river basins and in Kazakhstan, Uzbekistan, Iran, Iraq, Dubai, western China, and northwest Pakistan. Few human cases have been reported from Africa. This is a disease of adults tending domestic animals. Cases appear in April and peak during early summer. Vertebrate hosts for the virus include cattle, goats, hares, and hedgehogs. Transovarial tick transmission has been demonstrated. The incubation period is about one week, and nosocomial human infections have occurred repeatedly.

CLINICAL MANIFESTATIONS. Onset is typically abrupt with high, unremittent fever, chills, headache, and myalgia. There may be hyperemia of the upper trunk and neck, conjunctival effusion, vomiting, and diarrhea. Hepatomegaly is noted in about half the cases; splenomegaly is uncommon. Pronounced panleukopenia is almost invariably present, as is thrombocytopenia. Bleeding begins on about the fourth day of illness. Petechiae appear in the oral mucosa and skin, at times presenting as frank *purpura hemorrhagica.* Nose, gums, and intestinal tract are the most common sites of bleeding, and in this disease above all other viral hemorrhagic fevers, blood loss per se may be life threatening. Stiff neck, hyperexcitability, or coma occurs in about 10 per cent of cases, and these are grave prognostic signs. The cerebrospinal fluid, however, contains no leukocytes or increased protein. There may be proteinuria and microscopic hematuria, but renal function is rarely compromised. The fever and bleeding generally resolve by lysis at about the eighth day. Hypovolemic shock with a paradoxical rising hematocrit may appear just prior to the end of fever and is the most common cause of death.

DIAGNOSIS. Virus can be easily obtained from blood of patients during the first few days of illness. Specific complement fixation and neutralizing antibodies appear in the sera of most patients 30 to 60 days after onset of symptoms.

TREATMENT AND PROGNOSIS. Therapy is symptomatic. Management of fluid, electrolyte, and erythrocyte balance forms the continuous clinical challenge. Shock is a grave problem and should be anticipated and treated as outlined in Ch. 43 and 362. Whole blood transfusion may be necessary. Intercurrent bacterial infection is very common, especially pneumonia. Mortality in the Soviet Union ranges from 20 to 50 per cent. Patients surviving the acute illness generally recover completely, albeit quite slowly. Several instances of mono- or polyneuritis persisting for several months have been recorded.

PREVENTION. There is no vaccine yet available; thus avoidance of the disease in endemic foci depends on personal measures designed to prevent tick bites. Several nosocomial infections have occurred in the Soviet Union and Pakistan. Thus strict isolation of patients and use of protective clothing and respirators by medical personnel are indicated.

362. HEMORRHAGIC DISEASES CAUSED BY ARENAVIRUSES: ARGENTINE AND BOLIVIAN HEMORRHAGIC FEVERS AND LASSA FEVER*

Karl M. Johnson

DEFINITION. Argentine and Bolivian hemorrhagic fevers and Lassa fever are acute diseases caused respectively by Junin, Machupo, and Lassa viruses. Clinically, the diseases share the common features of fever, severe myalgia, leukopenia, hemorrhagic manifestations, shock, and neurologic abnormalities.

ETIOLOGY. The three viruses are serologically and morphologically related, and belong to the family Arenaviridae.

GEOGRAPHICAL DISTRIBUTION, INCIDENCE, AND PREVALENCE. Argentine hemorrhagic fever is localized to the provinces of Córdoba and Buenos Aires in northern Argentina, where several hundred to several thousand cases occur annually, principally among workers harvesting maize. Bolivian hemorrhagic fever has been reported only from Beni province of Bolivia, between the rivers Mamore and Branco. Infections are seen in inhabitants of certain of the small towns, as well as in rural populations. Lassa fever occurs in West Africa, notably Nigeria, Liberia, and Sierra Leone. Fatality rates in hospitalized cases of all three diseases range from 10 to 20 per cent.

EPIDEMIOLOGY AND PROBABLE MODE OF TRANSMISSION. The viruses have been isolated from wild rodents: Junin, most commonly from *Calomys musculinus*, *Calomys laucha*, and also *Akodon arenicola;* Machupo, from *Calomys callosus;* and Lassa, from *Mastomys natalensis.* An attractive current hypothesis is that infection is acquired by direct human contact (ingestion, inhalation, or entrance through mucous membranes or skin breaks) with virus-containing rodent excreta. For all three agents, persistent infection in rodents has been demonstrated, with viruria readily detectable for months. A similar pattern of chronic virus infection in rodents has been described for lymphocytic choriomeningitis virus.

PATHOLOGY. Few cases have received full study. Findings include irregularly focal diapedesis and capillary hemorrhage without much evidence of inflammatory reaction. Gross hemorrhages may be seen in the mucosa of the stomach and intestines and in the brain. Pulmonary infection, probably intercurrent, is frequently seen. Focal liver necrosis is prominent in Lassa fever.

CLINICAL MANIFESTATIONS. Although as many as half of all etiologically confirmed cases appear as acute undifferentiated fevers, the findings and clinical course of "full-blown" Argentine and Bolivian infections are so nearly identical as to justify joint description. The same holds for Lassa fever. Onset is usually gradual, with increasing fever, headache, diffuse myalgia, and anorexia. By the third day the temperature may be 39.5 to 40.5° C, with severe myalgia, particularly in the lumbar regions (or legs in Lassa fever). Conjunctival injection is present, a flush involving the upper trunk and face is frequently observed, and there may be a relative bradycardia. Beginning about the fourth day, scattered fine petechiae may appear on the face and neck, about the pectoral girdle, and/or in the buccal mucosa or palate. Aphthous ulcers of the oral mucosa and exudative pharyngitis have been a noteworthy feature of Lassa infections. The Rumpel-Leede test is frequently positive. Frank hemorrhages from one or more sites, including the stomach, intestines, nose, gums, and uterus, accompanied by microscopic hematuria, may occur. Hemorrhagic phenomena are not a common feature of Lassa infections. Although hemorrhage per se is rarely the precipitating cause, a hypotensive crisis frequently develops between the sixth and eighth days, coincident with a rapid return of temperature to normal after five or more days of sustained fever. Patients surviving this stress for 48 hours generally make a slow but complete recovery.

Perhaps a fifth of the patients with the Bolivian or Argentine disease develop neurologic signs. These are quite characteristic, and begin on about the fifth or sixth day with a fine intention tremor of the tongue. This may become so severe as to render speech unintelligible and to preclude oral ingestion of solid or even liquid food. If so, gross intention tremors of the extremities usually appear, occasionally accompanied by an intermittent nystagmus. Such patients often become delirious, and may experience generalized clonic and tonic convulsions. The cerebrospinal fluid appears normal, however, and contains neither leukocytes nor virus. Convalescence is marked by weakness and signs of autonomic nervous system lability such as postural hypotension, spontaneous flushing and blanching of the skin, and episodes of diaphoresis.

In addition to delirium and occasional coma, 5 to 10 per cent of Lassa fever patients suffer significant permanent damage to one or both eighth cranial nerves. Some Lassa fever patients have shown electrocardiographic evidence of myocardial involvement.

Transient loss of scalp hair and typical Beau's lines in the nails, particularly those of the fingers, are observed in a majority of cases several weeks after subsidence of the high sustained fever. Many patients are not able to resume full activity for at least one month after illness.

Leukopenia is almost invariably present, and cell counts may be as low as 1000 per cubic millimeter by the fourth or fifth day. All elements are reduced nearly equally, and there is often a mild to moderate thrombocytopenia during the first week. Usually the peripheral blood picture returns to normal rapidly after defervescence, although there may be transient relative lymphocytosis and mild anemia. During the latter portion of the febrile period, progressive increase in hematocrit similar to, but usually milder than, that of hemorrhagic nephrosonephritis (q.v.) is frequently observed. At about the same time, moderate proteinuria is common, although renal function is rarely compromised seriously, and frank azotemia and hyperkalemia are almost never present.

DIAGNOSIS. Fever, myalgia, and leukopenia in a patient having a history of rural contact in endemic areas should be interpreted as arenaviral disease until proven otherwise. Laboratory procedures are necessary. Virus can be recovered from blood of patients with Argentine hemorrhagic fever or Lassa fever. Specific antibodies appear within the first month of illness in Lassa fever. Diagnosis of Bolivian hemorrhagic fever may be difficult because virus is infrequently detectable in blood or other secretions and antibodies do not appear during the acute phase of illness.

These three agents have been responsible for several fatal laboratory infections, and work with the viruses should be carried out only with strictest precautionary measures, and complete isolation from other activities, in special high-risk laboratories.

TREATMENT. Careful measurement of fluid and electrolyte balance is mandatory. Frequent measurements of hematocrit and urinary protein excretion are crucial for recognition of incipient hypovolemic shock. Plasma expanders may be used to treat this condition, but often provoke intractable pulmonary

*The author wishes to express his thanks to Dr. Wilbur G. Downs for his considerable assistance in the preparation of this chapter, particularly with reference to the material on Lassa fever.

edema if treatment is delayed until frank clinical shock develops. Secondary bacterial infections must be recognized and promptly treated. Passive anti-Junin antibodies have been proved to reduce mortality in Argentine hemorrhagic fever if administered during the first eight days of illness, but are not of proven value in Lassa fever or the Bolivian disease.

PROGNOSIS. Although case mortality may reach 20 per cent in Argentine and Bolivian hemorrhagic fever, there are no early findings which aid prognosis. The onset of shock or neurologic abnormalities is an ominous sign, and at least half of such patients succumb. In Lassa fever admission levels of virus and glutamic oxalic transaminase in serum are highly and directly correlated with outcome of infection.

PREVENTION. Effective elimination of intimate human contact with certain wild rodents represents the only proven method for prevention of disease. This may be achieved by maintaining sound standards of personal and environmental hygiene. Campaigns to eliminate rodents, repair buildings, and clean rubbish near dwellings are highly successful when the disease is acquired mainly from peridomestic animals.

Hospital outbreaks involving medical staff have occurred several times with Lassa virus. Current evidence suggests that these are usually due to direct contact with blood and excreta rather than to infectious aerosols.

363. AFRICAN HEMORRHAGIC FEVER (Marburg-Ebola Disease)

Karl M. Johnson

DEFINITION. African hemorrhagic fever is an acute, highly fatal disease characterized by fever, prostration, rash, proteinuria, major hemorrhagic manifestations, pancreatitis, and hepatitis.

HISTORY. The disease was first described in Germany in 1967 and named Marburg disease. It was acquired through contact with green monkeys, *Cercopithecus aethiops*, imported from Uganda. Secondary nosocomial cases occurred. A few further cases occurred in South Africa (1975) and Kenya (1980). Major outbreaks with several hundred cases were recorded in Sudan (1976 and 1979) and Zaire (1976).

ETIOLOGY. This syndrome is caused by morphologically identical viruses, Marburg and Ebola, which are immunologically distinct.

EPIDEMIOLOGY. The ecology of Marburg and Ebola viruses is presently unknown. No evidence for Marburg infection was detected in green monkeys captured in Uganda subsequent to the original outbreak. The source of the index infection in the other outbreaks remains a mystery. Transmission is person-to-person, associated with close contact with patients. In Zaire contaminated needles were the source of many infections. Incubation period is about one week.

PATHOLOGY. These viruses attack the lymphoreticular system, the liver, and possibly the pancreas. Prominent hepatocellular necrosis without inflammatory reaction is a hallmark of infection. Large eosinophilic inclusions are found in liver cells, but the overall pattern of destruction is diffuse, rather than strongly mid-zonal as in yellow fever.

CLINICAL MANIFESTATIONS AND PATHOLOGIC PHYSIOLOGY. Onset is abrupt or insidious with headache and progressive fever. There is severe myalgia, and often vomiting and/or diarrhea occur. About the fourth day of illness sore throat and abdominal pain appear, and a day or so later many patients develop a fine maculopapular rash over the trunk and back which spreads to the limbs and may fade in two or three days. Bleeding, principally gastrointestinal, begins on the fifth to seventh day and is associated with rapid decompensation, ending in shock and death. Leukopenia, thrombocytopenia, and proteinuria are almost invariably present. There are extreme elevations of plasma transaminases and of amylase. In the few cases studied, definitive evidence for disseminated intravascular coagulation was found.

DIAGNOSIS. High persistent viremia is the basis for establishment of the diagnosis in acute cases. Virus is recovered by inoculation of blood into Vero cell cultures or guinea pigs that undergo a febrile infection. Immunofluorescent antibodies appear during the second week after onset and persist for several years. This method is more sensitive than the complement-fixation technique, which also has been used.

PROGNOSIS AND TREATMENT. With sophisticated medical management, mortality in Marburg infection is 25 to 30 per cent. Ebola virus infections treated in rural hospitals were 50 to 90 per cent fatal, the worst prognosis of any viral disease other than rabies. In addition to intensive supportive care, which should include continuous nasogastric aspiration to combat pancreatitis, intravenous heparin therapy may be of value to combat incipient intravascular coagulation.

PREVENTION. The secondary attack rate in African hemorrhagic fever rarely exceeds 10 per cent. Transmission can be interrupted by scrupulous isolation of patients, careful disposal of virus-contaminated excreta and fomites, and use of protective clothing and full-face respirators by medical personnel.

364. HEMORRHAGIC FEVER WITH RENAL SYNDROME (HFRS)

Karl M. Johnson

DEFINITION. Hemorrhagic fever with renal syndrome is an acute disease that occurs in northeastern Asia and, in milder form, in northern European USSR, Scandinavia, Czechoslovakia, Rumania, and Bulgaria. It is characterized by fever, prostration, vomiting, proteinuria, hemorrhagic manifestations, shock, and renal failure.

HISTORY. The disease was first described in the far east of the Soviet Union in the 1930's, with suggestive history as far back as 1913. An epidemic in United Nations troops in Korea, beginning in 1951, attracted much attention.

ETIOLOGY. The disease is caused by Hantaan virus, first recovered from the striped field mouse, *Apodemus agrarius*, in Korea. Strains also have been recovered from patients.

EPIDEMIOLOGY. The disease is rural, characterized by isolated cases widely separated in place. Environmental exposure in forests or fields near forests is invariably noted. Person-to-person transmission does not occur. Soviet workers believe that the disease is transmitted directly from asymptomatically infected rodents to man by means of virus-contaminated rodent excreta. Some outbreaks in Europe have coincided with population "explosions" of the redbacked vole *(Clethrionomys glareolus)*, involving invasion by rodents of fields, barns, and even houses. An urban form of the disease was recognized in Osaka, Japan, and several recent outbreaks in Japanese medical centers were traced to virus-infected colonized Wistar rats. Hantaan-related agents have been isolated from wild rats and voles, *Microtus*, in North America.

PATHOLOGY. Profound, protein-rich retroperitoneal edema is characteristic of early death in shock, but not of later deaths. Changes in various organs apparently have a similar pathogenesis and consist of widespread, often focal, congestion and hemorrhage, sometimes accompanied by necrosis, without significant inflammatory response. The "pathognomonic" lesion is found in the kidneys, which appear swollen and, when incised, exhibit extreme hemorrhagic congestion sharply localized to the medulla. Gross congestion or hemorrhage derived from dilated, congested small blood vessels is also found frequently in the right atrium, the pituitary, and the stomach, and less often in intestines, adrenals, lungs, and central nervous system. Liver and spleen are usually not grossly involved. Petechial hemorrhages may occur in the skin, heart, adrenals, brain, and serous surfaces.

CLINICAL MANIFESTATIONS AND PATHOLOGIC PHYSIOLOGY. Most patients exhibit fever, variable proteinuria, and isohyposthenuria. Only a minority of infections result in the severe clinically classic and highly unique hemorrhagic syndrome. This is initiated by a *febrile phase* lasting three to eight days, marked by severe myalgia and malaise, a flush over the face and neck, and conjunctival and palatine injection. Toward the end of this phase, thrombocytopenia, proteinuria, and petechiae appear and hematocrit increases, heralding a *hypotensive phase*, which develops rapidly and lasts one to three days. Effective blood volume decreases; hematocrit values may reach 70 per cent; nausea, vomiting, and abdominal or lumbar pain appear and have occasioned ill-advised laparotomy in misdiagnosed cases. Heavy proteinuria and oliguria occur, and clinical shock is an ever-present danger. Capillary hemorrhages are most common during this phase, and blood leukocytes now show a mild leukemoid reaction.

Patients surviving this acute clinical crisis proceed to an *oliguric phase*, with renal shutdown, hyperkalemia, secondary pulmonary infection, and, in some cases, pulmonary edema. There are biochemical changes associated with renal failure, and some patients exhibit a reactive hypertension related to functional hypervolemia which responds to phlebotomy. Patients who survive this phase must still endure a *diuretic phase*, which lasts for days to weeks. Management of fluid and electrolytes during this interval often proves extremely difficult, and bacterial pulmonary infections also are common. Nearly one third of all deaths occur during this period, and survivors often require one to three months for return of strength and normal urinary concentrating function.

DIAGNOSIS. Specific diagnosis is made by immunofluorescent technique, using cell cultures infected by Hantaan virus as source of antigen. Most patients already have low titers of antibody in acute phase sera, but diagnostic increases in titer regularly occur by the end of the second week of symptoms. The antibodies persist at least ten years. Retrospective serodiagnosis has now been confirmed in patients from the Soviet Union, China, Finland, and Japan, as well as Korea. Asymptomatic infections are unusual, but mild clinically apparent cases have been documented.

PROGNOSIS AND TREATMENT. Treatment is supportive and complex. Fluid management is critical. Plasma expanders are important in shock therapy. Hemodialysis may be required to cope with azotemia and hyperkalemia during the oligemic phase, and electrolyte balance requires delicate and precise handling during diuresis. Under optimal conditions mortality should not exceed 6 per cent.

PREVENTION. Avoidance of contact with rodent excreta is the only available method of prevention.

Barnes WJS, Rosen L: Fatal hemorrhagic disease and shock associated with primary dengue infection on a Pacific island. Am J Trop Med Hyg 23:495, 1974. *Clear evidence that severe hemorrhagic disease can result from first dengue virus infection. Whether host factors or a particular virus strain is responsible is not clear.*

Casals J, Henderson BE, Hoogstraal H, Johnson KM, Shelokov A: A review of Soviet viral hemorrhagic fevers, 1969. J Infect Dis 122:437, 1970. *A clinical, virologic, and epidemiologic report based on extensive travel of authors in Soviet Union. Data on hemorrhagic fever with renal syndrome (Korean) and Crimean hemorrhagic fever are of special value.*

Halstead SB, et al.: Observations related to pathogenesis of dengue hemorrhagic fever. Yale J Biol Med 42:261, 1970. *Epidemiologic case for secondary dengue infection as trigger for hemorrhagic fever.*

Halstead SB: In vivo enhancement of dengue virus infection in rhesus monkeys by passively transferred antibody. J Infect Dis 140:527, 1979. *Experimental data making secondary infection concept highly plausible.*

International symposium on arenaviral infections of public health importance. Bull WHO, 52:381, 1975. *Best single collection of articles on Lassa fever.*

Johnson KM, Halstead SB, Cohen SN: Hemorrhagic fevers of Southeast Asia and South America: A comparative appraisal. Prog Med Virol 9:105, 1967. *Extensive comparative review of dengue and South American arenavirus hemorrhagic fevers.*

Johnson KM, Webb PA, Lange JV, Murphy FA: Isolation and partial characterization of a new virus causing haemorrhagic fever in Zaire. Lancet 1:569, 1977. *Describes circumstances of initial recognition and depicts unique morphology of Ebola virus.*

Lee HW, Lee PW, Johnson KM: Isolation of the etiologic agent of Korean hemorrhagic fever. J Infect Dis 137:298, 1978. *Classic report of initial isolation of Hantaan virus, using convalescent human sera for immunofluorescent detection of agent in tissues of single wild rodent species.*

Mertens P, Patton R, Baum JJ, Monath PP: Clinical presentation of Lassa fever cases during the hospital epidemic at Zorzar, Liberia, March–April 1972. Am J Trop Med Hyg 22:780, 1973. *Excellent description of the most severe form of Lassa fever.*

Pantier R: Yellow fever. *In* Debré T, Celers J (eds.): Clinical Virology. Philadelphia, W. B. Saunders Company, 1970, pp 299-315. *A good review with summary of the clinical features of, and diagnostic procedures for, this disease.*

Pattyn SR (ed.): Ebola Virus Haemorrhagic Fever. Amsterdam–New York, Elsevier/North-Holland, 1978. *Proceedings of a symposium documenting events surrounding initial recognition of this disease in Sudan and Zaire.*

Sabattini M, Maiztegui JI: Fiebre hemorrágica argentina. Medicina (Buenos Aires) 30:Suppl 1, 111, 1970. *Definitive review of epidemiology of Argentine hemorrhagic fever. In Spanish.*

Simpson DIH, Knight EM, et al.: Congo virus: A hitherto undescribed virus occurring in Africa. Part I. Human isolation clinical notes. East Afr Med J 44:87, 1967. *First description of the agent indistinguishable from virus causing Crimean hemorrhagic fever. Hemorrhage was not a prominent feature of the cases reported here.*

Smorodintsev AA, Kazbintsev LI, Chudakov VG: Virus Haemorrhagic Fevers (Y Halperin, translator). Washington, D.C., Office of Technical Services, U.S. Department of Commerce, 1964. *Still the most comprehensive description of viral hemorrhagic fevers occurring in the Soviet Union.*

Strode GK: Yellow Fever. New York, McGraw-Hill Book Company, 1951. *A landmark volume documenting the work of the Rockefeller Foundation at home and abroad during the dawn of modern virology, the 1920's through 1940's.*

Symposium on epidemic hemorrhagic fever. Am J Med 16:617, 1954. *The definitive review on clinical pathophysiology of Korean hemorrhagic fever.*

WHO Expert Committee on Yellow Fever: Third report. WHO Tech Rep Ser No 479, 1971. *Thorough summary of continuing trends in patterns of occurrence of sylvan yellow fever worldwide. Recommendations for diagnostic approach to outbreaks and for use of yellow fever vaccines.*

Section Four THE MYCOSES

David J. Drutz

365. INTRODUCTION

Fungi differ from bacteria in three major respects:

1. Like mammalian cells, they are *eukaryotes*. That is, they possess a discrete nucleus bounded by a membrane containing several chromosomes. Bacteria are *prokaryotes*, possessing a single continuous chromosome and no true nucleus or nuclear membrane.

2. Fungi may reproduce sexually or asexually. When mating has taken place, the "sexual state" or *"perfect state"* is said to be present. Spores formed by the perfect state are of major importance in taxonomy. When the perfect form of fungi has not been identified, they are referred to as *deuteromycetes* or *fungi imperfecti* (e.g., *Coccidioides immitis, Candida albicans*).

3. Fungi may be *biphasic*, with one form in nature and a different form in the infected host. For example, *C. immitis, Histoplasma capsulatum, Blastomyces dermatitidis*, and *Sporothrix schenckii* are mycelia (molds) in the environment, but yeasts *(H. capsulatum, B. dermatitidis, S. schenckii)* or endosporulating spherules *(C. immitis)* in man. Because these fungi are basically soil saprophytes and do not appear to require mammalian hosts, it is not clear what benefit accrues to them by attacking man.

Fungal diseases are referred to as *mycoses*. Some mycoses are *endemic*. That is, susceptibility is conferred by living in a geographic area constituting the natural habitat of that fungus (e.g., coccidioidomycosis in California, Arizona, and Texas; paracoccidioidomycosis in South America). Most endemic mycoses (coccidioidomycosis, paracoccidioidomycosis, histoplasmosis, blastomycosis) are acquired by the respiratory route, are minimally symptomatic, and are recognized in retrospect by skin tests or serology. Occasionally pulmonary disease may be progressive, or systemic infection may occur. Race and hormonal factors appear to play some role (e.g., chronic pulmonary histoplasmosis is especially common in middle-aged white men with emphysema; disseminated coccidioidomycosis is most common in black or Filipino men, and in pregnant women regardless of race).

Some mycoses are chiefly opportunistic, occurring in a setting of immunosuppression (candidiasis, cryptococcosis, aspergillosis, mucormycosis) or diabetic ketoacidosis (mucormycosis). Certain other fungi may behave as opportunists in patients with depressed cell-mediated immunity (CMI) (*H. capsulatum, C. immitis,* and perhaps *Paracoccidioides brasiliensis* and *B. dermatitidis*). A separate phenomenon is the occurrence of anergy and depressed correlates of CMI in vitro that are seen in some patients with disseminated histoplasmosis, coccidioidomycosis, sporotrichosis, and paracoccidioidomycosis. Such defects may be associated with excessive suppressor T cell activity and are reversible with elimination of the pathogen.

Diagnosis of the mycoses is usually dependent on morphologic and cultural criteria. *Serologic tests* show cross-reactions and are often more confusing than helpful. However, there are outstanding exceptions: coccidioidomycosis complement-fixing (CF) antibody in the cerebrospinal fluid (CSF) is diagnostic of coccidioidal meningitis; detection of cryptococcal polysaccharide antigen in the blood or CSF is virtually diagnostic of systemic cryptococcosis. *Skin tests* are more useful in epidemiologic surveys than in diagnosis of individual infections. A positive skin test result indicates merely that infection has taken place in the past. Many skin tests are poorly standardized; some (e.g., blastomycin) are valueless for any purpose. The histoplasmin skin test stimulates antibody formation, thereby canceling the limited capabilities of histoplasma serology. Neither of the skin tests available for coccidioidomycosis (coccidioidin, spherulin) has an effect on coccidioidomycosis serology. Further, in a patient with known disseminated coccidioidomycosis a negative skin test result suggests a poor prognosis (especially if associated with a high CF titer), and return to positivity is a clue to therapeutic response.

Effective antifungal chemotherapy is limited. Amphotericin B has been in use for nearly three decades and remains the treatment of choice for most mycoses. Only *Petriellidium (Pseudoallescheria) boydii* is routinely resistant to amphotericin B. Dosage regimens are based more on clinical experience than on objective criteria, and therapy is limited by toxic side effects, principally azotemia. Flucytosine is an orally absorbed drug that serves as an adjunct to amphotericin B in cryptococcal meningitis and in some forms of candidiasis. Its therapeutic efficacy is limited by rapid development of resistance by fungi, and by bone marrow toxicity that appears at least partially related to its conversion to 5-fluorouracil in vivo. Miconazole is a parenteral imidazole with efficacy in coccidioidomycosis and several other mycoses. Its side effects include hyperlipidemia, hyponatremia, and pruritus. It is currently secondary in importance to amphotericin B, except in the treatment of *Pseudoallescheria* infection. Ketoconazole, an orally administered, broad-spectrum imidazole, has shown efficacy in chronic mucocutaneous candidiasis, *Candida* esophagitis, histoplasmosis, blastomycosis, paracoccidioidomycosis, and some forms of coccidioidomycosis. It covers essentially the same spectrum of mycoses as miconazole and can be administered on a long-term basis with minimal side effects (gastrointestinal distress; hepatitis; and interference with endogenous steroid synthesis, especially testosterone).

Dismukes WE, Stamm AM, Graybill JR, Craven PC, Stevens DA, Stiller RL, Sarosi GA, Medoff G, Gregg CR, Gallis HA, Fields BT Jr, Marrier RL, Kerkering TA, Kaplowitz LG, Cloud G, Bowles C, Shadomy S: Treatment of systemic mycoses with ketoconazole: Emphasis on toxicity and clinical response in 52 patients. Ann Intern Med 98:13, 1983. *The ease of ketoconazole administration and its low toxicity relative to that of amphotericin B has stirred major clinical interest in its use for diverse mycoses. This important paper provides a perspective for the likely efficacy of ketoconazole in a variety of mycoses. Additional data from this National Institute of Allergy and Infectious Disease collaborative study are eagerly anticipated.*

Drutz DJ: Newer antifungal agents and their use, including an update on amphotericin B and flucytosine. *In* Remington JS, Swartz MN (eds.): Current Clinical Topics in Infectious Diseases, 3. New York, McGraw-Hill Book Company, 1982, pp 97–135. *The clinical roles of amphotericin B, flucytosine, and miconazole are discussed in detail.*

366. HISTOPLASMOSIS

DEFINITION. Histoplasmosis is the most common endemic respiratory mycosis in the United States. The disease is noncommunicable and ordinarily self-limited, but reinfection, chronic pulmonary infection, and disseminated infection all may occur.

ETIOLOGY. *Histoplasma capsulatum* (perfect form: *Emmonsiella capsulata*) is a biphasic fungus, occurring in the mycelial phase in the environment, and in the yeast phase at 37° C and in infected hosts. The mycelial form produces two types of spores: tuberculate macroconidia (8 to 16 μm), and microconidia of a size (2 to 5 μm) more appropriate to be inhaled. The yeasts are ovoid (2 to 3 × 3 to 4 μm) and unencapsulated, bud singly from a narrow neck, and occur intracellularly in macrophages.

INCIDENCE AND PREVALENCE. Histoplasmosis occurs worldwide. Over 40 million people have been infected in the United States, and about 500,000 develop skin test positivity each year. Eighty to 95 per cent of persons in the Mississippi, Missouri, and Ohio River valleys are histoplasmin positive. *H. capsulatum var. duboisii* produces a disease restricted largely to central Africa ("African histoplasmosis") with slightly different clinical and histopathologic features.

EPIDEMIOLOGY. *H. capsulatum* is a soil saprophyte that prefers moderate temperatures and moist environments. Droppings from chickens, pigeons, starlings, blackbirds, and bats support its growth. Birds are not infected, but carry the fungi on their feathers. Bats are infected and excrete yeasts from an ulcerated intestinal mucosa. Histoplasmosis ("cave disease") may follow exploration of bat-infested caves. Although the fungus is found in greatest abundance in bat or bird-related microenvironments, microconidia are commonly present as "air pollutants" in endemic areas and probably account for the majority of sporadic infections. Focal outbreaks occur with disturbances that raise dust (e.g., demolition of old buildings where birds or bats have roosted), especially on the edge of an endemic zone where histoplasmin skin test reactivity is not universally present. Because histoplasmin reactivity may wane, persons who live in highly endemic areas are subject to reinfection.

PATHOGENESIS AND PATHOLOGY. Following the inhalation of microconidia, fungi replicate locally and disseminate hematogenously to the mononuclear phagocyte system. With the development of cell-mediated immunity, granuloma formation occurs, often with caseation necrosis, and the histoplasmin skin test becomes positive. Healing may be marked by exuberant calcification at pulmonary parenchymal and hilar loci (Ghon complex) and in the spleen. An exaggerated fibrotic response may lead to *fibrosing mediastinitis* with bronchial or vascular occlusion (e.g., superior vena caval obstruction). Layers of collagen may be deposited at the site of pulmonary coin lesions *(histoplasmomas),* their growth leading to thoracotomy for suspected malignancy.

H. capsulatum stains poorly with hematoxylin-eosin, but well with periodic acid–Schiff, Giemsa, or Gomori methenamine silver stains. Organisms are ordinarily found in macrophages, but large bizarre extracellular forms may be seen in endocarditis lesions or necrotic loci. The spectrum of host response is related directly to the effectiveness of cell-mediated immune mechanisms. With optimal immunity, fungi are rare, granuloma formation is well developed, and the disease is restricted in extent. With deficient immunity, macrophages, including those in circulating blood, are packed with intracellular yeasts, granuloma formation is poor, and disease is extensive. Granulocytes and serum factors play a secondary role in host defense.

In patients with centrilobular or bullous emphysema, histoplasmosis is opportunistic. Subintimal arterial proliferation leads to infarct-like pulmonary necrosis. In infants and older adults without obvious host defense defects, and in patients with chronic lymphocytic leukemia, Hodgkin's disease, steroid therapy, or other defects of cell-mediated immunity, progressive hematogenous dissemination may occur. Some of the manifestations (meningitis, adrenal insufficiency, intestinal ulceration) are attributable to an accompanying perivasculitis.

CLINICAL MANIFESTATIONS. ***Primary Histoplasmosis.*** At least 90 per cent of all respiratory encounters with *H. capsulatum* pass unnoticed or are attributed to "the flu." Manifestations include cough, fever, headache, myalgias, stomach cramps, and pleuritic pain. With heavier exposure, there may be dyspnea, cyanosis, deep chest pain, and pericarditis. Occasionally, there may be erythema nodosum, erythema multiforme, diffuse rash, or arthralgias—especially in white women. The chest roentgenogram may show patchy infiltrates; hilar lymphadenopathy is common, especially in children. Cavitation and pleural effusion may occur. Ghon complexes tend to be more highly calcified than in tuberculosis. Multifocal pulmonary lesions may heal with diffuse "buckshot" calcifications. These may erode into bronchi and be expectorated later as broncholiths.

Reinfection Histoplasmosis. The potential for re-exposure to microconidia is constantly present in endemic areas. Reinfection is characterized by a shorter incubation period (three to seven versus ten to eighteen days), miliary nodulation (rather than patchy bronchopneumonia), lack of hilar adenopathy, and a shorter and less severe disease course. However, very severe pulmonary disease with cyanosis and respiratory distress may also be seen.

Chronic Pulmonary Histoplasmosis. This disease occurs most commonly in middle-aged white men with pre-existing chronic obstructive pulmonary disease and centrilobular or bullous emphysema. Multiplication of inhaled *H. capsulatum* in an emphysematous bleb (characteristically in an apical-posterior location) results in antigenic spillage to contiguous lung areas and an acute segmental interstitial pneumonitis. Symptoms include cough, fever, and malaise. Microorganisms are sparse, and in 80 per cent of cases the disease resolves over two to three months with infarct-like necrosis, contraction of damaged tissue, and a fibrous residual. There may be later recurrences. In 20 per cent of patients, persistent infection leads to chronic cavitary disease. Thick-walled cavities expand by contiguity into the surrounding lung ("marching cavity"), and bronchogenic spread of their contents results in pneumonitis and fibrosis in dependent lung areas. Patients may have fever and a productive cough; one third have hemoptysis. Sputum cultures are positive in only 50 to 70 per cent. The patients usually pursue a declining course, less from actual infection than from progressive loss of functioning lung.

Disseminated Histoplasmosis. One third of cases occur in infants, the remainder predominantly in men over age 40. A clinically apparent pulmonary infection may precede dissemination in infants, but is less likely to do so in adults. Dissemination in adults may follow immunosuppression, with arousal of disease from latency. Infants have the poorest host response to infection, and the most fulminating course; disease in adults is usually subacute or chronic.

Clinical manifestations include weight loss, fever, weakness and malaise, hepatosplenomegaly, lymphadenopathy, and impaired bone marrow function (anemia, leukopenia, and thrombocytopenia). Oropharyngeal, nasopharyngeal, and laryngeal ulcerations, usually painful and often associated with dysphagia or hoarseness, constitute a major clue to the diagnosis. Gastrointestinal tract ulcerations (especially common in the ileocecal area) may present with bleeding, obstruction, perforation, or malabsorption. Adrenal insufficiency is common and may occur years after successful eradication of fungi. Chest roentgenograms may show evidence of primary or hematogenous infection. Endocarditis (aortic more than mitral or tricuspid valves) may present with emboli to large blood vessels. Central nervous system histoplasmosis may present with focal cerebritis or diffuse chronic meningitis with hypoglycorrhachia. The kidneys, prostate, and skin may also be involved, but osteomyelitis and arthritis are rare.

Ocular Histoplasmosis. Presumed ocular histoplasmosis syndrome (POHS) refers to a focal chorioretinitis in the macular area that is thought to be related to a hypersensitivity response to products of *H. capsulatum.* No direct relationship to fungal infection has been proved.

DIAGNOSIS. Histoplasmosis is as clinically diverse as tuberculosis. Particularly suggestive features include mucous membrane ulcerations, leukopenia, thrombocytopenia, adrenal insufficiency, buckshot pulmonary calcifications, and splenic calcifications. The diagnosis depends on demonstrating or culturing *H. capsulatum* from involved tissues, seldom a simple task. The roles of skin and serologic tests are limited. The *histoplasmin skin test* is seldom useful diagnostically because positive results are common in the endemic area. Conversely, disseminated disease is not necessarily associated with a negative result (unlike the situation with coccidioidomycosis). A positive skin test result also elevates titers of serum antibodies. The skin test should therefore be restricted to use in epidemiologic investigations. The *complement fixation test* (using mycelial or yeast phase antigen) may show cross-reactions with blastomycosis or coccidioidomycosis. Low level antibody titers may persist for years following primary histoplasmosis. A titer ≥1:32, or a four-fold titer rise, suggests but does not prove active histoplasmosis; nor does a negative titer rule out the disease. Titers do not parallel disease activity and are of little value in following therapy or estimating prognosis. Tests for antibody by the *immunodiffusion* method produce two bands (m, h) of potential diagnostic value. The occurrence of both bands in the serum of a patient who has not been skin tested with histoplasmin is highly suggestive of histoplasmosis. If only an m band is observed, early histoplasmosis may be present because the m band usually precedes the h band. The *latex agglutination test* with histoplasmin-sensitized latex particles is a useful aid to diagnosis of acute histoplasmosis, especially in titers ≥1:16. False positive and negative results may occur, and confirmatory diagnostic tests are required.

Primary pulmonary histoplasmosis is rarely diagnosed in the absence of a suggestive epidemiologic history or the investigation of a common-source outbreak. Most cases are probably overlooked or misdiagnosed as bacterial or viral processes. Sputum cultures are positive in only 20 per cent of cases. Skin test conversion is diagnostic, but seldom documented. Serologic tests may be helpful in diagnosis, as noted above.

Chronic pulmonary histoplasmosis is diagnosed on the basis of suggestive roentgenographic changes and positive sputum smears or cultures. Less than one third of cultures are positive in early, self-limited disease, whereas 70 per cent are positive in patients with marching cavities. Multiple cultures may be required before the fungus is found.

Disseminated histoplasmosis in one large series demonstrated positive cultures in the following distribution: oral lesions (91 per cent), lymph node (72 per cent), bone marrow (70 per cent), sputum (60 per cent), liver biopsy (57 per cent), blood (54 per cent), CSF (45 per cent), and urine (43 per cent). Organisms have also been cultured from the stool, prostatic secretions, and skin lesions. Fungi may be demonstrated directly by Wright, Giemsa, or methenamine silver stains of the buffy coat of blood, ulcer swabs or scrapings, sputum, or other infected materials.

TREATMENT. Primary pulmonary infection rarely requires treatment. Those with acute respiratory insufficiency following massive spore exposure may require a brief course of corticosteroid therapy, with or without accompanying antifungal therapy. Chronic pulmonary histoplasmosis resolves spontaneously in 80 per cent of cases, but resolution may be assisted by restriction of activity or bed rest. Progressive cavitary pulmonary histoplasmosis generally requires therapy with amphotericin B (approximately 2 grams over ten weeks), but repeated courses of treatment may be required. If pulmonary function permits, surgical resection of marching cavities should be considered. Patients with progressive disseminated infection should receive approximately 2 grams of amphotericin B over ten weeks (for infants, the dosage is 1 mg per kilogram per day for six weeks), although lower total dosages may be curative in some patients. Relapses can occur. Endocarditis may be more difficult to cure. Adrenal function should be evaluated at the time of diagnosis and monitored indefinitely thereafter. Adrenal insufficiency may occur years later, and patients should be warned of this possibility. Fibrosing mediastinitis is a manifestation of excessive host response rather than progressive infection. Antifungal chemotherapy is not necessarily indicated.

The role of the imidazoles (miconazole, ketoconazole) in histoplasmosis is currently unsettled. Recently studies suggest efficacy of ketoconazole in both pulmonary and disseminated histoplasmosis. However, caution is warranted in using this oral agent for immunocompromised patients with severe disease. In such patients, amphotericin B is clearly the drug of choice. Sulfonamides are of historical interest only.

PROGNOSIS. Chronic cavitary pulmonary histoplasmosis usually results in death from respiratory insufficiency. Progressive disseminated histoplasmosis (once uniformly fatal in those with poor host defenses) is curable, although relapses may occur.

PREVENTION. A 3 per cent solution of formalin sprayed on *H. capsulatum*–containing soil will destroy the fungi and control common-source outbreaks.

Goodwin RA Jr, Loyd JE, Des Prez RM: Histoplasmosis in normal hosts. Medicine 60:231, 1981. *When learning about histoplasmosis, this is the paper with which to begin.*

Goodwin RA Jr, Owens FT, Snell JD, Hubbard WW, Buchanan RD, Terry RT, Des Prez RM: Chronic pulmonary histoplasmosis. Medicine 55:413, 1976. *The definitive article on the subject by the group with the greatest clinical experience with this disease. There is a strong emphasis on immunopathogenesis.*

Goodwin RA Jr, Shapiro JL, Thurman GH, Thurman SS, Des Prez RM: Disseminated histoplasmosis: Clinical and pathologic correlations. Medicine 59:1, 1980. *An extensive review of experience with this disease in middle Tennessee. Immunopathogenesis is emphasized, but this paper is also an outstanding clinical contribution. Amphotericin B was usually curative.*

Wheat J, French MLV, Kohler RB, Zimmerman SE, Smith WR, Norton JA, Eitzen HE, Smith CD, Slama TG: The diagnostic laboratory tests for histoplasmosis: Analysis of experience in a large urban outbreak. Ann Intern Med 97:680, 1982. *This paper discusses the diagnostic usefulness of the complement fixation and immunodiffusion tests for histoplasmosis. Antibody responses differed among clinical syndromes, and titers were not necessarily elevated in patients with disseminated infection.*

367. COCCIDIOIDOMYCOSIS

DEFINITION. Coccidioidomycosis is a noncontagious respiratory mycosis of the southwest, and the second most common endemic mycosis in the United States, after histoplasmosis. It is usually self-limited, but may lead to chronic pulmonary infection or hematogenous dissemination.

ETIOLOGY. *Coccidioides immitis* is a biphasic fungus. The mycelial phase, a soil saprophyte of semiarid regions, fragments to release box-like arthroconidia (arthrospores) of a size suitable to be inhaled (2 to 5 μm). In the infected host, the fungus grows as large spherules, 10 to 80 μm in diameter, the cytoplasm of which segments to produce hundreds of endospores (2 to 5 μm diameter). Spherule rupture results in dispersal of endospores to surrounding tissues, where they mature to spherules, repeating the growth cycle.

INCIDENCE AND PREVALENCE. Coccidioidomycosis occurs in the southwestern United States and neighboring Mexico (the "Lower Sonoran life zone"), and in parts of Central and South America. Approximately 100,000 cases occur yearly. The *spherulin* (spherule-endospore) and coccidioidin (mycelial) skin tests detect approximately equal numbers of *C. immitis*-exposed patients. Each test misses 12 to 15 per cent of patients that the other test detects. Eighty to 95 per cent of the population is skin test positive in parts of California and Arizona. Infection is more common in those with outdoor activities. Extrapulmonary dissemination occurs in 1 of 2000 to 3500 white women, 1 of 500 white men, and 1 of 50 black men. The risk may be even greater in Filipinos. Pregnancy, depressed cell-mediated immunity, and corticosteroid therapy increase the risk of dissemination.

EPIDEMIOLOGY. *C. immitis* is distributed sporadically within the endemic zone. Arthroconidia are spread on the wind by any activity that raises dust; fomites may carry the spores outside the endemic area. Risk of infectivity drops dramatically once land is cultivated. Animals are commonly infected but pose no hazard for man. Newcomers to the southwest are at high risk for infection. A World War II study documented a 50 per cent skin test conversion rate within six months in airmen stationed in the Phoenix area. Skin test reactivity is associated with solid immunity; reinfection is almost unknown.

PATHOGENESIS AND PATHOLOGY. Coccidioidomycosis is characterized by suppuration (endospore response) and granuloma formation (spherule response). Cell-mediated immunity is the major host defense mechanism. In patients with extrapulmonary dissemination or chronic progressive pulmonary coccidioidomycosis, *C. immitis* skin test reactivity may never develop or may wane, and there is nonspecific suppression of reactivity to recall-type skin tests and tests of cell-mediated immunity in vitro. Most defects are reversible with therapy. Granuloma formation may be deficient, and suppuration may dominate. Antibody plays no apparent role in host defense.

CLINICAL MANIFESTATIONS. ***Primary Coccidioidomycosis.*** Sixty per cent of primary infections are asymptomatic. Symptoms in the other 40 per cent include cough, fever, headache, and pleuritic pain. Up to 5 per cent (predominantly white women) present with erythema nodosum or erythema multiforme and arthralgias ("valley fever"). Others may have "toxic erythema" resembling measles. Eosinophilia is common. The chest roentgenogram may show segmental or lobar infiltrates, often with hilar adenopathy. Pleural fluid is present in 5 to 20 per cent of cases, and fungi may be demonstrable by pleural biopsy. Cavitation may occur, usually without specific symptoms. Thin-walled cavities may persist and be discovered later on a routine roentgenogram. They are usually single, less than 4 cm in diameter, and seldom symptomatic, although the sputum may contain *C. immitis*. Up to one half of cavities will close spontaneously in two to four years. Rarely, they may lead to hemoptysis, become secondarily infected, or enlarge to encroach on normal surrounding lung.

Persistent coccidioidal pneumonia is manifested by persistence of the primary infection for six to eight weeks, with worsening pulmonary infiltrates, fever, chest pain, prostration, and productive cough. Resolution is slow; healing may result in fibrosis, bronchiectasis, and calcification. Fatality is especially common in immunosuppressed patients.

Chronic progressive coccidioidal pneumonia is an indolent disease process with weight loss, fever, hemoptysis, chest pain, and dyspnea. It is characterized by chronicity and biapical fibronodular lesions and cavities that resemble tuberculosis or histoplasmosis.

Pulmonary nodules (coccidioidomas) result from resolution of earlier infiltrative disease. Most are 1 to 4 cm in size and have semisolid centers that contain *C. immitis*. The lesions may cavitate, resulting in an "abscessing nodule."

Disseminated Coccidioidomycosis. Extrapulmonary dissemination usually occurs soon after primary infection, but diagnosis may be delayed, depending on the pace and sites of dissemination. The chest roentgenogram may or may not be abnormal. Dissemination may be unifocal or multifocal. The *skin and subcutaneous tissues* are the most common sites involved. Lesions are papular, verrucous, or ulcerative; subcutaneous abscesses may occur. *Osteomyelitis* occurs in 10 to 50 per cent of cases, involves single or multiple bones, and is most common in the vertebrae, tibia, skull, metatarsals, and metacarpals, especially at sites of tendon or ligament insertion. Complications include muscle abscesses or draining cutaneous fistulas. *Joints* may be involved by penetration from contiguous osteomyelitis or by hematogenous infection of the synovium. Large weight-bearing joints such as the knee and ankle are most commonly involved. There may be rapid joint destruction, or chronic nonerosive synovitis with progressive villous hypertrophy and pannus formation resembling rheumatoid arthritis. *Meningitis* occurs in 30 to 50 per cent of patients, often as the sole site of involvement. Most cases are hematogenous in origin; some reflect direct spread from skull or vertebral osteomyelitis. The disease process is subtle, with headache, lethargy, personality changes, and diverse neurologic abnormalities. The meningitis is predominantly basilar in location; intracerebral infection may be demonstrable by CT scan; hydrocephalus is common. Other manifestations of disseminated disease include *thyroiditis, tenosynovitis,* and *prostatitis.* Liver, spleen, lymph node, and kidney involvement is common but often clinically silent. Adrenal insufficiency may occur. Gastrointestinal tract involvement is rare.

DIAGNOSIS. Coccidioidomycosis may be confused with a variety of infections, including tuberculosis and other mycoses. Joint involvement may mimic primary rheumatologic disorders. Diagnosis is readily achieved by demonstrating endosporulating spherules in 10 per cent KOH wet mounts of sputum or inflammatory exudates. Biopsy specimens stained with hematoxylin-eosin, Gridley, periodic acid–Schiff or Gomori methenamine silver stains may demonstrate the fungi in diverse tissues. Cerebrospinal fluid (CSF) findings include pleocytosis, elevated protein, and hypoglycorrhachia; when present, eosinophils are a valuable clue to the diagnosis. *C. immitis* is not fastidious and can be recovered on most standard media. However, the mycelial phase is biohazardous and demands great care in laboratory handling. Fungi can be cultured from the CSF in only 20 to 40 per cent of instances. Urine cultures may disclose *C. immitis* in the absence of any abnormality of renal function or urinalysis. Bone marrow cultures may be positive, but blood cultures are rarely positive until disease is nearly terminal.

Serologic tests are extremely important in diagnosis and prognosis, and are uninfluenced by skin testing. Patients with symptomatic disease generally manifest an IgM antibody response that peaks by the second to third week of illness, and is replaced by an IgG response. The IgM antibody is demonstrable by tube precipitin, latex particle agglutination, or immunodiffusion (ID) techniques. The IgG response is detectable by complement fixation (CF) or ID methods. CF titers seldom exceed 1:8 to 1:16 in uncomplicated primary infection. Persistent elevations at 1:16 to 1:32 or more raise the likelihood of dissemination, particularly if associated with loss or absence of skin test reactivity. Minimal work-up for suspected dissemination includes wet mounts, biopsies and cultures from any suspicious lesions, lumbar puncture, bone scans, and cultures of concentrated morning urine. Patients with unifocal dissemination (particulary meningitis) may not show elevated CF titers in the serum or loss of skin test reactivity. CF antibody is present in the CSF in 75 to 95 per cent of cases of meningitis, however, and is diagnostic.

TREATMENT. Primary pulmonary infection seldom requires treatment, although a "prophylactic" course of 1 gram of amphotericin B may be given to patients at particular risk of dissemination (blacks, immunosuppressed patients). Isolated thin-walled cavities are usually asymptomatic, although surgical resection may be required for life-threatening hemoptysis or threatened rupture into the pleural space. Progressive pulmonary infection may benefit from a total course of 1 to 2 grams of amphotericin B; fungi are difficult to eradicate once significant destruction of pulmonary parenchyma has occurred. Disseminated coccidioidomycosis is characterized by spontaneous exacerbations and remissions, making therapeutic response difficult to interpret. Amphotericin B is often more likely to be ameliorative than curative. A total dose of 2 grams constitutes a minimal course of therapy; the goal is to produce clear clinical improvement and a persistent fourfold fall in the serum CF titer. Relapse is typical and necessitates retreatment. Meningitis must be treated by the intrathecal or intraventricular route; cure is elusive. Synovitis may require synovectomy or arthrodesis for cure.

Miconazole lacks nephrotoxicity, but is not clearly superior to amphotericin B in any other sense, and must also be given intrathecally for meningitis. Daily dosage ranges from 1800 to 3600 mg; treatment should be continued for two to three months. Major side effects include symptomatic hyponatremia, hyperlipidemia, and itching. The role of ketoconazole in therapy of coccidioidomycosis is controversial. It appears to be most useful in maintaining remissions induced by amphotericin B. However, it occasionally shows benefit in the primary management of infection that has disseminated to the skin and soft tissues. Optimal dosage and duration of therapy remain uncertain.

PROGNOSIS. Meningitis is usually fatal within two years without therapy. Even with therapy, mental deterioration or fatality may occur from hydrocephalus unless the complication is anticipated and managed by CSF shunting. Other forms of coccidioidomycosis tend to be more debilitating than lethal, although fulminating pulmonary infection may be fatal in the severely immunosuppressed.

PREVENTION. Partial control of *C. immitis* at dusty sites can be achieved by saturating the soil with 1-chloro-2-nitropropane. Patients from nonendemic areas who have risk factors for coccidioidal dissemination should be warned of the danger in working or residing in highly endemic areas.

Bouza E, Dryer JS, Hewitt WL, Meyer RD: Coccidioidal meningitis: An analysis of thirty-one cases and review of the literature. Medicine 60:139, 1981. *Coccidioidal meningitis is difficult to diagnose, harder to manage, and refractory to cure. This paper recounts the experience of UCLA-affiliated hospitals with coccidioidal meningitis between 1964 and 1976 and provides a valuable literature review.*

DeFelice R, Galgiani JN, Campbell SC, Palpant SD, Friedman BA, Dodge RR, Weinberg MG, Lincoln LJ, Tennican PO, Barbee RA: Ketoconazole treatment of nonprimary coccidioidomycosis: Evaluation of 60 patients during three years of study. Am J Med 72:681, 1982. *Although ketoconazole may produce clinical improvement in patients with various forms of coccidioidomycosis, relapse is not uncommon. Similar results are reported in a series of 29 patients (Catanzaro A, Einstein H, Levine B, Ross JR, Schillaci R, Fierer J, Friedman PJ: Ketoconazole for treatment of disseminated coccidioidomycosis. Ann Intern Med 96:436, 1982).*

Drutz DJ: Coccidioidal pneumonia. *In* Pennington JE (ed.): Respiratory Infections: Diagnosis and Management. New York, Raven Press, 1983, pp 353–373. *A thorough review of all aspects of pulmonary coccidioidal infection, including medical and surgical management.*

Drutz DJ, Catanzaro A: Coccidioidomycosis. State of the art. Am Rev Respir Dis 117:559, 727, 1978. *A review of all aspects of coccidioidomycosis and its treatment.*

Stevens DA (ed.): Coccidioidomycosis. A Text. New York, Plenum Medical Book Company, 1980, p 279. *An up-to-date compendium of the microbiology, epidemiology, immunology, serology, pathology, and clinical manifestations of coccidioidomycosis.*

368. BLASTOMYCOSIS (North American Blastomycosis, Gilchrist's Disease)

DEFINITION. Blastomycosis is a noncontagious, subacute or chronic endemic mycosis that follows inhalation of the conidia of *Blastomyces dermatitidis.* The organs most commonly affected are the lungs, skin, bones, and male genitourinary system.

ETIOLOGY. *B. dermatitidis* (perfect form: *Ajellomyces dermatitidis*) is a dimorphic fungus, occurring in the mycelial phase at ambient temperatures and as yeasts at 37° C or in the infected host. The yeast phase is characterized by cells of 8 to 15 (or more) μm in diameter that reproduce by single budding. Daughter cells are attached at a very broad (4 to 5 μm) base, and may reach the size of the mother cells before separating.

INCIDENCE AND PREVALENCE. Blastomycosis is encountered far less commonly than histoplasmosis and coccidioidomycosis. There is no diagnostic skin test or serologic test. Hence, the extent to which subclinical disease occurs is largely unknown, and endemic areas are defined in terms of clinical cases.

EPIDEMIOLOGY. Blastomycosis occurs most commonly in the southeastern United States, especially in the Ohio and Mississippi River valleys, and in areas of the United States and Canada adjacent to the Great Lakes. However, the disease is also encountered in Africa, Mexico, and Central and South America, so that "North American blastomycosis" is a misnomer. The ecologic niche for the fungus appears to be the soil, but its recovery has been sporadic and uncommon, and the factors governing its distribution are unknown. Persons at risk often have outdoor vocations or avocations. Clinical illness is most common in middle-aged men. However, studies during common-source outbreaks indicate that self-limited infection is independent of sex, age, or race. Dogs and horses are highly susceptible to blastomycosis, and the occurrence of veterinary cases helps to define endemic areas. In some instances hunters and their dogs have acquired blastomycosis simultaneously. Percutaneous inoculation of fungi has been documented in laboratory accidents, but in virtually all other circumstances cutaneous lesions result from hematogenous spread of apparent or inapparent pulmonary disease.

PATHOGENESIS AND PATHOLOGY. The factors governing host defense against *B. dermatitidis* are poorly understood. Human granulocytes kill yeast-phase organisms ineffectively in vitro; animal studies suggest that cell-mediated immunity contributes significantly to host defense. The serum of patients with blastomycosis contains an acquired heat-stable factor that impairs the locomotion of polymorphonuclear leukocytes, and may help to potentiate the disease. Disseminated disease may occur with greater frequency in the presence of immunosuppression.

Histopathologically, blastomycosis is marked by the simultaneous presence of suppurative and granulomatous foci. In fulminating infections, the suppurative component may predominate. Caseation necrosis is uncommon. Cutaneous and mucous membrane lesions are characterized by the presence of pseudoepitheliomatous hyperplasia. Identification of microabscesses and single budding yeasts helps in establishing the diagnosis.

CLINICAL MANIFESTATIONS. ***Pulmonary Blastomycosis.*** In most cases, respiratory infection is probably asymptomatic. In some cases, pleuritic chest pain, nonspecific "flu-like" symptoms, or arthralgias and erythema nodosum may mark the occurrence of acute infection. The correct diagnosis is probably seldom made in the absence of a specific search for a fungal etiology, as during a suspected common-source outbreak. Clinically apparent pulmonary blastomycosis has no distinguishing clinical or radiographic characteristics. Bronchitis is present in up to one third of cases and may contribute to rapid endobronchial spread. Cavitation, hilar adenopathy, and pleural involvement are all well documented. Fibrosis is common, but residual calcification is rare. Expanding mass-like lesions may be confused with malignancies. Miliary pulmonary lesions may be present in cases with fulminating hematogenous dissemination.

Disseminated Blastomycosis. Extrapulmonary disease may occur in the presence or absence of obvious lung disease, either during or after the initial pulmonary infection. Some cases may reflect late endogenous reactivation. The frequency of multisystem involvement is directly related to the thoroughness of diagnostic studies. The most common site of extrapulmonary dissemination is the skin, and skin lesions are often the presenting feature of blastomycosis. Lesions begin as papules, pustules, or subcutaneous nodules, and may involve exposed or unexposed areas. Some become verrucous and progress over weeks or months to produce an elevated, warty, crusted lesion with a serpiginous, indurated, dusky red or violaceous, abruptly sloping outer border. Prominent "black dots" at the surface mark the location of necrotic papillary blood vessels. Removal of crusts reveals a granulomatous base with numerous ulcers exuding bloody purulent material. Central healing and scarring may occur, with disease activity most prominent at the advancing borders. In some patients superficial ulcerative lesions may predominate. Disseminated papulopustular skin lesions have followed incision of pulmonary blastomycotic mass lesions at exploratory thoracotomy for suspected malignancy.

Bone lesions are encountered in 25 to 60 per cent of cases. They are most common in the axial skeleton (especially the vertebrae) and long bones, but may be detectable only by bone scan or radiographic bone survey. Lytic lesions with or without sclerotic margins may be seen. Draining sinuses without a verrucous appearance may mark underlying osteomyelitic foci. An acute arthritis, usually monarticular, occurs in three to five per cent of cases, either hematogenously or by direct bony spread. Involvement of the prostate, testis, and epididymis may be signaled by dysuria, pyuria, hematuria, urinary hesitancy, and tender intrascrotal mass lesions. Renal, hepatic, and splenic infections are common but usually clinically inapparent. Adrenal involvement may rarely cause Addison's disease. Central nervous system invasion occurs in about 5 per cent of cases, and may present as an intracranial mass, isolated meningitis, or spinal epidural granulomas or abscesses. Gastrointestinal involvement is rare.

DIAGNOSIS. Pulmonary blastomycosis may be confused with tuberculosis, other mycoses, bacterial pneumonia, or malignancy. Cutaneous blastomycosis is highly characteristic in appearance, but may be confused with chromomycosis, coccidioidomycosis, or some cutaneous malignancies. Diagnosis may be reached most quickly by direct microscopic examination of biologic specimens digested in 10 per cent KOH. Under these circumstances, characteristic single-budding yeasts may be seen in sputum, prostatic fluid, and other biologic specimens. Stains are not necessary. *B. dermatitidis* will grow on most standard culture media, but specimens should be held for at least one month. The myceliial phase is not sufficiently distinctive to permit a precise identification, so that conversion in vitro to the diagnostic yeast phase is required. Animal inoculation is not necessary. In fixed tissue specimens, hematoxylin-eosin staining reveals characteristic yeast cells with a doubly refractile cell wall, often accentuated by retraction of the protoplast from the outer cell wall. The periodic acid–Schiff stain preserves intracellular detail and helps differentiate *B. dermatitidis* (multinucleated) from *C. neoformans* and *H. capsulatum* (single nuclei). Fungi are easily seen with Gomori methenamine silver stain, but internal detail is lost.

Patients with blastomycosis should have complete evaluation for skin, bone, and genitourinary lesions, as the response to therapy may be monitored by observing the progress of disease in these sites. Adrenal function should also be evaluated as a few patients may go on to develop adrenal insufficiency.

The blastomycin skin test is valueless as a diagnostic or prognostic tool, and should not be used. The blastomycosis complement fixation test shows cross-reactivity with *H. capsulatum* and *C. immitis*, and is almost never clinically useful. An immunodiffusion test has shown more promising results.

TREATMENT. Most acute pulmonary infections are probably self-limited. In patients with progressive lung disease, extrapulmonary lesions, or immunosuppression, systemic antifungal therapy is indicated.

Amphotericin B and 2-hydroxystilbamidine reportedly provide similar rates of improvement in patients with noncavitary pulmonary disease or disseminated disease involving only the skin. However, amphotericin B (given in a total dose of at least 2 grams) is associated with fewer relapses, and is probably the choice for all forms of the disease. 2-Hydroxystilbamidine is given in a total dose of 4 to 15 grams (225 mg per day). Its side effects include nausea, vomiting, chills, fever, elevation of hepatic transaminase levels, and rare hypotensive or idiosyncratic reactions. Ketoconazole has shown promise in clinical trials, but treatment failures have occasionally been reported and experience is insufficient to warrant its recommendation as a drug of first choice, especially in severely ill patients.

PROGNOSIS. The natural history of extrapulmonary blastomycosis is that of a slowly progressive disease with a 20 to 90 per cent mortality, and severe disfigurement, depending upon the series reported. Case mortality with either amphotericin B or 2-hydroxystilbamidine is about 8 per cent. Most relapses occur within one year of treatment, but have been documented after as long as nine years. All patients with untreated pulmonary disease should be carefully observed for later evidence of disease activity.

Parker JD, Doto IL, Tosh FE: A decade of experience with blastomycosis and its treatment with amphotericin B. Am Rev Respir Dis 99:895, 1969. *The only published study comparing therapeutic effectiveness of amphotericin B and 2-hydroxystilbamidine. Except for noncavitary pulmonary disease and isolated cutaneous dissemination, amphotericin B was superior.*

Sarosi GA, Davies SF: Blastomycosis. State of the art. Am Rev Respir Dis 120:911, 1979. *A valuable review paper with a particular emphasis on pulmonary blastomycosis. An excellent companion piece to the Witorsch and Utz reference.*

Witorsch P, Utz JP: North American blastomycosis: A study of 40 patients. Medicine 47:169, 1968. *This paper contains a wealth of information concerning both pulmonary and systemic blastomycosis.*

369. PARACOCCIDIOIDOMYCOSIS

DEFINITION. Paracoccidioidomycosis (South American blastomycosis) is a noncontagious respiratory mycosis that may be acute and self-limited, or may produce progressive pulmonary disease or extrapulmonary dissemination. It is the most common systemic mycosis in South America.

ETIOLOGY. *Paracoccidioides brasiliensis* is a dimorphic fungus which in its mycelial phase is probably a soil saprophyte. In tissues or at 37° C the fungus is a spherical double-walled yeast cell, 6 to 60 μm in diameter, that has multiple buds on narrow necks, producing the appearance of "ship's wheels," "crown of buds," or "Mickey Mouse" figures.

INCIDENCE AND PREVALENCE. Paracoccidioidomycosis is limited to an area 20° N in Mexico to 34° S in Argentina. Brazil accounts for 70 per cent of the 5000 to 6000 reported cases, followed by Venezuela and Colombia. Natural infection in animals has not been documented, and common-source outbreaks in humans have not been reported.

EPIDEMIOLOGY. Equal numbers of men and women have positive paracoccidioidin skin tests, but clinical disease is 15 times more prevalent in men. Only 4 per cent of cases have been reported in children. Hormonal or occupational factors (especially agricultural work) may influence susceptibility. Asian and European immigrants often have more severe illness than patients who are native born. Whether this indicates a racial predisposition or merely exposure of a population with a lack of prior disease experience is uncertain.

Prominent oropharyngeal ulcerations in disseminated paracoccidioidomycosis led to the assumption that infection was acquired from contaminated vegetation introduced into the mouth. It is now clear that virtually all cases are acquired by the respiratory route. The vast majority of cases are probably self-limited, manifesting themselves by positive skin tests and minimal abnormalities of the chest roentgenogram.

PATHOGENESIS AND PATHOLOGY. The host response consists of a combination of suppuration and granulomas. In patients with impaired host defense, the suppurative response may dominate. The disease process is limited to the lungs in most cases, but lymphohematogenous dissemination may occur, especially in males beyond puberty and in immunosuppressed patients.

The spectrum of disease encountered clinically is a function of the integrity of cell-mediated host defense responses. In patients with progressive disease, there is secondary suppression of immunity with impaired skin test reactivity to paracoccidioidin and other recall-type skin test preparations. There is also an impairment of correlates of cell-mediated immunity in vitro (migration inhibition factor, lymphocyte blastogenesis). All these parameters commonly improve with treatment.

CLINICAL MANIFESTATIONS. Pulmonary paracoccidioidomycosis may be symptomatic or asymptomatic and may or may not be apparent when extrapulmonary disease is discovered. There is nothing distinctive about the acute pulmonary process. Progressive pulmonary lesions may be unilateral or bilateral, with or without hilar adenopathy. Chest roentgenograms may reveal cavitation (20 to 33 per cent of cases), infiltration, nodules, tumor-like masses, or fibrosis. Pulmonary paracoccidioidomycosis is commonly confused with tuberculosis but less often leads to residual calcification.

Extrapulmonary dissemination may occur acutely, especially in young persons, under which circumstance the disease process is dominated by lymphadenopathy, hepatosplenomegaly, and a miliary pattern on the chest roentgenogram. The disease may also disseminate after a period of years to decades. Many cases have been documented in persons who have long since emigrated from endemic areas so that continued exposure to the fungus is not an important predisposing factor. The clinical presentation is variable, depending on the sites of involvement. Oropharyngeal mucosal invasion is characteristic. Ulcerating lesions involve the gums, lips, tongue, palate, uvula, pharynx, tonsillar areas, or floor of the mouth. Lesions eventually become so painful that eating is extremely difficult. Gingival destruction may result in loss of teeth. Involvement of the epiglottis and larynx results in dysphonia. Ulcers of the nasal, conjunctival, and perianal mucous membranes may be encountered. There may be massive cervical and abdominal lymphadenopathy. Lymph nodes may break down to produce draining fistulas. A wide variety of crusted ulcerative, verrucous, and granulomatous skin lesions have been described, often on the face or at mucocutaneous borders. Ulcerating lesions of the intestinal tract may be encountered; the stomach is usually spared. Complications include malabsorption, protein-losing enteropathy, or intestinal perforation. There may be signs of adrenal insufficiency and involvement of the bones, testes, epididymis, heart, and pancreas. Central nervous system disease may present as a space-occupying lesion or meningitis. Hepatic, splenic, and renal involvement is common but usually clinically silent.

DIAGNOSIS. Paracoccidioidomycosis must be differentiated from tuberculosis, histoplasmosis, sporotrichosis, leishmaniasis, yaws, and syphilis.

Multiple-budding *P. brasiliensis* can usually be demonstrated in wet mounts or 10 per cent KOH preparations from sputum or infective foci. Characteristic fungus cells can also be seen in hematoxylin-eosin stained slides from biopsy material, but special stains (e.g., periodic acid–Schiff, Gridley, and Gomori methenamine silver) demonstrate the cells much more effectively. Fungi can be recovered in two to four weeks on blood agar at 37° C (tissue phase) or on Sabouraud's agar at 30° C (saprobic phase). Cultures of blood, urine, bone marrow, spinal fluid, and biopsy specimens (liver, lymph node, intestine) may be helpful in appropriate instances. In one study of 39 cases, diagnosis could be made from direct examination of biopsy material in 95 per cent and by culture of these materials or sputum in 85 per cent. Animal inoculation is not necessary for diagnosis.

Serologic tests are useful in following the course of established disease. Precipitins are the first antibodies to appear, and the first to disappear with successful therapy. Complement-fixing (CF) antibodies appear later in a titer proportional to the severity of infection. Sera from 85 to 95 per cent of patients with active disease demonstrate CF titers ≥1:32. Numbers of precipitin bands formed in the immunodiffusion (ID) test rather than the actual antibody titer indicate the degree of disease activity. (ID and CF tests are available at the Centers for Disease Control in Atlanta.)

There is still a need for a specific paracoccidioidin skin test. The present preparations appear to share antigens with *H. capsulatum* and *S. schenckii*. There is no commercially available paracoccidioidin skin test reagent in the United States.

TREATMENT. The largest therapeutic experience is with sulfonamides. Their low cost, relatively low toxicity, and good gastrointestinal absorption are partially offset by slow response, a 40 per cent failure and relapse rate, and the occurrence of sulfonamide resistance. The recommended dose of sulfadiazine for adults is 4 to 6 grams per day. Once clinical improvement has occurred (a matter of weeks to months), dosage is reduced by half and continued for three to five years. Amphotericin B produces a higher response rate and is considered the drug of choice for disseminated disease. However, relapses occur even after total doses of 2 grams, whether or not sulfonamides are added to the regimen. Therapy should be continued until CF titers stabilize at a low level and the number of precipitin bands is reduced. *P. brasiliensis* is extraordinarily susceptible to miconazole in vitro (MIC ≤0.001 per milliliter), and there is a good clinical response. Ketoconazole and trimethoprim-sulfamethoxazole also appear highly promising and have the advantage of oral administration. Iodides, flucytosine, and 2-hydroxystilbamidine are without benefit.

PROGNOSIS. Disseminated paracoccidioidomycosis is generally fatal in the absence of therapy, with death occurring from extensive pulmonary disease, central nervous system lesions, intestinal perforation, or adrenal insufficiency.

Londero AT, Ramos CF, Lopes JOS: Progressive pulmonary paracoccidioidomycosis. A study of 34 cases observed in Rio Grande do Sul (Brazil). Mycopathologia 63:53, 1978. *Emphasizes the pulmonary aspects of this respiratory mycosis.*

Restrepo A, Gomez I, Cano LE, Arango MD, Gutierrez F, Sanin A, Robledo MA: Post-therapy status of paracoccidioidomycosis treated with ketoconazole. *In* Graybill JR (ed.): Proceedings of a Symposium on New Developments in Therapy for the Mycoses. Am J Med 74 (#1B):53–57, 1983. *The promise of ketoconazole is emphasized in this paper as well as in the following reference, which is somewhat more difficult to obtain: Del Negro G: Ketoconazole in paracoccidioidomycosis. A long-term study with prolonged follow-up. Rev Inst Med Trop Sao Paulo 24:27, 1982.*

Restrepo A, Greer DL, Vasconcellos M: Paracoccidioidomycosis: A review. Rev Med Vet Mycol 8:97, 1973. *A thorough review of the disease; a classic article.*

Restrepo A, Robledo M, Giraldo R, Hernandez H, Sierra F, Guiterrez L, Londono M, Lopez R, Calle G: The gamut of paracoccidioidomycosis. Am J Med 61:33, 1976. *An excellent review with an emphasis on pulmonary and extrapulmonary clinical manifestations, and helpful photographs.*

370. CRYPTOCOCCOSIS

DEFINITION. Cryptococcosis is a noncontagious, often opportunistic mycosis characterized by respiratory tract colonization, acute or chronic pulmonary infection, or hematogenous dissemination, often with meningitis.

ETIOLOGY. Pathogenic cryptococci are budding yeasts, 4 to 20 μm in diameter with a characteristic polysaccharide capsule. Buds are usually single and narrow-necked. Serotypes A and D, and B and C, respectively, show mating compatibility, and their respective perfect forms are *Filobasidiella neoformans* and *F. bacillispora*. Pathogenic cryptococci produce characteristic pigmentation on agar containing phenolic substrates or extracted birdseed (niger seed: *Guizotia abyssinica*), and progressive neurologic infection when injected intracerebrally into mice. They are not found as laboratory contaminants.

INCIDENCE AND PREVALENCE. Because there is no skin test or epidemiologically useful serologic test, the incidence and prevalence of cryptococcosis are unknown. However, the disease occurs worldwide, with several hundred new cases yearly in the United States. Most pulmonary infections are probably overlooked. Cryptococcal meningitis, which accounts for some 90 per cent of reported disease, is dramatic and seldom overlooked. Cryptococcosis has increased in incidence as immunosuppression has become more common and diagnostic techniques have improved and has emerged as a particular problem in patients with acquired immune deficiency syndrome (AIDS).

EPIDEMIOLOGY. Serotype A causes most disease in the United States, serotype D in Europe. Disease caused by serotypes B and C is largely restricted to southern California. Serotypes A and D are most commonly found in avian habitats, especially in pigeon dung. Up to 5×10^7 viable *C. neoformans* per gram of pigeon feces has been recovered from urban environments. Although the feet, beaks, crops, and gut contents of pigeons may harbor cryptococci, the birds are not infected. High humidity and protection from weathering or soil contact promote survival of *C. neoformans* in the environment. Indoor sites may harbor cryptococci more frequently than outdoor sites. Serotypes B and C are rarely recoverable from the environment, suggesting that *C. bacillispora* occupies a unique ecologic niche.

Because most patients give no history of contact with pigeons, infection probably results from inhalation of airborne organisms. A few infections have been traced to air conditioners in which birds have nested. Ocular cryptococcosis has been transmitted by corneal transplantation. Many animals are infected with cryptococci, but pose no threat to man.

PATHOGENESIS AND PATHOLOGY. Cryptococci in the environment are unencapsulated. Either these forms or the basidiospores of *Filobasidiella* are small enough to be inhaled. Encapsulation takes place in the lung, and virulence is related to the presence, but not the amount, of encapsulation. (Occasional infections with unencapsulated cryptococci occur.) Phagocytes can kill unencapsulated cryptococci, but phagocytosis of capsulated fungi is impaired, apparently because attached opsonic antibody is masked from phagocytes by capsular material. Studies in athymic nude mice suggest that cell-mediated immunity (CMI) is crucial to host defense. Patients with defective CMI (Hodgkin's disease and other lymphoreticular malignancies, corticosteroid therapy) are especially susceptible to cryptococcal dissemination. Neutropenia appears to confer no additional risk.

The histopathology of cryptococcosis varies from a foamy, gelatinous process to a more granulomatous response. Caseation, calcification, and fibrosis are rare. Cryptococci are fragile and may collapse during fixation, leading to a crescentic appearance. They stain poorly with hematoxylin-eosin, but well with methenamine silver and periodic acid–Schiff. Mucicarmine specifically stains capsular mucopolysaccharide.

CLINICAL MANIFESTATIONS. Respiratory tract colonization usually occurs in patients with underlying lung disease and may be transient or persistent.

Pulmonary Cryptococcosis. Manifestations include fever, malaise, pleuritic pain, cough, scanty sputum, and hemoptysis. A pleural effusion or friction rub may be present. Solitary or multiple nodules or nodular-confluent infiltrates, tumor-like masses, or miliary densities may be found on chest roentgenograms; any lobe may be involved. Cavitation is present in 10 to 16 per cent of cases. Hilar adenopathy may occur with advanced disease. Chronic infection is common; slowly progressive pulmonary involvement over four to nineteen years has been documented. Many such cases are diagnosed at thoracotomy for suspected malignancy. Although some cases are associated with alveolar proteinosis, only 10 per cent of all patients with pulmonary cryptococcosis have evidence of immunologic deficiency.

Disseminated Cryptococcosis. Manifestations of central nervous system cryptococcosis reflect exudate over the base of the brain (meningitis and hydrocephalus), extension of infection along perivascular spaces with involvement of the gray matter (encephalitis), direct invasion of the optic pathways (visual impairment), focal ischemic damage related to brain stem vasculitis, and cryptococcomas in the brain or spinal cord. Meningitis is the most common manifestation of systemic cryptococcosis, and its principal symptom is headache. Associated findings include mental changes (confusion, lethargy, personality alteration, defective memory, agitation, or frank psychosis); ocular symptoms (blurred vision, retrobulbar pain, diplopia, and photophobia); stiffness of the neck and back; nausea and vomiting; and fever, nystagmus, ataxia, aphasia, hearing deficits, cranial nerve palsies, seizures, and paresthesias. Up to 50 per cent of patients have papilledema or optic neuritis. Deterioration of mentation may reflect the development of hydrocephalus. Cryptococcal meningitis may be quite chronic, with disease presenting over weeks to months, or very rarely even years. *Skin and mucous membrane* involvement is seen in 10 to 15 per cent of cases and can take the form of papules, pustules, abscesses, chancres, nodules, or cellulitis followed by vesiculation and ulceration. *Bone* involvement occurs in 5 to 10 per cent of cases and may be mistaken for malignancy. Joint involvement is extremely rare. Other sites of invasion may include the *liver* (hepatitis, hepatic necrosis), *kidneys* (urinary tract symptoms, pyelonephritis, papillary necrosis), *prostate* (prostatism), *adrenals* (adrenal insufficiency), spleen, lymph nodes, and testes.

DIAGNOSIS. The differential diagnosis of pulmonary cryptococcosis includes diverse infections and malignancies. Cryptococcal meningitis may be confused with various hypoglycorrhachic syndromes, including tuberculosis and coccidioidomycosis. A primary psychiatric disorder is often suspected.

Sputum cultures are positive in only 20 per cent of pulmonary infections. Sixty per cent of cases have been diagnosed by exploratory thoracotomy for suspected malignancy in older series. Patients with positive sputum cultures should be evaluated for systemic infection, with cultures of blood and urine; biopsy and culture of skin lesions; and a lumbar puncture, whether or not central nervous system disease is apparent. Bone marrow aspiration, liver biopsy, and prostatic massage may also be indicated. In a recent series of patients with cancer and disseminated cryptococcosis, 15 per cent of blood cultures and 27 per cent of urine cultures were positive. Positive blood cultures do not routinely predict a poor therapeutic outcome.

In patients presenting with meningitis, the chest roentgenogram may or may not be abnormal. Sputum cultures should be obtained along with a careful baseline evaluation for other foci of infection. Characteristic cerebrospinal fluid (CSF) findings include elevated pressure (90 per cent of cases); pleocytosis (usually lymphocytic, sometimes polymorphonuclear) with a total white blood cell concentration generally below 500 per cubic millimeter; and hypoglycorrhachia (CSF glucose level less than 50 per cent of a simultaneously obtained blood glucose) (55 per cent of cases). When spun CSF sediment (or other body fluid) is mixed with a drop of India ink or nigrosin and examined under high dry magnification, cryptococci stand out against the darkened background by their halo-like capsules. The India ink preparation is positive in only about 50 per cent of cases of cryptococcal meningitis, whereas CSF cultures are eventually positive in about 95 per cent. Diagnostic yield is improved by examining CSF by cytologic techniques, looking carefully for extracranial sites of infection, obtaining large volumes of CSF exclusively for culture (~10 ml, provided that there are no contraindications to removal of this volume), repeated lumbar punctures, and, in particularly refractory diagnostic situations, tapping the cisterna magna or lateral ventricles. Reports of elevated CSF alcohol concentrations reflect detection of the alcohol used to prepare the skin for lumbar puncture.

The latex cryptococcal agglutination test (LCAT) is based upon the agglutination of latex spheres coated with anticryptococcal antibody in the presence of capsular antigen. Cryptococcal antigen is found in the CSF in up to 93 per cent of proven cases of cryptococcal meningitis, and may also be found in the blood. Patients with AIDS tend to have particularly high blood lecithin:cholesterol acyltransferase titers. In some cases, the LCAT is positive when all other tests of CSF are nondiagnostic. Serum or pleural fluid LCAT determinations may be helpful in the differential diagnosis of pneumonia in immunosuppressed patients. Tests for cryptococcal antibody are seldom of diagnostic value.

TREATMENT. Patients with respiratory tract colonization or resolving pulmonary infection and intact immunity seldom require therapy. Patients whose pulmonary cryptococcosis is diagnosed at thoracotomy should have careful postoperative evaluation for extrapulmonary disease, including a lumbar puncture. If none is found, therapy may be safely withheld in those with intact host defenses, provided that there is careful follow-up evaluation. If long-term follow-up is unlikely, antifungal therapy should be administered because there may be a 3 to 10 per cent risk of meningitis occurring up to three years following surgery. Patients with progressive pulmonary infection, especially if immunosuppressed, and all patients with extrapulmonary infection require systemic antifungal therapy.

Therapy for pulmonary cryptococcosis is poorly defined, but an arbitrary total dose of 1 gram of amphotericin B delivered intravenously over five to six weeks (up to 50 mg on alternate days) would be expected to control most cases. Immunosuppressed patients may require more aggressive therapy.

Therapeutic guidelines for cryptococcal meningitis are more clearly defined. Combination therapy with amphotericin B and flucytosine is currently favored on three bases: (1) the two drugs are synergistic against cryptococci in vitro; (2) flucytosine reliably crosses the blood-brain barrier, whereas amphotericin B does not; and (3) a national cooperative study has demonstrated that a six-week treatment course with intravenous amphotericin B (0.3 mg per kilogram per day) plus oral flucytosine (150 mg per kilogram per day) cured or improved more patients, produced fewer failures or relapses, and was associated with less nephrotoxicity than amphotericin B given alone for ten weeks in a dose of 0.4 mg per kilogram per day. Potential problems relate to the added toxicity of flucytosine (bone marrow suppression, liver function abnormalities, diarrhea, and rash). Flucytosine induced marrow suppression is usually reversible.

In patients who fail to show clinical improvement with combination chemotherapy, or those whose CSF cultures remain persistently positive, consideration must be given to delivery of amphotericin B into the lumbar sac, cisterna magna, or a lateral ventricle via an Ommaya reservoir or similar device. Complications related to amphotericin B irritability or catheter placement are common. Patients must also be carefully evaluated for hydrocephalus, since therapeutic CSF shunting may be required.

Too few clinical data are available to warrant the use of miconazole except in unusual circumstances. Ketoconazole may have some value in the management of extrameningeal infection, but its penetration of the blood-brain barrier is insufficient to permit its use in cryptococcal meningitis. Flucytosine should never be used alone because of a high risk of acquired drug resistance by the fungi.

PROGNOSIS. Prior to the amphotericin B era, 80 per cent of cryptococcal meningitis patients died within two years. With current therapeutic regimens, 80 to 90 per cent of patients can be cured, although more than one treatment course may be required. Adverse prognostic factors include lymphoreticular malignancy or corticosteroid therapy; cerebrospinal fluid with high opening pressure, a low glucose level, less than 20 leukocytes per cubic millimeter, and positive India ink preparations; cryptococci isolated from the blood or extraneural sites; and high titers of cryptococcal antigen in CSF and serum. Treated patients with persistently elevated titers of cryptococcal antigen have a tendency to relapse. Elevated CSF protein concentrations and positive India ink preparations may persist for years following curative therapy, and have no apparent prognostic significance.

PREVENTION. Hydrated lime and sodium hydroxide may be used to control cryptococcal growth in droppings of pet pigeons, but are otherwise impractical. Control of pigeon populations in urban areas might be expected to reduce the risk of acquiring cryptococcosis in this setting.

Bennett JE, Dismukes WE, Duma RJ, Medoff G, Sande MA, Gallis H, Leonard J, Fields BT Jr, Bradshaw M, Haywood H, McGee ZA, Cate TR, Cobbs CG, Warner JF, Alling DW: A comparison of amphotericin B alone and combined with flucytosine in the treatment of cryptococcal meningitis. N Engl J Med 301:126, 1979. *This important paper provides the rationale for the combined therapeutic approach to cryptococcal meningitis used in the United States at this time.*

Diamond RD, Bennett JE: Prognostic factors in cryptococcal meningitis a study in 111 cases. Ann Intern Med 80:176, 1974. *An excellent review of the factors predictive of early death in cryptococcal meningitis, as well as those factors that influence response to therapy.*

Hermann KJ, Powell KE, Christianson CS, Huggins PM, Larsh HW, Vivas JR,

Tosh FE: Pulmonary cryptococcosis: Clinical forms and treatment. A Center for Disease Control Cooperative Mycoses Study. Am Rev Respir Dis 108:1116, 1973. *This interesting paper compares the presentation of pulmonary cryptococcosis in patients in chronic chest hospitals with that of patients in other settings. Colonization, infection, and treatment are discussed.*

Perfect JR, Durack DT, Gallis HA: Cryptococcemia. Medicine 62:98, 1983. *Cryptococcemia identifies patients with poor prognoses, largely because of underlying disease. However, some patients will respond to aggressive therapy with amphotericin B and flucytosine.*

371. SPOROTRICHOSIS

DEFINITION. Sporotrichosis is a subacute or chronic noncontagious mycosis of the skin and regional lymphatics that results from the percutaneous introduction of *Sporothrix schenckii.* In some cases, pulmonary disease results from inhalation of spores. Rarely, there is lymphohematogenous dissemination to joints, bones, and skin.

ETIOLOGY. *Sporothrix (Sporotrichum) schenckii* is a dimorphic fungus. In tissues and at 37° C in vitro it is yeast-like, appearing as spherical or cigar-shaped budding cells. In nature (25° C), the fungus exists as sporulating hyphae that produce conidia of a size (2 to 3 μm) suitable to be inhaled. *S. schenckii* is commonly found on vegetation or wood, or in the soil; it is related to *Ceratocystis stenoceras,* a plant pathogen.

INCIDENCE AND PREVALENCE. Sporotrichosis is especially common in Mexico, Central America, and Brazil, and occurs more frequently in the United States than in Europe. Susceptibility is less related to sex, age, or race than to opportunities for environmental exposure. Skin test data suggest that sporotrichosis may occur as a subclinical infection, especially in nursery workers.

EPIDEMIOLOGY. *S. schenckii* is a potential cause of infection in anyone who has frequent contact with vegetation (e.g., sphagnum moss, timber, hay, thorn bushes). Thus, it is an occupational hazard for farmers, gardeners, florists, greenhouse workers, timber cutters, and others. Some cases may be transmitted by insect or animal bite. The source of infection may be obscure in those with pulmonary or visceral involvement. In the most famous outbreak of sporotrichosis, nearly 3000 otherwise healthy South African gold miners acquired lymphocutaneous sporotrichosis from brushing past contaminated mine timbers. Spread from patient to patient, pulmonary disease and disseminated disease were notable by their absence. Epidemiologic proof that alcoholism predisposes to sporotrichosis ("syndrome of the alcoholic rose gardener") is lacking.

PATHOGENESIS AND PATHOLOGY. *S. schenckii* enters the skin through apparent or inapparent trauma. Strains that multiply well at 35° C but poorly at 37° C can produce cutaneous lesions, but not lymphatic spread or systemic involvement. Strains that multiply well at 35 or 37° C are capable of producing lymphocutaneous or visceral disease. Cell-mediated immunity is important in determining the extent of disease, and immunosuppressed patients appear more likely to develop multifocal systemic spread of infection. Patients with disseminated but not localized lymphocutaneous sporotrichosis show evidence of depressed cell-mediated immunity (delayed-type hypersensitivity and lymphocyte transformation) that reverses with treatment.

The basic histopathologic pattern is a combination of suppuration and granulomas, occasionally with caseation necrosis. Chronic cutaneous lesions demonstrate prominent pseudoepitheliomatous hyperplasia and may be confused with malignancies.

CLINICAL MANIFESTATIONS. In lymphocutaneous sporotrichosis, which accounts for 75 per cent of cases, a single lesion usually develops on an exposed skin surface, commonly following trauma. The pimple, wart, pustule, ulcer, abscess, or chancre fails to heal and typically spreads up the extremity over days to weeks, evoking a series of subcutaneous nontender nodular lesions along the thickened lymphatics. The nodules may ulcerate, releasing thin pus. Systemic signs and symptoms of infection are notably absent. Incision and drainage and antibacterial drugs are without benefit. The disease may slowly progress over months or even years; a few cases heal spontaneously.

In 20 per cent of cases, the process is strictly limited to the site of introduction in the skin ("fixed"). It is likely that this disease pattern is produced by *S. schenckii* strains that grow poorly at 37° C (see above). Lacking the diagnostic appearance of nodules following lymphatics, this form of sporotrichosis may be quite difficult to diagnose.

About 50 cases of pulmonary sporotrichosis have been reported. Disease may occur acutely, but more frequently presents as a chronic (thin-walled) cavitary process involving upper lobes and apices, and accurately mimicking pulmonary tuberculosis. Extracutaneous sporotrichosis is very rare. It may result from direct, deep implantation of fungi; from direct contiguous spread of lymphocutaneous disease; or by hematogenous spread from apparent or inapparent cutaneous or pulmonary loci. Common sites of dissemination include joints (especially knees, ankles, wrists, and small joints of the hands and feet) and bones (especially the tibia), sometimes with pathologic fractures. When joint disease occurs in the absence of a primary lymphocutaneous focus (as it does in more than 80 per cent of cases), it is classically confused with rheumatoid arthritis, sarcoidosis, villonodular synovitis, or gout. In immunocompromised patients with multifocal disease, there is often abrupt development of widespread subcutaneous nodules in a hematogenous distribution. Multiarticular joint disease may be present, and multifocal osteolytic foci may be visible roentgenographically. Cultures of the urine, bone marrow, and rarely even the blood may be positive. There are a few recorded cases of central nervous system sporotrichosis; chronic meningitis may be present.

DIAGNOSIS. The differential diagnosis of lymphocutaneous sporotrichosis includes sporotrichoid granulomas caused by atypical mycobacterial infections, other cutaneous mycoses, leishmaniasis, syphilis, anthrax, tularemia, cat scratch disease, and even furunculosis. Pulmonary sporotrichosis resembles pulmonary tuberculosis; sometimes the diseases coexist.

The diagnosis of lymphocutaneous sporotrichosis on histopathologic grounds is very difficult, as the fungi may not be easily demonstrable. Direct immunofluorescence or immunoperoxidase staining may be helpful, but is not generally available. *S. schenckii* is also difficult to identify directly in the sputum. In deep lesions, fungi may be demonstrable with special stains (e.g., methenamine silver, periodic acid–Schiff). Regardless of the locus of infection, diagnosis is made most accurately by recovering *S. schenckii* in culture. These fungi grow well on most standard media; cultures should be held at least four weeks before being discarded as negative. Conversion to yeast form in vitro or animal inoculation may assist in identification. Rarely, *S. schenckii* may be recovered from the sputum in the absence of any demonstrable disease process, thus reflecting the possibility of asymptomatic colonization.

Serologic tests are useful in establishing the diagnosis of extracutaneous or systemic forms of sporotrichosis when distinct clinical features are lacking. The yeast cell and latex particle agglutination tests are more sensitive than immunodiffusion or complement fixation techniques. In general, patients with extracutaneous disease have higher titers than those with lymphocutaneous involvement. A slide latex agglutination titer of 1:8 or above is considered presumptive evidence of sporotrichosis by the Centers for Disease Control, Atlanta. The test has limited prognostic value, since antibody levels may show little change during or after convalescence.

A sporotrichosis skin test is not commercially available.

TREATMENT. The treatment of choice for lymphocutaneous sporotrichosis is saturated solution of potassium iodide (SSKI). Its mechanism of action is unclear. Daily dosage is increased in dropwise fashion (usually 50 mg per drop) in a palatable vehicle until 3 to 5 grams or more is being administered each day. If signs of toxicity ensue (e.g., indigestion, rash, lacrimation, parotid swelling), dosage may have to be reduced. Amphotericin B is indicated when SSKI fails.

SSKI may be efficacious for noncavitary pulmonary sporotrichosis, but neither SSKI nor amphotericin B shows clear therapeutic superiority in cavitary infection. Resectional surgery may be indicated. Disseminated sporotrichosis is generally treated with intravenous amphotericin B (minimal dose, 2 grams), together with local intralesional therapy, arthrotomy, and other indicated drainage procedures. Amphotericin B appears substantially superior to SSKI in disseminated infection. Flucytosine, miconazole, and ketoconazole are poorly effective in any form of the disease.

PROGNOSIS. Cutaneous, lymphocutaneous, and mucocutaneous sporotrichosis commonly remit and relapse for years without therapy. Spontaneous cures are unknown in disseminated disease. The natural history and, indeed, the incidence and prevalence of pulmonary sporotrichosis are unknown. Cavitary pulmonary disease may be curable medically, but more often requires surgery. Untreated chronic pulmonary sporotrichosis is usually fatal.

Jung JY, Almond CH, Elkadi A, Tenorio A: Role of surgery in the management of pulmonary sporotrichosis. J Thorac Cardiovasc Surg 77:234, 1979. *A discussion of the disease process and the limitations of medical and surgical management.*

Kwon-Chung KJ: Comparison of isolates of *Sporothrix schenckii* obtained from fixed cutaneous lesions with isolates from other types of lesions. J Infect Dis 139:424, 1979. *Provides important information relating patterns of clinical disease with temperature optima for* S. schenckii.

Wilson DE, Mann JJ, Bennett JE, Utz P: Clinical features of extracutaneous sporotrichosis. Medicine 46:265, 1967. *Still the best reference concerning extracutaneous sporotrichosis.*

372. CANDIDIASIS (Candidosis)

DEFINITION. Candidiasis is a general term for a variety of local and systemic processes sharing in common colonization or infection by *Candida* species.

ETIOLOGY. The most common etiologic agent is *Candida albicans.* Others include *C. tropicalis, parapsilosis, stellatoidea, krusei, parakrusei, pseudotropicalis,* and *guilliermondi. Torulopsis glabrata* may be reclassified as *Candida glabrata. Candida* species are biphasic, but not in the usual sense (i.e., temperature or host dependent). Instead, yeasts (the usual colonizing form) may assume a pseudomycelial configuration, especially during tissue invasion. (*T. glabrata* remains yeastlike). Pseudomycelia result from the sequential budding of yeasts (blastospores), with resultant branching chains of elongated organisms, clearly delineated by constrictions. *C. albicans* can be readily identified in vitro by the production of unconstricted germ tubes within two to four hours of exposure to serum.

INCIDENCE AND PREVALENCE. Candidiasis occurs worldwide. Superficial infections such as thrush, paronychia, and intertrigo are universal. Invasive candidiasis has become a problem with the advent of antibiotics (destruction of normal inhibitory bacterial flora) and the use of myelotoxic or immunosuppressive agents, especially corticosteroids. Candidiasis is the most common opportunistic mycosis in the world.

EPIDEMIOLOGY. *Candida* species can be found in nature, but more commonly originate with man. *C. albicans* is found in the oropharynx, gastrointestinal tract, and vagina of a variable proportion of normal persons, but only rarely on the skin. Non-*albicans* species frequently colonize the skin. Vaginal colonization is increased by diabetes, pregnancy, and oral contraceptive agents. Carriage at all sites is increased by antibiotics. Unlike most other fungi, *C. albicans* is transmissible (e.g., from colonized birth canal to neonatal oropharynx, between sexual partners, by hands of medical attendants). Cutaneous infection generally requires skin trauma, maceration, and persistent moisture. Systemic candidiasis occurs most frequently in a hospital setting, among severely ill, antibiotic-treated patients with breaches of normal mucocutaneous barriers (e.g., indwelling intravascular lines or Foley catheters; gastrointestinal ulcerations from chemotherapeutic agents; burns or gastrointestinal surgery). Endocarditis may follow intravenous drug abuse, prolonged intravenous therapy, or placement of a prosthetic heart valve.

PATHOGENESIS AND PATHOLOGY. Candidiasis is a suppurative infection that sometimes has a granulomatous component. Both granulocytes and cell-mediated immunity are important in host defense. Polymorphonuclear leukocytes (PMNs) kill ingested yeasts by oxidative and nonoxidative mechanisms. *C. albicans* sometimes escapes the PMNs by germ tube penetration of the leukocyte wall. Pseudomycelia are attacked by apposition of PMNs, with exocytosis of lysosomal enzymes. Serum factors serve as opsonins and cause *Candida* clumping, assisting in bloodstream clearance. Neutropenia is a major risk factor for *Candida* dissemination. Patients with defective cell-mediated immune mechanisms (AIDS, the syndrome of chronic mucocutaneous candidiasis) are more susceptible to thrush and esophagitis than to hematogenous *Candida* dissemination.

CLINICAL MANIFESTATIONS. ***Mucocutaneous Infection.*** *Thrush* is characterized by a creamy to gray pseudomembrane, patchy or confluent, that covers the tongue, buccal mucosa, or other oropharyngeal surfaces. Ulceration and necrosis may be present. Membrane removal leaves a red, oozing base. Laryngeal involvement results in hoarseness. *Esophagitis* is often an extension of oropharyngeal disease, may be manifested by retrosternal pain and dysphagia, and has a highly suggestive appearance on barium swallow. *Intestinal candidiasis* is commonly asymptomatic, but is a major source of hematogenous invasion in the immunosuppressed. *Perianal* candidal overgrowth may follow antibiotic therapy, and produces or aggravates pruritus ani. *Intertrigo* involves the axillae, groins, inframammary folds, and other warm, moist areas. Lesions may be red and oozing or dry and scaly, with sharp scalloped borders and satellite vesicles, pustules, or bullae. *Paronychia* often follows chronic exposure of the hands or feet to moisture. The nails may become hardened, thickened, grooved, and discolored *(onychomycosis). Vulvovaginitis* is characterized by a variable discharge and pruritus. *Balanitis* is manifested by superficial penile erosions and pustules.

Chronic mucocutaneous candidiasis is a rare syndrome based upon limited T cell immunodeficiency. One fifth of patients show a familial tendency. In about half the cases, there is associated endocrinopathy (especially hypoparathyroidism, hypoadrenalism, hypothyroidism, or diabetes mellitus). Clinical features include persistent superficial *Candida* infection of the skin, scalp, nails, and mucous membranes, often in association with a dermatophyte infection. Disease may begin at any age and be extensive or very limited. Associated findings include alopecia, depigmentation, cheilosis, blepharitis, keratoconjunctivitis, and corneal ulcers. In the most severe cases, there is horn formation with thick, plaque-like, hyperkeratotic scales (*Candida* granuloma) involving the skin or nails. Immunologic abnormalities include decreased or absent response to *Candida* antigens by skin test or by tests of cell-mediated immunity in vitro.

Systemic Candidiasis. Most cases of systemic candidiasis are due to *C. albicans* and *C. tropicalis,* with an increasing number attributable to *C. glabrata.* Clinical manifestations of *C. albicans* and *C. tropicalis* infection tend to be apparent in three specific "target organs":

Eyes: A variable proportion of patients has *Candida* endophthalmitis, with single or multiple raised, white, fluffy chorioretinal lesions, in the presence or absence of overlying vitreous haze. Lesions are usually in the macular area within easy range of the ophthalmoscope and extend forward into the vitreous. They serve as a major clue to diagnosis and are a potential cause of blindness.

Kidneys: Renal involvement is attributable to the ability of bloodborne *Candida* to invade the renal tubules directly. Manifestations include diffuse renal abscesses, papillary necrosis, obstruction of the ureters by sloughed papillae or *Candida* balls (bezoars), and progressive renal insufficiency with flank pain and dysuria. *Candida* pyelonephritis must be differentiated from *Candida* cystitis, a benign infection often associated with prolonged catheterization or vaginitis.

Skin: Maculonodular skin lesions on an erythematous base may mark the occurrence of hematogenous *Candida* infection, sometimes with accompanying arthralgias or myalgias. The temptation to disregard these lesions as "pimples" must be overcome, lest a major clue to a lethal disease be overlooked.

Other manifestations of systemic candidiasis may include osteomyelitis (especially vertebral), arthritis, meningitis, and cerebral, myocardial, hepatic, splenic, and thyroid abscesses. Abscesses at the latter sites are seldom appreciated clinically. *Candida* pneumonia is rare. Although hematogenous involvement of the lungs is common, the miliary pulmonary lesions are usually too small to be seen on a chest roentgenogram.

Endocarditis. *C. albicans* endocarditis is most common in a setting of prolonged intravenous therapy, hyperalimentation, or a cardiac valve prosthesis. Non-*albicans* species are most frequent with intravenous narcotics abuse. Fungal valvular lesions are large and friable. Embolization and occlusion of large blood vessels are more common than in bacterial endocarditis; intracerebral lesions are common.

DIAGNOSIS. Superficial infections are diagnosed by examination of scrapings or swabs of infected lesions in the presence of 10 per cent KOH. *Candida* organisms can also be demonstrated by Gram stain. Endocarditis is diagnosed by blood cultures, echocardiographic demonstration of bulky valvular vegetations, or demonstration of fungi in an excised embolus. Systemic candidiasis may be difficult to diagnose. The presence of heavy colonization at usual carriage sites sets the stage for systemic disease, but does not prove that dissemination has occurred. The most reliable evidence of systemic candidiasis is biopsy demonstration of tissue invasion (hematoxylin-eosin or special fungal stains) or recovery of fungi from fluid in a closed body cavity (e.g., CSF, pleural or peritoneal fluid). Blood cultures are most likely to be positive when vented bottles and biphasic media are used. However, positive blood cultures or cultures from the tips of an intravenous line do not necessarily establish the diagnosis of systemic candidiasis, because fungemia may clear spontaneously with the removal of an intravascular focus of infection. Positive urine cultures may indicate cystitis or invasive upper urinary tract disease. The differentiation is not assisted by quantitative urine cultures (even 10^3 *Candida* per milliliter may be associated with pyelonephritis), fluorescent antibody coating studies, or the presence of pseudomycelia in the urine. Declining renal function and evidence of renal destruction (papillary necrosis), urinary tract fungal bezoars, and fungi from catheterized renal pelvis urine suggest that invasive disease is present. Positive sputum cultures usually indicate respiratory tract colonization; pneumonia is relatively rare and must be documented by invasive means. Meningitis is usually manifested by PMN pleocytosis, hypoglycorrhachia, and a positive CSF culture in 40 to 45 per cent of cases.

Skin testing is not helpful in diagnosing candidiasis, because delayed type hypersensitivity to *Candida* antigens is so common among normal persons that the test is used to screen for cutaneous anergy. *Serologic* studies based upon detection of antibodies (precipitins or agglutinins) may be falsely positive or negative, and do not clearly differentiate heavy colonization from systemic infection, although rising titers must be considered compatible with dissemination. Tests for specific cell wall carbohydrates (mannose or arabitol by gas liquid chromatography; mannan by various immunoassays) show great promise in the early diagnosis of invasive disease, and have the advantage of not relying on an immune response by an immunocompromised host.

TREATMENT. Topical preparations (nystatin, amphotericin B, clotrimazole, miconazole, haloprogin, gentian violet) may be used in the treatment of mucocutaneous infections. Chronic mucocutaneous candidiasis syndrome may respond to topical or systemic therapeutic agents (in particular, amphotericin B), but often relapses when medication is discontinued. Ketoconazole is particularly useful in this disease because it can be given indefinitely with relatively few adverse effects. Transfer factor and other immunologically active reagents have been used with variable success.

Systemic candidiasis should be treated with amphotericin B. The removal of precipitating factors (especially intravenous lines) is very important. Because removal of an intravascular focus does not guarantee that fungemia will be self-limited, treatment should be instituted in immunocompromised patients. In acutely ill patients, dosage should be raised quickly to 0.5 to 1.0 mg per kilogram of body weight per day, as tolerated. Alternate-day therapy can be employed and the dosage lowered once clinical improvement is apparent. The usual total dosage recommendation is 1.5 to 2.0 grams, but higher dosage or prolonged therapy may be required in refractory cases. Flucytosine may be added, using the same rationale as that employed for cryptococcosis (see Ch. 370). There are too few clinical data with either miconazole or ketoconazole to judge their value in systemic candidiasis; thus, amphotericin B remains the drug of choice.

Candida cystitis is often cured by Foley catheter removal and the substitution of intermittent ("straight") catheterization. Eradication of infection in those who must have an indwelling catheter, or those with non-catheter-related infection, may be attempted with amphotericin B bladder rinses; with low dose short-course intravenous therapy (amphotericin is excreted in the urine at a therapeutic level for days following intravenous dosing); or even with oral flucytosine, provided no catheter is in place. This is one of the few situations in which flucytosine may be used alone. Ketoconazole is largely metabolized by the liver; therefore, little active ketoconazole reaches the kidneys. There is an approximate 50 per cent failure rate when ketoconazole is used to treat candiduria.

Endocarditis is essentially incurable without valve replacement. Surgical treatment should be accompanied by a six- to ten-week course of amphotericin B and flucytosine, but cure is elusive. Endophthalmitis generally responds to amphotericin B and flucytosine. Local (sub-Tenon) treatment is employed in addition by many ophthalmologists.

PROGNOSIS. Chronic mucocutaneous candidiasis can be ameliorated, but rarely cured. Endocarditis patients often show evidence of disease activity after having been declared cured. Systemic candidiasis is curable, especially in those with intact immune mechanisms. Systemic candidiasis is common but difficult to document in febrile neutropenic patients. Empiric therapy with amphotericin B has led to an improved prognosis for recovery in these patients.

PREVENTION. Systemic candidiasis is avoided by adherence to sound principles of antibiotic use (avoidance of excessive dosage, duration, or breadth of antimicrobial spectrum) and avoidance of indwelling intravascular devices in favor of steel needles. If plastic cannulas are used, they must be changed at least every three days. In immunosuppressed patients, lowering colonization of the gastrointestinal tract with nystatin or ketoconazole is widely practiced, although its efficacy in preventing systemic spread has been questioned. Foley catheters should be avoided whenever possible.

Edwards JE Jr (moderator): Severe candidal infections. Clinical perspective, immune defense mechanisms, and current concepts of therapy. Ann Intern Med 89:91, 1978. *An up-to-date review of systemic candidiasis and chronic mucocutaneous candidiasis in the format of an Interdepartmental Clinical Case Conference from UCLA.*

Edwards JE Jr: Candida endophthalmitis. *In* Remington JS, Swartz MN (eds.): Current Clinical Topics in Infectious Diseases. Vol. 3. New York, McGraw-Hill Book Co., 1982, pp 381–397. *A timely review of this extremely important manifestation of hematogenous* Candida *dissemination.*

Edwards JE Jr, Foos RY, Montgomerie JZ, Guze LB: Ocular manifestations of *Candida* septicemia: Review of seventy-six cases of hematogenous *Candida* endophthalmitis. Medicine 53:47, 1974. *A review of this important complication of* Candida *septicemia.*

Eras P, Goldstein MJ, Sherlock P: *Candida* infection of the gastrointestinal tract.

Medicine 51:367, 1972. *An important paper that describes the types of lesions that occur in this frequent source of* Candida *sepsis.*
Fisher JF, Chew WH, Shadomy S, Duma RJ, Mayhall CG, House WC: Urinary tract infections due to Candida albicans. Rev Infect Dis 4:1107, 1982. *This paper provides valuable guidelines for the differentiation of renal and bladder* Candida *infection and recommends appropriate therapy for each.*
Kirkpatrick CH, Rich RR, Bennett JE: Chronic mucocutaneous candidiasis: Model-building in cellular immunity. Ann Intern Med 74:955, 1972. *A definitive review of this unique disease.*
Meunier-Carpentier F, Kiehn TE, Armstrong D: Fungemia in the immunocompromised host: Changing patterns, antigenemia, high mortality. Am J Med 71:363, 1981. *This paper documents the increasing importance of* C. tropicalis *as an opportunistic pathogen in immunocompromised patients.*
Pizzo P, Robichaud K, Gill F, Witebsky F: Empiric antibiotic and antifungal therapy for cancer patients with prolonged fever and granulocytopenia. Am J Med 72:101, 1982. *Premortem diagnosis of candidiasis in immunocompromised patients is accomplished in fewer than 40 per cent of cases. Hence, empiric antifungal therapy has become important in the management of persistently febrile leukopenic patients. This important paper explores the rationale and approach to therapy.*

373. ASPERGILLOSIS

DEFINITION. Aspergillosis is a poorly descriptive term encompassing a variety of disease processes that share an etiologic relationship with *Aspergillus* species. The dominant element may be any of the following:

1. *Colonization* of previously damaged respiratory tissues (aspergillary bronchitis, aspergilloma).
2. *Allergy* to inhaled spores or to fungi colonizing the bronchial tree (atopic asthma, allergic bronchopulmonary aspergillosis, extrinsic allergic alveolitis).
3. *Invasion* of (a) the lung, especially in immunocompromised hosts, with or without systemic spread, or (b) other loci, e.g. eyes, external ear canals, paranasal sinuses, burn wounds, prosthetic heart valves.
4. *Intoxication and/or neoplasm,* especially with ingestion of aflatoxin.

ETIOLOGY. *Aspergillus* species are ubiquitous and can be isolated from numerous sources (e.g., grains, leaves, grasses, soil, refrigerator walls, wet paint, construction and fireproofing materials). Their spores are frequently isolated from the air and are constantly being inhaled. The rarity of disease attests to the potency of normal host defenses. Although more than 300 *Aspergillus* species are known, only a few thermotolerant species are ordinarily pathogenic for man: *A. fumigatus* (the most common overall), *A. flavus* (especially in upper airway disease and sinusitis), *A. niger* (especially in external otitis), *A. nidulans, A. terreus, A. sydowi, A. clavatus,* and *A. glaucus.* In the tissues, *Aspergillus* hyphae are uniform, 2 to 7 μm in diameter, septate, and dichotomously branched with angles of ~ 45 degrees. These features are not diagnostic. There may be confusion with *Candida* pseudomycelia, *Pseudoallescheria* hyphae, or other fungi. *Aspergillus* species grow rapidly on most media and can be differentiated by their pattern of sporulation. They are rarely found in normal sputum or gastrointestinal contents.

INCIDENCE AND PREVALENCE. Aspergillosis is increasing in prevalence, particularly in patients with chronic respiratory disease or immunosuppression. Among the immunosuppressed, aspergillosis is second only to candidiasis as an opportunistic mycosis, and both are increasing in frequency because of better methods of controlling bacterial infection.

EPIDEMIOLOGY. *Aspergillus* infections occur worldwide, with no regard to age, sex, race, or occupation. Allergic bronchopulmonary aspergillosis is more common in the United Kingdom than in the United States, but is increasing in frequency in this country. Outbreaks of invasive aspergillosis in burned or immunosuppressed patients have followed exposure to spores released by hospital construction, contaminated air conditioning ducts and filters, and fireproofing materials above false ceilings. Filtration of hospital air results in lowered spore counts. Aflatoxin-related hepatotoxicity and malignancies have been documented in African tribes among whom spoiled peanuts are a major dietary component. *Aspergillus* infections are not considered transmissible from animals to man or from man to man.

SPECIFIC SYNDROMES (INCLUDING PATHOGENESIS, PATHOLOGY, CLINICAL MANIFESTATIONS, DIAGNOSIS, TREATMENT, AND PROGNOSIS). ***Colonization.*** *Aspergillary bronchitis* is characterized by the growth of sporulating mycelia on the surface of the bronchial mucosa, without tissue invasion. The mucosa shows only a mild inflammatory response. Bronchial casts containing mucus and mycelia may be expectorated.

Aspergillomas are fungal balls composed of tangled degenerating hyphae and amorphous debris that lie free in pulmonary cavities lined partially by modified bronchial epithelium. There is little surrounding inflammation. The cavities have generally been produced by other disease processes (tuberculosis, sarcoidosis, bronchiectasis, bullae, infarcts, necrotic neoplasms) and are particularly common in the upper lobes. The typical radiographic appearance is that of a freely movable intracavitary mass surrounded on its superior surface by a crescent of air (crescent sign, Monod's sign). This sign is not pathognomonic and may be mimicked by necrotizing tumors or pulmonary infarcts, echinococcal cysts, or other fungal balls. The natural history of aspergillomas is unknown, but some may undergo spontaneous liquefaction and absorption. Invasiveness is extremely rare, but may occur. Hemoptysis is encountered in 60 to 75 per cent of cases and is sometimes life threatening. Sputum cultures are often negative. Diagnosis may be established by bronchoscopy, bronchial brushing, or percutaneous transthoracic needle aspiration. Diagnosis may be assisted by the finding of elevated *Aspergillus* precipitins in the serum. Systemic antifungal therapy has been valueless. Intrabronchial amphotericin B therapy may occasionally be successful. Treatment is probably not indicated except with life-threatening hemoptysis. Under these circumstances, segmental resection or lobectomy is the treatment of choice. Selective bronchial artery embolization has been used in nonsurgical candidates.

Allergy. *Allergic bronchopulmonary aspergillosis* (ABPA) occurs in up to 20 per cent of patients with asthma and is related to the development of tissue hypersensitivity to antigens of *Aspergillus* species (usually *A. fumigatus*) that colonize the bronchial mucous membranes. Its immunopathogenesis includes type I hypersensitivity (IgE-mediated) with bronchospasm and type III (immune complex) and perhaps type IV (cell-mediated) hypersensitivity with permanent bronchial damage. The *Aspergillus* skin test is characterized by an early wheal and flare response (type I) and sometimes by a more delayed (four to six hours) Arthus (type III) reaction. Serum levels of IgE (both *Aspergillus*-specific and nonspecific) are significantly raised, and precipitating antibodies (involved in the type III response) are usually demonstrable in the serum. Clinical features include episodic bronchospasm, peripheral blood eosinophilia, history of transient or fixed pulmonary infiltrates (especially upper lobes), and central saccular bronchiectasis. Additional, less constant features include *Aspergillus* species in smears or cultures of sputum, eosinophils in the sputum, history of expectoration of brown plugs or flecks, and fever. Mucous impactions may result in segmental atelectasis or more generalized lung collapse. Irreversible complications of ABPA include pulmonary fibrosis, lung retraction, and bronchiectasis. In rare instances, aspergillomas may mimic some of the immunologic features of ABPA, and aspergilloma is a rare but recognized complication of the saccular bronchiectasis of ABPA.

Patients with a history of asthma and pulmonary infiltrates should be skin tested with *Aspergillus* antigen. If positive, serum should be obtained for determination of IgE and *Aspergillus* precipitins. The treatment of choice is prednisone in a dose of 0.5 mg per kilogram of body weight per day for two weeks, followed by the same dose on alternate days until the IgE serum level drops to a stable titer. At this point, steroid therapy is gradually withdrawn. The steroids appear to change the bronchial milieu to one unfavorable for colonization by *Aspergillus* species, as well as interfering with pulmonary hypersensitivity reactions. Some patients require no further therapy. Others will have recurrent attacks of ABPA (characteristically preceded by a jump in the IgE titer). These patients may require prednisone indefinitely.

In patients with *atopic asthma,* the inhalation of *Aspergillus* spores results in immediate bronchospasm based upon a type I immune response. There is no spore germination in bronchial passageways.

Extrinsic allergic alveolitis occurs predominantly in nonatopic patients who inhale *Aspergillus* spores, and is characterized by dyspnea, dry cough, malaise, myalgias, rales, diffuse micronodular infiltrates, and serum precipitins to *Aspergillus.* The skin test shows an Arthus response, with or without the preceding wheal and flare reaction. Similar processes include farmer's lung, maple bark stripper's disease, pigeon breeder's disease, and bagassosis.

Invasion. *Chronic necrotizing pulmonary aspergillosis* is an indolent cavitary process, often with mycetoma formation, that occurs predominantly in middle-aged patients with underlying pulmonary parenchymal disease. It is distinct from aspergilloma in that invasion of pulmonary tissue is clearly present. However, it is only semi-invasive when compared with the opportunistic form of infection described later. Patients have fever, productive cough, and pulmonary infiltrates with cavities. Demonstration of lung invasion by *Aspergillus* species and response to amphotericin B support the diagnosis, as does an elevated *Aspergillus* precipitin titer.

Opportunistic pulmonary aspergillosis occurs characteristically in patients with hematologic and lymphoreticular malignancy or organ transplants, generally in the face of intense immunosuppression, and often following the use of various antibacterial drug regimens for septic episodes. The basis whereby immunosuppression sets the stage for invasive pulmonary aspergillosis is unclear, since normal host defenses against this fungus are not fully understood. Apparently macrophages are responsible primarily for the killing of conidia, whereas neutrophils attack mycelia. Full-blown invasive disease occurs in settings in which there is damage to both arms of the immune system. However, even isolated neutrophil defects such as chronic granulomatous disease are characterized by an increased incidence of pulmonary infection and osteomyelitis caused by *Aspergillus* species.

Opportunistic pulmonary aspergillosis is characterized by widespread bronchial erosion and ulceration, followed by invasion of the pulmonary vasculature with thrombosis, embolization, and infarction. Clinical manifestations include a necrotizing patchy bronchopneumonia with or without signs and symptoms of accompanying hemorrhagic pulmonary infarction. The disease process may evolve slowly or rapidly, and abscesses may appear at the site of an apparently resolving pneumonia. In many instances, the abscesses have "crescent signs" and have been referred to as aspergillomas. However, they contain sequestra of infarcted lung tissue and invasive *Aspergillus* infection, and are thus distinct from the benign aspergillomas described earlier. In about 60 per cent of cases, the disease process remains confined to the lungs. In the others, there is hematogenous spread to the brain, liver, kidneys, gastrointestinal tract, thyroid, heart, skin, and other sites. Sometimes the pulmonary process itself is inapparent. In all infected loci, the disease is characterized by vascular invasion and tissue infarction and necrosis. Suppuration predominates; granulomatous response is rare. The differential diagnosis includes mucormycosis, nocardiosis, and necrotizing bacterial pneumonia. Any of these processes may also coexist with aspergillosis.

Invasive aspergillosis is commonly fatal. For patient survival, an aggressive approach to diagnosis and treatment is required. Patients whose therapy begins more than three to four days after the initiation of the infection seldom survive. Even with aggressive culturing, only one tenth to one third of patients have positive sputum cultures for *Aspergillus.* Recovery of *Aspergillus* species from the nasal mucous membrane may signal that deeper respiratory infection is taking place. If other conditions permit, diagnostic maneuvers should include transtracheal aspiration, fiberoptic bronchoscopy with brushing and transbronchial biopsy, percutaneous transthoracic pulmonary aspiration, or open lung biopsy. Fungi can be seen in impression smears and biopsies by Gomori methenamine silver or periodic acid–Schiff stains, but are also visible with hematoxylin-eosin. Identification may be hastened by immunofluorescent staining. Blood, urine, and CSF cultures are rarely positive. Skin tests and precipitin tests are of no value in diagnosis. Experiences with detection of circulating *Aspergillus* antigen by radioimmunoassay techniques provide hope that serologic methods may play a more useful role in diagnosis.

The treatment of choice is amphotericin B. The dosage should be raised rapidly to 0.5 to 1.0 mg per kilogram of body weight per day, as tolerated. Treatment may be given on alternate days once improvement is underway. Optimal total dosage is unsettled, but should probably be no less than 2 grams. Although some patients have received flucytosine or rifampin in combination with amphotericin B, proof of the superiority of such regimens is not available. The efficacy of granulocyte transfusions in leukopenic patients is unproven. Miconazole and ketoconazole are not useful in the management of aspergillosis.

Other loci: Aspergillosis is the most common fungal infection of the paranasal sinuses in otherwise healthy patients. Roentgenograms show opacification, with or without bony erosion. Surgery is usually sufficient for cure. Immunosuppressed patients may exhibit facial cellulitis and palatal necrosis reminiscent of mucormycosis. Aspergillosis is a rare but devastating complication of burn wounds. Antibiotics and local debridement are seldom effective. Amputation is often required for cure. *Aspergillus* infection of prosthetic cardiac valves is a rare but devastating complication of cardiac surgery. Blood cultures are virtually never positive. Antifungal antibiotics are ineffective, and valve replacement is necessary if there is to be any possibility of cure. Invasive cutaneous aspergillosis has occurred at the site of taping of extremities to boards used to stabilize intravenous infusions. Invasive eye disease may follow local trauma, surgery, or hematogenous spread of infection from other sites.

Binder RE, Faling LJ, Pugatch RD, Mahasaen C, Snider GL: Chronic necrotizing pulmonary aspergillosis: A discrete clinical entity. Medicine 61:109, 1982. *This paper calls attention to the fact that a form of limited invasive aspergillosis can occur in patients with underlying pulmonary parenchymal disease but little immunosuppression.*

Rinaldi MG: Invasive aspergillosis. Rev Infect Dis 5:1061, 1983. *A current review of the pathogenesis and pathologic and clinical features of this increasingly common infectious disease.*

Rosenberg M, Patterson R, Mintzer R, Cooper BJ, Roberts M, Harris KE: Clinical and immunologic criteria for the diagnosis of allergic bronchopulmonary aspergillosis. Ann Intern Med 86:405, 1977. *The best reference concerning allergic bronchopulmonary aspergillosis. Authors from the same group define aspects of management of this syndrome in Ann Intern Med 96:286, 1982.*

Weiner MH, Talbot GH, Gerson SL, Filice G, Cassileth PA: Antigen detection in diagnosis of invasive aspergillosis: Utility in controlled, blinded trials. Ann Intern Med 99:777, 1983. *This study indicates that radioimmunoassay for* A. fumigatus *antigen is a highly specific and moderately sensitive serodiagnostic test for invasive pulmonary aspergillosis.*

Young RC, Bennett JE, Vogel CL, Carbonne PP, DeVita VT: Aspergillosis. The spectrum of the disease in 98 patients. Medicine 49:147, 1970. Meyer RD, Young LS, Armstrong D, Yu B: Aspergillosis complicating neoplastic disease. Am J Med 56:6, 1973. *The best two references concerning invasive pulmonary and systemic aspergillosis.*

374. MUCORMYCOSIS (Phycomycosis, Zygomycosis)

DEFINITION. Mucormycosis is an acute suppurative opportunistic mycosis that produces predominantly rhinocerebral disease in patients with diabetic ketoacidosis; rhinocerebral, pulmonary, or disseminated disease in immunosuppressed patients; local or disseminated disease in patients with burns or open wounds; and gastrointestinal disease in patients with malnutrition or pre-existing intestinal disorders.

ETIOLOGY. "Phycomycosis" is an extremely broad term that includes mycoses attributable to fungi in the class Zygomycetes (zygomycosis). "Zygomycosis" includes diseases produced by fungi in the orders Mucorales (mucormycosis) and Entomophthorales (entomophthoromycosis). Entomophthoromycosis is due to infection with *Basidiobolus* and *Conidiobolus* species; occurs as a subcutaneous infection of normal young people, generally in the tropics; and is clinically and histologically distinct from mucormycosis. Mucorales known to produce mucormycosis include *Rhizopus, Mucor, Absidia, Mortierella, Cunninghamella, and Saksenaea* species. In the tissues, all these fungi appear as broad (6 to 50 μm), wavy, nonseptate (coenocytic), thick-walled hyphae with right-angle branching at haphazard intervals. They can be distinguished from one another only in vitro.

INCIDENCE AND PREVALENCE. Mucorales occur worldwide in soil and on decaying organic debris, and are economically important as food spoilage agents. Airborne spores may contaminate bacteriologic media. Colonization and infection are uncommon in normal persons. Mucormycosis is increasing in incidence because of expanding numbers of susceptible, immunosuppressed patients.

EPIDEMIOLOGY. Mucormycosis is acquired sporadically, by inhalation, by ingestion, or by contamination of wounds with spores. It is not communicable. Infection is unrelated to age, sex, race, or climate. Diabetics usually acquire their infections in the community; immunosuppressed patients, within the hospital. A recent outbreak of *Rhizopus* wound infections was related to the use of elasticized adhesive tape (Elastoplast, a nonsterile product), in direct contiguity with open wounds. The tape was found to be contaminated with spores of *R. oryzae* and *R. rhizopodoformis*. Mucormycosis of burn wounds may follow the use of topical mafenide, which suppresses other etiologic agents of burn wound infection.

PATHOGENESIS AND PATHOLOGY. Mechanisms of immunity are poorly understood. Evidence from various experimental models suggests roles for serum factors, polymorphonuclear leukocytes, and cell-mediated immunity, but in no consistent pattern. Acidosis appears more important than hyperglycemia in the susceptibility of experimental animals to rhinocerebral disease. This may relate to the acidic growth optima of the causative fungi, and the delay in polymorphonuclear leukocyte chemotaxis engendered by diabetic ketoacidosis.

The pathologic process in humans is characterized by suppuration with little granulomatous response. Invasion of blood vessels is characteristic, resulting in thrombosis, infarction, and embolization. Disease spreads by both direct and hematogenous extension, but the fungi are almost never recovered from the blood. Agents of mucormycosis stain readily with hematoxylin-eosin (eosinophilic hyphae). The Gomori methenamine silver stain is also useful, but results with the periodic acid–Schiff and Gridley stains are poor. Hyphae are generally surrounded by an acute inflammatory cell infiltrate, but sections with marked hyphal invasion sometimes show little or no cellular response.

CLINICAL MANIFESTATIONS. *Rhinocerebral mucormycosis* accounts for about half of all cases of mucormycosis. More than 75 per cent of cases of rhinocerebral mucormycosis occur in patients with acidosis, especially diabetic ketoacidosis. However, increasing numbers of cases are being seen in neutropenic patients with hematologic malignancies. It is one of the most rapidly fatal fungus diseases of man, death occurring within two to ten days of onset in untreated patients. Infection is presumably initiated by the germination of spores deposited on the nasopharyngeal mucous membranes. Early clinical manifestations include nasal stuffiness, blood-tinged nasal discharge, facial swelling, and facial or orbital pain. Examination of the nasal mucosa reveals dirty red or black necrotic turbinates—an appearance commonly mistaken for dried blood, and a major clue to the diagnosis. Facial cellulitis, palatal or nasal septal perforation, and signs of sinusitis may be present. Radiographs of the sinuses reveal nodular thickening of the mucous membranes, spotty destruction of the bony walls, and the absence of air-fluid levels. Spread of infection to the orbit results in orbital cellulitis, proptosis, and failing vision. Ultimately, there is a full-blown orbital apex syndrome reflecting the destruction of cranial nerves (III, IV, VI, and the ophthalmic branch of V) and blood vessels traversing the optic foramen and superior orbital fissure. Manifestations include complete ophthalmoplegia; a fixed, dilated pupil; corneal and upper facial anesthesia; chemosis and conjunctival hemorrhage; and blindness resulting from obstruction of the central artery of the retina. The disease commonly spreads to involve the internal carotid artery, and sometimes the cavernous sinus, cribriform plate, meninges, brain, and bones of the skull. Cerebral infarction caused by vascular compromise is common. The cerebrospinal fluid may disclose pleocytosis (≥50 per cent polymorphonuclear leukocytes) and elevated protein concentration, but hypoglycorrhachia is rare, and fungi are virtually never seen or cultured.

Pulmonary mucormycosis is nearly as common as rhinocerebral disease, and typically occurs as a complication of hematologic malignancy and cytotoxic or immunosuppressive therapy. Infection presumably follows inhalation of fungal spores. There are no characteristic clinical or roentgenographic findings, but the pattern of infarction and cavitation may resemble that of invasive pulmonary aspergillosis. Sputum cultures are rarely positive, and successful diagnosis usually requires invasive techniques such as open lung biopsy.

Gastrointestinal mucormycosis may result from the ingestion of fungal spores in patients with pre-existing gastrointestinal abnormalities or malnutrition. It is seldom suspected prior to laparotomy or autopsy.

Cutaneous mucormycosis: Local cutaneous infection may follow deep burns, application of contaminated wound dressings, or injections at contaminated skin sites.

Disseminated mucormycosis may follow pulmonary or burn wound infection. Cerebral involvement is common, but no organ is spared.

DIAGNOSIS. Rhinocerebral mucormycosis may be confused with midline granuloma, rhinoscleroma, thyroid disease, syphilis, tuberculosis, or nasal and orbital tumors. Pulmonary mucormycosis may be confused with a variety of opportunistic pulmonary infections in the immunosuppressed host, or with bland pulmonary embolization and infarction. The diagnosis of all forms of mucormycosis depends upon the *direct demonstration* of the characteristic hyphae in the tissues. Diagnosis is urgent and may be achieved by crushing fresh biopsy material between two slides, clearing with 10 to 20 per cent KOH, and examining for hyphae. Smears and swabs of sputum or wound exudate rarely disclose the fungus. Cultures are positive in less than 20 per cent of cases, and even positive cultures from superficial tissues might reflect the presence of fungal contaminants. No skin test is available, and there are no reliable serologic tests. Neither a negative tissue examination nor a negative culture rules out mucormycosis in the presence of a suggestive clinical picture, and collection of additional tissue specimens is indicated along with appropriate, aggressive therapy.

TREATMENT. Amphotericin B is the only drug with proven efficacy, and results of therapy do not necessarily correlate with results of tests of susceptibility to the drug in vitro. Successful therapy requires early diagnosis, control of the underlying disease process, aggressive debridement, and aggressive use of amphotericin B. Control of burn infection may necessitate amputation. The dose of amphotericin B should be rapidly increased to 0.5 to 1.0 mg per kilogram per day, in accordance with the patient's ability to tolerate the drug. Consideration should be given to local administration of drug into infected paranasal sinuses. With clinical improvement, amphotericin B can be given in an alternate-day regimen. A total dose of 2 to 4 grams is commonly suggested.

PROGNOSIS. The prognosis of mucormycosis is directly related to the rapidity of diagnosis and the aggressiveness of therapy. Prior to the advent of amphotericin B, rhinocerebral disease was fatal in 80 to 90 per cent of instances. Current data indicate that 75 per cent of patients with no systemic disease, 60 per cent of diabetics, and 20 per cent of patients with other underlying disorders survive rhinocerebral disease. Prognosis is poor in patients with hemiplegia, facial necrosis, or nasal deformity. Only about 15 patients have been reported to have recovered from pulmonary infection.

Blitzer A, Lawson W, Meyers BR, Biller HF: Patient survival factors in paranasal sinus mucormycosis. Laryngoscope 90:635, 1980. *An analysis of 179 cases of rhinocerebral infection with emphasis on significant prognostic factors.*

Lehrer RI (moderator): UCLA Conference Mucormycosis (part I). Ann Intern Med 93:93, 1980. *A thorough and up-to-date review of clinical, mycologic, and immunologic aspects of mucormycosis. The best reference on the subject.*

Meyer RD, Rosen P, Armstrong P: Phycomycosis complicating leukemia and lymphoma. Ann Intern Med 77:781, 1972. *The best reference available for pulmonary mucormycosis.*

375. MYCETOMA (Maduromycosis)

DEFINITION. A mycetoma is a localized lesion, usually of an exposed area such as the unshod foot (Madura foot), characterized by swelling and deep sinuses that discharge pus and grains (microbial colonies embedded in a host-derived proteinaceous matrix).

ETIOLOGY. Half of all mycetomas are produced by fungi (eumycetoma); the other half by actinomycetes (actinomycetoma). They resemble a syndrome produced by certain bacteria (botryomycosis). The etiologic agents originate in plant debris and soil, and are introduced by trauma. Etiologic agents of eumycetoma include (1) white to yellow grains—*Petriellidium (Pseudoallescheria) boydii* and *Acremonium (Cephalosporium), Trichophyton,* and *Microsporum* species; (2) yellow to brown grains—*Neotestudina (Zophia) rosatii;* and (3) black grains—*Madurella mycetomi* and *grisea (Pyrenochaeta romeroi), Phialophora (Exophiala) jeanselmei,* and *Leptosphaeria senegalensis* and *thompkinsii.* Etiologic agents of actinomycetoma include (1) white to yellow grains—*Nocardia asteroides, brasiliensis,* and *cavae* (tiny grains) and *Actinomadura madurae* (extremely large grains); (2) yellow to brown grains—*Streptomyces somaliensis;* (3) red grains—*Actinomadura pelletierii;* and (4) black grains—*Streptomyces paraguayensis.*

EPIDEMIOLOGY. Mycetomas are encountered worldwide, but especially in semitropical zones such as Sudan and Mexico. *P. boydii* is the most common cause of mycetoma in Europe and the United States, *N. brasiliensis* in Mexico.

The mycetomas occur most frequently in adult males from rural areas who work out of doors, experience repeated trauma, and care poorly for local wounds. The disease is not contagious, occurs in sporadic fashion, and is unrelated to animal contact. Mycetomas usually involve the feet or legs, but may involve the back, neck, or shoulders (in bearers of burdens), or the head (where *Trichophyton* and *Microsporum* eumycetomas are especially likely to occur).

PATHOGENESIS AND PATHOLOGY. The host-parasite interactions that foster the development of grains instead of free filaments by the weakly pathogenic organisms responsible for mycetomas are unknown.

Typical mycetomas consist of large granulomatous areas with a purulent center surrounded by a thick, fibrous capsule. Fistulous tracts that contain grains pass deep into underlying tissues, usually along fascial planes, and also drain at the skin surface. Focal areas of subcutaneous necrosis and intense fibrosis result in typical tumefaction. Tracts open and close over long periods of time. In actinomycetomas, the suppurative response tends to persist indefinitely, and there is a tendency to invade bones and muscles. Eumycetomas take on the character of foreign body granulomas.

CLINICAL MANIFESTATIONS. Mycetomas usually begin as a painless draining nodule at a site of trauma. Multiple secondary nodules develop over years and drain through sinus tracts. Lesions extend deeply into subcutaneous tissues, under the cover of thick fibrosclerous tissue. A common complaint is a sensation of deep itching. Disease may spread to bone (including medullary canal and epiphyses), joints, muscles, tendons,

and nerves. When extensive bony remodeling occurs, the process becomes painful. Blood and lymphatic vessels are damaged or interrupted, but regional lymphadenopathy is rare. In the typical "Madura fôot," the destruction of tarsal bones, nonimpairment of the tendons, and widespread plantar fibrosis give the foot a characteristic shortened and raised appearance. The sole is typically convex. The general health of the patient remains little affected. Rapid local or lymphohematogenous spread may occur when mycetomas involve the buttocks, chest, or trunk.

DIAGNOSIS. Mycetomas can be diagnosed by the presence of characteristic sinuses and grains. Collection of grains may be facilitated by gentle abrasion of lesions or overnight occlusion with saline-saturated gauze. Grains should be crushed, and wet mounts prepared in 10 to 20 per cent KOH. Examination of grains permits the broad differentiation of actinomycetoma (fine filaments), eumycetoma (broad hyphae), and botryomycosis (cocci or rods without filaments). Culture is necessary for etiologic diagnosis. Serologic tests are not routinely available.

TREATMENT. Treatment for actinomycetomas depends upon identification of the infecting agent and determination of its in vitro antibiotic susceptibility. Therapeutic responses have followed high dose penicillin regimens (e.g., 10 million units per day), with or without probenecid, 1 gram per day; sulfadiazine, 3 to 10 grams per day; or minocycline, 150 mg twice daily. *Nocardia brasiliensis* infections are especially likely to respond, perhaps because the smaller grains pose a less formidable barrier to drug penetration. Other useful drugs include diaminodiphenylsulfone (dapsone), 50 to 200 mg daily by mouth; co-trimoxazole (160 mg trimethoprim plus 800 mg sulfamethoxazole daily, by mouth); or streptomycin (3 grams intramuscularly per day for three weeks, then 2 grams daily for three weeks, then 1 gram daily). Prolonged streptomycin regimens carry the danger of vestibulotoxicity. Limb perfusion therapy and topical antimicrobial agents have also been used, together with judicious resectional surgery. Eumycetoma is considerably more difficult to treat. Amphotericin B given intravenously or locally has produced equivocal results. *P. boydii* may respond to miconazole, ketoconazole, or even thiabendazole. Unfortunately, eumycetoma often requires amputation.

PROGNOSIS. The mycetomas are often brought to medical attention late in the course of illness. Reasons include the absence of pain, the remote living conditions of patients, and the fear of amputation. In general, the prognosis for life is good, but the disease may be incapacitating.

Mariat F, Destombes P, Segretain G: The mycetomas: Clinical features, pathology, etiology and epidemiology. *In* Contributions to Microbiology, Vol 4, Host-Parasite Relationships in Systemic Mycoses; Part II, Specific Diseases and Therapy. Basel, Karger, 1977, pp 1-39. *A masterful, easily readable, and up-to-date review article with an emphasis on pathophysiology.*

Smego RA Jr, Gallis HA: The clinical spectrum of *Nocardia brasiliensis* infection in the United States. Rev Infect Dis 6:164, 1984. Nocardia brasiliensis *is a common cause of mycetoma throughout the world. It can also produce a variety of other skin, soft tissue, and systemic manifestations. This is an important review of the pathogenesis, diagnosis, and therapy of the gamut of* N. brasiliensis *infections.*

Tight RR, Bartlett MS: Actinomycetoma in the United States. Rev Infect Dis 3:1139, 1981. *A case report and review of 28 cases of actinomycetoma in the United States that emphasizes the importance of etiologic diagnosis, antibiotic susceptibility testing in vitro, identification of osteomyelitis, and protracted therapy in disease management.*

376. CHROMOMYCOSIS

Chromomycosis (dermatomycosis) is a general term for mycotic infections produced by dematiacious (brown-pigmented) fungi. There are three clinical forms: cutaneous, cystic, and cerebral.

CUTANEOUS CHROMOMYCOSIS

DEFINITION. Cutaneous chromomycosis (chromoblastomycosis, verrucous dermatitis), the classic form of chromomycosis, is a noncontagious chronic granulomatous infection, usually of exposed areas such as the extremities, and characterized by warty plaques, nodules, and cauliflower-like excrescences.

ETIOLOGY. Chromomycosis is produced by a variety of brown-pigmented saprophytic soil fungi that are genetically related, morphologically identical, and distinguishable only in vitro. They include principally members of the genera *Phialophora (Exophiala), Fonsecaea,* and *Cladosporium. Fonsecaea pedrosoi* is the most common etiologic agent.

INCIDENCE AND PREVALENCE. Cutaneous chromomycosis occurs worldwide, but is most common in tropical and subtropical areas, especially Brazil and Costa Rica. The first case report was from New England in 1915, and numerous cases have been documented in Texas and Louisiana.

EPIDEMIOLOGY. The etiologic agents reside in soil, decaying wood, or rotting vegetation. They are usually introduced by trauma, especially in barefoot persons. Cutaneous chromomycosis is most common in adult males who work out of doors, especially those with suboptimal nutritional or hygienic status.

PATHOGENESIS AND PATHOLOGY. There is pseudoepitheliomatous hyperplasia of the surface epithelium, and microabscesses with epithelioid and giant cell granulomas in the underlying dermis. Eventually, a chronic fibrosing inflammatory reaction supervenes. The characteristic tissue fungi develop as large, thick-walled, dark-colored rounded cells (4 to 12 μm in diameter), the so-called "sclerotic bodies." They multiply by septation and not by budding, and frequently remain attached to one another in clusters of two or more.

CLINICAL MANIFESTATIONS. Cutaneous chromomycosis starts as a small pink scaly papule, and slowly enlarges to a warty tumor that may spread to form a plaque. Mucous membranes are not often involved. Plaques may be verrucous with central scarring, extensively scarred with a serpiginous border, scaly, or indurated with fistulas. Some patients develop a papillomatous tumor reminiscent of a cauliflower. Ulceration may follow trauma or secondary infection, and local spread may occur by direct or lymphatic extension, or by autoinoculation through scratching. Regional lymphadenopathy is not common. It may take ten to fifteen years for a whole limb to be involved. Lymphedema and elephantiasis may result. Rarely the disease may be complicated by an epithelioid carcinoma. In some patients, widespread hematogenous dissemination occurs. Lesions have been documented in the pancreas, liver, bowel, lymph nodes, brain, and meninges. The organs may contain sclerotic bodies and/or hyphae.

DIAGNOSIS. Early lesions may be confused with malignancy, mycetoma, other mycoses, cutaneous tuberculosis, leishmaniasis, yaws, and "mossy foot" (lymphostatis verrucosis). Laboratory diagnosis is relatively easy. Although superficial crusts digested in 10 to 20 percent KOH may contain long brown branching hyphae, the diagnostic sclerotic bodies are more likely to be found intracellularly or extracellularly in pus, in granulation tissue obtained by curettage, or in biopsy specimens. The brown pigmentation of the fungi serves to identify them; special stains are seldom needed. Cultures may grow slowly and should be kept at least eight weeks. Serologic or skin tests are not available.

TREATMENT. Treatment is successful in inverse relation to the duration and extent of infection. Except when the lesions are small and early, surgery is nearly always followed by recurrence. Systemic amphotericin B may not produce fungistatic concentrations at the lesions. Intralesional amphotericin B has been tried with variable success, but is painful. Flucytosine* (150 mg per kilogram of body weight per day by mouth) cured 16 of 23 patients in a recent series. The other seven developed flucytosine-resistant fungi. Amphotericin B given simultaneously with flucytosine might retard emergence of flucytosine-resistant fungi. Thiabendazole (2 grams per day, orally), an anthelmintic, has given promising results, but is not approved for this use in the United States. Unpublished results suggest that ketoconazole, an orally administered imidazole, may be efficacious.

Response to therapy may be monitored by serial biopsies and cultures.

PROGNOSIS. Cutaneous chromomycosis usually remains localized and will not debilitate the patient if left untreated. Secondary infection resulting in lymphostasis and elephantiasis is disabling. There is a slight risk of hematogenous dissemination, probably increased by immunosuppression.

CYSTIC CHROMOMYCOSIS

Cystic chromomycosis (phaeosporotrichosis, phaeomycotic cyst, phaeohyphomycosis, hypodermomycosis) is characterized by the formation of a granulomatous cyst-like lesion, usually deep in subcutaneous or muscle tissue. The lesion, which is usually encapsulated, becomes necrotic and may ulcerate. The principal etiologic agent is *Exophiala jeanselmei.* Pigmented hyphae are present in exudate and in the abscess wall; sclerotic bodies are not seen. However, "yeast-like" cells of odd shapes and sizes have been reported.

Cystic chromomycosis must be differentiated from sebaceous cysts, tendon sheath granulomas, foreign body granulomas, or gummas. Hematogenous spread is rare. Treatment consists of surgical excision.

CEREBRAL CHROMOMYCOSIS

Cerebral chromomycosis (cerebral dermatomycosis, cladosporiosis, encephalomycosis) is a general term for any cerebral mycosis caused by a dematiacious fungus. The most important form, caused by *Cladosporium trichoides,* is characterized by the formation of abscesses containing pus, giant cells, and pigmented hyphae. Sclerotic bodies are not seen. Blood vessel invasion by hyphae occurs (reminiscent of aspergillosis or phycomycosis). Meningitis is present in about half the cases, sometimes as an isolated occurrence. The cerebrospinal fluid usually shows a polymorphonuclear leukocyte response; hypoglycorrhachia has not been reported. The site of primary infection may be the lung, but there is seldom evidence of pulmonary involvement. Cerebral chromomycosis is rarely diagnosed early enough to permit the evaluation of therapeutic regimens. Optimal management would seem to require surgical debridement and the use of flucytosine* or an imidazole, with or without amphotericin B.

---

*Investigational drug for this purpose.

Bennett JE, Bonner H, Jennings AE, Lopez RI: Chronic meningitis caused by *Cladosporium trichoides.* Am J Clin Pathol 59:398, 1973. *Comprehensive discussion of cerebral infection with dematiaceous fungi.*

Carrion AL: Chromoblastomycosis and related infections: New concepts, differential diagnosis, and nomenclatorial implications. Int J Dermatol 14:27, 1975.

Vollum DI: Chromomycosis: A review. Br J Dermatol 96:454, 1977. *Two brief, excellent reviews of the spectrum of disease produced by dematiaceous fungi.*

Part XX
DISEASES CAUSED BY PROTOZOA AND METAZOA

377. INTRODUCTION TO PROTOZOAN AND HELMINTHIC DISEASES

Adel A. F. Mahmoud

Human infections with parasitic protozoa and helminths account for a major proportion of the diseases caused by infectious agents. In spite of some worldwide efforts to control the spread and consequences of these infections, the associated morbidity and mortality have not been appreciably reduced. Furthermore, in the developed countries infection with protozoa and helminths is being seen with increasing frequency in immigrants and is also among the more important causes of disease in the growing number of patients with depressed immune responses.

The biology of the interaction between protozoa and helminths and their host is less well understood than that of other infectious agents. Most of these infections are prevalent in the developing countries in which limited attention has been paid to studies on pathogenesis, chemotherapy, or control. There are no reliable data on prevalence and morbidity caused by human protozoan and helminthic infections. Nevertheless, their magnitude is staggering; malaria infects 600 million, and ascariasis and trichuriasis one billion each, and 600 million are estimated to be infected with either schistosomiasis or filariases. Other infectious protozoa and helminths such as *Toxoplasma gondii, Entamoeba histolytica, Giardia lamblia, Pneumocystis carinii,* and *Strongyloides stercoralis* occur worldwide. Although the major burden of disease due to protozoan and helminthic infections falls on the developing world, some of these infections are becoming clinically recognized pathogens in the more developed countries. An additional dimension of the problem of protozoan and helminthic infections concerns the lack of effective chemotherapeutic agents in some instances and the excessive toxicity of these agents or the development of resistance to them in other instances.

BIOLOGY OF PARASITIC PROTOZOA AND HELMINTHS

This group of infectious agents belongs to the animal kingdom, unlike bacteria, viruses, or fungi. Such distinction led to restricting the term "parasite" to include only protozoa and helminths, and may have hampered our clinical as well as basic understanding of the mechanisms by which they cause disease and how to enhance host resistance effectively. The host-parasite relationship in protozoan and helminthic infections is complex because of the distinctive biological features of the organisms. Although protozoa are unicellular pathogens and are mainly microscopic in size, they are far larger than viruses and bacteria. A major biological feature of protozoa is their ability to multiply within mammalian hosts as do viruses, bacteria, and fungi. Protozoan infection, therefore, can be initiated by a relatively small inoculum of organisms, which then multiply within the host and reach the numbers that cause disease. A single infected mosquito bite, for example, can deliver enough malaria sporozoites to establish infection in the liver, where the organisms multiply and cause clinical disease upon invasion of red cells.

In contrast, helminths are multicellular organisms with well developed organ system structures. They vary in size from 1 cm to approximately 10 meters. Unlike other infectious agents, helminths do not multiply within mammalian hosts. Re-exposure is, therefore, necessary to increase the number of helminths in a host. This distinguishing feature has important clinical significance, as disease in most helminthiasis is closely related to intensity of infection. For example, anemia results from hookworm infection only if the individual is harboring a significant worm load or there are other reasons for nutritional deficiencies. In rare circumstances such as strongyloidiasis in the immunosuppressed, the worm can increase its population through an autoinfection cycle. This leads to life-threatening infection that necessitates aggressive medical attention.

Parasitic protozoa and helminths have developed elaborate mechanisms for evasion of host protective responses. One of the best studied is antigenic variation noted in African trypanosomiasis. Parasitemia in infected individuals declines with the development of a protective antibody response but is followed by the emergence of a new parasite variable antigen and an increase in their numbers. These organisms are capable of expressing at least 100 different variable antigens allowing a long chronic course of infection. The phenomenon of antigenic variation in trypanosomiasis is expressed through a surface glycoprotein of a molecular weight 65,000. The trypanosomes contain individual genes for all the different variable glycoproteins but only one is expressed at a time. The multiplicity of trypanosome variable glycoprotein genes and mechanisms for introducing mutations into them illustrate the degree of complexity and sophistication of these human pathogens.

The constantly changing nature of infectious disease is best illustrated in some parasitic protozoan and helminthic infections. For example, relatively unsuspected pathogens such as *Giardia lamblia* are now being recognized as the major identifiable cause of water-borne diarrhea in North America and several parts of the world. New human pathogens such as *Isospora* and *Cryptosporidium* species have been appreciated only recently as causes of diarrheal illness, particularly in the immunosuppressed. This group of patients, including those with acquired immune deficiency syndrome (AIDS), is particularly susceptible to several opportunistic Protozoan infections such as *Pneumocystitis carinii, Toxoplasma gondii,* and the coccidia. These new developments add to the difficulties experienced in the treatment and control of parasitic protozoa and helminths. For several, effective and safe chemotherapeutic agents are lacking (e.g., onchocerciasis and South American trypanosomiasis). In some circumstances the pathogen (e.g., *Plasmodium falciparum)* is rapidly developing resistance to the available drugs; insecticide resistance is also complicating vector control attempts. On the other hand, malaria vaccine may be a reality soon and new chemotherapeutic agents for onchocerciasis are to be introduced in the near future.

APPROACH TO THE PATIENT WITH PROTOZOAN OR HELMINTHIC INFECTION

Since most of the clinical manifestations of protozoan and helminthic diseases are not specific or pathognomonic, a high degree of suspicion is essential. The simple question "Where have you been?" and knowledge of the general geographic distribution of parasitic protozoa and helminth will often save exhaustive and costly diagnostic workups and may spare human lives.

The next phase in attempting to reach correct diagnosis

involves interpretation of the presenting symptoms and signs. Definitive diagnosis in most cases requires isolation and identification of the specific pathogen. Since the number of cases seen by any single laboratory in North America is limited, certain expertise is required for correct identification that may not be available to many practicing physicians. Consultations with the Centers for Disease Control are, therefore, helpful.

Schmidt GD, Roberts LS, eds.: Foundations of Parasitology, 2nd edition. C. V. Mosby Company, St. Louis, 1981. *A concise text for basic information on morphology and biology of protozoa and helminths.*

Warren KS, Mahmoud AAF, eds.: Tropical and Geographical Medicine. McGraw-Hill Book Company, New York, 1984. *Detailed description of the biology and molecular understanding of protozoa and helminths and the diseases they cause in individuals and in populations.*

Section One PROTOZOAN DISEASES

378. MALARIA

Louis H. Miller

DEFINITION. Malaria remains today one of the major health problems in the tropics. It is caused by four species of *Plasmodium, P. falciparum, P. vivax, P. ovale* and *P. malariae*, each of which produces disease with its own morphology and clinical characteristic (Table 378–1). The asexual erythrocytic parasite is the stage in the life cycle that causes disease, including the characteristic malarial paroxysm (fever, chills, and sweats). *P. falciparum* malaria causes the most morbidity and mortality and presents the therapeutic problem of chloroquine resistance. Since effective therapy is available for *P. falciparum* malaria, high mortality usually results from failure of the physician to include malaria in the differential diagnosis of a febrile patient who has traveled in the tropics or received a blood transfusion.

ETIOLOGY. Malaria parasites undergo a developmental cycle in female anopheline mosquitoes, the vector, and in humans. Mosquitoes, during a blood meal, inoculate *sporozoites* that rapidly enter liver parenchymal cells. The sporozoite surface is covered by a membrane protein with a multiply repeated epitope. Sporozoites may develop immediately in liver cells into thousands of individual merozoites (all types of malaria) or remain dormant as uninucleate hypnozoites for months to years before undergoing proliferation (the relapsing malarias, caused by *P. vivax* and *P. ovale*). Different strains of *P. vivax* produce their own characteristic timing patterns of relapse in patients who contract the disease. Some strains (e.g., from New Guinea) cause relapse monthly after the primary attack. Others cause relapse six months or longer after the primary attack or may not produce a primary attack.

Merozoites rupture from liver cells and pour into the bloodstream to invade erythrocytes. Development of the intraerythrocytic parasite follows one of the two pathways: asexual proliferation or differentiation into sexual parasites, the gametocytes, which await ingestion by the mosquito. In the mosquito they ultimately develop into infectious *sporozoites*. Asexual erythrocytic parasites develop from young ring forms through *trophozoites* to the dividing form, the *schizont*. Each mature schizont contains 6 to 24 merozoites, the number varying with the particular species. Merozoites, on rupture of infected erythrocytes, are released to invade other erythrocytes and thus continue the cycle.

Merozoites attach to erythrocytes by specific receptors. Erythrocytic determinants required for *P. vivax* and *P. falciparum* invasion are the Duffy blood group system and glycophorin, respectively. Blacks who are Duffy blood group negative *(FyFy)* are completely refractory to erythrocytic infection by *P. vivax*. En(a-) erythrocytes that completely lack glycophorin A have reduced susceptibility to invasion by *P. falciparum*.

The agents producing the three types of malaria, *P. vivax, P. ovale,* and *P. falciparum,* invade reticulocytes preferentially. *P. falciparum,* however, can infect erythrocytes of all ages and produces high parasitemias with resultant morbidity and mortality. *P. malariae* infects mature erythrocytes.

Each type of malaria induces characteristic morphologic changes on the infected erythrocyte membrane: knobs by asexual parasites of *P. falciparum;* knobs by sexual and asexual parasites of *P. malariae;* and *Schuffner's dots,* pink stippling of the infected erythrocyte, by sexual and asexual parasites of *P. vivax* and *P. ovale.* A histidine-rich parasite protein forms the knobs on the membrane of *P. falciparum*–infected erythrocytes, which mediate attachment to venular endothelium (sequestration) and may be a factor in obstruction of cerebral vessels leading to cerebral malaria. This sequestration explains the predominance of young parasites, ring forms, in the peripheral blood.

The asexual erythrocytic parasite has a haploid genome. Cloned populations of asexual parasites can change their expression of antigens on the erythrocyte surface (antigenic variation) in order to evade the host immune response.

EPIDEMIOLOGY. Most malaria patients seen in Europe and in the United States are infected in Africa, Asia, and Latin America (imported cases). Mosquito vectors capable of transmitting malaria still exist in countries where malaria has been eradicated (e.g., *Anopheles freeborni* in the Western United States). In these areas, rare episodes of transmission have occurred following infection of local mosquitoes by individuals infected in the tropics (introduced cases). Congenital infections occur; the clinical symptoms are not evident until weeks to months after delivery. Other causes of infection in nonendemic areas include blood transfusion and communal use of syringes by drug addicts. The single most important factor in preventing transfusion malaria is the exclusion of donors who have lived or traveled in endemic areas until their risk of infection is negligible, because chronic infections are often asymptomatic. Most

TABLE 378–1. CLINICAL AND DIAGNOSTIC DIFFERENCES AMONG THE FOUR SPECIES OF MALARIA

	P. falciparum	*P. vivax*	*P. ovale*	*P. malariae*
Clinical features	High parasitemia, severe anemia, renal failure, cerebral malaria, pulmonary edema, death	Splenic rupture, anemia		RBC infection persists for years; nephritis
Chloroquine resistance	Yes	No	No	No
Asexual cycle	48 hours	48 hours	48 hours	72 hours
Relapse	No	Yes	Yes	No
Characteristic on thin blood film	Rings predominate; multiply infected RBCs, rings with thread-like cytoplasm, double nuclei, banana-shaped gametocytes	Enlarged RBC with Schuffner's dots; trophozoite cytoplasm amoeboid; 12 to 24 merozoites in mature schizont	Oval RBC with fringed edges; Schuffner's dots; trophozoite cytoplasm compact; 6 to 16 merozoites in mature schizont	Trophozoite cytoplasm compact (band forms); 6 to 12 merozoites in mature schizont; RBC unchanged

P. falciparum–infected individuals undergo self-cure in three years; a rare case may persist for four years. Disease caused by *P. vivax* and *P. ovale* may last for three to five years. That from *P. malariae* may persist as an asymptomatic, erythrocytic infection for decades. Since infection by *P. falciparum* and *P. vivax* is most serious, blood donation should be excluded for four years after the traveler's return from the tropics.

The endemicity of malaria in the tropics is determined by vector capacity, host factors such as immunity, political stability and the commitment to malaria control, and the character of the parasite. The central concept in understanding malarial transmission in any part of the world is *vector capacity,* which is defined as the expected number of new infections produced per infective case per day. Vector capacity is determined by the interaction of the vector mosquito and its biology with the environment and the parasite.

INNATE RESISTANCE. Genetically determined host factors influence susceptibility to malaria. Certain polymorphisms have been associated with the distribution of *P. falciparum* in the world (e.g., hemoglobin S, thalassemia, and glucose-6-phosphate dehydrogenase [G-6-PD] deficiency). The evidence for a selective advantage of polymorphisms in malarious areas is most convincing for sickle trait (HB SA). Children who die of malaria in West Africa rarely have sickle trait, although the frequency of this phenotype is high in this region. In areas where the heterozygote has an advantage over either homozygote, a balanced polymorphism results. The mechanism of protection at the cellular level appears to be inhibition of growth in HB SA erythrocytes because *P. falciparum*–infected erythrocytes sequester along venules where O_2 tension is low.

Black Africans who have the Duffy blood group–negative genotype *(FyFy)* are resistant to infection by *P. vivax.* Elliptocytosis, a skeletal abnormality of erythrocytes, occurs throughout lowland tropical areas of Southeast Asia and Melanesia that are endemic for malaria; the erythrocytes are partially resistant to invasion by all types of malaria.

IMMUNITY. Immunity to malaria is primarily directed against the asexual erythrocytic parasite. Immunity to sporozoites occurs in adult populations of Africa but probably is of little importance in host survival. Immunity to the asexual erythrocytic parasite develops only after prolonged or repeated infection. Immunity usually does not prevent reinfection but reduces the severity of the disease or leads to an asymptomatic infection. The asymptomatic person, however, can infect mosquitoes and can transmit the infection directly to others through blood transfusion. Immunity wanes in a few years when the person is unexposed to reinfection. Recurrence of disease may occur in an immune person immediately after surgery or during pregnancy.

Immunity is species-specific (e.g., immunity to *P. falciparum* does not protect against *P. vivax*). Further, the immunity against *P. falciparum* is strain-specific, indicating variant antigens among strains. Passive transfer of antibody from hyperimmune adult West Africans to East or West African children reduced parasitemia.

The spleen is of primary importance in host survival against malaria. One mechanism may involve antibody and cells within the spleen. Alternatively, parasites may be killed by natural killer (NK) cells or other antibody-independent mechanisms.

PATHOGENESIS AND PATHOLOGY. The asexual erythrocytic cycle causes the symptoms and pathology. Fever and the associated symptoms of headache, nausea, and muscular pain occur at the time that schizont-infected erythrocytes rupture and new ring forms appear. Although pyrogens and other toxins may be released from ruptured schizonts to cause fever and symptoms of malaria, none has been identified to date.

Anemia is caused by hemolysis of infected erythrocytes and dyserythropoiesis. Coombs-positive hemolytic anemia occurs rarely and usually results from quinine sensitivity. Severe acute hemolytic anemia results in patients who are heavily infected with *P. falciparum.* African children with chronic low-grade *P. falciparum* parasitemia have severe anemia associated with dyserythropoiesis and a low reticulocyte count. Reticulocytosis occurs after antimalarial therapy. Drugs administered to patients with G-6-PD deficiency may cause severe hemolysis. Thrombocytopenia results from binding of malaria-specific IgG to malaria antigen adsorbed on platelets.

Renal failure and cerebral malaria occur in *P. falciparum* malaria. Mechanisms for renal failure include severe hemolytic anemia, hemoglobinuria, hypovolemia, and possibly splanchnic vasoconstriction.

Blackwater fever is severe hemolytic anemia and hemoglobinuria in a falciparum malaria patient; it may cause renal failure. Prior to the introduction of chloroquine in the 1940's, quinine was used for prevention and treatment of malaria. Because of this, Coombs-positive hemolytic anemia following quinine administration was the most common cause of blackwater fever. Today, blackwater fever results from high parasitemia.

P. falciparum malaria causes diffuse cerebral disease. The decreased deformability of infected erythrocytes and their tendency to adhere by knobs to vascular endothelium probably cause the plugging of capillaries in the brain. Ring hemorrhages develop around obstructed capillaries. The brain may become edematous, although usually the cerebrospinal fluid pressure is normal.

Unusual complications of severe falciparum malaria include centrilobular necrosis of the liver and pulmonary edema. The lungs have microvascular congestion, interstitual edema, and hyaline membrane formation as evidence of increased capillary permeability.

P. malariae produces chronic progressive nephritis. Immune complexes are deposited in the glomerular capillary wall. Antibody in the complexes is specific for *P. malariae.* The majority of kidneys with immune complexes contain the C3 component of complement; 25 per cent have *P. malariae* antigen.

CLINICAL MANIFESTATIONS. No sign or symptom is pathognomonic of malaria. *Fever* need not be accompanied by the characteristic *malarial paroxysm.* The paroxysm begins with a chilly feeling, bedshaking chills, and a rise in temperature. The skin appears pale, with cyanosis of the lips and nail beds. The patient experiences *headache* and *nausea,* and may vomit. Within one to two hours the temperature rises toward 39 to 40.5° C, the patient feels hot, and the skin is warm and dry. As the temperature falls, *sweating* begins and drenches clothing. The patient feels fatigued and weak and often sleeps. This description is most typical of benign malarias; fever may persist and symptoms are prolonged in *malignant falciparum malaria.* Fever is usually not periodic in malignant falciparum malaria, and during the initial attack of *P. vivax* malaria, when the infection is asynchronous. Periodicity of fever occurs only in synchronized infections when the majority of infected erythrocytes containing mature schizonts rupture at the same time. This occurs at intervals determined by the length of the asexual erythrocytic cycle. The cycle in *P. vivax* and *P. ovale* malaria takes 48 hours and thus the fever occurs every other day. *P. malariae* matures in 72 hours and causes fever every third day.

The pulse rate is elevated but not commensurate with the fever. A nonproductive cough may occur during fever. Orthostatic hypotension is common in falciparum malaria, and weakness may persist for weeks. Splenomegaly occurs frequently and hepatomegaly less frequently. Tenderness on palpation of liver and spleen may be due to sudden stretching of their capsules; splenic rupture, a potentially fatal complication, should be considered. The absence of hepatosplenomegaly does not exclude the diagnosis of malaria. Labial herpes simplex lesions are often present. Rashes and lymphadenopathy are uncommon and point to a diagnosis other than malaria.

Abnormalities in routine laboratory test results in uncomplicated malaria may include evidence of a hemolytic anemia, leukopenia caused by a decrease in granulocytes and lymphocytes, thrombocytopenia, and minimal albuminuria. The thrombocyte count returns rapidly to normal on treatment. Hyponatremia, which is seen frequently in *P. falciparum* malaria, is caused by salt depletion and water retention.

Asymptomatic Infection and Recrudescence. Partial therapy or immunity reduces parasitemia and symptoms may disappear. Despite persistent erythrocytic infection during these asymptomatic periods, parasites are difficult to locate on blood films. Periodic rises in parasitemia cause recurrent clinical attacks (recrudescence). The total duration of erythrocytic infection varies for each type of malaria. Most falciparum infections are eliminated in one year; a few persist for up to three years. *P. malariae* infection may persist as an asymptomatic infection for the life of the patient. How *P. malariae* evades the immune response for years while infecting new erythrocytes every 72 hours remains a mystery. The asymptomatic erythrocytic infection poses two potential risks to other individuals: first, donated blood induces malaria in the recipient; second, the asymptomatic patient can infect vector mosquitoes.

Relapse differs from recrudescence in that the infection that induces the relapse persists as a latent form in hepatic parenchymal cells. Relapses occur only in *P. vivax* and *P. ovale* malaria.

COMPLICATIONS. High parasitemia in *P. falciparum* infection accounts for the severe morbidity and mortality. When the parasitemia rises above 100,000 infected erythrocytes per cu mm and the hematocrit falls below 30 per cent, the patient may develop serious complications, which most commonly include severe hemolytic anemia, renal failure, and coma. Acute renal failure can be associated with hemolytic anemia and hemoglobinuria (blackwater fever). The hemolytic anemia may be caused by high parasitemia, quinine sensitivity, or oxidant drugs in patients with G-6-PD deficiency. Renal failure may occur in the absence of severe hemolysis and may be associated with hypovolemia. It may occur with normal urine volume. Blood urea nitrogen may rise rapidly in renal failure because of an increased catabolic rate.

Cerebral malaria presents as disturbances in consciousness ranging from somnolence to coma, major motor seizures, and organic psychosis. Since the signs and symptoms are not pathognomonic of malaria, other diseases should be excluded, even in patients with circulating malaria parasites. Marked hypoglycemia, especially during infusion of quinine and in pregnancy, may cause lapses in consciousness. Febrile seizures in young children are impossible to distinguish from seizures of malaria. Neurologic examination may reveal hyper-reflexion and bilateral Babinski's signs. Focal neurologic findings occur rarely. The cerebrospinal fluid pressure may be elevated and the concentration of protein increased. Pleocytosis is rare.

Greatly elevated bilirubin and transaminase occur rarely. Another unusual complication, pulmonary edema, may be associated with fluid overload. Since it is caused by increased capillary permeability, it is difficult to reverse and the outcome is often fatal.

Splenic rupture, a rare and serious complication, occurs most commonly in *P. vivax* infections.

Chronic infection with *P. malariae* in children may produce progressive nephritis that responds poorly to treatment with antimalarials or steroids.

Falciparum Malaria During Pregnancy in the Semi-immune. Parasites sequester in the vascular beds of the placenta. The primigravida, although previously immune, may have severe attacks of malaria and marked anemia. Consequently, chemoprophylaxis is indicated throughout the first pregnancy in the semi-immune. Malaria causes stillbirths and underweight newborns, especially in the primigravida.

Tropical Splenomegaly Syndrome. Patients living in regions of Africa and New Guinea endemic for falciparum malaria develop massive splenic enlargement, hepatic sinusoidal lymphocytic infiltrates, and elevated levels of serum IgM. They respond to chronic antimalarial chemoprophylaxis with decrease in spleen size and reversal of liver pathology. Mortality is high in patients who do not receive antimalarial therapy. Splenectomy is contraindicated because severe malaria may occur following splenectomy, even in a previously immune individual.

Burkitt's Lymphoma. This tumor occurs in areas of Africa hyperendemic for *P. falciparum* and is believed to be an atypical response to Epstein-Barr virus infection.

DIAGNOSIS. The high mortality from falciparum malaria in nonendemic areas results from the failure of clinicians to consider the diagnosis and to obtain malaria blood films. The diagnosis of malaria should be suspected in a febrile patient who has traveled in the tropics or who has received a blood transfusion. The incubation period—the time from inoculation of sporozoites by mosquito to the first symptoms—is about 10 to 16 days. Drug prophylaxis may suppress the initial attack of *P. falciparum* malaria for weeks to months and of the relapsing malarias caused by *P. vivax* and *P. ovale* for months to years. The definitive diagnosis is made from identification of malarial parasites on a Giemsa-stained thick and thin blood film. Blood examinations should be obtained immediately and repeated at 12-hour intervals, because the parasitemia may fluctuate. Parasites may be undetectable during the first few days of the initial attack and in asymptomatic, semi-immune persons. The clinician should not wait for a paroxysm to obtain a blood film, since delay in diagnosis and treatment of *P. falciparum* malaria increases the risk to the patient. If malaria is strongly suspected on clinical grounds in a patient with repeatedly negative blood films, a therapeutic trial may be instituted.

Well-prepared and properly stained thick and thin blood films simplify diagnosis. A cleaned slide should be labeled with the patient's name, the date, and the time. For the thick film, one drop of blood at one end of the slide should be evenly spread in a circular motion to a diameter of 2 cm with the edge of another slide. A second drop of blood should be spread on the slide for the thin film as for a routine blood cell examination. After the blood films are dry, the thick film should be lysed in water and the thin film should be fixed with absolute methanol. Both should be stained with Giemsa at pH 7.0 to 7.2.

Once malaria parasites are identified on the blood film, the most important distinction is whether the patient has *P. falciparum* malaria, because this will influence the initial therapy. Criteria suggestive of *P. falciparum* include predominant small ring forms and multiply infected erythrocytes, rings with double nuclei, rings as applique forms, and the diagnostic crescent-shaped gametocytes. Except during high parasitemia, trophozoites and schizonts are rarely seen; infected erythrocytes adhere to venular endothelium. *P. falciparum* does not cause enlargement or pink stippling (Schuffner's dots) of infected erythrocytes. If more than 5 per cent of the erythrocytes are infected, *P. falciparum* should be suspected. Diagnosis of a malaria other than that caused by *P. falciparum* does not exclude the diagnosis of *P. falciparum* malaria, since mixed infections may occur. Slides should be saved for evaluation by an expert. Inclusions in erythrocytes (e.g., Howell-Jolly bodies and siderocytes) and artifacts (e.g., platelets on erythrocytes, precipitated stain and dirt) may be confused with malarial parasites. *Babesia microti* resembles *P. falciparum* rings but can be differentiated by an experienced microscopist.

Serologic tests have no place in the diagnosis of the acutely ill patient. The indirect fluorescent antibody test is useful in identifying infected donors in cases of transfusion malaria.

THERAPY. ***P. falciparum.*** Prompt diagnosis and early treatment are essential. Delay in chemotherapy increases morbidity and mortality. All patients should be hospitalized and treated as a medical emergency. Patients whose condition appears stable on admission may have rapid worsening.

The decision on drug regimen will depend on the origin of the infection. Chloroquine resistance is widespread and will continue to appear in new areas. Therefore, every falciparum malaria case should be considered potentially chloroquine resistant. Resistance extends today from India through Southeast Asia to New Guinea and Vanuatu in the Pacific Islands, from

Panama to South America, and from East Africa to Zambia, Madagascar and the Comoros. *P. falciparum* malaria in patients from Central and West Africa should be treated with chloroquine and the response followed closely. Because partial resistance to quinine (i.e., response followed by recrudescence) occurs in Southeast Asia and other areas, quinine is usually not used alone in treatment. Resistance to Fansidar, a fixed-drug combination of pyrimethamine and sulfadoxine, has been reported in Southeast Asia and South America.

Since treatment failure may occur with any drug regimen, the course of parasitemia must be followed at 12-hour intervals. Failure to reduce parasitemia in the first 24 to 48 hours of treatment should raise the possibility of parasite resistance to that treatment. No asexual parasites should be detectable on smears four to five days after a course of chloroquine is completed; persistence after the fifth day indicates drug failure. A simple method for estimating parasitemia from the thin blood film is as follows: at low parasite densities, the number of infected erythrocytes in 25 oil emersion fields is counted; at high parasite densities, the number of infected erythrocytes per 500 erythrocytes is counted.

Gametocytes may persist in the blood for weeks after asexual forms have been successfully eliminated. Gametocytes do not cause disease and their presence does not indicate treatment failure.

Partially resistant parasites recrudesce up to two months after treatment in the nonimmune. The patient should be warned that any febrile episode weeks to months after treatment may indicate drug failure and requires evaluation for malaria.

SYMPTOMATIC AND SUPPORTIVE MEASURES. Treatment includes aspirin, sponging with tepid water, and fanning to increase evaporation. Orthostatic hypotension, usually observed early in infection, is an indication for complete bed rest.

Packed erythrocytes or whole blood should be infused slowly in severe anemia. Platelet transfusions are generally not indicated for thrombocytopenia, as the platelets rapidly return toward normal during specific chemotherapy. Uremia may progress rapidly because of the high catabolic rate and is an indication for early hemodialysis. Administration of excessive fluids may aggravate cerebral symptoms or precipitate pulmonary edema. Pulmonary edema is usually not associated with a rise in central venous pressure during intravenous fluid administration and often results in death despite treatment.

Although splenic tenderness is common in acute malaria, evidence of peritoneal and diaphragmatic irritation may indicate splenic rupture. This life-threatening complication is more common in *P. vivax* malaria.

TREATMENT OF CHLOROQUINE-SENSITIVE *P. falciparum*. Chloroquine-sensitive strains occur in Western India, Pakistan, West and Central Africa, and Central America (except Panama). These patients should be treated with chloroquine or amodiaquine unless they have high parasitemia, in which case they should be treated as described in the section on severe and complicated malaria. The recommended therapy for adults is either chloroquine phosphate, 1000 mg initially, 500 mg six hours later, and 500 mg on each of two succeeding days; or amodiaquine hydrochloride, 780 mg initially and 520 mg on each of the two succeeding days. The major acute toxicity occurs in Africans who experience severe itching of the palms of the hands and soles of the feet without any obvious skin abnormalities, but this is not an indication for discontinuing choloroquine unless the symptoms are severe.

Because of the possibility of chloroquine resistance, the parasitemia should be followed closely during treatment (see above) and alternative drugs instituted if indicated. Fever occurring weeks after therapy may indicate a recrudescence.

TREATMENT OF CHLOROQUINE-RESISTANT *P. falciparum*. The regimen combines three drugs given orally: quinine sulfate, 650 mg every eight hours for ten days; pyrimethamine, 25 mg twice daily for three days; and a sulfonamide (sulfisoxazole or sulfadiazine), 0.5 grams every six hours for five days. Occasionally, after treatment with this regimen, the patient may suffer a subsequent recrudescence. Recrudescent attacks may be treated either with a second course of quinine, pyrimethamine, and sulfonamide, or, alternatively, with the following regimen: quinine sulfate, 650 mg every eight hours for three days, plus tetracycline hydrochloride, 250 mg every six hours for ten days.

Cinchonism (nausea, vomiting, tinnitus, and vertigo) commonly results from treatment with quinine and is not an indication to alter or discontinue therapy. A rare complication of quinine therapy, Coombs-positive hemolytic anemia, is an indication for immediate withdrawal of the drug.

Mefloquine, a new experimental antimalarial drug, is highly effective against chloroquine-resistant *P. falciparum.* As more data become available on its relative safety, it may become the treatment of choice for *P. falciparum* malaria. Mefloquine alone or in combination with pyrimethamine and sulfadoxine is now undergoing extensive clinical trials. Mefloquine rarely causes disorientation, hallucinations, and lapses of consciousness two to three weeks after drug administration.

TREATMENT OF SEVERE AND COMPLICATED MALARIA. Patients with *P. falciparum* malaria who have parasitemia greater than 100,000 per cu mm, marked anemia, cerebral complications, or are vomiting repeatedly should be treated with intravenous quinine dihydrochloride. Quinine dihydrochloride, 600 mg dissolved in 250 ml of 5 per cent glucose in 0.075 M sodium chloride should be infused slowly over eight hours. This should be repeated every eight hours until oral medication is tolerated, at which time a combination of quinine, sulfonamide, and pyrimethamine should be administered orally. Since quinine is excreted by the kidneys and metabolized by the liver, the dosage in patients with renal failure and hepatic disease should be decreased by at least half.

Hypoglycemia is a life-threatening complication of severe malaria and occurs most commonly during intravenous quinine therapy and in pregnant women. Blood glucose should be monitored closely, especially in patients who have a change in the level of consciousness.

If quinine is not immediately available from the Centers for Disease Control and the patient is severely ill with high parasitemia, intravenous quinidine should be considered until quinine can be obtained. Although there is limited experience with intravenous quinidine in malaria, oral quinidine has been shown to be as effective as oral quinine against chloroquine-resistant *P. falciparum.* Quinidine does not have FDA approval for use in malaria; therefore, the physician should obtain informed consent. Quinidine gluconate (10 mg per kilogram maximum of 600 mg) should be infused slowly over four to six hours followed by a continuous infusion of quinidine gluconate (5 mg per kilogram over six hours maximum of 300 mg) until intravenous quinine becomes available. Quinidine is contraindicated in patients who have conduction disturbances, untreated cardiac failure, and hypotension. The patient should be monitored closely, although lengthening of the $Q\text{-}T_C$ interval is to be expected.

Exchange transfusions may improve survival in patients who have parasitemia greater than 15 per cent, although controlled studies have not been performed. Glucosteroids are contraindicated because they increase morbidity and mortality. Heparin is contraindicated even in patients with disseminated intravascular coagulation because of the risk of hemorrhage.

P. vivax, P. ovale, and P. malariae. Acute attacks with any of these species should be treated with chloroquine or amodiaquine (see regimen under treatment of chloroquine-sensitive *P. falciparum*).

P. vivax and *P. ovale* infections acquired by mosquito bites may have persistent hepatic forms and these must be eliminated to prevent relapses. After completion of chloroquine treatment, primaquine phosphate, 26.6 mg daily for 14 days, is administered. Primaquine causes hemolysis in patients with G-6-PD deficiency. Patients who have a mild G-6-PD deficiency may be treated under close supervision because the hemolysis is self-limited. Severe G-6-PD deficiency is a contraindication to the use of primaquine, each relapse requiring retreatment with chloroquine. Primaquine is not indicated in the treatment of transfusion malaria because erythrocytic parasites of blood-induced infections do not infect the liver.

Sites of Action of Antimalarial Drugs. Only the sites of action of pyrimethamine and sulfonamide are known. Pyrimethamine has a greater affinity for parasite than host dihydrofolate reductase and blocks folate metabolism. Pyrimethamine-resistant parasites have either a higher concentration of dihydrofolate reductase or an enzyme with a lower affinity for pyrimethamine. Sulfonamides block utilization of para-aminobenzoic acid (pABA). It has been suggested that chloroquine interferes with enzymatic digestion in the parasite's food vacuole or the processing of ferriprotoporphyrin into hemozoin pigment. It is proposed that unprocessed ferriprotoporphyrin is toxic to the parasite.

PREVENTION. ***Protection for the Individual.*** Ideal chemoprophylaxis is not available because of chloroquine-resistant *P. falciparum* in many areas of the world. In addition, chloroquine eliminates only the primary attack of *P. vivax* and *P. ovale* but has no effect on relapses that may occur months to years later. Therefore the patient should be warned that fever during or after travel in endemic areas may be caused by malaria, even though the patient was on drug suppression.

Prevention of malaria can usually be accomplished in adults by chloroquine phosphate, 500 mg orally once weekly, or amodiaquine hydrochloride, 520 mg orally once weekly. Long term use of chloroquine at recommended doses for malaria prophylaxis does not cause eye disease. The drug should be continued for six weeks after leaving an endemic area. Travelers who were heavily exposed to malaria and are not G-6-PD deficient should receive primaquine phosphate, 26.6 mg daily for 14 days, on return from an endemic area to eliminate hepatic forms of *P. vivax* and *P. ovale*.

Fansidar, each tablet of which contains pyrimethamine, 25 mg, and sulfadoxine, a long-acting sulfonamide, 500 mg, is effective for prevention of chloroquine-resistant *P. falciparum*, although Fansidar resistance occurs in Southeast Asia and Brazil. The dose is one tablet weekly. Long-acting sulfonamides, but not sulfadoxine, have been rarely associated with Stevens-Johnson syndrome. Chloroquine weekly prophylaxis should be taken with Fansidar because of strains of *P. vivax* resistant to this medication.

Because drug prophylaxis is not ideal, the traveler should be advised to prevent contact with night-biting *Anopheles*. The traveler should use netting over the bed, insecticides, and mosquito repellents such as Off (N,N-diethyltoluamide).

Chemoprophylaxis in Pregnancy and for Nursing Mothers. Drugs in pregnancy always present a potential risk to the fetus, especially for prolonged use as in chemoprophylaxis. Chloroquine is considered generally safe when used at the recommended dosage. Chemoprophylaxis in areas of chloroquine-resistant *P. falciparum* presents a more difficult problem. Fansidar, the drug of choice, contains pyrimethamine, which has exhibited teratogenicity in some animal experiments. Although there are no documented cases of fetal abnormalities during human pregnancy (e.g., during the treatment of toxoplasmosis in pregnant women), a low frequency of congenital defects could have been missed. In addition, sulfonamides may increase the risk of kernicterus in hyperbilirubinemic neonates, because sulfonamides displace unconjugated bilirubin from albumin. Therefore, short-acting sulfonamides should be used close to term, should be discontinued as soon as labor begins, and should not be given to a mother nursing a newborn.

Acute malaria because of its risk to mother and child should be treated according to the regimens outlined under Therapy. Primaquine should not be used during pregnancy for the treatment or prevention of relapsing malarias (*P. vivax* and *P. ovale*).

Eradication and Control in Endemic Areas. The major tools for the control of malaria have been directed against the vector. Antimalarial drugs, especially chloroquine, are used primarily to reduce morbidity and mortality. When malaria eradication was first instituted as a program of WHO in the 1950's, the program mainly emphasized spraying walls with residual insecticides, detecting malaria cases, and treating patients with antimalarial drugs. Insecticide resistance, avoidance by mosquitoes of sprayed surfaces, and outdoor feeding of mosquitoes have created major problems and led to the failure of malaria eradication in many areas. In addition, the spread of multidrug-resistant *P. falciparum* will probably increase morbidity and mortality in regions of resurgent malaria. There is no question that new tools such as vaccines and novel approaches to vector control will be sorely needed in the decades ahead.

Boyd MF (ed.): Malariology. Philadelphia, W. B. Saunders Company, 1949. *The best description of the course of each of the four human malarias in the nonimmune.*

Brown HW, Neva FA: Basic Clinical Parasitology. 5th ed. Norwalk, Appleton-Century-Crofts, 1983. *Color plates of malaria parasites for the inexperienced microscopist.*

Miller LH: Malaria. *In* Warren KW and Mahmoud AAF (eds.): Tropical and Geographical Medicine. New York, McGraw-Hill Book Company, 1983. *A general review of malariology with references.*

White NJ, Warrell DA, Chanthavanich P, Looareesurvan S, Warrell MJ, Krishna S, Williamson DH, Turner RC: Severe hypoglycemia and hyperinsulinemia in falciparum malaria. N Engl J Med 309:61, 1983. *A new complication of falciparum malaria.*

Udeinya IJ, Miller LH, McGregor IA, Jensen JB: *Plasmodium falciparum* strain-specific antibody blocks binding of infected erythrocytes to amelanotic melanoma cells. Nature 303:429, 1983. *An example of variant antigens in falciparum malaria.*

Development of mefloquine as an antimalaria drug. Bull WHO 61:169, 1983. *Review of data on an important, experimental antimalarial drug for chloroquine-resistant P. falciparum.*

379. AFRICAN TRYPANOSOMIASIS (Sleeping Sickness)

B. M. Greenwood

DEFINITION AND ETIOLOGY. Sleeping sickness, an infection caused by *Trypanosoma brucei*, occurs in two forms—West African or Gambian sleeping sickness and East African or Rhodesian sleeping sickness. Trypanosomes causing these diseases cannot be distinguished morphologically, but differentiation of isolates that are pathogenic for man from those that are not is often important. In general, nonpathogenic strains (*T. b. brucei*) lose their infectivity for laboratory animals when incubated in human serum, whereas strains pathogenic for humans (*T. b. gambiense* and *T. b. rhodesiense*) do not. These two subspecies can be differentiated by the electrophoretic pattern of their component enzymes.

On light microscopy *T. brucei* is seen to be an elongated trypanosome with a prominent nucleus, kinetoplast, and flagellum. Its length varies from 10 to 40 μ, slender and stumpy forms being found in the patient at the same time. Electron microscopy has revealed the detailed structure of the trypanosome. It is coated with an amorphous material which contains the variant antigens that are of vital importance to its survival.

EPIDEMIOLOGY. ***Distribution and Prevalence of Sleeping Sickness.*** Sleeping sickness is restricted to tropical Africa, where it has been recognized since the fourteenth century. Major epidemics, affecting several million people, occurred throughout the first half of the twentieth century. Sleeping sickness is now a less serious health problem, but many cases still occur in Zaire and in Uganda. Smaller foci persist in other countries such as the Ivory Coast.

Pathway of Infection. Tsetse flies are the natural vector of African trypanosomiasis. Intrauterine transmission has been recorded but is rare. Infections have followed accidental inoculation with trypanosomes in the laboratory.

When a tsetse fly bites an infected host, trypanosomes are sucked into the midgut with the blood meal. Here they pass around or through the peritrophic membrane, migrate forward between it and the gut wall, penetrate the gut wall, and reach the salivary glands, where development into new infective forms occurs. When a new host is bitten, trypanosomes pass down the proboscis with the saliva to start a new infection. Development within the fly takes two to five weeks.

Epidemiology of Gambian Sleeping Sickness. Humans are the main host of *T. b. gambiense*, but there is increasing evidence that animals such as the pig and sheep form an important reservoir of the infection. Gambian sleeping sickness is spread mainly by two species of tsetse fly, *Glossina palpalis* and *G. tachinoides*. These flies inhabit the shaded areas alongside rivers and streams, areas where their human victims can often be found. In some areas flies also rest and bite within a village. Thus, contact between humans and these tsetse flies is often very close, providing ideal conditions for transmission of the infection.

Epidemiology of Rhodesian Sleeping Sickness. *T. b. rhodesiense* differs from *T. b. gambiense* in being primarily a parasite of wild game, man acting only as an occasional and accidental host. Rhodesian sleeping sickness is spread by tsetse flies of the *G. morsitans* group, flies that can survive in open savanna. Rhodesian sleeping sickness is primarily an occupational disease, occurring mainly in those whose work takes them into areas of bush where wild game, especially the bushbuck, survives. Hunters, fishermen, honey-gatherers, and tourists are all at risk. This form of trypanosomiasis is usually a sporadic infection, but epidemics can occur. In the epidemic situation direct person-to-person transmission probably takes place.

PATHOLOGY. In the early stage of the disease the lymph nodes and spleen are enlarged and infiltrated with plasma cells and macrophages. Later, lymph nodes shrink and patchy fibrosis occurs. Lymphocytic infiltration of the pericardium and myocardium may be found, especially in the Rhodesian form of the disease. Characteristic changes are found in the brain and meninges once invasion of the central nervous system has occurred. These changes are most marked in long-standing cases of Gambian sleeping sickness. The meninges are thickened and infiltrated with lymphocytes, plasma cells, and morular cells. Morular cells are large cells with an eccentric nucleus displaced by numerous cytoplasmic vesicles which contain IgM. As the disease progresses, chronic inflammatory changes extend along the perivascular spaces to produce prominent perivascular cuffing. Finally, infiltration of the brain substance with lymphocytes, plasma cells, and morular cells takes place with accompanying neuronal degeneration and microglial proliferation.

PATHOGENESIS AND IMMUNITY. The immune response of the host plays an important part in the pathogenesis of sleeping sickness, but the nature of the immunopathologic reactions occurring in this infection has not been defined clearly. Patients with sleeping sickness have high serum immune complex levels and show laboratory abnormalities indicating activation of the complement and kinin systems. However, it is uncertain whether these immune complexes cause tissue damage; glomerulonephritis and arthritis are not usual features of the disease. Stimulation of the reticuloendothelial and B lymphoid systems may contribute to the lymphadenopathy and splenomegaly of the early phase of the infection. Large amounts of IgM are present in the serum and in the cerebrospinal fluid of patients with the infection. Only a small proportion of this immunoglobulin is parasite-specific antibody; the rest contains antibodies with a wide variety of specificities, including autoantibodies. Several aspects of lymphocyte function are impaired in patients with sleeping sickness. The resulting suppression of cellular and humoral immunity may contribute to the increased susceptibility of patients with sleeping sickness to other infections.

African trypanosomes possess surface and core antigens, both of which can induce an antibody response. Little is known about the role of cell-mediated immunity in this infection. In the presence of antibody to surface antigens, trypanosomes are lysed or taken up by cells of the reticuloendothelial system. However, successful eradication of the parasite is prevented by the process of antigenic variation. By progressive alteration of its surface antigens, the trypanosome is able to keep one step ahead of the host's immune response and thus to persist until the host eventually dies. The possible mechanisms of antigenic variation are of great interest to biologists. It is probable that each trypanosome possesses the necessary genetic information to synthesize several surface antigens, antigenic change being initiated by environmental factors such as contact with antibody.

CLINICAL FEATURES. Sleeping sickness passes through three pathologic and clinical phases: an initial phase in which trypanosomes are localized to the site of the tsetse fly bite; an early or systemic phase in which trypanosomes are widely distributed throughout the body; and a neurologic or advanced stage in which trypanosomes are largely restricted to the central nervous system. Rhodesian sleeping sickness is usually a much more rapidly progressive illness than Gambian sleeping sickness with less distinction between systemic and neurologic stages. However, this distinction is not an absolute one; in some outbreaks Gambian sleeping sickness has progressed rapidly, whereas occasionally Rhodesian sleeping sickness follows a more benign course.

Gambian Sleeping Sickness. Ten days after a bite by an infected tsetse fly, a small nodular lesion, a chancre, may develop at the site of the bite and persist for two to three weeks. This lesion, if it occurs, frequently passes unnoticed.

Months or even years after an infected bite, clinical features of systemic invasion with trypanosomes occur. Fever and lymphadenopathy are the main features of this early stage of the infection. Fever is usually intermittent and may be mild. Lymphadenopathy may be general, but the posterior cervical nodes are nearly always involved. Enlarged nodes are firm but not usually tender. Moderate splenomegaly may occur. Urticarial rashes, erythematous rashes, and localized edema may be seen. A variety of eye lesions have been recorded, but these are rare. Electrocardiograms are often abnormal, but clinical signs of heart disease are unusual. Mild normocytic anemia and mild thrombocytopenia are common. The serum IgM level is nearly always raised.

Months or years after the first appearance of symptoms, the clinical features of the early phase of the disease regress to be replaced by new symptoms and signs indicating invasion of the nervous system. Mild behavioral and personality changes are often the first signs of central nervous system involvement. Later, more florid psychologic changes may occur with hallucinations and delusions. Headache and backache are common

TABLE 379–1. SOME CONTRASTING FEATURES OF GAMBIAN AND RHODESIAN SLEEPING SICKNESS

	Gambian Sleeping Sickness	Rhodesian Sleeping Sickness
Causative organism	*Trypanosoma brucei gambiense*	*Trypanosoma brucei rhodesiense*
Distribution	West and Central Africa	East Africa
Source of infection	Humans (domestic animals)	Wild game (man)
Vector	*Glossina palpalis* or *tachinoides* (riverine tsetse)	*Glossina morsitans* (savanna tsetse)
Clinical features		
Lymphadenopathy	+ +	+
Heart failure	0	+ +
Neurologic	+ +	+
Disseminated intravascular coagulation	0	+
Diagnosis	Trypanosomes in lymph node juice or CSF	Trypanosomes in blood or CSF
Course of infection	Slow	Rapid

complaints. Drowsiness during the day, the feature from which the disease takes its name, may occur but is not invariable, and some patients are manic. If no treatment is given, the patient's level of consciousness progressively deteriorates until finally he lapses into stupor. Convulsions occasionally occur. Chorea and athetosis are the most frequently encountered localizing neurologic signs. Pyramidal tract involvement is less frequent and cranial nerve lesions are rare. Obesity and impotence or amenorrhea frequently occur and perhaps follow from damage to the hypothalamus. Severe itching is an unexplained symptom that may lead to skin changes. The cerebrospinal fluid shows an increase in cells and protein, much of which is IgM. Free immunoglobulin light chains may be present. Most of the cells are lymphocytes, but a few are plasma cells and morular cells. Trypanosomes may be present.

Rhodesian Sleeping Sickness. The clinical picture of Rhodesian sleeping sickness is similar to that described above, but on presentation the patient is usually more acutely ill than a patient with Gambian sleeping sickness, and the disease progresses more rapidly. Heart failure and jaundice occur more frequently than in Gambian sleeping sickness, but lymphadenopathy is usually less prominent. Neurologic features similar to those described above may be present, but sometimes death occurs before these have had time to develop. Anemia and thrombocytopenia are usual, and disseminated intravascular coagulation may occur. Liver function test results are often abnormal, and an abnormal electrocardiogram is usually obtained. Cerebrospinal fluid changes are the same as those described above.

DIAGNOSIS. The chancre of trypanosomiasis has no special features and is unlikely to be recognized unless there is a strong reason for suspecting trypanosomiasis. It must be differentiated from an allergic reaction to a tsetse fly bite. Trypanosomes are present in juice obtained from the lesion.

The clinical features of the early phase of sleeping sickness are similar to those of many infectious, neoplastic, and connective tissue diseases. Trypanosomiasis must be considered in the differential diagnosis of unexplained pyrexia or lymphadenopathy in any patient who has visited an endemic area, even if only for a short holiday. Diagnosis of Rhodesian sleeping sickness can usually be made by the demonstration of trypanosomes in a thick blood film. However, trypanosomes are found less frequently in the blood of patients with Gambian sleeping sickness even when concentration methods such as ion-exchange chromatography, culture, or animal inoculation are used. Diagnosis is made most readily in the early stage of Gambian sleeping sickness by the detection of trypanosomes in the juice obtained on puncturing an enlarged lymph node with a venipuncture needle.

Once invasion of the central nervous system has occurred, clinical diagnosis of sleeping sickness is usually not difficult. However, tragic misdiagnoses have been made in patients with predominantly psychologic features. Chorea may be so marked as to suggest Sydenham's chorea, and confusion with other extrapyramidal syndromes may occur occasionally. Diagnosis of the advanced stage of sleeping sickness is confirmed by examination of the cerebrospinal fluid. Trypanosomes can be found in most patients, provided both that the cerebrospinal fluid is examined immediately after collection and that scrupulously clean glassware is used. Measurement of the cerebrospinal fluid IgM level is often of great diagnostic help in patients in whom trypanosomes cannot be found. A high cerebrospinal fluid IgM in the presence of a modest increase in total protein is almost pathognomonic of sleeping sickness.

Many different serologic tests have been used to diagnose sleeping sickness. These tests have proved of great value in survey work but are of less value in the investigation of individual patients, as false-positive and false-negative reactions can occur.

TREATMENT. ***General Measures.*** Whenever possible, a patient with sleeping sickness should be treated in hospital. Lumbar puncture to determine the stage of the disease must be carried out before treatment is started. If abnormalities are found (a raised cell count or protein), the patient must be treated as having advanced disease, even if there are no clinical signs of central nervous system involvement. Poorly nourished patients may require dietary supplements. A search should be made for any associated infections, and these should be treated appropriately.

Many different drugs and dosage regimens have been used in the treatment of sleeping sickness, but few controlled trials have been undertaken and the treatment schedules currently in use were established empirically. All the drugs used in the treatment of sleeping sickness were developed many years ago, and all are toxic; there is still a great need for safer effective drugs.

Chemotherapy of Early Disease. Suramin is an effective treatment for early Gambian and Rhodesian sleeping sickness, but it is ineffective in advanced disease, since it penetrates poorly into the cerebrospinal fluid. Suramin* is a white powder that is made up in an aqueous solution immediately before use and given intravenously in a dose of 20 mg per kilogram of body weight. Occasionally it causes vomiting and collapse, so it is customary to start with a test dose of one fifth of this amount. A course comprises five to ten injections given at two- to five-day intervals. The drug can cause renal damage; because of this, the urine should be tested for protein and casts before each injection. Mild proteinuria can be ignored; but if heavy proteinuria develops or if casts are found, treatment should be stopped. Three injections of melarsoprol (see below) is an effective alternative form of treatment of early disease. Berenil is also effective but has been used less widely.

Chemotherapy of Advanced Disease. Melarsoprol (Mel B) is the treatment of choice for both Gambian and Rhodesian sleeping sickness once involvement of the central nervous system has occurred, even though the drug is very toxic. It is possible that toxicity is reduced by prior treatment with one or two injections of suramin, but melarsoprol should be started right away in patients who are very sick. Mel B is dispensed as a 3.6 per cent solution in propylene glycol. This is very irritating and is liable to produce thrombophlebitis. The full dosage of Mel B* is 3.6 mg (0.1 ml) per kilogram of body weight given intravenously up to a maximum of 5.0 ml. The following is an effective schedule of treatment for an adult: 2.5 ml on days 1 and 3, followed by 5.0 ml on day 5; rest for one week; 5.0 ml on days 15, 17, and 19; rest for a further week; and then 5.0 ml on days 29, 31, and 33 (total dose, 40.0 ml). Other schedules employ a more gradual build-up to full dosage. Treatment schedules should be kept flexible and slowed down if reactions occur. Febrile reactions are common after the first injection of Mel B, especially if suramin has not been given. Mel B can produce rashes, marrow depression, and renal damage, but its most serious side effect is an encephalopathy which occurs in about 5 per cent of patients. Encephalopathy occurs most frequently at the time of the third or fourth injection; it may develop very rapidly and has a mortality of about 50 per cent. It is uncertain whether it is due to arsenic poisoning or to an immunopathologic reaction. Dimercaprol (BAL) has been used to treat this complication of Mel B treatment, but its value has not been clearly established. It has been suggested that corticosteroids protect patients from Mel B encephalopathy, but this assertion has never been clearly documented.

Follow-up and Treatment of Relapses. The results of treatment of patients with early disease with suramin or melarsoprol are excellent, but occasional patients subsequently develop neurologic disease and require treatment with a full course of Mel B. Regular follow-up with clinical examination and lumbar puncture is therefore necessary for at least one year after treatment and preferably for longer.

---

*Available from the Centers for Disease Control (404–329–3670); (404–329–2888) evenings, weekends, and holidays.

Patients with neurologic disease also require regular follow-up, for treatment failures and relapses occasionally occur. Patients with a relapse of advanced disease should receive another full course of Mel B* (total dosage, 40.0 ml for an adult) together with nitrofurazone, for, despite the toxicity of this drug, there is an impression that relapsed patients treated with melarsoprol and nitrofurazone do better than those receiving melarsoprol alone. The adult dosage of nitrofurazone* is 0.5 gram given by mouth every six hours for five days, this course being repeated on two or three occasions. Nitrofurazone is a toxic drug causing peripheral neuropathy and hemolytic anemia, especially in those with glucose-6-phosphatase deficiency.

PROGNOSIS. Many patients with early Gambian sleeping sickness remain relatively well for months or years without treatment, and it is possible that a few recover spontaneously. Once central nervous system involvement has occurred, death is inevitable unless treatment is given. Death frequently follows a secondary infection, often pneumonia, in a stuporous and malnourished patient. Patients with Rhodesian sleeping sickness may die from heart failure.

The results of treatment of patients in the early phase of sleeping sickness are excellent, over 90 per cent making a complete recovery. However, a few patients subsequently develop central nervous system involvement and require further treatment. Mel B achieves a parasitologic "cure" in at least 90 per cent of cases of advanced disease, and many patients make a complete recovery. Unfortunately some patients are left with irreversible neurologic damage. These patients must be differentiated from those who have had a true relapse and require further treatment. About 5 per cent of patients die during the course of Mel B treatment.

An attack of sleeping sickness does not induce protective immunity, and reinfection may occur.

CONTROL AND PROPHYLAXIS. Many different approaches have been made to the control of sleeping sickness. In West Africa, survey teams have been used extensively to detect and treat asymptomatic patients early in the course of their disease, thus reducing the reservoir of infection. In East Africa, attempts have been made to reduce the reservoir of infection in wild game. A wide variety of techniques has been used to destroy tsetse flies, ranging from hand trapping to aerial spraying with insecticides. Currently, the potential control value of traps baited with animal odors is being evaluated.

Pentamidine* has been successfully used as a chemoprophylactic in Gambian sleeping sickness when given by a single intramuscular injection of 4 mg per kilogram every three to six months. However, its use carries the risk of producing cryptic infections, and the drug can cause diabetes. It should therefore be used only in those who are at considerable risk of being infected.

The occurrence of antigenic variation has been a major obstacle to the development of a successful vaccine. However, progress in culture of *T. brucei* in vitro and in analysis of the chemical structure of its variant antigens and the mechanisms underlying their expression holds out some hope for the future.

---

*Available from the Centers for Disease Control (404–329–3670); (404–329–2888) evenings, weekends, and holidays.

Apted FIC: Clinical manifestations and diagnosis of sleeping sickness. *In* Mulligan HW (ed.): The African Trypanosomiases. London, George Allen and Unwin, 1970, pp 661–683. *A comprehensive review of the clinical features of sleeping sickness.*

Ford J: The role of African Trypanosomiases in African Ecology. Oxford, Clarendon Press, 1971. *A very readable account of the social impact of human and cattle trypanosomiasis in Africa.*

Greenwood BM, Whittle HC: The pathogenesis of sleeping sickness. Trans Roy Soc Trop Med Hyg 74:716, 1980. *A review of the ways in which the immune response of the host may contribute to the pathology and clinical features of sleeping sickness.*

Lambert PH, Berney M, Kazyumba G: Immune complexes in serum and in cerebrospinal fluid in African trypanosomiasis: Correlation with polyclonal B cell activation and with intracerebral immunoglobulin synthesis. J Clin Invest 67:77, 1981. *An account of the possible role of immune complexes in the pathogenesis of sleeping sickness.*

Vickerman K: Antigenic variation in trypanosomes. Nature 273:613, 1978. *A concise and lucid review of this complex but very interesting biologic phenomenon.*

WHO and FAO: The African Trypanosomiases. Technical report series 635. Geneva, World Health Organization, 1979. *A short report covering various aspects of African trypanosomiasis in man and in cattle. Contains several tables with epidemiologic information.*

380. CHAGAS' DISEASE (American Trypanosomiasis)

Vanize Macedo

DEFINITION. Chagas' disease, an infection caused by *Trypanosoma cruzi* and named after its Brazilian discoverer, Carlos Chagas, is found only in the Western Hemisphere. A distinction must be made between infection and disease. The majority of infected patients develop no signs of clinically detectable disease. Chagas himself described the two main disease forms occurring years after the initial infection: a chronic cardiomyopathy often with intracardiac conduction defects, and dilatation of the esophagus or colon (the mega syndromes).

ETIOLOGY. The trypanomastigote is visible in peripheral blood films of man and the multitude of naturally or experimentally infected animals studied in the early or acute phase of the disease. It is polymorphic, 15 to 25 μ long, and has a large subterminal kinetoplast. Multiplication takes place only in an amastigote phase in host cells. The trypanomastigote penetrates a host cell (frequently a cardiac or smooth muscle cell), rounds up, and commences to replicate by binary fission every 12 hours. The time of rupture of this host cell will depend on its size. The amastigotes change into trypanomastigotes, which are released to circulate in the peripheral blood and penetrate new cells. After a period of weeks, the host immune response suppresses the trypanomastigote parasitemia to subpatent levels. Small numbers continue to circulate for years.

EVOLUTIONARY CYCLE. The insect vector of *T. cruzi* is a hemipteran, a reduviid bug of the subfamily Triatominae, of which about 100 species have been described. They are obligate blood suckers and withdraw a large blood meal rapidly by directly tapping a subcutaneous capillary with their stylet mouth parts. The great majority of these are sylvatic and maintain cycles among wild animals. Such bugs are found from within 200 miles of New York to the south of Argentina. For reasons that are unclear, a small number of species have become highly domesticated, and those cohabiting with man are the transmitters of Chagas' disease. The most important species in this respect are *Triatoma infestans, Panstrongylus megistus,* and *Rhodnius prolixus.*

EPIDEMIOLOGY. Transmission is usually at night, when the bugs are active. They feed mainly on the face and arms, the uncovered parts of sleeping man. As they engorge with blood, the rise in intra-abdominal pressure promotes defecation, and the trypanomastigotes in the feces can penetrate mucous membranes or small skin abrasions. The three main species of transmitting bugs all tend to defecate soon after feeding.

Congenital transmission and infection by blood transfusion can occur. More rarely, transmission may occur as a result of a laboratory accident. There exists the possibility of contamination by the digestive tract.

Chagas' disease has been described in all the countries of South America and Central America with the exception of Guyana and Surinam. In Mexico it is rare. Two autochthonous acute cases have been reported in Texas. The high standard of housing and the discrete nature of the sylvatic cycles makes transmission to man a very rare event in North America. Chagas' disease is a serious public health problem in South America, principally in Argentina, Brazil, Chile, Uruguay, and Venezuela. There are geographic differences in the disease; for example, cardiomyopathy is rare in Chile, and the mega syndromes are unknown in Venezuela. From some countries (e.g.,

Bolivia) there is little information on the status of Chagas' disease.

It is estimated that the prevalence of trypanosomiasis may reach 20 per cent in the rural zones of the countries where it is endemic. Socioeconomic conditions are bad in these areas and dwellings are of poor construction with mud and sticks, building materials which favor bug colonization. Chagas' disease is intimately linked with economic underdevelopment.

The medicosocial importance of the disease has not been determined, and we do not know for certain the role American trypanosomiasis plays in the economy of countries where it is endemic. Cardiopathy is the most important form of the disease, causing a significant mortality and inability to work in the most productive phase of life. Many employers in Brazil will not hire a worker with positive serology.

PATHOGENESIS. The local tissue inflammation promoted by rupture of nests of amastigotes of *T. cruzi* was the first interpretation of the pathology of the disease. This view explains the alterations that occur in the acute phase but not all those that occur in the chronic phase. In this phase amastigotes are rarely found.

There is evidence suggesting that an autoimmune process is at work in the chronic cardiomyopathy of Chagas' disease. Santos, Buch, and Teixeira have demonstrated that sensitized lymphocytes from rabbits chronically infected with *T. cruzi* are cytotoxic to normal cardiac cells. Cossio and colleagues have identified circulating autoantibodies to heart tissue in patients with chronic cardiomyopathy.

The importance of strains of the parasite or reinfection in the pathogenesis of Chagas' disease is still not clear.

PATHOLOGY. In the acute phase the infection is generalized, and amastigotes of *T. cruzi* can be found in cells of the reticuloendothelial system. Initially reticular cells are parasitized, and in a short time smooth and striated muscle cells, including cardiac muscle, glial and nerve cells, and fat cells, are invaded.

The inoculation lesion shows inflammation with infiltration of lymphocytes and plasma cells and fibroblastic proliferation. The heart is enlarged and flabby, with predominance of dilatation over hypertrophy. Hemorrhagic foci may be seen on the endocardium. Microscopically there is diffuse edema, both intestinal and interfibrillar congestion, and the presence of amastigotes in the cardiac fibers. The cardiac fibers show hyaline necrosis and degeneration (lesions of Margarino Torres). In the central nervous system there is mononuclear infiltration of the leptomeninges, congestive perivascular inflammation, and hemorrhage with glial proliferation and neurophagia. Amastigotes may be encountered in the cells of the central nervous system.

In the chronic cardiac form the heart is enlarged with both hypertrophy and dilatation, so that the apex is formed by the terminations of both ventricles. The epicardium is congested, and there may be a small pericardial effusion. There are no organic valvular lesions. The thinned myocardium of the apex may distend to form an apical aneurysm, a characteristic lesion of Chagas' disease. Mural thrombosis is frequent on the endocardium, particularly in the right atrium and the apex of the left ventricle. Thrombosis at the apex is an important finding in Chagas' myocarditis. These intracardiac thrombi are the source of emboli principally to the lungs, kidneys, cerebrum, and spleen. There is chronic passive congestion of the organs.

Microscopy demonstrates an intense diffuse myocarditis with focal areas of cellular infiltration containing mononuclear cells, lymphocytes, and plasma cells. There is hypertrophy of the cardiac fibers with small areas of focal necrosis, hemorrhage, and granular degeneration. A variable degree of fibrosis is associated with edema and vascular dilatation and congestion. Tissue amastigotes are rarely seen in chronic cases.

Andrade has shown that these inflammatory changes directly involve the conducting system of the heart, particularly the sinoatrial node, the inferior third of the atrioventricular node, the right half of the main bundle, the right bundle branch, and the anterior ramification of the left bundle branch. He established a good correlation between the electrocardiogram in life and these pathologic changes.

In the indeterminate form of Chagas' disease, active myocarditis with granuloma formation and neuronal destruction of Auerbach's plexus has been found, but in lesser degree than established cardiomyopathy. In megaesophagus and megacolon the organ is dilated with focal myositis associated with a diminution in the number of nerve cells in Auerbach's plexus.

In the congenital form a chronic placentitis with ischemia of the chorionic villi occurs. Edema and a histiocytic inflammatory infiltrate are present with small foci of necrosis in these villi. Amastigotes are visible in the cytoplasm of macrophages.

CLINICAL PRESENTATION. Chagas' disease has an acute and chronic phase. In endemic areas discrepancies exist between the prevalence of the chronic phase and the small number of cases diagnosed as acute disease.

Acute Phase. In areas endemic for Chagas' disease, the acute phase is diagnosed in about 1 per cent of patients. Probably in the majority of individuals the initial phase of the infection is not apparent. Seventy per cent of patients in this phase are children under ten years of age. Acute Chagas' disease is rare in adults.

The incubation period is 4 to 12 days. The signs at the portal of entry often call the attention of the physician to the possible diagnosis of the disease. Romaña's sign is present in half the patients in the acute phase. This is a unilateral, bipalpebral, firm, violaceous edema, frequently with conjunctivitis and enlargement of the preauricular gland. An inoculation chagoma may occur in exposed areas, such as the face or arms, where the bug has an opportunity of biting. This also is characterized by erythema and infiltrative tumefaction of the skin with satellite ganglion reaction, which, when it disappears, leaves hyperpigmentation. It is found in 25 per cent of patients in the acute phase. A minority of patients do not present signs of a portal of entry.

The disease is characterized by prolonged fever, asthenia, enlargement of lymphatic glands, edema of the face and legs, and hepatosplenomegaly. Tachycardia is frequently present even in the absence of fever. This is a sign of myocarditis, which is benign in the majority of cases and diagnosed only on electrocardiogram.

The signs of the acute phase disappear in two to four months. The so-called schizotrypanides are skin rashes that rarely occur in the acute phase. They may take the form of erythematous indurated plaques or may be morbilliform or urticarial in type, suggesting an allergic nature. Meningoencephalitis is also a rare complication, often occurring in children under one year of age and usually fatal. Clinical evidence of encephalitis may be complicated by convulsions.

Congenital Disease. Since this is rarely diagnosed, its prevalence in endemic areas cannot be estimated. Such newborns are underweight and afebrile, and have hepatosplenomegaly and often edema. Petechiae, bruising, and frank hemorrhage may be noted. Meningoencephalitis may produce convulsions and tremors of the face and limbs. If jaundice is present, it disappears in the third week. Metastatic chagomas have been described, with skin infiltration, infection, and even necrosis.

The Chronic Phase. INDETERMINATE FORM. After the acute phase, individuals can stay for many years or all their lives in a latent or indeterminate phase. These subjects do not have clinical, radiologic, or electrocardiographic signs. In endemic areas, approximately half of those infected show this form. It is probable that this number will diminish as more sophisticated methods for detecting disease are developed.

CARDIAC FORM. This is the most important clinical form of the chronic phase, and its prevalence can reach 30 per cent of individuals in an endemic area. The majority of patients have no cardiac symptoms or signs but only electrocardiographic evidence of disease.

Palpitations, usually the result of extrasystoles, are a frequent initial symptom. They may be accompanied by dizziness and precordial pain. Right-sided ventricular failure predominates, and dyspnea is infrequent.

Physical examination shows an irregular pulse and distant heart sounds, fixed splitting of the pulmonary second sound, gallop rhythm, and a functional regurgitant murmur in the mitral area. In advanced cases, tricuspid regurgitation can occur and cyanosis is present. Thromboembolic phenomena are very frequent and may precede symptoms of cardiac insufficiency. Total atrioventricular block is rare but is frequently accompanied by Stokes-Adams attacks.

DIGESTIVE FORM. The digestive form is characterized by dilatation and alteration in motility of the esophagus or colon. Rarely the stomach or small intestine shows similar changes.

In megaesophagus the principal symptom is long-standing dysphagia, which begins with difficulty with solid food and progresses until the patient can swallow only soft foods with the aid of frequent sips of water. In advanced cases, patients have pain on swallowing, regurgitation, and pyrosis with a sensation of suffocation. Hiccup, sialorrhea, and nocturnal cough are associated symptoms. Hypersalivation is accompanied by parotid gland enlargement. Marked weight loss is present, and aspiration pneumonias may occur in advanced cases.

Megacolon is manifested by retention of feces and gas and often progresses to fecaloma formation. Volvulus and intestinal obstruction are frequent complications. The majority of cases of megacolon are associated with megaesophagus. Half of the patients with digestive forms of Chagas' disease have abnormal electrocardiograms.

OTHER CLINICAL FORMS. Rare complications are megaureter, megabladder, megagallbladder, and bronchiectasis. The forms of central nervous system involvement in chronic infection, described by Chagas himself, are still debatable. The denervation process has been implicated in the dysfunction of various exocrine and endocrine glands.

DIAGNOSIS. *Acute Phase.* The acute phase is usually diagnosed by finding the trypanomastigote in the peripheral blood on direct examination of thick films. This is the best criterion for diagnosing the acute phase. Should this fail, simple concentration methods are usually positive, such as examination of the leukocyte cream after centrifugation or allowing the blood to clot and examining the supernatant (Strout's method). Biopsy of the calf muscle shows myositis and frequently nests of amastigotes.

The *xenodiagnostic test* is often positive before 30 days owing to the high number of circulating trypanosomes. Similarly, cultures (NNN) and subinoculation of mice recover the organism. The serologic reactions, usually positive in this early stage, are precipitins and agglutinins. There is a raised IgM. The complement fixation test result becomes positive four to six weeks after infection. The indirect immunofluorescent test becomes positive earlier than the hemagglutination and complement fixation tests. The white cell count shows leukocytosis caused by an intense lymphocytosis with atypical lymphocytes. The erythrocyte sedimentation rate is increased, as are the mucoproteins. Heterophil antibodies may appear in the serum, and the Paul Bunnell reaction may be positive. Protein electrophoresis reveals a slight hypoalbuminemia with a rise in gamma and alpha 2 globulins. The transaminases are slightly elevated. The electrocardiogram may show sinus tachycardia, low voltage complexes, first degree atrioventricular block, increased QT space, primary alterations in ventricular repolarization, and sometimes subepicardial ischemia. Alterations in cardiac rhythm are rare at this stage and a bad prognostic sign.

On x-ray examination, there may be enlargement of the cardiac shadow, which may be transitory. At times such enlargement is due to a pericardial effusion. Marked cardiomegaly indicates a bad prognosis.

Chronic Phase. Evidence of infection is established mainly by serologic tests such as complement fixation, hemagglutination, and immunofluorescence. Xenodiagnosis, using 40 bugs, will isolate an organism in about 50 per cent of cases. In the indeterminate phase, only these investigations will be positive.

A chest x-ray may be normal, but frequently a degree of cardiomegaly is seen progressing to marked global enlargement of the heart. The electrocardiogram is valuable, as conduction defects are common. In the endemic area of São Felipe, Brazil, the following abnormalities were present in a frequency of 15 to 20 per cent: complete right bundle branch block with anterior hemiblock, ventricular extrasystoles, first degree atrioventricular block, and alterations in ventricular repolarization. Total atrioventricular block or complete left bundle branch block occurred in only 0.2 per cent. There may be evidence of septal fibrosis. Digestive tract involvement is revealed by radiologic studies in a patient with a suggestive history. Both the esophagus and colon are dilated, with abnormal peristalsis and evidence of retained food residues.

DIFFERENTIAL DIAGNOSIS. Romaña's sign must be distinguished from conjunctivitis, orbital cellulitis, cavernous sinus thrombosis, insect bites, and trauma, all of which produce unilateral orbital edema. Clinically the acute phase may resemble typhoid fever, infectious mononucleosis, kala-azar, brucellosis, toxoplasmosis, and acute glomerulonephritis. Other types of acute myocarditis must be considered.

Congenital infections must be distinguished from syphilis, toxoplasmosis, and cytomegalic inclusion disease.

Chronic cardiomyopathy involves a differential diagnosis from the cardiomyopathies associated with alcohol, pregnancy, idiopathic cardiomyopathy, endomyocardial fibrosis, and ischemic heart disease. The absence of organic valvular lesions usually permits a distinction from rheumatic valvular disease. Carcinoma of the esophagus may mimic megaesophagus. The presence of positive serology and electrocardiographic changes assist in the differential diagnosis from megaesophagus and megacolon not caused by Chagas' disease.

EVOLUTION AND PROGNOSIS. Chagas' cardiomyopathy is variable in its course and of uncertain prognosis. In the acute phase 10 per cent of patients die of myocarditis or acute meningoencephalitis. The latter condition usually occurs in children under one year of age. The indeterminate phase can last a lifetime. The factors influencing the evolution of the disease are not clear. There is some evidence that reinfections could play a role in an endemic area. The strain of parasite and the host's response to it could be important. Cardiomyopathy begins in the second to fifth decade. Heart failure in these age groups leads to death one to five years after its initial appearance. The prognosis is poor if cardiac failure appears before 30 years of age.

A longitudinal study in São Felipe, Brazil, showed that each year the disease made a detectable progression in 5.5 per cent of patients. The mortality was 0.7 per cent per year. The principal cause of death was cardiac failure in 58.3 per cent. Sudden death from conduction defects occurred in 37.5 per cent. The following electrocardiographic changes were associated with a 50 per cent mortality in five years: total atrioventricular block, atrial fibrillation, left bundle branch block, multifocal extrasystoles, and septal fibrosis.

TREATMENT. Two drugs appear to kill circulating trypanosomes and may have value in the specific treatment of Chagas' disease. These are nifurtimox, a nitrofuran derivative (Bayer 2502 [Lampit]), and benznidazole, a nitroimidazole (RO7–1051 Rochagan).

Nifurtimox* is used in a dose of 8 mg per kilogram of body weight per day for a period of 120 days. With regard to eradicating parasitemia, it has given good results in patients in the acute and chronic phases in Chile, Argentina, and southern Brazil. In other areas of Brazil, such as Bahia, Goiás, and Minas

*Available from Centers for Disease Control (404–329–3670); (404–329–2888) evenings, weekends, and holidays.

Gerais, the results have been less satisfactory, only 40 per cent of individuals being uniformly negative on repeated xenodiagnosis after treatment. Experiments in animals infected with different strains of *T. cruzi* demonstrated different susceptibilities to nifurtimox. This reinforces the hypothesis that different strains of *T. cruzi* may be responsible for these variations in response to treatment. Benznidazole* is used in a dose of 5 mg per kilogram per day for 60 days and also eradicates parasitemia in a proportion of patients. Both these drugs have serious side effects and should be used only under direct medical supervision. The side effects include polyneuritis, dizziness, loss of weight, nausea, and insomnia. With use of benznidazole, exfoliative dermatitis and thrombocytopenic purpura have also been seen.

It is not known how important such specific treatment is in arresting the disease. If parasitemia is an important factor in the evolution of the disease, then certainly the acute phase should be treated. In the acute phase, both serologic tests and xenodiagnosis may remain negative after treatment. In the chronic phase, those in whom xenodiagnosis becomes negative remain positive serologically. It is still not clear whether such treatment is of value in the chronic phase.

When chronic myocarditis is associated with heart failure, the treatment is symptomatic. Digitalis must be used with care because of sensitivity of the damaged cardiac fiber, and the response is poor in relation to other cardiomyopathies. Extrasystoles, the most frequent arrhythmia, may be helped by procainamide. In ventricular tachycardia, procainamide and lidocaine are the drugs indicated. Beta-adrenergic blocking agents are dangerous in acute arrhythmias in Chagas' myocarditis, as they may produce bradycardia and shock. Deaths have been reported after the use of propranolol. In Stokes-Adams crises, isopropyl norepinephrine is useful. In patients with total atrioventricular block and a normal or slightly enlarged heart, implantation of a pacemaker is indicated. Marked cardiac enlargement carries a poor prognosis, because either the weak cardiac muscle cannot support the new rhythm or an intramural clot may become dislodged.

Initially megaesophagus is treated by balloon dilatation; in more advanced cases cardiotomy is often successful. Operations consisting of excision of the aperistaltic esophagus and replacement with a segment of colon or small intestine have been developed. In megacolon, evacuation of a fecaloma may be an emergency procedure. It has to be carried out with care, for rupture of the colon and septicemia can follow the procedure. Resection of the aperistaltic segment may relieve persistent constipation.

PROPHYLAXIS. The important prophylactic measures in the control of Chagas' disease are better housing, public health education, and application of insecticides in the house and its environs. Benzene hexachloride (BHC), the insecticide of choice, is applied in a suspension of 500 mg of the gamma isomer per square meter every six months.

In blood banks in endemic areas of Chagas' disease, 1:4000 gentian violet is added to stored blood 24 hours before use in order to kill the trypanosomes. To date, no results that can be applied to humans have been obtained with immunoprotection for Chagas' disease.

---

*Available from Centers for Disease Control (404–329–3670); (404–329–2888) evenings, weekends, and holidays.

American Trypanosomiasis Research. PAHO Scientific Publication 318, 1975. *A monograph with extensive reviews of many aspects of research.*

Andrade Z, Andrade SG: Chagas' disease (American trypanosomiasis). *In* Marcial-Rojas RA (ed.): Pathology of Protozoal and Helminthic Disease. Baltimore, Williams & Wilkins Company, 1971. *An account of the pathology of Chagas' disease.*

Chagas C: Processos patojênicos da tripanosomiase americana. Memórias do Instituto Oswaldo Cruz 8:5, 1916. *A classic account demonstrating Carlos Chagas' remarkable insight into the disease he discovered.*

Köberle F: Patologia y anatomia patológica de la enfermedad de Chagas. Bol Sanit Panam 51:404, 1961. *A paper examining the role of parasympathetic denervation in the pathogenesis of megasyndromes and cardiopathy.*

Laranja FS, Dias E, Nóbrega G, Miranda A: Chagas' disease—a clinical epidemiologic and pathologic study. Circulation 14:1035, 1956. *One of the first satisfactory accounts of the clinical cardiology.*

Prata A, Andrade Z, Guimarães A: Chagas' heart disease. *In* Shaper AG, Hutt MSR, Fejfar Z (eds.): Cardiovascular Disease in the Tropics. London, British Medical Association, 1974. *A review of Chagas' heart disease.*

World Health Organization: Chagas' Disease: Report of a Study Group. Technical Report Series No 202, 1960. *The first report published before the current wave of interest.*

381. LEISHMANIASIS

Franklin A. Neva

DEFINITION. Leishmaniasis is a protozoan infection caused by various species of the genus *Leishmania*. Paradoxically, the host cells for these intracellular parasites are macrophages, the very cells normally involved in defense mechanisms. The natural cycle of infection is usually a zoonosis, with phlebotomine sandflies as vectors transmitting the parasite among wild or domestic animals, especially rodents and canines. Humans are generally incidental hosts.

The traditional view that all human leishmanial infections result in either visceral or cutaneous involvement needs modification. Visceral involvement when it happens represents a severe systemic disease with parasites invading the reticuloendothelial system, and is characterized by hepatosplenomegaly, fever, weight loss, leukopenia, and ultimately death. The cutaneous disease is manifested by one or more indolent, ulcerative lesions that can heal spontaneously, but sometimes the disease later produces metastatic destructive lesions of the oronasopharynx—i.e., mucocutaneous leishmaniasis. While these concepts of visceral and cutaneous prototypes are useful, it is now apparent that clinical leishmaniasis is a spectrum of manifestations, especially as it involves the skin. There is increasing evidence that the clinical outcome of leishmanial infection is determined by the interaction of intrinsic characteristics of the infecting organism with immune response of the host. Unfortunately, nomenclature and speciation of *Leishmania* are still uncertain because of development of new technologies for classification.

ETIOLOGY. *Leishmania* exist in two morphologic forms, a motile flagellate or *promastigote*, and a smaller, nonmotile intracellular form, the *amastigote*. Promastigotes are found in the sandfly vector as well as in artificial cultures, both habitats requiring temperatures of about 22 to 26° C. Amastigotes, the form of the parasite in humans and other vertebrate hosts, are round or oval bodies of about $2 \times 5\ \mu$, without a free flagellum. Also called *Leishman-Donovan* or *LD bodies* after their describers, amastigotes contain a nucleus and a characteristic rodlike structure of extranuclear DNA, the *kinetoplast*. When stained by Giemsa or Wright's, the nucleus is reddish, the kinetoplast purple, and the cytoplasm a pale blue.

In the infected animal, leishmania are found only in macrophages where they multiply by binary fission, rupture out, and infect new cells. An appropriate sandfly vector becomes infected by ingesting infected cells from the skin or blood during a blood meal. In the gut of the sandfly, the parasites transform to promastigotes and multiply as spindle-shaped flagellates of 15 to 25 μ length and 2 to 3 μ width. In vectors ultimately capable of transmitting the parasite, promastigotes tend to migrate to a higher level in the gut of the fly, even into the pharynx and buccal cavity. At least seven days are needed before the sandfly becomes infective. The actual mechanism by which infective promastigotes are transferred to a new vertebrate host is not clear—possibly by regurgitation into the bite wound during a blood meal or perhaps even being rubbed into abrasions after a successful swat. Once inoculated, the promastigotes are taken up by macrophages; they are transformed into amastigotes and begin to multiply. Amastigotes that rupture from infected macrophages are taken up by adjacent cells; some infected cells may be transported to distant sites via the blood or lymphatics.

Classification of *Leishmania* was previously determined mainly by geographic origin of the parasite, and the nature of disease produced in the hamster. *L. donovani* was associated with visceral disease and produced fatal hepatosplenic disease in hamsters. This behavior in the hamster was consistent, even with isolates from different regions of the world. Strains causing cutaneous disease in the Old World produced only modest cutaneous lesions in the hamster and were called *L. tropica.* The situation with cutaneous strains from the Americas was more complicated, with isolates broadly separable into two groups, the *L. mexicana* and *L. braziliensis* complexes. Rapidity of growth in culture was considered an additional criterion for these two groups. In recent years, biochemical taxonomy based upon isoenzyme patterns and DNA peptide mapping has permitted a more detailed grouping of strains. In addition, immunologic reactivity to monoclonal antibodies and to membrane shed antigens (EF factors) is being used. In the final analysis, the most meaningful taxonomy of leishmania will probably come from correlating these biochemical and immunologic findings with biologic characteristics of the organisms. For example, the course of infection in genetically defined mice and sensitivity to heat appear to be two very useful biologic criteria.

PARASITE-HOST INTERACTION. Studies of leishmania with host cells under various conditions *in vitro* have illuminated clinically relevant issues in the host-parasite interaction. First, promastigotes are rapidly lysed by fresh serum, by activating the classical complement pathway. They are also destroyed by polymorphonuclear leukocytes. Since promastigotes often meet the same fate when ingested by macrophages, infection would seemingly be difficult or impossible to initiate. This paradox now appears to be explained by the recent finding that stationary phase leishmania are more infective than log phase organisms, from cultures as well as in the sandfly. Interestingly, the intracellular amastigotes are more resistant than promastigotes to the oxidative response of macrophages. However, if macrophages are activated by exposure to specific or nonspecific lymphokines, they are then capable of destroying most species of amastigotes.

When leishmania are ingested by macrophages they are enclosed in a phagocytic vacuole, whose membranes subsequently fuse with lysosomal vacuoles. Presence of acid hydrolases on the amastigote surface membrane is one of the features that protects the parasite from being destroyed.

Variation in temperature sensitivity of various species of leishmania is another critical factor that determines clinical expression of the disease. For example, *L. donovani* can survive and multiply in macrophages at higher temperatures than cutaneous strains. Among isolates causing cutaneous disease in the Americas, some members of the *L. mexicana* complex are inhibited to a greater extent at 37° C than are strains of the *L. braziliensis* complex. These differences in temperature tolerance probably explain why some varieties of cutaneous leishmaniasis can be treated successfully by local heat.

IMMUNOLOGY. The pattern of humoral and cell-mediated immune responses that normally develops during or after leishmanial infection varies with the clinical form of disease. Serum antibody can be demonstrated by a variety of tests, usually indirect immunofluorescence (IFA) or enzyme-linked immunosorbent assay (ELISA) in patients with established visceral or cutaneous leishmaniasis. Cell-mediated immunity in leishmaniasis can be evaluated by a delayed hypersensitivity skin test (leishmanin test, or Montenegro test) or by lymphocyte proliferation to leishmanial antigen. Positive skin test results and lymphocyte proliferation are normally present in patients with cutaneous disease, but only after recovery or effective treatment in patients with visceral disease. Cell-mediated immunity is absent or suppressed during active visceral infections.

Resistance to leishmaniasis is best correlated with presence of cell-mediated immunity. Its absence in visceral disease has already been noted, and it is dramatically demonstrated in a rare form of disease called *diffuse cutaneous leishmaniasis* (DCL). In patients with DCL, not only is there specific anergy to the skin test but parasites are very abundant in lesions, whereas lymphocytes are scanty, lesions do not ulcerate, and response to chemotherapy is poor. Antigen specific suppressor cells have been demonstrated in DCL. In contrast, a normal immune response in cutaneous leishmaniasis is generally associated with lesions that ulcerate and show relatively few parasites and abundant lymphocytes and even giant cells, plus a positive skin test. Thus, it is helpful to compare the clinical forms of leishmaniasis with the spectrum of disease response in leprosy.

Jaffe CL, McMahon-Pratt D: Monoclonal antibodies specific for *Leishmania tropica.* J Immunol 131:1987, 1983. *One of a series of papers on monoclonals for differentiating species.*

Kreutzer RD: Identification of *Leishmania* spp. by multiple isozyme analysis. Am J Trop Med Hyg 32:703, 1983. *One of the other main techniques being used in biochemical taxonomy.*

Neal RA, Hale C: A comparative study of susceptibility of inbred and outbred mouse strains compared with hamsters to infection with New World cutaneous leishmaniasis. Parasitology 87:7, 1983. *This provides comparative information on mouse vs. hamster susceptibility to leishmanial species, and also recent references to the extensive literature on inbred mice in leishmanial work.*

Sacks DL, Perkins PV: Identification of an infective stage of leishmania promastigotes. Science 223:1417, 1984. *Clarifies a previously suspected critical issue—that the parasite is infective for cells in stationary but not in log phase of growth, in the fly as well as in culture.*

Turk JL, Bryceson ADM: Immunological phenomena in leprosy and related diseases. Adv Immunol 13:209, 1971. *Provides the clinical and experimental bases for regarding leishmaniasis as a disease spectrum.*

VISCERAL LEISHMANIASIS (Kala Azar)

EPIDEMIOLOGY. The visceral form of leishmaniasis, caused by *L. donovani* and related organisms, has a worldwide distribution. Certain regions continue to be endemic areas of this disease. These include the following: northeast India, especially Assam and Bihar states; Kenya, Sudan, and Ethiopia in east Africa; northeast China; the shores of the Caspian Sea and Iran in south Asia; the countries of Europe, North Africa, and the Middle East surrounding the Mediterranean; and northeast Brazil. In addition to these macrofoci, smaller foci outside these extensions occur. In the western hemisphere, for example, visceral leishmaniasis is sporadically seen in southern Brazil, Paraguay, and northern Argentina, as well as in the vicinity of Belem at the mouth of the Amazon. Additionally, there are foci of transmission in Venezuela and Colombia, and extending north into Central America with isolated cases reported from El Salvador, Guatemala, Honduras, and even from Mexico.

With such a wide geographic distribution of the disease, it is not surprising that different species of phlebotomine flies are involved in the various regions. What is surprising is that the causative organisms from these widely separated regions are relatively uniform in their properties. Yet some investigators prefer to assign separate species designations to the parasites from certain geographic foci, such as *L. infantum* for the Mediterranean variety and *L. chagasii* for that from Brazil. While up to now such species designations have been based partly upon epidemiologic grounds, they are likely to be upheld by more discriminating analyses in current use of isoenzyme patterns and DNA characteristics.

FACTORS AFFECTING TRANSMISSION. Since *L. donovani* is usually transmitted as a zoonosis, consideration must be given to the various factors favoring natural transmission, and the manner in which humans become involved in the cycle. Since phlebotomine sandflies have a limited flight range, humans must come into their habitat to become infected, or the vector and reservoir host must both live close to people. The latter condition is fulfilled when dogs are reservoir hosts. The domestic dog, as well as wild canines such as the fox, develop a chronic systemic disease very similar to that of humans when infected with *L. donovani.* But an additional unique feature of leishmanial infection in canines is the frequent presence of organisms in the skin, including the nose and ears, which are favorite feeding sites of sandflies. An epidemiologic cycle of the parasite involving wild foxes, domestic dogs, and humans via the vector *Lutzomyia longipalpis* has been documented in northeast Brazil. The domestic dog has also been incriminated as an important reservoir host for visceral leishmaniasis of the Mediterranean region and in certain areas of China.

Rodents such as the Nile rat (*Arvicanthus niloticus*) are the likely reservoir in the Sudan, and the activity of the vector, *P. orientalis,* is high in clumps of acacia woodland near villages. In Kenya transmission of disease is associated with termite hills, which serve as resting places for the vector, *P. martini,* and around which village men gather in the evening. However, the animal reservoir in Kenya has not been identified. In some regions such as in northeast India, humans appear to be their own reservoir, and several factors serve to facilitate person-to-person transmission. The vector, *P. argentipes,* has a preference for human blood. The parasite is found in circulating monocytes in Indian cases of kala azar more frequently than usual. An additional source of parasites for the vector are dermal lesions containing large numbers of parasites that develop after the initial disease in Indian patients.

The last few decades have seen a resurgence of visceral leishmaniasis in regions where it had disappeared after the widespread use of DDT for malaria control. Phlebotomine populations were greatly reduced around houses, but zoonotic transmission was not affected. When use of residual insecticides was discontinued, transmission to people was re-established. This has occurred in the countries around the Mediterranean, with an epidemic reported in western Italy.

Outbreaks of visceral leishmaniasis have often followed famine, wars, and civil or political disturbances resulting in malnutrition and mass migration of people. It is not known whether this is due to greater exposure to infected vectors, defective immune response, reactivation of latent infection, or a combination of these and other factors.

PATHOLOGY. The organs mainly affected are the liver, spleen, bone marrow, and elements of the reticuloendothelial system in diverse sites. These organs and tissues hypertrophy, with the increased cells made up of parasitized macrophages and histiocytes, but little or no lymphocytic response. Generalized enlargement of lymph nodes is not a consistent finding (see below), but hyperplasia of lymphoid tissue in the nasopharynx and in the Peyer's patches of the gut is common. Endothelial proliferation occurs in certain organs such as within septae of pulmonary alveoli and in renal glomeruli.

The spleen is enlarged, sometimes to tremendous size, but is firm and has a thick capsule. While the splenic pulp is friable and there may be infarcts, the nature and chronic course of the enlargement make the spleen relatively resistant to tears from an aspirating needle. Enlargement of the liver is due to hyperplasia of the Kupffer cells, which are packed with amastigotes. Only rarely are parenchymal cells of the liver parasitized. There may be focal granulomas in the liver, with some fibrosis in chronic untreated cases.

The bone marrow is infiltrated with parasitized macrophages. Red cell and white cell production are normal initially but may be impaired late in the disease as the bone marrow is replaced by parasitized macrophages. Even in early disease, however, the peripheral blood shows leukopenia and anemia. Both of these are due to pooling and destruction of cellular elements in the enlarged spleen. There is a striking polyclonal B cell activation that results in high IgG and total serum protein values.

Some organs, most notably the kidneys, may show pathologic changes secondary to deposition of immune complexes. Connective tissues of various organs exhibit deposition of hyaline substance, probably related to elevated serum protein levels, with a distribution similar to that of secondary amyloidosis.

In the early stages of visceral leishmaniasis small nodules in the skin containing parasites have been described at or near the site of inoculation. There are scattered reports of parasites being demonstrated even in apparently normal skin. A more obvious type of skin involvement, although variable by geographic location, is post–kala azar dermal leishmaniasis. This is the development in some patients after recovery from disease of subcutaneous nodules of varying size that contain large numbers of parasites. For unknown reasons the lesions do not ulcerate in spite of their heavy load of organisms; thus they resemble the entity of diffuse cutaneous leishmaniasis (see below).

CLINICAL FEATURES. The incubation period is long, generally one to three months, but it may be as short as 10 to 14 days. There are well documented instances of activation of latent infection several years after exposure to the parasite, under conditions of immunosuppression. The onset is usually insidious and difficult to date, especially among people who regard intermittent fevers and lassitude as normal. The course may continue gradually, with intermittent fevers becoming noticeable, accompanied by sweats, weakness, and weight loss. These symptoms, perhaps including nonproductive cough and abdominal discomfort produced by an enlarging liver and spleen, may continue for months with the patient still up and about. In some patients the course of disease is more rapid, with high fever and chills, simulating typhoid fever or acute brucellosis. The most prominent physical findings are fever, splenomegaly, and cachexia, which is especially evident in the thorax and shoulder girdle. While the fever pattern can be variable, ultimately it often exhibits characteristic twice daily elevations to 38 to 40° C for some time. Generalized adenopathy is common in patients in some geographic areas, but it is seldom striking. In light-skinned patients hyperpigmentation of the abdomen and extremities may be noted; the term *kala azar* is Hindi for "black sickness." Splenic enlargement can be extreme in this disease, often reaching the iliac fossa, and the organ is firm and nontender. Some otherwise typical cases may involve only modest splenomegaly. The liver is also firm and nontender but not invariably palpable or enlarged.

COURSE AND COMPLICATIONS. Although there is strong indirect evidence from skin tests and serologic results that spontaneous recovery from visceral leishmaniasis can occur, it probably happens only early in the course of infection. As the disease progresses, weight loss, anemia, and other signs become clinically more apparent. Subcutaneous edema, ascites, and other evidences of hypoalbuminemia may develop. Bleeding from the nose or gums can occur. Finally, after a illness that may be as short as a few months or as long as a year, the patient becomes emaciated and exhausted. In the great majority of instances death is due to intercurrent infections such as pneumonia, tuberculosis, dysentery, and gangrenous stomatitis. Advanced cases are particularly susceptible because of leukopenia and undoubted impairment of cell-mediated immunologic function, although specific mechanisms have not been defined. Another cause of death is massive gastrointestinal bleeding.

Post–Kala Azar Dermal Leishmaniasis. As noted earlier, a small percentage of patients, after treatment or spontaneous recovery, develop skin lesions containing parasites. This is fairly common in India, less common in Africa, and quite rare in Brazil. The lesions begin as a hypopigmented or erythematous macular rash soon or late after treatment and are often located on the face. When the dermal lesions persist they are likely to become papular or nodular, especially on the forehead, cheeks, and earlobes, and closely resemble lepromatous leprosy. This syndrome combines clinical and parasitologic features of relapse of the visceral infection and a type of skin involvement seen in diffuse cutaneous leishmaniasis. Unfortunately, detailed assessment of immune response is not yet available in post–kala azar dermal leishmaniasis.

SPECIFIC LABORATORY DIAGNOSIS. Since other clinical states may mimic certain features of visceral leishmaniasis, demonstration of the parasite, preferably by culture, is essential before treatment is undertaken. In addition, presence or absence of the parasite can be used to monitor response to treatment. Organisms are most readily recovered by aspiration from bone marrow, spleen, liver, lymph nodes, or blood. Material obtained is:

1. Used to make thin smears on a slide, dried, fixed and stained with Giemsa or some other Romanovsky stain for examination under oil immersion for amastigotes. Parasitized macrophages often rupture on smearing so free parasites usually are present. Bone marrow aspiration is the method of choice because adequate material can be obtained. Splenic puncture in this disease is safe if the spleen is readily palpable below the costal margin, if prothrombin and bleeding times are normal, and if proper technique is used. A 21-gauge needle on a 10-ml syringe is inserted quickly; suction is applied and withdrawn in less than a second. The main disadvantage of splenic puncture is the small amount of material obtained, which must be kept sterile for dilution and culture after a few smears are made. Aspirates of lymph nodes are done similarly, but yield of positive results is much less than with bone marrow or spleen. Biopsies of either liver or lymph nodes could provide more material for culture. Buffy coat preparations of peripheral blood are seldom positive except in India.
2. Inoculated into NNN (Novy-MacNeal-Nicolle) medium, a blood agar slant made with 30 per cent defibrinated rabbit blood and overlaid with a liquid phase of balanced salt solution containing antibiotics (not amphotericin or Mycostatin). Schneider's insect culture medium containing 30 per cent fetal bovine serum (FBS) may be just as effective as NNN but can vary with strains and lots of FBS. Cultures are incubated at 22 to 25° C (not 37° C) and a few drops of material can be removed and examined fresh for motile promastigotes at intervals. A positive culture will usually show organisms within 10 to 14 days, but this may require up to 30 days.
3. Hamsters are very susceptible to *L. donovani* and can be inoculated. However, it may require three or four months before organisms are demonstrable in their liver or spleen, so this method is not very practical.

IMMUNOLOGIC TESTS. By the time patients with visceral leishmaniasis come to clinical attention they invariably have readily demonstrable antileishmanial serum antibodies. Although the IFA test with amastigotes as antigen has had the longest use, it now appears that ELISA using promastigotes for antigen is just as reliable and more practical. The ELISA test can be read visually if necessary, and has advantages for testing large numbers of sera, including eluted blood specimens collected in the field onto filter paper. Direct agglutination of fixed promastigotes is another test that can be used, but it requires treatment of serum samples to eliminate cross-reacting IgM and is not as specific as other tests. Serum from individuals infected with *Trypanosoma cruzi* will cross-react with leishmanial antigens; this is a problem only in certain areas of Latin America. The leishmanin skin test for delayed hypersensitivity is negative in cases of active visceral leishmaniasis but becomes positive after recovery. A low frequency of positive leishmanin reactors among certain populations residing in endemic areas but without a history of visceral leishmaniasis is generally interpreted as evidence for inapparent infections or spontaneous cures of the disease. Some investigators attribute otherwise unexplained positive leishmanin skin tests to human infections with nonpathogenic species of leishmania.

LABORATORY FINDINGS. Most of the laboratory abnormalities involve the hematopoietic system. Leukopenia, with absolute reductions in neutrophils and eosinophils and a relative increase in lymphocytes and monocytes, is characteristic. In one series the total white cell count was below 4000 in 90 per cent of cases by one month after onset of symptoms, and it frequently may be around 2000 or less per cu mm. Thrombocytopenia is also present, and the sedimentation rate is increased. A moderately severe normocytic and normochromic anemia, unless complicated by blood loss or deficiency states, is very common, caused by increased red cell destruction. In late stages of the disease prothrombin, bleeding, and clotting times are prolonged.

Total serum proteins are increased to levels of 9 to 10 grams per deciliter, virtually all IgG, because of polyclonal B cell activation. Serum albumin levels, especially in advanced cases, are normal or low. The striking hyperglobulinemia is the basis for the old recommended diagnostic tests, such as the formol-gel and Chopra reaction, before specific serodiagnosis was available. Evidence for circulating immune complexes, based upon C1q binding in the serum, is readily demonstrable. Liver function tests show only mild abnormalities, if any.

DIFFERENTIAL DIAGNOSIS. Chronic malaria in endemic regions may present some problems in differential diagnosis. In malaria-immune individuals the presence of malaria parasites in the blood does not rule out the additional diagnosis of leishmaniasis. Conversely, an enlarged spleen is hardly enough on which to base the diagnosis. Tropical splenomegaly syndrome (an exaggerated immune response to malaria) easily could be confused with the clinical picture of visceral leishmaniasis. Several different forms of schistosomiasis may also mimic visceral leishmaniasis; the acute disease with fever and hepatosplenomegaly, the severe chronic variety with Symmers' fibrosis and portal hypertension, and chronic relapsing enteric fever that can be a complication of schistosomiasis. Other diseases that may resemble kala azar include lymphoma, cirrhosis of the liver with hypersplenism, miliary tuberculosis, brucellosis, typhoid fever, and subacute bacterial endocarditis.

TREATMENT. The drug of choice for treatment has been and remains pentavalent antimony, even with novel approaches to possible use of other drugs. The antimony preparation available in the United States (from Centers for Disease Control, 404-329-3670, 8:00 A.M. to 4:30 P.M. EST Monday through Friday; 404-329-2888, evenings, weekends, and holidays) and some European countries is sodium stibogluconate (Pentostam), a preparation containing 100 mg antimony (Sb) per ml. The dose is 0.1 to 0.2 ml per kilogram of body weight, given daily by intramuscular or intravenous injection, not exceeding 1000 mg Sb per day. Another pentavalent antimony preparation used in Latin America, meglumine antimonate (Glucantime), is virtually identical but contains 85 mg Sb per ml. Children with this disease require more Sb than adults, and the total dosage required for cure varies in different parts of the world. In India ten daily doses are usually adequate, while the disease in Kenya requires 30 injections, and up to 30 per cent of cases may still relapse within six months. Pentavalent antimony is relatively nontoxic in comparison to the trivalent Sb, except for local pain at the injection site when given intramuscularly. Other side effects are cumulative with dose and include nausea, vomiting, slight elevation of liver enzyme values, and nonspecific T wave changes if electrocardiograms are taken.

Response to treatment is not dramatic and may not be apparent for several weeks. Useful indicators to follow are temperature, spleen size, hemoglobin, and white blood count. Weekly splenic aspirates were used by one group, with "cure" defined as two successively negative aspirates a week apart. Since relapse may occur up to a year after apparent cure, monthly follow-up for six months and then after a year is recommended.

Primary unresponsiveness to Sb, that is, little or no improvement during or after the first course, occurs in up to 10 per cent of cases. Resistance of *L. donovani* to Sb can be induced experimentally but has not been documented to occur in humans. Second-line drugs for unresponsive or relapsed patients are pentamidine or amphotericin B. The dose of pentamidine* is 4 mg per kilogram given intramuscularly three times weekly for ten doses, but severe pain at the injection site is common and sterile abscess formation can occur. Additional systemic side effects of anorexia, nausea, abdominal pain, hypotension, and development of diabetes in 10 per cent make the decision to use pentamidine a difficult one. The other second-line drug, amphotericin B, must be given intravenously on alternate days at 1 mg per kilogram each time over many weeks in order to achieve the recommended 1.5 to 2.0 gram total dosage. This drug regularly produces chills, fever, and nausea with each dose and a cumulative reduction of hemoglobin and renal function. New approaches to treatment include use of allopurinol or its derivatives and incorporation of drugs

*Available from Centers for Disease Control, Atlanta, GA.

in liposomes for more efficient and prolonged uptake by macrophages.

Supportive treatment can be very important, especially in the malnourished and debilitated. These patients are prone to develop complicating bacterial infections for which proper treatment must be instituted. Fluid and electrolyte balance must be corrected, and hemorrhagic complications may require blood transfusion. Good nursing care, attention to oral hygiene, adequate diet and correction of nutritional deficiencies are, of course, desirable.

PREVENTION. Since the epidemiology of kala azar varies between different geographic areas, the local conditions responsible for transmission must be understood in order to implement preventive measures. Where sandflies are in or around houses, vector control with insecticides is appropriate. If an animal reservoir such as the domestic dog is involved, destruction of infected dogs, especially strays, can be instituted. If focal sites of infected flies are known, they can be destroyed or avoided. Personal protection by wearing protective clothing in the evenings, use of insect repellents, and sleeping under fine mesh netting is applicable under some circumstances.

Chulay JD, Bhatt SM: A comparison of three dosage regimens of sodium stibogluconate in the treatment of visceral leishmaniasis in Kenya. J Infect Dis 148:148, 1983. *Report by a group with extensive experience in use of Pentostam. They used it in much larger doses than did others.*

Kager PA, Rees PH: Splenic aspiration; experience in Kenya. Trop Georg Med 35:125, 1983. *Report on large experience with this procedure in diagnosis of kala azar and response to treatment. Same tissue has review of literature on same topic.*

Most H, Lavietes PK: Kala azar in American military personnel. Medicine 26:221, 1947. *A classic paper, still one of the best on clinical aspects.*

CUTANEOUS LEISHMANIASIS OF THE OLD WORLD (ORIENTAL SORE) AND NEW WORLD INCLUDING MUCOCUTANEOUS OR ESPUNDIA

EPIDEMIOLOGY. Although basically the same disease, there are differences in epidemiology and clinical course in cutaneous leishmaniasis of the Old and New Worlds. In the Mediterranean basin, Middle East, and Southern Asia the disease tends to be clinically more benign and occurs in semiarid and desert climates; transmission can become established in villages and cities. Cutaneous leishmaniasis in the Americas is acquired by workers in the jungle or by farmers and their families living at its edges. The New World disease sometimes produces later metastatic and destructive lesions of the mucous membranes.

The epidemiology of cutaneous leishmaniasis is best understood in South Russia, Iran, and Middle Eastern countries where infected desert rodents (*Rhombomys opimus* and *Psammomys obesus*) live in burrows with phlebotomine vectors (often *P. papatasi*). People are infected with *L. tropica major* when they invade this environment to establish settlements, exacavate archaeologic ruins, or make war. If settlements are established, the parasite is likely to become involved in a new transmission cycle with dogs and humans as reservoirs and an urban sandfly such as *P. sergenti* as vector. Parasite species from such locations are often identified as *L. tropica*. The commonness of typical facial scars in adults in Iran, Afghanistan, Syria, and Iraq indicates the high frequency of cutaneous leishmaniasis in these countries.

The epidemiology of cutaneous leishmaniasis in West Africa and the sub-Sahara belt is less clear. Human cases are sporadic, with a rural transmission cycle, and the parasite species is often *L. tropica major*. In Ethiopia and Kenya, however, the animal reservoir is often the hyrax (*Procavia*), the vector is *P. longipes*, and the parasite species is *L. aethiopica*.

In the Americas cutaneous leishmaniasis occurs from Texas to northern Argentina, with only Chile free of the disease. Except for some areas of Peru, where the domestic dog is a reservoir, New World cutaneous leishmaniasis is a forest or jungle zoonosis with forest rodents or sloths serving as animal reservoirs. Western hemisphere sandfly vectors are now classified as members of the genus *Lutzomyia*.

The organism in Mexico and northern central America is classified as *L. mexicana mexicana*, an organism that does not produce mucocutaneous disease. The predominant organisms in the remainder of Central America, Panama, and northern South America are members of the *L. braziliensis* complex. These are considered capable of causing late mucous membrane involvement. Mucocutaneous leishmaniasis is generally believed to be associated with *L. braziliensis braziliensis*, occurring commonly in central Brazil, Bolivia, and tropical regions of Peru. However, this association of leishmanial species with clinical types of disease and with geographic distribution is still provisional. For example, a number of isolates of *L. b. braziliensis* have recently been reported from Belize, where *L. mexicana* was supposed to predominate, and members of the *L. mexicana* complex (*L. m. amazonensis*) have been recovered from classic mucous membrane lesions. It is likely that additional members of the two major complexes will be described as the newer methods of taxonomy are applied.

PATHOLOGY. The earliest changes at the site of inoculation have not been described. Established lesions show a large accumulation of macrophages containing amastigotes, with variable numbers of lymphocytes and plasma cells. There may be focal accumulations of polymorphonuclear cells, especially in areas of necrosis, but the exact mechanism for ulceration of the epithelium is not clear. With time, numbers of parasites diminish and the lesion heals. In other instances the lesion persists and a tuberculoid histologic reaction is seen with granulomas including multinucleated giant cells. This is the type of pathology seen in *chronic relapsing cutaneous leishmaniasis*, also known as the *lupoid* or *recidiva* form. Delayed skin test reactivity to leishmanial antigen is present in normally healing and recidiva leishmaniasis.

The unusual complication known as diffuse cutaneous leishmaniasis (DCL), associated with anergy to leishmanial antigen, has a different histologic picture. DCL lesions show a heavy infiltrate of foamy or vacuolated macrophages containing large numbers of amastigotes with only scant numbers of lymphocytes. Moreover, the overlying epithelium is not ulcerated.

The lesions of mucocutaneous leishmaniasis represent metastatic spread of organisms via the bloodstream to mucous membranes of the nose, mouth, and upper pharyngeal tissues. The histology is a confusing mixture of granulomatous inflammatory cell reaction with necrosis, fibrosis, and often response to secondary bacterial infection. Organisms are usually scanty. Tissue destruction involves cartilage with perforation of the nasal septum, loss of much of the nose and palate, and even involvement of the larynx.

CLINICAL MANIFESTATIONS. The lesion begins as a small erythematous papule on exposed areas, often the face or extremities, within two to eight weeks after infection. The papule may develop a tiny vesicle that opens and oozes some serous fluid and enlarges to several centimeters, with firm, raised, and reddened edges. The ulcer can remain relatively dry with a central crust (dry form) or may ooze (wet form). Lesions can be single or multiple; small satellite papules may occur at the edge of a larger lesion. Subcutaneous nodules in a centripetal alignment from an ulcer may develop (sporotrichoid form). Cutaneous leishmanial lesions will generally heal spontaneously, but the process can take a few months to a year or more. The result is a depressed, depigmented scar. *Recidiva* or *lupoid leishmaniasis* may sometimes develop, persisting for years. This lesion exhibits central healing with papules developing in the periphery or center of the scar. Regional adenopathy may or may not occur with cutaneous leishmaniasis; this finding is not helpful in differential diagnosis.

COMPLICATIONS. Metastatic spread of parasites and development of destructive naso-oropharyngeal lesions is a serious later sequel to cutaneous disease. This mucous membrane involvement occurs almost exclusively in the western hemisphere and is said to be associated primarily with *L. braziliensis*

braziliensis infections. Mucocutaneous disease due to *L. mexicana amazonensis* does occur, so until more data correlating parasite type with clinical disease are available, this complication can be equated with geographic region rather than parasite species. Thus, mucocutaneous leishmaniasis is most common in central Brazil and adjacent portions of Bolivia, Peru, and Ecuador, and relatively uncommon in Panama and Central America, for example. Mucosal involvement generally does not become manifest until the initial skin lesion has healed, even many years later, and presumably is more likely to occur if there has been no or inadequate treatment of the original ulcer.

Earliest signs and symptoms of mucosal disease commonly involve the nose, with epistaxis and obstruction. Perforation of the nasal septum is common, or the upper lip may be involved. The process can destroy cartilaginous structures of the nose and palate and extend to the larynx. Death may result from aspiration pneumonia or suffocation. Distinction should be made between the mucous membrane involvement that occurs as direct extension from a facial lesion, as in Ethiopia, and the late metastatic form seen in South America.

Diffuse cutaneous leishmaniasis (DCL) is a rare complication that offers insight into immunity to leishmaniasis because it features antigen-specific anergy and cell-mediated immunosuppression. DCL seems to occur more commonly in certain countries (Dominican Republic, Venezuela, and Ethiopia), and in the Americas is caused by organisms belonging to the *L. mexicana* complex. The disease begins with one or only a few nodular lesions that do not ulcerate but go on to metastasize to other cutaneous sites, primarily the face and extensor surfaces of the limbs. The subcutaneous nonulcerative nodular lesions are not associated with fever or other systemic symptoms and do not involve visceral organs. The appearance, distribution, and chronic nature of DCL has often led to the erroneous diagnosis of lepromatous leprosy. There is no mortality associated with DCL, but disfigurement and ulceration secondary to trauma at pressure points lead to morbidity, since this disease is notoriously unresponsive to the usual antileishmanial drugs.

DIAGNOSIS. Leishmaniasis can be suspected in anyone who develops one or more chronic ulcers on exposed areas of skin after recently visiting or working at archaeologic sites in the Middle East, at Mayan ruins, or in jungle or rural areas of Latin America. Ideally, diagnosis should be confirmed by culture of the organism in NNN or other appropriate media from a biopsy or aspirated specimen obtained from the edge of the lesion. Culture is the most sensitive method for detection of organisms. Excisional or punch biopsy offers an additional advantage of providing a portion of the specimen for histopathologic examination and routine bacteriologic, fungal, and acid-fast cultures in cases in which a wider differential diagnosis is required. Appropriate impression smears can also be made and stained from biopsied material, whether culture is possible or not. If biopsy is not possible because of circumstances or location of the lesion, scrapings from a slit made in involved skin or from the debrided base of an ulcer can be cultured or stained for organisms. The characteristic amastigotes in lesions appear larger and are more easily recognized in smears than in tissue sections. A recent technique that may permit direct and rapid species differentiation of leishmania, as well as diagnosis, is blotting with radiolabeled DNA probes. Numbers of parasites present and ease of culture vary with the strain, but the concentration of parasites in lesions tends to diminish with time as healing occurs, and they are also reduced if the ulcer is secondarily infected with bacteria. It is also usually difficult to culture or demonstrate organisms in the late lesions of mucocutaneous disease.

A positive leishmanin skin test and serum antibody can usually be demonstrated in patients by the time a cutaneous lesion has ulcerated. These tests remain positive in mucocutaneous disease. The most reliable serologic tests are the ELISA with promastigote antigen and indirect immunofluorescence with amastigote antigen. Cross-reactions with leishmanial antigens do occur in individuals with *Trypanosoma cruzi* infection and previous kala azar. It must also be remembered that positive skin and serologic tests can reflect a previous rather than a current leishmanial infection.

Cutaneous leishmaniasis must be differentiated from the following conditions, with decreasing likelihood of occurrence: nonspecific tropical or traumatic ulcers due to bacterial infection or stasis; fungal infections, especially sporotrichosis and blastomycosis; mycobacterial infections such as *M. marinum* and tuberculosis; syphilis and other treponematoses of the skin; sarcoidosis and neoplastic ulcers. Mucocutaneous leishmaniasis is especially likely to mimic infection with *Paracoccidiodes brasiliensis*, histoplasmosis, Wegener's mid line granuloma, or rhinoscleroma.

TREATMENT. As described earlier for visceral leishmaniasis, the standard and recommended treatment for cutaneous leishmaniasis is pentavalent antimony, available in the U.S. as Pentostam.* The dose is 0.1 to 0.2 ml per kilogram by intramuscular or slow intravenous injection, not exceeding 10 ml per dose. The drug is given daily for 10 to 15 days. Modest elevation of liver enzymes and/or mild nonspecific ST or T wave electrocardiographic changes may occur during therapy, especially after six or eight doses. These changes are generally not associated with symptoms, but it may be prudent to monitor them.

Old World cutaneous leishmaniasis, especially in patients from the Middle East, will often heal spontaneously within six months. Since leishmaniasis in this region does not metastasize to mucosal tissues, treatment may justifiably be withheld if the lesion is not extensive and appears to be healing.

In contrast, if the infection is known or suspected to originate from an endemic area of mucocutaneous disease, some authorities recommend that three courses of pentavalent antimony treatment be given for a cutaneous lesion. The possibility of later mucous membrane involvement, usually manifested by nasal obstruction and/or epistaxis, should be explained to the patient so that medical attention will be sought.

Regardless of the infecting species of parasite, it is not unusual for cutaneous leishmanial lesions to require a second course of antimony treatment. Two weeks of rest are generally allowed between courses of treatment. Although different strains of leishmania can vary in their susceptibility to antimony, naturally occurring resistance is very unusual. Yet the circumstances required to eliminate the organisms from a lesion are not fully understood, and probably a normal immunologic response on the part of the host is required.

Amphotericin B is indicated in cases in which antimonials have failed to control the disease. Side effects are severe and common. The effective total dose is lower than for many systemic mycoses, with a total dose of 1.5 to 2.0 grams for a 60 kilogram adult often being sufficient.

A number of other drugs with varying degrees of antileishmanial activity may be useful in treatment under certain circumstances. Cycloguanil pamoate,† an injectable repository, is moderately effective and popular among workers in camps who cannot afford to spend 10 to 15 days away from a distant workplace. Orally administered drugs such as rifampin, metronidazole, and ketoconazole have been touted on the basis of uncontrolled trials in a few patients, but they are clearly inferior to antimony. Innovative new approaches to therapy are under way with allopurinol analogues, liposome-encapsulated compounds, and even topically applied drugs; their ultimate usefulness remains to be established. The application of local heat (40 to 41° C) for 25 hours or more over a period of four or five days may be effective for lesions caused by the *L. mexicana* complex organisms.

PREVENTION. Transmission of leishmaniasis in cities can be prevented by control of sandfly populations with insecticides

*Available from Centers for Disease Control, Atlanta, GA.
†Investigational drug in the United States.

or destruction of breeding sites. Where reservoirs and vectors are sylvatic, other measures must be employed, such as insect repellents and use of protective clothing over exposed parts of the body. Vaccines should theoretically be effective since there is immunity to second episodes of cutaneous disease. However, the effectiveness of immunization with either viable or killed organisms has been difficult to evaluate.

Lainson R: The American leishmaniasis: Some observations on their ecology and epidemiology. Trans Roy Soc Trop Med Hyg. 77:569, 1983. *Perhaps heavier on taxonomy of parasites than justified, but excellent overview by a world's expert in ecology of this disease.*

Marsden PD, Nonata RR: Mucocutaneous leishmaniasis: A review of clinical aspects. Rev Soc Bras Med Trop 9:309, 1975. *This is a very good article, in English, with emphasis on Brazilian experience.*

Neva FA: Diagnosis and treatment of cutaneous leishmaniasis. *In* Remington JS and Swartz MN (eds.): Current Clinical Topics in Infectious Diseases. Vol. 3. New York, McGraw-Hill Book Company, 1982, p 364. *More detailed account of these aspects of the subject.*

Petersen EA, Neva FA: Specific inhibition of lymphocyte proliferation responses by adherent suppressor cells in diffuse cutaneous leishmaniasis. N Engl J Med 306:387, 1982. *Documentation of a basic immunologic defect in the diffuse cutaneous disease.*

382. TOXOPLASMOSIS

Henry Masur

Toxoplasmosis is a common disease of birds and mammals caused by the protozoon *Toxoplasma gondii*. The name *T. gondii* is descriptive of this arc-shaped protozoon, being derived from the Greek word *toxon*, meaning arc, and from the name of the North African rodent *gondi*, in which the organism was first recognized. *T. gondii* currently infects over 500 million humans around the world. This obligate intracellular organism can proliferate readily and cause clinically important disease in individuals with normal or abnormal immune function. A clear distinction must be kept in mind between *T. gondii* infection, which is defined by the presence of viable organisms in a patient, and toxoplasmosis, a relatively uncommon occurrence that indicates an active disease process.

HISTORY. In 1907 Nicolle and Manceaux first recognized this organism in the gondi. The first human case of congenital infection was described by Janku in Prague. The parasite was initially isolated from a case of congenital disease by Wolf, Cowen, and Paige in 1938. Three years later Pinkerton and Henderson recognized the first case of disease in adults. Frenkel subsequently suggested that retinochoroiditis might be caused by *Toxoplasma;* Wilder confirmed such an association in 1952. Epidemiologic studies over the last 40 years by Feldman, Jacobs, Thalhammer, and Desmonts led to the recognition that the infection is very common in most parts of the world including the United States. In 1967 Hutchison suggested that the cat played an important role in the life cycle of *T. gondii*. Subsequently, Wallace proved that there is a sexual cycle in the cat intestine that produces a newly recognized form, the *oocyst*. This provides an important link that explains the frequency of this infection in certain populations.

THE PROTOZOAN. Three forms exist in the life cycle of *T. gondii:* the *cyst*, the *trophozoite*, and the *oocyst*. The trophozoite has an arc or oval form and is about 3 to 4 μ in diameter and 6 to 7 μ in length. It is an obligate intracellular form that proliferates in acute infection. Trophozoites can enter vacuoles in any nucleated mammalian cell. They divide by endodyogeny, an asexual process whereby two daughter cells are formed within one parent cell. Division continues until the cell ruptures, releasing trophozoites to infect adjacent cells. As the host develops immunity, trophozoite proliferation slows.

Toxoplasma cysts are 10 to 200 μ forms that contain several thousand very slowly dividing organisms; these appear to develop within host cells. Cysts can be seen in any tissue, but they are most commonly found in brain, skeletal muscle, and cardiac muscle. Cysts are more resistant to environmental conditions than are trophozoites, and are able to remain viable after exposure to digestive enzymes.

Oocysts are 10 to 12 μ oval forms that exist uniquely in the intestinal mucosa of cats. Toxoplasma released from cysts or oocysts in the cat intestine enter epithelial cells where they proliferate and then mature by gametogony into micro- or macrogametocytes. A zygote is formed by the union of the gametocytes; this zygote matures in one to four days into an oocyst. Large quantities of oocysts (up to 10 million per day) are excreted by the cat for one to three weeks beginning three to five days after ingestion of the *Toxoplasma*-containing tissue. Cats also get a concurrent systemic infection. Oocysts are not infectious until they undergo sporogony outside the body, a process that requires 1 to 21 days depending on environmental conditions. Oocysts are quite hardy: they can exist outside the body for at least a year in warm moist soil. *Toxoplasma*-infected cats will probably excrete oocysts for a brief period when they are rechallenged orally with *Toxoplasma*.

EPIDEMIOLOGY. *Toxoplasma* infection is a world-wide zoonosis. Natural infection occurs by ingestion of cysts or oocysts and by transplacental transmission. In nature the cycle of infection is probably maintained by cats and birds and small mammals. Primary human infection usually occurs by accidental ingestion of infected cat feces or by consumption of inadequately cooked meat. The relative importance of these primary routes probably depends on the amounts of rare meat consumed, hygienic practices, and the proximity of a feline population. When cats consume infected animals or inadequately cooked meat scraps they become infected and excrete oocysts. Children are particularly likely to come into contact with contaminated cat feces when playing in sand, or to inhale aerosolized dried feces under dusty conditions. Cockroaches and flies have also been shown to transfer oocysts to uncovered food.

In North America and Western Europe where many cats are confined to the home and eat only processed foods, and where food is usually covered and refrigerated, the consumption of rare meat is probably of greater epidemiologic importance than contact with cats or insects. Pork and lamb are more likely to contain cysts than is beef. If meat is not cooked to 60° C, or frozen to -20° C (a temperature not reliably reached by most commercial freezers), the cysts will be infective.

Toxoplasma has been transmitted rarely by needle stick accidents involving laboratory workers, by accidental inoculation during autopsy procedures, and by transplantation of an infected heart or kidney. Since some immunodeficient patients (particularly those with chronic myelogenous leukemia) have parasitemia, and since persistent parasitemia for a year has been described in an apparently healthy individual, blood products could be a source of infection. However, a healthy blood donor has never been documented to transmit *Toxoplasma* infection and in general blood product transmission seems to be a very rare event.

Secondary *Toxoplasma* infection can occur by transplacental transmission. Such transmission occurs only if the mother acquires *Toxoplasma* infection during the pregnancy or perhaps during the few months prior to conception. The frequency of congenital toxoplasmosis is thus dependent on the frequency with which women of childbearing age acquire *Toxoplasma* infection. In the United States and Europe 0.5 to 1 per cent of women show high or rising antitoxoplasma titers during pregnancy. About 40 per cent of these infections are transmitted to the fetus, the likelihood of transmission increasing progressively during successive trimesters of pregnancy from 17 to 65 per cent.

The frequency of *Toxoplasma* infection in any population depends on a variety of sociologic, economic, and environmental factors. Among both men and women there is increasing prevalence of positive serologic results with increasing age. In the United States less than 1 per cent of infants have congenital *Toxoplasma* infection; there is an abrupt rise in prevalence during teenage years; and from age 15 to 50 years there is an increase of approximately 1 per cent per year. Thus, about 20 to 70 per cent of adults in this country have positive serologic tests for *Toxoplasma* infection, the precise number depending on the specific population studied. Individuals in cold, arid, or mountainous regions tend to have a lower frequency than those in tropical areas. There are isolated communities that have little or no *Toxoplasma* infection. The regional variations cannot all be explained on the basis of meat eating habits, the presence of felines, or climatic extremes.

PATHOGENESIS AND PATHOLOGY. *Toxoplasma* are liberated from cysts or oocysts in the gastrointestinal tract where they multiply in the mucosal cells. Trophozoites then disseminate via the bloodstream or lymphatics to infect any nucleated host cell. Multiplication of the trophozoites within host cell vacuoles does not appear to disturb host cell function until the dividing organisms cause the cell to rupture. As adjacent cells are infected and they are themselves ruptured, progressive tissue necrosis occurs and an inflammatory response is elicited. The inflammatory response typically consists of mononuclear cells, a few polymorphonuclear cells, and edema. How extensive the tissue necrosis and dissemination become depends on the effectiveness of both humoral and cellular immune mechanisms. Although any organ can be involved, small foci of infection are most often established in lymph nodes, skeletal muscle, myocardium, and brain. Even after effective immunologic response the organisms are not eradicated: a few cysts form in these organs as early as the first week of infection and remain dormant for the lifetime of the host unless host immunity is diminished, in which case active proliferation of the organisms can again cause substantial local disease and dissemination. In some patients primary infection can be associated with widely disseminated disease: most of these patients have defects in cell-mediated immune mechanisms.

Histopathologically the changes in lymph nodes are so characteristic of toxoplasmosis that they are virtually diagnostic even in the absence of a visualized or cultivated organism. The lymph node shows reactive follicular hyperplasia with irregular clusters of epithelioid histiocytes. These histiocytes have vesicular nuclei and abundant eosinophilic cytoplasm; they encroach upon the germinal centers and obscure their margins. The germinal centers have many mitoses and many necrotic cells. Monocytoid cells produce focal distention of subcapsular and trabecular sinuses. Trophozoites or cysts are rarely seen in lymph nodes, although promptly performed cultures will grow the organism in many cases.

When other organs are involved, the pathologic findings can vary from a few isolated cysts to a marked inflammatory response associated with extensive necrosis. In skeletal muscle or brain an isolated cyst can be found unassociated with any inflammatory response or with any clinical manifestations of organ dysfunction. In patients with disseminated disease, however, the heart, brain, liver, spleen, kidney, pancreas, or other organs can manifest an intense inflammatory response surrounding areas of necrosis that can vary greatly in size. The inflammatory response consists of lymphocytes, plasma cells, and monocytes in association with edema. Perivascular mononuclear inflammatory changes are often seen contiguous to the necrotic areas. Intracellular and extracellular trophozoites are usually found in the periphery of the lesion rather than in the necrotic center.

In the central nervous system the necrotic lesions with margins of mononuclear cell infiltrate may be single or multiple. Periaqueductal and periventricular necrosis in congenital infection may lead to obstruction of the aqueduct of Sylvius or the foramen of Monro, resulting in obstructive hydrocephalus. The necrotic areas may ultimately calcify. In the eye, single or multiple necrotic lesions in the retina are the first manifestations of *Toxoplasma* infection. Mononuclear cell infiltrates are seen in association with cysts or trophozoites. Granulomatous inflammation occurs secondary to the necrotizing retinitis. The disease involves the posterior chamber almost exclusively and may be complicated by iridocyclitis, glaucoma, or cataracts.

In immunocompetent patients primary *Toxoplasma* infection is associated with both a humoral and cellular immune response. Antibodies against various *Toxoplasma* antigens can be detected in the blood. Subsequently, lymphocytes become responsive to *Toxoplasma* antigens and produce lymphokines. These lymphokines enable mononuclear phagocytes to inhibit *Toxoplasma* replication and to kill the intracellular organisms. Even immunocompetent individuals are not able to eliminate all *Toxoplasma* organisms from the body: cysts characteristically form in brain and muscle and remain viable for the lifetime of the host. Outside of the retina these cysts do not cause disease unless host immune function is altered.

CLINICAL MANIFESTATIONS. ***Acquired Toxoplasmosis in the Immunocompetent Individual.*** The vast majority of individuals who are infected with *T. gondii* after birth have no apparent clinical symptoms. In the small number of individuals with a symptomatic illness lymphadenopathy (90 per cent), fever (40 per cent), and malaise (40 per cent) are the common manifestations. The lymphadenopathy classically occurs symmetrically in the posterior auricular, anterior cervical, or posterior cervical chains. Generalized lymphadenopathy or localized unilateral enlargement or enlargement of a solitary node can also be seen. The nodes are characteristically rubbery and nontender. Splenomegaly occurs in about 30 per cent of patients. The fever is usually low grade but on occasion can be high, rapidly fluctuating, and prolonged. Fatigue can be a prominent feature. A minority of patients has a sore throat, maculopapular rash, myalgias, arthralgias, urticaria, or headache. The sore throat presents as hyperemia rather than as an exudative pharyngitis. Thus, for most patients with clinically apparent disease toxoplasmosis manifests as either asymptomatic lymphadenopathy or as a mild disorder associated with malaise, fever, and lymphadenopathy, which is self-limiting over a period of several weeks. Toxoplasmosis can, however, be a prolonged, severely debilitating disorder that may prevent the patient from working for many weeks or months. The lymph nodes may fluctuate in size during the recovery period.

In immunocompetent individuals specific organ involvement can lead to clinically significant disease involving the lungs, myocardium, pericardium, liver, skin, brain, and skeletal muscle. These manifestations may dominate the clinical picture. Glomerulonephritis has been reported. Death due to toxoplasmosis in immunocompetent individuals is an extremely unusual event.

Laboratory evaluation reveals a normal leukocyte count with a slight lymphocytosis or monocytosis. When atypical lymphocytes are present they are found only in small numbers. The hemoglobin is usually normal, although a Coombs-negative hemolytic anemia has occasionally been reported. Serum transaminases are rarely elevated to more than twice normal. The chest radiograph is usually normal; hilar adenopathy is unusual. On the electrocardiogram ST and T wave abnormalities may be seen if myocarditis is present.

Ocular Involvement in the Immunocompetent Individual. *Toxoplasma* has been estimated to cause 20 to 35 per cent of cases of retinochoroiditis in children and adults. This ocular disease is almost always a consequence of congenital infection: there are very few well documented cases of eye disease caused by infection acquired by adults.

Symptoms of retinochoroiditis are usually noted initially during the second or third decade of life. Symptoms and the degree of visual loss depend on the location and the extent of retinal involvement. Patients may complain of blurred vision, scotomas, pain, or epiphora. Strabismus may be an early sign in children. The lesions appear acutely as white or yellow cotton-like patches that have indistinct, elevated margins. Inflammatory exudate in the vitreous may obscure visualization of the fundus. As the lesions age they become atrophic with whitish-gray plaques, more distinct borders, and black spots of choroidal pigment. Lesions may be peripheral, but characteristically they occur near the posterior pole of the retina. They are usually multiple and vary in age, but single lesions do occur. Panuveitis and papillitis with optic atrophy can occur, especially in association with central nervous system disease.

Exclusively anterior uveitis has never been proven to be caused by toxoplasma.

Patients with *Toxoplasma* retinochoroiditis have an unpredictable clinical course. Episodes of active disease may occur once or many times but usually stop after the age of 40. Recurrent episodes are often associated with progressive loss of vision.

Toxoplasmosis in the Immunodeficient Patient. Toxoplasmosis can occur as a disseminated disease in patients with immunodeficiencies, particularly those with defects in cell-mediated immunity. The majority of patients are those with hematologic malignancies (particularly Hodgkin's disease), organ transplants, and the acquired immune deficiency syndrome (AIDS). The clinical manifestations are variable. Fever, hepatosplenomegaly, pneumonitis, maculopapular rash, myositis, myocarditis, meningoencephalitis, and central nervous system mass lesions may be seen. The lymphadenopathy characteristic of acquired disease in the immunocompetent patient is often absent. This syndrome is usually fulminant and rapidly fatal. It is very difficult to distinguish from numerous other infectious and noninfectious processes that can present in a similar fashion. The most common presentation includes central nervous system involvement in which fever, headache, confusion progressing to coma, and focal neurologic signs occur. Seizures and signs of increased intracranial pressure may be present. The cerebrospinal fluid shows nonspecific changes that usually include pleocytosis and moderately elevated protein, and normal glucose content. Computerized tomography usually shows one or more lesions that are contrast-enhancing in a ring or nodular pattern.

Toxoplasmosis has been serologically associated with progressive polymyositis. It is unclear whether the association reflects the etiology of the muscular disorder or whether the disorder activates *Toxoplasma* infection. A few patients with polymyositis and high antitoxoplasma antibody titers have responded symptomatically to antitoxoplasma therapy.

Congenital Disease. Congenital toxoplasmosis is the result of acute infection acquired by the mother just before or during gestation. These *Toxoplasma* infections acquired by the mother are usually asymptomatic, as is *Toxoplasma* infection acquired by other immunocompetent hosts, and thus there is nothing to make the mother or her physician suspicious unless serologic testing is routinely performed. The likelihood that the fetus will become infected and the severity of the congenital infection are largely dependent on when during the gestation the infection is acquired. In cases in which the infection occurs late during gestation or involves very few organisms, the infant will probably have no clinical manifestations but will have positive humoral and cellular immune responses to *Toxoplasma*. Although the infant is asymptomatic, *Toxoplasma* trophozoites may continue to replicate after birth, causing more damage. Cysts of *Toxoplasma* will persist in the retina, brain, myocardium, and/or skeletal muscle for the infant's lifetime. If the infant remains immunocompetent during its lifetime, the only subsequent clinical manifestations that might occur are retinochoroiditis, which usually flares during the second or third decade of life; seizures; and mild retardation. In infants who are infected early during gestation or with large inocula, the clinical sequelae can be severe. Spontaneous abortion, stillbirth, and prematurity may result. The infant may be born with microophthalmia, microcephaly, seizures, cerebral calcifications, bilateral retinochoroiditis, rash, lymphadenopathy, pneumonitis, fever, or hepatosplenomegaly, which can result in severe incapacity. If the cerebral inflammatory response involves the aqueduct of Sylvius, hydrocephalus may result. Clinical manifestions of these complications may be apparent at birth or may become obvious several months later when the infant fails to reach normal milestones.

DIAGNOSIS. The diagnosis of toxoplasmosis can be based on serologic tests, lymph node histology, the demonstration of trophozoites in body tissues or fluids, or isolation of *T. gondii* from certain sites. Which diagnostic test is most appropriate depends on the clinical situation.

Serology. Measurement of antitoxoplasma antibody titers is the most commonly employed mechanism for diagnosing toxoplasmosis. The *Sabin-Feldman dye test* is a highly sensitive and highly specific dye exclusion test that uses live *T. gondii.* This test is the reference procedure with which other tests must be compared. The Sabin-Feldman dye test and the indirect fluorescent antibody (IFA) test give comparable titers: titers begin to rise one to two weeks after infection and reach a peak after two to eight weeks that is almost always ≥ 1:1000. Titers drift down slowly over several years and persist at low levels (1:16–1:64) for the patient's lifetime. The height of the initial peak does not correlate with severity of clinical disease. Sabin-Feldman dye test titers are positive at stable low levels in adults with reactivated ocular disease and in most immunoincompetent patients with disseminated toxoplasmosis. Titers in infants may be elevated because of passively transferred maternal antibodies. Sequential studies over four to six months must be performed to determine if the infant's titers are rising, suggesting that the infected infant is producing antibody, or if they are falling (usually by 50 per cent per month) and attributable to passively transferred maternal antibodies.

The IgM-fluorescent antibody (IgM-IFA) test is particularly useful for establishing recent *Toxoplasma* infection because titers appear early (as early as five days after infection) and disappear within several months. IgM-IFA tests have not been carefully standardized: the significance of specific titers needs to be evaluated by the laboratory performing the test. Detection of IgM antibodies by the double sandwich ELISA is more sensitive and specific than the IgM-IFA test but also has not been carefully standardized. The IgM-IFA titers are elevated in acute disease in immunocompetent individuals and in infants with congenital disease but are not elevated in adults with reactivated ocular disease or in most immunoincompetent individuals with disseminated toxoplasmosis.

The complement fixation test using soluble *Toxoplasma* antigen becomes positive three to six weeks after infection, rises for the succeeding two to eight months and falls to very low levels after one to two years. This test can be useful for documenting a titer rise in someone whose Sabin-Feldman dye test titer has already peaked and whose IgM-IFA or IgM-ELISA peak has already occurred, i.e., a patient whose infection occurred more than two to four months previously but less than six to eight months previously. Titers are often elevated in infants with congenital disease and in some immunologically abnormal patients with disseminated disease. Titers are not elevated in adults with reactivated ocular disease.

The indirect hemagglutination (IHA) test as performed in most laboratories measures antibodies that rise very late in the course of infection and persist for years. Titer rises occur so late that the test has very little clinical utility and is particularly poor for use as a screening device to identify pregnant women who have acquired *Toxoplasma* infection early during gestation and who might therefore elect abortion if still medically feasible. The indirect hemagglutination tests that are available in commercial kits are often poorly standardized and are therefore difficult to interpret.

False positive results are not known to occur with the Sabin-Feldman dye test. The IFA and IgM-IFA tests may produce false positive results if antinuclear antibody is present. Rheumatoid factor can also cause false positive IgM-IFA titers.

In summary, acute acquired toxoplasmosis is suggested serologically by Sabin-Feldman dye test or IFA titers ≥ 1:1000 and proven convincingly by the documentation of elevated IgM-IFA or IgM-ELISA titers, or the documentation of a two tube (or greater) titer rise in the Sabin-Feldman dye test, IFA test, complement fixation test, and perhaps the indirect hemagglutination test. Congenital toxoplasmosis in infants is documented by demonstrating elevated complement fixation or IgM-IFA titers, or by showing that Sabin-Feldman dye test or IFA titers are stable or rising over four to six months. Ocular toxoplasmosis or toxoplasmosis in the immunoincompetent host cannot be diagnosed with certainty by antibody testing: a negative Sabin-Feldman dye test or IFA test titer excludes *Toxoplasma* as a cause of the ocular disease.

Isolation of the Organism. *T. gondii* can be isolated from leukocytes, body fluids, or tissue by direct inoculation of the specimens subcutaneously or intraperitoneally into mice. The mice are then examined periodically for the presence of antibody to *Toxoplasma;* for the presence of trophozoites in the peritoneum; or for the presence of cysts in the brain. The isolation of *Toxoplasma* from leukocytes or body fluids is convincing evidence of acute infection, although parasitemia persisting for a year has been described. The isolation of *Toxoplasma* from tissue does not provide convincing evidence of acute infection because a tissue cyst may have been present for many years and may thus be irrelevant to the disease process active at the time of biopsy. *Toxoplasma* isolation requires several weeks to perform and is not a rapid diagnostic technique.

Histologic Diagnosis. The histologic findings in the lymph nodes of patients with acute toxoplasmosis, described earlier, are so characteristic as to be diagnostic. The inflammatory reaction in other tissues is much less specific diagnostically. In these other tissues free or intracellular trophozoites must be demonstrated for the diagnosis of toxoplasmosis to be established. The demonstration of *Toxoplasma* cysts proves that the patient was infected by *T. gondii* at some time in the past but does not document that the current clinical disease is related.

DIFFERENTIAL DIAGNOSIS. The differential diagnosis of a patient with lymphadenopathy includes lymphoma, Hodgkin's disease, acquired immune deficiency syndrome (AIDS), sarcoidosis, mycobacterial disease, cytomegalovirus disease, mononucleosis, brucellosis, tularemia, cat scratch disease, and many other infectious processes. Toxoplasmosis can be distinguished from mononucleosis by the absence of atypical lymphocytosis, exudative pharyngitis, elevated serum transaminases, and heterophile antibodies. Appropriate serologies, cultures, and lymph node biopsies are necessary to distinguish the other processes. Toxoplasmosis in immunosuppressed patients may mimic other disseminated infections: the central nervous system mass lesions need to be distinguished by biopsy from *Herpes simplex* infection, bacterial abscesses, fungal processes, and neoplasms.

Toxoplasma retinochoroiditis needs to be distinguished on the basis of lesion morphology, serology, and appropriate cultures from cytomegalovirus, herpes, tuberculosis, histoplasmosis, syphilis, and sarcoidosis. Congenital toxoplasmosis must be distinguished from cytomegalovirus disease, syphilis, *Herpes simplex* infection, rubella, erythroblastosis fetalis, and bacterial sepsis.

THERAPY. The need and duration of therapy depends on the clinical setting. Most immunocompetent adults with lymphadenopathic disease do not need specific antitoxoplasma therapy. Patients with severe or prolonged constitutional symptoms, patients with specific organ dysfunction, immunoincompetent patients, and probably patients infected by direct inoculation (laboratory workers and transfusion recipients) merit treatment. Treatment for patients with retinochoroiditis or for pregnant patients is more controversial.

A combination of pyrimethamine (Daraprim) and sulfadiazine has been shown to be effective in inhibiting the replication of trophozoites. There are no drugs that will kill trophozoites or eradicate the cyst form. Pyrimethamine can only be given orally: in adults an initial dose of 75 mg is given, followed by 25 mg daily. Infants should be given 1 mg per kilogram for three days followed by 0.5 mg per kilogram per day. Sulfadiazine 1 gram orally every six hours is the adult dose. Infants should receive 100 mg per kilogram per day. Triple sulfonamides can be substituted for sulfadiazine, but sulfisoxazole (Gantrisin) is ineffective. Good urine flow should be maintained by adequate fluid intake to prevent crystalluria. Since sulfa drugs and pyrimethamine inhibit folate synthesis, folinic acid (leucovorin) 3 to 9 mg should be administered two to three times weekly to prevent bone marrow toxicity. Platelet counts and white blood cell counts should be monitored at least twice weekly during therapy. Pyrimethamine is a potential teratogen and should not be used in pregnant women.

Evaluation of the effectiveness of sulfadiazine and pyrimethamine therapy has been limited by the marked variability in clinical course and the frequency of spontaneous improvement. There is considerable anecdotal experience, however, that specific therapy can shorten the symptomatic period of fever and fatigue (although not the lymphadenopathy) in immunocompetent patients with acquired disease and is probably effective in hastening the resolution of serious organ dysfunction. Often a four- to six-week course of therapy is given and then the clinical situation re-evaluated. In *Toxoplasma* retinochoroiditis primary therapy should be directed at controlling the hypersensitivity response with anti-inflammatory drugs such as corticosteroids if the lesions are extensive or central. Pyrimethamine and sulfadiazine should be used to prevent local proliferation of the organisms and potential dissemination during the period of drug-induced immunosuppression.

Sulfadiazine and pyrimethamine have been effective in a number of immunosuppressed patients in controlling systemic symptoms and specific organ dysfunction. Long-term therapy should be strongly considered for the duration of immunosuppression. Bone marrow toxicity is a major management problem in many of these patients, particularly those with AIDS or those treated with antineoplastic chemotherapy.

In pregnant women who plan to complete their pregnancy despite the acquisition of *Toxoplasma* infection during gestation, pyrimethamine is dangerous to give because of its teratogenic potential. There is some evidence that sulfadiazine alone may be effective therapy. In Europe spiramycin (not available in the United States) has been used but its efficacy has not been clearly established. Congenital toxoplasmosis should be treated aggressively whether or not the infant is symptomatic, because organism proliferation can continue after birth. Antitoxoplasma therapy will not reverse damage that has already occurred.

For patients who cannot tolerate sulfadiazine and pyrimethamine, there are no clearly effective alternatives. Studies in vitro and animal data suggest that trimethoprim, either alone or in combination with sulfa drugs, has some antitoxoplasma activity, although less than pyrimethamine. Clindamycin and spiramycin do not have an established role in the treatment of systemic human disease. There is some evidence suggesting that clindamycin may be useful for treating retinochoroiditis.

PREVENTION. Toxoplasmosis is usually transmitted by the consumption of undercooked meat or exposure to oocyst-infected cat feces, so effective prevention should be directed against minimizing exposure to these two sources. Meat should be cooked as mentioned earlier. Pet cats should be kept in the house and they should not be fed raw meat or have access to wild rodents or birds. Particularly susceptible individuals should avoid sandboxes or moist soil where outdoor cats may defecate.

Congenital toxoplasmosis can be largely avoided if pregnant women follow the aforementioned precautions carefully. Serologic testing at the time of the mother's first prenatal examination and again at 16 to 18 weeks of gestation permits recognition of mothers who have acquired toxoplasmosis early in pregnancy and allows consideration of therapeutic abortion.

There are no current guidelines for preventing *Toxoplasma* infection related to blood transfusions or organ transplantation, nor is it clear how reactivated disease can be prevented in immunodeficient patients.

Desmonts G, Couvreur J: Congenital toxoplasmosis. A prospective study of 378 pregnancies. N Engl J Med 290:110, 1974. *The risk of congenital toxoplasmosis is documented in this prospective study.*

Dorfman RF, Remington JS: Value of lymph node biopsy in the diagnosis of acute acquired toxoplasmosis. N Engl J Med 289:878, 1973. *The specific histologic characteristics of toxoplasma lymphadenitis are documented.*

Ruskin J, Remington J: Toxoplasmosis in the compromised host. Ann Intern Med 84:193, 1976. *The clinical manifestations in immunosuppressed patients are described.*

Schlaegel TF Jr: Ocular Toxoplasmosis and Pars Planitis. New York, Grune & Stratton, 1978. *This detailed volume comprehensively covers ocular toxoplasmosis.*
Wallace GD: The role of the cat in the natural history of *Toxoplasma gondii*. Am J Trop Med Hyg 22:313, 1973. *The sexual cycle of* T. gondii *in the cat is described.*
Welch PC, Masur H, Jones TC, Remington JS: Serologic diagnosis of acute lymphadenopathic toxoplasmosis. J Infect Dis 142:256, 1980. *The usefulness of different serologic techniques is assessed for diagnosing acute lymphadenopathic toxoplasmosis.*
Wilson CB, Remington JS, Stagno S, Reynolds DW: Development of adverse sequelae in children born with subclinical congenital *Toxoplasma* infection. Pediatrics 66:767, 1980. *An analysis of the sequelae that congenital* Toxoplasma *infection produced in 24 children.*

383. PNEUMOCYSTOSIS

Henry Masur

Pneumocystosis is a pulmonary disease characterized by dyspnea, tachypnea, and hypoxemia that occurs in immunodeficient patients and in malnourished or premature infants. It is caused by species of the genus *Pneumocystis*, organisms that are probably protozoa. *Pneumocystis* cause asymptomatic infection in healthy mammalian hosts and are seen extracellulary in the pulmonary alveoli.

HISTORY. In 1909, while studying the lungs of guinea pigs experimentally infected with *Trypanosoma cruzi*, Carlos Chagas described what he thought was a new sporogony stage of the trypanosome. In 1910, Carini noted an identical form in the lungs of rats infected with *T. lewisi*. Two years later, Delanoe and Delanoe recognized that this lung cyst of Carini was in fact a distinct organism. Numerous workers then identified *Pneumocystis* in the lungs of mice, rats, guinea pigs, rabbits, dogs, monkeys, and horses that had not been infected with trypanosomes. Subsequently, epidemics of interstitial plasma cell pneumonia of unknown cause were described in Europe. Although Chagas had recognized his sporogony stage in a human lung in 1911, it was not until 1953 that Vanek, Jirovec, and Lukes recognized the association between interstitial plasma cell pneumonia and *Pneumocystis*. Since that time, *Pneumocystis* pneumonia has been recognized with increasing frequency, particularly as the use of immunosuppressive therapies for malignant neoplasms and organ transplantation has increased, and as the life span of individuals with congenital immunodeficiencies has improved.

ORGANISM. The life cycle of *Pneumocystis carinii* is not known with certainty. Morphologic data suggest that a thick-walled cyst and a thinner-walled trophozoite are the major stages in the life cycle of this extracellular organism. The cyst is 5 to 6 μ in diameter, and usually contains a cluster of six to eight round sporozoites (1 to 2 μ in diameter). When the sporozoites are released by the cyst, they develop into the trophozoites (1 to 5 μ in diameter). Under certain conditions, the trophozoites undergo a series of changes, including loss of internal structure, appearance of villous projections on the outer membrane, and development of an unusual trilaminar membrane, changes which transform the trophozoite into the cyst stage. A trophozoite-to-trophozoite cycle may also occur. The intra-alveolar exudate contains a mixture of cysts and trophozoites, as well as cellular and microbial debris and plasma proteins. The cyst is the stage of the organism usually identified in clinical specimens by means of the characteristic outer membrane staining with methenamine silver nitrate (Color plate 5G), Gram-Weigert, or toluidine blue O stains. With Giemsa stain, sporozoites can be identified within the cyst, as can the trophozoites, especially in touch preparations of fresh lung tissue or in bronchial secretions.

EPIDEMIOLOGY. *Pneumocystis* species are widely distributed, infecting rodents, rabbits, dogs, goats, horses, sheep, and other mammals, including humans. There is no evidence that animals serve as a reservoir for infection of humans. Experimental animal models and epidemiologic investigations of human disease best support the theory that transmission is by a respiratory route via droplet spray. In a few cases, congenital transmission has appeared to be the most likely route of infection.

Epidemiologic data suggest that *Pneumocystis* is infectious, that healthy or diseased individuals can transmit the infection, and that infection is usually persistent and asymptomatic. Nude mice or cortisone-treated germ-free rats will not develop pneumocystosis unless they have respiratory contact with communally raised non-germ-free rats. Epidemics of human disease among institutionalized malnourished infants, outbreaks of pneumocystosis among hospitalized immunodeficient patients, family clusters of pneumocystosis, and the increased prevalence of antipneumocystis antibody among healthy medical personnel further support these concepts.

Pneumocystosis occurs most commonly in malnourished infants (especially in the second to fourth months of life when passively transferred maternal antibodies first reach low levels), patients with deficiency of immunoglobulins G or M, and patients with deficiencies in cell-mediated immune mechanisms. The vast majority of adult patients have either the acquired immune deficiency syndrome (AIDS) or have received chemotherapy for hematologic malignancies or organ transplantation.

PATHOLOGY AND PATHOGENESIS. In latent *Pneumocystis* infection, rare clusters of cysts unassociated with marked cellular response or alveolar exudate can be seen. In the rat model, latent *Pneumocystis* infection can develop into active pulmonary disease after corticosteroid or cyclophosphamide therapy, but not after irradiation, splenectomy, or neonatal thymectomy. In humans, the relative importance of specific predisposing factors is less clear. When the *Pneumocystis* organisms are able to multiply, the inflammatory response includes transudation of fluid into the alveoli and a mononuclear cell infiltrate of interstitial spaces. The alveoli become filled with a foamy, proteinaceous material that contains clumps of both trophozoites and cysts. In malnourished or premature infants with pneumocystosis, the interstitial spaces contain predominantly plasma cells and alveolar epithelial cells—hence the pathologic description, interstitial plasma cell pneumonia. In immunodeficient children and adults, however, the inflammatory response consists of lymphocytes, macrophages, and occasionally eosinophils. Polymorphonuclear leukocytes are not seen, even in patients with normal white blood cell counts. The lung is usually involved diffusely, although localized disease has occasionally been described. The lung is usually firm and rubbery in consistency. Other infections can be found in association with pneumocystosis, including generalized infections as well as viral or fungal or bacterial pneumonias. Rarely, *Pneumocystis* may occur outside the lungs, involving lymph nodes, spleen, or bone marrow.

CLINICAL MANIFESTATIONS. The major symptoms of pneumocystosis are dyspnea, tachypnea, and a nonproductive cough. Fever and cyanosis are often present. The clinical syndrome can progress rapidly over several days or can appear insidiously over weeks or months. The rapidly progressive form is characteristic of patients with malignant neoplasms, especially during corticosteroid withdrawal. The insidious form is typically seen in children with congenital immunodeficiencies and in adults with AIDS.

On physical examination, the patient usually shows signs of respiratory distress (tachypnea, dyspnea, and cyanosis) associated with fever, but some patients, particularly those with AIDS, may have a paucity of signs. Auscultation of the lungs usually reveals no abnormalities, although scattered rales and rhonchi may be heard.

Routine laboratory tests are not generally helpful in distinguishing pneumocystosis from other pulmonary processes that are common in immunodeficient patients. Leukocytosis can be seen, but most often the white blood cell count reflects the underlying disease or the effects of chemotherapy. Eosinophilia has been reported, especially in children with humoral immune deficiencies. The arterial blood gases will demonstrate decreased oxygen saturation and hyperventilation despite continuous oxygen therapy, consistent with alveolar capillary block. A mild respiratory acidosis may be seen. Early in the course of the disease the chest radiograph usually shows a perihilar interstitial or patchy reticulogranular infiltrate with peripheral sparing. At the time of presentation some patients, particularly those with AIDS, may have normal arterial blood gases and/or normal chest x-rays. As pneumocystosis progresses, diffuse alveolar infiltrates with air bronchograms usually involve the entire lung fields. Pleural reaction, pleural effusion, asymmetry of infiltrates, or nodular infiltrates are unusual manifestations of pneumocystosis alone, but can be seen in up to half of the cases, since more than one disease process is often present in the lungs.

COURSE. The course of untreated pneumocystosis is one of progressive pulmonary consolidation, hypoxemia, and death. After institution of appropriate specific therapy, improvement usually occurs in five to ten days. The radiologic findings may become transiently worse after institution of therapy, but will then improve over one to three weeks. An association of pneumocystosis with interstitial fibrosis or emphysema has been reported, but the etiologic role of pneumocystosis has been difficult to document in view of the many factors that could lead to pulmonary changes in these patients.

DIAGNOSIS. Once the suspicion of pneumocystosis is raised by the clinical setting of immune deficiency and progressive pulmonary symptoms, pulmonary secretions or lung tissue should be examined by methenamine silver, Gram-Weigert, Giemsa, or toluidine blue O stains. Sputum smears and transtracheal aspirates demonstrate the organism in fewer than 15 per cent of patients. Bronchoscopy can be diagnostic in the majority of patients if products of lavage and brushings are examined carefully. Percutaneous needle biopsy of the lung and transbronchial biopsy of the lung are also diagnostic in most patients, although sufficient lung tissue for satisfactory pathologic evaluation is not always obtained. Open lung biopsy provides the optimal chance for complete and accurate diagnosis. For most patients, the operative risk is justified by the need to distinguish *Pneumocystis* from other, clinically similar pulmonary processes that may be caused by viruses, fungi, bacteria; neoplastic disease, hemorrhage, or drugs. Definitive lung biopsy results permit specific therapy, thus avoiding the complications of prolonged broad-spectrum antimicrobials. If the biopsy must be delayed, or if surgery is contraindicated, a therapeutic trial with specific drugs against *Pneumocystis* should be instituted.

Reliable serologic techniques have not yet been developed for diagnostic purposes. Immunofluorescent antibody titers are significantly elevated in only about 30 per cent of patients with pneumocystosis, but are also elevated in some immunosuppressed patients without apparent pneumocystosis, and in some healthy contacts. These titers may be useful in the epidemic infantile form of pneumocystosis, and in epidemiologic investigations.

TREATMENT. If started early in the course of the disease, therapy for pneumocystosis is quite successful. Pentamidine isethionate was used to treat pneumocystosis in the United States for over a decade; its use decreased mortality from nearly 100 per cent to less than 50 per cent, particularly if the patient survived long enough to receive the drug for nine or more days. Pentamidine has now been supplanted by co-trimoxazole as the therapy of choice for pneumocystosis. Co-trimoxazole, the fixed combination of trimethoprim and sulfamethoxazole, appears to be as effective as pentamidine and less toxic. This drug combination interferes with the synthesis of folinic acid. Adults should be given at least a 14-day course of 20 mg per kilogram per day of trimethoprim and 100 mg per kilogram per day of sulfamethoxazole in four equal oral or intravenous doses. Serum concentrations should be monitored because critically ill patients may not absorb orally administered drugs optimally, and because factors such as abnormal renal function or unusual volumes of distribution may make levels unpredictable even after intravenous administration. Peak serum levels of 5 to 10 μg per ml trimethoprim and 100 to 150 μg per ml sulfamethoxazole, drawn 90 minutes after drug administration, have been documented in some successfully treated patients. Folinic acid can be administered orally or intravenously to prevent or to treat folate deficiency; the dose is 10 mg two to three times weekly. Hypersensitivity rashes and leukopenia are uncommon adverse effects in patients with malignant neoplasms but occur with unusually high frequency in AIDS patients.

If the patient is unable to tolerate co-trimoxazole because of hypersensitivity or an adverse reaction, or if the patient has not responded to seven to ten days of co-trimoxazole therapy, then the use of pentamidine should be considered. Pentamidine is available in the United States only from the Parasitic Drug Service, U.S. Public Health Service (404–329–3670, days; 404–329–2888, nights). The mechanism of action of pentamidine on *Pneumocystis* is unknown, but the drug inhibits incorporation of nucleotides into DNA and RNA, inhibits oxidative phosphorylation, and causes megaloblastic cell changes. Pentamidine is administered in one single daily intramuscular dose for 10 to 14 days. Pentamidine isethionate, the drug available from the Parasitic Drug Service in the United States, should be given at a dose of 4 mg per kg per day. In Canada and certain other countries the methylsulfonate salt of pentamidine is available; the dose is calculated differently since the product is labelled with the amount of pentamidine base present, rather than the amount of pentamidine salt: the dose is 2.3 mg of base per kg per day. In over 40 per cent of patients, pentamidine causes adverse effects, including renal insufficiency, abnormal liver function, and disturbances in bone marrow function or glucose metabolism (hypoglycemia or hyperglycemia). These adverse effects are usually reversible. Intramuscular administration often results in large and painful sterile abscesses. Intravenous administration has been associated with significant hypotension in the past and has thus been avoided. Recent experience suggests that slow infusion over 60 to 90 minutes of pentamidine diluted in 100 to 150 ml of fluid may be safe. Such an infusion must be considered experimental, however.

Repeat episodes of pneumocystosis have been documented after pentamidine and after co-trimoxazole therapy, particularly in patients with AIDS.

PREVENTION. Since the diseased patient may be able to spread the organism to other patients, to healthy medical personnel, and to family members, respiratory precautions should be maintained when the diagnosis is suspected. Such precautions may prevent hospital clusters of pneumocystosis. For certain highly susceptible patient populations such as children with acute lymphoblastic leukemia at institutions with high attack rates, and perhaps for patients with AIDS, continuous prophylactic treatment with co-trimoxazole is beneficial. The daily preventive dose is trimethoprim, 5 mg per kilogram per day, and sulfamethoxazole, 25 mg per kilogram per day, in two equally divided doses.

Burke BA, Good RA: *Pneumocystis carinii* infection. Medicine 52:23, 1973. *This thoroughly referenced review summarizes a large clinical experience as well as the literature to date, covering the biology, the clinical and pathologic aspects, and the epidemiology of pneumocystosis.*

Hughes WT, Kuhn S, Chaudhary S, Feldman S, Verzosa M, Aur RJA, Pratt C, George SL: Successful chemoprophylaxis for *Pneumocystis carinii* pneumonitis. N Engl J Med 297:1419, 1977. *This randomized, double blind study demonstrates the efficacy of co-trimoxazole for the prevention of pneumocystosis in a high risk pediatric population.*

Kovacs JA, Hiemenz JW, Macher AM, Stover D, Murray HW, Shelhamer J, Lane HC, Ormacher C, Hoenig C, Longo DL, Parker MM, Natanson C, Panillo JE, Fauci AS, Pizzo PA, Masur H: *Pneumocystis carinii* pneumonia: A comparison between patients with the acquired immunodeficiency syndrome and patients with other immunodeficiencies. Ann Intern Med 100:663, 1984. *The clinical presentation of pneumocystis pneumonia in AIDS is demonstrated to be more subtle than in other disease states, but response to therapy does not differ dramatically between the two groups.*

Singer C, Armstrong D, Rosen PP, Schottenfeld D: *Pneumocystis carinii* pneumonia: A cluster of eleven cases. Ann Intern Med 82:772, 1975. *An epidemiologic investigation of an outbreak of pneumocystosis. This article provides documentation about probable routes of transmission, with important implications for disease prevention.*

Walzer PD, Perl DP, Krogstad DJ, Rawson PG, Schultz MG: *Pneumocystis carinii* pneumonia in the United States. Epidemiologic, diagnostic, and clinical features. Ann Intern Med 80:83, 1974. *This article summarizes 194 confirmed cases of pneumocystosis in terms of information supplied to the Centers for Disease Control. Its data are useful and well organized.*

Winston DJ, Lau WK, Gale RP, Young LS: Trimethoprim-sulfamethoxazole for the treatment of *Pneumocystis carinii* pneumonia. Ann Intern Med 92:762, 1980. *The efficacy of intravenous co-trimoxazole in 11 adults with confirmed pneumocystosis is documented. Pharmacologic guidelines for therapy are provided.*

384. BABESIOSIS (Piroplasmosis)

Morton N. Swartz

DEFINITION. Babesiosis is a tick-borne malaria-like acute febrile illness caused by protozoa of the genus *Babesia* and usually occurring in sharply circumscribed endemic areas. Infection with *Babesia* was first recognized in animals, in which primary symptomatic illness (babesiosis) may be followed by persistent low-grade infection manifested only by the presence in blood of the parasites (babesiasis). Only recently has transmission of infection to humans been recorded—usually by ticks, rarely by transfusion of blood from an asymptomatic carrier.

HISTORY. Babès, in Romania in 1888, described an intraerythrocytic organism in cattle with fever and hemolytic anemia. Five years later, Theobold Smith identified a similar organism as a protozoan and the cause of Texas cattle fever, a disease that he went on to show was transmitted by ticks. The first human case of babesiosis, one which ended fatally, occurred in 1956 in a farmer in Yugoslavia who was exposed to tick infested cattle and who had undergone splenectomy 11 years earlier following an accident. However, babesiosis in humans may have been identified as early as 1904 when Wilson and Chowning noted organisms resembling those in piroplasmosis of cattle in the blood of several patients in Montana. Since these cases occurred in the endemic area of Rocky Mountain spotted fever, the findings were attributed to the latter disease. In the past 17 years 118 additional cases of infection with *Babesia* have been reported, a few from Europe but most from the northeastern United States.

PROTOZOAN AND VECTOR. Babesia is a protozoan that in mammalian hosts propagates only in erythrocytes and by a process of nonsynchronous budding. Different species of *Babesia* have been described in specific vertebrate hosts: e.g., *B. canis* (dogs); *B. bovis* (cattle); *B. equi* (horses); *B. microti* (rodents). The latter has been the etiology of most reported human cases, particularly those recently observed in the northeastern United States; rare cases in Europe have been due to *B. bovis* and *B. divergens*.

Ixodes dammini (northern deer tick) is responsible for the spread of babesiosis from rodents to humans. In development through its three stages (larva, nymph, adult) the tick requires three animal hosts (of the same or different species), each as a source of a blood meal. Deer are the usual hosts for the adult tick. The initial step in the cycle of transmission occurs when larvae feed on rodents (white-footed mice in endemic areas of Massachusetts and New York) and acquire *B. microti* in the process. Infection in this rodent population can be extensive in endemic areas (60 per cent of white-footed mice on Nantucket Island harbor this protozoan). Infection in the larvae ultimately involves the salivary glands. Nymphs, the next stage, are the most abundant ticks on rodent reservoir hosts and usually feed from May through September. When the nymph takes its blood meal from rodents or man (requiring a period of at least 48 hours of feeding during which sporozoites replicate, mature, and become infectious), human infection ensues. Although transovarial transmission of other babesial species in other tick hosts occurs, there is no evidence as yet that *B. microti* is transmitted in this way in *I. dammini*.

EPIDEMIOLOGY. Seven cases of babesiosis have been reported from Europe and over 100 additional human infections have been documented in the United States. The European cases have been caused by bovine *Babesia* (primarily *B. divergens*), have all occurred in splenectomized individuals, and have represented serious illness (57 per cent mortality). With the exception of two splenectomized patients in California who had infections thought to have been caused by equine *Babesia* and a patient in Georgia who harbored *Babesia* that were not defined as to species but were morphologically distinct from *B. microti*, the infections in the United States have all been caused by *B. microti*. The endemic area for human infection during the summer months includes circumscribed adjoining areas of Massachusetts (Nantucket Island, Martha's Vineyard, Cape Cod) and New York (Shelter Island, Fire Island, eastern Long Island).

Only about 5 per cent of nymphal *I. dammini* on Nantucket were found to be infected with *B. microti*. This finding, plus the fact that at least 48 hours of attachment and feeding are needed for transmission of infection, may account for the fact that infection is not more prevalent in endemic areas. However, the very high current frequency of parasitemia in white-footed mice in the offshore islands and the replacement of other rodent ticks by the newly dominant *I. dammini* may account for the increasing occurrence of human babesiosis (15 clinical infections in 1980) in the endemic areas of the Northeast.

Subclinical infection occurs in humans: 4 to 7 per cent of asymptomatic individuals spending time outdoors in endemic areas during the summer months had significant IFA antibody titers to *B. microti*, and seroconversion had occurred in most. This appreciable rate assumes importance in view of the occurrence of transfusion-induced babesiosis in four patients. In several instances asymptomatic blood donors had been in endemic areas and had significant IFA titers against *B. microti*; *B. microti* was isolated on intraperitoneal inoculation of hamsters with blood from one such donor.

CLINICAL MANIFESTATIONS. The incubation period following a tick bite is one to six weeks. However, since the engorged nymph is only 2 mm in diameter, its presence may be easily overlooked. The incubation period for blood (or platelet) transfusion-induced babesiosis has been long (six to nine weeks) in three cases. Unlike the European cases, which were very severe and uniformly occurred in splenectomized patients, 80 per cent of clinical cases from the United States have occurred in patients with intact spleens. Most patients have been over 50 years of age and, with two exceptions, all recovered.

The initial symptoms are nonspecific: malaise, fatigue, anorexia, headache, weakness. Fever (39 to 40° C), drenching sweats, chills, myalgias, and arthralgias then develop. Nausea and vomiting may occur; mental depression, mood lability, photophobia have been noted in some patients but meningeal signs have been absent. The onset may occur acutely over a period of a few days or may be more protracted over several weeks. Lymphadenopathy is absent, but splenomegaly is detected in some patients. Rash is not observed. However, simultaneous infection with Lyme disease (vector also *I. dammini*) has occurred.

More severe disease occurs in splenectomized patients. Of the 22 patients with reported cases, six died (including five Europeans with cases due to bovine strains) with prominent hemolytic anemia, hemoglobinuria, jaundice, and renal insufficiency.

Occasional asymptomatic cases of human babesiosis have been described (Mexico, Georgia, Massachusetts) in which the protozoan has been identified on blood smear or on animal inoculation of the individual's blood.

Hematologic changes consist of a hemolytic anemia with reticulocytosis, reduced serum haptoglobin level, normal or slightly reduced leukocyte count, and mild to moderate thrombocytopenia. Rarely, disseminated intravascular coagulation has developed in severe cases. In some patients with clinical babesiosis direct antiglobulin tests are positive on their red blood cells as in patients with malaria. Usually, from 1 to 10 per cent of erythrocytes on peripheral blood smears contain the parasite. Parasitemias well below 1 per cent and as high as 85 per cent have been reported in patients with clinical illness. Mild elevations of serum bilirubin, SGOT, and alkaline phosphatase are common. Urinalysis shows proteinuria and hemoglobinuria.

IMMUNITY. Babesiosis in humans caused by *B. microti* is a self-limited disease in most instances, presumably because of control exercised by the host immune defenses. IgM and IgG antibodies are detectable within a few days of the initial clinical manifestations, probably reflecting the relatively long prepatent period. However, parasitemia continues in the presence of such antibodies during the course of the clinical illness and after subsidence of symptoms. Considerable evidence indicates a role for the spleen in the host defense against *Babesia*: (1) increased severity of illness in asplenic humans, (2) increased level of parasitemia in experimental animals splenectomized before or during infection, and (3) recrudescent parasitemia following recovery from babesiosis in hamsters subsequently splenectomized.

The cellular immune response plays an important role in protection. Administration of antilymphocyte serum (ALS) to hamsters prior to infection with *B. microti* results in failure to induce specific antibody, exaggerated parasitemia, and death; in animals that have successfully handled infection, later administration of ALS results in recrudescent parasitemia and some mortality despite high serum antibody levels. Also, athymic mice are more susceptible to babesial parasitemia than normal mice. In humans with acute babesiosis T and B cell function is often suppressed on assay in vitro.

DIAGNOSIS. The diagnosis of babesiosis should be considered in a febrile patient from an endemic area in the tick season or who has received a blood transfusion (including platelet infusions or transfusions of frozen-thawed blood). The diagnosis is established by finding characteristic intraerythrocytic forms (pyriform, ring, tetrad) on thin or thick Giemsa-stained blood smears. Ring forms of *Babesia* (often several in a single red cell) may be mistaken for *Plasmodium falciparum* but can be distinguished by the presence of pigment in erythrocytes parasitized by older forms of the latter. Also, schizonts and gametocytes are absent in *Babesia* infection but may be present in blood smears of patients with malaria. Tetrad (maltese cross) forms are uncommonly present in human blood smears but are sufficiently distinctive when present to indicate babesiosis. With intense parasitemia extraerythrocytic parasites (merozoites) in clusters may be seen occasionally in blood smears. Since parasitemia may vary, smears should be repeated over several days in suspected cases. Confirmation of diagnosis can be made by demonstration of IFA antibody (Centers for Disease Control) to *B. microti* in sera of patients; titers rise to $\geq$ 1:1024 within the first few weeks of illness and then fall gradually over the next six months. Confirmation of the diagnosis can also be made by demonstration of parasitemia in blood smears of hamsters inoculated intraperitoneally with a patient's blood.

THERAPY. Patients with intact spleens, low level parasitemia, and mild symptomatology often recover without specific treatment. An effective treatment for this infection has not yet been established. Although chloroquine may produce symptomatic improvement, it has little activity against the parasite itself. The combination of quinine (650 mg orally every six hours) and clindamycin (300 mg intravenously every 6 hours) has been used successfully in treating two markedly symptomatic adults with prominent parasitemia. Pentamidine isethionate* (4 mg per kg intramuscularly daily) has been used in treatment but is of questionable benefit in eliminating parasitemia. Other antimalarial drugs (pyrimethamine-sulfadoxine, primaquine) have no effect on parasitemia in animals. Exchange transfusions have been very helpful in several severely ill patients with intense degrees (40 to 60 per cent) of parasitemia and hemolysis.

PREVENTION. Prevention consists of avoiding contact with nymphal *I. dammini* in endemic areas during May through September. If tick infested areas are to be entered, use of repellents containing diethyltoluamide is advisable. Also, careful daily examination for ticks should be performed, and any found to be attached should be removed by fine forceps placed close to the site of attachment. Asplenic patients particularly should avoid endemic areas where they might come in contact with ticks.

In view of the cases of transfusion-induced babesiosis, current policy is not to accept as blood donors anyone with a history of babesiosis or any permanent residents of endemic areas (Shelter Island, Nantucket, etc.).

---

*Available from Centers for Disease Control, Atlanta, GA.

Dammin GJ: Babesiosis. *In* Weinstein L, Fields BN (eds.): Seminars in Infectious Disease. New York, Stratton Intercontinental Book Corporation, 1978, p 169. *Comprehensive review of important aspects of babesiosis as a zoonosis and a disease of humans.*

Jacoby GA, Hunt JV, Kosinski KS, Demirjian ZN, Huggins C, Etkind P, Marcus LC, Spielman A: Treatment of transfusion-transmitted babesiosis by exchange transfusion. N Engl J Med 303:1098, 1980. *The role of exchange transfusion in the treatment of intense* B. microti *parasitemia.*

Rosner F, Zarrabi MH, Benach JL, Habicht GS: Babesiosis in splenectomized adults. Am J Med 76:696, 1984. *Helpful summary of the 22 reported cases of human babesiosis that have occurred in splenectomized patients.*

Ruebush TK II, Cassaday PB, Marsh HJ, Lisker SA, Voorhees DB, Mahoney EB, Healy GR: Human babesiosis on Nantucket Island. Ann Intern Med 86:6, 1977. *Good description of the clinical illness.*

Ruebush TK II, Juranek DD, Spielman A, Piesman J, Healy GR: Epidemiology of human babesiosis on Nantucket Island. Am J Trop Med Hyg 30:937, 1981. *Good overview of the epidemiology of babesiosis in a major endemic area.*

Sun T, Tenenbaum MJ, Greenspan J, Teichberg S, Wang RT, Degnan T, Kaplan MH: Morphologic and clinical observations in human infection with *Babesia microti*. J Infect Dis 148:239, 1983. *Detailed electron and light microscopic studies of* Babesia *infection in a patient with 85 per cent parasitemia.*

Wittner M, Rowin KS, Tanowitz HB, Hobbs JF, Saltzman S, Wenz B, Hirsch R, Chisholm E, Healy GR: Successful chemotherapy of transfusion babesiosis. Ann Intern Med 96:601, 1982. *An important paper describing a case of transfusion-induced babesiosis successfully treated with the combination of quinine and clindamycin.*

385. AMEBIASIS AND AMEBIC MENINGOENCEPHALITIS

Donald J. Krogstad

AMEBIASIS

DEFINITION. Amebiasis is defined as infection with the protozoan parasite *Entamoeba histolytica*.

ETIOLOGY. *E. histolytica* exists in both cyst and trophozoite forms. Motile trophozoites (12 to 50 μm) are typically found in the bloody and mucoid stools of patients with active disease. Cysts are smaller (10 to 20 μm) and nonmotile. They are the infectious form of the parasite and are characteristically found in the formed stools of asymptomatic patients and those with minimal disease. Their double cyst membrane is an adaptation that presumably protects them from desiccation and from gastric juice after ingestion. In contrast, trophozoites (which do not have this protective double membrane) disintegrate rapidly after excretion into the external environment and are not infectious on oral ingestion.

PREVALENCE. Available data suggest that less than 1 per cent of the United States population is infected with this organism (by stool examination) or has serologic evidence of previous infection (a positive antibody titer). The 5 to 10 per cent prevalence estimates of 50 to 70 years ago are no longer valid, although they may still be applicable in some developing countries.

EPIDEMIOLOGY. The epidemiology of amebiasis in most developed countries is a mixture of indigenous and imported disease. Because the organism does not require a soil phase in its life cycle, it is not restricted to warmer climates. Thus, it may be transmitted by the fecal-oral route in areas far from the tropics. For example, there have been well-described outbreaks of disease in the northern United States and Europe, including a recent outbreak that was transmitted by the practice of colonic irrigation. Amebiasis may also be transmitted by sexual activity and is an important public health problem among homosexual populations.

Imported disease may result from the immigration of infected persons or from foreign travel by tourists. Although many refugees who come to the United States are screened for amebiasis, most returning tourists and their physicians are unaware of this risk. Thus, these patients may be mistakenly diagnosed as having ulcerative colitis and inappropriately treated with steroids.

In developing countries, the lack of sanitation and the high prevalence of infection combine to produce a greater risk of transmission than in developed countries. In both developing and developed countries, patients severely ill with amebiasis are less likely to transmit the infection than relatively well or asymptomatic patients, because they excrete the more fragile trophozoite form in their stool. Thus, the epidemiology of amebiasis is complicated by the fact that the persons most important for transmission are minimally symptomatic or asymptomatic, and are thus less likely to seek medical help.

PATHOGENESIS AND MECHANISMS OF DISEASE. *Entamoeba histolytica* directly invades the intestinal mucosa to cause amebic colitis and may also travel via the bloodstream to produce metastatic infections in the liver and at other sites. Although the mechanism(s) by which *E. histolytica* produces disease is incompletely defined, contact-dependent killing of target cells may be an important pathogenetic factor. Ravdin and his colleagues have found that direct contact (between the parasite and the target cell) is necessary for the killing of mammalian target cells by amebae.

PATHOLOGY. Amebic colitis is characterized by flask-shaped ulcers that contain pus and amebic trophozoites. On histologic examination, trophozoites are usually identifiable with routine hematoxylin and eosin staining at the periphery of these ulcers. Except for the presence of *E. histolytica* and their characteristic flask shape, these lesions may be mistaken for the colitis of inflammatory bowel disease. In contrast, amebic abscesses in the liver and elsewhere usually contain few identifiable amebae, which tend to be at the border between the abscess and normal tissue.

CLINICAL MANIFESTATIONS. The vast majority of patients infected with *E. histolytica* have few or no detectable symptoms. In a minority of patients, this commensal relationship breaks down for unknown reasons and the organism becomes a pathogen. The manifestations of amebic colitis may be subtle or severe, and range from mild watery diarrhea to explosive, bloody dysentery with a fulminant course. In addition, it is not uncommon for the disease to wax and wane. The same patient may experience both exacerbations and remissions over a period of months to years without treatment.

Outside the gastrointestinal tract, amebic disease typically presents as a slowly expanding mass lesion. Abscesses are most frequently found in the liver, where right-sided lesions are much more common than left-sided ones (presumably owing to the vascular supply of the liver). For reasons that are not clear, amebic liver abscesses are much more common in males than females (6 to 7:1). Important clues to the presence of an amebic liver abscess include elevation of the right hemidiaphragm and right upper quadrant pain.

Although amebic abscesses are most common in the liver, the infection may also extend to the lung or pericardium and metastasize to other sites, including the central nervous system. Less frequently, lesions may present in the anogenital area. These have been confused with squamous cell carcinoma of the rectum, penis, and cervix on the basis of their macroscopic appearance, although histologic examination typically reveals *E. histolytica* trophozoites.

DIAGNOSIS. ***Stool Examination.*** Stool examination for *E. histolytica* is one of the most difficult tests to perform correctly in the clinical laboratory. False negatives are common because morphology is insensitive. In addition, false-positive results have been reported by inexperienced observers who have confused both white blood cells and other amebae with *E. histolytica*. *Entamoeba hartmanni* is a particular problem, because the only criterion by which it can be distinguished from *E. histolytica* is size. It tends to be smaller in diameter (cyst 5 to 8 μm, trophozoites 6 to 10 μm) than *E. histolytica*. This distinction is difficult for even experienced observers and is impossible without the use of an ocular micrometer to measure parasite size accurately.

In patients with severe intestinal disease, *E. histolytica* trophozoites tend to be large (25 to 50 μm in diameter) and actively motile. Another useful clue is the presence of ingested red blood cells, which are characteristic of *E. histolytica* but not the nonpathogenic protozoa. However, ingested red blood cells are not diagnostic of amebiasis. Macrophages may ingest red blood cells and have often been misdiagnosed as amebae on this basis in both shigellosis and salmonellosis. Although material should be preserved in polyvinyl alcohol fixative for a permanent record, the use of supravital stains such as methylene blue may be invaluable in defining the nuclear morphology of the parasite to distinguish it from white cells and other actively motile cells in the stool at the time of the initial stool examination.

The most important cause of false-negative stool examinations for *E. histolytica* is the presence of substances that interfere with the stool examination for parasites. These include particulate material that obscures the presence of the parasite (barium sulfate, bismuth, and kaolin compounds), agents that lyse trophozoites (soap and tap water enemas), and antimicrobials that decrease the number of parasites excreted in the stool (tetracycline, sulfonamides, antiprotozoal agents). After excluding the presence of these substances (for seven to ten days prior to stool examination), there are several additional procedures worth considering in patients with negative stool examinations who are suspected of having amebiasis. Because long delays in transporting specimens to the laboratory may produce false-negative results, the next step should be to obtain fresh material from the patient and to examine it directly. If these examinations are negative, one may often increase the yield by examining pus or exudate taken at proctoscopy or sigmoidoscopy. This material should be taken with a glass rod or metal spatula, because parasites tend to adhere to cotton swabs. If these results are negative, biopsy of a rectal valve is frequently diagnostic. Even if all efforts to make a morphologic diagnosis are unsuccessful, serology is often positive.

Serology. Because most patients develop symptomatic amebiasis over months to years, the usual two- to four-week delay for the development of antibodies is not a significant problem. In areas such as the United States where amebiasis is rare, a positive antibody titer is strong suggestive evidence for amebiasis. Most patients (≥ 80 per cent) with active intestinal disease have a positive indirect hemagglutination (IHA) test. The sensitivity of this test is even greater in extraintestinal (metastatic) disease, and 96 to 100 per cent of patients with liver abscess have a positive titer (≥ 1:128). Conversely, in areas where amebic infection is common, a positive titer is less useful because titers may remain elevated for years after resolution of the acute infection.

Recent studies by Pillai and colleagues suggest that many patients with active amebic disease have circulating immune complexes which contain amebic antigen, and that the titers of these immune complexes may decrease rapidly with treatment—in contrast to the IHA.

Radiology. Radiologic examination is often positive in amebic colitis. It may reveal mass lesions (ameboma), ulcerations, pseudomembranes, or toxic megacolon. These lesions are nonspecific and may readily be confused with either cancer or inflammatory bowel disease. Their lack of specificity emphasizes the need for a more specific diagnosis based on morphology or a positive serology.

A number of radiologic techniques have been used to demonstrate extraintestinal amebic disease. The most frequently used technique is the technetium 99 scan, which characteristically reveals an area of decreased uptake in amebic liver abscess. However, amebic liver abscesses have also been visualized by ultrasonography, gallium scan, and computed tomography. In selecting a radiologic technique, observer experience is a more important variable with ultrasonography than with the other techniques. We recommend the technetium scan as the initial radiologic test for liver abscess and computed tomography or ultrasonography if the technetium scan is negative, and for disease outside the liver.

TREATMENT. The treatment of amebiasis remains unsatisfactory. It is complicated because different forms of the infection require different treatment regimens (Table 385–1), and because several antiamebic drugs have significant toxicity. Emetine and dehydroemetine are cardiotoxic; metronidazole is mutagenic in bacteria and produces tumors in rodents.

Although susceptibility testing is not yet practical for individual patients, it is nevertheless important to individualize the treatment of patients with amebiasis. For instance, metronidazole penetrates the blood-brain barrier well, and is an excellent

TABLE 385–1. TREATMENT OF PATIENTS WITH AMEBIASIS*

Intestinal infection:	
Cysts on stool examination (patients with few or no symptoms):	
Diloxanide furoate (Furamide)†	500 mg three times a day for ten days
Diiodohydroxyquin‡	650 mg three times a day for twenty days
Metronidazole (Flagyl)	750 mg three times a day for five to ten days
Trophozoites on stool examination (patients with symptomatic disease):	
Metronidazole (Flagyl)	750 mg three times a day for five to ten days
Dehydroemetine†	1.0 to 1.5 mg per kilogram per day for ten days intramuscularly or subcutaneously
Extraintestinal infection:	
Metronidazole (Flagyl)	750 mg three times a day for five to ten days
Chloroquine plus diiodohydroxyquin‡	500 mg a day for ten weeks, plus 650 mg three times a day for twenty days
Dehydroemetine† plus chloroquine	As above, plus 500 mg a day for two to three weeks
Dehydroemetine†	As above

*Doses suggested are for adults: Unless otherwise noted, doses are for oral administration.

†Available from the Parasitic Disease Drug Service, Centers for Disease Control, Atlanta, Ga 30333 (404–329–3670; nights and weekends, 329–2888).

‡Now used less frequently because a close congener (iodochlorhydroxyquin-Enterovioform) has been associated with subacute myelo-optic neuropathy. Available from Panray Division of Orment Drug and Chemical, Englewood, NJ 07631, and Glenwood Laboratories, Tenafly, NJ 07670.

Reproduced with permission of The New England Journal of Medicine (from Krogstad et al., 1978).

choice for patients with suspected central nervous system involvement. Conversely, diloxanide furoate is the preferred agent for patients with minimal or no symptoms who are passing cysts in stool.

PROGNOSIS. The prognosis of amebic infection is usually excellent if it is recognized before the patient is critically ill. However, steroids have been shown to enhance the pathogenicity of *E. histolytica* in animals and may also interfere with the response to therapy in humans. In addition, peritonitis may result from colonic perforation in amebic colitis, or from rupture of an amebic liver abscess, and clearly results in a worse prognosis.

Although high IHA antibody titers are associated with active disease, patients whose titers fall more slowly after therapy do not necessarily have persistent disease. Therefore, we recommend that patients should be followed clinically and that those with persistently high titers should not be re-treated on this basis alone.

PREVENTION. Amebiasis can be prevented by careful hygiene. Because amebic cysts are killed by cooking, only uncooked foods such as salads or those contaminated after cooking can transmit the infection. In endemic areas, it is best to avoid fresh uncooked vegetables and fruits that cannot be peeled. The concentration of chlorine necessary to kill amebic cysts ($\geq$ 10 ppm) is substantially greater than the levels used for water purification (1 to 2 ppm) and is unpalatable. Therefore, most water systems depend on sedimentation and filtration to remove amebic cysts.

Adams EB, MacLeod IN: Invasive amebiasis. I. Amebic dysentery and its complications. Medicine 56:315, 325, 1977. *The extensive experience of these investigators with over 7000 cases documents the favorable outcome of uncomplicated amebic colitis and liver abscess (case-fatality rates of < 1 per cent) and the unfavorable outcomes associated with complications such as peritonitis and pericardial extension (case-fatality rates of 30 to 40 per cent).*

Cedeno JR, Krogstad DJ: Susceptibility testing of *Entamoeba histolytica.* J Infect Dis 148:1090, 1983. *With methods such as this one, it may ultimately be possible to perform susceptibility testing on isolates obtained from individual patients.*

Healy GR, Kraft SC: The indirect hemagglutination test for amebiasis in patients with inflammatory bowel disease. Am J Dig Dis 17:97, 1972. *Indirect hemagglutination antibody titers to* E. histolytica *are a reliable method of screening patients with inflammatory bowel disease for amebiasis.*

Istre GR, Kreiss K, Hopkins RS, et al.: Outbreak of amebiasis spread by colonic irrigation at a chiropractic clinic. N Engl J Med 307:339, 1982. *This outbreak demonstrates the potential danger of such practices (presumably including penile-rectal intercourse), which transfer colonic contents from one person to another.*

Krogstad DJ, Spencer HC Jr, Healy GR, Gleason NN, Sexton DJ, Herron CA: Amebiasis: Epidemiologic studies in the United States, 1971–1974. Ann Intern Med 88:89, 1978. *This study demonstrates that lack of diagnostic skill in the United States produces both false-positive and false-negative laboratory results that lead to inappropriate therapy and increased morbidity and mortality. It also emphasizes the difficulty of distinguishing clinically between inflammatory bowel disease and amebic colitis.*

Pillai S, Mohimen A: A solid-phase sandwich radioimmunoassay for *Entamoeba histolytica* proteins and the detection of circulating antigens in amebiasis. Gastroenterology 83:1210, 1982. *This report suggests that the disappearance of circulating immune complexes from the serum may be a clinically useful indicator of successful treatment.*

Ravdin JI, Croft BY, Guerrant RL: Cytopathogenic mechanisms of *Entamoeba histolytica.* J Exp Med 152:377, 1980. *These studies demonstrate that cell-to-cell contact is necessary for the killing of target cells by the parasite.*

AMEBIC MENINGOENCEPHALITIS

Amebic meningoencephalitis is an infection of the brain and meninges caused by free-living amebae. It has been associated with *Naegleria, Acanthamoeba, Hartmanella,* and other free-living amebae. (*Acanthamoeba* may also cause a keratitis that is similarly resistant to treatment.)

This is a rare disease; only 100 to 200 cases have been reported. However, its prevalence has probably been underestimated because of difficulty in making the diagnosis. There are two different forms of primary amebic meningoencephalitis. One occurs primarily in young, healthy individuals who have been swimming in artificial fresh water lakes and is typically caused by one of the free-living *Naegleria* species. The other is more subacute and is associated with immunocompromised hosts. It is usually due to *Acanthamoeba, Hartmannella,* or other free-living amebae, but not *Naegleria.*

In both of these infections, the morbidity and mortality are caused by meningitis and a hemorrhagic encephalitis. In disease caused by *Naegleria,* inflammatory and hemorrhagic changes along the olfactory tract are often prominent. This infection is thought to gain access to the central nervous system by crossing the cribriform plate from the nose during swimming exposure in fresh water. The pathogenesis of disease caused by *Acanthamoeba* and the other organisms not associated with fresh water exposure is less clear. However, several investigators have described other amebic infections at distant sites in these patients and have postulated hematogenous spread to the central nervous system.

Both types of amebic meningoencephalitis are characterized by fever, meningismus, and obtundation. The major distinctions between them are in the epidemiologic history and in the tempo of the disease. Infections caused by *Naegleria* tend to be more fulminant with a course of several days to a week and a half. In contrast, disease among immunosuppressed hosts tends to be more subacute.

The diagnosis of amebic meningoencephalitis is often missed because the organisms are mistaken for lymphocytes in the cerebrospinal fluid. In previously healthy young patients, the disease is also confused with viral infection. In compromised hosts, it may be confused with toxoplasmosis, cytomegalovirus infection, and other opportunistic pathogens. The diagnosis is best made by careful examination of spinal fluid wet mounts for motile trophozoites, 8 to 15 μm in size.

The outlook for patients with this infection is grim. There are only four known survivors. The limited data available suggest that intravenous and intrathecal amphotericin B and miconazole, plus oral rifampin, may be effective. However, serologic studies in areas with known cases suggest that subclinical illness and spontaneous recoveries do occur with this infection. Although the only preventive measure is to avoid swimming in lakes epidemiologically associated with this infection, the risk is low (probably less than one in a million).

Carter RF: Primary amebic meningoencephalitis—clinical, pathological and epidemiological features of six cases. J Pathol Bacteriol 96:1, 1968. *This early report describes cases associated with swimming exposure in Australia and identifies* Naegleria *as the responsible pathogen.*

Duma RF, Helwig WB, Martinez AJ: Meningoencephalitis and brain abscess due to a free-living ameba. Ann Intern Med 88:468, 1978. *This report documents a fatal case of amebic meningoencephalitis caused by a free-living ameba that could not be identified. It raises the possibility that an unknown number of the free-living amebae may be capable of causing this disease.*

Key SN III, Green WR, Willaert E, Stevens AR, Key SN Jr: Keratitis due to *Acanthamoeba castellani*: A clinicopathologic case report. Arch Ophthalmol 98:475, 1980. *This newly recognized entity may be amenable to treatment with topical polyenes such as pimaricin.*

Seidel JS, Harimatz P, Visvesvara VS, Cohen A, Edwards J, Turner J: Successful treatment of primary amebic meningoencephalitis. N Engl J Med 306:346, 1982. *The* in vitro *susceptibility studies in this report suggest that the combination of amphotericin B plus miconazole may be synergistic against* Naegleria.

386. OTHER PROTOZOAN DISEASES

David P. Stevens

The human host provides an ever-changing environment for protozoan infections. With the increasing prevalence of acquired immune deficiency, caused by either immunosuppressant drugs or the acquired immune deficiency syndrome (AIDS), protozoan infections that were previously considered rare or exotic are now observed more frequently. Notable examples are *Cryptosporidium* and *Giardia* infections in the presence of AIDS. With this changing epidemiologic setting, it will not be surprising in the future to find additional protozoa that play the opportunist's role as pathogenic agents.

These infections should be distinguished, however, from the numerous nonpathogenic protozoa that may be found in the stool of apparently healthy persons. Notable among them are *Entamoeba coli, Endolimax nana, Iodamoeba butschlii, Dientamoeba fragilis, Trichomonas hominis,* and *Chilomastix mesnili.* The clinician must rely on a skilled laboratory technician to differentiate these agents from pathogenic species such as *Entamoeba histolytica* and the organisms discussed in the following chapters.

GIARDIASIS

DEFINITION. Giardiasis is an infection of the small intestine caused by the flagellated protozoan *Giardia lamblia.* When symptomatic, it results in diarrhea, malabsorption, and weight loss.

INCIDENCE AND PREVALENCE. Giardiasis is present in all climates from the equator to the poles. Its prevalence is greater where community water supplies are chronically contaminated by human sewage. It is particularly prevalent in developing regions of the world where water supplies are not formally treated or where they overlap with sewage disposal systems such as local streams. Endemic giardiasis, however, is also found in certain areas of industrialized countries. Unexpected examples of the latter include the municipal water supply of Leningrad and many of the pristine streams of the Rocky Mountains. The prevalence of giardiasis in the United States was estimated from 24 published surveys to be 7.4 per cent. It is the most commonly identified cause of water-borne infectious diarrhea and the most frequently isolated stool parasite in the United States.

ETIOLOGY. Although van Leeuwenhoek was the first to observe *G. lamblia* when he peered at his own stool with his primitive microscope in 1681, several centuries elapsed before the pathogenicity of this small intestinal flagellate was appreciated. It was long thought to be a commensal. Only in the last several decades was its role as a cause of infectious diarrhea and malabsorption recognized.

The organism exists either as the motile, flagellated, pear-shaped trophozoite, 12 to 15 μm in length, or as the somewhat smaller, tough-walled oval cyst. Infection occurs in the small intestine of the host. Trophozoites either attach to the microvilli of the intestinal epithelium with single ventral foot-like sucking discs or move about in the unstirred layer of mucus just above the epithelial surface. The trophozoites, carried caudally by peristalsis, eventually encyst and are passed out into the environment. The cyst is resistant to many environmental stresses, including concentrations of chlorine normally found in treated municipal water supplies. It is ingested eventually by a subsequent host. Excystation occurs in the acid environment of the stomach, and infection is again established in the small intestine.

EPIDEMIOLOGY. *Giardia* spreads by two routes: water-borne infection, particularly in contaminated community water supplies, and direct person-to-person transmission. Over two dozen epidemics have been described in the United States consequent to breakdown of community water filtration systems. Epidemics in day-care centers for children and among promiscuous male homosexuals indicate that direct person-to-person spread can occur.

A possible role for animal reservoirs of infection has been suggested by the demonstration of *Giardia*-infected beaver upstream from communities where outbreaks of human infection have occurred. Although controversy remains about the possibility of cross-species transmission of human *Giardia,* it is now suspected that both beaver and dogs may carry *Giardia* species infectious for humans.

Giardia is a frequent source of diarrhea in travelers returning from endemic areas. Twenty-three per cent of North American travelers returning from Leningrad have been shown to have giardiasis. Typically, the infected traveler develops symptoms several weeks after returning home, and on this basis the infection may be distinguished from that caused by toxigenic *E. coli* and other forms of infectious traveler's diarrhea with shorter incubation periods.

Its presence in persons with humoral immune deficiency syndromes has long been recognized. It has been estimated that 80 per cent of persons with common variable immune deficiency and diarrhea—so-called immunodeficient sprue—improve when treated with anti-*Giardia* drugs.

PATHOGENICITY. Jejunal mucosal biopsies from infected persons range in appearance from normal to marked subtotal mucosal atrophy with submucosal inflammatory cell infiltration, reduced villous height, and elongated crypts. Electron microscopic observation of epithelial cells beneath overlying adherent trophozoites show deformation and blunting of the individual microvilli. The mechanisms for these changes remain unknown. Possible hypotheses include mechanical interference by *Giardia* overlying the epithelium, elaboration by the parasite of an unidentifiable soluble toxin, competition between the parasite and host for nutrients, direct damage of the epithelium by adherent trophozoites, concurrent abnormal small intestinal bacterial overgrowth, invasion of submucosa by *Giardia* trophozoites with consequent elicitation of cellular inflammation, and immunopathogenic mechanisms mediated by the host's immune system.

CLINICAL MANIFESTATIONS. The majority of infections with *Giardia* are asymptomatic. In those persons who are ill, disease ranges from mild diarrhea to severe debilitating malabsorption and weight loss. Reversible lactase deficiency as well as malabsorption of fat and vitamin B_{12} has been documented. The majority of symptoms result from malabsorption and include abdominal distention, cramps, nausea, flatulence, borborygmi, and frequent loose, bulky, foul, and urgent stools. Although some persons have a self-limited infection of several weeks' duration, many have a prolonged indolent illness with waxing and waning symptoms and progressive weight loss.

DIAGNOSIS. The diagnosis is established in the suspected patient by demonstration of cysts or trophozoites in stools, or trophozoites in small bowel contents. Because excretion of the organism in stool is episodic and its demonstration elusive, at least three stool specimens should be examined before a negative conclusion is drawn. If no organisms are seen, the small bowel contents should be sampled. This can be achieved by aspiration or passage of a string which will absorb sufficient jejunal fluid for examination. Microscopic examination of a wet preparation of jejunal contents will usually reveal motile organisms in the infected person. Small bowel biopsy may be reserved for situations when these measures are unsuccessful. The small bowel roentgenogram will usually show an edematous mucosa, but this finding is nonspecific. Hematologic studies are normal. Eosinophilia should not be expected, since this is a finding associated with infections by worms, not protozoa.

TREATMENT. All infected persons should be treated. Moreover, there is occasional justification for a trial of therapy in the rare patient with typical signs and symptoms of giardiasis but in whom exhaustive efforts to demonstrate the organism fail. Therapy is achieved with quinacrine hydrochloride, 100 mg three times daily for ten days. When this drug is contraindicated, metronidazole,* 250 mg three times daily for seven days, is an alternative. Treatment with either drug may be unsuccessful in 5 to 20 per cent of patients, requiring a second course of therapy. Resolution of symptoms is often slow, in spite of effective therapy.

Hoskins LC, Winawer SJ, Bortman SA, Gottlieb LS, Zamcheck N: Clinical giardiasis and intestinal malabsorption. Gastroenterology 53:265, 1967. *Virtually every aspect of the clinical presentation of giardiasis is described in this series of case reports.*

Mahmoud AAF, Warren KS: Algorithms in the diagnosis and management of exotic diseases. II. Giardiasis. J Infect Dis 131:621, 1975. *A succinct and critical outline for the process of evaluation and treatment of the patient with giardiasis. The bibliography is highly selective.*

Stevens DP: Giardiasis: Host-pathogen biology. Rev Inf Dis 4:851, 1982. *A detailed review of the sparse knowledge available on the pathogenesis of this infection.*

TRICHOMONIASIS

Trichomonas vaginalis is probably the only species of the trichomonads that is pathogenic for humans. It is a 10 to 20 μ motile flagellated organism that ordinarily inhabits the urethra, urinary bladder, vagina, and prostate. Nearly half of infections are asymptomatic. Recognized symptoms, however, include a yellow creamy vaginal discharge associated with itching and burning. Dysuria may be prominent. Infection in the male is almost always asymptomatic.

Diagnosis is made microscopically by identification of the organism in a wet preparation of the exudate. While long-term complications are unrecognized in otherwise healthy persons, treatment of both partners is required for cessation of symptoms of this sexually transmitted disease. Treatment is accomplished with a single 1 to 2 gram dose of metronidazole, although this is frequently associated with side effects of nausea, a metallic taste, or alcohol intolerance.

Fouts AC, Krause SJ: Trichomonas vaginalis: Re-evaluation of its clinical presentation and laboratory diagnosis. J Infect Dis 141:137, 1980. *An authoritative clinical report for further detailed study.*

BALANTIDIASIS

Balantidium coli is a large, motile, oval ciliate, some five to ten times the size of an erythrocyte. The trophozoite form resides as a facultative anaerobe in the colon. The great majority of infections in humans are noninvasive, asymptomatic, and self-limited. Infrequently a cause of disease, this protozoan can penetrate the colonic mucosa with formation of deep ulcers. Illness consists of dysentery, usually bloody, often with resulting dehydration and prostration. Complications include colonic perforation at the site of the ulcers. Infection may extend to mesenteric lymph nodes and, less commonly, the appendix and terminal ileum. Isolated reports of infection of vagina, liver, lung, and pleura have documented that extraintestinal migration of the organism is rare.

Balantidia infect numerous nonhuman reservoirs, particularly swine. It is said that 80 per cent of pigs in England carry this organism. The relevance of various other animal reservoirs, such as rats, to human infection is debated. The importance of porcine infections to human disease is borne out, however, by the documented high prevalence of balantidiasis in communities where swine and humans live together closely, e.g., in New Guinea, Micronesia, Peru, and southern Russia. Poor nutrition and debilitating illness seem to predispose to symptomatic balantidiasis. Person-to-person spread probably occurs in settings where crowding and poor hygiene exist.

Ingestion of *Balantidium* cysts leads to infection in the susceptible host. Excystation occurs at an unknown location in the gastrointestinal tract, and multiplication occurs in the colon. An immune response develops in humans when tissue invasion occurs and is demonstrated by the presence of circulating immunofluorescent antibodies. Encystation occurs in the distal colon or after expulsion into the environment. The cyst, resistant to drying and other environmental stresses, becomes again the infectious form for the subsequent host.

The diagnosis is confirmed in the suspected patient by microscopic demonstration of trophozoites in fresh wet preparations of liquid stool or scrapings of colonic ulcers. Cysts are less frequently observed in stool, and concentration techniques are usually required. Differentiation from amebiasis and idiopathic ulcerative colitis must always be considered.

Therapy is reserved for the patient with symptomatic infection and consists of tetracycline, 500 mg four times daily for ten days. Metronidazole, 250 mg four times daily for seven days, is probably effective and may serve as alternative therapy when tetracycline is not tolerated.

Knight R: Giardiasis, isosporiasis, and balantidiasis. Clin Gastroenterol 7:31, 1978. *There are few timely clinical reviews on balantidiasis; this is the best of the lot.*

COCCIDIOSIS (Cryptosporidiosis, Isosporiasis)

Coccidia may infect humans, usually with a short-lived infection characterized by diarrhea, malaise, and weight loss. Increasingly, these organisms have been found to cause chronic debilitating infections in human hosts suffering from immune deficiency states such as acquired immune deficiency syndrome.

The 4 to 6 μ oocysts of *Cryptosporidium,* a protozoa previously recognized exclusively as an animal parasite, have been found in stools of immune-compromised human hosts by the use of modified acid-fast staining techniques. The clinical presentation includes prolonged and debilitating diarrhea, weight loss, fever, and abdominal pain. Spread to the trachea and bronchial tree has been reported. Therapy including metronidazole, quinacrine, or antibiotics has been generally disappointing.

Infection with *Isospora belli,* the oocysts of which are 23 to 33 μ long and 12 to 14 μ wide, is often asymptomatic. Nevertheless, *I. belli* may result in malabsorption, diarrhea, weight loss, and even death. It is usually found in the tropics, often where uncooked meats are consumed. It is also spread directly by fecal-oral transmission. Consequently its presence in institutions where hygienic practices are poor should be suspected when the appropriate clinical presentation is observed. Microscopic examination of small bowel biopsy specimens show flattened mucosal villi accompanied by inflammatory cell infiltration. Several case reports describing *I. belli* infection in association with lymphoma suggest that it, too, should be suspected in immunosuppressed patients with diarrhea.

Pitlik SD, Fainstein V, Garza D, Guarda L, Bolivar R, Rios A, Hopfer RL, Mansell PA: Human cryptosporidiosis: Spectrum of disease. Report of six cases and review of the literature. Arch Intern Med 143:2269, 1983. *A detailed study of the clinical picture and timely review of available references.*

Treatment of cryptosporidiosis in patients with acquired immunodeficiency syndrome (AIDS). Morbid Mortal Wkly Rep 33:117, 1984. *A compendium of therapy administered to a total of 112 patients. The results were dismal.*

SARCOSPORIDIOSIS

Infections with *Sarcocystis hominis* (previously designated *Isospora hominis*) may be associated with abdominal pain, diarrhea,

*This use is not listed in the manufacturer's directive, but is recommended by the Centers for Disease Control.

and nausea. The human is the definitive host with sexual reproduction taking place in the small intestine; cattle are the intermediate host where the sarcocyst resides in the skeletal or cardiac muscle with little or no reaction. While infection in humans is relatively common in areas of the world where undercooked beef is ingested because of local custom, the definition of the precise role of this agent in human disease remains clouded by its frequent coincidence with other pathogenic agents.

Beaver PC, Gadgil RK, Morera P: Sarcocysts in man: A review and report of five cases. Am J Trop Med Hyg 28:810, 1979. *This reference provides a good starting point into the available clinical literature.*

Section Two HELMINTHIC DISEASES

387. INTRODUCTION

Adel A. F. Mahmoud

"Parasite" is an all-embracing definition for infectious causes of human disease and should include viruses, bacteria, protozoa, fungi, and helminths. Within this definition, a useful distinction between microparasites and macroparasites has been suggested. The former refers to all infectious agents that directly reproduce within the definitive or mammalian host (Ch. 377). On the other hand, macroparasites that include most helminthic infections have certain biologic characteristics that set them apart from other pathogens; these features are essential in understanding host-parasite relationship. Helminths or worms have no direct reproductive capabilities within their definitive host. Therefore, an increase in worm numbers in a particular host necessitates repeated exposures to the infective stage of the pathogen. Furthermore, worm infections are usually of long duration (mean life span varies from several months to several decades), and in most circumstances reinfection potential is abundant in endemic areas. In helminthiases, a majority of infected individuals harbor few worms; the resultant morbidity is therefore generally mild. In a minority of infected individuals, worm loads are high (infection is characteristically aggregated and not normally distributed in human populations); these subjects are at higher risk of developing significant pathologic sequelae. The multicellular nature of worms, their complex antigenic structures and their elaborate evasive mechanisms add to the complexity of host-parasite relationship. Unfortunately, there are as yet no clear approaches to induction of protective immunity in humans against worm infections.

Helminthiases are prevalent in many parts of the developing and developed countries. For example, *Ascaris lumbricoides* infects approximately one fourth of the world's population while *Enterobius vermicularis* is estimated to infect 40 million people in the United States. Some worm infections such as *Strongyloides stercoralis* are particularly important in the immunosuppressed host since hyperinfection may lead to grave morbidity and considerable mortality. A systematic clinical approach to individuals with suspected worm infections should include knowledge of the geographic distribution, mode of infection, and specific symptoms and signs, if any. Diagnosis is usually dependent on obtaining and handling appropriate samples to be examined by experienced laboratory personnel. Serologic tests may be of help in some specific circumstances, such as toxocariasis, when obtaining a definitive parasitologic diagnosis may be impossible or may expose the infected subject to unnecessary and potentially hazardous procedures.

Eosinophilia, when present, is a useful clinical manifestation of worm infections that migrate in host tissues. Worms that reside exclusively in body cavities such as adult *Ascaris lumbricoides* in the lumen of small intestines are not associated with eosinophilia. Increased eosinophil counts may be observed in peripheral blood or affected tissues of infected individuals. Specific chemotherapy is usually followed by an increase of cell count before it subsides to normal levels. Eosinophilia in helminthic infections results from a combination of specific worm components that are either chemotactic or that induce other host cells to release chemotactic, eosinophilopoietic, or activating factors. The cells obtained from individuals with helminthiases and eosinophilia exhibit more Fc and complement receptors on their surface, are metabolically activated, and may be more efficient than those from uninfected subjects in killing invading stages of worms. Because of the large size of most invading stages of worms, killing of these targets by eosinophils occurs extracellularly and is mediated by a combination of oxidative and nonoxidative mechanisms.

Chemotherapy of helminthic infections has changed drastically over the last few years. Currently, there are effective, safe, and orally administered chemotherapeutic agents for most worm infections. These agents are of great help to the clinician in treating individual cases and to the public health authorities in planning control programs.

Mahmoud AAF, Austen KF (eds.): The Eosinophil in Health and Disease. Grune & Stratton, New York, 1980, p 364.
Schmidt GD, Roberts LS (eds.): Foundations of Parasitology, 2nd ed. C. V. Mosby Company, St. Louis, 1981, p 795.
Warren KS, Mahmoud AAF (eds.): Tropical and Geographical Medicine, McGraw-Hill Book Company, New York, 1984, pp 345–541.

The Cestodes

Martin S. Wolfe

388. INTRODUCTION

More than 30 species of tapeworms, or cestodes, may infect man. They are dorsoventrally flattened and creamy white, and their habitat is the intestinal tract of vertebrates. With the exception of *Hymenolepis nana,* which can be passed directly from person to person, all the species that parasitize man require at least one intermediate host to complete their life cycle.

Adult cestodes range in size from the smallest, *Echinococcus* species of 2 to 9 mm long, to the largest, *Diphyllobothrium latum,* which ranges in size from 3 to 10 meters long. They all have characteristic morphologic and biologic features that differentiate them from other helminths and from each other. Most adult tapeworms consist of a head or scolex for attachment to the intestinal wall of the host. Behind this is an unsegmented narrow neck from which immature segments or proglottides develop progressively to fully developed mature proglottides. Most distal are the oldest and gravid segments, which are essentially a sac of eggs. The entire worm, from the scolex to and including the distal gravid proglottides, is called the strobila. Each mature proglottid has both sets of sex organs, nerve trunks, and an excretory canal. There is no alimentary canal in tapeworms, and food is absorbed directly from the cuticle, which has a microvillus surface similar to intestinal mucosa of vertebrates. Diagnosis of certain species can be made from the gravid segments, which may have particular branchings and shape of the uterus or position of the genital pore.

Eggs are passed from the bowel either in the segment or free in the stool, and contain a form infective for an intermediate host. Eggs may be operculate, an adaptation for hatching in water, or nonoperculate, which usually develop in soil. Operculate eggs, exemplified by *Diphyllobothrium latum*, are undeveloped when passed, and a free-swimming larva or coracidium hatches in 9 to 12 days. This is ingested by a copepod, in which further development takes place to a procercoid larva; this in turn is ingested by an appropriate fish, in whose flesh the infective or plerocercoid larva is found. When man ingests fish with a plerocercoid larva, the larva adheres to the small intestinal wall, where it develops. When nonoperculate eggs of other species are ingested by an appropriate intermediate host, an embryo or oncosphere is released, which has the capability of penetrating the intestinal mucosa. Oncospheres of *Taenia* species penetrate the intestinal wall of the intermediate host and develop into small fluid-filled structures called cysticerci, which are distributed in various tissues and cause the disease cysticercosis. *Hymenolepis nana* oncospheres penetrate only into the villi of the small intestine and develop into cysticercoids, which eventually break out into the lumen of the intestine and attach and develop into adults. With *Echinococcus granulosus* usually only one oncosphere develops into a cyst in the intermediate host, but this hydatid or echinococcal cyst is capable of producing daughter cysts, each containing many scoleces, from an internal germinating membrane.

Pathogenesis and symptomatology are determined by the various forms of development. Humans are the definitive host of adult *D. latum* and *Taenia* worms, but the most serious effects occur when man becomes an accidental intermediate host of *Taenia solium* and cysticerci lead to many small lesions in the muscle and brain. The cysticercoids and adults of *H. nana* and adults of *Taenia* species may cause irritation of the small intestine. *Echinococcus* and *Multiceps* species produce large space-occupying cysts with symptoms depending on their location.

In the following chapters, geographic distribution, essential biology, epidemiology, pathogenesis, symptomatology, diagnosis, and prevention will be described for each of the common and some less common related cestode species which parasitize man. A final chapter will deal with the treatment of tapeworms.

Beaver PC, Jung RC, Cupp EW: Clinical Parasitology, 9th Ed. Philadelphia, Lea & Febiger, 1984, Ch 25. *An encyclopedic review of both common and very rare tapeworms of man.*

Marcial-Rojas RA (ed.): Pathology of Protozoal and Helminthic Diseases with Clinical Correlations. Baltimore, Williams & Wilkins Company, 1971, pp 585–657. *A well-illustrated and very complete discussion of pathologic and clinical aspects of the major tapeworms.*

389. DIPHYLLOBOTHRIUM LATUM (The Fish Tapeworm)

This parasite is most prevalent in parts of the northern and southern temperate zones where fresh water fish are commonly eaten. The highest incidence of infection of humans is in the countries bordering the Baltic Sea, particularly Finland and Sweden. In North America, a high incidence of *D. latum* infection occurs in Alaska, Canada, and the smaller lake areas of northern Michigan and Minnesota. A related species carried by marine fishes, *Diphyllobothrium pacificum*, has recently been described from coastal Peru.

D. latum adults are the largest tapeworms of man and may reach 10 meters in length with up to 4000 proglottides. The scolex has two deep sulci or bothria, one dorsal and one ventral, for attachment to the wall of the ileum. The last four fifths of the worm consists of maturing and gravid proglottides. The mature proglottid is broader than it is long, and in its middle is a dark, rosette-shaped, coiled uterus, which is of diagnostic value. The distalmost proglottides gradually disintegrate and release eggs in the bowel lumen, rather than separating from the parent worm like *Taenia* segments. Eggs are yellowish-brown, ovoid, and operculated and measure 56 to 76 μ long by 40 to 56 μ wide. They contain immature embryos when discharged into the feces, and under favorable conditions they mature and hatch into a ciliated coracidium in 9 to 12 days. This is ingested by the first intermediate host, a freshwater copepod of the genus *Cyclops* or *Diaptomus*, wherein it develops into a procercoid larva. The copepod is in turn ingested by the second intermediate host, certain freshwater fish species, including pike, perch, and salmon. The procercoid larva develops into a plerocercoid larva (sparganum) within the muscle and viscera of the fish in 7 to 30 days. Man becomes infected by eating raw or insufficiently cooked fish. The sparganum adheres to the wall of the small intestine and reaches maturity in three to six weeks, and eggs begin to appear in the feces. Inadequate sewage disposal allows pollution by human feces of fresh water containing suitable intermediate hosts. The fishes of small lakes are more important sources of infection than those of the Great Lakes, since the cold deep waters of the latter inhibit the hatching of eggs. Women of particular ethnic groups, such as Jews, Russians, and Scandinavians, are more frequently infected, by eating raw or undercooked fish in the preparation of ethnic foods such as gefilte fish. *D. latum* may live for up to 20 years.

The great majority of infections are with a single worm in the ileum. Most infected persons are asymptomatic, but some may experience intestinal symptoms from mucosal irritation. A moderate eosinophilia may be present. The most harmful effect of the fish tapeworm is vitamin B_{12} malabsorption and, rarely, a megaloblastic anemia. The exact mechanism is not certain, but it is related to the absorption of vitamin B_{12} by the worm. This is reported primarily in Scandinavians.

Diagnosis can be made by recovering characteristic eggs in the feces, or from the typical proglottides which are broader than long and have a characteristic rosette-shaped uterus. There is no satisfactory serologic method of diagnosis.

Prevention is with adequate disposal of raw sewage. Fish from known or suspected infected lakes must be thoroughly cooked at 56° C for at least five minutes or frozen at −10° C for 72 hours to ensure destruction of the infective larvae.

SPARGANOSIS

Sparganosis is an uncommon infection of man with larval diphyllobothroid tapeworms closely related to *D. latum*. It is caused by the sparganum or plerocercoid larva of the genus *Spirometra*, which measures up to several centimeters in length. Most human infections have been encountered in the Orient and are caused by *S. mansonoides*. Very rarely, infection is with a budding larval tapeworm, *S. proliferum*. The life cycle is similar to that of *D. latum*. Adult worms are found in dogs and cats, and in man only the larval form occurs. Eggs hatch in water and develop into procercoid larvae in *Cyclops* species, which are swallowed by the secondary intermediate host—a frog, snake, bird, or mammal. A plerocercoid larva develops in the muscle and is finally ingested by the definitive host. Humans usually become infected by ingesting infected copepods containing the procercoid larvae. Infections in the Far East may occur from the ingestion of infected raw flesh of amphibians and reptiles or by the use of these animals' flesh for medicinal skin or eye poultices. After penetrating the intestinal wall, the larvae usually migrate through the tissues and localize in the subcutaneous or muscular tissues. When infected poultices are applied to the eye, localization and edema may occur around the eye. A slowly growing, pruritic nodule develops over a three- to ten-month period, eventually measuring up to 3 cm. Local indurations, periodic urticaria, edema, erythema, chills, fever, and marked peripheral eosinophilia may occur. The parasite should be considered in anyone with a localized subcutaneous swelling and a possible exposure history. Diagnosis is by finding the characteristic larvae in the removed nodules. Infection can be prevented by avoiding untreated drinking water in endemic areas and avoiding the ingestion of uncooked flesh of amphibians and reptiles or the use of this flesh for poultices in the Far East.

Editorial: Pathogenesis of tapeworm anemia. Br Med J 2:1028, 1976. *A brief update on this most intriguing aspect of fish tapeworm infection.*

Swartzwelder JC, Beaver PC, Hood MW: Sparganosis in southern United States. Am J Trop Med Hyg 13:43, 1964. *A number of interesting case reports.*

Von Bonsdorff B: Diphyllobothriasis in Man. London, Academic Press, 1977. *Written from a medical rather than parasitologic viewpoint. A useful reference book which covers developments in diphyllobothriasis since Birkeland's monograph of 1932.*

Weinstein P, Krawczyk HG, Peers JH: Sparganosis in Korea. Am J Trop Med Hyg 3:112, 1954. *Three case reports and discussion of snake eating among Koreans and its possible relationship to sparganosis.*

390. TAENIA SAGINATA (The Beef Tapeworm)

Cattle are the most important intermediate hosts. In Africa cattle are frequently and heavily infected, and human infection rates may exceed 10 per cent in some areas. The parasite occurs throughout Asia, there is a low level of endemicity in Latin America and Europe, and rare cases are indigenously acquired in the United States. *Taenia saginata* is one of the most frequently diagnosed tapeworms in the United States, usually being acquired abroad.

The adult worm ranges from 4 to 10 meters in length and consists of 1000 to 2000 proglottides. The scolex has four prominent muscular suckers for attachment to the small intestinal wall. Proglottides are usually detached singly and have muscular power that allows them to move through the anal sphincter, or they may be carried out with the feces. The eggs are liberated from the proglottid. They are yellow-brown and cannot be morphologically differentiated from those of *Taenia solium*. Eggs become mature in approximately two weeks, and are then infective to the intermediate hosts, primarily cattle. After hatching in the intestine, the oncospheres penetrate the intestinal wall and eventually localize in the skeletal muscles of cattle, where they develop in 60 to 75 days into small cysticerci having an opaque invaginated neck and a scolex with four suckers. In about 12 months the cysticercus degenerates and calcifies. Humans are the only definitive host and become infected by ingesting raw or undercooked beef containing cysticerci. The scolex evaginates and attaches to the jejunal mucosa, where in 8 to 12 weeks it develops into an adult worm. *Taenia* worms may live up to 25 years in man. Human infection is favored by the ingestion of meat in the form of beef tartare, rare steak, and undercooked shashlik or kabobs.

Usually only one worm is present, but multiple infections can occur rarely. In most cases the adult worms are in the upper jejunum and cause no damage or symptoms. Irritation, however, may cause flatulence, cramps, or diarrhea. Eosinophilia occurs in almost half of those infected and is usually less than 10 per cent. Infection is usually recognized by the spontaneous passage of gravid proglottides out of the anus or in the feces.

Diagnosis is made by pressing the passed proglottid between two large glass slides and counting the number of lateral uterine segments. *T. saginata* usually has 15 to 30 of these uterine segments, whereas the only other similar-appearing segment, that of *T. solium*, usually has less than 13 and an average of 9 uterine segments. Identification of lateral uterine segments can be made only on mature proglottides. In doubtful cases, diagnosis may require fixation and staining of the segments. Typical *Taenia* ova may be found on stool examination, but differentiation between *T. saginata* and *T. solium* cannot be made on egg morphology alone. Eggs may also be recovered from the perianal region with use of a scotch tape swab. Serologic tests have not proved useful in the diagnosis of *T. saginata*.

Infection can best be prevented by avoiding rare or raw beef in highly endemic areas such as Africa. Thorough cooking of beef at 56° C for five minutes or freezing at −10° C for ten days will kill cysticerci.

Pawlowski Z, Schultz MG: Taeniasis and cysticercosis (*Taenia saginata*). Adv Parasitol 10:269, 1972. *Detailed coverage of all aspects of this parasite.*

Penfold HB: The signs and symptoms of *Taenia saginata* infestation. Med J Aust 1:531, 1937. *Common and uncommon findings in 100 patients.*

391. TAENIA SOLIUM (The Pork Tapeworm; Human Cysticercosis)

Human infection is cosmopolitan but is especially prevalent where man commonly consumes raw or insufficiently cooked pork. Infections with both adult worms and tissue larvae are particularly common in India, Africa, Mexico, and Latin America, but are rare in the United States and western Europe where most recognized cases are imported.

The adult worm is smaller than *T. saginata*, measuring 2 to 4 meters long, and contains 800 to 1000 segments. The scolex has four cup-shaped suckers and differs from *T. saginata* in having a double crown of between 25 and 30 hooks on a low rounded rostellum. Mature proglottides are flabby, have less muscular action than those of *T. saginata*, and have 7 to 12 lateral branches. The ova are morphologically identical to *T. saginata* ova. Gravid proglottides or eggs are ingested by the usual intermediate host, the hog, and less frequently by other intermediate hosts, including wild boars, sheep, camels, and humans. Eggs must first be digested by gastric juice before they hatch and liberate oncospheres, which then penetrate the intestinal wall and are carried throughout the body. They typically are filtered out in the muscles but can also reach other organs. In 60 to 70 days cysticerci develop that contain an invaginated scolex with hooks and suckers. Cysticerci may remain viable in the hog for three to six years or, rarely, longer. Man is the only natural definitive host and becomes infected by eating raw or undercooked pork. The cysticerci are dissolved by gastric juices, and the larval worm attaches to the upper jejunum by its evaginated scolex. In 5 to 12 weeks it develops into an adult worm. Human infection with *Cysticercus cellulosae* occurs when people ingest eggs in contaminated food or water or eggs transferred from the anus to the mouth, or, rarely, by the regurgitation of ova into the stomach by reverse peristalsis associated with vomiting in the presence of an adult worm. Human infection is most common in populations with a preference for pork, thus being rare in Moslems and Jews. Infection is also related to general poor hygienic conditions in which hogs are allowed to have frequent contact with infected feces. As it often takes some years for cysticerci to develop, die, and lead to overt symptoms, most cases are recognized in adulthood.

Intestinal infection is usually with one adult worm, and this seldom causes anything more than local irritation and mild eosinophilia. Cysticerci may develop in any tissue or organ of the body. The cysticercus matures in man in a few months and forms a translucent cyst, which gradually becomes surrounded by a fibrous capsule. Eventually the larvae die and calcify. No serious effects result from cysticerci in their most frequent locations, the subcutaneous tissue and skeletal muscles, although palpable or visible subcutaneous nodules can be recognized in approximately half of those with established infections. These are more frequently felt in the pectoral and abdominal superficial tissues than in the limbs and may simulate neurofibromatosis. The invasive stage often causes no symptoms, but fever, eosinophilia, muscle aches, and fatigue have been described. In the brain cysticerci may be present in the cortex, meninges, ventricles, or substance of the cerebrum. Cysts in the ventricle may cause hydrocephalus. When parasites die in the brain, they provoke a severe inflammatory reaction that can lead to increased pressure symptoms. Calcification occurs after the parasite has been dead for some years.

Cerebrospinal changes occur more often in the presence of cysts in contact with the subarachnoid space rather than with parenchymatous cysts, and include pleocytosis, eosinophilia, increased protein, and decreased sugar. Patients with larvae in the brain may present with epilepsy, intracranial hypertension, and motor or sensory or personality changes many years after initial infection. *Cysticercus* is the most common larval tapeworm to invade the eye, which it reaches through the retinal artery. The unencapsulated larva is 6 to 14 mm in size and sausage shaped. It may lodge anywhere in the orbit, conjunctiva, or anterior chamber, but most commonly is subretinal in the vitreous. Reactions to live larvae are usually minimal, but dead parasites produce iridocyclitis, clouding of the vitreous, and severe retinal inflammation or detachment. Patients may present with intraorbital pain, light flashes, and blurred or absent vision. Cysts may rarely localize in all layers of the heart tissue and may produce myocarditis or congestive heart failure.

Diagnosis of adult worms can be made by finding *Taenia* eggs or characteristic segments in the stool. Cysticercosis is suggested by a history of infection with an adult worm, the presence of multiple subcutaneous nodules, typical symptoms, earlier residence in a highly endemic area where undercooked pork may have been eaten, and a moderate eosinophilia. Definitive diagnosis is by removal of subcutaneous nodules or brain cysts. After calcification of larvae, roentgenologic diagnosis from typical lesions may be made, but this is usually not possible until after five years of muscle infection or until after ten years of brain infection. Brain scan, EEG, and CT scan can confirm space-occupying lesions. With CT scan, different stages of development of the cysticerci may be seen in an individual patient. Cerebral cysticercosis must be differentiated from hydatid or coenurus cyst, brain tumors, and cerebral lues. An indirect hemagglutination test is presently the best available serologic test and is positive in a significant number of cases. However, a negative result cannot rule out cysticercosis. A complement fixation test may be positive on cerebrospinal fluid, particularly when inflammatory changes are present in the CSF.

Infection with adult worms can be prevented by heating pork from 49 to 53° C for at least a half hour, or freezing at −10° C for four days, which kills larvae. Pickling and smoking are usually not sufficient to destroy cysticerci. Proper hygienic measures and disposal of human excrement can prevent human cysticercosis.

Bickerstaff ER: Cerebral cysticercosis. Common but unfamiliar manifestations. Br Med J 1:1055, 1955. *Illustrative case reports and good discussion.*

Byrd SE, Locke GE, Biggers S, Percy AK: The computed tomographic appearance of cerebral cysticercosis in adults and children. Radiology 144:819, 1982. *The best available method for diagnosis of brain cysts.*

Dixon HBF, Lipscomb FM: Cysticercosis: An Analysis and Followup of 450 Cases. London Privy Council, Med Res Special Rept Ser No 299, 1961. *A classic review of 450 cases in British troops returned from India.*

Powell SJ, Proctor EM, Wilmot AJ, MacLeod IN: Cysticercosis and epilepsy in Africans: A clinical and serological study. Ann Trop Med Parasitol 60:152, 1966. *Clinical descriptions and value of hemagglutination test in diagnosis.*

Reddy PS, Satyendran DM: Ocular cysticercosis. Am J Ophthalmol 57:665, 1964. *Ten cases and general review of subject.*

392. HYMENOLEPIS NANA (The Dwarf Tapeworm)

Hymenolepis nana has a worldwide distribution but is most prevalent in warm, dry climates. It is common in southern and eastern Europe, the Middle East, Africa, and Latin America. In the United States it is particularly common in the southeastern and southwestern states and in institutional populations.

This parasite takes its name of the dwarf tapeworm from the very small size of the adult worm, which measures 25 to 40 mm long by 1 mm wide. It has a minute scolex with four cup-shaped suckers and a short rostellum armed with 20 to 30 small hooks. Individual segments are not seen in the stool, and mature proglottides are approximately 0.85 mm long by 0.22 mm wide. Eggs are set free by gradual disintegration of the distalmost proglottides. Eggs are characteristic in having a clear area between the shell and an inner envelope, and four to eight threadlike filaments arising from each of two polar thickenings of the inner envelope. They measure 45 by 35 μ. Eggs are immediately infective when passed in the feces. No intermediate host is required, and upon ingestion of the eggs by the definitive host (man, mouse, or rat) oncospheres hatch in the small intestine and penetrate into the villi, where they develop into cysticercoid larvae. In about four days these break out into the intestinal lumen and attach to villi in the upper two thirds of the ileum, where they become adults in 10 to 12 days. Internal autoinfection may lead to continued heavy infection. The life duration of the worm is only a few months. Infection is transmitted directly from hand to mouth and also by contaminated food and water. Children are infected more often than adults, as resistance increases with age.

Infections in man with over 1000 worms can occur. In most light infections no injury is caused to the mucosa and there are no symptoms, but mucosal irritation from heavy worm loads may lead to anorexia, abdominal pain, and diarrhea. Mild eosinophilia is often present.

Diagnosis is by the recovery of characteristic double membrane eggs in the stool. Personal hygiene, particularly in families and institutions, is the most effective method of prevention.

Otto GF: Human infestation with the dwarf tapeworm (*Hymenolepis nana*) in the southern United States. Am J Hyg 23:25, 1936. *Clinical aspects as seen in an earlier time in the United States.*

393. ECHINOCOCCOSIS (Hydatid Disease)

Three main species of *Echinococcus* infect man. *Echinococcus granulosus* is by far the most common with a worldwide distribution, especially in sheep-raising areas. Sheep are the main intermediate hosts, with dogs being the definitive host. Human infection rates are highest in southern Europe, the Mediterranean littoral, the Middle East, eastern Africa, Australia and New Zealand, and Latin America. The majority of cases in the United States are found in immigrants from endemic areas, but autochthonous cases are found in sheep-raising areas of western states. Another strain variant, *Echinococcus granulosus var. canadensis*, has a sylvatic cycle with wild animals as the main hosts and occurs in Alaska and Canada. Alveolar hydatid disease, caused by *Echinococcus multilocularis*, is restricted to the Northern Hemisphere, occurring in Europe, northcentral United States, Canada, and Alaska, with foxes as definitive hosts and rodents as intermediate hosts. A related species, *Echinococcus oligarthus*, with cats as normal hosts and small rodents as the main intermediate hosts, has been described in a few human cases in Panama and Colombia. The following discussion will refer primarily to *E. granulosus*.

Adult worms of the three species can be differentiated morphologically and are the smallest of the tapeworms, measuring from 2 to 9 mm long and consisting of a scolex, a neck, and usually three segments, the last of which is gravid. Adult worms inhabit the upper jejunum of the definitive host, principally dogs, wolves, coyotes, foxes, and cats. In dogs, their life span is three to six months. Ova, similar to those of *Taenia* species, are evacuated in the feces of the definitive host and are ingested by the intermediate host, primarily sheep and rodents, and less commonly by man. Eggs can live for some months in moist, shady soil. The shell is digested in the duodenum, and the freed embryo penetrates into the intestinal mucosa and is carried by the bloodstream until it is filtered out in a small capillary. This usually occurs in the liver, the first capillary filter; next most commonly in the lung; and less frequently in other tissues and organs of the body. The parasite then develops into a bladderlike cyst, which increases at a rate of approximately 1 cm per year. As the cyst grows, a fibrous connective tissue cyst wall is formed by reaction of the host. Inside this is a germinal layer from which budding secondary daughter cysts develop. Hydatid fluid fills the cyst, which in the case of *E. granulosus* is unilocular. With *E. multilocularis,* multilocular or alveolar cysts occur, owing to the very thin laminated membrane, which is not sharply separated from the surrounding tissue and allows for exogenous budding and malignant-like growth. Metastases may occur via the circulation. *E. oligarthus* cysts also tend to be multilocular. When dogs or other definitive hosts eat the infected flesh or offal of intermediate hosts, embryonic tapeworms within developed cysts are freed in the duodenum and attach by their scoleces to the intestinal wall, becoming adult worms.

Man is infected only by the larval or hydatid cyst stage through intimate contact with infected dogs or other definitive hosts. Infection of dogs and other reservoir hosts depends upon the dog-sheep (or rarely cattle), or wild animal-moose or rodent relationship, whereby reservoir hosts are infected by consuming infected carcasses or offal. Most *E. granulosus* infections occur in childhood by hand-to-mouth transmission of eggs picked up from the fur of dogs.

Pathology in man depends upon the location of the cyst. About 65 per cent of unilocular and 90 per cent of multilocular cysts occur in the liver, usually in the right lobe. *E. granulosus* cysts are multiple in about one quarter of patients. Lung cysts account for approximately 20 per cent of total *E. granulosus* infections, whereas the remaining 15 per cent may involve almost any other body organ or tissue. Physical signs and symptoms do not usually occur until cysts are at least 10 to 20 cm in diameter, about 10 to 20 years after initial infection. Rupture or leakage of viable cysts may lead to secondary multiple implantations of the peritoneum or other organs. Cysts may lead to compression or atrophy of surrounding tissue. Cysts may become inactive and calcify without ever causing symptoms, although there may still be some viability in a calcified cyst. There is less resistance to spherical growth in the lung than in the liver, and lung cysts may attain greater size more rapidly and rarely calcify. Brain cysts usually present at a younger age because of increased intracranial pressure, and they rarely calcify.

As many as 20 per cent of *E. granulosus* cysts may never cause symptoms. Symptoms related to liver cysts include right upper quadrant pain, hepatomegaly, and jaundice. Approximately half of patients with pulmonary cysts are asymptomatic, but cysts may cause chest pain, cough, and hemoptysis. Brain cysts may give signs of increased intracranial pressure and convulsions. With slow leakage of a cyst, urticaria and other allergic symptoms may occur, whereas rupture or needle puncture of a cyst may lead to anaphylaxis, which is often fatal. When eosinophilia is present, it is usually related to some leakage of fluid.

Echinococcosis must be suspected in anyone with a history of a slowly growing cystic tumor, particularly in the liver or lung, who has lived in an endemic area. A characteristic physical sign over a hepatic cyst on ballottement is the hydatid thrill. Liver function tests are usually normal with hepatic cysts except for a frequent elevation of alkaline phosphatase. Radiography may show older calcified lesions in the liver, spleen, or kidney. Echinococcal cyst is the leading cause of a round, reticulated calcified lesion in the liver, but the differential diagnosis includes calcified hemangiomas, metastases, and old amebic or bacterial abscesses. Radioactive or CT scans or sonography are useful in localizing noncalcified cysts. Invasive angiographic techniques are rarely required. Pulmonary cysts present as regular, well-defined, round shadows, which cannot be differentiated from a tumor. If a pulmonary cyst becomes detached from the adventitia, the so-called *water lily sign* is produced. Immunologic techniques are quite valuable and should always be employed preoperatively to alert the surgeon to the likely presence of a hydatid cyst. When the Casoni skin test, using an antigen with an appropriate nitrogen content, shows an immediate negative reaction, this is good but not absolute evidence of the absence of hydatid disease. False-positive test results may occur. Serologic procedures include indirect hemagglutination, bentonite flocculation, latex or complement fixation, and immunoelectrophoresis. Immunoelectrophoresis is the only one absolutely specific for hydatid disease, but it is presently not readily available. The diagnosis is confirmed by the finding at surgery of daughter cysts and scoleces in the cyst fluid. Closed needle aspiration of a lesion with any possibility of its being a hydatid cyst should never be performed before radiologic and immunologic studies have been done.

In endemic areas, infected dogs should be treated with a taeniafuge such as arecoline or niclosamide, and stray dogs should be destroyed. Dogs should be kept from eating uncooked carcasses or offal.

Gamble WG, Segal M, Schantz PM, Rausch RL: Alveolar hydatid disease in Minnesota. First human case acquired in the contiguous United States. JAMA 241:904, 1979. *Case report and literature review with particular reference to the disease in North America.*

Katz AM, Pan CT: *Echinococcus* disease in the United States. Am J Med 25:759, 1958. *A very thorough review of 556 cases diagnosed in the United States, the great majority of which were imported from highly endemic areas.*

Thatcher VE: Neotropical echinococcosis in Colombia. Ann Trop Med Parasitol 66:99, 1972. *A discussion of 11 cases from Colombia with this rare form of multilocular hydatid disease, which is also found in Panama.*

Wolcott MW, Harris SH, Briggs JN, Dobell ARC, Brown RK: Hydatid disease of the lung. J Thorac Cardiovasc Surg 62:465, 1971. *A series of 37 Tunisian cases treated by Hope Ship physicians. Emphasizes the need for surgery in diagnosis and treatment.*

394. OTHER, RARER TAPEWORMS

Hymenolepis diminuta, a common tapeworm of rats and mice, infrequently infects man. It has a cosmopolitan distribution worldwide, and the few cases reported in the United States have mostly been from the South. Various species of larval and adult insects are intermediary hosts and become infected by taking in eggs deposited in rodent stool. Man and dog are incidental hosts, becoming infected by ingesting one of the insects containing a cysticercoid larva, usually by eating stale grains or cereals infested with insects. The majority of human infections are in young children. Adult worms are 20 to 60 cm long and reside in the small intestine. No pathologic changes are recognized, but bowel irritation may cause minor gastrointestinal symptoms. The eggs resemble those of *H. nana,* differing in having no filaments at the pointed poles of the inner membrane. Diagnosis is by finding typical eggs in the stool.

Dipylidium caninum is the most common tapeworm of dogs and cats worldwide. Adult worms measure 15 to 80 cm in length and reside in the small intestine. Eggs, passed onto the ground in packets or in proglottides by infected animals or man, are ingested by larval fleas in which they hatch and develop into cysticercoid larvae. Humans having close contact with dogs or cats are infected by ingesting an infected flea. Human infection is infrequent, and small children are usually infected. The majority of cases are asymptomatic, but diarrhea, abdominal pain, restlessness, and eosinophilia have been reported. Diagnosis is by finding characteristic cucumber seed-shaped proglottides or characteristic eggs singly or in packets in the stool. Proglottides are motile and may migrate from the anus and can be mistaken for pinworms by history.

Coenurosis is a well-recognized disease of the central nervous system of animals. Humans are rarely infected. The adult tapeworm of the genus *Multiceps* is a common parasite of dogs and wolves. *Taenia*-like eggs are passed in the host's feces and are ingested by an intermediate host, a sheep or other ruminant, and occasionally by people. After hatching, larvae lodge primarily in the brain and central nervous system, but may also involve the eye or subcutaneous tissue, where they metamorphose into a coenurus, a bladder worm with multiple scoleces. Infections in temperate climates are probably due to *Multiceps multiceps,* usually involve the central nervous system, and may lead to increased intracranial pressure. The majority of subcutaneous cysts have been described from East Africa where the prevalent species is *Multiceps (Taenia) brauni*, and are manifested by a solitary tender subcutaneous nodule on the trunk or rarely by an eye cyst within the vitreous chamber, attached to the retina or choroid. Diagnosis is possible only with surgery. Both clinically and microscopically it is often difficult to distinguish coenurosis of the central nervous system from hydatid cyst or cysticercosis.

Cohen R, Mackey K: *Hymenolepsis diminuta* unresponsive to quinacrine. West J Med 127:340, 1977. *Case report of a symptomatic Mexican-American child.*

Hermos JA, Healy GR, Schultz MG, Barlow J, Church WG: Fatal human cerebral coenurosis. JAMA 213:1461, 1970. *The cerebral form of this disease seems to occur only in temperate climates and must be differentiated from hydatid cyst and cysticercosis.*

Templeton AC: Anatomical and geographical location of coenurus infection. Trop Geogr Med 23:105, 1971. *Review of 14 cases from Uganda involving subcutaneous nodules.*

Turner JA: Human dipylidiasis (dog tapeworm infection) in the United States. J Pediatr 61:763, 1962. *This tends to be primarily a disease of childhood but may not be as rare as earlier supposed.*

395. TREATMENT OF TAPEWORM INFECTIONS

The present drug of choice for *D. latum*, *Taenia* species, *Hymenolepis* species, and *D. caninum* is niclosamide (Niclocide). For *D. latum*, *T. saginata*, *T. solium*, and *D. caninum*, adults are given a single 2-gram dose. The tablets are chewed thoroughly in the morning and followed by water. No fasting or purging is necessary. The head and much of the worm disintegrate so that proof of cure depends on a negative stool examination for eggs at three months. For *H. nana* and *H. diminuta* the adult dose is 2 grams daily for five to seven days. Side effects are rare. Another effective drug against *D. latum*, *Taenia* species, and *H. nana* is paromomycin (Humatin), a poorly absorbed antibiotic that is considered an investigational drug for tapeworms in the United States. For *H. nana*, the adult dose is 45 mg per kilogram once a day for five to seven days, while for the other worms 1 gram every 15 minutes for four doses is administered. Quinacrine hydrochloride had formerly been used for these parasites but is most effective when administered through a duodenal tube, and cure rates are lower than with niclosamide. The anthelmintic drug mebendazole (Vermox) is effective against *Taenia* species in a dose of 300 mg twice daily for three days, but is not yet approved for this indication in the United States. Praziquantel, in a single dose treatment is very effective against intestinal *Taenia*, *Hymenolepsis*, and *Diphyllobothrium* infections in humans but is also not yet approved for cestode infections in the United States.

Praziquantel has also been shown to be effective against human cysticercosis of the brain and subcutaneous and muscle tissue. This has greatly improved the prognosis for this infection, formerly treated only surgically, with many cases being inoperable. To prevent potential immunologic reactions in the brain tissue caused by death of parasites, steroids are administred concurrently. Calcified cysticerci do not respond to this treatment, and when they cause seizures, anticonvulsants must be used for control. Successful treatment of neurocysticercosis in Mexico has been obtained by means of specific internal radiation with anti-*Cysticercus* antibodies labeled with iodine 131. Ocular cysticerci must be removed surgically; praziquantel is not recommended for treatment of ocular cysticercosis because of concern about ocular damage after parasite destruction in the eye.

Surgery is recommended for accessible symptomatic *E. granulosis* cysts. Sterilization of cysts should be performed at surgery by scolecidal solutions, such as hypertonic saline or a 10 per cent formaldehyde solution. Cysts may also be marsupialized, or cryosurgery may be used. For multiple cysts, poor surgical risk patients, and inaccessible cysts, mebendazole in large doses for several months has led to subjective improvement in most cases of *E. granulosis* and evidence of regression of cysts in some; in other patients, cysts continued to grow or were proved viable even after lengthy treatment. Hepatic lobectomy is the only operation for *E. multilocularis*, but complete removal is usually difficult. In patients with inoperable *E. multilocularis* cysts, the progressive course of the disease can be arrested by mebendazole, but treatment apparently has not killed the parasite. Related benzimidazole drugs, flubendazole, fenbendazole, and albendazole, also appear to be promising in inoperable hydatid infections.

Symptomatic coenurosis must be managed surgically. Complete surgical excision is the treatment of choice for sparganosis; if it is inoperable, injections of alcohol into the lesion will kill the parasite.

Groll E: Praziquantel for cestode infections in man. Acta Tropica 37:293, 1980. *Single-dose treatment of intestinal cestodes.*

Jones WE: Niclosamide as a treatment for *Hymenolepsis diminuta* and *Dipylidium caninum* infection in man. Am J Trop Med Hyg 28:300, 1979. *Effective treatment of these uncommon cestodes.*

Peña Chavarria A, Villaraejos VM, Zeledon R: Mebendazole in the treatment of *Taeniasis solium* and *Taeniasis saginata*. Am J Trop Med Hyg 26:118, 1977. *An alternative treatment for the commoner intestinal cestodes; not yet an approved indication in the USA.*

Perera DR, Western KA, Schultz MG: Niclosamide treatment of cestodiasis. Clinical trials in the United States. Am J Trop Med Hyg 19:610, 1970. *An early review of this drug, which has been further substantiated, showing it to be safe, simple, and effective.*

Sayek I, Yalin R, Savac Y: Surgical treatment of hydatid disease of the liver. Arch Surg 115:847, 1980. *A review of 100 surgically treated cases in Turkey.*

Schantz PM, Van den Bossche H, Eckert J: Chemotherapy for larval echinococcis in animals and humans: Report of a workshop. Z Parasitenkd 67:5, 1982. *Review of published literature and proceedings of a workshop on use of benzimidazoles against larval echinococcosis.*

Skromne-Kadlubik G, Celis C: Cysticercosis of the nervous system: Treatment by means of specific internal radiation. Arch Neurol 38:388, 1981. *Encouraging results in 500 patients in Mexico.*

Sotelo J, Escobedo F, Rodriguez-Carbajal J, Torres B, Rubro-Donnadieu F: Therapy of parenchymal brain cysticercosis with praziquantel. N Engl J Med 310:1001, 1984. *Promising new drug treatment of neurocysticercosis.*

Wittner M, Tanowitz H: Paromomycin therapy of human cestodiasis with special reference to hymenolepiasis. Am J Trop Med Hyg 20:433, 1971. *Successful treatment of various common cestodes with an alternative to niclosamide.*

The Trematodes

396. SCHISTOSOMIASIS (Bilharziasis)

Adel A. F. Mahmoud

DEFINITION. Schistosomiasis, a chronic worm infection, affects more than 200 million people in the world; several hundred million more live in endemic areas and are at risk of exposure to the parasites. In view of its prevalence and the morbidity it causes, schistosomiasis ranks among the most important public health problems of tropical and subtropical areas. The schistosomes are blood flukes that parasitize the venous channels of the definitive human host; infection is transmitted via freshwater snails. Man may be infected by one of three species: *Schistosoma haematobium*, *S. mansoni*, or *S. japonicum*. Each species is endemic in specific geographic areas of the world and results in defined clinical syndromes which, if left undiagnosed and untreated, may cause major morbidity or mortality. Other species that occasionally infect man include *S. intercalatum*, *S. mekongi*, *S. bovis*, *S. matthei*, and some avian schistosomes. In many parts of the world, enhancing agricultural productivity by developing and expanding water conservation schemes is an economic necessity. Inadvertently, these projects create ideal breeding places for the snail intermediate host, thus increasing prevalence of schistosomiasis in the population and possibly causing its spread to new areas. Currently, schistosomiasis is endemic in various areas of Africa, Asia, South America, and the Caribbean islands. In the United States, there are approximately 400,000 cases; these usually occur in Puerto Rican immigrants or travelers who have been infected while in endemic areas. Because of the absence of susceptible snails, the life cycle of the schistosomes cannot be established in this country.

Schistosomiasis has been the subject of much scientific and public health investigation, particularly over the past two decades. This has resulted in better understanding of the pathogenesis of disease syndromes and the development of new effective chemotherapeutic antischistosomal agents. Furthermore, a global strategy for schistosomiasis control is now emerging that could bring about its containment.

ETIOLOGY. The schistosomes are the most significant trematode parasites of man. Moreover, ancient Egyptian records and the presence of calcified *S. haematobium* eggs in mummies indicate that schistosomiasis existed as a human infection for several thousand years. The schistosomes differ from other trematode infections of humans in having separate sexes. The species of schistosomes that infect humans share some common features, although they are morphologically distinctive. Each worm has two suckers (anterior and ventral), and the bifurcate intestinal ceca unite posteriorly. The larger male (0.6 to 2.2 cm × 2 to 4 mm) has a ventral gynecophoric canal in which the female is held during copulation. The slender female worm (1.2 to 2.6 cm × 1 to 2 mm) has a rounded body with pointed ends.

The schistosome worms parasitize defined sites of the venous vasculature of humans. *Schistosoma haematobium* worms inhabit the venous plexus around the lower end of the ureters and the urinary bladder, whereas *S. mansoni* and *S. japonicum* are respectively located in the inferior and the superior mesenteric veins. Sexual maturity of female worms requires the presence of living mature males; when ready to deposit eggs, the worms move against the bloodstream toward the small venous radicles. The female schistosomes deposit ova singly or in bunches, depending on the species of the parasite, and retreat in the direction of blood flow. Egg deposition has been estimated at 300 per day for female *S. haematobium* and *S. mansoni* worms and 3000 per day for those of *S. japonicum*. The ova of each species have characteristic morphologic features, which are of diagnostic importance. Once deposited in the host, the eggs attempt to penetrate the venous capillaries and escape to the bladder or intestinal lumen; enzymatic secretions are thought to aid egg migration. The proportion of ova escaping from infected individuals varies in each species, and also may depend on the extent of pathology and state of resistance in the host. Eggs that fail to reach the lumen of urinary tract or gut are trapped in these organs or may be carried by portal blood to the liver; these ova result in inflammatory and immunopathologic changes which are a major cause of disease in schistosomiasis.

The schistosome eggs, upon deposition by female worms, contain immature miracidia; they take approximately 10 to 12 days to develop while migrating through the host tissues. Once mature, miracidia have a mean life span of 11 to 12 days, during which they must reach, via the bladder or intestinal lumen, the snail intermediate host. Promiscuous urination and defecation by infected individuals result in dissemination of the parasite eggs in the environment. In fresh water the schistosome ova hatch within a few hours. Miracidia escape head first and swim, usually near the surface of water; they remain infective to the snail intermediate host for approximately eight hours. On encountering the specific snail, the miracidia penetrate its tissues and undergo tremendous asexual multiplication and transformation into hundreds of cercariae. Schistosome infection of snails causes varying degrees of pathology in their liver and sexual organs and reduces their life span. Development of schistosomes inside the snail takes approximately four to six weeks, but it varies with the species of the parasite and mollusc and with changes in environmental conditions. Cercariae, the infective forms to man, emerge from the snails under specific conditions of light and temperature; they are elongate with a pear-shaped body and a long forked tail, and measure approximately 400 to 600 μm in length. They can survive in fresh water for almost 72 hours, but lose their infectivity considerably within the first 24 hours. Cercariae attach to skin of mammalian hosts by their oral or ventral suckers. Burrowing of the skin is helped by vertical vibratory movements of their bodies and secretions of the cephalic penetration glands; the process is usually completed within a few minutes. During penetration, the cercariae shake off their tails and change into the next stage of life cycle, the schistosomula, which lie in tunnels in the stratum corneum parallel to the skin surface. Schistosomula are anaerobic organisms with heptalaminar membrane (instead of the trilaminar cercarial membrane) and can no longer survive fresh water. They are thought to remain in the skin for one to three days before migrating to the lungs, finally reaching the liver in two to four weeks. The pathway of migration of the schistosomula inside the host is still controversial. They migrate via the venous circulation to the lungs, but how they reach the liver and their final habitat is still unclear. In the intrahepatic portal system the worms complete the major digestive and sexual stages of their development. Adult worms start their migration to their final habitat in two weeks and mate; viable eggs can be seen in the excreta five to nine weeks after cercarial penetration.

The mean life span of adult schistosome worms inside the human host is not exactly known. Several individual case reports indicate that worms may live 20 to 30 years. This, however, represents extreme cases, as examination of infected individuals who migrated to nonendemic areas and mathematic calculations indicate that the mean life span of the worms is much shorter, in the range of three to ten years. Such a mean duration of survival is still considerable in view of the capability of the worm to produce eggs continually and cause pathologic changes in the host.

EPIDEMIOLOGY. The endemicity of schistosomiasis in any specific area is dependent upon the unsanitary disposal of urine and feces, the presence of suitable snail hosts, and human exposure to cercariae-infected water bodies. Furthermore, the epidemiology of schistosomiasis is complex because of the existence of several stages of the life cycle of the parasite and the multitude of factors affecting each. These worms reach sexual maturity but do not multiply in the definitive host (man) whereas asexual division and extensive multiplication occur inside the snail intermediate host. Since adult schistosomes, like many parasitic worms and contrary to all other infectious agents, do not multiply in the human body, close correlation between worm load and fecal or urinary egg counts has been shown; estimates of intensity of infection can therefore be obtained by ova-enumerating procedures. Quantifying worm loads is important epidemiologically as well as for the individual patient, as it determines the extent of participation in transmission of schistosomiasis and predicts, to a large extent, the risk of morbidity and pathologic outcome.

In endemic areas, schistosomiasis prevalence and intensity show characteristic association with age and sex; infection is more common in the young and in males. Schistosomiasis is acquired early in childhood; prevalence and intensity gradually increase to a peak in the second decade of life. In older individuals, a modest reduction of prevalence may be seen in contrast to a sharp fall in intensity of infection. As schistosomiasis is acquired through contact with infected water bodies, the marked drop in intensity in adults may be due to a decrease in their water-related activities. Development of immunity may also explain age-related decrease in intensity, although there is not yet convincing evidence for acquisition of resistance against schistosomiasis in man. Intensity of infection in endemic communities shows another characteristic feature: most infected individuals harbor low worm loads, and only a small proportion acquire heavy infection. The underlying mechanism of this clustering of heavy infection in schistosomiasis is not known, but may be due to varying degrees of susceptibility and/or response of man to the parasites.

Determination of the incidence and rate of acquisition of schistosomiasis in the population of endemic areas is important for risk assessment and planning control strategies. The prevalence and intensity of infection peak in the age group 10 to 20 years in spite of the presumed multiple reexposures to the parasite. These observations suggest that the schistosomiasis transmission rate in endemic areas is slow. Several ecologic as well as host factors help maintain these features. For example, the prevalence of schistosomal infection in the snail intermediate host is usually low, ranging between 0.6 and 2 per cent. Cercarial dispersion in water bodies is considerable; they appear in significant numbers only during certain hours of the day and lose their infectivity shortly thereafter. Once on its way to invade a certain host, no more than 40 per cent of cercariae mature into adult worms. In addition, attempts to measure incidence rates in endemic areas confirmed the relatively slow rate of transmission, ranging from 2 to 4 per cent per year.

In some areas, the endemicity of schistosomiasis may be maintained by animal reservoirs; this is especially the case with *S. japonicum*, which infects dogs and cows. Although both *S. haematobium* and *S. mansoni* can infect primates and rodents, the role of these animals as reservoirs does not seem to be epidemiologically important.

PATHOGENESIS. Schistosomiasis is initiated by cercarial penetration of skin; inside the host three maturational forms of the parasite evolve: schistosomula, adults, and eggs. These stages are associated with morphologic, biochemical, and antigenic changes of the worm, which add to the complexity of host-parasite relationship. Disease caused by schistosomiasis occurs in only a small percentage of infected individuals, mainly those with high eggs counts. This relationship, however, is not exact, as the roles of other factors such as genetic background and immunologic modulatory mechanisms are now being elucidated.

Three distinct disease syndromes caused by schistosomiasis have been described; each corresponds roughly to a stage in the parasite development in the host. Cercarial dermatitis or swimmer's itch may be seen in infections with human schistosomes but more commonly when avian or other nonhuman cercariae penetrate the skin. Swimmer's itch caused by nonhuman schistosomes is commonly seen in the north central United States where some lakes are infected. The condition has also been reported in subjects exposed to *S. mansoni* or *S. haematobium* but rarely after exposure to *S. japonicum.* Primary exposure to these larvae results in either no reaction or immediate pruritic macular rash. On repeated exposures, sensitization occurs, and a more pronounced papular eruption develops with erythema, edema, and pruritus. Histopathologically, edema, round cell infiltrate, and eosinophila can be seen in the dermis and epidermis. Although the mechanism of this reaction is not known, it is probably due to host response to dying larvae and the subsequent development of humoral and cellular immunity.

Acute schistosomiasis or Katayama fever is a serum sickness–like syndrome which occurs three to nine weeks after infection. This period coincides with the onset of egg production and its associated increase in antigenic challenge to the host. Clinically significant acute schistosomiasis occurs more often with *S. japonicum* infections but has also been reported with the other two species. It is seen in previously unexposed individuals; the severity of symptoms and signs correlates with intensity of infection. There is very little known of the mechanism of this syndrome; it manifests itself as fever, abdominal pain, and headache with hepatosplenomegaly and eosinophilia. Elevations of serum IgG, IgM, IgE, and specific antischistosomal antibodies have also been observed, leading to the suggestion that the syndrome is a form of immune complex disease.

The basic pathologic lesion in chronic schistosomiasis is the egg granuloma. Although the schistosomes do not multiply in the definitive host, they continually produce eggs; some of these are trapped in the tissues. Enzymes and antigens are subsequently released from the eggs to facilitate their migration out of the body. These parasite products sensitize the host lymphocytes, which migrate to areas of egg deposition and recruit other cells through the secretion of lymphokines, and a compact cellular infiltrate "granuloma" is formed. Several cell types are prominent in the schistosome egg granuloma: lymphocytes, macrophages, eosinophils, and fibroblasts. Granuloma formation around the schistosome eggs leads to the development of lesions far bigger than the parasite ova. The extent of these granulomas along with the ultimate deposition of collagen results in most of the chronic fibro-obstructive lesions in schistosomiasis. In *S. haematobium* infection, granulomas at the lower end of the ureters impede urine flow and cause hydroureter and hydronephrosis. In *S. mansoni* infection, granulomas in the intestinal wall are associated with the abdominal manifestations of the disease, and those in the liver result in presinusoidal obstruction of portal blood flow, portal hypertension, splenomegaly, and esophageal varices. Similar lesions are seen in schistosomiasis japonica. Less commonly, eggs may be carried to almost any organ or tissue in the body eliciting granuloma formation and its pathologic sequelae. The mechanisms and control of granuloma formation and its modulation in schistosomiasis have been extensively studied; in *S. mansoni* and *S. haematobium*, cell-mediated immunologic reactions play a key role in granuloma production, whereas the etiology of *S. japonicum* granuloma is not yet clear. Furthermore, the size of the granulomatous response represents a delicate balance between sensitizing and modulating mechanisms. In chronic schistosomiasis, granulomas spontaneously modulate, i.e., their size decreases significantly, and may result in slow progression of disease manifestations. Modulation has been shown to be mediated by several arms of the host's immune system, including serum antibodies, immune complexes, suppressor lymphocytes, and macrophages. Functionally, granulomas serve to destroy the parasite eggs. Recent observations indicate that among the cells constituting the granulomatous response, eosinophils play a key role in egg destruction. The pathologic lesions seen in individuals infected with *S. intercolatum* are similar to those produced by *S. haematobium*, whereas infection with *S. mekongi* clinically closely resembles that with *S. japonicum.*

The immune response of individuals with schistosomiasis includes humoral as well as cellular components. The degree and extent of these responses provide the balance that may result in either asymptomatic infection or disease manifestations. Furthermore, mechanisms which control the host immune response such as genetic background have been demonstrated to influence the extent of granuloma formation and consequently disease. Recently, it has also been demonstrated that the host immune response to schistosome antigens also is inversely related to intensity of infection; impaired responses are seen only in those with heavy worm loads. These observations are similar to what has been demonstrated in other overwhelming mycobacterial or fungal infections. Whether the defect in immunity is a cause or consequence of infection is not yet clear. Another aspect of the host's immune response in schistosomiasis relates to the development of peripheral blood as well as tissue eosinophilia. Schistosomiasis, similar to other worm infections with tissue phases, results in significant increase of peripheral blood eosinophils; this is especially seen during the acute phase of infection. Later, in the chronic stage, eosinophil count may not be significantly elevated. Eosinophils are seen in subcutaneous tissues around the entry points of cercariae, and they constitute approximately 50 per cent of the cells in egg granulomas. The eosinophils have been shown to play a central role in host defenses against the invading stage of the parasite (schistosomula) and the phase (ova) retained in the tissues.

The occurrence of immunity to schistosomiasis in humans

has not convincingly been shown, as noted above. Although the drop of intensity and prevalence of infection in older individuals in endemic areas may reflect the development of resistance, these phenomena may be explained equally by the differences in patterns of contact with infected waters, or by changes in the rate of egg production by adult worms. Studies in vitro have demonstrated that several human cells—eosinophils, neutrophils, basophils, monocytes, and cytotoxic T lymphocytes—may alone or in combination with complement components or antischistosomal antibodies damage the larval stage of the parasite. The biologic relevance of these observations in man is not yet clear.

MANAGEMENT. Diagnosis of schistosomiasis must be based on the clinical presentation, positive geographic history, and finding the parasite eggs in the excreta or biopsy material. Quantification of infection and assessing viability of the eggs are important procedures not only for planning therapy but also for prognostic evaluation. Although tremendous advances have been made in serologic tests for schistosomiasis over the past decade, their diagnostic and prognostic value is not yet at the stage at which they can be used on a routine basis. Safe chemotherapeutic antischistosomal agents are now available and provide high cure rates. None of these drugs have any effect on cercarial penetration, on swimmer's itch, on the course of acute schistosomiasis, or as a prophylactic measure. Their major action is on the adult egg-producing worms. Appropriate management of patients with schistosomiasis must take into consideration the extent of disease and intensity of infection; measures directed against the parasite and those needed to alleviate the clinical, chronic manifestations of disease must be considered. Antischistosomal therapy, if given early enough during the course of disease, may lead to reversal of pathologic lesions. In late cases, chemotherapeutic measures may be useful only in preventing further damage resulting from the presence of the parasite.

CONTROL. The intimate relationship between humans and bodies of water in their environment leads to schistosomiasis endemicity. In addition, the lack of precise knowledge of the epidemiology of infection and disease in schistosomiasis has hampered efforts for its control. Recently, several developments such as single oral dose chemotherapeutic agents and better appreciation of transmission dynamics have led to clearer definition of strategies for control of schistosomiasis. Ideally, eradication of infection should be the target, but this is impossible to achieve with the currently available tools and the economic and social structure of the endemic areas. A more realistic approach, based on control of disease and reduction of transmission, may contain the infection and reduce its pathologic sequelae. The most cost-effective measure currently advocated is targeted mass chemotherapy, combined with focal mollusciciding if needed. Because of the specific features of infection dynamics, treated individuals remain with low egg counts for a few years. In addition, health education, attempts at raising socioeconomic standards, providing privies, and abandoning obsolete agricultural practices offer additional means for achieving progress in containing this infection.

Those traveling to endemic areas should be given proper advice. There are virtually no safe freshwater bodies in most of the areas endemic for schistosomiasis. Avoiding contact with these water sources is to be strongly recommended.

Butterworth AE, Vadas MA, David JR: Mechanisms of eosinophil mediated helminthotoxicity. *In* Mahmoud AAF, Austen KF (eds.): The Eosinophil in Health and Disease. New York, Grune & Stratton, 1980, pp 253–273. *Description of how human eosinophils destroy the schistosomula stage of the parasite.*

Ellner JJ, Olds GR, Osman GO, El Kholy A, Mahmoud AAF: Dichotomies in the reactivity to worm antigen in human schistosomiasis mansoni. J Immunol 126:309, 1981. *Demonstration of an inverse relationship between intensity of infection and immune response to schistosome antigens.*

Hofstetter M, Nash TE, Cheever AW, dos Santos JG, Ottesen EA: Infection with *Schistosoma mekongi* in Southeast Asian refugees. J Infect Dis 144:420, 1981. *Description of clinical and parasitological features of schistosomiasis mekongi.*

Iarotski LS, Davis A: The schistosomiasis problem in the world. Bull WHO 59:115, 1981. *An attempt to determine the global prevalence of schistosomiasis.*

Mahmoud AAF, Arap Siongok TK, Ouma J, Houser HB, Warren KS: Effect of targeted mass treatment on intensity of infection and morbidity in schistosomiasis mansoni. Lancet 1:849, 1983. *Evaluation of the clinical and parasitologic effects of targeting chemotherapy to those with hepatosplenomegaly and heavy infection.*

Mahmoud AAF, Warren KS, Peters PA: A role for the eosinophil in acquired resistance to *Schistosoma mansoni* infection as determined by anti-eosinophil serum. J Exp Med 142:805, 1975. *Demonstration of the in vivo protective function of eosinophils in animals with schistosomiasis.*

Olds GR, Mahmoud AAF: Role of host granulomatous response in murine schistosomiasis mansoni: Eosinophil-mediated destruction of eggs. J Clin Invest 66:1191, 1980. *Granuloma formation in schistosomiasis is a protective mechanism aimed at egg destruction. Ablation of eosinophils in the host leads to delay in egg destruction and exacerbation of disease.*

Warren KS: The immunopathogenesis of schistosomiasis: A multidisciplinary approach. Trans R Soc Trop Med Hyg 66:417, 1972. *Review of the sequence of events leading to disease in schistosomiasis.*

Warren KS: Regulation of the prevalence and intensity of schistosomiasis in man: Immunology or ecology? J Infect Dis 127:595, 1973. *A lucid discussion of the factors controlling transmission and regulation of infection in schistosomiasis.*

World Health Organization: Epidemiology and control of schistosomiasis. Technical report series 643, 1980. *Review of epidemiology, progress in some national control programs, and the different control strategies.*

SCHISTOSOMIASIS HAEMATOBIA
(Urinary Bilharziasis)

Schistosomiasis haematobia is due to human infection with the trematode *S. haematobium;* adult worms reside in the venous plexus around the urinary bladder, and their eggs are mainly found in urine of infected individuals. *S. haematobium* infection is endemic in Africa and some parts of the Middle East; it is highly prevalent in the Nile valley and extends along the Mediterranean coast of the continent. In West Africa it is more widely disseminated than *S. mansoni;* its distribution in East and South Africa is patchy. The parasite is endemic also on the islands of the Malagasy Republic. In southwest Asia, the endemic area includes most countries of the Middle East and Arabian peninsula. Clinically, infection with *S. haematobium* is the most significant of human schistosomes. Symptoms and signs of disease occur in over half of the infected individuals, including those with light worm loads. Because of the anatomic location of the pathologic lesions, gross urinary tract disease can result from a few granulomas at the lower end of ureters. In endemic areas, extensive hydroureters and hydronephrosis can be demonstrated in a considerable proportion of infected children; the natural history of these lesions and the course of disease in adults have not been clearly defined.

The adult male *S. haematobium* worms are distinguished by their finely tuberculate surface and by the presence of four to five large testes. The ovaries are found in the posterior half of the female body and contain 20 to 30 eggs. Mature *S. haematobium* eggs measure approximately 143×50 μm and are spindle shaped with a rounded anterior end and a conical posterior end which tapers to a terminal delicate spine. Eggs are mainly found in urine of infected individuals but may occasionally be seen in stools or rectal biopsies. The main intermediate hosts of *S. haematobium* in North Africa and the Middle East are freshwater snails of the genus *Bulinus;* in Africa south of the Sahara they belong to the subgenus *Physopsis.*

PATHOLOGY AND CLINICAL MANIFESTATIONS. The ova of *S. haematobium* pass from the venules of the vesical plexus into the bladder wall and the lower end of ureters, where most of the pathologic changes in infected individuals are seen. In the urinary bladder, the formation of egg granulomas leads to hyperemia, tubercles, ulcers, and polyps; as healing proceeds, sandy patches and scarring may be seen. Obstructive uropathy is the main functional disturbance caused by schistosomiasis haematobia. Other urinary tract lesions such as bacteriuria, calculi, and bladder cancer have been epidemiologically associated with *S. haematobium* infection, but no causal relationship has yet been confirmed. Ova of *S. haematobium* have occasionally been found in the lungs with subsequent focal pulmonary arteritis and diffuse hypertensive arteriolar changes; chronic cor pulmonale may occur in these patients.

Swimmer's itch and acute schistosomiasis have rarely been

described in *S. haematobium* infection. In contrast, symptoms caused by egg deposition in the urinary tract occur in a large proportion of infected individuals. In endemic areas, 50 to 90 per cent of infected subjects complain of dysuria, hematuria, or frequency. Hematuria is characteristically terminal, but with extensive ulceration the whole stream of urine may be bloody along with passage of clots. In late cases, symptoms related to secondary infection of the urinary tract, severe obstructive uropathy, or neoplasia may appear. Urine examination reveals proteinuria and hematuria; both signs are closely related to intensity of infection. An association between *S. haematobium* infection and bacteremia, mainly caused by *Salmonella* organisms, has been reported. Renal function may be compromised in patients with obstructive uropathy; both minimum urine osmolality and the ability to excrete an ingested water load are reduced, but there are nonspecific changes. Cytoscopic examination shows some degree of pathology in almost all infected individuals, the most common being hyperemia near the ureteral openings and the bladder trigone. Sandy patches, tubercles, ulcers, and polyps are less frequently seen. Radiographically, bladder calcification is a characteristic feature of urinary schistosomiasis; it is found in approximately 50 to 80 per cent of infected individuals. Other pathologic lesions are also frequently seen in 40 to 60 per cent of patients, including obstructive uropathy, hydroureters, hydronephrosis, and filling defects in the bladder and ureters. The severity of most of these symptoms and signs of schistosomiasis haematobia correlates with intensity of infection; however, in individuals with light infection, considerable pathologic changes can still be demonstrated.

DIAGNOSIS. Urine examination for *S. haematobium* eggs can be performed by direct or concentration methods. Excretion of the parasite eggs is maximal around midday, when samples should optimally be obtained. Diagnosis and quantification of infection can be achieved by filtering 10 ml of urine through Nucleopore membranes. Examination of more than one urine sample may be necessary to establish the diagnosis; rectal biopsy may alternatively be obtained in suspected cases with negative urine results. Once *S. haematobium* infection is diagnosed, assessment of urinary tract pathology by cystoscopy and intravenous pyelography is recommended. In addition, care must be taken in some endemic areas for early detection of bladder cancer by appropriate cytologic and histologic examinations.

TREATMENT. The drug of choice is metrifonate, an organophosphorus anticholinesterase compound that is highly effective against *S. haematobium* infections. Metrifonate is administered orally (7.5 mg per kilogram of body weight); the dose is repeated twice at weekly intervals. Cure rates are in the range of 60 to 90, with a more than 90 per cent drop in egg counts. Trials with a single oral dose of 10 mg per kilogram of body weight have shown high efficacy for field use; the percentage of reduction of egg counts was 96. No major side effects or contraindications to metrifonate use have been demonstrated. Following drug administration a few patients may complain of abdominal pain, nausea, or diarrhea. The main laboratory side effect is decrease of serum and red blood cell cholinesterase; however, it returns to normal within two to eight weeks. Praziquantel, a new broad-spectrum antischistosomal drug, is equally effective against *S. haematobium* infection. Antischistosomal therapy in schistosomiasis haematobia eliminates the parasites and reduces the extent of pathologic lesions. Residual urinary tract defects are treated medically; in rare cases surgical correction may be needed.

Davis A, Baily DR: Metrifonate in urinary schistosomiasis. Bull WHO 41:209, 1969. *A review of the therapeutic effect of metrifonate against* S. haematobium *infection.*

Lehman JS Jr, Farid Z, Smith JH, Basily S, El Masry NA: Urinary schistosomiasis in Egypt: Clinical, radiological, bacteriological and parasitological correlations. Trans R Soc Trop Med Hyg 67:384, 1973. *A complete clinical description of 200 individuals infected with* S. haematobium.

Mott KE, Dixon H, Osei-Tutu E, England EC: Relation between intensity of *Schistosoma haematobium* infection and clinical haematuria and proteinuria. Lancet 1:1005, 1983. *Correlation of proteinuria and hematuria to counts of* S. haematobium *eggs in urine.*

Peters PA, Mahmoud AAF, Warren KS, Ouma JH, Siongok TKA: Field studies of a rapid, accurate means of quantifying *Schistosoma haematobium* eggs in urine samples. Bull WHO 54:159, 1976. *Simple quantitative technique for urine examination.*

Smith JH, Kamel IA, Elwi A, von Lichtenberg F: A quantitative post mortem analysis of urinary schistosomiasis in Egypt. I. Pathology and pathogenesis. Am J Trop Med Hyg 23:1054, 1974. *Description of the pathology of schistosomiasis haematobia as it relates to egg counts and parasite load.*

Warren KS, Mahmound AAF, Muruka JF, Wittaker LR, Ouma JH, Siongok TKA: Schistosomiasis haematobia in Coast Province, Kenya. Am J Trop Med Hyg 28:864, 1979. *Correlation of morbidity with egg counts in schistosomiasis haematobia; even in lightly infected children disease manifestations are significant.*

SCHISTOSOMIASIS MANSONI
(Intestinal or Hepatosplenic Bilharziasis)

Schistosomiasis mansoni is due to human infection with the blood fluke *S. mansoni*, which parasitizes the inferior mesenteric venous channels. Parasite eggs are detected in stools of infected individuals, and far less commonly in their urine. Infection with *S. mansoni* is endemic in Africa, the Middle East, South America, and some Caribbean islands. The distribution of schistosomiasis mansoni in Africa overlaps with that of schistosomiasis haematobia; it is prevalent in the Nile delta in Egypt, in the Sudan, in Ethiopia, and in a broad belt across central Africa. In southwest Asia, it occurs in Yemen and Saudi Arabia. *S. mansoni* is sporadically distributed all over the northern part of South America and is endemic in several Caribbean countries and islands and in many parts of Puerto Rico.

Adult male *S. mansoni* worms have a grossly tuberculate surface and usually contain seven small testes. In the female, the ovary occupies the anterior half of its body, with a short uterus containing one to four ova. Mature eggs measure 155 × 66 μm, and are oval in shape with a lateral, long spine. *Schistosoma mansoni* infects man and primates and is found also in rodents such as mice and hamsters, but none of these animals play an important role as reservoirs for the infection. The intermediate snail hosts of *S. mansoni* are species of the genus *Biomphalaria* in Africa and *Australorbis tropicorbis* in the Americas.

PATHOLOGY AND CLINICAL MANIFESTATIONS. Cercarial dermatitis may occur following skin penetration by these larvae but is remarkably uncommon. Acute schistosomiasis mansoni appears between three and seven weeks after exposure; the presenting symptoms, in their order of occurrence, are fever, anorexia, abdominal pain, and headache. Less often, diarrhea, nausea, and vomiting may occur. Hepatosplenomegaly, eosinophilia, and elevated serum immunoglobulins are the main clinical signs. In a recent study, most of these manifestations correlated significantly with intensity of infection as evaluated by stool egg counts.

Schistosoma mansoni eggs are primarily deposited in the small veins around the large intestine of infected individuals; some of the eggs may be trapped in the gut wall or break loose into the portal circulation to be carried to the small intrahepatic portal venules. In patients with schistosomal hepatosplenomegaly, adult worms apparently move up to the veins surrounding the small intestine. On examination of the intestinal mucosa of infected subjects, it appears red and granular with pinpoint elevations surrounded by hyperemic zones. There may be minute hemorrhages and ulcerations. Sessile and pedunculated polyps, mainly in the rectosigmoid area, have been reported in Egyptians infected with *S. mansoni*, but not from other endemic areas. Pathologic examination of the liver in lightly infected individuals shows schistosome eggs with and without granulomas and mild portal inflammation. In advanced cases, the typical picture of Symmers' fibrosis is seen; the eggs are concentrated in and around large portal tracts with marked fibrosis and obstructive portal venous lesions. The lobular arrangement of liver parenchyma and its function are usually maintained. However, these structural changes lead to marked alteration of hepatic hemodynamics such as obstruction of portal blood flow through the liver and increase in number and size of intrahepatic arterial branches, thus shifting the blood flow through the liver from mainly portal to arterial sources. Portal hypertension leads to congestive splenomegaly and the formation of portosystemic venous shunts at the lower end of the esophagus and other sites. In these patients, the schistosome eggs may find their way to the pulmonary circulation, bypassing the obstructed portal blood flow. In the lungs, granulomas form around the trapped eggs, leading to arteriolar fibrosis and pulmonary hypertension.

Nervous system involvement in schistosomiasis mansoni is rare; the main clinical presentation, as in schistosomiasis haematobia, is transverse myelitis. The preferential involvement of the spinal cord may be due to the anatomic location of adult worms; both species rarely produce cerebral lesions. The underlying pathologic lesions are usually granulomas forming around eggs in the spinal cord.

Infection with *S. mansoni* does not have characteristic or specific symptomatology, in contrast to schistosomiasis haematobia. In several recent studies, infected individuals had a slightly higher incidence of crampy abdominal pain (21 to 48 per cent) and bloody diarrhea (4 to 28 per cent) than matched uninfected controls from the same endemic area. Examination of stools demonstrates an association between intensity of infection and the amount of blood detected. Other frequently mentioned nonspecific symptoms and signs, such as weakness, inability to work, or diarrhea, have not been convincingly demonstrated in any controlled studies. Significant enlargement of the liver is seen in 4 to 11 per cent of infected subjects, and splenomegaly occurs in 3 to 7 per cent. Patients with schistosomal hepatosplenomegaly present with a unique form of liver disease. The pathophysiologic changes are based on alteration of hemodynamics, fibrosis of large portal tracts, and very little derangement of liver function. Enlargement of the liver usually occurs in the left lobe, but later, in the course of infection and particularly in adults, uniform hepatomegaly may be seen. Simultaneously, gross enlargement of the spleen may occur; the organ is characteristically rubbery hard. Laboratory examination may show indications of anemia and a low degree of eosinophilia but no changes in liver function tests until late in the course of disease. Total serum proteins are usually normal, but gamma globulin elevations are common. An association between schistosomal hepatosplenomegaly and hepatitis B antigen and antibody presence has been described, but its pathophysiologic significance is not clear. Although hepatosplenomegaly usually occurs in heavily infected individuals, other underlying mechanisms may be involved. Recently, an association between HLA haplotypes and schistosomal hepatosplenomegaly has been demonstrated. In patients with pure schistosomal fibrosis uncomplicated by cirrhosis or viral hepatitis, liver function is preserved for a long time. These individuals often present clinically with an episode of hematemesis caused by rupture of esophageal varices without prior complaints. Bleeding may recur several times while the liver parenchyma maintains its normal functions. Finally, however, symptoms and signs of liver cell failure ensue, along with the development of stigmata of chronic liver disease and ascites.

Several less defined clinical syndromes have been associated with schistosomiasis mansoni. Formation of antigen-antibody complexes and their deposition in the kidney glomeruli have been demonstrated in infected laboratory animals as well as in individuals with chronic schistosomiasis mansoni. However, the prevalence of this syndrome and the rate at which it occurs in schistosomiasis are unknown, since proteinuria and nephrotic syndrome are not particularly prevalent in schistosomiasis-endemic areas. Schistosomiasis cor pulmonale is a better defined disease entity, although its incidence is not known. It usually occurs in patients with advanced hepatosplenic schistosomiasis mansoni or japonica because of the development of collateral circulation. In *S. haematobium*–infected individuals, the anatomic location of adult worms may help eggs reach the systemic circulation directly and become trapped in the pulmonary arterioles. Patients with schistosomal pulmonary hypertension present clinically with symptoms and signs similar to those in cor pulmonale of other causes. Aneurysmal dilation of the pulmonary artery and its branches, along with right ventricular hypertrophy, may occur. Other signs and symptoms of chronic schistosomiasis are usually detected, as well as parasite eggs in excreta or tissue sections.

DIAGNOSIS. Stool examination for the characteristic *S. mansoni* eggs is the definitive diagnostic procedure. Since assessing intensity of infection is essential, quantitative techniques are recommended. The Kato thick smear method involves examination of sieved 50-mg stool samples placed on glass slides and spread under a cellophane cover slip pre-soaked in 50 per cent glycerol. The slides should be left at least 24 hours to allow for clearing of fecal material; the embryo within the ova also clears, but the characteristic shape of the egg shell is retained. Rectal biopsy may be used for diagnosis of stool-negative cases, particularly in lightly infected individuals.

TREATMENT. The current drug of choice for treatment of schistosomiasis mansoni is oxamniquine. It is administered as a single oral dose of 15 to 20 mg per kilogram of body weight. In *S. mansoni* infections acquired in South America, this dose results in 70 to 100 per cent cure rates and a drop of 95 to 97 per cent in egg counts. If the patient to be treated was infected in Africa, higher doses are needed (60 mg per kilogram).* The drug is safe, and is associated with a few side effects such as dizziness and drowsiness. They occur in no more than 30 per cent of treated patients and disappear within six hours. Praziquantel, a new broad-spectrum antischistosomal drug, is equally effective against *S. mansoni*. In patients with advanced hepatosplenomegaly, antischistosomal chemotherapy may halt the advance of the disease process, but other medical measures are usually needed. Hematemesis and ascites should be treated medically; these patients do not require shunting surgery after their first bleeding episode. Although they are good surgical risks, postoperatively the incidence of portal encephalopathy is considerable.

Abdel Salam E, Ishaac S, Mahmoud AAF: Histocompatibility-linked susceptibility for hepatosplenomegaly in human schistosomiasis mansoni. J Immunol 123:1829, 1979. *The first demonstration of a relationship between defined HLA haplotypes (HLA-A1 and B5) and schistosomal hepatosplenomegaly.*

Cheever AW: A quantitative post mortem study of schistosomiasis mansoni in man. Am J Trop Med Hyg 17:38, 1968. *Correlation of worms loads with egg counts in tissues and feces, and detailed description of pathology of* S. mansoni *infection.*

Omer AHS: Oxamniquine for treating *Schistosoma mansoni* infection in man. Br Med J 2:163, 1978.

Peters PA, El Alamy M, Warren KS, Mahmoud AAF: Quick Kato smear for field quantification of *Schistosoma mansoni* eggs. Am J Trop Med Hyg 29:217, 1980. *Detailed description of the Kato thick smear technique for quantification of* S. mansoni *eggs.*

Siongok TKA, Mahmoud AAF, Ouma JH, Warren KS, Muller AS, Handa AK, Houser HB: Morbidity in schistosomiasis mansoni in relation to intensity of infection: Study of a community in Machakos, Kenya. Am J Trop Med Hyg 25:273, 1976. *Correlation of symptoms and signs of* S. mansoni *with fecal egg counts.*

SCHISTOSOMIASIS JAPONICA

Schistosomiasis japonica or Oriental schistosomiasis is due to human infection with the fluke *S. japonicum*. This schistosome species characteristically infects humans and domestic animals such as cats, dogs, and cattle, thus providing reservoir hosts which may contribute to its endemicity in certain areas of the Far East. On the main Asian continent, schistosomiasis japonica is prevalent in some parts of China, Thailand, Laos, Cambodia, and Malaysia. It is also endemic in Taiwan, Japan, the Philippines, and Celebes.

Adult *S. japonicum* male worms have a nontuberculate surface and seven medium-sized testes. The ovary occupies the middle part of the body of female worms and contains 50 to 100 ova. *S. japonicum* eggs are found in stools of infected individuals; they measure 89 × 67 μm and are oval or rounded with a lateral short, sometimes curved spine. The intermediate hosts

*This dose exceeds the manufacturer's recommended dosage.

for *S. japonicum* are snails of the genus *Onchomelania*. They are amphibious and have separate sexes, and each infected snail sheds an average of two cercariae daily. These organisms emerge in the evening and lie very close to the surface film of water; they can penetrate mammalian skin within a minute.

PATHOLOGY AND CLINICAL MANIFESTATIONS. *S. japonicum* infection results in pathologic lesions in the human definitive host which generally follow the same time course as described for schistosomiasis mansoni. Cercarial dermatitis is not a prominent feature of schistosomiasis japonica. Katayama fever, or acute schistosomiasis, was named after the district in Japan endemic for *S. japonicum* infections. Symptoms usually begin five to seven weeks after infection and are similar to those associated with schistosomiasis mansoni. The clinical features usually subside in a few days but may last for several months, and fatalities have been reported. The chronic manifestations of schistosomiasis japonica are related to ova deposited in the intestines and liver; adult worms produce ten times more eggs than those of *S. mansoni*. These ova are laid in aggregates and remain so in the intestinal wall or when carried to the liver by the portal blood flow. In addition, *S. japonicum* eggs differ from *S. mansoni* in their tendency to calcify in tissues. Schistosomiasis japonica granulomas vary in size tremendously and tend to show signs of necrosis.

The major pathologic lesions in schistosomiasis japonica are seen in the intestines, liver, lungs, and occasionally brain of infected individuals. Morphologically these lesions are initiated by the presence of eggs and proceed to granuloma formation and fibrosis as in schistosomiasis mansoni. Although it has always been assumed that, because of the ten-fold difference in egg productivity, disease in schistosomiasis japonica is more severe, there are no studies to confirm this suggestion. Individuals with chronic schistosomiasis japonica may present with no symptoms or several nonspecific complaints. Controlled surveys performed recently in endemic areas have shown no particular increase in complaints of weakness, abdominal pain, or diarrhea in infected individuals. Clinical signs of hepatosplenomegaly are more frequently seen in infected rather than uninfected individuals, but they were not uniformly correlated with intensity of infection. Severe hepatosplenic disease caused by schistosomiasis japonica may be seen in endemic areas, but its prevalence and relationship to intensity of infection and other complicating factors are unknown.

Cerebral schistosomiasis japonica is a unique syndrome reportedly occurring in 2 to 4 per cent of infected individuals in the endemic countries. *Schistosoma japonicum* infection of the central nervous system preferentially affects the brain. The lesions consist of large aggregates of eggs in the cerebral venous system, but adult worms have never been found in the brain. Cerebral schistosomiasis japonica presents clinically early in the course of the infection; the most frequent manifestation is focal jacksonian epilepsy; less commonly, generalized encephalitis may be the presenting feature.

DIAGNOSIS. Stool examination for *S. japonicum* eggs is the only reliable diagnostic procedure. The Kato thick smear technique provides both diagnosis and quantitative assessment of infection. Rectal biopsy may be used in individuals with light infections, particularly when a less common manifestation, such as cerebral schistosomiasis, is encountered.

TREATMENT. Currently, the drug of choice for treating schistosomiasis japonica is praziquantel. It is given orally as three doses of 20 mg per kilogram body weight. This dose of praziquantel has been shown to result in parasitologic cure in 70 to 80 per cent and to reduce fecal egg excretion by approximately 95 per cent. Praziquantel administration is associated with slight and clinically insignificant side effects such as abdominal pain. The same general medical recommendations outlined for advanced *S. mansoni* hepatosplenomegaly may be used in patients with late manifestations of schistosomiasis japonica.

Domingo EO, Tiu E, Peters PA, Warren KS, Mahmoud AAF, Houser HB: Morbidity in schistosomiasis japonica in relation to intensity of infection: Study of a community in Leyte, Philippines. Am J Trop Med Hyg 29:858, 1980. *A controlled study of the correlation between symptoms and signs of schistosomiasis japonica and fecal egg counts.*

Santos AT: Current chemotherapy of schistosomiasis japonica in the Philippines. SE Asian J Trop Med Public Health 7:306, 1976. *A review of the efficacy of niridazole and other schistosomal agents in schistosomiasis japonica.*

Santos AT, Blas BL, Nosenas JS, Portillo GP, Ortega OM, Hiyashi M, Boehme K: Preliminary clinical trials with praziquantel in *Schistosoma japonicum* infections in the Philippines. Bull WHO 57:793, 1979.

Warren KS, Su DL, Xu CY, Yuan HC, Peters PA, Cook JA, Mott KE, Houser HB: Morbidity in schistosomiasis japonica in relation to intensity of infection; study of 2 royal brigades in Anhui Province, China. N Engl J Med, 309:1533, 1983.

397. HERMAPHRODITIC FLUKES

S. K. K. Seah

The hermaphroditic flukes, unlike *Schistosoma* flukes, have male and female sex organs in the same worm, and self-fertilize. Those of medical importance are (1) flukes that parasitize the biliary tract, i.e., *Clonorchis sinensis*, *Opisthorchis* spp., *Fasciola hepatica*, *Dicrocoelium dendriticum*, and *Metorchis conjunctus*; (2) flukes that parasitize the intestinal lumen, i.e., *Fasciolopsis buski*, *Heterophyes heterophyes*, *Echinostoma ilocanum*, *Gastrodiscoides hominis*, and *Metagonimus yokogawai*; (3) flukes that parasitize the lung, i.e., *Paragonimus westermani* and other species; and (4) the mesocercarial stage of *Alaria americana*, which causes generalized systemic infection.

All of these flukes parasitize other mammals, and some of them, such as *Fasciola hepatica*, are of major importance in veterinary medicine. Most of these flukes have limited geographical distribution. However, with the migration of people around the world, human infections are often seen in nonendemic areas.

The hermaphroditic flukes are leaf-like, nonsegmented, and bilaterally symmetrical, ranging in size from a few millimeters to several centimeters. On one end is the anterior or oral sucker and just behind it the ventral sucker or acetabulum. The acetabulum acts as a holdfast to the epithelial tissue of the final host.

Eggs appear in bile and stool and, in the case of the lung fluke, in sputum and stool. The eggs are operculated. Some are fully embryonated when passed; others may require time for embryonation. The embryonated egg contains the first stage larva or miracidium. After hatching in fresh water the miracidium penetrates, or is ingested by, a suitable first intermediate host, a snail. In the snail the miracidium develops into thousands of cercariae, which are released into the water. The cercariae attach themselves to or penetrate into the second intermediate hosts, which, depending on the flukes, may be freshwater fish, crustaceans, frogs, or aquatic plants. The final definitive hosts (man or animals) acquire the infection by ingesting encysted metacercariae.

The treatment of digenetic trematodes is by the broad-spectrum anthelminthic praziquantel. Personal prevention of infection includes eating only well-cooked fish or crustaceans and avoiding raw watercress in endemic areas. Community prevention consists of cleaning up the environment and preventing infection of the intermediate hosts.

Seah SKK: Digenetic trematodes. Clin Gastroenterol 7:87, 1978. *A good review of all the hermaphroditic flukes; up to date and well referenced.*

HEPATIC HERMAPHRODITIC FLUKES

Clonorchiasis (Clonorchis Sinensis)

This infection is common in the Far East, especially southern China, Hong Kong, Taiwan, Japan, and Korea, where raw or undercooked fish have long been considered a delicacy. More than 40 species of freshwater fish, mainly the carp and salmon group, harbor metacercariae.

Clonorchis sinensis has a very long life span (probably up to 50 years), and this parasitic infection will likely be important in these areas for many years. Clonorchiasis occurs in all parts of the world where there are Asian immigrants from endemic areas.

After ingestion of the contaminated fish, the metacercariae excyst in the duodenum. Most of the larval flukes ascend the biliary tree directly, but some may pass via the portal circulation to the liver. During maturation of the fluke there is marked desquamation of biliary epithelium. The fluke matures in two to three weeks and begins to lay eggs. Flukes prefer to reside in the second order bile ducts, but in heavy infection they are found throughout the biliary system, including the gallbladder, and sometimes in the pancreatic duct. Adult flukes are grayish-brown, 15 × 3 mm. They feed on secretions from the bile duct mucosa. They cause low grade inflammatory changes of the biliary tree, proliferation of the biliary epithelium, and progressive portal fibrosis. As a rule there is no parenchymal damage and cirrhosis does not result from uncomplicated clonorchiasis.

CLINICAL MANIFESTATIONS. *Acute clonorchiasis* occurs one to three weeks after the ingestion of encysted metacercariae. There may be fever, chills, abdominal pain, diarrhea, tender hepatomegaly, and mild jaundice. The white blood cell count is raised with marked eosinophilia, and serum alkaline phosphatase, SGOT, SGPT, and bilirubin levels are elevated. The clinical presentation is often confused with acute viral hepatitis and seldom recognized. The ova of *C. sinensis* appear in the stool or bile three or four weeks after ingestion of the metacercariae. The history of eating raw fish in the endemic area and the eosinophilia should suggest the diagnosis.

The majority of people with ova of *C. sinensis* in their stools have no symptoms even when heavily infected. It is impossible to predict who will develop the complications of chronic clonorchiasis. *Acute suppurative cholangitis* is a severe febrile illness often associated with hypoglycemia and *Escherichia coli* bacteremia. The biliary system is blocked by numerous flukes and becomes secondarily infected. This condition carries a very high mortality rate. *Recurrent pyogenic cholangitis* is a recurrent febrile illness associated with clonorchiasis and intrahepatic bile duct calculi. During surgical operation or autopsy, *Clonorchis* flukes are not consistently found as in the case of acute suppurative cholangitis. With recurrent pyogenic cholangitis cirrhosis may eventually develop. The flukes occasionally block the pancreatic ducts and induce pancreatitis. Cholangiocarcinoma is a late complication of chronic clonorchiasis. Clonorchiasis has no causal relationship with hepatocellular cancer.

DIAGNOSIS. The diagnosis is made by finding the small operculated eggs in the stool or duodenal aspirate. The eggs average 29 × 16 μ; they are light brown and ovoid. Unfortunately the *C. sinensis* egg is almost identical to those of *Opisthorchis, Heterophyes,* and *Metagonimus.* To be absolutely certain of the diagnosis one must examine the adult fluke. However, geographic distribution may help in separating *Clonorchis* from *Opisthorchis.* Expulsion and eradication of the flukes by a course of bephenium hydroxynaphthoate will indicate whether the ova are *Heterophyes* or *Metagonimus.* In a patient with abdominal or other symptoms and *C. sinensis* eggs in the stool, it is often difficult to decide if the complaints are due to clonorchiasis. It is often necessary to eliminate other current illnesses before attributing the symptoms to clonorchiasis. As a rule in uncomplicated established clonorchiasis, there is no eosinophilia, elevation of sedimentation rate, anemia, or abnormal liver function test results, and radioisotope scan and ultrasound (B scan) of the liver are normal.

In acute clonorchiasis, leukocytosis, marked eosinophilia, and abnormal liver function test results are present. This condition must be distinguished from hepatic amebiasis and visceral larva migrans. In the former, eosinophilia is absent and serology for amebiasis is positive. In the latter, the serology for toxocariasis is positive. The presence of the flukes in the liver provokes irregular antibody response, and a large variety of serologic and skin tests is available in some centers. However, these are not sufficiently specific and sensitive for clinical use.

TREATMENT. Until recently there was no satisfactory treatment for clonorchiasis, but praziquantel has revolutionized the treatment of this condition. The recommended dosage is 75 mg per kilogram of body weight, divided into three doses on the same day. Praziquantel is well tolerated and no long-term toxicity has been shown. At the dose recommended there may be some gastrointestinal disturbance and transient headaches. Because this drug is safe, it is recommended that all cases of clonorchiasis whether symptomatic or not be treated. The cost of this drug may limit its use in mass chemotherapy in the endemic area.

The treatment of complications such as calculi, suppurative cholangitis, recurrent pyogenic cholangitis, and pancreatitis is both medical and surgical. Conservative treatment consists of broad-spectrum antibiotics and intravenous fluids. If this is not effective, a permanent and adequate drainage procedure, such as choledochoduodenostomy, is required. Suppuration usually kills many flukes, and medical treatment is not urgent. At surgery as many flukes as possible should be removed from the biliary tree.

PREVENTION. In the endemic areas, freshwater fish must be well cooked before eating.

Opisthorchiasis
(Opisthorchis Viverrini and Felineus)

Opisthorchis felineus is common in eastern Europe, the USSR, India, Japan, the Philippines, and Vietnam. *Opisthorchis viverrini* is common in northern Thailand and Laos. In northeast Thailand 90 per cent of the people over the age of ten have *O. viverrini* infection. The life cycles of these flukes are similar to those of *C. sinensis.* Infection is acquired by eating undercooked freshwater fish. Many animals, especially the cat, are natural reservoirs.

The pathology, clinical manifestations, and complications of opisthorchiasis are similar to those of clonorchiasis. Cholangiocarcinoma can also result from chronic opisthorchiasis. The eggs of *Opisthorchis* are almost identical to those of *Clonorchis.* This emphasizes the importance of geographic history, for the only other way of distinguishing the parasites would be by examination of the adult flukes. The treatment is the same as for clonorchiasis.

Dicroceliasis

Dicrocoelium dendriticum is a lancet-shaped fluke, measuring 10 × 2 mm, that normally inhabits the biliary tract of sheep and cattle. Man is occasionally infected by ingesting ants that have eaten slime balls containing cercariae secreted by the snail. This occurs in Europe, in Asia, and around the Mediterranean basin. Infection is usually asymptomatic, and there is little information on the pathologic changes in man. It is important for the physician to recognize the small (40 × 25 μ), fully embryonated, thick-shelled operculated eggs for what they are. This infection requires no treatment.

Fascioliasis (Fasciola Hepatica)

This is a common parasite in the biliary tract of sheep and cattle, but it may also infect all types of mammals, including man. Worldwide in distribution in sheep, it is prevalent in low wet pastures where suitable species of snails are present. The cercariae, discharged from the snails, attach themselves to the water plants and encyst as metacercariae. Man is infected mainly as a result of eating watercress and other aquatic plants gathered in these pastures. In the duodenum the immature fluke penetrates the mucosa, enters the abdominal cavity, and through some unexplained hepatotropism penetrates Glisson's capsule. The immature flukes migrate throughout the liver for some weeks until they reach the biliary tract, where they mature in about two months. The fluke measures 3 × 1.3 cm, and the eggs are large, ovoid, and operculated, measuring 140 × 75 μ.

CLINICAL MANIFESTATIONS. ***Acute Fascioliasis.*** Invasion and maturation occur during the first three months after ingestion of the metacercariae. The immature flukes produce small necrotic foci along the migration paths. There may be no significant symptoms, or there may be abdominal pain, hepatomegaly, fever, vomiting, and jaundice. Leukocytosis and marked eosinophilia are present, but *F. hepatica* eggs are not found in the stool at this stage.

Established Infection. The mature flukes now produce metabolites that irritate the biliary passages, resulting in hyperplasia. Obstruction and dilation of the biliary passage and cholecystitis may occur. There may be abdominal pain, hepatomegaly, recurrent urticaria, jaundice, irregular fever, diarrhea, and weight loss. Anemia from blood loss can be severe. The obstruction and irritation may produce thickening of the biliary tree, atrophy of the hepatic cells, and biliary cirrhosis. Cholelithiasis is common. The relationship of fascioliasis and biliary cancers is not proved.

Extrabiliary Fascioliasis. Ingestion of raw sheep and goat liver containing young flukes causes the condition called "halzoun" (suffocation). This pharyngeal fascioliasis is due to lodgment of flukes in the upper respiratory and digestive tracts. Inflammation and edema may lead to dysphagia, dyspnea, and even asphyxiation. Cutaneous fascioliasis, usually in the upper abdomen, presents as migratory nodules which are pruritic, painful, and inflamed, and vary in size from 2 to 5 cm. Rarely, the flukes may be found in the lung, peritoneum, muscles, eye, and brain.

DIAGNOSIS. In acute infection the diagnosis is made in an endemic area by a high index of suspicion and the clinical triad of fever, hepatomegaly, and marked eosinophilia. A history of ingestion of wild watercress supports the diagnosis. At this stage the stool does not contain eggs. Serologic tests, such as the complement fixation test, are helpful. In chronic infection the stool contains the characteristic large operculated eggs (140 × 75 μ). Duodenal and biliary aspirate will provide a higher yield than fecal examination. Liver function test results reflect the degree of hepatic cellular damage and biliary obstruction. Intravenous or percutaneous cholangiography may show abnormalities and filling defects. The diagnosis is often made during surgical operation for biliary disease. The diagnosis of halzoun in an endemic area is made by the history of ingestion of raw liver and the finding of a pharyngeal mass.

TREATMENT. In the past, bithionol, emetine, dehydroemetine, and chloroquine were used with some success in this condition. Praziquantel is now the drug of choice in fascioliasis. The recommended dosage is 75 mg per kilogram of body weight divided into three doses per day for two days. Ectopic flukes are removed surgically. Prevention consists of not eating raw watercress and raw sheep and goat liver in the endemic areas.

Fasciola Gigantica

This large fluke is a liver parasite of herbivorous animals and occasionally of man in Asia and Africa. The life cycle, mode of infection, clinical manifestations, and treatment are similar to those of *F. hepatica*.

Clonorchiasis

Flavell, DJ: Liver fluke infection as an aetiological factor in bile duct carcinoma of man. Trans Roy Soc Trop Med Hyg 75:814, 1981. *Reviews the evidence of liver flukes as factors in causing bile duct cancer.*

Gibson JB, Sun T: Clonorchiasis. *In* Marcial-Rojas RA (ed.): Pathology of Protozoal and Helminthic Diseases. Baltimore, Williams & Wilkins Company, 1971, pp 546-566. *Profusely illustrated; very good on all aspects, especially on epidemiology and pathology as seen in Hong Kong.*

Liu YH, Qiu ZD, Wang WG, Wang QN, Qu ZQ, Chen RX, Liu JB, Zhang CD, Qin SA: Praziquantel in clonorchiasis: A further evaluation of 100 cases. Chin Med J 95:89, 1982. *Describes the evaluation of this drug in China.*

Pearson RD, Guerrant RL: Praziquantel: A major advance in anthelminthic therapy. Ann Intern Med 99:195, 1983. *A good review of the pharmacology, toxicity, and usefulness of this drug in schistosoma, trematode, and cestode infections.*

Praziquantel—a new antiparasitic drug. Med Lett Drugs Ther 24:108, 1982. *A very good summary of this wonder drug.*

Rim HJ, Lyu KS, Lee JS, Joo, KH: Clinical evaluation of the therapeutic efficacy of praziquantel (Embay 8440) against Clonorchis sinensis infection in man. Ann Trop Med Para 75:27, 1981. *Describes the early use of this drug in large number of patients in Korea.*

Xu Z, Zhong H, Cao W: Acute clonorchiasis. Chinese Med J (Peking) 92:423, 1979. *Good description and documentation of the clinical course of the seldom recognized acute clonorchiasis.*

Opisthorchiasis

Viranuvatti V: Liver fluke infection and infestation in Southeast Asia. Progr Liver Dis 4:537, 1972. *Concise review of liver flukes, especially* Opisthorchis.

Fascioliasis

Jones EA, Kay JM, Milligan HP, Owens D: Massive infection with *Fasciola hepatica* in man. Am J Med 63:836, 1977. *Report of an unusual case with a prolonged course of illness. Illustrates many of the complications of this disease.*

Marcial-Rojas RA: Fascioliasis. *In* Marcial-Rojas RA (ed.): Pathology of Protozoal and Helminthic Disease. Baltimore, Williams & Wilkins Company, 1971, pp 490-497. *Good on the epidemiology and pathology of this disease.*

LUNG HERMAPHRODITIC FLUKES
(Paragonimiasis)

Paragonimiasis is due to infection with the adult *Paragonimus westermani* and other species. As a rule the infection is in the lung, where the flukes are encapsulated in the parenchyma. The disease is also called pulmonary distomiasis, endemic hemoptysis, and Oriental lung fluke disease. Human paragonimiasis occurs most commonly in the Far East, especially central China, Japan, Korea, Vietnam, Laos, Thailand, and the Philippines. It also occurs in the Indian subcontinent, Central and South America, and West Africa. In addition to *P. westermani*, over 30 species may affect man. Most of these flukes are parasites of mammals, especially of the cat family (cat, tiger, leopard), foxes, dogs, cattle, and pigs. *P. westermani* was first discovered in 1877 by Westerman in a tiger in the Amsterdam zoo.

The adult flukes live singly or in pairs encapsulated in the cystic spaces of the lung. They are ovoid, plump, and leaf-like, and measure about 1 × 0.5 × 0.4 cm. Oval yellowish-brown operculated ova (90 × 55 μ) are coughed up and expelled in the sputum or are swallowed and passed in the feces. The flukes have a life span of five to six years. In fresh water the miracidia escape from the ova and penetrate the first intermediate host, a suitable snail. After several weeks the cercariae emerge and penetrate the second intermediate host, the crayfish or crab. Man or animal acquires the infection by eating raw meat or viscera of the freshwater crustacean. In Korea and West Africa, fresh crab juice is used as a home remedy in the treatment of measles. In the duodenum the metacercariae excyst, enter the abdominal cavity, migrate through the diaphragm into the pleural space, and end up in the lung parenchyma, where they mature and begin to lay eggs about two months after ingestion of the crayfish. This circuitous route of migration explains the extrapulmonary cysts of *Paragonimus*.

PATHOLOGY. The migratory larval flukes tunnel into the lung at the periphery. This is accompanied by inflammatory reaction with many eosinophils. They finally encyst with a fibrous tissue wall. The cyst may communicate with a bronchus and may often be secondarily infected with abscess formation. The death of the fluke is followed by calcification. Flukes in the abdominal cavity may cause abscess and adhesion and intestinal ulceration, resulting in bloody diarrhea with mucus and ova. In the brain the temporal and occipital lobes are the favored sites of eosinophilic granulomas containing the flukes or ova. Lodgment of the flukes in the spinal cord causes transverse myelitis. Adult flukes have been found in other organs, including the genitalia and muscle. Some species are prone to cause ectopic paragonimiasis. Thus the characteristic feature of *P. skrjabini* is migratory subcutaneous nodules containing active flukes.

CLINICAL MANIFESTATIONS. In the rare case of acute paragonimiasis there may be fever, chills, and chest pain. The symptoms and physical findings are indistinguishable from those of bronchopneumonia. As a rule the onset is insidious and the symptoms are those of chronic bronchitis and bronchiectasis. Cough, especially in the morning, productive of thick, gelatinous, blood-tinged sputum, is the most prominent symptom. Exertional dyspnea and night sweats are common. Frank hemoptysis often occurs after a paroxysm of coughing. Chest pain and pleural effusion may be present, and clubbing of fingers may occur. The most characteristic physical finding is persistent moist, coarse rales over the area of involvement. Chest x-rays early in the disease show patchy, cloudy infiltrations, but later dense nodular opacities or ring shadows indicate the site of the cysts. Pleural thickening and calcification may be seen late in the disease.

Abdominal paragonimiasis occurs when the flukes localize in the abdomen. The symptoms are nonspecific dull ache, tenderness, and diarrhea, which may be bloody and accompanied by mucus. An abdominal mass with lung disease in a patient from an endemic area should raise this suspicion. On rare occasions the fluke localizes in the brain, resulting in a seizure disorder similar to cysticercosis. There may be pareses of varying degrees and optic atrophy with papilledema. The cerebrospinal fluid shows a raised protein concentration, and eosinophils are present. Children with cerebral paragonimiasis are usually mentally retarded. Subcutaneous localization of the fluke results in abscess formation.

DIAGNOSIS. This rests mainly on finding ova in the sputum. In more than half of the cases stools will also reveal the ova, especially after concentration. The main differential diagnoses in the chest x-rays are bronchopneumonia, bronchiectasis, tuberculosis, tumor, and the rarer fungal infections. In practice the most important differential diagnosis is tuberculosis. Active tuberculosis and paragonimiasis often are present in the same individual from the endemic area.

Abdominal paragonimiasis must be differentiated from intestinal parasitic and nonparasitic infections and other intra-abdominal disorders. The finding of the ova in the stool does not necessarily indicate abdominal paragonimiasis. The cerebral presentation must be differentiated from other causes of seizure disorder, space-occupying lesions, cysticercosis, hydatid disease, and meningoencephalitides.

Moderate eosinophilia is usual in the early cases, but in established cases there may be no abnormal hematologic findings. Serology, as a rule, is not useful in helminthic infections, and this is also true in paragonimiasis. The complement fixation test, using extract of the adult fluke as antigen, is positive when the fluke is alive, but the skin test may remain positive long after the fluke is dead.

TREATMENT. Praziquantel, because of its safety, ease of use, and high degree of efficacy, is replacing bithionol and niclofolan as the treatment of choice in pulmonary paragonimiasis. The recommended dosage of praziquantel in this infection is 75 mg per kilogram of body weight divided into three doses daily for two days.

Paragonimiasis of the central nervous system requires surgery. Praziquantel should be given before the operation. Subcutaneous flukes should also be surgically removed.

PREVENTION. In theory prevention is simple. Freshwater crustaceans must be well cooked before eating, and hands and utensils should be thoroughly washed after contact with raw crabs and crayfish. However, in endemic areas it is difficult to persuade people to relinquish long-established cooking and eating habits and the use of raw crab juice for medicinal purposes.

Chung CH: Human paragonimiasis. *In* Marcial-Rojas RA (ed.): Pathology of Protozoal and Helminthic Diseases. Baltimore, Williams & Wilkins Company, 1971, pp 504-535. *Very detailed description of the pathologic changes of this disease. Well illustrated.*

Monson MH, Koenig JW, Sach R: Successful treatment with praziquantel of six patients infected with the African lung fluke *Paragonimus uterobilateralis.* Am J Trop Med Hyg 32:371, 1983. *Describes the usefulness of this drug in the common Western African species of Paragonimus.*

Spitalny KC, Senft AW, Meglio FD, Moran J, Peter G: Treatment of pulmonary paragonimiasis with a new broad-spectrum antihelminthic, praziquantel. J Pediatr 101:144, 1982. *Report of an Indochinese refugee to America with pulmonary paragonimiasis successfully treated with this drug.*

Yokogawa M: *Paragonimus* and paragonimiasis. Adv Parasitol 7:375, 1969. *Good review of the finer parasitologic points on this fluke.*

INTESTINAL HERMAPHRODITIC FLUKES

Fasciolopsiasis (Fasciolopsis Buski)

Fasciolopsis buski is the largest intestinal fluke and is normally a parasite of pigs. Human infection is widespread in Southern China, Southeast Asia, and the Indian subcontinent. The eggs are passed in the feces, and the miracidia are released to penetrate a snail. The cercariae encyst as metacercariae on edible water plants. Often the infected plants are peeled by using the teeth to remove the "skin," and the metacercariae are swallowed in the process. The larvae attach themselves to the upper small intestine, where they mature in about four weeks. The adult fluke has an average size of 3 × 1.2 cm.

CLINICAL MANIFESTATIONS. Many light infections are asymptomatic, but heavy loads of flukes produce symptoms, especially in children. The worm load may be up to several thousand. The flukes attach themselves to the duodenal and jejunal mucosa and produce symptoms by trauma, obstruction, and toxin production. There may be abdominal pain, gastrointestinal hemorrhage, diarrhea, and intestinal obstruction. In severe cases there may be edema of the face, trunk, and legs, as well as ascites.

DIAGNOSIS. This rests on finding the large ova (135 × 80 μ), or recovery of characteristic adult flukes in the stool. Difficulty may be encountered in distinguishing the ova of *F. hepatica* and *F. buski.* Eosinophilia is common and may exceed 50 per cent of the white cell count. Serologic tests, such as the indirect fluorescent antibody test, are available in some centers. The specificity of serologic tests is unproved, and definitive diagnosis cannot be based on serologic tests alone. This is also true of skin tests. Facial edema may require differentiation of fasciolopsiasis from trichinosis or the nephrotic syndrome.

TREATMENT. In the past the drug of choice in endemic areas has been hexylresorcinol (Crystoid anthelmintic), given in a single dose of 1.0 gram by mouth. Tetrachloroethylene in a dose of 0.1 ml per kilogram is equally effective. These two inexpensive medications are not available in North America. Piperazine or bephenium hydroxynaphthoate can be used. Not all the flukes are eradicated in one treatment, but it may be repeated in one week. Praziquantel will probably emerge as the drug of choice in this condition. The dosage is 75 mg per kilogram of body weight divided into three doses per day for one or two days. Personal prevention consists of cooking aquatic plants before eating. Community prevention entails eradication of the snails with molluscacides, public education, and prevention of fecal contamination of ponds.

Other Intestinal Hermaphroditic Flukes

Heterophyes heterophyes and *Metagonimus yokogawai* are small flukes that are acquired by eating raw or undercooked fish that contain the metacercariae. The former is found in Egypt, Tunisia, south China, India, and the Philippines, and the latter in the Far East and Indonesia. The adult flukes are 2 to 3 mm long and attach themselves to the intestinal mucosa. Usually the infection is light and there are few symptoms. Very rarely the eggs gain access to the circulation and may be found in the organs. As a rule the eggs are passed in the stool; they closely resemble *Clonorchis* eggs. Both flukes can be treated with tetrachloroethylene as used for hookworm. Differentiation of the two species requires examination of the adult flukes by experts. Many species of the genus *Echinostoma* infect man in the Far East, but they rarely produce symptoms. *Gastrocoides hominis* occurs in India and Malaysia, and may cause diarrhea. In Western Canada the eggs of *Metorchis conjunctus,* which are somewhat similar to those of *Clonorchis,* are occasionally found in the stools of humans who eat raw fish. If treatment is called for, praziquantel (75 mg per kilogram of body weight in three divided doses for one day) is the treatment of choice.

Alaria americana is an intestinal trematode of carnivores, such as the fox, wolf, lynx, or skunk. Two cases of human infection by the mesocercariae of this fluke have been reported in Ontario. Mesocercaria is a stage of development between the cercaria and the metacercaria. The cercariae emerging from the snail penetrate tadpoles. As the tadpole grows into a frog the mesocercariae tend to concentrate in the hind legs. When the frog is eaten by a carnivore, the mesocercariae develop into metacercariae and adult flukes in the lung and the gut, respectively. When man, who is not the normal host, eats the frog the mesocercariae migrate all over the body. In the first reported case the mesocercaria was surgically removed from the retina of the eye. The second case was a fatal systemic infection manifested by severe respiratory distress, coma, a coagulation abnormality, and vasculitis. At autopsy mesocercariae were found in all organs. The diagnosis is by biopsy of affected organs. There is no known treatment, although praziquantel may be useful.

Faust EC, Beaver PC, Jung RC: Intestinal flukes. *In* Faust EC, Beaver PC, Jung RC: Animal Agents and Vectors of Human Disease. 4th ed. Philadelphia, Lea & Febiger, 1975, pp 134-141. *Emphasis is on the parasitology, life cycles, and morphology. A good reference for the lesser important parasites.*

Fernandes BJ, Cooper JD, Cullen JB, Freeman RS, Ritchie AC, Scott AA, Stuart PF: Systemic infection with *Alaria americana* (Trematoda). Can Med Assoc J 115:1111, 1976. *This is the first report of generalized infection with mesocercariae of this fluke. Good description of the clinical course and autopsy findings.*

The Nematodes

398. INTRODUCTION

Daniel S. Blumenthal

Nematodes are primitive, elongated, unsegmented worms, with a body cavity that is not lined with a peritoneum of mesodermal origin as is the body cavity of higher animals. The sexes are separate, but parthenogenesis occurs in some parasitic forms. The class includes half a million species; some are free-living, while others are parasitic for plants, invertebrates, and both wild and domestic vertebrates.

Eleven species are important parasites of humans. These may be classified as intestinal parasites or tissue parasites. The former include the hookworms *Ancylostoma duodenale* and *Necator americanus,* the large roundworm *Ascaris lumbricoides,* the whipworm *Trichuris trichiura,* the pinworm *Enterobius vermicularis,* and *Strongyloides stercoralis.* The adult *Trichinella spiralis* also inhabits the human intestine, but it is classified as a tissue nematode because its clinical manifestations are produced by larvae invading the tissues. The filariae are also tissue parasites; species commonly causing serious disease in humans include *Onchocerca volvulus,* the agent of river blindness; *Dracunculus medinensis,* the Guinea worm; *Loa loa;* and *Wuchereria bancrofti.* Several other nematodes are human parasites of lesser importance, and a variety of nematodes that ordinarily infect nonhuman species may occasionally infect people, sometimes causing serious disease.

The parasitic nematodes have evolved a great variety of mechanisms by which they are transmitted from one definitive host to another. Some (such as *Enterobius*) produce ova that may be passed from person to person, while the eggs of others (for instance, *Ascaris* and hookworm) must incubate in the soil before they become infective. Some, such as *Trichinella,* require an intermediate host that is eaten by the definitive host, whereas the intermediate hosts of some nematode parasites of animals release infective larvae. The filariae are transmitted by insect vectors.

Of the major nematode parasites of man, only *Strongyloides stercoralis* is capable of reproducing in the definitive host. This is true of most other helminthic infections as well, and distinguishes them from infections with viruses, bacteria, and protozoa. As a consequence, it is not usually necessary to seek total elimination of the parasite in a patient (or a community), since a light infection is not generally clinically significant. An exception is ascariasis, in which a single worm can cause serious morbidity or mortality.

It is hard to overestimate the amount of worldwide morbidity that is caused by parasitic nematodes. There are an estimated one billion cases each of *Ascaris* and *Trichuris,* a number equal to a quarter of the world's population. Approximately 600 million persons are infected with hookworm and 300 million with filariae. Nematode infections are still common in many communities in the United States. There are perhaps 4 million persons infected with *Ascaris* in this country; 2.2 million with *Trichuris,* 700,000 with hookworm, and 400,000 with *Strongyloides.*

In areas where soil and climatic conditions are suitable, nematode infections may be considered a marker of rural poverty. Only when this poverty, with its accompanying inadequate levels of sanitation and education, has been alleviated, will the prevalence of these parasites be reduced to unimportant levels.

Major nematode infections; other nematode infections. *In* Intestinal Protozoan and Helminthic Infections. Report of a WHO Scientific Group. Technical Report Series 666. Geneva, World Health Organization, 1981. *A comprehensive public health approach.*

Schultz MG: Parasitic diseases. N Engl J Med 297:1259, 1977. *Schultz discusses all parasitic disease, not just nematode infections, but speaks eloquently of the magnitude of the problem.*

Warren KS: The control of helminths: Nonreplicating infectious agents of man. Ann Rev Public Health 2:101, 1981. *A thoughtful commentary on efforts to control nematode and other helminth infections in developing countries.*

399. STRONGYLOIDIASIS

Daniel S. Blumenthal

DEFINITION. Strongyloidiasis is infection with the parasitic phase of *Strongyloides stercoralis.* Clinical manifestations may be caused by the adult worms in the small intestine or by the migrating filariform larvae.

ETIOLOGY AND LIFE CYCLE. The adult female *Strongyloides* is about 2 mm long and lives in the mucosal epithelium of the duodenum and jejunum, extending above or below this in the gastrointestinal tract in heavy infections. There is no parasitic male; reproduction in the parasitic phase is parthenogenic.

The life cycle of this parasite is complex and proceeds by several alternative pathways. Each worm produces fewer than 100 eggs daily. They hatch in the intestine of the host, and rhabditiform larvae are passed in the stool. These may metamorphose in the soil into infective filariform larvae or may mature into free-living adults that reproduce bisexually. They may then give rise to infective larvae in a later generation. The infective larvae invade the human host by penetrating the skin, travel through the venous circulation to the lungs, migrate through the alveolar capillary walls, ascend the respiratory tree to the epiglottis, and are swallowed to reach the small intestine, where they mature.

Alternatively, *Strongyloides* larvae may develop to the infective stage in the intestine, penetrate the intestinal wall to reach the circulation, and enter the cycle of infection. This process of *internal autoinfection* is unique to this species among nematodes. Infective larvae may also penetrate the perianal skin after being passed with the stool to enter the host by *external autoinfection.* These processes may enable an infection to persist 30 to 40 years in the absence of re-exposure of the host.

In immunosuppressed or malnourished patients, internal autoinfection may assume massive proportions with ectopic migration of the larvae, resulting in the *hyperinfection syndrome*.

EPIDEMIOLOGY. *Strongyloides* is found in warm climates throughout the world, but, except in institutions for the retarded, high community prevalence rates have not been reported. In the United States, strongyloidiasis is most common in Southern Appalachia, but occasional autochthonous cases have been found in northern cities. There is at least one report of transmission from dog to man. *Strongyloides fulbornii*, a parasite of monkeys, has been reported to infect people in Africa.

PATHOLOGY. As the larvae migrate through the lungs, they sometimes cause a pneumonic process similar to Löffler's syndrome in ascariasis.

In the small intestine, microscopic abnormalities include stunted, swollen, or fused villi; eosinophilic infiltration of the lamina propria; and mononuclear infiltration of the mucosa.

In the hyperinfection syndrome and in other severe cases of strongyloidiasis, intestinal changes are more pronounced. Parasites may be found in all layers of the intestinal wall, which is thickened by edema and fibrosis. An inflammatory response is seen, but without eosinophilia, and there may be micro- and macroscopic ulcerations. Pulmonary involvement in the hyperinfection syndrome is characterized by extensive larval migration and hemorrhagic pneumonia. Larvae may be found throughout the body, especially in the kidneys, brain, and heart.

CLINICAL MANIFESTATIONS. As the larvae penetrate the skin, particularly in cases of external autoinfection, they may cause a migratory pruritic eruption known as *larva currens*. Larvae migrating through the lung may cause pneumonia, with cough, dyspnea, and hemoptysis, but this is not common.

Mild intestinal infections are often asymptomatic. Moderate infections generally result in epigastric pain and intermittent diarrhea, whereas heavy infections may cause significant malabsorption with bulky, foul-smelling stools, abdominal distention, and hypoproteinemia with edema. In patients who are malnourished, the malabsorption may persist even after the infection is adequately treated.

COMPLICATIONS. The hyperinfection syndrome has been increasingly recognized in recent years in hosts with altered immune status, those with malignancies or malnutrition, and rarely those who are otherwise normal. The onset of symptoms in this complication is characteristically relatively abrupt, with fever and severe abdominal pain and distention, often accompanied by shock. Gram-negative sepsis frequently ensues; intestinal ulcerations caused by the parasite are thought to permit the entry of enteric pathogens into the circulation. When larval invasion of the lungs is severe, dyspnea and cough productive of blood-tinged sputum may be prominent.

DIAGNOSIS. *Strongyloides* ova do not appear in the stool; diagnosis is dependent on the identification of larvae. Multiple stool examinations, using concentration techniques, are generally necessary in light or moderate infections. Larvae may be identified in duodenal fluid when they cannot be found in stool specimens; the string test (Enterotest) is useful for obtaining samples of duodenal fluid for this purpose. In cases of hyperinfection, larvae may often be found in the sputum.

Eosinophilia is often present, but may be absent in cases of hyperinfection. Contrast media examination of the small bowel often demonstrates thickening and edema of the mucosal folds. Chest x-ray in patients with hyperinfection may show patchy infiltrates.

TREATMENT. The drug of choice, in both ordinary intestinal strongyloidiasis and hyperinfection, is thiabendazole, 25 mg per kilogram twice a day for two to five days. Nausea, vomiting, drowsiness, and vertigo are common side effects. Other drugs that have been used include pyrvinium pamoate, mebendazole, diethylcarbamazine,* and levamisole (not available in the United States). None of these drugs is recommended for pregnant women. A follow-up stool examination should be obtained two to six weeks following treatment, and stool examinations should also be obtained on other family members.

PREVENTION. This parasite, like the other soil-transmitted nematodes, is associated with rural poverty and its attendant conditions of poor sanitation and inadequate education. Alleviation of these conditions interrupts transmission. The wearing of shoes protects against infection.

Secondary prevention of the hyperinfection syndrome is important in persons from endemic areas who have altered immune status. Such patients should have studies appropriate to rule out *Strongyloides* infection, particularly when they exhibit suggestive gastrointestinal symptoms and/or eosinophilia.

Burke JA: Strongyloidiasis in childhood. Am J Dis Child 132:1130, 1978. *A comprehensive survey of this infection and review of the literature, complete with case studies.*

Igra-Siegman Y, Kapila R, Sen P, et al.: Syndrome of hyperinfection with *Strongyloides stercoralis*. Rev Infec Dis 3:397, 1981. *Reviews 103 cases of hyperinfection syndrome reported in the English language literature since 1964.*

Walzer PD, Milder JE, Banwell JG, Kilgore G, Klein M, Parker R: Epidemiologic features of *Strongyloides stercoralis* infection in an endemic area of the United States. Am J Trop Med Hyg 31:313, 1982. *Southeastern Kentucky is an area of particularly high prevalence of this parasite. This paper defines the epidemiology of* Strongyloides *in this area and points out that the infection is more common in geriatric patients than are other parasitic infections.*

400. CAPILLARIASIS

Daniel S. Blumenthal

Capillaria philippinensis infection was first observed in the north Philippines in 1963. Since then, it has also been found in Thailand. At least 1500 cases have been reported, with a case-fatality rate of about 10 per cent. This nematode is thought to parasitize birds, with fish and crustaceans serving as intermediate hosts. Humans are infected by eating the raw intermediate hosts. The ingested larvae mature and live in the crypts of the small intestine, where they reproduce. (*Strongyloides* is the only other nematode that reproduces in man.) The result is often a heavy infection; up to 40,000 adult worms have been recovered at one autopsy. The clinical syndrome is one of severe malabsorption and protein-losing enteropathy. The diagnosis is made by finding eggs or larvae in the stool; the eggs resemble those of *Trichuris*. An intradermal test is also available. The treatment of choice is mebendazole, 200 mg twice a day for 20 days; an alternative is thiabendazole, 25 mg per kilogram daily for 30 days. Fluid and electrolyte replacement and a high protein diet are also important.

Capillaria hepatica is a parasite of rats that occasionally infects the liver of man. The result is an acute or subacute hepatitis with eosinophilia. Diagnosis is made on liver biopsy; there is no known treatment.

Singson CN, Banzon TC, Cross JH: Mebendazole in the treatment of intestinal capillariasis. Am J Trop Med Hyg 24:932, 1975. *Little has been written about this parasite in the last 10 years. This study documents the value of mebendazole in treatment.*

401. HOOKWORM DISEASE

Daniel S. Blumenthal

DEFINITION. Two species of hookworm infect man: *Ancylostoma duodenale*, the so-called Old World hookworm, and *Necator americanus*, the so-called New World hookworm. Both species attach themselves to the mucosa of the small intestine and ingest blood. When this results in anemia, hypoproteinemia, and clinical symptoms, the condition is termed hookworm disease. If these findings are lacking, the host is said merely to have hookworm infection.

ETIOLOGY AND LIFE CYCLE. Hookworms are about 1 cm long; the female is slightly larger than the male, and *Ancylostoma* is

*Production of this drug in the United States has been discontinued.

slightly larger than *Necator*. *Ancylostoma* bears two pairs of upper teeth in its mouth, whereas *Necator* has a pair of upper and a pair of lower cutting plates.

The female *Ancylostoma* produces about 25,000 eggs per day; *Necator*, about 7000. These eggs are passed in the stool of the host and hatch in the soil within 48 hours. The emerging rhabditiform larvae molt twice within five to ten days and become infective filariform larvae. These may survive for several months in the soil.

Upon coming in contact with the skin of man, the filariform larvae penetrate, enter the venous circulation, and are carried into the lungs. There they migrate across the alveolar capillary walls, ascend the respiratory tree, and are swallowed to reach the small intestine. Infection with *Ancylostoma* may also be acquired by ingesting the filariform larvae; *Necator* is not infective by this route. The life span of *Necator* in the human host is two to six years; that of *Ancylostoma* is probably less.

EPIDEMIOLOGY. *Necator americanus* was once endemic throughout the southeastern United States, where it caused considerable disability among the rural poor. Its prevalence was greatly reduced by the work of the Rockefeller Sanitary Commission from 1910 to 1920, and has since continued to decline. *Necator* was originally imported to the New World from sub-Sahara Africa and has, in the past, been described as the predominant species in that part of the world, as well as in most of South and Central America. *Ancylostoma* was previously found exclusively in the Mediterranean basin, Asia, and parts of coastal South America. In more recent years, this distribution has become blurred.

In endemic areas, the highest prevalence rates are found in school-age children. During the time when hookworm was widespread in the southeastern United States, whites were noted to be more susceptible than blacks.

PATHOLOGY. A local inflammatory response occurs at the site of skin penetration by the filariform larvae, and as the larvae migrate through the lungs, an eosinophilic and mononuclear infiltration takes place along with local hemorrhages. A heavy passage of larvae through the lungs may cause a pneumonic process similar to Löffler's syndrome in ascariasis.

In the intestine, the adults attach themselves to the mucosa and actively suck blood. *Ancylostoma* ingests more blood (0.15 ml per worm per day) than *Necator* (0.03 ml per worm per day). The worms change sites of attachment at frequent intervals, leaving bleeding lacerations at their previous sites. The wall of the intestine becomes edematous, and a mononuclear and eosinophilic infiltrate surrounds each parasite.

CLINICAL MANIFESTATIONS AND COMPLICATIONS. Light infections, such as those generally found in the United States, are usually asymptomatic. In tropical countries, where worm burdens are often in the thousands, clinical manifestations of hookworm disease are frequent.

A pruritic vesicular or papular eruption, known as ground itch, may develop at the site of larval invasion. This is particularly pronounced after multiple exposures to the parasite. The passage of larvae through the lungs is sometimes associated with wheezing, dyspnea, and cough productive of blood-streaked sputum.

Abdominal pain and diarrhea may be caused by the adult worms in the intestine, particularly as the parasites attach themselves to the mucosa. The most important clinical manifestations, however, are those of anemia and hypoalbuminemia resulting from chronic blood loss. Weakness, fatigue, lassitude, and growth retardation are characteristic findings in patients with hookworm disease. Signs and symptoms of high-output congestive heart failure may be present, and peripheral edema may occur as a result of both the heart failure and hypoalbuminemia. The severity of anemia developed by the patient depends on the adequacy of dietary iron intake. Residents of communities endemic for hookworm often have inadequate diets and may be anemic independent of hookworm infection. On the other hand, an adequate diet may prevent anemia and hypoproteinemia despite significant infection.

DIAGNOSIS. The diagnosis of hookworm infection is made by the finding of characteristic ova in the stool. The ova of *Necator* and *Ancylostoma* are identical, but species differentiation is not necessary for appropriate treatment and follow-up.

Quantitation of hookworm ova by either the Stoll or Kato thick smear technique may be performed as an aid in estimating the intensity of infection. Egg counts greater than 2000 per milliliter of feces in women and children or greater than 5000 per milliliter of feces in men are considered clinically significant in infections with *Necator*.

Other laboratory findings associated with hookworm infection include eosinophilia, Charcot-Leyden crystals in the stool, and, in heavy infections, hypoalbuminemia and anemia as low as 2 grams of hemoglobin per 100 ml of blood.

TREATMENT. In holoendemic areas in the tropics, where resources are limited, it has generally been the practice to treat only moderate or heavy infections. In the United States, however, light infections should also be treated when discovered, and measures should be taken to prevent reinfection.

The drug of choice is pyrantel pamoate, which is given in a single dose of 11 mg per kilogram of body weight (maximum, 1 gram). Mebendazole, 100 mg twice a day for three days, is equally effective. Neither drug should be used in pregnant women; mebendazole should be used with caution in children less than two years old. The anemia should be treated with oral iron supplementation; in cases of severe anemia with hypoalbuminemia, transfusion may be necessary.

A follow-up stool examination should be performed two to six weeks after treatment; stool examinations should also be performed on other family members.

PREVENTION. Hookworm, like the other soil-transmitted nematodes, is prevented by alleviating the conditions of rural poverty with which it is associated. The most important factors in this regard are the construction of sanitary facilities for the disposal of human wastes and community education regarding the etiology of the infection. The wearing of shoes is also important. Iron supplementation of the diet in endemic areas will prevent most cases of anemia.

Gilman RH: Hookworm Disease: Host-pathogen biology. Rev Infec Dis 4:824, 1982. *A concise review of the topic.*

402. CUTANEOUS LARVA MIGRANS

Daniel S. Blumenthal

DEFINITION. Cutaneous larva migrans (creeping eruption) is infection with a larval nematode that wanders in the subcutaneous tissues. The most common agent is *Ancylostoma braziliense*, a hookworm of dogs and cats.

ETIOLOGY AND EPIDEMIOLOGY. In addition to *A. braziliense*, the larvae of several other nematodes can cause cutaneous larva migrans. These include *Ancylostoma caninum* (a dog hookworm) and several other species of hookworm and *Strongyloides* that oridinarily infect nonhuman hosts. The larvae of these species penetrate human skin if it is exposed to soil contaminated with the feces of infected animals. Rather than complete their life cycle, however, the larvae continue to migrate in the subcutaneous tissues.

The infection is most common in tropical and subtropical areas, particularly on beaches frequented by dogs. The coasts of the Gulf of Mexico and Florida are common locales in the United States. Children, farmers, plumbers (working under beach houses) and sunbathers are most often affected.

The larvae of *A. braziliense* tunnel in the epidermis just above the basal layer, rarely penetrating into the dermis. The tunnel is surrounded by eosinophil and round cell infiltration.

CLINICAL MANIFESTATIONS. An erythematous pruritic papule or nonspecific dermatitis occurs at the site of skin contact with the contaminated soil. In two or three days (occasionally weeks or months), this becomes a 2 to 3 mm wide, slightly elevated, serpiginous track or burrow. The patient experiences intense itching.

DIAGNOSIS AND TREATMENT. The diagnosis is clinical. There are no diagnostic tests and usually no eosinophilia.

Topical application, four times a day, of the commercially available 10 per cent suspension of thiabendazole appears to work as well as giving the drug orally. If the oral route is elected, the dosage is 25 mg per kilogram in two divided doses for two to five days.

Edelglass JW, Douglass CM, Stiefler R, Tessler M: Cutaneous larva migrans in northern climates. A souvenir of your dream vacation. J Am Acad Dermatol 7:353, 1982. *A good review with typical case presentations in United States tourists. The literature on topical and oral therapy is discussed.*

403. TRICHOSTRONGYLIASIS

Daniel S. Blumenthal

Several species of the genus *Trichostrongylus* infect both man and domestic ruminants. The infection is found widely in the Middle and Far East and Australia. Particularly high prevalence rates have been reported from Iran.

Ova are passed in the stool and hatch in the soil; larvae are ingested with leafy vegetables. The adult worms live in the intestines and suck small amounts of blood; heavy infections result in anemia. Diagnosis is made by identifying ova, which resemble those of hookworm, in the stool.

Treatment is with thiabendazole, 25 mg per kilogram twice a day for two days, or with pyrantel pamoate in a single dose of 11 mg per kilogram.

Ghadirian E, Arfaa F: Present status of *Trichostrongylus* in Iran. Am J Trop Med Hyg 24:935, 1975. *Documents the high prevalence of this parasite in Iran and discusses the reasons for this.*

404. GNATHOSTOMIASIS

Daniel S. Blumenthal

Gnathostomiasis is infection with the larvae of *Gnathostoma spinigerum,* an intestinal nematode of dogs and cats for which fish serve as an intermediate host. Infective larvae are ingested when raw or undercooked fish is consumed. The larvae do not complete their life cycle in humans but migrate through the body.

The infection is found throughout the Far East; the greatest number of cases has been reported from Thailand.

The larvae most often migrate to the subcutaneous tissues, where they are found in eosinophilic granulomata. In central nervous system gnathostomiasis, hemorrhagic tracks may be found in the brain. Fever, vomiting, and abdominal pain occur a few days after ingestion of the infective fish. A few weeks later, skin lesions appear; these consist of subcutaneous nodules or swellings that may be either pruritic or painful and are often migratory. Abscesses may form. In the CNS variety, there is paralysis of the extremities, encephalitis, and subarachnoid hemorrhage. Eye involvement with uveitis and orbital cellulitis represents a third variety. Gnathostome larvae have also been reported from many other parts of the body.

Peripheral eosinophilia is usual in cutaneous gnathostomiasis; the diagnosis is usually established by biopsy. In central nervous system infection, peripheral eosinophilia is an inconstant feature, but there are many eosinophils in the cerebrospinal fluid. This must be distinguished from the eosinophilic meningitis caused by *Angiostrongylus,* which is usually less severe. Diagnosis may be assisted by an enzyme-linked immunosorbent assay (ELISA), and an intradermal test has been described. Treatment of subcutaneous lesions consists of surgical removal. For central nervous system infection, mebendazole* 200 mg every three hours for six days may be given. The infection may be prevented by cooking fish thoroughly before eating.

*This use is not listed in the manufacturer's directive.

Boogird P, Phuapradit P, Siridej N, Chirachariyavej T, Chuahiran S, Vejjajiva A: Neurological manifestations of gnathostomiasis. J Neurol Sci 31:279, 1977. *A clinical and epidemiologic description of a series of 24 cases of CNS gnathostomiasis.*
Stowens D, Simon G: Gnathostomiasis in Oneida County. NY State J Med 81:409, 1981. *A typical case of cutaneous gnathostomiasis, with discussion.*
Daengsvang S: Gnathostomiasis in Southeast Asia. Southeast Asian J Trop Med Public Health 12:319, 1981. *A review of the literature on both human and animal gnathostomiasis.*

405. PRIMATE NEMATODIASES

Daniel S. Blumenthal

Several nematodes that ordinarily parasitize the intestine of monkeys occasionally infect man. *Oesophagostomum* sp. has been reported from Africa, Asia, and Brazil; it is responsible for the formation of granulomas in the intestinal wall. *Ternides deminutus* is sometimes found in the human colon in Africa and Asia; a heavy infection may cause anemia. *Physaloptera mordens,* also reported from Africa, may attach itself to the esophagus, stomach, or small intestine of humans.

Barrowclough H, Crome L: Oesophagostomiasis in man. Trop Geogr Med 31:183, 1979. *Presents a case, discusses the difficulties in diagnosis, and reviews the literature.*

406. ASCARIASIS

Daniel S. Blumenthal

DEFINITION. Ascariasis is infection with the large roundworm, *Ascaris lumbricoides.* Clinical manifestations may result from the migration of the larvae through the lungs, from the presence of the adult worms in the lumen of the small intestine, or from extraintestinal migration of the adults.

ETIOLOGY AND LIFE CYCLE. *Ascaris* is the largest of the intestinal nematodes. Adult females measure 20 to 45 cm in length; adult males are about three fourths as large. Worm loads in the intestine may range from only one or two to hundreds; the life span of the parasite averages about 18 months.

The female produces about 200,000 ova per day. These are passed by the host in the stool and become infective after an obligate period in the soil of about ten days. The eggs are killed by direct sunlight and temperatures above 45° C, but under proper soil and climatic conditions they may remain viable for years.

After ingestion by the host, the eggs hatch in the duodenum, and the larvae penetrate the intestinal wall, enter the venous circulation, and are carried to the lungs, where they migrate across the alveolar capillary walls. They then travel up the respiratory tree to the epiglottis and are swallowed, returning to the small intestine, where they mature. The worms reach maturity and begin producing eggs in about two months.

EPIDEMIOLOGY. It is estimated that a quarter of the world's population is infected with *Ascaris.* The parasite occurs throughout the world but is most common in warm climates. In the United States, ascariasis is common in many rural parts of the southeast. The prevalence of the infection is greatest in children 1 to 13 years of age.

PATHOLOGY. As the larvae pass through the lungs, they may cause an eosinophilic pneumonitis known as *Löffler's syndrome.* The pathologic process appears to be a combination of physical damage to the alveoli caused by the migrating larvae and an exudative interstitial pneumonia. The large numbers of eosinophils (and the scarcity of neutrophils) in the exudate suggest a hypersensitivity reaction, and previous exposure to the parasite may be important in the development of this response.

The adult worms in the small intestine do not invade the mucosa, but maintain their position by bridging across the lumen. Nonetheless, they may cause mucosal damage demonstrable on barium-contrast examination of the upper gastrointestinal tract. Microscopically, this damage is seen as broadening and shortening of villi, elongation of crypts, and round cell infiltration of the lamina propria. Mucosal disaccharidase deficiency has been described.

The adult worms may migrate to extraintestinal sites in response to drug administration, intercurrent illness in the host, or unknown causes, and in so doing may cause considerable damage.

CLINICAL MANIFESTATIONS AND COMPLICATIONS. The *Ascaris* pneumonia caused by the migration of the larvae through the lungs is characterized by cough, fever, and malaise and, in severe cases, by chest pain, dyspnea, and hemoptysis. Patchy pulmonary infiltrates are seen on chest x-ray.

Various nonspecific gastrointestinal symptoms have been described in association with the worms in the intestine. These include abdominal pain, diarrhea, vomiting, irritability, and anorexia.

Malnutrition in children has been associated with ascariasis, but the amount of malnutrition caused by the infection is controversial. Lowered serum vitamin A and C and protein values have been reported in infected children. Improvement in growth rates have also been reported following de-worming. The nutritional effects of ascariasis seem to stem more from the malabsorption of fats, protein, and carbohydrate caused by mucosal damage than from the ingestion of host nutrients by the parasite.

Serious and life-threatening complications of ascariasis include intestinal obstruction by a bolus of worms, intussusception, volvulus, appendicitis, intestinal perforation, hepatic abscess, aspiration of a worm, cholangitis secondary to bile duct obstruction, and pancreatitis secondary to pancreatic duct obstruction. Of these, intestinal obstruction is the most common; it occurs particularly in children under age six.

DIAGNOSIS. Infection is diagnosed by the finding of ova on microscopic examination of the stool. Often the patient will describe a typical worm passed in the stool; in endemic areas, this is sufficient evidence of ascariasis to warrant treatment.

Eosinophilia is an inconstant feature of intestinal ascariasis. Serologic tests are available, but do not reliably distinguish current from past infection, or *Ascaris lumbricoides* infection from visceral larva migrans.

Ascaris pneumonia is not associated with eggs in the stool unless adult worms are simultaneously present in the host intestine. A marked peripheral eosinophilia provides evidence for the etiology of the pneumonia, but may not be present until late in the course of the illness. Larvae may sometimes be identified in the sputum.

TREATMENT. Pyrantel pamoate is the drug of choice; it is administered in a single dose of 11 mg per kilogram (maximal dose, 1 gram). Mebendazole is equally effective and is particularly useful in mixed *Ascaris-Trichuris* infections; the dose is 100 mg twice a day for three days. It should be used with caution in children less than two years old. Piperazine citrate, in a dose of 75 mg per kilogram daily for two days (maximal daily dose, 3.5 grams), is another effective drug; it is contraindicated in persons with seizure disorders or impaired renal or hepatic function. Levamisole is also effective but is not available in the United States.

Because the goal in treatment of ascariasis is complete elimination of the parasite, a follow-up stool examination should always be obtained two to six weeks after treatment. Stool examinations should also be performed on other members of the patient's household.

No specific treatment is available for *Ascaris* pneumonia. Oxygen and steroids may be indicated in severe cases.

Intestinal obstruction caused by ascariasis should be treated conservatively with nasogastric suction, intravenous fluids, and the instillation of an anthelmintic via the nasogastric tube. Surgery is indicated only in the event of failure of medical management.

PREVENTION. *Ascaris,* like the other soil-transmitted nematodes, is a marker of rural poverty in areas of suitable soil and climatic conditions. Primary prevention is largely dependent on the alleviation of poverty with its accompanying inadequate levels of education and sanitation.

Secondary prevention is possible through the periodic mass treatment of all children or all persons in an endemic community. Such a program may result in the near-eradication of the infection; but in the absence of improved hygiene and education, it is likely that the parasite will eventually become reestablished.

Pawlowski ZS: Ascariasis: Host-pathogen biology. Rev Infec Dis 4:806, 1982.
Schultz MG: Ascariasis: Nutritional implications. Rev Infec Dis 4:815, 1982. *Two companion papers that together constitute a comprehensive review of the topic.*
Stephenson, LS: The contribution of *Ascaris lumbricoides* to malnutrition in children. Parasitology 81:221, 1980. *Argues that ascariasis negatively affects growth in children and that mass treatment of children should be undertaken in endemic areas.*

407. TOXOCARIASIS

Daniel S. Blumenthal

DEFINITION. Toxocariasis is infection with larvae of the dog ascarid, *Toxocara canis,* or less often, the cat ascarid, *Toxocara cati.* The larvae do not complete their life cycle in humans but migrate through the body, invading various organs and producing a syndrome known as *visceral larva migrans.* When the eye is involved, other organs are usually spared; this is known as *ocular larva migrans.*

ETIOLOGY. Humans become infected by ingesting soil contaminated with the feces of infected dogs or cats. Children with geophagia are at highest risk. Swallowed ova hatch in the small intestines and the larvae penetrate the intestinal wall to enter the circulation. When they reach a blood vessel with a diameter smaller than their own, they bore into the surrounding tissue. Larvae have been found in the liver, lungs, heart, and brain, as well as the eye.

EPIDEMIOLOGY. Toxocariasis is predominantly a childhood infection; fewer than 20 per cent of cases occur in adults. Visceral larva migrans tends to occur in younger children, while the ocular form of the infection tends to occur in older children. When both syndromes coexist, however, the patient is usually very young (under five years of age). Most cases are reported from the southern states. There is a strong association with the presence of a dog (especially a puppy) in the household. Serosurveys in the United States demonstrate a prevalence of antibodies to *Toxocara* of 15 to 25 per cent in black children age 1 to 11; white children have a prevalance of 4 to 5 per cent. This suggests that the vast majority of infections are asymptomatic.

PATHOLOGY. Migrating larvae leave tracks of hemorrhage, necrosis, and inflammatory cells. Eosinophilic granulomas or abscesses remain at the site of destruction of larvae; other larvae are walled off and may resume their migration up to years later.

CLINICAL MANIFESTATIONS. Common symptoms of visceral larva migrans are fever, coughing, wheezing, malaise, and weight loss. Physical findings commonly include wheezes, rales, and hepatosplenomegaly. Occasionally the central nervous system is involved, resulting in seizures or behavior disturbances. The white count may be greatly elevated (30,000 to 100,000) with 50 to 90 per cent eosinophils. Serum IgG, IgM, and IgE are usually elevated, as are isohemagglutinins.

In ocular larva migrans, the presentation may be one of visual loss, strabismus, or less often, eye pain. Funduscopic findings may range from a retinal granuloma to severe exudative endophthalmitis with retinal detachment. The condition often mimics retinoblastoma and must be distinguished by serologic testing to avoid needless enucleation.

DIAGNOSIS. Visceral larva migrans should be considered in any child with a persistent eosinophilia, especially if there is a history of pica and/or a household dog. Diagnosis may be confirmed by enzyme-linked immunosorbent assay (ELISA), which has a sensitivity of about 80 per cent and a specificity of about 90 per cent.

TREATMENT AND PREVENTION. Most cases of visceral larva migrans are mild and self-limited, and no treatment is indicated. In severe cases, thiabendazole in a dose of 25 mg per kilogram twice a day for five days may be given, although its benefits remain controversial. Corticosteroids should also be given in severe cases to alleviate symptoms and to limit eye damage in ocular larva migrans.

Household dogs should be examined by a veterinarian for intestinal nematodes and treated as necessary. Leash laws and control of stray dogs may reduce fecal contamination of public parks and playgrounds.

Glockman LT, Schantz PM: Epidemiology and pathogenesis of zoonotic toxocariasis. Epidemiol Rev 3:230, 1981. *An extensive review with emphasis on the seroepidemiology of toxocariasis.*

408. ANISAKIASIS

Daniel S. Blumenthal

Anisakiasis is infection with the larvae of an intestinal nematode of marine mammals. Several species of fish, including herring, serve as intermediate hosts, and human infection may be acquired when raw fish is eaten. The larvae of both *Anisakis* sp. and *Phocanema decipiens* have been implicated. Most cases have occurred in Japan or western Europe, particularly Scandinavia and the Netherlands. Fewer than 30 cases have been reported from the Western Hemisphere.

The larvae invade the wall of the small intestine, where they produce eosinophilic granulomata; intestinal obstruction or perforation may result. Living larvae are sometimes regurgitated. Serologic and intradermal diagnostic tests have been studied, but the diagnosis is generally made at laparotomy. Thiabendazole, 25 mg per kilogram twice a day for three days, may be given if surgical intervention is not required. The disease may be prevented by cooking or freezing fish prior to eating.

Smith JW, Wootten R: Anisakis and anisakiasis. Adv Parasitol 16:93, 1978. *An exceptionally complete review.*

409. TRICHURIASIS

Daniel S. Blumenthal

DEFINITION. Trichuriasis is infection with the whipworm, *Trichuris trichiura*. Clinical manifestations are caused by parasites in the cecum and large intestine; migration of larvae or adults elsewhere in the body has not been reported.

ETIOLOGY AND LIFE CYCLE. Both male and female adult *Trichuris* are about 30 to 50 mm long and have an elongated whiplike anterior portion which is embedded in the submucosa of the host's colon. The female produces 5000 to 10,000 eggs per day; these are passed in the stool and must incubate in the soil for at least three weeks. Embryonated eggs can survive in the soil for years.

Upon ingestion, the ova hatch in the small intestine, and the larvae proceed to the cecum and colon, where they mature. Egg production begins in two to three months. Adult worms survive for three to ten years in the host. Worm loads may number in the thousands.

EPIDEMIOLOGY. Trichuris is found in warm climates throughout the world. In the United States, it is estimated that 2.2 million persons are infected; over 40 per cent of children and adolescents in some rural communities in the southeastern United States harbor the parasite. Soil and climatic requirements for this parasite are similar to those for *Ascaris*, and infections with both worms often coexist in the same host.

PATHOLOGY. Pathologic findings are limited to the large intestine. Light infections cause little tissue reaction. Heavier infections cause edema and hyperemia of the mucosa; microscopically, there is a plasma cell, eosinophil, and polymorphonuclear infiltrate.

CLINICAL MANIFESTATIONS AND COMPLICATIONS. Light infections are often asymptomatic. Heavy infections are accompanied by abdominal pain and diarrhea, which may be severe and prolonged. Since the infection is limited to the large intestine, however, true malabsorption does not occur.

Rectal prolapse is a not infrequent complication of heavy infection. The visible white worms on the edematous mucosa have given the condition the name "coconut cake" prolapse. Worms have also been reported to obstruct the appendix and cause acute appendicitis. The question of whether trichuriasis causes intestinal bleeding is unresolved. Two studies using similar techniques have reached differing conclusions.

DIAGNOSIS. Characteristic eggs, with a mucous plug in each end, may be found on direct fecal smear. In light infections, stool concentration techniques are helpful in making the diagnosis.

Worms may be observed directly on proctosigmoidoscopy. An eosinophilia frequently accompanies infection.

TREATMENT. The drug of choice is mebendazole, 100 mg twice a day for three days regardless of body weight. Since side effects with this drug are very uncommon, even light asymptomatic infections may be treated. However, mebendazole should be used with caution in children under two years, and it should not be given to pregnant women. Oxantel is also effective; it is not available in the United States. A follow-up stool examination should be performed following treatment, and stool examinations should be obtained on other family members.

Reduction of rectal prolapse may be accomplished with a tissue-paper–covered finger; the tissue paper, which facilitates withdrawal of the finger, remains in the rectum and is later expelled. The buttocks may be taped together for a day or two after the prolapse is reduced.

PREVENTION. As with the other soil-transmitted nematodes, this parasite is associated with rural poverty. The provision of sanitary means for the disposal of human feces, combined with community education regarding the transmission of worms, is essential in prevention.

Chanco PP, Vidad JY: A review of trichuriasis, its incidence, pathogenicity and treatment. Drugs 15 (Suppl. 1):87, 1978. *A historical review.*
Greenberg ER, Cline BL: Is trichuriasis associated with iron-deficiency anemia? Am J Trop Med Hyg 284:770, 1979. *A slight reduction in hemoglobin levels was found in* Trichuris-*infected children compared to controls. Reviews the articles relevant to the controversy concerning trichuriasis and gastrointestinal blood loss.*

410. ENTEROBIASIS

Daniel S. Blumenthal

DEFINITION. Enterobiasis is infection with the pinworm, *Enterobius (Oxyuris) vermicularis*. This is a generally benign, although often symptomatic, parasitosis.

ETIOLOGY AND LIFE CYCLE. The adult female pinworm is about 1 cm long, the male, one fourth to one third as large. The parasites inhabit the cecum and colon. Gravid females emerge from the anus while the host sleeps, each female depositing several thousand eggs on the perianal skin. These are transmitted by person-to-person contact via the host's hands. Alternatively, they may be transmitted by bedclothes or become airborne. They remain viable in the environment only a few days. Swallowed eggs release larvae in the small intestine; these pass directly to the colon, where they mature.

EPIDEMIOLOGY. Pinworms are common throughout the world, in urban as well as rural populations and in the affluent as well as the poor. They are particularly common in group living situations, and their prevalence in institutions for the mentally retarded often exceeds 50 per cent. Adults are affected less often than children.

PATHOLOGY. The parasites in the intestine provoke little or no inflammatory response. Worms sometimes migrate into the appendix or fallopian tubes or escape into the peritoneum or elsewhere in the body, where they cause an inflammatory or granulomatous reaction.

CLINICAL MANIFESTATIONS. Many infections—perhaps the majority—are asymptomatic. The characteristic manifestation of symptomatic infections is pruritus ani caused by the deposited ova. This itch may result in restlessness or insomnia.

Nocturnal enuresis has been attributed to enterobiasis, and there are documented cases of bedwetting which resolved promptly upon treatment of concurrent pinworm infection. Most cases of enuresis are not associated with enterobiasis, however.

Numerous other symptoms in children have been attributed to this parasitosis, but no cause-and-effect relationship has been demonstrated. These include tooth-grinding, nose-picking, sleeping in the knee-chest position, anorexia, and abdominal pain.

COMPLICATIONS. Perianal scratching may result in excoriations or impetigo. Young girls may suffer bouts of cystitis or vaginitis caused by pinworms which enter the urethra or vagina during their nocturnal wanderings, carrying enteric bacteria. Thus, it is worthwhile to perform cellophane tape tests on girls with urinary tract infections. Pinworms have also been found in inflamed appendices. Rare manifestations of migrating pinworms include salpingitis, pelvic granulomas, and intestinal perforation. Syndromes resembling regional enteritis or carcinoma have been reported as resulting from enterobiasis.

DIAGNOSIS. Pinworm ova are usually not found in the stool but may be identified with a cellophane tape test. This test is performed by pressing the gummed side of a piece of cellophane tape to the perianal area, and then sticking the tape to a glass slide. The preparation is then examined microscopically for ova. At least three tests, performed on three different mornings before bathing, are necessary to attain a sensitivity of 90 per cent. On occasion, the worms may be seen if the suspected host's perianal area is inspected during sleep. Eosinophilia is not commonly associated with enterobiasis.

TREATMENT. A single-dose treatment with any of three drugs is effective in enterobiasis: pyrantel pamoate, 11 mg per kilogram (maximum, 1 gram); pyrvinium pamoate, 5 mg per kilogram (maximum, 350 mg); or mebendazole, 100 mg regardless of body weight. Patients should be warned that pyrvinium stains stools red. Mebendazole should be used with caution in children less than two years of age; none of these drugs should be given to pregnant women.

Treatment should be repeated in two weeks. Since this parasite is readily transmitted from person to person, it is best to treat the entire household in which a single case is identified. Treatment should be accompanied by the washing of bedclothes, but further environmental measures, such as the scrubbing of floors and toilet seats, should be discouraged. Parents should be reassured about the relative harmlessness of this infection.

PREVENTION. Residents of institutions should be examined periodically for this and other intestinal parasitoses. However, no effective measures for preventing enterobiasis in the general population have been described.

Sachdev YV, Howards SS: *Enterobius vermicularis* infestation and secondary enuresis. J Urol 113:143, 1975. *Describes several cases of nocturnal enuresis which resolved after treatment of pinworm infections.*

Simon RD: Pinworm infestation and urinary tract infection in young girls. Am J Dis Child 128:21, 1974. Kropp KA, Cichocki GA, Bansal NK: *Enterobius vermicularis* (pinworms), introital bacteriology and recurrent urinary tract infection in children. J Urol 120:480, 1978. *Two papers which provide evidence that pinworms play a role in causing urinary tract infections in girls.*

411. TRICHINELLOSIS (Trichinosis)

Donald W. Hoskins

DEFINITION AND ETIOLOGY. Trichinellosis is an intestinal and tissue nematode disease resulting from the ingestion of inadequately cooked meat containing larvae of *Trichinella spiralis*. The chief sources are pork, pork products, and bear or walrus meat. The enteral phase of the infection is largely unnoticed. Diffuse tissue invasion by *Trichinella* larvae, the result of the intestinal union of the adult worms, produces the trichinellotic syndrome of muscle pain and tenderness, fever, periorbital edema, and petechiae. The severity of an infection is directly related to the number and strain of *T. spiralis* larvae ingested, the duration of larval production, and poorly defined host factors.

The ingested larvae, resistant to acid-pepsin digestion, penetrate the villi of the small intestine, molt, and develop into mature adults within 48 hours. After fertilization, the gravid female burrows deep into the mucosa, discharging larvae (500 to 1500 per female) beginning 5 to 46 days after infection and continuing for two to four weeks or occasionally longer. Widely disseminated via lymphatics and bloodstream, *Trichinella* larvae (0.1 mm) enter most organs, but persist only in individual skeletal muscle fibers. Increasing almost ten-fold in size (to 1.0 mm) over succeeding weeks, larvae gradually become surrounded by a cyst wall of muscle origin. Although the capsules calcify within six months to two years, the larvae within remain viable for months to years, rarely for decades.

The adult worms are usually expelled from the intestinal tract after the third or fourth week of infection, the result of immunologic mechanisms, including mast cell degranulation and B and T lymphocyte activity.

The definitive hosts of this infection include numerous carnivorous and omnivorous mammals, although the hog remains the single most important source of human infection.

EPIDEMIOLOGY. Approximately 28 million people worldwide are infected with this parasite, close to 75 per cent of whom reside in the United States. The disease is most prevalent in the temperate zones. Most infections are mild and go unrecognized or misdiagnosed. At present, approximately 100 cases are reported annually in the United States; this represents a significant decrease (except for occasional outbreaks—Louisiana, 44 cases 1979–80) from earlier decades.

From 1940 to 1970, autopsy studies of human diaphragm revealed a drop in the prevalence (16.1 to 4.2 per cent) and severity of infection. The current infection rate is 1.6 to 2.2 per cent. This decline is largely attributable to laws prohibiting the feeding of raw garbage to swine. Currently, more than 98.5 per cent of swine in the United States are grain fed, and only 0.1 per cent are infected with *Trichinella;* garbage-fed swine have an infection rate of 0.5 per cent, down from 10 per cent in 1940.

Pork and pork products, especially sausage, account for 75 per cent of all human *Trichinella* infection; nonpork products account for 13 per cent, and in 12 per cent the source is undetermined. Ground beef contaminated by pork (e.g., in the meatgrinder) is a common source of nonpork-induced disease. Bear and walrus meat account for less than 6 per cent of the reported cases of trichinellosis in this country.

PATHOLOGY AND PATHOGENESIS. Microscopic ulceration, mucosal hyperemia, localized edema, punctate hemorrhages, and intestinal inflammation may result from the penetration of the adult *Trichinella* into the mucosa of the small intestine.

The larvae produce basophilic granular alteration of muscle fibers within 48 hours of invasion. The fibers enlarge, and edema, nuclear proliferation, and interstitial inflammation ensue. Later, fatty metamorphosis is followed by atrophy and fibrosis. Larvae may produce a severe myocarditis with focal necrosis and eosinophilic infiltration, but encystment does not occur in cardiac muscle. Eosinophilic infiltration of the endocardium with fibrosis has been reported in fatal trichinellosis. Nonpurulent encephalomeningitis with larvae in the cerebrospinal fluid, choroid, and retina may also occur.

CLINICAL MANIFESTATIONS. The vast majority of persons infected with *T. spiralis* exhibit few or no symptoms. Less than 12 per cent have gastrointestinal symptoms. Heavy infection may produce an acute enteritis (abdominal discomfort, diarrhea) one to two days following ingestion, with systemic symptoms occurring five to seven days later. The usual incubation period is seven to fourteen days, extending to three weeks or more in mild infections.

The onset of the trichinellótic syndrome is often acute with fever, muscle pain and tenderness, weakness, malaise, bilateral periorbital edema, and headache. Subungual, retinal, and subconjunctival petechiae and hemorrhage may be present, and a macular, petechial, or urticarial rash is not uncommon. Within the first two weeks of severe systemic disease, allergic phenomena such as edema, pneumonitis, and pleural transudate may occur.

Mild infection is characterized by fever of less than 38° C and symptoms of less than three weeks' duration; *moderate* infection persists for more than four weeks, and fever is usually greater than 38° C for one to two weeks. *Severe* infection persists for six weeks or more, fever is greater than 39° C for two weeks or more and serum albumin is usually less than 2.5 grams per deciliter.

Serious complications, including myocarditis, pneumonitis, and meningoencephalitis, occur most often in the third to ninth week of the disease. Mortality is less than 1.5 per cent and is almost always related to complications.

DIAGNOSIS AND DIFFERENTIAL DIAGNOSIS. Once considered, the diagnosis is not difficult. The trichinellotic syndrome coupled with marked peripheral blood eosinophilia (20 to 70 per cent), elevation of muscle enzymes (CPK, LDH, aldolase, and transaminases), and normal sedimentation rate should strongly suggest the diagnosis. Finding encysted larvae in any remaining suspected food source would be additional evidence.

Confirmation of the diagnosis is often accomplished by serologic testing, skin test, or muscle biopsy. Serologic testing is simple, highly sensitive, and specific. Antibodies are not detected, however, until three weeks or more after the onset of infection. Available tests include rapid screening counterimmunoelectrophoresis (CIE) and enzyme-linked immunosorbent assay (ELISA), passive hemagglutination (PHA), and indirect immunofluorescence (IF). The bentonite flocculation test is the most widely used; a titer of one to five or greater is considered positive, although a four-fold rise in the titer is more convincing. False positives do occur; 13.5 per cent of typhoid-paratyphoid sera may react positively. Two independent methods are often required to establish serodiagnosis of trichinellosis. Skin testing does not distinguish between past and present infection and therefore does not prove active disease.

Muscle biopsy may be positive as early as the second week of infection but is often not required. A small amount of muscle is excised under local anesthesia from a tender, painful, swollen muscle, a portion sent for routine pathologic examination, and a small amount crushed between glass slides and examined directly under a scanning or low power objective for motile larvae. Pepsin–hydrochloric acid digestion of 1.0 gram of muscle may also be performed and larvae sought microscopically.

The differential diagnosis in a disease with multisystem involvement is extensive. Common misdiagnoses include viral syndromes (influenza, gastroenteritis, various exanthems), collagen disease (periarteritis, dermatomyositis), sepsis (typhoid, pneumonitis, meningitis), allergic phenomena, and polymyositis.

TREATMENT. Rarely, infection with *T. spiralis* is suspected within hours or days of ingestion of infected meat. Treatment of the immature worms in the small intestine is usually successful and will abort or markedly inhibit systemic disease. Furthermore, given the relationship of the severity of infection to continued larval production by the adult female *T. spiralis* and the unknown duration of its fecundity, treatment of the intestinal phase in all cases up to six weeks after infection is advisable. Thiabendazole (Mintezol) 25 mg per kilogram twice daily (maximum 3.0 grams per day) for one week has been replaced by another benzimidazole, mebendazole (Vermox) 200 mg daily for four days, largely for improved patient tolerance. Alternatively, pyrantel pamoate (Antiminth) 10 mg per kilogram (maximum 1.0 gram per day) for four days has been used with similar results. Although none of these drugs is advocated during pregnancy, mebendazole is specifically contraindicated.

Mild to moderate systemic infection is treated with rest and analgesics; recovery may take weeks and complications are rare. All patients must be carefully observed, especially in the first two weeks following onset of systemic symptoms, for progression to a more acute and severe form of trichinellosis.

Acute severe trichinellosis will require corticosteroids in high doses (prednisone, 60 mg daily) for two or more weeks, primarily for inhibition of host response. Since the enteral phase of *T. spiralis* may be prolonged (and larval production extended) with the use of corticosteroids, the concomitant administration of a benzimidazole (mebendazole, 5 mg per kilogram daily for five to ten days) is advisable. The benzimidazoles (thiabendazole, mebendazole) have been used singly in the treatment of moderate to severe trichinellosis with improvement in well-being and defervescence of fever; the analgesic and anti-inflammatory properties of the drugs may account for the improvement seen rather than any tissue larvicidal properties in man. The risk of a hypersensitivity (Jarisch-Herxheimer) reaction on day three or four of treatment with benzimidazole therapy favors the combined corticosteroid-benzimidazole regimen in acute severe trichinellosis. Adverse effects of the benzimidazoles include headache, nausea, vomiting, dizziness, rash, and agitation.

PREVENTION. Thorough cooking of infected meat kills larvae; a temperature of 58.3° C throughout the meat is adequate. Freezing meat at −32° C for 24 hours or at −15° C (home freezer) for three weeks is also effective. Government inspection of meat in the United States does not exclude *Trichinella* infection, nor does the smoking, salting, or drying of meat.

The application of an enzyme-linked immunosorbent assay (ELISA) for the detection of antibody to *T. spiralis* in pooled hog sera at slaughter may be practical in the detection of infected sources.

Campbell WC (ed.): *Trichinella* and Trichinosis. New York, Plenum Press, 1983. *An expensive but highly valuable update on all aspects of parasite and pathogen. The practicing physician will especially appreciate the chapters on chemotherapy, clinical aspects, and immunodiagnosis. Extensively referenced work.*

Kim CW, Pawlowski ZS (eds.): Proceedings of the Fourth International Conference on Trichinellosis. University Press of New England, 1978. *This volume is strong in the clinical, pathologic, and therapeutic areas. Report of a symposium in Poland in 1976.*

Most H: Current concepts in parasitology. Trichinosis—preventable yet still with us. N Engl J Med 298:1178, 1978.

412. ANGIOSTRONGYLIASIS

Daniel S. Blumenthal

The larvae of two rodent parasites, *Angiostrongylus cantonensis* and *A. costaricensis*, may infect man. The pathology and clinical findings caused by the two species are quite different. The genus is also known as *Morerastrongylus*.

ANGIOSTRONGYLUS CANTONENSIS. Eosinophilic meningitis caused by larvae of the rat lungworm occurs in southeast Asia and many Pacific islands. The first cases in the Western Hemisphere were reported in 1981 from Cuba.

Humans are infected by ingesting, in an uncooked state, the snails, slugs, and crustaceans that serve as intermediate hosts. The infective larvae migrate to the capillaries of the meninges, where they cause an eosinophilic inflammatory response with granuloma formation. Clinically, there are signs of meningeal irritation, and there may be localizing neurologic findings, including paresthesias and cranial nerve palsies. There is a peripheral and cerebrospinal fluid eosinophilia. The eosinophilic meningitis of angiostrongyliasis must be differentiated from that caused by gnathostomiasis, cysticercosis, and other parasitoses. Most cases resolve uneventfully, but some result in permanent sequelae or death. There are no specific diagnostic tests available. Thiabendazole has been given for this infection, but there is no convincing evidence that it is effective. Steroids may control symptoms.

ANGIOSTRONGYLUS COSTARICENSIS. Human larval infection with this species has been reported in children in Central America, Mexico, and Venezuela. Adult *A. costaricensis* live in the mesenteric arteries of rats and other rodents; a slug serves as intermediate host. Larvae are shed in the slime of the slug, and children may become infected by handling slugs and then putting their hands in their mouths. Vegetables on which slugs have crawled may also be infective. Once ingested, the larvae travel to the mesenteric arterioles, where they cause edema of the wall of the cecum, appendix, and ascending colon. Yellow granulations of the subserosa and eosinophilic infiltrates are common pathologic findings. There may be ulcerations, peritonitis, and fistula formation. The clinical picture is similar to that of acute appendicitis, with fever and right lower quadrant pain and tenderness. A tumor-like mass may often be palpated in the right lower quadrant. There is usually marked eosinophilia. Contrast studies of the gastrointestinal tract may show abnormalities of the cecum, ascending colon, and terminal ileum. The diagnosis is usually established at surgery. If surgery is not required, thiabendazole may be tried, but its efficacy is in doubt.

Prevention of both types of infection is dependent on education and rodent control.

Chin-Yun Y: Clinical observations on eosinophilic meningitis and meningoencephalitis caused by angiostrongylus cantonensis on Taiwan. Am J Trop Med Hyg 25:233, 1976. *A series of 125 cases of this infection, including four deaths and three with permanent sequelae.*

Loria-Cortes R, Lobo-Sanahuja JF: Clinical abdominal angiostrongylosis. Am J Trop Med Hyg 29:538, 1980. *The largest series of* A. costaricensis *infection to date (116 children), with clinical and epidemiologic findings.*

Filariasis

413. INTRODUCTION

Eric A. Ottesen

Eight filarial parasites commonly infect humans (Table 413–1), but three are responsible for most of the pathology associated with these infections. There are the lymphatic dwelling filariae *Wuchereria bancrofti* and *Brugia malayi* and the subcutaneous filarid *Onchocerca volvulus.*

All eight species are transmitted by biting arthropods (Table 413–1) and go through complex life cycles that include a slow maturation phase of 3 to 18 months from the time infective larvae are introduced by the vector until the adult worms mature and reside in the lymph nodes, subcutaneous tissue, or body cavities. The offspring of these adults (microfilariae) are 200 to 250 μm long and 5 to 7 μm wide. They either circulate in the blood or migrate through the skin, awaiting ingestion by the appropriate arthropod in which they develop over one to two weeks to infective forms capable of initiating this life cycle again. Adult worms are long lived (probably 8 to 15 years), while microfilariae probably live about 6 months. Patent infection is generally not established unless exposure to infective larvae is intense and prolonged, and manifestations of disease usually develop slowly.

Diagnosis can be extremely difficult because it relies almost exclusively on parasitologic techniques to demonstrate microfilariae in the blood or tissue. At present, there are no completely satisfactory methods for making a definitive diagnosis in states of "amicrofilaremic filariasis" (before or after the microfilaremic state). When microfilariae circulate in the blood, they do so with or without a distinct periodicity (Table 413–1). Some are garbed in sheaths while others are sheathless. These two features, as well as other more subtle morphologic distinctions, are helpful diagnostically. Microfilariae can be identified either by direct observation of Giemsa-stained blood smears or, more sensitively, by concentration techniques using Knott's method (examination of centrifuged sediment after mixing 1 ml of blood with 9 ml of 2 per cent formalin) or membrane filtration of one or more ml of blood through a 3 μm- or 5 μm-pore Nucleopore membrane filter. Skin microfilariae are best sought by performing skin snips either as described in Ch. 422 or using a corneal-scleral (Holth) biopsy punch. Antibody detection, although helpful in certain situations, is generally nondiagnostic because it cannot differentiate current from past infection or exposure and because of antigenic cross reactivity between the filariae and other helminth parasites.

Diethylcarbamazine (DEC)* has been the single mainstay of treatment for all filarial infections since the late 1940's; however, it shows variable effectiveness for the different conditions. Suramin,† although extremely toxic, is also used for onchocerciasis. While little advance in the chemotherapy of these diseases has been made until recently, current prospects for more effective, less toxic drugs for filarial infection appear hopeful.

*Not commercially available in the United States but may be obtained in special circumstances from Lederle Laboratories.

†Available from the Centers for Disease Control, Parasitic Disease Drug Service, Atlanta, GA.

Hawking F: Diethylcarbamazine and new compounds for the treatment of filariasis. Adv Pharm Chemother 16:129, 1979. *A complete account of the most important drugs currently used to treat filarial infections.*

Ottesen EA: Filarisis and tropical eosinophilia. *In* Warren KS and Mahmond AA

TABLE 413–1. THE COMMON FILARIAL PARASITES OF MAN

Species	Distribution	Vector	Primary Pathology	Microfilariae: Primary Location	Microfilariae: Periodicity	Microfilariae: Presence of Sheath
Wuchereria bancrofti	Tropics worldwide	Mosquitoes	Lymphatic, pulmonary	Blood, hydrocele fluid	Nocturnal, subperiodic	+
Brugia malayi	Southeast Asia	Mosquitoes	Lymphatic, pulmonary	Blood	Nocturnal, subperiodic	+
Brugia timori	Indonesia	Mosquitoes	Lymphatic	Blood	Nocturnal	+
Onchocerca volvulus	Africa; Central and South America	Black fly	Skin, eye, lymphatic	Skin	None or minimal	−
Loa loa	Africa	Horse fly	Allergic	Blood	Diurnal	+
Mansonella perstans	Africa; South America	Midge	? Allergic	Blood	None	−
Mansonella streptocerca	Africa	Midge	Dermal	Skin	None	−
Mansonella ozzardi	Central and South America	Midge	Vague	Blood	None	−

(eds.): Tropical and Geographical Medicine. McGraw-Hill Book Co., 1983, pp 390–412. *Detailed clinical, parasitologic and epidemiologic discussions of filarial diseases.*

Sasa M: Human Filariasis. Baltimore, University Park Press, 1976, pp 819. *A book giving a global view of the epidemiology of filariasis.*

414. DRACUNCULIASIS

Donald R. Hopkins

Dracunculiasis, or guinea worm disease, is caused by infection with the parasite *Dracunculus medinensis.* It occurs mainly in the Indian subcontinent and West Africa, where up to about 10 million persons living in rural areas are thought to be affected.

Diagnosis of patent infections is easy. The thin white female worms, each up to 1 meter long, emerge directly through the skin, usually of the lower leg, ankle, or foot. The adult worms emerge 10 to 14 months after victims have drunk water containing infected *Cyclops,* a barely visible crustacean that serves as the parasite's intermediate host. When persons harboring such emerging worms enter a stagnant source of drinking water such as a step well or pond, larvae are released into the water. Some such larvae are ingested by *Cyclops,* where they undergo two molts before becoming infective to humans. When humans drink water containing *Cyclops* with infective larvae, the larvae penetrate the intestinal or stomach wall, mature, and mate, after which the male worms die.

The adult female worms emerge very slowly, over a period of weeks or months. Emergence may be preceded by generalized allergic symptoms and is usually accompanied by a burning sensation, then a blister that ruptures to form an ulcer at the site of emergence. Some worms present first as a serpentine cord just beneath the skin or at the center of an abscess. No immunity develops, so persons in endemic areas are infected year after year.

The great social and economic significance of dracunculiasis, which rarely is fatal, derives from the fact that emergence of the worm is very painful and is often associated with swelling, local arthritis, and secondary infection. Thus, victims are often unable to farm or sometimes even walk for weeks or months. Over half of the adults in a village may be crippled at the same time, and because the infection tends to be seasonal, these effects appear precisely when villagers need to harvest or plant their crops. School attendance is also affected.

Treatment is difficult because anthelmintics such as thiabendazole or metronidazole only marginally reduce the duration of emergence and associated pain. Aspirin can help relieve the pain. Emerging worms are best rolled around a small stick as their predecessors have been for centuries, care being taken not to break the worm (which would exacerbate the inflammation). Some worms can be removed surgically. Victims should be immunized against tetanus, which is an all too frequent complication caused by secondary infection of the ulcer around the emerging worm. Persons at risk should be taught to boil their drinking water or filter it through a piece of cloth, and to avoid entering sources of drinking water when the infection is patent.

Since the most effective intervention against this infection is to provide safe sources of drinking water, efforts are under way to take advantage of the International Drinking Water Supply and Sanitation Decade (1981–1990) to provide safe water to dracunculiasis-endemic areas as a priority, and thereby control or eliminate the disease.

Hopkins DR: Dracunculiasis: An eradicable scourge. *In* Epidemiologic Reviews. Vol 5. Baltimore, The Johns Hopkins School of Hygiene and Public Health, 1983, pp 208–219. *A recent review of all aspects pertaining to control and eradication of dracunculariasis.*

Muller R: *Dracunculus* and dracunculiasis. *In* Dawes B (ed.): Advances in Parasitology. Vol 9. New York, Academic Press, 1971, pp 73–151. *A thorough consideration of the parasite's biology, life cycle, and the disease it produces.*

415. LYMPHATIC FILARIASIS (Wuchereria bancrofti, Brugia malayi, and Brugia timori)

Eric A. Ottesen

ETIOLOGY. There are three lymphatic-dwelling filarial parasites of man, *Wuchereria bancrofti, Brugia malayi,* and *Brugia timori.* Adult worms are thread-like in form (2 to 10 cm long by less than 0.4 mm wide) and usually reside in the lymph nodes or afferent lymphatic channels. The female worms produce large numbers of microfilariae (175 to 300 μ long), which circulate in the peripheral blood awaiting ingestion by mosquito intermediate hosts, which are necessary to continue the parasite's life cycle. After about two weeks in these mosquitoes, the microfilariae develop into infective third stage larvae (L_3's). When infected mosquitoes feed, these L_3's leave the mosquito mouth parts and come to rest on the surface of the host's skin. If they then manage to penetrate the skin through the puncture wound at the site of the bite, transmission is successful; after a further developmental period lasting as long as 4 to 12 months, adult worms can again be found in the lymphatic tissues, where they mate and produce another generation of microfilariae. The adult parasites may remain viable in the human host for decades.

EPIDEMIOLOGY. For *W. bancrofti* man is the only definitive host and, thus, the natural reservoir for infection. Indeed, considerable experimental effort to establish the parasite in a wide variety of potential mammalian hosts has met with little success. *W. bancrofti* is found throughout the tropics and subtropics, including areas of South America and the Caribbean, Africa, Asia, and the Pacific. Two forms of the parasite are distinguished by the periodicity of their circulating microfilariae. Nocturnally periodic forms have microfilariae detectable in peripheral blood primarily at night, whereas in the subperiodic forms the microfilariae are usually present in the blood at all hours but with maximal levels often in the late afternoon. Generally, subperiodic bancroftian filariasis is found only in the Pacific islands east of 160° E longitude (including New Caledonia, Fiji, Samoa, Ellis and Cook Islands, Society Islands, and the Marquesas); elsewhere *W. bancrofti* is nocturnally periodic. The natural vectors are *Culex fatigans* in urban settings and usually anopheline or aedean mosquitoes in rural areas.

The distribution of brugian filariasis is much more restricted, being limited primarily to Malaysia, Indonesia, India, China, Korea, the Philippines, and Japan. Again, there are both nocturnally periodic and subperiodic forms of the parasite. The former is more common and is transmitted in coastal rice fields primarily by mansonian and anopheline mosquitoes; mansonian mosquitoes, found in swamp forests, are the major vectors of the subperiodic form. Unlike *W. bancrofti, B. malayi* can be a natural infection of cats and can be established in a number of laboratory animals. *B. timori* has been described only from two Indonesian islands.

PATHOLOGY. Most of the pathology of bancroftian and brugian filariasis is initiated in the lymphatics. Although details of the pathogenesis are lacking, the progression of pathologic changes is clear. Damaged lymphatics lead first to reversible lymphedema and then to chronic obstructive changes (elephantiasis) in the limbs, breasts, or genitalia, or to chyluria. The location of lymphatic damage determines the site and type of pathology expressed.

Adult worms, residing in the afferent approaches or cortical sinuses of the lymph nodes, incite local inflammatory reactions by undefined (probably immunologic) mechanisms. These reactions result in dilatation of the lymphatics and hypertrophy of the vessel walls. Endothelial and connective tissue proliferation leads to polypoid growths that protrude into the lymphatic lumen; but so long as the worm remains alive, the vessel appears to stay patent. Patency, however, does not assure normal lymphatic function, as lymphangiographic studies have clearly documented the development of a characteristic tortuosity of the lymph vessels with loss of valvular function and backflow of lymph leading to lymph stasis and lymphedema even during this "preobliterative phase."

Death of adult worms is accompanied by local necrosis and granulomatous reaction around the parasite with infiltration of plasma cells, eosinophils, and giant cells. Fibrosis occurs and the fragmented parasites are either completely resorbed or partially calcified. Lymphatic obstruction develops and associated endophlebitis may further complicate the lymphatic obstruction. Although there is subsequent formation of collateral lymphatics and some recanalization of obstructed vessels, lymphatic function remains compromised. Repeated infection with increasing host response to the parasite leads to the chronic changes of advanced elephantiasis.

CLINICAL MANIFESTATIONS. The three most common clinical presentations of the lymphatic filariases are asymptomatic microfilaremia, "filarial fever," and lymphatic obstruction. A fourth presentation, the tropical eosinophilia syndrome, is considered in Ch. 416.

Patients with asymptomatic microfilaremia rarely come to the physician's attention except through an incidental finding of microfilariae in the peripheral blood smear during mass surveys in endemic regions, or when blood eosinophilia leads to a diagnostic evaluation for filariasis. Such asymptomatic persons appear to be clinically unaffected by the parasites. It is likely that in some of these individuals the infections clear spontaneously, whereas the infections of others subsequently progress and become symptomatic, but what determines such clinical changes is unclear.

"Filarial fevers" are acute febrile episodes characterized by high fever (often with shaking chills), lymphatic inflammation (i.e., lymphadenitis and lymphangitis), and transient local edema. They occur as often as six to ten times per year in affected persons and usually last three to seven days before subsiding spontaneously. The factors that initiate these episodes are unknown, but they are definitely parasite related. The lymphangitis characteristically develops in a retrograde fashion, extending peripherally *from* the draining node where the adult parasites reside. Regional nodes are enlarged and painful, and the entire lymphatic tract often becomes indurated and inflamed. Concomitant local thrombophlebitis is common. In brugian filariasis especially, a single local abscess may form along the inflamed lymphatic and subsequently rupture to the surface, leaving a characteristic scar whose presence has been used epidemiologically as an indication of the clinical "activity" of filarial infection in *Brugia* endemic regions. Neither the lymphatic inflammation nor the characteristic abscesses appear to be bacterially induced. Such lymphadenitis and lymphangitis occur in the upper and lower extremities with both bancroftian and brugian filariasis, but involvement of the genital lymphatics is almost exclusively a feature of *W. bancrofti* infection. Thus, acute *bancrofti* episodes may also involve funiculitis, epididymitis, scrotal pain, and tenderness. Patients with filarial fevers may be microfilaremic but more often are not.

As lymphatic damage progresses, the edema and anatomic distortion that were initially transient develop into the permanent changes of elephantiasis. Pitting edema yields to brawny edema, and there is both thickening of subcutaneous tissue and hyperkeratosis. Fissuring of the skin develops along with nodular and papillomatous hyperplastic changes. Superinfection of these poorly vascularized tissues becomes a problem. In addition, in bancroftian filariasis, obstructed genital lymphatics may lead to scrotal lymphedema or hydrocele, whereas obstruction of the retroperitoneal lymphatics can increase hydrostatic pressure in the renal lymphatics, causing their rupture into the renal pelvis or tubules and leading to chyluria. Characteristically chyluria is intermittent, sometimes lasting for days or weeks before abating spontaneously and then recurring; often it is most prominent in the morning after the patient first arises.

DIAGNOSIS. Definitive diagnosis of filariasis can be made only by the demonstration of parasites, either adult worms associated with the lymphatics (rarely observed) or microfilariae in the blood, hydrocele fluid, or chylous urine. These fluids can be examined directly (20 cu mm on a slide with or without red blood cell lysis), after concentration of the parasites by centifugation in 2 per cent formalin (Knott's technique), or after filtration through a membrane (3- to 5-μm Nuclepore) filter. The time of blood collection should take into account the parasite's possible nocturnal periodicity.

Because many persons with filariasis (especially those with chronic pathology) are not microfilaremic, diagnosis must often be made clinically. The differential diagnosis is broad but in the acute episodes primarily includes thrombophlebitis, infection, and trauma. The edema and other lymphatic obstructive changes associated with chronic filariasis must be distinguished from the manifestations of congestive heart failure, malignancy, trauma, postsurgical scarring, and a number of less common congenital and idiopathic abnormalities of the lymphatic system. The many disorders associated with serum IgE and blood eosinophil elevations must be considered in evaluating asymptomatic filarial infections. Several specific points may help in this differential diagnosis: (1) Exposure to filariae must be prolonged or intense (for at least several months) before persons become infected; (2) the physical finding or history of *retrograde* lymphangitis can often aid in distinguishing filarial from bacterial lymphangitis; (3) although lymphadenopathy is characteristic of filariasis, alone it is never diagnostic; (4) lymphangiographic patterns of elephantiasis and chyluria are well defined so that, even though not always diagnostic, lymphangiography is sometimes useful in distinguishing filarial from congenital or neoplastic lymphatic abnormalities; (5) although total serum IgE and blood eosinophil levels are elevated in all filarial infections, they cannot distinguish filarial from other helminth infections except in the case of the tropical eosinophilia syndrome (see Ch. 416); and (6) because most residents of endemic regions have been immunologically "sensitized" to filarial antigens through years of bites by infected mosquitoes and because filarial antigens cross-react extensively with those of other nematode parasites, positive results in the numerous serologic and skin tests that have been developed are of little diagnostic value *except* in those who are not native to endemic areas.

TREATMENT. Available chemotherapy for lymphatic filariasis is both limited and inadequate. Diethylcarbamazine* (DEC, 5 mg per kilogram per day given in single or divided doses for two to three weeks) rapidly kills microfilariae in vivo, but its effect on adult parasites is not so clearly defined. Thus, following treatment with DEC, although the blood is temporarily free of microfilariae, the infection itself has often not been terminated, and several courses of DEC or long-term intermittent treatment with low doses of DEC are often required to kill the adult parasites. There are no other clinically useful drugs available for eradicating the infection.

Side effects of DEC treatment, although not so frequent or severe as those seen in onchocerciasis, can be troublesome, especially in brugian filariasis. These include fever, chills, headache, dizziness, nausea, vomiting, and arthralgias, all usually occurring in the first 24 to 36 hours. Both the likelihood of developing such reactions and the degree of their severity are directly related to the number of circulating microfilariae. Thus, the side effects of DEC administration at these dosage levels are due not to direct drug toxicity but to allergic or immunologic responses of the host to dying parasites. To avoid these reactions in highly parasitemic persons, one can initiate treatment with very small doses of DEC or premedicate the patients with steroids, as suggested for onchocerciasis (see Ch. 422). A very few patients may also develop filarial fever episodes with lymphangitis and lymphadenitis in the first days after DEC treatment. All of these side effects occur early in

*Production of this drug has been discontinued in the United States.

treatment and generally subside even with continued administration of the drug.

The results of severe chronic lymphatic damage generally are not reversible, but long-term low dose DEC has been shown to reverse early lymphedematous changes and careful attention to the management of lymphedema can minimize the development of further damage. Limb elevation, elastic stockings, and perhaps even diuretics are important, as well as local foot care to prevent damaging bacterial and fungal infection in these already compromised tissues. In the most extreme cases, surgical excision of redundant tissue can be performed. Hydroceles can be repeatedly drained or managed surgically. Chyluria also can sometimes be corrected surgically, but, interestingly, many cases have been reported in which diagnostic lymphangiography itself appears to have terminated the leak of chyle into the urine, probably as a result of its sclerosing effects.

PREVENTION. Because DEC kills developing preadult forms of many filarial species, it is used in veterinary practice as a prophylactic agent to prevent filarial infection of dogs. Its potential for prophylaxis in man, however, has not been evaluated. In public health programs DEC has been used successfully as a protective measure to reduce infection rates in selected populations. Because of its microfilaricidal effects, small doses administered intermittently to all residents of an endemic region (e.g., 3 mg per kilogram monthly) reduce the number of blood-borne microfilariae in the community to levels so low that successful transmission of the infection by mosquitoes cannot occur. Other approaches to filariasis control designed to eradicate the mosquito vectors have also proved effective.

Gooneratne BWN: Lymphangiography—Clinical and Experimental. London, Butterworths, 1974. *General description of lymphangiographic techniques, edited by a physician with great personal experience in the lymphangiography of filarial lymphatic obstruction. Three chapters are devoted exclusively to the lymphatic lesions seen in filariasis.*

Hawking F: Diethylcarbamazine and new compounds for the treatment of filariasis. Adv Pharmacol Chemother 16:129, 1979. *A thorough review of the pharmacology and clinical effects of the major chemotherapeutic agent used for treating filariasis. An evaluation of alternative drugs is also given.*

Ottesen EA: Immunopathology of lymphatic filariasis in man. Springer Semin Immunopathol 2:373, 1980. *Reviews the major immunologic findings in lymphatic filariasis and attempts to relate these findings to the pathogenesis of the various clinical syndromes associated with the infection.*

Sasa M: Human Filariasis: A Global Survey of Epidemiology and Control. Baltimore, University Park Press, 1976. *A fine compendium of epidemiologic observations, taxonomic detail, and host, parasite, and vector interactions. Techniques for detection of microfilariae in clinical specimens are described in detail.*

416. TROPICAL EOSINOPHILIA

Eric A. Ottesen

Tropical eosinophilia is a syndrome of acute and chronic lung disease first defined in the 1940's but not generally recognized as being of filarial etiology until the 1960's. Its main clinical features are a history of residence in a filaria-endemic region; paroxysmal cough and wheezing, which generally occur at night; scanty sputum production; occasional weight loss, low-grade fever, and adenopathy; and extreme blood eosinophilia (>3000 per microliter). It appears to be more common in Indians than in persons of other nationalities and more common in men than in women. Chest x-rays can be normal but generally show increased bronchovascular markings, diffuse miliary lesions, or mottled opacities primarily involving the mid and lower lung fields. Tests of pulmonary function almost always indicate restrictive abnormalities and often show obstructive defects as well. The association of the syndrome with filarial infection was first recognized by finding very high levels of antifilarial antibody in these patients and by noting the favorable response to treatment with antifilarial drugs (now diethylcarbamazine [DEC]* in doses of 5 to 6 mg per kilogram per day for two to three weeks). Later, several reports described microfilariae or their degenerating remnants in lung biopsy specimens. Most recently, extremely high levels of total serum IgE (usually 10,000 to 100,000 ng per milliliter) have been found in these patients, and an appreciable fraction of this IgE has been shown to be directed against filarial antigens.

Because of these and other findings, tropical eosinophilia is now considered to be a form of "occult filariasis" in which host immunologic hyperresponsiveness to the parasite results in such rapid clearance of microfilariae from the blood that this stage of the parasite is essentially never detectable. Generally this microfilarial clearance takes place in the lungs, and the clinical symptoms appear to result largely from the allergic and inflammatory reactions elicited by the cleared parasites. In some subjects, however, trapping of the microfilariae occurs predominantly in other organs of the reticuloendothelial system (liver, spleen, lymph nodes), and in these persons the major clinical manifestations are those resulting from hepatomegaly, splenomegaly, or lymphadenopathy. It has been postulated that infection with nonhuman filarial parasites is the major cause of tropical eosinophilia. More likely, however, the syndrome is caused not by an "abnormal parasite" but rather by an abnormal host response to those same parasites (*Wuchereria bancrofti* and *Brugia malayi*) that commonly cause lymphatic filariasis (see Ch. 415). In this respect, tropical eosinophilia is likely quite similar to another pulmonary eosinophilic disorder, allergic bronchopulmonary aspergillosis, both in its clinical expression and in its pathogenesis (see Ch. 373).

Diagnosis depends primarily on distinguishing tropical eosinophilia from the other important eosinophilic syndromes with pulmonary involvement, namely, Löffler's syndrome, chronic eosinophilic pneumonia, allergic aspergillosis, certain vasculitic syndromes, the idiopathic hypereosinophilia syndrome, drug allergies, and some helminth infections. Although there is no one clinical or laboratory criterion that will distinguish tropical eosinophilia from these other conditions, a history of residence in the tropics along with the presence of specific filarial antibodies and the response to DEC therapy are the most helpful differential points. Within three to seven days following administration of DEC, there is almost always marked improvement or disappearance of symptoms. Relapse may occur, however, months to years later and require retreatment. DEC will not, of course, reverse permanent pulmonary damage (primarily an interstitial fibrosis), which frequently develops prior to successful diagnosis and treatment of the disorder.

Neva FA, Ottesen EA: Tropical (filarial) eosinophilia. N Engl J Med 298:1129, 1978. *Concise review of historical, clinical, and pathogenetic aspects of the tropical eosinophilia syndrome.*

Udwadia FE: Pulmonary Eosinophilia. Progress in Respiration Research, Vol 7. Basel, S Karger, 1975. *Extensive review of tropical eosinophilia by a physician operating a chest clinic in Bombay, India, who has followed and studied over 450 patients with this disease. Rich in clinical detail and perspective.*

417. LOIASIS

Eric A. Ottesen

Loa loa is indigenous only to the rain forest belt of western and central Africa. Mature female parasites, about twice the size of the males, are 50 to 70 mm long and 0.5 mm wide. They live wandering through the subcutaneous tissue in humans, usually attracting attention only when they cross the eye subconjunctivally. The sheathed microfilariae produced by these females circulate with a diurnal periodicity that peaks about noon.

Clinical loiasis presents in two primary forms, one more common among individuals native to endemic regions and the other more common in visitors to these areas who acquire infection. Among the natives loiasis is often entirely asymptomatic until an adult worm appears moving across the eye or blood examination reveals microfilaremia. Such individuals may also have occasional episodes of "Calabar swellings." These are characteristic localized areas of erythema and angioedema (up to 5 to 10 cm in diameter) that occur primarily on the extremities and last one to three days before regressing spontaneously. These swellings appear to be a hypersensitivity

*Production of this drug has been discontinued in the United States.

reaction to the adult worm, whose presence can also be detected in some patients by either a subcutaneous crawling sensation or the appearance of a fine vermiform hive in the skin. When the inflammation extends to nearby joints or peripheral nerves, corresponding symptoms may develop. Rarely, nephropathy (probably immune complex mediated) and encephalopathy have been reported.

The major difference between this presentation and that seen in outsiders who acquire infection is the greater predominance of allergic or hyper-reactive symptoms in the latter. Episodes of angioedema are likely to be more frequent and debilitating, and patients are much less likely to have microfilariae in the blood. In addition, they often present with extensive blood eosinophilia (30 to 60 per cent of an elevated total leukocyte count) much like patients with tropical eosinophilia (Ch. 416). Diagnosis in these patients often cannot be made parasitologically and must be based on the characteristic history, clinical presentation, blood eosinophilia, and elevated filarial antibody titers. If untreated, a small (but undefined) percentage of such patients develops severe cardiomyopathy presumably secondary to the hypereosinophilia elicited by the infection.

Treatment is with diethylcarbamazine (DEC)* (6 to 10 mg per kilogram per day) for two to three weeks. The drug is extremely effective against microfilariae but less so against adult worms, so that multiple courses of treatment are often necessary before there is complete resolution of signs and symptoms. In cases of heavy microfilaremia (greater than several hundred microfilariae per ml of blood) allergic and other inflammatory side effects of treatment may be so severe that a regimen of 0.5–1 mg per kilogram DEC per dose (with or without simultaneous steroids) is safer for initiating treatment. Some evidence exists that DEC is effective in preventing loiasis when taken in doses of 5 mg kilogram per day for three days each month, but large trials of this prophylactic regimen have yet to be carried out.

Brockington IF, Olsen EGJ, Goodwin JF: Endomyocardial fibrosis in European residents in tropical Africa. Lancet i:583, 1967. *Description of the cardiomyopathy believed to result from the hypereosinophilia induced in some patients by loiasis.*

Duke BOL: Studies on the chemoprophylaxis of loiasis. II. Observations on diethylcarbamazine citrate (Banocide) as a prophylactic in man. Ann Trop Med Parasitol 57:82, 1963. *The only published experience on the potential chemoprophylactic effects of diethylcarbamazine in human loiasis.*

418. *MANSONELLA OZZARDI* INFECTION

Eric A. Ottesen

M. ozzardi is restricted in distribution to Central and South America and certain islands of the Caribbean. Adult worms have been recovered in humans only twice, both times from the peritoneal cavity. *Unsheated* microfilariae circulate in the blood with little or no periodicity.

Many investigators consider these parasites to be non pathogenic, but in one of the fullest clinical studies of an affected population it was asserted that the major clinical presentation is severe articular pain or dysfunction, especially in the arms and shoulders. Headache, fever, pulmonary symptoms, adenopathy, hepatomegaly, and pruritic skin eruptions also occurred in a small number of patients with a frequency greater than that in nonparasitized individuals in the same population. Diethylcarbamazine* has little or no effect on this infection.

Marinkelle CJ, German E: Mansonelliasis in the comisaria del Vaupes of Columbia. Trop Geogr Med 22:101, 1970. *A very complete and interesting account of clinical manifestations ascribed to* M. ozzardi *infections in South American Indians.*

Weller PF, Simon HB, Parkhurst BH, Medrek FF: Tourism acquired *Mansonella ozzardi* microfilaremia in a regular blood donor. JAMA 240:858, 1978. *Evidence for the ineffectiveness of diethylcarbamazine in* M. ozzardi *infections.*

419. PERSTANS FILARIASIS

Eric A. Ottesen

Mansonella perstans (formerly *Dipetalonema perstans, Acanthocheilonema perstans*) is distributed in a broad belt across the center of Africa and in northeast South America. Adult worms, up to 70 to 80 mm long, reside in the body cavities (pleural, peritoneal, and pericardial) and in the mesentery, perirenal, and retroperitoneal tissues. Microfilariae are liberated *unsheathed* from the females and circulate in the blood without regular periodicity.

M. perstans infection was long thought to be asymptomatic, because up to 90 per cent of individuals with the parasite appeared to have no difficulty with it. Subsequent studies, however, indicate clearly that *M. perstans* is capable of inducing a variety of symptoms including angioedematous swellings much like the Calabar swellings of loiasis; fever; headache; pain in bursae and/or joint synovia, in serous cavities, or over the liver; neurologic or psychologic symptoms, and extreme exhaustion. There is some evidence that symptoms are more prominent in "outsiders" coming to endemic regions, but in all series at least a quarter of the patients were asymptomatic despite persistent microfilaremia.

Treatment with diethylcarbamazine* (5-6 mg per kilogram per day for two to three weeks) is often ineffective, with multiple courses usually necessary to achieve cure. When the parasites are eliminated, however, patients characteristically lose their symptoms (no matter how vague), lose their eosinophilia, and regain a sense of well-being.

Adolph PE, Kagan IG, McQuay RM: Diagnosis and treatment of *Acanthocheilonema perstans* filariasis. Am J Trop Med Hyg 11:76, 1962. *Results from a series of patients evaluated in the United States after returning from doing missionary work in Africa.*

Clarke V deV, Harwin RM, MacDonald DF, Green CA, Rittey DAW: Filariasis: *Dipetalonemia perstans* infections in Rhodesia. Cent Afr J Med 17:1, 1971. *Discussion of the clinical expression of* M. perstans *filariasis in Africans and Europeans living in East Africa.*

420. DIROFILARIASIS

Eric A. Ottesen

Dirofilaria species are filarial parasites mostly of dogs, cats, and raccoons that sometimes infect man but almost never fully develop to complete their life cycles in this abnormal host. The distribution of cases is worldwide and reflects the distribution of the parasites in animals.

Two general types of clinical presentation predominate. Pulmonary dirofilariasis, caused by the dog heartworm *D. imitis*, usually presents as an asymptomatic solitary pulmonary nodule ("coin lesion") but occasionally with chest pain, cough, or hemoptysis. Microscopically there is local eosinophilia and granuloma formation accompanied by infarction and thrombosis around an impacted, immature worm. The second common clinical presentation is that of a subcutaneous nodule found anywhere on the body (or within the eye) that results usually from infection with the subcutaneous dwelling filarids of dogs (*D. repens*) or raccoons (*D. tenuis*) but occasionally from infection with *D. immitis*. Local lesions again are granulomatous and eosinophilic and are sometimes accompanied by bacterial superinfection.

Definitive diagnosis and treatment most often result from the same surgical (excisional) procedure. Blood eosinophilia is not a regular finding in these patients nor are detectable antifilarial antibodies. Furthermore, since the worms are usually incompletely developed, microfilaremia occurs only in the rarest of circumstances. These "abnormal" parasite infections do not respond to diethylcarbamazine and their treatment is primarily surgical.

Dissanaike AS: Zoonotic aspects of filarial infections in man. Bull WHO 57:349, 1979. *A scholarly, readable discussion of man's interaction with zoonotic filarial infections.*

Gershwin LJ, Gershwin E, Kritzman J: Human pulmonary dirofilariasis. Chest 66:92, 1974. *Description of the 35th of the more than 100 cases now reported, with a good discussion.*

*Not commercially available in the United States but available in special circumstances from Lederle Laboratories.

*Not commercially available in the United States but available in special circumstances from Lederle Laboratories.

421. POSSIBLE HUMAN MENINGONEMIASIS

Eric A. Ottesen

According to Orihel, microfilariae recovered from patients with neurologic disorders in Rhodesia (now Zimbabwe) resemble *Meningonema peruzzii* (which inhabit the leptomeninges of the brainstem in African monkeys) more closely than *Dipetalonema perstans*.

Orihel TC: Cerebral filariasis in Rhodesia—a zoonotic infection. Am J Trop Med Hyg 22:596, 1973. *Evidence that microfilariae recovered from the cerebrospinal fluid are* M. peruzzii.

422. ONCHOCERCIASIS (River Blindness)

Brian O. L. Duke

Onchocerciasis is a disease of the skin and eye which follows infection with the filarial worm *Onchocerca volvulus*.

ETIOLOGY. Infection comes from the bites of female blackflies (buffalo gnats) of the genus *Simulium*, which transmit the infective larvae of the parasite. Over some 10 to 20 months these larvae grow to threadlike adult worms (males 5 cm; females, 50 cm), which live for up to 15 years tangled together in fibrous nodules under the skin, in the intermuscular fascial planes, and against the capsules of joints or the shafts of long bones. The adult females produce a continuous supply of live embryos or microfilariae, which have a life span of 12 to 24 months in the subepidermal layer of the skin and which may invade the eye, lymph glands, or other organs. Skin microfilariae ingested by biting *Simulium* develop in seven to ten days to infective larvae and can be transmitted to a new host.

PREVALENCE AND EPIDEMIOLOGY. Some 20 to 40 million people are infected with *O. volvulus*, mostly in tropical Africa south of the Sahara; there are also foci in Yemen, Guatemala, Mexico, Venezuela, Ecuador, Colombia, and Brazil.

Infections are mostly found in communities located within 10 to 20 km of fast-flowing water courses in which *Simulium* flies breed. The main vectors are *S. damnosum* s.l. and *S. neavi* s.l. in Africa, and *S. ochraceum* in Guatemala and Mexico. In many communities almost all the people are infected, and in some West African savanna villages 10 to 15 per cent of the whole population may be blind from onchocerciasis.

PATHOGENESIS AND PATHOLOGY. The nodules arise from a granulomatous and fibrous reaction in the host's tissues produced in response to the adult worms. Apart from being unsightly or inconvenient, they seldom cause clinical manifestations. Dead microfilariae in the tissues produce small granulomas infiltrated with eosinophils and leading to fibrosis. In the skin in acute cases this produces an itchy papular rash. Prolonged heavy infection leads to fibrosis, scarring of the papillae, replacement of dermal collagen by hyalinized scar tissue, and atrophic changes. In the eye similar reactions around microfilariae give rise to the inflammatory and scarring lesions in the cornea, anterior uvea, chorioretinal tissues, and optic nerve head, any of which can lead to blindness.

Onchocerciasis is a cumulative infection. Repeated inocula of infective larvae lead to intense infections both in terms of adult worms and microfilariae. The more intense the infection, the greater is the risk of severe lesions. The host's immune response to the parasite also influences the clinical picture.

CLINICAL MANIFESTATIONS. Cases presenting in temperate climates are likely to be light infections, probably newly acquired, in persons who have recently resided in an endemic area. Commonly there is an adult worm(s) near the limb girdle on one side. The microfilariae from this invade the skin locally, giving rise to a persistent itchy rash, which typically has a lopsided distribution (e.g., one leg and buttock, or one arm and shoulder). The rash is composed of discrete red papules 1 to 3 mm in diameter, but wheals, vesicles, scratch marks, and secondary infection may be superimposed. The skin fold on the affected side is thickened, the draining lymph glands are slightly enlarged, and there may be deep aches and pains in the limb concerned. Seldom can a nodule be palpated. Sometimes there is no rash, but the skin is thickened and lichenified and may itch. Such patients are unlikely to have more eye involvement than a few fluffy opacities (punctate keratitis) around microfilariae dying in the cornea.

Heavy and chronic onchocercal infection is likely only among natives of the endemic area. Palpable nodules may be abundant over bony prominences. In the skin gross lichenification and hyperpigmentation occur, giving way later to atrophy, "lizard skin," and mottled depigmentation (especially over the shins). The femoral and inguinal lymph glands enlarge. They may come to lie in pockets of loose skin (known as "hanging groins"), which predispose to hernia. In the eyes severe visual loss or blindness can result from (1) sclerosing keratitis; (2) chronic iridocyclitis with acute exacerbations, leading to secondary glaucoma; (3) chorioretinal lesions (typically the Hissette-Ridley fundus); or (4) postneuritic optic atrophy.

DIAGNOSIS. Definitive diagnosis depends on finding an adult worm in an excised nodule, or microfilariae in a skin snip, which should be taken from an area of affected skin or, failing that, from the iliac crest or calf (in Africa) or from the scapula (in America). A cone-shaped fold of skin is raised with a needle point and sliced off with a razor blade to give a bloodless piece of skin 2 to 3 mm in diameter. This is placed in normal saline and examined under the microscope, at 20- to 100-fold magnification, for microfilariae, which usually emerge within a few minutes to a few hours. Microfilariae may also be seen in the cornea or anterior chamber with a slit lamp. In lightly infected cases in which no microfilariae can be detected, a presumptive diagnosis often has to be made on clinical grounds, and the Mazzotti test (50 mg of diethylcarbamazine citrate* by mouth produces an exacerbation of itching and rash in the affected parts within 24 hours) is very useful. Eosinophilia and a positive filarial indirect fluorescent antibody or skin test are suggestive but not specific.

Differential diagnosis includes scabies, prickly heat, insect bites (especially *Culicoides*), contact dermatitis, and, rarely, streptocerciasis (see Ch. 423).

TREATMENT. Nodules on the head should always be removed because of extra danger to the eye, but removal of all palpable nodules will not result in cure. Treatment depends on chemotherapy with diethylcarbamazine citrate (DEC-C)* to kill the microfilariae, followed by suramin† to kill the adult worms, and then more DEC-C to mop up the residual microfilariae. The full course of treatment lasts two to three months and requires regular knowledgeable medical supervision on account of (1) the severe systemic and local reactions (in skin and eye) which may supervene as the microfilariae are killed by DEC-C and (2) the intrinsic toxicity of suramin.†

In all but the lightest cases DEC-C* should be given under corticosteroid "cover" (betamethazone 1 to 2 mg t.d.s. started two days before the DEC-C)* since there is always a danger of doing damage to the posterior segment of the eye in infected persons. DEC-C* may be started at 50 mg for an adult on the first day and increased to 100 mg on the second day and then to 200 mg daily for one week. Suramin† is best given weekly by intravenous injection according to the schedule 0.2 gram, 0.4 gram, 0.6 gram, 0.8 gram, 1.0 gram, 1.0 gram for a 60-kilogram adult.

PROGNOSIS. In the absence of reinfection the parasites will die out within 15 years, but signs and symptoms of disease will persist and may get worse during this period.

PREVENTION. There is no chemoprophylaxis. Personal prophylaxis consists of avoiding the haunts of *Simulium* and of wearing clothing that reduces the area of skin exposed to bites.

The larvae of *Simulium* are highly susceptible to regular

---

*Production of this drug in the United States has been discontinued.

†Available from Centers for Disease Control (404–329–3670 8:00 A.M. to 4:30 P.M. Monday through Friday; 404–329–2888 evenings, weekends, and holidays).

intermittent application of insecticides (currently Abate is used) to their aquatic breeding sites. Control of transmission of *O. volvulus* has been achieved in this way in the Volta River Basin in West Africa.

Buck AA (ed.): Onchocerciasis: Symptomatology, Pathology and Diagnosis. Geneva, World Health Organization, 1974. *Provides excellent photographs of skin and eye lesions.*

Epidemiology of Onchocerciasis. Report of a WHO Expert Committee. Geneva, World Health Organization, Technical Report Series NO 597, 1976. *Full account of epidemiology and diagnostic methods.*

Ledingham JGG, Warrell DA, Wetherall JJ (eds.): The Oxford Textbook of Medicine. 13th ed. Oxford, Oxford University Press, 1981. *Section on onchocerciasis gives detailed, up-to-date account of treatment.*

423. STREPTOCERCIASIS

Brian O. L. Duke

Mansonella streptocerca is transmitted by midges, especially *Culicoides grahamii*. It occurs in the tropical forest belt of Africa from Ghana to Zaire. The adult worms are subcutaneous, especially over the torso; and the microfilariae, which have shepherd's-crook tails, are found in the skin (see Ch. 422 for skin-snipping technique).

Infection is usually symptomless, but the adult worms may produce hypopigmented macules (to be distinguished from leprosy), and the microfilariae occasionally cause itching papular rashes similar to those of onchocerciasis. Both adult worms and microfilariae are killed by diethylcarbamazine citrate* (e.g., seven to ten days of treatment at 2 mg per kilogram three times daily for an adult).

Meyers WM, Connor DH, et al.: Human streptocerciasis: A clinicopathologic study of 40 Africans (Zairians) including identification of the adult filaria. Am J Trop Med Hyg 21:528, 1972. *Covers the clinical aspects and gives references to other aspects.*

*Production of this drug in the United States has been discontinued.

Section 3 ARTHROPODS AND ANIMAL POISONS

424. ARTHROPODS AND LEECHES

William L. Krinsky

ARTHROPODS AS AGENTS OF DISEASE

Disease associated directly with arthropods results from toxic or allergic responses to the organisms or their products when humans are exposed by bites or stings, simple contact, or invasion through the skin or natural orifices. Arthropods most often involved in these types of exposure are listed in Table 424–1.

Physicians usually become aware of insects and their relatives (spiders, mites, ticks, scorpions, millipedes, and centipedes) when patients present with skin lesions caused by arthropods, when infestations of the creatures themselves are seen, when foreign bodies extracted from skin or sense organs are identified as arthropods, or when respiratory symptoms develop in response to arthropods or their products. Dermatoses associated with arthropods and human infestations with arthropods (e.g., lice, mites, fly larvae) are discussed in detail in this chapter. Arthropods as vectors are mentioned here; detailed discussions of arthropod-borne pathogens may be found elsewhere in this book. Arthropods as sources of respiratory and skin allergens are discussed in Ch. 434.

TABLE 424–1. ARTHROPODS CAUSING HUMAN PATHOLOGY

Human Exposure	Arthropod	Antigens or Toxins
Bites	Insects (lice, bed bugs and other true bugs; fleas; flies including mosquitoes, black flies, biting midges, sand flies, horse and deer flies, stable flies, tsetse flies, keds; ants)	Salivary secretions, venoms
	Arachnids (chigger and other rodent and bird mites; ticks; spiders)	
	Centipedes	
Stings	Insects (some ants, wasps, and bees)	Venoms
	Arachnids (scorpions)	
Invasion	Insects (fly larvae, *Tunga* fleas)	Salivary secretions, excretions
	Arachnids (scabies mites)	
Simple contact	Insects (caterpillars, pupae or adults of moths and butterflies; blister and some rove beetles)	Setae, spines, secretions (venoms) and excretions
	Arachnids (stored product mites)	
	Millipedes	

Disease associated with fear of insects (entomophobia) or a preoccupation with an imagined infestation (delusory parasitosis) falls within the realm of psychiatry. However, diagnosis of the latter requires careful, repeated examinations by a physician in consultation with an entomologist to rule out an unusual infestation or the presence of microscopic arthropods or their products.

Canizares O: Clinical Tropical Dermatology. Oxford, Blackwell Scientific, 1975. *This text includes detailed clinical information about cutaneous lesions caused by arthropods.*

Harwood RF, James MT: Entomology in Human and Animal Health. 7th ed. New York, The Macmillan Company, 1979. *This is a comprehensive textbook that provides detailed references to the diverse arthropod-associated problems discussed here.*

Biting Arthropods

Louse Infestations (Pediculosis)

Pediculosis is infestation of the body with lice (small wingless, dorsoventrally flattened insects in the order Anoplura). Pruritus is the primary symptom of pediculosis, although some infestations are asymptomatic. Infested persons may be irritable and restless as a consequence of physical discomfort and lack of sleep. Louse eggs (nits) seen cemented to hairs of the scalp or the observation of lice themselves confirms the diagnosis of head lice (*Pediculus capitis*). Nits (or lice) attached to the seams of clothing (often in undergarments) indicate the presence of body lice (*Pediculus humanus*), and nits or lice attached to pubic hairs indicate a pubic (crab) louse (*Phthirus pubis*) infestation.

The eggs are pearly yellow-white and opaque, elongate-oval, about 0.8 mm long and 0.3 mm wide and are attached singly to each hair or clothing fiber. After hatching, the nits appear translucent and opalescent. Although nits may be numerous, usually not more than 10 to 20 lice are found on or associated with most infested persons. The head louse egg is cemented on a hair about 1 mm above the scalp surface. Because hair grows 0.4 to 0.6 mm a day and most eggs hatch within five to ten days after deposition, generally it can be assumed that nits attached over 7 mm from the surface are nonviable. Pseudopediculosis is a condition in which other materials such as dandruff, hair casts, dried sebaceous secretions, or solidified hair spray droplets mimic head louse infestation.

Head and body lice are very similar in appearance. Adult head lice are 2.5 to 3.5 mm long and adult body lice are 3 to 4.5 mm long. Immature and adult head and body lice each have three pairs of about equal-sized legs bearing claws for gripping hairs or fibers. Adult pubic lice, somewhat crablike in appearance, are 1 to 2 mm long, about as broad, grayish-white or yellowish-brown, and have forelegs narrower than the other pairs; all pairs have strong claws for gripping coarse hairs. All louse immatures (three stages in each species) resemble their respective adults except in size, and all immatures and adults are obligate bloodsucking ectoparasites. The body louse is the only known natural vector of the pathogens of louse-borne typhus, trench fever, and louse-borne relapsing fever.

Head lice and their nits are found most frequently in the hair over the postauricular and occipital regions. Body lice, although occasionally found on the body, are usually seen in clothing with nits in the seams and creases in areas that contact the body. Crab lice and nits are found on hairs in the pubic and perianal regions, sometimes on hairs on the thighs and abdomen, less commonly on axillary hairs, beard, mustache, eyebrows, eyelashes, and rarely on the margin of the scalp. Pubic infestations are found only in postpubertal individuals.

The skin lesions produced by the bites of lice are erythematous papules that may be accompanied by urticaria or lymphadenopathy. Extensive erythema and pruritus result from hypersensitivity to louse saliva that develops after repeated feedings. Crab lice typically induce nonpruritic small gray-blue macules (0.3 to 1 cm diameter) with irregular borders (maculae ceruleae) that may persist for months. The lesions produced by any of the species may be covered with hair matted with eggs, dried serous secretions, and dark louse excrement. The latter, seen on the body or in underclothing, should trigger a physician's search for lice. Excoriations from scratching further disguise original bite lesions and may lead to impetigo, furuncular, or eczematous lesions. The possibility of louse infestation should be considered when pyoderma is seen. The lichenification and pigmentation seen in chronically infested individuals is called vagabond's disease (*morbus vagabondus*). A nondescript macular or papular erythematous rash on the trunk may be the presenting sign for an undiscovered head louse infestation. Similarly, postauricular and posterior cervical lymphadenopathy in the absence of other node enlargement should be suspected as a sign of head lice. Body louse infestation may be differentiated from scabies (see later discussion) by the absence of lesions on the hands and feet and the common occurrence of lesions in the intrascapular region. The differential diagnosis of louse-induced dermatitis from various mite-induced lesions or nonarthropod-associated dermatoses is made by finding nits or lice.

Treatment for lice includes shampoos, creams, and lotions containing insecticides. The most often used preparations contain lindane (gamma benzene hexachloride) or pyrethrins with piperonyl butoxide. Malathion lotion has recently been approved for use in the United States. One effective treatment for head lice is a four-minute shampoo with about 25 ml of 1 per cent lindane shampoo. This may not be ovicidal; therefore, to ensure that subsequently emerging lice are killed, the treatment may be repeated seven to ten days later, or only if lice are seen. Patients infested with body lice or pubic lice may apply lindane (1 per cent) lotion or cream to affected areas. This should be thoroughly washed off six to eight hours later. A repeat application may be necessary. Infested clothing and linen should be washed in hot water (60° C) for 20 minutes or dry cleaned.

After being treated, lice and nits can be removed with a metal comb with teeth 0.1 mm apart. Moisture or oil rinses may make removal easier. Mechanical removal is recommended for facial pubic lice infestations. Lice and nits may be removed from eyelashes with a trachoma (roller) forceps. This may be followed by treatment with one of various pediculicide ointments, such as yellow oxide of mercury (1 to 2 per cent), pyrethrin in Vaseline (1:8), or petrolatum, applied twice a day for seven to ten days. Blepharitis and other secondary infections associated with lice may require specific antibiotic therapy.

Prevention of recurrence involves treatment of infested human contacts and materials (fomites). Pillow cases, hats, scarves, and other items with which a person with head lice had contact should be washed or cleaned as recommended for clothing. Infested combs and brushes should be cleaned and boiled or soaked for one hour in lindane shampoo or Lysol (2 per cent). Head and body lice will survive only about three days (ten days maximum) away from the body. Sexual partners of persons with pubic lice should be treated, and bedding, towels, and clothing contacted should be washed or dry cleaned. Pubic lice will not survive longer than 24 hours away from a body; transmission via toilet seats is unlikely. Fumigation after any louse infestation is unnecessary, but vacuuming is helpful to remove stray lice and shed hairs with affixed nits.

Domonkos AN, Arnold HL, Odom RB: Andrews' Diseases of the Skin. 7th ed. Philadelphia, W. B. Saunders Company, 1982, pp 554–557. *This text has excellent photographs of nits, lice, and skin lesions seen in pediculosis.*

Raber IM: Pediculosis ciliaris. *In* Parish LC, Nutting WB, Schwartzman RM (eds.): Cutaneous Infestations of Man and Animal. New York, Praeger, 1983, pp 138–143. *This is a lucid description of the clinical aspects and treatment of pubic louse infestation of the eyelashes.*

Witkowski JA, Parish LC: Pediculosis. *In* Parish LC, Nutting WB, Schwartzman RM (eds.): Cutaneous Infestations of Man and Animal. New York, Praeger, 1983, pp 125–137. *A concise, well-documented discussion of clinical louse infestations.*

Flea Bites

Most fleas, unlike lice, do not infest the body. The common flea species that suck blood from humans visit the body for a few minutes to hours, during which time feeding occurs. As in louse infestations, flea bites generally cause pruritus, although some bites are asymptomatic. Each bite lesion is an erythematous papule with a hemorrhagic punctum. Sensitization of an individual to flea saliva may result in papular urticaria (common in affected children), bullous eruptions, or erythema multiforme–type lesions. Bites are usually multiple and irregularly grouped. Commonly seen bites in adults appear as widespread papules that become lichenified, or as grouped papules overlying erythema or edema. Persons entering a previously infested room that has been vacant for weeks or months often suffer from multiple bites on the ankles and legs as hungry fleas, stimulated by a warm-blooded host, emerge from pupal cocoons that have laid dormant in floor crevices, debris, or carpeting. As with louse bites, excoriated lesions may become infected and furuncular.

Fleas are small (about 1.5 to 4 mm long), wingless, laterally flattened, brown to black, obligate bloodsucking, temporary ectoparasitic insects (order Siphonaptera). The eggs are usually laid off the host, and larvae (resembling some fly larvae) live off the host, feeding on organic debris. Adults reach their hosts by jumping. Flea species that most often bite humans are the cat flea (*Ctenocephalides felis*), the dog flea (*C. canis*), and somewhat less commonly the so-called human flea (*Pulex irritans*). Occasional household infestations with these and other fleas may arise from abandoned wild animal nests built near houses.

Treatment of flea bites is usually symptomatic and involves the use of antipruritic and anti-inflammatory creams or lotions, or oral antihistamines. Secondary infections may require antibiotic therapy. Infested pets should be treated with specific insecticide powders, sprays, mists, or dips. Floors, carpets, upholstered furnishings, and pets' sleeping quarters should be sprayed or dusted with insecticides to kill larval, pupal, and adult fleas. Thorough cleaning, including vacuuming, of infested premises should eliminate the insects. Because fleas at all stages can live for weeks or months, a repeat insecticide application may be necessary.

Persons may protect themselves from fleas with repellents containing dimethyl phthalate or diethyl metatoluamide. Wild animal (especially rodent) fleas that may feed on humans present the greatest health risks because of their potential to transmit the bacilli of plague or tularemia, as well as the less virulent rickettsia of murine (flea-borne) typhus. Less commonly seen pathogens that are transmitted by accidental ingestion of fleas (mostly by children) are the dwarf tapeworm *Hymenolepis diminuta* and the dog tapeworm *Dipylidium caninum*.

Bagnall B, Rook A: Arthropods and the skin. *In* Rook A (ed.): Recent Advances in Dermatology. No. 4. Edinburgh, Churchill Livingstone, 1977. *This review includes information about the ecology of fleas and pathogenesis and clinical features of infestations.*

Smit FGAM: Siphonaptera (Fleas). *In* Smith KGV (ed.): Insects and Other Arthropods of Medical Importance. London, British Museum (Natural History), 1973. *This is a careful overview of the medical importance of fleas.*

Bed Bugs and Kissing Bugs

Bed bugs (Cimicidae) are flat, mahogany brown, wingless insects (5 to 7 mm long). Most of the species are bloodsucking ectoparasites of birds and bats. Two species (*Cimex lectularius* and *C. hemipterus*) feed almost exclusively on humans; the former is cosmopolitan, the latter has a tropical distribution. Both species may cause irritating, pruritic bite lesions in sensitized individuals. The bugs become engorged with blood in 3 to 15 minutes and feed only at night or in subdued light. They hide in crevices of bedding, beds, floors, and furnishings and in wood and paper trash accumulations during the day. The bites are often seen in short linear groups and vary from small urticarial lesions to large erythematous papules or bullae. The lesions are often excoriated, and eczematous reactions and pyoderma may be seen. Hypersensitivity reactions may include asthma, generalized urticaria, and arthralgia. While some affected persons complain of being awakened at night, most are troubled by the lesions on arising in the morning. Treatment is symptomatic. Prevention includes removal of debris that harbors the bugs, use of insecticides in crevices and hiding places, and cleaning of bedding and infested furnishings.

Triatomine kissing bugs (Reduviidae) that suck blood from a diversity of hosts are found in the New World subtropics and tropics and in Asia. Most of these cone-nosed bugs (8 to 38 mm long) are tan, brown, or black, with yellow or red spots around the dorsal edge of the abdomen. The bugs feed rapidly at night and, like bed bugs, these insects and their bites often go unnoticed. Sensitive individuals may develop papular lesions, small vesicles or, in the extreme, large urticarial or hemorrhagic nodular to bullous lesions. Generalized anaphylactoid reactions including shock and angioneurotic and laryngeal edema have occurrred. Despite the name, kissing bugs may feed not only near the lips but anywhere on the body. Domesticated species in the tropics are found most often in thatched houses or those with mud floors. In the southwestern United States, a species (*Triatoma protracta*) living in wood rat nests in desert areas occasionally invades homes. Unlike bed bug-infested dwellings, those affected premises harbor only one or a few bugs. Treatment of bites or severe allergic reactions is symptomatic. The major medical problems associated with triatomine bugs occur in Central and South America, where these insects are vectors of Chagas' disease trypanosomes.

Crissey JT: Bedbugs—an old problem with a new dimension. Int J Dermatol 20:411, 1981. *This review article discusses bed bug biology and the possible role of these bugs in human disease.*

Ryckman RE: Host reactions to bug bites (Hemiptera, Homoptera): A literature review and annotated bibliography. Parts I, II. Calif Vector Views 26:Nos. 1–2, 1979. *This is an excellent source of specific references about all bugs that prey on humans.*

Mosquitoes and Other Bloodsucking Flies

Mosquitoes (Culicidae) are found throughout the world, breeding wherever there is stagnant water. While biting, a female mosquito (3 to 6 mm long) induces a pruritic wheal that becomes an erythematous papule within 24 hours of the bite. In very sensitive persons, bullous lesions, cellulitis, or hemorrhagic necrotic reactions may follow the bites. Systemic anaphylactic reactions are rare. The most serious medical problems associated with mosquitoes relate to their transmission of the agents of yellow fever, dengue, arboviral encephalitides, malaria, and filariasis.

Biting midges (Ceratopogonidae), also called punkies or no-see-ums because of their minute size (most are 0.6 to 2 mm long), give a painful bite that feels like an ember on the skin. The resulting erythematous punctiform lesions may become papular and pruritic. Vesicles may develop that ooze fluid for days. These midges, especially *Culicoides* species, bite mostly on exposed parts of the body and may be pestiferous in sandy seashore or marshy areas where they breed. Biting occurs mostly at dawn or dusk.

Black flies (Simuliidae), also called buffalo gnats, are small (1 to 5 mm long), humpbacked, tan to black insects that breed only in running water. They are troublesome bloodsuckers in northern temperate regions where they harass woodland visitors. The bites may become hemorrhagic papules that ooze blood for hours. These lesions may be painful and cause recurrent pruritus as well. Lymphadenopathy is common in sensitive individuals, who may develop localized edema. Cephalalgia, fever, and nausea have occurred in persons receiving large numbers of bites. Black fly species found at high elevations in Central and South America and along rivers in Africa are of greatest medical importance because they transmit *Onchocerca volvulus,* the etiologic agent of river blindness.

Phlebotomine sand flies (Psychodidae) are delicate, small (2 to 3 mm long), hairy flies that are found mainly in subtropical and tropical areas. Various species are abundant in rain forests in the New World and in arid areas in the Mediterranean region and Asia. Biting occurs at night or in subdued light. The bites, which may be painful, occur usually on the extremities and cause pruritus and elevated pale urticarial lesions that become papular. Vesicular or bullous lesions may occur. Phlebotomine flies are of major medical importance as vectors of the pathogens of sand fly (pappataci) fever, bartonellosis, and leishmaniasis.

Other flies that may attack man and cause painful bites are the robust horse and deer flies (Tabanidae), stable flies, and tsetse flies. Tsetse flies, found only in Africa, should be avoided because they transmit the trypanosomes of African sleeping sickness. Sheep keds (wingless flies) that infest the wool of sheep occasionally bite sheep farmers and handlers of fresh wool.

Treatment of any of these fly bites is symptomatic and often includes the use of topical corticosteroids and oral antihistamines to reduce itching. Personal protection from biting flies mostly involves avoidance of the insects by use of screen enclosures, headnets, and insect repellents. Protective clothing and open mesh jackets impregnated with repellents are effective.

Allen JR: Mosquitoes and other biting flies. *In* Parish LC, Nutting WB, Schwartzman RM (eds.): Cutaneous Infestations of Man and Animal. New York, Praeger, 1983, pp 344–355. *This is a concise, clearly presented review of pathogenesis and clinical aspects of fly bites.*

Chiggers and Other Biting Mites

Chiggers are the larvae (six-legged stage) of trombiculid (itch or harvest) mites. These larvae (0.15 to 0.40 mm long), which are white to yellow or orange-red, are found on a diversity of vertebrates. Human infestation occurs following contact with grassy or shrubby vegetation inhabited by the mites. First exposure may not produce dermatitis or may produce only slightly irritating, transient erythematous macules or papules (1 to 2 mm). The more commonly seen skin reactions to chigger feeding are extremely pruritic, papular, papulovesicular or papulourticarial lesions (4 to 20 mm) that may persist with burning and itching for days to weeks. The lesions may fade and flatten or become hemorrhagic, purpuric, or vesicular. Diagnosis is dependent upon morphology and distribution of lesions, exposure history, and observation of the mites. Engorging chiggers may be apparent as minute reddish blebs embedded in hair follicles. The mites most often attach to skin covered by clothing, especially near belts, straps, or elastic bindings. Scrub itch (a misnomer) mites of Asia and South Pacific Islands usually do not cause dermatitis, but they are of major medical concern as vectors of scrub typhus rickettsiae.

Other mites that bite man but that are rarely recovered from the lesions they cause are pyemotid (straw, hay, or grain itch) mites, cheyletiellid (cat and dog fur) mites, and dermanyssoid (chicken, red, house mouse, tropical rat, fowl, and rodent) mites. All of these mites are extremely small (about 0.4 to 1 mm long) and, depending on the species, the six-legged larvae or eight-legged nymphs and adults may attack man. The resulting skin lesions may be extremely variable.

Differential diagnosis of mite-induced dermatitis from other forms of pruritic eruptions usually depends on associating the patient with a source of mites. Sources include wild and domestic animals, agricultural commodities, infested furniture, and, in chigger-associated cases, particular outdoor activities or habitats.

Treatment of dermatitis associated with biting mites is symptomatic. Antipruritic topical lotions and creams or oral antihistamines are useful. Secondary infections caused by excoriations may require antibiotic therapy. Rare allergic reactions, including edema and asthma, require emergency treatment (see Ch. 434).

Prevention of recurrences is dependent on destruction or fumigation of the mite source. Personal repellents (containing sulfur or diethyl toluamide) are helpful in preventing chigger infestation, although avoidance of infested areas is the best prevention. *Rickettsia tsutsugamushi* is the only pathogen of major medical importance specifically associated with mite transmission. *R. akari*, the etiologic agent of rickettsialpox, is transmitted by the house mouse mite.

Krinsky WL: Dermatoses associated with the bites of mites and ticks (Arthropoda: Acari). Int J Dermatol 22:75, 1983. *This review includes a list of mites causing human dermatitis and discusses clinical findings.*

Parkhurst HJ: Trombidiosis (infestation with chiggers). Arch Dermatol Syphilol 35:1011, 1937. *This is an extensive review of the biology and clinical importance of chiggers.*

Tick Bites and Tick Paralysis

Ticks, like mites, are arachnids that have six-legged larvae and eight-legged nymphs and adults. Ticks, found worldwide, are grouped in two major families, soft ticks (Argasidae) and hard ticks (Ixodidae). The former, which have rugose integuments, are associated with restricted habitats, such as rodent burrows and bird nests, and rarely feed on humans. When they do, most attach for only a matter of minutes and produce maculate, erythematous lesions (6 to 30 mm in diameter). Some species in Africa cause extensive ecchymosis; pain, pruritus, edema, ulceration, and necrotic lesions have also been observed. The pajaroello (talaja) tick (*Ornithodoros coriaceus*), found in Mexico, California, and Oregon, is known to produce hemorrhagic, painful lesions. In Europe, bites of the pigeon tick (*Argas reflexus*) have caused dyspnea, nausea, and loss of consciousness. Soft ticks are of primary medical importance as vectors of the borreliae of relapsing fevers.

Hard ticks have smooth, hard, shiny integuments and are found on a diversity of animals and in tall grass and forests. Ticks carried on dogs, cats, or other animals sometimes drop off and attach to man. Hard ticks remain embedded in the skin for days while becoming engorged with blood, and usually do not cause pain or discomfort. Engorging ticks, mistakenly identified as pedunculated moles or warts, are usually noticed only by chance observation. Typical tick bite lesions are small indurations with peripheral erythema. Unusual manifestations of hard tick bites include various forms of nonspecific dermatitis, acrodermatitis chronica atrophicans, necrotic ulcers, and alopecia. Most hard ticks attach, feed, drop off, and are never noticed. Nodular lesions that may persist for years at the sites of bites must be differentiated from malignancies, such as lymphomas. Hard ticks are of major medical concern as vectors of the etiologic agents of various arboviral hemorrhagic fevers and encephalitides, several kinds of tick-borne typhus (including Rocky Mountain spotted fever), tularemia, babesiosis, and Lyme disease. An engorging tick itself may induce tick paralysis (discussed below).

Attached soft ticks may be easily removed by gentle traction with a forceps. Hard ticks, usually more deeply embedded, require strong constant traction. Use of heat, flames, or caustic substances is ill-advised and may cause unnecessary damage to the patient. Hard ticks embedded in sensitive sites, such as the ear canal or genitals, may be covered with petrolatum. The ticks then detach within about two hours and can be gently removed. Complete extraction of the mouthparts lessens the chance of secondary infection. Persistent nodules that cause discomfort should be surgically excised.

Tick paralysis is an unusual form of ascending flaccid paralysis that may occur while a tick is attached to the body. Mostly children (especially girls) are affected. Tick paralysis in humans has been associated with only a small number of hard tick species but has been observed in North America, Europe, South Africa, and Australia. Most cases have been caused by female wood ticks, the Rocky Mountain wood tick (*Dermacentor andersoni*) in western North America, and the common dog tick (*D. variabilis*) in eastern North America, but only rare individuals, which are indistinguishable from other ticks of the same species, induce paralysis. Although nonspecific numbness or irritability may occur before the onset of paralysis, the initial consistent sign is *weakness in the legs*. Leg tendon reflexes are reduced or absent and Romberg's sign is often present. Sensory changes are rarely noted. Blood counts and lumbar puncture usually give no indication of the disease. Complete paralysis of the extremities may occur within a few days after a tick attaches. If the cause is unrecognized, paralysis usually progesses causing speech dysfunction, dysphagia, and ultimately death from aspiration or respiratory paralysis. If a tick is found, removal usually results in reversal of paralysis with a return to normal function in hours to weeks, depending on the severity of the neurologic deficit. The patient should be examined for other ticks, with special attention to concealed areas such as the scalp, ear canals, axillae, popliteal fossae, anus, and genitals. Even after all ticks are removed, death may occur in patients who exhibit bulbar or respiratory paralysis. A different form of paralysis is seen in Australia, where severe paralysis occurs about two days after the causative tick, *Ixodes holocyclus*, is removed. Supportive therapy usually leads to recovery after days to weeks.

The clinical presentation of tick paralysis may suggest poliomyelitis, Guillain-Barré syndrome, diphtheritic polyneuropathy, transverse myelitis, botulism, or other acutely developing neuropathies. The specific etiologic agent and mechanisms for the reduction in maximal motor nerve conduction velocities and decreased nerve action potentials seen in *Dermacentor* tick paralyses are unknown. A toxin isolated from *I. holocyclus* causes paralysis in dogs that is reversible with antiserum, but no substance or pathogen has been found in other tick species that induces paralysis in experimental animals or that is associated with human tick paralysis.

Prevention of tick bites and tick paralysis includes avoidance of tick-infested habitats. Individuals and their pets who enter such habitats should be thoroughly examined for crawling or attached ticks. Personal measures that may prevent ticks from reaching the skin include wearing long-sleeved shirts and long pants, tucking pants legs into socks, and using chemical repellents.

Gothe R, Kunze K, Hoogstraal H: The mechanisms of pathogenicity in the tick paralyses. J Med Entomol 16:357, 1979. *This review lists the tick species that have been associated with paralysis, general clinical aspects and experimental observations.*

Krinsky WL: Dermatoses Associated with the Bites of Mites and Ticks (Arthropoda: Acari). Int J Dermatol 22:75, 1983. *This is a review of skin lesions caused by acarines and epidemiologic and clinical factors helpful in diagnosis.*

Spider Bites

All spiders are eight-legged arachnids that use venom to immobilize their prey. Relatively few species have mouthparts (chelicerae) large and strong enough to inject venom into human skin. Among the better known spiders that cause moderate to severe reactions in man are the widows (*Latrodectus* species) of the Old and New Worlds, brown spiders (*Loxosceles* species) of the Americas, wandering spiders (*Phoneutria* species) and wolf spiders (*Lycosa* species) in South America, species of *Chiracanthium* in both hemispheres, funnel web spiders (*Atrax* species) in Australia, and *Harpactirella* species in South Africa.

The black widow (shoe button) spider (*Latrodectus mactans*) female may bite if it or its web is disturbed. Its abdomen is 6 mm wide and 9 to 13 mm long and is shiny black with a reddish hourglass marking or less well-defined markings on the underside. The spider lives in sheltered, dark, dry places such as corners of garages and in old stone walls and outhouses. The bite, which may not be felt, may become slightly swollen and appear as two erythematous puncture marks. Within a few hours, a bitten person develops intense muscle pains and commonly a tightening feeling in the chest. Abdominal (board-like) rigidity and waves of excruciating cramping pain are characteristic. Respiratory distress, nausea, vomiting, profuse perspiration, headache, vertigo, paresthesias of the extremities, and hyperactive reflexes are common. Speech difficulty and visual dysfunction may occur. The clinical presentation reflects the generalized neurotoxic effects of the venom that stimulates central, peripheral, and autonomic nerve activity. In untreated adults, the pathologic effects of the venom usually disappear within two to three days. Death from cardiac or respiratory arrest occurs mostly in very young children and elderly or hypertensive persons.

Differential diagnosis requires consideration of various abdominal and cardiovascular crises, such as perforated ulcer, acute appendicitis or pancreatitis, cholelithiasis, nephrolithiasis, splenic, renal, or mesenteric embolism, volvulus, porphyria, tetanus, and strychnine and lead poisoning. The generalized muscle pain, lack of abdominal tenderness, and the peripheral sensory changes help to differentiate widow spider bite from these other diseases.

Treatment with muscle relaxants, such as intravenous injection of 10 ml of 10 per cent calcium gluconate, temporarily relieves muscle pains. A specific antivenin available from Merck, Sharp and Dohme is effective against all *Latrodectus* venom and neutralizes the effects of the venom. Because the antivenin is derived from horses, horse serum sensitivity testing is required before the antivenin is administered.

The brown (violin or fiddleback) spiders, including *Loxosceles reclusa* (brown recluse) and *L. laeta* of the western hemisphere, are also secretive, living in secluded places in houses and nesting in clothing, and may bite when disturbed. They are 10 to 15 mm long and have a dark violin-shaped mark on the brown to gray cephalothorax. Their bites may cause only mild skin reactions but are most often recognized when a more serious condition, *necrotic arachnidism,* is the result. The sometimes painful lesion that develops two to six hours after a bite is a bulla or pustule surrounded by concentric rings of ischemia and erythema. Within 24 to 48 hours the lesion becomes cyanotic, and a central necrotic area begins to form. This area may slowly expand (up to 20 cm) over days to weeks. The resulting ulcer may not heal for weeks or months. Tissue destruction is thought to result from the enzyme activity of the venom and, possibly, venom activation of complement. Systemic reactions to the bite include fever, chills, edema, nausea, vomiting, dizziness, myalgias, and arthralgias; morbilliform and petechial eruptions may occur within 48 hours of the bite. A fatal complication, most often seen in children, is *intravascular hemolysis,* followed by hemoglobinuria and acute renal failure.

Treatment of necrotizing lesions is mainly symptomatic and may include surgical debridement and antibiotic therapy for secondary infection. Systemic corticosteroid therapy has been successful in reducing symptoms and skin destruction. Skin grafts may be needed to promote healing of chronic lesions.

Phoneutria (wandering) spiders often enter houses and may bite, causing intense pain, visual disturbance, tremors, profuse sweating, convulsions, priapism, tachycardia, and respiratory distress. Wolf spiders (*Lycosa* species) may produce painful but localized bite reactions. Specific treatment for *Phoneutria* and *Lycosa* bites is administration of antivenins available from the Butantan Institute, Sao Paulo, Brazil.

Chiracanthium species may bite producing erythema, edema, and pruritus. Necrotic lesions thought to be caused by these spiders may be confused with those of *Loxosceles* species. The mygalomorph funnel-web spiders (*Atrax* species) and *Harpactirella* spiders are aggressive and produce painful bites that have resulted in death.

Maretic Z, Lebez D: Araneism with Special Reference to Europe. Belgrade, Yugoslavia, Nolit Publishing House, 1979. *This book has extensive clinical information about* Latrodectus *envenomation and biological and clinical discussions relevant to other spider bites.*

Millikan LE: Loxoscelism and other arachnid problems. *In* Parish LC, Nutting WB, Schwartzman RM (eds.): Cutaneous Infestations of Man and Animal. New York, Praeger, 1983, pp 284–295. *This chapter includes excellent photographs of the necrotic lesions caused by recluse spider bites and a discussion of pathophysiology and treatment.*

Southcott RV: Arachnidism and Allied Syndromes in the Australian Region. Rec Adelaide Child Hosp 1:99, 1976. *This detailed review treats basic biology and clinical aspects of arachnid bites and infestations and is relevant to much of the world's fauna.*

Centipede Bites

Centipedes are multi-legged, elongated (up to 30 cm) arthropods with one pair of legs on each body segment. The first pair of legs is modified as poison claws that are used to inject venom into prey. Centipedes shun the light and are found under rocks and forest litter. The characteristic lesion resulting from a bite has two punctate hemorrhages in the center of an erythematous swelling. Centipede bites may cause severe (fiery) local pain that may be followed by inflammation, edema, and superficial necrosis. Systemic reactions may include headache, dizziness, and vomiting. The transient effects of a bite may be accompanied by irregular pulse, muscle spasm, or lymphadenopathy. There are a few reports of children dying from the bites of large tropical species, but their reliability has been questioned. Treatment is symptomatic and despite the venomous nature of these creatures, they rarely bite because of their nocturnal habits and tendency to escape when uncovered or disturbed during the day. In general, centipede bites cause few or no long-term pathologic effects.

Southcott RV: Arachnidism and allied syndromes in the Australian region. Rec Adelaide Child Hosp 1:99, 1976. *This includes a careful review (pp 174–177) of clinical aspects of centipede bites and some case histories.*

Stinging Arthropods

Bee, Wasp, and Ant Stings

Bees, wasps, and ants (order Hymenoptera) are insects that include solitary and social species that have females in which the egglaying tube (ovipositor) has been modified as a sting that secretes venom from abdominal glands. Solitary species rarely sting humans and their stings usually cause only minor pain or discomfort. The social bees that include honeybees and bumblebees all have two pairs of membranous wings, are stocky, hairy, and often colored with yellow and black or brown. The honeybee (*Apis mellifera*) and its various racial forms and close relatives are found worldwide and often are responsible for human sting reactions. Unlike other Hymenoptera, the honeybee has a barbed sting that becomes embedded in skin and, as the bee tries to escape, it leaves its venom apparatus and other abdominal organs and soon perishes. Social wasps include vespid wasps (yellowjackets, hornets, paper wasps) that are smooth insects sleeker than bees and often colored yellow and black, or with combinations of yellow, red, brown, or black. These wasps make the paper nests often found in trees, under eaves of houses, or underground. Honeybees and bumblebees may sting when accidentally disturbed while seeking nectar or pollen at flowers. Vespid wasps may become pestiferous around foodstuffs, being especially attracted to sweet or fermented liquids, fruit, and meats. Mutillid wasps (velvet ants, cow killers), which are hairy and wingless, sometimes sting persons in sandy, arid environments.

Human reactions to stings usually include intense local pain, followed by the appearance of a red punctum surrounded by a blanched area and erythema. A wheal forms and the swelling and erythema, accompanied by pruritus, may last for a few hours. Multiple stings, especially on the face, may cause more extensive edema, severe skin lesions such as multiple vesicles or bullae, or purpura that results from the hemolytic and anticoagulant properties of wasp venoms. Treatment includes gentle removal of the sting by scraping with a sharp blade (in cases of honeybee envenomation), application of ice, and topical hydrocortisone or oral antihistamines. Severe and sometimes fatal allergic reactions to stings of bees and wasps that occur in sensitized individuals are discussed in Ch. 434.

Ants (Formicidae) of some species can sting, causing severe pain. Two notable groups of New World stinging ants are the fire ants (*Solenopsis* species) and harvester ants (*Pogonomyrmex* species). Fire ants build ground nests that protrude as large mounds. Persons that encounter the ants are readily stung. Each ant grips the skin with its mandibles and then inserts its sting. The ant may pivot and sting many times. This behavior, compounded by the common occurrence of mass attacks, leads to a clustering of lesions. The usual reaction to the sting is fiery, sharp pain, followed by a wheal and flare response. Within hours, a clear vesicle appears that becomes pustular after about 24 hours. This sterile pustule may persist for three to ten days and dry as a crust that sloughs, leaving a macule, scar, or fibrous nodule. Systemic reactions such as dizziness, nausea, vomiting, profuse perspiration, cyanosis, and asthma usually occur in allergic individuals, but may also be seen in cases of multiple stings. Harvester ants also make mound nests and cause similar local sting reactions. Symptomatic treatment of local reactions is similar to that for bee and wasp stings. Treatment of allergic reactions is discussed in Ch. 434.

Harwood RF, James MT: Venoms, defense secretions, and allergens of arthropods. *In* Entomology in Human and Animal Health. 7th ed. New York, The Macmillan Company, 1979. *This is a review of the biology and clinical importance of stinging Hymenoptera.*

Rhoades RB, Schafer WL, Schmid WH, et al.: Hypersensitivity to the imported fire ant. A report of 49 cases. J Allergy Clin Immunol 56:84, 1975. *This is a detailed review of clinical data and treatment of fire ant stings.*

Scorpion Stings

Scorpions are mostly subtropical and tropical arachnids that have a pair of lobster-like claws (pedipalps) anteriorly and a curved spine posteriorly that is an outlet for the proteinaceous venom produced by a pair of venom glands. Scorpions are nocturnal predators and will sting man quickly and repeatedly when disturbed in their hiding places under rocks, lumber, vegetation or in materials such as shoes, bedding, or clothing left on the ground. In the United States only one scorpion species, *Centruroides sculpturatus*, of about 40 native species causes severe pathologic effects in humans. This small (about 6 cm long), straw-colored species is found only in Arizona. In Mexico, six species of *Centruroides* sting humans and cause serious envenomation. In Trinidad, *Tityus trinitatis* is of medical importance. In South America, this species and five others in the genus as well as one *Centruroides* species cause severe sting reactions. The arid regions that extend from North Africa to India are inhabited by the most abundant and dangerous scorpions.

The nature and severity of human reactions to scorpion stings are not consistent with the size, appearance, or aggressiveness of different species, so that closely related scorpion species may elicit disparate pathologic reactions. Intense and immediate pain at the site of a sting is common to all cases. When a mildly toxic scorpion such as *C. vittatus*, a common southern United States species, is involved, the pain may be followed by local swelling and perhaps skin discoloration, regional lymphadenopathy, pruritus, or paresthesias, and less commonly by nausea and vomiting. These reactions are transient, lasting for only minutes to as long as 24 hours. The more toxic species cause similar local pain but little or no skin response, and systemic effects are usually noted within a few minutes to 24 hours after the sting. The neurotoxic venoms of these species have cholinergic and adrenergic effects and may be hemolytic. Symptoms may include anxiety, drowsiness, syncope, increased salivation, lacrimation, and perspiration, diminished vision, photophobia, numbness and sluggishness of the tongue, vomiting, diarrhea or involuntary defecation and micturation, priapism, muscular fibrillations or spasms, and convulsions. Clinical signs may include hypotension or hypertension, irregular pulse, tachycardia and arrythmias, irregular respiration, rapid shifts in body temperature, oliguria or polyuria, and hemiplegia. Laboratory tests may reveal hyperglycemia, glycosuria, SGOT elevation, hematuria, and melena. Severe pathologic changes that may lead to death include myocarditis, pulmonary edema, and shock. Respiratory paralysis is the usual immediate cause of death. In the most toxic cases, death may occur within minutes of the sting or not for over 40 hours later, but most deaths occur in 2 to 20 hours after the sting. The mortality rate is highest in children. Close monitoring of affected patients is important because sudden relapses, often involving acute respiratory distress, may occur after a patient's condition seems to have stabilized.

Treatment of the least toxic stings is symptomatic and often includes application of ice and a local anesthetic to the sting site. The most important treatment for moderate to very toxic stings is administration of an antivenin. Antivenin to *C. sculpturatus* is available in Arizona from the Antivenom Production Laboratory, Arizona State University, Tempe, Arizona 85281 (602-965-3116; outside of business hours 602-965-3456; ask for Dr. William Northey). Antivenins against other species are available from laboratories in Mexico, Brazil, Turkey, Algeria, Egypt, and South Africa (addresses listed in Keegan, 1980).

Early treatment of these stings should include cooling of the sting site for up to two hours and, if the sting is on an extremity, use of a tourniquet for five to ten minutes. Oxygen administration or artificial respiration, sodium phenobarbitol injection, and parenteral solutions, including blood plasma, may be needed to treat respiratory distress, convulsions, and shock, respectively. Calcium gluconate (10 ml of 10 per cent solution) given as a slow intravenous injection will reduce muscle spasms. In the United States, morphine and meperidine are contraindicated because they enhance the toxic effects of *C. sculpturatus* venom. Morphine and barbiturates are not recommended for treatment of any scorpion stings because these drugs inhibit the bulbar respiratory centers.

Personal prevention against stings includes wearing heavy gloves and boots when reaching into hidden areas or when moving materials in which scorpions may hide. Shaking out shoes and other materials left on the ground before using them is essential. Removal of litter from around houses, sealing cracks in foundations, and selective use of pesticides are helpful means of preventing scorpions from inhabiting houses and gardens.

Keegan HL: Scorpions of Medical Importance. Jackson, University of Mississippi Press, 1980. *This book reviews scorpion morphology, taxonomy, biology, and geographic distribution, and clinical aspects and prevention of scorpion envenomation.*

Invasive Arthropods

Scabies

The scabies mite (*Sarcoptes scabiei*), unlike the other mites discussed, burrows into the skin and, because it reproduces on humans, can maintain a continuous infestation. Fertile female mites burrow into the skin and lay their eggs as they tunnel. Individuals of the resulting immature stages (larvae and nymphs) move out to the surface and rapidly enter hair follicles. Further development and mating takes place near the skin surface. The mite burrows are slightly raised, curved, or tortuous gray lines, 5 to 15 mm long, and at the end of each is a female, a minute pearly bleb. The burrows are restricted to the horny layer of the skin and occur most often in the sides of the fingers, the interdigital webs, flexor surfaces of the wrists, elbows, skin around the nipples, and penis. Other lesions, including erythematous papules, lichenified patches, and pustules, which occur in sites other than the burrows, may be seen on the abdomen, thighs, and buttocks. In infants and young children, burrows may occur in the palms and soles, and papular lesions may be seen on the scalp, face, and neck.

Intense pruritus that begins from two to six weeks after first exposure to the mite is presumably an allergic response to the mite or its products. Definitive diagnosis of the lesions is often difficult because of excoriations. In very clean individuals, few lesions may be present and burrows may not be clearly visible. Generalized urticarial papules may result from previous treatment with fluorinated corticosteroids. Some patients have pruritic inflammatory nodules ($\leq$ 12 mm in diameter) that occur on covered skin, especially the axillae, abdomen, scrotum, and penis. A severe form of scabies most often seen in immunologically compromised persons is called *crusted scabies* (originally called Norwegian scabies). As the name implies, warty plaques occur frequently on the hands and feet and extensive scaling covers the scalp to the trunk or below. Horny debris collects under the fingernails, which are usually distorted and thickened. Pruritus, erythema, and lymphadenopathy may occur to varying degrees.

Diagnosis of any scabies infestation depends on observation of a mite in skin scrapings of a burrow or in situ, by gently raising the top of a burrow with a sterile needle and looking with a magnifier. In most scabies cases, only 10 to 15 mites are present on the body. In crusted scabies, large numbers of mites (possibly more than a million) are present. To obtain a scraping of a burrow, an area suspected of infestation is scraped with a scalpel blade. The scraped material is examined at 50 to 100 times magnification. The movements of a living mite may be observed if the material is placed on a slide without any mounting media. Otherwise, the scraping may be cleared in a drop of potassium hydroxide (20 per cent) or suspended in mineral oil under a coverslip on the slide. The adult female mite is about 300 to 400 μm long, oval, with the dorsum convex and venter flattened. It has four pairs of legs, two pairs directed anteriorly and two posteriorly. Each anterior leg ends in an unjointed stalk with a distensible thin-walled sac at its tip; each posterior leg ends in a long, thick bristle. The size of the mite egg is about 100 × 150 μm.

Scabies lesions initially may be diagnosed as those of other skin conditions, e.g., neurodermatitis, dermatitis herpetiformis, lichen planus, and various other kinds of mite-associated dermatitis, such as that caused by *Cheyletiella* fur mites. The distribution of lesions and finally the observation of the mite will rule out these other diagnoses. Secondary infections appearing as pyoderma are common and nephrogenic strains of streptococci infecting the lesions may cause acute glomerulonephritis.

Treatment of uncomplicated scabies involves application of one of various acaricide lotions or creams. Lindane (1 per cent) is often used in a manner similar to that suggested for pediculosis; namely, a 6- to 12-hour treatment for adults and a 6-hour application for children, followed by thorough washing. The treatment should not be repeated more than once in seven days. Pruritus and dermatitis may persist for days after adequate treatment. Antipruritic medications such as antihistamines and Schamberg's lotion are often prescribed. Topical corticosteroids are contraindicated because of the urticarial reaction they sometimes cause.

Transmission occurs during contact with infested persons or with clothing recently worn by such persons. Transmission between bed partners is common and does not require bodily contact. All household and intimate contacts should be treated to prevent recurrence or continued transmission. The female mite will survive for only two to three days away from a host; therefore, as with louse infestations, fumigation of premises is unnecessary. Clothing, especially undergarments, bedding, and towels, should be laundered in hot water.

Scabies mites infesting domestic animals, including dogs and cats, occasionally cause dermatitis in man, but the lesions are usually limited to the areas that contact the animals. These mites are usually not recovered from humans.

Mellanby K: Scabies. Middlesex, England, E. W. Classey (1943), 1972. *This classic work available in this reprinted form is a comprehensive review of the basic biology, clinical evolution, and treatment of scabies.*

Parish LC, Nutting WB, Schwartzman RM (eds.): Scabies—Part II. *In* Cutaneous Infestations of Man and Animal. New York, Praeger, 1983, pp 53–109. *Several concise chapters give a clear and thorough review of the biology and clinical aspects of scabies.*

Myiasis and Tungiasis

Myiasis is the infestation of living vertebrate tissue by fly larvae. Many flies (order Diptera) that normally deposit eggs or larvae on carrion, manure, or decaying organic matter sometimes deposit their immature stages in open wounds or infected human tissues. These include blow flies, also called greenbottle or bluebottle flies (Calliphoridae), flesh flies (Sarcophagidae), and house flies (Muscidae). The larvae of some of these flies are attracted to draining infections, or clothing stained with urine or feces. The larvae crawl into lesions or natural orifices when an infected person sleeps on the ground or is otherwise exposed to flies. Individuals immobilized because of physical illness or old age who have such open lesions or infections, and especially those who are living in poor sanitary conditions, are particularly susceptible. Urogenital myiasis may cause dysuria, hematuria, and pyuria.

The sheep bot fly (*Oestrus ovis*) sometimes larviposits in the nose, ears, or eyes of sheep herders, who may develop external ophthalmitis from the migration of the larvae over the conjunctival surfaces. Other flies always oviposit in wounds. The screw worm fly (*Cochliomyia hominivorax*) of cattle in the southern United States and Mexico may oviposit on humans and is such a species. Other fly larvae always invade intact skin of domestic animals or man; species in this group include the human bot fly (*Dermatobia hominis*) found in Central and South America, the African Tumbu fly *Cordylobia anthropophaga*, and some species of *Wohlfahrtia* that have a predilection for the tender skin of infants. Larvae of cattle warble flies (*Hypoderma* species) and horse stomach bot flies (*Gasterophilus* species) may accidentally infest man and crawl about subcutaneously causing a creeping eruption that appears as erythematous, serpentine lesions or painful swellings.

Fly larvae that live in foodstuffs or organic detritus, e.g., vinegar flies (Drosophilidae) and cheese skippers (Piophilidae), are sometimes accidentally ingested and may cause gastrointestinal discomfort.

Wound or dermal myiasis often results in furuncular lesions, and an infested individual notices a swelling and feels pain or movement under the skin where the larvae are feeding on tissue fluids. Careful observation of the top of a lesion enables one to see two dark respiratory openings (spiracles) through which the larva breathes. Treatment consists of removal of the larvae by gentle compression of the swelling and pulling a larva out with a forceps. A local anesthetic may be helpful because the recurved spines that hold many larvae tightly under the skin may make removal difficult and painful. Topical antibiotics are used to control or prevent secondary infections. Removal of larvae that crawl into sensory openings or urogenital and anal orifices may require irrigation or surgical intervention, as may treatment of ophthalmomyiasis. Intestinal myiasis is usually self-limited, ceasing when the larvae are passed in the stool. Dermal myiasis of most kinds, if untreated, progresses until the mature larvae back out of the skin and drop to the ground to pupate. The physical and emotional distress caused by the presence of living larvae can be prevented if a physician considers the possibility of such an infestation and removes the larvae early in the infestation. Warble fly larvae, which normally migrate from the legs of cattle through the body to the back, in human infestations will also migrate dorsally and, unless they reach a cutaneous exit site, may cause extensive tissue damage that leads to chronic illness or death.

Prevention of myiasis requires use of frequently changed dressings on wounds and infections, and personal protection from flies such as screening or changes in behavior related to outdoor activities and eating habits. Use of eye protection in sheep bot fly areas is advisable.

Tungiasis is the infestation of vertebrate, including human, skin by the female flea *Tunga penetrans* (chigoe, jigger, or sand flea). This flea occurs in sandy soil in subtropical and tropical regions of the Americas, the West Indies, and Africa. It usually feeds between the toes, under a toenail, or in the sole of the foot, and becomes embedded as it gorges on blood. By eight to ten days after the flea begins feeding, it has grown to ≥5 mm from its original 1 mm size and it begins to release eggs through the skin opening. The flea, which remains embedded permanently, may cause irritation, pain, or pruritus, and the resulting swelling is often pustular. Secondary infections, including cellulitis and tetanus, are complications of infestations, and autoamputation of digits in Africans is apparently caused by inflammatory reactions to the flea.

Treatment of tungiasis includes removal of the flea with a sterile needle or pointed blade, tetanus vaccination, and application of topical antibiotics. Sometimes curettage is required to remove the flea, feces, or eggs retained in the skin. Personal protection against *T. penetrans* includes wearing footwear and using insect repellent. Because the flea is a poor jumper, sleeping above the ground surface usually prevents the flea from reaching the body.

Brothers W, Heckmann R: Tungiasis (*Tunga penetrans*) in Utah. J Parasitol 65:782, 1979. *This note succinctly describes the clinical problem and gives references to recent cases.*

Harwood RB, James MT: Myiasis. *In* Entomology in Human and Animal Health. New York, The Macmillan Company, 1979. *This is a thorough review of different clinical forms of myiasis.*

Arthropods and Contact Dermatitis

Various species of nonbiting mites found in stored products may cause dermatitis when they contact human skin. These microscopic foodstuff mites (Acaridae, Glycyphagidae) are found in various commodities including grains, cereals, seeds, bulbs, dried herbs, copra, dried vegetables, cured meats, mushrooms, humus, cheese, and animal and plant material used for stuffing furniture, pillows, and mattresses. Dried fruit mites (Carpoglyphidae) are found not only in various dried fruits but also in jams, jellies, spoiled fruit, wine, caramel, flour, and dried milk products. The skin reactions to these mites vary with the extent of exposure and host differences, but pruritic diffuse erythema with urticarial wheals or erythematous papular eruptions with each papule surmounted by a small vesicle are common. Laborers in granaries, food processing plants, and commercial kitchens and dockworkers are most susceptible.

Another form of pruritic dermatitis is caused by contact with various caterpillars, pupae, adults, and less often egg masses of moths and butterflies (order Lepidoptera). Urticating setae and spines on these life stages may cause mechanical irritation of the skin or may have toxic effects. Venomous materials are sometimes extruded from setae and spines connected to poison glands. Some of these toxins contain histamine and proteolytic enzymes. Mechanical or chemical irritation is often enhanced by barbs on the setae, which cause these structures to become tightly embedded in the skin. Dermatitis may result when setae or spines are touched or when people contact those that have become airborne around large infestations of the insects. Contact with setae, spines, or hairs from these caterpillars may cause intense stinging or fiery pain, followed by the formation of wheals, local edema, erythema, and pruritus. Less common reactions include lymphadenopathy, cephalalgia, shocklike symptoms, or convulsions.

Treatment of dermatitis caused by foodstuff and dried fruit mites or lepidopteran spines or setae is mainly symptomatic. Antipruritic substances including antihistamines, corticosteroids, and anesthetics have been used. Calcium gluconate (10 ml of a 10 per cent solution) given intravenously provides relief from the intense pain following contact with puss caterpillars (Megalopygidae). Specific treatment involves removal of the source of irritants. Commodities containing mites must be fumigated or destroyed. Spines or setae of lepidopterans may be removed from the skin with fine forceps. Use of protective clothing and thorough washing of exposed materials will help prevent continuation of these forms of dermatitis.

A third form of contact dermatitis results from vesicants produced by blister beetles (Meloidae) and some rove beetles (Staphylinidae). Cantharidin, first isolated from the meloid called the Spanish fly, is found in all species of blister beetles. This substance causes the mild to severe vesicular dermatitis that results when these beetles or their secretions are touched. The worldwide staphylinid genus *Paederus* contains more than 30 species that cause vesication.

Similar lesions, which usually follow a burning sensation and tanning of the skin, result from contact with defensive secretions of millipedes. Some species of these otherwise harmless herbivorous myriapods exude a fluid from pores along the length of the body. Secretions from the aforementioned beetles or millipedes will cause burning pain and conjunctivitis if they are rubbed into the eyes.

Treatment of toxic dermatitis associated with beetles or millipedes includes rapid washing of the skin or eyes, if affected, and use of local anesthetics. The dermal reactions caused by contact with mites, lepidopterans, beetles, and millipedes are usually transitory and do not have long-lasting effects.

Harwood RB, James MT: Vesicating Coleoptera. *In* Entomology in Human and Animal Health. New York, The Macmillan Company, 1979, pp 441–443. *This section discusses the nature of vesicant chemicals from beetles and reviews clinical cases.*

Radford AJ: Millipede burns in man. Trop Geogr Med 27:279, 1975. *Geographical distribution, toxicology, pathogenesis, clinical features, and treatment of millipede envenomation are carefully reviewed.*

Southcott RV: Lepidoptera and Skin Infestation. *In* Parish LC, Nutting WB, Schwartzman RM (eds.): Cutaneous Infestations of Man and Animal. New York, Praeger, 1983, pp 304–343. *This chapter gives a comprehensive review of worldwide lepidopterism, including pathogenesis and clinical presentations.*

PENTASTOMIASIS (Linguatuliasis)

Pentastomiasis is infestation with pentastomes, little-known invertebrates called tongue worms, which have been variously classified as arthropods or helminths. These bloodsucking endoparasites are found as adults in the lungs of reptiles and birds, or in the nasal cavity of carnivores, especially cats and dogs. Herbivores are normal intermediate hosts, but humans and other mammals can be dead-end aberrant hosts for the larvae. Ingested eggs hatch and the larvae burrow through the intestine and migrate to diverse tissues where they molt several times and become encysted as third stage larvae.

Human infestations have occurred in Europe, Africa, and North, Central, and South America. Two species account for most cases, *Armillifer armillatus,* found in pythons and other vipers in tropical Africa, and *Linguatula serrata,* found in canids in Europe and the Near and Middle East.

Infection occurs by accidental ingestion of tongue worm eggs contaminating food or drink, by ingestion of eggs picked up on fingers from handling infected snakes or lizards, or by ingestion of improperly cooked or raw reptiles. The third stage larvae (20 to 25 mm long) encysted in fibrous capsules occur most often in the liver and are rarely noted except incidentally at autopsy or as calcified cysts (3 to 6 mm in diameter) on x-ray examination. Rarely, a mass of cysts in the intestinal wall may cause obstruction. Cysts compressing vital structures such as bile ducts or bronchi may lead to infections or obstructions.

Linguatuliasis, the direct infection of humans with third stage larvae of *Linguatula* species, occurs most often in Lebanese people who eat raw or inadequately cooked liver or lymph nodes of goats and sheep. The ingested larvae migrate to the nasopharynx from the stomach. These larvae (5 to 10 mm long) cause Halzoun's syndrome, characterized by paroxysmal coughing, sneezing, nasal and lacrimal discharge, accompanied by pain and itching in the throat. Other symptoms may include hoarseness, dyspnea, dysphagia, and vomiting. Submaxillary and cervical lymph nodes may be enlarged. Recovery in most cases is spontaneous and occurs in seven to ten days; however, death from asphyxiation caused by tonsillar edema has been reported. A similar syndrome seen in Sudan, Turkey, and Greece is called Marrara's syndrome.

Prevention of pentastomiasis includes proper cooking of

exotic foods such as herbivore organs and reptiles, as well as improved hygiene of persons handling reptiles.

Hopps HC, Keegan HL, Price DL, Self JT: Pentastomiasis. *In* Marcial-Rojas RA (ed.): Pathology of Protozoal and Helminthic Diseases. Baltimore, Williams & Wilkins Company, 1971, pp 970–989. *This is a comprehensive review that includes basic biological and clinical information.*

LEECHES AS AGENTS OF DISEASE (Hirudiniasis)

Leeches of medical importance are bloodsucking annelid worms. Each has a ventral anterior or posterior sucker enclosing teeth that cut through the skin after the leech attaches. Feeding occurs within a half hour or more.

The leeches most often feeding on humans are aquatic (fresh water) species of *Hirudo,* the cosmopolitan medicinal leeches, *Limnatis,* the nasal leeches found from the Canary Islands east through Europe, Africa, and Asia, *Dinobdella,* found in Asia, and terrestrial species of *Haemadipsa,* found in Asia, Indonesia, Australia, Pacific Islands, and Central and South America. Humans are subject to attack by large leeches in tropical rain forests or infestation with aquatic species while wading or swimming.

Wounds produced by leeches are often painless and go unnoticed, except for the oozing blood or prolonged bleeding caused by an anticoagulant, hirudin. Pruritus is common at bite sites and although leeches are not known to transmit any human pathogens, secondary infections may occur. Immature aquatic leeches may be ingested with water and infest the upper respiratory and digestive tracts, or may invade the mouth, nose, eyes, vagina, urethra, or anus of swimmers.

Attachment of leeches to the nasal passages may cause epistaxis. Attachment to the larynx may cause hoarseness, dyspnea, and hemoptysis, and attachment to the pharynx or esophagus may cause dysphagia and hematemesis. Hemorrhaging from leech infestations may be so severe, especially in children, that anemia occurs that leads to death.

Techniques used for removing leeches from the respiratory and digestive tracts include a steady pull on the specimen with a forceps or hemostat, or narcotizing the leech with a spray of 5 per cent cocaine hydrochloride before removal. In genitourinary infestations, irrigation with a strong salt solution may cause the leeches to detach. A leech attached to skin, respiratory, or digestive tract surfaces may be induced to release its grip by holding it in a hemostat and touching the exposed part of the worm with a small flame or other cauterant.

Prevention of attack by aquatic and land leeches includes use of protective clothing and of insect repellents. Repellents applied to boots, trouser legs, and exposed skin are quite effective, but, because they are water soluble, must be reapplied every few hours in wet tropical regions where leeches are commonly found.

Keegan HL, Radke MG, Murphy DA: Nasal leech infestation in man. Am J Trop Med Hyg 19:1029, 1970. *This paper discusses two cases and reviews other clinical reports and treatment.*

425. SNAKE BITES

Jay P. Sanford

EPIDEMIOLOGY. Of the nearly 3500 species of snakes, fewer than one tenth are venomous. The poisonous varieties belong to five families (Table 425–1). Throughout the world, snake bites are estimated to account for 30,000 to 40,000 deaths annually. The largest number occur in Burma and Brazil. In the United States, the number of snakes bites is estimated at 8000 per year. Some 20 to 30 per cent of the bites by venomous snakes in the United States do not result in envenomation (poisoning). Most bites occur in the states bordering on the Gulf of Mexico. Despite the large number of bites with envenomation, fewer than 15 deaths occur and almost all of these are due to rattlesnake bites. This low case fatality ratio reflects the virtual absence of members of the species Elapidae and Hydrophidae in the United States.

Coral snakes, eastern and western varieties, are found in

TABLE 425–1. VENOMOUS SNAKES OF THE WORLD

Family	Common Varieties	Geographic Distribution
Crotalidae	Pit vipers (rattlesnakes, water moccasins, copperheads), fer-de-lance, bushmaster	Americas, Asia
Elapidae	Cobras, kraits, mambas, coral snakes, death adder	Worldwide except Europe
Colubridae	Boomslangs, bird snakes	Africa
Hydrophidae	Sea snakes	Indo-Pacific waters
Viperidae	True vipers, puff adder	Worldwide except Americas

southern and western states (North Carolina, South Carolina, Georgia, Florida, Alabama, Mississippi, Louisiana, Arkansas, Texas, New Mexico, Arizona). Their fangs are short and permanently erect. They envenomate through chewing movements. Since they are nocturnal and shy, they rarely bite humans.

The pit vipers (Crotalidae) are identified by a small depression between the eyes and nostrils. Their fangs are long and hinged, folding back when the mouth is closed and erect when open. Upon contact, venom is expressed by muscular contraction. The pit vipers are generally aggressive. The eastern (*Crotalus adamanteus*) and western (*C. atrox*) diamondback rattlesnakes are the largest and most dangerous in the United States. Their distribution includes the aforementioned states plus California, Nevada, and Oklahoma. Cottonmouths (*Agkistrodon piscivorus*), or water moccasins, are found along streams in the southern and southeastern states. They may inflict facial bites when disturbed while resting on tree branches. Contrary to lore, they can bite under water. Copperheads (*A. contortrix*), or highland moccasins, have a geographic distribution similar to the cottonmouths. Their bite is painful but rarely fatal.

PATHOGENESIS. Snake venoms are probably the most complex of all poisons. Due to the heterogenous composition and multiplicity of effects, snake venoms cannot be classified simply as neurotoxic, cardiotoxic, or hematotoxic on the basis of the snake family (Table 425–2).

Venoms from Elapidae and Hydrophidae contain basic polypeptides that produce a nondepolarizing neuromuscular block with resultant flaccid paralysis including respiratory paralysis. Cobra cardiotoxin, an additional basic polypeptide, depolarizes cell membranes of skeletal, cardiac, and smooth muscles, thus contributing to paralysis. Venom of the South American rattlesnake contains an acidic protein with nondepolarizing curare-like neuromuscular blocking effects. Viperatoxin isolated from the Palestine viper causes a peripheral nerve conduction block. A variety of enzymes, mostly hydrolases and phospholipase A, are present in most venoms. Bradykinin is released from bradykininogen by most crotalid and viperid venoms but not by Elapidae except the king cobra (*Ophiophagus hannah*). The venom of a single snake seldom contains all of the toxins. The composition and potency of venom is highly variable and differs not only among species but even among individual snakes.

SYMPTOMS AND SIGNS. ***Pit Viper Envenomation.*** In the United States, most patients reach a physician within 15 minutes to 3 hours. At that time it is essential to determine whether or not envenomation has occurred and, if it has occurred, to determine the severity; this has important therapeutic implications. The clinical effects are summarized in Table 425–3. The most important early findings of envenomation are swelling at the bite, usually occurring within ten minutes, and pain, although pain may be absent. Mild envenomation is characterized by local edema (one to five inches in diameter) and pain without systemic symptoms or signs. With moderate enven-

TABLE 425–2. BIOCHEMISTRY OF SNAKE VENOMS

Toxins	Family	Mechanism of Injury-Death
Neurotoxin (basic polypeptide)	Elapidae, Hydrophidae, South American rattlesnake *(Crotalus durissus terrificus)*, Palestine viper *(Vipera palestinae)*	Respiratory paralysis
Cardiotoxin	Elapidae	Cardiovascular depression
Enzymes	Elapidae, Hydrophidae, Crotalidae, Viperidae	Hemolysis
Phospholipase A		
5-Nucleotidase		
Phosphodiesterase		
Deoxyribonuclease II		
Ribonuclease		
Adenosine-triphosphatase		
Nucleotide pyrophosphatase		
Exopeptidase		
Hyaluronidase	(Absent in spitting cobra)	
l Amino acidoxidase		
Proteases	Crotalidae, Viperidae	Hypotension due to release
Acetylcholinesterase	Elapidae (absent in spitting cobra, mamba, coral)	
Alkaline phosphatase		
Acid phosphatase		

omation, local findings are more extensive—edema of 6 to 12 inches in diameter. Systemic findings occur: weakness, sweating, nausea, faintness, dizziness, ecchymoses, and tender regional lymph nodes. With severe envenomation systemic involvement includes tachycardia; tachypnea; hypothermia; hypotension; ecchymoses; paresthesias of the scalp, finger and toe tips; and muscle fasciculations. With very severe envenomations, gingival bleeding, hematemesis, hematuria, melena, oliguria, and coma occur.

Over the first 12 hours, the skin develops a tense discolored appearance and bullae, which may be either serous or hemorrhagic.

Coral Snake Envenomation. The bite wound usually resembles scratch marks and is somewhat painful, but there is little or no edema. The onset of systemic manifestations is usually delayed one to six hours. Paresthesias around the bite may occur within several hours. Systemic symptoms may include weakness, apprehension, giddiness, nausea, vomiting, excess salivation, and even a sense of euphoria. Bulbar and cranial nerve paralysis may develop with ptosis, diplopia, papillary dilatation, excess salivation, dysphagia, dysphonation, and respiratory failure.

LABORATORY FINDINGS. Proteolytic enzymes in venoms produce not only tissue damage but have a marked effect on coagulation, thrombin-like activity being most prominent. Within the first few hours there is a drop in platelets due to local consumption (occasionally to less than 10,000 per cu ml), a decrease in fibrinogen, and an increase in fibrin degradation products. Striking increases in prothrombin time and partial thromboplastin time occur with severe envenomation. Erythrocytes show a peculiar "burring" indicating membrane damage, and drops in hematocrit and hemoglobin concentration occur.

With pit viper envenomation, baseline laboratory tests should include complete blood count, platelet count, prothrombin time, partial thromboplastin time, bleeding time, urinalysis, and serum electrolytes. Blood should be obtained for typing and cross matching. In patients with envenomation of moderate or greater severity arterial blood gas determinations and an electrocardiogram are indicated. Hematologic studies should be repeated every four to six hours for the first day or until the coagulopathy has stabilized. With coral snake envenomation, repetitive coagulation studies are not indicated.

TREATMENT. ***First Aid.*** In general, too much emphasis has been placed on first aid at the expense of delay in definitive hospital care. The snake should be killed if this can be done quickly and safely and taken along with the patient to allow accurate identification; this may obviate unnecessary therapy. The dead snake must be handled with care since the head of an apparently dead snake can deliver a venomous bite for up to an hour after being severed. The value of incision and suction (I and S) has been questioned. It has been stated that if I and S is begun within three minutes after subcutaneous envenomation, 22 to 50 per cent of injected venom can be removed. Recovery is much less after intramuscular envenomation and if I and S is delayed. As a practical matter, if the patient cannot reach definitive care (antivenin) within one and one-half hours, prompt I and S is appropriate. If more than 15 minutes have elapsed since a bite, I and S should not be performed. Mouth suction should be used only if no other method is available. In the absence of oral lesions, mouth suction poses no risk to the first aider because ingestion of venom is harmless; however, mouth suction does result in the equivalent of a human bite to the victim. If a constricting band (not a tourniquet) is used, it should be placed immediately proximal to the wound. Linear incisions, 1 cm long and no deeper than 3 mm, should be made over each fang mark. If I and S is not to be used, the Australian Serum Institute recommends application of a broad firm constrictive bandage immediately over the bite, then bandaging of as much of the limb as possible. The affected part should be immobilized (splinted) promptly and the patient transported to the nearest medical treatment facility. The affected area should not be placed on ice. Cryotherapy results in greater tissue damage with the potential for necessitating amputation.

Hospital Care. On admission it is important to determine, if possible, if the bite was inflicted by a pit viper or a coral snake and whether envenomation has occurred. The mainstay of therapy is antivenom (antivenin), which is a horse serum product; hence it has a high potential of causing serum sickness later. There are two antivenoms: one polyvalent for North American pit vipers and another for eastern coral snakes. For minor envenomation, antivenin is not indicated. For more serious envenomation, antivenin should be administered. For mild pit viper envenomation, three to five ampules of antivenin should be diluted (10 ml each), then added to 500 ml of

TABLE 425–3. PIT VIPER ENVENOMATION: SYMPTOMS AND SIGNS (PERCENTAGE)

Local		Systemic: *Generalized*		Systemic: *Hematologic*		Systemic: *Neuromuscular*	
Fang marks	100	Weakness	70	Thrombocytopenia	42	Paresthesia scalp, fingertips	63
Edema	74	Tachycardia	60	Increased clotting time	37	Faintness, dizziness	57
Pain	65	Hypotension	54	Decreased hemoglobin	37	Paresthesias of affected part	57
Vesicles	40	Sweating	43	Burring of RBC	18	Fasciculations	41
Necrosis	27	Nausea/vomiting	42	Thrombocytosis	16		
		Hypothermia	42	Bleeding	15		
		Tachypnea	40				
		Regional adenopathy	40				

Adapted from Russell, FE: Ann Rev Med 31:247, 1980.

intravenous fluid. The patient should be skin tested for horse serum hypersensitivity. If the skin test is negative, the 500 ml should be given intravenously over 60 minutes. If the amount is adequate, the swelling will not progress and paresthesias will decrease. If progression occurs, the dose should be repeated. For moderate envenomation 5 to 10 vials, for severe envenomation 10 to 20 vials, and for very severe envenomation up to 40 vials (400 ml) may be required. In one series, the average dose required for adults with severe bites was 16 vials. Larger doses are required for bites in children and for those involving the fingers. Antivenin neutralizes both the local and systemic effects of the venom.

In coral snake bites, if any symptoms or signs develop within the first several hours, 3 to 5 vials of antivenin (Micrurus fulvius) should be given intravenously. Even in the absence of symptoms, patients should be observed in the hospital for approximately 48 hours because onset of symptoms may be delayed and insidious.

Antibiotics are usually recommended. Bacteriologic cultures of rattlesnake venom and fangs show growth from over 90 per cent. Aerobic gram-negative bacilli (*Enterobacter* sp., *Pseudomonas* sp., and *Citrobacter* sp.) and histotoxic clostridia (*C. perfringens*) are the predominant isolates. On the basis of the microbiologic results, administration of one of the newer beta-lactam antibiotics, piperacillin or azlocillin, is most appropriate. Such agents would also be effective against the human bite wound. Although *Clostridium tetani* were not isolated and there are only one or two reports of tetanus following snake bite, a tetanus toxoid booster is recommended.

In the severely envenomated patient, concurrent supportive measures include the management of shock and respiratory and renal failure. Pharmacologic doses of glucocorticords comparable with those used in "endotoxic shock" have been recommended, but benefits have not been demonstrated. Despite the hypofibrinogenemia and elevation of fibrin degradation products, heparin is not of benefit. Attention to early recognition and management of anaphylaxis is essential.

Decompressive fasciotomy is indicated if edema within closed muscular compartments is inadequately controlled and arterial blood supply is compromised. From the end of the first to the third week the majority of patients will develop serum sickness, the prevalence approximating 1 per cent per milliliter of horse serum administered.

PROGNOSIS. If adequate antivenom was administered intravenously, mortality is virtually nil. If cryotherapy was avoided, amputation or serious resultant deformities are uncommon.

Jimenez-Porras JM: Biochemistry of snake venoms. Clin Toxicol 3:389, 1970. *A detailed review of the enzymatic and toxic properties of snake venoms with an extensive bibliography.*

Ledbetter EO, Kutscher AE: Aerobic and anaerobic flora of rattlesnake fangs and venom. Arch Environ Health 19:770, 1969. *This is the only study available that addresses the potential microbiologic contaminants in snake bite wounds. It provides a reasonable basis for antibiotic selection.*

Medical Letter: Treatment of snake bite in the USA. The Medical Letter 24:87, 1982. *The process utilized by the Medical Letter results in a consensus among consultants. This provides a necessary balanced view in light of the facts that differences of opinion exist as to ideal management and that the number of annual cases is too few and dispersed to allow a prospective therapy trial.*

Russell FE: Snake venom poisoning in the United States. Ann Rev Med 31:247, 1980. *An excellent general review by one of the foremost authorities on the subject in the United States. An excellent source of clinical features.*

Simon TL, Grace TG: Envenomation coagulopathy in wounds from pit vipers. N Engl J Med 305:443, 1981. *This study on experimental envenomation in rabbits enables a sequential assessment of the clotting abnormalities that occur.*

Walt CH Jr: Poisonous snakebite treatment in the United States. JAMA 240:654, 1978. *A report on an extensive personal clinical experience utilizing the treatment approaches recommended by the Medical Letter.*

426. VENOMOUS AND POISONOUS* MARINE ANIMALS

John Williamson

The world's seas contain a formidable array of venomous and poisonous marine creatures capable of harming or even killing the human intruder. The story of their relationship to humankind dates from antiquity but their scientific study remains relatively neglected; for example, about 95 per cent of known marine biotoxins have scarcely been examined for their biological activity. The animals are found in greatest variety and profusion in warmer tropical and subtropical waters—the very seas that attract human activities. Communities dependent on the seas as a food source or as a tourist attraction are typically foremost in studying the subject. Current research is being conducted in Australia, French Polynesia, Japan, and the United States (including Hawaii). Although the subject has now emerged from the realm of folklore, lack of objectivity still causes misconceptions. Human injury by venomous marine creatures results from accidental or intentional human interference with the animal or its territory.

*The currently held view is that the administration of venoms requires mechanical penetration, whereas the term poison implies oral ingestion. The term toxins (here marine zootoxins) refers to both venoms and poisons.

Taxonomic Classification

Taxonomic classification is customary but is of limited practical value to those responsible for treatment and prevention of marine envenomation. The animals listed in Table 426–1 have accounted for the majority of human deaths and a significant number of the poisonings and injuries that are documented to date.

Animals Causing Human Fatalities

Table 426–1 lists invertebrates and vertebrates that cause fatalities by envenomation, and those animals responsible for fatal poisonings in humans.

BOX JELLYFISH. The box jellyfish (*Chironex fleckeri*), the world's only coelenterate known to be lethal to humans, has been responsible for 71 documented human deaths since 1884; many more reports remain unconfirmed. Found only in tropical West Indo-Pacific waters, it is a true jellyfish, carrying up to 60 extendable tentacles. These tentacles bear a vast number of nematocysts (stinging capsules, microbasic mastigophores) that discharge massively when a person blunders into them and becomes entangled. The animal is almost impossible to see under natural conditions. This massive envenomation produces rapid systemic absorption that is enhanced by struggling, and collapse occurs within minutes in serious cases. Seventy per cent of fatalities occur in women and children (small body mass and hairless skin). The venom is a high molecular weight protein mixture containing "lethal" and dermatonecrotic factors. The densely adherent tentacles produce whip wheals with a diagnostic ladder pattern on the envenomated skin. Treatment is immediate resuscitation on the beach, vinegar dousing, compressive bandaging, and injection of the specific antivenom, intravenously if possible, in a dosage large enough to be effective. The antivenom is sheep antiserum; therefore, appropriate precautions are necessary.

BLUE-RINGED OCTOPUS. At least two species (*Hapalochlaena maculosa* and *H. lunulata*) have produced morbidity and mortality. The venom is located in the salivary glands and is

TABLE 426–1. MARINE ANIMALS CAUSING HUMAN FATALITIES

- I. From Envenomation
  - A. Invertebrates
    1. Box jellyfish (*Chironex fleckeri*)
    2. Blue-ringed octopuses (Family *Octopodidae*)
    3. Venomous cone shells (Family *Conidae*)
  - B. Vertebrates
    1. Venomous sea snakes (Family *Hydrophiidae*)
    2. Scorpionfishes, including stonefishes (Family *Scorpaenidae*)
    3. Catfish (Suborder *Siluroidei*)
    4. Stingrays (Order *Rajiformes*)
- II. From Poisoning
  - A. Ciguatoxic fishes
  - B. Tetrodotoxic fishes
  - C. Shellfish
  - D. Sea turtles
  - E. Viscera of whales, porpoises, polar bears, walruses, seals

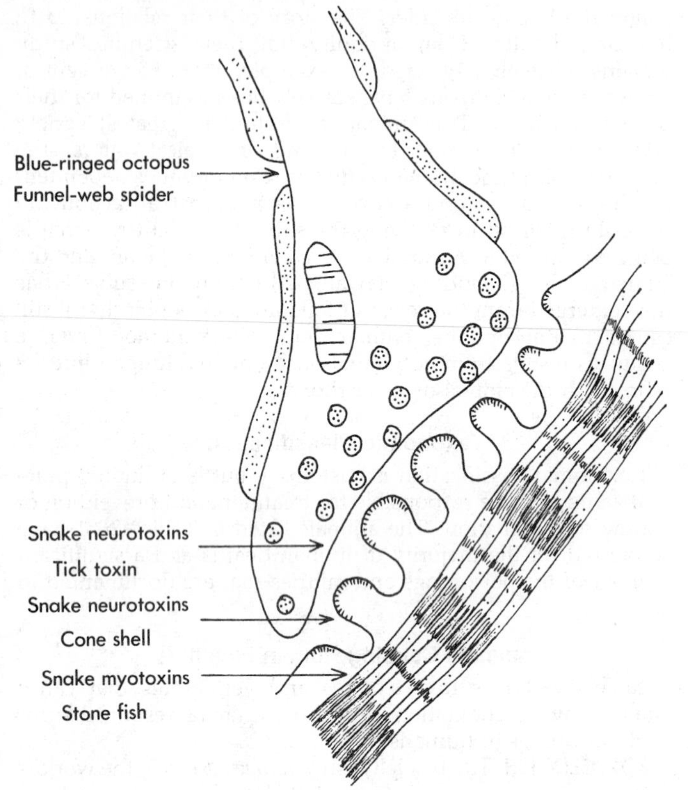

Figure 426–1. Scheme of a somatic neuromuscular junction, showing sites of action of a number of animal toxins (Courtesy of Dr. V. Callanan, Townsville).

injected by a bite that may be painless. The salivary toxin contains tetrodotoxin (M.W. 319), a unique biological material also found in the flesh of puffer fish (see below). It inhibits action potentials (Fig. 426–1) by specific blockade of sodium ion transport, and is thus in addition a valuable physiologic research tool. Clinically the danger is respiratory failure and hypoxia. Airway protection and expired air resuscitation will be life saving. There is no antivenom. First aid is as for snakebite (see Ch. 425).

VENOMOUS CONE SHELLS. There are 37 cases of cone shell envenomation in the literature, eight of them fatalities. Seven species of cone shells are considered dangerous. The injected venom produces postsynaptic neuromuscular blockade (Fig. 426–1) and thus death from hypoxia (respiratory failure). On-the-spot airway protection and expired air resuscitation will be life saving. No antivenom presently exists, but research is promising. First aid is identical to that for snakebite (see Ch. 425).

VENOMOUS SEA SNAKES. Apart from their predominance in warmer waters, the proven lethality of several species, and the availability of a specific antivenom (*Enhydrina schistosa* antivenom), the subject of sea snakebite can be considered in the same manner as land snakebite (see Ch. 425).

SCORPIONFISHES AND STONEFISHES. Deaths from zebrafish stings have been documented. No firm record of a fatality caused by stonefish (*Synanceja*) stings has been located from Australia, where these stings are not uncommon. In this group of animals dorsal spines inject the venom. The ensuing pain is a devastating experience, with intense local tissue swelling and discoloration. Immersion of the envenomated part in hot water offers partial pain relief. Medical management is concerned with pain relief (conduction anesthesia), prevention of wound infection, and in the case of stonefish stings specific antivenom injection with appropriate precautions. Tourniquets or compressive bandages should not be used.

CATFISH AND STINGRAYS. Despite their ubiquity, these animals rarely cause human death. A full account of their injuring and envenomating capabilities is given by Halstead (1978). Pieces of the brittle stingray spines not infrequently break off in wounds, necessitating careful exploration under anesthesia.

CIGUATERA (POISONING BY FISH IN THE TROPICS). This occurs in all tropical and subtropical seas and is a major public health and economic problem in the Pacific. About 1500 cases of ciguatera poisoning occur annually in the South Pacific alone. Deaths have been reported. The hoped-for simple chemical test of fish flesh to reveal the presence of ciguatoxin has not yet been developed. The most common symptoms are gastrointestinal (nausea, abdominal pain, vomiting, and diarrhea) and peripheral neurologic (paresthesiae, especially circumoral and intraoral, dental discomfort, and a classic reversal of peripheral temperature sense; that is, hot feels cold and vice versa). Ciguatoxin is believed to be passed along in the food chain, and at least one source has been traced to a dinoflagellate, *Gambierdiscus toxicus*. There is no antidote and treatment is symptomatic. Symptoms can persist for months. The chemical structure of ciguatoxin remains to be elucidated.

TETRODOTOXIC FISHES. These include toad fish and puffer fish. Ingestion of the toxin in the fish flesh produces symptoms and signs characteristic of tetrodotoxin's action potential blockade (Fig. 426–1), viz.: numbness, motor weakness, ataxia, and respiratory failure. Tetrodotoxin is one of the most toxic of known poisons and is the active component in blue-ringed octopus envenomation (see above). There is no specific antidote, so management of a patient is symptomatic.

SHELLFISH POISONING. Paralytic shellfish poisoning is due to the ingestion of saxitoxin and is associated with a fatality rate of about 8.5 per cent. This condition should be distinguished from the gastrointestinal and the allergic types of shellfish poisoning. Like ciguatoxin (see above), saxitoxin is thought to originate in dinoflagellate organisms, at the beginning of the marine food chain. Treatment is symptomatic. No specific antidote is known.

WHALES, PORPOISES, POLAR BEARS, WALRUSES, AND SEALS. Poisoning results from the ingestion of the viscera of these animals, notably liver or kidneys. The intoxication from such organs of polar bears, walruses, and seals is believed to be due to hypervitaminosis A.

Some Nonfatal Envenomations (Table 426–1)

These have occurred from true jellyfish (Class *Scyphozoa*), including *Carybdeid medusae* and the "hydroids" (Class *Hydrozoa*), including *Physalia* species (bluebottle, Portuguese man o'war), sea nettle (*Chrysaora quinquecirrha*), and mauve stinger (*Pelagia noctiluca*). Others have included corals and anemones (Class *Anthozoa*), and toxic sponges (Class *Demospongiae*).

A vast array of marine animals continues to be involved in less serious human envenomations, ranging from mild local itching to serious allergic manifestations. Certain treatment principles are becoming established.

1. Household vinegar inactivates undischarged nematocysts of several species of jellyfish (*Physalia, "Irukandji," Carybdia tamoya,* and *Cyanea*). Vinegar does nothing for the pain of the sting.
2. In general, ethyl alcohol should not be applied to marine stings.
3. Allergic phenomena can play a significant role in some marine envenomations such as jellyfish stings and toxic sponge contacts.
4. Immediate pain relief continues to be a problem. Local cooling (ice) helps in some jellyfish stings.

Bowerman M: Joint research on ciguatera. South Pacif Undw Med Soc J July to September: 24, 1980. *A useful summary of current research findings from the major centers in the Pacific.*
Burnett JW, Cobbs CS, Kelman SN, Calton GJ: Studies on the serologic response to jellyfish envenomation. J Am Acad Dermatol 9:229, 1983. *A controlled investigation of allergic reactions to sea nettle and Portuguese man-of-war stings.*
Edmonds C: Dangerous Marine Animals of the Indo-Pacific Region. Newport, New South Wales, Wedneil Publications, 1975. *A readable and well-illustrated overview of the subject.*

Halstead BW: Paralytic shellfish poisoning guide. Geneva, WHO Publication, 1982. *A good review of the subject.*

Halstead BW: Poisonous and Venomous Marine Animals of the World; Revised Edition. Princeton, Darwin Press, 1978. *The classic and encyclopedic reference text on the subject; an essential starting point.*

Hartwick R, Callanan V, Williamson J: Disarming the box jellyfish. Nematocyst inhibition in *Chironex fleckeri*. Med J Aust 1:15, 1980. *Demonstrates the value of vinegar and the problems of alcohol application in the first aid treatment of box jellyfish stings.*

Sutherland SK: Australian Animal Toxins. Melbourne, Australia, Oxford University Press, 1983. *This detailed and profusely illustrated work is the most recent hallmark in the subject of animal envenomation and poisoning, both marine and terrestrial. Destined to become a classic work. The definitive work on snake and spider bite management.*

Torda TA: Tetrodotoxic fish—clinical management. *In* Sutherland SK: Australian Animal Toxins. Cambridge, Oxford University Press, 1983, pp 458–459. *A recent update on a potentially dangerous clinical situation.*

Williamson J: Some Australian Marine Stings, Envenomations and Poisonings. 3nd ed., Brisbane, Surf Life Saving Association of Australia, Queensland State Centre, 1984. *A concise illustrated account at the level of first aiders and paramedics.*

Williamson JA, Callanan VI, Hartwick RF: Serious envenomation by the Northern Australian box jellyfish (*Chironex fleckeri*). Med J Aust 1:13, 1980. *A fully documented account of a near fatal sting that deals with all aspects of management.*

Part XXI
DISEASES OF THE IMMUNE SYSTEM

427. INTRODUCTION: THE IMMUNE SYSTEM

William E. Paul

The immune system consists of the recirculating pool of *lymphocytes* and *monocytes* and of cells in the bone marrow and in the organized lymphoid tissues, including the *lymph nodes, spleen, Peyer's patches,* and the *thymus.* The principal cells that comprise this system are the *B* and *T lymphocytes* and cells of the *monocyte-macrophage* lineage. These cells and their products, most notably *antibodies* and *lymphokines,* are responsible for the protective immunity that is so critical for survival of humans in the sea of potentially pathogenic microorganisms in which we live. The consequences of the failure to make an immune response or of major dysfunction in the immune system is graphically and tragically demonstrated by the fate of infants with severe combined immunodeficiency disease or of adults with acquired immune deficiency syndrome.

The immune response is initiated by introduction of an immunogenic substance into an immunocompetent individual. Such immunization results in activation and proliferation of T and B lymphocytes, which bear membrane receptors specific for antigenic determinants (epitopes) on the immunogen. This leads to the selective expansion of clones of specific lymphocytes that initially represented a very small fraction of the total lymphocyte population.

Stimulated B lymphocytes differentiate into antibody-secreting cells, of which plasma cells are a major morphologic type. Antibody-secreting cells produce *immunoglobulin* (Ig) molecules with antigen-combining sites that are identical to the antigen-combining sites of the membrane receptors expressed on their B lymphocyte progenitors. Ig's exist in a series of structurally distinct classes, including IgM, IgD, IgG, IgA, and IgE. Each of these types of Ig molecules has a distinctive function.

Stimulated T lymphocytes may differentiate into effector cells, such as specific cytotoxic T lymphocytes. Other members of the T cell population play critical roles in regulation of the immune system. Among these regulatory cells are *helper* T lymphocytes, which interact with B lymphocytes and aid them to develop into antibody-secreting cells, and *suppressor* T cells, which inhibit immune responses, principally by diminishing the action of helper T cells.

The negative regulatory aspects of the immune system, as exemplified by suppressor cells, are necessary to prevent the uncontrolled growth of individual B or T cells that might result as a consequence of continued antigenic stimulation. An equally critical need of the immune system is to limit the production of antibodies specific for *self* antigenic determinants and the appearance of effector T lymphocytes with self-specificity. Lymphocytes potentially capable of such self-specific responses are eliminated or their activation inhibited by the establishment of immunologic tolerance. Disorders in immunoregulation or of tolerance induction are a major feature of autoimmune diseases, such as systemic lupus erythematosus.

This Introduction will serve to describe briefly the principal cell types that participate in the immune response, the means through which these cells are activated, how they communicate with one another, the nature of the antibodies and other soluble products that they secrete, and how these cells mediate their immunologic functions.

B LYMPHOCYTES

B lymphocytes are precursors of antibody-secreting cells. They are found in all of the peripheral lymphoid tissues and in the recirculating pool of lymphocytes. In lymph nodes, B cells are mainly located in primary follicles within the subcapsular cortex. B cells bear membrane receptors through which they recognize foreign antigens. These receptors are Ig molecules, mainly of the IgM and IgD classes, that are specialized for expression within membranes. All of the membrane receptors of any individual B cell have the same binding specificity. When these cells differentiate into antibody-secreting cells, they produce antibodies with specificity identical to that of the membrane Ig (mIg) of the B cells. Thus, the extremely large number of distinct antibodies that may be produced in the course of immune responses represents the existence of a correspondingly large number of antibody-secreting cells, each of which produces antibody of only a single specificity.

ONTOGENY, MOLECULAR GENETICS, AND DIVERSITY OF B LYMPHOCYTES. B lymphocytes are derived from hematopoietic stem cells. These cells are found in embryonic life within the blood islands of the yolk sac, later in gestation within the liver, and in postnatal life principally within the bone marrow. The earliest identifiable member of the B lymphocyte lineage is the *pre-B* cell. This cell lacks mIg, but expresses in its cytoplasm one of the two constituent polypeptide chains of IgM molecules, the μ heavy (H) chain. Early pre-B cells rapidly cycle, but more mature pre-B cells are small and quiescent.

Within pre-B cells a series of remarkable genetic translocations occur, involving the genes coding for both of the polypeptide chains of Ig's (H and light [L] chains). Both H and L chains consist of amino-terminal regions, which are highly variable and which form the walls of the antigen-combining sites of Ig's, and of carboxy-terminal regions, which, for a given H chain class or L chain type, are essentially constant, except for allotypic variation (Fig. 427–1). These regions are designated the variable (V) and constant (C) regions of the H and L chains respectively. The H chain V region is encoded by three distinct genes, the *V, D,* and *J* genes (Fig. 427–2). In the germline DNA and in DNA of nonlymphoid cells, the H chain *V, D,* and *J* genes, which are on chromosome 14, are widely separated from one another, but in the course of pre-B cell development, two separate translocation events occur that bring these genes together to produce a single *VDJ* gene. This *VDJ* gene specifies an individual H chain V region. Germline DNA contains a large number (~300) of distinct V genes, a large but not yet determined number of *D* genes, and four functional *J* genes. It appears that these genes can be randomly combined, making possible the formation of a large number, probably more than 10,000, *VDJ* genes simply by combinatorial association. Furthermore, there are opportunities for somatic genetic changes, both in the translocation process and due to mutation and gene conversion events, so that the actual number of distinct *VDJ* genes that may be formed is much greater. Within any individual cell, only one functional set of *VDJ* translocation events appears to occur. The *VDJ* gene is initially assembled near the gene encoding the μ constant region (*Igh-C*μ gene). This leads to the expression within pre-B cells of μ H chains.

The L chain V region is also constructed by the translocation of distinct genes. L chain V regions are encoded by *V* and *J* genes, which are brought into apposition with one another; no *D* gene exists for L chains. L chains are of two different types, κ and λ. The *V* and *J* genes for κ (V_κ and J_κ) as well as the gene for the κ constant region (C_κ) are found on chromosome 2. The comparable λ genes (V_λ, J_λ, and C_λ) are on chromosome 22.

Translocation of H chain *V, D,* and *J* genes appears to precede translocation of L chain *V* and *J* genes; V_κ, J_κ translocation appears to precede translocation of V_λ, J_λ. In general, if V_κ and J_κ translocation events are successful and lead to an active κ gene, λ gene translocation events are not observed. Thus, an individual cell expresses only κ or λ chains but not both. Furthermore, a set of translocation events leading to the formation of active H or L chain genes generally occurs on only one of the two allelic chromosomes that specify H or L chains.

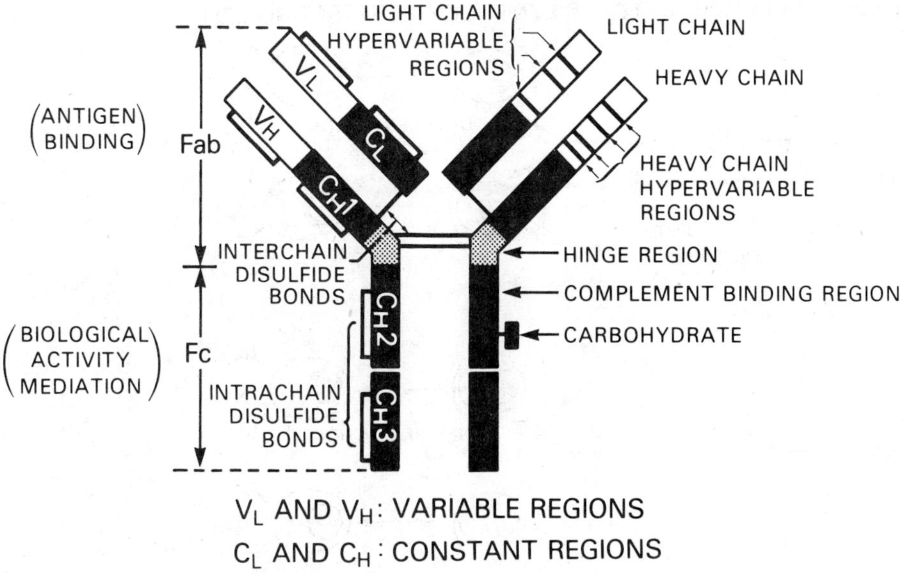

Figure 427–1. Structure of an Ig molecule. A schematic representation of an IgG molecule indicating the chain and domain structure of the molecule and the existence of hypervariable regions within variable regions of both H and L chains. *Fab* and *Fc* refer to fragments of the IgG molecule formed by papain cleavage. The former contains the V_H and C_{HI} H chain regions and an intact L chain; the latter consists of C_{H2} and C_{H3} region of two H chains, linked to one another by disulfide bonds. (From Wasserman RL, Capra JD: Immunoglobulins. *In* Horowitz MI, Pigman W (eds.): The Glycoconjugates. New York, Academic Press, 1977, pp 323–348.)

Thus, Ig H and L chains produced by any individual cell are derived from only one of the allelic chromosomes, resulting in the phenomenon of *allelic exclusion.*

The completion of functional H and L chain genetic translocation within a pre-B cell is associated with the appearance of mIg on the surface of the cell and thus with the differentiation of the pre-B cell into a B cell. Immature B cells express mIg only of the IgM class. As these cells mature further, they also express mIgD. This expression of mIgD, in addition to mIgM, by developing B cells appears to be associated with acquisition of new immune functions, such as resistance to tolerance induction and responsiveness to polysaccharide antigens.

Mature B cells express a series of other markers that have potential functional significance. These include receptors for the Fc portions of Ig's (*Fc receptors*), receptors for complement components (i.e., for the C3b and C3d fragments of C3), and class II *major histocompatibility complex* (MHC) molecules. (A complete discussion of the MHC is found in Ch. 436.) Although the precise physiologic roles of Fc and C3 receptors are still uncertain, class II MHC molecules on B cells are involved in the process by which helper T cells recognize and interact with B cells in the course of B cell responses to antigenic stimulation.

The events in pre-B cell and B cell development described thus far are antigen independent. Subsequent events in B cell development appear to require antigenic stimulation or stimulation by soluble factors made by antigen–activated T cells.

CONTROL OF B CELL RESPONSES. Resting, mature B cells can be activated as a result of cross-linkage of their membrane receptors by antigen or by anti-Ig antibodies (Fig. 427–3). B cells may also be activated by mitogenic agents such as the Cowan I strain of *Staphylococcus aureus*, bacterial lipopolysaccharide, and dextran sulfate. Responses to anti-Ig antibodies and to other mitogens are often used to assess B cell function. B cells activated by cross-linkage of their receptors enter the S phase of the cell cycle and then divide upon stimulation by a T cell-derived–B cell growth factor, now designated B cell stimulatory factor (BSF)-p1. This process also depends upon the presence of a macrophage-derived factor, *interleukin-1* (IL-1). B cells that are activated by receptor cross-linkage and that then proliferate following the action of BSF-p1 and IL-1 develop

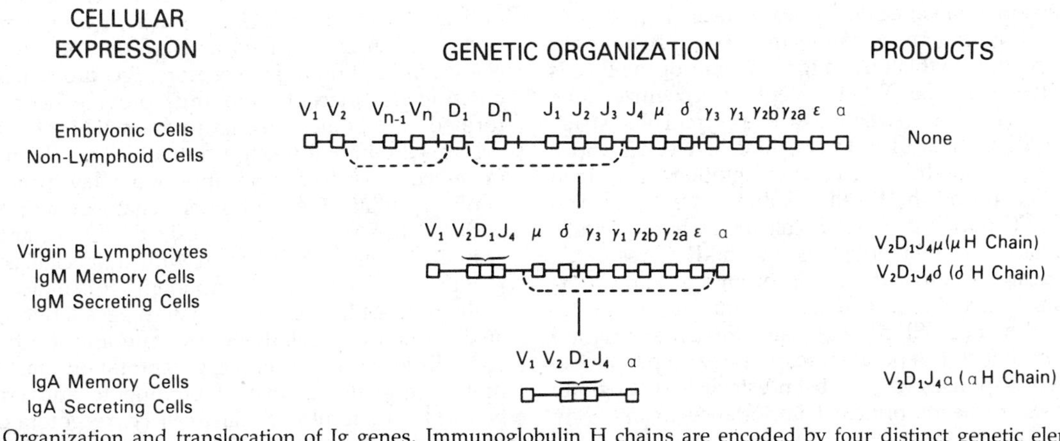

Figure 427–2. Organization and translocation of Ig genes. Immunoglobulin H chains are encoded by four distinct genetic elements: *Igh-V(V), Igh-D(D), Igh-J(J),* and *Igh-C* genes. The *V, D,* and *J* genes together specify the variable region of the H chain. The Igh-C gene specifies the C region. The same V region can be found in association with each of the C regions (e.g., in the mouse, μ, δ, γ3, γ1, γ2b, γ2a, ε, and α). A generally similar situation exists for human C region genes, but these genes have not been precisely ordered. In the germline genome, the *V, D,* and *J* genes are far apart, and there are multiple forms of each of these genes. In the course of lymphocyte development, a *VDJ* gene complex is found by translocation of individual *V* and *D* genes so that they lie next to one of the *J* genes, with the excision of intervening genes. This *VDJ* complex is initially expressed with μ and δ *C* genes, but may be subsequently translocated so that it lies near one of the other *C* genes (e.g., α) and in that case leads to the expression of a VDJα chain. (From Paul WE: The immune system: An introduction. *In* Paul WE (ed): Fundamental Immunology. New York, Raven Press, 1984, p 8.)

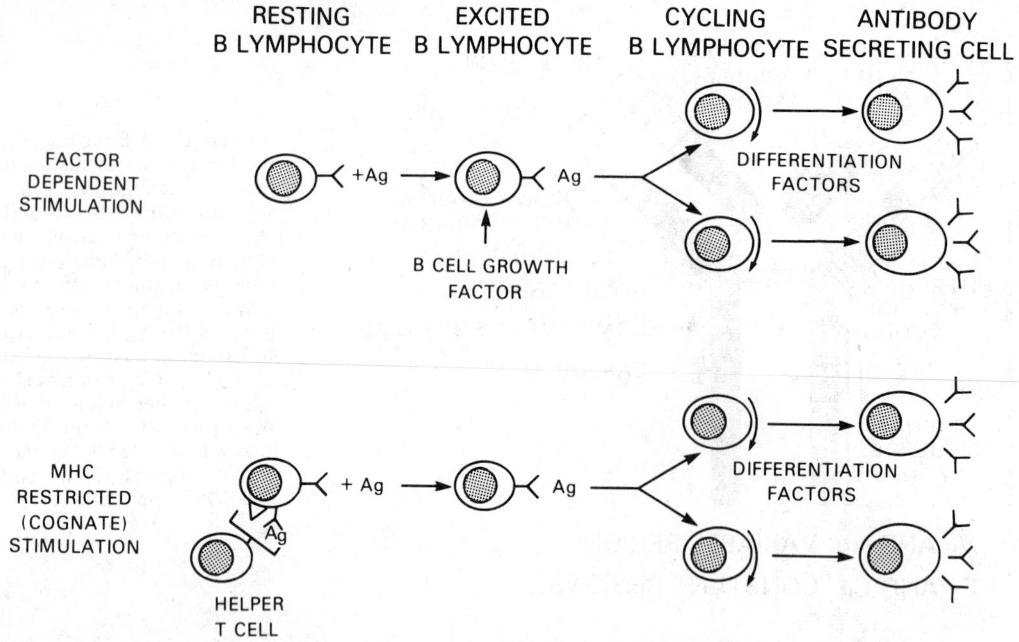

Figure 427–3. B cell stimulation. Resting B cells may be stimulated to proliferate and then to differentiate by two distinct mechanisms. One mechanism is designated factor-dependent activation. In this pathway, resting B cells are activated to an excited, or G_1, state by the action of agents that appropriately cross-link their receptors. Excited cells are acted upon by soluble factors, including B cell growth factor, and enter the S phase. Differentiation factors act upon these cells to cause them to synthesize and secrete Ig. The second major pathway involves the interaction of "histocompatibility-restricted" helper T cells with resting B cells. These T cells recognize antigen and class II molecules on the B cell surface and stimulate the cell to enter an excited state. This activation pathway is often designated cognate activation. The subsequent progress of the excited B cell may depend upon further interaction with helper T cells or soluble factors. Differentiation factors are probably necessary for differentiation of these into cells secreting Ig.

into antibody-secreting cells as a result of the action of B cell differentiation factors. This pathway of B cell responsiveness, which is controlled by the sequential action of a series of soluble T cell and macrophage products (lymphokines), is sometimes referred to as *factor-dependent* stimulation. Although detailed studies of the physiologic significance of factor-dependent activation in in vivo immune responses of humans have not yet been carried out, it seems most likely that it is mainly responsible for antibody responses to polysaccharides and to a related set of antigens designated type II antigens. Factor-dependent B cell stimulation would thus be critical to the development of immunity to the capsular polysaccharides of many pyogenic microorganisms, such as *Streptococcus pneumoniae*.

An additional way that resting B cells may be activated is through interaction with specific helper T cells (Fig. 427–3). Helper T cells bear membrane receptors that recognize epitopes on the same antigen for which the mIg molecules of the B cells are specific. However, the T cell receptors recognize such antigenic determinants in association with polymorphic structures of class II MHC molecules. Interactions between T and B cells that depend upon the T cell's corecognition of antigen and class II molecules on the B cell membrane are referred to as *cognate* or *MHC restricted* T cell–B cell interactions. B cells activated as a result of cognate interaction with MHC–restricted T cells also appear to require the action of growth and differentiation factors to proliferate and to develop into antibody-secreting cells. Whether BSF-p1, IL-1, and the differentiation factors important in factor-dependent responses also participate in cognate B cell responses has not been established. Cognate responses appear to be of principal importance in antibody responses to protein antigens.

IMMUNOGLOBULINS. Antibodies are Ig molecules. They exist in a series of classes that, as already noted, have distinct functions. Ig's are composed of one or more units, each of which consists of two identical H and two identical L chains. Both H chain and L chain polypeptides are divisible into a series of regions of 100 to 110 amino acids in length (Fig. 427–1). L chains consist of two such regions, an amino-terminal V region and a single carboxy-terminal C region. H chains consist of a V region and three or four C regions (C_{H1}, C_{H2}, . . .), depending on H chain class. Some classes of Ig's also have a hinge region, imparting segmental flexibility to the molecule. Hinge regions are located between C_{H1} and C_{H2} regions. The Ig's that consist of more than one unit of 2H and 2L chains (pentameric IgM and polymeric IgA) also contain one J chain per polymeric Ig molecule; the J chain is critical to maintaining such Ig's in their polymer form.

The various Ig classes have distinct functional properties (Table 427–1). IgM, in its membrane form, is one of the principal membrane receptors of B cells. In its secreted form and when cross-linked by antigen, IgM activates complement and thus is important in lysis and opsonization of bacteria and other foreign particles. IgG exists in a series of subclasses (IgG_1, IgG_2, IgG_3, and IgG_4). IgG_3 and IgG_1 are efficient complement-fixing antibodies when cross-linked and are the most efficient IgG subclasses in binding to Fc receptors. IgG molecules are capable of crossing the placenta and thus provide neonates with "preformed" antibodies during a period when their own immune systems are immature. IgA antibodies are the major Ig's found on mucosal surfaces and appear to play a major role in preventing initial access of microorganism to portals of entry. Secreted IgA is locally synthesized and is tranported through epithelial cells in association with a specialized 70,000-dalton polypeptide, secretory component. IgE molecules are principally responsible for immediate-type allergic reactions. They are secreted at a relatively low rate and are tightly bound to specialized Fc receptors (Fc_ϵ receptors) on mast cells and basophils. Antigens capable of binding to and cross-linking IgE bound to basophil and mast cell Fc_ϵ receptors cause the rapid release of vasoactive amines and other mediators from such cells; this mediator release is responsible for allergic and *anaphylactic* responses. IgD, as already mentioned, functions almost exclusively as a membrane receptor. Although it is secreted in small amounts, no specific function has been identified for IgD as a secretory Ig.

The initial Ig's expressed by any cell are mIgM and mIgD. The descendants of such cells may secrete antibody of any of

TABLE 427–1. PROPERTIES OF HUMAN IMMUNOGLOBULINS

	IgG	IgA	IgM	IgD	IgE
H chain class	γ	α	μ	δ	ϵ
H chain subclass	$\gamma1,\gamma2,\gamma3,\gamma4$	$\alpha1,\alpha2$	$\mu1,\mu2$		
L chain type	κ and λ	κ and λ	κ and λ	κ and λ	κ and λ
Molecular formula	γ_2L_2	α_2L_2* or $(\mu_2L_2)_2$SC†J‡	$(\mu_2L_2)_5$J‡	δ_2L_2	ϵ_2L_2
Molecular weight (approximate)	150,000	160,000 400,000§	900,000	180,000	190,000
Complement fixation (classic)	+	0	+ +	0	0
Serum concentration (approximate; mg/dl)	1,000	200	120	3	0.05
Serum half-life (days)	23	6	5	2–8	1–5
Placental transfer	+	0	0	0	0
Reaginic activity	?	0	0	0	+ +

*Monomeric serum IgA; † secretory component; ‡ J chain; § secretory IgA.
Adapted from Goodman JW: Immunoglobulins, I. *In* Stites DP, Stobo JD, Fudenberg HHY, Wells JV (eds.): Basic and Clinical Immunology. Los Altos, Lange Medical Publications, 1982, p 34.

the other Ig classes. Such Ig possesses the same V region as did the mIg of the progenitor B cell. The change in Ig class expression that occurs during B cell differentiation is known as "switching" and is dependent on a genetic translocation event, in which the chromosomal segment containing the assembled *VDJ* gene is moved from its location proximal to the C_μ gene into a new position proximal to the *C* gene for the Ig H chain constant region that will be expressed by the cell (i.e., $C_{\gamma1}$, $C_{\gamma2}$, $C_{\gamma3}$, $C_{\gamma4}$, C_α, C_ϵ) (Fig. 427–2).

T LYMPHOCYTES

T cells mediate both effector and regulatory functions. In general, these distinct functions are mediated by separate subpopulations of T cells. The principal T cell effector functions are the destruction of antigen-bearing target cells by specific "killer" T cells and the production of potent mediators. These mediators are responsible for induction of a variety of inflammatory phenomena, such as delayed-type hypersensitivity that is associated with activation of macrophages and with the chemotaxis of granulocytes and monocytes.

As regulatory cells, T cells function in a variety of distinct ways. They produce *interleukin-2* (IL-2), the T cell growth factor, which is critical to the development of cytotoxic T cell responses. They act as helper cells, collaborating with B cells and enabling them to produce antibodies to thymus-dependent antigens. Helper T cells play an important role in determining the class and idiotype of antibody produced in an immune response. A separate set of regulatory T cells, the suppressor T cells, inhibits both antibody synthesis and cell-mediated immune responses, including delayed-type hypersensitivity.

T lymphocytes can be identified and quantitated because they bear specific membrane molecules that can be detected with *monoclonal antibodies*. (Monoclonal antibodies are homogeneous populations of antibody molecules, generally produced by somatic cell hybrids between activated normal B cells and a plasmacytoma cell line. Such hybrids are referred to as hybridomas.) All peripheral human T cells bear a determinant recognized by the monoclonal antibodies OKT3 and Leu 4. This determinant is borne on a membrane molecule that appears to play an important role in the process through which T cells are activated. Mature T cells may be subdivided into two major groups, recognized by distinct monoclonal antibodies, OKT4 and OKT8. T4-positive cells generally include helper T cells, and T8-positive cells include cytotoxic and suppressor T cells, although exceptions to this generalization exist. Measurement of the numbers of T cells in each of these subpopulations and their responsiveness to several mitogenic lectins, such as phytohemagglutinin (PHA), concanavalin A (con A), and pokeweed mitogen (PWM), provides a convenient *initial* means to assess certain aspects of T cell function. More specific and complex in vitro assays can be performed to measure helper and suppressor function.

T CELL DEVELOPMENT. T cells originate from hematopoietic stem cells. In contrast to B cells, T cell precursors undergo critical aspects of their differentiation in a specific central lymphoid organ, the thymus (Fig. 427–4). T cell precursors enter the thymus where an extensive series of proliferative events occurs and in which these cells develop into mature, antigen-reactive T cells that are seeded into the peripheral lymphoid tissue. Much of the functional repertoire of possible T cell responses seems to be formed within the thymus. T cell receptors have a complex specificity pattern. Their receptors corecognize epitopes of foreign antigens in association with structures on class I or class II MHC molecules. These structures on MHC molecules are designated *histotopes*. A single T cell receptor molecule recognizes an epitope-histotope complex.

The mature T cells of an individual are principally specific for antigenic epitopes in association with the histotopes expressed on the individual's own class I or class II MHC molecules. This corecognition of antigen with *self*-MHC molecules is often referred to as *histocompatibility restriction* (Fig. 427–5). It appears that the intrathymic selection events that shape the T cell repertoire are based on the capacity of developing thymocytes to recognize histotopes of self-class I or class II MHC molecules on thymic epithelial cells or thymic macrophages. Such events lead to the development of mature populations of T cells that have partial specificity for self-MHC molecules. It also appears that tolerance to many self-antigens may be established within the thymus.

Upon leaving the thymus, T cells are found in all the peripheral lymphoid tissues and in the blood and lymph.

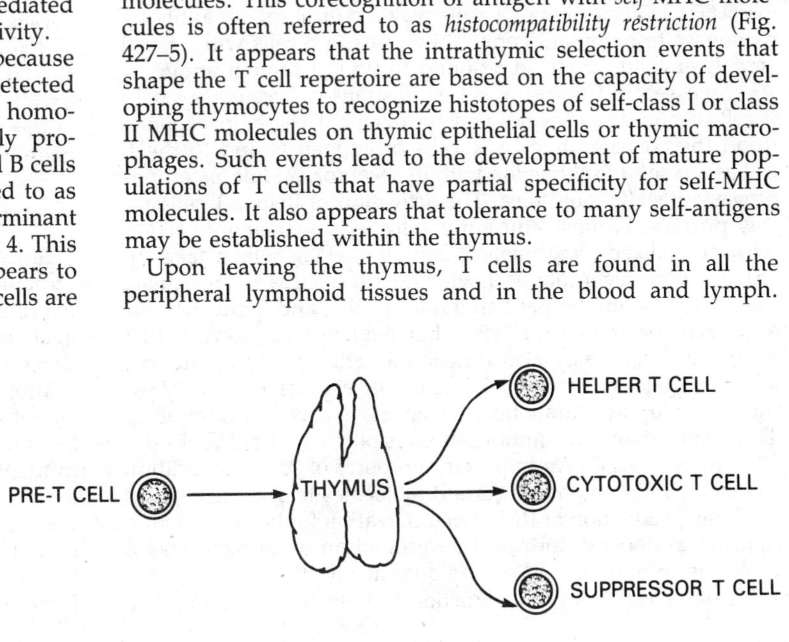

Figure 427–4. T cell differentiation. Precursors of T cells found in the hematopoietic tissue enter the thymus where they undergo differentiation and emerge into the periphery as cells of distinct function, bearing markers that allow their characterization. Whether a single pre-T cell can develop into each of the three T cell lines illustrated here or whether there are distinct sets of pre-T cells has not yet been elucidated.

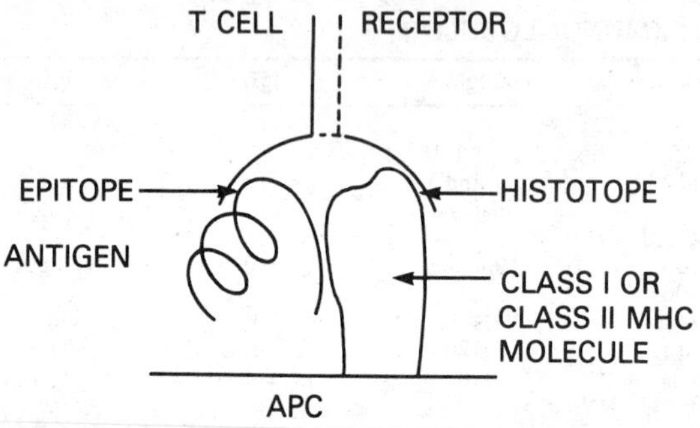

Figure 427–5. Corecognition of epitopes and histotopes by "MHC-restricted" T cell receptors. T cells that express histocompatibility-restriction in their interactions with B cells and macrophages have a complex antigen recognition system. These cells corecognize an antigenic determinant on a foreign molecule (an epitope) and a site on a self-MHC molecule (a histotope). Helper T cells generally corecognize epitopes with histotopes of class II MHC molecules. Cytotoxic T cells and their precursors generally corecognize epitopes with histopes of class I MHC molecules. The antigen recognition element of the T cell may be a single receptor with specificity for both the epitope and the histotope, or it may be two linked receptors, one specific for the epitope, the other for the histotope.

Within lymph nodes they tend to be principally found in the paracortex.

ANTIGEN-RECOGNITION BY T CELLS. Identification and characterization of the nature of the T cell receptor for antigen have been major goals of modern immunology. Recent work has provided very substantial insights into the nature of the T cell receptor. Monoclonal antibodies specific for unique structures on T cell clones block T cell activation by antigen. These antibodies, when polymerized onto polyacrylamide beads, can stimulate responses by the T cell clones for which they are specific. Such antibodies, designated *clonotypic* antibodies, appear to recognize epitopes on the antigen-binding receptors of T cells. The receptor molecule is a disulfide-linked heterodimer, consisting of two distinct chains (α chains and β chains), each of ~40,000 daltons. Both the α and β chains contain constant and variable peptides, suggesting that they may have a structure generally similar to immunoglobulins. A recently obtained complementary DNA clone appears to specify one of the two constituent polypeptide chains of the receptor. Detailed knowledge of the structure of the T cell receptor and of the genetic basis of antigen-binding repertoire of T cells will probably become available during the next several years.

HELPER T CELLS. Helper T cells play a critical role in antibody responses to many antigens. They provide B cells with critical signals enabling them to respond to typical protein antigens. As discussed in Control of B Cell Responses, T cells may help B cell responses in several ways. Cognate T cell help depends upon the corecognition by T cells of antigen bound to the B cell as a result of interaction with its receptor, and of histotopes of class II MHC molecules. The activation of helper T cells for this purpose is most efficiently achieved by their interaction with specialized *antigen-presenting cells* (APC), which take up antigen nonspecifically and which express class II molecules. Macrophages, epidermal Langerhan's cells, and dendritic cells appear to be important APC, but evidence is growing that activated B cells may also function as effective APC. Indeed, keratinocytes and endothelial cells can express class II MHC molecules upon stimulation by agents such as γ-interferon. These cells may have important physiologic and pathophysiologic roles as APC. An important property of APC, in addition to displaying antigen and class II molecules to T cells, appears to be the production of IL-1. T cell activation for helper function appears to depend both on the recognition of antigen-class II molecule complexes and on the presence of IL-1.

Helper T cells may also function to help B cells respond to antigen by producing BSF-p1, which is important in B cell proliferation, and by secreting a series of B cell differentiation factors.

Stimulated T cells produce IL-2 and thus play a critical role in proliferation of cytotoxic T cells. Recently the existence of T cell factors responsible for differentiation of precursors of cytotoxic T cells into active killer cells has been reported.

Whether the same T cells act as "cognate" helpers, as producers of B cell growth and differentiation factors, and as producers of IL-2 and cytotoxic differentiation factors is under current investigation. The means by which the production of these factors is regulated is poorly understood.

T cells also play an important role in regulating the class of Ig synthesized and in the selective expansion of clones of B cells that express certain unique antigenic determinants (*idiotopes*) on their receptors and on the antibodies that their descendants secrete. Such T cells appear to function by recognizing Ig determinants on the B cell rather than by recognizing antigen. Our understanding of the physiology and relative importance of "receptor-specific" helper T cells is much less complete than is that of cognate and factor-producing helper cells (see Idiotypic Networks).

SUPPRESSOR T CELLS. Suppressor T cells play important roles in the immune system both by inhibiting immune responses against self-components and by regulating responses to conventional antigens. The suppressor system is highly complex, consisting of a series of cell types that act sequentially. Several distinct suppressor systems have been described by investigators working with different experimental models and a consensus suppressor pathway has not yet been agreed upon. The sequential action of the cells that are members of suppressor pathways appears to have an important amplification effect; the final cell in the pathway inhibits the function of helper T cells. The action of such *suppressor-effector* cells on antibody-secreting cells and on cytotoxic T cells, or their precursors, has been less intensively studied, but evidence exists to suggest that these cells are also important sites of suppressor action.

CYTOTOXIC T CELLS. Cytotoxic T cells recognize, interact with, and destroy cells bearing specific foreign antigens. Cytotoxic T cells play a major role in the destruction of virally infected cells, which bear viral glycoproteins on their membranes. In addition, they may be very important in destroying tumor cells, which display unique tumor-associated antigens on their surfaces. Cytotoxic T cells generally corecognize foreign antigens together with histotopes on class I MHC molecules. Since essentially all cells express class I MHC molecules, cytotoxic T cells are capable of destroying cells of any type that express appropriate foreign antigens. The bulk of cytotoxic T cells are recognized by the OKT8 monoclonal antibody.

Cytotoxic T cells appear to lyse their target cells through a series of steps, including recognition and binding to the target cell and subsequent formation of "holes" in the membrane of the target cell. After this has been accomplished, the cytotoxic T cell may detach from its target and is free to attack other antigen-bearing cells. The cell in which membrane lesions have been induced will then undergo osmotic lysis (Fig. 427–6).

IDIOTYPIC NETWORKS

Since distinct antibodies have variable regions of different structure, it is hardly surprising that the antibodies themselves express unique antigenic determinants on their variable regions against which specific antibodies may be produced. These determinants are designated *idiotopes*, and the complement of idiotopes expressed by an individual Ig is its *idiotype*. The clonotypic antigenic determinants of T cells should be regarded as functionally equivalent to idiotopes of Ig. A provocative and influential theory holds that the immune system exists in a dynamic equilibrium in which members of each clone within the system are recognized by members of other clones (or by their products) through idiotope-antiidiotope interactions. A key postulate of this theory is that there is considerable structural similarity between many of the epitopes on exogenous

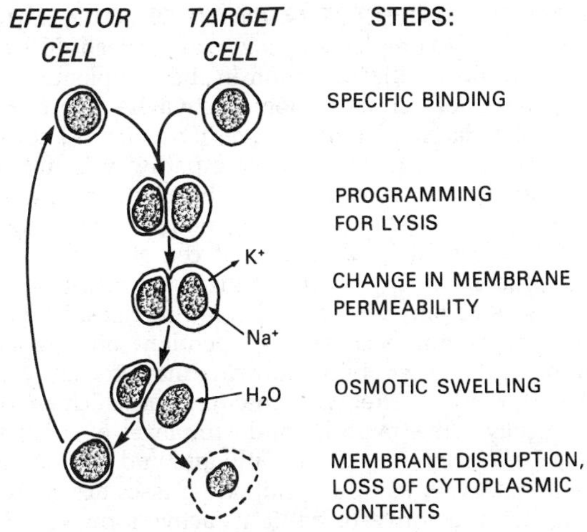

Figure 427–6. Stages in T cell-mediated lysis. (From Henry CS, Gillis S: Cell-mediated cytotoxicity. *In* Paul WE (ed.): Fundamental Immunology. New York, Raven Press, 1984, p 676.)

antigens and the idiotopes of Ig's or T cell receptors. Such idiotopes have sometimes been designated internal images of antigen. Thus, individual B cells and T cells may recognize internal images of antigen and may themselves be recognized by antibodies and T cells specific for the idiotopes they express. Such an interrelated system can allow an immune regulation based on recognition of receptors, without need for exogenous antigen, and can lead to dominance of a given immune response by cell types expressing particular idiotopes because of the action of idiotope-specific T cells or antibodies. Idiotopes that are dominantly expressed in immune responses because of such regulatory action have been designated *regulatory idiotopes*. The idiotope regulatory mechanism may offer opportunities for manipulation of the immune system to either enhance or suppress specific response. Furthermore, these idiotopes, as unique clonal markers, may also have value as specific markers of clonal malignant lymphoid disease. Therapy of human and experimental malignant lymphoid disease with idiotope-specific reagents appears to offer an exciting potential application of idiotypic network concepts.

MACROPHAGES

Cells of the monocyte-macrophage lineage play an important role in several aspects of the immune response. They have a critical function in (1) degrading complex structures, such as intact microorganisms, (2) processing the resulting antigens, and (3) presenting these antigens, in association with class II MHC molecules, to T cells that act as helper cells and that participate in cellular immune responses such as delayed hypersensitivity. This function depends upon the expression of class II MHC molecules on the macrophage. γ-Interferon, which is a product of activated T cells, can induce class II MHC molecules in macrophages. Thus, interactions between antigen-presenting macrophages and specific T lymphocytes are dynamic processes in which an initial activation step leads to the production of soluble factors capable of rendering many other macrophages competent to act as APC. A second important element in antigen presentation and T cell activation appears to be the production by macrophages of IL-1, a substance that has effects in many systems but that appears critical to activation of resting T cells.

Macrophages also function as phagocytic cells. They recognize and ingest foreign particles that are coated by antibodies or complement components (Ch. 148). Macrophages possess membrane Fc receptors, which bind avidly to the aggregated Ig found in antigen-antibody complexes; they also bear receptors for fragments of the third component of complement. These complement fragments are generated in the course of the activation of the complement cascade and are found on opsonized microorganisms and in association with immune complexes.

Whether phagocytosed microorganisms and tumor cells are destroyed depends on both the nature of the ingested particle and the state of activation of the macrophage. Phagocytosis itself appears to be associated with a respiratory burst that enhances the bactericidal activity of the macrophage. Furthermore, T cell products, such as macrophage-activating factor, increase the capacity of macrophages to destroy ingested microorganisms and cells.

NATURAL KILLER CELLS AND ANTIBODY-DEPENDENT CELLULAR CYTOTOXICITY

Natural killer (NK) cells are lymphoid cells from normal individuals that can lyse certain cell types, particularly members of certain long-term tumor cell lines. The NK cells in human peripheral blood are large lymphoid cells with prominent granules and are referred to as large granulocytic lymphocytes. However, their precise cellular lineage remains uncertain; they may be members of the T cell lineage, of the monocyte-macrophage lineage, or of an independent lymphoid lineage. Some patients with severe combined immunodeficiency have depressed NK activity while others display normal NK activity.

The cytotoxic mechanism employed by NK cells is probably very similar to that of specific cytotoxic T lymphocytes. It has been proposed that NK cells play an important role in surveillance mechanisms postulated to destroy emerging clones of malignant cells, but firm evidence for this view is still lacking.

Antibody–dependent cellular cytotoxicity (ADCC) is the destruction of antibody-coated cells by cytotoxic cells that possess Fc receptors. Evidence suggests that NK cells, or closely related cells, mediate ADCC. In general, the ADCC effector cells recognize the Fc region of IgG (Fc_γ) on the target cell, but Fc_μ- and Fc_ϵ-specific ADCC has been described.

ADCC almost certainly has immunopathologic significance. It appears to be important in autoimmune states in causing lysis of autoantibody-coated cells, in destruction of antibody-coated tumor cells, and in destruction of antibody-coated parasites.

CONCLUSIONS

The basic elements of the immune system, working together in a regulated manner, allow a rapid, specific and highly protective response against foreign substances such as those associated with pathogenic microorganisms and against neoantigens expressed by tumor cells. Disorders, both qualitative and quantitative, in this system can have profound effects. It is clear that deficient immune responses may expose the individual to potentially devastating consequences. Furthermore, much of the tissue damage that occurs in a wide range of diseases is due to abnormal action of immune mechanisms. The subsequent chapters of this part, Diseases of the Immune System, outline in detail the pathophysiology of the immune system itself, describing disorders that directly relate to its function. Chapters in Part XXII, Connective Tissue Diseases, describe many key examples in which disordered immune responses or, perhaps, normal responses to abnormal stimuli lead to profound disruption of normal function. Furthermore, immunologically mediated inflammation and tissue damage are key features of many diseases, affecting virtually every organ system. Progress in preventing and treating these disorders will require clear understanding of the nature of the immunologic abnormalities in each case. In turn, this will require a much deeper understanding of the normal physiology of the immune system than is now available to us.

Annual Review of Immunology, 1983–1984, Vol 1 & 2. *A yearly series of reviews on topics in fundamental and clinical immunology aimed at providing a means of keeping up with this rapidly developing field.*

Parker CW (ed.): Clinical Immunology. Philadelphia, W. B. Saunders Company, 1980. *A detailed discussion of the application of immunologic mechanisms in pathophysiologic situations and a discussion of immunologic aspects of many disease states.*

Paul WE (ed.): Fundamental Immunology. New York, Raven Press, 1984. *A general textbook of basic immunologic mechanisms.*

Samter MD (ed.): Immunologic Diseases. 3rd ed. Boston, Little, Brown & Company, 1979. *An extended discussion of immunologic diseases and the mechanisms that underlie them.*

Stites DP, Stobo JD, Fudenberg HH, Wells JV (eds.): Basic and Clinical Immunology. 4th ed. Los Altos, Lange Medical Publications, 1982. *A good introductory text.*

428. COMPLEMENT

Douglas T. Fearon

GENERAL CONSIDERATIONS. Complement functions as part of the immune system to protect the individual from microbial infection by mediating a variety of biologic reactions: opsonization, chemotaxis of leukocytes, increased vascular permeability, and cytolysis of target organisms. These activities of complement that promote an inflammatory reaction also carry the potential for damaging the host. Human disease related to complement may manifest either as defective resistance to infection secondary to impaired activation of the system or as hypersensitivity states caused by excessive complement activation.

The complement system consists of 18 proteins (Table 428–1) found in highest concentrations in plasma. These proteins are said to be in the "classic pathway" or "alternative pathway," names which arose from common usage rather than considerations of relative importance or phylogenetic priorities. The proteins of the classic pathway are designated by letter C and a number: C1 (which comprises three distinct proteins, C1q, C1r, and C1s, that are held together by calcium), C4, C2, C3, and C5 to C9. Proteins of the alternative pathway are designated by capital letters: B, D, P, H, and I. Although C3 has been found to be an essential constituent of the alternative pathway, it has retained its classic pathway nomenclature. Cleavage fragments of components are denoted by lower case letters, as in C3a, C3b, Ba, and Bb, and inactive components are signified by the letter i, as in C3bi and Bbi. An overbar, as in C$\bar{1}$, indicates that a component has been converted to its enzymatically active form.

TABLE 428–1. PROTEINS OF THE COMPLEMENT SYSTEM

Name*	Former Designation	Molecular Weight	Serum Concentration (μg/per Milliliter)
C1q	—	400,000	70
C1r	—	95,000	35
C1s	—	85,000	35
C4	—	209,000	400
C2	—	117,000	25
C3	—	185,000	1500
C5	—	200,000	85
C6	—	128,000	75
C7	—	121,000	55
C8	—	153,000	55
C9	—	80,000	200
B	C3 proactivator, glycine-rich β glycoprotein	95,000	250
D	C3 proactivator convertase	25,000	2
P	Properdin	160,000	25
C$\bar{1}$ inhibitor	—	105,000	180
C4-binding protein	—	$1.2-1.5 \times 10^6$	250
H	β1H	150,000	400
I	KAF, C3b inactivator	90,000	50

*This nomenclature for the alternative pathway proteins has been submitted by the Nomenclature Committee of the International Union of Immunology Societies to the World Health Organization for final approval and adoption.

ACTIVATING AND EFFECTOR PATHWAYS OF COMPLEMENT. The cleavage of C3 by complement enzymes, termed "C3 convertases," is the most critical reaction in the complement system for the elaboration of its biologic activities. There are two pathways, the classic and alternative, by which C3 convertase enzymes may be formed. The classic pathway is initiated by certain antigen-antibody complexes which confer immunologic specificity on this system. The phylogenetically older alternative pathway is activated by a variety of cell surfaces (including those of some bacteria, parasites, fungi, and mammalian cells) which possess certain biochemical characteristics. The alternative pathway is not necessarily dependent on antibody for recognition of the target. Both pathways may efficiently activate C3 and C5–C9 of the "effector" proteins from which are derived the biologically active peptides and complexes of complement.

Classic Pathway (Fig. 428–1). Only IgM and IgG can activate the classic pathway, as other antibody classes are not capable of binding C1 and converting it to its active form, C$\bar{1}$. Binding of the C1q subcomponent of C1 to the Fc regions of one IgM or of at least two adjacent IgG molecules within an antigen-antibody complex induces a conformational change in C1q that leads to conversion of C1r to active C$\overline{1r}$. This subcomponent then proteolytically activates C1s to C$\overline{1s}$. The C$\overline{1s}$ subcomponent of C$\bar{1}$ sequentially cleaves C4, whose major C4b fragment covalently binds to the immune complex, and C2 to generate C2a, which is taken up by C4b to form C4b,2a, the classic pathway C3 convertase. The site for proteolysis of C3 resides in C2a, which also acquires C5-cleaving activity after the major cleavage fragment of C3, C3b, covalently binds to adjacent sites on the target. The C4b,2a enzyme undergoes spontaneous decay of C3- and C5-cleaving activities by release of C2a, which immediately becomes inactive C2ai.

Three plasma proteins regulate activation of the classic pathway. The C$\bar{1}$ inhibitor (C$\bar{1}$INH) irreversibly binds to and blocks the enzymatic sites on C$\overline{1r}$ and C$\overline{1s}$, which prevents activation of C1s by the former and cleavage of C4 and C2 by the latter. C$\bar{1}$INH also retards spontaneous activation of C1. The C4 binding protein (C4bp) binds to C4b to prevent uptake of C2 or to dissociate C2a that is already complexed to C4b. Binding of C4bp also makes C4b susceptible to proteolytic inactivation by C3b/C4b inactivator (I), which yields two degradation fragments, C4c and C4d.

Alternative Pathway (Fig. 428-2). The alternative pathway is more complex than the classic pathway, since two C3 convertases are formed. The *"priming" C3 convertase*, C3,Bb, is assembled by the slow interaction in the fluid phase of C3 (in which the internal thiol ester has been hydrolyzed), B, D, and properdin regardless of the presence of activating substances, and

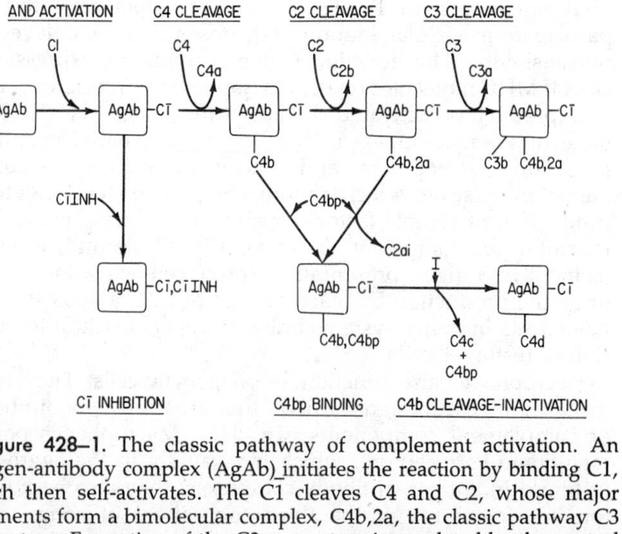

Figure 428–1. The classic pathway of complement activation. An antigen-antibody complex (AgAb) initiates the reaction by binding C1, which then self-activates. The C1 cleaves C4 and C2, whose major fragments form a bimolecular complex, C4b,2a, the classic pathway C3 convertase. Formation of the C3 convertase is regulated by the control proteins C1INH, C4bp, and I.

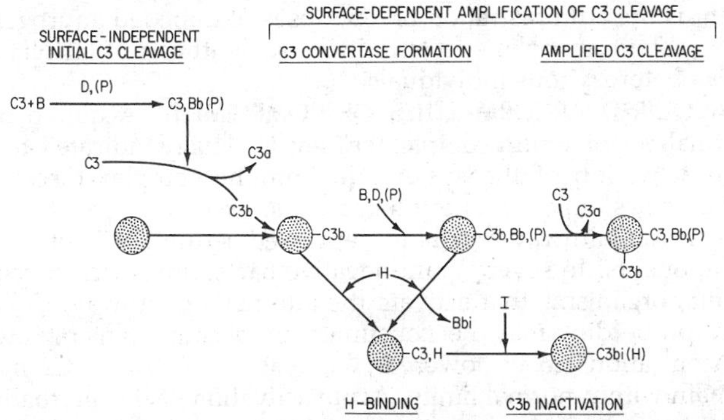

Figure 428–2. The alternative pathway of complement activation. C3b, which is slowly and continuously generated by a "priming" C3 convertase, C3b,Bb(P), may attach to bystander cells. If the cell is an activator of the pathway, the amplification C3 convertase, C3b,Bb(P), is formed and catalyzes cleavage and deposition of additional molecules of C3b. In contrast, C3b bound to a nonactivator binds the regulatory protein, H, and is converted to inactive C3bi by I. P is shown in parentheses to indicate that it augments C3 convertase activity but is not required for alternative pathway activation.

it continuously provides small amounts of C3b that can initiate formation of the *"amplification" C3 convertase*, C3b,Bb. This amplification C3 convertase is responsible for effective C3 cleavage by the alternative pathway, and the adjective "amplification" is used because C3b is both a subunit and a product of this enzyme. C3b that has attached covalently to cell surfaces binds B, and the latter is cleaved by D to uncover the C3 cleaving site on the Bb fragment. C3b,Bb rapidly loses activity by spontaneous dissociation of the catalytic Bb subunit, which becomes inactive Bbi. Properdin serves to stabilize C3 convertase activity by binding to the C3b subunit and retarding dissociation of Bb. C3b,Bb acquires C5 convertase activity after cleavage of additional C3 and deposition of C3b at an adjacent site on the activating target. Regulation of the amplification C3 convertase is essential because of its positive feedback potential and is effected by two control proteins, H and I. The capacity of H to bind to C3b endows it with three inhibitory effects: blocking formation of C3b,Bb, dissociation of Bb that is already bound to C3b, and increasing the susceptibility of C3b to proteolysis by I which yields C3bi, an inactive form of the protein.

The outcome of the competition between B and H for uptake by C3b on a cell membrane determines whether that cell activates the alternative pathway. C3b that is in the fluid phase or affixed to the surface of a nonactivator of the pathway binds H with almost 100-fold greater affinity than that with which it binds B, whereas C3b on the surface of an activator binds H less effectively, and uptake of the control protein is not favored relative to uptake of B. The latter circumstance results in formation of C3b,Bb on the surface of the activating cell and amplifies the reaction by cleavage of additional C3.

A biochemical characteristic of cell membranes that influences the affinity of cell-bound C3b for H is the relative amount of sialic acid that is present in membrane-associated glycoproteins and glycolipids. This carbohydrate increases the affinity of C3b for H but not for B so that its presence on a cell membrane prevents alternative pathway activation. Conversely, the absence of cell surface sialic acid permits activation to occur on a membrane.

The capacity of the alternative pathway to respond to cells that are deficient in sialic acid residues may be relevant to its role in natural resistance to infection, since most bacteria, some parasites, and all plants lack this carbohydrate. Moreover, some of the bacterial species having capsular sialic acid, such as Type III Group B *Streptococcus*, Groups B and C *Neisseria meningitidis*, and K1 *Escherichia coli*, are pathogenetic for man, suggesting that capsular sialic acid facilitates evasion of host defense. The capacity of antibody to enhance activation of the alternative pathway by bacteria and mammalian cells without involvement of classic activating components also has been demonstrated and may be related to alteration of the distribution of membrane structures capable of regulating the uptake and function of cell-bound C3b.

Effector Sequence (Fig. 428–3). Assembly of C5 convertases by the two activating pathways provides the enzyme specificity that is necessary to continue the complement reaction through the effector sequence. Proteolytic cleavage of C5 liberates the C5a peptide that has anaphylatoxic and chemotactic activities and yields the major C5b fragment that initiates assembly of the membrane attack complex of C5b–9. C6 and C7 bind to C5b to form a trimolecular complex with exposed hydrophobic regions that inserts partially into the membrane of the target cell bearing the C5 convertase. The uptake by membrane-associated C5b–7 of C8 and as many as five C9 molecules leads to further insertion of the complex into the membrane; formation of a transmembrane channel through which water, salt, and small molecules can pass; swelling of the cell; and, eventually, lysis.

Although the cytolytic function of complement may protect the host against certain organisms, many pathogenetic bacteria are resistant to the action of C5b–9. In these instances, the most critical reactions for host defense would be the proteolytic cleavages of C3 and C5, which generate activities that can recruit leukocytes to the extravascular focus of complement activation and enhance the capability of the cells for phagocytosis of the target. The C3a and C5a peptides release histamine from mast cells, increasing local vascular permeability. Another peptide derived from C3, C3e, promotes leukocytosis by releasing neutrophils from the bone marrow. C5a also causes accumulation of inflammatory cells at the site of complement activation by inducing adherence of neutrophils to endothelial cells and chemotaxis of polymorphonuclear leukocytes and monocytes. In addition, C5a increases the number of C3b receptors on neutrophils and monocytes. Once these cells have arrived, their capacity to ingest and kill the target organism is greatly enhanced by the presence of C3b on the complement-activating particle, as this opsonin attaches the target to the phagocyte via C3b receptors on the latter's plasma membrane. The functions of C3b receptors on B lymphocytes have not been entirely defined, although uptake of antigen, generation of B memory cells, and enhanced responses to pokeweed mitogen have been described. Thus, complement may kill cells directly by cytolysis or indirectly by recruitment of certain leukocyte functions.

INHERITED ABNORMALITIES OF COMPLEMENT (Table 428-2). ***Association with Increased Susceptibility to Infection.*** An increased incidence of bacterial infections in patients with homozygous deficiencies of C3, I, H, C5, C6, C7, or C8 has been

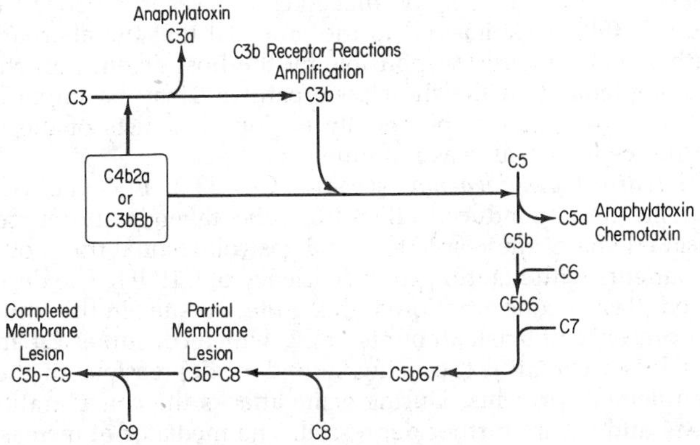

Figure 428–3. The effector sequence of complement, which is activated by the C3/C5 convertases of the classic and alternative pathways. Some of the prominent biologic activities associated with cleavage fragments and multimolecular complexes are shown.

TABLE 428-2. DISEASES ASSOCIATED WITH DEFICIENCIES OF COMPLEMENT

Deficient Component	Disease
Clq	SLE, vasculitis
Clr	Glomerulonephritis, SLE*
Cls	SLE
C1̄INH	HAE†, discoid LE, SLE
C4	SLE
C2	Glomerulonephritis, SLE, discoid LE, purpura, dermatomyositis, hemolytic anemia, JRA‡
C3	Pyogenic infections
I	Pyogenic infections
H	Pyogenic infections
C5	Neisserial infections, SLE
C6	Neisserial infections, Raynaud's phenomenon
C7	Neisserial infections, Raynaud's phenomenon
C8	Neisserial infections
C9	None
P	Neisserial infections

*Systemic lupus erythematosus.
†Hereditary angioedema.
‡Juvenile rheumatoid arthritis.

noted. Absence of C3 abolishes the capacity of serum to opsonize some pathogenetic bacteria, and prevents activation of C5–C9, from which are derived the chemotactic and cytolytic activities of complement. Thus, individuals with this deficiency have had multiple serious pyogenic infections. Two patients with homozygous deficiency of I or H and secondarily depressed serum concentrations of C3 and B also have increased susceptibility to bacterial infections. Absence of C5, which would impair both chemotactic and cytolytic activities of complement, was found in a patient with recurrent bacterial infections who also had systemic lupus erythematosus. Individuals with deficiency of C5, C6, C7, or C8 appear to have a selective propensity for developing disseminated neisserial infections without experiencing an increased incidence of infections with other pyogenic organisms, suggesting that cytolysis rather than phagocytosis is the primary host mechanism for defense against gonococci and meningococci.

Associations with Immunologic Disease. A variety of diseases with immunologic bases have been found in association with inherited deficiencies of Clq, Clr, Cls, C4, C2, and C3 components of the classic activating pathway. Also, patients with systemic lupus erythematosus have an inherited partial deficiency of C3b receptors on erythrocytes. Possible consequences of these deficiencies that may predispose to diseases associated with elevated levels of circulating immune complexes include impaired solubilization of immune complexes, impaired clearance of immune complexes, and lack of generation of peptide fragments of C3 that have immunoregulatory functions. The relatively low frequency of infectious diseases in persons lacking C1, C4, or C2 has led to the proposal that the alternative pathway is primarily responsible for the host defense function of complement, while the classic pathway may be important for the processing of potentially noxious products of the immune response, such as immune complexes.

Hereditary Angioedema (see also Ch. 431). Episodic, occasionally trauma-induced attacks of subcutaneous and submucosal edema of the respiratory and gastrointestinal tracts occur in patients with heterozygous deficiency of C1̄INH. The diminished plasma concentration of this protein results in the continual presence of small amounts of C1̄, which consumes C4 and, to a lesser extent, C2, causing secondary depressions of these complement proteins. During acute attacks the concentrations of C4 and C2 are further depressed. The mediator of increased vascular permeability is not known. As C1̄INH inhibits not only C1̄r and C1̄s of complement but also activated Hageman factor and kallikrein, regulation of several plasma protein enzyme systems is impaired in those patients. Current treatment is the administration of low doses of impeded androgens with potent anabolic effects to increase synthesis of C1̄INH in these heterozygous individuals.

ACQUIRED ABNORMALITIES OF COMPLEMENT. Acquired abnormalities of serum complement levels usually indicate excessive activation of the system. In immune complex diseases, such as systemic lupus erythematosus, excessive activation of the classic pathway results in depressed serum levels of these components. In severe gram-negative bacteremia or cryptococcemia, organisms that activate the alternative pathway, C3, B, and properdin, may be consumed in plasma, causing their concentrations to be lowered, whereas C1, C4, and C2 may remain within normal limits. Acute activation of the alternative pathway occurs also in patients undergoing hemodialysis with cellulosic membranes. The C5a that is generated during this procedure causes aggregation of neutrophils and their sequestration within the pulmonary vasculature. Some studies suggest this effect of C5a may have a role in the adult respiratory distress syndrome.

An unusual mechanism for alternative pathway activation occurs in some patients with membranoproliferative glomerulonephritis and in most patients with partial lipodystrophy with or without glomerulonephritis. Their sera have low levels of C3, normal concentrations of C1, C4, and C2, and an IgG autoantibody, termed C3 nephritic factor, which is specific for antigenic determinants on the amplification C3 convertase. Binding of this autoantibody to C3b,Bb creates a stable trimolecular complex that is resistant to dissociation of its catalytic Bb subunit by H, causing deregulated consumption of C3 by the alternative pathway. An IgG autoantibody to the classic pathway C3 convertase with analogous stabilizing activity has been described in a few patients with systemic lupus erythematosus.

CLINICAL MEASUREMENTS OF COMPLEMENT. Activation of a complement protein results in loss of its precursor, native activity, and in its accelerated clearance from plasma. If hypercatabolism is not compensated for by increased synthesis, the determination of depressed levels of complement protein in plasma or other body fluids may provide evidence for activation of the system. Complement can be measured by assaying the function of its components, by utilizing hemolytic assays which detect only native, unaltered proteins, or by immunochemical assessment of the protein concentration of individual components, usually by immunoprecipitation assays which do not discriminate between native and altered components. The most frequently employed functional assay of complement activity is the determination of the amount of serum or other body fluid required to lyse 50 per cent of a sample of sheep erythrocytes that has been sensitized with rabbit antibody, and is reported as CH50 units. The test measures the overall activity of C1–C9; is not influenced by the alternative pathway proteins B, D, or properdin; and is relatively insensitive to a modest decrease in the activity of a single component. However, the CH50 is useful as an initial screen to detect marked consumption of complement proteins or homozygous deficiencies of individual components. Specific functional assays for all components of both pathways require specialized reagents that are not available in most clinical laboratories, and individual components are usually measured by immunoprecipitation. For the evaluation of patients with hypocomplementemia, determination of the C4 and C3 protein concentrations is most informative. Low concentrations of C4 indicate that classic pathway activation has occurred, since C4 is extremely sensitive to C1̄. Depressed levels of C3 suggest that rather intense activation of either pathway is occurring, and, if found to be associated with normal levels of C4, indicate that exclusive activation of the alternative pathway is occurring. Recently developed radioimmunoassays for the peptide activation fragments of C4 and C3, C4a and C3a, may also be useful for determination of complement activation. Finally, the involvement of complement in a pathologic process is most directly assessed by immunofluorescent staining of individual complement proteins in the involved tissue.

Alper CA, Rosen FS: Inherited deficiencies of complement proteins in man. Springer Semin Immunopathol. In press. *Discussion of the clinical pathologic correlations of complement deficiency states.*

Fearon DT, Wong WW: Complement ligand receptor interactions that mediate biological responses. Ann Rev Immunol 1:243, 1983. *Review of cellular receptors for complement proteins, an aspect of complement that is the basis for many of the biologic effects of this system.*

Lachmann PJ, Peters DK: Complement. *In* Lachmann PJ, Peters DK (eds.): Clinical Aspects of Immunology. Boston, Blackwell Scientific Publications, Ltd., 1982, pp 18–49. *An excellent review of the basic biochemistry, biology, and clinical aspects of complement.*

429. PRIMARY IMMUNODEFICIENCY DISEASES

Rebecca H. Buckley

The first example of human immunodeficiency was described in 1952. Similar or related syndromes have subsequently been reported with increasing frequency. Immunodeficiency diseases may involve all components of the immune system, including lymphocytes, phagocytic cells, and the complement proteins. This chapter will focus on abnormalities of lymphocytes. Deficiencies of the complement system (see Ch. 428) are mentioned briefly. A review of the syndromes associated with neutrophil dysfunction is presented in Ch. 149 and an overall review of the compromised host is given in Ch. 257. The acquired immunodeficiency syndrome (AIDS) is described in Ch. 430.

Despite the large body of knowledge gained regarding functional derangements and cellular abnormalities in the various primary disorders of lymphocytes, the fundamental biologic errors for most of them remain unknown. Exceptions include two defects accompanied by purine salvage pathway enzyme deficiencies—adenosine deaminase in some cases of autosomal recessive severe combined immunodeficiency and purine nucleoside phosphorylase in some patients with Nezelof's syndrome. The genetic error in many other immunodeficiencies must, by definition, be located on the X chromosome. None of the primary defects studied have been found to have associated deficiencies of particular HLA antigens; thus they are unlikely to represent defects involving HLA-linked immune response genes on chromosome 6. Since trace amounts of immunoglobulins of all five isotypes can usually be found in the serum of even the most severely agammaglobulinemic patient, it is also unlikely that immunoglobulin deficiency states are due to deletions of genes encoding for immunoglobulin heavy chains. This does not, however, exclude the possibility of regulatory gene defects.

Various classifications of immunodeficiency disorders involving lymphocytes have attempted to postulate the cellular levels at which the defects occur. Cells with mature differentiation markers of both T and B lymphocytes, however, have been found in most of the known defects. In many cases, normal numbers of such cells have been found despite profound absences of T or B cell function or both. Thus, in most cases the suspect cell lineage is not missing but malfunctional. Table 429–1 lists the current state of knowledge of the most prominent functional deficits and the presumed cellular level of the defect in 18 primary immunodeficiency syndromes.

In contrast to the acquired immune deficiency syndrome (AIDS), which has a new case acquisition rate of 50 per week, primary immunodeficiency diseases are rare. The incidence of agammaglobulinemia is estimated at 1 in 50,000. Selective absence of serum and secretory IgA, the most common, has a reported prevalence of 0.03 to 0.97 per cent.

ANTIBODY DEFICIENCY DISORDERS

Antibody deficiency may occur either as an apparent congenital disorder or as an "acquired" abnormality. Most patients are recognized because they have recurrent infections, but some individuals with selective IgA deficiency or infants with transient hypogammaglobulinemia may have few or no infections. Table 429–2 lists some of the general features of these disorders.

X-LINKED AGAMMAGLOBULINEMIA. A majority of boys afflicted with this malady remain well during the first six to nine months of life, presumably by virtue of maternally transmitted immunoglobulin. Thereafter they repeatedly acquire infections with high-grade extracellular pyogenic organisms such as pneumococci, streptococci, and *Hemophilus* unless given prophylactic antibiotics or gamma globulin therapy. The most common types of infections include sinusitis, pneumonia, otitis, furunculosis, meningitis, and septicemia. Chronic fungal infections are usually not present, and *Pneumocystis carinii* pneumonia rarely occurs unless there is an associated neutropenia. Viral infections and live virus vaccines are also usually handled normally, with the notable exceptions of hepatitis and enterovirus infections. Several examples of paralysis after polio vaccine administration have occurred, presumably because of mutation of persistent vaccine virus to a more neurotropic form. In addition,

TABLE 429–1. CLASSIFICATION OF PRIMARY IMMUNODEFICIENCY DISORDERS*

Disorder	Functional Deficiencies	Presumed Cellular Level of Defect
X-linked agammaglobulinemia	Antibody	Pre-B cell
Common variable (B lymphocyte) hypogammaglobulinemia	Antibody	B lymphocyte
Selective IgA deficiency	IgA antibody	IgA B lymphocyte
Secretory component deficiency	Secretory IgA	Mucosal epithelium
Selective IgM deficiency	IgM antibody	T helper cells
Immunodeficiency with elevated IgM	IgG and IgA antibodies	IgG, IgA B lymphocytes
Transient hypogammaglobulinemia of infancy	None; immunoglobulins low, but antibodies present	Unknown
Antibody deficiency with near-normal immunoglobulins	Antibody	Unknown; ?B cell
X-linked lymphoproliferative disease	Anti–EBV nuclear antigen antibody	B cell; ?also T cell
DiGeorge's syndrome	T cellular; some antibody	Dysmorphogenesis of 3rd & 4th branchial pouches
Nezelof's syndrome (including with PNP deficiency)	T cellular; some antibody	Unknown; ?thymus; ?T cell; metabolic defects
Severe combined immunodeficiency syndromes (autosomal recessive; ADA deficiency; X-linked recessive; bare lymphocyte syndrome; reticular dysgenesis)	Antibody and T cellular; phagocytic in reticular dysgenesis	Unknown; metabolic defect(s); ?T cell; ?stem cell; ?thymus
Wiskott-Aldrich syndrome	Antibody; T cellular	Unknown
Ataxia-telangiectasia	Antibody; T cellular	B lymphocyte; helper T lymphocyte
Immunodeficiency with short-limbed dwarfism	T cellular	G1 cycle of many cells
Immunodeficiency with thymoma	Antibody; some T cellular	B lymphocyte; excessive T suppressor cells
Hyperimmunoglobulinemia E	Specific immune responses; excessive IgE	Unknown
Chronic mucocutaneous candidiasis	Variable cellular	?Antigen overload

*From Buckley RH: Immunodeficiency. J Allergy Clin Immunol 72:627–641, 1983.

TABLE 429–2. CLINICAL CHARACTERISTICS OF ANTIBODY DEFICIENCY DISORDERS

1. Recurrent infections with high grade extracellular encapsulated pathogens
2. Few problems with fungal or viral (except enterovirus) infections
3. Chronic sinopulmonary disease
4. Growth retardation not striking
5. Antibody deficiency in serum and secretions
6. May or may not lack B lymphocytes with surface immunoglobulins or complement receptors
7. Absence of cortical follicles in lymph node and spleen in X-linked agammaglobulinemia
8. Paucity of palpable lymphoid and nasopharyngeal tissue in X-linked agammaglobulinemia
9. Compatible with survival to adulthood or for several years after onset except for those with persistent enterovirus infections, autoimmune disorders, or malignancy

a dermatomyositis-like syndrome accompanied by chronic, eventually fatal central nervous system disease caused by various echoviruses has occurred in more than 20 patients. Approximately 20 per cent of patients have an arthritis resembling juvenile rheumatoid arthritis.

The diagnosis of X-linked agammaglobulinemia is suspected if serum concentrations of IgG, IgA, and IgM are below the 95 per cent confidence limits for appropriate age and race-matched controls (usually there is <100 mg per deciliter total immunoglobulin). The demonstration of antibody deficiency in serum and in external secretions is of great importance in distinguishing this disorder from transient hypogammaglobulinemia of infancy. Tests for natural antibodies to blood group substances, for antibodies to antigens given during standard courses of immunization, e.g., diphtheria, tetanus, or pneumococcus, and for antibodies to and ability to clear bacteriophage $\phi \times 174$ are markedly abnormal. Polymorphonuclear functions are usually normal, but some patients with this condition have had transient, persistent, or cyclic neutropenia.

Lymphopenia is uncommon, and the percentages of T cells and T cell subsets have been found to be normal or elevated in most instances. In contrast, blood lymphocytes bearing surface immunoglobulin, "Ia-like" antigens or the EBV receptor, or reacting with a specific anti-B cell serum are absent or present in very low number. Hypoplasia of adenoids, tonsils, and peripheral lymph nodes is the rule; germinal centers are not present, and plasma cells are rarely found (Fig. 429–1). Conversely, normal numbers of pre-B cells are found in the bone marrow. Mixed lymphocyte responsiveness and lymphocyte responses to antigens and mitogens are normal. Cell–mediated immune responses can be detected in vivo, and the capacity to reject allografts is intact. The thymus has appeared normal in all autopsied cases, and lymphoid cells are abundant in thymus-dependent areas of peripheral lymphoid tissues.

Except in those unfortunate patients who develop polio, persistent echovirus infection, or lymphoreticular malignancy (an incidence as high as 6 per cent has been reported), the overall prognosis is reasonably good if humoral replacement therapy is instituted early. Systemic infection can be prevented by administration of immune serum globulin (ISG; primarily IgG) by the intramuscular or intravenous route. Use of the traditional loading dose of 200 mg per kilogram and maintenance dose of 100 mg per kilogram every three to four weeks is currently under review; it is likely that higher or individualized doses, or both, will be recommended. Thus far, there have been no reports of the transmission of AIDS with ISG, and such preparations are also known to be free of hepatitis antigens. Use of random donor plasma as a source of Ig carries the risk of transmission of both of these, although plasma from a known safe donor is a valuable source (10 ml per kilogram will provide approximately 100 mg IgG per kilogram). Many patients go on to develop crippling sinopulmonary disease despite this therapy, since no effective means now exists for replacing secretory IgA at the mucosal surface. Intermittent or chronic antibiotic therapy is often necessary in addition for the management of such patients.

AGAMMAGLOBULINEMIA WITH IMMUNOGLOBULIN-BEARING B LYMPHOCYTES. This condition, also known as common variable agammaglobulinemia (CVAγ), may appear similar clinically in many respects to X-linked agammaglobulinemia. Although this disorder may occur in infants and young children, most patients present with a history of recurrent infection beginning several years after birth. This disorder is distinguished from X-linked agammaglobulinemia by later age of onset, somewhat less severe susceptibility to infections, and almost equal sex distribution. In contrast to patients with the X-linked form, patients with CVAγ may have normal-sized or enlarged tonsils and lymph nodes, and the latter may have cortical follicles. Additionally, such patients often have normal or near-normal numbers of circulating immunoglobulin-bearing B lymphocytes. Nevertheless, the serum immunoglobulin and antibody deficiencies are usually just as profound by measurement, and the bacterial etiologic agents are the same as in the X-linked disorder. Thus far no documented examples of fatal

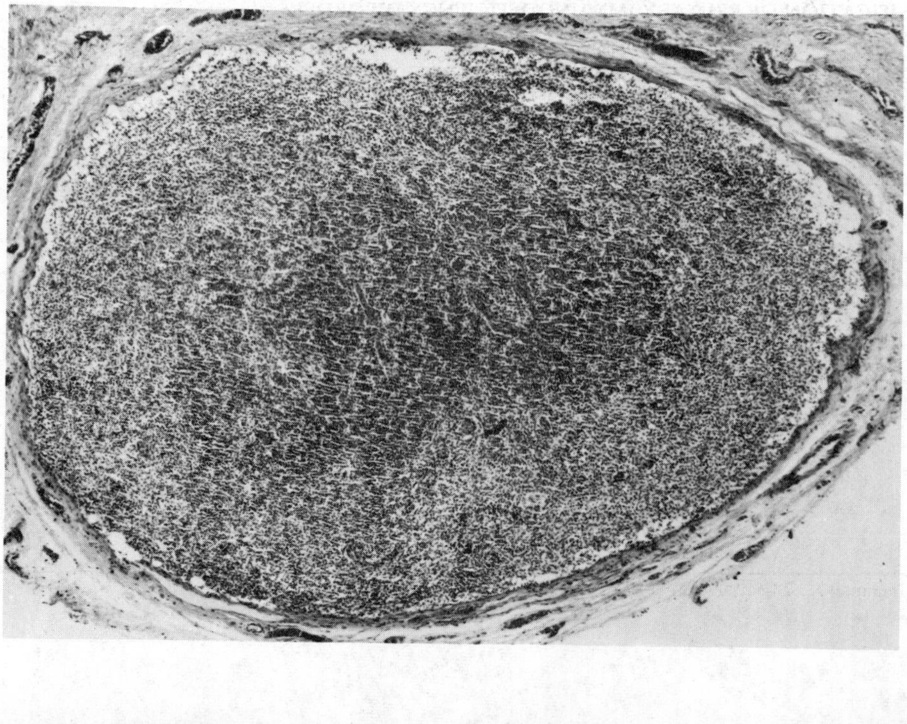

Figure 429–1. Section of lymph node from boy with infantile X-linked agammaglobulinemia, a classic example of an antibody deficiency disorder. Note absence of cortical follicles but relatively dense paracortical area. (From Buckley RH: *In* Middleton E, Reed CE, Ellis EF [eds.]: Allergy: Principles and Practice. St. Louis, C. V. Mosby Company, 1978, p 200.)

echovirus meningoencephalitis have occurred in patients with CVAγ.

This condition has been variably associated with a sprue-like syndrome, with or without nodular follicular lymphoid hyperplasia of the intestine; thymoma; alopecia areata; and autoantibody formation leading to hemolytic anemia, gastric atrophy, achlorhydria, and pernicious anemia. Frequent complications include giardiasis (seen far more often here than in X-linked agammaglobulinemia), bronchiectasis, gastric carcinoma, lymphoreticular malignancy, and cholelithiasis. Lymphoid interstitial pneumonia, pseudolymphoma, amyloidosis, and noncaseating granulomas of the lungs, spleen, skin, and liver have also been seen.

Despite normal numbers of circulating immunoglobulin-bearing B lymphocytes and the presence of lymphoid cortical follicles, the lymphocytes do not differentiate in vivo or in vitro into immunoglobulin-producing plasma cells, even in the presence of the polyclonal B cell activator, pokeweed mitogen. Although the primary biologic error responsible for this defect is unknown, in most patients it appears to be due to abnormal terminal differentiation of the B cell line. Because this disorder occurs in first-degree relatives of patients with selective IgA deficiency, and some patients with hyper-IgM have later become panhypogammaglobulinemic (or vice versa), it is possible that these diseases all belong to the same spectrum of B cell maturation arrests. The inconstancy of excessive suppressor T cell activity suggests that this mechanism is not etiologic for these disorders as a whole. The treatment of CVAγ is the same as for the X-linked disorder.

SELECTIVE IgA DEFICIENCY. An isolated near-absence (i.e., <10 mg per deciliter) of serum and secretory IgA is the most common immunodeficiency disorder so far detected, a frequency of 1:886 being reported among blood donors. Although IgA deficiency has been observed in apparently healthy individuals, it is commonly associated with ill health. The kinds of health problems experienced often reflect the type of clinic from which the patients are drawn. Among 75 from an allergy-immunology clinic, there were high frequencies of chronic or recurrent respiratory tract infection and atopic diseases. In contrast, 30 IgA-deficient patients drawn from a rheumatology clinic had a high frequency of autoimmune and/or collagen vascular disease.

IgA is the major immunoglobulin of external secretions. As would be expected, its deficiency is associated with infections occurring predominantly in the respiratory, gastrointestinal, and urogenital tracts. Bacterial agents responsible are essentially the same as in other types of antibody deficiency syndromes. A high incidence of viral hepatitis was noted in one group of IgA-deficient patients, but there is no clear evidence that patients with this disorder have an undue susceptibility to other viral agents. Children with IgA deficiency produce local IgM and IgG antipolio antibodies to killed vaccine given intranasally and IgM and IgG antirubella antibodies during convalescence from natural rubella. The compensating IgM seems to be locally synthesized and capable of combining with secretory piece for local secretion similar to IgA. Serum concentrations of other immunoglobulins are usually normal in patients with selective IgA deficiency, although an IgG_2 subclass deficiency has been reported in some, and IgM (usually increased) may be of the low molecular weight variety.

In addition to limiting the attachment of infectious agents to mucosal surfaces, secretory IgA antibodies probably act to prevent absorption of other foreign antigens, such as those in the diet. There is a high incidence of allergy and of IgG antibodies against cow's milk and ruminant serum proteins in patients with IgA deficiency. The antiruminant antibodies often present technical problems in immunoassays of IgA which employ goat (but not rabbit) antisera. Intestinal nodular hyperplasia has been seen in a few such patients. A sprue-like syndrome may occur in adults with selective IgA deficiency and sometimes responds to a gluten-free diet.

The basic defect leading to selective IgA deficiency is unknown. IgA–bearing blood B cells from most such patients also coexpress surface IgM and IgD, similar to cord blood B cells, suggesting maturation arrest. In addition, the B lymphocytes fail to secrete IgA in vitro. Some have exhibited excessive isotype-specific T suppressor cells. Studies of T cell function have been normal in most patients. The defect may not always be permanent. The author, in following over 150 such patients, has seen the spontaneous development of normal serum IgA concentrations in ten children documented for several years to have absence of or extremely low concentrations of IgA. The occurrence of IgA deficiency in both males and females and in families suggests autosomal inheritance.

Serum antibodies to IgA are found in as many as 44 per cent of such patients. This observation is of possible etiologic and great clinical significance. At least seven IgA-deficient patients have had severe or fatal anaphylactic reactions after intravenous administration of blood products. For this reason, only multiply washed erythrocytes or blood products from other IgA-deficient individuals should be administered to these patients; ISG (which contains a small amount of IgA) is contraindicated.

Currently the only treatment for IgA deficiency is vigorous treatment of specific infections with appropriate antimicrobial agents. Even if serum IgA could be replaced (in the face of anti-IgA antibodies), it would not be transported into the external secretions, since the latter is an active process involving only locally produced IgA.

SECRETORY COMPONENT DEFICIENCY. A patient with chronic intestinal candidiasis and diarrhea was found to lack IgA in his external secretions, despite having a normal concentration of serum IgA. This was traced to a lack of secretory piece, which prevented the normal secretion of locally produced IgA.

SELECTIVE IgM DEFICIENCY. If one uses a strict definition of a serum IgM concentration less than 10 mg per deciliter, there are very few well-documented cases of this entity. Fatal septicemia caused by meningococci and other gram-negative organisms has been noted in some such patients. Others have experienced bacterial infections of other types, including pneumococcal meningitis, tuberculosis, recurrent staphylococcal pyoderma, periorbital cellulitis, bronchiectasis, and recurrent otitis. There is no specific therapy; early and vigorous treatment with antibiotics is recommended to avoid the fatal septicemia that has occurred in some patients.

IMMUNODEFICIENCY WITH ELEVATED IgM. This disorder is characterized by very low serum concentrations of IgG and IgA but a markedly elevated concentration of polyclonal IgM. Some patients have low molecular weight IgM molecules. Similar to patients with X-linked agammaglobulinemia, those with this defect commonly become symptomatic during infancy with recurrent pyogenic infections, including otitis media, sinusitis, pneumonia, and tonsillitis. In contrast to patients with X-linked agammaglobulinemia, however, the frequent presence of lymphoid hyperplasia often leads away from a diagnosis of immunodeficiency. There is an increased frequency of autoimmune disorders, such as hemolytic anemia and thrombocytopenia, and transient, persistent, or cyclic neutropenia is common. Thymic-dependent lymphoid tissues and T cell functions are usually normal, but several have had partial T cell deficiencies. A sex-linked mode of inheritance has been proposed, but several examples of the disorder in females now seem to make this less certain.

The pathogenesis of the hyper-IgM syndrome has yet to be elucidated. Normal or only slightly reduced numbers of Ig-bearing B lymphocytes have been found in the blood; however, cultured B cell lines from such patients have shown the capacity to synthesize only IgM, suggesting a B cell maturation defect that prevents isotype switching. Plasma cells in lymph nodes contain only IgM.

Because these patients are unable to make IgG antibodies, the treatment is the same as for agammaglobulinemia.

TRANSIENT HYPOGAMMAGLOBULINEMIA OF INFANCY. This condition has been described as a prolongation and accentuation of the "physiologic" decline in serum immunoglobulin concentrations normally seen during the first three to seven months of life. Unlike patients with X-linked or common variable agammaglobulinemia, those with transient hypogammaglobulinemia can synthesize antibodies to human type A and B erythrocytes and to diphtheria and tetanus toxoids, usually by six to eleven months of age, well before immunoglobulin concentrations become normal. The finding of only eleven cases of transient hypogammaglobulinemia of infancy among over 10,000 sera tested by the author over a twelve-year period suggests that, contrary to popular opinion, this is not a common entity.

Gamma globulin replacement therapy is not indicated in this condition. In addition to the known risks of inducing anti-IgG allotype antibodies, passively administered antibodies could block endogenous primary antibody formation in the same manner that RhoGAM suppresses anti-D antibodies in Rh-negative mothers delivering Rh-positive infants.

ANTIBODY DEFICIENCY WITH NEAR-NORMAL IMMUNOGLOBULINS. Only scattered reports have appeared in the literature describing patients with deficient antibody responses despite apparently normal T cell function and normal or near-normal immunoglobulin concentrations. The author and her associates have studied the antibody-forming capacities of twelve such patients. Blood group antibody titers were absent in all but two, diphtheria titers were low in all, and tetanus titers were low in ten. Geometric mean antibody titers to thirteen pneumococcal serotypes were significantly lower than those of normal controls before and after immunization with tridecavalent pneumococcal polysaccharide vaccine. All patients cleared bacteriophage $\phi \times 174$ normally, but all primary immune responses were far below the normal range. Secondary responses to $\phi \times 174$ were also below the normal range in all but two, but, in both cases, most of the secondary response was IgM rather than IgG. This type of immune problem would not be detected unless functional tests of antibody-forming capacity are regularly conducted in the assessment of humoral immunity. Patients with this disorder are candidates for immunoglobulin replacement therapy.

X-LINKED LYMPHOPROLIFERATIVE DISEASE. This disorder, also referred to as *Duncan's disease* (after the original kindred in which it was described), is characterized by an impaired immune response to Epstein-Barr virus (EBV). Males affected with this condition are apparently healthy until they experience infectious mononucleosis. Two thirds of the 100 patients studied thus far died of overwhelming EBV–induced B cell proliferation during mononucleosis. A majority of the survivors developed hypogammaglobulinemia or B cell lymphomas or both. Such individuals have marked impairment in production of antibodies to the EBV nuclear antigen, whereas titers of antibodies to the viral capsid antigen have ranged from zero to markedly elevated. Antibody-dependent cell-mediated cytotoxicity against EBV-infected cells and natural killer function are depressed, and there is a deficiency in long-lived T cell immunity to EBV. Despite normal numbers of B and T cells, there is an elevated percentage of lymphocytes of the suppressor (T8) phenotype. In addition, lymphocyte immunoglobulin synthesis in response to polyclonal B cell mitogen stimulation in vitro is markedly depressed. Thus, both EBV-specific and nonspecific immunologic abnormalities occur in these patients.

CELLULAR IMMUNODEFICIENCY DISORDERS

Some important clinical characteristics of cellular immunodeficiency disorders are listed in Table 429–3. In general, patients with partial or absolute defects in T cell function have infections or other clinical problems for which there is no effective treatment or which are often of a more severe nature than in those with antibody deficiency disorders. It is therefore rare that such individuals survive beyond infancy or childhood.

TABLE 429–3. CLINICAL CHARACTERISTICS OF CELLULAR IMMUNODEFICIENCY DISORDERS

1. Recurrent infections with low grade or opportunistic infectious agents such as fungi, viruses, or *Pneumocystis carinii*
2. Delayed cutaneous anergy
3. Accompanied by growth retardation, short life span, wasting, and diarrhea
4. Susceptible to graft-versus-host (GVH) disease if given fresh blood, plasma, or unmatched allogeneic bone marrow
5. Fatal reactions from live virus or BCG vaccination
6. High incidence of malignancy

THYMIC HYPOPLASIA (DIGEORGE'S SYNDROME). This condition results from dysmorphogenesis of the third and fourth pharyngeal pouches, leading to hypoplasia or aplasia of the thymus and parathyroid glands. Other structures forming at the same age are also frequently affected, resulting in anomalies of the great vessels (right-sided aortic arch), esophageal atresia, bifid uvula, congenital heart disease (atrial and ventricular septal defects), a short philtrum of the upper lip, hypertelorism, an antimongoloid slant to the eyes, mandibular hypoplasia, and low-set (often notched) ears. The diagnosis is usually first suggested by the presence of hypocalcemic seizures during the neonatal period. DiGeorge's syndrome has occurred in both males and females, and there is little evidence that it is heritable.

A variable degree of hypoplasia is more frequent than total aplasia of the thymus and parathyroid glands. Some children with the features of this syndrome have little trouble with infections and show evidence of some cell-mediated immunity. They are often referred to as having partial DiGeorge's syndrome. Those with marked thymic hypoplasia may resemble infants with severe combined immunodeficiency in their susceptibility to infection with low-grade or opportunistic pathogens (i.e., fungi, viruses, and *Pneumocystis carinii*) and to graft-versus-host (GVH) disease from nonirradiated blood transfusions.

Serum immunoglobulins are usually normal for age, but some fractions, particularly IgA, may be diminished and IgE may be elevated. T cell numbers are decreased, and there is an increased number of B cells. Responses of peripheral blood lymphocytes following mitogen stimulation, like the intradermal delayed hypersensitivity response, have been absent, reduced, or normal. Careful postmortem studies have sometimes revealed tiny nests of thymic tissue containing Hassall's corpuscles and a normal density of thymocytes. Lymphoid follicles usually appear normal, but lymph node paracortical areas and thymus-dependent regions of the spleen show variable degrees of depletion, depending upon the degree of thymic hypoplasia. Because of variability in the severity of the immunodeficiency, it is difficult to evaluate claimed benefits of fetal thymus transplantation.

CELLULAR IMMUNODEFICIENCY WITH IMMUNOGLOBULINS (NEZELOF'S SYNDROME). This syndrome is characterized by lymphopenia, diminished lymphoid tissue, abnormal thymus architecture, and the presence of normal or increased levels of most of the five immunoglobulin classes. Children with this condition may have recurrent or chronic pulmonary infections, failure to thrive, oral or cutaneous candidiasis, chronic diarrhea, recurrent skin infections, gram-negative sepsis, urinary tract infections, severe varicella, progressive vaccinia, or combinations of these. An autosomal recessive pattern of inheritance has been suggested in some cases, but an X-linked mode seemed more likely in others. Other findings include neutropenia and eosinophilia. Serum immunoglobulins may be normal or elevated for all classes, but selective IgA deficiency and marked elevation of IgE occur not infrequently.

Studies of cellular immune function have shown delayed cutaneous anergy to ubiquitous antigens and low to absent in vitro lymphocyte responses to mitogens and allogeneic cells.

Such patients have profound deficiencies of total T cells and T cell subsets, with usually a normal helper (T4+) to suppressor (T8+) cell ratio, in contrast to patients with AIDS who characteristically have marked inversion of the T4:T8 ratio due to selective deficiency of T4+ cells. Peripheral lymphoid tissues demonstrate paracortical lymphocyte depletion. The thymuses are very small and have a paucity of thymocytes and usually no Hassell's corpuscles; however, again in contrast to AIDS, thymic epithelium is present. These could all be useful in distinguishing Nezelof's syndrome from AIDS in the pediatric age group, since it is the primary immunodeficiency disorder most likely to be confused with it. Fatal or serious infections have included varicella, vaccinia, *Pneumocystis carinii*, cytomegalovirus, rubeola, *Pseudomonas*, and *Mycobacterium kansasii*. Antibody-forming capacity has been apparently normal in roughly one third of the reported cases. Plasma cells are usually abundant in the lamina propria and lymph nodes. Although in one patient with this disorder reconstitution was successful by means of a matched sibling bone marrow transplant, most other forms of therapy have been unsuccessful.

With Purine Nucleoside Phosphorylase Deficiency. More than a dozen patients with Nezelof's syndrome have been found to have purine nucleoside phosphorylase (PNP) deficiency. In contrast to patients with adenosine deaminase (ADA) deficiency, serum and urinary uric acid are markedly deficient, and no characteristic physical or skeletal abnormalities have been noted. Three patients have suffered from a progressive neurologic disorder with spastic tetraplegia, two developed an autoimmune hemolytic anemia, and one has idiopathic thrombocytopenic purpura. Deaths have occurred from generalized vaccinia, varicella, lymphosarcoma, and GVH disease following a blood transfusion. In contrast to a majority of patients with Nezelof's syndrome, the thymuses of PNP-deficient patients have had some Hassall's corpuscles, reminiscent of some patients with ADA deficiency. Analyses of lymphocyte subpopulations with monoclonal antibodies in two such patients revealed marked deficiency of T cells and T cell subsets but increased numbers of cells with natural killer (NK) phenotype and function. Attempts to correct the immunologic and enzymatic deficiencies of PNP-deficient patients by enzyme replacement therapy, using normal erythrocyte transfusions or deoxycytidine, have not been very successful.

SEVERE COMBINED IMMUNODEFICIENCY (SCID) DISORDERS

The syndromes of SCID are distinguished by their apparent congenital absence of all adaptive immune function. Unless immunologic reconstitution can be achieved through immunocompetent tissue transplants or enzyme replacement therapy or unless gnotobiotic isolation can be carried out, death usually occurs before the patient's first birthday. For some time it has been assumed that an absence or a failure of proliferation and/or differentiation of the "primordial" stem cell was the basis of these syndromes. Unfortunately, this theory does not explain the great diversity of genetic, enzymatic, hematologic, and immunologic features observed. The major subcategories of this disorder are discussed below.

AUTOSOMAL RECESSIVE SEVERE COMBINED IMMUNODEFICIENCY DISEASE. Within the first few months of life, infants affected with this first-described SCID syndrome have frequent episodes of otitis, pneumonia, sepsis, diarrhea, and cutaneous infections. Growth may appear normal initially, but extreme wasting soon develops. Infections with opportunistic organisms such as *Candida albicans*, *Pneumocystis carinii*, vaccinia, varicella, measles, cytomegalovirus, and BCG frequently lead to death caused either by difficulties encountered in diagnosis or by a lack of effective treatment. These infants also lack the ability to reject foreign tissue and are therefore at risk for GVH disease. GVH reactions can result from maternal immunocompetent cells crossing the placenta or from the administration of blood products containing viable histoincompatible lymphocytes.

Immunologic evaluation reveals serum immunoglobulin concentrations to be diminished or absent, and no antibody formation occurs following immunization. There is a near-total lack of cellular immune function, with lymphopenia and absence of or extremely low lymphocyte responses to mitogens or allogeneic cells, delayed cutaneous anergy, and inability to reject foreign tissues. Marked heterogeneity of lymphocyte subpopulations exists among SCID patients, even among those with similar inheritance patterns. Despite the uniformly profound lack of T or B cell function, some patients have had low numbers of both B and T lymphocytes, whereas others have had elevated numbers of B cells; occasionally even normal numbers of both T and B cells have been found. Cytofluorographic studies with monoclonal antibodies to mature T cells and subsets have generally revealed some, albeit low, percentages of cells reacting with all such reagents; however, there is no increase in cells bearing the T6 antigen present on immature cortical thymocytes. Thus the lymphocytes present appear to have acquired surface markers characteristic of mature T cells. In contrast to similarly lymphopenic patients with AIDS, SCID patients rarely have an inverted ratio of helper (T4+) to suppressor (T8+) cells. Recently a new phenotype of SCID was characterized by the author in which virtually all of the lymphocytes of two infants with SCID were large granular lymphocytes with NK cell phenotype and function. NK function has been totally lacking in other SCID patients, again illustrating the striking heterogeneity at a cellular level. Typically, these patients have very small thymuses (less than 2 grams), which usually fail to descend from the neck, contain few thymic lymphocytes, lack corticomedullary distinction, and usually lack Hassall's corpuscles (see exception below). Despite the profound thymocyte depletion in SCID patients, thymic epithelium is present—in contrast to the situations in AIDS in which there is marked epithelial atrophy. Both the follicular and paracortical areas of the peripheral lymph nodes are depleted of lymphocytes. Tonsils, adenoids, and Peyer's patches are absent or extremely underdeveloped.

ISG fails to halt the progressively downhill course of SCID. Transplantation of bone marrow cells from HLA genotypically identical or D locus compatible donors has resulted in apparent complete correction of the immunologic defect in a number of these patients, with some 40 known long-term survivors. Fetal tissue transplants have been much less effective. Recently a major advance has allowed the use of haploidentical (half-matched) bone marrow cells for correction of the immunologic defect in SCID. In this technique, which takes advantage of the affinity of human T cells for soybean lectin and for sheep erythrocytes, post-thymic T cells are selectively and completely removed, leaving the stem cells intact for transplantation. To date, over 30 infants with SCID who would have otherwise died because of lack of an HLA-identical donor have been treated successfully with this approach, with virtually no signs of GVH reaction.

With Adenosine Deaminase (ADA) Deficiency. Absence of the enzyme ADA has been observed in some but not all patients with the autosomal recessive form of SCID; approximately 30 families have been identified in which ADA deficiency was associated with severe immunodeficiency. A marked accumulation of deoxyadenosine and its triphosphate may provide the biochemical mechanisms responsible for the immunodeficiency. Deoxyadenosine is an apparent suicide inactivator of the enzyme S-adenosylhomocysteine (SAH) hydrolase and could alter methylation in a manner which would lead to cell death. Although most such patients have had profound lymphopenia from the earliest age studied, a few have had early normal or fluctuating lymphocyte counts that declined by six weeks to two years of life. In marked contrast to "classic" SCID, some ADA-deficient patients have been found to have a few Hassall's corpuscles in their thymuses and changes suggestive of early differentiation. Other distinguishing features of ADA-deficient SCID disorders have included the presence of rib cage abnormalities similar to a rachitic rosary and multiple skeletal abnormalities of chondro-osseous dysplasia on radiographic examination.

Both matched sibling and haploidentical post-thymic T cell–depleted bone marrow transplants have resulted in lymphocyte chimerism and partial or complete correction of the immunologic defect in ADA-deficient SCID. Enzyme replacement therapy, consisting of the administration of 15 ml per kilogram of glycerol-frozen, irradiated, packed normal erythrocytes every two to four weeks, has resulted in temporary immunologic or clinical improvement or both in some such patients.

X-LINKED RECESSIVE SEVERE COMBINED IMMUNODEFICIENCY DISEASE. This is thought to be the most common form of SCID in the United States. There have been no examples of deficiencies of the purine salvage pathway enzymes ADA or PNP in association with SCID in pedigrees in which there has been proven X-linked inheritance. Clinically, immunologically, and histopathologically, these patients appear similar to those with the autosomal recessive form.

BARE LYMPHOCYTE SYNDROME. In this form of combined immunodeficiency there is a lack of expression of HLA antigens and the absence of B_2 microglobulin on lymphocytes. Nine examples of this defect have now been reported, all from the Mediterranean area. The associated defects of immunity and of HLA expression support the concept of a biologic role of HLA determinants in the development of functional T lymphocytes.

SEVERE COMBINED IMMUNODEFICIENCY WITH LEUKOPENIA (RETICULAR DYSGENESIS). In 1959, identical twin male infants were described who exhibited a total lack of both lymphocytes and granulocytes in their peripheral blood and bone marrow. Seven of eight infants reported died between 3 and 119 days of age from overwhelming infections; the eighth underwent complete immunologic reconstitution from a bone marrow transplant. The organisms responsible have been both bacterial and viral, including cytomegalovirus, *Pseudomonas*, *Klebsiella*, and pyogenic cocci. A genetic, probably autosomal, influence seems likely from reports of familial occurrences.

Serum immunoglobulins were very low and no lymphocyte responses to mitogens occurred in the four patients in whom immunologic evaluations were conducted. The thymus glands all weighed less than 1 gram, and no Hassall's corpuscles and few or no thymocytes were seen.

PARTIAL COMBINED IMMUNODEFICIENCY DISORDERS

IMMUNODEFICIENCY WITH THROMBOCYTOPENIA AND ECZEMA (WISKOTT-ALDRICH SYNDROME). This X-linked recessive syndrome is characterized clinically by the triad of eczema, megakaryocytic thrombocytopenic purpura, and undue susceptibility to infection. Often there is prolonged oozing from the circumcision site or bloody diarrhea during infancy. Atopic dermatitis and recurrent infections usually develop during the first year of life. Infections are caused by pneumococci and other bacteria with polysaccharide capsules, resulting in episodes of otitis media, pneumonia, meningitis, and sepsis. Later, as cellular immunity wanes, infections with *Pneumocystis carinii* and the herpesviruses become more frequent. Survival beyond the teens is rare; major causes of death are infections or bleeding, but a 12 per cent incidence of fatal malignancy also occurs in this condition. A papovavirus has been recovered from a reticulum cell sarcoma of the brain and from the urine of patients with this syndrome.

The earliest evidence of immunodeficiency is an impaired humoral immune response to polysaccharide antigens. Absent or markedly diminished isohemagglutinin titers are uniformly found, and poor or no responses are seen following immunization with polysaccharide antigens. Antibody titers to protein antigens also fall with time, and anamnestic responses are often poor or absent. Studies of immunoglobulin metabolism have shown an accelerated rate of synthesis, as well as hypercatabolism, of albumin, IgG, IgA, and IgM, resulting in highly variable immunoglobulin concentrations. The predominant dysgammaglobulinemia is a low IgM, an elevated IgA and IgE, and a normal or slightly low IgG concentration. Lymphocyte responses are moderately depressed, and cutaneous anergy is a frequent finding. Analyses of blood lymphocytes with monoclonal reagents have revealed low percentages of cells reacting with antibodies to all T cells and to the helper (T4+) and suppressor (T8+) subsets. However, as with the other primary cellular immunodeficiencies, there is usually no imbalance in the T4:T8 ratio.

The thrombocytopenia appears to be due to an intrinsic platelet abnormality, since antiplatelet antibodies are not usually demonstrated and survival times of homologous but not autologous ^{51}Cr-labeled platelets have been normal in these patients.

Treatment has been directed primarily toward control of bleeding with platelet transfusions, splenectomy, or both and of infections by intravenous administration of ISG. Several patients have had complete corrections of both the platelet and immunologic abnormalities by HLA-matched sibling bone marrow transplants after being conditioned with irradiation or busulfan and cyclophosphamide.

ATAXIA-TELANGIECTASIA. This is a complex syndrome with neurologic, immunologic, endocrinologic, hepatic, and cutaneous abnormalities. The most prominent clinical features are progressive cerebellar ataxia, oculocutaneous telangiectasia, chronic sinopulmonary disease, a high incidence of malignancy, and variable humoral and cellular immunodeficiency. Ataxia typically becomes evident soon after the child begins to walk and progresses until he or she is confined to a wheelchair, usually by ten to twelve years of age. Telangiectasias usually develop by three to six years of age. Recurrent, usually bacterial, sinopulmonary infections occur in roughly 80 per cent of these patients; common viral exanthems and smallpox vaccination have not usually resulted in untoward sequelae. However, varicella was fatal in one of the author's patients.

The malignant tumors reported have usually been of the lymphoreticular type, but others have been seen. Cells from such patients, as well as those from heterozygous carriers, have been reported to have increased sensitivity to ionizing radiation, defective DNA repair, and frequent chromosomal abnormalities. An autosomal recessive mode of inheritance seems operative.

The most frequent immunologic abnormality is selective absence of IgA, found in from 50 to 80 per cent of these patients. IgE concentrations are usually low, and the IgM may be of the low molecular weight variety. Specific antibody levels may be decreased or normal. In vivo, there is impaired but not absent cell-mediated immunity, as evidenced by delayed cutaneous anergy and prolonged allograft survival. Death from GVH disease has not been reported. Enumeration of blood T cells and subsets in five patients with this disorder revealed reduced percentages of total T cells and T cells of the helper (T4) phenotype, with normal or increased percentages of cells of the suppressor (T8) phenotype. In vitro studies of lymphocyte function have shown moderately depressed proliferative responses to mitogens, decreased T helper cell function, and an intrinsic defect in B cell IgA synthesis. The thymus is very hypoplastic and lacks Hassall's corpuscles. No satisfactory treatment has been found.

IMMUNODEFICIENCY WITH SHORT-LIMBED DWARFISM. An unusual form of short-limbed dwarfism with frequent and severe infections has been reported among the Amish; some affected individuals also had cartilage-hair hypoplasia. Features include short and pudgy hands; redundant skin; hyperextensible joints of hands and feet but an inability to completely extend the elbows; and fine, sparse light hair and eyebrows. Severe and often fatal varicella infections appear to be a particular hazard.

Progressive vaccinia and vaccine-associated poliomyelitis have also been observed.

The severity of the immunodeficiency varies; in one series, 11 of 77 patients died before age 20 but two were still alive at age 76. Three patterns of immune dysfunction have emerged: defective antibody-mediated immunity, defective cellular immunity, and severe combined immunodeficiency. The most striking abnormality appears to be one of defective cell proliferation due to an intrinsic defect related to the G1 phase, resulting in a longer cell cycle for individual cells. The trait appears to be autosomal recessive with variable penetrance.

IMMUNODEFICIENCY WITH THYMOMA. These patients are adults who almost simultaneously develop hypogammaglobulinemia, deficits in cell-mediated immunity, and benign thymoma (see Ch. 439). The thymomas are predominantly of the spindle cell variety. Eosinophilia or eosinopenia, aregenerative or hemolytic anemia, thrombocytopenia, or pancytopenia may also occur. Antibody formation is poor, although percentages of immunoglobulin-bearing B lymphocytes are normal, and progressive lymphopenia develops. Several patients with this disorder have been shown to have excessive suppressor T cell activity.

HYPERIMMUNOGLOBULINEMIA E SYNDROME. The hyper-IgE syndrome is a primary immunodeficiency characterized by recurrent staphylococcal abscesses and markedly elevated serum IgE concentrations. The disorder was first reported by the author and her coworkers in two young boys in 1972. These patients all have lifelong histories of severe recurrent staphylococcal abscesses involving the skin, lungs, joints, and other sites. Persistent pneumatoceles develop as result of their recurrent pneumonias. The pruritic dermatitis that occurs is not typical atopic eczema and does not always persist; respiratory allergic symptoms are usually absent. An autosomal dominant form of inheritance with incomplete penetrance seems possible. Laboratory features include exceptionally high serum IgE concentrations but usually normal IgG, IgA, and IgM concentrations; pronounced blood and sputum eosinophilia; abnormally low anamnestic antibody responses; and poor antibody and cell-mediated responses to neoantigens. In vitro studies have shown normal percentages of E rosette-forming, T3-, T4-, and T8-positive lymphocytes, and there is no increase in the percentage of IgE–bearing B lymphocytes. Lymphocyte responses to mitogens are normal, but responses to antigens or to related allogeneic cells have been absent or very low. Histologic sections of lymph nodes, spleen, and lung cysts show striking eosinophilia.

Phagocytic cell ingestion, metabolism, and killing mechanisms and total hemolytic complement have been normal in all patients. Defects of mononuclear and/or polymorphonuclear chemotaxis are present in some but not all patients, and thus are not the basic problem in this syndrome.

The most effective therapy is long-term administration of a penicillinase resistant penicillin, with the addition of other antibiotic or antifungal agents as required for specific infections.

CHRONIC MUCOCUTANEOUS CANDIDIASIS. This clinical syndrome, probably of multiple causes, is associated with chronic candidal infection of the skin and mucous membranes but only rarely life-threatening systemic infections of the types seen in patients with severe T cell dysfunction. Some patients have endocrinopathies involving the parathyroid, thyroid, adrenal, and/or pancreatic glands (see Ch. 240); however, many do not have either associated endocrinopathy or any demonstrable immunologic abnormality. Serum immunoglobulins are generally normal or increased, but IgA deficiency has been reported. Precipitating or agglutinating antibodies to *Candida* are usually present. Even in those patients who have had in vivo and/or in vitro evidence of deficient cell-mediated immunity, it is not clear whether it was primary or secondary to extensive fungal disease (e.g., an antigen overload mechanism). Ketaconazole (Nizoral) has been found to be the single most effective form of therapy. Nephrotoxicity prohibits continuous therapy with amphotericin B.

PRIMARY DEFICIENCIES OF THE COMPLEMENT SYSTEM

In addition to congenital or hereditary disorders of lymphoid cells, there are several well-defined primary immune defects involving the complement system. Genetically determined deficiencies have been described for all of the components of complement, and undue susceptibility to infection is a characteristic of certain of these, particularly for deficiencies of C2, C3, C5, C6, and C7. The types of infections experienced in C2, C3 and in some with C5 deficiency are generally similar to those of patients with antibody deficiency syndrome, whereas those in patients with deficiencies of the terminal components are usually of meningococcal or gonococcal causes. A normal CH50 would exclude all heritable complement deficiencies. The complement system is discussed in detail in Chapter 428.

Buckley RH: Normal and abnormal development of the immune system. *In* Joklik WK, Willett HP, Amos DB (eds.): Zinsser Textbook of Microbiology and Immunology. 18th ed. New York, Appleton-Century-Crofts, 1984, pp 317–340. *A concise review of ontogeny of the normal human immune system as well as the primary immunodeficiency disorders.*

Buckley RH: Immunodeficiency diseases. *In* Kelley WN, et al. (eds.): Textbook of Rheumatology. Philadelphia, W. B. Saunders Company, 1981, pp 1351–1377. *A comprehensive, extensively referenced chapter on primary immunodeficiency, with particular emphasis on the occurrence of collagen vascular and autoimmune diseases in certain of these disorders.*

Buckley RH, Sampson HA: The hyperimmunoglobulinemia E syndrome. *In* Franklin EC (ed.): Clinical Immunology Update. New York, Elsevier North Holland, 1980, pp 147–167. *A review of the clinical and immunologic features of 21 well-studied patients with the hyper-IgE syndrome.*

Purtilo DT, Sakamoto K, Barnabei V, et al.: Epstein-Barr virus–induced diseases in boys with the X-linked lymphoproliferative syndrome (XLP): Update on studies of the Registry. Am J Med 73:49, 1982.

Reisner Y, Kapoor N, Kirkpatrick D, Pollack MS, Cunningham-Rundles S, Dupont B, Hodes MZ, Good RA, O'Reilly RJ: Transplantation for severe combined immunodeficiency with HLA-A, B, D, DR incompatible parental marrow cells fractionated with soybean agglutinin and sheep red blood cells. Blood 61:341, 1983.

Rosen FS, Cooper MD, Wedgewood RJP: The primary immunodeficiencies. N Engl J Med 311:235, 300, 1984. *An excellent recent Medical Progress article which presents an overview of the basic biology and the clinical manifestations of these disorders. 260 references*

Stiehm ER, Fulginiti VA (eds.): Immunologic Disorders in Infants and Children. Philadelphia, W. B. Saunders Company, 1980. *The second edition of the only comprehensive textbook on pediatric immunology. Well referenced.*

Wedgwood R, Rosen FS, Paul NW (eds.): Primary Immunodeficiency Diseases. New York, Alan R. Liss Publishers, 1983. *Proceedings of the Fourth International Symposium on Immunodeficiency Diseases. Contributions by most authorities in the field. It is comprehensive and presents the state of the art as of 1982.*

430. ACQUIRED IMMUNO-DEFICIENCY SYNDROME (AIDS)

Anthony S. Fauci

DEFINITION. The acquired immunodeficiency syndrome (AIDS) has been defined by the Centers for Disease Control (CDC) as the presence of a reliably diagnosed disease that is at least moderately indicative of an underlying defect in cell-mediated immunity, for example, Kaposi's sarcoma in an individual who is less than 60 years of age, *Pneumocystis carinii* pneumonia, or other life-threatening opportunistic infections. Critical to the case definition is the absence of known causes of underlying immune deficiency and of any other host defense defects reported to be associated with the disease, such as immunosuppressive therapy or malignant lymphoreticular disease.

ETIOLOGY. AIDS is clearly caused by a transmissible agent. Although its precise etiology has not yet been conclusively proven, recent viral isolation and sero-epidemiologic studies have provided compelling evidence that the etiologic agent is a retrovirus of the human T cell leukemia/lymphoma virus (HTLV) family, which has been designated HTLV-III. This virus is lymphocytotropic, with a selective affinity for thymus-derived (T) lymphocytes that are of the inducer/helper subset defined by the T4 or Leu 3 phenotypic markers. Although other viruses such as the Epstein-Barr virus (EBV) and the cytomegalovirus (CMV) have been implicated by some investigators as being causal to the syndrome, it is now clear that they are either secondary infections or cofactors that result in immunosuppression and/or activation of lymphocytes, rendering them susceptible to infection with the primary etiologic agent.

INCIDENCE AND PREVALENCE. AIDS is either an entirely new disease or it existed in an epidemiologic setting whereby its incidence was low enough to remain unnoticed. The medical community first became aware of the syndrome in June and July, 1981, when CDC announced the unexplained occurrence of *Pneumocystis carinii* pneumonia in five previously well homosexual men in Los Angeles and Kaposi's sarcoma in 26 previously well homosexual men in New York and Los Angeles. By September, 1984, more than 5785 cases had been reported from at least 45 states and hundreds of additional cases worldwide. Since the incubation period is believed to be approximately one year, and in occasional cases it is felt to have been as long as four years, the full scope of the syndrome has not been realized, and it is difficult to project accurately the full impact and ultimate prevalence of AIDS. The epidemiologic pattern strongly suggests that sexual contact is the major means of transmission. The second most common mode of transmission appears to be via blood or blood products, as in individuals sharing needles for intravenous drug abuse or receiving a large number of transfusions of blood products. Thus the disease up to this point has remained largely confined within certain well-defined risk groups.

Clearly, homosexual or bisexual men constitute the largest risk group, accounting for over 70 per cent of all cases reported in the United States. Almost half of the reported cases in the world are from the New York City area, which has the largest concentration of male homosexuals in the United States. The next largest groups of patients are found in San Francisco and Los Angeles, cities that also have large concentrations of male homosexuals. Intravenous drug abusers with no history of homosexuality comprise the next largest group, with 17 per cent of the total patients. Haitian immigrants to the United States with no admitted history of homosexuality or intravenous drug abuse compose 5 per cent of cases. Recently it has become apparent that the disease is indeed seen in Haitians living in Haiti. However, it is unclear at this point what proportion of these fall into the first two risk groups of homosexuality and intravenous drug abuse. Lastly, hemophiliacs with no history of other risk factors compose almost 1 per cent of patients. Hemophiliacs are probably exposed to the transmissible agent of AIDS through the large numbers of transfusions of plasma products required for replacement of deficient clotting factors. This is especially true of individuals who receive large amounts of factor VIII concentrates. Almost 6 per cent of patients fall into none of the above categories. Within this group are several transfusion-related cases, infants born of mothers at risk for AIDS, and small numbers of women who are the heterosexual partners of individuals who either have AIDS or are at risk for AIDS. Others within this group with no known risk factors are a few patients who died before adequate information could be obtained and a very few others who truly have no apparent risk.

Physicians, nurses, and other health care or laboratory workers who deal with AIDS patients have not contracted AIDS unless they themselves fell into one of the recognized risk groups. This observation strongly suggests that casual or even close nonsexual contact will not transmit AIDS. Although AIDS is clearly epidemic in the risk groups mentioned, it seems likely to remain largely confined to these risk groups unless individuals in non-risk groups either have sexual contact with or are exposed to blood-borne transmission from someone with AIDS or incubating AIDS.

PATHOGENESIS AND IMMUNE DEFECT. The common denominator of AIDS is a profound acquired defect in cell-mediated immunity. Patients are anergic with a defect that is remarkably selective for the T lymphocyte. Most patients are lymphopenic with selective quantitative diminution in the inducer/helper T cell subset that is defined by the T4 or Leu 3 phenotypic markers. The suppressor/cytotoxic subset of T cell defined by the T8 or Leu 2 phenotypic marker is generally normal in number or only slightly increased or decreased, thereby resulting in marked decrease in the T4-T8 ratio within the peripheral blood. The T4 cells are not only quantitatively decreased but are also qualitatively defective in their functional capability. The selective defect in the T4 lymphocyte subset likely reflects the fact that HTLV-III is T4 lymphocytotropic. Natural killer cell and virus-specific T cell cytotoxicity are also defective in AIDS. This defect may well be due to the lack of induction of cytotoxic cells by the T4 cell or its soluble products. Finally, patients manifest hypergammaglobulinemia that reflects polyclonal hyperactivity of B lymphocytes. This B cell hyperactivity results in an actual B cell defect, as patients do not respond with an appropriate humoral response to in vivo antigen exposure as with immunizations.

The underlying defect in cell-mediated immunity leads to a dramatic decrease in host defenses, in turn leading to extraordinary susceptibility to recurrent opportunistic infections, one of the hallmarks of the syndrome. Patients are also susceptible to the development of Kaposi's sarcoma and, to a much lesser extent, of Burkitt-like lymphomas. It is unclear why patients develop Kaposi's sarcoma; furthermore, Kaposi's sarcoma is found to a much higher proportion in homosexuals with AIDS than in individuals in the other risk groups. AIDS patients who develop Kaposi's sarcoma have a significantly higher incidence of the HLA-DR5 haplotype.

Thus, the underlying pathogenesis of the syndrome itself relates to a profound defect in T-cell–mediated immunity caused by infection with a T lymphocytotropic virus. The subsequent manifestations of the syndrome result from this remarkable immune defect.

CLINICAL MANIFESTATIONS. Patients with AIDS exhibit a number of disease patterns. By strict definition, they must have either an opportunistic infection or Kaposi's sarcoma. In this regard, 50 per cent of patients have *Pneumocystis carinii* pneumonia without Kaposi's sarcoma, and approximately 26 per cent develop Kaposi's sarcoma without *Pneumocystis carinii* pneumonia. Smaller percentages of patients have both Kaposi's sarcoma and *Pneumocystis carinii* pneumonia or other opportunistic infections without Kaposi's sarcoma or *Pneumocystis carinii* pneumonia. The clinical manifestations reflect the particular opportunistic infection or the distribution of the neoplastic process. It is not uncommon for a given patient to have more than one opportunistic infection simultaneously.

Patients who develop *Pneumocystis carinii* pneumonia have the typical findings of this disease, with dyspnea and hypoxemia (see Ch. 383). The pneumonia may be abrupt and fulminant or insidious, with symptoms accelerating over weeks before the diagnosis is realized. CMV infections are manifest by fever and disseminated organ system involvement. Of particular importance is the chorioretinitis that often relentlessly progresses to total blindness. Herpes simplex virus may manifest as fulminant and life-threatening mucocutaneous dissemination. *Candida albicans* is commonly seen as oral thrush or esophagitis. *Cryptococcus neoformans* infections occur as meningitis or disseminated disease. Of particular interest are the disseminated infections with *Mycobacterium avium-intracellulare.* This infection is very rarely seen in individuals with iatrogenic immunosuppression or immunosuppression due to congenital cellular immunodeficiencies or spontaneous neoplasms. Yet this infection is relatively common in patients with AIDS. Disseminated *Mycobacterium tuberculosis* infection is seen to a lesser extent in AIDS, except in Haitian patients in whom it is relatively common. *Toxoplasma gondii* infections occur as intracerebral mass lesions or as chorioretinitis. Finally, a peculiar diarrheal syndrome has been linked to infection with the coccidial protozoa *Cryptosporium*. Many patients with AIDS have or develop intractable diarrhea for which no offending agent can be identified.

Another peculiar clinical syndrome associated with AIDS is a neurologic disorder that is characterized by progressive dementia with or without localizing signs. The etiology of this syndrome is unclear at present, and no etiologic agent has been identified, although biopsy specimens have revealed nonspecific inflammation, cerebral atrophy, or multifocal leukoencephalopathy.

Certain patients develop an unexplained syndrome of fever, weight loss, and wasting that is seemingly unrelated to the other manifestations of their disease, i.e., obvious opportunistic infections or Kaposi's sarcoma. However, in several patients these findings were ultimately explained by disseminated CMV or unrecognized *Mycobacterium avium-intracellulare* infections.

Kaposi's sarcoma in AIDS patients follows a significantly different pattern from Kaposi's sarcoma in nonepidemic groups, such as elderly men in the United States and Europe and organ transplant recipients. In these latter groups, the disease is generally indolent and confined to the skin, with only a 10 per cent incidence of extracutaneous organ involvement. In the Kaposi's sarcoma seen in children and young adults in certain areas of Africa, the incidence of extracutaneous involvement is 20 per cent, whereas in AIDS patients it is over 70 per cent. The most commonly involved organs are the lymph nodes, gastrointestinal tract, and lungs; however, virtually any organ system can be involved in this disseminated form.

Finally, a large number of male homosexuals have an unexplained lymphadenopathy syndrome that has been defined by the CDC as the presence for three months or longer of extrainguinal sites of lymphadenopathy with no recognizable cause for it. Biopsy, when available, reveals nonspecific lymphoid hyperplasia. Other individuals may have a wasting syndrome described above with or without lymphadenopathy. This constellation of signs and symptoms has been termed AIDS-related complex and even "pre-AIDS" by some. However, this terminology is not entirely appropriate, since it is unclear what proportion of these individuals will progress to full-blown AIDS. In this regard, HTLV-III has been isolated from over 80 per cent of such individuals.

DIAGNOSIS. The diagnosis of AIDS is made on the basis of the clinical criteria listed above. There are no laboratory tests that are diagnostic of the syndrome, although the selective diminution of the T4 lymphocyte subset in an otherwise well individual is strongly suggestive of the underlying immune defect. The presence of opportunistic infections or Kaposi's sarcoma in this setting confirms the diagnosis. It is of importance to realize that a mere reversal of the T4-T8 ratio of lymphocyte subsets does not of itself indicate that an individual is at risk to develop the full-blown syndrome. A number of common and relatively benign viral infections cause an increase in the T8 subset without substantially lowering the T4 subset, yet this will also result in inversion of the T4-T8 ratio. Since many homosexual males who do not have AIDS are frequently infected with viruses such as CMV and EBV, which cause reversals of T cell subset ratios, it would be inappropriate at this point to designate them as having a pre-AIDS condition.

TREATMENT AND PROGNOSIS. There is no known treatment for the underlying immune defects in AIDS, and there has been no report of spontaneous reversal of this defect. A number of attempts at immune reconstitution have been undertaken, including bone marrow transplantation, infusion of histocompatible lymphocytes, and administration of alpha interferon, gamma interferon, and interleukin 2. Despite the fact that some beneficial effects on the viral infections and Kaposi's sarcoma have been noted, there has thus far been no impressive and long-lasting reconstitution of immune function. However, extensive trials with these agents have not yet been completed. Kaposi's sarcoma has been treated with irradiation, chemotherapy, and certain of the immune reconstitutions mentioned above. Again, although partial and complete remissions of Kaposi's sarcoma have been effected in some patients, the underlying immune defect persists, and patients remain susceptible to repeated bouts of opportunistic infections or return of Kaposi's sarcoma or both. Several of the opportunistic infections such as *Pneumocystis carinii*, candidiasis, toxoplasmosis, cryptococcosis, typical tuberculosis, and herpes simplex can be effectively treated to a greater or lesser degree with antimicrobial agents, but there is no effective treatment for *Mycobacterium avium-intracellulare*, CMV and EBV infections, and cryptosporidosis.

The typical clinical course of the syndrome is one of repetitive and relentless attacks of a variety of opportunistic infections with or without Kaposi's sarcoma, ultimately leading to the death of the patient. The overall mortality of the syndrome is approximately 40 per cent. However, there are very few survivors among those who have had the disease since 1981, and given the fact that there are no reported cures, the true mortality of AIDS, at this point, may approach 100 per cent.

Fauci AS: The syndrome of Kaposi's sarcoma and opportunistic infections: An epidemiologically restricted disorder of immunoregulation. Ann Intern Med 96:77, 1982. *Description of the syndrome and discussion of potential scope and pathophysiologic mechanisms.*

Fauci AS, Macher AM, Longo DL, Lane HC, Rook AH, Masur H, Gelman EP: Acquired immune deficiency syndrome (AIDS). Ann Intern Med 100:92, 1984. *Detailed updated review and discussion of the epidemiology, clinical and pathologic manifestations, immune defect, potential etiologic factors, and currently utilized therapeutic approaches to AIDS.*

Gottlieb MS, Groopman JE, Weinstein WM, Fahey JL, Detels R: The acquired immunodeficiency syndrome. Ann Intern Med 99:208, 1983. *Extensive review of the syndrome with focus on the UCLA clinical experience.*

Murray JF, Felton CP, Garay SM, Gottlieb MS, Hopewell PC, Stover DE, Teirstein AS: Pulmonary complications of the acquired immunodeficiency syndrome: Report of a National Heart, Lung, and Blood Institute workshop. N Engl J Med 310:1682, 1984. *An excellent, recent, concise overview.*

Popovic M, Sarngadharan MG, Read E, Gallo RC: Detection, isolation, and continuous production of cytopathic retroviruses (HTLV-III) from patients with AIDS and pre-AIDS. Science 224:497, 1984. *Classic report providing compelling evidence that a retrovirus of the HTLV family (HTLV-III) is in fact the etiologic agent of AIDS.*

431. URTICARIA AND ANGIOEDEMA

Nicholas A. Soter

DEFINITION. Urticaria and angioedema are commonly encountered clinical entities that occur as evanescent areas of cutaneous edema. Urticaria appears as circumscribed elevated erythematous and usually pruritic areas of edema involving the superficial portions of the dermis. When the edema extends into the deep portions of the dermis or subcutaneous and submucosal tissues or both, it is designated angioedema and appears as large erythematous areas with diffuse borders. In addition to the skin, the respiratory and gastrointestinal tracts as well as the cardiovascular system may be involved singly or in any combination. The etiology of urticaria-angioedema is frequently unknown; however, its pathogenesis in many instances is believed to be related to activation of mast cells and/or basophils and release of their products, termed mediators of immediate hypersensitivity. Similar symptoms and signs may occur in association with activation of other inflammatory systems, such as the arachidonic acid metabolic pathways, the complement system (see Ch. 428), and the Hageman factor–dependent pathways of coagulation, fibrinolysis, and kinin generation with or without the participation of mast cells.

INCIDENCE AND PREVALENCE. Urticaria-angioedema may develop at any age. The highest incidence is in young adults, in whom it occurs in approximately 15 to 20 per cent. In patients with urticaria-angioedema, about 50 per cent will have both, 40 per cent urticaria alone, and 10 per cent angioedema alone. Approximately 50 per cent of patients with urticaria alone are free of lesions within one year, but 20 per cent continue to experience lesions for more than twenty years. Of patients with both urticaria and angioedema, 75 per cent experience symptoms for more than one year, 50 per cent for more than five years, and 20 per cent for more than twenty years. Age, race, sex, occupation, geographic location, and season of the year are involved as factors only insofar as they may contribute to exposure to an eliciting cause.

PATHOGENESIS AND PATHOLOGY. Urticaria-angioedema is often attributed to an immediate-type immunologic reaction (Type I, anaphylactic, or IgE-mediated hypersensitivity) produced by the antigen-induced release of biologically active materials from mast cells sensitized with specific IgE. Antigen-dependent activation and secretion in mast cells is initiated by bridging of pairs of adjacent IgE molecules and is dependent upon several subsequent intracellular events, including the activation of adenylate cyclase, membrane phospholipid methylation, and calcium flux (see Fig. 59–3). Urticaria-angioedema may also occur after mast cell degranulation induced by complement factors C3a and C5a, kinins, insect venoms, highly charged polyanions, or certain therapeutic and diagnostic agents. Physical stimuli such as trauma, pressure, cold, light, and heat may affect the mast cell via IgE or by unknown mechanisms.

The skin is rich in mast cells; the mean number is 7000 to 12,000 per cubic millimeter (see Fig. 438–1). The biologic effects of mast cells (described more fully in Ch. 438) are produced by the release of mediators, which alter venular permeability, contract smooth muscles, influence the motility of leukocytes, affect the generation and release of biologically active materials from other cell types, and enzymatically degrade complex substrates such as proteoglycans and collagen (see table in Ch. 438).

Urticaria-angioedema occurring after mast cell–mediated reactions is attributed primarily to the release of *histamine,* although other mediators, such as prostaglandin D_2, may play a role. Two tissue receptors, classified as H_1 and H_2, mediate the biologic activities of histamine. H_1-mediated effects include smooth muscle contraction, alterations in venular permeability, increases in airway resistance, and augmentation of motility of certain leukocytes. H_2-mediated effects include alterations in venular permeability, inhibition of T-lymphocyte function, depression of motility of certain leukocytes, suppression of basophil mediator release, increases in cardiac rate and force of contraction, and augmentation of gastric acid secretion. Inasmuch as the human skin vasculature contains both H_1 and H_2 receptors, vascular permeability may depend on the effect of histamine on both.

Skin biopsy specimens show edema involving the superficial portion of the dermis in the case of urticaria and the deeper dermis and subcutaneous tissue in the case of angioedema. Both urticaria and angioedema are associated with dilation of the venules with or without tissue infiltration by various numbers of lymphocytes and/or eosinophils and neutrophils. In some instances, necrotizing vasculitis with fibrinoid necrosis of the venule is present. In individuals with hereditary angioedema, examination of biopsy specimens from skin, larynx, and jejunum has shown subcutaneous or submucosal edema without infiltrating inflammatory cells.

CLINICAL MANIFESTATIONS. Urticaria and angioedema may occur together or individually in any location; however, angioedema most commonly affects the face. Episodes of urticaria-angioedema appear suddenly, usually persist fewer than 24 hours, and may recur. Recurrent episodes of fewer than four to six weeks' duration are considered acute, whereas those persisting longer are chronic.

Urticaria-angioedema can be classified into five groups that include those types which are IgE dependent or complement dependent, those which are due to a direct action on mast cells, those which occur after presumed alterations of the arachidonic acid metabolic pathways, and those which are idiopathic (see Table 431–1).

Idiopathic Urticaria-Angioedema. In at least 70 per cent of individuals with chronic episodes of urticaria-angioedema, the cause is unknown. Since this clinical condition is common, is easily recognized, and manifests a capricious course, it is often associated with concomitant events. Such attributions must be interpreted with caution. Although viral, fungal, bacterial, and helminthic infections, foods, medications, diagnostic agents, metabolic and hormonal abnormalities, malignant conditions, and emotional factors are frequently claimed as causes, proof of their etiologic relation often is lacking. Although idiopathic urticaria-angioedema is the most prevalent form, the diagnosis is one of exclusion and can be made only after the other types of urticaria-angioedema, discussed below, are eliminated. The laboratory studies to be considered in patients with urticaria-angioedema are noted under Laboratory Findings, below.

IgE-Dependent Urticaria-Angioedema. ATOPIC DIATHESIS. A history of acute episodes of urticaria-angioedema may be elicited in individuals with a personal or family history of asthma, rhinitis, or eczema. The prevalence of chronic urticaria, however, is not increased in atopic individuals. Moreover, in atopic persons urticaria-angioedema should not be too readily attributed to the atopic diathesis without a search for other causes.

SPECIFIC ANTIGENS. IgE-mediated urticaria-angioedema occurs after exposure to agents that include foods, diagnostic and therapeutic agents, pollens, and Hymenoptera venoms. In some instances, vasoactive substances or chemical additives may be responsible factors.

PHYSICAL STIMULI. Physical urticaria-angioedema occurs after a variety of stimuli, some of which are IgE dependent as demonstrated by passive transfer with serum of the cutaneous response to normal individuals (Prausnitz-Küstner reaction).

Dermographism. Dermographism occurs in 1.5 to 4.2 per cent of the normal population. It is usually recognized as a linear wheal appearing after the skin is briskly stroked with a firm object; however, its configuration depends on the eliciting stimulus. The transient pruritic wheal appears rapidly and fades within 30 minutes. Dermographism has been passively transferred to the skin of normal persons with both serum and its IgE fraction. Elevations in blood histamine levels have been detected after experimental scratching.

Pressure Urticaria-Angioedema. Pressure urticaria appears as erythematous, deep, often painful swelling that arises within minutes or up to six hours after sustained pressure, such as occurs under shoulder straps and belts, on the soles of the feet after running, and on the palms after manual labor. Although pressure urticaria-angioedema often occurs in individuals with dermographism or chronic idiopathic urticaria, an IgE-dependent mechanism has not been documented.

Vibratory Angioedema. Angioedema occurring after a vibratory stimulus has been reported with an autosomal dominant pat-

TABLE 431–1. CLASSIFICATION OF URTICARIA-ANGIOEDEMA

I. Idiopathic urticaria-angioedema
II. IgE-dependent urticaria-angioedema
    A. Atopic diathesis
    B. Specific antigen sensitivity
    C. Physical stimuli
    D. Contact urticaria
III. Complement-mediated urticaria-angioedema
    A. Hereditary angioedema
    B. Acquired C1 inhibitor abnormalities associated with angioedema
    C. Necrotizing venulitis
    D. Serum sickness
    E. Reactions to the administration of blood products
IV. Urticaria-angioedema due to agents with a direct action on mast cells
V. Urticaria-angioedema dependent on agents that alter the arachidonic acid metabolic pathways

tern of inheritance. It occurs also in association with cholinergic urticaria and after several years of occupational exposure to vibration. In the heritable form, the swelling appears rapidly, is transient, and is accompanied by facial flushing. A transient rise in plasma histamine was noted during experimental induction of vibratory angioedema both in the hereditary form and in those patients with acquired disease.

Cold-Induced Urticaria-Angioedema. There are both inherited and acquired forms of cold-induced urticaria-angioedema. The acquired form is more common. After exposure to changes in ambient temperature or direct contact with cold objects, patients experience a pruritic, urticarial eruption that may evolve into angioedema. Headaches, syncope, or wheezing may accompany an attack. If the entire body is cooled, as in swimming, hypotension and collapse, a potentially lethal event, may occur. Passive transfer with serum and its IgE fraction to the skin of a normal recipient has been documented, and the release into the serum of histamine and factors chemotactic for eosinophils and neutrophils has been detected after experimental challenge. Also, successful passive transfer with serum containing IgM antibody has been accomplished. In rare instances, acquired cold urticaria has been associated with underlying cryoproteins, notably cryoglobulins, cryofibrinogens, or cold hemolysins. The mechanism by which cryoproteins induce cold urticaria may be activation of the complement system.

Dominantly inherited cold urticaria has been described in immediate and delayed forms. In the immediate type, the eruption appears as erythematous macules or papules which manifest a burning sensation and which are accompanied by pyrexia, arthralgias, and a neutrophilic leukocytosis. In the delayed form, erythematous deep swellings develop 9 to 18 hours after cold challenge. This disorder is infrequently recognized, and its pathogenesis is unknown.

Light Urticaria. Idiopathic light or solar urticaria is a rare condition manifested by pruritus and urticaria-angioedema developing within minutes after exposure to the sun or to artificial light sources. Light urticaria also occasionally occurs in patients with systemic lupus erythematosus and erythropoietic protoporphyria. Classification of the urticarial response into subtypes is based on the reaction to specific portions of the light spectrum; however, individuals may respond to more than one portion of the spectrum. Histamine and factors chemotactic for eosinophils and neutrophils have been detected in serum after experimental exposure to UVB (290 to 320 nm), UVA (320 to 400 nm), or visible (400 to 700 nm) light. In some individuals the response has been passively transferred; in other subjects a serum factor induced by irradiation has been implicated in the development of the lesions.

Cholinergic Urticaria. Cholinergic urticaria is a distinctive eruption that develops after stimuli that allegedly raise core body temperature, such as a hot shower, exercise, or episodes of pyrexia. After an initial sensation of warmth, pruritic wheals 1 to 2 mm in size appear, surrounded by extensive areas of erythema. Wheezing has been noted, and obstructive alterations in pulmonary function have been documented during experimental induction of the clinical syndrome by exercise. Elevations in serum histamine and the appearance of factors chemotactic for eosinophils and neutrophils have been noted. Although injection of cholinergic agents such as methacholine into the skin has been employed as a diagnostic test, in only one third of individuals with cholinergic urticaria does this maneuver reproduce the skin lesions.

Heat Urticaria. Heat urticaria is a rare disorder in which urticaria-angioedema develops within minutes after exposure to locally applied heat. Elevations in plasma histamine levels have been noted after experimental challenge.

Aquagenic Urticaria and Aquagenic Pruritus. Contact of the skin with water of any temperature may result in pruritus alone or, more rarely, urticaria. The eruption consists of small wheals reminiscent of cholinergic urticaria. After experimental challenge, elevations of blood histamine have been noted in both aquagenic urticaria and aquagenic pruritus.

Contact Urticaria. Urticaria may occur after direct local contact with a variety of chemical substances. The eruption appears within minutes, is transient, and usually disappears within hours. Occasionally, systemic manifestations have been noted. Although passive transfer has been documented in some instances, agents such as stinging nettles, arthropod hairs, and chemicals may directly release histamine from mast cells.

Complement-Mediated Urticaria-Angioedema. HEREDITARY ANGIOEDEMA. Hereditary angioedema (HAE) occurs as episodes of edema of the skin and of the upper respiratory and gastrointestinal tracts. Episodes of swelling are self-limited, subside within 72 hours, and may occur over any area of the body, particularly on the face or an extremity. Urticaria alone is not a manifestation of HAE. Swelling of the face or buccal mucosa may progress to involve the larynx, with the danger of death by asphyxiation. The severity of the abdominal pain mimics surgical abdominal conditions.

HAE is transmitted as an autosomal dominant trait, and afflicted individuals are heterozygotes; however, the absence of a family history does not exclude the diagnosis. There are two forms of this inherited disease, each of which is characterized by the absence of function of the inhibitor (C$\overline{1}$INH) of the activated form of the first complement protein (C$\overline{1}$) of the classic activating pathway (see Ch. 428). Either the C$\overline{1}$INH protein and its function are lacking or normal levels of C$\overline{1}$INH protein without function are present. The absence of C$\overline{1}$INH provides a genetic marker for HAE and introduces the possibility that the lack of function of this complement factor is involved in pathogenesis of the clinical attacks. Levels of the fourth complement protein (C4) are also low, and levels of C4 and of the second complement protein (C2) diminish during clinical attacks. With the possible exception of post-traumatic attacks, the reasons for the episodic activation of C1 are unknown. In the absence of the C$\overline{1}$INH, the activation of Hageman factor after tissue trauma may lead to the conversion of plasminogen to plasmin, which subsequently activates C1. It is speculated that the angioedema is a result of a smooth muscle–contracting, heat-stable polypeptide derived by the action of plasmin on a complement fragment produced by the action of C$\overline{1}$ on C4 and C2. Urinary histamine levels are increased during attacks, presumably reflecting the degranulation of mast cells by C3a anaphylatoxin. Kallikrein has been found in the fluid of blisters induced over areas of edema, and increased bradykinin has been detected in plasma during attacks.

ACQUIRED C$\overline{1}$INH DEFICIENCY. The acquired depletion of the C$\overline{1}$INH sometimes associated with angioedema has been observed in patients with different types of lymphoproliferative disorders, in a patient with a rectal adenocarcinoma, and in some individuals with lupus erythematosus. In addition to low serum levels of C$\overline{1}$INH and C4, C1 and C1q levels are also reduced, thus permitting its differentiation from HAE. Abnormalities of complement in family members have not been reported.

NECROTIZING VENULITIS. Recurrent episodes of urticaria-angioedema may be manifestations of cutaneous necrotizing venulitis. An idiopathic clinical syndrome occurs primarily in women with associated transient arthralgia. The episodes of urticaria are chronic; individual lesions are transient, lasting fewer than 24 hours in many instances but occasionally up to three to five days. Most patients experience transient arthralgias of the peripheral joints. In some instances, diffuse glomerulonephritis has been noted as well as pyrexia, lymphadenopathy, obstructive pulmonary disease, and benign intracranial hypertension. These cases have been described under the terms erythema multiforme, lupus erythematosus–like syndrome, and hypocomplementemia-vasculitis-urticaria syndrome. Although some patients manifest serum hypocomplementemia with circulating C1q precipitins, many do not. Some patients with systemic lupus erythematosus or Sjögren's syndrome also manifest an urticarial form of cutaneous necrotizing venulitis.

SERUM SICKNESS. Serum sickness is a clinical symptom complex occurring after the administration of serum or drugs and lasting four to five days. The clinical manifestations include pyrexia, urticaria, lymphadenopathy, myalgia, and arthralgia. Urticaria is seen in over 70 per cent of patients with serum sickness, and often occurs at the site of injection.

REACTIONS TO BLOOD PRODUCTS. Urticaria-angioedema frequently occurs after the administration of blood products. Both the urticarial and the anaphylactic reactions noted after the transfusion of blood, serum, or IgG fractions are usually the result of immune complex formation with complement activation. Such immune complex reactions are especially prevalent in patients with IgA deficiency, in whom antibodies against IgA are present. Occasionally the urticaria may be due to the transfusion of IgE directed toward an antigen to which the recipient is subsequently exposed or to the transfusion of an antigen into a sensitized recipient. Activated Hageman factor has also been implicated in urticarial transfusion reactions.

Urticaria-Angioedema Due to Agents with a Direct Action on Mast Cells. The administration of opiates, polymyxin B, curare and tubocurarine, or radiocontrast media may be associated with the idiosyncratic release of histamine from mast cells. Between 5 and 8 per cent of individuals receiving radiocontrast media experience urticarial reactions, especially following intravenous administration.

Agents Which Presumably Alter Arachidonic Acid Metabolism. Urticaria-angioedema in response to administration of aspirin or nonsteroidal anti-inflammatory agents occurs commonly. Aspirin intolerance in patients with chronic urticaria is reported to be as high as 20 to 50 per cent. Patients intolerant to aspirin also react to indomethacin and to azo dyes, notably tartrazine, as well as to benzoates used as preservatives. Such reactions are often unrecognized, may serve to aggravate preexisting urticaria, and may occur from 15 minutes to 20 hours after ingestion. In patients intolerant to aspirin, reactions do not occur after exposure to structurally related compounds such as sodium or choline salicylate, whereas structurally unrelated agents such as indomethacin may precipitate the response.

LABORATORY FINDINGS. Laboratory evaluation is usually not helpful in patients with acute episodes of urticaria-angioedema. Historical information and physical findings offer better diagnostic clues. Acute urticaria may present as a manifestation of hepatitis B viral disease or serum sickness. In those patients whose acute urticaria-angioedema suggests an IgE-mediated allergic process, prick skin testing or assessment in vitro by radioallergosorbent test (RAST) of specific IgE antibody may be indicated; however, the likelihood of obtaining diagnostically relevant information from unselected prick skin tests or RAST is minimal. Prick skin testing is unreliable in the presence of dermographism.

Evaluation of chronic episodes of urticaria-angioedema requires more extensive laboratory analysis. The RAST has allowed the diagnosis of sensitivity to a variety of antigens, including foods, pollens, insect venom, and animal danders. Eosinophilia, when present, is a helpful feature in implicating a drug reaction or parasitic infestation as a cause of urticaria. Anti–hepatitis B surface antibody has been noted in some patients. Antinuclear antibody is helpful in detecting associated lupus erythematosus. Total serum concentrations of IgE in the absence of atopy are normal in patients with chronic urticaria-angioedema.

Assessment of the serum complement system is of value in detecting patients with hereditary and acquired forms of angioedema. In patients with HAE, immunochemical measurements of both C$\overline{1}$INH and C4 are low with normal levels of C1 and C3. If the C$\overline{1}$INH protein level is normal and the C4 low, functional assessment of C$\overline{1}$INH may be performed to confirm the diagnosis.

In patients with chronic idiopathic urticaria-angioedema the finding of an elevated erythrocyte sedimentation rate should prompt a biopsy of an urticarial lesion to search for underlying cutaneous necrotizing venulitis. In some patients with necrotizing venulitis hypocomplementemia may be detected. As not all patients with necrotizing venulitis manifest hypocomplementemia, the sedimentation rate has proved to be a more sensitive screening test than serum complement analysis.

DIAGNOSIS AND DIFFERENTIAL DIAGNOSIS. Urticaria and angioedema are easily recognizable. Urticarial eruptions are episodic and evanescent, with multiple lesions occurring in various stages of evolution and resolution. The differential diagnosis of urticaria includes papular urticaria, which consists of small wheals occurring after insect bites; the eruption of erythema multiforme that includes iris or target lesions; the early urticarial stages of the Henoch-Schönlein syndrome that evolve into palpable purpura; urticaria pigmentosa, which is a generalized, pigmented, papular or even nodular mast cell infiltration in which the skin lesions become urticarial upon rubbing (see Fig. 438–2); and the syndrome of perceptive deafness, fever with urticaria, and renal insufficiency consequent to amyloidosis.

Disorders included in the differential diagnosis of angioedema are contact dermatitis appearing as recurrent episodes of eyelid and facial swelling; cellulitis and erysipelas, which may at times resemble angioedema; lymphedema occurring after cutaneous pyoderma or surgery; and congestive heart failure, renal insufficiency, obstruction of the superior vena cava, myxedema, thrombophlebitis, and stasis, which may produce recurrent swelling. The Melkersson-Rosenthal syndrome consists of swelling of the lips, facial paralysis, and a fissured tongue.

TREATMENT AND PREVENTION. When urticaria-angioedema is due to a known agent, avoidance is the therapeutic choice. Since patients may respond to the administration of placebos and the disease tends to spontaneously remit, evaluation of therapeutic intervention is difficult. Avoidance of aspirin or food additives has been claimed to improve many patients. Recurrent episodes of idiopathic urticaria-angioedema are most effectively treated by the prophylactic administration of H_1 antihistaminic agents. A variety of H_1-type antihistamine preparations exist, which are used empirically. These agents are administered in divided doses; representative examples are chlorpheniramine maleate, 4 to 8 mg, or diphenhydramine hydrochloride, 25 to 50 mg, every four to six hours. The combination of H_2 antihistamines in combination with H_1 agents is of value in a small number of individuals. Epinephrine is rarely required, and the chronic systemic administration of corticosteroid preparations creates risks out of proportion to the therapeutic benefits. The treatment of physical urticaria includes avoidance of the precipitating stimulus and the empiric administration of antihistamines.

The treatment of HAE can be divided into management of the acute episode, preoperative prophylaxis, and long-term prevention of spontaneous attacks. Specific therapeutic measures to interrupt spontaneous attacks are not available. The primary maneuver is to maintain the airway. Preoperative preparation of patients with antifibrinolytic agents suppresses attacks of angioedema. Nonandrogenic or impeded anabolic steroids, such as oxymetholone, danazol, and stanozolol, are effective in prevention of spontaneous attacks. Toxicity caused by attenuated androgens is dose related; however, the adverse effects that occur with daily therapy subside with alternate-day therapy. Although statistically significant mean increases in the serum levels of C$\overline{1}$INH occur with both daily and alternate-day therapy, a significant mean rise in C4 levels occurs only on daily therapy. Thus clinical control can be achieved with therapeutic regimens of attenuated androgens that are not accompanied by immunochemical correction. Impeded androgens have also been used to treat acquired C$\overline{1}$INH deficiency with recurrent angioedema. There is no proven effective treatment for the urticaria-angioedema that occurs as a manifestation of underlying necrotizing venulitis although some patients benefit from the administration of prednisone or nonsteroidal anti-inflammatory agents.

Gigli I: Hereditary angioneurotic edema (hereditary angioedema). *In* Franklin EC (ed.): Clinical Immunology Update: Reviews for Physicians. New York, Elsevier Biomedical, 1983, pp 317–335. *A current review of hereditary angioedema, its pathogenesis, and treatment.*

Juhlin L: Recurrent urticaria: Clinical investigation of 330 patients. Br J Dermatol 104:369, 1981. *A recent epidemiologic study of a large number of patients with urticaria-angioedema.*

Monroe EW: Urticarial vasculitis: An updated review. J Am Acad Dermatol 5:88, 1981. *A review of patients with chronic urticaria-angioedema as a manifestation of necrotizing venulitis.*

Soter NA: Physical urticaria/angioedema as an experimental model of acute and chronic inflammation in human skin. Springer Semin Immunopathol 4:73, 1981. *A review of the types of physical urticaria and the use of such disorders to study mast cell participation in human cutaneous disease.*

Warin RP, Champion RH: Urticaria. London, W. B. Saunders Company, 1974. *The definitive monograph considering the entity urticaria-angioedema.*

432. ALLERGIC RHINITIS

John E. Salvaggio

DEFINITION. Allergic rhinitis is an IgE-mediated, inflammatory disease of the nasal mucous membranes, characterized by paroxysms of sneezing, itching of the nose, eyes, palate, pharynx, and conjunctivae, nasal stuffiness with partial or total obstruction of airflow, and mucous secretion often accompanied by postnasal drainage. The disease is often seasonal, depending on the pollination patterns of inhalant allergens that have direct impact on the respiratory mucosa. The condition may be perennial when due to nonseasonal allergens, such as dust, animal danders, some plant products, and molds.

ETIOLOGY. The most apparent seasonal allergens acting as etiologic agents in allergic rhinitis are pollens, such as ragweed, and mold spores. Tree pollens are usually released during the spring, and, in most parts of the country the height of the grass pollen season is late spring to midsummer. Much of the nasal symptoms caused by airborne weed pollens occur in late summer and the early fall months. Ragweed pollen is by far the worst offender in the eastern, midwestern, and southern United States. Many individuals with allergic rhinitis have an IgE-mediated response to crude house-dust antigen, which is a mixture of lint, danders, insect parts, fibers, and other particulate matter. In many geographic areas and household situations, mites, including *Dermatophagoides farinae* and *D. pteronyssimus,* appear to be the primary sources of antigen in house dusts. Animal danders, particularly cat dander, may be especially potent in inducing sudden, violent nasal symptoms, even when there is contact only with the dander, saliva, or urine of the animal. In certain patients, other inhalant allergens, including cottonseed and flaxseed, which may be constituents of animals feeds, fertilizers, and inexpensive upholstery, may cause perennial or sporadic symptoms. Mold spores may be very important perennial allergens, since they are found in both outdoor and indoor environments.

INCIDENCE AND PREVALENCE. Approximately 9 per cent of all patients seeking care at a physician's office do so for one of the common allergic diseases. It is estimated that 35 million Americans have allergic diseases: An estimated 8.9 million suffer from asthma with or without allergic rhinitis, 14.7 million have allergic rhinitis alone, and 11.8 million have other allergic manifestations, such as urticaria, angioedema, eczema, or food, drug, or insect hypersensitivity. Stated in another way, 17 per cent of all Americans have at least one common allergic disease, and 7 per cent of all Americans have allergic rhinitis alone. These incidence figures are deceptively low, since they approximate only the number of patients who, at the time of the particular study, are actually afflicted with the condition, and they do not include the large numbers of individuals who have had diseases such as allergic rhinitis in the past, but have since "recovered."

PATHOGENESIS AND MECHANISMS. Airborne particles (allergens) initially impact on the upper respiratory tract mucosa during inhalation. Many of the relevant allergens, which are water soluble, diffuse onto the respiratory epithelium, and a host IgE antibody response ensues with subsequent sensitization of respiratory tissues. Continued exposure of the appropriately sensitized upper respiratory tract mucous membranes to aeroallergens results in antigen-antibody interactions on the surface of submucosally located mast cells, with release of mediators of acute inflammation and production of clinical symptoms.

Both tissue mast cells and circulating basophils concentrate IgE on their surfaces, which may have up to 500,000 IgE molecules per cell. The IgE fixes to a glycoprotein receptor site on the membrane by its Fc fragment, resulting in an arrangement that permits exposure of the antibody combining sites (or Fab) to the surrounding milieu. Cross-linking of two IgE antibody molecules by specific antigen aggregates the corresponding receptor sites and results in initiation of a series of cellular biochemical events, culminating in the expulsion of secretory granule contents (Fig. 432–1). Among the important mast cell–derived mediators are histamine; bradykinin; thromboxanes; leukotrienes C, D, and E, which are derived from arachidonic acid released during the allergic reaction; eosinophil chemotactic factors of anaphylaxis (ECF-A), which are derived from the mast cell granule; heparin, which makes up 30 per cent of the dry weight of mast cell granules; superoxide dismutase (SOD), which is formed by the univalent reduction of oxygen; prostaglandins, which are C_{20} unsaturated fatty acid derivatives of arachidonic acid; platelet activating factor (PAF), a small phospholipid derivative of phosphoryl choline released from rabbit basophils; neutrophil chemotactic factor of anaphylaxis (NCF-A); inflammatory factors of anaphylaxis, which are constituents of the mast cell granules that induce a late–phase allergic inflammatory reaction; and a number of enzymes that are found in mast cell granules, such as chymotrypsin and trypsin. These enzymes may contribute to the tissue destruction accompanying various late–phase allergic reactions. There are immunologic as well as nonimmunologic triggers of this mast cell degranulation process. It is not uncommon for patients to note associations between symptoms and exposure to certain nonspecific irritants, such as strong odors, insecticides, and cigarette smoke.

CLINICAL MANIFESTATIONS. Common symptoms include *nasal stuffiness,* paroxysms of *sneezing,* profuse *mucous secretion,* and frequent *itching* of the nose, eyes, posterior pharynx, or conjunctivae. Soreness or inflammation of the conjunctivae, with excessive *tearing* and mucoid conjunctival discharge may be present in severe cases, and it is not uncommon for patients with recurrent symptoms to note a certain degree of fatigue, malaise, anorexia, and irritability. Many offending plants pollinate during the early morning hours. Thus, morning symptoms may be followed by improvement during the day, with a lessened degree of exposure. Repeated rubbing of the nose upward to relieve itching may cause a crease to develop across the nose, especially in children. Mouth breathing is common, as are typical dark, discolored infraorbital "shiners" (Fig. 432–2).

Examination of the nasal mucous membranes characteristically reveals bluish, edematous, boggy, pale nasal turbinates, often coated with clear secretion; but many persons with allergic rhinitis have an erythematous, boggy nasal mucosa, which can easily be confused with that seen in infectious rhinitis. At times the nasal airways may be completely obstructed, as a result of accumulation of mucus and turbinate swelling. Scleral and conjunctival injection and edema, plus periorbital swelling and tearing, may be noted. Nasal polyps are relatively uncommonly associated with uncomplicated rhinitis. They may, however, be associated with aspirin intolerance. Since asthmatics with aspirin intolerance often have severe disease, visualization of even small polyps in patients with rhinitis and asthma may provide important diagnostic leads.

In *seasonal rhinitis,* symptoms recur each year with regularity during the pollination season characteristic for a given area. IgE–mediated perennial rhinitis presents with a continuance of low-grade symptoms, which may improve only with removal

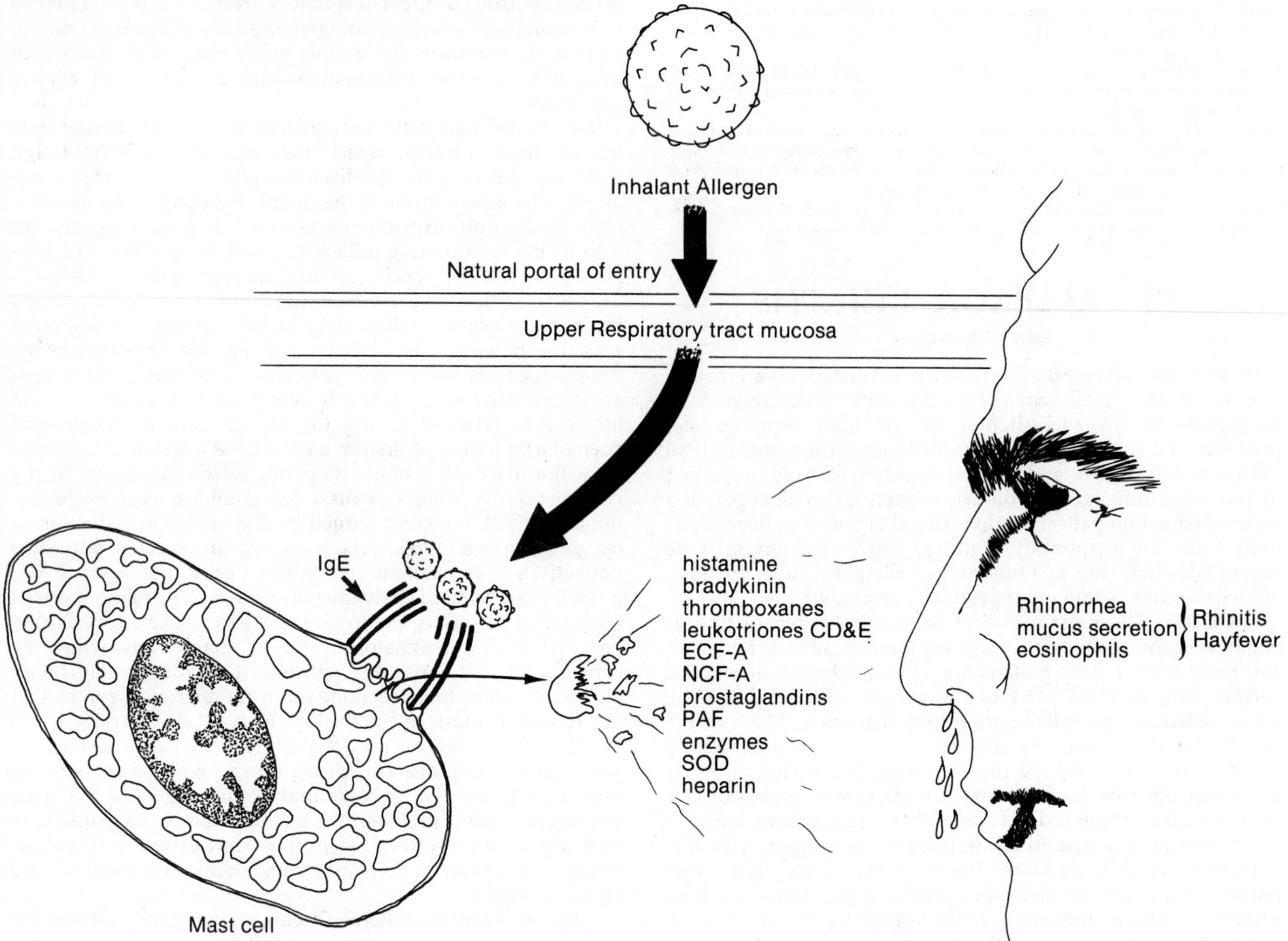

Figure 432–1. Pathogenesis of allergic rhinitis; antigen-antibody interaction and mediator release.

from the inciting causes. *Perennial rhinitis* of unknown cause (also called vasomotor rhinitis) also produces persistent symptoms without correlation to any specific allergen exposure. This type of perennial rhinitis is often worsened by changes in temperature or humidity or with exposure to irritants or other types of air pollutants. It is also often associated with profuse nasal discharge after the patient eats chilled, highly spiced, or heated foods, and such symptoms may be erroneously attributed to food allergy.

Serous otitis media may be superimposed upon the symptoms of seasonal or perennial allergic rhinitis. In many instances of serous otitis media, allergic factors cannot, however, be identified. Serous otitis can be an important complication in children, and may result from nasal obstruction or obstructive dysfunction of the eustachian tube as a result of mucosal edema and secretions. It can also lead to hearing loss with adverse effects on cognition or speech development in the young child. The diagnosis of serous otitis media is suggested by a history of symptoms such as delayed speech development or decreased auditory perception. The tympanic membrane on physical examination is frequently amber-colored and retracted, with decrease in motion if there is negative middle ear pressure, or no motion at all if there is a serous effusion.

Chronic sinusitis may be another complication, often manifested by the presence of chronic nasal discharge, nocturnal cough associated with postnasal discharge, pain, fever, headache, and recurrent otitis media. In adults, however, pain, headache, and low-grade fever are the most frequently recognized signs. Chronic sinusitis as a complication of seasonal allergic rhinitis should be considered whenever symptoms of allergic rhinitis are more protracted than expected, when the patient has severe dull-to-intense throbbing pain over the involved sinus area, or when prolonged or persistent cough develops that is suggestive of bronchitis that has failed to respond to appropriate therapy.

DIAGNOSIS (WITH DIFFERENTIAL DIAGNOSIS). A good history is most important in correctly diagnosing rhinitis. In addition to the history of classic physical signs and symptoms, careful skin testing with common inhalant preparations together with positive and negative control substances is a mandatory procedure in diagnosing specific allergic factors associated with rhinitis. Direct skin tests of the scratch, prick, and intradermal variety are the least expensive and time consuming. The intradermal test should never be performed without prior performance of negative scratch or prick tests. In general, negative skin test responses with common inhalant allergens indicate that rhinitis is of nonallergic origin. In vitro methods of detecting IgE antibodies have now been available for several years. In patients who are receiving medications that might prevent skin reactivity, or in those with extensive eczema or dermatographia that negate the use of skin tests, these in vitro assays for serum IgE antibodies can be of diagnostic aid. Total serum IgE levels

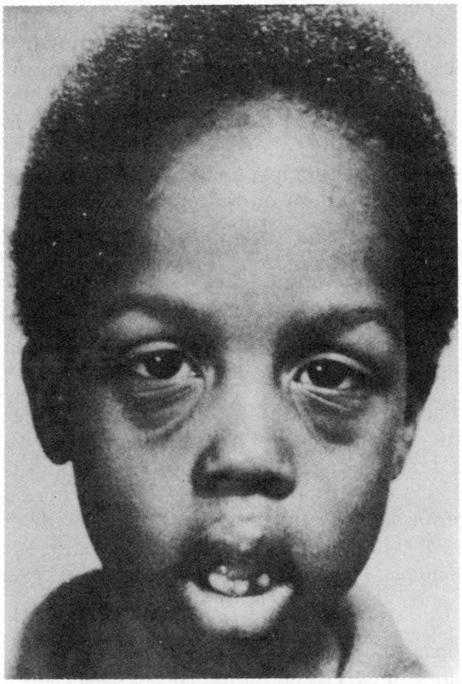

Figure 432–2. Typical appearance of highly allergic 6-year-old child. Note dark circles under eyes ("allergic shiners") and mouth breathing. Allergic nasal crease from constant "saluting" was also present. (Reprinted with permission from Mathews KP: Respiratory atopic disease. JAMA 248:2588, 1982.)

are elevated in only 30 to 40 per cent of patients with allergic rhinitis. They may also be elevated in many nonallergic conditions. Although frequently elevated in allergic rhinitis, the peripheral blood eosinophil count may be normal. A high peripheral eosinophil count may also be seen in nonallergic perennial rhinitis associated with nasal polyps, hyperplastic sinusitis, and idiopathic asthma. Of more significance is a smear of nasal secretions for eosinophils.

Clear-cut seasonal allergic rhinitis due to inhalant allergens seldom presents a differential diagnostic problem. Symptoms of the common cold may, however, be quite similar, although they usually last less than one week and are often associated with fever, pain, and the presence of considerable neutrophils in nasal secretions. Symptoms associated with structural abnormalities of the nasal area, such as polyps, deviated nasal septum, enlarged tonsils, or foreign bodies, are relatively constant rather than episodic as in classic seasonal allergic rhinitis. A suspected diagnosis of so-called rhinitis medicamentosa due to the rebound effects of nose drops, sprays, ovarian hormonal agents (such as oral contraceptives), reserpine derivatives, or hydralazine can often be confirmed when symptoms gradually improve following avoidance of the suspected agent. Nasal symptoms may accompany metabolic disorders such as hyperthyroidism or emotional states, but the relationship is unclear. During pregnancy and premenstrually, hormonally related rhinitis may occur. A condition known as nasal mastocytosis is associated with symptoms of perennial allergic rhinitis; the diagnosis can be made by nasal mucosal biopsy.

TREATMENT. Three basic principles are important in the treatment of rhinitis: avoidance of offending allergens of allergic rhinitis; use of symptomatic treatment, such as antihistamines, sympathomimetic drugs, and topical steroids; and allergenic extract immunotherapy.

Avoidance. When practical, avoidance of aeroallergens is the treatment of choice, since it removes the cause of difficulty and prevents symptoms. When a specific food, drug, occupational allergen, or animal dander is involved, it is the only measure that serves to both prevent and treat disease. All physicians should be familiar, for example, with standard antidust regimens for use in home environments. Although avoidance of outdoor exposure to ubiquitous seasonal and perennial pollens is virtually impossible, commonsense measures to avoid heavy exposure often help to prevent severe exacerbations of symptoms. For example, mold-sensitive patients should avoid barns, working with hay, raking leaves, or mowing grass. Simply keeping doors and windows closed significantly decreases indoor pollen and mold spore concentrations, and air conditioning makes a closed environment more tolerable. Although electrostatic air-purifying devices do not provide cooling or dehumidification, they are quite efficient in removing pollen grains and other large mold spores. In certain cases a patient may choose to leave an area of exposure during a particularly symptomatic season. Such measures may be applicable when well-defined seasons, such as the late-summer-and-early-fall ragweed season, are involved. Only rarely should consideration be given to making a permanent move from an area of exposure to particularly aggravating allergens, since, with time, allergic individuals generally tend to acquire new sensitivities to allergens in their adopted environment.

Symptomatic Treatment. Although, in general, antihistamines are only partially effective and are often associated with a side effect of drowsiness, they are often used alone or in combination with oral sympathomimetic agents, anticholinergics, cromolyn sodium, and topical corticosteroids. The H_1 antihistaminics often control symptoms of profuse nasal itching and sneezing. They act as competitive inhibitors for histamine at its H_1 receptor site. Since receptor sites can be effectively blocked prior to histamine release, better results are often obtained when these drugs are administered on a regular basis rather than intermittently. Antihistamines have been classified into six groups on the basis of chemical structure. These include the ethanolamines, such as diphenhydramine (Benadryl); the ethylenediamines, such as tripelennamine (Pyribenzamine); the alkylamines, such as brompheniramine (Dimetane); and chlorpheniramine (Chlor-Trimeton); the piperazines, such as hydroxyzine (Atarax, Vistaril); the phenothiazines, such as promethazine (Phenergan); and a miscellaneous group including cyproheptadine (Periactin), and azatadine (Optimine). In a typical case, one might start with one of the alkylamines such as chlorpheniramine maleate or brompheniramine maleate 4 mg three or four times a day in the adult (0.4 mg per kilogram per day in three or four divided doses in children). Both of these compounds are also available in long-acting preparations that can be given in 8- to 12-mg quantities two times a day.

The most commonly employed sympathomimetic nasal sprays and drops that contain alpha-adrenergic agonists are phenylephrine hydrochloride, a short-acting agent, and longer-acting preparations, such as oxymetazoline hydrochloride. In most cases, use of these compounds for more than a few days will result in progressively severe nasal obstruction secondary to rebound swelling of the nasal mucosa that may be a self-perpetuating process (known as rhinitis medicamentosa). Thus these agents are not recommended for long-term use in allergic rhinitis. Sympathomimetic agents administered orally, such as pseudoephedrine and phenylpropanolamine, may also reduce nasal congestion, although when used alone they may have significant CNS stimulatory effects, often leading to insomnia and nervousness. A 4 per cent solution of cromolyn sodium applied topically can also be of some benefit in the treatment of allergic rhinitis or conjunctivitis, or both, if administered frequently on a regular basis.

Topical corticosteroids are now widely used and highly successful in the symptomatic treatment and prevention of allergic rhinitis. These usually include the highly potent and rapidly metabolized corticosteroids such as beclomethasone dipropionate, flunisolide acetate, budesonide, and triamcinolone acetonide. These agents act primarily topically, and have a relative lack of systemic effects, which is most advantageous. Although of substantial value in treating seasonal allergic rhinitis, these agents may not work well in acute, severe cases associated with considerable nasal mucosal edema and obstruction. They also do not relieve ocular symptoms. If used intermittently on a regular basis, they can help in perennial allergic rhinitis and vasomotor rhinitis. In addition, they may be of some help in weaning patients from excessive use of vasoconstrictor nasal sprays. The rule for use of corticosteroids is "as much as necessary but as little as possible."

Dose response investigations in hay fever patients have shown total control of nasal symptoms in about 30 per cent of patients treated with 200 or 300 μg of beclomethasone dipropionate per day. This percentage is increased to 60 per cent when 400 μg per day are employed. Seasonal treatment on a daily basis with 400 μg per day is recommended and is considered to be quite harmless. (Each puff of beclomethasone dipropionate from a nasal inhaler is equal to approximately 42 μg of beclomethasone dipropionate, USP). Thus, one puff per nostril four times per day from the nasal inhaler would be a typical dose. Some attention should be paid to the frequency of prescription; for example, when 400 μg is recommended, one aerosol container will last approximately four weeks. In all cases, clinical improvement is usually apparent within several days, but symptomatic relief may not occur in some patients for as long as two weeks. In adults and children, the inhalation of 400 μg daily is without risk of systemic steroid side effects. There is also substantial evidence that this is the case in adults who use up to 800 μg daily (approximately 16 inhalations). In addition, cushingoid changes probably do not occur until the very large dose of approximately 1 mg (20 inhalations or more) is reached. When this drug is used it should be remembered that, in regard to therapeutic potency, eight inhalations is roughly equivalent to 7.5 mg of oral prednisone. These drugs should be used with caution in the presence of viral and fungal nasal diseases, such as ocular herpes or related diseases, in which there appears to be an associated defect in cell-mediated immunity.

Inhalant Allergen Immunotherapy (Desensitization or Hyposensitization). With this form of therapy, one attempts to alter the immunologic reactivity of an allergic inidividual so that there is less response upon natural reexposure to the offending allergen. The clinical decision to use immunotherapy in the patient with allergic rhinitis depends on several factors: (1) the existence of clinically important rhinitis should be confirmed; (2) maximum environmental control procedures should be utilized; and (3) the response to medication should be well defined. Immunotherapy is usually employed in patients who have substantial allergic components to their illness and who are not attaining satisfactory clinical improvement with environmental control and symptomatic treatment. The technique involves injecting increasing amounts of allergen subcutaneously, usually at weekly intervals, starting with a very low dose with gradual increases (usually a doubling of dosage) at each subsequent injection. One should always carefully monitor for the development of any untoward reactions. After incremental increases in the amount of allergen injected, a maintenance dose is achieved, the interval between subsequent maintenance injections varying from two to six weeks, depending upon individual patient reactivity and requirements. In most cases, a decrease in nasal symptoms following immunotherapy is usually obvious during the first six months to one year, and is maximum by three years of therapy. There are no universally accepted guidelines for the duration of therapy, and many physicians attempt trials of discontinuation after approximately four years of a successful program.

Symptomatic improvement with immunotherapy has been clearly shown in hayfever due to ragweed, grass, mountain cedar pollen, or birch pollen and asthma due to house dust mite, ragweed pollen, grass pollen, and cat dander. Beneficial results depend on an adequately high dosage of antigen; relapse may occur once continuing maintenance injections are abandoned. Results are specific for particular allergens employed. A variety of immunologic changes have been demonstrated following immunotherapy, but it is not known which are responsible for clinical improvement. Among these changes are a rise in serum IgG-blocking antibodies against the allergens employed; suppression in the usual seasonal rise in IgE antibodies, which normally follows environmental seasonal exposure; increase of blocking IgA and IgG antibodies in secretions; reduced basophil reactivity and sensitivity to allergens; reduced in vitro lymphocyte responsiveness to allergens; and an increase in specific T suppressor cells following immunotherapy.

New experimental approaches to the therapy of allergic rhinitis include the use of altered antigens (such as allergoids and polymerized forms of antigen) that ultimately result in a heightened degree of immunization, with considerably less chance to trigger sensitized mast cells and produce local or systemic reactions. The use of other routes of antigen administration (such as intranasally) has also been attempted, as have efforts to depress specific IgE antibody synthesis with or without effects on suppressor T cells, by linking allergens to certain agents such as polyethylene glycol, with subsequent production of tolerance. Still other efforts are directed toward such novel ideas as inhibition of IgE receptors on mast cells, basophils, and other IgE receptor–bearing cells.

Bellanti J (ed.): Immunology II. Philadelphia, W. B. Saunders Company, 1978. *A concise, well-illustrated text stressing simple fundamentals of clinical immunology.*

Middleton E Jr, Reed CE, Ellis EF: Allergy: Principles and Practice. 2nd ed. St. Louis, C. V. Mosby Company, 1983. *A multi-authored, two-volume reference work stressing immunologic, pharmacologic and clinical aspects of the common allergic diseases.*

Patterson R (ed.): Allergic Diseases. 2nd ed. Philadelphia, J. B. Lippincott Company, 1980. *A concise volume devoted to practical clinical aspects of the common atopic diseases.*

Parker C (ed.): Clinical Immunology. Philadelphia, W. B. Saunders Company, 1980. *A comprehensive two-volume text (basic and clinical) concentrating on experimental and clinical aspects of human diseases with strong immunologic overtones.*

Salvaggio J (ed.): Primer on allergic and immunologic diseases. JAMA 248:2579, 1982. *Compact article on the essentials of respiratory atopic disease, in a setting of other articles that stress the clinical implications of immunology for the medical student and resident.*

Stites D, Stobo J, Fudenberg H, Wells V (eds.): Basic and Clinical Immunology. 4th ed. Los Altos, Lange Medical Publishers, 1982. *A text outlining relevant features of basic immunology, immunologic laboratory tests, and clinical immunology. Clinical chapters focus on primary immunologic diseases and disorders with important immunopathologic characteristics.*

433. ANAPHYLAXIS*

Lawrence M. Lichtenstein†

Systemic anaphylaxis is the most dramatic example of an immediate hypersensitivity reaction. The first known report of this syndrome describes the sudden death of King Menes of Egypt, from the sting of a wasp, during the twenty-sixth century B.C. The experiments of Richet and Portier in the early 1900's, which gained them the Nobel Prize, showed that dogs who survived a large dose of sea anemone toxin died within a few minutes when given a minute dose some weeks later. They coined the term "anaphylaxis" to describe how this type of immunization led to a lack of protection rather than the expected immunity (i.e., prophylaxis).

Human anaphylactic reactions are uncommon, but have always received considerable medical attention because of their unexpected nature and occasionally fatal outcome. They occur in previously sensitized individuals after re-exposure to foreign antigens or low molecular weight substances that act as haptens. These reactions are mediated by IgE antibody, begin a few minutes after antigen exposure, and result from the release of basophil and mast cell mediators. Other "anaphylactoid" reactions probably involve the nonimmunologic release of the same chemical mediators. Systemic anaphylactic reactions involve the cutaneous, respiratory, circulatory, gastrointestinal, and hematologic systems. They range in severity from distress-

*Supported by Grant AI 08270 from the National Institute of Allergy and Infectious Diseases, National Institutes of Health.

†I would like to thank my colleague, Eugene R. Bleecker, M.D., for his aid in the preparation and writing of this chapter.

TABLE 433–1. AGENTS CAUSING ANAPHYLAXIS

Type	Common	Rare
Proteins	Venoms (Hymenoptera)	Hormones (insulin, ACTH, vasopressin, parathormone)
	Pollens (ragweed, grass, etc.)	Enzymes (trypsin, penicillinase)
	Foods (eggs, seafood, nuts, grains, beans, cottonseed oil, chocolate)	Human proteins (serum proteins, seminal fluid)
	Horse and rabbit serum (antilymphocyte globulin)	
Haptens and other low molecular weight substances	Antibiotics (penicillins, cephalosporins, tetracyclines, amphotericin B, nitrofurantoin, aminoglycosides)	Vitamins (thiamine, folic acid)
	Local anesthetics (lidocaine, procaine, etc.)	
Polysaccharides		Dextrans, iron-dextran

ing but self-limited, generalized urticarial reactions to sudden death.

ETIOLOGY. During the early part of this century, anaphylaxis was most often seen as a reaction to the proteins of horse serum, which was used in the preparation of diphtheria and tetanus antitoxins. Table 433–1 lists the inciting agents that are now most common. Proteins likely to cause these reactions are those in horse serum (now used to make antihuman lymphocyte globulin), hormones, enzymes, Hymenoptera venoms (in insect stings as described in Ch. 434), pollen extracts, and various foods (seafood, eggs, wheat products, nuts). Polysaccharides such as dextran are rarer causes of anaphylaxis. The most common etiologic agents are drugs, low molecular weight substances that are not antigenic in themselves but act as haptens, combining with native proteins to form an antigen. Antibiotics (penicillin, cephalosporins, tetracycline, nitrofurantoin), local anesthetics, vitamins, and some diagnostic agents are thought to act by this mechanism. Some substances (Table 433–2) that are administered by intravenous injection (iodinated radiopaque dyes or hypertonic solutions [mannitol]) as well as some nonsteroidal anti-inflammatory agents (acetylsalicylic acid, aminopyrine, indomethacin) may induce mediator release by nonimmunologic mechanisms that are poorly understood, or vascular shock by direct systemic vasodilatation. Although the parenteral administration of these agents is the cause of most reactions, oral and topical exposure can also cause systemic anaphylactic reactions in highly sensitive individuals.

In the two best-studied situations, penicillin and insect sting anaphylaxis, the incidence of sensitivity (e.g., a positive skin test) is not greater in patients with a familial or personal history of atopy. However, not all individuals with a positive skin test, indicating the presence of specific IgE antibody, are at risk of an anaphylactic reaction. Although the degree of risk in skin test–positive patients is very much higher than in skin test–negative patients, not all will react to any particular challenge.

PATHOGENESIS. In a susceptible individual, exposure to an antigenic agent causes the production of IgE antibodies. With repeat exposure, the antigen combines with IgE antibodies on the surface of basophils and mast cells to initiate a sequence of biochemical reactions that result in the active secretion of mediators such as histamine, arachidonic acid metabolites, and factors that attract and activate platelets, eosinophils, and neutrophils (see table in Ch. 438). These mediators constrict bronchial smooth muscle, increase vascular permeability, affect systemic and pulmonary vascular muscle tone, induce platelet aggregation and degranulation, attract inflammatory cells to the reaction site, and, in general, are responsible for the manifestations of anaphylaxis. Elevated levels of histamine have been measured during human anaphylactic shock and the intravenous injection of this mediator causes urticaria, bronchospasm, vasodilation, hypotension, and vomiting. It seems likely that other mediators are also involved. It is not yet possible, however, to describe the mechanisms involved in anaphylaxis in detail. The alterations in coagulability which have been reported, for example, may be due to platelet activating factors or to an enzymatic mediator which activates Hageman factor.

TABLE 433–2. AGENTS CAUSING ANAPHYLACTOID REACTIONS*

Curare
Hypertonic solutions (mannitol)
Nonsteroidal anti-inflammatory agents (acetylsalicylic acid, aminopyrine, indomethacin)
Radiopaque contrast material

*Reactions to these small molecular weight compounds may not be due to IgE-mediated immunologic mechanisms (see text).

CLINICAL FEATURES. The onset and clinical manifestations of systemic anaphylaxis vary, depending on the route of administration of the antigen or hapten. The physiologic features are also determined by the type, quantities, and sites of release of pharmacologic mediators, by factors that control releasability, and by differing sensitivity of the organs to the released mediators.

There is no universal response pattern or "shock" organ that is always involved in man. Individuals do, however, have a characteristic pattern of response which tends to repeat. This pattern is often preceded by an aura that is also characteristic and well recognized by the patient. Attention to these subjective symptoms, which precede the physiologic events by one to two minutes, may be valuable. The most common manifestations of systemic reactions are *cutaneous*: erythema, pruritus, urticaria, and angioedema, often of the eyes, lips, or tongue. In adults, the cutaneous symptoms are usually accompanied by one or more other features. There are two patterns of respiratory failure. The first is *upper airway obstruction* owing to edema of the larynx and/or epiglottis, which can cause acute distress and death by suffocation. The second involves *diffuse lower airway bronchoconstriction* similar to the respiratory abnormalities observed in status asthmaticus. Such airflow limitation is not relieved by endotracheal intubation and may lead to abnormalities of pulmonary gas exchange with subsequent hypoxemia and hypercarbia.

Perhaps the most severe clinical manifestation of anaphylaxis is *hypotensive shock*, which can develop with or without other symptoms. The cause is thought to be either peripheral vascular pooling of blood resulting from vasodilation or increased capillary permeability with functional loss of intravascular blood volume into the interstitial spaces. Electrocardiographic abnormalities, including conduction disturbances, arrhythmias, and ischemic or infarction patterns, have been noted during anaphylactic shock. These changes may reflect myocardial ischemia and arrhythmias caused by decreased coronary perfusion and oxygenation.

Rarely, other symptoms are associated with systemic anaphylactic reactions. These include gastrointestinal (vomiting, nausea, and diarrhea) and central nervous system symptoms. Prolonged hypotension or anoxia can, of course, cause a variety of secondary, more permanent changes.

Metabolic abnormalities in severe human anaphylactic shock include increased blood histamine levels, which correlate with the duration and severity of shock. There is also depletion of clotting factors V, VIII, and fibrinogen, activation of complement, and loss of high molecular weight kininogen. The utilization of these coagulation factors is consistent with acute intravascular coagulation and may account for clotting defects observed in clinical anaphylactic syndromes.

DIFFERENTIAL DIAGNOSIS. The diagnosis of systemic anaphylaxis is generally easy with a characteristic history of immediately antecedent exposure to foreign antigenic material and appropriate evidence of systemic involvement on physical examination. The presentation may, however, involve a patient unable to provide a history and suffering the secondary effects of shock, e.g., a myocardial infarction or an arrhythmia. Occasionally, this syndrome must be distinguished from other related clinical conditions, i.e., sudden acute bronchospasm in an asthmatic, vasovagal syncope, acute drug toxicity, hereditary angioedema, cold or idiopathic urticaria. Nonimmunologic "anaphylactoid" reactions to radiopaque dyes, hypertonic solutions, and nonsteroidal anti-inflammatory agents (indomethacin, aminopyrine, acetylsalicylic acid) have a similar clinical presentation and require an identical therapeutic approach, even though they may not be mediated by IgE antibody.

Because of the rapid onset of these reactions, initial laboratory testing is not helpful in making a diagnosis. The retrospective diagnosis of specific allergic sensitivity is by skin testing, or the measurement of specific IgE antibody by the radioallergosorbent test.

PREVENTION AND TREATMENT. The sudden, usually unexpected onset of human anaphylaxis with a rapid clinical course that leads to either swift recovery or death has provided little opportunity for prospective, controlled, therapeutic studies. Even when anaphylaxis is treated in an intensive care unit by trained personnel and a well-planned therapeutic approach, severe systemic reactions often do not respond to medical treatment. Therefore, every attempt must be made to prevent these reactions. A careful medical history should include inquiry about any previous allergic drug reactions. Patients who have previously experienced anaphylactic episodes should wear a Medic-Alert bracelet and be instructed in the importance of relating details of their specific drug allergies before taking medications; their medical records should prominently state the patient's allergic history. The physician should be aware of which medications, proprietaries, and foods contain allergens or cross-reacting antigens. Sensitization may occur in the absence of clinical symptoms; previous tolerance of a substance provides no guarantee that an anaphylactic reaction will not occur.

If diagnostic tests are not available, as with most drugs, it is appropriate to substitute another therapeutic agent for the treatment of a patient with a history of sensitivity to a particular drug. Again, knowledge of cross-reactivity is necessary. If, for example, cephalosporins are substituted for penicillin, there is a significant risk of reaction, since these agents share a common β-lactam ring. Penicillin causes more anaphylactic reactions than any other drug, but at least 80 per cent of patients with a history of a previous reaction will have negative skin tests (to penicilloyl-polylysine and a mixture of haptens [MDM]) and can tolerate the drug with impunity. This is an important consideration, since penicillin is a relatively nontoxic drug and most antibiotics that would be substituted have a significant incidence of side effects. (See Ch. 437 for a further discussion of penicillin allergy.) When penicillin or other allergens must be used in a sensitive patient, an effort can be made to desensitize the patient by the use of sequential low doses, initially intradermally, then subcutaneously, and finally intramuscularly into the peripheral part of an extremity. Such a procedure should be carried out by experienced personnel, and potentially allergenic substances should be administered in a setting where anaphylactic reactions can be effectively treated.

Early recognition of anaphylaxis is critical, since death or irreversible anoxic organ damage can occur rapidly. When an anaphylactic reaction is initiated by an injection into the arm or leg, a tourniquet should be placed around that extremity to stop antigen absorption. The initial pharmacologic treatment is the subcutaneous administration of 0.2 to 0.5 ml of a 1:1000 solution of epinephrine. This is the agent of choice. Antihistamines and corticosteroids play *no* role in the treatment of an acute reaction, although some physicians believe they limit late or recurrent cutaneous manifestations. Extrathoracic upper airway obstruction must be differentiated from diffuse bronchospasm, since severe laryngeal and epiglottic edema may require careful endotracheal intubation or an emergency tracheostomy to facilitate ventilation. Bronchospasm can be handled in a manner similar to the therapy for status asthmaticus, by the administration of inhaled B-2 sympathomimetics or by intravenous aminophylline (see Ch. 59). Hypoxemia should be treated with supplemental oxygen. Hypervolemic shock requires rapid intravenous fluid administration (normal saline and colloid) to maintain blood pressure. Additionally, epinephrine can be given intravenously in severe shock, and, if it is ineffective, an alpha-adrenergic vasoconstrictor (norepinephrine) should be tried. If severe vascular anaphylactic shock does not respond immediately to these measures, supportive treatment should be continued, preferably in an intensive care unit setting where vascular monitoring is available to guide additional therapy. Any patient who has had significant shock or airway obstruction should be hospitalized for at least 24 hours after the acute episode is handled, since these symptoms may recur many hours after an initial favorable response.

Bleecker ER, Lichtenstein LM: Systemic anaphylaxis. *In* Lichtenstein LM, Fauci AS (eds.): Current Therapy in Allergy and Immunology, 1983–1984. St. Louis, C. V. Mosby Company, 1983, pp 78–83. *A detailed description of how to treat this serious disorder.*

Parker CW: Systemic anaphylaxis. *In* Parker CW (ed.): Clinical Immunology. Philadelphia, W. B. Saunders Company, 1980, pp 1208-1218. *An up-to-date textbook review of what is known about etiology, pathogenesis and treatment.*

Smith PL, Sobotka AK, Bleecker ER, Traystman R, Kaplan AP, Gralnick H, Valentine MD, Permutt S, Lichtenstein LM: Physiologic manifestations of human anaphylaxis. J Clin Invest 66:1072, 1980. *Physiologic and biochemical changes monitored in human anaphylaxis occurring during a trial of therapy for insect allergy. Includes comments on therapy.*

434. INSECT STING ALLERGY*

Lawrence M. Lichtenstein†

The stings of insects of the order Hymenoptera have long been recognized as a potential cause of severe, often life-threatening reactions in susceptible individuals. These reactions are unrelated to the toxic chemicals in the venoms, being due to allergic sensitization. Insect sting allergy has recently become the most intensely studied model of anaphylaxis in man, resulting in important advances that have had rapid clinical application.

EPIDEMIOLOGY. The incidence of immediate hypersensitivity to insect stings based on history is 4 per cent; more than 20 per cent of the population, however, has positive skin test reactions to insect venoms without having had a reaction. Other allergies do not seem to predispose to insect sting sensitivity. The frequency varies with exposure and is therefore greater in children and males as well as those inclined to outdoor activities or beekeeping. Insect stings cause few fatalities, but the morbidity, fear, and change in life style caused by these reactions is significant. A large number of people suffer prolonged and unusually large local inflammatory reactions to insect stings, which are allergic in nature. As with other allergies, there appears to be an inherited predisposition, since multiple family members are often affected.

ETIOLOGY. The only insects possessing true stingers are those of the order Hymenoptera. There are two families of importance, the bees (honeybees, bumblebees) and the vespids (yellow jackets, hornets, wasps). The bees have barbed stingers which remain in the skin after a sting. Yellow jackets are the most common culprits, but honeybees are more commonly implicated in the western United States. Wasps are more common in the south central United States (especially Texas). The fire ant, common in the South and the Caribbean, is a

*Supported by Grant AI 08270 from the National Institute of Allergy and Infectious Diseases.

†I would like to express my thanks to my colleague, David B. K. Golden, M.D., for his aid in the preparation and writing of this chapter.

hymenopteran whose sting can also cause anaphylaxis. Sensitivity develops to antigens in the insect venom, most of which have enzymatic activity. A major allergen in both insect families is phospholipase, but they do not cross-react with one another.

PATHOGENESIS. The injection of foreign proteins commonly causes the production of specific antibodies of the IgE and IgG classes. Individuals may develop venom-specific IgE antibodies after any sting, this response persisting for less than three months to more than 25 years. Tissue mast cells and circulating basophils are sensitized by bound IgE, and a repeat encounter with the offending allergen will trigger release of the mediators of anaphylaxis (see Fig. 59–3). The initiation and persistence of this sensitization are related to inheritable and other unknown determinants. Sensitization may occur at any time in life, even after many uneventful stings. The sensitizing sting itself causes no unusual reaction, and is often so remote as to evade recollection.

Generalized mediator release from sensitized basophils and mast cells causes the many manifestations of anaphylaxis (see table in Ch. 438). Localization of symptoms to specific target tissues is not well understood. The pathology observed in fatal cases includes upper airway edema and obstruction, the visceral consequences of hypotension, or occasionally no discernible abnormality (see Ch. 433 for a discussion of anaphylaxis).

Large local reactions most often appear to be IgE dependent, but their prolonged time-course is not typical of immediate hypersensitivity. These reactions may involve a cascade of events beginning with mediator release from mast cells and culminating with local inflammation involving many cell types and numerous mechanisms. The potential roles of eosinophils, neutrophils, basophils, lymphocytes and lymphokines, complement, and mediators with prolonged release or activity have not been elucidated.

The venom-specific IgG antibody response to a sting is usually short lived, lasting only a few months. Repeated stings (as in beekeepers) are associated with high titers of IgG antibodies, which protect against allergic sting reactions. Beekeepers who do not have anaphylactic reactions have high IgG titers, as do affected individuals immunized with venoms. Passive transfer of these IgG antibodies protects sensitive patients from a sting. These protective antibodies are thought to block the allergic reaction by competing with IgE for the allergenic venom proteins and have therefore been termed "blocking" antibodies.

CLINICAL MANIFESTATIONS. Allergic reactions to insect stings are either generalized (systemic) or large local reactions. *Systemic sting reactions* present the classic manifestations of anaphylaxis described in Ch. 433. The observed frequency of the most common symptoms in adult patients is presented in Table 434–1. The risk of a fatal outcome increases, as might be expected, with age. Fatal anaphylaxis may occur without a past history of sting allergy.

The onset of systemic symptoms is rapid, within two to three minutes, and uncommonly occurs more than 30 minutes after a sting. Symptoms presenting hours later (except large local reactions) are not usually associated with immediate hypersensitivity or IgE antibodies. Unusual reactions such as vasculitis, nephropathies, encephalitis, and other neurologic manifestations have been reported, but no causal relationship has been established. Allergic respiratory symptoms may occur in beekeepers and their families owing to sensitization to the dust in the hives that contains bee body proteins. This sensitivity is unrelated to sting reactions.

Large local reactions are slow in onset and occur with or without concomitant early systemic reaction. The area of induration increases in size progressively for the first 24 to 48 hours, and then resolves gradually over several days. These reactions may be so large as to immobilize an entire limb, and are a significant cause of morbidity in sensitive individuals. Red streaks resembling lymphangitis may be observed and are often treated with antibiotics despite a lack of evidence for true cellulitis. Some individuals develop large local sting reactions

TABLE 434–1. SYMPTOMS REPORTED BY 245 PATIENTS

Symptom	%
Cutaneous only	14
Urticaria-angioedema	78
Dizziness-hypotension	61
Dyspnea-wheezing	53
Throat tightness-hoarseness	40
Loss of consciousness	33

in the absence of allergic sensitivity. These are exaggerated reactions to the toxic and inflammatory venom components, and often occur in persons who report similar large swellings to mosquito or fly bites, or who have cutaneous sensitivity to many irritants.

NATURAL HISTORY. The natural history of insect sting allergy has been incompletely documented. The incidence of venom sensitization in the general population was noted above, but the actual risk of reaction associated with sensitization is unknown. There is considerable variability in the reaction to a sting among those who are clearly allergic as demonstrated by positive skin tests and a history of previous reaction. In a small study 60 per cent of adults had a systemic reaction when stung by the appropriate insect. In children a repeat sting causes a reaction in only 8 per cent. The incidence in adolescents and young adults must lie between these extremes. This variability confounds the prediction of risk associated with sensitization.

Many patients and physicians believe that allergic sting reactions become progressively more severe with every sting. Although some patients progress from large local through mild systemic reactions to life-threatening anaphylaxis, most of those affected maintain a similar pattern of symptoms with every sting. Less than 10 per cent of those experiencing large local reactions will subsequently have systemic reactions. Factors favoring a systemic reaction include multiple stings, or stings in close temporal proximity (only weeks apart).

Sensitization may decrease or disappear in time, more commonly in children. However, resensitization has been observed upon resting.

DIAGNOSIS. The acute presentation of anaphylaxis may be easily diagnosed in the presence of classic symptoms and signs. The insect sting may be inapparent. Differential diagnosis is more difficult in localized reactions such as acute chest pain and dyspnea or syncope without urticaria or recognition of the sting.

The diagnosis of insect sting allergy currently rests on a convincing history and positive skin tests. Demonstration in vitro of venom-specific IgE by the radioallergosorbent test (RAST) is less sensitive than skin tests, but may be useful in equivocal cases.

Skin tests are performed intradermally with venoms diluted to concentrations in the range of 1 to 1000 ng per milliliter. Five venoms are used: honeybee (HB), yellow jacket (YJ), yellow hornet (YH), white-faced hornet (WH), and *Polistes* wasp (POL). Positive intradermal skin tests develop, within 20 minutes, a wheal greater than 5 mm in diameter with at least 20 mm of erythema. The degree of skin test sensitivity does not correlate with clinical sensitivity. Within a few months after a systemic sting reaction, skin tests are almost uniformly positive. Stings more remote in time are more commonly associated with an apparent loss of sensitivity (similar to the situation in penicillin-related anaphylaxis).

Honeybee venom sensitivity occurs independent of other venom allergies, but about 10 per cent of patients are sensitive to both bee and vespid venoms. The vespid venoms are highly cross-reactive, so that almost all vespid sensitive patients have positive YJ, YH, and WH skin tests even though most have been stung only by YJs. Half of these patients are also sensitive to POL venom. A few individuals are allergic to only one or two of the vespid venoms. In vitro RAST inhibition techniques are useful to distinguish cross-reactivity from specific sensitivity.

TREATMENT. The treatment of choice for anaphylactic reactions is subcutaneous epinephrine 1:1000, 0.5 ml initially and repeated twice at ten-minute intervals, if necessary, to reverse the progression of symptoms. Sublingual isoproterenol is probably ineffective. Antihistamines and glucocorticoids do not contribute to the management of life-threatening symptoms, but may reduce the duration and severity of cutaneous manifestations. Their use should not be considered until the termination of the acute episode. Intravenous volume expansion or airway maintenance may be necessary. In a few individuals, the process is resistant to epinephrine; in such instances an α-adrenergic agent (i.e., norepinephrine) may be tried. Affected persons not yet protected by immunotherapy are advised to carry, and are instructed in the use of, a kit containing a syringe device preloaded with one or two recommended doses of epinephrine.

Venom immunotherapy is successful in virtually all patients. Less than 3 per cent of those immunized have any systemic symptoms after a challenge sting, and these are uniformly less severe than their previous reactions. The indications for venom immunotherapy are currently based on an incomplete understanding of the natural history of the disease. Those with a history of life-threatening reactions should be treated. The risk of progression from strictly cutaneous to life-threatening respiratory or vascular reactions is uncertain. Cutaneous reactors who are more likely to be stung in their daily activities or who can, for a variety of reasons (location, age, cardiovascular disease), ill afford a more severe reaction should be treated. The cost and inconvenience of treatment may deter other cutaneous reactors from undergoing immunotherapy. Children, much more commonly than adults, have cutaneous symptoms only. These children may be left untreated. Venom immunotherapy is contraindicated in the absence of positive skin tests. Treatment is currently recommended using all venoms causing a positive skin test. While other mechanisms may contribute, the induction of increased serum levels of venom-specific IgG antibodies is the most apparent mechanism of protection for venom immunotherapy; about 5 μg per milliliter is required.

Rapid immunization in six to eight weekly visits is recommended, since it is associated with a significantly greater and more rapid immune response, and with fewer adverse reactions than a slower (more than 20 weeks) regimen. The maintenance dose of 100 μg of each venom is repeated monthly for at least six months, and is then continued at six- to eight-week intervals for an indefinite time. If treatment is interrupted for more than three months, it is likely that protection will diminish to inadequate levels. Although unusual in adults, loss of sensitivity during maintenance immunotherapy may occur. Skin tests should, therefore, be repeated every two years.

Adverse reactions to venom immunotherapy may be early or late. Immediate reactions include all the manifestations of anaphylaxis. During the initial course of treatment, 10 to 15 per cent of patients report systemic complaints, only half of which require epinephrine. At maintenance doses, systemic reactions occur rarely. After a systemic reaction, the dose should be reduced by up to 50 per cent on the subsequent visit, and then increased gradually toward 100 μg again.

Large local reactions occur frequently. Fifty per cent of treated patients experience at least one such reaction. These occur after 10 out of every 100 injections in the induction phase, most commonly in the midrange of doses (10 to 50 μg) and much less often at maintenance doses. Large local reactions do not presage systemic reactions and require a reduction of dose only for the most severe reactions. Long-term side effects have not been observed with venom immunotherapy or in beekeepers stung frequently for over 30 years.

Hunt KJ, Valentine MD, Sobotka AK, et al.: A controlled trial of immunotherapy in insect hypersensitivity. N Engl J Med 299:157, 1978. *A comparison of venom immunotherapy with whole body extract and placebo. Demonstrates efficacy of venom therapy and the clinical consequences of challenge stings.*

Lichtenstein LM, Valentine MD, Sobotka AK: Insect allergy: The state of the art. J Allerg Clin Immunol 64:5, 1979. *A review of diagnostic and therapeutic problems in insect allergy. Details the parameters which dictate the choice of patients for treatment.*

Schuberth KC, Lichtenstein LM, Kagey-Sobotka A, et al.: Epidemiologic study of insect allergy in children. II. Effect of accidental stings in allergic children. J Pediatr 102:361, 1983. *A prospective epidemiology study of repeat stings in children. Has implications for young adults.*

435. IMMUNE COMPLEX DISEASES

Charles G. Cochrane

DEFINITION. Immune complex diseases are caused by the deposition or formation of antigen-antibody complexes in tissues. Inflammation results and leads to acute or chronic disease of the organ system in which the immune complexes have been deposited. The antigen-antibody complex localizes in a particular organ by two major mechanisms: (1) when antigens of that organ are exposed to antibodies entering from the circulation; and (2) antigen-antibody complexes may form in the circulation, to be subsequently deposited in renal glomeruli, arteries, or venules, inducing inflammatory disease of each structure. Thus immune complexes are capable of causing severe inflammation in many organs of the body. For example, immune complexes may contribute to the pathogenesis of systemic lupus erythematosus, serum sickness, acute and chronic glomerulonephritis, rheumatoid arthritis, arteritis, vasculitis, and tissue injury associated with a wide spectrum of infectious agents. This chapter will examine the mechanisms by which the interaction of antigens and antibodies may form immune complexes and how this process may be injurious to the host.

PATHOGENESIS. The pathogenesis of immune complex diseases is best understood by examining several well-studied experimental models that closely mimic human diseases.

Immune Complex Disease with Tissue-Fixed Antigen. When the antigen is bound in an organ or is released locally from a tissue, the antibodies react with antigen at that locus to induce local inflammatory injury. As an example, antibodies in the circulation may react with antigens in the glomerular basement membrane of the kidney and result in inflammation of the glomerulus (glomerulitis) with acute or chronic injury. In human beings this takes the form of Goodpasture's disease. Similarly, when antigen-antibody complexes form in a joint space, synovitis results. This may play an important role in the pathogenesis of rheumatoid arthritis, in which antibodies have been found in the joint fluid complexed with many host proteins, especially IgG itself.

Immune Complex Disease Caused by the Deposition of Circulating Immune Complexes in Tissues. Acute immune complex disease, or serum sickness, can be produced in experimental animals by injection of serum protein antigens. The associated lesions are generally those of arteritis, glomerulonephritis, endocarditis, cutaneous rash, and synovitis. A mechanism for the production of immune complex disease is given in Figure 435–1. A chronic disease follows injections of the serum protein antigens for 30 days. In this form of the disease, chronic glomerulonephritis most characteristically results, often without the other lesions of the acute disease. In cases in which a large antibody response occurs, pulmonary inflammation and fibrosis of the lung result. The glomerular lesions of chronic immune complex disease contain lumpy deposits rich in antigen, immunoglobulin, and complement along the outer edge of the basement membrane (Figs. 435–2 to 435–4). These morphologic characteristics have formed the diagnostic features of immune complex glomerulonephritis of human beings. However, in contrast to the lesions of chronic serum sickness of experimental animals, the amount of the inducing antigen (when known, such as in poststreptococcal glomerulonephritis) is vanishingly small in concentration. By contrast, the IgG–

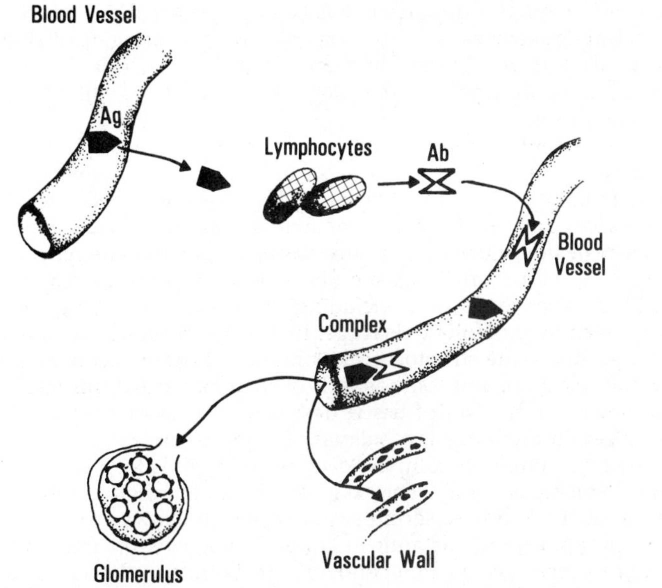

Figure 435–1. Schematic mechanism of the production of antibody by an antigen, the formation of antibody-antigen complexes in the circulation, and the localization of the complexes in tissues where inflammatory injury develops. Ag = antigen; Ab = antibody.

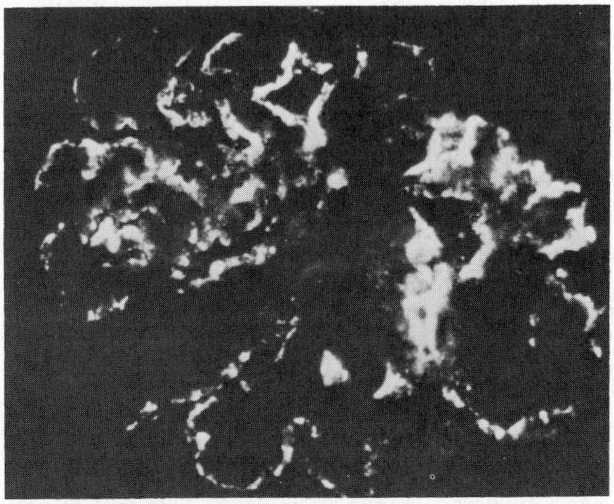

Figure 435–3. Fluorescent photomicrograph of a glomerulus similar to that in Figure 435–2, showing the presence of rabbit immunoglobulin along the glomerular basement membrane. The specific antigen and the third component of complement were localized in the same pattern.

anti-IgG complexes and cryoglobulins may dominate, suggesting that a nonspecific stimulation of the immune system followed the initial exposure to antigen. Possibly a polyclonal stimulation of B lymphocytes and diminished activity of immune-suppressor systems are important pathogenic mechanisms in these human autoimmune diseases. Some antibodies to IgG proteins are anti-idiotypic; they form complexes with the immunoglobulin of the appropriate idiotype.

The Mechanism of Deposition of Circulating Immune Complexes. Several factors determine the ability of circulating complexes to localize in the vessel walls of a particular organ. Important among these factors are the quantity of complexes and the size of the complex. No definite minimal concentration of the complexes in the circulation has been established, but there seems to be a requirement for the complex to be of a particular size (19S or greater) for its deposition in blood vessel walls. The size of the three-dimensional lattice of antigen-antibody complexes depends largely upon the affinity of the antibody for the antigen. For example, in experimental animals complexes of intermediate size circulate and cause tissue injury, whereas larger complexes are insoluble and are rapidly cleared from circulation by the reticuloendothelial system. Smaller complexes may fail to activate the mediator systems or be too small to be trapped in vessel walls. The small complexes may therefore circulate for long periods. Another factor that may play a role in the deposition of immune complexes is charge. By virtue of the overall anionic charge of the glomerular basement membrane, cationic immune complexes or free antigens possess an affinity for glomeruli and are retained longer than neutral or anionic molecules. Whether this plays a role in the development of glomerulonephritis, however, is unclear.

An increase in vascular permeability is required for circulating immune complexes to deposit in tissues and to initiate acute injury. The local release of vasoactive amines appears responsible for this increased permeability. Circulating antigen reacts with specific surface IgE on sensitized basophils to release an array of constituents, including histamine and a platelet acti-

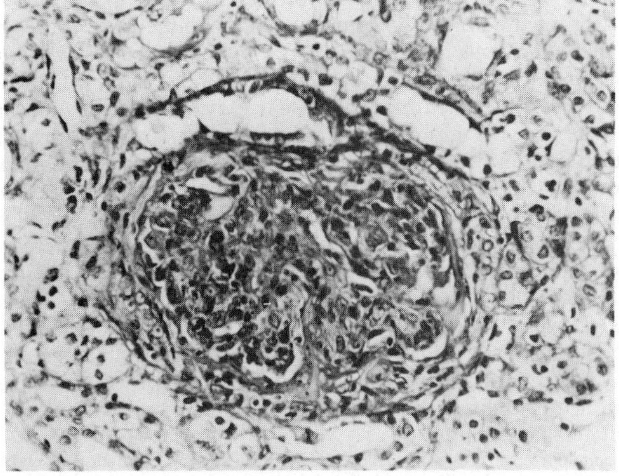

Figure 435–2. Glomerulus of a rabbit with subacute immune complex-induced glomerulonephritis. Inflammatory cells have accumulated, and injury of the glomerular basement membrane was evidenced by marked proteinuria. (× 150.)

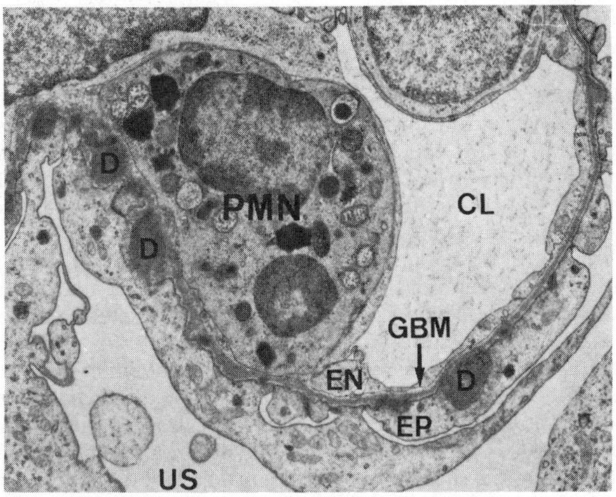

Figure 435–4. A polymorphonuclear leukocyte (PMN) is seen closely approximated along the glomerular basement membrane (GBM) in proximity to subepithelial (EP) electron dense deposits (D) in a rabbit with chronic serum sickness glomerulonephritis. The deposits are rich in antibody, complement, and, to a lesser extent, antigen by fluorescent antibody microscopy. Similar or identical deposits are observed in human immune complex glomerulonephritis. The endothelial cell (EN) has been displaced. Other abbreviations: CL = capillary lumen; US = urinary space.

vating factor (PAF). This latter factor causes clumping and degranulation of platelets and release of platelet histamine and serotonin. Thus an allergic reaction induces deposition of the circulating complexes in blood vessel walls. The anaphylatoxins C3a and C5a, generated by complement activation (see Ch. 428), also degranulate basophils and mast cells to liberate vasoactive amines and other substances. These may augment the increase in vascular permeability and facilitate the deposition of immune complexes along vascular basement membranes. In immune complex disease of man, the role of increased vascular permeability in the local deposition of circulating immune complexes has been documented in cutaneous vasculitis. In addition, in patients with active systemic lupus erythematosus, the circulating basophils undergo loss of granules and contain diminished levels of PAF. Basophils from patients with quiescent systemic lupus degranulate and release PAF upon exposure to DNA.

Host Factors Responsible for the Inflammation Caused by Immune Complexes. Immune complexes deposited in tissues activate mediator systems. These mediators are the cellular and humoral effectors of inflammatory injury—activated enzymes, biologically active peptides, oxidizing substances, polyamines, and prostaglandins—that are released in the tissues as a consequence of antigen-antibody complex deposition. The classic and, to a lesser extent, the alternative pathways of the complement system are activated by the complexed Ig molecule to initiate the complement cascade. This leads to the limited proteolytic cleavage of C3 and C5 to liberate small peptides, C3a and C5a and the fragment C3b, which rapidly bind to tissue structures such as vascular basement membrane. As noted, the peptides also degranulate basophils and mast cells releasing histamine, slow-reacting substance, and other substances that cause increased vascular permeability, smooth muscle contraction, and hypotension (see Table 438–1). C5a is also a potent chemoattractant for leukocytes. The remaining portion of the C3 molecule, C3b, binds white blood cells through the process of immune adherence, thus facilitating phagocytosis and discharge of lysosomal granules. Short-lived oxidants (usually free radicals of oxygen) are generated in vivo in inflammatory foci and produce injury through mechanisms that have not been clarified. Of particular interest, antioxidants have a profound therapeutic effect in experimental inflammatory disease.

White blood cells, platelets, and macrophages specifically bind the Fc portion of the antigen-antibody complex and in the process are stimulated to generate injurious oxidizing radicals (e.g., superoxide anion and H_2O_2) and to release their lysosomal granules containing proteolytic enzymes, peptides, and vasoactive amines into the surrounding fluid. The C5a peptide has a similar effect on leukocytes. The discharge of these effector molecules results in the inflammatory tissue injury characteristic of immune complex disease.

Acute immune complex–mediated injury depends, therefore, upon an interaction of the complement system and neutrophils at the local site. This has been clearly demonstrated in experimental studies of the Arthus reaction, pneumonitis, and arteritis in serum sickness; of immunologic synovitis; and of at least one form of experimental glomerulonephritis. In each reaction, an antigen-antibody complex is formed in the tissues, complement is rapidly activated, and neutrophils accumulate at the site. Inhibition of complement activation prevents the accumulation of neutrophils and prevents injury, suggesting that immune adherence by tissue-fixed C3b and stimulation of neutrophil chemotaxis by C5a are important functions in the genesis of these lesions. Production of neutropenia with specific antibody or by the use of nitrogen mustard also prevents the development of experimental immune complex injury even though complement is present. The release of mediators of inflammatory injury by neutrophils at the site of antigen-antibody complex deposition has been described above. Mononuclear leukocytes are also capable of generating oxidizing radicals and of releasing lysosomal constituents. C3e, a fragment derived from further degradation of C3b, stimulates leukocytosis.

Experimental immune complex disease is capable of destroying several tissues through these mechanisms. In joints, glycosaminoglycans and cartilage are destroyed; in blood vessels and glomeruli, the basement membranes are hydrolyzed. Fragments of the injured glomerular basement membrane may be excreted in the urine. Elastic fibers of arteries are destroyed, and connective tissues, including collagen in the lung, are damaged by proteolytic cleavage. In man the histologic features of arteritis, acute streptococcal glomerulonephritis, acute homograft rejection, and some aspects of rheumatoid arthritis imply a similar mechanism of tissue destruction. Loss of elastin and collagen in the lungs is a hallmark of emphysema.

Chronic immune complex disease may call into play other mechanisms of injury. For example, the glomerulonephritis of experimental chronic serum sickness, which shows the typical lumpy appearance of antigen-antibody deposits on immunofluorescence, occurs independently of both complement and neutrophils. Macrophages, which may be attracted by chemotactic factors from neutrophils and by other substances, probably play an important role in this lesion. Macrophages cause tissue injury by mechanisms similar to those described for neutrophils. They may also be stimulated to divide at the site of tissue injury by macrophage growth factors present in the inflammatory exudate. There is increasing evidence for an important role for the macrophage in both experimental models of chronic immunologic diseases and in immunologic lung disease in man. In a model of chronic membranous nephritis, marked by immune complex formation along the epithelial side of the glomerular basement membrane, complement appears to play an essential role in the development of proteinuria independently of leukocytes. In this lesion, which closely resembles membranous nephritis of humans, the immune complexes and activated complement components lie on or adjacent to the delicate slit-pore diaphragm that bridges the space between epithelial foot processes. This diaphragm may be an essential barrier to the passage of protein molecules, and its disruption by the membrane attack complex of complement may constitute a major cause of the glomerular dysfunction in chronic membranous nephritis.

Experimental myasthenia gravis is another interesting example of the role of mediators in the pathogenesis of diseases caused by antigen-antibody complexes. In this disease, antibodies react with motor end-plates (acetylcholine receptors); this reaction activates complement and stimulates the local accumulation of monocytes. If the activation of complement is prevented, the inflammatory destruction of motor end-plates and the loss of muscle function do not occur, despite the reaction of the antibody with the acetylcholine receptors.

The Significance of Circulating Immune Complexes in Human Disease. Circulating immune complexes have been detected in a wide variety of human diseases. Nevertheless, in diseases such as chronic glomerulonephritis, which is most probably caused by immune complexes, circulating complexes frequently cannot be detected. In other diseases in which immune complexes do not appear to play a role in pathogenesis, complexes may be readily measured in plasma. Thus the mere detection of circulating immune complexes does not necessarily imply that they play a role in the pathogenesis of the disease. Nevertheless, since the potential of immune complexes to deposit and establish inflammatory injury is established, their detection in the circulation should alert the physician to seek evidence of their pathogenicity in the individual patient.

Lambert PH, et al.: A WHO collaborative study for the evaluation of eighteen methods for the detection of immune complexes in serum. J Clin Lab Immunol 1:1, 1978. Theofilopoulos AN, Dixon FJ: The biology and detection of immune complexes. Adv Immunol 28:89, 1979. *These two references cover the mechanisms available for detecting immune complexes in the circulation of patients with a wide variety of disorders. The latter reference offers, in addition, useful information on the effects of immune complexes on the host's response.*

Salant DS, Belok S, Madaio MP, Couser WG: A new role for complement in experimental nephropathy in rats. J Clin Invest 66:1339, 1980. *This article reviews the finding that immune complexes can form on the epithelial side of the glomerular basement membrane and, through the activation of complement, produce injury.*

Schraufstatter IU, Revak SD, Cochrane CG: Proteases and oxidants in experimental pulmonary inflammatory injury. J Clin Invest 73:1175, 1984. *This article provides evidence that oxidants are generated in situ in inflammation, and reviews the available data on oxidants and proteases in human pulmonary inflammatory disease.*

436. THE MAJOR HISTOCOMPATIBILITY COMPLEX AND DISEASE SUSCEPTIBILITY

Hugh O. McDevitt

The major histocompatibility complex (MHC) in mouse and man was originally defined as a linked cluster of genes on one chromosome that determines the structure of a group of cell surface molecules that are the strongest antigenic barrier to tissue transplantation between two unrelated individuals of the same species. This genetic region was first identified by tumor graft and skin graft rejection experiments. Subsequently serologic analysis became feasible with antisera produced in one individual by application of skin grafts or injection of lymphocytes from another individual of the same species. With the development of sophisticated skin grafting techniques following World War II, and the advent of kidney transplants, interest in detailed analysis of the major histocompatibility system increased. Great progress was made in our knowledge of the structure of the human MHC, of the number of alleles at each locus in the system (genetic polymorphism), and of the structure of the gene products themselves.

All of this knowledge developed directly out of research in transplantation immunology, although a moment's reflection will make it obvious that this system could not have evolved to frustrate the transplant surgeon. Tissue compatibility systems are well described in plants and in invertebrates. These systems may have evolved in the transition from unicellular to multicellular organisms so that these gene products play a major role in the discrimination of self from nonself. The MHC regulates the recognition of antigenic foreignness at several levels by several different effector components of the immune system. This phenomenon has been amply documented and carefully analyzed at the cellular level, although the molecular mechanisms are not yet clear.

The genotype of several MHC gene products (MHC antigens) shows a striking association with susceptibility to a wide variety of human diseases as well as to a number of animal disease models. This presumably results from their role in regulating specific immune responses. A wide variety of diseases in almost every subspecialty of internal medicine, many of them autoimmune in nature, shows strong associations with particular alleles (alternate forms) of particular loci in the human MHC, as determined by typing MHC molecules on peripheral blood lymphocytes (human leukocyte antigens—HLA). An understanding of the MHC and of the functions of the MHC genes is therefore important in understanding the association with disease susceptibility, and may be vital in understanding the pathogenesis of these diseases.

This chapter will describe the genetic structure of the murine and human MHC, the biochemistry and molecular genetics of the MHC gene products, and the function of these genes at the cellular level. The chapter will conclude with a brief discussion of (1) the possible mechanisms of action of these gene products at the molecular level and (2) an attempt to relate these functions to regulation of the immune response and to the determination of susceptibility to particular diseases. Some or all of the MHC antigens are expressed on all cell types. They clearly play a major role at the cell surface in recognition of antigenic foreignness. This may be only one of several regulatory functions of a group of cell surface molecules whose evolutionary origins may extend much farther back than the appearance of vertebrates in evolution.

THE MAJOR HISTOCOMPATIBILITY COMPLEX IN THE MOUSE

Analysis of the major histocompatibility complex is most advanced in the mouse and in man. MHC genes, gene products, and the functions of the complex in these two species share extensive homology. The genetic organization of the MHC differs slightly in the two species. Unfortunately the nomenclature differs radically. Since the genetic analysis of the murine MHC is farther advanced, this system will be presented first, followed by a discussion of the corresponding genes in the human MHC. In this textbook of medicine, discussion of important and fundamental work in the mouse must of necessity be curtailed. The reader is referred to a more extensive discussion of this topic in the articles cited at the end of this chapter.

The mouse MHC was the second histocompatibility-determining locus described in the mouse, and therefore has been designated H-2.

Figure 436–1 is a linkage map of the seventeenth mouse chromosome. The histocompatibility-2 (H-2) region is approximately 15 centimorgans (cM) to the right of the centromere. (Genetic map units or distances are expressed as crossover frequencies. Two loci on the same chromosome that show genetic recombination, resulting from crossing over, 15 times in 100 matings are said to be 15 map units, or crossover units, or centimorgans, apart.) The H-2 complex is a small portion of the seventeenth mouse chromosome, and spans a genetic distance of 1.0 cM. Although this is small in terms of the size of the seventeenth chromosome, it is sufficient to encode for over 200 structural genes for polypeptides of approximately 20,000 daltons. The exact number of genes in the H-2 complex is not known. To date, over 50 genes have been mapped in the H-2 complex.

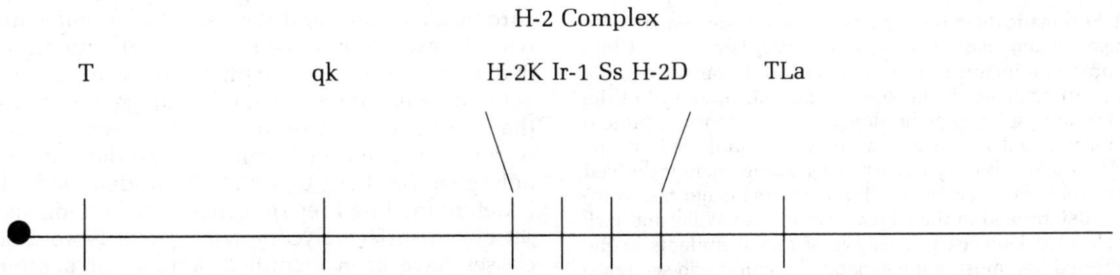

Figure 436–1. A schematic diagram of some of the genes on the seventeenth mouse chromosome. T is the short tail or brachyury locus. qk is the quaking locus. The H-2 complex is explained in detail in the text. TLa is the thymus leukemia antigen locus. (From McDevitt HO: *In* McCarty DJ [ed.]: Arthritis and Allied Conditions. 9th ed. Philadelphia, Lea & Febiger, 1979.)

TABLE 436–1. MAJOR PROPERTIES OF THE CLASS I (H-2K AND H-2D) GENE PRODUCTS OF THE MOUSE

Molecular weight: 45,000 dalton glycoprotein
Tissue distribution: Found on all nucleated cells, but especially on lymphocyte plasma membranes; constitutes 1 to 2 per cent of membrane protein of the lymphocyte
Polymorphism: Extremely high degree of genetic polymorphism
Biologic properties: Incompatibility of *H-2K* and/or *D* elicits rapid graft rejection, *strong* cytotoxic T cell reponse, *weak* mixed lymphocyte reaction, and production of IgG isoantibody

The MHC includes three major classes of genes and gene products that are also found in man (cf. Fig. 436–1). They will be discussed as a background for understanding the corresponding systems in man.

THE CLASS I GENE PRODUCTS ENCODED BY H-2K AND H-2D. ***Genetics and Biochemistry.*** The class I gene products are cell surface glycoproteins, molecular weight 45,000 daltons, that are present in the membranes of all nucleated cells as well as on red cells and platelets. These antigens were originally detected by isoimmunization to produce isoantisera. The presence or absence of H-2 incompatibility in a donor-recipient pair of mice is correlated with rapid versus subacute or chronic graft rejection. The structure of the class I histocompatibility antigens is determined by several genes, H-2K, H-2D, H-2L, and H-2R, and consists of a two-chain molecule in which each H-2K or H-2D polypeptide chain is tightly bound to a 12,000-dalton polypeptide known as β_2-microglobulin (Fig. 436–2). The β_2-microglobulin molecule is under the control of a structural gene on a separate chromosome. This two-chain structure, with a heavy and light chain, is reminiscent of the structure of immunoglobulins. In fact, β_2-microglobulin has a very marked amino acid sequence homology with a portion of the constant region of the IgG immunoglobulin heavy chain. In addition, H-2K and H-2D gene products also have partial amino acid sequence homology with some immunoglobulin molecules. This finding has led to speculation that immunoglobulins may have evolved from a primitive recognition system represented by the transplantation antigen system.

There is also marked amino acid sequence homology between the K and D gene products. This indicates that the two gene products probably arose by a process of tandem duplication from a single ancestral gene. The serologically different forms (alleles) of the K and D genes show multiple differences in amino acid sequence primarily in the first and second domains. As would be expected, the K and D gene products show remarkable amino acid sequence homology with their counterparts in the human MHC. The major characteristics of the H-2K and H-2D gene products are presented in Table 436–1.

The major histocompatibility antigens are unique among mammalian isoantigenic systems in their high degree of stable polymorphism. (Polymorphism is said to exist in a population when two or more different forms of the same gene and gene product are found in the population, both of which are present in more than 1 per cent of the individuals.) One of the most striking characteristics of the MHC is the enormous degree of genetic polymorphism for the class I genes. Each new population of wild mouse isolates from different geographic regions has shown at least one or two previously undetected H-2K or H-2D antigenic specificities. In man, a very high degree of polymorphism for the homologous loci is also seen.

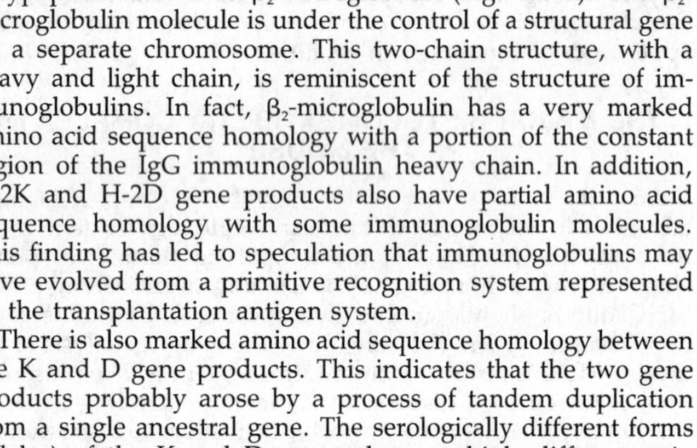

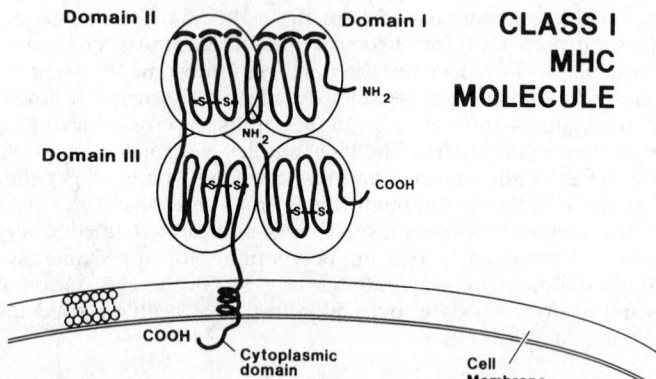

Figure 436–2. Schematic diagram of a class I major histocompatibility protein. The heavy chain (molecular weight 44,000) is organized into three globular protein domains labeled I, II, and III, a transmembrane domain, and a short cytoplasmic domain. Domains I, II, and III of the heavy chain and the β_2 microglobulin domain unite to form a protein composed of four globular domains arranged as indicated in the diagram with a two-fold axis of symmetry. This arrangement is derived from preliminary analysis of crystals of a human class I major histocompatibility protein determined in the laboratories of Don Wiley and Jack Strominger of Harvard University. Analysis of class I mutants in the mouse has suggested that most of the variation in amino acid sequence that results in an effect on immunologic recognition (see text) occurs in the first and second domains of the heavy chain of the class I histocompatibility protein. The sites of these variations are indicated by arcs, but their true position in space is unknown.

Function of the H-2K and H-2D Genes. The major biologic properties that can be attributed to the H-2K and D gene products are listed in Table 436–1. These gene products elicit a very strong cytotoxic T cell response, and a very weak or minimal mixed lymphocyte culture reaction. They are in some way involved in or influence the specificity of cytotoxic T cells for foreign antigenic molecules. The experimental findings are as follows. Following immunization with viruses, minor histocompatibility antigens, or haptens complexed to cell surface antigens, the cytotoxic T cells that subsequently develop are capable of killing target cells *only* when the target has on its surface both the foreign antigenic determinant (virus, minor histocompatibility antigen, or hapten) *and* molecules of the same H-2K or D gene products that were present on the immunizing cells originally injected. Two possible explanations for these findings have been considered: (1) cytotoxic T cells are differentiated to recognize only "altered self," and therefore recognize a foreign antigenic determinant on the cell surface only in combination with H-2K or D or both; or (2) the cytotoxic T cell carries two receptors, one of which is specific for self H-2K and D, and the other of which is specific for foreign antigens, the two receptors being in some way closely linked on the cytotoxic T cell surface.

The evidence presently available indicates that the T cell receptor is a single immunoglobulin-like molecule of 80,000 daltons, which is made up of two 40,000-dalton chains. This receptor "sees" a compound antigenic determinant created by the association of self H-2K or D with the foreign antigen on the cell surface.

THE CLASS II GENE PRODUCTS ENCODED BY THE H-2I REGION. ***Genetics and Biochemistry.*** The I region was initially identified because it was possible to show that genetic control of the immune response to a series of related synthetic polypeptide antigens was localized to a gene or genes mapping between the H-2K and S regions (Fig. 436–3). In closely related inbred strains of mice that were genetically identical for the other 19 chromosome pairs, and at most of the seventeenth chromosome with the exception of the I region itself, antisera were produced that reacted selectively with lymphocyte cell surface alloantigens. Because these cell surface antigens were associated with the I immune response region, they were given the name of I region associated, or Ia antigens. To date, Ia antigens are the only gene products that have been identified whose structure is determined by I region genes. The Ia antigens are a discrete set of cell surface glycoproteins. So far, two molecular weight classes have been identified—one a polypeptide of 33,000 to 34,000 daltons and the second a polypeptide of 28,000 to 29,000 daltons. These two chains form a heterodimer of 62,000 molecular weight (Fig. 436–4). The major characteristics of the Ia antigens are listed in Table 436–2. In the mouse there are only

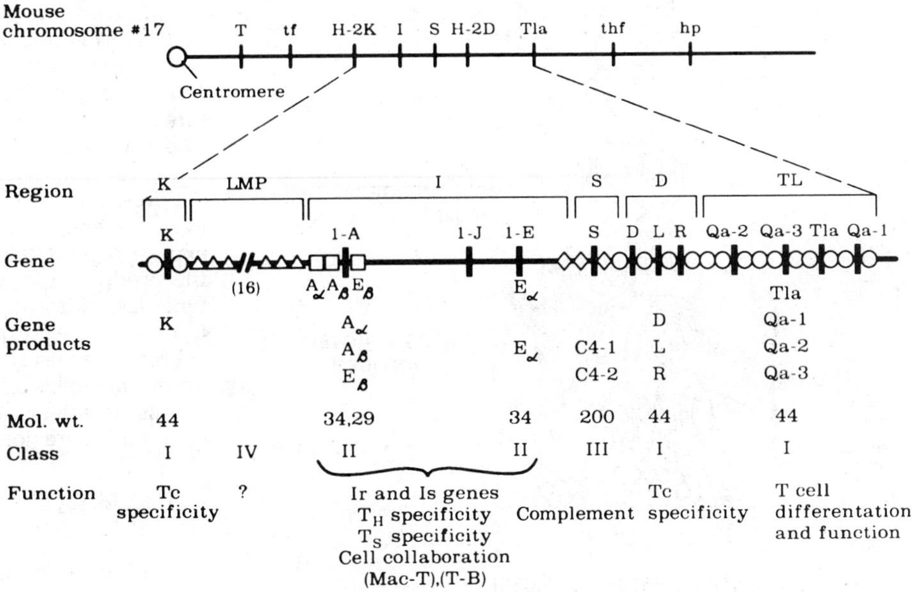

Figure 436–3. Schematic diagram of the genes of the murine major histocompatibility system. These genes are located on the seventeenth chromosome in the mouse, which is shown at the top of the diagram. The major histocompatibility system is shown in an expanded version in the second tier of the diagram in which it is broken up into subregions. Class I major histocompatibility genes are found in the K, D, and TL regions, while class II major histocompatibility genes (defined in the text) are found in the I region. Class III genes encoding several of the components of the complement system are found in the S region, and a set of 16 polypeptides is encoded by genes in the LMP region. The function of class I and class II genes is described in the text, and the function of class IV genes is unknown. ○ = class I genes; □ = class II genes; ◇ = class III genes; △ = class IV genes.

two class II molecules, I-A and I-E, encoded by four genes—A_α, A_β, E_α, and E_β.

The antigens eliciting the mixed lymphocyte culture reaction were also mapped to the I region. The mixed lymphocyte culture reaction is a proliferative response that occurs when lymphocytes from two unrelated individuals of the same species are cocultured together. T cell recognition of the allogeneic lymphocyte cell surface class II antigens results in rapid proliferation of a subpopulation of the T lymphocyte population from each donor.

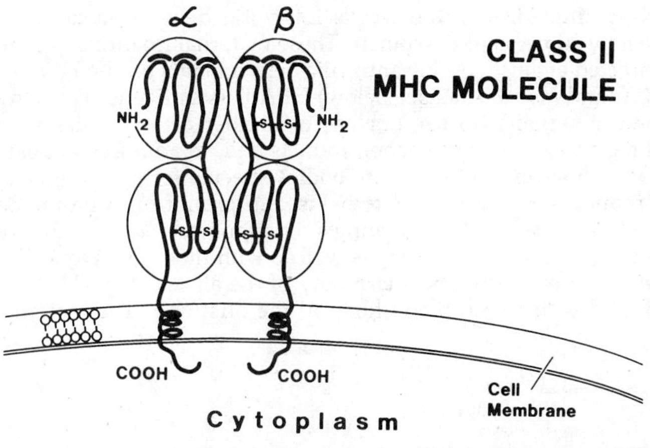

Figure 436–4. Schematic diagram of a class II major histocompatibility protein. This protein is composed of two polypeptide chains, an α chain of 34,000 molecular weight and a β chain of 29,000 molecular weight. As indicated in the diagram, three of these domains have intrachain disulfide loops with spacing reminiscent of immunoglobulin domains. Analysis of nucleotide sequence of complementary DNA clones of several different genetic forms (alleles) of the α chain by Mathis and Benoist in the author's laboratory, and of the β chains in John Seidman's laboratory at Harvard University, S. Tonegawa's laboratory at Massachusetts Institute of Technology, and the author's laboratory have shown that the major sequence differences between different alleles of the α and β chains occur in the first domain and that within the first domain, they occur in three "allelic hypervariable" regions that are positioned similarly to the hypervariable regions seen in immunoglobulin molecules. The position of these allelic hypervariable regions in space is as yet unknown but in the diagram is indicated as occurring at one end of the molecule (indicated by arcs) open to the aqueous environment in a manner similar to that seen in the three-dimensional folding of the antibody molecule.

The Functions of the I Region. The I-immune response region is defined primarily by the Ir genes—specific immune response genes that determine the ability of the individual's immune system to recognize an antigen as foreign and to mount an effective immune response, or to fail to recognize the antigen as foreign, in which case the animal is classified as a nonresponder to the antigen in question. More than 30 antigens have been shown to be under the control of Ir genes. Most of these antigens possess a restricted range of antigenic determinants available for recognition by the animal being immunized. For example, some of the antigens under Ir gene control are (1) simple synthetic polypeptides made up of two or three amino acids and therefore presenting a restricted range of antigenic determinants; (2) minor histocompatibility antigens, which presumably differ from the structure of the same antigen in the recipient by only a few amino acid residues; or (3) complex proteins for which Ir gene control operates only at a very low dose of antigen in which presumably one or a few antigenic determinants are "dominant." Although only 30 to 40 antigens have been shown to be under H-2 linked Ir gene control, it is likely that this control operates for most if not all foreign antigens.

I region genes appear to regulate immune reactivity by influencing the manner in which foreign antigens are seen by, or "presented to," T lymphocytes. One of the best examples of this comes from an analysis of the immune response of inbred guinea pigs to bovine insulin. Strain 2 guinea pigs respond primarily to antigenic determinants on the A chain of insulin, whereas strain 13 guinea pigs fail to recognize antigenic differences in the A chain of insulin but recognize antigenic differences in the insulin B chain. These two strains can then be crossed to produce an F_1 hybrid. When these hybrid animals

TABLE 436–2. MAJOR PROPERTIES OF THE CLASS II (I REGION) PRODUCTS (Ia ANTIGENS) OF THE MOUSE

Molecular weight: 34,000 and 29,000 dalton glycoprotein
Present in the cell membrane as a dimer between 34,000 and 29,000 dalton polypeptides
Tissue distribution: B lymphocytes, macrophages, some T cells, and epidermal cells
Polymorphism: High degree of polymorphism, not as great as *H-2K* and *D*
Biologic properties: Incompatibility at the *I* region elicits rapid rejection of bone marrow (lymphocyte), skin, and cardiac muscle grafts; *weak* cytotoxic T cell immune response; *strong* mixed lymphocyte culture reaction; and production of IgG isoantibody

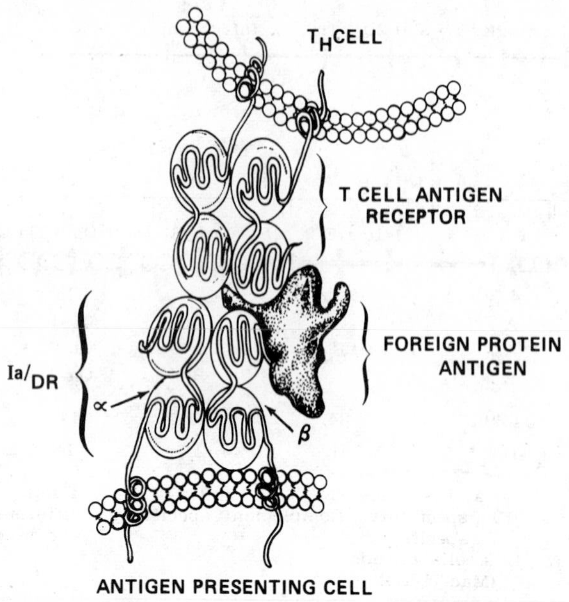

Figure 436–5. Schematic diagram of the interaction between the T helper lymphocyte (which is responsible for triggering proliferation and differentiation of B lymphocytes to produce antibody) and the foreign antigen on the surface of an antigen presenting adherent cell, or macrophage. The T lymphocyte is "restricted" in its ability to recognize a foreign antigen on the surface of the antigen presenting cell by the genotype of the class II histocompatibility protein on the antigen presenting cell. The T helper lymphocyte can recognize foreign antigen only if it is in association with a class II molecule of the same genotype as that present on the initial antigen presenting cell that induced the initial proliferation and differentiation of the T helper lymphocyte. This phenomenon of specificity of the T cell for both foreign antigen and class II histocompatibility antigen was initially described by Alan Rosenthal, Ethan Shevach, William Paul, and Ira Green at the National Institutes of Health.

are immunized to bovine insulin, their T lymphocytes will recognize antigenic differences in *either* the A chain or the B chain, when the insulin molecule is "presented" to the F_1 lymphocytes bound to the surface of F_1 macrophages. However, when the insulin molecule is presented to F_1 T lymphocytes on strain 2 macrophages, only A chain specific immune responses are elicited. When the insulin molecule is presented on strain 13 macrophages, only B chain antigenic differences are recognized. These findings are compatible with the possibility that class II determinants on the macrophages interact with foreign antigens. This interaction would influence the availability of particular foreign antigenic determinants for interaction with the helper T cell (T_H) receptor. This model postulates that Ia antigens engage in a wide variety of "specific" protein interactions with foreign antigens present on the macrophage cell surface. This interaction is similar to the interaction of class I molecules with foreign antigen that is the target of the cytotoxic T cell receptor. The only distinction is that helper T cells "see" foreign antigen in association with class II MHC molecules. This is diagrammed in Figure 436–5.

The I region determines the development of specific immune suppression as well as specific immune responsiveness. However, the effector cells mediating specific immune suppression express a genetically and functionally distinct Ia antigen that is the product of a gene mapping in a separate subregion (I-J). One class of Ia antigen determined by the I-J subregion appears to be selectively expressed on suppressor T cells.

I region genes also affect the efficiency of cell-cell interaction. Thus, the ability of T cells and macrophages, and T cells and B cells, to interact appears to require identity at the I region, or in one subregion (I-A or I-E) of the I region.

THE MAJOR HISTOCOMPATIBILITY COMPLEX IN HUMANS

The human MHC has been designated the *h*uman *l*eukocyte *a*ntigen or HLA system. The HLA system is found on the short arm of human chromosome 6 and spans a genetic distance of about 4.0 cM. A schematic diagram of the HLA system is presented in Figure 436–6.

HLA-A, B, AND C REGIONS. The HLA-A and B gene products of humans are homologous with the H-2K and D gene products of the mouse. The HLA-C gene product may be a tandem duplication of the HLA-B gene product. HLA-A, B, and C are the 44,000–dalton cell surface glycoproteins that are found on the surface of all nucleated cells in association with a 12,000–dalton β_2-microglobulin chain. Maternal isoantisera are routinely used to type for HLA-A, B, and C antigens. During the course of pregnancy, sufficient fetal lymphocytes leak into the maternal circulation to induce a significant titer of anti-HLA antibodies in the weeks following delivery in approximately 30 per cent of women. These maternal isoantibodies are directed against specific antigenic determinants on the HLA-A, B, C and (as we shall see below) HLA-D isoantigens. Thus any one maternal isoantiserum has a number of antibodies in it directed against these gene products and, in addition, appears to have several different antibodies specific for any one gene product, e.g., HLA-A. Maternal isoantiserum from a primipara will react with the offspring's lymphocytes, and with the lymphocytes of the father, as well as with those of anyone else in the population who shares any of the alleles of the HLA-A, B, and C loci with the father and the offspring. The maternal

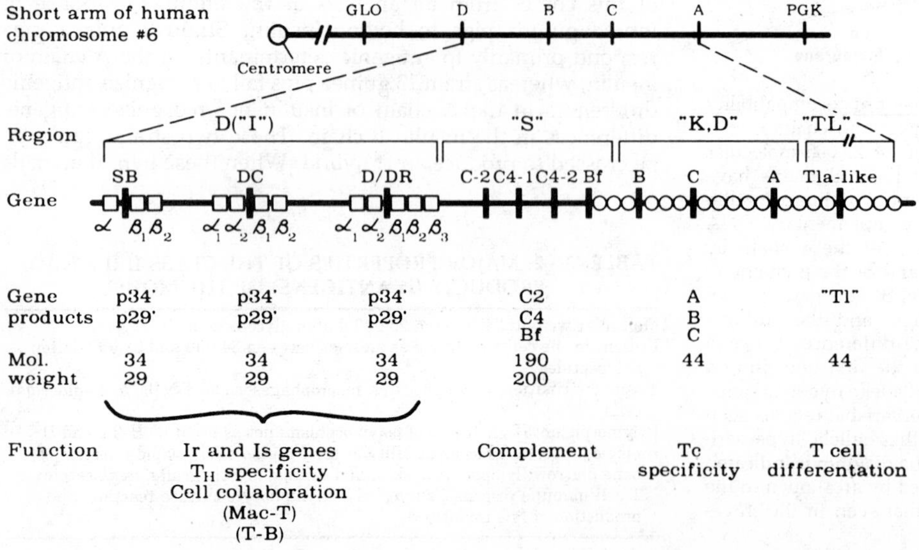

Figure 436–6. Schematic diagram of the human major histocompatibility complex on the sixth human chromosome. Aside from the difference in *position* and *number* of class II genes, the human and mouse systems are strikingly homologous. The symbols are the same as those given in Figure 436–3.

isoantiserum can thus be used to define the presence of these antigens in other members of the population.

By using a large number of different maternal sera, and a large panel of normal donor lymphocytes, combined with computer analysis of associations of reactions of paired sera with particular lymphocytes, many allelic antigenic specificities at the HLA-A, B, and C loci have been defined. There are approximately 20 different allelic antigenic specificities at the HLA-A locus, over 40 allelic antigenic specificities at the HLA-B locus, nearly 6 distinct antigenic specificities at the HLA-C locus. These allelic antigenic specificities have been assigned numbers; i.e., HLA-A1, A2, A3; HLA-B12, B16, B17, B27; and HLA-C1, C2, C3.

HLA-D REGION. The major difference in the genetic organization of the HLA system relative to the murine H-2 system is that the genes for determining the structure of the cell surface molecules eliciting the mixed lymphocyte culture reaction (MLR) map at a position *outside* of the region bounded by the two genes determining the class I histocompatibility antigens (HLA-A, B). The genetic region determining the structure of the antigens eliciting the MLR in the HLA system has been termed HLA-D. The HLA-D gene products in man were initially typed by using the mixed lymphocyte culture reaction. (By x-irradiating the lymphocytes of one of the two donors to a mixed lymphocyte culture reaction, it is possible to eliminate the responsiveness of that lymphocyte population. The mixed lymphocyte culture in this situation is termed a one-way mixed lymphocyte culture reaction, and measures only the ability of the responder lymphocytes to recognize alloantigens on the surface of the irradiated stimulator cells.) If stimulator cells are used that are homozygous at the HLA-D locus, then nonresponsiveness in the MLR in this situation is said to give a "typing reaction," and the responder lymphocyte population can be identified as possessing that particular HLA-D allele. Such homozygous typing cells (HTCs) were originally identified in the population, and at the Sixth and Seventh International Histocompatibility Testing Workshops were given provisional "workshop" or "w" designations as HLA-Dw1, Dw2, Dw3, and so forth. A total of ten HLA-D locus types or alleles have been identified by this method. Utilizing these homozygous typing cells, it is possible to identify somewhat more than 50 per cent, but less than 75 per cent, of the HLA-D genes (two genes for each individual) present in a normal population.

Differences at the HLA-D locus also elicit the production of isoantibodies in maternal sera, antibodies that are specific for B cell alloantigens whose structure is determined by HLA-D–linked genes. These sera show a distinct correlation with HLA-D locus types as determined by homozygous typing cells in the mixed lymphocyte culture reaction. These B cell alloantigens identified by maternal isoantisera have been provisionally identified as HLA-DR (for D-related) antigens. Since the HLA-D locus is analogous to the I region locus in terms of function in eliciting the mixed lymphocyte culture reaction, it is not surprising that HLA-D gene products are analogous to the I region polypeptides in the mouse. Indeed, HLA-D gene products are composed of two classes of polypeptide chains of 34,000 and 29,000 daltons displayed on macrophages, B cells, some T cells, and endothelial cells. The amino acid sequence of the human p34 polypeptide is homologous with the 34,000-dalton polypeptide of the I-E/C segment (E_α) of the I region of the mouse.

Murine Ia and human HLA-DR determinants are similar with regard to their ability to stimulate in a mixed lymphocyte reaction and in their tissue localization and structure. These genes also appear to function as immune response genes in man.

Despite these biochemical, structural, and functional similarities, there are marked differences in the genetic organization of the HLA-D genetic region when compared to the murine H-2I region. There are many more Class II MHC genes and gene products in man than in the mouse. There are three separate *types* of class II molecules in man, designated DR, DC, and SB (compared to two types, I-A and I-E, in the mouse). For each type there are multiple genes. In terms of genes expressed by gene products at the cell surface (in contrast to pseudogenes) there are: 1DR_α, 3DR_β, 2DC_α, 2DC_β, 2SB_α, and 2SB_β chains. This is a striking contrast with the mouse, and presumably results in much greater complexity in regulation of the immune response by class II molecules in man.

Population Genetics and Disease Associations

Specific combinations of particular alleles at the HLA-A, B, C, and D loci tend to occur together on the same chromosome in a particular combination more often than would be expected by chance. This phenomenon, known as *linkage disequilibrium,* is the opposite of linkage equilibrium. Equilibrium can be said to exist when any given allele of one gene is found on the same chromosome in combination with any specified allele of a second linked gene in a frequency determined by the product of the gene frequencies of the two specified alleles at the two loci. This linkage equilibrium develops because genetic crossing over will occur between the two loci and scramble any particular combination of specified alleles at the two loci. For a newly introduced (mutant) allele of one of the two genes, genetic equilibrium will develop more rapidly for genes that are farther apart. Even for closely linked genes, genetic equilibrium will ultimately develop, given sufficient numbers of generations and a random choice of breeding partners.

The HLA system constitutes one of the most remarkable examples of linkage disequilibrium in the human genome. There are several chromosomal combinations or haplotypes (a set of particular alleles of linked genes on one chromosome, the haploid number, is designated as a haplotype) that occur in a particular population at a frequency much higher than would be predicted by chance. Thus, in Caucasian populations, the A1,B8,Dw3 combination occurs much more frequently than would be predicted by the product of the gene frequencies of these three alleles in the population. The same is true for the A3,B7,Dw2 haplotype and for several other haplotypes. These alleles are thus said to be in linkage disequilibrium.

Linkage disequilibrium may reflect a selective survival advantage of a particular combination of alleles at linked loci. In most systems the precise mechanism of selective survival advantage is unclear. The same is true for the HLA system. There is clear evidence that HLA-A and B can influence cytotoxic T cell specificity, and presumptive evidence indicates that genes in the HLA-D region can dictate immune reactivity to a given antigenic determinant. This suggests at least one mechanism of selective advantage. Particular combinations of HLA-A, B, and D alleles might confer a very strong selective survival advantage in a population exposed to a particular selective force, such as a viral or bacterial infection. This would presumably vary with climate and environment, and similar variation in the occurrence of linkage disequilibrium has also been observed. Thus, the HLA-A3,B7,Dw2 haplotype is much more prevalent in Scandinavian countries and in temperate European areas than in Caucasian populations of European origin in Mediterranean countries and countries closer to the equator.

It must be kept in mind that an alternative mechanism may be operative in some cases, and has been documented in the mouse. This mechanism is suppression of crossing over due to an inversion in gene order on the chromosome exhibiting linkage disequilibrium.

Associations of the HLA Systems with Disease Susceptibility

Figure 436–7 indicates some of the more than 40 diseases for which it has been shown that susceptibility is associated with a particular HLA-A, B, or D locus type. Only a few diseases show primary association with an HLA-A or B type. Susceptibility to idiopathic hemochromatosis is associated with HLA-A3 in some populations, but is due to a linked gene influencing iron metabolism. Susceptibility to a wide variety of rheumatic

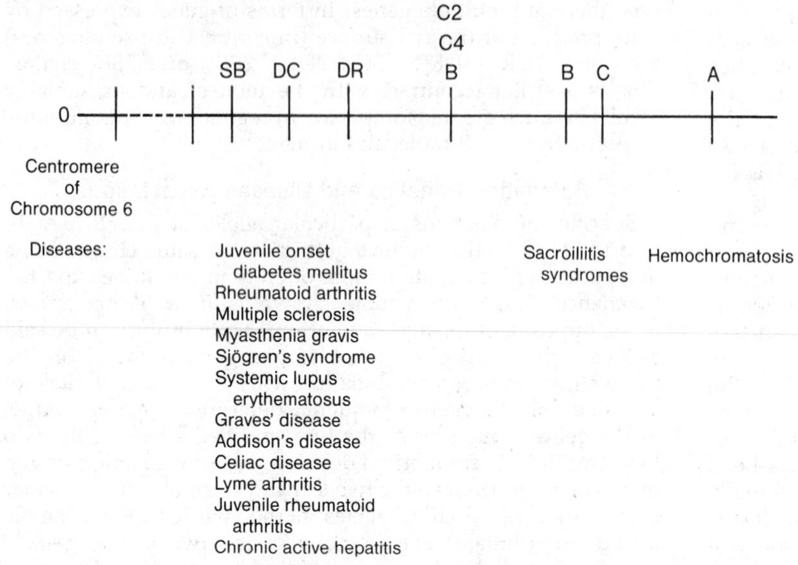

Figure 436–7. The HLA system and HLA-associated diseases.

diseases in which sacroiliitis and spondylitis are prominent features is associated with HLA-B27—one of the strongest associations between HLA and disease susceptibility. HLA-B27 occurs in approximately 5 per cent of the normal Caucasian population and in more than 90 per cent of patients with ankylosing spondylitis, more than 75 per cent of patients with Reiter's disease, and a majority of patients with psoriatic arthritis and inflammatory bowel disease in whom sacroiliitis occurs as a complication of their illness.

By far the largest category of HLA-associated diseases consists of those in which the primary association is with a particular HLA-DR or Dw type. Many of these diseases were originally reported to be associated with a particular HLA-B locus type, but subsequent studies have revealed that this is due to preferential combination of particular alleles of HLA-A, B, and D occurring together on the same chromosome more often than would be expected by chance owing to linkage disequilibrium.

The list of HLA-D locus–associated diseases is extensive and ranges from examples such as celiac disease, in which almost 100 per cent of the patients are HLA-Dw3, to thyrotoxicosis, in which slightly more than half of the patients are HLA-Dw3 (Dw3 occurring in the normal population in approximately 20 per cent of individuals).

In Caucasians the HLA-A1,B3,Dw3 haplotype is associated with a number of autoimmune diseases, including myasthenia gravis, thyrotoxicosis, Addison's disease, juvenile–onset diabetes mellitus, Sjögren's syndrome, and chronic active hepatitis. The A3,B7,Dw2 haplotype is associated with susceptibility to multiple sclerosis. A particularly intriguing example of this type is the frequent occurrence of the HLA-A10,B18,Dw2 haplotype with a deficiency in the structural gene for the second component of complement. Most of the cases of absolute deficiency of the second component of complement (a recessive defect) carry at least one dose of this haplotype. In addition, the A10,B18,Dw2 C2 deficiency haplotype in the heterozygote appears to be associated with a markedly increased incidence of autoimmune syndromes resembling systemic lupus erythematosus. This is one of several examples in which the C4,C2, properdin factor B genes of the HLA system may be playing a role in disease susceptibility.

The mechanism of the association of HLA-D type with susceptibility to this wide variety of diseases is unknown. However, four generalizations can be made from the available data: (1) Most of these diseases have a definite or suspected autoimmune pathogenesis. Examples of diseases in which an autoimmune pathogenesis is clearly established include myasthenia gravis, thyrotoxicosis, and systemic lupus erythematosus. Diseases in which an autoimmune pathogenesis is suspected but not yet clearly established include rheumatoid arthritis, multiple sclerosis, and juvenile–onset diabetes mellitus, as well as chronic active hepatitis, celiac disease, Sjögren's syndrome, and nontuberculous Addison's disease. (2) Susceptibility is a dominant trait, as is Ir gene–controlled immune responsiveness. (3) Only a minority of those carrying a susceptibility allele ever develop the disease, suggesting that environmental factors also play a role. (4) Not all individuals with a particular disease possess the allele associated with susceptibility, suggesting that other genes may influence disease occurrence, as has been shown for MHC-determined thyroiditis in chickens and myasthenia gravis in humans.

These four generalizations have a very major bearing on our attempts to understand the mechanism underlying the association between the HLA system and susceptibility to disease. Since the pathogenesis of these diseases is for the most part a mystery, any attempt to explain the mechanism of association with HLA must be, in part, speculative. Thus, the association of ankylosing spondylitis and Reiter's disease with HLA-B27 might be due to a direct effect of the B27 allele on the development of cytotoxic T cell responsiveness to an exogenous antigen that triggers an immune response to a cross-reacting self antigen. Alternatively, the association could reflect the effect of a gene closely linked to HLA-B27 and in very strong linkage disequilibrium with it. Definitive family studies to settle this point have not yet been carried out.

Similarly the association of a wide variety of autoimmune diseases, including rheumatoid arthritis, with the HLA-D locus raises the speculation that a hypernormal or hyponormal immune response to an exogenous antigen or to a self antigen might underlie the association. For example, the association of Graves' disease and myasthenia gravis with HLA-Dw3 might be due to a hypernormal immune response to an environmental agent that cross-reacts with either the thyrotropin receptor or the acetylcholine receptor, or alternatively might be due to a deficit in suppressor T cells that normally suppress what might otherwise be a damaging autoimmune response to the thyrotropin receptor or the acetylcholine receptor. Some of these possibilities are susceptible to experimental tests, but evidence is as yet lacking.

The existence of linkage disequilibrium in the HLA system, which has been referred to above, raises the possibility that none of the measured genes are responsible for the observed associations. The associations might in fact be due to other linked genes that are in linkage disequilibrium with the measured genes, including the DC and SB class II molecules. Our methods of genotyping for these molecules are at present imperfect. For example, the association of Graves' disease and juvenile-onset diabetes mellitus (as well as a number of other autoimmune diseases in Caucasians) with HLA-Dw3 might be due to a strong linkage disequilibrium between HLA-Dw3 and other genes predisposing to these diseases. In this situation none of the HLA-A, B, C, or D genes would be the true disease susceptibility genes.

It is clear that the HLA-D region is subdivided into several loci (at least 5_α and 7_β chain genes). Some of these loci might be of major importance in determining disease susceptibility. Typing methods specific for these additional D region subloci may reveal very strong disease associations, whereas current typing methods reveal only partial or weak association with DR type.

The possibility of gene complementation in disease susceptibility must also be taken into account. The relative risk of juvenile-onset diabetes in individuals who are HLA-DR3/DR3 or HLA-DR4/DR4 is very much less than that of individuals who are HLA-DR3/DR4. This is the first example suggesting gene complementation for susceptibility to a disease, and appears to be analogous to complementing Ir genes and Ia molecules described in the mouse. As our knowledge of the HLA-D region advances, our understanding and identification of the susceptible genotypes and of the mechanisms at work may well advance in parallel. Studies utilizing cDNA probes for the various class II α and β chain genes reveal a striking degree of genomic DNA restriction endonuclease fragment length polymorphism. Analysis of these polymorphisms, as well as DNA sequence analysis of class II α and β chain genes, will almost certainly refine and subdivide current HLA-DR haplotypes, and can be expected to refine and sharpen association of particular DR, DC, and SB genotypes with particular diseases. Application of these findings will undoubtedly have major impact on diagnostic approaches, prognosis, and ultimately on therapy.

Hood L, Steinmetz M, Malissen B: Genes of the major histocompatibility complex. Ann Rev Immunol 1:529, 1983.

Kaufman JA, Auffray C, Korman AJ, Shackleford DA, Strominger J: The class II molecules of the human and murine major histocompatibility complex. Cell 36:1, 1984.

Klein J: The Major Histocompatibility Complex. Chapter 8. *In* Immunology: The Science Of Self-Non Self Discrimination. New York, John Wiley & Sons, 1982.

Ryder LP, Svejgaard A, Dausset J: Genetics of HLA disease association. Annu Rev Genet 15:169, 1981.

437. DRUG ALLERGY

Charles E. Reed

An allergic cause of a drug reaction is suspected when an inflammatory lesion characteristic of those provoked by immunologic mechanisms follows administration of the drug. The variety of drug allergies gives the initial impression that any drug can cause any reaction; in fact, distinct patterns are the rule. Any particular drug tends to cause a similar reaction in different subjects. Typical examples include urticaria after penicillin G injection, lymphocytic pneumonitis after nitrofurantoin, or contact dermatitis from an ointment containing ethylenediamine. Allergic drug reactions need to be distinguished from expected side effects, idiosyncratic reactions of unknown cause, toxic reactions, psychophysiologic reactions, and also from immunologic manifestations of the underlying disease. A further distinction is made between allergic inflammation initiated by a ligand reacting with an antibody or a specifically reacting lymphocyte and similar inflammation initiated by some other chemical reaction. Unfortunately these distinctions are not always easy at the bedside, and there are few reliable clinical or laboratory tests.

Many patients relate a history of allergy to one or more drugs, often without an objective basis. Usually this history can be accepted and serves as a deterrent to excessive drug therapy. Sometimes, however, it is important to evaluate the possibility of allergy to a potentially lifesaving drug for which

there is no substitute, since many patients with a history of a reaction will tolerate the drug, particularly if several years have passed. If the allergy is still present, taking the drug can be disastrous with fatality from anaphylaxis, Steven-Johnson's syndrome, exfoliative dermatitis, interstitial pneumonitis, or vasculitis. A decision for a particular course of action often rests on judicious weighing of the potential benefits and risks rather than on a definitive diagnosis.

INCIDENCE AND PREDISPOSING FACTORS. Allergic reactions constituted only about 6 per cent of all adverse drug reactions in a 1968 study. The frequency is thought to be less today, except for reactions to radiographic contrast agents, which now account for about 60 per cent of drug-induced anaphylaxis and about 20 per cent of all cases of anaphylaxis. Radiographic contrast dyes do not cause anaphylaxis as a result of specific antibodies (see below). In one large study of drug reactions, which may have underestimated reactions in organs other than skin, the following distribution was found: erythematous and maculopapular rashes, 46 per cent; urticaria, 23 per cent; fixed eruptions, 10 per cent; erythema multiforme, 5 per cent; exfoliative dermatitis, 4 per cent; purpura, 2 per cent; anaphylaxis, 1 per cent; and vasculitis, 0.5 per cent.

Several predisposing factors exist. Previous drug allergy to the same or a related drug is most important, and the frequency of allergy is increased by multiple courses of treatment. Topical administration is the route most likely to sensitize, oral administration least, and parenteral intermediate. Parenteral administration provokes more severe reactions, especially anaphylaxis. Children are less likely than adults to react, and men less than women. Persons with history of atopic allergy may be at increased risk of anaphylaxis or urticaria but not of other kinds of allergic drug reactions. Indeed, subjects with atopic dermatitis are less easily sensitized than normal persons to antigens that cause contact dermatitis. The antigenic determinant in drug allergy is usually a metabolite rather than the drug itself; genetic differences in drug metabolism therefore influence allergic reactions. For example, persons with reduced acetyltransferase activity are more likely to develop drug-induced systemic lupus erythematosus from hydralazine.

MECHANISMS. Foreign macromolecules acting as complete antigens are the most likely to sensitize, eliciting an IgE or IgG antibody response that on a subsequent administration causes anaphylaxis, serum sickness, or vasculitis. Classic serum sickness that occurs after injections of large amounts of rabbit or horse serum requires large amounts of antigen and relatively high concentrations of circulating immune complexes. Most episodes of urticaria, fever, and arthralgia after the relatively small doses of macromolecules in current use probably involve a combination of IgE- and IgG-initiated events.

Low molecular weight drugs and diagnostic agents elicit an immune response only after reacting covalently with proteins. The hapten may be the drug itself, but is more often a drug metabolite. The hapten-protein carrier then functions as the complete antigen, both initiating sensitization and eliciting the reaction. An allergic reaction requires a multivalent ligand to cross-link antibody molecules either in fluid phase or bound to cell surface receptors. Univalent haptens actually inhibit cross-linking by occupying the antigen-binding sites. Some chemicals may react with host proteins in such a way that their tertiary structure is altered and the new antigenic determinant is not the hapten itself but the altered structure of the host protein. The allergic reaction may take any of the forms of allergic reaction described in Part XXI. The mechanisms of immune defense and hypersensitivity, like many other biologic functions, exhibit redundancy such that a drug reaction may involve more than one allergic mechanism at the same time. The fact that the hapten so often is a drug metabolite may explain the characteristic involvement of some particular organ where the metabolism occurs; alternatively, the hapten may react with a specific organ protein to account for the location of the reaction.

TABLE 437–1. ALLERGIC DRUG REACTIONS

- I. Systemic
  - A. Anaphylaxis
    - 1. Macromolecules
      - Allergenic extracts
      - Dextrans (including iron dextran)
      - Enzymes
        - Asparaginase
        - Chymopapain
        - Chymotrypsin
        - Trypsin
      - Heparin
      - Hormones (ACTH, insulin, etc.)
      - Human gamma globulin
      - Organ extracts
      - Protamine
      - Vaccines
      - Xenogenic sera
    - 2. Diagnostic agents
      - Fluorescein
      - Iodinated contrast media
    - 3. Antimicrobials
      - Aminosalicylic acid
      - Amphotericin B
      - Cephalosporins
      - Clindamycin
      - Ethambutol
      - Kanamycin
      - Lincomycin
      - Penicillins
      - Streptomycin
      - Sulfonamides
      - Tetracyclines
      - Vancomycin
    - 4. Other drugs
      - Aspirin
      - Bleomycin
      - Cisplatin
      - Colchicine
      - Cromolyn
      - Cytarabine
      - Dantrolene
      - Ethylenediamine
      - Indomethacin
      - Local anesthetics
      - Mephyton
      - Meprobamate
      - Organic mercurials
      - Niacin
      - Opiates
      - Pentamidine and stilbamidine
      - Probenecid
      - Sulfite
      - Tolmetin
      - Triamterene
      - Tubocurarine and other muscle-relaxing agents
      - Vitamin B_{12}
  - B. Serum Sickness
    - 1. Macromolecules
      - Dextrans
      - Heparin
      - Hormones (insulin, ACTH)
      - Vaccines
      - Xenogenic sera
    - 2. Antimicrobials
      - Cephalosporins
      - Griseofulvin
      - Lincomycin
      - Penicillins
      - Streptomycin
      - Sulfonamides
    - 3. Other Drugs
      - Barbiturates
      - Cholecystographic dyes
      - Hydantoins
      - Hydralazine
      - Mercurial diuretics
      - Phenylbutazone
      - Procarbazine
      - Thiouracils
- I. Systemic (*Continued*)
  - C. Drug Fever
    - 1. Antimicrobials
      - Aminosalicylic acid
      - Cephalosporins
      - Chloramphenicol
      - Erythromycin
      - Isoniazid-kanamycin
      - Nitrofurantoin
      - Penicillins
      - Pyrazinamide
      - Quinine
      - Streptomycin
      - Sulfonamides
      - Tetracyclines
    - 2. Other drugs
      - Allopurinol
      - Heparin
      - Hydantoins
      - Hydralazine
      - Iodides
      - Mercurial diuretics
      - Methyldopa
      - Penicillamine
      - Phenobarbital
      - Pneumococcal vaccine
      - Procainamide
      - Propylthiouracil
      - Quinidine
  - D. Vasculitis
    - Allopurinol
    - Busulfan
    - Colchicine
    - Diphenhydramine
    - Ethionamide
    - Furosemide
    - Hydantoins
    - Indomethacin
    - Iodides
    - Isoniazid
    - Meprobamate
    - Methamphetamine
    - Penicillins
    - Phenothiazines
    - Phenylbutazone
    - Propranolol
    - Propylthiouracil
    - Sulfonamides
    - Tetracyclines
    - Thiazide diuretics
    - Vaccines
  - E. Systemic lupus erythematosus syndrome
    - Chloroquine
    - Griseofulvin
    - Hydralazine
    - Isoniazid
    - Methyldopa
    - Oral contraceptives
    - Phenytoin
    - Procainamide
    - Tetracycline
    - Thiouracil
- II. Skin
  - A. Urticaria and angioedema
    - 1. Antimicrobials
      - Aminoglycosides
      - Cephalosporins
      - Isoniazid
      - Metronidazole
      - Miconazole
      - Nalidixic acid
      - Penicillin
      - Quinine
      - Rifampin
      - Spectinomycin
      - Sulfonamides
      - Suramin
    - 2. Other drugs
      - Aspirin and other nonsteroidal anti-inflammatory drugs
      - Calcitonin
      - Chloral hydrate
- II. Skin (*Continued*)
      - Cyclophosphamide
      - Doxorubicin
      - Ergotamine
      - Ethchlorvynol
      - Ethosuximide
      - Ethylenediamine
      - Methaqualone
      - Penicillamine
      - Phenothiazines
      - Procainamide
      - Quinidine
      - Tragacanth
  - B. Morbilliform-maculopapular rash
    - 1. Antimicrobials
      - Aminosalicylic acid
      - Ampicillin
      - Erythromycin
      - Gentamicin
      - Penicillin
      - Sulfonamides
    - 2. Other drugs
      - Allopurinol
      - Barbiturates
      - Gold salts
      - Hydantoins
  - C. Erythroderma and exfoliative dermatitis
    - Allopurinol
    - Carbamazepine
    - Chloral hydrate
    - Chlorpromazine
    - Ethylenediamine
    - Glutethimide
    - Gold salts
    - Hydantoins
    - Iodides
    - Penicillin
    - Phenobarbital
    - Sulfonamides
    - Trimethadione
  - D. Erythema multiforme
    - Acetaminophen-phenacetin
    - Ampicillin
    - Barbiturates
    - Chloroquine
    - Chlorpropamide
    - Clindamycin
    - Ethosuximide
    - Gold salts
    - Hydantoins
    - Hydralazine
    - Penicillins
    - Phenolphthalein
    - Phenylbutazone
    - Rifampin
    - Streptomycin
    - Sulfapyridine
    - Sulfonamides
    - Sulfonylureas
    - Trimethoprim-sulfamethoxazole
    - Vaccines
  - E. Photosensitive
    - 1. Topical
      - Fluorouracil
      - Halogenated salicylanilides
      - Hexachlorophene
      - Para-aminobenzoic acid esters
      - Promethazine
      - Sulfanilamide
    - 2. Systemic
      - Carbamazepine
      - Chlorpromazine
      - Griseofulvin
      - Imipramine
      - Lincomycin
      - Nalidixic acid
      - Phenothiazines
      - Quinethazone
- II. Skin (*Continued*)
      - Sulfonamides
      - Sulfonylureas
      - Thiazide diuretics
  - F. Fixed drug eruptions
    - Aspirin
    - Barbiturates
    - Gold salts
    - Iodides
    - Meprobamate
    - Penicillins
    - Phenacetin
    - Phenolphthalein
    - Phenylbutazone
    - Quinine
    - Sulfonamides
    - Tetracyclines
  - G. Erythema Nodosum
    - Bromides
    - Iodides
    - Oral contraceptives
    - Penicillin
    - Sulfonamides
  - H. Contact dermatitis
    - Ammoniated mercury
    - Ampicillin
    - Antihistamines
    - Bacitracin
    - Benzalkonium chloride
    - Benzocaine
    - Chlorpromazine
    - Ethylenediamine
    - Fluorouracil
    - Formaldehyde
    - Glucocorticoids
    - Glutaraldehyde
    - Hexachlorophene
    - Idoxuridine
    - Iodochlorhydroxyquin
    - Lanolin
    - Local anesthetics
    - Neomycin
    - Opiates
    - Para-aminobenzoic acid
    - Parabens
    - Penicillin
    - Phenothiazines
    - Propylene glycol
    - Streptomycin
    - Sulfonamides
    - Thimerosal
- III. Lung
  - A. Asthma
    - Aspirin and other nonsteroidal anti-inflammatory drugs
    - Cromolyn
    - Pituitary snuff
    - Sodium glutamate
    - Sulfite
    - Occupational exposures to:
      - Cephalosporins
      - Glutaraldehyde
      - Pancreatic enzymes
      - Papain
      - Penicillin
      - Phenylmercurials
      - Psyllium
      - Spiromycin
  - B. Eosinophilic pneumonitis
    - Aminosalicylic acid
    - Azathioprine
    - Carbamazepine
    - Chlorpropamide
    - Cromolyn
    - Gold salts
    - Mephenesin
    - Nitrofurantoin
    - Penicillin
    - Sulfonamides
  - C. Fibrotic and pleural reactions
    - Bleomycin
    - Busulfan

(*Table continues on facing page*)

TABLE 437–1. ALLERGIC DRUG REACTIONS (*Continued*)

III. Lung (*Continued*)
- Cyclophosphamide
- Ganglionic-blocking drugs
- Gold salts
- Hydrochlorothiazide
- Melphalan
- Methotrexate
- Methysergide
- Mitomycin
- Nitrofurantoin
- Procarbazine

IV. Liver
- A. Cholestatic
  - Chlorzoxazone
  - Erythromycin estiolate
  - Ethchlorvynol
  - Imipramine
  - Nalidixic acid
  - Nitrofurantoin
  - Phenothiazines
  - Sulfamethoxazole
  - Sulfonylureas
  - Troleandomycin
- B. Hepatocellular
  - Aminosalicylic acid
  - Amphotericin B
  - Ethacrynic acid
  - Furosemide
  - Gold salts
  - Griseofulvin
  - Halothane
  - Hydantoins
  - Isoniazid
  - Methyldopa
  - Monoamine oxidase inhibitors

IV. Liver (*Continued*)
  - Nitrofurantoin
  - Oxyphenisatin
  - Propylbutazone
  - Propylthiouracil
  - Pyrazinamide
  - Quinidine
  - Rifampin
  - Sulfonamides
  - Trimethadione
- C. Chronic Active Hepatitis
  - Methyldopa
  - Nitrofurantoin
  - Oxyphenisatin

V. Kidney
- A. Glomerulonephritis. See *Vasculitis*
- B. Interstitial nephritis
  - Cephalosporins
  - Diuretics
  - Furosemide
  - Nonsteroidal anti-inflammatory drugs
  - Penicillins, especially methicillin
  - Phenytoin
  - Rifampin
  - Sulfonamides
  - Thiazide

VI. Bone Marrow and Blood Cells
- A. Bone Marrow Aplasia
  - Chloramphenicol
  - Gold salts
  - Mephenytoin
  - Penicillamine
  - Phenylbutazone
  - Trimethadione

VI. Bone Marrow and Blood Cells (*Continued*)
- B. Anemia
  - Cephalosporins
  - Cisplatin
  - Penicillin
  - Acetaminophen
  - Aminosalicylic acid
  - Chlorpromazine
  - Insulin
  - Isoniazid
  - Melphalan
  - Phenacetin
  - Quinidine
  - Quinine
  - Rifampin
  - Stibophen
  - Sulfonamides
  - Sulfonylureas
  - Chlorpromazine
  - Hydantoins
  - Ibuprofen
  - Levodopa
  - Mefenamic acid
  - Methyldopa
  - Methysergide
- C. Thrombocytopenia
  - Acetaminophen
  - Acetazolamide
  - Acetylsalicylic acid
  - Aminosalicylic acid
  - Carbamazepine
  - Cephalothin
  - Chloramphenicol
  - Chlorpheniramine
  - Digitoxin
  - Ethchlorvynol
  - Gold salts

VI. Bone Marrow and Blood Cells (*Continued*)
  - Heparin
  - Hydantoins
  - Isoniazid
  - Levodopa
  - Meprobamate
  - Methyldopa
  - Penicillamine
  - Phenacetin
  - Phenylbutazone
  - Procainamide
  - Quinidine
  - Quinine
  - Rauwolfia alkaloids
  - Rifampin
  - Stibophen
  - Sulfonamides
  - Sulfonylureas
  - Thiazide diuretics
- D. Granulocytopenia
  - Chloral hydrate
  - Chlorpropamide
  - Dipyrone
  - Mercurial diuretics
  - Methimazole
  - Penicillins (Semisynthetic)
  - Phenothiazines
  - Phenylbutazone
  - Phenytoin
  - Procainamide
  - Propranolol
  - Sulfamethoxypyridazine
  - Sulfapyridine
  - Tolbutamide
- E. Lymphoid hyperplasia
  - Phenytoin
  - Mephenytoin

PREVENTION. The likelihood of serious drug allergy can be reduced by avoiding drugs with high sensitivity potential whenever possible. For this reason only a few macromolecules capable of acting as complete antigens remain in current use. Passive immunization with horse serum has been replaced with human serum except for anti-snake venoms. Egg-containing vaccines have either been replaced by tissue culture vaccines or are highly purified to remove most of the contaminating proteins. Reactions to highly purified vaccines like tetanus and diphtheria toxoids do occur occasionally, however. ACTH has been largely supplanted by glucocorticoids, and human insulin is available for the occasional patient who becomes allergic to beef or pork insulin. A few enzymes are still used, particularly asparaginase and chymopapain. Occasional reactions follow use of heparin and protamine. Dextran is avoided whenever possible because of its potential for causing anaphylaxis. Allergenic extracts are a special class of diagnostic and therapeutic materials carefully prepared to elicit allergy, and an excessive dose naturally can cause serious anaphylactic reactions.

The likelihood of serious drug allergy can be reduced by taking a careful history of drug allergy, by a high index of suspicion when fever, rash, or organ damage occurs during treatment, by careful recording of manifestation of drug reactions and diagnosis in the chart when they do occur and by proper instruction of the patient.

DIAGNOSIS. The history and physical examination provide the essential information for pattern recognition. A key point of the history is the time course of the reaction as well as the identity of the drug. Anaphylactic reactions follow within minutes, drug fever within an hour or two, contact dermatitis in a day or two, but cholestatic jaundice requires several days or a week. The character of the lesion is also important. Ampicillin characteristically causes a morbilliform rash that may be delayed for two days after the drug is stopped. All penicillins may cause urticaria within ten minutes, but the urticaria may not occur for several days. This distinction is important because the immediate reactions are more likely to be associated with anaphylaxis. A physician observing a drug reaction should record the physical findings for future use. For example, by history alone it is difficult to distinguish between laryngeal edema from anaphylaxis and the hyperventilation syndrome, but the presence of stridor and swelling of pharyngeal or laryngeal mucosa makes the distinction clear. Distinction between a drug reaction and an immunologic event from the underlying disease is important. For instance, many children with viral respiratory infections have transient urticaria that can be mistaken for a penicillin rash. Or, on the first or second day of penicillin treatment a patient with endocarditis may have a macular hemorrhagic rash and fever, reflecting a reaction to antigens released by antibiotic lysis of the bacteria rather than drug allergy.

Some of the most important patterns of drug reactions are summarized in Table 437–1.

Skin tests may be helpful in predicting anaphylaxis from macromolecules and are usually positive in patients with allergy to foreign sera, insulin, vaccines, and similar complex materials. With the important exception of penicillin, skin or in vitro allergy tests with low molecular weight drugs are not reliable for detecting anaphylactic (IgE-mediated) drug allergy, although positive skin tests have occasionally been reported after anaphylaxis from local anesthetics, cisplatin, and a few other drugs. Patch tests with single components are useful for identifying contact allergens. Ethylenediamine, one of the ingredients of many creams and ointments, is currently the most frequently encountered contactant. Attempts to adapt lymphocyte transformation tests for diagnosis of drug allergy have been unsuccessful. Deliberate trial of small doses of the drug strictly for diagnostic purposes is unwise and unnecessary, though it may be indicated as a precaution in situations in which the diagnosis of drug allergy is uncertain and no chemically unrelated substitute is available for an urgently needed drug.

MANAGEMENT. In addition to stopping use of the offending drug, the reaction itself may need symptomatic or supportive treatment appropriate to the specific situation. As a rule it is unwise to attempt to continue using the offending drug under a protective umbrella of antihistamines or glucocorticoids, although occasional desperate situations may justify an exception. The emergency treatment of anaphylaxis is described in Ch. 433.

SPECIFIC DRUG ALLERGIES. ***Penicillin.*** Penicillin is one of the most common drugs causing allergy, and as the most fully understood, it serves as a model for other drugs. Penicillin reactions include anaphylaxis, urticaria, vasculitis, dermatomyositis, maculopapular rashes, hemolytic anemia, drug fever, interstitial nephritis, pneumonitis, and contact dermatitis. Airborne penicillin can cause asthma in workers who produce or use it. The nature of the reaction is determined not only by the specific metabolite that becomes the hapten but also by the carrier molecule. For example, the penicilloyl determinant commonly evokes IgE antibody in cases of urticaria, but it also evokes IgG, and if it is combined with red cell membrane protein, it may be responsible for hemolytic anemia during the course of intravenous penicillin treatment. Many patients who claim to be allergic to penicillin tolerate it without adverse effect. In such patients, treatment with more expensive or toxic antibiotics would be unnecessary. Reliable tests are available for predicting which patients with a history of penicillin reactions will have a reaction. Cautious skin testing with dilute solutions of the antibiotic itself and with commercially available benzylpenicilloyl-polylysine (Pre-Pen) will provide guidance. If skin test reactions are negative to these reagents and to the "minor" determinants (the plain drug, penicilloate and penilloate), the probability of an allergic reaction is very low, no higher than in subjects receiving penicillin for the first time. The minor determinants are as yet available only in research settings, but only about 10 to 15 per cent of patients react to this reagent alone. Therefore, tests with the available reagents interpreted in the light of the history will usually allow appropriate treatment to proceed. The skin test with penicilloyl-polylysine begins with a prick of the 6.0×10^{-5} M solution, and if negative in 20 minutes, one proceeds to intradermal testing. Skin testing with the penicillin solution starts with a prick test with a solution containing 6000 units per milliliter of penicillin G or 4 mg per milliliter of other penicillins.

TABLE 437–2. ORAL DESENSITIZATION PROTOCOL FOR PENICILLIN

Dose*	Units	Route†
1	100	P.O.
2	200	P.O.
3	400	P.O.
4	800	P.O.
5	1,600	P.O.
6	3,200	P.O.
7	6,400	P.O.
8	12,800	P.O.
9	25,000	P.O.
10	50,000	P.O.
11	100,000	P.O.
12	200,000	P.O.
13	400,000	P.O.
14	200,000	S.C.
15	400,000	S.C.
16	800,000	S.C.
17	1,000,000	I.M.

*Interval between doses, 15 min.
†P.O. = oral; S.C. = subcutaneous; I.M. = intramuscular.
From Sullivan TJ, Yecies LD, Shaty GS, et al.: Desensitization of patients allergic to penicillin using orally administered β lactam antibiotics. J Allergy Clin Immunol 69:276, 1982.

Desensitization can be undertaken when skin test reactions are positive or when there are other reasons for suspecting an appreciable risk of anaphylaxis, but the patient has life-threatening infection with an organism for which no alternative antibiotics are available. Oral desensitization is preferred (Table 437–2).

Radiographic Contrast Agents. Iodinated contrast agents injected for radiographic examinations are now the most common cause of anaphylactic drug reactions. These reactions are not truly anaphylactic, for these materials do not combine with proteins to act as haptens but rather appear to act pharmacologically. As yet these reactions are not fully understood, but it is known that these drugs activate complement and release anaphylotoxin. Skin tests or small test doses do not predict reactivity. Persons who have had a previous reaction are at increased risk of a similar reaction from a subsequent injection. When a second examination is necessary, the patient should be given prednisone 50 mg every six hours for three doses, ending one hour before the procedure, and also an antihistamine shortly before.

Local Anesthetics. Most adverse reactions to local anesthetics are either toxic or psychophysiologic, but allergic reactions can occur. The most frequent is contact dermatitis; anaphylaxis is more serious though not as common. It has not yet been determined that skin testing with local anesthetics is useful in predicting anaphylaxis in patients with a history of reactions to local anesthetic. When local anesthesia is needed, an anesthetic as unrelated as possible to the one suspected of causing the reaction should be chosen, and a small test dose should be given first. Lidocaine seems to carry a low risk of allergy.

Aspirin and Other Nonsteroidal Anti-inflammatory Drugs. Shortly after its introduction in the late nineteenth century, aspirin was observed to provoke severe reactions in some patients with asthma. Such patients react in the same way to other nonsteroidal anti-inflammatory agents that inhibit cyclooxygenase, the key enzyme in the generating of prostaglandins from arachidonic acid. The typical reaction consists of acute bronchospasm, rhinorrhea, and occasionally urticaria. Most of the asthmatic patients who react to these agents also have nasal polyps and lack IgE-mediated allergy to common airborne allergens. In some patients with chronic urticaria but no respiratory disease, urticaria is the only manifestation of the reaction. The mechanism of this adverse response to aspirin is not allergic; extensive search for IgE antibodies has been unrewarding. Rather, it is presumably due to the inhibition of cyclooxygenase, but the precise mechanism is still undefined. Patients who have reacted to aspirin need not avoid other salicylates (except methylsalicylate), and salicylate-free diets are unnecessary. Five to ten per cent of aspirin-reactive subjects react similarly to tartrazine (FD&C yellow no. 5) added to foods or drugs. Skin tests to aspirin and similar agents are not useful and may be dangerous. No biochemical tests are available for diagnosis.

Sulfite. Sulfites, metabisulfites, and sulfur dioxide are added to foods to prevent discoloration and spoilage. Some asthmatic subjects develop acute severe reactions a few minutes after ingesting 10 to 100 mg. Though these reactions resemble those provoked by aspirin, they occur in different persons, and the biochemical pathway involved is presumably different. Lettuce and other salad ingredients prepared in restaurants in advance are often sprayed with sulfites to preserve freshness. This is perhaps the most common exposure. Other food sources include dried fruits, wine, some beers, and some soft drinks. Sulfites added as antioxidants to some medications for parenteral injection or aerosol administration can provoke similar reactions. No tests are available.

Parker CW: Drug allergy. N Engl J Med 292:511, 732, 957, 1975. *A masterful discussion of the principles of drug allergy that stresses immunologic mechanisms.*
Van Arsdel PW: Adverse drug reactions. *In* Middleton EJ, Ellis FF, Reed CE (eds.): Allergy Principles and Practice. 2nd ed. St. Louis, C. V. Mosby Company, 1983. *A detailed review and extensive listing of agents and reactions.*

438. MASTOCYTOSIS

Robert A. Lewis

DEFINITION. Mastocytosis is a rare disease of mast cell proliferation, which occurs in both cutaneous and systemic forms. The mast cell is a connective tissue cell normally found in most organs. It is not surprising, therefore, that systemic mastocytosis has been reported to involve virtually all tissues except the central nervous system, most commonly the skin, bones, gastrointestinal tract, liver, spleen, and lymph nodes. Mast cell leukemia and malignant transformation of solid tumors have been described in a few cases.

Mast cells are generally identifiable by their metachromatic granules (Fig. 438–1), which contain histamine, heparin, a tryptic protease, and a number of acid hydrolases, the last of which defines the granules as modified lysosomes. Mast cells, activated by either immunologic or nonimmunologic stimuli, secrete their lysosomal contents into the microenvironment and additionally liberate arachidonic acid from their membrane phospholipid stores, metabolizing it selectively to prostaglandin D_2 (PGD_2), and the sulfidopeptide leukotriene, LTC_4. LTC_4 is then further metabolized to its peptide cleavage products, LTD_4 and LTE_4, extracellularly. (A discussion of arachidonic acid metabolism is presented in Ch. 233.) Several of the clinical manifestations of mastocytosis as well as the choice of some therapeutic agents are based on the pathophysiologic actions of these substances, termed "mediators of immediate hypersensitivity," owing to their suspected roles in allergic disease (Table 438–1).

INCIDENCE AND PREVALENCE. Fewer than 1000 cases of mastocytosis have been reported, with equal occurrence in men and women. As the hallmark of this disease is based on cutaneous manifestations, mastocytosis is said to involve the skin in over 95 per cent of patients. The actual frequency with which mastocytosis involves other organs with sparing of the skin may thus be underestimated because of the bias of ascertainment. Cutaneous lesions begin more frequently in early childhood than after maturity. Visceral disease is not commonly associated with single isolated skin lesions, especially those arising in infancy or early childhood. However, approximately one quarter of adults with cutaneous lesions have visceral involvement.

TABLE 438–1. HUMAN MAST CELL–DERIVED PRODUCTS

Mediator	Function
Histamine	Increased vasopermeability; nonvascular smooth muscle contraction
Heparin	Anticoagulation; inhibition of complement activation
Prostaglandin D_2	Vasodilation; nonvascular smooth muscle contraction
Eosinophil and neutrophil chemotactic factors*	Eosinophil and neutrophil chemotaxis
Tryptase, arylsulfatase, N-acetyl-β-D-glucosaminidase, β-glucuronidase	Enzymatic degradation of proteoglycans and glycoproteins
Sulfidopeptide leukotrienes	Vasoconstriction; increased vasopermeability; nonvascular smooth muscle contraction (LTC_4) Vasodilation; increased vasopermeability; nonvascular smooth muscle contraction (LTD_4 and LTE_4)

*Evidence for association with human mast cell granule is indirect.

CLINICAL MANIFESTATIONS. Involvement of the skin in mastocytosis is termed *urticaria pigmentosa.* The lesions may be isolated mastocytomas or generalized and multiple (Fig. 438–2); they are usually reddish-brown and plaque-like or nodular. More rarely, telangiectatic or doughy-feeling erythrodermic forms of the skin lesions occur. When a cutaneous lesion is stroked firmly, it becomes pruritic and raised with surrounding erythema (Darier's sign). In many patients, stroking of seemingly uninvolved skin produces a wheal of dermographism, owing to microscopic dermal mastocytosis. Generalized pruritus and flushing may occur with or without cutaneous lesions.

Acute symptomatic episodes may occur, marked by systemic vasodilation with headache, dizziness, tachycardia, hypotension, syncope, and even frank shock. Rarely, such attacks may be fatal. These acute symptoms do not necessarily indicate systemic mastocytosis, since extensive cutaneous lesions are capable of releasing large amounts of the potent mediators

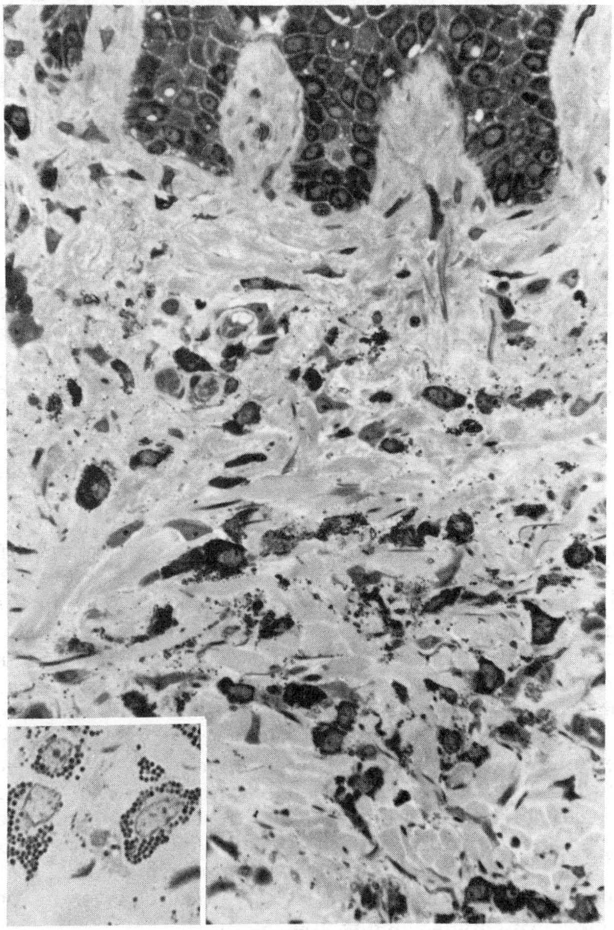

Figure 438–1. Mast cell proliferation in the dermis (Giemsa-stained lesional skin biopsy; × 520). Inset of dermal mast cells (× 1310). (Courtesy of J. Caulfield and A. Hein.)

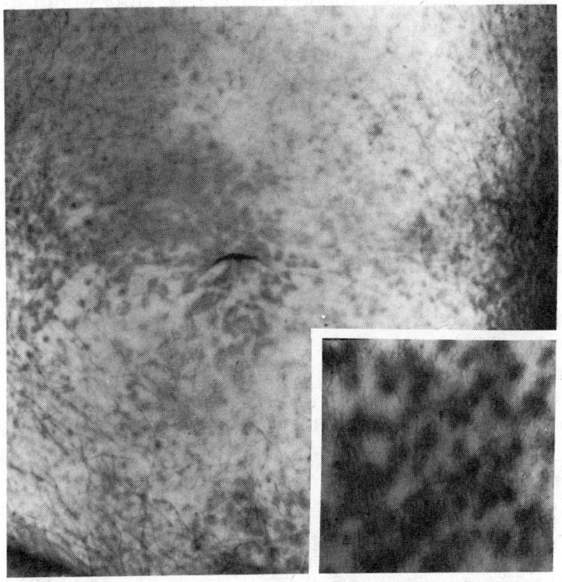

Figure 438–2. Skin lesions of mastocytosis (urticaria pigmentosa). Inset showing close-up view. (Courtesy of N. Soter.)

summarized in the table. Even the diagnostic test of stroking a cutaneous lesion to whealing may provoke systemic symptoms, especially those of flushing and colic in affected infants. Ingestion of alcohol may degranulate mast cells and set off acute symptoms.

Gastrointestinal symptoms may dominate the clinical picture. Anorexia, nausea, vomiting, diarrhea, and a possible predilection for peptic ulceration with or without hyperchlorhydria may complicate mastocytosis whether or not mast cells have proliferated in the gastrointestinal tract. Some patients have developed the malabsorption syndrome (see Ch. 103), which may be due to the release of mediators from mast cells infiltrating the small bowel mucosa and lamina propria. Hepatomegaly or hepatosplenomegaly may result from mast cell infiltration. The liver in mastocytosis may also be fibrotic and sometimes exhibits piecemeal inflammation. Rarely there is associated portal hypertension and gastroesophageal varices.

Osseous lesions occur in approximately 10 per cent of all patients with mastocytosis, or two thirds of those with systemic disease. These lesions, most commonly found in the pelvis, ribs, vertebrae, skull, and proximal long bones, may occasionally resemble Paget's disease radiologically. Bone pain may occur with or without pathologic fractures.

Occasionally rhinorrhea and rarely audible wheezing occur, reminiscent of the signs of allergic rhinitis and asthma, respectively. Ill-defined neuropsychiatric symptoms, ranging from malaise to decreased attention span and irritability, have been described. Anemia, leukopenia, thrombocytopenia, and even mast cell leukemia have been rarely reported in association with severe bone marrow infiltration by mast cells. Modest blood eosinophilia occurs occasionally, and the coagulation abnormalities of prolonged prothrombin and bleeding times related to heparin release, although uncommon, have also been reported.

DIAGNOSIS. The cutaneous lesions of urticaria pigmentosa in conjunction with Darier's sign are pathognomonic for mastocytosis. In their absence, additional criteria are necessary for the diagnosis. Osseous infiltration by mast cells may be suspected from radiologic lesions with adjacent areas of osteoporosis and mottled osteosclerosis. Bone marrow biopsy of involved areas demonstrates abnormally high numbers of mast cells and rarefaction of the spongiosa or, alternatively, myelofibrosis and sclerosis. In the absence of radiologic abnormalities, ^{99}Tc bone scans may define areas of increased radionuclide uptake to guide the site of the biopsy. Histaminuria two to three times greater than normal 24-hour levels (36 ± 14 μg) is common among patients with extensive cutaneous and/or visceral disease and useful when present, although both normal values and striking elevations up to 1300 μg per 24 hours have been reported. Two unique PGD_2 metabolites, which are, respectively, minimally present and undetectable in normal urine, have recently been described in urine specimens from patients with systemic mastocytosis. This observation, if confirmed and extended, may provide another sensitive diagnostic test.

For the patient with flushing, intermittent hypotension, diarrhea, tachycardia, and possibly hepatomegaly and peptic ulceration, the main differential diagnosis is with the carcinoid syndrome. The most direct criterion is a biopsy demonstrating mast cell proliferation as opposed to argentaffin cell infiltration in an involved organ. Failing this, the measurement of grossly elevated levels of histamine and its metabolites in the urine favors mastocytosis, whereas elevated urinary levels of 5-hydroxyindoleacetic acid (5-HIAA) are noted in the carcinoid syndrome. It must be recalled, however, that marked increases of urinary histamine may occur in gastric carcinoid (see Ch. 242), and elevated urinary excretion of serotonin metabolites may rarely occur in mastocytosis.

In addition to other clinical and laboratory manifestations, histopathology will differentiate the skin lesions of mastocytosis from those of histiocytosis X, myelomonocytic leukemia, cutaneous myelosarcoma, granular cell tumor, and dermatofibroma.

PATHOPHYSIOLOGY AND TREATMENT. When mast cells degranulate, they release their preformed granule-associated mediators and also generate newly formed PGD_2 and LTC_4. The mast cell in mastocytosis releases normal mediators in approximately normal amounts per cell. The most striking abnormalities seem to lie in the sensitivity of the degranulation response of the neoplastic cell to numerous physical stimuli, including not only gentle stroking (Darier's sign) but usually also moderate heat or cold. Once a skin lesion urticates, it requires up to three days to regenerate adequate granule histamine to form a second wheal.

In the past, the majority of the symptoms and signs of mastocytosis were ascribed to the effects of released histamine. Histamine is probably the major cause of local cutaneous whealing and pruritus as well as rhinitis. Vasodilation and gastrointestinal symptoms in this disease probably have a more complex pathogenesis. The combined use of antihistamines of both the H_1 antagonist group, such as chlorpheniramine maleate, and the H_2 antagonists, exemplified by cimetidine, has failed to control either the gastrointestinal symptoms or the hypotension in some patients with mastocytosis.

The identification of a vasodilating prostaglandin (PGD_2) formed by mast cells may therefore be relevant both to the pathophysiology of mastocytosis and to the development of effective therapy. Aspirin and other nonsteroidal anti-inflammatory compounds inhibit prostaglandin synthesis. It is therefore reasonable to try the use of such agents in mastocytosis. Aspirin therapy should be started in very small initial doses of 16 mg four times daily, with the dose doubled on each subsequent day for one week until either symptomatic relief is achieved or the side effects of salicylism supervene. The minimal therapeutic aspirin dose should then be maintained indefinitely. Aspirin should be given only after first initiating treatment with oral therapeutic doses of H_1 and H_2 antihistamines, such as 8 mg of chlorpheniramine maleate and 300 mg of cimetidine four times daily for an adult patient. The caution employed in initiating aspirin therapy follows from reports of a few patients with mastocytosis who have sustained precipitous hypotension after aspirin ingestion, suggesting the possibility that massive release of mediators may occur, including enhanced LTC_4 synthesis when nonsteroidal anti-inflammatory agents inhibit the cyclooxygenase pathway of arachidonate metabolism to prostaglandins.

The heparin released from islands of mast cells has been implicated in the prolonged local bleeding time at the sites of excised lesions, the occasionally reported purpura underlying cutaneous mastocytomas, and the rare incidence of significant gastrointestinal bleeding related to local mast cell infiltration. The development of osseous lesions that are both porotic and sclerotic may relate to the combined capacities of mast cell acid hydrolases and tryptase(s) for proteoglycan degradation which precedes collagenolysis, followed by tissue repair. Heparin has also been reported to cause osteopenia. Hepatic fibrosis when documented may also be a product of altered tissue repair in the presence of these enzymes. Therefore, drugs known to cause mast cell degranulation, such as alcohol, morphine, and codeine, are to be prohibited.

Disodium cromoglycate (cromolyn),* given as 100 mg orally four times daily, has been used successfully, particularly for the gastrointestinal symptoms. Cromolyn is thought to reduce mast cell degranulation by interfering with cellular calcium uptake. As little or none of the drug is absorbed, its local action on the gastrointestinal mast cells probably occurs without preventing histamine release from other mast cell infiltrated organs. Histaminuria is not modified by successful therapy with cromolyn. Less easily explained are the therapeutic effects of this agent in decreasing cutaneous symptoms of pruritus, whealing and flushing, as well as in relieving some of the neuropsychiatric complaints. Cromolyn may be given in combination with antihistamines and aspirin.

PROGNOSIS. Isolated cutaneous mastocytomas of infancy

*Approved for investigational use only.

commonly involute spontaneously. If this does not occur, the single lesions may be excised surgically. None of the suggested medical therapies reduce the number of mast cells in either cutaneous or visceral lesions.

Malignant mastocytosis is a very rare disorder with high mortality within two years of diagnosis. It may occur as either a cutaneous or a systemic disease and reportedly may appear by malignant transformation of a small minority of the clinically benign mastocytomas, especially of the systemic variety. Special histopathologic techniques may be necessary to detect the immature granules of malignant cells. Leukemia is associated with mastocytosis in fewer than 5 per cent of cases and may be monocytic, mastocytic, or myeloid, in approximately equal frequencies.

Lewis RA, Austen KF: Mediation of local homeostasis and inflammation by leukotrienes and other mast cell-dependent compounds. Nature 293:103, 1981. *A review of the biology of mast cell-derived mediators, including the leukotrienes.*

Parker CW, Cryer PE, Kissane JM: Clinicopathologic conference: Systemic mastocytosis. Am J Med 61:671, 1976. *An excellent review of the signs and symptoms of mastocytosis.*

Roberts LJ II, Sweetman BJ, Lewis RA, Folarin VF, Austen KF, Oates JA: Increased production of prostaglandin D_2 in patients with systemic mastocytosis. N Engl J Med 303:1400, 1980. *Important for future diagnostic and therapeutic considerations.*

Soter NA, Austen KF, Wasserman SI: Oral disodium cromoglycate in the treatment of systemic mastocytosis. N Engl J Med 301:465, 1979. *A prospective evaluation of cromolyn therapy for mastocytosis.*

439. DISEASES OF THE THYMUS

Daniel P. Stites

DEVELOPMENT, STRUCTURE, AND FUNCTION. The thymus is a central lymphoid organ which functions in the development and maintenance of immunologic competence. It arises embryologically from the third and fourth branchial clefts and then migrates caudad, as a bilobed organ, to the anterior mediastinum. Ectopic thoracic and cervical thymic rests are present in 30 per cent of normal individuals. The thymus enlarges until late puberty and then involutes, the lymphocytes and epithelial cells being nearly completely replaced with fat by the fifth or sixth decade. The normal thymus varies greatly in size. It is uniquely susceptible to marked involution within hours owing to the stress of serious illness or to treatment with glucocorticoids. The thymus is composed primarily of lymphocytes encased in a lattice of epithelial cells. It also contains a few myoid cells, macrophages, and plasma cells. The thymus is arranged into discrete lobules containing a cortex and medulla. Hassall's corpuscles are specialized aggregates of epithelial cells whose function is unknown.

The thymus begins to function by about ten to twelve weeks of gestation when immunocompetent T cells can first be detected. Undifferentiated stem cells migrate to the thymus from fetal liver and bone marrow prenatally and from the bone marrow postnatally. Local influences, probably from epithelial cells, induce maturation of thymic lymphocytes, which then divide in the cortex, migrate to the medulla, and emigrate to the peripheral lymphoid tissue as mature T cells. The cortex is also the site of intense lymphopoiesis. The thymus secretes a variety of incompletely defined hormones which maintain T cell competence in peripheral lymphoid organs. These substances are variously known as thymopoietin, thymin, and thymosin. The immunosuppressive effects of thymectomy vary with age, being most pronounced at younger ages (see below). The thymus also appears to play an important role in maintenance of tolerance to various antigens, in immune surveillance, and possibly in leukemogenesis (as judged by animal experiments).

THYMIC HYPOPLASIA. Hypoplastic thymus may be either congenital or acquired. In neonates and infants, *congenital thymic hypoplasia* is expressed as marked T cell and variable B cell immunodeficiency. Resulting diseases include reticular dysgenesis, severe combined immunodeficiency disease, DiGeorge's and Nezelof's syndromes, and ataxia-telangiectasia (see Ch. 429). Essentially all of these patients are diagnosed in childhood; the severity of the thymic lesion, if untreated, rarely allows survival beyond age ten to twelve years. Congenital thymic hypoplasia has been treated by thymic or bone marrow transplantation and by thymic hormone injections with variable success. *Acquired hypoplasia* or thymic involution occurs normally with age or results from stress (within hours or days), malnutrition, pregnancy, x-rays, glucocorticoids, or cytotoxic drugs. Acquired involution may be reversible after withdrawal of the offending cause.

THYMIC HYPERPLASIA. An enlarged thymus is very difficult to evaluate accurately because of its large normal variability in size. In the past, so-called status thymolymphaticus, a condition diagnosed with respiratory distress, and large thymic shadow on chest roentgenogram frequently led to unnecessary removal or radiation of normal thymuses. The concept of status thymolymphaticus has been abandoned. The thymus may rarely enlarge in thyrotoxicosis, Addison's disease, anencephaly, acromegaly, castration, cysts, or tumors (see below).

THYMUS AND MYASTHENIA GRAVIS. Myasthenia gravis is an autoimmune disease caused by the presence of antiacetylcholine receptor (AchR) antibodies (see Ch. 539). In myasthenia gravis there is a 10 per cent incidence of thymoma. In fact detectable enlargement of the thymus in myasthenia gravis usually heralds the presence of a thymoma. In 65 per cent of cases, the thymus is hyperplastic with increased numbers of germinal centers but not clinically enlarged. In the remaining 25 per cent of patients the thymus is normal. In large series of thymomas, 30 to 60 per cent of patients have myasthenia gravis. Rarely myasthenia gravis develops years after total thymectomy for thymoma, which militates against an absolute requirement for thymoma in the pathogenesis of this disorder. Neonatal myasthenia gravis occurs without any thymic abnormality, presumably owing to transplacental transfer of maternal antibody. There is little correlation with serum levels of anti-AchR antibody and clinical improvement in myasthenia following thymectomy. Damage to AchR antigen shared between muscles and thymic epithelial or myoid cells may explain the rather obscure relationship of the thymus to this autoantibody disorder.

EFFECTS OF THYMECTOMY. Total removal of the thymus during the neonatal period in rodents results in severe immunodeficiency, loss of T cells, and a wasting disease, a result of chronic unopposed infection. Thymectomy in adult animals, however, is associated with much subtler changes in T cell function. What is the effect of thymectomy in man? Because of the high incidence of extramediastinal thymic rests (30 per cent), thymectomy can rarely be considered total. Total thymectomy intentionally done during cardiothoracic surgery in children does not appear to result in compromised transplantation immunity. In patients with thymoma, a transient decrease in circulating lymphocytes and T cell functions is noted. Following thymectomy for myasthenia gravis, functional loss in some T cell populations occurs. However, the long-term effects of thymectomy either in immunologically normal patients during cardiac surgery or in cancer patients with thymomas is not known. These individuals should be carefully observed for development of autoimmune disease, infection, certain malignancies, or other signs of T cell deficiency.

THYMOMA. ***Definition.*** A thymoma is a neoplasm of thymic epithelial cells. This definition excludes other tumors that may affect the thymus such as lymphoma, germ cell tumors, and carcinoid. Thymomas are rare; fewer than 1000 cases have been reported. Nevertheless, it is the most common tumor of the anterior superior mediastinum (see Ch. 69).

Pathology. Thymomas contain various proportions of epithelial cells and lymphocytes. The latter are T cells and may constitute a large proportion of cellular content of the tumor; hence the term *lymphoepithelioma*. Although their significance is

TABLE 439–1. DISEASES ASSOCIATED WITH THYMIC TUMOR

Thymoma
- Myasthenia gravis
- Red cell aplasia
- Hemolytic anemia
- Neutrophil agranulocytosis
- Hypogammaglobulinemia (Good's syndrome)
- Systemic lupus erythematosus
- Polymyositis
- Pemphigus vulgaris
- Chronic mucocutaneous candidiasis

Carcinoid
- Cushing's syndrome
- Multiple endocrine neoplasia syndromes (see Ch. 240)

unknown, the activated appearance of these lymphocytes suggests a host reaction to neoplastic epithelial cells. These T cells all have the surface characteristics of thymocytes rather than peripheral blood T cells. Various histologic degrees of malignancy from minimal cytologic atypia to undifferentiated carcinoma exist. However, correlation of microscopic appearance with clinical malignancy is notoriously poor. In fact, local invasion of pleura, pericardium, vessels, and nerves is the major criterion for determining clinical malignancy of the tumor.

Clinical Manifestations. Median age of patients with thymoma is about 50 years, and no sex predominance is noted. About 30 per cent of patients present with myasthenia gravis; another 30 per cent are asymptomatic, and the diagnosis is suggested by an anterior mediastinal mass on chest roentgenogram. The remaining 30 to 40 per cent of patients have a variety of symptoms and medical syndromes associated with the tumor (Table 439–1). Symptoms and signs include cough, chest pain, dysphagia, dyspnea, hoarseness, neck mass, and superior vena cava syndrome.

A few patients with spindle cell thymomas have marked *hypogammaglobulinemia*. Whether the relationship is causal is not established. The rare occurrence of red cell aplasia with or without immunodeficiency and thymoma raises the possibility of T cell-mediated suppression of erythropoiesis or immunoglobulin synthesis. Direct evidence to support these notions is only fragmentary.

Diagnosis. The presence of a round or oval anterior mediastinal mass visualized in posteroanterior and lateral chest roentgenograms in the presence of myasthenia gravis or of some other known systemic manifestations is suggestive of thymoma. Computed tomographic (CT) imaging is useful in defining the size and location of thymomas and is occasionally useful in differentiating various thymic lesions. Thymic biopsy has no place in evaluation of anterior mediastinal masses, and mediastinoscopy is of little or no value. Some centers claim success with fine needle aspiration and cytology. Thoracotomy with adequate exposure to determine whether capsular invasion has occurred is needed for diagnosis of any thymic tumor. Differential diagnosis includes other primary or secondary thymic tumors (see below), cysts, post-traumatic hemorrhage, aneurysm or other abnormalities of the anterior mediastinal contents including metastatic tumors, giant lymph node hyperplasia, mesothelioma, thyroid and parathyroid tumors, and paragangliomas (see Ch. 69).

Treatment. Surgical removal of tumor followed by local irradiation if extracapsular extension has occurred is the treatment of choice. Distant metastases are rare; the tumor spreads mainly by local invasion of adjacent structures.

Prognosis. The prognosis is nearly entirely dependent on presence of local invasion and cannot be predicted by histologic appearance of the tumor. Noninvasive thymomas are usually cured by excision. Patients with invasive thymoma have about 50 per cent five-year survival.

OTHER TUMORS OF THE THYMUS. *Thymolipoma* probably represents a lipoma arising within normal thymus. This tumor is usually radiolucent and asymptomatic and has not been associated with myasthenia gravis. *Carcinoid tumor* of the thymus arises from neuroendocrine cells within the thymus (see Ch. 242). Fifty per cent produce ACTH-like molecules and cause Cushing's syndrome or hyperparathyroidism, or are associated with multiple endocrine adenomatosis; 30 per cent are malignant and metastasize. Surgery and radiotherapy are indicated. *Carcinomas*, particularly squamous cell types, may rarely occur. *Germ cell tumors* rarely occur: seminoma, teratoma, teratocarcinoma, choriocarcinoma, embryonal cell carcinoma, and yolk sac tumors. The thymus may be involved by *malignant lymphomas*. T cell lymphomas with acute lymphoblastic leukemia occur in the second decade. Cells from these tumors may have C receptors and are positive for terminal deoxynucleotidyl transferase. Hodgkin's disease usually is of nodular sclerosing type (see Ch. 158 and 160).

Baron RL, Lee JKT, Sagel SS, Levitt RG: Computed tomography of the abnormal thymus. Radiology 142:127, 1982. *This article delineates indications for CT scans in patients with clinical, surgical, and pathologic evidence of thymic diseases. It indicates that, on occasion, CT may suggest the specific nature of a thymic lesion.*

Namba T, Brunner NG, Grob D: Myasthenia gravis in patients with thymoma with particular reference to onset after thymectomy. Medicine 57:411, 1978. *Excellent review of literature on relationship of thymoma to myasthenia gravis with 72 locally studied cases.*

Pahwa R, Ikehara S, Pahwa SG, Good RA: Thymic function in man. Thymus 1:27, 1979. *Careful description of thymic physiology, with emphasis on role of thymic hormones.*

Salyer W, Eggleston JC: Thymoma. A clinical and pathological study of 65 cases. Cancer 37:229, 1976. *Clinicopathologic description of a large series of thymoma patients, annotating association with other medical syndromes.*

Part XXII
MUSCULOSKELETAL AND CONNECTIVE TISSUE DISEASES

440. APPROACH TO THE PATIENT WITH MUSCULOSKELETAL DISEASE*

James F. Fries

The rheumatic diseases present a major challenge to clinical judgment. The chronicity, variability, tendency to exacerbate and remit, biochemical and immunologic complexity, unknown pathogenesis, variable response to specific treatment, and myriad ways in which these diseases affect the patient's lifestyle, family relationships, self-image, and employability all combine to complicate the therapeutic equation. Difficult therapeutic decisions must be made for the most part without adequate experimental justification and evaluated against a poorly understood natural history.

Balanced against these tremendous uncertainties, contemporary management is relatively straightforward but has changed substantially. Present therapeutic strategy has shifted from dogma to flexibility. Good management now requires that therapeutic decisions be based upon individual circumstances rather than upon diagnosis per se. Further, treatment decisions are never final but are modified in a continuing feedback between application of treatment and observation of response. Decisions evolve and change over time as appropriate to the trends, tempo, and previous response of the particular patient. Clinical judgment is essential to good outcome. It is more than a truism to note that the art of medicine is reborn in the approach to a patient with a chronic disease. The broad principles underlying contemporary management strategy are set forth in this chapter and are divided into six major facets. The medical history, the physical examination, and the laboratory data, which are discussed in following chapters, are integrated into decisions regarding these six areas.

DETERMINING THE PATHOPHYSIOLOGY

Modern management individualizes therapy within diagnostic categories, based upon subgroups of patients with differing prognoses and different therapeutic requirements. Patients with the same diagnosis often should be managed very differently. Rheumatic disease patients frequently have features of several diagnostic entities at the same time.

Diagnosis is *not* the most important factor in selecting management in rheumatic disease. Management in musculoskeletal disease is more closely linked to the underlying pathophysiologic process than to the disease entity. Reversal of the pathophysiologic process (or negation of its impact) requires a clear visualization of that process. Even such a basic pathophysiologic concept as "inflammation" has different therapeutic implications. The inflamed synovial membrane (synovitis) typical of rheumatoid arthritis responds to a different spectrum of anti-inflammatory agents than does the inflammation of ligamentous insertions (enthesitis) typical of ankylosing spondylitis or the inflammation within the joint space induced by microscopic crystals.

Eight specific types of musculoskeletal pathology are readily distinguished by history and physical examination in most patients and provide a framework for pathophysiologic categorization. These categories are not mutually exclusive, but categorization of the predominant pathophysiology in a given patient is usually straightforward. The eight categories are discussed in the following paragraphs and are listed in Table 440–1 together with the prototype disease of the category, examples of the most useful laboratory tests for that category, and the typical treatments required. Management implications for each category are surprisingly distinct and provide guidelines for the ordering of laboratory investigations and the selection of initial treatment.

SYNOVITIS. Inflammation of the synovial membrane, with eventual damage to surrounding joint structures, is most strikingly manifested in the disease "rheumatoid arthritis." The synovium is tender, thickened, and palpable and may demonstrate warmth and, less often, redness. Joint destruction is caused by the enzymatic products of inflammation and develops slowly over many years. Management is based upon reducing the *rate* of damage to joint structures. The sedimentation rate is consistently elevated with significant synovitis, and the latex fixation or other tests for rheumatoid arthritis are often useful for further categorization. A wide range of pharmacologic and other treatments may be required, and many patients require sequential trials with a variety of agents. Some useful drugs, such as gold, penicillamine, and hydroxychloroquine, are not proven therapeutically effective in any other category, and others, such as aspirin, find their greatest use here.

ENTHESOPATHY. Inflammation in certain diseases is most marked at the enthesis, that transition region where ligament attaches to bone. Such inflammation is the hallmark of a family of rheumatic diseases of which the most common is ankylosing spondylitis. The distribution of musculoskeletal involvement in these diseases thus follows the location of regions of enthesis throughout the body. The marked predilection for the sacroiliac joints, heels, and spine identifies a process affecting areas characterized by ligament and tendon attachment. This specific pathophysiology has been recognized only in the last several years and provides a unifying basis for the observed clinical features of the diseases and their typical response to specific therapy. The HLA-B27 gene is usually present, and rheumatoid factor is predictably absent from the serum. Nonsteroidal anti-inflammatory agents, in particular indomethacin, phenylbutazone, and naproxen, are therapeutically effective and usually

*Adapted with permission from Kelley WN, Harris ED Jr, Ruddy S, Sledge CB: Textbook of Rheumatology. Philadelphia, W. B. Saunders Company, 1981, pp 353–358.

TABLE 440–1. CATEGORIES OF RHEUMATIC DISEASE

Pathology	Prototype	Most Useful Tests	Typical Treatment
Synovitis	Rheumatoid arthritis	Latex, erythrocyte sedimentation rate	Acetylsalicylic acid, gold
Enthesopathy	Ankylosing spondylitis	Sacroiliac radiographs, HLA-B27	Indomethacin
Cartilage degeneration	Osteoarthritis	Radiographs of affected area	Analgesic
Crystal-induced synovitis	Gout	Joint fluid crystal examination	Colchicine
Joint infection	Staphylococcal	Joint fluid culture	Antibiotics
Myositis	Dermatomyositis	Muscle enzymes, muscle biopsy	Corticosteroids
Focal conditions	Tennis elbow	None, radiographs of affected area	Localized
Generalized conditions	Fibrositis	Erythrocyte sedimentation rate	Conservative

are well tolerated over the long term. The spectrum of effective anti-inflammatory drugs used for enthesopathy is different from the spectrum effective in synovitis. Prednisone, for example, is neither indicated nor effective in most patients.

CARTILAGE DEGENERATION. Degenerative and other processes can cause fraying and destruction of the articular cartilage, with subsequent injury to the underlying subchondral bone. This occurrence is usually termed osteoarthritis (or osteoarthrosis), and a group of specific syndromes is recognized within this category. Narrowing of the apparent joint space and development of bony spurs make radiography the most useful investigative procedure; other ancillary tests are usually negative. Few patients have significant inflammation, and it is not surprising that anti-inflammatory treatment is not frequently useful. The analgesic effects of aspirin or nonsteroidal anti-inflammatory agents may be helpful; doses required for optimal effect are often considerably less than doses required for anti-inflammatory effects with the same compound. Treatment is symptomatic and is seldom dramatically effective.

CRYSTAL-INDUCED SYNOVITIS. Microcrystalline arthritis occurs when crystals forming in the synovial fluid (or injected therein) induce an acute inflammatory reaction in the joint fluid and the surrounding synovium. Gout is the prototype disease, with the inflammation in gout induced by crystals of monosodium urate. Similar syndromes may occur with crystals of several other types. The inflammatory response develops with a rather sudden clinical onset, increases to very intense inflammation within a period of hours, and spontaneously resolves without treatment over a period of a few days to a few weeks; this resolution is markedly accelerated with treatment. The physical factors underlying crystal formation determine that only one or, at most, a few joints are involved at a time. The crucial laboratory observation is inspection of the aspirated joint fluid for crystals under polarized light microscopy. Drugs inhibiting polymorphonuclear leukocytes are particularly effective, as exemplified by colchicine, a drug with little effect in any other rheumatic disease category.

JOINT INFECTION. The synovium encloses a body space that can be the site of direct infection by microorganisms. Critical to investigation of the patient with suspected joint infection is aspiration and culture of the joint fluid and, in many instances, culture of other body fluids as well. Treatment consists principally of prescribing an antibiotic specific for the microorganism involved. Drainage may be required.

MYOSITIS. Inflammation of muscle occurs in two closely related diseases, dermatomyositis and polymyositis, and in a distant relative, polymyalgia rheumatica. Determination of muscle enzyme levels and histologic examination of involved muscle may be the critical laboratory observations. In polymyalgia, the sedimentation rate is greatly elevated and is often the sole objective finding. Temporal artery biopsy may be useful when giant cell arteritis is demonstrated. Corticosteroids are almost always required in inflammatory muscle disease and, in contrast to every other rheumatic disease category, are usually required from the outset.

FOCAL CONDITIONS. A wide variety of conditions affecting the musculoskeletal system do not truly warrant the term "disease." Tendinitis, bursitis, low back strain, calcific tendinitis, and a variety of other entities can affect almost any area of the body and are among the most common of all medical problems. Laboratory aids are few, although radiography occasionally may be useful in locating calcium deposits or spurs or in ruling out fracture. The therapeutic imperative in localized problems (unfortunately often neglected) is to emphasize localized rather than general treatment measures. Treatment of the entire organism for a problem in one local area is seldom rewarding. Splints, slings, heat, and local injection are usually the most reasonable initial approach.

GENERALIZED CONDITIONS. A variety of ambiguous entities fall into this poorly defined category. Terms such as "fibrositis" or the "chronic muscle contraction syndrome" are sometimes used to indicate the likelihood of organic disease. The terms "psychogenic rheumatism," "nonarticular rheumatism," or "depressive equivalent" are frequently used to suggest an emotional component to such complaints. These patients are rich in symptoms but poor in objective evidence of pathology. The conditions may be extremely troublesome for the individual but are not progressive and do not result in physical crippling. Laboratory test results, such as the sedimentation rate, are normal and are employed only to rule out other categories of illness. Treatment is best termed "conservative." The therapeutic approaches listed for other categories are unlikely to be beneficial, and the physician who attempts pharmacologic intervention rather than reassurance, lifestyle counseling, and support often ends with a drug-dependent patient who gets no better.

These eight categories and the brief descriptions presented are supported by generalizations to which there are some exceptions. However, Table 440–1 suggests quite specific directions in which laboratory investigation and the therapeutic approach should begin. The experienced physician soon moves far beyond this table, but it provides a particularly useful framework upon which to place the more detailed clinical knowledge of following chapters.

USING THE LABORATORY SELECTIVELY

Laboratory tests in the rheumatic diseases usually provide confirmatory data rather than conclusive evidence. After the three exceptions of (1) the sacroiliac radiograph in ankylosing spondylitis, (2) the identification of specific crystals within the joint fluid, or (3) a positive bacteriologic culture from joint fluid, laboratory tests have varying degrees of lack of sensitivity and lack of specificity and, except in the unusual case, add relatively little to clinical assessment. As a result, the majority of patients presenting with musculoskeletal problems do not require any laboratory evaluation whatsoever. The key to appropriate use of the laboratory is selective use. Every test should have a specific indication, and blind "surveys" or "panels" should not be used.

One in six visits by a patient to a health professional is for a musculoskeletal complaint. The great majority of such physician visits occur for the common "focal conditions" of life. Low back pain, sprained ankles, tennis elbows, and other common musculoskeletal complaints account for most initial visits. The overwhelming majority of such problems are easily identified as self-limited. Optimal management includes ruling out more significant illness, advice about activity or rest, reassurance, occasionally symptomatic medication, and transmission of the expectation that the natural healing process will resolve the difficulty. The usual healing period for local musculoskeletal problems ranges from two to six weeks, depending upon the magnitude of the often inapparent injury, with the healing process beginning again from the start if there is reinjury during this period. Healing cannot be pharmacologically accelerated. Thus, optimal treatment usually requires "masterly inactivity," with confident reliance upon the natural healing process. Inappropriate rigor with test or treatment can lead to investigative mishaps, therapeutic side reactions, and an intensity of focus upon the problem entirely inappropriate to its magnitude. The careful rheumatic disease clinician uses time to establish the trends and tempo of the condition in the individual; time is used to remove the self-limited condition from the hazards of inappropriate response.

The critical initial decision, therefore, is whether the problem requires immediate action or whether the decision to investigate or treat can be postponed until the course of the disease and the magnitude of the appropriate response may be better estimated. A six-week "rule of thumb" is appropriate. In the absence of specific indication or immediate threat, a waiting period of six weeks from onset of symptoms serves to minimize inappropriate use of laboratory tests or treatment. Four major exceptions to the six-week rule obtain. First, a condition that is severe and involves a single joint (or, at most, a few joints) is much more likely, paradoxically, to require immediate attention than is a widespread polyarthritis. Acute gouty arthritis and infections, the usual causes of the "single hot joint," require immediate attention. In contrast, in rheumatoid arthritis, a period of six weeks is required even before the criteria for diagnosis can be met, and management in the first days of disease is most appropriately conservative. Many "possible rheumatoid arthritis" patients have minor problems that disappear as the viral or minor hypersensitivity reaction subsides. They need not be given the emotional burden of a "serious" diagnosis.

Secondly, a patient who is febrile, systemically ill, and otherwise showing signs of major disease deserves immediate attention. Endocarditis, neoplasm, tuberculosis, and other illnesses are frequently identified through musculoskeletal clues, and a connective tissue disease with systemic manifestations deserves immediate attention.

Third, if the problem is associated with significant trauma, the possible need for immediate orthopedic management should be considered. Fourth, an associated neurologic problem such as carpal tunnel syndrome, sciatic nerve compression, or cervical nerve root compression may be benefited by immediate attention. In practice, these four indications for action are relatively unusual. The large majority of patients with initial complaints of the musculoskeletal system are not found to have conditions requiring either intensive efforts at diagnosis or employment of hazardous therapy.

ESTABLISHING MANAGEMENT GOALS

Following current biomedical training, disease impact has often been defined in terms of numerically expressed test results. The level of autoantibodies, titer of rheumatoid factor, number of radiographic erosions, and sedimentation rate too often become the criteria for therapeutic success. The patient (and the patient's family) is much more directly interested in quite a different list of disease endpoints: in survival, in normal mobility and function, in absence from pain and other symptoms, and in the ability to remain solvent through the duration of a chronic illness. These five "D's" (death, disability, discomfort, drug toxicity, and dollar cost) are the major dimensions of patient outcome in the patient's own terms.

In some disease areas, such as oncology, consideration of the single outcome dimension of death suffices to dominate most clinical decisions. In contrast, in the rheumatic diseases value "trade-offs" among several outcome dimensions must be based upon the values of the particular patient, since different treatments may have contrasting effects on different outcome dimensions. For example, pain may be reduced by narcotics but disability increased; disability may be reduced by cyclophosphamide but a risk of death incurred; or short-term symptomatic relief by plasmapheresis may be obtained at very high cost.

Careful establishment of management goals must precede development of the individual management strategy. In some instances, a limited goal, such as regaining the ability to walk, may be dramatically useful to the patient and far more valuable to him or her than a modest reduction in the general severity of the disease. Some very worthy goals may not be achievable in the particular instance, and their pursuit may only increase the dimension of therapeutic toxicity. The question of what is desirable is usually subordinate to the question of what is achievable.

PLANNING FOR OPTIMAL LONG-TERM OUTCOME

Hospital-based training tends to focus attention on improving the patient's status at admission by the time of discharge. In chronic illness, such short-term benefits may be desirable but illusory. Corticosteroids, narcotic analgesics, and intra-articular injections often provide obvious short-term benefit. Unfortunately, the agent that provides the best initial response may lead to iatrogenic disaster over the longer term.

The basic therapeutic strategy holds that simple and nontoxic measures should be used first, and hazardous medications withheld unless the simpler approaches fail. But the individual patient frequently has special considerations requiring modification of such progressions. Thus, the tempo of disease may be such that joint destuction is developing over a short period of months; the therapeutic progression then requires acceleration. Or a major therapeutic attempt with gold, penicillamine, or an immunosuppressant agent may require months until the expected date of response. Meanwhile, the patient may have exhausted sick leave prior to forced retirement because of disability. Addition of a generally contraindicated agent, such as prednisone, might, under such circumstances, provide temporary support for the individual while more definitive therapy is taking hold. In a patient of advanced age, concern about the eventual hazard of malignancy secondary to a drug might well be small. In a vigorous and active male patient, there may be little concern about corticosteroid osteopenia. For a young patient, the expectation for patient outcome should perhaps be integrated over twenty to thirty years. In the older patient, both the risks and the benefits of treatment might be reduced, but not by the same amount. Again, the necessity for the individual program is seen.

The inexperienced clinician is often trapped by taking the short view of a chronic illness. The quack practitioner more intentionally follows the same strategy, that is, attempting to maximize immediate benefits while disregarding future problems. A chronic disease cannot be managed by short-term tactics; it requires a long-term strategy, shared and negotiated with the patient.

Such a strategy, it must be admitted, requires tactical modification at nearly every physician-patient encounter. At each visit, new information is always present, even if it is only the information about what has transpired in response to the last set of decisions. A decision is thus followed by observation, then by further decision, then by another period of observation. The decision strategy is flexible and, in the final analysis, frequently empiric.

USING A COMPLETE CLINICAL REPERTOIRE

Treatment of musculoskeletal disease is frequently discussed in terms of the available pharmacologic agents. This myopic view neglects the dominant contributions often afforded by reconstructive surgical procedures, by the use of appliances and devices to allow handicapped individuals to function more normally, by exercise to strengthen bones and tissues, or by personal interaction to increase the motivation and self-image of the patient.

A drug-based strategy tends to find its greatest use in early, systemic, inflammatory disease processes. Orthopedic approaches tend to have the greatest utility if the number of joints or regions involved is small, if major problems are concentrated in a single anatomic region, or after an inflammatory process has "burned out." Improvement after occupational therapy is often seen in patients with moderate to major disability who require adaptive devices to render the environment more friendly. The will to live a normal life sometimes can be more important to outcome than any specific therapy, and patient confidence (personal efficacy) is a useful therapeutic adjunct. Medical therapy that interferes with mental or emotional adaptation frequently appears to make things worse.

The novice at managing rheumatic diseases employs only a limited therapeutic repertoire. Typically, the patient requires a diverse program individualized to specific needs and frequently making use of a variety of individuals from different disciplines. Development of rational strategies requires intimate knowledge of the strengths and weaknesses of all available therapeutic modalities. The physician cannot manage chronic musculoskeletal diseases effectively without detailed knowledge of the techniques of complementary disciplines or a good working relationship with individuals who possess these skills.

ACHIEVING PATIENT UNDERSTANDING

The informed patient is the physician's greatest single asset in managing chronic illness. Consider even the recommendation that a patient should take aspirin. The lay media describe the hazards of aspirin, colloquialisms associate aspirin with physician neglect, and the over-the-counter availability suggests that aspirin is a minor remedy. Yet, for anti-inflammatory treatment with aspirin, the physician may aim for a narrow therapeutic range just below toxicity and far above the dose the patient expects. While establishing dosage, the patient is almost certain to encounter one or another side effect, even though the aspirin later may be well tolerated. The informed patient must know that anti-inflammatory and analgesic activities of aspirin are different, that a particular therapeutic range is important, that the drug is active against the inflammatory process itself, and that several weeks may be required to see the full effects of the drug. In the absence of such understanding, it is extremely unusual for a patient to do well on aspirin; patient education is a prerequisite for therapeutic success.

Most clinicians believe that patients with positive expectations have better outcomes. While causality is not established from this observation, it is reasonable to assume that restoration of hope and a positive self-image are beneficial parts of the treatment program. The patient with arthritis is under intense psychologic pressures. Self-image is threatened by diseases that may cripple and prevent remunerative employment. The possibility of dependence upon others is often present. Yet prognosis is generally better than that anticipated by the patient. The physician who is unaware that every patient with arthritis has significant fears may do great harm by inadvertently increasing those fears.

Additional considerations mandate careful patient education. The informed patient is more likely to comply with a particular therapeutic regimen. The patient's report of success or failure with previous recommendations is essential for the next clinical decision and must be as accurate as possible, again emphasizing the need for direct patient-physician communication. Unrealistic expectations followed by perceived therapeutic failures are a major cause of the burgeoning business in quack treatment of arthritis. The patient must be educated to recognize the falsity of overstated claims and the losses in courage, independence, and money that may result. The obscenity of the quack practitioner who makes a living by defrauding patients with arthritis focuses the attention of most physicians upon the outrage. At the more important level, however, the patient susceptible to the claims of the quack does not have a confident and informed relationship with his or her personal physician.

The management of musculoskeletal disease is directed in large part at maintenance of the independence of the individual. Most persons with arthritis can be independent and healthy individuals despite their musculoskeletal condition. This independence is the final goal of the individualized management strategy.

Fries JF: Education for outcome. J Rheum 5:1, 1978.
Fries JF, Holman HR: Systemic Lupus Erythematosus: A Clinical Analysis. Philadelphia, W. B. Saunders Company, 1975.
Fries JF, Mitchell DM: Joint pain or arthritis. JAMA 235:199, 1976.
Rodnan GP, Schumacher HR (eds.): Primer on the Rheumatic Diseases. Atlanta, Georgia, Arthritis Foundation, 1983.
Urowitz MB: SLE subsets—divide and conquer. J Rheum 4:332, 1977.

441. CONNECTIVE TISSUE STRUCTURE AND FUNCTION

Stephen M. Krane

Connective tissues are responsible for the form and shape of the animal body and, in addition, provide protection for vital organs and facilitate locomotion. The term connective tissue is also applied in a more restricted sense to structures such as dermis, tendons, fascia, bone, cartilage, and the capsules of the joint. All cells, however, make contacts with surrounding structures which involve connective tissues as components of the extracellular matrix. The matrix possesses chemical, physical, and mechanical properties uniquely suited to the function of tissues and organs of which the cells are a part. The extracellular matrix may be rigid (e.g., bone), elastic (e.g., blood vessel walls), compressible (e.g., cartilage), or liquid (e.g., synovial fluid). Most connective tissue matrices derive these properties by virtue of the content of fibrillar proteins, nonfibrillar macromolecules, and low molecular weight proteins and electrolytes. The properties of the matrix are therefore determined predominantly by the function of cells, specific for each tissue, which are responsible for synthesis of the matrix components. Many of the functions of the component cells, in turn, are influenced by the character of the extracellular matrix. The properties of connective tissues are also influenced by their relationships to the vascular system from which critical components are derived, such as water, electrolytes, and proteins. Indeed, the walls of blood vessels may themselves be considered as connective tissues. However, although some connective tissues are highly vascular (e.g., bone), others are essentially avascular (e.g., cartilage).

COMPOSITION OF EXTRACELLULAR MATRICES. The major components of the extracellular matrix are fibrillar proteins (collagens and elastin), globular proteins, complex carbohydrates, and, in the case of bone, the inorganic mineral phase. In most connective tissues the fibrillar proteins make up the bulk of the organic material. The *elastic fibers* consist of two distinct protein components. The most abundant is an amorphous protein (elastin) with no distinct periodicity by electron microscopy. The minor component associated with the elastin is a microfibrillar glycoprotein. Elastic fibers are most abundant in walls of large arteries and in some tendons and ligaments. In joints, however, collagens are the major fibrillar proteins. Collagens belong to a family of proteins which have similar chemical and structural properties. The term "collagen" is also used to refer to fibers or fiber bundles observed in tissue sections. The form of collagens in tissues is determined by the type of molecule that predominates and by interactions with other components of the matrix. Collagen fibers usually have diameters of 0.1 μm to 10 to 15 μm. The most abundant species, the interstitial collagens, such as those which predominate in tissues such as dermis, tendons, bone, and cartilage, have a characteristic banding pattern seen on electron microscopy with major periods of approximately 64 to 70 nm (Fig. 441–1). Some collagens such as those comprising basement membranes or others which are deposited pericellularly, appear amorphous and do not have a banded structure detected by electron microscopy. The collagen molecules of most collagens consist of three polypeptides (α chains) which have a characteristic and unique helical structure determined by the amino acid sequence. The collagen molecules of the interstitial collagens can be solubilized from some tissues. In solution these molecules behave as long, rigid rods with dimensions of approximately 300 × 1.5 nm. Each of the collagen polypeptide chains contains a glycine residue at every third position and is rich in amino acids such as alanine and proline. Collagens contain little phenylalanine and tyrosine and essentially no tryptophan, and, with the exception of type III collagen and the basement membrane collagens, usually lack cysteine in the body of the helical portion.

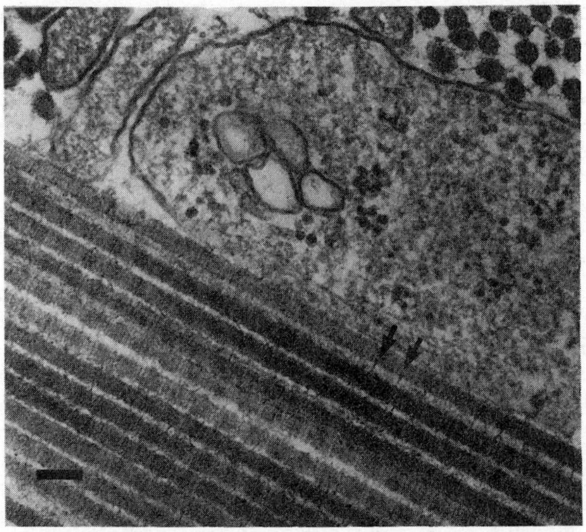

Figure 441–1. Electron micrograph of sections of 17-day-old chick Achilles tendon. Collagen fibrils are seen in longitudinal section in the lower left portion of the figure. These fibrils have a period of ~67 nm, as indicated by the distance between the two arrows. Fibrils seen in cross section at the upper portion of the figure have an average diameter of ~50 nm. Collagen fibers, which are made up of many fibrils, have diameters which range from 0.1 to 15 μm. Bar = 100 nm. (Courtesy of Dr. Romaine Bruns.)

Collagen chains in the course of synthesis also undergo unique post-translational modifications of several component amino acids. The most important of these modifications involves the introduction of a hydroxyl group in the 4 position of specific prolyl residues. The 4-hydroxyproline residues are considered to be responsible for stabilization of the collagen helix. In addition, there is a small amount of 3-hydroxyproline in most collagens, whose function is not known. Specific lysyl residues also are modified by hydroxylation in the 5 position to form hydroxylysine. The hydroxyproline and hydroxylysine of collagens liberated by proteolytic cleavage of the polypeptide chains in the course of physiologic remodeling or pathologic degradation are not reutilized for collagen biosynthesis. Quantitation of the urinary excretion of these amino acids therefore provides some index of collagen turnover. Certain ϵ-amino groups of lysines as well as hydroxylysines are oxidized to their respective aldehydes to form derivatives known as allysines and hydroxyallysines, respectively. Lysine, hyroxylysine, and their derivatives are involved in crosslinking between the chains that constitute the collagen molecules (intramolecular) as well as crosslinking one collagen molecule to another (intermolecular).

In the case of the interstitial collagens the characteristic banding pattern is accounted for by an ordered staggered arrangement of the collagen molecules within the collagen fibrils and the collagen fibers. The manner of molecular packing within the fibril in turn is determined by the amino acid sequence. The way the molecules are staggered in the fibril, however, gives rise to regions in which the molecules overlap and others in which there is no overlap (Fig. 441–2). It is probable that the mineral phase of bone is deposited predominantly within the voids or holes of the nonoverlap region. The

TABLE 441–1. GENETICALLY DISTINCT MAJOR TYPES OF COLLAGEN

Type	Chains	Form	Major Tissues
I	α1, α2	$[\alpha 1(I)]_2 2$	Bone, dermis, tendon fascia, arteries, parenchyma
I	α1	$[\alpha 1(I)]_3$	Embryo tendons
II	α1	$[\alpha 1(II)]_3$	Hyaline cartilage
III	α1	$[\alpha 1(III)]_3$	Dermis, arteries, uterus, parenchyma
IV	α1, α2	?	Basement membranes
V	α1, α2, α3 (A, B, C)	?	Basement membranes, pericellular, placenta, muscle

macromolecular structure of type IV collagen, the major fibrillar component of basement membranes, is very different from that of the interstitial collagens. Type IV collagen structure consists of a network of individual 390 nm-long molecules that are aggregated and crosslinked via identical ends to form a distinctive lattice.

These proteins with structural homologies make up the collagen family. The different homologous species are referred to as types, with each type the product of a different (nonallelic) genetic locus. The five most common and best characterized collagen types are listed in Table 441–1. These types do not have a unique tissue distribution, although some tissues are characterized by a marked predominance of one type—e.g., type II collagen in cartilage and type I collagen in bone. It is likely that each of these collagen types is largely responsible for the functional and morphologic properties of each connective tissue, although it has not yet been possible to relate function to a particular chemical modification. In addition to those types listed in Table 441–1, there are other less abundant collagens (at least five more types) described and partially characterized, each the product of a different gene. These include intima, long chain, endothelial cell, high molecular weight, and short chain collagens.

There is considerable information concerning the pathways of synthesis of various collagens. Even the genes from several animal species for the component polypeptide chains of several collagen types have been partially characterized, illustrating the enormous progress that has been made in the study of these molecules. Although the chains of the interstitial collagen molecules contain approximately 1000 amino acids, and the procollagen precursor contains additional polypeptide sequences at either end which would require a messenger RNA of approximately 4500 bases, the genes coding for each of the proα1 and proα2 chains have a length of approximately 38,000 bases. The enormous size of the genes is due to the presence of approximately 50 intervening DNA sequences (introns), which do not code for amino acid sequences of the mature collagen chains. A possible sequence of events in the course of synthesis of the collagen molecule is shown in Table 441–2. Further complexities are illustrated by the finding that, in the case of type I collagen, the genes coding for the constituent chains are not even on the same chromosome. In humans, the gene for the α1 chain is on chromosome 17 and that for the α2 chain on chromosome 7.

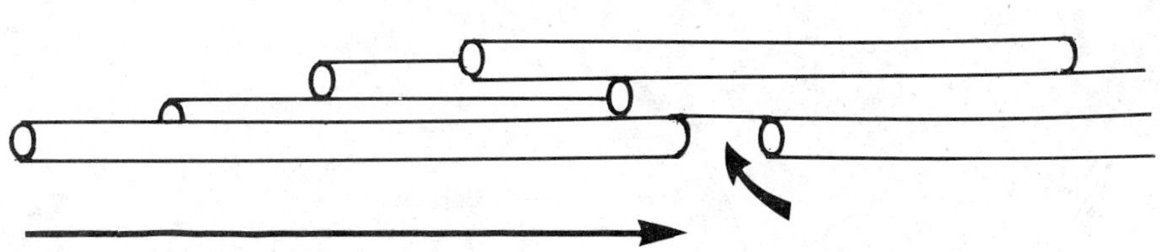

Figure 441–2. A model of the packing of the collagen molecules within the collagen fibril. The molecules, each consisting of three helical polypeptide chains, are depicted as long rigid rods and represented here by the cylinders. The length of the molecules is indicated by the long arrow. The structure gives rise to regions where adjacent molecules are in contact and others in which there are holes, indicated by the short arrow. It is suggested that the inorganic crystals of bone are located predominantly in these holes.

TABLE 441–2. SEQUENCE OF CELLULAR COLLAGEN BIOSYNTHESIS

1. Transcription of the gene for each collagen chain
2. Processing of collagen messenger RNA by removing ~ 50 noncoding sequences
3. Initiation of polypeptide α chain synthesis by formation of hydrophobic amino terminal leader sequence, followed by assembly of proregion and helix
4. Hydroxylation of prolyl residues begins on nascent chains
5. Hydroxylation of lysyl residues
6. Glycosylation of hydroxylysyl residues
7. Formation of –S–S– bonds at carboxyterminal extension
8. Formation of triple helix
9. Packaging for secretion
10. Amino terminal extension cleavage
11. Carboxyterminal extension cleavage
12. Formation of microfibril
13. Lysyl and hydroxylysyl oxidation
14. Formation of reducible crosslinks
15. Maturation and growth
16. Further crosslinking and interaction with other components

Despite the complexity of this synthetic process, there are several heritable disorders of connective tissue in which it is possible to demonstrate abnormalities in biosynthesis. Defects in synthesis of a particular type of collagen, type III collagen, have been demonstrated in a form of the Ehlers-Danlos syndrome (type IV), characterized by tissue friability and rupture of viscera and major blood vessels. Defects in hydroxylation of lysine have also been noted, which gives rise to another clinical form (type VI) of the Ehlers-Danlos syndrome. In addition, defects in processing of the procollagens have been demonstrated (Ehlers-Danlos syndrome type VII) as well as problems with crosslinking accounted for by failure to oxidize critical lysine and hydroxylysine residues (certain forms of cutis laxa). Insufficient synthesis of type I collagen has also been found in certain forms of osteogenesis imperfecta, particularly the classic dominant variety of moderate severity, associated with deafness and blue sclerae. In other cases of osteogenesis imperfecta, which fall into a different clinical and genetic grouping, additions or deletions of portions of the coding region for the procollagen extensions or the helical portions have been described. In one extraordinary case, no α2 chains are present in skin and bone nor are such chains secreted by fibroblasts. The defect lies in a portion of the extension peptides that does not permit normal assembly of the procollagen trimer. Thus, absence of α2 chains is not lethal; trimers of α1 chains can be formed.

Other major components of connective tissues include the *high molecular weight carbohydrates* that make up the so-called ground substance of the interfibrillar matrix. These macromolecules, formerly known as mucopolysaccharides, are composed of a glycosaminoglycan portion (the complex carbohydrate itself) linked to a core protein. The core protein with the glycosaminoglycans attached is termed the proteoglycan subunit. In articular cartilage, proteoglycans constitute approximately half the dry weight of the tissue. Another abundant complex carbohydrate present in many tissues and the major polysaccharide of synovial fluid is hyaluronic acid. The complex carbohydrates of cartilage are composed of high molecular weight polymers of the proteoglycan subunits, with the polysaccharide side chains of chondroitin sulfate and keratan sulfate linked to serine residues of the core protein. The polymeric components consist of these proteoglycan subunits bound to high molecular weight hyaluronic acid chains through interactions with another glycoprotein, called link protein. These proteoglycan aggregates are envisioned as occupying the spaces in cartilage surrounded by the collagen fibers and other components of the matrix. Both the proteoglycans and the collagens are synthesized by the articular chondrocytes.

In general, the cells of the connective tissues interact with the complex carbohydrates and the collagen fibers through glycoproteins, which are probably specific for each type of connective tissue. For example, the cell membranes of epithelial cells interact with a glycoprotein known as laminin, which by interacting with type IV collagen, a unique heparan sulfate glycoprotein, and another protein, nidinogen, together make up the structure of the basement membrane. Many connective tissue and other cells interact with collagens through the protein fibronectin. A protein similar to cellular fibronectin also circulates in plasma where it is known as cold insoluble globulin. Chondrocytes interact with their extracellular matrix through another glycoprotein called chondronectin.

STRUCTURE AND FUNCTION OF JOINTS. The structure and characteristics of the diarthrodial joints are determined by the

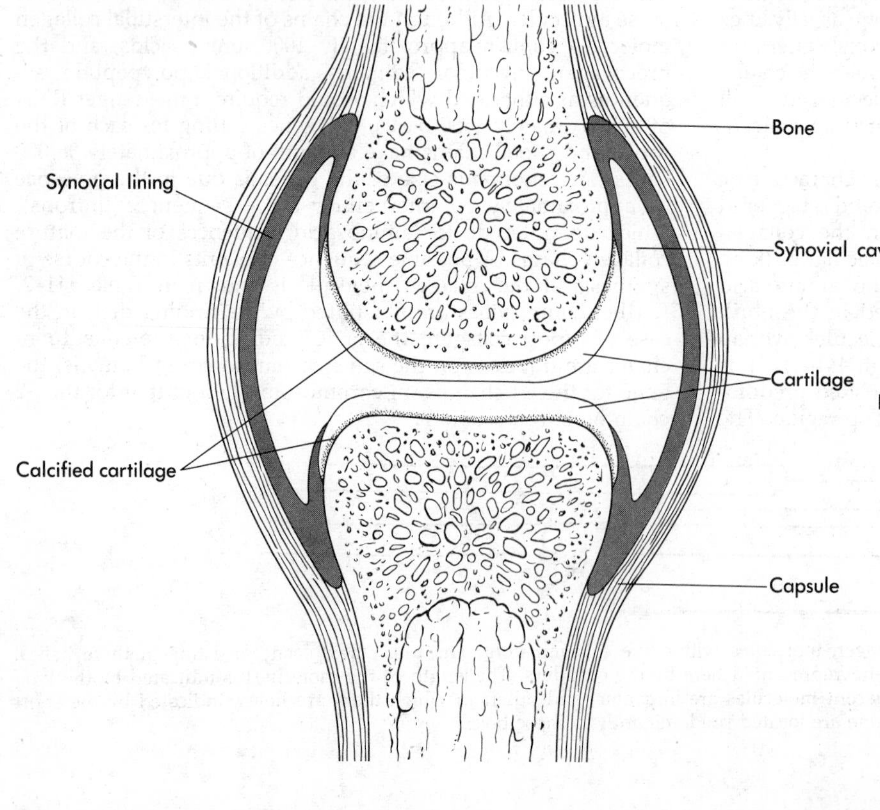

Figure 441–3. A schematic view of a diarthrodial joint.

function of specific cells which produce unique extracellular matrices. A typical joint such as that depicted schematically in Figure 441–3 has its characteristic components. The joint is ideally suited for the demands of weight bearing and motion, which must be operational with a minimum of wear over the lifetime of the individual. The functional properties of the joint are dependent upon a compressible, deformable cartilaginous surface which is properly lubricated and supported by relatively rigid subchondral bone. The stability of the joint, in turn, is determined by the connective tissue structure of the joint capsule, tendons, and ligaments, and is influenced by function of muscles concerned with movement or support of that joint. The joint cavity is lined by a synovial membrane, which normally consists of one or two layers of cells. Some tendency to piling up of the cells is observed at the margins of the joint where the synovium is reflected. The synovial lining cells are derived from connective tissue (they are not epithelial) and do not rest on a continuous basement membrane. In the normal synovium, at least two types of cells have been recognized. The type A cell is a phagocytic cell possibly related to macrophages; the type B cell is fibroblast-like.

The joint cavity contains a characteristic synovial fluid. Its high viscosity is due to the presence of hyaluronic acid, which is probably synthesized by the synovial lining B cells. Water, electrolytes, and some low molecular weight serum proteins such as albumin are derived by filtration from the subsynovial capillaries. Glucose and electrolytes are present in normal synovial fluid at concentrations similar to those in plasma. In inflammation of the synovium, glucose entry is impaired and utilization increased to account for the lower synovial fluid glucose concentrations in some forms of arthritis, such as rheumatoid and septic arthritis. The concentration of proteins in normal synovial fluid is inversely proportional to their molecular weights. Albumin is therefore the most abundant protein. Plasma α_2-macroglobulin, IgM, and fibrinogen are essentially excluded from normal fluids, possibly owing to molecular sieving effects of the hyaluronic acid in the interstitial regions of the synovium and the synovial fluid. In joint inflammation, there is increased entry of the high molecular weight proteins into the synovial fluid. These pathologic fluids may thus form a *fibrin* clot, whereas normal fluids do not. This is to be distinguished from the so-called *mucin* clot, which is composed of a protein–hyaluronic acid complex, which can be produced by the addition of dilute acetic acid to synovial fluid. A tight, ropy mucin clot is characteristic of normal or traumatic fluids, whereas inflammatory fluids tend to produce a fragmented clot or a dispersed sediment upon addition of acetic acid. The clinical diagnostic usefulness of the mucin clot test is not uniformly accepted, however.

The cartilage of the diarthrodial joint is avascular, and the chondrocytes must receive their nourishment from the synovial fluid; products of their metabolism are in turn disposed of through the synovial fluid. The function of the articular cartilage is critically dependent upon the interaction of the fibrillar collagenous matrix and the proteoglycans. By virtue of the highly negative charge on the proteoglycans, these molecules occupy a large domain. The extent to which articular cartilage is deformed on compression and the ability of the cartilage to regain its shape following release from compression is determined by interactions of the proteoglycan aggregates with the fibrillar matrix. It is envisioned that alternate compression and relaxation of the cartilage during motion and weight bearing are responsible for movement of fluid and electrolytes in and out of the cartilage interstitium and provide a mechanism for the nutrition of the chondrocytes. The properties of articular cartilage with its surface in contact with synovial fluid account for the extraordinarily low coefficient of friction upon movement of the joint. The viscous hyaluronic acid which serves a lubricating function for the synovial membrane is probably not responsible for lubrication of the articular cartilage itself. Other components such as lubricating glycoproteins interact with components on the surface of the articular cartilage, providing a so-called boundary type of lubrication. The very fact that the cartilage is capable of deforming under load and regaining its shape following release of the load also contributes to the low coefficient of friction of moving joints. This elastic, spongy nature of cartilage allows it to weep fluid when squeezed under high loads, which, in part, creates a film of lubrication at the head of the moving surfaces. It is also postulated that the highly ordered structure of the cancellous bone supporting the articular cartilage dissipates the shock of impact under loading and permits some of the mechanical forces to be dispersed away from the articular cartilage.

ALTERATION OF STRUCTURE AND FUNCTION OF JOINTS IN DISEASE. When joints are subjected to mechanical or chemical trauma, there are several predictable responses that occur in the articular cartilage and surrounding structures. Repeated mechanical trauma is associated with loss or decrease of the proteoglycan of the cartilage matrix, which can be appreciated histologically as a loss of the staining properties (e.g., metachromasia) attributed to this component. The mechanism for the proteoglycan loss probably involves the secretion of proteolytic enzymes, by the chondrocytes or by cells in the synovial fluid or the synovial lining, which, at neutral pH, cleave the core protein of the proteoglycans near the linkage region with the hyaluronic acid. Following cleavage of the core protein, the partially degraded proteoglycan is leached from the matrix. Alterations of this type have been observed following arthrotomy or bleeding into the joint. Since the articular chondrocytes have the capacity to resynthesize proteoglycans, if the mechanical injury is only temporary, some structure of the matrix can be restored. However, persistent deficiency of cartilage proteoglycan is accompanied by alteration in mechanical properties of the matrix manifested by an increased tendency of the cartilage to deform under load and a decreased ability to regain form following removal of the load. Only late in the course of injury is the collagenous component of the matrix affected. Although articular chondrocytes have retained the capacity for replication and to increase, often in clusters, in response to chronic injury, these cells have a limited capacity to resynthesize type II collagen and reconstitute the normal fibrillar matrix. The proliferation of cartilage cells in response to trauma and mechanical stress may also be followed by vascularization and activation of the endochondral sequence, resulting in formation of osteophytes, usually at the margin of joints. Trauma may also produce reactions in the synovium, probably mediated by altered vascularization in addition to increased numbers and activity of the synovial lining cells. These synovial reactions may in turn result in the formation of increased synovial fluid, manifested clinically as effusions. The composition of these synovial fluids closely resembles that of normal synovial fluid with respect to viscosity (the concentration of hyaluronic acid) and the type and relative concentration of the protein components (predominance of albumin and absence of high molecular weight plasma proteins such as fibrinogen, IgM, and α_2-macroglobulin). Thus, a mild degree of "synovitis" may be a component of either acute or chronic injury. Under these circumstances, however, few cells (100 to 500 per cubic millimeter) are present in the synovial fluid; lymphocytes and monocytes predominate, whereas polymorphonuclear leukocytes are scarce.

In almost all types of joint inflammation, however, whether acute, as in urate gout or pseudogout (calcium pyrophosphate deposition disease), or chronic, as in typical rheumatoid arthritis, there is an exudation of cells, particularly polymorphonulear leukocytes, into the synovial cavity. In these inflammatory joint diseases, the synovial fluid usually is characterized by a decreased viscosity, an inability to form a normal tight mucin clot, and an increased concentration relative to normal of macromolecules such as immunoglobulin, α_2-macroglobulin, and fibrinogen. Enzymes released from the inflammatory cells have the capacity to degrade the proteoglycan core protein and collagen of the articular cartilage and surrounding structures if their concentrations (activities) exceed those of inhibitors present in synovial fluid and synovial tissues.

The synovitis seen, for example, in rheumatoid arthritis may be particularly intense with chronic inflammatory cells present, especially at the margins of the joint where the synovial membrane is reflected. With persistent synovial inflammation, a mass of proliferating cells (pannus) may burrow beneath the articular cartilage and subchondral bone or appear to work its way over the surface of the articular cartilage, degrading matrix structures in its wake. These degradative processes are probably mediated by enzymes such as specific collagenases and elastase-like proteases capable of attacking matrix components. Alterations also occur in the subchondral bone in joint disease. In the noninflammatory forms, the subchondral bone may increase in mass by new bone formation (sclerosis). In contrast, in inflammatory joint disease, subchondral bone is frequently resorbed, producing the typical radiologic appearance of juxta-articular osteoporosis. Diaphyseal cortical bone is usually not thinned until late in rheumatoid disease; in some subjects, it may even be increased in thickness owing to periosteal new bone formation. When the inflammation subsides, bony erosions may heal, and some restoration of the diffuse juxta-articular bone loss may also occur. Defects or clefts in articular cartilage, on the other hand, generally do not heal with restoration of the original form because of the limited capacity of chondrocytes to resynthesize the specific collagenous fibrillar component of extracellular matrix.

Each of the extracellular components of the matrix of the joint structures has its unique pattern of composition with respect to the collagen type, proteoglycan, and glycoprotein component. The composition of these matrices must in turn determine their function. Return of function with healing of disease therefore requires restoration of the original composition, which, in turn, is dependent upon the ability of the tissue to undergo remodeling. The limited capacity for remodeling of some tissues, such as articular cartilage, therefore accounts for disability in several of the rheumatic diseases. Thus, in instances in which structure is sufficiently distorted and return of function impossible, the only alternative may be to use the artificial surfaces of joint prostheses to permit or regain motion and weight-bearing capacity and to alleviate pain.

Bornstein P, Sage H: Structurally distinct collagen types. Ann Rev Biochem 49:957, 1980. *The material discussed in this review complements that considered by Eyre and by Prockop et al.*

Brandt KD: Glycosaminoglycans. *In* Kelley WN, Harris ED Jr, Ruddy S, Sledge CB (eds.): Textbook of Rheumatology. Philadelphia, W. B. Saunders Company, 1981, pp 239–254. *This review on glycosaminoglycans extends and updates that of Lindahl and Höök.*

Eyre DR: Collagen: Molecular diversity in the body's protein scaffold. Science 207:1315, 1980. *An updated review of collagen structure and biosynthesis.*

Harris ED Jr: Biology of the joint. *In* Kelley WN, Harris ED Jr, Ruddy S, Sledge CB (eds.): Textbook of Rheumatology. Philadelphia, W. B. Saunders Company, 1981, pp 255–276. *A consideration of joint development, structure, and function as well as mechanisms proposed to account for the lubricating properties of joints. The formation of synovial fluid and its functions are also described.*

Hollister DW, Byers PH, Holbrook KA: Genetic disorders of collagen metabolism. Adv Human Genet 12:1, 1982. *A complete review of heritable disorders of collagen metabolism.*

Krane SM: Mechanisms of tissue destruction in rheumatoid arthritis. *In* McCarty DJ (ed.): Arthritis and Allied Conditions. A Textbook of Rheumatology. Philadelphia, Lea and Febiger, 1984. *A discussion relating the histologic features to the connective tissue degradation in rheumatoid arthritis.*

Kühn K: Chemical properties of collagen. *In* Furthmayr H (ed.): Immunochemistry of the Extracellular Matrix. Vol I. Methods. Boca Raton, CRC Press, 1982, pp 1–28. *Concepts of collagen composition as it relates to organization of the molecules in tissues are well-documented.*

Lindahl U, Höök M: Glycosaminoglycans and their binding to biological macromolecules. Ann Rev Biochem 47:385, 1978. *A review of the structure of the complex carbohydrates and their interactions with intracellular and extracellular macromolecules.*

Merlino GT, McKeon C, de Crombrugghe B, Pastan I: Regulation of the expression of genes encoding types I, II, and III collagen during chick embryonic development. J Biol Chem 258:10041, 1983. *A modern study of the regulation of collagen gene expression in which references to other applications are also given.*

Nimni M: Collagen: Structure, function and metabolism in normal and fibrotic tissues. Semin Arthritis Rheum 13:1, 1983. *A well-referenced review of collagen structure with particular attention to abnormalities in disease.*

Piez K, Reddi AH: Extracellular Matrix Biochemistry. New York, Elsevier-North Holland, 1984. *A comprehensive treatise on collagen biochemistry and metabolism as well as discussions of alterations in heritable and acquired diseases.*

Prockop DJ, Kivirikko KI, Tuderman L, Guzman N: The biosynthesis of collagen and its disorders. N Engl J Med 301:13,77, 1979. *A good review of what is known about the details of collagen biosynthesis and how this is disordered in certain diseases.*

Tsipouras P, Myers JC, Ramirez F, Prockop DJ: Restriction fragment length polymorphism associated with the proα2 (I) gene of human type I procollagen. J Clin Invest 72:1262, 1983. *An example of the kind of investigations that are currently being conducted in human beings using probes for the collagen genes.*

Wuepper KD, Holbrook KA, Pinnell SR, Vitto J: Supplemental issue: Structural elements of the dermis. J Invest Derm 79(Suppl 1):1, 1982. *Short reviews on most aspects of connective tissue function including adherence glycoproteins, elastic fibers, and proteoglycans.*

Yamada KM: Cell surface interactions with extracellular materials. Ann Rev Biochem 52:761, 1983. *Detailed discussion of how cells interact with the matrices in their environment with particular emphasis on fibronectin and laminin.*

442. MECHANISMS OF INFLAMMATION AND TISSUE DESTRUCTION IN THE RHEUMATIC DISEASES

Ralph Snyderman

Immunologic processes mediate the localization and rapid destruction of substances which, if disseminated, could disrupt the host's complex internal milieu. The immune system has several unique features which permit it to combat microbial invasion and provide resistance against the development and spread of cancer. Unlike other tissues, it consists not only of fixed structures (i.e., thymus, spleen, and lymph nodes) but also of motile cells which wander throughout the body, performing surveillance. It is also the only tissue which is able to destroy other components of the host. Both the protective and destructive abilities of immunologic processes relate largely to their inflammatory potential. Understanding how inflammation is initiated is thus essential for understanding the mechanisms of immunologically mediated resistance and for comprehending how tissue destruction occurs in the rheumatic disorders.

To fulfill its function of host defense, the immune system must differentiate self from nonself and then rapidly destroy substances recognized as nonself. An orderly progression of immunologic recognition, amplification of the immune reaction, accumulation of inflammatory cells, and finally destruction of the inciting agent is ordinarily an ongoing subclinical process. Inflammatory reactions can be initiated by either specific or nonspecific means (Table 442–1). Recognition of unique determinants (epitopes) on antigens by antibodies or by receptors on small lymphocytes initiates immunologically mediated in-

TABLE 442–1. COMPONENTS OF THE INFLAMMATORY RESPONSE

Function	Mediator
Recognition	
Specific	Immunoglobulins
	Lymphocytes
Nonspecific	Macrophages*
	Polymorphonuclear leukocytes
	Alternative complement pathway
	Hageman factor
Amplification	Complement
	Cytokines—lymphokines, monokines
	Kinin-forming system
	Arachidonic acid metabolites
	Mast cell products
Destruction of antigen	Macrophages
	Polymorphonuclear leukocytes
	Lymphocytes

*Macrophages are also involved in specific recognition since they are required for antigen presentation to lymphocytes.

flammation. Nonspecific recognition can be initiated by components of the immune system which bind to materials based on their charge, hydrophobicity, or lectin composition. Nonspecific recognition is mediated in part by phagocytic cells, such as polymorphonuclear leukocytes and macrophages, as well as by C3b, an initiator of the alternative pathway of the complement system (see Ch. 428), and by Hageman factor.

Following recognition of nonself, amplification systems are activitated and lead to the production of mediators of inflammation. The type of amplifier involved depends upon the recognition component and the nature and location of the inciting material. Amplification components of the immune system such as complement cleavage products, cytokines, and other phlogistic factors magnify the initial response to nonself. Inflammatory reactions can also be initiated by nonimmunologic means. For example, inflammation following tissue necrosis results from the direct cleavage of complement components by lysosomal proteases released by injured cells. This phenomenon may play a role in extending cardiac tissue damage following myocardial infarction. In gout or pseudogout, inflammation follows the phagocytosis, by polymorphonuclear leukocytes, of monosodium urate or calcium pyrophosphate dihydrate crystals. Ingestion of these agents by leukocytes leads to the release of lysosomal hydrolases as well as the synthesis of chemotactic factors, which attract other inflammatory cells into the joint.

Regardless of the type of inflammatory response, the accumulation of granulocytes and macrophages can result in the phagocytosis and degradation of the material that initiated the inflammatory event. The factors which determine whether an inflammatory response will be protective or destructive are poorly understood. They depend in part upon the nature and location of the inciting agent as well as its quantity and digestibility. The genetic makeup and the immunoregulatory competency of the host are also important. In general, when the antigen or other inciting agent is rapidly disposed of, the inflammatory process is protective and self-limited. When antigen persists or is excessive in amount, the inflammatory response can be locally destructive and become clinically apparent.

RHEUMATOID SYNOVITIS AS A MODEL OF INFLAMMATORY-MEDIATED TISSUE DESTRUCTION

A chronic, locally destructive inflammatory reaction in humans is exemplified by the synovitis present in some connective tissue disorders. The prototype disease is rheumatoid arthritis. The diarthrodial joint has several features that influence inflammatory processes which occur there. The synovial membrane is highly vascular and lines all intra-articular structures, except for cartilage. The synovial lining is devoid of a basement membrane and thus permits relatively free diffusion of soluble substances. Moreover, the synovium lines a closed cavity, the joint space; therefore any reactive materials gaining entrance to the joint space are difficult to remove.

Normal synovium is a thin layer of tissue whose lining is composed of two principal cell types supported by a loose connective tissue stroma (Fig. 442–1*A*). The Type A cell is rich in surface pseudopodia, and its cytoplasm has many lysosomes and prominent Golgi complexes but little rough endoplasmic reticulum. Type A synoviocytes have many characteristics of macrophages and are phagocytic, but ultrastructural studies have implied a secretory role for these cells as well. The Type B synoviocyte exhibits prominent rough endoplasmic reticulum, but few vacuoles, lysosomes, or cell processes. This cell is primarily a secretory cell, hyaluronic acid being an important product. Synoviocytes may, however, be multipotential, with their morphology reflecting the net result of stimuli present in the local milieu. Beneath the synovial membrane there are collagen fibrils, fatty tissue, and an extensive capillary network. Fibroblasts in this area produce Types I and III collagen. Lastly, the dense fibrous joint capsule provides a support for the

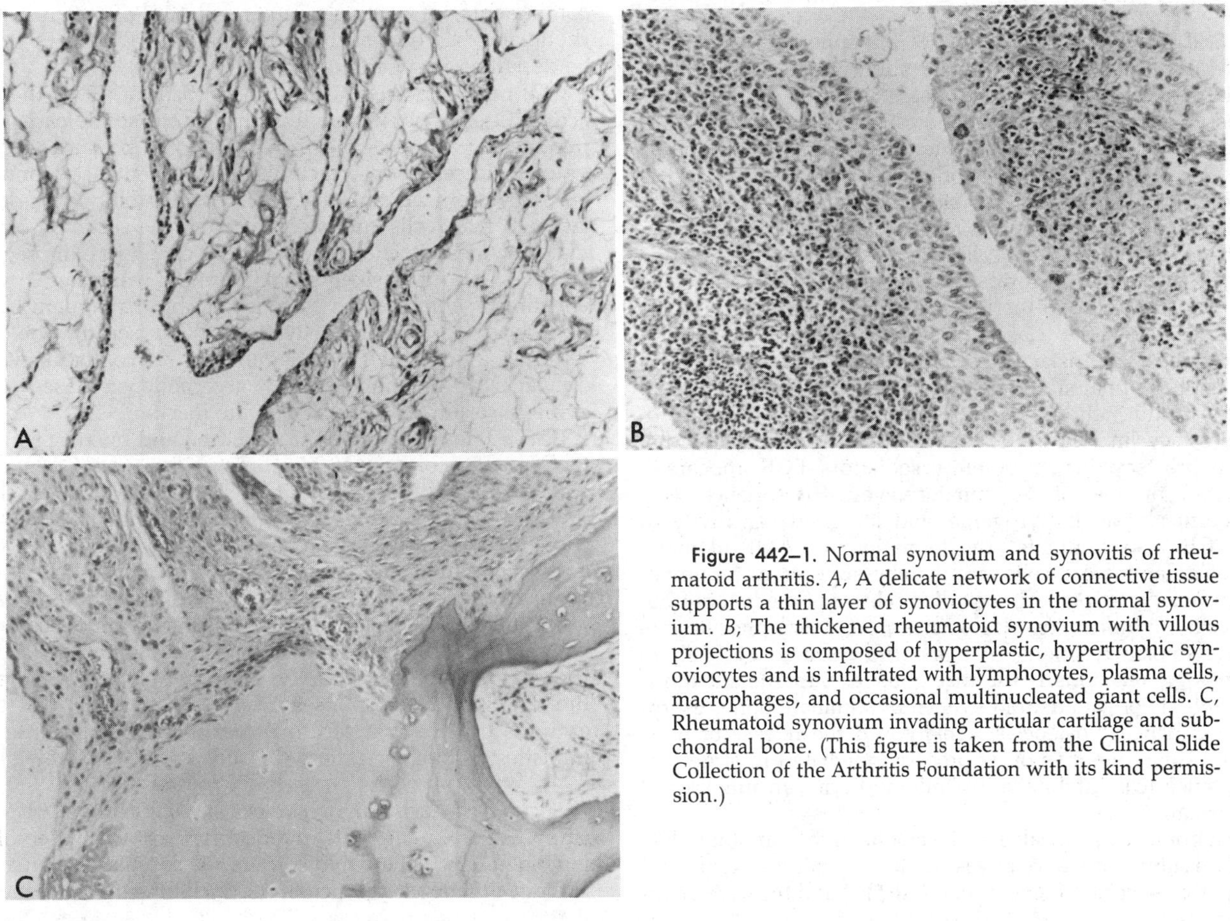

Figure 442–1. Normal synovium and synovitis of rheumatoid arthritis. *A*, A delicate network of connective tissue supports a thin layer of synoviocytes in the normal synovium. *B*, The thickened rheumatoid synovium with villous projections is composed of hyperplastic, hypertrophic synoviocytes and is infiltrated with lymphocytes, plasma cells, macrophages, and occasional multinucleated giant cells. *C*, Rheumatoid synovium invading articular cartilage and subchondral bone. (This figure is taken from the Clinical Slide Collection of the Arthritis Foundation with its kind permission.)

synovial lining membrane and separates the articular space from surrounding structures.

Rheumatoid synovitis exhibits three main components: inflammation, proliferation, and infiltration. In early stages, both Types A and B cells proliferate and increase in size. Fibrin deposits are frequently present on the inner synovial lining. Polymorphonuclear leukocytes predominate in the synovial fluid exudate, but cells are seen as infiltrates only in the superficial synovial layer. The supporting stroma beneath the lining cell layer becomes edematous and develops an increase in the number of small blood vessels. Concurrently, there are focal accumulations of inflammatory cells consisting of lymphocytes, plasma cells, macrophages, and occasionally mast cells. If the inflammatory synovitis persists, a proliferative lesion develops, characterized by synovial membrane thickening and projection of villous formations into the articular cavity (Fig. 442–1*B*). There is a concomitant increase in supporting connective tissue, small blood vessels, mononuclear cell infiltrates, and occasional multinucleated giant cells, as well as increased numbers of undifferentiated mesenchyme-like cells which have both phagocytic and synthetic potential. As the proliferative lesions progress, infiltration of surrounding structures develop as the fibrous-mesenchymal tissue (pannus) begins to invade and replace cartilage and bone at the periphery of the synovial reflection (Fig. 442–1*C*). The invasion of cartilage, subchondral bone, and tendon by inflammatory synovial tissue results in collagen destruction, degradation of proteoglycans in the cartilage matrix, and bony resorption.

MEDIATORS OF INFLAMMATION THAT PARTICIPATE IN THE RHEUMATIC DISEASES

Inflammatory reactions result from the local production of a number of mediators derived from humoral or cellular sources. A complex interplay of activation and suppression mechanisms modulates the type and magnitude of the inflammatory response which develops.

ARACHIDONIC ACID METABOLITES. Phospholipids are major constituents of cell membranes, including those of leukocytes and platelets, and are subject to degradation by cellular phospholipases under certain conditions such as exposure of cells to inflammatory or noxious stimuli. Cleavage of phospholipids results in the release of arachidonic acid, which can be further metabolized into a number of biologically potent mediators and modulators of inflammation. Prostaglandins (PG) are synthesized from arachidonic acid following the action of the enzyme cyclo-oxygenase, which forms PGG_2, which is then reduced to PGH_2. Depending upon the isomerase enzymes present in the particular tissue, the classic prostaglandins (PGE_2, $PGF_{2\alpha}$), thromboxanes, or prostacyclins will be formed. Leukocytes and explants of rheumatoid synovia produce predominantly PGE_2, platelets produce thromboxane A_2, and endothelial cells produce prostacyclin. Thromboxanes are potent vasoconstrictors, whereas prostacyclins are potent vasodilators. PGE_2 appears to modulate a number of inflammatory events. It enhances vascular permeability, is pyrogenic, and increases sensitivity to pain. PGE_2 also stimulates the formation of cAMP in many types of inflammatory cells and thereby suppresses a number of immunologic responses, including release of mediators from mast cells, lymphocyte blastogenesis, and lymphocyte-mediated cytotoxic reactions. An important source of PGE_2 in immunologic reactions is the macrophage. Supernatant fluids from explants of rheumatoid synovium stimulate bone resorption by enhancing osteoclast activity and the release of bone calcium. This phenomenon is probably mediated in large part by PG since it is inhibitable by indomethacin, an inhibitor of their formation.

Arachidonic acid can also be metabolized into another class of biologically active derivatives by the enzyme lipoxygenase. The hydroxy-eicosatetraenoic acids (HETEs) and the derivatives of 5-hydroperoxy-eicosatetraenoic acid (termed leukotrienes) are examples of these arachidonic acid metabolites and are synthesized by granulocytes, macrophages, and basophils. 5,12-HETE, also termed leukotriene B_4 (LTB_4), is a potent chemotactic factor, whereas leukotrienes C and D stimulate bronchoconstriction. LTB_4 has been identified in the synovial effusions of patients with rheumatoid arthritis and ankylosing spondylitis. Large amounts of LTB_4 are produced when granulocytes phagocytize monosidium urate crystals. This chemoattractant may, therefore, be important in the pathogenesis of gouty inflammation.

BIOLOGICALLY ACTIVE AMINES, HISTAMINE, AND SEROTONIN. Histamine is derived from the decarboxylation of histidine by the enzyme L-histidine decarboxylase. The majority of histamine is stored in mast cells and basophils and is complexed with mucopolysaccharides such as heparin. Stimulation of mast cells and basophils by a number of mechanisms causes secretion of histamine. This agent has diverse biologic activities, including constricting smooth muscle, enhancing vascular permeability, depressing leukocyte chemotaxis, blocking T lymphocyte function, and depressing further histamine release from mast cells and basophils. Histamine thus may modulate both acute and chronic inflammatory responses. Serotonin (5-hydroxytryptamine) is produced by the decarboxylation of 5-hydroxytryptophan. More than 90 per cent of body stores of serotonin are found in the gastrointestinal tract and the central nervous system; the remainder is present in the dense granules of platelets. The biologic role of serotonin in inflammation is not well understood, but it enhances the chemotactic responses of leukocytes and increases fibroblast growth in vitro. It also stimulates collagen formation.

BIOLOGICALLY ACTIVE PEPTIDES. ***Complement Cleavage Products.*** The complement (C) system functions as an important amplifier of inflammatory events initiated by immunoglobulins IgG and IgM as well as inflammatory reactions initiated by release of hydrolytic enzymes from traumatized cells or by leukocytes. The biology and biochemistry of this complex series of proteins are described in Ch. 428. Two complement cleavage products, C3a and C5a, derived from the third and fifth C components, respectively, are mediators of inflammation in rheumatic disorders such as rheumatoid arthritis and will thus be described in greater detail here.

C3a: Enzymatic cleavage of the α chain of C3 by the earlier-acting C components or by other proteases releases C3a, a peptide consisting of 77 amino acids. C3a mediates a number of biologic responses, including smooth muscle contraction, vasodilatation, enhanced vascular permeability, the degranulation of mast cells and basophils, and the secretion of lysosomal enzymes by leukocytes. C3a also has immunoregulatory effects and suppresses humoral immune responses in vitro by affecting T lymphocytes. C3a is the most abundant of the C peptides released upon activation of C in serum. The COOH-terminal arginine of C3a is required for its biologic activity, and cleavage of this amino acid by a carboxypeptidase-B–like enzyme in serum renders the peptide inactive.

C5a: C5a has a number of structural and biologic similarities to C3a. C5a consists of 74 amino acids, the COOH-terminal constituent also being arginine. C5a is derived from cleavage of the α chain of C5. In addition to having all the biologic activities of C3a, C5a is also an extremely potent chemoattractant for polymorphonuclear leukocytes, monocytes, and macrophages. C5a is the major source of chemotactic activity generated in serum treated with immune complexes or endotoxin and is also an important source of chemotactic activity in rheumatoid synovial fluids. In contrast to C3a, C5a potentiates humoral immune responses in vitro. Cleavage of the terminal arginine of C5a by a serum carboxypeptidase-B markedly diminishes its biologic activity but does not completely abrogate it.

Eosinophil Chemotactic Factors of Anaphylaxis (ECF-A). Eosinophil accumulation is characteristic of a number of rheumatologic and allergic disorders. Basophils and mast cells contain inflammatory mediators, including two tetrapeptides,

Val-Gly-Ser-Glu and Ala-Gly-Ser-Glu. Both of these substances are chemoattractants for eosinophils and to a lesser degree for neutrophils.

Crystal-Induced Chemotactic Factors. Leukocytes accumulate in the synovial fluid of individuals with gout or pseudogout following the ingestion by neutrophils of monosodium urate or calcium pyrophosphate dihydrate crystals, respectively. Incubation of neutrophils with these crystals in vitro results in the production by the cells of LTB_4 and a polypeptide chemoattractant with a molecular weight of 8400. The production of these chemoattractants are blocked by colchicine. A mechanism by which colchicine abrogates acute gouty arthritis may be its ability to inhibit the synthesis of chemoattractants by neutrophils.

Kinin-Forming System. An intimate association exists between the activation and regulation of the intrinsic clotting, fibrinolytic, and kinin-forming systems. Hageman factor (HF), factor XII of the clotting system, is central to the activation of all three systems. HF is activated nonspecifically by a number of agents, including exposure to crude preparations of collagen, vascular basement membranes, monosodium urate crystals, calcium pyrophosphate crystals, and endotoxin. Negatively charged surfaces also activate HF. Upon activation, HF (an 80,000 dalton β globulin) is cleaved, and its active form HF_A initiates the conversion of factor XI of the clotting pathway to XIa, and the conversion of prekallikrein to kallikrein. Kallikrein in turn activates plasminogen forming plasmin, an enzyme important in fibrinolysis. Kallikrein also cleaves a serum protein termed high molecular weight kininogen to form bradykinin, a nonapeptide with potent biologic activities. Interestingly, C1 esterase inhibitor (C1INH), a protein which functions as an inhibitor of activated C1, is also an important inhibitor of HF_A and kallikrein. Bradykinin and two other kinins produced by tissue kallikreins from kininogen induce smooth muscle contraction, increase vascular permeability, and induce pain. Cleavage of fibrinogen by plasmin results in the production of a number of products, including fibrinopeptide B, an agent which potentiates the action of bradykinin and has chemotactic activity for neutrophils in vitro.

Interleukins. Interleukins are immunoregulatory molecules synthesized by mononuclear leukocytes. Stimulation of macrophages by antigens as well as by factors from lymphocytes initiates the secretion of interleukin I (IL-1), a 15,000-dalton peptide with diverse biologic activities. Macrophages are required for many of the activities of lymphocytes, and certain of the "helper" functions of macrophages are mediated by IL-1. IL-1 may be identical to a factor termed mononuclear cell factor (MCF) which stimulates synovial cells to produce collagenase. IL-1 may also be identical to leukocytic pyrogen.

Interleukin 2 (IL-2), previously termed T-cell growth factor, is a 15,000-dalton polypeptide produced by T lymphocytes and stimulates the continuous proliferation of activated T lymphocytes in culture. Another class of mediators produced by stimulated lymphocytes is the lymphokines. These are discussed later in this chapter under the heading Inflammatory Reactions Initiated by Mononuclear Leukocytes.

LYSOSOMAL ENZYMES. Lysosomal enzymes are contained in a class of subcellular organelles termed lysosomal granules. One function of these enzymes is digestive in that they break down complex macromolecules. Lysosomal granules also contain antimicrobial constituents such as myeloperoxidase and lactoferrin. Leukocytes contain two types of lysosomal granules based on staining characteristics. These are termed the azurophilic and specific granules. Lysosomal enzymes play an important role in the digestion of antigens following phagocytosis. However, since these enzymes may also be released during phagocytosis or upon cell death, they can cause tissue destruction which sometimes accompanies inflammatory reactions. Lysosomal proteases found in leukocytes include collagenase, elastase, cathepsin D, and cathepsin G. These enzymes are capable of destroying extracellular structures and may thus participate in mediating tissue injury in the rheumatic diseases. Cathepsin D cleaves cartilage proteoglycan, whereas granulocyte collagenase is active in cleaving Type I and, to a lesser degree, Type III collagen substrates found in bone, cartilage, and tendon. The substrates of granulocyte elastase include collagen crosslinkages and proteoglycans, as well as the elastin components of blood vessels, ligaments, and cartilage. Lysosomal hydrolyases are also capable of producing mediators of inflammation through their direct action on C components such as C5, thereby producing C5a. Leukocytic hydrolyases can liberate kinin from kininogen. Plasminogen activator, an enzyme that converts plasminogen to plasmin (which stimulates fibrinolysis) is found in both granulocyte and macrophage lysosomes. Rheumatoid synovial collagenase is usually present as an inactive lysosomal proenzyme which requires plasminogen activator for conversion to its active form.

Regulation of the potent tissue destructive potential of the lysosomal proteases is mediated by protease inhibitors such as α_2 macroglobulin and α_1 antiprotease. These antiproteases are present in serum and in synovial fluids and inhibit protease enzymes by binding to them and covering their active sites.

PHYSIOLOGIC MECHANISMS OF INFLAMMATORY CELL ACCUMULATION

The accumulation of inflammatory cells at sites of antigen is central to the inflammatory process. Polymorphonuclear leukocytes and macrophages are motile cells which have many common physiologic characteristics. Both can perceive gradients of chemoattractant molecules and migrate directionally along such gradients. They also perform endocytosis (ingestion), secrete lysosomal enzymes, and generate superoxide anions (see Ch. 148). Polymorphonuclear leukocytes and macrophages perceive chemotactic factors by means of specific surface receptors. These cells have receptors for synthetic polypeptide chemotactic factors which may be analogous to bacterial products, as well as for C5a, CCF and LTB_4. Binding of chemoattractants to the surface of phagocytes results in orientation of the cells toward the source of the chemotactic gradient. Upon orientation, the cells lose their round configuration and become polarized in shape. The configuration of motile cells is triangular, with the base of the triangle facing toward the chemoattractant gradient (Fig. 442–2). This change in cell shape requires rearrangement of intracellular cytoskeletal elements. Microtubules provide a front-to-back polarization, whereas actin filaments accumulate at the front and back of the cells and provide the contractile forces required for movement. Chemotactic factors can also initiate other cellular responses by leukocytes, such as superoxide anion production and lysosomal enzyme secretion. The concentration of chemotactic factors required to initiate these latter processes approximately ten fold is greater than that required for the induction of chemotaxis. This phenomenon may prevent the release of potentially toxic products from the cells until they arrive at the inflammatory site where the concentration of chemoattractants is the greatest.

The mechanism by which chemotactic factors initiate their biologic responses in phagocytes is not entirely clear at present, but it is known that these factors induce transmembrane fluxes of calcium, sodium, and potassium which alter cellular transmembrane potential. Following exposure to chemotactic factors, there is a transient elevation of cAMP. Arachidonic acid is released from phospholipids in the phagocytic cell membrane through activation of phospholipases. Metabolism of arachidonic acid via enzymatic pathways involving cyclooxygenase and lipoxygenase results in the production of prostaglandins and leukotrienes. Transmethylation reactions mediated by S-adenosylmethionine are required for chemotaxis but methylation of phosphatidylethanolamine is inhibited by chemotactic factors in macrophages. This results in changes in the composition of newly synthesized phospholipids in cells exposed to chemoattractants. Alterations in the phospholipid composition

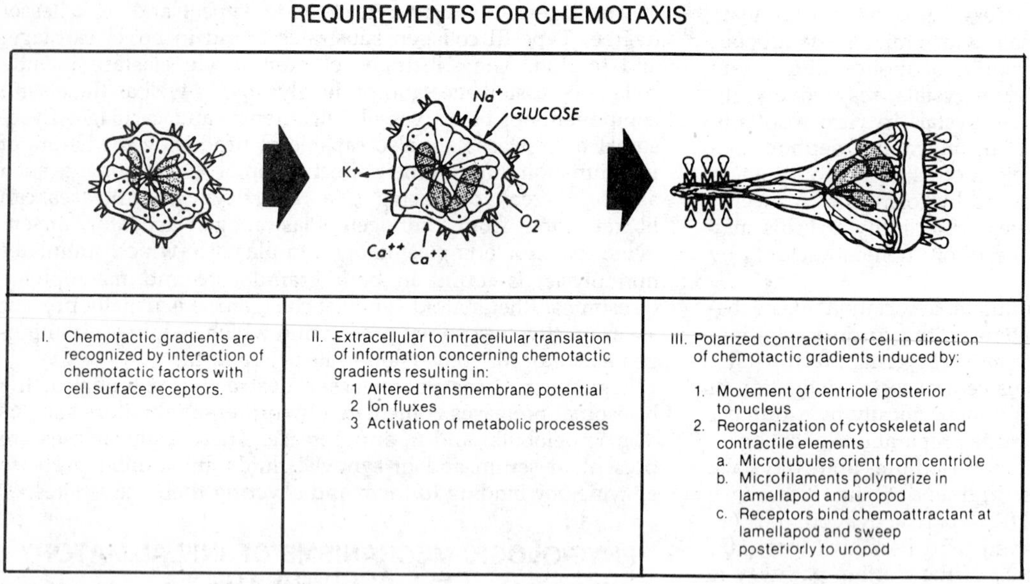

REQUIREMENTS FOR CHEMOTAXIS
Na+
GLUCOSE
K+
O2
Ca++ Ca++
I. Chemotactic gradients are recognized by interaction of chemotactic factors with cell surface receptors.
II. Extracellular to intracellular translation of information concerning chemotactic gradients resulting in:
1 Altered transmembrane potential
2 Ion fluxes
3 Activation of metabolic processes
III. Polarized contraction of cell in direction of chemotactic gradients induced by:
1. Movement of centriole posterior to nucleus
2. Reorganization of cytoskeletal and contractile elements
a. Microtubules orient from centriole
b. Microfilaments polymerize in lamellapod and uropod
c. Receptors bind chemoattractant at lamellapod and sweep posteriorly to uropod

Figure 442–2. The interaction of chemotactic factor receptors with chemotactic factors triggers the indicated cellular responses.

of the membrane at the leading edge of the chemotactically stimulated cells may be important for motility and for the activation of membrane associated enzymes such as protein kinase C. Lymphocytes are also highly motile cells but do not respond to the same chemotactic factors as do polymorphonuclear leukocytes and macrophages. The migration of lymphocytes is stimulated by specific antigens, mitogens, and by as yet undefined factors produced by lymphocytes.

Phagocytosis is initiated by binding of a particle to the surface of phagocytic cells. Particles carrying bound immunoglobulin or the complement fragments C3b or C3bi are more readily phagocytosed since they bind to Fc and C3b receptors on both polymorphonuclear leukocytes and macrophages. However, phagocytosis can occur in the absence of receptor involvement. Particle ingestion results from the envelopment and fusion of phagocytic cell membrane around the foreign material (Fig. 442–3). Intracellular lysosomes migrate to the phagocytic vesicle, fuse with it, and empty their contents, thus forming a phagolysosome. Within the phagolysosome, antigenic digestion and microbial killing generally occur. During the process of phagocytosis, lysosomal hydrolases and toxic oxygen radicals may be released.

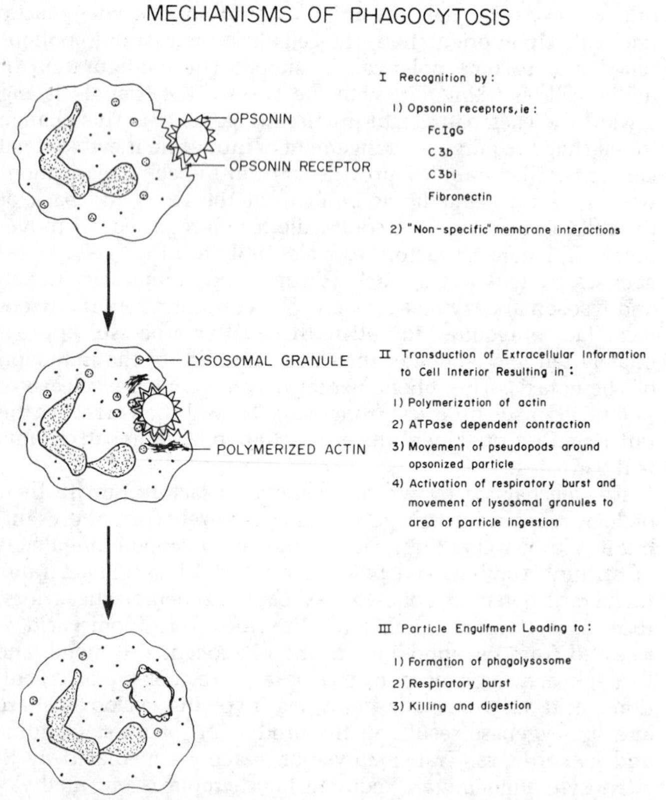

MECHANISMS OF PHAGOCYTOSIS
I Recognition by:
1) Opsonin receptors, ie:
FcIgG
C3b
C3bi
Fibronectin
2) "Non-specific" membrane interactions
OPSONIN
OPSONIN RECEPTOR
LYSOSOMAL GRANULE
POLYMERIZED ACTIN
II Transduction of Extracellular Information to Cell Interior Resulting in:
1) Polymerization of actin
2) ATPase dependent contraction
3) Movement of pseudopods around opsonized particle
4) Activation of respiratory burst and movement of lysosomal granules to area of particle ingestion
III Particle Engulfment Leading to:
1) Formation of phagolysosome
2) Respiratory burst
3) Killing and digestion

Figure 442–3. Requirements for phagocytosis. Particulate antigen binding to the membrane of phagocytic cells initiates cellular responses which lead to envelopment of the antigen. The process is enhanced when the antigens have bound opsonins.

IMMUNOLOGICALLY MEDIATED TISSUE INJURY

Inflammatory responses can produce adverse reactions in the host, ranging from minor local tissue irritation to selective destruction of organs or even sudden death. The nature of immunologically mediated inflammatory responses depends upon the immunologic recognition component which identifies the antigen. Four general types of immunologically mediated inflammatory reactions have been defined (Table 442–2). In clinical and experimental situations it is not infrequent to have more than one, and even all types, of these immune reactions operative simultaneously.

TYPE I REACTIONS: INFLAMMATION INITIATED BY REAGENIC (IgE) ANTIBODIES. IgE antibodies bind to mast cells and basophils by means of their Fc portion, which allows the Fab portion of the molecule to be available for binding to specific antigen. Shortly after the appropriate antigen binds, the cells degranulate and secrete their intracellular products, which include histamine, ECF-A, and heparin. Release of mediators from basophils or mast cells causes an increase in local vascular permeability within seconds and produces vascular stasis and smooth muscle contraction. Type I reactions are responsible for such allergic phenomena as urticaria, seasonal rhinitis, asthma, and systemic anaphylaxis (see Ch. 431 to 434).

TYPE II REACTIONS: TISSUE DESTRUCTION MEDIATED BY CYTOTOXIC ANTIBODY. The development of antibody to antigens on the surface of a host's own cells can lead to tissue destruction. Injury results from the binding of C-fixing antibodies to host tissue cells. Activation of the C cascade leads to the release of inflammatory mediators and the accumulation of inflammatory cells. Release of lysosomal enzymes and toxic oxygen radicals by inflammatory cells and direct cytolysis of target cells through C action contribute to tissue destruction. An example of a human disease resulting from the development of antibody directed toward self tissues is Goodpasture's syndrome (see Ch. 62). The result of antibody deposition is the explosive

TABLE 442–2. TYPES OF IMMUNOLOGICALLY MEDIATED INFLAMMATION

Type of Inflammation	Recognition Component	Soluble Mediator	Inflammatory Response	Disease Example
I. Reagenic, allergic	IgE	Basophil and mast cell products (i.e., histamine, SRS, ECF)	Immediate flare and wheal, smooth muscle constriction	Atopy, anaphylaxis
II. Cytotoxic antibody	IgG, IgM	Complement	Lysis or phagocytosis of circulating antigens, acute inflammation in tissues	Autoimmune hemolytic anemia, thrombocytopenia associated with systemic lupus erythematosus
III. Immune complex	IgG, IgM	Complement	Accumulation of polymorphonuclear leukocytes and macrophages	Rheumatoid arthritis, lupus erythematosus
IV. Delayed hypersensitivity	T lymphocytes	Cytokines	Mononuclear cell infiltrate	Tuberculosis, sarcoidosis, polymyositis, granulomatosis, vasculitis

onset of hemorrhagic pneumonitis and rapidly progressive glomerulonephritis. Spontaneous development of antibody to tissues is frequently seen in certain rheumatologic disorders, particularly systemic lupus erythematosus. Autoimmune hemolytic anemia occurs following the deposition of C-fixing antibodies plus C3 cleavage products on circulating red blood cells. As a consequence of this, the cells are rapidly destroyed either by macrophages in the reticuloendothelial system (particularly in the spleen) or, less commonly, by intravascular hemolysis mediated by C. Also common in individuals with systemic lupus erythematosus is idiopathic thrombocytopenic purpura, in which antibody develops against platelet antigens. This leads to thrombocytopenia owing to the rapid clearance of platelets by the reticuloendothelial system.

TYPE III REACTIONS: INFLAMMATION INITIATED BY IMMUNE COMPLEXES. The formation or deposition of certain types of immune complexes in local tissues produces an inflammatory response characterized by the accumulation of polymorphonuclear leukocytes within hours, followed by the influx of macrophages. Several mechanisms exist by which immune complexes initiate this reaction. The combination of IgM or IgG (subclasses 1, 2 or 3) antibodies with antigen leads to the binding and activation of the first component of C. As a result of this activation, C4 and C2 are cleaved and activated, and then C3 is cleaved into two fragments. The large fragment (C3b) binds to the immune complex; the small fragment (C3a) diffuses away from the immune reaction. C3a enhances vascular permeability, contracts venular smooth muscle, and degranulates mast cells and basophils. Diffusion of C3a from the site of the immunologic reaction toward nearby blood vessels initiates early events of the acute inflammatory response. Cleavage of the next component of complement, C5, releases the extremely potent inflammatory polypeptide C5a. Diffusion of C5a from the site of immunologic reactions establishes a gradient of this chemoattractant, the highest concentrations being at the site of the immune complex deposition itself. Polymorphonuclear leukocytes and macrophages detect this gradient by means of receptors for C5a and migrate to the site of immune complex deposition. Upon arrival at the site of immune complex formation, Fc and C3b receptors enhance complex binding to the phagocytic cells, and phagocytosis ensues (see Fig. 442–3).

If the amount of immune complex deposited locally is not great, the material can be phagocytized and digested by polymorphonuclear leukocytes and macrophages without tissue destruction. If the amount of immune complex formation is large or if a significant portion of the immune complexes is lodged in vessel walls, permanent tissue destruction can ensue. Polymorphonuclear leukocytes and macrophages contain abundant lysosomal enzymes and are capable of producing toxic oxygen radicals. In the process of phagocytizing immune complexes, particularly when these complexes are not easily internalized, the cells release their lysosomal enzymes and oxygen radicals externally. Cell death also results in enzyme release. The lysosmal enzymes are than capable of cleaving additional C5, thereby producing more C5a. These processes, when occurring within vessel walls, produce vasculitis and can lead to hemorrhagic necrosis and local tissue destruction.

Tissue damage initiated by C-fixing immune complexes can occur following the formation of antigen-antibody complexes in local tissue sites (an Arthus-type reaction) or in the circulation (a serum sickness reaction).

Serum sickness reactions occur when an individual develops C-fixing antibody to a circulating antigen. As antibody is produced, antigen-antibody complexes form in the circulation. During the early phase of antibody synthesis, the amount of antibody available for binding is small so that the complexes are formed in a setting of great antigen excess. Such complexes are not pathogenic. As antibody production increases, usually by seven days after antigenic exposure, the immune complexes become larger and the ratio of antigen to antibody decreases. When the complexes are in slight antigen excess, they tend to be deposited in the walls of small blood vessels, where they initiate inflammatory lesions. Palpable purpuric skin lesions (leukocytoclastic vasculitis), arthritis, glomerulitis, and fever, as well as depressed serum C levels, are common clinical manifestations. As antibody production continues, the remaining immune complexes in the circulation increase in size and are rapidly cleared by the reticuloendothelial organs. If the exposure to antigen ceases, the illness resolves. Examples of both types of inflammation initiated by immune complexes are common in rheumatic diseases such as rheumatoid arthritis and systemic lupus erythematosus (SLE).

Certain animals develop spontaneous immune complex diseases that bear striking similarities to human SLE. By studying such animals, a great deal has been learned about the immunopathology of human autoimmune diseases. The F_1 hybrid cross between New Zealand Black (NZB) and New Zealand White (NZW) mice (NZB/W F_1) develops an immunologic disorder characterized by the development of circulating antibody to nuclear proteins, glomerulonephritis, autoimmune hemolytic anemia, and vasculitis. In contrast to the NZB/W F_1 hybrids, NZB mice develop severe autoimmune hemolytic anemia but insignificant glomerulonephritis. NZW mice do not develop spontaneous autoimmune disease.

NZB/W disease illustrates the contribution of genetic, immunologic, and infectious factors to the production of a spontaneous immune complex disease. Genetically, multiple autosomal genes appear to be involved. Immunologically, the animals have heightened B cell responsiveness and depressed T cell suppressor function. The mice produce excessive levels of antibody to many experimental antigens and have a depressed ability to reject skin grafts. The disease itself appears to occur when the NZB/W mice begin to produce unusually large amounts of antibody to Gross leukemia virus, an agent that infects many normal mouse strains but usually produces no disease. In the NZB/W mice, however, antigen-antibody complexes develop and deposit in a granular "lumpy-bumpy" immunofluorescent pattern in the renal glomerulus, leading to immune complex–induced glomerulonephritis. The formation of circulating immune complexes causes a fall in the serum C titer, and a systemic vasculitis occurs.

Recently, mice with genetic backgrounds quite different from those of NZB/W have also been shown to develop spontaneous immune complex disease. MRL and BXSB animals develop an illness characterized by circulating immune complexes, depressed serum C, and immune complex nephritis. A single mutant gene termed lpr found in these mice appears to be responsible for autoimmune disease. As in the NZB/W mice, one of the antigens appears to be an oncornavirus protein. Interestingly, mice of the MRL strain differ from the NZB/W F_1 in that they produce antibody to a nuclear antigen termed Sm. This type of antibody has been previously found only in humans with SLE. The immune defect in MRL mice is associated with increased helper T cell activity and elaboration of a T cell factor that stimulates B cells.

The requirement for a genetic predisposition along with exposure to the appropriate infectious agent or other environmental factor is also likely in human SLE. Recent studies have demonstrated that humans with SLE usually share similar histocompatibility antigens at the DR locus. Moreover, abnormal T cell suppressor function is seen not only in patients with this disease but also in family members. There are numerous other examples of human illnesses that appear to occur secondary to the development of either circulating or localized immune complexes. These include certain adverse reactions to drugs, hypersensitivity pneumonitis, and reactions to viruses such as hepatitis B virus.

TYPE IV REACTIONS: INFLAMMATORY REACTIONS INITIATED BY MONONUCLEAR LEUKOCYTES. Recognition of antigen by lymphocytes initiates a different type of inflammatory reaction than does antibody, manifested in the kinetics of inflammation and in the types of cells that accumulate. Lymphocyte-initiated inflammatory reactions are termed "delayed hypersensitivity" because maximal inflammatory cell accumulation does not appear for 48 to 72 hours after secondary antigenic exposure. For example, if an individual previously sensitized to the tubercle bacillus is injected locally with antigen from this organism, a delayed type of inflammatory response ensues. The foreign material is encountered first by macrophages, which partially digest and alter the antigen. This altered form of antigen is recognized by small lymphocytes that contain specific surface receptors for the antigen. Exposure to the antigen initiates synthesis and release of cytokines (Table 442–3). Lymphokines diffuse from the lymphocytes to areas of the vessel wall closest to the immunologic event. Increased vascular permeability ensues; chemotactic gradients that attract macrophages and other lymphocytes result in inflammatory cell accumulation. Small numbers of granulocytes precede the mononuclear cell influx, but the number of these cells is far less than that seen in the inflammatory response mediated by immune complexes. Lymphokines also activate the macrophages, which become more metabolically active, develop higher levels of hydrolytic enzymes, and are better able to bind to and destroy tumor cells or many intracellular parasites.

TABLE 442–3. EFFECTOR MOLECULES (CYTOKINES) RELEASED BY MONONUCLEAR LEUKOCYTES

Lymphocyte Products (Lymphokines)	Function
Macrophage activating factor (MAF)*	Macrophage activation
Lymphocyte-derived chemotactic factors (LDCF)	Chemotactic factors for monocytes, granulocytes, and fibroblasts
Lymphotoxin	Target cell lysis
Interferon-δ	Antiviral activity, immunoregulation
Connective tissue activating peptide I (CTAP-I)	Enhances glycosaminoglycan synthesis by synovial cells
Osteoclast activating factor (OAF)	Bone resorption
Interleukin II (IL-II, T cell growth factor)	T lymphocyte replication
Monocyte Products (Monokines)	**Function**
Lymphocyte activating factor (LAF, interleukin I (IL-I)	Lymphocyte activation for blastogenesis, leukocytic pyrogen
Mononuclear cell factor (MCF), probably identical to IL-I	Stimulates synovial dendritic cells to produce collagenase
Monocyte-derived chemotactic factor	Leukocyte accumulation
Prostaglandins	Immunoregulation, bone resorption, enhances vascular permeability
Lysosomal hydrolases	Proteolytic functions
Complement components	Inflammatory mediators

*MAF is probably identical to interferon-δ.

Lymphocytes at the inflammatory site undergo blastogenesis and release lymphokines which recruit other nonsensitized lymphocytes, thus expanding the clones of cells capable of recognizing and responding to the specific antigen. If successful in complete destruction of the antigen, the inflammatory response resolves and produces no tissue necrosis. The inflammatory process continues, however, if the antigen is large in quantity or is difficult to digest, as are the waxes of the tubercle bacillus, or if the antigen is an organism resistant to phagocytic destruction. New cells arrive to replace the dying cells already present at the site, resulting in the release of proteolytic enzymes and toxic oxygen radicals. Lesions typical of delayed hypersensitivity reactions are seen in mycobacterial and fungal diseases, sarcoidosis, and a number of rheumatologic disorders, including polymyositis and the granulomatous vasculitides.

MECHANISM OF TISSUE DESTRUCTION IN RHEUMATOID ARTHRITIS

One can construct models which describe how the joint and its surrounding structures are injured by immunologic reactions in rheumatoid arthritis. Similar models can be devised for other rheumatic diseases, the differences largely relating to the location and type of the inflammatory reactions. In most instances a combination of types of immune reactions contributes to the tissue destruction.

The characteristic tissue reaction in rheumatoid arthritis is the development of synovitis, in which the normally thin, loose connective tissue is replaced by a rich infiltrate of lymphocytes, macrophages, and plasma cells (see Fig. 442–1*B*). In the synovial fluid, the predominant inflammatory cells are the polymorphonuclear leukocytes. The cells which have infiltrated the synovia are metabolically active; the plasma cells produce rheumatoid factors, and the mononuclear cells produce cytokines. Rheumatoid factors are immunoglobulins of the IgM, IgG, or, rarely, IgA class. These factors bind to the Fc portion of IgG antibodies, which either have combined with antigen or have been aggregated or denatured. Polymorphonuclear leukocytes taken from synovial fluids contain inclusions of immune complexes, many of which contain rheumatoid factors. Synovial fluid C levels are depressed in relation to the serum C level. The turnover of C components, particularly components of the classic pathway, is markedly enhanced in rheumatoid synovial fluid. Cleavage products such as C5a are present in rheumatoid synovial fluid, as are hydrolytic enzymes derived from inflammatory cells, kinins and LTB_4.

The sequence of events leading to the development of synovitis and destruction of surrounding structures in rheumatoid arthritis can be envisioned as follows: some as yet undefined antigen localizes in the synovium and is phagocytized by the Type A synovial cells. One can assume that the antigen is not completely destroyed, so that a partially digested form persists and diffuses into the synovial fluid. Binding of the processed antigen to B lymphocytes induces their differentiation to plasma cells, which then produce antibodies and rheumatoid factors upon chronic stimulation. Antigen activation of T lymphocytes triggers lymphokine synthesis followed by blastogenesis. The role of viruses as stimulators of the immune response in rheumatoid arthritis must be considered. Rheumatoid synovial explant cells established in permanent lines exhibit many characteristics of virally transformed lymphocytes. Cell lines of the

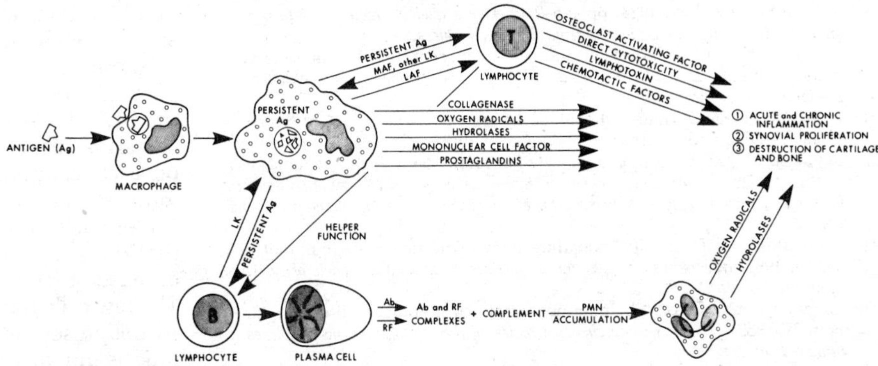

Figure 442–4. Model for the pathogenesis of articular inflammation in rheumatoid arthritis. Ab = antibody, LAF = lymphocyte activating factor, LK = lymphokines, MAF = macrophage activating factor, RF = rheumatoid factor.

B lymphocyte variety frequently contain antigens of the Epstein-Barr virus (EBV). This finding is interesting in that sera from approximately 65 per cent of patients with rheumatoid arthritis contain antibody, called a rheumatoid arthritis precipitin (RAP), which is directed at certain nuclear antigens present in human lymphoblastoid cell lines infected with EBV. The antigens have been termed rheumatoid arthritis nuclear antigens (RANAs). RANAs are found only in B lymphoblastoid cell lines, whose genomes contain the EBV genome, but no infectious viral particles are produced. RAPs are commonly present in the sera of patients who are rheumatoid factor positive but are also found in the sera of patients who are rheumatoid factor negative. The specificity of RAPs for rheumatoid arthritis has been questioned, as RAPs can be present in up to 20 per cent of normal individuals. In rheumatoid arthritis, there is no firm evidence to relate EBV causally to the disease, and serum antibody levels to EBV are not increased in the sera of rheumatoid arthritis patients. However, EBV does act as a polyclonal stimulator of antibody production and increases the mitogenic activity of lymphocytes. Regardless of the initiating agent, combination of antibody with antigen, as well as combination of antigen-antibody complexes with rheumatoid factors, or self-association of rheumatoid factors, activates C as well as the kinin-forming system by means of activating Hageman factor. This results in the production of inflammatory products such as C5a, arachidonic acid metabolites, kinins, and fibrinopeptides, which diffuse into the synovial fluid and to synovial blood vessels. These phlogistic agents enhance vascular permeability and attract polymorphonuclear leukocytes and macrophages. Polymorphonuclear leukocytes ingest the abundant immune complexes in the fluid, release lysosomal enzymes, and generate superoxide anions. This causes destruction of hyaluronate polymers in the joint fluid, as well as injury to cartilage. Cytokine production in the synovium leads to the further accumulation of macrophages, fibroblasts, and additional lymphocytes.

The unique structure of the joint space is important, as enzymes present in synovial fluid or released and synthesized locally by the cells constituting the proliferative synovial lesion contribute to the pathology evident in articular structures. The cartilage-degrading lysosomal enzymes collagenase and elastase are primarily derived from inflammatory cells. Proteinases released by dying cells may aid in superficial cartilage destruction by virtue of their role in uncrosslinking collagen fibrils, thus increasing their susceptibility to enzymatic degradation. Macrophages in the synovium produce prostaglandins, hydrolytic enzymes, collagenase, plasminogen activator, and IL-1. The synovial cell that is the most abundant source of collagenase in the rheumatoid synovium is one which has an unusual dendritic appearance and is adherent to glass but is nonphagocytic. Collagenase synthesis by this cell is greatly enhanced in the presence of IL-1 (mononuclear cell factor). With ongoing synovitis, early changes in cartilage involve the loss of proteoglycan content, often manifested microscopically as diminished metachromatic staining. In addition to collagenases, lysosomal proteinases can degrade aggregates of proteoglycans, and, once released from cartilage, these solubilized components are then sensitive to further enzymatic attack.

The final stage of the destructive process, demineralization of bone, may result from combined elements present initially in the inflammatory and later in the proliferative responses. Demineralization must occur in bone before this tissue is susceptible to collagenolytic enzymes. In rheumatoid synovitis, prostaglandins stimulate calcium release from bone matrix; other arachidonic acid metabolites are responsible for long-term leaching of mineral from bony matrix. In addition, bone demineralization is enhanced by heparin, which is released upon the degranulation of mast cells. Cellular mechanisms may also be operative in demineralization in that lymphocytes produce an osteoclast activating factor (OAF). In addition, connective tissue activating peptides (CTAPs) and specific lymphokines such as lymphocyte-derived chemotactic factor for fibroblasts (LDCF-F) attract and stimulate fibroblasts to produce collagen and may contribute to the ultimate fibrosis evident in the destroyed ankylosed joint.

The net effect, resulting from either persistence of antigen or disordered regulation of T and B cell activation, is a chronic inflammatory response in the synovium (Fig. 442–4). Continued cellular proliferation and influx lead to synovial proliferation and its invasion into surrounding structures. Diffusion of collagenase, PGEs, hydrolytic enzymes, and lymphokines into cartilage and bone results in erosion of these tissues. Rheumatoid arthritis thus illustrates the devastating local tissue destruction that results from chronic inflammatory reactions produced by the immune complex and delayed hypersensitivity types of immune responses.

Alspaugh MA, Tan EM: Serum antibody in rheumatoid arthritis reactive with a cell associated antigen. Demonstration by precipitation and immunofluorescence. Arthritis Rheum 19:711, 1976. *The initial description of rheumatoid arthritis precipitins.*

Bomalaski JS, Williamson PK, Zurier RB: Prostaglandins and the inflammatory response. Clin Lab Med 3(4):695, 1983. A detailed review of the role of prostaglandins in inflammation.

Dayer JM, Krane SM: The interaction of immunocompetent cells and chronic inflammation as exemplified by rheumatoid arthritis. Clin Rheum Dis 4:517, 1978. *An overview of cellular interactions in the generation of destructive rheumatoid synovitis.*

Kaplan AP: The intrinsic coagulation, fibrinolytic, and kinin-forming pathways of man. *In* Kelley WN, Harris ED, Ruddy S, Sledge CB (eds.): Textbook of Rheumatology, Vol. 1. Philadelphia, W. B. Saunders Co., 1981, pp 97–119. *A complete review of the Hageman factor–dependent pathways, including those that lead to kinin generation.*

McPhail LC, Snyderman R: Oxygen-dependent microbicidal activity of leukocytes. *In* Snyderman R (ed): Contemporary Topics in Immunobiology, Vol. 14. "Regulation of Leukocyte Function." New York, Plenum Press, 1984, pp 247–281. *A comprehensive overview of oxygen metabolism in phagocytes.*

Pisetsky DS, Caster SA, Roths JB, Murphy ED: *lpr* gene control of the anti-DNA antibody response. J Immunol 128:2322, 1982. *Evidence concerning the genetic regulation of anti DNA-antibody production and an autoimmune disease is presented.*

Samuelsson B: The leukotrienes: An introduction. *In* Samuelsson B, Paoletti R (eds.): Leukotrienes and Other Lipoxygenase Products. New York, Raven Press, 1982, pp 1–27. *An excellent review of the biochemistry of the leukotrienes and their potential biological roles.*

Smith HR, Steinberg AD: Autoimmunity—a perspective. *In* Paul WE, Fathman EG, Metzgar H (eds.): Annual Review of Immunology, Vol. 1. Palo Alto,

Annual Reviews Inc., 1983, pp 175–210. *A very readable review of human and animal autoimmune disease mechanisms. Many references.*

Snyderman R, Goetzl EJ: Molecular and cellular mechanisms of leukocyte chemotaxis. Science 213:830, 1981. *A thorough review of the mechanisms of leukocyte responses to chemotactic factors.*

Snyderman R, Pike MC: Transductional mechanisms of chemoattractant receptors on leukocytes. *In* Snyderman R (ed.): Contemporary Topics in Immunobiology, Vol. 14. "Regulation of Leukocyte Function." New York, Plenum Press, 1984, pp 1–28. *An up-to-date review of the biochemistry and biology of chemotactic factors and their receptors on leukocytes. Many references on inflammatory mechanisms.*

Theofilopoulos AN, Dixon FJ: Etiopathogenesis of murine SLE. Immunol Rev 55:179, 1981. *Interesting concepts and a good review of animal models of systemic lupus erythematosus.*

Theofilopoulos AN, Dixon FJ: Immune complexes in human diseases. Am J Pathol 100:531, 1980. *A comprehensive review of the role of immune complexes in human diseases.*

Wasserman SI: Mediators of immediate hypersensitivity. J Allergy Clin Immunol 72(2):101, 1983. *An exposition of the physiologic aspects of immediate types of hypersensitivity reactions.*

Weissmann G: Pathways of arachidonate oxidation to prostaglandins and leukotrienes. Sem Arth Rheu 13:123, 1983. *A recent review of arachidonate metabolism and its relevance to inflammation.*

Weissmann G, Smolen JE, Korchak HM: Release of inflammatory mediators from stimulated neutrophils. N Engl J Med 303:27, 1980. *A good update on the mechanisms of secretion by leukocytes.*

Wooley DE, Harris ED Jr, Mainardi CL, Brinckerhoff CE: Collagenase immunolocalization in cultures of rheumatoid synovial cells. Science 200:773, 1978. *This article stresses the importance of the dendritic cell as a source of collagenase in rheumatoid synovium.*

Ziff M: Pathophysiology of rheumatoid arthritis. Fed Proc 32:131, 1973. *A classic review of the pioneering work dealing with the immunology of rheumatoid arthritis.*

Zvaifler NJ: Pathogenesis of the joint disease of rheumatoid arthritis. Am. J. Med. 75:3, 1983. *A review of the role of various components of the immune response in rheumatoid arthritis.*

443. SPECIALIZED DIAGNOSTIC PROCEDURES IN THE RHEUMATIC DISEASES

Alan S. Cohen

An increasing number of specialized procedures are available for evaluation of patients with articular disease. Although many are useful, very few are diagnostic of a specific disorder. Laboratory data must be combined with clinical evaluation in order to arrive at a working diagnosis.

SYNOVIAL FLUID. In the patient with undiagnosed articular disease and an associated joint effusion, examination of the synovial fluid is mandatory. The preferred method of joint aspiration (most frequently the knee) is through the extensor surface, where major blood vessels and nerves are sparse and the synovial pouch is more superficial. If the synovial fluid sugar is to be measured, the patient should have fasted for at least six hours if possible. Careful sterile technique virtually precludes infection, the one very rare complication of arthrocentesis. The needle should be at least 19 gauge. After appropriate draping and intracutaneous instillation of 1 to 2 per cent procaine or Xylocaine, the needle is inserted through skin and subcutaneous tissue. It meets a small amount of resistance when it reaches the capsule and finally passes easily into the joint cavity. Although minimal amounts of fluid will suffice for basic studies, as a rule 10 to 15 ml will allow the necessary laboratory testing.

The synovial fluid is then ideally allocated as follows: (1) an aliquot (1 to 3 ml) in a sterile tube with heparin—for bacteriologic studies (cultures and Gram stain); (2) an aliquot (1 ml) in a clean nonsterile tube with heparin—for routine cytology, white cell count, and differential (can also be used for mucin test and crystal examination); (3) an aliquot (2 to 3 ml) without anticoagulant in a clean nonsterile tube—for color, viscosity, clot turbidity, mucin clot test, crystals, and inclusions (as well as proteins, rheumatoid factors, and complement if indicated); and (4) an aliquot (2 ml) in a clean nonsterile tube with preservative—for glucose analysis with parallel determination of serum glucose.

Cultures must be obtained on all synovial fluids, since indolent infections (bacterial, tuberculous) can mimic or be superimposed on well defined articular disease. Blood agar medium should be used; but if gonococcal infection is suspected, chocolate agar or its equivalent should be inoculated at the bedside. Appropriate cultures should be obtained if tuberculosis is suspected. A direct Gram stain should be performed on a concentrated specimen from the first tube, spun for 20 minutes in a clinical centrifuge.

Normal synovial fluid is a clear pale yellow viscous liquid that does not clot. It was appropriately named by Paracelsus because of its viscosity and physical resemblance to egg white. The few cells normally present (less than 200) are mononuclear. Although serous cavity fluids are plasma ultrafiltrates, synovial fluid is unique owing to the presence of hyaluronic acid (about 0.3 gram per deciliter) produced by the synovial lining cells. This large asymmetric molecule further influences the composition of synovial fluid, for because of its steric structure, some solute passage through the water surrounding the molecules may be hindered. Thus, according to the concept of excluded volume, the size and shape of the molecule plays a large role; i.e., large molecules such as fibrinogen and macroglobulin would be excluded, and small molecules would more easily enter the compartment. The state of hyaluronate (as roughly determined by the mucin clot test) may be a primary determinant of the nature of the synovial fluid in various pathologic conditions.

When a synovial membrane is inflamed for any reason, the white cell count in the synovial fluid increases. In a rough fashion one can classify such fluids into four groups (Table 443–1). Noninflammatory effusions (Group I) occur when the white cell count is normal or minimally increased, as in traumatic arthritis or degenerative joint disease. Only rarely will such fluid have white cell counts of over 2000 cells per cubic millimeter. Noninfectious mildly inflammatory effusions (Group II) with white cell counts rarely over 5000 occur in systemic lupus erythematosus and scleroderma. In noninfectious acute inflammatory effusions (Group III) characteristic of classic rheumatoid arthritis, gout, pseudogout, and rheumatic fever, the white cell count varies from 5000 to 25,000 but may exceed 50,000 or even 100,000 cells per cubic millimeter. Finally, in inflammatory effusions caused by infection (Group IV) the white cell count commonly varies from 25,000 to over 100,000 cells per cubic millimeter and in some instances resembles frank pus. As the white cell count becomes elevated, the percentage of polymorphonuclear leukocytes generally increases, the hyaluronate becomes degraded, and the synovial fluid sugar falls.

Normal synovial fluid does not clot owing to the absence of several clotting factors, including fibrinogen. Pathologic fluids do contain clots, and their size is roughly proportional to the degree of inflammation. Hyaluronate degradation can be roughly assessed by diluting 1 ml of joint fluid with 4 ml of 2 per cent acetic acid solution. When the mucin is normal, a tight ropy mass forms in a clear solution. This is termed a "good" mucin. A softer mass with shreds is a "fair" mucin, whereas a "poor" mucin shows shreds and soft small masses in a turbid solution.

Under normal conditions, the total synovial fluid protein is about one quarter that of the blood. Multiple studies have been performed to assess whether specific fractions might be related to specific disease states, but findings in general are nonspecific. One may conclude that if the synovial fluid total protein is over 2.5 grams per deciliter, the fluid is not normal, and that if it is over 4.5 grams per deciliter, there is significant inflammation.

Rheumatoid factors (antigamma globulins) are also found in the synovial fluid, occasionally when they are absent from the serum. Their presence and presumed local manufacture in the synovial membrane may be of diagnostic value. Antinuclear antibodies have been found not only in the synovial fluids of patients with systemic lupus erythematosus but also in those

TABLE 443–1. SYNOVIAL FLUID ANALYSIS

Diagnosis	Appearance	Total White Cell Count per Cubic Millimeter*	Polymorphonuclear Cells	Mucin Clot Test	Synovial Fluid-Blood Glucose Difference (Mean Milligrams per Deciliter)	Miscellaneous (Crystals, Organisms)
Normal	Clear, pale yellow	0–200 (200)	<10%	Good	No significant difference†	—
Group I (noninflammatory effusions)						
Degenerative joint disease; traumatic arthritis	Clear to slightly turbid	50–4000 (600)	<30%	Good	No significant difference	—
Group II (noninfectious, mildly inflammatory)						
Systemic lupus erythematosus; scleroderma	Clear to slightly turbid	0–9000 (3000)	<20%	Good (occasionally fair)	No significant difference	Occasional LE cell; decreased complement
Group III (noninfectious severe inflammatory effusions)						
Gout	Turbid	100–160,000 (21,000)	~70%	Poor	10	Monosodium urate crystals
Pseudogout	Turbid	50–75,000 (14,000)	~70%	Fair-poor	Not enough data	Calcium pyrophosphate dihydrate crystals
Rheumatoid arthritis	Turbid	250–80,000 (19,000)	~70%	Poor	30	Decreased complement
Group IV (infectious inflammatory effusions)						
Acute bacterial	Very turbid	150–250,000 (80,000)	~90%	Poor	90	Culture positive for gram-positive or gram-negative bacteria
Tuberculosis	Turbid	2500–100,000 (20,000)	~60%	Poor	70	Culture positive for *M. tuberculosis*

*Averages in parentheses.
†Less than 10 mg per deciliter difference.

of patients with rheumatoid arthritis and several other connective tissue diseases. Since DNA, especially in the native form, can be found free in synovial fluids from individuals with a variety of disorders, it is probable that its presence may reflect nonspecific tissue damage.

Complement levels in the synovial fluid depend upon rates of synthesis, catabolism, and local consumption. Analysis of complement components has been utilized not only for diagnosis but for evaluation of prognosis and for determination of the potential for immunologically related factors in the pathogenesis of the synovitis. The most severe depressions in complement factors have occurred in seropositive rheumatoid arthritis patients and in those with systemic lupus erythematosus (SLE). In rheumatoid arthritis the *serum* complement is not depressed, whereas in SLE it is low, in a fashion comparable to that of the synovial fluid. Although C4, C2, and C3 may be depressed in rheumatoid arthritis (when corrected for globulin in synovial fluid), and C3 particularly depressed in SLE, the fact that some persons with gout and bacterial arthritis also have depressed levels makes these determinations less specific. Elevated complement levels have been reported in Reiter's syndrome, gout, and ankylosing spondylitis. Cryoproteins, predominantly of fibrinogen but including cryoglobulins with DNA and IgG, are also found in synovial fluids of patients with rheumatoid arthritis and other types of synovitis, and rheumatoid fluids may contain complexes with Igs, rheumatoid factors, complement, and DNA.

The intense inflammatory activity of various synovial diseases is associated with the presence of a variety of enzymes in the synovial fluid. Some, but not all, investigators have implicated lysosomal enzymes (e.g., myeloperoxidase, lactoferrin, lysozyme, chymotryptic cationic protein) in the process of joint destruction. Collagenase, collagen, and antibodies to collagen have also been extensively studied. Such investigations have advanced our concepts of the pathogenesis of synovitis (especially rheumatoid), but generally measurements of these substances have not reached the routine clinical domain. Other proteins and peptides (C-reactive protein, plasminogen, vasoactive peptides, and oxygen-derived free radicals) have also been measured in synovial fluid, but their precise role in diagnosis is not clear.

Synovial fluid normally contains little lipid, but it demonstrates increased lipid content in rheumatoid effusions. Prostaglandin E_2 appears to be elevated in the fluid of patients with inflammatory synovitis. The glucose content of synovial fluid, which normally approximates that of serum, is markedly diminished in the presence of infection and may show a modest decrease (10 to 30 mg per deciliter) in other inflammatory effusions. Several of these nonspecific parameters are collectively useful in evaluating the degree and type of inflammatory synovitis (Table 443–1).

Several types of crystals have been found in synovial fluids. The two most important are monosodium urate, characteristic of gouty effusions, and calcium pyrophosphate dihydrate (CPPD), characteristic of the effusions of pseudogout (crystal deposition disease). Crystals that cause inflammation are usually 0.5 to 20 μm in length, sparingly soluble in water, and capable of being phagocytized. At the peak of inflammation most are intracellular. Other crystals such as calcium hydroxyapatite, calcium oxalate, cholesterol, and corticosteroid esters may also be associated with inflammatory effusions.

Crystals are demonstrated in synovial fluid (collected without oxalate) by examining a drop of synovial fluid placed on a slide and covered with a thin glass coverslip for examination in the polarizing microscope. Birefringent materials demonstrate two refractive indices when plane polarized light passes through them. The birefringence is termed positive when the crystals (which then appear blue) are aligned parallel to the slow rays of the retardation plate (first-order red plate compensator) and negative when the crystals appear yellow when in parallel alignment (blue when perpendicular). On polarization microscopy the monosodium urate crystals demonstrate strong negative birefringence and are usually long (8 to 10 μm) and needle-like in appearance. They may occur extracellularly or within polymorphonuclear or mononuclear cells. They are almost invariably in effusions associated with acute gout and are virtually diagnostic. They may, however, be present in gouty fluids between attacks. The CPPD crystals are often broader than urate crystals, may show a faint "line" down their center, appear parallelopiped, and in the polarizing microscope exhibit a weak positive birefringence. They have a significant association with acute attacks of arthritis in patients with chondrocalcinosis (articular cartilage calcification).

Under certain circumstances joint fluids, when nontraumatically aspirated, may demonstrate gross blood. One must consider bleeding disorders such as hemophilia, overdosage with anticoagulants, rare lesions such as pigmented villonodular synovitis and joint tumor, as well as neuropathic and traumatic forms of arthritis.

SYNOVIAL MEMBRANE HISTOPATHOLOGY. Synovial membrane is a non–basement membrane–lined, highly vascular structure consisting of several cell types (macrophages, fibroblasts, and possibly intermediate cells). It proliferates extensively during inflammation, such that synovial biopsy is often useful in establishing a diagnosis. The procedure is simple and may be an extension of the synovial fluid aspiration technique, using a wider bore Parker-Pearson needle. A specimen can also be obtained by arthroscopy or open surgical biopsy.

Although in the common rheumatic diseases (rheumatoid arthritis, degenerative joint disease, systemic lupus erythematosus) there are no common pathognomonic synovial membrane findings, the patterns of histologic involvement may be diagnostically useful. For example, severe synovial lining proliferation and especially the presence of lymphoid follicles are characteristic of rheumatoid arthritis, whereas the SLE membrane shows only minimal hyperplasia but may show dense surface fibrin and perivascular mononuclear infiltrates; rarely a pathognomonic hematoxylin body will be seen.

The procedure is very useful in the diagnosis of tuberculosis; the demonstration of an organism in section (or in culture) or a caseating granuloma with giant cells virtually establishes the diagnosis. Other instances in which the synovial biopsy could be helpful include hemochromatosis (in which iron is seen in the synovial lining cell), pigmented villonodular synovitis (villous hypertrophy, hemosiderin deposits with numerous giant cells), tumors (malignant cells in synovium), and ochronosis (fragments of pigmented cartilage in synovium). Although in properly fixed tissue (use of absolute alcohol) one can observe the crystals associated with gout on histologic examination, the procedure is not necessary to establish this diagnosis, since examination of synovial fluid so commonly demonstrates the crystals.

ACUTE PHASE PHENOMENA. The ancient Greeks observed the sedimentation of blood following venesection and used it as a basic diagnostic tool. It was reintroduced by Fahraeus and refined by Westergren, whose method is in common use today. The sedimentation rate is only one, albeit the most popular, of the acute phase phenomena utilized by rheumatologists to follow inflammation in their patients. Acute phase reactions refer to the increases in certain plasma proteins that occur after an extraordinary variety of tissue damage, i.e., toxic, chemical, infectious, inflammatory, or malignant. The functions of most of these proteins are not known, although presumably the damage led to increased protein synthesis in some cases. Only the sedimentation rate and C-reactive protein (CRP) will be briefly discussed here.

The basic measurement in the Westergren sedimentation rate is the rate of fall of erythrocytes in plasma; when rouleaux formation occurs owing primarily to increases in asymmetric proteins such as fibrinogen or macroglobulins (that alter the red cell zeta potential), the red cells sediment more rapidly. The original normal values are a 1 to 3 mm fall in one hour for men and a 4 to 7 mm fall in one hour for women. These levels may be elevated during menses or by certain drugs and appear to increase with aging. The cause of the last-named phenomenon is not clear despite several reports that seem to document it well. Many now accept sedimentation rates of 0 to 10 mm per hour for men and 0 to 15 mm per hour for women and suggest that the values may be as much as 10 mm per hour higher at age 50. Whether these represent changes in serum proteins with aging or undetected disease in the normal person is not yet clear. In the rheumatic diseases, however, the value of this determination is that when elevated (and it is often in the 30 to 100 mm per hour range), it can be an index for following the severity of inflammation and, when falling, for following the response to therapy. In addition, disorders such as temporal arteritis are characteristically associated with sedimentation rates of over 100 mm per hour.

One must be constantly aware, however, of the lack of specificity of this determination and that in selected series highly elevated sedimentation rates (over 100 mg per hour) are more commonly due to infections or malignancies. It is also documented that a small number of patients can have an active rheumatic disease (i.e., rheumatoid arthritis) with a normal sedimentation rate.

The CRP until recently has played little role in the evaluation of rheumatic diseases, although it has been the prototype acute phase reactant—virtually absent in normal conditions and appearing in large quantities in inflammation. It was named for its property of precipitating with pneumococcal cell wall polysaccharide. In recent years it has been isolated and characterized as a pentameric structure, and its molecular weight and primary structure have been determined. It has many homologies with a protein (AP) found uniquely in amyloid disease but is immunologically distinct. The existence and identification of these substances in phylogenetically distinct species add fascination to their role in man and their relation to one another. CRP rises under circumstances (infection, inflammation) similar to those that elevate the erythrocyte sedimentation rate.

The major differences between CRP and erythrocyte sedimentation rate are that CRP rises earlier (in hours), is a rapid indicator of tissue injury or infection, and tends to fall and reflect potential recovery faster. In addition, in uncomplicated systemic lupus erythematosus the CRP generally is only minimally elevated but becomes more clearly elevated in the presence of infection.

RHEUMATOID FACTORS. Fifty years ago, when Cecil and coworkers found high titers of "streptococcal agglutinators" in the sera of some rheumatoid patients, they were actually alluding to rheumatoid factors. Such factors are now defined as antibodies (present largely in the IgM fraction, but in other Ig fractions as well) to determinants of the Fc fragment of numerous animal (especially human and rabbit) IgGs. As antibodies they possess the characteristics of such proteins. They were named when their frequency in the sera of patients with rheumatoid arthritis (about 70 per cent) was observed. They lack both sensitivity and specificity in the detection of rheumatoid syndromes.

Most clinical tests depend upon the detection of IgM antibodies. In such assays particles (red blood cells or latex or bentonite particles) are coated with immunoglobulin G, mixed with the test serum, and observed for appropriate agglutination or flocculation. Various standardization procedures exist as well as different tube dilutions that are interpreted as positive. Internal standardization as well as the use of cross-reference laboratories is important.

The IgM antibody reacts with IgG to form a soluble complex which sediments in the ultracentrifuge with a coefficient of 22. In addition, IgG-IgG complexes sedimenting at an intermediate range can also occur, as well as larger, insoluble IgM-IgG complexes. In some instances the IgM rheumatoid factor is firmly bound to autologous IgG such that it is not detected on routine agglutination tests. Gel filtration under mildly acid conditions dissociates these IgG and IgM fractions. When the rheumatoid factor activity is found in such instances, the term "hidden rheumatoid factor" is sometimes applied.

Rheumatoid factors are uncommon in children with chronic arthritis. High titers have been correlated with severe progressive rheumatoid arthritis in patients with multiple rheumatoid nodules, vasculitis, skin ulcers, and other visceral manifestations. Rheumatoid factors are found in many diseases other than rheumatoid arthritis (other connective tissue diseases, leprosy, leishmaniasis, liver disease, tuberculosis). In some series of subacute bacterial endocarditis 50 per cent of the patients will transiently show rheumatoid factors in their sera. Although family studies of seropositive propositi suggest that there is a higher incidence in its members, epidemiologic use of rheumatoid factors has been of little help in determining the incidence of rheumatoid arthritis, since it may so often mark parasitic or infectious disease.

Since rheumatoid factors have been induced experimentally with bacterial antigens and since they are so commonly associated with chronic infectious diseases, the concept that an as yet unknown infectious agent or agents may play a pathogenetic role in rheumatoid disease is still under active investigation. Data thus far suggest that rheumatoid factor is an epiphenomenon and not a direct cause of rheumatoid arthritis.

The absence of rheumatoid factors in well defined groups of rheumatoid variants has led to the classification of seronegative spondyloarthritis for disorders such as psoriatic arthritis, ankylosing spondylitis, forms of juvenile chronic polyarthritis, and Reiter's syndrome.

ANTINUCLEAR ANTIBODIES AND THE LE CELL. The discovery of the LE cell by Hargraves in 1948 and subsequent studies demonstrating a lupus factor that reacted with nuclear material opened the door to a series of immunologic investigations that have led to new concepts of pathogenesis, diagnosis, and clinical course of systemic lupus erythematosus (SLE) and related disorders. The LE factor was initially regarded as a 7S immunoglobulin, but it is now known that this is only one of many autoantibodies in lupus sera, and that these occur in all immunoglobulin classes, although most are IgG's.

The evolution of this field is such that contradictory statements often appear concerning the role of autoantibodies in the immunopathogenesis of the disease, their diagnostic value, and clinical relevance in patient follow-up. The list of reported nuclear, cytoplasmic, and cell membrane antigens is long and somewhat confused by different methods of testing. We are concerned here only with those that are generally accepted and will take note of several new developments.

The prototype LE cell is a phagocytic polymorphonuclear cell containing (on Wright's stain) a homogeneous purple nuclear inclusion surrounded by a rim of cytoplasm and a compressed nucleus. It is produced in vitro from blood samples but can be found on direct examination of synovial, pleural, peritoneal, and pericardial fluid. It represents phagocytized deoxyribonucleoprotein (DNA-histone complex) and has as its tissue equivalent the isolated hematoxylin body. It has a high association with SLE. The LE cell can be present in other connective tissue diseases. However, it has a low sensitivity, is technically a time-consuming test and has been largely replaced by other immunologic procedures.

The next developments in the identification of antigen-antibody complexes involved complement fixation and precipitation tests, or particles (latex, bentonite, or red blood cells) coated with antigen which agglutinated on exposure to antibody. However, the fluorescence of isolated nuclear constituents or cells (especially the nuclei) on tissue slides after exposure to test sera was found to provide the most practical method for defining these antigen-antibody interactions (antinuclear antibodies) in a simple and reproducible fashion (Table 443–2). A homogeneous pattern of nuclear fluorescence indicates the presence of an antideoxyribonucleoprotein (LE cell factor), a peripheral (rim) pattern suggests the presence of anti-DNA antibody, and the speckled pattern reflects a variety of anti-acidic nuclear proteins. By appropriate dilution of sera, titers of antibody can be determined. Unfortunately the use of a variety of kits and of various substrates (mouse liver cells, buccal cells, tissue culture cells) has prohibited further standardization. Despite this, certain generalizations can be made, although the correlations are not absolute and exceptions occur. Indeed, there are patients with SLE in whose sera antinuclear antibodies cannot be identified. In addition to fluorescent methodology DNA binding assays, the *Crithidia* (a hemoflagellate with apparent specificity for nDNA antibody) assay, or commercial kits are increasingly employed.

TABLE 443–2. AUTOANTIBODIES TO DNA AND HISTONES

Antibody Reactive with	Clinical Association
Double-strand DNA only	SLE. Rare cases reported.
Double/single-strand DNA with reaction of immunologic identity	SLE (60–70%). Rarely in other diseases where it is usually in low titer
Single-strand DNA only. Antigenic determinants related to exposed purines and pyrimidines	SLE, other rheumatic diseases, and certain nonrheumatic diseases
Histones (H1, H2A, H2B, H3, H4)	Drug-induced LE (95–100%), rheumatoid arthritis (15–20%), and SLE (30%)

Reprinted with permission from: Tan EM: Autoantibodies to nuclear antigens (ANA): Their immunobiology and medicine. Adv Immunol 33:172, 1982.

From a pathogenetic point of view it is likely that multiple immunologic aberrations, seen particularly in SLE, do mediate certain aspects of the disease and may be responsible for renal and other tissue damage. However, in tissue culture, such antinuclear antibodies have been shown not to cause cell damage, and the IgG antibodies passed transplacentally have not been shown to cause permanent fetal damage. The closest association has been the presence of anti-nDNA antibodies in patients with SLE and active renal disease. These preparations usually contain some ssDNA antibody as well, but these are not highly specific and have been observed in a number of nonrheumatologic conditions associated with tissue damage, i.e., infection.

Antibodies to deoxyribonucleoprotein are present in many patients with SLE, but they also occur in other connective tissue diseases and in unaffected relatives and may be present in moderate titers for years in asymptomatic SLE patients.

The study of the extractable nuclear antigen (ENA), an acidic component, has led to the discovery that it contains several constituents. Antibodies against one, termed Sm antigen, are specifically associated with SLE but are found in only 20 to 30 per cent of such patients. Another, antiribonucleoprotein (anti-RNP), has led to the identification of mixed connective tissue disease—MCTD—either as a separate entity or a milder subset of lupus or scleroderma. Anti-RNP is found in SLE, scleroderma, and polymyositis, as well as in MCTD (Table 443–3). Even more recently, antigens associated with the sicca syndrome, SS-B, an acidic nuclear antigen (cross-reactive with Ro antigen of cytoplasmic extracts), and SS-A antigen, a similar antigen (cross-reactive with La cytoplasmic antigen), have been described. These antibodies and others appear to identify certain connective tissue diseases (i.e., anti-Scl-70 in scleroderma; anti-Jo-1 in polymyositis) but often have a low sensitivity. The accepted antigens and antibodies and an estimate of their incidence in disease are listed in Tables 443–2 and 443–3.

In addition to these, another nuclear antigen, termed RANA, has been found to have a close association with the Epstein-Barr (EB) virus and also a high association with rheumatoid arthritis. Whether this simply represents a marker for rheumatoid arthritis or implicates the EB virus in the pathogenesis of the disease remains to be seen.

Tests for cell-mediated immunity and for immune complexes are of interest, but currently their significance in the rheumatic diseases is not well defined.

RADIOGRAPHIC TECHNIQUES IN THE DIAGNOSIS OF ARTICULAR DISEASES. ***Clinical Radiology of Joints.*** Skeletal radiographs

TABLE 443–3. AUTOANTIBODIES TO NONHISTONE NUCLEAR PROTEINS AND RNA-PROTEIN COMPLEXES

Antibody Reactive with	Clinical Association
Sm antigen	SLE (30–40%). Marker antibody
Nuclear ribonucleoprotein (nRNP) or U1-RNP	MCTD (95–100%). Lower frequency in SLE, discoid LE, and scleroderma
SS-A/Ro antigen	Sjögren's syndrome (60–70%), SLE (30–40%)
SS-B/La antigen	Sjögren's syndrome (50–60%), SLE (10–15%)
Scl-70	Scleroderma (15–20%). Marker antibody
Centromere/kinetochore	CREST (70–90%). Marker antibody
RANA (rheumatoid arthritis associated nuclear antigen)	RA (90–95%)
Ma antigen	SLE (20%)
PCNA (proliferating cell nuclear antigen)	SLE (5–10%)
PM-1	Polymyositis/scleroderma overlap (87%) Dermatomyositis (17%)
Mi-1	Dermatomyositis (11%)
Jo-1	Polymyositis (31%)
Ku	Polymyositis/scleroderma overlap (55%)

Reprinted with permission from: Tan EM: Autoantibodies to nuclear antigens (ANA): Their immunobiology and medicine. Adv Immunol 33:173, 1982.

can contribute to the diagnosis of articular diseases because the bone and joint changes reflect the basic pathology. Proper integration depends upon an understanding of the pathophysiology of the various diseases and an appreciation of the typically affected areas. This discussion will highlight general patterns and differential diagnostic aspects of major diseases. The simplest classification is that used in assessing synovial fluid, i.e., inflammatory and noninflammatory articular disease.

General radiologic features of noninflammatory disease (such as degenerative disease) include uneven narrowing of the joint space, sclerosis of juxta-articular bone, and the presence of bone spurs and cysts. Target areas include the distal interphalangeal and first carpometacarpal joints, acromioclavicular joint, vertebral column, hip, and knee, with the appearance of genu varum.

Inflammatory joint disease (such as rheumatoid arthritis) is generally characterized by local bony demineralization, erosions, and narrowing of the joint space. The pattern includes bilateral symmetry with involvement of the metacarpophalangeal joints, ulnar styloid area, and glenohumeral and atlantoaxial joints, as well as metatarsophalangeal joints. Involvement of the knees leads to genu valgum.

In addition there are patterns of change that assist in the differentiation of several types of inflammatory articular disease. For example, in tophaceous gouty arthritis the eroded joint may demonstrate an "overhanging ledge," as opposed to the erosion of rheumatoid arthritis. It may show asymmetric intra- and extra-articular erosions, as opposed to the marginal intra-articular erosions of rheumatoid arthritis. Gout does not lead to osteopenia, and joint space narrowing will be a late phenomenon rather than an early manifestation as it is in rheumatoid arthritis.

In the seronegative spondyloarthropathies (e.g., psoriatic arthritis) the articular involvement is less likely to be symmetrical, the interphalangeal joints of the feet may be more involved than the metatarsophalangeals, osteopenia is uncommon, and periosteal new bone formation may be seen as well as bony ankylosis. Finally, evidence of sacroiliitis with narrowing, erosions, sclerosis, and obliteration of the sacroiliac joint, is common. Descriptions of specific changes, such as calcinosis in scleroderma and polymyositis and aseptic necrosis (osteonecrosis) associated with systemic lupus erythematosus, are detailed in the chapters devoted to the individual disease entities.

Several additional principles should be stressed in the radiographic examination of joints. First, films are of little value if they are not of good technical quality. Occasionally, for fine points, microradiography (high resolution magnification radiography) can clarify whether or not an erosion or lesion is present. Second, the use of radiography must be selective and usually can be limited both for safety and cost effectiveness. For example, in evaluating rheumatoid arthritis: (1) in the upper extremities the key films are those of the hands (including the wrists) in posteroanterior and 15 degree oblique views; (2) in the neck, a lateral view in flexion alone will give sufficient data; and (3) in the feet, posteroanterior and lateral views without the oblique will often suffice. To assess degenerative joint disease of the knee, it is vital to include a standing anteroposterior view of both knees in one frame. For examination of the patient with seronegative spondyloarthropathy, limited views of the spine—i.e., a posteroanterior view of the pelvis to visualize the sacroiliac joints, anteroposterior and lateral views of the lumbosacral spine, and a lateral view of the neck in flexion—may suffice.

Joint Scintigraphy—Radioisotopes in the Evaluation of Articular Disease. The use of labeled isotopes in tracer amounts to measure their accumulation over normal and pathologic joints for the assessment of articular disease was introduced in the 1960's. The isotope evaluated first was technetium-99m (^{99m}Tc) pertechnetate, which largely binds to serum protein and is localized in areas of increased tissue vascularity. These scans correlate well with clinical assessment of joints and routine radiography, and on occasion allow the earlier detection of inflammation (increased blood flow). However, they are nonspecific, usually do not add significantly to routine radiography, and add (albeit a small amount) to the total body exposure.

The introduction of the bone seeking isotope ^{99m}Tc-diphosphonate added a new dimension to scintigraphy, since this allowed better evaluation of the axial skeleton. In many centers this has become the scan of choice. It can on occasion localize early sacroiliac inflammation prior to routine radiography since new bone is laid down in the involved sacroiliac joint. However, it, too, gives nonspecific results (the lesions of degenerative joint disease are often not distinguishable from those of rheumatoid arthritis), and the other problems noted above pertain. A negative scintigram is believed to be predictive of the absence of serious articular disease. However, in assessments of normal individuals an occasional joint has appeared positive.

The routine history, physical examination, selected laboratory studies, and selected routine radiographs make the use of joint scintigraphy a procedure to be chosen by experts for a specific purpose rather than a routine part of the workup of a patient with arthritis.

Arthrography (Synoviography). The injection of a contrast medium, often together with air or carbon dioxide, to visualize a joint space has become an accepted diagnostic procedure. Its value lies in the assessment of internal derangements of a joint space (usually a knee or shoulder) rather than in diagnosing inflammatory disease. The usual contraindications are infection or a bleeding diathesis. The radiopaque dye is introduced and the radiograph obtained promptly to determine its dispersion.

Orthopedists use the technique widely (as well as arthroscopy) in the diagnosis of cartilage tears in the knee and rotator cuff injuries of the shoulder. It is of great value medically in assessing masses in the popliteal area. When the differential diagnosis of deep venous thrombosis versus a ruptured popliteal cyst arises, venography is almost always indicated as a prior procedure.

Synovial cysts in rheumatoid disease, e.g., popliteal (Baker's) cysts, may rupture and lead to pain and discomfort about the knee and in the gastrocnemius area. Often the differential diagnosis is between acute thrombophlebitis and ruptured synovial cyst. When thrombophlebitis has been excluded, arthrography can often define the medical problem. On occasion, large synovial cysts can be instrumental in the development of thrombophlebitis caused by the pressure effect. Synovial cysts can occur about other joints but usually are asymptomatic.

Arthroscopy. Arthroscopy is an endoscopic procedure that has widespread orthopedic use. Its major application is in injuries about the knee joint, especially meniscal tears. With advancing technology the procedure has also been utilized in other articular spaces.

It is occasionally used by the rheumatologist in undiagnosed monarticular knee disease as a method of obtaining a selective biopsy from a local area of the joint under direct observation. It is not, however, a routine procedure and should only be performed by those with appropriate expertise.

Miscellaneous. Other technologies have been applied to the diagnostic evaluation of articular disease. These include angiography (useful in defining synovial tumors), ultrasonic scanning (increasingly helpful in the assessment of intact popliteal cysts), and, most recently, computed tomography of the joint space. All these procedures have limited utility.

Allen JC, Kunkel HG: Hidden rheumatoid factors with specificity for native gamma globulin. Arthritis Rheum 9:758, 1966. *Early studies of rheumatoid factors (RFs) showed that IgM RFs existed in the serum complexed with autologous IgG for which they were specific. When the binding was strong, these RFs could go undetected in certain systems.*

Bartfield H, Epstein WV: Rheumatoid factors and their biological significance. Ann NY Acad Sci 168:1, 1969. *A volume devoted to clinical and investigative aspects of the nature of rheumatoid factors and their relevance to disease.*

Cohen AS (ed.): Laboratory Diagnostic Procedures in the Rheumatic Diseases. 2nd ed. Boston, Little, Brown & Company, 1975. *A definitive review of the methodology and interpretation of laboratory tests in rheumatology. Not included are radiologic aspects.*

Dixon AS, Rasker JJ: Synoviography. Clin Rheum Dis 2:129, 1976. *A fine exposition of synoviography (arthrography) of various joints and the information to be gleaned from these procedures.*

Goldenberg DL, Cohen AS: Synovial membrane histopathology in the differential diagnosis of rheumatoid arthritis, gout, pseudogout, systemic lupus erythematosus, infectious arthritis and degenerative joint disease. Medicine 57:239, 1978. *An analysis of synovial membrane histopathology in the common inflammatory articular diseases, pointing out patterns that are diagnostically useful even though individual pathognomonic findings are rare.*

Griffiths ID, Dick WC: Antibodies to DNA antigens: Their specificity and clinical relevance. Eur J Clin Invest 9:239, 1979. *An editorial that focuses on the many ways of determining anti-DNA antibodies. It stresses the current multiple sources of DNA used (12 different sources in a recent multicenter study) and points out that in using radiolabeled nuclear antigens the present binding activity is linearly dependent upon the DNA molecular weight.*

Hadler NM, Spitznagel JK, Quinet RJ: Lysosomal enzymes in inflammatory synovial effusions. J Immunol 123:572, 1979. *A useful study of lysosomal enzymes of synovial fluid that discusses both sides of the question as to whether these enzymes are major causes of articular tissue destruction.*

Harris ED Jr, Krane SM: Collagenases. N Engl J Med 291:557, 605, 652, 1974. *A scholarly review of an increasingly important enzyme (collagenase) that might itself (or through its inhibitor) play a role in cartilage destruction.*

Jackson RW, Dandy DJ: Arthroscopy of the Knee. New York, Grune & Stratton, 1976. *A simple text that outlines the advantages and hazards of arthroscopy.*

Kushner I, Volanakis JE, Gewurtz H: C-Reactive protein and the plasma protein response to tissue injury. Ann NY Acad Sci 389:1–482, 1982. *The latest update of the chemistry and significance of C-reactive protein.*

Ng KC, Brown KA, Perry JD, Holborow EJ: Anti RANA antibody: A marker for seronegative and seropositive rheumatoid arthritis. Lancet 1:447, 1980. *A new and interesting test for rheumatoid arthritis that may have pathogenetic significance.*

Resnick D, Niwayam G: Diagnosis of Bone and Joint Disorders with Emphasis on Articular Abnormalities, Vols 1–3. Philadelphia, W. B. Saunders Co., 1981. *An extensive review of the radiologic findings in articular diseases.*

Ropes MW, Bauer W: Synovial Fluid Change in Joint Disease. Cambridge, Mass., Harvard University Press, 1953. *The definitive work on synovial fluid analysis in various articular diseases. The data on synovial fluid white counts, differentials, mucin, clot, etc., of 30 years ago are still valid and represent the basis for most subsequent joint fluid analyses.*

Rosenspire KC, Kennedy AC, Russomanno L, Steinbach J, Blau M, Green FA: Comparisons of four methods of analysis of ^{99m}Tc pyrophosphate uptake in RA joints. J Rheumatol 7:461,1980. *One of the first critical comparisons of the value and limitations of various methods of joint scintigraphy.*

Sokoloff L (ed.): The Joints and Synovial Fluid I. New York, Academic Press, 1978. *A modern treatise on the development, ultrastructure, immunobiology, and macromolecules of joints.*

Tan E: Autoantibodies to nuclear antigens (ANA): Their immunobiology and medicine. Adv Immunol 33:167, 1982. *An authoritative review of antinuclear antibodies and their clinical significance by a major contributor.*

444. RHEUMATOID ARTHRITIS

J. Claude Bennett

Rheumatoid arthritis (RA) is a systemic inflammatory disorder of a chronic nature that is characterized primarily by the pattern of involvement of synovial joints. The inflammatory process may involve soft tissue such as tendons, ligaments, fascia, and muscle and may extend into bone. By virtue of the mediators of inflammation that are involved in the rheumatoid process, systemic involvement of a generalized inflammatory nature affecting many different organ structures may also be seen.

For purposes of classification of rheumatoid arthritis, for usefulness in the uniformity of diagnosis, and for adherence to investigative protocols, the American Rheumatism Association (ARA) has developed 11 criteria for the diagnosis of RA. Of these 11 criteria, 7 are needed for diagnosis of *classic RA,* 5 for diagnosis of *definite RA,* and 3 for diagnosis of *probable RA.* Also required is that criteria 1 through 5 be fulfilled by observation of the continuous presence of the signs or symptoms for at least 6 weeks. The following criteria have been developed: (1) morning stiffness; (2) pain on motion or tenderness in at least one joint (observed by a physician); (3) swelling in at least one joint (observed by a physician); (4) swelling (observed by a physician) of at least one other joint (any interval free of joint symptoms between the two joint involvements may not be more than three months); (5) symmetric joint swelling (observed by a physician) with simultaneous involvement of the same joint on both sides of the body; (6) subcutaneous nodules (observed by a physician) on bony prominences, extensor surfaces, or in juxta-articular regions; (7) roentgenographic changes typical of rheumatoid arthritis; (8) a positive agglutination test result to demonstrate the presence of rheumatoid factor; (9) a poor mucin precipitate from synovial fluid (with shreds and cloudy solution) obtained on adding synovial fluid to dilute acetic acid; (10) characteristic histologic changes in the synovium; (11) characteristic histologic changes in the nodules.

The ARA criteria also incorporate 20 exclusions that were developed in order to rule out the many other forms of rheumatic disease that might in their early stages mimic rheumatoid arthritis. It is not surprising, with the rheumatoid factor assay as the only quantitative criterion, that the ARA set of diagnostic criteria is somewhat cumbersome to use for diagnosis on a broad basis. A more rigorous set of criteria proposed at the Third International Symposium of Population Studies of the Rheumatic Diseases in New York City in 1966 tends to exclude the probable cases as defined by ARA criteria but still suffers from the same absence of a quantitative basis on which to make the diagnosis. Nevertheless, the ARA criteria have been extremely useful in terms of description of the disease, anticipation of its clinical course, and for allowing physicians to talk with each other in commonly agreed-upon terms regarding patients with this disorder. Rheumatoid arthritis has a worldwide distribution and seems to affect all racial and ethnic groups. There is a female to male preponderance of approximately 2:1 to 3:1. However, if one focuses on the more specific findings of the disease, such as the positive serologic test for rheumatoid factor and erosive changes on roentgenograms, the striking female preponderance becomes less obvious. Although the peak incidence of onset is between the fourth and sixth decades, there is an increasing prevalence with advancing age up to the seventh decade. There have been many determinations of prevalence in a number of different populations, and in general it varies from 0.3 to 1.5 per cent. For convenience it is acceptable to consider a frequency of rheumatoid arthritis of about 1 per cent in the general adult population.

ETIOLOGY

The etiology of rheumatoid arthritis remains elusive even after many years of intensive investigation along various lines of study. These avenues of research have involved studies of metabolic, endocrine, and nutritional factors, as well as those defined by family studies, geographic locations, occupation, and psychosocial variables. Currently the most promising approaches lie along two major avenues of research: (1) studies of abnormalities in the immune system and its regulation; and (2) a search for some infectious agent or agents.

The discovery of rheumatoid factors in the synovial inflammatory process has focused attention on the immune system for the past 30 years. There is clear evidence that rheumatoid arthritis is an autoimmune disorder in the sense that it involves antibodies against autologous immunoglobulin G (IgG). On the other hand, there is no compelling reason to believe that this has occurred de novo; rather, it may be a response to some specific initiating external agent. The immunologic factors that might play a role in the etiology are discussed in subsequent paragraphs.

For many years investigators have found evidence for the occurrence of polyarthritis in association with microbial organisms, including bacteria. These have included the streptococci, clostridia, diphtheroids, and mycoplasmas. The association of several viral diseases with inflammatory rheumatic syndromes has provoked the possibility that rheumatoid arthritis itself is caused by a virus. The striking synovitis sometimes seen following rubella infections and the arthritis that may precede the onset of jaundice in infectious hepatitis are interesting examples of viral associations with rheumatic syndromes. In addition, the Ross River virus can produce an epidemic syndrome that in many clinical respects resembles the systemic-onset form of juvenile chronic arthritis. The arboviruses, particularly those of the togavirus family, can cause profound joint manifestations (e.g., Chikungunya and O'nyong-nyong fever). However, direct experimental evidence for viral infection in RA has not been forthcoming in spite of extensive searches. Interestingly, Lyme arthritis, which is caused by a spirochete, has some features of chronic rheumatoid disease but is clearly separable from the usual form of RA. Perhaps the strongest reason investigators have pursued microbial organisms as primary inciting agents in RA is that a large number of animal models of RA exist that are caused by microorganisms or their products. These include particularly mycoplasma infections in rats, pigs, mice, and poultry and also *Erysipelothrix* infections in pigs. Other animal models involve the immunologic reactivity against adjuvant or against bacterial cell wall peptidoglycans. Both of these processes produce an erosive, destructive, and fibrosing picture of joint pathology.

Nevertheless, in spite of numerous investigations for an initiating event, there are no generally accepted scientific data for a causative organism in adult rheumatoid disease. There are, however, a number of immunologic abnormalities that develop in parallel with the inflammatory process and that will be described in the paragraphs that follow.

PATHOLOGY

It appears that the earliest events in the rheumatoid synovium involve microvascular injury and edema of the subsynovial tissues, leading to a mild synovial lining cell proliferation. However, there are some who believe that the first visible event is synovial cell proliferation followed by injury and inflammation. Polymorphonuclear leukocytes (PMNs) may develop in the superficial synovium, the small blood vessels may be involved by inflammatory cells, and tiny thrombi may often be seen. Phagocytic events occur in proliferating synovial tissues and involve large mononuclear cells. In established RA the synovium develops slender villous projections and appears edematous and proliferative as it protrudes into the joint cavity. At this time one may see hyperplasia and hypertrophy of the synovial lining cells, which increase in thickness two- to threefold in terms of cell layers. At this stage of synovial proliferation, segmental vascular changes may be seen, and there may also be venous distention and infiltration of the arterial walls by PMNs together with areas of thrombosis and perivascular hemorrhage. The subsynovial stroma, which in the normal state is acellular, becomes packed with inflammatory cells, largely mononuclear, which may collect into aggregates or follicles. Rarely one actually sees true germinal centers. Lymphocytes usually predominate in the follicles with a layer of plasma cells around the periphery. Although immunofluorescence demonstrates large numbers of immunoglobulin-producing cells (B-lymphocytes), the majority of lymphocytes in the rheumatoid synovium are T cells. Progression to chronicity is associated with an expansion of the synovial surface area. This growing synovium actually erodes into bone, causing roentgenographic changes, and into soft tissue (such as tendons and fascia), which ultimately give rise to the deforming qualities of the clinical picture of RA.

PATHOGENESIS AND IMMUNOLOGIC FEATURES

Researchers in the rheumatic diseases have generally tended to develop hypotheses of pathogenesis along one of two lines. One involves extravascular immune complex formation, which sets into process the inflammatory response. The other is that the disease itself may result from a cellular hypersensitivity. Proponents of the latter hypothesis would say that an accumulation of activated T-lymphocytes in the synovium is associated with the production of soluble factors (lymphokines) and that this stimulates the dramatic synovial proliferation and general inflammatory response. The observation of a rheumatoid-like arthritis in some agammaglobulinemic children may be cited as possible evidence for an important role of the cellular immune reaction in rheumatoid synovitis.

Nevertheless, the first concept, based on the formation of immune complexes, is the one currently adhered to by the greatest number of investigators. It implies that the immune response is triggered in a sufficient, and perhaps specific, way against some foreign antigen. Clearly the genetic makeup of the individual would be a determinant of this host response. Hence, one might expect to see characteristic association with histocompatibility markers as has been noted in seropositive RA with HLA-D4 and HLA-DR4. A local reaction ensues within the joint itself. RA seems to involve a multicentric immune response, that is, each synovial tissue reacts in its own way, and therefore one might see a different B-lymphocyte clonal reactivity in different locations within the same individual. Antigen-antibody complexes thus formed from this reaction within the joint cavity would then become trapped in hyaline cartilage and fibrocartilage and produce changes in matrix macromolecules. In addition, within the synovial fluid the immune response activates the complement system, kinins, phagocytic cells, and lysosomal enzyme release. Mediators produced through this mechanism would cause synovial cells to proliferate and to produce proteinases and prostaglandins. These products cause dissolution of the connective tissue macromolecules within the associated connective tissue and the articular cartilage. Mediators also activate fibroblasts to produce a denser, richer connective tissue matrix and further synovial proliferation.

The rheumatoid factors produced by subsynovial lymphocytes are perhaps a reaction to IgG that has become immunogenic because of its combination with an antigen or because of its alteration in some fashion. These complexes in the synovial fluid can fix and activate complement and perpetuate the inflammatory process. Finally, in order for progressive destruction of joint tissue to occur, the usual control mechanisms that inhibit inflammation, i.e., inhibit the degradative enzymes and their activators, must be overwhelmed. Presumably this occurs through saturation of the synovial fluid and the tissue inhibitors of specific enzyme systems. The evolution of these processes gives rise to a continuing and perpetuating proliferation of cells, stimulation of enzyme systems, and destruction of normal tissue matrices.

Much is now known about the ability of rheumatoid synovial tissue to produce large quantities of collagenase, elastase, cathepsins, and prostaglandins. Collagenase production seems to be markedly stimulated in synovial sites when they are exposed to interleukin I, derived from mononuclear cells and blood macrophages. This enzyme is generally inactive when released from synovial cells but may be activated by appropriate proteolytic enzymes. The important activator may be plasmin. Synovial cells produce a plasminogen activator that attacks plasminogen in the circulation and converts it to plasmin. Plasmin then activates the latent collagenase bound to collagen fibrils. This allows rapid destruction of collagen-containing tissues. These pathogenetic events may stop at any stage, but over the long, chronic evolution of the disease, it is their summation in conjunction with the mechanical forces of weight bearing that give rise to the clinical picture of arthritis and the production of the characteristic deformities.

Rheumatoid factors are specific antiglobulins that react against the Fc portion of IgG molecules. They are produced by B-lymphocytes in the blood and other tissues, including synovial tissue. Their presence has turned out to be a useful clinical test for RA, as they occur in the circulating blood in approximately 80 per cent of patients, the so-called seropositive group. It must be emphasized that a positive test result is not diagnostic and that it does occur in 1 to 5 per cent of normal subjects with an increasing incidence in older individuals. It also occurs in a variety of other diseases usually associated with hyperglobulinemic states such as cirrhosis, leprosy, schistosomiasis, and sarcoidosis.

High titers of rheumatoid factors generally are associated with more severe and active joint disease and more frequently are found in the presence of rheumatoid nodules. A variety of rheumatoid factor activities may be discerned. They may react only with autologous IgGs or with isologous ones and sometimes even with the IgG of other species (heterologous). IgM rheumatoid factor can react with five IgG molecules and produce very large components with sedimentation constants of 22S. Intermediate-size complexes (between 7S and 19S) containing only IgG molecules, some of which have rheumatoid activity against self and usually consist of three molecules, can be discerned. There is some evidence that these complexes occur to a greater extent in those individuals with widespread systemic disease and vasculitis.

The question arises as to why rheumatoid factors should be produced. It appears that they are in fact reacting to altered autologous IgG. The alteration in the IgG could be the result of its having bound to a specific antigen molecule. There is some evidence for this concept, primarily from the finding of rheumatoid factors in bacterial endocarditis and in other diseases associated with chronic antigenic stimulation. Associations have been made between RA and the Epstein-Barr virus, which is a polyclonal stimulator of B cells. It has been suggested that certain individuals may be stimulated to produce rheumatoid factor molecules because of their special host response to this virus. Although the association of rheumatoid factors with RA is overwhelming, they clearly do not cause the disease, since the transfusion of rheumatoid factors into normal volunteers does not initiate an inflammatory process. Nonetheless, this association bespeaks some fundamental process that must be taking place within the synovial tissues. The recent concept of multicentric immunoreactivity within various synovial tissues is of great importance to our understanding of the total clonal repertoires that might be involved. Perhaps the B-lymphocytes of individuals who are susceptible to RA react in special ways against a variety of antigens and subsequently stimulate the production of rheumatoid factors.

CLINICAL FEATURES

Rheumatoid arthritis has a highly variable clinical course. It could in fact be an expression of a heterogeneous group of diseases of diverse etiologies. The course may range from a mild disease of brief duration to a progressive, destructive, and crippling arthritis. Although there is no direct correlation among the extent of articular manifestations, joint destruction, and systemic manifestations, individuals who have very high titers of rheumatoid factors tend to have a more generalized systemic disease and a more erosive, destructive arthritic process.

Onset of Symptoms

The majority of patients, perhaps two thirds, have an insidious onset of their disease over weeks to months. During this period of time, malaise, fatigue, and perhaps diffuse musculoskeletal pain may be the predominant complaints. Only later do specific joints become involved with swelling, redness, pain, and tenderness. Frequently the onset of disease is symmetrical, involving especially the small joints of the hands, but also the elbows, the wrists, and the shoulders. As noted in the ARA diagnostic criteria, the symmetrical pattern is particularly useful in early disease in helping to differentiate RA from other forms of inflammatory arthritis. During this period of time, a frequent complaint is that of stiffness following inactivity. It can occur in the morning upon arising or following prolonged sitting. It is described by some as a "gelling" process and seems to be associated with edema within the inflamed tissues. So characteristic is this symptom that the duration of morning stiffness has been taken as a guide to the severity of the inflammatory process. In most clinical studies of RA, it is a useful bit of quantitative data that may be used to follow the activity of the disease. As the process evolves, the patient may have increasing difficulty with pain and stiffness. This limits the ability to move about, climb stairs, open doors, open jars, or to do detailed small movements, such as sewing. The patient may develop an associated psychologic depression and weight loss, and sometimes a low-grade fever may occur in association with the systemic manifestations of the disease.

An acute onset of disease is seen in about 20 per cent of patients. "Acute" refers to the rapid buildup of symptoms usually over a period of a few days. Occasionally an individual retires in the evening with no symptoms and wakes up the next morning with acute generalized RA. Such rapid onset of pain involving joints and surrounding soft tissues, as well as muscles, can present a difficult diagnostic picture. Such an acute onset of RA may be confused with acute myositis, viral syndromes, or, if focal, even septic arthritis.

Joint Manifestations

RA can affect any diarthrodial joint, and those most commonly involved are the small joints of the hands, wrists, knees, and feet. As the disease spreads, it may involve elbows, shoulders, sternoclavicular joints, hips, ankles, and, less commonly, the temporomandibular and cricoarytenoid joints. Spinal involvement in RA is generally limited to the upper cervical articulations, at least from the standpoint of clinically significant lesions.

Because of the synovial proliferation and inflammatory destruction of soft tissues, a laxity of ligaments and tendons develops, which, in conjunction with mechanical pressures and regular use, gives rise to typical deformities.

HANDS. One of the most common early signs of disease is swelling of the proximal interphalangeal (PIP) joints, giving the fingers a fusiform or spindle-shaped appearance. This is generally associated with bilateral and symmetrical swelling of the metacarpophalangeal (MCP) joints (Fig. 444–1). Although the distal interphalangeal (DIP) joints can be involved, they generally are not, and this is important in the differential diagnosis of RA and osteoarthritis. Soft tissue laxity gives rise to the appearance of an ulnar deviation of the fingers (Fig. 444–2*A*) that is frequently accompanied by palmar subluxation of the proximal phalanges. Swan neck deformities develop owing to hyperextension of the PIP joints in conjunction with flexion of the DIP joints (Fig. 444–2*B*). Flexion deformity of the PIP joints and extension of the DIP joints give rise to the boutonniere deformity. These changes are associated with loss of strength in the hands and frequently loss of the ability to maintain a

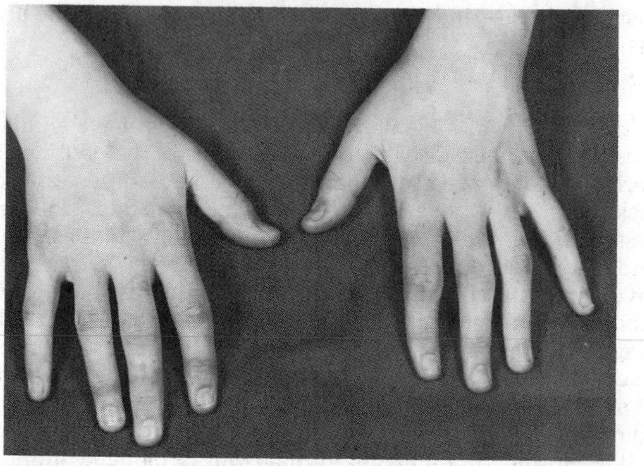

Figure 444–1. Early rheumatoid arthritis manifest as symmetrical swelling and slight flexion deformities of proximal interphalangeal joints of the hands. Roentgenograms were normal except for evidence of soft tissue swelling.

good pinch. Synovial erosions of tendons may lead to their rupture and sudden loss of the ability to extend the fingers.

WRISTS. The wrists are almost invariably involved in RA and frequently demonstrate easily palpable, boggy synovium. Such synovial proliferation on the volar aspect may compress the median nerve and produce the carpal tunnel syndrome. This consists of paresthesia and dysesthesia of the thumb and the second and third digits and the radial aspect of the fourth digit. It may also be accompanied by atrophy of the thenar eminence. Frequently, one of the first losses of motion in rheumatoid arthritis is the inability to dorsiflex the wrist fully. Normally the wrist should be able to move through nearly 180 degrees in its extremes of palmar and dorsiflexion.

KNEES. Synovial hypertrophy and effusion in this weight-bearing joint places it among the more frequently affected joints in RA. Effusions may be detected by ballotting the patella or by demonstrating a "bulge sign" along the patella when fluid is pushed into the suprapatellar pouch and then expressed back into the joint. One may expect to see quadriceps atrophy in association with chronic knee arthritis. Baker's cysts may form owing to enlargement of the semimembranous bursa into the popliteal space. Such synovial cysts may occasionally dissect and rupture and can give rise to symptoms mimicking acute thrombophlebitis. Sonargrams and arthrograms may be useful for confirmation of the diagnosis. Destruction of soft tissue about the knee can also give rise to marked joint instability.

FEET AND ANKLES. Arthritis is frequently present in the feet and may involve changes analogous to those described in the hands. Cock-up of the toes may produce subluxation of the metatarsal heads and finally a clawlike appearance.

NECK. Symptoms of neck pain are frequent in rheumatoid arthritis and may be associated with significant bony erosions because of involvement of the rheumatoid process in the cervical vertebrae. Although rare, continuous erosion may produce atlantoaxial subluxation, which can give rise to cervical dislocation and spinal cord compression, producing neurologic manifestations.

Extra-articular Manifestations

The occurrence of constitutional symptoms, occasionally a low-grade fever and minimal lymphadenopathy, are to be expected in RA. As the disease progresses, muscle atrophy, weakness, and sometimes the development of tremor can be seen. The latter is presumably caused by muscle fatigue and is usually associated with more severe disease and a poor prognosis.

SKIN. Subcutaneous nodules may develop at some time in approximately 20 to 25 per cent of patients. They are nearly always associated with seropositive disease and are found most frequently in the rapidly progressive and destructive form of the disease. Periarticular structures and areas subject to pressure, such as the elbows, the occiput, or the sacrum, tend to be the primary sites for subcutaneous nodules. They may occasionally break down or become infected but generally are asymptomatic. Another common skin manifestation in RA is the result of vasculitis. In the skin the vasculitic process often produces small brown spots, frequently in the nail folds or in the digital pulp. Larger areas of ischemic involvement may occur in the lower extremities with infarction of a toe or the development of skin sloughs over the malleoli. Histologic examination of the vasculitis may show only a mild venulitis with a relatively bland proliferation of affected digital vessels, or it may be a severe and widespread necrotizing vasculitis of the small and medium-size arteries, indistinguishable from polyarteritis nodosa. Rheumatoid vasculitis is frequently associated with high fever and other manifestations of systemic disease, including a depression of serum complement.

Another common skin manifestation is that of a tendency to easy bruisability and production of ecchymotic lesions. This seems to be caused by the general fragility of the skin in rheumatoid disease and is possibly associated with the systemic manifestations of the inflammatory process.

CARDIAC MANIFESTATIONS. Although symptomatic cardiac disease is not common in RA, a relatively frequent symptomatic lesion is acute pericarditis. It is unrelated to the duration of the arthritis and seems to appear most often in seropositive disease. The pericardial fluid characteristics include a low glucose concentration, increased lactic dehydrogenase (LDH) level, elevated immunoglobulin levels, and low complement activity. Pericardial disease may vary from a mild, fleeting process to a sizable effusion to cardiac tamponade and death. Some evidence of pericardial involvement with old fibrinous adhesions is found in about 40 per cent of RA patients at autopsy.

Lesions similar to rheumatoid nodules may be found involving the myocardium and the valves. Sometimes a focal inter-

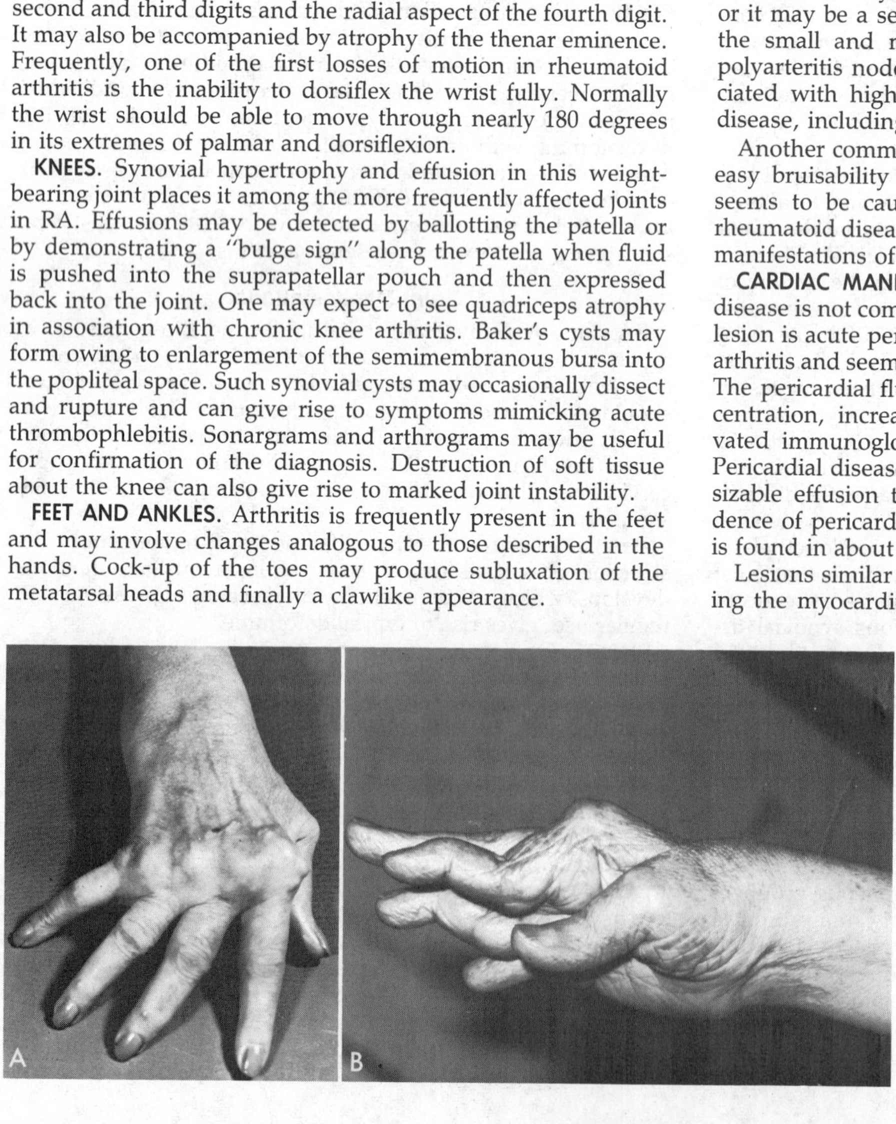

Figure 444–2. Hand deformities characteristic of chronic rheumatoid arthritis. *A*, Subluxation of metacarpophalangeal joints with ulnar deviation of digits. *B*, Hyperextension ("swan neck") deformities of proximal interphalangeal joints.

stitial myocarditis and arteritis of coronary vessels may be recognized. Occasionally valvular insufficiency, conduction abnormalities, and myocardial infarction secondary to these inflammatory lesions may be seen as clinical manifestations of rheumatoid heart disease.

PULMONARY MANIFESTATIONS. Rheumatoid pleural disease, though frequently found at autopsy, is most commonly asymptomatic. Occasionally a pleural effusion may be of sufficient size to cause respiratory limitation. Typically the pleural fluid is exudative, and white cell counts vary greatly but generally are less than 5000 per cu mm. Glucose levels tend to be low, and the LDH enzyme level is high. Total hemolytic complement, C3, and C4 levels are low. Immune complexes and rheumatoid factors are frequently found in the pleural fluid.

Intrapulmonary nodules may also be seen. Although they are usually asymptomatic, they may become infected and may cavitate or rupture into the pleural space with the production of a pneumothorax. Similar but distinct nodular infiltrates may also be seen in rheumatoid lungs in association with pneumoconiosis (Caplan's syndrome). Finally one may see a diffuse interstitial fibrosis and pneumonitis. This may progress to a honeycomb appearance on the roentgenogram, bronchiectasis, chronic cough, and progressive dyspnea. Pulmonary function tests show a diminished compliance and a restrictive ventilatory pattern.

NEUROLOGIC MANIFESTATIONS. Rheumatoid vasculitis is frequently associated with a mononeuritis multiplex syndrome in which there is patchy sensory loss in one or more of the extremities, frequently in association with foot drop or wrist drop. Biopsy of the sural nerve (when there is an abnormal conduction time) can confirm the diagnosis of vasculitis. As mentioned previously, neurologic complaints can also be produced in association with proliferating synovium, causing compression of nerves. This can result in conditions such as a median neuropathy (carpal tunnel syndrome) or a tarsal tunnel syndrome caused by an anterior tibial nerve palsy (resulting in foot drop). Although the central nervous system is usually spared, rheumatoid vasculitis and rheumatoid nodule-like granulomas have been known to occur in the meninges.

OPHTHALMOLOGIC MANIFESTATIONS. Episcleritis is a self-limited condition and may develop in association with mild pain and discomfort. Sjögren's syndrome can occur and cause corneal and conjunctival lesions associated with dryness of the eyes. Scleritis can be accompanied by severe pain and occasional visual impairment. Lesions may be found in the superior sclera as raised yellow nodules surrounded by hyperemia of the deep scleral vessels. If this progresses over a period of time, allowing the dark blue color of the choroid beneath to show through, it is termed scleromalasia perforans. The histologic picture is similar to that of the rheumatoid nodule.

FELTY'S SYNDROME. This syndrome is found in chronic RA associated with splenomegaly, lymphadenopathy, anemia, thrombocytopenia, and a selective leukopenia involving only the neutrophils. Although hypersplenism is proposed as one cause of the leukopenia, splenectomy fails to correct the abnormality in many patients. Gram-positive infections are common and frequently fail to respond to antibiotics. Interestingly, the incidence of infection may decline after splenectomy even when the neutropenia remains unaltered.

Clinical Laboratory Findings

A mild anemia, usually of the normocytic normochromic or hypochromic type, may be found. Sometimes there is a low serum iron level and normal or low iron binding capacity. The anemia, however, is generally resistant to iron therapy. The erythrocyte sedimentation rate tends to be elevated in most patients but only roughly parallels the disease activity. Although the white cell count and differential are usually normal, there may be a significant eosinophilia in association with systemic rheumatoid disease, especially vasculitis. The presence of rheumatoid factor by agglutination test is helpful in the clinical diagnosis of rheumatoid disease, and other serologic abnormalities, including antibodies against DNA and nuclear antigens in low titer, occur in a small percentage of patients. Although the finding of HLA-DR4 positivity by B cell typing is important for investigational purposes, it is not generally useful in the diagnosis of RA. Evidence now suggests that it is associated with a more aggressive disease, especially striking when found among seronegative RA patients.

Synovial fluid analysis generally shows white cell counts in the range of 5000 to 20,000 per cu mm with approximately 50 to 70 per cent as polymorphonuclear leukocytes. Synovial fluid complement is usually low, rheumatoid factors are usually present, and there is evidence of hyaluronate degradation, as shown by a poor mucin clot test.

Differential Diagnosis

The differential considerations in the diagnosis of RA are numerous. Although there is seldom confusion in classic rheumatoid arthritis, diagnosis can be more difficult in patients with early acute polyarthritis or those with involvement of only a few joints. One must consider osteoarthritis, gout, chondrocalcinosis, systemic lupus erythematosus (SLE), and progressive systemic sclerosis (PSS) as the more common diseases that might be confused with RA. In addition, a variety of systemic diseases, including sarcoidosis, inflammatory bowel disease, Whipple's disease, amyloidosis, chronic infection, and malignancies, can all present with arthritic syndromes mimicking RA. Therefore, a complete medical evaluation is indicated on all patients with joint manifestations. One must assess the patient for general systemic diseases and also for curable causes, such as bacterial infections. The careful analysis of synovial fluid is critical to differentiate rheumatoid arthritis from chronic gout and chondrocalcinosis. Critical evaluation of inflammatory joint effusions is useful not only for diagnosis but also as a guide for therapeutic responses.

COURSE AND PROGNOSIS

Although rheumatoid arthritis can follow several possible courses, most commonly the disease is initially intermittent but becomes more sustained with the passage of time. However, the course cannot be predicted, and although some patients show an unrelenting progression to deformity and occasionally even death, most patients will have episodes of relative or complete remission. An ARA committee has proposed criteria for clinical remission of rheumatoid arthritis in which five or more of the following requirements must be fulfilled for at least two consecutive months: (1) duration of morning stiffness not exceeding 15 minutes; (2) no fatigue; (3) no joint pain (by history); (4) no joint tenderness or pain on motion; (5) no soft tissue swelling in joints or tendon sheaths; and (6) erythrocyte sedimentation rate (Westergren method) less than 30 mm per hr for females or 20 mm per hr for males.

Remissions may be more frequent than generally appreciated, but a spontaneous remission is not likely beyond the first two years of the disease. It is usually helpful in chronic arthritis to establish an evaluation of functional capacity. Although there have been a number of suggested systems, a rough division would be the following:

Class I—No restriction of ability to perform normal activities.

Class II—Moderate restriction but adequate for normal activities.

Class III—Marked restriction, inability to perform most duties of the patient's usual occupation or self-care.

Class IV—Incapacitation or confinement to a bed or wheelchair.

THERAPEUTIC MANAGEMENT

The physician should recognize that RA is a chronic systemic disease that may be expected to have a prolonged course and an uncertain outcome. Therefore, one must remember that the majority of patients can continue to lead active lives with varying degrees of restrictions. In this setting of chronic disease, undue or excessive drug therapy, especially adrenocorticosteroids and immunosuppressive agents, can cause greater morbidity than the underlying disease itself. Objectives of management should include (1) relief of pain, (2) reduction of inflammation, (3) minimizing undesirable side effects, (4) preservation of muscle strength and joint function, and (5) as rapid a return to a normal lifestyle as possible. All patients with rheumatoid arthritis should begin with a basic program that includes (1) adequate rest, (2) adequate salicylate therapy, and (3) maintenance of joint function by physical measures.

Neither the patient nor the physician should be confused by the dual goals of balanced rest and exercise in rheumatoid disease. As has been noted for many years, it is only a rare patient with RA who does not improve significantly upon being hospitalized. From this we have learned that bed rest tends to decrease the general systemic inflammatory response. Most patients will soon learn that their fatigue, which occurs in the mid-afternoon, can be significantly reduced by a period of rest. This tends to give them a "second wind" for handling their functional requirements during the remainder of the day. Therefore, a regularly disciplined rest period in the mid-afternoon is most effective in maintaining the patient's overall sense of well-being. In acute exacerbations of disease, longer rest periods and perhaps even bed restriction are required to assist in suppression of the inflammatory process. Although it is clear that physical overexertion will increase synovitis and inflammation in the rheumatoid joint, it is also important that full range of motion be maintained. This can usually be accomplished by graded exercise programs for the patient. However, during acute phases, passive range of motion exercises by a physical therapist or an instructed lay person may be indicated.

Salicylate therapy is critical to this basic program. Salicylates are cheap, generally well-tolerated, and have a good track record of control of inflammation in RA. The patient needs to understand that salicylates should be taken in a continual daily dosage that provides a constant blood level of 20 to 30 mg per dl. For most people this will require between 3 and 6 grams of aspirin per day. If one expects to obtain anything more than analgesia from aspirin, this dose level must be reached. All patients should be monitored for toxicity, as indicated by blood tests, ototoxicity (deafness or ringing in the ears), or gastrointestinal intolerance. Because of the availability of buffered aspirin and coated aspirin, one can usually find a salicylate preparation for almost any patient.

Physical measures and various heat modalities such as shower, bath, warm pool, paraffin baths, hot packs, and so forth, should be employed to loosen the joints and to relieve stiffness. Exercise following these applications is designed to maintain motion of affected joints and to prevent muscle atrophy. These goals can generally be achieved without aggressive overactivity and can usually keep a patient fully mobile during the course of the disease. Acutely inflamed joints may need to be rested with either total body rest or splinting.

Drug Therapy

Even though the appropriate approach to aspirin therapy has been discussed previously, it should be pointed out that many salicylate preparations cause silent gastrointestinal bleeding. Fortunately, this is usually minimal and may not require a change of therapy. Overt gastrointestinal tract hemorrhage caused by aspirin is rare, but if gastrointestinal bleeding is contributing to a constant anemia, modification of the therapeutic regimen should be instituted.

Several nonsteroidal anti-inflammatory drugs (NSAIDs) are available, and many of them have effective analgesic, antipyretic, and anti-inflammatory activity in patients with rheumatoid arthritis. Indomethacin and phenylbutazone have been available for some time. Although they are more frequently used in osteoarthritis, they are also effective in some patients with RA. Newer nonsteroidals have recently been introduced in this country. They include the derivatives of phenylacetic acid (ibuprofen, fenoprofen), naphthalene acetic acids (naproxen), pyrrolealkanoic acid (tolmetin), indoleacetic acids (sulindac), a halogenated anthranilic acid (meclofenamate sodium), and, even more recently, piroxicam, zomepirac, and diflunisal. Most of these drugs are beneficial in patients with rheumatoid arthritis. They are generally no more effective than aspirin but may be better tolerated. Their major current disadvantage is their expense. The experience of physicians dealing with rheumatoid arthritis generally is that they will have to shift drugs occasionally in order to lessen side effects or to adjust to the needs of a given patient.

If the nonsteroidal anti-inflammatory drugs fail to control the disease, then one must consider the more slowly acting drugs, including antimalarials, gold, and penicillamine. Antimalarials are usually given as hydroxychloroquine 200 mg twice daily. This drug and chloroquine may cause retinal lesions and loss of vision; therefore the patient should be checked by an ophthalmologist at least twice a year. Gold salts are widely used and can produce remission in many cases. Because of the potential of gold toxicity on the kidney and bone marrow, frequent urinalysis and routine blood work (CBC) must be done, especially during the early phases of the therapeutic program. Treatment with gold is usually begun with a 10 mg test injection (Myochrysine or Solganal) for idiosyncrasy, then a 25 mg dose the second week, and a 50 mg injection weekly up to a total of about 1 gram. Usually during this period of time a therapeutic response occurs, and at that point the dose can be cut to alternate weeks and subsequently to every third or fourth week. Many patients have been on prolonged gold therapy for a number of years. However, side effects are common, with as many as 30 per cent of patients having to discontinue therapy because of them. The most common and the most annoying to the patient are pruritic skin rashes. More painful are mouth ulcers. Severe manifestations include bone marrow suppression, usually leukopenia or thrombocytopenia, and renal damage with proteinuria and rarely the nephrotic syndrome. Penicillamine is now available for the treatment of rheumatoid arthritis and is also quite effective in inducing improvements in the disease and sometimes even in inducing remissions. It suffers from some of the same problems as gold in that it affects both the bone marrow and the kidney. Therefore, patients must be carefully monitored for toxicity. Immunosuppressive agents such as azathioprine, cyclophosphamide, chlorambucil, and methotrexate have been used to treat especially severe and unremitting RA. Azathioprine has been given FDA approval for the treatment of rheumatoid arthritis, and large-scale cooperative studies are now under way to evaluate methotrexate therapy in specific cases of rheumatoid disease.

Other experimental approaches to the treatment of drug-resistant patients include plasmapheresis, leukapheresis, and total nodal irradiation. All of these procedures are experimental, and long-term effects are unknown.

One cannot ignore corticosteroids when considering the therapy of RA. Because of their side effects they are generally discouraged by most rheumatologists. Patients with active rheumatoid disease do not tolerate alternate-day steroids well, and therefore one quickly gets into a pattern of daily therapy. Although they can be useful in those patients who have neuropathy, vasculitis, pleuritis, pericarditis, scleritis, and related conditions, for the usual patient with only joint disease it is wise to avoid them. Local steroid injections can sometimes be helpful for the relief of persistent effusions or to get patients more mobile in preparation for appropriate physical therapy.

Finally, one must not overlook the very great importance of reconstructive orthopedic surgery. Perhaps the greatest contribution to the management of rheumatoid arthritis in the last 10 years has been the development of superb techniques for joint replacement therapy. The use of prosthetic devices for the patient with hip and knee disease has given excellent results, and the results for ankle, elbow, and shoulder replacement are improving rapidly. Reconstructive orthopedic surgery in patients who have had long-term destructive disease is a very major part of our total therapeutic armamentarium.

JUVENILE CHRONIC ARTHRITIS

Rheumatic diseases are not rare in children, but they differ somewhat from those in adults, and that difference is worth noting. Although the various subclasses of chronic arthritis in children have not yet been fully defined and although some still prefer the use of the term "juvenile rheumatoid arthritis," it is becoming increasingly popular to use the term "juvenile chronic arthritis." Currently, the disease is further subdivided into the following: systemic onset disease, polyarticular onset disease, and pauciarticular onset disease.

The first, systemic onset (Still's disease), accounts for about 20 per cent of patients. The disease can begin at any age. The rheumatoid factor and antinuclear antibody test results are generally negative. Clinical characteristics include a high intermittent fever, maculopapular rash, polyserositis, lymphadenopathy, hepatosplenomegaly, leukocytosis, and anemia. Although the disease is rarely life-threatening, it can be confused initially with leukemia or infection. A chronic polyarthritis usually develops in these patients within the first few months of the disease but sometimes not until years later.

Polyarticular onset disease without any extra-articular manifestations occurs in approximately 40 per cent of patients, and there is a female preponderance. The majority of these children are seronegative for rheumatoid factors. Those who are seropositive are generally older than eight years of age when the disease begins. Positive test results for antinuclear antibodies are often found. These patients may have malaise, low-grade fever, adenopathy, anemia, and growth retardation. With polyarticular disease one commonly sees cervical spine involvement, most typically at the C2-C3 apophyseal joints.

Pauciarticular onset disease affects another 40 per cent of children with juvenile arthritis, and there are several subgroups of this pattern. At least two can be identified. One subgroup is characterized by early onset with a female preponderance. The serum of these patients often is positive for antinuclear antibodies but negative for rheumatoid factors. Some tend to develop inflammation of the anterior uveal tract (iridocyclitis). This occasionally can be the major manifestation and can progress to blindness. Therefore, evaluation of these children for progressive ophthalmologic manifestations is important. The second subgroup of pauciarticular onset has a strong male preponderance, and many of these individuals are HLA-B27 positive, so they appear as young children with spondyloarthropathy.

Treatment is usually helpful for these children. Aspirin is a basic standby for therapy, and physical and psychosocial support are indicated. Although these subsets have many properties in common with adult rheumatoid disease, there are many distinctions, and one must be aware that there may be several different diseases with different etiologies grouped within this general category.

ADULT-ONSET STILL'S DISEASE

As indicated in the previous section, one of the subsets of juvenile chronic arthritis is the systemic onset form, which is Still's disease There have been several cases, now up to a total of 70 or more, of adult-onset Still's disease in which the clinical features are almost identical to those occurring in children. These patients exhibit high fevers, polyarthritis, tenosynovitis, and a salmon-colored maculopapular measles-like rash, particularly over the trunk and along pressure lines. Nodules sometimes occur in these patients, but the fever and rash are the most characteristic of the initial signs of disease and help to point toward the adult-onset form of Still's disease. Pericarditis and pleural effusions have been reported but are generally mild. Other systemic manifestations do occur. Acute symptoms generally respond to an adequate dose of salicylates, but occasionally nonsteroidal anti-inflammatory drugs or even prednisone may be necessary for short periods of time.

Alarcón GS, Koopman WJ, Acton RT, Barger BO: Seronegative rheumatoid arthritis: A distinct immunogenetic disease? Arth Rheum 25:502, 1982. *An interesting study of the association of histocompatibility markers and immunogenetic epidemiology in seronegative rheumatoid arthritis.*

Ansell B: Diagnostic criteria, nomenclature, classification. *In* Munthe E (ed.): The Care of Rheumatoid Children. Basel, EULAR, 1978, p 42. *A succinct description of the basis for diagnosis and classification of the juvenile chronic arthritides.*

Aptekar RG, Decker JL, Bujak JS, Wolff SE: Adult onset juvenile rheumatoid arthritis. Arth Rheum 16:715, 1973. *An excellent clinical discussion of the adult onset form of Still's disease.*

Bennett JC: The infectious etiology of rheumatoid arthritis. Arth Rheum 21:531, 1978. *A discussion of the various possibilities for the role of infectious agents in rheumatic diseases.*

Blumberg B, Bunim JJ, Calkins E, Pirani CL, Zvaifler NJ: ARA nomenclature and classification of arthritis and rheumatism. Arth Rheum 7:93, 1964. *The general outline of the ARA Diagnostic Criteria*

Hollingsworth JW: Local and Systemic Complications of Rheumatoid Arthritis. Philadelphia, W. B. Saunders Co., 1968. *An excellent and comprehensive discussion of the nonarticular complications of rheumatoid disease.*

Kotzin BL, Strober S, Engleman EG, Calin A, Hoppe RT, Kansas GS, Terrell CP, Kaplan HS: Treatment of intractable rheumatoid arthritis with lymphoid irradiation. N Engl J Med 305:969, 1981. *An interesting description of a current investigative approach to the treatment of rheumatoid arthritis.*

Krane SM: Aspects of the cell biology of the rheumatoid synovial lesion. Ann Rheum Dis 40:433, 1981. *Description of the biology of tissue destruction in the rheumatoid process dealing with both the enzymes involved and their regulation.*

Lewis JR: New antirheumatic agents. JAMA 237:1260, 1977. *A succinct description of the nonsteroidal anti-inflammatory agents.*

Pinals RS, Masi AT, Larsen RA: Preliminary criteria for clinical remission in rheumatoid arthritis. Arth Rheum 24:1308, 1981.

Schumacher HR: Synovial membrane and fluid morphologic alterations in early rheumatoid arthritis: Microvascular injury and virus-like particles. Ann NY Acad Sci 256:39, 1975. *An excellent description of the pathology of rheumatoid synovial tissue and synovial fluid.*

Short CL, Bauer W, Reynolds WS: Rheumatoid Arthritis. Cambridge-Harvard University Press, 1957. *A superb documentation of modes of onset and clinical features of rheumatoid arthritis throughout its entire natural history.*

Steinbrocker O, Traeger CH, Batterman RC: Therapeutic criteria in rheumatoid arthritis. JAMA 140:659, 1949.

Wees SJ, Sunwoo IN, Oh SJ: Sural nerve biopsy in systemic necrotizing vasculitis. Am J Med 71:525, 1981. *Description of a useful diagnostic procedure for vasculitis and peripheral neuropathy.*

Ziff M: Systemic rheumatoid disease: Immunological aspects. Adv Inflam Res 3:123, 1982. *A comprehensive review of the immunological mechanisms involving the pathogenesis of rheumatoid arthritis.*

445. THE SPONDYLARTHROPATHIES

Andrei Calin

The seronegative spondylarthritides are characterized by involvement of the sacroiliac joints, by peripheral inflammatory arthropathy, and by the absence of rheumatoid factor. Other features include (1) pathologic changes concentrated around the enthesis (i.e., the site of ligamentous insertion into bone) rather than the synovium. Nonenthesopathic changes may also develop in the eye, the aortic valve, the lung parenchyma, and the skin. (2) Clinical evidence of overlap among the various seronegative spondylarthritides. Thus, a patient with psoriatic arthropathy may well develop uveitis or sacroiliitis; a patient with inflammatory bowel disease may develop ankylosing spondylitis or mouth ulcers. (3) A tendency toward familial aggregation, with the suggestion that these entities "breed true" within families.

TYPES

The spondylarthropathies include the prototype disorder ankylosing spondylitis, as well as Reiter's syndrome (both the postvenereal, or endemic, and the postinfective, or epidemic, forms), the reactive arthritides (caused by infections with Yersinia and Salmonella), certain subsets of juvenile arthropathy (juvenile ankylosing spondylitis and the seronegative enthesopathic arthropathy syndrome), enteropathic sacroiliitis (ul-

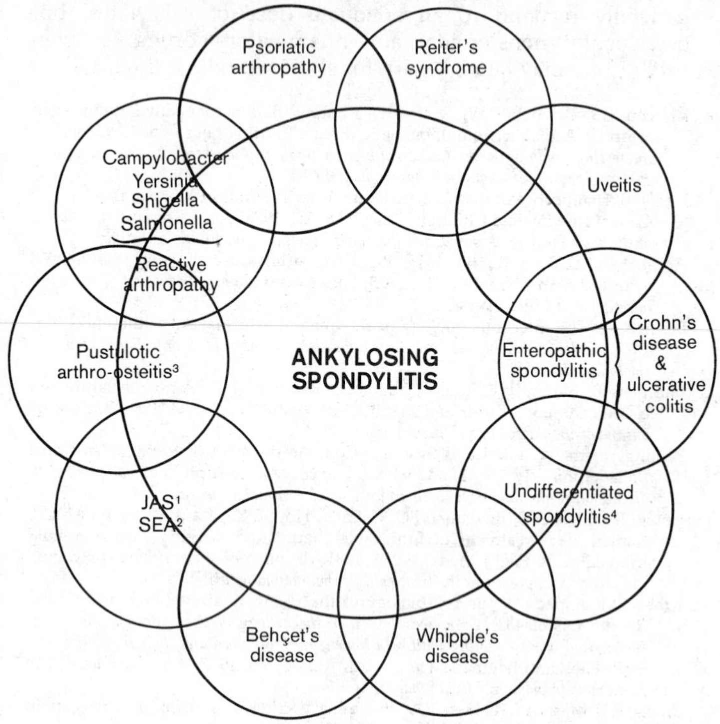

Figure 445–1. Individual conditions that overlap to form the spondyloarthritides. (1) Juvenile ankylosing spondylitis. (2) Seronegative enthesopathic arthropathy syndrome. (3) Considered by Japanese to be part of spondyloarthropathy spectrum (rare in United States and Europe). (4) Undifferentiated spondylitis (i.e., subset of patients who have spondyloarthropathic features but who fail to meet criteria for ankylosing spondylitis, Reiter's syndrome, or other condition, e.g., dactylitis, uveitis, plus unilateral sacroiliitis).

cerative colitis and Crohn's disease), psoriatic arthropathy, and perhaps a group of rarer disorders (Behçet's syndrome, Whipple's disease, and pustulotic arthro-osteitis) (see Fig. 445–1).

These disorders can be categorized according to the specific periarticular or articular involvement. The various spondylarthropathies can be distinguished from one another according to the particular peripheral joints involved, the associated clinical features (i.e., urethritis, conjunctivitis, skin involvement), and the manner in which the disease progresses (i.e., remission or relapse) (see Table 445–1).

HEREDITARY FACTORS

Hereditary factors play an important role in the development of the spondylarthropathies. Approximately 20 per cent of HLA-B27–positive individuals develop ankylosing spondylitis following an unknown environmental event or develop Reiter's syndrome after exposure to Shigella or other environmental agents. The offspring of an individual with HLA-B27 have a 50 per cent chance of carrying the same antigen and, thus, an overall 10 per cent chance of developing ankylosing spondylitis or Reiter's syndrome if exposed to a specific arthritogenic trigger.

The explanation for the link between HLA-B27 and the spondylarthropathies remains unknown. Hypotheses include (1) B27 acts as a receptor site for an infective agent; (2) B27 is a marker for an immune response gene that determines susceptibility to an environmental trigger; or (3) B27 may induce tolerance to foreign antigens with which it cross-reacts.

Patients with ankylosing spondylitis or Reiter's syndrome who lack HLA-B27 may be more likely to have a cross-reacting antigen such as B7, Bw22, or Bw42. We now know that the

TABLE 445–1. COMPARISON OF SERONEGATIVE SPONDYLOARTHROPATHIES

	Ankylosing Spondylitis	Reiter's Syndrome	Psoriatic Arthropathy	Enteropathic Spondylitis	Juvenile Arthropathy (JAS* subset)	Reactive Arthropathy
Sex	Male ≥ Female	Male ≥ Female	Female ≥ Male	Female = Male	Male > Female	Male = Female
Age at onset	20	Any age	Any age	Any age	<16	Any age
Uveitis	+	++	+	+	+	+
Conjunctivitis	−	+	−	−	−	+
Peripheral joints	Lower > Upper: often	Lower usually	Upper > Lower	Lower > Upper	Lower > Upper	Lower > Upper
Sacroiliitis	Always	Often	Often	Often	Often	Often
HLA-B27	95%	80%	20% (50% with sacroiliitis)	50%	90%	80%
Enthesopathy	+	+	+	?	+	?
Aortic regurgitation	+	+	?+	?	?	+
Familial aggregation	+	+	+	+	+	+
Risk for HLA-B27–positive individual	±20%	20%	?	?	?	20%
Onset	Gradual	Sudden	Variable	Gradual	Variable	Sudden
Urethritis	−	+	−	−	−	+/−
Skin involvement	−	+	++	−	−	−
Mucous membrane involvement	−	+	−	+	−	+
Symmetry (spinal)	+	−	−	+	+	−
Self-limiting	−	+/−	+/−	+/−	+/−	+/−
Remission, relapses	−	+/−	+/−	−	+/−	+/−

*JAS = Juvenile ankylosing spondylitis.

risk of developing ankylosing spondylitis for a B27-positive relative of a B27-positive patient is 25 to 50 per cent compared with about 5 per cent for a B27-positive subject. This argues for genetic differences between the two B27 groups.

ANKYLOSING SPONDYLITIS

Criteria for Diagnosis

The criteria for diagnosing ankylosing spondylitis have been evolving in recent years. The New York criteria have limitations. For example, precisely what constitutes reduced spinal mobility has not been adequately defined. Also, the criterion based on limitation of chest expansion is somewhat imprecise: it is difficult to measure chest expansion accurately, and the reduction below 2.5 cm occurs late in the course of the disease. A simpler approach defines ankylosing spondylitis as the presence of symptomatic sacroiliitis. A patient with back discomfort and radiologic evidence of sacroiliitis would be diagnosed as having ankylosing spondylitis. Symptomatic sacroiliitis is usually associated with a decreased range of spinal mobility.

Prevalence

Once considered a rare disease, the illness is now known to have a prevalence comparable to that of rheumatoid arthritis. Twenty per cent of HLA-B27–positive individuals have symptomatic sacroiliitis. Because the B27 antigen occurs in six to 14 per cent of white individuals, approximately 1 to 1.5 per cent of whites have ankylosing spondylitis. The distribution of this disease follows the population frequency of HLA-B27, and it is more common in whites than in blacks.

Ankylosing spondylitis has often gone undiagnosed; inappropriate diagnostic procedures lead to erroneous diagnoses (i.e., mechanical back disease). Such patients often receive incorrect therapy.

Although ankylosing spondylitis was formerly considered a predominantly male disease, several studies now suggest that there may be a more uniform sex distribution. Female patients are less frequently diagnosed, perhaps because physicians and radiologists may be reluctant to diagnose a disease that they consider to be rare in females. The disease may be milder in females and present with a greater number of peripheral joint manifestations. In the past, many women with ankylosing spondylitis were inappropriately diagnosed as having seronegative rheumatoid arthritis.

Clinical Presentation

A history of several of the following five features is suggestive of inflammatory spinal disease: insidious onset of discomfort, age less than 40 years, persistence for more than three months, association with morning stiffness, and improvement with exercise.

If this simple screening test is positive, radiologic evidence of sacroiliitis confirms ankylosing spondylitis. Many radiologists have been unfamiliar with rheumatologic joint disease and have diagnosed ankylosing spondylitis only when there was evidence of major ankylosis of the sacroiliac joints and spine. Ankylosing spondylitis can be diagnosed, however, in the presence of only minimal sacroiliitis. The severity of sacroiliitis is graded from 0 to IV, based on the amount of radiographically observed joint distortion. In many patients, the disease does not progress beyond Grade II or III.

Early change in the lumbar spine is manifested as squaring of the superior and inferior margins of the vertebral body. This phenomenon is caused by inflammatory disease at the site of insertion of the outer fibers of the anulus fibrosus (i.e., enthesopathy). Later changes result in the classic, though rare, bamboo spine. Comparable spinal changes are seen in primary ankylosing spondylitis and in the spondylitis associated with inflammatory bowel disease. In spondylitis associated with Reiter's syndrome and psoriatic arthropathy, however, the changes tend to be asymmetric and random.

Radionuclide scans, computed tomography, and other advanced radiologic techniques have been suggested to evaluate the condition of the sacroiliac joints, but a simple anteroposterior radiograph usually suffices.

Physical Examination

Examination of the spine may reveal muscle spasm and loss of the normal lordosis. In contradistinction to mechanical spinal disease, mobility is decreased symmetrically in both anterior and lateral planes. The degree of restriction of forward flexion can be documented by measuring the distraction, on flexion, of two points—the lower point at the level of the lumbosacral junction and the upper point 10 cm above this level. In a normal individual, the distraction of this 10-cm line is 5 to 12 cm, compared with 0 to 7 cm in an untreated spondylitis patient. Lateral spinal flexion is measured by the distraction, on contralateral flexion, of a 20-cm line drawn in the midaxillary plane. In this case, normal distraction varies from 5 to 12 cm, compared with 0 to 7 cm in spondylitis patients.

Peripheral joint involvement, especially in the lower limb, occurs at some stage in approximately 20 to 30 per cent of cases; the frequency increases with the severity of the disease. Inflammatory disease of the hip and shoulder may produce progressive disability. Enthesopathic features may include plantar fasciitis, costochondritis, and Achilles tendinitis.

Laboratory Findings

HLA-B27 testing should not be used as a routine screening procedure; it is expensive and usually unnecessary. A diagnosis of ankylosing spondylitis does require radiologic evidence of disease. B27 is present in over 95 per cent of white patients.

Other laboratory changes are less striking. Elevation of the erythrocyte sedimentation rate occurs in most patients but may be normal despite severe disease. Elevation of IgA levels and the presence of immune complexes suggest aberrant immunity. Serum creatine kinase and alkaline phosphatase activities may be elevated. Lymphocytes predominate in the synovial fluid, and synovial histologic findings are nonspecific.

Pathology

The synovial lesions of ankylosing spondylitis and rheumatoid arthritis share identical histopathologic characteristics: intimal cell hyperplasia; a diffuse lymphocyte and plasma cell infiltrate; formation of lymphoid follicles; and plasma containing IgG, IgA, and IgM. IgM is found less frequently in ankylosing spondylitis than in rheumatoid disease. Synovitis per se, however, does not explain the propensity toward ligamentous ossification and widespread new bone formation observed in ankylosing spondylitis. Inflammation at the enthesis accounts for the unique pathology, or enthesopathy, of ankylosing spondylitis; new bone formation appears to be a specific reparative process occurring at the enthesopathic site. Complications of severe spinal disease include fractures and spondylodiskitis after minimal trauma.

Extraskeletal Involvement

Extra-articular features include fatigue, weight loss, and low-grade fever. Cord compression resulting from spinal fractures or the cauda equina syndrome may cause neurologic symptoms. The negative effects of systemic involvement and of radiotherapy on the survival of patients with ankylosing spondylitis are well recognized.

EYE INVOLVEMENT. Uveitis develops in up to 25 per cent of patients during their illness. It occurs most often in HLA-B27–positive patients with peripheral joint disease but shows no correlation with the severity of the spondylitis. The visual episodes are usually self-limiting but may require local steroid therapy. Progressive visual impairment is more common in Reiter's syndrome than in ankylosing spondylitis.

PULMONARY DISEASE. Patients with severe disease may exhibit chronic infiltrative and fibrotic changes in the upper lung fields that mimic tuberculosis. Pulmonary ventilation is usually well maintained by the diaphragm, despite the chest wall rigidity. The pulmonary fibrosis is occasionally clinically silent, but most affected patients present with cough, sputum, and dyspnea. Cyst formation and subsequent *Aspergillus* invasion may cause hemoptysis.

CARDIOVASCULAR DISEASE. Aortic incompetence, cardiomegaly, and persistent conduction defects occur in 3.5 to 10.0 per cent of patients with severe spondylitic disease. Cardiac involvement may be clinically silent or may dominate the clinical picture. Thickened aortic valve cusps and scar tissue in the root of the aorta represent the major histologic changes.

AMYLOIDOSIS. Amyloid deposition is an occasional complication of ankylosing spondylitis, particularly in Europe. It may be present in up to 10 per cent of patients, although it appears to be of little clinical significance in most cases.

KIDNEY. In contrast with patients with rheumatoid arthritis who may show renal impairment as an expression of disease, renal glomerular function is apparently unimpaired in ankylosing spondylitis, despite recognized pathologic changes. An IgA nephropathy, however, has been described in patients with seronegative spondylarthropathy.

Treatment and Prognosis

Ankylosing spondylitis is a gratifying condition to recognize and treat early: much can be accomplished toward ameliorating symptoms and, perhaps, preventing spinal deformity. The primary objectives are to relieve pain, decrease inflammation, begin remedial strengthening exercises, and maintain good posture and function.

Anti-inflammatory agents relieve inflammation, pain, and spasm and permit patients to follow an adequate exercise program. There is some evidence that phenylbutazone decreases the rate of spinal fusion. Nevertheless, indomethacin is the drug of choice. Phenylbutazone, although more efficacious, may be more toxic. Indomethacin, started at a dosage of 25 mg three times a day, may be increased to a maximum of 150 mg daily. The dose should be titrated against response and side effects. Possible side effects include headache, vertigo, and depression, especially in older patients, and nausea, gastric discomfort, and diarrhea in all age groups. Phenylbutazone (100 mg t.i.d. or q.i.d.) is remarkably effective but must be used with caution. Dangerous side effects include agranulocytosis and aplastic anemia. Agranulocytosis is an idiosyncratic response, developing chiefly in young individuals within three to six weeks of the start of therapy. Aplastic anemia appears to be dose-related and occurs primarily in individuals more than 60 years of age.

Nonsteroidal anti-inflammatory drugs (NSAIDs) include ibuprofen (Motrin), naproxen (Naprosyn), fenoprofen (Nalfon), tolmetin (Tolectin), sulindac (Clinoril), meclofenamate sodium (Meclomen), and piroxicam (Feldene). If indomethacin is efficacious but not tolerated, one of these NSAIDs may be given. In general, these agents play a minor role in the management of the spondylarthritides. Phenylbutazone should be tried when indomethacin is ineffective.

Gold and penicillamine have not been adequately studied; radiotherapy, once the treatment of choice, is no longer practiced in view of the high risk of inducing leukemia.

The patient also needs remedial strengthening exercises and postural training. A firm mattress and small pillow are ideal when resting; attention to posture at work and at rest must be stressed. The best exercise regimen includes extension exercises and hydrotherapy; swimming is highly recommended.

In those few patients who, despite optimal management, develop an irreversible deformity, wedge osteotomy may be indicated. For those with destructive arthropathy of the hip, arthroplasty is useful despite the risk of postoperative reankylosis.

REITER'S SYNDROME

The most common cause of an inflammatory oligoarthropathy in a young male is Reiter's syndrome. This classic triad of urethritis, conjunctivitis, and arthritis represents the one chronic rheumatic disorder related to both a specific genetic background (HLA-B27) and a specific infection. Reiter's syndrome is often not self-limiting. Progressive disease may result in major disability. The disease may be defined as "an episode of arthropathy within one month of urethritis or cervicitis."

Whether a dysenteric (epidemic) or a venereal (endemic) infection is the most common precipitating event remains a matter of controversy. In young children, however, the former is the rule. In many cases, the distinction between urethritis as a precipitating factor and urethritis as an integral manifestation of the syndrome remains unclear; the association with venereal disease, however, creates a sense of guilt for the patient. In postvenereal Reiter's syndrome both *Chlamydia* and *Mycoplasma* have been implicated. In a patient with a specific predisposing genetic background, a variety of different organisms may be responsible.

Prevalence

The prevalence of Reiter's syndrome remains unknown. The disorder develops in at least one per cent of patients with nonspecific urethritis. *Shigella* dysentery is followed by Reiter's syndrome in one to two per cent of cases (i.e., 20 per cent of B27-positive patients).

The sex distribution of Reiter's syndrome is difficult to define because the syndrome is diagnosed only with difficulty in females, in whom urethritis is often clinically inapparent. Formes frustes of the syndrome are now being recognized. A woman presenting with uveitis and an inflammatory arthropathy of the knee in association with the HLA-B27 antigen may have Reiter's syndrome. Similarly, the disorder is difficult to recognize in children; a diagnosis is usually made only if an epidemic of dysentery is present and Reiter's syndrome has been recognized in other family members. Postdysenteric Reiter's syndrome almost certainly has an equal sex distribution.

Clinical Picture

Reiter's syndrome should be considered a symptom complex rather than the association of three specific features. The syndrome may present as a tetrad (i.e., with the addition of buccal ulceration or balanitis to the classic triad); alternatively, only two of the three cardinal features may be present. Several of the classic features may appear insignificant and be overlooked. For example, the urethritis may be mild, perhaps forgotten; the discharge may be minimal and remembered by the patient only after direct questioning. Balanitis may not be evident unless the prepuce is retracted and the glans penis closely inspected. Buccal ulceration is usually painless and apparent only after close inspection. A red eye may be forgotten or considered irrelevant, and the various skin lesions typified by keratoderma blennorrhagicum may be misdiagnosed.

Rheumatologic features include arthralgias, tenosynovitic episodes, plantar fasciitis, and other enthesopathies, as well as frank arthritis. The typical sausage-shaped digit is a frequent occurrence related to the disorder's enthesopathic nature.

Some 20 per cent of patients with Reiter's syndrome develop sacroiliitis and ascending spinal disease. Whether spondylitis should be considered a complication of the Reiter's syndrome or a manifestation of B27 disease remains unclear. Other radiologic evidence of Reiter's syndrome includes plantar spurs and periosteal new bone formation. Cardiac complications similar to those in ankylosing spondylitis occur late in Reiter's syndrome.

The hyperkeratotic skin lesions seen in Reiter's syndrome cannot be distinguished from those in psoriasis.

Formerly considered a self-limited process, Reiter's syndrome is now known to be a more or less persistent disease in many patients. About 80 per cent of patients have evidence of disease activity when they are re-examined after a five-year period.

Laboratory Evaluation

It is unclear whether the presence of HLA-B27 correlates with increased severity of Reiter's syndrome. A patient with severe Reiter's syndrome may have an erythrocyte sedimentation rate in the normal range or one as high as 100 mm per hour or more. Synovial fluid analysis is rarely diagnostic, apart from the fact that it reveals a relatively high complement level (reflecting a nonspecific inflammatory reaction), rather than the low level seen in rheumatoid arthritis (reflecting immune complex disease).

Occasionally, the diagnoses of ankylosing spondylitis and Reiter's syndrome may prove difficult to disentangle. Some patients who are diagnosed as having ankylosing spondylitis may have presented originally with Reiter's syndrome, but the episodes of urethritis have subsequently been forgotten by the physician and patient. Similarly, patients dignosed as having Reiter's syndrome may actually have ankylosing spondylitis with peripheral joint disease and a chance occurrence of urethritis.

Management

There is no cure for Reiter's syndrome. The patient's feelings of guilt and anxiety about sexual misconduct must be allayed. Although anecdotal evidence suggests that individuals with postvenereal Reiter's syndrome may develop a relapse following sexual activity, many individuals have spontaneous exacerbations. An explanation of allergic response may help the patient: asthma may develop on exposure to a known or unknown allergen in sensitive individuals; in the same way, Reiter's syndrome may flare up following an unknown allergic event.

Symptomatic management includes the use of indomethacin or phenylbutazone. Antibiotic therapy is controversial and probably unnecessary. Patients with severe recurrent uveitis may require steroid eye drops or subconjunctival preparations. The syndrome may remit, recur, or continue unabated despite steroid or even cytotoxic therapy.

THE REACTIVE ARTHROPATHIES

Reactive arthropathy refers to an inflammatory arthritis that follows an infection in which there is no microbial invasion of the synovial space. The B27-linked arthropathies following *Shigella, Salmonella, Yersinia,* and *Campylobacter jejuni* infection are in this group. Why some patients develop only an arthropathy whereas others have the full spectrum of Reiter's disease after exposure to one of these agents is unknown.

Yersinia Infection

Yersinia enterocolitica infection may produce the following: fever, mild gastrointestinal illness, and, after a latent period, polyarthropathy and erythema nodosum, especially in B27-positive individuals. The symptom complex may mimic acute rheumatic fever. The arthropathy may last for weeks or months, and in HLA-B27–positive individuals, sacroiliitis may occur.

Salmonellosis

An arthropathy associated with *Salmonella* infection mimics that caused by *Yersinia.*

Treatment of these disorders is the same as that of Reiter's syndrome.

JUVENILE CHRONIC ARTHROPATHY

Chronic arthritis in a child or teenager often persists into adulthood; therefore, an awareness of juvenile chronic arthropathy is relevant when attending adult patients. Until recently, the term juvenile rheumatoid arthritis was used, inappropriately, to describe all forms of childhood arthritis. As in adults, arthritis in children may be associated with psoriasis, inflammatory bowel disease, and other conditions. The acute systemic form, Still's disease, presents with fever, rash, and toxicity in young children who are negative for B27 and rheumatoid factor (IgM-anti-IgG). Still's disease is also recognized in adults. Another subset (in the spondylarthropathy group) consists largely of adolescent males who predominantly exhibit oligoarthropathy affecting the large joints of the lower limbs: such individuals are frequently positive for HLA-B27. This group may develop sacroiliitis or ankylosing spondylitis; the presence of B27 is associated with spinal disease involvement. Another group includes B27-negative individuals (usually females less than five years of age) presenting with an oligoarthropathy characterized by a positive fluorescent antinuclear antibody (FANA) test. These subjects are at risk for developing asymptomatic chronic iridocyclitis, in contrast with FANA-negative and B27-positive patients, who develop clinically obvious acute uveitis. A few older children (preponderantly females) develop a seropositive, nodular, and erosive disease that resembles adult rheumatoid arthritis. A B-27–related syndrome known as seronegative enthesopathy and arthropathy (SEA syndrome) is now also recognized in children.

THE ENTEROPATHIC ARTHROPATHIES

Two major clinical patterns of arthropathy associated with inflammatory bowel disease (ulcerative colitis and Crohn's disease) are peripheral arthropathy and spondylarthropathy.

Peripheral Arthropathy

Approximately 20 per cent of individuals with severe Crohn's disease or ulcerative colitis develop an acute migratory inflammatory polyarthritis, often of abrupt onset and involving the larger joints of the lower extremities. The arthritis resolves in weeks or months. Arthritis flare-ups usually parallel exacerbations of the underlying disorder. The pathogenesis of the joint complication is unknown. B27 antigen is not present. Treatment is directed at the primary disorder and is more effective in ulcerative colitis than in Crohn's disease.

Spondylarthritis

About one patient in five with inflammatory bowel disease develops sacroiliitis and, occasionally, severe ankylosing spondylitis. The spinal disease may precede the bowel disease or follow it. There is no correlation between the severity of the bowel disorder and the spondylitis, which mimics primary ankylosing spondylitis rather than the spondylitis associated with psoriasis or Reiter's syndrome. Therapy is the same as for classic ankylosing spondylitis. Despite the bowel disease, the nonsteroidal anti-inflammatory drugs are usually well tolerated.

About 50 per cent of individuals with both inflammatory bowel disease and ankylosing spondylitis are B27-positive, a percentage lower than that found in patients with primary ankylosing spondylitis.

A post–intestinal-bypass syndrome consisting of arthropathy and occasionally dermatitis is well recognized. Immune alterations have been described in these patients, and B27 is occasionally associated with this syndrome.

PSORIATIC ARTHROPATHY

Different subsets of psoriatic arthropathy are recognized, several forms of which appear to be enthesopathic rather than purely synovitic. Uveitis, sacroiliitis, and ascending spinal disease occur in up to 20 per cent of cases. Patients are seronegative for rheumatoid factor and exhibit sausage digits and characteristic radiologic changes. The disease may be markedly destructive.

Psoriasis itself is a genetically determined disease, associated with HLA-B13, HLA-Bw17, and HLA-Cw6. Moreover, HLA-B27 is present in approximately 20 per cent of individuals with psoriatic arthropathy even in the absence of sacroiliitis. HLA-Bw38, HLA-DR4, and HLA-DR7 appear to be genetic markers for patients with peripheral arthropathy. About 50 per cent of psoriatic spondylitis patients are B27-negative; thus, as with inflammatory bowel disease, other genetic or environmental factors are relevant.

Psoriatic arthropathy is a common disease, occurring in about 20 per cent of individuals with psoriasis, particularly in those patients with psoriatic nail disease. Women are affected only slightly more commonly than men, in contrast to the more marked sex distribution in rheumatoid disease. Several forms of psoriatic arthropathy, separated by indistinct boundaries, have been described.

1. Asymmetric oligoarthropathy. In general, there is little relationship between joint and skin activity. Patients with this common form of psoriatic arthropathy remain seronegative for rheumatoid factor. Asymmetric involvement of both large and small joints is seen; the sausage-shaped digit is common. A disparity is often observed between the clinical appearance and subjective symptoms. Any patient presenting with this form of arthropathy should be carefully examined for signs of psoriasis (scalp, umbilicus, gluteal region, and nails). In the past, many such individuals were considered to have seronegative rheumatoid arthritis.

2. Symmetric polyarthropathy resembling rheumatoid arthritis. Rarely, the pattern of arthritis may be indistinguishable from that seen in rheumatoid disease. This form may represent coincidental rheumatoid arthritis in a patient with psoriasis.

3. Arthritis mutilans. A resorptive arthropathy, arthritis mutilans is the severest form of destructive arthritis. The telescoping digits appear as the so-called opera-glass hand.

4. Psoriatic spondylitis. Approximately 20 per cent of subjects with psoriatic arthropathy have radiologic sacroiliitis (ankylosing spondylitis).

5. Psoriatic nail disease and distal interphalangeal joint involvement. Nail pitting, transverse depressions, and subungual hyperkeratosis often occur in association with distal interphalangeal joint disease. The relationship between the psoriasis and the arthritis remains unclear.

Laboratory Features

An elevated erythrocyte sedimentation rate, anemia, and rarely, hyperuricemia may occur. The frequency of positive tests for rheumatoid factor is the same as that found in the general population. The synovial tissue and fluid changes are nonspecific.

Radiologic Findings

Characteristic changes in this sometimes highly destructive disease include whittling of the distal ends of the phalanges, giving the joints a "pencil-and-cup" appearance; extensive bone resorption can result in an opera-glass hand. Erosions, ankylosis, periostitis, sacroiliitis, and ankylosing spondylitis are other typical radiologic findings.

Therapy

The skin and joints are treated separately. Improvement of the skin disease may be associated with amelioration of the joint inflammation. For mild arthropathy, indomethacin (25 to 50 mg t.i.d.) is the drug of choice. If this fails, phenylbutazone may be given. Gold and penicillamine may be useful, but few controlled studies have been done. Methotrexate is helpful in resistant cases.

Calin A (ed.): Spondylarthropathy. New York, Grune and Stratton, 1984, pp 1–427. *A multiauthored international text on spondylarthropathy including discussions on immunogenetics, the environment, and ethnic differences.*

Calin A, Marder A, Becks E, Burns T: Genetic difference between B27 positive patients with ankylosing spondylitis and B27 positive healthy controls. Arthritis Rheum 26:1460–1464, 1983. *An up-to-date analysis of the genetics of B27-associated disorders.*

Fox R, Calin A, Gerber R, and Gibson D: The chronicity of symptoms and disability in Reiter's syndrome: An analysis of 131 consecutive patients. Ann Intern Med 91:190–193, 1979. *A detailed evaluation of 131 consecutive patients with Reiter's syndrome.*

Wright V, Moll JMH: Seronegative Polyarthritis. Amsterdam, North Holland Publishing Company, 1976. *The best introduction to the concept of the spondylarthropathies.*

446. INFECTIOUS ARTHRITIS

Stephen E. Malawista

BACTERIAL ARTHRITIS

Bacterial arthritis usually results from bloodborne infection and much less commonly from direct penetration (e.g., needle aspiration) or contiguous osteomyelitis. Acute bacterial joint infections may be divided into two general groups, nongonococcal and gonococcal, based on their typically differing target populations, clinical characteristics, and ease of treatment. (This chapter emphasizes principles of diagnosis and management. Other areas of the text contain more detailed accounts of the problems and management of sepsis caused by specific bacteria.)

Nongonococcal Arthritis

Staphylococcus aureus heads the list of common infecting organisms in this group, followed by other gram-positive cocci (*Streptococcus pyrogenes, pneumoniae, viridans*) and gram-negative bacilli (*Escherichia coli, Salmonella* sp., *Pseudomonas,* etc.); *Hemophilus influenzae* is unusual except in children under four years of age, before protective immunity develops. Patients are often either very young or very old. Risk factors for bacterial arthritis during septicemia include debilitating chronic disease, immunosuppressive therapy, previous joint damage (e.g., rheumatoid arthritis, neuropathic arthropathy, joint surgery), sickle cell anemia, hypogammaglobulinemia, and intraarticular corticosteroid injections. After prosthetic joint replacement, an increasing problem has been late infection by organisms of low virulence, such as *Staphylococcus epidermidis.*

CLINICAL MANIFESTATIONS. A patient may present typically with the abrupt onset of a single severely tender red hot swollen joint, especially the knee or another weight-bearing joint; shaking chills and fever may occur. However, signs of inflammation may be masked in severely debilitated patients or in those given adenocorticosteroids or immunosuppressive agents. Bacterial arthritis superimposed on a noninfectious inflammatory joint disease may also be easily overlooked. For example, infection in one or a few joints of a patient with rheumatoid arthritis may be mistaken for a flare in the chronic disease. An infected joint in a gouty individual may go unrecognized for too long, even when the patient does not respond to his usual regimen for acute gouty arthritis (a good clue that something else is going on). A high index of suspicion is essential in these circumstances, because delay can lead rapidly to destruction of cartilage and bone and eventual fibrous or bony ankylosis.

DIAGNOSIS. When bacterial arthritis is suspected, prompt joint aspiration and both Gram stain and culture of synovial fluid are imperative; most nongonococcal bacterial will be recovered. Cultures for both aerobic and anaerobic organisms should be made. Synovial fluid leukocyte counts are frequently greater than 50,000 per cubic millimeter, and the glucose level low and lactate level high compared to those of serum, but these findings are not specific for infection. Bacteriologic studies should of course be extended to blood and other material (sputum, urine, etc.) from which the infection may have disseminated. On x-ray, only soft-tissue swelling is likely to be seen during the first week, but evidence of loss of articular cartilage and erosion of bone may appear rather soon thereafter in untreated patients.

MANAGEMENT. Successful management of bacterial arthritis depends primarily on early institution of appropriate antimicrobial therapy and effective drainage of the joint space. The selection of antimicrobial agents and recommendations regarding dose and duration of therapy are discussed in other areas of the text (Part XIX). Antibiotics are given parenterally, often in high doses, for two to four weeks, depending on the clinical situation and the patient's response. They generally attain adequate levels in joint fluid and need not be given intraarticularly; indeed, the latter procedure may induce a chemical synovitis. For drainage, daily (or even more frequent) closed joint aspiration through a large-bore needle is carried out until fluid no longer accumulates. Open surgical drainage usually can be avoided except when the hip or the shoulder is infected (difficult to evacuate completely by needle), when tissue debris or fibrin interfere with closed aspiration, or when loculations, gross joint destruction, or contiguous osteomyelitis is present. The affected joint should be at rest while inflamed, and mobilized to prevent atrophy when signs of acute inflammation have subsided.

Gonococcal Arthritis

Gonococcal infection is discussed in Ch. 302. The associated arthritis is by far the most common bacterial joint problem in generally healthy, sexually active teenagers and young adults, especially in urban populations. Gonorrhea is more likely to disseminate in women and in homosexual men, whose infections are often asymptomatic and therefore untreated. The risk of dissemination is particularly high during menses and pregnancy, in the post-partum period, and in individuals with genetic deficiency in the terminal components of serum complement (C5, C6, C7, or C8). Additional features that help to distinguish gonococcal from other bacterial arthritides include a high frequency of associated tenosynovitis and rash and of multiple joint involvement, especially in the wrists and hands. Diagnosis is frequently presumptive because synovial fluid smear and culture—which requires special media—are often negative, and corroborating cultural evidence from urethra, cervix, throat, rectum, blood, or skin may be lacking. Highly suggestive diagnostically is a history of fever and migratory polyarthralgias that progress to frank oligoarticular arthritis and are associated with tenosynovitis and skin lesions. The latter are either vesiculopustular on an erythematous base, often with necrotic centers, or hemorrhagic. Similar lesions are seen with arthritis caused by the meningococcus. Response to (even oral) antibiotic therapy (Ch. 302) and drainage is usually dramatic. Resistance to penicillin of gonococci that disseminate is known but is uncommon.

Tuberculous Arthritis

The general decline in the frequency of pulmonary tuberculosis in the western world is reflected in the relative rarity of tuberculous bone and joint disease. Infection usually reaches the joint from hematogenous dissemination to bone and direct extension from an osteomyelitic focus. Formerly, the classic presentation was chronic low back pain in a child because of involvement of lower thoracic or lumbar vertebrae, leading to collapse and sharp-angle kyphosis (Pott's disease). Currently, the typical target is a tuberculin-positive adult, often without evidence of pulmonary disease, who presents with chronic, insidious pain and swelling, usually in a single joint, especially the hip, knee, or wrist; this presentation is often mistaken for monoarticular rheumatoid arthritis. Tenosynovitis is common. Diagnosis depends upon culture of *Mycobacterium tuberculosis* from synovial fluid (positive in 80 per cent) or synovial biopsy (positive in 90 per cent). Sensitivities to chemotherapeutic agents must be determined; caseating granulomata and acid-fast bacilli are sometimes due to atypical mycobacteria resistant to the usual antituberculous drugs. Usual therapy for uncomplicated infections consists of long-term isoniazid and ethambutol or rifampin.

Masi AT, Eisenstein BI: Disseminated gonococcal infection (DGI) and gonococcal arthritis (GCA). Clinical manifestations, diagnosis, complications, treatment, and prevention. Semin Arthritis Rheum 70:173, 1981. *A careful review that satisfies its subtitle.*

Rosenthal J, Bole G, Robinson WD: Acute non-gonococcal infectious arthritis. Evaluation of risk factors, therapy and outcome. Arthritis Rheum 23:889, 1980. *Presentation of experience with 63 patients and general review.*

VIRAL ARTHRITIS

Many specific viral infections are associated with polyarthritis, notably hepatitis B and rubella, but also mumps and vaccinia (and formerly, smallpox) and occasionally adenovirus type 7, EB virus (in infectious mononucleosis) and other herpes viruses, and certain enteroviruses. Polyarthritis may dominate the picture of various mosquito-transmitted arbovirus infections, especially epidemic polyarthritis of Australia (Ross River virus) and the dengue-like illnesses, chikungunya and o'nyong-nyong.

In general, diagnosis is suggested by the exposure history (drug abuse for hepatitis B, immunization for rubella, epidemiologic considerations for arbo- or enteroviruses); recognition of the associated viral syndrome, which often includes fever, rash, and regional lymphadenopathy; brevity of the joint involvement (days to weeks); and changing antibody titers against specific antigens. Routine laboratory tests are nonspecific, and except for rubella, virus has rarely been recovered from synovial fluid. Little is known about pathogenesis, but studies of hepatitis B and rubella provide some clues.

Transient, often symmetrical polyarthritis or arthralgias resembling acute rheumatoid arthritis may be associated with both hepatitis B and rubella infections. In the case of *hepatitis B*, 10 to 30 per cent of patients have arthritis, often accompanied by urticaria, fever, and lymphadenopathy, all occurring days to weeks before the onset of frank hepatitis. This prodromal syndrome typically occurs when hepatitis B surface antigen (HBsAg) is in excess over antibody, hypocomplementemia is present, and serum contains immune complexes composed of HBsAg and anti-HB, other immunoglobulins, and complement components. Similar material has been found in affected dermal blood vessels, and the antigen has been seen in synovial tissue. With the development of antibody excess, complexes disappear, the arthritis and rash resolve, and frank hepatitis may supervene. The process resembles experimental serum sickness, and suggests an inflammatory pathogenetic mechanism driven by deposition of immune complexes. Joint symptoms may respond dramatically to salicylates.

Rubella arthritis is primarily a disease of adult women. It usually follows onset of the characteristic rash by a few days, but the rash may be absent and rheumatoid factor present, inviting diagnostic confusion. Arthritis is usually sudden in onset, symmetrical and polyarticular in distribution (fingers, knees, wrists), brief in duration (less than a month), and without residua. Salicylates are useful for pain and stiffness.

Arthritis may also occur within a few weeks of vaccination by attenuated rubella virus. Again, attacks are brief but may recur periodically for a few years without permanent joint damage. Rubella virus has been recovered from synovial fluid in both the natural and vaccine-induced disease and more recently in a few patients with various chronic joint syndromes. It seems capable of replicating in synovium; whether its new association with chronic disease is critical or coincidental remains to be determined.

Steere AC, Malawista SE: Viral arthritis. *In* McCarty D J (ed.): Arthritis and Allied Conditions. 10th ed. Philadelphia, Lea & Febiger (in press). *Survey of common and uncommon arthritides associated with specific viral illnesses.*

Wands JR, Mann E, Alpert E, Isselbacher KJ: The pathogenesis of arthritis associated with acute hepatitis B surface antigen-positive hepatitis. Complement activation and characterization of circulating immune complexes. J Clin Invest 55:930, 1975. *Clinical description and characterization of immunologic aspects of the syndrome.*

LYME DISEASE

Lyme disease (formerly Lyme arthritis) was recognized in 1975 because of unusual geographic clustering of children with inflammatory arthropathy in the region of Lyme, Connecticut. It is now known to be a complex immune-mediated multisystem disorder occurring at any age, in either sex, whose clinical hallmark is an early expanding skin lesion, *erythema chronicum migrans* (ECM), which may be followed weeks to months later by neurologic, cardiac, or joint abnormalities. Symptoms may refer to any one of these systems alone. Foci of Lyme disease have been found elsewhere along the northeastern coast of the United States, in many other states, in Europe, and in Australia. The disease is caused by a newly recognized spirochete, and transmitted by the minute tick *Ixodes dammini* or by related ixodid ticks.

In summer or early fall, days to weeks after a tick bite that may have gone unnoticed, a typical patient may present with ECM at the site and perhaps with systemic symptoms: chills and fever, malaise and fatigue, headache or stiff neck. Most such patients have circulating immune complexes. Those who also have elevated levels of serum IgM and cryoglobulins containing IgM are at high risk for subsequent organ involvement. This high-risk group tends to have the histocompatibility antigen DR2, which in turn correlates with the development of severe disease (but not with ECM alone). Within weeks, typical ECM expands to several inches in diameter with central clearing, then fades; secondary annular non–tick-associated lesions may occur.

Within weeks to months of ECM, there may be neurologic abnormalities (15 per cent of patients)—especially lymphocytic meningitis, cranial neuritis (including bilateral Bell's palsy), and motor and sensory radiculoneuritis—and cardiac abnormalities (8 per cent)—fluctuating degrees of A-V block and myopericarditis (but *not* valvulitis; cf. rheumatic fever). Early rheumatic complaints include migratory polyarthritis and arthralgias and tendinitis. Later (weeks to years), frank arthritis (without morning stiffness) may occur (60 per cent of patients) in a few large joints, especially knees, persist for weeks to months, and recur for years. Chronic joint disease, with erosion of cartilage and bone, is much less common.

Changes in synovium and synovial fluid resemble those in rheumatoid arthritis. Immune complexes are present, even when absent from blood. However, rheumatoid factor and antinuclear antibodies are lacking. Spirochetes have been isolated from blood (early), skin (ECM), and cerebrospinal fluid, but not yet from joints. Diagnosis, when ECM is lacking or missed, is facilitated by high or changing antibody titers against the *I. dammini* spirochete.

Oral tetracycline (or penicillin) eradicates ECM and usually prevents major complications. High-dose intravenous penicillin cures the meningitis and is currently used for complete heart block (with high-dose prednisone, when failure is present). The high-dose penicillin regimen has recently been shown to cure established arthritis in the majority of patients.

Steere AC, Malawista SE: Lyme disease. *In* Kelly WN, Harris ED Jr, Ruddy S, Sledge CB (eds.): Textbook of Rheumatology. 2nd ed. Philadelphia, W. B. Saunders Company (in press). *In depth presentation of the epidemiology, pathogenesis, natural history, immunology, diagnosis, and treatment of Lyme disease.*

Steere AC, Pachner AR, Malawista SE: Successful treatment of neurologic abnormalities of Lyme disease with high-dose intravenous penicillin. Ann Intern Med 99:767, 1983. *Meningitis, formerly treated with high-dose prednisone tapered over months, responds to penicillin in days.*

OTHER FORMS OF INFECTIOUS ARTHRITIS

Syphilitic Arthritis

Syphilis is discussed in Ch. 306. Joint disease associated with congenital and acquired syphilitic infections is now rare. In infants with congenital disease, musculoskeletal complaints are related to periostitis and osteochondritis. About the time of puberty, painless knee effusions (Clutton's joints) may be confused with rheumatoid or pyogenic arthritis. With acquired infection, arthralgias, arthritis, or tenosynovitis may accompany classic signs of secondary syphilis: rash, mucous plaques, alopecia, or lymphadenopathy. In tertiary lues, gummatous arthritis or periostitis (tibia, clavicles) may occur. Neuropathic arthropathy (Charcot joint) is reviewed in Ch. 497.

Fungal Arthritis

Any of the invasive mycoses can affect joints, usually by direct extension from bone. Frequent infectious agents include coccidioidomycosis and histoplasmosis—both of which may also be accompanied by erythema nodosum with joint involvement—sporotrichosis (often by direct penetration: rose thorns), blastomycosis, actinomycosis, and candidiasis. Clinically, the affected joint or joints resemble those in other forms of granulomatous arthritis (e.g., tuberculous). For diagnosis, the causative agent must be seen in appropriately stained synovial biopsy material or grown from synovial tissue or fluid.

447. SYSTEMIC LUPUS ERYTHEMATOSUS

Alfred D. Steinberg

Systemic lupus erythematosus (SLE) is a disease of unknown etiology characterized by inflammation in many different organ systems associated with the production of antibodies reactive with nuclear, cytoplasmic, and cell membrane antigens. Individual patients may have some, but not necessarily all, of the following: fatigue, anemia, fever, rashes, sun sensitivity, alopecia, arthritis, pericarditis, pleurisy, vasculitis, nephritis, and central nervous system disease. The course is often unpredictable with variable periods of exacerbations and remissions. There is no one clinical abnormality that definitely establishes the diagnosis, nor is there a single test for the disorder. As a result, criteria have been developed and modified in an attempt to include patients with SLE and to exclude patients with other disorders (see Table 447–1). Although these criteria have been developed for epidemiologic and research purposes, they are helpful in diagnosis as well. Nevertheless, it is possible to fulfill these criteria and not have SLE, and it is possible to fail to fulfill the criteria and still have SLE. Thus, a teen-age girl with a "butterfly" rash of the face, pleurisy, and large amounts of serum antibodies reactive with native DNA undoubtedly has SLE even if she does not yet manifest any other criteria. The disease derives its name (lupus = wolf) from the facial rash, which resembles the malar erythema of a wolf.

INCIDENCE. Although SLE can occur at any age (it has been diagnosed at birth and in individuals in the tenth decade of life), more than 70 per cent of patients experience the onset of disease between ages 13 and 40 years. Among children, SLE occurs three times as commonly in females as in males. In patients in their teens, twenties, and thirties, 90 to 95 per cent are female. Thereafter, the female predominance again falls to that observed before puberty.

The disorder is approximately three times more common among American blacks than American caucasians. Certain North American indian tribes (Sioux, Crow, Arapahoe) have an even greater predisposition toward SLE. Orientals have been less well studied; however, the data suggest that they are affected to approximately the same extent as American blacks. The overall annual incidence of SLE is about 6 new cases per 100,000 population per year for relatively low-risk populations and approximately 35 per 100,000 for relatively high-risk populations. The chance of a black female developing SLE in her lifetime is approximately 1 in 250.

These data suggest that both genetic factors and sex hormones may affect the probability of developing SLE. If a family member has SLE, the likelihood of SLE increases (approximately 70 per cent for identical twins and 5 per cent for other first degree relatives). Although males develop SLE less frequently than do females, their illness is not milder.

ETIOLOGY. The etiology of SLE is unknown. The signs and symptoms are thought to be due to the autoantibodies that react with self constituents and initiate inflammatory responses. The initiation of this process may be multifactorial (Fig. 447–1). Moreover, the factors may be different in different individuals with SLE. These factors are currently poorly understood. One or more genetic factors appear to be important in many individuals. These may be genes that allow augmented antibody responses following a variety of stimuli as well as genes that predispose to particular autoantibody responses. In addition, hormonal, metabolic, and environmental factors appear to act

TABLE 447–1. THE 1982 REVISED CRITERIA FOR CLASSIFICATION OF SYSTEMIC LUPUS ERYTHEMATOSUS*

Criterion		Definition
1. Malar rash		Fixed erythema, flat or raised, over the malar eminences, tending to spare the nasolabial folds
2. Discoid rash		Erythematous raised patches with adherent keratotic scaling and follicular plugging; atrophic scarring may occur in older lesions
3. Photosensitivity		Skin rash as a result of unusual reaction to sunlight, by patient history or physician observation
4. Oral ulcers		Oral or nasopharyngeal ulceration, usually painless, observed by a physician
5. Arthritis		Nonerosive arthritis involving two or more peripheral joints, characterized by tenderness, swelling, or effusion
6. Serositis	a)	Pleuritis—convincing history of pleuritic pain or rub heard by a physician or evidence of pleural effusion *OR*
	b)	Pericarditis—documented by ECG or rub or evidence of pericardial effusion
7. Renal disorder	a)	Persistent proteinuria greater than 0.5 grams per day or greater than 3+ if quantitation not performed *OR*
	b)	Cellular casts—may be red cell, hemoglobin, granular, tubular, or mixed
8. Neurologic disorder	a)	Seizures—in the absence of offending drugs or known metabolic derangements; e.g., uremia, ketoacidosis, or electrolyte imbalance *OR*
	b)	Psychosis—in the absence of offending drugs or known metabolic derangements, e.g., uremia, ketoacidosis, or electrolyte imbalance
9. Hematologic disorder	a)	Hemolytic anemia—with reticulocytosis *OR*
	b)	Leukopenia—less than 4000/mm³ total on two or more occasions *OR*
	c)	Lymphopenia—less than 1500/mm³ on two or more occasions *OR*
	d)	Thrombocytopenia—less than 100,000/mm³ in the absence of offending drugs
10. Immunologic disorder	a)	Positive LE cell preparation *OR*
	b)	Anti-DNA: antibody to native DNA in abnormal titer *OR*
	c)	Anti-Sm: presence of antibody to Sm nuclear antigen *OR*
	d)	False positive serologic test for syphilis known to be positive for at least 6 months and confirmed by *Treponema pallidum* immobilization or fluorescent treponemal antibody absorption test
11. Antinuclear antibody		An abnormal titer of antinuclear antibody by immunofluorescence or an equivalent assay at any point in time and in the absence of drugs known to be associated with "drug-induced lupus" syndrome

*The proposed classification is based on 11 criteria. For the purpose of identifying patients in clinical studies, a person shall be said to have systemic lupus erythematosus if any 4 or more of the 11 criteria are present, serially or simultaneously, during any interval of observation.

on the genetically conditioned immune substratum to predispose to or protect against disease expression. Androgens appear to protect against the development of SLE except in a subgroup of males who inherit a Y chromosome accelerating factor from their fathers. Estrogens probably predispose to SLE to a lesser extent than androgens protect against the expression of the illness. In general, factors that augment immunity favor disease expression whereas those that retard immunity, especially antibody production, tend to protect. Any of a variety of bacterial or viral infections may stimulate the immune system as may drugs or food additives.

The central role of immune regulations in the expression of illness has led to the concept that some patients may have a primary abnormality in the ability of their immune systems to perform normal self-regulatory functions. It is probably best to consider abnormal immune regulation as one of several factors that may contribute to illness. If any one is very abnormal, disease may occur. Under most circumstances, several defects probably combine to incite disease. However, once the process is initiated, impaired self-regulation would favor perpetuation of the disease-inducing abnormalities.

It has long been known that some individuals with SLE have disease exacerbations following exposure to ultraviolet light. Several different mechanisms are likely: UV light induces keratinocytes to secrete interleukin 1, which, in turn, stimulates B cells and induces T cells to produce growth factors (interleukin 2, B cell growth factors, B cell differentiation factors, interferon), which stimulate the immune system; UV light impairs processing of antigen and immune complexes, thereby increasing the load of pathogenic complexes on target organs; UV light induces cytosine and thymine dimer formation, which stimulates immune responses.

Certain drugs can cause an SLE-like illness in apparently healthy individuals. The drugs (Table 447–2) do not share common structural or chemical properties. The mechanisms of disease induction probably vary depending upon the structure of the drug. Even chemicals in foods may induce SLE. For example, alfalfa sprouts contain L-canavanine, which can induce an SLE-like illness. The extent to which "idiopathic" SLE is triggered by such specific environmental factors is unknown.

A variety of complement deficiencies have been associated with SLE. The most common is C2 deficiency. It is not clear whether the association is one of genetic linkage or predisposition because of the deficiency itself. The latter might occur if the deficiency led to increased susceptibility to infections that trigger illness.

For many years it has been thought that there might be a "lupus virus," a particular virus that induces disease. Patients with SLE have, in the endothelial cells of their kidneys and in their lymphocytes, structures that resemble viral nucleocapsids. In addition, retroviruses have been implicated in the immune-complex renal disease of animals with SLE-like disorders. Nevertheless, the evidence suggests that even if such a virus is important, it is only one of many factors critical to the development of disease.

AUTOIMMUNITY AND DISEASE IN SLE. In prior years it was believed that an anti-self response was harmful and that such responses did not occur normally. More recently it has become appreciated that normal immune responses involve self-self recognition. Moreover, many individuals produce nonpathogenic antibodies reactive with self antigens. As a result, disease occurs only when anti-self reactions are either excessive or productive of especially injurious immune responses. SLE is characterized by the production of large amounts of antibodies reactive with a great variety of different antigenic specificities. Some individual antibody molecules have been shown to cross-react with more than one antigen (DNA and cardiolipin or IgG and nucleoprotein). As a result, the true range of antibody molecules reactive with self-determinants may be less than the number of specificities as measured by the reactive antigens. Nevertheless, the range of determinants against which SLE antibodies may react is impressive (Table 447–3).

How could such self reactivity come about? It is believed that self-tolerance is a complex state brought about and maintained by several mechanisms. Very early in life, exposure to antigens tends to produce tolerance rather than immunity. Subsequently, several immune mechanisms tend to maintain self-tolerance. Although B lymphocytes and their progeny are

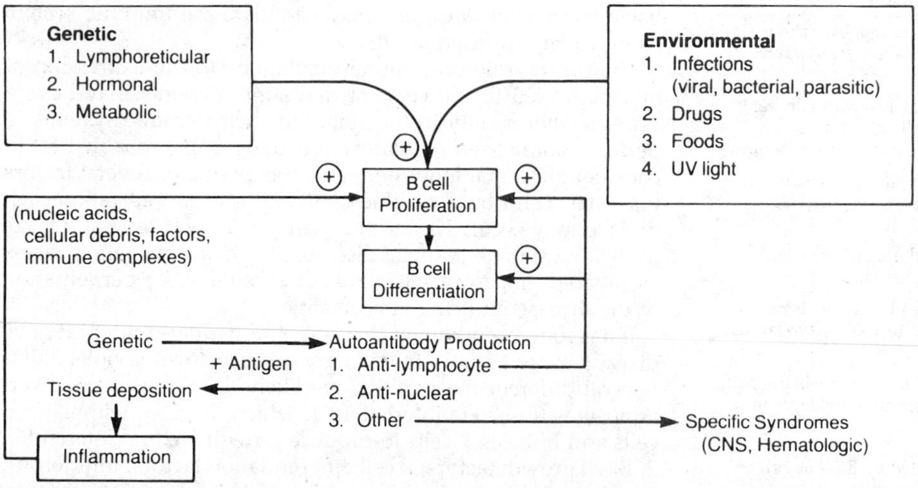

Figure 447–1. Initiation and perpetuation of systemic lupus erythematosus.

responsible for antibody production, under most circumstances they require helper T lymphocytes for activation, proliferation, and differentiation into antibody secreting cells. Moreover, specialized T cells (suppressor cells) appear capable of down-regulating immune responses. If the T cell population is self-tolerant, it may prevent B cells capable of differentiating into autoantibody producing cells from proliferating and differentiating. A defect in self-tolerance mechanisms could occur at any of several steps in the immune pathway. In addition, strong immune stimulation can overwhelm normal regulatory mechanisms rendering them incapable of function adequate to regulate the immune stimuli. Such strong immune stimuli as graft-versus-host disease (as after allogeneic bone marrow transplantation) or stimulation by any of a variety of powerful polyclonal immune activators (endotoxin) or even viruses that stimulate B cells (Ebstein-Barr virus) may drive B cells to produce antibodies and autoantibodies without the usual requirements for or regulation by T cells. Individuals with B cells capable of producing pathogenic autoantibodies that had been previously held in check by T cells may, under such circumstances, be driven to produce large amounts of injurious antibodies. Since it is often the quantity of autoantibody that determines whether or not disease occurs, quantitative aspects of immune regulation and immune stimulation may be critical to the balance between disease development versus relative health with minor immune abnormalities.

PATHOGENESIS. Systemic lupus is often classified as an immune complex type disorder. This designation is, at best, an oversimplification. SLE is a disease primarily mediated by antibodies; however, the details of pathogenesis are not proven for many of the clinical and pathologic findings. It is clear that patients with SLE produce autoantibodies and that many of these are injurious. This has been well demonstrated for the

TABLE 447–2. SOME DRUGS ABLE TO INDUCE FEATURES OF SLE

Related to Dose-Time Administration	More Idiosyncratic
Hydralazine	Aminosalicylic acid
Procainamide	D-Penicillamine
Alpha-methyldopa	Griseofulvin
Isoniazid	Penicillin
Chlorpromazine	Ampicillin
Chlorthalidone	Streptomycin
Phenytoin	Sulfonamides
Mephenytoin	Tetracycline
Trimethadione	Methylthiouracil
Primidone	Propythiouracil
Ethosuximide	Phenylbutazone
Carbamazepine	Oxyphenisatin
Phenylethylacetylurea	Practolol
	Tolazamide
	Methysergide
	Reserpine
	Quinidine
	Isoquinazepan
	Guanoxan

TABLE 447–3. AUTOANTIBODIES FOUND IN PATIENTS WITH SLE

Specificity	Comments
Nuclear	Present in most but not all patients
Native DNA	Essentially restricted to SLE
Denatured (single-stranded) DNA	May also cross-react with double-stranded DNA. High titers in SLE; lower titers in other diseases
Histones H1, H3-H4	SLE
Histones H2A-H2B	More common in drug-induced SLE
Sm	In a minority of SLE patients, but not found in other diseases.
Nuclear ribonucleoprotein	Found in SLE, but highest titers in "mixed connective tissue disease." Multiple small proteins and combined RNA have been discovered.
Nucleolar antigens	Scleroderma, SLE, Sjögren's Syndrome
SS-B (La, Ha)	Sjögren's Syndrome, SLE
SS-A (Ro)	Sjögren's Syndrome, SLE
Proliferating cell nuclear antigen	SLE
RANA	Especially in rheumatoid arthritis (Ebstein-Barr virus)
DNA-RNA hybrids, double-stranded RNA	SLE
Cytoplasmic	Less information available on these
Ribosomal ribonucleoprotein	SLE
Mitochondria	Primary biliary cirrhosis, SLE
Microsomal antigens	Chronic active hepatitis, malignancies
Lysosomes	SLE
Single-stranded RNA, tRNA	SLE
SS-B and SS-A	Sjögren's Syndrome, SLE
Cell membrane determinants	Common in SLE
Red cells	May occur without important hemolysis
White cells	Granulocytes, T cells, B cells
Platelets	Common without thrombocytopenia
Lipomodulin	SLE, RA, others ?
Receptors	Insulin, IL 2, others
Ia	Interferes with immune functions
Others	
Mitotic spindle and intracellular supporting proteins	SLE and other rheumatic diseases
Immunoglobulins	JRA, RA, SLE, Sjögren's Syndrome, others
Clotting factors	SLE and other diseases
Cardiolipin	May cross react with DNA
Thyroid antigens	Thyroid diseases, SLE, Sjögren's Syndrome

renal disease associated with SLE. Antibody reacts with antigen either in the circulation or in the glomerulus and complement is fixed, leading to release of chemotactic factors, attraction of leukocytes, and release of their injurious mediators of inflammation. The degree of pathology is determined, to a large extent, by the magnitude of the antibody deposition and the magnitude of the inflammatory process initiated. Continued deposition of antibody and continued induction of inflammation ultimately leads to irreversible renal damage. Similar processes occur in other organs. However, antibody and complement may be deposited in the skin or in the choroid plexus with or without an attendant inflammatory response. It must be presumed that the qualitative character of the antibody molecules (affinity, isotype, charge), the nature of the antigen or their combined properties (size, molecular configuration), or additional factors may be critical to pathogenesis.

It has long been taught that immunopathology of SLE results from the deposition of DNA–anti-DNA immune complexes. Although immune complexes may contribute to the immunopathology, it is likely that uncomplexed antibody may reach an organ where antigen is already present and there bind to antigen and initiate the inflammatory process. This idea is supported by demonstrations of DNA binding to basement membranes without antibody. Moreover, antibodies of other specificities appear to contribute to disease.

Antibody plays a role in SLE not only by depositing in vessels, but by binding to the surfaces of cells. Patients with SLE produce antibodies to erythrocytes, granulocytes, lymphocytes, and macrophages. These antibodies can cause such cells to be removed from the circulation by the reticuloendothelial system, killed by complement-mediated cytotoxicity, or more likely, by the mechanism of antibody-dependent cellular cytotoxicity (ADCC). In this non–complement-mediated killing, leukocytes recognize antibody-coated target cells and kill them. It is possible that ADCC may be responsible for some of the pathology initiated in the kidneys and other organs by other antibody-mediated mechanisms. In addition, antibody directed against renal antigens, for example renal tubular or glomerular basement membrane, may be generated as a result of immunization by fragments released from the inflammatory process. Such antibody induces additional renal pathology and may account for much of the disease in some patients.

It appears that many of the inflammatory lesions that occur in SLE are initiated by antibody and that the injury occurs in small vessels. Thus, any organ so affected could be a site of inflammation with the possibility of scarring, dysfunction, or both. Many of the central nervous system problems of patients (seizures, psychoses) as well as hematologic (anemia, thrombocytopenia, leukopenia), cardiac (coronary artery disease), dermal (alopecia, sun sensitivity), and other clinical and laboratory abnormalities have additional pathogenetic mechanisms. The hematologic abnormalities could all be explained by antibodies specifically reactive with the formed elements of the blood; however, many relate to suppression at the level of the bone marrow. The central nervous system disorders are multiple, and each may have its own pathogenetic mechanism. Because central nervous system involvement in SLE is not a single entity, individual patients may require different approaches to understanding and therapy.

PATHOLOGY. The pathologic abnormalities of SLE follow directly from the pathogenetic mechanisms; moreover, the same degree of variability is encountered. In organs affected by small vessel vasculitis, the first lesions are usually characterized by granulocytic infiltration and periarteriolar edema. This is usually (except in some cases of leukocytoclastic involvement of the skin) followed by round cell infiltration and ultimately a relatively acellular eosinophilic material composed of fibrin, immunoglobulins, and complement (fibrinoid) containing scattered hematoxylin bodies. These basophilic-staining bodies are nuclear debris, often associated with anti-nuclear antibody, and represent a correlate of the LE cell in vivo. Immunofluorescence analysis of affected areas demonstrates immunoglobulin and complement in the vessels in the affected areas. Arterioles, venules, and sometimes arteries and veins are involved.

Individual organs often have their peculiar abnormalities. The spleen has "onion skin lesions," concentric fibrosis of the walls and surrounding tissues of the central and penicilliary arteries. These lesions are thought to be diagnostic of SLE in patients with "idiopathic" thrombocytopenia. Nonbacterial verrucous endocarditis (Libman-Sacks) consists of vegetations on the heart valves or chordae tendineae; they can extend along the endocardium and become quite large.

The renal pathology varies from mild to severe glomerular inflammation and variable interstitial involvement. Most patients have relatively normal kidneys or a renal lesion consisting of minimal focal hypercellularity, thickening of the capillary basement membrane, and fibrinoid change. In clinically important glomerulonephritis, these lesions are more generalized and are usually a mixture of proliferative and membranous changes with increases in endothelial, mesangial, epithelial, and inflammatory cells, capsular inflammation leading to crescent formation, and focal thickening of the basement membrane and mesangial hypercellularity. Some kidneys are found to have membranous glomerulonephritis with considerable thickening of the basement membrane. Basement membrane thickening, when associated with fibrinoid changes, results in the so-called "wire loop" lesions. There may also be hyaline thrombi in glomeruli, focal necrosis, hematoxylin bodies, and sclerosis in healed lesions. Tubular degenerative changes and mixed inflammatory interstitial inflammation are common. Some patients have primarily mesangial disease; this carries a better prognosis than does capillary loop involvement. Extensive crescent formation and substantial glomerular or interstitial scarring are bad prognostic signs.

CLINICAL MANIFESTATIONS. SLE is a highly variable disease in terms of onset and course. A young woman may present with a butterfly rash, a history of recent sun sensitivity, pleuropericarditis, arthritis, fever, extreme fatigue, seizures, and nephrotic syndrome. This "typical" presentation, which is easily recognized as SLE, occurs in only a minority of patients. More commonly, patients may have only one or two signs or symptoms of SLE for a period of time, such as arthritis and fatigue. Only later do additional features of SLE occur. As a result, the initial presentation may not allow a definitive diagnosis nor insight into the organ systems that may become involved in the future. Many patients never develop major organ involvement. Some have kidney but not central nervous system involvement or vice versa. Thus, the clinical manifestations of one patient may be very different from those of another. Nevertheless, some associations between serologic findings and clinical features are valid on a statistical basis but may not hold for a given individual. Thus, patients with large amounts of anti-DNA, especially precipitating antibodies, are more likely to have renal disease. Those with antibodies to Ro (SS-A) and La (SS-B, Ha) are most likely to have sicca syndrome, muscle disease, lung disease, and inconsequential or no renal disease. In the paragraphs that follow, individual clinical features of patients with SLE are described (see also Table 447–4). Patients vary greatly in terms of organ system involvement and also in terms of the severity of disease when a given organ system is affected. Thus, most patients do not have many of the abnormalities described. In addition, SLE is characterized by periods of active disease followed by periods of less intense disease or even remission. In rare cases the patient has a rapidly progressive disease, but the majority can look forward to the time when the disease no longer interferes with their lives.

Constitutional Problems. The majority of patients have fatigue, fever, and weight loss at the time of diagnosis. However, before attributing these to SLE, a diligent search for other causes is necessary to rule out the concurrent presence of serious infection. Later in the illness, the recurrence of one or

TABLE 447–4. COMMON CLINICAL ABNORMALITIES IN PATIENTS WITH SLE

Abnormality	Approximate Frequency (%)*
Constitutional	
Fatigue	90
Fever	80
Weight loss, anorexia	60
Musculoskeletal	
Arthritis, arthralgia	90
Myalgia, myositis	30
Skin and mucous membranes	
Butterfly rash	60
Alopecia	50
Photosensitivity	40
Raynaud's phenomenon	30
Mucosal ulcers	30
Discoid lupus	20
Urticaria	10
Edema or bullae	10
Eye (conjunctivitis/episcleritis/sicca syndrome)	20
Gastrointestinal	30
Serosal (pleurisy, pericarditis, peritonitis)	50
Lymphoreticular	
Lymphadenopathy	50
Splenomegaly	30
Hepatomegaly	30
Hypertension	30
Bacterial infections	40
Pneumonitis (all)	30
"lupus"	10
Renal (all)	50
severe	20
Central nervous system	
Personality disorders	50
Seizures	20
Psychoses	20
Stroke or long tract signs	10
Migraine headaches	10
Cardiac	
Myocarditis	30
Murmurs and valvular disease	30
Coronary artery disease	20
Hematologic	
Anemia (all)	70
Hemolytic	10
Purpura (all)	50
Thrombocytopenia	10
Peripheral neuropathy	10

*Frequencies are compiled from a number of series and are rounded off to the nearest 10 per cent. There was some variation from series to series depending upon patient population, non-SLE therapy, and therapy for SLE. Some abnormalities are more common in younger patients than in older patients (e.g., splenomegaly and lymphadenopathy) and vice versa (e.g., muscle disease and sicca syndrome).

more of these findings often indicates an increase in disease activity. Fatigue, difficult as it may be to evaluate, often is the first sign that a flare is imminent.

Musculoskeletal Problems. Arthralgias are the single most common manifestation in SLE. They characteristically are much more transitory than in patients with rheumatoid arthritis (RA), lasting minutes to days in a given joint. With more longstanding or more severe disease, the pain may be constant and frank arthritis is observed. It is often symmetrical, the proximal interphalangeal joints of the hands, metacarpophalangeal joints, wrists, and knees being most commonly affected. Morning stiffness is reported by many patients with SLE and joint disease. Although the bony erosions characteristic of RA do not occur, deformities similar to those in RA develop in 10 to 15 per cent of patients and are thought to result from tendon disease. Occasionally patients experience rupture of the Achilles or quadriceps tendons. Myalgias occur in approximately 30 per cent of patients; only a portion of these have muscle tenderness. Many patients with SLE and muscle disease do not have elevations of creatine kinase activity; some of these have an elevated aldolase value. Muscle samples from such patients may be normal or show perivascular infiltration or atrophy. Some patients have a vacuolar myopathy that is also observed in corticosteroid-treated individuals.

Skin and Mucous Membranes. The typical butterfly rash varies from a slight blush to a clear-cut and somewhat edematous nonpapular erythematous covering of both cheeks and the bridge of the nose. Patients with a butterfly rash often look as though they have healthy rosy cheeks or have applied too much rouge. This lesion may occur in the absence of sun exposure, but is often exacerbated by the sun. It often precedes other manifestations of disease. A maculopapular erythematous eruption is also common. Indistinguishable from a drug eruption, it is often induced or exacerbated by sunlight and sometimes by a drug (Gantrisin and ampicillin are common offenders). The palms and soles are not always spared. Healing usually occurs without scarring. Urticaria and angioedema are more common than subepidermal bullae, which occur in only a few per cent of patients. Discoid lupus in SLE is indistinguishable from discoid lupus without systemic involvement; however, systemic disease may develop in patients with longstanding discoid lesions. In this rash, central atrophy, hyper- and hypopigmentation, telangiectasia, and follicular plugging accompany the usual stages of erythema followed by hyperkeratosis and then by atrophy. The hypopigmentation may be extensive and particularly disturbing to blacks.

Livedo reticularis occurs commonly in patients with SLE, but only rarely is it severe. Splinter hemorrhages, tender fingertip pulp lesions, and palmar erythema are sometimes remarkable. Purpura is more often secondary to vasculitis or capillary fragility (corticosteroid therapy is often responsible) than to thrombocytopenia.

Lupus profundus (relapsing nodular nonsuppurative panniculitis) occurs rarely in SLE patients. It may be limited to superficial panniculitis or may extend deeply into the thighs or buttocks. The overlying skin may ulcerate, and the deeper lesions often calcify.

One fifth of patients demonstrate vasculitic lesions of the skin. These can occur on the fingertips, forearms, lips, or lower leg (these latter may ulcerate). Although they are signs of disease activity, they do not usually imply impending disaster. The related mucosal ulcers are often painless and occur on the hard and soft palate, the nasal septum, other parts of the upper respiratory tract, and even the vagina. They are usually harmless, but occasional patients with involvement of the upper airway may require emergency tracheotomy.

Alopecia is usually diffuse; patients report increased hair on comb or brush or pillow. The hair will regrow in areas not scarred by discoid lesions.

Raynaud's phenomenon may be severe enough to cause digital gangrene and spontaneous amputation of the distal parts of the digits. More often it follows a more benign and variable course. Thrombophlebitis occurs in approximately 10 per cent of patients and may be accompanied by pulmonary emboli.

Eyes. Conjunctivitis or episcleritis or both are usually observed in younger patients at times of disease activity. Cytoid bodies (white exudates next to retinal vessels) are associated with active central nervous system involvement. Spasm of the retinal vessels may lead to transient or permanent blindness. Keratoconjunctivitis sicca occurs in 10 per cent of patients and is usually slowly progressive, but it often improves temporarily with therapy for other symptoms.

Gastrointestinal System. Anorexia, nausea, vomiting, and abdominal pain are observed in a minority of patients. Diffuse abdominal pain with or without rebound tenderness may be a manifestation of serositis or mesenteric arteritis. The latter can be complicated by intestinal infarct, which may lead to perforation and death. Corticosteroid therapy often improves symptoms in both situations; however, if perforation has already occurred, the symptoms may be blunted and therapy inappropriately delayed. Pancreatitis is occasionally due to SLE.

Dysphagia may be associated with reduced peristalsis, ulcerations of the esophagus caused by arteritis, or, more commonly, *Candida albicans* infection.

Liver. Liver enlargement occurs in about 30 per cent of patients with SLE. This is usually inconsequential. Fatty infiltration of the liver is common and rarely may be associated with hepatic insufficiency. Liver enzyme elevations often occur early in the illness in the absence of therapy. Aspirin treatment may induce such enzyme elevations. Chronic hepatitis is only occasionally observed in patients with SLE.

Heart. Pericarditis is usually symptomatic but without consequence; however, an occasional patient may experience tamponade. The most common EKG abnormality is nonspecific T wave changes. A prolonged P-R interval or evidence of ischemia or infarction may be found. Myocarditis may be manifested by unexplained tachycardia or mild dyspnea on exertion. More severe involvement is associated with frank heart failure. Coronary artery disease, most often atherosclerotic but occasionally arteritic, can lead to myocardial infarction, even in women in their early twenties.

Lung. Pleuritic chest pain occurs more commonly than x-ray evidence of effusion; however, massive effusions may occur. Pneumonitis in patients with SLE is often infectious; however a noninfectious syndrome occurs in SLE patients that varies from fleeting infiltrates (usually hemorrhagic) to marked consolidation and hypoxia. Diffuse interstitial pneumonitis also has been found in SLE.

Hematologic and Lymphoreticular Problems. Lymphadenopathy and splenomegaly may be sufficiently marked that it suggests a lymphoproliferative disorder. Moreover, polyclonal immune hyperactivity in the lymph node may be mistaken for giant follicular or other lymphomas. Hematologic abnormalities are almost invariably present in patients with active disease. The most common is the anemia of chronic disease—a normocytic anemia caused by impaired erythropoiesis. Hemolysis may occur in patients with or without a positive Coombs' test result, but significant hemolysis occurs in less than 10 per cent of patients. Iron deficiency often contributes to anemia. Many patients with lupus bruise easily; therapy and capillary fragility are more often the cause than a bleeding disorder. Mild thrombocytopenia occurs in a substantial proportion of patients with active disease; however, serious thrombocytopenia occurs in less than 10 per cent of patients. Two types of "anticoagulants" occur. One is a laboratory artifact caused by antibodies reactive with the phospholipids used in the partial thromboplastin time (PTT) test. This abnormality is not associated with prolonged bleeding and is not a cause of concern with regard to surgery or biopsies. Other antibodies may react with clotting factors (VIII, IX, XII, and others) and may be responsible for clinically important bleeding.

Nervous System. Peripheral neuropathies have been observed in about 15 per cent of patients with SLE, sometimes in the absence of other nervous system involvement. In addition to a sensory neuropathy, a mononeuritis multiplex picture (e.g., footdrop) is notable. Central nervous system involvement is quite variable. Psychological problems include personality disorders of every variety and numerous forms of frank psychosis (depression, paranoia, mania, schizophrenia). Differentiating that caused by lupus and that caused by corticosteroids is often a challenge.

Seizures, often grand mal, are common, especially in younger patients. Migraine headaches and cytoid bodies may be indications of disease activity. An organic brain syndrome with impaired mentation can progress to coma. Recovery may be complete, or there may be residual impairment. Movement disorders are more common in younger patients: chorea, athetosis, and hemiballismus are observed. Cerebellar abnormalities may occur independently or with other defects.

Transverse myelitis occurs in patients with SLE. Paralysis may also occur following intracerebral hemorrhage or thrombosis. Sterile meningitis may be observed. Despite the large variety of lupus-related nervous system problems, bacterial and other non-lupus causes must be sought and treated.

Kidney Disease. The great majority of patients have some degree of renal involvement. In many, the degree of abnormality is mild enough to escape clinical detection. In others, it is clinically detectable, but does not progress to functional impairment. Only a minority of patients have renal involvement that is threatening to the function of the organ. Hypertension and lupus renal involvement synergize in bringing about destructive changes. As a result, the presence of untreated hypertension poses a threat in patients with renal abnormalities.

Involvement in the kidney represents a multidimensional spectrum: rapidly progressive disease (a subacute glomerulonephritis picture), membranous involvement (usually with some mesangial hypertrophy) with nephrotic syndrome, a nephritic picture (mild to severe), and minimal abnormalities. Most patients have mesangial involvement. The progression to capillary loop pathology carries a worse prognosis. The biopsy picture can change from one form to another; as a result, the degree of active disease (e.g., necrosis) and scarring (glomerular hyalinization, interstitial) offers a much more useful measure than precise histologic classifications. The less scarring, the more there is to treat and preserve. If progression to renal failure occurs, chronic dialysis and renal transplantation are well tolerated. Most patients can be maintained with adequate renal function by modern therapy. Low-grade activity may be associated with slow progression to renal failure. Complete remissions of renal disease occur.

Menses and Pregnancy. Disease activity in menstruating women tends to be greatest in the period between ovulation and menses. Flares generally occur or worsen in this period. Menses are frequently irregular during active disease. Bleeding may be increased in patients with antibodies to clotting factors or with thrombocytopenia. Repeated spontaneous abortions are common in some women. Others, especially when in remission, carry to term without difficulty. Patients in remission at the time of conception tend to have relatively normal pregnancies. Advanced cardiac, central nervous system, or renal disease is a contraindication to pregnancy. The risk of a disease flare after induced abortion is the same as after delivery. Patients with active renal disease often experience exacerbation during pregnancy and may develop pre-eclampsia. Patients without renal involvement tend to have calmer pregnancies, but the disease often flares postpartum or postabortion. Increased dosage of corticosteroids during the time of delivery and for several weeks thereafter tends to reduce the likelihood of a disease flare. Babies of mothers with antibodies to SS-A may have congenital cardiac problems, including heart block.

LABORATORY FINDINGS. Specific tests for SLE are not available. The presence of large amounts of antibodies to native DNA is the single most useful diagnostic laboratory finding. A variety of abnormalities depend in large measure upon the organs involved. The lupus band test consists of a biopsy of nonlesional skin and staining for the presence of immunoglobulin and complement. This test is positive in about three fourths of patients with active SLE and one third of patients with inactive SLE; however, positive tests also occur in patients with rheumatoid arthritis, non-SLE renal disease, and certain dermatologic disorders. Many regard the test as not very helpful.

The LE cell consists of a nucleus that has been phagocytized. The phagocytosis requires antibodies reactive with DNA-histone and complement. In patients with extremely low complement, LE material that has not been phagocytized may be noted. About 80 per cent of patients with SLE are positive for LE cells. A small percentage of patients with related disorders are also positive: rheumatoid arthritis, especially with Felty's syndrome; Sjögren's syndrome; polymyositis-dermatomyositis. The fluorescent antinuclear antibody test (FANA or ANA) has been used as a screening test; however, many patients with related and unrelated diseases may also have positive tests. It is now possible to measure antibodies specifically reactive with various antigens (native DNA, Sm, various low molecular weight RNA species, SS-A, SS-B, etc.). These are much more informative than the FANA despite the improvement in usefulness of the FANA by virtue of analysis of patterns of staining.

Most patients with active SLE have impaired skin tests. Especially important is the common failure to respond to tuberculin in inactive patients as well.

Hematologic. Anemia usually is present in patients with active disease. Although leukopenia occurs in half of the patients, others may manifest leukocytosis. Corticosteroids may increase the white count. Infection in patients with SLE is to be suspected if there is an increase in percentages of granulocytes or immature granulocytes or both even in the absence of leukocytosis. Thrombocytopenia may precede other features of SLE. Antibodies to coagulation factors may be measured in coagulation abnormalities. Antibodies to phospholipids, which prolong the PTT, do not cause bleeding. A false-positive serologic test for syphilis is also observed in 15 per cent of patients.

Immune. The erythrocyte sedimentation rate (ESR) is usually elevated in patients with active disease; however, a minority of patients have normal ESR during periods of disease. Serum albumin levels are usually near normal except in patients with renal disease. Hypergammaglobulinemia may be marked in an untreated patient. Cryoglobulins may be increased in quantity. Rheumatoid factor occurs in low titer in patients with SLE. Reduced hemolytic complement levels (CH_{50}) are common in active disease, especially with renal involvement. Some patients have selected congenital complement deficiencies. Immune complexes may be found in the serum or plasma. Antibodies reactive with leukocytes (granulocytes, B cells, T cells) are found in the majority of patients. Platelet-bound immunoglobulin often occurs in the absence of thrombocytopenia as does a positive Coombs' test result in the absence of hemolysis. Antibodies are found that react with DNA, RNA, histones, nuclear ribonucleoprotein, and cytoplasmic antigenic determinants (see Table 447–3). Rarely, unusual antibodies have been found to react with histamine (inducing acquired Type I hyperlipoproteinemia), insulin receptors (exacerbating difficulties in sugar regulation), and other substances.

Renal. Proteinuria, granular or cellular casts, and cells (RBC, WBC) are found in the urine of patients with active kidney disease. Elevated serum creatinine levels may be reversible or fixed. Hypertension is common, even in the absence of renal failure. Renal biopsies are best used to determine therapy rather than to confirm the diagnosis.

Cardiac. Abnormal T waves are the most common EKG abnormality; evidence of coronary artery or hypertensive disease may be noted. Valvular abnormalities and pericardial fluid may be detected with echocardiograms.

Pulmonary. Pleural fluid may be seen on the x-ray. It is usually an exudate; however, the protein content may not be very high in patients with hypoalbuminemia. The glucose level is usually much higher than is observed in rheumatoid effusions. LE cells may be seen in the fluid. Pleural biopsies can show varying degrees of fibrosis and infiltration. Lung biopsies may show alveolar hemorrhage only; alveolar damage with interstitial edema and hyaline membranes; hypertrophy with or without vasculitis; or acute alveolitis. There is mild to severe hypoxemia. Patients with interstitial fibrosis show decreased vital capacity; others have disproportionately impaired diffusing capacities.

Nervous System. The EEG most commonly shows diffuse slowing. Seizures often occur in the absence of the typical patterns observed in patients with foci. The cerebrospinal fluid may be normal or have moderately elevated protein levels. The gammaglobulin levels are not increased. Granulocytes are indicative of infection; some patients have small numbers of round cells. Aseptic meningitis is occasionally found. A loss of brain substance may be noted in patients with chronic disease. Isolated loss of cortical or cerebellar neurones occurs.

DIAGNOSIS. SLE should be suspected in any person with a multisystem disease including joint pain. For epidemiologic and study purposes, four of the 11 criteria listed in Table 447–1 are required; however, the diagnosis may be made for other purposes with fewer criteria. SLE should be suspected if any of the criteria shown in Table 447–1 are present and unexplained. The disorder should be considered if any of the following are present: unexplained fever, purpura, splenomegaly, adenopathy, pneumonitis, myocarditis, or aseptic meningitis. The presence of a single symptom, such as serositis, and antibodies to native DNA in a young woman is highly suggestive of SLE.

Children are frequently misdiagnosed as having rheumatic fever or juvenile rheumatoid arthritis. Adults most commonly are misdiagnosed as having rheumatoid arthritis. Other diagnoses often applied to patients with SLE include Raynaud's disease, hemolytic anemia, idiopathic thrombocytopenia, thrombotic thrombocytopenic purpura, psychosis, vasculitis, progressive systemic sclerosis, lymphoma, autoimmune neutropenia, secondary syphilis, drug reaction, porphyria, multiple sclerosis, myasthenia gravis, polymyositis, glomerulonephritis, Henoch-Schönlein purpura, personality disorder, stroke, and seizure disorder.

In addition to those just listed, other diseases should be considered in patients suspected of having SLE: subacute bacterial endocarditis, bacterial peritonitis, gonococcal septicemia, meningococcal septicemia, tuberculosis, sarcoidosis, serum sickness, leukemia, leprosy, angioimmunoblastic lymphadenopathy, Wegener's granulomatosis, leptospirosis, Lyme arthritis, Rocky Mountain spotted fever, and acquired immune deficiency syndrome (AIDS).

Overlaps occur between SLE and other diseases such as progressive systemic sclerosis and Sjögren's syndrome. Some have defined these as "mixed connective tissue disease" or the "overlap syndrome;" others prefer less rigid categorizations.

THERAPY. The diagnosis of SLE often induces an emotional reaction. In addition, many patients with SLE have psychological problems that may be a result of the disease. Therefore it is necessary to provide effective emotional support. This includes an honest but optimistic assessment. Most patients with SLE can look forward to a normal lifespan, but with the requirement for periodic visits to the physician and treatment with various drugs. Many of the more serious problems do not affect most people. Renal failure can be handled by dialysis. Thus, although the patient must realize the presence of a serious and chronic disease, a dire prognosis should not be issued. Early involvement in educational programs and with physical therapists, dieticians, and occupational therapists may be helpful.

Patients with SLE usually need more than normal rest. Ten hours of sleep at night plus an afternoon nap would not be inappropriate. The more active the disease, the more rest needed. Ultraviolet light should be avoided: outdoor swimming should be limited to periods of reduced exposure (not at 1:00 PM ± 4 hours) and sunscreen should be used even for trips to the store. Drugs that augment the effects of UV light, such as tetracyclines and psoralens should be avoided. The same is true of foods containing large amounts of psoralens (celery, parsnips, figs, and parsley). Exercise should be appropriate to the clinical situation; however, exercise to the point of exhaustion should be discouraged. Stresses, including surgery, infections, childbirth, abortions, and psychological pressures may exacerbate the process and dictate additional treatment.

Although certain drugs can induce a lupus-like syndrome, there is little evidence that those drugs are detrimental to patients with SLE. Therefore, such drugs as alphamethyldopa and dilantin may be used without undue concern. However, sulfonamides are poorly tolerated by many patients; patients with active disease experience a rash up to one half of the time. Estrogens may worsen disease; therefore, birth control pills with minimum amounts of estrogens are preferred. Since hypertension is synergistic with immune-complex disease in bringing about pathology, the blood pressure should be kept in the middle of the normal range for age and sex.

Corticosteroids are frequently given. Short-acting drugs such as prednisone or methylprednisolone are preferred so that every other day therapy can be attempted and the hypothalamic-pituitary-adrenal axis not disrupted. The side effects of every other day steroids are much less than those of daily therapy. Low doses are less than 30 mg per 1.7 square meters per day of prednisone, and every attempt should be made to maintain patients on less than 25 mg per 1.7 square meters every other day. Moderate doses are 30–50 mg per 1.7 square meters per day. Higher doses may be necessary. Patients with marked multisystem involvement may temporarily require corticosteroids in divided doses. Heroic and experimental therapy includes boluses of very large doses of corticosteroids (1 gram or more of methylprednisolone) or of cyclophosphamide (0.5–0.75 grams per square meter) and plasmapheresis.

The role of prophylactic vigorous therapy has not been established for non–life-threatening situations. Total nodal irradiation may induce long-term suppression of disease as may monthly boluses of cyclophosphamide; however, these experimental procedures require further study. Azathioprine has long been used to treat patients with SLE; its usefulness may be limited to a subset of patients with moderate kidney disease or those with intractable skin disease or arthritis.

A major problem in the management of patients with SLE is not the acute treatment but the long-term management. The clinical picture (history plus physical exam) is usually a very good guide to the therapy of nonrenal and nonhematologic problems. In the latter two situations, the laboratory measures are helpful. Anemia, fatigue, and hypergammaglobulinemia tend to weigh in favor of more therapy. The long-term toxicities of corticosteroids (cataracts, asceptic necrosis of bone, infections) must always be balanced against the benefits of continued vigorous therapy. In tapering corticosteroids, it is generally advisable to drop rapidly to 30 mg per 1.7 square meters per day and then to reduce dosage more slowly. The lower the dose, the slower the tapering process should be. Rapid tapering can cause a disease flare, which requires re-institution of high doses.

The variable severity and extent of involvement in SLE dictate individualized treatment. It is helpful to divide problems into those of major organs, which therefore are life threatening, and those which are unpleasant but not life threatening (Table 447–5). The major exception to this division is a syndrome of acute toxic lupus observed primarily in pre-corticosteroid times: a young woman with high fever, serositis, rash, and arthritis might succumb to SLE in the absence of major organ involvement. This syndrome appears to be quite susceptible to therapy with corticosteroids in modest doses.

TABLE 447–5. MAJOR VERSUS NON-MAJOR ORGAN INVOLVEMENT IN SLE

Non-Major Organ SLE*	Major Organ SLE†
Alopecia	Glomerulonephritis
Fever	Central nervous system disease
Fatigue	Myocarditis
Anorexia	Pneumonitis
Arthritis	Thrombocytopenic purpura
Myalgia	Hemolytic anemia (marked)
Pleurisy	Severe granulocytopenia (rare)
Pericarditis	Mesenteric vasculitis
Peritonitis	
Rash	
Skin vasculitis	
Raynaud's phenomenon	
Mucosal ulcers	
Splenomegaly	
Lymphadenopathy	
Peripheral neuropathy	
Episcleritis	
Hepatitis	

*Usually does not require high-dose corticosteroids or other vigorous treatment. In all cases, a careful search for infection is carried out.

†Usually requires high-dose corticosteroids or other vigorous treatment. Individual patients vary greatly and some do not require vigorous therapy.

Non–major-organ involvements are best handled with symptomatic therapy: the less medicine the better. Hydroxychloroquine (200 mg–600 mg/d) is effective for skin involvement; it also may help treat arthritis and other manifestations. Nonsteroidal anti-inflammatory drugs (NSAIDs) such as aspirin and ibuprofen are useful for arthritis, serositis, and fever. Some patients tolerate one NSAID better than another—bizarre neurologic reactions may occur in SLE patients receiving ibuprofen; liver enzyme abnormalities may follow aspirin treatment; gastrointestinal tolerance varies. The combination of hydroxychloroquine + NSAID may be sufficient. The addition of low doses of corticosteroids may be necessary. Initial every other day therapy may not be possible; however, a subsequent switch to alternate day treatment reduces steroid-induced side effects. In patients with continued disease activity, symptoms may be prominent every other day, necessitating return to daily steroids. Even in the face of corticosteroid therapy, NSAID and hydroxychloroquine may add substantial benefit and allow a lower steroid dosage. Fevers occurring in spite of daily corticosteroids may respond to NSAIDs. Indomethacin may be especially effective in pericarditis.

The management of major organ involvement is usually directed at preservation of function and prevention of organ failure and disability or death. Myocarditis usually responds to the symptomatic treatment of SLE, but occasional patients may require specific treatment; moderate doses of corticosteroids are usually adequate. Thrombocytopenia and hemolytic anemia are treated more or less as they are in the absence of SLE. The hematologic parameters are followed. High-dose corticosteroids are instituted; if inadequate or they cannot be tapered to a reasonable dose, immunosuppressive drugs or splenectomy may be necessary. Plasmapheresis may be of temporary benefit. Plasma exchange may be helpful in patients with features of thrombotic thrombocytopenia (look for fragmented RBC on the peripheral smear). Patients with factor VIII deficiency caused by specific antibodies should be treated with plasmapheresis and immunosuppression. Mild pneumonitis usually responds to moderate doses of corticosteroids; severe disease requires heroic measures. Central nervous system involvement may require moderate to high corticosteroid therapy; in patients with severe involvement, intravenous cyclophosphamide (0.75–1.0 gram per 1.7 square meters) can be lifesaving. Seizures require treatment with both corticosteroids and anticonvulsants.

The most studied and controversial area is the treatment of SLE kidney disease. If there is active disease on biopsy and little scarring, high-dose corticosteroids or corticosteroids plus an oral immunosuppressive drug (azathioprine for example) may be sufficient. If there is active disease and more scarring, vigorous therapy may be considered. This includes the following choices: intravenous corticosteroids in large doses, intravenous cyclophosphamide, or plasmapheresis + cyclophosphamide. Randomized trials to determine the relative efficacy of these therapies are in progress. In the face of little disease activity and moderate scarring, aggressive therapy is usually not indicated.

Am J Kidney Dis 11(Suppl 1) (July, 1982). *Devoted to a symposium on SLE.*

Decker JL: Systemic lupus erythematosus: Evolving concepts. Ann Intern Med 91:587, 1979. *The experiences of a leading center for SLE research and patient care.*

DuBois EL: Lupus Erythematosus. Los Angeles, University of Southern California Press, 1978. *A lengthy monograph citing many case reports. Extensively referenced.*

Koffler D: Current perspectives on the immunology of systemic lupus erythematosus. Arthritis Rheum 25:721, 1982. *Devoted to a symposium on SLE.*

Ropes MW: Systemic Lupus Erythematosus. Cambridge, Harvard University Press, 1976. *Observations of a physician with over 40 years' experience with SLE patients.*

Rothfield NF: Systemic lupus erythematosus. Clin Rheum Dis Vol 1, Dec 1975. *Thirteen chapters dealing with systemic lupus.*

Smith HR, Steinberg AD: Autoimmunity—A perspective. Ann Rev Immunol 1:175–210, 1983.
Steinberg AD: Systemic lupus erythematosus. Insights from animal models. Ann Intern Med 100:714, 1984. *Up-to-date discussion of pathogenetic mechanisms of disease.*
Winchester RJ: New directions for research in systemic lupus erythematosus. Arthritis Rheum (Supplement to June 1978 issue). *Proceedings of a multicenter conference on systemic lupus.*

448. SYSTEMIC SCLEROSIS (Scleroderma)

Edward D. Harris, Jr.

Systemic sclerosis (Scl) is a generalized disorder of connective tissue characterized by thickening and fibrosis of the skin (scleroderma), prominent abormalities of the small arteries and microvasculature, and by distinctive patterns of involvement of internal organs including the gastrointestinal tract, heart, lungs, and kidneys. The initial manifestation of Scl is typically Raynaud's phenomenon which is eventually present in over 95 per cent of cases. Although Raynaud's phenomenon may be the only complaint for decades, skin involvement usually begins within two years, initially on the fingers and hands (acrosclerosis) but with variable extent and progression and in many cases involving the face, arms, legs, and trunk (diffuse or generalized scleroderma). Localized scleroderma, a term which includes morphea and linear scleroderma, involves the skin exclusively.

The diagnosis of Scl is most often made in patients between the ages of 35 and 55, yet all age groups may be affected. The disease is four times more common in females than in males and is found in all racial groups and geographic areas. The incidence of Scl remains uncertain with estimates of 4 to 12 cases per million population per year reported. Some observers feel many people are misdiagnosed as having Raynaud's syndrome alone or as having a related connective tissue disease. Although the cutaneous manifestations are clinically prominent, morbidity and mortality are related to the extent and severity of internal organ involvement.

PATHOGENESIS. The etiology and pathogenesis of Scl are unknown. Familial aggregation has been reported but is uncommon. Studies of HLA phenotypes have failed to reveal any consistent associations. Any hypothesis concerning the pathogenesis of Scl must explain a diverse body of findings including the heterogeneous patterns of disease; its progression and internal organ involvement; the high frequency of abnormal serologic and cellular immune reactions; the activated state of connective tissue; and the prominent vascular abnormalities.

Raynaud's phenomenon is the initial complaint in 70 per cent of patients with Scl. Histopathologically, the digital arteries reveal a distinctive accumulation of collagen and ground substance along with endothelial cell proliferation in the intima that leads to severe attenuation (greater than 75 per cent) of the arterial lumen in the majority of cases. Similar findings are evident in the small arteries of the heart, lung, kidney, and gastrointestinal tract. Nailfold capillaroscopy reveals distinctive abnormalities of enlarged, tortuous capillary loops interspersed with areas of capillary loss. While it is not clear whether these capillary abnormalities precede or develop concurrently with Raynaud's phenomenon in systemic sclerosis, the derangement of the capillary bed has been found to correlate with the degree and extent of internal organ involvement and is also felt to be a differentiating feature between Raynaud's disease and Raynaud's phenomenon as a manifestation of systemic sclerosis. Similar capillary lesions are evident in clinically unaffected muscle tissue and in the tissues of affected internal organs.

The factor or factors responsible for initiation of these vascular lesions is unknown. Patients with Scl sometimes have high levels of circulating immune complexes, yet there is little evidence of deposition of immunoglobulin and complement in involved tissues. A trypsin-like endothelial cytotoxic factor in serum has been reported, yet a similar activity has been found in other connective tissue diseases and its specificity for endothelium remains in doubt. The finding of increased von Willebrand factor activity and factor VIII/von Willebrand factor antigen in patients with Scl suggests that endothelial injury and repair are ongoing processes. Signs of platelet activation in vivo in Scl include moderate thrombocytosis, elevated plasma β-thromboglobulin levels, and increased numbers of circulating platelet aggregates.

The role of this platelet-endothelial interaction in the pathogenesis of the proliferative vasculopathy of Scl is unclear. The digital arteries of Scl have abnormal reactivity to cold and to serotonin but not to catecholamines. Recent studies have demonstrated cold-induced vasospasm in the circulation of the heart, lungs, and kidneys, suggesting that internal organ "Raynaud equivalents" may play a role in the visceral abnormalities of Scl as well.

Skin biopsies reveal dermal thickening secondary to increased collagen deposition and variable degrees of T lymphocyte accumulation. Although areas of recent fibrosis may have a higher ratio of Type III to Type I collagen, no significant abnormalities of physical properties, amino acid analysis, cross-linking, or solubility of collagen have been reported. Dermal collagenase activity appears normal.

Dermal fibroblasts from Scl cultured in vitro produce collagen and glycosaminoglycan at increased rates. This abnormality can be sustained for several generations of tissue culture. The cause of the increased collagen and matrix synthesis is unknown, but in vivo may be related to stimulation by monokines, lymphokines, or substances such as platelet-derived growth factor. The finding of dermal thickening and fibrosis in chronic graft-versus-host disease similar to Scl suggests that cellular immune factors may be fundamental elements in this process. Many patients with Scl have evidence of humoral immune abnormalities including serum antinuclear antibodies, rheumatoid factor, and hypergammaglobulinemia.

PATHOLOGY. Systemic involvement is characterized by sclerosis. Early findings in the *skin* in active scleroderma have revealed edema, plasma cell and/or lymphocyte infiltrates around eccrine sweat glands, loss of capillaries, and endothelial proliferation. Larger vessels may show fibromucinous accumulations in the intima. The *reticular dermis* is usually thickened. It may have a normal collagen-bundle pattern or may show broad, homogeneous, acellular deposits of collagen with indistinct bundle patterns. Other findings include atrophy of the rete pegs of the epidermis, atrophy of the hair follicles and sweat glands, perivascular lymphocytic infiltration, and hyalinization of arterioles. The subcutaneous tissue is replaced by thick collagen bundles which bind the dermis to deeper structures. Pathologic changes in the musculoskeletal system include acute and chronic inflammation in the *synovium* with no pannus formation but with more sclerosis than is found in rheumatoid synovium with an equivalent inflammatory response. Fibrin deposits are laid down around *tendons*, and *muscles* show a variety of abnormalities, the most common being fibrosis of the perimysium and epimysium, scattered cellular infiltrates, and atrophy and necrosis of muscle fibers similar to that seen in polymyositis.

In the internal organs, microvascular abnormalities (see Pathogenesis), mild inflammation, and edema in connective tissue are followed by increased deposition of fibrous tissue in both appropriate and inappropriate loci. This leads to distortion of the architecture of the tissues affected. In the *lungs*, a relatively low-grade interstitial pneumonitis is followed by interstitial fibrosis, most marked in lower lobes. After this, cyst formation and bronchiectasis may develop. Arteriolar thickening (concentric intimal proliferation or medial hypertrophy) is seen, particularly in those patients with clinical evidence of pulmonary hypertension. In the gastrointestinal tract, atrophy of the muscularis is more prominent than fibrotic replacement. The lower two thirds of the *esophagus* frequently is involved with muscle atrophy and fibrosis. Lesions secondary to reflux of gastric contents are present in 20 per cent of cases. Involvement of the *small bowel* begins with patchy subserosal fibrosis and may progress to almost complete replacement of smooth muscle with fibrous tissue. The small bowel may develop multiple sacculations, presumably at sites of weakness in the continuity of the wall. Dilation, muscle atrophy, and fibrosis are seen in the *colon;* the fibrosis is irregular, leading to the characteristic sacculations and diverticula. The *heart* is frequently enlarged and may be the only organ weighing more than predicted for the subject's body weight. Small patches of interstitial myocardial fibrosis commonly are found. In very severe cases, as much as 60 per cent of cardiac muscle is replaced by dense, relatively acellular and avascular fibrous tissue. Endocardial or valvular thickening is unusual and is rarely of hemodynamic significance. Fibrinous pericarditis is found quite often, even in the absence of uremia. *Kidneys* in Scl are normal in size when renal involvement has not been present clinically. In patients dying with uremia they may be small and frequently have small cortical infarcts. Histologically, fibromucinous intimal proliferation in the interlobular arteries, fibrinoid necrosis of small arteries and arterioles (including the glomerular tufts), and thickening of the basement membrane (the "wire-loop" lesions) may all be present. These changes are similar to those seen in kidneys from patients with malignant hypertension.

CLINICAL MANIFESTATIONS AND DIAGNOSIS. Paroxysmal vasospasm of the fingers with the characteristic sequential color changes of Raynaud's phenomenon is the typical initial manifestation of Scl. In individuals destined to develop generalized or *diffuse Scl,* Raynaud's phenomenon may be preceded by finger and hand edema, polyarthralgia or polyarthritis, or both, weakness, weight loss, or signs of specific internal organ involvement. Patients destined to develop more limited Scl may have Raynaud's phenomenon alone for many years prior to the development of other manifestations of disease. Confident diagnosis of early Scl is frequently confounded by the clinical resemblance to other connective tissue diseases or to idiopathic Raynaud's phenomenon alone.

Classification. Scl is variable in extent and progression but can be grouped into two principal syndromes of important prognostic and therapeutic implications. Individuals with *diffuse scleroderma* are at risk for rapidly progressive and generalized skin involvement and the full spectrum of visceral abnormalities. A nearly equal number of patients are characterized by slowly progressive and restricted skin changes—confined to the fingers, hands, and face—that have been termed the *CREST syndrome variant* (subcutaneous calcinosis, Raynaud's phenomenon, esophageal dysmotility, sclerodactyly, and telangiectasia). Patients with the CREST syndrome have a relatively benign and protracted course of disease and are at far less risk of involvement of the skeletal muscles, joints, heart, and kidneys.

Calcinosis, Raynaud's phenomenon, and telangiectasia are seen in both syndromes; thus accurate classification depends upon assessment of the extent of skin involvement, although other clinical and laboratory features should be considered (Table 448–1). Less commonly, patients may present with typical internal organ manifestations of Scl but without skin changes (systemic sclerosis sine scleroderma).

TABLE 448–1. CLINICAL CLASSIFICATION OF SYSTEMIC SCLEROSIS

	Diffuse Scleroderma	CREST Syndrome
Onset of Raynaud's phenomenon	Within 2 yrs	May be present alone for decades
Skin involvement	Acral and Trunk	Acral Only
Tendon friction rubs	60%	< 1%
Arthritis	40%	20%
Myositis	20%	< 5%
Interstitial pulmonary fibrosis	75%	Rare
Pulmonary hypertension	Rare	10%
Myocardial involvement	15–50%	5%
Renal involvement	25%	Rare
Esophageal dysmotility	90%	90%
Anti-centromere antibody	5–10%	50–70%
Anti-Scl 70 antibody	30–40%	Rare

Cutaneous System. The earliest change is painless pitting edema of the hands and fingers and occasionally more proximal locations. There may be symptoms of hand stiffness or of carpal tunnel syndrome. As the edema lessens, gradual tightening and thickening of the skin develop. The skin may appear shiny and taut with loss of normal skin folds. Joints become immobilized from tight encasement in thickened skin as well as from contractures of muscles, tendons, and palmar fascia. Generalized hyperpigmentation or spotty hypopigmentation may ensue. Recurrent traumatic ulcerations occur over the proximal interphalangeal joints. Chronic ischemic ulcerations may develop at the tips of the digits and the fingers themselves may shorten through progressive resorption of the terminal phalanges. Telangiectasia and subcutaneous calcinosis are common later findings. The skin of the face may appear smooth and waxy with a pinched immobile facies. Narrowing of the oral aperture may ensue, restricting lip movement and preventing adequate dental hygiene. Pruritus is uncommon, but scaling and erythema can be seen. Late in the course of illness, the skin tends to soften and atrophy.

The extent and severity of skin thickening typically worsen in the first several years of disease and thereafter many patients enjoy spontaneous improvement, an observation that complicates interpretation of long-term therapeutic trials. An individual patient with diffuse scleroderma may manifest rapidly progressive skin involvement or may have long intervals of stable or even spontaneously improving skin thickening, some of which may be due to waxing and waning of skin edema.

Musculoskeletal System. Almost half of patients with Scl present with joint pain or develop it during the first year of illness. Small joints are involved more often than large ones. Although an erosive synovitis can be seen, most joint deformity and immobility are best explained by periarticular soft tissue thickening and fibrosis. Tendons are frequently involved in *diffuse scleroderma,* mimicking arthritis. A leathery friction rub can be felt on active and passive motion of involved tendons. Muscle atrophy is often severe in areas such as the hands. Proximal muscle weakness indistinguishable from idiopathic polymyositis may be seen but is more typically a chronic and insidious process.

Gastrointestinal Tract. Of the internal organ systems, the gastrointestinal tract is the one most often involved in Scl. Oral symptoms include xerostomia and a progressive decrease in the size of the mouth. Sjögren's syndrome is seen often, and the frequency of its association with systemic sclerosis is probably underestimated. Symptoms referable to the esophagus, ranging from simple dysphagia to heartburn, nausea, and substernal fullness, are found in 45 to 60 per cent of cases. The dysphagia is related to absence of coordinated peristalsis, followed by loss of amplitude of esophageal body waves and incompetence of the lower esophageal sphincter. If reflex esophagitis becomes a persistent complication, stricture may develop. Vomiting, abdominal distention, and pain or diarrhea may indicate involvement of the small intestine. As in the esophagus, motility of the small bowel is decreased, and there may be malabsorption secondary to intraluminal stagnation with concomitant bacterial overgrowth. Functional bowel complaints secondary to pathologic changes in the colon are common. Disease of both large and small bowel may produce a clinical picture identical to paralytic ileus with incomplete obstruction at any level. An association between primary biliary cirrhosis and scleroderma with CREST syndrome is now recognized.

Heart and Lungs. Dyspnea is the most common cardiorespiratory symptom in Scl and is present in more than 50 per cent of patients. Fine, dry crackles at the bases of the lung are the first abnormality found on physical examination. In some patients, progression to respiratory insufficiency and death from hypoxemia are related to progressive pulmonary fibrosis. The earliest abnormality of pulmonary function is a decrease in pulmonary diffusion capacity. Those exposed in their occupation to silicate dust have a predilection to develop this form of the disease. Restriction of chest wall expansion by dermal fibrosis around the thorax rarely affects respiratory function. A few patients with severe cystic and fibrotic changes in the lungs have developed multifocal alveolar cell carcinomas.

Increasingly recognized as a prominent cause of late morbidity and a principal cause of mortality in patients with CREST syndrome is progressive pulmonary hypertension in the absence of significant pulmonary interstitial fibrosis. Rales are frequently absent but an increased pulmonic heart sound or signs of right ventricular failure may be seen. Pulmonary hypertension should be suspected if a severely reduced diffusion capacity is present.

Replacement of myocardium with fibrous tissue ("scleroderma heart disease") is an occasional primary cause of heart failure. In addition, impaired cardiac function can be attributed to right ventricular failure secondary to pulmonary hypertension. Fibrosis of the conducting system may lead to atrioventricular conduction defects and arrhythmias. The occurrence of angina-like pain and sudden death in patients with Scl associated with pathology showing ischemic reperfusion has suggested that a Raynaud's phenomenon in the heart is probably a true clinical event.

Kidneys. The sudden development of malignant hypertension resistant to therapy and uremia progressing rapidly to death is a dreaded complication of Scl. Most patients have had skin changes before development of abnormal renal function. Careful monitoring of blood pressure by the patient at home and search of peripheral blood smears for evidence of microangiopathic hemolyis may occasionally give warning that accelerated hypertension is developing. Progression to renal failure and death may follow quickly unless treatment is vigorous. Renal complications of Scl develop more often in cold months of the year.

Nervous System. Involvement of the nervous system is rare. Facial pain, questionably related to a trigeminal neuropathy, is seen occasionally and may be disabling. Significant reduction in mean conduction velocity of peripheral nerves has been reported.

LABORATORY FINDINGS. The erythrocyte sedimentation rate is elevated in most patients with Scl, and a mild anemia of chronic disease may be present. In addition, iron deficiency anemia may result from bleeding from esophagitis, and vitamin B_{12} and/or folic acid deficiency from overgrowth of organisms in an atonic bowel. Hemolysis is unusual, except for microangiopathic hemolytic anemia, which heralds severe accelerated hypertension. A number of serologic abnormalities link Scl to other connective tissue diseases. Mild hypergammaglobulinemia is present in 30 to 50 per cent of patients, rheumatoid factor in 25 to 35 per cent, antinuclear antibodies (often with a speckled or a nucleolar pattern) in sera of 40 to 80 per cent, depending on the assay used, and LE cells in less than 10 per cent of patients. Antinuclear antibody is directed against a soluble nuclear antigen, Scl-70 (particularly in patients with diffuse disease), nucleolar RNA, and the centromere of chromosomes (particularly in patients with CREST variant). DNA-binding activity in serum is absent.

The electrocardiogram shows nonspecific abnormalities in almost 50 per cent of patients. The pattern of conduction defects with very low voltage is seen only in those uncommon patients with marked myocardial replacement by fibrous tissue. Echocardiogram in these cases will reveal reduced ventricular wall motion. This technique is also useful in documenting small pericardial effusions. In general the electromyogram is normal; most patients have polyphasic waves of normal duration and size. Denervation potentials are seen only rarely.

Roentgenography. Roentgenograms are important for diagnosis and follow-up evaluation. The findings of soft tissue atrophy, subcutaneous calcinosis, and resorption of the tufts of the terminal phalanges without loss of apparent joint spaces between phalanges are virtually pathognomonic of Scl when seen on hand films. Upper gastrointestinal films reveal a dilated, atonic esophagus in about 60 per cent of patients. Small bowel studies may demonstrate segmental atony, dilation, and sacculation in the duodenum and jejunum. Linear or cystic pneumatosis (air in the wall of the gut) is occasionally seen in flat plates of the abdomen of patients with severe small bowel involvement. Barium studies of the colon reveal widemouth, asymmetrical diverticula in 20 to 40 per cent of patients; progression to a dilated, atonic megacolon rarely occurs. In patients with pulmonary involvement, chest roentgenograms reveal a diffuse reticular pattern with a honeycomb appearance in the lower lung fields. Serial films may document progression to dense interstitial fibrosis amid radiolucent cystic areas.

DIFFERENTIAL DIAGNOSIS. When Scl presents as persistent symmetrical polyarthritis involving the hands, as edematous puffy hands, or as Raynaud's phenomenon, a specific diagnosis may be impossible to make. Rheumatoid arthritis, systemic sclerosis, SLE, and dermatomyositis-polymyositis can all present in this fashion. If symptoms persist and the skin begins to appear thickened or bound down to underlying fascia, the physician should look for one or more of the following, which would help consolidate a diagnosis of Scl: (1) diminished numbers and dilation or tortuosity of nail-bed capillaries; (2) pitting scars in the distal digits below the nails; and (3) signs of systemic fibrosis such as bibasilar pulmonary fibrosis or disturbances of gastrointestinal (especially esophageal) motility. In a large multicenter study, *proximal* scleroderma itself was identified as the sole criterion necessary to make the diagnosis. The differential diagnosis of varied manifestations of Scl is listed in Table 448–2.

TREATMENT. Because so little is known about the pathogenesis of Scl, no specific treatment is available. Innumerable therapies have been attempted, but controlled trials have been few and outcome measures seldom uniformly applied. The inflammatory symptoms wax and wane as is characteristic of the connective tissue diseases. The tendency for skin involvement to improve spontaneously in late disease and the variability in progression of skin changes in early Scl confound the interpretation of uncontrolled trials and of long-term therapies.

TABLE 448–2. DIFFERENTIAL DIAGNOSIS OF SYSTEMIC SCLEROSIS

Raynaud's phenomenon
Raynaud's disease
Occupational trauma
Shoulder-hand syndrome
Heavy metal or ergot poisoning
Vascular disease (including SLE and polymyositis)
Hematologic abnormalities
Polycythemia vera
Cryoglobulinemia
Vinyl chloride toxicity
Skin changes
Werner's syndrome
Progeria
Chronic hypostatic edema
Lichen sclerosus et atrophicus
Porphyria cutanea tarda
Scleredema
Chronic graft-versus-host reactions
Bleomycin therapy
Fasciitis with eosinophilia
Carcinoid syndrome
Chronic insulin-dependent diabetes mellitus
Telangiectasia
Hereditary telangiectasia
Cirrhosis of the liver
Visceral disease
Idiopathic pulmonary fibrosis
Rheumatoid arthritis
Sarcoidosis
Infiltrative cardiomyopathies
Intestinal obstruction

In view of the prominent immunologic abnormalities of Scl, corticosteroids and immunosuppressants have been employed, but the consensus of this experience has been that neither affect significantly the natural history of Scl. Corticosteroids have been implicated in provoking Scl renal involvement, and their use should be reserved for patients with inflammatory muscle disease and some patients with rapidly progressive interstitial lung disease. Anti-platelet and vasodilator therapies including aspirin, dipyridamole, and calcium channel blockers have attracted recent interest, but results of preliminary trials have been disappointing. D-Penicillamine has been investigated in a number of trials for its known effect in inhibiting inter- and intramolecular cross-linkages of mature collagen. A recent large retrospective study suggested that patients receiving high doses ($\geq$ 750 mg per day) for prolonged periods of time (18 months) enjoyed lessening of skin thickening and a decreased incidence of new internal organ involvement, resulting in an improved survival when compared to a well-matched population not receiving this treatment. D-Penicillamine therapy was not associated with improvement of previously existing internal organ involvement nor with improvement in the vascular or immunologic aspects of Scl, and the rationale for such therapy in CREST syndrome remains unclear.

Previously refractory to all but the most desperate therapies (bilateral nephrectomy, renal transplantation), the accelerated hypertension, rapidly progressive renal insufficiency, and hyperreninemia of Scl renal crisis are now felt to respond to aggressive antihypertensive treatment. Dramatic successes have been reported with both captopril and minoxidil in which hypertension was controlled and renal damage reversible if treatment was begun at early stages (serum creatinine less than 4.0 mg/dl). Intriguingly, many of these patients have experienced reversal of skin involvement in a time course similar to that associated with D-penicillamine treatment, lending support to the concept of a vascular pathogenesis of Scl.

The mainstay of treatment of Scl is supportive. Many patients lead productive and useful lives. An important goal of therapy is to preserve function in and prevent injury to the hands. Vocational and occupational therapy can be important in maintenance of hand function. Digital ulcerations must be treated immediately with wound care, topical or systemic antibiotics, and vasodilators before they progress to substantial tissue damage. Antacids, cimetidine, and simpler maneuvers such as elevation of the head of the bed and avoidance of postprandial recumbency and tight clothing can lessen the symptoms of reflux esophagitis and delay or prevent secondary lower esophageal stricture. Esophageal dilatation is of help in certain patients but frequently must be repeated at regular intervals. Malabsorption and crampy diarrhea sometimes respond to broad-spectrum antimicrobials (e.g., tetracycline 0.25 gm twice daily) for presumed bacterial overgrowth. Constipation responds to agents that soften and increase the bulk of stool.

Symptomatic management of the vasospastic phenomena of Scl includes avoidance of cold, attention to proper dress, including both warm mittens and layered clothing for the trunk, and avoidance of emotional stress, nicotine, and caffeine. No drug therapy of Raynaud's phenomenon in Scl is universally effective or tolerated, but direct vasodilators such as nitroglycerin, calcium channel blockers, and prazosin appear better choices than sympatholytic drugs.

EOSINOPHILIC FASCIITIS. Eosinophilic fasciitis (EF) is a disorder characterized by rapidly developing symmetrical inflammation and scleroderma-like sclerosis of the deep fascia, lower subcutis, and dermis. Chiefly affected are the extremities and in many instances the face and trunk as well. In contrast to Scl, the fingers, hands and feet are typically spared; Raynaud's phenomenon, nailfold capillary abnormalities, and internal organ involvement are rarely present. Although the etiology of EF is unknown, some cases, especially in men, appear to have been precipitated by strenuous physical activity such as rapid assumption of physical fitness programs. All age groups are affected, but the majority of patients are between 30 and 60 years. Clinically, one finds erythema, edema, and severe induration of the skin and subcutaneous tissues. The overlying skin typically has an "orange-peel" appearance and exaggerated furrowing over the course of superficial veins is noted in anti-dependent postures. Arthritis is uncommon, but carpal tunnel syndrome is frequent and virtually all patients develop joint contractures. Muscle weakness secondary to disuse atrophy and occasionally occurring as an extension of inflammation deep to the fascia are seen.

Laboratory abnormalities include elevation of erythrocyte sedimentation rate, hypergammaglobulinemia, circulating immune complexes, and striking peripheral eosinophilia (typically over 2000/mm^3). Biopsy specimens should include skin to skeletal muscle; they reveal edema of the deep fascia and subcutis and infiltration with eosinophils, lymphocytes, and histiocytes in early disease. Later, tissue eosinophils are less conspicuous or are absent, and the predominant feature is fibrosis and thickening of the deep fascia, which can extend to the dermis.

Moderate corticosteroids (prednisone $\leq$ 20 mg/day) provide rapid symptomatic relief and readily obliterate the tissue and peripheral eosinophilia, athough they have not been demonstrated to speed the resolution of tissue fibrosis. The majority of patients experience clinical and biopsy resolution within three to five years, yet others have recurrences or persistent disease. The precise relationship of EF to Scl remains speculative. Many observers are struck by the clinical and laboratory resemblance of EF to acute generalized subcutaneous morphea.

OVERLAP SYNDROMES. Some patients with Scl present with simultaneous clinical and laboratory features of SLE, rheumatoid arthritis, polymyositis, or all three. The term "overlap syndrome" has replaced such colorful names as lupoderma and sclerodermatomyositis to describe patients with features of two or more connective tissue diseases. In general, patients with overlap syndromes tend to have less extensive Scl skin involvement, milder signs of digital ischemia, and less renal disease from either Scl or SLE.

Mixed connective tissue disease (MCTD) is recognized as a distinct overlap syndrome and describes patients with a positive antinuclear antibody test result with a speckled pattern and a high titer of serum antibody to extractable nuclear protein antigen (RNP) in a clinical setting of features of Scl, SLE, and polymyositis. Diffuse hand swelling, fever, and lymphadenopathy are frequent as well. Low levels of anti-DNA antibodies are sometimes found but antibody to Sm antigen is uncommon. Involvement of the kidneys and central nervous system occurs less frequently than in SLE, and the polymyositis responds to corticosteroids. In long-term follow-up of patients originally said to have MCTD, the majority were found to evolve toward more classic Scl, yet others had protracted clinical courses dominated by the features of SLE or polymyositis. Not all patients with clinical MCTD have antibody to RNP, and many patients with antibody to RNP have clinical manifestations consistent with diagnoses of SLE, Scl, or polymyositis alone. MCTD illustrates the ambiguities and the idiosyncratic nature of the clinical expressions of connective tissue diseases. Proper management requires close assessment of the features present in the individual patient. All patients presenting with an overlap syndrome should have tests of the presence and extent of muscle, renal, hematologic, and pulmonary involvement. A screening serologic profile, including serum rheumatoid factor, sedimentation rate, antinuclear antibody, anti-DNA antibody, and serum complement levels is appropriate. A high titer of speckled antinuclear antibody suggests that antibody to extractable nuclear antigen, either RNP or Sm, may be present, and in such instances these should be measured as well.

Follansbee WP, Curtiss EI, Medsger TA Jr, Steen VD, Mretsky BF, Owens GR, Rodnan GP: Physiologic abnormalities of cardiac function in progressive systemic sclerosis with diffuse scleroderma. N Engl J Med 310:142, 1984. *Abnormalities of myocardial perfusion are common in PSS and appear to be due to a disturbance of myocardial microcirculation of both ventricles.*

Fritzler MJ, Kinsella TD, Garbutt E: The CREST syndrome: A distinct serologic entity with anticentromere antibodies. Am J Med 69:520, 1980. *Anticentromere antibody was found in 26 of 27 CREST patients but only 8 of 115 with diffuse Scl and related connective tissue diseases.*

Haynes DC, Gershwin ME: The immunopathology of progressive systemic sclerosis (PSS). Sem Arthritis Rheum 11:331, 1982. *An extensively referenced review of the various immunologic aspects of Scl.*

Moore TL, Zuckner J: Eosinophilic fasciitis. Sem Arthritis Rheum 9:228, 1980. *A detailed literature review of 53 patients with illustrative case material.*

Nimelstein SH, Brody S, McShane D, Holman HR: Mixed connective tissue disease: A subsequent evaluation of the original 25 patients. Medicine 59:239, 1980. *In surviving patients, inflammatory disease manifestations (arthritis, serositis, fever, myositis) responded to steroid therapy and became less severe. Sclerodermatous manifestations (sclerodactyly, esophageal disease) persisted. There was a general evolution away from an MCTD picture toward Scl. Renal disease remained infrequent.*

Rodnan GP, Myerowitz RL, Justh GO: Morphologic changes in the digital arteries of patients with progressive systemic sclerosis (scleroderma) and Raynaud's phenomenon. Medicine 59:393, 1980. *This paper provides good examples of the histopathology of the arterial lesion of Scl as well as an excellent discussion of Raynaud's phenomenon in Scl versus Raynaud's disease.*

Steen VD, Medsger TA, Rodnan GP: D-Penicillamine therapy in progressive systemic sclerosis (scleroderma). Ann Rheum Dis 97:652, 1982. *A large and long-term retrospective experience with D-penicillamine treatment. Includes good clinical detail and a discussion of the difficulties inherent in treatment of Scl.*

Subcommittee for Scleroderma Criteria: Preliminary criteria for the classification of systemic sclerosis (scleroderma). Arthritis Rheum 23:587, 1980. *This large multicenter study has compiled the clinical and laboratory features of scleroderma and developed criteria for diagnosis of this disease.*

Traub YM, Shapiro AP, Rodnan GP, Medsger TA, McDonald RH Jr, Steen VD, Osial TA Jr, Tolchin SF: Hypertension and renal failure (scleroderma renal crisis) in progressive systemic sclerosis. Review of a 25-year experience with 68 cases. Medicine 62:335, 1983. *With renal dialysis and more effective treatment of severe hypertension, together with bilateral nephrectomy in selected patients, survivals of greater than one year were achieved in 11 patients treated in the past few years.*

Whitman HH, Case OB, Larugh JH, Christian LL, Botstein G, Maricq H, LeRoy EC: Variable response to oral angiotensin-converting-enzyme blockage in hypertensive scleroderma patients. Arthritis Rheum 25:241, 1982. *Experience with 12 patients emphasizing the need for early, aggressive intervention in Scl renal crisis.*

449. SJÖGREN'S SYNDROME

Norman Talal

DEFINITION. Sjögren's syndrome is a chronic inflammatory and autoimmune disease in which the salivary and lacrimal glands undergo progressive destruction by lymphocytes and plasma cells resulting in decreased production of saliva and tears. The term autoimmune exocrinopathy has been introduced. The spectrum of this illness includes a primary form (sicca complex), a secondary form accompanying rheumatoid arthritis (or occasionally another connective tissue disease), and a form characterized mainly by lymphoproliferation of either a benign infiltrative or a malignant nature. Females are involved ten times more commonly than males.

PATHOGENESIS. The several factors involved in the etiology of autoimmune diseases such as Sjögren's syndrome include genetic, immunologic, hormonal, and probably infectious (? viral). The discovery of the immune response (IR) genes, which exist in linkage disequilibrium with other genes in the major histocompatibility complex, has helped distinguish primary from secondary Sjögren's syndrome. The former is associated with HLA B8 DR3, whereas the latter is associated with DR4 (when rheumatoid arthritis is the accompanying illness). The Ia cell surface antigens, the presumed products of the IR genes, mediate the lymphocyte-lymphocyte and lymphocyte-macrophage interactions necessary for proper immune regulation. Autoimmune diseases probably arise as a consequence of disordered immunologic regulation. Although just how immune regulation becomes disturbed is not yet known, it seems likely that internal factors (such as sex hormones and latent viruses) as well as external factors (drugs or infectious agents) play a role. For example, the predominant female incidence of Sjögren's syndrome may relate to an ability of androgen to suppress and estrogens to accelerate autoimmune disease, as in the NZB/NZW F_1 mouse model.

CLINICAL MANIFESTATIONS. The symptoms of Sjögren's syndrome may be subtle and brought out only by careful and persistent questioning.

Ophthalmologic (Keratoconjunctivitis Sicca). The patient may notice accumulation of thick ropy secretions along the inner canthus owing to a decreased tear film and an abnormal mucus component. Related complaints include erythema, photosensitivity, eye fatigue, decreased visual acuity, and the sensation of a "film" across the field of vision. Desiccation can cause small superficial erosions of the corneal epithelium. Slit lamp examination may reveal filamentary keratitis (filaments of corneal epithelium and debris) in severe cases. Conjunctivitis caused by *Staphylococcus aureus* is a complication.

Salivary. Complaints resulting from dryness of the mouth are varied. The "cracker sign" describes the difficulties encountered in trying to eat dry foods without sufficient lubrication. Many subjects require frequent ingestion of liquids. They may resort to carrying water bottles or candy in purse or pocket. Additional features include oral soreness, adherence of food to buccal surfaces, fissuring of the tongue, and dysphagia. Angular cheilitis resulting from superimposed candidiasis may occur. Patients may lose the ability to discriminate foods on the basis of taste and smell. Dental caries are accelerated. The parotid gland enlarges in many patients secondary to cellular infiltration and ductal obstruction. Usually asymptomatic and self-limited, the enlargement can be recurrent and associated with pain or erythema. Focal infiltrates of lymphocytes are also found in the minor salivary glands of the lower lip. When biopsied, these lesions provide histologic confirmation and quantification of the degree of infiltration.

Other Symptoms. Dryness may also involve the nasal mucosa, leading to recurrent epistaxis, and may extend throughout the upper respiratory tract, causing hoarseness, recurrent bronchitis, and pneumonitis. Eustachian tube blockage can result in conduction deafness and chronic otitis. Dysphagia may be ascribed to several causes: decreased saliva, infiltration of the glands of the esophageal mucosa, esophageal webbing, and abnormal motility. Other exocrine gland functions may be affected, leading to loss of pancreatic secretions, hypo- or achlorhydria, dermal dryness, and lack of vaginal secretions.

Extraglandular Involvement. Extraglandular involvement occurs more frequently in patients with primary than secondary Sjögren's syndrome. Dependent nonthrombocytopenic purpura is generally associated with hyperglobulinemia. Raynaud's phenomenon is present in 20 per cent of patients. A diffuse interstitial pneumonitis resulting from lymphocytic infiltration may cause dyspnea. Obstructive disease (in the absence of smoking) may result from lymphocytic infiltration surrounding small airways. The most common renal abnormalities involve the tubules, particularly overt or latent renal tubular acidosis and hyposthenuria. The presence of glomerulonephritis should suggest coexisting systemic lupus erythematosus, cryoglobulinemia, or immune complex deposition. Peripheral and cranial neuropathy has been associated with vasculitis involving the vasa nervorum.

Lymphoproliferation and Lymphoma. The incidence of lymphoma is increased 44-fold in Sjögren's syndrome. Pseudomalignant or malignant lymphoproliferation may be present initially or may develop later in the illness. Most lymphomas belong to the B cell lineage, although the histologic appearance is variable. Many cases previously described as histiocytic lymphoma represent B cell lymphomas and remain sufficiently differentiated to synthesize monoclonal immunoglobulins. Other monoclonal immunoglobulin B cell proliferations in Sjögren's syndrome patients include Waldenström's macroglobulinemia, light chain myeloma, and non-IgM monoclonal gammopathies (IgG κ and IgA λ). A diminution of a previously elevated Ig class may signify malignant transformation. Pseudolymphoma is an intermediate stage in this transition from benign to malignant lymphoproliferation.

Other clinical indications of an increased risk of malignancy include persistent or greatly increased parotid swelling, generalized lymphadenopathy, and splenomegaly. Serial measurement of serum β-2 microglobulin offers another clue as to the clinical subset or course. β-2 microglobulin is elevated in the saliva of Sjögren's syndrome patients and in the synovial fluid of patients with rheumatoid arthritis. Salivary levels correspond with the degree of lymphocytic infiltration, and serum levels may be elevated in patients with renal and lymphoproliferative complications.

DIAGNOSIS. ***Clinical.*** The presence of dry eyes is suggested by a positive Schirmer test (less than 5 mm of wetting per five minutes, unanesthetized), but the frequency of both false-negative and false-positive results is high. The pattern and intensity of staining with rose bengal dye and slit lamp examination are more reliable in diagnosis. The presence of filamentary keratitis and corneal ulcerations indicates advanced keratoconjunctivitis sicca.

Diminution in stimulated parotid flow rate (PFR) (<5 ml per gland in ten minutes) is a sensitive indicator of xerostomia. Salivary scintigraphy, which measures the uptake, concentration, and excretion of ^{99m}Tc-pertechnetate by the major salivary glands, is a sensitive index of glandular function. Scintigraphy is expensive, however, and offers no advantage in diagnostic sensitivity over minor salivary gland biopsy. Lip biopsy is a sensitive and specific diagnostic procedure, is well tolerated by the patient, and causes no disfigurement. Further, biopsy offers more information; in addition to confirming the diagnosis, it allows quantification of the degree of lymphocytic infiltration and tissue damage. Aggregates of lymphocytes within the acinar tissue are scored, each aggregate of 50 or more cells representing a focus. The number of foci within 4 sq mm of glandular tissue is determined and constitutes the focus score. A focus score of more than 1 is characteristic of Sjögren's syndrome and is seen in less than 1 per cent of both normal and autopsy controls. The diagnosis of Sjögren's syndrome is based upon the presence of two of the following three criteria: (1) focus score of more than 1 in the labial salivary gland biopsy, (2) keratoconjunctivitis sicca, and (3) an associated connective tissue or lymphoproliferative disorder.

Clinically, a "sicca-like" syndrome may be caused by a number of other disease processes, including hyperlipoproteinemias IV and V, hemochromatosis, sarcoidosis, and amyloidosis. Use of anticholinergic drugs as well as a number of other medications may be the single most frequent cause of xerostomia. Thus, it is essential to establish the presence of focal lymphoid infiltrates and autoimmunity in a patient suspected of having Sjögren's syndrome.

Laboratory. Autoantibodies are common in Sjögren's syndrome. Rheumatoid factor may be found in 75 to 90 per cent; antinuclear antibodies may be positive in 50 to 80 per cent. Multiple organ-specific antibodies are noted, including antibodies directed against gastric parietal, thyroid microsomal, thyroglobulin, mitochondrial, smooth muscle, and salivary duct antigens.

An autoantibody to a nucleoprotein antigen called SS-B (also termed La) occurs in approximately 50–70 per cent of patients with primary Sjögren's syndrome and to a lesser extent in Sjögren's syndrome accompanied by SLE. Antibodies to a related nucleoprotein SS-A (also termed Ro) are less specific for Sjögren's syndrome, also occur in SLE, and are associated with vasculitis. An antibody (RAP) to an EB virus-related nuclear antigen (RANA) occurs in secondary Sjögren's syndrome with RA.

Antibodies to SS-A are less specifically associated with any one disease. A recent report identifies antibodies to SS-A in as few as 13 per cent of Sjögren's syndrome patients and as many as 46 per cent of systemic lupus erythematosus patients without Sjögren's syndrome.

Persons with Sjögren's syndrome manifest B cell hyperactivity. Evidence for this includes the polyclonal hyperglobulinemia seen in over 50 per cent of patients and the presence of numerous autoantibodies and circulating immune complexes. The lymphoid infiltrates in the salivary glands synthesize immunoglobulins locally. Serum hyperviscosity may result from either macroglobulinemia or polymerizing IgG with rheumatoid factor activity which forms intermediate complexes. Cryoglobulinemia may be present, as well as vasculitis and glomerulonephritis. A high proportion of patients with Sjögren's syndrome have circulating immune complexes as measured by C1q binding and Raji cell assays. Serum levels of complement are only infrequently low.

Peripheral blood T lymphocytes are decreased in about one third of patients. Immunoglobulin-positive lymphocytes in peripheral blood may be increased slightly. Abnormalities in T cell function may be present, particularly in patients with lymphoproliferative or other systemic features. These patients tend to have alterations in T cell subsets and decreased autologous mixed lymphocyte responses. Natural killer (NK) cell activity is also diminished as a consequence of immunoregulatory abnormalities rather than intrinsic deficits.

There is also a defect in reticuloendothelial clearance in patients with Sjögren's syndrome. In 12 of 19 patients, labeled IgG sensitized autologous red cells, which are usually cleared rapidly by splenic macrophages via surface membrane Fc receptor binding, persisted in the circulation for an abnormally long period. Eleven of the 12 patients had either extraglandular manifestations of Sjögren's syndrome or secondary Sjögren's syndrome.

TREATMENT. Treatment of Sjögren's syndrome is aimed at symptomatic relief and limiting the damaging local effects of chronic xerophthalmia and xerostomia. Ocular dryness responds to the use of artificial tears containing methylcellulose. Since staphylococcal blepharitis occurs in two thirds of patients, the lids should be cultured and infection eradicated. Soft contact lenses may be used to protect the cornea; this is controversial. Moisture may be maintained with frequent use of saline drops. Saran wrap occlusion or diving goggles may be worn at night in an attempt to prevent tear evaporation. Topical steroid use should be avoided unless specifically indicated, because corneal thinning and subsequent perforation may occur. The use of diuretics, many antihypertensive drugs, and antidepressants may further diminish lacrimal and salivary gland function. Xerostomia may respond to an increased fluid intake, use of a 2 per cent solution of methylcellulose, and sour sugar-free candies given as sialagogues. Scrupulous care of teeth is imperative; patients should avoid a high sucrose intake or the frequent use of sugar-containing candies to decrease oral dryness. Vigorous dental plaque control and topical application of fluoride should be used regularly. Oral candidiasis may be treated with mycostatin tablets for a prolonged course, with separate treatment of dentures. Vaginal dryness can be treated with propionic acid gels.

Only those patients with severe functional disability or life-threatening complications warrant corticosteroid or immunosuppressive therapy. Prednisone may suppress parotid swelling and improve the restrictive component of pulmonary disease. Immunosuppressive agents have decreased extraglandular lymphoid infiltrates and improved exocrine gland function in some individuals. Their use has been restricted to those patients with severe renal and pulmonary manifestations.

Strand V, Talal N: Advances in the diagnosis and concept of Sjögren's syndrome (autoimmune exocrinopathy). Bull Rheum Dis 30:1046, 1980. *This is an up-to-date and comprehensive review of clinical, laboratory, and pathogenetic features of Sjögren's syndrome.*

Talal N: Sjögren's syndrome and connective tissue disease with other immunologic disorders. *In* McCarty D (ed.): Arthritis and Allied Conditions. 10th ed. Philadelphia, Lea & Febiger, in press.

450. THE VASCULITIC SYNDROMES

Anthony S. Fauci

Vasculitis is a clinicopathologic process characterized by an inflammatory response within the blood vessel itself. Associated with this inflammation is a compromise of the vessel lumen with resulting ischemic changes in the tissues supplied by the vessel. Any size, location, and type of blood vessel may be involved, including large muscular arteries, medium-sized and small arteries, arterioles, capillaries, postcapillary venules, and veins. This heterogeneous category of diseases comprises unique syndromes as well as diseases with overlapping clinical and pathologic features. The vasculitis may be the primary process, or it may be a component of another underlying disease. Furthermore, vasculitis varies considerably in its clinicopathologic manifestations. Certain of the vasculitic disorders are rarely life threatening, e.g., the hypersensitivity vasculitic syndromes in which cutaneous involvement usually predominates. Other vasculitic syndromes may be fulminant and, if untreated, rapidly fatal diseases, e.g., Wegener's granulomatosis and polyarteritis nodosa.

The vasculitic syndromes are generally thought to result from immunopathogenic mechanisms; however, the evidence for this varies among the different syndromes. Among these mechanisms, the deposition of circulating immune complexes with subsequent vessel damage has emerged as the major immunopathologic event associated with most of the vasculitic syndromes. However, many individual patients with active vasculitis have not shown circulating or deposited immune complexes. This result could reflect an insensitivity of techniques in detecting certain types of immune complexes. In addition, complexes could be cleared at such a rapid rate as to preclude their detection. On the other hand, the presence of circulating immune complexes does not prove that the associated vasculitis is caused by them, since many nonvasculitic diseases are also associated with circulating immune complexes, and complexes per se need not result in vasculitis, even in diseases in which vasculitis is present.

In only a few diseases has the actual antigen involved in the immune complex been identified. The most noted of these is the hepatitis B surface antigen that has been demonstrated in the circulating immune complexes, cryoprecipitable serum components, and involved tissues of certain patients with hepatitis B antigenemia–associated vasculitis.

The mechanism of tissue damage from immune complexes is thought to be similar to serum sickness. In this model, soluble immune complexes are formed in antigen excess and deposited in blood vessel walls in areas of increased vascular permeability. The increased permeability is attributed to release of vasoactive amines from platelets or mast cells under the influence of specific IgE. Following deposition of complexes, various components of complement are activated, particularly C5a, which is strongly chemotactic for neutrophils. The neutrophils infiltrate the vessel wall at the site of immune complex deposition and release intracytoplasmic enzymes such as collagenase and elastase that directly damage the vessel wall. Compromise of the lumen occurs with resulting ischemic changes.

Certain of the vasculitides are characterized by granulomatous inflammation in and around the blood vessels. Although granulomatous responses are generally of the delayed hypersensitivity type, immune complexes themselves can trigger granuloma formation and thereby produce granulomatous vasculitis.

Why certain persons develop vasculitis and others do not is an extraordinarily complex issue and likely involves a number of host factors such as genetic predisposition, immunoregulatory mechanisms, and the integrity of the reticuloendothelial system, which clears the complexes from the circulation. In addition, the reasons why certain complexes cause vasculitis and why certain types of vessels and not others are involved probably relate to the size and physicochemical properties of the immune complex and to other physical factors such as turbulence of blood flow, hydrostatic pressure within vessels, and previously damaged vessel endothelium.

CLASSIFICATION OF THE VASCULITIC SYNDROMES

The remarkable heterogeneity and the obvious overlap among the vasculitic syndromes have led to difficulties in classification of this group of diseases. The first complete report of a vasculitic syndrome was in 1866 by Kussmaul and Maier who elegantly described the clinicopathologic features in a patient with what is now recognized as classic polyarteritis nodosa. Following this publication polyarteritis nodosa was the reference for all subsequently described vasculitides. It soon became evident that there were numerous vasculitis syndromes with diverse clinical and pathologic manifestations, but diagnostic criteria were controversial. More precise and accurate classification schemes now have emerged, based upon reexamination of clinical, pathologic, and immunologic features, as well as responses to certain therapeutic regimens. Table 450–1 illustrates one such classification scheme.

The first major group is the systemic necrotizing vasculitides. Within this group falls classic polyarteritis nodosa. This syndrome is described in detail in Ch. 451. It is the prototype of serious systemic necrotizing vasculitis and manifests certain features such as small and medium-sized muscular artery involvement, hypertension, visceral vessel involvement, and a noticeable lack of lung involvement. In the classic syndrome, eosinophilia, granulomatous reactions, and an allergic diathesis are not characteristic. Soon after the original description physicians recognized a systemic vasculitis which resembled classic polyarteritis nodosa except that lung involvement was a prominent feature. These patients generally manifested eosinophilia, granulomatous reactions, and a strong allergic diathesis, usually severe asthma. Most of these patients had what is now referred to as the allergic angiitis and granulomatosis of Churg-Strauss. This disease is quite similar to classic polyarteritis nodosa except for the divergent features mentioned above. Many systemic necrotizing vasculitides manifest clinicopathologic characteristics which overlap these two syndromes as well as the hypersensitivity group of vasculitis (discussed below). This subgroup has been referred to as the "polyangiitis overlap syndrome" of systemic necrotizing vasculitis, and is probably more common than either classic polyarteritis nodosa or Churg-Strauss disease.

In addition to the polyarteritis nodosa group of systemic necrotizing vasculitides, certain other vasculitides are systemic and involve multiple organ systems. However, they are referred to by different names, since they possess characteristic clinical and/or pathologic features. This is true of diseases such as Wegener's granulomatosis (see Ch. 452) and the giant cell arteritides. In the latter group, the two major subcategories—i.e., cranial or temporal arteritis (see Ch. 453) and Takayasu's

TABLE 450–1. THE CLINICAL SPECTRUM OF VASCULITIS

1. Systemic necrotizing vasculitis (polyarteritis nodosa group)
   - Classic polyarteritis nodosa
   - Allergic angiitis and granulomatosis (Churg-Strauss disease)
   - Polyangiitis overlap syndrome
2. Hypersensitivity vasculitis
   - Henoch-Schönlein purpura
   - Serum sickness and serum sickness–like reactions
   - Other drug-related vasculitides
   - Vasculitis associated with infectious diseases
   - Vasculitis associated with neoplasms (most lymphoid)
   - Vasculitis associated with connective tissue diseases
   - Vasculitis associated with other underlying diseases
   - Congenital deficiencies of the complement system
   - Erythema elevatum diutinum
3. Wegener's granulomatosis
4. Giant cell arteritides
   - Cranial or temporal arteritis
   - Takayasu's arteritis
5. Other vasculitic syndromes
   - Mucocutaneous lymph node syndrome (Kawasaki's disease)
   - Behçet's disease
   - Vasculitis isolated to the central nervous system
   - Thromboangiitis obliterans (Buerger's disease)
   - Miscellaneous vasculitides

arteritis (see Ch. 53) are systemic diseases involving large muscular arteries with mononuclear cell and often giant cell infiltration within the walls of the involved arteries. Despite the predisposition for certain vessels in these diseases (temporal artery in cranial arteritis and subclavian artery in Takayasu's arteritis), these are systemic diseases which involve multiple arteries. Lymphomatoid granulomatosis (see Ch. 452) is generally considered in the differential diagnosis of systemic necrotizing vasculitis with lung involvement such as Wegener's granulomatosis. However, it is not strictly speaking an inflammatory response in vessels, but an infiltration of blood vessel walls with atypical and often neoplastic appearing lymphoid cells.

The hypersensitivity vasculitides include a broad and heterogeneous group of disorders which have often caused confusion in categorization. These are discussed in detail in this chapter.

Other vasculitic syndromes can be considered under the category of "miscellaneous" for want of a better term. These include Behçet's disease, the major pathologic feature of which is a true vasculitis (see Ch. 464), and thromboangiitis obliterans, which is an inflammatory and occlusive disease of arteries and veins, although its true vasculitic character has been questioned. In addition to the granulomatous vasculitis of the central nervous system, which is seen in association with certain lymphoproliferative malignancies, there is also an uncommon syndrome of isolated vasculitis of the central nervous system that occurs in the apparent absence of systemic vasculitis or other systemic disease.

Finally, the coronary arteritis and myocardial disease of the mucocutaneous lymph node syndrome (Kawasaki's disease) will be discussed below.

HYPERSENSITIVITY VASCULITIS

Hypersensitivity vasculitis is a term applied to a heterogeneous group of disorders that are thought to represent a hypersensitivity reaction to an identifiable antigenic stimulus such as a drug or an infectious agent; hence the word "hypersensitivity." This immediately becomes a source of confusion, since many, or even all, of the vasculitic syndromes represent hypersensitivity reactions of one form or another. Although the antigenic stimuli associated with this group are heterogeneous, these disorders generally share the characteristic of involvement of small vessels. They can be subdivided into two basic groups. The vast majority of the patients manifest involvement of the postcapillary venules, and hence have a venulitis. A smaller group of patients falls into the second category, in which arterioles are predominantly involved (arteriolitis). Most importantly, there is a predominant and often exclusive involvement of the vessels of the skin. Confusion in the literature generally resulted from grouping this category of vasculitis with the more serious systemic varieties such as classic polyarteritis nodosa and related diseases. It is true that the hypersensitivity vasculitides may have variable degrees of organ system involvement other than of the skin. However, this is usually less severe than that of typical systemic vasculitis of polyarteritis nodosa and Wegener's granulomatosis. Most frequently, the skin is exclusively involved or, if other organ systems are involved, the cutaneous disease still dominates the clinical picture.

ETIOLOGY. As indicated by the terminology, the etiology is usually a recognizable antigenic stimulus such as a drug, microbe, toxin, or foreign or endogenous protein. From an etiologic standpoint the hypersensitivity vasculitides segregate into two distinct groups, depending on the source of the sensitizing antigen. In the classic original group, the antigen is foreign to the host. In the second group the antigen is endogenous. For example, certain connective tissue diseases may manifest a typical hypersensitivity small vessel vasculitis. These diseases are generally characterized by circulating immune complexes in which one of the components is an endogenous protein to which antibody is directed. This is true of patients with systemic lupus erythematosus who develop immune complexes composed of endogenous DNA and anti-DNA antibodies; in addition, patients with rheumatoid arthritis may develop immune complexes of rheumatoid factor with antibody activity against endogenous immunoglobulin. Thus, in most of the hypersensitivity vasculitides, the identity of the etiologic agent which triggers the formation of immune complexes is at least strongly suspected.

INCIDENCE AND PREVALENCE. It is difficult to determine an accurate incidence for the hypersensitivity group of vasculitides owing to the marked heterogeneity among these diverse syndromes. However, the hypersensitivity group of vasculitides is much more common than the group of systemic necrotizing vasculitides and other syndromes such as Wegener's granulomatosis and Takayasu's arteritis. The disease can be seen at any age and in both sexes; however, this varies considerably with the particular subgroup in question.

PATHOLOGY AND PATHOGENESIS. The histopathologic hallmark of the hypersensitivity vasculitides is a leukocytoclastic venulitis. The term leukocytoclasis refers to nuclear debris derived from the neutrophils that have infiltrated in and around the involved vessels. In skin biopsies, this type of involvement is most common in the postcapillary venules just beneath the epidermis. When biopsies are obtained in the acute phase of active disease, the typical pattern of neutrophil infiltration is readily observed. In the subacute or chronic stages, biopsies often reveal mononuclear cell infiltration. In certain of the subgroups, eosinophilic infiltration predominates. In the second and smaller category of hypersensitivity vasculitis, arterioles and capillaries are predominantly involved. In the typical case of hypersensitivity vasculitis with a predominance of cutaneous involvement, the lesions are usually found in the lower extremities or in the dependent areas such as the sacrum in supine patients. This is most likely due to the increase in hydrostatic pressure within the postcapillary venules in these areas.

Although immune complex deposition is widely considered to be the pathogenic mechanism of this group of vasculitis, not every case of hypersensitivity vasculitis has had immune complexes demonstrated, even when, carefully sought, as mentioned above.

CLINICAL MANIFESTATIONS. Just as this broad group is etiologically heterogeneous, so too are the clinical manifestations. However, the hallmark of the group is the predominance of cutaneous involvement. The skin lesions may appear as the classic palpable purpura which results from the extravasation of erythrocytes into the tissue surrounding the involved venules. In addition, one may see macules, papules, vesicles, bullae, subcutaneous nodules, ulcers, and even recurrent or chronic urticaria.

Even though skin lesions generally dominate, various organ system involvements can be seen. Certain constellations of clinicopathologic findings define relatively distinct syndromes. For example, in *Henoch-Schönlein purpura* the typical syndrome consists of palpable purpura (usually over the buttocks), arthralgias, gastrointestinal symptoms, and glomerulonephritis. Henoch-Schönlein purpura is usually seen in children; however, adults of any age may be affected. The disease usually remits spontaneously after one week. However, the disease is remarkable for its tendency to recur a number of times over weeks to months before remission is complete. The characteristic skin lesions are present in virtually all patients. The majority of patients also have arthralgias involving multiple joints, but frank arthritis is rare. The gastrointestinal involvement is usually manifested as colicky abdominal pain which may mimic an acute surgical abdomen. Patients may experience nausea, vomiting, diarrhea, constipation, and occasionally the passage of blood and mucus per rectum. In the more severe and rare case, bowel intussusception may occur. Renal disease is a glomerulitis (see Ch. 80), which is usually expressed as a microscopic hematuria without significant renal functional impairment. However, in rare cases renal failure can occur. Most frequently, patients recover spontaneously and completely.

Other groups within the hypersensitivity category include *serum sickness and serum sickness–like reactions*. The classic manifestations are fever, urticaria, arthralgias, and lymphadenopathy occurring seven to ten days after primary exposure to the antigen in question, which for serum sickness is usually a heterologous serum protein and for serum sickness–like reactions is usually a drug such as penicillin. Most of the manifestations of this disorder are not due to a vasculitis. However, in rare cases cutaneous vasculitis typical of the hypersensitivity group is documented. In addition, patients may rarely progress to a typical systemic necrotizing vasculitis involving multiple organ systems.

A number of disorders have vasculitis as a manifestation of an underlying primary disease. Included in these diseases are *systemic lupus erythematosus*, *rheumatoid arthritis*, *mixed cryoglobulinemia*, and *other connective tissue diseases*. In these disorders, the manifestations of the underlying disease usually predominate. When vasculitis is observed, it is generally of the small vessel cutaneous type, which is virtually indistinguishable from the vasculitis seen in the hypersensitivity group with recognized exogenous antigens. However, patients with these disorders, particularly systemic lupus erythematosus and rheumatoid arthritis, may also develop a systemic necrotizing vasculitis which closely resembles the polyarteritis nodosa group in manifestations and severity. Nevertheless, in the typical case, the cutaneous vasculitis usually dominates the clinical picture with respect to the vasculitic process.

Other diseases which may fall into this category of small vessel hypersensitivity vasculitis are the *vasculitis associated with congenital deficiencies of various complement components* such as C1r, C1s, and C2; *erythema elevatum diutinum*; *hypocomplementemic vasculitis*; the *vasculitis associated with certain neoplasms, particularly of the lymphoid type*; and the *vasculitis associated with other primary disorders such as ulcerative colitis, Crohn's disease, biliary cirrhosis, and retroperitoneal fibrosis*.

DIAGNOSIS. The diagnosis of hypersensitivity vasculitis rests on the demonstration of vasculitis on biopsy. Since the predominant organ involved is the skin, histopathologic material is usually readily available. Since cutaneous involvement is often present in severe systemic vasculitides, one should undertake a systematic workup of other organ systems in patients who present with apparently isolated cutaneous vasculitis.

TREATMENT AND PROGNOSIS. Therapy of the hypersensitivity group of vasculitides has in general been unsatisfactory. Since most cases resolve spontaneously, the lack of response to therapeutic regimens is of less importance. However, in those patients who go on to develop persistent cutaneous disease or serious organ system involvement, several regimens have been tried with variable results. In cases in which a recognized antigenic stimulus is present, the first order of therapy is to remove the antigen; e.g., to remove sensitizing drugs or responsible organisms by appropriate antibiotic therapy when possible. In situations in which disease appears to be self-limited, no specific therapy is indicated. However, when disease persists or results in organ system dysfunction, a glucocorticosteroid is the drug of choice. Prednisone is usually administered in doses of 1 mg per kilogram per day with rapid tapering when possible, in some instances directly to discontinuation or initially to an alternate-day regimen followed by ultimate discontinuation (see Ch. 29). In cases which prove refractory to corticosteroid therapy, cytotoxic agents such as cyclophosphamide have been used, as has plasmapheresis with or without cytotoxic drugs. The efficacy of these regimens has not yet been fully evaluated in hypersensitivity vasculitis. Thus, one should be reluctant to institute cytotoxic agents in persons with disease limited to the skin, particularly since the response of the cutaneous variety of hypersensitivity vasculitis to cytotoxic agents has not been as dramatic as the response of the systemic vasculitides such as Wegener's granulomatosis (see Ch. 452) and the polyarteritis nodosa group.

The prognosis of most of the diseases in this category is generally excellent, with spontaneous and complete remissions in most patients. However, certain patients may develop persistent and debilitating cutaneous disease, and others may evolve a typical systemic vasculitis with a serious prognosis.

MUCOCUTANEOUS LYMPH NODE SYNDROME
(Kawasaki's Disease)

The mucocutaneous lymph node syndrome is an acute febrile illness of infants and young children.

Patients manifest characteristic changes in the skin and mucous membranes with nonsuppurative lymphadenopathy. This disease is also discussed in Ch. 557. Although the course is generally benign and self-limited, a small percentage of patients (approximately 1 to 2 per cent) develop fatal complications. These complications almost invariably result from a vasculitic involvement of the coronary arteries. In fact, it is now generally agreed that many cases of "polyarteritis nodosa in children" were in fact the arteritic complications of unrecognized mucocutaneous lymph node syndrome.

The disease has occurred in almost epidemic proportions in Japan. Although the etiology is unknown, an infective agent is suspected. Clusters of cases have appeared throughout the United States.

Most fatalities occur as sudden deaths in infants and children in the convalescent stage of the disease (usually between the third and fourth week of illness). In virtually all autopsied cases, the coronary arteries manifested arteritis. Typically, bead-like aneurysms with thrombosis are noted along the main trunk and branches of the coronary artery. There is a typical vasculitic picture with intimal proliferation and infiltration of the vessel wall with mononuclear cells. Other manifestations include myocarditis, pericarditis, myocardial infarctions, and cardiomegaly.

One of the difficult questions is the extent to which one should examine a child with the syndrome for cardiac involvement. Since the coronary arteritis occurs in such a small percentage of patients, invasive cardiovascular procedures do not seem warranted. Noninvasive procedures such as echocardiograms and scanning techniques are currently being employed to detect incipient cardiac involvement.

The prognosis of Kawasaki's disease on the whole is excellent, and the vast majority of patients recover uneventfully. However, the consequences for those who develop coronary arteritis are often devastating, with sudden death the rule. Preliminary studies indicate that treatment with aspirin (30 mg per kilogram per day) has resulted in a lessening of the incidence of cardiac complications. There is some unconfirmed evidence that corticosteroids are not effective and may increase the incidence of cardiac complications. At present, it is recommended that children be treated with aspirin during the acute and convalescent phases of the disease.

Alarcon-Segovia D: The necrotizing vasculitides. Med Clin North Am 61:240, 1977. *A brief though rather complete coverage of a classification scheme of the necrotizing vasculitides. One of the latest well-organized attempts to categorize these syndromes appropriately.*

Christian CL, Sergent JS: Vasculitic syndromes: Clinical and experimental models. Am J Med 61:385, 1976. *Excellent review of the vasculitis syndromes with emphasis on the pathophysiologic mechanisms in several of the human diseases as well as in animal models of vasculitis.*

Cupps TR, Fauci AS: The Vasculitides. Philadelphia, W. B. Saunders Company, 1981, pp 1–211. *Comprehensive treatise on the entire spectrum of the vasculitic syndromes. Pathogenesis, clinicopathologic manifestations, and updated therapeutic approaches are discussed in detail.*

Fauci AS, Haynes BF, Katz P: The spectrum of vasculitis. Clinical, pathologic, immunologic, and therapeutic considerations. Ann Intern Med 89:660, 1978. *Review article which introduced an updated classification scheme of the vasculitis syndromes and which has employed this scheme to develop guidelines for an approach to a patient with vasculitis.*

Fauci AS: Systemic vasculitis. In: Current Therapy in Allergy and Immunology

1983–1984. Lichtenstein LM, Fauci AS (Editors), Philadelphia, B. C. Decker, Inc, 1983, pp 130–136. Detailed description of the various therapeutic modalities currently employed for the spectrum of systemic vasculitis with a practical guide for the use of these regimens.
Zeek PM: Periarteritis nodosa and other forms of necrotizing angiitis. N Engl J Med 18:764, 1953. *Classic article which represents the first well-organized approach to the rational classification of the vasculitic syndromes. It is still employed as the backbone of most classification schemes.*

451. POLYARTERITIS NODOSA GROUP

K. Frank Austen

DEFINITION. Kussmaul and Maier introduced the term periarteritis nodosa in 1866 to designate a morbid process manifested by numerous grossly visible or palpable nodules along the course of medium-sized muscular arteries. The lesions are segmental in distribution, have a predilection for the crotch of bifurcations and branchings, and involve all but the pulmonary arteries. The clinical manifestations are disparate and polymorphic, and result from partial or complete arterial occlusion, hemorrhage, and glomerulitis. In view of the necrotizing nature of the process, involving the entire arterial wall, Ferrari in 1903 suggested the alternative name of polyarteritis acuta nodosa; this entity is now termed *classic polyarteritis nodosa* to distinguish it from other entities falling within the polyarteritis nodosa group or syndrome (Table 450–1).

Pulmonary lesions, parenchymal and pulmonary arterial, are absent in classic polyarteritis but almost always precede the onset of polyarteritic lesions in other organs in the entity termed *allergic angiitis and granulomatosis* by Churg and Strauss. Such patients typically present with bronchitis, bronchial asthma, or pulmonary infiltration. The polyarteritic process in other organs is indistinguishable from that of classic polyarteritis nodosa, and thus Rose and Spencer have preferred the term *polyarteritis with pulmonary involvement* for this entity.

A polyarteritic process associated with hepatitis B antigenemia and extending from the medium-sized muscular arteries to arterioles and venules was recognized in 1970 by Gocke and colleagues and is now termed *polyangiitis* or *generalized necrotizing angiitis* to emphasize that the presentation of this polyarteritic process may include venulitis manifested in skin as palpable purpura or urticaria. Serous otitis media and amphetamine abuse are major associated events in the hepatitis B negative group with generalized necrotizing angiitis. On clinical grounds no criteria have been identified to distinguish between the hepatitis B positive and negative patients except that all positive hepatitis B antigenemia patients had abnormal liver chemistries. These were, however, occasionally minimal and then not different from those of the hepatitis B negative group.

Polyarteritis nodosa of childhood has a predilection for the coronary arteries and represents a fourth subgroup of the polyarteritis group or syndrome. In view of the recent evidence that approximately 1 to 2 per cent of children with the mucocutaneous lymph node syndrome (Kawasaki's disease) develop coronary arteritis, it may be that Kawasaki's disease or similar entities are the source of polyarteritis of childhood.

The incidence, age distribution, and male-to-female ratio of polyarteritis nodosa are difficult to determine because a diagnostic serologic procedure is lacking, and the spotty distribution of lesions makes biopsy uncertain. Nonetheless, the condition occurs from infancy to old age, with a peak incidence in the fifth and sixth decades of life, and the male to female ratio has been estimated at from 2 to 3:1.

PATHOLOGY. The lesions of polyarteritis involve arteries of medium and small caliber, especially at bifurcations and branchings. The segmental process involves the media, with edema, fibrinous exudation, fibrinoid necrosis, and infiltration of polymorphonuclear neutrophils and varying numbers of eosinophils, and extends to the adventitia and intima. Thrombosis and infarction or hemorrhage occur at this stage. Subsequently, the regions of fibrinoid necrosis are replaced by cellular granulation tissue, and the intima proliferates. Finally the involved segment is replaced by scar tissue with associated intimal thickening and periarterial fibrosis. These changes produce partial occlusion, thrombosis and infarction, and palpable or visible aneurysms with occasional rupture.

The glomerulitis is characterized by capillary microthrombi, focal fibrinoid necrosis, polymorphonuclear neutrophil infiltration, and capsular proliferation. With progression, the necrotizing feature of the glomerulitis is less apparent, and the process is difficult to distinguish from glomerulonephritis of other causes.

In allergic angiitis and granulomatosis and in polyangiitis, the acute fibrinoid necrosis with cellular infiltration involves arterioles and venules as well as medium-sized muscular arteries, whereas in classic polyarteritis such vessels are spared except in areas contiguous to involved medium-sized muscular arteries. It is characteristic of the polyarteritis nodosa group for the vascular lesions to be in different stages of evolution, i.e., acute, subacute, and healed. In allergic angiitis and granulomatosis the pulmonary granulomatous lesions in vascular and extravascular sites are accompanied by an intense eosinophilic infiltration. The granulomas often include an eosinophilic core of altered collagen and necrotic eosinophils surrounded by radially arranged macrophages, lymphocytes, plasma cells, and varying numbers of polymorphonuclear leukocytes, both neutrophilic and eosinophilic.

In patients with polyangiitis associated with hepatitis B antigenemia, the specific antigen has been recognized in immune complexes present in the circulation and deposited in affected vessels along with complement proteins. It is presumed that this pathogenetic mechanism prevails in the entire polyarteritis nodosa group, but the basis for arterial deposition is unknown. The deposition of immune complexes in venules and glomeruli is attributed to changes in permeability and to physical trapping.

CLINICAL MANIFESTATIONS AND DIAGNOSIS. The widespread distribution of the arterial lesions produces diverse clinical manifestations, which reflect the particular organ systems in which the arterial supply has been impaired. Among the early general symptoms and signs of polyarteritis nodosa are tachycardia, fever, weight loss, and pain in viscera and/or the musculoskeletal system so that the differential diagnosis is of fever of unknown origin. Striking and specific presenting signs may relate to abdominal pain, acute glomerulitis, polyneuritis, or myocardial infarction. Pulmonary manifestations, especially intractable bronchial asthma, would indicate allergic angiitis and granulomatosis rather than classic polyarteritis nodosa.

Renal. Renal involvement in two forms, renal polyarteritis and a glomerulitis, may occur separately or together. Renal polyarteritis is the most common lesion at postmortem examination (Table 451–1). Manifestations of the renal involvement include intermittent proteinuria and microscopic hematuria with occasional hyaline and granular casts. The glomerulitis is manifested by marked microscopic and even macroscopic hematuria, proteinuria, cellular casts, and progressive renal failure; survival of the acute phase is followed by progressive hypertension. Hypertension reflects healing renal polyarteritis, progressive glomerulitis, or both. Renal involvement is the cause of death in about two thirds of patients with classic polyarteritis nodosa and about one third of those with allergic angiitis and granulomatosis.

Gastrointestinal. Arterial lesions are commonly found in one or more abdominal viscera. The principal manifestation is pain, especially in the umbilical region or right upper quadrant; anorexia, nausea, and vomiting are less prominent. Impaired arterial supply to the bowel can produce mucosal ulcerations, perforation, or infarction with melena or bloody diarrhea. Involvement of appendix, gallbladder, or pancreas can stimulate appendicitis, cholecystitis, or hemorrhagic pancreatitis. Liver involvement can range from hepatomegaly with or without jaundice to the signs of extensive hepatic necrosis. Sple-

TABLE 451–1. INCIDENCE OF NECROTIZING ANGIITIS IN VARIOUS ORGANS AT NECROPSY*

	Polyarteritis Nodosa (Classic) (Per Cent)	Allergic Angiitis and Granulomatosis ("Polyarteritis with Pulmonary Involvement") (Per Cent)
Lungs (pulmonary arteries)	0	47
Heart	35	60
Kidneys: Glomerulitis	30	57
Renal polyarteritis	65	60
Stomach and intestines	30	40
Liver	54	37
Pancreas	39	17
Spleen	35	43
Brain	4	3
Periadrenal connective tissue	41	40
Voluntary muscle	20	33

*Reproduced in modified form from Rose GA, Spencer H: Quart J Med 26:43, 1957. There were 54 cases in the periarteritis group and 30 with the diagnosis of allergic angiitis and granulomatosis.

nomegaly is uncommon. There has been no consistent relationship between the development of necrotizing angiitis and the appearance of liver disease in patients with hepatitis B antigenemia. Some of the observed combinations include necrotizing angiitis as the initial clinical finding, superimposed upon chronic active hepatitis, or appearing simultaneously with an acute hepatitis. Death in this group can occur from liver failure but is more commonly due to the generalized necrotizing angiitis.

Central and Peripheral Nervous System. Neurologic manifestations are generally late occurrences in the course of polyarteritis nodosa, and their particular presentation reflects the specific brain area compromised. Headache, convulsive seizures, papillitis, and retinal hemorrhages and exudates occur with or without localizing signs referable to the cerebrum, cerebellum, or brainstem; meningeal irritation may occur as a result of subarachnoid hemorrhage. Multiple mononeuropathy, i.e., involvement of several or even many individual nerves at the same or different times, is a common finding and is attributed to arteritis of the vasa nervorum. The peripheral neuropathy is usually asymmetrical with both sensory and motor distribution. The former can be extremely painful, but the latter, with attendant muscular degeneration, has on occasion been so severe as to dominate the clinical presentation.

Articular and Muscular. Arthralgia and myalgia are frequent in polyarteritis nodosa. Arthralgia is migratory, generally without swelling, and apparently due to small localized arterial lesions rather than extensive synovitis. The interpretation of those rare instances of synovitis with deformity and arterial changes of periarteritis nodosa is difficult, but it seems preferable to consider such cases as rheumatoid arthritis. Muscle pain or weakness reflects either direct involvement of the arterial supply or a peripheral neuropathy from involvement of the vasa nervorum.

Cardiac. Polyarteritis of the coronary arteries and their branches has a frequency approaching that of renal polyarteritis, and heart failure is responsible for or contributes to death in one sixth to one half of the cases. An infantile form of polyarteritis nodosa, affecting children mainly under ten months of age, is manifested primarily by involvement of the coronary arteries. The clinical manifestations of cardiac involvement are those of partial or complete arterial occlusion as modified by the superimposition of renal hypertension and an appreciable incidence of acute pericarditis without effusion. Whereas the combination of infarction and hypertension commonly leads to left-sided failure, an occasional patient with allergic angiitis and granulomatosis will present with predominantly right-sided decompensation.

Genitourinary. Involvement of the ovaries, testes, and epididymis is frequent, though usually asymptomatic. Mucosal ulceration in the bladder can occasionally precipitate gross hematuria with dysuria.

Cutaneous. Cutaneous involvement of some form is believed to occur in over 25 per cent of those affected with polyarteritis nodosa. The acute cutaneous manifestations include polymorphic exanthemata—purpuric, urticarial, and multiform in character—and severe subcutaneous hemorrhage, resulting from necrotizing arteritis, with secondary gangrene. Ulcerations and a persistent livedo reticularis are associated with the more chronic stage of the disease. A most characteristic but uncommon finding is cutaneous and subcutaneous nodules; these occur at any time in the disease course. The nodules tend to group, appear in crops, are usually movable, may regress in days or persist for months, range in size from a pea to a walnut, and may cause the overlying skin to become reddened or to ulcerate.

Pulmonary. Although the bronchial arteries can be involved in classic polyarteritis, only allergic angiitis and granulomatosis which involves the pulmonary arteries and parenchyma with granulomatous lesions gives rise to clinical manifestations. Asthma, when present, is intractable and associated with a marked peripheral eosinophilia. Pneumonic episodes are transient or progressive and may be accompanied by hemoptysis and/or pleuritic pain. Respiratory involvement accounts for about one half of the mortality, with the remainder being due to the polyarteritic process in other organs.

COURSE UNTREATED. The course of polyarteritis nodosa is progressive with destruction of vital organs. Intermittent acute episodes resulting from thrombosis of vital or nonvital structures are prominent. Death is most frequently attributed to renal involvement in cases of classic periarteritis nodosa and to pulmonary lesions in those cases classified as allergic angiitis with granulomatosis. Cardiac failure caused by a combination of infarction and renal hypertension is an additional frequent cause of death in both groups, and acute vascular accidents in the gastrointestinal tract or central nervous system account for much of the remaining mortality. In the retrospective postmortem study of Rose and Spencer, the five-year survival rate was about 10 per cent in classic periarteritis nodosa, and about 25 per cent in allergic angiitis and granulomatosis if onset was dated from the start of respiratory symptoms. The more recent report of the British Medical Research Council in 1960 placed the 54 months' survival rate in polyarteritis nodosa at nearly 50 per cent. Rare patients with polyarteritis limited to nonvital sites have been reported to experience an unusually long course or even a lasting remission.

LABORATORY FINDINGS. Leukocytosis, predominantly polymorphonuclear, is apparent in over 75 per cent of the cases of polyarteritis nodosa or allergic angiitis and granulomatosis, eosinophilia often being marked in the latter group. The association of hepatitis B antigenemia with generalized necrotizing angiitis may be as high as one third of the cases, but probably this figure will prove to be smaller as experience widens. Hypocomplementemia, which has not been observed in classic periarteritis nodosa, has been present in patients with generalized necrotizing angiitis with or without hepatitis B antigenemia. The erythrocyte sedimentation rate is customarily elevated with or without some increase of the globulins. Abnormalities in the urine sediment, especially hematuria and proteinuria, reflect renal involvement. Abnormalities of the electrocardiogram and electroencephalogram are those expected on the basis of arterial occlusive disease or those secondary to the metabolic disturbances of uremia. Lesions apparent on chest roentgenograms are the rule in patients with allergic angiitis and granulomatosis. The findings range from transient or progressive infiltration to consolidation, cavitation, or scarring; upper and lower lobes are involved with equal frequency. As none of these findings is specific, antemortem diagnosis of polyarteritis depends upon biopsy. Since the arterial involvement is segmental and spotty in distribution, it is advisable to obtain tissue from a symptomatic site, and it is essential to section completely the entire specimen. A deep, open surgical biopsy, including subcutaneous tissue and underlying muscle, should be obtained whenever possible from a skeletal muscle exhibiting pain and tenderness. Involvement of the epididymis and testes is sufficiently common to make this a useful biopsy site if palpation reveals the typical nodularity of segmental vascular lesions. Needle and surgical biopsies of internal organs with clinical involvement, such as liver or kidney, are gaining in favor. As an alternative or additional procedure, angiography to detect aneurysms of medium-sized muscular arteries in renal, hepatic, or intestinal sites may be helpful.

DIFFERENTIAL DIAGNOSIS. The differential diagnosis of the polyarteritis group includes not only the constituent syndromes but also all those conditions associated with necrotizing angiitis. The key differences between classic polyarteritis nodosa and other causes of necrotizing angiitis include the absence of extravascular granulomas, sparing of the pulmonary arteries, failure of venous involvement except by contiguous spread, and predilection for medium-sized arteries. For allergic angiitis and granulomatosis the striking granulomatous response excludes all but Wegener's granulomatosis. The prominence of bronchial asthma, peripheral eosinophilia, and the usual absence of necrotizing lesions in the upper respiratory tract permit a tentative clinical distinction between allergic angiitis and granulomatosis and Wegener's granulomatosis. The relative absence of venular involvement, with or without hepatitis B antigenemia, separates classic periarteritis nodosa from the more common polyangiitis. The hypocomplementemia in some patients with polyangiitis is more characteristic of certain patients with hypersensitivity angiitis than of polyarteritis nodosa. Underlying connective tissue diseases are still recognized by their clinical characteristics even when necrotizing arteritis becomes prominent. For example, cases of rheumatoid arthritis with ulcerating cutaneous lesions and peripheral neuropathy often exhibit prominent rheumatoid nodules and a high titer of rheumatoid factor. The specificities of the immunoglobulins which accompany active systemic lupus erythematosus or mixed cryoglobulinemia are distinctive; in addition, in the presence of active renal disease both entities manifest a reduced serum complement level not generally observed in classic polyarteritis nodosa. Giant cell arteritis, in its limited form, cranial (especially temporal) or aortic arch (Takayasu's) arteritis, or in its disseminated state lacks the glomerulitis, peripheral neuropathy, and cutaneous manifestations notable in polyarteritis nodosa. The combination of progressive nephritis and pulmonary hemorrhage seen in Goodpasture's syndrome is unlike polyarteritis nodosa. The drug-induced hypersensitivity angiitis group may be difficult to separate on purely clinical grounds, although the history of antecedent drug administration, the frequency of pulmonary involvement, infrequency of gastrointestinal manifestations, and absence of nodules along arteries are useful points. The clinical presentation in Henoch-Schönlein purpura, mostly in children and with a relatively good prognosis, is distinctive. Necrotizing vasculitis with or without renal disease in C2 deficiency, hypergammaglobulinemic purpura, and other syndromes listed under hypersensitivity angiitis are differentiated by the unique features responsible for designating the entity.

Additional entities to be considered in the differential diagnosis are certain microbial and occlusive diseases with diverse manifestations, notably chronic meningococcemia, subacute infective endocarditis, trichinosis, and certain rickettsial diseases. A few vascular occlusive diseases, including Degos' disease and thrombotic thrombocytopenic purpura, must also be considered. Necrotizing papulosis of Degos, with its occlusive arterial lesions of the skin, gastrointestinal tract, and brain, is best characterized by the cutaneous manifestations. These lesions typically involve the trunk and extremities, begin as pink to gray papules, undergo central umbilication, and persist for variable periods with depressed (porcelain-like) centers covered with a removable scale and surrounded by a red elevated margin. The absence of both thrombocytopenia and intravascular hemolysis distinguishes periarteritis nodosa from thrombotic thrombocytopenic purpura. Additional points of help in the differential diagnosis of periarteritis nodosa in general are the rarity of Raynaud's phenomenon, the absence of the nephrotic syndrome, and the lack of lymphadenopathy.

TREATMENT. The commonly employed anti-inflammatory agents such as salicylates or phenylbutazone have little or no clear effect on the polyarteritis group, and thus corticosteroids have been employed most widely. Large doses, in the range of 40 to 60 mg of prednisone per day, afford symptomatic relief and apparently do improve the one-year survival statistics. On the other hand, the study by the Medical Research Council of England did not reveal a better 54 months' survival period in a steroid-treated group as compared with a control series, whereas early steroid treatment was considered efficacious in the Mayo Clinic series. In a series of 17 patients falling within the polyarteritis group, including two with allergic angiitis and granulomatosis and six with hepatitis B–associated polyangiitis, 14 experienced dramatic remission with the introduction of cyclophosphamide at a dose of 2 mg per kilogram per day. It was subsequently possible to reduce the cyclophosphamide and to taper the steroids to every other day and yet maintain a remission state by clinical criteria and in some instances by resolution of microaneurysms on repeat celiac axis angiography. Although this experience is uncontrolled, the historical outcome and time course of response to the addition of a cytotoxic agent justify the approach.

Churg J, Strauss L: Allergic granulomatosis, allergic angiitis, and periarteritis nodosa. Am J Pathol 27:277, 1951. *This is the classic reference to the polyarteritis nodosa subgroup termed allergic angiitis and granulomatosis, and describes the cardinal clinical and pathologic manifestations.*

Collagen Diseases and Hypersensitivity Panel: Report to Medical Research Council. Br Med J 1:1399, 1960. *This is the classic reference on the natural history of the polyarteritis nodosa group, untreated and with steroid intervention.*

Cupps TR, Fauci AS: The Vasculitides. Philadelphia, W. B. Saunders Company, 1981. *An excellent and up-to-date general review of differential diagnosis, classification, and treatment.*

Fauci AS, Katz P, Haynes BF, Wolff SM: Cyclophosphamide therapy of severe systemic necrotizing vasculitis. N Engl J Med 301:235, 1979. *A most important contribution dealing with the effectiveness of cyclophosphamide therapy in the management of a series of patients falling within the polyarteritis group and including such subgroups as allergic angiitis and granulomatosis and hepatitis B–associated polyangiitis.*

Moore PM, Fauci AS: Neurologic manifestations of systemic vasculitis. A retrospective and prospective study of the clinicopathologic features and responses to therapy in 25 patients. Am J Med 71:517, 1981. *An up-to-date analysis of the beneficial effects of therapy.*

Mowrey FH, Lundberg RA: The clinical manifestations of essential polyangiitis (periarteritis nodosa) with emphasis on the hepatic manifestations. Ann Intern Med 40:1145, 1954. *A useful description of the gastrointestinal manifestations observed in patients with the polyarteritis nodosa group.*

Reza JJ, Dornfeld L, Goldberg LS, Bluestone R, Pearson CM: Wegener's granulomatosis. Long-term follow-up of patients treated with cyclophosphamide. Arthritis Rheum 18:501, 1975. *The introduction of cyclophosphamide therapy altered the natural history not only of Wegener's granulomatosis but subsequently also of the polyarteritis nodosa group, and thus this is an important reference article.*

Rose GA, Spencer H: Polyarteritis nodosa. Quart J Med 26:43, 1957. *This classic article argued most effectivly that allergic angiitis and granulomatosis was not a distinct entity from classic polyarteritis nodosa but could most easily be considered polyarteritis nodosa with pulmonary involvement. This is the current interpretation, and from a clinical point of view nothing need be added to the clinical and pathologic material contained herein.*

Sergent JS, Lockshin MD, Christian CL, Gocke DJ: Vasculitis with hepatitis B antigenemia. Long-term observations in nine patients. Medicine 55:1, 1976. *This represents the five-year experience of the group which originally described the association of hepatitis B antigenemia with necrotizing vasculitis and contains important information with regard to the natural history and clinical course of the disease.*

452. WEGENER'S GRANULOMATOSIS AND MIDLINE GRANULOMA

Anthony S. Fauci

WEGENER'S GRANULOMATOSIS

DEFINITION. Wegener's granulomatosis is characterized by the classic clinicopathologic features of necrotizing granulomatous vasculitis involving the upper and lower respiratory tracts, glomerulonephritis, and variable degrees of systemic, small vessel vasculitis.

ETIOLOGY. The cause is unknown, although it is generally considered to represent an aberrant hypersensitivity reaction to an unknown antigen. There have been no associations with allergic diatheses, geographic location, travel, or domestic or occupational exposure.

INCIDENCE AND PREVALENCE. Although an uncommon disease, Wegener's granulomatosis is no longer thought of as being extremely rare, as it is now recognized earlier and more frequently in clinical practice. The male:female ratio is approximately 1.3:1. The disease can be seen in any age group from infancy to old age. The mean age of onset is 40.6 years.

PATHOLOGY AND PATHOGENESIS. The characteristic histopathologic feature of this disease is necrotizing vasculitis of small arteries and veins together with granuloma formation.

The upper airway disease most often involves the paranasal sinuses and nasopharynx with necrotizing granuloma, with or without demonstrable vasculitis. Pansinusitis with erosion of adjacent bone may occur, as well as nasal septal perforation and saddle nose deformity.

Almost all patients have lung involvement (see Ch. 62). The infiltrates are usually multiple, bilateral, and nodular, with a tendency to cavitate. Endobronchial disease may result in airways obstruction and atelectasis.

Histopathologically, the renal lesion begins as a focal and segmental necrotizing glomerulitis which may lead to rapidly progressive glomerulonephritis and renal failure (see Ch. 80).

In addition to these classic features, virtually any organ can be involved with granuloma, vasculitis, or both.

The immunopathogenesis of the disease remains an enigma. Circulating immune complexes and immune complex–like renal deposits have been demonstrated in some patients. In contradistinction, the extensive granuloma formation in various organs is suggestive of delayed type hypersensitivity or cellular immune mechanisms. It is possible that there is an overlap of more than one type of immunologic mechanism, or that there is a granulomatous response to a particular type of immune complex in this disease.

CLINICAL MANIFESTATIONS. Wegener's granulomatosis is a multisystem disease manifesting a variety of signs and symptoms. However, in most patients the upper airway and, less frequently, the pulmonary symptoms dominate the presenting clinical picture.

Patients usually complain of severe upper respiratory symptoms and signs such as paranasal sinus pain, drainage, and purulent or bloody nasal discharge. Nasal mucosal ulceration and septal perforation may occur, as well as the classic saddle nose deformity. Serous otitis media commonly results from eustachian tube blockage, and variable degrees of hearing impairment may occur.

Eye involvement occurs in up to 60 per cent of patients and may range from mild conjunctivitis to severe episcleritis, granulomatous sclerouveitis, ciliary vessel vasculitis, and proptosis.

Pulmonary manifestations may include cough, hemoptysis, chest discomfort, and shortness of breath. However, it is not uncommon that asymptomatic pulmonary infiltrates are discovered on chest x-ray during workup for other problems.

Nonspecific symptoms such as weakness, malaise, arthralgia, anorexia, and weight loss are common. Fever may result from the underlying disease, but often reflects secondary infection in paranasal sinuses.

Skin disease resulting from vasculitis with or without granuloma is seen in 45 per cent of patients. Heart involvement is infrequent and usually appears as pericarditis or coronary vasculitis. Nervous system involvement, seen in up to 20 per cent of patients, may be exhibited as cranial neuritis, mononeuritis multiplex, or cerebral vasculitis and/or granuloma.

Renal disease usually determines the course and ultimate outcome of generalized Wegener's granulomatosis. Proteinuria with variable degrees of hematuria, red blood cell casts, and other sediment abnormalities may indicate smoldering disease activity. However, once renal function abnormalities appear, evidence of rapidly progressive glomerulonephritis usually ensues, leading to renal failure if appropriate therapy is not instituted. A limited form of Wegener's granulomatosis without renal involvement has been described. However, it most likely constitutes part of the spectrum of the generalized disease.

There are no diagnostic laboratory findings in this disease. The erythrocyte sedimentation rate is invariably markedly elevated. Mild anemia and leukocytosis may be seen, but eosinophilia is not characteristic. Mildly elevated rheumatoid factor titers are common, as is mild hypergammaglobulinemia, particularly of IgA.

DIAGNOSIS. The diagnosis can be strongly suspected when the classic picture of upper and lower airway disease together with renal involvement is present. It is confirmed by the histopathologic demonstration of necrotizing granulomatous vasculitis in appropriate tissues such as nasal or sinus mucosa. The pulmonary infiltrates are the source of tissue with the highest diagnostic yield. Percutaneous renal biopsy is extremely important in documenting glomerulonephritis, particularly in early disease or when the diagnosis is unclear.

Recognition of the classic clinicopathologic complex of Wegener's granulomatosis should make differentiation from other similar disorders relatively easy. However, differential diagnosis should include the vasculitides, connective tissue diseases, infectious and noninfectious granulomatous diseases, and tumors of the upper airway or lung. Goodpasture's syndrome is differentiated by the demonstration of antiglomerular basement membrane antibody. Idiopathic midline granuloma (see below) is a localized destructive disease which mutilates the upper airway and facial tissues. Wegener's granulomatosis does not erode through facial tissue, and idiopathic midline granuloma does not include lung or renal disease. Of particular interest in the differential diagnosis is a disease called *lymphomatoid granulomatosis*. It involves predominantly lungs, skin, central nervous system, and kidney. It is clearly different from Wegener's granulomatosis. It is not a classic inflammatory vasculitis, but an invasion and destruction of vessels by atypical lymphocytoid and plasmacytoid cells resembling a lymphoma; the renal disease is not a glomerulonephritis but a nodular infiltration of the kidney by these bizarre lymphoid cells; and upper airway disease is quite uncommon. Up to 40 per cent of cases of lymphomatoid granulomatosis may evolve into a frank lymphoma.

TREATMENT AND PROGNOSIS. The treatment of choice in this disease is cytotoxic agents, and of the cytotoxic agents cyclophosphamide* is clearly the most effective. It should be given in daily oral doses of 1 to 2 mg per kilogram per day. In initiation of treatment in fulminant cases, the drug may be given intravenously in doses of 4 to 5 mg per kilogram per day for a few days with subsequent change to the lower oral dosage regimen. A therapeutic response can usually be induced and maintained without causing severe leukopenia. Leukocyte counts should be closely monitored during therapy, and dosages of cyclophosphamide should be adjusted to maintain the leukocyte count above 3000 per cubic millimeter and the neutrophil count no less than 1000 to 1500 per cubic millimeter in order to avoid risk of infection. Cyclophosphamide should be continued for 1 full year following remission. In patients who cannot tolerate cyclophosphamide, azathioprine* in similar doses may be used.

Corticosteroids should be used initially, together with cyclophosphamide. Prednisone, 60 mg per day for a brief period of time, is recommended until the cyclophosphamide becomes effective (usually within 2 to 3 weeks). The prednisone should then be converted to an alternate-day regimen, tapered, and discontinued after approximately 6 months.

The disease was formerly universally fatal, usually within months after onset of renal disease. With cyclophosphamide

*Investigational drug for this purpose.

use, the prognosis is quite good, and long-term remissions have been achieved in over 90 per cent of patients. Several patients have maintained remission for years following discontinuation of cyclophosphamide. Several patients in drug-induced remissions, but with residual irreversible renal failure, have undergone successful renal transplantation.

Fauci AS: Granulomatous vasculitides: Distinct but related. Ann Intern Med 87:782, 1977. *An editorial which outlines the distinctions and overlaps among the various granulomatous vasculitides.*

Fauci AS, Haynes BF, Katz P: The spectrum of vasculitis. Clinical, pathologic, immunologic, and therapeutic considerations. Ann Intern Med 89:660, 1978. *Comprehensive review article which describes the entire spectrum of the vasculitides and places Wegener's granulomatosis in perspective in relation to the other systemic vasculitides.*

Fauci AS, Haynes BF, Katz P, Wolff SM: Wegener's granulomatosis: Prospective clinical and therapeutic experience with 85 patients for 21 years. Ann Intern Med 98:76, 1983. *Clinicopathologic features of the disease are discussed and detailed information on use of the combined cyclophosphamide-alternate day prednisone regimen is provided. Complete remissions were achieved in 93 per cent of patients.*

Liebow AA, Carrington CRB, Friedman PJ: Lymphomatoid granulomatosis. Hum Pathol 3:457, 1972. *Original description of the newly recognized entity of lymphomatoid granulomatosis. Extensively details the cases from a restrospective standpoint. An important paper, but overly long and cumbersome to read.*

Steinman TI, Jaffe BF, Monaco AP, Wolff SM, Fauci AS: Recurrence of Wegener's granulomatosis after kidney transplantation. Successful re-induction of remission with cyclophosphamide. Am J Med 68:458, 1980. *Wegener's granulomatosis recurred four years after renal transplantation and responded to cyclophosphamide after failing to respond to azathioprine.*

MIDLINE GRANULOMA

DEFINITION. Midline granuloma is a rare disease manifested by a relentlessly progressive, localized destructive process that predominantly involves the nose, paranasal sinuses, and palate, with erosion through contiguous structures such as the orbit and face. It is characterized by nonspecific acute and chronic inflammation and necrosis with or without granuloma formation.

ETIOLOGY. The cause of midline granuloma is unknown. Since the tissue reaction is suggestive of a hypersensitivity or immunologically mediated process, a localized fulminant response to an unidentified antigen has been proposed. No etiologic connections have been made with prior allergic rhinitis, chronic sinusitis, or infection. Certain upper airway tumors can result in inflammatory and granulomatous responses with necrosis. The underlying histopathology of the neoplasm is masked and the process closely resembles midline granuloma. However, true midline granuloma is a distinct entity in which no identifiable cause can be found despite multiple deep biopsies, long-term follow-up, and postmortem examination. This entity should appropriately be referred to as idiopathic midline granuloma, as opposed to the inflammatory and granulomatous responses associated with upper airway neoplasms.

PATHOLOGY. The typical histopathologic features are nonspecific acute and chronic inflammation with necrosis. The tissue is infiltrated with neutrophils, monocytes, lymphocytes, plasma cells, and, in some cases, eosinophils. True granuloma formation with or without typical Langhans giant cells may not be present in every case. Thrombosis of small vessels, perivascular cellular infiltration, and secondary involvement of vessels resulting from the inflammatory process may occur, but true primary vasculitis is rarely seen. If neoplastic cells are identified, the process can no longer be considered idiopathic midline granuloma. Secondary pyogenic infection of the involved tissue with its added inflammatory response is frequent.

CLINICAL MANIFESTATIONS. The disease can occur in all age groups, but most patients are in the fifth and sixth decades. It is slightly more common in women than men and occurs in all races.

The clinical presentation can vary, but in most cases symptoms are first related to the nose and paranasal sinuses with rhinorrhea and nasal stuffiness, followed by purulent nasal discharge resulting from superimposed infection. Nonhealing ulcerations of the nasal mucosa occur, and perforation of the nasal septum is frequent. Some patients present with disease in the oral cavity with or without nasal and paranasal sinus involvement. This usually occurs as ulcerations of the buccal mucosa, gums, or hard and soft palate. Some patients present with relatively painless perforation of the palate noted by the regurgitation of food or saliva into the nasal cavity. Occasionally, patients initially complain of symptoms related to the eye. The disease may be relatively indolent or fulminant, but it is always progressive. Relentless destruction of soft tissue, cartilage, and bone occur. Erosion of paranasal sinus walls occurs, with spread into contiguous structures such as the orbit. Destruction of the soft and hard palate, the nasal septum, and even the entire nose occurs. The destructive process may erode through the skin, resulting in dramatic mutilation of facial structures. The necrotic tissue and paranasal sinus cavities frequently becomes infected, usually with *Staphylococcus aureus*. The necrotic tissue can be quite malodorous, although the patients themselves frequently lose their sense of smell. Local lymphadenopathy occurs rarely and is suggestive of an underlying malignancy.

There are no characteristic laboratory findings except those related to the inflammatory process such as leukocytosis, elevated erythrocyte sedimentation rate, mild anemia of chronic disease, and hyperglobulinemia. Roentgenographic studies reveal pansinusitis with destruction of various cartilaginous and bony structures of the upper airways. Since this is a localized disease, laboratory abnormalities related to other organ systems should prompt one to investigate other possible causes.

Surgical procedures in the involved areas can lead to rapid acceleration of the disease, although, following appropriate treatment, debridement may benefit healing. Death usually occurs from secondary systemic infection or from inanition. Other causes are erosion into a major blood vessel with exsanguination or erosion into the central nervous system and subsequent meningitis.

DIAGNOSIS. The diagnosis of midline granuloma is made by the characteristic clinical presentation together with characteristically nonspecific histopathologic findings, but, most important, after other diseases with similar findings have been ruled out.

Midline granuloma is sometimes confused with Wegener's granulomatosis. They are clearly distinct entities. Wegener's granulomatosis is a systemic disease characterized by necrotizing granulomatous vasculitis of the upper and lower respiratory tracts with glomerulonephritis (in the generalized form). Midline granuloma rarely manifests true primary vasculitis in the lesions and by definition is a localized disease without pulmonary or renal involvement. Furthermore, Wegener's granulomatosis rarely if ever causes palatal perforation and does not erode facial tissues.

The greatest difficulty arises in distinguishing true idiopathic midline granuloma from neoplasms of the upper airways, particularly midline malignant reticulosis and certain lymphomas, whose malignant histopathology can be masked by the intense inflammatory reaction. Careful search for disseminated malignancy as well as complete examination of multiple adequate biopsy specimens often either reveal the neoplastic disorder or confirm midline granuloma.

Other diseases which must be ruled out are infectious diseases such as tuberculosis, syphilis, lepromatous leprosy, histoplasmosis, blastomycosis, coccidioidomycosis, mucocutaneous leishmaniasis, and rhinoscleroma (caused by a *Klebsiella* species). Pseudotumor of the orbit must also be ruled out.

TREATMENT. Corticosteroid therapy is ineffective and can worsen infection. Cytotoxic agents have been used with variable results, most of which were ultimately failures.

The treatment of choice is local radiation therapy. High dose (5000 rads) radiotherapy to the involved areas results in a high percentage of remissions.

PROGNOSIS. If untreated, the disease is uniformly fatal. Since the use of high dose local radiotherapy, the prognosis for survival is excellent, with greater than 70 per cent remission rate and even cures after up to 15 years of follow-up. Hence the disease should no longer be referred to as "lethal" midline granuloma. High dose radiotherapy is associated in some cases with serious complications and side effects. However, the risk is outweighed by the fatal alternative. The mutilation and disfigurement that result from far advanced disease are often a source of great psychologic difficulty. Reconstructive plastic surgery and prostheses have resulted in dramatic functional and cosmetic improvements in some patients.

Fauci AS, Johnson RE, Wolff SM: Radiation therapy of midline granuloma. Ann Intern Med 84:140, 1976. *Prospective, 15-year study of ten patients with idiopathic midline granuloma which establishes the efficacy of high dose local irradiation therapy. Discusses differential diagnosis as well as the salient features that distinguish midline granuloma from Wegener's granulomatosis.*

Fechner RE, Lamppin DW: Midline malignant reticulosis. A clinicopathologic entity. Arch Otolaryngol 95:467, 1972. *Important paper pointing out that certain types of destructive upper airway neoplasms can closely mimic midline granuloma.*

Friedmann I: Midline granuloma. Proc R Soc Med 57:289, 1964. *Classic description of many of the clinicopathologic features of midline granuloma.*

Stewart JP: Progressive lethal granulomatous ulceration of the nose. J Laryngol 48:657, 1933. *Original complete description of midline granuloma with firm establishment of the disease as a distinct clinicopathologic entity.*

Tsokos M, Fauci AS, Costa J: Idiopathic midline destructive disease (IMDD). A subgroup of patients with the "midline granuloma" syndrome. Am J Clin Pathol 77:162, 1982.

453. POLYMYALGIA RHEUMATICA AND GIANT CELL ARTERITIS

Louis A. Healey

POLYMYALGIA RHEUMATICA

Polymyalgia rheumatica is a syndrome consisting of pain and stiffness in pelvic and shoulder girdles, very rapid erythrocyte sedimentation rate, and a prompt response to a small dose of corticosteroid. For reasons unknown, it is a disease of older patients. The diagnosis is made with reluctance in anyone less than 50 years old, and most patients are over age 60. It is seen more often in women than in men (2.5:1). Almost all patients affected are Caucasian. Both polymyaligia and giant cell arteritis show statistical association with HLA determinants CW_3, DR_3, and DR_4.

Patients experience pain in the neck, back, shoulders, upper arms, and thighs. The onset may be gradual but at other times is so abrupt that patients go to bed well and awaken in the morning stiff and sore as if they had chopped wood or shoveled snow. Morning stiffness and jelling after prolonged sitting are essential features of the history. Patients graphically describe how a spouse has to pull them out of bed or, if they are alone, how it is necessary for them to wiggle like a snake and then push themselves up from a kneeling position. Although such a story may initially suggest weakness, the limitation is actually due to pain and stiffness rather than lack of strength. Some patients experience widespread symptoms and complain that they hurt all over. In others the pain and stiffness is in either shoulders or hips, but in all it is symmetrical. Low grade fever, malaise, apathy, and weight loss are sometimes present. Carpal tunnel syndrome has been noted.

Despite the severity of complaints, the physical examination of these patients is surprisingly normal. Tenderness or limitation of shoulder and hip motion may be detected; effusions are present in the knees at times. Muscle strength is normal when tested. Radiographs are unremarkable. The clue to the diagnosis is the erythrocyte sedimentation rate, which is always elevated, usually very high, and may exceed 100 mm per hour (Westergren method). Unless this test is performed, the diagnosis is easily missed. Fibrinogen and alpha II globulins are both high. Slight anemia may be present. Rheumatoid factor and antinuclear antibodies are not present, serum complement is normal, and circulating immune complexes have not been consistently detected. Serum levels of muscle enzymes, electromyograms, and muscle biopsies are normal. Evidence from scans, biopsies, arthroscopy, and synovial fluid cell counts suggests that the symptoms of pain and stiffness may stem from synovitis.

Although polymyalgia rheumatica appears to be a distinct clinical entity, it is obvious from this description that it is not a specific one, and as such it is often necessary to exclude other diseases in order to make the diagnosis. The sedimentation rate indicates that this is an inflammatory disease and serves to separate it from osteoarthritis or the functional musculoskeletal pain of fibrositis. Difficulty in getting out of bed or rising from a chair may suggest the weakness of polymyositis, but, as mentioned, muscles are normal. The common diagnostic problem is to differentiate polymyalgia rheumatica from the onset of rheumatoid arthritis. Patients with rheumatoid arthritis tend to have synovitis of the distal joints—wrists, metacarpophalangeal, and metatarsophalangeal. When present, the rheumatoid factor is helpful, but at times, the diagnosis only becomes evident with follow-up visits.

The response of the pain and stiffness of polymyalgia rheumatica to 10 to 20 mg of prednisone may truly be described as dramatic. Many patients are well by the next day; improvement is so invariable that if it does not appear within one week, the original diagnosis should be questioned. After two to four weeks, the dose can be tapered and patients remain free of symptoms on 5 to 7.5 mg of prednisone daily, without risk of steroid side effects. The duration that therapy will be required is uncertain. Some patients can stop after one year, but others will have to continue. The duration can be determined only by attempting to withdraw the drug and observing for a recurrence of stiffness and pain. Aspirin and other nonsteroidal anti-inflammatory drugs provide partial relief but are not so effective as even small doses of steroid.

GIANT CELL ARTERITIS

Since the recognition that any of the larger arteries may be involved, the term *giant cell arteritis* has been preferred to the original names *temporal* or *cranial arteritis.* In contrast to polyarteritis, smaller arterioles are not affected; thus pulmonary and renal complications are not seen, and stroke or myocardial infarction does not occur more frequently than would be expected in this age group.

Clinical manifestations may conveniently be divided into localized or systemic. Local manifestations depend on the artery involved. Inflammation of the temporal artery produces severe headache, most often in one temple. The artery may be tender and swollen. Sudden unilateral blindness is due to occlusion of the terminal branches of the ophthalmic artery. Since blindness is irreversible, this is the most dreaded complication of the disease. Pain in the masseter muscles with chewing is attributed to involvement of the facial artery. This "jaw claudication" is a pathognomonic symptom of giant cell arteritis. Transient diplopia from ischemia of extraocular muscles is important to recognize, since it may lead to early diagnosis, steroid treatment, and preservation of vision. Arteritic involvement of the aorta can cause aortic arch syndromes with claudication in the arms and unequal pulses or, rarely, aneurysm formation. Systemic manifestations include fever, anemia, weight loss, malaise, and polymyalgia rheumatica. Some or all of these may be present in varying degree. If headache and other cranial symptoms are either not present or minimal and systemic symptoms predominate, the patients may present such diagnostic problems as fever of unknown origin, unexplained anemia, or possible occult carcinoma.

As with polymyalgia rheumatica, the only laboratory abnormality is the rapid erythrocyte sedimentation rate. Anemia is usually mild but can be more significant with hematocrit as low as 28 per cent. Red blood cell indices are normal, and there is a failure to utilize iron despite the presence of normal stores in the marrow. Tests of liver function, particularly the alkaline phosphatase, may show slight to moderate abnormalities, but biopsy of the liver shows normal tissue or slight fatty changes.

The diagnosis is established by biopsy of the temporal artery, which is safe and convenient to perform as an office procedure. The characteristic histologic picture shows zones of inflammatory infiltrate composed of histiocytes, lymphocytes, and giant cells surrounding markedly fragmented internal elastic lamina with intervening segments of normal artery. When headache, visual symptoms, or other signs of cranial artery involvement are present, the diagnosis may be suspected and the biopsy is usually positive. However, the characteristic arteritis has also been found in some patients with polymyalgia rheumatica, fever, or other systemic symptoms even when the temporal artery appears clinically normal.

Giant cell arteritis responds well to steroid treatment, but higher doses are needed to suppress the inflammation. When cranial arteritis is diagnosed or even suspected, treatment should be started immediately with at least 50 mg of prednisone in order to preserve vision. If the diagnosis is proved by biopsy, this dose should be continued for four weeks before gradual reduction is instituted with the aim of achieving the same maintenance dose and duration of therapy as described for polymyalgia rheumatica. Such a program carries a risk of steroid toxicity, particularly osteoporosis and vertebral collapse, which must be balanced against the risk of blindness. Symptoms are a better guide to titrating the steroid dose than the sedimentation rate. If the patient has been treated with high-dose steroid for one month, it is preferable to follow the clinical response as the dose is tapered. The risk of steroid toxicity from treating the sedimentation rate is greater than the risk of a complication of arteritis in a patient whose sedimentation rate increases somewhat as the steroid dose is lowered.

The exact nature of the relation between polymyalgia rheumatica and giant cell arteritis is uncertain, in large part because the etiology of both diseases is not known. Both are diseases of older patients, the vast majority of whom are Caucasian. Both frequently are seen in the same patient. Sixty per cent of patients with giant cell arteritis experience polymyalgia rheumatica either as a prodrome or at some time during their illness. Conversely, of patients with polymyalgia rheumatica and normal-appearing temporal arteries, only 10 per cent show arteritis on biopsy. The majority of polymyalgia patients respond well to low-dose prednisone and never develop clinical evidence of arteritis.

Chuang T-Y, Hunder GG, Ilstrup DM, Kurland LT: Polymyallgia rheumatica. A 10-year epidemiologic and clinical study. Ann. Intern Med 97:672, 1982. *Based on an entire county population, this study gives the best information on incidence. The 10-year follow-up provides a look at the course of the disease, response to treatment, outcome, and complications.*

Healey LA, Wilske KR: The Systemic Manifestations of Temporal Arteritis. New York, Grune & Stratton, 1978. *This 140-page monograph describes clinical manifestations, histology, and treatment. English language references are critically reviewed. Research and possible etiology are discussed.*

454. DERMATOMYOSITIS AND POLYMYOSITIS

Ronald P. Messner

DEFINITION. Polymyositis is an inflammatory disease of skeletal muscle of unknown etiology, characterized by symmetrical weakness of the limb girdles, neck, and pharynx. Patients with this illness can be divided into five clinical categories:

Type I —Adult polymyositis
Type II —Dermatomyositis
Type III—Myositis with malignancy
Type IV—Childhood myositis
Type V —Myositis associated with other connective tissue diseases (overlap syndromes)

In this chapter the term polymyositis is used to characterize the whole group of patients, while adult polymyositis is used to denote Type I patients.

Proposed criteria for diagnosis of polymyositis are (1) symmetrical proximal muscle weakness, (2) elevation of muscle enzyme activities in serum, (3) typical EMG abnormalities, (4) positive muscle biopsy, and (5) typical rash of dermatomyositis. Patients are classified as having definite disease with four, probable disease with three, and possible disease with two criteria. The use of this system has helped to standardize the diagnosis and has greatly facilitated comparision of different reported series of patients.

INCIDENCE. Polymyositis has an annual incidence of approximately 7 cases per 1 million population. There is no relationship to birth order, family size, socioeconomic level, or geographic location. Familial cases are unusual. Age distribution is bimodal, with a small peak between ages 10 and 14 and a larger peak around age 50. Patients with myositis associated with malignancy have a mean age just over 60, whereas those with overlap syndrome have a mean age around 35. In adult and childhood polymyositis, females outnumber males by two to one. In cases associated with overlap syndromes the female dominance is even more pronounced. The sex ratio is nearly equal in dermatomyositis and myositis associated with malignancy.

PATHOLOGY AND PATHOGENESIS. The characteristic features of polymyositis on muscle biopsy include (1) degeneration of individual fibers, sometimes with vacuolation; (2) regeneration indicated by sarcoplasmic basophilia, large vesicular nuclei, and prominent nucleoli; (3) necrosis of part or all of a muscle fiber (moth-eaten fibers) and phagocytosis of the debris by macrophages; (4) increased variation in fiber size without hypertrophy of individual fibers; (5) interstitial and/or perivascular mononuclear cell infiltrate; (6) perifascicular atrophy; and (7) interstitial fibrosis. These findings may vary from patient to patient and even on multiple biopsies of a single patient. Approximately 15 per cent of initial muscle biopsies are normal, and the full picture of typical changes can be expected in about 50 per cent. Biopsy should be performed on a muscle that is involved but not totally weakened. Electromyography may aid in localizing an involved area, but the biopsy should not include the exact site of the electromyograph needle puncture, for these areas may show focal fiber destruction.

Skin biopsy should be done in an area of clinical dermatitis rather than relying on that obtained at muscle biopsy without regard for the condition of the skin. Marked dermal edema, basal vacuolation, and colloid bodies occur in the skin in both dermatomyositis and systemic lupus erythematosus, but in dermatomyositis the basement membrane is normal in thickness and does not stain for immunoglobulin or complement in indirect immunofluorescence studies.

One leading theory of the pathogenesis of polymyositis attributes muscle damage to cell-mediated autoimmunity. Evidence that supports this hypothesis includes the presence of lymphocytes and macrophages in the inflammatory infiltrate, sensitivity of lymphocytes to muscle antigens in vitro, and direct cytotoxicity of lymphocytes to cultured muscle cells. Recent information has, however, cast doubt on the ability of polymyositis lymphocytes to kill muscle cells. Although cell-mediated immune damage remains an attractive explanation, the exact mechanisms responsible for muscle injury are unknown.

There is little evidence to support the idea that antibodies participate in the pathogenesis of polymyositis. Antibodies to crude muscle extracts or myosin are no more frequent in polymyositis than in muscular dystrophy. Antibodies reactive with intact muscle are absent. Antimyoglobin antibodies occur in about two thirds of patients, but it is unclear whether they are primary or secondary factors in the disease process. A subset of children with polymyositis experiences cutaneous ulceration and intestinal infarction suggestive of necrotizing vasculitis, but examination of tissue reveals primarily noninflammatory endarteropathy and lymphocytic perivasculitis. Direct evidence of immune complex deposition is lacking in these children and in most adults, but a growing body of evidence suggests that ischemic damage caused by capillary abnormalities may be important in the pathogenesis. Replication of the capillary basement membrane and alterations in endothelial cells are frequent findings on electron microscopy, and the area of muscle served per capillary is increased. Loss of capillaries characteristically starts in the periphery of the fascicles and is more pronounced in children than in adults. These changes are probably not due to muscle atrophy, because the ratio of capillary lumina to muscle cell area does not change in Duchenne dystrophy and increases in denervation atrophy.

Infection caused by a virus or an organism such as *Toxoplasma gondii* has also been postulated as a cause of polymyositis. The incidence of IgM *anti-Toxoplasma* antibodies is increased in patients with polymyositis, and *Toxoplasma* organisms have been identified in a few cases of adult polymyositis, but treatment for toxoplasmosis has had little effect on the muscle disease. Whether these cases represent secondary infection with *Toxoplasma* or true toxoplasmic myositis is unclear. Coxsackievirus has been isolated from a few cases of polymyositis, and the incidence of antibodies to coxsackie B virus is increased in children with dermatomyositis. A good animal model has not been available for study of this disease. The recently described myositis that occurs in newborn mice after injection with coxsackie B1 virus might provide a system to study both the role of infection and the role of cell-mediated immunity in muscle damage.

CLINICAL MANIFESTATIONS. Weakness of the proximal muscles occurs in nearly all patients and is the presenting complaint in 70 per cent. The typical case begins with gradual onset of weakness in the hip girdle and proximal leg muscles. Muscle pain and tenderness are absent or mild. Weakness of the shoulders, proximal arm muscles, and neck flexors follows. Involvement of the pharyngeal muscles may occur with dysphagia, dysphonia, and dysarthria. Early symptoms include inability to rise from a low chair, climb stairs without the use of a railing, or raise the arms above the head to comb the hair. In advanced cases, the patient may be unable to lift the limbs against gravity. Muscular wasting is variable and frequently minimal until late in the disease. Contractures are almost exclusively associated with longstanding disease. The ocular muscles are almost never involved, and weakness of distal muscles occurs in less than 20 per cent of cases. Asymmetric weakness, weakness of isolated muscle groups, and acute onset with global weakness are unusual. Deep tendon reflexes are normal or slightly reduced. Muscle symptoms of childhood polymyositis are similar to those of the adult form, but fever, weight loss, rash, contractures, and subcutaneous calcification are more common.

Arthralgias occur in about one quarter of patients with adult polymyositis or dermatomyositis. True arthritis is usually mild; begins prior to or coincident with weakness; involves the hands, wrists, and knees; and responds quickly to steroid treatment. Synovial fluid has good viscosity and mononuclear cells. Synovial biopsy reveals fibrin deposition, focal loss of lining cells without proliferation, and mild inflammation. Patients with myositis and overlap syndromes may have joint involvement typical of rheumatoid arthritis or systemic lupus erythematosus. A peculiar arthritis of the hands with erosions, periosteal calcification, and instability of the interphalangeal joints of the thumb has also been described.

An erythematous skin rash occurs on the forehead, neck, shoulders, trunk, and arms of about one third of the patients with polymyositis. A lilac or heliotrope rash occurs on the upper eyelids and face in 15 per cent and is highly suggestive of the diagnosis of dermatomyositis. The rash may be associated with edema. Reddened, elevated, scaly patches are characteristically seen over the extensor surfaces of the small joints of the hands, the elbows, the knees, and the medial malleoli. Nailfolds may show periungual telangiectasia, dilated and distorted nailfold capillary loops alternating with avascular areas, or thickening and roughening without redness. In some patients, the finger pads become shiny and atrophic with constant peeling. Patients with myositis and overlap syndromes may display the whole spectrum of dermatologic changes associated with connective tissue diseases. Raynaud's syndrome occurs in one half of the patients with overlap syndrome and one fifth of those with adult polymyositis and dermatomyositis. It is less common in children and in patients with malignancy.

Dysphagia in polymyositis is primarily due to weakness of the striated musculature of the posterior pharynx. Dysfunction of the esophagus occurs, but is usually overshadowed by pharyngeal dysfunction. Hypomobility and poor absorption in the small intestine have been seen in a few patients without symptoms of frank scleroderma. Vasculitis associated with the childhood form of the disease may lead to mesenteric thrombosis.

Asymptomatic electrocardiographic abnormalities are common in polymyositis, but cardiac involvement manifested by congestive heart failure or heart block occurs in only 5 per cent of patients. Inflammatory cardiomyopathy, fibrosis, and small vessel disease have been found in some of these patients at autopsy. Interstitial pneumonitis occurs in 5 to 10 per cent of the patients. Cough and dyspnea precede muscle weakness in one half of the cases of interstitial pneumonitis. No relationship is apparent between the severity of the lung and muscle involvement. Vasculitis is not characteristic of this lesion, and pleurisy is uncommon. The presence of active inflammation on lung biopsy correlates well with steroid responsiveness. Renal involvement is rare. When renal failure occurs, it is most often attributable to myoglobulinuria. A few renal biopsies have revealed mesangial proliferation, suggesting that immune complexes may play a role in some cases.

About 10 per cent of patients with polymyositis have coexistent malignancy. The incidence of tumors is highest, 15 per cent, in dermatomyositis. It is also increased in adult polymyositis, but not in childhood polymyositis. Females are affected as frequently as males. Patients with associated malignancy are older than the average patient with polymyositis. Myositis precedes or occurs simultaneously with the diagnosis of malignancy in two thirds of patients, and in most instances the two diagnoses are made within the span of a year. Tumors of the breast and lung are the most common. Those of the ovary and stomach occur more frequently than in the general population, whereas tumors of the colon and rectum are less frequent. Polymyositis associated with malignancy has no clinical features that differentiate it from polymyositis alone. Extensive undirected radiographic screening of these patients for cancer has proved unrewarding. Clues to the coexistence of a malignancy are almost always present on history, physical examination, or routine laboratory tests.

CLINICAL COURSE AND PROGNOSIS. The five-year survival rate of patients followed over the last 20 years is approximately 80 per cent. The best survival rate occurs in children, and the worst in adults with malignancies. Death within the first year is usually due to pneumonia associated with dysphagia and aspiration. The leading causes of death are malignancy, infection, and cardiovascular disease. Deaths from muscular weakness are relatively rare. About half of the surviving patients will attain almost complete recovery of muscle strength.

LABORATORY DATA. Serum levels of muscle-derived enzymes, principally creatine kinase (CK), transaminases (SGOT, SGPT), lactate dehydrogenase (LDH), and aldolase, are elevated at some time during the course of the disease in 99 per cent of the patients and will be normal at any one time in about 10 per cent. The CK may be normal in as many as 36 per cent of cases at the time of presentation. Diagnostic accuracy can be improved by obtaining a battery of enzyme assays. The levels of these enzymes correlate reasonably well with disease activity and can be used as guides to therapy. Serum levels of myoglobin are elevated in approximately half of the patients and also correlate with clinical activity.

The incidence of rheumatoid factors and fluorescent antinuclear antibodies is remarkable only in patients in the overlap category. Antibodies to the Sm antigen are absent, but anti-RNP antibodies have been reported. Polymyositis patients have a number of antibodies directed against antigens present in calf thymus nuclear extracts that are separate from the Sm, nRNP, SS-A, and SS-B systems found in other autoimmune disorders. The JO-1 system occurs exclusively in polymyositis and defines a subset of patients with a high incidence of pulmonary fibrosis. The JO-1 antigen has been identified as histidine tRNA synthetase. Children with polymyositis have an increased incidence of HLA-B8 and DR3.

Anemia may be present but is rarely severe. The erythrocyte sedimentation rate is abnormal on initial evaluation in only half of the patients and cannot be relied upon as an index of disease activity. Gamma globulins are normal or elevated. With few exceptions total hemolytic complement and C3 are normal. Radionuclide scanning with ^{99m}Tc-polyphosphate may reveal increased uptake in areas of active myositis.

The electromyogram (EMG) is abnormal in almost all patients. The most common abnormalities, reduction in amplitude and duration of motor unit potentials, occur in 90 per cent of cases but are not specific for polymyositis. Evidence of membrane irritability, including fibrillation, positive sharp waves, and increased insertional activity, occur in half to three quarters of the EMGs. Spontaneous bizarre high frequency discharges are also characteristic. Electromyographic patterns do not differ among the clinical types of disease. In some patients the characteristic pattern is present only in certain muscle groups. The paravertebral musculature is frequently involved and should be included in diagnostic electromyography.

DIAGNOSIS AND DIFFERENTIAL DIAGNOSIS. Polymyositis is but one of a variety of diseases that may be present with muscle weakness and pain.

Neurologic disease is a primary concern in the evaluation of these patients. The history and physical examination will usually establish the neurologic origin, and EMG will show neuropathic changes. In muscular dystrophy a family history is often present and the symptoms progress over years rather than months. The CK may be elevated and may decrease on treatment with corticosteroids, but clinical improvement does not occur. The early involvement of the ocular and facial muscles helps differentiate myasthenia gravis.

Steroid myopathy begins insidiously in the proximal leg and hip muscles and spreads to involve the shoulders and arms. Other signs of glucocorticosteroid excess are usually present, but there is a poor correlation between the actual dose of corticosteroids and this syndrome. Raising the dose over a previously tolerated level may induce myopathy, and decreasing it to the previous level may relieve the symptoms. Muscle biopsy is normal. The combination of elevated urinary creatine and normal serum enzyme activities has been suggested as a useful differential point in favor of steroid myopathy. Other drugs that may cause myopathy include alcohol, clofibrate, penicillamine, azathioprine, phenytoin, polymyxin, chloroquine, and emetine.

Both hyper- and hypothyroidism may cause proximal muscle weakness. Thyrotoxic myopathy is usually insidious in onset and occurs most often in men. Muscle biopsy shows mild atrophy without inflammation. The electromyogram is nonspecific, and muscle enzymes are not elevated. In hypothyroidism, however, serum creatine phosphokinase may reach exceptionally high levels, and the electromyogram may be identical to that in polymyositis. Hyperparathyroidism may also cause proximal muscle weakness, an abnormal electromyogram, and muscle atrophy without an inflammatory infiltrate.

Weakness and myalgia may occur after exercise in McArdle's syndrome, carnitine palmityltransferase deficiency, myoadenylate deaminase deficiency, or renal tubular acidosis. A syndrome closely mimicking polymyositis may be seen in phosphate depletion, which is most often due to the use of nonabsorbable antacids. Muscle enzymes are not elevated. The electromyogram may be normal or show a pattern of denervation. Weakness disappears upon restoration of body phosphorus.

Direct invasion of muscle by an infectious agent may also mimic polymyositis. Trichinosis is characterized by a history of an antecedent gastrointestinal infection and coexisting symptoms of fever, edema of the eyelids, an urticarial rash, and eosinophilia. Muscle biopsy and positive serologic tests for trichinosis will confirm the diagnosis. Tropical pyomyositis is caused by *Staphylococcus aureus* in 90 per cent of patients. The onset is usually subacute with pain in the gluteal, quadriceps, or trunk muscles. Abscesses develop deep within the muscle and result in an initial hard woody swelling. Serum muscle enzymes are normal, and blood cultures are usually negative. Treatment requires antibiotics and surgical drainage.

Acute exertional rhabdomyolysis is characterized by muscular pain, swelling, induration, and weakness. It occurs after strenuous exercise in apparently healthy individuals. The urine contains heme pigment but not erythrocytes. Serum levels of muscle enzymes are elevated.

Patients with hypereosinophilic syndrome may have proximal muscle weakness, muscle tenderness, elevated serum enzymes, and a myopathic electromyogram, but muscle biopsy shows striking eosinophilic infiltrate. Eosinophilia is also present in the blood, and systemic features such as congestive heart failure and peripheral neuropathy are prominent. Eosinophilia also occurs in diffuse fasciitis with eosinophilia. These patients have sore and tender muscles and a peculiar puckering and thickening of the skin, and may develop contractures over a few weeks' time. They can be identified by the characteristic thickening of the fascia between the subcutaneous fat and muscle on biopsy.

Microemboli from atheromatous plaques in the aorta, or from nonbacterial endocarditis associated with carcinoma may produce a syndrome described as monomyositis multiplex. Pain usually involves the legs. It is sudden in onset and lasts for a short time, only to recur in a different site. Serum levels of muscle-derived enzymes and the erythrocyte sedimentation rate may be elevated and a myopathic pattern is present on electromyography, but the muscle biopsy is diagnostic. Diabetic amyotrophy may cause asymmetrical pain, weakness, and wasting in the proximal lower limbs, but the electromyogram and muscle biopsy are those of a neuropathy rather than a myopathy.

Polymyalgia rheumatica occurs in the elderly and is characterized by proximal muscle pain and stiffness without weakness. The only laboratory abnormality is a striking elevation of the erythrocyte sedimentation rate. Prompt relief after treatment with a small dose of corticosteroid is a helpful differentiating point. Other rheumatic connective tissue diseases may have myositis as part of the symptom complex. These patients should be labeled as having polymyositis only if they meet the independent criteria for the diagnosis.

TREATMENT. Bed rest is necessary during the active stage of the disease. Active physical therapy should be reserved until the inflammation has subsided.

In spite of a lack of adequately controlled therapeutic trials, corticosteroids are generally accepted as the drug of choice. Prednisone, 50 to 100 mg, is given daily in divided doses, and continued until definite improvement occurs. Serum enzymes typically decrease to half their pretreatment values one month after initiation of therapy, and reach normal values in two to three months. Muscle strength usually shows definite improvement in two months. Attempts to decrease steroid dosage rapidly or discontinue treatment prematurely may lead to a recurrence of the disease. A single daily dose or alternate-day steroid therapy may be tried in order to decrease the side effects, but should be attempted only when the disease is in good control. Maintenance therapy will be necessary for years in many cases. Failure to respond to steroids occurs in about 20 per cent of the patients. Immunosuppressive drugs such as methotrexate or cyclophosphamide or plasma exchange may be beneficial in these instances, but controlled studies to substantiate their efficacy are not available. Combined therapy with azathioprine and prednisone has been shown to reduce steroid requirements and improve function in long-term treatment compared to steroid alone. Polymyositis associated with malignancy may occasionally undergo a dramatic remission when the tumor is removed.

Bohan A, Peter JB, Bowman RL, Parson CM: A computer-assisted analysis of 153 patients with polymyositis and dermatomyositis. Medicine 56:255, 1977. *Presents data on which the classification and diagnostic criteria recommended in this chapter are based.*

Bunch TW: Prednisone and azathioprine for polymyositis. Arthritis Rheum 24:45, 1981. *A three-year controlled study suggesting the addition of azathioprine to conventional treatment with prednisone may have long-term benefits.*

Callen JP: Dermatomyositis and malignancy. Clin Rheum Dis 8:369, 1982. *Contains practical advice on the question of how extensively polymyositis patients should be investigated for malignancy.*

Crowe WE, Bove KE, Levinson JE, Hilton PK: Clinical and pathogenetic implications of histopathology in childhood polydermatomyositis. Arthritis Rheum 25:126, 1982. *Contains a clear description of the vascular lesions present in biopsies of the childhood form of polymyositis.*

Kagen LJ: Approach to the patient with myopathy. Bull Rheum Dis 33:2, 1983. *A concise discussion of the use of various tests and grading systems in diagnosis of muscle disease.*

455. CALCIUM CRYSTAL DEPOSITION ARTHROPATHIES

H. Ralph Schumacher, Jr.

At least three different calcium-containing crystals are now known to deposit in joints and to be associated with a variety of patterns of arthritis in much the same way as urate crystals cause the various features of gouty arthritis. Calcium pyrophosphate and occasionally calcium oxalate crystals produce linear or punctate calcifications in menisci and articular cartilage that can be readily seen on roentgenograms. These calcifications are termed chondrocalcinosis. Both these crystals and calcium apatite can also deposit diffusely in synovium and periarticular tissues, giving a soft tissue pattern on roentgenograms. X-rays may not show obvious calcifications when crystals are relatively few. Definitive diagnosis is only made by aspiration of synovial fluid for identification of the crystal type.

CALCIUM PYROPHOSPHATE DIHYDRATE (CPPD) CRYSTAL DEPOSITION DISEASE (Pseudogout Syndrome)

This is defined by the identification of rod or rhomboid-shaped weakly positively birefringent crystals (2 to 25 μ long) in synovial fluid or articular tissue. This is a common cause of arthritis; it is most frequent in the elderly. Up to 27 per cent of nursing home patients in their 80's have x-ray evidence of chondrocalcinosis on this basis. Familial cases have been described in populations of various ethnic origins. Both sexes are affected.

The cause of CPPD crystal deposition is not established, but deficiency of phosphatases and local connective tissue changes are probably important. CPPD crystals deposit only in joints and adjacent tendons or bursas, where they produce hematoxyphilic clumps replacing the normal tissue. Virtually any joint can be involved, but knees, wrists, and second and third metacarpophalangeal joints are the ones most commonly involved, so that chronic cases can be confused with rheumatoid arthritis. Acute bouts of crystal-induced arthritis in one or more joints can mimic gout, which led to the early term "pseudogout." CPPD crystal deposition often complicates osteoarthritis; crystals were seen in 42 per cent of osteoarthritic knee effusions in one series. Whether crystals contribute to cartilage degeneration in osteoarthritis is not yet clear. Occasionally, severe arthritis mimics the destruction seen in neuropathic joints. Radiographic evidence of calcification can be present in some patients for years without producing any symptoms.

Synovial effusions are generally inflammatory with leukocyte counts up to 100,000 per cu mm and contain 80 to 90 per cent neutrophils during acute attacks. Between attacks crystals can be seen in clear, noninflammatory joint effusions.

CPPD deposition can be an important clue to a number of associated diseases, many of which have specific treatments that can control systemic features if not the arthropathy. Diseases seen in association with CPPD include hyperparathyroidism, hemochromatosis, myxedema, ochronosis, hypophosphatasia, hypomagnesemia, and perhaps acromegaly and Wilson's disease. CPPD deposition frequently is seen as a complication of other advanced arthritides such as gout and rheumatoid arthritis. Septic arthritis can complicate CPPD deposition.

Treatment of inflammatory episodes with thorough aspiration and use of nonsteroidal anti-inflammatory agents is generally successful. Intra-articular steroid injections may provide relief for refractory involvement of individual joints. Intravenous colchicine may also be helpful. No long-term preventive measures are known, and the prognosis is slow progression punctuated by inflammatory bouts. Chronic use of nonsteroidal agents can be tried in patients with chronic or recurrent inflammation.

McCarty DJ: Proceedings of a conference on pseudogout and pyrophosphate metabolism. Arthritis Rheum 19(Suppl), 1975 (275 pages). *Multiple authors discuss clinical picture, pathogenesis, and management.*

Schumacher HR, Gibilisco P, Reginato A, et al.: Implications of crystal deposition in osteoarthritis. J Rheum (Suppl 9), 40, 1983. *The association of crystals with osteoarthritis is reviewed.*

APATITE CRYSTAL DEPOSITION DISEASE

Individual apatite crystals can be seen only by electron microscopy (EM), but clumps of these crystals appear as shiny (but not generally birefringent) globules 2 to 15 μ in size that can suggest the diagnosis. Apatite crystal deposition and crystal-induced inflammation are common findings in bursitis and periarthritis. Apatite also occurs in some otherwise unexplained acute arthritides and like CPPD is common in osteoarthritic joint effusions. Most joints or bursas can be involved, but the more common sites include shoulders, hips, knees, and digits. X-rays can show soft-tissue calcifications with or without bony erosions and occasionally with severe destruction. Calcium stains such as Alizarin red can help suggest the presence of apatite. Definitive diagnosis of the crystal type can only be made by EM with electron probe elemental analysis, x-ray diffraction, or infrared spectroscopy. Synovial or bursal effusions can have many or only a few leukocytes. Serum studies are generally normal, except that phosphate levels are often elevated in renal dialysis patients, who are at high risk of apatite deposition.

Apatite deposition can also be associated with scleroderma and the other connective tissue diseases. In most instances the cause of soft-tissue apatite deposition is not known. Treatment for acute arthritis or periarthritis is with nonsteroidal anti-inflammatory agents or colchicine. Aspiration of crystals and local injection with depot corticosteroids can also be effective.

Paul H, Reginato AJ, Schumacher HR: Alizarin red S staining as a screening test to detect calcium compounds in synovial fluid. Arthritis Rheum 26:191, 1983. *This describes a simple office screening test for apatite and other calcium-containing crystals.*

Pinals RS, Short CL: Calcific periarthritis involving multiple sites. Arthritis Rheum 9:566, 1966. *This recurrent calcific periarthritis is related to apatite crystals.*

Schumacher HR, Somlyo AP, Tse RP, et al.: Arthritis associated with apatite crystals. Ann Intern Med 87:411, 1977. *Clinical picture, diagnostic evaluation, and review.*

OTHER CALCIUM-CONTAINING CRYSTALS

Calcium oxalate deposition can occur in joints of renal failure patients on chronic hemodialysis, producing x-ray evidence of soft tissue calcification and chondrocalcinosis. Acute or chronic joint effusions can be seen. Diagnosis is made by identification of typical bipyramidal crystals. When less characteristic crystals are seen, other techniques as described under apatite deposition can be used. Calcium hydrogen phosphate dihydrate (brushite) and octacalcium phosphate have also been described in synovial fluids and tissues; their relationship to joint disease is not yet defined.

Hoffman EC, Schumacher HR, Paul H, et al.: Calcium oxalate microcrystalline-associated arthritis in end stage renal disease. Ann Intern Med 97:36, 1982. *Three cases with oxalosis and arthritis are described. Methods to identify oxalate crystals are included.*

456. RELAPSING POLYCHONDRITIS

H. Ralph Schumacher, Jr.

This uncommon disease is characterized by recurrent inflammation and destruction of cartilaginous and other connective tissue structures. Commonly involved cartilages are the pinnae of the ears, nasal cartilages, and tracheal rings. Polychondritis occurs nearly equally in both sexes and at any age but with a peak of onset between the ages of 30 and 50.

The pathologic lesion seen by light microscopy consists of loss of matrix staining, predominantly superficial infiltration with polymorphonuclear neutrophils or lymphocytes, and eventual destruction of normal structures followed by fibrosis. Electron microscopy in addition shows alterations of superficial chondrocytes, matrix, and elastic fibers. The cause of polychondritis is unknown, but the location of lesions and the frequency of associated systemic diseases suggest the importance of systemic factors. Antibodies to type II collagen and the presence of cell-mediated immunity to proteoglycan are evidences of immunologic aberrations.

The most common initial clue to the diagnosis is inflammation of the cartilaginous structures of the ears. There is generally rather acute onset of pain and tenderness with erythema and swelling of one or both helices. The lobe is spared. Inner and middle ear involvement can occur, causing hearing loss or vertigo. Nasal cartilage involvement can produce a saddle nose. Laryngeal and tracheal disease can cause hoarseness or life-threatening upper respiratory obstruction. Ocular manifestations are common and include conjunctivitis, episcleritis, iritis, and rarely other problems such as optic neuritis. Antigens in the eye that are cross-reactive with cartilage proteoglycans and their link protein have been identified.

Cardiac involvement, especially of the aortic root with aortic insufficiency, is seen in up to one fourth of cases. There may also be aortic aneurisms. Arthritis is reported in about three fourths of cases. This is nondestructive. It is not clear whether articular cartilage is involved in the same way that other cartilages are or whether other factors account for the arthritis. Fever, rashes, and neurologic and renal disease can occur.

There are no diagnostic laboratory tests for relapsing polychondritis, although the erythrocyte sedimentation rate is often elevated. There may be anemia and leukocytosis. Roentgenograms can detect the tracheal narrowing.

Relapsing polychondritis is associated with other diseases in one third or more of cases. These include rheumatoid arthritis, systemic lupus erythematosus, Sjögren's syndrome, thyroid disease, ulcerative colitis, vasculitis of various types, cryoglobulinemia, diabetes mellitus, biliary cirrhosis, malignancies, sinusitis, mastoiditis, and occasionally other diseases.

In mild cases, nonsteroidal anti-inflammatory agents can be used for symptomatic treatment, although adrenocorticosteroids are generally needed for acute inflammatory episodes and severe respiratory involvement. There is no evidence that steroids alter the long-term course of the disease. Immunosuppressives have been used with apparent benefit. Dapsone has recently been used with success in several series.

The course is unpredictable. Deaths have occurred from cardiac or respiratory involvement, and aortic valve disease has required surgery. Remissions do occur; some patients have chronic or relapsing disease over many years.

Conn DL, Dickson ER, Carpenter HA: The association of Churg-Strauss vasculitis with temporal artery involvement, primary biliary cirrhosis and polychondritis in a single patient. J Rheum 9:744, 1982. *Vasculitis and other associated diseases are common.*

Ebringer B, Rook G, Swana T, Bottazzo GF, Doniach D: Autoantibodies to cartilage and type II collagen in relapsing polychondritis and other rheumatic diseases. Ann Rheum Dis 40:473, 1981. *Immune mechanisms are described and discussed.*

Martin J, Roenigk HH Jr, Lynch W, et al.: Relapsing polychondritis treated with dapsone. Arch Dermatol 112:1272, 1976. *The interesting beneficial effects of dapsone.*

McAdam LP, O'Hanlan MA, Bluestone R, et al.: Relapsing polychondritis: Prospective study of 23 patients and a review of the literature. Medicine 55:193, 1976. *The best general review.*

Ruhlen JL, Huston KA, Wood WG: Relapsing polychondritis with glomerulonephritis: Improvement with prednisone and cyclophosphamide. JAMA 245:847, 1981. *Renal involvement can occur. Drug therapy can include immunosuppressives.*

Shaul SR, Schumacher HR: Relapsing polychondritis. Electron microscopic studies of ear cartilage. Arthritis Rheum 18:617, 1975. *Pathologic findings and their implications are described and reviewed.*

457. OSTEOARTHRITIS (Degenerative Joint Disease)

David S. Howell

Osteoarthritis (OA) is a complex response of joint tissues to aging and to genetic and environmental factors, characterized by degeneration of cartilage, bony remodelling, and overgrowth of bone. Idiopathic osteoarthritis refers to the common variety encountered during aging that is unrelated to known systemic or local diseases and includes certain hereditary and erosive subsets. *Secondary* osteoarthritis refers to the form indistinguishable from the idiopathic (primary) type on a pathologic basis but clearly provoked by antecedent events, such as an inflammatory, metabolic, endocrine, developmental, or heritable connective tissue disorder (Table 457–1). Effects of a macrotrauma, repeated microtrauma, or prolonged immobilization

TABLE 457–1. ETIOLOGIC CLASSIFICATION OF OSTEOARTHRITIS*

Idiopathic (primary)
Localized
Hands: Heberden's nodes, erosive interphalangeal arthropathy
Feet: hallux valgus, hammer toes; talonavicular osteoarthritis
Knees: medial, lateral, patellofemoral compartments
Hips: sites of cartilage loss—eccentric (superior), concentric (axial, medial), diffuse
Spine: zygoapophyseal joints, osteophytes, intervertebral discs (spondylosis); ligaments, e.g., disseminated idiopathic skeletal hyperostosis
Other single sites: shoulder, temporomandibular, carpometacarpal joints
Generalized—Includes three or more areas listed above (described by Kellgren and Moore)
Mineral deposition diseases
Calcium pyrophosphate deposition disease
Hydroxyapatite arthropathy
Destructive disease (e.g., Milwaukee shoulder)
Secondary
Post-traumatic
Congenital or developmental
Legg-Calvé-Perthes hip dislocation
Epiphyseal dysplasias
Disturbed local tissue structure by primary disease, e.g., ischemic necrosis, tophaceous gout, hyperparathyroid cysts, Paget's disease, rheumatoid arthritis, osteopetrosis, osteochondritis
Miscellaneous additional diseases
Endocrine: diabetes mellitus, acromegaly, hypothyroidism
Metabolic: hemochromatosis, ochronosis, Gaucher's disease
Neuropathic arthropathies
Miscellaneous: frostbite, Kashin-Beck disease, caisson's disease
Mechanical: obesity, unequal lower extremity length; valgus/varus deformities, ligamentous laxity

*Compiled by Osteoarthritis Diagnostic Criteria Committee. American Rheumatism Association, 1983.

on normal joints may dispose the joints to secondary osteoarthritis.

When bony hypertrophy estimated by roentgenographic changes is used as a criterion, the majority of the population over 50 years of age is afflicted with osteoarthritis. By the eighth decade there is evidence of disease in 90 per cent of persons. It is the leading cause of joint pain and related disablements in middle-aged and elderly patients.

PATHOLOGY. Minor cartilage softening in non–weight-bearing sites and hypertrophic bony changes may persist a lifetime without producing symptoms. Osteoarthritis depends on development of progressively deepening clefts and erosions typically in weight-bearing sites. The disease advances over a period of years but rarely reaches the level of severity seen in rheumatoid arthritis, i.e., there is rarely joint fusion or pannus formation, and major subluxations are uncommon.

The earliest histologic changes may be documented in the surface, subsurface, and deep zones of articular cartilage. These changes include loss of staining reactions for proteoglycans, with areas of cell injury, or loss followed by proliferation. On electron microscopic views, lipid accumulations, reduced cartilage collagen fibril size, edema, and surface irregularities are found. Clefts, microcysts, and erosions arise at the site of these changes. Aggressive lesions consist usually of vertical clefts in cartilage, which progress to deep erosions and exposure of subchondral bone. Bony thickening, eburnation, cysts, and bone-on-bone contact across the joint surface typifies end-stage disease.

ETIOLOGY. The most accepted premise is that primary changes in articular cartilage underlie development of osteoarthritis. Nevertheless, in a substantial subset of patients, biomechanical deficiencies arising from dysplasias of major or minor nature are causative. Similar biomechanical deficiencies may arise related to adolescent and adult remodelling of bones and abnormal distribution of weight-bearing forces (Table 457–1).

Repeated industrial or sports-invoked macro- and microtraumatic events may produce excessive wear and hypertrophic remodelling responses. Evidence has been obtained for reduced biomaterial properties of cartilage as a function of aging and for possible metabolic disturbances in cartilage metabolism, as in diabetes mellitus, acromegaly, and ochronosis.

The subchondral bone table is disturbed by tissue remodelling early in the disease or by such afflictions as Paget's disease or hyperparathyroidism with subchondral cysts. Hyperlaxity of ligaments per se or as part of certain overt (heritable) disorders of connective tissue can lead to osteoarthritis.

PATHOGENESIS. As a result of a multiplicity of etiologic factors, an apparent final common pathway of disease expression involves breakdown of cartilage both by direct physical injury and enzymatic degradation resulting from injury to chondrocytes and indirectly by subchondral bone stiffening from remodelling. Most important in this context is injury of the collagen network or framework that holds together articular cartilage. This network retains in a semi-dehydrated conformed state the abundant, intensely hydrophobic, charged, proteoglycan macromolecules. The latter exert an osmotic pressure of several atmospheres against the network. Ungluing or cleavage of the collagen network by maldistributed or excessive weight-bearing forces, or degradation of the network by enzymes elaborated by injured cartilage cells may occur. This response to various precipitating events leads to loss of essential elastic properties.

In early osteoarthritis, repair responses by local chondrocytes are usually of a poor quality, leading to almost no replacement of lost tissue. From advanced erosions penetrating the marrow, tissue repair is more effective and consists of mixtures of fibro- and hyaline cartilage. Normal rugged biomaterial properties are never recovered by the repair cartilage. As degeneration proceeds, wear particles break off from both original and repair cartilages. These fragments are carried to the synovial lining membrane where a phagocytic response engenders low-grade inflammation and synovial effusion, proliferation of synovial cells, and thickening of the synovial membranes. In some cases, it is speculated that membrane-engendered inflammatory factors may then amplify cartilage breakdown.

Several biochemical abnormalities have been noted in osteoarthritic cartilage: increased water content, decreased aggregation and content of proteoglycans, decreased chain length and altered profiles of glycosaminoglycans, and increased proteolytic enzyme levels.

CLINICAL MANIFESTATIONS. The clinical presentation may be divided into early and late stages. Throughout these stages, there is deep, aching pain in the afflicted joints, morning stiffness of short duration, and variable joint thickening and effusion. Early stages are dominated by pain on motion with stiffness, night pain, and responsiveness to anti-inflammatory medication. The late stages are dominated by joint instability, predominance of pain at rest accentuated on weight-bearing, and failure of responsiveness to anti-inflammatory agents. The present description of clinical features is developed largely on an anatomic basis inasmuch as signs and symptoms reflect regional patterns of involvement. Roentgenographic and laboratory workup and treatment are discussed later.

Hands. Heberden's nodes refer to the osteoarthritic disfigurements of distal interphalangeal joints, and Bouchard's nodes signify equivalent lesions of the proximal interphalangeal joints of the hands (Fig. 457–1). Early Heberden's nodes have a soft consistency and may be associated with prominent inflammatory signs. In the chronic stage, they are characterized by bony enlargement and angular deformities with variable symptom-

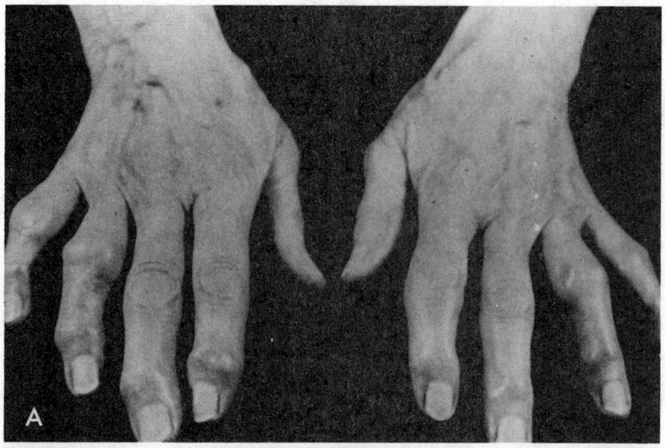

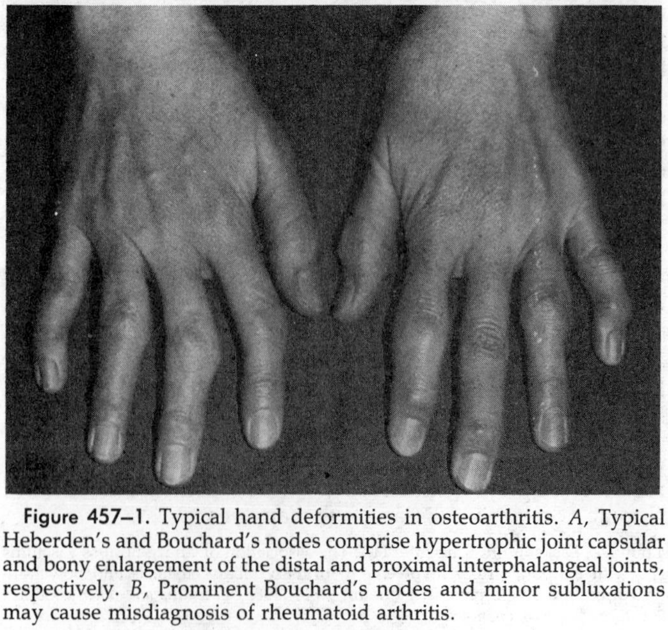

Figure 457–1. Typical hand deformities in osteoarthritis. *A,* Typical Heberden's and Bouchard's nodes comprise hypertrophic joint capsular and bony enlargement of the distal and proximal interphalangeal joints, respectively. *B,* Prominent Bouchard's nodes and minor subluxations may cause misdiagnosis of rheumatoid arthritis.

atology. Heredity and sex, in addition to microtrauma, are prominently involved in the development of Heberden's nodes, which are more common in women at menopause or late middle age. The only other common hand lesion involves the first carpometacarpal joint. Such lesions are associated with pain in the radial side of the wrist, intensified by physical activities such as golf, tennis, and knitting.

Knees. The commonest source of major disability in osteoarthritis is from knee involvement. At any one time, heat, synovial thickening, or effusions have been documented in at least 50 per cent of cases. Elicitation of crepitus, which persists on repeated flexion and extension of the knee, bony marginal overgrowth, mediolateral instability (in the late stages), and synovial effusion are important diagnostic aids. Degenerative changes are usually more prominent in the medial compartment of the knee, leading to varus (bowleg) deformities. Developmental defects, i.e., knock knee or bowleg deformity, predispose to OA.

Degenerative alteration of the patellofemoral joint is termed chondromalacia patellae. This syndrome of mild effusion and knee pain is usually associated with trauma and occurs predominantly in young adults. It is usually preceded by developmental biomechanical disturbances influencing knee flexion. There is often spontaneous remission of symptoms, but some cases progress to irreversible patellofemoral osteoarthritis.

Malum Coxae Senilis (Coxarthrosis). Clinical manifestations of primary hip joint disease appear usually in late middle or old age. Perhaps one third or more of cases arise from acetabular dysplasia, as well as growth or maturational disturbances in the femoral neck and head. Altered bone growth as well as developmental thickening at the zenith of the acetabulum may be causative in less than 5 per cent of cases. Beyond these factors, there is a background of adult bone remodelling and altered joint incongruity, which may further compromise normal weight-bearing patterns and chondrocyte nutrition. In addition, a variety of acquired disorders such as rheumatoid arthritis and ischemic necrosis of the femoral head are important etiologically.

Groin pain on weight-bearing or motion is a dominant symptom and is usually referred to the anterior aspect of the thigh above the knee. Over a period of months or a few years, invalidism from severely restricted mobility and pain is a common outcome of untreated disease.

Spinal Osteoarthritis (Including Herniated Disc Syndrome). Throughout the spine, weight-bearing compressive forces are largely supported by one set of articulations—the intervertebral discs. These are elastic organs similar to articular cartilage in respect to the fact that they depend on properties of the semidehydrated proteoglycan molecules. A high osmotic pressure at rest results from proteoglycan confinement by cartilage endplates in two dimensions and the annulus fibrosis in the third. An additional important elastic component is provided by the annulus fibrosis. Rotary motions in the back and neck depend upon the zygoapophyseal joints. All of these joints undergo osteoarthritic changes almost identical in nature to those of the peripheral joints (see Ch. 459 for specific clinical features). Ordinarily, the former joints protect the latter against severe torsional trauma; under certain conditions, especially flexion of the lumbosacral spine, the rotary joints are of much less protectional value, and annular tears may occur under these (and several other) conditions. Resultant displacement of discal products into the spinal foramen adjacent to nerve rootlets and/or spinal canal occurs, depending on the conditions of damage. Injury of these structures both by mechanical trauma and activated inflammatory pathways comprises one of several causes of neural dysfunction leading to symptoms. The relationship of the posterior zygoapophyseal joints in the cervical, thoracic, and lumbar spines to their respective nerve roots as they traverse the intervertebral foramina, and the proximity of an additional set of *joints of Luschka* in the cervical spine (segment C2 to C7) have similar importance because of potential damage to nerves by inflammation secondary to mechanical irritation.

Notably, symptoms of osteoarthritis in the cervical spine depend upon the neural segment involved. Pain, aggravated by motion, often radiates into the supraclavicular and upper trapezius regions, as well as the occiput and distal upper extremities. Overgrowth of bone in either the cervical or lumbar spine can cause narrowing of the spinal canal and encroachment on the spinal cord rather than the nerve roots. In the neck, a myelopathy of a painless nature may result. Constriction of the spinal cord by surrounding bone, disc, or ligamentous thickening, leads to the syndrome of spinal stenosis most common in the lumbosacral spine. Neurogenic claudication pain (resembling vascular claudication) is an important symptom in this condition and must be differentiated from vascular insufficiency (see Ch. 459 for management of discogenic claudication).

Diffuse Idiopathic Skeletal Hyperostosis. This is characterized by a flowing ligamentous calcification along the anterolateral aspects of vertebral bodies. There is usually only minor symptomatology, and the thoracic spine is most often affected without intervertebral disc narrowing.

LABORATORY FINDINGS. There are no specific abnormalities in osteoarthritis. The sedimentation rate is usually within normal limits, synovial fluid is clear and exhibits a normal range of viscosity, and there is a negative mucin clot test result. Leukocyte counts in synovial fluid generally vary from 150 to 1500 per cu mm; wear particles including whole fragments containing proteoglycans and collagen fibers as well as mineral particles are often identified in the fluid.

ROENTGENOGRAPHIC FEATURES. There is usually narrowing of the radiolucent interosseous joint space resulting from destruction of articular cartilage. Bony cysts varying in size may be seen in subchondral or denuded bone, which may be densely sclerotic. Osteophyte formation at the margins of affected joints is the basis for the most striking roentgenographic findings. Degeneration of lumbar and cervical intervertebral discs results in narrowing of the interspaces. A vacuum sign or marked translucency in the disc may be seen. Evidence for disc degeneration is usually documented in anteroposterior and lateral roentgenograms. For visualization of osteophytes blocking foramina, particularly in the cervical spine, oblique views are mandatory. Oblique views are also valuable for defining bony sclerosis and joint-space narrowing of the zygoapophyseal joints of the lumbar spine.

DIFFERENTIAL DIAGNOSIS. Osteoarthritis and rheumatoid arthritis are readily distinguished in terms of their usual clinical presentation. The latter is generally associated with prominent signs of joint inflammation, characteristically afflicting the hands and wrists symmetrically, especially the metacarpophalangeal joints. These joints almost never are affected in osteoarthritis.

Differentiation of these disorders is more complicated when seronegative rheumatoid arthritis involves only (or predominantly) the lower extremities. The presence of a normal erythrocyte sedimentation rate, negative serum rheumatoid factor test result, and minimal synovial fluid change support the diagnosis of osteoarthritis. Despite severe deformities, occasionally seen with Heberden's and Bouchard's nodes, the lack of ulnar drift and metacarpophalangeal and diffuse wrist involvement help to rule out rheumatoid arthritis. Erosive osteoarthritis characteristically shows bony destruction and inflammatory changes in the proximal and distal interphalangeal joints but not in the metacarpophalangeal joints.

Secondary osteoarthritis must be considered in the presence of joint hypermobility, chondrocalcinosis, heritable disorders such as the Ehlers-Danlos syndrome, mechanical derangements of the joints, metabolic bone disorders, ochronosis, neuropathies, and hemochromatosis. Spinal involvement in osteoarthritis is distinctly different from that in ankylosing spondylitis; the latter predominantly afflicts young men and has characteristic and distinctive roentgenographic features involving sacroiliac sclerosis and fusion, calcification and ossification of the annulus fibrosus and adjacent paravertebral ligaments, and formation of bridging syndesmophytes (bamboo spine).

TREATMENT. Although treatment depends in large measure on the site and severity of joint involvement, the outlook with a multidisciplinary long-term management program is relatively optimistic for functional restoration and symptomatic improvement.

Early disease with signs of mild to moderate inflammation but without joint instability can usually be managed successfully with a combination of measures: (1) Relief of pain with mild analgesics (e.g., acetaminophen 500 mg three or four times a day) or nonsteroidal anti-inflammatory agents (e.g., aspirin 2400 to 3600 mg daily) or both. Indomethacin, ibuprofen, naproxen, fenoprofen, and tolmetin are alternative agents, advantageous as substitutes for aspirin. Where possible, intermittent rather than continuous usage is encouraged to avoid gastrointestinal side effects, especially acid peptic disease; (2) Revision of daily schedule of activities, increased joint rest, and selected avoidance of activities unfavorable to the symptomatic joints; (3) Protection of joints with relevant devices, i.e., splints, crutches, walkers, canes, etc.; (4) Use of weight-reducing diets; (5) Diazepam, 5 mg three to four times daily or another suitable agent may be used sparingly for acute episodes of muscle spasm; (6) Application of moist heat or cold packs may help; (7) Symptomatic response, in refractory cases, to intra-articular or para-articular injections of small amounts of corticosteroid at infrequent intervals is useful; (8) Once pain and muscle spasm have been relieved, a formalized program of physical therapy followed by a prolonged home exercise program is often recommended in the hope of retarding further joint deterioration.

In the case of cervical osteoarthritis, hyperextension and hyperflexion should be avoided. The patient should sleep flat on one pillow and employ intermittent traction devices available for home use. A cervical collar restricts motion and minimizes pain (see Ch. 459 for treatment of osteoarthritis in the lumbar spine).

The principal anatomic regions that are most benefited by orthopedic surgery are the knee, hip, and spine. Several surgical procedures are appropriate for patients with severe hip involvement, including osteotomy, mold arthroplasty, total joint replacement, and arthrodesis. For the knee, debridement, either through an arthroscope or via open surgery, osteotomy, and a variety of partial or complete arthroplasties are used for treatment. Tibial or femoral osteotomies may be of long-term benefit by realigning weight-bearing forces, but considerable follow-up rehabilitation is required. Otherwise, joint replacement is the treatment of choice for many cases of advanced osteoarthritis of the knees characterized by intractable pain, loss of function, instability, or all three. Some indications for spinal surgery are: (1) advancing intractable nerve deficits, (2) spinal instability, and (3) spinal stenosis affecting bladder or rectal function because of autonomic nerve involvement.

Bland JH, Cooper S: Osteoarthritis: A review of the cell biology involved and evidence for reversibility; management rationally related to known genesis and pathophysiology. Semin Arthritis Rheum. In press. *Emphasis is on practical management as influenced by cell biology, physiology, and what is known concerning etiology and pathogenesis.*

Howell DS, Talbott JH: Osteoarthritis symposium. Semin Arthritis Rheum 11:1, 1981. *Studies of fundamental and clinical nature relating to inflammatory components of osteoarthritis. For those not daunted by scientific data.*

McCarty DJ (ed.): Arthritis and Allied Disorders. Osteoarthritis, Section IX. Philadelphia, Lea and Febiger, 1979, pp 1135–1189. *A useful reference with chapters amplifying all topics discussed in this chapter, but not at a level too burdensome for the internist.*

458. THE PAINFUL SHOULDER

David S. Howell

Shoulder pain is a common source of incapacitation and can result from numerous causes. Intrathoracic, diaphragmatic, and cervical pathologic lesions all can cause pain referred to the shoulder, a fact that deserves early consideration and strong emphasis. A characteristic of intrinsic painful disorders is that they often originate in periarticular soft structures—synovial membranes, tendons, and associated muscles. These structures have a unique role in joint stabilization. Loading forces are attenuated by the action of muscles across the coordinated bearings—glenohumeral, acromioclavicular, and sternoclavicular joints—as well as across the scapulothoracic surfaces. Multiple bursae and tendons near their attachment sites, particularly the rotator cuff tendons, are subject to microinjury and inflammation. Secondary recurrent pain and muscle spasm occur, followed by atrophic or reflex dystrophic responses or both. The most common disorders afflicting these structures are briefly reviewed in this chapter.

CALCIFIC TENDINITIS. A frequently encountered cause of painful shoulder is focal injury or degeneration of the rotator cuff tendons. Roentgenograms reveal calcium-containing minerals in the tendons of the rotator cuff in roughly 3 per cent of middle-aged persons, usually from prior insults. Mineral deposits in tendinous sites may engender bursal inflammation of variable intensity. Acute shoulder pain with radiation into the upper arm and neck is common. Associated muscle hypertonicity with limitation of shoulder motion and guarding, exquisite local tenderness over the inflamed site, and pain on motion or during prolonged rest are prominent. Most often roentgenograms show linear densities in the supraspinatus, infraspinatus, or subscapularis tendons. Occasionally, a diffuse calcific pattern in the subacromial bursa is seen. Evidence of acute inflammation usually subsides within one week, but subacute rotator cuff tendinitis may persist or recur for months to years.

Management is conditioned by the duration and intensity of attacks. Adequate early pain relief is of paramount importance and is usually attainable by use of moist heat or ice compresses, rest, including arm support, analgesics, and a nonsteroidal anti-inflammatory agent. Newer agents are discussed in Ch. 444. In most patients, pain and muscle spasm subside with variable reduction of mineral deposits. Injection of an adrenocorticosteroid derivative commonly hastens symptomatic recovery.

Follow-up evaluation is important to assess completeness of recovery. Residual loss of strength or joint motion or chronic pain deserves a conscientious program of active exercises, including both supervised therapy in a physical medicine facility and a home program of daily exercise. Long-term physical therapy or surgical excision of mineral deposits is seldom necessary.

BICIPITAL TENDINITIS. Inflammation of this tendon and synovial sheath is a frequent cause of shoulder pain. The tendon through attrition may subluxate from the bicipital groove or rupture. Localized tenderness on palpation with accentuation of pain by flexion or extension of the elbow against resistance or by internal rotation and abduction distinguishes the diagnosis clinically.

Treatment includes moist heat or ice compresses, rest, and nonsteroidal anti-inflammatory agents in the acute stages, and frequently the instillation of corticosteroids. Chronic recurrent disease is suggestive of the aforementioned mechanical derangements or an additional rotator cuff tear. Surgical transfer of the tendon may lead to satisfactory recovery.

ROTATOR CUFF TEARS. After heavy work, sports, or accidental injury, degenerative lesions in the rotator cuff often engender breakdown with moderate to major tendinous and ligamentous tears, predominantly in middle-aged persons. Complete rupture of the rotator cuff renders the arm incapable of abduction to 90 degrees. With mild tears, there is pain between 60 and 90 degrees abduction. Either preceding or following these tears, an impingement syndrome frequently occurs at the coracoacromial arch. Often this is associated radiographically with cysts or sclerosis of the greater tuberosity of the humerus, osteophytes at the anterior margin of the acromion, and narrowing of the distance between the humeral head and acromion. These changes are related to trauma from impingement of the aforementioned bones. Since the rotator cuff forms, in part, the roof of the glenohumeral joint and floor of the subacromial and subdeltoid bursae, tears in the cuff permit synovial joint fluid extrusion into these bursae—demonstrable by arthrogram.

Primary treatment of rotator cuff tears consists of heat and aspirin, 2.4 to 3.6 gm per day, or other nonsteroidal anti-inflammatory agents such as ibuprofen, 1200 to 2400 mg per day. Partial immobilization and exercise programs are indicated for incomplete tears. When these measures fail, surgical repair is often required.

ADHESIVE CAPSULITIS. This (frozen shoulder) disability of middle-aged persons develops more commonly in women than in men and is of unknown etiology. The diagnosis is suspected when persons with no primary shoulder disease develop active and passive restricted motion of the glenohumeral joint attended by increasing pain in the shoulder over a period of weeks to months, and it is more certain when an arthrogram shows a contracted joint capsule. Fibrosis is seen on pathologic study. Rotator cuff tears, hemarthroses, anterior shoulder capsule tear, psychophysiologic shoulder dysfunction, and shoulder-hand syndrome can all cause immobile painful shoulders and may be confused with adhesive capsulitis.

The key feature of management is prevention of severe pain through early use of heat, analgesics, range of motion exercises, and, if these are unsuccessful, the judicious use of intra-articular or systemic corticosteroids.

Manipulation mobilization under general anesthesia followed by a course of intensive physical therapy rarely is required for advanced disease.

SHOULDER-HAND SYNDROME. Shoulder pain and stiffness concurrent with pain, swelling, and vasomotor changes in the hands, wrists, and arms of various intensity and duration characterize this syndrome. Thickening of the skin and edema may follow, resembling Sudeck's atrophy. A small per cent of cases eventually develop adhesive capsulitis and sclerodactyly. This syndrome, which affects patients over age 50 years and follows acute severe illness such as cerebral vascular accident, myocardial infarction, and trauma to the distal upper extremity, is believed to be caused by reflex sympathetic stimulation. Associated changes of cervical osteoarthritis probably have a minor role if any. When the disease is bilateral, the differentiation from acute rheumatoid arthritis or polymyalgia rheumatica may be difficult. The most important feature of treatment is aggressive physical therapy assisted by analgesics and prednisone in a short moderate dosage trial of 20 to 30 mg per day for three weeks, tapered at the end of the course. Stellate ganglion blocks and local corticosteroid injections are sometimes employed.

AMYLOID ARTHROPATHY. In two thirds of patients, there is shoulder involvement usually secondary to myeloma. There is para-articular infiltration with amorphous amyloid fibers causing the "shoulder pad sign." Acute inflammatory signs are usually absent (see Ch. 210).

ISCHEMIC NECROSIS. This disease is half as common in the humeral head as in the hip. Diffuse shoulder pain precedes conventional radiologic changes, the most helpful of which is an irregular translucent band localized in subchondral bone.

POLYMYALGIA RHEUMATICA. This syndrome is often characterized by severely painful shoulders and upper arms in aged persons with anemia, high sedimentation rates, and negative rheumatoid factor test, and in a small percentage of cases temporal arteritis and retinal ischemia threatening to vision (see Ch. 548). Dramatic response of shoulder pain to low-dose corticosteroid administration (prednisone 10 mg per day) is characteristic.

MILWAUKEE SHOULDER. This syndrome consists of a painful, destructive, bilateral arthropathy in middle-aged and elderly patients with capsular calcification, joint effusions, and a high frequency of eroded rotator cuff tendons. Synovial fluids are virtually free of inflammatory cells despite a reported high collagenase activity.

Kozin F: Painful shoulder and the reflex sympathetic dystrophy syndrome. *In* McCarty DJ (ed.): Arthritis and Allied Conditions. Philadelphia, Lea and Febiger, 1979, pp 1091–1120. *An extremely concentrated and detailed coverage, especially useful as a reference for differential diagnosis.*

Post M: The painful shoulder. Clin Orthop 173:2, 1983. *A symposium by multiple authors on various clinically important syndromes and discussion of current management.*

459. THE PAINFUL BACK

David S. Howell

Among degenerative disease, low back pain is the leading cause of industrial absenteeism and chronic disablement in some studies. The back is a complex structure serving weight-bearing and locomotor functions. It provides for major support of body structures and transmission of loading forces through the sacroiliac joints to the lower limbs. The fundamental functioning unit is an articular triad composed of two zygoapophyseal joints posteriorly and the intervertebral disc anteriorly. The disc is comprised of a nucleus pulposus encompassed by the annulus fibrosis. These structures are arranged in a series and stabilized throughout the spine by ligaments. The spinal bones also encase the spinal cord and the cauda equina, and through successive foramina rootlets connect the spinal cord with peripheral neural pathways (see Ch. 457 for detailed discussion of the cervical spine and Ch. 445 for the Spondyloarthropathies).

ETIOLOGY OF BACK PAIN. In Table 459–1, the numerous causes of back pain are displayed according to disease subgroups. Although all vertebral levels can be affected, pain

TABLE 459–1. ETIOLOGY OF BACK PAIN

- Mechanical or Traumatic
  - Paraspinal ligaments and musculature
    - Myofascial syndrome, sacroiliac strain
  - Spondylogenic
    - Osteoarthritis-related lesions-zygoapophyseal joints
    - Degenerative lesions—intervertebral discs
    - Mechanical insufficiency, congenital and acquired, of ligaments and bones
    - Spondylolisthesis
    - Spinal stenosis
    - Fractures
- Metabolic
  - Vertebral bodies, partial collapse and distortion—osteoporosis; osteomalacia—Paget's disease—often with secondary osteoarthritis
- Tumors
  - Neural tumors, osteosarcoma, metastatic tumors, e.g., from breast, thyroid, kidney
  - Myeloma, lymphoma, leukemia
- Systemic Inflammatory Disease
  - Spondylitis (ankylosing)—Reiter's disease; psoriatic or enteropathic arthropathy
  - Disseminated ankylosing skeletal hyperostosis
- Infections
  - Pyogenic, fungal, tuberculous disc infection, *Herpes zoster* infection, paraspinal abscesses
- Referred Pain
  - Vascular—aneurysms, sclerosis of aorta and branches
  - Tumors or inflammation of pleural, pulmonary, pericardial, cardiac, or neck origin
  - Viscerogenic disease of gallbladder, pancreas, stomach, intestines, kidneys, ureters, bladder, prostate, uterus
  - Pelvis or retroperitoneal tumors or inflammation
- Non-Organic Components
  - Hysterical conversion
  - Learned painful behavior
  - Psychosis
  - Litigation neurosis, malingering
  - Chronic pain syndrome
  - Substance abuse

in the low back is most prevalent. The majority of patients present with problems relating to functional or mechanical disturbances, and these must be distinguished from a wide variety of diseases either of focal origin or referred from multiple organ systems.

MEDICAL HISTORY. *Sex.* Compression vertebral fractures from osteoporosis have their highest prevalence in postmenopausal women. Gynecologic pathology such as endometriosis is the basis for some referred patterns of back pain. Reiter's disease, ankylosing spondylitis, and back injuries are found more commonly in males.

Age. Young people with back pain most commonly suffer with congenital abnormalities, injury, spondyloarthropathies, and herniated disc syndromes. In middle and old age, osteoporosis, vertebral collapse, degenerative states, including spinal stenosis, and malignant lesions are common.

Family History. Familial patterns of segregation are often detected in respect to spondyloarthropathies and uncommonly in respect to spinal degenerative conditions.

Nature of Pain. A review of events or conditions that accelerate or retard symptoms should be gathered. The chronic inflammatory diseases (spondyloarthropathies) are associated with increased pain and stiffness on inactivity. Patients with lumbar disc protrusion and radicular pain generally are relieved by lying flat with the knees flexed and are uncomfortable sitting. Sudden or acute onset of symptoms is suggestive of a mechanical or infectious origin of symptoms respectively. Constitutional symptoms such as fever, weight loss, and fatigue are important clues to infectious, inflammatory, or neoplastic disorders.

In regard to localization, the dorsal segment suggests osteoarthritis, vertebral fracture, neoplasm, herpetic radiculitis, or referred pain from the viscera (see later paragraph). Localization of pain in the low back is usually of little help in regard to differential diagnosis.

Claudication-type pain, with onset after sustained walking, suggests either spinal stenosis or arterial insufficiency. The former condition often refers pain to the thigh and is poorly relieved by standing still. Usually neurogenic claudication is relieved by sitting, whereas vascular claudication is reduced by standing.

Referred Pain. A deep aching pain referred to various sites in the upper and midback may be engendered by lesions in the upper gastrointestinal tract. Pain of malignancy (whether local or referred) is typically severe and unrelieved by change of position or mild analgesics.

In respect to neuropathic symptoms, alteration of the structure of the vertebral foramina may lead to radicular dissemination of pain. In such instances, compression or traction of nerve rootlets or extension of inflammation to them can lead to sensory and motor nerve symptoms and signs, i.e., paresthesias, hypoesthesias, and muscle weakness.

Symptomatology. Discogenic pain is characteristically aggravated by cough or sneeze. Rarely, loss of bowel or urinary sphincter function can result from cord compression or bilateral involvement of sacral nerve roots from spinal stenosis, tumors, or infectious lesions.

PHYSICAL EXAMINATION. General examination of the back is discussed in Ch. 440. Descriptions here are confined to vertebral compression fractures, degenerative disc disease, and lumbosacral strains and sprains.

Lumbosacral Strain. This and related myofascial syndromes are the most common ailment seen in office practice. A history of injury is often followed by prompt or delayed low-back pain. Transient disc prolapse, subluxation of facet joints, and injury to muscles or ligaments are diagnostic considerations. Physical signs are usually limited to paravertebral muscle spasm, tenderness, and restricted lower back motion without evidence of nerve root involvement.

Vertebral Compression Fractures. These are the most common complication of osteoporosis with resultant traction or compression of rootlets adjacent to collapsed vertebrae. Sudden onset of severe pain associated with the postural strain of lifting heavy objects or hyperflexing the trunk is found. Major physical findings consist of localized tenderness and muscle spasm related to the level of the nerve roots affected. Poorly localized back pain may be associated with osteoporosis in the absence of vertebral collapse. Metastatic tumor, myeloma, and metabolic bone disease, especially osteopenia of aging, are common underlying conditions.

Discogenic Disease. The commonest form of low back pain with radiculitis is associated with prolapse, protrusion, or extrusion of intervertebral disc substance. Usually the onset of acute symptoms is preceded by chronic intermittent low-back pain, although a discrete injury may precipitate an attack. Ninety per cent of disc herniations are localized at L4–L5 or L5–S1 levels. A proprioceptive neuromuscular disturbance may engender a fixed forward flexion or lateral list of the spine. Discs involving the L4 nerve root or above may cause pain referred along the course of the femoral nerve with hip extension and knee flexion. Knee extension may be weak and the patellar reflex reduced or absent. Patients with L5 nerve root disturbance complain of classic sciatic distribution of pain, i.e., radiating to the posterior thigh and the anteromedial leg and foot, in association with weakness of the toe extensors. First sacral radiculopathy is associated with pain over the posterior thigh, calf, and heel, weakness of the ankle and toe flexors, and reduced or absent achilles tendon reflex. Frequently, loss of neurologic function is subtle and requires repeated testing to document. A positive response to straight leg-raising is most frequently indicative of L4–L5 or L5–S1 disc protrusion. Usually there is elicitation of pain on hip flexion with the knee extended and absence of pain on repetition of hip flexion with the knee flexed (positive Lasègue's sign). The cauda equina syndrome is a form of spinal stenosis and is an uncommon but an important complication of massive disc prolapse. In the cauda equina syndrome, central midline disc displacement causes paralysis of the sacral root with bladder and bowel dysfunction. It is characterized by severe bilateral leg pain, urinary retention, weakness of the anal sphincter, and bilateral nerve root abnormalities. Once complete neurologic block has occurred, deceptively pain is often alleviated, and the patient will require a neurologic examination to verify the need for emergency surgery.

Spondylolisthesis. This term, which refers to forward displacement of one vertebra on another, commonly involves the L4–L5 and L5–S1 levels. Bursts of segmental severe girdle pain are typical, often worse on activity and relieved by rest.

LABORATORY PROCEDURES. Tests performed are dictated by the results of medical history and physical examination. Simple x-rays of the back may suffice if a traumatic injury is causative. In instances of suspected metabolic disturbance, appropriate screening tests such as serum calcium, phosphorus, and alkaline phosphatase measurements should be obtained. Complete blood counts, sedimentation rate, urinalysis, and automated serum chemical profiles are sometimes justified to clarify the diagnosis. Anemia and an elevated sedimentation rate should prompt a more extensive search for infectious, inflammatory, and neoplastic diseases.

X-RAY STUDIES. *Routine X-ray Studies.* These include frontal, lateral, and oblique films of the lumbosacral spine, which can demonstrate foraminal encroachment, compression fractures, degenerative changes, and subluxation of zygoapophyseal joints, as well as interspace narrowing (see Ch. 457). There may be severe degenerative changes by x-rays with few or no relevant symptoms, and severe back pain may occur in the absence of significant radiographic signs and be of discogenic origin.

Additional Imaging Procedures. When surgical intervention is planned or a diagnosis remains questionable and requires an imperative answer and high resolution, cat scans (noninvasive) are increasingly preferred to myelography, although the latter may be necessary. It is not usually necessary to perform a discogram (injection of radiopaque dye directly into the disc). When osteomyelitis or neoplastic involvement is likely, radionuclide bone scans are helpful. A percutaneous vertebral biopsy under fluoroscopic guidance may be performed to establish histopathologic diagnosis or bacteriologic diagnosis at highly suspicious sites obvious from scans or x-rays. Epidural venography scans have become an additional useful tool in precisely delineating sites of discogenic disease. Electromyography can confirm the presence of nerve root deficits.

MANAGEMENT. Conservative therapy for mechanical disorders of the spine and disc herniation focuses on bedrest, analgesics, muscle relaxants, and anti-inflammatory medication. Pelvic traction is also of benefit in some patients. Application of moist heat, e.g., hydrocollator packs wrapped with a wet towel, may relieve pain and muscle spasm. Cyclobenzaprine (10 mg) or diazepam (5 mg) three to four times daily serves as a useful muscle relaxant. The amount of bedrest is dependent on the severity of symptoms. After enforced bedrest for about a two-week period, gradual ambulation and a program of exercises together with back protection including a lumbosacral support are recommended. Most cases of disc herniation respond to conservative therapy; those unresponsive require further measures, including intrathecal and epidural steroids, nerve root or sleeve infiltrations with steroids, and injections of chymopapain into the disc space. This latter treatment is now approved for general use by the FDA. Before surgery is indicated, a psychological assessment, a thorough program of muscle relaxants, and exercises emphasizing back stretching and abdominal strengthening should be attempted.

Progressive muscular weakness and progressive neurologic deficit despite bedrest and other aforementioned measures, as well as the cauda equina syndrome, are indications for surgery. Relative indications for laminectomy are severe pain, unrelieved by bedrest, and recurrent episodes of incapacitating pain. Ninety to ninety-five per cent improvement following surgery is anticipated, although 70 per cent of patients experience relief of pain whether or not the disc is removed.

Following either conservative therapy or laminectomy, a program of prophylactic management thereafter includes postural education, performance of daily exercise program to strengthen the lumbar and abdominal muscles, and avoidance of lower spine stress. Besides laminectomy, joint fusion for spondylolisthesis and discogenic disease or unroofing procedures for spinal stenosis are sometimes necessary. Myelography or cat scans are indicated preoperatively to establish definitively the nature and extent of disease as well as the level of vertebral involvement.

Acute symptoms from compression fractures require appropriate rest and relief of pain with analgesics. Activities must be selected to avoid additional compression fractures. (See Ch. 249 for management of osteoporosis.)

Brown MD (ed.): Intradiscal Therapy: Chymopapain or Collagenase. Chicago, Year Book Medical Publishers, Inc, 1983. *Clinical research results on an important alternative procedure to laminectomy. Results are cautiously interpreted.*

Lipson SJ: Low back pain. *In* Kelley WN, Harris ED Jr, Ruddy S, Sledge CB (eds.): Textbook of Rheumatology. Philadelphia, W. B. Saunders Company, 1981, pp 451–471. *A useful reference; concisely written orthopedic diagnostic and therapeutic steps.*

MacNab I: Backache. Baltimore, Williams & Wilkins Company, 1977. *This monograph reviews practical aspects of diagnosis and management of backache. Excellent philosophic concepts and relevant classification of backache by a pioneer innovator in orthopedic surgery.*

Quinet RJ, Hadler NM: Diagnosis and treatment of backache. Semin Arthritis Rheum 8:261, 1979. *Detailed exposition of diagnosis and management tailored for the internist.*

460. DISEASES WITH WHICH ARTHRITIS IS FREQUENTLY ASSOCIATED

Giles G. Bole

Arthritis can be a significant feature of each of the diseases discussed in this chapter. Description of the disorder is brief and limited to the rheumatic manifestations of the disease.

More detailed discussion of each entity is found in other chapters devoted to these diseases.

SARCOIDOSIS

The most common rheumatic manifestation of sarcoidosis is an acute, symmetric polyarthritis associated with erythema nodosum and hilar adenopathy (Löfgren's syndrome). The ankles are most frequently involved, followed by the wrists, the proximal interphalangeal joints, and the elbows. Arthritis and the other acute manifestations usually resolve spontaneously within a few weeks without sequelae. Circulating immune complexes and an increased frequency of HLA-B8 are found in these patients. Treatment with salicylates, oral colchicine, or corticosteroids has been symptomatically beneficial in individual cases. Chronic granulomatous sarcoid synovitis is an uncommon form of oligoarthritis that can cause joint destruction. It is less responsive to drug treatment and follows a variable clinical course.

HEMOCHROMATOSIS

Joint involvement has been observed in approximately half of the patients with idiopathic hemochromatosis. Joint swelling with bony enlargement is particularly common in the small joints of the hands, but the wrists, hips, and knees may be affected. The clinical and roentgenographic features resemble osteoarthritis more than they do inflammatory joint disease. There is roentgenographic evidence of narrowing of the joint space with subchondral erosions and sclerosis. Chondrocalcinosis is present in about 50 per cent of patients with arthropathy and may lead to acute episodes of crystal-induced synovitis (see Ch. 485). Management of this arthropathy includes the use of a nonsteroidal anti-inflammatory drug and prosthetic weight-bearing joint replacements in advanced disease.

SICKLE CELL DISEASE AND OTHER HEMOGLOBINOPATHIES

Severe polyarthralgia is a frequent manifestation of the crises of sickle cell disease. Occasionally the pain is accompanied by transient joint effusions. Skeletal abnormalities result from widening of bone marrow spaces and focal sickle cell thrombosis in bone. The most common bony lesion is avascular osteonecrosis of the femoral head; less commonly the humerus and vertebral bodies are involved. This complication is also associated with sickle cell trait, hemoglobin C disease, sickle cell disease, and sickle cell–thalassemia disease. In children, periostitis may result in transient diffuse swelling of the hands and feet (dactylitis). Sickle cell disease is associated with an increased incidence of bacterial arthritis and osteomyelitis, especially those caused by gram-negative organisms. Arthropathy in patients with the thalassemia syndromes is attributed to stress fractures of weakened subchondral bone.

HYPERLIPOPROTEINEMIA

In familial hypercholesterolemia (Type II hyperlipoproteinemia) recurrent episodes of acute migratory polyarthritis occur in homozygous cases. In heterozygous patients achilles tendonitis, monoarthritis, or polyarthritis of brief duration and variable severity can involve both large and small joints. Tendinous xanthomas appear in late stages of this disease. In some individuals with hypertriglyceridemia (Type IV hyperlipoproteinemia) a mild asymmetric oligoarthritis of chronic or recurrent type has been observed. Several of these patients have had periarticular bone cysts identified in joint radiographs. Certain of the reported cases may have occurred in association with familial combined hyperlipidemia, which includes individuals with both of these plasma lipoprotein profiles. Several authors have reported gradual reduction in the severity and frequency of articular symptoms after correction of the plasma lipid abnormalities by appropriate dietary and drug therapy.

HYPOGAMMAGLOBULINEMIA

A polyarthritis, rarely deforming in character, has been observed in as many as one third of patients with congenital or acquired hypogammaglobulinemia. The pattern of joint involvement resembles that of rheumatoid arthritis; in addition, other connective tissue diseases such as systemic lupus erythematosus, systemic sclerosis, and dermatomyositis have been associated with immune deficiency states. A variety of autoimmune phenomena and connective tissue syndromes, including juvenile arthritis, have been observed in patients with selective IgA deficiency. Regression of arthritis has been observed following institution of gamma globulin therapy. (See Ch. 429.)

HYPERPARATHYROIDISM

Patients with hyperparathyroidism are subject to a variety of associated rheumatic disorders that may occur singly or in combination. These include hyperuricemia and gouty arthritis, chondrocalcinosis with episodes of calcium pyrophosphate dihydrate crystal-induced synovitis (CPPD disease), and osteoarthritis resulting from deformation of atrophic subchondral bone. Rheumatic symptoms, particularly those associated with CPPD disease, may be the first manifestations of hyperparathyroidism.

ACROMEGALY

The majority of patients with acromegaly develop an atypical form of osteoarthritis. Increased levels of growth hormone result in hypertrophy of articular cartilage, subchondral bone, and periarticular tissues. Hypermobility of joints, a common manifestation, may contribute to degenerative change. The fingers and knees are most frequently affected. Pathognomonic radiographic features include overgrowth of bone and cartilage. Median nerve entrapment (carpal tunnel syndrome) secondary to wrist synovitis is common.

FAMILIAL MEDITERRANEAN FEVER

Joint involvement is second only to peritonitis as the most common manifestation in this disease. The arthritis is usually monoarticular and acute in onset and most commonly affects the large weight-bearing joints. The articular attacks remit in a few days, and only in a few cases do joint symptoms persist for weeks to months. Arthritis, like other manifestations of this syndrome, is recurrent, but permanent damage to joints other than the hip is rare. (For a more complete discussion, see Ch. 209.)

WHIPPLE'S DISEASE

This disease is now recognized as an unusual host response to a bacterial infection. It is characterized by diarrhea, malabsorption, fever, anemia, increased skin pigmentation, and migratory polyarthralgia or polyarthritis. Permanent joint damage is rare, and the disease is suppressed by chronic antibiotic therapy (see Ch. 103).

461. MISCELLANEOUS FORMS OF ARTHRITIS

Giles G. Bole

NEUROPATHIC JOINT DISEASE (Charcot Joints)

This chronic progressive degenerative arthropathy can be a complication of a variety of neurologic disorders. Impairment of proprioceptive and pain sensations deprives the affected joint of the normal protective reactions that ordinarily modulate the forces of weight bearing and motion. Diabetic neuropathy is now the most common and syphilitic tabes dorsalis the second most common cause of this joint disorder. Syringomyelia, myelomeningocele, and congenital indifference to pain are less frequent causes of neuropathic arthropathy. The basic neurologic lesion determines the distribution of the affected joints. In tabes dorsalis, the knees, hips, ankles, and vertebrae are frequently involved. In diabetic neuropathy, the changes are limited to the distal lower extremities, and in syringomyelia the shoulder and elbow joints are most commonly affected.

Although pain is generally present, discomfort tends to be disproportionately mild relative to the degree of joint destruction. Clinical, pathologic, and roentgenographic features of chronic neuropathic joint disease reflect severe degrees of destruction and disorganization of the involved joints. Synovial fluid is usually noninflammatory, but it can be hemorrhagic and contain destructive debris (fragments of cartilage or bone). In the early stages, the differentiation from other causes of joint derangement depends upon the demonstration of a sensory neuropathy.

Management includes immobilization of affected joints and restriction of weight-bearing activities with crutches, splints, and braces. Surgical arthrodesis, although frequently unsuccessful, is indicated in selected individuals. Total joint replacement has been attempted, but success has been severely limited and most consider this approach contraindicated at the present time.

HEMARTHROSIS

Recurrent or chronic hemarthrosis is the most common complication of a group of heritable disorders of blood coagulation (see Ch. 167). Hemarthrosis can be a complication of anticoagulant therapy or severe trauma to a normal joint.

In hemophilia, joint bleeding usually begins before the age of five and tends to recur repeatedly during childhood in response to even minor injury. The most common sites are the knees, elbows, and ankles, but any joint can be involved.

Acute hemarthrosis usually results in marked local inflammation and joint symptoms that can last for days to weeks. Approximately half of the patients with hemophilia develop chronic deformities in one or more joints. Some of them develop a chronic progressive synovitis, restricted to one or a few joints, which clinically and roentgenographically resembles rheumatoid arthritis. In chronic cases there is marked synovial membrane hyperplasia, destruction of articular cartilage, and erosions of subchondral bone. This chronic progressive pattern probably results from a low level of continuous or intermittent bleeding into involved joints. Joint fluid, in chronic cases, usually contains blood and very high levels of leukocyte-derived proteases. Other musculoskeletal manifestations of hemophilia include bleeding into muscle and bone. The resolution of large hematomas can produce chronic cysts within these tissues.

The first principle in management is to prevent trauma, a goal not easily achieved in children. Acute hemarthrosis should be managed by immobilization, analgesic therapy, and the administration of appropriate plasma concentrates that contain the required coagulation factor. Aspirin and other nonsteroidal analgesics that alter platelet function should be avoided. If there is marked distention of a joint or bursa, aspiration can be accomplished after the defect in coagulation has been corrected. When pain and acute inflammation have subsided, an exercise program to restore joint range of motion should be initiated. For the patient with severe chronic deforming joint disease, the availability of potent plasma concentrates has made it possible to perform synovectomy and arthroplasty in selected instances.

HENOCH-SCHÖNLEIN PURPURA

Polyarthralgia and a nondeforming arthritis, most frequently affecting knees and ankles, are common manifestations of this disorder. Other features include nonthrombocytopenic purpura, abdominal pain, and glomerulonephritis. The syndrome is rare in adults. (For a more detailed discussion see Ch. 166.)

MULTICENTRIC RETICULOHISTIOCYTOSIS (Lipoid Dermatoarthritis)

This rare disorder usually begins in the middle decades of life and affects females three times more frequently than males. It is characterized by the development of multiple histiocytic nodules in the skin and severe polyarthritis that may simulate rheumatoid arthritis. The firm reddish-brown or yellow papular nodules are most commonly found on hands, forearms, head, neck, and chest. Mutilating joint destruction, especially in the interphalangeal joints, occurs in approximately half of the patients with this syndrome. Diagnosis is made by demonstration of histiocytes and multinucleated giant cells, containing PAS-positive material, in skin or synovium. Similar infiltrates have been observed in other organs. Reports of apparent benefit from adrenocorticosteroid or immunosuppressive therapy are difficult to interpret because of the tendency for spontaneous remission in this disorder.

HYPERTROPHIC OSTEOARTHROPATHY

This term refers to a syndrome that includes clubbing of fingers and toes, periostitis at the ends of long bones, arthritis, and in some cases signs of autonomic dysfunction such as flushing, blanching, and profuse sweating of the extremities. The syndrome occurs with a wide variety of underlying disease states. There is a rare hereditary and idiopathic (pachydermoperiostosis) form of this disorder. The fully expressed pattern is usually associated with intrathoracic disease: lung carcinoma, lung abscess, emphysema, bronchiectasis, chronic interstitial pneumonitis, or mesothelioma. Clubbing, usually without periostitis, can be seen with cyanotic heart disease, cystic fibrosis, bacterial endocarditis, biliary cirrhosis, ulcerative colitis, regional enteritis, or thyroid disease.

The distal joints (wrist, elbows, ankles) and long bones of the forearms and legs are most frequently affected. There are inflammatory changes in the periosteum, synovial membrane, and periarticular structures. The periosteum is "lifted" by the deposition of new bone matrix and subsequent mineralization. Clubbing results from edema, cellular infiltration, and connective tissue proliferation in the nailbeds.

Pain, tenderness, and enlargement of the distal portions of extremities may be accompanied by an acute polyarthritis that superficially resembles rheumatoid arthritis. Correct diagnosis of the acute polyarthritis syndrome is established by the recognition of digital clubbing and roentgenographic evidence of periostitis and intrathoracic disease.

The production of a humoral substance that mediates increased vascularity or connective tissue proliferation or both has long been suspected as the pathogenic factor in hypertrophic osteoarthropathy, but no such factor has been demonstrated. Evidence that neural factors are involved is derived from observations of striking resolution of signs and symptoms after denervation of the hilum or vagotomy on the same side as the thoracic lesion. Regression of osteoarthropathy has also been observed after resection of pulmonary neoplasms.

Aside from therapy directed at the associated disease, there is no effective treatment of hypertrophic osteoarthropathy. Symptomatic benefit may be obtained from salicylates, other analgesics, or adrenocorticosteroids.

PALINDROMIC RHEUMATISM AND INTERMITTENT HYDRARTHROSIS

These terms describe two different constellations of clinical findings in which no pathogenic mechanism or mechanisms have been defined and in which the symptoms are often the prodrome of another rheumatic disease. *Palindromic rheumatism* is a term applied to a recurrent pattern of polyarthritis that in individual cases is quite constant. The episodes are usually of brief duration. Many patients eventually develop typical features of rheumatoid arthritis. *Intermittent hydrarthrosis* is typified by recurrent joint effusions usually occurring in young females at menstruation and involving the knee. Like palindromic rheumatism, there is a strong tendency for cases to evolve into rheumatoid arthritis. Diagnostic arthrocentesis is justified in each condition based upon the local joint findings during an acute attack. Since each of the disorders remits spontaneously for variable periods of time, there is no uniform opinion regarding treatment, which is strictly symptomatic.

462. NONARTICULAR RHEUMATISM

Giles G. Bole

This term designates a group of painful disorders resulting from involvement of tendons, bursae, and other periarticular structures. Conditions causing shoulder pain are considered separately in Ch. 458.

BURSITIS

Bursae are closed synovial spaces located at sites of friction between skin, ligaments, tendons, muscles, and bones. Trauma is the most common cause of acute bursitis, but almost any illness characterized by joint synovitis can be associated with inflammation in the lining of bursae. Bursae commonly involved include the following: subdeltoid, trochanteric, olecranon, and prepatellar. Septic or gouty bursitis can be documented by appropriate studies of aspirated fluid. Protection of an inflamed bursa from friction and trauma is the most important aspect of treatment, but moderate doses of salicylates or other nonsteroidal anti-inflammatory drugs can be helpful. Local injection with an adrenocorticosteroid preparation is indicated if symptoms are severe or refractory to other treatment.

TENOSYNOVITIS

Tendon sheaths, like bursae, have synovial linings and can be involved by any process capable of inducing joint synovitis. Transient tenosynovitis in the hand or foot is a frequent manifestation of gonococcemia. Calcific tendinitis, a common source of shoulder pain (see Ch. 458), can be associated with severe inflammation and simulate acute gout. Focal thickening of a tendon sheath and adjacent tendon can result in "locking or trigger" phenomena. This problem, termed stenosing tenosynovitis, is most common in the flexor tendons of the fingers. Involvement of the abductor pollicis longus and extensor pollicis brevis tendons of the thumb (De Quervain's syndrome) produces pain and tenderness at the radial aspect of the wrist. There are few generalizations regarding management, since tenosynovitis can be a manifestation of various disease states, including rheumatoid arthritis and other connective tissue syndromes, infection, crystalline synovitis, or hyperlipidemia. The most common form of tenosynovitis, unassociated with systemic disease, often subsides with rest of the part. If symptoms are severe or recurrent, local injections of adrenocorticosteroid preparations are usually effective. Surgical excision of the affected tendon sheath is indicated for those patients with persistent disability.

TENNIS ELBOW (Epicondylitis)

This common disorder is characterized by pain over the lateral aspect of the elbow. Tenderness is localized at the site of origin of the extensor communis apparatus at the lateral epicondyle. The problem, most common in middle-aged males, is related to sports activities or occupations that involve repetitive wrist extension or pronation-supination. Pain is accentuated by resisted wrist extension. If symptoms fail to respond to rest, local injection of an adrenocorticosteroid preparation is usually successful. An exercise program designed to stretch and strengthen the forearm extensor muscles may also be required.

Medial epicondylitis, sometimes referred to as golfer's elbow, is associated with pain and tenderness over the medial aspect of the elbow, at the site or origin of the wrist flexors. Therapy is similar to that for tennis elbow.

CARPAL TUNNEL SYNDROME

This problem results from entrapment of the median nerve as it passes deep to the transverse carpal ligament at the wrist. Inflammation of the adjacent flexor tendons and their sheaths, the most common basis for median nerve entrapment, can be a feature of rheumatoid or other forms of arthritis; but in most patients the tenosynovitis is localized and unassociated with systemic disease. The syndrome can be seen in endocrine disorders, granulomatous infections, amyloidosis, and pregnancy. The most consistent symptoms are dysesthesia, paresthesia, and hypesthesia in the middle three digits of the hand. Referred pain to the more proximal upper extremity is common. Symptoms are usually intermittent, occurring most frequently during the night. Forced flexion of the wrist or nerve compression locally (Tinel's sign) can induce characteristic symptoms. In a minority of patients, there is progressive wasting of the muscles of the thenar eminence. Conservative management consists of fitting a removable wrist splint and the local injection of an adrenocorticosteroid preparation. Surgical release of the transverse carpal ligament is indicated for patients with persistent disability.

TIETZE'S SYNDROME

This anterior chest wall disorder is characterized by painful enlargement of the upper costal cartilages. It is usually unilateral and limited to a single costochondral juncture. Occasionally the manubriosternal and sternoclavicular joints are affected. The disease may be recurrent, but remission is the rule. If discomfort is severe or recurrent, analgesics, heat, or local infiltration (adrenocorticosteroid or local anesthetic agents) may be beneficial. The condition is distinct from costochondritis, which occurs at multiple sites lower in the anterior rib cage and is unattended by local palpable swelling of a costochondral junction.

FIBROSITIS

This term has been applied to a poorly defined symptom complex that is characterized by pain and stiffness in varying areas, most commonly in the neck, shoulder girdle, and posterior aspect of the trunk. Physical signs except for questionable nodules or thickening of the deep fasciae are lacking, and results of laboratory and roentgenographic studies are normal. Localized areas of tenderness, commonly in the paravertebral areas medial to the scapula, have been termed tender or "trigger points." The syndrome usually begins in the middle years of life and is most common in females. Because the majority of patients appear tense and anxious and have no recognizable objective basis for their symptoms, the syndrome is often considered psychogenic. Patients with fibrositis frequently report difficulty with sleep, and electroencephalographic studies have demonstrated disturbances in slow wave non-REM sleep in some cases. Since pain and stiffness can be manifestations of a variety of musculoskeletal, neurologic, and systemic disorders, the diagnosis of fibrositis requires the exclusion of more specific disease entities. Patient and physician tend to share an unhappy experience in efforts to control symptoms. The results of strong reassurance that serious disease is lacking are variable, as are the results of therapy with salicylates, sedatives, tranquilizers, and muscle relaxants. Some authors favor the use of moderate doses of one of the tricyclic antidepressants to control the patient's reported sleep disturbance and other symptoms.

463. SYNOVIAL TUMORS

Giles G. Bole

Primary malignant tumors of joints are rare. Synovioma is a highly malignant fibroblastic sarcoma which usually originates in the knee or periarticular structures of the thigh. This neoplasm is most common in late childhood or early adult life. The recommended therapy is wide excision (frequently requiring amputation), irradiation, or systemic chemotherapy or all three. Synovial chondrosarcoma is a rare neoplasm that may simulate synovial chondromatosis. It most frequently involves the knee and is slow in producing distant metastases. Radical excision or amputation is the treatment of choice.

Benign tumors arising within joints include lipoma, chondroma, hemangioma, and xanthoma. These neoplasms are rather uncommon and are most frequently found in or about the knee.

Synovial chondromatosis is uncommon. It is characterized by multiple foci or cartilage metaplasia in the synovial tissues. The metaplastic growths form nodules and can detach and grow as loose bodies in the joint space. The lesions can also undergo ossification. The latter condition is referred to as synovial osteochondromatosis. The knee is the most common site of involvement; the disease is rarely polyarticular. Symptoms include crepitation, swelling, limitation of motion, and intermittent locking of the affected joint. Treatment is surgical synovectomy.

Pigmented villonodular synovitis is the most common term applied to a disorder characterized by villous or nodular growths that invade the synovial lining of joints, bursae, or tendons. It has a characteristic histopathologic picture, i.e., presence of inflammatory granulomas that contain hemosiderin, cholesterol crystals, and multinucleated giant cells. Authorities disagree about whether the condition should be classified as a form of chronic synovitis or as a true neoplasm. The knee is most frequently involved, but it can occur in the hip, elbow, ankle, or foot. Synovial fluid is usually hemorrhagic or xanthochromic. The inflammatory granuloma frequently invades the cartilage, subchondral bone, and periarticular structures. Localized pigmented villonodular synovitis can affect extra-articular bursae or tendon sheaths or occur as a solitary nodule in a single joint. The treatment of choice for each of these conditions is synovectomy or local excision of the tumor masses. Recurrence is uncommon.

464. BEHÇET'S DISEASE

Ralph Snyderman

DEFINITION. Behçet's disease is an inflammatory disorder of unknown etiology characterized by recurrent oral and genital aphthous ulcers, ocular inflammation, and skin lesions of erythema nodosum and acneiform eruptions. Behçet's disease also frequently involves the joints, the central nervous system, and the gastrointestinal tract.

INCIDENCE AND PREVALENCE. Behçet's disease is common in northern Japan, Turkey, and Israel. In Japan the current prevalence is 1 per 10,000. The frequency in the United States is far less. An annual incidence of 1 per 300,000 was determined for Olmstead County, Minnesota. The disease does not occur frequently in Japanese-Americans, perhaps suggesting environmental factors in addition to genetic predisposition in the etiology of this illness.

ETIOLOGY AND PATHOGENESIS. No infectious agent has been consistently isolated. Sera frequently contain circulating immune complexes of the IgA and IgG variety, as well as elevated levels of chemotactic activity for leukocytes. Antibodies reactive against oral mucosal cells have been found, and factors produced by patients' lymphocytes are toxic for oral mucosal cells. However, these findings are also present in individuals with recurrent aphthous stomatitis alone. Serum complement levels in Behçet's disease are usually elevated, particularly levels of C9. Most patients with neurologic involvement have demyelinating antibodies in their sera. There is a strong association of HLA-B5 with Behçet's disease in Japan and in the Mediterranean area. Heavy metal exposure, certain foods (particularly English walnuts), and toxic factors such as organophosphates have initiated attacks in some individuals.

PATHOLOGY. Behçet's disease is primarily an inflammatory disorder involving small blood vessels, particularly venules. Areas of ulceration initially show an intense mononuclear cell infiltration around blood vessels. As the lesion evolves, polymorphonuclear leukocytes and plasma cells predominate. The early lesions resemble a delayed hypersensitivity reaction, the later lesions an immune complex–Arthus-type reaction. The role of immune complexes in causing the venulitis is, however, questionable, since immunoglobulins are not routinely found in vessel walls.

CLINICAL MANIFESTATIONS. Behçet's disease can occur in many forms, but recurrent oral aphthous ulcers are present in 99 per cent of patients, and in almost 70 per cent these are the initial symptoms. Ocular symptoms occur in 90 per cent, skin lesions in 85 per cent, and genital ulcerations in nearly 70 per cent. Arthritis is present in approximately half of the patients with Behçet's disease. The onset is usually in the third or fourth decade. Behçet's disease affects men and women approximately equally. Indicators of poor prognosis include neurologic and posterior uveal tract involvement. In the absence of these, the disease tends to be unpredictable and remitting. In Japan, the mortality is approximately 4 per cent, with blindness occurring in as many as 65 per cent of untreated individuals. Young males have the worst prognosis.

The diagnosis of Behçet's disease is based upon the criteria listed in Table 464–1. Complete Behçet's syndrome is associated with all four major criteria. Persons with three major sites of involvement, or ocular lesions plus one other major site, have incomplete Behçet's disease. The diagnosis should be suspected when two major sites are affected. Since all manifestations need not appear, some investigators have grouped this illness into subtypes based upon the primary tissue involvement (i.e., neuro-Behçet's, oculo-Behçet's).

The oral aphthous ulcers are painful, unlike those of Reiter's syndrome, and occur singly or multiply on the lingual, gingival, buccal, or labial mucosal membranes. In Reiter's and Stevens-Johnson syndromes, the ulcers occur on the palate, pharynx, and tonsils, structures rarely involved in Behçet's disease. The aphthae of Behçet's disease usually last for approximately a week and may heal with or without scarring. Ulcers can also appear on the scrotum, vulva, penis, vaginal mucosa, or perianal areas. These lesions may be painless in women. Their gross appearance is similar to that of the oral aphthous ulcers. Vulvar lesions frequently occur premenstrually. Other types of cutaneous involvement are common. Painful, recurrent lesions of erythema nodosum may appear in crops over the tibia. Superficial thrombophlebitis can occur in the upper or lower extremities. Skin eruptions resembling acne vulgaris frequently appear on the upper thorax and face.

TABLE 464–1. DIAGNOSTIC CRITERIA OF BEHÇET'S DISEASE (SYNDROME)*

Major criteria
1. Recurrent oral aphthous ulcers
2. Eye lesions
   a. Recurrent hypopyon, iritis, or iridocyclitis
   b. Chorioretinitis
3. Genital ulcerations
4. Skin lesions
   a. Erythema nodosum-like eruptions
   b. Superficial thrombophlebitis
   c. Pustular skin lesions
   d. Hyperirritability of the skin (pathergy)

Minor criteria
5. Arthritis
6. Gastrointestinal lesions
7. Epididymitis
8. Vascular lesions (occlusion of blood vessels, aneurysms)
9. Central nervous system involvement
   a. Brainstem syndrome
   b. Meningoencephalomyelitic syndrome
   c. Organic confusional states

*Modified from the recommendations by the Behçet's Syndrome Research Committee of Japan (1972).

Approximately 40 per cent of patients with Behçet's disease exhibit a cutaneous phenomenon termed "pathergy." Venipuncture or injection of sterile saline into the skin of these patients results in the formation of a pustule. This phenomenon is not pathognomonic for Behçet's disease.

Ocular lesions may consist of anterior or posterior uveitis. Anterior uveitis frequently produces hazy vision as an initial manifestation. The development of a hypopyon is not unusual. Recurrent posterior uveitis is an ominous expression of Behçet's disease which, if untreated, frequently leads to bilateral blindness. Choroidal exudates and bleeding may be seen.

Articular manifestations consist of arthralgias and arthritis. The involvement is usually asymmetrical, affects one to several large joints such as the knees, ankles, elbows, and wrists, and resolves during remissions. Permanent joint damage is rare.

Gastrointestinal involvement during acute attacks, present in approximately 50 per cent of patients, is most commonly manifested by vomiting, abdominal pain, diarrhea, flatulence, or constipation. More specific for Behçet's disease are erosions or superficial ulcers in the terminal ileum or colon. Intestinal ulcers occasionally perforate. Differentiation of Behçet's disease from ulcerative colitis or regional enteritis may be difficult.

Nervous system involvement occurs in approximately 10 per cent of patients and can be extremely severe, explosive, and associated with a poor prognosis. Manifestations include hemiplegia, paraplegia, cerebellar dysfunction, and psychologic changes.

Superficial venous occlusions, perhaps related to abnormalities in the blood fibrinolytic system, occur in up to 40 per cent of patients. Inferior or superior vena caval obstructions can lead to death. Occlusive lesions have also occurred in the aorta and other large arteries. Epididymitis occurs in approximately 6 per cent of male patients.

TREATMENT. No therapy has been proved uniformly effective. Since the illness is unpredictable and frequently remitting, long-term continuous therapy with potentially dangerous drugs is not justified except in specific situations. Chlorambucil (0.1 to 0.2 mg per kilogram per day) has been reported to prevent blindness in patients with posterior retinal involvement. Other immunosuppressive agents such as azathioprine, cyclophosphamide, and 6-mercaptopurine have also been used. Since neuro-Behçet's syndrome is life-threatening, immunosuppressive agents are frequently used for this manifestation. Corticosteroids are strictly palliative for the inflammatory lesions (i.e., anterior uveitis) and should not be used except during acute flares of the disease. Avoidance of factors known to precipitate attacks (i.e., particular foods or toxic materials) should be encouraged. Colchicine (0.6 mg orally twice a day) is sometimes effective in treating the mucocutaneous and cutaneous lesions. Transfer factor has not been effective in double-blind clinical trials. In patients with gastrointestinal manifestations, a trial of sulfasalazine (2 to 4 gm per day) is warranted. Sulfasalazine may also be useful in patients without obvious gastrointestinal complaints. Fibrinolytic agents have been recommended for patients with occlusive vascular disease. Because the disease is remitting in nature, the efficacy of therapy is difficult to evaluate.

Chajek T, Fainaru M: Behçet's disease. Report of 41 cases and a review of the literature. Medicine 54:179, 1975. *Concise but thorough review of clinical features in a large number of patients with Behçet's disease.*

Lehner T, Barnes CG: Behçet's Syndrome. London, Academic Press, 1979. *Book devoted to Behçet's disease. Good review of the immunologic findings and clinical manifestations of the illness.*

Marquardt JL, Snyderman R, Oppenheim JJ: Depression of transformation and exacerbation of Behçet's syndrome by ingestion of English walnuts. Cell Immunol 9:263, 1973. *An immunologic study of Behçet's disease with a potential clue for pathogenesis.*

Michelson JB, Chisari FV: Behçet's disease. Surv Ophthalmol 26:190, 1982. *An up-to-date review of Behçet's disease, particularly good for ocular manifestations.*

Shimizu T, Ehrlich GE, Inaba G, Hayashi K: Behçet disease (Behçet syndrome). Semin Arthritis Rheum 8:223, 1979. *Comprehensive review of clinical features, pathology and potential pathogenic mechanisms of Behçet's disease.*

465. PANNICULITIS AND DISORDERS OF THE SUBCUTANEOUS FAT

Gerald S. Lazarus

INTRODUCTION. The subcutaneous tissue is a fibrofatty layer spread between the flexible skin and the rigid muscles. It functions not only as a thermal and mechanical insulator but also as an active metabolic organ. The mature lipocyte contains an eccentric nucleus and a single large vacuole. The characteristic signet ring lipocytes are organized into lobules by fibrous septa, which are continuous with the dermis and contain the blood and lymph vessels and reticuloendothelial cells.

The diagnosis of panniculitis frequently requires skin biopsy. The most important histologic characteristic of the deep skin biopsy is the location of the inflammatory process. Inflammation primarily in the septa is designated *septal panniculitis,* whereas the presence of inflammatory cells primarily in the fat lobules is designated *lobular panniculitis.* The presence or absence of vasculitis further differentiates panniculitis into the four major groups.

LOBULAR PANNICULITIS WITHOUT VASCULITIS. ***Nodular Panniculitis—Weber-Christian Disease.*** Nodular panniculitis describes a group of syndromes or diseases characterized by subcutaneous nodules and inflammatory cells in the fat lobules. The term Weber-Christian disease is applied when cutaneous lesions are associated with systemic complaints.

The etiology of this group of diseases is unknown. In the early stages the fat lobules are infiltrated with polymorphonuclear leukocytes. Later, macrophages appear and ingest fat, producing the characteristic lipophagic granuloma. The lesions heal with lobular fibrosis. Uncommonly, minimal septal vasculitis may be observed.

Lobular panniculitis most commonly presents in females between the ages of 30 and 60, although cases have been reported in all age groups. The lesions begin as red, slightly tender nodules deep in the skin. They appear more or less in symmetrical crops on thighs and lower legs, but lesions may also occur on arms, trunk, and face. The number of lesions may vary enormously. The lesions become firmer, less red, and less tender over a period of weeks. They heal, leaving a depressed hyperpigmented scar. *Liquefying panniculitis* is a variant in which the lesions become necrotic and drain an oily, yellow-brown fluid. *Rothmann-Makai syndrome* is a very rare variant of lobular panniculitis, affecting children with numerous large lesions; the lesions do not liquefy, and healing usually occurs within 12 months.

Systemic nodular panniculitis or *Weber-Christian disease* is a widespread process affecting cutaneous and visceral fat. Patients usually present with unequivocal cutaneous nodules and arthralgias, malaise, fatigue, weight loss, and abdominal pain. Involvement of the bone marrow may produce anemia, leukocytosis or leukopenia, and bone pain. Hepatomegaly, steatorrhea, and intestinal perforation have also been reported. Inflammation may occur in other internal organs such as lungs, pleura, pericardium, spleen, kidney, and adrenal glands. Visceral involvement may be confined to the retroperitoneal space, producing abdominal pain, nausea, and vomiting. Alpha$_1$-antitrypsin deficiency and lymphoma have occasionally been reported in association with nodular panniculitis.

The prognosis of nodular panniculitis is good in patients with only cutaneous involvement. There are frequent remissions and exacerbations of the lesions. Some cases recover after a few months, and permanent remission is usual after several years. On rare occasions visceral involvement may be fatal.

There is no specific therapy for this disease. Saturated potassium iodide, increasing from 5 drops three times daily by 1 drop per day to 30 drops three times daily, has been suggested. Hydroxychloroquine, 200 mg twice per day, has also been advocated as treatment. High dose prednisone, 40 to 60 mg for one to two weeks with gradual tapering over six to eight weeks, has also been reported to be of value in patients with severe disease; steroids should be used only for acute attacks and for limited periods of time.

Lobular Panniculitis Associated with Pancreatic Disease. The diagnosis is made by skin biopsy, which reveals acute fat necrosis with characteristic ghost cells. These patients often have associated arthritis, ascites, and eosinophilia. Acute pancreatitis, trauma to the pancreas, chronic pancreatitis, pancreatic cysts, and pancreatic carcinoma have been reported to be associated with this syndrome. Diagnosis depends upon the histologic findings at skin biopsy and documentation of a specific pancreatic abnormality. Therapy is directed at the underlying pancreatic disease.

Poststeroid Lobular Panniculitis. Children who receive large doses of steroid for a short period of time, followed by abrupt discontinuance, may develop lobular panniculitis. Lesions may occur in the viscera, and a fatal case has been reported.

Physical Lobular Panniculitis. Physical trauma of any kind and cold injury, especially in children, can produce lobular panniculitis. A unique traumatic panniculitis occurs in the obese breasts of women in their 50's. Injection of silicones or other foreign materials into female breasts or buttocks and into the male genitalia may induce a granulomatous foreign body nodular panniculitis. Similar inflammatory lesions may be seen following injections of Talwin.

Lobular Panniculitis Associated with Systemic Disease. Lupus erythematosus, sarcoidosis, granuloma annulare, and infections including deep fungi and pyogens may present as lobular panniculitis. Lymphoma or leukemia may also present as panniculitis; histologically, these lesions demonstrate malignant cells in the fat lobules. Lupus erythematosus confined primarily to the fat is known as lupus profundus. The skin may be exclusively involved, or the panniculitis may be associated with systemic disease. Granuloma annulare, a disease characterized by ring-shaped lesions of the skin, may also involve the fat.

LOBULAR PANNICULITIS WITH VASCULITIS. This category of disease includes *nodular vasculitis* and *erythema induratum.* The eruption consists of recurring, tender, painful nodules on the calves, which often ulcerate and heal with scarring. It is much more common in females than in males. Increased erythrocyte sedimentation rate and hypertension have been associated with this syndrome. Bazin gave the name erythema induratum to this disease when histologic examination revealed caseation necrosis and the lesions were associated with tuberculosis.

There is no specific therapy for this syndrome. Most patients have remission of lesions with bed rest. Severe cases have been successfully treated with nonsteroidal anti-inflammatory drugs, dapsone, and prednisone. In the very rare case of nodular vasculitis associated with tuberculosis, appropriate antituberculous therapy is indicated.

SEPTAL PANNICULITIS WITHOUT VASCULITIS. This histology in a patient with nodular, painful, tender lesions, especially on the anterior leg, is diagnostic of *erythema nodosum,* which is discussed in Ch. 556. A chronic disease similar to erythema nodosum clinically and histologically except that the lesions spread peripherally over months, forming rings, is called *sub-*

acute migratory panniculitis. This disease responds to therapy with increasing doses of saturated potassium iodide as described for nodular panniculitis. Septal panniculitis without vasculitis can also be seen in scleroderma, eosinophilic fasciitis, and necrobiosis lipoidica diabeticorum.

SEPTAL PANNICULITIS WITH VASCULITIS. *Thrombophlebitis* may present with subcutaneous nodules. Histology reveals inflammation of veins with adjacent panniculitis (see Ch. 54).

Cutaneous polyarteritis is a chronic and recurring, painful nodular eruption, primarily of the legs. There is often an associated mottled livedo vascular pattern. Cutaneous polyarteritis is associated with myalgias, arthralgias, and increased erythrocyte sedimentation rate. Histologic examination demonstrates leukocytoclastic vasculitis of medium-sized arterioles. This disease is usually not associated with systemic involvement. It has a benign course, but lesions may recur for years.

Therapy includes nonsteroidal anti-inflammatory agents and short courses of corticosteroids. Cutaneous polyarteritis associated with granulomatous bowel disease has responded to short courses of Cytoxan.

LIPOATROPHY. Loss of subcutaneous tissue can occur as a consequence of healing in almost any of the panniculitides described previously. The most common diagnosable cause of lipoatrophy is recurrent insulin injection. Insulin lipoatrophy is usually associated with repetitive injections of high doses of insulin in exactly the same location in females. Talwin injections may also produce panniculitis and severe lipoatrophy.

Total lipoatrophy associated with diabetes may occur in children and adults. The clinical picture is dramatic, and there is almost complete loss of subcutaneous fat. Partial lipoatrophy usually begins in children or young adults. It is five times more common in females than in males. Patients often lose the fat in the face and the upper half of the body. In some cases, there is hypertrophy of the fat on the lower half of the body. Patients with partial lipodystrophy often develop progressive mesangiocapillary glomerulonephritis and hypocomplementemia. Diabetes develops in one third of these patients. Retinitis pigmentosum has also been reported with this disease. The prognosis depends upon the severity of the renal disease.

Ackerman AB: Panniculitis. *In* Ackerman AB: Histologic Diagnosis of Inflammatory Skin Diseases. Philadelphia, Lea & Febiger, 1978, pp 779-826. *An outstanding review of the classification and histopathology of panniculitis.*

Bennett WM, Bardana EJ, Wuepper K, Houghton D, Border WA, Gotze O, Schreiber R: Partial lipodystrophy, C3 nephritic factor and clinically inapparent mesangiocapillary glomerulonephritis. Am J Med 62:757, 1976. *Description of the association of lipodystrophy with glomerulonephritis.*

Bondi EE, Lazarus GS: Panniculitis. *In* Fitzpatrick TB, Eisen AZ, Wolff K, Freedberg IM, Austen KF (eds.): Dermatology in General Medicine. 3rd ed. New York, McGraw-Hill Book Company, In press. *A complete overview of panniculitis, emphasizing clinical description, mechanisms, and treatment.*

Epstein EH Jr: Lipodystrophy. *In* Fitzpatrick TB, Eisen AZ, Wolff K, Freedberg IM, Austen KF (eds.): Dermatology in General Medicine. New York, McGraw-Hill Book Company, 1979, pp 795-797. *Concise review of the lipodystrophy syndromes with appropriate pertinent references.*

Parks DL, Perry HO, Muller SA: Cutaneous complications of pentazocine injections. Arch Dermatol 104:231, 1971. *Good discussion of the cutaneous complications of pentazocine injections.*

Winkelman RK, Bowie BM: Hemorrhagic diathesis associated with benign and systemic histiocytosis. Arch Intern Med 140:1460, 1980. *A review of severe systemic lobular panniculitis.*

466. MULTIFOCAL FIBROSCLEROSIS (Multicentric Fibrosclerosis, Fibrosing Syndromes)

H. Ralph Schumacher, Jr.

In rare instances the delicate fibrous areolar tissue in a certain anatomic region becomes the site of a chronic low-grade inflammatory process, leading to deposition of dense sclerotic plaques, which may obstruct or limit the movement of adjacent viscera. When the process is in the active phase, there are characteristic findings of chronic or granulomatous inflammation, with mononuclear cell infiltration and occasional giant cells. In the end-stages the pathologic lesion is simply that of scar tissue, so that by the time this process causes clinical manifestations there may be little evidence of the initial inflammatory reaction. In at least some cases there is an accompanying vasculitis. As a general rule the process tends to originate in the midline, around the great vessels, then spreads laterally. In most cases a clue to the inciting mechanism is lacking; hence the frequent use of the term "idiopathic" in describing the various syndromes.

Syndromes that have been considered as manifestations of multifocal fibrosclerosis include retroperitoneal fibrosis, mediastinal fibrosis, sclerosing cholangitis (see Ch. 129), Riedel's thyroiditis (see Ch. 228), pseudotumor of the orbit, Peyronie's disease (a sclerotic induration of the corpora cavernosa of the penis), and practolol peritonitis. Other sites of a similar fibrosis, such as the testes, vagina, and suprasellar area, have also rarely been reported. A case of retroperitoneal fibrosis occurring with scleroderma has been described. The toxic syndrome following ingestion of adulterated rapeseed oil in Spain exhibits vascular disease and multiple areas of fibrosis but apparently does not include the sites seen with multifocal fibrosclerosis. Pulmonary and myocardial fibrosis syndromes have generally not been seen as related to multifocal fibrosclerosis.

The fibrosing pattern of response in multifocal fibrosclerosis may follow different kinds of injury. For example, there is an association between therapy with methysergide and some cases of retroperitoneal fibrosis, and the suggestion has been made that fibrosing mediastinitis can occur as a sequel to infection with *Histoplasma capsulatum.* In a number of instances the disease has developed concurrently with a neoplastic process such as reticulum cell sarcoma or carcinoid tumor. Sclerosing cholangitis is sometimes associated with ulcerative colitis or with Crohn's disease. Other associated factors have been retroperitoneal or intraabdominal surgery, several infectious agents, drugs, and systemic vasculitis.

Although most of these syndromes have been described as separate entities, depending on the clinical manifestations and the interests of the writers who have reported them, it should be emphasized that several anatomic areas may become affected in one person. For example, retroperitoneal fibrosis and sclerosing mediastinitis may be present at the same time. Even more interesting is the report by Comings and his associates of two brothers, offspring of a consanguineous marriage, who exhibited varying combinations of retroperitoneal fibrosis, mediastinal fibrosis, sclerosing cholangitis, Riedel's thyroiditis, and pseudotumor of the orbit. This brings up the possibility of a genetic predisposition to disease of this character, but of course does not exclude other precipitating factors, e.g., common exposure to some chemical. The former possibility is given support by the description of an association between the occurrence of fibrosing syndromes and alpha$_1$-antitrypsin deficiency. Some reports also have described an association of familial mediastinal or retroperitoneal fibrosis with seronegative spondyloarthropathies.

Comings DE, Skubi KB, Van Eyes J, Motulsky AG: Familial multifocal sclerosis. Ann Intern Med 66:884, 1967. *Description of multiple sites of fibrosis in two brothers.*

Goldbach P, Mohsenifar Z, Salick AI: Familial mediastinal fibrosis associated with seronegative spondyloarthropathy. Arthritis Rheum 26:221, 1983. *Two siblings with both diseases but HLA-B27 negative.*

RETROPERITONEAL FIBROSIS

In retroperitoneal fibrosis the process usually begins over the promontory of the sacrum and extends laterally across the ureters and up as high as the level of the second or third lumbar vertebra. Less commonly the lesion develops in other extraperitoneal areas, for example, contiguous with the kidneys, duodenum, descending colon, or urinary bladder. In some cases there has been an associated vasculitis in the skin and subcutaneous tissue, manifested by the formation of nodules, erythematous discolorations, and ulcerations. Similarly, inflammatory changes in small vessels at the sites of the sclerosis have been noted. Glomerulonephritis has been seen in a few patients.

The occurrence of retroperitoneal fibrosis in patients taking methysergide for migraine has been reported with greater frequency than could be due to chance. Occasional cases have been reported in association with use of various beta-adrenergic blocking agents, hydralazine, or methyldopa.

The disorder is about twice as common in males, and the peak age incidence is in the fifth and sixth decades. Cases have been reported in children. The manifestations are variable, depending on the anatomic location of the process. Pain is the most common symptom; it is vague, tends to be located in the low back, and may be accompanied by symptoms referable to the gastrointestinal tract. The patient is likely to lose weight and have low-grade fever. There may be some anemia and elevation of the erythrocyte sedimentation rate. Although the ureter is the structure most often affected, symptoms referable to the urinary tract are uncommon until obstructive uropathy has led to azotemia and other clinical manifestations of renal insufficiency. The fibrosing process may surround the inferior vena cava, but signs of obstruction of that vessel are relatively uncommon. Thromboembolism and hypertension can be complications. Arterial invasion has been described. Retroperitoneal fibrosis occasionally develops in association with abdominal aortic aneurysm.

Diagnosis of retroperitoneal fibrosis is difficult because of the lack of localizing manifestations. It is most often suggested by the findings at intravenous pyelography: displacement of the ureters toward the midline and evidence of obstruction, usually at the level of the pelvic brim. One or both ureters may be affected. In rare instances a mass can be palpated in the pelvis or on the posterior abdominal wall. Ultrasound, computed tomography (CT) scans, and nuclear magnetic resonance (NMR) imaging can also identify the fibrosing masses. Once the presence of a mass has been disclosed, the main problem in differential diagnosis lies in distinguishing retroperitoneal fibrosis from retroperitoneal tumor. For that reason multiple deep biopsies should be made at the time of laparotomy.

Surgical treatment, if employed before there has been severe renal damage, is often highly successful. Inasmuch as the fibrosing process is seldom invasive, the constricted organ can usually be freed by blunt dissection so that normal movement or flow is restored. Relief of ureteral obstruction is usually achieved simply by dissecting this structure free of its fibrous encasement and bringing it out on the anterior surface of the sclerotic mass. Occasionally, however, the obstruction recurs months or years after such treatment. Some surgeons wrap the ureters in omentum to try to decrease recurrent obstruction. Steroid therapy may be helpful, but the evidence for this is limited, and prompt surgical relief should usually be attempted whenever significant obstruction is present. Steroid treatment may be employed as an adjunct to surgical measures. When the inferior vena cava is obstructed, surgical relief is technically difficult and risky; here it may be preferable to temporize, in the hope that development of collateral pathways may alleviate the circulatory block.

The long-term outlook is fairly good if the disease is recognized and if its obstructive consequences can be treated suitably by surgical means. The disease often tends to run its course and subside. Most deaths have been caused by renal failure.

Hricak H, Higgins CB, Williams RD: Nuclear magnetic resonance imaging in retroperitoneal fibrosis. Am J Radiol 141:35, 1983. *Documentation of the increasing value of CT scans and NMR in diagnosis.*

Littlejohn GO, Keystone E: The association of retroperitoneal fibrosis with systemic vasculitis and HLA-B27: A case report and review of the literature. J Rheum 8:665, 1981. *Vasculitis has been documented histologically in 37 of 500 cases reviewed and may be much more common. An association with HLA-B27 and sacroiliitis is seen in this case.*

MEDIASTINAL FIBROSIS

Taut bundles of collagenous tissue form in the superior and anterior mediastinum with impingement on the aorta, trachea, esophagus, and pericardium, but the predominant manifestations are those caused by obstruction of the superior vena cava: puffy, suffused appearance of the face and conjunctivae; non-pitting edema of the face, neck, and upper extremities; and distended veins in the neck and upper extremities. Rarely the principal vessels affected are the pulmonary arteries, causing pulmonary hypertension. More frequently the pulmonary veins are involved, and here severe hemoptysis may be the most prominent manifestation. The main task in differential diagnosis is to distinguish this relatively benign condition from obstruction caused by tumor. Roentgenographic examination of the chest may reveal little or no abnormality, but angiographic studies show obstruction of the affected vessels. Thoracotomy may be required for histologic diagnosis.

As already mentioned, histoplasmosis, and possibly tuberculosis too, may be a cause of mediastinal fibrosis; therefore these should be considered. Some patients with this syndrome have shown gradual improvement over months or years, presumably because of development of collateral circulation. Successful superior vena cava bypass surgery has been described.

Doty DB: Bypass of superior vena cava: Six years experience with spiral vein graft for obstruction of superior vena cava due to benign and malignant disease. J Thorac Cardiovasc Surg 83:326, 1982. *Superior vena cava syndrome relieved for up to six years. Four patients had fibrosing mediastinitis.*

Dye TE, Saab SB, Almond MD, Watson L: Sclerosing mediastinitis with occlusion of pulmonary veins. J Thorac Cardiovasc Surg 74:137, 1977. *An unusual and serious but treatable cause of hemoptysis.*

Goodwin RA, Nickell JA, Dez Prez RM: Mediastinal fibrosis complicating healed primary histoplasmosis and tuberculosis. Medicine 51:227, 1972. *Excellent review, certainly implicating histoplasmosis.*

PRACTOLOL PERITONITIS

An unusual fibrotic syndrome has been observed in patients treated with the beta-adrenergic blocking drug practolol. This drug closely resembles propranolol in chemical structure, but the risk of fibrotic reaction in the peritoneum is far smaller, perhaps nonexistent, with propranolol.

Practolol peritonitis seldom manifests itself in less than 12 months after beginning treatment. Some cases have developed a year or longer after cessation of therapy. Thus, although practolol has been withdrawn from use, occasional late occurring cases might still be seen. The peritonitis consists of a thick fibrous encasement of the small intestine, and the symptoms are those of subacute obstruction. It has usually been possible to relieve the symptoms by surgery, with blunt dissection to peel away the fibrous tissue. Some improvement occurs with time. A few patients have developed apparently related respiratory disease.

Part XXIII
NEUROLOGIC AND BEHAVIORAL DISEASES

Section One CLINICAL STUDY OF THE PATIENT WITH NEUROLOGIC SYMPTOMS

467. APPROACH TO THE PATIENT, INCLUDING GENERAL MANAGEMENT

Fred Plum

Patients with symptoms and signs referable to the nervous system place special requirements on the physician's clinical approach. The most immediate task is to consider whether the symptoms are merely the nonspecific signals of a systemic disorder or reflect intrinsic neurologic disease. Pain, headache, nausea, dizziness, fatigue, and weakness all lack specificity until taken in context with the rest of the history and physical findings; as often as not, such symptoms can reflect the emotional ravages of disturbed psychologic adjustment. To understand and treat human beings requires that the doctor know *who* is sick as much as or more often than *what* is sick. Put in Peabody's words, "The secret of the care of the patient is caring for the patient."

A second major consideration is to realize that although all patients are to some degree frightened of illness, concern over the possibility of paralysis, severe pain, or mental impairment instills an especial terror which requires the doctor's attention and reassurance. When examining such patients, if at all possible follow Osler's dictum: "Do the kind thing and do it first."

The third major consideration stems from the nervous system's vulnerability to damage and its inability to repair itself. In a broad sense, the purpose of the practice of medicine is to protect the brain. Man's brain makes him human. Damage it and life loses its meaning in direct proportion, no matter what other physiologic benefits may accrue in the process. The brain cannot be regenerated, repaired, or homotransplanted. It accumulates no metabolic debts, and, unless supplied continuously by an effective circulation carrying a large volume of oxygen and substrates, it digests itself promptly and irreparably. The doctor's mandate is clear: in seriously and acutely ill patients with neurologic abnormalities, life- or brain-threatening complications must be treated even while proceeding with diagnostic procedures which may take several more minutes, hours, or days to complete.

Wise and sensitive management of the neurologic patient requires attention to both disease and humane need. In general, the more specific and acute the illness, the less immediately important become the broad concerns of the patient. By contrast, patients whose diseases lack quick and specific remedies (e.g., most degenerative diseases, most residua of severe trauma) usually need far more from the doctor than the local pharmacy can supply. Three important maxims apply to all treatment situations: protect the brain first, no matter what successive steps must follow; relieve pain even while proceeding with diagnosis; and give reassurance, hope, and explanation at every step along the way. To plan long-term management effectively and economically, try to construct an accurate prognosis as early as possible. In acute, self-limited illnesses, such as meningococcal meningitis or most acute inflammatory polyneuritis, for example, one knows the probable outcome within a few days of onset. One even knows for most such patients the difference in convalescent time required before they will return to their former occupations. However, with diseases with intermediate outcomes such as multiple sclerosis, full recovery is less certain and the risk of relapse or chronic disability may require the physician to appraise all aspects of the patient's life in order to give proper guidance. At the third extreme are patients who become severely aphasic and hemiplegic from stroke or demented from Alzheimer's disease. They may never recover independence, and their proper early management requires that one guide whole families through major social and financial readjustments in planning for the future. How the doctor manages such complexities determines to a considerable degree his effectiveness as a physician.

Bennett AE: Communication Between Doctors and Patients. London, Oxford University Press, 1976. *A series of essays with a particularly good chapter by Maguire and Rutter on interviewing techniques for medical students.*

DeJong RN: The Neurological Examination. 4th ed. Hagerstown, MD, Harper & Row, 1979. *A comprehensive and detailed explanation of the technique and physiology of the examination.*

Elstein AS, Shulman LS, Sprafka SA: Medical Problem Solving. An Analysis of Clinical Reasoning. Cambridge, MA, Harvard University Press, 1978. *An excellent description of how clinical problems are solved.*

Emerson CP: Reminiscences of Sir William Osler. Int Assoc Med Museums Bull 1926, p 294. *A volume of gems on teaching, care, and scholarship by America's greatest clinician.*

Mayo Clinic and Foundation: Clinical Examinations in Neurology. Philadelphia, W.B. Saunders Company, 1981. *A useful compendium of clinical and electrophysiologic approaches to neurologic diagnosis.*

Peabody FW: The care of the patient. JAMA 88:877, 1927. *A thoughtful and compassionate statement about the doctor-patient relationship.*

468. PRINCIPLES OF DIAGNOSIS

Fred Plum

Two major, alternative strategies underlie the way that most physicians approach the process of diagnosis. One, *pattern recognition,* is the classic technique of putting together the symptoms and signs into a syndrome and determining that the result conforms to a condition that the doctor has read about, has previously observed, or can ferret from the medical literature. The method profits by experience and specialization and relies relatively less on an analytic consideration of basic mechanisms in disease. The other, *logic and probability,* consists of analyzing signs and symptoms as manifestations of disordered physiology and deducing their meaning in terms of the anatomic structures involved and the way diseases affect these structures. The reliability of the resulting diagnostic hypothesis is tested by estimating the probability that certain abnormalities in bodily mechanisms will accompany one another and by the knowledge of the frequency with which such involvements occur. History, physical examination, and laboratory tests serve as constant back-checks and extensions of the deductive process. Skillful physicians utilize both pattern recognition and logic-probability in varying measure. The pattern-recognizing qualities of astute clinicians can reach legendary quality, but even the most experienced doctors usually mentally test their diagnostic impressions against a physiologic benchmark to see if the implied pathophysiology "makes sense" (i.e., fulfills physiologic probabilities). For the young physician, especially as scientific knowledge grows in medicine, a logical approach based on deductions from pathophysiology is imperative, for it focuses attention on the patient's main problem and avoids the pitfall of treating minor symptoms or laboratory perturbations that provide no threat to the patient's health. Particularly in neurologic diagnosis the strong communicative power of the nervous system and its reflections of the patient's inner self mean that information derived from the history and neurologic examination usually lends itself to logical analysis and probability testing (e.g., is it likely that *this* patient would have *this* disorder at *this* time with *this* combination of symptoms?).

Armed with a provisional diagnostic formulation in anatomic and physiologic terms, the physician then should require only a limited number of laboratory tests to establish the precise mechanism of disease or to rule out the presence of some other, unsuspected condition or illness. One should recall, however, that the complexity of disease is such that even the most exhaustive efforts accurately diagnose only about 85 per cent of first time admissions to major medical centers. The number of relatively trivial uncertainties and errors probably rises higher in ambulatory patients with self-limited problems which inherently receive less attention or disappear without causing serious disability.

The first step in neurologic diagnosis is anatomic. To arrive at a regional diagnosis one asks: Does the patient have a structural disease (i.e., is the process organic, physiologic-functional, or psychiatric)? If a disease is present, is it monofocal or diffuse? Given the likelihood that a neurologic disorder is present, one asks in succession: Are the lesions peripheral (i.e., at the receptor, muscle effector, synapse, or nerve) or central (i.e., in the spinal cord or brain)? If central, does the disease affect structures above or below the foramen magnum, above or below the tentorium, on the right or the left side? Is the process static, worsening, or improving? Given the answer or answers to these questions, one can then formulate a pathologic-etiologic diagnosis according to whether the evidence suggests a disorder that is genetic, developmental, traumatic, environmental-toxic, infectious, immunologic, degenerative, neoplastic, metabolic, nutritional, physiologic (e.g., epilepsy, migraine), or psychophysiologic (e.g., tension backache, vasodepressor syncope). One then proceeds to nonspecific and specific laboratory tests in order to confirm the clinical diagnostic hypotheses.

469. THE NEUROLOGIC HISTORY

Jerome B. Posner

In most respects, the neurologic history is similar to the general medical history. The purpose (to supply diagnostic information that will direct the physical and laboratory examinations and lead to an appropriate diagnosis) and the format (e.g., chief complaint, present illness, past history, social history, review of systems) are the same. However, the neurologic history usually supplies a greater proportion of the diagnostically relevant information than does a medical history; many neurologic diseases are not accompanied by abnormal physical or laboratory findings, and in these instances the physician must depend solely on the history to reach an appropriate diagnosis. Even when the patient suffers from a neurologic disease marked by physical signs and/or laboratory abnormalities, the history usually supplies about 80 per cent of the total diagnostic information. Furthermore, because neurologic abnormalities affect such important functions as thinking, moving, and feeling, it is unusual for patients to have significant abnormal signs which have not been perceived as symptoms by the patient. (Exceptions occur in demented patients and those with lesions of the nondominant parietal lobe, characterized by denial of disability. In these instances, abnormal behavior is recognized by family and friends.) Thus, findings on examination not recognized by the patient (or his family) are likely to be irrelevant or even misleading. By contrast, symptoms complained of by the patient, such as mild weakness or alterations of sensation, are probably significant even if too subtle to be detected by the most meticulous neurologic examination. (For example, a patient who complains of horizontal diplopia on extreme left lateral gaze is probably suffering from weakness of the left lateral rectus even if the finding is absent at the time of examination, e.g., myasthenia gravis, or too subtle for the physician to detect. On the other hand, the physician's finding by "red glass test" of horizontal diplopia in extreme lateral gaze in a patient who does not complain of diplopia probably represents congenital weakness of the muscle and is of no consequence.) Finally, because neurologic symptoms are so keenly appreciated by the patient, a meticulous history often allows a physician to localize the disease anatomically and to understand its pathophysiology even before he begins the physical examination.

Taking the neurologic history does (or should) occupy the majority of time spent with a patient suffering a neurologic disorder. At the completion of the history, the physician should be able either to make a definite diagnosis or to formulate three or four hypotheses which can be tested by the physical and laboratory examinations. Because there are an almost infinite number of potential questions which might be asked of a patient with a neurologic disorder, the physician must develop a strategy that allows him to achieve the maximal useful information in a reasonable period of time. Elements of that strategy are listed below. (Specific questions which might elicit useful diagnostic information in patients suffering from neurologic disease may be found in standard texts on the neurologic history and evaluation and, in this textbook, under the descriptions of specific diseases.) In taking a neurologic history, the physician must observe the following guidelines:

BE INTERESTED AND SUPPORTIVE. The purpose of the neurologic history is not only to gain diagnostic information but also to learn enough about the patient's psychologic and social background to establish a satisfactory doctor-patient relationship, and thus to be able to manage the patient's illness satisfactorily. Diagnostic information is often lost when the patient does not volunteer symptoms that he believes would not interest the physician or that are too intimate or embarrassing to tell to an "unsympathetic stranger." Such information will be volunteered to the physician who demonstrates by his attitude his interest, reassurance, and support.

BE ALERT TO NONVERBAL CUES. What the patient does is often as important as what he says. The patient's overall appearance and demeanor, his tone of voice, or a sigh or a tear in discussing what appear to be relatively trivial symptoms may be important clues to an underlying depression or severe anxiety over those symptoms.

REQUIRE PRECISION. Interviewers should not accept jargon or names of diseases from the patient. Jargon terms such as "dizziness" or diagnostic appellations such as "sinus headache" require a thorough exploration of the exact nature of the symptom and its effect on the patient. For example, a patient who complains of dizziness may mean vertigo (a vestibular symptom), lightheadedness (potentially caused by cardiovascular disease), syncope, ataxia, diplopia, or psychogenic dissociation—all symptoms which have very different physiologic meanings. "Sinus headache" is a diagnostic term often given to or used by patients to describe headaches which in fact are rarely caused by sinusitis but are usually migraine or tension headache.

MAINTAIN A BALANCE BETWEEN LISTENING AND ASKING. Physicians should elicit the history in the patient's own words and, whenever possible, should allow the patient to tell the story without interruption. Excessive interruptions indicate to the patient that the physician is in a hurry or disinterested, and may lead the patient to exclude vital information. By hearing the patient out, the physician often gains important information concerning the patient's fears and anxieties. However, the physician must ask direct questions to encourage relevance, achieve precision, and place each symptom in its correct context. If the patient does not volunteer it, the physician must ask about the intensity and frequency of the complained symptoms, their duration, events and factors that precipitate or relieve them, and any other symptoms associated in time with the patient's major complaint. For example, a patient with "cluster headaches" (see Ch. 477) may complain only of severe, disabling headache, but careful questioning may reveal that the headaches occur in two- to three-month clusters once or twice a year, characteristically appear three times a day, are always localized in and around the left eye, last no more than 30 to 40 minutes, are the most intense pain the patient has ever experienced, frequently awaken him at night, and can always be precipitated by alcohol intake during the cluster period. Such a precise history allows no other diagnosis.

FORM HYPOTHESES. The physician cannot be a passive recipient of the patient's story. The patient supplies too much information, much of it not diagnostically relevant, for the physician to recall at a later time, even with notes. Thus, the physician, while taking the history, must sift and distill the information as he receives it in order to retain what is relevant and be allowed to forget irrelevant information. Concurrently, he must form hypotheses about the nature of the patient's symptoms as they are presented, and test those hypotheses by asking pertinent questions. Hypotheses are tested and refined during the course of taking the history, so that by the end of the history the physician has three or four potential diagnoses to guide his physical and laboratory examinations. The best hypotheses are broad explanations of the patient's symptoms in anatomic and/or pathophysiologic terms, which are gradually refined into etiologic terms as the history develops. (For example, in a patient complaining of weakness of the right arm and leg, the hypotheses might include a left hemispheral structural lesion or a cervical cord lesion. As the physician elicits a history of weakness in the face and difficulty with language, the cervical cord hypothesis can be discarded and the left hemispheral lesion accepted. Additional history of slowly progressive weakness accompanied by headache and lethargy will lead the physician to hypothesize a mass lesion of the left hemisphere, possibly hematoma, tumor, or abscess, and a history of heavy smoking with recent cough could lead him to consider a metastatic lung tumor. At the end of the history, the physician has arrived at the conclusion that the patient has a mass lesion in the left hemisphere and has hypothesized several etiologic entities.) Hypotheses should give preference to those illnesses that are probable (i.e., common diseases are more likely than rare diseases), serious (e.g., brain tumors should be considered before tension headache), treatable (e.g., combined systems disease and spinal cord meningioma should be ruled out before making a diagnosis of multiple sclerosis), and novel (some patients do indeed have rare diseases, and these should not be forgotten in taking the history).

ALWAYS TAKE A COMPLETE HISTORY. Even if the diagnosis seems clear from the chief complaint and the present illness, other aspects of the patient's history must be elicited to ensure that other physical or psychologic disabilities are not playing a role in the patient's discomfort. In particular, inquiry must be made about the patient's mood (e.g., is he depressed or suicidal?), his usual daily activities (and whether the illness interferes with them), his sexual activities, the nature of psychologic and physical support at home, and his view of the illness and how it affects him.

END BY SUMMARIZING. At the end of the history it is useful to summarize the history as the physician understands it, asking the patient if the summary is correct and if anything has been missed. Such a summary gives the patient a chance to supply information which may have been left out in the initial history and to correct any misunderstandings. It also allows the patient to present new data on areas concerning him.

OBTAIN FURTHER HISTORY FROM THE PATIENT'S FAMILY AND FRIENDS. If the history appears incomplete, and particularly if part of the patient's illness involves changes in mental state or episodic unconsciousness, the patient's family, friends, and colleagues should be asked to corroborate the history and to supply missing elements, giving their views on how the signs and symptoms affect the patient's daily life.

GEAR THE NEUROLOGIC EXAMINATION TO THE HYPOTHESES. It is neither possible nor desirable to perform all elements of the neurologic examination on every patient. Thus, the hypotheses generated during the course of the history determine which of the nonroutine neurologic maneuvers the physician will carry out during the course of his examination. For example, olfactory sensation need not be tested routinely, but if the physician has hypothesized a frontal lobe tumor, significant head injury, or pernicious anemia, all of which may affect olfactory sensation, then this function must be tested. A complaint of intermittent numbness in an upper extremity should lead the physician to test for compromise of the thoracic outlet, even though that is not part of the routine neurologic examination. In similar fashion, hypotheses generated during the history direct the laboratory examination even in the presence of a normal neurologic examination. For example, if the history gives strong evidence of a left hemispheral mass lesion, failure to find a hemiparesis on examination does not rule out a brain tumor, and a computed tomographic scan must be performed. Even if the tests are initially uninformative, a strongly suggestive history requires that the doctor follow the patient closely.

470. THE NEUROLOGIC EXAMINATION

Fred Plum

Several texts can be consulted for the detailed techniques of bedside neurologic examinations. The necessary length of the complete examination and the potentially bewildering complexity of detailed neuroanatomy sometimes intimidate students and general physicians. This is unfortunate, because an understanding of a few fundamental principles about the nervous system plus the mastering of a relatively brief but systematically thorough approach to the examination can give a working knowledge that allows for the reliable and effective practice of medicine. The secret is to learn a relatively rapidly applied approach that covers the main elements of nervous system function and to be familiar with how to apply more exhaustive evaluations to selective functions if and when material in the history or the baseline examination suggests abnormalities in special parts.

An effective neurologic examination proceeds from general to specific in its principles and rostral to caudal in its anatomy. Such an examination checks on the integrity of major functions and yet avoids bogging down in details which do not relate to the complaints of most patients. In awake and talking patients, listen to them as they give their histories. Begin at that point to evaluate mental status and language (inconsistencies? vagueness on important points? word-blocking? circumlocutions? paraphasias? agrammaticisms?). Apply at least a brief mental examination on everyone, but be gentle and understanding: "How has your memory been? Can I just check a couple of points with you?" Check orientation. Examine memory for recent events, for public figures, and for three unrelated words at five minutes. Review the capacity to handle abstractions (boy—dwarf, small tree—bush, proverbs). Provide a problem in simple arithmetic (nickels in $1.35). Check serial sevens. Have the patient repeat five numbers backwards or the spelling of "world." But be patient and remember that anxiety can occlude the performance of even a normally good mind. Have the patient stand and walk; remember that the nervous system is the organ of communication and behavior, and that one learns most about man while watching him attempt natural tasks. Watch the patient at least partially dress and undress (apraxia); remark on alertness-dullness; hyperactivity-apathy; adventitious movement–akinesia; visible deformities, asymmetries, or weaknesses in functional tasks; hypertrophies-atrophies; cutaneous abnormalities (pox, birthmarks, café au lait spots, pigmented or hair spots over spinal defects); a straight, flat, or crooked spine. In other words, learn to observe constantly and closely, comparing always what you see with what you already have seen in thousands of people living everyday lives.

Examine cranial functions, screening certain structures and

innervations in every patient. Palpate the skull and test the neck gently for suppleness and length. Then examine in everyone vision (rough fields and acuity), the optic fundi, pupillary activity, ocular movements, corneal reflexes, jaw movement, facial movement, bilateral hearing, swallowing, speaking, and breathing. One can omit or defer from most routine examinations such tests as those of smell, taste, facial sensation, labyrinthine-vestibular activity, sternocleidomastoid function, or the integrity of detailed tongue movements unless symptoms suggest the involvement of these bodily areas. Examine in everyone the extremities and trunk for symmetry (hypertrophy or atrophy), size, at least grossly for strength, muscle tonus, adventitious movements (e.g., tremors, fasciculations, tics), coordination (rhythmic movements and point-to-point tests), and reflexes. If the patient has no sensory symptoms, he is unlikely to have abnormal sensory signs. Nevertheless, make a brief check of the distal extremities for the threshold perception of vibration and pin prick before deciding that things are normal. Examine the plantar responses. Evaluate autonomic and sphincter functions as part of the general medical examination. Get in the habit of examining the neck over the carotid arteries for bruits that may herald partial stenoses. Above all, be systematic and consistent in the approach and *do not jump at diagnosis until all the evidence is in.* Doctors often make diagnoses too quickly and surrender wrong ones reluctantly. By contrast, they view even partial unknowns as challenging problems. Try to choose the latter approach until matters become certain.

USE OF LABORATORY TESTS. Advances in laboratory methods during recent years have remarkably increased the accuracy of diagnosis and physiologic evaluations. At the same time, excessive technology raises the costs of medical care unnecessarily. More than anything else, the physician's ordering practices influence this aspect of health care costs. The doctor must recognize the precise advantages for both positive and negative knowledge that derive from each test, and order only those which add substantially to the patient's evaluation and treatment. To give an example: when managing an adult with recent onset of headache, the results of a computed tomographic scan, whether normal or abnormal, commonly help the doctor's management and provide the patient with great reassurance. However, to repeat the scan just to intensify reassurance for a querulous patient or an insecure physician wastes the time and resources of all concerned.

471. NEUROLOGIC DIAGNOSTIC PROCEDURES

Samuel Rapoport

LUMBAR PUNCTURE

With the advent of modern brain imaging devices, lumbar puncture is performed far less often currently than in the past. Nevertheless, sampling the cerebrospinal fluid (CSF) remains an indispensable step in diagnosing several infectious diseases and is an emergency procedure in cases of suspected bacterial meningitis. Table 471–1 gives other indications and contradications. Other considerations of when and when not to do lumbar puncture can be found in Ch. 476. Postlumbar puncture headache is discussed in Ch. 475.

TABLE 471–1. INDICATIONS AND CONTRAINDICATIONS FOR LUMBAR PUNCTURE

Diagnostic:	Known or suspected meningitis-encephalitis Acute: Bacterial, viral Subacute: Tuberculous, syphilitic, fungal, neoplastic Chronic: Syphilitic, granulomatous, neoplastic Intracranial-intraspinal hemorrhage (when no CT is available)
Useful:	Multiple sclerosis Acute polyneuropathy Suspected benign intracranial hypertension (CT negative)
Contraindicated:	Noninfectious states of undiagnosed increased intracranial pressure Thrombocytopenia or anticoagulated states Local skin or epidural infections
Therapeutic:	Antimicrobial or anticancer therapy

IMAGING TECHNIQUES

Brain, Dura, and Skull

COMPUTERIZED TOMOGRAPHY. Computerized tomography (CT) is performed by measuring transmission of an x-ray beam across the brain and computing density differences in two dimensions based on the amount of radiation that is transmitted across a tomographic slice of variable thickness. The resulting image displays density of tissue on a black and white scale. Water produces the least dense reference and is portrayed as black. Relatively more dense tissue appears progressively whiter, with bone and metallic objects being the whitest. A typical scan depicts the spinal fluid in the cerebral ventricles and subarachnoid spaces as black, the calvarium as dense white, the cortical gray matter as light gray, and the cortical white matter as a darker gray. Masses of blood within brain tissue appear as circumscribed white or gray-white images, while areas of encephalomalacia, such as result from cerebral infarcts, emerge as dark gray. Resolution with current instruments yields excellent images of the cerebrum, differentiating among cortical mantle, white matter tracts, deep nuclei, and cerebral ventricles. Shifts of intracranial structures caused by mass lesions are readily detectable. CT is currently the most accessible way of accurately and safely evaluating structural lesions of the brain and surrounding dural and osseous structures. The 5 mm spatial resolution of present techniques, as well as the ability of many machines to calculate the volume of a desired brain area, makes it easy to determine changes in the size of lesions as a function of time or treatment. Intravenously administered iodinated x-ray contrast agents leak across the abnormally permeable capillary beds of certain intraparenchymal brain lesions, providing an increase in the scan density of the desired areas. Such enhancement becomes particularly useful in detecting lesions that are isodense with normal surrounding brain on routine CT scans, as well as lesions whose small size falls below the spatial resolution of the instument.

Advantages. The general availability of CT scans, as well as the short time required for a complete examination, renders it a most valuable emergency diagnostic procedure. In victims of head trauma with neurologic abnormalities, CT scanning allows immediate determination of whether hemorrhage has occurred intraparenchymally or in one of the dural compartments, thus guiding therapy. In patients with acute stroke, CT readily distinguishes hemorrhage from ischemia, guiding decisions for anticoagulant therapy. Brain tumors usually can be differentiated from their surrounding edema, and the response of intracranial abscesses to antimicrobial therapy can be monitored. The degree of cerebral atrophy can be assessed. The ratio of ventricular size to the size of the cortical subarachnoid spaces provides a useful index of hydrocephalus, and the density of the white matter surrounding the ventricies often gives an indication of how recently the process has arisen. Most abnormalities of the skull, orbits, neural foramina, and cranial sinuses can be detected, making obsolete most skull x-rays and almost all nuclide brain scans.

Disadvantages. CT scans cannot detect lesions smaller than 5 mm in diameter, and they often visualize posterior fossa structures poorly because of artifacts generated by surrounding bone. Subacute subdural hematomas sometimes generate an image isodense with surrounding brain, rendering them undetectable. Small brain tumors located superficially on the cortex are often difficult to detect, even after contrast injections, because of averaging artifact from the surrounding bone. Small, low-grade infiltrating brain tumors may have a density very close to that of surrounding brain tissue and possess too little blood-brain barrier permeability to be detected. Almost no nonstructural brain diseases disfigure the CT scan. The technique often cannot differentiate between tumor and infarct, or among metastatic tumor, primary tumor, and brain abscess. The resolution of CT is insufficient to detect any but giant cerebral aneurysms. Assessment of the cerebral vasculature requires angiography.

NUCLEAR MAGNETIC RESONANCE (NMR). NMR measures the energy required to align the nuclear dipoles of hydrogen protons so that they point in the same direction when tissue is placed in a magnetic field. The technique provides a density map of hydrogen protons that can be processed to generate a video image that reproduces the cross-sectional anatomy of the brain with very high spatial detail and contrast resolution.

Indications. NMR, unlike CT, is unaffected by the artifact of x-rays reflected from bone, so that it generates better images of the structures of the posterior fossa. For similar reasons, better assessment of the intrasellar contents can be achieved. NMR has the unique ability to image the longitudinal axis of the brain and cervical spine, and it depicts both the normal and abnormal anatomy of the craniocervical and spinomedullary junctions more clearly than does any other diagnostic procedure. Owing to substantially better resolution powers, down to a millimeter or less with powerful magnets, NMR can detect plaques of multiple sclerosis and post-traumatic contusions far better than can CT. NMR is clearly superior to CT scanning in detecting intra-axial brainstem tumors. It is not yet fully established whether one technique is more sensitive than the other for detection of the majority of brain tumors, strokes, and other structural lesions. Instrumentation of NMR is advancing so rapidly that any conclusions at this juncture would be premature.

Disadvantages. NMR is not suitable for emergency situations, since life-support equipment can be drawn vigorously and violently into the magnet. Similarly, patients with surgical clips or metallic prostheses cannot be introduced into the magnetic field. The procedure currently requires 45 minutes to complete fully satisfactory images. The long-term risks of exposure to a large magnetic field are believed to be negligible; the technique is totally noninvasive and free of exposure to x-rays.

Spine, Spinal Cord, and Cauda Equina

Bony abnormalities of the spine, including primary or metastatic tumors and vertebral collapses, usually can be detected by conventional x-rays. Radiographs of the cervical spine are indispensable for evaluating abnormalities of the foramen magnum and displacement of the odontoid due to fractures. Demonstration that such abnormalities are impinging on neural tissue requires myelography. When one suspects root compression alone, such as with herniated discs, myelography performed with water-based contrast agents provides superior resolution to other agents, especially in the region of the cauda equina, and outlines the configuration of individual roots. Water-based agents, however, frequently cause nausea, vomiting, headache, and transient encephalopathy; since these agents are absorbed from the spinal fluid into the systemic circulation and excreted through the kidney, they can trigger allergic reactions in susceptible individuals. Rarely, they may cause renal insufficiency. These side effects are seldom observed with oil-based myelographic dyes such as Pantopaque. In patients with metastatic cancer it is advisable to perform myelography with Pantopaque so that the effects of treatment can be evaluated later by flouroscopy. NMR can provide longitudinal views of the spine, epidural space, and neural tissue, outlining bony abnormalities and intervertebral discs as they impinge on neural tissue.

Myelography demonstrates intrinsic spinal cord abnormalities such as tumors or syrinxes as circumscribed narrowings of the contrast column in the subarachnoid space. CT scanning through areas of such abnormalities reveals their tissue density, differentiating solid tumor from cyst. Longitudinal images of the spinal cord on NMR permit one to visualize the total length of the tumor or syrinx as well as cross-sectional views through the abnormality. Conventional CT scanning fails to provide longitudinal views of the spine and spinal cord, and to be certain of the total length and of the level of the spinal abnormality one must perform multiple transverse CT cuts. The spinal cord is not well visualized by CT scan, which must be enhanced with subarachnoid contrast material for adequate evaluation of intraspinal lesions. Intervertebral disc protrusion can be confirmed with conventional transverse CT scans, but clear definition of impingement on spinal roots or cord similarly requires the injection of subarachnoid contrast material.

NEURAL PLEXUS. In patients in whom soft tissue masses are suspected of impinging on the brachial or the lumbosacral plexus, CT scanning through the area provides the most valuable available technique for delineating the lesion and the local extent of its spread.

ELECTRODIAGNOSTIC STUDIES

Electroencephalography (EEG)

The electroencephalogram is a record of the electronically amplified dendritic activity of the superficial layers of the cerebral cortex. The instrument is indispensable for documenting the presence and type of epileptiform discharges, aiding the diagnosis of seizure disorders. In patients with altered states of consciousness, EEG helps differentiate seizures from metabllic encephalopathy and aids in distinguishing between organic and psychogenic causes of unresponsiveness. When seizures develop in comatose or theraputically paralyzed patients, the EEG can delineate the response to treatment, making it possible to titrate anticonvulsant dosage against cessation of epileptiform discharges. Absence of EEG activity supports the diagnosis of brain death.

Sensory Evoked Potentials

Measurement of the EEG time-locked to a visual, auditory, or somatosensory stimulus generates modality-specific potentials that are highly reporducible and provide information on the integrity of the pathway carrying the signal.

VISUAL EVOKED POTENTIALS (VEP). VEP usually are performed by haveing the subject fixate on a reversing black-white checkerboard pattern. Electrodes placed over the scalp record a positive potential, the latency of which is related to conduction in the optic nerve and central visual pathways. The method is

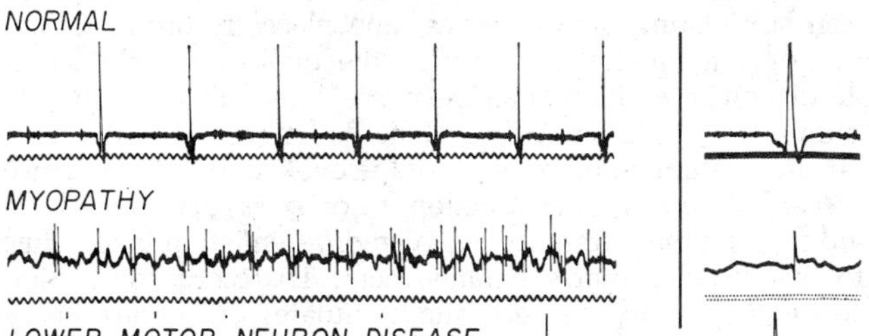

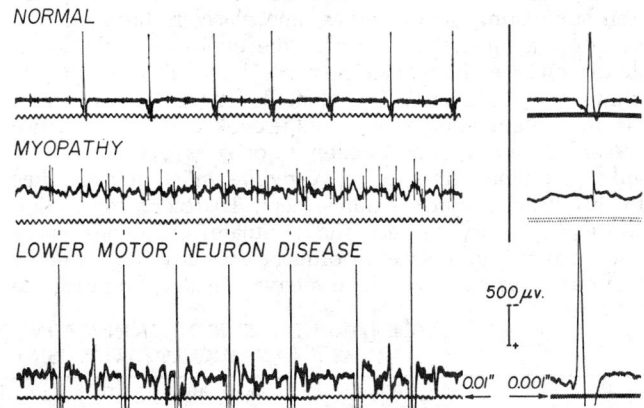

Figure 471–1. Diagram of muscle electrical activity showing motor action potentials during weak voluntary contraction of the biceps brachii. Note the normal amplitude and duration of the potentials on the top line compared to small, short duration potentials in muscular dystrophy and the enlarged amplitude and duration in amyotrophic lateral sclerosis. (From Aronson AE, Anger RG, et al.: Clinical Examinations in Neurology, 5th ed. Mayo Clinic and Mayo Foundation, 1981.)

TABLE 471–2. PATTERN OF EMG AND NERVE CONDUCTION ABNORMALITIES IN MONONEUROPATHY, POLYNEUROPATHY, RADICULOPATHY, AXONOPATHY, AND MOTONEURON DISEASE

	EMG Abnormality	Nerve Conduction Abnormality
Mononeuropathy	Limited to muscles innervated by damaged nerve	Limited to damaged nerve
Polyneuropathy	Diffuse	Diffuse
Radiculopathy	Limited to muscles innervated by damaged root	Usually none
Axonopathy/Motoneuron Disease	Diffuse	None

highly sensitive for detecting demyelination of the optic nerve, whether produced by compression, toxic agents, metabolic abnormalities, or multiple sclerosis.

BRAINSTEM AUDITORY EVOKED POTENTIALS (BAEP). Presentation of a white noise click stimulus to the ear generates a series of potentials from the brainstem auditory relay pathway, which can be recorded over the scalp at the vertex. The clinically relevant potentials occur within the first 10 milliseconds following the stimulus. The first potential recorded is generated by the auditory nerve, and subsequent potentials are generated, respectively, in the superior olive, lateral lemniscus, and inferior colliculus. Thus, a measure of conduction between various points along the auditory pathway between eighth nerve and inferior colliculus is provided. BAEPs detect abnormalities due to demyelinative, destructive, or compressive lesions affecting brainstem auditory pathways.

SOMATOSENSORY EVOKED POTENTIALS (SEP). Stimulation of a peripheral nerve by pulse of constant voltage or constant current gives rise to potentials that can be recorded over the spine and scalp. The median or peroneal nerves are most often stimulated. Stimulation of a lower extremity nerve, such as the peroneal, gives rise to a volley whose transit can be recorded at all levels of the spine. If bipolar electrode arrays are placed over the spine, the latency of the recorded potential increases progressively from lumbar to cervical spine and brain. Measurement permits calculation of a conduction velocity that is thought to reflect conduction in the posterior columns of the spinal cord. The time interval between the potential recorded at the cauda equina and over the scalp measures total conduction time in the somatosensory pathway. Any lesion, whether demyelinative, nutritional, compressive, or destructive, that affects this ascending pathway in spinal cord or brainstem can delay the total conduction time.

Electromyography and Nerve Conduction Studies

Appropriate percutaneous electrical stimulation of a peripheral nerve excites the nerve to generate an action potential. When stimulating motor nerves, one places recording elelctrodes over a muscle and records the evoked muscle action potential on an oscilloscope. The nerve innervating that muscle is stimulated at various points along its length. The time from each site of stimulation to onset of the evoked muscle response is recorded and the conduction velocity is determined by dividing the time difference between different stimulation sites into the distance that separates them. To record conduction velocity in sensory nerves, one stimulates cutaneous nerve branches distally and places recording electrodes over the nerve at various proximal sites. Time interval divided into distance again provides the conduction velocity. The *F-response* gives an indication of conduction in motor nerves from the site of stimulation antidromically to the motoneuron and orthodromically back to the site of recording; when analyzed in conjunction with the conduction velocity of the more distal portions of the nerve, it provides a measure of conduction in the proximal portions of a motor nerve and ventral root. The *H-reflex* provides the electrical equivalent of the stretch reflex by stimulating sensory fibers of the posterior tibial nerve in the popliteal fossa at low intesnsities and recording the muscle evoked action potential from the soleus muscle. These peripheral nerve and muscle electrophysiologic studies assist in determining whether disease involves nerve, muscle, or both and in determining the distribution of abnormality. They facilitate the differentiation of demyelinating neuropathy from axonal neuropathy, neuropathy from radiculopathy, and primary muscle disease from disease of the motor unit. Demyelinating neuropathies affect mainly large fibers and slow the conduction velocity. When disease damages axons in addition to myelin, there is a decrease in the number of axons that can be electrically activated, resulting in a diminution in the size of the compound action potential.

Electromyography (EMG) is performed by inserting a needle electrode into the muscle to record the structure's electrical activity (Fig. 471–1). Under normal circumstances muscle at rest is silent, but in denervated or diseased states muscle membranes become spontaneously excitable, generating fibrillation potentials of small amplitude. When the nerve itself is diseased, entire motor units may become spontaneously active. The resulting fasciculations are often visible percutaneously and can be detected by the electrode. Furthermore, when damaged axons cease to innervate muscle fibers, remaining axons gradually sprout collaterals that reinnervate the denervated fibers; consequently, the size of the few remaining motor units increases. As a result, in partially denervated muscles one records during voluntary contraction a decrease in the number and an increase in the size of the electrical potentials generated by the activated motor units. By contrast, as muscle fibers degenerate in primary disease of muscle, the size of motor units decreases, since each nerve now innervates fewer fibers: during voluntary contration the number of activated units is normal but their amplitude is smaller. The anatomic distribution of abnormalities helps differentiate a mononeuropathy from a generalized neuropathy and a radiculopathy from a neuropathy. In primary myopathies, the distribution of abnormality helps in characterizing the myopathy itself. Tables 471–2 and 471–3 provide guides to the usefulness and pertinent changes in electrophysiologic tests in various neuromuscular disorders.

TABLE 471–3. DIFFERENTIATION AMONG MYOPATHY, AXONOPATHY, MYELINOPATHY, AND RADICULOPATHY USING ELECTROPHYSIOLOGIC STUDIES

	Myopathy	Axonopathy	Myelinopathy	Radiculopathy
Nerve conduction velocity	Normal	Normal	Slow	Normal
F-response	Normal	Normal	Delayed/absent	Delayed/absent
H-reflex*	Normal	Normal	Delayed/absent	Delayed/absent
EMG				
Voluntary contraction	Predominance of small motor units	Predominance of large motor units	Normal	Normal/some large motor units
Spontaneous activity	Fibrillations	Fibrillations, fasciculations	Normal	Fibrillations, fasciculations

*Usually studied with posterior tibial nerve stimulation, recording the soleus contraction, thus providing an index of S1 root function only.

NEUROMUSCULAR TRANSMISSION STUDIES

Diseases of the neuromuscular junction (myasthenia gravis, Eaton-Lambert myasthenic syndrome, botulism) are characterized by normal nerve conduction velocity and usually a normal EMG. Repetitive electrical activation of the neuromuscular junction, however, will produce either an abnormal diminution or an abnormal facilitation of the evoked muscle action potential. In myasthenia gravis repetitive stimulation of a peripheral nerve most often causes a rapid progressive decrement of the amplitude of the muscle evoked action potential owing to rapid saturation of the small number of post-synaptic receptors by the released acetylcholine. In botulism and Eaton-Lambert myasthenic syndrome, where the defect is on the presynaptic membrane, repetitive stimulation of the nerve overcomes the presynaptic blockade of acetylcholine release and usually elicits an increase in the size of the muscle evoked action potentials.

Bradbury M, Radda GK, Allen PS: Nuclear magnetic resonance techniques in medicine. Ann Intern Med 98:514, 1983. *A well-written summary of this rapidly advancing field.*

Chiappa KH: Evoked Potentials in Clinical Medicine. New York, Raven Press, 1983. *This and the below-mentioned three texts provide excellent summaries and current references for the field.*

Goodgold J, Eberstein A: Electrodiagnosis of Neuromuscular Disease. Baltimore, William and Wilkins, 1983.

Johnson EW: Practical Electromyography. Baltimore, Williams and Wilkins, 1983.

Mayo Clinic: Clinical Examinations in Neurology. 5th ed. Philadelphia, W. B. Saunders Company, 1981.

Spehlmann R: EEG Primer. New York, Elsevier, 1981. *An excellent general reference on electroencephalography.*

Weisberg LA: Computed tomography in the diagnosis of intracranial disease. Ann Intern Med 91:87, 1979. *A useful summary article.*

Section Two DISORDERS OF CEREBRAL FUNCTION

472. DISTURBANCES OF CONSCIOUSNESS AND AROUSAL

472.1 Sustained Impairment of Consciousness

Jerome B. Posner

PATHOGENESIS

DEFINITIONS. From the medical standpoint, consciousness include two interdependent but separate functions: wakefulness and psychologically recognizable mental activity. Its antithesis, *coma,* is a state of complete mental unresponsiveness with eyes closed and no evidence of psychologically or physiologically appropriate responses to stimulation. Between these antipodes lie a series of abnormal states of mentation and arousal that reflect the effects of different degrees, loci, and acuteness of brain dysfunction damage. *Obtundation* and *drowsiness* describe states of impaired alertness or wakefulness wherein patients continue to respond to verbal stimuli. *Stupor* is a state wherein subjects arouse when vigorously stimulated but immediately sink back to unresponsiveness as soon as external stimuli are withdrawn. Amnesia, asphasia, and dementia are conditions in which the content of consciousness is reduced but relatively normal arousal and sleep-wake cycles remain. The *vegetative state* describes a usually chronic or semichronic condition wherein patients with severe forms of brain damage sleep and awaken but have no recognizable psychological functions. Brainstem and autonomic functions are retained. Vegetative states may follow severe acute brain injuries caused by head trauma or cardiac arrest, for example. Chronic vegetative states also comprise the terminal stages of progressive organic dementias such as Alzheimer's or Huntington's disease. The *locked-in state* describes patients who are awake and retain mental content but owing to paralysis of descending motor pathways, cannot express themselves because of paralysis of the muscles that control speach or facial expression or move the limbs. The site of the lesion usually involves motor pathways in the base of the pons or, less often, midbrain. Sparing of the brainstem tegmentum in these structures explains why consciousness is retained.

MECHANISMS OF CONSCIOUSNESS AND UNCONSCIOUSNESS. The physiologic basis of consciousness depends on close interaction between the intact cerebral hemispheres and activating mechanisms located in the central gray matter of the upper brainstem. The cerebral hemisphere contribute the substrate for most of the specific psychologic components, including language, memory, intellect, and learned responses to sensory stimuli. However, in order for the cerebrum to function and to integrate its component psychologic activities, the hemispheres must be aroused or activated by structures that originate in the thalamus, hypothalamus, midbrain, and tegmentum of the upper pons. An important component of this arousal mechanism is located within what Magoun, Morruzzi, and their colleagues called the ascending reticular activating system; other brainstem systems lying along the deep central gray matter core of the brainstem also influence cerebral cortical activity and the state of consciousness. In addition, conscious behavior is heavily influenced by the activity of intra- and interhemipsheric interconnecting neural pathways.

The relation of the cerebral cortex to consciousness is both quantitative and qualitative. All hemispheric lesions of any great size interfere with both specific somatosensory areas (e.g., vision, cutaneous sensation, movement control) and association cortex. Lesions of the latter alter the integrative aspects of consciousness, and the sudden total loss of the cortex or its connections to the deeper nuclei causes several days or weeks of coma even if the brainstem remains intact. Between the extremes of alert, intelligent consciousness and a state of unresponsive coma lies a continuum along which the size and location of the lesion and the impairment of mind, memory, wit, and personality are roughly proportional to one another.

GENERAL CAUSES AND MANIFESTATIONS OF DELIRIUM, STUPOR, AND COMA

As indicated above, to produce an alteration of consciousness, disease or dysfunction must damage or depress either the two cerebral hemispheres or the upper brainstem or both.

TABLE 472–1. THE COMMON CAUSES OF STUPOR AND COMA

Supratentorial lesions (causing upper brainstem dysfunction)
Cerebral hemorrhage
Large cerebral infarction
Subdural hematoma
Epidural hematoma
Brain tumor
Brain abscess (rare)
Subtentorial lesions (compressing or destroying the reticular formation)
Pontine or cerebellar hemorrhage
Infarction
Tumor
Cerebellar abscess
Metabolic and diffuse lesions (see also Table 472–2)
Anoxia or ischemia
Hypoglycemia
Nutritional deficiency
Endogenous organ failure or deficiency
Exogenous poison
Infections
Meningitis
Encephalitis
Ionic and electrolyte disorders
Concussion and postictal states
Psychogenic unresponsiveness

A potentially bewildering series of individual disorders can have one or both of these effects, as may be seen in Table 472–1. However, if one examines the mechanisms by which neurologic diseases cause coma, real or apparent, these maladies fall into four categories that can be distinguished by their anatomic distribution and the resulting signs and symptoms they produce. These are (1) supratentorial mass lesions, (2) subtentorial compressive or destructive lesions, (3) metabolic brain diseases, and (4) psychogenic unresponsiveness.

Supratentorial Mass Lesions

Supratentorial masses impair consciousness because as they expand they shift and squeeze the contents of the supratentorial compartment and, in so doing, compress the diencephalon. The expanding process can originate anywhere in the hemisphere and ultimately produces this reaction because the fibrous tentorium and the bones of the base of the skull resist movement except toward the tentorial opening. As a result, the diencephalic tectum and adjacent midbrain become compressed, and the diencephalon may be displaced downward through the tentorial notch (transtentorial herniation).

How do supratentorial masses progress so that these reactions occur? The brain has certain common responses to injury, including edema, vascular dilatation, and the invasion of leukocytes and proliferation of glial cells. The intensity and tempo of these individual pathologic responses vary according to the nature of the original lesion and the rate at which it appears, but the end result of neoplasms, infection, and infarcts is often the same: the original lesion gradually enlarges and, ripple-like, its effects expand outward to impair structures ever more remote from itself in the inexpansible intracranial cavity. Effects that lie remote from the primary lesion are due partly to edema spreading away from its edges and partly to an actual shift of the brain within the skull, compressing normal tissues and blood vessels against rigid structures such as the falx cerebri and the tentorium. At this stage, clinical signs of increased intracranial pressure are common and imply that an intracranial lesion is already exerting generalized deleterious effects.

The clinical picture of supratentorial mass lesions producing stupor or coma has several distinctive features. Localizing symptoms such as frontal headache, focal seizures, or other changes consistent with hemispheric disease almost always precede the development of unconsciousness. Physically, most patients demonstrate a combination of *focal* hemispheral signs, e.g., sensorimotor defect, aphasia, and visual field defect, reflecting the site of the original pathologic process, plus *diffuse* signs of supratentorial dysfunction, indicating that the lesion is exerting remote effects on the opposite hemisphere and the deep-lying diencephalon. An important negative finding is that, unless the patient is in the terminal stages of illness, no evidence of direct subtentorial brainstem dysfunction can be found: pupillary and oculovestibular reflexes remain intact. As a supratentorial lesion progresses, the neurologic signs and symptoms evolve in a characteristic, orderly, rostral-caudal pattern. The more rostrally located neurologic functions disappear first, followed by more caudal impairment, first in the diencephalon and then down the brainstem almost as if the structures were being progressively transected from above downward, each plane of function being removed before the next becomes greatly impaired.

The aforementioned description needs amplification to be complete. Some supratentorial masses that begin and enlarge in neurologically silent areas such as the frontal lobes or the subdural space can lack a focal signature. Lesions of this type may be revealed only when the patient develops signs of diffuse forebrain dysfunction plus, perhaps, headache and evidence of increased intracranial pressure.

Stupor or coma with supratentorial lesions is ominous because it implies that the deeply located upper brain stem is already compressed or distorted and that the much more serious complication of herniation of the forebrain into the tentorial notch threatens to occur. Such herniation begins either with direct downward displacement of the diencephalon (central herniation) or with the uncus of the temporal lobe squeezing into the tentorial notch and against the midbrain (uncal herniation). Either way, if the hernia develops fully, it usually impacts itself upon the midbrain and nearly always results in permanent brain damage or death. A characteristic constellation of symptoms heralds each of these patterns of transtentorial herniation. With impending *central* herniation, stupor becomes gradually deeper, and the subjects sigh, yawn, or develop periodic respirations. The pupils shrink to 1 to 2 mm in diameter, but retain their light reflexes. Oculocephalic reflexes (doll's eye maneuver) are brisk and oculovestibular responses (cold caloric test) are marked by tonic deviation of the eyes toward the stimulated side rather than by physiologic nystagmus. The extremities stiffen into bilateral rigidity or spasticity, combined with extensor plantar responses. With *uncal* herniation, signs are in many ways similar to the above except that as the uncus slides over the tentorial edge, it often compresses the third nerve ahead of it, even before the diencephalon is squeezed. The result is that the pupil on the side of the herniation begins to dilate more than its fellow. Eventually, the pupil dilates widely and becomes light-fixed, and the patient declines into stupor. Shortly afterward, oculomotor functions of the third nerve are usually impaired, and the involved eye turns outward. If the herniating process continues, the opposite third nerve becomes involved, and then the brainstem. To initiate effective treatment one must recognize the process before this advanced stage and halt it with osmotic jecompressing agents or surgical treatment. Otherwise, when conditions progress this far, few subjects recover without residual neurologic injury.

Subtentorial Mass or Destructive Lesions

The subtentorial regions critical to consciousness extend along the paramedian tegmentum from the level of the rostral midbrain down to roughly the middle of the pons. Destruction or compression of this critical area causes stupor or coma, and partial damage to it impairs cognition. Expanding lesions of the posterior fossa produce a similar effect if they compress the upper brainstem. Compression of the medulla oblongata by the cerebellar tonsils causes stiff neck, along with irregularities of respiratory and cardiac rhythm, but does not directly impair consciousness.

The characteristic clinical feature of subtentorial destruction or compression causing coma is evidence of focal brainstem dysfunction, usually asymmetrical, which frequently can be anatomically pinpointed by the clinical findings. The pupils are almost always abnormal, because either pontine or medullary sympathetic pathways or third nerve nuclei or fibers are destroyed. Dysconjugate eye movement are common, and bizarrely or independently moving eyes, ocular bobbing, or rotating ocular deviation usually means primary brainstem dysfunction. Unilateral facial anesthesia involving both the brow and lower face, absent caloric responses to one side, and eye deviation toward the paralyzed arm and leg all suggest a subtentorial lesion. The combination of flaccidity in the arms and flexor responses in the legs signifies pontine-midbrain damage. Seldom do the signs indicate complete brainstem transection. This restricted, discrete localization is unlike metabolic lesions causing coma in which the signs commonly indicate incomplete dysfunction at several different levels of the brain, and also is unlike the secondary brainstem dysfunction and coma that follow supratentorial herniation, in which *all* function at any given level tends to be lost as the process progressess from rostral to caudal along the neuraxis.

Purely compressive lesions of the posterior fossa rarely cause coma until late in their course when the patient is near death. The pathologic process involved is usually a hemorrhage, abscess, or tumor of the cerebellum or fourth ventricle. In such instances, occipital haadache, nystagmus, diplopia, nausea, vomiting, cranial nerve signs, and ataxia usually precede unconsciousness. Important points in distinguishing destructive and compressive posterior fossa lesions from metabolic depression of the brainstem are that in metabolic depression, other than that caused by sedative drugs, oculovestibular responses are generally preserved until the advanced stages, and pupillary light reflexes are nearly always preserved with both endogenous and exogenous metabolic depression. By contrast, structural brainstem lesions causing coma always disrupt the oculovestibular responses, and those involving the midbrain also interrupt the pupillary reflexes.

Delirium and Exogenous Metabolic Brain Disease

DEFINITIONS. Metabolic encephalopathy is a term applied to the behavioral changes which result from diffuse or wide spread multifocal failure of cerebral metabolism. The disorder usually begins acutely or subacutely and often subsides with time and/or treatment. The clinical picture is one in which confusion, thinking errors, behavioral abnormalities, disorders of consciousness, and abnormal motor activity predominate. In some instances (e.g., vitamin B_{12} deficiency or hypothyroidism) metabolic encephalopathy is more insidious in onset. The usual clinical findings then resemble dementia (see definition below) rather than delirium. However, the brain disorder remains reversible by appropriate treatment. Some causes of metabolic encephalopathy are listed in Table 472–2. The table also includes some primary disorders of the central nervous system such as encephalitis, meningitis, concussion, and seizures disorders, because these develop acutely, are reversible with appropriate treatment, and clinically resemble acute metabolic brain disease.

Metabolic brain disease is common and often misdiagnosed. When mild, it produces intellectual dullness, social indifference, and vague perplexity easily mistaken by observers for psychogenic depression or simply low intelligence. More severe

TABLE 472–2. SOME CAUSES OF METABOLIC BRAIN DISEASE

I. Deprivation of oxygen, substrate, or metabolic cofactors
  *A. Hypoxia (interference with oxygen supply to the entire brain—cerebral blood flow normal)
    1. Decreased oxygen tension and content of blood
      Pulmonary disease
      Alveolar hypoventilation
      Decreased atmospheric oxygen tension (e.g., high altitude)
    2. Decreased oxygen content of blood—normal tension
      Anemia
      Carbon monoxide poisoning
      Methemoglobinemia
  *B. Ischemia (diffuse or widespread multifocal interference with blood supply to brain)
    1. Decreased cerebral blood flow resulting from decreased cardiac output
      Stokes-Adams syndrome, cardiac arrest, cardiac arrhythmias
      Myocardial infarction
      Congestive heart failure
      Aortic stenosis
      Pulmonary embolism
    2. Decreased cerebral blood flow resulting from decreased peripheral resistance in the systemic circulation
      Syncope: orthostatic, vasovagal
      Carotid sinus hypersensitivity
      Low blood volume
    3. Decreased cerebral blood flow due to generalized or multifocal increase in cerebrovascular resistance
      Hyperventilation syndrome
      Increased blood viscosity (polycythemia, cryo- and macroglobinemia, sickle cell anemia)
      Bacterial meningitis and encephalitis
      Subarachnoid hemorrhage
    4. Decreased local cerebral blood flow due to widespread small vessel occlusion or tissue necrosis
      Disseminated intravascular coagulation
      Systemic lupus erythematosus
      Subacute bacterial endocarditis
      Cardiopulmonary bypass
      Small emboli (fat, fibrin, platelets)
      Acute viral encephalitis
    5. Alterations of blood flow due to failure of autoregulation
      Hypertensive encephalopathy
  *C. Hypoglycemia
      Resulting from exogenous insulin
      Spontaneous (endogenous insulin, liver disease, etc.)
  D. Cofactor deficiency
      Thiamine (Wernicke's encephalopathy)
      Niacin
      Pyridoxine
      B_{12}
      Folate
II. Diseases of organs other than brain
  *A. Diseases of nonendocrine organs
      Liver (hepatic coma)
      Kidney (uremic coma)
      Lung (CO_2 narcosis)
      Pancreas (exocrine pancreatic encephalopathy)
II. Diseases of organs other than brain (*Continued*)
  *B. Hyper- and/or hypofunction of endocrine organs
      Pituitary
      Thyroid (myxedema-thyrotoxicosis)
      Parathyroid (hyper- and hypoparathyroidism)
      Adrenal (Addison's disease, Cushing's disease, pheochromocytoma)
      Pancreas (diabetes, hypoglycemia)
  C. Other systemic diseases
      Diabetes
      Cancer
      Porphyria
      Sepsis
III. Exogenous poisons (see also Ch. 25)
  *A. Sedative drugs
  B. Acid poisons or poisons with acidic breakdown products
      Paraldehyde
      Methyl alcohol
      Ethylene glycol
  C. Psychotropic drugs
      Tricyclic antidepressants and anticholinergic drugs
      Amphetamines
      Lithium
      Phenothiazines
      LSD-mescaline
      Monoamine oxidase inhibitors
  D. Others
      Penicillin
      Anticonvulsants
      Steroids
      Cardiac glycosides
      Cimetidine
      Heavy metals
      Organic phosphates
      Cyanide
      Salicylates
IV. Abnormalities of fluid, ionic, or acid-base environment of CNS
  A. Water and sodium (hyper- and hyponatremia) (hypo- and hyperosmolality)
  B. Acidosis (metabolic and respiratory)
  C. Alkalosis (metabolic and respiratory)
  D. Magnesium (hyper- and hypomagnesemia)
  E. Calcium (hyper- and hypocalcemia)
  F. Phosphorus (hyper- and hypophosphatemia)
  G. ? Trace metal deficiency or excess
V. Disordered temperature regulation
  A. Hypothermia
  B. Heat stroke, fever
VI. Infections or inflammation of CNS
  A. Leptomeningitis
  B. Encephalitis
  C. Acute "toxic" encephalopathy
  D. Parainfectious encephalomyelitis
  E. Cerebral vasculitis
  F. Subarachnoid hemorrhage
VII. Miscellaneous diseases of unknown cause
  A. Seizures and postictal states
  *B. "Postoperative" delirum
  C. Concussion
  *D. Acute delirious states
      Sedative drug withdrawal
      "Postoperative" delirium
      Intensive care unit delirium
      Drug intoxications

*Alone or in combination, the most common causes of delirium seen on medical or surgical wards.

encephalopathy elicits either a florid picture of tremulous agitation, rich and frightening hallucinations, and periods of seemingly complete loss of contact with the environment, or a more quiet, withdrawn, akinetic state which may fade into stupor or coma. The former, often called *delirium* or *toxic psychosis,* may be confused with a functional psychosis, and the latter, often called *acute* or *subacute confusional state,* is likely to be mistaken for structural brain disease or psychological depression. Although certain specific systemic disorders characteristically cause one or another of the aforementioned syndromes, each can occur with any of the metabolic brain diseases; thus the terms "delirium," "toxic psychosis," and "confusional state" are used interchangeably in this chapter to describe the wakeful stage of metabolic encephalopathy.

The term *dementia* is used operationally to describe an irreversible loss of memory and cognitive functions, usually insidious in onset, irreversible, and often, but not always, resulting from intrinsic disease of the brain. Demented patients usually do not have the clouding of consciousness associated with deliriuim. However, an insidiously developing, quiet delirium may be clinically indistinguishable from the early stages of dementia.

CLINICAL FEATURES OF METABOLIC BRAIN DISEASE. The purpose of the physical and laboratory examination in a patient with suspected metabolic brain disease is two-fold: first to determine if the observed changes in consciousness are due to metabolic brain disease (i.e., to rule out structural brain disease or psychiatric dysfunction); and second, to determine exactly the type of metabolic defect causing the delirium. In general, evaluation of the state of consciousness, motor activity, and autonomic acitivity, as detailed below, helps answer the first question, whereas the general physical examination, examination of ventilation, and laboratory examination (the latter two detailed below) help answer the second question. It cannot, however, be overemphasized that, despite the difficulties of examining a delirious patient, a thorough and systematic general physical, neurologic, and laboratory examination *must* be undertaken if a definitive diagnosis is to be established and definitive treatment to be applied. Some principles of the examination are outlined in Table 472–3.

State of Consciousness and Mental Content. Disorders of attention are the earliest sign and the hallmark of metabolic brain disease. The patient may appear quietly perplexed or preoccupied and be unable to concentrate sufficiently to deal with significant stimuli in the environment. Conversely, he may appear hypervigilant and distractible, attending briefly to each new environmental stimulus no matter how trivial or irrelevant. Attentional defects may be subtle at onset and are easily mistaken for normal if slightly odd behavior. At about the same time, restlessness or lethargy, emotional lability, insomnia or drowsiness, and vivid nightmares may appear. Patients often appear fearful and anxious, or depressed, and may express the fear that they are "going crazy." They may be restless, irritable, and easily distracted. Conversely, they may lie quietly or sleep when left alone, and rarely read or attend to the world around them. With more severe metabolic disturbances, patients become drowsy and finally stuporous or comatose. The particular affect that prevails in patients with metabolic encephalopathy depends partly on the nature of the illness and partly on the rapidity of its development; previous personality often has suprisingly little influence. Thus, barbiturate- or alcohol-withdrawal syndromes, acute liver necrosis, and porphyria often cause an agitated delirium, whereas uremia, pulmonary encephalopathy, and anoxia usually produce a more quit illness. Rapijly developing metabolic abnormalities are more likely to produce agitated delirium than those that develop more slowly.

Disturbances in cognition appear along with altered alertness and awareness and are characterized by difficulties with immediate recall and the ability to abstract. Normal subjects readily recall and repeat 6 or 7 digits forward and 5 or 6 backward and can identify the common denominator between such pairs as an apple and an orange or a fly and a tree, but delirious patients cannot. However, innate intelligence and education also determine cognitive abilities and, unless the physician has examined the patient previously, it is difficult to attribute mild disturbances to a metabolic defect. An early sign of delirium, although usually not as early as altered alertness and cognition, is impairment of memory and orientation. Loss of memory for recent events is a hallmark of metabolic and other organic brain disease and is tested by asking the patient about the names of his doctors, some important current events, and his recent activities. Orientation to place and time should be specifically tested by asking the date and year, the day of the week, and the present location. Orientation for time, particularly the year, is lost early in patients with delirium and orientation for place a little later.

Perceptual errors, e.g., mistaking the physician for an old friend or family member, illusions and hallucinations are common accompaniements of delirium. They frighten and agitate some patients, but are quietly tolerated by others. The nature of the illusions and hallucinations seems to reflect the individual's personality, and often the same hallucinations accompany separate episodes of delirium. A quiet, withdrawn patient must be specifically asked about hallucinations, because he often fails either to volunteer the information or to behave as if he were hallucinating. Hallucinations of metabolic origin may be visual, auditory, tactile, or a combination, contrasting with those of schizophrenia, which are usually auditory only.

Fluctuations of the mental status are common in metabolic encephalopathy. Patients may be totally out of contact one moment and lucid the next. Lucid intervals appear unpredictably and last for minutes or hours. Some of the fluctuation is environmentally related. Thus delirious patients characteristically become more disoriented at night, in unfamiliar surroundings, and in situations in which restraints and background noise and unfamiliar activity replace familiar sensory stimuli. One study demonstrated a higher incidence of postoperative delirium in patients treated in a windowless intensive care unit than in those treated in a similar one with windows.

Motor Activity. Tremor, asterixis, and multifocal myoclonus are characteristic of metabolic brain disease, and the specificity of the latter two makes them the most important physical signs that distinguish metabolic encephalopathy from psychiatric illness or from structural brain disease.

TABLE 472–3. PHYSICAL EXAMINATION OF PATIENTS WITH SUSPECTED METABOLIC BRAIN DISEASE

- History (from relatives or friends)
  - Previous medical illness (diabetes, uremia, heart disease)
  - Previous psychiatric history
  - Access to drugs (sedative, psychotropic drugs)
  - Recent complaints (headache, depression)
- General physical examination
  - Evidence of trauma
  - Evidence of chronic or acute systemic illness
- Neurologic examination
  - Mental status
    - Affect (agitated, depressed, apathetic)
    - Alertness (delirium, obtundation, stupor, coma)
    - Memory (recent events, recall of objects)
    - Orientation (time, place, person)
    - Perceptual abnormalities (illusions, delusions, hallucinations)
    - Psychomotor activity
  - Motor examination
    - Focal weakness
    - Tremor
    - Asterixis
    - Myoclonus
    - Seizures
  - Autonomic examination
    - Pupillary size and responses
    - Temperature
    - Heart rate and rhythm
    - Diaphoresis
    - Ventilation

The *tremor* of delirious patients is coarse and irregular at a rate of about eight to ten per second. It is usually absent at complete rest. It is best seen in the fingers of the outstretched hands. It is less specific than asterixis and multifocal myoclonus, and may affect patients with psychiatric disease as well as those with systemic illness not associated with delirium.

Asterixis is an abnormal, involuntary jerking movement elicited in the hands by asking patients to dorsiflex the wrist and spread the extended fingers. Its mildest form involves irregular random lateral jerking movements of the fingers at the metacarpophalangeal joints. With fully developed asterixis there is sudden palmar flexion of the fingers at the metacarpophalangeal joints and of the wrist. The movements are asynchronous in the two hands and nonrhythmic. They occur every 2 to 30 seconds, recover quickly, and cannot be controlled by the patient, even when he is aware of their presence. Asterixis may also involve the feet and tongue. In the obtunded patient the same movement can sometimes by evoked by passively dorsiflexing the wrist or the ankles. Bilateral asterixis almost universally accompanies metabolic encephalopathy at some stage of the illness. It is absent in patients with spychiatric disorders unless they are taking large amounts of drugs, and is encountered rarely, and then unilaterally, in patients with structural brain disease such as decompensating subdural hematomas or deep hemispheral infarcts, especially involving the basal ganglia.

Multifocal myoclonus consists of sudden nonrhythmic, nonpatterned gross muscle contractions in a resting person. The movements are most common in the face and shoulders but occur anywhere in the body. Multifocal myoclonus can often be elicited, if not present at rest, by passive movements of the shoulder and upper arm. It occurs in a later and more severe stage of metabolic illness than does asterixis, and may physiologically represent a more intense and widespread manifestation of that abnormal movement. Multifocal myoclonus makes its most frequent appearance in uremia, hypercarbic-anoxic encephalopathy, and penicillin overdose, but can occur in virtually all metabolic encephalopathies.

Psychomotor activity ranges from extreme hyperactivity to total immobility. Delirious patients may be unwilling or unable to stay in bed, pacing the halls, in constant movement, with outbursts of aggressiveness which may culminate in attacks on others. With more severe delirium, there may be groping movements, picking at the bedclothes, and constant tossing and turning. Such patients may fall out of bed and injure themselves. Increased psychomotor activity is typically observed in acute deliria such as delirium tremens and drug withdrawal states. More commonly, delirium is manifested by reduced activity, with the patient lethargic, drowsy, and generally bradykinetic. The same patient may run the gamut from psychomotor overactivity to reduced activity during the course of the delirium. *Speech* is often abnormal. Patients with increased psychomotor behavior often speak rapidly, with a muttering or slurred speech which, because of its speed, is incomprehensible. Patients with reduced psychomotor activity may speak slowly, monotonously, and so softly as not to be clearly heard.

Seizures, hyperactive stretch reflexes, and *focal signs* frequently accompany severe metabolic brain disease. The seizures are usually generalized and the motor abnormalities usually symmetrical. However, focal paresis and focal seizures are not rare, especially with anoxia, hypoglycemia, or hyperosmolality. Signs of focal disturbance make it more difficult to distinguish between metabolic and structural brain disease. However, in metabolic brain disease the focal signs are usually mild and fleeting, and they are accompanied by more widespread neurologic dysfunction than occurs with gross structural disease.

Autonomic Activity. *Pupillary light reactions are always preserved in metabolic coma with the few exceptions to be mentioned, and absence of the pupillary light reaction strongly suggests a structural lesion.* The exceptions are glutethimide intoxication, which may produce mid-position or slightly dilated fixed pupils; anticholinergic drug administration, which produces fixed, dilated pupils; and exposure to severe anoxia, or asphyxia, which produces fixed dilated pupils and, if sustained, probably implies irreversible brain damage. The pupils, whatever their size and reaction to light, are usually symmetrical in patients comatose from metabolic brain disease, but often asymmetrical in patients comatose from structural brain disease.

TABLE 472–4. LABORATORY EVALUATION OF METABOLIC BRAIN DISEASE

Test	Reason for Test
Immediate:	
Glucose	Hypoglycemia, hyperosmolar coma
Na^+	Osmolar abnormalities
Ca^{++}	Hyper- or hypocalcemia
BUN	Uremia
Arterial blood pH, P_{CO_2}, P_{O_2}	Acidosis, alkalosis, hypoxia
Lumbar puncture	Infection, hemorrhage
Later:	
Liver function tests	Hepatic coma
Sedative drug levels	Overdose
Blood and CSF culture	Sepsis, encephalitis, meningitis
Full electrolytes, including Mg^{++}	Electrolyte imbalance
Coagulation profile	Intravascular coagulation
EEG	

Hypothermia is common in delirious patients with myxedema, hypoglycemia, and barbiturate intoxication. Hyperthermia with profuse perspiration and tachycardia accompanies most agitated deliria and is especially common with delirium tremens. Hyperthermia without perspiration suggests anticholinergic drug ingestion or infection. Hyperthermia also marks salicylate and occasionally phenothiazine overdosage.

LABORATORY TESTS. The causes of metabolic coma are legion, and a final diagnosis usually depends on extensive laboratory tests. The tests which should be performed immediately to establish the presence of life-threatening metabolic defects are listed in Table 472–4, along with those whose results are not available immediately but should be done as soon as possible if the diagnosis is unclear.

PSYCHIATRIC DISORDERS

Psychiatric dysfunction may mimic alterations in consciousness. Patients with psychiatric disorders may complain of memory loss, confusion, and/or hallucinations. Patients with psychiatic amnesia, unlike those with metabolic or structural brain disease, often claim disorientation for self (i.e., they deny that they know who they are), even though they may be oriented for place and time. Furthermore, if the patient's cooperation can be elicited, recent memory and cognitive functions are usually preserved. Hallucinations are auditory rather than visual or tacitile, and asterixis and multifocal myoclonus are never present. Patients with extreme anxiety may hyperventilate, producing respiratory alkalosis and a diffusely slow electroencphalogram. Except for that problem, however, the physical and laboratory evaluations are generally normal.

In patients with psychiatric unresponsiveness, the segmental neurologic examination is likewise normal. Breathing is eupneic or voluntarial hyperpneic. Such patients are quietly unresponsive, with all their limbs flaccid. Eye are usually closed and frequently resist eyelid opening. In some patients, the eyes may deviate toward the bed when the patient is turned on his side. The eyelids are incapable of the slow closure of the passively opened eyelids that accompanies true coma. Pupils are briskly responsive or, if psycho-plegics have been self-instilled, widely dilated. Oculocephalic responses are unpredictable, but if the diagnosis is doubtful, irrigating the tympanum with 50 ml of cold water produces physiologic nystagmus rather than the tonic eye deviaiton of the comatose patient with structural or metabolic disease. At times the diagnosis may be difficult because psychiatric delirium or unresponsiveness is superimposed on underlying physical illness (e.g., a patient hospitalized with a severe medical or neurologic illness may be so anxious that he is unable to cope with his environment and thus develops delirium or unresponsiveness). In instances in which there is serious doubt about the diagnosis, slow infusions of small amounts of sodium amobarbital (Amytal interview) may allow thucphysician to establish contact and rapport with the psychiatrically withdrawn patient. The drug may be similarly used to awaken patients rendered unconscious by continuous focal seizures.

GENERAL MANAGEMENT OF ALTERED CONSCIOUSNESS

HISTORY. Several questions must be asked and answered by the physician when he attempts to diagnose and manage the patient with severe brain dysfunction of unknown cause. First he must determine if the disease is focal (i.e., structural) or multifocal-diffuse. If focal, is it (1) supra- or subtentorial in distribution? (2) arrested, improving, or worsening? (3) best treated medically or surgically? If apparently multifocal-diffuse, is the disorder due to (1) exogenous drugs, (2) endogenous metabolic error, (3) CNS infection or hemorrhage, or (4) psychogenic unresponsiveness? Given the answers to these questions, what is the specific etiologic diagnosis? However, even before pursuing this logical approach, the physician must ensure that the brain and other vital organs receive no further injury while he obtains whatever history, examination, or laboratory data are required. This means that in critical situations, lifesaving measures should be underway while clinical and laboratory steps are undertaken to reach an accurate diagnosis and initiate definitive treatment.

It requires considerable restraint to approach a patient with altered consciuosness methodiccally, for the urge to act without delay is understandably strong but potentially dangerous. Inquiry into both the past medical history and the circumstances under which the patient lost ocnsciousness generally discloses more of diagnostic value than any other maneuver. Is there any suggestion that head trauma could have occurred recently? Is chronic renal, hepatic, or myocardial disease? Could a seizure have preceded the present unconsciousness? Has the subject been taking insulin? Have there been recent changes in mood, behavior, or neurologic function to suggest an evolving intracranial process? Was the subject "blue," depressed, or moody, and did he have access to depressant drugs? Is he a "spree" drinker? These and other questions must be covered comprehensively with relatives, past physicians, friends, police, or ambulance personnel. One should always remember that most cases of "coma of unknown cause," whether found at home or in the emergency room of a busy hospital, are due to self-induced drug intoxication.

PHYSICAL FINDINGS. One must perform both a meticulous neurologic examination and a thoughtful physical review of every body system, because disease in remote organs often causes or accentuates dysfunction in the brain.

Fever implies infection, inflammation, or neoplasm. On the other hand, hypothermia, (30 to 36° C) in a patient not severely exposed to cold suggests depressant drug poisoning, hypoglycemia, or severe lower brainstem injury, as by infarction. Hypertension may be the cause of hypertensive encephalopathy or the underlying cause of cerebral hemorrhage. Conversely, an elevated blood pressure can be a symptom of subarachnoid hemorrhage in a subject not previously hypertensive. Hypotension in a supine patient implies low blood volume (hemorrhagic or traumatic shock, severe nutritional and fluid depletion), low cardiac output (myocardial infarction), or low peripheral resistance (depressant drug poisoning). Extreme tachycardia (over 180 per minute) can mean that unconsciousness is the result of lowered cardiac output from a supraventricular cardiac arrhythmia. Bradycardia suggests heart block and the Adams-Stokes syndrome or a myocardial infarct.

The pattern and depth of respiration are often informative in evaluating both neurologic function and acid-base balance. A rapid evaluation of the patient's ventilatory status, coupled with an estimate of blood acid-base balance, frequently narrows the range of possible causes of metabolic coma. A careful clinical examination of the respiratory rate and depth usually allows the physician to estimate whether his patient is hyperventilating, eupneic, or hypoventilating. Caution must be excerised in evaluating patients with severe emphysema whose respiratory effort is increased and who may be tachypneic but nevertheless hypoventilating because of ineffective lungs. Caution must also be used in evluating patients poisoned with depressant drugs who appear to be hypoventilating but are actually eupneic because their metabolic needs are so low. Unexplained abnormalities in the respiratory pattern demand rapid determination of blood gas and acid-base status. A delirious and clinically *hyperventilating* adult with a low serum pH probably has diabetic ketosis, uremia, lactic acidosis, or poisoning with an acidic product. Severe metabolic acidosis, if not treated, is rapidly lethal. Uremia, diagetes, and Addison's disease can be treated specifically (see Ch. 78, 230, and 229), and the others often respond to prompt and urgent treatment of the acidosis by infusion of bicarbonate. If, however, the serum pH is elevated in the delirious and hyperventilating adult, pulmonary disease, cardiac disease, hepatic coma, or neurogenic hyperventilation probable cause. Pneumonia is probably the most common cause of mild respiratory alkalosis in unconscious patients; the others can be evaluated by appropriate laboratory tests. When the serum pH is elevated and the bicarbonate is between 10 and 15 mEq per liter (mixed respiratory alkalosis and metabolic acidosis), sepsis, especially with Gram-negative organisms, salicylism severe hepatic coma are the probable causes.

A similar analysis can be applied to *hypoventilating* patients. In these, the severe problems are depressant drug poisoning, which produces a low serum pH with a normal bicarbonate, and chronic pulmonary failure, which produces a low serum pH and usually a high serum bicarbonate. (The serum bicarbonate level indicates the duration of hypoventialtion.) Both situations demand ventilatory support.

The skin should be searched for petechiae (thrombocytopenic or nonthrombocytopenic purpura, meningococcemia, and bacterial endocarditis), bruises, evidence of nutritional deficiency, icterus, angiomatous spiders, and the bright pinkness of carbon monoxide poisoning. Fleshy or clubbed fingertips suggest carcinoma of the lung, or less often, lung abscess or congenital heart disease (with brain embolism or abscess). A meticulous examination of the optic fundi is imperative but should be completed without cycloplegics, the use of which destroys the potential diagnostic value of pupillary reactions in coma. In the fundus oculi, the pathologic changes of many diseases causing coma can be viewed directly: increased intracranial pressure, hypertensive vascular diase, diabetes, blood dyscrasias, tuberculosis, sarcoidosis, bacterial endocarditis, cryptococcosis, collagen vascular disease, and even subarachnoid hemorrhage producing subhyaloid bleeding.

Chest examination has two potentially rewarding findings: cardiac murmurs suggest bacterial endocarditis with consequent focal, embolic encephalitis; the wheezes and obstructive sounds of the pulmonary cripple suggest CO_2 retention causing narcosis. In the abdominal examination, the presence of masses suggesting polycystic kidneys increases the chances that subarachnoid hemorrhage has occurred, whereas liver enlargement (hepatic coma is common with hepatomas) or splenic enlargement (both blood dyscrasias and infectious mononucleosis can cause encephalitis-like illness) can provide valuable leads.

During the neurologic examination, certain potentially informative steps are sometimes overlooked. The skull should always be palpated and isnpected meticulously. Edema of the scalp commonly overlies fresh fracture lines, and basal skull fractures predispose to blood pigment stains behind the ear (Battle's sign) and about the orbit (raccoon eyes). Blood also may escape from basal fractures into the ear canals, the middle ears, or the nostrils. The skull should be percussed, because focal or unilateral skull tenderness, manifested by grimacing or withdrawal in a stuporous subject, often overlies an intracranial mass lesion. The neck should be tested carefully: stiff neck can reflect meningitis, cerebellar tonsillar herniation, or, occasionally, simply skeletal muscle spasticity. The stiff neck of acute bacterial meningitis is rarely equivocal; that of impending herniation is commonly less severe and lacks accompanying signs of infection or a prominent Kernig sign. It usually requires several hours or a day or more for stiff neck to develop after subarachnoid bleeding.

Table 472–5 gives a profile of neurologic functions useful for evaluating patients with acute brain dysfunction. As the table indicates, certain signs discriminate among normal, impaired, or absent cerebral hemispheric functions, whereas others point toward the presence of moderate or severe brainstem dysfunction. This fundamental examination is easily completed within a few minutes in most patients and can be employed both for immediate anatomic diagnosis and for indicating whether the patienimproving or worsening as time and treatment transpire.

Laboratory Tests. A *CT scan* often resolves much of the issue of the diagnosis of impaired consciousness, particularly in potentially lethal but surgically treatable diseases. If the diagnosis is in doubt, an emergency CT scan should be obtained whenever possible. An abnormal CT scan which identifies supratentorial or subtentorial mass lesions indicates that urgent treatment must be applied. A negative CT scan reassures the physician that he can safely perform a lumbar puncture and informs him that no mass lesion exists, greatly narrowing the choices and suggesting metabolic brain disease.

When to do a lumbar punture is always a serious question. All physicians are aware that in patients with increased intracranial pressure the procedure sometimes induces fatal herniation of the brain through the tentorium or foramen magnum. For this reason, lumbar puncture is best avoided if the physician strongly suspects his patient of having an expanding intracranial mass, particularly in the posterior fossa. Such forbearance is particularly advisable when CT scanning is immediately available. There are certain treatable diseases such as meningitis, however, that can be diagnosed only by lumbar puncture, and many others such as encephalitis or subarachnoid hemorrhage in which the procedure yields valuable preliminary diagnostic informaiton. When the advice of neurologic specialists is unavaialble, the doctor has no choice but to proceed with lumbar puncture if the diagnosis is in doubt and he believes

TABLE 472–5. THE NEUROLOGIC EXAMINATION OF THE PATIENT WITH ACUTELY ALTERED OR CHANGING CONSCIOUSNESS*

Verbal function—oriented, syntactically normal; confused; aphasic; incomprehensible sounds only; mute
Spontaneous eye movements—conjugate pursuit; roving conjugate; dysconjugate; none
Eye opening—spontaneous; in response to verbal stimuli; in response to noxious stimuli; none
Corneal response to stimulation—present; *absent*
Pupillary (note size) response to light stimulation—brisk; *unequal* (test directly and consensually); *sluggish; absent*
Oculocephalic-oculovestibular responses—quick phase nystagmus present; tonic conjugate; *dysconjugate; absent*
Motor response to noxious stimulation—appropriate; stereotyped withdrawal; asymmetrical; abnormal flexor ("decorticate"); abnormal extensor ("decerebrate"); *flaccid*
Breathing pattern—eupneic; rhythmic hyperpnea or hypopnea; regularly irregular (Cheyne-Stokes); *ataxic or bizarrely irregular; absent*

*Each function is subdivided in best-worse order and roughly indicates the rostral-caudal level of impairment. Signs of impaired or absent brainstem function are italicized. (For details consult Plum F, Posner JB: Diagnosis of Stupor and Coma. 3rd ed. Philadelphia, F. A. Davis Company, 1980.)

†Note that eye opening reflects only the state of arousal and not necessarily the presence of psychologic awareness or interaction.

the procedure has a reasonable chance of offering valuable information. Certain steps minimize the risk. One is to use a small (No. 20 or 22) needle. Another is to attach the manometer to the needle before releasing fluid, a technique that prevents sudden subarachnoid pressure shifts. Jugular manometrics should *never* be performed, for they offer little useful data and increase the risk of impacting potential intracranial herniations.

The *electroencephalogram* (EEG) is moderatley useful in evaluating patients with alterations in consciousness. In patients with metabolic brain disease, the EEG is usually slow but symmetrical, and bilateral synchronous paraxysmal bursts of 1 to 3 per second (Hz) activity are frequently superimposed upon the slow background. The degree of slowing roughly parallels the severity of the encephalopathy. Patients with agitated delirium are often exceptions and particularly those suffering from drug withdrawal may have rapid rather than slow EEGs. Normal 8 to 13 Hz activity, however, is usually absent. In patients with supratentorial structural disease, the slow activity is usually more prominent on the side of the lesion. In some patients, alteration of consciousness is caused by a continuosly discharging focal lesion (focal status epilepticus), and such abnormalities may be detected by the presence of focal spikes or sharp waves.

EMERGENCY MANAGEMENT OF COMA

The definitive treatment of altered states of consciousness requires removing, correcting, or halting the specific process responsible to whatever degree possible. Often, however, accurate diagnosis and specific therapy require time to carry out and become effective. In the meantime one must move immediately to protect the brain against permanent damage.

Certain general therapeutic measures apply to the care of all patients:

1. *Assure an adequate airway and oxygenation.* Immediately check and clean out the upper airway. If the patient is entirely unresponsive, arragne for the skillful insertion of an endotracheal airway, but first give 1 mg of atropine intravenously to guard against hypoxigenic vagal cardiac arrest. Be sure that no neck fracture exists before extending the head for intubation. Ausculate both lung bases after inserting the tube to assure that lower airway is open. If a ventilator is used, a rate less than 16 per minute and adjust the volume to give arterial blood gases of Pa_{O_2} >80 mm Hg and Pa_{CO_2} 30 to 35 mm Hg. It is difficult to avoid leaving the patient supine while diagnosis is pursued; but once the diagnosis of metabolic encephalopathy is made, place the patient in mild Trendelenburg position and turn from side to side each hour.

2. *Maintain circulation.* Check the blood pressure and pulse frequently (insert a venous line immediately to replace volume loss), and infuse vasoactive agents to keep mean blood pressure at 80 to 90 mm Hg or more.

3. *Give glucose.* Draw bloods for emergency blood gas and chemical determinations (see Table 472–4) and, if hypoglycemia is a possible diagnosis, immediately give 50 ml of 50 per cent glucose. The glucose will not appreciably intensify hyperosmolality, but there is evidence that hyperglycemia may enhance ischemic brain disease, and thus glucose should be given with caution. However, it is potentially too dangerous to the brain to wait. (Bloods are drawn first in order not to lose evidence for the diagnosis.)

4. *Stop generalized seizures.* Repetitive convulsions can result from either intracranial mass lesions or metabolic-diffuse encephalopathies. In either event, status epilepticus can cause coma and within a short period of time produces irreversible brain damage as well. Start treatment with intravenous diazepam, 10 mg, keeping ventilator available to treat depressed breathing. As soon as convulsions stop, give between 500 and 1000 mg of phenytoin intravenously at a rate of less than 50

TABLE 472–6. COMMON DRUG POISONINGS, SIGNS OF TOXICITY, AND TREATMENT

Drug	Signs and Symptoms		Diagnostic Test	Treatment
	Mild	*Severe*		
Opiates Heroin Morphine Meperidine Methadone Hydromorphone Oxycodone Levorphanol	"Nodding" drowsiness, small pupils, urinary retention, slow and shallow breathing; skin scars and subcutaneous abscesses; duration 4–6 hours; with methadone, duration to 24 hours	Coma; pinpoint pupils, slow irregular respiration or apnea, hypotension, hypothermia, pulmonary edema	Response to naloxone Urine	Naloxone, 0.4 mg intravenously or intramuscularly; repeat at 15-minute intervals not more than twice; repeat in 3 hours if necessary; if no response by second dose, suspect another cause; treat shock; find and detect infection
Depressants Alcohol Barbiturates Chloral hydrate Glutethimide (Doriden) Meprobamate (Equanil)	Confusion, rousable drowsiness, delirium, ataxia, nystagmus, dysarthria, analgesia to stimuli	Stupor to coma; pupils reactive, usually constricted; oculovestibular response absent; motor tonus initially briefly hyperactive, then flaccid; respiration and blood pressure depressed; hypothermia; with glutethimide, pupils moderately dilated, can be fixed; with meprobamate, withdrawal seizures common; with methaqualone, coma, occasional convulsions, tachycardia, cardiac failure, bleeding tendency	Blood, urine, breath Blood Blood Blood	Intubate, ventilate, gavage; drainage position; antimicrobials; keep mean blood pressure above 90 mm Hg and urine output > 300 ml per hour; avoid analeptics; hemodialyze severe phenobarbital poisoning
Methaqualone (Quaalude, Sopor, Mandrax)	Hallucinations, agitation, motor hyperactivity, myoclonus, tonic spasms		Blood	
Benzodiazepines (Librium, Valium, Tranxene, Ativan, Dalmane, etc.) Ethchlorvynol (Placidyl)	Usually taken with another sedative if poisoning is attempted		Blood	As above; diuresis of little help
Stimulants Amphetamines Methylphenidate	Hyperactive, aggressive, sometimes paranoid, repetitive behavior; dilated pupils, tremor, hyperactive reflexes; hyperthermia, tachycardia, arrhythmia Acute torsion dystonia	Agitated, assaultive and paranoid excitement; occasionally convulsions; hypothermia; circulatory collapse	Blood	Chlorpromazine
Cocaine	Similar but less prominent than above; less paranoid, often euphoric	Twitching, irregular breathing, tachycardia, occasionally convulsions	None: clinical appraisal only	Sedation
Psychedelics (LSD), mescaline, psilocybin, phencyclidine, STP)	Confused, disoriented, perceptual distortions, distractable, withdrawn or eruptive, leading to accidents or violence; wide-eyed, dilated pupils; restless, hyperreflexic; less often, hypertension or tachycardia	Panic		Reassure; diazepam satisfactory; avoid phenothiazines
Scopolamine-atropine (knockout drops, Transderm delirium)	Agitated or confused, visual hallucinations, dilated pupils, flushed and dry skin	Florid toxic disoriented delirium, visual hallucination; later, amnesia, fever, dilated fixed pupils, hot flushed dry skin, urinary retention		Reassure; sedate lightly; (1) avoid phenothiazines; (2) do not leave alone
Antidepressants Tricyclics (Tofranil, Elavil, Desipramine, etc.)	Restlessness, drowsiness, tachycardia, ataxia, sweating	Agitation, vomiting, hyperpyrexia, sweating, muscle dystonia, convulsions, tachycardia or arrhythmia	Clinical	Symptomatic; gastric lavage; inject physostigmine for coma or arrhythmia. Intensive care, anticonvulsants, and antiarrhythmics for severe cases
MAO inhibitors (Parnate, Nardil, Eutonyl, etc.)	Hypertensive crises, agitation, drowsiness, ataxia	Hypotension; headache; chest pain; agitation; coma, seizures and shock	Clinical	Symptomatic; gastric lavage

Table continued on opposite page

TABLE 472–6. COMMON DRUG POISONINGS, SIGNS OF TOXICITY, AND TREATMENT (*Continued*)

Drug	Signs and Symptoms: *Mild*	Signs and Symptoms: *Severe*	Diagnostic Test	Treatment
Phenothiazines	Acute dystonia, somnolence, hypotension	Coma; convulsions (rare); arrhythmias; hypotension	Clinical	Symptomatic; gastric lavage
Lithium	Mild lethargy	Lethargy; muteness with appearance of distraction; coma; multifocal seizures; slow or fluctuating course	Blood	Hydrate if mild; hemodialyze for coma or convulsions
Acid-forming intoxicants				
Methanol (formic); ethylene glycol (oxalic and hippuric); other organic alcohols	Inebriation with hyperpnea	All produce progressive hyperventilation, drunkenness, stupor, eventually convulsions and death. Early blindness with methanol	Blood shows increasingly severe anion-gap acidosis	Inhibit hepatic alcohol dehydrogenase by giving alcohol until acidosis controlled, Treat acidosis vigorously
Salicylate				
Aspirin	Tinnitus, dyspnea	Older persons: confusional state or toxic delirium leading to stupor, convulsions, coma	Blood salicylate > 60 mg/dl	Alkaline diuresis

mg per minute. IF seizures continue, give more diazepam or resort to barbiturate general anesthesia. Repetitive focal seizures and myoclonus are potentially less damaging to brain, and their continuation does not require that one resort to anesthesia.

5. *Restore blood acid-base and osmolar balance.* Extremes of either acidosis or alkalosis usually reflect profound metabolic problems, severe circulatory insufficiency, the postictal state (muscular lactic acidosis), or hyperadrenocorticism. Since secver metabolic acidosis can precipitate cardiovascular irregulalarity and alkalosis depresses breathing, they should be corrected. Extreme hypo- and hyperosmolality are equally dangerous to brain and should be corrected, the first with hypertonic saline and the second with fluids (and insulin for hyperglycemia). Beware of too rapid reversal, however, because osmotic delays across the blood-brain barrier during treatment can lead to large fluid shifts in or out of brain. A reasonable goal is to correct blood by about 15 to 20 mOsm in 24 hours.

6. *Treat infection.* Several kinds of infection cause or intensify delirium and coma. Obtain nose, throat, blood, and would cultures, and perform lumbar puncture if indicated. With any sign of infection, begin antimicrobial treatment after obtaining the cultures cited above, based on either the results of smears or the most probable organism.

7. *Treat extreme body temperatures.* Hyperthermia above 40° C or hypothermia below 34° C should be brought to within 2° C of normal.

8. *Give thiamine, 50 to 100 mg intravenously.* Many patients admitted to emergency rooms in stupor or coma are malnourished and therefore vulnerable to Wernicke's encephalopathy if loaded with glucose.

9. *Consider specific antidotes.* Most patients admitted to emergency rooms in coma have taken an overdose of drugs, often in combination. For narcotic overdose, give 0.4 mg of naloxone intravenously every five minutes until the subject awakens. If the subject may be an addict, dilute the dose in 10 ml of saline and give slowly, trying to avoid withdrawal phenomena. Remember that naloxone's duration of action of two to three hours is shorter than that of several narcotics, and the dose may require repeating.

10. *Control agitation,* avoiding barbiturates but employing diazepam or haloperidol as necessary.

11. *Protect the corneas against abrasions,* using ophthalmic ointment and, if necessary, taping the lids shut.

472.2 Acute Central Nervous System Poisoning

Fred Plum

This portion of the chapter briefly discusses the diagnosis and treatment of the most frequent forms of self-induced and accidental poisoning that produce acute severe neurologic dysfunction. At one time sedative drugs, especially the barbiturates, were the chief offenders, but patients and industry recently have become more imaginative in their choices and the list of common agents has lengthened. To find descriptions of poisons not included in this section, especially chronic neurotoxic agents, the reader should consult the textbooks listed in the references.

Table 472–6 lists the most common acute neurotoxic poisonings in the United States, gives their principal signs of toxicity, and outlines their treatment. Antidepressants, benzodiazepines, phenothiazines, barbiturates, opiates, and alcohol either alone or in combination cause the great majority of coma-inducing poisonings. Clinical appraisal must be used to diagnose the agent causing several of these reaction patterns, specific chemical tests being either unavailable or impractically slow. Nevertheless, when any doubt exists, one should keep admission serum samples for possible later analysis. Blood levels or size of the dose are unreliable guides to the potential depth of coma or other risks with most of the drugs because tolerance develops to chronic ingestion, making individuals react differently to similar doses. The mixing of drugs and alcohol adds to the unreliability. Only the opiates and some of the sedatives create an immediate risk of death; concurrent alcohol ingestion enhances both these risks. Opiate poisoning is discussed in more detail in Ch. 481.

PATHOGENESIS. All sedative drugs depress the central nervous system, although not equally on a gram-molecular weight basis, and not to the same degree so far as different central structures are concerned. The duration of action varies widely and depends largely on how the particular drug is detoxified or eliminated. The short-acting barbiturates, pentobarbital, secobarbital, and amobarbital, are detoxified by the liver, as is methaqualone. They exert their maximal effects promptly after being absorbed and, even in huge doses, seldom cause neurologic depression lasting longer than three to five days. Barbital and phenobarbital are partially detoxified by the liver and partially excreted in the urine. Severe poisoning with the latter agent can cause coma lasting 10 to 14 days. Glutethimide has a short duration of action comparable to that of secobarbital, but it is poorly absorbed from the gut and may generate more long-lasting neurotoxic metabolites. Meprobamate has an intermediate duration of effect lasting for days. Bromide rarely causes full coma, but, once it reaches high levels, it replaces chloride in the blood and tissues and persists for weeks to cause symtoms without further ingestion.

Although the sedatives have few important effects outside the nervous system, barbiturates, glutethimide, and meprobamate in toxic doses tend to produce hypotension. Also, glutethimide possesses anticholinergic properties and is the only sedative that predictably produces lightfixed pupils in anesthetic doses.

A withdrawal syndrome consisting of tremulousness, agitation, and sometimes delirium, and convulsions can develop after prompt withdrawal of any of the hypnotic sedatives. Convulsions are a particular problem after withdrawal from meprobamate and methaqualone.

CLINICAL MANIFESTATIONS. Stupor or coma caused by depressant drug poisoning presents the characteristic picture of severe metabolic brain disease. The depression of the central nervous system tends to be bilateral and symmetrical, and the drug affects simultaneously many levels, including the spinal cord. Respiratory and circulatory controlling mechanisms in the lower brainstem are affected only with very high doses or not at all, and, except with glutethimide or extremely large, smooth muscle-paralyzing doses of the barbiturates, the pupillary light reflexes are preserved. Early in the course of acute poisoning, patients can demonstrate muscular hypertonus or even spasticity as the result of uneven depression of different neurologic levels. Within a short time, usually an hour or less, flaccidity supervenes, and the stretch reflexes tend to disappear. Even moderate degrees of drug depression can depress or block the oculovestibular reflexes.

As mentioned, blood levels are a poor index to the depth of coma. Generally speaking, however, blood levels of short-acting barbiturates of more than 2.5 mg per deciliter and phenobarbital blood levels of more than 12 mg per deciliter are associated with very deep coma to the level at which apnea and hypotension become management problems. Apnea rarely supervenes with the benzodiazepines.

DIAGNOSIS. The combination of unresponsiveness, preserved or sluggish pupillary reactions, absent oculovestibular reactions, motor areflexia, hypothermia, and depression of respiration and circulation is clinically diagnostic of sedative-anesthetic drug poisoning. Only infarction or hemorrhage of the pons resembles this clinical state, and with lesions of the pons the pupils are usually small or pinpoint, the stretch reflexes are generally preserved or hyperactive, and the plantar responses are extensor. Specific chemical tests will detect barbiturates, glutethimide, meprobamate, methaqualone, and bromides in blood or urine, and can be done as emergency measures.

MANAGEMENT OF COMA. Treat the patient first, not the drug. First comes general physiologic support. There are no specific antidotes, but certain precautions must be taken. Patients with drug overdose can sink rapidly and unexpectedly to deeper levels of anesthesia and should never be left alone with unskilled attendants.

Assure the Airway First and Throughout. Depressant drugs suppress the cough reflex and the ciliary action of the tracheal and bronchial mucosa. Give atropine, 1 mg intravenously, and place a cuffed endotracheal tube fefore attempting gastric lavage. Subsequently, deflate the endotracheal cuff hourly, replace the tube at 48 hours, and consider tracheostomy at 96 hours if no signs of awakening have occurred.

To empty the stomach in still arousable subjects, give apomorphine subcutaneously, 6 mg for adults and 1 to 2 mg for children. If not available, ipecac 20 ml may be given orally, followed with glasses of water to induce vomiting. Place vomiting subjects prone to avoid aspiration. For patients already in coma once the endotracheal tube is in place, gavage the stomach until clear, using a large double-barreled tube and plain water or half-normal saline for the irrigating solution. To absorb remaining drug in the gut, instill 2 tablespoons of activated charcoal before withdrawing the tube. Repetitive dosing with charcoal may accelerate phenobarbital elimination if coma lasts longer than 12 hours.

Start moistened oxygen 25 per cent via a suitable nonobstructing airway connector. Treat any evidence of hypoventilation immediately with an automatic ventilator. Shallow breathing in a deeply comatose patient frequently reflects no more than the subject's depressed metabolism; if the rate falls below 12 per minute or the physician entertains serious doubts as to the adequacy of ventilation, artificial respiration is indicated. Measure arterial blood gases and initiate artificial respiration in any case if the arterial Po_2 falls below 100 mm Hg on 25 per cent oxygen or if the Pco_2 climbs above 45 mm Hg. High concentrations (greater than 30 per cent) of oxygen therapy should be confined to patients receiving artificial respiration, for such treatment increases the risk of CO_2 retention in nonventilated subjects.

Treat the Circulation. Maintain the blood pressure, but avoid overhydration. Shock is rare with depressant posioning, but the action of the drugs on smooth muscle commonly produces moderate hypotension, which in turn impairs glomerular infiltration and renal clearance of drugs. Beware of patients with tricyclic antidepressant poisoning. These drugs cause bizarre and sometimes fatal arrhythmias whose treatment may require an experienced cardiologist. A widened QRS or QT interval may particularly predispose to ventricular tachycardia.

For all patients with depressant poisoning give fluids and pressor agents so as to maintain mean blood pressure at 80 to 90 mm Hg and a urine flow approaching 300 ml or more per hour. Dopamine will be sufficient to attain perfusion in many patients. Norepinephrine can be used cautiously if less vigorous pressor agents fail to maintain ideal systemic pressures. Judge fluid intake by urine output, after first inserting a catheter for accurate collections. If hour-by-hour fluid excretion does not match intake by the third hour of treatment, try raising the blood pressure rather than first loading in more fluids. Oliguric renal failure almost never occurs except in patients who have been in profound shock. Remember, however, that patients who have been in coma for several hours before reaching hospital may have shifted enought of their blood volume into extravascular compartments to be seriously hypovolemic. Nevertheless, avoid fluid overload. Check electrolytes at intervals of 12 hours; once diuresis is attained, replace sodium with half-normal saline and potassium at a rate of 80 to 120 mEq or more per day. Digitalis or other cardiac drugs are useful only for patients with heart disease.

Monitor blood pressure, pulse, and respiration every half hour. In the unventilated patient, the presence of a respiration rate above approximately 20 implies either pneumonitis or, less often, incipient pulmonary edema. Most patients with drug poisoning are hypothermic, and body temperatures above 37.5° C generally imply infection. Hypothermia above 33° C requires no special treatment.

Prevent Complications. Keep unconscious patients semiprone in the drainage position and change their position from side to side, but never place them fully supine. Treat potential pulmonary infection with a broad-spectrum antibiotic. These patients will be unconscious for only a few days, and the risk of emergence of drug-resistant bacterial infections is of less concern than is pneumonia caused by already aspirated material.

Hemodialysis is not necessary to treat poisoning with the short-acting hypnotics. However, hemodialysis may shorten the duration of coma for patients who have ingested large amounts of long-acting barbiturates such as barbital or phenobarbital, or who are in very deep coma from glutethimide overdose. Dialysis also is indicated for severe lithium or bromide poisoning.

Analeptics and pharmacologic stimulants are contraindicated for coma caused by depressant drug poisoning. Most carry the risk of overstimulating or producing convulsions in lightly poisoned patients.

RECOVERY AND PROGNOSIS. Patients recovering from coma require close medical supervision. Severe pneumonitis can develop as late as three to four days after recovery. If antimicrobial drugs were started during coma, they are best continued for at least 48 hours after it ends. Permanent physical sequelae are rare. Among 356 of our own such cases, residual brain injury was observed only once (in a patient who suffered an acute cardiac arrest). Peripheral nerve injuries from pressure developed in 6 subjects, and 14 subjects had pressure skin lesions leaving scars. Thre were no other physical residua.

Later management varies according to the patient's underlying psychiatric disorder and his attitudes upon recovery. Serious suicide attempts are never accidents, and reports of near-fatal ingestion caused by misunderstanding the dose or forgetting previous doses carry little validity. The expert opinion of a psychiatrist should be sought before deciding whether to release or to institutionalize a patient. The immediate prognosis is good, but there is a high incidence of recurrent attempts over the years.

Gilman AG, Goodman LS, Gilman A (eds.): The Pharmacological Basis of Therapeutics. 6th ed. New York, Macmillan, 1980. *The bible of its field.*

Hulten BA, Heath A: Clinical aspects of tricyclic antidepressant poisoning. Acta Med Scand 213:275, 1983 *A study of laboratory findings, complications, and treatment of 225 severely ill patients with a 2 per cent mortality.*

Spencer PS, Schaumberg HH: Experimental and Clinical Neurotoxicology. Baltimore, Williams and Wilkins, 1980. *A valuable compendium to nervous system poisons, mostly of the chronic variety.*

472.3. Prognosis in Severe Brain Damage and Diagnosis of Brain Death

Fred Plum

An important part of the physician's responsibility includes forecasting the outcome of illness. Modern medical advances save many lives that only a few years ago would have been lost to severe disease or trauma. Unfortunately, however, when severe brain dysfunction accompanies acute illness, it creates the risk that if the brain does not recover, vigorous treatment may be followed by an unwanted outcome. Several surveys conducted among both laymen and professionals have indicated that most persons would prefer death over a life of overwhelming and permanent neurologic disability. These considerations have resulted in the development of several empirically based guidelines to help the physician predict between possibly good and almost certainly very poor neurologic outcomes following severe illnesses causing severe brain damage or coma.

Nontraumatic Coma

The outcome from severe medical coma depends upon its cause and, with the exception of depressant drug poisoning, upon the initial severity and extent of neurologic damage as revealed by certain clinical neurologic signs obtainable at onset and within the first few days of illness.

At the onset it must be emphasized that depressant drug poisoning, no matter how deep the coma, reflects a state of general anesthesia; barring severe complications, almost all such patients who survive to reach medical attention can recover physically unscathed. This favorable prognosis applies even when coma is so profound that normal brainstem reflexes and the EEG temporarily disappear. Since most coma of unknown origin leading to emergency house calls or emergency room visits will be due to drug ingestion, such initially undiagnosed patients should receive maximal treatment unless direct evidence points to severe structural brain damage or systemic disease and the use of drugs by ingestion or for therapy has been ruled out.

TABLE 472–7. NEUROLOGIC TESTS THAT BEST INDICATE THE COURSE OF COMA AND ITS PROGNOSIS

Verbal responses	Ocular movements
Eye opening	a. Spontaneous
Pupillary reactions	b. Vestibular reflex
Corneal responses	Motor responses to noxious stimulation

Aside from drug poisoning, the acute or subacute development in the course of medical illness of loss of consicousness lasting more than a very few hours carries a poor prognosis in which only about 15 per cent of patients are likely to make a good recovery. The major problem in making early treatment decisions lies in attempting to discriminate between patients who have a chance of reaching a good outcome and those whose chances of a self-rewarding neurologic recovery are extremely small. In making such early decisions, clinical signs of abnormal foregrain and/or upper brainstem function have been found to be the most powerful available prognostic indicators. The nature of the underlying illness has secondary influence on whether or not a good outcome occurs but does not modify the accuracy of predictions between the extremes of good and bad prognosis as indicated by early signs. No laboratory determinants have been found accurately to predict outcome, nor does age significantly influence the quality of survival of adults in medical coma.

The clinical tests most valuable for estimating the capacity for recovery after medical coma are identical with those used in making the initial diagnosis and in following the later course of the patient in coma (Table 472–7). Verbal responses and eye opeining reflect mainly forebrain functions whereas tests of pupils, corneals, eye movements, and motor activity reflect the state of brainstem activity. In most instances, one cannot reliably estimate the outcome of coma immediately after the event, a time when rapid improvement often occurs. After about six hours, however, so long as the patient has not received heavy doses of sedative drugs or alcohol, certain neurologic findings begin to correlate increasingly strongly with teh potential for neurologic recovery and also confidently predict the outcome of about one third of those patients who ultimately will do badly. By the end of the first day, clinical signs accurately predict about two thirds of the patients who actually will do well. With each successive day, the signs develop greater predictive power. When considered appropriate, treatment can be adjusted accordingly.

Figure 472–1 provides a series of algorithms that describe the actural outcome of 500 patients in medical comas as related to their neurologic findings at 6 hours and on days one, three, and seven following onset. Reference to the charts discloses that signs of brainstem dysfunction (absent pupillary or corneal responses, imperfect or absent oculocephalic responses, or abnormal motor responses to stimulation) worsened the prognosis and, in combination, made it essentially hopeless when they persisted beyond the third day.

A few patients following an acute diffuse brain injury such as follows cardiac arrest, become immediately vegetative following the ictus and remain so as the days pass into weeks. Most who regain verbal abilities later than the end of the second week are left with prominent intellectual defects, especially in recent and anterograde memory, even if sensorimotor activities return to normal. No recorded example exists of an adult who has regained independent recovery after spending more than three weeks either in coma or a vegetative state. Care must be taken in such instances, however, to rule out a locked-in state (Ch. 472.1).

Traumatic Coma

Coma following head injury enjoys a somewhat more favorable outcome than that associated with medical illness. About

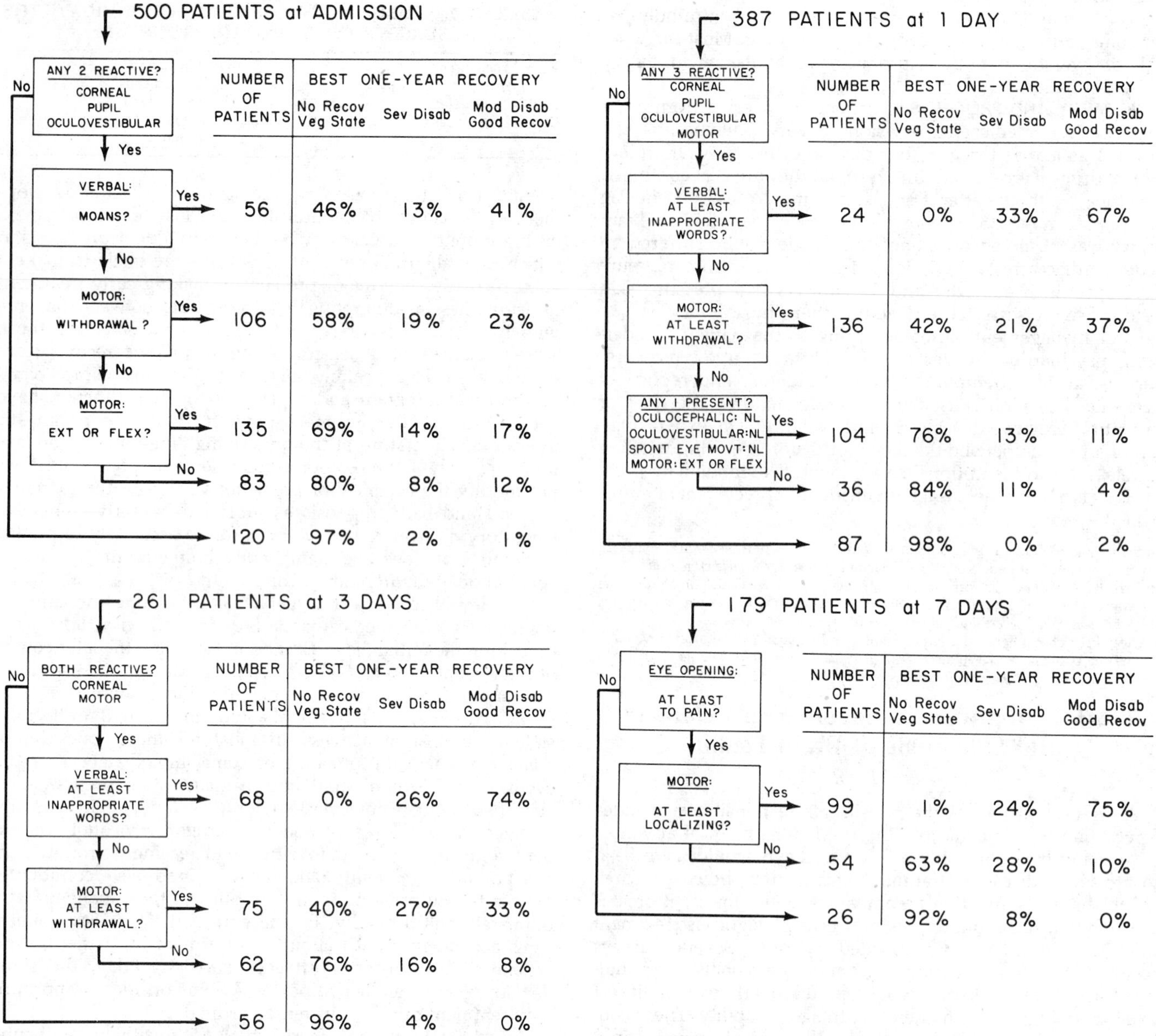

Figure 472–1. The best one-year outcome for 500 optimally treated patients in coma from nontraumatic causes. For each time period following onset, the diagram correlates the degree of recovery with clinical signs observed at that point. Although the diagrams describe actual events in a specific population, the numbers in most instances are sufficiently large to provide a basis for estimating prognosis among similarly affected patients in the future. (From Levy DE, Bates D, Caronna JJ, Cartlidge NEF, Knill-Jones RP, Lapinski RH, Singer BH, Shaw DA, Plum F: Prognosis in nontraumatic coma. Ann Intern Med 94:293, 1981, with permission.)

50 per cent of patients in coma from head injury die, and neurosurgeons debate whether treatment greatly affects that figure. Recovery is closely linked to age: the younger the better. As with medical coma, abnormal neuro-ophthalmologic signs reflecting brainstem dysfunction carry from the start a prognosis for death or disability with approximately 90 per cent of such patients either dying or remaining in near-vegetative states.

Brain Death

Modern resuscitative devices can maintain the functions of the heart, lungs, and visceral organs for hours or days after the life-maintaining brainstem dies. The modern emergence of this hopeless condition has led countries worldwide to adopt the principle that death of the person occurs whenever either the brain or the heart irreversibly fails in its functions. In the United States the time of brain death has been accepted as the time of the person's death in all instances in which the matter has been brought to judicial attention. Many states accept the brain death concept by statute, and in none has judicial review overturned it. The advantages to making the diagnosis and acting upon it are several. Proper medical preparations in such instances may preserve vital organs for transplantation so that other may live. Furthermore, the highly expensive hospital care of an artifically maintained corpse both offends humanity and adds to already burdensome medical costs. The Presidential Commission sets as the criterion for brain death the "irreversible cessation of all functions of the entire brain, including the brainstem." Criteria for the practical application of these principles are listed in Table 472–8.

Certain points in the diagnosis of brain death must be emphasized. *Recoverable drug depressant poisoning can in all ways resemble brain death and must be explicitly ruled out.* In any doubtful case, any evidence of EEG activity or of reflex activity of the

TABLE 472–8. CRITERIA FOR DIAGNOSIS OF BRAIN DEATH

1. Nature and duration of coma is known
   a. Known structural disease or irreversible systemic metabolic cause
   b. No chance of drug intoxication or hypothermia; no paralyzing or sedative drugs recently given for treatment
   c. Six-hour observation of no brain function is sufficient in cases of known structural cause when no drug or alcohol is involved in cause or treatment; otherwise, 12 to 24 hours plus negative drug screen required
2. Absence of cerebral and brainstem function
   a. No behavioral or reflex response to noxious stimuli above foramen magnum level
   b. Fixed pupils
   c. No oculovestibular responses to 50 ml ice water calories
   d. Apneic during oxygenation for ten minutes
   e. Systemic circulation may be intact
   f. Purely spinal reflexes may be retained
3. Supplementary (optional) criteria
   a. EEG isoelectric for 30 minutes at maximal gain
   b. Brainstem-evoked responses reflect absent function in vital brainstem structures
   c. No cerebral circulation present on angiographic examination

brainstem means that the brain is not dead and contravenes immediate discontinuation of life support. However, purely spinal reflex activity can persist after brain death, including reflexes of the limbs and even some upper cervical-controlled trunk movements.

In these controversy-laden and litigious times, it is recommended that physicians faced with applying and acting upon the diagnosis of brain death familiarize themselves with the additional pertinent material listed in the references.

Abrams MB, et al: Deciding to Forego Life-Sustaining Treatment. A Report on the Ethical, Medical, and Legal Issues in Treatment Decisions. President's Commission for the Study of Ethical Problems in Medicine and Biomedical and Behavioral Research. Washington, D.C., United States Government Printing office, March, 1983. *A long and thoughtful report on the problems associated with the terminally ill and the neurologically hopelessly damaged patient.*

Arena JM: Poisoning: Toxicology, Symptoms, Treatment. 4th ed. Springfield, IL, Charles C Thomas, 1979. *A detailed, classic text on all aspects of poisoning.*

Barber J, et al.: Guidelines for the determination of death: Report of the medical consultants on the diagnosis of death to the President's Commission for the Study of Ethical Problems in Medicine and Biomedical and Behavioral Research. Neurology 32:395, 1982. *The detailed report describing that cardiac death and brain death are equivalent and giving criteria for each.*

Driesbach RH: Handbook of Poisoning. 10th ed. Los Altos, CA. Lange Medical Publishers, 1980. *Succinct and handy, an excellent and up-to-date quick source to consult in emergencies.*

Levy DE, Bates D, Caronna JJ, Cartlidge NEF, Knill-Jones RP, Lapinski RH, S.INGER BH, Shaw DA, Plum F: Prognosis in nontraumatic coma. Ann Intern Med 94:293, 1981. *Provides detailed information correlating nature of illness and early clinical neurologic signs with best one-year outcome in 500 patients with loss of consciousness due to medical illness.*

Plum F, Posner JB: Diagnosis of Stupor and Coma. 3rd ed, revised printing. Philadelia, F. A. Davis Company, 1982. *Comprehensively discusses pathogenesis, diagnosis, prognosis, and emergency management of patients with acute severe brain dysfunction. Extensive references, especially to mechanisms and metabolic-diffuse brain diseases.*

472.4. Brief Loss of Consciousness

Fred Plum

Brief, not immediately explained loss of consciousness is a frequent complaint of patients entering any hospital emergency room. The cause of most such attacks, if diagnosable at all, can be determined on the basis of an accurate history alone. Routine physical and simple laboratory procedures, including blood work and ECG, are the most important additional diagnostic measures. Vasovagal reflex syncope is by far the most frequent cause of brief loss of consciousness (Table 472–9). Among patients with unwitnessed attacks, however, the cause of as many as one third eludes exact diagnosis even after comprehensive laboratory evaluation and a year or more of follow-up.

TABLE 472–9. PRINCIPAL CAUSES AND APPROXIMATE FREQUENCIES OF BRIEF LOSS OF CONSCIOUSNESS

Syncope	
Vasovagal/psychophysiologic	55%
Cardiovascular	10%
Central nervous system	
First seizure	10%
Other	5%
Drug-metabolic	5%
Undiagnosed, including hysteria	15%

Certain immediate guidelines aid empirically in differential diagnosis and prove valuable in deciding whether and to what extent further laboratory investigations will be necessary or fruitful. Among patients younger than age 40 years, brief loss of consciousness is almost always either vasodepressor syncope or undiagnosable unless the history or physical findings explicitly indicate the presence of severe heart disease, systemic illness, a seizure disorder or epileptiform movements during the attack, or alcohol-drug abuse. Among patients older than age 40 years, cardiac causes of syncope increase in frequency; but even among older patients, if the history, physical, and standard laboratory evaluation disclose no evidence of severe cardiac, systemic, or neurologic illness, the symptom most often has benign implications. Cryptic thrombophlebitis producing pulmonary infarction is a threat at any age; hypoglycemia or other metabolic perturbations are rare causes of brief loss of consciousness in the absence of strongly suggestive associated symptoms.

Neurologic causes of brief loss of consciousness other than syncope are comparatively few and are usually diagnosable by history: CT scans and EEGs almost never provide the diagnosis in patients unsuspected of neurologic disease. Drugs contribute importantly to loss of consciousness, producing hypotension in cardiacs and other older persons and predisposing to withdrawal seizures at any age over about 25 years. Head injury, while a common cause of brief concussion-amnesia, seldom represents a diagnostic problem unless neither witnesses nor evidence of surface trauma are present. Malingering-hysteria is a possible explanation for unexplained loss of consciousness, but the diagnosis should be considered only when social circumstances are appropriate, when history reveals evidence of previous similar difficulties, or when the examiner witnesses an obviously factitious attack. Even then, underlying associated physical disease should be ruled out.

SYNCOPE

Syncope is the commonest cause of brief unconsciousness and results, by definition, from an acute, global reduction in cerebral blood flow (CBF) sufficient to deprive cerebral-reticular neurons of substrate. Among otherwise healthy young persons syncope almost always carries a benign prognosis except for the associated inconvenience or specific attack-related dangers that future episodes may carry. Among persons in older age groups, cardiac causes for syncope become more common and must be meticulously searched for, as studies in some groups of patients with cardiogenic syncope show a one-year mortality as high as 30 per cent. Syncope rarely results from focal cerebral vascular disease, the only exception to this maxim being in patients in whom more than one of the four internal carotid-vertebral arteries are occluded so that any further arterial flow reduction globally affects brain perfusion.

With any cause of syncope, the degree of impaired unconsciousness depends upon (1) the severity of reduction of CBF and (2) its duration. Table 472–10 lists the major causes and the following paragraphs discuss the principal mechanisms and disorders following the order of the table.

SYNCOPE DUE PRIMARILY TO IMPAIRED RIGHT HEART FILLING (Mainly Reflex Syncope). Most examples of syncope resulting from a failure of right heart filling are associated with abnormalities in the neural feedback loop that reflexly controls the systemic circulation. The normal heart rate and blood pressure are regulated by efferent parasympathetic and sympathetic projections that originate from nuclei in the lower pons and medulla. Limbic forebrain and hypothalamic influences modulate cardiac action and the circulation mainly by acting on these medullary areas. Parasympathetic influences act predom-

TABLE 472–10. PRINCIPAL MECHANISMS OF SYNCOPE

I. Impaired right heart filling, cardiac rate slow and abnormal (mainly reflex)
  A. Vasodepressor syncope (vasovagal)
    1. Psychophysiologic (including hyperventilation)
    2. Visceral reflex (micturition, pain, gastrointestinal dilatation, acute vertigo)
    3. Carotid sinus, type 2
  B. Orthostatic hypotension
    1. Reduced blood volume (hemorrhage, acute salt and water loss, protein loss, enteropathy, burns)
    2. Hypotensive drugs
    3. Neurogenic and idiopathic
  C. Mechanically impaired right heart venous return (cough syncope, acute pulmonary infarction, fainting lark, near-term pregnancy, pericardial tamponade)

II. Impaired cardiac output
  A. Vagovagal attacks (transient sinus arrest)
    1. Psychophysiologic (uncommon)
    2. Visceral trauma (glossopharyngeal neuralgia, swallow syncope, tracheal stimulation, dilatation of hollow viscus)
    3. Carotid sinus, type 1
  B. Cardiac arrhythmia or asystole
    1. Extreme tachycardia > 160–180/minute
    2. Severe bradycardia < 30–40/minute
    3. Heart block: Morgagni-Adams-Stokes syndrome
    4. Ventricular fibrillation

III. Cerebral ischemia (rare)
  A. Severe cervical arterial obstructive disease plus transient ischemic attack (TIA) in remaining single carotid or vertebral artery
  B. Transient acutely increased intracranial pressure (plateau waves)
  C. Basilar migraine

inantly to slow the heart; they exert a minimal influence on the blood vessels. Postganglionic sympathetic fibers originate in the paravertebral cervical and thoracic sympathetic ganglia. They innervate the heart as well as both the arterial (resistance) and venous (capacitance) vascular beds of the viscera, trunk, and extremities. Closing the peripheral sympathetic reflex loop on the afferent side are fibers that arise in the baroreceptors of the aortic arch, other arteries, and, especially, the carotid sinus: their stimulation reduces the descending sympathetic outflow of the medullary pressor area.

Syncope resulting from failure of right heart filling nearly always reflects pooling of blood in the venous, capacitance vessels of the lower extremities or the splanchnic abdominal circulation. Relaxation of arterial resistance vessels plays a lesser role. Since gravitational factors contribute importantly to the impaired venous return, fainting caused by impaired right heart filling almost always occurs in the erect or, occasionally, sitting positions.

Acute Vasodepressor (Vasovagal) Syncope. This is the most common cause of fainting and typically is marked by a diphasic course. During an initial brief period of apprehension and anxiety, heart rate, blood pressure, total systemic resistance, and cardiac output all may increase. *This initial sequence,* however, often is *lacking*. The vasodepressor phase follows, during which heart rate and blood pressure fall, cardiac output declines, and the CBF eventually drops. Both sympathetic and parasympathetic abnormalities are involved, since atropine prevents the bradycardia but not the depressor response. Symptoms of palpitation, salivation, and anxiety characteristically mark the first phase, whereas progressive sensations of lightheadedness, giddiness, abdominal sinking sensations, nausea, urinary urgency, and finally "gray-out" or faintness accompany the vasodepressor component. Occasionally the reflex suppression of sympathetic tone comes so rapidly that the affected subject topples like a log. Rarely, with a severe attack of vasodepressor syncope, as with other forms of profound reduction of cardiac output and cerebral ischemia, brief tonic convulsive movements result.

Vasodepressor syncope most often is precipitated by conscious or unrecognized feelings of fear, disgust, and especially anxiety that precipitate discharges from the forebrain limbic system to activate medullary vasodepressor centers. During the course of the faint, such subjects appear pale rather than cyanotic, and the accompanying parasympathetic hyperactivity characteristically induces piloerection and sweating. Awareness and normal cardiovascular reflexes usually return promptly once the subject becomes supine. Occasionally dysautonomic influences on the heart are so profound as to induce arrhythmia. Engel and others have speculated that this is one mechanism causing sudden death, associated with sudden grief or fright.

Fainting is more likely in hungry subjects, in a warm moist environment, and after prolonged standing. A few individuals give a history of lifelong susceptibility to fainting attacks, and rarely one gets a history of multiple family members in several generations who have been susceptible to recurrent vasodepressor syndope.

Visceral reflex syncope acts via the same medullospinal pathways as the examples cited above. Afferent small myelinated pain fibers project directly on depressor and parasympathetic centers in the medulla. Thus a sense of faintness or even complete syncope can follow immediately after any of the following: emptying a full bladder from the standing position (micturition syncope), acute visceral pain (as occurs with a suddenly distended gut or an abrupt joint or ligament injury), or an attack of severe vertigo (as occurs with Menière's disease).

Carotid Sinus Syncope Type 2 describes a severe vasodepressor response to carotid sinus massage. The condition is rare and seldom a practical consideration except with neoplasms of the neck that directly irritate afferent glossopharyngeal fibers.

The diagnosis of vasodepressor syncope is made largely by history; rarely are the events medically witnessed. Among young persons who lack histories of neurologic or cardiovascular disease and have normal physical examinations, laboratory examinations beyond routine blood work and an ECG are almost always uninformative and therefore unnecessary. Treatment is symptomatic. Impending sensations of faintness should be treated promptly by placing the subject supine. Placing the head far forward in a sitting position is customary but less effective, because it fails to drain the enlarged pool of blood located in the muscles and veins of the lower extremities. If the heart rhythm is regular, no further resuscitative measures are needed. With severe irregularities or asystole, cardiopulmonary resuscitation is in order, but this is a rare requirement. Subjects who have fainted should be mobilized slowly, because the reflex abnormality occasionally can persist for as long as two hours. Prophylactic treatment has little value except when fainting occurs in response to disease or injury which requires attention.

Orthostatic Hypotension. Acute orthostatic hypotension occasionally can occur in normal persons after acute blood loss or following prolonged standing; affected subjects undergo a sudden collapse of sympathetic reflex tone, e.g., as with soldiers at parade rest in a hot sun. Recurrent symptoms of syncope or faintness accompanying the erect position, however, usually can be traced to the presence of the chronic use of vasodepressor drugs or to neurologic disorders involving the peripheral or central nervous system. Increased age tends to intensify the effects of the neurologic disorder; in a few instances, autonomic failure appears to be attributable entirely to blunting of central autonomic reflex control. Many drugs accentuate tendencies to orthostatic hypotension, including almost all of the antihypertensive agents and a large proportion of the antidepressants, phenothiazines, and sedatives. Bed rest deconditions sympathetic vasomotor reflexes and predisposes to orthostatic hypotension. Any tendency to impaired sympathetic reflex control is accentuated by a reduced blood volume such as is caused by Addison's disease, protein loss, or enteropathy. The combination of chromic diuretic use and vasodepressant medication outnumbers all other causes combined.

Orthostatic hypotension sufficient to cause cerebral symptoms can occur either rapidly upon standing or develop insidiously over seconds or minutes. Although symptoms of faintness and giddiness predominate in some patients, others lack such warnings, presumably because of the absence of strong efferent parasympathetic activity. When patients in this latter group sit for long periods or stand, they may become confused or tremulous without the usual sensations of faintness. Mental cloudiness, staggering, or falling is more common than complete unconsciousness. Diagnosis comes from observing an acute or progressive decline in the mean blood pressure of more than 10 to 15 torr in the erect position. Autonomic insufficiency can be inferred by observing an unchanging pulse rate despite the hypotension, and confirmed by establishing other evidence of autonomic impairment. The simplest way to evaluate sympathetic tone at the bedside is to take the pulse while the supine patient performs a vigorous Valsalva maneuver; the normal response consists of a palpable post-Valsalva slowing of pulse and a 10 to 30 torr rise in mean blood pressure. Other autonomic changes are discussed in Ch. 478 on Autonomic Disufficiency.

Treatment of orthostatic hypotension depends upon the cause. Symptomatic treatment requires eliminating drugs that cause hypotension, searching for and correcting causes of blood volume depletion, and applying elastic stockings to the lower extremities. When other measures fail, an increased salt intake and, subsequently, administering the salt-retaining steroid fludrocortisone, 0.3 to 0.8 mg per day in divided doses, can be cautiously initiated. The chronic use of vasopressor agents seldom helps. Just as vasomotor reflexes can be deconditioned by excess bed rest, they can be at least partially reconditioned by erect activity. Every effort should be made to keep affected patients up and walking.

Most other instances of syncope caused by *mechanical impairment of right heart filling* result from conditions in which the diagnosis and mechanism are fairly self-evident, as noted in Table 472–10. Treatment is directed at the underlying cause.

SYNCOPE DUE PRIMARILY TO IMPAIRED LEFT HEART OUTPUT (Mainly Cardiac Syncope). *Vagovagal attacks* consist of reflexly induced changes in the cardiac rhythm, including nodal or sinus arrest, atrioventricular asystole, atrioventricular block, sinoatrial block, and ventricular arrhythmias. Usually these are accompanied by relatively minor vasodepressor changes in the peripheral vasculature, implying a lesser sympathetic component. Most but not all patients with vagovagal attacks belong to the older population and have associated heart disease. Most vagally induced cardiac arrhythmia or arrest represents an abnormally intense cardiac response to a relatively normal degree of increased parasympathetic stimulatioc or sympathetic inhibtion. Vagal bradycardia or arrest occasionally is induced by sudden emotional stimuli, but more commonly follows acute noxious or abnormal visceral stimulation. Severe bradycardia or arrest especially accompanies glossopharyngeal neuralgia, swallowing in patients with mechanical esophageal lesions, sudden painful dilatations of a hollow viscus, prostatic manipulation, tracheal stimulation, or visceral wounds. *Carotid sinus syncope Type 1* is a rare phenomenon in which massage or pressure of the sinus induces transient asystole.

Cardiac-related syncope represents less than 10 per cent of all patients who present to emergency or outpatient facilities complainint of brief loss of consciousness. The symptom has medical importance far beyond that number, however, because of its implications of serious disease or sudden death if not effectively prevented or treated.

Cardiac syncope almost always reflects serious heart disease. Analyses of large series of patients show that serious associated risk factors include severe hypertension; a history of, respectively, myocardial infarction, congestive heart failure, or severe valvular disease (especially arotic stenosis); and electrocardiographic monitoring abnormalities on laboratory testing. With cardiac patients, even extensive laboratory studies often fail to disclose the specific reason for asystole-syncope, but major associated abnormalities on prolonged electrocardiographic monctoring include episodes of sinus pauses lasting more than 8 seconds, sinus bradycardia less than 40 per minute, atrial fibrillation with a slow ventricular rate, sustained supraventricular tachycardia, and Mobitz type II atrioventricular block. In the absence of specific predisposing abnormalities discovered by history, physical examination and ECG monitoring, direct electrophysiologic studies of the heart, cardiac catheterization, coronary or cerebral angiography, brain CT scanning, and electroencephalography seldom add diagnostically helpful information. Management of cardiac syncope depends upon the nature of the underlying heart disease, although affected persons should be considered for pacemaker insertion.

OTHER CAUSES OF BRIEF LOSS OF CONSCIOUSNESS

Hyperventilation is closely related to syncope in its mechanisms in that a globally reduced cerebral blood flow gives rise to sensations of giddiness, faintness, and other distress. Full unconsciousness rarely occurs without some additional abnormal maneuver. The abnormal state is most often part of an anxiety response, and often is accompanied by sensations of suffocation, pressure on the chest, and a sense of being unable to obtain the satisfaction of a lung-filling deep breath. Extreme or prolonged hyperventilation can produce feelings of unreality with anxiety bordering on panic.

In healthy subjects, only a modest increase in respiratory rate and depth is required to drop Pa_{CO_2} levels within a very few minutes to 25 mm Hg or less; once a new steady state develops, little more than the normal level of breathing is sufficient to match bodily CO_2 production and maintain hypocapnia. Accordingly, casual inspection may show no more than a respiratory rate of 16 to 18 per minute, interrupted perhaps by occasional sighs. Hypocapnia induces cerebral vasoconstriction, which reduces the amount of oxygen delivered to the brain and is the presumed basis of many of the accompanying sensations.

Symptoms and signs include feelings of unreality, difficulty in concentrating, and several hard-to-explain sensory complaints, such as unilateral or bilateral chest pain or paresthesias involving the body and extremities. Symptoms of facial twitching, carpal spasm, and perioral paresthesias are more easily understood as part of alkalotic tetany.

Diagnosis is easy when otherwise structurally healthy patients complain of the aforementioned symptoms in settings of anxiety dyspnea, but often is conjectural when made in retrospect. Some patients can reproduce their symptoms by voluntarily overbreathing, and insights gained from the maneuver can be helpful in guiding treatment. Most often the symptoms are observed as part of a larger pattern of anxiety and must be treated accordingly.

Hyperventilation occasionally precipitates syncope under special circumstances. Children sometimes voluntarily hyperventilate, then perform a vigorous Valsalve maneuver to induce syncope in the already partially oxygen-deprived brain (fainting lark). Athletes may unconsciously repeat a similar sequence when competing in contests such as weight lifting or squat jumps. More dangerous is a pattern wherein underwater swimmers hyperventilate before diving, then exhaust their oxygen reserves by exercise before producing sufficient carbon dioxide to result in dyspnea. The ensuing cerebral hypoxia can induce submersion syncope, which is sometimes fatal.

SEIZURE DISORDERS. Seizure disorders, discussed fully in Ch. 510, produce a diagnostic problem under four principal circumstances:

1. *Rapid, profound syncope* may induce a single brief tonic seizure or series of clonic twitches as a result of abrupt cerebral ischemia. The response is somewhat more frequent with severe episodes or when the subject has made maximal effort to stand or sit despite premonitory symptoms. Differential diagnosis rests on identifying the following as more consistent with syncope: the attendant psychologic circumstances and physical

appearance, the associated medical conditions and body position, the brief quality of the seizure, and the presence of a normal neurologic examination and interictal EEG.

2. *Akinetic seizures* in children consist of attacks of suddenly falling or pitching to the ground. Similar seizures occur in the supine position and are marked by psychologic unresponsiveness accompanied by generalized muscular hypotonia or brief body spasm. Diagnosis rests on the typical history, the absence of pallor during witnessed episodes, the age and frequency of onset, and the presence of an abnormal interictal EEG. *Absence (petit mal) seizures* rarely provide a diagnostic problem, since the child, although out of contact during the attacks, neither falls nor turns pale and usually has no memory of the episode. The EEG is abnormal.

3. *Partial complex (psychomotor) seizures* sometimes include brief behavioral automatisms in which the subject recalls only being out of contact and may retrospectively consider himself to have suffered a state of unconsciousness. Usually the presence of a characteristic, self-recognized aura or set of incipient symptoms indicates the diagnosis. Falling to the ground rarely occurs unless a generalized seizure develops. Witnessed attacks and the EEG usually are typical and, in any event, not syncopal in their appearance.

4. *Postictal unresponsiveness* from grand mal attacks produces unconsciousness for five to thirty minutes, the duration usually depending on the severity of the preceding convulsion. Diagnosis is a problem only if the seizure was unwitnessed, in which case the state may look like concussion or profound fainting. However, the postictal state is marked initially by flushing (cyanosis), giving way to pallor, hyperpnea, and deep unresponsiveness.

HYPOGLYCEMIA (see Ch. 231). Hypoglycemia, usually caused by excess exogenous insulin, less often by insulin secreted from endogenous tissues, can produce a variety of relatively brief episodes of neurologic dysfunction. These can consist, variably, of brief confusional episodes, seizures of a variety of types, narcoleptic-like syndromes, and focal or tetraparetic weakness with or without coma. The condition is rare except in insulin-receiving diabetics. Diagnosis depends on suspicion plus the detection of blood sugars of less than 30 to 40 mg per deciliter during an attack or following induced fasting.

DRUG OR ALCOHOL BLACKOUTS. Drug or alcohol blackouts consist of episodes of such severe intoxication that they anesthetize memory for the event, leaving the subject with an episode of focal amnesia. Many are accompanied by "passing out," a condition with a clinical appearance that differs in no way from deep, barely arousable sleep.

CONCUSSION-POSTCONCUSSION AMNESIA. Variable periods of memory loss for immediate sugsequent events can follow brief periods of concussive unconsciousness. The usual question is whether an intrinsic malady caused the fall or whether the fall represented the whole illness. Only diagnostic diligence can solve the issue.

ACUTE INTRACRANIAL HYPERTENSION. This condition occasionally produces brief episodes of loss of consciousness that may resemble syncope. The classic, but rare, example occurs with colloid cysts of the third ventricle which intermittently obstruct that cavity or produce plateau waves (Ch. 472.1). More frequently, brief unconsciousness may accompany the onset of acute subarachnoid hemorrhage. The unconscious episode, which is syncopal in its abruptness and often accompanied by either a tonic extensor spasm or brief clonic jerks, is most often due to an acute cardiac arrhythmia accompanying the onset of bleeding. Cerebral hemorrhage with intraventricular rupture can produce similar intracranial events.

CONDITIONS SOMETIMES RESEMBLING LOSS OF CONSCIOUSNESS

DROP SPELLS. These are poorly understood attacks affecting mainly women of middle age or older. The legs of affected subjects suddenly and unexplainedly give way, and the women fall, often injuring themselves but experiencing no observed interruption of consciousness. The cause is unknown, although basilar artery ischemia has been postulated. There is no known effective treatment.

TRANSIENT GLOBAL AMNESIA (see Ch. 493 to 495). This name is applied to attacks lasting usually one to six hours, rarely longer, wherein the subject loses knowledge of all immediate and many recent past events but retains knowledge of self, the distant past, and the maenities of behavior. The episodes affect the middle-aged or elderly, and are suspected but not proved to represent the effects of vascular disease. During the attack, patients have not associated neurologic deficits and recover spontaneously and completely, but with no memory for the content of the episode. Consciousness is not lost and only if the patient was entirely unattended during the episode would the diagnosis be in question.

CONVERSION REACTIONS OR MALINGERING. Hysterical or other psychogenic unresponsiveness is almost impossible to diagnose in retrospect from the history. If such a condition occurs during the physical examination, however, the diagnosis is based on the absence of physiologic abnormality and the presence of additional, often bizarre features. Most subjects awaken with gentle but firm confrontation. A few do so only when advised that psychiatric admission lies in store. Mutilating stimuli are unjustified and often unsuccessful as ways to prove the diagnosis.

Day SC, Cook ET, Funkenstein H, Goldman L: Evaluation and outcome of emergency room patients with transient loss of consciousness. Am J Med 73:15, 1982. *An analysis of 198 patients, giving differential diagnosis, identifying low- and high-risk groups, and indicating relative value of laboratory tests.*

De Bono DP, Warlow CP, Hyman NM: Cardiac rhythm abnormalities in patients presenting with transient non-focal neurological symptoms: A diagnostic gray area? Br Med J 1:1437, 1982. *An evaluation of 89 patients versus controls. Only arrhythmias in young patients and bradyarrhythmia at any age were considered relevant. Monitoring contributed to diagnosis in less than one third.*

Engel GL: Psychological stress, vasodepressor (vasovagal) syncope and sudden death. Ann Intern Med 89:403, 1978. *Must reading for the internist by one of the pioneers in understanding of both the physiology and emotion of cardiovascular responses.*

Evans DW, Lum LC: Hyperventilation: An important cause of pseudoangina. Lancet 1:155, 1977. *A clinical article, emphasizing the often misleading symptoms of the disorder.*

Kapoor WN, Karpf M, Maher Y, Miller RA, Levey GS: Syncope of unknown origin. The need for a more effective approach to its diagnostic evaluation. JAMA 247:2687, 1982. *Among 121 older patients with syncope, cardiac monitoring, cardiac electrophysiologic studies, and cardiac catheterization provided diagnostic evidence in only 13. Glucose tolerance tests, head CT, brain scans, lumbar puncture, and skull x-ray aided diagnosis in none.*

Kapoor WN, Karpf M, Wieand S, Peterson PA, Levey GS: A prospective evaluation and follow-up of patients with syncope. N Engl J Med 309:197, 1983. *Among 204 mainly older patients with syncope, 40 per cent of whom were hospitalized from the start, diagnosis could be made in 53 per cent. Twenty-six per cent had a cardiovascular cause. At one year half the cardiovascular group had died, compared to 12 per cent with noncardiovascular causes and 6 per cent in the idiopathic group.*

472.5. Sleep and Its Disorders

J. Allan Hobson

Modern research supports three important changes in our common-sense orientation to sleep:

First, sleep is a complex biologic function with extremely variable length and depth. Individuals may vary in their baseline sleep need between four and ten hours. Short sleepers tend to be hyperactive but productive and well-adjusted, whereas long sleepers tend to be low-key, underachieving, and mildly depressed. Experiments in animals show marked differences in sleep length in genetically different strains; given the existence of a bell-shaped distribution of sleep length, the duration variable cannot, per se, be taken as an index of pathology, and the physician should beware of pushing patients against powerful biologic gradients.

Second, sleep is variable *within* individuals. Marked, built-in changes take place over the life span. The neonate sleeps two thirds of the time. At sexual maturity, this duration has fallen by half, but the capacity for deep, fulfilling sleep is still robust. By age 40 the sleep of fully productive humans is normally more shallow, and by age 60 sleep length may have decreased further. There is a linear positive correlation between age and the number of awakenings.

Third, sleep is also variable within individuals from one sleep-wake cycle to the next. There is a dynamic relationship between waking state variables and sleep characteristics over both the short and long term. Hence, during highly productive periods, sleep need may decrease; sleep length may also undergo unwanted but normal shortening during periods of anxiety and stress. Within limits—to be judged by the individual's adaptive responses—these should be regarded as signals to be heeded, understood, and dealt with during the awake state rather than symptoms of disease needing to be extinguished via the chemical manipulation of sleep.

Activity patterns also influence sleep variables. Few farmers complain of insomnia during the haying season, and animal experiments indicate that moderate exercise reduces sleep latency while also increasing sleep length and depth. These points should be brought home to the sedentary city dweller. Another point is that sleep is not only variable and responsive but carefully regulated. Thus good sleep can often be expected to follow poor. And, despite highly publicized initial results, sleep deprivation studies have not revealed specific or long-lasting ill effects, so that conservative management is not likely to be dangerous even to the patient who may ultimately need pharmacologic treatment.

PHYSIOLOGY AND PHARMACOLOGY OF SLEEP. The metabolism of all organisms is temporally ordered. Cosmic forces synchronize circadian rhythms, endogenous oscillations of slightly more than 24 hours in length, which are reset each day by light and other time cues. In all mammals, including man, the circadian oscillator appears to include the suprachiasmatic nucleus of the hypothalamus. The hypothalamus receives a direct input from the optic tract, which presumably delivers the light pulses that reset the rhythm each day. Lesions of the posterior hypothalamus produce hypersomnia, whereas lesions of the anterior hypothalamus produce insomnia.

As all who have crossed time zones in jet airplanes can testify, the circadian rhythm is a powerful, persistent, and plastic determinant of when we sleep and wake. Whether its action is mediated by the sleep-inducing peptides that have been isolated from the spinal fluid of sleep-deprived animals or by conventional neurotransmission is not yet clear, but it is certain that the EEG sleep cycle is under its control.

Each sleep period consists of a series of biphasic 90- to 100-minute cycles. The non–rapid eye movement (NREM) phase, which initiates sleep and each subsequent cycle is also called slow wave or synchronized sleep. It is characterized by progressive EEG slowing and by corresponding decreases in muscle tone, heart rate, respiratory rate, and blood pressure. When this deactivation process is maximal—at about mid-cycle—subjects are difficult to rouse and may be disoriented or even confabulate when asked to report their mental activity.

The rapid eye movement (REM) phase of the cycle, which follows NREM and ends each cycle, is also called fast wave or desynchronized sleep. It is characterized by progressive reactivation of the EEG and autonomic functions. Paradoxically, however, muscle tone is even further depressed in REM; this is caused by active inhibition which finally obliterates tonus and effectively paralyzes all but the ocular musculature. Silently signaling the intense internal activation of many neuronal systems of the brain, the eyes execute spectacular runs of nystagmiform movement behind the still-closed lids. Heart and respiratory rates quicken and blood pressure rises, especially during the clusters of REM. Upon awakening from REM sleep, subjects are easily aroused and often report detailed and vivid dreams.

This NREM-REM cycle repeats itself, usually without interruption, four or five times each night. Since the later cycles have shallower NREM troughs, relatively more time is devoted to REM toward morning. Major shifts in posture—of which the subject is generally unaware—occur at NREM-REM phase transitions, hence at least eight or ten times per night. The important point for the physician to grasp is that the physiologic systems underlying mentation, movement, and cardiorespiratory control are all undergoing dynamic and dramatic changes in their operating properties throughout the night.

Lesion and ablation studies in animals indicate that the system controlling the EEG sleep cycle is located in the pontine brainstem. Single cell recordings suggest that this pontine clock is composed of two interconnected neuronal populations whose activity levels fluctuate periodically and oppositely. Their out-of-phase oscillation appears to be due to the reciprocal interaction of their excitatory and inhibitory neurotransmitters.

During waking the resting activity level of aminergic inhibitory neurons is high. The nuclei containing these "waking" cells include the noradrenergic locus ceruleus and the serotonergic dorsal raphe, which have been implicated in control of sleep state, mood, and learning. As a consequence of aminergic inhibition, the resting activity level of cholinergic neurons in many brainstem reticular nuclei is actually low in waking. During the non-REM phase of the sleep cycle, aminergic inhibition gradually declines; simultaneously, cholinergic excitation gradually increases so that at mid-cycle the balance between aminergic inhibition and cholinergic excitation shifts. The REM period occurs when aminergic inhibition has fallen to its low point and cholinergic excitation becomes maximal. The microinjection of either cholinergic agonists *or* aminergic antagonists into the pontine brainstem is capable of converting an animal's state from awake to REM sleep. Unfortunately, the drugs used in clinical practice and in most research studies are administered by parenteral routes and may thus affect multiple peripheral and central systems with confusing, contradictory, and uninterpretable results.

A PATHOPHYSIOLOGIC APPROACH TO THE SLEEP DISORDERS. *A static shift* in net drive on one or both of the opposing brainstem populations will result in an increasing propensity for one state or the other to occur. Thus insomnia (or too much waking) will occur if there is either aminergic overactivity or cholinergic underactivity, or both. Examples are stress, anxiety, and amphetamine-induced insomnia; all are characterized by aminergic overactivity and all are countered by aminergic antagonists. Reciprocally, hypersomnia (or too little waking) will occur if there is either aminergic underactivity or cholinergic overactivity, or both. Examples are boredom, characterologic depression, and narcolepsy—all characterized by aminergic underactivity and all countered by aminergic agonists. The probability of waking or sleep is thus a function of the set-point of the controlling oscillator. Set-point level is susceptible to environmental influences: exogenous (e.g., noise) and endogenous (e.g., cortical or muscular) inputs both play their part.

The *dynamics* of the system are such that timing errors may occur, resulting in a temporal dissociation of sleep-wake state components. For example, if the subsystems controlling mentation and motor activity are not precisely coordinated, we may see hallucinosis (hypnagogic hallucinations) when falling asleep, or persistent immobility (sleep paralysis) when aroused from REM—as in narcolepsy; conversely, we may see motor activity emerge from deep NREM sleep—as in somnambulism, sleep talking, or enuresis.

The dynamic shifts in level of activity of the multiple neuronal subsystems that are integral to state regulation by reciprocal interaction also have predictable autonomic manifestations. Thus the decreasing aminergic drive on brainstem reticular neurons that is integral to sleep onset may be associated with cessation of breathing (as in central sleep apnea) if the set-point of the respiratory oscillator—which itself is a reticular system—is suddenly changed. Similarly, the deactivation (probably a disfacilitation) of motor systems that is integral to sleep onset may compromise a marginal airway via decreasing tonus of glossal and hypoglossal muscles (as in obstructive sleep apnea).

THE EVALUATION OF SLEEP COMPLAINTS. Until recently, sleep was neither directly observed nor measured, so that the physician was literally groping in the dark in his diagnostic efforts. Sleep laboratory studies indicate that there are two kinds of errors in subjective reporting: overestimation of time spent awake in insomnia, and underestimation of the physiologically important respiratory disturbances that occur in sleep. Thus an insomniac patient perceives his one or two hours of sleep loss as three or four, whereas a severely apneic patient can be unaware of the hundreds of arousals that occur causing recurrent cyanosis with oxygen saturations of 50 per cent or less! This irony is compounded by the fact that the anxious insomniac may put great pressure on the physician for a prompt, uncritical, and even potentially dangerous therapeutic program, whereas the apneic patient, urgently needing tracheostomy, remains lethargic and uncomplaining.

Objective observation can be accomplished in several direct and simple ways prior to referral for sleep laboratory evaluation. One is the sleep log, which should be kept for at least two and preferably for four weeks following an initial visit. On a single sheet, each line of which represents 24 hours, are recorded the times of retiring, falling asleep, arousals, awakening, and arising. Dated entries, corresponding to the lines, indicate subjective state and behavioral data for the intervening waking periods.

The sleep log can be more reliable if there is a cooperative bed partner or roommate. Since the bed partner is not only a potential investigative collaborator but often the plaintiff, it is important that he or she be invited to the follow-up visit, if not the intake. Because of the snoring (sleep apnea) or kicking (nocturnal myoclonus) of the patient, it may be the bed partner who is the more insomniac!

Obstructive apneic episodes can be documented by the bed partner, using an audio cassette recorder. The tape recorder is also useful in the characterization of sleep talking, sleep walking, bruxism, night terrors, and nightmares.

So sensitive is sleep to situational variables that even more vigorous efforts should be made to increase our capability of documenting both normal and abnormal sleep in its natural habitat. New techniques capable of clinical adaptations include actigraphic movement recording and visual monitoring by time-lapse photography or video of the posture shifts that normally accompany the NREM-REM stage shifts of the sleep cycle. These relatively simple, home-based recording techniques give values which correlate with subjective estimates of good and poor sleep and even provide measures of sleep latency, a critical variable in the documentation of insomnia and its therapeutic management.

At present, sleep laboratory studies provide the only definitive means of documenting the diagnostic signs of the specific sleep disorders. If narcolepsy, nocturnal myoclonus, or sleep apnea cannot be ruled out by the simple means described above, referral to a sleep laboratory is indicated.

CLASSIFICATION OF SLEEP DISORDERS. The balance of this chapter follows a simple, complaint-ordered scheme: too little sleep (insomnias), too much sleep (hypersomnias), or abnormal sleep behavior (parasomnias) (see Table 472–11).

The Insomnias. Sleep is so variable and complaints of insomnia are so common as to raise serious questions about the point at which complaints of too little sleep should be regarded as abnormal (in a statistical sense) or pathologic (in a medical sense). In the absence of objective data, considerable judgment is required in making these decisions. Current trends, spurred by the discovery of side effects of sedative medication, are toward a conservative, behaviorally oriented management approach of disorders of initiating and maintaining sleep. To be successful, this approach must first emphasize careful diagnostic study to determine specific underlying causes. In the most common, nonspecific cases, patients need education in the multifactorial determinants of sleep quality and duration, support in their behavioral and pharmacologic potentiation, and close follow-up monitoring of these interventions.

TABLE 472–11. CLASSIFICATION OF SLEEP DISORDERS BY COMPLAINT

- Too little sleep (the insomnias)
  - Specific
    - Circadian rhythm shifts
    - Nocturnal myoclonus
    - Sleep apnea syndromes (see below)
  - Secondary
    - Medical
      - Fever
      - Pain
      - Cardiopulmonary disease
    - Psychiatric
      - Anxiety, stress
      - Alcohol and drugs
      - Depression
      - Schizophrenia
- Too much sleep (the hypersomnias)
  - Specific
    - Narcolepsy
    - Kleine-Levin syndrome
    - Sleep apnea syndromes
  - Secondary
    - CNS lesions
    - Pickwickian syndrome
    - Depression
- Abnormal sleep behavior (the parasomnias)
  - Motor
    - Enuresis
    - Sleep walking
    - Sleep talking
    - Night terrors
    - Bruxism
  - Respiratory
    - Sleep apnea syndromes—central, peripheral, mixed types

Usually the primary care physician is the person who most possesses the proximity, continuity, and credibility necessary for success in this area in which time, knowledge, and care are the only effective substitutes for the illusion of magical cure. In addition to the conditions discussed here, it should be recognized that the sleep apnea syndrome is an important part of the differential diagnosis of insomnia.

MEDICAL INSOMNIA. Specific and nonspecific effects on the sleep cycle oscillator are exerted by many medical conditions. These include diseases producing fever (which immediately suppresses REM sleep) and pain (which produces a general increase in arousal level). Sleep loss is common in hospital settings, where sleep-disruptive procedures combine with anxiety to make night life miserable for many patients. Patients with coronary or pulmonary insufficiencies may decompensate during the autonomic storm of REM sleep. The patient with congestive heart failure or emphysema may be aware or unaware of the frequent interruptions of sleep which are caused by anoxic stimulation of the reticular formation and which may be lifesaving. Before prescribing sedatives, specific treatment of the underlying medical disease and manipulation of environmental variables must be vigorously pursued.

PSYCHIATRIC INSOMNIA. A variety of neurotic and psychotic disorders, all known to be associated with disturbances in balance of central sympathetic and cholinergic activity, are characterized by difficulty falling asleep and staying asleep. Anxiety and obsessional neuroses, the schizophrenias, and the manic-depressive syndromes are now postulated to be mediated by abnormal neurotransmission in the same central adrenergic systems as those which regulate sleep.

The management of chronic anxiety, always notoriously difficult, is now further complicated by the discovery of three undesirable properties of the class of agents called benzodiazepines. One is a subtle but pernicious addiction syndrome, associated with the long-term use of diazepam. As in other cases of drug dependency, insomnia may be a presenting complaint and the physician must, by careful history-taking and restraint, avoid compounding or aggravating an already iatrogenic disorder of sleep. Another is rebound insomnia, a worsening of sleep following intermediate term use of nitrazepam, flunitrazepam, temazepam, and triazolam. The third is an interference with daytime functioning caused by the cumulative build-up of active metabolites of such "long-acting" agents as flurazepam, diazepam, and flunitrazepam, whose products have half-lives of 36 to 48 hours. Short-acting agents, with half-lives of ten to twelve hours, are less liable to suppress daytime effectiveness (lorazepam, triazolam, and temazepam).

GUIDELINES FOR PRESCRIBING SEDATIVES. A versatile and flexible approach to sedative prescription is needed to exploit the assets and minimize the liabilities of the medication used. For example, when the desired relief of acute anxiety and insomnia has been obtained from a diazepine such as diazepam (Valium), 2 to 5 mg at bedtime, patient and physician can expect some temporary worsening of sleep when the drug is withdrawn. One should not attempt to suppress this time-limited effect of the treatment itself by increasing drug administration. The other agents (e.g., triazolam [Halcion], 0.25 to 0.5 mg at bedtime) tend not to produce rebound and are effective hypnotics. They do not suppress REM, but, like their short-acting congeners, they do suppress Stages III and IV of NREM sleep. In cases of persistent or recurrent insomnia, intermittent and alternating drug use reduces the problems of habituation and withdrawal. Recent suggestions that barbiturates can be reconsidered seem ill advised in view of the low margin of safety and addictive potential of these agents.

Enthusiasm has been expressed for tryptophan sedation (1 to 5 grams at bedtime) but the efficacy of this naturally occurring amino acid has not been proved. The old standby chloral hydrate (0.5 to 1.0 gram at bedtime) still deserves consideration. Amitriptyline (50 mg at bedtime) has been reported to be sleep enhancing even in patients who are not depressed, and the tricyclic antidepressants also improve the sleep of severely depressed patients who may complain of sudden worsening of sleep when effective treatment is stopped. During such withdrawal, frightening hypnopompic hallucinations may mislead both patient and doctor into thinking that psychosis is recurrent when, in reality, a time-limited and transitory pharmacodynamic intensification of REM sleep is the cause. As with rebound insomnia, this complaint demands reassurance, not reinstitution of medication.

Alcohol is a self-administered CNS depressant with profound short- and long-term effects on sleep. The REM phase of the cycle is suppressed during the first part of the night when sleep may be unusually sound. An associated suppression of normal posture shifts may explain the Saturday night paralysis that results from nerve compression occurring in alcoholic sleep. Later in the night, when metabolic breakdown products accumulate, sleep is fitful and more REM deprivation is incurred. Hangover includes a feeling of sleepiness and fatigue which alcohol may temporarily reverse only to perpetuate and intensify. Long-term REM deprivation may be an intervening variable in the ultimate development of alcoholic hallucinoid syndromes; in fact, delirium tremens develops at the peak of REM rebound on about the third day of withdrawal.

NOCTURNAL MYOCLONUS. In late middle age and elderly patients, rhythmic muscle twitches may cause sleep-disturbing involuntary movements of the extremities. The benzodiazepine clonazepam (0.5 to 1.0 mg at bedtime) is reported effective, probably because of a combination of anticonvulsant, sedative, and muscle relaxant effects.

The Hypersomnias. The conditions to be considered as possibly responsible for the complaint of excessive sleep or sleepiness include sleep disorders (narcolepsy) and specific medical disorders (e.g., pickwickian syndrome, CNS lesions). They also include conditions in which the excessive sleepiness is secondary to the disturbed sleep of the parasomnias (sleep apnea syndromes) or a manifestation of underlying mood or personality disorder (depressive and passive dependent types).

NARCOLEPSY. Narcolepsy is a syndrome which is best understood as an increased excitability of the REM generator. Patients complain of persistent drowsiness and one or more of a tetrad of specific signs: (1) *Sleep attacks,* which occur suddenly, are often REM sleep attacks. (2) *Cataplexy* is an equally sudden muscle weakness akin to the atonia which normally occurs only in nocturnal REM. Cataplexy is often precipitated by surprise, mirth, or anger. (3) *Hypnagogic hallucinations* are the subjective accompaniment of sleep-onset REM periods. (4) *Sleep paralysis* is an abnormal extension of REM sleep atonia into the waking state. Thus the narcoleptic patient demonstrates both kinds of sleep pathophysiology: a low set-point level of the REM oscillator—which explains the direct precipitation of REM sleep from waking (the sleep attacks and the sleep onset REM periods); and a dissociation of the ascending (conscious state) and descending (muscle tone) components of REM sleep—which explains the sleep attacks without cataplexy, the cataplexy without sleep attacks, and the sleep paralysis.

Polygraphic studies of narcolepsy demonstrate increased sleepiness (multiple sleep latency test), identify the sleep attack as REM sleep, and disclose REM periods at nocturnal sleep onset. Since narcolepsy is vocationally disabling and sometimes life threatening, it is important that every effort be made to establish the diagnosis objectively. It is equally important not to label all patients who complain of drowsiness as narcoleptic, since many may have sleep apnea syndrome or a nonspecific sleep disorder. Because of stigmatization of affected individuals as "lazy" and because of the legal problems of long-term management with amphetamines, the existence of self-help groups is a welcome innovation.

The set-point of the pontine oscillator can be raised—and the narcolepsy syndrome prevented—by either decreasing cholinergic excitatory drive or increasing aminergic inhibitory drive, or both. The second mechanism best accounts for the traditional effectiveness of the amphetamines, which increase the efficacy of noradrenergic synapses by mimicry. The more recently described beneficial effects of the antidepressants, especially upon cataplexy, are probably due both to blockade of norepinephrine reuptake and/or monamine oxidase inhibition, both of which enhance noradrenergic inhibition by increasing the duration of physiologically released norepinephrine, and to the anticholinergic effects of these drugs. Because they produce fewer long-term problems, the amine reuptake blockers, if effective in a given patient, are the agents of choice.

KLEINE-LEVIN SNYDROME. This extremely rare disorder occurs primarily in adolescent males and is characterized by episodic periods of excessive sleep and overeating, lasting up to several weeks. The cause is unknown. There is no specific treatment, but the condition remits in adulthood.

DEPRESSION. Not only do asymptomatic long-sleepers tend to be depressed, some clinically depressed patients also tend to hypersomnolence (as well as to difficulty falling asleep). Markedly shortened REM latency, increased REM percentage, and increased REM density allow depressive sleep disturbance to be distinguished from that of the insomniac and of normal individuals. This depressive sleep disorder is best treated with amine reuptake blockers (which are also anticholinergic) and is aggravated by physostigmine.

PICKWICKIAN SYNDROME. Hypersomnia is integral to the pickwickian syndrome and a primary result of the anoxemia and hypercarbia consequent upon waking state hypoventilation. It should be emphasized that waking arterial oxygen levels are normal in the sleep apnea syndromes and that the hypersomnia seen in those conditions is, in part, secondary to the sleep disturbance.

The Parasomnias. All the parasomnias share the feature of loss of control of some neural subsystem during sleep. All appear to be age, sex, and sleep stage dependent.

ENURESIS. Bedwetting is a troublesome sleep disorder occurring predominantly in preadolescent males. (Roughly 10 per cent of boys aged four to fourteen are affected.) Because the full bladder does not trigger an awakening, enuresis has been conceived of as a disorder of arousal. The beneficial effects of imipramine (25 to 50 mg given at bedtime) have been attributed mainly to peripheral anticholinergic effects on the bladder. Because of the risks of using drugs and even behavioral treatment in children, only the most persistent and severe cases should be treated.

NIGHT TERRORS, NIGHTMARES, SLEEP WALKING, SLEEP TALKING, AND BRUXISM. Dissociation of sensory and motor integration during NREM sleep characterizes all of these conditions. In night terrors, there is a partial arousal, in panic, from Stages III and IV of NREM sleep, associated with tachycardia and tachypnea. Although capable of coordinated motor behavior and responsive to sensory input, the affected child may hallucinate and thus terrify his parents as much as himself. Fortunately night terrors are benign and short lived, so that reassurance is both appropriate and adequate. Nightmares also occur in older subjects. They can be precipitated from NREM sleep when they are characterized by pure fear (without visual hallucinoid imagery) or REM sleep (when vivid frightening dreams are reported). In both types, intense autonomic storm is measurable. Nightmares of the NREM type have been reported to respond to benzodiazepines with Stages III and IV suppressing properties (such as diazepam, 2 to 5 mg). Age is also helpful here, since Stage IV declines markedly in the fourth decade. The REM type of nightmare (or bad dream) may persist and may present as sleep interruption insomnia. No specific treatment has been reported.

In sleep talking and sleep walking, automatic motor activity begins in Stages III and IV of NREM sleep without full arousal and without accompanying mental activity; bruxism occurs in Stage I of NREM sleep. Sleep talking is entirely benign and should not be treated; disturbed roommates may have to make adjustments. Preventive measures are indicated in bruxism and sleep walking; a boxer's mouthpiece prevents enamel destruction by the persistent and automatic tooth grinding (in bruxism), and a child's stairway gate or other physical restraint may avoid embarrassment and injury to the sleep walker (in somnambulism). There is no evidence that any of these conditions are psychologically determined, and all are age related.

THE SLEEP APNEA SYNDROMES. The respiratory neurons of the brainstem constitute a reticular oscillator of similar design and close proximity to the sleep cycle clock. It is therefore little wonder that this system shows such dramatic state dependency. It may even turn out that some neurons, especially those of the so-called pneumotaxic center, are common to both systems.

At sleep onset and increasingly throughout the NREM phase of sleep, respiration slows and deepens as if the excitatory drive on the medullary respiratory oscillator were decreasing; in contrast, the advent of REM is associated with an increase in variability of both rate and depth of respiration. Hence, one may see a marked hyperpnea—a series of rapid short shallow breaths—or an apneic pause, or both, in association with the clusters of eye movement that punctuate REM and give this curious sleep phase its name.

The respiratory neural oscillator moves air through a complex peripheral system (the airway and lungs) and is influenced by a variety of feedback influences. All of these peripheral factors are also subject to the vicissitudes of the sleep-wake cycle via the autonomic and spinal pathways affecting smooth and skeletal muscle. Thus the decreases in muscle tone that are part of NREM sleep onset, and the further active inhibition of muscle tone that is an intrinsic part of REM, may render a marginal airway nonpatent, so that air cannot be moved even if the consequent changes in blood gases signal the sleep-depressed respiratory oscillation to increase its output. Upon such a background the terms central, peripheral, and mixed type of sleep apnea assume logical and lucid order. In fact, physiology suggests that all state-dependent respiratory changes, from the normal to the pathologic, must involve *both* central and peripheral factors.

Middle-aged male patients complaining of either excessive daytime sleepiness or incapability of staying asleep at night should be considered as possibly suffering from the sleep apnea syndrome. If they are obese and snore, then descriptions on tape recordings of their obstructive apneic spells—which occur on the order of 300 times per night—may be obtained from a bed partner. These peripherally mediated events are due to collapse of a fat-compromised airway by the negative intrathoracic pressure of inspiration; the situation is only made worse by the vigorous compensatory respiratory effects which ensue, accompanied by the strained grunting of the Müller maneuver, and which are often noted by the observant bed partner. Observable cyanosis may be a sign of the oxygen desaturation (50 per cent is not unusual). Recovery occurs only when arousal restores both the set-point of the respiratory oscillator and the tonus of the tongue and pharyngeal musculature. The frequent awakenings contribute to the excessive daytime sleepiness.

Even the peripheral obstructive type of apnea, which is often relieved by tracheostomy or a continuous positive-pressure nasally delivered airstream, probably has a central component because neither surgery nor weight loss eliminates the sleep apnea episodes. Furthermore, some men who are neither obese nor airway obstructed show only the apneas. These individuals may reflect most purely the CNS pathophysiology common to all the sleep apnea syndromes. Such cases are uncommon and difficult to diagnose—an important point, since sedative medication, prescribed as a well-intentioned response to the complaint of insomnia, may depress the sensitivity of the respiratory reticular formation which translates hypoxia into a life-saving arousal. Patients suspected of having sleep apnea syndrome are best referred for diagnosis and treatment to a sleep laboratory with pulmonary recording capability.

Cardiac abnormalities can complicate the pickwickian syndrome and the sleep apneas. Marked sinus arrhythmias may accompany the apneic spells, and extreme bradycardia, asystoles, second degree atrioventricular block, premature ventricular contractions, atrial flutter, and ventricular tachycardia have all been reported. The abnormalities clear if night-time apnea and its associated hypoxemia are prevented.

CONTRIBUTING FACTORS AND CLINICAL VARIANTS OF SLEEP APNEA SYNDROME. At all ages males are more prone than females to intrinsic sleep abnormalities. The tendency to snore, to stop breathing, and to collapse and/or obstruct the airway in sleep has a genetic component and is greater in men of the same family. The times in life at which pathologic consequences are most likely to emerge are infancy (sudden infant death syndrome), puberty (chubby puffer syndrome), and late middle age (sleep apnea syndrome).

Cardiorespiratory arrest is a likely cause of *sudden "crib" death* in infancy. In those infants who are "near-miss" for sudden infant death, apneas occur with increasing frequency at four and one half months of age, predominantly during NREM sleep. The period of greatest risk for fatal accidents is between birth and six months of age, and respiratory infection is thought to be a contributing factor. Home-monitoring systems have been developed to detect apneas and alert parents to the need for resuscitative maneuvers.

In the *chubby puffer syndrome*, obese prepubescent males may resemble adult pickwickians whose symptoms are ascribed to primary alveolar hypoventilation, and this sign may persist after temporary relief has been provided by adenotonsillectomy. These facts imply a central respiratory abnormality whose neural basis is as yet obscure. Treatments designed to increase central respiratory drive with aminophylline and progesterone have not been generally effective. Recent reports claim that the antidepressant tricyclic agent protriptyline has been effective.

Physiology and Pharmacology

Hobson JA, Brazier MAB (eds.): The Reticular Formation Revisited. New York, Raven Press, 1980. *This book covers the most recent basic research on the neurobiology of the reticular formation, including its role in control of respiration, muscle tone, and the states of consciousness.*

Hobson JA, Steriade M: Neuronal basis of behavioral state control. *In* Handbook of Physiology, Section on Neurophysiology, Volume on Intrinsic Regulatory

Systems of the Brain. American Physiological Society, 1984. *A comprehensive and critical review of cellular level studies of sleep phenomena and a detailed account of the neurophysiologic and neuropharmacologic basis of the reciprocal interaction model of sleep cycle control.*

Lader M (ed.): New perspectives in benzodiazepine therapy. Arz Forsch/Drug Res 30:851, 1980. *This set of papers provides an up-to-date survey of a rapidly developing area of neuropharmacologic research with important clinical applications.*

Sleep Disorders

Guilleminault C, Dement WC (eds.): Sleep Apnea Syndromes. New York, A. R. Liss, 1978. *A symposium addressing the clinical and physiologic aspects of the disorders.*

Hauri P: The Sleep Disorders. 2nd ed. Kalamazoo, MI, Upjohn, 1982. *A concise, complete, and sensible summary with excellent illustrations; for medical students, house officers, and practitioners.*

Hobson JA: Sleep: Order and disorder. Behav Biol Med Monogr 1:1, 1983. *A detailed and extensively referenced discussion of sleep pathophysiology.*

Roffwarg H: Diagnostic classification of sleep and arousal disorders. Sleep 2:1, 1979. *A comprehensive diagnostic inventory which constitutes an invaluable reference for the sleep disorders specialist.*

Sullivan CE, Issa EG, Berthon-Jones M, Eves L: Reversal of obstructive sleep apnea by continuous positive airway pressure applied through the nares. Lancet 1:862, 1981. *Description of a new, effective, nonsurgical treatment with a diagram of the effective nasal adapter.*

473. REGIONAL DIAGNOSIS OF CEREBRAL DISORDERS

Fred Plum

Localizing diagnosis is an important part of the evaluation of neurologic diseases. Although radiographic methods for examining the brain safely and painlessly have advanced a great deal during recent years, they commonly fail to detect the early stages of many tumors, some regional infections, and most degenerative diseases. The regional diagnosis of most epileptogenic foci also lies below the discriminatory powers of conventional radiography or imaging methods. Since therapy in epilepsy often depends on the anatomic locus of the seizure focus, clinical judgment becomes crucial. Regional diagnosis helps in differentiating neurologic from psychiatric disease and provides the additional reward that it tells the observer something about how the brain works, a philosophic interest that has increasingly drawn human inquiry for the past two centuries.

Several general principles influence the accuracy of regional clinical diagnosis. First, lesions that damage the corticospinal, somatosensory, or special sensory pathways generally can be localized earlier and more precisely than those that affect the brain's association cortex. Second, the rate at which a lesion appears and enlarges and the degree to which it irritates surrounding brain tissue influences not only how rapidly signs and symptoms develop but their severity as well. Slowly growing intracranial tumors, for example, sometimes can reach the size of small oranges before they produce notable signs and symptoms, even when they impinge on primary motor or sensory pathways. By contrast, pea-sized metastatic growths can in some instances produce incapacitating disabilities. Third, certain individual behavioral symptoms can reflect perturbed functions in any of several of the cerebral association areas; inattention, for example, can accompany disease in either the frontal or parietal lobe, and the distinction of its regional cause must be made by identifying additional signs that accompany it. Finally, by shifting soft tissues against the unyielding skull and dural meninges, large lesions of the brain sometimes produce functional changes in neural structures that lie at a distance from the lesion itself. Such remote effects especially accompany acutely arising lesions such as brain infarcts, hemorrhages, or malignant tumors. Sometimes, however, they can lead the unwary observer to errors of clinical localization even when slowly enlarging masses are at fault.

Frontal Lobes

The frontal lobes influence two principal functions, motor control and expressive behavior. The neurons constituting the primary motor area reside in the precentral gyrus and are arranged somatotopically along that structure in a manner that gives especially large representation to the fine movements regulating phonation and distal limb control, especially of the upper extremity. The adjacent, postcentral gyrus of the parietal lobe provides the cortical receiving area for sensory perceptions and is arranged with a similar somatotopic representation. The two cortical areas work interdependently, and the pre- and post-Rolandic banks often are described together as the primary sensorimotor cortex. Immediately anterior to the primary motor strip lies the premotor cortex on the lateral surface and the supplementary motor area on the medial frontal cortex. Cerebellar, basal ganglia, and cortical association projections feed into this premotor area, which provides prefinal integration of motor acts before the motor cortex synthesizes their final coordination and transmits the signal via the corticospinal tract. Within the prefrontal areas lie the principal zones influencing voluntary, saccadic control of eye movements. Broca's speech area is found along the inferior prefrontal region of the dominant hemisphere. The remainder of the lateral and medial surface, plus almost all of the inferior surface of the frontal lobes, contains neural mechanisms regulating behavior, emotion, and autonomic function, especially as these activities relate to motor expression.

Motor symptoms of frontal lobe disease (Table 473–1) are most prominent when lesions directly intrude on the Rolandic motor strip or its descending corticospinal pathways in the corona radiata or internal capsule. Selective premotor signs and symptoms occur when a lesion in that region either stimulates seizures or reaches a relatively large size.

Two major behavioral syndromes result from frontal lobe damage. Both usually reflect the presence of relatively large lesions directly or indirectly producing bilateral frontal lobe dysfunction; unilateral abnormalities, unless they produce seizures, often remain asymptomatic in their early stages. As an example, unilateral prefrontal lobe amputation can be carried out to remove localized tumors, often leaving no discernible change in personality or behavior. Similarly, minor effects have attended efforts to relieve or alter abnormal psychiatric traits by unilateral anterior frontal lobe removal. Such procedures, to cause a change in behavior, usually must interrupt limbic frontal pathways.

SYNDROME OF THE BASAL FOREBRAIN. This clinical constellation accompanies large, usually bilateral lesions involving the septal area and adjacent basal forebrain extending forward into the orbitofrontal cortex toward the frontal pole. Affective patients are apathetic, inattentive, hypokinetic, and hypophonic or mute. Many show an autonomic apraxia, being unable to initiate deep breathing or to micturate on command. There may

TABLE 473–1. MOTOR SYMPTOMS OF FRONTAL LOBE DISEASE*

	Paralysis	Seizure
Precentral gyrus	Focal distal weakness, maximal in lower face, hand, sometimes foot. Distribution occasionally resembles glove or stocking. Hyperactive reflexes, mild spasticity, Babinski if foot involved.	Jacksonian: focal onset of face, thumb, foot with "march" toward proximal limb and trunk.
Corona radiata or internal capsule	Increasingly spastic hemiplegia.	
Prefrontal area	Slow, hypokinetic, sometimes ataxic movements; ocular ipsiversion; paratonic resistance to passive stretch; palmar or plantar grasping; Broca's syntactic aphasia, occasionally mutism.	Adversive: ocular contraversion, elevated arm, body turning, speech arrest.

*All arise contralateral to the brain lesion.

be incontinence because of indifference. The lesions often displace more posteriorly located structures so as to produce corticospinal tract dysfunction with hyperactive deep tendon reflexes and extensor plantar responses on one or both sides of the body.

FRONTAL POLAR AND PREFRONTAL SYNDROMES. Small lesions often cause no measurable behavioral abnormalities. Large ones produce the frontal lobe syndrome of classic repute. Affected patients are distractible, euphoric, and facetious, and are unable appropriately to plan ahead or to judge the future implications of present acts or experiences. Lesions affecting the medial prefrontal cortex may result in urgency incontinence. Seizures, if they occur, include adversive or grand mal attacks. Enlarging lesions may eventually encroach upon premotor function to cause hypokinesia, contralateral inattention, paratonia, and grasp reflexes.

Parietal Lobe

The postcentral gyrus contains the neural mechanisms that abstract somatosensory stimuli into stereoperception and stereognosis. The more posteriorly located association cortex receives heavy afferent projections from somatosensory and visual receiving areas and progressively abstracts the information to create an internal map by which the subject gives attention to the spatial world of his body and the outer world that surrounds it. Several perceptual and cognitive functions of the parietal association cortex are predominantly lateralized to one or the other hemisphere. The nondominant hemisphere especially relates to recognition of external space, sometimes on both sides of the body, while the dominant parietal lobe abstracts right-sided body space but also influences the capacity for arithmetic calculation and for right-left orientation. Both hemispheres contribute importantly to the advanced programming of complex motor acts (praxis).

The *syndrome of the postcentral primary somatosensory cortex* includes impaired or absent capacities to recognize the form, texture, relative size, and weight of objects, especially of complex items producing multiple spatial-morphologic stimuli. The integration of morphologic perception into memory must also be coded in this area, since patients with only partial cortical sensory loss still have great difficulty in naming a palpated object even when they possess some residual capacity to describe its form. For example, one of our otherwise intelligent patients with a post-Rolandic parietal lesion was able to identify a block in her left hand as being "an edged, partly flat lump" but was unable to synthesize this into calling it either a block or a cube. Lesions confined to the primary cortical sensory area do not affect cutaneous thresholds for vibration, pain, temperature, or simple touch.

Small lesions affecting the posterior parietal areas produce few abnormal symptoms. Limited evidence from man plus physiologic analyses in the monkey suggests that the dorsal posterior region functions largely to make beginning abstractions of somatosensory perceptions and relate them to visual perception. The inferior parietal region, located where the parietal, occipital, and temporal lobes converge, serves a multimodal function in which somatosensory, spatial, visual, and auditory perceptions are integrated and related to the memory, limbic, and language functions of the temporal lobes. Most so-called parietal lobe syndromes reflect damage predominantly to this posterior inferior area.

Nondominant posteroinferior parietal lobe syndromes include symptoms whose severity and extent depend directly upon the size and acuteness of the lesion. Most frequent is constructional apraxia, really a spatial defect, reflected by difficulties in either drawing simple figures such as a clock face or in copying the outlines of a cube or intersecting hexagons. Selective spatial disorientation sometimes is striking. One of our patients, a milkman with a small neoplasm in this region, remained capable in all dimensions of his job except that he was no longer able to recall automatically the pattern of his delivery route. Dressing apraxia similarly may be a relatively isolated symptom of the nondominant parietal lobe. With larger lesions in this area, patients develop inattention to contralateral space, a phenomenon sometimes called neglect, which may extend to include the failure to perceive left-sided tactile or visual stimuli when such stimuli are presented to both sides of the body or visual field simultaneously (the phenomenon of extinction). With very large lesions extending deeply to involve the thalamus or forward to impair the descending corticospinal pathways, patients may fail to recognize the presence of the sensory defect and even deny that a hemiparesis exists (anosagnosia). Acutely, patients with such large lesions may suffer a protracted confusional delirium. Later or sometimes from the start some exhibit a remarkable emptiness of affect and a degree of inattentiveness that suggests that neither their bodies nor the world contralateral to the damaged hemisphere any longer exists in either their attention or their memory. Almost always the cause of such severe "parietal lobe" syndromes lies in cerebral infarcts that damage a substantial fraction of the territory of the middle cerebral artery, with the tissue injury extending well beyond the parietal lobe. Most specific agnosias or apraxias also can be traced to the presence of similarly large lesions or bilateral disturbances of the hemispheres.

Left-sided, dominant hemisphere parietal lesions produce symptoms somewhat different from the above. The effects of very large lesions usually cannot be judged because they nearly always are associated with severe aphasia. Constructional apraxia accompanies restricted left posterior inferior parietal lobe damage more frequently than right-sided damage. Patients with lesions in this area commonly have great difficulties making arithmetic calculations (acalculia) even of a simple nature. Some authorities attribute a combination of acalculia, right-left disorientation, agraphia, and finger agnosia (Gerstmann's syndrome) to damage of the left inferior parietal lobe, but it is doubtful that it occurs with lesions isolated to that area.

Temporal Lobes

The temporal lobes contain neural structures critical to auditory perception, memory, language, and emotion. Each auditory cortex receives projections from both ears so that hearing itself rarely is disrupted by cerebral lesions. The memory and language functions of the temporal lobes are discussed in Ch. 474. The inferior loop of the geniculocalcarine radiation passes through the temporal lobe, where its injury may give rise to characteristic visual field defects as described in Ch. 479.

The parahippocampal region and the hippocampus of the temporal lobe contribute to the phylogenetically ancient "limbic lobe" of the cerebral cortex, which rims the upper brainstem and together with certain subcortical nuclei makes up the *limbic system.* The limbic system integrates emotions and their expressions with memory and with the polymodal sensory input that converges upon the temporal lobe. The system projects to efferent motor and other areas of the cortex and via the hypothalamus to autonomic and reticular structures in the brainstem and spinal cord.

In monkeys, removal of the temporal lobes bilaterally gives

TABLE 473–2. ICTAL MANIFESTATIONS OF TEMPORAL LOBE EPILEPTIC FOCI

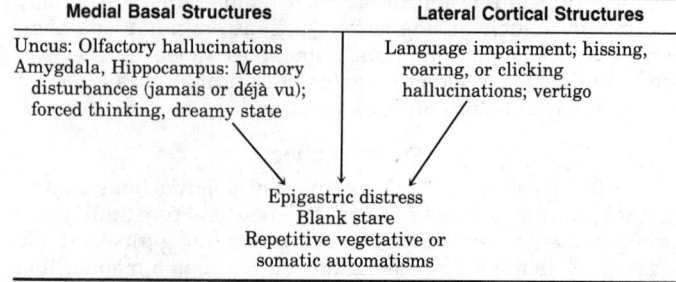

Medial Basal Structures	Lateral Cortical Structures
Uncus: Olfactory hallucinations Amygdala, Hippocampus: Memory disturbances (jamais or déjà vu); forced thinking, dreamy state	Language impairment; hissing, roaring, or clicking hallucinations; vertigo

↓ (both)

Epigastric distress
Blank stare
Repetitive vegetative or somatic automatisms

TABLE 473–3. COMMON INTERICTAL TRAITS OF PATIENTS WITH TEMPORAL LOBE EPILEPTIC FOCI

Humorless
Obsessional
Dependent
Philosophical
Sad
Hyposexual

rise to a remarkable behavioral disorder termed the Kluver-Bucy syndrome, marked by amnesia, excessive orality, distractibility, placidity, and indiscriminate sexuality. A somewhat similar constellation of symptoms, usually accompanied by more extensive behavioral changes, has been reported in humans, most often following diffuse brain injuries or in one of the degenerative dementias. More restrictive visceral and emotional aberrations mark the ictal and to some degree interictal behavior of patients with temporal lobe epilepsy (Ch. 510). Tables 473–2 and 473–3 list some of these major symptoms.

Controversy has surrounded the question of whether patients with temporal lobe or limbic system lesions or temporal lobe epilepsy are more given to violence or psychosis as a direct result of their lesions. Present evidence is inconclusive. If restrained during an attack, patients with temporal lobe epilepsy often will lash out physically. Unprovoked violence, however, probably is no more frequent among patients with temporal lobe epilepsy than among the remainder of the population. It seems doubtful that epilepsy or specific brain lesions can be regarded as a medically satisfactory explanation for aggressive crime.

Occipital lobe functions are discussed with disorders of the visual system (Ch. 479–2).

Baer D: Hemispheric specialization and the neurology of emotion. Arch Neurol 40:195, 1983. *Several studies are reviewed that suggest that the right hemisphere may be "dominant" for certain emotions.*

Baer DM, Fedio P: Quantitative analysis of interictal behavior in temporal lobe epilepsy. Arch Neurol 34:454, 1977. *An important effort to quantify differences in personality traits between epileptics and controls.*

Biemond A, Vinken PJ, Bruyn GW: Localization in Clinical Neurology. Handbook of Neurology. Vol 2. Amsterdam, North Holland, 1969. *A compendium of classic observations on the topic.*

Delgado-Escueta AV, Mattson RH, King L, et al.: The nature of aggression during epileptic sezures. N Engl J Med 305:711, 1981. *An NIH committee reports that the phenomenon is rare.*

Hier DB, Mondlock J, Caplan LR: Behavioral abnormalities after right hemisphere stroke. Neurology 33:337, 1983. *A careful analysis of large series of patients with damage to the right parietal lobe and more.*

Lilly R, Cummings JL, Benson DF, Frankel M: The human Klüver-Bucy syndrome. Neurology 33:1141, 1983. *Twelve patients with severe bilateral anterior temporal lobe damage are described with rather mixed syndromes.*

Mesulam M-M: A cortical network for directed attention and unilateral neglect. Ann Neurol 10:309, 1981. *A thoughtful synthesis of the sensory integrative functions of the parietal association areas.*

Pritchard PB, Lombroso CT, McIntyre M: Psychological complications of temporal lobe epilepsy. Neurology 30:227, 1980. *A confirmation of the high incidence of behavioral-personality difficulties in these patients.*

Roland PE: Astereognosis. Arch Neurol 33:543, 1976. *Empirical confirmation that stereognosis depends on mechanisms that arise in the immediate postcentral cortex.*

Roland PE, Larsen B, Lassen NA, Skinhøj E: Supplementary motor area and other cortical areas in organization of voluntary movements in man. J Neurophysiol 43:118, 1980. *Preprogramming of hand movement is associated with increased blood flow in supplementary motor areas, while during actual movement blood flow increased bilaterally in these areas as well as in the bilateral premotor and motor areas of the cortex. A classic in the physiologic substrate of behavior.*

Stevens JR, Hermann BP: Temporal lobe epilepsy, psychopathology, and violence: The state of evidence. Neurology 31:1127, 1981. *A vigorous defense against the view that psychopathology and temporal lobe epilepsy are directly linked.*

474. FOCAL DISTURBANCES OF HIGHER FUNCTION

Fred Plum

LANGUAGE AND APHASIA

Verbal language represents the process by which the forebrain applies symbolic terms to objects and concepts in order to formalize its knowledge of sensory perceptions, memories, emotional responses, and the stream of preverbal inner thoughts. The neuroanatomy of the mechanisms that accomplish language is known, albeit imprecisely, from three sources. One is the postmortem study of patients who have been carefully evaluated for language impairment. The second is the change produced in language by stimulating various regions of the cerebral cortex by skilled surgeons in the process of operating on appropriate patients. The third is radiography, including CT, NMR, and PET scans, which allow one to study the anatomy of language in the intact patient.

Although wide areas of both hemispheres contribute to language function, the critical regions are concentrated in two principal cortical zones, a posterior, predominantly receptor–integrative zone and an anterior region devoted predominantly to language expression. The principal posterior portion of the language cortex occupies the posterior superior temporal gyrus extending from approximately the transverse auditory gyrus back to the end of the Sylvian fissure. This, the Wernicke area, represents the region where sensory perceptions appear to be integrated with inner thought and memory so as to generate the fundamental abstractions of language. The region of the adjacent angular and supramarginal gyri, as well as of the superiorly adjacent parietal operculum and, perhaps, the pulvinar nucleus of the thalamus, contributes importantly but in a clinically less predictable manner to the fundamental synthesis of language. More anteriorly, *Broca's area,* lying in the inferolateral frontal lobe just anterior to the primary motor cortex and extending under the surface into the frontal operculum, is critical to the normal verbal or written expression of speech. Lesions surrounding the Wernicke area, interrupting pathways projecting into it but not the speech cortex itself, disrupt selective aspects of posterior language function, while peri-Brocal lesions somewhat similarly produce partial impairments in the expression of language. Evidence obtained by Penfield and others, who have removed tumors or epileptogenic lesions from Broca's area, indicates that in some of these patients most or all of verbal and written expression may return following damage to or even removal of parts of this region. Normal language function, however, rarely returns to the adult who suffers severe damage to the Wernicke area of the dominant hemisphere.

Language function is strongly lateralized in most human brains. Anatomically, the left hemisphere usually contains a longer Sylvian fissure than the right, and the planum of the left temporal lobe (the area lying in the Sylvian fissure in back of the posterior edge of the transverse (Heschl's) auditory gyrus) is larger than the right in two thirds of brains. The anatomic changes are found in infants and fetuses as well as in adult brains. Clinically, language laterality in patients can be estimated in two major ways: by correlating the side of temporofrontal brain lesions with the presence or absence of an aphasia and, in persons with normal speech, by observing the effect of injecting amobarbital sodium into the ispsilateral or contralateral carotid artery. The anesthetic briefly anesthetizes the ipsilateral hemisphere, including its language activities, and gives important preoperative knowledge of the risks of surgery to the particular area of brain. Both kinds of studies indicate that in almost all right-handed persons the left hemisphere is heavily dominant for speech and that aphasia resulting from damage to the left posterior language areas seldom fully recovers. Among the left-handed and the strongly ambidextrous, about 70 per cent show a left hemisphere language dominance or predominance. Of the remaining 30 per cent, about half show strong language representation in each hemisphere, while the remainder are right dominant. A feature of many left-handed and ambidextrous persons is that damage to the major language area on either side may produce acute symptoms of aphasia, but a higher percentage recover than do right-handed persons with comparable left hemispheric lesions.

Language function in children represents a special case. Most youngsters who suffer a severe hemispheric brain injury when less than six years of age recover normal or nearly normal language capabilities whether or not aphasia accompanies the early postinjury period. Even among such children, however, transient aphasia occurs nine times more often following damage to the left temporal frontal area than to the right.

Aphasia or dysphasia describes an impairment or loss of language function as a result of damage to the specific language areas of the cerebrum. The condition must be distinguished from *dysarthria*, a disturbance in the articulation of speech, as well as from defects in sensory systems that prevent perceptions from reaching the language cortex. Persons deaf and blind from peripheral causes can learn a language as long as the brain is intact, while disease of the motor system, the cerebellum, or the vocal apparatus can cripple or halt the outflow of words but does not produce aphasia.

The pattern of an aphasia depends on the part or parts of the speech brain that are damaged. Language represents the integration and expression of many aspects of brain function and injuries to its mechanisms can result in a number of somewhat varying symptom complexes. Among the properties of a language are (1) the comprehension of symbols, (2) the ability to transform perceptions or inner thoughts into words, and (3) the ability to express symbols. Geschwind (Table 474–1) has found that most aphasic disorders can be classified by testing comprehension of language, fluency of output, and ability to repeat phrases.

Lesions damaging the dominant posterior superior temporal gyrus and its adjacent area characteristically destroy the capacity to recognize the sensory symbols of language or to transform inner thoughts into meaningful words. The classic result is *Wernicke's aphasia*. Affected patients cannot recognize spoken, written, or symbolic instructions except, perhaps intermittently, the simplest verbal commands (e.g., "Stop!"). Despite the severe injury to comprehension, the brain preserves a memory storehouse of words so that expressed words often are chosen correctly. Patients with Wernicke's aphasia speak fluently with a natural rhythm, although the result possesses neither understandable syntax nor meaning. Insight is lost and prognosis for total recovery is poor. Posterior lesions outside the immediate Wernicke area tend to produce more restricted disturbances. Lesions of the parietal operculum may give rise to conduction aphasia, a disorder in which the patient speaks fluently but makes many errors similar to those of Wernicke's aphasia. However, comprehension is relatively normal.

Other strategically placed focal lesions of the posterior dominant hemisphere can destroy selectively one or another dimension of language perception. *Alexia* (inability to comprehend written language while retaining relatively good general vision, especially in the left visual field) without *agraphia* (the inability to write language despite the preservation of related motor function) results when a lesion destroys the left visual cortex and, in addition, extends to involve the splenium of the corpus callosum. The placement cuts off the projection that otherwise connects the unaffected right visual cortex to the language areas of the left. Such patients, despite their inability to comprehend the written word, can speak and write normally, in contrast to those with a combination of *alexia with agraphia*, in whom normal auditory comprehension, thought, and speech remain, but the comprehension of both visual and written language symbols is lost. The abnormality is rare and has been stated to follow lesions of the left angular gyrus. *Pure word deafness* describes the circumstance in which auditory language perception selectively is lost despite intact hearing and the preservation of other language capabilities. This rare phenomenon follows bilateral selective damage to the auditory cortex of the superior temporal gyrus or, reportedly, can accompany subcortical white matter damage in the left temporal lobe that injures the adjacent left auditory cortex and disconnects the transcallosal fibers from the right temporal lobe destined for Wernicke's area.

Broca's aphasia is characterized by severe disturbances in the output of either spontaneous or commanded speech and writing. Comprehension is relatively well preserved, although things spoken usually are understood better than things read. Largely because of vascular distributions, many patients with Broca's aphasia also have an associated right hemiparesis or hemiplegia, but this is the result of an independent internal capsular lesion. Enlargement of the lesion into the adjacent premotor cortex is believed to explain an associated motor apraxia observed in some such patients. A more restricted lesion may cause aphasia characterized by slow, effortful, dysarthric speech with normal syntax and preserved ability to write normally.

Global aphasia describes the combined severe loss of all major aspects of language function. Affected patients acutely are often mute and most have an accompanying right hemiplegia. Shortly thereafter it becomes apparent that they can neither comprehend nor express language except, perhaps, in the form of brief expletives or phrases. Insight, as judged from other behavior, is poor, as is prognosis for full recovery.

A group of aphasic disorders is characterized by the ability of the patient to repeat after the examiner phrases and often long sentences. Such ability to repeat implies that Wernicke's and Broca's areas as well as the primary connections between them must be intact and that the responsible lesions must be near to but not involving the primary speech areas. Geschwind has divided these aphasias with good repetition into those called (1) transcortical motor (similar to Broca's), (2) transcortical sensory (similar to Wernicke's), and (3) the isolation syndrome

TABLE 474–1. CLASSIFICATION OF APHASIAS

	Expression	Comprehension	Repetition	Other Signs	Localization
Broca's (expressive)	Nonfluent	+	−	Right hemiparesis worse in arm; mood depressed	Lower posterior frontal
Wernicke's (receptive)	Fluent	−	−	Often none; may be euphoric and/or paranoid	Posterior superior temporal area
Conduction	Fluent	+	−	Often none; cortical sensory loss in right arm; depressed	Usually parietal operculum
Global	Nonfluent	−	−	Right hemiparesis worse in arm; flat affect	Massive peri-Sylvian lesion
Transcortical motor	Nonfluent	+	+		Anterior to Broca's area or supplementary speech area
Transcortical sensory	Fluent	−	+		Surrounding Wernicke's area posteriorly
Transcortical mixed (isolation syndrome)	Nonfluent	−	+		Both of the above
Anomic	Fluent	+	+		Lesion of angular gyrus or second temporal gyrus

*After Geschwind, 1970.
+ = relatively or fully intact.
− = definitely impaired.

(caused by a large lesion producing a global type of aphasia except for normal repetition). Included in this group of disorders is *anomic aphasia*, associated with a lesion of the angular gyrus and characterized by rambling, lengthy, empty, and poorly focused speech, with transparent circumlocutions—talking around forgotten words. However, the diagnosis of anomic aphasia deserves a word of caution. Nonspecific difficulties in word-finding are common in the elderly and may accompany diffuse disorders of the brain that produce delirious or confusional states, only to disappear largely or entirely when the general illness subsides.

Mutism, the inability to speak, occurs in several forms. Acutely, it appears in association with vascular lesions of the left frontal lobe involving either part of Broca's area or its conducting pathways. Under such circumstances, mutism coupled with right hemiplegia, as indicated above, reflects the presence of a relatively large brain lesion and gives way to a less complete language disturbance within a few days. As an isolated symptom of a vascular lesion, however, acute mutism characteristically carries a benign prognosis and disappears within a few days to a week or so without leaving residual expressive symptoms. Acute mutism also occurs paroxysmally with epileptic attacks involving the left inferior premotor area, the commonest underlying cause being a neoplasm. More sustained mutism develops as a symptom of bilateral frontal lobe damage (Ch. 473) and is accompanied by apathy, inattention, and hypokinesia. Sustained mutism and behavioral withdrawal also can accompany severe psychiatric disorders. Such illnesses can be recognized by their lack of signs, symptoms, or laboratory findings of structural frontal lobe disease. *Anarthria*, the inability to speak because of abnormal innervation or mechanical disease of the vocal apparatus, differs from mutism in that affected patients make sounds and usually express vividly their frustration over being unable to speak. Occasionally, anarthria will reflect an hysterical disorder, in which case the alert, attentive subject usually displays insouciant indifference to the lack of vocal capacity. Neurogenic causes of anarthria include either severe bulbar or pseudobulbar palsy, conditions readily diagnosed by the presence of other signs and symptoms of nuclear or supranuclear paralysis.

Although brief disturbances in language function can result from seizures or transient attacks of vascular insufficiency, the development of a true aphasia, i.e., a selective disturbance in language function that is not part of a global decline in the intellect and lasting for more than a few hours, almost always reflects a focal structural lesion of the brain. The commonest cause is vascular damage, either from infarction or from hemorrhage, in the distribution of the middle cerebral artery or, less often, the posterior or anterior cerebral arteries. Occlusions of the latter may damage the pulvinar or disconnect right hemispheric sensory perceptions from the language areas in the left hemisphere. The second most frequent cause of aphasia is severe head trauma, neoplasms and other space-occupying lesions making up most of the remaining causes. None of these causes of aphasia typically produce very discrete brain lesions and several, such as vascular disease, are prone to generate either multifocal brain damage or large lesions whose effects extend considerably beyond the language zones. Language represents an exclusively human function, so that aphasia can be studied only in the damaged human brain. The anatomic variability of the lesions that cause aphasia necessarily leads to an equally inconsistent patterning of its major symptoms. The examiner must constantly recall these principles when trying to analyze a language defect in an effort to localize its anatomy and diagnose its cause.

APRAXIA

Apraxia refers to a disturbance of or an inability to perform learned motor acts despite retention of sufficient sensory and language function to understand the command and the motor capacity to carry it out (praxis). Students of brain function are inconsistent in their views about the mechanism of the phenomenon. Those disposed toward precise localizationist views of the brain postulate apraxia to occur under the following circumstances: (1) *Ideational apraxia*. Visual and receptive functions of the language areas of the left hemisphere are relatively preserved, but the propositional ideas of motor activity are lost, so that commands to carry out skilled acts cannot be executed. Imitation is also impaired and both sides of the body can be affected. Tools of daily living such as pencils, combs, and eating utensils can sometimes be recognized and even named by the affected subject but cannot accurately be utilized. The defect traditionally has been inferred to result from damage to the dominant posterior inferior parietal lobe area. (2) *Ideomotor apraxia*. Visual, receptive, and ideational functions of the dominant hemisphere are preserved, but the subject is unable to perform an act to command despite understanding the task, retention of the ability to move the involved body part, and ability to imitate the act. Affected patients tend to have insight into their motor incapacity and may shrug or smile hopelessly as their tentative efforts fail accurately to carry out the command. The condition is considered to reflect a conduction defect that interrupts commands that emanate from the posterior language area and are intended for Broca's area in the dominant hemisphere. We find the phenomenon rare except as an inconstant accompaniment to moderately severe posterior aphasias. (3) *Limb-kinetic, kinetic, or motor apraxia*. Patients with expressive aphasia may have great difficulty carrying out motor commands involving the face or hand of either side, despite their apparent ability to understand what is said. The defect is considered to reflect damage to a premotor area in the dominant hemisphere, which retains the command map (engram) for learned motor functions. Affected patients appear to understand instructions and may even haltingly repeat them verbally but are unable to imitate with either hand acts such as combing the hair, using a toothbrush, waving, and saluting. By contrast, some of these functions may be carried out in automatic settings, such as in performing the morning toilet. In our experience motor apraxia is uncommon except with frontal lobe lesions that are either large, bilateral, or only part of a more widespread forebrain dysfunction. (4) *Callosal apraxia*. Lesions producing destructive damage to the anterior portion of the corpus callosum or interrupting the transcallosal motor pathway that connects the left frontal lobe to the right can result in apraxia of the left hand to verbal but not to visually mediated commands. The disorder has been attributed to disconnection of the pathway that connects verbally released motor engrams putatively located in the left, dominant premotor area from reaching the premotor areas of the right hemisphere.

Except for the rare example of anterior callosal apraxia, we seldom have encountered motor apraxia as a distinct neuropsychologic deficit unaccompanied by wider functional impairments of aphasia or dementia, complications that make mechanistic interpretations difficult. The value of apraxia as a sign of specific physiologic impairment or anatomic localization has been commensurately small.

Constructional apraxia and *dressing apraxia* are disorders of skilled movements that relate more to damaged perceptual mechanisms than to motor impairments. Constructional apraxia describes difficulty in arranging or copying objects in accordance with their normal spatial relationships. Dressing apraxia refers to the inability properly to relate the shape and parts of garments to the appropriate part and form of the body so as to clothe oneself. In isolation, both constructional and dressing apraxia relate to large lesions that destroy or damage the spatial integrating functions of the posterior parietal lobe, especially the right, and its transcortical-subcortical connections. Alternatively, they tend to be prominent features of the bilateral temporoparietal abnormalities that accompany Alzheimer's disease. Constructional apraxia is the more common of the two defects and affects interpretations of material presented to either visual field or carried out by either side of the body. Dressing apraxia is less common and when associated with severe left somatosensory defects or denial tends more selectively to affect that side of the body. Both abnormalities tend to clear during convalescence. Their occurrence with acute damage to the parietal lobe suggests that they depend upon dysfunction in areas outside the immediate area of tissue destruction. We have observed a few instances of sustained bilateral dressing apraxia apparently related to single, focal, and only moderately large neoplasms involving the junctional area between the occipital and parietal cortex on the right side.

Several motor abnormalities sometimes have been called apraxia that are more appropriately considered to be combinations of pseudobulbar palsy and the effect of abnormal supranuclear reflexes. *Gait apraxia* due to a combination of bilateral pyramidal and extrapyramidal weakness of the lower extremities with paratonic rigidity and plantar grasping falls into this category (Ch. 480.2). Similarly, *oculomotor apraxia,* a term applied to complete or partial inability to look conjugately in particular directions on command is best understood as a bilateral interruption of the descending supranuclear oculomotor pathways from the frontal eye fields. The supranuclear defect of frontal pathways impairs but does not necessarily totally interrupt voluntary control of the direction of gaze and is enhanced by the sparing of an uninhibited, occipitally originating, visual fixation reflex. Characteristically, patients affected with the disorder must blink to block fixation before they can voluntarily redirect gaze toward the new point. They easily follow fixated objects.

AGNOSIA

Agnosia, at least as separated from a more global dementia with its attendant visual spatial defects, is an uncommon psychologic phenomenon characterized by the inability to recognize a complex sensory stimulus despite the preservation of elemental perceptions and the absence of a defect in language. The distinct existence and mechanisms of the disorder as an isolated neurologic event have been controversial, but all workers agree that agnosia requires bilateral impairment of the primary or association-cortical areas of the affected perception. The disorder is best considered as a form of monomodal amnesia or an interruption in the connection between the involved sensory area and the memory mechanisms of the hippocampal formation.

Visual agnosia is the most frequently encountered disturbance of this genre. It consists of the failure to recognize and name familiar objects, pictures, or faces despite, for example, the ability to describe or copy them. The phenomenon has been associated with bilateral posterior occipital-temporal-parietal lesions or with right-sided posterior parietal lesions plus dementia. Mechanistically, one can regard the disorder as a selective defect in the progressive abstraction of visual symbols into memory. Insight usually is lacking. *Auditory agnosia,* or pure word deafness, is extremely rare and has been described with the aphasias. The inability to recognize objects or events by the sounds they make also has been reported, but it too is rare except with direct damage to both transverse auditory gyri. *Tactile agnosia* exists only as a part of the astereognosis that results from damage to the primary postcentral sensory cortex.

MEMORY AND ITS IMPAIRMENT

Memory is the process by which the brain encodes, stores, and retrieves its sensory perceptions, ideas, and motor skills. The process is identical to learning. Disturbances of memory-learning include two dimensions: defects in past memory, called *retrograde amnesia,* and the inability to form new memories from ongoing events, called *anterograde amnesia.*

PATTERNS OF MEMORY FAILURE. The components of memory can be grouped into three major epochs—immediate, intermediate, and remote. *Immediate memory or recall* consists of holding in the mind material just heard or read with no necessary intervening process of memory storage. The capacity to register and repeat received stimuli lasts until the subject's mind is interrupted by some other stimulus and is reflected by such simple tests as repeating after the examiner a series of numbers. Except for grossly confused or delirious subjects, patients with organic brain disease usually show little or no defect in immediate memory.

Intermediate memory covers the time span beginning within a few seconds past and extending backward for 24 to 48 hours or more. It is tested by asking about knowledge of current events or the content of recent meals or asking the subject to repeat three unrelated words two to five minutes after having been given them. As with immediate memory, inattention may impair the answers. *Long-term memory* begins beyond that epoch, but this too has its gradations, for childhood memories tend to be singularly well recalled even as more recent ones begin to fade. As a result, standard I.Q. tests that examine primarily words and functions learned before the age of 14 years often give normal or nearly normal scores even in adults who have suffered from diseases that severely damage or destroy recent and anterograde memory.

MEMORY MECHANISMS. Memory has both nonspecific and specific substrates. Many regions of the cerebral hemispheres nonspecifically process the initial stages of learning about one's outer and inner world. Subcortical regions involved in translating events into memory are only partly known but relate closely to the limbic system. Structures located in the medial thalamic and probably hypothalamic regions as well as in the ascending brainstem reticular formation and basal forebrain activating systems are known to play an important role. Reflecting these widespread processings, at least some memory deficits accompany large lesions affecting any lobe of the brain.

Specific structures make especially important contributions to the anatomy of adult memory. In experimental primates, both the hippocampus and amygdala have been implicated in this regard. In humans, evidence suggests that at the cortical level, the hippocampus appears to play the major role in the retrieval of recent memories and the laying down of new ones. Unilateral damage to the human hippocampus results in relatively subtle defects, left hippocampal damage being followed by modest impairments in verbal memory while right hippocampal damage may produce difficulties in visual spatial memories and the recognition of musical tones. Occasional patients with inferomedial left temporal lobe damage develop transient, fairly severe amnesia for places, events, and verbal memories. If the opposite hemisphere is spared, this subsides in three to four days, leaving no clinically detectable residuals. In contrast to these mild or evanescent effects of unilateral injury, bilateral damage or surgical removal of the hippocampus in the adult is devastating and results in profound and usually permanent deficits in intermediate memory affecting especially the verbal-visual-spatial spheres. The degree of retrograde amnesia is proportional to the extent of hippocampal damage but rarely extends back beyond late adolescence. Proportional defects in anterograde learning accompany the retrograde loss. At the subcortical level, bilateral damage to the dorsal-medial nuclei of the thalamus and, less consistently, the ventral-medial hypothalamus, including the mammillary bodies, results in humans in a profound multidimensional disturbance of memory. The prominent memory loss that accompanies Huntington's disease suggests that striatal mechanisms may contribute to the normal memory process.

Understandings of the cellular physiology and molecular

biology of the memory-learning process are just beginning. Cerebral cortical memory mechanisms depend in an incompletely understood way on cholinergic projections that link the subcortical basal forebrain with the hippocampus and the association cortex of the temporal, parietal, and frontal lobes. Degeneration of these projections affects the memory functions of experimental animals and is a prominent accompaniment of the dementia of Alzheimer's disease. Anatomic studies have shown that an increase in neuronal connections in the hippocampus accompanies the learning process, while a reduction of dendritic synapses accompanies the memory failure of human dementia with Alzheimer's disease. Kandel, working with simple invertebrate nervous systems, has found that genetically regulated influences predispose to presynaptic increases in neurotransmitter output during the development of classic conditioning. These beginning steps may lead to better future understanding and treatment of the human amnesias.

CLINICAL MEMORY DISORDERS. Many middle-aged and elderly persons report an increasing but isolated difficulty in recalling proper names and recent events of minor importance. This "benign forgetfulness" bears no consistent relationship to the progressive dementias and is best treated with prompt and vigorous reassurance.

As discussed in Ch. 475, the most frequent causes of severe memory loss are the degenerative dementias, severe head trauma, brain anoxia or ischemia, nutritional impairment, encephalitis, and, less frequently, intracranial mass lesions.

Korsakoff's syndrome is a severe disturbance of recent memory that occurs most often as a sequel to acute and frequently repeated attacks of severe thiamine deficiency. The fully developed disorder includes profound recent memory loss, lack of insight, disorientation to time and place, and confabulation. In Western countries, nutritional Korsakoff's syndrome most frequently affects alcoholics and often accompanies or follows the florid signs and symptoms of acute Wernicke's encephalopathy (Ch. 482) or delirium tremens (Ch. 17). The condition, however, can follow any circumstance in which thiamine-free calories provide the major or only sustained source of nutrition. The memory failure in thiamine deficiency is accompanied consistently by bilateral damage to the dorsal medial nucleus of the thalamus. Other structural abnormalities affect the mammillary bodies as well as various areas of the cortex, including the hippocampus.

Severe retrograde and anterograde memory loss producing a Korsakoff syndrome can follow global cerebral anoxia-ischemia, status epilepticus, and subarachnoid hemorrhage. All of these conditions selectively damage vulnerable neurons in the hippocampus that normally relate to the functions of learning and memory. Even modest head trauma temporarily interrupts memory-mediating neural connections in the hippocampus and diencephalon: concussive injuries frequently produce an initially severe degree of retrograde and a lesser degree of anterograde amnesia; in most instances the retrograde memory loss almost fully disappears with time. Concurrently, anterograde learning increasingly improves. A less fortunate prognosis accompanies prolonged post-traumatic coma. When this lasts more than two to three weeks, most patients, particularly those over 25 years old, never fully recover from the memory loss.

Permanent or prolonged amnesia occasionally can follow bilateral cerebral infarction, large brain tumors, or surgical operations. Such cases have shown bilateral damage of either the hippocampus, the medial diencephalon, or both structures. Herpes simplex encephalitis characteristically leaves severe and often permanent amnesia in its wake. The disease has a predilection to produce necrotic-inflammatory lesions that destroy the limbic system lying along the medial surfaces of the temporal lobes.

Transient global amnesia (TGA) is a condition marked by fully alert periods lasting from several minutes to as long as 12 hours or so of acute confusion during which the affected person can identify himself but is severely disoriented for time and place. A severe deficit in retrograde memory accompanies the beginning of the attack and gradually disappears as it wears off. Status epilepticus with partial complex or nonconvulsive generalized (petit mal) seizures can produce a somewhat similar amnesic state. Attacks of such "minor status" are distinguished by dull, slow-witted, and inattentive behavior. Most TGA attacks come on in middle-aged or elderly persons and appear to reflect temporary vascular insufficiency affecting hippocampal memory areas or their immediate neural connections. Patients with TGA usually remain bright, attentive, and alert and are distressed by their acute confusion. They tend repeatedly to ask where they are and what is going on until, within a few hours, the disorientation gradually disappears. Most TGA attacks neither leave residual limitations nor carry a strong risk of recurrence.

Psychogenic memory impairment can affect either recent or remote recall, usually in clinically recognizable patterns. Preoccupation, forced inattention, or reduced arousal may result in inconsistent responses to testing, some answers to current events being given accurately and others not at all. Severe depressive illnesses may reduce language to near muteness or incomprehensible monosyllables. In general, organic disturbances in memory are marked by variability in what is remembered, emotionally reinforced material being recalled better than neutral events. With organic memory loss, disorientation is worst for time, less for place and persons, and never for self. In most instances, events of the recent past are unevenly forgotten more than remote memories, and the providing of cues often improves recall. By contrast, psychogenic amnesia tends to be greatest for emotionally important events, may elide from the patient's memory well-defined blocks of past events while leaving intact the recall of preceding or following material, may affect remote memories equally with recent ones, resists improvement with cues, and sometimes even includes disorientation to self. "Who am I? What's my name?", unless spoken during obvious delirium or a proved epileptic seizure, always reflects malingering.

TREATMENT. Patients with acute post-traumatic amnesia show a high rate of spontaneous recovery. Improvement of memory loss from other organic disorders is less predictable except when the amnesia can be traced to an excess use of medication or a temporary systemic disorder such as hepatic, renal, or pulmonary insufficiency. Memory loss with depression (pseudodementia) improves with the treatment of the psychiatric illness. A few patients with memory loss due to herpes simplex encephalitis enjoy a slow, spontaneous recovery, but most retain at least some permanent incapacity. Memory loss from thiamine deficiency or subarachnoid hemorrhage has an unpredictable prognosis; some patients improve, others do not, depending largely on the severity of the initial amnesia. Similar principles guide prognosis for recovery from postanoxic amnesia. In adults within these groups, whatever improvement occurs usually takes place within three to six months of onset. Permanent, incapacitating retrograde and anterograde amnesia affects patients with known bilateral destructive lesions of the hippocampus or the anterior-medial thalamic area. To date, neither neuroactive peptides, neurotransmitter precursors, neurotransmitters, nor dietary agents have achieved clinically useful benefits in the treatment of either the severe fixed amnesias or those that accompany the progressive dementias.

Beecher WB, Milner B: Loss of recent memory after bilateral hippocampal lesions. J Neurol Neurosurg Psychiatr 20:11, 1957. *Removal of the uncus and underlying amygdaloid complex in 31 patients resulted in little behavioral change beyond improved tractability, mentioned in several instances. When the hippocampus was bilaterally damaged as well, memory impairment resulted.*

Geschwind N: The apraxias. Neural disorders of learned movement. Am Sci 63:188, 1975. *A hard-line localizationist interpretation of the apraxias.*

Geschwind N: Disconnection syndromes in animals and man. Brain 88:237, 585, 1965. *A long and thoughtful review of the subject.*

Geschwind N: The organization of language and the brain. Science 170:940, 1970. *A summary of the organization of language areas and the syndromes that follow their damage.*

Guberman A, Stuss D: The syndrome of bilateral paramedian thalamic infarction. Neurology 33:540, 1983. *A review of vascular lesions in this area producing the amnesic syndrome.*

Heilman K, Valenstein E (eds.): Clinical Neuropsychology. Oxford, Oxford University Press, 1979. *A multiauthored collection of essays on major aspects of disorders of higher brain function.*

Kandel ER, Schwartz JH: Molecular biology of learning: Modulation of transmitter release. Science 218:433, 1982. *A well-written review of efforts to establish at the cellular level the fundamentals that underlie learning and memory.*

Penfield W, Roberts L: Speech and Brain Mechanisms. Princeton, Princeton University Press, 1959.

Victor M, Adams RD, Collins GH: The Wernicke-Korsakoff Syndrome. Philadelphia, FA Davis Co., 1971. *The classic monograph on the subject links the medial thalamus to memory.*

Woods BT, Schoene W, Kneisley L: Are hippocampal lesions sufficient to cause lasting amnesia? J Neurol Neurosurg Psychiatr 45:243, 1982. *The evidence from a well-studied case shows that they are.*

475. AMENTIA AND DEMENTIA

Fred Plum

GENERAL CONSIDERATIONS

DEFINITION AND PREVALENCE. Dementia is a clinical term describing a sustained or permanent decline in several dimensions of intellectual function so as to interfere with the individual's normal social or economic activity. The condition must be differentiated from *amentia,* or mental retardation, in which normal intellectual function fails to develop, and *delirium,* a reversible state of diffuse mental impairment usually unaccompanied by permanent neuropathologic abnormalities.

The symptom of a *static dementia* can follow any disease that permanently structurally damages large portions of the association areas of the cerebral hemispheres. Thus, for example, single episodes of severe head injury, global brain ischemia from cardiac arrest, large intracranial neoplasms or hemorrhages with their surgical removal, or infections such as severe encephalitis or meningitis each can injure the brain sufficiently to prevent intelligence from ever returning to a pre-illness level. Such conditions, however, represent but a fraction of the problem compared to the *progressive dementias* that affect increasing numbers of persons as the average life span grows longer. In the United States alone estimates indicate that close to a million persons are incapacitated by a fixed or progressive dementia. One can predict from present population age trends that this number will double or triple by the early twenty-first century unless scientific research slows or halts the epidemic.

Table 475–1 indicates the most common causes of the progressive dementias and provides rough estimates of their frequencies drawn from several sources. The figures emphasize the relatively greater problem of the progressive, "primary" dementias, especially of the Alzheimer type.

EARLY CLINICAL MANIFESTATIONS. The component symptoms of dementia vary as broadly as do the underlying components of the damaged mind whose worsening they reflect. The diagnosis of dementia implies the deterioration of several aspects of the intellect; monosymptomatic neuropsychologic defects such as aphasia or a circumscribed amnesia usually are classified separately. Acute, static dementia seldom provides a problem in diagnosis. Almost as soon as the acute illness passes, family, employers, and sometimes even the patient usually recognize that something is wrong, that things are different. Problems with social relationships or employment soon follow, and when no improvement takes place within weeks or months, the diagnostic problem becomes not whether a mental decline has occurred but to what degree and how the patient can restructure his world to his new, possibly permanent limitation.

TABLE 475–1. MAJOR CAUSES AND APPROXIMATE FREQUENCIES OF PROGRESSIVE DEMENTIA

1. Senile dementia, Alzheimer type	50%
2. Multi-infarct (arteriosclerotic) inflammatory	20%
3. Combination of 1 and 2	
4. Communicating hydrocephalus	5%
5. Alcoholic–post-traumatic	5%
6. Huntington's	5%
7. Intracranial mass lesions	5%
8. Uncommon or mixed with above:	10%
Chronic drug use; Creutzfeldt-Jacob; metabolic (thyroid, liver, nutritional); degenerative (spinocerebellar, amyotrophic lateral sclerosis, parkinsonism, multiple sclerosis, Pick's, Wilson's, epilepsy); static dementia	

Early diagnosis in the progressive dementias is less certain and more difficult. Initial symptoms especially involve deterioration in mood, personality, recent memory, judgment, and the capacity to form abstractions, none of which is easily quantified, especially in the elderly. In general, families or work associates notice a change before the patient does, and persons who live by intellectual efforts show their limitations earlier than do those with routine or manual jobs. Danger signals in mood and behavior consist of a loss of vitality, of curiosity, and of mental energy—of "sparkle." Some patients become so apathetic as to seem depressed, while in others great anxiety or increased irritability disrupts a once pleasant personality. Affective responses lose their depth; some early dements become paranoid. Loss of recent memory is a universal feature of the progressive dementias. One notes in affected patients an increasing tendency to make lists, then to forget where they left the lists. Appointments are missed, plans forgotten, stories of recent events become narrated repeatedly with no insight. Eventually orientation fails, first for days, then years, then months and finally for place but never for self. Interest lags—first in papers, books, and new challenges, later in work, and eventually in friends and family. Debts may be accumulated silently, property unwisely sold, accounts lost, meals cooked twice over or served half-cold. In a curious, even startling way mental capacities may fluctuate suddenly and widely without apparent relationship to external events. In Alzheimer's disease and some of the other primary progressive dementias social amenities tend to be retained until late in the course. Incontinence, soup on the shirt, and a disheveled appearance are more characteristic of frontal lobe disease and intracranial mass lesions than of the diffuse cortical and subcortical cellular diseases that produce progressive dementia.

DIAGNOSIS AND DIFFERENTIAL DIAGNOSIS. The three principal questions are (1) Does a true decline in intellect exist? (2) If so, what is its probable cause? (3) Can any aspect be treated effectively? Bedside testing answers the first, while the second and third require laboratory assistance.

The clinical examination of any patient with subacute or chronic central nervous system disease should include at least a brief evaluation of mental function. The test should be given gently and the results interpreted with due allowance for the patient's social background, schooling, innate capacities as judged by life attainments, and probable anxiety provoked by admission to hospital and fear of failure. The standard bedside examination measures orientation, language, and memory-retention by identifying recent major current events, the spelling of w-o-r-l-d backwards, and recalling three unrelated words at five minutes. Asking the subject to perform serial sevens backwards tests attention span, while proverbs and definitions (e.g., river from canal) give some idea of abstract capabilities.

As with other functions in medicine, quantitation of mental capacity is desirable and for this the Minimental Status examination (Table 475–2) provides valuable help. To obtain the evaluation usually requires considerably less than 10 minutes. Normals score 27 to 30, while clinically demented persons usually score less than 20. Psychologically depressed patients generally have intermediate scores.

When a quantitative baseline is desired against which to compare the effects of treatment or the rate of future deterioration, the Weksler Adult Intelligence Scale (WAIS) provides useful information but requires the assistance of a trained

TABLE 475–2. OUTLINE OF MINIMENTAL STATUS EXAMINATION

Test	Score
What is the *year, season, date, day, month*	5
Where are you: *state, county, town, place, floor*	5
Name three objects: State slowly and have patients repeat (Repeat until patient learns all three)	3
Do reverse serial 7's (five steps) or spell "WORLD" backwards	5
Ask for the three unrelated objects above	3
Name from inspection a pencil, a watch	2
Have patient repeat "No ifs, ands, or buts"	1
Follow a three-stage command (1 pt each) ("Take a paper in your hand, fold it, and put it on the floor.")	3
Read and obey, "Close your eyes"	1
Write a simple sentence	1
Copy intersecting pentagons	1

*From Folstein MF, Folstein SE, McHugh PR: Minimental state. A practical method for grading the cognitive state for the clinician. J Psychiatr Res 12:189, 1975. The authors found that out of a possible score of 30, mean score for dementia was 9.7, depression with cognitive impairment was 19.0, and uncomplicated affective depression was 27.6.

psychologist. In mild to moderate dementia the verbal score of the WAIS provides an index of learning capacity, while the performance part reflects current mental abilities. A discrepancy of more than 15 points between the two provides a strong indication of structural brain damage.

The laboratory evaluation of dementia depends on the combined results of the history, general physical and neurologic examinations, and preliminary laboratory results. In the absence of important leads from these sources (e.g., signs of chronic liver disease, uremia, severe vascular disease, bacterial endocarditis, a space-occupying intracranial lesion, etc.), the laboratory tests listed in Table 475–3 are in order and will detect nearly all of the treatable causes of dementia that would not quickly be suspected from the clinical examination. The yield will be low in suspected degenerative cases, but the seriousness of the problem deserves the dignity of careful evaluation.

Pseudodementia is a term applied to reversible states in which reduced cognitive functions appear to indicate progressive organic brain disease but instead are caused by chronic drug intoxication (usually prescribed) or depressive illness. The aging brain is especially susceptible to both conditions. Diagnosis in the first instance comes by taking a meticulous history of medications and reducing all potential offenders gradually so as to judge their effects on symptoms. Barbiturates, benzodiazepines, butyrophenones, tricyclic antidepressants, MAO inhibitors, anticholinergics, corticosteroids, and digitalis are most often responsible.

Psychologic depression (Ch. 476) is a common response to the physical and emotional deprivation of elderly life. The associated apathy, semi-mutism, akinesia, anxiety, and indifference often can suggest a mistaken diagnosis of dementia. Careful evaluation, however, quickly brings out differences. In contrast to demented patients, those with depression complain repeatedly of their poor memory. Patients with depression commonly eat little, often are severely constipated, sleep less than normal, and tend to behave best at night. They may answer questions slowly or reluctantly, but when they do, they respond to factual queries relatively well, revealing proper general orientation and understanding of commands. Errors occur because of indifference or obstinate refusal rather than poor comprehension. Depressed patients may stumble over tests requiring attention, but they rarely forget major recent events or political figures, and when they cooperate, they do not fail either simple tests of language or two- or even three-stage verbal commands. By contrast, patients with incapacitating dementia are disoriented, their nights are more agitated and confused than their days, they have difficulty following commands, both attention and recent memory are severely impaired, and many of them suffer difficulties in language and specific learned motor functions. Differences on mental status examinations usually are readily apparent. Laboratory tests add differentiating points. Brain imaging procedures show anatomic abnormalities in many of the dementias, and the EEG is slow in most of the dementias but not in depression.

TABLE 475–3. LABORATORY TESTS MOST USEFUL IN DEMENTIA OF UNKNOWN ORIGIN

Blood: CBC and ESR, serologic test for syphilis (STS)
Metabolic screen (SMA 12–16)
Serum thyroxine, B_{12} level
Chest x-ray and head CT scan
Lumbar puncture: cells (cytologic analysis if present), protein, STS

Depression sometimes accompanies dementia, especially that associated with multiple strokes, head trauma, and Huntington's disease, all conditions in which insight tends to be relatively preserved. One reaches the diagnosis of an associated psychologic problem by clinical sensitivity to the patient's mood and complaints and by observing behavior that is disproportionally withdrawn and mute for the degree of testable cognitive loss.

ALZHEIMER'S DISEASE

This commonest of the progressive dementias affects both men and women, beginning in rare instances as early as the late teens or 20's and increasing in frequency progressively with age to affect approximately 5 per cent of persons over age 65 years and over 20 per cent of those who reach 80 or more. In past years, patients younger than age 65 were classified as having Alzheimer's presenile dementia, while older ones were believed to have a different illness termed senile dementia. Clinical and biologic evidence, however, indicates that both terms describe the same disease, irrespective of age.

ETIOLOGY. The cause of Alzheimer's disease (AD) is unknown. The disease exists worldwide, and no evidence suggests a relationship to nutritional factors, infection, exposure to toxins, or other environmental factors. A history of affected family members occurs in about a quarter of cases. This plus the fact that patients with trisomy 21 (Down's syndrome) almost all develop Alzheimer's changes in the brain at about age 30 years suggests a genetic factor, with susceptibility transmitted perhaps as an autosomal dominant trait. Other influences, however, must be important, since identical twins show less than 50 per cent concordance for the illness, and when such cases have appeared, several years have separated their appearance within the affected pair.

PATHOLOGY AND PATHOPHYSIOLOGY. AD produces a progressive neuronal degeneration of selective cells in the association and memory areas of the cerebral cortex, combined with similar abnormalities in certain subcortical nuclei. Some of the latter, in turn, cause a secondary degeneration of the ascending cholinergic pathways that diffusely connect the basal forebrain with the cerebral hemispheres. The locus ceruleus degenerates in many, but not all, cases, reducing noradrenergic influences on the forebrain and brainstem.

When viewed at autopsy examination, the temporal lobe in AD is usually smaller than in brains of similarly aged normals. Gross, more generalized atrophy sometimes is seen in younger, chronic victims of the disease. Histologic examination usually discloses characteristic abnormalities. Neuronal loss affects especially the large pyramidal cells of the parietal and frontal association areas, the hippocampus, and the amygdala. This change may account for the decline in somatostatin found in most areas of the cortex. The basal forebrain nucleus of Meynert, which gives rise to the major cholinergic projection to the cortex, suffers severe degeneration. Silver-staining plaques containing degenerating neuronal products are scattered prominently in the cortex and subcortex. Many of the degenerating nerve cells contain tangles of twisted intracellular fibrils of a unique protein configuration.

The pathologic changes of AD are more quantitatively than

qualitatively different from other brains. Somewhat similar abnormalities occur in other disorders, and neuronal loss, plaques, and tangles can be found in the brains of many intellectually intact old persons, although in substantially lesser concentrations than in most AD victims. The reduction in cholinergic innervation appears to be a more specific alteration, although its functional impact remains unclear. Cell loss in the hippocampus and amygdala correlates with the prominent amnesia of the disease. The pyramidal cell dropout in areas of association cortex explains many of the early psychologic symptoms and correlates with recent research studies that show that brain metabolism is moderately reduced in early cases of AD, with the temporal-parietal-occipital association areas suffering the greatest decline.

SIGNS AND SYMPTOMS. Failure of recent memory is the earliest prominent symptom. Amnesia is followed in frequency by disturbances in emotional behavior consisting most often of either a reduction in affect or an increase in anxiety. Focal psychologic deficits are prominent, demonstrated by difficulty in managing spatial relationships or in initiating motor skills, and by a nominal memory loss that may become so severe as to resemble a specific aphasia. Disorders of descending motor pathways almost never occur, so that strength and reflexes remain unscathed. No defects arise in somatosensory or special sensory functions. Social amenities are preserved until very late; even with moderately advanced, incapacitating dementia almost all AD patients continue to dress well, to maintain neat appearances, and to avoid incontinence. Only in very rare instances do either myoclonic or generalized convulsions mark either the early or intermediate stages of the illness.

The onset of AD usually is insidious, although hints of abnormal behavior sometimes appear several years before sustained clinical changes allow a firm diagnosis. Among older victims a suddenly unexpected delirious or paranoid reaction associated with a minor febrile illness or an operation such as cataract extraction may be the first harbinger. The early progressive loss of recent memory can be difficult to distinguish from the "benign forgetfulness" for names and trivial events that affects many older persons in their sixth or seventh decade. When the defect extends to a failure to keep appointments, to initiate or keep track of important business or domestic matters, or becomes coupled with a progressive loss of interest, early AD should be suspected. Less frequently, isolated psychologic deficits producing spatial disorientation, apraxia, syntactic aphasia, or acalculia may be prominent. The time course of evolution varies widely from patient to patient. In younger individuals a period of years sometimes separates the first suggestions of "peculiar" behavior from the advent of a readily diagnosed dementia.

Except for the signs of abnormal mental status, the physical and neurologic examinations remain normal in early or intermediate stage AD. Laboratory tests are not helpful except in a negative sense. CT scans of the brain may or may not show moderate cortical atrophy but are otherwise unremarkable; blood and CSF studies are uninformative. The EEG usually is moderately but nonspecifically slow.

DIFFERENTIAL DIAGNOSIS. Diagnosis in AD is made by exclusion and largely on clinical grounds. No specific laboratory determinants exist, and brain biopsy is unjustified. The main problem occurs when laboratory tests show no abnormality. Early multi-infarct dementia, psychologic depression, drug intoxication, some of the diffuse angiopathies, metabolic deficiency, chronic meningitis, Pick's disease, or diffuse primary or metastatic brain tumor sometimes may create diagnostic errors. Within a matter of weeks to a very few months, however, clinical diagnosis proves accurate in about 80 per cent of cases, the exceptions being mainly neuropathologic rarities or another form of primary degenerative dementia such as the rare Pick's disease or an unclassifiable neuropathologic change.

MANAGEMENT. There is no specific treatment of AD. Dietary efforts aimed at increasing acetylcholine levels in the brain have resulted in no discernible benefit. Research workers have given prostigmine orally or by injection, but any ensuing mental-behavioral changes have been too small to suggest this as a practical approach.

The brunt of the care usually falls on family or social agencies during the early and intermediate stages of illness. Institutionalization often is required in the late stages when patients may sink to a purely vegetative level. Occasionally depression is a prominent early symptom; it responds to small doses of the usual antidepressants. Sedatives or tranquilizers tend only to make matters worse. With restless, agitated patients, tasteless liquid haloperidol can be given in doses of 0.5 to 1 mg two to three times daily as needed. The Alzheimer's Disease Foundation can provide the family with useful advice. Mace and Rabin's valuable guide is listed in the references.

OTHER PRINCIPAL DEMENTIAS

MULTI-INFARCT DEMENTIA (MD). This term describes diffuse mental impairment resulting from cerebral vascular disease. The condition is much less common than Alzheimer's disease and usually is readily distinguishable clinically. A general decline in intellectual function results from multifocal occlusion of cerebral arteries and arterioles either from remotely arising emboli or from intrinsic cerebral arteriolar occlusive disease. The condition appears most often in association with diabetic or hypertensive vascular disease, producing infarcts large and small that involve specific sensorimotor areas as well as areas of association cortex dealing with specific and nonspecific cognitive functions. As a result, disturbances in gait, station, and skeletal motor function accompany abnormalities in language, praxis, gnosis, mood, abstract thinking, and attention. Lesions can affect any area of the brain but are most frequent in the distribution of the middle and anterior cerebral arteries. Pseudobulbar palsy is common, as is pathologic crying and laughing and abnormal motor reflexes. A high incidence of frontal lobe infarction is accompanied by a reduction in attention as well as emotional lability, often coupled with a disregard for neatness and social niceties. Insight often is retained and accompanied by depression of mood. Many patients develop urinary incontinence. Multi-infarct dementia characteristically progresses in steps, with each new bite out of the brain accompanied by an abrupt minor or major worsening, sometimes with modest improvement between. Occasionally, the individual infarcts of hypertensive arteriolar disease may be so small (lacunae) that the effect of their successive appearance gives the impression of an insidiously developing and gradually progressing process. Nevertheless, the presence of prominent motor changes and abnormal motor reflexes almost always differentiates the process from Alzheimer's disease; radiographic studies rule out a space-occupying lesion or communicating hydrocephalus and CSF analysis eliminates infection as the mechanism of the mental decline. Signs of systemic vascular disease are almost invariably present.

HYDROCEPHALIC DEMENTIA. Chronic communicating hydrocephalus, sometimes called normal pressure hydrocephalus, occasionally produces an insidiously beginning and gradually progressive dementia, with forebrain functions becoming especially impaired by the abnormal hydrodynamic process. Affected persons may give a history of remote subarachnoid hemorrhage, recurrent head trauma, or meningeal infection, but the cause of the hydrocephalus often lies in the remote past and remains unknown. The condition is most frequent in late middle-aged or elderly men. In hydrocephalic dementia, CT scans or other imaging studies show marked enlargement of the cerebral ventricular system, especially the lateral and third ventricles. Sometimes one finds narrowing of the aqueduct of Sylvius, but more frequently there is dilatation of all of the ventricles with reduced or absent sulcal markings over the surface of the brain, especially at the vertex. The periventricular white matter often appears abnormally lucent owing to increased water content. The cerebrospinal fluid pressure usually lies in the range of 180 to 220 mm H_2O, but lower levels often are found. CSF contents are normal and the presence of an elevation of cell count or protein immediately suggests a more active meningeal abnormality. With such chronic obstructive hydrocephalus, the periventricular white matter of the cerebral hemispheres, especially of the frontal lobes, undergoes gradual atrophy, resulting in progressive signs and symptoms of frontal lobe dysfunction.

The typical signs and symptoms of hydrocephalic dementia comprise a triad of frontal-type dementia, broad-based ataxia, and urinary incontinence. Attention declines, abstract reasoning and the capacity to anticipate future events decays in parallel, and patients become careless in appearance and attire. Motor dysfunction is prominent and consists of a rigid-spastic increased resistance to passive movement of the extremities, especially the lower, coupled with a stiff, broad-based, hesitating, small-stepped, tottering gait, often accompanied by palmar and plantar grasp reflexes. Diagnosis depends principally on the clinical picture and the characteristic CT scan. Surgical CSF-shunting procedures are followed by intellectual and motor improvement in about half the cases. The operation is more often successful when the cause of the meningeal obstruction is evident or improvement follows a brief trial of spinal drainage by lumbar puncture.

HUNTINGTON'S DISEASE. Huntington's disease (HD), an inherited disorder transmitted as an autosomal dominant trait with close to complete penetrance, produces a combination of a choreiform movement disorder and dementia, as discussed in Ch. 485. The brain at autopsy shows prominent gross atrophy of the caudate, putamen, and, to a lesser degree, globus pallidus, with loss of the small neurons of the caudate and putamen being the most prominent cellular change. Studies of brain oxidative metabolism of asymptomatic family members at risk for HD have shown selective hypofunction in the region of the caudate possibly heralding onset of the disease. Early symptomatic patients show hypometabolism in both caudate and putamen but not at the cortical level. Postmortem pharmacologic studies of the striatum and its connections in HD have shown prominent decreases in the content of the synthesizing enzymes for GABA and acetylcholine, as well as decreases in the peptide neurotransmitters, substance P, enkephalin, and cholecystokinin. These changes relate more firmly to our understanding of the pathophysiology of the movement disorder than to the dementia, which currently lacks a satisfactory mechanistic explanation. The recent apparent identification of the locus of the Huntington gene suggests that preclinical diagnosis and genetic counseling may soon be a 100 per cent accurate opportunity for family members.

The earliest certain abnormalities in HD are usually those of the movement disorder. Early cognitive changes consist of a difficulty in anticipating and planning the future combined with a patchy memory loss, especially for serial tasks or memorization. Word memory and language functions are relatively well retained, as is spatial recognition. Later, the dementia takes on a more general quality. Prominent psychiatric symptoms mark the early stages in about two thirds of cases. Depression or schizophreniform behavior is common, and approximately 10 per cent of patients with HD commit suicide.

CREUTZFELDT-JAKOB DISEASE. Creutzfeldt-Jakob disease (CJD) is an infrequent disorder transmitted by a submicroscopic agent of unknown type ("slow virus") (Ch. 504). The brain is marked by a diffuse involvement of gray matter, with all affected areas showing neuronal loss, astrocytic proliferation, and a spongy appearance on histologic examination. The cardinal clinical features are the early appearance and rapid progression over several months of signs of upper motor neuron dysfunction coupled with increasing dementia, focal motor or myoclonic convulsions, and prominent changes in the EEG. CT scans are normal. These features distinguish CJD from the other dementias described in this chapter.

PICK'S DISEASE. This is a rare cortical atrophy of unknown cause with an age incidence that overlaps that of AD. The illness usually develops insidiously and progresses slowly for

a period of three to ten years or more. Severe atrophy affects the cortical mantle, especially in the frontal and temporal regions, including the hippocampus. Microscopic examination shows neuronal loss, extensive gliosis, and characteristic swollen, pear-shaped "Pick cells." Plaques and tangles are unusual. The caudate, globus pallidus, and thalamus show less consistent cellular losses. Physiologic studies during life disclose a reduction in cerebral blood flow and, by implication, metabolism in the frontotemporal areas, maximally frontally. CT scans reveal frontotemporal atrophy. In keeping with the pathologic findings, early clinical signs and symptoms include prominent disturbances in memory and in the anticipation and regulation of planned activities. Affected patients are apathetic, slovenly, and hypoactive and tend to forget the purpose of their acts, yet they retain spatial orientation and direction. Incontinence develops early and vocal productivity declines, often to the level of mutism. Signs of extrapyramidal and corticospinal motor dysfunction develop late, adding further distinction from the clinical picture of AD, the alternate diagnosis most likely to be considered. There is no treatment.

Blackwood W, Corsellis JAN: Greenfield's Neuropathology. Chicago, Arnold-Yearbook, 1976. *The standard reference for the classic morphology of the dementias.*

Chase TN, Foster NL, Fedio P, Brooks R, Mansi L, DiChiro G: Regional cortical dysfunction in Alzheimer's disease as determined by positron emission tomography. Ann Neurol 15:S170, 1984. *The greatest reduction in metabolism affected posterior association cortex.*

Coyle JT, Price DL, DeLong MR: Alzheimer's disease: A disorder of cortical cholinergic innervation. Science 219:1184, 1983. *Construction of the cholinergic hypothesis of AD by the group that discovered the abnormality of the basal forebrain projection to the cortex.*

Cummings JL, Benson DF: Dementia: A clinical approach. Boston, Butterworths, 1983. *The best current monograph on the subject.*

Hachinski VC, Iliff LD, Zilhka E, DuBoulay GH, McAllister VL, Marshall J, Ross RW, Symon L: Cerebral blood flow in dementia. Arch Neurol 32:632, 1975. *A validation of the vascular defect in multi-infarct dementia, together with helpful scales aimed at defining the presence of dementia and the criteria for suspecting stroke as its cause.*

Katzman R, Terry R: The Neurology of Aging. Philadelphia, FA Davis, 1983. *This recent monograph discusses many aspects of the needs of the aging patient, including conditions that must be differentiated from dementia.*

Kuhl DE, Phelps ME, Markham CH, Metter EJ, Riege WH, Winter J: Cerebral metabolism and atrophy in Huntington's disease determined by ^{18}FDG and computerized tomographic scan. Ann Neurol 12:425, 1982. *Caudate metabolism is shown to be reduced both in patients with HD and in some at-risk offspring.*

Mace NL, Rabin PV: The 36-hour Day. A family guide to caring for persons with Alzheimer's disease, related dementing illnesses, and memory loss in later life. Baltimore, Johns Hopkins University Press, 1981. *An invaluable book for families and friends of the affected.*

Sulkava R, Haltia M, Paetau A, Wikstrom J, Palo J: Accuracy of clinical diagnosis in primary degenerative dementia: Correlation with neuropathological findings. J Neurol Neurosurg Psychiatr 46:9, 1983. *Clinical criteria accurately predicted autopsy findings in 22 of 27 patients, two of whom showed no diagnosable morphologic abnormality.*

Terry RD, Katzman R: Senile dementia of the Alzheimer type. Ann Neurol 14:497, 1983. *A summary of the most recent scientific information about the disorder.*

476. PSYCHOLOGIC ILLNESS IN MEDICAL PRACTICE

Paul R. McHugh

FUNCTIONAL PSYCHOSES

The psychoses gather together several different clinical entities. To be placed within the category an entity must produce disturbances in thinking and perception that are inexplicable solely as responses to experience and are severe enough to distort the patient's appreciation of the world and the relationship of events within it. The category psychosis has no uniform foundation as in somatic pathology nor any more objective aspect of psychopathology to mark its distinction from other collections of psychiatric symptoms. It is thus a term difficult to use with precision. Sometimes psychosis is used as a euphemism for insanity, sometimes as a synonym for schizophrenia, one of the entities within the category, and sometimes to draw an elusive distinction as between neurotic and psychotic depression.

The unmodified term can be qualified by a differentiation into organic and functional psychoses. Here the term psychosis means only severe mental illness. The organic psychoses, delirium, dementia, and Korsakoff's syndrome, are produced by a variety of cerebral pathologies. The functional psychoses, schizophrenia and manic-depressive disorder, lack a recognizable neuropathology.

This differentiation is practical. It draws a distinction in kind that affects treatment and prognosis, and it indicates the character of the clinical problem. For the organic psychoses the central problem is the cause of the pathologic changes. For the functional psychoses the central problem is consistent diagnosis.

Schizophrenia and manic-depressive disorder are clinical disease entities. The criteria for their diagnosis are their symptoms alone. There are no objective tests verifying a diagnosis. Only the natural history or response to empirically discovered treatments can confirm a diagnostic opinion. Since they lack a recognized neuropathology and are by definition inexplicable as responses to experience, there are no comprehensive etiologic explanations for these disorders. Treatment therefore is symptomatic rather than fundamental. Both prevention and radical cure await a chance discovery or a major scientific advance in understanding the biologic foundations of human behavior.

McHugh PR, Slavney PR: The Perspectives of Psychiatry. Baltimore, The Johns Hopkins University Press, 1983. *The authors discuss theconcept of disease as it arises in psychiatric thinking and address the methodologic problems of psychiatry as a medical discipline.*

Schizophrenia

Schizophrenia is a devastating disturbance of mind and personality appearing in clear consciousness and characterized by several distinctive alterations in mental experiences, modes of thinking, and mood that are seldom completely resolved. The most characteristic features occur during the active phases of the disturbance, and take the form of hallucinations, delusions, and altered behavior toward others. Specific intellectual and affective disabilities varying from minimal to severe can develop insidiously or remain after an attack. A crucial element of the definition is that all these symptoms occur in a patient free of any relevant and discernible pathologic change in his nervous system.

CLINICAL MANIFESTATIONS. The symptoms of schizophrenia can begin at almost any stage in life, but most commonly occur during adolescence and early adulthood and then either insidiously or as an acute attack followed by a series of attacks, each leaving behind personality defects of increasing severity.

In some patients it is possible to recognize a particular premorbid personality. They may have seemed more timid or seclusive than others. They may have been bookish, unsociable, and preoccupied with philosophic and religious ideas to the exclusion of friendships and community experiences. But this so-called *schizoid personality* is not found in most patients who develop schizophrenia. *At least half of schizophrenic patients had premorbid personalities indistinguishable from normal.*

Among the mental changes that mark the onset of a schizophrenic illness, only some are specific to this disorder. Emotional unrest, uncertainty, perplexity, and confusion can be found in many disorders other than schizophrenia, and therefore a diagnosis of schizophrenia cannot rest on them. There are, however, a number of mental changes that are more or less diagnostic. These can be usefully divided into abnormal mental experiences and disturbed modes of expression. The abnormal mental experiences seem somewhat more reliable evidence of the illness simply because they are easier to elicit with confidence and less dependent upon interpretation than disturbances in expression.

Hallucinations and delusions are the outstanding schizophrenic mental experiences. Although hallucinations can occur in many disorders such as delirium, dementia, and occasionally manic-depressive disorder, certain forms of hallucinations are more specific for schizophrenia. Thus auditory hallucinations are the most common hallucinations in schizophrenia, and certain kinds of auditory hallucinations are almost diagnostic. Thus hearing one's thoughts aloud or hearing voices commenting about one's every action or several voices engaged in a conversation in which derogatory and praising remarks are passed with the patient discussed in the third person are the most typical schizophrenic hallucinations.

Although delusions, i.e., false beliefs that are incorrigible, idiosyncratic, and preoccupying, also can be found in many disorders other than schizophrenia, in this illness delusional experiences are dramatic and well developed. They can begin as vague, fearful interpretations and "half-beliefs" and develop into firm incorrigible convictions. A delusion coming on suddenly, not prompted by any hallucination or previous delusion, nor related in any obvious way to the patient's mood, is called a "primary delusion" and is highly suggestive of schizophrenia. Many other schizophrenic experiences are of delusional form, but have such individual characteristics that they have been named for themselves.

Commonly schizophrenics have delusions about bodily control, the so-called passivity experiences. The patient feels as though he were under the control of some outside force or power making him behave as an automaton without a will of his own. He may feel hypnotized and feel forced to make particular movements, speak with a special voice, or walk to certain areas. The patient may believe these feelings come to him as penetrating waves from electronic or telephonic equipment.

The schizophrenic patient may experience changes in his thinking. Particularly he may feel that his thoughts are disrupted by some outside agency, that his thoughts are withdrawn from his mind, or that other thoughts are inserted into it. He may believe that people can hear his thoughts, which are leaving his mind as waves broadcast to others.

In contrast to these abnormalities of experience are the disturbances in the patient's mode of expression. Particularly noticeable is his abnormal language. Characteristically, he is difficult to understand. His thinking is expressed in a vague and awkward fashion with words poorly chosen and ideas poorly related to one another. Strikingly, the patient makes no effort to correct the vagueness of this thinking or to improve the clarity of his talk. Often, asking a question of the patient, the examiner receives a reply that is off the point and that goes into unnecessary details. Although the questions of the interview seem to start the patient toward a particular answer, it is never reached, but the patient takes up abstract and unnecessary ideas and must be redirected toward his goal. The examiner, laying the responsibility for the confusion on himself, may work to express himself more clearly, and only after considerable effort recognize that the difficulty in communication rests with the odd replies from the patient.

Another prominent disturbance is emotional expression of these patients. They seem distant, unresponsive, and cold. On some occasions the patient's emotional attitude seems incongruous, particularly for the thoughts he is expressing. Thus he may laugh while saying that he is in mortal danger. This cold or incongruous attitude and manner give the schizophrenic patient his most striking features, and even when at their mildest can be baffling and distressing symptoms to his family.

Other abnormal modes of expression of the schizophrenic patient are disturbances in stance and mobility called catatonic symptoms. Gestures may seem stiff, slow, and mannered. Some schizophrenic patients make repetitive movements or facial grimaces. Others may become totally immobile and mute. Still others may assume unnatural postures and hold them for long periods.

During the active phases of the schizophrenic illness the flamboyant subjective experiences are most prominent. During the chronic phase of schizophrenic illness expressive disturbances in thought and emotion are more evident, varying from mild to severe. Although at times some patients seem free of symptoms, whether a careful examination does reveal mild residual disturbances in thinking and emotional responsiveness is debated and difficult to disprove.

DIAGNOSIS. The diagnosis of schizophrenia rests on recognition of the distinctive clinical symptoms of this disorder and the exclusion of other conditions which may produce similar symptoms.

Many disorders of brain function can imitate schizophrenic symptoms; but with the exception of the three schizophrenia-like disorders to be discussed, patients with the other brain disturbances also manifest disturbed consciousness, disorientation, and disruption of cognitive abilities, particularly recent memory function, that are not found in schizophrenia.

Mania or depression can be confused with schizophrenia (to the considerable embarrassment of the diagnostician when the patient recovers completely on receiving treatment appropriate for these conditions). A source of difficulty is the occurrence of delusions, which are common enough in mania and depression but usually spring directly from the mood and the attitudes of self-confidence or self-blame that are so prominent in those disorders.

In schizophrenia disturbances in experience, including the auditory hallucinations and delusions just described, form the most secure basis for diagnosis. Thus, in a person free of brain disease or drug intoxication, recognition of auditory hallucinations with voices commenting on the patient in the third person, primary delusional experiences, passivity experiences, or disturbances in "thought control" permit the diagnosis of schizophrenia to be made with some confidence. In fact, Kurt Schneider has referred to these as "first rank symptoms" of schizophrenia because of the diagnostic confidence their discovery brings.

If these symptoms cannot be found, then diagnosis must rest upon recognition of manifest disturbances in thought and emotional expression. It should be pointed out, however, that opinion holding a person's thought to be illogical and vague, or his affective responses to be inadequate or incongruous, is an evaluative judgment and must be held with somewhat less confidence, if the difficulties are minimal or inconstant, than opinion resting on recognition of delusions and hallucinations.

Catatonic symptoms of immobility, posturing, and grimacing, along with the disturbances in behavior described as negativism or reluctance to cooperate, must be carefully interpreted. Only in those patients in whom no evidence of a prominent mood change can be found should a diagnosis of schizophrenia be made. Motility changes in the direction of psychomotor retardation are prominent features of depressive disorder, a condition as common as schizophrenia and more common than the catatonic variety of schizophrenia.

Symptoms of emotional unrest, anxiety, withdrawal, and hostility can be found in schizophrenic patients, but these are common to many other psychiatric disorders, and therefore can never form the basis for a secure diagnosis of schizophrenia. However, that diagnosis is rendered more likely if it can be established that the patient was developing normally without an apparently vulnerable personality, and if these symptoms appeared without a change in the patient's mood or the pattern of his life. Since these more general symptoms can be found in both schizophrenia and many other psychiatric disturbances, it is important to search carefully for the more basic symptoms of hallucinations and delusions from which emotional unrest and unpredictable behavior may stem. Often repeated efforts are required to gain cooperation of the patient so that he will divulge the existence of those basic symptoms that make a diagnosis of schizophrenia certain.

ETIOLOGY. There is no neuropathology or consistent pathophysiology that can be observed to develop with progression of the disorder and that might give some hint of causation. An approach to a consideration of etiology has to be more circuitous and the opinions derived held with somewhat less assurance than is true of other clinical entities. Two aspects of etiology can be conveniently separated for the purpose of organizing the information we have. One aspect is "cause," that is, any prerequisite element needed to set in motion a train of events leading to the entity. The other is "mechanism," that is, the particular nature of the train of events, be they psychologic, neurologic, or biochemical, that produce the symptoms. For schizophrenia there is some information relating to "cause" and also to "mechanism," but it is far from conclusive.

"Cause" or Prerequisite Elements in Schizophrenia. The genetic constitution has been decisively demonstrated to be one of the "causes" of schizophrenia. The risk of schizophrenia increases with the closeness of genetic relationship to a schizophrenic patient. Thus only 1 per cent of very distant relatives of a schizophrenic patient will themselves suffer from the disorder. This is no higher than the risk in the general population. But 5 to 6 per cent of siblings and 40 to 50 per cent of monozygotic twins of schizophrenic patients will have schizophrenia.

The possible objection that these data merely reflect the increasingly common environment of progressively closer relatives has been refuted by observations on monozygotic twins brought up apart who continue to show an identical high risk. Heston made the same point in a different fashion by studying a group of offspring of schizophrenic mothers. These particular children were raised from earliest infancy in foster homes by normal, nonschizophrenic mothers and fathers. The incidence of schizophrenia in these children was exactly the same as that reported for children raised by a schizophrenic parent. They thus resembled their biologic mother although reared apart from her.

It has nevertheless been impossible to fit schizophrenia into a clear mendelian pattern of dominant or recessive inheritance. Some students of the disease would describe the hereditary contribution to schizophrenia as polygenic, i.e., the sum of a number of contributions from the genes no one of which is solely responsible. The polygenic concept might permit environmental factors to play a large role in causation. Thus a mild genetic vulnerability might express itself in a schizophrenic phenotype only in those who face injurious environments, whereas those carrying a more severe genetic vulnerability might show the disorder in any environment. It is difficult at the moment to propose a test that would exclude the polygenic hypothesis as a possibility.

The same studies that have established a genetic contribution to the etiology of schizophrenia have also given evidence of the inadequacy of genetics as a sufficient cause for the disorder. That 50 per cent of monozygotic twins of schizophrenic patients are free of this illness means one of the following: (1) Although the genetic constitution is necessary and sufficient to produce schizophrenia, the symptoms employed to define a case fail to provide an adequate means of recognizing all examples of the disorder, and 50 per cent are mistakenly called normal. (2) The defining symptoms encompass a mixed group of disorders, and in only 50 per cent of these disorders are genetic features necessary. (3) A genetic vulnerability for schizophrenia is necessary but not sufficient. It must be combined with certain life experiences that need not be common for genetically identical individuals.

The present inadequacy of the genetic hypothesis to provide a complete description of the "cause" for schizophrenia reinforces a search for environmental and experiential causes. It has proved just as difficult to determine an environmental contribution as to define the genetic contribution. Thus the experiences of being raised by a cold and distant mother, or of receiving insistent, simultaneous, but incompatible directions from the parents, or of simply living in a disharmonious family incapable of providing a healthy environment for psychologic growth have all been considered causes of schizophrenia.

Such disturbed experiences have been found in the lives of some schizophrenic patients when viewed retrospectively after the onset of the illness. But none has proved to be a common experience in all schizophrenic people. Nor has it been possible to predict an increased incidence of schizophrenia among individuals living in comparably disturbed situations. At present the most economical view of the role of life experiences in the "cause" of schizophrenia holds that *any* adversity, be it a psychologic shock, abnormality in critical relationships, or physical injury (particularly brain injury) may provide a partial contribution in causing schizophrenia, but that most of these adversities are exerting their causal effects upon a genetically vulnerable individual.

"Mechanism" of the Schizophrenic Syndrome. This is the other aspect of etiology. Given that some combination of genetic and environmental attributes is probably prerequisite for the illness, by what derangements are the symptoms produced? Are they produced by some change in a psychologic function that might have been learned or developed through experience, or are they produced by some morbid change in the nervous system that alters the normal capacity to perceive, integrate, and respond? There have been proposals for each of these "mechanisms."

It has been proposed that the mechanism of the disturbance has been through the production of a particular psychologic change fundamental to the whole syndrome and from which all the symptoms can be explained. Thus Federn has proposed a "loosening of ego boundaries" as the essential feature mediating this illness, whereas Bleuler proposed a basic disturbance in associational thinking. A crisis of identity has been proposed by proponents of existential psychiatry. These views have a ring of plausibility perhaps derived from their resemblance to experiences common to all people, part of which can seem to be reflected in the behavior of schizophrenic patients. But they depend on concepts that are difficult to define except in terms of what they purport to explain.

Other studies have attempted to demonstrate the possibility that the mechanism is a change in the central nervous system. No such change has been demonstrated in schizophrenia as yet, so supporters of this possibility have had to reason by analogy.

Three well-documented conditions affecting the brain can give rise to a mental disturbance resembling schizophrenia. The most familiar is the syndrome found with *chronic amphetamine intoxication.* In this condition the patient is alert and oriented but preoccupied by auditory hallucinations and delusional ideas indistinguishable from those seen in schizophrenia. The disturbance may last from several days to a few weeks, but disappears eventually after the withdrawal of the stimulant.

Slater, Beard, and Glithero have demonstrated that among patients suffering from *psychomotor epilepsy,* caused by an irritative lesion in the limbic portions of the temporal lobe, a certain number develop a paranoid schizophrenia-like syndrome after 10 to 15 years of epilepsy. This condition displays all the classic delusional and hallucinatory symptoms of schizophrenia, but there is less tendency toward deterioration of thinking and personality.

Finally, certain patients, *withdrawing from excessive alcohol ingestion,* suffer from a period of auditory hallucinations. Although in most of these patients the hallucinatory experience clears within 24 to 48 hours, in a small proportion a chronic condition of persisting auditory hallucinations associated with delusional beliefs, incongruous affect, and disturbed thought develops. This chronic condition may be indistinguishable from the schizophrenic syndrome, and may persist for many years.

For all these schizophrenia-like conditions the possibility exists that the pertinent features might be the expression of a latent predisposition for schizophrenia in the affected individuals. But there is no evidence of a predisposition. The relatives of these patients do not have an increased incidence of schizophrenia, and the patients themselves do not have schizoid traits in their premorbid personalities.

The existence of these conditions demonstrates that the symptoms of schizophrenia are capacities of the damaged human brain. Yet we are ignorant of any common pathologic feature of these brain disorders that could by implication be the fundamental mechanism for schizophrenia. One possibility is that each of these disorders represents an extraexcitatory arousal of the brain, particularly of the reticular formation and limbic system, either directly via amphetamine or epileptic discharge or in rebound from long-continuing action of the depressant ethanol. It may be that the condition of schizophrenia itself is thus produced by some excessive activity in these or related brain regions evoked by the genetic-environmental "causes" discussed above. Mednick and Schulzinger have also found some evidence suggestive of hyperarousal in children of schizophrenic mothers who go on to develop the disease themselves.

Another proposed mechanism for producing schizophrenia is through some change in body metabolism or chemistry that could itself alter cerebral and psychologic functions. In fact the difficulties in establishing a role for biochemistry in the etiology of schizophrenia rest not with chemical methodology but with such issues as defining the group being studied, avoiding chemical artifacts related to dietary habits or medications given chronically hospitalized people, and deciding what biochemical change to look for. The papers of Kety should be consulted for a more thorough discussion of these difficulties.

New methods for imaging the brain are being employed in an effort to discern a neuropathology of schizophrenia. Computer axial tomography (CAT) has demonstrated that some patients with schizophrenia have enlarged ventricles and an apparent loss of brain tissue. This change may be more obvious in patients with prominent expressive changes as defined above, rather than those with the acute symptoms of hallucinations and delusions.

Any brain change in schizophrenia will likely be chemotransmitter specific. The most likely candidate for this transmitter problem is dopamine. The hypothesis that some functional excess of dopamine is present in schizophrenia was proposed by Snyder from observations that the therapeutic potency of phenothiazines parallels their capacity to block dopamine receptors. This hypothesis has provoked postmortem chemical studies of the brains of schizophrenics and the employment of positron emission tomography (PET). Both methods have provided suggestive, but as yet inconclusive evidence for an increase in dopamine receptors in schizophrenia. Complications of diagnosis, drug treatment, and age effects remain to be sorted out. However, we seem closer to defining a pathologic basis and mechanism for at least some forms of this disease.

Thus our knowledge of "mechanism," as much as our knowledge of "cause," is still fragmentary and provisional. But on the bits of evidence at hand, the view that seems easiest to defend is that schizophrenia will prove to be due to some deranged neural mechanism that can occasionally be produced by brain disease but more often is the outcome of an anomaly of the genetic constitution.

TREATMENT. The treatment for any schizophrenic patient is complex and should not be attempted by the inexperienced. A period of hospitalization will usually be required. There a program to include drug therapy, psychologic treatment, and social evaluation can be planned.

The sheet anchor of treatment now for schizophrenia is the *phenothiazine* drugs, discovered in the 1950's almost by accident. To date there is no secure explanation for their effectiveness. Clearly they are not simply acting by virtue of their sedative effect, since their remarkable action is not mimicked by other sedatives. They can remove the symptoms of schizophrenia, including the delusions, hallucinations, and disordered thought, and are not restricted to relieving excitement or anxiety as the term tranquilizer might imply.

The most versatile phenothiazine preparation is the original: chlorpromazine. The dose required to treat acute symptoms varies widely from patient to patient, and amounts from 200 to 2000 mg per day may be necessary. Maintenance dosage is similarly an individual matter, but 100 to 200 mg per day is usually an effective range. Since cessation of treatment results in the reappearance of symptoms in 60 to 70 per cent of patients within six months, drug therapy is often given over years. This practice, however, must be evaluated in light of a movement disorder (tardive dyskinesia) that may appear with prolonged use of phenothiazines. Tardive dyskinesia is a chronic choreoathetotic disorder affecting primarily the faciobulbar musculature but in some examples the extremities as well. It is resistant to most pharmacologic treatment with the exception of giving larger doses of the phenothiazines that provoked it originally. Since it is a particular danger of chronic high dose phenothiazine treatment, the attempt should be to employ as small a dose as possible in chronic administration. The report of Crane gives details.

The *psychotherapy* suitable for the schizophrenic patient has been a subject of intense controversy. The more radical approaches based on psychologic and particularly psychoanalytic views of the genesis of schizophrenia have not achieved their optimistic goals of curing the patient by relieving some basic psychologic conflict. More modest psychotherapy is indispensable when it is intended to help the patient in his everyday affairs, taking advantage of those personal assets that persist despite his illness, and establishing a relationship of friendly rapport in order to guide him in his management of personal and social issues, which, if mishandled, can be demonstrated to provoke distress and further illness. In fact, Vaughn and Leff have shown that the social setting in which a schizophrenic patient is placed after hospitalization is as crucial for his outcome as is his medication. Placement in a household in which intense emotional engagement by some family member with the patient is the rule can be shown to provoke new symptoms regardless of the medication regimen. Thus his psychiatrist, usually at first with the help of a psychiatric social worker, must strive to find a domestic arrangement that is calm and supportive but not too emotionally demanding, and a daily routine that combats the tendency to withdraw from all social contacts into an isolated and perhaps fantasy-ridden existence. Efforts made to instruct the family members on the nature of the symptoms of schizophrenia and on the need to avoid an excess of expressed emotion over the patient have been usedful in reducing both medication requirements and relapses. To accomplish these goals is one of the most challenging exercises in medical treatment. The growth of "halfway houses" as residences for previously hospitalized schizophrenic patients has been prompted by recognition of the need for stable and structured social environments for schizophrenic patients once they have improved enough to leave the hospital.

PROGNOSIS. Prognosis for any patient diagnosed as schizophrenic is always guarded. Certain features carry a good prognosis: high intelligence, a normal premorbid personality, an acute onset, catatonic features in the illness, and a family history of affective disorder. Other features carry a poor prognosis: low intelligence, schizoid premorbid personality, insidious onset of the illness, symptoms of thought disorder, affective blunting in the illness, and a family history of schizophrenia.

The use of phenothiazines has considerably improved the prognosis of schizophrenia, 30 to 50 per cent of patients having complete remissions on follow-up over five years. Another 30 to 40 per cent show some residual symptoms but are able to live in the community, and only 10 to 20 per cent require further hospitalization if phenothiazine treatment is begun and maintained after their first attack of the illness.

Crane GE: Persistent dyskinesia. Br J Psychiatry 122:395, 1973. *Definitive study of the neuroleptic-induced movement disorder with epidemiologic and therapeutic implications.*

Fish FJ: Schizophrenia. Bristol, John Wright & Sons, 1976. *Still the best introduction to the clinical issues and methods of reasoning about this disorder.*

Heston LL: Psychiatric disorders in foster home reared children of schizophrenic mothers. Br J Psychiatry 112:918, 1966. *The original paper on the method of adoption study for discerning a genetic element in schizophrenia.*

Kety, SS: Biochemical theories of schizophrenia, I and II. Science 129:1528, 1590, 1969. *Still the best summary of the pitfalls and findings of biochemistry in the search for a mechanism and cause for schizophrenia.*

Slater E, Beard AW, Glithero E: The schizophrenia-like psychoses of epilepsy. Br J Psychiatry 109:95, 1963. *The classic demonstration of the important relationship between a schizophrenia syndrome and the brain.*

Snyder SN: The dopamine hypothesis of schizophrenia: Focus on the dopamine receptor. Am J Psychiatry 133:2, 1976. *The best described hypothesis offering some hope for the eventual comprehension of this condition.*

Tune LE, Creese I, DePaulo JR, Slavney PR, Coyle JT, Snyder SH: Clinical state and serum neuroleptic levels measured by radioreceptor assay in schizophrenia. Am J Psychiatry 137:2, 1980. *The demonstration that neuroleptic levels in blood have a clear relationship to their therapeutic effectiveness in schizophrenia. An indication that very soon such measurements will be standard for the proper care of these patients.*

Vaughn CE, Leff JP: The influence of family and social factors in the course of psychiatric illness. Br J Psychiatry 129:125, 1976. *An empirical demonstration with crucial therapeutic implications of the role of emotional and situational elements in provoking relapses in schizophrenia.*

Manic-Depressive Psychosis

The essential feature of this psychosis is an excessive disturbance of mood and self-appraisal from which its other mental symptoms seem to arise. This disturbance can be in the direction of elation and self-confidence or sadness and self-blame. The course tends to be episodic, even periodic, with attacks of elation (mania) or sadness (depression) interspersed with periods of apparent mental health varying in length from weeks to years. Individual patients may suffer attacks of only one kind throughout their lifetime. Single or repetitive attacks of depression seem to be the most common manifestation, but attacks alternately manic and then depressive or even repetitively manic are not unusual.

CLINICAL MANIFESTATIONS. *Depression.* During an attack of depression the patient complains of feeling miserable and uncertain of himself. He may give evidence of his sadness by a dejected appearance and by restlessness and distractibility. Some patients are slowed in their activity, and this can progress to a psychomotor retardation of such severity that the patient seems totally unresponsive.

Mental examination of the depressed patient usually brings to light not only his feelings of sadness or misery but also a lowered self-esteem that can vary in intensity from feelings of inadequacy and incompetence to convictions of personal worthlessness, blameworthiness, and evil. This combination of depressed mood with self-blame is the diagnostic sign of this condition. It will also explain most of the other symptoms, modes of behavior, and dangers faced by the depressed patient.

Other symptoms include delusional extrapolations of the attitudes of self-blame. These can increase to a belief that the patient's guilt is notorious, that he is to be arrested, and that he will be condemned to die or to suffer some extraordinary punishment either in this world or the next. Suspiciousness and fear of mistreatment based on these delusional beliefs may be difficult to distinguish from similar attitudes in the paranoid schizophrenic patient. A useful if not cast-iron distinction is the depressive's belief that the suspected ill treatment comes as a justified punishment and not, as with the schizophrenic, as an undeserved persecution.

In some severely depressed patients delusional ideas can become bizarre and even grandiose in concept. Thus they come to believe that they have been the cause of cosmic disasters, that the sun is darkened by them, that whole cities have been deserted because of their presence, or that they and their progeny are accursed in the sight of the Divinity. Delusions of bodily change may take the form that their brains are rotting, their bowels totally blocked, or their bones fractured and dislocated.

Delusional ideas may concern the relationship of the patient to the world and to others. He may believe that he has lost all his money, that he has become a burden to others, that he is universally despised, or even that he gives off such a bad odor that people cannot stand his presence. Again, these beliefs are usually reflective of the patient's inner attitude of self-blame, self-contempt, and hopelessness.

The point about these opinions is that they are delusional

and not just false. They are unshakable opinions held in the face of all contrary evidence. Only treatment of the depressive disorder will remove them.

The most worrisome symptom of the depressed patient is *inclination to suicide.* It is easily appreciated that attitudes of such hopelessness and despair as have been described could prompt self-destruction. But it is not necessary to have such exaggerated delusions for suicide to be a distinct risk. Vigilance for suicidal intentions must be maintained throughout the course of the depressive disturbance. The physician should ask any depressed patient about thoughts of self-injury. A series of questions useful in estimating suicidal risk is provided in the discussion of Depression (below). Often this simple action will reveal both the severity of the mood disturbance and the need to bring the patient into hospital for his own protection.

Homicide is also a possibility for the depressed patient, and is particularly likely in those who harbor beliefs that their family shares in their guilt and accursed characteristics. Any suggestions by the patient that he might prefer death should be most seriously believed.

Along with these psychologic symptoms the depressed patient will often suffer from disturbances in his sleep, particularly waking early in the morning and being unable to return to sleep. Other physical disturbances include bodily aches and pains, loss of appetite, constipation, and weight loss. These features may combine with the retardation to give the appearance of chronic physical ill health. In fact, many depressed patients will first consult internists complaining of such physical symptoms. Helpful to the differentiation of the patient whose somatic symptoms are part of a depressive illness is a discovery of the features of depressed mood, and attitudes of self-blame or hopelessness when these features are combined with complaints of poorly localized pains, with loss of appetite or weight loss, or even with preoccupations about the state of the inner organs.

Mania. Symptoms that are almost the exact opposite of those seen during an attack of depression appear during an attack of mania. Now the patient says that he is in excellent spirits, that he feels well, and in fact has never felt better. He is active and restless, and appears energetic, confident, and quick-witted. These characteristics tend to worsen, and it is in their more extreme form that they become recognized as symptoms. The restlessness and energy become overactivity, with the patient moving constantly and planning progressively less plausible projects. His speech becomes incessant, rapid, and disjointed, one idea following another with little connection between them. His attitude of confidence becomes grandiose self-satisfaction. He may be overbearing and pompous. He often will be irritated by his surroundings, easy to anger, and perhaps suspicious that the efforts being made to control him are unjust.

Although a manic patient can usually be recognized by his overactivity, ebullience, and great self-confidence, he can develop as well ideas of resentment and feelings that he is being in some way unfairly noticed or persecuted. These ideas, on investigation, are found to derive from his own delusional opinion that he is so important that he must be under scrutiny by forces such as foreign powers. Occasionally, these persecutory ideas are so prominent that a diagnosis of schizophrenia is entertained. It is, however, the direct connection of these ideas to the attitude of self-confidence that allows a diagnosis of mania to be made.

With the mental changes manic patients exhibit disturbed social behavior. They may have increased sexual interest and may become promiscuous. They tend to overspend and be reckless with money. They may insult their employers and so be fired from their jobs. In the first attack of mania and before the severe restlessness and disorganization of thought appear, these activities may not be recognized as the products of mental illness, but may be construed as actions for which the patient can be held accountable. Thus the patient can be subjected to severe losses, to legal actions, or to moral criticism that can hamper his life long after his manic attack is over. To protect him from these consequences hospitalization of the manic patient may be required.

ETIOLOGY. ***"Cause" or Prerequisite Elements in Manic-Depressive Disorder.*** As with schizophrenia, an important genetic contribution to the etiology of the manic-depressive disorder seems certain. There is a progressive frequency of incidence with increasing blood relatedness so that with monozygotic twins the concordance rate is over 50 per cent. It is likely that genetic constitution is a necessary but not sufficient cause for this disorder. Certain other features of the illness require consideration. First, the illness does appear in attacks interspersed with periods in which the person appears to be normal. Second, the attacks are somewhat seasonal, appearing more frequently in the spring and fall than in summer and winter. Third, although many attacks occur spontaneously, many seem to be precipitated by some disturbing event. Presumably some other elements must combine with the genetic vulnerability to explain these features. Again, the most easily defended position would hold that a necessary cause for manic-depressive disorder is the genetic constitution of the patient, but that any of a large number of environmental disturbances can bring out the disorder.

Mechanism in Manic-Depressive Disorder. As with schizophrenia, a pharmacologically induced disorder has enhanced confidence that, whatever the "cause," the mechanism for affective disorder is a neural one. Treatment with reserpine for hypertension produced depression in up to one of four patients, and this depression was accompanied by the typical delusional attitudes of the manic-depressive psychosis. The discovery that reserpine depleted brain neurons of biogenic amines, particularly norepinephrine and serotonin, has prompted a variety of hypotheses that propose some lack of norepinephrine, serotonin, or other biogenic amines at synaptic sites in the brain for emotional control. That many effective antidepressant agents also influence these same amines has been a further support to these hypotheses.

TREATMENT. The first rule in managing either manic or depressed patients is that most of them should be in a hospital. Their conditions can bring catastrophe to themselves and their families in the form of financial mismanagement in mania and suicide in depression. If these diagnoses are strongly suspected, then psychiatric opinion should be immediately sought so as to determine whether hospitalization should be imposed. It is critical to have expert help, because the patient can often hide the severity of the disorder in a mass of explanations which may appear quite plausible. In the hospital the suicidal patient must be closely supervised and definitive treatment should not be long deferred.

It is crucial to diagnose these patients and separate them from those with other conditions, because new drug treatments have proved effective for them and are specific to the affective disorders. Two classes of pharmacologic agents are effective in *depression.* Seemingly more effective are the so-called *tricyclic antidepressants,* the prototype of which is imipramine. This drug, given in doses of from 75 to 300 mg per day, will relieve a depressive attack in 50 per cent of patients. The recent development of the means for measuring plasma levels of tricyclic antidepressants has revealed a partial explanation for failures to respond. A narrow range (50 to 170 ng per milliliter) encloses therapeutic plasma nortriptyline levels. The failure to reach this level or the exceeding of it inhibits a full response. A rational pharmacology for these medications will soon require plasma measurements to be available as a routine. Maintenance therapy of 100 to 150 mg per day should be continued for six to eight months after recovery. If tricyclics are ineffective, the logical practice should be to switch to the other class, which includes the drugs that have as their primary action the capacity to inhibit the enzyme monoamine oxidase. These drugs, in doses of 45 to 75 mg per day, have also proved useful in depression.

If *monoamine oxidase inhibitors* are used, the patient must be warned to avoid foodstuffs such as cheese, broad beans, and some yeast extracts, which have pressor amines of the phenylethylamine group that includes tyramine. If absorbed by patients whose monoamine oxidase enzyme is depleted, they can cause sudden elevation of blood pressure with headache, blurred vision, and even cerebrovascular hemorrhage.

The mainstay of treatment for severe depression is *electroconvulsive treatment* (ECT). In contrast to the drugs which relieve the symptoms of depression, ECT will terminate an attack of depression usually in four to eight treatments. This treatment can produce the most dramatic and quick recovery from the depths of a life-threatening depression, and should not be withheld from a delusional patient or any seriously depressed patient who has failed to respond to drug treatment after three to four weeks. Maintenance with imipramine, 100 to 150 mg per day for six months, is recommended after ECT for the avoidance of relapse shortly after successful treatment.

The *treatment of mania* is often very difficult, particularly if the patient is suspicious about medicines. Haloperidol in doses of 2 to 10 mg thrice daily taken orally has proved effective. This compound is liable to produce severe extrapyramidal side effects which can be combated with antiparkinsonian drugs and with Benadryl. Chlorpromazine in doses of 300 to 1000 mg per day can also be tried.

An effective measure for controlling mania is the use of lithium ion in the form of lithium carbonate. This compound is available in 300 mg tablets, and daily intake of 900 to 2400 mg per day can relieve manic excitement. It is, however, essential to follow plasma lithium concentration in these patients, because toxic signs of disorientation, tremor, anorexia, and diarrhea can appear if plasma lithium concentration rises above 2 mEq per liter. The therapeutic level and the toxic level of lithium are close, and therefore the medication must be started when the patient can be carefully supervised in a hospital. Maintenance lithium treatment can be recommended, because there is fair clinical evidence that in this fashion some further attacks of mania may be avoided.

Maintenance lithium treatment is not without problems, however. It can produce several renal complications—in particular, nephrogenic diabetes insipidus and, rarely, a nephrotic syndrome secondary to an interstitial nephropathy.

These problems appear to increase with the duration as well as the dose of lithium given (DePaulo, 1980). No patients have had renal failure produced by lithium, but it would seem prudent to make some measure of glomerular filtration rate prior to beginning lithium treatment and annually as long as the treatment is maintained. A creatinine clearance test is an adequate screening test.

The diabetes insipidus, if severe, can be a serious problem if the patient being treated with lithium nonetheless falls ill with mania or depression and fails to sustain a fluid intake either because of the distractions of mania or the delusions and psychomotor retardation of depression. The patient in such circumstances can become dangerously dehydrated or can develop a severe lithium intoxication. The patient and family should be counseled about this problem and the need to maintain the fluid intake.

In the face of such complications, the decision on whether a given patient should be sustained on lithium is a judgment. The complications of the treatment must be weighed against the frequency and psychosocial impairments of subsequent attacks of affective disorder.

PROGNOSIS. The prognosis for a single attack of mania or depression is excellent. Even without treatment patients tend to recover completely within six months. With antidepressant treatment the medication can be withdrawn after six to eight months with fair assurance that symptoms will not recur at this time.

The longer-range prognosis is not so favorable. Eighty per cent of people who have suffered one attack of affective disturbance will have another at some time in their lives, but this may not be for many years. Some patients, however, will have recurrent attacks of mania or depression interrupted by only brief intervals of normal behavior.

The best advice to give patients who have suffered from their first affective attack is that they will very likely be quite well for years, but that they and their family should be aware that their mood changes are to be considered seriously, and they should seek psychiatric attention promptly if such a mood change tends to persist or worsen. Prien's work indicates that individuals who suffer recurrent attacks of any form of manic-depressive disorder are best maintained on lithium for an extended, even an indefinite, period.

Akiskal HS, McKinney WT: Overview of recent research in depression. Arch Gen Psychiatr 32:285, 1975. *A masterful consideration of ten possible models for the etiology of depression, ranging over psychoanalytic, behavioral, biologic, sociologic, and existential concepts. The authors attempt to be comprehensive, critical, but reconciling.*

Kragh-Sorensen P, Hasen CE, Asberg M: Plasma levels of nortriptyline in the treatment of endogenous depression. Acta Psychiatr Scand 49:444, 1973. *The definitive article indicating the need for plasma levels of antidepressants because it demonstrates an optimal level below which and above which the patients do not improve. A most clear demonstration of a therapeutic "window."*

Lewis A: Melancholia. J Ment Sci 80:1, 277, 1934; 82:488, 1936. *The classic triad of papers on the history, symptoms, and course of endogenous depression, written before the advent of effective physical treatments.*

Prien R, Klett J, Caffey E: Lithium prophylaxis in recurrent affective illness. Am J Psychiatry 131:198, 1974. *A clear indication of the utility of lithium in treatment.*

Winokur G, Clayton PJ, Reich T: Manic-Depressive Illness. St. Louis, C.V. Mosby Company, 1969. *This is the definitive monograph on the subject.*

PERSONALITY DISORDERS AND NEUROTIC SYMPTOMS

GENERAL CONSIDERATIONS. The concept of disease entities that supports our understanding of the functional psychoses does not suit all psychologic disturbances and particularly those that are described as personality disorders or neurotic symptoms. There is uncertainty both in terms and in concept here. For example, the designation neurosis is ambiguous in that it seems a name for a clinical entity with some sharp distinction from normal, but a cardinal symptom of one neurosis, *anxiety*, is an experience of all people at some time and is an appropriate mood in certain circumstances. What then is abnormal in *anxiety neurosis*? Is this abnormality of a quantitative or a qualitative nature? To what kind of patient can the term anxiety neurosis be applied? Should we use it only for patients in the emotional "state" of anxiety, or is it suitable regardless of the present state if a patient has "traits" that make him prone to this emotion?

The term *personality* and particularly its extension, *personality disorder*, can be just as troublesome. Personality seems a word similar to such terms as character or temperament, words intended to describe aspects of human psychologic variation distributed in a smoothly graded fashion in the population. But if that is true, then the distinction personality disorder can seem an arbitrary, socially contrived, or judgmental decision, since no sharp dividing line is to be expected in smoothly graded characteristics. In later sections of this chapter, an attempt is made to dispel some of these ambiguities while considering several emotional disturbances often called neurotic that occur in a general medical setting.

Although many mental changes and emotional disturbances in patients can be ascribed to known or presumed pathologic changes in brain function, certain varieties of human psychologic constitution and certain life experiences can themselves provoke emotional disturbance and disrupted behavior. The terms personality disorder and neurotic symptoms are intended to describe the disturbances that result from variation in human constitution and experience by invoking the concepts of potential and response. Personality always means *potential*. It encompasses and describes the abiding and distinctive traits or tendencies of an individual to react to circumstances in a particular fashion. Thus by "optimistic personality" is meant an individual who can be expected to respond with cheerfulness and optimism in situations in which others are less likely to do so. An individual's personality is the sum of numerous traits, and a comparison with others is implicit in the description of each trait. Thus every trait can be conceived as a dimension of variation along which people can be dispersed in a fashion similar to their dispersal along the dimensions of height, weight, or intelligence. Any definition of an individual's personality is an attempt to place him in relationship to others in respect to one or more traits. An individual can be said to have a disorder of personality if he deviates to such an extreme along the range of variation for some trait that either he or others complain of its effects.

Whereas personality and personality disorder indicate potential, the neurotic symptoms are emotional *responses* displayed when the individual is troubled by circumstances. For anyone certain environments and life events are conducive to anxiety, others to depression, and still others to suspiciousness. People with a disorder of personality have an increased potential for these responses and are provoked to them by less extreme circumstances and less specific stimuli. Thus paranoid personality disorder is a term used to describe an individual who tends to show attitudes of suspiciousness and feelings of persecution (the neurotic symptoms) in settings so minimally threatening that they will seldom provoke such attitudes in others. If, however, his life is relatively free of threatening features, these feelings will be diminished and, despite his personality traits, symptoms may be avoided.

Before such concepts can be used in the evaluation and management of a particular patient, that patient must be well known to the doctor, and the possibility of other conditions that could produce similar symptoms must be excluded. For this a detailed psychiatric history, mental status, and physical examination are needed. The latter two can be obtained during the first interview, but historical information about the patient's family background, developmental milestones, sexual adjustment, scholastic and occupational achievement, habits, and medical problems may require several hours of examination. Observations from his relatives improve the accuracy of such information, and their descriptions of his personality are indispensable. All these data, combined with the knowledge of the patient's present condition, form the basis for diagnosis, treatment, and prognosis, and to embark on such matters without this information is to commit a capital error. The result is often failure of treatment, because the patient has been misunderstood and emphasis given to minor rather than major features of his problem.

As it becomes clear that a given patient's disturbance is the outcome of the kind of person he is and the situations that he faces, the data of the psychiatric history and the mental status examination can usually be divided into three categories which, although closely related, are usefully distinguished: (1) the predisposing factors for the disturbance, including personality traits and formative life experiences; (2) the precipitating factors; and (3) the symptoms themselves and their effect on the patient.

PREDISPOSING FACTORS. Predisposing factors are those features special to an individual that make him vulnerable to emotional disturbance. The most critical factor is personality, the traits of which are distinguished in the patient's temperament, attitudes, and predictable responses. But personality is the outcome of genetic constitution, intellectual endowment, and lifetime experiences, and each of these is a predisposing factor in itself. Predisposing factors often overlooked are the patient's social status and cultural situation.

Finally, the state of health is an important predisposing feature, because physical illness, through the distress it produces or by direct effects on the central nervous system, interferes with a person's capacity to cope with circumstances and thus leads to psychologic symptoms.

PRECIPITATING FACTORS. The precipitating factors are events or experiences that have disrupted emotional equilibrium and bear a close temporal relationship to the disturbance for which the patient seeks help. The common-sense expectations that personal illness, or conflict produced by changes in family or occupational circumstances, could precipitate psychologic distress have been confirmed in studies reviewed recently by Wing. Holmes has attempted to grade life events in a hierarchy of emotional stressfulness, and many workers have found his scale useful for estimating the relative distress different patients have endured. Some psychologic precipitants are more recondite, because they depend on a special meaning an individual gives events, perhaps a symbolic meaning derived from the particular patient's early life experiences. Before emphasizing these more abstruse precipitants of a unique character, it is usually wise to consider the more immediate and obvious ones that may be present.

SYMPTOMS. Later in this chapter the symptoms of anxiety, depression, and hysterical reaction are discussed, because they are common in the general practice of medicine. These conditions do not exhaust the neurotic disorders, but are the most common seen in medical practice. For a comprehensive consideration of the neurotic reactions, reference can be made to the text by Goodwin and Guze.

All neurotic symptoms emerge as complaints either of the patient himself or of others who must deal with him. They are symptoms in the sense that they disturb the patient's sense of well-being or they interfere with his behavior and his adaptability to circumstances. They can vary from mild to severe, and they can be acute or chronic.

In the assessment of these symptoms the patient should be encouraged to describe how he feels, how the symptoms developed, what seems to make them worse or better, what they are like when compared with previous emotional reactions, and how they disturb him now. *The aim is to come to appreciate these symptoms as understandable responses of this particular person to his particular circumstances.* The overall principle is that we are considering here not classes of patients suffering from distinct disease entities, but individuals troubled by their special life circumstances and needing assistance tailored to their particular personal nature and situation. The specific symptoms, their characteristic predisposing and precipitating factors, their effects on behavior, and modes of treatment will be considered in the balance of this chapter.

A comprehensive consideration of the psychotherapy of neurotic reactions can be found in the monograph of Frank and his associates.

Frank, JD, Hoehn-Saric R, Imber SD, Liberman BL, Stone AR: Effective ingredients of successful psychotherapy. New York, Brunner/Mazel, 1978. *A thoughtful, practical, and scholarly approach to psychotherapy based on 25 years of painstaking empirical research. This book is the outstanding work in a field of many entries. Its documentation of (1) demoralization as the central issue for the patient, (2) those characteristics of patient and therapist conducive to successful treatment, and (3) the equal effectiveness of different therapeutic schools of thought is noteworthy.*

Goodwin DW, Guze SB: Psychiatric Diagnosis. 2nd ed. New York, Oxford University Press, 1979. *A brief but thorough text describing the psychiatric syndromes. A good introduction to the approach to psychiatry exemplified in the American classification of psychiatric disorder DSM III.*

Holmes TH, Rahe RJ: The social readjustment score. J Psychosomat Res 11:213, 1967. *The presentation of a scoreable approach to stressful life events that has helped take some of the subjectivity out of this awkward assessment.*

Wing JK: Innovations in social psychiatry. Psychol Med 10:219, 1980. *A thorough and up-to-date review of concepts and research into the precipitants of psychiatric disorders.*

Anxiety

DEFINITION. Anxiety is an unpleasant mood of tension and apprehension. It is fear's first cousin, and like fear it has prominent autonomic effects when severe, but fear is an emotion sharply focused on immediate dangers. Anxiety is usually imposed by the anticipation of future danger, distress, or difficulties. As an emotional response common to people, anxiety is useful. Activities that arouse it are avoided and those that diminish it are sustained. Although anxiety may spur people to perform difficult tasks skillfully and admirably, when excessive it is a hindrance, as some well-prepared students demonstrate when facing a critical examination. Anxiety is a medical problem when it is excessive, inappropriate, or without obvious cause.

FORMS OF ANXIETY AND THEIR PREDISPOSING AND PRECIPITATING FACTORS. Anxiety can occur (1) as an affective response of anyone under circumstances of threat or danger; (2) as a symptom of another psychiatric disorder, such as delirium, dementia, or schizophrenia; or (3) as a psychopathologic state in which excessive anxiety is the prominent feature.

It is not difficult to appreciate the predisposing and precipitating factors of anxiety as an affective response to danger. Anxiety is a psychologic reaction to anticipated troubles of all sorts. But people and troubles vary. Some—the timid, the inexperienced, the excessively conscientious—are frequently anxious in situations that seem not to affect others. Most people are at least mildly anxious whenever they seek medical advice; when threatening dangers are intense or prolonged as in chronic painful illness or in battle, even the most resistant individuals can develop an incapacitating anxiety. Resistance to anxiety varies with physical condition. When tired, sick, or injured, people are more easily threatened.

Common precipitants of anxiety in daily life are circumstances of conflict in which an action is demanded but the correct action may be difficult to discern. Thus, a person may be anxious over difficult decisions on which rest his economic and social future or because the decisions produce an unpredictable response in an inconsistent superior.

Laboratory models for this kind of conflict and its effects on the emotional state have been produced. Pavlov trained dogs to respond to the picture of a circle by rewarding such responses with food. He did not reward responses to an ellipse. Then by simply compressing the ellipse so that it gradually approached a circle in shape, he made a discrimination progressively more difficult. The emotional response of these dogs was remarkable. They became agitated when put into harness for the experiment. They tore at their restraints, barked, and refused to attempt the discrimination. In this state, they not only made many mistakes but they became unable to make discriminations that had previously been easy. It is not difficult to see analogies in both situation and behavior between these dogs and people in situations of conflict.

An emotional state of anxiety can, as mentioned, be a symptom of any of a number of neurologic and psychiatric disorders. The person with brain damage may become anxious in situations that do not seem immediately threatening, but appear so to him because of his disturbed capacity for analysis and discrimination. In fact, one of the first indications of a dementia can be an attack of severe anxiety without obvious provocation.

A prolonged, irritable anxiety state can follow a head injury, as one of the symptoms of the so-called postconcussional syndrome. Gronwall and Sampson demonstrate that it may be due to a mild disturbance in cognitive capacity subjectively evident to the patient but demonstrable objectively only with difficulty.

A mood of tension and agitation can occur in the delirious states, such as those that follow withdrawal from alcohol or barbiturates. It can also sometimes be produced by the hallucinogenic drugs such as LSD 25. In these situations it may be disturbed perceptions and misinterpretations that arouse anxiety, but occasionally the anxiety appears as one of the several symptoms of psychologic arousal and seems independent of anything that the patient experiences or understands.

The conditions in which anxiety can be recognized as a psychopathologic state are several. Included here are the phobic states in which the patient suffers an excessive fear of some object, animal, or situation such as the dark or thunder and lightning. These monosymptomatic phobias usually commence in childhood and are of less clinical importance because they are well encapsulated and seldom lead to medical attention.

It is the condition sometimes referred to as *agoraphobia with panic attacks* that should be distinguished from these other conditions. This disorder has carried many names, including neurasthenia, effort syndrome, neurocirculatory asthenia, and, most recently, *panic disorder*. The condition is a familial disorder, as first noted by Cohen and his associates. A careful family survey by Crowe et al. of first degree relatives of patients with panic disorder found a morbidity risk of 42 per cent among female relatives and 22 per cent among male relatives. In fact, familial morbidity risk for panic disorder is as high as any in the psychiatric genetics literature.

The precipitating event for panic attacks can be a calamitous emotional experience, such as a bereavement, separation, or injury, but it can be a more trivial distressing event superimposed upon a chronic state of some tension and uneasiness. The precipitating event then triggers off the panic attack, which will recur irregularly and unpredictably in the future.

These spontaneously occurring panic attacks that seem so inexplicable to the patient lead to the development of an anticipatory anxiety as the patient begins to fear the recurrence of another attack. In fact, this can lead to the phobic avoidance of any situation which can be thought to provoke these panic attacks, and this avoidance can grow to such an extreme that the patient is housebound; hence the term agoraphobia. But agoraphobia is probably a misnomer, in that what the patient is fearing is not open spaces but being away from familiar surroundings and entering settings where the inexplicable but very distressing panic attacks occur. The term panic disorder is preferable.

MANIFESTATIONS OF ANXIETY. Regardless of the cause of anxiety, its manifestations are divisible into three groups: (1) The inner feelings of tension, apprehension, and dread that form the anxious mood itself. (2) A disturbance of the intellectual power. The anxious patient is unable to think clearly and to use proper judgment, to learn efficiently, or to remember accurately. (3) The somatic and autonomic symptoms that accompany tension, anxiety, and fear. These include tension headache, tremor, giddiness, dyspnea, heart palpitation, gastric distress, urinary frequency, backache, and general feelings of weakness.

A model anxiety state is to be seen among combat soldiers. The infantryman is a prepared subject for anxiety. He is threatened with death or mutilation. He must go without sleep, remain exposed to the weather, and often be hungry. He is usually unable to understand all that is happening around him. He is repeatedly frightened by gunfire and distressed by the death of comrades. If he is exposed to such circumstances long enough, he develops a severe and persisting anxiety state, sometimes called combat exhaustion or battle fatigue. Swank, in his classic studies of combat exhaustion in the European campaign of World War II, described all the features. Soldiers complained of emotional tension and were easily startled, had difficulty sleeping, reported mental confusion and memory deficits, and complained of headache, back pain, palpitations, weakness, and fatigability. The complaint of persistent fatigue was found in all of the men.

Swank documented that this condition develops after severe or prolonged combat. The character of the individual symptoms and the sequence of the development were stereotyped but they appeared earliest among units with the highest casualty rates. All men apparently, though, will develop this condition if exposed to battle long enough. Wolff reported that the average man in the Army of the United States during the Korean conflict reached this point after 85 days of combat.

The symptoms of anxiety that physicians see in patients in circumstances that are threatening to them or as symptoms of other diseases are not different. The patients all have the same three groups of symptoms but may report that one is more prominent than the others, such as emphasizing the tension and fatigue, the intellectual difficulties, or the somatic and autonomic difficulties.

Panic attacks are distinct from the chronic tension and anxiety found in these circumstances and can be recognized by their characteristic features. They occur usually on a background of some persistent, generalized anxiety or apprehension, but the attacks occur at times when there appears to be no obvious threatening circumstance. Although the panic attack can occur at any time, a most favorite time is when the person is in a situation in which rapid exit would be difficult, such as traveling in a bus, train, or elevator; standing in a crowded store or restaurant; or waiting in a supermarket line.

The attacks are experienced as episodes of uneasiness that start without any identifiable precipitant and build up over ten to fifteen minutes to a level of severe panic, only to subside again by the end of an hour. As the feeling of anxiety increases, the patient may notice dyspnea, choking sensations, sweating, flushing, paresthesias, trembling or shaking, heart palpitations, weakness, or lightheadedness. A common complaint in an anxiety attack is the sensation of tightness in the chest, as though the lungs could not be adequately filled. The patient responds to this sensation by deep and sighing respirations, sometimes to the point of producing a respiratory alkalosis that adds to the feelings of giddiness with tingling of the fingertips and even tetany with carpopedal spasms. This is the *hyperventilation syndrome* that adds its symptoms to the panic feelings. The patient may act upon his symptoms by trying to flee from the situation and may in the future avoid the situations in which the panic attack appeared. This avoidance may get so extreme that the patient becomes essentially housebound.

A chronic anxiety may be provoked by a chronic situation of conflict and threat, or it may be the outcome of repeated panic attacks in which the anxiety is now focused particularly on the fear of further attack. With the chronic condition symptoms are less intense, although not different in quality from those of acute anxiety. The patient is tense and on edge. He may also report some feelings of sadness or hopelessness along with his anxiety. He will have a number of somatic complaints, particularly frontal or occipital headache, anorexia, and weight loss, and on examination he may have physical signs of tension, a fine tremor of the extended hands, brisk tendon reflexes, rapid heartbeat, and pupillary dilatation.

That there is a clear genetic vulnerability to panic disorder implies that there may be a biologic foundation to this condition distinguishing it from anxieties that can be understood as graded responses of an individual to varying threats. Certainly its stereotyped presentvation, its response to medication, and its tendency to remissions and exacerbations, as well as this genetic predisposition, encourage a search for a biologic system that can be provoked into action by some ordinarily nonthreatening event. The recent recognition that receptors for the benzodiazepine class of drugs are to be found naturally in the brain leads to proposals that there may be some natural "tranquilizer" ligand, with the implication that a pathophysiology of such a system of ligands and their receptors might prove to be a basis for this particular disorder. If such a system were discovered, it would also most likely illuminate the other anxieties generated by more obviously threatening circumstances and treatable with exogenous benzodiazepines.

DIAGNOSIS. Usually the recognition of anxiety is not difficult. The patient's voiced complaint is his distressing emotional state. His associated disturbances in thinking and autonomic functions serve to confirm the diagnostic impression. Most often the major issue is not the diagnosis of anxiety but rather the question of why the patient is anxious now. This question must be answered from knowledge of the circumstances of the onset of anxiety, the signs and symptoms that accompany it, and the personality of the patient. The decision as to whether this patient's anxiety is a response to circumstances, a symptom of some underlying psychiatric or neurologic disorder, or a psychopathologic state of its own can be made on the basis of this knowledge.

It is crucial, though, to recognize the panic disorder, since it will have a specific treatment. It can occasionally be presented by a patient who focuses his complaints on the physical symptoms that accompany the attacks, such as his cardiac palpitations or his giddiness and vertigo. Then the condition can be confused with episodic cardiac or neurologic conditions. Most helpful to the proper diagnosis is the discernment that the episodes are always accompanied by intense anxiety and by several autonomic reactions. A search for such particular symptoms as air hunger, tremulousness, and hyperventilation is diagnostically helpful. It is sometimes necessary to exclude other conditions with appropriate laboratory tests. As with all psychologically disturbed patients, laboratory studies should not be delayed or protracted, but should be decided upon, and this phase of the examination should be finished as promptly as possible. Knowledge of the existence of panic disorder as a specific condition is most helpful to its recognition.

TREATMENT. Treatment will vary with the cause and severity of the anxiety. Many mildly anxious patients whose anxiety is a response to threat or conflict can be helped by a physician who is willing to listen carefully to their difficulties and offer some support and occasional advice. These patients have disturbances that are transient and are based on some particular problem or self-doubt that can eventually be resolved.

Those with more severe anxiety but from the same source can be aided by a combination of pharmacologic treatment and repeated compassionate discussions of their difficulties. The pharmacologic agent to be recommended for this form of anxiety is chlordiazepoxide (Librium), which can be given in doses of 10 mg three to four times a day.

Only occasionally is it necessary to bring such patients into hospital. This is done in an effort to remove them from some pathogenic setting that has provoked a vicious circle of anxiety, decompensation, failure, and more anxiety. Yet such hospitalization is often remarkably effective in bringing such patients relief. Again some sedation as well as psychologic support can be given to them, and again chlordiazepoxide can be recommended in combination with a milieu of support and understanding that allows the patient to regain emotional balance.

Patients with chronic anxiety can be referred with confidence to specialists in psychotherapy. Jerome Frank and his associates have documented that certain personality features have prognostic significance in the psychotherapy of anxiety, and their monograph on the ingredients of successful psychotherapy can be consulted.

As emphasized, though, panic attacks must be specifically recognized. This is because (1) it is clear that they are distinct from other anxieties in family history, course, and phenomena, and (2) they do *not* respond to the sedatives such as chlordiazepoxide but do respond well to tricyclic antidepressants or monoamine oxidase inhibitors. The tricyclic antidepressant imipramine has proved particularly useful. Often patients respond at a relatively low dose of 25 to 50 mg per day, but it can be gradually raised until panic attacks abate. Doses that have been effective have ranged from 5 to 300 mg of imipramine. The monoamine oxidase inhibitor phenelzine in doses of 30 to 60 mg per day has also been demonstrated to be effective in this condition. These medications interrupt the panic attacks but may leave the patient with some continuing chronic tension. For this a small dose of chlordiazepoxide can be recommended. The medication for the panic attacks should be maintained until the patient is attack free for six to twelve months.

Psychologic management in the panic disorder does form a useful adjunctive treatment. It is particularly important to explain the nature of this condition to patients, because often they fear that the panic attacks indicate that they have some progressive mental disorder. Simply discovering that it is a recognized entity with an established treatment has been comforting to many patients through the period of adjusting medication and establishing a plan for managing the attacks. It is also helpful to remind the patient that recovery will not be immediate, that relapses can occur, and that, since it is the panic symptom that is being treated, panic will be experienced several times before it is controlled, but that in about 80 per cent of patients this control will ultimately be achieved.

The patient can aid in his own recovery if he tries not to flee from a situation in which he experiences a panic attack. To help the patient do this, he can be told truthfully that the panic will not lead to mental disruption or total loss of control but customarily will reach some peak intensity and then gradually abate over a period of ten to fifteen minutes. If the patient can simply sustain himself in the setting until some abatement occurs, the next occasion will often be less severe. Along with the medications that tend to suppress their occurrence, this behavioral management of the individual attacks gradually gives the patient a sense of control of the panic experience and with this a capacity to free himself from the constraints on his activity that he previously used to avoid panic.

Cohen ME, Badal DW, Kilpatrick A, Reed EW, White PD: The high familial prevalence of neurocirculatory asthenia (anxiety neurosis, effort syndrome). Am J Hum Genet 3:126, 1951. *The classic description of the panic attack syndrome and its familial occurrence. Most useful also for its consideration of differential diagnosis.*

Crowe RR, Pauls DL, Slymen DJ, Noyes R: A family study of anxiety neurosis. Arch Gen Psychiatry 37:77, 1980. *A recent confirmation of the familial prevalence of panic disorder.*

Gronwall DA, Sampson H: The Psychological Effects of Concussion. London, Oxford University Press, 1975. *An elegant demonstration of a deficit in information-processing capacity in patients after concussive injuries.This deficit is often inapparent to routine examination but can have profound effects on emotional reactivity. A model of neuropsychiatric research.*

Marks IM: Fears and Phobias. New York, Academic Press, 1969. *A readable and thorough discussion of various anxiety states, with particular consideration of treatment and prognosis.*

Rohs RG, Noyes R: Agoraphobia. Newer treatment approach. J Nerv Ment Dis 166:701, 1978. *A good review of psychologic and psychopharmacologic treatments of panic disorder.*

Swank RL: Combat exhaustion. J Nerv Ment Dis 109:475, 1949. *The classic description of the causes, symptoms, and signs of situation-specific anxiety. Still rewarding to study.*

Depression

DEFINITION. Depression is a term for a mood of sadness and gloom. It can be a symptom of manic-depressive psychosis (see above for a complete consideration of the subject). Here we are dealing with depression that occurs as a response to troubled life circumstances. Such depression can usually be given a more specific name, such as discouragement, demoralization, or grief—terms that carry specifically the connotation of an emotional reaction.

The troubled mood is usually not hard to recognize. The patient appears miserable, his face expressive of sadness and perhaps tension. He may move without confidence or purpose and report that his energy is decreased and his thinking slow and difficult. Appetite is usually lessened, often with weight loss, and sleep is restless and diminished. Sexual interest will be greatly reduced. The patient may also say that he is irritable and fearful. Depending on the severity of his depression, the patient will seem socially disorganized, proving inefficient in work, failing in duties, and neglectful of appearance. His acknowledged inadequacies in these respects may add to his sense of misery and may prompt thoughts of resigning from work, leaving his family, or even committing suicide.

Although various troubles can provoke depression, there is a specific response that illustrates features common to many depressive reactions. That response is *grief,* well studied by Dr. C. M. Parkes.

Grief is an experience in almost every lifetime and is the response that follows the loss, usually by death, of some relative or friend. The severity of the reaction and its duration depend upon many factors, but the most important is the closeness of the relationship and degree of dependence of the mourner on the lost individual.

Grief is a state that follows a pattern of development in which certain stages can be recognized even though the transition from one to the next is not possible to define exactly and features from one can persist in the others. The *first stage,* which lasts several days, begins upon learning of the death. The mourner feels stunned and appears bewildered, does not seem to grasp his loss fully or to relate its implications to his feelings coherently. He may appear irritable, tearful, or anxious, but can also seem calm and capable. Although his emotions and behavior may be unpredictable, they are often culturally modified as he carries out such customs as funeral rituals. He himself will usually report afterward that his emotions were blunted and his thinking uncertain, and that his depressed mood was not fully experienced. Parkes refers to this period as the stage of numbness, blunting, or shock.

This stage ends gradually but usually within one week of the bereavement, when there is an increase in the emotion of sadness and the appearance of an intense sense of loss that comes in waves, called pangs of yearning or pining by Parkes. In this *second stage,* between these surges of distressing feelings, which are so frequent at first as to be almost continuous, the patient is usually irritable and sad, with sleep and appetite diminished. Activity, which often takes the form of aimless moving about rather than productive work, may be increased, particularly so during a depressive surge, a point Parkes uses to support his analogy of this stage of grief to the searching behavior of animals separated from their mates. It is the phenomenon of *surges of misery,* however, that is most characteristic of grief and usually aids in its recognition. With time these occur less often, but it is common experience to have such a wave of depressive feelings sweep over a person following a reminder of the loss years after the bereavement.

The *third period of grief* appears with a diminution in the attacks of yearning and the anxious restlessness. This phase, usually entered into within several weeks of bereavement, customarily lasts the longest. It is a stage of depressed feelings with apathy and a disinclination to find purpose or interest in work. The patient is no longer restless, sleepless, or without appetite, but his emotional state is one of gloom and discouragement and his capacity for enjoyment or for physical or intellectual work is greatly reduced. Parkes refers to this as the stage of disorganization when the patient seems withdrawn, may complain of ill health, and fails to plan ahead. This state may last over a year and only gradually be replaced with more customary feelings. Recovery may be brought about in part by the natural but chance occurrence of new integrative activities and friendships, and can be facilitated by efforts of the mourner to expose himself to the opportunities for these restorative experiences.

Depressions that are responses to difficulties in life other than bereavement are very similar to this third stage. Symptoms like those in the first two stages of grief can appear briefly in distressing situations that have a sudden onset, such as being informed of an unexpected personal misfortune. But these are usually transient features and are soon replaced by a mood of sadness and discouragement very like that of the third stage.

PRECIPITATING FACTORS. In this form of depression it is usually not difficult to recognize the change as a response to some difficulty, for the patient is often preoccupied with the trouble itself and is ready to draw the link between it and his present mood. Precipitating situations can be of many kinds. They can be sudden and specific events in which something is lost, such as a relationship or a job. Other provocations are situations chronically thwarting to the sense of achievement and mastery, as in an education program in which students are confronted with their errors but given little effective teaching to overcome them. Moving away from home can provoke the very unpleasant depressive reaction, homesickness, especially in persons who depend a great deal on the support of friends and family. In general, circumstances that disturb a person's sense of stability, security, effectiveness, or worth provoke depressive responses.

The more such a precipitant is prolonged or accompanied by a growing realization of his difficulties, the more likely the person is to show a depressive response. A paradigm of these features for a precipitant is found in debilitating physical illnesses such as cancer. Here the protracted and continually worsening clinical situation provides constant reminders of losses suffered and brings more each day. That depression is a universal occurrence in such circumstances has been demonstrated by Hinton in his study of the dying.

For reasons not fully understood, there are some physiologic states and physical illnesses that commonly provoke depressive moods. Patients with hepatitis or any severe viral illness are particularly prone to report a depressive mood and to find reasons for it in trifles that did not trouble them when they were well. Endocrine alterations such as the postpartum state, Cushing's disease, or Addison's disease are also precipitants of depressive feelings that can be very distressing to the patient and of such profound degree as to occasionally promote a suicidal action. Certain brain diseases, particularly stroke, may also precipitate a prolonged and distressing depressive state. In all these circumstances the mood of depression may rest on some disturbed physiologic mechanism in the central nervous system as yet unknown. Their possible relationship to manic-depressive disorder is discussed above.

PREDISPOSING FACTORS. Given that situations of difficulty can lead to depression, there are features of personality that can make an individual more vulnerable to this response, perhaps by making him assess losses and difficulties more acutely and by inhibiting his power to resolve them. Especially vulnerable are those insecure and sensitive individuals who perceive criticism when none is intended and find a source of depressive feelings in their self-doubting.

Another depressive predisposition is that of the self-dramatizing and emotionally unstable and immature individual who tends to amplify emotional reactions of all sorts. When such an individual finds himself in situations of discomfort in which his feelings may be neglected, he seems more prone than others to develop a sense of dissatisfaction, distress, and depression. Slavney and McHugh present empirical evidence of this predisposition in their report of depressive symptoms in 80 per cent of patients hospitalized with the diagnosis of hysterical personality.

Finally, individuals limited in their capacity to cope with difficulties are predisposed to depressive responses. Particularly vulnerable for this reason are the mentally retarded. Even modest impairment in intellectual endowment will interfere with the person's ability to find solutions to situations that present him problems, and his failure and uncertainty tend to provoke a depressive mood. Borderline mental retardation is often overlooked in the search for predisposing factors, and a history of poor occupational and scholastic performance in a depressed patient warrants formal intelligence testing.

Social factors have been considered important in depression since Durkheim. Brown and Harris have documented in a careful epidemiologic study a group of predisposing features for depression among women in an urban setting. It was more frequent in working class than in middle class women and was highly related to threatening life events. Whether the woman suffered a depressive response to these events seemed to depend on four other vulnerability factors. These were the presence of three or more children under 14 at home; no employment for the woman outside the home; absence of a confiding, intimate relationship, as with the husband; and loss of the woman's mother before age 11. Such predisposing features emphasize the isolated life experience of young mothers and the importance of efforts to help them with these aspects as well as to aid them over more acute crises.

DIFFERENTIAL DIAGNOSIS. The differential diagnosis of depressive states can be difficult, particularly if it is not carried out methodically. The most important distinction to draw is that between depression as a response to troubled circumstances and depression as a symptom of manic-depressive disorder. This important discrimination rests on clinical grounds and cannot be made with certainty in all situations. Thus, although the depressions of the widow, the homesick, and the patient with a fatal illness can all be recognized as responses, the trap is in making this understandable connection with every depression and explaining it always as being due to some recent difficulty. If the family of the patient says he is more depressed than they would expect him to be under the circumstances, the diagnosis of a depressive response might be questioned. Also, the presence in the patient of remarkable changes in self-attitude such as the appearance of beliefs that he is a criminal or deserves punishment for minor transgressions, or that he is infectious and filled with physical corruption, are not seen in the usual depressive response and should lead to the consideration of manic-depressive psychosis. Finally, a previous history of mania or of depression, or a family history of affective disorder, should influence the interpretation of depression and sway the diagnosis away from the depressive response (see above).

TREATMENT. Although the depressive response is characteristic enough to be recognized easily again and again, the particular predispositions, precipitants, and interactions are never exactly the same from one patient to another. Treatment is based on these particulars and is thus unique to some extent to each occasion. It is therefore hard to describe the treatment of depression without some sense of dissatisfaction because, although the principles are simple, no list of them applies to every patient.

An important early decision in treatment is the need for hospitalization. This is usually determined by how severely the mood disturbance interferes with self-care, by the availability of a supportive and protective environment at home, and particularly by the presence of suicidal features. To assess the last, the patient must be asked if he has been considering self-injury. Although judgment is required in evaluating his answers, a sequence of questions probing for suicidal thoughts should be routine for every patient with depression. A proportion of the patients will deny all thought of self-injury and can be assumed to be of lesser suicidal risk. Those who admit to such thoughts should be asked if they have any means in mind. To that question still more patients will reassure the doctor that their thoughts on suicide have not reached so severe an intensity. Those patients, however, who admit to having considered a means (pill, gas, shooting) must be considered of higher risk, and thought must be given to protecting them, perhaps by hospitalization or by guaranteeing that they are under the supervision of friends or relatives. Finally, the patients should be asked if they have acquired any means or done anything to try them out. Again a proportion of patients will say that they have not been that despondent, but those who say that they have done such things are at very high risk and should in most cases be hospitalized.

Once a decision is made about the site of treatment, in a hospital or on an outpatient basis, the act of reaching a secure diagnosis of a depressive reaction in a patient is the first step in its treatment, because this judgment requires that the doctor has come to understand the patient and his predicament. To gain this understanding the doctor's first meetings should be devoted to listening to the patient's description of his circumstances, of his emotional changes, and of the connections he draws between his experiences and his depressive mood. If appropriate, other informants such as relatives can amplify on the patient's statements and give details of his past modes of coping with trouble. All these efforts are intended to bring the doctor an appreciation of this particular individual and the circumstances that he faces. Such knowledge, combined with the relationships of trust, respect, and empathy that develop naturally in its acquisition, provides the resources for treatment.

The therapeutic efforts from this foundation are directed toward re-engaging the patient in life experiences in which success can be found, replacements for losses enjoyed, and a sense of integrity and control regained. Usually the first need of the patient is some help in simple tactics for the management of his current troubles and for the avoidance of their repetition in the future.

At this stage a sense of helplessness often prompts the patient to abandon many of his activities and efforts, but if at all possible he must be encouraged not to give in to these promptings, because doing so tends to perpetuate the disturbed mood by holding him from opportunities to reassess his situation and to try out solutions. His daily work, even when less efficiently performed, is often helpful in directing his attention to matters other than his troubles.

With assistance in simple matters of personal management, the patient can be helped to some success in his circumstances, bringing him encouragement and promoting a willingness to maintain his efforts and to plan for the future. Educating the patient in how certain circumstances strike his particular vulnerabilities and so provoke depressive responses can be helpful.

The most useful ingredient of the treatment is the support and interest of the doctor. This is particularly true for those depressive feelings that emerge in the context of chronic or progressive medical illness. Patients report that the supportive information and sense of planning together provided by the physician managing such an illness are major sources of encouragement and relief. Such support encourages the patient to express his feelings and discuss his circumstances. In this way not only is the physician provided with more information about assets and vulnerabilities of the patient, but often there is spontaneous recognition by the patient of causal features for his difficulties that brings both relief to his mood and self-perceived tactics for their resolution. If this supportive relationship can be maintained and developed, improvement of depression can be expected. For the occasional patient with whom such a relationship fails or who succumbs frequently to depressive reactions because of some intractable predisposition, more prolonged treatment by specialists in psychotherapy can be recommended.

Finally, treatment with pharmaceutical agents may help. Chlordiazepoxide, 10 mg three times daily, may relieve agitation somewhat in the bereaved or otherwise reactively depressed. A sleeping medication, flurazepam hydrochloride (Dalmane), is helpful for the sleeplessness. The *antidepressant medications,* although most useful in the manic-depressive psychoses, can be tried in some patients with a prolonged depressive response. Imipramine in a dose of 150 to 250 mg a day or the monoamine oxidase inhibitor phenelzine, 15 mg three times daily, has helped individual patients, but this symptomatic relief should be considered a minor part of the treatment plan in patients with this form of depression.

Brown G, Harris T: Social Origins of Depression. London, Tavistock, 1978. *A readable account of several years of painstaking research on the psychosocial causes of depression in women.*

Durkheim E: Suicide: A Study in Sociology. (Translated by George Simpson.) Glencoe, IL, Free Press, 1951. *An excellent translation of this classic study by one of the fathers of sociology.*

Parkes CM: Bereavement: Studies of Grief in Adult Life. London, Tavistock, 1972. *A comprehensive and invaluable book for this universal human problem.*

Hysteria

DEFINITION. Hysteria is a disturbance of behavior in which symptoms and signs of physical ill health are imitated more or less unconsciously for some personal advantage. As the phrase "more or less unconsciously" implies, hysteria may be hard to distinguish from "malingering," in which the imitation of illness is a well-appreciated fraud. Frank malingering is rare, though, because the power of human self-deception is usually adequate to persuade a person of the validity of his own symptoms. The only ones who can be called malingerers with any confidence are some self-mutilating patients and the remarkable pathologic liars, picturesquely called examples of the *Munchausen syndrome,* who travel from hospital to hospital gaining admission by means of dramatic acts of illness.

PREDISPOSING AND PRECIPITATING FACTORS. Hysterical symptoms are to be seen as responses to distressing experiences. They can occur in almost any person facing danger or difficulty, especially if, as with soldiers in battle or prisoners, the distress is intense and prolonged and physical symptoms can provide a viable escape. Dull-witted or immature persons with inadequate powers of introspection and self-control may produce transparently hysterical symptoms in response to milder distress, such as school difficulties or family problems. Some of the exaggerations and elaborations of medical symptoms common in hospitalized patients may be similarly interpreted as responses to the distress of illness by persons whose capacity for self-control has been weakened by somatic illness. Hysterical symptoms can be the first manifestations of a dementing illness or of a depressive or schizophrenic psychosis, and these disorders must be considered when a previously well-balanced adult develops a suspiciously hysterical symptom.

Commonly, though, hysteria is a disturbance in the behavior of a person predisposed by an attention-seeking, emotionally unstable, and egocentric personality. In fact, these characteristics form what has become known as the "hysterical personality" even though hysteria can occur in other types of people, and these characteristics do not invariably produce hysterical symptoms. Most easily recognized in such people is their flair for the dramatic, and thus the recent term *histrionic personality* has been applied to them in the new American psychiatric classification (DSM III). They show this tendency in flamboyant dress and in exaggerated, even melodramatic, responses to questions about their symptoms. They are never so happy as when they are the center of attention. Karl Jaspers characterized the hysterical personalities as those who "crave to appear, both to themselves and others, as more than they are and to experience more than they are capable of." The zeal of these patients for exaggeration and drama renders them more liable to hysterical symptoms. But other kinds of people can have these symptoms. In all of them usually a discouraged, depressive mood has been prompted by difficulties in life, and the hysterical symptoms then emerge from this mood state.

As implied by the concept of gain from imitation of illness, there are social predisposing factors here. Perhaps most fundamental is the social advantages that derive in our society from what Parsons has called the "sick role." The sick are relieved of certain obligations such as working and self-sufficiency with the assumption that sickness is a state that is of itself unpleasant, that the patient is involuntarily victim to sickness, and that he will do all that is required to escape from it. For certain circumstances and certain people the "sick role" may offer such attractions that the illness-imitating behavior that we call hysterical appears. It is likely that the irritation some doctors feel for these patients derives from the belief that the patients are gaining unfair advantages and wasting resources needed by others. It is perhaps helpful to employ Pilowski's concept of "abnormal illness behavior" for these patients and so extricate ourselves from an inappropriate, judgmental, and ineffective approach toward them.

SYMPTOMS AND SIGNS. Many of the phenomena of somatic illness can be imitated by hysteria. The accuracy of the imitation depends on the medical sophistication of the patient. A doctor or nurse is more likely to produce a convincing imitation than is an unqualified person.

Common hysterical symptoms are vague subjective disorders, such as generalized weakness, dizziness, indigestion, or pain. Hysterical pain can occur in any part of the body, but the head and neck, the region over the heart, and the low back are particularly favored. Hysterical pain can be of any character, from dull aching to sharp and stabbing pain, but it is often described by the patient in vivid similes such as "like a bullet," "like a bolt of lightning," "aches like an abscessed tooth," or "sore as a hot boil." Usually, hysterical pain is not confined to a local area as around a pathologic lesion, nor is it referred into the distribution of a particular nerve or dermatome. Rather, hysterical pain is felt in a general region of the body and spreads, sometimes in bizarre ways, into contiguous areas without regard to neuroanatomic boundaries. Thus pain beginning in the face may spread along the side of the head and into the back, crossing from the region of the trigeminal nerve into the upper cervical nerve regions. Hysterical pain often varies in its character, intensity, and distribution, changing considerably with attention or suggestion. Occasionally it can be remarkably improved by a small amount of intravenous amobarbital sodium when analgesics do not help.

Although vague symptoms of a subjective kind such as pain or dizziness are the present vogue in hysteria, crude and gross symptoms are still seen. These may be psychologic, such as the amnesia or fugue states, in which memory is partially lost, often in situations in which the patient is depressed or anxious. Other psychologic symptoms shown occasionally include auditory and visual hallucinations and even flamboyant delusions. These must be carefully judged, but appear most commonly in young people who have read popular books on psychology and psychiatry and are apparently suggested into these symptoms by their reading at a time when they are distressed over other matters.

Motor disturbances in the form of abnormal movement, disturbed gaits, seizures, or paralyses are occasionally hysterical symptoms. Hysterical seizures can usually be distinguished from epileptic ones. The patients only rarely injure themselves, bite their tongues, or lose their urine. They do not have the typical tonic and then clonic phases of a seizure, but tend to show a dramatic flailing of the limbs. Consciousness is partially retained, and seizures hardly ever occur when the patient is alone. The EEG is normal.

Sensory disturbances are particularly favored hysterical symptoms. Thus, *blindness* or *deafness* is common, often developing dramatically at a time of emotional distress. Loss of sensation over one side of the body to pin prick or light touch is frequently found after a susceptible patient has been examined by a neurologist.

DIAGNOSIS. Diagnosis of hysteria is seldom easy and never popular. Ideally, it should rest on three supports: first, the *form* of the hysterical manifestation; second, the *personality* of the patient; and third, the *setting* in which the symptoms developed. Often it is not possible to find all three supports to a diagnosis, but all should be sought.

Commonly, hysterical symptoms are vague and variable. In fact, the more definite and consistent a patient's description of the onset, location, nature, and duration of his symptoms, the less likely the symptoms are to be hysterical. Hysterical symptoms and signs are also usually incompatible with what is known of anatomy and physiology. Thus sensory losses do not conform to patterns of nerve distribution; reflexes remain intact and unchanged in the palsies of arm and leg; seizures of the entire body do not disturb consciousness; total blindness appears without a disturbance of pupillary reflex or of opticokinetic nystagmus. The hysterically mute person can phonate on coughing. The hysterically deaf person speaks louder to be heard over increased ambient noises. Many other hysterical symptoms have been analyzed for such inconsistencies by Head.

Knowledge of the personality and past history of the patient is helpful to a diagnosis of hysteria. The recognition that the symptoms are occurring in an hysterical personality should prompt an observer to look very closely at the symptoms before embarking on extensive laboratory tests or upon surgery. Similarly, knowledge of a previous vague and poorly understood medical disturbance can lend weight to an opinion that a new symptom that has eluded diagnosis is occurring in an individual prone to hysteria. Conversely, hysteria can usually be eliminated as an explanation for symptoms in an emotionally stable, middle-aged person. People who have passed through adolescence and young adulthood without resorting to hysterical behavior are unlikely to employ it when older.

The setting in which the symptoms develop should be carefully scrutinized, and a search made for a distressing event that may have provoked an hysterical reaction or for any purpose that the hysterical symptoms may serve. Occasionally, a clear association between the symptoms chosen and a particular recent disturbance in the life of the subject can be found, such as an amnesia developing in a person who has done something shameful or criminal, or weakness and pain persisting in a person who is seeking financial compensation for an injury. Often, though, motivations behind hysterical symptoms are vague and uncertain. It is usual to find that the patient is unhappy or anxious about some aspect of his life circumstances and that the hysterical symptoms serve to call attention to his distress. Also, it may be possible to demonstrate that the development of particular symptoms has been prompted by suggestion: weakness of legs, for example, developing in a nurse caring for a paraplegic patient, or peculiar falling attacks after the patient has witnessed an epileptic seizure.

Guzé and his associates have pointed out a subgroup of patients with a chronic hysterical disorder who have had recurrent complaints of symptoms involving almost every bodily system. These patients, with what Guzé terms *Briquet's syndrome,* present diagnostic difficulties to many specialists as their complaints change, worsen, and improve in unpredictable ways. They usually have undergone multiple medical and surgical procedures. The same criteria that lead to the diagnosis of single hysterical symptoms can be applied to this group. Additionally they can be reliably differentiated from most medical patients by the sheer number of systems that have been involved in their past complaints.

A careful study of the symptoms, the personality, and the life setting of a patient usually allows a reasonably certain differentiation of hysterical symptoms from those of a medical illness. There are, however, certain medical problems that are notoriously easily confused with hysteria. These are the diseases that produce vague and changing symptoms that seem to vary with the patient's motivation and, at least in their early phases, lack convincing physical signs. If such an illness occurs in a patient who has features of the hysterical personality and who will therefore describe the symptoms in a dramatic and flamboyant fashion, physicians may be even more persuaded to believe that the illness is only deceptively physical. Examples of diseases frequently confused with hysteria because of their subtle clinical features are the first attack of multiple sclerosis, particularly if sensory changes alone are produced; the weakness of arms and legs seen early in acute idiopathic polyneuritis of the Guillain-Barré type; the difficulty in swallowing of bulbar myasthenia gravis; the attacks of muscular weakness in periodic paralysis; the tonic posturings and oculogyric crises of postencephalitic parkinsonism; the pain of a cauda equina tumor; and the abdominal pain of acute intermittent porphyria.

MANAGEMENT OF HYSTERIA. The management of hysterical patients is difficult. No one method can be recommended unqualifiedly. But there are certain principles that can be followed. To help hysterical patients it is essential to have sympathy for them. Many doctors find these patients irritating. It is just as possible to see them as individuals displaying an intriguing aspect of human behavior that has profound implications in their lives. It is pointless to argue with these patients about the validity of their symptoms. A useful approach is to agree that they have had an illness producing their symptoms, but that they are now improving even though total recovery has not arrived.

It is important to diagnose hysteria promptly. Hesitation in diagnosis leading to several hospital admissions for extensive laboratory investigations is a good way to solidify hysterical symptoms in a patient. Among other things, the uncertainty of doctors helps persuade a patient that the symptoms are real. Repeated examinations increase the consistency with which symptoms are reported. Long hospitalization, mounting bills, and the inconvenience caused to others make it difficult for a patient to abandon symptoms without embarrassment. The gratifying attention given to the patient in the hospital, perhaps as an example of an intriguing diagnostic problem, can feed the self-dramatizing tendencies and so encourage the behavior.

There is always a risk of error in any diagnosis, because diagnosis is only a weighing of probabilities. The diagnosis of hysteria, though, depends purely on a physician's judgment and, before relief of symptoms is accomplished, can be confirmed in the laboratory only by evidence of health. Physicians, for obvious reasons, fear more the error of calling a physically sick patient hysterical than the error of mishandling hysteria. They often prefer to exclude, by laboratory examination, progressively more unlikely diseases than to study carefully the symptoms and the individual who has produced them, even though this would lead more directly to a definite diagnosis as well as an understanding of the response. It may be unwise to counsel too strongly against this behavior because medical diagnosis is never easy. A compromise can be found in the admonition to perform immediately the laboratory tests that seem necessary for a patient but, when hysteria is suspected, to bring the period of investigation as quickly as possible to a close so that management of the specific symptom can be begun.

Treatment of the specific symptoms rests basically upon persuasion. The doctor is persuading the patient to perform the functions that the patient claims are disabled. Intravenous amobarbital sodium given to the point at which the patient is mildly intoxicated and his speech slurred is particularly helpful in making and establishing a persuasion. Usually, some ingenuity is required for success. The hysterically blind person can, for example, be persuaded first that he can distinguish light from dark and then gradually to distinguish forms, to read large print, and, finally, small newspaper type. The person who claims he cannot walk can be encouraged first to move his legs in bed, and then to stand, to make a few tentative shuffles, and finally to stride out. The hysterically deaf person can be persuaded to hear through a stethoscope and then gradually that he can hear without it. A dramatic show of some kind is often helpful in removing these symptoms. If a physician has success in partially removing hysterical symptoms, he should persist in his treatment without interruption in order to bring about as much improvement as possible and even to restore full function. When there is recovery of function, the patient should perform his recovered skills in public—before his family, other patients, and several doctors—to prevent his relapsing immediately into his former state.

The fear that sudden removal of hysterical symptoms will result in a disastrous psychologic collapse is exaggerated. Rarely, a depressed patient with hysterical symptoms has an increase in depression, but it is clear that in those situations a depression was overlooked and the more secondary hysterical symptoms were emphasized.

Some hysterical disorders are refractory to treatment. Among these are the disorders assumed for some material gain, such as compensation. They usually are not improved until some settlement is made. Episodic disorders such as hysterical seizures can be hard to control. Sometimes, however, a statement to the patient that they will not recur, given with full authority by a physician whom the patient trusts and respects, may eliminate these symptoms. The longer the patient has hysterical symptoms, the harder they are to remove. This is a corollary to the aforementioned observation that hysterical symptoms produced for transparent reasons and bordering on malingering are more difficult to eliminate than are the ones produced by an attention-seeking personality in some emotional distress.

Simultaneously with treatment of the specific symptoms, the emotional state and present life of the patient should be studied to discover any distress that may have precipitated the hysterical symptoms. Then advice, social assistance, or guidance can be offered to aid the patient in resolving these difficulties. This aspect of their psychologic treatment depends on developing a relationship of friendship and mutual respect identical to that found necessary in treating an anxious or depressed person.

Long-term management of hysterical patients is much more difficult than treatment of individual symptoms. It is not wise to have the average hysterical patient embark on depth psychotherapy, because he tends to produce more symptoms and to recount involved sexual and other fantasies in order to maintain the interest of his doctor. If possible, these patients should be followed by one physician who understands them and the behavior that they are liable to produce and is also competent to recognize physical illness should it arise. This physician can save these patients from needless surgery and long hospitalization. He can remove hysterical symptoms promptly by being alert to the diagnosis and providing help for the difficulties that precipitate them.

Guzé S: The validity and significance of the clinical diagnosis of hysteria (Briquet's syndrome). Am J Psychiatry 132:138, 1975. *This paper demonstrates the means and clinical utility of distinguishing patients with a chronic hysterical disorder.*

Head H: The diagnosis of hysteria. Br Med J 1:827, 1922. *A valuable description of a variety of hysterical manifestations that can be confused with neurologic disorders.*

Pilowski I: Abnormal illness behavior. Br J Med Psychol 42:347, 1969. *A most intriguing way of looking at hysteria as a socially provoked abnormal behavior.*

477. DRUG ABUSE AND DEPENDENCE

Robert B. Millman

Drug abuse results from the complex interaction of an individual, his social and cultural environment, and the pharmacology and availability of particular drugs. Frequently no sharp line distinguishes appropriate use from misuse of any drug. Drug abuse may therefore be defined as the use of any substance in a manner that deviates from the accepted medical, social, or legal patterns within a given society. These substances may be grouped into six major classes: (1) opiates; (2) central nervous system depressants, including alcohol, hypnotics, and tranquilizers; (3) central nervous system stimulants, including the amphetamine group and cocaine; (4) cannabis; (5) psychedelics; and (6) miscellaneous inhalants.

Abuse of some drugs may be intermittent and lead to little physical, psychologic, or social deterioration. In other cases, the user may become dependent on the drug in order to function at what he perceives to be a satisfactory level. This *psychologic dependence*, or habituation, varies in intensity and may culminate in *compulsive drug abuse*, in which the supply and use of particular drugs become primary concerns of living. In addition, certain drugs have the capacity to produce *physical dependence*. This is an altered physiologic state induced by the repeated administration of a drug that requires the continued administration of the drug to prevent the appearance of a syndrome characteristic for each drug, the *withdrawal*, or *abstinence, syndrome*. The term *"addiction"* should be reserved for a pattern of compulsive drug use that includes an overwhelming involvement with the acquisition and use of a drug, loss of control, and a tendency to relapse after withdrawal.

ETIOLOGY AND PATTERNS OF ABUSE. Initially, drugs may be taken to satisfy curiosity, to reduce pain, to influence mood, to change activity levels, to reduce tension and anxiety, to decrease fatigue and boredom, to facilitate social interaction, to heighten sensation and awareness, and for many other reasons. If caffeine, nicotine, alcohol, and prescription and over-the-counter depressants and stimulants are included, few people in the United States would be found who take no psychoactive drugs. Patterns of abuse vary from the experimental or intermittent use of a particular drug or combination under defined circumstances, such as the use of marijuana and alcohol at a party, to a compulsive "polydrug-abuse" pattern, in which a variety of drugs are taken in a disorganized and dangerous manner on a daily basis.

SOCIOLOGIC FACTORS AND EPIDEMIOLOGY. Social and cultural factors determine initial drug-experimentation patterns and define acceptable drug-abuse behaviors for a given group. The use of alcohol is condoned and even encouraged in many segments of society. Cocaine and depressant use have become an integral part of membership in some urban upper-middle-class groups. During the past several years, the use of heroin by the upper classes also has increased.

Drug-use trends may be broadly summarized. Large increases in the prevalence of marijuana use occurred in the mid-1960's among adolescents and young adults, particularly males and those living in metropolitan areas. This trend continued in the late 1960's, accompanied by increased involvement by other age groups, those living in rural areas, and females. Increased use of other drug classes occurred during this period as well. Currently (1984), the prevalence of marijuana and depressant use is remaining stable; heroin and cocaine use is increasing, and amphetamine and hallucinogen use has declined.

PSYCHOBIOLOGIC FACTORS. Personality and constitutional factors, in part, determine the individual's psychoactive responses and influence the choice of drugs and patterns of abuse. Amphetamines may produce tranquility in some people. Alcohol and barbiturates impair behavior control in others and may permit certain personality types to act in a hostile and violent manner. Genetic factors have been strongly implicated in the development of alcoholism.

No predictive test or system will determine whether or not a person will become a compulsive user, or which people will use which drugs. It is generally agreed that the experimental or intermittent abuse of drugs is not necessarily an indication of psychopathology. Compulsive drug use is frequently associated with psychopathology. In some people the drug use may be an attempt at *self-medication* of painful feelings of anxiety, shame, inadequacy, loneliness, guilt, and depression. Others may be seeking to allay unacceptable aggressive or sexual drives or to control psychotic symptoms. At the same time, some severely disturbed people have experimented with alcohol, opiates, and other drugs and have not become compulsive users.

Conditioned learning is an integral part of the development and maintenance of compulsive drug-abuse patterns. This may occur in the presence or absence of physical dependence. The drug-craving and withdrawal syndrome that long abstinent ex-addicts experience when they return to a site of former drug use is, in part, a reflection of this conditioning process. Learning also influences the nature of the subjective drug experience. The prolonged use of psychoactive drugs to treat medical illness sometimes induces addiction.

PHARMACOLOGIC FACTORS. *Tolerance* refers to the decreased effect obtained from repeated administration of a given dose of a drug or to the need for increased amounts to obtain the effects that occurred from the first dose. Tolerance may be either *drug disposition* (metabolic) in type, in which there is more rapid inactivation or excretion of a drug, or *pharmacodynamic* (cellular), in which cells in the nervous system adapt to drug concentrations. Both may occur with the same drug. The physical dependence that develops concurrently with tolerance to opiates, barbiturates, and alcohol is poorly understood and may be related to pharmacodynamic tolerance mechanisms. *Cross-dependence* refers to the ability of one drug to suppress abstinence symptoms produced by withdrawal of another. Cross-dependence may be complete or partial, as with alcohol and the barbiturates.

DIAGNOSIS. To provide adequate treatment, one must characterize the specific problems of drug abuse and dependence, the psychologic set, and the social situation. The nature and degree of drug-induced psychoactive effects and any abstinence symptoms and signs should be assessed. Drug abusers are often poor historians and may minimize or exaggerate the extent of their drug use, depending on their perception of the situation, their needs, and the attitude of the examiner. It is likely that an opiate user will exaggerate the extent of his use so as to obtain more opiates during the detoxification process and perhaps suffer decreased abstinence symptoms. A college student may minimize his diazepam dependence, since the extent of his use might be considered evidence of weakness or serious psychopathology.

Evaluation of the mode of administration and the adverse effects of the drugs is important in diagnosis. Signs of repeated intravenous injections ("tracks") suggest heroin, amphetamine, or cocaine abuse. These drugs are also "sniffed," whereby the material is inhaled and absorbed through the mucous membranes of the nasopharynx and respiratory tract, a route suggested by chronic sinusitis or perforation of the nasal septum.

Routine qualitative procedures for the detection in urine of morphine (the major metabolite of heroin), methadone, amphetamines, cocaine, marijuana, and the most frequently abused general depressants are currently available in many laboratories. Agents usually are detected if a dose sufficient to produce pharmacologic effects has been taken within 24 hours prior to the urine sample. Since results are not immediately available ordinarily and since false positives occur, these tests should be used to confirm the clinical impression. They are most useful as an adjunct to the continuing evaluation of patients already in treatment. In emergency situations, blood levels of suspected drugs can usually be obtained immediately.

TREATMENT AND PREVENTION. Treatment of specific addictions is given in subsequent sections. Drug abusers are often faced with prejudice and hostility on the part of treatment personnel; e.g., "They did it to themselves." Since many of their personality characteristics and behavior patterns occur in response to the attitudes of society, an inquiring, compassionate stance is crucial in the treatment of this group of patients.

Drug abusers often relapse after detoxification and varying periods of abstinence. This tends to frustrate the physician or the treatment team, who may give up on particular patients. The problem may be conceptual; physicians often regard substance abuse as an acute illness, not unlike pneumonia, and liable to complete cure after detoxification. This is an unrealistic assumption given the chronic nature of most psychologic and social difficulties. Then, too, the pharmacologic dependence may be more protracted than previously imagined. Patience and continuing enthusiasm are as essential as in most other branches of medicine.

Drug-abuse prevention programs have focused on educational efforts, in which the risks of drug abuse are publicized, and on legal sanctions. Both approaches have serious deficiencies. Perhaps more important than either of these would be the provision of reasonably attractive vocational, recreational, and educational alternatives to drug abuse in those most at risk, namely, the young and psychosocially disadvantaged. Physicians must be extremely prudent in prescribing potentially abusable drugs.

Jaffe J: Drug addiction and drug abuse. *In* Gilman AG, Goodman LS, Gilman A (eds.): The Pharmacological Basis of Therapeutics. 6th ed. New York, Macmillan, 1980, pp 535–584. *Overview of pharmacologic and clinical aspects of drug use and abuse.*

Lowinson JH, Ruiz P. (eds.): Substance Abuse: Clinical Problems and Perspectives. Baltimore, Williams and Wilkins, 1981. *Exhaustive compendium of substance abuse–related subjects considered from multiple perspectives.*

Pradhan SN, Dutta SN (eds.): Drug Abuse, Clinical and Basic Aspects. St. Louis, C. V. Mosby Company, 1977. *Comprehensive textbook on the pharmacology and clinical aspects of the drugs of abuse.*

OPIATES

Opiates or narcotic analgesics refer to natural or synthetic drugs that have pharmacologic actions similar to those of the derivatives of opium. Opium is obtained from the poppy plant *Papaver somniferum* and contains more than 20 alkaloids, of which morphine and codeine are relevant to this discussion. Heroin, the principal opiate of abuse in the United States, is converted from morphine by the addition of two acetyl groups (diacetyl-morphine). Meperidine and methadone are synthetic narcotic analgesics. Pentazocine is a synthetic analgesic compound that has actions similar to both the opiates and the narcotic antagonists.

INCIDENCE. People have used opium for medical, religious, or recreational purposes since ancient times. The use of patent medicines containing opiates was widespread in the United States during the period from 1850 to 1906, when the labeling requirements of the Pure Food and Drug Act caused many preparations to be withdrawn. The Harrison Narcotics Act of 1914 and Supreme Court decisions in the 1920's made possession of narcotics without a prescription a crime and created a climate in which addicts were considered to be criminals and in which physicians could not prescribe narcotics to addicts. The number of oral opiate users declined, and the primary remaining group were those who injected heroin or morphine. Illegal dealers became the only source of opiates. Prices rose precipitously, and addicts frequently resorted to criminal activity to finance their addiction. The growth of urban ghettos and the development of efficient production and delivery systems ushered in the present era of extensive heroin use associated with a pervasive street culture that supports the heroin-dependent life.

Heroin use reached epidemic proportions in the United States in the mid- to late 1960's. The majority of users were members of urban ethnic minority groups. Males predominated over females, and the population was quite young. After a decline in heroin use during the mid-1970's, there has been a resurgence of the problem. People of diverse socioeconomic and cultural groups are involved, including the urban affluent. A similar phenomenon is occurring in western Europe and appears to be related to increased supplies of more pure forms of heroin from southwest Asia and Iran. Estimates vary widely, although between 5 and 10 per cent of the youthful and young adult population in the United States are reported to have used the drug. Heroin addiction is a leading cause of death in urban males aged 15 to 35.

PATTERNS OF ABUSE. Street heroin ("smack," "scag," "junk," "dope") is adulterated ("cut") with quinine, lactose, mannitol, maltose, and other substances as it passes from the importer to the user. The purity of the final package varies enormously, from 4 to 70 per cent. Initial street use is generally by "sniffing." A user's first experience with the drug is often somewhat unpleasant because of nausea, vomiting, and anxiety; these symptoms abate with subsequent use. Effects may then be perceived as a sense of relaxation and peace with relief of worry and tension, a euphoric state in which all things are as they should be. At the outset, use may be intermittent and separated by weeks or months. It is not known how many people experiment with the drug and stop using it. Those who do continue to use heroin develop tolerance to its euphoric effects and begin to inject the drug subcutaneously and eventually intravenously ("mainlining"). Intravenous injection produces a warm flushing of the skin and pleasurable bodily sensations described as similar to sexual orgasm and called a "rush" or "kick." Chronic intravenous use of opiates and other drugs may occlude available veins, necessitating a return to subcutaneous injection.

As tolerance increases and physical dependence becomes manifest, more drug must be used more often; the street addict now devotes all his time and energy to supporting his addiction ("habit"). Involvement in the "junkie" subculture, with its own language and behavioral systems, ensures his supply of drug and provides the social structure that makes it possible to live as an addict. Any source of money is acceptable; males engage in theft and forgery, whereas females become prostitutes and shoplifters. Every user is a potential "dealer" of drugs, since this is the most efficient way of making money. Food, clothing, sexual desires, and dignity subordinate themselves to the ever-present need for opiates. In addition, an unknown number of heroin addicts are able to maintain employment and their families and avoid the behavior patterns of the street "junkie."

If heroin is not available or is in poor supply, addicts will use other opiates, particularly illicitly obtained ("street") methadone because of its long duration of action, to allay their withdrawal symptoms. Compulsive use of illicit methadone occurs, although usually after an initial period of heroin dependence. Most narcotic addicts also abuse alcohol, sedatives, stimulants, and marijuana, and mixed addictions are frequent.

Opiate addicts demonstrate appreciable psychopathology, including high levels of neurotic, personality, and psychotic characteristics, although no common pattern is apparent. Personality characteristics and behavior patterns result in part from the interaction of the addict and the drug in the sociocultural environment of addiction. Inner-city minority-group addicts are often remarkably stable given their difficult living situations and the high degree of personality integration and intelligence required to survive as a street addict. Middle-class people may be more severely disturbed, and the drug use may represent an attempt at self-medication for symptoms that reflect borderline or psychotic personality disorders.

PHARMACOLOGY. Morphine and heroin lose much of their analgesic potency when taken orally, whereas codeine and meperidine remain active, and methadone retains most of its analgesic efficacy after oral administration. Heroin is hydrolyzed to morphine in the body and, except for its greater potency and more rapid onset of action, has pharmacologic properties similar to those of morphine. Morphine is concentrated in parenchymatous tissues, skeletal muscle, and, to a lesser extent, brain. It is conjugated with glucuronic acid and excreted primarily in the urine and secondarily in the feces. Traces of morphine can be found in urine for 48 hours, although 90 per cent or more is excreted within the first 24 hours.

Administered subcutaneously, methadone and morphine exert approximately equal analgesic effects; heroin is three times stronger, whereas meperidine and codeine are approximately one tenth as potent. Morphine or heroin taken intravenously is effective almost immediately; duration of action varies from three to six hours. Oral administration prolongs the action of all the opiates, particularly that of methadone, in which the onset of effect occurs within 30 minutes and the duration of action in nontolerant individuals is four to ten hours.

Morphine or heroin administred to a nontolerant individual induces analgesia through a reduction in the anxiety and tension that result from the perception of pain. Related to this is a feeling of well-being or euphoria. Mental clouding, characterized by an inability to concentrate, sleepiness, or "nodding," also occurs. Opiates cause pupillary constriction, depression of respiration and body temperature, and stimulation of central nervous system centers to produce nausea and vomiting. Other acute effects include decreased motility of the stomach, diminished pancreatic and biliary secretions, decreased propulsive contractions of the small and large intestine, and increased tone of the anal sphincter, leading to constipation. Increased tone of the detrusor muscle leads to a sensation of urgency; increased tone of the vesical sphincter may result in urinary retention. Antidiuretic hormone release is stimulated while ACTH, corticotropin-releasing factor, and gonadotropin are inhibited. Peripheral vasodilatation produces pruritus and an increase in perspiration.

ADDICTION AND WITHDRAWAL PROCESSES. Repeated use of narcotic analgesics produces tolerance to most of the acute narcotic effects, and the lethal dose is markedly increased. Whereas a 10-mg dose of morphine may produce euphoria in a nontolerant individual, some addicts can consume as much as 5 grams daily. Tolerance to all the opiate effects does not occur equally; highly tolerant users will continue to demonstrate pupillary constriction and constipation. Cross-tolerance occurs with all narcotic analgesics. Tolerance to narcotics is primarily due to some form of cellular adaptation to the drug's action, with increased metabolism of lesser importance.

Physical dependence develops concurrently with tolerance and can emerge after only a few exposures on succeeding days. The syndrome varies according to the particular drug and its usage. With heroin, the first withdrawal signs are generally seen shortly before the next scheduled dose. They are purposive in nature and include feelings of anxiety, depression, restlessness, irritability, and drug craving. Lacrimation, rhinorrhea, yawning, and perspiration become apparent eight to fifteen hours after the last dose of narcotic. A restless sleep may intervene ("yen sleep") interrupted by more severe withdrawal symptoms and signs, including dilated pupils, sneezing, coryza, anorexia, nausea, vomiting, diarrhea, abdominal cramps, bone pains, myalgias, tremors, weakness, insomnia, goose flesh, and, very rarely, convulsions or cardiovascular collapse. With morphine and heroin, withdrawal symptoms peak at 36 to 48 hours, and most symptoms subside over the next five to ten days. With methadone, the onset of withdrawal symptoms is more gradual, the peak is less pronounced and later, and the duration may be more than two or three weeks. The abstinence syndrome may be precipitated within minutes in opiate-dependent persons by administration of a narcotic antagonist such as nalorphine, levallorphan, or naloxone, although there are no medical indications for this diagnostic procedure.

Pentazocine (Talwin), a drug with weak opiate-antagonist effects and moderate opiate-agonist effects, elicits morphine-like subjective effects in nontolerant individuals. Higher doses produce dysphoric effects, including nervousness, anxiety, and, infrequently, bizarre alterations in perception and behavior. To speed the onset of action of pentazocine and to lengthen the duration of psychoactive effects, pentazocine is frequently abused in combination with the antihistamine tripelennamine ("t's and blues"). Tolerance, physical dependence, and addiction can occur. Abrupt withdrawal of the drug from persons taking 500 to 700 mg daily results in irritability, abdominal cramps, nausea, vomiting, hyperthermia, lacrimation, and drug-seeking behavior. When pentazocine is administered to opiate-dependent patients, its antagonistic actions may precipitate withdrawal symptoms.

Subsequent to the termination of abstinence symptoms or after a course of detoxification, most addicts experience recurrent urges for narcotics and generally resume their use of these drugs. Psychologic factors play a role, however. Evidence is accumulating that metabolic and neurophysiologic changes persist long after the detoxification process is completed, as does some tolerance. Protracted abstinence signs, as indicated by alterations in blood pressure, pulse rate, body temperature, respiratory rate, and pupillary size, and symptoms, particularly depression and anxiety, have been documented for up to 30 weeks and may relate to the high incidence of relapse. The associations ex-addicts experience when they are exposed to their old neighborhoods and friends intensify the persistence of drug craving.

MECHANISM OF OPIATE ACTION. Structurally and sterically specific receptors for the opiates are located in areas of the nervous system associated with the integration of sensory information and emotion, particularly the limbic system. The presence of these receptors led to the discovery of naturally occurring morphine-like peptides in the brain and gastrointestinal tract (enkephalins) and pituitary gland (endorphins). The endogenous morphine-like compounds elicit analgesia, produce tolerance and physical dependence, and compete with radioactive opiates for the receptor. All the peptides so far identified except one have amino acid sequences present in the pituitary hormone, β-lipotropin. The enkephalins have been implicated in the control of pain, affective states, and appetitive drives. A model that includes a neurohumoral feedback mechanism has been postulated to play a part in the opiate addiction syndrome. If, under resting conditions, opiate receptors are exposed to a basal level of the morphine-like substances, when exogenous opiate is administered, the overloading of the receptors might suppress the synthesis or release of endogenous opioid. Termination of the exogenous opiate administration might deprive the receptor because of endogenous opioid deficiency, generating changes responsible for the immediate or protracted abstinence syndrome. The anxiety and panic of the opiate abstinence syndrome have been proposed to result from noradrenergic hyperactivity and have led to treatment of the state with adrenergic agonists (see below).

MEDICAL COMPLICATIONS. The patterns of use, unknown and markedly variable opiate dose, lack of hygienic administration techniques, and the variety of adulterants used to dilute the opiate produce an extensive morbidity and mortality (estimated to be about 1 to 3 per cent per year) associated with opiate abuse and dependence.

Acute heroin reactions secondary to the intravenous use of street drug are responsible for one half to four fifths of all fatalities from narcotics. Formerly thought of as true pharmacologic overdoses with respiratory depression, these reactions may also be due to opiate-induced cardiac arrhythmias or hypoxia by unexplained mechanisms. Acute reactions to adulterants, including quinine, allergic reactions, and synergistic effects from multiple-drug use, may also be implicated. The syndrome is marked clinically by the rapid development of cyanosis, pulmonary edema, respiratory distress, and varying levels of consciousness progressing to coma. Increased intracranial pressure and occasionally convulsive seizures are seen. Fever to 40° C may occur initially and may persist for 48 hours in association with leukocytosis. The pupils are usually pinpoint, although dilated, nonreactive pupils may occur with hypoxia or multiple-drug use. The pathologic picture includes pulmonary congestion and edema and frequently cerebral edema.

Skin abscesses, cellulitis, and *thrombophlebitis* are the most frequent complications of heroin addiction. Pentazocine injection causes characteristic chronic ulcers in areas of severe "woody" induration. *Septicemia* and *acute* and *subacute bacterial endocarditis* with involvement of either or both sides of the heart are seen. *Staphylococcus aureus* is frequently the causative organism in right-sided lesions. Peripheral and pulmonary embolic phenomena occur. Osteomyelitis occurs infrequently. The introduction of quinine as an adulterant and the eradication of malaria in this country have decreased the incidence of this complication.

Viral hepatitis transmitted by the communal use of contaminated needles is a frequent complication of intravenous drug use. Persistent abnormal liver function tests, hypergammaglobulinemia, and increased serum immunoglobulins are due in some cases to variants of chronic hepatitis, but may also be due to effects produced by alcohol, malnutrition, allergic phenomena, adulterants, and recurrent or chronic infections. False-positive serologic tests for syphilis and AIDS appear with appreciable incidence.

Pulmonary complications include pneumonia, abscess, infarction, and tuberculosis. Disseminated extrapulmonary tuberculosis has been reported. Angiothrombotic pulmonary hypertension and granulomatosis result from the intravenous injection of foreign bodies, including talc or cotton. Vascular lesions include local arterial occlusion, phlebitis, mycotic aneurysms, and necrotizing angiitis.

Neurologic complications of street heroin use include transverse myelitis, acute inflammatory polyneuropathy, peripheral nerve lesions, toxic amblyopia secondary to quinine, and muscle disorders, including acute rhabdomyolysis with myoglobinuria and a fibrosing chronic myopathy. Septic states may lead to bacterial meningitis and brain, subdural, and epidural abscesses. Narcotism is a leading cause of tetanus, particularly when the drugs are injected by the intramuscular route. Mortality rates lie in the 50 to 75 per cent range.

Pregnant addicts have a high incidence of toxemia and premature babies. Withdrawal symptoms are noted in a variable percentage of the newborns. Sexual difficulties, including decreased libido, impotence, and delayed ejaculation, are frequent in male heroin addicts.

Homicide, suicide, and *accidents* account for between 20 and 40 per cent of narcotic-related deaths. In any given case, it is often difficult to distinguish among the three.

TREATMENT. Methods of treatment of narcotic dependence vary, depending on the treatment goals, factors in the etiology of the addiction, and the characteristics of individual patients. The magnitude of the addict's desire to stop using opiates is an important factor in the selection of the appropriate treatment modality as well as in the outcome. These motivational factors are difficult to assess, since, within one or two years after the onset of the addiction, most addicts express the wish to terminate it. Nevertheless, many continue the compulsive use of heroin for many years and suffer repeated treatment failures. Approaches are primarily psychosocial, pharmacologic, or combinations of these. Since addiction has physical, psychologic, and social determinants, treatment is best provided by a well-organized team approach. Individual practitioners should be prepared to make an accurate diagnosis, treat the acute and chronic sequelae of the drug use, and effect the appropriate referral.

ACUTE OPIATE REACTIONS (OVERDOSE). If an acute opiate reaction is suspected, immediate nonspecific supportive, resuscitative measures should be instituted, and 0.4 mg of the narcotic antagonist naloxone should be given intravenously or intramuscularly. A positive response, consisting of pupillary dilatation, increased respiratory rate and minute volume, and increased alertness, should occur within one to two minutes after intravenous injection. If a positive response does not occur, a second 0.4-mg dose may be administered in five to ten minutes. If a positive response again fails to ensue, the existence of an acute opiate reaction is doubtful. If a response occurs, the patient's respiratory rate and volume and level of consciousness should be monitored for the next 24 hours, since the antagonistic actions of naloxone persist for only two to three hours, whereas the agonistic effects of large doses of heroin or morphine may last longer and the effects of methadone may persist for 24 to 36 hours. Naloxone administration may be repeated after two to three hours as necessary. If it is anticipated that the patient is physically dependent on narcotics, the initial intravenous injection of 0.4 mg of naloxone should be diluted to 0.1 mg per milliliter and given slowly and in the smallest amounts necessary, to minimize the precipitation of a violent abstinence syndrome. Evidence of infection or trauma should be sought and treated as necessary.

WITHDRAWAL TECHNIQUES. Withdrawal of narcotics is most effectively accomplished by inpatient or outpatient substitution of oral methadone for any of the natural or synthetic narcotic analgesics (detoxification). Doses ranging from 20 to 40 mg daily are instituted, followed by a gradual reduction of dosage over the course of 14 days or more. Detoxification with decreasing doses of propoxyphene napsylate, a mild analgesic, has been effective, particularly when the degree of dependence is minimal or methadone is not available. Clonidine,* an alpha-2-adrenergic agonist, has shown promise in suppressing the abstinence syndrome. After tapering and cessation of narcotic use, clonidine is given in divided doses of 0.1 to 0.2 mg. The dose is then increased over the course of the next four to ten days to a maximum of 1 to 1.5 mg daily in three divided doses. The clonidine is then tapered over a four- to five-day period. Clonidine can cause postural hypotension and sedation, necessitating close observation, frequent blood pressure checks, and dosage adjustment. Acupuncture has also been reported to be effective in reducing opiate withdrawal symptoms. As mentioned previously, however, whatever the treatment, the relapse rate remains high.

METHADONE MAINTENANCE. In the United States, methadone maintenance has been the most widely used approach in the treatment of opiate dependence. This mode of therapy emphasizes social and emotional rehabilitation rather than abstinence. The treatment is based on the two major properties that distinguish methadone from other narcotics: good oral efficacy and long duration of action. After oral ingestion in tolerant individuals, the duration of action of methadone is extended to 24 to 36 hours owing to a reservoir of drug in tissues. Initially, oral methadone is administered daily in doses that will allay symptoms of abstinence. The dose is gradually increased until a stabilization level is reached at which patients will be tolerant to the euphoric effects of the drug and will experience no persistent craving for opiates. If the stabilization level is high enough (60 to 100 mg), there is a good degree of cross-tolerance to the effects of other narcotics, such that the effects of even large doses of intravenous opiates will not be felt. Approximately 65 per cent of patients in well-run programs remain in treatment. Improvement has been noted in the work and school records of patients retained in the program, and their criminal activity has declined markedly. Long-term methadone maintenance has been shown to be medically safe, with no toxicity when properly administered. Performance and learning are normal in methadone-maintained subjects. Medication should be dispensed in a clinic situation that provides medical care and extensive rehabilitative services so as to facilitate satisfactory re-entry into non-drug-dominated ("straight") society. Late methadone detoxification is sometimes possible.

Many former addicts, although they may be heroin free, are unable to acquire the necessary skills and education to make a social adjustment. They continue to abuse alcohol and other drugs. Illicit diversion of methadone doses by clinic patients has led to the availability of the drug for the street-addict population.

NARCOTIC ANTAGONISTS. Naltrexone, a long-acting narcotic antagonist, should shortly become available for the treatment of detoxified addicts. This agent blocks the euphoriant effects of opiates and prevents the development of physical dependence in patients who continue to use opiates. Unfortunately, while naltrexone has proven to be effective in some patients when administered on a three-times-a-week basis, it does not relieve chronic opiate hunger, and patients tend to cease its use and relapse to heroin. Clinical trials are under way with buprenorphine, a drug that combines potent and long-term opiate agonist and antagonist properties. This promising new agent appears to suppress the opiate abstinence syndrome and blocks the effects of high doses of opiates. In contrast to methadone maintenance, abrupt termination of high-dose buprenorphine maintenance results in a mild, almost negligible withdrawal syndrome.

PSYCHOSOCIAL APPROACHES—ABSTINENCE PROGRAMS. A number of programs exist that emphasize abstinence from opiates and other drugs as a primary component of treatment. These take the form of either voluntary groups or supervised institutionalization.

Voluntary groups are generally self-regulatory in nature and staffed predominantly by former drug users. The individual remains in a closed, drug-free environment for variable periods of time, frequently one to two years, and is encouraged to develop a new set of social and living skills that will enable him to remain drug free upon completion of the program. Outpatient programs are also under way. Some of the well-known therapeutic communities are Daytop Village, Phoenix House, and Project Return. Therapeutic communities are valuable for many people, although only a small percentage of heroin addicts are motivated to enter a community, and follow-up studies of individuals who have returned to society are disappointingly few.

Results of traditional psychotherapy has been disappointing for most compulsive opiate abusers. Specialized forms of group psychotherapy may help some patients. After variable and sometimes prolonged periods of addiction, an unknown number of addicts spontaneously cease opiate use. This "maturing-out" process may be related to advanced age and the difficulty of obtaining drugs, a decline of internal psychologic conflicts, and the cumulative effect of various treatment programs.

Dole VP, Nyswander M: A medical treatment for diacetyl morphine (heroin) addiction. JAMA 193:646, 1965. *First description of methadone maintenance treatment.*

Gold MS, Rea WS: The role of endorphins in opiate addiction, opiate withdrawal and recovery. Psychiatr Clin North Am 6(3):489, 1983. *Data and theoretical framework relative to the role of endogenous opioids in addiction, and treatment implications. Extensive references.*

Sternbach G, Moran J, Eliastam M: Heroin addiction: Acute presentation of medical complications. Ann Emerg Med 9(3):161, 1980. *Review of the acute presentation of medical sequelae of heroin abuse and treatments. Extensive references.*

Stimmel B: Heroin Dependency: Medical, Economic and Social Aspects. New York, Stratton Intercontinental Medical Book Corporation, 1975. *Comprehensive discussion of heroin dependency and treatment.*

CENTRAL NERVOUS SYSTEM DEPRESSANTS

All central nervous system depressants are subject to abuse. The most frequently abused drugs in this category are the benzodiazepines, particularly diazepam (Valium) and chlordiazepoxide (Librium); the short-acting barbiturates, particularly pentobarbital (Nembutal) and secobarbital (Seconal); assorted other hypnotics such as glutethimide (Doriden), methyprylon (Noludar), and methaqualone (Quāālude); and amitriptyline (Elavil), an antidepressant with sedative properties. Bromide abuse has become rare.

INCIDENCE AND PATTERNS OF ABUSE. A continuum of depressant use extends from appropriate use to compulsive abuse and addiction. Depressants in general and the benzodiazepines in particular have become the most widely prescribed drugs throughout the world. Currently in western society, about one in five adult females and one in ten adult males take benzodiazepines or other depressants in the course of one year. Approximately 30 per cent of general practitioners and internists prescribe these drugs. The pattern of abuse may begin intermittently at night to decrease anxiety and ensure sleep, progress to nightly use with increased doses, and culminate in prolonged daily use to maintain an adequate level of function. Whereas the risk of serious dependence on the benzodiazepines is lower than with the hypnotics, the prevalence of tranquilizer use has led to substantial drug dependence, particularly in women. An individual may obtain drugs from several physicians at one time, none of whom is aware of the magnitude of the patient's use. Alcohol is frequently used in association with the depressants.

Hypnotic and tranquilizer use also involves the drug subcultures.

*This use is not listed in the manufacturer's directive.

Illicit sources of drugs are most often employed, and a wealth of street names have evolved, including "ludes" (methaqualone), "reds" (secobarbital), "yellows" (pentobarbital), and "double trouble" (amobarbital and secobarbital). Most use is oral, although some individuals inject the drugs intravenously or intramuscularly. The amounts taken vary, but some individuals ingest as much as 30 hypnotic doses of the short-acting barbiturates or benzodiazepines daily over many months.

Surveys suggest that 20 per cent of adolescents and young adults abuse depressants. Patterns and extent of use vary markedly, but generally depressants are taken in association with other drugs. Intermittent users may take several times the therapeutic dose, possibly in addition to marijuana, alcohol, and cocaine, to get "high" enough to enjoy a concert or party.

The "high" that the user obtains from abuse of depressant drugs has been characterized as the sense of tranquility or peace that occurs just prior to sleep in normal individuals. Inhibitions and anxiety are blunted, and there may be a feeling of aggressiveness, freedom, and pleasant numbness. Sexual pleasure and ability are said to be enhanced at low doses of these drugs; higher doses lead to a decreased ability to perform sexually. Violent and antisocial behavior frequently serves to isolate depressant abusers ("down heads") from other groups of drug abusers.

PHARMACOLOGY. Depressants are absorbed rapidly after oral administration and are distributed throughout the body. They are general depressants of nerves and of skeletal, smooth, and cardiac muscles, although at low doses the central nervous system is primarily affected. Central nervous system effects vary from mild sedation to coma, depending on the particular drug, the dose, the route of administration, the degree of excitability of the nervous system, and tolerance. In some individuals under certain circumstances, small doses produce an initial stimulation not unlike that produced by alcohol. Barbiturate-induced sleep is similar to physiologic sleep except for a reduction in the proportion of rapid eye movement (REM) sleeping time; benzodiazepines suppress REM sleep less. Duration of action varies with the particular depressants. Aftereffects, including drowsiness, depression, impairment of judgment and performance, and occasionally hyperexcitability, may persist for many hours.

Both drug-disposition and pharmacodynamic tolerance to the depressants develop rapidly with repeated administration. Drug-disposition tolerance in the short-acting barbiturates and some other depressants results from the activation of drug-metabolizing liver-enzyme systems and is characterized by the more rapid degradation of the drug and a decrease in sleeping time. The range of tolerance is narrow, and individuals tolerant to the sedating and intoxicating effects of 1 gram of pentobarbital may become intoxicated for prolonged periods upon the addition of 0.1 gram. Although the lethal dose of barbiturates varies in individuals, in distinction to the opiates, tolerance does not increase this dose significantly from that of nontolerant individuals. Severe poisoning is likely to occur when more than ten times the hypnotic dose is ingested at one time. Acute barbiturate poisoning may thus be superimposed on chronic intoxication at any time. The combination of sublethal doses of depressants with opiates or alcohol may also result in acute poisoning. Cross-tolerance develops to all barbiturates as well as to paraldehyde, meprobamate, and benzodiazepines. Partial cross-tolerance between alcohol and the depressants occurs.

CLINICAL MANIFESTATIONS. Acute depressant poisoning may occur either accidentally or incident to a suicide attempt. Approximately 25 per cent of all drug-related deaths are due to barbiturates and related hypnotics; few deaths have been ascribed to the benzodiazepines alone. Accidental overdoses may be due rarely to "drug automatism"; an individual may fail to fall asleep after several hypnotic doses, become confused, and ingest an overdose. Upon recovery, there may be no memory of the excessive drug ingestion. The clinical manifestations and treatment of severe poisoning are discussed in Ch. 472.2. The acute and chronic signs and symptoms of mild depressant intoxication resemble those of intoxication with alcohol. The individual shows general sluggishness, difficulty in thinking, slowness of speech and comprehension, poor memory, faulty judgment, emotional lability, and narrowed attention span. Neurologic signs include thick, slurred speech, nystagmus, diplopia, strabismus, vertigo, ataxic gait, hypotonia, dysmetria, and decreased superficial reflexes. Sensation, deep-tendon reflexes, and pupillary responses are unaltered. Skin rashes have been reported. Unexplained seizures in adults should always prompt one to consider chronic depressant drug abuse. Adverse effects of chronic depressant use include decreased psychomotor efficiency, anterograde amnesia, changes in interpersonal style, rebound insomnia, and drowsiness. Neurologic damage and permanent memory deficits have been reported but are poorly documented.

ABSTINENCE SYNDROME. A characteristic *general depressant withdrawal syndrome* occurs and is similar to the symptoms of withdrawal from alcohol. It varies in severity, depending on the drug, dose, and frequency of use. *In contrast to the opiate withdrawal syndrome, that from depressants may be life-threatening.* The first manifestation of this syndrome might be considered the rebound increase in nightly rapid eye movement sleep, associated with nightmares and a sense of having slept badly, that occurs after discontinuation of use of only therapeutic doses of barbiturates or benzodiazepines for several nights. In general, the time required to produce physical dependence is shorter with the short-acting depressants, and the withdrawal symptoms are more abrupt in onset and more severe than with the longer-acting sedatives.

When short-acting hypnotics are abruptly withdrawn, signs and symptoms of the intoxication clear over the initial 12 to 16 hours, and the patient appears to improve. Restlessness, anxiety, tremulousness, and weakness then occur, which may be accompanied by cramps, nausea, vomiting, and orthostatic hypotension. These symptoms progress, and coarse hand tremors, muscle twitching, hyperactive deep reflexes, and increased blink reflex appear within 24 hours. Symptoms generally attain their peak during the second and third days, and convulsions may occur then or before. Most patients who have seizures subsequently improve, but some develop typical delirium tremens, which potentially can lead to fatal cardiovascular collapse. The abstinence syndrome generally clears by about the eighth day, usually leaving no serious residua. Clearing is frequently preceded by a period of prolonged sleep. With longer-acting barbiturates and benzodiazepines, seizures may not occur until the seventh or eighth day. Irritability, anxiety, sleep disturbances, and severe psychiatric symptoms may persist for many months, but may be related to pre-existing psychopathology.

As with the opiates but not the barbiturates, specific receptors for the benzodiazepines have been found in all vertebrates studied. The binding sites are found in highest concentrations in the cortex, the cerebellum, and the amygdala and appear to relate to inhibition of central nervous system function.

TREATMENT. Treatment is composed of acute withdrawal procedures and long-term rehabilitation. Outreach and educational programs aimed at intermittent abusers of depressants before they become addicted may be important.

If physical dependence is determined or strongly suspected, hospitalization and close observation are indicated. A long-acting general depressant with which the physician is familiar should be administered after the intoxication clears but before major withdrawal symptoms have begun. Diazepam is widely used, since the agent produces measurable blood levels and protection against the development of either withdrawal symptoms or dangerous intoxication. Patients who are taking large amounts of lesser known sedatives should be withdrawn from the original drug of abuse. If the patient will not tolerate the oral administration of diazepam or more rapid sedation is required, intramuscular injections of the same doses may be used. Patients may usually be switched to oral drugs after a few intramuscular injections. With oral medications, an initial dose of 20 to 40 mg of diazepam should be administered and the patient carefully observed for signs of intoxication or withdrawal. Succeeding doses should be adjusted to provide a mild but manageable level of intoxication marked by inconstant, slow nystagmus on lateral gaze, slight dysarthria, and ataxia. A rough approximation of the dosage of depressant to be given daily is calculated by substituting 15 mg of diazepam for each 100 mg of the short-acting barbiturate the patient reports using. Most patients will require between 60 and 100 mg daily for stabilization, to be given in four divided doses; higher doses may be required in the case of severe tremulousness or hallucinations. This "stabilization dose" should be carefully controlled to prevent signs of increased intoxication. Patients should be maintained on this dose for 24 to 48 hours, after which the dose of diazepam can be reduced by 15 to 20 mg or less daily. The patient should be observed carefully for signs of insomnia, tremulousness, increased deep tendon reflexes, and orthostatic hypotension, at which point withdrawal should be suspended for one to two days. If severe symptoms emerge, diazepam should be administered parenterally. Delirium, convulsions, or fever should be treated as an emergency, with increased doses until the patient is able to sleep for eight to twelve hours, after which the stabilization dose is determined, as described above. Once a withdrawal delirium develops, increased doses of diazepam may only partially restore equilibrium; agitation and disorientation may persist for several days.

Satisfactory care requires that fluid and electrolyte losses be replaced and complicating medical and surgical conditions treated. Increasing fever without evidence of infection necessitates additional sedation, antipyretics, sponging, or cooling blankets. Phenothiazines, butyrophenones, and phenytoin are not indicated. In general, the substitution program may take from ten days to three weeks. It should not be hurried. During the process, patients should be as active as possible, eat regularly, and take part in group activities. Patients who are concurrently dependent on opiates should be withdrawn from the general depressant first, while being maintained on suitable doses of methadone. Opiate withdrawal procedures may then be effected.

Anxiety, irritability, depression, and insomnia often persist for weeks or months after withdrawal is completed and are associated with the danger of relapse or suicide. Provision must be made for inclusion of patients in well-structured, supportive, long-term therapeutic programs on either an inpatient or an outpatient basis.

Physicians must be cautious when prescribing depressants for the relief of anxiety and insomnia. Attempts should be made to diagnose and treat the source of these symptoms without medication. If necessary, benzodiazepine tranquilizers may be used in low doses for well-defined, short periods or on an intermittent basis.

BROMIDES. Chronic bromide intoxication (bromism) has become rare. However, the agent is still found in some proprietary headache remedies, and the daily ingestion of small doses can result in an accumulation of this long-acting drug to toxic levels over a period of weeks. Central nervous system symptoms and signs are variable and include drowsiness, impaired thought and memory, dizziness, and irritability, leading in severe cases to confusion, hallucinations, lethargy, and coma. Neurologic disturbances include tremors, thick speech, motor incoordination, and decreased superficial reflexes. Various types of skin eruptions, ranging from acneiform lesions to proliferative nodular lesions similar to those of tertiary syphilis, are found in 25 per cent of patients with mental symptoms. The diagnosis is established by serum bromide levels above 9 mEq per liter (75 mg per deciliter) in association with the aforementioned clinical picture.

Treatment consists of sedation when necessary and the daily administration of 200 mEq of either sodium or ammonium chloride, together with sufficient fluids to ensure a large urine output. This reduces the half-life of bromide to three or four days. Diuresis with chloruretic drugs may be useful if more rapid displacement of bromide is indicated. Hemodialysis rapidly clears bromides and may be indicated in treating comatose patients.

Tyrer P, Owen R, Dawling S: Gradual withdrawal of diazepam after longterm therapy. Lancet 1:1402, 1983. *A double-blind, placebo-controlled study of the incidence and characteristics of the diazepam withdrawal syndrome with relevant background and references.*

Wesson PR, Smith DE: Barbiturates: Their Use, Misuse and Abuse. New York, Human Science Press, 1977. *Comprehensive treatment of patterns of use, adverse consequences, and treatments.*

CENTRAL NERVOUS SYSTEM STIMULANTS

Central nervous system stimulants or sympathomimetics that are subject to abuse include cocaine, the amphetamines, methylphenidate (Ritalin), phenmetrazine (Preludin), and diethylpropion (Tepanil). This discussion will consider primarily cocaine, an alkaloid of the coca plant, which is indiginous to the mountain slopes of Central and South America, and the amphetamine group, including amphetamine, dextroamphetamine, and methamphetamine.

INCIDENCE AND PATTERNS OF ABUSE. Mountain-dwelling Indians in Bolivia and Peru have been chewing coca leaves to alleviate fatigue, suppress appetite, and increase productivity since pre-Incan times. The cocaine alkaloid was isolated in Europe in the mid-nineteenth century and was recommended briefly as a treatment for depression and other emotional disorders and even as a cure for morphine and alcohol addiction, before its usefulness as a local anesthetic was appreciated.

During the past 20 years, in association with the profound increases in other illicit drug use in American society, the prevalence of cocaine use has increased remarkably. Current estimates suggest that 25 to 30 per cent of youthful and young adult populations have used the drug, with about one-fourth of this number being current users. The affluent have been particularly at risk because of the expense of the drug, although users cut across all socioeconomic and demographic lines.

Cocaine is available through illicit channels as a variably adulterated white powder, with a "gram" costing between $100 and $125. The drug may be sniffed, ingested orally, smoked, administered intravenously or applied to mucous membranes. Upon insufflation, the primary mode of use in the United States, effects are perceived within minutes and persist for 20 to 40 minutes. Psychoactive effects include a feeling of increased energy, intensity, confidence, and alertness, coupled with irritability and often some anxiety. Increased activity, planning, and talking occur.

There is a continuum of abuse from the rare or occasional use of the drug to luxuriously punctuate a variety of occasions to a pattern of compulsive use in which it becomes the dominant concern of living. Regular users often use the drug continuously, and the higher the dose the more powerful is the compulsion to repeat the experience. During a "run" of varying duration, 1 to 10 grams of the drug or more may be used daily; at this stage the user is often irritable, nervous, and suspicious and unable to function. There may be intense involvement in complicated and often unnecessary tasks such as reorganizing a room or disassembling a television set. Alcohol, sedative-hypnotics, opiates, and marijuana are often taken concurrently to alleviate anxiety and irritability. When the supply of drugs is depleted or users become too disorganized or debilitated to continue, the "run" ends. Cessation of cocaine use is marked by apathy, fatigue, depressed mood, and often a period of deep sleep ("crashing"). Symptoms are reported to persist for days or weeks and serve as a powerful reinforcement to resumption of the drug use pattern.

Upon intravenous use, effects are perceived as a "rush" of intense euphoria and power, and the compulsion to repeat the experience is intense. Injections may be repeated at 10- to 20-minute intervals for many hours. A recent phenomenon is the marked increase in the smoking of "free base," an alkaline extraction of cocaine that is more volatile than the hydrochloride form and more rapidly absorbed in the lungs. Blood levels and psychoactive effects approach those of intravenous injection.

Most of the psychoactive effects of the *amphetamines* are similar to those of cocaine with regard to elevation of mood, decreased need for food and sleep, and hyperactivity. When amphetamines were prescribed by physicians for a variety of conditions, many people became dependent, finding that they had to continue to ingest the drug in order to prevent depression and maintain optimal levels of performance. The advent of tolerance necessitated increased doses, occasionally five to ten times the original 5- to 10-mg amount prescribed. A significant decline in use has occurred recently as a result of federal and state regulations that severely limit prescribing and manufacturing practices with respect to the amphetamines.

Patterns of use of amphetamines in chronic drug-abusing populations, particularly the young, resemble those of cocaine. Whereas any amphetamine or other sympathomimetic agent may be used, methamphetamine ("speed," "crystal," or "meth") is preferred because it has more pronounced central effects and fewer peripheral ones. The drugs are "sniffed," administered intravenously, and taken orally. Use may be intermittent and limited to special occasions such as a party or journey or may be continuous for several days or even longer. As tolerance develops, the dose is increased and the drug taken more frequently, such that 1 gram may be injected every two to four hours.

PHARMACOLOGY. Systemic effects of cocaine and amphetamines include increased cardiac contraction, increased blood pressure and heart rate, dilated pupils, constriction of peripheral blood vessels, rise in body temperature, relaxation of the bronchial musculature, increased contractility of the urinary bladder sphincter, and increased venous pressure, pulmonary arterial pressure, and renal blood flow. Central effects include stimulation of the cerebrospinal axis and the brainstem respiratory centers. In low doses these drugs increase alertness and physical and cognitive ability, particularly when performance has been compromised by lack of sleep. Appetite depression occurs and probably derives from a combination of factors, including an inhibitory effect on the lateral hypothalamus as well as the improvement in mood that occurs. Cocaine is an effective topical local anesthetic and vasoconstrictor of mucous membranes.

Tolerance develops to both the peripheral and central effects of the amphetamines. Tolerance to the psychoactive effects of cocaine does not occur; there may be some psychologic tolerance to the euphoric effects. Tolerance to the respiratory and cardiac stimulant effects of cocaine does occur. Cross-tolerance exists among the amphetamines, but no cross-tolerance has been demonstrated between the amphetamines and cocaine.

Cessation of cocaine or amphetamine use does not generally produce major physiologic symptoms. The depression, anxiety, increased appetite, lassitude, and prolonged sleep that ensue might be considered an abstinence syndrome and evidence of physical dependence. During the subsequent sleep, the EEG characteristically shows a marked increase in the percentage of REM sleep, and nightmares may occur. Rarely, withdrawal has been marked by headaches, profuse sweating, muscle cramps, disorientation, and confusion. Cocaine and the amphetamines are among the most powerful reinforcers of continued drug-taking behavior.

ADVERSE EFFECTS. The chronic intranasal administration of cocaine or amphetamines commonly causes irritation or ulceration of the nasal mucosa and may lead to perforation of the nasal septum. Corneal ulcers also occur. Chronic users may be debilitated and subject to infections as a result of lack of sleep and poor nutrition. A sensation of something crawling under the skin is described ("cocaine bugs") such that compulsive users will frequently have excoriations and open sores from constant scratching and pinching. The intravenous use of these drugs is associated with the expected complications that result from nonsterile conditions. A necrotizing cerebral angiitis with resulting stroke has been associated with methamphetamine abuse. *Acute cocaine toxicity* is dose related and is characterized by initial sympathomimetic effects including tachycardia, hypertension, hyperthermia, arrhythmias, and convulsions, followed by brainstem depression leading to respiratory failure and cardiovascular collapse. *Acute amphetamine toxicity* is also marked by extensions of the sympathomimetic effects. Stroke, coma, and sudden death remain rare but are increasing in association with the use of high doses of cocaine. Deaths have occurred as a result of the accidental breaking of bags containing large quantities of cocaine ingested in smuggling attempts. The lethal dose of cocaine is estimated to be about 1.2 grams; that of the amphetamines varies depending upon the extent of tolerance.

Compulsive cocaine and amphetamine abusers suffer from a variety of preexisting psychiatric problems and the abuse engenders even more. Depression, anxiety, irritability, insomnia, and decreased libido occur frequently. Paranoid ideation and stereotyped compulsive behavior are common. Chronic users are frequently aware of these characteristics of the drugs and will not act on ideas of persecution. Antisocial or violent behavior may occur when this insight is lacking. Continued use frequently leads to a well-described cocaine or amphetamine psychosis that is often indistinguishable from acute paranoid schizophrenia. The reactions appear to be inevitable if the dose and frequency of use are continually increased or high doses maintained. Psychotic episodes have been precipitated in some individuals after a single small dose. The syndrome is marked by paranoid ideation; stereotyped compulsive behavior; visual, auditory, and tactile hallucinations; and loosening of associations occurring in a setting of clear consciousness and correct orientation. The psychotic episodes invariably appear while the patients are under the influence of the drug and generally abate within a few days to several weeks after cessation of drug use. Subsequently, affected individuals have a lower threshold for precipitation of psychotic episodes even after long intervening periods. Prolonged psychotic episodes may relate to the premorbid personality of the user. A toxic hallucinatory state and dyskinetic and dystonic reactions occur rarely.

TREATMENT. Amphetamine and cocaine abusers demonstrate markedly diverse patterns of drug use. Accordingly, treatment must be flexible. Treatment of the medical complications is considered elsewhere in this textbook. Treatment of anxiety reactions marked by hypertension and tachycardia may be accomplished with benzodiazepines or similar agents. Withdrawal from these drugs requires a safe, supportive atmosphere, much reassurance, and benzodiazepines when necessary for extreme anxiety. Detoxification with decreasing doses of the sympathomimetics is not indicated, although many users will be addicted to alcohol or sedatives. Treatment of psychotic symptoms may require hospitalization. Phenothiazines or other major tranquilizers may be necessary for prolonged psychotic reactions. After recovery, depressive symptoms and the possibility of suicide must be considered.

Physicians should prescribe amphetamines and related drugs with great caution. Some authorities suggest that the childhood hyperkinetic disorders and narcolepsy are the only acceptable indications for their use.

Mule SJ (ed.): Cocaine: Chemical, Biological, Clinical, Social and Treatment Aspects. Cleveland, CRC Press, 1976. *Comprehensive review of the subject, with extensive bibliography.*

Wetli CV, Wright RK: Death caused by recreational cocaine use. JAMA 241:2519, 1979. *An analysis of deaths associated with cocaine use.*

CANNABIS (Marijuana and Hashish)

INCIDENCE AND PATTERNS OF ABUSE. Cannabis has been used extensively in many societies since antiquity as a form of folk medicine and for recreational purposes. The prevalence of cannabis use has increased explosively in the United States and Western Europe during the past 20 years. More than two thirds of people from 18 to 25 are estimated to have used the drug, with 35 per cent being current users. Increased use is being noted in younger and older age groups as well. Whereas geographic, social, and cultural considerations are determinants of whether a person will use cannabis, personality characteristics are important in determining the frequency and pattern of use.

The drug is peripheral to the life of the occasional user, and frequently there is no other drug use. Others demonstrate a compulsive abuse pattern, with lives dominated by the acquisition and use of cannabis and other drugs. Occasional users generally smoke in groups, where the ritual of preparation and sharing of the cigarette is an integral part of social interaction. Chronic smokers frequently smoke alone.

Marijuana is usually smoked in homemade cigarettes ("joints"). Hashish is smoked in a wide variety of small pipes. Both preparations may be ingested in combination with food or drink, although this is less common.

PHARMACOLOGY. Cannabis preparations are three to four times more potent when smoked than when taken orally. After inhalation, effects begin within minutes, peak within one hour, and are dissipated within three hours. After ingestion, effects begin in 30 minutes to two hours, peak at three hours, and persist for four to six hours. The effects of cannabis correlate with the appearance in plasma of active polar metabolites of delta-9-THC. Kinetic interactions have been described between several of the cannabinoids in marijuana, suggesting that, in accordance with popular belief, the pharmacologic and psychoactive effects of different strains may vary apart from the differences in delta-9-THC content.

The acute physiologic effects of cannabis are dose related and include an increase in heart rate, conjunctival vascular congestion, decreased intraocular pressure, bronchodilatation, increased airway conductance, and peripheral vasodilatation. Dryness of mouth and throat, fine tremors of fingers, ataxia, nystagmus, nausea, and vomiting have been noted. Orthostatic hypotension and loss of consciousness occur infrequently. Sleep patterns may be altered.

Psychoactive effects depend on the dose, the route of administration, the personality of the user, and the environmental and social setting in which the drug is used. Enhanced perception of colors, sounds, patterns, textures, and taste is reported. Mood changes are complex; a sense of increased well-being is frequently experienced, although anxiety and depression may be increased by the drug as well. Drowsiness or hyperactivity and hilarity may occur. Time seems to pass slowly, and short-term memory is impaired. Motor performance is variably impaired. It is probable that alterations in attention are responsible for some of the reported decrements in performance and cognitive function. *Driving performance is significantly impaired by marijuana intoxication.*

Inexperienced users of cannabis report fewer subjective effects than experienced users but demonstrate more decrement in perceptual and psychomotor performance. A social learning process may be involved in the initial perception of psychoactive effects. A varying degree of tolerance develops to some of the psychologic and physiologic effects of the drug, particularly the subjective "high" and the effects on heart rate. A mild withdrawal syndrome, marked by irritability, restlessness, sleep disturbances, sweating, tremor, nausea, and vomiting, occurs under experimental conditions of heavy use but has not been a clinical problem.

Cannabis preparations have been shown to reduce the nausea patients experience incident to cancer chemotherapy and to be effective in reducing intraocular pressure in glaucoma. Research continues on the therapeutic indications for the drug.

ADVERSE EFFECTS. There are no documented fatalities caused by an overdose of cannabis. The increased workload of the heart may pose a threat to patients with hypertension, cerebrovascular disease, and coronary atherosclerosis. Decreased pulmonary function, including vital capacity, has been reported in chronic users, with an increased incidence of bronchitis, sinusitis, and nose and throat inflammation. Marijuana smoke contains 50 to 100 per cent more benzopyrine and other hydrocarbons, as well as more tar, than cigarette smoke. Some of these compounds are considered to be carcinogenic, although an increased incidence of cancer in marijuana smokers has not been reported. The reported in vitro reduction in thymus-dependent lymphocytes and inhibition of DNA, RNA, and protein synthesis require clarification. Reduced gonadotropin and testosterone levels, altered characteristics and decreased production of sperm, compromised ovulation, decreased fertility, and increased fetal loss have been reported in animals, but the clinical significance of these findings is unclear.

Adverse reactions are generally psychologic in nature, infrequent, and dependent on the dose, the personality of the user, and the setting. The most common adverse effects are simple depression, acute panic reactions, and paranoid ideation. These symptoms usually abate in several hours. An acute toxic psychosis, transient in nature, with confusion, disorientation, and auditory and visual hallucinations, occurs infrequently. There is disagreement as to whether cannabis may precipitate a psychotic episode in a stable, well-structured personality, although prolonged psychotic episodes certainly arise in people with borderline psychologic adjustment.

The chronic, heavy use of marijuana may cause diminished goal-directed activity, apathy, and an inability to master new problems, particularly in workers who are engaged in complex tasks or for whom mental operations predominate —"amotivational syndrome." In populations involved in simpler tasks or with high motivation, work performance did not decline. There is no evidence that cannabis use leads to criminal activity.

TREATMENT. Treatment of the frequently seen depressive and panic reactions should be personal, supportive, and reassuring. The patient must be continually reminded of the drug-induced nature of his difficulty. Tranquilizers are sometimes indicated in violent or aggressive states. Psychotherapy and hospitalization may be indicated in more severe or chronic disorders.

Marijuana and Health. Report of a study by a Committee of the Institute of Medicine: Division of Health Sciences Policy. Washington DC, National Academy Press, 1982. *Comprehensive analysis of the impact of marijuana on health and behavior.*

Tashkin DP, Calvarese BM, Simmons MS, Shapiro BJ: Respiratory status of seventy-four habitual marijuana smokers. Chest 78(5):699, 1980. *Controlled study of the long-term effects of marijuana on respiratory status and lung function.*

PSYCHEDELICS

The psychedelic drugs characteristically produce distinctive alterations in perception, thought, feeling, and behavior. They are among the oldest known psychoactive drugs, having long been used as an adjunct to religious practices in some societies. They are sometimes classified as hallucinogens, psychotogens, or psychotomimetics. In this country, the most frequently abused drugs in this category are related either to the indolealkylamines such as the synthetic *lysergic acid diethylamide (LSD, "acid")*, *psilocybin* ("magic mushrooms"), *psilocin, dimethyltryptamine (DMT)*, and *diethyltryptamine (DET)*, or to the phenylethylamines such as *mescaline*, which is derived from the peyote cactus, and the substituted amphetamines such as 2,5-dimethoxy-4-methylamphetamine *(DOM, "STP")*. Since the pattern of physiologic and psychologic effects produced by other agents is similar to that seen with LSD, this discussion will center on LSD. By virtue of their ability to produce bizarre alterations in behavior, anticholinergic compounds and the general anesthetics *phencyclidine* ("angel dust," PCP) and *ketamine* are included with the psychedelics.

PHARMACOLOGY. LSD is the most potent psychedelic known. It is more than 100 times more potent than psilocybin and 4000 times more potent than mescaline in producing psychologic effects. The usual illicit street dose is probably around 200 μg, but doses as low as 20 μg produce psychologic effects in susceptible individuals. The drug is generally taken orally, although it has been injected on occasion. Central sympathomimetic stimulation occurs within 20 minutes after ingestion, characterized by mydriasis, hyperthermia, tachycardia, elevated blood pressure, piloerection, increased alertness, and facilitation of monosynaptic reflexes. Nausea and occasionally vomiting occur.

Psychoactive effects are evident within one to two hours; these vary within and among subjects depending upon conditions of dose, mood, expectation, setting, and time. Perceptions are heightened and may become overwhelming. Afterimages are prolonged and overlap with ongoing perceptions. Objects may seem to move in a wavelike fashion or melt. Illusions and synesthesias, the overflow of one sense modality to another, are common. There may be a sense of unusual clarity, and one's thoughts may assume extraordinary importance. Time seems to pass slowly, and body distortions are commonly perceived. True hallucinations with loss of insight may occur in susceptible individuals. Mood is highly variable and labile, and may range from expansive reactions characterized by euphoria and self-confidence to a constricted reaction marked by depression and panic.

The syndrome begins to clear after 10 to 12 hours, and fatigue and tension may persist for an additional 24 hours. The duration of action of mescaline is about 12 hours, that of psilocybin is 4 to 6 hours, that of DOM is 6 to 8 hours, and that of phencyclidine is 4 to 6 hours. DMT must be injected or sniffed, and effects last less than 2 hours.

Tolerance to LSD develops rapidly. Repeated daily, doses become ineffective in three to four days. Recovery is equally rapid, so weekly use of the same dose is possible. Cross-tolerance has been demonstrated between LSD, mescaline, psilocybin, and the amphetamine-based psychedelics, but not between LSD and amphetamine. Some tolerance occurs with chronic PCP use. Physical dependence does not occur with LSD or any of the psychedelic drugs.

Mechanisms of action are unknown but may depend on a complex interaction of serotonin and norepinephrine systems in the central nervous system. LSD lowers the threshold for reticular arousal via sensory input and may influence the processes concerned with the filtration and integration of sensory information.

ADVERSE EFFECTS. Acute physiologic toxicity of the LSD-related psychedelic drugs is low at doses that produce marked psychologic effects. No deaths directly attributable to the use of these drugs have been reported. Evidence suggests that pregnant women exposed to illicit LSD have an elevated rate of spontaneous abortions. LSD may inhibit antibody formation and disrupt the body's immune system.

The acute panic reaction ("bad trip," "freak-out") is the most frequent complication of psychedelic use. These vary in intensity and rarely have led to suicide attempts and accidents. Fear of death or insanity and sensations of breathlessness or paralysis are common. In most cases, this acute reaction subsides as drug effects are dissipated. Other complications include prolonged psychotic disorders, acute and chronic paranoid reactions, and depressive states. Adverse psychologic reactions are most frequent in emotionally disturbed individuals in crisis situations or insecure environments who take the drug in unsupervised settings. High doses of psychedelic drugs lead to an increased incidence of these complications.

At low doses, the *acute toxic effects of phencyclidine* resemble those of LSD, although violent and psychotic reactions are reported more frequently. At higher doses, the drug produces severe physiologic toxicity, and deaths have been reported. Common features include emotional lability, excited intoxication, nystagmus, gross incoordination, elevated blood pressure, and increased deep-tendon reflexes which may progress to a state of extreme muscular rigidity. High doses may lead to arrhythmias, convulsions, and coma. A chronic dementia has been described in phencyclidine abusers, marked by memory gaps, disorientation, and visual and speech disturbances.

ANTICHOLINERGIC COMPOUNDS. Ingestion of the alkaloids *atropine, hyoscyamine,* and *scopolamine* in their natural plant forms occurs incident to the ingestion of "herbal teas" and a variety of proprietary medications, and several deaths have occurred. Excessive use of *antihistaminic* compounds with anticholinergic effects also occurs. Symptoms of the potent peripheral effects of intoxication include dilated, fixed pupils, dry skin and mouth, flushing, hyperthermia, and tachycardia. Psychoactive effects are those of an acute toxic delirium, with clouding of consciousness and loss of memory for the period of intoxication. Vivid sensory phenomena are not prominent, although hallucinations may occur.

TREATMENT. Treatment of the acute panic reaction may usually be accomplished by ensuring a supportive environment with someone in constant attendance and a minimum of other external stimuli. The user should be reminded continually that the effects he is experiencing are due to the drug and will pass in time. In particularly agitated patients, diazepam or haloperidol orally or intramuscularly may be used. In the event of precipitation of prolonged psychosis, hospitalization with supportive care may be required. Flashbacks are treated with reassurance and/or psychotherapy when these are severe. In general, the duration and severity of these decrease with time if psychedelic drug use ceases.

Treatment of the acute intoxication caused by low doses of phencyclidine is similar to that for the other psychedelics, particularly with respect to reduction of external stimuli and tranquilization. Toxic reactions from higher doses may require hospitalization and intensive supportive care.

Gastric lavage is indicated in the severely obtunded patient. To enhance the excretion of phencyclidine, acidification of the urine may be accomplished acutely by the intravenous administration of ammonium chloride, 75 mg per kilogram per day in four divided doses, or ascorbic acid, 500 mg every four hours, with repeated monitoring of blood pH, blood gases, BUN, blood ammonia levels, and electrolytes. If symptoms are mild, cranberry juice and 1 or 2 grams of ascorbic acid given orally four times daily may be sufficient.

Treatment of anticholinergic poisoning is symptomatic and consists of protecting the patient from self-injury, providing fluids, and reducing the fever. Administration of cholinesterase inhibitors and suitable tranquilizers may be indicated; phenothiazines are contraindicated because of their anticholinergic effects.

Arronow R, Done A: Phencyclidine overdose: An emerging concept of management. J Am Col Emerg Phys 7(2):56, 1978. *Summary of physical and psychologic symptoms of acute phencyclidine reactions and suggested treatment.*

Grinspoon L, Bakalar JB: Psychedelic Drugs Reconsidered. New York, Basic Books, 1979. *Comprehensive discussion of the use and abuse of psychedelics, with an extensive bibliography.*

INHALANTS

ORGANIC SOLVENTS. The inhalation of a wide range of organic solvents, particularly the toluene in glue, has become popular among young persons during the past 20 years. The drugs are easily available, inexpensive, and convenient to use. The material is usually squeezed into a plastic bag and the vapors inhaled. As used recreationally, these solvents produce intoxication and dizziness not unlike that experienced with alcohol. Few adverse effects have been reported, although suffocation caused by the plastic bag has apparently occurred. Prolonged exposure or overdose, as in the case of addicts or industrial workers, may have serious adverse effects on a variety of organ systems. Cerebral degeneration has been reported in sniffers, as have been deaths secondary to the inhalation of the anesthetic agent halothane, a halogenated hydrocarbon. The inhalation of aerosol sprays containing fluorocarbon propellants is also occurring. The rare occurrence of toxicity and death may be via the induction of cardiac arrhythmias or upper-airway obstruction and hypoxia.

AMYL NITRITE. Amyl nitrite ("amies," "poppers") inhalation has become quite prevalent in youthful and young adult populations, particularly as a sexual aid. A variety of other volatile nitrites, marketed as deodorizers or "aromas" under a variety of exotic brand names, are similarly used. Use is intermittent and characterized by an instantaneous feeling ("rush") of flushing, dizziness, hilarity, and activity. Effects persist for minutes. Adverse effects include palpitations, postural hypotension, and headache, occasionally progressing to loss of consciousness. Prolonged adverse effects have not been reported.

NITROUS OXIDE. Recreational inhalation of nitrous oxide alone or in combination with oxygen is a rarely reported phenomenon that occurs in some youthful populations. Psychoactive effects occur in 15 to 30 seconds and persist for less than five minutes. The experience is described as one of intoxication, euphoria, and hilarity. Adverse effects have not been reported.

TREATMENT. Since the effects of the inhalants are evanescent, specific acute treatments are generally not indicated. When inhalant use is chronic or associated with psychopathology, appropriate long-term treatments should be provided.

Lazar RB, Ho SU, Melen O, Daghestani AN: Multifocal nervous system damage caused by toluene abuse. Neurology 33:1337, 1983. *A recent description of cases, supplemented with a thorough bibliography.*

Sharp CW, Brehm ML (eds.): Review of Inhalants: Euphoria to Dysfunction. NIDA Research Monograph 15. US Department of Health, Education and Welfare, October 1977. *Comprehensive review of the preclinical and clinical data on the various inhalants.*

Section Three PATHOPHYSIOLOGY AND MANAGEMENT OF MAJOR NEUROLOGIC SYMPTOMS

478. AUTONOMIC DISORDERS AND THEIR MANAGEMENT

Fred Plum

THE NONENDOCRINE HYPOTHALAMUS

To survive in a constantly changing, often threatening environment, humans must continuously and automatically adjust the activity of both their internal organs and their outward behavior. The task of maintaining a stable internal environment in the face of minor potential perturbations falls largely to the autonomic nervous and endocrine systems. Major or more sustained challenges, however, must be met by emotional drives or reflex emergency motor acts, both mediated by the limbic system. The hypothalamus (HT) stands between these biologically comprehensive, internally and externally directed regulatory mechanisms, serving as a kind of command post that receives afferent signals of visceral, somatic, and emotional need or sufficiency, then integrates the sum and translates the message to coordinate internal homeostasis with outward behavior. Chapters 222, 224, and 226 further discuss the neuroendocrine role of the HT.

To accomplish its astonishingly complex functions, the hypothalamus has evolved into a neuroendocrine structure in which interneuronal connectivity, in addition to being mediated by conventional neurotransmitters, is modulated and sometimes mediated by endocrine-like peptides. Many of the latter substances spread diffusely from their secreting neurons, either through the HT itself or to remote points in the brain after entering the cerebral ventricles or blood. Anatomically the HT is tightly packed with fibers of passage interlaced among what, by conventional histologic stains, appears to be a diffuse reticulum of nerve cells. Only after applying modern immunocytochemical methods to discern specific nuclei and pathways does the remarkable anatomic richness of the structure and its connections emerge.

The tightly packed, interwoven contents of the hypothalamus make it difficult or impossible to assign specific signs and symptoms to any but a few local areas (Table 478–1). Ventromedial and posteriorly located lesions tend to produce greater functional abnormalities than those located elsewhere, because their position inevitably interrupts fibers leading to the endocrine and descending autonomic nervous systems, respectively. Except when they affect unilateral descending sympathetic projections, clinically detectable changes in autonomic function due to HT disorders always imply the presence of bilateral lesions. Table 478–2 lists the principal diseases that attack the structure.

COGNITIVE AND BEHAVIORAL ABNORMALITIES. Severe retrograde and anterograde memory loss and even a chronic delirium can accompany ventromedial hypothalamic destruction in man. Outbursts of fear and rage sometimes accompany lesions in this region, whereas lateral-posterior damage tends to be associated with apathetic hypoactivity. Disorders of specific neurotransmitter systems have not, as yet, been linked successfully to these functional changes. Loss of libido in the male frequently accompanies structural HT disease but usually reflects associated gonadotropic or autonomic deficiency.

DISTURBANCES OF SLEEP AND AROUSAL. In animals, stimulation of the anterior hypothalamus produces behavioral sleep, whereas destruction of that area results in chronic insomnia, findings consistent with the cholinergic-aminergic theory of sleeping-waking behavior (Ch. 472). Limited evidence suggests that similar effects apply in humans. Selective anterior HT destruction in man is too uncommon to permit conclusions, but posterior hypothalamic destruction or inflammation frequently produces sleep disorders, the most frequent causes being stroke, neoplasm, or encephalitis. Hypersomnolence and chronic sleeplike stupor or coma lasting longer than three to four weeks are pathognomonic for damage or dysfunction in this area. No evidence supports the suggestion that the *Kleine-Levin syndrome,* a condition marked by episodic hypersomnia and hyperphagia in young boys, reflects primary hypothalamic dysfunction (Ch. 472).

HEAT REGULATION. The preoptic anterior HT contains separate receptors for warmth and cold as well as for pyrogens. Diurnal changes in central excitability and in the level of circulating ovarian hormones provide additional nonspecific stimuli. In turn, the HT activates varying combinations of behavioral autonomic and endocrine responses that conserve or dissipate body heat. Diseases in the region can be responsible for hypothermia or, rarely, hyperthermia.

Hypothermia. RELATIVE POIKILOTHERMIA. Poikilothermia, defined as a fluctuation in body temperature of greater than 2° C with changes in ambient temperature, is the most common central abnormality of heat regulation in man. Most such cases are detected by a lowered body temperature. Poikilothermia results from damage to the posterior hypothalamus and rostral mesencephalon. Damage to this area impairs not only autonomic heat-regulating pathways but those that control the sense of thermal discomfort and the behavioral regulation of body temperature as well. As a result, many patients with poikilothermia are unaware of their condition and do little to avoid it. At ordinary ambient temperatures of 20 to 25° C, the degree of hypothermia tends to be proportional to the degree of functional hypothalamic impairment. Relative poikilothermia resulting from impaired hypothalamic-autonomic function frequently affects elderly persons (*senile hypothermia*), making them dangerously susceptible to lowered environmental temperatures. Chronic poikilothermia also accompanies several degenerative disorders that affect the HT in children and adults.

TABLE 478–1. REGIONAL SYNDROMES OF THE HYPOTHALAMUS*

	Preoptic Anterior Hypothalamus	Tuberal and Ventromedian Hypothalamus	Posterior Hypothalamus
Integrates	Endocrine, thermal, parasympathetic autonomic	Cognition; endocrine; sympathetic autonomic caloric balance; fluid balance	Consciousness; cognition; complex endocrine; autonomic; thermal
Contains	Sleep-inducing mechanism; forebrain parasympathetic paths; thermal sensing areas	Final common endocrine paths	Reticular activating system; regulatory and outflow autonomic effectors
Acute lesions	Insomnia; hyperthermia; diabetes insipidus; inappropriate ADH	Hyperthermia; diabetes insipidus; hypothalamic-endocrine disorders	Hypersomnia; poikilothermia; autonomic storm
Chronic lesions	Insomnia; complex endocrine changes (e.g., precocious puberty); endocrinotropic abnormalities; hypothermia; hypodipsia	Medial: memory loss; emotional disorders; hyperphagia and obesity; endocrinotropic abnormalities Lateral: emotional disorders; emaciation	Memory loss; apathy; hypersomnia; poikilothermia; autonomic incoordination; complex endocrine disorders (e.g., precocious puberty)

*As indicated in the text, functional localization is more precise for some activities than for others.

TABLE 478–2. PRINCIPAL CAUSES OF HYPOTHALAMIC DISEASES IN ADOLESCENTS AND ADULTS

Congenital midline brain defects, e.g., agenesis of corpus callosum
Stroke: Basilar artery occlusion, subarachnoid hemorrhage
Tumors: craniopharyngioma, glioma, hamartoma, dysgerminoma, dermoid, lipoma, lymphoma or leukemia, meningioma
Trauma
Encephalitis
Granulomas: sarcoid, tuberculosis, histiocytosis X
Wernicke's polioencephalopathy (thiamine deficiency)
Progressive idiopathic degeneration (rare, childhood)

Poikilothermia regularly follows extensive damage to the posterior hypothalamus or midbrain by stroke, trauma, neoplasm, encephalitis, or thiamine deficiency. Such central hypothermia must be differentiated from that caused by metabolic disorders such as acute or chronic sedative drug ingestion, hypoglycemia, and myxedema.

PAROXYSMAL HYPOTHERMIA. Sustained hypothermia (as opposed to relative poikilothermia) is rare in humans. Less uncommon is paroxysmal hypothermia consisting of attacks of lowered body temperature that vary widely in frequency from daily to more than a decade apart. Such attacks usually begin abruptly, last from minutes to days, and are characterized by sweating, flushing of the skin, and a fall in body temperature, usually to 32° C or lower. Fatigue, decreased mental responsiveness, hypoventilation, hypotension, cardiac arrhythmias, ataxia, lacrimation, and asterixis may accompany the temperature drop. The attacks subside either slowly (hours to days) or rapidly with shivering and peripheral vasoconstriction. During hypothermia, mechanisms for both heat production and heat dissipation respond normally, but around a lower temperature set-point. Most affected patients have had direct evidence for hypothalamic disease; several have suffered from congenital agenesis of the corpus callosum. In some instances anticonvulsant therapy stops the attacks.

Hyperthermia. Chronic fever never results from HT disease, and even acute neurogenic fever is rare. The most frequent causes of acute neurogenic hyperthermia include gross head injury, surgical trauma or spontaneous bleeding into the region of the anterior hypothalamus, and hemorrhage in the adjacent meninges or the third ventricle. With neurogenic hyperthermia, the body temperature can rise to potentially fatal levels of 42° C or higher as a result of active heat production unbalanced by heat dissipation. The cardiovascular changes that normally accompany fever are disproportionately lacking. If standard cooling measures fail, small (2 mg) doses of morphine can ameliorate dangerously high neurogenic fevers.

DISORDERS OF FEEDING BEHAVIOR AND CALORIC BALANCE. Influences generated by the forebrain, especially the limbic system, provide the major influences on feeding behavior in man; primary hypothalamic error accounts for no more than a tiny fraction of human obesity or emaciation, making it all the more important to recognize when it occurs.

In experimental animals, stimulation of the ventromedian region of the HT inhibits feeding, whereas lesions destroying this region produce hyperphagia and a weight gain that later stabilizes at a new elevated set-point. Evidence suggests that the changes are mediated by autonomic influences on the digestive tract and on insulin secretion to enhance appetite. Conversely, stimulation of the lateral hypothalamus induces feeding in excess of caloric requirement, whereas damage to the region results in a temporarily severe aphagia that slowly recovers to maintain a chronically lowered body weight. Both hyperphagia and hypophagia due to HT dysfunction occasionally can be observed in man.

Hypothalamic Obesity. Most patients with hypothalamic obesity have shown at autopsy diffuse or large lesions of the structure. A few, however, have suffered from precisely placed abnormalities of the ventromedian hypothalamus. Examples include leukemic infiltration, with the most severe damage localized in the ventromedian region; others have consisted of discrete tumors in this area. Affected patients have experienced remarkable combinations of food-seeking behavior, including ravenous hyperphagia, decreased motor activity, and sometimes enormous obesity.

The hypothalamus integrates a set-point that roughly regulates the individual's body weight. In patients who develop hypothalamic obesity, whether or not hyperphagia continues or disappears depends upon whether (a) the neurologic abnormality is fixed and (b) the new disease-related set-point for weight has been reached. Patients with obesity following surgical procedures or severe closed head trauma that affects the hypothalamus illustrate this principle. Characteristically, such persons eat ravenously and gain weight quickly following the injury until they reach their new set-point, at which point they become normophagic and stabilize at a new, higher weight.

Emaciation sometimes accompanies hypothalamic disease in man, but the associated lesions usually have been large and their specificity uncertain. Efforts to link hypothalamic disease and anorexia nervosa have been unsuccessful.

WATER BALANCE. The HT controls body water content and osmolality via coordinated mechanisms regulating affective thirst, drinking behavior, and the release of antidiuretic hormone (ADH) via the paraventricular (PV) and supraoptic (SO) nuclei. HT or limbic system disease can produce four principal disorders of water balance, including ADH deficiency (diabetes insipidus), inappropriate ADH secretion, neurogenic (essential) hypernatremia, and episodic hyperdipsia. Chapters 76 and 226 discuss much of the pathophysiology of these disorders. Important from the neural standpoint is to understand that osmoreceptors and volume receptors appear to reside in different areas of the hypothalamus. Osmoreceptors and central thirst receptors have been identified within the preoptic region. These respond to afferent stimulation from peripheral thirst receptors as well as to local sodium concentrations and circulating levels of the peptide angiotensin. Volume receptors appear to lie more laterally in the HT and project to the PV and SO nuclei by pathways different from those that carry osmoreceptor signals. Peripherally, thirst is stimulated or quenched by signals arising from receptors lying within the mouth and interstitial fluids, while different receptors arising from heart, large capacitance systemic veins, and carotid baroreceptors signal volume control needs. Differential peripheral stimulation of the two systems or selective damage to the central osmoreceptor-thirst area explains some examples of inappropriate ADH secretion and most if not all cases of neurogenic (essential) hypernatremia.

Neurogenic (Essential) Hypernatremia. This disorder is marked by four features: (1) elevated serum sodium unaccompanied by circulating volume deficiency, (2) a preserved renal tubular responsiveness to ADH, (3) an inadequate secretion of ADH in response to osmotic stimuli, and (4) the absence or deficiency of appropriate thirst (hypodipsia) despite otherwise relatively normal conscious behavior. True essential hypernatremia is rare; most cases of serum hyperosmolarity accompanying intracranial disease result from a nonspecific combination of dehydration and stupor-impaired drinking behavior.

Essential hypernatremia in its milder and more chronic forms often elevates the serum sodium only modestly, and such patients characteristically lack symptoms except for a remarkable lack of thirst. Close attention often discloses considerable fluctuation in daily serum sodium values above the 150 mmol per liter mark. When sodium levels climb to the 160 to 170 mmol per liter range, affected patients develop weakness and sometimes fever as well as muscle tenderness and cramping that may progress to fatigue, ataxia, and even myoglobinuria. Mental symptoms include lethargy, anorexia, depression, and irritability. With elevations of serum sodium above 180 mmol per liter, most patients become confused or stuporous, and some will die. Patients with essential hypernatremia fail to experience thirst, but many retain persistent habitual drinking, although at a volume insufficient to maintain a normal serum osmolality. They commonly lack clinical evidence of dehydration; only mild hypovolemia or even normovolemia can accompany serum sodium levels as high as 200 mmol per liter or more. An associated hypokalemia usually contributes to the muscular symptoms. Urine volumes may be low or normal but are always more dilute than appropriate for the serum hyperosmolality. The administration of exogenous ADH induces a more concentrated urine. Either an acute water load or a hypertonic saline load, however, can produce an increase in free water clearance, reflecting the failure of central osmoreceptors to respond to the latter stimulus.

The hypothalamic defect that produces essential hypernatremia is inexactly localized. Almost all affected patients have had associated neurologic or endocrine abnormalities, but many have lacked radiographic evidence of central nervous system abnormalities. Some give a history of diffuse head trauma, while in others space-occupying lesions destroy the entire hypothalamic region by the time of death. In a few patients, restricted tumors have involved the preoptic and tuberal region. The mechanisms of essential hypernatremia remain unsettled. The absence of thirst is critical, and this, along with direct measurements showing that serum vasopressin levels fail to increase when sodium levels rise but fall when blood volume increases, indicates either that osmoreceptor function is selectively uncoupled from the behavioral and hormonal control of water balance or that mechanisms that regulate natriuresis are distinct from ADH control.

Treatment consists of lowering the serum sodium and raising the potassium by manipulating the diet and conditioning the patient automatically to drink several liters of water each day regardless of thirst. Spironolactone, chlorpropamide, and the thiazide diuretics may help to achieve fluid balance. Treatment of hypernatremic crises must be initiated slowly: symptoms of water intoxication can develop if serum sodium is reduced by more than 20 mEq per deciliter per day.

Hyperdipsia and Self-induced Water Intoxication. Excessive water drinking in the absence of either hypovolemia or serum hyperosmolality is termed primary hyperdipsia and must be differentiated from the compensatory hyperdipsias of conditions such as diabetes insipidus, diabetes mellitus, or polyuric renal failure. In the absence of inappropriate ADH secretion, symptoms of severe hyperdipsia, i.e., hypervolemia, hyponatremia, and clinical water intoxication accompanied by stupor, delirium, and convulsions, are infrequent. The problem never arises, to our knowledge, as the result of primary central nervous system disease. Most severe hyperdipsia occurs in persons with acute psychiatric disorders who drink excessively to overcome delusional fears. Occasionally, acute water intoxication occurs in alcoholics with gastritis or in youngsters drinking huge amounts of fluids on a dare, e.g., during ritual hazing or tea-party games.

DISORDERS OF PERIPHERAL AND CENTRAL AUTONOMIC FUNCTION

Centripetal parasympathetic influences emanate largely from the anterior HT, whereas sympathetic descending pathways take their origin mainly in the posterolateral reticulum of the structure. Autonomic control extends to almost every organ of the body and perturbations in these regulatory systems probably take more American patients to doctors than all other conditions combined. The large number of autonomic drugs annually prescribed for cardiovascular, gastrointestinal, pulmonary, and genitourinary disorders affirms this premise.

Most *psychosomatic disorders* produce their symptoms at least partly and often predominantly through the limbic-autonomic system. As John Hunter said of his angina pectoris, "My life is in the hands of any rascal who chooses to annoy and tease me." (He subsequently died during an argument at a hospital board meeting.) Autonomic influences act in subtle ways, and abnormal responses to life stress are often highly individual matters, not easy to separate from the nervous system's routine adjustments to living. Clinical sensitivity to the possibility that the brain rather than the target organ sometimes causes the symptoms represents perhaps the most important first step in detecting pathologic autonomic adjustments to life stress.

Diffuse, moderate sympathetic-parasympathetic dysfunction can accompany occasional cases of otherwise typical parkinsonism and is seen as a component to several of the late-life cerebellar or olivopontocerebellar degenerative disorders. Similarly, many elderly patients gradually lose the briskness of their autonomic reflexes and suffer an insidious decline in orthostatic circulatory control, sexual function, heat regulation, urinary and rectal sphincter continence, and bowel motility, all of which must be treated symptomatically. More severe diffuse autonomic dysfunction occurs in two major forms: one is observed chiefly in association with chronic or acute disease of the peripheral nerves; the other consists of diffuse autonomic dysfunction accompanied by degeneration of corticospinal, extrapyramidal, or cerebellar pathways.

Peripheral Autonomic Insufficiency

Involvement of autonomic fibers is prominent in several axonal diseases and peripheral neuropathies, including, especially, acute poliomyelitis, acute inflammatory neuropathy, diabetic neuropathy, tabes dorsalis, and poisoning with the toxic chemical acrylamide. Autonomic impairment with predominantly sympathetic dysfunction accompanies the peripheral neuropathy of inherited amyloid disease.

A small number of patients have been recorded as suffering from a variably complete degree of acutely or subacutely developing failure of the major parts of peripheral sympathetic and parasympathetic function without accompanying somatomotor or sensory changes (*acute pandysautonomia*). Most cases have been in children, although the first reported example was in a middle-aged male. Recovery has been the rule, and the disorder generally is regarded as a selective variant of idiopathic inflammatory neuropathy, a condition in which more restricted autonomic signs and symptoms in the form of tachycardia, hypertension, sweating impairment, and gastrointestinal atony commonly accompany the more prominent motor and sensory changes. Similarly restricted adrenergic abnormalities also accompany the motor polyneuropathy of acute intermittent porphyria. The treatment in all instances is symptomatic.

FAMILIAL DYSAUTONOMIA. This disorder, also called Riley-Day syndrome, is a rare autosomal recessive disorder that predominantly affects Ashkenazi Jewish children and is characterized by several developmental defects, prominently including abnormalities in peripheral and probably central adrenergic and cholinergic neurotransmission.

Idiopathic Autonomic Insufficiency (Idiopathic Orthostatic Hypotension, Shy-Drager Syndrome)

This is a rare degenerative disorder of unknown etiology that strikes during middle age, causing progressive autonomic dysfunction; severe debility or death may occur within 5 to 15 years of onset. Associated extrapyramidal abnormalities and lesions of pigmented brain nuclei may play a prominent role in the genesis of symptoms.

Pathogenesis and Pathology. Histologic examination at autopsy has disclosed various changes, ranging from the severe to the barely detectable. Degenerative abnormalities may affect autonomic ganglia in the periphery, the preganglionic intermediolateral cell column in the spinal cord or autonomic centers in the hypothalamus, nigrostriatal system, pontine nuclei, and globus pallidus. Postmortem biochemical studies have revealed marked depression of dopamine-β-hydroxylase, which converts dopamine to norepinephrine, in sympathetic ganglia, whereas tyrosine hydroxylase, the rate-limiting enzyme in catecholamine biosynthesis, is decreased in locus ceruleus. In parkinsonian patients, tyrosine hydroxylase may be depressed in substantia nigra. The pathogenesis of the disease is unknown.

Several observers have suggested that at least two entities

may constitute idiopathic autonomic insufficiency. The first may consist of autonomic insufficiency alone, whereas the second may be characterized by autonomic insufficiency in association with a variety of neurologic signs, including movement disorders resembling Parkinson's disease. The degree of clinical overlap between these groups, however, is consistent with the existence of a broad continuum rather than distinct entities.

Clinical Manifestations. Symptoms of autonomic dysfunction predominate early in the course. Characteristically, initial difficulties consist of sexual impotence; urinary hesitancy, urgency, or incontinence; and/or anhidrosis. These early symptoms are frequently unrecognized and undiagnosed. Within months to years, the hallmark of the disorder, postural hypotension, appears. This may be manifested as dizziness, giddiness, or frank syncope upon standing. Less frequently, patients complain of generalized weakness, cervico-occipital discomfort, or leg weakness upon standing. Attendant autonomic symptoms include intermittent diplopia, dysphagia, and diarrhea, fecal incontinence, or constipation. A parkinsonian disorder, consisting of bradykinesia, coarse tremor, and rigidity, is common, and tends to progress inexorably. Myoclonus, gait disturbance, and signs of olivopontocerebellar dysfunction may also occur.

Physical signs of autonomic dysfunction parallel the aforementioned symptoms. Orthostatic hypotension, a greater than 30/20 mm Hg fall in blood pressure upon assumption of the erect position, constitutes the fundamental sign. Other signs include absence of sinus arrhythmia and absence of the normal overshoot in diastolic pressure during phase IV of the Valsalva maneuver. Autonomic dysfunction may express itself in Horner's syndrome, in parasympathetic pupillary changes, or as anhidrosis even with elevated ambient temperature. Muscle wasting, fasciculation, and extensor plantar responses occasionally have been observed.

A variety of clinical laboratory tests may be employed to evaluate autonomic function, and only the simplest will be delineated here. *Miosis* in response to ocular administration of dilute solutions of methacholine, or *mydriasis* after instillation of dilute epinephrine, suggests respectively parasympathetic or sympathetic denervation supersensitivity. On the other hand, absence of mydriasis after ocular instillation of cocaine or hydroxyamphetamine suggests that endogenous norepinephrine stores are defective. Absence of sweating with elevation of the ambient temperature and absence of the axon reflex after intradermal histamine suggest denervation of cutaneous structures. The presence of an abnormally accentuated blood pressure response to the intravenous infusion of norepinephrine is consistent with widespread denervation supersensitivity.

Differential Diagnosis. Orthostatic hypotension itself may accompany intravascular hypovolemia (as with massive hemorrhage or adrenal insufficiency), vasodepressor syncope, acute cardiac failure from a variety of causes, familial hyperbradykininism, and intracranial posterior fossa mass or vascular lesions. However, in these conditions other signs of autonomic dysfunction are absent. On the other hand, autonomic insufficiency, including orthostatic hypotension, may occur with any disease that alters peripheral or central autonomic pathways. Many disorders conform to this description. A variety of peripheral neuropathies may be accompanied by dysautonomia, including the acute Guillain-Barré syndrome; the chronic neuropathies of diabetes mellitus, amyloidosis, Wernicke's disease, and porphyria; and the congenital Riley-Day syndrome. Ganglion dysfunction may result from ingestion of ganglioplegic agents. Tabes dorsalis is commonly accompanied by autonomic signs. Autonomic dysfunction may result from interruption of descending pathways in the spinal cord, as observed with syringomyelia, trauma, or spinal tumor. Pontine hemorrhage may interrupt descending sympathetic pathways in the brainstem, thereby causing sympathetic dysfunction. Differentiation from these diseases is readily accomplished by suitable history, examination, and laboratory tests.

Course and Treatment. Although treatment does not alter the underlying pathologic process, it may allow an otherwise bedridden invalid to lead a considerably improved life. Orthostatic hypotension may be treated with a variety of measures, dictated by the severity of the problem. The first line of defense consists of antigravity stockings, which prevent pooling of blood in the lower extremities upon standing. In moderately severe cases, intravascular volume expansion may be achieved by using the mineralocorticoid desoxycorticosterone acetate or 9-α-fluorocortisone and sodium chloride, with potassium supplementation. In severe cases, oral sympathomimetic agents, including ephedrine or hydroxyamphetamine, may be added. Indomethacin may be effective in selected patients for the treatment of orthostatic hypotension. The use of monoamine oxidase inhibitors may be potentially hazardous in those patients who are subject to denervation suprasensitivity. Although the diet may be rigorously regulated in the hospital setting, this is rarely possible on an outpatient basis. For example, such foods as cheese, broad beans, Chianti, raisins, bananas, and aged or smoked meat contain significant quantities of vasoactive amines. Inadvertent ingestion of microgram quantities of vasoactive amines in the diet may result in alarming elevation of blood pressure in patients being treated with monoamine oxidase inhibitors for widespread sympathetic denervation.

Parkinsonian signs and symptoms may be successfully treated with L-dopa and the customary anticholinergic agents.

ABNORMALITIES OF SWEATING. *Anhidrosis*, a relatively uncommon complaint, occurs as part of a rare, probably autosomal recessive disorder in which it is associated with congenital insensitivity to pain. Anhidrosis due to congenital absence of the sweat glands is similarly rare. Anhidrosis also follows pre- or postganglionic sympathetic denervation produced by disease or surgical procedures and can occur in the appropriate territorial distribution of any diseased or damaged peripheral nerve.

Hyperhidrosis, defined as sweating in excess of apparent thermal requirements, is a common response to anxiety, especially among persons less than 30 years old. Longstanding severe hyperhidrosis causing constantly dripping hands and feet is an uncommon but socially troublesome disorder of unknown cause. Emotional factors seem to contribute little. Severe cases can be relieved by sympathectomy directed at the upper extremities. The procedure is best limited to either the upper or lower extremities, since compensatory accentuation of pre-existing sweating tends to affect nondenervated parts. Total sympathectomy produces too many undesirable side effects to be recommended. Hyperhidrosis localized to a particular body part occasionally occurs in association with irritation of the related preganglionic fibers or ganglia by an infection or neoplasm and deserves careful attention from that standpoint.

Urinary Bladder Control

Abnormalities in micturition, collectively termed *dysuria*, arise from four principal causes: local disease in the bladder and urethra, neurologic disorders, drug effects, and psychologic perturbation. Table 478–3 outlines a differential diagnosis of these conditions based on the predominant symptoms, while the following paragraphs briefly discuss neurogenic mechanisms.

The bladder is a hollow pelvic structure composed of the interlacing smooth muscle fibers of the detrusor covered by its internal mucous membrane and outer serosa. The bladder is smooth muscle and its resistance to stretch is determined predominantly by the viscoelastic properties of its wall rather than by direct neurogenic mechanisms. With progressive filling, the normal intravesical pressure rises slowly, remaining below about 15 cm of water until average capacities are reached, between 400 and 600 ml, at which point the intravesical pressure rises either abruptly owing to the onset of the micturition reflex or more gradually owing to reaching the elastic limits of the wall itself. Normal adult micturition volumes average between 200 and 400 ml, but with acute urinary retention the structure can stretch abnor-

TABLE 478–3. MECHANISMS OF DYSURIA

Painful Urination
- Cystourethral inflammation (Ch. 85)
- Urethral stricture
- Psychogenic

Increased Frequency-Urgency
- Increased fluid intake of any cause (e.g., diabetes, alcoholism)
- Cystourethral inflammation
- Psychogenic
- Partial outlet obstruction (e.g., prostatic hypertrophy)
- Neurogenic
  - Damage to prefrontal or spinal inhibitory pathways
  - Spinal reflex facilitation

Incontinence
- Stress: Small volumes, brief urgency, women more than men
  - Normal in 50 per cent of giggling girls
  - Multiparas with cystocele, other outflow damage
  - Increases with normal aging
- Retention-overflow: Dribbling or small volumes, pain in pelvis or flanks, palpable bladder
  - Causes as listed with retention
  - Severe cystitis (small bladder volume)
- Confusional: Small or large volumes, usually shameless
- "Spastic": Large volumes, sporadic occurrence, prominent urgency, emptying complete
  - Prefrontal lesions
  - Extramedullary advanced spinal compression
  - Occasionally partial outlet obstruction
  - Circumstance: bedridden or crippled elderly with facilities remote
- Spinal: Moderate volumes, brief urgency, frequent occurrence, high residual urine
  - Intramedullary cervical-thoracic-lumbar lesions (multiple sclerosis, neoplasms, etc.)
  - Occasionally with partial peripheral denervation

Retention
- Acute or chronic outflow obstruction
- Acute neurologic disease
  - Peripheral: Autonomic polyneuropathy, pelvic trauma, cauda equina compression, conus lesions
  - Central: Poliomyelitis, spinal transection
- Drugs (usually plus local structural problems)
  - Anticholinergics, antidepressants, opiates
- Psychogenic
- Postanesthetic

mally to accommodate one or more liters, while chronic infection and hypertrophy may contract it to a capacity of no more than 60 to 100 ml.

Urine enters the bladder from the paired ureters and normally leaves via the membranous urethra. In both sexes the lower detrusor musculature joins with elastic tissue to form an involuntary internal sphincter that normally can resist passively induced intra-abdominal–intravesical pressures as high as 150 mm Hg. The more distal urethra is encircled by voluntarily controlled striated muscle innervated by the somatomotor pudendal nerve. More competent in men than in women, this external sphincter can withstand briefly the intraurethral detrusor-induced pressure of normal micturition but is unnecessary to normal urinary continence.

The act of voiding represents a stretch-induced parasympathetic reflex of smooth muscle facilitated by brainstem and spinal mechanisms, normally inhibited or released by forebrain regulatory influences. The actual neuromuscular sequence consists of an initial voluntary relaxation of the skeletal muscle of the pelvic floor followed by the disinhibited reflex discharge, which contracts the detrusor, assimilates and relaxes the musculoelastic tissue of the internal sphincter, and empties the organ by a fusion of successive detrusor contractions.

The complete reflex mechanism for micturition exists within the spinal cord. The afferent route of the arc depends upon fibers that originate in stretch receptors in the bladder wall and travel centrally via sacral roots 2 to 4. Efferent preganglionic fibers arise in the lateral columns of the sacral segments of the conus medullaris, whence they travel in the cauda equina to and through the lower sacral foramina to synapse with their final ganglia over the outer surface of the bladder and the region of the proximal urethra. Centrally, afferent proprioceptive signals travel rostrally via the lemniscal system while descending inhibitory influences originate in the paramedian prefrontal cerebral cortex. These latter pathways are joined in the brainstem and upper spinal cord by reflex-facilitating fibers that enhance complete reflex bladder emptying. The pathway descends in the spinal cord within the lateral funiculus to synapse upon the sacral preganglionic neurons.

CEREBRAL DISTURBANCES IN MICTURITION. Damage to the bilateral prefrontal area lowers the micturition reflex threshold, resulting in a proportionately smaller bladder capacity. The chief symptoms are sudden, sometimes uncontrollable urgency with moderately large volumes, usually of less than 250 ml, but complete bladder emptying. The cystometrogram shows a normal bladder pressure-volume filling curve but a reduced micturition reflex threshold, with a comparably reduced threshold to filling sensation. Clinical evaluation or CT scanning of the head readily discloses evidence of structural frontal lobe disease.

Dementia leads to an incontinence of indifference (a loss of bladder training) in which visceral physiology remains intact but social restraints depart. Patients with severe physical disabilities such as hemiplegia, advanced arthritis, etc., may develop *pseudoincontinence* due to difficulty in reaching the toilet or, occasionally, as a depressed, angry, and frustrated response to the limitations of their condition.

SPINAL DISTURBANCES OF MICTURITION. Gradual *extramedullary* spinal cord compression produces few changes in bladder function until late in the course when the reflex is facilitated along with somatic motor reflex pathways. Urgency with moderately reduced voiding volumes results. Incontinence occurs only with advanced or sudden cord compression. *Intramedullary* spinal lesions can directly affect the descending parasympathetic pathways, releasing the reflex from higher inhibition and impairing brainstem-originating pathways that facilitate complete detrusor emptying. The reflex threshold drops and urgency-frequency with moderate volumes results, often leaving a high postvoiding residual volume. Sporadic reflex incontinence is common.

Acute spinal transection produces reflex inhibition in the distal segment ("spinal shock"), with loss of voiding reflexes as well as of somatomotor ones. Acute retention develops, stretching the smooth muscle wall and producing a flat pressure-volume curve with no reflex. Overflow dribbling incontinence ensues. Reflex recovery is marked by increasingly large, randomly spaced, reflex partial bladder emptyings that in many instances can be trained by skill and patience into complete self-stimulated reflex voidings.

PERIPHERAL (PREGANGLIONIC OR SOMATIC AFFERENT) DEFECTS IN VOIDING. These can result from disease of either efferent or afferent peripheral nerves (e.g., occasional inflammatory neuropathy, diabetic neuropathy, tabes dorsalis, pelvic carcinoma), of the cauda equina, or of the conus medullaris. Depending upon the rate of neuritic progression, the bladder gradually dilates, with sensations of fullness disappearing commensurately with the degree of mechanical stretching. Normal sensations of urgency disappear, and the reflex progressively loses its effectiveness. Residual urine volumes increase. Ultimately, moderate to severe retention occurs, with or without spontaneous dribbling or occasionally spurting, small-volume overflow incontinence. In the absence of cystitis, the cystometrogram shows a flat filling curve on which, in time, autonomous ganglion-induced local detrusor contractions increasingly become superimposed. Spontaneous parasympathetic activity eventually leads to nearly continuous autonomous local detrusor activity, producing a hypertrophied bladder wall with a decreased bladder capacity and a steep pressure-volume curve.

TREATMENT OF NEUROGENIC BLADDER DIFFICULTIES. This varies according to the anatomic distribution of the cause. Urinary tract infections intensify all neurogenic functional abnormalities and should be treated promptly and effectively. Urgency or urgency-incontinence due to cerebral lesions or spinal extramedullary compression sometimes is aided by antispasticity drugs such as baclofen or parasympathetic blocking agents such as oxybutynin chloride 5 mg bid or tid. Often such symptoms are relatively minor and can be treated by addressing the neurologic abnormality and forcing fluids in an attempt to stretch the bladder wall so as to raise the threshold for the voiding reflex. Urgency-retention-incontinence due to intramedullary spinal lesions can be difficult to manage, especially when a high residual urine volume leads to recurrent urinary tract infection. Many women and some men can be taught clean self-catheterization to assure complete bladder emptying every four to six hours, thereby minimizing infection. Effective control is more difficult to attain in persons who suffer damage to the conus or peripheral micturition pathways; they usually require the assistance of an experienced urologist to develop effective bladder care.

Male Sexual Function

Organic disturbances of male sexual function are limited almost entirely to loss of libido, failure to attain an erection of sufficient strength to carry out sexual intercourse (impotence), and failure to attain normal ejaculation-emission. Masters and Johnson define impotence somewhat generously as greater than a 25 per cent failure during attempted intercourse. Failure to reach orgasm or the presence of premature or delayed ejaculation with normal libido and erectile capacity almost always reflects a psychogenic rather than an organic problem.

Neural control over male sexual activities arises within forebrain limbic areas, generating sexual drives that, in turn, are chronically stimulated by the effects of circulating androgens. Descending pathways travel with the parasympathetic outflow. Parasympathetic sacral efferents control penile tumescence by inducing vascular engorgement and also stimulate a large proportion of the severally originating pelvic contractions that initiate ejaculation and lead to the sensation of orgasm. Sympathetic stimulation contracts the seminal vesicles and closes the bladder neck to prevent retrograde emission, thereby guaranteeing anterograde ejaculation. Genital sensory fibers reach the spinal cord via the S2 to S4 dorsal roots and thenceforth ascend in the lemniscal system. Considerable evidence gained from the study of sexual function in paraplegics with a lesion producing an isolated, distal thoracic and lumbosacral spinal cord indicates that the cord contains all the necessary reflexes to complete sensory-induced erection and ejaculation.

Male impotence is common and increases with age to affect at some time almost half the population over 55 years; at that age psychogenic causes appear to be primary in only about 25 per cent. Therapeutic drugs and alcohol excess represent the most frequent causes of male impotence. Aging itself, however, eventually becomes a cause, and about 25 per cent of males of 70 years or more have erection failure attributable to aging alone.

Impotence has several possible causes, as indicated in Table 478–4, and more than one can operate in a given patient. In perhaps 10 per cent of cases no satisfactory explanation can be found. Psychologic factors are always important. They account for as many as half of the overall cases and must be inquired into carefully even when adequate organic reasons appear to exist.

Differential diagnosis begins with a careful history. Does the patient's complaint reflect a recent change in libido and performance or a longstanding pattern that has finally proved more troublesome to a sexual partner than to self? Longstanding absence or low level of libido can reflect either psychologic factors, chronic temporal lobe disease, or primary or secondary androgenic failure. If the disease is recent in origin, does it relate entirely to a specific partner? Such instances are usually psychogenic and best managed by a sex therapist if a careful history, physical examination, and tumescence studies provide no suggestion of the organic disorders listed in Table 478–4. If recent in onset, did libido remain high as potency declined? The latter pattern is more common among drug-induced or neurologic disorders than among endocrine ones.

Specific drugs most often causing impotence are listed in Table 478–5. Among the endocrine disorders, most that are severe enough to cause impotence are readily recognized. Pituitary tumors and hypothalamic lesions impairing gonadotropic release usually give prominent additional symptoms (Ch. 225). Hypo- or hyperthyroidism similarly generates other systemic symptoms. In doubtful cases, measurement of serum prolactin, testosterone, thyroxin, and triiodothyronine should settle the question. Borderline changes of a single serum hormone value, however, seldom provide evidence for a disorder of potency that will be reversed by giving hormone therapy.

Neurologic disturbances cause only about 10 per cent of all cases of impotence, although the symptom affects patients with a number of neurologic diseases and deserves compassionate inquiry. Temporal lobe disease affecting limbic systems is associated with reduction in male libido, while structural lesions involving descending parasympathetic systems commonly interfere with the capacity to gain and maintain an erection. Peripheral neurologic disorders, as Table 478–4 indicates, are the commonest neurologic offenders and should be approached as indicated in Ch. 526 to 531.

Aside from a record of sexual inadequacy limited to a specific partner, little in the history alone guarantees psychogenic causes. Since patients with physical illness may suffer psychogenic impotence (e.g., postmyocardial infarction or post-stroke sexual failure) while others with prominent psychiatric disorders may have unsuspected physical illness (e.g., depressives with diabetic neuropathy), objective testing measures are valuable in differential diagnosis. Useful in this regard is the measurement of nocturnal penile tumescence (NPT), which, taken during sleep monitoring, records the frequency and intensity of the erections that normally accompany rapid eye movement sleep. When matched suitably for age with normal controls, the results correlate highly although not completely with psychogenic (no appreciable decline in NPT) versus organic (moderate to marked decline in NPT) impotence.

Treatment of male impotence depends upon the cause. Drug avoidance or readjustment can benefit many cases, as can substitution therapy when endocrine failure is demonstrated.

TABLE 478–4. PRINCIPAL ORGANIC CAUSES OF MALE SEXUAL FAILURE

Drugs
Endocrine
Secondary: pituitary adenoma; idiopathic or acquired hypogonadotropic hypogonadism; hyperprolactinemia
Primary gonadal failure
Advanced diabetes mellitus
Hypothyroidism, hyperthyroidism (rare)
Chronic Systemic Illnesses
Cirrhosis
Chronic renal failure
Disseminated malignancy, etc.
Neurogenic
Temporal lobe disorders: trauma, epilepsy, neoplasm, stroke
Intramedullary spinal lesions: paraplegia; demyelinating disorders; neoplasms; syrinx; Shy-Drager dysautonomia
Peripheral nerves. Somatic or autonomic neuropathies; pelvic neoplasms, granulomas, trauma; structural lesions of cauda equina or conus medullaris
Urologic
Complete prostatectomy; priapism; local trauma or neoplasms; Peyronie's disease; rectosigmoid "cleanouts"
Vascular
Severe aortic atherosclerosis; lower aortic bypass

TABLE 478–5. DRUGS OFTEN REPORTED TO INTERFERE WITH MALE POTENCY

Alcohol	Guanethidine
Anticancer chemotherapy	Immunosuppressives
Anticholinergics	Lithium
Antiparkinson agents	Opiates
Barbiturates and congeners	Phenothiazine
Benzodiazepines	Several antihypertensive ganglionic blockers
Bethanidine	Several diuretics
Cannabis	Tricyclic and MAO-inhibitor antidepressants
Cimetidine	

Local genital abnormalities should be approached surgically. A variety of surgically implantable prostheses to assist erection have become available in recent years to aid the patient affected with impotence caused by neurogenic or locally severe vascular disease. Thus far, attempts at revascularizing the penis have met with only limited success. Testosterone therapy given in the absence of a demonstrated androgen deficiency almost never provides more than placebo benefit and creates a carcinogenic risk as well.

Hypothalamus and Its Disorders

Greenberg HS, Rocher LL, Clavin DB, Ehren Kranz JRL: Episodic hyperhidrosis, hypothermia, and agenesis of the corpus callosum. Neurology 33:1122, 1983. *The most recent comprehensive review of this uncommon condition, with the addition of new material.*

Martin JB, Lourdis DMD: Potential implications of brain peptides in neurologic disease. *In* Martin JB, Reichlen S, Bick KL (eds.): Neurosecretion and Brain Peptides. New York, Raven Press, 1981. *Covers the known and possible associations of these newly identified neuromodulators with neurologic disease, some of the hypothalamus.*

Plum F, Van Uitert R: Non-endocrine diseases and disorders of the hypothalamus. Res Publ Assoc Res New Ment Dis 56:415, 1977. *A comprehensive review of the clinically important autonomic functions of the hypothalamus written at the dawn of the peptide era. Extensively referenced.*

Peripheral and Central Autonomic Functions

Appenzeller O: The Autonomic Nervous System. 2nd ed. New York, Elsevier, 1976. *The only available comprehensive monograph of recent origin.*

Bannister R, Oppenheimer DR: Degenerative diseases of the nervous system associated with autonomic failure. Brain 95:457, 1972. *A description of various autonomic syndromes associated with degenerative disease, with an attempt to classify the disorders tentatively.*

Black IB, Petito CK: Catecholamine enzymes in the degenerative neurological disease idiopathic orthostatic hypotension. Science 192:910, 1976. *An analysis of biochemical deficits in autonomic failure, with specific reference to catecholamine biosynthetic enzymes.*

Bradbury S, Eggleston C: Postural hypotension: A report of three cases. Am Heart J 1:73, 1925. *The first definitive report of idiopathic orthostatic hypotension.*

Hines S, Houston M, Robertson D: The clinical spectrum of autonomic dysfunction. Am J Med 70:1091, 1981. *An analysis of 297 patients with various forms of autonomic insufficiency of both secondary and primary causes.*

Kochar MS, Itskovitz HD: Treatment of idiopathic orthostatic hypotension with indomethacin. Lancet 1:1011, 1978. *The first report of the use of indomethacin, a potentially useful agent, in the treatment of postural hypotension.*

Nass R, Chutorian A: Dysesthesias and dysautonomia: A self limited syndrome of painful dysesthesias and autonomic dysfunction in childhood. J Neurol Neurosurg Psychiatr 45:162, 1982. *A description of three children with a self-limited selective sensory and autonomic neuropathy, presumably of the inflammatory type.*

Petito CK, Black IB: Ultrastructure and biochemistry of sympathetic ganglia in idiopathic orthostatic hypotension. Ann Neurol 4:6, 1978. *Correlation of ultrastructural and enzymatic deficits in one form of autonomic insufficiency.*

Shy GM, Drager GA: A neurological syndrome associated with orthostatic hypotension. Arch Neurol 2:511, 1960. *The definitive clinicopathologic analysis of autonomic insufficiency associated with generalized neurologic degeneration.*

Young R, Asbury A, Corbett J, Adams R: Pure pandysautonomia with recovery. Description and discussion of diagnostic criteria. Brain 98:613, 1975. *A detailed description of the entitled disorder.*

Ziegler MG, Lake CR, Kopin IJ: The sympathetic-nervous-system defect in primary orthostatic hypotension. N Engl J Med 296:293, 1977. *A clinical study using circulating catecholamines and metabolites to analyze the pathogenesis of idiopathic orthostatic hypotension.*

Urinary Bladder Control

Andersson K-E, Sjögren C: Aspects on the physiology and pharmacology of the bladder and urethra. Prog Neurobiol 19:71, 1982. *Describes bladder-urethral innervation and comprehensively lists drugs that have been used to treat bladder dysfunction.*

Boyarsky S, Labay P, Hanick P, Abramson AS, Boyarsky R: Care of the Patient with Neurogenic Bladder. Boston, Little, Brown and Company. 1979. *A well-balanced monograph describing all aspects of this difficult subject.*

Williams ME, Pannill FC: Urinary incontinence in the elderly. Physiology, pathophysiology, diagnosis and treatment. Ann Intern Med 97:895, 1982. *A thorough, highly practical guide with an extensive bibliography.*

Male Sexual Function

Bennett AH (ed.): Management of Male Impotence. Baltimore, Williams and Wilkins, 1982. *A useful multiauthored monograph that covers the organic causes of the problem.*

Kaplan HS: Disorders of Sexual Desire. New York, Bruner/Meizel, 1979. *A detailed review of the most frequent psychogenic sexual dysfunctions.*

Kolodny RC, Masters WH, Johnson VE: Textbook of Sexual Medicine. Boston, Little, Brown and Company, 1979. *A good textbook of sexual medicine designed for students and general physicians.*

Slag MF, Morley JE, Elson MK, et al.: Impotence in medical clinic outpatients. JAMA 249:1736, 1983. *Among 1181 men attendees at a VA Hospital, 34 per cent with a mean age of just over 60 years had erectile dysfunction.*

Spark RF, White RA, Connolly PB: Impotence is not always psychogenic. Newer insights into hypothalamic-pituitary-gonadal dysfunction. JAMA 234:750, 1980. *Thirty-seven of 105 consecutive patients evaluated for impotence in an endocrine clinic had previously unsuspected hypogonadism, hyperprolactinemia, or hyperthyroidism. Appropriate treatment restored potency in 33 cases.*

479. THE SPECIAL SENSES AND RELATED FUNCTIONS

479.1. Smell and Taste

Fred Plum

OLFACTION

The capacity to detect odor provides humans with both strong limbic system signals and potential safety warnings. Smell contributes importantly to the anticipation and ingestion of food, since much of what we "taste" derives from olfactory stimulation during the ingestion and chewing of food. Most humans can recognize and identify a thousand or more different odors; efforts to reduce this large repertory into the compoundings of a limited number of elemental aromas have been unsuccessful.

Olfactory receptors lie in a roughly dime-sized area of specialized pigment epithelium that archs along the superior aspect of each side of the nasal mucosa. Constantly regenerating bipolar sensory cells in this area thrust short receptor hairs into the overlying mucus to detect aromatic molecules as they dissolve. Central afferent fibrils traverse the cribriform plate to reach the olfactory bulb on the ventral surface of the frontal lobe whence second and third order neurons project directly and indirectly to the prepyriform cortex and parts of the amygdaloid complex of the same and opposite side of the brain, representing the primary olfactory cortex.

Olfactory sense can be reduced (hyposmia), absent (anosmia), or distorted (dysosmia). Dysosmia usually results from the products of local disease but occasionally represents a psychiatric symptom. Anosmia can be partial or complete, inherited or acquired. Thus, anosmia or hyposmia for specific selective odors occurs rarely an as autosomal or recessive inherited trait. Congenital anosmia accompanies certain autonomic and endocrinopathic disorders, notably hypogonadotropic hypogonadism (Kallman's syndrome).

Most acquired disturbances of smell result from transient or sustained disease of the nasal mucous membranes that deadens or dries out the receptor membrane. The disorder seldom is complete and commonly responds to local treatment. More severe and often permanent anosmia results from basal skull fractures, frontal fossa brain tumors affecting the olfactory pathways, and, much less often, herpes zoster, B_{12} deficiency, and multiple sclerosis. Sudden, idiopathic anosmia usually associated with loss of taste as well has been reported, possibly the result of a local neurotropic viral infection. No satisfactory treatment has been found for such neurogenic anosmias. Affected patients must be warned explicitly to avoid gas heating and to install smoke alarms to compensate for the life-threatening hazards of the defect. *Parosmia* is a distortion of olfactory perception (normal odors perceived as a foul smell) that may occur without prior anosmia or during recovery from anosmia.

Hallucinations of smell, usually of a foul quality, occur with epileptogenic lesions affecting the region of the amygdala and are termed uncinate fits.

GUSTATORY FUNCTION

Taste, like smell, has both vegetative and survival values, the latter perhaps more necessary among our primitive ancestors. The impairment or loss of taste is a serious complaint with a variety of illnesses, in some of which a concurrent olfactory loss is actually at fault.

The brain abstracts its specific sense of taste from signals fed from tastebuds and associated receptors that lie on the dorsal surface of the tongue and in the adjacent faucial areas. Fungiform papillary buds on the anterior tongue respond mainly to sweet and sour stimuli, while foliate and valate papillae located along the base of the tongue and adjacent areas detect predominantly bitter qualities. The distribution of selective taste receptors may vary from time to time within the individual so as partly to guide food selection according to nutritional need. The anterior two thirds of the tongue is innervated by branches of the chorda tympani division of the intermediate and facial nerves, making it especially susceptible to injuries or infections that affect the latter nerve on its route through the middle ear and petrous bone. Glossopharyngeal nerve fibers supply the taste receptors of the posterior two thirds of the tongue and fauces. Both innervations project to the nucleus tractus solitarius of the medulla and then via a series of relays to reach the postcentral somatosensory cerebral cortex. Taste receptors on the tongue have an innately relatively high threshold that increases further with age, often making specific testing difficult for diagnostic purposes.

Taste loss or reduction is termed *ageusia* or *hypogeusia*, distortion being *dysgeusia*. The reference by Schiffman provides a long list of specific disorders that sometimes can reduce or alter taste or smell sensations. Chief specific offenders from the neurologic standpoint are Bell's palsy, which reduces perception; epileptic aurae, which occasionally include gustatory sensations; and depressive or paranoid delusions, which more distort the sense of taste or smell than destroy them. Among systemic problems, aging, hepatitis, cancer, and various forms of drugs are the main causes of symptoms of taste reduction or distortion. Investigation for the symptom of taste loss or abnormal taste involves first a clinical search for local mucous membrane or neurologic disease, followed by a systematic review of medications being taken, possible exposure to toxic fumes, and, if still necessary, a more exacting inquiry into possibly hidden systemic illness.

As with defects in smell, there is no specific treatment for taste loss except giving attention to the underlying illness. Dietary zinc supplements provide no proven advantage. Nontoxic odorants and spices commonly increase the palatability of food, as does switching from one substance to another during meals.

Doty RL: A review of olfactory dysfunctions in man. Am J Otolaryngol 1:57, 1979. *A comprehensive basic review, extensively referenced.*

Howe JG, Gibson JD: Uncinate seizures and tumors, a myth re-examined. Ann Neurol 12:227, 1982. *Most patients with such seizures lack radiographic evidence of structural brain abnormalities.*

Schiffman SS: Taste and smell in disease. N Engl J Med 308:1275, 1337, 1983. *A two-part, well-referemced review of an often neglected medical problem.*

Smith M, Smith LG, Levinson B: The use of smell in differential diagnosis. Lancet 2:1452, 1982. *An amusing index to disease-produced odors useful to the clinician.*

479.2. Neuro-ophthalmology

Fred Plum

The mechanistic understanding of visual impairment, along with disturbances of pupillary and oculomotor control, lies close to the heart of diagnosing neurologic disorders. Diseases of the eye itself are further considered in Part XXIV.

ANATOMY OF THE VISUAL PATHWAYS

Light entering the eye falls on the retinal rods and cones, which transduce the stimulus into neural impulses to be transmitted to the brain. What each eye "sees" is termed its *visual field*. The geometry of the system dictates that the nasal side of the left eye and the temporal side of the right see the left side of the world and vice versa and, similarly, that the upper half of each retina sees the lower half of the world (Fig. 479–1) and vice versa.

Retinal sensitivity to light stimulation increases centrifugally toward the cones of the central macular area, which transmit a distinctive

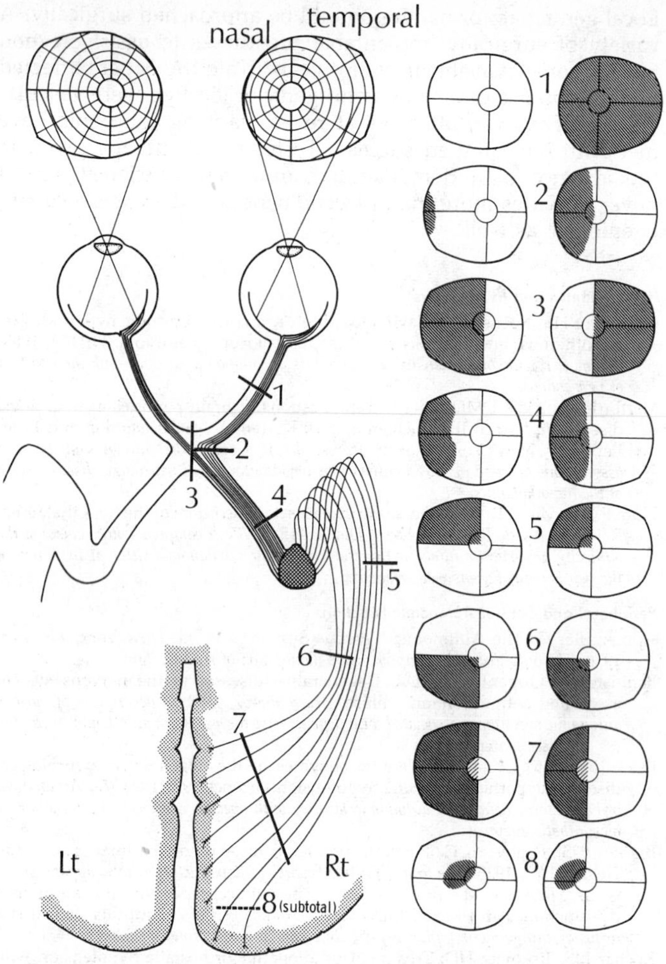

Figure 479–1. Visual fields that accompany damage to the visual pathways. 1. Optic nerve: Unilateral amaurosis. 2. Lateral optic chiasm: Grossly incongruous, incomplete (contralateral) homonymous hemianopia. 3. Central optic chiasm: Bitemporal hemianopia. 4. Optic tract: Incongruous, incomplete homonymous hemianopia. 5. Temporal (Meyer's) loop of optic radiation: Congruous partial or complete (contralateral) homonymous superior quadrantanopia. 6. Parietal (superior) projection of the optic radiation: Congruous partial or complete homonymous inferior quadrantanopia. 7. Complete parieto-occipital interruption of optic radiation. Complete congruous homonymous hemianopia with psychophysical shift of foveal point often sparing central vision, giving "macular sparing." 8. Incomplete damage to visual cortex: Congruous homonymous scotomas, usually encroaching at least acutely on central vision.

maculopapillary bundle that enters the temporal-lateral one third of the optic disc. Other nerve fibers from the retina lie axially within the optic nerve in a pattern that largely repeats their retinal distribution.

The arterial supply to the optic nerve and retina both derive from branches of the carotid-born ophthalmic artery. The *central retinal artery* approaches the eye along each optic nerve, and pierces the inferior aspect of the dural sheath about 1 cm behind the globe to enter the center of the nerve. The artery emerges in the fundus at the center of the nerve head whence it irrigates most of the retina by superior, medial, inferior, and lateral branches. Anastomotic branches derived from the choroidal and posterior ciliary arteries supply the nerve head itself and the macular region. Venous drainage from the retina and nerve head flows primarily via the central retinal vein, whose course of exit from the eye parallels that of the entry of the artery. The venous anatomy explains why inflammatory lesions of or adjacent to the optic nerve head cause venous distention and ipsilateral papilledema (optic neuritis), whereas inflammation lying posterior to the point where the vein leaves the nerve produces only visual loss without swelling of the nerve head (retrobulbar neuritis).

Behind the eye the optic nerve passes through the orbital foramen and sphenoid bone to reach the optic chiasm. In the chiasm, nerves from the nasal half of each retina decussate and join the fibers from the temporal half of the contralateral retina (see Fig. 479–1). From the chiasm, the *optic tracts* pass around the cerebral peduncles to reach the lateral geniculate ganglia of either side. At the level of the geniculate, fibers serving corresponding points in each retinal half visual field lie adjacent to each other, and this proximity is maintained in the subsequent relay to the calcarine cortex. The geniculocalcarine radiation initially fans out into superolateral and inferolateral projections, the latter passing around the lateral ventricle and for a short distance into the temporal lobe (Meyer's loop) before turning posteriorly to head for the striate cortex of the occipital lobe. At the occipital pole, the striate cortex (area 17) lies along the superior and inferior banks of the calcarine fissure, with macular fibers projecting most posteriorly to the occipital pole, and more peripheral retinal projections lying more anteriorly. Each occipital pole "sees" the opposite half world. Fibers serving the superior retinal quadrants project to the superior bank of the calcarine fissure, and those from the inferior quadrants project to the inferior bank. No satisfactory evidence indicates that the macula enjoys bilateral anatomic representations in the striate cortex.

DIAGNOSIS OF VISUAL IMPAIRMENT

DEFINITIONS. *Amblyopia* refers to dimness or partial loss of vision, *amaurosis* to blindness. *Scotomas* are errors of relative or complete visual loss circumscribed within a comparatively better total field of vision for the particular eye.

Abnormalities affecting structures lying anywhere from the retina to the occipital pole produce distinctive abnormalities in the visual field. Visual field defects impairing half or nearly half of a field are termed *hemianopic.* Those affecting less than this extent are termed partial field defects, often with the additional designation of *quadrantic* or *altitudinal* (superior or inferior), according to the abnormality. A visual defect that affects similar parts of the right or left half field in both eyes is called *homonymous;* identical errors of involvement from the two eyes are termed *congruent.* Scotomas may reflect abnormalities anywhere from the retina or its projecting pathways to the striate cortex. Most frequently they result either from prechiasmatic lesions of the optic nerve or retina, less often from partial lesions of the occipital cortex. Involvement of the macular area or its projections produces *central* scotomas. Scotomas that lie near the macular visual area are sometimes called *paracentral,* whereas those that extend into macular vision from the more peripheral field may be termed *cecocentral.* Central scotomas always interfere with visual acuity. An uncorrectable reduction in acuity below 20/50 indicates either a central scotoma or a diffuse impairment of the visual pathway of that eye.

Difficulty seeing may arise as a result of local disease in the eye as well as from neurologic disorders that affect tissues extending anywhere from the retina to the occipital cortex. Essential to understanding is a careful examination of the globes themselves, together with ophthalmoscopy and measurements of visual acuity and visual fields.

OPHTHALMOSCOPIC EXAMINATION. One should use bright tangential ophthalmoscopic light to detect any corneal, lenticular, or vitreous opacities. Ophthalmologists routinely dilate the pupil to examine the fundus, but this step should be avoided in acutely ill patients or those suspected of neurologic diseases until one is certain that intrinsic pupillary abnormalities will not be important in reaching a diagnosis or in following the patient's course.

VISUAL ACUITY. Visual function for neurologic purposes consists of the *best corrected visual acuity.* It is best tested quantitatively with refractive errors corrected and for each eye separately. The normal reference is a recognition of letters at an idealized 20 feet, and acuity charts are designed with ever larger letters that normally are recognized at proportionately greater distances. Thus if one reads at 20 feet letters no better than those normally perceived at 40 feet, vision is recorded as 20/40. Small visual charts that are easily carried in the physician's case permit quick and fairly accurate bedside appraisals of acuity.

Visual fields can be tested at the bedside by confrontation, and rough estimates of their integrity can be made even in patients with reduced alertness. With practice and a cooperative subject, accurate confrontation fields can be obtained that even outline scotomas. The examiner should place the test object, e.g., a red match head, midway between his eye and the patient's and test the patient's unilateral visual field against his own. The field should be tested individually for each eye, since the finding of an asymmetrical (incongruous) or symmetrical visual field change represents an important localizing sign.

PATHOLOGIC DIAGNOSIS OF VISUAL IMPAIRMENT

LESIONS OF THE EYE. Corneal, lenticular, or vitreous opacities large enough to produce visual symptoms almost always can be detected by inspection or funduscopic examination. Refractive errors can be distinguished from neurologic abnormalities by the pin hole test. Patients with uncorrected myopia or presbyopia will correct vision to normal by gazing at the test chart through a pin hole in a card held immediately over the eye. The tiny aperture overcomes any aberration created by the failure of the lens to accommodate.

Glaucoma caused by impaired absorption of the aqueous humor results in a high intraocular pressure that usually produces gradual visual loss with reduced night-time vision, "haloes" seen around illuminated lamps, and, often, pain in the affected eye. Uncommonly, rapid visual loss can occur with few premonitory symptoms. Diagnosis comes from the tonometric measurement of a high intraocular pressure and may be suspected by palpating an abnormally firm globe and observing a deep, pale optic cup and attenuated blood vessels.

Retinal tears and detachment give rise to unilateral distortions of the visual image, seen as sudden angulations or curves of objects containing straight lines *(metamorphopsia).* Hemorrhages into the vitreous humor or unilateral infectious or inflammatory lesions of the retina can produce scotomas that in all ways resemble those resulting from primary disease of the central visual pathway.

Serious visual losses due to abnormalities affecting the lower visual pathways tend to affect the two eyes asymmetrically or separately, produce non-homonymous visual field defects, and are prone to interfere with the pupillary light reflex.

Monocular visual loss is due to a lesion of one eye, its retina, or optic nerve. Ocular and retinal lesions can usually be detected with the ophthalmoscope. Most acute or subacute optic nerve disease is due to demyelinating-inflammatory illness, vascular obstruction, or neoplasm. Demyelinating disease of the nerve head (*optic neuritis* or "papillitis") produces papilledema along with loss of central vision only in the affected eye; subjectively unrecognized scotomas sometimes may be found in the other eye. Demyelination in the optic nerve behind where the retinal vein emerges (retrobulbar neuritis) initially leaves a normal-looking disc but a central or paracentral scotoma. Vascular lesions produce either total amaurosis or a sector field defect consistent with an intraocular arterial occlusion *(ischemic optic neuropathy).* Funduscopic appearances are characteristic. Tumors invading the nerve or space-occupying lesions compressing it anywhere between the orbit and the chiasm cause gradually declining unilateral impairment of either central vision (intrinsic or far advanced lesions), or a sector defect of the peripheral visual field. With such chronic lesions, the affected optic nerve becomes visibly atrophic. In doubtful cases, fluorescein ocular angiography, visual evoked responses, or electroretinography can assist in the localizing diagnosis of a prechiasmal or retinal lesion.

Binocular visual loss can result from disease located anywhere along the central visual pathways from the retinas to the occipital poles. Retinal, prechiasmatic optic nerve or chiasmatic lesions are the most common cause of bilateral global visual loss, i.e., amblyopia that involves both halves of the visual fields of each eye. Degenerative diseases of the postgeniculate radiations as well as traumatic, vascular, and rarely neoplastic disorders involving both occipital lobes serve as less frequent causes of such bilateral visual impairments. Most *bilateral retinal disease* producing visual failure in younger subjects is due to heredodegenerative conditions. Vascular diseases, diabetes, idiopathic (senile) macular degeneration, and bilateral retinal detachments are causes in older age groups. In the pigmentary retinal degenerations, visual loss begins peripherally and proceeds centrally and often very slowly before acuity (central vision) is impaired. By contrast, pigmentary macular degenerations affect mainly younger children and impair central vision early in their course. Most of the retinal degenerations produce characteristic and recognizable ophthalmoscopic appearances. With the pigmentary degenerations the visual fields shrink progressively in size. With the macular degenerations, on the other hand, the fields show noncongruent central scotomas.

Acute *bilateral optic nerve* disease with visual loss, although less common than unilateral disease, is caused most often by inflammatory-demyelinating illness, less frequently by optic nerve or retinal vascular disease, or by toxic or nutritional optic neuropathies. In younger persons and those lacking a clear history of toxic exposures, demyelinating lesions overwhelmingly predominate. Symptoms are of an abrupt or subacute onset with visual blurring or loss of acuity which may progress rapidly to blindness within hours or days. There may be pain about the eyes, particularly on eye movement.

Papilledema resulting from increased intracranial pressure occasionally causes visual loss under one of three circumstances: (1) Acute transient episodes of amaurosis lasting a few seconds and attributed to acute rises in intracranial pressure (plateau waves) that interfere with retinal venous drainage into the cavernous sinus or with vascular irrigation of the occipital lobe. (2) Acute bilateral sustained amaurosis following abrupt surgical relief of longstanding severely increased intracranial pressure. This is rare. (3) Progressive loss of peripheral vision with longstanding severe papilledema, presumably owing to pressure atrophy of the most peripherally lying fibers in the tightly sheathed optic nerve. Table 479–1 gives the main differential points between papilledema and optic neuritis.

Subacute or chronic optic nerve disease results mainly from toxic-nutritional causes and the inherited optic atrophies. The latter sometimes accompany spinocerebellar degeneration or selectively affect the optic nerves in both juvenile and adult (Leber's) forms. With either cause, visual loss is moderate or severe and affects primarily or initially central vision; ophthalmoscopy shows mild to moderate primary optic atrophy. (*Primary optic atrophy,* that caused by primary degeneration, retrobulbar compression or demyelination of the optic nerve, is characterized by a pale white optic disc, a reduced vascularity, and a sharply demarcated edge that separates the disc margin from the relatively normal-appearing surrounding retina. *Secondary optic atrophy* follows chronic papilledema and is characterized by pallor of the disc plus superimposed papilloretinal scarring: the disc looks atrophic but more gray, the vessels are attenuated, and the margin between the disc and the surrounding retina lacks clear demarcation.)

Lesions involving or compressing the *optic chiasm* produce nonhomonymous visual abnormalities that affect the unilateral visual fields incongruously (e.g., bitemporal hemianopia). Intrinsic or extrinsic neoplasms and parachiasmal arterial aneurysms are the common causes. Gliomas that arise in the chiasm are rare in adulthood but, when they occur, impair central vision early. Extrinsic space-occupying lesions compressing the chiasm can arise from its superior lateral or inferior aspect and include dysgerminomas, craniopharyngiomas, pituitary adenomas, meningiomas arising from the sphenoid bone, and large aneurysms of the carotid artery. Asymmetrical, lateral (bitemporal) inferior or superior visual field impairments combined with subtle primary optic atrophy are early signs. The patient often is unaware of visual impairment until the deficit encroaches on central vision in one or both eyes.

TABLE 479–1. DIFFERENTIATION OF OPTIC NEURITIS FROM PAPILLEDEMA

	Optic Neuritis	Papilledema
Central-cecocentral visual loss	Present	Absent
Distribution	Usually unilateral	Usually bilateral
Ocular pain on movement	Present	Absent
Direct light reflex	± Reduced	Intact
CT scan of head	Normal	Often abnormal
Visual evoked responses	Abnormal	Normal
Lumbar puncture pressure	Normal	Elevated

Optic tract abnormalities are comparatively rare but produce characteristic visual changes. The fibers serving identical points in the homonymous half fields do not fully commingle in the anterior optic tract so that lesions encroaching on this structure produce incongruous and usually incomplete homonymous hemianopias. Mild and sometimes subtle optic hemiatrophy accompanies longstanding tract lesions. Pupillary reactions usually appear normal by bedside testing.

LESIONS OF THE GENICULATE GANGLIA, VISUAL RADIATION, OR OCCIPITAL CORTEX. These most often result from vascular damage, traumatic injuries, neoplasms, or, rarely, inflammatory or degenerative disorders involving the cerebral white matter. Their localization can be deduced by the resulting visual field defects (see Fig. 479–1), most of which are fully congruent, occasional exceptions being observed in the horizontal margins of field defects occurring with temporal lobe lesions. Postgeniculate damage to the visual radiations can go long unrecognized unless hemianopia intrudes on macular vision. Even then, psychophysical adjustments shift the foveal point so that few patients with occipital lesions permanently split the visual image unless the adjacent parastriate cortex is involved.

Bilateral damage to the visual radiation or occipital cortex produces *cortical blindness.* Postgeniculate amaurosis can be differentiated from pregeniculate causes by (1) a normal funduscopic appearance, (2) intact direct and consensual pupillary light reflexes, and (3) the presence of anatomically appropriate lesions by CT scan. When the injury to the visual radiation concurrently involves the right parietal lobe, such patients may be unaware of or even deny the existence of visual loss. Visual evoked response studies will distinguish cortical visual loss from hysteria or malingering if any doubt exists following the CT scan.

Partial damage involving adjacent areas of the superior and inferior banks of the calcarine cortex is relatively rare, but occasionally can follow traumatic or ischemic injuries. Those at or near the occipital pole result in central or paracentral scotomas that are usually but not always hemianopic. Aside from the history and CT findings, differentiation from an optic nerve defect depends on the congruity of the resulting field defect, the absence of pupillary reflex abnormalities, and, often, the results of testing visual evoked responses.

PUPILLARY FUNCTIONS

Neural mechanisms controlling the pupil travel widely through the nervous system, making changes in pupillary activity a frequent clue to neurologic diagnosis.

ANATOMY AND DIAGNOSIS OF PUPILLOMOTOR ABNORMALITIES. The size of the pupil is governed by a tonic balance between sympathetic and parasympathetic innervation of the pupillodilator (sympathetic) and pupilloconstrictor (parasympathetic) muscles of the iris. Sympathetic stimulation widens the pupil *(mydriasis);* parasympathetic stimulation narrows it *(miosis).* Paralysis of either of the innervations results in a near maximal response in the unopposed direction. In the normal resting state, light entering the eye provides the major stimulus governing the size of the pupil; sympathetic mydriasis occurs characteristically as part of the more brief "fight or flight" defense reaction.

Retinal influences on the pupil take origin in the retinal rods and cones with maximal sensitivity in the macular area. The fibers follow the crossed and uncrossed visual pathways to the pregeniculate portion of the optic tracts where the light receptor fibers diverge to the pretectal area located at the midbrain diencephalic junction. Interneurons project from this region to the Edinger-Westphal nuclei atop the midbrain third nerve complex of either side. From that point, paired parasympathetic efferents leave the midbrain with the third nerves to travel in the interpeduncular space across the petroclinoid ligament and edge of the tentorium whence, after traversing the cavernous sinus, they enter the superior orbital fissure. In the orbit, the parasympathetic efferents synapse in the ciliary ganglion from which short ciliary nerves enter the eye to reach the pupillary muscles.

The principal sympathetic control of the pupil originates in the ventrolateral hypothalamus (first order neuron), whence fibers descend ipsilaterally to the lower brainstem tegmentum and then the cervical cord, where they lie superficially and synapse with the preganglionic neurons in the intermediolateral cell column of the upper three thoracic segments. Preganglionic fibers (second order neurons) emerge with the ventral roots of C8, T1, and T2, and ascend in the neck to synapse in the superior cervical ganglion adjacent to the base of the skull. Postganglionic (third order neurons) pupillary fibers accompany the internal carotid artery through the skull, leaving it to follow the ophthalmic branch of the trigeminal nerve to reach the pupillodilator muscles of the eye.

Topologic diagnosis of pupillary abnormalities follows anatomic principles. Lesions of one retina or prechiasmatic optic nerve produce no pupillary abnormalities at rest, but light stimulation of the affected nerves evokes an impaired or absent pupillary constriction with an impaired consensual constriction in the opposite eye *(the afferent pupil)*. The affected pupil may be slightly larger than its fellow. By contrast, stimulation of the opposite, normal eye elicits a brisk consensual response in the amaurotic eye. Chiasmal lesions produce pupillary defects proportional to the degree that they encroach on fibers of the maculopapillary bundles; pupillary changes are a late sign. Lesions compressing or damaging the tectal region interrupt the afferent light reflex bilaterally to produce midposition or moderately wide (greater than 5 mm) and light-fixed pupils. Pupillary constriction on accommodation is preserved until late stages. Damage to the midbrain tegmentum and third nerve nuclei destroys the preganglionic parasympathetic pupillary control but interrupts descending sympathetic pathways at the same time. The result is irregular, often unequal and fixed, midposition pupils of 3 to 5 mm diameter. Interruption of the emerging third nerve in the ventral midbrain or along the proximal part of its course produces a mid-dilated pupil 6 to 7 mm in diameter. For unclear reasons, injury to the third nerve in the cavernous sinus or anterior to it sometimes misleadingly spares the pupil.

Sympathetic paralysis of the eye with ptosis and miosis (Horner's syndrome) can result from lesions anywhere along the course of the pathway. Topical diagnosis is made best by identifying associated signs in the brainstem or neck or along the carotid artery. Failure of the affected eye to dilate after instilling hydroxyamphetamine 1 per cent indicates a postganglionic (third order neuron) lesion.

Certain pupillary problems may occur in relative isolation. These include *essential anisocoria,* a lifelong difference in the size of the two pupils with normal reflex reactions; the disparity remains constant during constriction and dilatation. *Adie's tonic pupil* is a medium to large (3 to 6 mm) pupil that constricts little or not at all to light and slowly to accommodation but constricts with the instillation of dilute pilocarpine (0.02 per cent) or mecholyl 2.5 per cent. The abnormal pupil is associated with diminished to absent deep tendon reflexes in the extremities. The condition usually affects one eye or occasionally both, is more frequent in women 25 to 45 years of age, and carries no serious implications. Its cause is unknown. *Argyll Robertson pupils* are small, 1 to 2 mm, unequal, irregular, and fixed to light, and constrict to accommodation.Their principal cause is tertiary neurosyphilis, although partial Argyll Robertson changes occur with diabetes and certain of the autonomic neuropathies. Unexplained unilaterally or bilaterally dilated pupils as an isolated finding can result from the accidental or intentional instillation of mydriatics. The recent widespread use of scopolamine skin pads has increased the problem. Failure of the pupil to constrict promptly with pilocarpine 1 per cent gives the diagnosis if the history is withheld.

DISTURBANCES OF OCULAR MOVEMENT

DEFINITIONS. Abnormal, disjunctive eye movements can result from disturbances at several levels. These include abnormalities in the action of the individual ocular muscles, the oculomotor myoneural junctions, the oculomotor nerves and their three paired nuclei in the brainstem, and the internuclear medial longitudinal fasciculus that yokes the eyes in parallel movements. The term strabismus describes an involuntary deviation of the eye from its normal physiological position. *Nonparalytic strabismus* is due to an intrinsic imbalance of ocular muscle tone and is usually congenital. *Paralytic strabismus* results from defects in ocular muscle innervation. Strabismus is called *comitant* when the relationship between the two ocular axes remains constant in all directions of gaze, *noncomitant* when they change, and *latent* when the imbalance is brought out only by covering one eye to prevent fixation. Latent strabismus can become manifest during great fatigue or in association with high fever and systemic illness. Congenital comitant strabismus present at birth or soon thereafter carries with it the strong risk that, if uncorrected, the subject will suppress vision in the nondominant eye during the developmental period when it usually forms its connections with the visual cortex. The result is unilateral, permanent reduction of vision in the nondominant eye *(amblyopia ex anopia)*. Strabismus beginning after binocular fusion is developed produces sudden diplopia, which gradually disappears as the subject automatically suppresses the image from the misaligned eye. Postinfancy visual suppression does not lead to permanent visual loss.

Defects in ocular movement resulting from faulty action of the eye muscles or their peripheral innervation from the third (oculomotor), fourth (trochlear), or sixth (abducens) cranial nerves or their nuclei in the brainstem are called *ocular paralyses* or palsies. This contrasts with abnormalities in eye movement on conjugate gaze owing to abnormalities of the medial longitudinal fasciculus or supranuclear structures, which are called *gaze paralyses.*

OCULAR PARALYSES. The *abducens nerve* serves the external rectus muscle. Beyond the nucleus, selective involvement of the abducens nerve anywhere along its pathway inside or outside the brainstem leads to isolated weakness of abduction of the affected eye. Destruction of the specific area of the abducens nucleus in the brainstem damages not only the area that controls abduction in the ipsilateral eye but also the neurons that control lateral conjugate gaze to that side. The *trochlear nerve* serves the superior oblique muscle which intorts the eye and moves it down. Patients with superior oblique weakness often tilt the head in the opposite direction. One usually observes a slight upward deviation of the involved eye in vertical down gaze accentuated by adducting the affected globe. Involvement of the third nerve nucleus in the midbrain always produces at least some bilateral oculomotor weakness; either a nuclear or subnuclear lesion of the third nerve within the brainstem can be identified by the presence of other central neurologic defects that arise concomitantly. Peripheral third nerve paralysis can result from lesions damaging the structure anywhere from its origin from the ventral midbrain to where it enters the orbit via the superior orbital fissure. Depending upon its completeness, third nerve palsy produces a widely dilated pupil, severe ptosis, and an externally deviated eye held in position by the unopposed contraction of the external rectus muscle. In such conditions, the continued trochlear action reveals itself by intorsion of the eye as the subject fixes on an object brought from above to below the horizontal meridian.

ABNORMALITIES OF CONJUGATE GAZE. Conjugate movements of the eyes are regulated by supranuclear pathways that descend from the forebrain to reach the lower and upper ends of the medial longitudinal fasciculus (MLF) in the brainstem. The forebrain pathways direct gaze in response to voluntary action and visual reflex tracking, whereas the brainstem MLF yokes the two globes by reciprocal innervation and inhibition so as to assure normal fusion of the visual image.

Pathways descending from the frontal lobes regulate rapid voluntary and saccadic eye movements. *Saccades* are quick (up to 700° per second), ballistic movements that rapidly change fixation. Stimulation in humans of one frontal gaze area conjugately directs the eyes to the opposite side; acute damage to the same region (e.g., by hemorrhage or infarct) results in 24 to 72 hours of inability to direct the eyes contralaterally. Combined activity of both frontal lobes moves the eyes up or down. Bilateral damage to the gaze areas of both frontal lobes or their descending pathways may produce an inability to move the eyes voluntarily despite preserved visual reflex tracking movements, a condition termed oculomotor apraxia.

Pathways descending from the parieto-occipital region of the two hemispheres subserve slow visual tracking or *pursuit movements*. Visual pursuit movements cannot track faster than 50° per second (vestibulo-ocular reflex movements can track up to 400° per second). Loss of parieto-occipital function impairs smooth following movements reflected in a loss of opticokinetic nystagmus toward the diseased hemisphere.

Best present evidence indicates that pathways from the frontal eye fields descend initially in the ipsilateral internal capsule, then decussate to synapse in the para-abducens conjugate gaze area of the opposite side of the pons. Parieto-occipital eye fields send their impulses via the pretectal area to descend in the brainstem tegmentum and reach the pontine para-abducens region. Pathways from both cerebral areas that regulate vertical eye movements enter the MLF at both the lower pontine and the upper midbrain levels. In clinical situations, lesions at midbrain level more often affect vertical gaze than do those at the pontine level. This is especially seen in *Parinaud's syndrome*, in which lesions impinging on the pretectal area and the midbrain tegmentum interrupt incoming pathways from the light reflex and the cerebral eye fields. The result is wide, light-fixed pupils and a loss of upward gaze, which is at first voluntary and later reflex as well. Damage to either para-abducens area paralyzes lateral conjugate gaze to the side of the lesion. Thus with conjugate gaze paralysis of forebrain origin the eyes "look" toward the lesion, whereas with conjugate gaze paralysis of brainstem origin the eyes look away from the lesion.

The pathway for the MLF lies in the brainstem immediately ventral to the periaqueductal gray matter and decussates just rostral to the abducens nucleus. Lesions of the MLF characteristically produce an *internuclear ophthalmoplegia* (INO) with which the eyes in the primary position at rest may either be parallel or show a mild skew deviation, but move disjunctively in lateral gaze. (Skew results from any of a number of lesions involving the brainstem and has little localizing value.) Characteristic of a fully developed INO is that during lateral gaze toward the side of the interrupting lesion, the ipsilateral eye abducts and shows nystagmus, whereas the contralateral, adducting eye partially or completely fails to move nasally because of failure of ascending impulses to reach the opposite third nerve nucleus. Classically, adduction for near vision convergence is relatively well preserved. Internuclear ophthalmoplegia may be unilateral or bilateral, partial or complete, depending upon the location of the lesion and the degree of damage to the paired MLF structures. Demyelinating and small vascular lesions (e.g., systemic lupus erythematosus, hypertension) are the most common cause of a unilateral INO isolated from other ocular palsies or brainstem signs. Larger brainstem lesions that damage one or more oculomotor nuclei plus the MLF, often produce bizarre combinations of disjunctive eye movements coupled with nuclear oculomotor paralyses. Partial ophthalmoplegia from myasthenia gravis can sometimes resemble an inconstant INO and that disease should be tested for in doubtful cases.

NYSTAGMUS. Nystagmus, a rhythmic to-and-fro movement of the eyes, can be of two types. *Pendular nystagmus* oscillates at equal rates between the extremes of movement, whereas *jerk nystagmus* consists of a slow phase away from the visual object, followed by a quick saccade back toward the target. The two are not always easily differentiated, even with the aid of electronic recordings of eye movement. The deviation of jerk nystagmus is defined by the quick phase. Nystagmus should be described by its direction, relation to direction of gaze, and intensity (i.e., amplitude times frequency).

Nystagmus reflects a disorder or imbalance in a complex neural network that involves the visual pathways, the labyrinths, proprioceptive influences arising from neck muscles, the vestibular and cerebellar nuclei, the reticular formation of the pontine brainstem, and the oculomotor nuclei. The references at the end of this chapter give more detailed consideration. For most clinical purposes the discriminations to be made about nystagmus are whether it is congenital or acquired; if acquired, whether peripheral or central in origin; and if central, whether structural or metabolic in cause.

Congenital nystagmus is present by birth or early infancy and most often but not always relates to primary central visual loss. It may last into adult life, manifests itself equally in the two eyes, appears mainly pendular and horizontal, and produces a diagnostically characteristic wave form on ocular recordings. In most instances the head oscillates reciprocally with the eyes.

Acquired pendular nystagmus in adults most often reflects cerebellar or brainstem disease and frequently possesses a chaotic, multidirectional quality in which the eyes may move independently. Most jerk nystagmus in adults reflects dysfunction of the vestibular end-organ (the labyrinth), the vestibular nerve, or the vestibular nuclei in the brainstem.

Knowledge of the normal responses to *caloric irrigation* of the tympanum aids in understanding labyrinthine influences on eye movements. Warm water irrigation stimulates the ipsilateral labyrinth; cold water irrigation inhibits it (i.e., mimics disease or destruction). In the awake subject, cold water induces fast beating nystagmus away from the irrigation; in the subject with depressed forebrain but intact brainstem function, the eyes move slowly, tonically toward the irrigation but nystagmus is absent. Table 479–2 gives some criteria that help differentiate between nystagmus of peripheral and of central origin.

Purely horizontal fine nystagmus at the extremes of gaze is

TABLE 479–2. CLUES TO THE ORIGIN OF VESTIBULAR NYSTAGMUS*

Symptom or Sign	Peripheral (End-Organ)	Central (Nuclear)
Direction of nystagmus	Unidirectional, fast phase opposite lesion	Bidirectional or unidirectional
Purely horizontal nystagmus without rotary component	Uncommon	Common
Vertical or purely rotary nystagmus	Never present	May be present
Visual fixation	Inhibits nystagmus and vertigo	No inhibition
Severity of vertigo	Marked	Mild
Direction of environmental spin	Toward slow phase	Variable
Direction of past-pointing	Toward slow phase	Variable
Direction of Romberg fall	Toward slow phase	Variable
Effect of head turning	Changes Romberg fall	No effect
Duration of symptoms	Finite (minutes, days, weeks) but recurrent	May be chronic
Tinnitus and/or deafness	Often present	Usually absent
Common causes	Infectious (labyrinthitis), Ménière's disease, neuronitis, vascular, trauma, toxic	Vascular demyelinating, neoplastic

*Reprinted, with permission of the publisher and author, from Glaser JS: Neuro-ophthalmology. Hagerstown, MD, Harper & Row, 1977.

a common finding without pathologic significance. It is more common with fatigue or poor lighting. When bidirectional gaze-evoked nystagmus is prominent or involves vertical as well as horizontal movements to an equal degree, excessive sedative or anticonvulsant drug ingestion is probably the cause.

Several unusual forms of nystagmus have neurologic localizing qualities: *Dissociated nystagmus,* i.e., unequal in the two eyes, implies a brainstem lesion. *See-saw nystagmus* involves the eyes reciprocally rising and falling, then reversing their reciprocal directions. The phenomenon accompanies parasellar tumors or, less often, upper brainstem damage. *Convergence* or *retractory nystagmus* accompanies mesencephalic lesions. *Periodic alternating nystagmus* consists of a horizontal jerk nystagmus that changes its direction periodically. A typical sequence would be jerk nystagmus 90 seconds to the left, followed by a 10-second inert pause, followed by jerk nystagmus 90 seconds to the right, with the sequence then repeating itself. The finding has been associated with a variety of posterior fossa abnormalities, especially those involving the region of the craniocervical junction. *Down-beat* nystagmus produces downward jerks with the eyes in the primary gaze position; it often reflects a craniocervical abnormality such as the Arnold-Chiari malformation, but can occur with parenchymal lesions such as multiple sclerosis. Some subjects have the capacity to induce *voluntary nystagmus,* which is extremely rapid, occurs in short bursts of 10 to 15 seconds or so, is present on the extremes of gaze, and may be unequal in the two eyes. It is doubtful whether cervical disease produces clinically significant nystagmus.

Other abnormalities of conjugate eye movements include *ocular bobbing,* consisting of fast conjugate downward eye jerks followed by a slow return to the primary gaze position. The phenomenon accompanies severe displacement or destruction of the pons or, much less often, metabolic CNS depression. *Ocular myoclonus* consists of continuous rhythmic, pendular oscillations, most often vertical with a rate of two to five beats per second. Often it accompanies palatal myoclonus and has a similar pathogenesis. *Ocular flutter* consists of brief, intermittent, horizontal oscillations arising from the primary gaze position. It blends into *opsoclonus,* a pattern of rapid, chaotic, conjugate, repetitive saccadic eye movements ("dancing eyes"). Both of these disorders usually reflect cerebellar dysfunction, but can emerge as a remote effect of systemic neoplasm, especially neuroblastoma in children. *Ocular dysmetria* consists of saccadic overshoots or undershoots of conjugate eye movement during rapid following of a visual object. It reflects cerebellar dysfunction.

Glaser JS: Neuro-ophthalmology. Hagerstown, MD, Harper & Row, 1977. *An excellent one-volume didactic introductory text.*

L'Esperance FA (ed.): Current Diagnosis of Chorioretinal Disease. St. Louis, The C. V. Mosby Co., 1977. *A well-written and referenced text to diseases of the eye producing visual loss.*

Walsh FB, Hoyt WF: Clinical Neuro-ophthalmology, 3 vols. Baltimore, Williams & Wilkins Company, 1969. *An encyclopedic reference work. Although over a decade old, it provides the most comprehensive analysis to most aspects of the field.*

Zee DS, Leigh RJ: Disorders of Ocular Movement. Philadelphia, F. A. Davis Company, 1983. *An up-to-date monograph that gives the clinical and physiological details of modern investigations on ocular control.*

479.3. Hearing and Equilibrium

Jerome B. Posner

The neural pathways subserving hearing and those most important for equilibrium and spatial orientation are anatomically proximate through much of their course, from their end organs in the inner ear to their termination in the superior portion of the temporal lobe. Because of the close anatomic linkage, disorders that affect hearing often affect equilibrium as well, and vice versa. For this reason, they are considered together here. Despite their major anatomic similarities, there are substantial pathophysiologic differences that make clinical examination of the two systems quite different: (1) The auditory system is physiologically relatively isolated, so that its function and dysfunction can be tested independently of other neural systems. (2) The vestibular system, on the other hand, has many close physiologic linkages with the motor system (particularly the cerebellum, oculomotor system, and the autonomic nervous system) and can be tested only indirectly by noting secondary effects on oculomotor and cerebellar functions. (3) Abnormalities of the auditory system lead only to a few well-defined and unique symptoms, i.e., hearing loss or distortion and/or tinnitus. (4) Abnormalities of the vestibular system may cause symptoms that mimic disorders of other neural structures. Such symptoms include dizziness or vertigo, ocular abnormalities (nystagmus), motor abnormalities (including ataxia or sudden falls), and autonomic abnormalities (including nausea and vomiting and even syncope).

HEARING

Anatomy and Physiology of Hearing

In normal hearing, sound waves are transmitted from the tympanic membrane via the three ossicles of the air-filled middle ear (air conduction) to the oval window, to which is attached the basilar membrane of the fluid-filled cochlea. The ossicles serve to increase the gain from tympanum to oval window about 18-fold, compensating for the loss that sound waves moving from air to fluid would otherwise suffer. In the absence of this system, sound may reach the cochlea by vibration of the temporal bone (bone conduction) but with much less efficiency (approximately 60 db loss). Hair cells lying along the cochlear basilar membrane detect the vibratory movement of that membrane and transduce vibration into nerve impulses. The nerve impulses are relayed via nerve cells that synapse at the base of hair cells and have their bodies in the spiral ganglion to the cochlear nucleus of the ipsilateral pontine tegmentum. Auditory frequency receptors are distributed unevenly along the basilar membrane. Hair cells sensitive to higher frequencies (above 2000 to 4000 Hz) are localized along the basilar turn of the cochlea, while lower frequency receptors are distributed along the full length of the structure. For this reason, partial deafness characteristically affects the perception of higher more than lower frequencies. Within the brainstem, auditory signals ascend from the ventral and dorsal cochlear nuclei to reach the superior olivary nuclei of both sides. Thus, nervous system lesions central to the cochlear nucleus do not cause monaural hearing loss and, conversely, unilateral lesions do not cause deafness. From these structures, the pathway projects by way of the lateral lemnisci to the inferior colliculi. Each inferior colliculus transmits to the other and to its ipsilateral medial geniculate body which, in turn, sends the final projection to the transverse auditory gyrus lying in the superior portion of the ipsilateral temporal lobe.

The normal ear can detect sound frequencies ranging between about 20 and 20,000 Hz, with the upper range dropping off fairly rapidly with advancing age. The ear is most sensitive between 500 and 4000 Hz, in part because the middle ear has a resonant frequency of about 3000 Hz. Normal speech resonates at frequencies of 2000 Hz and below. Standard clinical audiograms test hearing frequencies only below 8000 Hz. The intensity of sound is quantified by decibels (db), a logarithmic abstraction calculated from the smallest perceptible difference in intensity that the normal ear can discriminate. A 30 to 40 db loss (about 100-fold decrease) impairs normal conversation; an 80 db loss is deafness.

Symptoms of Auditory Dysfunction

Only two symptoms result from disease of the auditory system: The first is hearing impairment, sometimes associated with a distortion as well as a decrease in the intensity of sound, and the second is tinnitus, a sound heard in the ear or head not arising from the external environment. Hearing loss is termed *conductive* (external and middle ear), *sensorineural* (cochlea and auditory nerve), or *central* (brainstem and cerebral hemispheres), according to the anatomic location of the abnormality. Most deafness is conductive or sensorineural.

Conductive hearing loss is characterized by equal loss of hearing at all frequencies and by well-preserved speech discrimination once the threshold for hearing is exceeded. With sensorineural hearing loss, the hearing levels for different frequencies are usually unequal, typically resulting in better hearing for low than for high frequency tones. Patients with sensorineural hearing loss often have difficulty hearing speech that is mixed with background noise and may be annoyed by loud speech.

Three important manifestations of sensorineural lesions are diplacusis, recruitment, and tone decay. Diplacusis and recruitment are common with cochlear lesions; tone decay usually accompanies eighth nerve involvement. With diplacusis the tonal quality of a pure tone is distorted so that it may sound like a complex mixture of tones. Binaural diplacusis occurs when the two ears are affected unequally so that the same frequency has a different pitch in each ear, i.e., the patient hears double. Monaural diplacusis occurs when two tones or a tone and noise are heard simultaneously in one ear. With recruitment there is an abnormally rapid growth in the sensation of loudness as the intensity of a sound is increased so that faint or moderate sounds cannot be heard, whereas there is little or no change in the loudness of intense sounds. The inability to maintain perception of a continuous tone presented above auditory threshold is called tone decay. Patients with conductive or cochlear lesions can usually hear a continuous tone for at least 60 seconds, whereas the perception of the tone rapidly decays in patients with eighth nerve lesions.

HEARING TESTS. Hearing may be examined either at the *bedside* or in the *laboratory*. The examiner can test for hearing loss in the speech frequencies by observing the patient's response to spoken commands at different intensities. Higher frequencies can be tested by noting the distance at which the patient can hear a watch tick. Loss of watch tick sound out of proportion to whisper or low speech suggests sensorineural hearing disorders, which often involve only higher frequencies. With the speech and watch tick tests the physician uses his own hearing level as a standard. With tuning forks, the physician can test hearing in each ear at different frequencies and distinguish conductive from sensorineural hearing loss. In the Rinne test, nerve conduction is compared to bone conduction by holding a tuning fork (256 or 512 Hz) against the mastoid process until the sound can no longer be heard. It is then placed one inch from the ear and, in normal subjects, can be heard about twice as long by air as by bone. If bone conduction is better than air conduction, the hearing loss is conductive, but care must be taken to assure that the bone conduction is not heard in the normal ear. In the Weber test, a 512 tuning fork is placed on the patient's forehead or upper teeth. Normally this sound is referred to the center of the head. If it is referred to the side of unilateral hearing loss, the hearing loss is conductive; if it is referred away from the side of unilateral hearing loss, the loss is sensorineural. The Weber test is often unreliable in conductive hearing loss because the patient cannot accept the fact that he hears better in what he knows to be the diseased ear. Hyperacusis and recruitment (see below), two components of sensorineural hearing loss, can often be tested for at the bedside by having the patient compare the pitch and intensity of the tuning fork tone in each ear as it is struck with progressively harder blows.

Although bedside tests are useful in screening hearing loss, more sophisticated audiometric hearing tests are necessary to localize the degree and site of hearing loss with certainty. These tests include audiometry, impedance measurement, and auditory evoked responses.

Pure Tone Audiometry. Pure tones at selected frequencies are presented via either earphones (air conduction) or a vibrator pressed against the mastoid portion of the temporal bone (bone conduction). The minimal level that the subject can hear is determined for each frequency. The *speech reception threshold* (SRT) is the intensity at which the patient can correctly repeat 50 per cent of the words presented. The SRT is a test of hearing sensitivity for speech and should reflect the hearing level for pure tones in the speech range. The *speech discrimination test* measures the ability to understand speech when it is presented at a level that is easily heard. In patients with eighth nerve lesions, speech discrimination can be severely reduced even when pure tone thresholds are normal or nearly normal, whereas in patients with cochlear lesions discrimination tends to be proportional to the magnitude of hearing loss.

Recruitment is usually measured by the alternate binaural loudness balance (ABLB) test (if the hearing loss is unilateral). This test compares the loudness for tones of varying intensity as perceived by the pathologic ear and the normal ear. Recruitment is present if smaller increases in stimulus intensity are required in the poorer ear than in the better ear to maintain equal loudness. *Tone decay* is usually tested by presenting a tone at a prescribed suprathreshold level and asking the patient to respond as long as he hears the tone. Special tests for central auditory lesions assess the patient's ability to understand *distorted speech* or speech that is presented to one ear with a *competing message* in the other ear.

Impedance Measurement. By inserting a probe in the external canal that both presents and measures the sound pressure level of a tone, the acoustic impedance of the middle ear can be assessed. Two types of impedance measurements are routinely used: *tympanometry* and *stapedius reflex measurement*. Tympanometry, the measurement of impedance as a function of ear canal air pressure, is primarily useful for detection of middle ear disorders; stapedius reflex measurements are particularly useful for identifying lesions of the eighth nerve and/or brainstem. The stapedius muscle contraction is measured indirectly by determining the impedance-change induced at the tympanic membrane when the muscle contracts. The reflex consists of (1) auditory nerve, (2) brainstem interneurons, and (3) facial nerve. If the middle ear structures are intact, loss of the stapedius reflex suggests a lesion in this reflex arc.

Auditory Evoked Responses. These can be recorded from scalp electrodes at 0 to 10 msec (early), 10 to 50 msec (middle), and 50 to 500 msec (late) following a click stimulus. The early potentials reflect electrical activity at the cochlea, eighth nerve, and brainstem, whereas the later potentials reflect cortical activity. Computer averaging of the responses to 1000 to 2000 clicks separates the evoked potential from background noise. Evoked responses may be used to estimate the magnitude of hearing loss and to differentiate among cochlear, eighth nerve, and brainstem lesions.

CAUSES OF HEARING LOSS

Conductive Hearing Loss

Conductive hearing loss arises from abnormalities of external or middle ear and can raise hearing threshold no more than 60 db, since bone conduction persists intact. Obstruction in the external auditory meatus (the most common cause of conductive hearing loss) impairs air transmission to the tympanum. This benign condition, caused by *impacted cerumen*, is usually first noticed after bathing or swimming, when a droplet of water closes the remaining tiny passageway. A *fluid-filled middle ear* reduces movement of the ossicles against the oval window. The most common serious cause of conductive hearing loss is inflammation of the middle ear, *otitis media*. Either infected (suppurative otitis) or noninfected (serous otitis) fluid accumulates in the middle ear, impairing the conduction of airborne sound. Since the air cavity of the middle ear is in direct connection with the mastoid air cells, infection can spread through the mastoid bone and occasionally into the intracranial cavity. Chronic otitis media with perforation of the tympanic membrane can result in an invasion of the middle ear and other pneumatized areas of the temporal bone by keratinizing squamous epithelium (cholesteatoma). Cholesteatomas can produce erosion of the ossicles and bony labyrinth, resulting in a mixed conductive-sensorineural hearing loss.

Otosclerosis is a process in which the annular ligament that attaches the stapes to the oval window overgrows and calcifies. It reduces ossicular transmission via the window to the cochlear basement membrane. Seventy per cent of patients with clinical otosclerosis notice hearing loss between the ages of 11 and 30, and there is a positive family history in approximately 50 per cent of cases. The hearing loss is typically conductive, although in some individuals the cochlea may be invaded by foci of otosclerotic bone, producing an additional sensorineural hearing loss. Otosclerosis usually stabilizes when the hearing level reaches 50 to 60 db and rarely progresses to deafness. Other common causes of conductive hearing loss include trauma, congenital malformations of the external and middle ear, and glomus body tumors.

Sensorineural Hearing Loss

Genetically determined deafness, usually from hair cell aplasia or deterioration, may be present at birth or develop in adulthood. The diagnosis of *hereditary deafness* rests on the finding of a positive family history. In many instances the inheritance is through a recessive gene or a dominant gene with low penetrance, making it difficult to determine the genetic nature of the disorder. *Intrauterine factors* resulting in congenital hearing loss include infection (especially rubella); toxic, metabolic, and endocrine disorders; and anoxia associated with Rh incompatibility and difficult deliveries.

Acute unilateral deafness usually has a cochlear basis. Bacterial or viral infections of the labyrinth, head trauma with fracture or hemorrhage into the cochlea, or vascular occlusion of a terminal branch of the anterior-inferior cerebellar artery all can damage extensively the cochlea and its hair cells. An acute, idiopathic, often reversible, unilateral hearing loss strikes young adults and is presumed to reflect either a viral infection or a vascular disorder of the cochlea. Sudden unilateral hearing loss, often associated with vertigo and tinnitus, can result from a perilymphatic fistula. Such fistulae may be congenital or may follow stapes surgery or severe or mild trauma to the inner ear.

Drugs cause sudden bilateral hearing impairment fairly often. Salicylates, furosemide, and ethacrynic acid potentially produce transient deafness when taken in high doses. More toxic to the cochlea are the aminoglycoside antibiotics (gentamicin, tobramycin, amikacin, kanamycin, streptomycin, and neomycin). These agents can destroy cochlear hair cells in direct relation to their serum concentrations and the cumulative duration of drug exposure, causing permanent hearing loss. Some anticancer chemotherapeutic agents, particularly cisplatin, cause severe ototoxicity.

Subacute, relapsing cochlear deafness occurs with *Ménière's syndrome*, a condition associated with fluctuating hearing loss and tinnitus, recurrent episodes of abrupt and often severe vertigo, and a sensation of fullness or pressure in the ear. Recurrent endolymphatic hypertension (hydrops) is believed to cause the episodes. Pathologically, the endolymphatic sac is dilated and the hair cells become atrophic. The resulting deafness is subtle and reversible in the early stages but subsequently becomes permanent and characterized by diplacusis and loudness recruitment. The disorder is usually unilateral. When bilateral (less than 20 per cent of cases), it begins in one ear before the other.

Gradually progressive hearing loss with age is known as *presbycusis*. Presbycusis reflects deterioration in the cochlear receptor system with degeneration of the hair cells, especially at the base. As a result, higher tones are lost early, with audiograms showing a characteristically sharp decline at each successive frequency above 2000 Hz. The recurrent trauma of noise-induced hearing loss affects approximately the same cochlear region and is almost as frequent, particularly among those with exposure to loud military or industrial noises. Loud, blaring modern music has become a recent offender. The increasing tone loss starts initially above a slightly higher threshold of about 4000 Hz but moves down toward speech frequencies with repeated exposure.

Hearing loss from direct damage to the acoustic nerve in the petrous canal occasionally results from abscesses within or trauma to the surrounding bone; severe, abruptly beginning deafness marks the event and is usually associated with acute vertigo due to concurrent vestibular nerve injury. Progressive unilateral hearing loss that arises insidiously and worsens by almost imperceptible degrees is characteristic of benign neoplasms of the cerebellopontine angle, such as acoustic neurinomas. Bilateral gradual eighth nerve deafness is uncommon, but when it occurs it suggests the angle tumors of neurofibromatosis.

Central Hearing Loss

Central hearing loss is unilateral only if it results from damage to the pontine cochlear nuclei on one side of the brainstem. Such can occur with ischemic infarction of the lateral brainstem, e.g., due to occlusion of the anterior-inferior cerebellar artery, a plaque of multiple sclerosis or, rarely, invasion or compression of the dorsal lateral pons by a neoplasm or hematoma. Bilateral degeneration of the cochlear nuclei accompanies some of the rare, recessively inherited disorders of childhood.

Because of the extensive cross innervation of the supranuclear auditory pathways, clinically important unilateral hearing loss never results from neurologic disease arising rostral to the cochlear nucleus. Bilateral hearing loss could in theory result from bilateral destruction of central hearing pathways anywhere along their course. In practice, involvement of neighboring structures in brainstem or hemisphere would usually lead to such severe neurologic disability that the hearing loss becomes an unimportant additional sign. Two exceptions occur: In rare instances, bilateral hearing loss has been reported as an early sign of pineal region tumors, presumably from compression of the inferior colliculi. Most affected patients also have other signs of brainstem tectal dysfunction, including loss of upward gaze. Bilateral infarctions of the anterior transverse gyrus of the temporal lobe may also cause central deafness, but usually it is accompanied by aphasia as well as some involvement of the nearby Wernicke's area in the dominant hemisphere. *Spatial orientation* for sound depends upon the integrity of several of the neural structures and pathways carrying auditory information in the brainstem to, as well as in, the auditory cortex itself. Lesions lying anywhere along this path can impair the function.

Diagnosis and Treatment of Hearing Loss

The physician should perform bedside tests of hearing in all patients, regardless of complaint. Many patients can gradually develop hearing loss in one ear without being aware of it. In others, hearing loss is detected only by some activity that requires a single ear, such as using the telephone. The tuning fork test can usually distinguish conductive from sensorineural hearing loss. Inspection of the external auditory canal and tympanic membrane can often identify the cause of conductive hearing loss. The presence of associated symptoms of vertigo, tinnitus, or pressure or fullness in the ear suggests cochlear damage, whereas those of ataxia and nystagmus may suggest eighth nerve or central damage. A complete evaluation of the patient's hearing loss requires testing by a skilled otolaryngologist using modern techniques of audiometry and evoked potential measurement. Such an evaluation should be carried out whenever the cause of hearing loss is not immediately apparent. The physician is likewise responsible for the monitoring of hearing in patients undergoing treatment with potentially ototoxic agents. Vestibular function should also be monitored, since many of the ototoxic agents damage the vestibular system before or in addition to the auditory system.

The treatment of most hearing loss is usually unsatisfactory and is best left to skilled specialists. If an underlying disorder has not yet destroyed the auditory system and can be ameliorated medically or surgically, hearing may be improved or preserved. Some patients with otosclerosis respond to stapedectomy. Closure of a perilymphatic fistula may improve hearing. Antibiotic and decongestive treatment of otitis media may be useful. The surgical treatment of Ménière's syndrome is still controversial. Some patients with nonreversible damage to their hearing can be assisted by hearing aids. Patients with conductive hearing loss require simple amplification, but those with sensorineural hearing loss often need frequency-selective amplification in order to make hearing aids useful.

TINNITUS

Tinnitus is the term applied generally to noises that arise spontaneously in one or both ears. Tinnitus may be classified as either *objective,* i.e., the patient is hearing a sound arising externally to the auditory system, a sound that can usually be heard by the examiner with a stethoscope, or *subjective,* i.e., the sound arises from an abnormal discharge of the auditory system and cannot be heard by the observer. *Objective tinnitus* usually has benign causes such as noise from temporomandibular joints, opening of eustachian tubes, or repetitive contraction of the stapedius muscle. Sometimes in a quiet room the patient can hear the pulsatile flow in the carotid artery or a continuous hum of normal venous outflow through the jugular bulb. The latter can easily be obliterated by gentle compression of the jugular vein. Pathologic objective tinnitus occurs when patients hear turbulent flow in arteriovenous anomalies or tumors (e.g., glomus jugulare tumor). Objective tinnitus may also be an early sign of increased intracranial pressure. Such tinnitus, which can be obliterated by pressure over the jugular vein, probably arises from turbulent flow of compressed venous structures at the base of the brain. The symptom is also transiently relieved by decreasing intracranial pressure, as for example by lumbar puncture.

Subjective tinnitus can arise from anywhere in the auditory system. The sounds most frequently complained of are metallic ringing, buzzing, blowing, roaring, or, less often, bizarre clangings, poppings, or nonrhythmic beatings. A degree of tinnitus, heard as a faint, moderately high-pitched metallic ring, can be observed by almost everyone if they concentrate their attention on auditory events in a quiet room. Sustained, louder tinnitus accompanied by audiometric evidence of deafness occurs in association with both conductive and sensorineural disease. The phenomenon can be a manifestation of salicylate, quinine, or quinidine toxicity. Tinnitus observed with otosclerosis tends to have a roaring or hissing quality, while that associated with Ménière's syndrome often produces sounds that vary widely in intensity with time and quality, sometimes including roarings or clangings. Tinnitus with other cochlear or auditory nerve lesions tends to be higher pitched and ringing in quality.

Tinnitus without observable deafness appears sporadically and for variable lengths of time in many persons without other evidence of an ongoing pathologic process. In many such instances, one suspects that the auditory experience is no more than an anxious preoccupation with normal auditory physiology. Beyond a careful audiologic examination, audiometric testing, and checking for a history of ingested medications, few diagnostic measures prove useful. Tinnitus may be a very distressing symptom to some patients. Masking sounds (white noise) delivered to the involved ear may give some patients relief, but no treatment removes the symptoms.

EQUILIBRIUM

Anatomy and Physiology of the Vestibular System

The paired vestibular end organs lie within the temporal bones proximate to the cochlea. Each end organ consists of three semicircular canals that detect angular acceleration and two otolithic structures, the utricle and saccule, that detect linear (gravitational) acceleration. Like the cochlea, these organs possess hair cells projecting into a fluid-filled (endolymph) membrane. The hair cells of the three semicircular canals, each of which is oriented at right angles to the others, are concentrated in the ampulla, where they are embedded in a gelatinous mass called the cupula. Movement of the head causes the endolymph to flow either toward or away from the cupula, distorting the hair cells and, depending on the direction of endolymphatic movement, either stimulating or inhibiting their firing. Since the hair cells of the semicircular canal are tonically active, both excitation and inhibition change the rate of discharge. Furthermore, the two sets of semicircular canals are approximately mirror images of each other, so that rotational movement of the head that excites one canal will inhibit the analogous canal on the opposite side. The hair cells of the otolith apparatus, the utricle and saccule, are concentrated in an area called the macula. The macula of the utricle lies approximately in the plane of the horizontal canal and the macula of the saccule is essentially vertical. The hair cells are imbedded in a membrane that also contains calcite masses or otoliths; the density of otoliths is considerably greater than that of the endolymph. As the head is moved, the force of gravity on the otoliths distorts the hair cells, producing firing of these organs.

A discharge of hair cells from either semicircular canals or otoliths is detected by nerve fibers at the base of the hair cells. These fibers have their cells of origin in Scarpa's ganglion. The nerve fibers travel in the vestibular portion of the eighth nerve contiguous with the acoustic nerve. The vestibular portion of the eighth nerve is divided into superior and inferior vestibular nerves. The fibers of the horizontal and vestibular canals as well as the utricle and anterior saccule compose the superior vestibular nerve, while those of the posterior canals compose the inferior vestibular nerve. Nerve fibers from various portions of the semicircular canal terminate in different vestibular nuclei at the pontomedullary junction. There are also direct connections between the semicircular canals and many portions of the cerebellum with the greatest representation in the floculonodular lobe, the so-called vestibulocerebellum. Efferent fibers from the brainstem travel through the vestibular nucleus to reach the hair cells of the semicircular canal and utricles. Efferent fibers are inhibitory in nature and may, like the efferent fibers of the cochlea, have as their function selecting input to which the brain will attend. From the vestibular nuclei, second order neurons make important connections to the vestibular nuclei of the other side, to the cerebellum, to motor neurons of the spinal cord, to autonomic nuclei in the brainstem, and, most importantly for the examining clinician, to the nuclei of the oculomotor system. Fibers from the vestibular nuclei also ascend through the brainstem and thalamus to reach the cerebral cortex, where the representation of the vestibular system is bilateral. The exact site of cortical representation is unclear. Clinical evidence points to both superior temporal and inferior parietal lobes as possible sites.

Symptoms and Signs of Vestibular Dysfunction

The vestibular system is a finely tuned tonically discharging system. Any imbalance in discharge between the paired peripheral vestibular end organs or their primary receiving areas in the vestibular nuclei, if not caused by a true movement of the head or body, produces a mismatch between vestibular input and other sense organs (such as the eyes and proprioceptive apparatus) and leads to an illusory sensation of movement in space called vertigo. Vertigo is the only direct symptom of a vestibular abnormality, but because the vestibular system influences other neural systems, vertigo may be accompanied by autonomic symptoms (nausea, vomiting, diaphoresis), motor symptoms (ataxia, past pointing, falling), or ocular symptoms (oscillopsia—a visual sensation that the environment is moving). Also because of the close interconnection among neural systems, the sensation of vertigo can be produced by abnormalities of the visual or somatosensory system as well as, much more commonly, the vestibular system.

Vertigo may be mild or severe, physiologic or pathologic. *Physiologic vertigo* occurs when there is a mismatch among the vestibular, visual, and somatosensory systems induced by an external stimulus. Common examples of physiologic vertigo include motion sickness, height vertigo (the sensation that occurs when one looks down from a great height), and visual vertigo (the sensation sometimes felt when one visualizes a motion picture of a roller coaster or other violent movement). *Pathologic vertigo* usually arises from an abnormality of the vestibular system but less commonly can be produced by visual or somatosensory disorders. *Severe vertigo* is a sensation usually well described by the patient and easily recognized by the physician. *Milder vertigo*, however, may easily be confused with the lightheadedness of syncope, the unsteadiness of ataxia, and the psychogenic symptoms of anxiety or dissociation.

The major clinical *sign* of a disordered vestibular system is *nystagmus*. Nystagmus, like vertigo, can be physiologic or pathologic. Examples of physiologic nystagmus include optokinetic nystagmus, which occurs when watching telephone poles from a moving train, and rotational nystagmus, such as occurs when one rotates himself in space. Like vertigo, nystagmus can originate from sites other than the vestibular system, particularly the visual or cerebellar systems, and may occur either with or without vertigo. Vestibular nystagmus arises when there is unbalanced input from the two vestibular systems. For example, stimulation of the horizontal canal on the left side increases the output from the left horizontal canal relative to the right and causes a reflex movement of the eyes toward the right. There is a rapid compensatory (non-vestibular) movement of the eyes back to the midline, so that in the awake patient the net movement of the eyes is only a few degrees. In the comatose patient, vestibular stimulation may produce full conjugate lateral deviation of the eyes with only slow return to the midline. Nystagmus is named for the direction of the rapid component. Thus, stimulation of the left horizontal canal which drives the eye slowly to the right with a compensatory movement to the left is called left beating nystagmus.

Tests of Vestibular Dysfunction

Most vestibular problems presenting to the physician are episodic, and there are neither symptoms nor signs when the physician examines the patient. The best test of vestibular dysfunction, therefore, is a careful *history*. The history should attempt to distinguish vertigo (the illusion of movement in space) from lightheadedness (syncope) and ataxia (dysequilibrium of the body without a true movement in space) and from psychogenic symptoms (the feeling of dissociation). If the history is not clear, bedside *provocative tests* to mimic the symptom may assist the physician in making a pathophysiologic diagnosis. *Hyperventilation*, which lowers the P_{CO_2} and decreases cerebral blood flow, causes a "light-headed" sensation associated with syncope. Ask the patient to *hyperventilate* maximally for three minutes to cause lightheadedness. If the episode exactly mimics the patient's symptoms, it suggests that anxiety and hyperventilation may be playing an important role. In addition, during the course of hyperventilation the patient may suffer dry mouth, chest tightness, and paresthesias, which he may then recognize are part of his spontaneous attacks, thus helping in the diagnosis. *Tandem walking* (heel to toe) with eyes opened or closed will reproduce the sensation of dysequilibrium. The *Bárány rotation maneuver* (rotating the patient about a vertical axis 10 times over 20 seconds), caloric tests (see below), and positional tests (see below) can reproduce the symptoms of vestibular vertigo. The physician should also examine the patient carefully for nystagmus. The patient should fix a light in both horizontal and vertical gaze and in both the erect and supine positions. Sustained nystagmus suggests pathology of the vestibular system, and vertical nystagmus suggests that it is central rather than peripheral. Nystagmus and vertigo can sometimes be precipitated by rapid movements of the head in space (*Nylen-Bárány test*). The examiner tilts the seated patient so that the head is hanging 45 degrees below horizontal, with first one ear and then the other dependent. He observes for nystagmus and vertigo. Bedside *caloric tests* in a patient without vertigo or nystagmus at the time of the examination can often reproduce the patient's symptoms and identify the site of the pathology. With the patient lying supine and the head elevated approximately 30 degrees, water 7° C above or below body temperature is douched against the tympanic membrane. In the normal situation, cold water produces nystagmus away from the side of stimulation (because of inhibition of the horizontal semicircular canal) and warm water nystagmus to the side of stimulation (because of stimulation of the semicircular canal). An astute patient suffering from labyrinthine vertigo can often tell which stimulation reproduces the symptoms, thus assisting in the localization of the lesion. Absence of response on one side suggests labyrinthine failure on that side. Because most peripheral nystagmus is partially inhibited by the visual fixation of the open eyes, accurate quantitative evaluation requires electrical recording of the eye movement with the eyes closed. *Electronystagmography* can be performed in the resting position, with the head rotated into various positions to provoke nystagmus, and before, during, and after caloric stimulation. Electronystagmography is often helpful in identifying the pathology of the vestibular system and localizing it when identified.

Causes of Vertigo

PHYSIOLOGIC VERTIGO. Table 479–3 lists some of the physiologic causes of vertigo. In almost all instances, the diagnosis is clear from the history. One exception may be head extension vertigo, a sensation of vertigo or postural imbalance induced with the head maximally extended while the patient is standing. This vertigo is abruptly terminated when the head is flexed to a neutral position. The symptoms may mistakenly be attributed to vertebral artery insufficiency. Physiologic head extension vertigo does not occur when the head is extended in the lying position and occurs only rarely when the patient is sitting. If physiologic vertigo becomes a clinical problem, it is best treated by supplying sensory cues that help to match the various sensory systems. Thus, motion sickness, which is often exacerbated by sitting in a closed space or reading, giving the visual system the miscue that the environment is stationary, may be relieved by looking out at the environment and watching it move. Height vertigo caused by a mismatch between sensation of normal body sway and lack of its visual detection can often be relieved by the patient's either sitting or visually fixing a nearby stationary object.

PATHOLOGIC VESTIBULAR VERTIGO. Vertigo can be caused by disease of either the peripheral or central vestibular apparatus (Table 479–4). In general, peripheral vertigo is more severe, is more likely to be associated with hearing loss and tinnitus, and often leads to nausea and vomiting. Nystagmus associated with peripheral vertigo is frequently inhibited by visual fixation. Central vertigo is generally less severe than peripheral vertigo and is often associated with other signs of central nervous system disease. The nystagmus of central vertigo is not inhibited by visual fixation and frequently is very prominent when vertigo is mild or absent.

PERIPHERAL VERTIGO. *Benign positional vertigo* is an extremely common disorder of middle age that accounts for at least 25 per cent of patients presenting to the physician complaining of vertigo. Typically, the patient first experiences severe whirling vertigo when turning over or first lying down in bed at night. Less commonly, the patient may experience similar symptoms when he sits up from a lying position or when he turns suddenly while standing or walking. Usually the symptoms are most severe when the patient lies on the side of the affected

TABLE 479–3. TYPES OF PHYSIOLOGIC VERTIGO

Motion sickness
Height vertigo
Visual vertigo (e.g., motion pictures)
Somatosensory vertigo
Auditory vertigo
Head extension vertigo
Bending vertigo
Space sickness

TABLE 479–4. CAUSES OF VESTIBULAR VERTIGO

Peripheral Causes	Central Causes
Peripheral vestibulopathy	Brainstem ischemia
Labyrinthitis and/or vestibular neuronitis	Cerebellopontine angle tumors
Acute and recurrent peripheral vestibulopathy	Demyelinating disease
"Benign" positional vertigo	Cranial neuropathy
Ménière's syndrome	Seizure disorders (rare)
Vestibulotoxic drugs	Heredofamilial disorders
Post-traumatic vertigo, metastatic tumor, etc.	Spinocerebellar degenerations
Other focal peripheral disease	Friedreich's ataxia
Infection	Olivopontocerebellar atrophy
Ischemia	Other central causes
Otosclerosis	Brainstem tumors
Perilymphatic fistula	Cerebellar degenerations
Cervical arthritis	Paraneoplastic syndromes

ear. The vertigo is sudden in onset, very severe, and may be accompanied by nausea or vomiting. The patient usually reports that the vertigo ceases when he moves out of the position that causes it, but in fact if he remains in that position, it rarely lasts more than a minute. About 15 per cent of patients with benign positional vertigo report that it followed a head injury, often mild; in most patients there is *no* pre-existing illness. The pathophysiology of the disorder is not established, but some investigators have postulated that debris from otoliths may enter the posterior canal and artificially stimulate that canal when it is in the dependent position. The diagnosis is made by the characteristic history and the reproduction of the attack by the Nylen-Bárány maneuver: With the affected ear dependent, there is a latent period of several seconds during which the patient has no abnormal sensation, followed by the sudden onset of severe vertigo accompanied by rotatory nystagmus when the patient looks toward the dependent ear, and vertical nystagmus when the patient looks away from that ear. The vertigo and nystagmus usually last 30 to 50 seconds and then cease. When the patient sits up there may be brief milder vertigo, with nystagmus in the opposite direction. If the maneuvers are repeated, each subsequent attack becomes less lengthy and less severe until attacks fatigue completely. The illness usually runs a course of several weeks and then resolves but may recur several times over many years. If the patient has the classic history and physical findings, no further evaluation is necessary. If the history or findings are atypical, the condition must be distinguished from other causes of vertigo and nystagmus (see below) and may occur with tumors or infarcts of the posterior fossa. Typical benign positional vertigo is very rarely associated with such conditions. The treatment for most patients is simple reassurance. Since the vertigo can be fatigued, many patients find that repetitively producing the vertigo each day gives them prolonged relief.

PERIPHERAL VESTIBULOPATHY. This disorder, also called acute labyrinthitis or vestibular neuronitis, may occur as a single bout or may recur repeatedly over months or years. Characteristically, the patient has the acute onset of severe vertigo, often associated with nausea and vomiting. This may follow a respiratory infection, but often there is no preceding illness. The vertigo may be so severe that the patient is unable to sit or stand without vomiting or ataxia and prefers to lie absolutely still in bed with the involved ear uppermost, often refusing to move. Nystagmus is invariably present, usually horizontal or rotatory, and directed away from the involved labyrinth. The severe symptoms usually improve substantially within 48 to 72 hours, allowing the patient to be up and about. However, the patient often notes for weeks or months following the episode that sudden movements of the head produce mild vertigo or nausea. The pathogenesis of the illness is not entirely known. Although the disorder is called *acute labyrinthitis,* suggesting a viral infection of the labyrinth, recent EEG and evoked potential studies suggest that in many patients there are accompanying eighth nerve or brainstem abnormalities, leading some to refer to the disorder as *vestibular neuronitis.*

In some patients, attacks (usually less severe) of acute vestibulopathy occur over many months or years. There is no way of predicting whether an individual with a first attack will have repetitive attacks. In the patient suffering from repetitive attacks, the differential diagnosis includes Ménière's syndrome (see above) and otosclerosis. At least 25 per cent of patients with otosclerosis suffer from vertigo. In both of these disorders, hearing tests will be abnormal as well. Labyrinthine fistulae have been reported to produce episodic vertigo. Fistula testing by a skilled otolaryngologist should establish that diagnosis.

MÉNIÈRE'S SYNDROME. Ménière's syndrome is also described on page 2039. The disorder accounts for about 10 per cent of all patients with vertigo. The diagnosis is established primarily on the basis of the hearing tests.

VESTIBULOTOXIC DRUG-INDUCED VERTIGO. Several drugs that damage the auditory system (see page 2039), such as the aminoglycosides, may also damage the labyrinth. The patient may suffer acute vertigo, either along with or independent of hearing loss and tinnitus. Unfortunately, many patients being treated with the drug are bedridden and are unaware of labyrinthine failure until they recover from their acute illness and attempt to ambulate. Then they discover that they are unsteady on their feet, the environment tends to jiggle in front of their eyes (oscillopsia), and they feel vertiginous. Younger patients adapt after weeks to the labyrinthine failure; older patients may be permanently disabled. Usually there is no nystagmus, but the patient is ataxic. Caloric tests may demonstrate absence or hypoactivity of the labyrinth, and the Bárány rotation test may fail to elicit either vertigo or nystagmus. The best treatment is prevention. If the drug is discontinued early during the course of symptoms, the disorder may stabilize or improve.

POST-TRAUMATIC VERTIGO. Head injury may lead to benign positional vertigo (see above) or may produce a more vaguely described, rather constant feeling of dizziness or vertigo, usually associated with anxiety, difficulty in concentrating, headache, and phonophobia. Vertigo in this complex of symptoms called the *post-traumatic syndrome* is probably peripheral in origin, but its exact pathogenesis is unknown. The post-traumatic syndrome often follows a mild head injury, and the vague vertiginous feelings may persist for weeks or months. Reassurance that the patient has no substantial brain damage may help. Vestibular suppressants (see page 2043) can diminish the symptoms.

OTHER PERIPHERAL CAUSES OF VERTIGO. Vertigo may be an additional symptom in patients suffering from *sudden hearing loss.* The pathogenesis of the disorder is unknown but may be vascular. Bacterial infection of the labyrinth or occasionally otitis media causes vertigo. Degenerative and genetic abnormalities of the labyrinthine system can cause vertigo. *Cervical vertigo* is the term given to the vertiginous feelings associated with head movement in patients with cervical osteoarthritis or spondylosis. The disorder probably is caused by unbalanced input from cervical muscles to the vestibular apparatus. Acute neck strain may occasionally be associated with vertigo. Local anesthetics injected into one side of the neck can produce vertigo and ataxia by a similar lack of balanced input. There is no nystagmus in these disorders.

Central Vertigo

Central causes of vertigo, less common than peripheral causes, are usually characterized by less severe vertigo than that resulting from peripheral lesions, no hearing loss or tinnitus, and concomitant neurologic signs of brainstem or cerebellar dysfunction. When central vertigo is usually accompanied by other neurologic signs or symptoms, the localization is strongly suggested by history and physical examination.

CEREBROVASCULAR DISEASE. If ischemia, infarction, or hemorrhage affects the brainstem or cerebellum, vertigo accompanied by nausea and vomiting is a relatively common symptom. Occipital headache usually accompanies the vertigo, and nystagmus as well as other neurologic signs suggesting brainstem or cerebellar dysfunction will be found. Rarely, vertigo is the sole symptom of *transient ischemic attacks* of the brainstem, but most patients suffering such attacks will, if carefully questioned, report headache, diplopia, facial or body numbness, and ataxia as well. However, even in the absence of other symptoms, elderly patients with risk factors for cerebrovascular disease, such as hypertension, diabetes, heart disease, or hyperlipidemia, should be evaluated for posterior fossa vascular disease: Caloric testing and auditory evoked potentials may provide evidence of central vestibular and auditory dysfunction. CT scans with fine cuts of the posterior fossa may reveal evidence of infarction, and digital venous angiography can rule out surgically correctable lesions of the posterior fossa vasculature. For further discussion of the diagnosis and treatment of cerebrovascular disease, see Ch. 494.

CEREBELLOPONTINE ANGLE TUMORS. Most tumors growing in the cerebellopontine angle (e.g., acoustic neuroma, meningioma) grow slowly, allowing the vestibular system to accommodate and thus usually producing a vague sensation of dysequilibrium rather than acute vertigo. Frequently the patient complains of tinnitus, hearing loss, and a sensation that he is being pulled or pushed when he walks. Occasionally episodic vertigo or positional vertigo will herald the presence of a cerebellopontine angle tumor. In virtually all of the patients, retrocochlear hearing loss is present, and responses to caloric tests are decreased or absent on the involved side. Careful CT scans through the temporal bone and posterior fossa usually reveal the tumor. Nuclear magnetic resonance may be an even more sensitive test in these disorders.

DEMYELINATING DISEASE. Acute vertigo may be the first symptom of *multiple sclerosis,* although only a small percentage of young patients with acute vertigo eventually develop multiple sclerosis. Such central vertigo is often accompanied by nystagmus and other signs of brainstem dysfunction. A past history of transient neurologic deficits suggests multiple sclerosis, and CT scan or, if available, nuclear magnetic resonance scan may reveal demyelinating plaques. Oligoclonal bands in the cerebrospinal fluid strongly suggest the diagnosis. Vertigo in multiple sclerosis is usually transient and often associated with other neurologic signs of brainstem disease, in particular internuclear ophthalmoplegia or cerebellar dysfunction. Vertigo may also be a symptom of *parainfectious encephalomyelitis* or, rarely, *parainfectious cranial polyneuritis.* In this instance, the accompanying neurologic signs establish the diagnosis.

CRANIAL NEUROPATHY. A variety of acute or subacute illnesses affecting the eighth cranial nerve may produce vertigo as an early or sole symptom. The most common such disorder is *herpes zoster.* The *Ramsay-Hunt syndrome (geniculate ganglion herpes)* is characterized by vertigo and hearing loss associated with facial paralysis and sometimes pain in the ear. The typical lesions of herpes zoster, which may follow the appearance of neurologic signs, are found in the external auditory canal and sometimes over the palate. Whether herpes zoster is ever responsible for vertigo in the absence of the full-blown syndrome is not certain. *Granulomatous meningitis* or *leptomeningeal metastases* and cerebral or systemic *vasculitis* may involve the eighth nerve, producing vertigo as an early symptom. In these disorders, cerebrospinal fluid analysis usually suggests the diagnosis.

SEIZURE DISORDERS. Patients suffering from temporal lobe epilepsy occasionally suffer vertigo as the aura. Vertigo in the absence of other neurologic signs or symptoms is never caused by epilepsy or other diseases of the cerebral hemispheres.

OTHER CENTRAL CAUSES. Many structural lesions of the brainstem or cerebellum, particularly if rapid in onset, may cause vertigo. In a few instances, *paraneoplastic brainstem or cerebellar degeneration* may present with vertigo, and, as with *brainstem tumors, cerebellar degenerative diseases,* and other structural disease of the brainstem and posterior fossa, there are usually other neurologic symptoms and there are almost always signs of brainstem or cerebellar dysfunction in addition to the vertigo and nystagmus.

Evaluation of the "Dizzy" Patient

1. Try to determine by history (see page 2040) whether the patient is suffering from vertigo or nonvestibular dizziness, e.g., syncope (Ch. 480), ataxia (Ch. 472), diplopia, or anxiety (Ch. 476).

2. Perform a standard physical and neurologic examination, with special attention to heart and blood pressure (orthostatic hypotension or cardiac arrhythmias) for suspected syncope, cerebellar or peripheral nerve dysfunction for ataxia, visual and oculomotor examination for visual vertigo, and nystagmus and past pointing for vestibular causes.

3. Try to elicit the symptoms by provocative tests (dizziness simulation battery).

4. Laboratory evaluation including routine blood studies and chemistries, 24-hour cardiac monitoring, electroencephalography, audiometry, and electronystagmography may be required to establish the cause of the dizziness.

5. If the symptoms are vestibular, decide by the above tests whether the abnormality is physiologic or pathologic. Physiologic abnormalities require little more than reassurance and the use of vestibulosuppressive drugs in appropriate circumstances (see below), whereas pathologic vertigo requires more careful vestibular evaluation.

6. The above examinations should also have indicated whether, if the vertigo is pathologic, it is peripheral or central. Peripheral vertigo that is not typically benign positional or Ménière's disease requires careful otolaryngologic examination, including hypocycloidal tomography and CT scanning of the temporal bones. A search for perilymphatic fistulae should be made. Most peripheral disorders are, however, benign and self-limited.

If the disorder is *central,* neuro-otologic evaluation should include CT scanning of the brain, with particular attention to the posterior fossa. It is likely that in the future nuclear magnetic resonance scanning will be superior to CT scanning in defining lesions of the posterior fossa. Spinal fluid evaluation may also be required. In most instances, careful attention to history, physical examination, and provocative tests will establish the diagnosis.

Treatment

The best treatment of symptomatic vertigo is successful treatment of the underlying disease. In many instances that is not possible and the physician can prescribe symptomatic treatment only. In acute vertigo, such as occurs with labyrinthitis, patients should be, and in fact will insist on being, at bedrest. Vestibulosedative drugs such as meclazine 25 mg 4 times daily or diazepam 5 mg 4 times daily may also be helpful. If the patient is vomiting, 25 mg prochlorperazine suppositories may be helpful. In more chronic vertiginous disorders, the vestibulosuppressive drugs such as meclazine are often helpful. Scopolamine 0.4 to 0.8 mg together with methylphenidate 5 mg orally may give relief of vertigo, particularly motion sickness. Recently transdermal scopolamine paste-on units placed behind the ear have been reported to be effective in the treatment of the vertigo of motion sickness for up to 72 hours. These, like all scopolamine products, may produce anticholinergic side effects. If head or neck movement precipitates vertigo, a cervical collar may relieve the symptoms.

Baloh WR: Dizziness, Hearing Loss and Tinnitus: The Essentials of Neurotology. Philadelphia, F. A. Davis Company, 1984. *A new monograph with sections on anatomy and physiology, clinical examination, and treatment.*

Brandt T, Daroff RB: The multisensory physiological and pathological vertigo syndromes. Ann Neurol 7:195, 1980. *An excellent clinical review of the pathophysiology of vertigo and the clinical findings in patients with that disorder.*

DeWeese DD, Saunders WH: Textbook of Otolaryngology. 6th ed. St. Louis, The C. V. Mosby Co., 1982. *A recent edition of an excellent text, with good chapters on hearing loss, tinnitus, dizziness, and vertigo. The bibliography is good.*

Rudge P: Clinical Neuro-Otology. Clinical Neurology and Neurosurgery Monographs, Vol. 4. Edinburgh, Livingstone, 1983. *A thorough and comprehensive discussion of the anatomy and physiology, clinical assessment, and specific diseases of the auditory and vestibular system.*

480. DISORDERS OF MOTOR FUNCTION

480.1. Asthenia, Fatigue, and Weakness

Fred Plum

The closely related symptoms of asthenia, fatigue, and weakness relate to motor activity in different ways. *Asthenia* is anticipatory, occurring in advance of the act. It consists of an inner sense of usually subacute or chronic lassitude in which persons feel weak before they start or expect that greater than normal effort will be required to perform tasks. Affected persons hesitate to undertake motor activity, fearing that strength or endurance may be insufficient to the requirement. Small reductions in motor power or impaired endurance can be difficult to measure, so that asthenia sometimes reflects the presence of clinically undetectable motor weakness as in mild myasthenia gravis or in the early course of acute polyneuropathy. Similarly, asthenia can be an early, prominent symptom of thyrotoxicosis. The symptom can accompany acute lateral cerebellar dysfunction, presumably due to impairment of neocortical long loop feedback control, and emerges with the complex difficulty in initiating movement that accompanies parkinsonism. Most asthenia, however, is non-neurogenic and accompanies several psychologic and systemic disorders.

Most organically based asthenia has a relatively recent onset and arises in association with other symptoms, signs, or laboratory findings of physical illness. Subacute or chronic asthenia (neurasthenia, formerly called "effort syndrome") contributes prominently to the symptoms of anxiety or depression. Its physiology is little understood. The symptom may be accompanied by signs of autonomic imbalance, including tachycardia, recurrent sighing, multifocal blushing, and inappropriate sweating. Neurasthenia is difficult to treat; affected patients often tenaciously regard their symptom and its accompaniments as expressions of some still-undiscovered organic disease rather than as a reflection of psychologic maladjustment.

Fatigue refers to an abnormal rate or degree of exhaustion during or following motor activity. Abnormal fatigue can be local or generalized and either acute, subacute, or chronic. Many systemic illnesses produce at least briefly a sense of generalized lassitude, purposelessness, and easy exhaustion, including bacterial and influenzal infections, hepatitis, infectious mononucleosis, myocardial infarction, endocrine disorders (e.g., Addison's disease, panhypopituitarism, and hypo- or hyperthyroidism), severe anemia, malnutrition, disseminated malignancy, and anticancer chemotherapy. Fatigue is a prominent symptom of certain chronic neurologic disorders such as parkinsonism and multiple sclerosis. A distressing sense of purposelessness, easy tiring, and lack of initiative characterize the postconcussion syndrome and states of chronic sedative drug ingestion. The managment of such complex mixtures of psychic and somatic reactions provides a major challenge for the physician. It is best to approach the matter directly, as the symptoms are common and easily self-reinforced if not managed effectively in their early stages. *Local* fatigability with a rapid decline in strength after repeated movement of a particular group of muscles is characteristic of myasthenia gravis. Less easily measurable feelings of muscle tiredness also accompany local peripheral motor neuropathy or radiculopathy. Chronic fatigue that remains unexplained by a careful search for systemic or neuromuscular causes often has a psychogenic basis.

Most acute fatigue states have a metabolic or musculoskeletal origin and can be related to a recent illness or to episodes of unusual exercise or muscular hyperactivity. Almost all kinds of muscular or neuromuscular weakness lower the threshold for the exercised part to tire, but persistent somatic fatigue rarely can be attributed to mere chronic overwork. Organically engendered fatigue states are worse in the evening than in the morning. They are accentuated by further activity and typically relieved by sleep. Psychogenic fatigue follows the opposite pattern, being maximal in the morning and declining in the evening as the social pace increases.

Weakness refers to a specific loss of strength in voluntary muscle movement, usually complained of as an inability to complete a specific and familiar act. The symptom can be subtle. Patients sometimes ignore even prominent degrees of weakness until noticed by friends or family ("your foot drags" or "why are you limping?") or brought out by the examiner's tests. The presence of weakness can reflect disease or dysfunction at any level of the nervous system: muscle, neuromuscular junction, peripheral nerve or root, anterior horn cell, descending motor systems, basal ganglia or cerebellum, and even hysteria or malingering. Muscular weakness can develop from locomotor indirect involvement with generalized metabolic dysfunction as with hyponatremia, hyper- or hypothyroidism, certain drug intoxications, and in the setting of starvation or cancer. Painful areas of bone and joint inflammation can induce local, non-neurogenic weakness as a protective response against the further discomfort of movement.

480.2. Ataxia and Related Gait Disorders

Fred Plum

Any neurologic illness that affects sensorimotor functions in the lower extremities can interfere with the coordinated act of walking. Accordingly, an introductory analysis of the differential features of certain gait abnormalities may prove helpful in diagnosis. Other chapters provide descriptions of the well-known abnormalities that characterize parkinsonism, chorea, athetosis, spastic paraparesis, and various forms of poly- and mononeuritic motor weakness.

ATAXIA. Ataxia is a failure of muscular coordination expressed as irregularity or awkwardness of movement. Common usage has applied the term most often to an unsteadiness of walking, but the same principles apply to disturbances in coordinated movements affecting the upper extremities, the speech mechanisms, or even the eye movements. In the literal sense, ataxia can result from any abnormality in motor function, whether induced by faulty peripheral sensory mechanisms or by disturbances of descending corticospinal, basal ganglion, or cerebellar control. Most often the analysis of ataxia as a diagnostic problem lies in distinguishing disturbances in proprioceptive control from those caused by weakness, cerebello-vestibular abnormalities, or the influence of toxic drugs.

PROPRIOCEPTIVE (SENSORY) ATAXIA. Proprioceptive ataxia can result from diseases of the large afferent fibers of the peripheral nerve, dorsal root, or the dorsal spinal funiculus, and less often from lesions of the brainstem lemniscal system or the sensory projection from the thalamus to the parietal lobe cortex. The functional defect results from a variable loss of knowledge of the location of the body part combined with relatively preserved strength in the member. Afferent peripheral nerve, dorsal root, and spinal lesions most often result from inflammatory-demyelinating neuropathy, diabetic neuropathy, syphilitic tabes dorsalis or meningomyelopathy, and any of several inherited forms of spinocerebellar degeneration. Cyanocobalamin (B_{12}) deficiency involves both the peripheral nerve and the dorsal column of the cord, whereas multiple sclerosis and allied demyelinating diseases affect the cord alone.

Nerve or root lesions cause a bilateral defect that characteristically (1) affects the lower more than the upper extremities; (2) involves position as much as or more than vibratory sensation but may sometimes be difficult to verify; (3) shows absent or greatly reduced deep tendon reflexes; and (4) produces a broad-based, weaving gait that with severe sensory loss becomes lurching, sometimes leg flinging, or pounding, and is worse in the dark (rombergism). Spinal dorsal column lesions produce similar symptoms except that position loss may be more profound, the signs may be less equally symmetrical, the tendon reflexes can be preserved, and pathologic reflexes may be present if the abnormality also involves the descending corticospinal tract. Brainstem lemniscal involvement resembles spinal impairment but is seldom bilateral. Position sense loss may outstrip vibratory impairment. Patients with peripheral or spinal sensory ataxia are subjectively well aware of their deficits. They are also aware that their lack of coordination is not due to "dizziness," which distinguishes them from patients with vestibular disorders. Parietal or thalamoparietal proprioceptive impairment produces an ataxia that is usually unilateral and (1) affects the contralateral upper extremity as severely as the lower, (2) disproportionately impairs position sense more than vibration, and (3) may go partially unrecognized or be denied by the patient (anosognosia).

CEREBELLAR ATAXIA. The motor abnormality associated with cerebellar lesions depends on the localization of the abnormality in the cerebellum and on whether or not adjacent or related neural structures are involved. Thus midline, lateral hemispheric, and cerebellar outflow lesions each tend to produce somewhat distinct syndromes. These differences become less typical and more individualized when cerebellar tumors compress the adjacent brainstem to produce additional dysfunction or when diseases such as disseminated sclerosis or spinocerebellar degeneration affect neurologic structures that lie remote from the cerebellum

Spinocerebellar disorders produce a predominantly sensory ataxia superimposed on which is a variable degree of cerebellar dyssynergia, depending on the extent to which specific cerebellar inflow and outflow pathways are affected in the particular disease in question.

Midline cerebellar dysfunction results principally from degenerative (nutritional-alcoholic, remote effects of carcinoma) or neoplastic (medulloblastoma, hemangioblastoma, metastasis) disease. The gait is characteristic with legs thrust widely apart and extended, the arms extended in compensatory balance, and walking accomplished by short steps. Affected patients usually look at the ground for additional sensory stabilization and turn en bloc. With extension into the anterior midline cerebellum, stretch reflexes become hyperactive. In the early stages of the illness, the upper extremities and cranial nerves can be affected little or not at all, even in the presence of substantial lower extremity ataxia. As the disorder advances, truncal titubation appears, as can difficulty in rhythmic movements of the upper extremities and, eventually, even nystagmus. Posterior midline space-occupying lesions may add retropulsion to this symptom complex. It is difficult to be sure whether this last-mentioned symptom emanates from cerebellar or underlying brainstem dysfunction.

Lateral cerebellar hemispheric abnormalities produce ipsilateral hypotonia and incoordination marked by an irregular swaying gait and a tendency to drift toward the side of the lesion. The feet are spread apart, although not so broadly as with midline lesions, and patients characteristically cannot manage close-footed tandem walking. Rombergism is absent, but, as with all ataxias, distorted vision or closing the eyes moderately accentuates the patient's unsteadiness. Rhythmic movements and point-to-point tests are impaired in both the upper and lower extremities. If classic intention tremor appears, it implies that the abnormality includes the outflow from the dentate nucleus or its projection through the superior cerebellar peduncle to the red nucleus of the midbrain.

DRUNKENNESS. Drunkenness, whether due to alcohol or depressant drug intoxication, results mainly from bilateral labyrinthine-vestibular dysfunction and is accompanied by sensations of both vertigo and dizziness. Few patients with cerebellar disease walk the streets with as much incapacity as a severe alcoholic. Severely intoxicated patients reel, lurch, twist, and fall. Lesser degrees of intoxication produce unsteadiness, a tottering, cautious gait with the feet placed moderately widely apart, clumsiness, dysarthria, and nystagmus in all directions.

VESTIBULAR ATAXIA. Chronic unilateral impairment of the vestibulosensory system can occur with lesions anywhere along the peripheral pathway, including labyrinthine destruction by disease or drugs, eighth nerve damage from cerebellopontine angle tumor, or compression, injury, inflammation, or neoplasms damaging the vestibular complex in the brainstem. Patients with such abnormalities tend to drift toward the side of impairment and then quickly correct the deviation in the opposite direction. Turning accentuates their unsteadiness and induces missteps. Bilateral damage to the vestibular nuclei in the brainstem results in a narrow-based ataxia with poor compensating movements in the limbs, drifting or falling to either side, and a tendency to retropulsion and falling backward. Patients with vestibular dysfunction depend heavily on visual proprioception so that closing the eyes accentuates the gait disorder.

SPASTIC ATAXIA. Combined abnormalities of the spinal dorsal columns and cortical spinal tracts produce a characteristic broad-based tottering and sometimes pounding gait with the knees held high but the legs moving stiffly. The condition occurs with demyelinating diseases and other intrinsic spinal disorders such as vascular malformations, cyanocobalamin deficiency, arachnoiditis, and, occasionally, neoplasms.

FRONTAL LOBE GAIT DISORDERS. Patients with frontal lobe disease can suffer any of several gait disorders, depending upon the anatomic distribution of the lesions. Unilateral injury to the foot-leg area of the somatosensory cortex produces a focal monoparesis, whereas bilateral motor-premotor damage results in a relatively narrow-based, stiff-legged impairment, sometimes with scissoring of the legs. More anteriorly placed premotor and prefrontal abnormalities arise in association with deep bilateral tumors, multiple cerebral infarctions, or communicating, "low pressure" hydrocephalus. The ensuing ataxia sometimes (and probably erroneously) is called "gait apraxia." It consists of a severe difficulty in walking or otherwise using the lower extremities so long as the patient is in the erect position. The feet appear glued to the floor (magnet reaction), and attempts to walk often consist of short shuffles or even hops, before the legs get moving. Walking, once (or if) it begins, proceeds as a halting and broad-based movement made easier by guidance or support. Advanced cases may be unable to get underway and, unless supported, increasingly tend to retropulse or fall backward, even from a sitting position. A degree of clinically obvious dementia accompanies the gait disorder.

Patients with frontal ataxia of this type show a greater ability to move their legs on command when lying supine than when standing. Examination of the lower extremities discloses an increased paratonic resistance to passive movements coupled with bilateral plantar grasp responses, extensor thrust responses, and usually accentuated tendon reflexes. These reflex abnormalities and physiologic dysfunctions, rather than the elusive mechanisms of an ill-defined apraxia, best explain the difficulty in movement.

HEMIPARESIS. Both pyramidal-corticospinal and extrapyramidal motor disorders sometimes have a hemiparetic pattern and in their early stages can be confused with one another clinically. Severe spastic hemiplegia from damage to the corticospinal tract or the full-blown stooped, festinating, semishuffling gait of parkinsonism is so well known and readily recognized as to require no discussion. More subtle hemiparesis, however, can easily be overlooked, especially when it reflects the akinesia of early parkinsonism. In their initial stages, both pyramidal and extrapyramidal disorders produce mild or inconstant weakness, a susceptibility to easy fatigue in the affected member, and a sense of stiffness. Both corticospinal and parkinsonian hemiparesis incipiently produce a gait disorder marked by a slack arm and a reduction of other automatic accessory movements on the affected side, a tendency to scuff the toe, and a measure of bodily akinesia. Both may result in an increase in muscular resistance to passive stretch on the involved side; in the early stages it may be difficult clinically to distinguish between pyramidal spasticity and extrapyramidal rigidity. The following points help in differential diagnosis. Patients with early pyramidal tract dysfunction tend to have unilaterally increased reflexes on the affected side. When walking, they flex the wrist and fingers, circumduct the lower extremity, and hold the foot in an equinovarus position. Patients with early hemiparetic parkinsonism, on the other hand, tend to have greater facial and bodily hypokinesia, to stoop, and to show at least some cogwheel resistance on rotary movements of the elbow or wrist. They extend the affected wrist and step the weak foot forward rather than circumducting it. The foot itself is held in simple varus position. The deep tendon reflexes may or may not be slightly asymmetrical.

GAIT DISTURBANCES IN THE ELDERLY. Any of several specific visual, somatosensory, or motor diseases may impair walking in elderly persons. Less easily classified but fairly typical walking difficulties include a tendency to walk with slow, short, mincing, and unsteady steps (marche à petits pas). Fairly common is a stooped position coupled with a moderately broad-based, unsteady gait, sometimes associated with CT evidence of a chronic communicating hydrocephalus (see Ch. 515).

RETROPULSION. A tendency to step backward from the standing position or to fall backward while sitting can be a symptom of several serious, acquired midline abnormalities of the brain. The physiology of the disorder is poorly understood. It accompanies midline tumors of the posterior cerebellum as well as degenerative disorders affecting the central vestibular mechanisms bilaterally, and has been reported in association with bilateral lesions affecting the sides of the third ventricle, the basal ganglia, and the frontal lobes. Occasionally the abnormality is associated with large, unilateral frontal lobe neoplasms that produce an increase in intracranial pressure and intracranial shift. Retropulsion of posterior fossa origin is especially dangerous, as it often comes on suddenly and is accompanied by a loss of the normal postural protective mechanisms that guard against injury during falling.

HYSTERICAL GAIT. Hysteria can mimic a variety of hemiparetic, steppage, or ataxic gait disorders. With a hemiparetic type, the pattern usually gives itself away by an atypical dragging behind of the affected leg during a series of hops or supported steps. The most obviously factitious hysterical disorder is a lurching, irregularly based, sometimes bent-forward walk in which the patient grasps any object in reach for support and reels from side to side inconsistently. Such patients may sink to the floor, but almost never endure an unsupported, self-injuring fall. Signs of altered muscular tonus or abnormal reflexes are absent, and the bizarre movements not only differ from the expected pattern of sensory or cerebellar dysfunction but often change from examination to examination.

De Jong RN, Magee KR: The Neurological Examination. 4th ed. Hagerstown, MD, Harper & Row, 1979. *A comprehensive text with detailed references.*

Garcin R: Coordination of voluntary movement and the ataxias. *In* Vinken PJ, Bruyn GW, Garcin R (eds.): Handbook of Clinical Neurology, Vol 1, Disturbances of Nervous Function. Amsterdam, North Holland, 1969, pp 293, 309. *A detailed and thoughtful exposition of clinical and physiologic principles.*

Kremer M: Sitting, standing and walking. Br Med J 2:63, 1958. *A succinct and readable analysis.*

480.3. Episodic Loss of Motor Function

Jerome B. Posner

Motor disorders cause paralysis, usually accompanied by alterations in muscle tone. In most instances, the weakness is either persistent or progressive. Sometimes, however, patients report episodic loss of motor function affecting one or more extremities which, although severe, is brief in duration and followed by a return to normal. Such episodic loss of motor function can be caused by a variety of pathophysiologic abnormalities. Because the symptoms are episodic, the patient is usually entirely normal when he presents to the physician; therefore, preliminary diagnosis depends on obtaining an accurate description of the event. The paragraphs below describe the potential causes of episodic loss of motor function. Individual disorders are described in detail under pertinent headings in other chapters.

Drop Attacks

PATHOPHYSIOLOGY. The most perplexing diagnostic problem associated with episodic loss of motor function is the so-called drop attack. A patient, usually in the later decades of life, who is standing or walking suddenly falls to the ground. In a classic drop attack, the patient does not lose consciousness, has not tripped or otherwise lost his balance, and is able to resume normal activity immediately or shortly following the fall. Affected persons suffer no accompanying neurologic signs but often fall with sufficient suddenness and force to cause injury.

Pathophysiologically, drop attacks without loss of consciousness occur when tonic, long loop, posture-controlling discharges from the central nervous system to extensor muscles of the leg transiently cease. The sudden loss of anterior horn or corticospinal tract function may result from direct damage to these structures, leading to transient paralysis, or from removal of tonic facilitation of these structures, leading to sudden failure of muscle tone. *Transient ischemia* can produce drop attacks when motor pathways are involved bilaterally. Such an event is likely only when the transient ischemia occurs in the distribution of either the anterior spinal or the vertebrobasilar arterial system. Episodic spinal cord ischemia is usually accompanied by sensory as well as motor changes, and the patient may be able to report a level of sensory change that localizes the dysfunction to the thoracic or lumbar spinal cord. Vertebrobasilar insufficiency may cause drop attacks as the only symptom, but more commonly the patient suffers other signs of brainstem ischemia (Ch. 494). The only detailed autopsy report of a patient with drop attacks shows infarction affecting the corticospinal tracts in the lower pons and upper medulla.

All drop attacks, however, do not have the implication of severe spinal or brainstem ischemia. *Cryptogenic drop attacks* occur in many middle-aged and elderly individuals whose evaluation reveals no evidence of either cardiac or central nervous system vascular disease. The attacks may occur episodically for months or years without the development of other nervous system disease. Although they are not rare, nothing is known of the pathophysiology of these drop attacks.

Cataplexy, the sudden loss of motor tone without paralysis or change in consciousness, is an occasional cause of drop attacks. The fall to the ground is usually slower than with the classic drop attack, and the patient rarely hurts himself. Cataplexy is thought to be a fragment of the loss of motor tone that occurs normally during REM sleep and usually occurs as a part of the narcolepsy syndrome (Ch. 472.5). Occasionally cataplexy occurs as an isolated symptom of the sudden rises of intracranial pressure (*plateau waves*) that sometimes accompany brain tumors or hydrocephalus (Ch. 515). Because there are important connections between the vestibular system and pathways controlling muscle tone, sudden *vestibular failure* can cause drop attacks. Such episodes are almost always accompanied by vertigo and usually by nausea and vomiting as well. *Akinetic* or *myoclonic seizures* causing drop attacks are common in childhood but rare in the adult. However, drop attacks occasionally have been reported in adults that appear to be epileptic in origin and respond to anticonvulsant drugs.

DIAGNOSIS. The first task for the physician in the differential diagnosis of drop attacks is to determine whether the patient was truly unconscious at any time throughout the episode. If unconsciousness is known or reasonably suspected, the first diagnosis should be syncope and the diagnostic evaluation directed toward that disorder (Ch. 472.4). If it is clear that the patient is conscious throughout the episodes and that the disorder cannot be attributed to tripping or loss of balance, the physician should probe carefully for accompanying symptoms or signs that may help to localize the cause. Back pain, lower extremity paresthesias or sensory loss, or sudden changes in bladder or bowel function accompanying the drop attacks suggest spinal cord dysfunction. Headache, diplopia, and dysarthria accompanying the attack suggest brainstem dysfunction, probably caused by vertebrobasilar arterial insufficiency. Tinnitus or vertigo suggests vestibular dysfunction. Severe headache, particularly if accompanied by nausea and vomiting, suggests plateau waves from increased intracranial pressure.

A CT scan will rule out a brain tumor or hydrocephalus leading to plateau waves. In the absence of demonstrated syncope or a cause of increased intracranial pressure, the most serious potential diagnosis is vertebrobasilar transient ischemic attacks. Patients in whom no other diagnosis can be made should be considered to have cerebral vascular disease and be so treated until proved otherwise (Ch. 493). In many patients, however, no diagnosis can be made and no definitive treatment prescribed. Elderly patients with drop attacks not due to cerebral vascular disease sometimes benefit by carrying a cane, which may prevent or lessen the force of the fall. Patients in whom no diagnosis can be made should probably be evaluated by electroencephalography and be considered for a trial of anticonvulsant agents.

Other Transient Paralyses

Episodic loss of motor function in one or more extremities can be a perplexing problem. Affected patients may complain of sudden or rapid loss of motor function involving an arm or a leg or both, with or without associated sensory symptoms, but without abnormal motor movements of either the arm or the leg. Several pathophysiologic abnormalities can cause such symptoms, and these abnormalities may be clinically indistinguishable from each other. The first and most common is a *transient ischemic attack* from vascular insufficiency in the distribution of the internal carotid artery. All patients suffering episodic loss of motor function on one side of the body should be considered to be suffering from transient ischemic attacks until proved otherwise. Other, less common, causes of transient loss of motor function include *plateau waves* associated with increased intracranial pressure, *nonconvulsive epileptic attacks*, and *late-life complicated migraine*. In transient ischemic attacks and plateau waves, there is usually sudden loss of motor function lasting 5 to 15 minutes and, in the instance of plateau waves, often an accompanying headache and sometimes some clouding of consciousness; with atonic seizures and migraine, the onset of motor dysfunction is usually but not always slower, but it too persists for 5 to 20 minutes. The motor weakness in late-life migraine may or may not be accompanied by a contralateral headache that appears as the motor change disappears. Patients with transient ischemic attacks or plateau waves also may have headaches at times indistinguishable from migraine.

Since the four entities may be clinically indistinguishable from each other, all must be considered in the differential diagnosis of episodic weakness. A CT scan establishes the presence and causes of increased intracranial pressure and plateau waves; digital venous angiography often establishes the initiating cause of transient ischemia as lying in the carotid or basilar artery distribution; electroencephalography may assist in the diagnosis of a seizure disorder, but the EEG is often normal between episodes. A past or family history of migraine assists in the diagnosis of late-life migraine but is not diagnostic. Therapeutic trials directed successively at treatment of the several causes of these episodic attacks sometimes help in reaching a definitive diagnosis.

481. DISORDERS OF SENSATION

Jerome B. Posner

MAJOR SENSORY PATHWAYS AND SYMPTOMS

An organism perceives its environment through its sensory systems. The sensory systems can be divided roughly into three physiologic entities: *special sensation,* including smell, vision, hearing, equilibrium, and taste (see Ch. 479); the *exteroceptive* or somatosensory system, which perceives environmental influences directly contacting the organism, including the sensations of pressure, touch, temperature, and pain; and the *enteroceptive* system, which senses the internal environment, including both consciously perceived pressure and pain sensation and unconsciously perceived alterations of osmolality, chemistry (aortic and carotid chemoreceptors, glycoreceptors, etc.), and pressure (cardiovascular baroreceptors). *Proprioception,* only some of which is perceived consciously, includes special sensation (vestibular system), exteroceptive receptors (joint position sense), and enteroceptive receptors (muscle sensation). When portions of the sensory system are diseased, the organism no longer accurately perceives its environment and thus cannot interact with it to full effect.

When the sensory system is disordered, sensation may be diminished, increased, or distorted. In the exteroceptive system, diminution or absence of function is called *hypesthesia* or *anesthesia*, respectively. Diminution or loss of pain sensation is called *hypalgesia* or *analgesia*; diminution or loss of temperature sensation, *thermhypesthesia* or *thermanesthesia,* etc. Hyperfunction of the exteroceptive sensory system is characterized either by a lowered threshold to stimulation (hyperesthesia), a phenomenon that occurs in some instances of physical (e.g., sunburn) or chemical abnormalities of cutaneous receptors, or by spontaneous discharge, leading to pins and needles or burning sensations that may or may not be painful (*paresthesias*). Distortion of sensory input leads to *dysesthesias,* usually an unpleasant or painful sensation produced by a stimulus that is ordinarily painless, or to hyperpathia. *Hyperpathia* follows damage to the sensory system that elevates the threshold of perception of noxious stimuli, but once that threshold is exceeded, a severely painful or unpleasant sensation is the response to what would normally be only a modestly unpleasant stimulus. *Causalgia* is a condition in which both painful paresthesias and hyperpathia exist and are characterized by a sense of burning pain.

Anatomy and Physiology of Sensory Pathways

Two major sensory pathways subserve both exteroception and conscious proprioception. The first pathway subserves the sensations of pain, temperature, and crude touch. It begins as free nerve endings of small myelinated and unmyelinated fibers. "Free nerve endings" have never been identified microscopically, nor is there complete agreement on the adequate stimulus for discharging these receptors, but current studies suggest that mechanical deformation and hot and cold are the important stimuli.

The receptors are connected to small (5 μ), thinly myelinated, "A delta" fibers, which conduct at about 35 meters per second, and to unmyelinated "C" fibers (1 to 2 μ), which conduct at about 0.5 meter per second. This dual set of fibers explains the phenomenon of "double pain." A noxious stimulus elicits first a sharp, pricking, well-localized pain mediated by the more rapidly conducting fibers, and the C fibers mediate a burning, poorly localized, exceedingly unpleasant "second pain."

All primary sensory afferents have their cell bodies in the dorsal root ganglion, but the small fibers of the first pathway enter the spinal cord via the dorsal root, lateral to the large myelinated (touch and proprioception) fibers, and then ascend or descend for one or two segments in the medial portion of Lissauer's tract to enter the more ventrally placed dorsal horn.

After synapsing in the dorsal horn, the ascending pain pathways in the spinal cord divide into two groups: the neospinothalamic tract, which is believed to subserve the perception of intensity and localization of pain, temperature, and crude touch, and the phylogenetically older paleospinothalamic tract, which is believed to subserve the arousal and emotional components of pain. The axons of the neospinothalamic tract arise from the dorsal horn, cross the anterior commissure, and ascend in the anterolateral quadrant of the spinal cord. The axons terminate in the ventral basal complex of the thalamus, principally within the ventral posterolateral nucleus (VPL) ipsilateral to the side of their ascent. The thalamic terminations of these fibers coincide to a large extent with those of the dorsal column, and the pathway shows somatotopic localization at the thalamic level, the face and upper body being represented most medially. Third order neurons from the thalamus project to somatosensory area 1 (sensorimotor cortex), with the same somatotopic localization as other sensory modalities. Lesions at the thalamic level often lead to chronic so-called "thalamic pain." The paleospinothalamic tract, whose cells of origin in the dorsal horn receive C fiber input, also crosses in the anterior commissure and ascends in the spinal cord closely applied to but more ventral than the neospinothalamic tract. Many of the fibers of the paleospinothalamic tract send collaterals to the reticular formation of the brainstem, but some reach the thalamus, terminating in several nuclei, particularly the nucleus centralis lateralis and the intralaminar nuclei.

The second system consists predominantly of larger myelinated fibers and subserves the functions of light touch, position sense, and tactile localization. The anatomy and physiology of the peripheral portion of this second pathway is described in Ch. 525. The central nervous system part begins where these large fibers enter the spinal cord via the dorsal root ganglion, lying in a position medial to the smaller fibers that subserve pain and temperature. Most of the large fibers ascend without synapsing in the posterior and to a lesser extent lateral columns of the spinal cord to reach the gracile and cuneate nuclei in the low brainstem. Second order neuron fibers then decussate and ascend in the medial lemniscus through the brainstem to reach the contralateral ventral posterior lateral nucleus of the thalamus. Third order neurons projected from the thalamus terminate in the cerebral cortex, prodominantly in the sensorimotor strip surrounding the Rolandic fissure. Lesions of this system lead to loss of sense of position of the limbs and body in space, inability to localize tactile stimuli or to distinguish between one and two closely placed stimuli (two-point discrimination), and inability to describe accurately the size, shape, and texture of objects (stereoanesthesia). Subcortical lesions of the system also cause loss of the ability to recognize vibratory sensation (pallesthesia).

The two major exteroceptive systems are anatomically separated through much of their course, particularly in the spinal cord, and they differ physiologically as a result of fiber size. Thus, lesions at different sites in the nervous system and lesions of different physiologic natures cause unique sensory syndromes that assist in localizing the site and nature of the disorder. Some of these syndromes are described in detail in other chapters. The paragraphs below describe the symptoms that help physicians localize sensory disorders, and the next section details the pathophysiology and clinical findings of common pain problems.

Localization of Sensory Disorders

PERIPHERAL NERVES. Sensory perception begins when a physical or chemical stimulus alters the activity of a *sensory receptor* in such a way that the stimulus is transduced into an electrical potential (receptor potential). If the potential is large enough, the nerve to which the receptor is connected will discharge and the stimulus will eventually reach the central nervous system. There are a wide variety of receptors, each of which transduces one of the physical and chemical stimuli that the organism is capable of perceiving. These receptors range from free nerve endings in the skin (touch, pressure, pain) to the highly specialized photoreceptors of the retina and the hair cells of the auditory and vestibular system. Certain degenerative diseases can affect the receptors in the eye or the ear, but no known disorders exist that affect receptors of the somatosensory system. Thus, the most peripheral disorders of the somatosensory system occur either in the axon itself (axonal neuropathy) or in the myelin sheath encasing the axon (Ch. 525). Many diseases of peripheral nerves affect both large and small fibers, leading to a diminution of all sensory modalities to approximately equal degree. In some disorders of peripheral nerves, however, small or large fibers can be involved preferentially, leading to a "dissociated sensory loss." When small fibers are predominantly affected, one finds pin and temperature sensation involved out of proportion to light touch, vibration, and position sense. Because autonomic fibers are also small, trophic changes in skin and joints may accompany such a small fiber peripheral neuropathy, but because motor fibers and the afferent portion of the stretch reflex are subserved by large fibers, these functions are relatively preserved despite sometimes profound loss of pain and temperature sensation. Such selective small fiber damage is sometimes encountered in diabetes and is common in some of the hereditary neuropathies as well as in toxic-nutritional neuropathies (Ch. 528 to 530). Large fiber loss is more common in demyelinating neuropathies and may lead to profound loss of localizing touch and proprioception, with relative preservation of crude touch, pin, and temperature sensation. Such disorders are commonly accompanied by paresthesias and sometimes spontaneous pain. The deep tendon reflexes are absent because of damage to large afferent fibers from muscle, and there is usually weakness as well. The diagnosis of a peripheral neuropathy involving sensory fibers is established by the distribution of the sensory loss, which may be in the distribution of a single nerve, multiple individual nerves (mononeuritis multiplex), or a symmetrical distal stocking-and-glove distribution (polyneuropathy). Polyneuropathies are distributed distally because longer axons are more vulnerable to disease than shorter ones. In general, mononeuropathies are caused by local disease (e.g., compression entrapment), mononeuritis multiplex by vascular disorders (e.g., polyarteritis), and polyneuropathies by immunologic or metabolic disorders (e.g., demyelination-inflammatory neuropathy, diabetes, uremia, nutritional neuropathy).

SPINAL CORD. True dissociation of sensory loss is more common in spinal cord disorders than in those originating in peripheral nerves or roots. Lesions of the posterolateral columns produce profound loss of position and vibration sense with normal crude touch, pin, and temperature sensation. Usually corticospinal tracts are involved as well as sensory pathways, and thus most such patients often have hyperactive reflexes and extensor plantar responses. Lesions of the spinothalamic tract or of crossing fibers from the posterior horn to the spinothalamic tract cause loss of pain and temperature sense with preservation of vibration, position, and localizing touch. Such dissociated sensory loss is common in syringomyelia and may occur with infarction of the anterior portion of the spinal cord from occlusion of the anterior spinal artery. In both of these disorders, motor function may be relatively well preserved. When only one side of the spinal cord is involved, one finds loss of proprioceptive sensation on the ipsilateral side and loss of pin and temperature sensation on the contralateral side, both below the level of the lesion. There is usually a small band of decreased sensation to all modalities resulting from damage to the posterior horn at the level of the lesion. This so-called Brown-Séquard syndrome is sometimes seen with tumors either compressing or invading the spinal cord and is a common presenting syndrome in radiation myelopathy. Lesions of the spinal cord are rarely confused with those of peripheral nerves, even when the latter show dissociated sensory loss, because the sensory loss in spinal cord lesions is usually proximal as well as distal and restricted to those segments below the spinal cord level damaged. Thus, by the time a polyneuropathy causes substantial sensory loss above the knees, nerve fibers supplying the fingertip are usually involved as well, whereas with a thoracic spinal cord lesion the arms are always spared. Furthermore, motor signs of upper motor neuron disease, particularly extensor plantar responses, usually correctly identify the central nature of a spinal cord disorder rather than pointing to a peripheral disturbance.

BRAINSTEM. In the lower brainstem, spinothalamic and proprioceptive pathways remain separated, lateral lesions of the medulla causing loss of pin and temperature sensation on the ipsilateral side of the face (a result of damage to the descending root of the trigeminal nerve) and the contralateral side of the body. This sensory abnormality is usually accompanied by other signs of lateral medullary damage (Wallenberg's syndrome) and spares proprioceptive pathways. Higher in the brainstem, as the two pathways converge in their route toward the thalamus, damage causes contralateral sensory loss to all modalities, usually accompanied by cranial nerve palsies, ataxia (from the cerebellar outflow), and motor weakness.

CEREBRUM. In the thalamus, damage to the ventral posterolateral nucleus causes decreased sensation of all modalities on the contralateral side of the body and face. Sensory loss is often accompanied by dysesthesias. A curious *thalamic syndrome* often appears four to six weeks after acute thalamic damage and has been attributed to denervation hypersensitivity of sensory neurons in the midbrain reticular formation. The patient develops spontaneous pain in the distribution of the sensory loss, usually associated with a dysesthetic response to touch and a hyperresponsiveness to pinprick once threshold is exceeded. The thalamic syndrome is rare but causes a particularly unpleasant pain intractable to most therapeutic endeavors. Conversely, surgical lesions of the intralaminar nuclei, which receive fibers from the paleospinothalamic tract, often decrease pain without affecting sensory thresholds.

Damage to the cerebral cortex causes sensory loss in which the synthetic qualities of sensation are involved out of proportion to crude sensation. Pain sensation is usually preserved, although the patient may describe a pin as feeling less sharp on the involved side. The distribution of sensory impairment follows the sensory homunculus. Depending on the cortical location of the lesion within that distribution, touch and vibration are usually relatively preserved as well. Position sense loss is often profound; the patient is unable to distinguish between one and two points touching the finger or foot, and cutaneous sensations, even though identified, may not be localized. Patients may be unable to identify the nature of an object placed in their hands, even though they are able to describe certain of its qualities (astereognosis). Patients with large cortical sensory lesions are often relatively inattentive to sensation from the contralateral side of the body, particularly if there is a distracting stimulus to the ipsilateral side. Thus, the patient presented with two symmetrical cutaneous sensory stimuli may fail to identify the one contralateral to the cortical lesion even though the strength of the stimulus exceeds threshold (extinction). With less severe damage, if two nonhomologous stimuli are presented (as, for example, to left hand and right face), the patient may perceive the stimulus on the involved side as occurring homologous to the stimulus on the uninvolved side ("You touched both sides of my face"). Such extinction phenomena are characteristic of parietal lobe lesions, particularly in the nondominant hemisphere. Smaller or more restricted lesions of the parietal lobe may lead to subtle changes in sensory function, with only synthetic modalities such as stereognosis, two-point discrimination, and graphesthesia (ability to identify numbers or letters traced on the palm or fingertip) involved.

PAIN

Pain is the most common symptom for which patients seek medical assistance, and chronic pain is among the most vexing problems which physicians face. Pain can have no precise definition because only the individual suffering it, not the observer, perceives it. Sir Thomas Lewis described the situation exactly when he said pain is "known to us by experience and described by illustration." Pain always has two aspects: the first is an emotionally neutral perception of a stimulus which is usually sufficiently strong to produce tissue damage; the second is an affective response to the perception of that stimulus. Pain implies damage to the organism, either physical or psychologic, and chronic pain, if untreated, will itself damage the organism. It is the physician's two-fold therapeutic task to discover and treat the cause of pain and also to treat the pain itself, whether or not the underlying cause is treatable.

Diagnosis of Painful Disorders

Pain is either "acute" or "chronic." The point at which acute pain becomes chronic pain varies, but pain of over six months' duration is usually considered chronic. Several clinical features differentiate acute from chronic pain. Patients suffering from severe acute pain can usually give a clear description of its location, character, and timing. Furthermore, objective signs, particularly of autonomic nervous system hyperactivity, with tachycardia, hypertension, diaphoresis, midriasis, and pallor, are present. Acute pain usually responds well to analgesic agents, and psychologic factors often play a minor role in its pathogenesis. By contrast, in patients suffering from chronic pain, the localization, character, and timing of the pain are more vague, and because the autonomic nervous system adapts, signs of autonomic hyperactivity disappear. Furthermore, chronic pain usually responds less well to analgesic agents, and psychologic factors are more important than in acute pain. All of these factors may lead the physician to believe that the patient's complaints are exaggerated. Since there are no reliable objective tests to assess chronic pain, the physician *must* believe the patient's report, taking into consideration his age, his cultural background, his environment, and other psychologic circumstances known to alter reaction to pain. *In general, the physician is wise to accept at face value the patient's report of the severity of his pain unless there is overwhelming evidence to the contrary.*

For purposes of classification by pathogenesis, chronic pain can be divided into three categories, although the physician should realize that there is much overlap among these categories. The first is chronic pain associated with structural disease. Such pain occurs with rheumatoid arthritis, metastatic cancer, or sickle cell anemia, and may be characterized by prolonged episodes of pain alternating with pain-free intervals, or by unremitting pain waxing and waning in severity. Psychologic factors may play an important role in exacerbating or relieving pain, but treatment of the pain by analgesics or therapy directed to the underlying disease is usually more helpful. The second group of patients suffers from psychophysiologic disorders causing pain. In these patients, structural disease such as a herniated disc or torn ligaments may once have been present, but psychologic factors have engendered chronic physiologic alterations such as muscle spasm, which produces pain long after the underlying deficit has healed. Such patients tend to respond poorly to analgesic drugs, but often respond well to combination therapy directed at the end-organ (e.g., injection of trigger points in muscles) and at psychologic factors which are disturbing them. The third group of patients complains of pain which appears to be caused by neither structural nor physiologic disorders. These patients are suffering from somatic delusions. Such patients usually have profound psychiatric disorders such as psychotic depression or schizophrenia, and the history of the pain is so vague and bizarre and its distribution so unanatomic as to suggest the diagnosis. These patients respond *only* to psychiatric therapy.

A thorough history, general physical examination, and careful neurologic examination are imperative in any patient complaining of pain. Often the description of the nature and distribution of the pain is so characteristic (e.g., trigeminal neuralgia or tabetic lightning pains) that it allows no other diagnosis. Inquiry should be made concerning (1) the temporal pattern of pain, (2) its distribution, (3) exacerbating factors, and (4) relieving factors.

For example, headache beginning early in the morning before arising suggests increased intracranial pressure, whereas headache occurring late in the day is more suggestive of tension. Back pain and sciatica made worse by sitting or walking suggest disc disease, whereas back pain and sciatica which are worse while in bed suggest intraspinal tumor. Back pain and sciatica exacerbated by cough or sneeze suggests intraspinal disease, whereas similar pain not exacerbated by cough or sneeze suggests disease in the pelvis. Pain in the back or legs exacerbated by straight leg raising suggests disease of the nervous system, whereas a similar pain exacerbated by rotating the hips suggests pelvic or hip disease. All pain is relieved to some extent by distraction and a pleasurable environment, and exacerbated by anxiety or psychologic stress.

A careful psychiatric history, looking particularly for signs and symptoms of depression, should be elicited from all patients. Specifically, physicians should inquire about the degree to which pain has interfered with the patient's activities, whether he is having difficulty sleeping, and whether there is a change in appetite or bowel habits. Early morning awakening, anorexia, and constipation are somatic manifestations of depression and may either be caused by chronic pain or exacerbate the effects of the pain.

A general physical examination must be performed. Both the physical and laboratory examination should begin with the assumption that the site of pathologic change is at the site of pain. The painful areas should be examined for swelling and redness as well as for any obvious deformity. (The pain of herpes zoster usually precedes the rash, and occasionally on examination one may note only the faintest reddening of the skin in a dermatomal distribution.) The areas reported as painful should be palpated, the temperature estimated, and points of tenderness sought. (If the site of pain is in a soft tissue, bone, or joint, it should be tender to palpation as well as spontaneously painful.) Joints should be taken through a full range of motion and the effect of movement on the pain assessed. Nerve trunks going to the extremities should be palpated and stretched by movement of that extremity (e.g., straight leg raising; abduction and extension of the arm). Inflamed and compressed nerve roots and nerve plexuses are more painful when stretched. A careful neurologic examination must also be performed. If there are neurologic abnormalities (e.g., weakness, sensory loss, reflex changes) in the painful part, one can infer that nervous system disease is responsible for the pain. The absence of specific neurologic abnormalities on first examination does not guarantee, however, that the nervous system is free of disease, because the process may simply not have advanced beyond the stage of selectively involving pain pathways. For example, a Pancoast tumor may produce pain in the shoulder and arm before other signs of neural involvement, such as Horner's syndrome or motor or sensory loss, appear.

Finally, laboratory examinations are performed. If the site of disease appears to be in bones or joints, x-rays of those structures or radioisotope scans may localize it. First attention should be paid to the local site of pain, but the physician should acquaint himself with the common referred patterns of pain (e.g., hip disease commonly causes knee pain, cardiac pain is frequently referred to the ulnar aspect of the arm and forearm, the pain of renal colic may be felt primarily in the groin and testicle, and pain resulting from disease of the throat may be referred to the ear).

Referred pain is pain perceived at a site remote from the source of the disturbance. Usually, referred pain is cutaneous and evoked by disease of deep structures innervated by the same dermatome. Referred pain may be associated with cutaneous hyperalgesia and even relieved by procaine injection into the area of referral. When pain is referred to the same dermatome or myotome as innervates the diseased structure (e.g., pain down the medial aspect of the arm [T1-T2] produced by myocardial infarction or angina pectoris), it is often helpful in diagnosis. However, pain is sometimes referred at a great distance from the primary site to segments not similarly innervated, and there the mechanism is perplexing (e.g., anginal pain referred to the jaw). Various theories have been suggested to account for referred pain. Such theories as division of the same nerve into deep and superficial branches, release of chemical mediators in the nervous system, and convergence of cutaneous and visceral nerves into common synaptic pools at the spinal cord all explain the dermatomal referral of pain but fail to explain pain at remote sites.

Management

In some patients, pain is best managed by treating the underlying disorder (e.g., steroids for giant cell arteritis relieve headache and muscle pain promptly; radiation therapy for bone pain caused by cancer is often helpful). In others, a particular kind of pain has a particular treatment (see Specific Pain Syndromes below), but in many patients the pain is chronic and the physician is able neither to treat the underlying disturbances nor to offer specific therapy for that type of pain. In treating this type of chronic and severe pain, certain general principles should be followed:

1. The pain should be treated by the simplest effective means, but all efforts should be made to relieve it. Pain, especially when chronic, is both physically debilitating and psychologically demoralizing. It should be considered by the physician as a serious symptom and treated to the extent that the patient is made comfortable.

2. Pain should be treated early. There is both clinical and experimental evidence that if pain goes untreated for an extended period of time, abnormal excitatory states arise in the central nervous system so that treatment directed toward peripheral structures which initially would have relieved the pain are no longer effective. In general, the earlier one undertakes to treat pain, the more successful one is.

3. Pain should be treated promptly. Clinical evidence suggests that if analgesic drug doses are spaced so far apart that severe pain recurs, the analgesic becomes less effective. Thus patients should be encouraged to take analgesic agents when the pain first reappears rather than wait until it becomes unbearable.

4. More than one treatment should be utilized. Various treatments of pain are additive and should be used together rather than separately. Combinations of narcotic and non-narcotic analgesics are often more effective than either alone and adjuvant analgesics such as the phenothiazines and butyrophenones (see Table 481–1) may enhance analgesic effect. Non-pharmacologic methods of pain control, including hypnosis, relaxation techniques, biofeedback, and "cognitive coping skills," can often help in selected patients with chronic pain.

5. Narcotic drugs should be used with discrimination, but they should not be withheld if no alternative therapy is effective. Long-term use of narcotics produces tolerance and physical dependence. These effects should not be confused with drug habituation or "addiction," which implies both a psychologic dependence and drug abuse for effects other than analgesia. The percentage of patients who actually become psychologically dependent on narcotics given to treat medical illness is unknown. Many physicians are impressed that narcotic psychologic dependence is unusual in patients treated for pain if the pain is later relieved by other means. The side effects of narcotic drugs include *tolerance,* which requires gradually increasing doses to maintain analgesia; *physical dependence,* which means that narcotics must be withdrawn gradually if they are to be discontinued after prolonged use; *constipation,* which requires careful attention to bowel function, including the use of stool softeners, laxatives, and enemas; and at times *somnolence.* All narcotic drugs produce some degree of somnolence; in individual patients, if somnolence is a problem, lower doses should be given more frequently, amphetamines added, or several different narcotics tried, because the patient may tolerate a particular drug better than another in comparable doses. Other than those mentioned, the side effects of narcotic drugs are few. Methadone maintenance programs as well as other long-term studies have proved that patients can take narcotics in large doses over long periods of time without physical damage and continue to function usefully in society. Rarely, multifocal myoclonus and seizures may occur following repetitive doses of meperidine from accumulation of the metabolite

normeperidine. Substitution of an alternative narcotic alleviates the seizures.

6. Psychogenic factors always play a role in chronic pain—the pain is more severe when the patient is anxious and stressed and less severe when he is relaxed. The physician must assess the psychologic factors in any patient with pain. However, no patient should be diagnosed as having "psychogenic pain" until an exhaustive examination has ruled out structural disease. Depression, whether endogenous or reactive, should be treated with antidepressant drugs. Tricyclic antidepressants have analgesic properties, and may be effective in relieving pain by themselves; more frequently they are effective as analgesic adjuvants. Psychiatric consultation is necessary if psychogenic factors are causing the pain.

7. Placebo effects are important. In most clinical studies, about one third of patients report relief of pain when given a placebo, although the extent of relief is rarely equal to that achieved by analgesic drugs. The physician can utilize a patient's desire to be free of pain by approaching the therapy in an enthusiastic and reassuring manner. It is less important whether it is the placebo or the drug which was effective than that the patient be relieved of his pain.

8. Multidisciplinary pain clinics which diagnose and treat intractable pain exist in many centers and should be utilized to evaluate and treat severe and chronic problems.

ANALGESIC AGENTS. Analgesics are drugs which decrease pain without causing loss of consciousness. Analgesics (see Table 481–1) can be divided clinically into those which are suitable for mild pain, generally non-narcotic agents; those suitable for moderate pain, usually narcotics or narcotic antagonists with low addiction potential; and those which are suitable for severe pain, generally narcotic agents except for methotrimeprazine, a phenothiazine. The mild analgesics appear to act peripherally by blocking the pain chemoreceptors and perhaps by relieving inflammation. There is also evidence for a central effect of some of these drugs as well.

The physician's strategy in treating chronic pain should begin with the mildest agents and add stronger agents or analgesic adjuvants only when mild agents fail to work. Drugs should always be given in sufficient amounts and at sufficiently short intervals to achieve relief of pain. Treatment should begin with aspirin or acetaminophen, 600 mg every three to four hours. If the pain is due to musculoskeletal spasm or if anxiety is prominent, one of the mild tranquilizers (diazepam or meprobamate) can be added. If the pain fails to respond to this mild regimen, one adds drugs used for the treatment of moderate pain (e.g., codeine, oxycodone). If the pain is still unrelieved

TABLE 481–1. ANALGESIC AGENTS

		Usual Dose*		
Type	**Generic Name (Proprietary)**	*Oral (mg)*	*Subcutaneous or Intramuscular (mg)*	**Comment**
Some agents used for mild to moderate pain	Aspirin	600 q 3–4 h		Side effects of dyspepsia and GI bleeding
	Acetaminophen (Tylenol)	650 q 3–4 h		Equal to aspirin but without GI side effects; less anti-inflammatory effect
	Dextropropoxyphene (Darvon)	65 q 3–4 h		Weak narcotic related to methadone
	Ibuprofen (Motrin)	200 q 6 h		Useful for pain associated with inflammation; less GI toxicity than aspirin
Some agents used for moderate to severe pain	Codeine	1 tab q 4–6 h	130 q 4–6 h	Narcotic with low addiction potential; additive effect if used with mild analgesics
	Oxycodone (with acetaminophen = Percocet)	5 q 4–6 h		Preferred over codeine by many patients
	Pentazocine (Talwin)	30–50 q 4–6 h	60 q 4 h	Narcotic antagonist (produces withdrawal in patients physically dependent on narcotics); hallucinations and dysphoria at higher doses; not recommended for general use
Some agents used for severe pain: narcotics and antagonists	Levorphanol (Levodromoran)	2 q 3–4 h	10 q 3–4 h	Potent oral narcotic; long plasma half-life†
	Morphine		2 q 3–4 h	The standard narcotic agent for treatment of pain
	Meperidine (Demerol)	50–100 q 3–4 h	75 q 2–4 h	More rapid onset and shorter duration of action than morphine; can cause CNS hyperirritability with chronic administration
	Methadone (Dolophine)	10–20 q 4 h	10–15 q 3–4 h	Potent oral narcotic; long plasma half-life
	Hydromorphone (Dilaudid)	7 q 3 h	1 q 3 h	Potent, short-acting
Non-narcotic agents	Methotrimeprazine (Levoprome)		20 q 4–6 h	Phenothiazine; no tolerance; produces sedation and postural hypotension
	Dextroamphetamine	10 q 6 h		Enhances narcotic effect and decreases somnolence in postoperative pain
Some agents used as analgesic adjuvants (probably little or no analgesic properties per se but used to relieve anxiety and/or depression)	Minor tranquilizers—muscle relaxants:			
	Diazepam (Valium)	5 qid		Useful with mild analgesics for acute or subacute pain associated with muscle spasm and/or anxiety
	Meprobamate (Miltown)	200–400 qid		
	Antidepressants:			Reported useful in pain associated with depressive symptoms (esp. atypical facial pain); may be useful when combined with analgesic agents for chronic pain of many kinds; may cause over-sedation or anticholinergic symptoms
	Amitriptyline (Elavil)	25–75 qd		
	Imipramine (Tofranil)	25 qid		
	Phenothiazines:			Reported useful in pain associated with anxiety or depression and in some specific pain syndromes (e.g., thalamic pain, postherpetic pain); these drugs may have analgesic properties or potentiate analgesics; fluphenazine and amitriptyline have been reported to relieve postherpetic pain; may cause oversedation, depression, Parkinson-like syndrome, hypotension, or urinary retention
	Chlorpromazine (Thorazine)	25–50 qid		
	Fluphenazine (Prolixin)	1–3 qd		
	Butyrophenones:			
	Haloperidol	2 mg tid		

*Intramuscular dose of narcotics is equivalent to 10 mg of morphine. Since tolerance develops to these drugs, doses must be increased with continued use. Oral doses are not equivalent to intramuscular doses but represent usual starting doses.

†Analgesic "half-life" differs from plasma half-life.

and the physician satisfies himself that psychogenic factors are not responsible, the agents used for moderate pain should be discontinued, and agents used for severe pain should be added to the mild analgesic. Levorphanol, 2 mg, methadone, 10 mg, or hydromorphone, 4 mg, every three to four hours, are the agents of choice if oral drugs are to be used, and morphine, 10 mg every three to four hours, if a subcutaneous or intramuscular agent is necessary. If the pain continues as a chronic and unremitting problem not relieved by these drugs, or if anxiety and depression appear to be the major contributors to the pain, a major tranquilizer (phenothiazine) or antidepressant agent, or both, may be added to the mild analgesics and narcotic agents. At times a satisfactory resolution of an intractable problem may be achieved by the combined use of a narcotic and non-narcotic analgesic with a tranquilizer or an antidepressant. The physician must be careful to adjust the doses of each so as to produce maximal pain relief with minimal sedation and unpleasant side effects. The physician should be prepared to increase the dose of those particular drugs to which tolerance develops as necessary to control pain. No tolerance develops to non-narcotic analgesics.

Non-Narcotic Mild Analgesics. Aspirin and acetaminophen (Tylenol, Tempra) are the most useful of the mild analgesics. However, acetaminophen differs from aspirin in that it does not have aspirin's anti-inflammatory properties. Either aspirin or acetaminophen may be given in doses of 600 mg every three to four hours, either alone for relief of mild pain or in conjunction with more potent drugs for relief of severe pain. Ceiling effects and unpleasant side effects prevent the use of increasing doses of these drugs to treat more severe pain. The side effects of aspirin (clotting disorders, dyspepsia, and gastrointestinal bleeding) make acetaminophen a safer drug and probably the drug of choice at usual therapeutic doses. However, acute overdose of acetaminophen can cause severe hepatotoxicity, and there is evidence that alcohol ingestion increases its toxic effects on the liver. Aspirin and acetaminophen taken together may be more effective than either one alone. Aspirin or acetaminophen plus codeine is more effective than codeine alone.

Narcotic Analgesics. Tolerance develops to all narcotics. Thus there is no set dose of these drugs, and with continued use dosage must increase. *The physician is wise to learn to handle two or three drugs and use those consistently rather than using all the drugs occasionally.* The physician must be prepared to use more than one, because some patients find that side effects of the drugs make one preferable to another. Morphine, 10 mg intramuscularly, is the standard by which other narcotic analgesics are judged. Intramuscular morphine has its maximal effect in 60 to 90 minutes and lasts between three and six hours. It requires 60 mg or more of morphine orally to give the same analgesic effect as 10 mg intramuscularly. Levorphanol has a relatively high oral/parenteral ratio for analgesia; 2 mg given intramuscularly is equal to 10 mg of morphine intramuscularly, and 4 mg given orally is equal in total effect to 10 mg of morphine given intramuscularly. Methadone also has a relatively high oral/intramuscular potency ratio; 10 mg intramuscularly or 20 mg orally equals 10 mg of morphine intramuscularly. Codeine and dihydrocodeine are also effective orally and are generally used in doses of 50 to 60 mg as a mild analgesic. They often cannot be used to relieve severe pain, because side effects preclude high doses. Pentazocine is a mild analgesic when given in doses of 30 mg and is equal to morphine if given in intramuscular doses of 60 mg. It is a mixed narcotic agonist-antagonist, and thus can produce withdrawal in a physically dependent patient. Pentazocine is not included in the Federal Controlled Substances Act. However, dysphoria, hallucinatory effects, and toxic psychoses are frequent side effects and limit its use. Like the other narcotics it can produce respiratory depression.

Other Agents. The phenothiazine methotrimeprazine (Levoprome) is a potent analgesic agent. Given intramuscularly in doses of 20 mg, it is equivalent to 10 mg of morphine intramuscularly. The drug is an effective antiemetic and does not suppress cough or respiration but does produce sedation and postural hypotension, making it useful only for hospitalized patients.

Anticonvulsant drugs are probably useful only in pain associated with spontaneous neuronal firing such as trigeminal neuralgia. Low doses of amitriptyline (25–75 mg daily) produce an analgesic effect independent of any antidepressant effect and the drug is useful in efforts to manage patients with chronic neurogenic pain syndromes.

Dextroamphetamine has been reported to enhance the effectiveness of narcotic agents in postoperative patients while counteracting the undesirable side effects of sedation and possibly respiratory depression. Whether the drug may also be an effective adjuvant for chronic pain remains to be established.

PHYSICAL METHODS OF PAIN RELIEF. There are a bewildering variety of physical methods designed to relieve pain. These vary from simply rubbing a partially denervated area with a soft towel to placing radiofrequency lesions stereotactically in the thalamic and hypothalamic reticular formations. The simpler procedures can be carried out by the general physician or even by the patient; the more complicated ones, depending on their nature, demand the expertise of a skilled anesthesiologist or neurosurgeon.

The physician's approach to the use of physical methods for intractable pain should embody certain general principles:

1. Nondestructive procedures should be tried first. Cutaneous stimulation, either by hand or by battery-driven electrodes, or local anesthetic blocks in conjunction with analgesic drugs may be effective in relieving pain. If these simple procedures fail, the services of an anesthesiologist or neurosurgeon should be procured and a treatment plan embodying the use of analgesics and physical procedures outlined.

2. The least destructive procedure should be tried first. In general, the procedure should be directed first at the peripheral nervous system, and only if this fails, at the spinal cord, brainstem, or cerebrum. Quantitative data on the incidence of pain relief and its duration are sketchy for most of these procedures and seem to vary from center to center, depending on the skill and enthusiasm of the investigator reporting.

3. Thus, the choice of a particular procedure often depends not only on the nature of the patient's disease but on the particular skills, experience, and bias of the physician.

4. If and only if a full trial of analgesic drugs has failed should destructive procedures for relieving pain be tried. These destructive procedures can and should be used in conjunction with analgesic drugs, because, even if the drugs have failed to relieve pain on their own, they may act synergistically with physical methods. Nerve blocks and surgical procedures often yield only temporary relief in patients with chronic pain. Thus many of the enthusiastic reports in the literature refer to patients followed for only a short period of time. When the patients are followed over months or years, the pain which was relieved shortly after the procedure often returns and is as bad as or worse than it was prior to the operation. For this reason, patients with cancer who are not expected to live a long time are often better candidates for surgical destructive procedures than are patients with pain originating from more benign conditions.

5. Patients with chronic pain being considered for destructive procedures must be thoroughly evaluated psychiatrically. If psychogenic factors play a major role in the genesis of pain, surgical procedures will not help, and often the pain will be exacerbated after surgical intervention.

Cutaneous Stimulation. Cutaneous stimulation of a painful area, particularly one which has been partly denervated, is often effective in relieving pain. This procedure, which probably has its greatest use in the treatment of postherpetic neuralgia, consists of rubbing the painful area with a soft cloth or terrycloth towel, almost constantly at first but then with gradually lengthening intervals of rest between rubbing periods. Often a period of rubbing will yield relief which long outlasts the stimulus, and continued intermittent rubbings may totally relieve the pain. The "gate theory" offers an explanation of the rubbing phenomenon, i.e., rubbing stimulates large fiber afferents which may close the gate against incoming pain fibers. Whatever the explanation, the procedure is often useful in the treatment of painful phantom limbs and in chronic cutaneous or extremity pain after surgery. Battery-powered electrical stimulators which give one control over the frequency and intensity of the cutaneous stimulation can also be used. The electrodes of the stimulator may be placed over the painful area or over the peripheral nerve supplying the painful area, and stimulation using an intensity and frequency which produces a vibratory sensation is applied.

Acupuncture Analgesia. Acupuncture analgesia has become increasingly popular in the past several years, but few carefully controlled studies attest to its usefulness. A needle is placed under the skin, often in a place remote from the painful site but at times into the painful site, and the area is stimulated either by twirling the needle or by electrically vibrating it. Recent experiments in animals and man suggest that the analgesic effect of acupuncture is partially reversed by naloxone, leading to the hypothesis that one mechanism of acupuncture analgesia is through release of endogenous analgesic substances. The usefulness of acupuncture in Western medicine is still not clear.

Nerve Blocks. Direct block of peripheral nerves, using either anesthetic agents (lidocaine) or neurolytic agents (phenol), has been popular in the treatment of thoracic and abdominal pain, particularly that pain which follows surgery. Blocks may be dangerous if used in the extremities, because they may paralyze as well as anesthetize; but in areas where they can be used, relief of pain sometimes long outlasts the period of anesthesia. The procedure is a simple one when performed by a skilled anesthesiologist.

Subarachnoid injection of anesthetics or neurolytics directed at nerve roots has been utilized in patients with widespread and intractable pain. Phenol can likewise be injected into the subarachnoid space and directed at particular nerve roots by positioning the patient. The mechanism of action is destruction of nerve fibers; if material spills into the cauda equina, bladder and bowel dysfunction are common. The relief of pain may be only transient. Spinal opiate administration with small doses (2 mg) of morphine given into the epidural or subarachnoid space may produce prolonged analgesia without substantial side effects. This technique is useful in the management of patients with postoperative pain. Continuous epidural infusions of opiates, using implantable infusion pumps, in cancer patients with chronic pain has been reported to be useful.

Other Procedures. Several nondestructive procedures directed at the affective component of pain are currently in use. These include not only psychotherapy and hypnotism but also more recently developed techniques of biofeedback, operant conditioning, relaxation techniques, and cognitive behavioral methods. These approaches have been gaining in popularity as our understanding of the psychologic components of chronic pain has improved. Preliminary studies suggest that stimulation of the medial thalamus following stereotactic placement of electrodes is effective in relieving some chronic neurogenic pain. Tolerance does not develop to this stimulation-produced analgesia.

Each nonsurgical procedure directed at the *peripheral nervous system* has its surgical counterpart. In patients with chronic pain such as that which follows herpes zoster, the skin has been undercut in an attempt to totally denervate it. Postoperative infection is a complication at times and the pain relief is transient, thus contraindicating this procedure. Peripheral nerves can be cut, particularly in the thorax and abdomen, but this should not be done unless prior nerve blocks have indicated that it will be effective and sustained. The peripheral nerves regenerate after a time, and often the pain returns. Dorsal root ganglia in the thorax and abdomen can be removed for chronic pain or the dorsal roots themselves cut. This procedure also should not be done unless nerve blocks have indicated that it will be effective. Several roots must be cut off either side of the painful area if one is to achieve long-term pain relief.

Surgery of the Central Nervous System. There are four kinds of surgical procedures directed at the central nervous system for the relief of pain. The *first type* involves the placement of electrodes on the skin, along peripheral nerves, and along spinal cord pathways. A few years ago there was some enthusiasm about electrodes surgically placed on the dorsal columns with a subcutaneous power pack which would allow the patient to control frequency and intensity of stimulation. Failure of this method to give prolonged relief and the morbidity of the procedure have led many neurosurgeons to abandon it. More recently, electrodes have been placed stereotactically in the periventricular gray matter, again using a power source controlled by the patient. Total body analgesia with increase in pain threshold has been observed for three to eight hours following stimulation, but tolerance develops to the analgesic effect. This procedure is still an experimental one, and its effectiveness requires further evaluation.

The *second type of procedure* destroys pain pathways in the spinal cord, brainstem, or brain. Spinothalamic tracts can be destroyed either surgically, after a laminectomy (open cordotomy), or by the placement of a radiofrequency lesion through a needle (percutaneous cordotomy). These procedures are particularly effective in relieving pain in the lower extremities and have the advantage that, although pain and temperature sensations are lost, cutaneous sensation and motor power remain intact. At times the level of anesthesia approaches within one or two cord segments of the level at which the destructive lesion is placed, but often there is a drop to about five segments below the placement of the lesion. Thus, the lesion must be placed considerably higher than the site of pain. If the lesion is placed unilaterally, pain often reappears on the other side of the body, necessitating another lesion. Bilateral lesions considerably enhance the risk of motor weakness and bladder and bowel dysfunction, but in skilled hands these risks are low. Occasionally patients with bilateral percutaneous lesions in the cervical cord suffer loss of automatic respiratory function (Ondine's curse). Percutaneous spinothalamic tract cordotomy, when done by a skilled technician, produces satisfactory pain relief in 70 to 90 per cent of patients, with a small mortality (1 to 5 per cent) and morbidity rate. The procedure is particularly useful in patients with terminal cancer, because the pain relief is usually sustained until death and the procedure does not require a major operation. An analogous lesion in the low brainstem placed in the descending tract of the trigeminal nerve has been reported useful in relieving facial pain. Pain and temperature sensation are lost, but cutaneous sensation remains intact. Lesions have been placed in the spinothalamic tract of the midbrain, so-called mesencephalic tractotomies. The dangers of this lesion are considerably greater than those of spinal cord lesions, and most centers have abandoned the procedure. Several neurosurgeons have placed lesions in the thalamus, both in the ventral-basal complex and in the interlaminar nuclei. Although good results are occasionally reported for both, the ventral-basal lesions appear only to produce transient relief of pain, whereas those placed in the intralaminar nuclei at the end-point of the paleospinothalamic tract appear to be more successful. There are rare reports of removal of sensory portions of the parietal lobe in relieving chronic pain, but the rarity of the reports implies the ineffectiveness of the treatment.

The *third surgical method* directed at pain relief is to place lesions in the frontal lobe, particularly the limbic projection to the frontal areas, in an attempt to alter the patient's psychologic response to pain rather than alter the pain pathways themselves. Several different surgical procedures, including frontal lobotomy, frontal leukotomy, and cingulotomy, have been tried with varied success. These procedures, which alter the patient's personality as well as his suffering, probably deserve trial only when all other procedures have failed.

The *fourth procedure* is directed at ablating the pituitary gland and is reported to be particularly effective in the treatment of pain from bony metastases from hormonally sensitive tumors such as those of breast or prostate. However, it has also been reported effective in pain caused by nonhormonally sensitive tumors. The pituitary may be ablated either surgically or by injection of destructive chemicals into the sella turcica (chemical hypophysectomy). In some series, 30 to 50 per cent of patients with pain from metastatic tumors have reported pain relief.

Good statistical data comparing the various surgical procedures for pain are difficult to come by. The best extant data indicate that initial relief of pain occurs with almost all procedures in 50 to 80 per cent of patients, with spinothalamic tract cordotomies yielding the best results. Longer-term follow-up suggests that considerably less than 50 per cent of patients achieve lasting relief, in many series the figure being as low as 20 per cent. Patients with malignant disease seem to have greater pain relief even initially than those with more benign conditions, probably because selection of patients with benign conditions often includes many with psychogenic pain.

Bonica JJ: The Management of Pain. Philadelphia, Lea & Febiger, 1953. *A classic monograph.*

Bonica JJ, Lindblom U, Iggo A (eds.): Proceedings of the Third World Congress on Pain, Edinburgh. Advances in Pain Research and Therapy. Vol 5. New York, Raven Press, 1983. *An up-to-date multi-authored monograph describing new developments in the physiology, pharmacology, and management of pain.*

Sternbach R: Pain Patients: Traits and Treatment. New York, Academic Press, 1974. *Important monograph on the psychology of chronic pain.*

Twycross RG, Lack SA: Symptom Control in Far Advanced Cancer: Pain Relief. London, Pitman Books Ltd., 1983. *An up-to-date monograph describing in detail the control of pain in patients with cancer. Many of the concepts are equally applicable to other chronic diseases causing pain.*

HEADACHE AND OTHER HEAD PAIN

Headache is one of man's most common afflictions. It ranks ninth among the causes of visits to physicians and is a major source both of time lost from work and of medical diagnostic procedures. The frequency of disabling headache is explained in part by the rich nerve supply to the head (including afferent nerve fibers from trigeminal, glossopharyngeal, vagus, and upper three cervical nerves) and in part by the psychologic significance of head pain, causing anxiety about even modest headache, whereas a pain of equal severity elsewhere in the body might be ignored. Head pain can result from distortion, stretching, inflammation, or destruction of pain-sensitive nerve endings as a result of intra- or extracranial disease in the distribution of any of the aforementioned nerves. However, most head pain arises from extracerebral structures and carries a benign prognosis. The physician's twofold task is first to distinguish the commoner, benign head pain from more serious causes and then to administer appropriate treatment. The diagnosis can usually be established by history and physical findings alone; skull x-rays, CT scans, and other diagnostic tests are seldom required. Table 481–2 is a simplified classification of the pathogenesis of head pain; the overwhelming majority of headaches are either muscle contraction or common migraine headaches, with both abnormalities frequently playing a role in a given individual. The other forms of headache are much less common.

Migraine and Other Vascular Headaches

The term *vascular headache* applies to a group of clinical syndromes of unknown etiology in which the final step in pathogenesis of the pain appears to be dilatation of one or more branches of the carotid artery, leading to stimulation of nerve endings supplying that artery. There may be a release of noxious substances by either the arterial wall or the nerve ending, causing a substantially lowered pain threshold. Such substances as serotonin, substance P, bradykinin, histamine, and prostaglandins alone or in combination have all been implicated in the pathogenesis of vascular headache. Most vascular headaches are unilateral in distribution and often but not always throbbing in quality, and they recur over months or years. Individual headaches are frequently precipitated by identifiable environmental or psychologic factors. During the course of a vascular headache, the involved arteries may be tender to the touch, and pain may be relieved temporarily by compression of the carotid artery, only to return with increased severity when compression is released. Most vascular headaches can be relieved by prompt administration of vasoconstrictive agents, and many recurrent headaches can be prevented by one of several vasoactive drugs. So-called "common migraine" may affect as many as 25 per cent of the population. Other vascular headache syndromes are less common, but each has distinctive clinical findings.

TABLE 481–2. PATHOPHYSIOLOGIC CLASSIFICATION OF HEADACHE

Vascular Headache
Migraine Headache
Classic migraine
Common migraine
Complicated migraine
Variant migraine
Cluster Headache
Episodic cluster
"Chronic" cluster
Chronic paroxysmal hemicrania
Miscellaneous Vascular Headaches
Carotidynia
Hypertension
Hangover
Toxins and drugs
Occlusive vascular disease
Muscle Contraction (Tension) Headache
Common tension headache
Depressive equivalent
Conversion reaction
Temporomandibular joint dysfunction
Atypical facial pain
Cervical osteoarthritis
Traction-Inflammation Headache
Cranial arteritis
Increased or decreased intracranial pressure
Extracranial structural lesions
Pituitary tumors
Cranial Neuralgias

Classic Migraine

Classic migraine is distinguished by well-defined symptoms of neurologic dysfunction that precede or less often accompany the headache. Neurologic symptoms are usually visual, consisting of bright flashing lights (scintillation or fortification scotomata) beginning in the center of a homonymous visual half-field and radiating over 10 to 30 minutes outward toward the periphery. Less commonly, the visual abnormalities are monocular (retinal) or consist of hemianoptic loss of vision in place of or following the scintillating scotomata. Other neurologic disturbances that can occur in classic migraine include unilateral paresthesias, usually involving the hand and perioral area, aphasia, hemiparesis, and hemisensory defects. An uncommon variant named *basilar artery migraine* occurs predominantly in children and adolescents and is characterized by vertigo, ataxia, and diplopia, along with hemiparesis or hemisensory changes. Rarely, confusion, stupor, or even coma may develop. Neurologic symptoms of classic migraine usually last no longer than 30 minutes and generally clear before the headache phase begins. However, in some instances neurologic signs may persist for hours or, rarely, for days, throughout and even beyond the headache phase of the illness.

The pathogenesis of the neurologic dysfunction is not fully understood. Measurements of regional cerebral blood flow during episodes of classic migraine have shown a wave of focal hyperemia followed by abnormally low flow (oligemia) spreading from posterior to anterior over the cerebral cortex. The degree of oligemia is not sufficient in and of itself to produce the neurologic symptoms, nor is it always accompanied by neurologic symptoms. One explanation is that there may be a wave of physiologic depression that spreads across the cortex, accounting for both the neurologic symptoms and the changes in blood flow. Changes in brain blood flow do not accompany common migraine, even though the headache phase of the illness is similar. Thus, it is likely that if "spreading depression" is the cause of the neurologic symptoms of migraine, it is only one of several precipitating factors that may produce the headache.

The syndrome of classic migraine has four parts: (1) The *prodromal phase* occurs in a minority of patients and consists of an alteration of mood, often occurring for 24 or more hours before the headache. Patients may complain of increased hunger or thirst, drowsiness, euphoria, or depression. In some patients, known precipitants such as red wine commonly induce an attack. (2) The second phase consists of the *neurologic symptoms* described above. The neurologic symptoms may occur without subsequent headache (termed migraine equivalent), particularly in older people. (3) The third phase usually begins as the neurologic symptoms clear and characteristically consists of a unilateral throbbing frontotemporal *headache* on the side opposite the neurologic symptoms. The headache is frequently accompanied by nausea, photophobia, vomiting, diarrhea, phonophobia (noise intolerance), and a general feeling of being unwell. The headache commonly lasts four to six hours but may persist for one or more days. If the headache is prolonged, it may change into a dull, aching, bilateral pain extending back into the neck and shoulders. The headache phase is often terminated either by vomiting or by a period of sleep. (4) The *post-headache* phase is characterized by a feeling of exhaustion, tenderness of the scalp at the site of the headache, and recurrence of headache on sudden head movement.

The diagnosis of classic migraine is made by history; physical findings are absent, and laboratory evaluation is not helpful. When the attacks are atypical, particularly when neurologic disability is severe or prolonged, CT scans or digital intravenous angiography (DIVA) may be required to rule out structural lesions of the brain or its vasculature (brain tumors, particularly meningiomas, or arteriovenous anomalies). However, such instances are rare. The treatment of classic migraine is similar to that of common migraine (see below), except that classic migraine attacks usually occur no more than four or five times a year and rarely more than once a month.

Common Migraine

Common migraine is similar to classic migraine except that neurologic symptoms are absent. Many patients with classic migraine also have episodes of common migraine. Common migraine is characterized by recurrent headaches, often severe, frequently beginning unilaterally, and usually associated with malaise, nausea and/or vomiting, and photophobia. The disorder often begins in childhood, affects women more often than men, and runs in families (70 per cent of patients give a family history). Characteristically, the headache affects individuals with perfectionistic and "driven" personalities. Identifiable factors that often precipitate individual headaches are holidays and weekends, menstrual periods, foods (especially red wine, chocolate, nuts, and aged cheese), environmental stimuli (such as bright sunlight, too much sleep, and undue emotional stress or resentment). Medical conditions and their treatment may also precipitate attacks. Vasodilators such as nitroglycerin and antihypertensives and serotonin releasers such as reserpine, as well as estrogens and oral contraceptives, have been reported to cause migraine attacks in susceptible individuals. The diagnosis of common migraine is usually made by the history. Important historical points that help distinguish migraine from the equally common tension headaches (see below) include their unilaterality, their association with nausea or vomiting, the tendency of migraine to awaken one from sleep, a positive family history, and a positive response to ergot preparations. When the diagnosis is in doubt, treatment of the patient for common migraine often clarifies the issue.

TREATMENT. The best treatment for migraine is prevention. Whenever possible, the patient should avoid precipitating factors. Medications known to cause migraine should be withdrawn if others can be substituted. Foods commonly implicated may also be withdrawn and, if withdrawal is effective, replaced one at a time to determine the specific precipitant. The patient should attempt to avoid undue stress or fatigue and not to sleep excessively on weekends. If these methods fail and severe headaches occur frequently (once a week or more), pharmacologic prophylaxis is indicated. Several agents have been reported effective in the prophylaxis of migraine, but not every patient responds to each agent. Perhaps the safest and most effective class of drugs are the beta-adrenergic blockers, particularly propranolol. The drug is begun at a dose of 80 mg a day in divided doses, and increased as tolerated until headaches are controlled. Recent reports suggest that calcium channel blockers such as verapamil* (80 mg three to four times daily) are also effective. Methysergide, a serotonin antagonist, is effective at a dose of 2 mg three to four times daily. Methysergide must be employed cautiously because it can cause serious side effects, including vascular insufficiency, retroperitoneal or pleural fibrosis, and fibrotic thickening of heart valves. The side effects can be minimized by gradually withdrawing the drug for one month after every four to six months of treatment. Amitriptyline in gradually increasing doses from 25 to 125 mg daily may be useful if the above drugs fail.

Acute attacks, if mild, often respond to analgesic agents and bedrest. More severe attacks are best treated by ergot preparations such as ergotamine tartrate. The drug, given parenterally, is sufficiently effective (85 to 90 per cent) to be useful as a diagnostic test. Oral ergot 1 to 2 mg given at the onset of a headache is effective in about 50 per cent of patients. However, during the headache, absorption of the oral form of the drug is often poor, and better results can be achieved with sublingual or rectal ergot preparations. The best nonparenteral results are generally achieved by the insertion of half of a 2-mg ergotamine rectal suppository. The side effect of *ergotism* makes it unwise to treat frequent migraine headaches in this way, and therefore one should switch to prophylaxis if the headaches occur more than once a week.

Migraine Variants

There are several migraine syndromes that differ sufficiently from classic and common migraine to earn separate names. *Ophthalmoplegic migraine* is the name given when an ocular motor palsy develops during the course of a severe migraine attack. Ophthalmoplegic migraine usually begins in childhood and is characterized by unilateral pupillary dilatation, ptosis, and paralysis of ocular muscles occurring 12 to 24 hours *after* the beginning of an attack of severe migraine. The ophthalmoplegia usually clears within hours to days but frequently recurs. Angiography (usually DIVA) may be required to rule out a carotid aneurysm. *Hemiplegic migraine* is a familial syndrome in which aphasia, confusion, and hemiparesis or hemiplegia precede or more often accompany the migraine attack. Repetitive episodes alternating from side to side may occur over many years. *Complicated migraine* is a term applied to attacks of migraine prodromes in which the focal neurologic defects may last for the entire headache attack and may even leave permanent residua. The few available anatomic studies of such patients have shown ischemic brain infarction involving the functionally impaired region.

Cluster Headache

Cluster headaches are short-lived attacks of severe, acute, and intense unilateral head pain that occur in clusters lasting

*This use is not listed in the manufacturer's directive.

several weeks, only to disappear for months or years on end. The disorder affects men much more than women and usually first begins between the third and sixth decades. Clusters characteristically occur in the spring and fall and last three to eight weeks. The individual headaches occur one to several times a day, particularly at night, and frequently with a predictability that allows one to set his clock by them. Each attack, which lasts 30 minutes to two hours, is characterized by rapid onset of a knife-like pain in the nostril or behind the eye which spreads to involve the forehead. During the attack, the ipsilateral nostril may be stuffy or water, and the eye may tear. In about 20 per cent of instances, a homolateral Horner's syndrome develops. During the course of the headache, the patient is usually unable to lie still (the opposite of the situation with migraine) and restlessly paces the floor. The pain may be so severe that the patient bangs his head against the wall or threatens suicide. The headache disappears as abruptly as it came, usually leaving no residua. Unlike the patient with migraine, the patient with cluster headaches does not feel systemically ill, and there is no nausea, vomiting, or feeling of exhaustion when the headache ceases. During the time when clusters are occurring, but not between such periods, alcohol will invariably induce an attack. When the headaches occur frequently, the Horner's syndrome may outlast the head pain.

The pathogenesis of cluster headache is unknown, although it is believed to be a vascular headache related to migraine. The diagnosis is established by the characteristic history. Treatment of an acute attack is usually not worthwhile, since by the time the patient absorbs the analgesic agents the attack is over. In some patients the headache rapidly responds to oxygen inhalation. Several drugs prevent attacks of cluster headache. Ergotamine tartrate given prophylactically in a dose of 1 mg four times a day, or 2 mg at bedtime if the attacks are all nocturnal, is often effective. The drug should be withdrawn every seventh day to prevent the symptoms of ergotism and to see if the cluster has ceased. Methysergide 2 mg three to four times daily is also often effective; since the cluster rarely lasts more than eight weeks, the drug can be discontinued and thereby is safe. Prednisone 40 mg daily in divided doses may also work and can be added to methysergide if the former is only partially effective. Lithium carbonate in daily doses of 0.9 to 1.5 grams sometimes works.

Cluster Variants

Several variants of cluster headache should be recognized by the physician, since their treatment may be different. The most striking is *chronic paroxysmal hemicrania,* a rare disorder consisting of painful episodes similar to cluster headaches that appear many times a day and recur unremittingly for years. There may be as many as 10 to 20 headaches daily, each lasting 10 to 30 minutes. Indomethacin orally in doses of 75 to 150 mg daily has relieved all subjects. A cluster variant characterized by daily cluster headache without remission, multiple brief jabs of pain in the head, and a background of continuous unilateral headache of variable severity exacerbated by exertion has recently been described and is said to respond to indomethacin in most instances. Patients who did not respond to indomethacin did so to tricyclic antidepressants.

Other Vascular Headaches

Several vascular headache variants deserve mention so that the physician may recognize them as benign and treat them appropriately. Included are *orgasmic headaches,* severe short-lived bilateral throbbing headaches occurring in either sex and appearing abruptly at orgasm. The attack can be differentiated from subarachnoid hemorrhage because the headache usually disappears within minutes to an hour or more and may recur repetitively. Usually the illness is self-limited, but if not it may respond to 1 mg of ergot given an hour before sexual activity. *Exertional headache* occurs, as the name implies, during active exercise. Like orgasmic headaches, these are usually bilateral and throbbing, and may last several hours. They respond well to indomethacin. Vascular headaches have been reported to follow minor *trauma* to the carotid artery in the neck and to *carotid endarterectomy*. These headaches are unilateral, recurrent, and severe and usually respond to prophylaxis with propranolol. *Carotidynia* is the name given to spontaneous vascular headaches associated with unilateral anterior neck pain and/or carotid tenderness. They usually respond to the same treatment as vascular headaches. When attacks of carotid pain and/or headache recur, the diagnosis is not difficult, but the first attack must be distinguished from a spontaneous dissection of the carotid artery and may require intravenous angiography for diagnosis.

Hangover headache is part of a larger syndrome, usually including premature awakening from an evening of overindulging and often accompanied by a fine tremor of the extremities and mild gastric distress or nausea, mental dulling, and mild incoordination. The pathogenesis is related to alcohol withdrawal, dehydration, and the toxic effect of various congeners found with different intoxicants. *Nitrites* can induce pulsating headache and, occasionally, facial flushing, most often after the ingestion of processed foods ("hot dog" headache). *Monosodium glutamate* has been blamed for the "Chinese restaurant syndrome," characterized by postprandial headache, tight sensations about the face and head, and, less often, giddiness and diarrhea.

Hypertensive headaches occur only in patients with very severe or episodic hypertension. They are characterized by early-morning, usually throbbing, occipital headache that responds to the treatment of the hypertension.

Muscle Contraction (Tension) Headache

Muscle contraction or tension headaches are characterized by a steady, non-pulsatile, unilateral or bilateral aching pain, usually beginning in the occipital regions but also often involving frontal or temporal regions as well. The headaches are so named because they are frequently accompanied by tight and tender muscles at the site of the most severe pain. They are probably the commonest cause of headache in the adult. In one clinic series of 726 consecutive headache patients, 279 were classified as due to tension and 181 as suffering from migraine; in 221 patients no exclusive diagnosis could be made. Tension headaches are recurrent, often present every day, and usually begin in early afternoon or evening, with a dull occipital or frontal pain that may spread to grip the entire head "in a vise." Unique among headaches, the pain may be constantly present for days, weeks, or months and is often associated with severe tenderness in the posterior cervical, temporalis, or masseter muscles. The pain may be quite severe, but patients rarely complain of nausea, vomiting, or malaise, although modest dizziness, blurring of vision, and sometimes tinnitus may occur. These headaches are more frequent in women, in individuals who are tense and anxious, and in those whose work or posture requires sustained contraction of posterior cervical, frontal, or temporal muscles. There is much overlap between the symptoms of common migraine and tension headaches, and many patients suffer from both. The distinguishing features favoring tension headaches include pressure or tightness, which is worst at the back of the neck, increased severity of pain as the day progresses, and pain that is preceded by or associated with clear anxiety-producing situations. Tension headaches are less commonly unilateral than migraine and less commonly associated with nausea and vomiting, do not usually awaken the patient from sleep, and do not respond to ergot preparations.

The pathogenesis of tension headaches is unclear. They are commonly accompanied by skeletal muscle contraction about the neck, face, and jaw, and palpation of those muscles may reveal sharply localized painful areas or nodules, injection of which with local anesthetics transiently relieves the headache. Sometimes massage has a similar effect. Patients are frequently aware that sustained contraction of muscles leads to headache. The contracting muscles or the nerves supplying them may release vasoactive substances such as lactate, serotonin, bradykinin, and prostaglandins, which lower pain threshold. Thus, some of the same substances implicated in migraine may also play a role in tension headache and explain the frequent overlap between the two syndromes. Muscle contraction headache may also be a result of sustained contraction of the head as a consequence of structural disease of the eye, ear, nose, paranasal sinuses, teeth, scalp, or intracranial contents.

TREATMENT. The first step in treatment is to identify causal factors. If these include abnormalities of posture leading to sustained muscle contraction, these should be corrected. Many patients with tension headache, particularly chronic ones, are depressed and respond to treatment with antidepressant agents such as amitriptyline. Others are tense and anxious and respond to anti-anxiety agents such as diazepam. This drug, in a dose of 15 to 20 mg a day for two to three weeks, is often effective as a diagnostic test. The relief of chronic headache establishes the diagnosis for the physician and helps to convince the patient that tension and anxiety are playing a major role in the headache, thus making the patient more amenable to psychotherapeutic endeavors. In addition, these drugs frequently break up a cycle of anxiety–muscle tension–anxiety, so that a short course may give prolonged relief.

An individual headache may be treated with aspirin. This drug is probably more useful for tension headaches than acetaminophen because of its anti-prostaglandin properties. Vasoactive agents used for the treatment of migraine have no role in this disorder unless vascular headaches are concomitantly present. Some clinics report that biofeedback treatments effectively relieve muscle contraction and thus the headache.

Tension Headache Variant

There are several rather characteristic headache syndromes of unknown cause that may have muscle contraction and psychologic tension as part of their pathogenesis. The syndrome most clearly related to muscle contraction headache is the so-called "temporomandibular joint syndrome." Patients complain of unilateral or bilateral head pain, usually in the temporal region and in the jaw, often radiating into the ear. The pain is often associated with tenderness of the masseter and temporalis muscles and may be exacerbated by chewing. Patients characteristically are tense and anxious individuals. Accompanying symptoms often include limitation of full movement at the temporomandibular joint when opening the jaw, bruxism, and malocclusion. The disorder sometimes responds to dental manipulation, particularly use of a mouth guard that prevents bruxism. However, for most patients analgesics and anti-anxiety manipulation effectively treat muscle contraction head pain. *Post-traumatic headaches* are dull, generalized, aching head pains that follow head injury. The injury is often mild, indeed sometimes trivial. The patient suffering the "post-traumatic syndrome" complains of headache often coupled with unsteadiness, giddiness, difficulty concentrating, insomnia, and fatigue. Contrary to popular belief, the syndrome is no more common in patients seeking compensation for the injury than not. It often persists for months or years. Treatment, like that of muscle contraction headaches, consists of psychologic support and reassurance and the use of mild analgesics and sometimes anti-anxiety agents. Patients should be encouraged to return to work as soon as possible and to try to live a normal life despite the symptoms. The disorder can blend into *depressive headache,* a chronic generalized headache, usually vaguely described, sometimes associated with giddiness and unsteadiness, that occurs as a frequent and sometimes predominant manifestation of depression. The headache may have muscle contraction and tension as its pathogenesis or may be a *somatic delusion* in a severely depressed patient. In either event, the treatment of choice is an antidepressant drug.

Atypical Facial Pain

Atypical facial pain or atypical facial neuralgia is a term used to describe a syndrome characterized by steady aching facial pain, usually unilateral, localized to the lower part of the orbit, maxillary area, and sometimes the jaw. The pain begins without a known precipitating episode and may last for hours to days. It may spread to involve the head or neck, and muscles of the jaw and neck are often tender. Sometimes autonomic symptoms including sweating, flushing, a nidus, and pallor are present. The disorder usually affects women, often in early middle age. Patients affected with the disorder are tense, anxious, and often chronically depressed. The pathogenesis of the illness is unknown. The autonomic changes have led some to suggest that the syndrome is a migraine variant, and the muscle tenderness and depression have led others to suggest that it be classified with musculoskeletal tension pain. Patients suffering from atypical facial pain should be examined carefully for local pathology of the eyes, nose, teeth, sinuses, and pharynx, but such is rarely found. Careful psychologic evaluation will often reveal a masked depression. Treatment is usually unsatisfactory. Analgesic agents are usually not helpful, and patients respond poorly to routine psychotherapy. In some patients, ergot preparations or propranolol appears to be effective, and others respond to physical methods such as massage and biofeedback. Antidepressants are sometimes helpful. It is important to recognize that the syndrome is not caused by structural disease and that patients require no invasive diagnostic or therapeutic procedures. Dental extraction does more harm than good.

Traction/Inflammation

Cranial Arteritis

This condition receives detailed consideration in Ch. 451 but deserves mention here as an important cause of headache in the elderly. The illness almost always appears after age 60 and usually later. The onset is usually with unilateral or bilateral temporal, occipital, or fronto-occipital head pain of variable intensity, often coupled with tenderness of the painful areas. Many patients have pain in the jaw muscles, making chewing uncomfortable. Nodules occasionally are palpable on affected vessels. The great risk is occlusion of retinal arteries secondary to untreated inflammation. Diagnosis depends on suspicion and usually on the presence of an elevated erythrocyte sedimentation rate. Diagnosis should be confirmed by arterial biopsy because definitive steroid treatment, once started, often must be maintained for many months. Since migraine-vascular headaches and depressive headaches also can have their onset in the elderly, a confirmed diagnosis is essential.

Meningitis and Subarachnoid Hemorrhage

Acute and subacute meningitis cause gradually developing headache resulting from inflammation of pain-sensitive structures surrounding the brain. The headache is usually generalized, throbbing, and very severe. It may be rapid or gradual in onset, and by the time it is fully developed is associated with nuchal rigidity. The diagnosis is established by lumbar puncture. In patients suspected of harboring an intracranial mass lesion, CT scan of the brain should be performed first and lumbar puncture deferred, unless the physician suspects that the patient is suffering from acute bacterial meningitis, in which case lumbar puncture must be done immediately. In *subarachnoid hemorrhage,* the initial sudden headache is caused by alteration of intracranial pressure. This headache is succeeded by a chronic persistent headache, often accompanied by nuchal rigidity that results from inflammation of the meninges caused by the blood. In a patient suspected of having suffered a subarachnoid hemorrhage, a CT scan should be performed first. The presence of extravascular blood establishes the diagnosis and obviates the need for lumbar puncture, which may exacerbate the bleeding by altering intracranial dynamics. The absence of identifiable hemorrhage on CT scan, however, does not rule out a small subarachnoid hemorrhage, and lumbar puncture then must be performed to establish or rule out the diagnosis definitively.

Alterations of Intracranial Pressure

Headache from altered intracranial pressure is caused by compression or traction of pain-sensitive vascular and neural structures over the apex and base of the brain. In the instance of *intracranial hypotension,* the loss of spinal fluid decreases the buoyancy of the brain so that the organ descends when the upright position is assumed, exerting traction on structures at its apex and compression on structures at its base. (In rare instances, the small bridging veins that enter the sagittal sinus may rupture and cause subdural hematomas.) In *intracranial hypertension,* the source of pain is probably compression of vascular and neural structures at the base of the brain by tumor or edematous brain.

INTRACRANIAL HYPERTENSION. Increased intracranial pressure per se does not lead to headache unless pain-sensitive structures are distorted. Many patients with high intracranial pressure from brain tumors, jugular venous obstruction, hydrocephalus, or pseudotumor cerebri do not suffer headache. If headache is present, it may be mild or severe, throbbing or steady, localized or generalized. When localized, it usually overlies the site of the lesion, but posterior fossa lesions may cause bifrontal headache. The headache is characteristically at its worst early in the morning, although it usually does not awaken the patient from sleep. It is exacerbated by stooping, coughing, moving the head suddenly, or straining at stool. Many patients prefer to sleep in the sitting position. The headache is rarely continuously intense. Reflecting transient rises of intracranial pressure, there are often waves of intense headache, sometimes accompanied by nausea, vomiting, or other neurologic signs. These "pressure or plateau waves," lasting 5 to 20 minutes, commonly are precipitated by assuming the upright posture.

The treatment of headache related to increased intracranial pressure is the treatment of the underlying disease (Ch. 513). Mild analgesics produce temporary relief; narcotic analgesics should not be used because of their tendency to produce respiratory depression and further raise the pressure in neurologically compromised individuals.

INTRACRANIAL HYPOTENSION (see Ch. 512). Intracranial hypotension usually follows a lumbar puncture and is due to continued leakage of cerebrospinal fluid through a rent in the dural sheath. (Rarely, a dural tear may occur spontaneously or follow mild trauma, producing the syndrome of *spontaneous* intracranial hypotension.) The syndrome develops 12 hours to several days after the lumbar puncture and is characterized by headache that occurs on assuming the upright position. There is no evidence that a period of recumbency after a lumbar puncture prevents subsequent development of the headache. The headache usually begins as a dull ache in the posterior cervical area, radiating laterally out toward the shoulders and cephalad toward the frontal area. It persists, often growing more severe, as long as the patient is in the upright position, and when most severe it may be associated with perspiration, nausea, and vomiting. Persistent headache of intracranial hypotension can lead to diplopia, probably a result of traction on the abducens nerves. The diagnosis of post–lumbar puncture headache is made by history; spontaneous intracranial hypotension is suspected by the history of positional headache and confirmed by low (<30 mm H_2O) or even negative CSF pressure on attempted lumbar puncture. The fluid is usually normal, but there may be an elevated protein concentration if the needle has entered a subdural or epidural fluid collection. Analgesics relieve the mildest headaches; the most severe ones can be controlled only by assuming the recumbent position. The headaches usually clear within a few days to a few weeks; in rare instances, surgical repair of the torn dura is necessary.

Extracranial Structural Lesions

Nasal and Sinus Headache

Although acute or chronic inflammation and neoplasms of the paranasal sinuses can cause headache, most patients who have been physician- or self-diagnosed as having sinus headaches are in fact suffering from either vascular or muscle contraction headache. Most true paranasal sinus headaches result from acute inflammation of the paranasal sinuses, which produces pain localized over the involved sinus and is associated with the stigmata of acute infection, including fever, swelling, and tenderness over the sinus and engorgement of the turbinates, ostia, nasofrontal ducts, and superior nasal spaces. Most of the discomfort comes from the ostia, which are many times more sensitive than the poorly innervated walls of the sinuses. Typically, "sinus" headache commences in the morning (frontal) or early afternoon (maxillary) and subsides in the early or late evening. The pain is dull and aching, is made worse by changing head position, and is seldom associated with nausea and vomiting. Sinus headache is best treated with decongestants and analgesics. Persistent purulent discharges should be cultured and appropriate antimicrobial drugs employed. Chronic suppurative disease in the frontal, ethmoid, and sphenoid sinuses, or in the mastoid air cells, may result in osteomyelitis and inflammation of adjacent cranial tissues. Headache persisting after surgical drainage of the diseased sinus is evidence for extradural and possibly subdural infection. More chronic inflammation and neoplasms, particularly when they occur in the sphenoid sinus, may not be accompanied by the usual physical signs of sinusitis. In such instances, sinus x-rays or CT scan may be required to establish the diagnosis.

Dental Pain

Noxious stimuli in a tooth usually evoke local toothache, but severe dental pain can be extremely difficult to localize. Afferent fibers for sensation in the teeth are contained in the second and third divisions of the trigeminal nerve. Headache in the areas supplied by the latter is, in rare instances, associated with prolonged, intense toothache or follows a tooth extraction. More commonly, in association with toothache, tooth extraction, or a tender, diseased tooth, distant tissues exhibit surface hyperalgesia, tenderness, and vasomotor reactions, such as tender eyeballs, reddening of the conjunctivae, and tenderness of the auricular and temporal tissues. Because of secondary muscle contraction, other sites of tenderness and pain may be noted behind the ears, behind the lower border of the mastoid process, and in the muscles of the occiput, neck, and shoulders. The upper teeth frequently hurt in association with disease of the nasal and paranasal structures. Occasionally, in coronary insufficiency, pain is experienced in the lower jaw. One should beware of ascribing bizarre pains in and around the jaws to a dental origin unless unequivocal acute inflammatory dental lesions are present. Dental extraction rarely ameliorates neuralgias or atypical facial pain. However, hysterical or delusional face pain is often attributed by the patient to prior dental work. Headache may not be attributed to a diseased tooth unless the injection of procaine into the tissues about the suspected tooth greatly reduces the intensity of, or eliminates, such headache.

Aural Pain

Severe pain in the vicinity of the ear can be caused by disease of the teeth, acute tonsillitis, inflammatory and neoplastic disease of the larynx and nasopharynx, temporomandibular joint disorders, tumors, inflammation in the posterior fossa, and disease of the cervical spine and its soft tissues. Pain in the ear is also associated with vascular headaches, atypical facial pain, and herpes zoster of the fifth and seventh cranial nerves and, rarely, the glossopharyngeal nerve. True glossopharyngeal neuralgia causes severe pain radiating from the tonsil into the ear. It has the usual timing feature of "tic."

Primary ear disease is relatively infrequent—but important—as a source of headache, because it almost always indicates inflammation or destructive disease. Acute otitis media (purulent or nonpurulent), furunculosis of the ear canal, traumatic rupture of the tympanum, and fracture of the anterior wall of the bony canal all cause pain in the ear associated with sustained tender contraction of adjacent skeletal muscles. Osteomyelitis of the mastoid bone may be associated with inflammation of the nearby periosteum as well as of dura and adjacent tissues (epidural abscess)—both sources of pain in or behind the ear. Pain in this region also accompanies tumors of the acoustic nerve and inflammation and thrombosis of the lateral sinus.

Eye Pain and Headache

Errors of refraction (hypermetropia, astigmatism, anomalies of accommodation), disturbances of ocular muscle equilibrium, and glaucoma are universally described as causing headache. Refractive errors are also said to give origin to such other symptoms as aching of the eyes, "sandy" feeling in the eyes, pulling sensations in and about the orbit, and conjunctival congestion. Headache is mild in degree and usually starts around and over the eyes and subsequently radiates to the occiput and back of the head.

The pain of glaucoma at first remains localized in the eyeball, then extends along the rim of the orbit and, finally, throughout most of the area supplied by the ophthalmic division of the trigeminal nerve. Nausea and vomiting sometimes accompany such headaches, which can become prostratingly severe if not treated promptly.

Simple myopia does not evoke headache because the myope, in attempting to improve his vision by the contraction of his eye muscles, actually makes his vision worse and soon abandons the attempt.

With inflammation of the iris and ciliary body, light may cause intense pain in the eye and adjacent areas because of movement of the inflamed iris. When the iris is immobilized, pain is allayed.

Pituitary Pain

Headache caused by pituitary tumors is the result of compression and distortion of pain-sensitive structures at the base of the skull, particularly the diaphragma sella. Pain is generally referred to the frontal or temporal regions bilaterally and may on occasion be referred to the vertex or occipital regions. Because the pain is not related to intracranial pressure, it does not have the same temporal characteristics of most brain tumor headaches and instead can occur at any time and is frequently chronic and unremitting. The headache is usually accompanied by evidence of endocrine failure, particularly loss of libido and impotence in the male. The combination of loss of libido and chronic headache may lead the physician to suspect depression rather than a pituitary lesion. The diagnosis can be established by endocrine examination and by CT scan of the pituitary fossa. Acute headache occurring with known pituitary lesions (*pituitary apoplexy*) usually results from infarction or hemorrhage into the tumor. Sudden expansion of the tumor may compromise the overlying optic chiasm, leading to visual loss, or invade the laterally lying cavernous sinus, producing ocular palsies. Pituitary apoplexy should be treated surgically by emergency drainage of the hemorrhagic or infarcted material.

Cranial Neuralgias

The term cranial neuralgias refers to several distinctive head pains that appear to result from sudden and excessive discharge from the involved nerve. The best-known cranial neuralgia is trigeminal neuralgia. The concept of cranial neuralgias has been expanded to include the chronic burning pain that frequently follows herpes zoster infection of the nerve. Some also include atypical facial pain and temporomandibular joint syndrome under the cranial neuralgias, but these probably have muscle contraction or vascular disturbances as their pathogenesis and in this chapter are included under those headings.

TRIGEMINAL NEURALGIA. Trigeminal neuralgia (tic douloureux) is a disease characterized by sudden, lightning-like paroxysms of pain in the distribution of one or more divisions of the trigeminal nerve. Most observers believe that most trigeminal neuralgia is caused by compression of the trigeminal nerve by arteries or veins of the posterior fossa. In some patients there is no identifiable structural disease. Occasionally trigeminal neuralgia may be a symptom of a gasserian ganglion tumor, of multiple sclerosis, or of a brainstem infarct involving the descending root of the trigeminal nerve.

The history is diagnostic. The pain occurs as brief, lightning-like stabs, frequently precipitated by touching a trigger zone around the lips or the buccal cavity. At times, talking, eating, or brushing the teeth serves as a trigger. The pains rarely last longer than seconds, and each burst is followed by a refractory period of several seconds to a minute in which no further pain can be precipitated. The pains, however, often occur in clusters so that the patient may report that each pain lasts for hours. The pain is limited to the distribution of the trigeminal nerve, usually affecting the second and third division or both. Spontaneous remissions and exacerbations are common, the exacerbations tending to occur in spring and fall. Between paroxysms of pain, the patient is asymptomatic. Tic pain rarely occurs at night. In idiopathic trigeminal neuralgia, the neurologic examination is entirely normal. In symptomatic trigeminal neuralgia, there may be sensory changes in the distribution of the trigeminal nerve, and such a finding should prompt a careful search for structural disease of the nervous system.

Carbamazepine is the drug of choice for the treatment of trigeminal neuralgia. The anticonvulsant drug is given in doses varying from 400 to 800 mg a day, but because of its sedative properties the initial dose is 100 mg twice daily, gradually increased to the required maintenance dose. No more than 1200 mg should be taken daily. The drug is not an analgesic and is only effective for specific kinds of pain such as trigeminal neuralgia, glossopharyngeal neuralgia, and the lightning pains of tabes dorsalis. Rarely, aplastic anemia has been reported, and complete blood counts are procured prior to the initiation of therapy and at intervals thereafter. Other side effects include dizziness and sedation. Phenytoin* in doses of 400 mg a day is also effective in trigeminal neuralgia but less so than carbamazepine. Occasionally the two drugs appear to be synergistic. Baclofen* 60 to 80 mg daily has also been found to be a useful agent. If medical treatment fails, surgical intervention is necessary. The most popular operations are radiofrequency lesions of the gasserian ganglion (radiofrequency gangliolysis) and posterior fossa craniotomy to relieve the trigeminal nerve of compression by vascular structures. The first operation can be done under local anesthesia and is generally effective initially, but has a high relapse rate. The second operation is as effective as the first, and appears to have a lower relapse rate. Both operations produce either mild or no loss of sensation in the face, and thus are preferable to such operations as section of the nerve root proximal to the ganglion, which, however, affords permanent relief. Local anesthesia of the ganglion or the peripheral branches of the nerve at some time prior to surgery is desirable because some patients find the anesthesia produced by nerve section less tolerable than the pain itself.

GLOSSOPHARYNGEAL NEURALGIA. Glossopharyngeal neuralgia is characterized by pain similar to that of trigeminal neuralgia but in the distribution of the glossopharyngeal and vagus nerves. The trigger zone is usually in the tonsil or posterior pharynx, and the pain spreads toward the angle of the jaw and the ear. Occasional patients suffer cardiac slowing or arrest during these attacks as a result of the intense afferent discharge over the glossopharyngeal nerve. Carbamazepine is often effective, but if it fails, glossopharyngeal nerve roots are sectioned in the posterior fossa. Symptomatic glossopharyngeal

*This use is not listed in the manufacturer's directive.

neuralgia is occasionally the presenting complaint in a patient with a tonsillar tumor, and careful examination of the pharynx and tonsillar fossa for mass lesions must be carried out.

OTHER NEURALGIAS. Similar but much rarer disorders than trigeminal or glossopharyngeal neuralgia have been reported to involve the greater occipital nerve and the nervus intermedius portion of the facial nerve. The clinical features and treatment of these rare disorders are similar to those for trigeminal neuralgia.

POSTHERPETIC NEURALGIA. Postherpetic neuralgia refers to severe and prolonged burning pain with occasional lightning-like stabs in the involved dermatome after an attack of herpes zoster. The disorder commonly affects the first division of the trigeminal nerve. Its treatment is discussed in Ch. 501.

Diagnostic Evaluation

Headache is an extremely common disorder, and the excessive application of expensive and highly technical laboratory procedures to the diagnosis and management of benign head pain has been a substantial cause of unnecessary medical costs. Set against this truism is the fact that in some instances a timely CT scan or lumbar puncture can give lifesaving information about an otherwise undiagnosable problem. Given these antitheses, the following principles may help in the management of the individual patient:

1. Patients with chronic classic or common migraine or with chronic tension headache rarely require more than a careful history and examination. Even when the unilateral prodromes and headache of longstanding, classic migraine consistently affect the same side, the incidence of associated intracranial lesions remains so low that CT scan is unnecessary and arteriography unjustified.

2. Headaches that are of recent origin or progression deserve investigation by CT scan. This principle especially applies to headaches that have a consistently focal distribution, follow trauma, or begin after the age of 30 years.

3. The EEG is almost never useful in the diagnosis of diseases causing headache and can be omitted. Skull x-rays are useful in diagnosing headache only (a) when searching for abnormalities involving the base of the brain such as sellar and suprasellar lesions or (b) immediately following head trauma. CT scans have superior discriminating capacities to plain x-rays and, when available, make x-rays unnecessary.

4. Diagnostic lumbar puncture should be performed with any acute headache that (a) is accompanied by fever or (b) is explosive or the most severe headache ever suffered (a history typical of acute subarachnoid hemorrhage). Lumbar puncture should, if possible, be deferred until after CT scanning with other forms of acute headache, especially if stiff neck but no fever is present. (This combination may indicate partial herniation of cerebellar tonsils into the foramen magnum secondary to an intracranial mass lesion.)

5. If CT scanning is available, radioisotopic brain scanning almost never adds useful information and is expensively superfluous.

Diamond S, Dalessio DJ: The Practicing Physician's Approach to Headache. 3rd ed. Baltimore, Williams & Wilkins, 1982. *This short, up-to-date monograph describes the practical approach to the management of headache. The book is beautifully illustrated.*

Headache and Cephalgia. *Two journals which publish original articles concerning new developments in the diagnosis and management of headaches and other types of head pain.*

Packard RC: Symposium on Headache. Neurol Clin Vol 1, No 2, May, 1983. Philadelphia, W. B. Saunders, 1983. *A comprehensive and up-to-date review of headache and its management.*

Saper JR: Headache Disorders. Current Concepts and Treatment Strategies. Boston, John Wright, PSG Inc., 1983.

NECK AND BACK PAIN

Neck and/or back pain, whether localized or radiating into the extremities, is one of man's most common afflictions. Low back pain is believed to affect about 80 per cent of all individuals at some time during their lives. Neck or back pain is a major cause of time lost from work. Most neck or back pain is transient and neither life-threatening nor associated with obvious pathologic abnormalities. Because the pathophysiology of most such pain is poorly understood, the physician often encounters patients for whom he can neither make a certain diagnosis nor prescribe rational therapy. Fortunately, most patients suffering neck or back pain recover within a few weeks no matter what the treatment. Estimates are that 70 per cent of patients recover within one month and 90 per cent within three months. Only 4 per cent of patients suffering neck or back pain are disabled longer than six months. In those patients who suffer transient episodes of neck or back pain, the cause is rarely established. Some authorities believe that the majority suffer from bulging or herniated intervertebral discs (see Ch. 519). Others believe that disc disease is a minor cause and that most neck and back pain is caused by lesions of other pain-sensitive structures in and around the spine, especially the facet joints, paravertebral musculature, sacroiliac joints, or vertebral bodies themselves.

A small number of patients develop chronic pain or neurologic dysfunction that portends serious disease. In this small number, meticulous diagnostic evaluation and vigorous therapy often prevent or reverse serious or potentially lethal neurologic sequelae. Most patients with chronic pain and neurologic dysfunction suffer from mechanical lesions compressing the nerve roots, paravertebral nerve plexuses, or spinal cord. The lesions are described in Ch. 518. The following provides a general discussion of the management of the patient who complains of acute or subacute neck or back pain.

ANATOMY AND PHYSIOLOGY OF THE SPINE. The functional unit of the spine is composed of two segments: The anterior segment contains two adjacent vertebral bodies separated by an intervertebral disc. The function of the anterior segment is to bear weight and cushion the shock to the spine from such activities as walking and running. The posterior segment is composed of the vertebral arches, the transverse processes, the posterior spinous processes, and the paired articulations known as "facets," with the facet joint between them. The posterior segment is a non–weight-bearing structure that has the function of protecting the contained spinal cord and nerves as well as allowing the spine to be mobile both in extension and in rotation. Not all of the structures of this unit are pain-sensitive. The vertebral body, at least its periosteum, is pain-sensitive (therefore, compression fractures are, at least initially, painful), whereas the intervertebral disc is not in itself pain-sensitive. However, if the intervertebral disc bulges and compresses the posterior longitudinal ligament, pain may result even if the nerve root itself is not involved. Posteriorly, the synovium-lined facet joints are pain-sensitive, although the intraspinal ligaments holding the posterior elements together are not. The paravertebral muscles surrounding and supporting the spine are pain-sensitive, particularly when they are overstretched or when they go into spasm. In the neutral position, the nerve root occupies only a small portion of the intervertebral foramen from which it exits the spinal canal. However, when the spine is extended, i.e., when it is in the hyperlordotic posture, the intervertebral foramen becomes smaller, potentially causing impingement on a nerve root and also leading to overlap of the facet joints, the latter allowing for irritation of the pain-sensitive synovial membranes. This is the reason that on examination of patients with intervertebral disc disease or with pain originating from the facet joints, the pain may be relieved somewhat by flexion of the spine and exacerbated by extension or lordosis. It is also the reason that hyperlordosis, a common postural abnormality, sometimes leads to chronic low back pain and why most back exercises have as their goal the production of a flat or slightly flexed but certainly not hyperlordotic lumbar spine.

Another anatomic finding of clinical importance in evaluating low back pain is that lumbar roots exit through that portion of the intervertebral foramen that is above the intervertebral disc. Thus, even though the L4 root exits between L4 and L5, a herniated disc between these vertebral bodies occurs just below the exit of the L4 root and thus will usually compress the L5 and not the L4 root. A herniated disc between the fifth lumbar and the first sacral vertebral body will usually compress the S1 root and not the L5 root. If, however, the disc protrudes more medially, an occurrence much less common than laterally protruding disc, an L4-L5 disc may involve the caudally directed sacral roots rather than the L5 lumbar root. Only if the disc completely extrudes into the vertebral canal will an L4-L5 disc compress the L4 root. In the cervical spine, the roots exit above a vertebral body with the same number (i.e., C4 root exits between C3 and C4). Thus, a herniated C4-C5 disc may compress the C6 or C5 root, but not the C4.

Neck or back pain may be severe and disabling and can originate from any of the pain-sensitive structures in the spine or surrounding muscles, the description giving no sure clue as to its etiology. Only if pain radiates in a clear dermatomal distribution can the physician infer that a nerve root has been damaged or compressed by the process.

EXAMINATION OF THE PATIENT. The task for the physician is to separate those patients with potentially serious disease who require extensive diagnostic evaluation from those with more common, if unknown, causes of neck and back pain who need only reassurance, sometimes coupled with bedrest, analgesics, and physical therapy.

The diagnostic evaluation begins with the history. Get a complete description of the pain. Most benign back pain is of acute or subacute onset, and frequently follows by minutes to hours some unaccustomed physical activity, particularly lifting or bending. Often patients awaken stiff and sore the morning after unusual exercise. Sometimes low back pain begins acutely, frequently on arising in the morning, without any obvious precipitating event. Most neck pain begins as a stiff neck, often on awakening in the morning, without a history of any unusual activity. In many patients neck or low back pain recurs episodically over many years. Most benign neck or back pain is dull and aching in quality, exacerbated by movement and relieved by rest. The majority of patients with benign neck or back pain are comfortable when they are recumbent and immobile, or are able to find at least one position that relieves the pain. Pain that is present when the patient is immobile and cannot be relieved by positional manipulation should lead the physician to search for a more serious disorder. Ask if the pain radiates from the neck or back, around the chest or abdomen, or into an extremity. If the radiation is in a dermatomal distribution, and particularly if it is accompanied by paresthesias or loss of sensation, there is probably mechanical compression of the root supplying that dermatome, and more likely than not the patient will have identifiable structural disease of the nervous system. However, radiating pain into an extremity may not follow a strict dermatomal distribution and may not be accompanied by paresthesias. Instead, there is diffuse aching often associated with muscle tenderness in a distribution different from and more widespread than a dermatome. The distribution labeled sclerotomal does not necessarily imply compression of a root. The pathogenesis of such sclerotomal pain is poorly understood, but has been produced by injection of noxious substances such as hypertonic saline into the posterior longitudinal ligament of the spinal canal, into facet joints, and into paravertebral muscles. Many believe the source of the pain is muscle spasm resulting from irritation of nerve endings in ligamentous and muscular structures.

Take additional history. A past history of serious systemic illness may suggest disease of vertebral bodies. For example, carcinoma of the breast or thyroid may cause back pain from bony metastases years after the primary tumor has been successfully treated. A previous systemic infection may lead to delayed onset of vertebral osteomyelitis or an epidural abscess. A family history may also give clues to the etiology of back pain. For example, neurofibromas causing neck or back pain by compressing nerve roots or the spinal cord may be associated with neurofibromatosis. Rheumatoid arthritis and ankylosing spondylitis are causes of familial back pain.

A careful general physical examination is mandatory. The examination may reveal evidence of systemic disease such as cancer or infection, indicating a similar process causing low back pain. Urinary tract infections, pelvic disease, abdominal aneurysms, and other intra-abdominal or intrathoracic processes may cause back pain by impinging on vertebral bodies or paravertebral structures. Peripheral nerves can be easily palpated at several sites (e.g., ulnar nerve at the elbow, peroneal nerve at the head of the fibula, sacral roots by pelvic or rectal examination). Palpable thickening may lead to a diagnosis of neurofibromatosis. Special attention should be paid to mobility of the spine and paravertebral structures. In most patients who complain of a stiff neck there is some limitation of movement of the cervical spine, but if gradual movement of the cervical spine causes intense pain, if pain on neck flexion is referred to the thoracic or lumbar area, or if neck flexion causes paresthesias radiating into the arms, legs or back (Lhermitte's sign), spinal cord compression should be suspected. Most low back pain not caused by a herniated disc is exacerbated by forward flexion and relieved by lying down. The paravertebral muscles are often in spasm, straightening the normally lordotic lumbar spine, and are often tender to palpation. Sometimes the palpating finger encounters nodule-like thickenings that, when pressed, produce pain radiating into an extremity in a sclerodermal distribution. In most people with severe low back pain, particularly if it radiates into a lower extremity, the pain increases when the extended leg is raised from the bed (straight leg raising sign). However, pain referred to the contralateral back or leg when the nonpainful leg is raised (crossed straight leg raising) implies root compression within the spinal canal. Point tenderness over a spinous process raises the suspicion of involvement of that vertebra by either tumor or infection.

The neurologic examination is important. Sensory loss, reflex diminution, and weakness all suggest serious structural disease and require further evaluation. The distribution of neurologic abnormalities localizes the lesion. Remember, however, that patients in severe pain are reluctant to move the painful part, particularly against resistance, and often appear to be weak when the neuromuscular structures are in fact normal. Likewise, guarding can affect deep tendon reflexes, either increasing or decreasing them with respect to the normal side. Such reflex alteration may mislead the observer into believing that the patient has nervous system disease. Repeating the neurologic examination after pain has been relieved by analgesics usually clarifies whether or not there is neurologic dysfunction. Clear and reproducible neurologic signs, particularly sensory loss in a dermatomal distribution or a diminished stretch reflex, imply root compression.

SIGNS AND SYMPTOMS OF NERVE ROOT AND SPINAL CORD COMPRESSION. The spinal cord and its attached motor, sensory, and autonomic nerve roots are the primary occupants of the spinal canal. The spinal cord itself extends in the adult from the first cervical to the first lumbar vertebral body, and the spinal roots continue in the subarachnoid space to the second sacral vertebra. The caudal portion of the spinal cord is called the conus medullaris, and the bunched roots below the cord the cauda equina. Within the spinal canal, the spinal cord and its roots can be subjected to mechanical compression and deformation by several processes. The resulting signs and symptoms depend on the location of the pathologic process, its speed of development, and whether it affects the nerve roots or the spinal cord alone.

Acute compression of nerve trunks and nerve roots is not generally painful. Pressing on the median nerve at the wrist or the ulnar nerve at the elbow is rarely painful. A sharp blow may cause the nerve to discharge, causing paresthesias in the distribution of that nerve but not severe pain. However, once a root or nerve is damaged, as when chronic compression produces edema, demyelination, and inflammation, the root becomes tender to compression or stretch. Then pain occurs, usually both at the site of compression and in part or all of the dermatomal distribution of that root (radicular pain). The symptoms of chronic compression of nerve roots are pain, paresthesias, sensory loss, weakness, atrophy, and hyporeflexia. These abnormalities are confined to the tissues supplied by the root(s) involved, thus localizing the lesion. Knowing the myotomal and dermatomal distribution of spinal roots (see Table 518–1) often allows one not only to localize the lesion but also to suggest its etiologic diagnosis, since involvement of a single root is more likely to occur with intervertebral disc herniation (see Ch. 519), whereas multiple root dysfunction is likely to be caused by tumor or chronic inflammation. However, myotomal and dermatomal localization must be utilized cautiously. In the first place, not everyone obeys the standard maps (e.g., in about 5 per cent of patients intrinsic muscles of the hand are supplied exclusively by the median or ulnar nerve rather than shared between the two). Also, there is much overlap between contiguous dermatomes and contiguous myotomes, and the apparent size of a dermatome may vary from day to day or even hour to hour, depending on the excitability of the central nervous system. Excepting these caveats, however, the localizing diagnosis of root lesions is usually quite accurate.

In most instances, pain is the prominent symptom of root compression. Pain is experienced in the overlying spine, deep in certain muscles supplied by the compressed root, and in the cutaneous distribution of the injured root. Pain is usually least severe when the patient is in a position that minimizes compression of the root and most severe in positions that compress or stretch the root. With intervertebral disc herniations, lying down may be very comfortable and sitting up uncomfortable, whereas with tumors within the spinal canal compressing nerve roots, the opposite may be true. With both disc herniation and tumor, pain is exacerbated by increasing intraspinal pressure, e.g., coughing, sneezing, and straining.

Pain, both local and radicular, is also an early complaint in patients with spinal cord compression. As with root disease, the pain of spinal cord compression is usually exacerbated by movements that stretch the cord (neck flexion, straight leg raising) or that increase intraspinal pressure (coughing, sneezing, straining). In addition, patients harboring compressive spinal cord lesions are often tender to percussion over the vertebral body at the site of compression. Other clinical signs of spinal cord compression depend on the speed with which the compression develops, the transverse and longitudinal site of the lesion, and the vulnerability of the individual spinal fibers. The spinal cord accommodates fairly well to gradually developing compression (as, for example, from meningiomas and neurofibromas), and these disorders may cause the gradual onset of painless paraparesis or paraplegia. Because the cord has accommodated to the evolution of a compressing lesion, subsequent decompression, even when patients are severely paraparetic, often leads to complete resolution of neurologic symptoms. On the other hand, rapidly developing lesions such as epidural hematomas, acute midline herniated discs, or epidural spinal cord compression from metastatic tumor cause rapidly developing neurologic signs that respond poorly to therapy once severe paraparesis has developed. The site of compression in the transverse plane also determines clinical signs, particularly when the compression develops slowly. For example, lateral lesions compressing one side of the spinal cord may cause Brown-Séquard's syndrome (ipsilateral hemiparesis and vibration and position sense loss, with contralateral pain and temperature loss); compression of the posterior portion of the cord may cause bilateral position and vibratory loss, with preservation of pin and temperature sensation and of motor power. However, because mass lesions twist the cord as they compress it and also interfere with the vascular supply to sites beyond the compression, one can depend only in a general way on the neurologic signs to evaluate the exact transverse site of spinal cord compression. The longitudinal location of the lesion is likewise important. Cervical lesions cause quadriplegia; thoracic lesions, paraplegia; and upper lumbar lesions, normal motor function with bowel and bladder dysfunction and extensor plantar responses (conus medullaris syndrome). Lesions below the first lumbar vertebral body compress the cauda equina, causing loss of bowel and bladder function with lower motor neuron leg weakness and normal plantar reflexes. Certain spinal tracts appear to be more vulnerable to compression than others. The corticospinal tracts and posterior columns appear particularly vulnerable, the spinothalamic tracts and descending autonomic fibers less so. As a result, weakness, spasticity, and reflex hyperactivity tend to be the earliest signs of spinal cord compression, with paresthesias and vibratory and position sense loss occurring soon thereafter. Loss of pain and temperature sensation and of bladder and bowel function usually occur late in the course of spinal cord compression. The spinocerebellar pathways are also sensitive to compression, and at times ataxia mimicking cerebellar disease may be the only sign of spinal cord compression.

LABORATORY AIDS TO INVESTIGATION. In most patients with benign neck or back pain no laboratory tests are required. However, if, after a careful history and examination, the physician suspects structural disease of the spine or root or spinal cord compression, laboratory tests will help confirm the clinical diagnosis and identify the site and nature of the disorder. Plain x-rays of the spine should be the first test in patients suspected of harboring structural disease. For suspected cervical lesions, frontal, lateral, oblique, and open-mouth odontoid views are required. If the patient has a short neck, the lower cervical area on lateral view may be obscured by the shoulders and require tomography. Flexion and extension views of the neck are often helpful to determine if subluxation is present. If the *patient* is allowed to control the degree of flexion and extension, these tests are not harmful. For the thoracic and lumbosacral spine, frontal and lateral views are usually sufficient. Flexion and extension views assess subluxation. Review the x-rays with the radiologist to assure that all potential lesions of the site in question have been assessed. Pay particular attention to the sagittal diameter of the cervical and lumbar canal (see Ch. 519), to the pedicles (see Ch. 520), and to the presence of osteophytes and loss of height in disc spaces (see Ch. 519). Congenital anomalies (see Ch. 523) should also be searched for, but the physician should recognize that congenital anomalies of the spine are common and most do not cause pain or other symptoms. Similarly, most patients of middle age or older have evidence of cervical and/or lumbar osteoarthritis. Such abnormalities do not prove that the radiologic defect is responsible for the symptoms. However, changes such as significant spondylolisthesis, marked multiple disc narrowings, stenosis of the lumbar canal, or vertebral destruction from tumor or infection are likely to be responsible for pain and often for neurologic disability. If back pain is referred to the lower extremities, x-rays of the pelvis and femora may reveal unsuspected abnormalities.

Computed tomography (CT scan) can detect erosion of vertebral bodies not identified on plain x-rays or bone scan, can identify paravertebral masses, dumbbell tumors growing through the intervertebral foramen, and herniated discs. With high resolution CT scanners, tumors and syrinxes within the cord can sometimes be identified. Thus, the CT scan is now the best radiologic test for the diagnosis of spine, nerve root, and spinal cord disease. Nuclear magnetic resonance (NMR) for scanning of the spinal cord and canal promises to identify intramedullary lesions such as tumor and syrinxes not currently seen by other techniques. NMR with or without CT may eventually replace more invasive diagnostic tests such as myelography.

X-ray tomography is useful in defining bony lesions in some areas of the spine, particularly at T1 and the sacrum where obscuration of the vertebral canal by overlying shadows makes plain films hard to interpret. Tomography is also useful in assessing minor degrees of bone destruction when plain x-rays are normal. It may sometimes be more sensitive than CT. A *radionuclide bone scan* is a more sensitive but less specific method of identifying lesions of the vertebrae. Destruction of bone by tumor may be identified by bone scan before plain x-rays become positive. Unfortunately, trivial traumatic, arthritic, and inflammatory lesions may also produce a positive bone scan. Occasionally the bone scan is normal even when plain x-rays reveal obvious bone destruction.

Myelography, using either lipid- or water-soluble radiopaque contrast material, will reliably outline compressive lesions. Myelograms must be viewed in both the frontal and lateral planes to determine if lesions are extradural, intradural, or intramedullary. If a complete block to the passage of the contrast material is encountered after lumbar injection, a cisternal or upper cervical injection of contrast material will determine the upper extent of the lesion. *Lumbar puncture* is useful to detect the presence of malignant cells or infecting organisms in the spinal fluid. When a mass lesion is suspected, a lumbar puncture should be performed only in conjunction with myelography. *Spinal angiography* is a specialized technique, sometimes essential for the detailed investigation of tumors and vascular malformations within the spinal cord. The technique is particularly useful to the surgeon who requires preoperative knowledge of the vascular supply. *Discography* is a controversial technique for identifying clinically important herniated discs. Under fluoroscopic control, less than 1 ml of contrast material is injected into the nucleus pulposus. Leakage of contrast material through the anulus fibrosis indicates disease of the disc space. More importantly, if the patient's spontaneous pain pattern is exactly reproduced, one can infer that it is that damaged disc which is producing the patient's symptoms. Unfortunately, at times asymptomatic discs may yield positive discograms.

Electromyography also helps in diagnosis. When the level of nerve root or spinal cord compression cannot be determined clinically, electromyographic evidence of lower motor neuron dysfunction restricted to a particular myotome strongly suggests root or anterior horn cell involvement at that level. Caution in evaluating lower motor neuron dysfunction in spinal cord compressive lesions is essential because tumors of the upper cervical spinal cord occasionally cause atrophy with fasciculations and fibrillations in the hand, probably from ischemia of anterior horns in the lower cervical cord. The paraspinous muscles are supplied by the posterior ramus of each emerging nerve root, and electromyographic evidence of denervation in those muscles implies a lesion close to the vertebral body before anterior and posterior rami diverge. In some patients with back pain but without clinically definable root symptoms, denervation of paraspinous muscles points to root involvement at the level of back pain. *Somatosensory evoked potentials* can be recorded along the spinal cord or in the brain after a peripheral nerve is stimulated. Abnormalities sometimes identify the site of a spinal cord lesion. Evoked potentials diminish or disappear with posterior column dysfunction. Their exact role in the diagnosis and prognosis of spinal cord lesions is still unresolved.

MANAGEMENT OF NECK AND BACK PAIN. If there are no clinical findings to suggest serious structural disease of the spine, nerve roots, or spinal cord, patients should be treated as if they suffered from an acute neck or back strain, without further diagnostic evaluation. Because most patients recover within a few weeks without specific therapy, it is difficult to assess various therapeutic regimens. For severe pain, the best treatment probably consists of bedrest on a firmly supported mattress in the position most comfortable for the patient. The best positioning for low back pain is usually semi-Fowler's position (head slightly elevated with pillows under the knees). Bedrest should be combined with analgesic agents (usually aspirin or acetaminophen) and with local heat. Patients should be encouraged to stay in bed except to go to the bathroom until they are free of pain. When the patient is free of pain, he should gradually ambulate and then start a program of strengthening exercises for the paravertebral muscles of the neck and back in order to prevent recurrence of the pain (see references). Other treatment modalities, including physical therapy, traction, procaine or saline injection into trigger points, and spinal manipulation, have not been shown to be more efficacious than the regimen described above. Manipulation of the neck is potentially dangerous because the vertebral arteries can be occluded as they enter the skull by excessive or unskilled manipulation. Using standard therapy, 70 to 80 per cent of patients will become free of pain within a four-week period and able to return to full activity. During the period of bedrest, repeated physical and neurologic examinations are unwise, since vigorous movement of the neck, back, and extremities often exacerbates the pain and delays improvement. A small minority of patients continue to have chronic pain, and these patients, along with those whose initial examination has suggested more serious disease, need further evaluation. For neck pain, a soft cervical collar often is as effective in immobilizing the neck as is bedrest.

The management of some specific causes of nerve root and spinal cord compression is considered in Ch. 519. Other causes of neck and low back pain, such as ankylosing spondylitis, rheumatoid arthritis, multiple myeloma, spinal tuberculosis, and Paget's disease, are discussed elsewhere in this text.

Cailliet R: Low Back Pain Syndrome. 3rd ed. Philadelphia, FA Davis, 1981. *A well-written monograph with schematic drawings illustrating the anatomy, physiology, causes, and treatment of low back pain.*

Cailliet R: Neck and Arm Pain. 2nd ed. Philadelphia, FA Davis, 1981. *This short monograph describes the clinical anatomy and physiology of the cervical spine and the causes of pain originating from disorders of that area.*

Keim HA, Kirkaldy-Willis WH: Low back pain. Clinical Symposia, Vol 32, No 6, 1980. Summit, NJ, Ciba-Geigy Corporation. *Beautifully illustrated monograph on the anatomy and pathophysiology of low back pain. Drawings demonstrate the physical examination of the back and therapeutic exercises.*

SOME SPECIFIC PAIN SYNDROMES

Some disorders causing pain produce a specific constellation of signs and symptoms that sets them apart from other and more common causes of pain. Moreover, many of these pain syndromes often respond completely to treatment with nonanalgesic medications. Thus, it behooves the physician to recognize these disorders and to prescribe appropriate treatment. Those disorders that particularly affect the head, neck or back are discussed above. Others are discussed in the paragraphs below.

LIGHTNING PAINS OF TABES. The lightning pains of tabes are acute, short-lived pains in the trunk or lower extremities which occur with structural lesions of the dorsal roots and particularly with tabes dorsalis. Lightning pains are analogous to trigeminal and glossopharyngeal neuralgia. Like those two disorders, the pain usually responds to carbamazepine. There is no surgical therapy.

"REFLEX SYMPATHETIC DYSTROPHIES." This is a term that applies to pain, hyperalgesia, hyperesthesia, and autonomic changes, usually after injury to an extremity. If the injury has involved a peripheral nerve, particularly the sciatic or median nerve, the syndrome is called *causalgia* (hot pain). If the injury has not involved a peripheral nerve, such terms as post-traumatic painful osteoporosis, Sudeck's atrophy, post-traumatic spreading neuralgia, minor causalgia, shoulder-hand syndrome, and reflex dystrophy have been applied, the particular term depending on the outstanding symptom. Whatever the term, the pathophysiology of all these disorders appears to be the same, as do their clinical manifestations and response to therapy.

The disorder may follow either a major or a minor injury to an extremity, after which severe pain, usually of a burning quality, develops in the extremity. The pain is continuous but exacerbated by emotional stress and is associated with severe hyperpathia, so that moving or touching the limb is often intolerable. At first the pain is localized to the site of the injury or the distribution of the nerve injured, but with time it spreads, often to involve the entire extremity. Along with the pain there are vasomotor changes, first of vasodilatation (warm and dry skin) but later a change to vasoconstriction (edema, cyanosis, cool skin). Other autonomic disturbances include either hyperhidrosis or hypohidrosis; trophic changes in the skin, subcutaneous tissue, and muscles; and osteoporosis. The entire symptom complex is rarely present in any one patient, and one sign or symptom usually predominates. Untreated, severe reflex sympathetic dystrophy leads to muscle atrophy, fixation of joints, osteoporosis, and a useless extremity. The exact mechanism of the pain and sympathetic changes is not understood.

Treatment should be undertaken as early as possible, because there is evidence that the earlier the treatment, the more effective it will be. Treatment begins with local anesthetic infiltration of the painful site, using 2 to 5 ml of 0.5 per cent lidocaine, repeated frequently enough to maintain relief of pain. When local measures fail, most patients are relieved by sympathetic block with lidocaine. This procedure often gives permanent relief, but if repeated local anesthetics produce only transient benefit, surgical sympathectomy should be considered.

POSTHERPETIC NEURALGIA. Postherpetic neuralgia refers to severe and prolonged burning pain with occasional lightning-like stabs in the involved dermatome after an attack of herpes zoster. Severe postherpetic neuralgia is usually a disease of elderly patients and, like most chronic pain, is exacerbated by emotional upset and relieved to some degree by distraction. Touching the involved area usually exacerbates the pain. Treatment of postherpetic neuralgia is not entirely satisfactory, but the initial treatment should be directed toward stimulating the painful area. Brisk rubbing for many hours a day with a terrycloth towel or stimulation of the dermatome with a cutaneous electrical stimulator often brings relief which long outlasts the stimulus. Initially, when therapy is undertaken, the hyperpathia may be so severe that the patient is unwilling to have the area stimulated. One can then spray the area with a local anesthetic (e.g., ethyl chloride) before stimulation is undertaken. During the first 48 to 72 hours, stimulation should be done as often as possible when the patient is awake and then decreased gradually. Care must be taken to keep the rubbing light so as not to excoriate friable skin. Relief of pain may take several weeks. Analgesic drugs are sometimes beneficial, and psychotropic drugs (amitriptyline, 75 mg daily, and fluphenazine, 1 to 3 mg daily) have been reported to be useful. The results of surgical therapy are usually poor. Recent evidence suggests that nerve blocks using agents injected paraspinally or epidurally may relieve postherpetic neuralgia if given early in its course. There is also some evidence that adrenocorticosteroids and interferon used for the treatment of acute herpes zoster may diminish the incidence of postherpetic neuralgia. In many patients the disease runs its course, and after a year or two the pain disappears spontaneously. Thus mutilating surgical procedures are probably not indicated.

PHANTOM LIMB PAIN. Phantom limb pain is a chronic and severe pain appearing to be localized in an amputated or totally denervated limb. All patients suffer phantom sensations after amputation, but in only about 10 per cent is it painful, usually when there has been severe pain prior to operation. The pain is frequently similar to that suffered before amputation, or at times it may resemble muscle pain with the phantom seeming to be in a cramped or uncomfortable position. In most instances, the pain lessens and disappears with time, but in occasional patients it is a chronic and severe problem. Therapy is difficult. A search should be made for painful neuromas, but these are an uncommon cause of phantom pain, and even if small neuromas are found and removed, the pain is not usually relieved. Surgical procedures directed at the central nervous system are often not helpful. The pain may be triggered by touching the amputation stump, but over the passage of time healthy areas of the body when touched may also trigger pain in the phantom. Phantom pain is sometimes permanently abolished by cutaneous stimulation, either rubbing or electrical stimulation, or by repeated anesthetic blocks of peripheral nerves proximal to the stump. Narcotic analgesics may be helpful; other analgesic agents are usually not helpful. Sympathetic blocks have been reported to relieve pain in some patients for prolonged periods, but sympathectomy rarely produces relief as lasting as with causalgia. The mechanism of phantom pain is unknown.

MYOFASCIAL PAIN SYNDROMES. Pain arising from skeletal muscle is common. Unaccustomed exercise causes soreness and tenderness in the involved muscles but is rarely a source of patient complaint. Prolonged tonic contraction of skeletal muscles, however, has an underlying pathogenesis of psychologic tension, resentment, and anxiety, and may produce pain in which the cause is not immediately apparent to the patient. Examples are tension headache arising from chronic contraction of paraspinous muscles at the base of the skull, anterior chest pain from contraction of pectoralis major, posterior thoracic or lumbar pain from paraspinous muscle contraction, and abdominal pain from rectus muscle retraction. The pain is initially localized over the area of muscle contraction but may spread widely into a distribution characteristic for the muscles involved. The muscles are usually tender to palpation, and there is often a particular tender area somewhere in the muscle, called a trigger area, which, when palpated, reproduces the entire distribution of the spontaneous pain. When the pain is acute, it may be treated with rest, local heat, and mild analgesic drugs, along with muscle relaxant drugs such as diazepam or meprobamate. When the pain is chronic or severe, particularly when a trigger area is found, local anesthesia with ethyl chloride spray or local injection of 0.2 per cent lidocaine or physiologic saline sometimes affords relief. At times, a single injection breaks the pain–muscle tension–pain cycle and permanent relief is achieved. At other times, repetitive injections with the addition of analgesic agents and muscle relaxants are required.

Section Four ALCOHOL-RELATED AND NUTRITIONAL DISORDERS OF THE NERVOUS SYSTEM

482. ALCOHOL-RELATED AND NUTRITIONAL DISORDERS OF THE NERVOUS SYSTEM

Ivan Diamond

Alcohol-related neurologic disorders usually occur in patients who have abused the agent for a long time on a regular basis. Such patients should be distinguished from "binge" drinkers, who resume adequate diets after brief bouts of drinking; instead they tend to be chronic alcoholics who often suffer poor nutrition over months to years. It is not known why some alcoholics develop neurologic complications while others do not. Genetic factors are suspected to play a role in alcoholism, and certain individuals within the susceptible population may carry an inherent risk for neurologic disease when nutrition is inadequate. The individual alcohol-related neurologic disorders described below often occur together in the same patient. The consequences of nonalcoholic malnutrition and specific vitamin deficiencies are discussed in Ch. 214 and 217.

WERNICKE'S ENCEPHALOPATHY

Wernicke's encephalopathy is an acute disorder that occurs most commonly in chronic alcoholics. It also develops in other

TABLE 482–1. CONDITIONS ASSOCIATED WITH WERNICKE'S ENCEPHALOPATHY

Chronic alcoholism
Starvation
Persistent vomiting
Hyperemesis gravidarum
Gastric malignancy
Gastritis
Intestinal obstruction
Digitalis intoxication
Systemic diseases
Malignancy
Hepatic failure
Disseminated tuberculosis
Uremia
Iatrogenic
Inadequate parenteral nutrition
Chronic hemodialysis

conditions listed in Table 482–1. This is the only alcohol-related neurologic disorder that can be corrected by a specific vitamin—thiamine.

CLINICAL MANIFESTATIONS. A clinical triad of ophthalmoplegia, ataxia, and global confusion is characteristic. Affected patients may complain of double vision or difficulty with balance. There is almost always horizontal nystagmus on lateral gaze. Vertical nystagmus, usually on upward gaze, occurs in about 50 per cent of cases. Bilateral, often asymmetric, lateral rectus palsies are characteristic and may develop rapidly. Defects in conjugate gaze are common. Bilateral ptosis and total external or an apparent internuclear ophthalmoplegia occurs rarely. Occasionally, one observes a diminished pupillary reaction to light, but light-fixed pupils should suggest an alternate or additional diagnosis.

Virtually all patients have an ataxic gait due to cerebellar involvement. This can be so mild that it is demonstrable only by tandem walking or rapid turning, or it can be so severe that the patient cannot stand. Peripheral neuropathy and vestibular dysfunction frequently complicate Wernicke's encephalopathy and contribute to the ataxia. Intention tremor is less common, and speech disturbances are rare.

Most patients have an acute confusional state characterized by inattention, disorientation, and sleepiness. Stupor or coma occurs but is rare. Sometimes patients may be hyperactive and agitated (alcohol withdrawal, see Ch. 17) but usually are apathetic, indifferent, and amnesic for new information.

Associated physical abnormalities related to chronic alcoholism or poor nutrition are often present. These include signs of liver disease and portal hypertension (see Ch. 121) as well as lesions of the skin and mucous membranes (see Ch. 552). Tachycardia and orthostatic hypotension are common. Hypothermia occurs less frequently; any fever should prompt a search for concomitant infection. Patients with Wernicke's encephalopathy do not develop beriberi heart disease (see Ch. 217).

PATHOLOGY. The distribution of lesions in the brain is unique and appears to account for the clinical findings. The major lesions occur in the periventricular regions of the diencephalon, mid-brain, and brain stem, and in the superior vermis of the cerebellum. The lesions of Wernicke's encephalopathy may vary in severity and age in the same patient. They consist of areas of demyelination and glial proliferation. Microglia are prominent in acute lesions and fibrous astrocytes in older ones. Acute lesions show capillary dilation with occasional petechial hemorrhages. In experimental animals, accompanying defects in serotonergic transmission can be demonstrated in affected areas.

TREATMENT. Thiamine is the only factor that produces sustained improvement in Wernicke's encephalopathy. Because intestinal absorption is impaired in malnourished alcoholics, thiamine (50 to 100 mg) is given parenterally before starting infusions. One must avoid administering glucose prior to giving thiamine, as it can precipitate or worsen the encephalopathy in thiamine-depleted patients. Recovery begins promptly. In most cases, ophthalmoplegia and gaze palsies begin to resolve rapidly during the first day; nystagmus, gait ataxia, and confusion may show improvement within days to weeks. After recovery from the acute encephalopathy, however, many patients are left with nystagmus and gait ataxia. This residual cerebellar disorder is clinically and pathologically identical to the sometimes independently arising syndrome of alcoholic cerebellar degeneration described below. Nearly all patients with Wernicke's encephalopathy recover from the global confusional state, but many are left with a residual, more circumscribed disorder of memory—Korsakoff's amnestic syndrome.

KORSAKOFF'S AMNESTIC SYNDROME

CLINICAL MANIFESTATIONS (see also Ch. 478). There is a characteristic defect in forming new memories (anterograde amnesia) and in summoning previously established memories (retrograde amnesia). Recent memories tend to be most severely affected. Patients are usually disoriented for place and time. Immediate recall is intact, but patients are unable to remember the same items several minutes later. Confabulation often occurs early in the course. Affected patients are usually unaware of their memory deficits and blissfully unconcerned. Other aspects of cognitive function, including arousal, language, praxis, and judgment, are spared.

PATHOLOGY. The pathologic findings of active or remote Wernicke's encephalopathy may be present. Consistent damage to the dorsal medial nucleus of the thalamus probably accounts for the memory deficits.

TREATMENT. Unlike the acute motor abnormalities of Wernicke's encephalopathy, Korsakoff's amnestic syndrome often does not improve after thiamine treatment. About 20 per cent of patients recover completely, but more than half show little or no change. If improvement occurs, it may take one to three months to be recognizable. All patients with Korsakoff's syndrome should be given thiamine to treat possible coexistent Wernicke's encephalopathy and to prevent progression of the amnesia.

METABOLIC CONSIDERATIONS. Thiamine (vitamin B_1) in human tissues is derived entirely from dietary sources and is absorbed in the small intestine (Ch. 217). A saturable, energy-dependent transport system regulates uptake of thiamine into the brain and CSF. A series of reactions produces phosphorylated thiamine derivatives, and thiamine pyrophosphate (TPP) is a required co-factor for certain enzymes in carbohydrate and amino acid metabolism. The four principal thiamine-dependent enzymes are pyruvate dehydrogenase, α-ketoglutarate dehydrogenase, transketolase, and branched-chain α-ketoacid dehydrogenase. A report that patients with the Wernicke-Korsakoff syndrome may have a genetic defect in transketolase activity awaits confirmation. In addition to its role as a co-factor, thiamine and thiamine triphosphate (TTP) may also be important in the electrical function of neural membranes. Defects in some of these thiamine-dependent activities may underlie the acute symptoms of Wernicke's encephalopathy or Korsakoff's syndrome. However, there is no proof that they are directly responsible for the findings in these disorders.

The confusional state and oculomotor disturbances seen in Wernicke's encephalopathy respond to thiamine treatment, and it is said that recovery may proceed during thiamine therapy whether or not alcohol consumption continues. However, calorie-containing ethanol appears to be an important contributing factor to the neurologic deficits. Malnourished prisoners of war who developed Wernicke's encephalopathy rarely exhibited the irreversible amnestic syndrome. Moreover, nystagmus, ataxia, and the memory deficits often fail to improve after thiamine therapy, indicating that some areas of the brain have become irreversibly damaged. The molecular metabolic defect that precedes tissue damage in Wernicke's encephalopathy and Korsakoff's amnestic syndrome is not known.

ALCOHOLIC CEREBRAL ATROPHY

Many chronic alcoholics develop cerebral atrophy that increases with age and that can be visualized on CT scans of the brain. There is usually symmetrical enlargement of the lateral ventricles and an increase in the size of cerebral sulci and the width of interhemispheric and sylvian fissures. The abnormalities may disappear if drinking is discontinued. Many chronic alcoholics also show deficiencies on psychometric examination. However, the CT scan abnormalities do not correlate well with such specific cognitive defects. The specific mechanisms of these cerebral abnormalities are not known.

ALCOHOLIC NEUROPATHY

CLINICAL MANIFESTATIONS. Polyneuropathy is common among alcoholic patients. The most typical complaints are weakness, pain, and paresthesias in the hands and especially the feet. Symptoms usually begin insidiously in the legs and progress proximally and symmetrically. Abnormal motor and sensory signs develop concomitantly. Patients may complain of burning pain and heat sensations on the plantar surfaces of the feet and aching pain in the calves. Dysesthesias can become so severe that light touch and deep pressure are intensely unpleasant. Burning pain made worse by contact can interfere with walking despite adequate strength.

On examination muscle weakness and wasting are usually more prominent distally, affecting legs more than arms and never the latter exclusively. The muscles may feel flabby and tender to pressure. Weakness can be so severe that contractures develop at the ankles and knees. Sensory abnormalities usually involve all modalities, but especially the pain and temperature modalities early in the course, and are more prominent distally. The deep tendon reflexes are usually absent to diminished in a distal to proximal distribution. Even asymptomatic patients often show mild sensory loss in the feet and absent Achilles tendon reflexes.

Involvement of the vagus nerve and thoracoabdominal sympathetic chain occurs rarely and can produce hoarseness, dysphagia, vocal cord paralysis, and hypotension. Cerebrospinal fluid protein levels are usually normal.

PATHOPHYSIOLOGY AND TREATMENT. The classic pathologic findings in alcoholic neuropathy are axonal degeneration and demyelination. Some investigators propose that alcoholic peripheral neuropathy, since it first affects smaller sensory fibers, is characterized by axonal degeneration with electromyographic signs of denervation and normal nerve conduction velocities being found at that stage. By contrast, superimposed nutritional neuropathies are prone to produce segmental demyelination of large fibers as well as axonal degeneration. This may result in slow nerve conduction velocities.

A specific vitamin deficiency has not been documented in alcoholic neuropathy. Treatment consists of a balanced diet with supplemental B vitamins. Recovery is always slow and often incomplete. Several weeks may be needed for motor improvement to begin, and it may take a year before patients with marked weakness begin to walk.

ACUTE AND CHRONIC ALCOHOLIC MYOPATHY

ACUTE MYOPATHY. This is a dramatic and life-threatening condition that develops in chronic alcoholics during prolonged heavy drinking. Symptoms begin abruptly with pain, cramps, tenderness, weakness, and swelling of the legs. Muscle involvement may be generalized or confined to one limb. Creatine phosphokinase activity in blood is elevated, and muscle biopsy shows acute rhabdomyolysis. Myoglobinuria often occurs and may lead to acute renal failure, hyperkalemia, and death. Electromyography usually shows evidence of a primary myopathy (Ch. 539). Recovery usually follows days to weeks of abstinence, occasionally leaving residual proximal muscle weakness in its wake.

CHRONIC MYOPATHY. This is a chronic, painless disorder of proximal muscle weakness and atrophy that occurs rarely in alcoholics. It can be mild or severe. Muscles of the pelvic girdle and thighs are involved most frequently; weakness of shoulder girdle muscles is less common. Improvement usually occurs within two to three months after ethanol withdrawal. A coexistent alcoholic peripheral neuropathy may contribute to the weakness.

ALCOHOLIC CEREBELLAR DEGENERATION

Cerebellar cortical degeneration occurs frequently in chronic alcoholics. About half the patients have an associated peripheral neuropathy. Men are affected more often than women. Most patients give a history of episodic binge drinking superimposed on heavy consumption extending back over many years. Some complain of progressive unsteadiness and difficulty in walking, but these more insidiously developing symptoms often reflect a superimposed peripheral neuropathy that may clear with treatment. Abnormalities of gait and station are the most common findings. Initially, unsteadiness is demonstrated when the patient turns rapidly, and tandem walking is difficult or impossible. Gradually, the feet become more widely based, walking becomes hesitant, and truncal ataxia is added. Ataxia of the legs may be demonstrable on heel to shin tests, but nystagmus, dysarthria, and tremor are rare. Often the cerebellar syndrome develops abruptly or rapidly over several weeks and then remains stable. Sometimes the disorder evolves more slowly, with exacerbation following a binge or during an intercurrent illness. The most prominent pathologic abnormality is degeneration of the neurons of the anterior and superior cerebellar vermis with loss of Purkinje cells. CT or NMR scans confirm cerebellar vermis atrophy. Abstinence and treatment with a balanced diet and supplemental B vitamins may produce moderate improvement in the gait ataxia as peripheral neuropathy recovers.

NUTRITIONAL AMBLYOPIA

This is a condition of retrobulbar neuritis involving the maculopapillary fibers. It is caused by a nutritional deficiency and is encountered primarily in alcoholics. The patient complains of dim or blurred vision that evolves gradually over weeks to months. Decreased visual acuity occurs in one or both eyes, accompanied by bilateral symmetrical central or centrocecal scotomas. Peripheral visual fields are usually unaffected, and funduscopic examination is usually normal. Treatment consists of abstinence and a balanced diet with supplemental B vitamins. The extent of recovery varies inversely with the severity of impairment before therapy.

CENTRAL PONTINE MYELINOLYSIS

Central pontine myelinolysis (CPM) is a rare disorder that affects alcoholics primarily but also occurs in children and adults with severe electrolyte disorders, liver disease, malnutrition, anorexia, burns, cancer, Addison's disease, sepsis, and Wilson's disease.

PATHOPHYSIOLOGY, SIGNS, AND SYMPTOMS. The signs and symptoms relate closely to the pathologic change, which consists of a varying extent of symmetrical focal myelin destruction involving the basal central pons, with similar lesions occasionally affecting extrapontine areas. There is no associated inflammation or nerve cell destruction, and the lesions appear to be reversible with time and proper nutritional and fluid balance.

Typically CPM evolves within days or weeks in severely ill patients, often in association with acute post-alcoholic complications. Almost always the condition follows by one to three days a period of profound hyponatremia followed by rapid osmolal correction of greater than 20 mEq per liter. Mental symptoms often are prominent and consist of clouded consciousness or an increase in a post-alcoholic delirious state. Reflecting interruption of corticospinal pathways in the pons, a flaccid or spastic quadriparesis ensues, accompanied in many instances by bulbar difficulties of speaking and swallowing. Some patients develop a supranuclear ophthalmoplegia and the mortality is high. Reflecting the sparing of the pontine tegmentum, sensory abnormalities usually fail to develop. Formerly, most cases were discovered at postmortem examination, but the characteristic story has recently led to many cases being diagnosed during life, confirmed by characteristic abnormalities on CT scan. Complete recovery can take place in patients whose underlying illness makes this possible. Treatment consists of meticulous maintenance of electrolytes, especially sodium balance and adequate nutrition. The exact pathogenesis is unknown but has been attributed to edema of the basis pontis associated with the rapid electrolyte changes.

MARCHIAFAVA-BIGNAMI DISEASE

This is a rare disorder consisting of symmetrical demyelination of the corpus callosum and adjacent white matter. Although at one time described in Italian men who drink red wine, the disorder affects mainly severely alcoholic middle-aged men addicted to various kinds of alcoholic beverages. The clinical features are variable, and diagnosis is seldom made before death. Patients may have a progressive dementia over several years accompanied by agitation or apathy, hallucinations, and emotional disorders until seizures, stupor, and coma supervene. Clinical findings such as rooting and sucking responses, grasp reflexes, paratonic rigidity, incontinence, and a slow hesitant gait suggest bilateral frontal lobe involvement. Recovery is rare. Symmetrical demyelination in the corpus callosum may be seen on CT scans. The specific etiology is unknown.

VITAMIN B_{12} DEFICIENCY

Vitamin B_{12} deficiency causes subacute degeneration of white matter in the dorsal and lateral columns of the spinal cord, peripheral nerves, optic discs, and cerebral hemispheres. The neurologic findings usually accompany a macrocytic (pernicious) anemia, but anemia need not be present. Hematologic and pathophysiologic considerations of vitamin B_{12} deficiency and details of treatment are discussed in Ch. 217.

CLINICAL MANIFESTATIONS. Neurologic symptoms develop in most patients with long untreated pernicious anemia, especially those in whom anemia has been masked by folate ingestion. Patients first complain of paresthesias in the hands or legs, such as tingling, numbness, and "pins and needles" sensations. Stiffness and weakness of the legs with unsteadiness in walking may be bothersome, particularly in the dark. Neurologic symptoms progress relentlessly if untreated; ataxia and stiffness eventually are followed by paraplegia and dysfunction of bowel and bladder. Psychologic symptoms are frequent and include apathy and depression, irritability and paranoid tendencies, nocturnal confusion, and dementia. Intellectual deterioration does not usually develop in the absence of other neurologic signs. Failing vision with central scotomas occurs rarely.

Initially one may find few objective changes despite complaints of paresthesias. Later, symmetrical distal impairment of vibratory sensation occurs, usually first in the legs but eventually reaching the trunk and arms. Position sense is affected less prominently, although Romberg's test may be positive. The earliest changes are those of a peripheral neuropathy. The patellar and Achilles tendon reflexes are diminished or absent, and there may be decreased perception of touch, pain, and temperature in the feet and ankles. In the intermediate advanced case, one finds symmetrical weakness in the legs associated with spasticity, clonus at the knees and ankles, increased or decreased deep tendon reflexes, and extensor plantar responses. Tingling distal paresthesias may follow flexion of the neck (Lhermitte's sign).

PATHOLOGY. The most prominent early findings are in the peripheral nerves and dorsal and lateral columns of the spinal cord. Fragmentation and spongy degeneration of myelin usually begin in the lower cervical and upper thoracic regions; in untreated patients the disease progresses up and down the spinal cord and reaches into the ventral columns. Myelin sheaths and axons are destroyed, and Wallerian degeneration is found in the spinal cord funiculi. Cerebral white matter is affected late. Peripheral nerves may show distal degeneration.

DIAGNOSIS. Serum vitamin B_{12} levels are low and appear to correlate with the severity of the neurologic findings. In pernicious anemia this is due to impaired absorption of vitamin B_{12}, which is the basis of the commonly used Schilling test. There is diminished or absent intrinsic factor, usually in association with gastric achlorhydria. Vitamin B_{12} deficiency can also result from intestinal malabsorption syndromes, gastrectomy, or inadequate diet. These are discussed in Ch. 217. Methylmalonic acid is increased in blood and CSF and its increased excretion in the urine is regarded as a sensitive and specific indicator of vitamin B_{12} deficiency. The CSF protein concentration may be increased slightly. Neurologic disorders that can be confused with vitamin B_{12} deficiency include multiple sclerosis, cervical spondylosis, spinal cord tumors, and syphilitic meningomyelitis. A virtually identical syndrome has been reported after chronic abuse of nitrous oxide (Ch. 481).

PATHOGENESIS. The molecular pathogenesis of the neurologic lesion in vitamin B_{12} deficiency is unknown. Vitamin B_{12} exists in different forms, some of which are required for at least two enzymes: N5-methyltetrahydrofolate homocysteine methyltransferase, which catalyzes the synthesis of methionine and regeneration of tetrahydrofolate, and methylmalonyl-CoA mutase, which generates succinyl-CoA. The activities of both enzymes are reduced in vitamin B_{12} deficiency. Methionine is a substrate for protein synthesis and is a precursor for transmethylation reactions in neurotransmitter, phospholipid, and protein metabolism. Prolonged exposure to nitrous oxide, which produces a neurologic disorder resembling combined system disease, also inhibits methionine synthesis. Reduced activity of methylmalonyl-CoA mutase probably accounts for the increased excretion of methylmalonic acid because methylmalonate is not converted to succinyl-CoA.

TREATMENT. Intramuscular administration of vitamin B_{12} is the only treatment for vitamin B_{12} deficiency due to pernicious anemia. Therapy should be started immediately and continued throughout the patient's lifetime as described in Ch. 217. Early neurologic changes can be rapidly and completely reversed if treatment with vitamin B_{12} is begun promptly within the first few weeks of the illness. If the neurologic manifestations have reached the stage of producing spinal cord dysfunction, therapy will halt progression of the disease but improvement cannot be guaranteed.

Charness ME, Diamond I: Alcohol and the nervous system. Current Neurology 5:383, 1984. *A discussion of recent advances in many alcohol-related neurologic disorders.*

Dreyfus PM, Geel SE: Vitamin and nutritional deficiencies. *In* Albers RW, Siegel GJ, Katzman R, Agranoff BW (eds.): Basic Neurochemistry. 3rd ed. Boston, Little, Brown and Company, 1981. *A clear discussion of the basic neurochemistry of the vitamins.*

Greenberg DA, Diamond I: Wernicke-Korsakoff syndrome. *In* Tartar RE, Van Thiel DH (eds.): Alcohol and the Brain: Chronic Effects. New York, Plenum Publishing Corp., 1984. *A discussion of recent advances.*

Norenberg MD, Leslie KO, Robertson AS: Association between rise in serum sodium and central pontine myelinolysis. Ann Neurol 11:128, 1982. *In 12 hyponatremic patients a rise in serum sodium of greater than 20 mEq per liter was followed by the disorder, which did not appear in other hyponatremic patients treated more cautiously. A good bibliography accompanies.*

Victor M, Adams RD, Collins GH: The Wernicke-Korsakoff Syndrome. Philadelphia, F. A. Davis Co., 1971. *A classic clinical-pathologic description of the disorder.*

Vinken PJ, Bruyn GW: Handbook of Clinical Neurology. Vol. 28, Metabolic and Deficiency Diseases of the Nervous System. Amsterdam, North Holland Publishing Co., 1976, Ch. 1–14. *A comprehensive review of nutritional diseases of the nervous system.*

Section Five THE EXTRAPYRAMIDAL DISORDERS

Stanley Fahn

Extrapyramidal disorders are associated with abnormalities of the basal ganglia and are characteristically manifested by a combination of abnormal involuntary movements, alterations in muscle tone, and disturbances in postural stability. Included are the syndromes of parkinsonism, tremor, chorea, athetosis, dystonia, and hemiballism, collectively referred to as *movement disorders,* a heading which also encompasses the syndromes of myoclonus and tics, maladies that probably arise from sites outside the basal ganglia. As a general rule, diagnosis of the particular abnormal involuntary movement depends more on careful clinical observation than on laboratory study. The age and mode of onset, genetic traits, exposure to drugs and toxins, progression of symptoms, and development of other neurologic features (e.g., dementia) usually provide the most important clues.

ANATOMIC, PHYSIOLOGIC, AND BIOCHEMICAL CORRELATES. The basal ganglia comprise five paired nuclei: caudate nucleus, putamen, globus pallidus (or pallidum), subthalamic nucleus, and substantia nigra (Fig. 1). The first three lie deep within the cerebral hemispheres and collectively are referred to as the corpus striatum. The subthalamic nucleus is in the diencephalon, and the substantia nigra is located in the midbrain.

Although separated by the internal capsule, the caudate and putamen are similar microscopically, chemically, and physiologically, and are considered collectively as the neostriatum or striatum. The striatum serves as the main site of neural input into the basal ganglia, receiving afferents from all parts of the cerebral cortex and from the nucleus centrum medianum of the thalamus. The major output of the striatum is to the pallidum and the zona reticulata portion of the substantia nigra. The pallidum and zona reticulata are also separated by the internal capsule, but are similar microscopically, chemically, and physiologically. These two regions serve as the major site of neural output from the basal ganglia, with the principal neural efferent pathway going to the ventral anterior (VA) nucleus of the thalamus and thence to the premotor cortex. The premotor cortex is one source of the corticospinal tract (pyramidal tract), the major descending cortical efferent pathway controlling motor function.

The subthalamic nucleus receives afferents from the pallidum and sends its efferents back to the pallidum. Thus, it can be considered to function as a modulator of the globus pallidus and probably regulates the basal ganglia output to the VA nucleus of the thalamus. In an analogous fashion, the substantia nigra can be considered to modulate the neostriatum. The dorsal part of the substantia nigra (zona compacta) sends efferents to the neostriatum (the dopaminergic nigrostriatal pathway), and the ventral part of the substantia nigra (zona reticulata) receives fibers from the neostriatum.

Considerable progress has been made in identifying and understanding the neurotransmitters of some of the neuronal pathways in the basal ganglia. The nigrostriatal pathway contains dopamine and may inhibit the striatum. The other inputs to the striatum (the thalamostriatal pathway and the glutamate-containing corticostriatal pathway) are excitatory. The GABA-containing efferents from the striatum to the pallidium and substantia nigra are inhibitory. Lesions of the substantia nigra with resulting loss of dopamine in the striatum result in the bradykinetic syndrome of parkinsonism. Drugs that deplete dopamine (e.g., reserpine) and drugs that block striatal dopamine receptors (e.g., phenothiazines) can also cause parkinsonism. By contrast, excessive dopamine activity (e.g., levodopa overdosage) produces the hyperkinetic state of chorea. A lesion of the subthalamic nucleus produces contralateral hemiballism. It is generally believed that such a lesion removes an inhibitory influence on the pallidum (disinhibition). Lesions in the corpus striatum produce inconsistent patterns of dyskinesias, depending on particular sites and mode of involvement. Athetosis and dystonia can follow trauma and vascular lesions of the striatum, whereas chorea accompanies degenerative loss of neurons in this structure (e.g., Huntington's chorea).

The basal ganglia serve as a major input to the pyramidal tract motor system. In fact, a lesion of the pyramidal tract sufficient to cause paralysis will eliminate existing dyskinesias, such as tremor and chorea. The term extrapyramidal system was originally coined to denote a motor system operating in parallel with and independent from the pyramidal tract. This is incorrect, but the long use of the term "extrapyramidal" in clinical medicine has embedded it as synonymous with the basal ganglia system.

Phylogenetically, the extrapyramidal system is ancient and serves as the predominant motor system for reptiles and birds. In higher animals it is believed to be involved in automatic movements (e.g., walking, swinging arms when walking, feed-

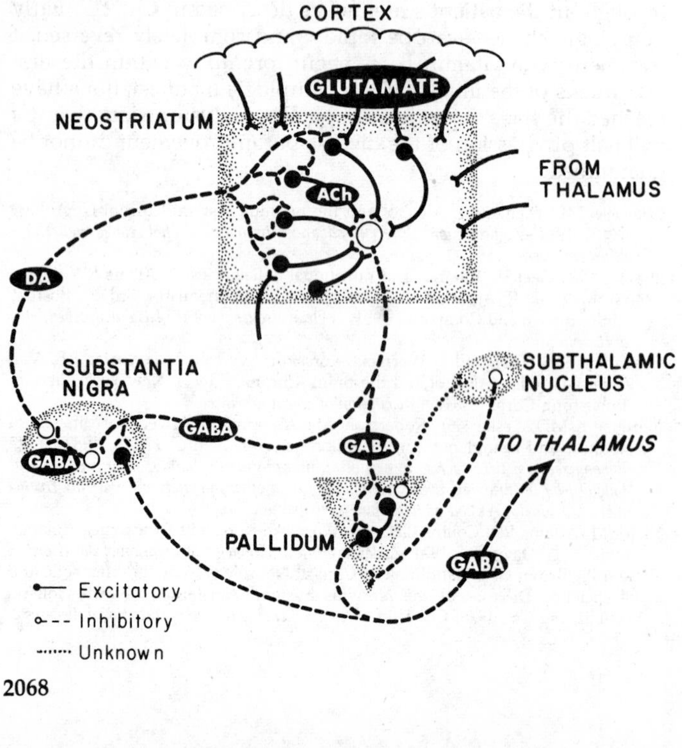

Figure 1. A simplified scheme of the neuronal pathways in the basal ganglia, depicting their function and suspected neurotransmitters. DA = dopamine; ACh = acetylcholine; GABA = gamma-aminobutyric acid.

ing), control of muscle tone, and maintenance of posture. Much of our knowledge of the function of the basal ganglia has been derived from clinicoanatomic correlations in humans.

ABNORMAL INVOLUNTARY MOVEMENTS. Movement disorders can be divided into *bradykinesia* (or *akinesia*), a paucity of automatic and spontaneous movement, and *hyperkinesia* (or *dyskinesia*), which is excessive or abnormal involuntary movements. Bradykinesia is a feature of parkinsonism and is virtually specific for that syndrome, whereas the dyskinesias are subdivided into specific types, depending on their rhythmicity, speed, duration, repetitiveness, and other characteristics. As a general rule, dyskinesias are absent during sleep, reduced with relaxation, and increased with stress.

Tremor refers to relatively rhythmic oscillatory movements. These can result from alternating contractions of opposing muscle groups (e.g., parkinsonian tremor) or from simultaneous contractions of agonist and antagonist muscles, with one group more forceful than the other (e.g., essential tremor). Clinical examination of tremor can aid in the etiologic diagnosis (Table 1). One should seek for (1) tremor at rest (hands in lap when patient is sitting or at side when patient is lying supine), (2) postural tremor (arms outstretched in front of body), (3) action tremor (when patient is moving arms or using hands to write or lift a cup of water to the mouth), and (4) intention tremor (finger-to-nose maneuver).

The classic parkinson tremor is present at rest. In the limbs, it is almost always distal, being present in the hands (pill-rolling) and feet. Tremor can also involve the tongue, lips, and chin, but rarely the head or neck. The rate of parkinsonian tremor is usually from 3 to 7 Hz. Characteristically, the tremor at rest transiently disappears when the patient initiates movement of the involved part. Some patients with parkinsonism may have an action tremor in addition to or instead of tremor at rest.

Postural and action tremors are more rapid than tremor at rest (rate between 7 and 11 Hz) and are also more severe distally than proximally. Drugs, metabolic illnesses, and essential tremor are common causes. These tremors can usually be suppressed by beta-adrenergic blockers such as propranolol and metoprolol. Intention tremor is a manifestation of cerebellar pathology, especially in the major outflow pathway, the superior cerebellar peduncle. The most common cause is multiple sclerosis; unfortunately, no effective drug is available for this problem. Thalamotomy may bring relief of all types of tremor.

Chorea refers to brief, irregular, nonrhythmic contractions that can involve any or all parts of the body. In disorders such as Huntington's disease and Sydenham's chorea, the choreic movements are not repetitive; instead, they flow from one muscle to another. This can be an important distinction from tardive dyskinesia, in which the brief movements are rhythmic and repetitive (stereotypic). In chorea, patients frequently try to mask the abnormal jerks by carrying out voluntary movements, so-called semipurposeful movements. Patients with chorea cannot maintain a sustained, even contraction, as manifested by "milkmaid" grips, inability to keep the tongue protruded, stuttering gait, and clumsiness with dropping of objects.

Ballism is a form of chorea in which the brisk, involuntary contractions affect proximal muscles and are of large amplitude, causing wild, flinging movements of the limbs. These movements usually occur unilaterally (hemiballism).

TABLE 1. A CLASSIFICATION OF COMMON ABNORMAL TREMORS

I. Tremor at rest
  A. Parkinsonism
II. Postural and action tremor
  A. Essential tremor
  B. Accentuated physiologic tremor
    1. Epinephrine, amphetamines
    2. Thyrotoxicosis
    3. Anxiety, fatigue
    4. Lithium, tricyclics
    5. Alcohol withdrawal
III. Intention tremor
  A. Multiple sclerosis
  B. Wilson's disease
  C. Phenytoin toxicity

Athetosis refers to continual slow, writhing movements that can involve limbs (distal and proximal), trunk, head, face, and tongue. When the movements are brief, the term choreoathetosis is commonly applied; when sustained contractions occur at the end of an athetotic movement, the term athetotic dystonia can be used. It is common to see an increase of athetotic movements when the patient carries out voluntary movements or is speaking (overflow phenomenon).

Dystonia refers to involuntary movements with sustained contractions at the end of the movement. The positions can be prolonged (dystonic postures) but usually last only a second or less (dystonic movements). Dystonic movements are usually of a twisting nature; hence the term torsion dystonia. They may be brisk from the beginning to peak of the contraction, and a misdiagnosis of chorea is not uncommon. However, if a twisting aspect is present, a diagnosis of dystonia is appropriate even if sustained contractions are not obvious. Action dystonia refers to dystonic movements that occur only when the affected part of the body is in voluntary motion. For example, twisting movements of a leg or foot may appear only when the patient attempts to walk. As the dystonia becomes more severe, the involuntary contractions appear at rest as well. Another peculiar but characteristic feature of dystonia is the lessening of abnormal contractions by tactile or proprioceptive input. For example, patients with torticollis will frequently place a hand on the mandible to provide some relief from the involuntary muscular contractions. Dystonic movements may be generalized or limited to only one part of the body. The focal dystonias include spasmodic torticollis, writer's cramp, blepharospasm, and spastic dysphonia.

Myoclonus refers to shock-like or lightning-like movements due to muscular contractions or inhibitions (the latter is referred to as negative myoclonus). Myoclonic jerks can involve a single muscle or a group of muscles, with the amplitude ranging from a small muscular flicker to a large body-moving synchronous jerk. The myoclonus that accompanies the initial stage of sleep is an example of the latter and represents a normal physiologic form. Asterixis, which resembles a tremor, is an example of negative myoclonus. It occurs in metabolic encephalopathies and is due to brief periods of electrical silence in muscles.

Tics are complex coordinated movements that appear suddenly and transiently. Head shaking, eye blinking, shoulder shrugging, and complex facial contortions are examples. In addition to motor tics, vocal tics are common, and when present indicate a diagnosis of Tourette's syndrome (Ch. 486).

ALTERATIONS IN MUSCLE TONE. Increased muscle tone (rigidity) and decreased muscle tone (hypotonia) are common components of extrapyramidal disorders. Tone is determined by the examiner who manipulates the passive limb, neck, and trunk of the patient. Rigidity is most commonly encountered in parkinsonism, and must be differentiated from spasticity. The latter accompanies corticospinal tract lesions and is manifested by increased tone in either flexion or extension of a limb, with sudden relaxation as the muscle continues to be stretched (clasp knife phenomenon). Spasticity is also associated with weakness, increased tendon reflexes, and a Babinski sign. In contrast, rigidity is present in both flexion and extension and continues throughout the length of muscle stretch. Most often it is jerky (cogwheeling) owing to an underlying tremor rhythm, but it can be smooth (lead-pipe rigidity). Electromyographic recordings reveal that the agonist and antagonist muscles contract simultaneously, even when the patient attempts to relax. Hypotonia occurs characteristically in chorea and may also be present in patients with torsion dystonia at a time when the muscle is not involuntarily contracting.

DISTURBANCES OF POSTURAL REFLEXES. Normally, an individual can recover balance quickly if thrown off his center of gravity. However, such postural reflexes tend to be lost in parkinsonism, Huntington's disease, and Wilson's disease. The effect leads to falling when the patient attempts to walk or stand. Such reflexes can be tested by pulling the standing patient backward or forward toward the examiner with a quick tug on the shoulders. One must prepare to catch the patient should he not be able to recover owing to loss of postural reflexes.

Postural changes, such as stooping and kyphosis, are encountered in parkinsonism. Torsion dystonia can lead to postural deformities such as scoliosis, tortipelvis, and lordosis. Eventually, fixed postures develop as a result of contractures.

Carpenter MB: Anatomy of the corpus striatum and brain stem integrating systems. *In* Handbook of Physiology. The Nervous System II. 2nd ed. Bethesda, MD, American Physiological Society, 1982, pp 947–995. *A detailed review of basal ganglia anatomy.*

DeLong MR, Georgopoulos AP: Motor functions of the basal ganglia. *In* Handbook of Physiology. The Nervous System II. 2nd ed. Bethesda, MD, American Physiological Society, 1982, pp 1017–1061. *A review of basal ganglia physiology in terms of motor behavior.*

Jankovic J, Fahn S: Physiologic and pathologic tremors: Diagnosis, mechanism, and management. Ann Intern Med 93:460, 1980. *An etiologic classification of tremors and their mechanisms and treatment.*

Kita ST: Electrophysiology of the corpus striatum and brain stem integrating systems. *In* Handbook of Physiology. The Nervous System II. 2nd ed. Bethesda, MD, American Physiological Society, 1982, pp 997–1015. *A review of the physiology of the neuronal pathways within the basal ganglia.*

Martin JP: The Basal Ganglia and Posture. Philadelphia, J. B. Lippincott Company, 1967. *An outstanding discussion of the role of the basal ganglia in postural mechanisms in normal and disease states.*

Penney JB Jr, Young AB: Speculations on the functional anatomy of basal ganglia disorders. Ann Rev Neurosci 6:73, 1983. *A review of neurotransmitter pathways within the basal ganglia and speculations on their role in movement disorders.*

483. PARKINSONISM

Parkinsonism is a clinical syndrome consisting of four cardinal signs: tremor at rest, rigidity, bradykinesia, and loss of postural reflexes. Not all patients have all four cardinal signs. Bradykinesia refers to a paucity of automatic and spontaneous movements and difficulty in initiating voluntary movement. Bradykinesia is almost always present in parkinsonism and is virtually synonymous with this diagnosis. Bradykinesia accounts for the majority of parkinsonian symptoms and signs: a general slowing down of movement, masked face (hypomimia), decreased frequency of blinking with a staring expression, decreased swallowing resulting in drooling of saliva, soft voice (hypophonia), loss of speech modulation, impaired handwriting with micrographia, decreasing amplitude in performing rapid repetitive movements (such as opening and closing the hand or tapping the foot), difficulty in arising from a chair and turning in bed, loss of armswing on walking with a tendency to take short steps or shuffle, and loss of spontaneous gesturing when speaking.

Parkinsonism is the most common extrapyramidal disorder, and indeed is one of the most prevalent neurologic conditions, along with epilepsy, stroke, and dementia. Its prevalence has been placed at close to 1 million individuals in the United States, with the addition of 50,000 new cases each year. It is a prominent cause of disability.

Parkinsonism can be categorized into three etiologic groups (Table 483–1): (1) the primary or idiopathic disorder referred to as Parkinson's disease, (2) secondary or acquired parkinsonism, and (3) "parkinsonism-plus" syndromes, in which additional neurologic findings are present. A history of encephalitis, exposure to drugs or toxins, surgical removal of the parathyroid glands, or previous strokes suggests one of the secondary forms of parkinsonism. The presence of impaired ocular movements, orthostatic hypotension, cerebellar ataxia, or dementia suggests one of the "parkinsonism-plus" syndromes.

In parkinsonism, dopamine activity in the striatum is deficient. In Parkinson's disease, there is a loss of pigmented neurons in the substantia nigra and locus ceruleus with subsequent loss of their dopamine and norepinephrine neurotransmitters. In postencephalitic parkinsonism, the midbrain is particularly affected, with loss of substantia nigra neurons. In these two conditions degeneration of the dopaminergic nigrostriatal pathway leads to striatal dopamine deficiency. Reserpine depletes striatal dopamine, and antipsychotic drugs (e.g., phenothiazines and butyrophenones) block dopamine receptors. In other conditions (e.g., lacunar infarcts, hypoparathyroidism, striatonigral degeneration, and progressive supranuclear palsy), it is suspected that striatal dopamine receptors are directly affected. Involvement of the dopamine receptor renders treatment with levodopa or dopamine agonists ineffective.

TABLE 483–1. A CLASSIFICATION OF COMMON FORMS OF PARKINSONISM

I. Primary
  Idiopathic parkinsonism (Parkinson's disease)
II. Secondary
  A. Infectious: postencephalitic parkinsonism
  B. Toxins: manganese, carbon monoxide
  C. Drugs: antipsychotics, reserpine
  D. Hypoparathyroidism
  E. Vascular
III. Parkinsonism-plus
  A. Striatonigral degeneration
  B. Progressive supranuclear palsy
  C. Shy-Drager syndrome
  D. Normal pressure hydrocephalus
  E. Alzheimer's disease
  F. Wilson's disease
  G. Huntington's disease

PRIMARY PARKINSONISM (Parkinson's Disease)

The incidence of Parkinson's disease increases with age, but, because the population declines with age, the peak age at onset is in the sixth and seventh decades of life. Idiopathic parkinsonism can occur in younger adults and, rarely, in children. (Although juvenile parkinsonism can represent primary parkinsonism, it is often a feature of Wilson's disease, Huntington's disease, or rarer forms of pallidal degeneration.) Both sexes are affected, males more than females by a ratio of 3:2. Familial parkinsonism sometimes occurs.

Parkinson's disease begins insidiously, most commonly with tremor or bradykinesia in one limb. The symptoms then involve the other limb on the same side and tend to remain unilateral for several years before spreading to the opposite side. Rigidity, masked face, and soft voice appear early, and the patient reports a slowness in carrying out the day's activities. The gait becomes short stepped and shuffling. Loss of postural reflexes with unsteadiness on turning and festination (the need to walk faster and faster to avoid falling forward) appears as the disease progresses. Postural deformities appear: the head is flexed forward, the trunk is stooped and may be tilted to one side, the hands develop ulnar deviation with flexion at the metacarpophalangeal joints and extension at the interphalangeal joints, and the arms are adducted at the sides with elbows flexed. This characteristic posture plus masked face often allows first inspection to make the diagnosis even if tremor is not present.

As the disease progresses, patients develop gait hesitation ("freezing") on initiating gait (start-hesitation), when approaching a target (terminal-hesitation), and when trying to walk in a crowded area, as if the feet are glued to the ground. With progressive bradykinesia and loss of postural reflexes, the patient eventually becomes wheelchair bound. Swallowing difficulty with choking becomes a problem. Parkinson's disease is not lethal, but increased mortality occurs because of debility, aspiration pneumonia, urinary tract infections, and decubitus ulcers. The rate of progression varies. Disability seldom ensues until 10 to 15 years after onset.

Other symptoms include personality changes: the patient becomes less assertive and more passive, dependent, fearful, and indecisive, disabling qualities for persons in an executive position. Depression is common, and dementia may ensue as the disease progresses. Some patients complain of pain, tingling, numbness, and burning sensations, usually on the side of initial symptoms. These are frequently misdiagnosed as arthritis or bursitis. Primitive reflexes, such as Myerson's sign (repetitive blinking on repetitive tapping of the glabella), snout reflex, and palmomental reflex, are commonly found.

Pathologically, depigmentation of the normally pigmented brainstem nuclei is characteristic, and cytoplasmic eosinophilic inclusions (Lewy bodies) are seen microscopically in substantia nigra and locus ceruleus neurons. The cause of Parkinson's disease is unknown.

SECONDARY PARKINSONISM

This category comprises numerous disorders in which parkinsonism provides the predominant symptoms or in which it plays a smaller role in the clinical picture. The list includes poisonings with manganese, carbon monoxide and a synthetic opiate by-product (MPTP), brain tumors affecting basal ganglia function, cerebral trauma, intoxication with neuroleptic drugs, encephalitis, hypoparathyroidism and basal ganglia calcification, chronic hepatocerebral degeneration, and cerebrovascular disease. Most frequent are drug-induced parkinsonism, postencephalitic parkinsonism, and vascular parkinsonism.

DRUG-INDUCED PARKINSONISM. Drug-induced parkinsonism rivals idiopathic parkinsonism as the most common form of this syndrome. High dosages of both reserpine and the antipsychotic drugs (e.g., phenothiazines and butyrophenones) cause parkinsonism. Reserpine is now usually used only in low dosage to treat hypertension, making the antipsychotic agents the predominant offending agents. Reserpine depletes the storage of dopamine in the dopaminergic nerve terminals in the striatum; the antipsychotic agents block postsynaptic dopamine receptors in the striatum. The latter produce several extrapyramidal syndromes: (1) Acute *akathisia* (motor restlessness) can occur as the dosage is increased; sometimes anticholinergics relieve this symptom. (2) Acute *dystonic reactions* can appear with the initial doses, especially in children and young adults. These dystonic postures can be relieved with parenteral administration of anticholinergics (benztropine, 2 mg intramuscularly), antihistamines (diphenhydramine, 50 mg intravenously), or diazepam (5 to 7.5 mg intravenously). (3) *Oculogyric crisis,* in which the eyes are deviated in a fixed posture for minutes to hours, is a form of dystonia, but occurs in adults as well as children. It can be relieved by the drugs described above. (4) *Parkinsonism* can appear as a toxic reaction and resembles idiopathic parkinsonism in all the cardinal signs of the syndrome. Levodopa will not reverse this complication, probably because the dopamine receptors are blocked and occupied by the antipsychotic agent. Oral anticholinergic drugs are effective (e.g., trihexyphenidyl, 2 mg three times a day). If the antipsychotic drug is withdrawn, the symptoms will clear over several weeks to months. (5) *Tardive dyskinesia,* a chorealike disorder presenting predominantly as an oral dyskinesia, can appear after long-term use of antipsychotic drugs. The condition may be irreversible and can worsen when the drugs are withdrawn.

POSTENCEPHALITIC PARKINSONISM. The pandemics of encephalitis lethargica (von Economo's encephalitis) that occurred between 1919 and 1926 left in their wake a variety of extrapyramidal disorders (chorea, dystonia, oculogyric crises, and parkinsonism). The onset of parkinsonism can occur years after the encephalitis and even after mild, subclinical cases. Although a viral etiology is suspected, the causative agent has never been established. An influenza strain is suspected, but serum antibody titers in patients with postencephalitic parkinsonism have been normal.

Clinically, postencephalitic parkinsonism is a more slowly progressive disorder than Parkinson's disease and may stabilize. Affected patients may have oculogyric crises and a variety of neurologic deficits, such as hemiplegia, ocular palsies, dystonia, chorea, tics, or behavioral disorders. Postencephalitic parkinsonism is more sensitive to levodopa therapy than is Parkinson's disease, and patients with the former may require approximately one half the usual dosage needed in the latter.

Rarely, other types of encephalitis may be followed by parkinsonism. The condition has been reported in association with coxsackieviruses, Japanese B encephalitis, and western equine encephalitis. In most cases, the parkinsonian syndrome either improves or remains stable.

VASCULAR PARKINSONISM. Most parkinsonism among persons over age 70 is of the idiopathic variety. However, vascular or arteriosclerotic parkinsonism does occur infrequently and can appear in middle life as well as in old age. Occasionally it follows a stroke, but more often it appears as a complication of multiple small infarctions involving the striatum. Gait disturbance is the most frequent complaint, with short steps, "freezing," and unsteadiness on turning common. Increased muscle tone and loss of postural reflexes are present, but tremor is rare, as are masked facies and classic bradykinesia. Dementia may be present, as well as hyperactive tendon reflexes and Babinski signs. Antiparkinson drugs have little benefit.

PARKINSONISM-PLUS (Multisystem Degenerations)

The clinical signs of parkinsonism can accompany other neurologic deficits in several multisystem degenerative diseases including striatonigral degeneration, olivopontocerebellar degeneration (with cerebellar ataxia), progressive supranuclear palsy (with ophthalmoplegia), and Shy-Drager syndrome (with orthostatic hypotension). Parkinsonism with profound dementia can occur in patients in whom cerebral pathology reveals features of both Alzheimer's disease and Parkinson's disease. The parkinsonism-dementia complex is also seen in some patients with normal pressure hydrocephalus, which typically presents as a triad of gait disturbance, dementia, and urinary incontinence. Rarely, parkinsonian features, with or without associated dementia, accompany otherwise typical amyotrophic lateral sclerosis.

STRIATONIGRAL DEGENERATION. First described in 1961, striatonigral degeneration presents clinically as Parkinson's disease. As the disease progresses, however, signs of cerebellar ataxia and laryngeal stridor may appear. Loss of neurons occurs predominantly in the substantia nigra and putamen, with additional degeneration in other basal ganglia and the cerebellum. This disorder may be one of the many types of the olivopontocerebellar degenerations (see Ch. 490). The diagnosis can be suspected clinically by its failure to respond to levodopa, explained by the loss of dopamine receptors with the neuronal loss in the striatum.

PROGRESSIVE SUPRANUCLEAR PALSY. Well delineated in 1964 by Steele, Richardson, and Olszewski, progressive supranuclear palsy can resemble Parkinson's disease, but tremor is rare. Additional distinguishing features are external ophthalmoplegia, nuchal dystonia (especially neck hyperextension), and a dystonic facial smile with deep nasolabial folds (rather than the flattened folds seen in Parkinson's disease). The presence of ophthalmoplegia is required for the diagnosis. Initially vertical eye movements are lost. Whereas upward gaze alone is limited in Parkinson's disease, downward gaze is also impaired in progressive supranuclear palsy. Eventually, horizontal eye movements become limited. The ophthalmoplegia is supranuclear, and a full range of reflex eye movements can be detected by the doll's eyes test. Pathologically, basal ganglia, brainstem, and cerebellum contain neuronal loss and neurofibrillary tangles. There is no effective treatment, but dopamine agonists help some patients.

MANAGEMENT OF PARKINSONISM

GENERAL PRINCIPLES. The overall goals of therapy should be directed toward keeping the patient functioning independently as long as possible. Athough symptoms can often be suppressed, at least for a short period of time, the consequences of chronic drug administration must be considered, since long-term levodopa use may be accompanied by disabling adverse effects. It is best to individualize therapy in such matters as when to start drugs, which ones to utilize, and regulation of medications. The last-named point is a continual process in treating parkinsonism; one must constantly adjust drug dosage and timing to achieve the optimal balance between amelioration of symptoms and avoidance of unacceptable adverse reactions.

Parkinsonism is frequently accompanied by fearfulness, passivity, dependence, and depression, and affected patients need repeated encouragement and reassurance in meeting the stresses of everyday life and their all-too-realistic fears of the future.

PHYSICAL THERAPY. Parkinsonism inherently produces immobility. Patients must be encouraged to be as active as possible; the family must participate in this as well. Maintaining employment as long as feasible, taking long walks, gardening, and becoming active in hobbies are among the possibilities. As the disease advances, more formal home exercise programs with a physiotherapist can be arranged. Appropriately placed hand bars enable patients to get up unassisted from toilet seats or beds. Patients should be encouraged to carry out activities of daily living as independently as possible. For gait difficulty and unsteadiness, a cane is not useful but may serve as a warning that the patient is handicapped, thereby avoiding unnecessary jostling and preventing falls and fractures, a common complication. Pain from rigid cervical muscles may be relieved by heat and massage.

DRUG THERAPY. When the disease is mild and symptoms not troublesome, drugs are not necessary. The physician can explain that the symptoms may progress very slowly in the first few years, that drugs can be utilized at the appropriate time, and that regular evaluations will be carried out. As symptoms become annoying or restrict activities, drug therapy becomes necessary. Levodopa combined with a peripheral dopa decarboxylase inhibitor (carbidopa, benserazide) is the most potent agent available. However, in many patients the best response to levodopa occurs in the first two to three years of use; furthermore, clinical fluctuations ("on-off" and "wearing-off" phenomena) occur in many patients with chronic administration. Therefore, it is reasonable to initiate drug therapy with less potent antiparkinson agents (anticholinergics and amantadine) and to reserve levodopa for annoying or disabling symptoms that are no longer suppressed by these agents.

The antiviral agent amantadine HCl (Symmetrel) has an antiparkinsonian effect in approximately two thirds of patients. The usual dosage is 100 mg twice a day, and any benefit becomes evident within two to three days. If the disease is mild, effectiveness may persist, but in more advanced stages it decreases unless levodopa has been given concomitantly. Amantadine is believed to act by enhancing the release of dopamine stored in presynaptic terminals. As the storage supply is depleted, amantadine loses it effect. If the stores are replaced by administered levodopa, the effect can be prolonged. The most common adverse effect is livedo reticularis, a medically unimportant reddish mottling of the skin present around the knees. If pronounced erythematous edema of the ankles occurs, amantadine should be discontinued. Amantadine also can cause nonfrightening visual hallucinations, usually of people and animals. Lowering the dosage usually provides relief. If amantadine is not effective within three days, it should be discontinued.

Anticholinergics are particularly useful as adjuncts to levodopa, especially to suppress tremor. They can also be used in the mild stages of parkinsonism before levodopa is administered, and are the agents of choice in drug-induced parkinsonism. Commonly employed anticholinergics are trihexyphenidyl (Artane), available in 2- and 5-mg tablets; benztropine mesylate (Cogentin), as 1- and 2-mg tablets; ethopropazine (Parsidol), as 50- and 100-mg tablets; cycrimine (Pagitane), as 1.25- and 2.5-mg tablets; procyclidine (Kemadrin), as 2- and 5-mg tablets; and biperiden (Akineton), as 2-mg tablets. Treatment should be initiated with small doses (e.g., trihexyphenidyl, 2 mg three times daily), and gradually increased until further increases yield no additional benefit or side effects occur. Peripheral anticholinergic adverse effects include blurred vision, dry mouth, anhidrosis, hyperthermia, constipation, and urinary urgency or sometimes retention. The major symptoms of central anticholinergic effects are mental disturbances, including forgetfulness, confusion, delusions, hallucinations, somnolence, and rarely coma. The last of these can be treated with physostigmine, 0.5 to 2 mg intramuscularly. Anticholinergics tend to produce mental disturbances in the elderly and can be bypassed and levodopa used instead in older patients.

When parkinsonian symptoms cannot be adequately suppressed by amantadine or anticholinergics (alone or in combination), levodopa is employed. Peripheral adverse effects (anorexia, nausea, vomiting) can be largely avoided if levodopa is taken concomitantly with a peripheral dopa decarboxylase inhibitor. In the United States this combination is marketed as Sinemet, which contains carbidopa and levodopa. The combinations available are 10/100-mg, 25/100-mg, and 25/250-mg (carbidopa/levodopa) tablets. In other countries, both carbidopa/levodopa and benserazide/levodopa combinations are available, the latter being marketed as Madopar in 20/100-mg and 50/200-mg tablets. The more decarboxylase inhibitor used, the less likely are peripheral adverse effects. However, the potency of levodopa is enhanced, increasing the possibility of central adverse effects such as abnormal involuntary movements (chorea and dystonia), confusion, hallucinations, delusions, somnolence, and postural hypotension. One method is to begin treatment with carbidopa/levodopa, 10/100 mg three times daily. If peripheral adverse reactions appear, change to 25/100-mg tablets. There is usually a latency period before maximal benefit at a given dose is encountered. The dosage can be increased gradually, utilizing half-tablets in the incremental build-up of doses, in order to "fine tune" the patient's response. A general concept is that low dosage may prevent complications seen with chronic use, including clinical fluctuations and loss of efficacy. Therefore, the patient who is retired from his occupation can be brought to a level approximately 80 to 85 per cent free of symptoms, rather than totally free, which may require higher dosages. Still-employed persons may need higher dosages to stay at work. Concomitant administration of amantadine and anticholinergics may allow for smaller doses of levodopa, and may be especially valuable to control certain symptoms, such as tremor. Levodopa can control tremor, but is especially effective in eliminating rigidity and reducing bradykinesia. Loss of postural reflexes may be ameliorated in the early but not advanced stages of the disease. With long-term treatment central adverse effects are usually more troublesome than peripheral ones. In such situations, it may be necessary to change from carbidopa/levodopa to levodopa alone. Levodopa is available in capsules and scored tablets in strengths of 100, 250, and 500 mg. Since the potency of levodopa is increased about four-fold if given as carbidopa/levodopa, levodopa alone allows for finer adjustments of the central effects of the drug.

Levodopa is contraindicated in patients with a history of malignant melanoma and in those with psychosis or profound dementia. In the presence of cardiac arrhythmias, as much as 200 mg per day of carbidopa (available as Lodosyn from Merck, Sharp and Dohme) should be given to block peripheral formation of dopamine; in addition, antiarrhythmic agents or digoxin should be used as indicated. Levodopa can be administered safely in hepatic, renal, and hematopoietic disorders. With a history of peptic ulcer, carbidopa/levodopa is preferred over levodopa alone.

In more advanced stages of parkinsonism or with chronic administration of levodopa, central adverse effects may appear with doses that are insufficient to control the symptoms of the disease. Since levodopa dosage must be reduced in this situation, adjunctive medications may be useful. In addition to amantadine and the anticholinergics mentioned above, drugs with mild anticholinergic properties can be employed. These include diphenhydramine (Benadryl), orphenadrine (Disipal), and chlorphenoxamine (Phenoxene). They are available in 50-mg strength, and a dosage of 50 mg three times daily may prove helpful. In contrast to the more powerful anticholinergic agents, these three drugs tend to be free of producing mental disturbances.

Tricyclic antidepressants are commonly employed to relieve the depressive symptoms that often accompany parkinsonism. Amitriptyline, 50 to 75 mg at bedtime, and imipramine, 25 mg three times daily, are commonly used. For tremor incompletely relieved by antiparkinson drugs and aggravated by stress or anxiety, anxiolytic agents such as diazepam provide some relief.

Direct-acting dopamine receptor agonists have less antiparkinsonian effect than Sinemet but more than amantadine and anticholinergics. Bromocriptine (Parlodel) is commercially available; other agonists (pergolide, lisuride, mesulergine) are limited currently to investigational studies. Bromocriptine is used as an adjunct to levodopa, preferably in low dosages (up to 40 mg per day), since higher dosages are frequently accompanied by adverse reactions. The most serious toxic effects are hallucinations, delusions, and confusion, and these tend to be more severe and longer lasting than those induced by levodopa. Other adverse effects seen with levodopa also occur with bromocriptine, including anorexia, nausea, vomiting, postural hypotension, and abnormal involuntary movements. In addition, erythromelalgia (St. Anthony's fire) can occur in the extremities, probably related to an ergot effect of bromocriptine, which is an ergot derivative. Erythromelalgia disappears when the drug is discontinued. Bromocriptine unfortunately tends to lose its effect with long-term use. It is probably best employed when the patient has clinical fluctuations from levodopa or when adequate dosages of levodopa are not possible.

Clinical fluctuations from levodopa therapy usually begin to occur after the drug has been administered for two years or longer and appear in at least 40 per cent of patients on long-term therapy. These troublesome fluctuations may prevent patients from working and are resistant to control. There are two predominant forms: the "on-off" phenomenon and the "wearing-off" or "end-of-dose" effect. The on-off phenomenon consists of sudden loss of the antiparkinson effect of levodopa. Symptoms of severe parkinsonism may produce immobility from severe bradykinesia and rigidity. The "off" states appear irregularly and may last up to several hours. They may occur several times daily and disappear ("on" effect) as suddenly as they occur, even without another dose of levodopa. Higher dosages of levodopa or bromocriptine can prevent these on-off episodes, but usually induce continuous and distressing dyskinesias.

The wearing-off phenomenon comes on gradually, as plasma levels of levodopa fall to low levels. The phenomenon is a pharmacokinetic effect due to reduced bioavailability of levodopa as a result of its short half-life in plasma (30 to 45 minutes). Spacing the doses more closely is a partial remedy, and some patients take levodopa every three hours, every two hours, or even more frequently to prevent the "off" periods. Unfortunately, the price is to cause a state of continual dyskinesia. Perhaps longer-acting dopamine agonists will solve this problem. Some patients with severe wearing-off phenomena are unable to miss a single dose of levodopa without being in an "off" state, and if awakened in the middle of the night are immobile. These "dopa addicts" require levodopa before retiring for the night and perhaps during the night. Patients who are free of clinical fluctuations do not usually require bedtime medication and can be maintained on three doses a day.

Drug holidays from levodopa can temporarily reverse clinical fluctuations and loss of drug efficacy. The concept is that the abstinence restores sensitivity of dopamine receptors, making them once again respond to the drug. The risks and discomfort are serious. Because of immobility and the possibility of aspiration, such levodopa withdrawal must be done in a hospital. Usually a patient is too uncomfortable to be off levodopa for longer than a few days, although ten days is the goal. Swallowing difficulty should terminate this withdrawal period in order to avoid aspiration. It is not certain that the long-term benefit from a drug holiday is sufficient to justify the risks involved.

Treatment of postencephalitic parkinsonism usually requires smaller dosages of levodopa than does idiopathic parkinsonism. Drug-induced parkinsonism responds well to anticholinergics. Striatonigral degeneration may respond to levodopa in the early stages of the disease, but then becomes resistant to therapy, as does progressive supranuclear palsy. In such diseases, in which striatal dopamine receptors are not responsive to levodopa or dopamine agonists, anticholinergics are the drugs of choice. Unfortunately, these agents offer only modest relief of symptoms compared to the usually dramatic relief of idiopathic parkinsonism by levodopa.

SURGICAL MEASURES. Stereotactic lesions of the ventrolateral thalamus can alleviate tremor and rigidity of the contralateral limbs. This approach is not useful for bradykinesia and loss of postural reflexes, which are the predominant causes of disability, nor does it halt progression of the disease. Moreover, bilateral surgery to relieve tremor on both sides usually results in impaired speech. With the introduction of levodopa therapy, surgical therapy has almost entirely been discontinued.

COURSE OF THE PARKINSONIAN SYNDROME. Although levodopa and other drugs do not alter the progression of the disease, they do increase survival time because of improved functional capacity. The mortality rate, which was three times that of the normal population, has been reduced by half since the introduction of levodopa. The symptom that becomes least responsive is loss of postural reflexes, and falling with resultant hip fracture is a potential consequence. Although chronic levodopa therapy may bring troublesome adverse effects of clinical fluctuations, dyskinesias, mental disturbances, and loss of efficacy, many patients continue to have a substantial response to the drug for a decade or more.

Earnest MP, Fahn S, Karp JH, Rowland LP: Normal pressure hydrocephalus and hypertensive cerebrovascular disease. Arch Neurol 31:262, 1974. *Discusses concept of arteriosclerotic (vascular) parkinsonism and its possible mechanism via normal pressure hydrocephalus.*

Fahn S: Secondary parkinsonism. *In* Goldensohn ES, Appel SH (eds.): Scientific Approaches to Clinical Neurology. Philadelphia, Lea & Febiger, 1977, pp 1159–1189. *A classification and review of causes of parkinsonism other than Parkinson's disease.*

Fahn S, Duffy P: Parkinson's disease. *In* Goldensohn ES, Appel SH (eds.): Scientific Approaches to Clinical Neurology. Philadelphia, Lea & Febiger, 1977, pp 1119–1158. *Thorough review of this illness.*

Hoehn MM, Yahr MD: Parkinsonism: Onset, progression and mortality. Neurology 17:427, 1967. *Provides the best data on the progression of parkinsonism prior to the introduction of levodopa therapy.*

Langston JW, Ballard P, Tetrud JW, Irwin I: Chronic parkinsonism in humans due to a product of meperidine-analog synthesis. Science 219:979, 1983. *A report describing young adults who developed acute parkinsonism after self-injection of a toxic substance known as MPTP.*

Marsden CD, Parkes JD, Quinn N: Fluctuations of disability in Parkinson's disease—clinical aspects. *In* Marsden CD, Fahn S (eds.): Movement Disorders. London, Butterworth Scientific, 1982, pp 96–122. *A detailed account of the varieties of clinical fluctuations seen in patients with parkinsonism due to the disease and due to levodopa therapy.*

Mayeux R: Depression and dementia in Parkinson's disease. *In* Marsden CD, Fahn S (eds.): Movement Disorders. London, Butterworth Scientific, 1982, pp 75–95. *A review of the literature documenting the prevalence of symptoms of depression and dementia in patients with Parkinson's disease.*

484. ESSENTIAL TREMOR (Familial or Senile Tremor)

Essential tremor is a monosymptomatic disorder, expressed as tremor of the hands, head, and, least frequently, voice. The tremor in the hands is usually more rapid than that encountered in parkinsonism and occurs with volitional movement instead of at rest. It is aggravated by handwriting and suppressed by the use of alcohol. The age of onset is variable, typically beginning at least mildly before the age of 25 and persisting throughout life with some increase in intensity and spread to other body parts. Physical and social disability may result. There is a strong familial incidence distributed as an autosomal dominant trait. With late-life onset, the tremor is commonly called *senile tremor*. No specific pathologic lesion has been reported in the nervous system in this condition. An occasional patient may develop Parkinson's disease on top of a longstanding history of essential tremor. Beta-adrenergic blocking agents are useful in some patients, but dramatic relief of tremor is not achieved with these drugs. Propranolol* in a dosage of 120 to 240 mg per day in three or four divided doses has been most commonly used. The selective beta-1 adrenergic blocker metoprolol seems to be equally effective in doses of 50 mg three times daily. This drug has the advantage that it can be used in patients with bronchospasm or asthma. Beta-adrenergic blockers should be avoided in patients with congestive heart failure or heart block. It is probably safer to avoid the use of drugs in the elderly population. Some wine with meals offers sufficient relief while the hands are engaged in feeding. The major differential diagnosis is parkinsonism, but the lack of bradykinesia, rigidity, and postural abnormalities, as well as the presence of tremor with action instead of at rest, rules out that disorder.

Fahn S: Differential diagnosis of tremors. Med Clin North Am 56:1363, 1972. *Describes the clinical approach in diagnosing tremors and presents a useful classification.*

Newman RP, Jacobs L: Metoprolol in essential tremor. Arch Neurol 37:596, 1980. *Reports the successful use of metoprolol to control tremor in the presence of asthma.*

Young RR, Shahani BT: Pharmacology of tremor. Clin Neuropharmacol 4:139, 1979. *Reviews pharmacologic evaluations of tremor.*

485. THE CHOREAS

A large number of disorders may present with choreic movements (Table 485–1), having in common brief, involuntary contractions. It is important to determine whether the movements are fluid-like (flowing from one location to another), as in classic choreic disorders, or whether they are rhythmically repetitive in the same site (stereotypy), as in tardive dyskinesia. The presence of other neurologic deficits (gait disturbance, dementia) can assist in the diagnosis of Huntington's disease, and a detailed family history and drug history are essential for reliable diagnosis. A difficult diagnostic problem is encountered in the patient with Huntington's disease who has been treated with antipsychotic drugs. Such patients can present with a mixed picture of tardive dyskinesia and Huntington's disease.

*This use is not listed in the manufacturer's directive.

TABLE 485–1. A CLASSIFICATION OF COMMON CAUSES OF CHOREA

I. Hereditary
  A. Huntington's disease
  B. Wilson's disease
  C. Ataxia-telangiectasia
  D. Lesch-Nyhan syndrome
  E. Chorea-acanthocytosis
II. Secondary
  A. Infections
    1. Sydenham's chorea
    2. Encephalitis
  B. Drugs
    1. Levodopa
    2. Estrogen (oral contraceptives)
    3. Phenytoin
    4. Antipsychotic drugs
  C. Metabolic and endocrine
    1. Chorea gravidarum
    2. Thyrotoxicosis
  D. Vascular
    1. Lupus erythematosus
    2. Polycythemia vera
    3. Hemichorea-hemiballism
III. Unknown
  A. Senile chorea

HEREDITARY CHOREA (Chronic Progressive Chorea, Huntington's Disease)

Huntington's disease is the most common of the hereditary choreas. It is a progressive degenerative disorder predominantly affecting the basal ganglia and the cerebral cortex. Clinically, it is manifested by a triad consisting of choreic movements, intellectual decline leading to dementia, and emotional disturbances. The disease is transmitted as an autosomal dominant trait with complete penetrance. Both sexes are equally affected, and each offspring has a 50 per cent chance of becoming affected. In the United States the prevalence ranges from 4 to 8 per 100,000 population. The disease usually begins in adulthood after childbearing, with a peak age at onset of 40 years; it can begin at any age, however, and in approximately 10 per cent onset occurs before the age of 20 (juvenile Huntington's disease). As a general rule, juvenile cases exhibit bradykinesia and rigidity, rather than chorea and hypotonia. The presence of a movement disorder is essential to the disease; emotional disturbances and cognitive disorders are common problems in the general population and hence are not sufficient by themselves for the diagnosis. Motor symptoms begin with clumsiness and the dropping of objects. The choreic movements then become apparent, typically consisting first of brief, low amplitude movements of the fingers, but spreading to involve all parts of the body (arms, legs, trunk, neck, and face). The movements can be proximal as well as distal in the limbs, and flow from one site to another. In the face they are more common in the forehead than around the mouth (the latter being more common in tardive dyskinesia). It is difficult for the patient to keep the tongue protruded for 20 seconds and to maintain a steady tight grip (causing a milkmaid grip). The chorea is more pronounced on standing and walking, and abnormal gait is characterized by hesitation and stuttering steps. Postural instability develops, often with subsequent falls. Choking is a common and sometimes fatal symptom.

Emotional disorders are common in Huntington's disease and may precede choreic movements. Personality changes, mania, hallucinations, delusions, paranoia, schizophrenia, impulsiveness, hostility, and agitation can develop, sometimes as the first sign of involvement. Most common are apathy and withdrawn behavior with a decrease in conversation and inattention to personal hygiene. Depression is frequent and leads to an increased incidence of suicide. These personality disturbances are especially troublesome for the family of the affected person. Cognitive changes tend to appear later. There is impairment of recent memory and judgment, loss of capacity to plan and organize, and intellectual decline. Dementia leads to urinary and fecal incontinence and an inability to handle activities of daily living (see also Ch. 479).

Pathologically, there is loss of neurons with reactive gliosis in many regions of the brain, particularly in the striatum and cerebral cortex. Cell loss is accompanied by depletion of neurotransmitters, the most consistent effect being a marked reduction of GABA and its synthesizing enzyme, glutamic acid decarboxylase, in the basal ganglia. There is also a loss of acetylcholine neurons and of dopamine, acetylcholine, and serotonin receptors. Treatment with GABA agonists or cholinergic agonists has not led to clinical improvement.

The differential diagnosis of chorea is long (Table 485–1), but the triad of chorea, progressive dementia, and emotional disturbances strongly suggests Huntington's disease. The diagnosis is readily apparent if a positive family history is obtained, but such a history may be lacking because a parent is unavailable, has disappeared, or has died before symptoms appeared. The lack of a positive family history in the presence of longevity and good health of the parents raises questions of paternity, spontaneous mutation, or incorrect diagnosis. Computed tomography of the head eventually will reveal atrophy of the caudate nuclei; this may assist in the diagnosis. Accurate diagnosis of affected persons and carriers is now possible by identifying a genetic marker linked to the Huntington gene.

The technique has great promise for both diagnosis and prevention by confident genetic counseling.

Treatment of Huntington's disease should extend to the family as well as the patient, since this is a hereditary disorder with potential involvement of offspring and since the mental symptoms create enormous family stress. Explaining the disease and offering nondirective genetic discussion of the inheritance pattern are important and will enable family members who are at risk for the disease or are known carriers to reach a decision about having children. Therapy is available for many of the symptoms. Presynaptic dopamine-depleting agents (reserpine and tetrabenazine) and postsynaptic dopamine antagonists (antipsychotic agents) can reduce chorea, although the latter drugs are less effective than the former and may cause tardive dyskinesia. Reserpine therapy should begin with a small dose (0.25 mg per day); the daily dosage is then increased weekly by 0.25 mg until chorea declines. As much as 8 to 10 mg per day may be required. A slow buildup in dosage will usually avoid nasal stuffiness and depression. Postural hypotension and increased apathy can occur and necessitate a reduction in dosage. Dementia is not treatable, but emotional disturbances can be ameliorated. Tricyclic antidepressants are useful for depression, and antipsychotic agents can treat psychosis.

Chorea-acanthocytosis is much less common in the United States than is Huntington's disease but is more common in Japan. It is manifested by mild chorea and tics, self-mutilation (usually of lips and tongue), loss of tendon reflexes, elevated serum creatine phosphokinase, presence of acanthocytes in the blood, and atrophy of the caudate nuclei. Other hereditary disorders that can manifest chorea are covered elsewhere: Wilson's disease in Ch. 205, ataxia telangiectasia in Ch. 492, and Lesch-Nyhan syndrome in Ch. 196.

Barbeau A, Chase TN, Paulson GW (eds.): Huntington's chorea, 1872–1972. Adv Neurol, Vol 1, 1973. *The first monograph summarizing previous studies and presenting new data, including the observation of reduced GABA levels.*

Chase TN, Wexler NS, Barbeau A (eds.): Huntington's disease. Adv Neurol, Vol 23, 1979. *Provides an update of the voluminous research that has been conducted on Huntington's disease since 1972.*

Gusella JF, Wexler NS, Conneally PM, et al.: A polymorphic DNA marker genetically linked to Huntington's disease. Nature 306:234, 1983. *Reports the localization of the gene for Huntington's disease to chromosome 4.*

Kuhl DE, Phelps ME, Markham CH, Metter EJ, Riege WH, Winter J: Cerebral metabolism and atrophy in Huntington's disease determined by 18-FDG and computed tomographic scan. Ann Neurol 12:425, 1982. *Positron emission tomography reveals hypometabolism of striatum in patients with Huntington's disease and in some at-risk individuals.*

Sakai T, Mawatari S, Iwashita H, Goto I, Kuroiwa Y: Chorea-acanthocytosis: Clues to clinical diagnosis. Arch Neurol 38:335, 1981. *Descriptions of the clinical features of chorea-acanthocytosis, which is more common in Japan than in the United States.*

Shoulson I: Care of patients and families with Huntington's disease. *In* Marsden CD, Fahn S (eds.): Movement Disorders. London, Butterworth Scientific, 1982, pp 277–290. *Describes a practical approach to the diagnosis, genetic counseling, and management of families with Huntington's disease.*

SECONDARY CHOREA

Acquired chorea has many causes (Table 485–1), which the history, examination, and laboratory studies can usually distinguish. Clinically, the choreic movements are similar in the different disorders except for tardive dyskinesia.

SYDENHAM'S CHOREA (St. Vitus' Dance). This is an acute chorea encountered primarily during childhood, with the greatest incidence between the ages of five and fifteen. Later occurrence is uncommon, but it can be associated with pregnancy (chorea gravidarum). There is a female preponderance after the age of ten. A close relationship exists with rheumatic fever, and the condition has declined substantially in recent years.

The choreic movements in this disorder are usually generalized, and only 20 per cent of patients have hemichorea. The brief, involuntary movements flow from site to site, and the patient has difficulty sitting quietly. Fidgety behavior, clumsiness, dropping of objects, dysarthria, and an awkward gait are common. Other neurologic symptoms are infrequent.

Sydenham's chorea is not fatal, and recovery occurs in two to six months. Pathologic studies have been few and have disclosed scattered lesions of vasculitis in the cortex, basal ganglia, cerebellum, and brainstem. There are no specific laboratory abnormalities. The differential diagnosis depends on eliminating other causes of chorea by appropriate history and laboratory studies.

Recurrence, with as many as two or three attacks over a period of years, occurs in almost one third of the patients. Since the disease is self-limited, specific drugs may not be necessary. If the chorea is disabling and interferes with school work, antichoreic drugs are used. Short-term treatment with perphenazine (12 to 16 mg per day in divided doses) or haloperidol (3 to 6 mg per day in divided doses) can be effective. Some patients with Sydenham's chorea may have residual deficits of valvular heart disease, behavioral problems, mild motor abnormalities, and a poor performance in psychometric testing.

HEMIBALLISM. Hemiballism is a forceful, violent form of hemichorea manifested by flinging movements of the limbs on one side of the body. The most common cause is a vascular lesion, either a hemorrhage or an infarct involving the opposite subthalamic nucleus. Tumors rarely are involved. Most often hemiballism or hemichorea develops on recovery from a hemiparesis and hemisensory deficit secondary to stroke. Occasionally the sensorimotor deficits are minor, and ballism occurs as the initial event. Like other abnormal involuntary movements, hemiballism disappears during sleep. In most instances, the intensity of hemiballism decreases gradually to hemichorea and then fades away after several weeks, but in some patients the movements persist. Severe movements can be exhausting but can be controlled with drugs such as reserpine or antipsychotic agents. Because of the self-limiting nature of hemiballism, it is reasonable to use antipsychotics for their rapid onset of action and then slowly withdraw the drug to avoid producing tardive dyskinesia.

SENILE CHOREA. Occasional patients, usually older than 60 years, present with generalized chorea resembling Huntington's disease, but with no associated dementia, emotional disturbance, positive family history, or evidence of other etiologies. Postmortem studies reveal striatal pathology identical to that of Huntington's disease. It has been speculated that such so-called senile chorea is a late-onset form of Huntington's disease in which cognitive symptoms have not developed because of the advanced age of onset. No definitive genetic studies are available.

Aron A, Freeman J, Carter S: The natural history of Sydenham's chorea. Am J Med 38:83, 1965. *One third of patients evaluated an average of 29 years after the initial episode of chorea were found to have valvular heart disease.*

Bird MT, Palkes H, Prensky AL: A follow-up study of Sydenham's chorea. Neurology 26:601, 1976. *An average of an eight-year follow-up evaluation revealed that some individuals have behavioral disorders, abnormal electroencephalograms, and poorer performance on psychometric testing.*

Johnson WG, Fahn S: Treatment of vascular hemiballism and hemichorea. Neurology 27:634, 1977. *Reports on the effectiveness of the antipsychotic drug perphenazine in eight cases of hemiballism.*

Klawans HI, Moses H, Nausieda PA, Bergen D, Weiner WJ: Treatment and prognosis of hemiballism. N Engl J Med 295:1348, 1976. *Report on the effectiveness of haloperidol and chlorpromazine in 11 cases.*

Nausieda PA, Grossman BJ, Koller WC, Weiner WJ, Klawans HL: Syndenham's chorea: An update. Neurology 30:331, 1980. *This survey points out the marked decrease in the incidence of the disorder in recent years.*

TARDIVE DYSKINESIA

This most feared complication of antipsychotic drug therapy can persist indefinitely. The disorder is associated with chronic administration of these drugs (hence the name "tardive"), but there are reports of its occurring after exposure of only several weeks. Tardive dyskinesia is more common in women and the elderly, and is more likely to occur with exposure to high dosages and longer duration of treatment. The drugs themselves mask the symptoms so that onset is not clearly recognized. Withdrawal of the drug exposes the dyskinesia, which consists of rhythmically repetitive, rapid movements that can occur in most parts of the body. The lower part of the face is involved most often; this oral-lingual-buccal dyskinesia resembles continual chewing movements, with the tongue intermittently darting out of the mouth ("fly-catcher" tongue). In the trunk the movements usually assume a repetitive flexion and extension pattern ("body-rocking"). The distal parts of the limbs may show incessant flexion-extension movements ("piano-playing" fingers and toes), whereas the proximal muscles are usually spared. On standing the patient may have repetitive movements of the legs ("marching in place"). Superficially, the gait may appear unaffected, but the arms tend to swing to a larger degree than normal and the stride may elongate. The patient may be unaware of the movements unless there is an associated akathisia (a subjective feeling of restlessness), characterized by the need to move about and walk back and forth. Sometimes patients describe feeling as if they were going to jump out of their skin. This is the most distressing symptom in the tardive dyskinesia syndrome, and resembles the acute akathisia that sometimes accompanies an initial administration of antipsychotic drugs, but disappears when the drug is withdrawn. In contrast, akathisia as it occurs in tardive dyskinesia is a chronic form that is made more severe by drug withdrawal; hence it is analogous to the dyskinesia. Both tardive akathisia and tardive dyskinesia can be suppressed by antidopaminergic drugs.

The major differential diagnoses are Huntington's disease and a focal form of facial and mandibular dystonia referred to as Meige's syndrome. Huntington's disease is particularly difficult to differentiate from tardive dyskinesia because choreic movements and emotional disturbances occur in both disorders. However, several helpful signs serve to distinguish between these two conditions (Table 485–2). Patients with known Huntington's disease also may develop tardive dyskinesia if antipsychotic drugs are used in its treatment. Meige's syndrome causes long-lasting facial movements (sustained dystonic movements), compared to the rapid, brief, and repetitive movements in tardive dyskinesia. A drug-free history eliminates tardive dyskinesia by definition.

In addition to the classic form of tardive dyskinesia described above, there are two clinical variations. One is the self-limiting "withdrawal emergent" syndrome, in which choreic movements resembling those seen in Sydenham's chorea or Huntington's disease appear when the antipsychotic drug is suddenly discontinued. There are flowing, rather than repetitive, choreic movements. The withdrawal emergent syndrome is most common in children. Reintroducing the antipsychotic drug and tapering it slowly may eliminate the symptoms. The other variant is the presence of sustained dystonic movements rather than choreic movements. This variant (tardive dystonia) is more common in young adults than in the elderly population.

TABLE 485–2. DIFFERENTIAL DIAGNOSIS OF TARDIVE DYSKINESIA AND HUNTINGTON'S DISEASE*

Clinical Features	Tardive Dyskinesia	Huntington's Disease
Akathisia	Present	Absent
Body-rocking	Present	Absent
Marching-in-place	Present	Absent
Oral-lingual-buccal dyskinesia	Present	Sometimes present
Darting tongue	Present	Rarely present
Repetitive movements	Present	Absent
Flowing movements	Absent	Present
Forehead chorea	Absent	Present
Saccadic eye movements	Normal	Abnormal
Protrusion of tongue	Maintained (normal)	Not maintained
Milkmaid grip	Absent	Present
Postural stability	Normal	Impaired
Walking	Reduces chorea	Increases chorea
Gait	Normal	Stuttering, ataxic

*Although the tabulated clinical features may be found in any individual patient, they are not always present in every patient.

Tardive dyskinesia is believed to be caused by the development of supersensitive dopamine receptors as a result of chronic blockade by antipsychotic drugs. There is no satisfactory explanation of why the disorder is often permanent. Some patients who remain drug free for several months to years have a resolution of the syndrome, and withdrawal of the offending agents is the treatment of choice. But many patients, particularly those with psychosis or severe tardive akathisia, must continue to take antidopaminergic drugs to suppress these disabling symptoms. Antipsychotic drug therapy may be required to treat psychosis. If the patient does not have psychosis, then dopamine-depleting drugs (reserpine and alpha-methylparatyrosine) that act presynaptically are the preferred agents and can relieve both the dyskinesia and akathisia. The dosages are increased slowly, as in the treatment of Huntington's chorea. The approach to treatment is diagrammed below.

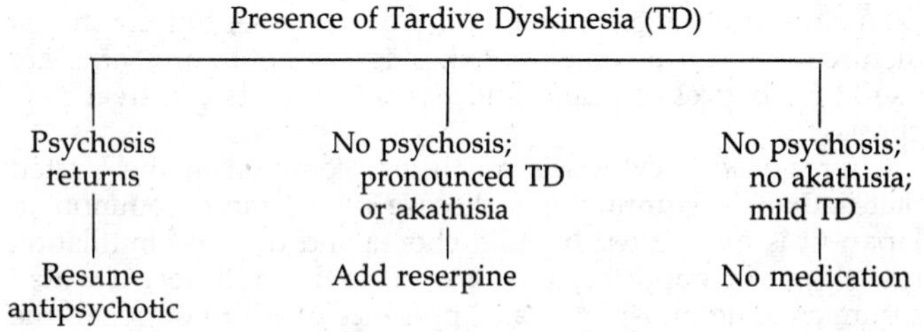

Levodopa administration for a few months to desensitize the dopamine receptors, followed by its withdrawal, is being evaluated as a therapeutic agent.

The incidence of tardive dyskinesia appears to be increasing owing to widespread administration of antipsychotic drugs. It is important to consider this complication before prescribing these agents. Such drugs should be used only in clinical situations in which no satisfactory alternatives exist.

Alpert M, Friedhoff AJ, Diamond F: Use of dopamine receptor agonists to reduce dopamine receptor number as treatment for tardive dyskinesia. Adv Neurol 37:253, 1983. *Report of partial success in treating tardive dyskinesia with levodopa, followed by its withdrawal after eight weeks.*

Baldessarini RJ, Tarsy D: Tardive dyskinesia. *In* Lipton J, DiMascio A, Killam KF (eds.): Psychopharmacology. A Generation of Progress. New York, Raven Press, 1978, pp 993–1004. *A concise review of the clinical features and the pharmacology of tardive dyskinesia.*

Fahn S: Treatment of tardive dyskinesia: Use of dopamine-depleting agents. Clin Neuropharmacol 6:151, 1983. *Report of control of tardive dyskinesia and tardive akathisia with the use of reserpine and alpha-methylparatyrosine.*

486. OTHER EXTRAPYRAMIDAL DISORDERS

MYOCLONUS

Myoclonic jerks are sudden, shock-like muscular contractions or inhibitions (the latter are called negative myoclonus). They can be singular or repetitive, rhythmic or arrhythmic, symmetrical or asymmetrical, synchronous or asynchronous, and generalized, segmental, or focal. Typically, myoclonic jerks occur unpredictably and irregularly. However, a form of regular and rhythmic myoclonus exists, *palatal myoclonus,* which results from infarction or degeneration involving some of the anatomic triangle that links the dentate nucleus, red nucleus, and inferior olivary nucleus. This form is categorized as myoclonus (rather than tremor) because of its synchronous (instead of alternating) contractions. Lesions in many parts of the nervous system, including spinal cord, brainstem, cerebellum, and cerebral cortex, can give rise to myoclonus. Myoclonus is most often a symptom of an irritable nervous system. It is present in many diseases (Table 486–1) but can also occur as an isolated phenomenon (essential myoclonus). When associated with objective neurologic findings, it is usually progressive. In contrast, essential myoclonus (familial or sporadic) tends to be stable and nonprogressive. Nocturnal myoclonus, now called "peri-

TABLE 486–1. A CLASSIFICATION OF COMMON FORMS OF MYOCLONUS

I. Benign myoclonic jerks
  A. Physiologic: sleep jerks, anxiety
  B. Essential myoclonus: familial or sporadic
  C. Periodic movements of sleep
  D. Associated with petit mal or grand mal seizures
II. Symptomatic myoclonus
  A. Myoclonus epilepsy
  B. Dementias: Creutzfeldt-Jakob, Alzheimer's
  C. Infectious: subacute sclerosing panencephalitis
  D. Lipidoses
  E. Cerebellar degenerations
  F. Hypoxia
  G. Toxins: methyl bromide, strychnine
  H. Drugs: levodopa, tricyclics
  I. Systemic illnesses: uremia, hepatic, dialysis encephalopathy
III. Rhythmic myoclonus
  A. Palatal myoclonus
  B. Ocular myoclonus

odic movements of sleep" because of its regularity, may awaken patients from sleep; it is often associated with "restless legs syndrome," dysesthesias, and mild dyskinesias while awake.

To treat myoclonic syndromes, especially posthypoxic action myoclonus, clonazepam is the drug of first choice. Because drowsiness and ataxia are common adverse effects, the dosage of clonazepam should be increased gradually until improvement or adverse effects are encountered. A dosage as high as 8 mg per day (in four divided doses) may be necessary. Valproate is another useful drug; the dosage should be increased gradually until it is effective or toxic. As much as 3000 mg per day may be necessary. The combination of clonazepam and valproate can be particularly effective. Other useful drugs include carbamazepine (up to 1000 mg per day), diazepam (up to 40 mg per day), and the serotonin precursor 5-hydroxytryptophan. The last-named drug is not available commercially in the United States.

Marsden CD, Hallett M, Fahn S: The nosology and pathophysiology of myoclonus. *In* Marsden CD, Fahn S (eds.): Movement Disorders. London, Butterworth Scientific, 1982, pp 196–248. *Most recent review of myoclonus. It presents a classification scheme based on etiology.*

TICS (Habit Spasms, Gilles de la Tourette's Syndrome)

A tic is a sudden rapid series of involuntary movements that are usually complex and coordinated. For example, an irregular sequence of movements can contain such diverse movements as eye blinking, head shaking, shoulder shrugging, and limb and facial gestures. In some instances patients describe a compelling need to make these movements. Tics can be voluntarily controlled for brief intervals, but such conscious efforts are usually followed by more intense and frequent contractions. Stress and anxiety aggravate tics, and psychotherapeutic management may diminish them.

In some individuals tics reflect recurrent nervous mannerisms appropriately called habit spasms. Other tics are caused by neurologic disorders. They may be present in the acute phase of encephalitis or as a sequela of encephalitis. Most tics are of unknown etiology and are sometimes familial. Tics can be considered in a spectrum, from transient tics of childhood, through persistent tics, to the most severe type in which vocal tics are also present. This last form is known as Gilles de la Tourette's syndrome. Vocalizations occur as various involuntary and compulsive sounds (barking, sniffing, throat clearing, yelping noises) and words or fragments of words, often obscene (coprolalia). Motor tics in Tourette's syndrome may also include obscene gestures (copropraxia). The age of onset is usually between two and fifteen years. As a general rule, there are periods of remissions and exacerbations, and the tics move from one part of the body to another. Many patients show a tendency for the tics to become less severe and more controllable with age. The presence of vocal tics, especially coprolalia, adds a new dimension to the patient's problem of adjusting in society. Patients are hesitant to be seen in public, and avoid areas where silence is required (cinema, theater, library). They are frequently misunderstood, teased, or insulted by schoolmates, teachers, and strangers. No anatomic abnormalities have been observed in the brain, but the consistency of the clinical syndrome gives every evidence that Tourette's syndrome is an organic disorder.

Haloperidol appears to be the most effective drug for treating tics and is given in divided doses up to 20 mg or more a day. Treatment is begun with a small dosage and increased slowly until control is achieved or adverse affects are obtained. Unfortunately, haloperidol affects personality ("zombie" effect) and school performance. Furthermore, there is a danger of inducing tardive dyskinesia or its variants. Other drugs should be tried initially, such as clonazepam (3 to 6 mg a day) and clonidine (up to 0.6 mg daily) in divided doses.

Friedhoff AJ, Chase TN (eds.): Gilles de la Tourette syndrome. Adv Neurol, Vol 36, 1982. *The proceedings of the first international symposium on this subject. It provides reports of many studies on tic disorders.*
Golden GS: Tics and Tourette's: A continuum of symptoms? Ann Neurol 4:145, 1978. *Describes families in which some individuals have only motor tics and others have both motor and vocal tics (Tourette's syndrome) and suggests a continuum of tic syndromes.*
Shapiro AK, Shapiro ES, Bruun RD, Sweet RD: Gilles de la Tourette Syndrome. New York, Raven Press, 1978. *Thorough review of the literature and an analysis of the large number of cases personally observed by the authors.*

ATHETOSIS (Mobile Spasms)

Clinically, athetosis falls between the rapid movements of chorea and the sustained movements of dystonia. The term is applied to constant writhing and twisting movements without fixed postures. Yet as the spectrum of torsion dystonia becomes better appreciated, athetosis increasingly seems to be part of the dystonic syndromes; athetotic dystonia may therefore be a more appropriate name. Athetosis is most frequently encountered in patients who suffered perinatal brain injury, usually from hypoxic damage (athetotic cerebral palsy). Athetosis has also been reported in kernicterus, in rare childhood degenerative diseases of the basal ganglia, in glutaric aciduria, and after hemiplegia secondary to strokes in childhood. Athetosis thus appears to be the expression of torsion dystonia caused by basal ganglia damage at an early, still developing age. In athetotic cerebral palsy pathologic studies reveal either status marmoratus of the striatum or status dysmyelinatus of the globus pallidus.

Athetosis involves the limbs (distal and proximal), trunk, neck, face, and tongue. The movements are enhanced when the patient attemps to speak ("overflow"). Speech is impaired with poor articulation, in part becuse of continual tongue movements and facial movements. Stress and attempted voluntary movements also bring out an overflow of writhing movements throughout the body. This increase of athetotic movements makes it difficult for the patient to handle daily tasks. There is no satisfactory treatment. Diazepam or anticholinergic agents may provide a little amelioration.

Dooling EC, Adams RD: The pathological anatomy of posthemiplegic athetosis. Brain 98:29, 1975. *Describes pathologically documented cases of unilateral athetosis following childhood hemiplegia.*
Leibel RL, Shih VE, Goodman SI, Bauman ML, McCabe ERB, Zwerdling RG, Bergman I, Costello C: Glutaric acidemia: A metabolic disorder causing progressive choreoathetosis. Neurology 30:1163, 1980. *A newly described metabolic error and a cause of infantile athetotic dystonia.*
Spiegel EA, Baird HW: Athetotic syndromes. *In* Vinken PJ, Bruyn GW (eds.): Handbook of Clinical Neurology, Vol 6. Amsterdam, North-Holland, 1968, pp 440–475. *The best and most thorough clinical review of athetosis in a relatively sparse literature on this subject.*

487. THE DYSTONIAS

TORSION DYSTONIA (Dystonia Musculorum Deformans, Torsion Spasms)

The torsion dystonias comprise a group of disorders in which twisting movements (torsion spasms) are characteristic. Slow torsion spasms are called athetotic dystonia or athetosis, but more often torsion spasms are rapid and are mistakenly called chorea. One characteristic feature of torsion spasms is their propensity to be maintained at the end of the movement for a second or so (dystonic movements) and even for minutes to hours (dystonic postures). Ultimately contractures can occur, leading to permanent deformity, especially in the still-growing child. Both agonist and antagonist muscles contract simultaneously in dystonia. Dystonia can be present when the patient is at rest or in the process of a volitional movement (action dystonia). In carrying out a voluntary movement, inappropriate muscles contract when they should be quiescent. Dystonic movements are sometimes broken up into a tremor pattern (dystonic tremor), which may be due to the patient's attempt to resist the abnormal pulling and maintain a more normal posture. Dystonia varies with change of posture, worsens with stress, decreases with relaxation or hypnosis, disappears with sleep, and is modified by tactile or proprioceptive input.

The torsion dystonias can be etiologically divided into primary and secondary types (Table 487–1). The first is more common and includes hereditary forms (both autosomal recessive and autosomal dominant) and those that are sporadic or idiopathic. The autosomal recessive form is found most often in Ashkenazic Jews and commonly begins between the ages of five and fifteen. The legs are typically affected first, starting with action dystonia. At rest the patient may seem normal, but when he stands or walks, one or both feet assume an equinovarus posture and the leg executes a bizarre stepping twisting movement. As the disease progresses, the other leg and other parts of the body become involved. Lordosis, scoliosis, tortipelvis, and torticollis can appear. Because of modification by proprioceptive input, walking backward may be less abnormal than walking forward. Action dystonia of the arms interferes with handwriting and other manipulations. Dystonic movements appear when the patient is at rest, and eventually dystonic postures may develop. When dystonic movements are absent, muscle tone is normal or hypotonic; hypertonia accompanies dystonic movements. Mentation, sensation, strength, and tendon reflexes remain normal. Not all patients show progression. Many tend to plateau after a period of progression.

Autosomal dominant and sporadic dystonia each follow the same pattern as the recessive form, except that the age of onset tends to be somewhat older and the disease is usually less progressive. Penetrance is usually incomplete, and there are many formes frustes in other members of the family: club foot, scoliosis, torticollis, writer's cramp, and essential tremor.

As a general rule, the younger the age of onset of dystonia, the more likely the disease is to begin in the feet and legs and to become progressive and generalized: juvenile onset tends to begin in the hands and arms and plateaus after involving several segments; adult onset tends to remain focal, the neck being the most common site (spasmodic torticollis). Other common varieties of focal dystonia are blepharospasm, facial and mandibular dystonia (Meige's syndrome), spastic dysphonia, and writer's cramp. Primary dystonia with childhood onset is also referred to as dystonia musculorum deformans.

TABLE 487–1. A CLASSIFICATION OF COMMON DYSTONIC STATES

I. Primary
  A. Hereditary
    1. Autosomal dominant trait
    2. Autosomal recessive trait
  B. Idiopathic
II. Secondary
  A. Associated with other neurologic syndromes
    1. Wilson's disease
    2. Huntington's disease
    3. Hallervorden-Spatz disease
  B. Environmental causes
    1. Perinatal cerebral injury
    2. Encephalitis
    3. Head trauma
    4. Focal cerebrovascular injury
    5. Toxins: manganese, carbon monoxide
    6. Drugs: phenothiazines, levodopa

No clear-cut pathologic lesions have been discerned in the brain in primary torsion dystonia. It is assumed that the lesion is of a chemical and physiologic nature, affecting the basal ganglia, especially the striatum, since this is the area of pathology in secondary or acquired forms of dystonia. Moreover, drugs that affect the basal ganglia (i.e., levodopa, antipsychotic agents) can induce dystonic movements and postures.

A variety of drugs have been proposed to treat torsion dystonia, but none has been consistently effective. High dosage anticholinergics are often effective and are well tolerated in children if the daily dose is increased gradually. A recommended schedule is to begin with trihexyphenidyl (Artane), 2.5 mg twice daily, and increase the daily dosage at a rate of 2.5 mg weekly. The dosage should be increased until there is satisfactory improvement or intolerable adverse effects. As much as 50 mg per day in four divided doses may be necessary. Unfortunately, most adults cannot tolerate high dosages of anticholinergics. Common adverse effects are dry mouth, blurred vision, forgetfulness, and confusion. Other compounds that may provide some benefit are carbamazepine (Tegretol, 400 to 800 mg per day), diazepam (Valium, 30 to 60 mg per day), and, rarely, levodopa (500 to 1500 mg per day). Dorsal column stimulation may help some patients. Stereotactic thalamotomies can be effective for limb dystonia, but several repeat procedures may be necessary, and bilateral surgery entails a high risk of producing a major speech deficit. Patients should not undergo such surgery unless they are well aware of the risks, have had an adequate trial of pharmacologic agents, and have intractable, disabling symptoms.

SPASMODIC TORTICOLLIS

Spasmodic torticollis is the most common of the various forms of focal torsion dystonia. It usually begins in adulthood and remains limited to this region of the body. Occasionally there is spread to involve the vocal cords (spastic dysphonia) and one or both arms (segmental dystonia). The patient notices a pulling sensation in the neck musculature turning the chin toward one shoulder. Usually that shoulder is elevated as well. When the symptom is mild, the patient can easily straighten the neck; when severe, the head may be held in prolonged twisted postures. In some patients the head may be flexed (antecollis), extended (retrocollis), tilted, or shifted instead of rotated or twisted. These are all examples of the same disorder and carry the name of spasmodic torticollis. A concomitant head tremor is frequent. In many patients the tremor is most pronounced when the patient attempts to keep the head straight (i.e., a dystonic tremor); in others tremor persists irrespective of the position of the head, and therefore represents essential tremor that may also be present in the hands. Placing a hand on the jaw tends to provide some relief of the torticollis.

In spasmodic torticollis, multiple and bilateral neck muscles, including the sternocleidomastoids, trapezius, and scalenus muscle, are involved in the involuntary contractions. In most patients, spasmodic torticollis persists and can be painful. In addition to pharmacologic therapy (discussed above under Torsion Dystonia) sensory biofeedback therapy has had some success in patients with spasmodic torticollis. Dorsal column stimulation is sometimes helpful. Surgical section of the spinal accessory nerve produces inconsistent relief. Initial therapy should utilize anticholinergics along with other drugs, if necessary, such as diazepam and carbamazepine. Most patients improve only mildly with drug therapy.

CRANIAL DYSTONIA

Cranial dystonia (blepharospasm, Meige syndrome) is the second most common form of adult-onset focal dystonia. It usually begins with increased blinking and then worsens, and forced contractions of the orbicularis oculi eventually develop. Frequently, other muscles innervated by the facial nerve are also involved, including those around the lips. The contractions sometimes spread to involve mandibular muscles and even the tongue and neck. When the dystonia spreads to involve the jaw muscles, the "blepharospasm-plus" has been called Meige syndrome. Bright light usually aggravates the blepharospasm, and many patients wear dark glasses, even indoors. When severe, blepharospasm can result in functional blindness, preventing many activities, such as reading, driving, watching movies, and shopping. Pharmacotherapy is frequently unsuccessful. Some patients will improve with baclofen, anticholinergics, clonazepam, or antipsychotic agents. Surgical therapy, such as sectioning or making radiofrequency lesions of the branches of the facial nerve, can be helpful; regrowth of the nerve branches frequently leads to eventual return of symptoms.

Couch JR: Dystonia and tremor in spasmodic torticollis. Adv Neurol 14:245, 1976. *Report of an analysis that indicates spasmodic torticollis to be a feature of torsion dystonia and that tremor is a forme fruste of the disease in family members.*

Eldridge R, Fahn S (eds.): Dystonia. Adv Neurol Vol 14, 1976. *Summarizes the state of the art up to the date of publication.*

Fahn S: High dosage anticholinergic therapy in dystonia. Neurology 33:1255, 1983. *Reports the successful use of very high dosage of anticholinergic agents in children with dystonia.*

Jankovic J, Ford J: Blepharospasm and orofacial-cervical dystonia: Clinical and pharmacological findings in 100 patients. Ann Neurol 13:402, 1983. *A thorough review of the clinical features of blepharospasm and associated dystonic movements.*

Lal S, Hoyte K, Kiely ME, Sourkes TL, Baxter DW, Missala K, Andermann F: Neuropharmacologic investigation and treatment of spasmodic torticollis. Adv Neurol 24:335, 1979. *Study revealed that anticholinergic drugs can be effective in reducing torticollis.*

Marsden CD: Dystonia: The spectrum of the disease. *In* Yahr MD (ed.): The Basal Ganglia. New York, Raven Press, 1976, pp 351–367. *Discusses the different forms of dystonia.*

Section Six INHERITED, CONGENITAL, AND IDIOPATHIC DEGENERATIVE DISEASES OF THE NERVOUS SYSTEM

Roger N. Rosenberg

The classic eponymic neurologic diseases discussed in this section produce characteristic pathologic changes in specific nuclei and fiber tracts in brain, spinal cord, and peripheral nerve. The disorders are usually progressive and symmetrical in their pathologic and clinical expression, and many have a clear genetic basis of inheritance or suggestion of familial involvement. The disorders involve specific regions or systems of the nervous system such as cerebellar nuclei and fiber tracts or the corticospinal or extrapyramidal motor system, resulting in specific neurologic symptoms and signs referred to as system degenerations. In most of the inherited degenerative disorders to be discussed the primary impact of disease involves the neuron, changes produced in astrocytes and oligodendrocytes being presumably of a reactive and secondary nature.

488. STRIATONIGRAL DEGENERATION

Striatonigal degeneration (Joseph's disease) is a rare disease of the nervous system inherited as an autosomal dominant disorder in persons of Portuguese or Azorean ancestry. A nongenetic form of striatonigral degeneration that resembles parkinsonism also has been described.

PATHOLOGY. The major pathologic findings are a loss of neurons and glial replacement in the corpus striatum and the zona compacta portion of the substantia nigra. The thoracic spinal cord shows degeneration of the posterior and lateral fiber tracts. There is also a moderate loss of neurons in the dentate nucleus of the cerebellum and in the nucleus ruber of the midbrain.

CLINICAL MANIFESTATIONS. The disease affects adults over 25 years old. The main neurologic findings in type I disease include extremity weakness and spasticity of all extremities, especially the legs, often with associated dystonia of the face, neck, trunk, and extremities. Patellar and ankle clonus are common, as are extensor plantar responses. The gait is slow and stiff, with a slight increase in base and lurching from side to side caused by spasticity. Affected persons have no truncal titubation. Pharyngeal weakness and spasticity cause difficulty with speech and swallowing. Of note are prominent horizontal and vertical nystagmus, the loss of the fast saccadic eye movements, hypermetric and hypometric saccades, and impairment of vertical gaze. Facial fasciculations, facial myokymia, and lingual fasciculations without atrophy are common and early manifestations. Signs of cerebellar dysfunction are prominent in cases with a late-life onset.

DIAGNOSIS. Autosomal dominant striatonigral degeneration should be considered in persons with an appropriate family history developing progressive dystonia, rigidity and spasticity of pharynx, trunk, and extremities, and associated hyperreflexia, clonus, and extensor plantar responses. The entity is distinguished from Huntington's disease by the preservation of intellect.

489. MOTOR NEURON DISEASES

The term motor neuron disease refers to a group of chronic neurologic disorders that selectively affect with varying combination and rapidity the anterior horn cells of the spinal cord and lower brainstem, plus, in some cases, those large motor neurons of the cerebral cortex that give rise to the corticospinal tract. Clinically significant sensory change or cerebellar dysfunction is absent in all instances. Cases in which upper motor neuron changes are prominent in addition to muscle fasciculation, atrophy, and weakness are called *amyotrophic lateral sclerosis* (ALS). *Progressive bulbar palsy* is a variant of ALS that produces relatively rapidly advancing upper and lower motor neuron involvement of the muscles of the jaw, pharynx, and tongue. Cases lacking signs of upper motor neuron disease and producing only a slow, progressive muscle wasting and weakness often are termed *progressive muscular atrophy* (PMA). A variety of clinical subtypes of PMA occur, some of which can produce restricted motor involvement that progresses extremely slowly over a period of many years. *Werdnig-Hoffmann disease* of infancy and young children and the *Wohlfart-Kugelberg-Welander disease* of older children and adolescents represent other variants of motor neuron disease. *Primary lateral sclerosis* is a very rare condition in which the corticospinal tracts degenerate in association with some loss of cortical neurons but no impairment of anterior horn cells. The disorder produces progressive spasticity of the extremities and bulbar muscles, unaccompanied by other neurologic abnormalities. Most autopsy studies of primary lateral sclerosis have shown disseminated sclerosis, spinal cord compression, other degenerative disorders, or high spinal neoplasms, but a few examples of the true condition do exist.

AMYOTROPHIC LATERAL SCLEROSIS

Amyotrophic lateral sclerosis (ALS) can first affect bulbar muscles, a single limb, the extremities on one side of the body, the lower or upper extremities symmetrically, or all four limbs simultaneously, depending upon the individual case. The disorder occurs mainly in the fifth, sixth, and seventh decades of life and runs a progressive course lasting from two to seven years. The bulbar form runs a more malignant course. ALS usually occurs sporadically, but familial groupings have occurred, indicating either a genetic predisposition for disease or common exposure to an unknown causative agent. Familial cases tend to come on younger and progress more rapidly than do sporadic ones. Despite extensive searches to establish ALS as an autoimmune or slow virus disease, no firm leads exist, and the cause of the motor neuron diseases remains unknown.

PATHOLOGY. The neuropathologic findings in ALS consist of degenerative changes and loss of the Betz cells in layers 3 and 5 of the precentral cerebral cortex, Brodmann's areas 4 and 6. These are absent in the more benign cases of progressive muscular atrophy. Neuronal loss also occurs in the motor cranial nuclei and the motor neurons in the anterior horns of the spinal cord. There are no characteristic features associated with the neuronal loss, and the musculature innervated by the affected motor cranial nuclei and anterior horn cells undergoes neurogenic atrophy as a result of denervation.

CLINICAL MANIFESTATIONS. ALS produces a variety of clinical patterns, all of which show muscle weakness and wasting but which vary in their rate of progression, the distribution of the major weakness, and the rapidity with which signs of upper motor neuron dysfunction occur. Patients develop a slowly progressive impairment of motor function affecting distal more than proximal structures, as evidenced by muscle atrophy involving the intrinsic muscles of the hand. Over a period of six months to a year, the process results in symmetrical muscle atrophy involving the hands, forearms, and shoulder girdle muscles. The disease may develop quite asymmetrically in some patients. Prominent and early in most patients is the occurrence of fasciculations resulting from acute and widespread denervation of entire motor units. The patient may have muscle cramps, but rarely any sensory symptoms. The deep tendon reflexes are usually preserved in the upper extremities in the early phase of disease. Signs of upper motor neuron involvement may develop at any time but almost always by the time muscle involvement has lasted as long as a year. These include spasticity, particularly in the lower extremities with associated hyperreflexia, clonus, and extensor plantar responses on one or both sides. Characteristically, the superficial abdominal reflexes and the cremasteric reflexes as well as the bladder and anal sphincters remain normal. Generalized fasciculations and muscle atrophy in most instances involve the lower extremities later than the upper. These combinations of upper and lower motor neuron deficits are characteristic of ALS. Occasionally, spasticity predominantly involves the pharynx, larynx, and extremities, and signs of muscular atrophy and fasciculations are hard to detect. In such instances, EMG testing may give the answer. The loss of the gag reflex, pharyngeal paralysis, lingual atrophy and fasciculations, and diffuse extremity atrophy and fasciculations with reduced myotatic reflexes indicate a severe bulbospinal variant of ALS (progressive muscular atrophy almost always spares the cranial nerves). ALS spares the extraocular muscles. Patients may show signs of emotional lability. Intellectual functions deteriorate in approximately 5 per cent of patients. The cerebrospinal fluid is normal. Changes of muscle denervation can be confirmed by electromyography (EMG). The motor nerve conduction velocities remain normal, however, even in the presence of severe atrophy, a finding that separates this disorder from the peripheral motor neuropathies, in which conduction velocities are reduced.

DIFFERENTIAL DIAGNOSIS. Conditions to be differentiated are primary muscle disease, peripheral nerve disorders, spinal cord compression, or tumors and conditions damaging the corticospinal tracts. None of these conditions, however, fully imitates the characteristic combination of painless, diffuse neurogenic muscle impairment plus spasticity and absent sensory change that marks severe motor neuron disease. Muscle disease can be separated by changes in serum enzymes, EMG, and biopsy. Most peripheral nerve disorders produce sensory impairment. They do not cause fasciculation, and they do cause slowing of nerve electrical conduction velocity. Cervical spinal cord or ventral spinal root compression from spondylosis or tumor often causes pain, and usually produces a combination of weakness and atrophy restricted to the arms, plus spasticity and sensory changes in the legs.

Multiple sclerosis can result in spasticity, but not muscular atrophy or fasciculation, and sensory changes are usual. Intracranial disorders can produce bilateral spasticity, but other signs of brain involvement easily distinguish the condition.

TREATMENT. This must be symptomatic and supportive, as there is no specific therapy.

WERDNIG-HOFFMANN DISEASE

Werdnig-Hoffmann disease is a progressive impairment of the motor system occurring in infancy and early childhood. The lower motor neuron is exclusively involved, paralyzing musculature innervated by motor cranial nuclei and anterior horn cells of the spinal cord. Infants and young children may present with this syndrome at birth or in the first few months of life with diffuse flaccidity, muscular atrophy, muscle fasciculations, and reduced to absent myotatic reflexes with associated respiratory and swallowing difficulties. There may be prominent lingual fasciculations and atrophy in the first few months of life. A muscle biopsy indicates neurogenic atrophy, and the cerebrospinal fluid is normal. Electromyography shows acute denervation with normal peripheral nerve conduction velocities. The disorder is inherited as an autosomal recessive trait. The cause is not known.

WOHLFART-KUGELBERG-WELANDER DISEASE

Wohlfart-Kugelberg-Welander disease is an autosomal recessive disorder in which symptoms begin during late childhood, adolescence, or early adulthood and include progressive proximal muscle atrophy, weakness, and fasciculations. It is very slowly progressive and is usually compatible with a life span into the third or fourth decade. Typical examples have been described in families in which other children have Werdnig-Hoffmann disease. Thus varying penetrance of a single gene mutation inherited in an autosomal recessive manner may produce either an aggressive form of motor neuron disease in childhood (Werdnig-Hoffmann disease) or a more benign form of motor neuron disease in later childhood and early adulthood (Wohlfart-Kugelberg-Welander disease). The onset in the first and second decades of life of proximal weakness and atrophy with fasciculations but a very slow progression without evidence of upper motor neuron involvement separates this disorder from amyotrophic lateral sclerosis. The presence of denervation without the insertional irritability characteristic of polymyositis can be determined by electromyography. Both Wohlfart-Kugelberg-Welander disease and polymyositis may present with progressive proximal weakness and atrophy; if fasciculations are not prominent, electromyography and muscle biopsy are of important differentiating value. Neurogenic denervation can be identified in biopsied muscle, thus separating it from the acquired or inherited myopathies. The cause of the disorder is unknown, and specific therapy is not available.

490. SPINOCEREBELLAR DEGENERATIONS

This term applies to a group of progressive degenerative disorders in which ataxia and dysmetria resulting from predominant involvement of the cerebellum and its pathways are combined to greater or lesser degrees, with impairment of other sensory and motor systems. All represent system degenerations, and many of the specific entities have a well established genetic basis. Although clinical signs of cerebellar involvement predominate, the extension of the disorders to involve other regions of the nervous system can produce more complex neurologic symptoms. The important and common inherited spinocerebellar degenerations include (1) Friedreich's ataxia; (2) olivopontocerebellar degeneration; (3) Roussy-Lévy syndrome; (4) Bassen-Kornzweig syndrome; (5) Refsum's syndrome; (6) Marie's ataxia; and (7) dyssynergia cerebellaris myoclonica (Table 490–1).

As classified by Greenfield, the spinocerebellar degenerations can be grouped into predominant spinal forms, spinocerebellar forms, and cerebellar forms. Further subclassification exists in the olivopontocerebellar degenerations, with at least five subtypes identified by Konigsmark and Weiner with both autosomal dominant and autosomal recessive forms of inheritance. The spinocerebellar degenerations have common neuropathologic features from the peripheral nerve through the spinal

TABLE 490–1. THE COMMON INHERITED AND ACQUIRED SPINOCEREBELLAR DEGENERATIONS

Syndrome	Age of Onset	Rate of Progression	Reflexes	Sensory Change	Cerebellar Deficit	Other Important Clinical Features
			Spinal Syndromes			
Friedreich's syndrome	First decade	Slowly progressive	Absent myotatic DTRs, extensor plantar response	Moderate loss	Severe	Dysarthria, nystagmus, moderate mental retardation; arched feet; scoliosis; cardiomegaly with fibrosis; autosomal dominant or recessive or sporadic
Hereditary spastic paraplegia	First or second decade	Slowly progressive	Hyperreflexia, clonus, extensor plantar response	Minimal loss	None	Paraplegia; impaired bowel and bladder function; may occur in families with typical Friedreich's syndrome or olivopontocerebellar degeneration; autosomal dominant or recessive or sporadic
Roussy-Lévy syndrome	First or second decade	Slowly progressive	Absent myotatic DTRs, extensor plantar response	Moderate loss	Moderate	Absence of dysarthria, peroneal muscular atrophy; intermediate between Friedreich's and Charcot-Marie-Tooth diseases; autosomal dominant or recessive
			Polyneuropathy			
Charcot-Marie-Tooth disease	First or second decade	Slowly progressive	Absent	Moderate loss	None	Predominant peroneal muscle atrophy; nerves may be hypertrophic; optic-acoustic nerve involvement occurs; usually autosomal dominant
Dejerine-Sottas disease	First or second decade	Slowly progressive	Absent	Moderate loss	None	Dysarthria, nystagmus, tremor; hypertrophic nerves; scoliosis; elevated CSF protein; usually sporadic or autosomal recessive
Ataxia telangiectasia	First decade	Slowly progressive	Reduced	Minimal loss	Severe	Telangiectatic lesions involving sclerae, face, pinna, and neck; pulmonary infections; increased incidence of lymphoma; hypogamma-IgA; autosomal recessive
Bassen-Kornzweig syndrome	First decade	Slowly progressive	Absent	Moderate loss	Severe	May have mental retardation; acanthocytosis; steatorrhea; pigmentary retinal degeneration; abetalipoproteinemia; autosomal recessive
Tangier disease	First decade	Slowly progressive	Reduced	Moderate loss	None	Enlarged, yellowish-appearing tonsils; defect in high density lipoproteins; autosomal recessive
Refsum's disease	First decade	Slowly progressive	Absent	Severe loss	Severe	Nyctalopia; pigmentary retinal degeneration; ichthyosis; cardiac conduction defects; deafness, elevated serum phytanate; defect in lipid alpha oxidase activity; autosomal recessive
			Cerebellar Syndromes			
Olivoponto-cerebellar degeneration	Third to fifth decade	Slowly progressive	Hyperreflexia, clonus, extensor plantar response	Moderate loss	Severe	Late development of optic atrophy and muscle atrophy; may develop a moderate dementia; CT scans show pontine and cerebellar atrophy; may be autosomal dominant or recessive
Carcinomatous cerebellar degeneration	Adult	Less than 10 years	Reduced	Moderate loss	Truncal	Truncal greater than extremity ataxia; dysarthria and nystagmus minimal; lung carcinoma most common association
Alcoholic cerebellar degeneration	Adult	Slowly progressive	Reduced	Moderate	Lower extremities and trunk	Lower extremities affected more than upper; dysarthria and nystagmus minimal; peripheral neuropathy present
Dyssynergia cerebellaris of Ramsay Hunt	Adult	Slowly progressive	Reduced	Normal	Moderate	Induced myoclonic jerks with intention; generalized seizures; sporadic

TABLE 490–2. BIOCHEMICAL DEFECTS IN THE INHERITED ATAXIAS

Associated Biochemical Defect	Clinical Type	Age of Onset	Clinical Features
		Lipid Disorders	
Autosomal recessive			
1. Storage of phytanate due to defect in alpha oxidase	Refsum's disease	20–30 years	Ataxia; retinitis pigmentosa; deafness; ichthyosis; cardiac arrhythmia; polyneuropathy
2. Abetalipoproteinemia	Bassen-Kornzweig syndrome	5–10 years	Ataxia; acanthocytosis; retinitis pigmentosa; polyneuropathy; malabsorption of fat
3. Arylsulfatase A deficiency	Juvenile onset metachromatic leukodystrophy	5–20 years	Ataxia; mild mental retardation; polyneuropathy
4. Storage of G-M2 ganglioside due to hexosaminidase A deficiency, alpha locus type	Juvenile onset atypical spinocerebellar ataxia	3 years	Progressive ataxia, spasticity, dysarthria; muscle atrophy; pes cavus; dystonic features; normal intelligence
5. Storage of G-M2 ganglioside due to hexosaminidase A deficiency, beta locus type	Juvenile onset atypical ataxia with cherry-red spots	2 years	Progressive ataxia and intention tremor; macular cherry-red spots
6. Partial deficiency of hexosaminidase A and B	Adult onset spinocerebellar degeneration	20 years	Gait and limb ataxia; head titubation; dysarthria; tremor; grimacing; chorea
X-linked recessive			
1. Storage of long chain (C24-30) fatty acids	Adrenoleukomyelo-neuropathy (Nixon-Blaw disease)	5–20 years	Cortical blindness and spasticity; skin pigmentation; childhood onset of adrenal cortical insufficiency; adult onset with ataxia and polyneuropathy
		Carbohydrate Disorders	
Autosomal recessive			
1. Pyruvate carboxylase or pyruvate dehydrogenase deficiencies or inhibitor of thiamin triphosphate formation in brain (inhibitor of thiamin pyrophosphate–ATP phosphotransferase)	Leigh's disease (subacute necrotizing encephalopathy)	Birth–5 years; rare adult form	Acute episodic extraocular muscle palsies; optic atrophy; hypotonia; ataxia; mental retardation; somnolence; hyperreflexia; extensor plantar responses; elevated serum pyruvate and lactate
2. Mitochondrial malic enzyme	Friedreich's ataxia	5–15 years	Progressive gait and limb ataxia; dysarthria; nystagmus; areflexia; extensor plantar reflex; distal sensory loss
3. Oxidative metabolism with elevated serum lactate and pyruvate	Adult onset neuromyopathy with ataxia—Kearns-Sayre syndrome	20–50 years	Retinitis pigmentosa; neuromyopathy; ophthalmoplegia; ataxia; cardiac arrhythmias; muscle biopsy shows ragged red fibers
		Disorders of Amino Acid Metabolism	
Autosomal recessive			
1. Deficiency in branched chain keto acid decarboxylase	Maple syrup urine disease and variants	Birth–5 years	Mental retardation; seizures; failure to thrive; irritability; anorexia; ataxia; maple syrup odor to urine; excretion of branched chain amino acids and keto acids
2. Hyperglycinemia	Spastic paraparesis with muscular atrophy and arm dysmetria	2–10 years	Spastic paraparesis; peroneal muscle atrophy; distal sensory loss; pes cavus; optic atrophy; arm dysmetria
3. 5-Oxoprolinuria due to deficiency of glutathione synthetase	Ataxia and defect in gammaglutamyl cycle (I) (reduced glutathione synthesis)	10 years	Progressive mental retardation; spasticity; limb and gait ataxia; tremor; hemolytic anemia with intermittent jaundice
4. Generalized aminoaciduria due to deficiency of gamma-glutamylcysteine synthetase	Ataxia and defect in gamma-glutamyl cycle (II) (reduced glutathione synthesis)	20 years	Hemolytic anemia; areflexia; gait and limb ataxia; distal sensory loss; staccato speech; acute psychosis
5. Defect in tryptophan absorption from gut; aminoaciduria	Hartnup disease	5–25 years	Intermittent ataxia; episodic, pellagra-like skin rash; progressive mental retardation; spasticity; choreoathetosis
6. Deficiency in glutamate dehydrogenase	Olivopontocerebellar degeneration	20–40 years	Progressive gait and limb ataxia; spasticity; mild extrapyramidal features; late distal amyotrophy and sensory loss; rare mental changes
		Disorder of Urea Cycle Metabolism	
Autosomal recessive			
1. Argininosuccinate synthetase deficiency	Citrullinemia, subacute type	Infancy	Vomiting; somnolence; tremor; ataxia; seizures; delay in mental and physical development; hyperammonemia
		Disorder of Immunologic Function	
Autosomal recessive			
1. Reduced serum immunoglobulins (IgA, IgG, and IgM); lymphopenia	Ataxia telangiectasia (Louis-Barr syndrome)	5–12 years	Telangiectasia of face and sclerae; Friedreich's phenotype with ataxia; dysarthria; areflexia; extensor plantar responses; oculomotor apraxia
		Disorder of Protein Metabolism (Increased Amounts of Glial Proteins)	
Autosomal dominant			
1. Increased glial acidic filamentous protein and a complex of 40,000 mw proteins in cerebellum and basal ganglia seen on 2-D gels	Joseph's disease	20–65 years	Gait ataxia often with either corticospinal and extrapyramidal findings or late onset polyneuropathy

cord and up to the cerebellum with its attendant connections. Although these disorders are well described both clinically and pathologically, only in Friedreich's syndrome, Refsum's disease, and the Bassen-Kornzweig syndrome do molecular insights exist into the cause. The similarity of neuropathologic findings in the Bassen-Kornzweig syndrome and Friedreich's syndrome despite very different molecular defects indicates the vulnerability of the spinocerebellar system to different chemical abnormalities as well as its limited neuropathologic response. A survey of biochemical defects in the inherited ataxias is presented in Table 490–2.

FRIEDREICH'S ATAXIA

This commonest form of spinocerebellar degeneration begins in childhood and is inherited mainly as an autosomal recessive or dominant disorder. Sporadic cases presumably represent "spontaneous" examples of the recessive trait. Friedreich's ataxia comprises a syndrome including several subtypes with common clinical features and pathologic changes. Established or possible causes (Table 490–2) include several inborn errors of metabolism, including disorders of lipids, diseases of oxidative metabolism, aminoacidurias, and the partial deficiency of serum immunoglobulin levels.

Blass et al. have described children in whom pyruvate oxidation was low in muscles from 4 of 7 patients with Friedreich's syndrome, in 4 of 12 patients with other ataxias, and in 8 of 19 patients with familial or idiopathic neuropathies. In those studies the degree of pyruvate dehydrogenase complex activity correlated with the severity and rapidity of the spinocerebellar disease process. For example, patients with less than 15 per cent of normal pyruvate dehydrogenase activity but with normal oxoglutarate dehydrogenase generally had severe neurologic disease and lactic acidosis beginning in infancy. Severe deficiencies of both complexes have been described in one infant with severe disease. Several patients with 20 to 30 per cent of normal pyruvate dehydrogenase activity had a milder illness in which ataxia was the most prominent sign. The patients with Friedreich's syndrome had the mildest defect, with 40 to 50 per cent of normal pyruvate dehydrogenase activity together with 50 per cent of normal oxoglutarate dehydrogenase activity. Most recently, Stumpf et al. have reported a marked reduction in activity in fibroblast cultures of the mitochondrial malic enzyme. Despite these biochemical abnormalities in some patients, in the vast majority of typical Friedreich's ataxia patients no biochemical abnormality is found.

PATHOLOGY. Demyelination with secondary gliosis affects the spinocerebellar tracts, the lateral corticospinal tracts, the posterior columns, and the peripheral nerves. Neuronal loss involves the primary sensory neurons in dorsal root ganglia as well as the cells of Clarke's column which give rise to the spinocerebellar tracts. Less often, neuronal loss affects the anterior horns of the spinal cord and cell layers in the cerebellar cortex and deep cerebellar nuclei. A diffuse and major loss of myocardial fibers with subsequent replacement by fibrosis may occur in some patients.

CLINICAL MANIFESTATIONS. Midline ataxia appears first with impairment of gait, poor coordination, and frequent falling. Gait problems may be the only sign of disease for many years, but eventually dysarthria and ataxia of arm and hand emerge. By the midpart to end of the second decade of life most patients require assistance in walking. Nystagmus is an early and prominent feature, as is the loss of fast saccadic eye movements. A few patients develop optic atrophy during the later stages of the disease. Progressive skeletal deformities include kyphoscoliosis, pes cavus, and, less consistently, a deformed and high arched palate. Distal sensory deficits, especially in the legs, develop after several years and include impairment in position sense and vibratory sensation as well as, less prominently, a reduction in pain and temperature perceptions. Additional expressions of motor dysfunction include extensor plantar responses with normal or reduced tone in trunk and extremities and absent deep tendon reflexes. Moderate weakness and the occurrence of atrophy of the extremities and occasional fasciculations are late developments. About half the patients develop cardiomegaly, murmurs, bundle branch block, T wave inversions, and complete heart block on electrocardiograms. Cardiopulmonary arrest and congestive heart failure may occur. A small percentage of patients are mentally retarded and few reach high intelligence.

DIAGNOSIS. The presence in childhood or young adolescence of insidiously beginning and slowly progressing truncal and extremity ataxia, with dysarthria and subsequent nystagmus, extensor plantar responses, and areflexia, is typical. When one adds the findings of scoliosis, pes cavus, and proprioceptive and vibratory loss in the lower extremities, hardly any other diagnosis is possible. Motor nerve conduction velocities are normal in the common neurogenic form of the disorder, but electromyography may detect denervation potentials, especially in the legs. In the hypertrophic neuropathic form of ataxia, the motor nerve conduction velocities are slowed and the peripheral nerves may be palpably enlarged with demyelination noted in peripheral nerve biopsies. The cerebrospinal fluid protein is normal. Muscle biopsies often show neurogenic atrophy but are unnecessary for diagnosis. The electrocardiogram may contain abnormalities as recorded above and the chest roentgenogram may show cardiomegaly.

DIFFERENTIAL DIAGNOSIS. Diagnosis of Friedreich's syndrome is not difficult if the case meets the aforementioned criteria. Multiple sclerosis and subacute combined degeneration of the spinal cord caused by vitamin B_{12} deficiency differ in both age of onset and clinical characteristics. Cerebellar or spinal tumors produce a more rapid course and, usually, pain. The *Roussy-Lévy syndrome,* which may not be a distinct disorder, is recognized by most authorities as having an autosomal dominant pattern. The onset occurs in childhood with ataxia, areflexia, pes cavus–clubfoot deformity, and kyphoscoliosis. It differs from Friedreich's ataxia in sparing position and vibratory sensation and by the absence of extensor plantar responses as well as of nystagmus and dysarthria. Patients with *Refsum's disease* caused by elevated serum phytanate as a result of a defect in lipid alpha-oxidase suffer the additional defects of optic atrophy, pigmentary retinal degeneration, ichthyosis, and deafness. Patients with the *Bassen-Kornzweig syndrome* have spinocerebellar signs but also prominent steatorrhea, abetalipoproteinemia, and acanthocytosis of the red blood cells.

Hereditary spastic paraplegia expresses an autosomal dominant, recessive, or sex-linked recessive trait by the occurrence of peroneal muscular atrophy, skeletal deformities, nystagmus, and prominent spastic paraplegia. The syndrome overlaps with other forms of spinocerebellar degeneration in some families.

OLIVOPONTOCEREBELLAR DEGENERATIONS

The olivopontocerebellar atrophies represent a group of adult-onset disorders manifested clinically by progressive involvement of cerebellar functions and pathologically by a reduction in neurons in the inferior olivary nuclei of the medulla, the basis pontis, the cerebellar cortex, and the deep cerebellar nuclei. Closely related are at least some examples of autonomic insufficiency of the Shy-Drager type (Ch. 478).

PATHOLOGY. Grossly, atrophy involves the cerebellum, cerebellar peduncles, and basis pontis. Microscopically, Purkinje cells, granule cells of the cerebellar cortex, and neurons from the dentate nucleus and other deep cerebellar nuclei all are severely reduced.

CLINICAL MANIFESTATIONS. Olivopontocerebellar atrophy has several variants whose principal clinical manifestations vary with the phenotype. Sporadically arising cases outnumber those with abnormal familial histories, but the pathologic changes are similar. Essential features include the development in mid-adult life of progressive ataxia, dysarthria, dysmetria, dysdiadochokinesia, nystagmus, and loss of fast saccadic eye movements. Subsequently, patients develop spasticity, optic nerve atrophy, distal sensory involvement, and late intellectual dysfunction.

In general, truncal ataxia develops initially in the second or third decades of life, and extremity ataxia and dysmetria and prominent dysarthria follow within a decade. After several years, perhaps a third of affected patients show spasticity with associated hyperreflexia, clonus, and extensor plantar responses. Nystagmus, optic nerve atrophy, and loss of fast saccadic eye movements occur frequently. A small fraction of patients display the late occurrence of muscle atrophy with fasciculations, including the facial muscles, muscles of mastication, and lingual musculature. Palatal myoclonus is an uncommon but almost pathognomonic accompaniment when it occurs. Variations in the illness include sensory deficits in a distal distribution, intellectual deterioration, signs of extrapyramidal dysfunction, external ophthalmoplegia, and early visual loss.

The olivopontocerebellar degenerations described by Holmes, Sanger-Brown, and Marie represent phenotypic variants of this general class of disease. The syndrome of *Ramsay Hunt's* dyssynergia cerebellaris myoclonica is perhaps a rare variant beginning in childhood and includes prominent, progressive ataxia and myoclonic seizures inherited as an autosomal dominant trait.

DIAGNOSIS. The olivopontocerebellar atrophies are characterized by the development early in adult life of progressive symmetrical involvement of cerebellar functions, followed in many instances by progressive and symmetrical development of spasticity in the legs. Abnormalities of eye movement, intellectual impairment, and muscle atrophy with distal sensory loss complete the clinical picture, sometimes with the addition of palatal myoclonus. Computed tomography demonstrates cerebellar atrophy, pontine atrophy, and, late in the disease, cerebral atrophy and large lateral ventricles. Motor nerve conduction velocities may be slow, and muscle denervation may be detected by electromyography. The cerebrospinal fluid is normal. Neither specific diagnostic laboratory tests nor specific treatments exist for most patients. A few patients with recessively inherited disease have had a moderate reduction in leukocyte glutamate dehydrogenase activity, as reported by Plaitakis et al. Progressive cerebellar deficits, which include truncal ataxia, nystagmus, and dysarthria, are also produced as a result of chronic malnutrition and as a remote effect of cancer, and these possibilities must be considered when a family history of cerebellar disease is lacking.

491. SYRINGOMYELIA

Syringomyelia is derived from the Greek word syrinx, which means tube, and refers to the occurrence of a cavity within the spinal cord. Such cavities usually are located in the central region at the cervical level; they often extend into the medulla (syringobulbia) and may extend inferiorly into the thoracic and lumbosacral regions of the cord. Most instances of syringomyelia occur in association with acquired spinal congenital malformations or with spinal intramedullary neoplasms, of which perhaps 25 per cent produce an associated syrinx.

PATHOLOGY. The syringomyelic cavity is usually associated with the central canal of the spinal cord but may be independent of it as well. The cavity may extend over many segments of the cervical cord and may be in direct anatomic communication with the fourth ventricle. The term hydromyelia is often used to describe those cavitary lesions of the spinal cord which do communicate with the fourth ventricle. The syringomyelic cavity dissects into and progressively replaces the gray matter of the posterior and anterior horns of the spinal cord, as well as disturbing the decussating spinothalamic pain-carrying fibers in the anterior commissure. The cavity wall is maintained by astrocytic glial and fibroblastic membranes and blood vessels. Most often, syringomyelia is associated with other congenital malformations at the cranial cervical junction, including the Arnold-Chiari malformation with herniation of the cerebellar tonsils, fusion of the cervical vertebrae (Klippel-Feil syndrome), or malformations at the lumbosacral region, including spina bifida and associated meningomyelocele. Hydrocephalus resulting from cranial cervical malformations or stenosis of the aqueduct of Sylvius occurs in some patients.

CLINICAL MANIFESTATIONS. Symptoms of syringomyelia most often begin in the second or third decade with a typically "dissociated," selective impairment in pain and temperature sensation with the preservation of the sense of touch. Earliest detected sensory changes are usually in the hands, but examination commonly discloses a similar loss in the neck, shoulders, upper chest, and back. Sensory loss is accompanied by progressive atrophy of the musculature in the upper extremities with skeletal malformations, principally kyphoscoliosis. Progressive analgesia results in severe painless ulcers, burns, and Charcot joints. Atrophy of arm, forearm, and intrinsic hand musculature, fasciculations, and areflexia develop progressively. Later upper motor neuron signs arise in the legs owing to encroachment of the syringomyelic cavity into the lateral columns of the cord. Late involvement of vibratory and position sensations in the lower extremities and an associated Romberg sign indicate that the syrinx is extending into the posterior columns of the spinal cord. A preganglionic Horner syndrome may develop owing to dissection of the syrinx into the intermediolateral cell column of the lower cervical and first thoracic segment of the spinal cord containing sympathetic neurons. The kyphoscoliosis that sometimes heralds the disease results from the asymmetrical denervation and atrophy of paravertebral muscles. The disease process is progressive, usually symmetrical, and clearly evident in adult life.

Syringobulbia refers to the development of the syringomyelic cavity into the medulla with resultant destruction of the medullary structures in the lateral tegmentum. Dissociated impairment of pain and temperature over the face, nystagmus, pharyngeal and vocal cord paralysis, and lingual atrophy are most typical. Syringobulbia is always associated with syringomyelia and is not a separate process.

DIAGNOSIS. Lepromatous neuropathy, certain rare congenital and acquired peripheral neuropathies, and intramedullary destructive lesions of the spinal cord and brainstem are the only conditions causing insidiously developing and progressive, widespread, dissociated loss of pain and temperature sensation. Leprosy can be considered if the subject has grown up in an endemic area, but neither it nor other peripheral neuropathies produce signs of spinal cord involvement. When the dissociated sensory loss is coupled with signs of long tract disease in the lower extremities or is decidedly asymmetrical in distribution and dermatomal in pattern, the differential consideration lies between congenital syrinx and intramedullary neoplasm. Pain is more frequent with tumors. Myelography, CT, or NMR imaging usually can make the distinction.

TREATMENT. Treatment generally is unsatisfactory. Surgical decompression of the distended syrinx by a laminectomy and drainage of the cavity has been claimed to slow the disease progression. Some surgeons state that the placement of muscle tissue at the junction of the fourth ventricle and the upper cervical canal with or without a ventriculocardiac shunt has stabilized the neurologic status of patients. Syrinx associated with spinal tumor is treated by treating the tumor appropriately.

492. THE PHAKOMATOSES OR NEUROCUTANEOUS SYNDROMES

NEUROFIBROMATOSIS
(Von Recklinghausen's Disease)

Von Recklinghausen's disease or neurofibromatosis is a genetic disorder inherited as an autosomal dominant trait and characterized by the occurrence of pigmented skin lesions, multiple tumors of spinal or cranial nerves, tumors of the skin, and the associated occurrence of gliomas and intracranial meningiomas. There is an increased association with pheochromocytomas, cystic lung disease, renal vascular lesions causing hypertension, fibrous dysplasia of bone, gastrointestinal neurofibromas with chronic blood loss, and medullary thyroid carcinoma and other tumors of endocrine glands.

PATHOLOGY. The characteristic feature of the disease is the occurrence of multiple "neurofibromas" associated with nerves in their peripheral, intraspinal, or intracranial segments. Electron microscopic studies indicate that these tumors represent proliferation of fibroblasts or neurilemmal sheath cells (Schwann cells) in peripheral nerve. The tumors may become confluent in the region of the brachial or sacral plexus and produce large plexiform neuromas which can evolve into malignant sarcomas. Intracranial astrocytomas, ependymomas, glioblastomas, and meningiomas are also encountered with increased frequency, as are optic nerve gliomas in childhood. Stenosis of the aqueduct of Sylvius with noncommunicating hydrocephalus is also observed in this disease. The skin manifestations include pedunculated polyps, lightly colored pigmented lesions with sharp edges (referred to as café au lait spots), and depigmented lesions. Neoplasms of endocrine organs, including medullary thyroid carcinomas and pheochromocytoma with associated hypertension, have been reported in a number of patients.

Replacement of normal bone with fibroblasts and fibrocytes in a pattern similar to that of fibrous dysplasia in some patients results in overgrowth of bone with the occluding of cranial foramina and rarefaction and cyst formation. The congenital absence of a portion of the sphenoid bone resulting in pulsating exophthalmos, congenital vertebral anomalies, bone cysts, pseudoarthrosis of the tibia, local gigantism of an extremity, and scoliosis all can be encountered. Histologic abnormalities of the cerebral cortex, ectopic islands of gray matter, and focal gliosis are described and may be the basis for the increased incidence of mental retardation.

Zelkowitz et al. reported on what may be the primary basis for loss of cell contact inhibition and thus benign tumor formation. In careful studies reduced epidermal growth factor binding sites on the surface of neurofibromatosis fibroblasts were documented and may be a useful assay for genetic counseling purposes.

CLINICAL MANIFESTATIONS. Neurofibromatosis can present in a variety of ways, but the presence of multiple cutaneous neurofibromas and café au lait pigmented skin lesions represents the hallmarks.The pigmented skin lesions occur most commonly over the trunk and in the axilla. If greater than 1.5 cm in diameter and more than six in number they indicate neurofibromatosis. Nerve involvement can be solitary, involving individual nerves of the extremities, or multiple and diffuse. Multiple cranial nerves are affected as well, resulting in facial weakness, facial numbness, deafness, and visual loss with optic nerve atrophy. Multiple confluent tumors and fibrosis of the affected parts result in elephantiasis neuromatosa. A marked increase in the proliferation and overgrowth of skin and subcutaneous tissues of the skull, neck, and trunk can result in gross asymmetrical hypertrophy. Neurofibromas associated with the nerve root can invade the intervertebral foramen and result in compression of spinal cord or brainstem. Large neurofibromas of a cranial nerve can produce increased intracranial pressure resulting from hydrocephalus. Some such lesions present as a cerebellopontine angle mass lesion with ipsilateral cerebellar signs. The fifth, seventh, eighth, and tenth cranial nerves are commonly involved with neurofibromas, producing facial muscle weakness, facial numbness, weakness and atrophy of the muscles of mastication, deafness, and vertigo. Rarely, spontaneous fractures of vertebrae or long bones result because of fibrodysplasia or cystic bone formation.

The cerebrospinal fluid protein is elevated in patients having large tumors that result in cord compression. Roentgenograms of the skull and internal auditory meatus show erosion caused by adjacent tumors.

DIAGNOSIS. Neurofibromatosis is diagnosed readily by the occurrence of the characteristic neurofibromas and skin pigmented lesions. The tumors are often multiple and vary considerably in size. Most tumors are smooth, soft, and multilobulated, and can be palpated along the course of a peripheral nerve. Hypertensive patients must be evaluated for the possibility of renal artery stenosis as well as for pheochromocytoma with urinary determinations of catecholamines. Cranial nerve palsies and hydrocephalus signal the presence of an intracranial neoplasm and the need for CT brain scans or angiography for precise definition. Cerebellopontine angle meningiomas and cranial nerve or spinal nerve tumors are usually resectable and must be considered in patients manifesting progressive brainstem or spinal cord deficits. There is no treatment for neurofibromatosis other than resection of symptomatic tumors and decompression of hydrocephalus.

TUBEROUS SCLEROSIS (Bourneville's Disease)

Tuberous sclerosis (Bourneville's disease or epiloia) is a neurocutaneous disorder inherited as an autosomal dominant trait. Its triad of findings includes facial nevi (adenoma sebaceum), epilepsy, and mental retardation.

PATHOLOGY. The gross brain has many firm nodules on the surface and in the deep layers of the cortex, the underlying white matter, the basal ganglia, spinal cord, brainstem, and cerebellum. They line the lateral ventricles as projections referred to as "candle gutterings." The histologic appearance of the nodules shows a proliferation of primitive glia with multinucleated giant cells. Vascular malformations, meningiomas, gliomas, and hamartomas of the brain also occur.

The cutaneous lesions include characteristic facial "nevi" that take their origin from terminal nerves in the subcutaneous region of the skin and include a hyperplasia of connective tissue and blood vessels. Funduscopic examination can disclose similar nodules or phakomas consisting of glial elements, fibroblasts, and ganglion cells arising from the retina. Rarely an optic nerve glioma develops. Rhabdomyomas of the heart can occur, as can renal tumors and neoplasms of endocrine organs, including testis, pancreas, ovary, and thyroid.

CLINICAL MANIFESTATIONS. The clinical appearance is characteristic. Patients develop mental retardation and epilepsy during the first decade of life. The occurrence of mental retardation is evident by six years of age. Several years after the development of seizures the characteristic cutaneous facial lesions first develop in a symmetrical distribution on the malar and nasal regions and appear to be yellow or orange-red, varying in size from several millimeters to 1 cm. The occurrence of areas of roughening of the skin (shagreen patches) in the shape of small spheres caused by fibrous hyperplasia, café au lait spots, areas of depigmented nevi, and, rarely, subungual neurofibromas are characteristic of tuberous sclerosis and link it genetically to von Recklinghausen's neurofibromatosis. The concurrent neoplasms in other organs rarely cause clinical complications. Papilledema and other focal neurologic deficits signal the occurrence of a large intracranial tumor.

STURGE-WEBER DISEASE

Sturge-Weber disease produces a port wine–colored capillary hemangioma on the face, accompanied by a similar vascular malformation of the underlying meninges and cerebral cortex. The cause is unknown. No clear evidence of a hereditary cause has been established.

PATHOLOGY. The cutaneous hemangioma follows the distribution of one or more divisions of the trigeminal nerve. The underlying meninges contain a similar vascular lesion, and the capillaries of the cortex may show thickening and calcification, especially in the second and third cortical layers. The cerebral cortex may undergo atrophy with loss of nerve cells and a proliferation of glia. Cerebral calcification clearly outlines the cortical mantle in an undulating manner.

CLINICAL MANIFESTATIONS. The presence of a port wine facial nevus following the sensory dermatomal distribution of the first, second, or third portions of the trigeminal nerve is diagnostic. Generalized or focal motor seizures may occur with or without associated mental retardation. Affected patients can develop hemiplegic atrophy with shortening of the extremities contralateral to the calcified atrophic hemisphere. Exophthalmos, glaucoma, buphthalmos, optic atrophy, and other cutaneous port wine nevi and retinal angiomas can be present. There is no specific treatment; seizures are managed with anticonvulsant drugs. The stain deserves cosmetic repair, if possible.

HIPPEL-LINDAU DISEASE

Hippel-Lindau disease is a familial disorder inherited in a simple autosomal pattern producing hemangioblastomas of the cerebellar hemispheres with associated angiomas of the retina and cystic change in the kidney and pancreas. It presents in the fourth to sixth decades of life, usually not associated with cutaneous vascular lesions. The disorder can present with signs of cerebellar mass lesion, cerebellar hemorrhage, brainstem vascular malformations, or hemangioma of the retina. A clinical association with pheochromocytomas and polycythemia has been noted, especially in the patients with cerebellar hemangioblastomas. The diagnosis should be suspected in any patient with cerebellar brain tumor or cerebellar hemorrhage, especially in association with an elevated hematocrit. Diagnosis and treatment are as for other such mass lesions.

ATAXIA TELANGIECTASIA

Ataxia telangiectasia is a neurocutaneous disorder that begins in the first decade of life with prominent telangiectatic lesions involving the bulbar conjunctivae, malar eminences, ear lobes, and occasionally upper neck regions, associated with cerebellar ataxia and nystagmus. The condition is an autosomal recessive disorder. A chromosome translocation involving chromosome 14, increased chromosome breakage, and reduced lymphocyte response to phytohemagglutinin have been described and represent the only molecular clues to the pathogenesis.

PATHOLOGY. Neuropathologic changes include loss of Purkinje, granule, and basket cells in the cerebellar cortex as well as of neurons in the deep nuclei of the cerebellum. Neuronal loss is also present in the inferior olives of the medulla. The posterior columns of the spinal cord undergo demyelination, and there is a loss of anterior horn cells in the spinal cord and ganglion cells of the spinal ganglia. The most consistent defect of the lymphoid system is a poorly developed or absent thymus.

CLINICAL MANIFESTATIONS. The onset of the telangiectatic lesions occurs in the first decade of life and is associated with progressive deficits in cerebellar functions with early onset nystagmus. Truncal ataxia, extremity ataxia, dysarthria, extensor plantar responses, myoclonic jerks, areflexia, and distal sensory deficits occur in a pattern somewhat resembling that of Friedreich's syndrome. The patients have a high incidence of recurrent pulmonary infections and neoplasms of the lymphoreticuloendothelial system.

DIAGNOSIS. Ataxia telangiectasia is diagnosed by the characteristic telangiectatic lesions in association with a truncal ataxia, other cerebellar deficits, and abnormal eye movements. Serum protein electrophoresis documents a deficiency of gamma globulins, especially IgA and IgE. Cellular immune abnormalities include lymphocytopenia, a reduced response to skin test antigens, and lack of sensitization to dinitrochlorobenzene (DNCB).

Barnett HJM, Foster JB, Hudgson P: Syringomyelia. London, W. B. Saunders Company, 1974. *Comprehensive review of clinical manifestations, neuropathology, and treatment. A classic book.*

Blass JP, Kark RAP, Menon NK: Low activities of the pyruvate and oxoglutarate dehydrogenase complexes in five patients with Friedreich's ataxia. N Engl J Med 295:62, 1976. *Description of a new biochemical defect in patients with Friedreich's ataxia. First clear correlation between clinical syndrome and a defined enzyme defect.*

Brady RO: Inherited metabolic diseases of the nervous system. Science 193:733, 1976. *Excellent, comprehensive metabolic and biochemical review of genetic diseases of the nervous system.*

Crowe FW, Schull WJ, Neel JV: A Clinical Pathological and Genetic Study of Multiple Neurofibromatosis. Springfield, Ill., Charles C Thomas, 1956. *Classic clinical and neuropathologic study of the variations encountered in dominantly inherited neurofibromatosis.*

Gilman S, Bloedel J, Lechtenberg R: Disorders of the Cerebellum. Philadelphia, F. A. Davis Company, 1981. *Comprehensive book describing physiology and clinical syndromes of the cerebellum.*

Greenfield JG: The Spinocerebellar Degenerations. Springfield, Ill., Charles C Thomas, 1954. *Definitive review of the inherited and noninherited syndromes producing degeneration of the cerebellum and its pathways.*

Horton WA, Eldridge R, Brody J: Familial motor neuron disease. Neurology 26:460, 1976. *Description of genetic patterns in motor neuron disease.*

Konigsmark BW, Weiner LP: The olivopontocerebellar atrophies. Medicine 49:227, 1970. *Classic paper classifying and describing dominantly and recessively inherited degeneration of the cerebellum and its pathways.*

McFarlin PE, Strober W, Waldmann TA: Ataxia telangiectasia. Medicine 51:281, 1972. *Detailed comprehensive review of ataxia telangiectasia.Clinical and neuropathologic features are emphasized. A good background in clinical immunology is required.*

Plaitakis A, Berl S, Yahr M: Neurological disorders associated with deficiency of glutamate dehydrogenase. Ann Neurol 15:144, 1984. *Twelve of 88 tested patients with degenerative diseases producing basal ganglia or cerebellar abnormalities had 48 per cent reduction of GDH when compared with controls.*

Refsum S: Heredopathia atactica polyneuritiformis: Phytanic acid storage disease (Refsum's disease). *In* Vinken PJ, Bruyn GW (eds.): Handbook of Clinical Neurology, Chap 10, Vol 21, Part I. Amsterdam, North Holland Publishing Company, 1975, pp 181, 229. *Authoritative description of patients with Refsum's disease, including clinical, neuropathologic, and biochemical data.*

Rosenberg RN: Biochemical genetics of neurologic disease. N Engl J Med 305:1181, 1981. *Review of specific biochemical or molecular defects in inherited neurologic diseases.*

Rosenberg RN: Dominant ataxias. *In* Kety S, Rowland L, Sidman R, Matthysse S (eds.): Genetics of Neurological and Psychiatric Disorders. New York, Raven Press, 1983. *Review of clinical and basic science mechanisms in the dominant ataxias.*

Rowland LP (ed.): Human Motor Neuron Diseases. New York, Raven Press, 1982. *A good multiauthored review of the topic.*

Schwartz JF, Rowland LP, Eder H, Marks PA, Osserman EF, Hirschberg E, Anderson H: Bassen-Kornzweig syndrome. Deficiency of serum beta-lipoprotein. Arch Neurol 8:438, 1963. *Classic description of the clinical, neuropathologic, and biochemical abnormalities in Bassen-Kornzweig syndrome.*

Stumpf D, Parks J, Eguren L, Haas R: Friedreich ataxia: III. Mitochondrial malic enzyme deficiency. Neurology 32:221, 1982. *A new biochemical finding in the Friedreich syndrome.*

Zelkowitz M, Edmiston K, Stambouly J: Reduced epidermal growth factor binding sites in neurofibromatosis fibroblasts. Neurology 30:374, 1980. *New finding of epidermal growth factor binding sites as an explanation for altered tissue growth in neurofibromatosis.*

Section Seven CEREBROVASCULAR DISEASES

H. J. M. Barnett

493. INTRODUCTION

Vascular stroke represents the most common devastating disease affecting the central nervous system. In developed countries it is the third leading cause of death, ranking behind heart disease and cancer. Among white populations in the U.S. and Canada the annual incidence rate is between 1 and 2 per 1000, the death rate is between 0.5 and 1 per 1000, and the prevalence is between 4 and 6 per 1000. Blacks have an increased incidence. Encouragingly, in both North America and Western Europe the incidence of stroke is declining at a rate approaching 5 per cent per year, a change attributed to the improved control of hypertension and rheumatic fever.

Vascular stroke occurs as a result of two major causes: *ischemia* and *hemorrhage.*

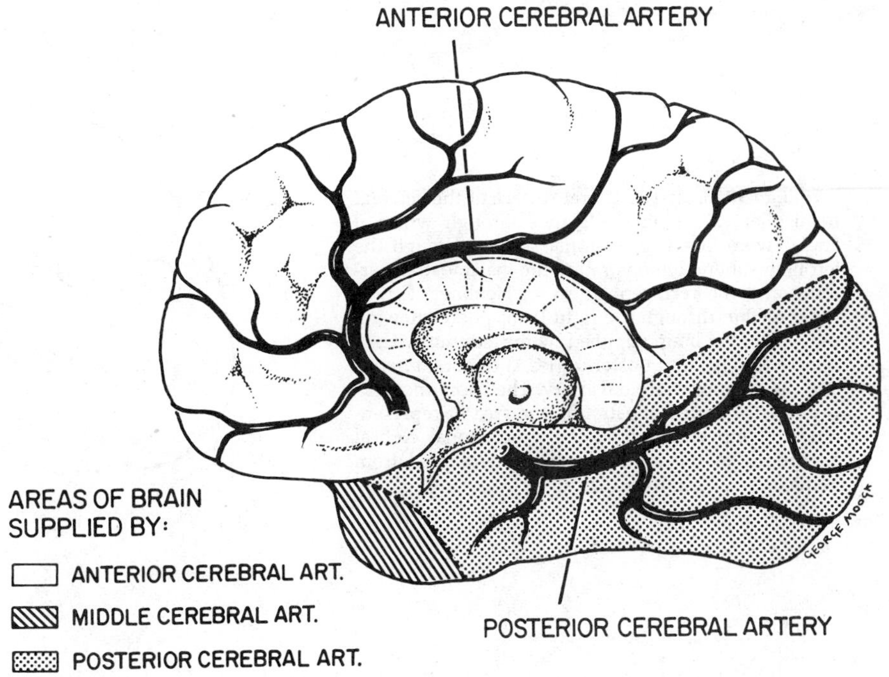

Figure 493–1. The medial surface of the cerebral hemisphere, showing the course of the anterior and posterior cerebral arteries and the medial area of brain supplied by them and the small area of medial supply of the middle cerebral artery.

ANATOMY AND SUPPLY OF THE MAJOR CEREBRAL ARTERIES

Interference with the blood supply to the brain by occlusion and stenosis, and to some degree as a consequence of arterial rupture, produces neurologic syndromes related to arterial territories rather than to specific neuroanatomic and physiologic systems. The interpretation of vascular syndromes is based on a working knowledge of these arterial territories.

Four large arteries supply the brain, the two common carotid and the two vertebral arteries. The left common carotid artery arises from the aortic arch and the right from the innominate artery in the upper thorax. The two vertebral arteries originate from the right and left subclavian arteries respectively. Each common carotid artery bifurcates in the neck at the level of the upper border of the thyroid cartilage forming the internal and external carotid arteries. No branches arise in the extracranial course of the internal carotid artery. Each internal carotid artery enters the skull through the ipsilateral foramen lacerum, passes through the cavernous sinus, and gives off the ophthalmic, anterior choroidal, and posterior communicating arteries and terminally bifurcates into the anterior and middle cerebral arteries.

ANTERIOR CEREBRAL ARTERY. As Figures 493–1 and 493–2 show, the anterior cerebral artery supplies the medial and superior surfaces of the cerebral hemisphere and the whole of the most anterior portion of the frontal lobes. This area contains the motor and sensory cortex for the foot and leg and the supplementary motor cortex. The anterior cerebral artery, through medial lenticulostriate and Heubner's arteries, also supplies several deep structures of importance, including the anterior nucleus of the thalamus with contributions to the corona radiata, the anterior limb of the internal capsule, the head of the caudate nucleus, and the putamen. The first part of either of the paired anterior cerebral arteries is vestigial or absent in 3 to 4 per cent of normal individuals, its cortical portion being supplied from the opposite normal side by the anterior communicating artery.

MIDDLE CEREBRAL ARTERY. The middle cerebral artery (Figs. 493–2 and 493–3) irrigates most of the lateral surface of the

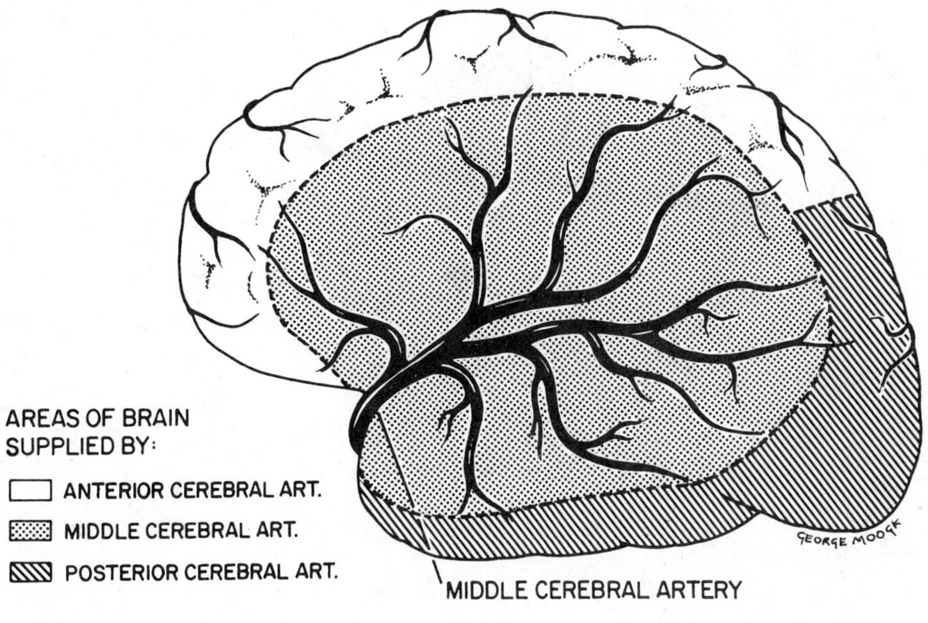

Figure 493–2. The lateral surface of the cerebral hemisphere and the course of the middle cerebral artery. The middle cerebral artery has been elevated from the Sylvian fissure to better illustrate its course. (For clarity the shadings differ from those in Figure 493–1.)

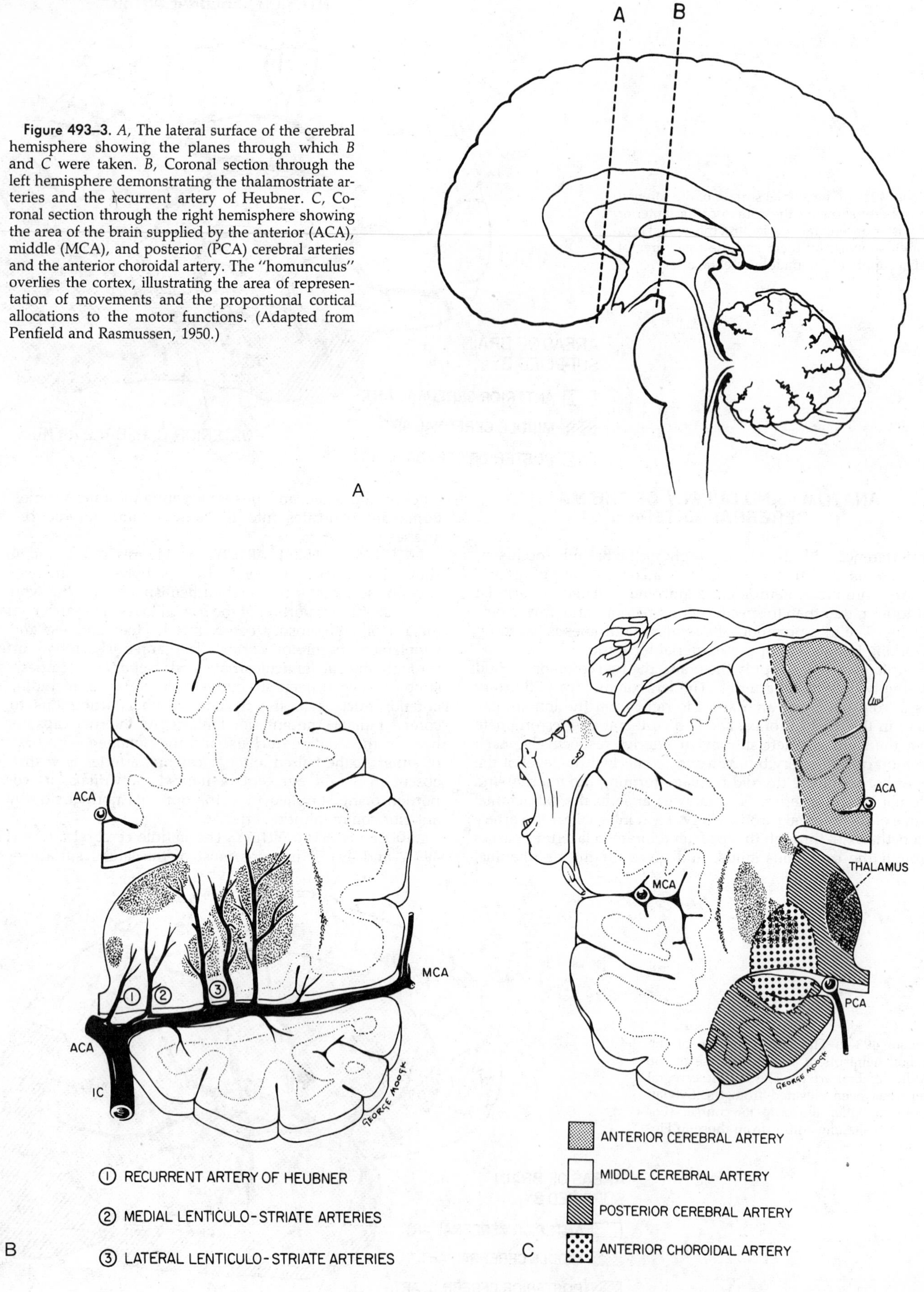

Figure 493–3. *A,* The lateral surface of the cerebral hemisphere showing the planes through which *B* and *C* were taken. *B,* Coronal section through the left hemisphere demonstrating the thalamostriate arteries and the recurrent artery of Heubner. *C,* Coronal section through the right hemisphere showing the area of the brain supplied by the anterior (ACA), middle (MCA), and posterior (PCA) cerebral arteries and the anterior choroidal artery. The "homunculus" overlies the cortex, illustrating the area of representation of movements and the proportional cortical allocations to the motor functions. (Adapted from Penfield and Rasmussen, 1950.)

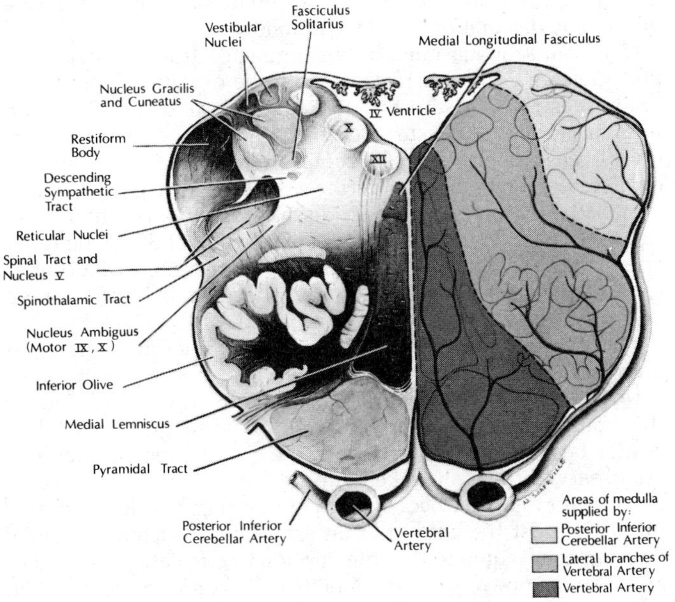

Figure 493–4. Cross-section of the medulla oblongata at the level of the hypoglossal nuclei. Short branches of the vertebral and anterior spinal arteries supply the medial medulla. Longer circumferential branches, including the posterior inferior cerebellar artery, supply the lateral portions of the medulla.

cerebral hemisphere with the exception of the occipital and frontal poles. The cortex supplied includes the primary motor and sensory areas for the face, throat, hand, and arm; the optic radiations; and, in the dominant hemisphere, the cortical areas for speech. The perforating (lenticulostriate) branches of the middle cerebral artery reach the depths of the cerebral hemisphere and contribute to the supply of the posterior limb of the internal capsule, basal ganglia, and corona radiata.

VERTEBRAL AND BASILAR ARTERIES. The vertebral arteries arise from the subclavian arteries and after a short, free course traverse the bony canals in the transverse processes from the sixth to the second cervical vertebrae and then enter the skull through the foramen magnum. The vertebral arteries have numerous branches in the neck, which anastomose with branches of the occipital artery and with the ascending and deep cervical arteries from the costocervical and thyrocervical arteries. Individual variations are common, and in approximately 10 per cent of cases one of the vertebral arteries is vestigial with the result that a single vertebral artery provides the main source of blood for the basilar artery. Immediately after entering the skull, each vertebral artery gives off a medial branch, which unites with its opposite to form the anterior spinal artery. Rostral to this point, the posterior inferior cerebellar arteries arise.

At all levels of the brainstem the ventral medial portion is supplied by short paramedian vessels. The ventrolateral portion is supplied by short circumferential branches from the vertebral or basilar arteries. The dorsal-lateral portion and the cerebellum are supplied by long circumferential branches: the posterior inferior, the anterior inferior, and the superior cerebellar arteries.

The vertebral artery lies on the lateral surface of the medulla oblongata ventrally, and from it and the anterior spinal artery short paramedian branches supply the pyramids, the inferior olives and medial lemnisci, the medial longitudinal fasciculi, and the emerging fibers of the hypoglossal nerve, as shown in Figure 493–4.

The more dorsal and lateral portion of the medulla includes the spinothalamic tract, the vestibular nuclei, the sensory nucleus of the fifth cranial nerve, descending fibers of the sympathetic nervous system, the restiform body, and the emerging fibers of the vagus and glossopharyngeal nerves; these structures are supplied by longer branches from the vertebral artery and the branches from the posterior inferior cerebellar artery. The most cephalad and dorsal segment of the medulla includes the vestibular and cochlear nuclei, which, along with the posterior portion of the cerebellum, are supplied by the posterior inferior cerebellar artery.

At the lower borders of the pons, the two vertebral arteries unite in the ventral midline to form the basilar artery. The basilar artery extends along the ventral aspect of the pons and the midbrain in the midline. From this artery short perpendicular branches enter the pons to supply paramedian structures, including the corticospinal tracts, the pontine nuclei, the medial lemnisci, the medial longitudinal fasciculi, and the pontine reticular nuclei (Fig. 493–5). The anterior inferior cerebellar artery, the long circumferential branch at this level, supplies the lateral portion of the pons, which includes the emerging seventh and eighth cranial nerves, the trigeminal nerve root, the vestibular and cochlear nuclei, and the spinothalamic tracts. It also gives branches to the most dorsal and lateral of these structures as it runs dorsally to irrigate the cerebellum.

At the midbrain level the basilar artery lies in the midline in the peduncular fossa (Fig. 493–6). Short branches pass laterally and dorsally to both sides to supply the cerebral peduncles, the emerging fibers of the third nerve, medial portions of the red nuclei, the medial longitudinal fasciculus, the oculomotor nuclei, and the midbrain reticulum. Branches of the posterior cerebral artery supply the lateral portions of the peduncles, the

Figure 493–5. Cross-section of mid-pons. The medial portion receives blood supply from short perforating basilar artery branches. More laterally, the blood supply comes from lateral basilar artery branches.

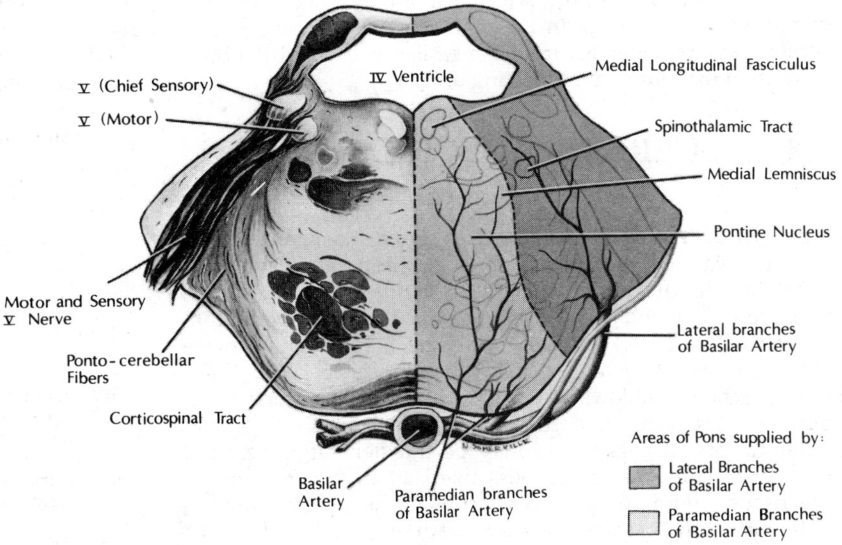

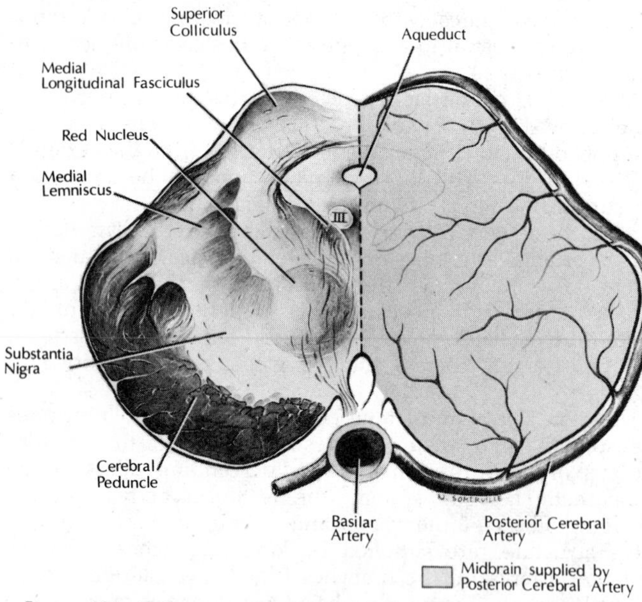

Figure 493–6. Cross-section of the midbrain. The posterior cerebra artery passes around the midbrain and gives off short branches supplying the medial, lateral, and dorsal regions.

red nuclei, and the medial lemnisci. The superior cerebellar arteries contribute to the supply of the dorsal portions of the midbrain, including the colliculi and the superior portion of the cerebellum on each side.

POSTERIOR CEREBRAL ARTERY. As shown in Figures 493–1 and 493–2, the cortical branches of the posterior cerebral artery supply the posterior pole of the lateral surface of the cerebral hemisphere and the posterior portion of the medial and inferior surfaces of the hemispheres. The cortical supply includes the calcarine cortex (the primary visual receptive area) and the hippocampus. Short perforating branches of the posterior cerebral artery supply the midbrain, including the cerebral peduncle and red nucleus, as well as the subthalamic area, the thalamus, and the posterior portion of the internal capsule, and contribute to the optic pathways and part of the hypothalamus.

Anatomic variation is common in the origin of the posterior cerebral artery. In approximately 70 per cent of cases, the origins of both posterior cerebral arteries arise from the apex of the basilar artery and small posterior communicating arteries connect to the carotid arteries. In 5 to 10 per cent of cases, the major supply of blood to the posterior cerebral arteries derives from the internal carotid artery via more robust posterior communicating arteries. In the remaining cases, one posterior cerebral artery originates from the basilar artery and the other from the posterior communicating artery.

494. CEREBRAL ISCHEMIA AND INFARCTION

DEFINITIONS AND ETIOLOGY. The signs and symptoms of ischemic vascular stroke result from interference with the circulation to the brain owing to a generalized or localized reduction of blood flow. Ischemia results from conditions interfering diffusely or locally with the blood supply to the brain, and its many causes are outlined in Table 472–2 of Ch. 472.1. Ischemia follows upon general or local reductions in perfusion pressure which deprive brain tissue of oxygen and other metabolites. Ischemia may be transient; if ischemia is incomplete and persists for less than ten to fifteen minutes, the tissue commonly survives. More prolonged or complete ischemia results in infarction, i.e., death of the tissue. Depending on the site and extent of the infarction, mild to severe neurologic disability or death will follow.

Cerebral ischemia must be distinguished from hypoxia. Hypoxia relates to the interference with the oxygen supply to the brain, despite a relatively normal cerebral blood flow and normal perfusion pressure. Cerebral hypoxia occurs for a variety of reasons, including a general reduction of atmospheric oxygen tension, pollution of the atmosphere (e.g., by carbon monoxide), chronic pulmonary disease, pulmonary emboli, and reduced or altered oxygen-carrying capability of the blood (e.g., anemia, methemoglobinemia). Ischemic infarction will occur as a consequence of severe hypoxia, although it is uncommon and relative ischemia usually is required.

The causes of cerebral ischemia are numerous. The most important are shown in Table 494–1.

NEUROPATHOLOGY OF ISCHEMIA. With prolonged ischemia the brain softens and the margins between gray and white matter become indistinct. Under the microscope the neurons are observed to be shrunken and necrotic. Frequently the area of infarction is pale, occasionally hemorrhagic. A hemorrhagic infarct is most frequent after an embolic obstruction, but may develop as a sequel to the interruption of circulation in a major artery and appears in the watershed or border zone between branches of the artery supplying the cortex or the deeper structures. An example would be the watershed infarct at the margins of the anterior and middle cerebral artery supply which may follow occlusion of the internal carotid artery. As infarcts age, the necrotic central core breaks down and is removed by phagocytic action. The area of previous necrosis (or hemorrhage) may be represented by a cavity filled with yellow fluid and a lining of glia and fibrovascular tissue, sometimes stained with hemosiderin. Areas of infarction are not unusual in postmortem examinations performed on older patients who have died of other causes. They may be numerous and exist in the absence of previous clinical symptoms.

Cerebral edema, variable in amount and dependent on the extent of the infarction, accompanies cerebral infarction. If edema is extensive, it produces distortion of the hemisphere or cerebellum with a shift medially beneath the falx, downward or upward through the tentorium cerebelli, or downward through the foramen magnum. The effects of such compression shifts are visible on CT scanning and are discussed in Ch. 472.1.

Edema and swelling resulting from infarction in the cerebellum can impede the circulation of cerebrospinal fluid and at times leads to obstructive hydrocephalus.

DEGREES OF ISCHEMIA. Partial interference with the cerebral circulation produces neither tissue ischemia nor abnormal symptoms and signs if compensatory mechanisms operate efficiently. With altered systemic blood pressure, even to hypotensive levels, autoregulation by the cerebral arteriolar bed usually is sufficient to adjust the circulation quickly and preserve the vitality and function of brain tissue. Alternatively, ischemia may be sufficiently prolonged and collateral circulation sufficiently inadequate that a major catastrophic stroke results. Between these extremes, gradations of severity may be identified:

A transient ischemic attack (TIA) is defined as a loss of neurologic function caused by ischemia, abrupt in onset, persisting

TABLE 494–1. CAUSES OF CEREBRAL ISCHEMIA

1. Arterial disease: (a) Atherothrombosis in the intra- and extracranial arteries; (b) emboli from the extracranial and larger intracranial arteries
2. Emboli of cardiac origin
3. Cardiac disease causing reduced cerebral blood flow
4. Lacunar infarction
5. Generalized cerebral hypoxia
6. Cerebral artery thrombosis due to nonarteriosclerotic vasculopathies
7. Cerebral artery thrombosis due to coagulation abnormalities (polycythemia, thrombocytosis)
8. Cerebral arterial spasm following subarachnoid hemorrhage
9. Cerebral arterial vasoconstriction associated with migraine
10. Cerebral vein and sinus thrombosis

for less than 24 hours, and clearing without residual signs. Most such TIAs last only a few minutes. If disability persists for more than 24 hours but is attended ultimately by no persisting symptoms or signs, it is conventionally called a *reversible ischemic neurologic disability* (RIND). The study of patients who have experienced TIA or RIND indicates that in approximately 15 per cent of them CT scans will detect a persistent lesion in the appropriate arterial supply. The pathogenic process by which TIA or RIND occurs is the same as that which produces clinical signs of persistent stroke, only the size of the lesion making the difference.

An ischemic event that is sufficiently severe and in an appropriate location to leave persistent disability but is short of a calamitous stroke, is defined as a *partial nonprogressing stroke* (PNS). The ultimate in severity of ischemia produces a more major degree of permanent neurologic disability, *a completed stroke.*

The disability from an ischemic event most often reaches its maximum in a few minutes. Not infrequently, however, the disability will worsen gradually or stepwise over a matter of hours to as much as a week or more: a *progressing stroke* or a *stroke-in-evolution.* When progress ceases and the clinical condition stabilizes, a PNS or a completed stroke will persist.

ATHEROTHROMBOTIC STROKE. ***Sites of Occlusion.*** Arteriosclerosis of the major extracranial arteries to the brain accounts for most strokes. The most common site for obstructive disease of the carotid artery is the region of the carotid sinus, followed by the portion within the cavernous sinus. In Caucasians, the carotid artery is responsible for atherothrombotic stroke six to seven times more frequently than is the main trunk of the middle cerebral artery. In those of Oriental race, the ratio of carotid to middle cerebral disease is reversed.

The extracranial course of the vertebral artery commonly evidences disease at its origin and at the C1–C2 level just prior to entry into the cranium. Intracranially, the most common site for vertebral artery disease and occlusion is within 1 to 2 cm of the termination of the artery, most commonly just beyond the origin of the posterior inferior cerebellar artery. Disease in the basilar artery has a predilection to involve its mid-portion (Fig. 494–1).

Anastomotic Circulation. The manifestations of stroke commonly are described in terms of the arterial territories supplied by branches of the internal carotid and vertebral-basilar arteries, i.e., as syndromes of the anterior, middle, and posterior cerebral artery, as well as of the vertebro-basilar tributaries. It is now recognized that obstruction in the more proximal, commonly the extracranial, part of the arterial supply to the brain often presents a picture indistinguishable from that of more distal obstructions. Internal carotid artery occlusion, for example, can produce no symptoms if intracranial anastomoses compensate for the obstruction. Without such protection, carotid occlusion commonly results in ischemia distributed in some part of the middle cerebral artery territory.

Collateral supply for the internal carotid artery has several potential sources: the ipsilateral basilar circulation via the posterior communicating artery; ipsilateral leptomeningeal communications between the cortical branches of the posterior cerebral artery and those of the middle and anterior cerebral arteries; the ipsilateral external carotid artery by retrograde flow through the ophthalmic artery and, of less importance, through the middle meningeal and ascending pharyngeal arteries; and, contralaterally, through the anterior communicating artery.

The vertebral artery forms anastomoses with branches of the occipital artery and branches of the ascending and deep cervical arteries arising from the thyrocervical and costocervical arteries. Vertebral artery occlusion near its origin commonly results in no symptoms because of the development of an extensive cervical anastomotic network. More serious effects are expected when the vertebral artery is occluded more distally. At any level, obstruction to one or even both vertebral arteries may be asymptomatic. Commonly a modified ischemic syndrome emerges because of the protective effect exerted by the collateral circulation.

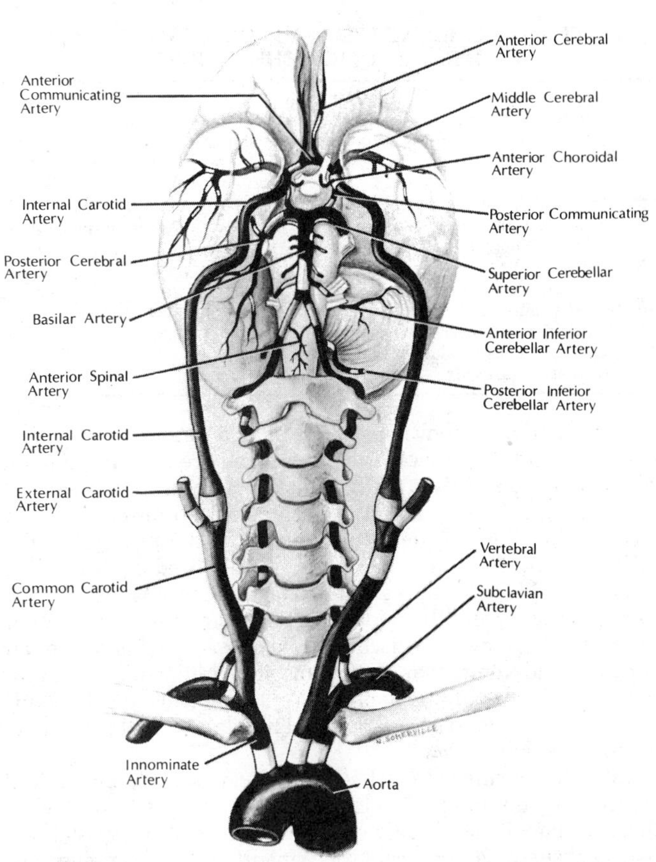

Figure 494–1. The light bands around the arteries indicate the sites of predilection for atheroma. The two most common sites to cause symptoms are the region of the carotid sinus and the intracranial portion of the carotid artery.

Basilar artery occlusion usually produces serious consequences, but the extent of the ischemia can be modified by collateral supply. In rare instances this will be sufficient to allow asymptomatic basilar artery occlusion. Mid-basilar artery occlusion or serious stenosis results in a reduction of pressure in the artery such that there is a reversal of flow with blood coming from the anterior circulation via the posterior communicating artery. The potential exists for collateral communication between the large branches of the vertebral and basilar arteries, particularly the superior, anterior inferior, and posterior inferior cerebellar arteries.

"Watershed" Infarction. Infarcts often occur in the territory where the cortical arteries overlap. The anterior and middle cerebral arteries are the major terminal branches of the internal carotid artery, and circulation may be least effective in the "marginal" or "boundary" zone or "watershed" between these branches following an occlusion of the internal carotid artery. Severe impairment of cerebral perfusion, such as occurs with cardiac arrest, tamponade, and exsanguination, especially results in infarction in these border zones. As the circulation becomes restored, blood passes into the surrounding tissues through capillaries damaged by hypoxia. Watershed infarcts tend, therefore, to be hemorrhagic.

STROKE DUE TO EMBOLI OF CARDIAC ORIGIN. Technologic advances in the past decade permit more accurate identification of cardiac sources for emboli (Table 494–2). Instead of the estimated 3 to 5 per cent of 20 years ago, the estimated incidence of stroke caused by thromboembolism originating from the heart has risen to 20 per cent. The mural thrombus forming on the endocardium in conjunction with myocardial infarction is an important source and accounts for 8 to 10 per cent of strokes. At least 5 per cent of patients with a myocardial infarction have clinical evidence of cerebral embolization. Postmortem studies

TABLE 494–2. CARDIAC LESIONS PRODUCING CEREBRAL THROMBOEMBOLIC ISCHEMIC EVENTS

1. Myocardial infarction—mural thrombosis
2. Postinfarction aneurysms and akinetic segments—stasis thrombi
3. Postinfarction atrial fibrillation—atrial thrombi
4. Mitral stenosis with or without atrial fibrillation—atrial and auricular thrombi
5. Atrial fibrillation of any cause—persistent or paroxysmal thrombi
6. Mitral regurgitation with atrial mural "jet lesions"—small mural thrombi
7. Bacterial endocarditis—valvular mycotic thrombi
8. Nonbacterial thrombotic endocarditis—valvular thrombi
9. Prolapsing mitral valve—valvular thrombi
10. Mitral annulus calcification—? degenerate valve fragments
11. Calcific aortic stenosis—? degenerate valve fragments
12. Atrial myxoma–neoplastic tissue—? attached thrombi
13. Prosthetic heart valve—attached thrombi

of patients dying from myocardial infarction identify systemic emboli in 45 to 60 per cent, half of which are cerebral. Emboli after myocardial infarction are most common in the second week. In one large series 84 per cent occurred in the first four weeks; 6 per cent in the second month, and 8 per cent in the third month. The left hemisphere is embolized slightly more often than the right, the carotid circulation more often than the vertebrobasilar, and the middle cerebral artery more than other intracranial arteries. Postischemic akinetic segments of the left ventricle and ventricular aneurysms are additional but uncommon sources of thromboembolism. Occasionally postischemic rhythm disorders, particularly atrial fibrillation, will precipitate embolic strokes.

Since the incidence of rheumatic fever is declining, mitral stenosis is no longer as common a cause as formerly of thromboembolic stroke. Once the diagnosis of mitral stenosis is established, 20 per cent of patients will suffer systemic embolism within five years, approximately half of which will involve the brain. Of those with such emboli, half will have recurrent emboli, most commonly within the first year after the initial event. The association of atrial fibrillation increases the risk of stroke. The Framingham Study disclosed that atrial fibrillation with rheumatic heart disease results in a 17-fold increase in stroke risk. Atrial fibrillation alone, without rheumatic heart disease, produces a six-fold increase in risk of stroke.

Careful cardiac history and physical examination, supplemented when indicated by ECG monitoring, two-dimensional echocardiography, wall-motion studies, and, in certain selected cases, ventricular angiocardiography, identify the less common cardiac conditions associated with cerebral thromboembolism listed in Table 494–2.

Certain valvular and mural lesions cannot be identified with certainty by physical examination, ECG, and routine radiography. These include atrial myxoma, mitral annulus calcification (a degenerative process in older subjects), and the myxomatous degeneration of the mitral valve which is the most common cause of the "ballooning" or *"prolapse"* of the *mitral valve* (PMV). Such lesions are identified by echocardiography and are being recognized increasingly as causes of ischemic events, in younger patients in the case of PMV, and in older subjects with mitral annulus calcification. The principal clinical challenge is to know when a condition like PMV, which occurs asymptomatically in 6 to 8 per cent of normal persons, is a cause of serious but common symptoms. An epidemiologic study indicated that in patients under the age of 45 who are afflicted with cerebral or retinal ischemic events, 30 per cent had no other recognizable causal factor than PMV, whereas controls matched for age and sex and without cardiac or cerebral symptoms had only a 6 to 8 per cent incidence of PMV. Familial PMV is well known, and several families are on record with strokes in younger members. Marfan's syndrome is accompanied by an increased incidence of PMV, and juveniles with this disorder have been observed with stroke when PMV was the only recognizable causative factor.

CARDIAC DISEASE CAUSING REDUCED CEREBRAL BLOOD FLOW. Disorders of cardiac output and serious hypotension result in diffuse disturbances of brain function. The most common manifestation is the syncopal Stokes-Adams attack caused by heart block, but similar clinical pictures can accompany sinoatrial node disorders, intermittent ventricular arrhythmias, or a variety of conditions producing severe orthostatic hypotension. Failing circulation produces clinical signs reflecting a diffuse reduction of cerebral perfusion, characterized by syncope, convulsions, visual blurring, nonspecific dizziness, and occasionally vertigo. Discrete focal hemispheric events, characteristic of thromboembolic ischemia, are uncommon with these hemodynamic occurrences.

LACUNAR INFARCTION. Lacunar infarction is a condition most commonly associated with longstanding hypertension in which multiple small infarcts occur in the region of the corona radiata, internal capsule, striatum, thalamus, basis pontis, and cerebellum. The distribution of the infarcts favors the territory of the penetrating branches of the middle and posterior cerebral arteries and the median branches of the basilar artery. The infarcts soften, are absorbed by phagocytosis, and leave small (1 to 3 mm diameter) residual cavities (lacunes). Similar lesions occasionally result from emboli passing distally from atheromatous lesions in the large arteries, but in most instances the pathologic cause is fibrosing hyaline degeneration ("lipohyalinosis"), followed by thrombotic occlusion in distal arteries 50 to 150 μm in diameter. The lesions are in the same small arteries which rupture in primary spontaneous intracerebral hemorrhage. It is not known why these vessels develop thrombosis in some hypertensive individuals while they become necrotic and rupture in others.

The incidence of lacunar infarction is uncertain. The Harvard Stroke Registry, a prospective study of stroke in the Boston region, estimated that 19 per cent of strokes were of lacunar origin. A decline of such cases is now evident as part of the reduction in deaths resulting from hypertension.

NONARTERIOSCLEROTIC VASCULOPATHIES. *Fibromuscular hyperplasia* is the most common nonarteriosclerotic disorder affecting the large arteries, predominantly in their extracranial course. It is of unknown etiology, first described in the renal arteries with a predilection to affect females of middle age. Although it is most commonly asymptomatic, minor or major thromboembolic events occur; the long-term prognosis is good and late recurrence of ischemic events is uncommon. An increased incidence of berry aneurysm is reported with the condition.

Dissecting aortic aneurysm consequent upon the medial necrosis related to hypertension and occurring in middle life rarely may cause obstruction to the innominate, common carotid, and subclavian arteries. Stroke developing in association with crushing pain in the chest radiating to the back and possibly into the abdomen, with obliteration of some upper or lower limb pulses, suggests this diagnosis. Affected patients who are normotensive and under middle age should be examined for features of Marfan's syndrome.

Traumatic and spontaneous dissection of carotid and vertebral-basilar arteries is a disorder distinct from aortic dissection. Dissections have been described as a sequel to trauma, including direct blows to the neck, fracture dislocations that injure the vertebral artery in its bony canal, and indirect damage such as follows neck manipulations or other violent twisting or severe cervical hyperextension movements. Most dissections develop spontaneously without recognizable disease in the arterial wall. In a minority there is detectable medial degeneration, fibromuscular dysplasia, or advanced atheroma. The condition occurs in both sexes from childhood to middle life. Internal carotid artery dissection is most common and is characterized by neck, ear, face, or head pain. A bruit is frequently audible, sometimes noted by the patient. Horner's syndrome occurs. Minor intermittent hemispheric TIAs or major strokes develop. The dissection may be bilateral, and at times is accompanied by a similar condition in the vertebral artery. Angiography reveals a long, remarkably narrowed segment of the upper cervical portion of the artery. This stenosis may persist or be combined with segmental fusiform dilatation of part of the diseased artery. In some patients, a return to near-normal or normal appearances has been noted in repeat arteriograms. A similar condition of even rarer occurrence involves the basilar artery and presents with evidence of basilar artery ischemia with or without evidence of subarachnoid hemorrhage.

Pulseless disease or *Takayasu's arteritis* is a granulomatous angiitis, involving fibrous proliferation, mononuclear infiltration, and occasional giant cells. There is a predilection for the condition to involve the media and adventitia of the arch of the aorta in young Japanese females. Occlusion or severe narrowing develops in the cranial as well as the subclavian arteries; branches of the abdominal aorta may be involved. Another inflammatory arteriopathy, particularly common in Japan, *moyamoya,* results in a progressive obliteration of the intracranial carotid arteries. In affected subjects, an extensive vascular network develops with dilatation of many small branches beyond the stenoses, and abundant small collaterals develop from the ascending pharyngeal and meningeal branches of the external carotid artery. The angiographic appearance resembles a "puff of smoke" (moyamoya). Progressive and stepwise neurologic disability is the rule, and many patients suffer abrupt worsening or death from rupture of one of the many anastomotic arteries.

A variety of uncommon pathologic processes can involve the smaller intracranial arteries and arterioles (Table 494–3).

CEREBRAL ARTERY THROMBOSIS DUE TO COAGULATION ABNORMALITIES, POLYCYTHEMIA, OR THROMBOCYTOSIS. *Coagulation abnormalities* are implicated in a variety of conditions which produce cerebral hemorrhage; they are less often associated with thrombotic events in the cerebral circulation. Some of these, such as consumption coagulopathies and thrombotic thrombocytopenic purpura (TTP), can produce combinations of hemorrhage and thrombosis in the same individual. The phenomena are confined to patients with serious systemic illness.

There are a variety of less devastating clinical states in which abnormalities of the coagulation process may be accompanied by cerebral ischemic events and stroke. Table 494–4 lists the more common conditions, none of which have been correlated with specific coagulation abnormalities. Venous thrombosis is more common in some of these conditions than is arterial occlusion. Nevertheless the gamut of ischemic phenomena, varying from TIA to devastating stroke with massive infarction, may complicate any of these conditions.

The angiographic study of patients with these conditions tends to indicate branch arterial occlusions rather than large extracranial artery lesions. However, the initiating thrombus that eventually produces the thromboembolic intracranial occlusion may begin in the large aortic branches or in the pulmonary veins and pass cephalad from these sites.

Thrombocytosis, whether alone or with other features of polycythemia, is a rare but recognized platelet abnormality sometimes accompanied by transient and major persistent cerebral and retinal ischemia.

TABLE 494–3. NONARTERIOSCLEROTIC ANGIOPATHIES CAPABLE OF CAUSING TIA AND STROKE

Large Arteries
1. Fibromuscular hyperplasia
2. Dissecting aortic aneurysm
3. Traumatic and spontaneous carotid and vertebral-basilar artery dissection
4. Takayasu's arteritis (pulseless disease)
5. Moyamoya
Smaller Arteries and Arterioles
6. Collagen vascular disease
7. Giant cell ("temporal") arteritis
8. Meningovascular syphilis
9. Allergic vasculitis
10. Congophilic angiopathy
11. Vasculitis with homocystinuria
12. Vasculopathy resulting from drug abuse
13. Vasculitis with Behçet's disease
14. Granulomatous angiitis

TABLE 494–4. CONDITIONS WITH POTENTIAL FOR ALTERED BLOOD COAGULATION PRODUCTIVE OF CEREBRAL ISCHEMIA

The postpartum period
Pregnancy
Ingestion of oral contraceptives
Manifest and occult cancer
Postoperative and post-traumatic states
Paroxysmal nocturnal hemoglobinuria
Hyperviscosity syndromes
Polycythemia rubra vera
Sickle cell disease
Macroglobulinemia

INTRACRANIAL VENOUS AND SINUS THROMBOSIS. In the era prior to antibiotic therapy, retrograde extension of septic thrombosis from the face to the cavernous sinus and from the mastoid and middle ear to the lateral sinus occurred relatively frequently. The results were devastating and the outcome generally fatal.

Septic venous and sinus thrombosis complicates infections of the middle ear, sinuses, and face. Lateral sinus thrombosis presents with headache and tenderness localized to the mastoid area. Extension of the inflammatory process to the jugular foramen results in dysfunction of cranial nerves IX, X, and XI. Extension toward the tip of the petrous bone results in diplopia from sixth cranial nerve involvement and in facial numbness from trigeminal nerve involvement. Thrombi from the jugular vein may produce fatal pulmonary emboli. Extension occurs into the sagittal sinus and, if sufficiently extensive, impairs venous drainage as well as absorption of cerebrospinal fluid and can result in increased intracranial pressure, papilledema, vomiting, and impaired consciousness. Persistent functional failure of the arachnoid granulations within the longitudinal sinus may be complicated by ventricular dilatation, a conditon called "otitic hydrocephalus."

Septic thrombophlebitis may spread from the nasal sinuses or infections of the face and involve the cavernous sinus. The condition is rare nowadays. The clinical features of cavernous sinus thrombosis include painful proptosis, at times bilateral, with progressive ophthalmoplegia and involvement of the first sensory division of the trigeminal nerve. Meningitis commonly occurs with coma and death in cases that are severe or far advanced prior to therapeutic intervention.

Aseptic thromboses of cerebral veins and sinuses have become more common than the septic variety since the introduction of antibiotics. Even so, the condition is uncommon but may occur spontaneously or with any of the conditions listed in Table 494–4.

Premonitory headaches and transient ischemic events herald more florid signs and symptoms in intracranial venous thromboses. Focal or generalized seizures occur in half of the cases. Major focal neurologic deficits develop and in some instances are bilateral. Mild and occasionally marked evidence of subarachnoid hemorrhage is present, and the cerebrospinal fluid may be sufficiently bloody to suggest the possibility of the rupture of an intracranial aneurysm. This subarachnoid blood comes from hemorrhagic infarction, characteristic of venous thrombosis in the brain just as it is in the retina. Diagnosis can be confirmed from the venous phase of cerebral arteriography with a failure to fill all or part of a major sinus, particularly the sagittal or the lateral sinus. The finding on head CT scan of the "delta sign," a visualization of a dark opacity in the contrast-enhanced posterior portion of the sagittal sinus at the torcula, is diagnostic. This appearance results from the stationary blood (thrombus) within the sinus.

The prognosis for aseptic cerebral phlebothrombosis is usually favorable. Even major neurologic deficits usually resolve completely, although some patients develop future epilepsy and a few develop major permanent disability or death.

SYNDROMES AND SYMPTOMS OF CEREBRAL ARTERIAL ATHEROTHROMBOSIS AND THROMBOEMBOLISM. The clinical features of ischemic infarction from intrinsic arterial disease and from embolic arterial obstruction are similar. The variability of collateral circulation makes it difficult, in the presence of a partial stroke, to state from history and physical examination alone that a main artery is occluded as opposed to one of its branches. Characteristic features of each vascular territory will be given separate consideration.

Internal Carotid Artery. The most common site for atheroma leading to stroke or threatening stroke is the carotid sinus where the common carotid artery bifurcates. Minor lesions, smooth or ulcerative stenosis, and sometimes complete occlusions can be present without any symptoms.

Internal carotid artery stenosis is frequently accompanied by transient events (TIA or RIND). The most characteristic symptom is ipsilateral monocular visual loss. Common symptoms are episodic weakness and/or sensory disturbance of the contralateral arm, leg, or face, at times causing a transient hemiplegia and hemisensory defect that returns to normal within minutes, hours, or days. The speech may be slurred, or, if the dominant hemisphere is involved, dysphasia may be present. Since an embolus may be carried from a stenosis in the proximal internal carotid artery to obstruct an important retinal or cerebral artery branch, persistent and severe signs and symptoms may occur. Consciousness is preserved during an ischemic event in carotid territory unless the ischemia initiates an uncommon convulsive episode. Vertigo, diplopia, and simultaneous bilateral visual loss are not symptoms of carotid artery disease.

Carotid artery occlusion may occur with no symptoms or signs or with no more than a single transient event, or it may be ushered in by a series of transient or minor persisting events followed by a major hemisphere stroke. Fifty per cent of cases of major strokes from carotid artery occlusion occur with no warning episodes. The motor and sensory cortex may be involved with impaired motor and sensory function of the face, arm, and leg. Speech will be lost if the dominant hemisphere is implicated. Large infarcts can cause severe brain edema with serious secondary consequences.

Approximately one third of patients with an internal carotid occlusion complain of mild to severe ipsilateral or, occasionally, contralateral frontal and orbital pain coincident with the onset. The cause is probably a consequence of distention of collateral arterial channels. Approximately 15 per cent of patients with internal carotid artery occlusion develop an ipsilateral Horner's syndrome. Some of these occur without significant evidence of cerebral ischemia, and may reflect an involvement of the vasa nervorum to the periarterial sympathetic fibers. An alternative explanation in some cases is ischemia of the cells of origin of the sympathetic pathway in the hypothalamus.

Palpation of the internal carotid artery is diagnostically inconclusive and potentially misleading. Below the upper border of the thyroid cartilage the palpable pulse is that of the common carotid artery; above this level the superficial pulsation is that of the external carotid artery. Even in the presence of a known complete occlusion of the internal carotid artery, it is often difficult to judge pulse differences. The external carotid pulse may be more apparent than usual as a result of compensatory anastomotic flow to the intracranial portion of the internal carotid artery. Total absence of the carotid pulse indicates an occlusion of the common carotid artery. This may be confirmed by noting the absence of facial and superficial temporal artery pulsations.

Bruits are common over an internal carotid stenosis and are heard loudest at the bifurcation, i.e., at the level of the upper border of the thyroid cartilage. *To identify a bruit as being of carotid origin, one must trace its disappearance down the artery, thereby separating it from transmitted heart sounds.* Carotid bruits, once identified, can subsequently disappear, reflecting a normalization of previously high blood pressure or the occlusion of a stenotic lesion. Harsh bruits usually reflect severely stenotic arteries and may be accompanied by localized palpable thrills. External carotid artery stenosis can produce a local bruit despite internal carotid occlusion. Severe intracavernous carotid stenosis may result in an orbital bruit; such bruits can also accompany severe stenosis or occlusion of the ipsilateral or contralateral internal carotid arteries, possibly from dilatation of anastomotic arteries. The absence of a bruit is not helpful as a negative finding: substantial stenosis and ulcerative disease as well as complete occlusion may be present without audible bruit.

Stenosis of an internal carotid artery is more likely to be associated with recurrent ischemic events than is an occluded artery. Nevertheless, with occlusion, recurrent ischemic events may continue from thromboembolism from the distal soft "tail" of the thrombus in the cavernous sinus portion of the carotid artery; from ulcerative atheroma in the ipsilateral, common, or external carotid arteries; or from a residual "stump" of the occluded internal carotid artery. If such a "stump" remains open, it provides a site for turbulent flow, predisposing to the accumulation of platelet-fibrin thrombus material. From these neck sources the intracranial circulation is embolized through retrograde flow in the ophthalmic artery or through meningeal and ascending pharyngeal anastomoses.

Middle Cerebral Artery. The middle cerebral territory is the most common site for cerebral infarction. The main trunk of the middle cerebral artery is occasionally the site of severe atheroma out of proportion to the other intracranial or extracranial arteries, at times in excess of that affecting the internal carotid artery. Perhaps most often, however, occlusion of the main stem of the middle cerebral artery and of its major branches reflects embolic disease. Experimental emboli placed in the carotid artery or the aorta have a predilection to lodge in the middle cerebral as opposed to other intracranial arteries. In a young person with a middle cerebral artery occlusion or occlusion of one or more of its branches, a cardiac source should be sought. In older patients, either a cardiac or an internal carotid source for thromboembolism is more probable than intrinsic disease of the middle cerebral artery. Recurrent ischemia, persistent or transient, may involve the middle cerebral artery distribution in both hemispheres or in one hemisphere and the posterior circulation, within a reasonably short period of time. Such symptoms may reflect atherothrombotic disease of two arterial systems or alert the examiner to the possibility of emboli from the heart.

The cortical distribution of the middle cerebral artery supplies the areas representing movements and higher sensory functions for the upper limb and face, sparing the leg. Dominant hemisphere involvement produces aphasia. Posterior parietal lesions may result in a lower quadrantanopia. The capsular and ganglionic branches, including particularly the lenticulostriate branches, supply a major amount of the posterior limb of the internal capsule, and infarcts in this territory produce hemiplegia with variable sensory components and with the possibility of an accompanying homonymous hemianopia—all contralateral to the lesion.

Anterior Cerebral Artery. The clinical presentation of occlusion of the anterior cerebral artery depends on the involved segment of the artery and on the availability of collateral circulation. Proximal occlusions may produce no symptoms because of adequate flow through the anterior communicating artery. At the opposite extreme, occlusion of an artery responsible for the complete supply to both anterior cerebral arteries because of a vestigial proximal portion of the opposite anterior cerebral artery results in the rare syndrome of bilateral leg paralysis, urinary incontinence, and serious personality change. Intermediate between these extremes is the usual picture of an occlusion producing partial contralateral leg weakness and sensory loss, minimal arm involvement, and a sparing of face and speech function. Voluntary control of urination is commonly disturbed; mental confusion and behavioral disorders may be encountered. Since the ganglionic branches contribute to the supply of the subcortical white matter beneath the motor speech area, dysphasic symptoms may result from occlusion of the proximal part of the anterior cerebral artery.

Vertebral-Basilar (Posterior) Circulatory System. Occlusion of one vertebral artery and even of both arteries near their origin may sometimes be accompanied by no tissue damage or symptoms because of good collateral circulation. More often, the clinical picture from unilateral vertebral artery occlusion is the lateral medullary syndrome (Wallenberg's syndrome), caused by ischemia in the supply of the posterior inferior cerebellar artery. The ipsilateral findings include limb ataxia; Horner's syndrome; loss of appreciation of facial pain and temperature (trigeminal nerve); paralysis of larynx, pharynx, and palate (tenth nerve); and nystagmus. Intense vertigo and vomiting are common at the outset. Contralateral findings consist of impaired pain and temperature sensations, sparing only the face (see Fig. 493–4).

If one vertebral artery is vestigial, the remaining one becomes the main supply of the medulla. Depending on the condition of the posterior communicating artery, it may be the origin of much of the basilar artery flow. Under these anatomic circumstances, more serious brainstem infarction can result from a single vertebral artery occlusion.

The subclavian artery is most commonly occluded proximal to the origin of the vertebral artery. When an arteriogram is done in this condition, and the opposite vertebral artery is injected with contrast, the flow in the vertebral artery in the side of the subclavian occlusion will be reversed. Contrast material flows down the vertebral artery and into the subclavian artery. Most patients tolerate this diversion without symptoms, but in occasional patients the diversion may produce symptoms of brainstem ischemia aggravated by arm exercise, a phenomenon called the "subclavian steal." It is rare and almost always associated with evidence of extensive occlusive and stenotic arterial disease in the other arteries to the brain.

Basilar Artery. Occlusion of the basilar artery results in variable amounts of infarction of pons, midbrain, cerebellum, and occipital and medial temporal lobes. Asymptomatic basilar occlusion is rare. Most such occlusions, whether thrombotic or embolic, result in patchy infarction of the anatomic structures within the artery's territory of supply. As elsewhere in the brain, the availability and adequacy of collateral circulation determine the degree and extent of infarction. The usual and frequently fatal presentation of basilar artery occlusion includes the sudden development of sustained coma from ischemia of the midbrain reticular activating system, accompanied by bilateral third nerve palsies proceeding to fixed and dilated pupils and paralysis of the face, bulbar muscles, tongue, and all extremities. Incomplete clinical pictures include combinations of bilateral corticospinal tract involvement to any or all four limbs, usually more on one side than another; ataxia in the limbs; variable sensory loss; and a variety of cranial nerve lesions which frequently are on the side opposite the major weakness ("crossed" syndromes). Horner's syndrome may be seen.

On occasion, the basilar collateral circulation is sufficient that infarction will be confined to the ventral structures on one side with a hemiparesis difficult or impossible to distinguish from a more rostral capsular or cortical lesion. Such partial brainstem lesions may result from total occlusion of the main trunk of the basilar artery but more often are the consequence of occlusion of the median and short circumferential branches of the basilar artery by atherothrombotic, lacunar, or embolic obstructions.

Posterior Cerebral Artery. The site of occlusion, anatomic variations, and the availability or lack of collateral supply determine the clinical syndromes arising from posterior cerebral artery atherothrombosis or embolism. Infarctions from proximal branch obstruction include the "thalamic syndrome" and complex midbrain syndromes, including several of the eponymic "crossed syndromes." Hemiballismus or hemichoreoathetosis, intention tremor, and ataxia may be encountered. Conjugate gaze palsies may be added to the third nerve abnormalities and may include upward gaze paresis, skew deviation, and retraction nystagmus.

Cortical branch arterial lesions result most often in homonymous hemianopia, but an upper quadrantanopia may result from interference with the lower fibers of the optic radiation in the temporal lobe. Dyslexia and a variety of visual hallucinations and distortions follow ischemia of visual association cortex.

Bilateral cortical lesions produce cortical blindness and in confused subjects are commonly accompanied by denials that the blindness exists. Sometimes central vision is preserved if the macula is represented in the posterior part of the calcarine cortex and receives leptomeningeal collateral supply from the anterior and middle cerebral cortical arteries.

Amnestic strokes result from bilateral interruptions of the posterior cerebral arteries, producing ischemia in the hippocampal formations of the temporal lobes.

Lacunar Strokes. Several acute stroke syndromes have been delineated that are associated with small vessel disease producing areas of infarction and subsequent cavitation ("lacunes"). The lacunar lesions are less than 3 mm in diameter but may be multiple and occasionally coalesce to form larger areas visible by CT scanning. The most important of the clinical syndromes related to these lacunar infarcts are "pure motor hemiplegia"; "pure sensory stroke" involving face, arm, and leg; and an "ataxic hemiparesis syndrome." Motor hemiplegia results from small discrete infarcts in the internal capsule or the basis pontis. Pure sensory stroke indicates lacunar infarction of the thalamus. Ataxic stroke indicates thrombotic obstruction of the small penetrating basilar artery branches supplying the basis pontis involving the cerebellar peduncle, as well as the corticospinal tracts in this portion of the pons. At times a distinction cannot be made between a primary motor hemiplegia from a capsular lesion and a similar picture produced by a discrete lesion in the basis pontis producing no more damage than to the corticospinal tract.

PATHOGENESIS OF THREATENED STROKE. Stroke prevention has become a realistic goal; thus it is very important to have an appreciation of the way in which stroke presents. A "threatened stroke" may be regarded as any ischemic cerebral or retinal event that causes a TIA, RIND, PNS, or progressing stroke (see previous discussions), each being conditions that can proceed to a devastating stroke. Since it is common for patients with early TIA to go on to develop RIND or PNS prior to a complete stroke, we will discuss together the pathogenesis of all the earlier warning conditions. Such warning ischemic events result from a variety of conditions, which are listed in Table 494–5.

The relative importance of these conditions in producing focal and/or generalized cerebral ischemia remains under active investigation. At the moment the order in which they are listed in Table 494–5 appears to be close to an accurate ranking of their importance.

Artery-to-Artery Emboli. The retina, in which the arterioles are visible at the bedside, provides a microcosm reflecting the circulatory dynamics and pathology of the cerebral arterioles and arteries. Patients under study for recurrent unilateral visual

TABLE 494–5. PATHOGENETIC MECHANISMS OF THREATENED STROKE

Artery-to-artery emboli
Cardiac emboli
Lacunar infarction
Hemodynamic factors
Nonarteriosclerotic vasculopathies
Mechanical interference with arteries
Coagulation abnormalities
Thrombocytosis
Cerebral venous and sinus thrombosis

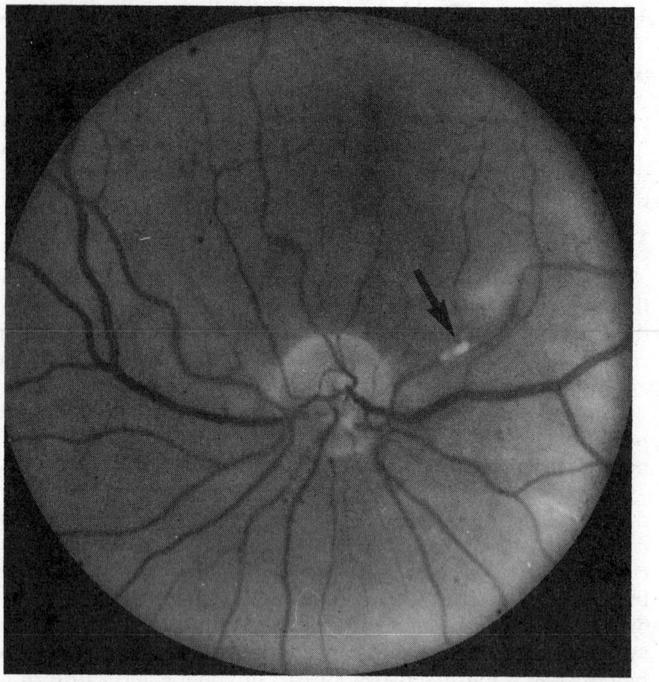

Figure 494–2. Atheromatous debris ("bright plaque") lodged in retinal arteriole in patient with history of attacks of amaurosis fugax. (From Barnett HJM: Med Clin North Am 63:649, 1979.)

loss *(amaurosis fugax)*, a particular variety of TIA, have been observed with three kinds of material located in the retinal arterioles coincident with the development of this symptom. First, grayish-white material composed of platelets and fibrin has been noted passing in the arterioles from the central disc region out to the periphery over a 5- to 45-minute period. Second, fragments of atheromatous debris in the form of bright yellowish amorphous material have been noted. These "bright plaques" may pass through reasonably quickly or lodge and be visible for days or weeks before disappearing (Fig. 494–2). They may persist and become surrounded by white fibrous scar. Finally, pure crystals of cholesterol may be visualized, caught at the bifurcation of a retinal arteriole.

The source of platelet-fibrin emboli is to be sought in the heart valves and chambers or attached to its walls, or in the arteries which lead from it to the brain and retina. Emboli of atheromatous debris and pure cholesterol crystals come from the arteries but not from the heart. Surgeons at operation have observed both types of emboli lodging in the operative field of the exposed cortex in patients known to have irregular and ulcerative atheroma of the internal carotid or middle cerebral arteries. At postmortem examination, pathologists have identified atheromatous debris lodged within thrombi obstructing cortical and deep arteries and arterioles.

The onset of symptoms from major arterial disease may reflect the fact that the narrowing has become great enough to lead to platelet deposition in the area of turbulence beyond the stenosis. An alternative triggering mechanism is the occurrence of hemorrhage into an atheromatous plaque with a rupture into the lumen triggering off thrombosis and embolism or resulting in the formation of a roughened surface upon which platelets and fibrin are deposited. Close scrutiny of patients affected with symptoms of threatened stroke reveals that many have atheromatous lesions in the arteries leading to the territory of the threatening symptoms. Whether the significance of such emboli to TIA in the carotid artery is greater than in the vertebral-basilar territory remains an open question. One of the difficulties in proposing a difference in pathogenesis in the two major arterial systems lies in the fact that vertebral-basilar symptoms are sometimes initiated by cardiac and other systemic circulatory phenomena, and by a number of nonvascular conditions. Despite these limitations, in one study 78 per cent of cases with threatening stroke in the carotid artery territory and 82 per cent of vertebral-basilar cases had arteriographically detectable lesions appropriate to the symptoms.

Emboli of Cardiac Origin. In all age groups one must consider the heart as a source for symptoms and signs of threatening stroke. The common heart lesions resulting in major strokes also can produce minor ischemic events. Most common are mural thrombi from myocardial and endocardial infarction, mitral stenosis with and without atrial fibrillation, and atrial fibrillation from any cause. Any of these can be the ultimate cause of cerebral ischemic symptoms. More attention to the heart and improved capability of examining it adds to the number of conditions recognized to produce cerebral thromboembolism (see Table 494–2).

Lacunar Infarction. Lacunar infarcts (lacunes) are preceded by transitory symptoms in about one quarter of the cases. It is not easy to distinguish such transient events from the more usual artery-to-artery emboli, since many hypertensive individuals develop atheroma in the major arteries.

Hemodynamic Factors. Transient hemodynamic events such as cardiac arrhythmias tend to produce diffuse cerebral ischemic symptoms rather than focal ones. The evidence to support this statement comes from a variety of sources. In one study a series of 37 patients who had experienced focal TIA were exposed to a drop in blood pressure by pharmacologic and postural changes sufficient to induce syncope. Only one patient experienced focal symptoms. In a series of patients dying several days following global ischemia caused by cardiac arrest, the associated areas of cerebral infarction did not correspond to the sites of major atheromatous lesions. By contrast, old infarcts from previous cerebral events corresponded to arteriosclerosis in the appropriate arteries. A study of 290 patients who required a pacemaker because of heart block indicated that although 231 patients had suffered neurologic symptoms, only two had experienced focal ischemic events. Despite this, one sometimes encounters patients in whom a sudden impairment of cardiac output or an episode of severe hypotension (idiopathic cases, autonomic system dysfunction and disease, iatrogenic orthostatic hypotension, pulmonary emboli, carotid sinus hypersensitivity) has been accompanied by a focal ischemic event or a major stroke. Occasionally in the presence of a previously occluded major artery (internal carotid or basilar), a postural drop in blood pressure will result in symptoms that revert to normal when the patient reclines. When this happens, one usually finds that other major arteries are severely stenosed or occluded as well.

Nonarteriosclerotic Vasculopathies. Nonarteriosclerotic vasculopathies are so diverse as to make a generic description of little value. None are common, but collectively they must be recalled, especially when threatened or developed stroke takes an unusual pattern. Table 494–3 lists the conditions. Minor events in all of these disorders may precede major hemisphere or brainstem ischemic infarction. Repetitive and multiple events involving more than one hemisphere should always draw attention to the possibility of a widespread vasculopathy or to a cardiac source.

Mechanical Interference with the Course of the Cerebral Arteries. The location of the common and internal carotid arteries renders them liable to direct trauma with rupture and hemorrhage and even more to injury and subsequent thrombosis. Occasionally violent hyperextension neck injuries can stretch the carotid arteries abruptly in their extracranial course, producing intimal damage, medial dissection, and thrombosis. Similar injury can damage the vertebral artery before its entry at the C6 level into its protective bony canal in the transverse processes of the cervical vertebral bodies. At the C1-2 level, the artery is more mobile and may be levered into a hyperextended and rotated position by athletic injury, motor vehicle accident, or violent chiropractic manipulations. The trauma can lead to early thrombotic occlusion and the clinical picture of a vertebral artery ischemia, or may be followed by recurrent transient ischemic events reflecting a damaged endothelium with an irregular surface attracting thrombi and subsequent thromboembolic events.

Within the canal of the vertebral artery, there may be encroachment on the lumen of the vessel by osteophytes forming at the uncovertebral fissures, or "neurocentral joints" of the spine developing because of cervical spondylosis. Such conditions rarely cause symptoms, even when the artery must deviate around a large osteophyte. There is little movement at this site, and what there is requires lateral flexion to produce further narrowing of the affected artery. The popular concept of cervical spondylosis being a common cause of symptoms such as dizziness and vertigo is erroneous. At most this is a rare cause of ischemic events, and as a rule it occurs only after a severe neck injury.

The internal carotid artery below and adjacent to the cavernous sinus rarely may be distorted and encroached upon by tumors such as "en plaque" meningioma or extensions of nasopharyngeal cancer. Occasionally an odontoid dislocation, of traumatic origin or secondary to rheumatoid disease, will produce brainstem ischemic symptoms related to neck movement by compressing the lumen of the vertebral artery. Similarly, on very rare occasions benign tumors extending into the foramen magnum produce intermittent symptoms of vertebral artery insufficiency.

With routine activities involving neck hyperextension, elderly subjects may complain of episodes of blurred or lost vision, syncope, vertigo, or ataxia. Some of these effects may reflect vertebral artery compromise, but the mechanism is not clear.

TRANSIENT CAROTID AND VERTEBRAL-BASILAR ISCHEMIA. ***Symptoms and Signs.*** TIA, RIND, and PNS forewarn the possibility of a more significant stroke. There are some differences between the management of carotid compared with vertebral-basilar disease, and both may mimic other nonvascular conditions. Thus it is essential for the physician to be aware of the various expressions of TIA symptomatology. It must be recognized that at times a distinction cannot be made between symptoms arising from insufficiency of the internal carotid versus the vertebral-basilar arteries. Since cardiac emboli can produce similar symptoms, the occurrence of transient symptoms must not be construed as final evidence of an arterial abnormality in the carotid or the vertebral-basilar territory. The initial symptoms experienced by 311 patients with associated internal carotid disease are given in Table 494–6.

Amaurosis fugax is highly suggestive of carotid disease. The patient must be observant enough to ensure that a hemianopic disturbance is not mistaken for a monocular visual loss. The patient should be asked to cover one and then the other eye during subsequent attacks to make this distinction. Frequently the description is of a window blind coming down over the vision, obliterating the sight. Flashing or shimmering sensations only seldom emanate from retinal ischemia.

When a patient describes ipsilateral visual loss and on other occasions experiences transient loss of feeling or strength in

TABLE 494–6. SYMPTOMS OF CAROTID ARTERY DISEASE*

Symptoms	TIA AND RIND (208 Cases) (%)	PNS (103 Cases) (%)
Monocular visual	34	21
Paresis (mono-, hemi-)	59	88
Paresthesia (mono-, hemi-)	57	62
Facial paresis	22	43
Facial paresthesia	30	26
Dysphasia	21	30
Dysarthria	14	18
Headache	11	11
Binocular visual (hemianopsia)	7	10
"Dizziness"—nonspecific	6	2
Mental change	1	—
Convulsions		
Focal	—	—
Grand mal	1.5	2
Loss of consciousness	—	1
Visual hallucination	1	—

*From Barnett HJM: Clin Neurosurg 23:543, 1976.

TABLE 494–7. SYMPTOMS OF VERTEBRAL-BASILAR ARTERY DISEASE*

Symptoms	TIA or RIND (78 cases) (%)	PNS (46 Cases) (%)
Binocular visual	50	30
Vertigo	51	35
Diplopia	44	48
"Dizzy"	22	13
Ataxia	41	46
Paresthesia	44	54
Paresis	33	59
Dysarthria	21	37
Headache	18	33
Nausea and vomiting	14	17
Hearing loss	3	7
Mental change	8	8
Dysphagia	4	4
Dysphasia	3	4
Visual hallucinations	5	2
"Drop attacks"	4	4
Convulsions	—	2
Drowsiness	1	2

*From Barnett HJM: Clin Neurosurg 23:543, 1976.

the opposite limbs or face, there is little doubt about the carotid artery origin of the symptoms. It is rare for ocular and limb symptoms to occur simultaneously.

Vertebral-basilar symptoms are more varied. Binocular visual loss is exceeded as a symptom only by vertigo and diplopia. The symptoms described in a series of 124 vertebral-basilar cases are outlined in Table 494–7.

The binocular visual symptoms frequently involve the entire vision, and descriptions vary from a complete blackness to a haziness of vision. At times a description is obtained of a veil over the vision with a random preservation of normal islands. Flashing and shimmering may occur as in migrainous aura. Loss of consciousness is uncommon and did not appear in our patients. Syncope, however, is a common expression of cardiac arrhythmia producing diffuse reduction in cerebral perfusion.

Motor or sensory symptoms simultaneously involving both sides of the body are highly suggestive of vertebral-basilar ischemia; so, also, is unilateral weakness or sensory loss along with evidence of cranial nerve symptomatology, especially vertigo or oculomotor dysfunction producing diplopia. The variety of symptoms experienced by patients with vertebral-basilar disease reflects the anatomic substrate subserved by the vertebral and basilar arteries and their branches. A guide to the origin of common and uncommon symptoms is given in Table 494–8.

Certain symptoms cannot be accurately localized if they occur in isolation. For example, a transient monoplegia or even a hemiplegia may arise from dysfunction of the hemisphere, either cortical or capsular, but might originate from the corticospinal tract in the ventral brainstem. Corresponding sensory phenomena may be equally difficult to localize. The occurrence or recurrence of dysarthria may be from the involvement of corticobulbar fibers coming from the nondominant hemisphere and proceeding from this area of carotid supply down to their location in the brainstem with its vertebral-basilar supply. In general, such isolated dysarthria is more likely to result from carotid than vertebral-basilar insufficiency.

Five to 10 per cent of patients with TIA experience symptoms that reflect abnormalities in both the carotid and vertebral-basilar arterial territories. Careful analysis of characteristic carotid symptoms such as amaurosis fugax or dysphasia, or of vertebral-basilar symptoms such as simultaneous bilateral long tract involvement and dysfunction of cranial nerve nuclei, helps clarify the coincidence of anterior and posterior symptomatology.

Drop attacks, in which a fully conscious older person loses the ability to remain standing, have been attributed at times to vertebral-basilar ischemia. If they are within the framework of

TABLE 494–8. CORRELATION OF VERTEBRAL-BASILAR ISCHEMIC SYMPTOMS WITH ANATOMIC STRUCTURES

Symptom	Anatomic Structure
Common symptoms:	
Bilateral visual blurring	Visual cortex—occipital lobe
Diplopia	Oculomotor nuclei—midbrain and pons
Vertigo	Vestibular nuclei—medulla and pons
Bilateral, alternating, or "crossed" motor and sensory symptoms	Long motor and sensory tracts, cranial nerve nuclei
Ataxia	Cerebellum or cerebellar connections
Less common symptoms:	
Episodic unconsciousness, drowsy state	Reticular activating structures of midbrain and rostral connections
Tinnitus and deafness	Cochlear nuclei
Dysphagia	Tenth nerve nuclei
Nausea and vomiting	Vagus nerve area
Confused episodes	Bilateral temporal lobe, upper brainstem
Amnestic episodes, transient global amnesia	Bilateral temporal lobe
Visual hallucinations	Parietal-occipital region
Symptoms less readily localized:	
Isolated monoplegia or hemiplegia and similar sensory phenomena	? Possibly carotid ? Possibly vertebral-basilar
Dysarthria	? Possibly in brainstem ? Possibly nondominant hemisphere
Drop attacks	? Pontine reticular structures ? Ventral corticospinal tract

an otherwise typical constellation of vertebral-basilar symptoms, this is an acceptable explanation for the phenomenon. It is not certain whether the symptom reflects ventral brainstem ischemia or an ischemia of the pontine portion of the reticular activating structures responsible for the regulation of postural tone. Drop attacks that recur in isolation from other symptoms cannot be ascribed to arterial disease and they provide a diagnostic enigma. Akinetic seizures and cardiac arrhythmic events enter into the differential diagnosis.

Transient global amnesia (see Ch. 478) occurs fairly frequently in older persons. When the episodes occur in conjunction with typical vertebral-basilar ischemic phenomena, their cause may be assigned properly to an ischemic origin. When impaired circulation accounts for these occurrences, it is probable that the ischemia affects bilaterally the medial temporal lobes. Less global or "transient partial amnesia" sometimes occurs and appears to be an incomplete manifestation of a similar disturbance.

Headache is common in cerebrovascular disease. It may accompany TIA and also stroke. It is most common on the side of the ischemia, frontotemporally, but may lie on the opposite side or in the occiput. As a rule such headaches are mild and nonthrobbing, lasting from a few minutes to a few hours. Thomas Willis in 1664 described a violent headache in association with an asymptomatic occlusion of the carotid artery. The designation of "Willis' headache" for the pain associated with cerebral ischemia is appropriate and, as he suggested, may be due to dilatation of anastomotic arteries.

A number of symptoms in combination with others which are appropriately attributed to carotid and vertebral-basilar disease cannot be so designated if they occur or recur in isolation. They may reflect the earliest evidence of ischemia; but if they are not accompanied by other symptoms, their exact origin must remain in doubt. More common and prosaic conditions may be the cause. The list of such indeterminate isolated symptoms includes headache, episodic loss of consciousness, amnestic episodes, drop attacks, attacks of vertigo, deafness, diplopia, and dysarthria. Even in patients with known arterial disease, with neck and orbital bruits, such isolated symptoms cannot be assigned confidently to ischemia. Frequent but stereotyped recurrence of a single symptom speaks against ischemia and requires a search for alternative mechanisms.

DIFFERENTIAL DIAGNOSIS OF TIA. Transient episodes of hemispheric, brainstem, or retinal dysfunction cannot be equated automatically with ischemia. Other conditions may mimic circulatory disturbances by exhibiting recurrent symptoms of equally abrupt onset.

Every patient presenting with the symptom of amaurosis fugax requires close scrutiny for an alternative cause other than thromboembolism. Primary ocular conditions such as muscae volitantes ("floaters"), vitreous hemorrhage, glaucoma, and retinal detachment may be mistaken. Papilledema may be associated with transient visual obscurations, as may the early phases of the ischemic optic neuropathy secondary to giant-cell ("temporal") arteritis. Migrainous auras tend to be scintillating and hemianopic, but patients often mistakenly assume they are of monocular origin. Only occasionally does migraine produce truly monocular visual symptoms.

Localized sensory ischemic events may be difficult to distinguish from focal sensory seizures. Both may occur in the same subject, since a local area of ischemia may become an epileptogenic focus. The lack of a "march" in the ischemic episode is helpful in distinguishing it from sensory epilepsy.

Benign and malignant as well as primary and metastatic brain tumors, arteriovenous malformations, subdural hematomas, and on rare occasions multiple sclerosis may produce short-lived symptoms, coming and going and mimicking ischemia. A postictal paralysis (Todd's paralysis) must not be mistaken for a transient paresis of ischemic origin. Thrombi can develop in aneurysms, and some embolize to the territory of the involved artery with carotid or vertebral-basilar symptoms indistinguishable from those resulting from arteriosclerotic lesions.

Benign positional vertigo, Menière's disease, and other peripheral vestibular causes of vertigo can be mistaken for hindbrain ischemia, since there may be accompanying ataxia. Such patients often describe visual blurring in association with severe vertigo, and they may be syncopal, increasing the resemblance of their symptoms to those of a central lesion. The occurrence and aggravation of tinnitus and deafness with vertigo are useful in alerting the physician to a peripheral vestibular origin.

Vertigo, diplopia, slurred speech, and loss of consciousness may be manifestations of "basilar artery migraine." In such patients, motor and sensory phenomena may be marked because of hemisphere involvement—"hemiplegic migraine." The diagnosis of these uncommon varieties of florid migraine must be made cautiously and seldom in the absence of an accompanying family history. The other family members must manifest an equally striking aura, with accompanying hemicrania, usually developing in late adolescence and early adult life. An important distinction is that migraine of this dramatic type rarely has its onset during the late adult years. Structural lesions are to be suspected and "hemiplegic migraine" becomes a diagnosis by exclusion in middle-aged or older subjects.

Of special importance in the differential diagnosis of vertebral basilar insufficiency are cardiac and circulatory hemodynamic crises producing diffuse disturbances of cerebral perfusion. Most patients who develop complete heart block, as well as some afflicted with a sick sinus syndrome and a variety of tachyrhythmias, experience neurologic symptoms. Sudden loss of consciousness, convulsions, vertigo, and nonspecific dizziness are the common events. Confusion, amnesia, and diplopia may be described. Focal events mimicking TIA are uncommon.

COURSE AND PROGNOSIS. ***The Prognosis of Threatened Stroke.*** Prognosis for threatened stroke patients depends on a number of factors, especially on the particular pathogenesis of the threatening symptoms. Available data are drawn largely from the group of TIA patients and indicate that after the first warning symptoms there is a 5 to 6 per cent chance per year thereafter of stroke recurring and an equal possibility of death, more often from myocardial infarction than from stroke or nonvascular causes. Some evidence indicates that the first three months after the onset of TIA carries a slightly higher risk than subsequent time periods. The prognosis for patients with TIA, RIND, and minor stroke (PNS) is nearly identical. Figures are available from the Canadian Cooperative Study with respect to the specific variety of threatening stroke caused by atherothrombosis with artery-to-artery emboli. Among the 289 patients not given effective treatment, the probability of stroke and death in the first year after diagnosis was 13 per cent, by the end of the second and third years the cumulative stroke and death figures were 22 and 30 per cent, respectively. The outlook for untreated males was worse than for untreated females.

The Prognosis of Completed Stroke. About one fourth to one fifth of patients with either thrombotic or embolic cerebral infarction die with their first attack. This figure varies somewhat with the cause of the infarction and especially with other factors such as age, cardiac status, and the degree of neurologic disability. The mortality rises sharply with increasing age: for patients over the age of 70 and those with marked neurologic defects, coma, or extensive systemic vascular disease, the initial mortality approaches 50 per cent. Infarction of the ventral portions of the brainstem after basilar artery occlusion, especially with quadriplegia, carries a poor outlook, although good medical and nursing care may preserve a vegetative or severely disabled existence for long periods.

The prognosis for cerebral infarction is better in younger patients; in those with the least evidence of vascular disease at other sites, especially cardiovascular disease; and in those who do not have hypertension, diabetes, or severe neurologic defects.

About one fifth of patients who survive a cerebral infarction from atherosclerotic vascular disease suffer another stroke within the next 12 to 24 months. However, the most significant limiting factor on survival is not recurrent stroke but cardiovascular disease. Thus in the Cornell-Bellevue stroke series, fully half of the patients who survived the initial cerebral infarction died at a later date from myocardial infarction or cardiac failure.

Recurrence of cerebral infarction is common with cerebral emboli of any cause. Estimates made over varying time periods indicate the rate of recurrent strokes caused by cerebral emboli from rheumatic heart disease to be between 30 and 70 per cent. Including extracerebral sites, nearly all patients have more than one embolus. In rheumatic heart disease, 40 per cent of the recurrences take place within the first month of the original episode and 50 to 60 per cent within the first year. Each cerebral recurrence carries a strong chance of causing death or further neurologic disability.

Course of Completed Stroke. During the first 72 hours gradual worsening of neurologic deficits and incipient or increasing impairment of consciousness are frequent. The worsening is sometimes due to extension of the cerebral infarction because of progressive and extending thrombosis or because of further emboli breaking off from a proximal arterial or cardiac source. In many instances, however, worsening is caused by the spread of edema around the necrotic area. Nowadays edema can be visualized readily by the CT scan. Other causes of lethargy and stupor in patients with cerebral infarction are the presence of fever; the injudicious use of sedatives, tranquilizers, or narcotics; circulatory failure; respiratory embarrassment; electrolyte imbalance; or combinations of these.

Patients whose course is not complicated by severe cerebral edema usually show an early improvement in neurologic function. If some voluntary movement is preserved, a good chance exists for return of more. When function improves rapidly after the onset, the outlook for a good recovery is excellent. A slow return of function over weeks or months is associated with a less complete recovery. If flaccid paralysis persists from the onset with no return of voluntary movement after 30 to 60 days, the outlook for useful recovery is poor. Substantial sensory loss impairs the chances of recovery of motor function and interferes with the process of rehabilitation. With brainstem infarction, the course is usually one of gradual improvement if the infarct is localized in the lateral medullary area. Symptoms of nausea, vertigo, diplopia, difficulty in swallowing, hoarseness of voice, and ataxia lessen and many times disappear. Recovery from cerebral infarction and return of limb function and speech may continue slowly for as long as one to two years, but most of the improvement takes place within the first two to three months.

MANAGEMENT OF CEREBRAL ISCHEMIA. ***Investigation of Stroke, PNS, RIND, and TIA.*** The investigation as well as the treatment program is influenced by a number of factors. Patients with complete and major strokes need not be submitted to the rigorous investigation required in patients with TIA, RIND, or PNS in whom worsening can still occur. The particular variety of ischemic stroke (atherothrombotic, cardiac emboli, lacunar infarction, hemodynamic, venous infarction) influences decisions regarding treatment, as does the location in carotid as opposed to vertebral-basilar arteries. Age, the condition of the other arteries in the body, the presence of other morbid conditions, and the presence or absence of any major organ failure affect the vigor with which the physician pursues investigation and treatment.

The general examination must evaluate the condition of the systemic arteries, especially those to the lower extremities, by palpation and auscultation of the femoral pulses, evaluation of pedal pulses, and the condition of the integumentary structures of the feet. The comparability of upper limb pulses and bilateral blood pressure readings is essential, since differences may betray serious subclavian disease compromising the origins of the vertebral arteries. Bruits located over the clavicular region and the course of the carotid arteries in the neck, the mastoid area, or the orbits suggest the presence of widespread arterial disease. One must carefully evaluate the heart, including its rhythm and ECG analysis, in order to exclude a recent myocardial infarction, mitral or aortic valve disease, and atrial fibrillation.

Evidence for heart disease should be pursued extensively if there is no overt evidence of vascular disease and particularly in younger normotensive individuals with cerebral ischemia. Twenty-four-hour cardiac ECG monitoring, echocardiography, and wall-motion studies using gated acquisition techniques can be valuable. These studies carry the greatest yield in patients with a history or physical signs suggestive of heart disease. In patients lacking symptoms or signs of heart disease these studies are useful most often in patients under the age of 45 years.

Lumbar puncture is required in a few cases of stroke or TIA, particularly if meningovascular syphilis is a serious consideration. It is not a part of a routine workup in most cases of cerebral ischemia. Electroencephalography (EEG) will be useful only if seizures occur at the onset or during the subsequent course of what appears to be cerebral ischemia. In TIA the EEG is of little practical value, and with a devastating stroke the procedure contributes little to the evaluation of the patient. Doppler sonography of the carotid arteries is a noninvasive technique to detect obstructive or seriously stenotic disease. The method is prone to error. The information it imparts rarely influences the immediate management of an acute stroke but is useful as a preliminary screening test in patients with TIA, RIND, and PNS. Its use in asymptomatic disease is discussed later in this chapter. The development of computer analysis of venous-bolus angiography, a safer method of visualizing the arteries than is routine arteriography, will replace many noninvasive studies, particularly when this new technology is improved to the point of yielding better resolution.

Risk factors should be evaluated in victims of stroke, especially in those with TIA, RIND, and PNS. The presence of hypertension, fasting cholesterol and triglyceride levels, hematocrit, and cigarette smoking habits should be ascertained. Diabetes is important, and recent evidence suggests that hyperglycemic patients suffer larger and more serious cerebral infarctions than do normoglycemic patients.

Cerebral angiography should be carried out if there is diagnostic doubt and the illness cannot be differentiated from an arteriovenous malformation or a giant aneurysm by clinical criteria. Usually, however, the CT scan is more valuable in diagnosing neoplasms. Carotid angiography is indicated to search for surgically treatable lesions if the clinical picture suggests disease in the territory of the carotid artery and the general condition of the patient or the severity of the stroke does not preclude consideration of endarterectomy. Angiography is not indicated in the evaluation of most patients with stroke arising in the vertebral-basilar territory.

All cases with stroke and threatened stroke ideally should receive a CT scan. The technique distinguishes among small unsuspected hemorrhages, old and recent infarctions, and hemorrhagic infarctions and excludes unsuspected space-occupying lesions whose symptoms may imitate vascular ischemia. A negative CT scan obtained several days after the onset of persisting signs of ischemia suggests a location in the brainstem or a lacunar infarction, especially in the hypertensive patient. CT scanning has made isotope brain scanning obsolete in the study of stroke and threatened stroke.

Treatment of Threatened Stroke (TIA, RIND, PNS). Once an accurate individualized decision regarding the pathogenesis of the ischemia has been made, the possibilities for preventive treatment include risk factor management, antispasmodic drugs, antithrombotic drugs, and surgical therapy.

Risk factors are not always amenable to successful manipulation. Heredity cannot be altered. It is not certain that the reduction of high blood lipids alters the outlook once symptoms have been experienced. No data indicate that the elimination of hyperglycemia by rigid diabetic regulation reduces stroke in patients with TIA, RIND, or PNS. Control of both hyperlipidemia and diabetes mellitus is indicated, however, despite the lack of satisfactory supportive data. Cigarette smoking should be eliminated. Hypertension demands therapy, and in all age groups and both sexes the systolic and diastolic pressures must be kept at or below 160 and 90 mm Hg. An increase in hematocrit with an accompanying increase in blood viscosity has been identified as an added risk factor if above 50 and probably should be controlled with the judicious use of phlebotomy. Cardiac abnormalities, whenever amenable to therapy, require careful attention. Carotid bruits are a recognized risk factor for stroke, but evidence to date fails to prove that their investigation and surgical treatment are justified.

Antispasmodics, vasodilators, and "vasoactive" drugs have been widely used and extensively promoted, but no evidence indicates that these preparations have any value in treatment.

Antithrombotic drugs, first introduced as heparin and Coumadin derivatives, remain controversial in stroke prevention. In cases of threatened stroke from emboli arising in mural thrombi following myocardial infarction, and in mitral stenosis with and without atrial fibrillation, their use has received fairly wide acceptance. In the former instance they need not be utilized after eight weeks. In the latter condition prolonged use is customary, since most cases of rheumatic heart disease with emboli have a high incidence of recurrent events over a long period of time, particularly within the year after the initial embolus.

Many authorities advise the use of anticoagulants for recently developed TIAs in carotid and vertebral-basilar territory, recommending them for two to three months or longer if a flurry of TIAs recur and are not relieved by platelet antiaggregant therapy. The data upon which this treatment is based are equivocal and the therapy is empirical. In progressing stroke, many workers advise the use of heparin followed by a few weeks of Coumadin treatment. Controlled studies with convincing data are lacking to establish this as a scientifically proven approach, and its use remains empirical. Anticoagulants alone or combined with platelet antiaggregant agents are usually recommended in the prevention of embolization following the insertion of a prosthetic heart valve. Anticoagulants are not of value in patients with a completed stroke. The administration of anticoagulants carries a risk of fatal intracerebral or other hemorrhage, and their administration always must be rigidly controlled.

Two large and several smaller clinical trials have evaluated platelet antiaggregants in TIA, RIND, and PNS. The weight of evidence indicates that aspirin is effective in preventing stroke and death in a significant number of patients threatened with atherothrombotic stroke. The benefit to females is uncertain: one of the large trials detected a male benefit only, while the other large trial appeared to indicate no particular difference in responsiveness by gender. No benefit has yet been demonstrated for the other known platelet antiaggregants, sulfinpyrazone and dipyridamole. Theoretical evidence, however, supports the hypothesis that the combination of aspirin with dipyridamole may be superior to either drug alone. Trials are underway to establish or disprove this possibility. The optimal dosage of aspirin is unsettled. Clinical studies in stroke prevention have employed 1 to 1.5 grams daily. The balance between the dose of aspirin that suppresses the production of the aggregating thromboxane A_2 from platelets, through cyclooxygenase inhibition, and the dose that suppresses the production of antiaggregating prostacyclin by the vascular endothelial cells, through similar cyclooxygenase inhibition, is under active study. Theoretical evidence indicates that lower doses of aspirin may affect the platelet and spare the inhibition of the more beneficial prostacyclin production. In time the problem of optimal dosage will be settled by clinical trial. For the moment, the best that can be stated is that present evidence from clinical trials favors the use of 1300 mg of aspirin daily. Little information exists on the use of platelet antiaggregants in patients threatened with stroke from cardiac emboli. Some preliminary data from patients with rheumatic heart disease encourage further study.

Special consideration for anticoagulant therapy is required for cerebral vein and sinus thrombosis. Because it is an example of thrombus formation in a slow-flowing venous system, the coagulation cascade is particularly operative. In addition there is a good possibility of accompanying crural thrombosis, and a hazard exists for spread of thrombus to other veins and sinuses and for extension down the jugular vein to produce fatal pulmonary embolism. The therapeutic dilemma is that cerebral venous infarction, as in the retina, is hemorrhagic. When the diagnosis is established by a combination of clinical evidence and whatever supporting radiologic information is available, a CT scan should be employed to exclude a gross amount of blood in the subarachnoid space or in the infarcted area. If CT scanning is not available, a brisk subarachnoid hemorrhage should be excluded by a lumbar puncture. If blood is not present, heparin therapy followed by Coumadin therapy is recommended for 8 to 12 weeks. If blood is found by either technique, anticoagulation should be withheld for 72 hours. These recommendations must be accepted as empirical because no better evidence is available.

Role of Surgery in Cerebral Atherothrombotic Disease. The realization that many patients with cerebral ischemia are afflicted with disease of the extracranial arteries, combined with the development of acceptably safe cerebral angiographic procedures and the development of surgical capability to operate on arterial lesions, culminated in the first carotid endarterectomy being carried out in 1952. The role of surgery in the management of lesions of the cerebral arteries continues to be under active study. The answers are not easily obtained, and it is well to weigh the decision carefully in all cases with the following guidelines:

1. Carotid endarterectomy has become common practice for patients with specific neurologic symptoms appropriate to a stenosed and/or ulcerated atheromatous lesion in the lower cervical portion of the internal carotid artery.

2. A single major randomized study was carried out to determine the benefit of carotid endarterectomy and found no advantage for surgery. However, the study was completed

before the improved skills in angiography and surgery of the past decade were available. The results of such a study might be improved if the controlled trial were repeated.

3. Cerebral angiography and carotid endarterectomy carry a small but definite risk even in the most expert hands. If the combination of morbidity and mortality from these two procedures in a given institution exceeds 3 per cent, it is likely that the patient will fare as well by medical management alone. The risk-benefit ratio is too low to place either of these procedures in inexperienced hands.

4. A carotid endarterectomy at the usual level of the carotid sinus will be a dubious advantage if there is evidence of a stenotic or ulcerated lesion intracranially that equals or exceeds in size that in the neck area.

5. Patients with vertebral artery symptoms are not considered candidates for surgery at present. Proximal lesions in the vertebral artery may be accessible, but there is little evidence that such patients benefit by endarterectomy. Patients with vertebral-basilar symptoms do not benefit from surgery on simultaneously stenosed but asymptomatic carotid lesions.

6. Whether or not surgery is performed in suitable candidates, risk factor management and the utilization of appropriate antithrombotic treatment must not be overlooked. No controlled study to determine the benefit of endarterectomy has been pursued since the benefits of risk factor management and antihypertensive treatment have been established.

7. Carotid endarterectomy in the presence of a completed stroke or in the presence of a complete arterial occlusion appropriate to the symptoms has no demonstrated value.

Final conclusions about the role of carotid endarterectomy in extracranial symptomatic vascular disease await careful future observations. In the interim patients should be subjected to this procedure only after careful analysis of the appropriateness and significance of the symptoms and a full awareness of the angiographic and surgical risks in the particular institution concerned.

Operations purporting to revascularize the brain have been perfected technically and are being applied in a preliminary way in stroke prevention. Some enthusiasts are utilizing the procedures in the treatment of developed stroke. The operation of superficial temporal to middle cerebral artery anastomosis is innovative, but its physiologic or clinical benefits are unproven. A multicenter collaborative trial is attempting to evaluate the benefit of such anastomoses in preventing stroke in susceptible patients. No major trial is being conducted to evaluate the procedure as a means of improving the neurologic condition of the patient with a developed infarction. This is of dubious potential benefit.

The Asymptomatic Carotid Lesion. A bruit detected on routine physical examination, or stenosis revealed by carotid angiography in an artery from which no symptoms have arisen, presents unresolved management questions that are the subject of strong difference of opinion. Long-term surveillance of several large series of patients with neck bruits has determined that a bruit frequently is an index of widespread arterial disease and that such bruits are associated with an increased risk of stroke. However, the resultant stroke often develops in arteries other than the one in which the bruit exists. Bruits are more common in females than in males, but the risk for stroke in males with bruits is greater than that in females. The incidence of bruits increases with age and with the existence of hypertension. Prophylactic endarterectomy has been practiced by some surgeons as a prelude to open heart and aortic surgery if asymptomatic carotid disease is detected in the preliminary arteriograms. The weight of present evidence argues against this practice. Cerebral ischemic events after these major procedures are most often due to emboli initiated by the cardiopulmonary bypass procedure rather than to hypotension and hemodynamic focal ischemia. Until carefully conducted studies reveal convincing evidence to the contrary, we recommend not operating on asymptomatic carotid lesions and bruits.

Treatment of Completed Stroke. Treatment of cerebral infarction is designed to preserve life, limit the extent of the infarction, reduce disability, and prevent recurrences.

Stroke victims present with the same life-threatening circumstances as do patients with other serious neurologic illness. The principles of therapy are the same: the maintenance of a proper airway; adequate fluid, electrolyte, and caloric intake; and adequate urinary output. Constant vigilance is required to prevent aspiration pneumonitis and avoid necrotic skin lesions at pressure points.

The development of cerebral edema threatens to extend the brain damage. Many programs have been recommended to control its development and spread in the ischemic brain but with little success. The results of treatment with osmolar agents are disappointing, unpredictable, and short lived. Nevertheless if patients with large hemispheric infarcts deteriorate, especially if they develop reduced brainstem function, hypertonic mannitol is administered quite often despite the lack of evidence for convincing benefit. The use of corticosteroids either alone or with mannitol has been largely discredited.

Experimental evidence in animals has suggested that deep barbiturate coma given immediately after stroke onset may reduce the ultimate neuronal damage from cerebral infarction. Clinical results have not shown any advantage for the procedure, and this drastic form of treatment cannot be recommended.

Efforts to increase cerebral blood flow to limit the amount of ischemic infarction have been attempted. Vasopressor as well as vasodilator regimens have been attempted by hyperoxygenation or by producing hypercarbia, neither with evidence of benefit.

Treatment in the later and convalescent stages of stroke should be directed toward lessening the deformity and disability and requires daily passive exercise of paretic limbs, and early ambulation with appropriate assistance.

Rehabilitation. Recovery from stroke depends mainly on spontaneous neurologic recovery. It may be assisted by learning to improve function and utilize alternatives, and this requires an active rehabilitation program. Programs of retraining should begin as soon as there is no longer evidence of increasing infarction. Stabilization of the neurologic findings for 12 to 24 hours is usually sufficient evidence to permit the start of rehabilitation. All programs have as their goal the retraining of the remaining functions for maximal effectiveness. Although a few patients require and benefit from special hospital facilities for rehabilitation, most such programs can be carried out on medical services without the aid of extensive equipment. An internist or general physician who is interested in rehabilitation can direct programs of activity and exercise, and can achieve results in rehabilitating hemiplegic patients which are about as effective as those of specialized centers.

The first requirement is to increase the patient's tolerance to sitting and standing, both of which are impaired by weakness and by changes in the sense of balance. Patients are allowed to sit up and then stand for increasingly long periods, beginning with five to ten minutes several times a day. During this period daily active and passive exercises of the weakened extremities are carried out. When patients begin to stand they need firm support and often splinting or bracing of the knee on the weakened side; marked quadriceps weakness may occasionally demand a long leg brace. Ambulation is one of the main goals of rehabilitation. Gait training should begin as soon as the patient can comfortably stand for 15 to 20 minutes without fatigue. The support of parallel bars or a walker should be depended upon at first. After ambulation begins, it may be necessary to brace the foot to avoid the foot drop and inversion that commonly occur after hemiplegia. At the same time that the patient is relearning to walk, he should be trained to develop new skills with his unaffected arm and to improve the strength and function in the paretic arm. This is done by an active program of exercise and by retraining the patient in the activities of daily living such as eating, dressing and undressing, and personal hygiene. Usually the maximal effect of rehabilitation and recovery is gained in three to four months, but some patients continue to show improvement over periods lasting as long as two years. Passive exercise must be continued indefinitely for severely paralyzed patients if contractures are to be avoided.

A painful shoulder resulting from periarthritic changes is common after hemiplegia and may develop despite early passive motion of the member. Continued passive movements combined with heat and, if persistent, with subacromial steroid injection or a short course of systemic steroids will avoid additional pain and permanent fixation of the shoulder adduction movements.

For patients with cerebral infarction who have mild to moderate dysphasia, speech therapy may be helpful. It encourages patients and their families to be aggressive about the need to practice talking and gives considerable encouragement. Speech therapy does not help severe dysphasia.

HYPERTENSIVE ENCEPHALOPATHY. Hypertensive encephalopathy is an uncommon acute neurologic disorder characterized by attacks of headache, nausea, vomiting, visual impairment, focal or generalized seizures, and drowsiness, which may proceed to stupor and coma. Transient focal deficits, including hemiparesis, dysphasia, and hemianopia, may occur. The blurred vision reflects cortical or local retinal ischemic changes, but it is not necessarily associated with retinal hemorrhage or papilledema. Although the latter retinal findings are present in many of the patients, in others the only abnormality is that of narrowing, often segmental, of the arterioles. The blood pressure as a rule is severely elevated. Some patients have had longstanding raised blood pressure with recent further elevation, whereas in others a markedly elevated pressure is a new development.

Hypertensive encephalopathy can complicate acute nephritis, chronic renal disease, eclampsia, and pheochromocytoma. Hypertensive crises and encephalopathy can follow the ingestion of a combination of monamine oxidase inhibiting drugs with food high in tyramine content. The crises can result from the abrupt withdrawal of antihypertensive therapy, particularly clonidine. Excessive autonomic stimulation by bladder or gastrointestinal distention can precipitate hypertensive encephalopathy in patients with acute and chronic spinal cord injuries that can be fatal if not promptly treated.

The brain at postmortem examination in hypertensive encephalopathy sometimes appears grossly normal. In others, the organ is swollen, with evidence of tentorial and cerebellar pressure cones. The average weight of the brain may not be above normal, and edema is not a universal finding even with a history of increased intracranial pressure and papilledema. Cut section reveals small petechial hemorrhages and sometimes larger hypertensive hemorrhages. Microscopically, one finds scattered small areas of infarction accompanied, in patients with longstanding hypertension, by hyaline necrosis of the arteriolar walls.

The pathogenesis of hypertensive encephalopathy is thought to be due to a breakdown in the normal process of cerebral autoregulation, the process whereby cerebral blood flow is maintained at relatively stable levels by arteriolar changes, despite fluctuations in the mean systemic arterial pressure. The intensity and speed of elevation of blood pressure in this condition exceeds the tolerance of the regulatory mechanisms, and a combination of segmentally narrowed and segmentally dilated arterioles results. It appears that the blood-brain barrier is disturbed and that through the segmentally dilated portions of the arterioles brain edema develops. Necrotic arterioles may lead to the creation of petechial and larger hemorrhages.

Uremia closely resembles hypertensive encephalopathy in its symptoms. Once that condition is ruled out by determining that the BUN is below 100 mg per deciliter, the differential diagnosis includes the more usual complications of severe hypertension, including isolated intracerebral hemorrhage, ischemic infarction related to atherothrombosis in large arteries, and lacunar infarction. These conditions are more likely to exhibit focal clinical signs which are florid and persistent. By contrast, the focal neurologic deficits in hypertensive encephalopathy tend to be transient, mild, and multifocal. Sudden increases in intracranial pressure from obstructive hydrocephalus, brain tumor, and subdural hematoma may precipitate severe hypertension, as may acute lead encephalopathy in children. All these conditions also cause papilledema and convulsions. A careful history and attention to the condition of the retinal arterioles, heart size, and the associated conditions in which hypertensive encephalopathy develops will be valuable in differential diagnosis.

Hypertensive encephalopathy is a medical emergency. Its treatment consists of the prompt lowering of the blood pressure, taking great care to avoid dropping it to hypotensive levels. The drug of choice is sodium nitroprusside administered parenterally. The goal of the treatment is to reduce the blood pressure to acceptable levels within 30 to 60 minutes by careful titration of the parenteral drug. Although the intracranial pressure is commonly raised, it will respond to lowering of the systemic pressure and separate therapeutic measures are not required. Hypercapnia can aggravate or precipitate hypertensive encephalopathy and is to be avoided. Convulsions should be treated with intravenous diazepam, 10 to 20 mg, repeated every 30 minutes if need be until the seizures stop, taking care not to suppress respirations. The maximal dosage should be kept between 100 and 150 mg in 24 hours. An alternative is to give phenytoin (Dilantin) through a duodenal tube or intravenously in a dose of 0.5 to 1 gram per day, although that drug is less useful for immediately terminating seizures. Oral phenytoin, 300 mg daily, can be given prophylactically for a few weeks after the acute stage has passed.

Provided that the blood pressure is manageable, that other organs are not in end-stage failure, and that the cause of the hypertension is remediable, the long-term prognosis for the patient promptly recognized and treated for hypertensive encephalopathy is good. Strict, continuing supervision and regulation of the blood pressure are mandatory. Hydrochlorothiazide, beta-blockers, and alpha-methyldopa, alone or in combination, are usually the most effective drugs.

Barnett HJM: Pathogenesis of transient ischemic attacks. *In* Scheinberg P (ed.): Cerebrovascular Diseases. New York, Raven Press, 1976, pp 1-21. *The varieties of this clinical phenomenon are delineated.*

Barnett HJM: Heart in ischemic stroke—a changing emphasis. Neurol Clin 1:291, 1983. *A description of the traditional and the more recently recognized cardiac sources for cerebral ischemia.*

Bousser MG, Eschwege E, Haguenau M, Lefaucconnier JM, Thibult N, Touboul D, Touboul PJ: "AICLA" controlled trial of aspirin and dipyridamole in the secondary prevention of athero-thrombotic cerebral ischemia. Stroke 14:5, 1983. *The second large controlled trial of aspirin in stroke prevention, demonstrating a 50 per cent risk-reduction in stroke for both sexes.*

Brice JG, Dowsett DJ, Lowe RD: Haemodynamic effects of carotid artery stenosis. Br Med J 2:1363, 1964. *A landmark study which indicates that a residual lumen of the carotid artery above 2 mm does not compromise blood flow or produce a pressure gradient.*

Canadian Cooperative Study Group: A randomized trial of aspirin and sulfinpyrazone in threatened stroke. N Engl J Med 299:35, 1978. *The controlled trial which indicated the efficacy of aspirin in stroke prevention in males.*

Chester EM, Dimitris P, Agamanolis DP, Banker BQ, Victor M: Hypertensive encephalopathy: A clinicopathologic study of 20 cases. Neurology 28:928, 1978. *A detailed study of the cerebral and systemic vascular changes found in patients dying with longstanding hypertension culminating in renal failure.*

Corrin LS, Sandok BA, Houser OW: Cerebral ischemic events in patients with carotid artery fibromuscular dysplasia. Arch Neurol 38:616, 1981. *A natural history study of patients with fibromuscular dysplasia indicative of a reasonably benign prognosis.*

Easton JD, Sherman DG: Progress in cerebrovascular disease. Management of cerebral embolism of cardiac origin. Stroke 11:433, 1980. *An excellent review of the risk of stroke from cardiac lesions with a discussion of therapeutic strategies for management.*

Fisher CM: Lacunes: Small, deep cerebral infarcts. Neurology 15:774, 1965. *A paper which led to the recent revival of interest in this important complication of hypertension.*

Genton E, Barnett HJM, Fields WS, Gent M, Hoak JC: Cerebral ischemia: The role of thrombosis and antithrombotic therapy. Stroke 8:150, 1977. *A review article on antithrombotic therapy of threatened stroke.*

Heyman A, Wilkinson W, Heyden S, Helms MJ, Bartel AG, Karp HR, Tyroler HA, Hames CG: Risk of stroke in asymptomatic persons with cervical arterial bruits. A population study in Evans Country, Georgia. N Engl J Med 302:838, 1980. *A long-term surveillance study of asymptomatic carotid bruits indicates that they predict an increased risk of stroke.*

Hypertension Detection and Follow-Up Program Cooperative Group: Five-year findings of the hypertension detection and follow-up program. 1. Reduction in mortality of persons with high blood pressure including mild hypertension. JAMA 242:2562, 1979. *The importance of mild to severe untreated hypertension carefully assessed in the best study to date.*

Mohr JP, Caplan LR, Melski JW, Goldstein RJ, Duncan GW, Kistler JP, Pessin MS, Bleich HL: The Harvard cooperative stroke registry: A prospective registry. Neurology 28:754, 1978. *The report of a prospective registry to determine the incidence of the varieties of stroke in the Boston Hospitals.*

Ross Russell RW: How does blood pressure cause stroke? Lancet 2:1283, 1975. *A thoughtful commentary on the modern concepts of the pathogenesis of the arteriolar reaction in the cerebral complications of hypertension.*

Sherman DG, Hart RG, Easton JD: Abrupt change in head positon and cerebral infarction. Stroke 12:2, 1981. *An updated report on the risk of vertebral artery lesions producing stroke from neck manipulation.*

Skinhoj E, Strandgaard S: Pathogenesis of hypertensive encephalopathy. Lancet 1:461, 1973. *A good introduction to modern concepts about the pathophysiology leading to the clinical picture of hypertensive encephalopathy.*

Soltero I, Liu K, Cooper R, Stamler J, Garside D: Trends in mortality from cerebrovascular diseases in the United States, 1960 to 1975. Stroke 9:549, 1978. *A discussion of the declining incidence of stroke and the probable factors responsible for the phenomenon.*

Wiebers DO, Whisnant JP, O'Fallon WM: Reversible ischemic neurologic deficit (RIND) in a community: Rochester, Minnesota, 1955–1974. Neurology 32:459, 1982. *Describes the incidence, prevalence, and prognosis of reversible ischemic neurologic deficit (RIND) and notes the lack of substantial difference from TIA.*

Wolf PA, Kannel WB, Gordon T, McNamara PM, Dawber TR: Asymptomatic carotid bruit and risk of stroke: The Framingham Study (abstract). Stroke 10:96, 1979. *An important reference for decision-making in regard to asymptomatic carotid bruit management.*

495. INTRACRANIAL HEMORRHAGE

Intracranial hemorrhage constitutes approximately 15 per cent of acute cerebrovascular disorders, usually with drastic consequences, since it results in an abrupt increase in the intracranial contents. Perhaps a majority of patients lose consciousness at least briefly, and many die without recovering awareness. Although there are many causes of intracranial hemorrhage, the anatomic locations of the bleeding importantly influence the clinical picture, and these fall into the following general categories: (1) *Subarachnoid hemorrhage* for the most part results from bleeding from arteries on the surface of the brain, and is limited to the space between the pial and the arachnoid membranes which contains the cerebrospinal fluid. (2) *Intracerebral hemorrhage* results from rupture of vessels within the substance of the brain. (3) Surface bleeding may extend into the brain, producing a combination of *subarachnoid hemorrhage and intracerebral hemorrhage*. (4) *Intraventricular hemorrhage* results from the extension of intracerebral hemorrhage or subarachnoid blood into the ventricles.

ETIOLOGY. Bleeding from aneurysms of arteries composing the circle of Willis and bleeding from arterioles damaged by hypertension or arteriosclerosis are the two most common causes of intracranial hemorrhage. Traumatic intracranial hemorrhage, which is also common, is discussed in Ch. 516. Table 495–1 lists the usual causes of spontaneous intracranial hemorrhage.

TABLE 495–1. CAUSES OF SPONTANEOUS INTRACRANIAL HEMORRHAGE

1. Arterial aneurysms
   a. "Berry" aneurysm
   b. Fusiform aneurysm
   c. Mycotic aneurysm
   d. Aneurysm with vasculitis
2. Cerebrovascular malformations
3. Hypertensive-atherosclerotic hemorrhage
4. Hemorrhage into brain tumor
5. Systemic bleeding diatheses
6. Hemorrhage with vasculopathies
7. Hemorrhage with intracranial venous infarction

Arterial Aneurysms. "BERRY" ANEURYSMS. These are round or saccular dilatations characteristically found at arterial bifurcations on the circle of Willis and its major branches or connections. The cause of berry aneurysms is unsettled. Muscle and elastic tissue defects in the media, possibly of congenital origin, are subjected to the physical effects of pulsatile arterial pressure aggravated by turbulence in the circulation through the aneurysm. The result is a gradual distention and thinning of the weakened segment until the wall is no longer able to contain the blood under arterial pressure. Aneurysms under 4 to 5 mm in diameter rarely rupture, whereas most aneurysms that reach 5 to 7 mm are likely to bleed, usually from the dome. Some reach a size of 2 to 3 cm or more ("giant aneurysm") before rupturing, or never rupture at all and act as a mass lesion compressing adjacent structures. Atheromatous plaques form in some aneurysms and may contribute to weakening of the wall. Larger aneurysms develop thrombi which may calcify. This process thickens the wall and may account for the growth of some to giant size without rupture.

Aneurysms and subarachnoid hemorrhage are more common in association with hypertension whether idiopathic or associated with coarctation of the aorta and polycystic renal disease. Aneurysms are known to rupture under conditions associated with sudden rise in blood pressure, including severe emotional excitement, violent argument, and physical exertion (e.g., athletic competition or coitus).

Intracranial aneurysms occur in all age groups but most commonly rupture in the fifth, sixth, and seventh decades. They are slightly more common in women than in men (3:2). Approximately 85 per cent of congenital berry aneurysms develop in the anterior part of the circle of Willis derived from the internal carotid artery and its major branches (Fig. 495–1). The most common site is at the origin of the posterior communicating artery from the internal carotid artery, followed in frequency by the middle cerebral and the anterior communicating arteries. Fifteen per cent of aneurysms arise from the vertebral or basilar arteries and their branches. Aneurysms are multiple in 15 to 20 per cent of patients and are associated with arteriovenous malformation (AVM) in a small number. In subjects examined in the Cooperative Aneurysm Study, 8 per cent of the AVMs were associated with single or multiple aneurysms.

FUSIFORM ANEURYSMS. These are spindle-shaped dilatations of arteriosclerotic origin arising along the course of the large arteries. They occur most commonly on the basilar artery and less frequently on the carotid artery. When small, fusiform aneurysms are asymptomatic, but they can enlarge sufficiently to interfere with the function of surrounding structures, including the cranial nerves at the base of the brain; some compress the brainstem, others mimic cerebellopontine angle tumors, and still others simulate pituitary and suprasellar neoplasms. The underlying arteriosclerotic disease may be associated with ischemic attacks or infarction in the territory supplied by the artery and its branches. Occasionally embolism may result from thrombi forming within a large fusiform aneurysm. Fusiform aneurysms are less frequently a site of hemorrhage than are berry aneurysms; when rupture occurs, it is more often fatal since it is not amenable to direct surgical management. Extreme arteriosclerotic elongation (ectasia) of the basilar artery may be the precursor to a fusiform aneurysm. Rarely, ectasia or fusiform basilar aneurysm has been described in association with communicating hydrocephalus in which the dilated tip of the elongated basilar artery interferes with the normal cerebrospinal fluid outflow from the third ventricle and along the subarachnoid space.

MYCOTIC ANEURYSMS. Septic emboli from acute and subacute bacterial endocarditis result in arterial necrosis, which may lead to thrombosis or aneurysm formation at the site of lodgment. Such aneurysms tend to arise in a diagnostically characteristic location along the distal branches of the middle and anterior cerebral arteries rather than at the base. Frequently they are multiple.

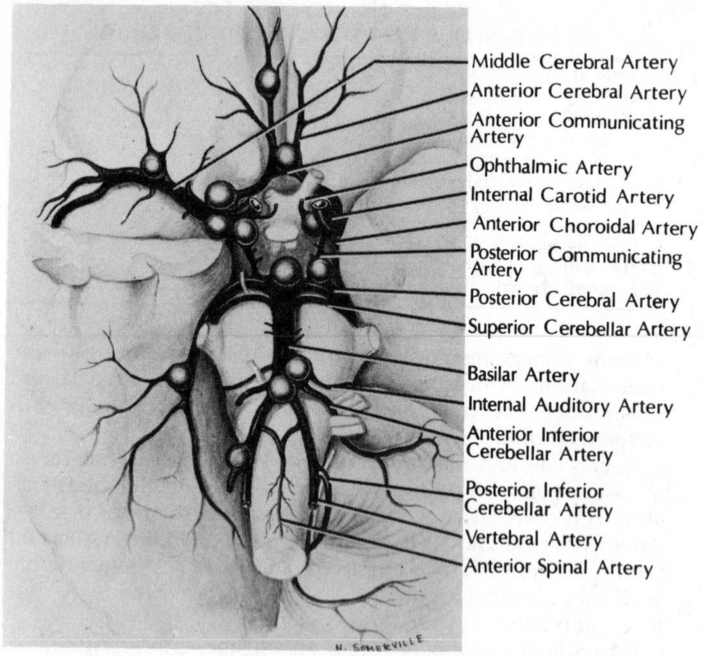

Figure 495–1. The common sites for berry aneurysms to develop at the bifurcation of arteries on the undersurface of the brain.

ANEURYSMS WITH VASCULITIS. A rare form of aneurysm is associated with collagen vascular disease, usually polyarteritis nodosa. Recently a vasculitis has been described in individuals practicing drug abuse, particularly the abuse of amphetamines. The resultant arteriopathy produces irregularly dilated segments, one of which may rupture to produce subarachnoid and intracerebral hemorrhage.

Cerebrovascular Malformations. Vascular malformations within and on the surface of the brain parenchyma constitute about 7 per cent of cases with subarachnoid hemorrhage. Four varieties are recognized: capillary telangiectasia, cavernous angioma, venous angioma, and arteriovenous malformation (AVM). Capillary telangiectasias are found most commonly as incidental postmortem findings in the brainstem; occasionally they cause bleeding into the brainstem. Venous angiomas often are the cerebrovascular abnormality associated with the Sturge-Weber syndrome. Most commonly they present with seizures; less often, with hemorrhage. Cavernous angiomas are the cause of many examples of cryptic intracerebral hemorrhage—"cryptic" since the vessels are not outlined by angiography. These lesions may be discovered at postmortem examination or during the excision of a hematoma. Their usual location is in the subcortical white matter. For unknown reasons cavernous angiomas occur twice as commonly in females as in males.

AVMs produce symptoms more commonly than the other types of cerebral vascular malformations. The malformations consist of tangled, interconnected networks of vessels in which arterial blood passes directly to the draining veins without intervening capillaries. They range in size from barely detectable lesions up to huge networks large enough to occupy an entire lobe of the brain, or to cover most of one cerebral hemisphere. They occasionally involve the cerebellum and brainstem. AVMs tend to be supplied by more than one parent artery, and the draining veins may be as large as 1 cm in diameter. It is uncertain how often AVMs rupture, but at least small bleedings appear to occur in more than 50 per cent of cases. Others declare themselves with recurrent unilateral headache of migraine type (an unusual cause for migraine, however), with epileptic seizures, or by producing a slowly increasing neurologic defect. Most AVMs do not increase much in size once they have been detected. When enlargement occurs, it is in association with small hemorrhage or with thrombosis of draining veins. Progressive neurologic disability may occur because of pressure of the abnormal arteries upon the underlying brain or possibly from shunting of blood into the malformation rather than to the underlying brain (an "intracranial steal").

Hypertensive-Arteriosclerotic Hemorrhage. At least two thirds of parenchymatous cerebral hemorrhages in adults are accompanied by clinical or pathologic evidence of systemic hypertensive vascular disease. Most of the remainder occur in subjects showing atherosclerotic vascular changes. With the increase in availability of CT scanning, small intracerebral hemorrhages in all lobes have been identified more often than were previously suspected. Most such lobar hemorrhages present as minor strokes in hypertensive or elderly patients and are initially misdiagnosed as ischemic lesions.

Hemorrhage into Brain Tumor. Primary and metastatic tumors of the brain may be the site of hemorrhage. Apoplectic onset is encountered with tumors that are benign or malignant, primary or metastatic. Hemorrhage is most common in rapidly growing malignant gliomas and very vascular secondary tumors (e.g., melanotic carcinoma; renal, thyroid, chorionic, and bronchogenic carcinoma). Bleeding complicates the clinical course in some benign brain tumors, including meningioma and pituitary adenoma, and in some slowly growing gliomas, including oligodendroglioma.

Systemic Bleeding Diatheses. Intracerebral hemorrhage complicates leukemia, aplastic anemia, thrombocytopenic purpura, hemophilia, and a variety of less common bleeding diseases. Usually there is evidence of bleeding elsewhere. The hemorrhage in the brain involves more locations than is usual in hypertensive hemorrhage, including superficial cortical areas. Multiple hemorrhages may occur, particularly in thrombotic thrombocytopenic purpura and with the consumption coagulopathies. Thrombotic infarction may accompany the hemorrhagic tendency in some instances. The primary process may lie in the vessel wall rather than in the circulating blood.

Anticoagulant therapy can be complicated by intracerebral as well as extradural, subdural, and subarachnoid hemorrhage. In the case of the intracranial surface clots, trauma is a major precipitant, but in many instances no history of injury can be obtained. When the intracerebral hematomas are in the usual locations for hypertensive hemorrhages, the relation to the anticoagulation will be uncertain and possibly incidental. By contrast a subcortical location of a hematoma is uncommon in spontaneous hypertensive hemorrhage. Extension through the pia into the subarachnoid space is common in hematoma complicating anticoagulation therapy and uncommon in spontaneous hypertension cases.

Hemorrhage with Vasculopathies. Polyarteritis nodosa is the most significant nonarteriosclerotic degenerative disease of arteries producing intracerebral hemorrhage. It may do so by causing an aneurysmal dilatation or by producing necrotic disruption of the artery. Cerebral hemorrhage with systemic lupus erythematosus is usually secondary to accompanying hypertension. Congophilic (amyloid) angiopathy is associated with intracerebral hemorrhage and occurs in older nonhypertensive patients. The usual presentation is by a sudden apoplexy with signs of cerebral hemorrhage in a patient with a recent history of progressing dementia. Such hemorrhages are often multiple and affect sites not common in hypertensive intracerebral hemorrhage. "Lobar" (white matter) hematomas in older patients are more often associated with this vascular lesion than with any other pathologic entity. When, in patients over 60 years of age, more than one lobar hematoma develops within a few days or weeks of the initial hemorrhage, the diagnosis of hemorrhage from congophilic angiopathy is reasonably certain. This amyloid degeneration of the cerebral arterioles is six times more common in women than in men and is not associated with systemic amyloidosis. Drug abuse, particularly the use of amphetamines, is associated with intracerebral hemorrhage. These hemorrhages are frontal, are occasionally ganglionic, may extend into the subarachnoid space or the ventricles, and are the accompaniment of a vasculitis in most of the cases that have been examined in detail.

Hemorrhage with Intracranial Venous Infarction. This presents most commonly in association with the complex findings described for septic or nonseptic lateral, sagittal, and cavernous sinus thrombosis (see Ch. 494). The finding of blood in cerebrospinal fluid coupled with seizures at the onset sometimes makes it difficult to distinguish between this condition and an aneurysmal rupture on clinical examination alone.

PATHOLOGIC CONSEQUENCES OF ANEURYSM RUPTURE. Aneurysms lie within the subarachnoid space, and their rupture introduces blood into this space under arterial pressure. The bleeding may be minimal and emerge through a very small tear in the sac. At the other extreme there may be sufficient bleeding to fill the basal cisterns, or to produce a hematoma locally distorting the subarachnoid space and the overlying brain. Such hemorrhages can be under sufficient pressure to cause reflux into the fourth ventricle through the foramina of Magendie and Luschka and to fill and distend the ventricles with blood. Also, aneurysms in any of the usual locations commonly send their jet of blood directly into the parenchyma of the brain. Anterior communicating artery aneurysms lying adjacent to the medial surface of the frontal lobes, and middle cerebral artery aneurysms lying within the sylvian fissure adjacent to the frontal and temporal lobes, are particularly prone to rupture into the brain. Anterior communicating aneurysms may rupture into both frontal lobes. Basilar artery aneurysms may rupture into the diencephalon or midbrain. Such intracerebral hemorrhages commonly extend through the brain substance and rupture secondarily into the ventricles.

Aneurysm rupture may include hemorrhage into the adjacent cranial nerves. The most common cranial nerve to be implicated is the third nerve, owing to rupture of an aneurysm at the point of origin of the posterior communicating artery from the internal carotid artery. Much less commonly, third nerve palsy is due to a basilar artery aneurysm. The optic nerve commonly is involved with ophthalmic artery aneurysms, and carotid aneurysms in the cavernous sinus involve the three cranial nerves acting on the muscles of the eye (III, IV, VI) and the first division of the trigeminal nerve. The distortions resulting from increased intracranial pressure commonly result in unilateral or bilateral sixth nerve palsies. Most cranial nerve palsies developing in patients with aneurysm result from bleeding in the nerve and not from compression of the nerve by the aneurysm. Large aneurysms, acting as space-occupying lesions, may damage cranial nerves progressively by compression.

Adherence of the dome of the aneurysm to the arachnoid may result in rupture into the subdural space, and a substantial quantity of subdural blood is present at postmortem examination in approximately 10 per cent of patients who die of ruptured aneurysm. Rarely, such a subdural hematoma occurs with little or no subarachnoid bleeding.

Rupture of an aneurysm produces a sudden increase in the intracranial pressure. Several mechanisms are involved. In the first place, an expanding hematoma, whether intracerebral, intraventricular, subdural, or subarachnoid, represents an abruptly enlarging space-occupying lesion. Also, blood in the basal cistern interrupts the natural flow of cerebrospinal fluid. Finally, if the pacchionian granulations become distended with blood, the reabsorption of the spinal fluid is impeded. Papilledema and subhyaloid hemorrhage in the retina follow, with coma and deterioration of brainstem function, and secondary hemorrhages develop within the midbrain.

As a late sequel to subarachnoid hemorrhage, hydrocephalus may develop or persist. The cerebrospinal fluid pressure measurements, although moderately elevated, tend to approach normal—an example of so-called "normal-pressure" hydrocephalus. Some examples of this complication are known to be sequelae to a fibrosing reaction in the basal cisterns, in particular the cisterna ambiens, producing, in effect, an extraventricular obstructive phenomenon. Others may be associated with ventricular ependymal damage and a change in the hydrodynamics of cerebrospinal fluid circulation, with accumulation of interstitial fluid in the subependymal tissue. Both causes create a form of communicating hydrocephalus.

Ischemic infarction of the brain is common in patients with subarachnoid hemorrhage. This is rarely due to arterial or venous thrombosis but is associated with segmental and at times extensive reactive narrowing of the intracranial arteries, termed vasospasm. As observed in arteriograms, cerebral vasospasm usually appears four to ten days after subarachnoid hemorrhage and develops in more than one third of patients suffering a ruptured aneurysm. In the absence of a further hemorrhage, vasospasm causes focal neurologic deterioration of 20 per cent of individuals following subarachnoid hemorrhage. Vasospasm is most marked in the territory of arteries adjacent to the bleeding point and tends to be less when the bleeding is slight. Vasoactive substances, including prostaglandins, serotonin, catecholamines, and methemoglobin, are released by the blood in the subarachnoid space and are believed to precipitate this vasospastic response. Desquamation of the endothelial cells, followed by platelet-fibrin thrombogenesis in the affected arteries, has been described. Edema, necrosis of the media, and intimal proliferation have been described as sequelae to the initial chemically induced vasospasm.

CLINICAL FEATURES OF SUBARACHNOID HEMORRHAGE. The location of the bleeding is the main determinant in the clinical presentation: aneurysms that rupture entirely into the subarachnoid space present with features of meningeal irritation or transiently increased intracranial pressure; with the formation of an intracerebral hematoma or when the blood ruptures into the ventricles, more devastating signs develop. Direct involvement of adjacent cranial nerves produces specific focal features (e.g., a third nerve palsy with posterior communicating and basilar aneurysms). Vasospasm and obstruction of the cerebrospinal fluid pathways impose new clinical signs. The most common symptom of subarachnoid hemorrhage is the sudden development of a violent headache. At the onset many patients localize the headache frontally or temporally. Soon it becomes occipital, spreads to involve the entire head and neck, and at times radiates down the spine and the backs of the legs. Arterial distortion and injury produce the first head pain, and the spreading discomfort is due to increased intracranial pressure and meningeal irritation.

The initial hemorrhage may be minor, a "warning leak" characterized by the sudden development of a headache usually severe but sometimes only moderately intense, with or without associated neck stiffness. This type of headache in an adult not prone to headache may disappear in two to three days, but demands that subarachnoid hemorrhage be considered. If hemorrhage is suspected, a diagnostic lumbar puncture must be done, since subsequent rupture is often more devastating, and in many instances fatal. The initial hemorrhage often is preceded by no other warning symptoms, but some patients complain of minor neurologic symptoms in the days or weeks prior to the major event. Although emotional excitement and physical exertion are known to precipitate the hemorrhage in some patients, they occur as well during sleep. Possibly this is because surges of increased blood pressure occur during the REM phases of sleep.

Brief loss of consciousness or seizures are common at the onset, preceded by an awareness of dizziness or vertigo and by vomiting. Persistent coma usually means massive intracerebral or intraventricular bleeding. Recovery of consciousness in a few minutes is the rule if the bleeding is confined to the subarachnoid space or is localized as a small intracerebral hematoma. The development of brainstem signs commonly indicates transtentorial compression, but occasionally indicates a posterior fossa aneurysm with rupture into the brainstem.

Neck rigidity is the most common physical sign; if severe bleeding has occurred, it produces retraction of the neck into hyperextension. Small, round hemorrhages observable by funduscopic examination over or near the optic nerve head have a "subhyaloid" or preretinal location and may be associated with the early development of papilledema. These changes reflect the fact that the optic nerve sheath is surrounded by an extension of the subarachnoid space, and an abrupt rise in the cerebrospinal fluid pressure interferes with venous return from the retina.

Cranial nerve palsies are usually the result of direct hemorrhage into the particular nerves. Secondary distortions from the mass effect of a hematoma can impair the function of cranial nerves emerging from the brainstem. Hemorrhages occurring within the brainstem account for some cranial nerve palsies.

When lateralizing signs, including hemiplegia, develop at the beginning or within a few hours, an intracerebral hematoma, a large subdural hematoma, or occasionally a subarachnoid hematoma is the usual cause. If such signs develop after several days without a fresh and violent headache, one suspects the presence of vasospasm producing ischemia and infarction. Delirium is a common and nonspecific symptom with subarachnoid hemorrhage; gradual deterioration of consciousness, after three or four days with or without an accompanying worsening of pre-existing neurologic deficits, suggests the development of hydrocephalus with increasing intracranial pressure.

Systemic signs include low-grade fever, glycosuria, albuminuria, and a peripheral white blood cell count up to 15,000. A massive outpouring of systemic catecholamines may cause multifocal micronecrosis of the myocardium, which can produce ECG abnormalities that simulate the changes of myocardial infarction. An occasional patient with subarachnoid hemorrhage develops acute pulmonary edema. Others develop the syndrome of inappropriate antidiuretic hormone secretion (SIADH).

Little other than the past history clinically distinguishes the symptoms of subarachnoid hemorrhage resulting from the rupture of an AVM from those that emanate from a ruptured aneurysm. Intracerebral bleeding is more common with AVMs since most of them lie within the brain. Accordingly, focal neurologic signs and evidence of the sudden development of a mass lesion are frequent accompaniments of a rupture. The presence of an AVM as the cause of subarachnoid hemorrhage is suggested by a history of previous focal seizures, by indolently or slowly stepwise progressing focal neurologic signs, and occasionally by recurrent unilateral throbbing headache suggesting migraine. In addition to meningeal irritation and focal neurologic signs reflecting bleeding, one finds a bruit over the orbit or skull in approximately 40 per cent of patients. Apart from occasional giant aneurysms, bruits are not audible with berry aneurysms.

LABORATORY INVESTIGATION OF SUBARACHNOID HEMORRHAGE. Cerebrospinal fluid examination by lumbar puncture is indicated in all patients with suspected subarachnoid hemorrhage unless computed tomography (CT) has been carried out and identifies blood in the subarachnoid space and/or brain and ventricles. With blood identified by CT scan little is gained by cerebrospinal fluid examination, and angiography becomes the next step in diagnosis. Furthermore, in the presence of an intracerebral hematoma lumbar puncture adds an unnecessary risk of inducing pressure coning. Small subarachnoid hemorrhages often fail to cast their shadow on the CT scan. Accordingly, in spite of a negative CT examination, if the history or signs suggest subarachnoid bleeding, a lumbar puncture is obligatory. If a CT scan is not available, lumbar puncture should be done whenever there is reasonable cause to suspect subarachnoid hemorrhage and provided that there are no signs of a mass lesion. The CT scan evidence of bleeding diminishes rapidly after the first week and should be supplemented with a lumbar puncture seeking discolored fluid, increased cells, or protein.

Confusion may result when bloody cerebrospinal fluid is encountered after a "traumatic" lumbar puncture. Even the most careful insertion of a lumbar puncture needle sometimes causes local bleeding. Usually when this occurs, the fluid dripping from the needle hub is streaked with blood and, as the fluid is collected, the amount of blood decreases in each successive tube. It is imperative, whenever cerebrospinal fluid is obtained, to compare it to water in an identical tube. Normal cerebrospinal fluid is as crystal clear and colorless as tap water. If the fluid is pink or bloody, it should be immediately centrifuged for five minutes and the supernatant visually recompared with water. Pink or yellow discoloration (xanthochromia) of the supernatant, caused by blood or the degradation of hemoglobin in the hypotonic cerebrospinal fluid, is a certain sign of subarachnoid hemorrhage. The supernatant of a freshly spun tube of blood from a traumatic tap will be clear and colorless. A repeat lumbar puncture several hours after a traumatic tap may exhibit xanthochromia. Since fresh blood left standing in cerebrospinal fluid on the way to a hospital laboratory will undergo lysis and discolor the supernatant, one should centrifuge the obtained specimen immediately.

Immediately after a subarachnoid hemorrhage, the proportion of white to red blood cells in the cerebrospinal fluid is the same as in the peripheral blood. After the lapse of 12 hours or more, the white blood count rises from the meningeal irritation; in a few days, when the red cells have become crenated, there may be as many as 500 polymorphs and lymphocytes, followed a few days later by lymphocytes alone. The protein content slowly increases to as high as 80 to 100 mg; the glucose content declines slightly at most. During the first two weeks or so, the cerebrospinal fluid pressure commonly rises to levels of 200 to 300 mm, and at times readings as high as 500 mm will be recorded owing to an associated communicating hydrocephalus.

COMPUTED TOMOGRAPHY. Immediate CT examination demonstrates blood in the subarachnoid space in about 95 per cent of cases of ruptured aneurysm or AVM. The technique will not demonstrate the high density of blood in cases in which the CT scan is delayed. Less than 30 per cent of cases of ruptured aneurysms show blood in the subarachnoid space four days after the hemorrhage. The CT scan is invaluable in the detection of intracerebral, intraventricular, subdural, and occasional subarachnoid hematomas, and has become an essential part of the optimal study of patients with subarachnoid hemorrhage. The finding of a subarachnoid clot in the CT scan in the first 24 hours following a subarachnoid hemorrhage greatly increases the likelihood that vasospasm will complicate the patient's course. Aneurysms larger than 5 mm in diameter often are directly visualized by this technique, particularly after contrast enhancement. Serial CT studies help determine whether new symptoms are related to rebleeding, ischemia secondary to vasospasm, the development of edema surrounding previous intracerebral bleeding, or hydrocephalus.

ARTERIOGRAPHY. The cerebral angiogram remains the definitive procedure to identify aneurysms and AVMs. The procedure is performed in all cases of subarachnoid hemorrhage that are considered reasonable operative risks or when diagnostic doubt exists. Four-vessel angiography is mandatory because 15 per cent of aneurysms occur in the posterior circulation, because multiple aneurysms occur in another 15 per cent of patients, and because of the association of aneurysm with AVM in a small but important number of patients. When aneurysms are multiple, the largest and most irregular is usually the source of the hemorrhage. Angiography is essential to identify areas of local or general vasospasm and occasionally may have to be repeated pre- and postoperatively when new signs develop requiring the physician to differentiate between fresh bleeding and the development of vasospasm. The CT scan complements this investigation in determining whether most of the blood is subarachnoid, intracerebral, or subdural in location.

PROGNOSIS IN SUBARACHNOID HEMORRHAGE. Subarachnoid hemorrhage from ruptured aneurysm carries a grave prognosis. It has been estimated that 28,000 individuals per year in the United States experience a subarachnoid hemorrhage caused by a ruptured aneurysm and that 10,000 die or are disabled from the initial event without referral for treatment, 9,000 die or are disabled despite treatment, and 9,000 survive without major disability. In a 30-year survey of morbidity from Rochester, Minnesota, extending from 1945 to 1975, the probability of survival for 30 days from the onset of the first subarachnoid hemorrhage was only 42 per cent. Only 39 per cent of patients survived for six months, and of these 25 per cent were disabled. The first two weeks after the initial bleeding are the most hazardous for recurrence. Very late recurrences have been described as long as 20 years after the initial bleeding. Long-term studies of prognosis, involving at least a ten-year follow-up period, indicate that if patients survive six months from subarachnoid hemorrhage, rebleeding occurs at a rate of 3.5 to 4 per cent per year and the mortality from such rebleeding is about 65 per cent.

The prognosis for bleeding from AVMs is better than that for aneurysm. Initial mortality is 10 per cent, and subsequent rebleeding occurs in approximately 20 per cent at a rate for fatal recurrence of 1 per cent per year in one major series followed for 35 years. There is a slight increase in mortality for recurrent compared with initial bleeding. Neurologic disability in the patients who have bled is higher than in surviving aneurysm patients because of the usual intracerebral location of the malformations.

TREATMENT OF BERRY ANEURYSM. The goal of aneurysm treatment is to prevent further rupture of the aneurysm while maintaining normal cerebral perfusion. The logical approach to the management of a patient with a ruptured aneurysm is to exclude the thin-walled sac from the pressure of the arterial blood while concurrently maintaining the normal patency of the parent and adjacent branch vessels. This is best accomplished by surgically placing a small metal clip or ligature across the neck of the sac. Unfortunately, it has proved to be hazardous to submit a patient to immediate or emergency surgery following subarachnoid hemorrhage. At this point in time the brain is bruised and swollen, the normal arterial autoregulation is impaired, and surgical manipulation may hasten and aggravate the evolution of vasospasm. Accordingly, many surgeons delay eight to ten days before performing craniotomy, meanwhile reducing the patient's risk of rebleeding by the judicious control of blood pressure and the giving of antifibrinolytic agents. Collaborative investigation is under way in an effort to identify patients for whom early operation appears to be the correct approach. If the aneurysm cannot be directly obliterated, surgical ligation of a proximal vessel may be effective in reducing the risk of recurrent hemorrhage by reducing the pressure and turbulence within the sac. In the anterior circulation aneurysm, where the common or the internal carotid artery or one of the major intracranial branches must be ligated, some surgeons employ a preliminary superficial temporal to middle cerebral artery anastomosis to protect against the ischemic infarction that might otherwise be expected to develop.

Recent advances in technique, including the development of the operating microscope, improved angiography, the CT scan, improved anesthesia, controlled hypotension, and the modern management of vasospasm, have reduced the morbidity and mortality of patients considered appropriate for surgery. Nevertheless, many patients die first or never become suitable candidates for surgery so that subarachnoid hemorrhage from ruptured aneurysm retains a distressingly high morbidity and mortality. The risk of dying in the first eight weeks after rupture remains at 40 per cent. The following points are important in deciding on the management of these patients:

1. The best results from direct clipping of the neck of an aneurysm are obtained in patients who have no focal neurologic signs, have had no evidence of focal bleeding for seven to ten days, and have no evidence of vasospasm in an arteriogram performed immediately prior to surgery. Unfortunately by this time about 20 per cent of hospitalized patients have died or become disabled by rebleeding, infarction, or other complications.

2. A patient deteriorating from a hematoma or hydrocephalus may require urgent surgery to remove the mass and reduce the raised intracranial pressure. Usually the aneurysm will be dealt with at the same time. Patients already in stupor or coma, however, rarely do well with surgical treatment.

3. The presence of vasospasm requires delay of surgery until the spasm disappears or it is apparent that it is causing no further neurologic worsening. Blood volume expanders such as albumin or dextran with crystalloid are recommended to treat patients with evidence of spasm so as to improve intracranial blood flow.

4. During the period of delay prior to surgery careful pharmacologic control of the blood pressure and complete rest in a quiet environment must be sought. Epsilon-aminocaproic acid,* an inhibitor of fibrinolysis, administered in a dosage of 30 to 40 grams per day intravenously is believed by many to reduce the chance of rebleeding.

5. Occasional patients develop SIADH. Fluid and electrolyte intake should be monitored appropriately. The commonest electrolyte imbalance is the result not of excess antidiuretic hormone output but of excessive administration of 5 per cent dextrose solutions, causing iatrogenic hyponatremia.

6. Patients with subarachnoid hemorrhage are best treated in centers possessing experienced teams of neurologists, neurosurgeons, and radiologists rather than by inexperienced and occasional operators. In the hands of skilled surgeons most aneurysms can be dealt with successfully, provided that the complications of vasospasm, intracerebral hemorrhage, hydrocephalus, or continuing comatose states can be prevented.

7. Giant aneurysms rebleed in 30 per cent of cases. Removal is more hazardous than with berry aneurysms even in the hands of skilled and experienced surgeons. However, no other treatment can assuredly prevent progressive and disabling neurologic signs or fatal hemorrhage.

TREATMENT OF ARTERIOVENOUS MALFORMATION. Large AVMs should not be removed if they have not bled, especially if they are in an area of the brain where a surgical approach might damage vital neurologic function. Some malformations can be dissected out and removed. Those located in the frontal or occipital poles can sometimes be safely excised by lobectomy. Ligation of the feeding vessels coupled with balloon catheter embolization and the injection of plastic polymers into the vessels of the anomaly is being carried out in a few centers. Serious complications can occur, and its indications are regarded as uncertain and its value as unproved.

---

*This use is not listed in the manufacturer's directive.

PATHOLOGY OF SPONTANEOUS HYPERTENSIVE-ARTERIOSCLEROTIC INTRACEREBRAL HEMORRHAGE. Intracerebral hemorrhage as a consequence of arteriolar hypertensive disease tends to occur in five locations. The first two are the most common: external capsular–putaminal hemorrhage and internal capsular–thalamic hemorrhage. Central pontine hemorrhages and cerebellar hemorrhages are less common. Least common are hemorrhages in the subcortical white matter and centrum ovale, remote from the vital structures involved with the more usual varieties.

Hypertension hastens the progress of arteriosclerosis in the larger arteries, but in many patients it produces its most devastating effects on the arterioles. The arterioles of the capsular and ganglionic (lenticulostriate) branches of the middle and posterior cerebral arteries, those supplying the central pontine structures (penetrating branches of the basilar artery), and those lying in the central cerebellum are the sites of predilection for the characteristic arteriolar changes. These distinct changes affect the small intracerebral arteries 50 to 150 μm in diameter. Microaneurysms (Charcot-Bouchard aneurysms) form with loss of lining endothelium, media, and elastic tissue, and all are replaced by fibrous tissue. Fibrin and fat constitute the hyaline tissue within the walls, and the process is described by various names, including fibrinoid necrosis and lipohyalinosis. The penetrating arteries subject to these changes are peculiar in that they do not divide into smaller branches, and the suggestion has been made that they are more vulnerable to the direct transmission of marked fluctuations of blood pressure. These same penetrating small arteries develop necrotic degeneration leading to rupturing in some hypertensive patients, whereas in others a less necrotic process leads to lipohyalinosis with thrombi and lacunes.

Hypertensive-arteriosclerotic intracerebral hemorrhages tend to be catastrophic despite their origin from an arteriole of small size. It is postulated that one arteriole ruptures, producing a small hemorrhage, and that this in turn compresses surrounding tissues. Ischemia from this compression is thought to speed the process of necrotic degeneration of adjacent arterioles, producing a "cascade" effect and an expanding area of hemorrhage. Hemorrhages in the cerebral hemisphere tend to dissect along fiber pathways and rupture into the ventricles. Relatively few extend directly into the subarachnoid space, although secondary drainage into the subarachnoid space from the ventricles is common. Pontine and cerebellar hemorrhages extend into the subarachnoid space either by direct extension or indirectly through the fourth ventricle. Massive intracerebral hemorrhage often shifts the brain tissue under the falx or downward through the tentorium, leading to secondary brainstem hemorrhage, attributed to a combination of venous obstruction and arterial ischemia. Many smaller hemorrhages remain circumscribed but may be associated with extending edema of the surrounding brain.

CLINICAL MANIFESTATIONS OF SPONTANEOUS INTRACEREBRAL HEMORRHAGE (Fig. 495–2). Intracranial bleeding develops abruptly and evolves over a period of minutes to hours. The ictus usually occurs while the patient is awake and active as compared to thrombotic obstructions, which more commonly occur during sleep. With a typical onset the patient cries out with the intensity of head pain or complains of distressing dizziness. Frequently there is a history of hypertension, and with the onset of bleeding the blood pressure can rise to excessively high levels. Cardiomegaly is common, and retinal arteriolar changes, although not always impressive, are observed within minutes to hours; 75 per cent of patients with a large hemorrhage (greater than 2 to 3 cm diameter by CT scan) will lose consciousness (Fig. 495–3). The associated physical findings depend on the size and site of the bleeding.

External Capsular–Putaminal Hemorrhage. Affected patients are likely to lose consciousness within minutes to hours and quickly develop evidence of hemiplegia. With smaller lesions there may be drowsiness without loss of awareness and the rapid evolution of a hemiplegic stroke. Conjugate deviation of the eyes to the side opposite the paretic limbs is common, but deviation toward the paralysis can occasionally reflect the irritative effects of the blood. Larger lesions compress the upper brainstem so that coma deepens, with dilated and fixed pupils, bilateral motor hypertonus, Babinski signs, and intermittent or irregular respirations.

Internal Capsular–Thalamic Hemorrhage. The onset is often not distinguishable from the more laterally located hemorrhage described above. In some instances there will be an awareness of sensory disturbances. If the patient is examined while still alert, a homonymous hemianopia may be detected because of the involvement of the optic radiation in the posterior limb of the internal capsule. The medial location of this hemorrhage and its compression of the tectal-midbrain area produce a variety of conjugate gaze palsies, including defective vertical and lateral gaze, fixed downward deviation of the eyes, unequal pupils briefly nonreactive to light, skew deviation, and retraction nystagmus.

Pontine Hemorrhage (Fig. 495–4A). Coma, accompanied by quadriplegia, decerebrate rigidity, and breathing irregularities, occurs early. The usual oculomotor sign is the finding of tiny pupils that are reactive to light; oculovestibular responses rapidly disappear. The majority of patients die after a few hours or days, but with the advent of CT scanning a larger number of nonfatal lesions are being diagnosed than were previously recognized. Most who survive are quadriparetic and severely disabled.

Cerebellar Hemorrhage (Fig. 495–4B). The clinical picture is ushered in with sudden occipital headache, diplopia, and incoordination. Early difficulty is experienced with stance and gait without prominent lateralizing ataxic signs. Vertigo is uncommon. The development is not as rapid as in pontine hemorrhage and usually evolves over several hours. Sixth nerve or conjugate lateral gaze palsies are common eye signs, but ocular bobbing and skew deviation can ensue, as can facial weakness, dysarthria, and dysphagia.

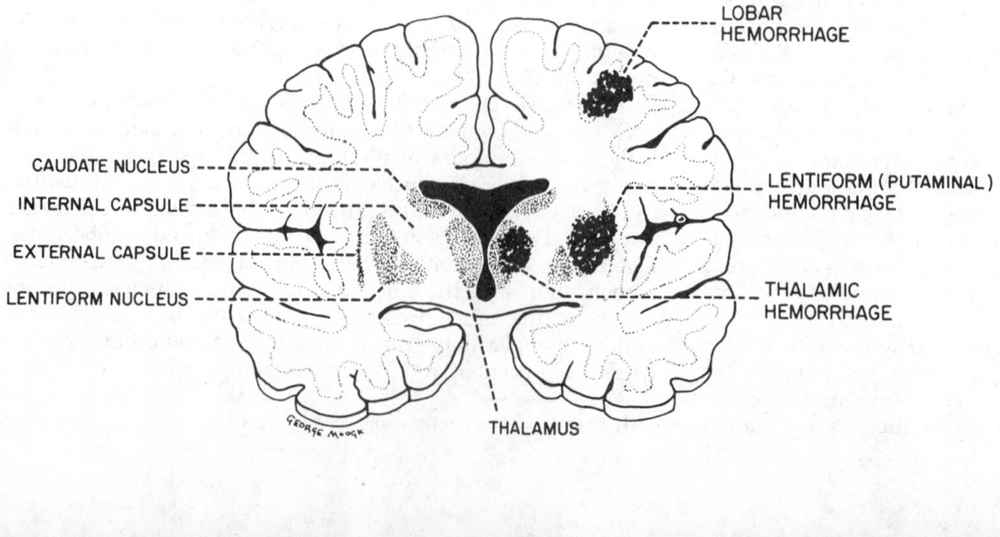

Figure 495–2. A coronal section through the cerebral hemispheres illustrating thalamic, putaminal, and lobar subcortical hemorrhages.

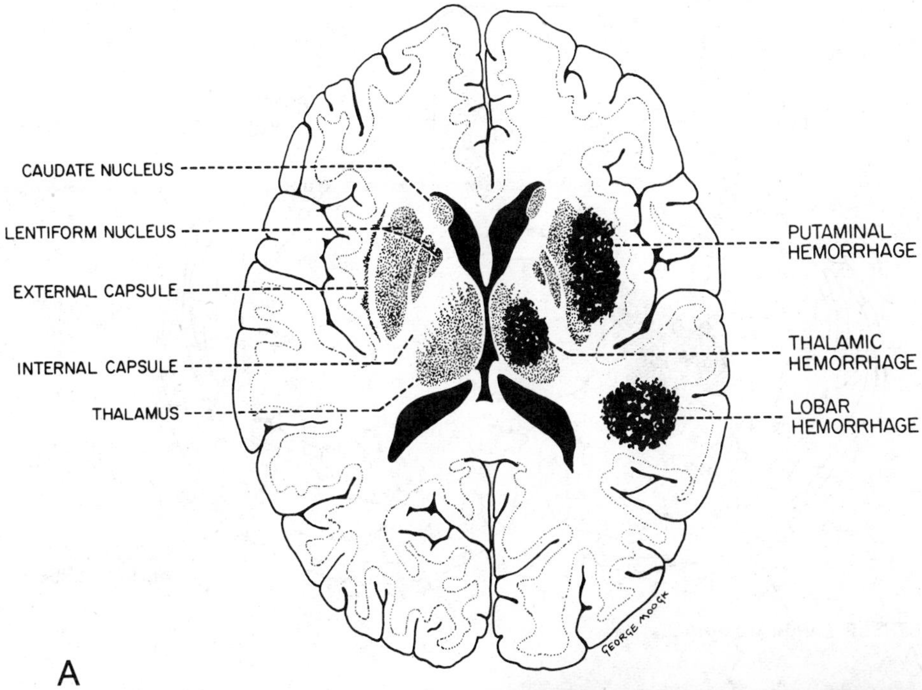

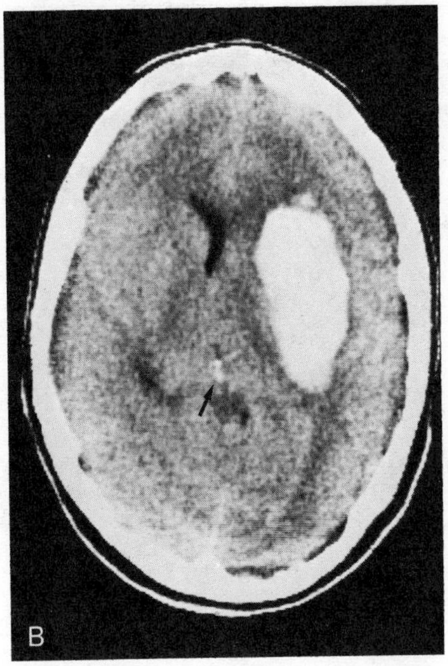

Figure 495–3. *A,* A horizontal section through the cerebral hemispheres illustrating thalamic, putaminal, and lobar hemorrhages. *B,* CT scan showing a putaminal hemorrhage. The ipsilateral lateral ventricle is obliterated by the mass effect and some blood is visible in the third ventricle (arrow).

Progressive worsening in these patients can occur either from enlargement of the hematoma and edema in surrounding tissue, producing pressure on the brainstem, or from obstruction by the mass of the fourth ventricle, leading to a subacute hydrocephalus with equally serious implications. Recognition of the condition is crucial, since surgical treatment can be lifesaving, as noted later in this chapter.

Hemorrhage in Subcortical White Matter. A small number of intracerebral hemorrhages in hypertensive individuals occur in less vital areas of the brain, generally in the centrum ovale. Such small white matter hemorrhages can produce the picture of progressing stroke. Spread of surrounding edema or further bleeding leads to clinical signs, including the development of drowsiness. However, many patients remain alert and do not develop evidence of subarachnoid bleeding. Spontaneous recovery with little or no disability is common. CT scans establish the diagnosis.

DIFFERENTIAL DIAGNOSIS OF HYPERTENSIVE HEMORRHAGE. In establishing a diagnosis of hypertensive intracerebral hemorrhage, the sudden onset and the evolution over a few minutes to hours are important. Such abrupt onsets also occur, however, with thrombosis and embolism. Headache is the predominant feature at the onset in at least one half of hemorrhages and in less than one fourth of cases of thromboembolism. Vomiting is prominent as an early symptom. Funduscopic examination will indicate extremely reduced arteriolar caliber and probably periarteriolar hemorrhages. Nuchal rigidity is common with primary intracerebral as well as subarachnoid hemorrhage. It disappears as the depth of coma increases. Restlessness and vomiting are more common with hemorrhage than with infarction. Convulsions are common with intracerebral hemorrhage, are less frequent with subarachnoid hemorrhage, and are uncommon (<10 per cent) with cerebral infarction. The most important clues to the diagnosis of hypertensive hemorrhage are the explosive onset, the history of high blood pressure, an early decline of the level of consciousness, and the detection

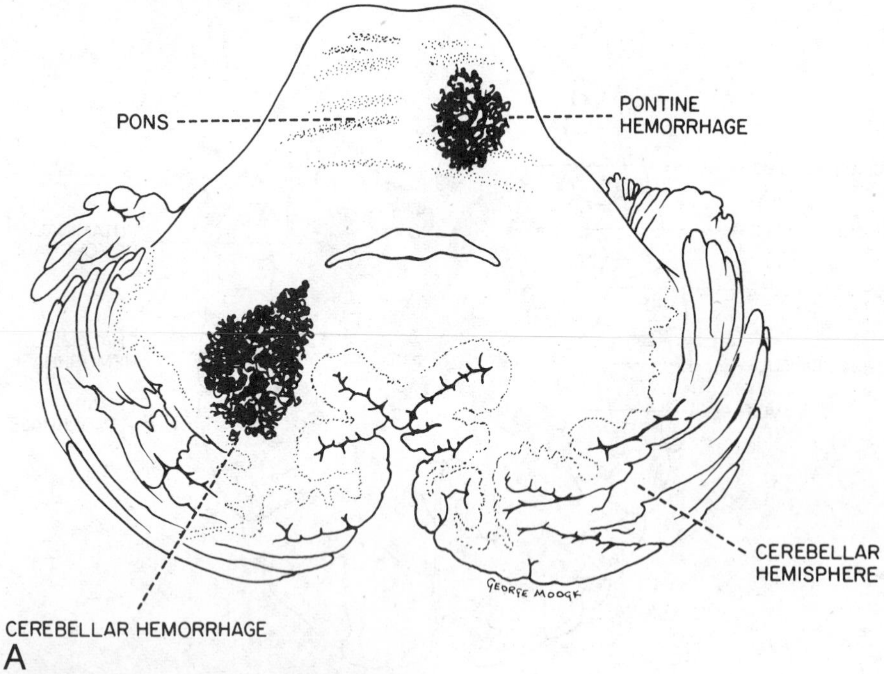

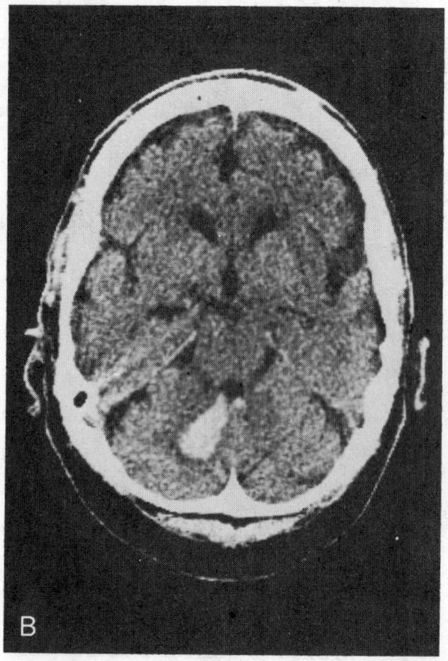

Figure 495–4. *A,* A horizontal section through the pons and cerebellum illustrating pontine and cerebellar hemorrhages. *B,* CT scan illustrating a hemorrhage in the right cerebellar hemisphere approaching the midline.

of meningeal irritation and blood in the cerebrospinal fluid (by CT scanning preferably) with the evidence of a focal lesion in the areas described.

INVESTIGATION OF INTRACEREBRAL HEMORRHAGE. The introduction of the CT scan has revolutionized the safety and sureness with which this diagnosis can be established. CT will identify the size and exact location of the hemorrhage, as well as the degree of surrounding edema and the amount and location of any distortion of the brain. Lumbar puncture is potentially hazardous and should be avoided. Angiography should be performed only when a surgical lesion such as aneurysm, AVM, or a brain tumor might exist, and in certain carefully selected cases in which surgical drainage might be considered. The possibility of a bleeding disorder requires that routine blood counts and platelet counts be performed and bleeding and prothrombin times obtained.

COURSE AND PROGNOSIS OF HYPERTENSIVE HEMORRHAGE. Hypertensive intracerebral hemorrhage carries a grave immediate prognosis. Some patients die on the day of the ictus, and 50 to 75 per cent succumb within one month. Coma at the onset is a poor prognostic sign, and most affected patients never recover consciousness. Mortality is slightly lower (40 per cent) in patients up to the fifth decade and increases in later decades.

Death occurs when a hemorrhage of sufficient size ruptures into the ventricles, causing them to become distended, or into the hemisphere, resulting in compromise of brainstem function. Pontine and cerebellar hematomas interfere most quickly with vital brainstem functions.

If the patient survives, subsequent recovery of considerable function is a good possibility. The hemorrhage resorbs slowly, and the compressed neural tissue commensurately regains much of its previous functional activity. With larger hemorrhages in which the brainstem is secondarily disrupted, functional restoration is not expected and will be accompanied by permanent sequelae. Subsequent bleeding is rare with appropriate blood pressure control.

TREATMENT OF INTRACEREBRAL HEMORRHAGE. The treatment of intracerebral hemorrhage is mostly unsatisfactory. The principles involved in the care of seriously disabled, stuporous, or comatose patients apply, with attention to the airway, fluids, and electrolytes.

Localization of the clot by history, physical signs, and, if available, CT scanning will determine the need to consider some cases for a surgical evacuation. Evacuation can benefit the small number of cases with *cerebellar hematoma* recognized before the onset of coma. If CT is available, such patients should have daily or more frequent CT scans. If signs of clinical worsening progress after admission, prompt ventricular shunting or direct removal of the clot is indicated. Signs of bilateral corticospinal tract dysfunction or reduction in level of consciousness imply that severe brainstem dysfunction has already occurred and that action has been delayed too long. Smaller intracerebellar hematomas less than 3 cm in diameter usually resolve without surgical evacuation.

Evacuation of the occasional supratentorial hematoma is considered when the lesion is larger than usual and is in the subcortical white matter, and the patient is not afflicted with calamitous hemiplegia and aphasia but is showing signs of progression with evidence of incipient deterioration of the level of consciousness. However, evacuation of most examples of hypertensive intracerebral hematoma is a futile pursuit. The most satisfactory recoveries occur in patients who have not been submitted to operation.

Too rapid lowering of the level of blood pressure while attempting to reduce the amount of bleeding may be dangerous. In the hypertensive patient the uninvolved brain requires a higher than normal perfusion pressure because of the intraluminal resistance of the widespread arteriolar disease. A dramatic reduction of blood pressure puts the patient at risk to the development of additional neurologic disability from ischemia. If the patient survives the ictus, gradual restoration of normal blood pressure and its maintenance at normal levels are mandatory.

Cole FM, Yates P: Intracerebral microaneurysms and small cerebrovascular lesions. Brain 90:759, 1967. *A study of the arteriolar changes found in hypertensive and elderly persons.*

Drake CG: Giant intracranial aneurysms: Experience with surgical treatment in 174 patients. Clin Neurosurg 26:12, 1979. *Combined with the paper by Sundt and Piepgras, a comprehensive statement is provided on the surgical approach to an uncommon but distressing clinical condition.*

Drake CG: The treatment of aneurysms of the posterior circulation. Clin Neurosurg 26:96, 1979. *A review of a very large experience in this area.*

Drake CG: Cerebral arteriovenous malformations: Considerations for and experience with surgical treatment in 166 cases. Clin Neurosurg 26:145, 1979. *A comprehensive review of the clinical features and treatment possibilities.*

Fields WS, Maslenikov V, Meyer JS, et al.: Joint study of extracranial arterial occlusion. JAMA 211:1993, 1970. *The survival data from the only major randomized trial to evaluate carotid endarterectomy in stroke prevention. Should be read with Kurtzke's critique.*

Gilbert JJ, Vinters HV: Cerebral amyloid angiopathy: Incidence and complications in the aging brain. I. Cerebral Hemorrhage. Stroke 14:915, 1983. *An update on these subcortical hemorrhages that occur in the aging brain*

Heyman A, Wilkinson W, Heyden S, Helms MJ, Bartel AG, Karp HR, Tyroler HA, Hames CG: Risk of stroke in asymptomatic persons with cervical arterial bruits. A population study in Evans County, Georgia. N Engl J Med 302:838, 1980. *A long-term surveillance study of asymptomatic carotid bruits indicates that they predict an increased risk of stroke.*

Kassell NF, Drake CG: Review of the management of saccular aneurysms. Neurol. Clin. 1:73, 1983. *A contemporary discussion on the diagnosis of saccular aneurysm, the prevention of rebleeding, the problem of vasospasm, and early versus later surgical intervention.*

Kurtzke J: Formal discussion. *In* Whisnant JP, Sandok BA (eds.): Cerebral Vascular Diseases. New York, Grune & Stratton, 1974, pp 190–193. *A succinct and impressive critique of the joint study of extracranial carotid surgery.*

Ojemann RG, Heros RC: Spontaneous brain hemorrhage. Stroke 14:468, 1983. *A recent article on spontaneous brain hemorrhage and its management.*

Ott KH, Kase CS, Ojemann RG, Mohr JP: Cerebellar hemorrhage: Diagnosis and treatment. A review of 56 cases. Arch Neurol 31:160, 1974. *A comprehensive review of a condition which must be recognized early for optimal management.*

Ropper AH, Davis KR: Lobar cerebral hemorrhages: Acute clinical syndromes in 26 cases. Ann Neurol 8:141, 1980. *A description of a series of patients with intracerebral hemorrhage located outside the usual locations common to the hypertensive patient. This paper reflects part of the new understanding of brain hemorrhage in normotensive and hypertensive patients diagnosed by CT scanning.*

Sahs AL, Perrett GE, Locksley HB, Nishioka H (eds.): Intracranial Aneurysms and Subarachnoid Hemorrhage. A Cooperative Study. Philadelphia, J. B. Lippincott Company, 1969. *The report of a cooperative study with valuable data respecting the problems of subarachnoid hemorrhage. As the preface indicates, not designed as a recipe-book for definitive therapy.*

Shenkin HA, Zavala M: Cerebellar strokes: Mortality, surgical indication and result of ventricular damage. Lancet 2:429, 1982. *A recent summary of the condition.*

Sundt TM Jr, Piepgras DG: Surgical approach to giant intracranial aneurysms. Operative experience with 80 cases. J Neurosurg 51:731, 1979.

Sundt TM Jr, Whisnant JP: Subarachnoid hemorrhage from intracranial aneurysms. Surgical management and natural history of disease. N Engl J Med 299:116, 1978. *A report of the progress being made to improve by surgery on the natural history of subarachnoid hemorrhage. The disease remains serious.*

Wolf PA, Kannel WB, Gordon T, McNamara PM, Dawber TR: Asymptomatic carotid bruit and risk of stroke: The Framingham Study (abstract). Stroke 10:96, 1979. *An important reference in decision-making respecting asymptomatic carotid bruit management.*

Section Eight INFECTIOUS AND INFLAMMATORY DISORDERS OF THE NERVOUS SYSTEM

Bacterial Diseases

496. PARAMENINGEAL INFECTIONS

Donald H. Harter

Central nervous system infections caused by pyogenic bacteria other than acute meningitis include brain abscess, collections of pus enclosed within membranes covering the brain and spinal cord (subdural empyema, cerebral epidural abscess, spinal epidural abscess, spinal subdural empyema), and dural sinus infection and thrombosis. Most of these paracranial diseases are secondary to adjacent infections of the ear, sinuses, or bones of the skull or migrate from an infection elsewhere in the body.

Availability of newer techniques, such as CT and radionuclide scans, has greatly improved the early diagnosis and, therefore, treatment of localized central nervous system infections. The new imaging techniques also permit monitoring the progress of the infection during treatment. Correct use of these methods should further reduce the mortality and morbidity from these infections in years ahead.

BRAIN ABSCESS

DEFINITION. Brain abscess describes encapsulated or free pus in the substance of the brain. Abscesses may vary in size from a microscopic focus of inflammatory cells to a major encapsulated area of necrosis occupying a major part of a cerebral hemisphere. They may be single or multiple and caused by local extension or hematogenous spread.

INCIDENCE. Brain abscess is about one sixth as frequent as bacterial meningitis and constitutes approximately 0.7 per cent of all neurosurgical operations. The condition occurs two to three times more frequently in males than in females.

PREDISPOSING FACTORS. The causes of brain abscess can be classified into those in which a primary focus of infection can be identified and those in which no extracranial focus can be found. In the majority of cases a primary focus can be found at the time of initial presentation or at necropsy. Brain abscess can arise by extension from infections within the cranium, by introduction of bacteria at the time of head trauma, or as a metastatic infection from other parts of the body. The site of primary infection can be classified into otolaryngologic causes (middle ear disease and sinus infections), metastatic infections (sepsis, pulmonary disease, and cardiac disease), or trauma.

Otogenic Abscess. About 0.5 per cent of patients with acute otitis media and 0.3 per cent of patients with chronic otitis media will develop brain abscess. Middle ear infection, even in the antibiotic era, remains the most common single causative disease. Otogenic brain abscesses are usually located in the temporal lobe or cerebellum.

Infection spreads along the path of bony erosion; final intracranial spread is precipitated by an acute exacerbation of a chronic process. Spread to the posterior fossa may be through the lateral sinus or through the internal ear with erosion of the bony labyrinth and necrosis of the horizontal semicircular canal, oval window, or promontory. Involvement of the posterior fossa occurs quickly once labyrinthine fluid is infected. Alternatively, a cholesteatoma in the mastoid antrum and attic erodes through the antral roof, leading to infection. In cerebellar abscess there is often evidence of retrograde thrombosis from the lateral, petrosal, or superior petrosal venous sinuses, but the importance of such retrograde thrombosis in the origin of otogenic abscess is uncertain. The duration of otorrhea preceding brain abscess caused by middle ear disease may vary from one month to as long as 20 years.

Infection of Paranasal Sinuses. Paranasal sinus infection accounts for about 5 to 10 per cent of all brain abscesses, usually extending directly from the frontal sinus into the anterior part of the frontal lobe. Rarely, infection of the ethmoid sinus can cause a deep temporal lobe abscess in the region of the uncus. Infection may erode the sinus wall and invade the brain directly or may spread by veins communicating with the cavernous sinus or brain.

Trauma to the Face and Skull. Brain abscess secondary to trauma is usually due to an unrepaired dural laceration in association with a compound depressed skull fracture. The abscess is always directly related to the site of injury. Penetrating gunshot wounds are often responsible for brain abscesses. In post-traumatic brain abscess a bone fragment or other foreign body may be found in the devitalized tissue. Sometimes the injury may be seemingly trivial and unsuspected. For example, penetration of the orbital roof and temporal bone by pencil tips has given rise to brain abscess. Brain abscess may also follow otolaryngologic or neurosurgical operations.

Metastatic Brain Abscess and Hematogenous Spread. Hematogenous brain abscesses usually originate from the heart, lungs, or pleura. Less frequently, septic foci in the skin, teeth, abdomen, or surgical wounds may be the origin. The incidence of metastatic abscess is always less than that of otogenic or rhinogenic abscess.

The single most important cause of metastatic brain abscess is chronic infection of the pleura or lungs, including bronchiectasis, empyema, and lung abscess. Brain abscesses metastatic from the lung often lie in frontal, parietal, or deep cortical regions but are seldom in the cerebellum. They follow a more chronic course than abscesses of cardiac origin. Metastatic abscess is believed to originate from a transient bacteremia with release of infected material into the pulmonary venous and systemic circulations. A number of these patients have had thoracic surgery.

About 10 per cent of brain abscesses are associated with congenital heart disease. Affected patients often present with the sudden onset of a focal neurologic deficit in a stroke-like manner. Paradoxical infected embolism, bacterial endocarditis, and primary thrombosis with secondary bacteremic infection have all been held responsible for the development of brain abscess. The mortality of brain abscess in association with pulmonary or cardiac disease is higher than that from abscesses of other causes.

Metastatic brain abscess of pure dental origin is rare. There is often intervening cellulitis, sinusitis, and osteomyelitis of the mandible and base of the skull, permitting direct rather than hematogenous spread. Intrauterine contraceptive devices have been incriminated as an occasional source of metastatic brain abscess.

ETIOLOGY. Comprehensive statements about the bacteriology of brain abscesses are difficult to make because of diversity in the isolation methods used. Many bacteria, notably anaerobic species, have peculiar or particular growth requirements, making them difficult to cultivate. A lack of attention to detail can lead to a failure to isolate the responsible bacteria or microorganisms in as high as 60 per cent of cases. In many instances more than a single bacterial species is isolated from a brain abscess.

For best results a gram-stained smear should be studied at the time of surgery. Aerobic and anaerobic bacterial and fungal cultures should be planted. Ideally, the bacteriologist should be on hand when the abscess is tapped in the operating room. If this is not possible, the neurosurgical team should know precisely how to inoculate suitable media as soon as the aspirate is available. Aspirated purulent material should be rapidly transported to the bacteriologic laboratory. Blood cultures should also be taken at the time of operation. Samples should be collected into a liquid anaerobic culture medium containing antibiotic inactivators.

The most common microorganisms isolated from brain abscesses are aerobic or anaerobic streptococci. Nontraumatic brain abscess has become largely a disease of streptococci, more particularly of anaerobic or microaerophilic strains. *Bacteroides* and enteric bacteria are still recovered in a number of cases. *S. pneumoniae* is now a rare cause unless the abscess is the sequel to occult cerebrospinal fluid rhinorrhea or occurs in an elderly person in association with pneumococcal pneumonia. Staphylococcal abscesses are usually due to penetrating head trauma or bacteremia. Clostridial infections are post-traumatic. Gram-negative bacilli very rarely occur alone.

Rarely *Actinomyces* and *Nocardia* species may be recovered from an abscess cavity. Actinomycotic brain abscess may be secondary to infection elsewhere, particularly the chest and oropharynx. *Nocardia asteroides* is a rare cause of cerebral abscesses which are often multiple, multilocular, and thick walled. They almost invariably are associated with pulmonary infection. Cerebral infection with *Candida albicans* can also lead to abscess formation.

PATHOLOGY. The factors leading to the development of intracerebral abscess with encapsulation in some cases and not in others are poorly understood. Localized inflammatory changes with necrosis and edema, thromboses of vessels, and collections of degenerating leukocytes represent the early response to bacterial invasion. The histologic appearance of brain abscess includes an inner layer of pus surrounding a zone of inflammatory granulation tissue, which varies in thickness. In the early acute stage, granulation tissue may be absent and the limits of the abscess defined by a zone of infiltration by polymorphonuclear leukocytes and plasma cells. Foci of perivascular cuffing are present. There is often surrounding edema of the white matter.

The acute area of local suppuration is followed in several weeks by encapsulation of the liquefied brain and accumulated pus. There is still no satisfactory explanation for the variation and progression of encapsulation from patient to patient. Virulence of the organism and ability to make granulation tissue may be involved, but what controls these factors is unknown. As encapsulation proceeds, a layer of granulation tissue merges with surrounding collagenous tissue in which there is evidence of continuing fibroblastic activity and reticulin fibers. Active fibroblasts appear to infiltrate the surrounding brain, and a zone of avascular necrosis forms. The macroscopic appearance of a dormant smooth capsule at the time of excision is not confirmed histologically, because there is active vascular hyperplasia and perivascular cuffing about the capsule. Meninges adjacent to the abscess are often infiltrated by inflammatory cells.

Multiple satellite abscesses may develop and communicate with the principal cavity. Because abscess cavities may spread through the central white matter, they often extend through the ventricular wall, producing meningitis, and may rupture into the cerebral ventricles.

CLINICAL MANIFESTATIONS. Brain abscess may happen at any time of life, but the highest incidence of the disease occurs between the second and fifth decades.

General Features. The symptoms of brain abscess are generally those of a space-occupying intracranial lesion. The illness may be acute with fever, headache, nausea or vomiting, increasing obtundation, seizures, and localizing neurologic findings. As noted, occasional cases produce a stroke-like onset. One should suspect brain abscess in the presence of chronic middle ear disease, congenital heart disease, sinusitis, or bronchiectasis. The diagnosis should also be considered in the presence of other forms of sepsis such as osteomyelitis, surgical wound infections, dental and periodontal disease, and pneumonia. Absence of a focus of infection, however, never excludes the possibility of brain abscess.

Symptoms of acute infection are often lacking unless the focus giving rise to the abscess is still active. Chills and fever at the onset of nervous system invasion may accompany an embolic lesion in the brain secondary to acute endocarditis. The body temperature may be elevated, normal, or subnormal. Approximately one third of patients lack a history of fever and remain afebrile during their illness. Most do not have fever when admitted to hospital.

Increased intracranial pressure usually develops rapidly. Headache, nausea, and vomiting are common early symptoms. Seizures, more often generalized than focal, are present in one quarter to one third of patients. The diagnosis of brain abscess can often be inferred because of past or present evidence of otitis media or sinusitis. Unexplained headache in a child with cyanotic congenital heart disease should be regarded as being due to brain abscess until proved otherwise. Headache may be localized to the side of the abscess, but it is often generalized and increases in severity as the abscess expands. Signs attributable to meningeal irritation may be present.

Increased intracranial pressure may lead to bradycardia, confusion, drowsiness, and stupor. Papilledema may be a relatively late event, but develops eventually in about half of cases. Signs of damage to the third or sixth cranial nerves may reflect an increased intracranial pressure and may not have localizing value. The course of untreated brain abscess is usually fulminating, ending fatally in five to fifteen days. In certain patients, however, the course may be prolonged and misdiagnosed as a brain tumor. Although the use of CT scanning has made localization on clinical grounds less important in many parts of the world, several distinct presentations can be recognized.

Temporal lobe abscesses tend to cause language difficulties, visual field abnormalities, or signs of uncal herniation, while *frontal lobe abscesses* are more prone to produce behavioral abnormalities or focal seizures. Both frontal and parietal lobe abscesses tend to cause contralateral motor or sensory dysfunction. Deep-lying hemispheric abscesses may be difficult to differentiate, without biopsy, from malignant brain tumors. *Cerebellar abscesses,* almost all of which extend from middle ear infections, produce ipsilateral cerebellar dysfunction, stiff neck, and, often, signs of increased intracranial pressure. Brain stem abscesses are rare and cause signs consistent with their anatomic location.

LABORATORY DIAGNOSIS. Elevation of the white blood cell count is of limited value, being above 20,000 per cubic millimeter in about 10 per cent of brain abscess patients. Lumbar puncture is unjustified when brain abscess is suspected, especially if CT scanning is available. If a lumbar puncture is inadvertently performed, cerebrospinal fluid pleocytosis greater than 5 cells per cubic millimeter is found in about two thirds of patients, a protein content greater than 100 mg per deciliter in two fifths, and a cerebrospinal fluid glucose level less than 40 mg per deciliter in about one fifth. Pressure usually is moderately elevated, and the fluid usually is sterile.

X-ray studies of the skull, including mastoids and sinuses, may disclose evidence of otitic or paranasal sepsis.

The CT scan is the most valuable test for diagnosis, and its application has had a remarkable effect in reducing the mortality of brain abscess. The most frequently observed CT appearance is a lucent area surrounded by a faint dense rim with a second lucent zone outside the rim. After intravenous administration of contrast material; dense ring enhancement is seen around an area of low attenuation with a lucent area of edema peripheral to the enhanced ring. Varying degrees of compression or shift of the ventricular system indicate mass effect (Fig. 496–1). The CT scan of patients with suspected brain abscess should be performed with and without contrast enhancement. Occasionally, one observes a patchy, nonuniform enhancement pattern consistent with preliquefactive inflammation, "cerebritis." The differential diagnosis includes septic infarcts, tumors with cyst formation, or metastatic tumors.

Ring formation represents an area of hypercellularity and hypervascularity with varying amounts of fibrous tissue. Ring enhancement is neither synonymous with a well-formed capsule nor relates to the patient's clinical condition. Ring formation may be seen in the stage prior to capsule formation and may persist after complete surgical excision and in clinically stable patients.

Arteriography adds little to the CT diagnosis of brain abscess.

In the absence of a CT scan, radionuclide brain scanning is the most reliable method of detecting supratentorial brain abscess. The scan may become positive in the early stages of focal cerebritis before true abscess or pus formation. Cerebral abscess has also been identified by radionuclide scanning after the injection of the patient's leukocytes labeled with indium-111. The EEG in brain abscess is almost always abnormal, usually indicating only the presence of a space-occupying lesion.

TREATMENT. Early diagnosis and prompt initiation of antimicrobial therapy are crucial. Once antimicrobial agents are started, parenteral corticosteroids may be used to reduce brain edema, although in any but late cases their benefit is problematic. During the stage of acute focal suppuration or cerebritis, surgical intervention is not indicated.

Recent evidence indicates that many brain abscesses can be treated by nonsurgical means if carefully monitored by CT scans. Treatment with antibiotics and other medical supportive measures alone is indicated before capsule formation has occurred or when a capsulated abscess is small and produces no shift or compression of intracranial structures. Patients who improve on medical treatment alone all show a decrease in enhancement of ring formation on CT scan and, gradually, a shrinking and disappearance of the lesion.

In all likelihood an increasing number of brain abscess patients will be nonsurgically managed in years to come. Because penicillin-susceptible organisms predominate in brain abscesses, the optimal antimicrobial regimen consists of giving 10 to 20 million units of penicillin intravenously daily in divided doses. If there is reason to suspect the presence of another organism not susceptible to penicillin, chloramphenicol or another drug can be given concurrently. If there is evidence for staphylococcal infection, adequate amounts of a penicillinase-resistant penicillin or a cephalosporin drug should be given. Antimicrobial drug therapy can be modified after the antibiotic sensitivity of the microorganism identified in abscess pus has been determined. Treatment should be continued for six weeks.

If, despite medical treatment, the patient's clinical status changes for the worse and/or the CT scan shows an increase in the size of the abscess and an increase in the intensity of ring enhancement, surgical treatment is mandatory. However, heightened ring enhancement may occur after steroids have been discontinued; if the patient shows continued clinical improvement on antibiotic therapy, close, nonsurgical observation can continue.

Possible operations include initial aspiration of the abscess cavity, followed in some cases by excision at a second operation, or primary total excision of the abscess. If the abscess is superficial and encapsulated, primary excision is the operation of choice. Persistence of a ring sign on CT scan after primary abscess excision does not imply that a residual abscess has formed. If the abscess is deep or affects a neurologically critical area, aspiration and injection of antimicrobial agents is the only operative possibility.

PROGNOSIS AND OUTCOME. Mortality from all brain abscesses remained at 30 to 40 per cent after the use of antibiotics had become common practice. The use of the CT scan to assist in diagnosis and to monitor treatment appears to have reduced this rate. Although results are still incomplete, some place current mortality as low as 5 per cent. Mortality is greatest in patients with reduced consciousness at the time of admission.

Residual neurologic damage is frequent in survivors of brain abscess. Convulsive seizures are frequent and require continuous anticonvulsant medication (see Ch. 510).

SUBDURAL EMPYEMA

DEFINITION AND CAUSE. Subdural empyema refers to an intracranial collection of pus located between the inner surface of the dura and the outer surface of the arachnoid. The most common causes are infections of the paranasal sinuses or middle ear. Other causes include rupture of an intracerebral abscess, cranial osteomyelitis, infection of a subdural hematoma, penetrating wounds of the skull, leptomeningitis, and septicemia. An acute exacerbation of sinusitis just prior to the development of subdural empyema is common.

PATHOLOGY. Infection may enter the subdural space by direct extension following erosion of osteitic areas or by indirect extension through progressive thrombophlebitis of mucosal veins and subsequent spread to dural veins, venous sinuses, and cerebral veins. The first route is more common in otitic infections, the second in paranasal infections. When the infection enters the subdural space, it elicits a prompt inflammatory response with rapid pus formation. Extension of pus depends on the primary site of infection. Dorsolateral and interhemispheric collections are common; those beneath the cerebral hemispheres are uncommon. After paranasal infection, subdural pus usually forms at the frontal poles and extends posteriorly over the convexity of the frontal lobe. It may reach into the parietal and occipital areas and along the falx and sylvian fissure. When a subdural collection occurs after ear infection, it passes posteriorly and medially over the falx to the tentorium. Pus climbs above the tentorium and extends over the occipital poles.

Thrombosis or thrombophlebitis of superficial cortical veins is a common complication, and produces hemorrhagic infarction of the area drained by the diseased vessels. The cerebral hemisphere under the pus collection is depressed and indented. Superficial layers of the cerebral cortex undergo ischemic necrosis. Microscopic studies disclose various degrees of organi-

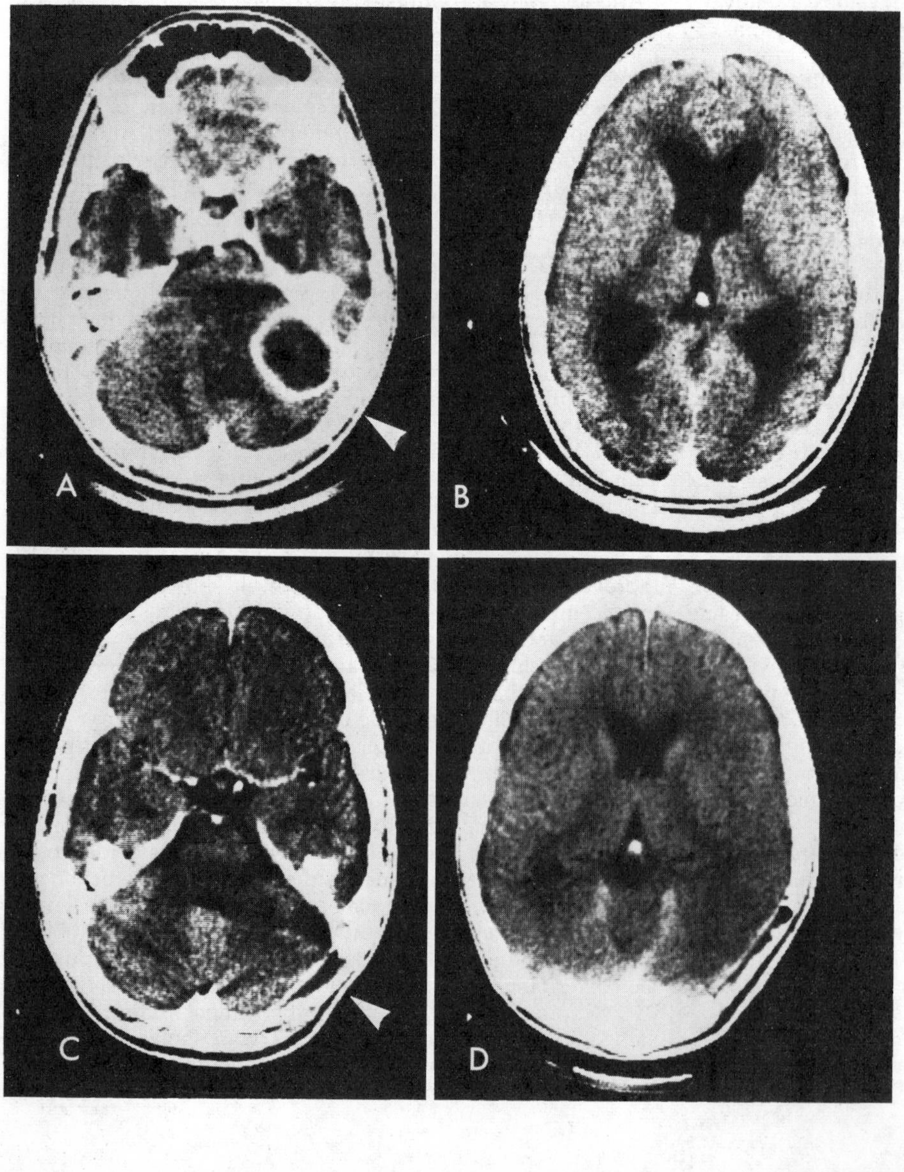

Figure 496–1. CT scan of cerebellar brain abscess in a 16-year old boy with chronic otitis media.

Initial findings: *A*, Characteristic ring appearance of the acute, untreated abscess after intravenous contrast injection. *B*, Moderate associated dilation of the lateral ventricles (hydrocephalus) due to partial obstruction of the aqueduct and fourth ventricle.

Re-examination twelve days later (after twelve days of antimicrobial therapy and ten days after removal of the well-encapsulated 3.5 cm diameter abscess): *C*, Area of abscess removal. *D*, Normal-sized lateral ventricles. The boy subsequently recovered completely.

zation of the exudate on the inner surface of the dura and infiltration of the underlying pia with inflammatory cells.

ETIOLOGY. The most common organism isolated from subdural pus is the streptococcus, often an anaerobe. Other frequent pathogens include staphylococci and gram-negative enteric organisms.

CLINICAL MANIFESTATIONS. Symptoms and signs of antecedent sinusitis, otitis, or osteomyelitis often blend into those of subdural empyema. The usual clinical onset is with high fever, headache, and vomiting, followed by impaired consciousness and signs of meningeal irritation. The patient gradually or rapidly becomes irritable and drowsy. Stiff neck and Kernig's sign are present, and the area of the abscess is characteristically tender to percussion. Progression of the infection leads to confusion, stupor, or coma. Focal neurologic signs appear, including convulsions, hemiparesis, and aphasia, and may be the result of compression of the cerebral cortex underneath the pus collection or cortical thrombophlebitis and cerebral infarction. In the later stages, the intracranial pressure may rise. The entire clinical picture may evolve in as little as a few hours or as long as ten days or more. Without treatment, death usually occurs within a few days after the onset of focal neurologic findings.

LABORATORY DIAGNOSIS. A marked peripheral leukocytosis is usually present. X-rays of the skull may show infection of the mastoid or nasal sinuses or osteomyelitis of the skull. The cerebrospinal fluid is under increased pressure and usually contains a few hundred to 1000 or more cells, an increased protein content, and a normal or near normal glucose level.

Spinal fluid is typically free of bacteria. There is potential danger in the performance of a lumbar puncture in patients with subdural empyema who have evidence of increased intracranial pressure, and the procedure should be avoided if the diagnosis can be reached or is strongly suggested by other procedures.

CT scan of the head characteristically depicts a crescent-shaped area of increased density at the periphery of the brain and mass displacement of the cerebral ventricles and midline structures. Contrast enhancement demonstrates a rim-like crescent adjacent to the cortex or a collection of pus near the falx. CT scan may be of greater reliability in showing the subdural empyema which develops in patients after drainage of a chronic subdural hematoma than in subdural empyema of other causes.

In the absence of a CT scan, cerebral arteriography is the most reliable method for detecting a subdural mass lesion. The combination of CT scanning and cerebral angiography is the current procedure of choice for demonstration of subdural empyema.

Radionuclide scan in subdural empyema is rarely sensitive enough to visualize small bilateral or parafalcial collections. It can be of help, however, in diagnosing an associated brain abscess.

TREATMENT. Subdural empyema requires prompt surgical drainage of pus by burr holes or craniotomy. Vigorous systemic therapy with penicillin (10 to 20 million units daily) and other antimicrobials as indicated is begun before surgery and continued until the infection is brought under control. Antibiotics are commonly instilled into the subdural space at the time of operation. Surgical treatment of the accompanying sinusitis, frontal osteomyelitis, or mastoiditis is usually postponed until the intracranial infection has subsided.

OUTCOME. Mortality from subdural empyema remains at between 25 and 40 per cent, usually because of delayed diagnosis. The main causes of death are thrombophlebitis associated with dural venous sinus thrombosis and massive cerebral infarction, fulminant meningitis, and multiple intracerebral abscesses. Progressive and uncontrollable cerebral edema contributes to a lethal outcome.

CEREBRAL EPIDURAL ABSCESS

Cerebral epidural (or extradural) abscess is a collection of purulent material localized to the outer layer of the dura. It occurs in relationship to adjacent osteomyelitis, mastoiditis, or paranasal sinusitis. Epidural abscess may lead to sinus thrombophlebitis, subdural empyema, leptomeningitis, or brain abscess.

Signs and symptoms are nondistinctive and apt to be masked by primary disease of the ear, nasal sinuses, or skull, or by secondary complications. There may be ipsilateral headache, fever, localized pain, tenderness on local percussion, and swelling with pitting edema. Evidence of increased intracranial pressure is rarely present. Focal neurologic signs are uncommon. In most cases the cerebrospinal fluid is sterile, contains a few lymphocytic cells, and has a mild elevation of protein content. Many cerebral epidural abscesses are diagnosed at the time of operation for a subdural empyema or a brain abscess. Treatment is with surgical drainage plus appropriate systemic antibiotic therapy.

MAJOR DURAL SINUS THROMBOSIS

The large dural sinuses may become thrombosed spontaneously, when they are infected, or when there is infection in the adjacent epidural or subdural spaces. Although any dural sinus may be involved in intracranial infection, the paired sinuses (lateral, cavernous, and petrosal) are affected most often. Spontaneous or primary sinus thrombosis tends to favor unpaired sinuses. Venous sinuses may become infected by contiguous spread from otorhinogenic foci of infection, by periphlebitis leading to the direct spread of infection through the sinus wall, by an infected draining vein, or by septic venous embolization. Inflammation may also spread from infected dural sinuses to the extradural and subdural spaces by direct extension or venous radicles, to the leptomeninges and adjacent brain, to the bloodstream, and to distant sites by embolism.

Thrombosis of major dural sinuses may result in increased intracranial pressure, multifocal regions of brain ischemia, or cerebral infarction, all because of obstruction to venous drainage from the brain.

LATERAL SINUS THROMBOSIS. Lateral sinus thrombosis is almost always a complication of acute or chronic otitis media, mastoiditis, or cholesteatoma formation. Infants and children are most commonly affected. The thrombosis may coincide with the acute attack of middle ear disease or may be delayed until the chronic stage of ear infection.

The classic symptoms of lateral sinus thrombosis are fever, headache, nausea, and vomiting. An increase of pain in the ear or cessation of aural discharge may point to sinus thrombophlebitis. Local venous distention and swelling, pain, redness, and tenderness indicate involvement of the mastoid emissary vein and may extend into the neck over the jugular vein. Pain in the neck with restriction of movement accompanies jugular vein involvement.

The intracranial pressure is typically increased and more apt to be high when the right lateral sinus is occluded, since it normally is the larger of the two. Papilledema is usually bilateral, but may be unilateral because of extension of the process to the ipsilateral cavernous sinus. Drowsiness and coma are common. Convulsive seizures occur, but focal neurologic findings are unusual.

Spread to the inferior petrosal sinus may lead to abducens nerve paralysis and trigeminal nerve involvement (Gradenigo's syndrome). Involvement of the ninth, tenth, and eleventh nerves may occur because of damage to the jugular bulb and related structures. The symptoms produced include pain on swallowing, dysphagia, dysarthria, hoarseness, weakness or spasms of the sternocleidomastoid and trapezius muscles, and changes in pulse and respiration. The incidence and mortality of lateral sinus thrombosis have been greatly reduced since the introduction and use of antibiotics for middle ear and mastoid infections. The differential diagnosis of lateral sinus thrombosis includes a flare-up of mastoiditis; a perisinus, subdural, or brain abscess; and leptomeningitis.

CAVERNOUS SINUS THROMBOSIS. Cavernous sinus thrombosis is usually due to a suppurative process in the orbit, nasal sinuses, or upper half of the face. Infection may reach the cavernous sinus by the anterior route (ophthalmic veins from orbit, frontal sinus, nasal cavity, and upper face), by the middle route (sphenoid sinus by direct spread or the pharyngeal and pterygoid plexuses from pharynx, upper jaw, and teeth), and by the posterior route (petrosal sinuses and occasionally ear and lateral sinuses). Spread by the anterior route follows the most acute course, and that by the posterior route the most protracted course. The initial infection is usually a furuncle, acute sinusitis, or ear infection. Most infections are due to *Staphylococcus aureus*.

Cavernous sinus thrombosis usually produces an illness of desperate severity with high fever, headaches, malaise, prostration, nausea, vomiting, convulsions, tachycardia, and leukocytosis. Characteristically, the sensorium remains clear until late in the infection. Local changes include chemosis, edema, and cyanosis of the upper face, particularly of the eyelids and base of the nose. These are due to obstruction of the ophthalmic vein as it enters the cavernous sinus. Superficial veins over the forehead may be distended. Swelling of the lids, haziness of the cornea, local pain, and photophobia may make examination of the eyes difficult. Ophthalmoplegia, often first affecting the sixth nerve, is common. The pupil may be dilated from parasympathetic paralysis or small and immobile if both parasympathetic and sympathetic fibers are involved. Involvement of the first division of the trigeminal nerve may lead to eye pain and hyperesthesia of the forehead. Retinal hemorrhages and papilledema are late events. Visual acuity may be normal or moderately impaired. When the infection originates in the throat, sphenoids, or ear, the evolution of the disease is less acute, and the orbit becomes less engorged.

The differential diagnosis of cavernous sinus thrombosis includes orbital tumors, meningiomas and other tumors in the region of the sphenoid, trichinosis, malignant exophthalmos, and arteriovenous aneurysms.

SUPERIOR SAGITTAL SINUS THROMBOSIS. The superior sagittal sinus is less commonly involved in septic thrombosis than the lateral or cavernous sinuses. Infections may reach the superior sagittal sinus by extension from the nasal cavities, by secondary spread from the lateral or cavernous sinuses, or by extension from osteomyelitis or an epidural or subdural infection. The site of initial thrombosis depends on the source and route of infection.

General signs of superior sagittal sinus thrombosis are prostration, fever, headache, and papilledema. Local signs include edema of the forehead and anterior part of the scalp. At times, there is engorgement of the scalp veins. The neurologic symptoms include convulsive seizures and motor paralysis. Focal seizures which alternatively involve one and then the other side of the body are characteristic. One or both legs may be weak or paralyzed, but the motor loss may be hemiplegic in distribution with the leg and proximal arm involved. Some patients develop homonymous hemianopsia or quadrantanopsia, paralysis of conjugate ocular movements, visual disorientation, alexia, apraxia, or aphasia.

DIAGNOSTIC TESTS. X-rays of the skull may provide evidence of middle ear disease, sinusitis, osteomyelitis, fracture, or other conditions associated with dural sinus thrombosis. Radionuclide dynamic and static scans sometimes show termination of radionuclide activity in the mid-portion of the sinus. CT brain scan most frequently discloses a high-density lesion (static blood) in the involved sinus on the pre-contrast scan and a filling defect in the sinus after contrast enhancement.

Cerebral angiography is the most specific diagnostic test for the demonstration of venous sinus thrombosis. Particular attention must be paid to the late filling of the venous sinuses and veins. Sagittal sinus thrombosis has been demonstrated by digital subtraction angiography.

TREATMENT. Appropriate antimicrobial drugs in high dosage and surgical drainage with the removal of infected bone and extradural or intrasinus abscess constitute the proper treatment of major sinus thrombosis secondary to infection. Ligation of the jugular vein in lateral sinus thrombosis to prevent the spread of septic emboli is usually unnecessary. Because of the frequent isolation of penicillinase-producing staphylococci, semisynthetic penicillins should be used until culture results are reported. Anticoagulants should not be used because venous thromboses tend to produce hemorrhagic brain tissue. Prognosis for recovery is fairly good when optimal treatment is given expeditiously, but residual neurologic deficits are frequent.

MALIGNANT EXTERNAL OTITIS

Malignant external otitis begins as an infection of the external auditory canal due to *Pseudomonas aeruginosa.* It affects mainly elderly patients with diabetes mellitus. The infection spreads from the outer ear to the soft tissues below the temporal bone and invades the parotid gland, temporomandibular joint, masseter muscle, and temporal bone. Necrotizing osteitis of the temporal bone develops. The high mortality rate originally reported for the condition (about 40 per cent) led to the use of the adjective "malignant" for this form of temporal bone infection.

The symptoms and signs include rapidly evolving pain in the ear, with or without purulent discharge, swelling of the parotid gland, trismus, and paralysis of the sixth to twelfth nerves. Death is usually caused by the development of meningitis.

Patients with malignant external otitis should be treated with intravenous carbenicillin and gentamicin. Minor surgical debridement is helpful. Antimicrobial treatment should be continued for about a week after apparent cure in order to avoid recurrent disease.

CEREBRAL MANIFESTATIONS OF BACTERIAL ENDOCARDITIS

Neurologic symptoms and signs occur in 25 to 30 per cent of patients with subacute bacterial endocarditis. The most common neurologic manifestation is cerebrovascular disease, which occurs in about half of the patients. Cerebral infarction, hemorrhage, or transient focal ischemic attacks are all seen and behave like similar lesions from other kinds of emboli. Another presentation consists of a subacute toxic encephalopathy, producing confusion, delirium, hallucinations, confabulation, disorientation, paranoid ideation, and other mental disturbances. Milder manifestations include drowsiness, insomnia, apathy, irritability, and personality changes. Autopsy studies suggest that these mental changes reflect the effects of multiple thromboemboli.

Mycotic aneurysms represent about 5 per cent of the neurologic manifestations. These aneurysms usually arise in the distal portion of the middle cerebral artery. They typically present with subarachnoid or intracerebral hemorrhage. Occasional mycotic aneurysms have been observed to disappear after antimicrobial therapy, but late rupture of a mycotic aneurysm after bacteriologic cure may occur. Infected embolic material carried to the nervous system may erode blood vessel walls and cause brain abscess or meningitis. There is a higher incidence of meningitis in acute bacterial endocarditis than in the subacute form. Brain abscess and embolic infarction of cerebral tissue may also complicate acute bacterial endocarditis.

SPINAL EPIDURAL ABSCESS

DEFINITION. Spinal epidural abscess describes a collection of purulent material located outside the dura mater within the spinal canal.

INCIDENCE. Epidural abscesses account for approximately one of every 20,000 admissions to United States hospitals. They make up two thirds of surgically treatable infections of the spinal cord and canal. Epidural abscesses occur at all ages, most affecting adults between 20 and 50 years of age.

PREDISPOSING FACTORS. Infections may reach the spinal epidural space by direct extension from an inflammatory process in adjacent tissues, by metastasis through the bloodstream from infections elsewhere in the body, or by perforating wounds. Bacteremia and resultant hematogenous dissemination appear to account for about one third of acute cases. Furuncles, urinary tract infections, dental infections, chronic pulmonary disease, and decubitus ulcers all have been implicated. Contamination of the epidural space by direct spread accounts for another third of acute cases and approximately one half of chronic cases in adults. The usual focus is an adjacent vertebral osteomyelitis with direct extension into the anterior epidural space. Surgical wounds, retroperitoneal abscesses, and lumbar punctures represent other potential causes. In children the usual sources of bacteremia are perineal skin infections, urinary tract infections, pharyngitis, and endocarditis.

Chronic debilitating diseases, diabetes mellitus, immunosuppressive therapy, and heroin abuse are common contributing factors. About one quarter of patients give a history of recent back trauma.

ETIOLOGY. *Staphylococcus aureus* is the most common cause and accounts for 50 to 60 per cent of epidural abscesses. Other bacteria responsible for the infection include *E. coli* and other gram-negative organisms. Hemolytic and anaerobic streptococci have also been recovered.

PATHOLOGY. Infection in the epidural space may be acute or chronic. In acute cases, there is a purulent necrosis of the epidural fat extending over several segments, or the entire length of the cord. The pus is almost always posterior to the spinal cord, but may extend to the anterior surface as well. The epidural fat is hyperemic and infiltrated with numerous polymorphonuclear leukocytes. If the infection is of low virulence, the abscess may be circumscribed and have a granulomatous appearance. Necrosis in the periphery of the cord may result from pressure of the abscess; myelomalacia of one or several cord segments may occur when spinal veins or arteries are thrombosed. Ascending and descending degeneration of the spinal cord can extend above and below the level of the necrotic lesion. In chronic infections, the dura is thickened and gray. The epidural fat is missing and replaced by granulation tissue. In the absence of pus, the granulation tissue may be mistakenly identified as a neoplasm.

CLINICAL MANIFESTATIONS. The clinical course of spinal epidural abscess proceeds in four phases: back pain, radicular pain, muscular weakness, and paralysis. Back pain is characteristically present at the level of the major pathologic process. It is usually severe and localized to a small region of the spine. Movement of the spine in the anteroposterior direction is limited, and the spinous projections overlying the disease process are tender to percussion. Fever and malaise are usually present.

Two to four days later, irritation of nerve roots leads to radicular pains in the trunk or extremities. An erroneous diagnosis of neuritis may be made at this time. Meningeal signs evolve, and headache becomes a common symptom.

The illness then progresses to cause neurologic impairment at and below the level of the lesion. If the abscess compromises the spinal cord, paraparesis and sensory loss occur, accompanied by urinary and fecal incontinence. Abscesses in the lumbosacral spine compress the cauda equina and produce painful sensations in nerve root distribution, eventually resulting in weakness, depressed stretch reflexes, and sensory impairments. There is often erythema and swelling in the area of back pain and tenderness. If appropriate treatment is not initiated, paralysis occurs within hours or at most a few days. Immediate surgery is indicated when any degree of weakness is detected, since most patients who become completely paralyzed will remain so permanently.

Evolution of a chronic epidural abscess is much slower. Fever and malaise are unusual. Weakness and paralysis may not develop for weeks or months.

LABORATORY DIAGNOSIS. The white blood cell count and erythrocyte sedimentation rate characteristically are elevated. X-rays of the spinal column may show osteomyelitis or a contiguous abscess, but are usually normal.

If spinal cord or cauda equina compression is suspected, it is wise to proceed directly with myelography. Lumbar puncture should be performed with caution when acute epidural abscess is suspected. The needle should be introduced slowly and suction applied with a syringe as the epidural space is approached. If the infection has extended to the level of the puncture, pus may be encountered; the needle should be withdrawn immediately at that point without entering and possibly infecting the subarachnoid space. Spinal fluid obtained from below the level of the abscess is xanthochromic or cloudy in appearance, with a cell count varying from a few to several hundred cells per cubic millimeter. The protein content is often between 100 and 1500 mg per deciliter. The spinal fluid sugar content is normal, and cultures of the fluid are usually sterile unless meningitis has developed. Chronic epidural abscess usually produces a complete or almost complete spinal block with an inconstant pleocytosis and an elevation of the protein content.

Myelography is abnormal in all cases. Complete extradural block is found in 80 per cent and the remainder have a partial block. Myelography should be performed by cervical subarachnoid puncture in patients in whom complete block or a lumbar abscess is suspected. Every effort should be made to define the entire extent of the abscess. Spine CT scans may someday be useful in the diagnosis of spinal epidural abscess but presently are less useful than myelography.

Acute spinal epidural abscess must be differentiated from acute or subacute meningitis, acute poliomyelitis, acute transverse myelitis or multiple sclerosis. The clinical and spinal fluid findings usually permit differentiation of these conditions. Chronic adhesive arachnoiditis and tumors within the epidural space may be confused with chronic epidural abscess; the myelogram should clarify the diagnosis.

TREATMENT. The treatment of spinal epidural abscess is immediate surgical decompression preceded and followed by appropriate antibiotic therapy. Aerobic and anaerobic cultures should be obtained at operation. The area of acute suppuration should be irrigated with an antibiotic solution. Large doses of penicillin are begun prior to surgery and continued postoperatively unless bacterial cultures and sensitivities indicate otherwise.

PROGNOSIS AND OUTCOME. Mortality from epidural abscess is near 30 per cent. The most important determinant for recovery is the patient's neurologic status at the time of operation. Total recovery occurs in patients who have no total paralysis or whose weakness has lasted less than 36 hours. One half of patients paralyzed for 48 hours or more progress to permanent paralysis or death.

SPINAL SUBDURAL EMPYEMA

Infection beneath the dura, but outside the spinal cord, is called spinal subdural empyema. The condition is very rare and has a predilection for the cervical and thoracic spinal cord. The symptoms and signs are indistinguishable from spinal epidural abscess. Coexisting meningitis is common. There is often a greater degree of spinal tenderness than in spinal epidural abscess. Sudden transverse myelitis occurs, attributable to spinal cord infarction from vascular compromise caused by the pus collection. The lesion is best demonstrated by myelography. *Staphylococcus aureus* is the most commonly isolated microorganism. Prompt antimicrobial and surgical treatment is mandatory.

Brain Abscess

Brewer ND, MacCarty CS, Wellman WE: Brain abscess: A review of recent experience. Ann Intern Med 82:571, 1975. *Describes diagnosis, microbiology, and treatment in 60 patients.*

deLouvois J: Bacteriological examination of pus from abscesses of the central nervous system. J Clin Pathol 33:66, 1980. *Discussion of the often elusive bacteriology of these conditions.*

Gruszkiewicz J, Doron Y, Peyser E, Borovich B, Schachter J, Front D: Brain abscess and its surgical management. Surg Neurol 18:7, 1982.

Nielsen H, Gyldensted C, Harmsen A: Cerebral abscess: Aetiology, and pathogenesis, symptoms, diagnosis and treatment: A review of 200 cases from 1935–1976. Acta Neurol Scand 65:609, 1982. *This and the above article emphasize the sharp reduction in mortality since CT scanning has allowed better diagnosis and monitoring.*

Rosenblum ML, Hoff JT, Norman D, Edwards MS, Berg BO: Nonoperative treatment of brain abscesses in selected high-risk patients. J Neurosurg 52:217, 1980. *Reports successful treatment by antimicrobial agents alone in eight high-risk patients followed closely by serial CT scans.*

Shaw MDM, Russell JA: Cerebellar abscess: A review of 47 cases. J Neurol Neurosurg Psychiatry 38:429, 1975. *A review of one of the largest available series, 90 per cent secondary to otogenic disease. Effective treatment required adequate radical mastoidectomy plus appropriate treatment of the abscess itself.*

Subdural Empyema

Kaufman DM, Miller MH, Steigbigel NH: Subdural empyema: Analysis of 17 recent cases and review of the literature. Medicine 54:485, 1975. *A thorough consideration of the subject.*

Kaufman DM, Litman N, Miller MH: Sinusitis: Induced subdural empyema. Neurology (New York) 33:123, 1983. *Reviews experience in 17 patients, only 5 of which had a history of sinusitis. CT exams missed the abscess in 2 of 7 patients.*

Luken MG III, Whelan MA: Recent diagnostic experience with subdural empyema. J Neurosurg 52:764, 1980. *Reviews radiographic and therapeutic aspects of primary and secondary subdural empyemas.*

Cerebral Epidural Abscess

Morello A, Hoen TI: Chronic epidural abscess and condensing osteomyelitis of the skull. Neurology 4:633, 1954. *Describes well mechanisms and pathogenesis of the condition.*

Sharif HS, Ibrahim A: Intracranial epidural abscess. Br J Radiol 55:81, 1982. *Points up potential value of CT imaging in detecting this uncommon disorder before serious neurologic damage occurs.*

Major Dural Sinus Thrombosis

Brown P: Septic cavernous sinus thrombosis. Bull Johns Hopkins Hosp. 109:68, 1961. *One of the few papers dealing directly with infected thromboses.*

Kalbag RM, Woolf AL: Cerebral Venous Thrombosis. London, Oxford University Press, 1967. *The classic monograph on the subject.*

Rao KCVG, Knipp HC, Wagner EJ: Computed tomographic findings in cerebral sinus and venous thrombosis. Radiology 140:391, 1981. *In all patients, CT revealed unusual or small ventricular hemorrhages, low density areas, and increased density of dural sinuses and tentorium.*

Malignant External Otitis

Damiani JM, Damiani KK, Kinney SE: Malignant external otitis with multiple cranial nerve involvement. Am J Otolaryngol 1:115, 1979. *A good discussion of the subject.*

Strauss M, Aber RC, Conner GH, Baum S: Malignant external otitis: Long-term (months) antimicrobial therapy. Laryngoscope 92:397, 1982. *Six patients with this often fatal syndrome were treated successfully with long-term antimicrobials plus (in two) extensive surgical debridement.*

Cerebral Manifestations of Bacterial Endocarditis

Churchill MA Jr, Geraci JE, Hunder GG: Musculoskeletal manifestations of bacterial endocarditis. Ann Intern Med 87:754, 1977. *Outlines the muscular, arthritic, and myalgic manifestations of the disorder. In 27 per cent of patients, musculoskeletal complaints were among the first symptoms.*

Pruitt AA, Rubin RH, Karchmer AW, Duncan GW: Neurologic complications of bacterial endocarditis. Medicine 57:329, 1978. *The most recent comprehensive review on the subject.*

Spinal Epidural Abscess

Altrocchi PH: Acute spinal epidural abscess vs. acute transverse myelitis. Arch Neurol 9:17, 1963. *A classic paper emphasizing the differential diagnosis of these disorders.*

Baker AS, Ojemann RG, Swartz MN, Richardson EP Jr: Spinal epidural abscess. N Engl J Med 293:463, 1975. *Reviews course and treatment of 39 patients treated in the antimicrobial era.*

Kaufman DM, Kaplan JG, Litman N: Infectious agents in spinal epidural abscesses. Neurology (New York) 30:844, 1980.

Spinal Subdural Empyema

Fraser RAR, Ratzan K, Wolpert SM, Weinstein L: Spinal subdural empyema. Arch Neurol 28:235, 1973. *A case report and review of ten examples from the literature of this uncommon disorder that can be cured only if recognized and treated early.*

497. SYPHILITIC INFECTIONS OF THE CENTRAL NERVOUS SYSTEM

Kenneth P. Johnson

A general exposition of *T. pallidum* infection is presented in Ch. 306. The following presentation is restricted to a discussion of neurosyphilis.

Neurosyphilis is the invasion and persistent infection of the leptomeninges and, in some cases, brain parenchyma with the spirochete *Treponema pallidum*. Such persistent infection may be asymptomatic or may cause a wide spectrum of neurologic abnormalities.

PATHOLOGY. A meningitis of varying severity and extent is present in every case of active neurosyphilis regardless of the neurologic syndrome. The cerebrospinal fluid (CSF) reflects this involvement even in cases of asymptomatic neurosyphilis.

Study of a few cases of *acute syphilitic meningitis* has shown a meningeal inflammatory reaction in which lymphocytes and plasma cells predominate primarily about blood vessels, often with evidence of early arteritis, although cerebrovascular accidents are rare in this stage of the disease. Reactive arachnoiditis, especially about the base of the brain, is also seen. This accounts for the cranial nerve palsies and for an impairment of CSF circulation that can sometimes result in increased intracranial pressure. A granular ependymitis is commonly present which rarely may obstruct CSF flow through the aqueduct.

In *meningovascular syphilis*, typically a more chronic disorder occurring months or a few years after the primary lesion, the inflammatory response is usually prominent. An associated arteritis (usually small vessels) predisposes to arterial occlusion and consequent infarction of neural tissue. When larger arteries become occluded, infarction of brain or spinal cord may be extensive.

In *general paresis* there is direct invasion of neural tissue by the spirochete, in addition to the meningitis. The cortical architecture is often markedly disordered. One finds meningeal thickening, atrophy of cerebral tissue (especially of frontal and temporal lobes), enlargement of ventricles, and a granularity of the ependymal surface. Microscopically, diffuse destruction and loss of neurons, especially in the cortex, are found. Special stains may demonstrate the presence of *Treponema pallidum*. Reactive gliosis with pleomorphic microglia is characteristic. Inflammation of the meninges is prominent with varying degrees of arteritis.

In *tabes dorsalis* and primary optic atrophy, the pathogenesis of the neurologic lesion is unclear. Direct invasion by the spirochete and an immunologic reaction affecting the meninges may both occur. Grossly the dorsal roots and the dorsal aspect of the spinal cord appear wasted. Secondary demyelination of dorsal columns is readily demonstrated. Involvement of anterior roots with resultant amyotrophy occurs rarely. Why the syphilitic process shows a predilection for dorsal roots is unknown.

Focal granulomatous accumulations *(gummas)* are rare; they may reach the size of clinical brain tumors and extend into the brain parenchyma from a meningeal origin. More diffuse granulomas of the dura (hypertrophic pachymeningitis) sometimes compress neural structures, especially the spinal cord.

CLINICAL SYNDROMES IN NEUROSYPHILIS. ***Asymptomatic Neurosyphilis.*** This is the most common form of neurosyphilis; it generally follows the acute infection within one to three years. As the term suggests, affected patients lack symptoms or signs of neurologic disease. The diagnosis rests on the finding in the CSF of a low-grade meningitis plus the immunologic abnormalities of syphilis. Adequate treatment prevents the development of neurologic symptoms.

Atypical Neurosyphilis. As of 1980, primary syphilis occurs in 70,000 or more persons per year in the United States and secondary syphilis in perhaps 13,000. The spirochete is known to invade the central nervous system (CNS) frequently during these early phases of infection, even though detectable neurosyphilis is rare. Probably the organism is cleared by normal host defenses. Large numbers of persons frequently receive antibiotics to which *T. pallidum* is sensitive for other conditions, but in doses inadequate to cure neurosyphilis. Therefore, many investigators fear that atypical forms of neurosyphilis may be developing following partial antibiotic therapy. Such partial treatment may also modify CSF and serologic reactivity, impairing diagnostic efficiency. Therefore, unusual or bizarre neurologic syndromes accompanied by some CSF abnormalities should at least raise the possibility of neurosyphilis. This is especially important in high risk groups such as homosexual males, in whom syphilis appears with increased frequency.

Symptomatic Neurosyphilis. MENINGITIS. An acute meningitis develops only rarely, although it seems likely that some patients with mild or even moderate symptoms go unnoticed. Symptomatic syphilitic meningitis usually occurs during the early weeks or months after infection, often during the period of the secondary rash or concurrently with a mucocutaneous relapse in a patient previously but inadequately treated. The full-blown illness usually lasts less than one month, but symptoms may persist for longer periods. Headache, vomiting, malaise, and irritability are prominent. Kernig's and Brudzinski's signs develop. Occasionally, confusion, delirium, seizures, and cranial nerve palsies (seventh and eighth nerves most common) occur. Argyll Robertson pupils do not occur in acute syphilitic meningitis. Acute syphilitic hydrocephalus with increased intracranial pressure, including papilledema, may lead to confusion with other inflammatory and neoplastic conditions. The CSF always contains an increased number of white blood cells (average about 500 per cubic millimeter—usually mononuclear, rarely polymorphonuclear), an elevated total protein (average, about 100 mg per deciliter), and normal sugar concentrations (reduced rarely). An elevated gamma globulin concentration develops in 70 per cent of cases. The serum serologic tests for syphilis (VDRL and FTS-ABS) are usually but not always positive.

The response to therapy is generally prompt, although an occasional patient will subsequently develop some other form of neurosyphilis.

MENINGOVASCULAR SYPHILIS. The incidence of this form of neurosyphilis is low, a figure of 3 per cent of syphilitic patients being recorded. Men are affected more often than women (3:1). Meningovascular syphilis occurs most commonly from two to ten years after the primary lesion. Symptoms and signs of meningitis are lacking, although headache is a frequent complaint. The neurologic deficits may develop slowly, or abruptly upon occlusion of a major vessel. Depending upon the distribution of infarction, the patient may develop hemiplegia, hemisensory defect, dysphasia, or homonymous hemianopia. Focal cerebral seizures develop occasionally. A transverse myelopathy may produce varying degrees of paraparesis, sensory loss, and impaired function of bladder and bowel. Infarction of the anterior two thirds of the cord, with resultant paraplegia and loss of pain sensation below the lesion, can follow occlusion of the anterior spinal artery. Sensory functions subserved by the posterior columns are usually preserved. Hydrocephalus and various cranial nerve palsies have been described.

A CSF lymphocytic pleocytosis (up to 100 cells per cubic millimeter) and an elevated protein concentration are characteristic. The CSF gamma globulin content is often elevated. Syphilitic reagins (VDRL) are nearly always present in the CSF as well as in the blood.

The progress of meningovascular syphilis can usually be halted by specific antibiotic treatment, but the degree of functional recovery depends upon the extent and location of the infarcts.

GENERAL PARESIS (DEMENTIA PARALYTICA, GENERAL PARALYSIS OF THE INSANE). General paresis can develop at any time from 2 to 30 (usually 10 to 25) years after the primary lesion. It appears more often in men than in women (3:1). About 60 per cent of paretics present with a progressive simple dementia; less than 20 per cent display manic symptoms and megalomania. Often faulty judgment, impaired memory (recent memory affected first), disturbed affect (depression or euphoria), or paranoia develops and progresses. The patient may complain of "nervousness," but characteristically lacks insight into the nature of his difficulty. Fine or coarse tremors, often affecting facial muscles and tongue, are present in about two thirds of the patients with fully developed general paresis. Abnormal pupillary responses, including Argyll Robertson pupil (see Tabes Dorsalis, below), impassive facies, slurred or dysarthric speech, exaggerated stretch reflexes, and extensor plantar responses are additional abnormal neurologic signs. Convulsions occur in 10 per cent of patients, and strokes may develop secondary to vasculitis.

The CSF is always abnormal, containing a modest (15 to 100) increase in mononuclear cells and an elevated total protein concentration (greater than 50 mg per deciliter in 75 per cent, and 100 mg per deciliter or higher in about 20 per cent of cases). An elevated CSF gamma globulin level is routinely found in general paresis as well as the presence of oligoclonal IgG bands. Nearly every patient has a positive VDRL and RPR (see below) test for syphilis in the CSF, and more than 90 per cent of patients have a positive blood serologic test. Incomplete, prior treatment may modify the CSF abnormalities.

General paresis, once established, evolves rapidly. If untreated, the disease is universally fatal, usually within three years. If paresis is recognized early and treated vigorously, about 80 per cent of patients will improve, but only about one half completely recover neurologic function.

TABES DORSALIS (LOCOMOTOR ATAXIA). Tabes dorsalis develops in less than 5 per cent of patients with untreated syphilis, and symptoms usually appear 10 to 20 years after the primary infection. Men are more often affected.

Dysfunction of affected posterior roots develops insidiously, usually first in the lower limbs. Impaired joint position sense results in stumbling and progressive sensory ataxia, especially in the dark when visual compensation is imperfect. Hypotonia, secondary to a lack of modulation of muscle tension by afferent fibers, accentuates the slapping gait. Paresthesias usually appear early in the disease.

Lightning pains are characteristic of tabes dorsalis but are nonspecific, occurring also in other diseases affecting dorsal roots, e.g., diabetic neuropathy. Lightning pains develop in at least 75 per cent of patients and migrate from one area of the body to another, although they are most common in the lower extremities. They are brief, sharp, burning, or aching jabs, sometimes flitting from one body region to another without predictable pattern. Involvement of thoracoabdominal nerve roots gives rise to visceral pains (gastric or visceral crises), which may simulate intrinsic visceral disease and can lead to misdiagnosis of abdominal surgical disease; in one series an estimated 25 per cent of tabetic patients had undergone inappropriate operations for tabetic pain. However, one must occasionally be wary, for the impairment of pain sensation in tabetics or the too quick assignment of lightning pain can induce disregard for true surgical emergencies.

As tabes advances, pain sensation is progressively lost and recurrent peripheral trauma goes unnoticed. Indolent ulcers of the skin develop; the toes and balls of the feet are especially vulnerable. Weight-bearing joints and adjacent bone, deprived of pain sensation, are destroyed by the constant trauma of use in 5 to 10 per cent of tabetic patients (Charcot joints).

Unless general paresis coexists, as it does in a small percentage of cases (taboparesis), tabetic patients are mentally normal. Optic atrophy complicates tabes dorsalis in about 10 per cent of cases or occurs as an isolated disorder. Argyll Robertson pupils that are small, irregular, and unequal, and respond poorly to light but constrict with accommodation, are present in most cases. Occasionally, other oculomotor functions are involved as well. Hypotonia, ataxia, and a slapping broad-based gait are common. Affection of the sensory arc accounts for the greatly diminished or absent stretch reflexes, especially the Achilles reflex. The plantar responses are normal in most cases. Loss or diminution of position and vibratory sensation is found in every case. Increased swaying when the eyes are closed and the patient is standing with feet together (Romberg's sign) results from the impaired position sense. Variable degrees of hypoesthesia and hypalgesia occur in nerve root distribution. Isolated areas of hypalgesia (Hitzig zones) sometimes affect the trunk or shoulders. Delayed perception (from one to several seconds) of pain stimuli delivered to a distal extremity provides a classic sign. Urinary bladder and bowel impairment produces incontinence and constipation in up to one third of cases. Male impotence and orthostatic hypotension are major complaints. Cystitis, hydronephrosis, and pyelonephritis are common complications of a hypotonic bladder.

The course of tabes dorsalis is unpredictable, and the response to antisyphilitic therapy varies. Patients who have had symptoms for a few months or at the most a few years, with prominent CSF abnormalities and no prior therapy, often improve with treatment. Patients with severe degeneration of dorsal roots and who suffer from painful complications usually retain many of their troubles but progress relatively little after antisyphilitic therapy ("burned out" tabes). Partial relief of pain may be achieved by analgesics, but narcotics carry a high risk of producing addiction. Benefit has been reported with anticonvulsant doses of phenytoin or carbamazepine. Urologic assistance may be required to deal effectively with uropathy. Penetrating skin ulcers and Charcot joints may similarly require surgical treatment.

OPTIC ATROPHY. Visual impairment in syphilis may result from iritis, choreoretinitis, increased intracranial pressure, or primary optic atrophy. Optic atrophy occurs in 1 per cent of patients with untreated syphilis and is five times more common in males than in females.

Because the outer portions of the optic nerve are first affected, the initial visual impairment tends to be peripheral. Ultimately, however, the papillomacular bundle becomes involved, and impaired visual acuity with central and paracentral scotomas develops. It has been estimated that, without treatment, 50 per cent of patients go blind in two years and 90 per cent in ten years. One eye is typically affected before the other. Optic pallor is usually present by the time symptoms appear, but in the early stages it is recognizable only by the reduced vascularity. The optic atrophy of syphilis is indistinguishable from that caused by other diseases. The CSF is abnormal in most patients with active disease of the optic nerve. Intensive antisyphilitic therapy may arrest the disease process and preserve what vision remains, but return of vision cannot be anticipated.

GUMMA. This rare complication of syphilis usually presents as an intracranial or intraspinal mass lesion and behaves as a slowly growing neoplasm. The correct diagnosis may be suspected from a positive serum serologic test for syphilis or from CSF abnormalities. Removal of the tumor mass, supplemented by antimicrobial therapy, alleviates symptoms and prevents spread of the disease.

CONGENITAL NEUROSYPHILIS. Syphilis acquired in utero after the first trimester of pregnancy tends to be a fulminant disease. Miscarriages and stillbirths are common, and a wide spectrum of clinical manifestations may be recognized in the infant or child who survives. *Neurosyphilis* develops in an estimated 10 to 20 per cent of infants and children with congenital syphilis. *Asymptomatic neurosyphilis* may be diagnosed in the early months or years of life by routine CSF examinations on children of syphilitic mothers. But, as with the acquired disease, symptoms and signs of active neurosyphilis develop only after a latent period, which in the case of *juvenile paresis* may be as long as 20 years. More often, symptoms first appear late in the first decade or during adolescence. Clinical syndromes and CSF findings mirror those found with the acquired disease, except that *tabes dorsalis* is exceedingly rare and *chorioretinitis* more common. Hydrocephalus, cranial nerve palsies (eighth cranial nerve especially), and seizures may complicate congenital syphilitic meningitis. Syphilis should be considered as a potential cause of cerebrovascular accidents in children. More than a third of all children with juvenile paresis have been retarded mentally from early life.

Non-neurologic stigmata of congenital syphilis include dental deformities (Hutchinson's teeth), saddle nose, frontal bossing of the skull, saber shins, and interstitial keratitis (usually developing during the second decade). These signs are not seen in acquired syphilis. Fortunately, the current practice of obtaining routine serologic tests on all pregnant women and on infants of syphilitic mothers has almost eliminated congenital neurosyphilis in many areas of the world. It should be remembered that the mother can acquire syphilis at any time during pregnancy and that negative serologic studies obtained early do not exclude the possibility of active syphilis later in pregnancy. Some institutions routinely test blood from the umbilical cord for the reagin of syphilis.

Early and intensive treatment of infants with congenital syphilis materially reduces the morbidity (see Treatment) from neurologic complications. Results from even optimal treatment of patients with juvenile paresis remain poor.

LABORATORY DIAGNOSIS OF NEUROSYPHILIS. Laboratory studies can be of considerable aid in the diagnosis of neurosyphilis and in the evaluation of therapy. Nevertheless, both false-positive and false-negative results may occur with all assays currently available, so that the final diagnosis requires a consideration of clinical as well as laboratory data.

Cerebrospinal Fluid Changes. Neurosyphilis always includes meningeal inflammation and its accompanying abnormalities in the CSF. Because of the chronic nature of the meningitis, the CSF changes are usually mild. A modest increase in cells, predominantly lymphocytes, numbering from 6 to 100 per cubic millimeter, is noted. The cytologic identification of plasma cells may be useful. The total CSF protein is usually elevated moderately to between 40 and 100 mg per deciliter. The CSF glucose is almost always normal.

The presence of treponemes within the CNS stimulates a local immunologic response, including the production of immunoglobulins which leak into the CSF. This is expressed as an increase in the CSF immunoglobulin G (IgG) level, which can be measured either as the IgG percentage of total protein (usually above 12 per cent) or, more specifically, by an IgG index. The index formula

$$\frac{\text{CSF IgG}}{\text{Serum IgG}} : \frac{\text{CSF albumin}}{\text{Serum albumin}},$$

which requires assessment of albumin and IgG in both serum and CSF, can be used to determine a specific increase in CSF IgG, considered by most workers to be a measure of IgG synthesis within the CNS compartment. In most laboratories an IgG index above 0.7 is considered abnormal. Specific elevation of CSF IgG is almost always noted in neurosyphilis.

In addition to quantitative IgG abnormalities, a qualitative CSF change is generally noted in neurosyphilis when concentrated CSF is assayed by agarose electrophoresis. This method demonstrates the presence of oligoclonal IgG bands which appear in perhaps 70 per cent of cases of confirmed neurosyphilis. Spirochetes have been demonstrated directly in CSF of patients with secondary syphilis by immunofluorescent methods.

Serologic Tests. The serologic tests for syphilis can be divided into two groups: those which are nontreponemal, and those which measure specific serologic reactivity to treponemal antigens. The nontreponemal tests use purified cardiolipin, which reacts with an antibody (formerly called reagin) in the serum or CSF to produce a serologic reaction. Presently, two flocculation tests, the Venereal Disease Research Laboratory (VDRL) and the rapid plasma reagin (RPR) tests, are routinely available and both can be accurately quantitated. Both are inexpensive and readily adapted to screening large numbers of specimens. Neither of these tests is as sensitive as the specific treponemal tests, and both may react in several nonsyphilitic disease states, especially the autoimmune disorders such as systemic lupus erythematosus. The specific treponemal serologic tests include the treponemal immobilization test (TPI), which is expensive, difficult to assay, and not routinely available, and the readily available indirect immunofluorescence assay, the fluorescent treponemal antibody–absorbed (FTA-ABS) test. The FTA-ABS test uses inactivated treponemes reacted with the patient's serum, which has been previously absorbed with an extract of nonpathogenic Reiter treponemes to remove nonspecific reactants. The other increasingly useful specific test is the treponemal hemagglutination test, which employs sheep or turkey erythrocytes coated with antigens of *T. pallidum.*

In practice, the nontreponemal tests are used for screening purposes and the specific treponemal tests for confirmation of diagnosis. It should be noted that the nontreponemal assays may be incorrectly reported in 5 to as many as 25 per cent of cases; therefore, if a negative result is obtained in a suspected case of neurosyphilis or a positive result is unexpectedly found, the test should first be repeated. Following confirmation of the nontreponemal assays, a specific treponemal test can be used to confirm the diagnosis.

Both the nonspecific and the specific treponemal antibody assays are positive in serum by the secondary stage of syphilis when acute meningitis and meningovascular syphilis appear. In the majority of late asymptomatic cases as well as in tabes dorsalis and general paresis, the tests are also often positive, although late CNS involvement sometimes has been reported with negative serology. The serum FTA-ABS is usually reactive even if the VDRL is negative in these late cases.

The serologic assay of CSF in neurosyphilis is still controversial. Most authorities advocate the use of the CSF VDRL test, both as an aid in the diagnosis of neurosyphilis and as a rough evaluation of therapy. The CSF VDRL is rarely falsely positive during nonsyphilitic disease states. If the test is positive, it is assumed that the patient does have invasion of the CNS by *T. pallidum,* especially if there is confirmatory clinical or CSF evidence of neurosyphilis. Usually the CSF VDRL titer falls with adequate treatment, although it may remain positive for prolonged periods. Accordingly, therapy must also be monitored by the clinical response and by a decrease in the number of CSF cells, total protein, or IgG level. The specific serologic tests often remain reactive for long periods after an apparent cure.

The specific treponemal tests, especially the CSF FTA, have yielded conflicting results in the diagnosis of neurosyphilis. Contamination of CSF with a minute amount of blood has been shown to convert a negative CSF sample to a positive one, so that CSF containing any red blood cells cannot be reliably used in a CSF FTA test. Some investigators believe that because of the extreme sensitivity of the test, even moderate amounts of antibody in the serum may cross to the CSF in the absence of true neurosyphilis. In the absence of elevated cells, protein, or IgG, no diagnostic conclusion can be made from finding a positive CSF FTA assay.

The need for evaluation of CSF during late (over one year after contact) asymptomatic syphilis remains unclear. Most authorities advocate CSF examination in all cases of a positive serum FTA-ABS test with an unclear treatment history. One recent study showed a very small yield of positive CSF findings in such patients. Nevertheless, in view of the differing treatment recommendations for late asymptomatic versus neurosyphilis patients, a CSF examination prior to therapy should probably be performed. Of course, evaluation of any patient with a positive serum FTA-ABS and any neurologic abnormality, even if not typical of the classic neurosyphilis syndromes, requires CSF assay to rule out atypical neurosyphilis.

TREATMENT OF NEUROSYPHILIS. Penicillin is the antibiotic of choice for all forms of syphilis, and no resistant strains of *T. pallidum* are known. Because the organism divides slowly and penicillin is effective during the dividing stage, prolonged therapeutic blood and CSF levels are necessary to accomplish a cure. Aqueous procaine penicillin G, 9 million units total given intramuscularly in 15 daily 600,000-unit doses, or benzathine penicillin G, given intramuscularly in three 2.4 million–unit doses at weekly intervals, has been advocated. However, some cases of neurosyphilis have progressed after such therapy, and other studies have failed to detect penicillin in CSF, especially after recommended weekly benzathine penicillin. Therefore, several authorities advocate hospitalization of all patients with neurosyphilis and treatment with 2 to 4 million units of aqueous crystalline penicillin G intravenously every four hours (12 to 24 million units per day) for ten days. As mentioned above, therapy is monitored clinically and when repeating the CSF evaluation two to six months later. CSF leukocytes should decline, as should total protein and IgG levels and, usually, the CSF VDRL titer. If CSF cell, protein, or IgG abnormalities persist unchanged, retreatment should be considered.

In cases of penicillin allergy, tetracycline HCl or erythromycin, 500 mg four times a day orally for 30 days, is usually curative.

Felman YM, Nikitas JA: Syphilis serology today. Arch Dermatol 116:84, 1980. *A detailed, comprehensive review of currently used serologic tests to detect infection with* T. pallidum *during each phase of disease.*

Holmes MD, Brant-Zawadzki MM, Simon RP: Clinical features of meningovascular syphilis. Neurology 34:553, 1984. *A short review of an acute form of neurosyphilis.*

Jaffe HW, Kabins SA: Examination of cerebrospinal fluid in patients with syphilis. Rev Infect Dis 4(Suppl.): 5842, 1982. *Current review of the assays available to analyze cerebrospinal fluid for evidence of neurosyphilis.*

Jones JE Jr, Harris RE: Diagnostic evaluation of syphilis during pregnancy. Obstet Gynecol 54:611, 1979. *Diagnosis and treatment of syphilis are necessary to prevent late maternal complications as well as congenital syphilis. A rational diagnostic approach is advocated.*

Merritt HH, Adams RD, Solomon H: Neurosyphilis. New York, Oxford University Press, 1946. *A classic lucid text on neurosyphilis, written when the various syndromes were still common and readily observable.*

Traviesa DC, Prystowsky SD, Nelson BJ, Johnson KP: Cerebrospinal fluid findings in asymptomatic patients with reactive serum fluorescent treponemal antibody absorption tests. Ann Neurol 4:524, 1978. *A study of the variations in the laboratory diagnosis of syphilis between different laboratories testing the same specimen. Text includes a helpful discussion of the use of lumbar puncture to detect neurosyphilis in asymptomatic patients.*

Venereal Disease Control Advisory Committee, Center for Disease Control, Atlanta, Georgia: Syphilis: recommended treatment schedules, 1976. Ann Intern Med 85:94, 1976. *Current official recommendations for treatment of all forms of syphilis.*

Wiggelinkhuizen J, Mason R: Congenital neurosyphilis and juvenile paresis. A forgotten entity? Clin Pediat 19:142, 1980. *A useful discussion of congenital and juvenile neurosyphilis, a disease fortunately rare but unfortunately underdiagnosed.*

Viral Infections of the Nervous System

498. INTRODUCTION

Richard T. Johnson

Most viral infections of the nervous system represent uncommon but important complications of systemic infections. With a few exceptions such as rabies or B virus *(herpes simiae),* nervous system infections are caused by agents that often infect humans. Some of these viruses, such as polioviruses and arthropod-borne encephalitis viruses, cause clinically significant disease only on the rare occasion when the nervous system is involved. Others, such as herpes simplex and mumps virus, are frequent causes of mild disease that assumes a more serious form when the central nervous system is infected.

Experimentally, viruses have been shown to invade the nervous system by centripetal movement in peripheral nerves, by penetration across the olfactory mucosa, or by a viremia. In man most viruses that infect the nervous system spread to the brain and meninges from blood, although neural spread appears to be important in rabies, B, herpes simplex, and varicella-zoster virus infections. The infrequency of nervous system involvement can be attributed to a variety of host defense mechanisms, including cellular and humoral responses, interferon production, anatomic barriers of nonsusceptible cells, and the activity of the reticuloendothelial system, which clears viruses from the blood. Youth, severe nutritional deficiency, and defects of cellular immunity have been shown to increase the risk of nervous system infection with some viruses, but in most patients the factors that have permitted central nervous system invasion are not evident.

Viral infections of the nervous system can lead to diverse clinical signs and symptoms, varied clinical courses, and protean pathologic changes. This diversity can be explained by the following two principles: (1) the varied cell populations of the nervous system have different susceptibilities to different viruses; and (2) viral infections can have varied effects on susceptible cells. If infection is limited to the meninges covering the nervous system, signs of viral meningitis may be the only clinical manifestations. If the infection spreads to the parenchymal cells of the brain, in addition to signs of meningeal irritation, signs of encephalitis develop. Some viruses cause even more selective involvement of specific cell populations in the brain and spinal cord and thus evoke characteristic clinical symptoms and signs. For example, in poliovirus infections the selective vulnerability of anterior horn cells leads to a characteristic clinical finding of acute meningitis with lower motor neuron paralysis. On the other hand, rabies virus infections in animals tend to spare the cortical neurons involved in most types of encephalitis and infect neurons of the limbic system. Therefore, instead of obtundation, seizures, and motor or sensory deficits, the infected animal shows alertness, loss of timidity, aberrant sexual behavior, and aggressive activity. This selective infection of cells of the limbic system appears to be a diabolic adaptation of the rabies virus to specific cell populations, so that the clinical disease in animals can drive the host to transmit the virus to another host by biting. Glial cell populations may also be selectively involved, such as in progressive multifocal leukoencephalopathy in which virus infection and cell lysis appear limited to the oligodendrocytes, causing a slowly progressive demyelinating disease.

The virus-cell interaction may be quite varied. There may be *acute lysis* of the infected cell, transformation of the cell with production of neoplasm, or *chronic infection* causing cellular dysfunction, cellular degeneration, or no abnormality. In acute viral infections the clinical and pathologic abnormalities may result either from an acute viral destruction of cells, as in acute viral meningitis or encephalitis, or from the host's immunologic response to the infection, as has been postulated in postinfectious encephalomyelitis. A *latent infection* is a virus-host relationship in which the virus remains present in some form in the host without giving rise to any signs of infection, but which can, when some trigger mechanism comes into play, emerge as an acute infectious process. This appears to occur in herpes zoster and in the majority of cases of herpes simplex encephalitis. *Chronic viral infections* are those in which there is an ongoing active infection, which may give rise to a somewhat irregular or unpredictable course extending over many months or years. Chronic inflammatory disease of the central nervous system is seen with fetal infections by rubella and cytomegaloviruses. In these indolent infections virus can be recovered for long periods of time postnatally and may or may not cause continuing or evolving clinical signs of disease. *Slow infections* have a more predictable course than chronic infections. They are defined as infections with an incubation period lasting for months to years, followed by a protracted but predictable clinical course ending in death. Slow viral infections of the nervous system in man include kuru, Creutzfeldt-Jakob disease, subacute sclerosing panencephalitis, progressive rubella panencephalitis, and progressive multifocal leukoencephalopathy (see Ch. 504).

499. VIRAL MENINGITIS AND ENCEPHALITIS

Richard T. Johnson

DEFINITIONS. *Viral meningitis* is a benign, self-limited illness with clinical signs of headache, fever, and meningeal inflammation. *Viral encephalitis* is a more severe illness in which fever, headache, and meningeal inflammation are complicated by depression of the state of consciousness, seizures, and/or focal neurologic deficits suggesting inflammation within the parenchyma of the brain.

The clinical syndrome of viral meningitis is also called *aseptic meningitis* or *serous meningitis,* since some bacterial infections and chemical irritants can cause identical clinical symptoms and cerebrospinal fluid changes. Encephalitis is also called *meningoencephalitis* or *encephalomyelitis,* the latter indicating concurrent signs of spinal cord involvement.

ETIOLOGY. A variety of viruses have been associated with meningitis and encephalitis (Table 499–1). The two syndromes represent a clinical continuum and are caused by the same spectrum of viral agents. However, some viruses tend to cause predominantly benign disease such as the coxsackie- and echoviruses, which cause about half of all cases of viral meningitis but are only rarely associated with encephalitis. Other viruses tend to cause more severe disease such as arthropod-borne viruses (arboviruses) and herpes simplex virus, which are the major causes of fatal encephalitis (Table 499–2).

Enteroviruses are small, nonenveloped RNA viruses of the picornavirus family, and include polioviruses, group A and B coxsackieviruses, and echoviruses. Over 50 serotypes have been associated with meningitis and encephalitis; the serotypes most frequently recovered from patients with viral meningitis are echoviruses 3, 4, 6, 9, 11, 18, and 30, coxsackievirus A9, and coxsackieviruses B1 through 5. Echovirus 9 has been associated with the largest epidemics.

Mumps virus is a large, enveloped RNA virus of the paramyxovirus family. Mumps is the single most common cause of

TABLE 499–1. VIRUSES ASSOCIATED WITH ACUTE CENTRAL NERVOUS SYSTEM INFECTIONS IN THE UNITED STATES

RNA Viruses
Enteroviruses
Polioviruses
Coxsackieviruses, groups A and B
Echoviruses
Togaviruses
Eastern encephalitis*
Western encephalitis*
Venezuelan equine encephalitis*
St. Louis*
Powassan*
Rubella
Reovirus
Colorado tick fever*
Bunyavirus
California encephalitis*
Arenavirus
Lymphocytic choriomeningitis
Rhabdovirus
Rabies
Myxoviruses and paramyxoviruses
Influenza
Parainfluenza
Mumps
Measles
DNA Viruses
Herpesviruses
Herpes simplex, types 1 and 2
Varicella-zoster
Epstein-Barr
Cytomegalovirus
Adenoviruses

*Arthropod-borne viruses (arboviruses).

TABLE 499–2. FREQUENCY OF ASSOCIATION OF AGENTS WITH ASEPTIC MENINGITIS AND ENCEPHALITIS*

Etiologic Agent	Percentage of Cases	
	Aseptic Meningitis	*Encephalitis*
Enteroviruses	40	10
Mumps	12	14
Lymphocytic choriomeningitis	6	9
Leptospira	3	2
Herpes simplex	1	10
Arboviruses	1	11
Other†	2	4

*Data from Johnson, 1982.
†Includes Epstein-Barr virus, measles, influenza, *Mycoplasma pneumoniea*, Rocky Mountain spotted fever, and fungal infections.

viral meningitis and mild encephalitis. Lymphocytic choriomeningitis virus is a small, enveloped RNA virus of the arenavirus group, which also causes both meningitis and mild encephalitis.

Herpesviruses are large, structurally complex, enveloped DNA viruses that cause a variety of neurologic diseases. Type 1 herpes simplex virus is associated with severe encephalitis in adults and represents the most common cause of endemic fatal encephalitis. Type 2 herpes simplex virus, a major cause of fatal neonatal encephalitis, seldom causes severe encephalitis in adults but has been associated with cases of meningitis. Headache and pleocytosis often accompany herpes zoster infections, but it is not known whether meningitis without radicular pain or cutaneous eruptions can be a manifestation of recrudescences of latent varicella-zoster virus infections (see Ch. 501). The Epstein-Barr virus has been related to meningitis and encephalitis, complicating approximately 1 per cent of cases of infectious mononucleosis. Cytomegalovirus, like rubella virus, is associated primarily with chronic congenital infections. However, cytomegalovirus causes encephalitis in immunocompromised patients and rarely in immunocompetent adults.

The acute neurologic disease associated with measles, vaccinia, rubella, and primary varicella (chickenpox) infections in most cases represents postinfectious encephalomyelitis. This may also be true of the encephalitis that has occasionally been reported with influenza and parainfluenza virus infections.

The arboviruses include viruses of several families (togavirus, bunyavirus, and reovirus) that are transmitted by mosquitos or ticks. More than 15 different arboviruses have been associated with encephalitis in varied geographic areas of the world; seven cause meningitis or encephalitis in the United States (Table 499–1). Over 100 cases of California virus encephalitis are reported annually over a wide geographic area. Eastern, western, St. Louis, and Venezuelan equine encephalitis viruses cause localized epidemics; St. Louis virus is the predominant cause of major epidemics.

Adenoviruses are respiratory viruses that only rarely cause meningitis or severe childhood encephalitis. Nonviral agents that cause clinical syndromes indistinguishable from viral meningitis or mild encephalitis include *Leptospira*, *Treponema pallidum*, the *Treponema* of Lyme disease, *Mycoplasma pneumoniae*, and *Rickettsia*.

EPIDEMIOLOGY. Over 5000 cases of aseptic meningitis and over 2000 cases of encephalitis are reported to the Centers for Disease Control annually, but this represents only a small fraction of the total number of cases per year in the United States. Both viral meningitis and encephalitis are reported with greater frequency during the later summer and early fall, and this increase results, in large part, from the seasonal dissemination of enteroviruses and arboviruses.

Epidemiologically the viruses causing meningitis and encephalitis in man fall into three categories: (1) Viruses that spread from man to man; these agents generally cause disease during a particular season of the year and often in epidemics. (2) Viruses acquired from infected animals (zoonoses); these agents may have distinct geographic distributions, and a history of animal contact in patients is often obtained. (3) Viruses spread by hematophagous arthropods and necessitating a cycle in the arthropod host; these viruses have very specific seasonal and geographic limitations.

The enteroviruses are spread by hand-to-mouth contact and to a lesser extent by respiratory spread or by fecal contamination of fomites or vectors. Virus growth is primarily in the intestinal tract. Although enteroviral infections occur throughout the year, the incidence of these infections increases dramatically in summer and early fall, often reaching epidemic proportions. Because of the mode of spread, family outbreaks are common, and the spread of virus is facilitated in families or communities with preschool children.

Mumps virus is spread by the respiratory route. Mumps occurs throughout the year, but there is a marked increase in incidence during the spring. Although the incidence of infection with mumps virus is equal between the sexes, males develop meningitis three times more frequently than females.

Lymphocytic choriomeningitis virus is the major zoonotic virus causing meningitis and encephalitis. The natural host of this virus is *Mus musculus*, the common house mouse, and the virus is present in its excreta. Man acquires the infection by contact with contaminated dust or food. Human disease is more common in winter, when the natural host tends to move indoors, increasing human exposure. Recently, lymphocytic choriomeningitis virus has also been found in hamsters, and human infections have been traced to laboratory and pet hamsters. Leptospiral infections are also acquired from both domestic and wild animals. These spirochetes are excreted in urine and contracted by man through contact with animal tissue, contaminated soil, or water polluted by animal urine.

Each of the arboviruses has a different epidemiologic cycle (see Ch. 356). In the United States, eastern, western, St. Louis, California, and Venezuelan equine encephalitis viruses are transmitted by mosquitos. Powassan virus and Colorado tick fever virus are transmitted by ticks. The seasonal occurrence of these infections is limited to seasons when the vectors are feeding. Eastern encephalitis virus is limited largely to the Atlantic and Gulf coasts and normally circulates between birds and salt marsh mosquitos, which do not bite humans. When ecologic changes alter the bird-mosquito balance, the virus can overflow into other mosquitos that feed on mammals. Regional deaths of horses or pheasants usually herald the rare human outbreaks. Western encephalitis virus is limited to the western two thirds of the country and normally circulates between mosquitos and birds; horses and humans become inadvertent hosts when bitten by infected mosquitos. This virus causes many more human infections than does eastern encephalitis virus, but only 1 in 100 of those infected develop encephalitis. St. Louis encephalitis virus causes both rural and urban disease over a large area of the United States. In the rural areas the virus has the same pattern as western encephalitis virus, but in urban areas more explosive outbreaks can occur when the virus is introduced into urban breeding mosquitos and urban birds become the intermediate hosts. California virus has a different cycle involving woodland mosquitos and small animals; birds are not involved. In recent years the virus has been related to encephalitis every year over a wide geographic area of the eastern half of the United States. Disease is confined almost entirely to children. Venezuelan encephalitis is transmitted from mosquitos to animals, and the virus has recently spread into Florida and the southwestern states. Most people infected with the virus have an influenza-like illness, but about 3 per cent develop acute meningitis or encephalitis. Powassan virus has been found in ticks in Canada and along the northern border of the United States; it is a rare cause of encephalitis in man. Colorado tick fever is found in ticks in the Rocky Mountain area; about 18 per cent of infected patients develop meningitis; encephalitis is rare.

PATHOGENESIS AND PATHOLOGY. Viruses usually replicate in cells at the site of entry. For example, after oral ingestion enteroviruses grow in the gastrointestinal tract; after respiratory spread viruses grow in the respiratory tract; or after subcutaneous or intravenous inoculation arboviruses grow in local subcutaneous, vascular endothelial, or muscle cells. Following local replication, dissemination of virus usually occurs via the blood. Despite the longstanding belief that the blood-brain barrier was impervious to viruses, it is now evident that the majority of viruses invade the central nervous system from the blood. The cerebral capillary endothelium is nonfenestrated, has tight junctions, and is surrounded by a dense basement membrane with astrocytic processes apposed to the outer surface. These structures do constitute a relative barrier to virus invasion, but experimentally viruses are found to invade the nervous system both by infection of the vascular endothelial cells with subsequent infection of surrounding glia and neurons and by passage of virus through endothelial cells. Experimentally viruses have also been found to grow in the choroid plexus and to seed virus into the cerebrospinal fluid.

Since viral meningitis by definition is a benign disease, its histopathologic correlates are unknown. In fatal encephalitis an inflammatory reaction is usually prominent in the meninges and in a perivascular distribution within the brain. Although the perivascular inflammatory reaction is composed predominantly of mononuclear cells, polymorphonuclear cells may be evident. Neural cells may show degenerative changes, and apparent phagocytosis of neurons by macrophages or microglial cells (neuronophagia) is often found.

Pathologic changes in encephalitis cannot unequivocally distinguish the agent involved. Topographic localization of lesions is of little value except in distinguishing poliomyelitis, rabies, and herpes simplex virus infections. Intranuclear inclusions are seen in herpesvirus infections and in measles virus infections, and in the latter cytoplasmic inclusions may also be found. Cytomegalovirus infections produce a characteristic pathology with the induction of cytomegalic cells containing inclusion bodies. Although fatal cases of mumps virus encephalitis are rare, pathologic studies have shown both the acute inflammatory lesions usually seen in virus encephalitis and perivenular demyelination characteristic of postinfectious encephalomyelitis.

CLINICAL MANIFESTATIONS. *Viral Meningitis.* The major clinical manifestations of viral meningitis are headache, fever, and nuchal rigidity. Signs and symptoms are often abrupt in onset and may persist from three days to two weeks. Other symptoms may include general malaise, sore throat, nausea and vomiting, drowsiness, abdominal pain, and chills and fever. The headache is often frontal or retro-orbital and associated with photophobia. Fever is seldom elevated above 40° C. Nuchal rigidity may not be as severe as that seen in bacterial meningitis and may be detectable only with extreme flexion.

Viral meningitis caused by several of the enteroviruses is often associated with rashes. The eruption usually appears at the same time as the fever and persists for four to ten days. In coxsackievirus A5, 9, and 16 and echovirus 4, 6, 9, 16, and 30 infections the rash is typically maculopapular and nonpruritic, and may be confined to the face and trunk or may involve extremities, including the palms and soles. In echovirus 9 infections the rash may be petechial, causing confusion with meningococcal infections. In group A coxsackievirus infections herpangina may develop, characterized by grayish vesicular lesions on the tonsillar fossae, soft palate, and uvula. In coxsackievirus A16 and rarely other group A serotype infections a vesicular rash may involve hands, feet, and oropharynx (hand-foot-and-mouth disease; see Ch. 345).

Mumps virus meningitis and encephalitis are associated with parotitis in approximately half the cases. However, the parotitis may precede or follow the meningitis by as much as a week. Evidence of parotitis associated with meningitis is not diagnostic of mumps virus infection, because parotitis has also been reported with group B coxsackievirus and lymphocytic choriomeningitis virus infections. Orchitis is seen in one third of postpubertal males, and tenderness of mammary tissue can be found in one third of postpubertal females with mumps virus infections. Oophoritis, pancreatitis, and thyroiditis may also be seen.

Aseptic meningitis caused by the type 2 herpes simplex virus may coincide with the eruption of genital lesions. In some cases this meningitis has been associated with radicular pain simulating lumbar or sacral root compression.

Viral Encephalitis. In addition to headache, fever, and nuchal rigidity, alterations of consciousness characterize encephalitis; mild lethargy may progress to confusion, stupor, and coma. Focal neurologic signs usually develop, and seizures are common. Motor weakness, accentuated deep tendon reflexes, and extensor plantar responses may be observed. Abnormal movements are seen in some cases of encephalitis, and rarely a tremor characteristic of Parkinson's disease may develop. The hypothalamic-pituitary area may be involved, causing severe hyperthermia or poikilothermia, diabetes insipidus, and inappropriate antidiuretic hormone secretion. Involvement of the spinal cord can lead to flaccid paralysis, depression of tendon reflexes, and paralysis of bowel and bladder. Increased intracranial pressure can cause third and sixth cranial nerve palsies.

In herpes simplex virus encephalitis, signs often include bizarre behavior, hallucinations, and aphasia, suggesting the temporal lobe localization typical of that infection (see Ch. 500).

LABORATORY FINDINGS. Blood count may be normal, show moderate leukopenia, or show a moderate leukocytosis. Epstein-Barr virus infections are suggested by large numbers of atypical mononuclear cells, as well as by positive heterophil reactions. Serum amylase may be elevated with mumps virus infections. Lymphocyte choriomeningitis virus infections are frequently associated with pulmonary infiltrates.

Cerebrospinal fluid examination is essential to establish the diagnosis of aseptic meningitis and encephalitis, but it is of little help in determining the specific virus involved. The cerebrospinal fluid may be under normal or moderately elevated pressure. The fluid is usually clear but may show xanthochromia if the protein content is over 100 mg per deciliter. Cell counts are variable, but 10 to 1000 cells are usual with a predominance of mononuclear cells. If the fluid is examined early in the course of disease, there may be no cells or a preponderance of polymorphonuclear cells. Repeat examination in 24 hours will usually show the characteristic presence of mononuclear cells. The protein content is usually elevated, and percentage of IgG may be high, suggesting intrathecal antibody synthesis. Gel immunoelectrophoresis may show oligoclonal bands of IgG, indicating the limited heterogeneity of antibody, and these bands may persist for six months or more after recovery. The glucose content in the cerebrospinal fluid is generally normal, although mild depressions are seen, particularly with mumps and lymphocytic choriomeningitis virus infections.

The electroencephalogram usually shows diffuse slowing, but shifting foci, marked asymmetry, and seizure activity may be evident in encephalitis. Diffuse slowing is not a grave sign in viral meningitis, because this abnormality can persist briefly even after the patient is asymptomatic.

Cerebral angiography, radioisotopic scans, and computed tomography of the brain may show localization of lesions of the temporal lobes in herpes simplex virus encephalitis, but these studies are of no value in differentiating other forms of encephalitis.

DIAGNOSIS AND DIFFERENTIAL DIAGNOSIS. The most important aspect of differential diagnosis is to exclude those treatable diseases which may masquerade as viral infections. These include tuberculous and fungal meningitis, parameningeal infections, brain abscess, partially treated bacterial meningitis, subacute bacterial endocarditis, amebic encephalitis, and other illnesses that may present headache, fever, and nuchal rigidity. The differential diagnosis of encephalitis is important, as specific therapy is now recommended for herpes simplex virus encephalitis (see Ch. 500).

A definitive etiologic diagnosis can be determined only by appropriate virologic laboratory studies. However, an educated clinical guess regarding the cause can be based on public health information concerning agents currently being disseminated in the area; on knowledge of the agents endemic to the area and the season of the year; and on the patient's history, including past immunizations and illnesses, possible insect bites, place of residence, travel in areas where particular infections are prevalent, health of the family, and type of dwelling place.

The coxsackievirus and echovirus infections occur sporadically throughout the year but reach epidemic proportions in the late summer and fall. Furthermore, they cause family outbreaks and protean manifestations. Thus the patient with aseptic meningitis occurring in late summer or fall who gives a history of other family members with nonspecific illness, rash, pleurodynia, or other enterovirus-associated disease probably has meningitis caused by a coxsackie- or echovirus. Transient lower motor paralysis reminiscent of poliomyelitis is also occasionally seen with these infections.

Mumps virus infections tend to occur in the spring, and a history of exposure is commonly obtained. Since there is no evidence that reinfection with mumps virus can occur, a clear-cut past history of parotitis during a mumps virus epidemic is good evidence against the patient's having mumps meningitis.

Patients with lymphocytic choriomeningitis virus infections often provide a history of living in mouse-infested houses or working in barns or other places frequented by mice. Alternatively, a history of exposure to or recent acquisition of a pet hamster should be sought. Lymphocytic choriomeningitis virus often causes a biphasic illness, with rather severe respiratory symptoms or pneumonitis preceding the abrupt onset of meningitis or encephalitis.

The mosquito-borne virus infections characteristically occur only in late summer and early fall before the frost. They vary in prevalence from year to year, depending on rainfall or other factors influencing mosquito, bird, and wildlife populations. Public health data regarding the dissemination of eastern, western, and St. Louis viruses in the population may be helpful in suggesting the diagnosis. California encephalitis virus shows little variation in frequency from year to year. Since this infection is usually acquired by children after exposure to woodland mosquitos, a history of preceding recreational woodland exposure may be obtained.

Herpesvirus infections show no seasonal distribution. In type 1 herpes simplex virus infection, a past history of cold sores, exposure to herpes labialis, or presence of labial lesions at the time of encephalitis is of no help in ruling out or suggesting the diagnosis. The diagnosis is suggested by the severity of the encephalitis and signs of localization to the temporal lobes. In contrast, onset of type 2 herpes simplex virus meningitis may coincide with the appearance of genital lesions.

Reaching a specific etiologic diagnosis in the laboratory necessitates obtaining acute and convalescent phase serum specimens. It is also useful to obtain specimens for isolation of virus (cerebrospinal fluid, stool, blood, and throat washings). Convalescent serum alone is of little value, as antibodies to most of the agents causing meningitis or encephalitis are widespread. Disease can be associated with a specific agent serologically only if a four-fold or greater increase in antibody is demonstrated between the early phase of disease and convalescence. Therefore blood should be drawn in the first few days of disease, and a subsequent serum specimen should be obtained two to six weeks later. The optimal specimens for viral isolation are dependent on the virus being sought. Arboviruses and enteroviruses can be isolated from the blood but are seldom recoverable at the time of clinical meningitis or encephalitis. During the acute disease coxsackie- and echoviruses are most readily isolated from stool or cerebrospinal fluid and, in some cases, throat washings. Lymphocytic choriomeningitis virus is most readily isolated from blood or cerebrospinal fluid. Mumps virus may be isolated from saliva, throat washings, or cerebrospinal fluid. Type 2 herpes simplex virus may also be isolated from the cerebrospinal fluid or blood. Unfortunately, type 1 herpes simplex virus can seldom be isolated from blood or cerebrospinal fluid, and definitive serologic studies require antibody determinations on spinal fluid. An early diagnosis of type 1 herpes simplex virus encephalitis still requires a brain biopsy.

TREATMENT. With the exception of vidarabine, now recommended in treatment of herpes simplex virus encephalitis, specific antiviral therapy is not available for viral meningitis or other forms of encephalitis. Treatment consists of supportive therapy and the management of the complications of encephalitis, including coma, seizures, and increased intracranial pressure.

In both viral meningitis and encephalitis bed rest is indicated. Strict isolation procedures are not essential, as most of the viruses causing meningitis and encephalitis are common in our environment. If an enteroviral infection is suspected, precautions in handling of stools and handwashing should be instituted. If measles, chickenpox, rubella, or mumps virus infections are evident, the usual isolation from susceptibles is recommended.

The headache and fever of meningitis can usually be managed with judicious doses of aspirin. Severe hyperthermia may develop in encephalitis, necessitating the use of more vigorous therapy, but it should be remembered that viruses are thermolabile. Therefore modest temperature elevations may serve as a natural defense mechanism, and attempts to reduce mild temperature elevations to normal or subnormal levels may be ill advised.

Patients with severe encephalitis are often in coma. Since these patients may make remarkable recoveries even after prolonged periods of coma, vigorous supportive therapy and avoidance of complications are essential. The airway must often be maintained by intubation or tracheostomy, and mechanical respiration may be necessary. Although intravenous fluids may suffice for brief periods, prolonged coma necessitates feeding with a nasogastric tube. Blood glucose and electrolytes should be checked frequently, because water, glucose, and salt control are frequently compromised during encephalitis. The respiratory tract, urinary tract, intravenous site, and skin are common sites of infection in comatose patients, and infections should be sought assiduously, treated vigorously, and avoided by skillful nursing, maintenance of bronchial drainage, frequent turning to avoid decubitus ulcers, and meticulous catheter care.

Although seizures frequently complicate encephalitis, prophylactic anticonvulsants are not usually recommended. If seizures develop, they can usually be managed with phenytoin and phenobarbital. If status epilepticus develops, more vigorous therapy should be instituted, remembering to treat the hypoxia and hyperthermia that complicate and aggravate status epilepticus.

Modest increases in intracranial pressure can be treated with glycerol given orally or by rectal tube. This osmotic agent is probably preferable to urea or mannitol, because it can be given over a longer period of time. Steroids should be avoided in the routine treatment of encephalitis because of their inhibitory effects on host-immune responses. However, when increased intracranial pressure is severe, the use of dexamethasone is indicated.

PROGNOSIS. Viral meningitis is a benign disease, and full recovery usually occurs within 5 to 14 days of onset, although some patients describe persistent fatigue, lightheadedness, and general asthenia that may persist for months.

The prognosis of encephalitis is dependent on the etiologic agent. The mortality rate of untreated herpes simplex virus encephalitis is approximately 70 per cent, with a high rate of sequelae in survivors. Arbovirus encephalitides have variable mortality rates; the mortality rate with eastern encephalitis is approximately 50 per cent; with St. Louis, 10 per cent; with western, 10 per cent; with Venezuelan equine, 1 per cent; and with California, less than 0.5 per cent. The mortality rates for western encephalitis are greater in children under one year of age, and for St. Louis encephalitis they are greater in the elderly. Nonfatal encephalitis caused by eastern, western, and St. Louis viruses leaves a relatively high rate of neurologic sequelae.

Encephalitis associated with mumps or lymphocytic choriomeningitis viruses is very rarely associated with death, and sequelae are infrequent. However, hydrocephalus has been reported as a late sequela of mumps meningitis and encephalitis in children.

Evans AS: Viral Infections of Humans. Epidemiology and Control. 2nd ed. New York, Plenum Medical Book Company, 1982. *A well-organized and up-to-date text with good chapters covering the epidemiology of enteroviruses, mumps, herpesviruses, arenaviruses, and arboviruses.*

Grist NR, Bell EJ, Assaad F: Enteroviruses in human disease. Prog Med Virol 24:114, 1978. *A comprehensive and well-referenced review of enteroviral diseases.*

Johnson RT: Viral Infections of the Nervous System. New York, Raven Press, 1982. *A current monograph that covers pathogenesis, epidemiology, and clinical features of acute central nervous system infections.*

Johnstone JA, Ross CAC, Dunn M: Meningitis and encephalitis associated with mumps infection. A 10 year survey. Arch Dis Child 47:647, 1972. *A concise report of clinical and laboratory data on 137 patients with mumps meningitis and encephalitis.*

500. HERPES SIMPLEX ENCEPHALITIS

Richard T. Johnson

DEFINITION. Herpes simplex encephalitis is the commonest nonepidemic fatal encephalitis. Unlike other viral encephalitides, herpes simplex encephalitis in children and adults shows unusual clinical and pathologic features of temporal and frontal lobe localization, epidemiologic and serologic evidence that most episodes represent reinfection or activation of latent infection, and unique problems of laboratory diagnosis. Early diagnosis is critical, since this is the one form of encephalitis for which effective antiviral drugs are now available. Herpes simplex encephalitis was formerly called *acute necrotizing encephalitis* or *acute inclusion-body encephalitis*.

ETIOLOGY. Encephalitis can be caused by either of the two distinct serotypes of herpes simplex virus: type 1, oral herpes; or type 2, genital herpes. Most cases of localized encephalitis are caused by type 1, with only a few caused by type 2 virus. In contrast, the diffuse, nonlocalized acute encephalitis of newborns is usually caused by a genital strain acquired during passage through the birth canal, but occasionally may be caused by type 1 virus. Aseptic meningitis and radiculitis caused by type 2 virus in adults are described in Ch. 499.

Herpes simplex viruses are large complex viruses containing double-stranded DNA coiled around core proteins. This mass is surrounded by a capsid 100 nm long, a tegument composed of fibrillar material, and finally an envelope derived from host cell nuclear membrane containing viral glycoproteins. The virion diameter is 180 nm. Since types 1 and 2 have approximately 50 per cent nucleic acid sequence homology, they share a number of common antigenic sites and biologic properties but can be differentiated by their monospecific antibodies. Herpes simplex viruses are naturally infectious only in man, but in the laboratory they have a wide host range in animals, embryonated eggs, and a variety of primate and nonprimate cell cultures.

INCIDENCE AND PREVALENCE. One thousand to two thousand cases of herpes simplex encephalitis are estimated to occur each year in the United States. The disease is seen worldwide. There is no seasonal distribution, and no sex-related preference. The disease develops at all ages, but a diphasic age distribution is evident, with persons under 20 and over 40 affected more frequently than those in the third and fourth decades of life. Predisposing factors are unknown. Most patients are otherwise in good health, although the disease can occur in immunocompromised patients.

EPIDEMIOLOGY, PATHOGENESIS, AND PATHOLOGY. Type 1 herpes simplex virus is a ubiquitous agent. Antibody develops in half the human population by age 15 and in 90 per cent by adulthood. Primary infection usually occurs during childhood by salivary or respiratory contact. This primary infection may be asymptomatic or cause gingivostomatitis, pharyngitis, or respiratory disease. During the primary infection, the virus is thought to be transported along the local sensory nerves and to establish latency in the corresponding sensory ganglia. In the case of type 1 herpes simplex virus, this is usually the trigeminal ganglia or in some persons the upper cervical or vagus ganglia. Type 2 herpes is usually acquired by venereal contact, and latency has been documented in the sacral ganglia. This latency appears to persist for life. Free infectious virus cannot be recovered from latently infected ganglia of humans or experimental animals, but virus is activated in cultures of the ganglion cells. Virus is probably sequestered as viral nucleic acid.

Activation occurs frequently. About 25 per cent of the population have activation of trigeminal ganglia infections manifested by herpes labialis or cold sores. In other asymptomatic individuals, virus can be intermittently recovered from the nasopharynx. Patients who develop encephalitis have a similar frequency of antecedent herpes labialis. This fact and serologic evidence of past infection in acute-phase sera indicate that most cases of encephalitis do not represent primary infections but are either reinfections or activations of the latent infection, with involvement of the brain.

The pathology of herpes simplex encephalitis shows a remarkable localization. The orbital surface of the frontal lobe, temporal lobe structures, and insular cortex develop hemorrhagic necrosis with inflammation and inclusion bodies. The involvement can be strikingly asymmetric. Selective vulnerability of a specific subgroup of cells fails to explain the localization, since both types 1 and 2 herpes cause diffuse encephalitis in neonates and the cells involved in localized encephalitis include both neurons and glia over a contiguous area. The findings suggest that the virus spreads from cell to cell along the base of the brain within the middle and anterior fossae.

The unique localization might be explained by the route of virus entry into the central nervous system with subsequent limitation of spread by antibody. Two such routes have been suggested. One is that primary infection or reinfection might occur across the olfactory bulbs with infection of the orbital-frontal lobes and subsequent spread to the temporal area. Alternatively, encephalitis might result from activation in the trigeminal ganglia, with spread along fibers from the ganglia that innervate pial and dural vessels.

CLINICAL MANIFESTATIONS. Herpes encephalitis can have an insidious or a fulminant course. Fever is almost invariably present, and headache is a prominent early symptom. Characteristically, 90 per cent of patients develop symptoms or findings that suggest a local lesion in one or both temporal lobes. Personality changes, hallucinations, or bizarre behavior may be evident for several days or even a week before other signs evolve, and in some cases this has led to initial hospital admission for psychiatric services. Memory may be impaired out of proportion to other cognitive functions, reflecting bilateral involvement of hippocampal systems. Generalized or focal seizures ensue in 40 per cent of patients. Hemiparesis develops in one third, frequently with a greater involvement of face and arm corresponding to the inferior frontal localization. Aphasia, superior quadrantal visual field defects, and paresthesias reflect the temporal lobe localization. In some patients there is rapid deterioration from stupor to coma without localizing signs.

DIAGNOSIS. Cerebrospinal fluid often shows increased pressure. Mononuclear cell pleocytosis usually ranges from 10 to 500 cells per milliliter, but occasionally there are either no cells or a high number of neutrophils. Red blood cells are frequent, but their presence does not indicate the diagnosis of herpetic encephalitis, nor does their absence exclude it. Protein content is usually elevated, and sugar content is usually normal or is only mildly decreased. The virus can rarely, if ever, be recovered from spinal fluid. Thus the spinal fluid examination suggests a viral encephalitis but does not differentiate a herpetic cause.

The most sensitive early test to suggest herpes encephalitis is the electroencephalogram (EEG). Unilateral or bilateral periodic discharges from the temporal leads occur in many patients, and slow wave complexes at regular two to three per second intervals are highly suggestive of the disease. Radionuclide scans may show uptake in one or both temporal lobes. Cerebral angiography usually demonstrates temporal swelling, prolonged arterial filling, and localized hypervascularity in one or both temporal lobes. Computed tomography (CT) frequently shows low-density temporal lobe lesions that may be accompanied by uptake of contrast material in the Rolandic fissure and opercular areas as well as the temporal lobe. However, the CT changes may develop later than those in the EEG or radionuclide scans.

Early definitive diagnosis of herpes simplex encephalitis depends on cerebral biopsy. To be useful in management, the biopsy should be taken as soon as clinical findings or laboratory tests indicate a viral encephalitis with frontal-temporal localization. The biopsy should be taken from an abnormal area. One cause of false negative results has been the sampling of frontal lobes or of the nondominant temporal lobe when clinical signs indicate disease in the dominant temporal lobe. Virus may be recovered from one area when it is not recoverable from others. Needle biopsy through a burr hole is probably more hazardous than craniotomy and open biopsy. In view of the frequent increase in intracranial pressure, craniotomy with decompression of the affected temporal lobe may have a therapeutic effect. This procedure also allows direct visualization of the affected area and selection of an optimal biopsy specimen. Tissue should be fixed for routine histology, frozen for immunocytochemical staining, inoculated into cell cultures for virus isolation, and possibly prepared for electron microscopy. Routine histologic studies can confirm the diagnosis of inflammatory encephalitis and rule out many other diseases, but characteristic inclusion bodies are recognized in only about one half of the biopsy virus-positive specimens. Immunocytochemical staining and electron microscopy can be done rapidly and usefully by experienced microscopists. However, both procedures are limited by a high yield of false negative results (30 per cent and 55 per cent, respectively) and a small number of false positive results because of nonspecific staining or inability to distinguish particles of Epstein-Barr virus. Virus isolation studies seldom yield false negative results but never false positive results.

A serologic diagnosis of herpes simplex encephalitis can be made with cerebrospinal fluid studies, but this cannot be sufficiently timely to guide effective antiviral therapy. Patients with herpes simplex encephalitis usually but not always develop a four-fold or greater increase in antibody to virus between acute and convalescent phase sera, but similar increases may result from nonspecific activation of virus associated with other infections. Increases in antibody in cerebrospinal fluid and elevated IgG and oligoclonal bands develop late in disease. A distorted ratio of antibody in spinal fluid and serum indicates intrathecal synthesis of virus-specific antibody. This is helpful in establishing a retrospective diagnosis of herpes simplex encephalitis and in detecting false negative biopsy results.

When herpes simplex encephalitis is suspected because of clinical findings or laboratory studies, biopsies show that only one third to one half of patients have the disease. A variety of other viruses have also been found sporadically to cause a similar localization. In 20 per cent of cases in which biopsies are done, other diseases have been found for which other treatments are indicated, including arteriovenous malformations, abscess, fungal and tuberculous infections with focal inflammation, and tumor. The cerebral biopsy is necessary to establish early diagnosis and for optimal patient management. No noninvasive diagnostic study has yet proved effective.

TREATMENT. Vidarabine is the approved drug for treatment of biopsy-proven cases of herpes simplex encephalitis. Its efficacy was originally established in a small placebo-controlled study that showed a reduction of mortality from 70 to 28 per cent. Subsequent open studies of large numbers of patients continue to show mortality of approximately 30 per cent, in contrast to mortality of 70 to 80 per cent in untreated patients or patients treated with cytosine arabinoside, an ineffective drug. When the diagnosis of herpes simplex encephalitis is suspected, biopsy should be performed and intravenous vidarabine administration started at a dose of 15 mg per kilogram daily for ten days. If there is surgical delay, the drug can be started within 24 hours prior to biopsy.

Vidarabine is a relatively nontoxic drug, but it does produce immunosuppression, is relatively insoluble, requires a fluid load, and has some degree of neurotoxicity. For these reasons the drug is contraindicated in patients with other encephalitides, and the morbidity and mortality of encephalitis patients without proven herpes infections appear to be increased if vidarabine is given indiscriminately. If the biopsy shows that the patient does not have encephalitis, vidarabine administration can be discontinued immediately. If encephalitis is found but immunocytochemical, immunocytologic, or isolation methods prove negative after five days, vidarabine should probably be discontinued. In addition to vidarabine, the other supportive treatment for acute viral encephalitis must be instituted (see Ch. 499).

Despite the efficacy of vidarabine, morbidity and mortality remain high, and the drug has undesirable side effects. Other drugs are currently being tested. Studies of vidarabine monophosphate, a more soluble derivative of the parent compound, have been halted because of unexplained greater mortality. Acyclovir is an acyclic nucleoside that has unique features for an antiviral agent because it is a selective substrate for herpes virus thymidine kinase. The drug is phosphorylated to the active compound largely in infected cells and is retained there. Once activated, the drug selectively inhibits the virus-specific DNA polymerase 10 to 20 times more than it inhibits cellular DNA polymerases. In theory, acyclovir appears superior and less toxic. Whether it is as effective as or more effective than vidarabine in treatment is being determined in controlled studies.

PROGNOSIS. For patients treated with vidarabine, the outcome depends on age and level of consciousness when therapy is begun. Ninety per cent of patients survive who are under age 30 years and only lethargic when treated, while among patients who are in coma when therapy starts mortality approaches 60 per cent, regardless of age.

Approximately half of patients who survive herpes simplex encephalitis retain debilitating sequelae, including motor and sensory deficits, aphasia, or Korsakoff's psychosis. Age and level of consciousness at the time of initiation of therapy are the major determinants. Fifty-eight per cent of patients under 30 years of age and 32 per cent of those over age 30 recover fully if treatment is initiated when they are only lethargic. In contrast, only 8 per cent survive without sequelae if therapy is delayed until after the onset of coma.

Adams H, Miller D: Herpes simplex encephalitis: A clinical and pathological analysis of twenty-two cases. Postgrad Med J 49:393, 1973. *A detailed study of a large series of patients with a careful correlation between postmortem findings and the clinical course and laboratory abnormalities.*

Baringer JR: Herpes simplex virus infection of nervous tissue in animals and man. Prog Med Virol 20:1, 1975. *A detailed review of the biology of these infections, describing their behavior in nervous tissue, their latency, and their relation to acute illness.*

Davis LE, Johnson RT: An explanation for the localization of herpes simplex encephalitis? Ann Neurol 5:2, 1979. *Speculation on the pathogenesis of the localized disease.*

Nahmias AJ, Whitley RJ, Visintine AN, Takei Y, Alford CA, the NIAID Collaborative Antiviral Study Group: Herpes simplex virus encephalitis: Laboratory evaluations and their diagnostic significance. J Infect Dis 145:829, 1982. *A current evaluation of virus identification methods and serologic tests.*

Whitley RJ, Soong SJ, Dolin R, Galasso GJ, Ch'ien LT, Alford CA, the NIAID Collaborative Antiviral Study Group: Adenine arabinoside therapy of biopsy-proven herpes simplex encephalitis. N Engl J Med 297:289, 1977. *A model placebo-controlled study showing a reduction of mortality from 70 to 28 per cent with no or only moderately debilitating neurologic sequelae in more than 50 per cent of survivors.*

Whitley RJ, Soong SJ, Hirsch MS, Karchmer AW, Dolin R, Galasso G, Dunnick JK, Alford CA, the NIAID Collaborative Antiviral Study Group: Herpes simplex encephalitis: Vidarabine therapy and diagnostic problems. N Engl J Med 304:313, 1981. *The data suggest that young patients who are only lethargic when therapy is begun have the best prognosis and that brain biopsy is rarely associated with serious complications.*

Whitley RJ, Soong SJ, Linneman C, Liu C, Pazin G, Alford CA, the NIAID Collaborative Antiviral Study Group: Herpes simplex encephalitis: Clinical assessment. JAMA 247:317, 1982. *The necessity of brain biopsy for early diagnosis is documented.*

501. HERPES ZOSTER

Richard T. Johnson

Herpes zoster is an acute viral infection of sensory ganglia and the corresponding cutaneous areas of innervation. The disease is characterized by localized pain along the distribution of the nerve and a vesicular skin eruption over a single or adjacent dermatomes. The disease is due to the same virus that causes chickenpox (varicella) (Ch. 339) and is thought to represent an acute localized recrudescent infection by the varicella virus that has remained latent in the sensory ganglia since the primary attack of chickenpox. Herpes zoster is also called shingles or zona.

ETIOLOGY. The varicella-zoster virus is a herpesvirus. The virus core measures 45 to 50 mμ and contains deoxyribonucleic acid. This is surrounded by a capsid with a diameter of 50 to 100 mμ and an outer envelope, giving a total diameter of the virion of 150 to 250 mμ. Morphologically, varicella virus resembles herpes simplex virus, with which it shares some common antigens, but it is markedly different from herpes simplex virus in its limited host range and in its loss of infectivity in most cell-free preparations. The virus is naturally pathogenic only for man, although chickenpox has been seen in anthropoid apes in zoos. There is some evidence of experimental transmission of the virus to several species of monkeys. The virus can be grown in a variety of cell cultures of human and primate origin but not in nonprimate cells. The virus is avidly cell-associated and can usually be transmitted in the laboratory only by the inoculation of infected cells, although the virus is stable in a cell-free form in the vesicular fluid.

INCIDENCE. Herpes zoster occurs at a rate of three to five cases per thousand persons per year. The disease is rare in childhood and is most frequently seen in persons over the age of 50 years. It is estimated that half the people reaching 85 years of age have suffered from at least one attack of herpes zoster. Both initial attacks and recurrences are more frequent in persons with malignancies or diabetes mellitus and in patients receiving immunosuppressant drugs or radiation therapy.

EPIDEMIOLOGY, PATHOGENESIS, AND PATHOLOGY. Chickenpox may develop after exposure to a patient with zoster, although this is less likely than development of chickenpox after exposure to chickenpox. In contrast, zoster rarely develops after exposure to chickenpox or other cases of zoster. Furthermore, chickenpox is a seasonal disease occurring mainly in the winter and spring and in epidemic proportions every two to four years. In contrast, zoster is neither seasonal nor epidemic in incidence.

The precise pathogenesis of herpes zoster is unknown, but the following hypothesis is widely accepted. Chickenpox is transmitted from man to man by respiratory spread, and in the susceptible person the virus probably disseminates throughout the body by viremia. Infection of the skin occurs through the blood, and vesicles develop most prominently over the face and trunk. It is postulated that virus then spreads centripetally via sensory nerve fibers to reside dormantly in the sensory ganglia. Virus replication is later activated. In some cases activation is associated with the development of malignancy, local x-irradiation, immunosuppressive therapy, trauma, treatment with arsenicals, neurosyphilis, or tumor entrapment of the dorsal root ganglia or nerve root. Nevertheless, in most patients there is no obvious exciting cause, and it is thought that the decline of immunity with age may promote reactivation. When virus multiplies in the ganglia, an active ganglionitis develops, causing pain along its sensory distribution. Virus then passes down the nerve and multiplies again in the skin, causing characteristic clusters of vesicles. The localized zoster lesions are most common over trigeminal or thoracic dermatomes corresponding to the areas of major eruption during the primary chickenpox infection. The more rapid secondary immune response may prevent hematogenous dissemination. Resolution and limitation of the rash of herpes zoster do not correlate well, however, with the development of antibody but appear to correlate with the collection of inflammatory cells and the presence of interferon in the vesicular fluid.

Pathologic studies of herpes zoster show an acute ganglionitis with an intense inflammatory response, cell necrosis, and occasionally hemorrhages within the ganglia. In addition, there is predominantly unilateral inflammation in the adjacent segments of the cord or brainstem, involving the posterior more than the anterior horns. Oligodendrocyte infection with focal demyelination has been described. A mild leptomeningitis is generally found that is most intense over the segments of involvement. Inflammation in the roots distal to the ganglia is also present, representing a true peripheral mononeuritis.

The skin innervated by the nerve shows degeneration of the basal and deep prickle cell layers of the epidermis. Ballooning degeneration of these cells causes the formation of the intradermal vesicles. Giant cells and eosinophilic intranuclear inclusions are found in the base of the vesicles.

CLINICAL MANIFESTATIONS. The eruption of herpes zoster is often preceded by malaise and fever for two to four days. Pain or dysesthesia along the segmental dermatome also precedes the rash by four to five days. The pain often has a superficial tingling or burning quality, but may vary from severe deep pain, suggesting appendicitis, cholecystitis, or pleurisy, to very mild itching. The pain may be intermittent or constant. Tenderness or hypesthesia may be detected along the dermatome during this pre-eruptive stage. The cutaneous lesions arise first as small, red macules, which rapidly vesiculate, becoming tense, clear vesicles on an erythematous base. On about the third day, the vesicular fluid becomes turbid as inflammatory cells collect within. Within five to ten days, the vesicles dry and crusts develop. However, in severe cases the vesicles may become confluent with a gangrenous appearance, and healing may be delayed for many weeks. During the course of the rash, the regional lymph nodes usually enlarge, and a few vesicles spread to adjacent dermatomes but seldom to the other side of the body. Pain or dysesthesia usually persists for one to four weeks; approximately 30 per cent of patients over age 40 have pain that persists for months to years. This postherpetic neuralgia is more common in the elderly when there has been a prolonged period of pain prior to cutaneous eruption and a more severe rash.

The distribution of lesions of herpes zoster corresponds to the areas of most intense rash of varicella. Although any sensory nerve distribution can be affected, two thirds of all lesions occur along thoracic dermatomes, and most of the remaining one third affect sensory branches of cranial nerves. Cranial nerve involvement tends to be more severe with greater pain, more meningeal irritation, and more serious neurologic complications. The ophthalmic division of the trigeminal nerve is the most common site of cranial involvement, accounting for 10 to 15 per cent of all cases. Usually the rash spares the eye, but occasionally keratoconjunctivitis develops. The maxillary and mandibular branches may be involved, with painful lesions involving the gums and oral epithelium. During varicella, vesicles are frequent on the buccal mucosa, which can lead to ascending infection of the petrosal as well as trigeminal ganglia. With later activation, glossopharyngeal zoster may develop with posterior pharyngeal pain and lesions in the tonsil, posterior tongue, and posterior pharyngeal wall. Similarly, the sensory fibers of the facial nerve near the external auditory meatus may carry virus to the geniculate ganglia. With activation, pain and vesicles develop in the external auditory meatus, with loss of taste in the anterior two thirds of the tongue and an ipsilateral facial palsy (Ramsay Hunt syndrome). The facial palsy is presumably due to inflammation or compression of the motor fibers of the facial nerve as they pass through the ganglion. However, with cranial zoster signs often implicate multiple cranial nerves or ganglia and suggest localized involvement of the brainstem. Ophthalmic zoster is frequently associated with abnormalities of oculomotor function, ptosis, or paralytic mydriasis and otitic zoster with severe vertigo and hearing loss.

Motor function may also be affected with herpes zoster in cervical, thoracic, and lumbar segments. The motor paralysis usually occurs within the dermatome involved by the rash, but occasionally is dissociated. Diaphragmatic paralysis with cervical zoster is usually unilateral. Asymptomatic paralysis of intercostal muscles may be found if sought. Thoracic lesions occasionally are accompanied by constipation, hypomotility, and even paralytic ileus. Urinary retention or urinary and fecal incontinence has been described with herpes zoster of sacral dermatomes. Signs of severe diffuse encephalitis, acute transverse myelitis, cerebellar ataxia, or ascending myelitis are rare and occur primarily in patients who have been receiving immunosuppressive therapy. Fatalities are infrequent.

An unusual complication of herpes ophthalmicus has recently been recognized. Days to months after the onset of vesicular lesions a sudden contralateral hemiplegia develops. Angiography may demonstrate a segmental narrowing of the carotid or cerebral arteries, scans show multifocal infarctions, occasionally bilateral angiitis develops, and in fatal cases a granulomatous arteritis with giant cells is found. The vasculitis appears to develop near the ganglia and spread distally. Whether direct viral infection or an allergic reaction causes the angiitis during convalescence from zoster is unknown.

Since the primary lesion even in uncomplicated herpes zoster is in the nervous system, cerebrospinal fluid commonly shows a pleocytosis and elevation of protein even in the absence of signs of meningeal irritation. These findings per se in the spinal fluid should not be a matter of concern.

Zoster sine herpete is typical pain in an appropriate sensory area that is not followed by the development of the characteristic vesicles. How often common transient intercostal or cranial pains represent activation of varicella virus in ganglia without spread to the skin is uncertain. An antibody response to varicella virus has been demonstrated in the absence of a rash in patients with transient intercostal pain or facial pain resembling trigeminal neuralgia and in patients with facial palsy (Bell's palsy). However, the vast majority of cases of trigeminal neuralgia and Bell's palsy are associated neither with serologic evidence of activation of the varicella nor with any other known viral infection.

Cutaneous dissemination is rare, occurring in less than 2 per cent of the cases. Dissemination is more common in patients with underlying malignancies, and about one quarter of the patients with Hodgkin's disease show a progressive spread of vesicles beyond the original one or two dermatomes of involvement. Such cutaneous dissemination, however, generally does not progress for more than six days, and spontaneous recovery occurs in most patients.

DIAGNOSIS. Characteristic development of pain and vesicular eruptions over single or adjacent dermatomes served by a segmental or cranial nerve branch usually presents no problem in differential diagnosis. However, similar zosteriform lesions can be caused by herpes simplex virus in infants.

Multinucleated giant epithelial cells with intranuclear inclusions can be found in Giemsa-stained scrapings from the base of an early vesicle, and virions can readily be found in vesicular fluid by electron microscopic examination. Neither of these tests, however, differentiates zoster from herpes simplex virus infections, although they can differentiate zoster or chickenpox from smallpox infections. Varicella and herpes simplex virus infections can be differentiated by fluorescent antibody staining of cells in scrapings from vesicles.

Virus can be isolated from vesicular fluid and, in some cases, from cerebrospinal fluid by inoculation of fluid onto cultures of human or primate cells. Serologic diagnosis can also be made, but in human sera some cross-reactions are found with herpes simplex virus, so that simultaneous serologic tests should be carried out against both viruses.

TREATMENT. Optimal treatment of acute eruption of herpes zoster is still unclear. Previously advocated treatments such as administration of protamine, vitamins, x-irradiation, vasodilators, antimicrobials, and gamma globulin are useless. In a controlled study corticosteroids decreased the incidence of postherpetic neuralgia, although they failed to alter the rate of healing or shorten the period of acute pain. However, this benefit must be weighed against the potential hazard of corticosteroids enhancing dissemination. Conversely, in controlled studies vidarabine and acyclovir have been shown to shorten the duration of acute pain and speed the healing of vesicles but not to decrease the incidence of postherpetic neuralgia.

In the young immunocompetent patient, little should be done to treat the acute eruption other than symptomatic application of powder or calamine lotion to the rash and use of analgesics for pain. In the immunocompromised patient, vidarabine or acyclovir should be given intravenously for at least five days to decrease the threat of cutaneous or visceral dissemination. In nonimmunocompromised elderly patients the risk-benefit ratio of corticosteroids is undefined, and antiviral drugs are of limited usefulness because of the need for intravenous treatment and the failure to decrease postherpetic neuralgia, the most dreaded complication in the elderly. Studies of the efficacy of oral administration of acyclovir and a re-evaluation of corticosteroids are currently in progress; these may clarify the indications for these drugs for the elderly immunocompetent patient.

There are no data to indicate the efficacy of vidarabine or acyclovir in zoster encephalomyelitis or granulomatous angiitis. Their use is rational with these potentially fatal complications, but since both conditions develop late in disease, antiviral drugs may not be effective. Because granulomatous arteritis may represent an allergic response, corticosteroids have been used in some cases but without clear-cut results.

Postherpetic Neuralgia. The development of prolonged postherpetic neuralgia after recovery from herpes zoster presents a difficult problem in management. Although the pain usually abates over a period of months to years, it is refractory to the usual analgesics. Application of cold to the area by use of an ethyl chloride spray may give transient relief. Tranquilizers or sedatives can sometimes be of help. Carbamazepine, an analgesic and anticonvulsant chemically related to the tricyclic antidepressants, is the drug of choice for postherpetic neuralgia but may be more effective when combined with other tricyclic compounds, such as amitriptyline, which more specifically block serotonin reuptake. A recent study of carbamazepine in conjunction with a similar drug, clomipramine, showed more effective pain relief than did transcutaneous nerve stimulation. Local injection of nerve root or nerve section should be avoided, since the origin of the neuralgia is in the ganglia. Surgical intervention, therefore, requires proximal nerve section or cordotomy, and results are often disappointing. In general, the patient is better served by protection from addiction or destructive surgery, treatment with analgesics and tricyclic antidepressants, and reassurance that pain usually abates with time.

PROGNOSIS. There is a popular misconception that herpes zoster does not recur. However, zoster does not give immunity to further attacks, and the likelihood of a second attack is about the same as, if not slightly greater than, that of having suffered the first. Most patients recover uneventfully, although severe vesiculation may lead to permanent scarring. Scarring of the cornea after ophthalmic involvement may result in permanent visual impairment. Motor paralysis of the local nerves recovers to adequate function levels in over 75 per cent of cases. Even in patients with encephalomyelitis, the mortality rate appears to be less than 10 per cent, and permanent sequelae are rare. The prognosis, however, must be more guarded in patients who have underlying neoplastic disease, in whom both the disease and the chemotherapeutic agents used in the treatment may increase the possibility of cutaneous and visceral dissemination.

PREVENTION. A vaccine to prevent primary chickenpox is being evaluated, but no method is known to clear latent virus from ganglia. Sera obtained from patients recuperating from herpes zoster can prevent chickenpox in children if given within 72 hours of the time of exposure. This zoster immune globulin is recommended for children on immunosuppressive therapy or with leukemia who have been exposed to chickenpox or herpes zoster. Similar measures are not recommended for disabled adults exposed to chickenpox or to zoster, although contact should be avoided in immunocompromised adults because it is in this group that occasional cases of zoster have been thought to be related to exposure to chickenpox or zoster.

Bean B, Braun C, Balfour HH: Acyclovir therapy for acute herpes zoster. Lancet 2:118, 1982. *A double-blind study of the efficacy of intravenous acyclovir therapy for zoster in otherwise healthy adults. Acyclovir did not appear to affect postherpetic neuralgia.*

Eaglstein WH, Katz R, Brown JA: The effects of early corticosteroid therapy on the skin eruption and pain of herpes zoster. JAMA 211:1681, 1970. *A double-blind study showing decrease in incidence of postherpetic neuralgia when herpes zoster in patients over age 60 is treated with corticosteroids.*

Gerson GR, Jones RB, Luscombe DK: Studies of the concomitant use of carbamazepine and clomipramine for relief of post-herpetic neuralgia. Postgrad Med J 53:104, 1977. *A controlled study showing greater efficacy of tricyclic compounds over transcutaneous stimulation in relief of pain in postherpetic neuralgia.*

Hilt DC, Buchholz D, Krumholz A, Weiss H, Wolinsky JS: Herpes zoster ophthalmicus and delayed contralateral hemiparesis due to cerebral angiitis: Diagnosis and management approaches. Ann Neurol 14:543, 1983. *A recent report of four cases with review of the English literature and thoughtful consideration of pathogenesis and therapy.*

Hope-Simpson RE: The nature of herpes zoster: A long-term study and a new hypothesis. Proc Roy Soc Med 58:9, 1965. *A classic. Simple observational data collected over 16 years from a general practice is beautifully presented to formulate the hypothesis of sensory ganglion latency and to speculate on man's evolving interrelationships with viruses.*

Jamsek J, Greenberg SB, Taber L, Harvey D, Gershon A, Couch RB: Herpes zoster-associated encephalitis: Clinicopathologic report of 12 cases and review of the literature. Medicine 62:81, 1983. *A recent article providing references on unusual neurologic complications.*

Juel-Jensen BE, MacCallum FO: Herpes Simplex, Varicella, and Zoster. Philadelphia, J. B. Lippincott Company, 1972. *This book contains a wealth of clinical data on herpes zoster, some of which has not been published elsewhere.*

McCormick WF, Rodnitzky RL, Schochet SS Jr, McKee AP: Varicella-zoster encephalomyelitis. Arch Neurol 21:559, 1969. *The best description of the neuropathology of fatal herpes zoster infections.*

502. ACUTE ANTERIOR POLIOMYELITIS

Richard T. Johnson

DEFINITION. Paralytic poliomyelitis is an acute febrile illness producing signs of meningeal irritation and flaccid motor paralysis. The term poliomyelitis means inflammation of the gray matter of the spinal cord. The disorder is characteristic of central nervous system infections with polioviruses. Mild forms of the syndrome are now often recognized with other enterovirus infections. Paralytic poliomyelitis is also called *infantile paralysis* or *acute anterior poliomyelitis*.

ETIOLOGY. Polioviruses are small, 28-nm-diameter, nonenveloped ribonucleic acid viruses that are members of the enterovirus group of the picornavirus family. There are three distinct serotypes, but they cross-react serologically, particularly types 1 and 2. Polioviruses have a restricted host range; most strains can be transmitted experimentally only to primates and cell cultures of primate origin. The host range of the polioviruses appears to be related primarily to specific cellular receptor sites for the virus; in human cells the coding for the receptor has been localized to chromosome 19. The coxsackieviruses, groups A and B, echoviruses, and related enteroviruses also can cause paralytic poliomyelitis, but unlike the polioviruses, other enteroviruses are also associated with a variety of clinical symptoms (see Ch. 341 to 347), and the resultant paralysis tends to be mild and transitory.

EPIDEMIOLOGY. Polioviruses have three distinct epidemiologic patterns. The first is endemic poliomyelitis, which occurred throughout the world until the end of the nineteenth century and is similar to the endemic disease still seen in tropical areas and developing countries. The second is the epidemic polio seen in economically advantaged countries during the first half of the twentieth century. The third is the pattern of sporadic cases seen in these countries since widespread immunization.

Descriptions of sporadic cases in children appeared in the eighteenth and early nineteenth centuries. Epidemic disease was first seen among small children in Scandinavia in the late nineteenth century and in North America and the remainder of Northern Europe in the early twentieth century. The age of patients developing paralytic poliomyelitis increased from epidemic year to epidemic year. In the great epidemic of 1916 in New York City, 9000 cases of paralysis were reported, and 80 per cent involved children under five years of age. During the epidemics of the 1950s, the peak incidence of paralysis was in children from five to nine years of age, and one third of the cases and two thirds of the deaths occurred in persons over age 15. These temperate-zone epidemics were seasonal, usually occurring in late summer and early fall. Even during epidemics when more virulent strains were circulating, the ratio of inapparent infection to disease ranged from 50:1 to 500:1.

Serologic surveys show that all three polioviruses have a worldwide distribution, and children even in population isolates have evidence of past infection with all virus types. Paralysis is age-dependent and is more frequent with advancing age. In virgin population epidemics, adults and adolescents with primary infections are ten times more likely to develop paralysis. In such epidemics almost all deaths are of patients over 20 years of age. Thus, prior to immunization programs, essentially all individuals experienced infections with all three types of virus. It is assumed that as sanitation improved virus dissemination among the very young declined, exposing a more susceptible population of older children and adults to primary infection. Quite possibly, during the time preceding epidemics of poliomyelitis children were infected with all three strains of virus at a period of infancy when they still had passive maternal antibody protection. Changes in living patterns and sanitation delayed acquisition of infection and led to an increase in the number of nonimmune persons and the appearance of the epidemic paralytic disease. As sanitation continues to improve in the developing world, more cases of paralytic poliomyelitis are seen. These cases, as expected, primarily occur in infants under three years of age. In developing tropical and semitropical countries, infections occur throughout the year, and outbreaks of disease are infrequent. Facilitation of spread in high humidity and the prevalence of other enterovirus infections that may cause interference may inhibit epidemics in these areas.

With widespread introduction of poliovirus vaccines in temperate-zone countries, the epidemic chain has been broken. In the past ten years, only 5 to 32 cases of paralytic poliomyelitis have been reported each year in the United States. Small outbreaks have occurred with the introduction of virus along the Mexican border and among religious groups where immunization is not practiced. Of the 208 cases of paralytic poliomyelitis reported between 1969 and 1982, 91 were related to vaccine viruses. Such cases occur primarily in adults in contact with children excreting vaccine virus or in children with hypogammaglobulinemia.

PATHOGENESIS AND PATHOLOGY. Humans are the only

known natural hosts of polioviruses. Virus is spread from person to person by hand-to-mouth contamination, although respiratory spread or passive transmission by insects or fomites may have a minor role. Virus is introduced orally, and initial replication occurs in lymphoid cells of the pharynx and gut. Virus can be found in the throat for several days and is excreted in feces for several weeks. After its initial replication, a viremia develops, with probable invasion of the central nervous system from the blood. There also may be neural spread from gut to spinal cord. Within the central nervous system there is selective vulnerability of motor neurons. Virus may spread from neuron to neuron by axonal transport. A possible explanation for the greater susceptibility of adults to severe paralytic and bulbar poliomyelitis is the more rapid axonal transport with maturation. Other host factors influencing paralysis include (1) excessive physical activity during the period of asymptomatic infection, which appears to favor paralysis of the exercised limbs; (2) pregnancy, which increases the risk of paralytic paralysis; (3) local injections during preceding weeks, which increase the risk of paralysis in the injected extremity; and (4) tonsillectomy, which heightens the risk of bulbar paralysis.

In fatal cases of acute poliomyelitis, inflammatory lesions are found primarily in the spinal cord when perivascular cuffing and diffuse infiltrates of mononuclear cells are present. The anterior horn cells of the spinal cord and the motor nuclei of the lower brain show the most marked abnormalities, with chromatolysis of motor neurons. Inflammatory reaction often spreads to the intermediate and posterior columns. Lesions are also found in the hypothalamus, thalamus, and brainstem, particularly in the vestibular nuclei, the deep nuclei of the cerebellum, and the reticular formation that regulates autonomic, respiratory, and circulatory functions. Lesions of the cerebral cortex are usually confined to the motor area.

CLINICAL MANIFESTATIONS. Replication of polioviruses in the intestinal tract often is not associated with any clinical signs but may cause the so-called *minor illness,* with fever, malaise, headache, and mild gastrointestinal symptoms of anorexia, nausea, vomiting, or diarrhea. This minor illness may or may not be evident three to ten days prior to obvious central nervous system involvement. Central nervous system involvement may be associated with asymptomatic meningitis, referred to as *nonparalytic poliomyelitis,* or with paralytic disease. Preceding the paralysis there are usually stiff neck, intense muscle aches, and headache with fever ranging from 38.5 to 40° C. Muscle pain and cramps may be accompanied by diffuse transient fasciculations. Paralysis may develop with great rapidity, proceeding from barely evident weakness to tetraplegia in only a few hours, or it may have a more indolent course, with additional weakness appearing over a four- to five-day period. The spread shows no consistent pattern, but paralysis is nearly always asymmetrical and at times widely scattered in its distribution. Lower extremities and lower trunk are involved most frequently. In the initial phases there may be hyperreflexia, but this is followed by flaccid paralysis with reduced or absent deep tendon reflexes. Although dysesthesias are frequent, sensory loss is rare. More than 50 per cent of adults have at least transient urinary retention.

Involvement of the brainstem is an ominous sign. This may be heralded by agitation, fear, or delirium. The ocular motor nerves are usually spared, but nystagmus with peripheral vision frequently occurs on extremes of gaze. Facial paralysis is usually restricted to one or more muscles and rarely is manifested as total facial paresis. Paralysis of swallowing is the most frequent abnormality of cranial nerve function but is usually transient. Muscle paralysis of the larynx may cause respiratory obstruction, but the greater dangers are autonomic abnormalities usually seen in adults with involvement of the reticular formation. Fulminating elevations of blood pressure, tachycardia, acute pulmonary edema, and cardiac arrhythmias are frequent with bulbar paralysis. Respiration may be ataxic, and potentially fatal sleep apnea may occur.

DIAGNOSIS AND DIFFERENTIAL DIAGNOSIS. Diagnosis in paralytic poliomyelitis is dependent on the typical clinical presentation and cerebrospinal fluid findings that document inflammation. The spinal fluid usually has a modest pleocytosis of 10 to 1000 mononuclear cells per milliliter, although early in the course of the disease there may be fewer than 10 cells or a preponderance of polymorphonuclears. Protein concentration is usually modestly elevated, and sugar content remains normal. These findings are important in the differentiation from *acute polyneuritis (Guillain-Barré syndrome).* In Guillain-Barré syndrome pleocytosis is absent or mild, and protein concentration often rises over 100 mg per deciliter, an unusual finding in poliomyelitis. More importantly, patients with polyneuritis are seldom systemically ill or febrile, and the paralysis tends to be symmetrical, in contrast to the patchy paralysis in poliomyelitis.

Paralytic poliomyelitis caused by most coxsackieviruses and echoviruses tends to have a more benign course with less serious and more transient paralysis. However, in countries with successful vaccine programs these other enteroviruses are the commonest cause of the paralytic poliomyelitis syndrome. Spinal fluid changes are similar, and definitive differentiation can only be made by isolation of virus or demonstration of antibody increases between sera from acute and convalescent phases. Furthermore, paralysis caused by nonpolio enteroviruses seldom occurs in epidemic outbreaks, with the exception of coxsackievirus A7 and two recently isolated enteroviruses.

Coxsackievirus A7 was related to several local outbreaks of paralytic disease in the Soviet Union in the 1950s and in the United Kingdom and France in the 1960s. Enterovirus 70 is the major cause of acute hemorrhagic conjunctivitis, a disease first observed in Africa in 1969. Subsequent epidemics in both Africa and Asia have probably affected more than 80 million people. Smaller outbreaks have also been reported in South and North America. Unlike other enteroviruses, this agent appears to be spread from eye to eye, and after an incubation period of only one to two days causes a febrile illness characterized by severe conjunctivitis with hemorrhage. In a small percentage of the cases a lower motor neuron paralysis resembling poliovirus infections has occurred, but curiously this paralysis usually develops several weeks after the acute illness and is often heralded by severe radicular pains. Paralysis is more common in adult males. The virus has shown a neural virulence in monkeys similar to that observed with polioviruses. Enterovirus 71 was first associated with aseptic meningitis but has shown different manifestations in different epidemics. A strain of this virus has been implicated in several outbreaks with paralytic poliomyelitis in Eastern Europe, primarily affecting young children. Fatal cases of bulbar paralysis were seen.

Epidemic neuromyasthenia (benign myalgic encephalomyelitis, Iceland disease, Royal Free disease) has some clinical similarities to poliomyelitis. Over the past 40 years, approximately 20 outbreaks have been observed of this curious disorder. Most outbreaks have involved residential communities, half of them affecting hospital staffs. The majority of cases occur in persons in the third decade of life, with women outnumbering men, although the sex ratio has been variable between outbreaks. Most outbreaks have occurred during the summer months with rapid spread, suggesting an epidemiology similar to that of poliomyelitis. However, attack rates have been higher than those seen in epidemics of paralytic poliomyelitis; for example, nearly 200 were affected at Los Angeles County Hospital in 1934 and over 300 at the Royal Free Hospital in London in 1955.

The disease begins abruptly with headache and severe muscle pains; posterior cervical lymphadenopathy and fever are variable findings. Muscle paralysis is seen in 10 to 80 per cent of patients, depending on the outbreak, but this paralysis differs from poliomyelitis since atrophy does not develop and hyperreflexia rather than hyporeflexia is found. Sensory symptoms are common, but objective sensory loss is rare. Occasionally painful muscle spasms, myoclonus, and other involuntary movements are seen, and objective signs of focal brainstem disease may be present, such as diplopia, facial paralysis, acute vertigo with nystagmus, deafness, and palatal paresis. Acute urinary retention has been described. Laboratory findings are remarkably normal. In some cases abnormal lymphocytes or an increased excretion of creatinine has been reported. The cerebrospinal fluid is usually entirely normal; 95 per cent of the cases show no pleocytosis. Variable nonspecific abnormalities have been reported on the electromyogram. The disease tends to have a protracted course. Although most patients show complete recovery within three months, relapses of weakness and myalgias are frequent, and emotional disturbances—particularly complaints of memory loss, depression, and emotional lability—may be prolonged.

Several of the early outbreaks of epidemic neuromyasthenia occurred during epidemics of paralytic poliomyelitis. An emotional etiology has been suggested by this correspondence, the high rates among young women, and the paucity of objective clinical or laboratory findings. However, something more than mass hysteria appears to be involved; the outbreaks, although widely distributed over time and place, have been remarkably stereotyped, and objective findings have been present in a significant percentage of the patients. The broad spectrum of symptoms and variable findings would make sporadic cases very difficult to diagnose, whereas in closed communities where epidemic spread of the infectious agent is facilitated, the disease would be more readily recognized. Certainly, the failure to find a pleocytosis in the spinal fluid, the inconsistency of fever, and the uniformly negative virologic studies are not conclusive evidence against a possible viral etiology.

TREATMENT. There is no specific treatment for paralytic poliomyelitis. Symptomatically, patients are treated with bed rest, aspirin, and other nonnarcotic analgesics for fever and pain and with hot packs for muscle spasm. The complications of bulbar poliomyelitis, including swallowing paralysis, respiratory failure, and cardiac abnormalities, are managed for the most part as they are in other diseases.

PROGNOSIS. During the acute illness it is impossible to predict the precise outcome. Fewer than 5 per cent of patients with paralytic poliomyelitis die with acute disease. Those over age 40 and those with bulbar involvement are at greatest risk. Muscle groups that maintain partial function at the end of the acute illness usually show good recovery. Recovery in areas of total paralysis is less certain.

Many years after paralytic poliomyelitis, a few patients, usually in their fifth or sixth decades, notice increasing weakness that is sometimes associated with muscle loss and fasciculations. The weakness is often in the area of the original paralysis. The more benign course and lack of upper motor neuron signs differentiate this late *postpoliomyelitis motor neuron disease* from *primary motor neuron disease*. It has been postulated that postpoliomyelitis disease may result from the persistence of polioviruses, but it more likely represents an aging process superimposed on a depleted anterior horn cell neuron population that may have been overloaded by the sprouting and reinnervation of larger motor units during recovery from the paralysis years before.

PREVENTION. Both live and killed poliovirus vaccines have proved successful for almost 30 years. Inactivated poliovirus vaccine used in the United States from 1955 to 1961 was effective in controlling epidemic polio, and its use has been continued with good disease control in several Northern European countries. The attenuated live oral poliovirus vaccines have been used in most of the world since 1961. Currently in the United States a trivalent oral polio vaccine (TOPV) is given in early childhood. The TOPV confers humoral and intestinal immunity similar to that of the natural infection, can be administered without trained personnel, and is inexpensive and easy to prepare. The vaccine virus is excreted in stools, and therefore inadvertent immunization is provided to many who fail to receive the vaccine. The disadvantage of TOPV is that a large percentage of paralytic poliomyelitis cases now seen in the United States are vaccine-related, either in hypogammaglobulinemic children or in adults who have been in contact with vaccine recipients. This risk has led to cogent arguments for return to use of the killed vaccine, but poor compliance and a dwindling supply of monkeys for tissue cultures and safety testing make this change impractical.

The advantages of the killed vaccine are that new preparations now produce very good and sustained immune responses and that it poses no danger of paralytic accidents. In developing countries where endemic poliomyelitis remains a problem, both vaccines have unique drawbacks. The TOPV often fails to confer immunity in tropical countries, presumably because of interference by other enteroviruses in the gut, but the killed polio vaccines pose problems in cost of production and delivery.

If an adult is traveling in areas of high endemicity or has special occupational risks and has not acquired past immunity, the killed polio vaccine is preferable. It is also indicated for immunodeficient children and their siblings.

Lyle WH, Chamberlain RN (eds.): Epidemic neuromyasthenia 1934–1977. Current approaches. Postgrad Med J 54:705, 1978. *Proceedings of a comprehensive symposium held at the Royal College of Medicine.*

Mulder DW, Rosenbaum RA, Layton DP: Late progression of poliomyelitis or forme fruste amyotrophic lateral sclerosis? Mayo Clin Proc 47:756, 1972. *A description of the problem based on the findings in 34 patients.*

Nathanson N, Martin JR: The epidemiology of poliomyelitis: Enigmas surrounding its appearance, pathogenicity, and disappearance. Am J Epidemiol 110:672, 1979. *A thoughtful essay, analyzing why poliomyelitis appeared and then disappeared as an epidemic disease in the United States during this century. The authors conclude that any change in present United States immunization practices carries considerable risk of reappearance of the disease.*

Paul JR: A History of Poliomyelitis. New Haven, Yale University Press, 1971. *A vividly told story of the social and scientific effects of one of the major "diseases of civilization."*

Robbins RC, Fox JP, Hopps HE, Horstmann DM, Quinn TC: International symposium on poliomyelitis control. Rev Infect Dis 6(Suppl 2):S301, 1984. *Proceedings of a recent conference posing the question of whether poliomyelitis can be eradicated worldwide. The disease in developing countries, current use and merits of live and killed vaccines, and the potential for better vaccines are discussed.*

Wadia NH, Katrak SM, Misra VP, Wadia PN, Miyamura K, Hashimoto K, Ogino T, Hikiji T, Kono R: Polio-like motor paralysis associated with acute hemorrhagic conjunctivitis in an outbreak in 1981 in Bombay, India: Clinical and serologic studies. J Infect Dis 147:660, 1983. *Also discusses novel modes of enterovirus transmission, problems in virus isolation, and neurovirulence in monkeys.*

503. RABIES

Michael A. W. Hattwick

DEFINITION. Rabies is an acute viral disease of warm-blooded animals, which may incidentally affect man, almost always as the result of a rabid animal bite. Human rabies is characterized by a variable incubation period, an acute neurologic illness leading rapidly to coma, and complications involving neurologic, pulmonary, and cardiovascular systems.

ETIOLOGY AND PATHOGENESIS. The rabies virus is a member of the rhabdovirus group, which includes more than 70 viruses, only three of which are reported to affect man: rabies, Duvenhage, and mokola virus. The virions are approximately 75 × 180 to 200 nm in length, contain single-stranded RNA, and are cylindrical with one conical and one flat end, giving rise to the characteristic bullet shape. Rabies virus is inactivated by drying, heating to 56° C for one hour, sunlight, ultraviolet light, and many chemical agents, including formalin, 50 to 70 per cent ethanol, strong acids, 0.1 to 1 per cent quaternary ammonium compounds, and 20 per cent soap. The virus is composed of four proteins: a glycoprotein, which is responsible for the induction of neutralizing antibodies, and is concentrated in spikes attached to the nucleocapsid core; a nucleocapsid protein, which produces complement-fixing but not neutralizing antibodies; and two membrane proteins, which are closely associated with the nucleocapsid.

Rabies virus obtained from the nervous tissue of animals which have developed the disease under natural conditions is referred to as "street virus" and is characterized by relatively long incubation periods after intracerebral inoculation (15 to 30 days or more), high infectivity after peripheral inoculation, and production of either "furious," or "dumb" (paralytic) rabies. Virus after serial passage in the brains of laboratory animals is referred to as "fixed" rabies virus and is characterized by a short incubation period after intracerebral inoculation (six to eight days), and production of paralytic rabies. Antigenic variations exist between strains of rabies virus and between rabies virus and serologically related rhabdoviruses.

After introduction by inoculation or animal bites, the virus remains near the site of inoculation for a variable time, during which replication in muscle cells may occur. Unless inactivated by natural or induced defense mechanisms, the virus subsequently enters the axoplasm of peripheral nerves, from where it travels to spinal ganglia and brain. The rabies virus spreads centrifugally soon after it reaches the central nervous system, is present in neurons throughout the body, and may be demonstrated by fluorescent antibody staining of corneal cells or skin biopsies. The virus is present in saliva in many but not all cases, and has also been identified in urine and cerebrospinal fluid. Concentrations in the brain are highest in the brainstem, basal ganglion, hippocampus, and cerebellum. Histologic examination shows perivascular lymphocytic infiltration, edema, vascular congestion, and relatively intact nerve cells. Characteristic oval cytoplasmic Negri bodies containing nucleocapsids are found in ganglia and in pyramidal cells, particularly of Ammon's horn or the cerebellum, but may be absent in 20 per cent or more of both human and animal cases.

EPIDEMIOLOGY. Rabies normally persists as an enzootic disease in warm-blooded animal species, in which it is maintained by bite transmission and possibly by transmission from mother to offspring. In areas where domestic animal rabies has been inadequately controlled, dog and cat rabies accounts for more than 90 per cent of reported cases. In other regions the majority of animal rabies cases are in wild animals. The virus is known to be maintained as an enzootic in only a few wild animal species, including, in the United States, skunks, foxes, bats, raccoons, and, elsewhere in the world, mongooses, wolves, and vampire bats. Epizootics of rabies in wild animals appear at intervals, most recently in raccoons in southeastern United States. In the United States during the 1950's, intensive dog and cat rabies control programs, including vaccination and stray animal elimination, reduced the number of annually proved rabid dogs from more than 7000 to less than 700. About 30 countries are classified as rabies free, largely because of geographical isolation and strict animal control and importation programs.

The epidemiology of human rabies closely parallels that of animal rabies; where dog rabies is inadequately controlled, most human cases result from rabid dog bites. In the United States from 1970 to 1984 27 human cases have occurred associated with a wide variety of exposures: dogs (2), a cat (1), skunks (2), bats (5), laboratories working with rabies (2), corneal transplant (1), and rabid animals in other countries (8). Six had no known exposure.

CLINICAL RABIES IN ANIMALS. Rabies virus may be present in the saliva of presymptomatic rabid animals for periods that vary with the animal species and with the rabies virus strain endemic in the area. The periods may last up to seven days for American dogs, one day for cats, four days for skunks, ten days for insectivorous bats, and possibly longer for vampire bats. Whenever a presymptomatic secretor of rabies virus has been killed and adequately examined, the brain has also contained rabies virus. Clinical rabies in animals may present either as hyperactivity (furious rabies) or as paralysis (paralytic rabies). Most animals die relatively rapidly after the onset of symptoms, although nonfatal rabies occurs.

CLINICAL RABIES IN MAN. Clinical rabies may be divided into five phases: incubation period, prodrome, acute neurologic phase, coma, and recovery.

Incubation Period. The incubation period normally ranges from 20 to 60 days, but periods as short as 10 days and as long as 19 years have been reported. Cases of rabies without any known exposure also occur. Incubation periods tend to be shorter in children than in adults, when the site of the bite is on the head rather than on the extremities, and in persons who have received postexposure treatment, possibly because of the elimination of long incubation rabies in the latter series. During the incubation period the person is asymptomatic except for symptoms related to local wound healing or postexposure treatment. Steroids have been reported to increase rabies mortality in mice and to decrease the immune response to rabies vaccine and should not be used in treating persons exposed to rabies.

Prodrome. The initial symptoms consist of malaise, anorexia, fatigue, headache, and fever. About half the patients have pain or paresthesias at the site of exposure. Apprehension, anxiety, agitation, irritability, nervousness, insomnia, and depression may be prominent; less commonly, cough, chills, sore throat, abdominal pain, nausea, vomiting, diarrhea, dysuria, pyuria, and priapism have been reported.

Acute Neurologic Phase. Two to ten days following the first symptoms, signs of nervous system involvement develop, including hyperactivity, hallucinations, disorientation, bizarre behavior, seizures, nuchal stiffness, or paralysis. Most patients develop hyperactivity, consisting of intermittent agitation, thrashing, biting, or other bizarre behavior, lasting up to five minutes. The episodes may occur spontaneously or may be precipitated by tactile, auditory, visual, or olfactory stimuli. Between episodes the patient is usually relatively lucid and cooperative, although often anxious. In half or more cases attempts to drink are followed by severe pain from spasms of the pharynx or larynx, inducing choking, gagging, and fear (hydrophobia). Hyperventilation and cardiac arrhythmias may be prominent.

Unless the patient dies abruptly, paralysis ensues and heralds impending coma. In about 20 per cent of cases paralytic symptoms dominate the clinical course (dumb rabies). Paralysis may be diffuse and symmetrical; may be maximal in the bitten extremity; or may ascend. Paralytic rabies appears to be particularly frequent after exposure to rabid bats or in persons who have received postexposure vaccination. During this period the mental status fluctuates, with increasing periods of confusion, disorientation, stupor, and finally coma. Nuchal rigidity may be present, but lumbar puncture reveals an increased number of cells in only about 50 per cent of cases. The acute neurologic phase lasts two to ten days with a longer duration in the paralytic forms and ends either with an abrupt death or with the onset of coma.

Coma Phase. In untreated cases the patient typically develops respiratory arrest shortly after the onset of coma and expires.

Recovery Phase. Intensive medical management can avert many of the complications in clinical rabies, and three cases of recovery have now been reported. In each the person had received either pre- or postexposure prophylaxis before the onset of clinical illness. In two of the three patients, a six-year-old boy and a 45-year-old woman, recovery was reported to be complete. The third case developed in a laboratory worker and the patient recovered with residual neurologic defects of speech and motor function.

COMPLICATIONS. A variety of complications have been reported, including increased intracranial pressure, cerebral edema, inappropriate secretion of ADH, diabetes insipidus, hypertension, hypotension, cardiac arrhythmias, and hypothermia. Seizures may be generalized or focal and are often accompanied by cardiac arrhythmias, cardiac arrest, or respiratory dysfunction. Hyperventilation and respiratory alkalosis are characteristic of the prodrome and early neurologic phase, whereas progressive hypoxia, hypoventilation, irregular respirations, respiratory arrest, and decreased pulmonary compliance develop later. Pneumonia, cardiovascular complications, vascular thromboses, gastrointestinal bleeding, and urinary tract infections are common late complications.

DIFFERENTIAL DIAGNOSIS. The diagnosis of clinical rabies is not difficult given a history of exposure and characteristic symptoms. If a history of exposure is not obtained, the differential diagnosis includes all forms of encephalitis. In recent years rabies has occurred after corneal transplants, and in six individuals without known history of exposure to possibly rabid animals other than hunting or working in wooded areas.

The diagnosis of rabies can be confirmed by isolation of virus from human saliva, human brain tissues, human cerebrospinal fluid, and/or urine. Attempts to isolate the virus late in the clinical course may be unsuccessful due to the development of neutralizing antibodies. Diagnosis of rabies during life occasionally can be made by utilizing fluorescent antibodies to stain rabies-infected cells obtained from corneal smears or skin biopsy specimens, although both false-positive and false-negative results occur. Diagnosis during life may also be made by measuring serum and cerebrospinal fluid antibody titers, a characteristic response occurring during the second and third weeks of illness. In unvaccinated patients neutralizing antibodies are absent until 6 to 12 days after onset and then rise rapidly to very high titers. In vaccinated patients a similar sharp rise occurs 6 to 12 days after clinical onset. Cerebrospinal fluid antibody levels rise later than do serum antibodies and are present in titers much higher than would be expected by passive transfer from the serum.

TREATMENT. Treatment of human clinical rabies consists of meticulously applied medical intensive care. Reports of human-to-human spread of rabies are rare except in the instance of corneal graft transmission. Nevertheless, rabies may be present in human saliva, cerebrospinal fluid, and urine, and treatment of persons possibly exposed to rabid patients should follow the same guidelines given for exposure to any rabid animal, as indicated below. Therapy of clinical rabies using rabies immune globulin, rabies vaccine, and human interferon has been tried, with no evidence of benefit.

PREVENTION. The most important aspect of rabies prevention is control of rabies in domestic animals. When it is not possible to prevent exposure of individuals to rabid animals or to environments containing rabies virus, prevention relies on local wound care and immunoprophylaxis. Two forms of immunoprophylaxis exist, pre- and postexposure. Both trace back to Pasteur, who showed that vaccination with inactivated rabies virus would protect against subsequent challenge with virulent rabies virus. Modern vaccines are based on growth of the virus in tissue culture, avian embryos, or suckling mice and harvested with methods that eliminate the presence of myelin components that are believed to be responsible for neurologic reactions. In the United States the only vaccines presently available are prepared on human diploid cells (HDCV), but vaccines prepared from infected mature nervous tissue (NTV) are still used in some countries.

The effectiveness of pre-exposure prophylaxis has been well established. Available studies generally indicate that individuals who have responded to pre-exposure prophylaxis with an adequate antibody response are protected against subsequent challenge by peripheral inoculation. A recent case of nonfatal rabies in an immunized laboratory worker exposed by an aerosol suggests that this protection may not extend to nonbite exposures. Protection against rabies following exposure requires both early and long-lasting immunity. The early immunity can be produced by passive antibodies or by induction of interferon. The lasting immunity must be produced by a potent vaccine. A number of studies have demonstrated that the combination of passive antibodies and active immunization with rabies vaccine is effective. In the absence of postexposure prophylaxis, the risk of human rabies following a bite on the arm or hand has been estimated as about 15 per cent for rabid dog bites and 40 per cent for rabid wolf bites. The combination of serum and vaccine prophylaxis reduces this incidence to less than 1 per cent. Both serum and vaccine are now recommended for all confirmed rabies exposures.

Pre-exposure Prophylaxis. Human diploid cell vaccine is sufficiently safe to justify immunization of individuals at high risk, such as veterinarians, animal handlers, some laboratory workers, and persons who vocationally or avocationally are likely to come in contact with rabid animals. Pre-exposure prophylaxis with HDCV consists of three 1-ml injections given intramuscularly on days 0, 7, and 21 or 28. Adequate antibody responses to this regimen have been demonstrated in all vaccinees studied. HDCV can also be given intradermally in a dose of 0.1 ml on days 0, 7, and 28. Individuals receiving intradermal pre-exposure prophylaxis should have serum tested for rabies antibodies two to three weeks following the last dose in the series. When antibody response is inadequate, an additional booster dose should be given and antibodies rechecked. Serologic testing is not required following a three-dose regimen by the intramuscular route. A person with continuing risk of inapparent or unavoidable exposure and no history of hypersensitivity reactions should have booster doses at two-year intervals. Type III hypersensitivity reactions may occur frequently after HDCV boosters, and booster doses should be given only when clearly indicated.

Postexposure Prophylaxis. Prevention of rabies in exposed individuals who have not received or responded to pre-exposure prophylaxis requires local wound therapy, passive immunization with hyperimmune rabies globulin, and rabies vaccination. The decision to initiate postexposure prophylaxis is based on the type of exposure (bite or nonbite), the animal species involved, and the condition of the animal at the time of exposure. Treatment is recommended for any bite by a known or suspected rabid dog, cat, skunk, bat, fox, coyote, raccoon, bobcat, or other carnivore unless the animal is proved nonrabid by laboratory tests. A healthy dog or cat which is available for observation should be confined for ten days, and rabies treatment given only if the animal develops rabies during the holding period. Treatment recommendations for persons exposed to a dog or cat that has escaped depend on information regarding the epizootiology of rabies in the area, which is available from local public health officials. Bites by rodents, rabbits, and hares almost never require postexposure prophylaxis. Recommendations regarding other exposures such as to livestock, laboratory specimens, or aerosol should be individually evaluated, and consultation with public health officials may be needed.

An important part of postexposure prophylaxis is local wound treatment. Rabies virus can be inactivated by soap, quarternary ammonium compounds, alcohol, and other viricidal chemicals. Local wound cleansing alone can markedly reduce the incidence of rabies in laboratory animals. Tetanus prophylaxis and appropriate antibiotic treatment for infected local wounds should be given as indicated.

Rabies immune globulin (RIG) should be administered once as soon after the exposure as possible. Up to one half of the dose of RIG should be infiltrated into the area around the wound and the rest administered intramuscularly. Human rabies immune globulin is available in 2- and 10-ml ampules containing 150 IU per milliliter and is given in a dose of 20 IU per kilogram.

Human diploid cell rabies vaccine (HDCV) is more potent than previous vaccines and is given as five 1-ml doses, 1 ml each day on days 0, 3, 7, 14, and 28. For a person who has received adequate pre-exposure prophylaxis with HDCV or has a documented adequate antibody response to another rabies vaccine, postexposure vaccination with two 1-ml doses of HDCV intramuscularly on days 0 and 3 is recommended. Serum antibody titers should be determined at the time of the last dose in persons who may be immunosuppressed due to a disease process or steroid use, who have received rabies prophylaxis with vaccines other than HDCV, or who have not had one of the above recommended regimens. If a titer of greater than 0.5 IU per milliliter of serum is not found, additional doses of vaccine should be given and the titer rechecked.

Minor complications are commonly associated with HDCV. Local pain, swelling, erythema, or induration occur in 50 per cent of vaccines. Systemic reactions including headache, malaise, fever, lymphadenopathy, nausea, or abdominal pain have been reported in 20 per cent. More serious complications with HDCV appear uncommon. Between 1974 and 1984, when nearly 2 million doses of HDCV were distributed worldwide, only two cases of associated neurologic reactions were reported. Both were Guillain-Barré–like illnesses, and the patients recovered fully. Anaphylaxis, urticaria and other allergic reactions have also occurred, but no fatal complications have been reported. Neurologic complications following vaccination with nervous tissue vaccines occur with an estimated incidence of 1 per 1630 vaccinees, and have a 15 per cent mortality rate. In most areas these complication rates are higher than the risk of rabies, and have led to the discontinuation of NTV use. Steroids should not be used to treat adverse reactions to rabies vaccine unless the reaction is life threatening, or the risk of rabies has been ruled out.

CONTROL MEASURES. The most important aspect of control is the prevention of spread between domestic animals by a combination of active vaccination and elimination of stray animals. Both killed virus and modified live rabies vaccines are available for animal use, and rabies programs can be highly effective in reducing both dog rabies and the number of associated human cases. Control of rabies in wild animals has not yet proved practical. In the absence of wild animal reservoirs and with favorable geographic conditions, rabies control programs can eradicate rabies, as has occurred in England and Japan. In such rabies-free areas preventing reintroduction of rabies requires strict importation control, including a six-month quarantine of animals with vaccination at the time of entry.

Anderson LJ, Nicholson KG, Tauxe RV, Winkler WG: Human rabies in the United States 1960–1979. Epidemiology, diagnosis, and prevention. Ann Intern Med 100:728, 1984.

Baer GM (ed.): The Natural History of Rabies, Vols I and II. New York, Academic Press, 1973. *Most comprehensive general review.*

Bernard KW, Hattwick MAW: Rabies virus. *In* Mandell GC, Douglas RC, Bennett JE (eds.): Principles and Practice of Infectious Disease. 2nd ed. New York, John Wiley & Sons, 1984. *Most current review.*

Centers for Disease Control: Rabies prevention: Recommendations of the Immunization Practices Advisory Committee. Morbid Mortal Wkly Rep 29:265, 282, 1980; updated recommendations: Morbid Mortal Wkly Rep 31:279, 1982; 32:601, 1983. Supplementary statement on pre-exposure prophylaxis by the intradermal route, 33:185, 1984. *Systemic allergic reactions following immunization with human diploid cell rabies vaccination.*

Hattwick MAW: Human Rabies. Public Health Rev 3:229, 1974. *Detailed review of human rabies.*

Hattwick MAW, Weiss TT, Stechshulte CJ, Baer GM, Gregg MB: Recovery from rabies: A case report. Ann Intern Med 76:931, 1972. *First documented nonfatal human case.*

504. SLOW VIRAL INFECTIONS OF THE NERVOUS SYSTEM

Richard T. Johnson

Slow viral infections have been related to several chronic and subacute neurologic diseases in which clinical signs of infection are lacking and in which the pathologic changes are those of degenerative or demyelinative processes. The term slow infection was originally coined in the veterinary literature to describe several transmissible diseases of sheep. Two of these sheep diseases, *scrapie* and *visna*, are the prototypes of slow infections of the nervous system. Both are transmissible. After inoculation of sheep with tissue from an affected sheep, a latent period of one to four years ensues during which the sheep appear well. This is followed by the insidious onset of neurologic signs that progress without fever for one to six months and lead inevitably to death. Scrapie is clinically characterized primarily by ataxia and visna by progressive paralysis. Pathologically the diseases are very different. The lesions of scrapie are confined to the nervous system, where there is marked proliferation of astrocytes and degeneration of neurons with vacuolization of their cytoplasms. By contrast, central nervous system lesions of visna are characterized by marked inflammation and demyelination. The agents responsible for these two slow infections of sheep are also very different. The scrapie agent has been transmitted to a variety of other animals, but the agent does not cause cytopathic changes in cell culture, and no virus-like particles have been found in infectious tissue by electron microscopy. The infectivity of this tissue remains remarkably stable on exposure to physicochemical treatments that inactivate classic viruses. Furthermore, animals naturally or experimentally infected with scrapie fail to develop any evidence of an immune response against the agent. In contrast, the visna virus is an enveloped RNA retrovirus. Although transmissible from sheep to sheep, it has not been transmitted to other animals but can be grown in a variety of tissue cultures. Of the five slow infections of the human central nervous system described below, kuru and Creutzfeldt-Jakob disease resemble scrapie pathologically, and the agents responsible for these diseases have properties similar to those described for the scrapie agent. Therefore scrapie, kuru, and Creutzfeldt-Jakob disease have been classified together as the subacute spongiform encephalopathies. Subacute sclerosing panencephalitis, progressive rubella panencephalitis, and progressive multifocal leukoencephalopathy, like visna, are due to classic viruses. These viruses have been visualized by electron microscopy, are antigenic in natural and experimental hosts, and can produce rapid cytolytic infection in some cell cultures even though they are capable of causing slow infections in man.

KURU

Kuru is an endemic disease of Melanesian tribal people inhabiting a remote area of the Eastern Highlands of central New Guinea. The disease has been seen only among the Fore linguistic group and neighboring groups with whom they have intermarried. Within this limited area, kuru, until recently, was the most common cause of death. The disease predominantly affected adult women and children over age five. Adult males were least involved. The disease begins insidiously with unsteadiness of stance and gait. A progressive symmetrical cerebellar ataxia develops over a period of months and follows a relentless, afebrile course until the patient is unable to make the slightest movement without violent ataxic tremors. Late in the course of the disease, abnormalities of extraocular movement and mental changes develop. The disease invariably leads to death in 3 to 20 months. Extensive laboratory examinations have failed to show systemic abnormalities, and the cerebrospinal fluid remains normal. Pathologic changes are confined to the brain where a marked diffuse noninflammatory increase of astrocytes and degeneration of neurons with cytoplasmic vacuolization are found. The findings are most prominent in the cerebellum and pons and, to a lesser degree, in the hypothalamus and basal ganglia.

When brain tissue from patients dying of kuru was inoculated into chimpanzees for long-term observations, a similar disease developed after incubation periods of 18 months to four years. This disease has subsequently been transmitted from chimpanzee to chimpanzee and to several other species. The agent can be transmitted with serial dilutions, proving that it replicates within the primate host. However, like scrapie, the agent of kuru has not been seen by electron microscopy, does not induce cytopathic changes in cell culture, is resistant to physical and chemical treatments that usually inactivate viruses, and fails to evoke a demonstrable immune response in humans or experimentally infected primates.

In recent years there has been a striking decline in the incidence of kuru, and the disease has disappeared among children. This decreasing incidence has coincided with the suppression of cannibalism in this primitive culture, providing circumstantial evidence that kuru was transmitted during the practice of ritual cannibalism.

CREUTZFELDT-JAKOB DISEASE

Creutzfeldt-Jakob disease is an uncommon form of rapidly progressive dementia accompanied by myoclonus, upper motor neuron paralysis, and other neurologic signs. The disease usually develops between ages 40 and 65, is worldwide in distribution, and usually occurs sporadically. However, a familial history is obtained in 10 to 15 per cent of patients, with a pattern of autosomal dominant inheritance. The dementia develops rapidly, so that deterioration from day to day or week to week is evident. Myoclonic jerks usually develop early in the disease, and often massive symmetrical myoclonic jerks of the limbs occur when the patient is startled by unexpected light or sound. Pyramidal tract signs, cerebellar ataxia, visual disturbances, and muscle wasting with fasciculations are common but inconstant features. The disease is inexorably progressive, usually reducing the patient from good health to helplessness or death in less than a year. The cerebrospinal fluid shows no abnormality, but the electroencephalogram becomes abnormal early in the disease, showing diffuse slowing with superimposed bursts of sharp waves.

Neuropathologic findings include diffuse noninflammatory loss of cortical neurons with a remarkable increase in fibrous astrocytes. Vacuoles are present in neurons and astrocytes, and this may give a spongiform appearance to the cerebral cortex. Inclusion bodies are absent. The pathologic findings are very similar to those of kuru and scrapie.

A similar disease develops in chimpanzees inoculated with brain tissue of most patients with Creutzfeldt-Jakob disease after an incubation period of 11 to 71 months. The pathologic changes in the brain resemble those of Creutzfeldt-Jakob disease. The disease has also been transmitted from chimpanzee to chimpanzee, to Old and New World monkeys, to domestic cats, to guinea pigs, and to mice. Little information is available on the agent of Creutzfeldt-Jakob disease, but the absence of virus-like particles on electron microscopic examination of infectious tissues, the failure to demonstrate cytopathic changes in cell cultures, and the absence of a demonstrable immune response suggest that the agent is similar to those causing kuru and scrapie.

The mode of spread is unknown, but the ability to transmit disease with tissues from familial cases suggests the importance of genetic factors or the possible vertical transmission of the agent. The failure to find increased incidences in medical personnel, laboratory investigators, or spouses of patients suggests a lack of significant communicability by respiratory, enteric, or sexual contact. Furthermore, the agent has not been detected in blood, sputum, or urine of patients, although it is present in extraneural tissue. On the other hand, apparent person-to-person transmission has been documented with the development of Creutzfeldt-Jakob disease in a patient 18 months after receiving a corneal transplant from another patient who proved to have the disease; by the occurrence of the disease in two young patients less than two years after cerebral corticography using the same implanted electrodes previously used in a patient with Creutzfeldt-Jakob disease; and by the occurrence of the disease in a number of patients within two years after undergoing intracranial surgery. In view of these observations, isolation of patients with Creutzfeldt-Jakob disease does not appear indicated, but careful disposal of needles and special sterilization of surgical instruments used on these patients appear mandatory. Medical personnel should avoid contamination of open sores or the conjunctiva with tissue, and no organs or corneas from patients with ill-defined neurologic diseases should be used for transplantation purposes.

No known treatment alters the relentless course of Creutzfeldt-Jakob disease.

SUBACUTE SCLEROSING PANENCEPHALITIS
(Dawson's Encephalitis, Subacute Inclusion Body Encephalitis)

This is an uncommon, subacute encephalitis that affects children or young adults between the ages of 4 and 20 years. The onset is usually insidious and is characterized by deterioration in schoolwork and behavioral disorders. This is followed in weeks or months by mental deterioration and neurologic signs, the most characteristic of which is myoclonus. The disease usually terminates after a third stage of stupor, blindness, dementia, and decorticate rigidity, which may last months to years. The cerebrospinal fluid is under normal pressure and shows no pleocytosis but an increased concentration of gamma globulin, corresponding in large part to antibodies against measles virus. During the stage of active myoclonus, the electroencephalogram usually shows a typical pattern of general suppression of activity, with periodic (8 to 15 seconds) synchronous bursts of high-voltage slow and sharp waves. Occasionally an apparent arrest of the disease process or even transient clinical improvement is seen.

In the brain perivascular infiltrates of mononuclear cells are characteristic, and eosinophilic intranuclear inclusion bodies are found in neurons and glial cells. Electron microscope studies of cerebral biopsies show virus-like particles resembling the nucleocapsids of paramyxoviruses. Astonishingly high levels of antibodies against measles virus can be demonstrated in the serums of most patients, and measles virus antigen is present in the brain. The measles virus associated with the disease is apparently defective.

The pathogenesis of subacute sclerosing panencephalitis is obscure. This disease bears little resemblance clinically or pathologically to the fulminating forms of measles virus infections, in which virus dissemination may lead to giant-cell pneumonia. Furthermore, it is distinct from parainfectious encephalomyelitis that occasionally complicates measles virus infections, in which acute neurologic disease occurs and perivascular demyelination is found in the brain and spinal cord. Epidemiologic studies have shown that subacute sclerosing panencephalitis is more common in males than females, in children of rural than of urban origin, and in patients with a history of measles during the first two years of life. These findings suggest that environmental factors and presence of residual transplacental passive immunity may play roles in inducing defective infection or precipitating disease.

Empirical treatments of patients with antiviral agents, interferon inducers, and immunosuppression and immunoenhancement therapies have provided no convincing evidence of beneficial effects. The sharp decline in cases five to seven years after the widespread use of measles vaccine attests to its preventive effect.

Rubella virus on rare occasions produces a similar chronic encephalitis called progressive rubella panencephalitis. The majority of patients bear stigmata of congenital rubella virus infections. However, after normal development or development within the limitations of the static congenital abnormalities, a chronic neurologic disease develops at 8 to 19 years of age. As in subacute sclerosing panencephalitis, the disease begins with the insidious deterioration of intellectual function, but myoclonus is variably present and cerebellar ataxia is a more prominent early finding. The disease follows an afebrile course over a period of years. Cerebrospinal fluid usually shows a mononuclear cell pleocytosis and mild protein increase with elevated gamma globulin. Antibodies to rubella virus are greatly increased in serum and cerebrospinal fluid. Neuropathologic findings include meningeal and perivascular inflammation, demyelination and gliosis in white matter, and mineralization around vessels similar to the mineralization seen in congenital rubella encephalitis. Rubella virus has been recovered from brain.

PROGRESSIVE MULTIFOCAL LEUKOENCEPHALOPATHY

This is a rare demyelinating disease of the central nervous system. It usually develops in patients having pre-existing disorders of the reticuloendothelial system such as leukemia, lymphoma, or sarcoidosis, or in those who have an acquired immune deficiency syndrome or who are immunosuppressed therapeutically or after organ transplantation. The neurologic abnormalities develop rather suddenly and follow a subacute progressive course until death. The findings usually suggest multifocal disease. Abnormalities of motor function, sensation, vision, or speech are common, and dementia frequently develops. The cerebrospinal fluid shows little if any abnormality, and the electroencephalogram shows only nonspecific slowing. Computed tomography may show multiple lucencies in the subcortical white matter. Pathologic lesions in the brain consist of multiple foci of demyelination in various stages of evolution. Oligodendrocytes are depleted within the foci, but surrounding the foci they are enlarged and contain eosinophilic intranuclear inclusions. The astrocytes within the demyelinated areas are often bizarre and contain mitotic figures. Inflammatory cells are usually not prominent.

Electron microscopic examination in almost all cases of progressive multifocal leukoencephalopathy has shown particles in the oligodendrocyte inclusions resembling small papovaviruses. Two small deoxyribonucleic acid viruses related to simian-virus 40 have been isolated from brain tissue of patients dying from progressive multifocal leukoencephalopathy. The JC virus, a new human papovavirus to which most persons have antibody since childhood, appears to be the causative agent in most cases. Viruses antigenically indistinguishable from simian-virus 40 have been related to a small number of cases. Neither of these viruses has been associated with any disease in man except progressive multifocal leukoencephalopathy. The disease apparently results from opportunistic infection of the brain by normally nonpathogenic agents. The viruses appear selectively to infect and lyse oligodendrocytes, the glial cells that maintain the myelin sheaths, and cause demyelination. The disease occurs in patients with impaired cellular immune responses, but it is not known whether it represents a primary infection of an immunologically incompetent patient or a reactivation of a latent or persistent papovavirus infection.

Evaluation of possible therapeutic agents has not been possible because of the rarity of cases and the infrequency of diagnosis during life.

OTHER NEUROLOGIC DISEASES

Since viruses can cause disease after a long incubation period, can produce disease with a subacute or relapsing course, and can give rise to noninflammatory pathologic changes, the possible role of slow or latent virus infection in a variety of neurologic diseases has been entertained.

In several chronic or relapsing inflammatory diseases of the nervous system, a viral cause has been suspected. *Chronic focal epilepsy* (epilepsia partialis continua, Kozhevnikov's epilepsy) is, in some cases, associated with a chronic focal inflammatory process in the brain. In several Soviet laboratories, tick-borne encephalitis virus has been isolated from surgically removed cerebral epileptogenic foci years after the acute encephalitis. No viruses have been isolated from similar cases in other countries. Chronic focal epilepsy can be a manifestation of focal disease processes such as neoplastic, vascular, or traumatic lesions, but chronic infection may play a role in some cases.

Recurrent acute meningitis or encephalitis occurs in three clinical syndromes of unknown cause in which latent viral infection has been suspected. *Mollaret's meningitis* is a rare, recurrent meningitis characterized by repeated attacks of headache, fever, and nuchal rigidity. Each attack is abrupt in onset and lasts for two to three days; the patient is entirely well between episodes. During attacks, the cerebrospinal fluid may contain large numbers of both polymorphonuclear and mononuclear cells and also large, poorly staining "epithelial cells," characteristic but not pathognomonic of this disease. More severe recurrent neurologic involvement can occur in *Behçet's syndrome* and in the *Vogt-Koyanagi-Harada syndrome.* Behçet's syndrome is a chronic disease characterized by recurrent oral and genital ulcers and inflammatory ocular lesions, usually taking the form of acute recurrent iritis. In about one quarter of the patients neurologic signs develop, consisting either of cranial nerve palsies, focal seizures, hemiparesis, or other focal signs or of severe depression of consciousness, coma, or meningeal signs, suggesting more diffuse neurologic involvement. Neurologic deficits usually remit and relapse but may be progressive. Neuropathologic findings include meningeal inflammatory reactions, perivascular inflammation, and focal areas of necrosis. The Vogt-Koyanagi-Harada or uveoencephalitic syndrome is characterized by depigmentation of skin and hair, inflammatory ocular lesions (usually consisting of iridocyclitis or exudative retinal detachment), and meningitis. Unlike Behçet's syndrome, neurologic involvement occurs in all cases, often precedes the ocular inflammation, and usually consists only of headache, nuchal rigidity, and a mononuclear cell pleocytosis. However, transient decrease in hearing and tinnitus may accompany the meningitis, or a severe encephalitis may develop, leaving permanent neurologic deficits. Neuropathologic findings have consisted only of a chronic arachnoiditis. Reports have been made of isolations of unidentified viruses from patients with Mollaret's, Behçet's, and Vogt-Koyanagi-Harada syndrome, but none of these claims has been entirely convincing. An allergic cause has also been postulated in each of these disorders, and consequently treatment with corticosteroids has been advocated.

Considerable interest in a possible viral cause of *multiple sclerosis* has been stimulated by epidemiologic data that indicate the role of a common exposure factor, serologic studies showing higher antibody levels against measles virus in patients with multiple sclerosis, observation of viral-like particles in brains, and unconfirmed claims of virus isolations. These data are still inconclusive. A notion that Parkinson's disease might have a viral cause has been entertained ever since the observation was made that a form of parkinsonism was a frequent sequela of encephalitis lethargica (von Economo's disease). Similarly, the possible role of a slow infection in amyotrophic lateral sclerosis and in a variety of other demyelinating and degenerative diseases has also been postulated. Although the spectrum of neurologic disease that can be potentially attributed to slow, latent, or chronic viral infections has greatly broadened in recent years, evidence is still scant for incriminating a transmissible agent in these chronic neurologic diseases.

Gajdusek DC: Unconventional viruses and the origin and disappearance of kuru. Science 197:943, 1977. *This Nobel Prize lecture recounts the story of kuru and discusses the interrelationships of the spongiform encephalopathy agents.*

Johnson RT: Selective vulnerability of neural cells to viral infections. Brain 103:447, 1980. *A review of the varied mechanisms by which viruses can cause chronic degenerative and demyelinative diseases as well as malformations and tumors of the brain. The major emphasis is on experimental diseases in animals, but chronic human diseases are covered.*

Johnson RT: Viral Infections of the Nervous System. New York, Raven Press, 1982. *This monograph summarizes known slow infections as well as the possible role of viruses in multiple sclerosis, amyotrophic lateral sclerosis, Parkinson's disease, and recurrent meningitis and encephalitis.*

Masters C, Harris JO, Gajdusek C, Gibbs CJ Jr, Bernoulli C, Asher DM: Creutzfeldt-Jakob disease: Patterns of worldwide occurrence and the significance of familial and sporadic clustering. Ann Neurol 5:177, 1978. *Recent collection of epidemiologic data on 1435 patients with Creutzfeldt-Jakob disease.*

Narayan O, Penney JB Jr, Johnson RT, Herndon RM, Weiner LP: Etiology of progressive multifocal leukoencephalopathy. Identification of papovavirus. N Engl J Med 289:1278, 1973. *This paper reports identification of papovaviruses in brains of 13 patients with progressive multifocal leukoencephalopathy. Rapid diag-*

nostic methods using fluorescent antibody staining and electron microscopic agglutination techniques are employed.
Padgett BL, Walker DL: New human papovaviruses. Prog Med Virol 22:1, 1976. *Virologic studies of JC and BK viruses are comprehensively reviewed, including discussion of the role of JC virus in progressive multifocal leukoencephalopathy.*
Roos R, Gajdusek DC, Gibbs CJ Jr: The clinical characteristics of transmissible Creutzfeldt-Jakob disease. Brain 96:1, 1973. *A summary of the clinical signs and symptoms of patients with Creutzfeldt-Jakob disease. The studies focus on transmissible cases and define the syndrome on this basis.*
Wolinsky JS: Progressive rubella panencephalitis. *In* Vinken PJ, Bruyn GW (eds.): Handbook of Clinical Neurology. Amsterdam, North-Holland Publishing Company, 1978, pp 331-341. *This chapter consolidates the limited data on the cases of progressive rubella panencephalitis. The clinical and pathologic data are particularly well covered.*

Section Nine NEUROLOGIC DISORDERS ASSOCIATED WITH ALTERED IMMUNITY OR UNEXPLAINED HOST-PARASITE ALTERATIONS

505. ACUTE TRANSVERSE MYELITIS

H. Richard Tyler

CLINICAL SYNDROME. "Transverse myelitis" refers to a clinical syndrome most often affecting the mid to upper thoracic level of the cord. There is a relatively rapid onset of severe paraparesis or paraplegia usually affecting all motor and sensory pathways distal to the lesion. It has a sharp segmental distribution, with the "clinical" lesion extending over one to three spinal segments. It occurs as a sporadic illness at any age without any seasonal incidence. About half of the patients give a history of a preceding infection or mild trauma. About one third run a low grade fever. Rarely "warning" phenomena consisting of transient paresthesias in the lower extremities precede the major syndrome by one to four weeks.

The most common presentation is initiated by radicular or localized back pain, usually affecting the thoracic region. Pain is quickly followed by bilateral paresthesia of the feet and toes and a rapidly rising sensory loss and weakness until a total paraplegia develops. Urinary and fecal incontinence and retention are prominent. Less commonly, progressive weakness of the lower extremities or retention of urine may precede other symptoms. The syndrome usually takes hours to a few days to develop. Some progression may continue in episodic or stepwise fashion for up to two weeks.

Rarely an acute spinal lesion can develop apoplectically, producing an initial flaccid state (spinal shock), which slowly evolves into a spastic paraplegia. Some patients will remain flaccid, suggesting that funicular necrosis has affected the spinal cord, not only involving the segmental level but producing descending damage in the gray matter, especially of the anterior horns.

Following this acute or subacute onset most patients enter a stable phase with no change taking place for a number of days to a few weeks. About half of the patients then undergo partial improvement, although at least some residuum, usually spastic paraparesis, is found in most. Occasionally a residual partial Brown-Séquard–like lesion with crossed sensory loss and ipsilateral motor weakness and spasticity is seen. About 50 per cent of the patients do not recover and are left with a severe spastic paraplegia. Those who recover usually have done so by three months.

"Partial" syndromes occur. One important group has an abrupt onset of symptoms and signs related to the anterior portion of the cord in the distribution of the anterior spinal artery, suggesting a vascular mechanism. In this group there can be relative preservation of the posterior column function.

In general, patients who have a rapid progression to a total paralysis and develop flaccidity below the level of the lesion have a more ominous prognosis than those who develop their syndrome subacutely over 5 to 12 days.

DIAGNOSIS. There may be enough swelling of the spinal cord in severe lesions to produce a spinal subarachnoid block acutely. Myelographically this appears as intramedullary swelling and can be difficult to distinguish from intramedullary tumor or hemorrhage. This development usually disappears in three to four weeks, but may be associated with a very high protein content and xanthochromia. The spinal fluid usually is acellular, but some cases contain up to 200 cells, usually lymphocytes. Rarely when necrosis affects the cord, a polymorphonuclear excess can be seen. Less commonly the destruction is so severe that it elicits an associated meningeal inflammation with secondary fibrosis and obliteration of the subarachnoid space. This can cause the appearance of a block by myelogram and abnormal spinal fluid and dynamics two to three months after the acute lesion. Patients who develop either an acute or delayed block may require surgical exploration to guarantee that no treatable situation is present.

PATHOLOGY. There is a destruction of all tissues of the spinal cord at the level involved. There is subsequent liquefaction of the tissue, invasion with macrophages, and scarring of the meninges to the residual tissue. Inflammatory cells, including polymorphonuclear leukocytes, and plasma cells can be seen in some of the more acute cases.

ETIOLOGY. Because of the "acute" nature of the syndrome, the suggestions as to its nature have included vascular, demyelinating, and infectious causes. In individual cases each has something to suggest its role. In most instances no cause is found and the disorder must be regarded as a "syndrome" (rather than a "disease") and capable of being produced by multiple causes. Why the thoracic cord is so selectively susceptible is unknown, but the vascular supply to the cord is probably most vulnerable in this area.

Some patients develop an acute transverse myelitis in association with segmental viral infections such as herpes zoster. With such infections the spinal cord shows a massive infiltration of inflammatory and plasma cells and an arteritis showing active inflammatory changes. Extensive tissue destruction produces a poor prognosis. In milder forms of the illness, inflammatory changes without arterial damage affect the tissue, and prognosis is better.

Because spinal cord lesions are common in multiple sclerosis, some authorities suggest that acute transverse myelitis may often represent the initial attack or a severe attack of demyelinating disease. Although the disorder is sometimes recurrent, less than 10 per cent of patients with transverse myelitis later develop signs of disseminated demyelinating disease. It should be noted that spinal lesions of multiple sclerosis rarely cause severe destructive lesions of both gray and white matter and can usually be suspected by their more gradual onset, asymmetry, and partial nature.

A vascular cause has been suggested largely because damage to a critical blood vessel supplying the spinal cord can result in the segmental destruction of the cord. In the lower thoracic area there is usually one larger radicular artery (artery of Adamkiewicz), surgical damage to which in renal, aortic, or thoracic operations can result in a syndrome of "transverse myelitis." There is an appreciable incidence of transverse myelitis in patients with systemic lupus erythematosus, which is ascribed to infarctions secondary to vascular compromise. However, in most autopsied cases of transverse myelitis, no vascular lesion has been demonstrated. Sometimes this may be a result of the failure to dissect the blood supply from its origin at the aorta to the spinal cord. Nevertheless the spinal lesion is consistent with infarction and liquefaction necrosis.

DIFFERENTIAL DIAGNOSIS. The differential diagnosis of spinal disorders that can mimic acute transverse myelitis is based on features of the illness which indicate the location, mode of progression, completeness of the transverse lesion, its symmetry or lack thereof, and any evidence of disseminated or associated lesions. Laboratory tests on spinal fluid and radiologic studies are crucial.

The most important diagnosis to consider with rapid progression of spinal symptoms is an epidural space infection of the spinal cord (acute epidural abscess) (see Ch. 496). This condition produces a surgical emergency that, if not appropriately treated, can lead to irreversible damage. Characteristically, epidural abscess occurs in a febrile patient with a warning of severe local back or radicular pain. An obvious source of infection exists in perhaps 50 per cent of cases. The onset is followed rapidly by symptoms of spinal cord dysfunction, including bladder incontinence and paraparesis. X-rays may show bone changes of osteomyelitis in as many as 20 per cent. The peripheral white count is usually elevated with a shift to the left. The sedimentation rate is almost always elevated. Spinal fluid examination usually shows an increased number of polymorphonuclear cells and a complete block. Since many of these features accompany "transverse myelitis," often myelograms and occasionally exploratory surgery must be carried out to arrive at proper diagnosis.

Spinal cord compression from other causes such as metastatic or primary tumor usually develops at a pace slower than transverse myelitis, with symptoms present over a longer period of time. Such compressions are more likely to present with asymmetrical findings and a partial Brown-Séquard syndrome. Occasionally, tumors may compress the cord rapidly over a period of hours, making differential diagnosis more difficult. However, the presence of known tumor, radiographic vertebral lesions, and findings by myelography usually resolve the problem.

Demyelinating disease, i.e., multiple sclerosis and its variants, frequently produces myelopathic findings. When these develop, they usually are painless, generally spare sensory pathways, tend to come on over two to six days rather than over hours, and rarely completely affect the cord. A rare form of demyelinating disease called Devic's disease combines severe spinal lesions with severe optic nerve lesions. This particular combination of findings has an ominous prognosis and frequently causes permanent cord dysfunction.

A partial, predominantly motor spastic paraparesis sometimes follows a known viral infection, especially measles (rubeola) or chickenpox (varicella), less often rubella and variola. The spinal signs are usually part of a more widespread perivenous demyelinating reaction.

In large poliomyelitis epidemics occasional patients present with signs of transverse myelitis accompanying other evidence of active polio infection. These patients are often left with the same severe spinal lesions, including sensory loss, that one sees with transverse myelitis. Transverse myelitis must be differentiated from the myelopathy caused by granulomatous infectious processes such as tuberculosis, coccidioidomycosis, and nocardiosis. Intramedullary abscess with actinomycosis, nocardiosis, aspergillosis, and cryptococcosis can damage the cord and produce myelitic phenomena.

Vascular diseases such as syphilis and dissecting aneurysm of the aorta have also been associated with acute spinal cord damage by affecting segmental arteries going to the spinal cord.

In patients with cancer and chronic infections such as tuberculosis, focal damage to the cord, especially in its dorsal aspect, has been described as causing myelopathy.

Subacute necrotic myelopathy of Foix and Alajouanine is characterized by a month-long progressive stepwise course. It is caused by successive infarctions associated with spinal arteriovenous malformations.

A rapidly progressing myelopathy over hours in a previously healthy person should always raise the question of spontaneous epidural or subdural bleeding. This usually occurs without known cause. In a patient taking coumarin anticoagulants or with a blood dyscrasia, one is necessarily more aware of this potential complication. The diagnosis may be made by computed tomographic body scan, which can demonstrate the mass of blood, or by exploration. Decompression of the cord is usually indicated.

Radiation myelopathy is discussed in Ch. 562.

TREATMENT. Treatment of acute transverse myelitis is supportive. The initial concern is to rule out treatable disease. Once this is done, the major concern is to prevent complications. Steroids are contraindicated because they have no beneficial effect and increase complications.

To prevent skin breakdown patients should be turned frequently, and every effort made to protect pressure points. Mattresses that distribute pressure over wide areas are preferable.

Most patients have urinary retention. A regular program of intermittent catheterizations by experienced personnel is preferable to an indwelling catheter. Fluid intake should be kept high and urinary infections treated promptly. There may be an ileus acutely. Prevention of fecal impaction is desirable. Patients with lesions that ascend into the cervical area may require mechanical ventilation.

Bed rest provides no advantages, and patients should be mobilized after the first few days if possible. Complicating venous thrombosis of the legs is common and best avoided by mobilization and passive movement.

Although some physicians give ACTH or steroids, no satisfactory evidence supports their routine use.

Berman M, Feldman S, Alter M, Zilbar N, Kehang E: Acute transverse myelitis: Incidence and etiological considerations. Neurology 31:966, 1981. *A retrospective review of the syndrome in a well controlled population with probably the best statistics available.*

Plum F, Olson ME: Myelitis and myelopathy. *In* Baker AB, Baker CH (eds.): Clinical Neurology, Vol 3. Hagerstown, Md., Harper & Row, 1978. *A complete review of the entities that can cause spinal cord damage, e.g., infection, toxins, radiation, as well as idiopathic disorders. Very complete reference list.*

Ropper AH, Poskanzer DC: The prognosis of acute and subacute transverse myelopathy based on early signs and symptoms. Ann Neurol 4:51, 1978. *An excellent review of the experience of a large general hospital with a good description of the clinical findings and follow-up of patients.*

506. CENTRAL NERVOUS SYSTEM COMPLICATIONS OF VIRAL INFECTIONS AND VACCINES

Jerry S. Wolinsky

Central nervous system (CNS) symptoms and signs arising in the course of systemic infections usually reflect direct CNS invasion by the inciting organism. Less frequently, systemic infections, especially viral infections, or the administration of certain vaccines give rise to CNS abnormalities that do not appear to depend on direct invasion of the brain but rather to reflect dysfunction as the result of presumed autoimmune or toxic mechanisms selectively. Several reasonably distinct patterns of involvement have been delineated. Two of these, *acute disseminated encephalomyelitis* and *acute hemorrhagic encephalomyelitis,* appear to be mediated by immune mechanisms and have a peripheral nervous system counterpart, *acute inflammatory polyneuropathy* or the *Guillain-Barré syndrome* (see Ch. 526). The remainder, *Reye's syndrome, acute toxic encephalopathy,* and *acute cerebellar ataxia of childhood,* are likely to be toxic in origin.

ACUTE DISSEMINATED ENCEPHALOMYELITIS (ADE)

DEFINITION. Acute disseminated encephalomyelitis (*parainfectious* or *postinfectious encephalomyelitis, acute demyelinating encephalitis, immune-mediated encephalomyelitis*) is an acute disease of the CNS that most commonly occurs in association with viral infections or as a complication of vaccination. Involvement of brain and spinal cord is usually widespread but may be limited to discrete areas such as the optic nerves, as in optic neuritis or papillitis, or to a single spinal cord level, as in acute transverse myelitis (see Ch. 506).

ETIOLOGY AND PATHOGENESIS. Predisposing factors to ADE include infection by such common agents as measles virus, herpes varicella-zoster virus, influenza virus, rubella virus, mumps virus, nonspecific upper respiratory infections, mycoplasmal pneumonia, and possibly Epstein-Barr virus. ADE also has been well documented to follow immunization for smallpox (classic *postvaccinal encephalomyelitis*), measles, and formerly rabies. Other vaccines are less well implicated in the genesis of ADE.

The neurologic complications usually occur six to ten days after the appearance of the exanthem or onset of other specific symptoms. However, ADE can occur prior to or concomitantly with systemic symptoms of infection. Characteristically, ADE begins ten days to three weeks after initiation of the vaccination regimen. Perhaps the most easily understood form of ADE is that which at one time followed vaccination against rabies with inactivated inoculum of fixed rabies virus propagated in animal brain. These early vaccines were undoubtedly contaminated with CNS proteins, including the antigens associated with myelin. Both complement-fixing antibody and specific lymphocyte blast transformation responses to crude and purified CNS antigens have been measured in blood of rabies vaccinees, and these responses were highest in those whose course of vaccination was complicated by ADE. The incidence of neuroparalytic accidents has been reported to be as high as 1:600 to 1:6000 persons vaccinated with such vaccines. Current rabies vaccines derived from virus grown in human diploid cells appear to be essentially free of neural complications (Ch. 503).

The analogy between ADE related to rabies vaccination and the animal model CNS autoimmune disease, *experimental allergic encephalomyelitis (EAE),* is compelling. In EAE, crude brain homogenates, selected highly purified myelin components, or peptides containing the encephalogenic sequences of myelin basic protein (MBP) can, under proper conditions, induce an acute CNS perivascular inflammatory and demyelinative reaction that is histologically identical to ADE. In affected animals, clinical disease begins 10 to 14 days after sensitization and is associated with both humoral and cellular immune reponses directed against the inciting CNS antigen(s). Furthermore, EAE can be adoptively transferred to naive animals by T lymphocytes. This fact suggests that this cell type is of primary importance in the pathogenesis of the immune-mediated disorder.

The occurrence of ADE following viral infections is more difficult to understand. Encephalitis is relatively frequent following measles (1:1000 cases), but there is little evidence to implicate invasion of the CNS by measles virus as an obligate prerequisite and no compelling data available to support cross-reactivity between the antigens of measles virus and CNS proteins such as MBP. Nonetheless, very early in the course of measles ADE, specific blast transformation responses to MBP are apparent in children when the peripheral blood lymphocytes are tested in vitro and, as would be expected with any type of acute CNS demyelination, measurable quantities of MBP are released into the cerebrospinal fluid (CSF). These findings support the hypothesis that acute measles transiently alters the immune system, which in some persons results in a breakdown of tolerance to CNS antigens. This process appears to occur frequently, as reflected by a high incidence of abnormal appearing electroencephalograms (EEGs). Only occasionally is the process expressed symptomatically. Both EEG abnormalities and clinical ADE can occur after vaccination with live attenuated measles virus but at a markedly lower frequency, with ADE arising in about 1:1,000,000 persons vaccinated for measles.

INCIDENCE. Valid incidence figures for ADE are difficult to derive because clinical diagnosis is often uncertain and pathologic diagnosis the exception. Encephalitis complicates about 1:1000 cases of measles. ADE following induced vaccinia (vaccination for smallpox) is only of historical interest but occurred in the United States with a reported incidence of 2.9 per million primary vaccinations. Higher frequencies of occurrence have been reported in other countries. ADE following other childhood viral illnesses or vaccinations is distinctly uncommon. In adult cases, most examples of ADE have no identifiable antecedents.

PATHOLOGY. Neuropathologic changes consist of perivenular infiltration by lymphocytic and mononuclear cells and variable amounts of primary demyelination extending in centripetal manner from involved vessels of the white matter. The axons are relatively spared. This primary lesion can occur throughout the neuraxis but tends to be most prominent in the centrum semiovale of the cerebrum and in the pontine white matter. Attendant edema may impart a swollen appearance, but otherwise the brain appears grossly normal. The primary perivascular demyelination appears to be a potentially reversible lesion. Repair occurs through remyelination. In certain cases, large confluent lesions take on a superficial resemblance to the plaques of multiple sclerosis, differing primarily in that all lesions reflect a similar age of onset.

CLINICAL MANIFESTATIONS. The clinical disorder can resemble almost any of the acute encephalitides. In adults neurologic symptoms often first suggest the illness. With the childhood exanthemata, CNS symptoms usually begin about five days after the onset of the rash (range 0 to 24 days, with rare examples of ADE preceding the rash). The course of the preceding illness is in no way typical for patients who subsequently develop ADE. Fever or recrudescence of fever is nearly universal. Headache, with or without meningismus, and lethargy occur in from 20 to 80 per cent of cases. In about half of the cases there is one or more generalized seizure. Usually the onset of altered consciousness is abrupt, occurring within a few hours, but CNS symptoms sometimes evolve over several days. Stupor, delirium, or coma develops in severe cases. Multifocal motor and sensory deficits of varied severity are common and often asymmetrical.

The EEG is abnormal in appearance, with widespread slowing of background rhythms. The CSF in children almost invariably shows a modest mononuclear pleocytosis of 20 to 200 cells per cubic millimeter and occasionally higher. Adult CSF is sometimes acellular. The fluid contains a slight elevation of protein content, a normal glucose level, and a raised myelin basic protein level. After several days, computed tomographic scans may show scattered low density lesions in white matter, at least some of which enhance with contrast during the acute phases of the disease.

The duration of active CNS disease varies from days to weeks. The overall mortality is about 20 per cent. About 90 per cent of survivors recover completely or nearly completely, although severe residual deficits can occur. Even among the patients who recover, convalescence can be protracted for many months.

DIAGNOSIS. Diagnosis in ADE is by exclusion. First encephalitis, meningitis, or meningoencephalitis must be excluded as a direct effect of a virus or other infectious agent. In the setting of a recent exanthematous illness or vaccination, ADE is more readily implied. However, in pathologic series of clinically diagnosed ADE occurring in the course of mass vaccination programs, postmortem examination proved the majority of patients to have had other illnesses, including potentially treatable CNS infections. Differentiation of an initial severe episode of multiple sclerosis can be challenging, but subsequent recurrences eventually make the proper diagnosis clear.

TREATMENT. Treatment consists of supportive care, including the use of anticonvulsants and, when necessary, intensive care monitoring. Neither corticosteroids nor other immunosuppressive drugs have any proved benefit.

ACUTE HEMORRHAGIC LEUKOENCEPHALITIS

Acute hemorrhagic leukoencephalitis is a fulminant and fatal syndrome believed to have an immunopathogenesis similar to that of ADE. Typically, the illness arises either spontaneously or following an uneventful upper respiratory illness. Sudden headache precedes the neurologic symptoms, which include seizures and rapid progression from lethargy to coma in a matter of a few hours to several days. Major focal neurologic abnormalities are common and may suggest lateralized cerebral involvement. Systemic signs and symptoms include fever and marked peripheral leukocytosis. The accompanying CSF pleocytosis usually shows a preponderance of polymorphonuclear cells and sometimes evidence of minor degrees of hemorrhage into the subarachnoid space. More than 80 per cent of all recognized cases of acute hemorrhagic leukoencephalitis are fatal, although these findings may be biased by selective reports of postmortem studies. The brain is usually swollen, and examination shows bilateral but asymmetric abnormalities with petechial hemorrhages scattered throughout the white matter. Microscopic lesions consist of small ball and ball-ring hemorrhages with perivascular polymorphonuclear cell infiltrates and fibrin deposition in and about involved vessels, features reminiscent of hyperimmune forms of EAE. The clinical differential diagnosis includes ADE and acute viral encephalitis, especially herpes simplex encephalitis (see Ch. 500). Computed tomography may be diagnostically helpful in selected cases. Therapy is supportive, and although corticosteroids are often used they have no proved benefit.

Fenichel GM: Neurological complications of immunization. Ann Neurol 12:119, 1982. *A critical review of neurologic complications of vaccination including those reported to follow pertussis vaccines.*

Johnson RT, Griffin DE, Hirsch RL, Wolinsky JS, Roedenbeck S, de Soriano IL, Vaisberg A: Measles encephalomyelitis—Clinical and immunological studies. N Engl J Med 310:137, 1984. *A multifaceted study of ADE complicating natural measles which emphasizes possible mechanisms of disease pathogenesis.*

507. REYE'S SYNDROME

Jerry S. Wolinsky

DEFINITION. Reye's syndrome is a well delineated biphasic disease in which one of several common viral illnesses is followed by an acute and sometimes fatal encephalopathy associated with fatty infiltration and dysfunction of the liver.

ETIOLOGY AND PATHOGENESIS. Reye's syndrome most commonly occurs following influenza A, influenza B, and herpes varicella-zoster virus infections. Many other common viral illnesses have been implicated, each at a much lower frequency. Little evidence links the precipitating viral infection directly to either the central nervous system or hepatic involvement. A toxic origin is proposed for both types of involvement. The hepatic dysfunction appears to be the primary error and the direct result of a mitochondrial disturbance that causes secondary metabolic derangements including hyperammonemia, lactic acidemia, and elevated levels of serum-free fatty acids. The latter derangements have been implicated in the pathogenesis of the brain swelling and increased intracranial pressure that dominate the clinical course of severe cases. What causes the mitochondrial impairment and whether aspirin plays a potentiating role in inducing the syndrome remain to be clarified.

INCIDENCE. Reye's syndrome occurs most commonly among suburban white children between 1 and 15 years of age but has been reported in adolescents and rarely in adults. However, inner-city black infants may be especially at risk for the disease. Prospectively derived incidence figures for susceptible age groups are as high as 6.2 per 100,000 children when the syndrome is defined rigorously by highly predictive criteria.

PATHOLOGY. The liver shows a noninflammatory, panlobular, hepatocellular accumulation of lipid droplets and both histochemical and ultrastructural evidence of inflammation. At postmortem examination, swelling of astrocytic foot processes and ultrastructural changes in mitochondria similar to those seen in hepatic mitochondria may be found in the greatly swollen brain.

CLINICAL MANIFESTATIONS AND COURSE. Reye's syndrome is a biphasic disorder. As symptoms of the initial viral illness begin to wane or clear, the dramatic features of Reye's syndrome begin, usually with intractable vomiting associated with lethargy or delirium. Early diagnosis is confirmed by the findings of nonicteric hepatic dysfunction, an elevated arterial blood ammonia level, and serum transaminase levels that exceed three times normal levels. Hepatic enlargement is present in about one half of the cases. Children under one year of age often show hypoglycemia. Signs of central nervous system deterioration include the development of generalized seizures, deepening obtundation, and the emergence of signs of central herniation (see Ch. 472). The cerebrospinal fluid is under increased pressure but is acellular, with otherwise normal constituents.

DIAGNOSIS. Diagnosis rests on the clinical findings and appropriate biochemical abnormalities. Liver biopsy may be useful in atypical cases but usually is not necessary. Central nervous system infection or the presence of known toxins, particularly salicylate, must be actively excluded.

TREATMENT. Falling mortality rates in Reye's syndrome (now approximately 10 per cent) probably reflect both better recognition and reporting of the disease and improved early supportive treatment. Affected patients require intensive care monitoring until the course of the disease is well established. Hypoglycemia and electrolyte abnormalities must be corrected. Many authorities suggest hydration with solutions of high glucose content. Conservative measures to control hyperammonemia appear warranted.

ACUTE TOXIC ENCEPHALOPATHY OF CHILDREN

A syndrome distinguishable from Reye's syndrome only by the absence of hepatic involvement and a high incidence of acute convulsions can follow both banal viral infections and vaccination. A noninflammatory brain swelling accounts for the cerebral symptoms. The findings of cerebrospinal fluid examination are normal except for increased intracranial pressure. This syndrome sometimes arises de novo and sometimes is associated with common respiratory infections. It is the most common of the central nervous system complications of rubella and occurs in about 1:6000 cases. The pathogenesis is unknown. There is no evidence to directly implicate an abnormality of cellular immune mechanisms.

Lichtenstein PK, Heubi JE, Daugherty CC, Farrell MK, Sokol RJ, Rothbaum RJ, Suchy FJ, Balistreri WF: Grade I Reye's syndrome: A frequent cause of vomiting and liver dysfunction after varicella and upper-respiratory-tract infections. N Engl J Med 309:133, 1983. *A prospective study of the incidence and course of Reye's syndrome.*

508. NEUROLOGIC COMPLICATIONS IN THE IMMUNOLOGICALLY COMPROMISED HOST

Jerry S. Wolinsky

Modern treatment of several previously fatal conditions in many instances leads to an immunocompromised state that is associated with opportunistic infections of the central nervous system (CNS). Such treatments include organ transplantation for renal, bone marrow, and cardiac failure; chemotherapy and radiotherapy of carcinoma, leukemia, and lymphomas; and immunosuppressive treatment of autoimmune diseases. The epidemic emergence of the acquired immune deficiency syndrome (AIDS) also has been associated with a marked increase in the number of unusual CNS infections likely to be encountered in routine practice.

CENTRAL NERVOUS SYSTEM INFECTIONS IN TRANSPLANT RECIPIENTS. Renal transplantation is now commonplace, and bone marrow and cardiac transplantations are performed with increasing effectiveness. Hospital-acquired bacterial species predominate in early infections in transplant recipients. Immunosuppression, especially lethal irradiation used in preparation for marrow transplantation from nonidentical donors, almost predictably gives rise to reactivation of herpes viruses: first herpes simplex viruses types 1 and 2 (HSV), then herpes varicella-zoster virus (HVZ), and finally cytomegalovirus (CMV). The systemic manifestations of each can be overwhelming, but symptomatic CNS dissemination has so far been remarkably infrequent. However, encephalitis or meningitis can complicate either HSV or HVZ infections. Also, while electroencephalographic, computed tomographic, and brain scan findings evolve as anticipated in the intact host, the characteristic cerebrospinal fluid (CSF) pleocytosis is often absent, especially in patients with severe leukopenia. CNS involvement by CMV has been pathologically documented in transplant patients but has not been associated with a recognizable clinical syndrome. At present such involvement often appears to be asymptomatic. The availability of effective antiviral chemotherapy now makes it imperative to attempt early diagnosis in cases of suspected HSV or HVZ meningoencephalitis (see Ch. 500 and 501).

Transplant patients are at greatest risk of infection by opportunistic agents after the second month of the transplant. They remain at risk while they are on most immunosuppressive regimens, if they are azotemic, and when there are ongoing graft versus host or chronic rejection reactions. *Listeria monocytogenes, Cryptococcus neoformans,* and *Aspergillus fumigatus* account for the overwhelming majority of infections. *Toxoplasma gondii, Candida* species, *Nocardia asteroides,* the rhinocerebral phycomycoses, and *Coccidioides immitis* are less frequently encountered.

The acute or subacute development of fever in the transplant patient should suggest *Listeria* meningitis even in the absence of meningeal signs. The CSF has the characteristics of a purulent meningitis, although occasionally patients with *Listeria* infection have misleading mononuclear pleocytosis (see Ch. 271). Otherwise unexplained headache of acute to chronic duration, even in the absence of a febrile response or confusion, should suggest the possibility of cryptococcal meningitis. A mononuclear pleocytosis with or without a low glucose content are the characteristic CSF findings (see Ch. 370). India ink preparations can provide immediate confirmation of diagnosis and tests for cryptococcus antigen can be more helpful than direct culture of the organism from the CSF. Since both listerial and cryptococcal meningitis represent some of the most frequently encountered and more manageable infections that affect the immunocompromised host, careful attention must be given to symptoms that suggest infection of the CNS.

Aspergillis fumigatus infections of the CNS usually are manifested as acute fulminant disease with seizures, obtundation, and frequently apoplectic onset of focal neurologic deficits. The propensity of *Aspergillis* to invade and destroy blood vessels underlies the frequent stroke-like appearance of infected patients. Low density lesions with ill-defined, poorly contrast-enhancing borders may be seen on computed tomography, but diagnosis depends on brain biopsy in the absence of systemic disease. Current diagnostic and therapeutic approaches to this CNS infection are inadequate (see Ch. 373).

CENTRAL NERVOUS SYSTEM INFECTION IN PATIENTS WITH LYMPHOMA, LEUKEMIA, OR CHRONIC IMMUNOSUPPRESSIVE THERAPY. Splenectomy, often used in the staging of Hodgkin's disease, places patients at increased risk for conventional bacterial infections that may be complicated by meningitis. In community-acquired infections, *Hemophilus influenzae* and *Streptococcus pneumoniae* species predominate. Metastatic spread from various systemic sites by a wide spectrum of bacterial organisms is a continual threat for all immunosuppressed patients. The usual signs and symptoms of CNS infection can be obscured by the anti-inflammatory effect of therapy. The use of chronic immunosuppressive therapy for leukemia, lymphoma, or presumed autoimmune disorders can be complicated by *Listeria monocytogenesis* in a manner similar to that described for transplant patients. The emergence of listerial meningitis often follows an increase in the intensity of the immunosuppressive regimen.

Cryptococcal meningitis and *Aspergillus* meningoencephalitis are significant sources of morbidity for this group of patients. Their clinical appearances parallel those seen in organ-transplant patients. Segmental zoster, occasionally with dissemination, is a well recognized problem among these patients, and CNS toxoplasmosis is occasionally encountered. Of special interest is *progressive multifocal leukoencephalopthy (PML),* which may account for up to 10 per cent of all CNS infections in this patient group. Progressive deterioration in mental status and the evolution of focal neurologic deficits in the absence of meningismus or CSF abnormalities characterize the clinical symptomatology of PML. Serial computed tomographic scans are usually diagnostic, but the recent observation that some patients with CNS infections by HVZ can have a clinical course similar to that of PML must be considered because HVZ is potentially responsive to antiviral chemotherapy.

ACQUIRED IMMUNE DEFICIENCY SYNDROME (AIDS). Recently, a new syndrome has been described characterized by the presence of severe acquired cell-mediated immune deficiency, opportunistic infections, and in some cases the development of Kaposi's sarcoma or lymphoma in selected, otherwise healthy population groups. Neurologic symptoms occur in about 30 per cent of cases, and an opportunistic CNS infection may be the mode of initial presentation for 10 per cent of all AIDS patients.

CNS toxoplasmosis is particularly prominent, accounting for about one third of all CNS infections in AIDS patients. Single or multiple toxoplasma abscesses give rise to a clinical picture that usually consists of progressive focal deficits associated with abscess location. Less frequently, confusion and lethargy with or without seizures suggest more global CNS dysfunction. Computed tomography usually shows a typical abscess pattern of a low density lesion surrounded by a well defined capsule. The appearance of the capsule usually is enhanced by contrast administration. CSF findings are variable and often normal. Serologic evidence of toxoplasmosis is often present, but specific antibody and antibody isotype titer levels frequently fail to confirm active disease. Brain biopsy, directed by CT localization, is often indicated. The presence of an abscess in an AIDS patient by itself, however, may be an adequate basis for beginning extended therapy with sulfadiazine and pyrimethamine.

A slowly progressive global deterioration of cognitive function is probably the commonest neurologic complication of AIDS. This process sometimes culminates in marked dementia with urinary incontinence in the absence of significant motor signs. The severe form may affect 10 per cent of AIDS patients. Milder degrees of deterioration are even more common. Serial CT scans often disclose increasing cerebral atrophy, and most patients show CSF pleocytosis. Postmortem findings in 50 per cent of patients are consistent with viral infection. Inclusion cells typical of CMV can be identified in some instances, but a definitive cause has not been established.

Pulmonary and systemic infections with *Mycobacterium avium-intracellulare* are frequent among AIDS patients. Instances of CNS meningoencephalitis caused by this agent should be anticipated, but so far cases have been reported infrequently. Otherwise typical PML complicates the course of about 2 per cent of AIDS patients. Cryptococcal meningitis, *Candida albicans* abscesses, coccidioidomycosis meningoencephalitis, and other infections by opportunistic agents that can invade the CNS occur at low frequencies.

As with renal transplant recipients, AIDS patients develop primary CNS lymphomas at rates far exceeding those of the normal population. These usually are immunoblastic lymphomas with variable clinical manifestations. Serial computed tomographic scans may be necessary to define abnormalities related to these diffusely infiltrating tumors. Despite the associated severe cell-mediated immune deficiency, a Guillain-Barré–like syndrome also has been recognized to complicate the courses of several AIDS patients.

Hooper DS, Pruitt AA, Rubin RH: Central nervous system infection in the chronically immunosuppressed. Medicine 61:166, 1982. *Analysis of ten years' experience with opportunistic CNS infections at a major hospital and comprehensive literature review.*

Snider WD, Simpson DM, Nielsen S, Gold JWM, Metroka CE, Posner JB: Neurological complications of acquired immune deficiency syndrome: Analysis of fifty patients. Ann Neurol 14:403, 1983. *Analysis of the experience with neural complications of AIDS at a major referral center.*

Section Ten THE DEMYELINATING DISEASES

509. THE DEMYELINATING DISEASES

Donald H. Silberberg

The demyelinating diseases are disorders that affect myelin to a greater extent than other nervous system components. In this section disorders that primarily affect central nervous system (CNS) myelin are discussed; analogous diseases of the peripheral nervous system, the demyelinating peripheral neuropathies, are discussed in Ch. 524 through 536. A few disorders, such as the neurologic complications of vitamin B_{12} deficiency and some of the leukodystrophies, affect both central and peripheral myelin.

Since central myelin is an extension of the oligodendrocyte, which manufactures the myelin sheath, most demyelinating diseases include alterations in or disappearance of this glial cell. An oligodendrocyte process wraps around a segment of an axon in a concentric fashion to form myelin. One oligodendrocyte sends processes to segments of from several to 20 or 30 axons within an area of several millimeters surrounding the oligodendrocyte. Each segment of axon myelinated by one oligodendrocyte process is 1 mm or less in length. The most active synthesis of myelin starts in utero and continues for the first two years of life; however, synthesis continues as part of brain and spinal cord growth until the adult CNS weight is achieved.

Each tightly compacted layer of mature myelin is a bimolecular lipid leaflet between parallel layers of hydrated protein, which is in close apposition to the polar groups of the lipid molecules. The lipids, which constitute about 75 per cent of the dry weight of myelin, include cerebroside, phospholipids, and cholesterol. Proteins include the distinctive molecule, myelin basic protein (the antigen capable of eliciting experimental allergic encephalomyelitis in experimental animals), proteolipid proteins, and many others detectable by electrophoretic separation but not yet well characterized. Turnover of the components of mature myelin continues at a slower rate than the rate of exchange which characterizes myelin during development. The relative contribution of the oligodendrocyte, the axon, or perhaps even nearby astrocytes to the maintenance of mature myelin is not known. What is clear is that both developing and mature myelin are readily susceptible to injury by many disease mechanisms. Myelin is commonly injured as part of many disease processes which ultimately damage neurons and other cells; the focus of this section is on those disorders which primarily damage or result in the failure of the normal development of myelin.

TABLE 509–1. DISORDERS SELECTIVELY AFFECTING MYELIN

I. Demyelinating diseases (acquired destruction of preformed myelin)
- A. Multiple sclerosis
  - 1. Uniphasic events presumably related to multiple sclerosis
    - a. Optic neuritis
    - b. Acute transverse myelopathy
- B. Parainfectious disorders
  - 1. Acute disseminated encephalomyelitis
  - 2. Acute hemorrhagic leukoencephalopathy
- C. Viral infections
  - 1. Progressive multifocal leukoencephalopathy
  - 2. Subacute sclerosing panencephalitis
- D. Nutritional disorders
  - 1. Combined systems disease (B_{12} deficiency)
  - 2. Demyelination of the corpus callosum (Marchiafava-Bignami)
  - 3. Central pontine myelinolysis
- E. Anoxic-ischemic sequelae
  - 1. Delayed postanoxic cerebral demyelination
  - 2. Progressive subcortical ischemic encephalopathy

II. Dysmyelinating diseases (developmental failure to form or maintain myelin)
- A. The leukodystrophies
  - 1. Metachromatic leukodystrophy
  - 2. Sudanophilic (Pelizaeus-Merzbacher disease)
  - 3. Globoid cell (Krabbe's disease)
  - 4. Adrenoleukodystrophy (Schilder's disease)
  - 5. Others (e.g., Alexander's, Canavan's, Seitelberger's disease)
- B. Aminoacidurias (e.g., phenylketonuria)
- C. Neonatal hypothyroidism

CLASSIFICATION. Definitive classification awaits an understanding of the causes of these disorders. Failing that, a mixed temporal-etiologic-descriptive classification must serve as the scaffold. A useful distinction is to separate what seem to be acquired disorders from those which are errors in development (Table 509–1). Multiple sclerosis will be discussed first, since it is by far the most common of these problems.

MULTIPLE SCLEROSIS

DEFINITION. Multiple sclerosis (MS) is a disorder of unknown etiology which is defined both by its clinical characteristics and by the typical scattered areas of brain, optic nerve, and spinal cord demyelination which the disease produces. Clinical diagnosis requires evidence on neurologic examination of two or more CNS white matter lesions, preferably with at least a month's interval between symptoms, in a patient of the appropriate age, in whom evidence is lacking of any other explanation for the signs and symptoms. MS usually produces its first clinical symptoms between ages 15 and 50 years. Occasional cases occur beyond these extremes, but the average age of onset is 33. Most patients recover clinically to some extent from individual bouts of demyelination, producing the classic remitting and exacerbating course, particularly early in the disease. Except for autopsy findings, presently available laboratory data may support the clinical diagnosis but cannot be used to define MS.

ETIOLOGY. Despite recognition and description of MS for over 150 years, its cause remains unknown. The tissue response has features of an immunopathologic process, with perivenular mononuclear cell infiltration and absence of any overt histopathologic evidence of an infection. Two other lines of evidence point to either an immunologic cause or immunologic participation in the MS process: (1) the frequent elevation of cerebrospinal fluid (CSF) gamma globulin, apparently synthesized by the plasma cells in areas of demyelination, and (2) changes in the proportion of lymphocyte subclasses and reactivity in the peripheral blood and CSF. These changes are, however, nonspecific and may be the consequence of demyelination induced by some other disease mechanism, rather than the cause of the demyelination.

Epidemiologic studies suggest an infectious etiology. Perhaps the best evidence for this is the outbreak of MS which occurred in the Faroe Islands during the 20 years following the start of World War II. The Faroes were occupied by British troops during the war. No cases of MS had occurred prior to the occupation. The sudden appearance of MS starting several years after the arrival of the troops strongly suggests the presence of an infectious agent. In those geographic areas where MS is prevalent, it is more common farther from the equator, which suggests the presence of an environmental factor, presumably an infectious agent. Efforts continue to recover a virus from MS tissues: to date, no reported isolation has been duplicated by others. MS is among the diseases with a strong linkage to certain HLA haplotypes. The particular haplotype varies from one population group to another. In North America, haplotype DW-2, a D locus marker, is found in about 65 per cent of MS patients, as compared with 15 per cent of control subjects. Additional evidence for an immunogenetic component in the etiology of MS is the increase in frequency of MS among close relatives of patients with MS and the fact that MS is rare among Orientals, even after emigration to the United States. A possible synthesis is that MS is an unusual consequence of infection by a common virus, or any of several viruses, with subsequent immunologic alterations in genetically susceptible individuals.

INCIDENCE AND PREVALENCE. The prevalence of MS in the northern United States and Canada and in northern Europe is about 60 per 100,000 population (Table 509–2). In Denmark the chance of an individual developing MS in a lifetime is 1 in 500. The risk is somewhat higher for women. MS is almost unknown among Orientals and among African blacks. There is no evidence for changing incidence or prevalence, except where population patterns are undergoing changes as the result of immigration.

EPIDEMIOLOGY. The epidemiology of MS has fascinated observers since the 1930's, when neurologists in northern Europe reported to their Mediterranean colleagues that MS was more common in northern cities (Table 509–2). This gradient by latitude has also been shown in the United States. In Australia and New Zealand MS is more common in the southern latitudes. Migration from high incidence areas, such as England and northern Europe, to low incidence areas, such as South Africa or Israel, permitted the observation that the immigrant who moves during childhood acquires the lower incidence of the new country. For those moving after puberty, the chance of developing MS remains what it would have been in the country of origin and follows presumptive exposure to an environmental agent by about 15 years.

The regional population figures are punctuated by many reports of clusters of an unusual number of cases in a small area, such as particular cantons in Switzerland. Many of the population studies were done before the availability of HLA typings, so that some of the observed regional differences may prove to have a genetic basis. Multiple sclerosis occurs in both members of about 50 per cent of monozygous twin pairs when the disease has been identified in one. This supports the concept that genetic susceptibility may increase the chances of developing MS, but is not sufficient to cause it and may not be required for its development.

TABLE 509–2. THE PREVALENCE OF MULTIPLE SCLEROSIS*

Area	Latitude	Prevalence per 100,000
Iceland	65° N	72
Shetland Islands	61° N	129
Oslo, Norway	60° N	80
Göteborg, Sweden	58° N	120
Carlisle, England	55° N	82
Hamburg, Germany	54° N	73
Winnipeg, Manitoba	50° N	40
Bas-Rhin, France	49° N	41
Rochester, Minnesota	44° N	64
Marseilles, France	49° N	21
Sappuro, Japan	43° N	2
Boston, Massachusetts	42° N	41
Denver, Colorado	40° N	38
San Francisco, California	38° N	30
Seoul, Korea	38° N	2
Israel	31° N	15
New Orleans, Louisiana	30° N	6
Bombay, India	18° N	2
Cairns, Australia	17° S	7
South Australia	30° S	38

*Modified from Alter M, Loewenson R, Harshe M: J Chron Dis 26:755, 1973.

PATHOLOGY. The lesions of MS consist of scattered areas of dissolution of CNS myelin, within which the axons remain intact. The border between histologically normal myelin and myelin dissolution is often sharp, or may shade from normal to thinning of myelin before bare axons occur. Some areas may show only partial myelin destruction. Lesions range in size from 1 mm to several centimeters in diameter, and occur throughout the brain, optic nerves (which are central tracts of white matter), and spinal cord. Although plaques may occur anywhere within CNS myelin, there are predilections for involvement of the optic nerves, periventricular regions within the cerebrum, and cervical spinal cord. Most if not all plaques occur near blood vessels.

Oligodendrocytes disappear from within plaques. Astrocytes proliferate and fill much of the volume vacated by myelin and oligodendroglia, forming the scar that lent the term "sclerosis" to multiple sclerosis. This produces an area that is firm to palpation on cut sections, and plaques can be seen as grayish depressed areas in fresh autopsy sections. One always finds many more plaques at autopsy than could have been suspected on the basis of the clinical history and examination. Similarly, the sensitivity and resolution provided by nuclear magnetic resonance (NMR) imaging often reveal clinically unsuspected plaques. Occasionally, typical plaques of MS are found in individuals who gave no history of neurologic abnormalities (benign MS). The acute lesion of MS may produce considerable edema, visible as cord swelling on myelography or optic nerve enlargement on computed tomography (CT scan). Electron microscope examination of plaques shows evidence of attempts at remyelination. However, this is not nearly so complete as to explain the remissions of neurologic dysfunction that characterize MS and remain unexplained.

Perivascular and mononuclear cells collect within and around plaques. Macrophages which engulf myelin breakdown products are present. Plasma cells appear to synthesize much of the excess of gamma globulin which is found in and around plaques and in CSF. Plasma cells occur throughout affected tissue, and persist in large numbers throughout a patient's lifetime, correlating with the observation that once CSF gamma globulin elevation appears, it persists. It is not known whether plasma cells and other mononuclear cells precede, accompany, or follow myelin and oligodendrocyte destruction.

LABORATORY ABNORMALITIES. *Cerebrospinal Fluid.* CSF gamma globulin elevation occurs in about 75 per cent of MS patients, more commonly after the first year following the appearance of symptoms. Normal CSF gamma globulin is less than 13 per cent of total CSF protein by most testing methods. The gamma globulin is mostly IgG, but often contains IgA and IgM as well. Separate discrete "oligoclonal" bands are seen in the gamma region on agarose or polyacrylamide gel electrophoresis in about 90 per cent of patients, including some with normal total IgG levels. These abnormalities are helpful when other causes of the phenomenon are excluded; these include CNS syphilis, subacute sclerosing panencephalitis, chronic meningitis, and any disease associated with a peripheral blood paraproteinemia. Other CSF abnormalities in MS can include elevation in total protein, usually to no more than 100 mg per deciliter, and an increase in the number of mononuclear white cells, usually to 5 to 15 per cubic millimeter, rarely to more than 50 per cubic millimeter. Myelin destruction releases myelin basic protein (MBP) into the CSF, which can be detected by radioimmunoassay. The amount present correlates with disease activity and lesion size and location; none is detectable normally, or during quiescent periods in MS patients. MBP levels rise in association with acute attacks or rapid progression. This serves as a valuable index of disease activity, but is not specific to MS. Myelin destruction from any other cause, such as acute infarction, causes a similar elevation of MBP.

Alterations in the ratio of subclasses of peripheral blood and of CSF lymphocytes occur at the time of acute exacerbations. These changes, which may indicate abnormalities of immunoregulation, are of interest to those investigating the pathogenesis of MS; at present they do not contribute to differential diagnosis.

Neurophysiologic Function Studies. The presence of myelin enhances the propagation of the nerve impulse along the axon. Loss of myelin, from any cause, slows conduction velocity. This alteration in conduction velocity can be measured by timing the appearance of an evoked potential (visual, auditory, or somatosensory) after an appropriate stimulus. Measurement of the latency of the visual evoked response (VER) is used most widely. The patient's visual system is stimulated by viewing a changing checkerboard pattern or flash stimulus with one eye at a time, and the evoked response is recorded with electroencephalogram scalp leads over the occipital cortex. The normal latency from stimulus to evoked response in most laboratories is less than 102 to 105 milliseconds. A prolonged latency indicates an abnormality in the visual system, most commonly within the optic nerve in patients with MS. An abnormality of the visual, auditory, or somatosensory evoked response is used to detect dysfunction (prolonged conduction velocity) either as an objective measurement of what has already been detected clinically or for detection of a presumed subclinical abnormality. The abnormalities detected are not specific for MS (see Role of Laboratory Aids, below).

CT and NMR Scans. Hypodense areas seen with the CT scan reflect the presence of lesion in various stages, ranging from inflammation with edema to various degrees of demyelination. Edema, which may resemble a mass lesion, often occurs acutely. During this stage, leakage of intravenously injected contrast material into the lesion area reflects abnormal leakage of the blood-brain barrier. Atrophy is seen in those instances of severe demyelination.

NMR imaging provides an even more sensitive method for detecting hypodense areas of demyelination and is becoming an important supportive aid in diagnosis.

CLINICAL MANIFESTATIONS. ***Onset.*** The random distribution of MS lesions leads to a great variety of initial symptoms and signs, alone or in combination. Further, it must be kept in mind that lesions occur in clinically silent areas of CNS white matter so that the first lesion that announces itself clinically may not be the first that has occurred in an individual. Common initial problems include weakness of one or more extremities, unilateral visual loss (optic neuritis), incoordination, and paresthesias (Table 509–3). Urinary frequency, incontinence, hesitancy, or retention; vertigo; hearing loss; facial, extremity, or truncal pain; dysarthria; and changes in intellectual function occur less commonly. Weakness most often affects the lower extremities and may produce a range of dysfunction from slight fatigability to paraparesis. The arm and hand may be involved alone or with the legs. Patients who develop paraparesis often develop urinary urgency and constipation. Incoordination as the result of cerebellar lesions, or loss of position sense, may occur independently of weakness and often leads to gait impairment or to tremor-like, clumsy movements of the arms and hands. Paresthesias range from the spontaneous perception of vague pins-and-needles discomfort, or girdle-like pressures, to the pain of classic trigeminal neuralgia. Loss of perception of vibration and position at the ankle and toes is common; loss of pain and touch perception is less frequent. Impairment of two-point discrimination over the palmar surface of the fingertips often accompanies cervical cord lesions.

TABLE 509–3. FIRST SYMPTOMS OF MULTIPLE SCLEROSIS IN 937 PATIENTS*

Symptom	Per Cent†
Weakness	48
Paresthesias	31
Visual loss	25
Incoordination	15
Vertigo	6
Sphincter impairment	6

*Combined series of Carter et al., 1950; Poser, 1972; and McAlpine et al., 1972.
†Many patients experience more than one symptom at onset.

Visual loss varies in degree from slight blurring with a small central scotoma, slight decrease in acuity, and a slight impairment of color perception, to no light perception. The patient often reports pain on eye movement acutely. Other visual symptoms include blurring secondary to nystagmus on primary gaze with continuing movement of the visual axis, or explicit perception of nystagmus as spontaneous movement of objects (oscillopsia). Diplopia often occurs as the result of involvement of the pontine white matter. Horizontal nystagmus of the abducting eye on lateral gaze with paresis of the adducting eye, termed *internuclear ophthalmoplegia,* is common. It is often unilateral at first, and is due to lesions involving the median longitudinal fasciculus in the pons. In rare instances, extensive midline lesions lead to alterations of consciousness.

The speed of onset of symptoms varies from minutes to days, and in patients with a chronic progressive course symptoms may appear to increase gradually over many months. The rate of recovery (remission) varies enormously, but usually occurs over the course of two to eight weeks following an acute bout.

Clinical Course. At least 70 per cent of patients experience some improvement in the days to months following their initial bout. Such recovery ranges from slight to virtual disappearance of the dysfunction which heralded the existence of a problem. Whether or not a particular patient will improve, and to what extent, is as unpredictable as whether or not more lesions will occur and when. Overall, 70 per cent or more will report typical exacerbations and remissions early in their course. However, in many patients as time goes by, the recovery from individual bouts decreases, disability results from accumulated failures to improve, and the course becomes chronically progressive.

About 30 per cent of patients develop successive disabilities without remission, often with long periods of clinical stability between periods of deterioration. This course occurs more commonly in patients experiencing their first neurologic manifestations after age 45. As a result, older onset patients seem to compress the course of events, and often develop the same degree of dysfunction within a few years that takes decades to occur in a younger onset patient.

Most patients experience additional difficulties at some time after their initial symptoms; subsequent acute bouts or chronic progression may produce signs and symptoms in any combination. Several generalizations are of interest, but help little when counseling the individual patient. Ten years after onset about 50 per cent of patients are still able to carry out their household and/or employment responsibilities. Twenty years after onset about 25 per cent have these capacities. However, a fortunate few patients never develop significant disabilities, whereas others are bedridden within months after onset. One of the major psychologic burdens which patients with MS must bear is the total uncertainty about their future, and most neurologists find it useful to emphasize the hopeful possibilities, allowing the patient's course to reveal its own manner of progression.

The average interval from clinical onset to death is 35 years. If premature death occurs, it is usually due to bacterial infection resulting from urinary retention, decubiti, or inability to handle pulmonary secretions. More rarely, primary respiratory failure from lower medullary lesions spells the terminal event.

FACTORS POSSIBLY AFFECTING THE CLINICAL COURSE. Elevation of body temperature by as little as 0.5° C will noticeably reduce neurologic function in some patients, particularly if the patient has experienced recent disease activity. Reduction in visual acuity, incoordination or weakness, and sensory or bladder dysfunction can be affected. This is the result of slowed axonal conduction induced by heating, and the alterations disappear within hours of regaining normal body temperature. For this reason, many patients' conditions worsen with the fevers of an intercurrent illness (a pseudobout). In addition, some patients seem to experience true exacerbations concomitantly with an intercurrent infection. Patients should be instructed to rest and respond to respiratory infections with more care than they might otherwise and to use aspirin to reduce fever.

There is no evidence that pregnancy makes exacerbations or progression of MS more likely. Decisions regarding childbearing should be made on the basis of the patient's overall situation, rather than on the basis of this concern alone.

DIAGNOSIS. Multiple sclerosis remains as a clinical challenge; despite the availability of increasingly complex laboratory aids, the diagnosis of clinically definite MS rests on evidence garnered from the history and physical examination alone. Physical signs on examination providing solid evidence for two or more lesions of central white matter occurring at least a month apart in a patient between age 10 and the early 50's, in the absence of any other possible etiology, are required. If the evidence for a second lesion is history alone, the diagnosis should be considered possible or probable, rather than clinically definite MS. The differential diagnosis includes cervical cord compression resulting from tumor or cervical spondylosis; cerebral, cerebellar, brainstem, and pituitary tumors; familial spinocerebellar degenerations; acute systemic lupus erythematosus (SLE); sarcoidosis; brainstem atherosclerotic cerebrovascular disease; vitamin B_{12} deficiency; chronic barbiturate or other intoxications; and psychogenic disturbances.

If all of the patient's signs can be attributed to a lesion in a single area of the nervous system, the working assumption must be that one is not dealing with MS. In patients with a persistent headache, seizures, persistent and progressive unifocal signs, or papilledema (without a central scotoma), the CT brain scan is the most sensitive screening procedure. In addition, the CT or NMR scan may show hypodense areas or mild generalized atrophy, consistent with MS. High resolution CT scan examination of the spinal canal may obviate the need for myelography to exclude cervical mass lesions.

Spinocerebellar degenerative diseases differ from MS by having associated abnormalities (such as the areflexia commonly seen with Friedreich's ataxia), by progressing slowly within a given neuroanatomic system, such as the cerebellum and its connections, and by having an abnormal family history. However, MS occurs more commonly in first degree relatives of patients with MS, so that family history alone is not sufficient to make the distinction. Neurologic presentation of SLE in young women can be distinguished by appropriate immunologic testing. The neurologic manifestations of B_{12} deficiency may precede the peripheral red blood cell abnormalities by several years; the deficiency is detected by the serum B_{12} level or Schilling test. The correct diagnosis of brainstem arterial disease in patients in their 50's can sometimes be difficult; absence of the CSF abnormalities associated with MS helps, as does the fact that all the abnormalities can be localized to a small anatomic area. The clinician's suspicion of chronic drug intoxication, often accompanied by nystagmus and ataxia, may be substantiated by appropriate blood levels, or other evidence of disturbed behavior.

The total absence of objective neurologic signs at any time, together with symptom patterns or apparent weakness or sensory loss that does not conform to known neuroanatomic systems, raises the suspicion of psychogenic illness. However, one must be wary, for many patients with urinary retention, urgency, or incontinence; ataxia; or vague sensory symptoms occurring in the early stages of MS have been misdiagnosed as psychoneurotic. Evoked response or CSF abnormalities will help exclude purely psychogenic disturbances, but must not be overinterpreted.

Role of Laboratory Aids. The rational use of laboratory abnormalities requires an awareness of their limitations. Elevation of the total CSF gamma globulin, or the appearance of an oligoclonal pattern within the gamma region on electrophoresis, is not specific for MS, although the non-MS causes can usually be readily excluded. However, these abnormalities fail to appear in 10 to 20 per cent of patients with clinically definite multiple sclerosis. Further, many patients who experience a single episode of neurologic abnormality, such as optic neuritis or transverse myelopathy, may exhibit CSF gamma globulin abnormalities, but do not develop a second clinically visible lesion after long follow-up. Thus it is not appropriate to make the diagnosis of MS with a first neurologic attack, even when one encounters CSF gamma globulin abnormalities.

Similarly, although evoked potential abnormalities serve to suggest the possibility of a lesion in that part of the CNS tested, the nonspecific nature of the electrophysiologic alterations makes it unwise to base a diagnosis on such data. A patient with paraparesis and prolonged latency of the VER may have MS, but could possibly have two tumors, pernicious anemia, systemic vasculitis, or a spinal cord tumor plus an uncorrected refractive error. Also, multiple lesions detected on CT or NMR scan may reflect another disease process. Despite these cautions, the discovery of CSF abnormalities commonly associated with MS, evoked potential evidence of a second lesion, or multiple lesions on CT or NMR scan helps greatly to focus on MS as a possible or probable diagnosis.

TREATMENT. Management of the patient with MS requires a combination of an understanding of the personal problems posed by an unpredictable disorder of unknown etiology, an awareness of the measures available to alleviate spasticity, urinary incontinence, and other dysfunctions, and a skeptical approach to "definitive" treatments which are proposed to alter the course of the illness. The fact that over 70 per cent of patients experience spontaneous improvement following an acute bout makes evaluation of proposed treatment difficult, time consuming, and expensive. Nevertheless, carefully conducted controlled trials are the only means for deciding whether or not an agent helps patients with MS. Testimonial-style reports should not be accepted as evidence until a controlled study has confirmed the findings. At present, no method for prevention of MS is known.

Dealing with patients affected by a chronic, sometimes disabling disease for which there is no specific treatment is frustrating to many physicians. Patients with MS often report that they must help alleviate their physician's depression by denying problems. Most patients respond well to an explanation of the disease, a discussion of those things which can be done, and assurance that vigorous research is underway to develop better treatment.

Acute bouts of neurologic dysfunction may be treated with short-term administration of corticosteroids. There is evidence that administration of ACTH for 10 to 14 days somewhat shortens exacerbation, although the ACTH (or other corticosteroid) does not alter the long-term course of MS. From 40 to 80 units of ACTH per day may be used; prednisone, 40 to 60 mg per day, or equivalent doses of other oral corticosteroids are often employed as alternatives. The period of treatment should not exceed three or four weeks, with appropriate precautions to avoid steroid complications. It must be emphasized that there is no evidence that corticosteroids (or any other agent) modify the MS pathogenic process. Beneficial effects are most probably due to antiedema and anti-inflammatory effects. Many responsible clinicians choose not to treat patients in this manner, believing that minimal evidence favors steroid use.

Therapeutic trials to evaluate various immunosuppressants, immunoenhancing agents, plasmapheresis, and other treatments are underway; none can be recommended at present.

Physical therapy plays an important role in several aspects of patient management, including developing alternative muscle strengths, preventing contractures, improving daily living, and providing supportive psychotherapy. A cool bath or swimming pool improves neurologic function transiently by lowering body temperature and improving axonal conduction. Occupational therapy is often a key to the patient's adjustment to MS.

Spasticity and flexor spasms can be alleviated with baclofen, or with diazepam, which inhibits central synaptic transmission. Individual responses vary sufficiently that one must start with very low doses and increase slowly if needed. Many patients depend on spasticity for support while walking, so that removal of this aid or induction of weakness or drowsiness as temporary side effects limits treatment. Occasionally, leg contractures occur despite physical therapy, and require orthopedic surgical relief for ease of handling the patient.

Bladder dysfunction is usually the result of incomplete emptying, accumulation of residual urine, and overflow frequency or incontinence and infection. Rational treatment requires careful urologic evaluation, often including urodynamic studies, in order to plan appropriate pharmacologic therapy. Uninhibited bladder contraction leading to urinary frequency or incontinence may be alleviated by controlling infection and restricting fluid intake prior to trips or several hours before sleep. Imipramine, oxybutynin chloride, or propantheline may help patients who cannot initiate urination, or cannot fully empty their bladder. Attempts to void at fixed intervals and the Credé maneuver often help. If catheterization becomes necessary, many women can learn self-catheterization in order to avoid the complications of an indwelling catheter. Long-term urinary bacterial suppressant therapy is helpful in minimizing infection in patients carrying residual urine. The possibility of an ascending urinary tract infection must be sought and treated appropriately in any patient with recurrent cystitis.

Constipation usually responds to stool softeners and laxatives. Many patients must be reassured that no harm arises from the lack of a daily bowel movement.

Painful paresthesias and dysesthesias may occur, and fortunately are usually transient. Carbamazepine, diazepam, or phenytoin will usually provide relief. Prevention of decubiti in the paraplegic or desensitized patient requires constant vigilance.

Specific psychiatric support is often needed to aid patients and their families. The incidence of marital breakup, changes in roles within the family, and financial problems is exceeded only by the frequency of frustration over the unpredictability of MS. The physician often must call on a range of associates, including social workers, community agency workers, and psychiatrists, in order to help these patients cope.

Brown FR, Beebe GW, Kurtzke JF, Loewenson RB, Silberberg DH, Tourtellotte WW: The design of clinical studies to assess therapeutic efficacy in multiple sclerosis. Neurology 29:1, 1979. *A thorough review of the many factors which must be taken into consideration in designing a study to determine whether or not a proposed treatment benefits patients with multiple sclerosis.*

Carter S, Sciarra D, Merritt HH: The course of multiple sclerosis as determined by autopsy proven cases. Res Publ Assoc Nerv Ment Dis 28:471, 1950. *A description of the clinical features of a well-characterized group of patients who came to autopsy.*

Cohen SR, Herndon RM, McKhann GM: Radioimmunoassay of myelin basic protein in spinal fluid: An index of active demyelination. N Engl J Med 295:1455, 1976. *This paper presents the first large series of patients in whom measurement of myelin basic protein in CSF was correlated with disease activity.*

Compston DA, Batchelor JR, Earl CJ, McDonald WI: Factors influencing the risk of multiple sclerosis developing in patients with optic neuritis. Brain 101:495, 1978. *An excellent study of the correlation between HLA type in patients with optic neuritis and subsequent development of multiple sclerosis.*

Hallpike JF, Adams CWM, Tourtellotte WW (eds.): Multiple Sclerosis. Pathology, Diagnosis, and Management. Baltimore, Williams & Wilkins, 1983. *A good compilation of current information and concepts.*

Kurtzke JF, Hyllested K: Multiple sclerosis in the Faroe Islands: 1. Clinical and epidemiological features. Ann Neurol 5:6, 1979. *A lucid description of the remarkable, seemingly limited epidemic of multiple sclerosis in the Faroe Islands.*

McAlpine D, Lumsden CE, Acheson ED: Multiple Sclerosis. A Reappraisal. 2nd ed. Edinburgh, Churchill Livingstone, 1972. *The major currently available monograph on multiple sclerosis. Excellent clinical and epidemiologic descriptions.*

McDonald WI, Halliday AM: Diagnosis and classification of multiple sclerosis. Br Med Bull 33:4, 1977. *An up-to-date discussion of the problems of correct diagnosis and classification of multiple sclerosis.*

Poser C, Presthus J, Horstal O: Clinical characteristics of autopsy-proved multiple sclerosis. Neurology 16:791, 1966. *A valuable analysis of the presentation and signs and symptoms which developed among a large series of patients in whom MS was proved by autopsy.*

Poser S, Raun E, Wikstrom J, Poser W: Pregnancy, oral contraceptives, and multiple sclerosis. Acta Neurol Scand 59:108, 1979. *The largest study of the possible effect of pregnancy or oral contraceptives on the course of MS; this study shows no relationship.*

Reinherz EL, Weiner HL, Hauser SL, Cohen JA, Distaso JA, Schlossman SF: Loss of suppressor T cells in active multiple sclerosis. N Engl J Med 303:125, 1980. *The first report of the use of monoclonal antibody typing of human lymphocytes in multiple sclerosis. The references include previous analyses of lymphocyte abnormalities in MS.*

Williams A, Eldridge R, McFarland H, Houff S, Krebs H, McFarlin D: Multiple sclerosis in twins. Neurology 30:1139, 1980.

MULTIPLE SCLEROSIS VARIANTS

Neuromyelitis Optica (Devic's Disease)

Neuromyelitis optica describes a syndrome characterized by the occurrence of partial or complete transverse myelopathy and optic neuritis. Loss of vision and paraplegia may occur in either disorder, and days or weeks may elapse between the onsets of the two symptom complexes. It is best considered a syndrome, in that it may occur as the result of multiple sclerosis, acute disseminated encephalomyelitis, systemic lupus erythematosus, or sarcoidosis. When this symptom complex occurs in the course of multiple sclerosis, its clinical and pathologic features are indistinguishable from those of MS.

Diffuse Sclerosis, Transitional Sclerosis

These terms describe a group of progressive neurologic disorders occurring primarily in young patients who manifest severe neurologic deficits of various types with progressive visual and mental deterioration. These are pathologists' terms, which were first used in the late nineteenth century. Schilder described three cases of what came to be known as Schilder's cerebral sclerosis, or Schilder's disease. It is likely that three separate conditions have been included as Schilder's disease, and that this eponymic designation should be discarded. Some cases represent the result of severe confluent extensions of large lesions of multiple sclerosis. Some represent white matter disease of known viral origin, such as subacute sclerosing panencephalitis and progressive multifocal leukoencephalitis (see Ch. 504). A third group includes the leukodystrophies (see later discussion). It is probable that adrenoleukodystrophy was the disorder identified by Schilder in one of his early cases.

Possibly Related Monophasic Disorders

ACUTE DISSEMINATED ENCEPHALOMYELITIS. This disorder is characterized by varying degrees of perivenous mononuclear cellular infiltration and demyelination. It appears most commonly after viral infections that do not normally affect the nervous system, or as a complication of immunization. Since an episode of acute disseminated encephalomyelitis (ADEM) closely resembles an acute attack of multiple sclerosis, it may be impossible to make the distinction until sufficient time has elapsed to determine whether or not a second bout occurs. By definition, ADEM describes those patients in whom further attacks do not occur. The distinction between ADEM and MS is blurred by the not infrequent occurrence of typical exacerbations in the course of MS, concomitant with intercurrent viral infection.

OPTIC NEURITIS. Optic neuritis denotes partial or complete loss of vision in one or both eyes, attributable to one or more optic nerve lesions of unknown etiology. If a cause is known, it is more precise to describe, for example, syphilitic optic neuropathy, or optic neuritis or neuropathy secondary to multiple sclerosis. Retrobulbar neuritis describes a lesion in the posterior two thirds of the optic nerve. The term "papillitis" indicates a lesion in the anterior portion of the optic nerve, leading to an ophthalmoscopic appearance indistinguishable from that of acute papilledema, but differing from the papilledema of increased intracranial pressure by being associated with reduction of visual acuity early in its course. The visual loss usually, but not always, includes macular vision with appearance of a central scotoma and a reduction in color perception. Pain on eye movement is frequent during the first few days of the event. Unless the patient has papillitis, ophthalmoscopic examination is normal for the first two to three weeks, after which disc pallor with loss of small vessels on the disc or more severe atrophy may develop.

Visual loss occurs over the course of hours to several days, and almost always recovers to some degree within several weeks. Blindness as the result of the optic nerve demyelination of MS rarely occurs. Optic neuritis can occur as the presenting sign of MS (see Table 509–3) or at any time during the course of the disease. Practically all MS patients exhibit optic nerve demyelination at autopsy, which underlies the usefulness of the visual evoked response. Approximately one third of patients who develop idiopathic optic neuritis will go on to develop the clinical manifestations of MS. The presence of the CSF abnormalities associated with MS makes this course somewhat more likely, but does not have firm predictive value; certainly MS may develop in the absence of CSF gamma globulin abnormalities.

The illnesses which can mimic idiopathic optic neuritis include optic nerve compression on any basis, neurosyphilis, ischemic optic neuropathy (in older patients), pernicious anemia, Leber's optic atrophy (which is hereditary), tobacco-alcohol amblyopia, and chronic papilledema with optic atrophy and visual loss, associated with prolonged increased intracranial pressure.

ACUTE TRANSVERSE MYELOPATHY. Like optic neuritis, acute transverse myelopathy may occur in isolation, or as the first sign of MS, or at any time in the course of MS. It describes partial to complete paralysis of the legs or of all four extremities, usually accompanied by sensory loss and bowel and bladder dysfunction. As described in Ch. 505, acute transverse myelopathy may be the result of any of a number of disease processes. The same cautions regarding the use of laboratory aids in attempting to predict the later development of MS apply to acute transverse myelopathy as to optic neuritis.

LEUKODYSTROPHIES

These disorders are diseases of dysmyelination, rather than demyelination, in that the normal formation of myelin is interfered with by a genetically determined biochemical defect. The classification of leukodystrophies is based on their histopathology. A biochemical defect is known for several of these disorders, but they all remain relatively rare, incurable disorders, affecting individuals from the first months of life to the 20's.

Metachromatic Leukodystrophy

This, the most common of the leukodystrophies, describes diffuse dysmyelination, usually starting in the first ten years of life. It produces personality changes leading to dementia, convulsions, cranial nerve abnormalities, and finally severe spasticity or rigidity. Death usually occurs in from two to four years, although longer survival is reported. Juvenile and adult onset cases have been reported.

The appearance of metachromatic material (staining red with toluidine blue) in the urinary sediment and in peripheral nerves usually allows diagnosis during life. The metachromatic material also collects in the liver, gallbladder, kidneys, and spleen. The CSF protein is usually elevated above 100 mg per deciliter.

Metachromatic leukodystrophy is usually inherited as an autosomal recessive trait. The pathogenesis of the widespread loss of normal myelin is accumulation of sulfatides in glial cells, in Schwann cells, within myelin lamellae, and in the cytoplasm of some nerve cells. The underlying biochemical defect is abnormally low activity of arylsulfatase A, an enzyme in the system which normally reduces the concentration of cerebroside sulfate.

Sudanophilic Leukodystrophy

This subset includes a heterogeneous group of diseases which have in common only the fact that extensive CSF myelin destruction occurs, associated with products of myelin breakdown, cholesterol esters which stain bright red with the usual fat stains. This staining quality distinguishes these diseases from the metachromatic leukodystrophies and led to the term "sudanophilic." These pathologic characteristics are found in aminoacidurias, adrenoleukodystrophy, and Pelizaeus-Merzbacher disease.

ADRENOLEUKODYSTROPHY. This disorder describes the combination of diffuse dysmyelination and myelin breakdown associated with idiopathic adrenocortical insufficiency. It occurs exclusively in males, inherited as a sex-linked recessive trait. The onset of the disorder occurs most often in childhood, but has been reported in adults, and it produces a similar progression of symptoms as described for metachromatic leukodystrophy. One of the original patients described by Schilder most probably had adrenoleukodystrophy. CSF protein is elevated in most patients. Endocrine testing reveals primary adrenal failure. Instances of adrenal failure alone have been reported in relatives of patients with adrenoleukodystrophy.

Pathologic examination reveals widespread changes in CNS myelin, and also peripheral nerve demyelination, with numerous lipid lamellar inclusions throughout the tissue. The underlying biochemical defect is not known.

PELIZAEUS-MERZBACHER DISEASE. This rare leukodystrophy affects males primarily, is inherited as a sex-linked recessive trait, and starts in early infancy. It progresses slowly, producing extensive, diffuse, symmetrical disturbances of myelin staining associated with gliosis within the cerebrum and cerebellum. The peripheral nervous system is not affected. The underlying biochemical defect is unknown. No treatment is available.

Globoid Cell Leukodystrophy (Krabbe's Disease)

This affects infants in the first two to three months of life, initially producing irritability and unexplained episodes of crying, sensitivity to light and noise, and failure to achieve developmental milestones. During the second year these children become opisthotonic, developing myoclonic jerks and atypical seizures, and optic atrophy begins. Rarer instances occur in late infancy, between two and six years of age, or in adulthood.

Neuropathologic examination reveals marked loss of myelin throughout the brain with the presence of globoid cells. These occur either as round or oval mononuclear cells the size of large glia or as larger irregular multinucleated cells. Their cytoplasm stains positively with PAS. These globoid cells contain the material which accumulates in abnormal quantities, galactocerebroside (galactosyl ceramide). The major enzymatic defect is deficiency of galactocerebroside-galactosidase. It is believed to be transmitted as an autosomal recessive trait. No treatment is known.

Spongy Degeneration of White Matter

Many disorders can produce the pathologic changes leading to this label, including aminoacidurias and other metabolic disturbances. Those instances in which no underlying metabolic defect is apparent are often called Canavan's disease. It produces the onset of weakness in early infancy, leading to spastic paraplegia, severe mental retardation, optic atrophy, and enlargement of the head. Death usually occurs by 18 months. The brain is usually larger than expected for that age. Central nervous system myelin does not stain, and there is a honeycomb-like appearance (status spongiosus) of the deeper layers of the cerebral cortex and white matter near the cortex. The majority of infantile cases occur among those descending from eastern European Jewish families. It is inherited as an autosomal recessive trait. Rarer juvenile cases are more likely to be sporadic and less likely to be from Jewish families. Spongiform degeneration is also produced by exposure to large amounts of hexachlorophine in infancy and by Creutzfeldt-Jakob disease (see Ch. 504), and can be produced experimentally in animals by intracerebral injection of ouabain, a selective blocker of ATPase.

Austin J: Metachromatic form of diffuse cerebral sclerosis: II. Diagnosis during life by isolation of metachromatic lipids from urine. Neurology 7:716, 1957. *Description, clearly written, of methods for identifying metachromatic urinary sediment in children with this disorder.*

Schaumberg H, Powers J, Raine C, Suzuki K, Richardson E: Adrenoleukodystrophy. Arch Neurol 2:577, 1975. *A thorough review of the clinical and neuropathologic features which characterize this entity, including a discussion of its relationship to "Schilder's disease."*

Seitelberger F: Pelizaeus-Merzbacher's disease. *In* Vinken P, Bruyn G (eds.): Handbook of Clinical Neurology, Vol 10. Amsterdam, North-Holland, 1970, p 150. *An excellent review of this and related degenerative diseases of myelin.*

Suzuki K, Suzuki Y: Globoid cell leukodystrophy: Deficiency of galactocerebroside-galactosidase. Proc Natl Acad Sci USA 66:302, 1970. *This report describes the detection of the enzyme deficiency underlying this rare form of leukodystrophy.*

Section Eleven THE EPILEPSIES

510. THE EPILEPSIES

Jerome Engel, Jr.

DEFINITION AND PREVALENCE. Epilepsy is the term applied to a group of disorders, perhaps better called the epilepsies, that are characterized by recurrent, spontaneous, transient paroxysms of hyperactive brain function resulting in epileptic seizures. The epileptic attack or seizure, the common denominator of all of these conditions, may appear as impaired consciousness, involuntary movement, autonomic disturbance, or psychic or sensory experiences. Epileptic disorders can be considered either primary, conditions of intrinsic nonprogressive presumably hereditary cerebral hyperexcitability, with seizures as the only manifestation of disordered brain function, or secondary, wherein the epileptic attacks are symptoms of some known pathologic process affecting the brain.

Epileptic disorders most commonly begin in early childhood but can appear at any time. Epidemiologic surveys indicate that 0.5 per cent of the United States population have active seizures, 3 per cent have had a recurrent seizure disorder at some time in their life, and 9 per cent have experienced at least one epileptic seizure. These figures may represent an underestimation since the stigma attached to epilepsy causes many individuals to deny or hide their disorder. Prevalence is greater in areas of the world where there are high rates of infection, poor perinatal care, frequent head trauma, and other opportunities for increased brain injury.

PATHOGENESIS. Most investigators now believe that the fundamental abnormality in all epileptic conditions can be traced to the cerebral cortex, including the limbic cortex (hippocampus). In chronic epilepsy, the recurrent neuronal paroxysms that underlie ictal (seizure) events are transient expressions of a more permanently physiologically disordered cortex. Even though epileptic seizures are intermittent, the epileptogenic cortical abnormality persists throughout the interictal (between seizures) period.

Epileptogenic cortex in the interictal state is characterized by the appearance of brief high-amplitude electrical discharges that usually can be recorded from the scalp by *electroencephalography (EEG).* The typical interictal EEG discharge consists of a sharp negative transient wave followed by a slower wave, referred to as a *spike-and-wave complex.* Studies of well localized cortical epileptogenic lesions (epileptic foci) in animals indicate that the EEG spike-and-wave complex reflects the summation of highly synchronized abnormal alterations in neuronal membrane potentials. These abnormal membrane events consist of large paroxysmal depolarization shifts followed by prolonged after-hyperpolarizations. The depolarization shift results in enhanced neuronal excitation, while the after-hyperpolarization represents inhibition that may prevent ictal development. Neurons in cortical areas adjacent to the epileptic focus may demonstrate paroxysmal hyperpolarization only, forming an inhibitory surround that appears to prevent epileptic spread during the interictal state. It is unclear to what degree these abnormal membrane events recorded from epileptic foci reflect inherent pathologic properties of individual epileptic neurons as opposed to disturbances in interconnections of groups of neurons.

When seizures begin in an epileptic focus, the interictal EEG spike-and-wave complex is replaced by ictal low voltage, fast, rhythmic electrical discharges. At the cellular level this change represents a breakdown of the inhibitory after-hyperpolarization and the onset of a more continuous hyperexcitable depolarized state. If the inhibitory surround is also overcome, adjacent more normal cortical areas are recruited into the ictal process by nonsynaptic means. This *ephaptic spread* can proceed in a slow and orderly fashion across the cortex to produce a gradual progression of ictal symptoms that reflect functions of the involved cortical structures. Consciousness is preserved when ictal discharges are confined to a relatively discrete area of cortex in one hemisphere.

Ictal propagation to distant brain areas can occur via long fiber tracts, leading to the development of additional symptoms. Propagation to the contralateral hemisphere, particularly to limbic structures such as the hippocampus, the amygdala, and their projections, leads to impaired consciousness. Propagation to frontal lobes and subcortical motor systems can result in progression to a tonic-clonic convulsion.

Partial seizures begin with symptoms that reflect ictal discharges in an epileptic focus involving a part of the cerebral cortex and adjacent subcortex. *Generalized seizures* begin bilaterally from the start and are caused by widespread or multiple cortical epileptogenic foci or diffusely epileptogenic cortex related to primary hereditary, toxic, or metabolic disturbances. Some seizures may be precipitated by normal synchronizing afferent influences from subcortical centers. This may be the predominant mechanism of seizure initiation in the hereditary primary generalized seizure disorders, but it appears to be the cortex and not the deeper nuclei that is primarily abnormal. For this reason, the term *corticoreticular* has replaced centrencephalic or subcortical epilepsy for these conditions.

The fundamental neuronal defects that account for epileptogenesis appear to vary from one condition to another. Common causes of acute experimental partial and generalized convulsive seizures in animals include toxic and metabolic alterations that produce membrane instability; drugs that block the action of inhibitory transmitters; and electric currents that create polarizing fields. Although these findings may explain why epileptic seizures occur in association with certain clinical conditions, they are probably not relevant to mechanisms that spontaneously generate recurrent seizures in chronic epileptic disorders. Studies of chronic epileptic foci from animals and patients and investigations of naturally occurring primary generalized epileptic disorders in animals have revealed inconsistent biochemical and anatomic disturbances at the cellular level but no definitive explanations for the ultimate epileptogenic properties.

Mechanisms responsible for the termination of epileptic seizures are even less well understood than those that start them in the first place. Seizures do not stop merely as a result of neuronal exhaustion but rather appear to self-activate inhibitory mechanisms. Neuronal function is depressed after a seizure, and there may be prominent postictal symptoms. Tonic-clonic convulsions and partial seizures with impaired consciousness are followed by diffuse EEG suppression and periods of confusion and fatigue lasting minutes to hours. Other partial seizures may be followed by transient localized EEG suppression and focal neurologic deficits, known as *Todd's paralysis,* caused by postictal dysfunction of cortical structures involved in the ictal event.

It is likely that the pathophysiologic processes discussed apply to both partial seizures and generalized tonic-clonic convulsions. The different ictal manifestations of these conditions may merely reflect the localization and extent of the cortical disturbances. However, this does not appear to be the case for all epileptic conditions. For instance, in some nonconvulsive generalized seizures (absences) ictal and interictal EEG spike-and-wave discharges are indistinguishable and respond to drugs that are different from those used to treat partial and convulsive seizures. Certain myoclonic jerks, infantile spasms, neonatal seizures, and forms of partial continuous epilepsy are unassociated with specific ictal EEG patterns and demonstrate still another spectrum of drug responsivity. Some of these latter disorders may reflect subcortical disinhibition with pathophysiologic mechanisms more similar to extrapyramidal movement disorders than to epilepsy.

ETIOLOGY. The causes of epilepsy are many, and several factors may coexist in the same patient. Commonly, it is the combination of a cerebral lesion and a genetic predisposition that determines the appearance of epileptic seizures. Systemic illness or trauma may uncover a latent epileptic condition.

Genetic factors may contribute to the development of epilepsy in three ways: (1) an individual may inherit a low threshold for seizures; (2) genetic traits underlie certain specific primary epileptic conditions; and (3) many inherited diseases of the brain are associated with structural disturbances that produce seizures.

A number of poorly understood genetic factors determine the susceptibility of individual brains to develop generalized convulsions in response to nonspecific stresses such as sleep deprivation, fever, and alcohol withdrawal. Persons who experience such convulsions do not have epilepsy as such, but they do have lowered convulsive thresholds that make them more likely to develop chronic recurrent seizures of all types if brain injury occurs for other reasons. Consequently, patients with seizures caused by pathologic processes that are clearly not familial may have family histories of epilepsy or isolated seizures.

Benign inherited primary epileptic disturbances, presumably as a result of biochemical defects and unassociated with other neurologic dysfunctions, account for 30 per cent of chronic epileptic disorders. Specific autosomal dominant genetic traits have been identified as responsible for the characteristic EEG patterns of three-per-second spike-and-wave complexes seen in the generalized disorder *(petit mal epilepsy)* and for the centrotemporal spikes seen in the partial disorders *(sylvian* or *rolandic epilepsy)*, but not all individuals with these traits have seizures. Other benign familial primary generalized epilepsies have been described with faster spike-and-wave EEG discharges and bilaterally synchronous myoclonic jerks.

Inherited neurologic diseases also can produce chronic recurrent epileptic seizures that are secondary to specific pathologic processes within the brain. These include inborn errors of metabolism such as phenylketonuria and the lipoidoses; other degenerative diseases, not only those that affect gray matter, such as the progressive myoclonus epilepsies, but also the leukodystrophies; and syndromes such as tuberous sclerosis and neurofibromatosis that are associated with the development of cerebral ectopic or alien tissue.

Congenital lesions due to pre- and perinatal injuries are commonly encountered in epileptic patients. Minor focal lesions that can give rise to partial seizures include microgyria, porencephalic cysts, areas of calcification, and atrophy. More severe trauma, anoxia, and infections such as toxoplasmosis, cytomegalic inclusion disease, rubella, herpes, and syphilis also can produce diffuse neocortical and hippocampal damage and secondary generalized seizure disorders.

Head trauma with cicatrix formation is an important cause of epileptic seizures. Chronic recurrent seizures occur in 30 per cent of patients with acute hematomas, 15 per cent of those with depressed skull fractures, and 5 per cent of those hospitalized for severe closed head trauma. Epilepsy is rare, however, after head trauma without loss of consciousness. Seizures occurring at the time of injury (contact seizures) or within the first week thereafter do not necessarily herald development of a recurrent epileptic disorder. Chronic posttraumatic seizures usually have a delayed onset, most often beginning 6 to 12 months following injury and occasionally starting even many years later.

Infectious processes involving the brain and its coverings can produce acute and chronic seizures. As with trauma, generalized seizures that occur during active meningitis and encephalitis may not indicate a recurrent epileptic condition. Acute and chronic recurrent generalized and partial seizures are seen with slow virus infections and are common late sequelae when adhesions or scars result from purulent meningitis, fungal infections, or destructive viral processes such as herpes simplex encephalitis. Partial seizures may be the first sign of focal bacterial encephalitis or abscess formation, lesions especially likely to produce chronic epilepsy. Other focal inflammatory processes such as tuberculomas and parasitic infestations, particularly cysticercosis and schistosomiasis, are common causes of partial seizures in many countries and because of increased international travel are sometimes found outside their endemic areas.

About half of all *brain tumors* located in the anterior and middle cranial fossae produce epileptic symptoms. Gliomas are most often implicated, but any neoplasm that impinges on the cortex can produce seizures. Partial seizures are common with *Sturge-Weber syndrome* and often result from small cryptogenic hamartomas, ectopias, and angiomas.

Cerebral vascular diseases produce seizures in many ways. Partial seizures are rare during acute strokes and usually reflect embolic events with bleeding into the cortex rather than thrombosis. Completed strokes, however, often produce scar tissue that can become epileptogenic months or years later. Such a process is presumed to be the most common cause of unexplained recurrent partial seizures in the elderly. Partial and generalized seizures are early symptoms of cerebral venous thrombosis, cerebral arteritis, and hypertensive encephalopathy (now rare). Partial seizures often occur with arteriovenous malformations (AVMs), and small cortical hemorrhages of any cause can produce refractory partial seizures or focal myoclonic jerks.

Systemic toxic and metabolic disturbances caused by exogenous and endogenous substances that lower seizure thresholds or produce neuronal membrane instability as well as ionic imbalance, such as hyponatremia, can give rise to generalized convulsions, but these are not considered epileptic conditions. Nevertheless, such metabolic causes occasionally can lead to status epilepticus with subsequent brain damage or death. It is important to recognize the rare reversible metabolic causes of seizures in infancy, such as hypocalcemia and pyridoxine deficiency, that can be treated easily by replacement therapy. Toxic or metabolic disturbances may occasionally cause partial seizures because of associated unsuspected focal cerebral lesions from old head injuries. These occur most commonly in alcohol and drug abusers who are undergoing withdrawal. Hyperosmolar conditions such as nonketotic hyperglycemia and uremia may also give rise to partial seizures, presumably because of brain shrinkage that tears bridging vessels and produces small areas of hemorrhage into the cortex.

Miscellaneous disorders that can cause seizures include gray matter degenerative diseases such as allergic encephalopathies and very rarely the presenile and senile dementias. Demyelinating diseases occasionally produce lesions adjacent to cortex that cause epileptic attacks: seizures occur in 3 per cent of patients with multiple sclerosis.

Mesial temporal sclerosis, consisting of largely unilateral neuronal loss often accompanied by astrocytic proliferation in the hippocampus and adjacent limbic structures, is found in over half the patients who have undergone temporal lobe resection for complex partial seizures. This may be the most common pathologic finding in epilepsy, but it remains uncertain whether the lesion is the cause or the result of seizures. Prolonged convulsive seizures are known to produce cell loss in the hippocampus, the neocortex, and the cerebellum. Some authorities believe that prolonged convulsions (lasting more than 30 minutes), such as those that occasionally accompany fever in infancy or childhood exanthems, can produce mesial temporal sclerosis and that this lesion becomes epileptogenic later in life. In any event, this form of epileptic brain damage suggests that in some situations epilepsy itself becomes a cause of progressive symptoms. Even if mesial temporal sclerosis does not actually cause seizures, it may alter their manifestations and account for some interictal behavioral disturbances. For this reason convulsive seizures should be controlled as promptly as possible.

CLINICAL MANIFESTATIONS AND CLASSIFICATION. At present epileptic seizures are classified by their clinical manifestations (Table 510–1), since precise anatomic and pathophysiologic correlates of specific ictal behaviors are still largely unknown. The classification plays an essential role in the diagnosis and management of epileptic disorders for four major reasons:

1. The diagnosis of epilepsy is often difficult because of the similarity between certain epileptic attacks and intermittent symptoms of nonepileptic disorders. Recognition that a patient's complaints are consistent with a known epileptic seizure pattern determines whether the true nature of the condition has been identified or even suspected. The classification of epileptic seizures by specific symptoms is particularly useful for this purpose.

2. Differentiation between partial and generalized seizures is of great clinical value. Partial seizures indicate the presence of a focal brain disturbance that may be a curable cause of epilepsy, such as a surgically resectable scar, or a focal progressive process that requires specific attention, such as an infection or neoplasm. Because the exact expression of a partial seizure is determined by the site of ictal onset and spread and not by the causative agent, additional clinical information is necessary to identify the nature of the underlying lesion.

3. The choice of antiepileptic drugs is determined by the seizure type rather than by the specific cause or anatomic substrate. Certain generalized seizures in particular are effectively treated by classes of pharmacologic agents that are different from those used to treat partial or generalized convulsive seizures. Consequently, the differential diagnosis between absence attacks and complex partial seizures and between myoclonus and convulsions is essential for determining appropriate drug therapy.

4. A number of epileptic syndromes have been defined on the basis of seizure manifestations and other clinical features. Although pathophysiologic mechanisms or underlying disease processes have yet to be identified for most, diagnosis of a specific syndrome usually has important therapeutic and prognostic implications. In particular, recognition of the benign inherited primary epileptic conditions such as true petit mal, juvenile epileptic myoclonus, and sylvian epilepsy may facilitate prompt control with the proper medication, spare the patient unnecessary tests, and relieve anxiety by assurance of an excellent outcome. A diagnosis of temporal lobe epilepsy in a medically intractable patient suggests that complete cure may be possible by surgical resection.

TABLE 510–1. CLASSIFICATION OF EPILEPTIC SEIZURES*

Partial seizures (focal, local)
- Simple partial seizures
  - With motor signs
  - With somatosensory or special sensory symptoms
  - With autonomic symptoms or signs
  - With psychic symptoms
- Complex partial seizures
  - Simple partial onset followed by impairment of consciousness
  - With impairment of consciousness at onset
- Partial seizures evolving to generalized tonic-clonic convulsions (secondarily generalized)

Generalized seizures (convulsive or nonconvulsive)
- Nonconvulsive seizures
  - Absence seizures
  - Atypical absence seizures
  - Myoclonic seizures
  - Atonic seizures
- Convulsive seizures
  - Tonic-clonic seizures
  - Tonic seizures
  - Clonic seizures

Unclassified epileptic seizures

*Modified from Commission on Classification and Terminology of the International League Against Epilepsy: Epilepsia 22:489, 1981.

Partial Seizures. Although the expression of partial seizures depends on the areas of cerebral cortex that are involved, the precise anatomic origin of specific seizures cannot always be accurately inferred from ictal symptoms, since functional localization within the brain remains inexact. Moreover, epileptic manifestations may reflect dysfunction produced by propagation away from the primary lesion as much or more than from the area where the focus lies.

Partial seizures are classified as simple when consciousness is preserved. *Simple partial seizures* reflect an ictal discharge that is localized within one hemisphere. The ictal symptoms can take many forms.

Motor symptoms begin with clonic or tonic movements of a discrete body part. Areas of the body with large representation in the motor cortex, such as the face and hand, are involved most frequently. When spread occurs in an orderly fashion along the precentral gyrus, there is a progression of clonic motor symptoms from thumb or face, for example, referred to as a *Jacksonian March.* More commonly, however, ictal discharges in frontal cortex activate multiple muscle groups to produce complex versive movements such as turning of the head, eyes, or body to one side and posturing with one or more extremities. Involvement of the supplementary motor cortex classically results in adversive seizures with turning of the head and eyes away from the epileptic focus and elevation of the contralateral arm. The arm position can vary, however, and the direction in which the head turns is not a good localizing or lateralizing sign. Other simple motor manifestations include speech arrest or vocalizations when language areas are involved; eye or lid twitching, which is most often initiated from frontal or occipital foci; and inappropriate laughter unassociated with humor *(gelastic epilepsy).* Simple partial clonic or tonic motor seizures can be followed by a transient *Todd's paralysis* of involved muscles, but suspicion of an underlying progressive lesion is justified when postictal focal deficits persist after 48 hours.

Sensory symptoms occur with lesions in or connected to primary sensory cortex. Thus, localized paresthesias or numbness arise with seizures emanating from the parietal lobe, unformed luminous visions occur with lesions of the occipital lobe, and unpleasant olfactory and gustatory sensations, vertigo, and sounds result from lesions of appropriate areas of the temporal cortex. Postictal Todd's phenomena such as blindness, deafness, and anesthesia may occasionally follow simple partial seizures with sensory symptoms.

Autonomic symptoms often are due to ictal involvement of limbic structures in the mesial temporal and frontal lobes that project to the hypothalamus and brainstem and include feelings of epigastric rising or distress, nausea, or vague lightheadedness. Brief paroxysmal epigastric symptoms, including vomiting, can be the sole manifestation of an epileptic disorder *(abdominal epilepsy).* This condition has most often been identified in children, but it is rare and probably greatly overdiagnosed. In other autonomic seizures ictal signs and symptoms such as pallor, flushing, sweating, piloerection, pupillary dilatation, cardiac arrhythmia, and incontinence may be apparent.

Psychic symptoms can occur with ictal discharges in limbic and association cortex and mimic features of psychiatric disorders. These include dysmnesic symptoms such as feelings of familiarity (deja vu) and unfamiliarity (jamais vu) and forced thinking; cognitive disturbances such as dreamy states, depersonalization, and time distortion; affective symptoms such as fear and rage, which often are associated with appropriate autonomic changes, depression, and on rare occasion elation; illusions such as multiple images (polyopsia) or distortions of size (micropsia and macropsia); and hallucinations consisting of stereotyped mixed sensory experiences such as visions of well-formed recognizable faces or specific scenes accompanied by voices that can be understood, familiar smells, and emotional responses. Persistent psychic symptoms in epileptic patients may also be postictal.

Simple partial seizures are usually brief and do not interfere with daily living unless they occur frequently or evolve into other types of attacks. Simple partial seizures that consist only of experiential phenomena may be referred to as *auras* when the patient perceives them as a warning of impending more noticeable epileptic symptoms. Patients who complain only of simple partial seizures may report having many seizures a week or many a day, with each lasting a few seconds.

Partial seizures are classified as complex when they impair consciousness. Approximately 40 per cent of patients with epilepsy experience *complex partial seizures* with impaired consciousness ranging from a complete loss with unresponsiveness to mere amnesia for the ictal event. Complex partial seizures are presumed to reflect bilateral ictal involvement of limbic structures, particularly the hippocampus, amygdala, and their connections. The seizure may begin with impaired consciousness from the start, or spread of ictal discharge may result in evolution from a simple into a complex partial event. This evolution occurs most often when the simple partial seizure is caused by a lesion involving the mesial temporal lobe or a region of cerebral cortex directly connected to mesial temporal limbic areas. Autonomic auras most commonly precede complex partial seizures and include epigastric rising or distress and psychic experiences. Complex partial seizures that are preceded by olfactory auras are called *uncinate fits.* These fits may be more consistently associated with brain tumors than are other types of seizures.

The term complex partial seizure is not synonymous with *temporal lobe, psychomotor,* and *limbic seizures.* These designations have more specific anatomic implications and may involve ictal symptoms resulting from unilateral activation of mesial temporal limbic structures without impaired consciousness. Some complex partial seizures that manifest themselves solely as brief lapses in consciousness or that are associated with atypical behavior may not reflect primary activation of the limbic system. The complex partial seizure that typifies the temporal lobe or psychomotor attack begins with a motionless stare at the time consciousness is impaired, followed by purposeless movements called *automatisms.* Alimentary automatisms, such as chewing, swallowing, sucking, and lip smacking, are most common and presumably reflect amygdala involvement. Other examples of automatisms include verbal utterances of sounds or words; gestural movements such as fumbling, posturing, and picking at clothing; expressions of emotion; and ambulation. Ongoing activities such as washing dishes or even driving a car may continue automatically. Patients may undress, run, respond to commands, and demonstrate a variety of complicated automatisms that indicate a residual ability to relate to the environment despite the ictal state. In complex partial seizures that emanate from structures outside the temporal lobe, patients can display irregular thrashing movements of the extremities, scream, fall, or exhibit bizarre behavior that can be difficult to differentiate from hysteria.

Complex partial seizures usually last from a few seconds to a few minutes and are followed by confusion and amnesia for the ictal event, although most patients remember an aura. Postictal anterograde amnesia and automatisms are common, and aphasia often occurs when seizures begin in the dominant hemisphere. Other cognitive deficits and headache may be present during the postictal period. In cases of unusually prolonged or recurrent complex partial seizures, postictal anterograde memory disturbance may persist for hours or days.

Complex partial seizures and postictal symptoms can severely disrupt daily life. While it is not uncommon for patients to have many complex partial seizures a week and several auras a day, even one or two seizures a year may prevent them from driving a car or destroy a chosen career.

Both simple and complex partial seizures can evolve into *secondarily generalized tonic-clonic convulsions.* Most patients with partial seizures experience at least some secondarily generalized seizures, but generalization usually occurs infrequently and is more easily controlled by drugs than are partial ictal symptoms. Some patients, particularly those with lesions in the frontal lobes, have partial seizures that always secondarily generalize. When such secondarily generalized partial seizures begin in a silent area of the brain, initial focal symptoms may be overlooked by both the patient and observers. When neither ictal symptoms nor signs provide a clue that a seizure is secondarily generalized, postictal focal or lateralizing signs and symptoms such as reflex asymmetry, focal weakness, or aphasia may indicate a partial seizure disorder. Differentiation from true generalized convulsions in these cases is important to identify potentially progressive or treatable focal lesions.

Generalized Seizures. *Absences* are brief losses of consciousness that can be of two types. Both begin almost exclusively in childhood and take the form of a blank stare, which can also be associated with mild clonic movements of eyelids and face, more generalized jerks, alterations in motor tone, and simple automatisms. *Petit mal absences* affect about 10 per cent of epileptic children, last less than ten seconds, demonstrate a typical EEG pattern consisting of symmetrical, synchronous, and regular three-per-second (or slightly faster) spike-and-wave discharges, and begin and end abruptly without pre- or postictal EEG or clinical disturbances. These seizures are characteristic of benign genetic epileptic disorders of the primary generalized type. *Atypical absences* also occur in about 10 per cent of epileptic children, can last longer than ten seconds, demonstrate asymmetrical, asynchronous, and irregular three-per-second (or slower) spike-and-wave discharges on the EEG, and produce some degree of postictal confusion and EEG disturbance. Atypical absences often occur in patients who have other types of generalized seizures, as well as neurologic deficits, mental retardation, and a characteristic slow spike-and-wave (less than 2.5 per second) EEG pattern. This symptom complex is called the *Lennox-Gastaut syndrome* and results from multiple or diffuse brain lesions. True petit mal and atypical absences must not be confused with each other or with complex partial seizures consisting only of brief lapses of consciousness, since cause, prognosis, and treatment differ for the three seizure types.

Absences can occur spontaneously hundreds of times a day. Petit mal absences respond well to appropriate medications, tend to disappear during adolescence, and are rarely disabling. Atypical absences may be refractory to therapy and can disrupt normal function. Children with atypical absences, however, are usually hampered more by other seizures and by neurologic and mental deficits.

Myoclonic seizures are single, rapidly recurrent, bilaterally synchronous shock-like jerks of the face, trunk, and extremities that are not associated with loss of consciousness. A single myoclonic jerk that occurs while a person is falling asleep is a normal physiologic event. More frequent myoclonus implies a more serious problem. In most patients with myoclonic seizures, these events cluster shortly after waking or when falling asleep. A prolonged attack can terminate in a generalized tonic-clonic convulsion. Myoclonic seizures occur in certain rare benign genetic epileptic disorders of the primary generalized type such as *juvenile epileptic myoclonus (impulsive petit mal)* and respond well to drug therapy.

In contrast to myoclonic seizures, there are many other types of myoclonic jerks that are not generalized and should not be considered epileptic. These include (1) the asymmetrical or sporadic (involving first one area of the body and then another) jerks that are spontaneous or induced by movement or sensory stimulation and that result from anoxic, toxic, and metabolic disturbances and (2) the *progressive myoclonus epilepsies* that are associated with lesions of the diencephalon, brainstem, and cerebellar nuclei. Other myoclonic phenomena that are not epileptic seizures include regular rhythmic *palatal myoclonus* and *segmental myoclonus* that are caused, respectively, by medullary and spinal cord lesions and *benign familial (essential) myoclonus* of unknown origin.

Tonic-clonic (grand mal) convulsions occur at least once in 80 per cent of epileptic patients. Occasionally, such seizures can be epileptic responses of a normal brain to nonspecific physiologic stress or systemic disturbances. More often they represent the final form taken by partial seizures that secondarily generalize or are a manifestation of a generalized epileptic disorder. Convulsions that are not secondarily generalized from partial seizures never have auras, although patients may occasionally recognize nonspecific affective changes or experience a flurry of bilaterally synchronous myoclonic jerks some hours before a seizure occurs. The typical generalized convulsion begins with a sudden cry accompanied by loss of consciousness, falling, and bilateral tonic extensor rigidity of the trunk and extremities. After several seconds of rigidity, recurrent clonic muscular contractions are produced for one or two minutes, until the seizure ends, leaving the patient flaccid and unconscious. Cyanosis results from breath-holding during the tonic phase, and autonomic hyperactivity is prominent. The blood pressure increases abruptly, the body temperature rises, and the patient salivates and may have urinary and fecal incontinence. The tongue and the inside of the mouth often are bitten. Occasionally generalized convulsive attacks consist of either tonic or clonic activity alone.

Postictal depression can last many minutes, occasionally hours, and rarely a day or more. During this period patients gradually regain consciousness but feel exhausted, frequently complain of headache, and wish to sleep. A few remain partially confused. Focal or lateralized postictal symptoms do not occur following true generalized tonic-clonic convulsions.

Grand mal convulsions rarely occur more than a few times a year in primary generalized epileptic disorders but can occur daily in severe secondary generalized disorders. In both situations, however, the generalized seizures tend to respond well to antiepileptic drugs.

Atonic seizures (drop attacks), considered to be minor motor epileptic events, begin almost exclusively in childhood and are usually associated with diffuse lesions of the brain. The ictal episode consists of a sudden loss of tone that is too brief to determine whether alteration of consciousness has occurred. In its simplest form, the child's head drops for a second or less. In more severe forms, the patient loses tone in the entire body, collapses to the floor, and often incurs serious injuries such as concussion, broken bones, and lost teeth. This characteristic drop should be distinguished from the more gradual slump that can accompany partial seizures, the more rigid loss of balance that occurs during tonic or tonic-clonic convulsions, and the sudden impulsive falls that result from myoclonic jerks. Atonic seizures occur many times a day, are refractory to therapy, and can be the most debilitating ictal manifestation of the Lennox-Gastaut syndrome. Brief *tonic seizures* also occur as minor motor symptoms of secondary generalized epileptic disorders.

Unclassified Seizures. *Infantile spasms* begin in the first year of life as brief intermittent ictal events that take a variety of forms, ranging from subtle twitches of the mouth or nose to violent jackknife or salaam movements. They result from severe diffuse disturbances of brain function from a variety of causes, are often associated with a severely abnormal interictal EEG pattern called *hypsarrhythmia,* and have a poor prognosis. Because infantile spasms may reflect subcortical disturbances similar to myoclonus or movement disorders, they have been removed from the current classification of epileptic seizures. However, children with this EEG and clinical symptom complex *(West's syndrome)* usually develop recurrent epileptic seizures as they get older, and their illness often evolves into the Lennox-Gastaut syndrome.

Because of an immature brain, *neonatal seizures* almost never generalize. Rather, they manifest themselves subtly as jitteriness, focal or multifocal twitches, clonic movements, and posturing. The cerebral cortex in the neonatal period may not be sufficiently well developed to sustain epileptic activity, and often no correlation exists between electrographic abnormalities and behavioral seizure activity. Consequently, many of these events could also reflect disturbances that are primarily subcortical and not epileptic. Benign as well as severely disabling forms of neonatal seizures occur.

Patterns of Seizure Occurrence. Appreciation for precipitating factors and temporal patterns of certain epileptic seizures can influence approaches to management. In some of the primary generalized epileptic disorders, seizures may be induced by specific sensory stimuli, most commonly flashing light *(photosensitive epilepsy).* Reading, video games, music, and other specific complex stimuli may activate seizures in patients with rarer forms of *reflex epilepsy.* The seizures themselves range from brief absences through synchronous myoclonic jerking to occasional generalized convulsions. It is unusual for partial seizures to be induced by specific sensory stimuli, although they can be provoked by emotional stress and drowsiness. *Hyperventilation* is a potent activator of petit mal and atypical absence seizures and sometimes will precipitate other types of ictal events as well. Possibly the associated respiratory alkalosis may explain why some patients report an increased incidence of seizures during exercise. Sleep deprivation and withdrawal from alcohol and sedative drugs are well established precipitants of partial and generalized convulsive seizures in patients with chronic epilepsy. Some patients have seizures that occur only at night or only during the day. Others exhibit regular cycles of seizures over days or months or patterns of seizure clusters followed by prolonged seizure-free periods. The term *catamenial epilepsy* is used when seizures regularly recur in women around the menstrual period. Women with all forms of epileptic disorders commonly experience more frequent seizures at this time of the month, and seizures may worsen or disappear during pregnancy.

Status Epilepticus. Rapidly recurring or continuous ictal events are referred to as status epilepticus. *Epilepsia partialis continua* is a state of simple partial seizures that can last hours, days, or weeks. The focal clonic motor form resembles myoclonic jerks, while the rarer sensory and psychic forms may be difficult to differentiate from psychiatric disorders. Ictal EEG changes may be difficult to identify.

Complex partial status epilepticus is a rare condition of rapidly recurring seizures characterized by a fluctuating level of consciousness, automatic behavior, and ictal EEG discharges recorded over the temporal lobe. The condition may be confused clinically with a psychosis or metabolic disturbance and must be included in the differential diagnosis of altered states of consciousness; failure to treat it promptly can be followed by prolonged memory deficits.

Absence status or *spike wave stupor* consists of a continuous state of dulled mentation, which often has a subtle appearance. Eye blinking and other associated movements can occur, and there is a characteristic EEG pattern of diffuse spike-and-wave discharges. The condition occurs fairly often in patients with atypical absences and is also seen with a juvenile form of primary generalized petit mal epilepsy. A rare type of absence status of unknown cause also affects older adults with no previous history of epilepsy. Absence status is not a medical emergency, since no secondary brain damage occurs. The benign and adult forms respond well to antiepileptic drugs, but atypical absence status associated with diffuse lesions of the brain may be extremely difficult to control.

Major motor status epilepticus exists when generalized tonic-clonic convulsions recur so frequently that consciousness is not regained between them. This can occur with the generalized disorders but is more commonly a result of partial seizures that secondarily generalize. In the latter instance, the partial onset often is not recognized because of the severity of the attacks. Toxic and metabolic disturbances, including drug and alcohol withdrawal, can precipitate major motor status epilepticus in epileptic patients as well as in nonepileptic individuals with genetically low seizure thresholds. Major motor status epilepticus can also be a presenting symptom of acute intracranial hemorrhage and infections, as well as brain tumors and other focal processes, especially in the frontal lobes. Major motor status epilepticus is a life-threatening situation demanding immediate treatment.

Epileptic Syndromes. A number of epileptic syndromes have already been mentioned, and some of the more clinically distinctive ones are listed in Table 510–2. It is particularly valuable to recognize those syndromes that respond well to specific treatment and that are associated with a good prognosis. In this group should be included several familial conditions and temporal lobe epilepsy.

Sylvian or *rolandic epilepsy* (benign partial epilepsy of childhood with centrotemporal spikes) is a familial disorder that may be the cause of as many as 20 per cent of childhood seizures. It is characterized by nocturnal generalized convulsions and simple partial seizures that occur during the day. Typically, the partial seizures begin with perioral or lingual paresthesias, although other sensory or motor symptoms may occur, especially involving the face. The EEG demonstrates centrotemporal interictal spikes that may be unilateral or bilaterally independent. Associated neurologic deficits are lacking, and the seizures respond well to medication. The disorder almost always disappears during adolescence.

A rare benign partial epilepsy of childhood with occipital spike-and-wave discharges is characterized by seizures with visual symptoms followed by headache. This disorder may be a form of migraine.

One or more *febrile convulsions* occur in 3 to 4 per cent of otherwise healthy children between the ages of six months and five years and consist of brief tonic-clonic generalized seizures. Although febrile convulsions can be recurrent, the syndrome is so benign that it is usually not considered an epileptic disorder, and treatment is usually not necessary. A genetic basis is certain but poorly defined. Affected children outgrow their vulnerability between three and five years of age, although 5 per cent develop seizures without fever later. Against the diagnosis of benign febrile convulsions are the following: seizures lasting longer than ten minutes, focal abnormalities during or after the seizure, or an abnormal neurologic or mental status examination result. In such instances an underlying neurologic disorder is likely and treatment is required.

The primary generalized epileptic conditions of the petit mal type, mentioned earlier, account for 10 per cent of childhood epilepsies. Several varieties are recognized depending on the age of onset, frequency of EEG spike-and-wave discharges, and occurrence of myoclonic seizures. Infrequent grand mal seizures can occur in all forms, or they may occur alone. Response to appropriate medication is usually excellent, especially when onset is in early childhood. These disorders often remit in adolescence; a juvenile onset or myoclonic seizures tend to worsen the prognosis.

True petit mal absences and grand mal seizures should not be confused with similar ictal events that occur in children with the Lennox-Gastaut syndrome as the result of diffuse or multiple lesions of the brain. Patients with primary generalized epilepsy are otherwise neurologically normal, with brief absences accompanied by regular synchronous EEG spike-and-wave discharges. Although patients with the Lennox-Gastaut syndrome can have absences identical to the primary generalized type, usually they also have or develop additional neurologic impairment, mental subnormality, multiple seizure types including drop attacks, irregular asymmetrical paroxysmal EEG discharges, and abnormal baseline EEG rhythms. In contrast to the excellent prognosis for the primary generalized epilepsies, seizures associated with the Lennox-Gastaut syndrome and other secondary generalized epileptic disorders are difficult to control. The patients often become severely handicapped by the frequent attacks as well as other static or progressive interictal neurologic deficits.

Juvenile epileptic myoclonus is a primary generalized epileptic disorder that begins in mid to late childhood with bilaterally synchronous myoclonic seizures. The paroxysms can be completely controlled with appropriate medication, and there are no other associated disturbances. The condition should not be confused with the myoclonic disorders characterized by sporadic, often stimulus-sensitive, myoclonic jerks, such as postanoxic myoclonus and the progressive myoclonus epilepsies. These last-mentioned sporadic myoclonic events are not epileptic, are extremely difficult to treat, and are usually associated with other evidence of diffuse cerebral injury.

The *progressive myoclonus epilepsies* comprise a group of familial cerebral degenerative disorders that affect both cortical and subcortical gray matter, leading to progressive neurologic deficits, dementia, sporadic multifocal myoclonic jerks, occasional epileptic myoclonus, and tonic-clonic convulsions. Whereas the epileptic myoclonus and convulsions respond well to medication, patients are severely disabled by the nonepileptic sporadic myoclonus and other handicaps. The course may be rapid with severe neurologic and mental impairment *(Lafora type)*, intermediate *(Unverricht-Lundborg type)*, or relatively slow with little mental impairment or EEG disturbance *(Ramsay-Hunt syndrome*, which is associated with cerebellar disturbances and may be considered a separate entity). A benign familial myoclonic syndrome *(essential myoclonus)* also exists.

Temporal lobe (psychomotor, limbic) epilepsy is the most common chronic epileptic syndrome and may account for 40 per cent of adult epilepsies. It is characterized by auras and complex partial seizures involving temporal lobe limbic structures either initially or occasionally by spread from other areas. Typically there are unilateral or bilateral independent anterior temporal EEG spikes. Patients may also have memory deficits and psychiatric symptomatology. Complex partial seizures, as described earlier, are often difficult to control medically but can be abolished by surgical resection. Patients with complex partial seizures that do not respond to appropriate medical therapy should be referred to a surgical facility for evaluation.

Epilepsia partialis continua also often is unresponsive to medication. This disorder occurs in adults after severe cerebral injury, such as anoxia or stroke—occasionally with brain tumors. It also can be seen in young children, particularly those with a rare unilateral chronic cerebral inflammatory disorder of unknown cause. The continuous focal motor seizures reflect widespread or multiple rather than single lesions that usually are not amenable to localized surgical resection. Seizures can be abolished by large resections such as in hemispherectomy,

TABLE 510–2. CLINICALLY DISTINCTIVE EPILEPTIC SYNDROMES

	Partial Epilepsies	Generalized Epilepsies
Primary (without structural lesions; benign, genetic)	Benign partial epilepsy of childhood with centrotemporal spikes (sylvian, rolandic) Benign partial epilepsy of childhood with occipital spike waves (may be migraine)	Benign febrile convulsions (should not be considered a chronic epileptic disorder) Petit mal epilepsies; many forms, including: true petit mal, juvenile forms Juvenile epileptic myoclonus Reflex epilepsies
Secondary (with structural lesions and associated neurologic disturbances)	Temporal lobe epilepsy Epilepsia partialis continua Epileptic acquired aphasia	Lennox-Gastaut syndrome Infantile spasms Progressive myoclonus epilepsies (many forms)

and this may be indicated in some children who already have hemiatrophy and hemiparesis.

Epileptic acquired aphasia syndrome is a rare partial seizure disorder of unknown cause that appears as language deterioration in young children and is associated with bilateral temporal epileptiform EEG spikes. The disorder resolves spontaneously.

DIAGNOSIS. Diagnosis in epilepsy involves searching for treatable causes when possible and recognizing epileptic conditions that indicate a specific prognosis and therapy. When a treatable cause of epilepsy is not revealed, management of the seizures is determined by correct diagnosis of the type of epileptic disorder.

History. The history is usually the most important part of the diagnostic evaluation. In order to obtain an accurate description of the typical ictal events, it is essential that someone who has witnessed the seizures accompany the patient to the interview.

The patient's own description of any auras should be recorded as well as the ictal behavioral changes observed by others. The occurrence of an aura or other focal symptoms at onset, during progression, or in the postictal period indicates a partial rather than a generalized seizure disorder. If more than one type of seizure occurs, each should be described separately. Often patients will report several seizure types, which after careful questioning are revealed to be variations of the same ictal phenomenon and not evidence for multiple lesions. For instance, when auras are not followed by further symptoms they may be recognized as one event, while the same aura that spreads to become a complex partial seizure may be reported as another phenomenon. If on occasion there is evolution to a secondarily generalized seizure without postictal recall of the aura, a careful description of the initial ictal events by an observer often will verify that the generalized convulsion is a manifestation of the same epileptogenic lesion. When patients report only seizures that are generalized from the start, an attempt should be made to determine whether convulsive and nonconvulsive ictal manifestations resemble those of benign genetic disorders, generalized disorders caused by diffuse or multiple brain lesions, or secondarily generalized partial seizures caused by a focal lesion. Clues to the differential diagnosis derive from the circumstances and age at onset of seizures and how they may have changed with time or treatment.

Drug regimens and other treatment plans can be influenced by knowledge of how often seizures occur, whether they are more common at certain times of the day or month, or whether they are related to certain precipitating factors. If the patient has been treated previously, it is important to know what drugs have been used and the specifics of their therapeutic and toxic effects.

The history can provide crucial etiologic information. In children, patterns of early development may delineate the difference between a progressive degenerative disorder and a static lesion. There may be evidence of specific predisposing factors such as perinatal injury, intracranial infections, or reactions to immunizations. A history of a prolonged childhood convulsion preceding the onset of complex partial seizures raises the possibility of mesial temporal sclerosis causing the subsequent chronic epileptic disorder. In older patients there may be hints of cerebral vascular disease or systemic cancer. A history of head trauma at any age can be relevant but must be evaluated carefully because parents and patients often recall trivial injuries of no importance occurring days or weeks prior to the first seizure. In addition, a specific injurious event such as a fall may be mistakenly interpreted as having generated traumatic epilepsy when it actually represented the first seizure.

The family history can reveal important genetic factors. The existence of relatives with similar seizures or other neurologic symptoms suggests a specific primary epileptic disorder. A family history of individuals with isolated seizures or varied epileptic conditions may indicate the inheritance of a lowered threshold for seizures. Absence of left-handedness in the family of a left-handed patient may hint at early injury of the left cerebral hemisphere.

The psychosocial history both gives important clues to diagnosis and indicates needs for more specific evaluations. Patients with benign inherited epileptic disorders should have normal school and work histories and no evidence of mental disturbance. A history of specific cognitive deficits suggests a focal lesion, while more generalized mental impairment suggests a diffuse abnormality. When the latter is progressive, more detailed laboratory, EEG, and psychometric examinations can determine whether the patient has an underlying degenerative disease, increasing dysfunction because of recurrent seizures, or toxic symptoms of overmedication.

Physical Examination. The general medical examination can uncover systemic diseases responsible for seizures. In addition to searching for toxic, metabolic, infectious, neoplastic, and cardiovascular diseases, stigmata of tuberous sclerosis, neurofibromatosis, hemangiomas, and other predisposing congenital disorders should be sought. Asymmetry (hemiatrophy) in the size of hands, feet, and face may indicate a long-standing lesion in the contralateral hemisphere.

The neurologic examination can provide evidence for a specific diagnosis or reveal focal disturbances that differentiate between partial and generalized seizure disorders. In the absence of focal features, findings of minimal brain dysfunction, such as clumsiness, posturing, and hyperreflexia, or more marked diffuse impairment indicate a secondary rather than a primary generalized seizure disorder.

The mental status examination can distinguish specific cognitive deficits caused by focal lesions from more general mental retardation or dementia. Poor attention span in patients on drug therapy may indicate medication side effects rather than structural lesions. Increasing degrees of fixed neurologic and mental impairment confer a poor prognosis for both seizure control and psychosocial adaptation.

If possible, patients should be observed during a seizure. Status epilepticus usually lasts until hospitalization, absences can be provoked by hyperventilation, reflex seizures are easily induced (it is unwise to attempt to induce tonic-clonic convulsions), and spontaneous seizures may occur in the examining room. The initial manifestations and early development should be noted. Consciousness should be assessed by repeating a phrase to determine whether the patient can recall it after the seizure is over. Even if the seizure appears to be generalized at the start, postictal examination of neurologic and mental status may reveal focal deficits that indicate a partial seizure disorder. When circumstances make direct examination impossible, try to find a reliable witness who can describe the attack.

Laboratory Studies. Epilepsy provides no diagnostic hematologic or chemical laboratory tracers, but such tests can help to diagnose underlying disease processes that give rise to seizures. One or more generalized epileptic attacks can mildly increase protein content and white cell count in the cerebrospinal fluid for 24 to 48 hours. Although up to 100 white cells per cubic millimeter have been reported after major motor status epilepticus, a lumbar puncture revealing more than 10 white cells per cubic millimeter should initiate a search for an intracranial inflammatory process. In infants and young children with seizures, it is wise to test blood and urine for metabolic disorders. In older patients with refractory focal motor seizures, hyperosmolar syndromes such as hyperglycemia and uremia should be considered. Complete blood count, liver function tests, blood urea nitrogen, and urinalysis are necessary in all patients about to begin antiepileptic drug therapy to establish a baseline for evaluating possible subsequent toxic side effects.

Radiologic Studies. A computed tomographic (CT) scan is necessary for adolescents and adults with the recent onset of seizures but may be avoided in younger children when history and other examinations indicate a primary generalized disorder or a nonprogressive lesion. Cerebral angiography should be confined to cases in which surgery is considered or a primary vascular disorder is suspected.

Psychometric Studies. Psychometric testing, including standard tests of attention, performance and verbal IQ, memory, language, and personality can help verify the existence of a focal or diffuse brain disturbance. When there is evidence that mental function is deteriorating, serial testing can quantify the change and evaluate subsequent trends of disease or therapy. An astute psychometrician should also be able to offer advice for improving psychosocial adaptation.

Electroencephalography. The EEG is the single most useful diagnostic laboratory test for epilepsy. However, overinterpretation of the EEG often generates an unwarranted diagnosis of epilepsy. A number of spike-like EEG events can be normal, and 2 per cent of the nonepileptic population may have true epileptiform spike-and-wave complexes on their EEGs but never develop seizures. Conversely, 20 per cent of patients with epilepsy do not demonstrate epileptic abnormalities on a routine interictal EEG. Whereas an EEG can help verify a clinical diagnosis of epilepsy, interictal epileptiform EEG abnormalities alone should be considered neither necessary nor sufficient information for arriving at this diagnosis. However, if a seizure occurs in the EEG laboratory, the association of an ictal EEG pattern with observed ictal clinical behavior makes possible a definitive diagnosis.

The pattern of interictal EEG abnormalities may help determine the type of epileptic disorder. Focal spike-and-wave discharges or slow waves indicate a partial epileptic disorder. A diagnosis of benign Sylvian epilepsy may be confirmed by characteristic centrotemporal spikes that are easily differentiated from the anterior temporal EEG transients of temporal lobe epilepsy. While bilaterally synchronous EEG discharges may also reflect a focal lesion (secondary bilateral synchrony), especially in the frontal lobes, such activity more often indicates a generalized epileptic disorder. Focal or diffuse slowing of baseline EEG rhythms and irregular or asymmetrical spike-and-wave complexes at a frequency of 2.5 per second or less indicate that the generalized epileptic disorder is secondary rather than primary.

Activation procedures used in the EEG laboratory include hyperventilation for absences, photic stimulation for photosensitive epilepsy, and sleep. But there are major pitfalls: hyperventilation in children and some normal adults can induce high amplitude slowing resembling spike-and-wave discharges; photomyogenic responses of facial muscles to photic stimulation can occur in normal individuals and during drug and alcohol withdrawal and should not be considered evidence of epilepsy; a number of normal sharp transients that occur during sleep and on arousal often are misinterpreted as epileptic spikes.

Nonstandard techniques, available in some laboratories, may offer additional diagnostic advantages. Nasopharyngeal and sphenoidal electrodes can clarify interictal EEG spike patterns originating in mesial temporal structures, but the same information usually can be obtained more easily from ear lobe electrodes. Special epilepsy centers exist throughout the country that offer prolonged EEG telemetry and television monitoring to provide a more precise description of specific ictal events when diagnosis is in doubt. Ambulatory EEG monitoring is being developed for outpatient evaluations.

A repeat EEG may be indicated to determine whether behavioral deterioration is due to an increase in subclinical seizure activity, an increase in drug side effects, or a progressive underlying lesion. If necessary, EEG telemetry combined with frequent antiepileptic drug level determinations or ambulatory monitoring can improve medical management by allowing dose schedules to be tailored to individual patients' needs.

The EEG is also essential for monitoring the progress of therapy for status epilepticus when clinical behavior is not a reliable guide. This is often true in stupor related to spike-and-wave discharge patterns and in complex partial status epilepticus and is always the case when anesthesia or paralysis is used to control major motor status epilepticus.

DIFFERENTIAL DIAGNOSIS. The diagnosis of epilepsy should be made only on firm clinical evidence. Such a diagnosis can have irreversible psychosocial effects resulting in the loss of a driver's license, a job, independence, and self-esteem. Consequently, a physician often does more harm by making an unjustified diagnosis than by reserving judgment until the nature of the disorder has declared itself adequately. When doubt exists injury can be minimized by warning the patient to avoid the conditions that might have precipitated the event and to be aware of potentially dangerous situations should another event occur.

Systemic Disturbances. Syncope is the most common systemic disturbance confused with epilepsy. Syncope can be associated with motor twitches and in rare instances may produce a tonic-clonic convulsion in susceptible individuals. This condition must be treated as syncope, not as epilepsy. Because cardiogenic syncope can cause a convulsion while seizures may be associated with cardiac arrhythmias, diagnostic monitoring of blackout spells should ideally include both ECG and EEG recordings. Other intermittent systemic disorders that can be mistaken for epilepsy include breath-holding spells in early childhood, hyperventilation syndrome, alcoholic blackouts, intermittent porphyria, hypoglycemia, pheochromocytoma, tetanus, and toxic-metabolic abnormalities.

Neurologic Disturbances. Nonepileptic episodic neurologic disturbances are most often of vascular origin. Transient ischemic attacks must be considered when intermittent neurologic symptoms occur in older patients. Drop attacks beginning in adulthood usually are caused by posterior fossa vascular disturbances or cataplexy and are almost never epileptic. Transient global amnesia also is more likely to have a vascular rather than an epileptic cause. Prodromal migraine symptoms can resemble epileptic seizures, and the subsequent headache can be mistaken for a postictal headache. The distinction between migraine and epilepsy is not always completely clear.

Sleep disorders are also commonly mistaken for epilepsy. Narcolepsy is easily diagnosed when all four of the classic symptoms are present; however, if sleep attacks, cataplexy, sleep paralysis, or hypnogogic hallucinations occur alone, they can be confused with epileptic seizures. Careful questioning usually will elicit evidence for some of the other symptoms as well. Hypersomnia, as seen in Klein-Levin and sleep-apnea syndromes, as well as dyssomnias such as somnambulism, night terrors, and enuresis must be differentiated. On rare occasions epileptic seizures can be manifested as nocturnal ambulation, fear, and urinary incontinence; all-night sleep EEG recordings may be necessary to make the correct diagnosis in such instances.

Other neurologic symptoms that can masquerade as epilepsy include intermittent vertigo from a variety of causes and the episodic uncontrolled movements that occur with *Gilles de la Tourette's syndrome,* hemiballismus, chorea, athetosis, and other extrapyramidal disorders. Although the involuntary movements of paroxysmal choreoathetosis are not epileptic, they can often be successfully treated with antiepileptic medication. The myoclonic disorders discussed earlier also should not be confused with epilepsy.

Behavioral Disturbances. It is extremely important to differentiate between true epileptic seizures and conversion reactions. Hysterical seizures (*pseudo seizures*) may be manifested in ways that have psychologic significance such as with pelvic thrusting, may involve motor symptoms that do not fit with known anatomic spread patterns, and only rarely result in injury to the patient despite risk. Nevertheless, it is impossible to make this diagnosis definitively from a description or even from observation of a seizure. Virtually any paroxysmal behavior, no matter how bizarre, could be a true epileptic seizure. The diagnosis of hysterical seizures may be made with some confidence, however, when ictal events are suggestive for the reasons just stated, EEG recordings are normal, antiepileptic medication is ineffective, and evidence of secondary gain is obtained during psychiatric interview. EEG telemetry and television monitoring of ictal events may help to substantiate the diagnosis.

There are several considerations, however, which limit conclusions drawn from telemetry. Simple partial ictal events may have no EEG correlates that can be recorded from the scalp, EEG changes that accompany motor seizures may be obscured by muscle artifact (but postictal EEG suppression is evidence that a true epileptic seizure has occurred), and repeated bilaterally synchronous myoclonic jerks unassociated with loss of consciousness may be mistaken for psychogenic events. Even if a definite diagnosis of hysterical seizure disorder can be made, many such patients have epileptic seizures as well. When hysterical seizures and real seizures coexist, EEG and television monitoring may help to differentiate the two types and provide a basis for independently assessing the results of psychiatric and medical treatment.

Some true epileptic symptoms can be confused with behavioral disturbances. Frequently occurring absences in children can be mistaken for attentional deficits, learning disabilities, and disciplinary problems, but the EEG should provide the correct diagnosis. Certain simple partial seizures with sensory or psychic symptoms may be interpreted as psychotic hallucinations. Although these epileptic experiences can have an emotional content, they usually are more strereotyped and more likely to have visual components than are psychotic hallucinations. Rarely, *fugue states* may represent continuous epileptic seizures *(poriomania)* or prolonged periods of postical confusion.

Episodic dyscontrol is a poorly defined entity consisting of intermittent periods of inappropriately violent, occasionally destructive behavior. Confusion with epilepsy is compounded by the fact that some patients with this syndrome have epileptic seizures as well. If the episodic behavior lasts only several minutes, is uncharacteristic of the patient's interictal personality, and there is amnesia for the event with appropriate remorse afterward, this may possibly reflect an epileptic disturbance. Although ictal EEG recordings have not supported this contention, an occasional patient with episodic dyscontrol may be helped by antiepileptic medication. Organized and directed violence is not seen during the epileptic seizures described earlier, and epilepsy is never the cause of premeditated criminal acts.

Epileptic Seizures That Are Not Epilepsy. Under certain circumstances generalized tonic-clonic convulsions can occur entirely as a natural reaction to physiologic stress or transient systemic injury and should not be considered evidence of an epileptic illness. These include single isolated convulsions resulting from documented precipitating events such as sleep deprivation, alcohol or sedative drug withdrawal, use of convulsant drugs, fever, and acute head trauma and recurrent convulsions induced by reversible infectious, toxic, or metabolic processes and limited to the period of systemic illness. However, a chronic epileptic condition probably exists if there is an indication of focal ictal or postictal features; if there is evidence of an intracerebral lesion; or if seizures recur in the absence of the presumed cause.

TREATMENT. Treatable causes of epileptic seizures include intracerebral mass lesions that can be surgically removed and toxic, metabolic, infectious, and vascular diseases that require medical management. A treatable cause cannot be found in most patients with chronic recurrent seizures, however, and the objective of therapy is then to maximize useful function, ideally by complete eradication of seizures without introduction of additional unwanted side effects. Adequate control is usually possible with appropriate pharmacologic, surgical, and psychosocial management. Only about half of patients treated for chronic epilepsy can expect to become seizure free indefinitely.

Pharmacologic Therapy. Although many antiepileptic drugs are available, it is prudent to become familiar with and use the few that are most effective for each of the various seizure types (Table 510–3). Pharmacologic therapy is based on obtaining an accurate diagnosis of seizure type or epileptic syndrome, selecting the single most appropriate drug for that diagnosis (monotherapy), and correlating measurements of drug levels in the serum with patient reports in order to adjust dosages and dose schedules for the best control and fewest side effects. The best control does not necessarily mean the greatest reduction in seizure frequency. In certain patients, the disability caused by some continued seizures may be less than limitations induced by therapy. For example, a few absences a day for a child is preferable to an alternative of no seizures on a dose of antiepileptic medication that produces continuous sedation and impairs school performance. Similarly, aggressive therapy is not justified for a patient with refractory epilepsy when high drug levels exacerbate existing physical and mental handicaps without producing a worthwhile improvement in the seizure pattern.

Pharmacokinetic Principles. Dose planning for individual antiepileptic drugs depends on the pharmacokinetic factors that determine the amount of available drug in the blood. The therapeutic ranges for individual antiepileptic drugs refer to the ranges of steady state levels of each drug that are effective in controlling seizures. Average or approximate pharmacokinetic variables for the commonly used antiepileptic drugs appear in Table 510–4.

The proper dose schedule for a newly introduced drug depends on balancing the need for rapid control of seizures against the avoidance of side effects. If a patient has been warned about the possible occurrence of another seizure and takes appropriate precautions, it usually is not necessary to build a drug level rapidly at the risk of producing severe side effects. It is more important that the patient accept the drug of first choice. Patients can be encouraged to remain on medication by beginning a drug regimen slowly, taking the medication with meals when nausea is anticipated, using higher doses at bedtime when sedation is anticipated, and reducing doses transiently when untoward side effects occur. Most unpleasant dose-related side effects are temporary, and an appropriate regimen eventually can be instituted. A loading dose can be given practically for some drugs (phenytoin and phenobarbital) when the risk of repeated seizures requires therapeutic levels to be rapidly achieved despite side effects. A loading dose of 1.5 (rather than 2) times the calculated total daily dose may be an adequate compromise between obtaining rapid seizure control and producing minimal side effects if the planned maintenance schedule is begun less than one half-life after the loading dose.

Although a maintenance steady-state level of a drug can be achieved with an interdose interval of approximately one half-life time, in this situation drug levels will fall below the protective range if a single dose is missed. However, a dose schedule that requires a drug to be taken too frequently may be inconvenient and reduce compliance. An interdose interval of 0.5 half-lives, which amounts to one to four times a day for the commonly used medications, is usually recommended. Therapeutic failure using recommended dose schedules may result from aberrant absorption and metabolism in some pa-

TABLE 510–3. THERAPEUTIC CLASSIFICATION OF EPILEPTIC SEIZURES

Seizure Type	Preferred Drugs
Partial seizures and generalized convulsions	Carbamazepine Phenytoin Phenobarbital Primidone Valproic acid
Absences	Ethosuximide Valproic acid Clonazepam
Myoclonus	Clonazepam Valproic acid

tients, and dose schedules must then be determined individually from measurements of serum drug levels.

The recommended therapeutic range for a given drug is based on average measures. One should use these values as a guide rather than a goal; therapeutic drug levels in individual patients may be well above or well below the average. Once an effective maintenance schedule has been achieved, determinations of trough serum drug levels, drawn just before the morning dose, provide a reliable record of long term alterations in steady state conditions. Such measurements are useful when recurrence of seizures or side effects result from decreases or increases in available drug.

ENZYME INDUCTION AND INHIBITION. The most common reasons that subtherapeutic antiepileptic drug serum levels occur after an effective maintenance schedule has been achieved are failure of patients to comply with the dose and enzyme induction. Enzyme induction refers to the increased metabolism of a drug by the liver as a result of chronic administration of that drug or addition of another drug. Because of enzyme induction, the steady state serum levels of a drug may gradually decline with time on the same dose schedule. If seizures recur and serum drug determinations reveal lower steady state levels, the amount of drug given should be increased. A common error at this point is to add a second drug that produces further enzyme induction and leads to subtherapeutic levels of both drugs. Because the antiepileptic effects usually are not cumulative but the toxic side effects are, there is an increase in both seizures and toxic symptoms.

Enzyme inhibition can also occur with addition of a new drug. Consequent reduction in metabolism causes an increase in the serum level of the first drug. In this situation, side effects that may be ascribed to the newly added second drug are actually related to toxic levels of the first. When a patient must use more than one drug, measurements of serum drug levels are essential to determine how these drugs are interacting and which may be responsible for altering seizure frequency or increasing side effects.

The best strategy for pharmacologic management is to choose the single best drug for the condition and gradually to increase the dosage over weeks or months until seizure control or intolerable side effects occur. The end point of this process must be determined clinically for each patient. If a drug is ineffective, it should be replaced with another by gradually reducing the first drug while increasing the second. An exacerbation of seizure frequency may be a transient response to withdrawal of the first drug and does not indicate that the second is ineffective. To obtain optimal control when multiple seizure types are present, the use of two drugs may be unavoidable.

Selection of Antiepileptic Drugs. PREFERRED AGENTS. While specific types of seizures respond to specific drugs (Table 510–3), many factors determine the choice of the best single drug for an individual patient. The trend today is to treat generalized convulsive and partial seizures first with either carbamazepine or the hydantoin phenytoin. The idiosyncratic hematologic side effects of carbamazepine, which were generally feared when this drug was initially introduced, have proved to be rare, and carbamazepine often is preferred over phenytoin by epileptologists. While both drugs offer the same protection, phenytoin use is associated with a high incidence of disturbing cosmetic side effects.

The barbiturates primidone and phenobarbital are also used for convulsive and partial seizures. They are less effective than carbamazepine and phenytoin, but some authorities prefer to begin with phenobarbital because it is the least expensive of the available antiepileptic drugs and has the fewest dangerous side effects. Sedation is common but may not be a problem at lower doses and may subside over time even at higher doses. Furthermore, both carbamazepine and phenytoin can dull mentation at high doses. Barbiturates are a problem in children, since these drugs commonly engender hyperkinetic activity and other undesirable behavioral disturbances. Most epileptologists now generally prefer carbamazepine for this age group because it does not seriously alter behavior. Phenobarbital should not be given to patients with depressive tendencies. It can exacerbate psychologic depression and is the most common mechanism of suicide in the epileptic population.

The drug of choice for absence seizures remains ethosuximide, since it is safer than valproic acid. Valproic acid can produce serious idiosyncratic hepatic side effects that laboratory tests may not predict. Fortunately, mortality from this complication is rare (1 per 35,000), and valproic acid is effective against a variety of seizure types. Valproic acid is the drug of choice for mixed seizure disorders because of its broad spectrum of action and for juvenile epileptic myoclonus. Valproic acid may be more effective than ethosuximide for atypical absences and also is used widely as a second choice drug for other types of seizures. Enzyme inhibition occurs with valproic acid, which greatly increases serum levels of other antiepileptic drugs. This is a particular problem with the barbiturates and sometimes results in inadvertent sedation or even coma.

The drug of choice for nonepileptic forms of myoclonus is the benzodiazepine clonazepam, although valproic acid is also effective against most myoclonic phenomena. In progressive myoclonus epilepsy, where myoclonic jerks and seizures are both present, valproic acid may be the best hope for control with monotherapy. If this is unsuccessful, clonazepam plus carbamazepine or phenytoin may be required. Clonazepam and valproic acid given together may interact to make seizures worse and produce unpleasant side effects.

SECOND LINE ANTIEPILEPTIC DRUGS. Clonazepam is a benzodiazepine currently used as an adjunctive medication for convulsive and partial seizures, although it may also be an effective

TABLE 510–4. COMMONLY USED ANTIEPILEPTIC DRUGS

Drug	Seizure Type	Adult Dose (mg/kg)	Therapeutic Range (μg/ml)	Half-life (hours)	Peak Time (hours)	Daily Doses
Carbamazepine (Tegretol)	P, GC	15–25	8–12	12	2–6	4
Phenytoin (Dilantin)	P, GC	3–8	10–30	24	4–8	2
Primidone (Mysoline)†	P, GC	10–20	5–15	12	2–4	4
Phenobarbital	P, GC	2–4	15–40	96	6–18	1
Chlorazepate (Tranxene)	P, GC	0.7–1.0	1–2*	30*	1*	2
Mephobarbital (Mebaral)	P, GC	4–10	10–30*	96*	6–18*	1
Mephenytoin (Mesantoin)	P, GC	2–10	10–40	100*	27*	1
Ethosuximide (Zarontin)	A	10–30	40–100	30‡	2–3	2
Trimethadione (Tridione)	A	20–40	500–1200*	240*	120–240*	1
Clonazepam (Clonopin)	A, M	0.03–0.3	0.01–0.05	30	1–2	2
Methsuximide (Celontin)	P, A	10–25	20–40*	40*	<3	2
Valproic acid (Depakene)	All	15–60	50–100	8	1–4	4

Modified in part from Leal KW, Troupin AS: Clin Chem 23, 1964, 1977.
*For derived metabolite.
†Substantial antiepileptic effect is obtained from derived phenobarbital.
‡For children (60 hours for adults).
Key: P = partial; GC = generalized convulsive; A = absence; M = myoclonus.

primary antiepileptic. Other drugs that may be of value if first line drugs fail include the hydantoin mephenytoin and the barbiturate mephobarbital for convulsive and partial seizures and clonazepam and trimethadione for absences. Methsuximide is effective against absence and atonic and partial seizures and can be used alone or as an adjunctive medication. Acetazolamide may be a useful adjunctive medication, particularly for ten days premenstrually through the end of menses for women with catamenial accentuation of epilepsy. Adrenocorticotropic hormone (ACTH) and adrenocorticosteroids have been found useful in the treatment of infantile spasms but not in other epileptic conditions.

SIDE EFFECTS. Almost all antiepileptic drugs potentially produce undesirable side effects, and physicians should consult the *Physicians' Desk Reference* or a current textbook before first use. Common dose-related side effects of carbamazepine and the hydantoins include nausea, dizziness, diplopia, and ataxia. Sedation, impaired mentation, and hyperactivity occur most often with the barbiturates and benzodiazepines. These symptoms may abate with time. Drug-induced folic acid deficiencies may reach symptomatic levels in some patients and require vitamin supplements. Idiosyncratic side effects that usually affect skin, blood, liver, and kidneys are potentially more serious. When a new drug is introduced, complete blood counts and appropriate blood chemistry analyses should be obtained every four weeks for several months, and then monitored every 3 to 12 months as long as therapy continues. Leukopenia as low as 3000 commonly occurs with carbamazepine and does not necessarily indicate impending agranulocytosis. Moreover, an elevated serum alkaline phosphatase level alone does not indicate a hepatotoxic reaction. Mild pruritus may be treated medically. Evidence of blood dyscrasias, liver or kidney damage, or more serious skin rash requires prompt discontinuation of medication and referral to the proper specialist. Cosmetic side effects commonly associated with phenytoin include hirsutism, gingival hyperplasia, and coarsening of features; weight gain and alopecia are occasionally seen with valproic acid therapy. Carbamazepine can cause water retention and is not used for patients with congestive heart failure. A paradoxic increase in seizure frequency may result from elevated drug levels, particularly with phenytoin, and can cause seizures to recur after a period of control.

Pregnancy presents certain problems for women with epilepsy. Seizures may become more frequent, and antiepileptic drug clearance may increase, requiring higher doses of medication. Hemorrhagic disease of the newborn occurs with phenobarbital and phenytoin and can be treated with vitamin K. A two- to three-fold drug-related increase in the incidence of birth defects has been documented for phenytoin, but the nature of all antiepileptic drugs is such that they may have teratogenic effects. Phenytoin is not recommended for women of childbearing age; however, there is little to be gained from discontinuing effective medication once pregnancy has been determined, especially after the first trimester has been completed. The risk to mother and fetus from seizures may be greater than the risk of teratogenicity. Maternal drug levels can cause sedation and withdrawal in newborns but do not present a problem for breast-fed infants.

Surgical Therapy. Resective surgery has proved safe and beneficial and can cure a chronic epileptic condition when all else fails. Most surgical facilities will consider epileptic patients potential candidates for resective surgical therapy if (1) a partial seizure disorder has been documented, (2) seizures continue at a frequency that seriously interferes with daily living despite adequate levels of appropriate antiepileptic medication, and (3) there is not substantial interictal mental retardation or psychosis. Patients with complex partial seizures of temporal lobe origin are ideal candidates for surgery. Worthwhile improvement occurs in 85 per cent of such patients, and as many as two thirds may become seizure free after anterior temporal lobectomy. Common postoperative deficits include a visual superior quadrantanopsia and minor memory disturbances, the latter being more noticeable with resection in the dominant hemisphere. Local resection of an extratemporal focal epileptogenic lesion is also possible if the area of cortex can be identified precisely and removed safely. A history of generalized convulsions, a focus in the dominant hemisphere, or the presence of bilateral independent temporal spike foci on EEG do not contraindicate surgery.

Presurgical evaluation varies from center to center but generally involves localization of an epileptogenic lesion responsible for all or most of the patient's habitual seizures and determination that the abnormality can be removed without producing unacceptable neurologic deficits. Localization by surface EEG alone is possible if confirmed by independent tests of focal dysfunction such as neuropsychologic evaluations, analysis of baseline and barbiturate-induced EEG rhythms and more recently positron emission tomography. Stereotaxic depth electrode recordings can identify resectable epileptogenic lesions in some patients with complicated presentations who would not otherwise be considered surgical candidates. When necessary, the extent of the cortical excision is determined by intraoperative electrocorticography.

Section of the corpus callosum has been particularly effective in controlling drop attacks, and patients with other secondary generalized and partial seizure patterns have experienced improvement from this operation. While *hemispherectomy* is the most effective surgical procedure for epilepsy, it is only justified for children who have severely incapacitating unilateral seizures and hemiparesis. Destructive lesions and cerebellar stimulation are no longer routinely recommended.

Other Therapeutic Considerations. Patients with some types of seizures may benefit from special management. Reflex seizures induced by specific stimuli can be treated by avoiding the stimuli. For example, epileptic photosensitivity can be abolished by patching one eye or wearing colored glasses, and desensitization is possible for many forms of reflex seizures. Spread of some simple partial seizures may be aborted by strong or painful sensory stimulation administered at onset. Operant conditioning (biofeedback) sometimes can reduce seizures in some patients, but the approach is generally impractical. When seizures occur only at specific times of the day, medications can be adjusted to insure maximum levels at those times, and daily schedules can be altered so that the patient is home or in a safe environment when at risk.

Patients with all types of seizures should remain active and maintain daily habits that insure regular meals, adequate sleep, and a reduction in unnecessary stress. Alcohol or sedative drugs can be taken sparingly, but excessive use can provoke seizures during withdrawal. Patients who have seizures associated with an alteration in consciousness, particularly those that occur without warning, should be counseled to avoid hazardous situations: they should not swim alone, should shower rather than bathe, should not climb to unprotected heights, and should not operate potentially dangerous power-driven machines, including automobiles.

A *ketogenic diet* has been used as a last resort to treat children with medically intractable generalized seizures, but this does not replace antiepileptic drugs and usually has minimal or no effect on seizure frequency and severity.

Emergency Treatment. First aid for a generalized tonic-clonic convulsion consists of protecting the patient from self-injury. Clothing should be loosened, sharp objects removed from the area, and the patient's head cushioned from impact. Hard objects or fingers must not be inserted into the patient's mouth: patients do not choke on their own tongues. When the seizure is over, turn the patient's head to drain oral secretions. Have someone stay with the patient during the postictal period until full consciousness has returned. It is not necessary to call an ambulance unless the patient has never had a seizure before, the seizure lasts longer than ten minutes, another attack occurs before consciousness is regained, or there is evidence of injury, respiratory distress, or pregnancy. Patients should not be forcibly restrained during complex partial seizures but protected from surrounding hazards until ictal and postictal symptoms cease and they can care for themselves.

Major motor status epilepticus is a medical emergency requiring immediate intervention to prevent permanent brain damage or death. A recommended approach appears in Table 510–5. As soon as the airway is secured, a quick neurologic examination should be performed to appraise critical forebrain and brainstem functions. There may be evidence of an acute intracerebral lesion with herniation or other life-threatening conditions. Because the effects of diazepam are short-lived, it should be administered simultaneously with a longer-acting antiepileptic drug. Phenytoin usually is preferred, since it produces no sedative effects. This allows the patient to regain consciousness when seizures are terminated and facilitates neurologic evaluation. If seizures have not stopped 60 minutes after the institution of therapy, high intravenous doses of phenobarbital or general anesthesia are recommended; some physicians prefer to use a 4 per cent intravenous solution of paraldehyde in normal saline solution, which can be titrated to maintain the desired therapeutic effect. If these latter approaches are necessary, intubation and ventilation should be used and the progress of treatment followed with EEG recordings.

Once status has been controlled, maintenance drug therapy is instituted. The most common cause of major motor status epilepticus is a sudden reduction or discontinuation of antiepileptic drugs in patients with known seizure disorders.

Psychosocial Considerations. To some extent, psychosocial disturbances among epileptics are situational. Because most seizures occur spontaneously and unpredictably, many patients spend their lives anticipating inappropriate behavior, embarrassment, or serious injury. When patients have a sufficient warning, they may be able to remove themselves from public view or from potentially dangerous situations. In many cases, however, the fear of seizures may cause conscious or unconscious major restructuring of life patterns, with some patients almost becoming reclusive. Epileptics are frequently unable to find work if they admit to a seizure disorder, so that their opportunities for rewarding social relationships are reduced and a sense of worthlessness ensues. In most states, patients with seizures that impair consciousness are not allowed to drive. They are advised to undertake activities that could result in serious injury with caution and never alone, so that their self-confidence is further damaged. Depression and suicide are more common among epileptics than in the general population.

Although the evidence is controversial, a high incidence of aberrant personality traits, affective disorders, and psychoses are suggested among patients with epilepsy, particularly those with complex partial seizures of limbic origin. The literature variably describes *"the epileptic personality"* with words such as aggressive, emotional, overinclusive, sober, hypermoral, and hyposexual. However, the findings are by no means consistent. Even if such traits can be attributed to certain epileptic patients, it is unclear how much of this behavior results from functional disturbances caused by the underlying pathologic lesions or specific seizure activity, how much can be attributed to the effect of long-term antiepileptic drug therapy, and how much relates to the patient's long overprotection and the stigmata of being epileptic. Several authors have reported a paranoid schizophreniform psychosis in patients who have had epilepsy for many years, but the specificity of this syndrome is also debatable.

Only about one in four patients with uncontrolled epilepsy is handicapped by seizures alone. The others have physical, intellectual, and/or psychiatric disabilities that disrupt their daily lives. Epileptic seizures, perhaps more than any other neurologic symptom, are modified by internal and external influences that are under the control of the patient and other persons. For these reasons, treatment of the epileptic patient requires more than manipulation of anticonvulsant drugs, and outcome depends upon more than just seizure control. The physician must come to know the patient and the patient's family, their psychologic interactions, and their social situation. Furthermore, improving psychosocial adaptation itself often leads to a reduction in seizure frequency. To provide the comprehensive care required by patients with seizure disorders, the physican must attend to the patient as well as to his neurological disorder. The doctor must be friend as well as therapist.

TABLE 510–5. MANAGEMENT OF CONVULSIVE STATUS EPILEPTICUS

Treatment Goal	Cumulative Time Since Arrival in Emergency Room (Minutes)
Restore homeostasis	
Check for airway obstruction; check blood pressure, nasal O_2; intubate as needed	0–15
Draw blood sample for glucose, blood urea nitrogen, electrolytes, complete blood count, drug level determination	0–15
Start administering isotonic saline solution, 1000 ml, IV	
Administer glucose 50%, 50 ml, IV; thiamine, 100 mg, IM	0–15
Stop convulsive seizures	
Give diazepam, 10 mg. IV; repeat administration of 10 mg with every seizure, up to 50 mg*	15–60
Give phenytoin, 20 mg/kg, IV (< 50 mg/minute)	15–60
If seizures do not stop by 1 hour, give high doses of phenobarbital IV or general anesthesia	60–120

Modified from Wasterlain CG. *In* Engel J Jr, et al.: Ann Intern Med 97:584, 1982.

*Exceeds manufacturer's recommended dosage.

Commission on Classification and Terminology of the International League Against Epilepsy: Clinical and electroencephalographic classification of epileptic seizures. Epilepsia 22:489, 1981. *The currently accepted classification of epileptic seizures and definition of relevant terms.*

Dreifus FE, Lee SI: Epilepsy Case Studies. Garden City, Medical Examination Publishing Company, 1981. *A brief introduction to the clinical approach to epilepsy, followed by a large number of case histories illustrating specific points with questions, answers, discussions, and appropriate references.*

Engel J Jr, Crandall PH, Rausch R: The Partial Epilepsies. *In* Rosenberg RN, et al. (eds.): The Clinical Neurosciences. New York, Churchill Livingstone, 1983. *A discussion of surgical therapy for epilepsy, including presurgical evaluation and operative techniques.*

Engel J Jr, Troupin AS, Crandall PH, Sterman MB, Wasterlain CG: Recent developments in the diagnosis and therapy of epilepsy. Ann Intern Med 97:584, 1982. *A concise review of modern approaches to the management of epileptic patients. Includes recent references.*

Epilepsy Abstracts 1947–present. *Published first by* Excerpta Medica, *this monthly journal contains abstracts of all epilepsy-related papers and is an easy entrance into the literature on any subject.*

Gastaut H, Broughton R: Epileptic Seizures. Springfield, Charles C Thomas, 1972. *Complete descriptions of almost all epileptic phenomena.*

Gumnit RJ: The Epilepsy Handbook, The Practical Management of Seizures. New York, Raven Press, 1983. *An excellent practical guide for the diagnosis and treatment of patients with epilepsy. Does not include references.*

Penfield W, Jasper H: Epilepsy and the Functional Anatomy of the Brain. Boston, Little Brown, 1954. *A classic by pioneers of modern epileptology; describes epileptic phenomena and applications of clinical data to the understanding of normal brain functions.*

Schwartzkroin PA, Wyler AR: Mechanisms underlying epileptiform burst discharges. Ann Neurol 7:95, 1980. *A Review of basic research on epileptic mechanisms and an attempt to synthesize conflicting data from various experimental models.*

Solomon GE, Kutt H, Plum F: Clinical Management of Seizures. Philadelphia, W. B. Saunders Company, 1983. *This small handbook is packed with information for the practicing physician, including many illustrations, tables, and references.*

Spehlmann R: EEG Primer. Amsterdam, Elsevier/North Holland, 1981. *A simple straightforward introduction to clinical EEG.*

Temkin O: The Falling Sickness: A History of Epilepsy from the Greeks to the Beginnings of Modern Neurology. Baltimore, Johns Hopkins University Press, 1945. *A detailed account of epilepsy facts and fiction throughout history.*

Woodbury DM, Penry JK, Pippenger CE (eds.): Antiepileptic Drugs. New York, Raven Press, 1982. *A multiauthored compendium of recent concepts of pharmacologic therapy of epilepsy.*

Section Twelve INTRACRANIAL TUMORS AND STATES OF ALTERED INTRACRANIAL PRESSURE

511. INTRACRANIAL TUMORS

William R. Shapiro

Intracranial tumors include neoplasms, both benign and malignant, and space-taking lesions of chronic inflammatory origin (granulomas) that develop in brain, meninges, or skull. The present chapter concerns neoplasms; granulomas are covered elsewhere. Neoplastic tumors frequently affect the nervous system. Primary tumors of the central nervous system are the second most common cancer in children, and in adults are more common than systemic Hodgkin's disease. In 1983 in the United States there were approximately 12,000 new cases of primary central nervous system cancer. About 15 per cent of deaths from systemic cancer are directly associated with metastases of the nervous system, mostly from primaries in lung or breast, malignant melanoma, lymphomas, and leukemias.

PATHOGENESIS. ***Intracranial Neoplasms as a Form of Cancer.*** The cause of brain tumors is unknown, although genetic factors appear to be important in tumors such as hemangioblastoma, neurofibroma, and some gliomas. When a patient develops systemic cancer, his body must deal with a "cancer burden" consisting of a population of neoplastic cells in the blood or bone marrow (leukemia) or in a solid, single mass or in multiple metastatic masses (carcinoma or sarcoma). For the average adult, it is thought that a 1-kg burden of systemic tumor is lethal. In contrast, a brain tumor shares its space in the skull with the brain, which already occupies 1200 cc, and in this confined space 100 grams of tumor is almost always lethal. By the time a patient develops neurologic symptoms, the tumor is usually 30 to 60 grams in size. Benign intracranial tumors are slow growing, with few mitoses, no necrosis, and no vascular proliferation. They may arise in the meninges or as neuroectodermal tumors. Malignant tumors are characterized by more rapid growth, invasiveness, frequent mitotic figures, necrosis, vascular proliferation, and endothelial hyperplasia. However, "benign" brain tumors that cannot be entirely excised will be lethal, and "malignant" brain tumors rarely metastasize out of the central nervous system. Thus, the distinction between benign and malignant is less important for intracranial tumors than for systemic cancer.

Intracranial tumors differ from systemic cancers in several other ways. Primary neuroectodermal tumors tend to infiltrate the brain, whereas secondary metastatic brain tumors are partly encapsulated. The microenvironment of tumors in the brain—the blood-brain barrier—influences both diagnosis and therapy. The blood-brain barrier in normal brain retards entry of many compounds, including radiologic contrast agents and chemotherapeutic drugs. The blood-brain barrier appears to be intact in most benign neuroectodermal tumors, but it becomes progressively disrupted in malignant brain tumors. The breakdown of the barrier allows the entry of contrast agents and radioisotopes that permit the tumor to be perceived separately from the brain in scanning techniques. Both experimental and clinical studies suggest that the disruption of the barrier in malignant tumors also permits the entry of chemotherapeutic agents. It is not yet clear to what degree the blood-brain barrier breaks down at the growing edge of an infiltrative malignant brain tumor or within very small brain tumors; in both circumstances, the barrier may be only minimally disrupted. A second factor that distinguishes brain tumors from systemic cancer is the absence of a lymphatic system in the brain. Fluid that accumulates from leaking capillaries within the brain tumor cannot be removed except via slow diffusion toward the cerebrospinal fluid (CSF) pathways. This fluid, or "cerebral edema," itself produces symptoms by adding to the mass effect of tumors. Central nervous system tumors are also distinguished from systemic cancer by the rarity with which they metastasize to the rest of the body. Instead, they tend to infiltrate within the brain, and some have a predilection to spread along CSF pathways, producing obstruction and hydrocephalus. Perhaps the most important difference between central nervous system neoplasms and systemic cancer is that "cancer operations" are not possible in the brain. Removing generous margins of normal tissue along with such visceral tumors as lung or colonic cancer interferes with normal function to only a moderate degree. On the other hand, attempting to remove normal tissue margins in brain tumor can produce irreparable neurologic dysfunction. The surgeon removing visceral cancer operates in the surrounding normal tissue. The neurosurgeon attempting to remove a primary neuroectodermal tumor must stay within the confines of the tumor if he is to spare brain tissue. Often, he must leave tumor-infiltrated brain tissue because its removal would produce unacceptable neurologic dysfunction. Such considerations weigh heavily in the management of patients with intracranial neoplasms.

CLASSIFICATION AND PATHOLOGY. Tumors of the nervous system may be classified by pathology and by location. Table 511–1 depicts a classification of intracranial tumors by both pathology and location. Pathologically tumors are defined in terms of their tissues of origin. Neuroectodermal tumors are the most common primary parenchymal tumors of the central nervous system and occur at any age. About half are relatively benign, infiltrating astrocytomas, but they may be cystic. Neuroectodermal tumors can arise in the cerebrum in the form of astrocytomas, oligodendrogliomas, and the more malignant glioblastoma multiforme. Childhood astrocytomas tend to lie in the cerebellum and are frequently cured by surgical extirpation. Juvenile astrocytomas occur around the third ventricle, and most brainstem gliomas are infiltrating astrocytomas. Adult astrocytomas may be calcified, and some undergo malignant degeneration. The oligodendroglioma is often calcified but only rarely becomes malignant. The classic malignant parenchymal brain tumor is the glioblastoma multiforme. This tumor may arise de novo or by progressive malignant degeneration of an astrocytoma. About half of all intracranial gliomas are glioblastomas; 20 per cent are astrocytomas. In children, astrocytomas represent half of the cerebellar tumors, medulloblastomas and ependymomas making up the rest of the intracranial tumors.

Older classifications defined astrocytomas in four grades from the histologically most benign (grade I) to the most malignant (grade IV). However, a simpler classification has been shown in trials of brain tumor therapy to correlate more predictably with prognosis. *Astrocytomas* are characterized histologically by increased numbers of uniform cells resembling fibrillary gemistocytic or, less commonly, protoplasmic astrocytes; mitoses are absent. Patients harboring this tumor commonly survive four to seven years or longer. *Anaplastic astrocytomas* contain astrocytic elements with considerable nuclear pleomorphism, markedly increased cellular density, increased mitotic figures, endothelial hyperplasia, but no necrosis. These tumors are associated with survival of 1.5 to 2.5 years. *Glioblastoma multiforme* is characterized by heterogeneous cell populations with bizarre pleomorphic nuclei that make it difficult to identify their astrocytic origin. There is prominent endothelial hyperplasia and areas of focal necrosis that often resemble palisades. Survival with this tumor exceeds a year in only a minority of patients.

Intracranial ependymomas occur primarily in children as fourth ventricle masses that obstruct the CSF pathways. Medulloblastomas arise from a primitive neuroectodermal cell, usually in the cerebellum, and may seed throughout the CSF. They are highly malignant, although sensitive to radiation therapy and chemotherapy.

Mesodermal tumors are represented most commonly by the benign meningioma. Meningiomas arise in certain favored sites: along the dorsal surface of the brain, the base of the skull, the

TABLE 511–1. CLASSIFICATION OF INTRACRANIAL TUMORS

	Location and Macroscopic Characteristics	Microscopic Characteristics
Neuroectodermal		
Astrocytoma	Diffuse infiltration, especially cerebrum and brainstem; microcystic or macrocystic, especially in cerebellum; occasionally calcifies	Astrocytic proliferation and infiltration; may convert to glioblastoma multiforme
Oligodendroglioma	Circumscribed, globular mass, often cystic and often calcifies	Diffuse, cellular, wide perinuclear halos; rarely becomes malignant
Glioblastoma multiforme (malignant astrocytoma)	Variegated, infiltrative; occasionally cystic, necrotic, or hemorrhagic	Cellular pleomorphism, necrosis, palisading; endothelial hyperplasia, mitoses present
Ependymoma	Most often fourth ventricle, demarcated	Regular, polygonal cells that form rosettes; rarely malignant
Medulloblastoma	Most commonly arises in vermis of cerebellum in children	Highly cellular, hyperchromatic nuclei; seeds the meninges via CSF
Mesodermal meningioma	Arises from dura on dorsal surface, along base of brain, from falx, sphenoid ridge	Benign, variable pattern; rarely converts to malignant tumor
Cranial nerves		
Acoustic schwannoma (acoustic neurilemoma), trigeminal neurilemoma	Nodular mass on cranial nerve	Benign, Schwann cell proliferation
Neurofibroma	Nodular mass on cranial nerve	Schwann cell and fibroblast proliferation
Pituitary tumors		
Adenomas	Sellar and suprasellar masses of various sizes	Chromophobic, acidophilic, and basophilic; all may be secretory or nonsecretory
Craniopharyngioma	Sellar or suprasellar, often calcified and cystic	Derived from Rathke's pouch
Pineal tumors	Germinomas, may produce endocrinopathy	May seed via CSF
Metastatic tumors	Parenchymal, skull, meningeal	Depends on nature of primary tumor
Vascular tumors	Arteriovenous malformation	Non-neoplastic
	Hemangioblastoma (von Hippel-Lindau syndrome)	Neoplastic
Congenital tumors	Craniopharyngioma, chordoma, dermoid, teratoma	
Granuloma and parasitic cysts	Tuberculoma, toruloma (cryptococcosis), sarcoidosis, cysticercosis	

falx cerebri, the sphenoid ridge, or within the lateral ventricles. Although these tumors are benign, they often reach large size before they are discovered and may be difficult to remove. The most common cranial nerve tumor is the acoustic schwannoma (neurilemoma, neuroma). Such tumors have been discovered earlier in recent years through the advent of refined auditory tests and computed tomographic (CT) scans and are frequently removable via a translabyrinthine approach. The pituitary tumors include the adenomas and the craniopharyngiomas. Pituitary adenomas may appear as intrasellar masses extending into an extrasellar location. The advent of advanced radiologic techniques has made it easier to diagnose microadenomas of the pituitary. Craniopharyngiomas are developmental tumors derived from Rathke's pouch and may be intrasellar or suprasellar in location; they are frequently calcified and often cystic. Pineal tumors occur primarily in children and rarely truly originate from the pineal gland; most commonly they are germinomas and may produce endocrinopathies. Metastatic tumors may invade the brain parenchyma, the skull, or the meninges; their pathology depends on the primary tumor. The benign colloid cyst usually grows in the anterior third ventricle. Vascular tumors include arteriovenous malformations, which are not truly neoplastic, and the hemangioblastomas, which are. The latter tumors, when located in the brainstem or cerebellum, may be part of the von Hippel–Lindau syndrome that includes hemangioblastomas elsewhere in the body. Congenital tumors include the craniopharyngiomas, chordomas (that arise from the primitive notochord), dermoids, and teratomas. Granulomas and parasitic cysts come from tuberculomas, cryptococcosis (toruloma), sarcoidosis, and cysticercosis.

PATHOPHYSIOLOGY. Brain tumors produce *generalized symptoms* because of their expanding size and *focal symptoms* by direct compression on or infiltration into specific areas of the brain. As tumors grow, they raise the intracranial pressure because the volume of the intracranial cavity is fixed. The total mass effect is a sum of both the tumor size and the cerebral edema the tumor produces. Large tumor masses obstruct the CSF pathways, producing enlargement of the upstream ventricular system. As the primary or secondary mass produced by the tumor enlarges, brain tissue may be displaced through the fixed intracranial openings, producing various herniation syndromes as discussed in Ch. 472.

Focally, the mass of the tumor compresses and infiltrates the surrounding brain tissue. Edema, produced within a parenchymal brain tumor, increases the total size of the mass. Cerebral edema may also be produced by compression by an extra-axial tumor, in which case the edema comes from the brain itself. Focal symptoms occur as the tumor compresses surrounding brain, producing distortion and ischemia; such symptoms may be reversible if the pressure is relieved before tissue necrosis occurs. In addition, tumor tissue may infiltrate along nerve fiber tracts, interfering with neurologic function. Cyst formation within tumors provides another mechanism that compresses adjacent normal brain.

CLINICAL MANIFESTATIONS. The symptoms and signs of intracranial tumor depend on the size of the tumor and on its rate of growth. The characteristic clinical feature of intracranial neoplasms is that they produce progressive symptoms. The rate of progression ranges from an acute apoplectic onset such as follows hemorrhage into an intracranial neoplasm, or a seizure disorder associated with cortical stimulation to a slowly progressive mental deterioration associated with slower growing neoplasms.

Headache occurs frequently as a general manifestation of an intracranial neoplasm and most commonly accompanies rapidly growing tumors. Of special importance are headaches that have recently begun or changed in character, are worse in the morning or awaken the patient at night, or are of a recurrent nature. The occurrence of a headache in a patient not otherwise prone to headaches or a recent change in headache pattern in patients known to have headaches should alert the physician to a possible intracranial expanding lesion.

Papilledema occurs in only about one fourth of patients with intracranial neoplasms, and its absence does not exclude such pathology. It is more likely to accompany tumors that obstruct CSF flow and may be accompanied by visual phenomena, especially acute visual obscurations and "graying out." Papilledema is part of the "pseudotumor cerebri" syndrome described below.

Generalized convulsions, along with focal seizures (see below), occur in 35 per cent of patients with cerebral tumors. They are more likely to accompany slower-growing tumors than the more rapid malignant neoplasms. They are more likely to occur following alcohol use or withdrawal of barbiturates or other sedative drugs. The onset of generalized convulsions in the adult or focal seizures at any age should alert the physician to the possibility of a structural lesion. Intracranial tumors produce generalized major motor seizures and various forms of focal seizures. Minor temporal lobe seizures that occasionally resemble petit mal attacks may accompany temporal lobe tumors. Other lesions of the temporal lobe may give rise to psychomotor seizures that may be associated with olfactory hallucinations (uncinate fits), disorders of visual or auditory perception, or episodes of "déjà vu" phenomena or of automatic behavior. Jacksonian seizures usually imply a lesion of the motor or sensory cortex.

Mental changes are frequent manifestations of intracranial tumor. They are often subtle in quality and gradual in onset and may not attract the attention of coworkers or family members until the patient's behavior changes substantially. Mental changes may include impersistence in routine tasks, increased irritability, emotional lability, inertia, faulty insight and forgetfulness, reduction in the range of mental activity, indifference to social practices, reduced initiative and spontaneity, and blunted affect. The patient may complain of fatigue, tiredness, dizziness, and lethargy. If the tumor continues to grow, such symptoms progress to confusion, dementia, and eventually stupor. Changes in personality may be described in psychologic terms but should be recognized as symptoms of structural brain disease rather than functional anxiety or depression.

Nausea and vomiting may occur as a result of direct or reflex stimulation of the emetic center of the medulla. This most often accompanies increased intracranial pressure, particularly with brainstem displacement secondary to herniation or bleeding into the CSF. Vomiting that occurs without preceding nausea may be projectile.

Vasomotor and autonomic changes that accompany expanding intracranial tumors include bradycardia and hypertension, as well as respiratory abnormalities associated with brainstem compression. Rarely, patients with brain tumor may have gastric ulceration (Cushing's ulcer) that may produce hemorrhage. Fortunately, however, the adrenal corticosteroids used for treating the edema of brain tumors rarely contribute to such hemorrhages. Other autonomic changes associated with hypothalamic compression include fever, hypothermia, hyperthermia, disturbances in eating and drinking, and occasionally more specific abnormalities such as diabetes insipidus, inappropriate antidiuretic hormone secretion, hypopituitarism, and precocious puberty.

False localizing signs may accompany prolonged elevation of intracranial pressure. They include unilateral or bilateral lateral rectus palsy from sixth nerve traction and compression, hemiplegia ipsilateral to a cerebral tumor from compression of the opposite cerebral peduncle against the tentorium, and visual field defects ipsilateral to the tumor from compression of the opposite posterior cerebral artery.

Focal clinical manifestations of intracranial tumors depend on localized impairment of nervous tissue function, and therefore vary with the location of the process. Of specific interest are focal seizures which sometimes accompany cerebral tumors. They imply specific cortical irritation from either a benign or a malignant condition. Visual loss—reduced visual acuity, field defects, or diplopia—implies involvement of the visual apparatus from a local eye problem to the occipital cortex or to the oculomotor nerves. Hearing impairment may mean reduced auditory acuity or the occurrence of tinnitus, and may be associated with vertigo. Speech disturbances may be transient or progressive and include dysphasia and dysarthria. Motor signs include postural disturbances, incoordination, weakness, and tremor. Sensory disturbances include unusual pains, paresthesias, or numbness. Ataxia may accompany local tumors in the posterior fossa or occasionally in the frontal lobes. Anosmia may be associated with infrafrontal meningiomas. Neuroendocrine disturbances may accompany pituitary and pineal tumors. Cerebral hemorrhage into a tumor, usually choriocarcinoma, testicular tumors, melanomas, glioblastomas, and, more rarely, other primary tumors, may produce an associated subarachnoid hemorrhage.

TUMOR SYNDROMES. Tumors of the cerebral hemispheres are characterized by progressive, focal neurologic deficits and commonly by generalized or focal convulsive seizures. Tumors of the *frontal lobe*, being in a "silent area," often first cause impairment of judgment and of intellectual function. Tumors involving the motor pathways produce contralateral hemiplegia. A tumor of the medial surface of the frontal lobe may cause urinary urgency or, occasionally, precipitate incontinence. Mental changes and ataxic gait are common when the tumor spreads across the corpus callosum to both frontal lobes. Tumors of the dominant hemisphere are frequently associated with disturbances in language.

Parietal lobe tumors may produce either generalized convulsions or sensory focal seizures. Cutaneous tactile, pain, and temperature senses are usually spared, but stereognosis and the cortical sensory modalities (position sense, two-point discrimination) are impaired contralaterally. Contralateral homonymous hemianopia, apraxia, and anosognosia (nonrecognition of bodily defects) may also be present with tumors in the nondominant hemisphere. Denial of illness is characteristic, especially if obtundation is present. Speech disturbances, agraphia, and finger agnosia may occur when the tumor involves the dominant hemisphere. Thalamic invasion produces contralateral cutaneous sensory impairment.

Temporal lobe tumors, particularly in the nondominant hemisphere, are often relatively "silent" except when they cause convulsive seizures. A tumor deep in the temporal lobe may cause contralateral hemianopia, psychomotor seizures, or convulsive seizures, preceded by an olfactory aura or visual hallucinations of complex formed images. Tumors involving the surface of the dominant temporal lobe produce mixed expressive and receptive aphasia or dysphasia, chiefly anomia.

Occipital lobe tumors usually cause contralateral quadrantic defects in the visual field or a hemianopia with sparing of central vision. Associated seizures may be preceded by an aura of flashing lights, but not formed images.

Cranial, extradural, or subdural metastatic tumors, by compression or invasion of the underlying brain tissue, produce the same localizing signs as those caused by primary tumors.

Tumors of the *pituitary* and suprasellar region produce neurologic and endocrinologic abnormalities. Pituitary adenomas may present as intrasellar secretory or nonsecretory masses, or masses with extrasellar extension. Secretory adenomas produce hormones that cause specific endocrinopathies. For example, adenomas that overproduce growth hormone lead to gigantism prior to puberty and acromegaly after puberty. Basophilic adenoma produces ACTH, leading to Cushing's syndrome. Chromophobe adenomas once were believed not to secrete hormones, but now are known to be responsible for most of the endocrinopathies caused by pituitary tumors. The most common endocrine hypersecretion is prolactin, producing amenorrhea and galactorrhea in women and, less frequently, impotence and gynecomastia in men. Many secretory tumors are microadenomas found only after an endocrine abnormality is discovered.

Enlarging pituitary adenomas cause headache; as the tumor grows out of the sella, it compresses the optic chiasm, nerve, or tracts and the hypothalamus. The most common visual field defect is bitemporal hemianopia, but unilateral optic atrophy, contralateral hemianopia, or any combination of the three may occur. Hypothalamic compression usually causes diabetes insipidus from injury to the supraoptic-pituitary tract. The tumor may destroy functioning glandular tissue and cause pituitary deficiency. Skull x-rays show a characteristic balloon-shaped appearance of the sella, but microadenomas may produce no more than laterally placed focal bulging of the sellar floor, visible only on x-ray tomograms.

Other tumors in the region of the sella turcica (e.g., meningiomas, craniopharyngiomas, metastases, dermoid cysts) or aneurysms may compress the optic chiasm, invade the sella, and produce symptoms similar to those of chromophobe adenoma.

Pineal tumors (usually germinomas) occur at any age but are most common in childhood. Precocious puberty may result, especially in boys. The tumor compresses the aqueduct of Sylvius, causing hydrocephalus, papilledema, and other signs of increased intracranial pressure. The pretectum rostral to the superior colliculi is also compressed, resulting in paralysis of upward gaze, ptosis, and loss of pupillary light and accommodation reflexes.

Gliomas of the brainstem are usually astrocytomas, of which about one half eventually become anaplastic. Symptoms result from destruction of nuclear masses or unilateral or bilateral paralysis of the fifth, sixth, seventh, and tenth cranial nerves and paralysis of lateral gaze. Damage to the motor or sensory pathways causes hemiplegia, hemianesthesia, or cerebellar disturbance (ataxia, nystagmus, intention tremor). Increased intracranial pressure appears late in brainstem tumors.

Posterior fossa tumors: Tumors of the fourth ventricle and cerebellum (usually medulloblastomas, ependymomas, or occasionally a metastasis) interfere with CSF circulation, and symptoms of increased pressure appear early. Ataxic gait, intention tremor, and other signs of cerebellar dysfunction follow.

Cerebellopontine angle tumors, particularly acoustic schwannomas, are characterized by tinnitus, unilateral hearing impairment, and sometimes vertigo. Pressure on the adjacent cranial nerves, brainstem, and cerebellum produces loss of corneal reflex, facial palsy and anesthesia, palatal weakness, signs of cerebellar dysfunction, and, rarely, contralateral hemiplegia or anesthesia. Loss of vestibular response to caloric stimulation, enlargement of the porus acusticus as shown by skull x-ray, and a high CSF protein content suggest an acoustic schwannoma.

Diffuse meningeal neoplasm (meningeal carcinomatosis): Carcinomas, gliomas, sarcomas, melanomas, and lymphomas may diffusely infiltrate the leptomeninges and subarachnoid space to produce a syndrome of chronic meningitis, which may simulate chronic meningitis caused by fungi, tuberculosis, sarcoidosis, and meningovascular syphilis. Characteristically, there is involvement of more than one central nervous system region, i.e., brain, cranial nerves, spinal cord and nerves. Common manifestations include headache, mental changes, cranial nerve palsies, weakness and areflexia, and minimal or no signs of meningeal irritation. The CSF findings generally establish the diagnosis. The pressure may be normal or elevated, sugar content is often below 45 mg per deciliter, protein content is usually elevated, and cell counts may reveal an increased number of mononuclear cells or cytologic evidence of malignant cells. Cultures are negative. Biochemical tumor markers (β-glucuronidase) are frequently present.

Optic nerve gliomas may develop in the intraorbital, retro-orbital, or chiasmatic region of the optic nerve, the first being most common. These tumors usually occur in early childhood, with uniocular loss of vision as the most common presenting symptom. Proptosis is seen in about a third of the cases. Uniocular optic atrophy or papilledema may be noted. X-ray evidence of enlargement of the optic foramen is common. The tumor is most often a slowly growing astrocytoma, may be associated with neurofibromatosis, and will occasionally invade the hypothalamus.

Tumors of the skull: Benign osteomas rarely reach a size sufficient to compress underlying brain. Malignant tumors arising in the paranasal sinuses or nasopharynx directly invade the base of the skull and cause chronic facial pain and multiple cranial nerve involvement. Tumors of the glomus jugulare (nonchromaffin paraganglioma) arise near the jugular bulb and often lead to progressive deafness and a bloody discharge in the external auditory canal. Other lesions that give x-ray evidence of bone destruction and that must be differentiated include Paget's disease, Hand-Schüller-Christian disease, eosinophilic granuloma, and cholesteatoma (epidermoids). As noted, metastases are common to the skull and will occasionally invade through the dura to produce subdural effusions indistinguishable in their manifestations from subdural hematoma.

DIAGNOSIS. Computed tomography and now nuclear magnetic resonance (NMR) scanning permit the diagnosis of most intracranial tumors at a level of safety not achievable by invasive techniques. Such tumors produce abnormalities in the normal structures and may be visualized directly or after the intravenous infusion of iodide-containing contrast material (see Fig. 511–1). Skull tumors are seen as eroded regions of bone. Parenchymal lesions may distort the normal ventricular structures and produce cerebral edema visible as low density regions in the brain's parenchyma. After intravenous contrast enhancement, the tumor may be visualized as a hyperdense region, frequently ring-like, around a central radiolucent area. The more malignant the tumor, the more densely enhanced will it appear. The degree of enhancement is a function of the breakdown of the blood-brain barrier rather than of the presence of tumor cells themselves, and therefore is much more likely to occur with more malignant tumors. Low density lesions may imply cysts, necrotic tumor, or cerebral edema. Ventricular enlargement occurs secondary to obstruction of CSF pathways. CT has almost eliminated the need for pneumoencephalography in the diagnosis of brain tumor, although contrast-enhanced arteriography may be necessary as an aid to guiding surgical treatment. In the latter technique, the tumors are visualized as displacing normal blood vessels and often demonstrate abnormal vasculature within the tumor itself.

Routine skull x-rays are usually not needed when high-quality CT scanning is available. Similarly, electroencephalography and isotope encephalography have been largely replaced by CT scanning as a screening test for brain tumor.

Lumbar puncture and examination of CSF rarely contribute to the diagnosis of intracranial neoplasm except for diffuse meningeal carcinomatosis. Lumbar puncture is contraindicated in the presence of raised intracranial pressure associated with a mass lesion producing incipient herniation. A CSF examination for meningeal carcinomatosis should be deferred until after CT is used to search for solid intracranial neoplasms.

DIFFERENTIAL DIAGNOSIS. The characteristic clinical feature of intracranial neoplasm is progressive neurologic dysfunction traceable to a focal neurologic origin. The onset may be abrupt, as when a hemorrhage or seizure occurs, or may be insidious as the brain tumor grows. Any neurologic disease producing similar symptoms can be confused with intracranial neoplasm; a neoplasm should be ruled out while considering other diagnoses. Computed tomography is the procedure of choice. The importance of considering other neurologic syndromes in differential diagnosis lies in emphasizing the clinical differences that should lead the physician to search for intracranial neoplasm.

Benign intracranial hypertension is described in detail elsewhere (Ch. 513). Patients develop headache and papilledema but usually have no focal signs, and CT demonstrates no mass lesions. Patients with stroke characteristically present with acute onset of neurologic dysfunction, although occasionally a "stuttering" onset may be confused with the insidious history of tumor. Patients with subdural hematoma may have headache, drowsiness, papilledema, and hemiparesis; the diagnosis can be suspected on clinical grounds but requires CT or arteriography for certainty. Patients with dementia from Alzheimer's disease usually have minimal motor abnormalities. The problem of differentiating tumor from granuloma or abscess is more difficult. Cysticercosis is suggested by exposure to an endemic area and by the presence of eosinophilic pleo-

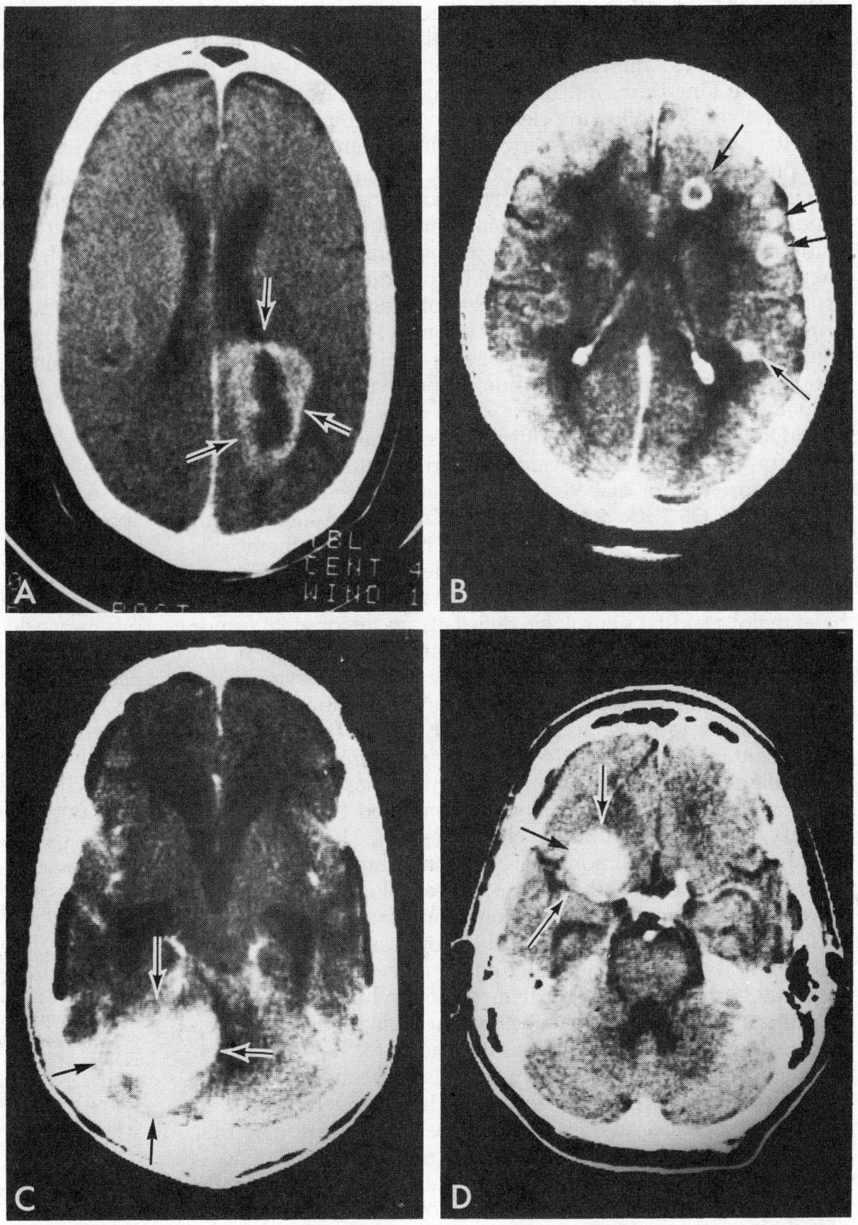

Figure 511–1. Computed tomographic scans of patients with intracranial tumors. *(A)* Glioblastoma multiforme of the medial parieto-occipital lobes. Note the ring enhancement with central region of hypodensity (arrows). *(B)* Multiple metastatic brain tumors from carcinoma of the lung. Each enhanced mass represents a brain tumor (arrows). *(C)* Medulloblastoma of the right and mid-cerebellum. Note the displacement and encroachment of the fourth ventricle and hydrocephalus (arrows). *(D)* Sphenoid wing meningioma. The lesion is diffusely contrast enhanced (arrows).

cytosis in the CSF. Although CT scans are usually characteristic, a differential diagnosis between tumor and brain abscess can sometimes be difficult and may require biopsy.

TREATMENT. ***Surgery.*** The principles of treating intracranial neoplasm include its removal if possible, its palliation if unresectable. Surgery for intracerebral tumors has several goals: (1) diagnosis, which can be established in life only by surgical tissue removal; (2) treatment of symptoms, especially those arising from increased intracranial pressure; (3) debulking of tumor as a form of anticancer therapy; and (4) permitting time for radiation and early chemotherapy. Surgery for meningiomas should be aimed at total removal and cure if possible, and subtotal removal to relieve symptoms if total removal is not possible. For infratentorial parenchymal tumors, surgery is necessary for diagnosis and to open CSF pathways. Surgery for benign cerebellar or acoustic schwannomas is potentially curative. For acoustic schwannoma, surgery may be accomplished by a translabyrinthine approach if the tumors are small, or by suboccipital craniectomy if the tumors are larger. Surgery for metastatic brain tumors should be considered in selective circumstances if the metastatic tumor is single or if systemic disease is minimal or well controlled. Pituitary tumors are usually removed by transsphenoidal resection, although, if they are large, a transfrontal craniotomy may be necessary.

Radiation Therapy. Radiation is utilized primarily for malignant tumors. The radiation therapy is delivered through whole-head or large-field ports for a total dose of up to 6000 rads in six to seven weeks. Radiation therapy has been recommended as a form of treatment in low grade astrocytomas and oligodendrogliomas, although the efficacy of such therapy has not been demonstrated by prospective trials. For such tumors, the radiation is usually limited to the region of the tumor at total doses of 5000 to 5500 rads. Radiation therapy is the therapy of choice for most metastatic brain tumors. Radiation therapy is frequently recommended for large pituitary tumors after surgery.

Medical Therapy. Corticosteroid hormone therapy usually will relieve cerebral edema if present. Steroids almost always improve general clinical manifestations, but are less effective against specific clinical manifestations. Dexamethasone in doses of 16 to 32 mg per day is recommended, although attempts should be made to reduce the doses slowly to a level of relatively stable symptoms. Anticonvulsants are given to patients who have seizures, and any patient who develops generalized or focal seizures should be placed on anticonvulsants for three to five years or permanently, if attacks continue postoperatively. Patients who do not have seizures usually do not require long-term anticonvulsant therapy. Since the likelihood of a seizure following clean neurosurgical intervention is low, it is usually not necessary to maintain such patients on anticonvulsants. Seizures occurring late after primary therapy for intracranial neoplasms imply recurrence of tumor and should immediately lead to re-evaluation of the patient's status. National cooperative trials have demonstrated that several chemotherapeutic agents are useful in the adjunctive treatment of malignant astrocytomas. Two examples are bis-chloroethyl-nitrosourea (BCNU) and methyl-cyclohexyl-chloroethyl-nitrosourea (methyl-CCNU). These agents are highly toxic and should only be administered under the direction of physicians trained in their use.

Endocrine replacement is often necessary after treatment of pituitary adenomas and includes anterior pituitary hormones and vasopressin for diabetes insipidus as required.

OUTCOME OF THERAPY AND PROGNOSIS. For *malignant neuroectodermal tumors,* e.g., glioblastoma multiforme, therapy is palliative, almost never curative. Patients are often able to return to gainful employment for a year or two, unless they have major residual neurologic deficits from the original tumor or from the surgery. Late radiation damage to the brain can occur and may be responsible for the return of symptoms, although tumor recurrence accounts for most patient worsening. Chemotherapy is immunosuppressive and bone marrow depressant, and may lead to systemic infection and bleeding. For malignant astrocytomas, most recent studies give a median survival time of 52 weeks following combined treatment with surgery, radiation, and BCNU chemotherapy; 25 to 30 per cent of patients survive 18 months. Factors favoring longer survival include age younger than 50, histopathology of anaplastic astrocytoma rather than glioblastoma multiforme, and minimal postoperative neurologic deficit. The prognosis for more benign intracerebral neuroectodermal tumors is better than for the malignant tumors. Radiation therapy is often helpful. Although patients may have minimal residual neurologic deficits, they frequently return to gainful employment for several years. Seizures are likely, but control is usually obtained. Patients may survive for three to seven years with relatively preserved neurologic deficit until tumor recurrence or progression occurs. Childhood medulloblastoma carries a much better prognosis with the advent of whole neuraxis radiation therapy; five-year survival rates of 50 to 60 per cent are now being reported.

Following therapy of *metastatic brain tumors,* short-term results are often good. With a combination of steroids and either radiation therapy alone or a combination of surgery and radiation therapy, two thirds to three fourths of patients show substantive amelioration of presenting symptoms. Many patients are able to return to work for short periods of time. The median survival of such patients is approximately six months, with survival at a year limited to 10 to 15 per cent of the patients. Most patients do not die of their metastatic nervous system disease but rather of their primary or systemic cancer. There are occasional long-term survivors of more than two years. *Meningeal carcinomatosis* treated with combination radiation therapy and intrathecal chemotherapy often responds when the primary tumor is lymphoma or carcinoma of the breast. Both neurologic deficits and the CSF may improve for periods of up to a year or more. Affected patients usually die of their systemic disease.

Meningiomas are often curable. There may be residual neurologic deficits, including seizures, but overall the prognosis for survival is excellent, and that for neurologic recovery is good to very good. After surgery for meningiomas, most patients return to full-time employment. Meningiomas rarely recur and rarely become malignant, and most patients can be expected to survive a normal lifespan. The prognosis of patients with *acoustic schwannomas* depends on the size of the tumor. For small acoustic schwannomas and especially those removed by translabyrinthine approach, the results are excellent, with a low mortality and a high percentage of cures. Eighth nerve deficits, including hearing loss and some vestibular difficulty, may hinder overall functional capacity. Facial paresis is common, and occasionally functionally disturbing. In contrast, there is a 10 to 20 per cent mortality with surgical resection for large tumors and considerable morbidity. Many patients have residual neurologic deficits, including hearing loss, facial paresis, and hydrocephalus.

Pituitary tumors and *craniopharyngiomas* carry a fairly good prognosis. Fifty to 60 per cent of macroscopically obvious pituitary adenomas come to attention because of visual failure, whereas in 20 per cent headaches are the initial symptom. Less commonly, an endocrine abnormality is noted, although microadenomas, occurring primarily in women, are usually diagnosed because of infertility, galactorrhea, or amenorrhea. Rarely, pituitary apoplexy can occur. Adult craniopharyngiomas similarly have a good prognosis, although recurrence is somewhat more common than in children following therapy of such tumors. Pituitary tumors may be removed by transsphenoidal microsurgery or craniotomy. They may also be treated by irradiation alone or irradiation after surgery. Surgery is indicated if vision is threatened, but the method of treatment of microadenomas is controversial. Hyperprolactinemia from pituitary adenomas may be effectively treated with bromocriptine, but resection or irradiation is necessary to treat the tumor itself.

Other intracranial tumors generally have a good prognosis, depending on their location. *Cholesteatomas* and *colloid cysts* are usually easily removed with little neurologic deficit, although some tumors may not be resectable because of danger to surrounding normal brain.

Bloom HJG: Medulloblastoma in children: Increasing survival rates and further prospects. Int J Radiat Oncol Biol Phys 8:2023, 1982. *A concise review of the problem of therapy in this disease by a recognized authority. Well referenced.*

Cairncross JG, Kim J-H, Posner JB: Radiation therapy for brain metastases. Ann Neurol 7:529, 1980. *One of the largest series of such cases yet reported.*

Fishman RA: Brain edema. N Engl J Med 293:706, 1975. *An excellent review of the mechanisms of cerebral edema.*

Russell DS, Rubinstein LJ: Pathology of Tumours of the Nervous System. 4th ed. Baltimore, Williams & Wilkins Company, 1977. *An excellent, well illustrated textbook of tumors of the nervous system.*

Shapiro WR: Treatment of neuroectodermal brain tumors. Ann Neurol 12:231, 1982. *A review of the treatment of adult primary brain tumors; includes results of national cooperative trials of surgery, radiation therapy, and chemotherapy.*

Walker MD: Brain and peripheral nervous system tumors. In Holland JF, Frei E (eds.): Cancer Medicine. 2nd ed. Philadelphia, Lea & Febiger, 1982, p 1603. *A good review of the clinical presentation of central nervous system tumors.*

Wasserstrom WR, Glass JP, Posner JB: Diagnosis and treatment of leptomeningeal metastases from solid tumors: Experience with 90 patients. Cancer 49:759, 1982. *A definitive review of wide-ranging experience with this disease, including its diagnosis and treatment.*

512. INTRACRANIAL HYPOTENSION

David A. Rottenberg

Cerebrospinal fluid (CSF) pressure measured at lumbar puncture in the lateral decubitus position normally ranges from 70 to 200 mm CSF (5 to 15 mm Hg). Low (or zero) lumbar CSF pressure may be recorded in patients with chronic subdural hematoma or spinal subarachnoid block. Such low pressure recordings may be associated with normal or raised intracranial pressure in the absence of free communication between the ventriculocisternal and lumbar CSF compartments. Intracranial hypotension with low lumbar CSF pressure is usually a consequence of prior lumbar puncture, craniospinal CSF fistula, or profound dehydration. The term *aliquorrhea*—spontaneous or "primary" intracranial hypotension—has been used to describe those rare cases in which, in the absence of known or discernible CNS injury or disease, self-limited symptoms and signs of low spinal fluid pressure develop.

The clinical syndrome of low spinal fluid pressure is characterized by severe throbbing frontal and occipital headache, which appears within 30 seconds after the patient assumes an erect posture and which subsides completely when he lies down. Associated complaints may include dizziness, nausea, stiff neck, and photophobia. The disorder often arises 3 to 21 days after lumbar puncture, and the symptoms described are uncommonly followed by diplopia and a rapidly evolving (unilateral or bilateral) abducens palsy. In most instances, the palsy resolves completely within six weeks to six months. Rarely, auditory symptoms such as buzzing, popping, humming, roaring or frank hearing loss may supervene.

Symptoms and signs of intracranial hypotension probably result from CSF leakage, loss of the normal CSF "cushion," and caudal displacement of the brain within the cranial vault. Traction on pain-sensitive intracranial structures, including cerebral veins and venous sinuses dilated in a compensatory manner, and stretching of the abducens nerve over the apex of the petrous temporal bone probably account for the observed headache and diplopia. Auditory symptoms and signs may reflect a functionally important fall in intralabyrinthine pressure. Treatment is largely symptomatic, since the manifestations of the low spinal fluid pressure syndrome are almost always transient. When symptoms are persistent, disabling, or both, an *epidural "blood patch"* may be indicated. This procedure involves the injection of 10 ml of the patient's own blood into the epidural space to seal a presumed dural leak. Rarely, in very long-lasting cases surgical exploration has exposed the dural leak and closed it. As regards symptomatic intracranial hypotension following lumbar puncture, the use of a small (22-gauge) needle diminishes the risk of headache and abducens paralysis. Contrary to popular belief, bed rest has no effect on the incidence or duration of post-lumbar-puncture headache.

MacRobert RG: The cause of lumbar puncture headache. JAMA 70:1350, 1918. *A classic description of lumbar puncture headache. No better illustrations of the causative mechanism have ever been published.*

Vandam LD, Dripps RD: Long-term follow-up of patients who received 10,098 spinal anesthetics. JAMA 161:586, 1956. *This prospective study of over 10,000 spinal anesthetizations documents the incidence of headache associated with lumbar puncture and describes the syndrome of decreased intracranial pressure.*

513. INTRACRANIAL HYPERTENSION

David A. Rottenberg

Cerebrospinal fluid (CSF) pressure in excess of 250 mm CSF is usually a manifestation of serious underlying neurologic disease. Although intracranial hypertension is most often observed in the setting of a rapidly expanding intracranial mass lesion, CSF outflow obstruction or cerebral venous congestion as well as a variety of systemic and central nervous system disorders may be pathophysiologically associated with increased intracranial pressure (ICP) (Table 513–1). It should be emphasized that lumbar CSF pressure may not accurately reflect ICP. In patients with intracranial mass lesions and brain hernias, lumbar CSF pressure may be normal or low despite grossly elevated supratentorial CSF pressure. Kinking of the aqueduct of Sylvius or impaction of the temporal lobes into the tentorial incisura or of the cerebellar tonsils into the foramen magnum can prevent the transmission of ICP into the lumbar subarachnoid space.

There are no pathognomonic symptoms or signs of intracranial hypertension. Nevertheless, the observation of frequently associated symptoms and signs such as headache, papilledema, unilateral pupillary dilatation, oculomotor or abducens paresis, irregular respirations, and so forth should indicate possible raised intracranial pressure. Most of the signs and symptoms traditionally associated with intracranial hypertension are related to traction on cerebral blood vessels, distortion of pain-sensitive dura mater, impending herniation with intermittent vascular compression, midline shifts, or axial distortion of the brainstem and are not caused by increased ICP per se. Papilledema, when present, is the most reliable sign of intracranial hypertension; however, many patients with raised ICP fail to develop papilledema, and in some patients with pseudotumor cerebri (see later discussion), papilledema develops and then subsides spontaneously although CSF pressure remains elevated. Moreover, papilledema is not synonymous with raised ICP. Ocular hypotony, bilateral optic neuritis, orbital venous stasis, retrobulbar tumors, and granulomatous inflammation or cystic lesions of the optic nerve sheath may produce papilledema in the absence of intracranial hypertension. Retinal venous pulsations, when present, imply that CSF pressure is normal or not significantly elevated, but the absence of spontaneous venous pulsations is not helpful diagnostically. A variety of nonepileptic paroxysmal phenomena (crescendo headache, visual obscurations, photopsia, chalastic-hypertonic fits, impairment of consciousness, sensory hallucinations) have been described in relation to spontaneous elevations of ICP, often referred to as *plateau waves.* The occurrence of plateau waves during sleep may explain why nighttime deterioration and early morning headache are frequently reported by patients with raised ICP.

The initial treatment of any patient with increased ICP whose neurologic status is deteriorating is aimed at reducing the volume of the intracranial contents in an attempt to prevent irreversible brain damage (Table 513–2). Once the patient's condition has stabilized, additional treatment modalities are employed in an effort to consolidate the gains of emergency therapy and to allow the physician ample opportunity to deal with the underlying pathologic process. Almost always, ICP is not the actual cause of the patient's distress but a reflection of a pre-existing pathologic process; the definitive treatment of intracranial hypertension is ultimately determined by the nature of the underlying pathologic process.

TABLE 513–1. PATHOGENESIS OF INCREASED INTRACRANIAL PRESSURE

Perturbation	Proximate Cause	Clinical Example
Increased dural sinus venous pressure	Sinus compression or occlusion	Sagittal sinus thrombosis Otitic hydrocephalus Brain tumors
	Increased sinus blood flow	CO_2 retention Arteriovenous malformation
	Increased peripheral venous pressure	Internal jugular vein occlusion Superior vena cava syndrome Congestive heart failure
Increased CSF outflow resistance	Ventricular outflow obstruction	Brain tumors Aqueductal stenosis
	Obliteration of the cisternal and/or convexity subarachnoid space	Meningitis Extra- or subdural masses Cerebral masses or edema
	Plugging of the arachnoid villi	Subarachnoid hemorrhage Infectious polyneuritis Spinal cord tumors
Increased rate of CSF formation	Increased choroidal CSF formation	Choroid plexus papilloma
	Increased extrachoroidal CSF formation	Hypo-osmolality Cerebral edema

TABLE 513–2. EMERGENCY TREATMENT OF IMPENDING HERNIATION IN ACUTELY DECOMPENSATING PATIENTS

Therapy	Dosage or Procedure
Osmotherapy	Mannitol, 0.5 to 2.0 grams per kilogram intravenously over 15 minutes followed by 25 grams as needed
Corticosteroids	Dexamethasone, 100-mg intravenous push followed by 100 mg daily in divided doses
Hyperventilation	Lower P_{CO_2} to 25 to 30 mm Hg

Ethelberg S, Jensen VA: Obscurations and further time-related paroxysmal disorders in intracranial tumors; syndrome of initial herniation of parts of the brain through the tentorial incisure. Arch Neurol Psychiatr 68:130, 1952. *A fascinating account of pseudoparoxysmal phenomena in patients with intracranial tumors.*

Lundberg N: Continuous recording and control of ventricular fluid pressure in neurosurgical practice. Acta Psychiatr Neurol Scand (Suppl) 149:1, 1960. *An encyclopedic account of ventricular CSF pressure measurement and monitoring. The clinical significance of plateau waves is nowhere better discussed.*

Rottenberg DA, Posner JB: Intracranial pressure control. *In* Cottrell JE, Turndorf H (eds.): Anesthesia and Neurosurgery. St. Louis, C. V. Mosby Company, 1980, pp 89–118. *This well-referenced chapter provides a quantitative description of the CSF system. Some familiarity with the subject is helpful.*

514. PSEUDOTUMOR CEREBRI

David A. Rottenberg

DEFINITION. Pseudotumor cerebri is a syndrome of increased intracranial pressure in the absence of localizing neurologic signs, intracranial mass lesion, or cerebrospinal fluid (CSF) outflow obstruction in an alert, otherwise healthy appearing patient. Pseudotumor (also called *benign intracranial hypertension, serous meningitis,* or *otitic hydrocephalus*) can be associated with a variety of systemic and iatrogenic disorders. The illness is usually brief and benign, lasting weeks to several months. However, recurrent and chronic cases have been reported, and permanent visual loss rarely may occur in spite of vigorous medical or surgical treatment. Chronically increased intracranial pressure may give rise to the "primary empty sella syndrome," which refers to a globular enlargement of the sella turcica caused by an incompetent diaphragma sellae.

CLINICAL MANIFESTATIONS. Pseudotumor cerebri may be manifested as asymptomatic papilledema. More common early symptoms include headache, nausea and vomiting, visual disturbances (blurring, obscurations of vision, scotomata), retro-ocular pain, diplopia, tinnitus, and vertigo. Bilateral papilledema, the cardinal feature, is almost invariably present and may be associated with peripapillary retinal hemorrhages, exudates, or both. Visual loss, the only serious complication of pseudotumor, may occur either early or late in the course of the disease. Hypertension may be a risk factor for visual loss, but obscurations of vision do not predict subsequent visual failure. Characteristically, visual field testing reveals enlarged blind spots. Generalized constriction of the peripheral isopters and inferior nasal quadrantopsia are less frequently observed, as are central and paracentral scotomata. Diplopia, caused by unilateral or bilateral abducens palsy, may develop as a false localizing sign. The remainder of the neurologic examination results are normal. As regards the diagnosis of papilledema, it is important to distinguish *pseudopapilledema*—defined as an anomalous elevation of the optic disc—from true papilledema, which is prima facie evidence of increased intracranial pressure. Anomalous elevation of the optic papilla, which may be associated with identifiable hyaline bodies *(drusen),* should suggest the diagnosis of *retinitis pigmentosa.* In patients with ophthalmologically visible hyaline bodies, static perimetry frequently reveals a range of visual field abnormalities, including enlargement of the blind spot, nerve fiber bundle defects (particularly in the inferior nasal field), and general constriction.

PATHOPHYSIOLOGY. Pseudotumor cerebri is generally believed to be a self-limited disease in which CSF pressure returns to normal as clinical symptoms remit. However, clinical improvement is not always accompanied by a reduction in CSF pressure, and there is a subgroup of pseudotumor patients whose pressure remains persistently elevated after neurologic signs and symptoms have resolved. The course of such cases implies that clinical symptoms may be independent of the absolute magnitude of CSF pressure and that chronically raised intracranial pressure may be totally asymptomatic. Also, despite persistently elevated CSF pressure, most patients with chronic pseudotumor do not become hydrocephalic. This observation suggests that whatever mechanism "resets" CSF pressure above normal does not necessarily predispose to the development of communicating hydrocephalus. Although pseudotumor cerebri may occur without obvious precipitants in the setting of general good health, its occasional relationship to drug administration and steroid withdrawal and its reported association with a variety of endocrine disorders suggest the existence of a final common mechanism rather than a multitude of distinct pathogenetic mechanisms.

Chronically increased intracranial pressure necessarily implies an increase in dural sinus venous pressure, an increase in CSF outflow resistance, an increase in the rate of CSF formation, or some combination of these factors. One or more of these mechanisms must elevate CSF pressure in pseudotumor patients. Pathogenetic hypotheses that postulate an increase in brain bulk consequent to an increase in cerebral blood volume or in brain water content (interstitial brain edema) do not provide an adequate explanation for the intracranial hypertension of pseudotumor.

ASSOCIATED DISORDERS. The typical patient with pseudotumor is 20 to 40 years old, female, and obese. The frequency of menstrual irregularities in obese female pseudotumor patients may simply reflect the increased incidence of menstrual irregularities in obese females of child-bearing age. The association of pseudotumor with head trauma, middle ear disease, internal jugular vein ligation, oral contraceptive use, pregnancy, and polycythemia vera can be explained on the basis of cerebral venous sinus thrombosis and/or increased sagittal sinus venous pressure. Corticosteroid therapy, steroid withdrawal, hypoparathyroidism, hypervitaminosis and hypovitaminosis A, and a variety of commonly prescribed drugs (nalidixic acid, nitrofurantoin, tetracycline, and sulfonamides) have been considered as precipitating causes. In some cases an effect on the arachnoid villi and CSF outflow resistance has been postulated.

DIAGNOSIS. The diagnosis of idiopathic pseudotumor cerebri in a patient with papilledema but without localizing neurologic signs is one of exclusion. Intracranial masses (tumors, hematomata, infections) and CSF outflow obstruction must be ruled out by appropriate neuroradiologic studies, including transmission computed tomography (CT) or nuclear magnetic resonance scanning (NMR), or both. Cerebral angiography is occasionally necessary in order to rule out dural venous sinus or cortical venous thrombosis. Skull films, electroencephalography and/or pneumoencephalography are seldom indicated. Lumbar puncture, which is usually deferred until CT or NMR scanning has revealed a normal or small ventricular system, is required in order to confirm the diagnosis of increased intracranial pressure. Lumbar spinal fluid pressure is elevated, frequently above 300 mm CSF, but the composition of the fluid is normal; the protein content is usually in the low normal range, below 20 mg per dl. Laboratory evidence of hypothalamic-hypophyseal insufficiency may be present, but the diagnostic significance of subclinical endocrinopathy in obese patients with increased intracranial pressure remains to be established. Pseudopapilledema can be distinguished from true disc edema by means of stereoscopic color fundus photography and fluorescein angiography.

TREATMENT. Whereas papilledema may persist for many years without visual impairment, visual failure may occur without warning, often early in the course of the disease. Thus, if the aim of treatment is to prevent visual loss, all pseudotumor patients ideally should be treated from the time of diagnosis. Unfortunately, there is no convincing evidence that any of the frequently recommended treatment modalities are efficacious, and the high rate of spontaneous remission complicates the evaluation of various therapies. At present, four general approaches to symptomatic treatment are used: (1) repeated lumbar puncture, (2) ventriculosystemic shunting, (3) medical treatment (with corticosteroids, glycerol, diuretics, acetazolamide), and (4) incision of the optic nerve sheath.

Although repeated (weekly) lumbar puncture may provide transient relief of symptoms and document the occurrence of remission, there is no convincing evidence that this therapeutic approach is beneficial. Subtemporal decompression, once the mainstay of neurosurgical treatment, has been abandoned because of significant morbidity and mortality in the absence of established benefit. This procedure has been replaced by ventriculosystemic or lumboperitoneal shunting, the efficacy of which has not been determined. The use of glycerol, chlorthalidone, and acetazolamide has been advocated by various authors. Corticosteroids (especially prednisone) have been the mainstay of medical treatment in many clinics, although there is evidence to suggest that systemic corticosteroid administration, by raising intraocular pressure, may increase the risk of visual loss. Incision of the optic nerve sheath for the relief of papilledema is of unproved value and is performed infrequently because of the risk of postoperative blindness.

In conclusion, repeated lumbar puncture and the administration of diuretics (such as furosemide) are relatively safe and may provide temporary symptomatic relief. The use of corticosteroids, which can provoke pseudotumor cerebri in susceptible individuals and may raise intraocular pressure, seems to be contraindicated. The normal or small ventricles of patients with pseudotumor provide difficult targets for shunt catheters; thus, lumboperitoneal shunting is preferable to ventriculosystemic shunting and should be considered the treatment of last resort in patients with disabling symptoms or failing vision, or both.

Ahlskog JE, O'Neill BP: Pseudotumor cerebri. Ann Intern Med 97:249, 1982. *A critical review of the clinical syndrome of pseudotumor cerebri. The section on patient management is particularly noteworthy.*

Bulens C, De Vries WAEJ, Van Crevel H: Benign intracranial hypertension. J Neurol Sci 40:147, 1979. *A careful clinical evaluation of 36 pseudotumor patients with long-term follow-up.*

Corbett JJ, Savino PJ, Thompson HS, Kansu T, Schatz NJ, Orr LS, Hopson D: Visual loss in pseudotumor cerebri. Arch Neurol 39:461, 1982. *This paper provides a detailed and definitive discussion of the only serious complication of pseudotumor cerebri, visual loss.*

515. HYDROCEPHALUS

David A. Rottenberg

Hydrocephalus refers to the net accumulation of cerebrospinal fluid (CSF) within the cerebral ventricles and the consequent enlargement of the ventricles. Although acute obstructive hydrocephalus usually produces a sudden increase in intraventricular pressure, CSF pressure is frequently normal (or low) in patients with chronic hydrocephalus. It is useful to distinguish between "noncommunicating" and "communicating" hydrocephalus; the former is produced by lesions that obstruct the CSF circulation at or proximal to the foramina of Luschka and Magendie, the latter by obstruction of the basal cisterns or convexity subarachnoid space such that the ventricular system communicates with the spinal subarachnoid space. It is also useful to distinguish hydrocephalus associated with cerebral atrophy ("hydrocephalus ex vacuo") from congenital or acquired disorders of the cerebrospinal fluid system

DIAGNOSIS. Ventriculomegaly is readily diagnosed by means of computed tomographic (CT) or nuclear magnetic resonance (NMR) scanning. The diagnosis of hydrocephalus, however, must take into account the increase in ventricular volume that accompanies normal aging and the presence or absence of cerebral atrophy. Enlargement of the temporal horns and an inability to visualize the sylvian and interhemispheric fissures or cerebral sulci, plus the presence of periventricular lucencies, favor the diagnosis of hydrocephalus. A normal or small fourth ventricle in the presence of enlarged lateral and third ventricles suggests aqueductal stenosis.

ACUTE HYDROCEPHALUS. Sudden complete ventricular outflow obstruction leads to acute hydrocephalus, coma, and death. Partial obstruction is more common and only moderately less dangerous. Acute obstructive hydrocephalus may arise as a complication of head injury, spontaneous subarachnoid hemorrhage, cerebellar hemorrhage or infarction, acute exudative meningitis, viral encephalitis, colloid cyst of the third ventricle, and decompensation of large intracranial tumors or hematomas. Chronic hydrocephalus in the adult is most frequently caused by aqueductal stenosis or the complications of subarachnoid hemorrhage; other reported causes and associations include hindbrain (Chiari) malformations, spinal cord tumors, ectasia and elongation of the basilar artery, granulomatous meningitis, and meningeal carcinomatosis. In many instances, the cause of chronic symptomatic hydrocephalus ("normal-pressure hydrocephalus") cannot be determined. It should be noted that unequivocally asymptomatic hydrocephalus may be found in approximately 4 per cent of patients over the age of 60 who consult a neurologist for assorted neurologic complaints and undergo CT scanning.

CLINICAL MANIFESTATIONS. The patient with acute hydrocephalus has severe headache, lethargy, signs of increased intracranial pressure (papilledema and/or abducens palsy), and signs of the causative lesion. Hyperactive reflexes and bilateral extensor plantar responses are almost invariably present. Ventricular CSF pressure is markedly increased, but this increase may not be transmitted to the lumbar subarachnoid space. Patients with chronic communicating hydrocephalus, including normal-pressure hydrocephalus, have a progressive dementia, characterized by forgetfulness and psychomotor retardation, an unsteady gait, and urinary incontinence. Apathy, hypophonia, and bilateral pyramidal and extrapyramidal signs may be present. The lumbar CSF pressure is usually normal or near normal in range.

TREATMENT. Acute hydrocephalus responds dramatically to ventricular drainage and CSF diversion. Treatment of the primary lesion is the treatment of choice. Temporary ventricular decompression or ventriculosystemic shunt may be necessary in some cases. Medical treatment (with acetazolamide) for long-term symptomatic hydrocephalus is not efficacious. Ventricular shunting also has been employed for patients with chronic communicating hydrocephalus. Unfortunately not all respond, and there are no reliable clinical or neuroradiologic predictors of shunt response. Absence of cerebral atrophy and temporary psychomotor improvement after lumbar puncture seem to correlate with, but do not guarantee, benefit from a shunt operation.

Adams, RD, Fisher CM, Hakim S, Ojemann RTG, Sweet WH: Symptomatic occult hydrocephalus with "normal" cerebrospinal-fluid pressure. N Engl J Med 273:117, 1965. *This classic account of normal pressure hydrocephalus is still worth reading.*

Milhorat TH: Acute hydrocephalus. N Engl J Med 283:857, 1970. *A concise account of an uncommon but serious and eminently treatable illness.*

Vassilouthis J, Richardson AE: Ventricular dilatation and communicating hydrocephalus following spontaneous subarachnoid hemorrhage. J Neurosurg 51:341, 1979. *A retrospective study of 210 patients in whom subarachnoid hemorrhage was confirmed by lumbar puncture. The authors distinguish between early and delayed ventricular enlargement and discuss the clinical consequences of both syndromes.*

Section Thirteen INJURY TO THE HEAD AND SPINE

Donald P. Becker

516. HEAD INJURIES

GENERAL CONSIDERATIONS

Head injuries in Western nations are a major contributing factor in half of the deaths that result from physical trauma. Trauma is the leading cause of death in Western nations in persons of ages 1 to 44 years, and head injury clearly is a major medical problem. While 50,000 Americans die each year as a direct consequence of traumatic brain injury, another 50,000 to 60,000 survive severe head injury with varying degrees of disability. Each year about a million Americans seek medical care for a head injury that involves the brain.

The brain injury represents the most serious sequel to head trauma. Brain injuries from head trauma range from mild, in which a person is momentarily stunned and sees "stars," to severe, in which extensive brainstem damage rapidly leads to death. Brain injuries produce various degrees of pathologic damage, ranging from cellular and subcellular reversible injury to shearing and tearing of brain cells and even disruption of brain tissue by contusion, brain hemorrhage, or laceration. The lesions vary in location and degree from patient to patient. Following the initial brain damage, the brain may be further damaged by secondary hypoxemia from respiratory embarrassment, cerebral ischemia from elevated intracranial pressure, or brain shift caused by accumulation of an intracranial hematoma or brain swelling. The physician must seek to define, in each patient, the locations, extent, and nature of the brain damage and plan management accordingly.

MECHANISMS OF BRAIN INJURY AND TRAUMATIC UNCONSCIOUSNESS

DIFFUSE BRAIN MOVEMENT INJURY. The most common mechanism is brain movement and deformation within the skull—the "acceleration-deceleration" injury. In deceleration injury, the rapidly moving head is suddenly stopped, as in an auto-tree collision. The skull movement is immediately arrested but the gelatinous and viscoelastic brain continues to move during a 20-millisecond time period. The brain may also rotate in the skull around the axis of the brainstem. Different loci of the brain substance are deformed to different degrees, and internal shearing and stress forces can traumatize and disrupt cells and their processes in depths of the brain. If blood vessels are not disrupted, there may be no intracerebral hemorrhage, even with severe injury leading to early death. The immediate loss of consciousness results from the deformation affecting the brainstem and its reticular activating system.

In acceleration injury, the head is suddenly accelerated, as occurs, for example, during the boxer's upper cut when the head jolts back and inertial forces strike the still unmoving brain against the accelerating skull. If the brainstem cells have been severely traumatized, he may remain unconscious for days or longer. If the brainstem trauma was mild, he may be unconscious for just a few seconds or less than a minute. In this case most of the traumatized brain cells are presumed to recover.

CONCUSSION. This term describes head trauma associated with brief unconsciousness but no physical signs in sensorimotor systems or by radiographic test to indicate residual structural brain damage. Brief vegetative paralysis may occur at the moment of impact, as noted in the later discussion. The physiologic basis for the loss of consciousness and rapid recovery is not well understood, but sudden diffuse neurotransmitter release has been postulated.

DIRECT BRAIN INJURY. The other major mechanism of brain damage is direct tissue injury under the site of impact. Extensive local brain injury can occur even among patients who remain alert. For example, a crushing injury to the fixed head can drive a large plate of skull inward, destroying the right posterior parietal and occipital lobes, yet the patient need not lose consciousness despite a left homonymous hemianopsia and neurologic signs of injury to the right sensory associative cortex. With the head fixed, only the directly traumatized cerebrum is damaged; the brainstem is not deformed, and there is no loss of consciousness.

Gunshot wounds cause brain damage along the tract of the missile and extending radially outward from the path in proportion to the size and velocity of the missile. The shock wave will cause loss of consciousness if it reaches the brainstem with sufficient force.

CLINICAL APPEARANCE OF THE PATIENT

MILD BRAIN INJURY. Most are caused by acceleration or deceleration brain movement. The mildest form is represented by visual disturbance ("seeing stars") and a sensation of being dazed or stunned that lasts seconds to several minutes. The next degree is immediate unconsciousness. Boxers present a classic example. With a clean knockout blow there is prompt flaccidity, accompanied by apnea and bradycardia, with widely dilated pupils that are unresponsive to light. Rarely, a generalized seizure follows the blow. Oculovestibular reflexes may be lost transiently. In experimental animals given this "mild" injury, there are simultaneous transient arterial hypertension and slowing of the electroencephalogram. The signs and symptoms usually resolve over 30 to 60 seconds, and the individual progressively becomes oriented.

The duration of postconcussion signs and symptoms is variable and related to the intensity of the blow and degree of brain deformity. Recovery from mild injury takes place in 3 to 5 minutes. With stronger blows the physiologic response can be prolonged, and apneic periods lasting 8 to 12 minutes following the blow have been recorded in humans, with subsequent excellent recovery. Nevertheless, a major cause of death from acute head injury is prolonged apnea leading successively to hypoxemia, arterial hypertension, hypotension, and cardiac arrest. Early artificial respiration by a well-trained rescue worker undoubtedly saves some lives.

Most persons who lose consciousness probably suffer at least some irreversible injury to brain cells. Although most of the traumatized cells rapidly regain normal function, some recover only over a protracted period of time and others never. The "punchdrunk" boxer shows evidence of the cumulative effect of recurrent brain damage, part of which is a progressive communicating hydrocephalus. Affected persons are dysarthric, absent-minded, and argumentative. They have difficulty concentrating and a poor memory for recent events and walk on a wide base, with a stiff, spastic gait.

Within minutes after the injury, patients with mild brain trauma are characteristically alert and oriented. They can usually describe what they were doing up to the moments before the injury and have little or no retrograde amnesia. They rarely remember the blow itself and often cannot remember events that occurred for up to ten minutes after the accident. This period of memory loss following the injury is called the time of *antegrade amnesia* or *post-traumatic amnesia*.

MODERATE BRAIN INJURY. Patients with moderate brain injury characteristically remain lethargic or stuporous after emerging from periods of unconsciousness lasting five to ten minutes or more. They are often intermittently restless and sometimes combative but return to sleep if undisturbed. They may speak in short sentences or phrases or repeatedly say the same word. Most are sufficiently in contact to follow at least a simple single-stage command. Some have symptoms of a mild to moderate delirious reaction. Although a mild focal neurologic deficit such as a hemiparesis or visual field defect may exist, these patients do *not* show signs of motor posturing such as decorticate or decerebrate positioning of the limbs spontaneously or in response to noxious stimuli.

Patients with moderate brain injury usually make a reasonably satisfactory recovery, even when they have suffered subarachnoid hemorrhage, cerebral contusions, or a small intracerebral hematoma. A few have reduced mental performance, reflecting the presence of permanent brain damage.

Over a period of several days to one to two weeks, such patients gradually recover orientation and alertness. Mild focal neurologic deficits usually disappear. However, during the acute stages these patients are potentially vulnerable to secondary brain insults from respiratory insufficiency and hypoxemia, the growth of an intracranial blood clot, or development of brain edema, and they require close observation and carefully applied medical care.

SEVERE BRAIN INJURY. Such patients do not regain consciousness for at least 20 minutes and often much longer after injury. When seen at hospital, they do not speak understandable words or follow simple commands. This state remains after cardiopulmonary resuscitation. Other serious neurologic signs are common, and prognosis is related largely to evidence of brainstem injury. Motor posturing (decorticate and decerebrate responses) indicating extensive deep cerebral injury occurs in 30 per cent. Decerebrate (extensor) posturing carries a poorer prognosis than decorticate posturing. Impaired eye movements to the doll's head maneuver (oculocephalic test) or ice water irrigation of the ear canal (oculovestibular test) are seen in 40 per cent of patients in this group and represents brainstem damage or, less often, inner ear or cranial nerve III, IV, VI, or VIII injury. Bilateral pupillary unresponsiveness to light also signifies brainstem damage. Bilateral decerebrate (extensor) posturing with impaired or absent oculocephalic responses implies a very extensive brain injury involving both the hemispheres and brainstem. Most such patients (80 per cent) die, and the survivors can be expected to remain severely disabled or vegetative, even in the absence of an intracranial hematoma or elevated intracranial pressure.

Patients with decerebrate motor posturing but *normal* eye movements have a less extensive brain injury and sometimes make a good recovery. Likewise, patients with normal motor responses to noxious stimuli, but who have impaired eye movements or fixed pupils, occasionally make a good recovery because of the more limited extent of the brain damage. Patients with severe head injury who have normal withdrawal or normal flexor response of their limbs to noxious stimuli can be expected to make a good recovery *unless* they harbor an intracranial mass lesion that causes a major brain shift or elevates intracranial pressure to levels over 40 mm Hg for a prolonged period or unless they develop systemic complications such as septic shock or pulmonary edema.

The presence of flaccidity or paralysis of all four limbs to noxious stimuli may be caused by a concomitant spinal cord injury, but even if related to the brain injury, flaccidity is an ominous sign.

About 40 per cent of patients with severe brain injury harbor an intracranial hematoma causing brain compression and displacement as well as a high intracranial pressure. Such patients almost always require prompt surgery to evacuate the mass lesion. If the physician waits for signs of neurologic deterioration, further permanent brain damage will usually occur. Patients who show with bilateral decerebrate posturing, impaired eye movements, and pupils fixed to light can, on rare occasions, recover if they are harboring a subdural or epidural hematoma and the clot is quickly evacuated.

PATIENTS SHOWING PROGRESSIVE NEUROLOGIC DETERIORATION. The conditions of patients with mild, moderate, or severe brain injury may progressively worsen. If the vital signs and blood oxygen levels are satisfactory, such early deterioration usually comes from an expanding intracranial hematoma, usually in the subdural or epidural space, but sometimes from an intracerebral hematoma. A less frequent cause is progressive brain swelling. Unless checked by prompt treatment, such expanding masses threaten to produce potentially fatal uncal or central transtentorial herniation with signs and symptoms as outlined in Ch. 472. It is imperative that the signs of impending transtentorial herniation be recognized because rapid appropriate treatment with osmotic diuretics and surgical evacuation of a mass can save life and, perhaps more important, brain function.

SKULL FRACTURES

Fractures of the calvarium may indicate the general site and severity of the blow, but their occurrence often bears little relationship to the severity of the underlying brain injury. Autopsy demonstrates an intact skull in 30 per cent of patients who die from severe head injury. Patients with no fracture may have extensive brain injury. Linear, nondisplaced skull fractures may gain clinical importance if the crack extends across the groove of the middle meningeal artery in the temporal bone. Bleeding from this artery is a common cause of an *extradural hematoma*. This clot commonly causes brain compression within a few hours of injury. However, most patients with a linear fracture of the temporal bone do not develop an epidural hematoma, and some patients who accumulate epidural blood clots do *not* have radiographically visible fractures of the temporal bone. Thus knowledge of the presence or absence of a linear fracture is of limited help in directing the care of the individual patient. Modern diagnostic facilities with computed tomographic (CT) scanning have largely replaced plain skull x-rays in the evaluation of head injuries.

Fractures across the base of the skull produce a potential for complications. The dura over the base of the skull is thin and firmly adherent to the bone and can be easily lacerated. If the fracture traverses an air sinus or the middle or external ear canal, external communication risks producing intracranial infection, particularly meningitis. Clinical signs of communication include cerebrospinal fluid (CSF) rhinorrhea or otorrhea or the presence of intracranial air visible on radiography. When a fracture occurs on the floor of the anterior fossa, blood usually seeps into the loose periorbital tissue, producing the appearance of "raccoon eyes." With fractures of the floor of the middle fossa, subcutaneous blood may accumulate over the mastoid bone just behind the ear (*Battle's sign*). Although opinions differ, the evidence indicates that antibiotics used prophylactically do not reduce the incidence of meningitis. Traumatic CSF rhinorrhea or otorrhea usually stops spontaneously or after treatment with repeated lumbar punctures. CSF leaks that persist for longer than seven to nine days should be surgically repaired.

The cranial nerves exit via the skull base and any may be traumatized by a basal skull fracture. Post-traumatic cranial nerve palsies involving II, III, IV, VII, and VIII almost invariably reflect the presence of a fracture. A fracture may damage the olfactory and abducens nerves, but these cranial nerves have a long intracranial course and also can be traumatized by brain movement and deformation.

In *depressed skull fracture* the outer table of one or more of the segments is displaced below the level of the inner table of the surrounding intact skull. The bone position on x-ray represents the end point; the fragments usually have penetrated more deeply at the moment of impact and then "bounced" back. Open depressed fractures require cleansing and debridement of the wound to prevent infection. Post-traumatic epilepsy can be a problem. When such fractures are complicated by a lacerated dura mater, a seizure in the first week after injury, or a period of post-traumatic antegrade amnesia for over 24 hours, the incidence of chronic epilepsy reaches 60 per cent. Patients who have a dural laceration but a short period of post-traumatic amnesia and no early seizures have a 15 per cent chance of developing post-traumatic epilepsy.

CLINICAL PATHOLOGY, INTRACRANIAL PRESSURE (ICP), AND CEREBRAL BLOOD FLOW

With severe brain injury rotational brain movement is so great that grossly visible intracerebral hemorrhagic lesions can be created at the moment of trauma. Contusions and lacerations occur for the most part on the anterior and inferior surfaces of the frontal lobes and in the anterior and middle portions of the temporal lobes. Memory deficits resulting from temporal lobe injury, emotional deficits from the frontal lesions, and intellectual and behavioral impairment from both are common residual abnormalities. Focal motor, cortical sensory, or visual defects are less common. Intracerebral hematomas in the depths of the brain can develop from vascular disruption. Large hematomas in the brainstem are usually fatal.

Following brain trauma, further damage can occur because of a growing blood clot or brain swelling. The brain almost always swells around a contusion and in some cases diffusely in both hemispheres, a process thought to be caused by impairment of normal cerebrovascular autoregulation. When vascular autoregulation is impaired, the cerebral vessels lose their normal resistance tone and dilate in response to the head of arterial blood pressure, which passes downstream toward the capillary bed. In the face of normal or elevated arterial blood pressure, the brain becomes full and engorged with blood, much like an erectile organ.

Cerebrovascular engorgement, brain edema, or a growing blood clot or contusion can, alone or in combination, raise ICP well above the normal level of up to 10 mm Hg, and the pressure can eventually reach levels that impair blood flow. If cerebrovascular autoregulation is preserved, ICP must reach levels of 60 mm Hg or more before blood flow is reduced to levels that hamper tissue nutrition. In patients with severe head injury, autoregulation is usually impaired to at least some degree. In this situation, brain tissue flow may fall to critical levels when the ICP reaches only 20 to 30 mm Hg. If cerebral blood flow declines below 20 ml per 100 grams per minute, neurologic worsening follows, producing gradual or abrupt deterioration of neurologic signs. Such deterioration can occur with ICP values as low as 25 or 30 mm Hg. Although opinions differ, many neurosurgeons believe that brain ischemia stemming from elevated ICP is an important problem in severe head injury. Most patients who have a large intracranial mass have elevated ICP during their postoperative course.

Expanding intracranial hematomas can cause neurologic deterioration, because they elevate ICP, cause diffuse reduction in brain blood flow, and cause shifts, distortion, and local compression of brain tissue. Other delayed brain insults result from systemic complications, including hypoxemia from pulmonary or upper respiratory airway insufficiency, arterial hypotension from septic shock or sudden gastrointestinal hemorrhage, severe hyponatremia, and myocardial infarction. Most comatose patients who die after arriving at hospital do so because of severe elevation of ICP or as an immediate result of one of the systemic insults.

MANAGEMENT

Patients with mild to moderately severe head injuries require close monitoring to prevent medical complications and to guard against the potential delayed effects of intracranial hemorrhage or cerebral edema. With severe mechanical brain injury, carefully planned treatment in experienced hands appears to reduce mortality by 20 per cent and to improve recovery. The rapid transfer of the patient from the accident scene to an appropriately equipped hospital is equally important. Delays in transport or at a receiving hospital can be devastating. Patients with subdural hematoma who arrive at their final hospital in less than two hours fare twice as well as those who are admitted five or more hours after the accident.

IMMEDIATE MANAGEMENT. On arrival in the emergency room, approximately 35 per cent of comatose patients with severe head injury are hypoxemic (Pa_{O_2} <60 mm Hg), 15 per cent are hypotensive (systolic pressure <95 mm Hg), and 10 per cent are anemic (hematocrit <30 per cent). These abnormalities can worsen the already damaged brain and should be corrected during emergency care.

At the Scene of the Accident. Care must be taken to avoid flexing the patient's spine while moving the patient. The patient should be placed promptly in the supine, horizontal, neutral position. The three-quarter prone position should *not* be used. In the supine position, the patient can be examined and the airway dealt with directly. The mouth should be cleared.

If the patient is apneic or hypoventilating, assisted ventilation is indicated, using mouth-to-mouth assistance or positive pressure ventilation with an oral airway and Ambu bag. When the rescue team arrives, face mask positive pressure, an esophageal occlusive airway, or endotracheal intubation can be applied, depending on local expertise. One hundred per cent oxygen should be administered and continued during transportation to the hospital. Serious scalp bleeding can usually be controlled with firm pressure against the bone. Rescue workers can be taught to use the *Glasgow Coma Scale (GCS)* to assess the level of brain function (Table 516–1). Painful stimulus is administered by firmly pressing one of the victim's fingernails at the base. The GCS assessment plus examination of pupil size and reactivity to light provides an adequate emergency measure of brain function.

Transport. Provided that one has a skilled emergency crew, the patient should be transferred without delay to an optimal care hospital where CT scanning and neurosurgical care are available. Distance traveled is not the primary consideration. The only indication for transport to a local receiving hospital is profound shock (blood pressure <60 to 70 mm Hg).

For ideal care during transport of comatose patients, the following steps should be followed: insert an intravenous catheter, 16-gauge, for the possible administration of agents to maintain circulation. Initially, use a saline solution, Ringer's lactated solution, 100 ml per hour. Administer nasal oxygen at 3 to 5 liters per minute. If the patient is intubated, deliver oxygen at 100 per cent concentration. Place a nasogastric tube and empty the stomach by suction. Place a cervical collar or sandbags to protect the neck. Many recommend administration of a single intravenous dose of steroids equivalent to 50 mg of dexamethasone or 250 mg of methylprednisolone, but there is little evidence that this has a beneficial effect. Make repeated assessment of pupils, eye opening, and motor and verbal response during transport. Repeatedly check the pulse, blood pressure, and breathing. Osmotic agents such as mannitol should be given when there is progressive neurologic deterioration consistent with a growing mass and tentorial herniation.

Emergency Room Care. VENTILATION. Patients not talking and not following commands should be intubated. Respiratory insufficiency in the comatose patient can occur suddenly and unexpectedly from upper airway obstruction, generalized sei-

TABLE 516–1. GLASGOW COMA SCALE

Eye opening	
Spontaneous	4
To sound	3
To pain	2
None	1
Motor response	
Obeys commands	6
Localizes pain	5
Normal flexion (withdrawal)	4
Abnormal flexion (decortication)	3
Extension (decerebration)	2
None	1
Verbal response	
Oriented	5
Confused conversation	4
Inappropriate words	3
Incomprehensive sounds	2
None	1

zures, or soft tissue swelling in the neck. When positive pressure ventilation is initiated early, progressive respiratory failure only rarely occurs, although ventilation often must be maintained for several days. Also, CT scanning and other diagnostic procedures are improved with patient immobility; an intubated, ventilated patient can be temporarily paralyzed with pancuronium bromide.

CIRCULATION. If the patient is hypotensive, the arterial blood pressure should be brought into the normal range (mean pressure, 80 to 100 mm Hg).

Acute hypotension may result from the primary brain insult, but this should be transient or should promptly reverse with administration of intravenous fluids. Most often, hypotension reflects blood loss, and the blood volume must be rapidly expanded with appropriate agents.

A central venous pressure line should be inserted and blood drawn for a coagulation screen, blood count, and availability for typing and cross-matching, determination of electrolyte levels, SMA 12, blood alcohol, and arterial Po_2, Pco_2, and pH. A serum and urine toxicology screen is done if drug overdose or abuse is suspected.

If the circulation is satisfactory, administration of intravenous fluids is begun at 125 ml per hour of 5 per cent dextrose in 0.45 per cent saline solution. The patient should be kept well hydrated and not hemoconcentrated. As long as the serum sodium level does not fall, normal or even excessive hydration will not cause brain edema. Hyponatremia, however, can accentuate brain edema and intracranial hypertension.

EXAMINATION. The emergency room examination should include visual observation of the entire body, the extremities for possible fractures, and the pelvis for stability, as well as an evaluation of the abdomen, chest, and cardiovascular system.

Neurologic examination includes the GCS, plus appropriate evaluation of brainstem function. The pupils are evaluated for size, reactivity, shape, and position. If the cervical spine is in proper alignment, the oculocephalic reflexes are tested; otherwise, oculovestibular reflexes (cold calorics) are obtained. The motor system is evaluated for weakness and muscle tone, reflexes are tested for symmetry and response, a sensory examination is attempted, and the superficial reflexes are tested. (See Ch. 472 for evaluation of the comatose patient.)

TRIAGE ACCORDING TO SEVERITY OF INJURY. For purposes of defining initial management, patients can be grouped as having mild, moderate, or severe injury, as described earlier.

Mild Injury (Grade I). The concern is that Grade I patients may develop delayed damage from extradural or subdural hematoma. Most such patients can be observed at home if results of their initial examination are normal, with warnings to the family to awaken the patient during the first night to check responsiveness. If there is severe headache, vomiting, or lethargy, a 24-hour period of hospital observation is advisable. CT scan rather than skull films is the procedure of choice.

Moderate and Severe Injury (Grades II and III). Standard radiographs are obtained in the emergency room and include skull: anteroposterior and lateral (cross table); cervical spine: lateral (cross table); and chest: anteroposterior (semi-upright if possible). Other x-rays are taken as indicated by the physical examination. A diagnostic peritoneal lavage to detect cryptic abdominal hemorrhage is recommended if the patient has been hypotensive, hemoglobin level is below 10 grams per deciliter, or the patient has had violent body trauma.

A CT head scan is recommended in all Grade II and III patients, promptly in those with Grade III status. Assignment to the operating room or intensive care unit can then be made on the basis of the findings.

Because up to 40 per cent of comatose patients with severe brain injury show a major intracranial mass, the radiographic indications for surgical evacuation are important. If there is a clearly identifiable extra-axial lesion of increased (or decreased) density and the midline can be seen to be shifted on the CT scan, by 5 mm or more, many neurosurgeons believe that surgery is indicated. Intra-axial hematomas producing comparable shifts also are considered surgical problems. Small intra- or extra-axial lesions without midline shift and no contralateral balancing lesion can be managed without surgery. However, frequent neurologic examinations are recommended in order to guide therapy and determine if evacuation of a mass is ultimately required. Some surgeons believe that all such patients deserve ICP monitoring.

If immediate access to CT is not available, Grade III patients should have an angiogram or a ventriculogram. A ventriculogram provides rapid information about the position of the midline and the ICP level. Midline shifts of 5 mm or more are an indication for craniotomy.

INTENSIVE CARE AND MEDICAL MANAGEMENT. *Neurologic Monitoring and General Graphic Display.* A 24-hour clinical chart describing the neuro-ophthalmologic findings and the status of motor responses and voluntary motor strength provides an excellent graphic description of the brain-injured patient's course. The same side of the graphic neurologic examination sheet can contain graphs or spaces for recording hourly pulse rate, arterial blood pressure, ICP (when appropriate), body temperature, respiratory state and rate, and central venous pressure. Indications and techniques for intracranial pressure recording are discussed in the references.

Other important variables include hemoglobin and hematocrit levels, white blood counts, arterial blood gases, serum electrolytes, and other pertinent metabolic measurements. A radial arterial indwelling catheter can be used to monitor arterial blood pressure and to obtain blood samples. A transducer will keep the system patent, and this method can usually be used for three to five days. Urine specimens, CSF specimens (when available), and tracheal aspirate should be sent for bacterial culture at regular intervals.

Fluid and Electrolyte Management. Central venous pressure should be maintained at 8 to 12 cm H_2O or pulmonary wedge pressure at 5 to 10 cm H_2O. Urinary output measured via an indwelling bladder catheter should be about 30 ml per hour. Higher or lower outputs imply either improper fluid administration or some other specific medical abnormality. Fluid therapy usually recommended is dextrose, 5 per cent in 0.45 per cent saline solution, plus 20 mEq of KCl per 1000 ml. About 3000 ml per day is usually given to adults, but gastric, third space, and diarrheal losses must be replaced. Serum and urine electrolyte levels should be checked daily.

Many patients with head injuries transiently develop hyponatremia caused by inappropriate secretion of antidiuretic hormone (ADH). This may occur as early as the second day after injury. The treatment is fluid restriction and slow administration of 5 per cent dextrose and isotonic saline solution. Severe hyponatremia may require hypertonic intravenous saline solution; sometimes steroid hormones that cause sodium retention are used. If the central venous pressure is low and the patient is volume depleted, then the hyponatremia may be caused by inappropriate antidiuretic hormone release. Treatment consists of giving hypertonic saline solution and *no* fluid restriction.

If the patient cannot eat after five days, feeding via nasogastric tube can usually begin. Earlier efforts risk producing aspiration or vomiting. Total parenteral nutrition (TPN) can be started the day following injury. There is preliminary evidence that TPN, given to match metabolic needs, can reduce nitrogen loss and muscle wasting, can stimulate recovery of the immune system, and may reduce mortality. Since hyperglycemia may predispose to a potentially harmful cerebral lactic acidosis, blood sugar concentration should be maintained below 180 milligram per cent.

Ventilation. Most authorities recommend using controlled ventilation for all comatose head injury patients, employing a volume respirator initially set in adults at a rate of 12 per minute with a tidal volume varying between 750 and 900 ml (13 ml per kilogram of body weight). The slow rate permits adequate venous blood return to the heart, and the large volume helps re-expand collapsed alveoli. Minute volume is adjusted to bring the $Pa{CO_2}$ in a range of 25 to 30 mm Hg and oxygen flow to maintain a $Pa{O_2}$ above 70 mm Hg. To "phase" the patient onto the ventilator and avoid respiratory distress, intramuscular chlorpromazine, intravenous morphine, or pancuronium bromide (Pavulon), 2 to 4 mg intravenously, can be used as needed. Ventilator control is continued until the patient begins to follow commands or becomes neurologically stable. Most patients are maintained on this regimen for three to four days, but it can be used successfully for as long as two to three weeks.

Medications and General Care. Although seizures are infrequent following closed head injury, convulsions can precipitate a second brain insult by increasing ICP, causing respiratory distress, or increasing cerebral metabolism. To reduce this risk, phenytoin sodium and phenobarbital are usually begun on admission. Despite the lack of evidence that steroids are beneficial, they are often given to severely head-injured patients as dexamethasone or methylprednisolone every six hours. Cimetidine, 300 mg every six hours to inhibit gastric acid secretion, and antacids can reduce the likelihood of serious gastric bleeding.

Elevation of the head 10 to 20 degrees, turning and changing position every hour, frequent pulmonary toilet, pulmonary physical therapy, long-leg antiembolic stockings, standard catheter care, connecting a nasogastric tube to suction, instilling artificial tears every four hours, oral hygiene, and range of motion exercises of all extremities are all standard.

The role of ICP management and the controversial question of using barbiturate anesthesia in management are discussed in the appropriate references.

RECOVERY FROM HEAD INJURY

Most recovery from traumatic brain injury occurs in the first six months, but some neurologic improvement can continue for 12 to 18 months. Improvement thereafter is usually due to retraining or learning of special skills. Few patients with severe brain injury fully recover their neurologic and psychologic faculties. Even patients with mild brain injury frequently have annoying subjective symptoms that last up to one to two years or longer.

The location and extent of the initial and secondary brain injuries determine the quality of the ultimate outcome. Focal residual neurologic deficits such as hemiparesis or hemianopsia are relatively uncommon. Unfortunately, deficits and alterations in intellectual function, memory, and behavior are frequent and reflect injury to the frontal and temporal lobes and limbic structures. Most patients who survive severe brain injury recover independence; 80 per cent are able to function without assistance in daily living. Of the remainder, 15 per cent end up severely disabled, and a further 5 per cent are severely demented or vegetative.

Rehabilitation after head injury should include neuropsychologic testing and therapy tailored to specific handicaps in the motor, emotional, behavioral, and mental spheres. Endogenous depression is common and may be related to a reduced level of brain biogenic amines. Drug treatment with antidepressants is often effective. Family counseling is critical.

POSTCONCUSSIVE SYNDROME. Many patients who suffer brain injury experience annoying symptoms that may last for months and, rarely, years. Those who had a mild or moderate injury and are thus expecting an early complete recovery complain the most. Often, there are no obvious abnormal neurologic signs, and the physician is at a loss to explain the complaints. The symptoms usually include headache, irritability, and a feeling of lightheadedness or dizziness but not true vertigo. Other complaints include difficulty with concentration, worry and apprehension, a preoccupation with self, a lack of interest in others' affairs, mild difficulty with memory, intolerance to loud noises and alcohol, insomnia, and loss of sexual interest. Quick movements or turning the head up or sideways may bring on lightheadedness or a dazed, weak feeling. Perhaps as many as half of these patients show mild, subtle neurologic signs such as abnormal electronystagmography.

The anatomic basis for the postconcussive syndrome is not known. Presumably, many patients have had an injury to the vestibular apparatus. Associated neck injuries (whiplash) are often a part of the complex. Neural connections between damaged neck muscles and the brainstem may be a contributing cause. Minimal brainstem injury could conceivably be responsible for some of the symptoms. The syndrome is so frequent and the complaints so consistent that it must have a consistent biologic substrate, but whether this is structural, neuropharmacologic, or psychologic remains a mystery. The symptoms are not merely a reflection of compensation claims or pending litigation, although such concerns undoubtedly influence the length and degree of the complaints. The most important aspect of treatment is firm and immediate reassurance that the symptoms are not unusual, have no serious implications, and will eventually disappear. The patient who is told there is no reason for his complaints becomes even more preoccupied with his symptoms. Diazepam, 5 mg three or four times a day, helps some patients. Recovery is the rule but may take as long as several years in some cases.

CHRONIC SUBDURAL HEMATOMA

Chronic subdural hematoma presents a problem apart from acute traumatic brain injury. The clinical syndrome develops remotely in time from the original trauma. The effects of the lesion on the brain relate primarily to brain shift, although focal cortical compression, elevated ICP, and cerebral vascular insufficiency with brain ischemia occasionally contribute to the pathogenesis of the symptoms. Subdural hematoma is a disorder that follows mild more often than severe head injury and occurs more frequently among the alcoholic, the elderly, and those receiving anticoagulants. The minor head injury may not be remembered by the patient or his family. Headache is common and may be present almost from the time of injury. After two or three weeks subtle mental changes may occur and the patient may become somewhat lethargic with a loss of initiative. Following this stage, at about six weeks after injury, the patient may develop waxing and waning of the level of consciousness. A slight paresis with a Babinski sign may be seen. If untreated, patients may then progressively develop signs and symptoms of tentorial herniation (see Ch. 472). Obtundation, somnolence, confusion, and memory loss are the most frequent early signs. The clinical diagnosis can be difficult. Before the days of widely available radiographic contrast studies, many patients thought to be psychotic and confined to mental institutions were found at autopsy to have chronic subdural hematomas. Seizures are uncommon and are associated with a poor outcome.

The clinician must consider chronic subdural hematoma in the differential diagnosis of any new mental disturbance or focal neurologic deficit in the patient who is 40 years or older and in all patients with chronic alcoholism. CT scanning will clarify the diagnosis in nearly all instances. The hematoma will appear less dense than brain in most cases. However, early in development some chronic subdural hematomas may be isodense with brain on CT, and all that may be seen is a shift of the ventricular system. Smaller hematomas may resolve spontaneously, but for larger lesions surgical drainage by twist drill or burr holes is the treatment of choice.

Becker DP, Miller JD, Young HF: Diagnosis and treatment of head injury in adults. *In* Youmans JR (ed.): Neurological Surgery. 2nd ed. Philadelphia, W. B. Saunders Company, 1982. *This chapter presents a comprehensive, detailed, and practical description of head injury management.*

Bricolo A, Turazzi S, Feinotto G: Prolonged post-traumatic unconsciousness: Therapeutic assets and liabilities. J Neurosurg 52:625, 1980. *Coma and emergence from unconsciousness is a complex phenomenon. This article is the most well documented modern view on unconsciousness after head injury. The references are well selected.*

Gadisseux P, Ward JD, Young HF, Becker DP: Nutrition and the neurosurgical patient. J Neurosurg 60:219, 1984. *Fulfilling nutritional requirements in comatose traumatized patients can make a difference in outcome. Contains an excellent bibliography.*

Jennett B, Teasdale GM: The Management of Head Injuries. Philadelphia, F. A. Davis Company, 1981. *A comprehensive manuscript giving detailed statistics on the relation of outcome to early signs and to varied treatments.*

Russell RR: The Traumatic Amnesias. London, Oxford University Press, 1971. *A short, lucid, and delightfully written treatise covering brain injury mechanisms and memory loss in head injury.*

Rutherford WH, Merrett JD, McDonald JR: Sequelae of concussion caused by minor head injuries. Lancet 1:1, 1977. *This brief paper places the postconcussive syndrome into perspective. The authors discuss the interplay between symptoms from organic brain damage and post-traumatic neurosis.*

517. INJURIES TO THE SPINE

GENERAL CONSIDERATIONS

The spinal column surrounds and encases the spinal cord, nerve roots, and cauda equina. This part of the anatomy, made up of the vertebral bodies, intervertebral discs, ligaments, and vertebral joints, provides the major support for the body as well as flexibility for the neck and back. Injury to the spine can cause severe pain, impair spinal support and flexibility, and create deformity. It is, however, potential or actual injury to the nervous system so intimately enclosed by the spinal column that presents the greatest hazard.

Spinal cord injury has a low incidence but a high residual morbidity. Each year in the United States, approximately 8000 new cases are admitted to hospital. There are about 200,000 individuals who have survived traumatic spinal cord injury living in America today, half quadriplegic and half paraplegic. Slightly more are rendered quadriplegic at the time of injury, but a higher, early death rate renders the ratio equal. Half of the initially quadriplegic and 60 per cent of the paraplegic patients remain completely paralyzed below the level of their spinal lesions. Only 17 per cent recover enough function to walk. Eighty per cent are under age 40, and half of the injuries occur in the 15- to 25-year age group.

MECHANISMS OF INJURY TO SPINE AND SPINAL CORD

Physical forces generally deform the spinal column in one of four ways: flexion injuries can fracture the vertebral body and cause acute disc rupture; extension deformation often fractures posterior bony elements (laminae and spinous processes) and disrupts the strong and stabilizing longitudinal ligaments that run along the anterior and posterior surfaces of the vertebral bodies; compression injuries cause explosion fractures of the vertebral body and tear surrounding ligaments; and rotational injuries can disrupt the entire ligamentous structures. Flexion or extension injuries usually have a major rotational element which combines to produce extensive ligamentous and bony injury.

If there is deformation and dislocation of the spinal column at the time of injury, the spinal cord can be injured at that moment. If the spinal column remains dislocated, an additional insult of continuing pressure on the spinal cord and nerve roots may compound the problem. The maximal vertebral displacement that actually occurs at the moment of impact is greater than that seen on the initial x-ray, since the bone rebounds back toward normal position.

The cervical spine is the least protected and most flexible portion of the vertebral column. It is relatively fixed to the thoracic spine below and its top end supports the head. This makes it vulnerable, and only moderate trauma can cause a fracture or fracture dislocation. The cervical spinal canal normally is at least 30 per cent larger in diameter than the spinal cord. Individuals who have normal or large canals can often tolerate a considerable vertebral dislocation and show no spinal cord deficit. In contrast, patients with narrow canals or older individuals with osteoarthritic ridging causing a narrow canal can develop major spinal cord deficits from flexion or extension injury with minimal or no spinal column malalignment. Relatively low energy forces can displace the cervical spinal column. The result is that a relatively larger number of partial or reversible cord injuries occur in the cervical region. In contrast, the vast majority of thoracic cord injuries are complete and irreversible. The thoracic spine has additional fixation from the ribs and is the least flexible area of the spine. Tremendous force is required to malalign the thoracic spine; if dislocation occurs, the spinal cord is subjected to a major impact. Additionally, the thoracic canal is normally small in relation to the spinal cord diameter, and malalignment that does not relocate is likely to cause continued compression of the cord.

The lumbar column is heavily constructed and gains additional support from the bulky paraspinal muscles. Here, also, massive energy forces are required to dislocate the spine. The lumbar canal widens relative to the neural structures it contains. The spinal cord usually ends opposite the top of the L2 vertebra. Below this level are the cauda equina, which can tolerate much higher levels of trauma and compression than the spinal cord. So, although incomplete neural lesions of the thoracic cord are a rarity, incomplete neural lesions at the thoracolumbar junction and lumbar and cervical region are fairly common.

COMPLETE AND INCOMPLETE SPINAL CORD INJURY

Whether the neurologic deficit came on *immediately* and whether it is *complete* below the level of injury are the most notable factors in spinal cord injury. Patients with complete functional transection rarely recover, especially if they remain transected upon arrival at the hospital and stay so after realignment of the spinal canal. A patient may be rendered immediately "transected" from a cervical injury and then begin to recover function within minutes of the injury. This is considered to be a *concussive,* reversible membrane injury to the cervical cord. Such patients invariably show recovering neurologic function by the time they reach the hospital. An even rarer patient may be completely functionless on admission with a malaligned cervical spinal fracture dislocation and may begin to recover almost immediately after early spinal realignment. In such a case the cord injury was mild and the compressive forces were at the threshold of irreversible injury.

An *incomplete* spinal cord injury is one in which the patient shows *any voluntary* movement or preserved sensation below the level of the lesion. This may include no more than touch or pin sensation in the perianal region (termed sacral sparing; the sacral sensory fibers run in the most peripheral aspect of the spinal cord at the cord equator). The distinction is important because some patients with incomplete lesions eventually show remarkable functional improvement in motor and sensory function. All the compact bundles of ascending and descending long fiber tracts in the white matter of the spinal cord tend to be damaged to the same degree. If one bundle or part of a fiber tract retains function across the injury site, there is a good chance that the remaining tracts have only been severely concussed and not disrupted or contused. Reports in the literature and elsewhere of spectacular recoveries following "complete" lesions with no distal normal neurologic function even after 6 to 24 hours probably represent failure of the examiners to test sensory function sufficiently, especially perianal function. Retained distal reflex function does *not* define an incomplete lesion. Bulbocavernous reflex, full penile erection in males, anal wink, cremasteric reflex, reflex leg withdrawal, or downgoing toe movement to noxious stimuli can all represent reflex activity in an isolated cord. Spinal shock, defined as loss of all reflex activity below the lesion, is usually present for three to six weeks after complete lesions, but in civilian spinal cord trauma, it may not develop at all. This is especially true with cervical cord damage.

The center gray matter is the most sensitive and vulnerable to physical blows to the spinal cord. As the force of the blow increases, increasing damage extends radially outward into the more lateral ascending and descending long white matter fiber tracts that carry information from brain to body and vice versa.

SPINAL CORD INJURY NEUROLOGIC SYNDROMES

The *central cord syndrome* represents the clinical correlate of the cord damage from injury force just above the concussive blow. With increasing trauma, the lesion extends from central gray matter into the medial portion of the cord white matter. This medial location is where voluntary myelinated motor fibers to the arms are located (motor fibers to the legs are more peripheral). The characteristic clinical syndrome is identified by lower motor neuron changes in the arms combined with spasticity in the legs, with the arms being weaker than the legs. Sensory modalities are variably involved, depending upon extent of injury into the posterior columns and anterolateral columns, but pain and temperature sensation is characteristically reduced in the hands. Urinary retention incontinence is often present (voluntary urinary bladder function is also transmitted in medially placed myelinated fibers). Striking neurologic recovery may be seen over time, although some permanent handicap in arm and hand function often remains.

In the *anterior cord syndrome,* voluntary motor function and pain and temperature sensation are absent, but distal position sense, light touch, and vibratory sensation remain. The anterior and lateral columns of the cord are dysfunctional, but the posterior columns are intact. Anterior cord compression or a lesion involving the anterior spinal artery may be the culprit. Prognosis for good recovery in these cases is less common than that in the *posterior cord syndrome,* in which the opposite clinical picture is present.

Recovery with *Brown-Séquard's syndrome* lies between the aforementioned extremes. Affected patients have dysfunction of half of the cord (the meridian defined in the sagittal plane), with distal motor weakness ipsilateral to the lesion and distal pain and temperature loss contralateral to the lesion. They may also have ipsilateral loss of position and vibratory sense if the injury represents a true "hemisection" of the cord. Improvement is the rule, but some permanent deficit almost always remains.

All the syndromes seen with incomplete spinal cord lesions may be associated with continuing compression of the cord from bony spicules, herniated discs, or displaced vertebrae that remain dislocated after the initial blow.

Most patients with incomplete lesions show progressive improvement, but on occasion neurologic worsening develops. Early after injury progressive loss of function is almost always due to continued or increased compression of the spinal cord by a protruded disc, bone spicules, or distortion of the spinal canal.

The level of the injury is critical. Complete lesions involving the cervical spine cause quadriplegia. If the lesion is above the C4 cord level, the mortality rate is high because diaphragmatic breathing control (via C3–5 cervical roots to the phrenic nerve) is impaired. Patients with complete lesions in the C6 cord region may retain some biceps function but can lack important arm extension, wrist extension, and finger flexion. If the injury is at C7–T1 spine level (C8 cord level), hand intrinsic function is impaired, but since the patient usually retains wrist extension, linkage splints applied to the wrist and fingers will give finger pincer function. Spinal cord injuries that are complete after 24 hours do not show distal motor or sensory functional improvement, but neurologic function related to the level of injury may improve. Thus, a patient with a complete injury at C7 cord level might initially lack wrist extension and finger movement and have weak triceps functions, yet over time may regain improved triceps function and recovery of wrist extension.

PATIENT MANAGEMENT

EMERGENCY AND EARLY MANAGEMENT. Careful placement of the patient in a neutral supine position at the accident site and maintenance of that position during transport are now being employed by most rescue teams. During transport, the head should be kept in alignment with the spine and the spine not flexed during any movement. Nasal oxygen should be administered and artificial ventilation and cardiovascular support provided as needed.

In the emergency room cardiorespiratory resuscitation is often required. Tracheostomy should be avoided; if intubation is necessary, nasotracheal or endotracheal intubation should be performed. Following a major cervical or upper thoracic cord injury, signs of peripheral sympathetic nervous system denervation are common. Characteristically, patients have bradycardia, hypotension, and perhaps hypothermia. Immediately following the impact, there occurs a brief and temporary three- to four-minute episode of marked arterial hypertension secondary to cord sympathetic massive discharge. The hypotension that then follows the initial hypertensive phase can be reversed with alpha-adrenergic agonists such as metaraminol, and also responds to intravenous fluid administration. Hypoxemia is common after cervical and upper thoracic cord trauma. The thoracic intercostal muscles are paralyzed, and diaphragmatic breathing initially may be inadequate to support adequate ventilation. Associated lung, chest, and abdominal injuries are frequent. After resuscitation a baseline neurologic examination can be completed and appropriate spine x-rays obtained. The goals of treatment are to realign the spinal column, restore spinal canal diameter, stabilize the spine, and prevent a secondary or delayed cord injury.

Cervical Spine Injuries. Fracture-dislocations should be promptly reduced. These injuries often are unstable and threaten to produce worse cord damage. Skull tongs that can be placed without the necessity of a scalp incision or skull drill holes are now available. These metal tongs (prototype, Gardner-Wells) with sharp points are placed just above the pinna, and fix firmly to the skull. Initially, weights are applied at 5 pounds per interspace (a C3–4 dislocation would have 15 to 20 pounds). Weights are increased progressively under x-ray control (a radiograph and neurologic examination are checked after each 5- to 10-pound addition of weight). With careful and judicious use of diazepam (Valium) or, in unusual cases when ventilation is controlled, neuromuscular junction blockade, most dislocations can be reduced with less than 60 pounds. Following reduction, further management concerning the need for restoration of canal diameter is controversial. Patients whose neurologic deficits remain complete do not ordinarily improve with surgical decompression of the spinal cord, and those whose are incomplete generally improve. All agree that the patient who demonstrates neurologic worsening should have the canal diameter defined and restored. The modern view that many specialists espouse is that the canal diameter should be defined radiologically in *all* cases and any pressure on the cord removed surgically so as to give the spinal cord maximal chance for recovery. Clinical evidence to support this aggressive approach is not available.

Myelography with or without CT will define diameter and cord position. If extrinsic cord compression is present and surgery is to be performed, the operation must be tailored to the location of the intraspinal pressure and the type of ligamentous rupture. Anterior compression is best removed via an anterior approach to the spine.

Thoracolumbar Injuries. An open operation is almost always required to reduce thoracic and lumbar fracture dislocations. This should usually be preceded by myelography and possibly CT. Surgical reduction and stabilization can often be accomplished with intraoperative traction on the laminae, using Harrington metal rods. Permanent fusion is accomplished with intraoperative bone grafting at the injury site in operated cases.

MEDICAL CARE. Over 40 per cent of patients with spinal cord injury have serious medical complications. Cardiovascular-pulmonary complications are the most lethal, urinary complications the most common, and skin breakdown from pressure the most intractable to treatment. Prompt diagnosis and treatment of complications are the predominant factors in early management. Medical care during the acute phase should follow the principles defined in Ch. 516.

Cardiorespiratory. Because the intercostal muscles are paralyzed with higher lesions, vital capacity is impaired, and breathing is diaphragmatic-abdominal. Pressure on the abdomen must be avoided when the patient is prone. Patients often hyperventilate and reduce their $Pa{CO_2}$. Ventilatory reserve is reduced, and a small pulmonary insult can cause hypoxemia.

The cardiovascular system may be very unstable. Arterial tone is diminished because of the traumatic sympathectomy, and venous tone decreased because of muscle paralysis. Peripheral pooling in the vascular compartment is profound. Severe bradycardia can be life threatening. Anticholinergics such as atropine will help reverse this, but occasionally a cardiac pacemaker is temporarily needed. Although the hypotension will temporarily respond to alpha agonists such as norepinephrine, volume expansion with colloids and saline is imperative. Monitoring of the central venous pressure or wedge pressure and heart rate helps one gauge requirements. Venous stasis is responsible for a high incidence of venous thrombosis and pulmonary embolism. Antiembolic stockings, continuous passive leg movement, and subclinical heparinization may reduce this complication.

Gastrointestinal. Paralytic ileus is common, and nasogastric suction is advisable for a minimum of 48 hours. Hyponatremia is common secondary to high sodium loss via nasogastric suction, diarrhea and urinary loss, or loss into the gut in association with the adynamic ileus. Total parenteral nutrition, begun early, may minimize the complications of inanition. With extensive paralysis, metabolic and caloric requirements may be reduced below normal. Once eating begins, daily stool softeners and laxative suppositories given every other day will help the patient develop spontaneous reflex defecation.

Skin. After two hours of pressure, anesthetic skin begins to develop ischemic changes that can lead to ulcer formation. Skin over the sacrum, ischial tuberosities, trochanters, and heels is prone to pressure sores. A program designed to prevent skin pressure should begin as soon as possible after admission.

Spinal Cord Injury Beds. Rotating bed frames that incorporate traction devices are commonly used to change patient position. Recently, a bed that moves continuously and essentially places the patient in perpetual motion has been introduced. It is expensive and has not yet been widely applied, but the reported reduction of pulmonary complications, decubitus ulcers, and venous thromboembolism is impressive and attests to the need for frequent turning, pulmonary toilet, range of motion passive exercises to extremities, and early mobilization. Halo traction for external cervical spine stabilization has permitted earlier mobilization for many patients.

Genitourinary Tract. A Foley catheter should remain in the urinary bladder for ten days, during which time chemoprophylaxis is recommended. After the tenth day, it is a good policy to discontinue straight drainage and begin an every-four-hour intermittent catheterization program, preferably done by the patient. Reflex spontaneous voiding may sometimes be achieved, but one must monitor the patient for possible ureteral reflux, which can lead to hydroureter, hydronephrosis, and renal damage. In the male, reflex penile erections are not uncommon, and can often be brought on by tactile stimulation. Ejaculation can also be induced in some patients. Both males and females can often participate in satisfying sexual activity and, on occasion, become parents.

Pain, Spasticity, and Reflex Dysautonomia. Severe pain and spasticity with flexor spasms may affect the lower extremities. Baclofen, a gamma-aminobutyric acid analogue, dantrolene, and diazepam alone or in combination often control these symptoms. Surgical procedures such as rhizotomy, myelotomy, and neurectomy are seldom required. Reflex dysautonomia characterized by acute onset of sweating above the injury level, hypertension, headache, and leg spasms may occur spontaneously, but more often reflect an overdistended urinary bladder, gastric dilatation, sexual activity, or an infected hypertrophic spastic bladder.

REHABILITATION. Direct and straightforward discussions with patient and family should begin immediately regarding the diagnosis and prognosis. Early, honest communication usually creates an optimal attitude for expeditious institution of a rehabilitative program. The common psychologic response to spinal cord injury is initial denial, followed by anger and then depression. The patient must be encouraged to cope and move quickly to retraining. Physical therapy, occupational therapy, and respiratory therapy should begin early. Physical restoration is not the only goal of a rehabilitative program. The total process includes psychologic, social, sexual, and vocational rehabilitation. Most patients can be brought back into competitive society. Life expectancy following spinal cord transection for those who survive the initial hospitalization period is just 10 per cent less than for the population at large, but lifelong follow-up care is a necessary part of the medical program. The major impediments to success are renal failure, decubitus ulcers, and psychosocial problems.

Cooper PR, Maravilla KR, Sklar FH, et al.: Halo immobilization of cervical spine fractures. Indications and results. J Neurosurg 50:603, 1979. *Halo immobilization is now in common use. Indications, complications, and contraindications are clearly outlined.*

Guttmann L: Spinal Cord Injuries, Comprehensive Management and Research. 2nd ed. Oxford, Blackwell Scientific Publications, 1976. *This is the most comprehensive publication on spinal cord injury. Sir Ludwig pioneered the development of spinal cord injury centers, which deal with care from injury through rehabilitation. The clinical descriptions of medical syndromes and ultimate results are superb.*

Maynard FM, Reynolds GG, Fountain S, et al.: Neurological prognosis after traumatic quadriplegia. J Neurosurg 50:611, 1979. *A careful assessment of how patients recover with modern care. The neurologic findings and recovery in patients are well documented.*

Yashon D: Spinal Injury. New York, Appleton-Century-Crofts, 1978. *Modern diagnosis and management as practiced in the United States are clearly outlined in a practical manner. Common complications are discussed lucidly, and each chapter is well referenced.*

Young HF, Becker DP: Complications of spine surgery and trauma. *In* Greenfield LJ (ed.): Complications in Surgery and Trauma. Philadelphia, J.B. Lippincott Company, 1984. *Complications of spinal trauma and their management are covered in a comprehensive yet concise fashion.*

Section Fourteen MECHANICAL LESIONS OF NERVE ROOTS AND SPINAL CORD

Jerome B. Posner

Several lesions of the vertebral column, its contents, or its surroundings cause symptoms by distorting or compressing the spinal cord or its exiting nerve roots. With the exception of herniated intervertebral discs, these mechanical lesions of nerve roots or spine are not common, but their most frequent symptom, neck or back pain, is very common indeed, and the physician must consider these lesions in the differential diagnosis of many patients. Furthermore, if untreated, many of these disorders lead to more serious symptoms of sensory loss, paralysis, and incontinence—abnormalities that can often be reversed by early diagnosis and appropriate treatment. A general approach to the patient suffering from neck or back pain is considered in Ch. 481. This section begins with a discussion of the differential diagnosis of muscle, nerve root, and spinal disorders and proceeds to consideration of mechanical lesions of spine and nerve roots. Individual disorders of the peripheral nerves are considered in Section Fifteen and those of the muscle and neuromuscular junction in Section Sixteen.

518. DIFFERENTIAL DIAGNOSIS OF MUSCLE, NERVE ROOT, AND SPINAL DISORDERS

INTRODUCTION. In order for an organism to move, perceive its environment, and maintain homeostasis in a changing environment, signals from peripheral receptors must reach the brain, and signals originating in brain effectors must reach appropriate end-organs. Three different *peripheral common pathways* subserve the functions of motion, sensation, and homeostasis. Some knowledge of the anatomy and physiology of these three common pathways (motor, sensory, and autonomic) is required for the physician to make an intelligent differentiation among lesions of the individual elements of these pathways.

ANATOMY AND PHYSIOLOGY. The *lower motoneuron* is anatomically and physiologically the most well defined of the peripheral common pathways. It consists of the cell body of an anterior horn cell of the spinal cord and its axon that travels through a nerve root, a nerve plexus, and a peripheral nerve to end at the myoneural junction and innervate a number of voluntary muscle fibers. The anterior horn cells consist of large alpha motoneurons destined to innervate extrafusal skeletal muscle fibers that control motion and small gamma motoneurons that innervate intrafusal muscle fibers that control tone. The anterior horn cells of a spinal segment and their emerging axons form a nerve root arranged so that each segment innervates a specific group of muscles called a myotome. In the thoracic and abdominal area, the nerve roots continue as peripheral nerves to innervate intercostal and abdominal muscles in the myotomal pattern. Elsewhere, however, as the nerve roots leave the spinal canal, they intermix and rearrange themselves to form nerve plexuses and later peripheral nerves, both of which innervate muscles in a pattern different from that of a single nerve root (see accompanying table). Branches to specific muscles leave the nerve trunk at specific points along its course, allowing one to determine the site of a nerve lesion by the pattern of muscles paralyzed or spared. For example, damage to the radial nerve in the humeral groove (a common site of compression) paralyzes the brachioradial muscle and the wrist and finger extensors but spares the triceps muscle. A lesion of the radial nerve in the axilla involves the triceps muscle as well. When a motor nerve reaches the muscle that it will innervate, each large heavily myelinated alpha motoneuron fiber (12 to 20 μ in diameter) breaks up into several small, nonmyelinated twigs, each twig reaching an individual extrafusal muscle fiber. Each nerve fiber innervates between 10 (in the ocular muscles) and 1000 (in proximal limb muscles) muscle fibers. The muscle fibers innervated by an individual nerve fiber are scattered throughout the muscle bundle, but become grouped because of reinnervation if there is longstanding disease of the lower motoneuron (see Ch. 471 and 489).

The peripheral common pathway for sensation, the *lower sensory neuron,* is less well defined. It begins with either specialized or nonspecialized receptors that supply a small area of tissue (pacinian corpuscles that measure mechanical deformation are an example of a specialized receptor, and free nerve endings in the skin are examples of unspecialized ones). The receptors transduce mechanical, chemical, and other forms of energy into a depolarization of the sensory nerve ending, which generates an action potential in the peripheral sensory axon. The pattern of the peripheral sensory axon recapitulates that of the motor axon in that it travels first in a peripheral nerve, rearranges itself into nerve plexuses (except in the abdomen and thorax), and then enters the spinal canal as a sensory root. The area of skin supplied by each sensory root is called a dermatome (see Table 518–1). The cell body of the peripheral sensory neuron, unlike the lower motoneuron, is not in the spinal cord but in the dorsal root ganglion, usually lying within the intervertebral foramen. Sensory neurons range in size from the large, heavily myelinated I-A fibers (12 to 22 μ), afferent from muscle spindles; through type II fibers (5 to 12 μ) that subserve light touch and proprioception, and the small, myelinated type III fibers (2 to 5 μ) that subserve temperature and sharp, pricking pain; to the small unmyelinated C-fibers (0.1 to 1.3 μ) that subserve poorly localized noxious, burning pain (see Ch. 481). Each dorsal root ganglion cell possesses a branched axon, the first branch reaching the periphery and the second branch extending from the dorsal root ganglion to enter the dorsolateral portion of the spinal cord. Many large myelinated axons ascend in the dorsal columns without synapsing to reach the cuneate and gracile nuclei of the lower brainstem. These long ascending axons often send branches to synapse at segmental levels as well. Other large, myelinated axons synapse in the posterior gray matter of the spinal cord and then ascend in the spinocerebellar tracts to bring sensory information to the cerebellum. Small, unmyelinated axons synapse in the posterior horn of the spinal cord and then cross in the anterior commissure to ascend in the spinothalamic tract.

Lower autonomic neurons are of two types, sympathetic and parasympathetic. (Strictly speaking, lower autonomic neurons as defined here are not the same as lower motor and sensory neurons, since the sympathetic and parasympathetic fibers which leave the spinal cord synapse once in the periphery before reaching their end-organ. However, the analogy is useful in determining differential diagnoses in patients with disease of the autonomic nervous system.) *Lower sympathetic neurons* begin in the interomediolateral cell column of the spinal cord from T1 through L3. They exit the spinal cord in the ventral root but leave the spinal nerve in the paravertebral region to enter the paravertebral chain of ganglia that extend from the base of the skull to the coccyx. Sympathetic fibers may either synapse in a paravertebral ganglion or travel farther from the spinal cord to synapse in a prevertebral ganglion (e.g., the celiac or superior mesenteric). The synaptic mediator is acetylcholine. From both the paravertebral and prevertebral ganglia, long postganglionic axons travel along either spinal nerves or blood vessels to reach and synapse on the effector organ. The synapse may be on smooth muscle (e.g., pupillary fibers, blood vessels, respiratory tree, gut, and urinary bladder) or on glandular structures such as lacrimal, salivary, and adrenal glands. The synaptic mediator in most postganglionic sympathetic fibers is norepinephrine, but in some, such as sweat glands, the mediator is acetylcholine. Other mediators have been postulated.

Parasympathetic neurons arise either in the special visceral nuclei of the brainstem (including the oculomotor complex, the superior and inferior salivary nuclei, and the vagus nuclei) or in the lateral horns of the second, third, and fourth sacral spinal segments. They exit the central nervous system with cranial nerves (the oculomotor, facial, glossopharyngeal, and vagus) or sacral roots 2, 3, and 4. The preganglionic parasympathetic fibers travel with cranial or spinal nerves until they synapse in a ganglion near the organ they will innervate (e.g., the ciliary ganglion of the eye). Postganglionic fibers then synapse on smooth muscle or glandular structures of the organ destined for innervation. Both the preganglionic and the postganglionic parasympathetic fibers are cholinergic.

GENERAL CHARACTERISTICS OF PERIPHERAL COMMON PATHWAY LESIONS. Lesions of the peripheral common motor, sensory, and autonomic pathways have characteristics that distinguish them from lesions of their respective supranuclear pathways of the brain and spinal cord. Lesions of individual portions of each pathway (particularly with respect to the motor system) also have characteristics that distinguish them from lesions elsewhere in the same pathway. The former characteristics are considered first and the latter in succeeding paragraphs. As a general rule in neurology, when the nervous system is involved at several levels, only the most distal level can be discerned reliably by clinical examination. For example, in the presence of severe muscle disease, one usually cannot determine if the motor nerves supplying these muscles are normal, and in the presence of motor nerve disease one often cannot determine if the corticospinal tracts or motor areas of the brain are intact.

The general characteristics of primary muscle and lower motoneuron dysfunction include weakness, atrophy (rarely pseudohypertrophy [see Ch. 524 and 537]), diminished muscle tone (myotonia is an exception), hypo- or areflexia, and relatively preserved dexterity. The last is particularly important in distinguishing upper from lower motoneuron lesions; with lower motoneuron lesions, skilled movements are preserved until the patient becomes profoundly weak. With upper motoneuron lesions, skilled movements are invariably involved to a greater extent than is gross strength. Patients with lower motoneuron lesions are fully cognizant of the fact that they are weak. Patients with upper motoneuron lesions, particularly when proprioceptive functions are also impaired, may be unaware of their deficit.

The general characteristics of involvement of the lower sensory neuron include loss of one or more primary modalities of sensation (touch, pain, temperature, proprioception), with relative preservation of the integrative sensory modalities, i.e., stereognosis, graphesthesia. In lower sensory motoneuron disorders, stereognosis and graphesthesia may be impaired, but only in proportion to the loss of primary modalities. The opposite is sometimes true with upper sensory neuron lesions. In lower sensory neuron lesions caused by local mechanical disease of a root, plexus, or nerve, all primary sensory modalities are usually lost to a similar degree. (There are exceptions: during the development of compressive nerve lesions, the largest fibers suffer disproportionately, leading to early light touch and proprioceptive loss with *relative* preservation of pain; local anesthetic injection into a nerve affects small pain fibers first.) In some metabolic or inflammatory lesions of the lower sensory neuron (e.g., nutritional neuropathy, Guillain-Barré polyneuropathy), individual fiber types may be selectively involved, leading to the loss of one modality of primary sensation and preservation of the others, but in these instances the pattern of sensory change is almost always bilateral, symmetrical, and of a distal stocking-glove or dermatomal distribution. Sensory loss involving one half of the body if organic in origin always implies an upper sensory neuron lesion.

Only a few features distinguish lower autonomic neuron lesions from upper autonomic neuron lesions. The outstanding one is *denervation hypersensitivity*, the response of a denervated target organ to concentrations of transmitter or transmitter-like substances lower than necessary to stimulate an innervated organ. For example, a parasympathetically denervated pupil constricts when exposed to 0.125 per cent pilocarpine, a parasympathetic agent; a normal pupil will usually not respond. Denervation hypersensitivity is most marked when the lesion involves postganglionic fibers; it is less when preganglionic, lower autonomic neuron fibers are impaired; the response is virtually nonexistent when upper autonomic neuron fibers are damaged.

A second feature of postganglionic lower autonomic neuron lesions is failure of the end-organ to respond to a chemical substance which promotes release of transmitter from nerve terminals. For example, in sympathetically denervated pupils, if the lesion is in the postganglionic fibers, hydroxyamphetamine hydrobromide 1 per cent, which acts at the presynaptic nerve terminal to stimulate release of norepinephrine, will fail to dilate the pupil; a normal pupil will dilate when exposed to this drug.

CHARACTERISTICS OF MUSCLE LESIONS. These diseases are discussed in Ch. 537 to 539. Like lower motoneuron lesions, disease of muscle is characterized by weakness, atrophy, and diminished tendon reflexes. In general, diseases of muscle affect proximal muscles more profoundly than distal ones, and deep tendon reflexes are preserved until the patients become quite weak. Muscle disease, particularly if it is acute and inflammatory, can be accompanied by pain and tenderness in the muscles, but other sensory symptoms or signs are absent. The electromyogram of muscle disease is characteristic in that the potentials are of small amplitude and short duration, with a normal number of motor units recruited on attempted volitional movement (complete interference pattern). Fibrillation potentials, which are characteristic of nerve disorders, may occasionally be seen in muscle disease, particularly polymyositis (see Ch. 451). The intracellular muscle enzyme creatine phosphokinase may be elevated in the serum. Muscle biopsy is also characteristic, demonstrating random loss of muscle fibers with central migration of nuclei. Sometimes specific histochemical changes characterize a particular muscle disorder.

DISEASES OF THE MYONEURAL JUNCTION. These diseases are discussed in Ch. 537 to 539. In general, myoneural junction diseases are characterized by intermittent and fluctuating weakness (particularly in myasthenia gravis, but also in the myasthenic syndrome), by fatigability, and by a characteristic muscle distribution (bulbar and respiratory muscles are predominantly affected by myasthenia gravis and botulism, proximal extremity muscles by the myasthenic syndrome). Responses to cholinergic test substances or electrical studies of neuromuscular transmission are necessary to establish the diagnosis. There are no sensory changes, although some patients with the myasthenic syndrome complain of paresthesias.

DISEASES OF THE PERIPHERAL NERVES. These diseases are discussed in Ch. 524 to 536. Lesions of peripheral nerves are characterized by the distribution of sensory loss, motor weakness, and autonomic dysfunction, as well as by the early loss of deep tendon reflexes. Because most peripheral nerves are mixed sensory and motor, patients with lesions of peripheral nerves usually suffer both sensory loss and motor dysfunction. Some exceptions occur if the nerve or the portion of the nerve involved is exclusively or almost exclusively sensory or motor. (For example, radial nerve palsies may produce weakness alone when the autonomous area of sensory distribution is so small that the overlap from other nerves allows normal sensation; carpal tunnel syndromes may produce solely sensory changes in the median nerve distribution because the motor twig is not compressed.) If autonomic fibers travel with the nerve, autonomic changes may also develop in the same distribution. These can consist of signs of autonomic hyperactivity (e.g., hyperhidrosis, decreased temperature) or reduced activity (e.g. hypohidrosis, warmth, swelling, discoloration, shiny skin, and failure of wrinkling on immersion in water). Involvement of peripheral nerves can be of several types, each of which has characteristic pathologic and electrographic changes (see Ch. 471). In general, when peripheral nerves or more proximal portions of the lower motoneuron are involved, the electromyogram is characterized by long duration, high amplitude action potentials with a reduced number of motor units recruited on volitional movement, and by spontaneous activity in the muscle, consisting of fibrillations and fasciculations. Muscle biopsy in peripheral nerve involvement reveals grouped atrophy, but several months are usually required for these changes to become evident.

PLEXUS AND ROOT INVOLVEMENT. Involvement of nerve plexuses and roots is distinguished from dysfunction of muscle by the same characteristics that distinguish peripheral nerve from muscle lesions. Plexus and root lesions differ from peripheral nerve lesions by the distribution of sensory and autonomic changes. Knowledge of the differences among root, plexus, and peripheral nerve innervation of various structures is required to make this distinction (see Table 518–1).

SPINAL CORD LESIONS. Spinal cord lesions can be distin-

TABLE 518–1. DIFFERENTIAL DIAGNOSIS OF LESIONS OF NERVE ROOTS AND PERIPHERAL NERVES*

Nerve

	C2–3	C5	C6	C7	C8	T1
Pain	Back of head, lateral face, behind ear	Lateral border of arm and medial scapula	Lateral forearm, thumb, and index finger	Posterior arm, lateral hand, mid-forearm, and medial scapula	Medial forearm and hand	Deep aching in shoulder and axilla to olecranon
Sensory loss	Posterior scalp, pinna, lateral face	Lateral border of upper arm	Lateral forearm, including thumb	Mid-forearm and middle finger	Medial forearm and little finger	Axilla down to olecranon
Reflex loss	None	Biceps	Supinator	Triceps	Finger stretch	None
Motor deficit	Usually none	Deltoid, supraspinatus, infraspinatus, rhomboids	Biceps, brachioradialis, brachialis (pronators and supinators of forearm)	Latissimus dorsi, pectoralis major, triceps, wrist extensors, wrist flexors	Finger flexors, finger extensors, flexor carpi ulnaris (thenar muscles in some patients)	*All* small hand muscles (in some thenar muscles via C8)
Some causative lesions	Tumor, injury	Brachial neuritis, cervical disc or spondylosis, upper plexus injury	Cervical disc or spondylosis	Cervical disc or spondylosis	Pancoast tumor, rare in disc lesions or spondylosis, metastatic tumor, thoracic outlet syndrome	Pancoast tumor, cervical rib, outlet syndromes, metastatic carcinoma in deep cervical nodes
Autonomic changes	Gustatory sweating					Horner's syndrome

Peripheral

	Axillary	Musculocutaneous	Radial	Median
Pain	Across shoulder tip	Lateral forearm	Dorsum of thumb and index finger	Thumb, index and middle finger, often spreads up forearm
Sensory loss	Small area over deltoid	Lateral forearm	Dorsum of thumb and index finger (if any)	Lateral palm and lateral fingers
Reflex loss	Nil	Biceps jerk	Triceps jerks and supinator jerk	Finger jerks (flexor digitorum sublimis)
Motor deficit	Deltoid (teres minor cannot be evaluated)	Biceps, brachialis (coracobrachialis weakness not detectable)	Triceps, wrist extensors, finger extensors, brachioradialis, supinator of forearm	Wrist flexors, long finger flexors (thumb, index and middle fingers), pronators of forearm, abductor pollicis brevis
Some causative lesions	Fractured neck of humerus, dislocated shoulder, deep intramuscular injections	Very rarely damaged	Crutch palsy, Saturday night palsy, fractured humerus in supinator muscle	Carpal tunnel syndrome, direct trauma to wrist

*Modified from Patten JT: Neurological Differential Diagnosis. New York, Springer-Verlag, 1977.

TABLE 518–1. DIFFERENTIAL DIAGNOSIS OF LESIONS OF NERVE ROOTS AND PERIPHERAL NERVES (*Continued*)

Roots

T4	*T10*	*L2*	*L3*	*L4*	*L5*	*S1*	*S2–4*
Anterior chest and/or upper back	Midback and/or anterior abdomen	Across thigh	Across thigh	Down to medial malleolus	Back of thigh, lateral calf, dorsum of foot	Back of thigh, back of calf, lateral foot	Buttocks, genitalia, back of thigh
Usually none (upper back and chest at nipple level)	Usually none (midback and abdomen at umbilicus level)	Often none	Often none	Medial leg	Dorsum of foot	Behind lateral malleolus	Buttocks, genitalia
None	Decreased abdominal reflex	None	Adductor reflex	Knee jerk	None	Ankle jerk	Bulbocavernosus
Not discernible	None	Hip flexion, adduction of thigh	Knee extension, adduction of thigh	Inversion of foot	Dorsiflexion of toes and foot (latter L4 also)	Plantar flexion and eversion of foot	Bladder and bowel
Intravertebral or paravertebral tumor, herpes zoster	Intravertebral and paravertebral tumor, herpes zoster	Neurofibroma, meningioma, neoplastic disease; disc lesions very rare (except L4 < 5 per cent *all*)			Disc lesions, metastatic malignancy, neurofibromas, meningioma		Tumor, midline disc
Chest wall, piloerection, hyperhidrosis, unilateral gynecomastia, galactorrhea	Chest wall, piloerection, hyperhidrosis, retrograde ejaculation	Alterations in temperature and color of all or parts of the leg or thigh					Incontinence, impotence, urinary retention

Nerves

Ulnar	*Obturator*	*Femoral*	*Sciatic, Peroneal Division*	*Sciatic, Tibial Division*
Ulnar supplied fingers and palm distal to wrist, pain occasionally along course of nerve	Medial thigh	Anterior thigh and medial leg	Often painless	Often painless
Medial palm and fifth and medial half of ring finger, but often none at all	Often none		Often just dorsum of foot	Sole of foot
Nil	Adductor reflex	Knee jerk	None	Ankle jerk
All small hand muscles excluding abductor pollicis brevis, flexor carpi ulnaris, long flexors of ring and little fingers	Adduction of thigh	Extension of knee	Dorsiflexion, inversion and eversion of the foot (plus lateral hamstrings)	Plantar flexion and inversion of foot (plus medial hamstrings)
Elbow: trauma, bedrest, fractured olecranon; wrist: local trauma, ganglion of wrist joint	Pelvic neoplasm, pregnancy	Diabetes, femoral hernia, femoral artery aneurysm, posterior abdominal neoplasm, psoas abscess	Pressure palsy at fibula neck, hip fracture or dislocation, penetrating trauma to buttock, misplaced injection	Very rarely injured, even in buttock; peroneal division more sensitive to damage

guished from lesions of the rest of the final common pathway in part because spinal lesions are usually accompanied by signs of upper motoneuron disease as well as lower motoneuron disease and in part because of the relatively unique signs of lower motoneuron disease of the spinal cord. In the motor system, involvement of the anterior horn cells produces not only weakness, atrophy, and reflex diminution but also fasciculations (i.e., spontaneous firing of individual bundles of muscle that can be observed through the overlying skin). Fascicular twitchings occur with other lesions of the lower motoneuron as well, but less commonly than in anterior horn cell disease. In addition, in most spinal cord disease, the corticospinal tracts are involved, leading to spasticity, hyperactive reflexes, and extensor plantar responses. Extensor plantar responses may be present even when other signs of corticospinal tract disease are masked by the concomitant lower motoneuron disease.

In the sensory system, because the spinothalamic tract subserves pain and temperature sensation on the contralateral side of the body and the dorsal columns subserve proprioception on the ipsilateral side, dissociation between pin and temperature sensation on the one hand and proprioception and vibration on the other suggests spinal cord disease. When the spinocerebellar pathways are involved selectively, ataxia is the prominent complaint. If other pathways are spared, deep tendon reflexes may be normal or even hyperactive. The crossing of several pathways in the spinal cord gives additional clues that localize disease processes to the spinal cord. Lower and upper motoneuron disease confined to one side of the body, whether or not accompanied by vibratory and position sense loss, with absence of pain and temperature sensation on the contralateral part of the body (so-called *Brown-Séquard's syndrome*) suggests disease of one half of the spinal cord. Bilateral lower and upper motoneuron disease dysfunction, with bilateral loss of pain and temperature but sparing of light touch and position sense, suggests involvement of the anterior two thirds of the spinal cord, probably by occlusion of the anterior spinal artery or one of its branches. Profound absence of position sense, more marked in the upper than the lower extremities, with relative preservation of vibration sense suggests a posteriorly placed lesion of the upper cervical cord compressing the posterior columns. Anterior compressive lesions of the cord such as occur with herniated discs often produce bilateral and symmetrical upper motoneuron corticospinal tract dysfunction accompanied by profound loss of vibratory sense, relative sparing of position sense, and almost total sparing of pain, temperature, and touch sensation. The explanation for these findings is not certain. Some have suggested that the effect is due to mechanical deformation of the heavily myelinated fibers of the posterior columns and corticospinal tracts when the spinal cord is pushed but still tethered by the denticulate ligaments.

PAIN. Pain is a common but not an invariable accompaniment of lesions of peripheral common pathways. Pain and tenderness in muscles may appear with polymyositis and other inflammatory diseases of the muscle. They are generally absent from most myopathies and the dystrophies. Peripheral nerves that are compressed or entrapped often cause pain both locally and in the distribution of that nerve. Pain may also precede other symptoms of sensory change in nutritional neuropathy. Pain is a prominent finding in mechanical compressive lesions of nerve plexuses and roots, and may be present long before clinical sensory or motor findings indicate dysfunction of the neural structure. Such pain is commonly constant and relatively severe, but frequently can be relieved by postural maneuvers which serve to decompress the neural structure. Thus, patients with lumbar discs may be free of pain when they are lying down or standing and bending forward, because both positions make the intervertebral foramen larger. The same patient may be uncomfortable when sitting or standing in a hyperlordotic position, because both of these positions increase the pressure in the disc and make the intervertebral foramen smaller.

MANAGEMENT OF PERIPHERAL COMMON PATHWAY LESIONS. In patients presenting with symptoms of peripheral common pathway dysfunction, particularly weakness, atrophy, loss of tendon reflexes, and signs of lower sensory and autonomic neuron dysfunction, appropriate management depends on diagnosis. The physician should first endeavor by history and physical examination to localize the lesion to one of the structures of the peripheral common pathway. Such a localization is usually made clinically, on the basis of the history and neurologic findings, but may require the support of laboratory tests. The most important tests for diagnosing abnormalities of peripheral structures are electrodiagnostic studies and muscle and nerve biopsy; the most important tests for examining central structures are CT scan and myelography. Once the lesion is localized, the physician should consider in a systematic fashion the lesions that may involve that structure. These are detailed in later chapters. Each disease of each of the structures of the final common pathway produces characteristic signs, symptoms, and pathologic changes.

When a definite diagnosis has been made, appropriate treatment can be instituted if the disorder diagnosed has an appropriate treatment, e.g., thymectomy, steroids, possibly plasmapheresis, and anticholinesterase agents for myasthenia gravis. In the absence of an appropriate treatment, the physician must attempt to keep the patient as functional as possible given the degree of disability. This includes the use of analgesic drugs to relieve pain if present, the use of assistive devices such as short leg braces in patients with foot drop, a wheelchair for patients who cannot walk, scrupulous attention to skin and joint care in patients with sensory loss in areas subject to trauma, and a fairly active program by skilled physical therapists who can train the patient not only to strengthen the muscles that remain but to learn to substitute one muscle for another. With appropriate training, many otherwise bedridden patients can lead a full life in a wheelchair, using other assistive devices. Since many of the diseases of the lower motoneuron are progressive, frequent monitoring of the patient's neurologic status, with special attention to respiratory function, may help in planning activities that he is capable of carrying out. These disorders are usually disabling but do not affect cognitive functions, and patients frequently become desperate, demanding the latest "cure" that has appeared in the newspapers or that is being tried in some distant clinic around the world. The physician has an important role to play in helping the patient evaluate the likelihood that the new therapy will be effective and in continuing to give supportive therapy so that the patient does not feel abandoned. Paradoxically, it might seem, this approach is much easier for patients with terminal cancer than those with neuromuscular disease. In cancer, a variety of new and experimental drugs are available that even to the scientist appear to have a rational basis. In many of the neuromuscular diseases, the nature of the illness is so obscure that one has no rational basis for choosing even an experimental drug. It is in this setting that unlikely remedies (such as snake venom) appear and the physician's emotional support can be particularly helpful.

Aids to the Investigation of Peripheral Nerve Injuries. London, Her Majesty's Royal Stationery Office, 1953. *A paperback pictorial essay that should be carried in every physician's bag. Photographs demonstrate how to test muscles, and drawings illustrate the sensory and motor distribution of nerve roots and nerves.*

Patten J: Neurological Differential Diagnosis. New York, Springer-Verlag, 1977. *A monograph describing with schematic drawings the localization and differential diagnosis of common neurologic lesions.*

519. INTERVERTEBRAL DISC DISEASE

HERNIATED DISC. Herniated intervertebral discs are the most common identifiable cause of neck or low back pain (see Ch. 481). Between each two vertebral bodies is a fibrocartilaginous intervertebral disc. The disc consists of a soft inner nucleus pulposus (a remnant of the notochord) surrounded by thicker fibrous tissue (the anulus fibrosus). The nucleus pulposus is gelatinous in structure and acts as a shock absorber between adjacent vertebral bodies. With advancing age, the nucleus pulposus loses fluid, volume, and resiliency, and the entire disc structure becomes more susceptible to trauma and compression. Tears develop in the anulus fibrosus as a result of repeated minor trauma, and eventually, if the tears become large enough, a portion of the soft nucleus pulposus herniates through the anulus. Asymptomatic herniation may occur into the center of the vertebral bodies bordering the disc (Schmorl's nodules). However, if the disc material herniates into the vertebral canal, it compresses nerve endings and nerve roots, causing pain and other symptoms. Generally, the disc herniates lateral to the posterior longitudinal ligament, thus compressing spinal roots as they enter the intervertebral foramen. Occasionally the disc herniates more centrally, compressing either the spinal cord in the cervical or thoracic area or the cauda equina in the lumbar area. Some authors use the term herniated disc to mean that the disc maintains continuity with the nucleus pulposus, and extruded disc to mean that the disc fragment within the spinal canal has lost continuity with the disc itself. The signs and symptoms of herniated discs are caused by compression of the disc on either nerve roots or the spinal cord. The specific signs and symptoms depend in part on whether the predominant compression is spinal cord or nerve root, and in part on the level at which the neural structures are compressed. The most common sites of disc herniation are in the lumbar area, between L4 and L5 and between L5 and S1. The L5 and S1 roots are those commonly compressed by lumbar disc herniation. (Because of the anatomy of the exiting roots, a laterally herniated disc between L4 and L5 compresses the L5 root, and a disc between L5 and S1, the S1 root.) L3–L4 herniations are less common. In the cervical area, the common herniations occur between C5 and C6 (C6 root) and C6 and C7 (C7 root). Less commonly, herniations appear between C3 and C4, C4 and C5, and C7 and T1. The C7 root is the one most commonly compressed by cervical disc herniation. Thoracic discs are rare, but when they occur they usually compress the spinal cord as well as the emerging root because most of the thoracic vertebral canal is occupied by spinal cord. Although clinical localization in diagnosis of disc disease is usually quite accurate, at times an extruded disc fragment may be large enough to affect several roots, or may migrate from the disc space in which it herniated, causing signs at a distance from the original herniation.

The most common symptom of a herniated disc is pain. The pain from disc disease is of two types: local and radicular. Local pain is felt as a dull aching in the neck or back, with an associated stiffness of those structures, frequently occurring episodically in response to minor trauma (or no discernible trauma at all) months or years prior to the development of radicular pain. The exact pathogenesis of the local pain in disc disease is not known, but some believe that it results from compression of the sinu-vertebral nerve, a recurrent branch of the nerve root that supplies the dura mater. Radicular pain may occasionally be the first sign of disc disease, but is far more likely to follow repetitive bouts of local pain. Radicular pain is generally sudden in onset, often following minor trauma such as a twist, turn, or unusual bend. Radicular pain is perceived as sharp and well localized, and may radiate from the back along the entire distribution of the involved root or affect only a portion of the root. Both local and radicular pain have the characteristics of being exacerbated by activity and relieved by rest.

With cervical disc herniation, most patients hold their necks stiffly and resist passive movement. Lateral bending either to or away from the side of the herniated disc frequently exacerbates both the local and radicular pain. The patient may be more comfortable with his neck slightly flexed but is usually comfortable only in the recumbent position. Patients with lumbar disc disease are most comfortable lying, most uncomfortable sitting, and a little less uncomfortable standing. The back is held stiffly, so that the normal lumbar lordotic curve is no longer apparent, and pain is usually exacerbated by extension of the back. Slow forward bending sometimes relieves the pain. Muscle spasm is prominent with both cervical and lumbar disc disease. Raising the intraspinal pressure, as by coughing, sneezing, or straining, increases the pain sharply. Stretching the compressed root also aggravates the pain. In the upper extremities, extending the arm and laterally flexing the neck away from the extended arm often reproduces radicular pain. In the lower extremities, raising the extended leg with the patient in the recumbent position frequently reproduces the pain of an L5 or S1 radiculopathy and, if the pain is felt on the opposite side as well (crossed straight leg raising), the sign is very suggestive of herniated disc disease. Symptoms of L4 radiculopathy can often be reproduced by extending the hip (stretching the femoral nerve) when the patient is lying in the prone position. Often tenderness is present along the entire distribution of the nerve(s) supplied by the compressed root as well as in muscles supplied by the root. In patients with cervical disc disease, palpation or light percussion of the brachial plexus and the supraclavicular fossa or axilla often causes pain. In patients with lumbar disc disease, palpation over the femoral nerve (L4) in the groin or over the sciatic nerve (L5–S1) in the calf, thigh, or buttocks often causes severe pain. Occasionally tenderness in the calf (the posterior tibial nerve) is so striking as to suggest that the patient is suffering from thrombophlebitis rather than disc herniation. Other neurologic signs that commonly accompany disc disease include paresthesias and sensory loss in the distribution of the involved root and motor weakness in the myotome supplied by that root. The most important single sign is a diminished or absent reflex, giving objectively verifiable evidence of neurologic disease.

If an intervertebral disc herniates medially rather than laterally, it may spare the root and involve the spinal cord directly. When this occurs, there may be little or no pain or pain in a bilateral radicular distribution. Sometimes the pain is felt at a site far distant from the disc herniation as a result of compression of long sensory tracts in the spinal cord. The signs and symptoms of cord involvement are the same as those of compression of the spinal cord by other mass lesions. The corticospinal tracts are involved early, leading to spastic weakness and hyperreflexia below the site of the compression. Large myelinated dorsal column fibers are more sensitive than spinothalamic fibers, leading to an early loss of position and particularly vibration sense, with relative sparing of pin and temperature sensation. In contradistinction to diseases that arise within the spinal cord themselves, compressive lesions tend to spare bladder and bowel function until late. (The exception is when the compression occurs either at the conus medullaris or in the cauda equina.)

The diagnosis of herniated disc is deduced from the characteristic clinical symptoms and findings. In many patients with radiculopathy, findings are minimal and it is the history that must establish the diagnosis. The differential diagnosis of herniated disc disease when there are signs of spinal cord or root dysfunction includes the several mass lesions that can compress roots or spinal cord; these are described in Ch. 518. When the patient complains of back pain, with or without a radicular component, but has no motor, sensory, or reflex changes to suggest the site of a radiculopathy, the differential diagnosis includes pain arising from pain-sensitive nerve endings in the muscles, ligaments, and joints of the vertebral bodies and the paravertebral structures. These structures must be examined carefully to determine which of them is responsible. A high-resolution computed tomographic (CT) scan often establishes the diagnosis.

There is controversy about the management of herniated discs. Most physicians believe that the first step is bedrest. Some investigators have reported that adrenocorticosteroids, either taken orally or injected into the epidural space, may hasten resolution of pain and other symptoms. A short course of oral steroids is safe, but there is no unequivocal evidence that it is efficacious. Steroids injected into the epidural or subarachnoid space, particularly those in depot form, may produce severe inflammatory reactions and are inadvisable. Surgery is indicated when (1) bedrest fails, and the patient is incapacitated by severe, intractable pain; (2) a centrally placed lumbar disc compresses the cauda equina, producing urinary dysfunction; (3) motor weakness, e.g., foot drop, is severe and progresses on bedrest; or (4) acute cervical or thoracic discs cause substantial myelopathy. Myelography may be performed before surgical extirpation to localize the site of disc herniation and to determine whether other disc lesions or tumors are present as well, but in many cases the CT scan alone suffices. The best operation removes the involved disc, leaving as much bone as possible intact. Fusion of the lumbar spine is rarely necessary. Lumbar disc operations are done posteriorly via a laminotomy. Cervical disc operations may be done either posteriorly to decompress the cord or anteriorly to remove the disc without disturbing posterior bony elements. The surgical approach for myelopathy should probably be anterior if the disc is in the cervical area and lateral if the disc is in the thoracic area.

A relatively new technique of disc dissolution by the injection of the enzyme chymopapain directly into a lumbar disc space has received enthusiastic support from some centers. The technique is still being subjected to clinical trials, and what role it will play in the therapeutic armamentarium remains uncertain.

SPONDYLOSIS. Spondylosis is a term applied to chronic degenerative disease of intervertebral discs associated with reactive changes in the adjacent vertebral bodies. Spondylotic changes in the neck and low back increase with increasing age and are almost invariably present in the elderly. Spondylosis is usually asymptomatic except when the reactive tissue compresses a nerve root or the spinal cord. When this occurs, the signs and symptoms are similar to those of herniated disc disease, but the onset is less abrupt and the treatment often more difficult. In both the cervical and lumbar areas, spondylosis is more likely to produce spinal cord or cauda equina symptoms if the sagittal diameter of the spinal canal is congenitally narrow. The symptoms are much more likely to develop in middle life if a marginally adequate canal is further impinged upon by osteophytes. The signs and symptoms of *cervical spondylosis* result from compression either of the spinal cord or its emerging roots and are thus similar to those of herniated discs. Most patients suffer either radiculopathy or myelopathy, but not both. Pain is common in patients with spondylotic radiculopathy but usually less acute and severe than that with herniated discs. Because the onset is more insidious, pain may not be a prominent feature, and muscle spasm may be absent. However, the vertebral degenerative changes in the neck lead to limitation of movement in all directions. The classic picture of cervical spondylotic myelopathy is one of little or no pain but slowly developing weakness, atrophy, and fasciculations in the upper extremities, particularly the small muscles of the hand, and spastic paraparesis with decreased proprioception in the legs. At first the findings may suggest a diagnosis of amyotrophic lateral sclerosis. However, in cervical spondylosis there are sensory changes, particularly vibration loss in the lower extremities, and in amyotrophic lateral sclerosis there are fasciculations in areas different from the anterior horn cells compressed at the cervical level (e.g., the tongue). The differential diagnosis also includes other compressive lesions of root and spinal cord.

Plain x-rays of the cervical spine confirm the presence of cervical spondylosis, but many patients without symptoms have similar x-ray findings. Evidence that spondylosis is symptomatic is found by measuring the sagittal diameter of the cervical canal. When the diameter is less than 10 mm, cord compression is almost a certainty. If the diameter is over 13 mm, it is unlikely that cord compression is occurring, but a soft disc or tumor not seen on the x-ray may be impinging on the cord. The CT scan sometimes helps to delineate accurately the size of the cervical canal, and myelography determines the site of the lesion and the degree of obstruction.

The natural history of cervical myelopathy and radiculopathy is not well established. It is known that many patients experience long periods of pain relief and remission or stabilization of neurologic symptoms. Such spontaneous improvement often makes it difficult to evaluate the effect of a particular treatment. Many physicians prefer, once having established the diagnosis, to begin conservative treatment with a period of bedrest accompanied by cervical traction and stabilization of the neck with a soft collar. If these approaches are successful, they should be continued. However, if the patient develops progressive neurologic signs in the face of conservative treatment, surgical therapy is indicated. Most neurosurgeons believe that if the spinal cord compression occurs at one or two segments, anterior removal of the disc material with spinal fusion is the preferred course. If more than a few segments are involved, laminectomy with foraminotomy is preferred.

In some patients with cervical spondylosis (or with congenital narrowing of the cervical spinal canal, or both), neurologic symptoms are exacerbated by exercise, with pain, numbness, and weakness appearing when a particular extremity is exercised. The pathogenesis is thought to be compression of the spinal cord so severe that the blood supply to the area cannot increase during its activity, leading to ischemia of cord and root structures (pseudoclaudication).

The considerations described above under cervical spondylosis also apply to *lumbar spondylosis*. The symptoms of lumbar spondylosis are similar to those of herniated disc, often occurring at multiple levels. One outstanding difference is the frequent presence of pseudoclaudication from cauda equina compression in patients with spinal stenosis from either spondylosis or congenital narrowing. Typically, symptoms and signs are evoked or accentuated by walking, and include pain, paresthesias, and weakness in the lower extremities. All of the symptoms may disappear when the patient ceases walking, even though he remains in the standing position. At times, however, the symptoms may be exacerbated by prolonged standing and relieved only by sitting or lying down. Pseudoclaudication of the cauda equina may be distinguished from intermittent vascular claudication in several ways. In vascular disease, the pulses in the lower extremities are usually absent or become absent as the patient begins exercise. With vascular disease, the symptoms are usually reproducible and stereotypic, i.e., the patient can predict the exact distance he can walk at a given speed before symptoms develop. Symptoms of cauda equina pseudoclaudication are less stereotypic, so that on some days patients can walk much longer distances than others. The reason for this variability is not known. In patients with pseudoclaudication the neurologic examination may be normal when the patient is at rest, but neurologic signs, particularly reflex absence, may appear as the patient exercises. In patients with pseudoclaudication the lumbar canal is narrowed on either lateral x-ray or CT scan, and there is a substantial block to the passage of myelographic dye. With severe lumbar stenosis, conservative treatment usually fails and decompressive laminectomy is the treatment of choice.

520. NEOPLASMS OF THE SPINAL CANAL

Neoplastic growths that cause nerve root or spinal cord compression can be paravertebral, extradural, intradural, or intramedullary. The majority of neoplasms that cause spinal cord compression are extradural and metastatic. Most extradural neoplasms originate in the vertebral body surrounding the spinal cord and compress spinal roots or cord without invading them. Most intradural neoplasms also cause symptoms by compressing spinal roots or cord without invading, but unlike extradural neoplasms the majority are benign and slow growing. Intramedullary neoplasms cause symptoms by both invading and compressing spinal structures; the tumors may be either benign or malignant.

PARAVERTEBRAL TUMORS. Neoplastic lesions that begin in or metastasize to the paravertebral space often cause serious and perplexing neurologic problems. The tumor may extend longitudinally within the paravertebral space, progressively compressing nerve roots as it grows. At times, the tumor may grow through an intervertebral foramen and compress not only the nerve root but also the spinal cord. Rarely, spinal cord symptoms may be caused by paravertebral tumors compromising radicular arteries that supply the spinal cord. If the tumor is more lateral than the immediate paravertebral space, the brachial, lumbar, or sacral plexus may be compressed, causing symptoms similar to root compression but with a different pattern of sensory and motor loss. The symptoms of extravertebral tumor begin insidiously with severe, unremitting pain, often with a burning quality and usually localized just lateral to the spine, radiating in a band-like pattern in the distribution of the involved dermatome(s). If the lesion involves abdominal or thoracic roots, motor and sensory changes are usually not appreciated by either the patient or the examiner. Autonomic changes may be a prominent or the only neurologic sign. Hyperhidrosis occurring in a band coinciding with the site of the pain strongly suggests the diagnosis. When the tumor involves cervical or lumbar roots, the pain may be soon followed by numbness in fingertips or toes, with accompanying weakness and reflex diminution, depending on the roots involved. Autonomic changes, including anhidrosis or hyperhidrosis, may affect the arm or leg. Horner's syndrome and/or diaphragmatic paralysis often accompany cervical or upper thoracic paravertebral tumors. The diagnosis is best established by computed tomographic (CT) scan at the level suggested by the clinical findings. The CT scan can also determine whether the lesion has grown through the intervertebral foramen or has eroded vertebral bodies. Myelography should also be performed to assess the extent of intravertebral tumor.

The differential diagnosis of paravertebral tumor includes a variety of other disorders that cause paravertebral pain with or without compression of nerve roots. *Psychophysiologic muscle tension syndromes* often cause low back or neck paravertebral pain. In some instances, there may be radiation of the pain, usually in a nondermatomal distribution. On examination there is often marked tenderness of muscles, and sometimes one can find trigger points identified by either their hardness to palpation or their ability to reproduce patients' symptoms when they are compressed. Relief of pain in these instances can be produced by injecting the trigger point with saline solution or a local anesthetic. Temporary relief of pain after such injection does not imply that structural disease is absent; the trigger points may be a reaction to spinal or nerve root disease. In muscle tension syndrome, autonomic, sensory, or motor changes are never present. Disease of kidneys and other viscera lying in the retroperitoneal space may cause pain similar to that of paravertebral tumors, but the pain usually does not radiate and is not associated with autonomic, motor, or sensory changes. Percussion of the involved viscera reproduces the pain that is described as a dull ache rather than a neurogenic burning pain. Spontaneous or induced *entrapment neuropathies* not caused by tumor occasionally mimic the symptoms of paravertebral tumor. Chronic pain after a thoracotomy *(post-thoracotomy pain)* probably results from entrapment of nerve roots at the time of surgery, perhaps with neuroma formation. The pain characteristically appears shortly after surgery and may be unremitting for many years. Motor, sensory, or autonomic changes are rare. The pain can sometimes be relieved by paravertebral anesthetic blocks.

The management of paravertebral masses depends on the diagnosis. In patients known to have cancer, particularly lymphomas or carcinomas of the breast or lung, the tumor can be assumed to be metastatic and should be treated with radiation therapy and, if available, chemotherapy. If the patient has no history of cancer, a biopsy is required and, depending on the site of the lesion, resection may be attempted both to establish a diagnosis and to decompress the nerve roots. Once the diagnosis is established by biopsy, further therapy such as radiation or chemotherapy may be indicated.

EXTRADURAL TUMORS. Extradural neoplasms compress spinal roots and cord in one of three ways. Either they arise in vertebrae surrounding the spinal cord and grow into the epidural space or they arise in the paravertebral space and grow through the intervertebral foramen to compress the cord laterally. Rarely, tumors may arise in the epidural space itself, without involving either vertebral or paravertebral structures. Most extradural neoplasms are metastatic from carcinomas of the breast, lung, prostate, or kidney or from malignant melanoma. Some extradural neoplasms arise de novo in the vertebral bodies (e.g., chordoma, osteogenic sarcoma, myeloma, chondrosarcoma). A minority of extradural neoplasms are benign (e.g., chordoma, osteoma, osteoid osteoma, angioma). Because extradural neoplasms usually arise in and destroy bone before producing spinal cord compression, local pain is the first symptom and may precede the development of either radicular pain or other symptoms of spinal cord compression by weeks or months, depending on the rate of growth of the tumor. Rarely, extradural neoplasms may be painless and the first symptoms may be those of spinal cord dysfunction. The first spinal cord symptoms other than pain are usually those of corticospinal tract disease with weakness, spasticity, and hyperreflexia, followed by paresthesias and loss of vibration and position sense. Unless the lesion compresses the conus medullaris or the cauda equina, bladder and bowel dysfunctions are late signs. As with other causes of spinal cord compression, extradural neoplasms cause symptoms first distally and later proximally. Thus, even thoracic and cervical neoplasms generally cause weakness and numbness in the legs before trunk and upper extremity muscles are involved. The diagnosis of extradural spinal cord compression must be suspected by the history of pain followed by signs and symptoms of spinal cord dysfunction and confirmed by radiographic study. In about 85 per cent of patients suffering from extradural spinal cord compression, there are bone lesions at the site of compression on plain radiographs. In the few patients with negative plain radiographs, x-ray tomography, radionuclide bone scan, or CT scan may demonstrate a bone lesion. The diagnosis of extradural spinal cord compression and its localization require myelography. A myelogram not only establishes the site of cord compression but also determines that the compression is extradural rather than intradural or intramedullary. The differential diagnosis of extradural neoplasms includes inflammatory disease of bone and epidural abscess (e.g., vertebral tuberculosis, bacterial osteomyelitis), acute or subacute epidural hematomas (see Ch. 505), herniated intervertebral discs, spondylosis, and, very rarely, extramedullary hematopoiesis (in patients with severe and chronic anemias) or epidural lipomatosis (in patients on chronic steroid therapy). Often a definitive diagnosis can be made only by biopsy of the lesion either during the course of a decompressive laminectomy or by percutaneous needle biopsy of the involved vertebral body.

The treatment of extradural neoplasms depends on the cause. Most neoplasms that cause extradural spinal cord compression are malignant and progress rapidly. Once spinal cord symptoms begin, paraplegia may develop in a matter of hours to days. Complete paraplegia is irreversible, whereas patients with mild to moderate spinal cord signs often can maintain or regain spinal cord function. Thus, the early diagnosis and vigorous emergency treatment of extradural spinal cord compression is mandatory. The diagnosis and localization are established by myelography. The treatment of patients known to be suffering from cancer who develop typical signs and symptoms of spinal cord compression from extradural metastases is radiation therapy. Therapy should begin with corticosteroids (dexamethasone, 16 to 100 mg daily) to decrease spinal cord edema, and radiation therapy should begin immediately upon establishing the diagnosis. If chemotherapeutic agents are available, they should be used in conjunction with steroids and radiation therapy for the treatment of metastatic or primary malignant tumors of the extradural space. In patients not known to be suffering from a primary cancer, metastatic disease is the most common cause of extradural spinal cord compression, but in these instances a definitive diagnosis must be made by biopsy. Such patients should begin corticosteroid therapy followed by surgery with removal of as much tumor as possible for both diagnostic and therapeutic purposes. If a malignant neoplasm is encountered at operation, radiation therapy should be begun as soon after the surgery as is practical. In a few patients in whom radiation therapy and chemotherapy are ineffective, resection of the vertebral body involved by tumor may delay the development of paraplegia. In some patients with extradural tumors and destruction of the vertebral body, subluxation may compress the cord and may be relieved by surgery. Benign extradural tumors require surgery.

INTRADURAL EXTRAMEDULLARY TUMORS. Most intradural tumors are benign. Meningiomas and neurofibromas are the two most common types. Teratomas, arachnoid cysts, and lipomas are less common causes. *Meningiomas* occur in middle-aged and elderly women, predominantly in the thoracic region of the spinal cord. Another common site of meningiomas is at the foramen magnum. Meningiomas are benign, slow growing, and usually located on the posterior aspect of the spinal cord. Pain is the first symptom in the majority of patients, but in about 25 per cent the meningioma is painless, the first symptom being gradually developing signs of spinal cord compression. Because they are often located on the posterior aspect of the cord, paresthesias and sensory changes beginning distally in the lower extremities are a frequent early symptom and are often mistaken for peripheral neuropathy. As the disease progresses, however, corticospinal tract signs indicate the spinal origin of the symptoms. Even when spinal cord signs and symptoms are obvious, the lack of pain may lead one to suspect a degenerative or demyelinating disease such as multiple sclerosis rather than a neoplasm. In patients with meningiomas, the lumbar puncture reveals an elevated spinal fluid protein content higher than that in degenerative or demyelinating diseases. Myelography usually establishes the diagnosis of a tumor. When the tumors are located posteriorly, if small or near the foramen magnum, they may be difficult to identify on the usual prone myelogram. If a meningioma is suspected and routine myelography is negative, the spinal needle should be removed and the patient fluoroscoped in the supine position in order to visualize adequately the posterior aspect of the subarachnoid space. The treatment of spinal cord compression from meningiomas is surgical removal. Because the tumor grows so slowly and the cord has an opportunity to adapt to compression, even patients with severe neurologic disability often make a full recovery after the lesion is removed.

The second common cause of intradural spinal cord compression is *neurofibroma.* Because these tumors usually arise from the dorsal root, radicular pain is often the first symptom preceding signs of spinal cord compression by months or years. When spinal cord compression develops, it progresses slowly. Some patients with spinal neurofibromas suffer from neurofibromatosis. That diagnosis may be suspected either by a positive family history or by the cutaneous stigmata of the disease. A neurofibroma may extend on either side of the intervertebral foramen, involving the root both in the paravertebral space and within the spinal canal. As neurofibromas grow through the intervertebral foramen, they enlarge it, a finding appreciated by an appropriately positioned radiograph. The cerebrospinal fluid protein is almost always elevated. The diagnosis is established by myelography, and surgical extirpation of the lesion usually leads to complete recovery.

Occasionally *metastatic tumors* involving the leptomeninges present with intradural extramedullary mass lesions. Pain is almost always a prominent early symptom, and spinal cord compression develops more rapidly than it does with the more benign intradural tumors. In addition, malignant cells are frequently encountered in the spinal fluid. Spinal fluid glucose may be low in addition to the protein being elevated. The treatment of intradural malignant neoplasms is radiation therapy and chemotherapy, since complete surgical extirpation is almost always impossible. Because the tumor has almost always seeded the entire subarachnoid space, radiation therapy, if it is to have more than temporary effect, must be supplemented by chemotherapy or be delivered to the entire neuraxis.

INTRAMEDULLARY TUMORS. The most common intramedullary spinal tumors are astrocytomas (usually benign) and ependymomas. Other tumors which occasionally cause intramedullary spinal lesions are hemangioblastomas, lipomas, and hematogenous metastases. Pain is an early symptom of most intramedullary tumors, and signs of spinal cord dysfunction progress rapidly or slowly, depending on the growth characteristics of the tumor. Intramedullary tumors are often associated with syringomyelia, the syrinx sometimes being at a distance from the primary tumor and producing its own symptoms of spinal dysfunction. The so-called characteristic signs of intramedullary spinal cord lesions (dissociated sensory loss, sacral sparing, and early onset of bladder and bowel dysfunction) are not reliable enough clinically to distinguish intramedullary from extramedullary lesions; that diagnosis must be established by myelography and in the future probably by nuclear magnetic resonance scan. In some patients with long-standing benign intramedullary lesions, plain radiographs of the spine may show widening of the spinal canal and erosion of the pedicles. Myelography reveals an enlarged spinal cord, sometimes with complete block to the passage of myelographic contrast material. If a syrinx is suspected, a CT scan performed six hours after myelography with water-soluble contrast material usually reveals contrast material in the syrinx. The differential diagnosis of intramedullary tumors includes intramedullary abscesses and syringomyelia without tumor. A definitive diagnosis is established by biopsy. Successful surgical removal of intramedullary tumors is possible, particularly with ependymomas and hemangioblastomas but sometimes with gliomas as well. Highly skilled and experienced surgeons are necessary for tumors to be removed without increasing neurologic symptoms. If the tumor cannot be totally excised, postoperative radiation therapy often delays recurrence.

Ependymomas have a predilection to involve the lower end of the spinal cord and the filum terminale. An unusual symptom sometimes produced by such tumors is hydrocephalus. The patient may present with headache, papilledema, and enlarged cerebral ventricles without cauda equina signs or with only minor signs such as mild sacral sensory loss or an absent ankle jerk. The pathogenesis of the hydrocephalus is believed to be the plugging of pacchionian granulations by protein exuded from the tumor into the spinal fluid. The diagnosis is suspected in a patient with papilledema and hydrocephalus because the spinal fluid protein is very high; myelography establishes the diagnosis.

521. INFLAMMATORY DISEASES OF THE SPINAL CANAL

Inflammatory diseases that compress nerve roots and spinal cord can arise in extradural, intradural, or intramedullary areas. Extradural inflammatory lesions include tuberculosis or other bacterial osteomyelitis with extradural extension and primary extradural bacterial abscesses. These entities are discussed in Ch. 496. Intradural but extramedullary inflammatory diseases include bacterial, fungal, and parasitic meningitis; inflammatory disease of the leptomeninges of unknown cause such as sarcoidosis or Behçet's syndrome; and reactions to foreign substances such as myelographic contrast material, spinal anesthetics, or steroids. Occasionally, leptomeningeal infiltration with tumor or subarachnoid hemorrhage causes an inflammatory response of the leptomeninges that mimics subacute or chronic infection. All of these inflammatory intradural lesions can lead to spinal arachnoiditis. *Spinal arachnoiditis* is characterized by neck and back pain and by radicular pain in the distribution of the roots involved in the inflammatory process. Dysfunction of multiple roots, particularly in the lumbosacral area, is common; occasional patients go on to develop signs of spinal cord dysfunction, which may progress to paraplegia. The diagnosis of spinal arachnoiditis is established by myelography. A myelogram reveals spotty and irregular collections of contrast material with impairment of the flow through the subarachnoid space. Sometimes there is a complete block to the passage of the myelographic contrast material. The spinal fluid may contain an increased cellular response and a decreased glucose concentration. The protein concentration is usually elevated. Sometimes a specific infectious organism can be identified either by microscopic examination or by culture. There is no treatment for spinal arachnoiditis unless a specific infective agent is identified that can be treated with appropriate chemotherapy.

Intramedullary infectious processes include bacterial and parasitic abscesses and acute transverse myelitis. These entities are discussed under the appropriate chapter headings.

522. VASCULAR DISORDERS OF THE SPINAL CANAL

Extradural, intradural, and intramedullary vascular disorders all can cause spinal cord compression. The most common and most serious extradural vascular disease is *spinal epidural hematoma.* Hemorrhage into the spinal epidural space may occur spontaneously or be associated with trauma, a bleeding diathesis, or a vascular malformation. It is particularly common in patients being treated with anticoagulants. It may occasionally follow lumbar puncture, particularly in patients with bleeding abnormalities. Hemorrhage usually arises from the epidural venous plexus and tends to collect over the dorsum of the spinal cord covering several segments. The clinical picture is characterized by the sudden onset of severe localized back pain and the rapid development of spinal cord dysfunction, often leading to complete paraplegia in several hours. If the patient has a known bleeding disorder, the clinical diagnosis is easily established. In patients without known bleeding or clotting disorders the differential diagnosis includes acute epidural abscess and acute transverse myelopathy. Although occasional patients recover from paraparesis related to epidural spinal cord compression spontaneously, the majority require emergency surgical evacuation if the spinal cord function is to be saved. The more rapidly the paralysis develops and the longer the delay in decompression, the less likely is the patient to recover.

Intradural but extramedullary vascular lesions are usually caused by hemorrhage from *vascular malformations* on the surface of the spinal cord. Spinal subarachnoid hemorrhage is characterized by the sudden onset of back pain, often with a radicular component with or without the development of signs of spinal cord compression. A lumbar puncture reveals evidence of subarachnoid hemorrhage with red cells, xanthochromic spinal fluid, and usually an elevated protein concentration. In the absence of spinal cord signs, the differential diagnosis includes spontaneous intracerebral subarachnoid hemorrhage. The diagnosis of spinal subarachnoid hemorrhage is usually suspected clinically because symptoms begin with back pain in spinal subarachnoid hemorrhage and headache in intracerebral hemorrhage. Arteriovenous anomalies of the subarachnoid space and spinal cord can often be identified on myelography by the characteristic worm-like appearance of the surface of the spinal cord. Supine myelography may be necessary. More direct identification of the vascular anomaly requires selective spinal angiography. Because spinal angiography can be risky, it should be considered only if surgery is contemplated. Some subarachnoid vascular malformations can be successfully removed after their feeding vessels are identified by angiography.

Vascular malformations may be present within the substance of the spinal cord as well as on its surface. They may thus give rise to intramedullary hemorrhage (hematomyelia) as well as subarachnoid hemorrhage. The sudden development of partial or complete transverse myelopathy is the most common onset. If there is bleeding into the subarachnoid space, pain in the neck and back and other signs of meningeal irritation occur.

Arteriovenous malformations may also compress the spinal cord or give rise to hemodynamic changes that result in spinal ischemia. In such cases, distortion and compression of the cord by enlarged, abnormal vessels occur only gradually, and patients present with slowly progressive symptoms of spinal cord dysfunction. Transient exacerbation of symptoms may occur in association with menstrual periods or pregnancy.

Complete or partial recovery of function can follow episodes of spinal cord ischemia or even small hemorrhages. The unchanging localization of the attacks and the prominence of pain help differentiate those symptoms caused by arteriovenous malformations from other recurrent neurologic disorders such as multiple sclerosis. In some patients a spinal bruit may be heard by auscultation over the site of the malformation. Angiography with regional catheterization of radicular vessels is necessary to establish the diagnosis and as a preliminary step to surgical treatment. Advances in microsurgery have increased considerably the chances for satisfactory removal of spinal vascular malformations. Embolization of the malformation or ligation of feeding arteries has been performed when the lesion cannot be removed surgically.

523. CONGENITAL ANOMALIES OF THE CRANIOVERTEBRAL JUNCTION, SPINE, AND SPINAL CORD

Congenital anomalies of the spine are common and are often encountered on radiographs of patients suffering from neck or low back pain. Some congenital anomalies such as *spina bifida occulta* are so common as to be considered variants of normal and are probably never responsible in and of themselves for low back pain. Other congenital anomalies such as the *Klippel-Feil syndrome* (congenital fusion of two or more cervical vertebrae) are not responsible for neck pain or other neurologic symptoms except when associated with coexisting congenital anomalies of the central nervous system. Congenital abnormalities of the spine that are common and usually asymptomatic but that must be considered potential causes of neck or back pain include *facet tropism* (misalignment of the facets on the two sides of the corresponding vertebral body; several authorities believe that this increases rotational stress on the facet joints and may cause back pain); *transitional vertebrae,* such as in sacralization of a lumbar vertebra or lumbarization of a sacral vertebra, altering spinal mechanics and resulting in instability and stress and sometimes producing back pain; and *spondylolisthesis* (forward slipping of one vertebral body onto another, caused by a defect between the articular facets). A third group of congenital anomalies of the spine consists of those that are likely to cause not only neck or back pain but also neurologic disability. These include *basilar impression,* which is often associated with *Arnold-Chiari malformation* (see later discussion). Severe spinal *scoliosis* or *kyphosis,* congenital *stenosis* of the lumbar or cervical spinal canal, anterior and lateral spinal *meningoceles,* and *diastematomyelia* are other causes of back pain and neurologic disability. Diastematomyelia is a bony abnormality that divides the spinal canal, leading to duplication of the spinal cord. It is usually associated with evidence of spina bifida on plain x-rays, and sometimes the bony septum can be identified as well. Patients who become symptomatic in adulthood almost always have some cutaneous abnormality, especially hypertrichosis over the sacral area. The disorder may be associated with other congenital abnormalities of the central nervous system as well.

ARNOLD-CHIARI MALFORMATION

INFANTILE FORM. The Arnold-Chiari malformation is characterized by downward displacement of the cerebellum through the foramen magnum of the skull and by similar caudal elongation of the medulla. The infantile form is commonly associated with other midline defects such as spina bifida and meningocele, hydrocephalus caused by aqueductal or fourth ventricular obstruction, and other congenital malformations of the brain and cord. The infantile form of the Arnold-Chiari malformation usually occurs because of hydrocephalus in the early months of life, with evidence of spina bifida or frank paraparesis resulting from meningomyelocele. Therapy is directed toward surgical relief of the hydrocephalus with a ventricular shunting procedure and repair of the meningomyelocele. Prognosis is poor for patients with extensive defects.

ADULT FORM. The malformation may be asymptomatic until adult life, when the patient gradually develops symptoms and signs of dysfunction of the cerebellum, lower cranial nerves, pyramidal tracts, and posterior columns. Downbeat nystagmus is a characteristic sign. At times the initial signs may be those of hydrocephalus secondary to obstruction of the cerebrospinal fluid pathways or to coexisting syringomyelia of the cervical spinal cord and medulla (see Ch. 491 and 513). Commonly, there is x-ray evidence of fusion of the cervical vertebrae, platybasia, or basilar impression, but computed tomographic or nuclear magnetic resonance scans can establish the diagnosis even when there are no coexisting bony abnormalities. The Arnold-Chiari malformation in adults may simulate syndromes produced by tumors near the foramen magnum and by multiple sclerosis. Surgical enlargement of the foramen magnum and decompression of the cervicomedullary junction are beneficial in selected cases.

BASILAR IMPRESSION AND PLATYBASIA

Basilar impression refers to abnormal invagination of the cervical spine into the base of the posterior fossa of the skull. The diagnosis is made from lateral roentgenograms of the skull when there is excessive protrusion of the tip of the odontoid process of the axis above Chamberlain's line, that is, a line drawn from the back of the hard palate to the posterior margin of the foramen magnum. Other radiologic criteria are also useful. *Platybasia* refers to flattening of the base of the skull, wherein lateral roentgenograms of the skull reveal flattening of the angle between the orbital plates of the anterior fossa and the clivus, the sloping anterior floor of the posterior fossa. The angle is normally 135 degrees and becomes 145 degrees or more in platybasia. Platybasia alone is asymptomatic.

These malformations, which commonly coexist or may exist alone, are usually developmental in origin, and there may be hereditary transmission. Occasionally, these deformations of the base of the skull may result from metabolic bone diseases such as rickets, osteitis deformans, osteomalacia, or osteogenesis imperfecta. The congenital form may be associated with the Klippel-Feil syndrome, Arnold-Chiari malformation, and other congenital malformations of the altas and axis, such as fusion of the atlas to the base of the skull, malpositioning of the odontoid process, or atlantoaxial subluxation. Minor degrees of deformity of the base of the skull give rise to no symptoms. The neck appears shortened, and its movements may be limited. With more severe invagination, there may be signs of impaired function of the cerebellum, lower cranial nerves, pyramidal tracts, and posterior columns. Syringomyelia and syringobulbia may also be present. Increased intracranial pressure may develop owing to obstruction of the foramina of the fourth ventricle and the basal cisterns. The clinical manifestations must be differentiated from those caused by neoplasms in the region of the foramen magnum and multiple sclerosis. When neurologic signs are progressive, surgical decompression of the posterior fossa and upper cervical cord may be indicated.

Aminoff MJ: Spinal Angiomas. Oxford, Blackwell Scientific Publications, 1976. *A comprehensive text on spinal vascular anomalies.*

Austin GM (ed.): The Spinal Cord. 3rd ed. New York, Igaku-Shoin, 1983. *The third edition of a comprehensive, multi-authored monograph describing the clinical findings and management of many disorders of the spinal cord, including lumbar and cervical disc disease.*

Vinken PJ, Bruyn GW: Tumours of the spine and spinal cord, I & II. Handbook of Clinical Neurology, Vol. 19, 20. New York, American Elsevier Publishing Company, 1975, 1976. *Comprehensive descriptions of benign and malignant tumors and herniated discs.*

Vinken PJ, Bruyn GW: Congenital malformations of the spine and spinal cord. Handbook of Clinical Neurology, Vol 32. New York, American Elsevier Publishing Company, 1978. *Comprehensive essays on congenital anomalies of the spine and spinal cord, including chapters on stenosis of the lumbar and cervical spinal canal and spondylodysplasia.*

Section Fifteen DISEASES OF THE PERIPHERAL NERVOUS SYSTEM

524. INTRODUCTION AND BASIC TERMINOLOGY

Herbert H. Schaumburg

The structure and function of the peripheral nervous system (PNS) appear deceptively simple when compared with the central nervous system (CNS). Actually, however, PNS diseases represent a confusing jumble of conditions whose only common thread appears to be PNS dysfunction. Thus, while the anatomic diagnosis of peripheral neuropathy is readily established in nearly 100 per cent of cases by symptoms and signs, the correct cause is determined in less than one half of cases except in a few special centers. Recent clinical and experimental studies suggest a simple, anatomic classification of most PNS disorders (see Ch. 525) insuring that a working knowledge of the common peripheral neuropathies can be easily mastered. However, since common diseases (diabetes or malignancy) produce more than one type of anatomic reaction in the PNS and most physicians are "etiology oriented," this chapter is organized according to individual diseases, stressing their common anatomic and pathophysiologic features whenever possible.

Certain terms associated with peripheral nerve disease have, by common usage, acquired set connotations. These include:

Neuropathy (peripheral neuropathy). This is the usual term for any disorder of peripheral nerves and replaces the term *peripheral neuritis.*

Polyneuropathy (symmetrical polyneuropathy). This designates a generalized process resulting in widespread and symmetrical effects on the peripheral nervous system.

Focal or multifocal neuropathy (mononeuropathy, mononeuropathy multiplex). These terms indicate local involvement of one or more individual peripheral nerves.

Dysesthesia. This term, like paresthesia, is poorly defined; it is commonly used to describe an unpleasant sensation produced by an ordinarily painless stimulus.

Paresthesia. This term indicates a spontaneous aberrant sensation such as pins and needles or tingling.

Hypoesthesia. This term refers to diminished sensation.

Hyperesthesia. This condition is an excessive response to sensory stimulus, even when the sensory threshold is elevated.

525. ANATOMIC CLASSIFICATION OF NEUROPATHY

Herbert H. Schaumburg

SYMMETRICAL GENERALIZED NEUROPATHY (POLYNEUROPATHY)

DISTAL AXONOPATHY (dying-back neuropathy). This is the most common morphologic reaction of the peripheral nervous system (PNS) to toxins and probably underlies many metabolic and hereditary neuropathies.

The pathologic features include initial degeneration of the distal ends of large and long axons; the myelin sheath breaks down concomitantly with axonal disintegration. Axonal degeneration appears to advance slowly proximally toward the nerve cell body. Schwann cells and their connective tissue tubes remain in distal nerves, facilitating appropriate peripheral regeneration (Fig. 525–1).

Many prominent clinical phenomena closely correlate with the morphologic profile. Gradual onset reflects chronic metabolic disease or prolonged intoxication, stocking-glove sensorimotor loss reflects distal axonal degeneration in long nerves (sciatic, ulnar), normal cerebrospinal fluid protein reflects the sparing of proximal sited nerve roots, and slow recovery corresponds to the indolent rate of axonal repair.

MYELINOPATHY. The term myelinopathy, when applied to the PNS, refers to conditions in which the lesion primarily affects myelin or the myelinating (Schwann) cell. The Guillain-Barré syndrome is the only frequently encountered disease that primarily affects PNS myelin. It is likely that the demyelination of spinal roots and nerves in this disorder results from an immune-system–mediated attack on PNS myelin.

The cardinal pathologic features, depicted in Figure 525–2, include primary destruction of the myelin sheath with the axon usually left intact. Demyelination initially affects multiple sites in nerves. The Schwann cell subsequently divides and rapidly remyelinates the axon to restore function.

Many prominent clinical findings correlate closely with the morphologic profile. Onset and recovery are rapid, reflecting the speed of demyelination and remyelination. Initial changes may be distal or proximal or may affect cranial nerves. Generalized weakness and reflex loss are dominant features, reflecting the vulnerability of long myelinated fibers, and the cerebrospinal fluid protein is usually elevated because inflammation in spinal roots results in leakage of protein into the surrounding subarachnoid space.

NEURONOPATHY. This term describes conditions in which the initial morphologic or biochemical changes occur in the neuron cell body. If the changes are intense, the affected neuron dies and there is permanent total motor or sensory dysfunction in the affected segment. The neuronopathies are a heterogeneous, poorly understood group of conditions and, in the broadest sense, include many disorders of motor, sensory, and autonomic neurons. Infectious neuronopathies include familiar conditions such as poliomyelitis (motor neuronopathy) and herpes

TABLE 525–1. CLASSIFICATION OF PERIPHERAL NEUROPATHY

A. Symmetrical generalized polyneuropathy
   - Distal axonopathy (associated with drugs, industrial chemicals, metabolic diseases, deficiency syndromes)
   - Myelinopathy (associated with diphtheria, Guillain-Barré syndrome, genetic leukodystrophies)
   - Neuropathy (associated with motor neuron diseases, herpes zoster neuronitis, carcinomatous sensory neuronopathy)

B. Focal and multifocal neuropathies (mononeuropathy)
   - Ischemia
   - Trauma
   - Infiltration (granulomatous, malignancy)

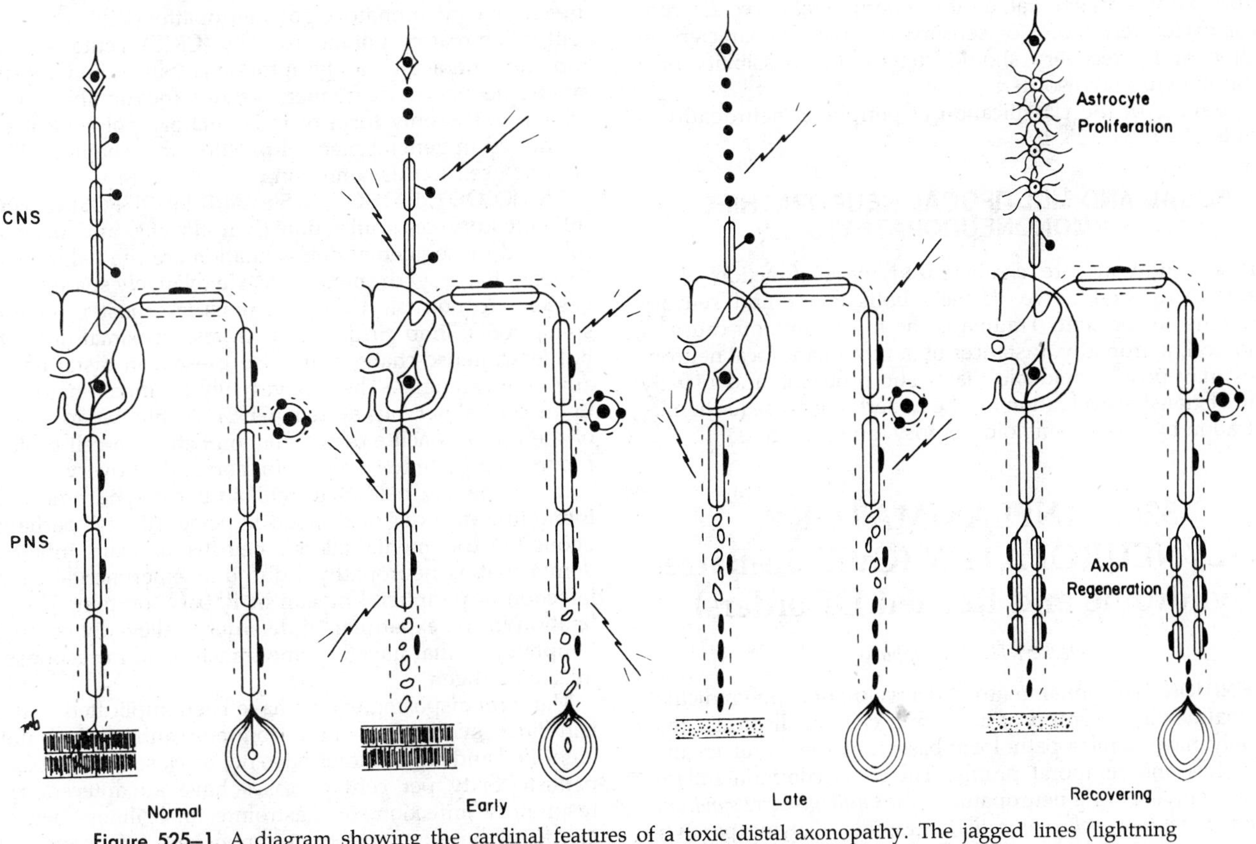

Figure 525–1. A diagram showing the cardinal features of a toxic distal axonopathy. The jagged lines (lightning bolts) indicate that the toxin is acting at multiple sites along motor and sensory axons in the PNS and CNS. Axon degeneration has moved proximally (dying-back) by the late stage. (From Schaumburg, et al., with permission.)

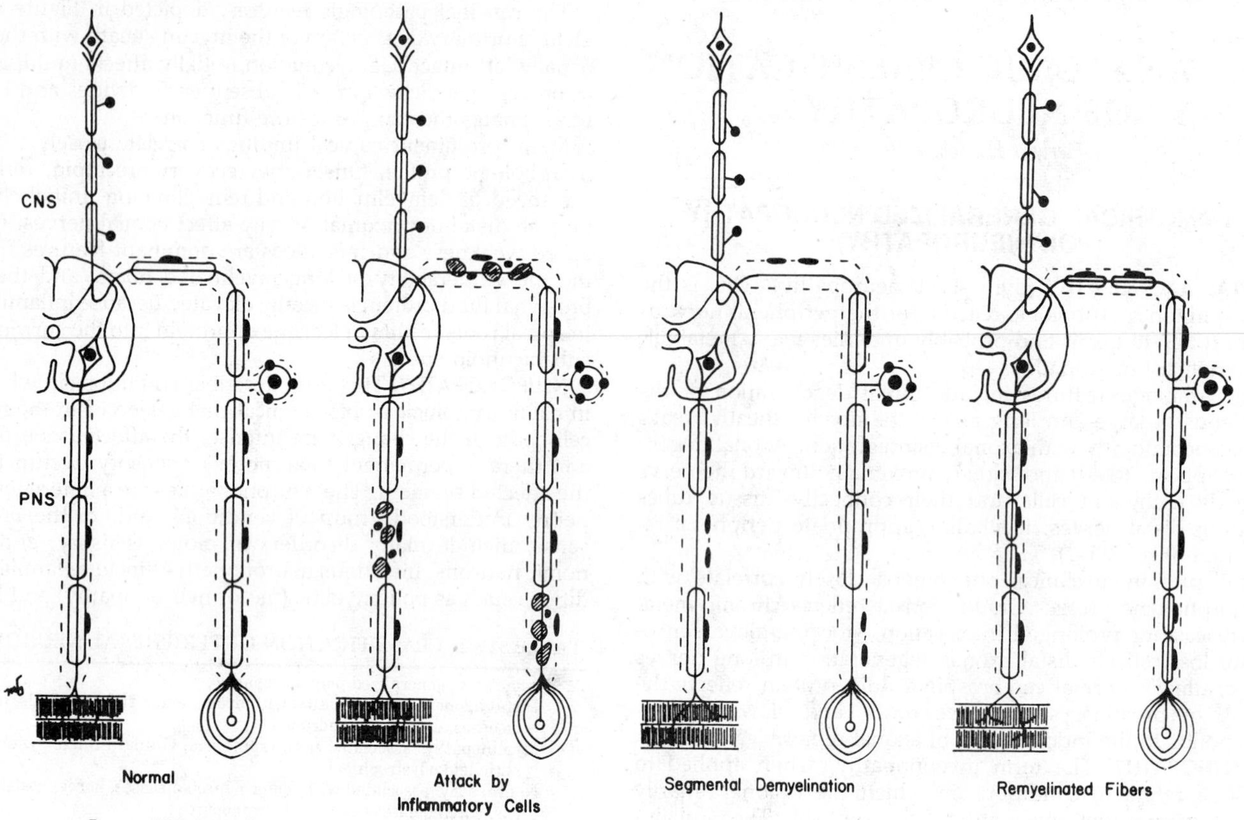

Figure 525–2. A diagram of the cardinal pathologic features of an inflammatory myelinopathy. Axons are spared as is CNS myelin. After the attack, the remaining Schwann cells divide and remyelinate the denuded segments of axons. (From Schaumburg, et al., with permission.)

zoster ganglionitis (sensory neuronopathy). Some hereditary and toxic neuropathies probably are best conceptualized as neuronopathies. In general, a diffuse peripheral nerve disorder that is exclusively motor or sensory and that is characterized by little or no recovery should suggest the possibility of a primarily neuronal disorder.

An outline of the classification of peripheral neuropathy is provided in Table 525–1.

FOCAL AND MULTIFOCAL NEUROPATHIES (MONONEUROPATHY)

These conditions are characterized by dysfunction of an isolated peripheral nerve. Usually both motor and sensory symptoms are present. Trauma is the most common cause of monofocal neuropathy. Instances of nontraumatic focal neuropathies may pose formidable diagnostic problems and usually require extensive evaluation for the underlying cause (ischemia, infiltration by tumor, amyloid, leprosy, among others).

526. INFLAMMATORY POLYNEUROPATHY (Guillain-Barré Syndrome and Related Disorders)

Herbert H. Schaumburg

DEFINITION. The inflammatory demyelinating polyradiculoneuropathies are a group of acute and chronic disorders that probably have similar pathologic bases but can differ in anatomic sites and temporal profile. The most common inflammatory demyelinating neuropathy is the *Guillain-Barré syndrome (acute postinfectious polyneuropathy)*, a rapidly evolving paralytic illness of unknown origin. Its salient morphologic feature is widespread inflammatory peripheral nervous system (PNS) demyelination, presumably secondary to a hypersensitivity reaction. Other less common forms of inflammatory neuropathy are chronic inflammatory polyneuropathy (CIP), chronic recurrent inflammatory polyneuropathy (CRIP), acute sensory neuropathy, and acute pandysautonomia. Since the Guillain-Barré syndrome, the most frequent acute paralytic illness in young adults, is the only form of inflammatory polyneuropathy encountered in general medical practice, this chapter will largely confine itself to this condition.

PATHOLOGY, PATHOGENESIS, AND PREDISPOSING FACTORS. Inflammatory cell infiltration (lymphocytes and plasma cells) followed by segmental demyelination are the hallmarks of the Guillain-Barré syndrome. Axons are relatively spared and blood vessels are normal. These reactions are most pronounced in spinal roots, limb girdle plexuses, and proximal nerve trunks, but less intense changes are also present in distal nerves and autonomic ganglia. There is virtually no inflammatory change in the central nervous system (CNS). Within two to three weeks of the onset of acute demyelination Schwann cell proliferation occurs as a prelude to remyelination and recovery.

It is generally held that Guillain-Barré syndrome is an autoimmune disorder of delayed hypersensitivity, perhaps analogous to experimental allergic neuritis, an acute inflammatory demyelinating neuropathy induced in experimental animals by injection of peripheral myelin or P_2 basic protein. The demyelination in the experimental disorder is allegedly controlled by lymphocytes that have become transformed in response to the injected antigen.

Many predisposing events have been implicated in the Guillain-Barré syndrome, but a common antigen has not been identified and HLA studies have not disclosed any predisposing pattern. Sixty per cent of cases have an antecedent upper respiratory infection or gastrointestinal illness within one month of onset; a host of common viral infections including infectious mononucleosis, hepatitis, and Epstein-Barr virus have been implicated. Other alleged predisposing factors include vaccination against rabies and swine flu, surgery, pregnancy, and malignancy (especially lymphoma).

CLINICAL FEATURES. This is a worldwide illness and occurs throughout the year. It has a bimodal age distribution, with the majority of cases in young adults and a second lesser peak in incidence in the 45 to 64 age group.

The Guillain-Barré syndrome is a rapidly progressive, largely reversible, predominantly motor neuropathy. The cardinal clinical features are progressive and usually symmetrical weakness, combined with hyporeflexia. Weakness usually begins in the distal lower limbs and spreads upward (ascending paralysis); however, this pattern is not inevitable and patients may have weakness of the proximal upper limbs or face. Most weakened individuals do not appear systemically ill, and constitutional signs such as fever, chills, and weight loss are unusual.

The eventual degree of paralysis varies, encompassing a broad spectrum that includes the occasional individual who never progresses beyond a mild footdrop to others with extreme weakness of all extremities and of the face. Severe involvement may lead to flaccid quadriplegia with inability to breathe, swallow, speak, or move the eyes. Limb weakness is generally symmetrical and early muscle atrophy uncommon. Tendon reflexes are usually absent.

The presence of facial weakness helps to distinguish the Guillain-Barré syndrome from most other neuropathies, apart from those related to sarcoidosis. Rarely, limb ataxia, paralysis of eye movements, and diffuse hyporeflexia may be the sole manifestations (*Miller Fisher syndrome*). Central nervous system involvement is not part of this illness. Increased intracranial pressure and papilledema may rarely occur late.

Sensory symptoms, usually distal paresthesias, are present in most cases, rarely persist or progress (in contrast to the weakness), and generally are not accompanied by signs of a profound loss of sensation. Mild impairment of distal position and vibration sensation and slight loss of pinprick sensation over the toes are common.

Autonomic dysfunction accompanies many cases and probably reflects involvement of the myelinated preganglionic fibers and the ganglia. Orthostatic hypotension and hypertension are frequent, may result from denervation supersensitivity, are difficult to treat, and can complicate the management of patients with respiratory compromise. Individuals who appear otherwise clinically stable can die suddenly following unexplained fluctuation in blood pressure or cardiac dysrhythmias.

Cerebrospinal fluid (CSF) and electrodiagnostic studies are helpful. The CSF protein concentration is usually normal during the first three days of illness; it then steadily rises and may reach levels in excess of 500 mg per deciliter. The CSF protein level may remain elevated for several months, even after recovery is underway. Mononuclear cells, usually less than 10 per millimeter, are present in up to one half of the cases.

Early in the illness, distal motor nerve conduction may be normal. Presumably, in such cases the disease process is confined to spinal roots and proximal nerves. If the demyelination affects distal nerves as well, more profound slowing of motor conduction, characteristic of segmental demyelination, occurs. Analysis of the F response, a measurement of proximal motor conduction, may be of value in patients suspected to have Guillain-Barré syndrome who display normal distal motor conduction.

Differential diagnosis is not difficult, especially since the decline of poliomyelitis and diphtheria in North America. Hypokalemia, tick paralysis, botulism, acute myelitis, and cervical spine fracture should be ruled out rapidly.

COURSE AND PROGNOSIS. Rapid progression of weakness is characteristic of the Guillain-Barré syndrome. Paralysis is maximal by one week in more than half, by three weeks in 80 per cent, and by one month in 90 per cent. In the remaining 10 per cent of cases, weakness may progress for variable intervals up to eight weeks.

Recovery usually begins with two to four weeks after progression ceases. The pattern is variable, normally proceeding at a steady pace. Within six months 85 per cent of patients are ambulatory. Occasionally individuals experience more rapid recovery and are able to return to work within two months following quadriparesis. Rare cases show little or no improvement.

Although in time most patients recover almost complete function, the illness is not benign. The overall mortality is 5 per cent, and more than 50 per cent of all patients retain evidence of damage to the peripheral nervous system. Sixteen per cent remain significantly handicapped by weakness. Few features of the initial clinical illness are of help in predicting the eventual outcome. In general, individuals who experience only mild distal extremity weakness and subsequently improve within weeks of the first signs do best.

TREATMENT. Patients suspected of having the Guillain-Barré syndrome must be admitted to the hospital even if the involvement is minimal, since the neuropathy may evolve rapidly and unpredictably. In general, such patients should be admitted to a unit where respiratory care is available, to remain until their condition stabilizes or improves. The tidal volume, oxygen saturation, vital capacity, blood pressure, and ability to cough and swallow should be closely monitored, since they can change without warning.

If a need for mechanical ventilation is anticipated (as determined by the degree of respiratory effort, the vital capacity, and the blood gases), it should be instituted early without waiting for decompensation.

Autonomic dysfunction may produce pupillary disturbances, neuroendocrine disturbance, peripheral pooling of blood, poor venous return, cardiac arrhythmias, and low cardiac output. Beat to beat (R-R) variation of the heart rate during normal and deep breathing is a reliable index. Pharmacologic manipulation of blood pressure in Guillain-Barré syndrome patients is perilous and should be avoided unless absolutely necessary.

Some patients will be unable to swallow or to gag. Feeding should be done through a small nasogastric tube. The patient should be sitting when food is given and for 30 to 60 minutes thereafter to minimize the risk of aspiration.

If patients with the Guillain-Barré syndrome can be carried through the acute stage of progressive paralysis (usually two to three weeks), strength will gradually return. Since most patients achieve good recovery after months of weakness, the importance of extremely fastidious supportive care in the acute stage cannot be overstressed. Glucocorticoids and plasmapheresis are not indicated.

ACUTE INFLAMMATORY SENSORY POLYNEUROPATHY (Postinfectious Sensory Neuropathy or Neuronopathy)

This disorder is presumed to represent a sensory polyradiculopathy and is probably the counterpart of the motor polyradiculoneuropathy of Guillain-Barré. There are no histopathologic studies; it is suggested that inflammatory demyelination of the dorsal roots has also involved adjacent dorsal root ganglion cells. Thus this disease may be conceptualized as a combined myelinopathy-neuronopathy disorder to explain the rapid onset and poor recovery of many cases.

As in the motor variety of the disease, a preceding infection may antedate the neurologic syndrome by several weeks. Typically the onset is acute or subacute and marked by combinations of sensory dysfunction and pain. The sensory dysfunction is most commonly described as unsteadiness in gait or clumsiness in the use of the hands. Even more incapacitating are painful dysesthesias that develop in some patients. Varying combinations of lancinating pain, prickling hyperesthesia, constricting bandlike sensations, and burning or coldness of skin may be described. Any region of the body may be affected, and the disorder involves proximal as well as distal dermatomes. Lower limbs tend to be affected more than upper, and the various modalities of sensation may be affected to different degrees. Patients often exhibit sensory ataxia, and because of the severe impairment of joint position the limbs may be held in distorted positions. Tendon reflexes are often diminished or absent.

Concurrent minor involvement of motor and autonomic function may occur. Cerebrospinal fluid changes are similar to those in the motor variety of the illness. Motor nerve conduction velocity may be within normal limits; by contrast, nerve action potentials cannot be elicited from stimulation of sensory nerve fibers, either because the afferent fibers have degenerated or because the action potential is so dispersed.

Prognosis for recovery in sensory polyneuropathy is poor. Symptoms of cutaneous hyperpathia often persist or recur for many years. Sensory ataxia usually improves but may not recover completely. This persistence of the neurologic deficit probably reflects irreversible damage of spinal ganglion neurons.

ACUTE INFLAMMATORY AUTONOMIC NEUROPATHY (Postinfectious Pandysautonomia)

Acute inflammatory autonomic neuropathy is a poorly understood, rare condition that may be the autonomic counterpart of the motor and sensory varieties already described. Pathologic studies are unavailable. The onset and time course are similar to those in the motor and sensory neuropathies. Principal symptoms include postural hypotension, cramping abdominal pain, and varying amounts of diarrhea and constipation. Hypotension may be so severe that the patient cannot sit up without losing consciousness. Affected subjects reportedly improve with time, but few long-term follow-up studies are available.

CHRONIC RELAPSING INFLAMMATORY NEUROPATHY (CRIP) AND CHRONIC INFLAMMATORY POLYNEUROPATHY (CIP)

DEFINITION, PATHOLOGY, AND PATHOGENESIS. Affected individuals initially have an illness similar to the Guillain-Barré syndrome, although usually with a more gradual onset, but subsequently undergo either a chronic relapsing (CRIP) or a chronic progressive course (CIP). The salient histologic features of both chronic forms are remarkably similar to those of the Guillain-Barré syndrome. It is claimed that onion-bulb formation (concentric rings of Schwann cell processes around a demyelinated axon) is a prominent feature of CRIP and that lymphocytic infiltration is more common in CIP. It is generally considered that CRIP and CIP represent clinical variants of the same condition and may have a pathogenetic mechanism in common with the Guillain-Barré syndrome.

CLINICAL FEATURES. Both conditions are rare. The temporal relationship to antecedent infections is much less frequent than for the Guillain-Barré syndrome.

The cardinal symptoms and signs reflect predominant motor involvement. Weakness of the extremities, intercostal muscles, and lower cranial nerves all occur in CIP and CRIP.

Sensory complaints are almost as common as weakness, and objective signs of sensory loss are more frequent in the chronic disorders than in the Guillain-Barré syndrome. Hyporeflexia or areflexia have been observed in almost all patients.

The development and course of illness are considered the salient features that distinguish between CRIP and CIP. CRIP and CIP generally each have a protracted onset and an indolent progression. The occurrence of subsequent relapsing episodes suggests CRIP, while steady progression suggests CIP. In many instances these guidelines become blurred. For example, it may be impossible to distinguish between a fluctuation in the course of progressing CIP and a relapse in the course of CRIP. This factor, in concert with the histopathologic similarities, suggests that CIP and CRIP are variants of the same condition.

The course of CRIP may vary considerably in the interval between relapses, the severity of episodes, and the rate and degree of recovery. Subsequent attacks usually resemble the initial one, and disability varies considerably. With treatment, improvement is generally good between episodes. Life-threatening episodes with respiratory insufficiency are more common early in the illness. The degree of disability following repeated attacks is variable, and the attacks often cease after a few years.

The course of CIP is usually stepwise but may be gradual. If untreated, this condition may become disabling or fatal; the prognosis is uncertain.

The CSF protein level is elevated at some stage of the illness in almost every case of CIP or CRIP but may fluctuate to normal levels in either condition. Slowed nerve conduction, sometimes profound, in both motor and sensory nerves is characteristic of CIP and CRIP, although this is not always present. Nerve biopsy may be extremely helpful in diagnosis if a diseased area can be located. The histologic picture is characteristic for these disorders. The differential diagnosis of CRIP is seldom a problem after several episodes have occurred. The differential diagnosis of CIP is sometimes extremely difficult. Unless a nerve biopsy displays characteristic changes, CIP may be indistinguishable from some hereditary disorders (see Ch. 530).

TREATMENT. Glucocorticoids are often efficacious in both disorders. Plasma exchange may produce marked improvement in CRIP but does not appear effective in CIP. This technique offers a useful alternative for individuals who cannot tolerate long-term corticosteroids or other immunosuppressive therapy.

527. THE DIABETIC NEUROPATHIES

Herbert H. Schaumburg

A variety of peripheral nerve disorders may occur in diabetes mellitus, reflecting the multiple causes of nerve degeneration in this disorder. Diabetic neuropathies may be classified as either mononeuropathies or symmetrical polyneuropathies, but neuropathy is frequent in diabetes and mixed syndromes often occur. For instance, an individual with symmetrical sensory polyneuropathy may develop acute third nerve palsy (a mononeuropathy). See Table 527–1.

SYMMETRICAL POLYNEUROPATHY

PATHOLOGY AND PATHOGENESIS. Pathologic studies in individuals with advanced distal sensory neuropathy show nonspecific changes that include mixtures of axonal loss and segmental demyelination. The pathogenesis of the symmetrical polyneuropathies and the clinical features, which often selectively involve particular fiber types, favor a metabolic basis, but the inconsistent relationship of severity of neuropathy to control of blood glucose does not support this hypothesis. Other biochemical mechanisms currently suggested endorse either accumulation of nerve sorbitol or depletion of nerve myoinositol.

CLINICAL FEATURES AND TREATMENT. ***Distal Primary Sensory Neuropathy.*** This is the commonest type of diabetic peripheral nerve disorder, estimated to be present in about 40 per cent of individuals with diabetes of 25 years' duration. It is present in less than 10 per cent of patients at the time of diagnosis (which it may antedate) and is uncommon in children.

It may be asymptomatic, with abnormal signs first detectable

TABLE 527–1. CLASSIFICATION OF DIABETIC NEUROPATHIES

Symmetrical polyneuropathies
Distal primary sensory neuropathy
Autonomic neuropathy
Rapidly reversible neuropathy
Mononeuropathy and multiple mononeuropathies
Cranial neuropathies
Focal nerve lesions (other than cranial)
Proximal painful lower limb neuropathy (diabetic amyotrophy)

on routine examination, or there may be a variety of symptoms. There appear to be three consistent patterns:

1. A "large-fiber" pattern with paresthesias in legs, absent ankle jerks, and impaired senses of light touch, vibration, and position in the lower limbs. Slight distal weakness is common and the hands may become involved.

2. A "small-fiber" pattern with dull aching pain and impaired senses of cutaneous pain, touch, and temperature sensation. Position and vibration sense, deep tendon reflexes, and strength are usually spared. Autonomic nervous system dysfunction may accompany this variant.

3. A rare "pseudotabetic" pattern associated with long-term diabetes. Severe impairment of cutaneous and deep senses permits ulceration of the feet and distal joint deformity. Romberg's sign is present, tendon reflexes are absent in the legs, and hypotension and Argyll Robertson pupils may be observed.

The course is variable in sensory neuropathy. Most often it fluctuates and then plateaus at a steady level. The pseudotabetic variety of the illness has an especially bad prognosis. Electrodiagnostic tests usually reveal changes in sensory conduction and variable alteration in motor conduction. The cerebrospinal fluid protein level is usually elevated, sometimes to a very high level.

There is no specific treatment. Diabetic neuropathies of all types are more likely to develop and patients recover less well if the metabolic state is poorly supervised. Simple analgesics rarely help the severe pain that accompanies sensory neuropathy. Trial treatment with phenytoin, carbamazepine, phenothiazine, and tricyclic antidepressants is advocated. Persons with pain and temperature insensitivity of hands and feet are vulnerable to many injuries that potentially can cascade into ulceration, cellulitis, lymphangitis, osteomyelitis, and osteolysis. Similar abnormalities are seen in syphilitic tabes, leprosy, inherited amyloidosis, and other inherited and acquired neuropathies, with the aforementioned sensory loss. The goal in treatment is to prevent the onset of tissue damage or, when it has occurred, to promote healing and prevent further damage. Persons with loss of pain and temperature sensation should not engage in most forms of manual labor or perform potentially bruising tasks with the hands and feet. Repeated inspection of hands and feet is necessary. If any bruise or ulcer appears, weight bearing or rough use should be stopped until healing occurs. Shoes should be wide and well constructed. The insides of the shoes must be inspected to remove retained objects or nails. Such patients should soak the feet in lukewarm water for 15 minutes twice daily and cover them lightly with petrolatum lotion to retain moisture in the softened skin.

Autonomic Neuropathy. Diabetic autonomic neuropathy generally is associated with symmetrical sensory neuropathy and occasionally predominates. Autonomic involvement may be asymptomatic or can cause incapacitating disability. Three types of dysfunction are prominent: gastrointestinal, cardiovascular, and genitourinary. The common gastrointestinal disturbances are gastroparesis, episodic nocturnal diarrhea, and colonic dilatation. Cardiovascular manifestations include impaired vasomotor reflexes (postural hypotension), elevated heart rate, and loss of respiratory sinus arrhythmia. Genitourinary disturbances are especially distressing and include disordered micturition with large residual volume, retrograde ejaculation, and impotence. Impotence is sometimes the initial manifestation of autonomic neuropathy. It usually steadily worsens and rarely, if ever, is improved by control of hyperglycemia, the use of testosterone, or penile implants.

Treatment of autonomic disturbances is difficult. Diabetic diarrhea may be helped by codeine phosphate or diphenoxylate, but not all cases respond favorably. A single 250-mg dose of tetracycline, if given at the outset, sometimes aborts the attack. Simple cases of postural hypotension may be helped by support stockings. More severe cases may require supplemental sodium in the diet plus sodium-retaining steroids.

Rapidly Reversible Neuropathy. Newly diagnosed untreated diabetics may display asymptomatic slowing of nerve conduction velocity. This slowing is rapidly reversed by lowering blood sugar concentration to normal levels. It seems unlikely that this phenomenon is associated with structural breakdown in peripheral nerve fibers, and it is not known whether such individuals are at greater risk of developing persistent symptomatic neuropathy.

MONONEUROPATHY AND MULTIPLE MONONEUROPATHY

PATHOLOGY AND PATHOGENESIS. It is widely held that isolated peripheral nerve lesions in diabetics have a vascular basis. Several clinical facts support this notion: they have an abrupt onset, often recover spontaneously, and are most common in the elderly. Three autopsy studies, two of oculomotor palsy and one of femoral neuropathy, have demonstrated focal vascular lesions within the area of nerve damage.

CLINICAL FEATURES AND TREATMENT. ***Cranial Nerve Lesions.*** Isolated or multiple palsies of extraocular muscle nerves or lower cranial nerves may be the first indication of diabetes in asymptomatic older adults. The third nerve is most frequently affected. Onset is usually abrupt and is associated with an intense, retro-orbital aching sensation. Sparing of the pupillomotor fibers in diabetic third-nerve palsy helps distinguish this condition from lesions that compress the nerve, such as aneurysm. Satisfactory recovery of nerve function usually occurs within several weeks.

Isolated Peripheral Nerve Lesions (Other Than Cranial). Almost every isolated peripheral nerve can be affected by diabetic mononeuropathy. Lesions of the ulnar, radial, sciatic, peroneal, tibial, and lateral cutaneous nerves of the thigh are especially common. Diabetic nerves are especially vulnerable to compression, and lesions frequently appear at such sites. Onset is abrupt and usually painful. Recovery is usually good in distally sited lesions and less satisfactory if the lesions are proximal. Treatment includes physical therapy and use of appropriate orthotic devices.

Proximal Lower Extremity Motor Neuropathy (Diabetic Amyotrophy). This syndrome usually appears after middle age. Cardinal findings include progressive, painful, asymmetrical weakness of thigh muscles, loss of knee jerks, and a few sensory abnormalities. The spinal fluid protein level is usually elevated, and the motor changes are usually bilateral, differentiating the condition from acute nerve root disease. Recovery is gradual. There is considerable variation in all of the clinical features, and many patients display distal weakness as well. As a result, the term diabetic amyotrophy has come to encompass a spectrum of illnesses that range from ischemic femoral or lumbar plexus neuropathy to symmetrical proximal metabolic neuropathy. Treatment includes major analgesics for relief of the severe self-limited pain and physical therapy directed at the thigh and hip flexor muscles.

528. NEUROPATHY ASSOCIATED WITH UREMIA

Herbert H. Schaumburg

DEFINITION AND ETIOLOGY. Uremic polyneuropathy can be associated with chronic renal insufficiency of any cause. The cause is unknown. It is widely held that uremic neuropathy is related to dialyzable toxins or metabolites normally excreted by the kidneys. The responsible agent has a molecular weight exceeding that of urea or creatinine.

PATHOLOGY. Axonal degeneration is characteristic of this disorder, and the distribution suggests that it is a distal axonopathy. The nature of the axonal change is nonspecific.

CLINICAL FEATURES. Initially, sensory symptoms predominate, with especially frequent tingling paresthesias of the leg. Occasionally a "burning foot" or "restless leg" syndrome accompanies uremic polyneuropathy. Muscle cramps in the distal extremities are common. Diminished sensation in distal limbs is the most consistent feature, usually in combination with hyporeflexia and moderate weakness.

Uremic neuropathy has an insidious onset, and subclinical cases are common. Most cases progress over several months to reach a plateau despite worsening of the renal state. The prognosis of untreated uremic neuropathy is poor.

TREATMENT. Successful renal transplantation both prevents and reverses uremic polyneuropathy. Patients with mild cases display prompt relief of paresthesias and a steady return of strength. Recovery is more prolonged in advanced cases and is not always complete. Chronic hemodialysis is less helpful and often ineffective in reversing the neuropathy.

529. NEUROPATHY ASSOCIATED WITH ENDOCRINE DISEASES (OTHER THAN DIABETES)

Herbert H. Schaumburg

Hypothyroidism is associated with both mononeuropathy and symmetrical polyneuropathy. Clumsiness and limb ataxia of uncertain origin are common and usually are attributed to cerebellar disease. Thyroid replacement therapy ameliorates the carpal or tarsal tunnel syndrome and the diffuse symmetrical neuropathy.

Acromegaly produces entrapment neuropathies at wrist and elbow and a distal symmetrical polyneuropathy. Proximal muscle weakness occurs independently of the peripheral neuropathies and may make the clinical profile confusing. The carpal tunnel syndrome presumably results from compression by acral soft-tissue hyperplasia and osteoarthritis. Improvement follows removal of the pituitary tumor, and surgery of the carpal ligament is seldom necessary. Symmetrical polyneuropathy usually occurs late in the illness and bears no relationship to plasma levels of growth hormone. No studies have been made of the effect of removal of the pituitary adenoma on neuropathy.

530. HEREDITARY NEUROPATHIES

Herbert H. Schaumburg

GENERAL. These represent a group of slowly progressive disorders probably caused by inborn errors of metabolism. They are characterized by the type of inheritance, by their natural history, and by which population of neurons is involved. Predominant involvement of lower motor neurons (progressive muscular atrophy) is called *inherited motor neuropathy;* involvement of sensory neurons is *hereditary sensory neuropathy (HSN);* involvement of both motor and sensory neurons is *hereditary motor and sensory neuropathy (HMSN);* and involvement of autonomic neurons is *dysautonomia.*

Expression of clinical symptoms in inherited neuronal disorders varies widely from patient to patient. Functional disability is frequently less than might be expected from the neurologic signs. Certain of these disorders (HMSN Type I, HMSN Type II) are common and probably account for many cases of cryptogenic neuropathy. The number of correct diagnoses increases considerably when the patient's asymptomatic relatives are examined clinically and by nerve conduction studies.

HEREDITARY MOTOR AND SENSORY NEUROPATHY

These disorders, previously described by various eponyms (Charcot-Marie-Tooth disease, Roussy-Lévy syndrome, Dejerine-Sottas disease) are now numerically subdivided into Types I, II, and III. Table 530–1 outlines the salient features of these conditions.

TABLE 530–1. THE HEREDITARY MOTOR AND SENSORY NEUROPATHIES (HMSN)

Nomenclature	Heredity	Clinical Features	Pathology and Pathogenesis
HMSN Type I (peroneal muscle atrophy) (hypertrophic form of Charcot-Marie-Tooth disease)	Autosomal dominant	Common; many mild cases; childhood onset; slow progression; predominantly motor; deformed feet (pes cavus); extreme distal lower limb atrophy; very slow motor nerve conduction	Possibly a distal axonopathy but much segmental demyelination and remyelination ("onion bulbs"); nerves may be enlarged
HMSN Type II (neuronal form of Charcot-Marie-Tooth disease or peroneal muscle atrophy)	Autosomal dominant	Less common than Type I; onset in second decade; nerve conduction almost normal; otherwise, identical to Type I	Possibly a motor and sensory neuronopathy syndrome; loss of fibers; little remyelination (no "onion bulbs")
HMSN Type III (Dejerine-Sottas disease)	Autosomal recessive	Rare; infantile onset; short stature, scoliosis, pes cavus; steady progression to severe disability; very slow nerve conduction	Few studies; enlarged nerves; many "onion bulbs"; pathogenesis unclear

DISORDERS OF PERIPHERAL SENSORY NEURONS

Patients with disorders of peripheral sensory neurons characteristically suffer from pain, cutaneous injury from lack of sensation, unsteady movement from kinesthetic sensory loss, or combinations of these conditions. Frequently they also have autonomic dysfunction. The nature of these symptoms and the associated sensory loss correspond reasonably well with the populations of fibers affected. Thus patients with loss of pain and temperature sensation and with autonomic impairment have degeneration mostly of unmyelinated and small myelinated fibers, whereas patients with loss of touch-pressure sensation have degeneration of large myelinated fibers of cutaneous nerves. In advanced disease this selectivity of involvement by fiber size tends to be lost.

HEREDITARY SENSORY NEUROPATHY, TYPE I. Hereditary sensory neuropathy, Type I, is a dominantly inherited sensory radicular neuropathy. It has been variously termed as perforating ulcers of the feet, mutilating acropathy, acrodystrophic neuropathy, and hereditary sensory radicular neuropathy. The severity varies widely. Sensory loss is usually more severe over the feet and legs than in the hands and forearms, and some patients have lancinating pains. Pain and temperature sensation are affected more than touch-pressure sensation. Nerve conduction of motor fibers is usually normal, as is life expectancy in most cases. Late in the disorder, perforating ulcers of the foot may develop, especially in patients with poor foot care.

HEREDITARY SENSORY NEUROPATHY, TYPE II. This is a recessively inherited disorder, also called congenital sensory neuropathy, that usually manifests itself in infancy or childhood with a mutilating acropathy characterized by paronychia, whitlows, ulcers of the fingers and plantar surfaces of the feet, and, frequently, unrecognized fractures of the extremities. Sensory loss affects all types of cutaneous and sometimes kinesthetic sensation and is most marked distally in all four limbs. Tendon reflexes are usually absent.

HEREDITARY SENSORY NEUROPATHY, TYPE III (DYSAUTONOMIA OF RILEY-DAY). Familial dysautonomia is a recessively inherited disorder of Jewish infants and children. It affects peripheral autonomic neurons, peripheral sensory neurons, peripheral motor neurons, and probably other central nervous system neurons. Characteristics are onset in infancy, poor feeding, repeated episodes of vomiting and pulmonary infections, autonomic disturbances, and premature death. Autonomic abnormalities include defective lacrimation, defective temperature control, skin blotching, excessive perspiration, hypertension, and postural hypotension. There is also insensitivity to pain, areflexia, corneal insensitivity, and absence of the fungiform papillae of the tongue. A congenital abnormality of nerve growth factor is postulated.

531. TOXIC NEUROPATHY Pharmaceutical Agents

Herbert H. Schaumburg

GENERAL. New pharmaceutical agents are constantly being implicated as causes of peripheral neuropathy. Except for isoniazid, pyridoxine, and vincristine, few careful experimental studies of these substances have been conducted. Clinical reports are the sole basis for many of the alleged drug-induced neuropathies. Since following prolonged use most agents appear to produce an insidious-onset distal axonopathy, there is frequently little in the clinical diagnostic profile that helps to identify the offending agent. The most important diagnostic factor in these disorders is a meticulous history of drug use. Table 531–1 lists pharmaceutical agents that are associated with generalized neuropathy. Treatment consists of withdrawing the drug if symptoms are prominent or progressive.

TABLE 531–1. PHARMACEUTICAL AGENTS ASSOCIATED WITH GENERALIZED NEUROPATHY

Chloramphenicol
Dapsone*
Disulfiram
Dichloracetate
Ethionamide
Gold
Gluthethimide
Hydralazine
Isoniazid†
Lithium
Metronidazole-misonidazole
Nitrofurantoin*
Nitrous oxide
Platinum (cis-platinum)†
Pyridoxine†
Sodium cyanate
Thalidomide†
Vincristine

*Predominantly motor.
†Predominantly sensory.

532. TOXIC NEUROPATHY Occupational, Biological, and Environmental Agents

Herbert H. Schaumburg

GENERAL. Many potential toxic chemicals are deployed in the work place and general environment, and several have been implicated as causes of peripheral neuropathy, usually of the distal axonopathic type. Since the various agents result in similar clinical syndromes, a careful occupational and environmental history is often the most important clue for diagnosis. The various agents are listed in Table 532–1, with prominent clinical features included in parentheses. *Buckthorn* and *diphtheritic neuropathies,* which are demyelinating conditions, are listed as the sole examples of diseases in which biologic toxins are consistently associated with neuropathy. Diphtheria is further discussed in Ch. 276.

TABLE 532–1. AGENTS CAUSING SYMPTOMS ASSOCIATED WITH TOXIC NEUROPATHY

Acrylamide (truncal ataxia)
Arsenic (sensory, brown skin, Mees' lines)
Buckthorn toxin
Carbon disulfide
Cyanide
Dimethylaminopropionitrile (urinary complaints)
Dichlorophenoxyacetic acid
Biologic toxin in diphtheritic neuropathy (pharyngeal neuropathy)
Ethylene oxide
n-Hexane
Lead (wrist drop, abdominal colic)
Lucel-7 (cataracts)
Methyl bromide
Organophosphates (cholinergic symptoms, delayed onset of neuropathy)
Thallium (pain, alopecia, Mees' lines)
Trichlorethylene (facial numbness)

533. MISCELLANEOUS DISEASE-SPECIFIC NEUROPATHIES

Herbert H. Schaumburg

NEUROPATHY ASSOCIATED WITH MALIGNANCY AND DYSPROTEINEMIA

Direct compression of nerves by metastic tumors occurs within the spinal canal or invertebral foramina and behind tight fascial sheaths. Bronchogenic, renal, prostatic, and breast carcinomas are especially prone to such metastases. The direct and nonmetastatic neurologic effects of cancer are described in Ch. 174.

Polyneuropathy is more common in multiple myeloma than in most other malignancies; furthermore, subclinical neuropathy appears to be frequent. Recent evidence has made it increasingly apparent that the benign gammopathies are also associated with polyneuropathy. Accordingly, the gradual development of a painful sensorimotor or sensory neuropathy in a male in middle age or later should lead to the suspicion of dysproteinemia or myeloma. These conditions are described in Chapter 174.

AMYLOID NEUROPATHY

Extracellular deposition of the fibrous protein amyloid is associated with peripheral neuropathy in both hereditary (nonimmunoglobulin-derived) amyloidosis and nonhereditary (immunoglobulin-derived) amyloidosis.

Hereditary amyloidosis is frequent only in endemic regions such as Portugal and Japan. Rare variants have also been described in Iowa and Indiana. In the Portuguese variety, which is inherited as an autosomal dominant trait, the disorder usually begins in the third, fourth, and fifth decades and affects predominantly small sensory and autonomic fibers. Lumbosacral dermatomes show a syringomyelia-like loss of pain and thermal discrimination with preservation of touch-pressure sensation. Loss of potency in the male, postural hypotension, and bladder and bowel incontinence are common in advanced stages. The disorder tends to progress over a decade or so. Biopsied sural nerves show an endoneurial reduction in unmyelinated and small myelinated fibers with nodular deposits of amyloid among the nerve trunks.

Nonhereditary amyloidosis may be divided into primary and secondary varieties. The peripheral neuropathy of primary amyloidosis also affects the distal aspects of the lower extremities more than the upper and includes small fibers as much as or more than larger ones. When typical symptoms of neuropathy are associated with enlargement of the heart, nephropathy, and enlargement of the tongue, the diagnosis of primary amyloidosis should be strongly suspected and can be confirmed by histologic examination of rectal mucosa, kidney, carpal ligament, muscle, gingivae, nerve, or bone marrow. No effective treatment for the neuropathy is available.

Patients with multiple myeloma who develop a symmetrical carpal tunnel syndrome should be investigated for systemic amyloidosis.

NEUROPATHY ASSOCIATED WITH NECROTIZING ANGIITIS AND RHEUMATOID ARTHRITIS

No fewer than nine disorders are associated with vasculitis and ischemic neuropathy. These include: polyarteritis nodosa, rheumatoid arthritis, systemic lupus erythematosus (SLE), hypersensitivity angiitis, allergic granulomatosis (Churg-Strauss syndrome), Sjögren's syndrome, Wegener's granulomatosis, and cranial arteritis (temporal arteritis).

Only polyarteritis nodosa, rheumatoid arthritis, and lupus erythematosis are encountered with any frequency in clinical practice. Although the fundamental expression of these conditions varies considerably, they all produce similar clinical and pathologic syndromes of ischemic mononeuritis multiplex. The pathogenesis of nerve fiber destruction in each condition presumably relates to focal ischemia from arteriolar occlusion. The clinical features are similar to those depicted for the mononeuropathies associated with diabetes (Ch. 527).

Rheumatoid arthritis, in addition to producing a vascular mononeuropathy, may also cause entrapment neuropathy (reflecting prolonged immobilized postures and nerve compression by articular deformity) and a chronic symmetrical sensory neuropathy. This latter disorder develops with long-term rheumatoid arthritis and is characterized by mild, distal, symmetrical sensory loss. Although frequently painful, the condition is generally benign and improves spontaneously. Corticosteroid treatment is not indicated.

INFECTIOUS AND GRANULOMATOUS NEUROPATHY (HERPES ZOSTER, LEPROSY, AND SARCOIDOSIS)

HERPES ZOSTER. This viral disorder affects sensory ganglia of cranial or spinal nerves to produce characteristic disorders, which are discussed in Ch. 501.

LEPROSY. This remains one of the most common neuropathies on a worldwide scale. It is discussed in Ch. 300.

SARCOIDOSIS. Peripheral neuropathy of uncertain pathogenesis develops in 5 per cent of cases. Both multiple mononeuropathy and symmetrical polyneuropathy occur. A mixture of localized granulomatous infiltration and vascular compromise is probably the cause.

Mononeuropathy can affect either the spinal or the cranial nerves. Most cranial neuropathy with sarcoid involvement occurs as an acute facial (Bell's) palsy that is indistinguishable from the idiopathic variety unless it causes an isolated bilateral facial paralysis that is almost pathognomonic. Simultaneous bilateral involvement is rare. Lower cranial nerves are less commonly involved. Severe paralysis is common and incomplete recovery the rule, even with corticosteroid therapy.

Distal symmetric polyneuropathy is a rare complication of sarcoidosis. Little is known about the specific cause, prognosis, or natural history of this neuropathy. Paradoxically, this form of neuropathy is usually not accompanied by prominent evidence of systemic disease.

ACUTE PHYSICAL INJURY. The results of recent experimental studies suggest a simple classification for acute nerve injury in which the clinical features, including prognosis, closely approximate the nature of the acute injury. Basically there are three different types (classes 1 through 3). In mild injury (class 1) axonal integrity is maintained but myelin may be damaged. In more severe injury (class 2) axonal continuity is lost but the connective tissue framework of the nerve is maintained. In the most severe injuries (class 3), nerve fibers and connective tissue are damaged to varying degrees. Table 533–1 depicts the types of nerve injury and their corresponding anatomic and clinical features.

NEUROPATHY ASSOCIATED WITH ALCOHOLISM, NUTRITIONAL DEFICIENCY, AND MALABSORPTION

See Ch. 482.

TABLE 533–1. TYPES OF NERVE INJURY

Type	Anatomic Lesion	Clinical Features	Course and Prognosis
Class 1	Either (A) transient conduction block due to ischemia or (B) demyelination	(A) Mild sensory loss and weakness (ischemic type) from transient abnormal posture (legs crossed) (B) Prolonged compression (Saturday night palsy) with paralysis and moderate sensory loss below site of lesion	(A) Rapid complete recovery (B) Gradual (lasting weeks) complete recovery
Class 2	Axonal interruption; connective tissue intact	Closed crush and percussion injury; loss of motor, sensory, and autonomic function below site of lesion; surgical exploration not indicated	Very slow recovery; prognosis best with distal lesions
Class 3	Transection of axons and connective tissue sheaths	Severe stretch injuries (heavy blows, motorcycle accidents) or penetrating wounds; total loss of all motor, sensory, and autonomic function; surgical intervention indicated for penetrating wounds	Little recovery even with surgical repair; poor prognosis

534. ACUTE PHYSICAL INJURY AND CHRONIC COMPRESSION-ENTRAPMENT NEUROPATHIES

Herbert H. Schaumburg

The pathophysiologic features of chronic compressions and entrapment are still debated. It is widely held that demyelination initially occurs and, if the condition persists, axonal destruction may follow. Several clinical forms are common, including carpal tunnel syndrome, ulnar palsy, meralgia paresthetica, and cervical rib form.

CARPAL TUNNEL SYNDROME. The median nerve becomes compressed at the wrist as it passes deep within the tissue to the flexor retinaculum. The usual symptoms include numbness, tingling, and burning sensations in the hand and fingers. The pain sometimes radiates up the forearm as far as the elbow or even as high as the shoulder or root of the neck. These sensations are occasionally restricted to the radial fingers but may affect all the digits. Pain and paresthesias are most prominent at night and often wake the patient from sleep. They may be relieved by shaking the hand. The hand tends to feel numb and useless on waking in the morning, but these sensations subside after brief use. The symptoms may recur following use or when the patient is sitting with the hands immobile. Such symptoms may persist for many years without objective signs of median nerve damage. In other patients, weakness of the thumb muscles develops in association with atrophy of the lateral aspect of the thenar eminence. Sensory loss may appear over the tips of the fingers. Occasionally, patients have motor symptoms of median nerve deficit in the hand without paresthesias, or motor and sensory signs may be discovered incidentally in the absence of symptoms, particularly in older individuals.

Most cases of carpal tunnel compression occur in middle-aged and often obese females. In younger women it is commonly associated with excessive use of the hands, and it may develop in males after unaccustomed use of the hands, such as in house-painting. The disorder may be caused by tenosynovitis at the wrist, by involvement of the wrist joint in rheumatoid arthritis, or as a consequence of osteoarthritis of the carpus, perhaps in relation to an old fracture. Other predisposing causes are pregnancy, myxedema, acromegaly, infiltration of the transverse carpal ligament in primary amyloidosis, and chronic hemodialysis treatments. Diagnosis is based on clinical symptoms, the finding of Tinel's sign over the median nerve in the tunnel, and demonstration of conduction block at the wrist by motor nerve velocity studies. Individuals with muscle weakness and wasting or prominent sensory loss should undergo decompression of the nerve by section of the transverse carpal ligament. In patients with paresthesias alone or when the cause is probably tenosynovitis at the wrist, a reduction in hand activity may be sufficient to allow the symptoms to subside. Injection into the carpal tunnel of a long-acting corticosteroid preparation sometimes gives temporary relief, as does splinting of the wrist to reduce movement. When troublesome symptoms persist, decompression is advisable.

For most patients with paresthesias, symptoms are relieved by decompression. Sensory impairment and cutaneous hyperesthesia, however, may persist postoperatively, and there may not be recovery after prolonged denervation of the thenar muscles.

ULNAR PALSY. The ulnar nerve may be injured at the elbow, especially in persons with a shallow ulnar groove, those who rest their weight on their elbows excessively, and those who are cachectic and lie in bed. Injury may occur years following a previously malunited supracondylar fracture of the humerus with bony overgrowth *(tardive ulnar palsy).* Contrary to the findings in the carpal tunnel syndrome, muscle weakness and atrophy characteristically predominate over sensory symptoms and signs. Patients notice atrophy of the first dorsal interosseous muscle or difficulty in performing fine manipulation. There may be numbness of the small finger, the contiguous half of the proximal and middle phalanges of the ring finger, and the ulnar border of the hand. Treatment in mild cases consists of prevention of further injury. A doughnut cushion for the elbow may be helpful. Mobilizing and transplanting the nerve to a position in front of the medial epicondyle sometimes prevents further progression.

LATERAL CUTANEOUS NERVE OF THE THIGH. *Meralgia paresthetica* is an entrapment neuropathy resulting from compression of this nerve as it passes under the inguinal ligament. Although the cause often remains unexplained, obese persons wearing tight girdles, individuals with gun belts, and those with pendulous abdomens are especially prone to develop numbness or burning sensations over the lateral thigh. Sometimes prolonged standing or walking provokes the symptoms. Weight reduction may help, and in many cases the condition subsides spontaneously. Surgical decompression is rarely necessary.

CERVICAL RIB AND THORACIC OUTLET SYNDROME. Angulation of the brachial plexus over an abnormal rib or fibrous band can damage its lower fibers and lead to weakness and wasting of the small hand muscles. Numbness and pain may occur along the inner border of the forearm and hand. Surgical removal of the rib or fibrous band sometimes abolishes the pain and paresthesias, but the small muscles of the hand often fail to recover strength. Cervical rib compression is uncommon, and most patients with paresthesias of the fingers prove to have either root compression from a cervical disc or a carpal tunnel syndrome.

535. BELL'S PALSY, BRACHIAL NEURITIS, AND TRIGEMINAL NEUROPATHY

Herbert H. Schaumburg

BELL'S PALSY (Idiopathic Facial Paralysis)

PATHOLOGY AND PATHOGENESIS. Neither the pathology nor the pathogenesis of this common illness are known. It is likely that mild cases with rapid recovery represent segmental demyelination and that axonal degeneration occurs in instances with prolonged dysfunction.

CLINICAL FEATURES. Idiopathic unilateral facial paralysis may develop rapidly within a few hours or evolve over one or two days and is often accompanied by pain behind the ipsilateral ear and excess tearing. Numbness of the face is a common complaint but inevitably refers to a proprioceptive sensation that accompanies weakness. Global facial muscle weakness is the hallmark of this condition. Hyperacusis, diminished lacrimation, and abnormal taste sensation are present to variable degrees. Untreated, 80 to 85 per cent of all patients with Bell's palsy recover completely or almost so. In a smaller number, persistent facial weakness ensues. Rarely, motor recovery fails completely. Aberrant regeneration is frequent. There may be embarrassing synkinetic movements (chewing producing eye winking) or excessive lacrimation.

Patients who are going to recover completely usually begin to show improvement during the first two weeks, while those destined to have permanent residual disability show no changes in status for three or more months. Except when paralysis is incomplete, there is little in the acute clinical profile to indicate prognosis. In patients who have complete paralysis from the onset, reliance must be placed on careful observation and electrodiagnostic tests of nerve excitability (performed at about one week after the onset).

Most authorities recommend treatment with prednisone, 1 mg per kilogram daily in two divided doses for four days, with dosage tapered to a total of 5 mg per day within ten days. It is claimed that prednisone therapy should be instituted as soon as possible if it is to have an effect in decreasing residual paralysis and synkinetic movements. In any event, pain usually subsides promptly. The unusual residual of a severe facial paralysis has a distressing cosmetic effect. Hypoglossal-facial nerve anastomosis will restore facial tone and is the operation of choice.

ACUTE BRACHIAL NEURITIS (Idiopathic Brachial Plexus Neuropathy)

PATHOLOGY AND PATHOGENESIS. There have been no thorough pathologic examinations of this condition, and the pathogenesis is unknown. Biopsy of cutaneous nerves has revealed nonspecific axonal degeneration. In most cases there is no common antecedent illness, immunization, or toxic exposure; some cases follow surgical procedures. The clinical profile is identical to that in certain serum vaccine paralyses, and a common immunologic basis has been suggested.

CLINICAL FEATURES. The condition arises as an acute, painful, and usually monophasic illness characterized by brachial plexus dysfunction. It is especially common in males aged 18 to 40. A cardinal feature is sudden severe shoulder girdle-scapular pain, occasionally extending into the arm or hand. The pain persists for a few days to a week and then subsides concomitantly with or shortly after the appearance of weakness, although it sometimes persists for several weeks. The serratus anterior is the single most commonly affected muscle. Distal weakness occurs less frequently. Rarely, the entire arm and ipsilateral diaphragm are affected. Uncommonly, weakness may appear in the other arm. Tendon reflexes are diminished in the involved extremity, but sensory loss is slight or negligible, being most commonly found at the apex of the shoulder. Involvement is usually restricted to muscles innervated by the brachial plexus. Weakness and atrophy of involved muscles lasts for months in many cases, but total recovery occurs in 90 per cent within two or three years. Treatment consists of physical therapy and orthotic devices to prevent joint damage. Corticosteroid therapy has no demonstrated value. There are occasional recurrences.

TRIGEMINAL NEUROPATHY

Rare cases are encountered of a slowly progressive bilateral sensory loss confined to the territory of the trigeminal nerve. This may lead to tissue destruction, particularly around the nostrils, as a result of repeated picking and scratching. Drug toxicity with trichloroethylene or stilbamidine may cause this syndrome. Sjögren's syndrome, systemic sclerosis, and trigeminal neurilemomas should be excluded. Some cases have been found at autopsy to have infiltration of the trigeminal ganglion with amyloid. The explanation for other cases is obscure.

536. NERVE BIOPSY IN PERIPHERAL NERVE DISEASE

Jerry G. Kaplan

Nerve biopsy is most useful in identifying the cause of multiple mononeuropathy syndromes (amyloidosis, sarcoidosis, leprosy, and vasculitis) and demyelinating neuropathies. Conditions readily diagnosed on clinical grounds, such as diabetic neuropathy and Guillain-Barré syndrome, do not require biopsy. Biopsy is seldom helpful in distal axonopathies, since most display similar nonspecific findings.

Either the sural nerve at the ankle or the radial nerve at the wrist may be sampled under local anesthesia. Tissue should be processed for routine histopathologic study, electron microscopy, and nerve fiber teasing. The latter technique is especially useful because it allows the rapid examination of long segments of individual fibers. Ideally, nerve biopsy should be performed only in institutions with considerable experience in using these techniques by a surgeon accustomed to handling such tissues.

Chapter 471 gives a description of diagnostic electrical studies in nerve or muscle disease.

Asbury AK, Arnason BG, Adams RD: The inflammatory lesion in idiopathic polyneuritis: Its role in pathogenesis. Medicine 48:173, 1969. *The classic comprehensive description of the role of the inflammatory cell in Guillain-Barré syndrome.*

Asbury AK, Johnson PC: Pathology of Peripheral Nerves. Philadelphia, W. B. Saunders Co., 1970. *A concise, clearly written book covering the salient aspects of peripheral neuropathy.*

Dyck PJ, Oviatt KF, Lambert EH: Intensive evaluation of unclassified neuropathies yields improved diagnosis. Ann Neurol 10:222, 1981. *A description of the increased diagnostic yield when a patient with neuropathy is studied in a special center.*

Dyck PJ, Thomas PK, Lambert EH: Peripheral Neuropathy. Philadelphia, W. B. Saunders Company, 1984. *A multiauthored and authoritative reference for peripheral nerve disease.*

Moore PM, Cupps T: Neurological complications of vasculitis. Ann Neurol 14:155, 1983. *A comprehensive review of the protean neurologic complications of these disorders, especially the neuropathies.*

Raff MC, Asbury AK: Ischemic mononeuropathy and mononeuropathy multiplex in diabetes mellitus. N Engl J Med 279:17, 1968. *A paper that clearly demarcated the role of small-vessel disease in diabetic mononeuropathy.*

Schaumburg HH, Spencer PS, Thomas PK: Disorders of Peripheral Nerves. Philadelphia, F. A. Davis Company, 1983. *A short lucidly written monograph providing a good introduction to this complex subject.*

Spencer PS, Schaumburg HH: Experimental and Clinical Neurotoxicology. Baltimore, Williams & Wilkins, 1980. *A multiauthored comprehensive text with special emphasis on the peripheral nervous system.*

Sunderland S: Nerves and Nerve Injuries. New York, Churchill Livingstone, Inc., 1978. *A monumental monograph on nerve injury; the standard reference.*

Section Sixteen DISEASES OF MUSCLE AND NEUROMUSCULAR JUNCTION

Lewis P. Rowland

537. INTRODUCTION

DEFINITIONS. The *motor unit* comprises four elements: the motor neuron, its peripheral axon, the terminal branches and corresponding neuromuscular junctions, and the many muscle fibers innervated by the particular nerve cell. The major symptom of most diseases of the motor unit is *weakness*.

The word *atrophy* means, literally, "lack of nourishment." It has come to mean wasting of muscle, or loss of muscle bulk from any cause, and it is also used to denote single muscle fibers that are smaller than normal when viewed microscopically. When used in the name of a disease, atrophy always implies that the muscle wasting is secondary to a neural disorder, e.g., infantile spinal muscular atrophy, progressive spinal muscular atrophy, or peroneal muscular atrophy. To avoid ambiguity, it is therefore appropriate in examining patients to use "wasting" rather than "atrophy" to describe diminution in muscle bulk unless the cause is known to be neurogenic. *Myopathies* include disorders characterized by weakness or some other symptom of muscle dysfunction that is not due to emotional or neurogenic cause. Some authors speak of "primary" or "secondary" myopathies, but there is little evidence that any muscle disease is really "primary," in the sense that there is an abnormality in muscle and nowhere else. In some myopathies, as in thyrotoxic myopathy, the fundamental disorder is elsewhere, and this could be true even in genetically determined diseases. The *dystrophies* are a subgroup of myopathy with three special characteristics: heritable transmission, progressive weakness, and histologic evidence of degeneration of muscle with no evidence of abnormally stored material or structural abnormality of the fibers.

DIFFERENTIAL DIAGNOSIS OF MUSCLE DISEASE

The differential diagnosis of muscle disease can be broken down into several considerations: (1) the nature of the symptoms, (2) combinations of muscles affected, (3) age of the patient, (4) findings on examination, (5) tempo of disease, (6) genetics, and (7) results of laboratory studies.

SYMPTOMS. *Weakness* implies lack of normal strength or power. However, patients with pathologically weak muscles usually complain of the consequences of weakness, not weakness itself. That is, they have difficulty walking or rising from low seats if leg muscles are affected. They may lose manual dexterity for buttoning clothes or writing, or have difficulty lifting or raising the arms. Or, if cranial muscles are affected, there may be *dysarthria* (slurred speech), *dysphagia* (difficulty swallowing), *diplopia* (double vision), or *ptosis* (a droopy eyelid). In contrast, explicit complaint of loss of strength is less likely to be a manifestation of disease; a fading athlete may be growing older, losing prowess, but he or she is not sick. Complaints of fatigue, constant tiredness, and an urge to rest are likely to be manifestations of emotional depression but not muscle disease.

In muscle diseases, it has also been traditional to explain the weakness in solely morphologic terms; many muscle fibers show evidence of degeneration and are ultimately replaced by fat and connective tissue. However, clinical weakness often seems disproportionately more severe than the histologic evidence indicates. Conversely, many fibers may be morphologically abnormal (for instance, muscle fibers may be severely distorted by stored glycogen in McArdle's disease), but the patient may not be weak at all. Therefore, we presume that functional alterations of muscle, as well as the morphologic changes, also contribute to the weakness of muscle disease.

Other symptoms of muscle disease are less common than weakness. Aching muscles *(myalgia)* may result from vigorous exercise of specific muscles that are "untrained" or "out of condition," or may occur more diffusely in patients with polymyositis or dermatomyositis, or during attacks of myoglobinuria. Myalgia is attributed to stimulation of pain-sensitive nerves within muscle by edema or toxic metabolites but has not been formally studied. In *myoglobinuria,* the red muscle pigment is released from muscle into blood serum in amounts sufficient to darken the urine overtly. Oxidized myoglobin appears rust-colored or brown, rather than red. Limb weakness, myalgia, and malaise often accompany attacks of frank myoglobinuria, the causes of which will be discussed later. *Myotonia* refers to a painless condition of impaired relaxation of muscle after a forceful contraction; for instance, patients may have difficulty letting go after trying to unscrew a bottle cap or turn a recalcitrant doorknob. Myotonia occurs in several different diseases, but the common physiologic abnormality seems to be repetitive depolarization of muscle fibers. It is most common in specific genetic disorders but may affect otherwise normal individuals who are taking diazacholesterol or other drugs that affect the lipid composition of muscle cell membranes.

Muscle cramps are another kind of involuntary and sustained muscle spasm, but differ from myotonia in that sustained voluntary effort is not a precipitating factor and because the sudden forceful shortening of a cramp is painful.

When any one of these symptoms (other than weakness) is prominent, the differential diagnosis is narrowed to a relatively few conditions. The differential diagnosis of weakness, however, involves much of clinical neurology. We are not here concerned with cerebral causes of weakness (likely to be expressed by hemiparesis) or other upper motor neuron disorders (which may cause weakness or incoordination of all four limbs) because they are immediately separated from diseases of the lower motor neuron or motor unit by the characteristic exaggeration of tendon reflexes, clonus, and Hoffmann and Babinski signs. Neurogenic and myopathic diseases of the motor unit, however, must be distinguished from each other, and the distinction is not always easy. The following criteria help.

CHARACTERISTIC COMBINATIONS OF MUSCLES AFFECTED IN DIFFERENT SYNDROMES. A few conditions can be recognized at a glance because of the characteristic appearance of the patient, imparted to some extent by the particular set of muscles affected. Perhaps the most specific is the long, lean face of myotonic dystrophy—long and lean because the temporalis and masseter muscles are small; the appearance is made even more characteristic because there may be ptosis of the eyelids (caused by weakness of the levators) and eversion of the lips (caused by weakness of facial muscles). Dysarthria (resulting from weakness of oropharyngeal muscles) and thin neck (resulting from smallness of sternomastoid muscles) contribute to the appearance.

In myasthenia gravis, many of the same muscles are affected. Ptosis of the eyelids, facial weakness, dysarthria, and dysphagia are common but the appearance differs. In contrast to those with myotonic dystrophy, patients with myasthenia are more likely to have diplopia and ophthalmoparesis, asymmetric ptosis (often unilateral), and do not have the long, lean face or thin neck. The only other myopathic conditions likely to be confused with these disorders of cranial muscles are the *ocular myopathies,* described later. Among neurogenic diseases, only motor neuron disease causes diffuse and symmetrical weakness of cranial muscles, but the eyelids and ocular movements are spared, and only oropharyngeal muscles are affected prominently.

When limb muscles are affected predominantly, there are few characteristic combinations that distinguish neurogenic from myopathic disease, a distinction that often must be made by laboratory tests. Even when specific combinations are engrafted in the names of conditions (such as "facioscapulohumeral muscular dystrophy" or "scapuloperoneal syndromes"), the cause may be either neurogenic or myopathic. In both of these sets of disorders, *"winging of the scapula"* (visible protrusion of the scapula away from the chest wall) is prominent.

In general, two rules apply: (1) Distal limb weakness is more likely to be due to neurogenic disorder, but some cases are myopathic. (2) Proximal limb weakness is more likely to be myopathic, but this is an even less reliable criterion because there are so many exceptions. Probably the only syndromes of proximal limb weakness that are evident on inspection are facioscapulohumeral muscular dystrophy and Duchenne dystrophy. In the latter, however, it is not just the distribution of weakness that identifies the disorder, for the patient is always a young boy and the severity of weakness is appropriate to his age; by about age 12 he will not be able to walk. Before he stops walking, his calves are likely to appear disproportionately large *("pseudohypertrophy").*

AGE AT ONSET OF WEAKNESS. Duchenne dystrophy is not the only diagnosis that depends on age. In the neonatal period, at least three neuromuscular disorders may appear: neonatal myasthenia gravis (in children of myasthenic mothers), myotonic muscular dystrophy, and botulism. "Congenital myasthenia gravis" and "congenital myopathies," despite the names, usually become evident later in the first year or two of life. In the first year of life, almost all cases of limb weakness of neuromuscular origin (not cerebral) are due to infantile spinal muscular atrophy (Werdnig-Hoffmann disease); peripheral neuropathy and early-onset myopathies are only rarely expressed before age two years.

After infancy, children and adults experience the gamut of neuromuscular diseases, involving areas from the motor neuron through the peripheral nerve and neuromuscular junction to muscle, although the names and tempo may differ at different ages. Among the diagnostic clues that depend upon age are the following: (1) Among the muscular dystrophies, the Duchenne form is one of early childhood, almost always evident before age three years. Facioscapulohumeral and limb-girdle forms usually begin in adolescence. The only muscular dystrophies that begin after age 35 are some cases of the autosomal dominant forms (myotonic muscular dystrophy, facioscapulohumeral dystrophy, and ocular myopathies). (2) Dermatomyositis occurs in children (and with roughly equal frequency in all decades of life into old age). Polymyositis, in contrast, rarely occurs before adolescence. (3) Charcot-Marie-Tooth disease and other hereditary neuropathies begin in childhood or adolescence, rarely later.

SIGNS ON EXAMINATION. When there is solely proximal limb weakness, both neurogenic and myopathic disorders can cause the same triad of manifestations: weakness, wasting, and loss of reflexes. Some signs are indicative of neurogenic disease: (1) *Fasciculation,* visible twitching of portions of a muscle, occurs in chronic motor neuron diseases, rarely in peripheral neuropathy, and probably never in myopathy (with the possible exception of a severe form of thyrotoxic myopathy that is no longer seen in these days of prompt diagnosis of hyperthyroidism). (2) *Glove-stocking patterns of cutaneous sensory loss* imply peripheral neuropathy. (3) *Combinations of upper and lower motor neuron signs* in the same limbs are virtually pathognomonic of amyotrophic lateral sclerosis. Similarly, the combination of distal limb weakness, fasciculation, and other lower motor neuron signs in the arms or cranial muscles with upper motor neuron signs in the legs bespeaks amyotrophic lateral sclerosis.

When, as is too often the case, there are no clear signs of neurogenic disease and there is only chronic proximal limb weakness, the differential diagnosis depends upon laboratory tests, as described below.

Few signs can be regarded as pathognomonic of myopathy. *"Pseudohypertrophy"* of the calves, or disproportionate enlargement of these or other muscles, is characteristic of Duchenne dystrophy but occurs occasionally in other myopathies and also in some cases of neurogenic disease. Myotonia is characteristically myopathic, but other disorders (that are different electromyographically) may be similar clinically. The combination of myotonia and muscular enlargement is restricted to myotonia congenita. Only the concomitant appearance of myoglobinuria and weakness or the entire constellation of signs that indicate myotonic muscular dystrophy can be regarded as definitely myopathic.

TEMPO OF DISEASE. Recognition and definition of neurogenic and myopathic diseases are often based upon tempo. For instance, periodic paralysis is just that—attacks of weakness that come on in moments or hours and last for hours or days. Between attacks, the patient may be normal or there may be chronic weakness that is less severe than in the periodic attacks.

The periodic pattern differs from the fluctuations seen in myasthenia gravis, which may be of three kinds: (1) There may be minute-to-minute variation, especially for ptosis of the eyelids. (2) There may be variations during the course of a single day, or from day to day. (3) There may be longer and more dramatic fluctuations in severity, exacerbations or periods of improvement. The extremes are represented by "myasthenic crisis," which is defined by the need for respiratory assistance, or "remissions," in which symptoms disappear for weeks, months, or years, only to return again. No other neuromuscular disease fluctuates the way myasthenia gravis does.

Both myasthenia and periodic paralysis, when first starting, may appear to be acute illnesses, but there are not many other acute neuromuscular disorders. Among the myopathies, polymyositis may become severe in a few days or weeks, and attacks of myoglobinuria may be accompanied by severe weakness in a day or two. But most myopathies are chronic. Among neurogenic diseases, the Guillain-Barré syndrome usually reaches peak severity in a few days or within two weeks. A similar pattern is followed by brachial plexus neuropathies, toxic neuropathies, and botulism, but most acquired neuropathies are slower in evolution, taking months to reach maximal severity, and most genetic neuropathies progress for years.

GENETICS. Genetic patterns influence diagnosis in two ways. First, a family history of affected relatives may alert the clinician (or the patient) to a known diagnosis, or the pattern of inheritance may suggest the diagnosis. Second, when a diagnosis of genetic disorder is made, other members of the family may then be identified as carriers of recessive genes (by biochemical markers) or as affected by a dominant disorder (by clinical examination). In the near future, it is expected that the application of recombinant DNA techniques will aid in the identification of specific heritable diseases in individual patients and their relatives.

LABORATORY TESTS. Many diseases can be identified without recourse to any laboratory test. Other conditions may also be diagnosed clinically, but laboratory tests are used to confirm the diagnosis, to be certain that some other condition is not masquerading. That is why muscle biopsy and EMG are done in myotonic disorders or Duchenne dystrophy, for example, although these procedures are essentially superfluous for diagnosis if the serum creatine kinase (CK) concentration is very high.

Some conditions are virtually defined by laboratory tests. For instance, changes in muscle biopsy define the "structurally specific" congenital myopathies (such as central core disease or nemaline disease), mitochondrial myopathies, and lipid-storage myopathies, all of which are named after the specific abnormal structure. Changes in muscle biopsy may also aid in the diagnosis of sarcoid, amyloidosis, toxoplasmosis, trichinosis, or periarteritis nodosa. But all of these are rare, and the most common use of both muscle biopsy and EMG is to determine whether or not weak muscle is denervated.

In general both EMG and biopsy give concordant results. Discordant or contradictory results occur in 5 to 10 per cent of cases and are of two types: (1) If the EMG is consistent with denervation but the biopsy shows "myopathic" changes, most centers would give primacy to the EMG because the muscle biopsy may show myopathic changes in unequivocally denervating disorders, as in survivors of paralytic poliomyelitis. (2) If the reverse is found—"myopathic EMG" and denervating changes in the biopsy—no diagnosis is possible, a conflict only rarely experienced.

Several pairs of diseases are defined by EMG and muscle biopsy. In each of these pairs the clinical syndromes are similar, and, unless there is overt fasciculation, the clinician cannot distinguish the neurogenic and myopathic forms. In assigning a diagnosis to any of these pairs, EMG signs of denervation make one diagnosis, and either lack of these neurogenic signs or a "myopathic" EMG pattern makes the other diagnosis (Table 537–1).

Diagnostic Use of Muscle Biopsy. SIGNS OF DENERVATION. Normally, histochemical stains show two major types of muscle fibers. One type stains strongly for glycolytic enzymes, the other for oxidative enzymes. In some muscles there is only one fiber type, but in most human muscles both types are represented in a "checkerboard" pattern. This biochemical differentiation parallels physiologic differences of fast- and slow-twitch fibers. Furthermore, all of the muscle fibers innervated by the same neuron are of the same fiber type. Studies have shown that the muscle fibers of a normal single motor unit are not usually grouped together but the fibers of several units are intermingled.

The diagnostic signs of denervation in human biopsies are based upon these principles and concepts of "collateral sprouting" in reinnervation. In partially denervated muscle, surviving terminal axons send branches to adjacent muscle fibers which have lost the original innervation. By this process, the size of functioning units is larger than normal, and contiguous muscle fibers are of the same histochemical type (fiber-type grouping) instead of the normal checkerboard appearance. Atrophic fibers may also appear in groups (group atrophy), and this may be a consequence of later denervation of an augmented motor unit. Another histochemical sign of denervation, defined by its appearance, is the "target fiber," which is found only in neurogenic disorders but is not understood. All of these histologic signs tend to affect muscle focally so that lack of morphologic change in a small sample does not exclude a neurogenic disorder.

SIGNS OF MYOPATHY. In contrast to the group lesions of denervation, myopathic changes often occur randomly. More specifically "myopathic" changes include evidence of degeneration and regeneration of muscle fibers. Degenerating fibers lose their normal striations and become fragmented and subject to invasion by macrophages. Early in the process, there is disproportionate variation of fiber size. The smaller fibers are thought to be recently regenerated or to result from fiber-splitting. The large fibers are larger than usual, occur more often in chronic disorders, and may be due to compensatory

TABLE 537–1. PAIRS OF DISEASES THAT ARE DISTINGUISHED BY EMG AND MUSCLE BIOPSY

Age	Neurogenic	Myopathic
Infancy	Infantile spinal muscular atrophy	Severe congenital myopathy
Childhood and adolescence	Juvenile spinal muscular atrophy	Limb-girdle muscular dystrophy Facioscapulohumeral muscular dystrophy Quadriceps myopathy
Adults	Motor neuron disease	Distal myopathy

work hypertrophy of surviving fibers when diseased fibers cannot participate in the work of the muscle. In muscular dystrophies, macrophages are few, except in scattered fibers, and there is little perivascular monocytic response, but these signs of "inflammation" may be prominent in polymyositis. In both the dystrophies and polymyositis, regeneration is heralded by a basophilic appearance in sections stained with hematoxylin and eosin, presumably because of increased content of RNA in newly formed fibers that are actively making new proteins. In advanced myopathy, muscle fibers are replaced by fat and connective tissue; this may be evident earlier in some dystrophies, but the end-stage is similar in either neurogenic or myopathic disease.

OTHER HISTOCHEMICAL ALTERATIONS. The "congenital myopathies" are identified by, and defined by, physical structures such as nemaline rods, fingerprint structures, and central cores. These structures are "specific" only in appearance, since little is known about the pathogenesis of any of them. Histochemical methods also allow the identification of accumulations of glycogen or lipid, observations that may lead to specific biochemical diagnosis by appropriate biochemical tests on muscle homogenates.

SPECIFIC DIAGNOSIS BY MUSCLE BIOPSY. None of the preceding uses of muscle biopsy is definitive; even accumulations of glycogen or lipid require further biochemical analysis. The only truly specific diagnoses that can be made from a biopsy are sarcoid, periarteritis nodosa, amyloidosis, and parasitic infestation (trichinosis, cysticercosis, toxoplasmosis). By using special histochemical stains, it is possible to identify conditions caused by genetic lack of phosphorylase or phosphofructokinase, but these and other specific enzyme disorders should be verified by enzyme assay of homogenates. Special studies may aid in the diagnosis of Lafora's disease and neuronal ceroid lipofuscinosis.

ROLE OF ELECTRON MICROSCOPY. Ultrastructural study of muscle has engaged a major research effort, but the electron microscope has no role in routine diagnosis.

RESEARCH APPLICATIONS OF MUSCLE BIOPSY. Research laboratories throughout the world are using biopsied muscle specimens for biochemical analysis, physiologic study, or muscle culture. Muscle diseases are almost all resistant to specific therapy and hope for ultimate treatment lies in this kind of research. Because of this, because diagnostic biopsy provides only limited information that is not likely to affect therapy, and because it is difficult to justify more than one standard biopsy, it seems reasonable to make a plea for regional muscle biopsy centers. At present, biopsies are done in most community hospitals, and by the time the patient reaches a research center it is difficult to suggest a second biopsy for purely research purposes.

Electromyography. The distinction between neurogenic and myopathic disease depends upon the electrical activity of a muscle at rest and during weak contractions. Attention is paid to the frequency, amplitude, and duration of motor unit potentials. Details of the electromyogram and its diagnostic usefulness in muscle disorders are given in Ch. 471.

Biochemical Studies. The most common biochemical test used in the diagnosis of muscle disease is the measurement of serum activity of sarcoplasmic enzymes, especially CK, but also other enzymes. In myopathic diseases, these enzyme activities are characteristically high; the enzyme proteins in serum are thought to enter blood from necrotic muscle or because of altered permeability of muscle surface membranes. CK determination is often regarded as the most sensitive, and it may be—in the sense that CK is often abnormal when other enzymes are normal. However, the increased sensitivity in detecting myopathies comes at a price, because CK is also often abnormal in chronic motor neuron diseases, thus losing the ability to discriminate myopathic and neurogenic diseases. In most hospitals, routine blood chemistry determinations are now automated and include other enzyme activities such as GOT, GTP, and LDH. The concentrations of these serum enzymes also rise in patients with muscle disease and only rarely in neurogenic disease. When there is no obvious heart or liver disease, therefore, these other enzymes may be useful in neuromuscular diagnosis. Still other enzyme assays (such as aldolase or pyruvate kinase) or radioimmunoassay for myoglobin are favored in some institutions but have no special advantage in the diagnosis of muscle disease. Similarly, isoenzyme analysis has no particular advantage; even the MB or "cardiac" isoenzyme of CK may appear in the serum in Duchenne dystrophy or polymyositis, not because the heart is involved but presumably because this isoenzyme dominates in immature muscle skeletal muscle fibers, and regenerating fibers are plentiful in these diseases.

Specific biochemical diagnosis is restricted to the glycogen and lipid storage diseases and the analysis of myoglobinuria, as discussed later. These biochemical studies are indicated when histochemical stains show accumulation of fat or glycogen in syndromes of limb weakness, and in all cases of nontraumatic myoglobinuria.

Brooke MH: A Clinician's View of Neuromuscular Diseases. Baltimore, Williams & Wilkins Company, 1977. *A favorite of students because of the lively and accurate descriptions of clinical syndromes.*

Buchthal F, Schmallbruch H: Motor unit of mammalian muscle. Physiol Rev 60:90, 1980. *A modern statement of the organization of the motor unit, with attention to physiology and morphology.*

Dubowitz V: Muscle Disorders in Childhood. Philadelphia, W. B. Saunders Company, 1978. *A comprehensive review of common and rare syndromes by a single author who is an experienced clinician. The many excellent illustrations include instructive photographs of patients and muscle biopsies.*

Goodgold J, Eberstein A: Electrodiagnosis of Neuromuscular Diseases. 3rd ed. Baltimore, Williams & Wilkins Company, 1983. *A popular, well-illustrated, and clear introduction to the theory and practice of electromyography and nerve conduction studies.*

Mastaglia FL, Walton JN: Skeletal Muscle Pathology. Edinburgh, Churchill-Livingstone, 1982. *Lucid descriptions and beautiful illustrations cover the common and the exotic conditions.*

Vinken PJ, Bruyn GW, Ringel SP (eds.): Diseases of Muscle. Handbook of Clinical Neurology. Vols. 40, 41. Amsterdam, North-Holland Publishing Company, 1979. *Individual chapters by different authors cover every conceivable disorder in great detail.*

Walton JN (ed.): Diseases of Voluntary Muscle. 4th ed. Edinburgh, Churchill-Livingston, 1981. *A multiauthored and authoritative book, with attention to basic science as well as clinical aspects. The four editions attest to the book's status as the standard reference.*

538. INHERITED DISEASES

MUSCULAR DYSTROPHIES

DEFINITION. Muscular dystrophies are inherited myopathies, characterized primarily by progressively severe weakness. In the absence of known biochemical abnormality, they are distinguished from similar diseases by lack of histologic evidence of any metabolic storage material, or by changes other than those of degeneration and regeneration of muscle or tissue reactions to these processes.

ETIOLOGY. Although it is generally believed that inherited diseases must be due to a missing or structurally abnormal protein (either an enzyme or a structural protein), this abnormality has not been identified in any form of dystrophy. Increasing biochemical and ultrastructural evidence implicates the muscle surface membrane as the site of fundamental disorder. There is evidence of dysfunction of enzymes that are an integral part of the membrane, and there are gaps in the plasma membrane that permit the entry of large molecules such as horseradish peroxidase, a protein, or procion yellow, a dye. Biochemical study of isolated membranes has been limited, however, because only small amounts of tissue are available in a biopsy and the membrane preparations include fat and connective tissue. In red blood cell membranes and cultured fibroblasts no consistent abnormality has been discovered.

Pathologic and biochemical abnormalities can be detected in muscle, and there is no clear evidence of neural abnormality in traditional terms. There is still debate about the possible role of altered motor neurons, and some writers postulate a debatable vascular cause, functional ischemia of muscle.

CLASSIFICATION. No classification of the muscular dystrophies is entirely satisfactory, but clinical and genetic analysis provides the best approach at present. The classification in Table 538–1 is based upon the clearly identifiable features of Duchenne dystrophy, facioscapulohumeral dystrophy, and myotonic muscular dystrophy. Limb-girdle dystrophy is probably not a single disease but encompasses cases that do not fall into the other categories. The techniques of molecular genetics should give more precise classifications.

INCIDENCE. None of the muscular dystrophies is common. Incidence rates vary from 5 per million births for facioscapulohumeral dystrophy to about 250 per million for Duchenne dystrophy. The mutation rate of Duchenne dystrophy is high, 7×10^{-5}, and about two thirds of the cases appear sporadically, with no other affected individual in the family.

PATHOLOGY. Pathologic abnormalities are restricted to skeletal muscle, sometimes involving cardiac muscle. The brain, spinal cord, and peripheral nerves are devoid of histologic change, although some authors have implicated the brain because of a seemingly high incidence of mental retardation in children with Duchenne dystrophy. Terminal pneumonia may cause changes in the lungs, and there may be a variety of associated diseases not directly linked to the dystrophy. In myotonic muscular dystrophy, baldness and testicular atrophy are integral parts of the disease in men, and corneal opacities affect both sexes.

The abnormalities in muscle seem to involve all fibers in random fashion. Early, there is scattered evidence of necrosis and regeneration, with prominent variation in fiber size, including many fibers much larger than normal and many fibers that appear hyalinized. Later, fibers disappear, to be replaced by fibrous connective tissue and fat. "Pseudohypertrophy" is probably due to both "true" hypertrophy (large fibers) and increased accumulation of fat and connective tissue. In myotonic dystrophy, unusual figures form "ring fibers" (with one fiber running at right angles, encircling the other fibers in the same bundle) and "sarcoplasmic masses," or accumulations of sarcoplasm that are free of myofilaments. However, these abnormalities occur occasionally in other diseases and are not pathognomonic of myotonic dystrophy. In Duchenne dystrophy, the myocardium may be affected by similar changes, but cardiac symptoms are rarely evident in life, a discrepancy that has been attributed to the sedentary life imposed upon the patients by advanced muscular weakness. Myopathic changes in the heart are common in myotonic dystrophy. There is no good evidence that smooth muscle is regularly affected in any form of dystrophy.

Ultrastructural investigations suggest an early, and perhaps primary, abnormality of the muscle surface membrane, but it is not clear how this might be related to the progressive degeneration of muscle. The postulated abnormality of the surface membranes may allow an inappropriate influx of calcium, and this could have several deleterious effects, including local hypercontraction of myofilaments near the sites of calcium entry (overstretching and disrupting myofilaments in adjacent sarcomeres), stealing of intracellular ATP (because mitochondrial calcium uptake is an energy-dependent process), or activating of intracellular proteases. The initiating event in the degenerative process is not known; disruption of myofibrillar structure, alterations of mitochondria, and degeneration of tubules and sarcoplasmic reticulum all seem to proceed together.

CLINICAL MANIFESTATIONS. The symptoms and signs of all forms of the muscular dystrophies are related to weakness alone, except that additional systems are involved in myotonic dystrophy. In other forms, the symptoms depend upon the distribution of weakness and the age at onset. In *Duchenne dystrophy* weakness is primarily proximal at onset, and symptoms begin early. By definition, girls are not affected. (However, girls with chromosomal abnormalities may have the disorder; study of these unusual cases identified the location of the Duchenne gene as Xp21.) There are no symptoms in the first year of life, but walking may be somewhat delayed beyond 18 months. Once the child walks, some abnormality is usually evident to an experienced observer (either a parent with a previously affected child or a skilled physician). The boys tend to waddle or walk on their toes, or fall frequently and have difficulty rising. They are probably never able to run, because they have difficulty raising their knees. These symptoms become more evident as the children grow older, and even the most unsuspecting parent becomes aware of some abnormality by age five. Teachers sometimes may detect the difficulty when the child starts school. Some cases are averred to start between ages five and ten, but these must be exceptional. It is difficult to examine individual muscles of a young child, but the waddling gait, the typical method of rising from the ground by "climbing up" himself (*Gowers' sign*), enlargement of calf or other muscles, and inability to run are characteristic. Myotatic reflexes may be normal at first, but by three years the knee jerks are usually lost, and later the ankle jerks disappear. As the child grows, increased growth and coordination may com-

TABLE 538–1. CLASSIFICATION OF HUMAN MUSCULAR DYSTROPHIES

	Duchenne Dystrophy	Facioscapulohumeral Dystrophy	Limb-Girdle Dystrophy	Myotonic Dystrophy
Genetic pattern	X-linked, recessive	Autosomal, dominant	Autosomal, recessive	Autosomal, dominant
Age at onset	Before age 5	Adolescence	Adolescence	Early or late
First symptoms	Pelvic	Shoulders	Pelvic	Distal; hands or feet
Pseudohypertrophy	+	0	0	0
Predominant weakness, early	Proximal	Proximal	Proximal	Distal
Progression	Relatively rapid; incapacitated in adolescence	Slow	Variable	Slow
Facial weakness	0	+	0	Occasional
Ocular, oropharyngeal weakness	0	0	0	Occasional
Myotonia	0	0	0	+
Cardiomyopathy	0 or late	0	0	Arrhythmia, conduction block
Associated disorders	None (?mental retardation)	None	None	Cataracts; testicular atrophy and baldness in men
Serum enzymes	Very high	Slight or no increase	Slight or no increase	Slight or no increase
Prevalence (per million population)	38	5	20	25
Incidence (per million births)	251	5	47	–
Mutation rate	9×10^{-5}	5×10^{-7}	3×10^{-5}	10×10^{-6}

pensate temporarily for the concurrent progressive weakness and wasting, but the disease always prevails. There is increased difficulty walking. Going up grades or stairs first requires aid, then becomes impossible. Weakness of the trunk muscles leads to increased lordosis and a protuberant abdomen. Then the arms become weak. Finally, in early adolescence, the child becomes unable to walk. This may be accelerated by a period of inactivity after an injury or an orthopedic operation. Contractures appear, at first in the feet, as the gastrocnemius muscles tighten. When the child stops walking, flexion contractures limit motion of the knees, and scoliosis becomes more a problem with prolonged sitting. Ultimately respiration becomes shallow and the child is increasingly subject to pulmonary infection. Sooner or later, one of these infections is fatal, usually in the third decade. Although muscles are ravaged from the neck down, the cranial muscles are entirely spared. Congestive heart failure and abnormalities of cardiac rhythm are rare.

Becker dystrophy has manifestations similar to those of Duchenne dystrophy, including X-linked inheritance, but the onset is later in childhood or in adolescence, and the tempo is slower and more variable. This form may also be devastating, but some patients are able to function, albeit with limitations, well into adult life. The clinical similarities include pseudohypertrophy of calf muscles and increased serum content of creatine kinase (CK) and other sarcoplasmic enzymes. However, although the two forms are similar, they are genetically separate; there are no mildly affected individuals in typical Duchenne families, nor are young children affected severely in Becker families. In some sporadic cases and in some families it is difficult to decide whether the disorder is Duchenne dystrophy of relatively late appearance or Becker dystrophy of relatively early appearance. The distinction awaits recognition of the specific genes or specific biochemical abnormalities in the two or more forms.

Still a third X-linked recessive form is called *Emery-Dreifuss muscular dystrophy*. It differs from the Duchenne type in later age at onset and benign course and from both Duchenne and Becker types because pseudohypertrophy is not found and serum enzymes are normal or only minimally increased. Additionally, the Emery-Dreifuss form has two characteristics that are not found in either of the other X-linked dystrophies: cardiac arterial standstill and contractures at knees, elbows, and neck. The cardiac disorder poses a threat of sudden death and requires treatment by pacemaker.

The manifestations of *limb-girdle dystrophy* are also similar because weakness of muscles of the pelvic girdle usually initiates the syndrome, but symptoms start in late childhood or adolescence. Girls are affected as often as boys, and pseudohypertrophy is rare. Waddling gait, difficulty in walking and climbing, and frequent falls are common. Occasionally, symptoms begin in the shoulder girdle. In either case, there is usually weakness in all four limbs by the time the patient seeks medical attention. Severity, age at onset, and rate of progression vary considerably, suggesting that this category contains more than one disease.

Facioscapulohumeral dystrophy is distinct. Symptoms vary in severity so that some affected individuals never have any disability (but can be recognized by the signs), whereas others become incapacitated early; there are all grades in between. The first symptoms are apt to be related to difficulty in raising the arms or to prominence of the scapulae. Weakness of the legs may affect pelvic girdle muscles, or equally prominent weakness of the anterior tibial muscles may lead to a steppage gait. Weakness of trunk muscles may lead to prominent scoliosis. The face is always involved on examination; the perioral muscles may be more affected than those of the upper face, but ultimately patients have difficulty in closing the eyes. The sternal head of the pectoral muscle is affected earlier than the clavicular head, a selectivity that can be detected on testing the individual muscles, and leads to a peculiar appearance of the axillary folds when the arms are dependent, because the anterior axillary fold of normal people is formed by the sternal portion of the pectoral muscle. As a result, the anterior axillary fold normally extends upward and outward from the chest to the head of the humerus, but in patients with this form of muscular dystrophy the anterior fold may seem to rise straight up or even reverse, rising medially toward the clavicle. Winging of the scapulae can be seen when the patient leans against a wall with the arms extended, and the weakness of shoulder girdle muscles leads to an unusual appearance because, viewed from the front, the superior margin of the scapula is higher than the clavicle.

Myotonic muscular dystrophy diverges from the preceding types in several respects. (1) The distribution of weakness differs in that cranial muscles are often affected and limb weakness is initially more marked in distal muscles. Thus weakness of the hands precedes shoulder weakness, and footdrop or steppage gait precedes symptoms of pelvic muscle weakness. *Ptosis, facial weakness,* and *dysarthria* are signs not seen in the other forms of dystrophy. Moreover, there is almost always selective weakness and smallness of the sternomastoids. The masticatory muscles either are poorly developed or waste early (even when not symptomatically weak), causing a characteristic long, lean facial appearance. (2) Myotonia, or difficulty in relaxation, may be symptomatic, and after a firm grip the patient may have difficulty letting go. Myotonia may cause other symptoms in patients with myotonia congenita (see below), but in the dystrophy only the hands are affected by this kind of stiffness. Myotonia of grip may be evident on examination, and can also be elicited by percussing the thenar eminence. In normal persons this evokes a rapid twitch, whereas in patients with myotonia, a sustained contraction of the adductor pollicis muscle persists for several seconds, only gradually relaxing. Similar responses to percussion may be elicited in the finger extensors or tongue but the response is difficult to demonstrate in other muscles. Although myotonia is a dramatic sign and a symptom that can be relieved by drugs, it is not the symptom that causes the major disability in myotonic dystrophy; weakness is the problem. (3) Other systems are involved in this pleomorphic disorder; cataracts appear sooner or later in all patients, and are sometimes the only sign of the disease; most of the men (but not the women) have frontal baldness; testicular atrophy affects most of the men, but often after they have already sired children to perpetuate the disease (there is no definite evidence of gonadal insufficiency in affected women); the basal metabolic rate is often low, but other tests of thyroid function are normal (extrathyroidal hypometabolism). The incidence of diabetes mellitus may be increased. Glucose metabolism is often abnormal but analysis has been difficult and controversial; insulin resistance may be due to decreased affinity of insulin receptors. (4) Conduction defects are common in the electrocardiogram and may lead to clinically significant arrhythmia or congestive heart failure.

Certain rare forms of muscular dystrophy are named after the prominent manifestations. *Ocular muscular dystrophy* is a slowly progressive disorder in which ptosis of the eyelids and progressive immobility of the eyes are the cardinal features. The pupils are spared, and both eyes are usually affected symmetrically so that diplopia is uncommon. Other muscles of the head, neck, and limbs may also be affected, varying from family to family. This syndrome raises problems of definition; some cases probably are myopathic in origin, but this kind of ophthalmoplegia is often associated with other manifestations that are clearly neurogenic (such as spinocerebellar degeneration or peripheral neuropathy). The final distinction is often difficult or impossible to make because, in ocular muscles, the conventional electromyographic and biopsy criteria of myopathy are not valid. In some patients with myopathic ophthalmoplegia, structural and biochemical abnormalities may be found in limb muscles. Abnormally large mitochondria are present in increased numbers; this can be seen dramatically in electron microscopy, and the numbers are sufficient to stain fibers red in the trichrome stain for light microscopy, leading to the appellation "ragged red fibers." In these cases there is apt to be an accumulation of glycogen, but the biochemical cause of this has not been ascertained.

Distal myopathy, as the name implies, affects distal leg and hand muscles first. It is probably the rarest form of dystrophy, and can be identified only by characteristic signs of myopathy in electromyography and muscle biopsy.

In the *scapuloperoneal syndrome* distal weakness in the legs resembles that of neurogenic peroneal muscular atrophy, but sensory loss is lacking, and there is proximal weakness in the shoulder girdle similar to that of facioscapulohumeral dystrophy. Some of these cases are myopathic and some neurogenic as distinguished by electromyography, muscle biopsy, and serum enzymes. In either case, autosomal dominant inheritance and a relatively slow progression seem characteristic.

DIAGNOSIS. The clinical picture of Duchenne dystrophy entails little diagnostic confusion. In its first stages, some children are merely regarded as clumsy, and some receive orthopedic care because of toe-walking; otherwise the diagnosis becomes obvious. As noted, the trait is transmitted as a sex-linked recessive, and once a case is recognized, members of the family rapidly detect the signs in subsequently affected youngsters. Once a family is known, affected individuals can be identified in the neonatal period because the serum enzymes are already markedly abnormal. Limb-girdle and facioscapulohumeral dystrophy must be differentiated from neurogenic diseases, from congenital myopathies, and from polymyositis, as will be discussed below. Myotonic dystrophy may be confused with endocrine disorders or, because of the distal weakness, with neuropathy or amyotrophy, or with hypothyroidism or gonadal disorders. Ocular myopathy must be differentiated from myasthenia gravis; there is no fluctuation of symptoms in the myopathy, and the weakness does not respond to cholinergic drugs.

The familial cases of progressive ophthalmoplegia (ocular muscular dystrophy) also have to be distinguished from an unusual syndrome that seems to be sporadic and has only once been reported to affect siblings. This form, *the Kearns-Sayre syndrome*, is identified by the triad of progressive ophthalmoplegia, pigmentary degeneration of the retina, and onset before age 15. Almost all patients with these three features will be found to have evidence of heart block on the electrocardiogram and cerebrospinal protein content of more than 100 mg per deciliter. More than half of these patients also have short stature, hearing loss, and evidence of corticospinal tract or cerebellar disease.

The differential diagnosis of the myopathies also depends upon the age of the patient. In childhood and adolescence, the major problems involve peroneal muscular atrophy (Charcot-Marie-Tooth) and "muscular atrophy simulating muscular dystrophy" (Wohlfart-Kugelberg-Welander). In adults, amyo trophic lateral sclerosis is the major problem. At all ages, polyneuritis must be considered.

MOLECULAR GENETICS. The chromosomal site of the gene for Duchenne dystrophy is known to be on the short arm of the X chromosome, and flanking probes are already available. It is anticipated that even closer probes will be available in 1985. The method then could be used for prenatal diagnosis and for precise identification of carriers.

The gene for Becker dystrophy was long thought to be on the long arm of the X chromosome because it seemed to be linked to the gene for colorblindness. However, molecular probes suggest that the Becker gene is allelic to the Duchenne gene; this would account for the similarity of these diseases. With better probes, it should be possible to identify young boys while they are still walking, and this would give more accurate prognosis.

The gene for myotonic muscular dystrophy is on chromosome 19, as determined by linkage studies and molecular probes. If better probes can be found, it would be possible to identify which at-risk members of the family will have the disease and which will be spared. It will also be possible to determine whether the syndrome is heterogeneous and comprises more than one form.

TREATMENT. There is no specific treatment for any form of dystrophy. Physical therapy, exercises, splints, braces, and corrective orthopedic surgery are applied in different centers with varying degrees of enthusiasm. Some claim that walking can be prolonged into late adolescence in Duchenne dystrophy. The most poignant decisions concern the use of antimicrobial drugs or supported respiration for young men paralyzed from the neck down and with no hope of ultimate recovery. The myotonia of myotonic dystrophy can be relieved by phenytoin (0.3 to 0.6 gram daily) or by quinine (0.3 to 1.5 grams daily), but this is rarely the problem, and nothing can be done for the weakness. Cataracts are treated surgically upon appropriate indication, and cardiac arrhythmias and congestive heart failure are managed accordingly.

PROPHYLAXIS. Genetic counseling offers the only possibility to control muscular dystrophy at present. Carriers of Duchenne dystrophy may often but not always be identified by abnormally increased serum enzyme activity (higher than normal, but not as high as in affected boys). In some centers, antenatal detection of sex allows selective prophylactic abortion. There is presently no way to determine whether a male fetus is affected, however. The development of methods to measure CK in fetal blood unfortunately did not predict reliably whether the fetus was affected. Fetal blood sampling may ultimately provide the way to identify the true biochemical abnormality in the fetus, assuming that it will be the same in both muscle and erythrocytes, an assumption that is not proved. Birth control ought to be effective in dominantly inherited diseases such as facioscapulohumeral and myotonic dystrophy, but many cases are relatively mild and the risk is acceptable to some families. The high rates of mutation do not encourage optimism that genetic restriction can be the ultimate goal.

Bradley WG: The limb-girdle syndromes. Handb Clin Neurol 40:433, 1979. *A thoughtful review of a common syndrome that illustrates the difficulty of separating myopathies from neurogenic disorders.*

Harper PS: Myotonic Dystrophy. Philadelphia, W. B. Saunders Company, 1979. *A modern classic; thorough in coverage, thoughtful in analysis, and written in a lively style.*

Munsat TL: The classification of human myopathies. Handb Clin Neurol 40:275, 1979. *Overview of the problem of identifying different muscle diseases, introducing a multiauthored summary of all of the dystrophies.*

Roses AD, Pericak-Vance MA, Yamaoka LH, Stubblefield E, Stajich J, Vance JM, Roses MJ, Carter DB: Recombinant DNA strategies in genetic neurological diseases. Muscle Nerve 6:339, 1983. *A primer of modern genetic approaches to muscular dystrophies and other diseases in which the gene product is not known.*

Rowland LP: Biochemistry of muscle membranes in Duchenne muscular dystrophy. Muscle Nerve 3:3, 1980. *A detailed review of the evidence for and against the theory that the genetic lesion in this disease affects muscle surface membranes.*

Rowland LP, Layzer RB: X-linked muscular dystrophies. Handb Clin Neurol 40:349, 1979. *A review of the four different forms of X-linked muscular dystrophy.*

Stuart CA, Armstrong RM, Provow SA, Plishker GA: Insulin resistance in myotonic dystrophy. Neurology 33:679, 1983. *A review and study of an unresolved endocrine problem in myotonic muscular dystrophy.*

OTHER INHERITED BIOCHEMICAL DISORDERS: METABOLIC MYOPATHIES, MITOCHONDRIAL MYOPATHIES, AND FAMILIAL MYOGLOBINURIA

DEFINITION. The muscular dystrophies may ultimately prove to be disorders of metabolism, but that is speculative and the term "metabolic myopathy" is now used only for diseases in which there are more or less clearly defined abnormalities of glycogen, lipid, or energy metabolism. Although some of these conditions are described in greater detail in other chapters, it is necessary to mention them here because they enter into the differential diagnosis of syndromes of proximal limb weakness or myoglobinuria.

GLYCOGEN STORAGE MYOPATHIES

These diseases, described in detail in Ch. 179, were the first heritable diseases of muscle in which the biochemical defect was discerned. Of the several forms, the only ones that do not affect muscle are type 1 (lack of glucose-6-phosphate dehydrogenase) and type 6 (lack of liver phosphorylase).

Pompe's disease, the infantile form of glycogen storage disease type 2, is associated with *lack of acid maltase.* It affects both motor neurons and muscle, causing a clinical disorder that resembles Werdnig-Hoffmann disease, from which it is distinguished by glossomegaly and cardiomegaly with congestive heart failure. It is uniformly fatal by one year of age. In another group of acid maltase deficiencies the disease starts later in childhood or even in adult years. The syndrome is one of proximal limb and diaphragm weakness that resembles either limb-girdle dystrophy or polymyositis. The only clinical clues to the nature of the disease are the prominence of respiratory failure and the presence of myotonic discharges in the electromyogram (although there is no clinical myotonia). Histologically, there is a vacuolar myopathy, which can be shown to be due to deposition of glycogen in skeletal muscle. In the infantile form, but not in late-onset forms, cardiac muscle is affected and motor neurons in the brain and spinal cord are also swollen and distorted by abnormal accumulation of glycogen. Lack of acid maltase is demonstrated by biochemical assay of muscle homogenates or in the urine.

Type 3 glycogen storage disease, caused by *lack of the debrancher enzyme system,* is usually manifest by hepatomegaly and hypoglycemia, but skeletal muscle may be involved with the liver, or even alone. This disorder may also resemble limb-girdle dystrophy or polymyositis. Diagnosis is suspected on the basis of histochemical study of muscle and proved by biochemical analysis. Types 5 and 7, resulting from *lack of phosphorylase (McArdle's disease)* or *phosphofructokinase (Tarui's disease)* are causes of recurrent myoglobinuria, as described earlier and in Ch. 179.

LIPID STORAGE AND MITOCHONDRIAL MYOPATHIES

There is no adequate classification of mitochondrial myopathies because the specific biochemical abnormalities are unknown. For the same reason it is not known how many of these disorders are inherited and how many are acquired. For convenience, they may be separated into four categories: (1) a group identified only by morphologic abnormality, (2) abnormalities of muscle lipid metabolism, (3) abnormalities of pyruvate oxidation or electron transport, and (4) myoglobinuria. See Table 538–2.

MORPHOLOGICALLY ABNORMAL MITOCHONDRIA. In these conditions the mitochondria are too numerous, too large, or contain abnormal crystalline inclusions. Histochemical examination with the light microscope reveals a colorful pattern in muscle fibers as a result of accumulations of large mitochondria. In trichrome stain, the muscle fibers are blue and the mitochondria at the periphery are a striking red, giving rise to the popular term *"ragged red fibers."* The histologic abnormality is associated with a diversity of clinical syndromes, and there is no apparent relationship between the mitochondrial abnormality and the symptoms. For instance, the histologic changes are seen in both congenital and later-life syndromes of proximal limb weakness. The same changes are almost always present in patients with two very different kinds of ocular myopathy, including those with the specific constellation of manifestations that characterize the Kearns-Sayre syndrome (described earlier) and those with nothing more than restricted external ophthalmoplegia. Even vague fatigue states or cramps may be associated with abnormal mitochondria. In some of these nonspecific syndromes, there may be a persistent but slight increase in venous blood lactate content, not enough to cause acidosis. In others, there is profound lactic acidosis, as described below in disorders of pyruvate metabolism. Results of biochemical studies of mitochondria are either normal or show minor and nonspecific deviations from controls. There is no effective therapy.

LIPID STORAGE MYOPATHIES. In some syndromes of proximal limb weakness, there is gross accumulation of lipid *within* muscle fibers (in contrast to the fat that is deposited *between* fibers in Duchenne dystrophy), which can be identified by simple histochemical stains. Usually there are mitochondrial abnormalities as well. The accumulation of lipid in some cases can be attributed to very low levels of muscle carnitine, a compound necessary for the esterification and transport of long-chain fatty acids into mitochondria. Fatty acid oxidation

TABLE 538–2. MITOCHONDRIAL MYOPATHIES

Common Name	Clinical Manifestations	Morphologic	Biochemical Abnormality
Morphologic abnormality			
Nonspecific mitochondrial myopathy	Proximal limb weakness (early or late), cramps, fatigue syndrome	Ragged red fibers, giant mitochondria, increased number of mitochondria, crystalline conclusions	Slight or no increase in venous lactate
Ocular myopathy	Progressive ophthalmoplegia with or without limb weakness	Same	Same
Kearns-Sayre syndrome	Ophthalmoplegia, pigmentary degeneration of retina, heart block, high CSF protein, neural disorders	Same	Same
Lipid storage myopathy			
Muscle carnitine deficiency	Limb weakness	As above, plus lipid storage	Carnitine low in muscle, normal in serum
Systemic carnitine deficiency	Limb weakness plus hepatic encephalopathy	Same, plus lipid storage	Carnitine low in muscle, serum, and liver
Triglyceride storage disease	Ichthyosis, steatorrhea, limb weakness	Lipid storage in muscle, white blood cells	No specific abnormality
Disordered energy metabolism			
Pyruvate dehydrogenase deficiency Cytochrome deficiencies	Limb weakness plus encephalopathy in infants	Lipid storage, ragged red fibers	Lactic acidemia; lack of one of three components of PDH or cytochrome
Luft's disease	Euthyroid hypermetabolism	Same	Partial uncoupling of mitochondrial respiration and phosphorylation
MELAS*	Myopathy, encephalopathy, strokes in childhood	Same	Lactic acidosis, biochemical disorder not known
Fukuhara syndrome	Ataxia, myoclonus, seizures	Same	Lactic acidosis, biochemical disorder not known
Myoglobinuria			
DiMauro's disease	Recurrent myoglobinuria	Usually normal	Lack of carnitine palmityl transferase
Malignant hyperthermia	Fever, muscle stiffness, lactic acidosis, myoglobinuria, cardiac arrhythmia	Normal	Abnormal muscle response to caffeine; increased muscle adenyl cyclase

*MELAS = mitochondrial encephalomyopathy, lactic acidosis, and stroke.

is impaired and triglycerides accumulate. There is no predictable clinical pattern except that progression may be slightly more rapid than in most muscular dystrophies or there may be periods of improvement or worsening, or respiratory muscles may be affected—all characteristics that might lead to suspicion of polymyositis rather than muscular dystrophy. There are at least two types of carnitine deficiency. In one *(muscle carnitine deficiency)*, the content of carnitine in muscle is about 10 per cent of normal, but the serum content of carnitine is normal and symptoms are confined to limb weakness. In the second type *(systemic carnitine deficiency)*, serum and liver carnitine contents are reduced in addition to muscle, and symptoms include attacks of hepatic encephalopathy that may be fatal. Oral carnitine therapy has helped some patients, and, for unknown reasons, prednisone may help. Some cases are familial in a pattern that suggests an autosomal recessive trait; the sporadic cases could also be inherited, but some may be acquired. In the third syndrome of proximal limb weakness and lipid storage in muscle, carnitine determinations are normal and the cause of lipid accumulation is not known.

One other lipid storage myopathy can be recognized by four characteristics that seem to go together: congenital ichthyosis, lifelong steatorrhea, lipid storage myopathy, and accumulation of triglycerides in white blood cells and cultured fibroblasts or cultured muscle. The cause is not known.

DISORDERS OF PYRUVATE METABOLISM OR ELECTRON TRANSPORT. A block in the oxidation of pyruvate would affect such a fundamental metabolic process that it ought to be incompatible with life. In fact, genetic lesions affecting each of the three component enzymes of the pyruvate dehydrogenase complex have been identified. These syndromes usually appear in the newborn period and affect brain as well as muscle; the resulting encephalopathy and severe lactic acidosis are rapidly fatal. Less severe but similar syndromes affect older children with encephalopathy, proximal limb weakness, lactic acidemia, and lipid storage myopathy. Although a disorder of mitochondrial oxidation of pyruvate is suspected, the nature of the disorder is not clear because the pyruvate dehydrogenase enzymes are normal.

There are also infantile syndromes of severe myopathy that seem to be due to inherited abnormalities of the cytochromes.

A most dramatic mitochondrial disorder is *Luft's disease*, described in only two unrelated adults with euthyroid hypermetabolism. Heat intolerance was manifest by constant sweating and fever that resulted from uncoupling of mitochondrial respiration and phosphorylation of unknown cause, with no satisfactory treatment.

FAMILIAL MYOGLOBINURIA. Sporadic myoglobinuria is described in Ch. 539. In some persons, however, repeated attacks from childhood suggest a genetic disorder, and sometimes more than one individual in a family is affected. Some of these familial cases are due to lack of muscle phosphorylase or phosphofructokinase. The patterns of myoglobinuria are similar in both disorders, but phosphofructokinase deficiency is accompanied by hemolytic anemia as well as the myopathy. These disorders can be recognized by the ischemic work test in which contracture is induced and venous lactate fails to rise, by histochemical evidence of glycogen accumulation in muscle, and finally by biochemical assays for the appropriate enzymes (see Ch. 179).

In three recognized disorders of glycolysis, there is no storage of glycogen, but recurrent myoglobinuria is seen. The affected enzymes are phosphoglycerate kinase (DiMauro), phosphoglycerate mutase (DiMauro), and lactate dehydrogenase (Kanno). They are distinguished from other forms of recurrent myoglobinuria only by biochemical analysis.

In the most common form of inherited myoglobinuria (*DiMauro's disease*), the missing enzyme is carnitine palmityl transferase, which plays a vital role in the oxidation of long-chain fatty acids. It might be expected that lack of this enzyme would result in the same syndrome that accompanies carnitine deficiency. However, in DiMauro's disease, there is neither persistent limb weakness nor consistent lipid storage; the only symptoms are recurrent attacks of myoglobinuria. In still other cases of familial recurrent myoglobinuria, no abnormality has been found in either lipid or glycogen metabolism.

In all of these familial syndromes, episodic myoglobinuria is the main and usually the only manifestation. Permanent proximal limb weakness is rare. Renal failure, however, may complicate an attack of myoglobinuria of any cause. The only way to prevent attacks is to limit physical activity, avoiding prolonged or unusually vigorous exercise. The limits are soon learned by affected individuals.

MALIGNANT HYPERTHERMIA. Malignant hyperthermia is a rare problem defined by a catastrophic reaction to general anesthesia. In the course of preparing for surgery, the patient receives a muscle relaxant (usually succinylcholine) and a general anesthetic (usually halothane). Soon the muscles become very stiff and body temperature begins to rise rapidly. Severe metabolic acidosis caused by lactic acidemia follows, and there may be myoglobinuria. Cardiac arrhythmias and renal failure may ensue. When the syndrome was first recognized, the incidence was said to be about 1 in every 50,000 general anesthesias, and the mortality rate was about 75 per cent. Now, however, anesthesiologists are alert to the possibility. By stopping the operation, ending anesthesia, cooling rapidly, neutralizing the acidosis, and, perhaps, giving dantrolene, the malignant element can be removed. Similar syndromes are seen in patients who take psychoactive drugs (*malignant neuroleptic syndrome*) and in heat stroke, but these syndromes are not seen in families with malignant hyperthermia.

In some families, the condition seems to be inherited as an autosomal dominant trait, but in most cases the event is sporadic and there is likely to be more than one kind of susceptibility. Patients with central core disease and Duchenne muscular dystrophy may be at special risk. It is suspected that patients inherit an abnormal susceptibility to either succinylcholine or halothane (or other agents), to which they react by excessive and prolonged release of calcium in muscle and that this is followed by the other manifestations.

Treatment of the acute attack requires prompt intervention to institute symptomatic measures. Prevention is difficult because it is so hard to identify those at risk. Some patients who have actually had attacks have congenital structural abnormalities (such as cryptorchidism or pedal abnormalities), or they may have high serum creatine kinase activity between attacks, or there may be minor abnormalities of nonspecific nature in muscle biopsy. Several patients have had histologic evidence of central core disease. However, none of these characteristics has proved a reliable guide, and immediate relatives of patients should have physiologic tests of excised muscle with caffeine or biochemical studies of adenylate cyclase or phosphorylase activity. If either physiologic or biochemical test results are abnormal, a warning bracelet should be worn by the individual. Even if these tests give normal results, all immediate relatives of patients who have had attacks should be identified to anesthesiologists before elective surgery. Patients with central core disease or Duchenne dystrophy also require caution for elective surgical procedures, especially in early childhood.

Prophylaxis may be possible. If there is sufficient evidence of risk, the individual may be given dantrolene by mouth for 24 hours before elective surgery. In a multicenter study, the mean dose was 2.5 mg per kilogram of body weight, but this does not guarantee protection.

DiMauro S: Metabolic myopathies. Handb Clin Neurol 41:175, 1979. *Clearly written review of myopathies resulting from disorders of glycogen or lipid metabolism and mitochondrial abnormalities.*

DiMauro S, Trevisan C, Hays A: Disorders of lipid metabolism in muscle. Muscle Nerve 3:369, 1980. *Review of a rapidly evolving field.*

Gronert GA: Malignant hyperthermia. Anesthesiology 53:395, 1980. *Comprehensive review of a clinical problem of growing importance.*

Penn AS: Myoglobin and myoglobinuria. Handb Clin Neurol 41:259, 1979. *A thorough review of the many causes of myoglobinuria.*

Rowland LP, DiMauro S: Glycogen storage diseases of muscle: Genetic problems. Res Proc Assoc Nerv Ment Dis 60:239, 1983. *A review of the heterogeneity of these syndromes.*

Scarlato G, Cerri C (eds.): Mitochondrial Pathology in Muscle Diseases. Padua, Piccin Medical Books, 1983. *Chapters cover this evolving field, including infantile disorders of pyruvate metabolism, other identified biochemical abnormalities of mitochondrial function, and clinically identified disorders such as the Kearns-Sayre and Fukuhara Syndromes.*

Willner JH, Nakagawa M: Controversies in malignant hyperthermia. Semin Neurol 3:275, 1983. *A critical review of the methods used to detect susceptibility to this baffling syndrome.*

CONGENITAL MYOPATHIES

DEFINITION. These are rare diseases characterized by weakness that is usually mild but persists throughout life, usually remaining stationary or progressing imperceptibly.

ETIOLOGY. The cause is not known. A few of these disorders are familial and suspected of having a genetic basis, but so many cases are sporadic that other causes are not excluded, and there are no clear clues.

PATHOLOGY. These diseases are defined in terms of pathology, and most of them have been delineated within the past 20 years since the introduction of histochemical techniques to study muscle biopsy. The names of the diseases reflect the predominant anatomic disorder.

In *central core disease,* the central portion of the muscle fiber appears rather amorphous, in contrast to the fibrillar appearance of the surrounding normal portion. In cross-section, the central portion appears blue when stained with Gomori's trichrome, in striking contrast to the red periphery. The central areas lack all oxidative enzyme activity, and there are no mitochondria in this region. In *nemaline myopathy* or *rod myopathy,* small threadlike or rod bodies are scattered throughout the fiber. The rods are barely visible in conventional hematoxylin and eosin stains, but can be seen readily in phase contrast or with the trichrome stain. In electron microscopy the structures seem to originate in the Z-band, and circumstantial evidence suggests that they are composed of tropomyosin. *Myotubular myopathy* designates the appearance of myofibers that resemble a stage in the early development of fetal muscle, with nuclei located centrally rather than at the periphery and surrounded by a halo of apparently empty space. Because the pathogenesis of this appearance is uncertain, some investigators prefer the name *centronuclear myopathy.* As indicated above, some *mitochondrial myopathies* are associated with only morphologic abnormalities of these organelles (with no recognizable functional abnormality) in a syndrome of congenital and static limb weakness.

CLINICAL MANIFESTATIONS. Some congenital myopathies lack specific morphologic signs; such disorders have been called *severe nonspecific congenital myopathy* or, if associated with severe mental retardation, *congenital muscular dystrophy of Fukuyama.* (Because the syndrome is not progressive, "myopathy" may be the preferable word.) Nonspecific myopathic changes are also seen in patients with multiple congenital abnormalities of joints, *arthrogryposis multiplex congenita.* Some cases of arthrogryposis show histologic changes that imply a neurogenic cause.

These disorders are only exceptionally symptomatic in the first year of life, except that the onset of walking may be delayed. Later, symptoms of proximal limb weakness become evident: waddling gait, difficulty in climbing stairs, frequent falls, scoliosis, and weakness of the arms. Sometimes, onset of the syndrome in adults makes it unlikely that the morphologic changes were congenital, and some acquired but unknown cause is suspected. In none of the structurally defined congenital myopathies is it possible to link the morphologic abnormality to a biochemical or physiologic cause of the weakness.

The hallmark of arthrogryposis is congenital fixation of joints, often with other skeletal abnormalities. The disorders may be mild or severe but are always static.

GENETICS. Most cases of congenital myopathy are sporadic, but some patterns of inheritance suggest autosomal dominant or autosomal recessive transmission. Arthrogryposis syndromes are likely to be autosomal dominant if there is more than one case in a family, but most are sporadic.

DIAGNOSIS AND TREATMENT. Proximal limb weakness in a young child is usually myopathic in origin, but must be distinguished from the neurogenic Wohlfart-Kugelberg-Welander syndrome and from polyneuritis. Myopathic abnormalities in the electromyogram, an abnormal family history, an incidence in girls, and especially the histologic abnormalities define the individual entities. The serum enzymes may be normal or slightly increased. In some clinics most cases of apparently congenital myopathy fail to meet the specific histologic criteria, showing only nonspecific myopathic changes in biopsy. There is no better designation for these cases than "congenital myopathy," but it is likely that there is more than one cause.

In infancy, the major cause of weakness is a form of motor neuron disease (*Werdnig-Hoffmann disease*). Among infants with multiple congenitally fixed joints (arthrogryposis multiplex), some prove to have myopathic disease as defined by muscle biopsy and electromyography. In some cases, neonatal difficulty in swallowing is followed by delayed onset of walking, possibly persistent weakness, obesity, childhood diabetes, mental retardation, and a characteristic facial appearance (*Prader-Willi syndrome*), but there is no abnormality on muscle biopsy or electromyogram.

Bender, AN: Congenital myopathies. Handb Clin Neurol 41:1, 1979. *A thorough review of the congenital myopathies that are identified by morphologic abnormality.*

Brooke MH, Carroll JE, Ringel SP: Congenital hypotonia revisited. Muscle Nerve 2:84, 1979. *A skeptical view of the practice of "defining" disease solely on the basis of morphologic change.*

Brown LM, Robson MJ, Sharrard WJW: The pathophysiology of arthrogryposis multiplex congenita neurologica. J Bone Joint Surg 62-B:291, 1980. *A clinical analysis, with discussion of orthopedic treatment.*

Dubowitz V: Muscle Disorders in Childhood. Philadelphia, W. B. Saunders Company, 1978. *Congenital myopathies are placed in the perspective of other neuromuscular diseases of childhood by an experienced clinician and investigator.*

Edstrom L, Wroblewski R, Mair WGP: Genuine myotubular myopathy. Muscle Nerve 5:604, 1982. *Detailed analysis of one dramatic form of congenital myopathy.*

Hall JG, Reed SD, Greene G: The distal arthrogryposes: Delineation of new entities—review and nosologic discussion. Am J Hum Genet 11:185, 1982. *An interesting attempt to classify hereditary arthrogryposis syndromes according to association with other congenital malformations.*

Mastaglia FL, Walton JN: Skeletal Muscle Pathology. Edinburgh, Churchill-Livingstone, 1982. *Illustrations and discussion of the congenital disorders are provided in this excellent text.*

MYOTONIA CONGENITA
(Thomsen's Disease)

DEFINITION. Myotonia congenita is a rare disorder characterized by difficulty in relaxation of skeletal muscle after forceful contraction, present from early childhood.

There are occasional sporadic cases, but most are inherited in a pattern corresponding to an autosomal dominant trait. In a few families, the disease seems to be autosomal recessive. The abnormality must be inherent within the muscle, because myotonic phenomena may be elicited after all neural influences are abolished by spinal anesthesia, block of motor nerves by local anesthesia, or blockade of the neuromuscular junction by intra-arterial injection of d-tubocurarine. Myotonia is abolished by the intramuscular administration of procaine. In human myotonia congenita, as in a genetic myotonia of goats, there seems to be an abnormality of chloride conductance in muscle, and this could account for the tendency to discharge repetitively. The disorder in myotonic muscular dystrophy seems to differ, and it is possible that the biochemical abnormality is different in each of the several forms of inherited human myotonia.

CLINICAL MANIFESTATIONS. The difficulty in relaxation is widespread. Difficulty in relaxing the grip may lead to prominent and sometimes embarrassing symptoms. Ocular muscles may be affected, so that the eyes seem momentarily "stuck" in one position, or the eyelids may remain closed after forceful closure. Sometimes oropharyngeal muscles are affected, with difficulty in speaking or swallowing. Startle reactions may induce stiffness of the legs, thwarting sudden attempts to catch a bus or run from home plate. There is no weakness, and one characteristic is the unusual muscular development of many patients, causing a Herculean appearance. The myotonia can be elicited by tapping any muscle in severely affected cases. Reflexes are unaltered.

DIAGNOSIS. The major problem is in distinguishing the disorder from myotonic muscular dystrophy. Here the only symptoms and signs are related to myotonia. There is no weakness, cataract, baldness, or gonadal atrophy. So-called "transitional cases" are probably patients in families with myotonic muscular dystrophy who are only mildly affected and show only myotonia before the other manifestations.

TREATMENT. For many years, quinine was the staple treatment in doses of 0.3 to 1.5 grams daily. Recently, phenytoin has proved equally effective and less apt to cause disagreeable side effects in therapeutic doses of 0.3 to 0.6 gram daily. Procainamide has also been used, in doses of 4 to 6 grams daily, but this drug is prone to induce lupus erythematosus and is therefore avoided.

Harper PS: Myotonic Dystrophy. Philadelphia, W. B. Saunders Company, 1979. *The standard reference for this multisystem disorder and related conditions.*

Howeler CJ, Busch HFM, Bernini LF, Van Loghem E, Khan PM, Nijienhuis LE: Dystrophia myotonica and myotonia congenita concurring in one family. Brain 103:497, 1980. *These two disorders are ordinarily distinct and only rarely occur in the same family—a paradox awaiting the techniques of molecular genetics for solution.*

Lipicky RJ: Myotonic syndromes other than myotonic muscular dystrophy. Handb Clin Neurol 40:533, 1979. *Analysis of myotonic syndromes by a leading physiologist who has been investigating the basic mechanisms.*

Roses AD, Harper PS, Bossen EH: Myotonic muscular dystrophy. Handb Clin Neurol 40:485, 1979. *Comprehensive review of clinical and biochemical aspects.*

FAMILIAL PERIODIC PARALYSIS

DEFINITION. Periodic paralysis is characterized by recurrent attacks of flaccid weakness usually associated with abnormally high or low serum potassium concentrations. Many cases are familial. In sporadic cases the abnormality may be due to aberrations of potassium metabolism.

ETIOLOGY AND PATHOGENESIS. Familial cases are distributed in a pattern consistent with autosomal dominant inheritance. Hypokalemia during attacks was the first metabolic abnormality to be recognized, with no loss of potassium in urine. It was presumed that potassium shifted from extracellular to intracellular compartments, especially muscle. This has been difficult to prove, and the anticipated hyperpolarization of the muscle membrane potential has not been substantiated by direct measurement with intracellular electrodes. Abnormalities of glucose metabolism have been suspected, because attacks can be precipitated by infusions of glucose and insulin, by eating a large meal, or by administration of epinephrine. However, biochemical studies have failed to pinpoint the abnormality.

In other families, the serum potassium rises during attacks, which can be induced by ingestion of potassium. This variety is therefore called *hyperkalemic periodic paralysis* and is generally considered to be the mirror image of the hypokalemic type, with potassium presumably shifting out of muscle and into blood during attacks. There are clinical differences between the two forms of periodic paralysis, but there are so many areas of overlap and so many common features that it is difficult to decide just how many genetically distinct forms there really are.

PATHOLOGY. In both forms of periodic paralysis there may be vacuoles within muscle fibers. These may be numerous or scanty, and it is not clear whether they are more frequent in paralyzed muscle. Most electron microscopists believe that the vacuoles are derived from the sarcoplasmic reticulum, but others think they originate in the T-system in areas of necrotic muscle. Glycogen seems to be increased in amount in ultrastructural studies, but the results of biochemical analysis have been inconsistent. There is no evidence that other organs are affected in either form of the disease. The heart is usually spared pathologically.

CLINICAL MANIFESTATIONS. In the hypokalemic variety, attacks tend to start in late childhood or adolescence, frequently occur at night, are apt to be severe, and last for a day or more. In the hyperkalemic variety, attacks start at an early age, occur much more frequently, tend to be milder, and may last minutes or hours. Moreover, patients with hyperkalemic periodic paralysis usually have some evidence of myotonia, often limited to percussion myotonia of the tongue. Lid-lag and Chvostek's sign are identified with the hyperkalemic type. These clinical distinctions may break down in application to individual cases and are only crude guides. Moreover, many features are common to both types: dominant pattern of inheritance, susceptibility to attacks during periods of rest after vigorous exercise, ability to ward off attacks by mild exercise after a mild attack has begun, persistent weakness between attacks, vacuoles in muscle, lack of clear relation between serum potassium concentration and severity of paresis, induction of local weakness by cooling, and protection against attacks by acetazolamide. Some patients are affected by attacks in which the serum potassium may be either high or low.

Typical attacks start with weakness of the legs, followed by weakness of the arms. Cranial muscles are affected in severe attacks only, and respiratory insufficiency is exceptional. The attacks may be mild and brief, or severe and prolonged, with all gradations in between. During severe attacks, the myotatic reflexes are lost, and the muscles are electrically inexcitable. Attacks are rarely apoplectic in onset and usually take an hour or more to develop, except that attacks beginning in sleep may be fully developed when the patient awakes. Paresthesias and myalgia may be prominent at the onset, or may be completely lacking. Some patients are aware of oliguria during the attack and diuresis afterward.

The serum potassium is in the range of 2.5 to 3.5 mEq per liter in hypokalemic attacks, and 5.0 to 7.0 mEq per liter in the hyperkalemic type. Between attacks serum potassium values may be normal. The electrocardiogram is altered as would be predicted from the serum values, with low T waves in hypokalemia and peaked T waves in hyperkalemia.

In the hyperkalemic form, some members of the family may be found to have myotonia without any history of periodic paralysis.

In both types of the disease, there may be persistent weakness between attacks, most often proximal, sometimes distal. Experience with acetazolamide therapy indicates that even long-lasting weakness may be reversible, regardless of pathologic changes in muscle. A few patients with intermittent normokalemic or hyperkalemic paralysis have had persistent cardiac arrhythmia, especially bigeminy, and bouts of ventricular tachycardia. The cardiac disorder is neither temporally related to attacks of limb weakness nor related to serum potassium content.

DIAGNOSIS. Periodic paralysis can be recognized by the history of typical attacks; no other disease causes this pattern of recurrent weakness. In myasthenia gravis, weakness may come and go, but less abruptly and with a duration of weeks rather than hours or days; remissions are less frequent so that it is less "periodic." Polymyositis may be transient, but episodes are rarely shorter than several weeks or months. Attacks of myoglobinuric weakness could conceivably be confusing if the pigmenturia were not recognized, but myalgia and malaise are so prominent that it is rarely mistaken for periodic paralysis. Hysterical attacks might be confusing.

If the patient is seen during the attack and the serum potassium level is abnormal, other causes of hypo- or hyperkalemia must be considered. Low serum potassium concentrations with paralysis are also encountered in hyperaldosteronism; potassium-losing nephritis; potassium depletion caused by laxative abuse, diuretics, or diarrhea; and thyrotoxicosis. *Thiazide* and *thalidone diuretics* are likely to be an increasingly frequent cause of hypokalemic weakness; in one series, about 25 per cent of randomly chosen patients receiving these drugs had serum potassium content below normal. Hyperkalemia is most often due to renal insufficiency, but may also occur in adrenal insufficiency, after administration of spironolactone, or as a manifestation of aldosterone deficiency.

Thyrotoxicosis can cause a variant of periodic hypokalemic paralysis closely resembling the familial variety. The condition especially occurs in young Chinese and Japanese men in their third or fourth decade, but other Asians and women have occasionally been affected. The clinical manifestations of hyperthyroidism are usually not prominent, although tachycardia and even cardiac arrhythmias are frequent. Attacks are commonly precipitated by exercises or heavy carbohydrate meals. Serum potassium is low. Effective treatment of the thyrotoxicosis abolishes this form of periodic paralysis.

A family history of periodic paralysis is useful in diagnosis, but sporadic cases may be indistinguishable from the familial disorder. If the patient is not having a spontaneous attack when studied, the only way to distinguish the two forms is to provoke an attack. The techniques to be described have been used in numerous centers with many patients, without serious complications. But induced attacks may be frightening to patient and physician, and should be left to experienced investigators. Facilities for supported respiration should be immediately available. Appropriately informed consent is mandatory. Because of the uncertainty of clinical distinction, it is advisable to start with glucose (100 grams) given intravenously in one hour with 20 units of regular insulin either in the infusion or given subcutaneously. Hypoglycemic symptoms should be anticipated, and the electrocardiogram should be monitored. Hypokalemia is induced as the blood sugar falls, usually within one hour after the infusion is completed. If an attack is induced, it can be terminated with administration of 7 to 10 grams of potassium chloride (KCl) or about 90 to 130 mEq of mixed potassium salts by mouth. Whether or not an attack is induced by glucose and insulin, but especially if it is not, the patient should then be challenged with potassium. This poses problems because it is not clear how much potassium constitutes an adequate challenge. The author starts with 3 grams of KCl by mouth (or 40 mEq of mixed potassium salts). If this fails, the dose is gradually increased on successive days to a maximum of 8 or 10 grams of KCl (about 100 or 125 mEq of potassium salts). Patients with hyperkalemic paralysis have attacks with serum potassium levels between 5 and 8 mEq per liter.

Other members of the family should be investigated clinically and electromyographically for evidence of myotonia.

TREATMENT. Acute attacks of hypokalemic paralysis are best treated with oral KCl, 5 to 10 grams (65 to 130 mEq of potassium). Relief of weakness usually commences within 30 minutes but may take several hours, and some attacks are peculiarly refractory.

Hyperkalemia may be relieved by infusions of glucose and insulin. Chlorothiazide and calcium gluconate have also been reported to be effective. In severe attacks, weakness may persist even after the serum potassium has returned to normal concentrations.

The traditional method used to protect patients against hypokalemic paralysis was, until recently, a low-sodium diet supplemented by oral KCl, or perhaps by spironolactone or dexamethasone. Then, acetazolamide in small doses, sometimes only 250 per mg daily, sometimes more, was found to be effective prophylaxis in the hyperkalemic type. Subsequently, it was found that similar doses of acetazolamide were equally effective in the hypokalemic variety, so a single drug is beneficial in both forms. How it exerts this effect is not known. The best-known effects of this compound relate to its ability to inhibit carbonic anhydrase, but muscle lacks this enzyme, and no definite systemic effects of the drug have been recognized in the doses used, but respiratory acidosis may be responsible.

Engel AG: Hypokalemic and hyperkalemic periodic paralysis. *In* Goldensohn ES, Appel SH (eds.): Scientific Approaches to Clinical Neurology. Philadelphia, Lea & Febiger, 1977, pp 1742–1761. *Research on this interesting problem has not progressed rapidly. This is still a valid statement of what is known about the disordered physiology, with a comprehensive review of clinical aspects.*

Griggs RC, Resnick J, Engel WK: Intravenous treatment of hypokalemic periodic paralysis. Arch Neurol 90:539, 1983. *Intravenous therapy is rarely necessary; when it is, mannitol solutions are preferred instead of glucose for administered potassium.*

Riggs JE, Griggs RC: Diagnosis and treatment of the periodic paralysis. *In* Klawans H (ed.): Clinical Neuropharmacology, Vol 4. New York, Raven Press, 1979, pp 123–138. *Practical guidelines for diagnosis and treatment.*

MYOSITIS OSSIFICANS

This rare disorder is most dramatic in its consequences, producing the "stone man" of circus sideshows. Symptoms usually begin in early childhood, with transient and localized swellings of the neck and back. Ultimately there is progressive rigidity of the neck, trunk, and limbs. Palpable plates are discernible beneath the rigid parts. Severely affected patients may be able to stand and walk, and yet unable to bend so that they must be raised from bed with assistance. The bars beneath the skin are visible roentgenographically. Microscopically, muscle is replaced by bone and connective tissue. Whether the primary disorder is in the fibroblasts (leading to abnormal ossification) or in the muscle itself is not resolved. Muscle biopsy early in the disease may show widespread necrosis and inflammation, but serum enzymes are not always elevated, nor is the electromyogram always myopathic. Few cases are familial, but the disorder is believed to be inherited because digital abnormalities are almost always present in both the patients and other members of the family in a pattern suggesting an autosomal dominant inheritance. Microdactyly commonly affects the great toe, and clinodactyly (curved digits) may affect the hands. There is no detectable systemic abnormality of calcium and phosphate metabolism, and there has been no effective therapy.

Bassett CAL, Donath A, Macagno F, Preisig R, Fleisch H, Francis MD: Diphosphonates in the treatment of myositis ossificans. Lancet 2:845, 1969. *Evaluation of this treatment still fails to prove its worth.*

Connor JM, Smith R: The cervical spine in fibrodysplasia ossificans progressiva. Br J Radiol 55:492, 1982. *Fusion of cervical vertebrae, a congenital anomaly, may be a universal finding in these patients, even when there is no ossification of adjacent muscle.*

Smith R: Myositis ossificans progressiva. A review of current problems. Semin Arthritis Rheum 4:369, 1975. *The most modern and detailed review of this condition.*

539. SPORADIC DISORDERS

ACQUIRED MYOPATHIES

Several acquired myopathies, particularly when they present with little or no systemic symptoms or evidence of inflammation, enter the differential diagnosis of the muscular dystrophies. Most common are dermatomyositis and polymyositis, but the other disorders listed in the following paragraphs require consideration as well.

DERMATOMYOSITIS-POLYMYOSITIS. Polymyositis without cutaneous lesions is the commonest syndrome likely to be confused with muscular dystrophy. The syndrome probably has several causes and is discussed in Ch. 454. In the absence of a telltale rash, the criteria listed in Table 539–1 help to differentiate the disorder from the primary myopathies. The following paragraphs describe several additional acquired myopathies that must be distinguished from polymyositis.

TABLE 539–1. FEATURES SUGGESTING POLYMYOSITIS RATHER THAN DYSTROPHY

No family history of similar disease
Rapid onset, with weeks or months to maximum disability
Any spontaneous unequivocal improvement
Dysphagia and neck weakness common
Arthralgia or Raynaud's symptoms common
Inflammatory reaction in muscle biopsy
Signs of irritability (spontaneous activity) in the EMG
Age over 35 at onset

CARCINOMATOUS MYOPATHY. Muscle weakness without rash may occur in patients with carcinoma of the lung or of any other primary site. Myeloma, macroglobulinemia, and other gammopathies may also be associated with myopathy. The tumor itself may or may not be symptomatic, and treatment of the tumor may or may not affect the muscular symptoms.

COLLAGEN DISEASES. Proximal limb weakness may occur in the course of systemic lupus erythematosus, progressive systemic sclerosis, rheumatoid arthritis, Sjögren's syndrome, or rarely, periarteritis nodosa or giant cell arteritis. In these circumstances, the myopathy is treated as part of the general disorder.

ENDOCRINE DISEASE. *Thyrotoxic myopathy* is a well-recognized but now rare syndrome. Usually there is clinical evidence of hyperthyroidism, but not always ("apathetic hyperthyroidism"). Signs of hypermetabolism are especially apt to be lacking in elderly patients. The myopathy disappears when the patient is rendered euthyroid by treatment. Similarly, weakness may complicate *hypothyroidism*, and sarcoplasmic enzyme levels in serum may rise so much that polymyositis is suspected. Another muscle syndrome of hypothyroidism is *Hoffmann's syndrome*, a peculiar difficulty in relaxing muscles that lack the characteristic electromyographic abnormalities of myotonia, that is therefore called *"pseudomyotonia."* This, too, disappears with appropriate replacement therapy.

Hyperparathyroidism and hyperadrenocorticism may also be responsible for weakness that looks like any other proximal myopathy. Weakness may be part of hyperpituitarism, but acromegalic features always overshadow the myopathy. Myalgia, with or without weakness, may be a prominent symptom in patients with osteomalacia, and the muscular disorder may respond dramatically to administration of vitamin D. If the endocrine disorder is not clinically overt and the myopathy is pronounced, the condition may simulate polymyositis. However, serum enzyme levels are not usually increased.

INFECTIONS. Structures resembling viral particles have been seen with the electron microscope in cases of polymyositis, and sometimes there are acute myopathic disorders in individuals with serologically proved influenza or other viral infections, or with encephalomyelitis assumed to be viral in origin. In one special form, children with congenital agammaglobulinemia develop dermatomyositis, and echovirus can be isolated from cerebrospinal fluid. Other infections or infestations that can be associated with clinical polymyositis are trichinosis, toxoplasmosis, cysticercosis, schistosomiasis, and trypanosomiasis.

SARCOIDOSIS. Sarcoidosis is a significant cause of polymyositis. Usually there is other evidence of the disease, but sometimes the first symptoms are due to weakness, and in a few cases only muscle seems to be involved. Myalgia may be severe in these patients.

DRUGS. A variety of drugs used to treat more common disorders may themselves cause muscular weakness, especially triamcinolone and other fluorinated adrenal steroids (but probably all steroids), vincristine, chloroquine, bretylium, emetine, ipecac, carbenoxolone, guanethidine, thiazide diuretics and other kaluretics, epsilon-aminocaproic acid, penicillamine, and clofibrate. Repeated injections of narcotics and other drugs may lead to fibrosis of muscle that simulates a diffuse myopathy.

ALCOHOLIC MYOPATHY. The clearest myopathic disorder in alcoholic persons is acute myoglobinuria. Some of these individuals, and some who never have an attack of pigmenturia, also suffer from proximal limb weakness, especially affecting the legs. The serum creatine kinase is often elevated. The problem in some of these patients, however, is that they also suffer from the typical polyneuritis of alcoholism, and it then becomes difficult to prove that the muscular weakness is not also secondary to a neurogenic disorder. Too few patients have been evaluated to know whether abstinence and a good diet will reverse the persistent weakness.

CHRONIC HYPOKALEMIA. Chronic hypokalemia from any cause may be associated with the syndrome of polymyositis: weakness of relatively abrupt onset, muscle necrosis in biopsy, and high serum enzymes. This is most commonly seen in patients taking thiazide diuretics, but may also occur in hypokalemic states caused by chronic diarrhea. Hypokalemia may also contribute to some cases of alcoholic myopathy.

Alpert JN, Groff AE, Bastian FO, Blum MA: Acute polymyositis caused by sarcoidosis: Report of a case and review of the literature. Mt Sinai J Med 46:486, 1979. *Description of one cause of polymyositis.*

Askari A, Vignos PJ Jr, Moskowitz RW: Steroid myopathy in connective tissue disease. Am J Med 61:485, 1976. *Paradoxically, steroid therapy of muscle disease may also cause weakness. This paper reviews the problem but may underestimate the difficulty of resolving it.*

Bohan A, Peter JB, Bowman RL, Pearson CM: A computer-assisted analysis of 153 patients with polymyositis and dermatomyositis. Medicine 56:255, 1977. *A standard reference for questions about the controversial classification of these diseases.*

Callen JP: The value of malignancy evaluation in patients with dermatomyositis. J Am Acad Dermatol 6:253, 1982. *There appears to be little value if there is no evidence of malignancy on physical examination or from blood counts, chest films, and stool guaiac tests.*

Floyd M, Ayar DR, Barwick DD, Hudgson P, Weightman D: Myopathy in chronic renal failure. Q J Med 43:509, 1974. *The standard discussion of the problem.*

Gamboa ET, Eastwood AB, Hays AP, Maxwell J, Penn AS: Isolation of influenza virus from muscle in myoglobinuric polymyositis. Neurology 29:1323, 1979. *First description of viral isolation in polymyositis.*

Lane RJM, Mastaglia FL: Drug-induced myopathies in man. Lancet 2:562, 1978. *Comprehensive listing of iatrogenic causes of muscle disease.*

Magid SK, Kagen LJ: Serologic evidence for acute toxoplasmosis in polymyositis-dermatomyositis. Am J Med 75:313, 1983. *Toxoplasmosis is a documented cause of acute polymyositis. Whether it is a common cause of chronic syndromes, as suggested by serologic data, is uncertain.*

Perkoff GT: Alcoholic myopathy. Ann Rev Med 22:125, 1971. *The best review of the subject.*

Rowland LP, Clark C, Olarte M: Therapy for dermatomyositis and polymyositis. Adv Neurol 17:63, 1977. *A critical review of reported therapies.*

Schott GD, Wills MR: Muscle weakness in osteomalacia. Lancet 1:626, 1976. *A clear description of an often unrecognized problem.*

Stern LA, Fagan JM: The endocrine myopathies. Handb Clin Neurol 40:235, 1979. *Thorough review of myopathies associated with endocrine disorders.*

Whitaker JN: Inflammatory myopathy: A review of etiologic and pathogenetic factors. Muscle Nerve 5:573, 1982. *A thorough review of reported cellular and humoral abnormalities in these syndromes, emphasizing the paucity of definitive evidence.*

SPORADIC MYOGLOBINURIA

DEFINITION. Sporadic myoglobinuria comprises a group of disorders characterized by injury of muscle and excretion of myoglobin in the urine in amounts sufficient to discolor the urine. *Rhabdomyolysis* has been proposed as a more precise term, but it is never used except when there is gross myoglobinuria and is therefore of dubious value.

PATHOGENESIS. Sensitive radioimmunoassays for myoglobin show small amounts of myoglobin in normal serum. Like serum enzymes, the serum content of myoglobin may increase in myopathies or after myocardial infarction, and under these circumstances myoglobin may pass into the urine, although not in amounts sufficient to darken. (Oxidized myoglobin in the urine is more likely to appear brown than red.) The clinical syndrome of "myoglobinuria" refers to gross pigmenturia and implies more acute and more massive destruction of muscle.

Sometimes the cause of overt myoglobinuria is evident, as in *crush injuries.* Similar pressure injuries may occur in comatose persons who lie on one side without moving for prolonged periods. This kind of injury is perhaps more apt to occur when there are other causes of *metabolic depression;* for instance, in coma after suicidal ingestion of barbiturates or carbon monoxide intoxication, or prolonged unconsciousness in the snow. A similar effect may be induced by *arterial occlusion* by tourniquet or embolism, or even by prolonged knee-chest posture under anesthesia.

In other patients, the cause is less discernible. In every series of patients with myoglobinuria, a disproportionate number are *alcoholics*, but why this should occur is not known. Sometimes there has been exposure to a known *membrane toxin,* such as the bite of the Malayan sea snake. In some addicts, heroin (or an adulterant) seems to cause myoglobinuria. Or there may be *metabolic alterations* that do not ordinarily cause this kind of trouble, such as diarrhea with hypokalemia; potassium depletion caused by diuretics, amphotericin, or licorice; diabetic acidosis; or systemic infection with fever. In many attacks, however, not even these clues prevail.

The most common cause of myoglobinuria is probably unusually *vigorous exercise* by an otherwise normal person. Most cases have been reported by military physicians, and designations include such titles as the "squat-jump syndrome" or "march hemoglobinuria." When large numbers of recruits endure these tortures, a certain number will have attacks of myalgia followed by pigmenturia. Why these individuals have attacks and others are spared is not clear, but this seems to be a "normal" variation. In civilians, cases have been caused by the excess muscular activity of an initiation rite into a club or fraternity, and isolated attacks have occurred after the vigorous muscular activity induced by succinylcholine before it achieves relaxation. With the spread of running for fun and health, cases of myoglobinuria have been reported in joggers and marathon athletes.

In *malignant hyperthermia,* there is a rapid rise in temperature, widespread muscular rigidity, hyperkalemia, and metabolic acidosis, with a fatal outcome in about 75 per cent. The offending agents are usually halothane and succinylcholine. Increased serum activities of sarcoplasmic enzymes are the rule, and often there is myoglobinuria. The intense muscular contraction may be the proximate cause of myoglobinuria in this syndrome, but the widespread metabolic disorder probably contributes. Spontaneous convulsions and electroconvulsive therapy have also been followed by myoglobinuria. The only genetic causes presently recognized are deficiencies of phosphorylase, phosphofructokinase, carnitine palmityl transferase, phosphoglycerate kinase, phosphoglycerate mutase, or lactate dehydrogenase.

CLINICAL MANIFESTATIONS. In attacks other than those caused by local crushing or arterial occlusion, the clinical picture is similar. Affected muscles are apt to be the ones subject to greatest physical strain (the legs in squat-thrusts, the arms after chinning or push-ups, the arms and legs after wrestling matches). The muscles ache, may be swollen, and are weak. Sometimes there is so much edema that local vascular abnormalities are suspected. There may be fever and considerable malaise. Symptoms persist for several days even though pigmenturia rarely lasts more than 48 hours. Recovery may be gradual. Cranial muscles are rarely involved, and although respiratory failure is uncommon it is a hazard. The most important threat to life is renal injury due to excretion of heme. There may be red cells or myoglobin in the urine as well as casts. Oliguria is followed by azotemia and hyperkalemia.

DIAGNOSIS. The diagnosis of myoglobinuria can be made on clinical grounds and with relatively simple tests, but precise identification of the pigment depends upon either absorption spectrophotometry and electrophoresis on starch gel, acrylamide, or cellulose acetate, or more recently, immunochemical methods. The urine may appear red-brown because of hemoglobin, myoglobin, or porphyrins. The latter would not give a positive test result with benzidine (or other heme-reacting reagents), and would give a positive Watson-Schwartz test result for porphobilinogen. Besides, the neurologic disorder of porphyria is neuropathy, not an acute myopathy. If the urine gives a positive test for heme and contains no or few erythrocytes, the pigment is either myoglobin or hemoglobin. If it is hemoglobin, the serum would be pink (after a hemolytic reaction), whereas the color of the serum in myoglobinuria is normal. (This distinction depends upon the affinity of serum haptoglobin for hemoglobin and not for myoglobin. Hemoglobin is not excreted until haptoglobin is saturated by visible amounts of the pigment, whereas myoglobin is excreted at much lower concentrations.) Furthermore, in attacks of myoglobinuria, the muscular weakness and myalgia are distinctive, and serum enzymes are greatly increased, whereas they are not in hemolysis.

Myoglobinuria should be considered a possible cause in all cases of acute renal failure of uncertain etiology. If the serum content of sarcoplasmic enzymes is very high (e.g., creatine kinase values to 10,000 to 50,000 units, with a method giving normal maximal values of 50 units), myoglobinuria must be the cause.

TREATMENT. If there is no renal injury, myoglobinuria is not threatening. The hazards of renal injury are not directly correlated to the amount of pigment excreted, and other factors are probably involved. Once an attack starts, it is useful to encourage excretion of dilute urine by administration of mannitol or other osmotic diuretics; some authorities favor alkalinizing agents, although it has not been clearly demonstrated that these treatments protect the kidneys. Few patients are left with residual weakness, but in some the syndrome is characterized by prolonged weakness punctuated by attacks of myoglobinuria.

Gabow PA, Kaehny WD, Kelleher SP: The spectrum of rhabdomyolysis. Medicine 61:141, 1982. *A thorough review of myoglobinuria from the view of the nephrologist.*

Gamboa ET, Eastwood AB, Hays AP, Maxwell J, Penn AS: Isolation of influenza virus from muscle in myoglobinuric polymyositis. Neurology 29:1323, 1979. *Viral infections may cause myoglobinuria.*

Knochel JP, Barcenas C, Cotton JR, Fuller TJ, Haller R, Carter NW: Hypophosphatemia and rhabdomyolysis. J Clin Invest 62:1240, 1978. *Detailed analysis of metabolic abnormalities that may cause myoglobinuria in alcoholics.*

Rowland LP: Myoglobinuria. Can J Neurol Sci (in press), 1984. *A review of contemporary problems from the view of a neurologist focusing on muscle rather than on the kidney.*

MYASTHENIA GRAVIS

DEFINITION. Myasthenia gravis is a disease of unknown cause, due to circulating antibodies to acetylcholine receptors, and manifested by weakness that has special characteristics: predilection for ocular and other cranial muscles, tendency to fluctuate in severity, no signs of neural lesion, and amelioration of weakness by cholinergic drugs.

ETIOLOGY. Although the initiating event is not known, it seems clear that myasthenic weakness results from the presence of circulating antibodies to acetylcholine receptor (AChR). Rabbits and other species can be immunized with purified AChR. When antibodies appear in the blood, weakness results, which has all the essential properties found in the human disease. Also, as in human myasthenia, there are morphologic changes at the neuromuscular junction, especially simplification of the postjunctional folds, with loss of functional AChR sites, and antibody can be demonstrated on the postjunctional membrane by immunocytochemical methods. As a result, the postjunctional membrane becomes less sensitive to the application of acetylcholine or other agonists.

Soon after experimental autoimmune myasthenia gravis was discovered, similar antibodies to AChR were found demonstrated in the blood of patients with myasthenia gravis. In a transient syndrome of infants born to myasthenic mothers, the symptoms disappeared when the antibodies disappeared. When purified IgG from patients was injected into mice, characteristics of myasthenia were induced in the animals, and if the plasma (but not lymphocytes) of patients was removed by plasmapheresis or thoracic duct drainage, the symptoms were ameliorated. For all these reasons, the antibodies seem to be responsible for the symptoms of the disease.

Some questions remain. Foremost is the nature of the events that initiate the formation of the antibodies. Also, it is not clear what role sensitized lymphocytes play, for there is evidence of altered cellular immunity, too. There are questions about the antibodies themselves, for they seem to be directed to antigenic sites on the AChR other than the combining site for acetylcholine. Simple blockade of AChR by steric hindrance is one possible mechanism, but the antibodies also seem to accelerate the loss of AChR, and other mechanisms of interference are possible. In intercostal muscle from patients with the disease, miniature end-plate potentials are reduced in amplitude and there is decreased sensitivity to cholinergic agonists.

Other evidence of an autoimmune disorder includes the following: abnormalities of the thymus gland in most patients, either germinal centers or thymoma; accumulation of lymphocytes in muscle and other organs; increased coincidence with other autoimmune diseases; and increased frequency of nonspecific autoantibodies against nuclear antigens (ANA), striation-binding muscle antigens, and thyroid antigens.

NEUROMUSCULAR DISORDER. The symptoms of myasthenia gravis resemble those of curare intoxication. This observation led to the use of curare antagonists in treatment, and several drugs currently in use are inhibitors of the enzyme cholinesterase. These drugs also partially repair a physiologic defect that can be detected in patients by relatively simple techniques. When the ulnar nerve of normal individuals is stimulated at rates of 20 per second or less, the action potential of the hypothenar muscles is sustained at a constant amplitude. In patients with myasthenia, however, there is a rapid decline in the height of the evoked potentials. If the patient is then given neostigmine, the amplitude of the evoked potentials is restored to normal. This abnormality has been regarded as characteristic and is consistent with the reduced amplitude of miniature end-plate potentials found in intercostal muscle. Microelectrode studies of excised intercostal muscle have also demonstrated reduced sensitivity of the end-plates to cholinergic agonists.

The use of repetitive stimulation for diagnostic purposes has disadvantages because it causes some discomfort to the patient and because decrementing responses can be encountered in diseases other than myasthenia gravis. Attention has therefore been given to single-fiber electromyography (SFEMG), but this technique may be neither more convenient for the examiner nor more comfortable for the patient. In SFEMG, the intervals are measured between discharges of different fibers within the same motor unit. These intervals vary normally, a variation called "jitter," and the temporal limits have been defined. In myasthenia, jitter increases; when the intervals are very long, expected potentials do not appear, a phenomenon called "blocking," and the number of blockings increases in myasthenia. These abnormalities are attributed to slowing of and uncertainty of neuromuscular transmission.

INCIDENCE AND PREVALENCE. The prevalence of myasthenia gravis is about 33 per million population and the annual incidence of new cases is about 2 to 5 per million. Cases occur in all decades of life, most frequently at about age 40. Among young adults, the disease affects women about three times more frequently than men. Among children and older persons, however, men and women are affected equally. There are a few familial cases, perhaps somewhat more than by chance, and there may be increased incidence of thyroid or other autoimmune disease in relatives of patients with myasthenia. Some genetic predisposition is suggested by a disproportionate frequency of particular transplantation antigen haplotypes in affected individuals, and these may differ in those with thymoma and in younger patients with no tumor.

PATHOLOGY. Pathologic changes in myasthenia gravis are limited to muscle and thymus. Skeletal muscles may appear normal but often contain collections of lymphocytes around blood vessels. Some cases show degeneration of muscle fibers, and the inflammatory cellular response may be extensive. Rarely, similar lesions are encountered in the myocardium. With the electron microscope, there is simplification of the postjunctional folds and widening of the synaptic cleft. Using labelled α-bungarotoxin, loss of AChR sites can be demonstrated and, with immunocytochemical methods, IgG and complement are seen on postsynaptal membranes.

The thymus gland is often abnormal. Encapsulated tumors (thymoma) occur in about 15 per cent of cases, almost all after age 30. About 25 per cent of these tumors invade locally, but distant metastases are virtually unknown and local invasiveness is rarely a cause of symptoms. Lymphocytic proliferation, in the form of germinal centers, is seen in thymus glands of almost all other patients, but sometimes the gland appears normal, and in some older individuals the gland is so involuted that it cannot be found. Patients dying of this disease usually have some pulmonary disorder (edema, atelectasis, infection) resulting from the terminal events. It has not been shown that myasthenia occurs more frequently in patients with cancer than might be expected on the basis of chance.

CLINICAL MANIFESTATIONS. The most common presenting symptoms relate to weakness of eye muscles, causing ptosis or diplopia. At the onset these symptoms may last only a few days, then disappear, only to return weeks or months later. Ptosis frequently varies even in the course of a single day. Diplopia may be noted in particular directions of gaze. Difficulty in chewing, dysarthria, and dysphagia are common. Limb weakness is often proximal, so that patients have difficulty climbing stairs, rising from chairs, or lifting heavy objects or raising the arms overhead. However, distal weakness is not uncommon, and the initial symptoms may be related to the strength of the hands or fingers. Selective respiratory weakness is unusual. There is no alteration of consciousness, no pain, and, in untreated patients, no cramps or muscular twitching. Difficulty in chewing and swallowing may lead to loss of weight, but specific wasting of muscle occurs only in patients with severe chronic weakness.

On examination there is evidence of weakness of the appropriate muscle groups. If any sensory abnormality is found, there must be some other disorder, alone or in combination with myasthenia. Similarly, hyperactive reflexes and Babinski signs imply some other disorder, as does complete loss of reflexes. Weakness is responsible for all the signs of myasthenia. Ptosis may be unilateral or bilateral. Most often, there is asymmetrical weakness of several ocular muscles in a pattern that cannot be explained by disorder of a particular ocular motor nerve. In addition, there is frequently weakness of eye closure because of paresis of the orbicularis oculi. Muscles of the lower face are involved later. Lingual and palatal weakness is evident in patients with dysarthria, causing a nasal twang and indistinct speech. In advanced cases, patients support the chin with one hand to help them talk, a maneuver almost pathognomonic of myasthenia. Neck weakness may be mild or severe enough to cause difficulty in holding the head erect. Limb weakness may be mild or so severe that the patient cannot walk or even turn in bed. Ventilatory insufficiency occurs only in severely affected patients and usually in generalized disease, but some patients with oropharyngeal weakness may be unable to breathe unassisted even though limb muscles are strong. A normal neurologic examination is inconsistent with the diagnosis of myasthenia gravis if the patient is symptomatic at the time and is not taking anticholinesterase drugs.

COURSE. The nature of the disease in a given patient is established within weeks or months of onset, with fluctuations afterward. If after one year, or certainly after two years, myasthenia is still restricted to ocular muscles, it is unlikely to become generalized; purely ocular myasthenia may account for 20 per cent of all cases.

SPECIAL FORMS OF MYASTHENIA. ***Neonatal Myasthenia.*** Infants born to myasthenic women may have a transient syndrome of weakness. The most prominent symptom is difficulty in sucking and swallowing. This may be the sole manifestation, or there may also be noticeable reduction in spontaneous movement and in the vigor of the baby's cry. Only rarely is there respiratory difficulty, but unrecognized neonatal myasthenia has been fatal in exceptional cases. The condition can be identified by the intramuscular injection of neostigmine (0.1 to 0.25 mg), followed by improved sucking, a louder cry, better response to the Moro reflex, and stronger spontaneous movements. Small doses of cholinergic drugs may be administered therapeutically, but more often all that is needed is a nasogastric tube to ensure adequate nutrition. Symptoms subside within a week or, at most, a month.

Congenital Myasthenia. Myasthenia gravis may commence at any age. But a few children seem to have had ophthalmoplegia from birth, with or without other signs of myasthenia. The mothers do not have symptoms of myasthenia (in contrast to mothers of children with neonatal myasthenia). Although presumably congenital, this disorder rarely causes concern until after the first year of life, when the ophthalmoplegia is recognized as having always been present. Many children with congenital myasthenia have no demonstrable antibodies to AChR. Some investigators therefore believe this is a distinct syndrome of "hereditary myasthenia," which they distinguish from the more common "acquired autoimmune" form. Whether this is a reliable distinction is not certain. With standard tests, congenital myasthenia behaves physiologically and pharmacologically like forms of later onset, and it fluctuates in typical fashion. Moreover, antibodies are not found in all cases of later onset, and some familial cases are not congenital, beginning in adolescence or later.

Thyrotoxicosis. About 5 per cent of patients with myasthenia have thyrotoxicosis at some time. Usually the two disorders occur simultaneously, but sometimes hyperthyroidism is evident for weeks or months before there are myasthenic symptoms. Only rarely does myasthenia come long before the thyrotoxicosis, and patients who appear euthyroid do not ordinarily have laboratory evidence of thyroid overactivity. Treatment of the two disorders is directed according to the usual indications for each.

DIAGNOSIS. The diagnosis of myasthenia usually is obvious by history and examination and is immediately confirmed by the response to cholinergic drugs. For adults, 10 mg of edrophonium is given by vein, 2 to 3 mg at a time. If there is no increase in muscle strength within 30 seconds, a second dose of 3.0 mg is given and the patient's condition re-evaluated. If there is still no response, the remainder of the dose is given. This drug is preferred when cranial muscles are being tested because the response is prompt and dramatic. Cranial weakness cannot be simulated voluntarily, and placebo injections are unnecessary.

If it is desired to evaluate limb strength, the injection of neostigmine has advantages because the effect lasts longer, permitting more leisurely testing. The adult dose is 1.5 mg intramuscularly, and it is usually combined with atropine, 0.5 mg, to avoid the muscarinic symptoms of abdominal cramps and sweating. When limb strength is evaluated, it is sometimes advisable to evaluate placebo responses by giving the atropine 30 minutes before the neostigmine. In all cases of myasthenia gravis there is some response to these drugs, but the response is sometimes slight, and the test may have to be repeated on several occasions to provide convincing evidence.

To provide confirmatory evidence, the electromyographic response to nerve stimulation may be studied. The characteristic decline in amplitude of the evoked potential may be normal when the disease is restricted to the eyes. As noted above, SFEMG is finding increasing use in diagnosis. Rarely, it is desirable to administer d-tubocurarine, but this involves hazards and should probably be left to research centers; d-tubocurarine should never be given without appropriate precautions to support respiration.

Detection of antibodies to AChR has become an important diagnostic criterion, but also has limitations. With the most sensitive assay (using human antigen), about 85 per cent of patients are "positive" and there are virtually no false positives. With other commonly used antigens (such as denervated rat muscle), even more test results are negative in patients with unequivocal myasthenia. There are no special characteristics of the patients with negative antibody test results, except perhaps that patients with ocular and congenital forms are more likely to lack antibodies. A negative test result does not exclude the diagnosis.

In evaluating patients with known or suspected myasthenia, it is useful to perform a standard series of laboratory studies. In addition to repetitive nerve stimulation and tests for AChR antibodies, the possible presence of thymoma is assessed. These tumors are almost always evident in standard radiograms of the chest supplemented by oblique views. Lateral laminagrams are even more revealing, but still not quite 100 per cent accurate. Computed tomography (CT) invariably shows the tumor, but it is also prone to false-positive interpretations of soft tissue images that are not thymomas. Invasive studies such as thymic venography, mediastinal pneumography, or isotope scans have no additional value. Thyroid function should be tested, and it is useful to evaluate immunologic disorders by serum protein electrophoresis, LE cell preparation, latex fixation test for rheumatoid factor, and antinuclear antibodies. Tests for muscle antibodies or lymphocyte sensitivity are performed in special centers.

The differential diagnosis requires special consideration. Probably the most frequent error in diagnosis concerns patients with emotional fatigue states and hysterical weakness. There are no cranial muscle symptoms in these patients (except globus hystericus), whereas cranial muscles are involved in virtually all myasthenics. Their symptoms are not those of weakness but of exhaustion, and in tests of strength against resistance there is apt to be marked variation in effort, or dramatic giving way.

Acute oculomotor paralysis occurs in four diseases: myasthenia gravis, botulism, acute cranial polyneuropathy, and acute Wernicke's encephalopathy. Each has its special hazards and treatments and deserves thoughtful consideration in such cases. Amyotrophic lateral sclerosis and peripheral neuropathy may be confused with myasthenia when these disorders affect cranial muscles, but signs indicative of a neurogenic disorder distinguish them from myasthenia. Polymyositis may be confusing, but ocular muscle paresis is not found. There is some debate about the specificity of the therapeutic effect of cholinergic drugs, but for practical purposes it may be taken that an authentic (not placebo), convincing (not equivocal), and reproducible (not seen by one examiner only) effect is found only in myasthenia gravis.

TREATMENT. Therapeutic efforts fall into two categories: those which affect symptoms without influencing the course of the disease (cholinergic drugs), and those designed to induce remission of the disease itself (thymectomy, steroids, immunosuppressive drugs). Plasmapheresis can be considered an intermediate form of therapy, with effects lasting longer than those of cholinergic drugs but not as prolonged as, for instance, the optimal effect of thymectomy. Management starts as soon as the diagnosis is made, using cholinergic drugs. Then decisions are made regarding other forms of treatment.

In treating myasthenia, the clinician is faced with a variety of choices that include anticholinesterase drugs, corticosteroids, immunosuppressive drugs, thymectomy, and plasma exchange. Authorities disagree about the preferred sequence of choices, but the following guidelines may be useful:

1. Treatment should start with anticholinesterase therapy because improvement is prompt and use of these drugs entails little risk. However, cholinergic drugs alone rarely restore normal function, and, except in very mild cases or those restricted to ocular muscles, some other form of therapy is also indicated.

2. For all patients, the severity of symptoms and risks of therapy must be weighed in considering thymectomy or the use of steroids or immunosuppressive drugs. For this reason, thymectomy is rarely performed in patients with solely ocular myasthenia. For the same reason, some authorities hesitate to use steroids or immunosuppressive drugs in ocular myasthenia, in which risks might outweigh advantages. However, for some individuals (police officers, actors, or those who work on roofs or other heights), the disabling effects of ocular myasthenia might warrant the risks of steroid therapy.

3. Because of the advances in surgical technique, anesthesia, and respiratory support, the risks of thymectomy in major centers have been reduced to almost nil. Additionally, complete remission or significant improvement is seen in about 85 per cent of patients after thymectomy. Therefore, the operation is done increasingly for all patients with generalized myasthenia.

It seems logical to refer these patients to centers where sufficient numbers are seen to deal with specific questions of myasthenic management.

4. Although some investigators have recommended treatment with steroids before thymectomy (so that the resulting improvement would make postoperative care easier), this policy has been contested and may be supplanted by use of plasma exchange to prepare patients for thymectomy.

5. If these guidelines prove to be appropriate, steroid therapy would be reserved for patients with severe disability after thymectomy, or who are otherwise not candidates for thymectomy. Although it has not been demonstrated that the risks of immunosuppressive drugs (azathioprine, cyclophosphamide) are actually greater than the risks of steroids, most authorities in this country reserve these drugs for patients who fail to improve after both thymectomy and steroid therapy.

Cholinergic Drug Therapy. The major drugs used to treat myasthenia gravis are inhibitors of cholinesterase, neostigmine and pyridostigmine. It is best to use only one drug; there is no benefit from combinations of two or more. Neostigmine is provided in 15 mg tablets, and pyridostigmine in 60 mg tablets; these are essentially interchangeable. The choice is arbitrary because there is no evidence that the maximal benefit achieved by one is more than that of the other. Most patients prefer pyridostigmine because it is less apt to cause abdominal cramps and diarrhea or noticeable peaks and valleys of strength. Pyridostigmine is also provided in a slow-release capsule (Timespan) of 180 mg, said to provide 60 mg immediately and the remainder in 8 to 12 hours. Some clinicians use the prolonged-action preparation throughout the day, but because of uncertainties of release, it seems advisable to use this only at bedtime for patients who would otherwise have to awaken at night or who are very weak on waking in the morning. (For patients who cannot swallow pills, both drugs may be administered parenterally, and pyridostigmine may be given as a syrup. The intramuscular dose is about one tenth of the oral dose, and the intravenous dose is one thirtieth of the oral dose.) Decisions about optimal dosage are sometimes difficult. Some authorities advocate the use of edrophonium to evaluate oral drug therapy; a test dose of 2 mg is given intravenously. If the patient's condition improves, oral therapy has been too little. If there is aggravation of weakness, oral therapy has been too much. Other authorities find this an unreliable guide, and we do not use this technique. If edrophonium is not used, there is nothing but clinical observation to guide the therapist. For mild cases, two tablets of either neostigmine or pyridostigmine three times daily, with meals, is useful. If there is inadequate response, the dose may be increased, first by shortening the interval between doses, then by increasing the quantity of drug with each dose. Problems arise because these drugs never completely reverse symptoms. Therefore the dose should be increased only so long as there is clear-cut response, and it should not be increased beyond the amount giving some perceptible benefit. Doses exceeding 120 mg every two hours are almost never necessary.

Overtreatment itself can cause weakness; cholinesterase inhibitors may cause a depolarizing block at the neuromuscular junction. This probably does not occur with oral treatment in the amounts recommended.

Drugs advocated as "adjuvants" include potassium chloride, ephedrine, and guanidine, but their true value is unproved and guanidine may cause aplastic anemia.

Steroids and Immunosuppressive Drugs. Prednisone now enjoys widespread popularity in the treatment of myasthenia, but it has never been put to an adequately controlled prospective therapeutic trial. Some investigators report improvement in as many as 80 per cent of patients treated, with virtually no side effects. Others are less enthusiastic about beneficial effects and are more concerned about deleterious effects. Some treat virtually all patients; others restrict therapy to those with incapacitating disease. It is agreed that the minimal early dose should be about 50 mg daily for an adult, often given as 100 mg on alternate days. For patients who are seriously ill, larger doses may be used. Initiation of steroid therapy may cause an exacerbation of myasthenia. Therefore, in less emergent situations, it seems advisable to start with a prednisone dosage of 25 mg on alternate days and gradually increase to the full dose in a week or two. Some use prednisone preparation for thymectomy; others reserve steroids until some interval after thymectomy. If there is no beneficial response, it is not clear how long prednisone should be continued before deeming the trial a failure; a minimum of three months at full dosage seems reasonable. No matter how used, steroid drugs should be initiated with close supervision and probably in hospital because of the danger of temporarily increasing the weakness.

The mechanism of action of steroids in myasthenia is not known, but current theories favor an immunosuppressive role. More specific immunosuppressive drugs such as azathioprine, methotrexate, or cyclophosphamide have also been used. There is no indication that these drugs are any better than prednisone, and evaluation of them is probably best performed in research centers.

Surgical Treatment. Thymectomy is followed by significant improvement in about 85 per cent of patients with myasthenia and no tumor. Patients with thymoma fare worse whether the tumor is excised or not.

All patients with generalized myasthenia may be considered for thymectomy, but most clinicians are reluctant to recommend the operation for patients with solely ocular symptoms, for preadolescent children, or for the elderly. However, in each of these categories individual circumstances might warrant thymectomy. Because the effects of thymectomy are not seen for months or years, it should not be regarded as an emergency procedure.

In preparing patients for operation, the usual oral dosage cholinergic medication is maintained until the day of surgery, and then stopped abruptly. Endotracheal intubation is used throughout the thymectomy and maintained for assisted respiration in the immediate postoperative period. Induction of anesthesia requires no special precautions, but many anesthesiologists prefer to dispense with muscle relaxants. Parenteral steroids in appropriate dosage should be given to patients who have been taking prednisone in the preoperative period.

After the operation, depending upon circumstances, the endotracheal tube may be removed in a few hours or the next day. If there are any complications and the endotracheal tube must remain in place, it ultimately becomes necessary to consider tracheostomy, but this is necessary in few cases. Specific cholinergic drug therapy is withheld if there is postoperative fever or any other obvious complication; when these complications have been controlled, pyridostigmine therapy may be restarted at a level of one half the preoperative dose.

Plasmapheresis. Plasmapheresis is safe, and beneficial effects are seen in almost all patients. However, plasma exchange is expensive because of the instruments, supplies, and personnel involved. It requires several hours and a trip to the hospital. The benefits may be slight or great and may last days or months without relation to antibody titer. It is not clear that concomitant use of prednisone or azathioprine enhances or prolongs improvement. Conversely, it has not been shown that the long-range effects of steroids or immunosuppressive therapy are enhanced or accelerated by plasma exchange. To determine whether plasma exchange can shorten the duration of myasthenic crisis or neonatal myasthenia would require a controlled clinical trial. For all of these reasons, the ultimate role of plasma exchange in treating myasthenia remains to be clarified; it is being evaluated in many centers, and guidelines may soon be forthcoming. In the meantime it is being used only for patients with severe symptoms that have resisted other therapeutic approaches or in preparation for thymectomy.

Crisis. Patients with myasthenia gravis may suddenly develop difficulty breathing that is severe enough to require artificial ventilation. This may be induced by systemic infection or major surgical procedures, but often there is no apparent cause. Patients with oropharyngeal weakness are especially liable to this threat, perhaps because of aspiration. Whenever there is doubt about the adequacy of ventilation or the state of the airway, endotracheal intubation should be used for short periods of respiratory support. The insertion of a cuffed tube makes intermittent positive pressure breathing feasible and also reduces the hazard of aspiration. Patients are best transferred to a respiratory intensive care unit. Cholinergic drugs are stopped. After several days, usually after fever (a common concomitant of crisis) has started to subside, drugs may be started once again, at half the precrisis dosage. The cause of crisis is not clear, but it is usually transient and will subside if the patient can be kept alive. The mortality rate of crisis was formerly about 50 per cent, but since the advent of intensive care units, few patients die, and these are mostly elderly persons with complicating cardiac and renal disease.

A few patients require assisted ventilation for prolonged periods. For these patients, a trial of either plasmapheresis or steroid therapy seems warranted.

PROGNOSIS. The course of myasthenia is variable. The disease may be restricted to ocular muscles for many years, with no threat to life. Other patients are disabled to a variable degree by oropharyngeal or limb weakness, and a few are crippled. Crisis occurs in about 10 per cent of the cases. The overall mortality from myasthenia itself is probably less than 5 per cent, and although myasthenia was formerly the main hazard, intercurrent and unrelated disease is now more often the cause of death.

Drachman DB: The biology of myasthenia gravis. Ann Rev Neurosci 4:195, 1981. *Thoughtful review of the pathogenesis of myasthenic manifestations.*

Engel AG: Myasthenia gravis. Handb Clin Neurol 41:95, 1979. *Comprehensive discussion of clinical aspects and pathophysiology of myasthenia.*

Grob D (ed.): Myasthenia gravis. Pathophysiology and management. Ann NY Acad Sci 277:1, 1981. *Covers every conceivable aspect of the pathogenesis and treatment of myasthenia.*

Keesey J, Bein M, Mink J, Sample F, Sarti D, Mulder D, Herrmann C Jr, Peter JB: Detection of thymoma in myasthenia gravis. Neurology 30:233, 1980. *Discussion of the value and limitation of computed tomography in detecting thymoma.*

Lindstrom J, Dau P: Biology of myasthenia gravis. Ann Rev Pharmacol Toxicol 20:337, 1980. *Detailed review of the immunology of myasthenia.*

Lindstrom JM, Lambert EH: Content of acetylcholine receptor and antibodies bound to receptor in myasthenia gravis, experimental autoimmune myasthenia gravis and Eaton-Lambert syndrome. Neurology 26:130, 1978. *A detailed review of the pathophysiology of these disorders.*

Lisak RP, Barchi RL: Myasthenia Gravis. Philadelphia, W. B. Saunders, 1982. *An immunologist and a neuroscientist combine efforts to give a lucid and comprehensive review of theory and practice.*

Pascuzzi RM, Coslett HB, Johns TR: Long-term corticosteroid treatment of myasthenia gravis: Report of 116 patients. Ann Neurol 15:291, 1984. *A review of extensive clinical experience.*

Rodriguez M, Gomez MR, Howard FM, Taylor WF: Myasthenia gravis in children: Long-term follow-up. Ann Neurol 13:504, 1983. *Therapeutic decisions may be especially difficult in children with myasthenia; guidelines are presented in this analysis.*

Rowland LP: Controversies about the treatment of myasthenia gravis. J Neurol Neurosurg Psychiat 43:644, 1980. *Intended to be an impartial but critical review of the controversies that influence clinicians in the choice of therapy.*

EATON-LAMBERT SYNDROME (Myasthenic Syndrome)

DEFINITION. The Eaton-Lambert syndrome is a "facilitating" disorder of neuromuscular transmission in which the amplitude of the first muscle action potential evoked by stimulation of the nerve is reduced, and with repetitive stimulation the amplitude of the action potential increases to more than three times the original height.

PATHOGENESIS. The first cases were associated with oat-cell carcinoma of the lung, but cases have been found with other tumors, with other diseases, and sometimes with no complicating disorder. Microelectrode studies indicate that the defect is due to impaired release of acetylcholine at the nerve terminals. Antibodies to components of nerve terminals may be responsible.

CLINICAL MANIFESTATIONS. The first evidence may be prolonged apnea after curarization for surgery. Formal testing with d-tubocurarine also indicates that patients are unduly sensitive. Other patients may have symptoms of limb weakness, but cranial muscle weakness is never prominent. The response to cholinergic drugs is usually equivocal at best. Pain in the limbs and dry mouth may be prominent. Movements may be peculiarly slow, and tendon reflexes may be lost. In tests of strength the patient may seem to get stronger with continued effort. Myotatic reflexes are frequently depressed.

DIAGNOSIS. The signs listed above diverge sufficiently from myasthenia to avoid confusion; only limb weakness and curare sensitivity are similar. The remainder of the syndrome resembles polymyositis, and polyneuritis would also have to be considered. The diagnosis is made by the response to repetitive stimulation. Antibodies to AChR have not been found in typical cases. When the diagnosis of Eaton-Lambert syndrome has been established, special efforts should be made to find the underlying tumor.

TREATMENT. Guanidine promotes the release of acetylcholine, and the drug is effective in daily doses of 35 mg per kilogram of body weight, given orally. This drug may suppress bone marrow, however, and great caution must be taken so that guanidine should probably not be used unless the neuromuscular disorder is disabling. 4-Aminopyridine is also effective in promoting release of acetylcholine, but it is also hazardous and may cause seizures. Steroid therapy may be beneficial. Plasmapheresis may be beneficial. Any tumor should be treated appropriately.

Eaton LM, Lambert EH: Electromyography and electric stimulation of nerves in diseases of motor unit: Observations in myasthenic syndrome associated with malignant tumors. JAMA 163:1117, 1957. *The classic description of the Eaton-Lambert syndrome.*

Elmqvist D, Lambert EH: Detailed analysis of neuromuscular transmission in a patient with myasthenic syndrome sometimes associated with bronchogenic carcinoma. Mayo Clin Proc 43:689, 1968. *The original electrophysiologic analysis of the Eaton-Lambert syndrome.*

Lange DJ: The Eaton-Lambert syndrome: Current concepts of pathogenesis and treatment. Neurol Neurosurg Update 4:1, 1983. *A comprehensive review of pathogenesis, diagnosis, and treatment.*

Newsom-Davis JN, Murray NMF: Plasma exchange and immunosuppressive drug treatment in the Lambert-Eaton myasthenic syndrome. Neurology 34:480, 1984. *Treatments based on the theory that the syndrome is caused by autoantibodies.*

UNUSUAL CAUSES OF NEUROMUSCULAR BLOCK

Botulism and *tick paralysis* are described in Ch. 279 and 424. Both cause a syndrome of flaccid quadriplegia with paresis of cranial muscles and must be differentiated from polyneuritis, myasthenia gravis, and periodic paralysis. In neither is there a sensory disorder, but autonomic fibers may be affected in botulism, especially pupilloconstrictor fibers (resulting in a dilated, fixed pupil). The electromyogram in botulism may resemble that in the Eaton-Lambert syndrome, an observation that may be diagnostically important.

Several *aminoglycoside antimicrobial drugs* interfere with the release of acetylcholine, and may cause clinical syndromes. The offending drugs include neomycin, streptomycin, colistin, polymyxin, and kanamycin. The most common manifestation is postoperative apnea without other evidence of paralysis. This is most apt to occur in patients with renal failure, presumably with unusually high blood levels of the antimicrobial drug. In occasional cases, however, there may be flaccid quadriplegia. Administration of calcium and guanidine may be helpful, but the essence of management is supportive treatment and use of a safer antimicrobial.

Cornblath DR, Sladky JT, Sumner AJ: Clinical electrophysiology of infantile botulism. Muscle Nerve 6:448, 1983. *Analysis of 25 cases in one hospital.*

Swift TR: Disorders of neuromuscular transmission other than myasthenia gravis. Muscle Nerve 4:334, 1981. *A comprehensive review of theoretical and practical aspects of these syndromes.*

SYNDROMES OF MUSCULAR OVERACTIVITY: CRAMPS AND RELATED DISORDERS

Cramps, caused by painful, abrupt shortening of muscle, affect almost everyone at some time or other. Electromyographic investigation indicates that motor units fire at a rate of about 300 per second, much higher than the most vigorous voluntary contraction. It is presumably the high rate of discharge that causes the palpable muscle tautness and the pain. The pain can be relieved by stretching the affected muscle, or by massage. The stimulus responsible for cramps is not known; relief by stretching suggests that some central mechanism is involved, since this is the stimulus for receptors in muscle that inhibit discharge of the motor neuron to the same muscle. Certain conditions are associated with a propensity to cramps: denervation (especially amyotrophic lateral sclerosis), pregnancy, and electrolyte disorders (especially water intoxication and hyponatremia). Cramps attributed to hypo-osmolarity are seen in some patients treated with maintenance hemodialysis and respond to treatment with hypertonic solutions of glucose or sodium.

Cramps occur most commonly in otherwise normal individuals, and some people are more susceptible than others for unknown reasons, with or without a family history of cramps. Others occur only at night, and can be prevented by quinine sulfate, 0.3 gram orally at bedtime. Others occur frequently during the day, occasionally so often that the individual is effectively crippled. Phenytoin, 0.3 to 0.6 gram daily, may be helpful to these patients, but some are resistant to this and to other drugs that may be tried, including diazepam and diphenhydramine. Patients with "*benign fasciculation*" (lacking weakness, wasting, or other signs of motor neuron disease) seem especially prone to have frequent cramps.

Tetany is a special form of cramp, identified by its predilection for flexor muscles of the hand and fingers, its association with laryngospasm, and its relationship to hypocalcemia. Tetany can be painful. It differs from other cramps electromyographically because of the characteristic rhythmic grouping of discharging potentials. Hyperventilation tetany is likely to be overlooked as a cause of cramps or laryngospasm.

Contracture is the term reserved for the painful shortening of muscles in glycogen storage diseases, in which the muscles are electrically silent although maximally shortened.

Myokymia has been used to describe a variety of apparently different disorders characterized by cramps in association with spontaneous twitching of muscle. In some cases there are prolonged trains of spontaneous potentials, whereas in others there is grouping of potentials. Some of these patients have difficulty in relaxing grip, but, unlike myotonia, the muscular activity is abolished by neuromuscular blocking agents, indicating a neural rather than a muscular origin. Hyperhidrosis is prominent in some patients and is secondary to the increased muscular activity.

Continuous shortening of the muscle would lead to abnormal postures and abnormally increased resistance to passive movement. These abnormalities, of course, are often due to central neurologic disorders. In recent years, however, an increasing number of patients have been described because of fluctuating rigidity of axial and limb muscles. For want of a better name, and lacking understanding of the pathogenesis, this has been called the *stiff man syndrome.* The diagnosis requires that there be no signs of cerebral or spinal cord disease, and there must be continuous electromyographic activity despite authentic attempts to relax. Ordinary cramps may be superimposed upon the persistent stiffness. Diazepam, 30 to 60 mg daily, may bring dramatic relief.

A variety of other names have been applied to these syndromes, including *Isaac's syndrome, quantal squander, armadillo disease, neuromyotonia,* and *continuous muscle fiber activity.* Some cases of brief duration may be related to mild cases of tetanus. It will take some time to sort out the variety of causes. If these unusual forms can be analyzed, we may yet understand why an otherwise normal individual occasionally has a cramp.

Auger RG, Daube JR, Gomez MR, Lambert EH: Hereditary form of sustained muscle activity of peripheral nerve origin causing generalized myokymia and muscle stiffness. Ann Neurol 15:13, 1984. *A description of an unusual form of the syndrome with an excellent discussion of differential diagnosis.*

Gordon EE, Januszko DM, Kaufman L: A critical survey of stiff man syndrome. Am J Med 42:582, 1967. *Whatever this disease is, this paper describes it.*

Hudson AJ, Brown WF, Gilbert JJ: The muscular pain–fasciculation syndrome. Neurology 28:1105, 1978. *Review of an old problem; also called "benign fasciculation."*

Layzer RB: Motor unit hyperactivity states. Handb Clin Neurol 40:259, 1979. *Comprehensive and lucid description of cramps and related disorders.*

Milutinovich J, Graefe V, Follette WC, Scribner BH: Effect of hypertonic glucose on the muscular cramps of hemodialysis. Ann Intern Med 90:926, 1979. *Cramps are common in patients treated with hemodialysis; this describes one approach to management.*

Sheehy MP, Marsden CD: Writers cramp—a focal dystonia. Brain 105:461, 1982. *A comprehensive discussion and description of the problem.*

Van den Bergh P, Bulcke JA, Dom R: Familial muscle cramps with autosomal dominant transmission. Eur Neurol 19:207, 1980. *Familial susceptibility to cramps is being recognized more frequently.*

Part XXIV
EYE DISEASES

John W. Gittinger, Jr.

540. INTRODUCTION

Because many systemic diseases manifest in the eyes, ophthalmoscopy is a necessary skill for the physician. The pupil of the eye is a window opening onto the arterioles and venules of the retina, the optic disc, and the pigmented tissues of the fundus. In addition, the pupil, innervated by both sympathetic and parasympathetic nerves, provides an index of autonomic function.

The second, third, fourth, fifth, sixth, and seventh cranial nerves subserve vision. Ocular motility is the most precisely documented of complex motor acts. Similarly, the intracranial visual pathways—optic nerve, chiasm, and tract, geniculate body, superior colliculus, optic radiations, striate cortex, and visual association areas—are the paradigm of sensory processing in the nervous system.

The discussion that follows highlights the interrelationship between ocular and systemic disease, beginning with a brief review of the two common ophthalmic disorders—cataract and glaucoma—and then turning to ocular entities and ocular manifestations of medical disorders likely to present to nonophthalmic physicians.

Leigh RJ, Zee DS: The Neurology of Eye Movements. Philadelphia, F. A. Davis Company, 1983. *The current understanding of neural control of eye movements.*

Moses RA: Adler's Physiology of the Eye; Clinical application. 7th ed. St. Louis, C. V. Mosby Company, 1981. *A clinically oriented review of basic physiologic mechanisms.*

541. CATARACT

A cataract is an opacity of the lens that manifests as painless, gradual loss of vision. Cataracts are described according to their location—nuclear (deep in the lens), cortical (more superficial), and subcapsular (immediately beneath the capsule). Cataracts are classified as immature, mature, or hypermature. An immature cataract has some clear cortex; a mature cataract is totally opaque: the pupil appears white—leukocoria. A hypermature cataract has liquefied cortex that leaks through the capsule and may excite destructive inflammation. Immature cataracts are usually removed for visual reasons. A mature or hypermature cataract in an eye with potential for useful vision should be removed to prevent irreversible damage.

Etiology

Congenital cataracts are a feature of rubella embryopathy and often are associated with other congenital malformations. Acquired cataracts may result from trauma, radiation, or metabolic disorder. In some cases of Wilson's disease, orange copper deposits appear on the anterior capsule—the sunflower cataract. Chlorpromazine administration may result in a brown or white dusting on the anterior lens surface. Red, green, and blue opacities in the lenticular cortex characterize myotonic dystrophy but are occasionally encountered in its absence. All of these colorful cataracts have diagnostic, but little visual, significance.

Hypocalcemia may be cataractogenic. Cataracts occur in disorders of carbohydrate metabolism: hypoglycemia, galactosemia, and diabetes mellitus. Diabetics do not necessarily have an increased incidence of cataracts, but theirs progress rapidly, perhaps because of variations in lens hydration as the result of changing sugar concentrations in the aqueous humor.

Systemic corticosteroids promote formation of posterior subcapsular cataracts. Because of the path light takes through the lens, posterior subcapsular cataracts reduce vision more than similar, eccentric opacities. Central posterior opacities get in the way of light most often when the pupil is small, as in bright light or with near work. Difficulties with driving and reading are the first complaints of patients with posterior subcapsular cataracts.

Most cataracts have no known etiology. The common nuclear sclerotic cataract, or senile cataract, is often familial, but no specific factors have been proven to accelerate or retard its development.

Treatment

The treatment for cataract is surgical removal. With the exception of mature and hypermature cataracts and of immature cataracts that have swollen sufficiently to threaten to precipitate angle-closure glaucoma (see below), most cataracts are removed for visual reasons. Considerations in planning cataract extraction are the patient's visual needs, the potential for visual improvement, and the risks of surgery. A person who drives will require surgery when the better eye is worse than 20/40, the legal minimum for a driver's license in most states. By contrast, an elderly patient with 20/200 vision and limited visual needs may be perfectly happy without intervention. Care must be taken to identify intercurrent ocular disease; removal of the lens of an eye with advanced glaucoma or macular degeneration does not necessarily improve vision.

The risk of cataract surgery itself is relatively small. Despite the possibility of intraocular hemorrhage, postoperative infection, corneal decompensation, or problems with wound healing, the chances for a good visual outcome are excellent. Even successful cataract surgery increases the likelihood of subsequent retinal detachment, and a small percentage of eyes develop prolonged cystoid macular edema with reduced acuity.

General anesthesia constitutes a major portion of the risk when it is used. Cataract surgery can usually be performed under local anesthesia, and this should be considered the method of choice in medically fragile patients.

Spaeth GL: Ophthalmic Surgery; Principles and Practice. Philadelphia, W. B. Saunders Company, 1982. *A clear and concise presentation of the current state of ophthalmic surgery. Indications, techniques, and complications are discussed.*

542. GLAUCOMA

Glaucoma is a group of disorders in which elevated intraocular pressure damages the optic nerve. The major types of glaucoma are open-angle, angle-closure, congenital, and secondary.

The dynamics of aqueous humor control intraocular pressure. The aqueous humor is derived from blood by a process of secretion and ultrafiltration in the ciliary body. Aqueous humor then passes from the posterior chamber through the pupil to fill the anterior chamber, the space between the back of the cornea and the plane of the iris and pupil. The aqueous humor is reabsorbed through the trabecular meshwork, located in the angle between the cornea and the iris, to enter Schlemm's canal, which connects with the venous system.

Open-angle Glaucoma

In chronic open-angle glaucoma, the most common glaucoma, a block in aqueous humor reabsorption exists at the level of the trabecular meshwork. Intraocular pressure rises above its normal maximum of 21 mm Hg and gradually destroys axons and supporting tissue on the optic disc.

The prevalence of open-angle glaucoma varies with the population studied and the diagnostic criteria employed. A conservative estimate of unequivocal glaucoma in American and European adults is 0.5 per cent. A much larger percentage of these adults sustains increased intraocular pressure without signs of optic nerve damage—*ocular hypertension*. The patient with ocular hypertension is considered a glaucoma suspect.

Open-angle glaucoma is ordinarily asymptomatic until well advanced. Only rarely does the elevated intraocular pressure cause corneal edema, with the attendant perception of halos around lights. Pain is not characteristic of open-angle glaucoma. Initial visual loss in chronic open-angle glaucoma is confined to the peripheral field, especially in the nasal area and the area surrounding fixation. Visual acuity remains normal until late in the course of the disease.

Diagnosis is made by measurement of intraocular pressure, examination of the optic disc, and testing of the visual fields. Gonioscopy, the visualization of the angle structures under high magnifications with special contact lenses, allows distinction of an angle-closure from an open-angle mechanism.

The treatment of open-angle glaucoma is primarily medical. Topical administration of parasympathomimetics (pilocarpine and carbachol), beta-adrenergic blockers (timolol), and sympathomimetics (epinephrine) decreases intraocular pressure. When these medications—individually and in combination—are ineffective in arresting progressive disc damage and visual field loss, indirect parasympathomimetics (echothiophate) and carbonic anhydrase inhibitors (acetazolamide and methazolamide) are prescribed.

If maximum tolerated medical therapy fails to halt progression, surgery is indicated. *Laser trabeculoplasty* opens aqueous outflow channels by burning the surface of the trabecular meshwork. If all else fails, a surgical fistula can be created between the anterior chamber and the subconjunctival space, allowing direct absorption of aqueous humor by subconjunctival and episcleral vessels. This operation is called a filtering procedure.

The management of open-angle glaucoma and that of systemic hypertension have many similarities. In both, the prevention of complications depends upon early recognition, careful follow up, and patient compliance with therapeutic regimens. Routine measurement of intraocular pressures (*tonometry*) at general physical examinations is often advocated, but careful ophthalmoscopy with referral of patients whose central excavation ("cup") exceeds one-third of the disc's area may be an equally effective screen.

Angle-closure Glaucoma

When aqueous outflow is mechanically impeded owing to a shallow anterior chamber, the resulting increase in intraocular pressure is angle-closure glaucoma. Intraocular pressure is normal until resistance to aqueous flow through the pupil—pupillary block—bows the iris forward to obstruct the resorptive surfaces in the angle. The pressure then rises precipitously, often to above 50 mm Hg.

Acute angle-closure glaucoma is generally monocular. The eye is red and painful, and the pupil about 6 mm and fixed. Vision is decreased. The patient is diaphoretic and nauseated and often vomits.

Typical angle-closure glaucoma is easy to recognize. Occasionally, chronic or subacute angle-closure mimics open-angle glaucoma. Gonioscopy is then necessary to distinguish between the two mechanisms. The elderly often do not develop the full set of clinical signs and symptoms. One should always consider angle-closure glaucoma when the patient presents with a fixed, mid-dilated pupil and decreased vision.

Angle-closure can be precipitated in predisposed eyes by dilating the pupils. The risk of pharmacologic dilation is assessed by noting the depth of the anterior chamber. Eyes with shallow anterior chambers are at risk for angle-closure. This distinction is not always easy to observe, and in some cases an experienced ophthalmologist may not be able to determine whether an angle will close with dilation. The risk of dilation increases with age, and everyone over the age of 50 whose anterior chamber is less than full depth should be considered to have the potential for angle-closure. This does not mean, however, that most patients should not be dilated, but rather that dilation should be performed with a relatively short-acting mydriatic agent such as tropicamide or hydroxyamphetamine. The patient should then be observed until the effects of the mydriatic are known.

A nonophthalmologist should probably not routinely dilate adult outpatients. Children and inpatients should be dilated if there is no other contraindication such as recent head trauma, an iris-fixated intraocular lens, or impending general anesthesia. With these exceptions, the diagnostic benefits of dilation outweigh the risk of precipitating angle-closure. Should angle-closure glaucoma develop, it can be recognized and promptly treated.

An acute angle-closure attack is a medical emergency. Initial management consists of administration of parenteral acetazolamide, oral glycerol or intravenous mannitol, and topical pilocarpine, and perhaps timolol. Once the attack has been broken, the anatomic predisposition can be effectively eliminated by creating a communication between the posterior and anterior chamber through the peripheral iris, either with a laser—*laser iridotomy*—or with surgical iridectomy. The anterior segment abnormality that underlies angle-closure glaucoma is bilateral, and prophylactic surgery on the other eye is usually indicated.

Congenital Glaucoma

Congenital glaucoma is an open-angle glaucoma that is the result of dysgenesis of the angle structures. Increased intraocular pressure enlarges the immature eye (*buphthalmos*), and a corneal diameter greater than 12 mm suggests congenital glaucoma. Progressive corneal enlargement ruptures the deeper layers of the cornea, with resulting corneal edema and loss of transparency. The cornea of a child with advanced congenital glaucoma is enlarged, with a ground-glass translucency.

Treatment of congenital glaucoma is both surgical and medical. Congenital glaucoma is fortunately rare; the prognosis for preservation of vision is only fair.

Secondary Glaucoma

Secondary glaucoma develops as the consequence of another ocular disease. Examples of secondary glaucomas are angle-closure glaucoma precipitated by intumescence of the lens, glaucoma developing as a result of formation of new vessels in the angle, and glaucoma in a chronically inflamed eye. Severe blunt trauma to the eye damages angle structures, predisposing to the subsequent development of open-angle glaucoma.

The treatment of secondary, lens-induced angle-closure glaucoma is surgical removal of the lens. Most other secondary glaucomas are managed in much the same way as primary open-angle glaucoma. Neovascular glaucoma is difficult to treat, and most eyes ultimately lose all useful vision. If the stimulus to neovascularization is ischemia, ablation of ischemic tissues by photocoagulation may halt progression. If neovascularization continues, medical control will become ineffective. Filtering procedures generally fail because exuberant tissue growth closes the surgical fistula, a problem that may be circumvented by the implantation of a plastic valve connecting the anterior chamber and the subconjunctival space. Destruction of the ciliary body by an externally applied liquid nitrogen probe—*cyclocryotherapy*—controls intraocular pressure, but seldom preserves useful vision.

Any glaucoma where all light perception has been lost is called *absolute glaucoma*. Enucleation is the definitive treatment for a blind, painful eye.

Chandler PA, Grant WM: Glaucoma. Philadelphia, Lea & Febiger, 1979. *A well-written exposition of one approach to glaucoma. Glaucoma syndromes are especially well covered.*

Kolker AE, Hetherington J Jr: Becker-Shaffer's Diagnosis and Therapy of the Glaucomas. St. Louis, The C. V. Mosby Company, 1983. *The best one-volume compendium on this subject. The illustrations are numerous and clear.*

543. DISC SWELLING AND OPTIC ATROPHY

The optic disc marks the transition from retina to optic nerve. The central retinal artery and vein pass through the disc and bifurcate on its surface. There is considerable variation in the disc's ophthalmoscopic appearance. Vessels enter the interior of the eye through the nasal half of the disc. A central excavation or cup occupies a variable portion of its substance; vessels are often seen curving over the edge of this cup.

Over one million axons originate in the ganglion cells of the retina and pass through each optic disc. Although these axons are nearly transparent, in the light of a bright ophthalmoscope they form fine reflective striations on the disc's surface and the immediately surrounding retina. Disc swelling is a consequence of ischemia, infarction, infiltration, or local changes in tissue pressures.

Papilledema

Disc swelling from increased intracranial pressure is termed papilledema; nevertheless, it does not represent purely extracellular edema. Instead, the increased intracranial pressure results in an accumulation of axoplasm, the cytoplasm of the axons, in and around the disc. Normally the axoplasm circulates along the axon—axoplasmic flow. Increased intracranial pressure causes axoplasmic stasis at the level of the lamina cribosa, the perforated plate of sclera through which the axons leave the eye. This stasis appears ophthalmoscopically as a protrusion of the disc, with swelling most obvious just adjacent to the disc's normal borders. When the increase in intracranial pressure is rapid, the veins are engorged, and hemorrhages appear on the disc or adjacent retina.

Papilledema is usually bilateral, but may be asymmetrical. Visual acuity remains normal in acute papilledema. Only in long-standing papilledema does secondary optic atrophy, with decreased vision, ensue (see below).

Pseudopapilledema

Because the common causes of papilledema include intracranial tumor and hemorrhage, its recognition and differential diagnosis are important. Various other disc appearances may be confused with papilledema. Hyperopic (farsighted) eyes are small, with axonal crowding at the disc. Drusen of the optic nerve, which are depositions of hyaline material in the prelaminar optic nerve, appear as swollen discs in young persons. Such anomalous discs are often discovered incidentally. One clue to their nature is the frequent absence of the physiologic cup, for in true papilledema the cup is preserved until the disc swelling is far advanced.

Papillitis

Papillitis is an anterior form of optic neuritis. In the majority of acute optic neuritides the disc appears normal—*retrobulbar optic neuritis.* In papillitis, the disc is swollen and may be hemorrhagic, an appearance ophthalmoscopically indistinguishable from papilledema. Unlike papilledema, however, acuity is characteristically reduced, and papillitis is often truly unilateral.

Ischemic Optic Neuropathy

Papillitis is largely a disease of the young. In older persons, disc swelling and loss of vision suggest infarction—ischemic optic neuropathy. Often only the superior or inferior half of the disc is involved, with consequent loss of function in the inferior or superior visual field. Most instances of ischemic optic neuropathy are idiopathic, but the disorder may be the initial manifestation of giant cell or temporal arteritis, a disease of the elderly. In such cases the erythrocyte sedimentation rate is usually elevated; symptoms of this generalized arteritis include malaise, fever, headache, scalp tenderness, and painful chewing.

Other Causes of Disc Swelling

Another cause of disc swelling is severe hypertension. The relative roles of local vascular changes and of increased intracranial pressure in the pathogenesis of the disc swelling that defines malignant hypertension are uncertain. Decreased intraocular pressure, encountered after ocular surgery or injury, also produces disc swelling. The disc is rarely swollen during an attack of angle-closure glaucoma, because the sudden increase in intraocular pressure allegedly obstructs axoplasmic flow.

Infiltration of the optic nerve heads is encountered in leukemia, metastatic carcinoma, and sarcoid. Cryptococcal invasion of the optic nerve is associated with disc swelling in some cases of cryptococcal meningitis.

Optic Atrophy

Optic atrophy results from death of the axons in the retina and optic nerve. Disc pallor and optic atrophy are not synonymous; some pallor is a feature of normal discs. The optic nerve's axons originate in the ganglion cell layer of the retina, pass through the optic disc, nerve, chiasm, and tract, and terminate in the lateral geniculate body and brain stem. A large majority of these axons synapse in the lateral geniculate body of the thalamus; axons subserving the pupillary light reflex leave the optic tract to synapse in upper brain stem centers. A lesion anywhere from the retina through the optic tract will cause optic atrophy. Lesions behind the lateral geniculate in early life may cause trans-synaptic degeneration and optic atrophy.

Optic atrophy may be classified as primary, secondary, and glaucomatous. *Primary optic atrophy* refers to progressive pallor without loss of disc substance, a sign of wallerian degeneration as the result of compression, vascular injury, or axonal death from toxic or metabolic disturbances. *Secondary optic atrophy* develops after disc swelling, as in chronic papilledema. Vascular and glial changes may give the disc an irregular, milky gray appearance with ill-defined borders. The distinction is not absolute; some cases in which the process is clearly "secondary" have a crisp, white disc. *Glaucomatous optic atrophy* denotes loss of disc substance, already referred to as increased cupping. Again, nature rejects arbitrary classifications, and enlarged cups are occasionally observed with compressive optic neuropathy.

Optic atrophy is difficult to recognize in children, in whom the discs may have a pale appearance normally. In adults with nuclear sclerotic cataracts, the pallor is masked by the lens acting as a yellow filter. The diagnosis of optic atrophy should not be made unless there is evidence of alteration in visual function: decreased acuity or field—or, in infants, nystagmus.

In the final analysis, optic atrophy is not a clinical finding but a pathologic entity. In retinitis pigmentosa there is a primary dystrophy of the rods and cones. The ganglion cells remain intact, but there are secondary vascular and gliotic changes with a waxy pallor of the disc, but not a true optic atrophy. Disc pallor is a finding to be evaluated in the context of the entire ophthalmologic and neurologic examination.

Miller NR: Walsh and Hoyt's Clinical Neuro-Ophthalmology. 4th ed. Baltimore, Williams & Wilkins Company, 1982, Vol 1, pp 175–271, 329–342. *The most recent revision of a classic monograph. The pages cited contain a comprehensive review of the entities discussed briefly here.*

544. OCULAR INFLAMMATION

Uveitis

Uveitis is any inflammation of the uveal tract—the iris, ciliary body, and choroid. There are two major clinical types of uveitis: anterior and posterior. Anterior uveitis, also known as *iritis* or *iridocyclitis,* has as its hallmark cells in the anterior chamber. Curiously, it is the rare case of iritis that displays any recognizable iris abnormality. Posterior uveitis may take the form of *chorioretinitis.* The choroid and retina are so intimately connected that it is difficult to have inflammation of one without the other.

Acute anterior uveitis presents with congestion of the eye, often in a perilimbal distribution described as ciliary flush. Frequently, the eye is painful, vision reduced, and the pupil small and poorly reactive. The diagnosis is confirmed on slit lamp examination by the presence of free cells in the aqueous humor, visible as bright points as the slit beam passes through the anterior chamber. In more severe inflammation, *keratitic precipitates,* cellular aggregates on the back of the cornea, appear. The slit beam itself is seen passing through the normally optically empty anterior chamber, its light dispersed by the protein and other solutes leaking into the aqueous from inflamed vessels, a phenomenon called *flare.*

Most cases of anterior uveitis are idiopathic. Rarely, anterior uveitis can be a manifestation of a systemic inflammatory disease such as sarcoid, or an infection such as syphilis or tuberculosis. In such cases the inflammation may be marked, with large, oily keratitic precipitates classically described as resembling mutton fat. This variant of anterior uveitis is *granulomatous iritis.*

Uveitis and Arthritis

Juvenile rheumatoid arthritis and ankylosing spondylitis are especially apt to be associated with uveitis. The uveitis of ankylosing spondylitis is an acute, usually self-limited, anterior uveitis. Young men with this disorder may have recurrent episodes that respond to standard treatments (see below). A great majority are HLA-B27 positive. By contrast, the uveitis accompanying juvenile rheumatoid arthritis is chronic and may initially be subclinical. The young women with the pauciarticular form of juvenile rheumatoid arthritis who develop uveitis often have white and quiet eyes. With time, however, adhesions, called posterior synechiae, form between the iris and lens, leading to a potential secondary pupillary block glaucoma or occlusion of the pupil. The inflammation may cause cataract formation and ectopic calcification in the corneal epithelium—band keratopathy. Physicians treating seronegative pauciarticular arthritis should schedule slit lamp and dilation examinations several times a year. Posterior synechiae are visible with a hand light after instillation of mydriatics as the pupil does not fully dilate and has an irregular, scalloped border.

Reiter's Disease

The triad of arthritis, urethritis, and conjunctivitis suggests Reiter's disease. This develops most often in men between the ages of 20 and 40 as a nonbacterial urethritis followed by polyarthritis and ocular inflammation. The initial ocular manifestation is usually a mucopurulent conjunctivitis, followed in many cases by an anterior uveitis. Keratitis and episcleritis also occur. As in ankylosing spondylitis, with which it shares similarities, HLA-B27 is often positive. Reiter's disease is usually self-limited.

Behçet's Syndrome

Uveitis (or retinitis) is also a cardinal feature of Behçet's syndrome. Behçet's original description of oral and genital ulceration combined with ocular inflammation has been expanded to include many other manifestations of Behçet's syndrome. In some cases a layer of white cells forms in the lower portion of the anterior chamber (*hypopyon*). Hypopyon iritis is characteristic of Behçet's syndrome. In other patients the primary manifestation may be a retinal vasculitis and vitritis. Rarer neuro-ophthalmic manifestations such as cranial nerve palsies or homonymous hemianopias are part of a wider central nervous system involvement.

Uveomeningitis—The Vogt-Koyanagi-Harada Syndrome

Another systemic disease with characteristic ocular inflammation is uveomeningitis (the Vogt-Koyanagi-Harada syndrome). This disease affects the uvea, retina, meninges, and skin and is especially common in Orientals. Manifestations include meningeal signs, alopecia, poliosis, vitiligo, tinnitus, and dysacousis. There may be an anterior or a posterior uveitis with exudative retinal detachment.

Reticulum Cell Sarcoma

A steroid-responsive exudative process simulating uveitis occurs in adults over the age of 40 and represents a lymphoreticular neoplasia (variously called reticulum cell sarcoma, histiocytic sarcoma, or—when the brain is involved—microglioma). Diagnosis may be made from the cytology of a vitreous aspirate, and treatment with radiation has palliative value.

Leukemia

An apparent iritis developing during a course of treatment for leukemia may represent infiltration of the anterior segment. Diagnosis and therapy are similar to reticulum cell sarcoma.

Treatment

The treatment of uveitis consists largely of topical or, when the inflammation is prolonged or severe, systemic immunosuppression. Prednisolone or dexamethasone topically, or prednisone orally, is the preferred drug. Cytotoxic immunosuppressive agents are sometimes used in chronic, intractable uveitis. Mydriatic-cycloplegics in anterior uveitis reduce discomfort and retard posterior synechiae formation.

James DG, Spiteri MA: Behçet's disease. Ophthalmology 89:1279, 1982. *A review of Behçet's disease's multiple manifestations with excellent color illustrations.*

Kanski JJ: Anterior uveitis in juvenile rheumatoid arthritis. Arch Ophthalmol 95:1794, 1977. *A description of the ocular findings in 160 children with seronegative rheumatoid arthritis and uveitis evaluated in a rheumatology unit.*

Ohno S, Char DH, Kimura SJ, O'Connor GR: Vogt-Koyanagi-Harada syndrome. Am J Ophthalmol 83:735, 1977. *An analysis of 51 patients with uveomeningitis.*

Rosenthal AR: Ocular manifestations of leukemia: A review. Ophthalmology 90:899, 1983. *This paper covers the retinal, orbital, optic nerve, and uveal manifestations of leukemia.*

Sloas HA, Starling J, Harper DG, Cupples HP: Update of ocular reticulum cell sarcoma. Arch Ophthalmol 99:1048, 1981. *A case report occasioning a thorough review.*

Smith RE, Nozik RM: Uveitis: A Clinical Approach to Diagnosis and Management. Baltimore, Williams & Wilkins Company, 1983. *The most current of the monographs on uveitis. Many entities are briefly discussed.*

545. OCULAR INFECTIONS

Ocular infections (or inflammations) are most sensibly grouped according to their locations. The most common and most superficial infection is a *blepharoconjunctivitis.* Infection of the lacrimal gland is a *dacryoadenitis;* infection of the lacrimal drainage system, a *dacryocystitis.* When the cornea is involved, the infection is called *keratitis. Uveitis, scleritis,* and *episcleritis,* which are seldom infectious, are discussed elsewhere. Infection or inflammation inside the eye is an *endophthalmitis.* An infectious *vitritis* is usually called an endophthalmitis, e.g., *Candida* endophthalmitis. Some *chorioretinitis* is infectious.

Conjunctivitis

Inflammation of the mucous membranes of the eye is conjunctivitis. Isolated lid involvement is blepharitis. Most often these contiguous structures are both inflamed—blepharoconjunctivitis—but the term conjunctivitis is conventionally applied (just as iritis is for iridocyclitis). The etiologies for the conjunctivitides include allergic, viral, bacterial, chlamydial, and chemical. Mild acute viral conjunctivitis, with a watery discharge and lids that are sealed closed upon awakening, usually requires only symptomatic treatment—warm or cool compresses and a topical vasoconstrictor to whiten the eye. Antibiotics have no clear efficacy. Any severe or chronic conjunctivitis should be managed by an ophthalmologist.

Gonococcal Conjunctivitis

Purulent conjunctivitis is usually bacterial and amenable to antibiotics. An important variety is gonococcal conjunctivitis, a disease of the newborn (*gonococcal ophthalmia neonatorum*) and of sexually active adults. The eye is markedly inflamed with a copious discharge and swollen lids, a picture described as hyperpurulent conjunctivitis.

The discharge should be Gram stained and cultured on Thayer-Martin medium. Treatment consists of parenteral penicillin, or an equivalent antibiotic, and saline lavage of ocular secretions. There is debate as to the necessity and efficacy of topical antibiotics. Untreated gonococcal infection can penetrate the intact eye and destroy it; treatment should be immediately initiated if there is a reasonable suspicion of the diagnosis.

Chlamydial Conjunctivitis

In some parts of the world, chronic chlamydial conjunctivitis leads to conjunctival scarring and corneal vascularization, a disease known as *trachoma*. The resulting corneal blindness is an important international public health problem. In developed countries, chlamydial infection manifests as a subacute conjunctivitis, frequently with associated urethritis. Although a keratitis may be present, severe corneal damage does not ensue. Chlamydial conjunctivitis, also called *inclusion blennorrhea* because of the cytoplasmic inclusions found in Giemsa-stained conjunctival scrapings, is difficult to eradicate in adults unless treated with systemic tetracycline or erythromycin.

Herpesvirus hominis Keratitis

Viral keratitis is a common and potentially serious consequence of infection with *Herpesvirus hominis*. The corneal involvement may be recognized by the characteristic *dendrite*, a branching epithelial ulcer. Topical antivirals promote healing, but recurrence is frequent, with increasing risk of corneal stromal involvement and scarring. Topical steroids activate epithelial herpes infections and should not be used without ophthalmological consultation.

Corneal Ulcers

Bacterial and fungal infections of the cornea are a serious threat to vision. Corneal ulcers tend to develop in the context of ocular trauma or contact lens wear, after surgery, or with pre-existing corneal disease. Corneal ulceration appears as an area of white, gray, or yellow infiltrate that stains with fluorescein. Such patients should be referred promptly to an ophthalmologist for further evaluation and treatment.

Endophthalmitis

Infection inside the eye is seen most often following accidental or surgical perforation of the eye. Epidemics have been reported following use of contaminated solutions in intraocular surgery. Only rarely do infections elsewhere metastasize to the eye.

Bacterial endophthalmitis must be treated very aggressively if there is to be any chance of preserving vision. When the infection is recognized, cultures and smears are taken from the anterior chamber and vitreous cavity by aspiration, and a course of systemic, topical, and periocular antibiotics is begun. The choice of antibiotics depends upon what organisms, if any, are found on the Gram stain.

Candida Endophthalmitis

Candida albicans is the most prevalent organism causing metastatic (endogenous) endophthalmitis. Fungemia after prolonged use of intravenous catheters or parenteral drug abuse results in colonization of the eye, with multiple white, fluffy chorioretinal infiltrates. These often involve the macula, reducing central vision. Careful direct ophthalmoscopy through a dilated pupil is indicated in patients at risk. Most *Candida* endophthalmitis requires systemic administration of antifungal agents, although spontaneous resolution has been observed.

Infectious Chorioretinitis

CONGENITAL TOXOPLASMOSIS. A common type of infectious chorioretinitis is *toxoplasmosis*, acquired in utero. This protozoan parasite can remain dormant in large, pigmented chorioretinal scars for many years and then become active, with white infiltration at the border of the scar and an overlying vitritis. If a previously uninvolved macula is threatened, treatment with pyrimethamine and sulfa or with clindamycin may be indicated.

CYTOMEGALOVIRUS CHORIORETINITIS. Cytomegalovirus chorioretinitis appears in immunosuppressed hosts as a discrete area of white or yellow retinal opacification with associated hemorrhage or vascular sheathing. The ophthalmoscopic picture may resemble that of a branch retinal vein occlusion (see below), but in this instance, one eye often has multiple foci and there is a tendency for bilaterality.

Diagnosis can be made clinically and by culture of throat and urine. Dosages of immunosuppressive drugs should be reduced, if possible. The efficacy of treatment with the antiviral agent adeninine arabinoside is uncertain.

OTHER INFECTIOUS CHORIORETINITIDES. Syphilis and tuberculosis are now rarely encountered as chorioretinitis. *Herpesvirus* retinitis resembles that of cytomegalovirus. Cryptococcal meningitis may have an associated chorioretinitis.

Parke DW II, Jones DB, Gentry LO: Endogenous endophthalmitis among patients with candidemia. Ophthalmology 89:789, 1982. *A prospective study of 38 patients with fungemia. Over one third of patients with* Candida *had ocular lesions.*

Pollard RB, Egbert PG, Gallaher JG, Merigan TC: Cytomegalovirus retinitis in immunosuppressed hosts. I. Natural history and effects of treatment with adenine arabinoside. II. Ocular manifestations. Ann Intern Med 93:655, 1980. *Reports of a large case series. The possible role of adenine arabinoside in treatment is discussed.*

Vastine D: Infections of the ocular adnexa and cornea. *In* Peyman GA, Sanders DR, Goldberg MF (eds.): Principles and Practice of Ophthalmology. Philadelphia, W. B. Saunders Company, 1980, pp 281–355. *This well-referenced and comprehensive review appears in one of the recently published major textbooks of ophthalmology.*

546. ORBITAL DISEASE AND TUMORS

Graves' Orbitopathy

The orbitopathy of Graves' disease consists of inflammation and infiltration of orbital tissues, with characteristic enlargement and scarring of the extraocular muscles. The varied clinical manifestations include lid retraction, exophthalmos, and limitation of eye movement.

Graves' orbitopathy frequently develops in persons previously treated for hyperthyroidism. When the orbitopathy first appears, the patient may be hyperthyroid, euthyroid, or hypothyroid. A classic Graves' orbitopathy in the absence of a demonstrable thyroid abnormality, even to sophisticated testing, is referred to as *ophthalmic Graves' disease*. Computed tomography demonstrating enlarged ocular muscles is probably the most sensitive diagnostic maneuver.

Graves' orbitopathy is the most frequent cause of both unilateral and bilateral exophthalmos. Retraction of the upper lid to expose sclera above the cornea exaggerates the appearance of exophthalmos and predisposes to a major complication, corneal exposure. Tethering of the eye by fibrotic muscles produces a mechanical ophthalmoplegia. Movement up and out is often restricted; pure loss of abduction mimicking sixth nerve palsy occurs. Ophthalmoplegia is not necessarily accompanied by obvious exophthalmos.

Enlargement of the ocular muscles at the apex of the orbit may lead to another major complication of Graves' orbitopathy—compressive optic neuropathy. Severe exposure or major visual loss from compressive optic neuropathy is an indication for treatment. Systemic steroids will reduce exophthalmos and relieve optic nerve compression temporarily. Surgical decompression of the orbit by one of several routes is one definitive therapy; orbital irradiation is also used. Direct surgery on the ocular muscles relieves diplopia and permanent lid retraction.

Pseudotumor of the Orbit

Orbital pseudotumor is an idiopathic inflammation that falls within the spectrum of lymphoproliferative disorders. Its clinical manifestations are pain, exophthalmos, and limitation of eye movement. There may also be erythema and swelling of the lids. Orbital pseudotumors thus mimic orbital infection, true tumors, and the orbitopathy of Graves' disease. The major site of inflammation is muscle (myositis), nerve (perineuritis), sclera (scleritis), or lacrimal gland (dacryoadenitis).

If the inflammation is posterior to the orbital apex in the walls of the cavernous sinus, the painful ophthalmoplegia that results is called the *Tolosa-Hunt syndrome*. Orbital pseudotumor merges pathologically and clinically with orbital lymphoma, which in turn merges with systemic lymphoma.

Initial evaluation of a patient with clinical signs and symptoms of orbital pseudotumor should include orbital ultrasonography and computed tomography. A trial of high dose systemic corticosteroids is usually indicated prior to biopsy. Orbital biopsy is not a trivial undertaking and should be reserved for steroid-unresponsive or recurrent processes. Some histologically benign infiltrations do not respond to corticosteroids. Biopsy in such cases reveals fibrous tissue—*sclerosing pseudotumor*. Occasionally, a patient with a histologically benign pseudotumor subsequently develops a systemic lymphoma.

A necrotizing vasculitis, Wegener's granulomatosis, must also be included in the differential diagnosis of orbital pseudotumor, especially when the inflammation is bilateral. Most cases of Wegener's granulomatosis involve contiguous sinus structures, but local ocular forms of the disease have been reported. The combination of progressive proptosis and sinus disease also suggests orbital aspergillosis, especially in residents of warmer climates.

Rhabdomyosarcoma

Rhabdomyosarcoma is the commonest malignant tumor of the orbit during the first decade of life and occurs during the second and third decades. The initial presentation is usually ptosis with lid infiltration and proptosis. Progression may be extremely rapid, the clinical picture mimicking trauma or cellulitis. Biopsy and prompt treatment with irradiation and chemotherapy results in a high percentage of survival, although vision in the eye on the side of the tumor is seldom preserved.

Other Orbital Tumors

The variety of primary, secondary, and metastatic tumors in the orbit is large. Most present with exophthalmos, visual loss, and limitation of eye movement. High degrees of malignancy are rare with meningiomas, gliomas, hemangiomas/lymphangiomas, and dermoids. Carcinomas of the lacrimal or meibomian glands represent a serious threat to life, and some cases require the most terrible of all ophthalmologic surgery—*exenteration*, removal of the orbital contents. Carcinoma from contiguous sinuses invades the orbit, and breast carcinoma is especially likely to metastasize to the orbit.

Rootman J, Nugent R: The classification and management of acute orbital pseudotumors. Ophthalmology 89:1040, 1982. *A personal series detailing the presentation and management of 17 cases of acute pseudotumor. The value of computed tomography and the effectiveness of steroids are emphasized.*

Sergott RC, Glaser JS: Graves' ophthalmopathy. A clinical and immunologic review. Surv Ophthalmol 26:1, 1981. *A comprehensive review of the subject.*

547. INTRAOCULAR TUMORS

Retinoblastoma

Retinoblastoma, a malignancy of the retina, is the most common intraocular tumor of childhood (and one of the more common tumors at any site). One third are bilateral. About 6 per cent of retinoblastomas are inherited as an autosomal dominant disease; half of these are bilateral. Ninety per cent of retinoblastomas are discovered before the child is three.

Retinoblastomas present in several ways. Perhaps the most important is as childhood strabismus, a condition ordinarily considered benign. Any child with strabismus should have a fundus examination to rule out retinoblastoma. The most common presentation is *leukocoria*, a white pupillary reflex. This manifestation is shared with mature cataract, retinopathy of prematurity, toxoplasmosis, *Toxocara* endophthalmitis, and other anomalies and disorders of the interior of the eye. Retinoblastoma should also be considered in a child with a detached retina and glaucoma, or with neovascularization of the anterior segment (suggested by spontaneous hyphema). Retinoblastomas tend to calcify, and CT and ultrasound scans help in making the differential diagnosis.

Early treatment improves survival and approaches 100 per cent if the tumor is small and unilateral. Enucleation (removal of the eye and attached optic nerve) and radiation are the primary therapeutic modalities. Children with a history of retinoblastoma have an increased incidence of osteosarcomas and other tumors, which are not necessarily found in the fields of previous radiotherapy.

Malignant Melanoma

Primary melanomas develop in the conjunctiva or choroid, and skin melanomas have a predilection for metastasis to the eye and orbit. Malignant melanomas of the choroid are the most common primary intraocular tumor of adulthood. Most occur in middle-aged Caucasians.

The prognosis of malignant melanoma of the choroid depends upon size, cytology, and the presence or absence of extrascleral extension. Choroidal malignant melanomas often metastasize to the liver.

The differential diagnosis of a pigmented intraocular mass includes benign choroidal nevus, senile disciform macular degeneration (also known as central exudative hemorrhagic retinopathy), peripheral exudative hemorrhagic chorioretinopathy, choroidal hemangioma, and hypertrophy or hyperplasia of the retinal pigment epithelium. Many eyes have been removed because of the suspicion of malignant melanoma when the pathology revealed a benign condition.

Enucleation is the traditional treatment for malignant melanoma of the choroid. Many pigmented choroidal tumors are now followed without intervention, especially when they are found incidentally in the seeing eyes of elderly patients. The effect of enucleation on life expectancy is currently being debated.

Metastatic Carcinoma to the Eye

Once considered rare, metastatic cancer is now the most common ocular malignancy of adulthood, with an incidence exceeding that of choroidal melanoma. Most are carcinomas invading the choroid, the commonest being carcinoma of the breast. Although ocular metastases appear late in the course of breast carcinoma, they may be the first sign of disseminated disease. Next in frequency are carcinomas of the lung, followed by kidney, gastrointestinal tract, testis, and prostate. With lung or renal carcinoma, the primary site may be inapparent at the time the metastasis is detected.

If tumor is identified elsewhere, removal of the eye is seldom indicated. Enucleation should be performed only if the eye is completely blind and painful, as palliative radiotherapy often preserves vision.

Abramson DH, Notterman RB, Ellsworth RM, Kitchin FD: Retinoblastoma treated in infants in the first six months of life. Arch Ophthalmol 101:1362, 1983.

Lennox EL, Draper GJ, Sanders BM: Retinoblastoma: A study of natural history and prognosis of 268 cases. Br Med J 3:731, 1975. *Two reviews of large series treated in Great Britain and the United States.*

Mewis L, Young SE: Breast carcinoma metastatic to the choroid. Ophthalmology 89:147, 1982. *The current status of detection and treatment.*

Yanoff M, Fine BS: Ocular Pathology; A Text and Atlas. 2nd ed. Philadelphia, Harper Medical, 1982. *A comprehensive textbook with many clinicopathologic correlations.*

548. RHEUMATOID AND CONNECTIVE TISSUE DISEASES

To a neurologist, the eye is an anterior extension of the brain; to a rheumatologist, the eye is a joint. Medicine and ophthalmology come together in the diagnosis and management of rheumatoid and connective tissue disorders. Uveal manifestations are discussed in conjunction with uveitis; the toxicity of drugs used in treatment, in a chapter on drug side effects; and the retinal changes, under ocular vascular disease. This chapter will deal with scleritis and episcleritis and keratoconjunctivitis sicca.

Episcleritis and Scleritis

Inflammation of the collagenous shell of the eye is divided into superficial (*episcleritis*) and deep (*scleritis*). The transparent, avascular cornea is continuous with the opaque, vascular sclera and may be secondarily involved.

Episcleritis resembles a localized conjunctivitis. The inflammation is deeper, however, and the dilated vessels do not blanch with topically applied phenylephrine 2.5 per cent, as in a pure conjunctivitis. Episcleritis usually is self-limited (although it may be recurrent) and does not permanently damage the eye. Most episcleritis is idiopathic, but it may be encountered in rheumatoid arthritis, polyarteritis nodosa, Wegener's granulomatosis, systemic lupus erythematosus, dermatomyositis, progressive systemic sclerosis, and relapsing polychondritis.

Scleritis is more likely than episcleritis to accompany a systemic disease, although the list of associations is about the same for the two disorders. Any portion of the sclera may be affected. The differential is especially difficult with posterior scleritis, which may present as ocular pain or as an exudative retinal detachment. Anterior scleritis is often a prolonged, indolent inflammation with eventual permanent structural alteration of tissues. Pain, which may be severe, is often a prominent feature.

In the initial phase the inflammation is localized and may be nodular or diffuse. With prolonged inflammation, scleral thinning results in a localized bluish discoloration as the underlying choroid becomes visible. Scleral necrosis with perforation is possible; this is especially frequent in rheumatoid arthritis. The adjacent cornea may melt away.

Management of scleritis is difficult. Local steroid injections may predispose to perforation. Systemic corticosteroids and other antirheumatic drugs are useful in some patients. The ocular process often closely parallels the activity of the underlying disease, and the best approach to the patient is a systemic one.

Keratoconjunctivitis Sicca

Corneal inflammation as the result of drying is referred to as *keratoconjunctivitis sicca.* Keratoconjunctivitis sicca, a dry mouth (xerostomia), and a connective tissue disorder constitute *Sjögren's syndrome.* The underlying pathophysiology appears to be an autoimmune reaction in the lacrimal and salivary glands. Sjögren's syndrome is common in patients, especially middle-aged women, with rheumatoid arthritis. The possibility of a dry eye should be considered with complaints of burning, irritation, or excessive secretions. Unfortunately, these symptoms are notoriously nonspecific.

Diagnosis depends upon demonstration of tear hyposecretion (usually by decreased wetting of a strip of litmus or filter paper placed between the lower lid and the eye in the inferior cul-de-sac) and corneal and conjunctival epithelial damage. Once epithelial cells start to slough, the corneal surface will take up the vital dye fluorescein instilled into the conjunctival sac. Devitalized cells that have not yet been sloughed stain with rose bengal, making this dye even more sensitive than fluorescein as a test for keratitis sicca.

Treatment consists of tear replacement and reduction of tear turnover. Various preparations of artificial tears are available. All share the disadvantage that they must be instilled very frequently to be effective. Longer lasting ointments blur vision. Other therapeutic maneuvers include occlusion of the lacrimal puncta to reduce tear outflow and placement of contact lenses, moisture chambers, or goggles over the eyes to decrease evaporation. Such measures are reserved for severe keratitis.

Watson PG, Hazleman BC: The Sclera and Systemic Disorders. London, W. B. Saunders Company Ltd., 1976. *A monograph on the subject.*

549. OCULAR VASCULAR DISEASE

Systemic Hypertension and Arteriosclerosis

Despite widely held notions to the contrary, the retinal vascular abnormalities in hypertension are nonspecific and variable. They can, nonetheless, be important both diagnostically and therapeutically. The effects of blood pressure on the retinal vessels depend upon both its absolute level and its duration. Although essential hypertension is a disease of arterioles, the retinal vascular bed lacks sympathetic innervation, and the fundus changes must be considered secondary.

Arteriolar narrowing is both the commonest and the most difficult hypertensive change to differentiate as abnormal. The normal ratio of the diameters of the arteriolar and venous blood columns is 2:3 or 3:4. A decrease in this ratio can best be appreciated in the smaller branches away from the disc.

Other findings include microaneurysms, hemorrhages, lipid deposits, and edema. Retinal and disc edema usually follows a rapid increase in systemic blood pressure. Disc edema defines the entity *malignant hypertension.* By contrast, opacification (or sclerosis) of the vessel walls—described ophthalmoscopically as copper or silver wiring—occurs with longstanding hypertension.

Thickening of the arteriolar wall explains arteriovenous crossing changes—AV nicking and venous dilation distal to the crossing. Cotton-wool spots are signs of local ischemia; hemorrhages and hard exudates are signs of vascular leakage. Microaneurysms indicate irreversible structural alterations in the capillary beds. Vascular occlusions (see below) and ischemic optic neuropathy are potential consequences of hypertensive vascular changes.

Some classifications distinguish arteriosclerotic from hypertensive changes, but this division is difficult to justify clinically or pathophysiologically. The only pure arteriosclerotic change is atheroma of the retinal arterioles. This is seen as a yellow-white plaque in the central retinal artery or its first branches, where the arteries still have an internal elastic lamina. These plaques must be differentiated from calcific or lipid emboli, which are usually smaller or more peripheral. Hypertension accelerates atherosclerosis, but atherosclerosis does not require hypertension.

Diabetic Retinopathy

The retinal vessels react in a limited number of ways. Diabetic retinopathy shares many features with hypertensive retinopathy. Diabetes is simply the most common of the vascular retinopathies.

The pathophysiologic defect in diabetic retinopathy appears to be at the level of the retinal capillaries. Progressive degeneration of the cells of the capillary walls results in leakage, diffuse and focal expansion (microaneurysms), and closure of these small vessels. The ischemic retina in the focal areas of nonperfusion probably elaborates factors stimulating new vessel and fibrous ingrowth. (A retinopathy similar to that of diabetes is produced by radiation, usually radiotherapy given as part of the treatment for head and neck cancers. The radiation damages capillary cells.)

Diabetic retinopathy is classified as *background* or *proliferative.* Background retinopathy is further subdivided into *simple* background—with microaneurysms, dot/blot hemorrhages, and hard exudates—and a *preproliferative* form. In preproliferative background retinopathy there is beading of veins, cotton-wool spots, and many hemorrhages. Also characteristic is intraretinal new vessel pathology, so-called *intraretinal microvascular anomalies* (IRMA).

In proliferative retinopathy, neovascularization appears on the disc and elsewhere, especially along the major vascular arcades. There may be fibrovascular proliferation and vitreous hemorrhages. Proliferative diabetic retinopathy confers a poor visual prognosis.

Background retinopathy alone reduces visual acuity when there is edema or exudation in the macula. There are more new cases of blindness from background retinopathy with macular edema than from proliferative retinopathy, because backround retinopathy is so much more prevalent. The incidence of diabetic retinopathy increases with the duration of the disease. Background retinopathy with macular edema is common in adult-physiology diabetics over age 50.

Treatment

Good control appears to retard the progression of diabetic retinopathy. There is now proof that ablation of ischemic retina by panretinal photocoagulation helps preserve central vision in patients with early proliferative retinopathy, making this the current treatment of choice. Advanced proliferative retinopathy may require major intraocular surgery—*pars plana vitrectomy.* In such cases the visual prognosis is guarded even with intervention, but an estimated 50 to 75 per cent of operated patients experience some visual improvement.

Other Vascular Retinopathies

RETINOPATHY OF COLLAGEN VASCULAR DISEASE. Retinopathy in systemic lupus erythematosus is common but nonspecific. The most frequent findings are retinal hemorrhages and cotton-wool spots. Cotton-wool spots are localized areas of axoplasmic stasis caused by ischemia, which may indicate active vasculitis. Although occasionally referred to as "soft exudates," cotton-wool spots are not exudations. Patients with lupus often have hypertensive retinopathy (see above).

Central nervous system involvement in lupus may be associated with optic and chiasmal neuropathy, papilledema, ocular motor cranial nerve palsies, and hemianopias. A migraine-like syndrome is also a feature of CNS lupus.

RETINOPATHY OF HEMATOLOGIC DISEASE. Anemia and thrombocytopenia predispose to retinal and subconjunctival hemorrhages. When these are the result of leukemia, the hemorrhages often have a white center—the classic *Roth spot.* Roth spots are encountered in a number of situations, including septic embolism from subacute bacterial endocarditis, and are therefore nonspecific.

Leukemia is one cause of hyperviscosity retinopathy, characterized by venous tortuosity and dilation, retinal hemorrhages, and vascular occlusions. A chronically elevated leukocyte count also predisposes to capillary drop out and microaneurysm formation, but proliferative retinopathy is rare. Other causes of hyperviscosity retinopathy are Waldenström's macroglobulinemia, multiple myeloma, polycythemia, and sickle cell anemia. In extreme cases sludging of blood in the veins is visible ophthalmoscopically.

PERIPHERAL RETINAL NEOVASCULARIZATION. Diabetic retinopathy affects largely the posterior pole of the eye. The retinopathy of prematurity (retrolental fibroplasia) and sickle cell disease have their major impact on the peripheral retina. The etiology of the retinopathy of sickle cell disease is multiple occlusions of capillaries by abnormal blood constituents. In the retinopathy of prematurity, high levels of oxygen prevent the normal growth of vessels into the retinal periphery of the developing eye, resulting in an ischemic stimulus when ambient oxygen levels return to normal. High levels of oxygen are also directly toxic to vessels.

The ocular and systemic manifestations of sickling hemoglobinopathies correlate poorly. In patients with sickle cell anemia, proliferative retinopathy is rare. Peripheral neovascularization is more common in sickle cell hemoglobin C disease (SC) and sickle cell thalassemia (S-thal). Patients with sickle cell trait usually have no ocular symptoms, although hypoxia encountered at high altitudes may precipitate hemorrhages and vascular occlusions.

The ocular findings in sickle hemoglobinopathies include small, dark red, comma-shaped conjunctival vascular segments, best seen on the inferior bulbar conjunctiva after instillation of a topical vasoconstrictor. Ischemic infarction of iris segments is also observed. In addition to the "sea fan" peripheral neovascularization, other characteristic retinal findings include hemorrhages that have a salmon pink coloration from hemoglobin breakdown products—salmon patch hemorrhages—and black chorioretinal scars with irregular borders in the equatorial periphery—the black sunburst sign.

Treatment of Peripheral Neovascularization

About one fifth of proliferative sickle retinopathy regresses spontaneously. The rest, if untreated, will progress to retinal detachment and vitreous hemorrhage. Treatment consists of photocoagulation or transscleral cryotherapy or diathermy.

Retinal Vascular Occlusions

CENTRAL RETINAL ARTERY OCCLUSION (CRAO). The central retinal artery is a branch of the ophthalmic artery, in turn a branch of the internal carotid artery. Occlusion of the central retinal artery causes sudden, usually nearly complete, visual loss in one eye. Ophthalmoscopy reveals arteriolar narrowing and venous stasis (most obvious as segmentation of the venous blood column—"boxcar" pattern).

Within hours the fundus picture changes as the infarcted superficial layers of the retina lose their normal transparency to assume a milky-white translucency. Because the thin retina over the fovea receives its oxygen from the underlying choroid, this region retains its normal reddish-pink color. This contrasts with surrounding tissue, producing an appearance described as a cherry red macula. (A similar appearance is encountered in certain lipid storage diseases, where abnormal metabolic products partially opacify the ganglion cell layer.)

Eventually arterial flow is restored, the edema resolves, and the fundus appearance returns to near normal. The disc, which is initially normal because it derives its blood supply from the surrounding choroid, gradually becomes pale and atrophic. After several weeks it is difficult to distinguish a central retinal artery occlusion from other causes of optic atrophy.

Acute central retinal artery occlusion is an emergency. Prompt action may dislodge an embolus and restore circulation in time to prevent retinal death and to preserve vision. For a nonophthalmologist this action consists of firm, intermittent pressure on the globe. This ballotment alternately raises and lowers intraocular pressure. Ophthalmologists use other measures: retrobulbar injection of anesthetic and anterior chamber paracentesis to lower the pressure in the ocular vascular bed. Inhalation of a mixture of 95 per cent oxygen and 5 per cent carbon dioxide is recommended by some. Rarely does any treatment save vision.

In a number of eyes, portions of the retina are supplied by vessels arising from the choroidal circulation. Retina supplied by such cilioretinal arteries will be spared if the central retinal artery alone is occluded. In a few eyes, the island of spared retina encompasses the disc, macula, and intervening retina; visual acuity remains normal even in the presence of a CRAO. Most eyes with CRAO are deprived of useful vision.

CRAO's are the result of emboli (atheromatous, myxomatous, and material from diseased or artificial heart valves), of local small vessel disease, or of carotid occlusion. A CRAO is sometimes the initial sign of giant cell arteritis or polyarteritis nodosa. CRAO has been reported in patients with sickle cell trait after trauma or other stress.

BRANCH RETINAL ARTERY OCCLUSION (BRAO). Branch arterial occlusions present as sudden visual loss that leaves only a portion of the field affected. Ophthalmoscopically there is a wedge-shaped area of infarcted retina spreading outward from an arteriolar bifurcation.

In contrast to central retinal artery occlusions, branch retinal artery occlusions are almost always embolic in origin. By far the commonest source of emboli in older adults is the ipsilateral carotid artery. In children and young adults, migraine, coagulation abnormalities, increased intraocular pressure, and oral contraceptives may predispose to vascular occlusions.

CENTRAL RETINAL VEIN OCCLUSION (CRVO). The dramatic ophthalmoscopic findings of dilated, tortuous veins, extensive retinal hemorrhages, and disc swelling in one eye have classically been called a central retinal vein occlusion. Actually there is evidence that such *hemorrhagic retinopathy* is the consequence of both arterial ischemia and venous disease.

A CRVO presents as sudden unilateral visual loss in older adults, but unlike a CRAO, a CRVO is not an emergency, as there is no accepted immediate therapy. There are also no specific accompanying diseases, although hypertension and diabetes are loosely associated, and hypercoagulable states must be considered.

Visual prognosis varies. In the fully developed form usually encountered in older persons, vision is poor and generally remains so. Panretinal photocoagulation appears to decrease the risk of subsequent neovascular glaucoma. A less severe ophthalmoscopic picture is encountered in younger patients. Acuity in such *partial central retinal vein occlusion* or *venous stasis retinopathy* is only slightly reduced, and the visual prognosis is good. Ischemic oculopathy after carotid occlusion produces a similar retinopathy; retinal arterial pressures measured by ophthalmodynamometry or ocluopneumoplethysmography will be low in such cases.

BRANCH RETINAL VEIN OCCLUSIONS. Patients with branch vein occlusions complain of blurred vision. In the fundus, hemorrhages and cotton-wool spots spread out in a wedge from an arteriovenous crossing. As in CRVO, there are few specific systemic associations. Neovascular glaucoma is rare, but vision may be persistently reduced by macular edema. Branch retinal vein occlusion must be distinguished from viral retinitis.

Asdourian GK: Peripheral retinal neovascularization—differential diagnosis. *In* Peyman GA, Sanders DR, Goldberg MF (eds.): Principles and Practice of Ophthalmology. Philadelphia, W. B. Saunders Company, 1980, pp 1277–1298. *A clear review of clinical manifestations and pathogenesis.*

Brown GC, Magorgal LE, Shields JA, et al.: Retinal arterial obstruction in children and young adults. Ophthalmology 88:18, 1981. *A report of 27 cases of BRAO or CRAO in patients under 30 years of age.*

Gold D, Feiner L, Henkind P: Retinal arterial occlusive disease in systemic lupus erythematosus. Arch Ophthalmol 95:1580, 1977. *A discussion of the retinal findings.*

Kearns TP: Differential diagnosis of central retinal vein obstruction. Ophthalmology 90:475, 1983. *This paper is one of four in the same issue that describes the work-up, differential, and management of CRVO.*

Lessell S: The neuro-ophthalmology of systemic lupus erythematosus. Docum Ophthalmol 47:13, 1979. *This paper is hard to find but well worth the effort. The most complete review of the ocular manifestations other than retinopathy.*

Little HL, Jack RL, Patz A, Forsham PH: Diabetic Retinopathy. New York, Thieme-Stratton Inc., 1983. *A collection of 31 position papers on various aspects of diabetic retinopathy.*

550. THE EYE AND MEDICATIONS

Drugs with Ocular Side Effects

ANTICHOLINERGICS. A variety of systemic drugs have ocular side effects. Any medication with anticholinergic properties can dilate the pupil and diminish accommodation (the ability to focus at close range). The possibility of angle-closure is the basis for the caution that such medications are contraindicated in glaucoma. Patients on therapy for open-angle glaucoma are at little risk, as mydriasis will not usually affect intraocular pressure. If the patient has known angle-closure, previous iris surgery all but eliminates the danger of dilation. Only when there is a potential for angle-closure are such drugs contraindicated, and this is usually unrecognized. Of the systemic anticholergic drugs, transdermal scopolamine alone can dilate and fix pupils and paralyze accommodation even in young persons.

CORTICOSTEROIDS. Systemically administered corticosteroids are cataractogenic. Prolonged administration of high dosages of corticosteroids often leads to the formation of posterior subcapsular cataracts. Topical corticosteroids increase intraocular pressure in genetically predisposed persons. Topical steroids also activate *Herpesvirus* keratitis and should be administered only under the supervision of an ophthalmologist.

QUININE AND CHLOROQUINE. Quinine—used for malaria and muscle cramps, as an abortifactant, and to dilute street heroin—may cause acute blindness, with narrowing of the retinal arterioles. An overdose increases the probability of toxic effects, but rare persons are sensitive even to therapeutic doses. The symptoms of quinine toxicity include dizziness, tinnitus, and hearing loss. Central vision may improve, with persistent constriction of peripheral field and evolution of optic atrophy.

The synthetic antimalarials chloroquine and hydroxychloroquine, used for the treatment of systemic lupus erythematosus and rheumatoid arthritis, have a specific retinal toxicity. This usually appears only after prolonged administration of the drugs in doses exceeding 250 mg per day for chloroquine and 400 mg per day for hydroxychloroquine. Reduced visual acuity is the usual initial symptom, but the parafoveal retina is most affected. The chloroquine binds to pigmented tissues, exerting a toxic effect on the retinal pigment epithelium with loss of pigmentation in a target-like or bull's eye pattern around the fovea. Discontinuation of the drug may result in improvement, but if the process is moderately advanced, visual loss may be progressive.

Chloroquine and hydroxychloroquine also cause whorl-like corneal epithelial deposits, which reduce acuity and produce halos around lights. Such deposits bear no direct relationship to the retinal toxicity and disappear after discontinuation of the drug.

THIORIDAZINE. Phenothiazines are potentially toxic to retina and retinal pigment epithelium, producing a coarse pigmentary degeneration. Of those now in common use, only thioridazine has clinically significant toxicity, and then only with dosages exceeding 1 gram per day for prolonged periods.

ETHAMBUTOL. Various drugs have been implicated in optic neuropathies. Only with ethambutol is the incidence of such side effects high enough that monitoring is considered mandatory. The physician administering ethambutol should perform monthly checks of acuity and color vision, especially when dosages exceed 15 mg per kilogram.

Oculocutaneous Disorders

A variety of related disorders (including erythema multiforme, Stevens-Johnson syndrome, and toxic epidermal necrolysis, or Lyell's syndrome) arise as idiosyncratic responses to drugs or infections. Their ocular manifestations are a bullous conjunctival eruption followed by a cicatricial conjunctivitis. Adhesions, called symblepharons, may obliterate the conjunctival sacs. The alterations in conjunctival architecture prevent the normal production and distribution of tears. A severe dry eye may be the most disabling sequela of these disorders.

Early treatment with topical steroids (and perhaps antibiotics to prevent secondary infection) is sometimes effective in limiting damage. Sweeping the conjunctival fornices several times a day with a sterile glass rod inhibits symblepharon formation.

Systemic Side Effects of Topical Ocular Medications

Medications in solution are easily absorbed from the nasal mucosa, and systemic side effects are more likely with drops than ointments. Dilation of the pupil with 10 per cent phenylephrine solution has been known to precipitate severe hypertension, especially in infants and the elderly. Topical epinephrine increases ventricular extrasystoles in some patients. Timolol maleate causes bronchospasm in asthmatics.

Topical anticholinergics such as atropine, scopolamine, and cyclopentolate may contribute to confusional states in the elderly. Cyclopentolate is occasionally a cause of acute hallucinations and even psychosis in the young. Pilocarpine, used in large doses in the treatment of acute angle-closure glaucoma, has resulted in cholinergic overdose—nausea, vomiting, salivation, and gastrointestinal cramps. As these are also symptoms of the angle-closure attack itself, such toxicity may not be immediately recognized, leading to continued administration and cardiovascular collapse.

Echothiophate iodide, an organophosphate used in the treatment of some forms of childhood strabismus and of open-angle glaucoma, predisposes to cholinergic crisis, mimicking an acute surgical abdomen. Also, patients receiving echothiophate have impaired metabolism of succinylcholine. Use of succinylcholine during the induction of general anesthesia in a patient receiving echothiophate has caused death.

Carbonic Anhydrase Inhibitors

Acetazolamide and methazolamide inhibit aqueous production and are used systemically to reduce intraocular pressure when topical medications are inadequate. Most patients experience paresthesias; their absence is thought by some to indicate noncompliance. Carbonic anhydrase inhibitors also induce a systemic acidosis, with a syndrome of malaise and anorexia, depression, and weight loss that responds to concurrent administration of sodium bicarbonate. Acetazolamide increases the incidence of urolithiasis. The combination of a carbonic anhydrase inhibitor and a thiazide diuretic depletes body potassium. Carbonic anhydrase inhibitors should not be given to people with known allergy to sulfonamides.

Adler AG, McElwain GE, Merli GJ, Martin JH: Systemic effects of eye drops. Arch Intern Med 142:2293, 1982. *A brief review that serves as a cautionary tale.*

Fraunfelder FT, Meyer SM: Drug-Induced Side Effects and Drug Interactions. 2nd ed. Philadelphia, Lea & Febiger, 1982. *A compendium based on a collection of reports of side effects.*

Grant WM: Toxicology of the Eye. 2nd ed. Springfield, Charles C Thomas, 1974. *An enormous review with component parts that are still coherent and readable.*

Part XXV
SKIN DISEASES

Marie-Louise Johnson

551. INTRODUCTION

The skin is our interface with the world, and more. It is the glassine bag through which physiologic and chemical changes are perceived; the self-substance that is invaded and traumatized from within and without; an organ that responds and repairs, that shares the burdens of growing up and growing old, of environmental insults, and of systemic disease.

As an organ system it is unique. It stretches before the examiner patently obvious with significant data waiting to be read. The student attuned to palpating and auscultating forgets to look. He misses basic physiologic facts about his patient, perhaps significant signals of serious disease. Further, when the patient draws attention to a skin change, the student is uncertain as to what it may be or its importance. If the patient is sufficiently persistent, or the examiner sufficiently compulsive, a consultation can be obtained, usually with dispatch during medical school and house staff training. But later, when the examiner is removed from the medical center and the logistics and economics of the consultation must be reckoned, decisions are made on shaky foundations. The risk of ignoring the mortal and promoting morbidity is increased as much as is the cost of care through unnecessary referral. Such decisions are not infrequent; some 30 per cent of Americans have a dermatologic problem that should be seen by a physician; further, 52 per cent of all problems related to the skin present to internists, pediatricians, and generalists.

This is not to say that every practicing physician needs to be a dermatologist. It does suggest that every doctor involved in patient care should be comfortable recognizing and treating *common* skin problems, ten of which constitute 76 per cent of the burden of skin disease as established by population survey (Table 551–1).

Part XXV reviews pathophysiologic mechanisms that will prepare the observer for an informed assessment of the skin. Once there is confidence in identifying the morbid processes observed, the facts can be interpreted and the diagnosis elaborated. Without awaiting a confirmed impression, however, the patient can be made more comfortable; thus Ch. 554 will emphasize principles of therapy as well as precautions and proscriptions. Finally, the more common dermatologic conditions will be reviewed, as well as those that have implications for systemic illness, and those which in their management utilize medications and modalities of therapy uncommon to other disciplines. Our aim is to ensure an ease of recognition and management for the common dermatoses; to provide a useful guide to the identification and assessment of cutaneous signs of systemic disease; and, finally, to sharpen suspicion and enhance understanding of the risk and challenge of the more significant dermatologic diagnoses as judged by morbidity and mortality. In no way are the following chapters an attempt to substitute for a text in dermatology; hence frequent reference will be made to the literature, especially to selected texts and review articles, where the reader can further his knowledge.

TABLE 551–1. PREVALENCE OF COMMON DERMATOLOGIC DISEASE IN THE UNITED STATES*

	Rate per 1000	Numbers (in 1000's)
Fungus infections	81.1	15,733
Tinea pedis	38.7	7509
Tinea unguium	21.8	4232
Tinea versicolor	8.4	1623
Tinea cruris	6.7	1301
Acne vulgaris	68.1	13,217
Cystic acne	1.9	375
Acne scars	1.7	321
Seborrheic dermatitis	28.2	5476
Verruca vulgaris	8.5	1684
Folliculitis	8.0	1553
Atopic dermatitis	6.9	1332
Lichen simplex chronicus	4.5	882
Hand eczema	1.6	311
Dyshidrotic eczema	2.1	405
Psoriasis	5.5	1070
Vitiligo	4.9	957
Herpes simplex	4.2	824

*Persons 1 to 74 years of age—noninstitutionalized.

Johnson ML, Roberts J: Skin conditions and related need for medical care among persons 1–74 years, United States 1971–1974. Vital and Health Statistics Series II, No 212 (1979). *Because this study had by direct examination gathered data on a large and representative sampling of the noninstitutionalized American population, it provides the most extensive and reliable source for information about the prevalence and morbidity of dermatologic problems.*

Stern RS, Johnson ML, DeLozier J: Utilization of physician services for dermatologic complaints. Arch Dermatol 113:1062, 1977. *A good look at who goes where for dermatologic services based on national survey data.*

General Dermatology Reference Texts

Braverman IM: Skin Signs of Systemic Disease. 2nd ed. Philadelphia, W. B. Saunders Company, 1981. *An excellent review of cutaneous signs that should evoke from the internist or generalist concern of systemic disease.*

Fitzpatrick TB, Eisen AZ, Wolff K, Freedberg IM, Austen KF (eds.): Dermatology in General Medicine. 2nd ed. New York, McGraw-Hill Book Company, 1979. *A solid, readable, complete text with great strength in pigmentation.*

Fitzpatrick TB, Eisen AZ, Wolff K, Freedberg IM, Austen KF (eds.): Dermatology in general medicine. Update. New York, McGraw-Hill Book Company, 1983. *An expansion and "tidying up" of the text of the same title.*

Moschella SL, Pillsbury DM, Hurley HJ Jr: Dermatology, 2 vols. Philadelphia, W. B. Saunders Company, 1975. *A detailed text with historical insights and helpful treatment advice.*

Rook A, Wilkinson DS, Ebling FG: Textbook of Dermatology, 2 vols. 3rd ed. Oxford, Blackwell Scientific Publications, 1979. *With the greatest detail and finest prose, the Rook book is quite "compleat."*

552. PATHOPHYSIOLOGY

The skin is an essential organ. Deprived of significant amounts, as by burn and trauma, we cannot survive. Excessive losses of fluid and electrolytes are difficult to replace, and without the natural barrier to organisms infection is hard to contain.

But the disruptions of the integument are not always so gross. To understand challenges that have targeted effects, to interpret disease processes that show characteristic anatomic change or deposits of immune proteins at selected sites, some detailed information about the structure and function of the skin is required.

ANATOMIC CONSIDERATIONS

The living envelope which enfolds us contributes 16 per cent or so to the body weight of the average adult. It is composed of two mutually dependent layers of distinct developmental origin: the outer *epidermis* from the ectoderm and the inner *dermis* from the mesoderm, both cushioned on the fat-containing subcutaneous tissue, the *panniculus adiposus* (Fig. 522–1). Mesenchymal structures such as collagen, blood vessels, and fat originate from the mesoderm.

The stratified cellular epidermis is derived by a division of a basal layer of cells which forms successive sheets moving outward as keratinocytes synthesizing the insoluble protein keratin. From the *stratum germinativum* the columnar basal cell resting on a basement membrane generates, by mitosis, daughter cells, one or both of which progress to the surface, becoming more polyhedral as they go; still nucleate, they are bound at the tufts called desmosomes, to which are fixed cytoplasmic filaments constituting by their quill-like appearance the *stratum spinosum* (Fig. 552–2). In the course of 14 days the matured daughter cell will have flattened from a polyhedral form to a pancake, acquiring keratohyaline granules that in the aggregate

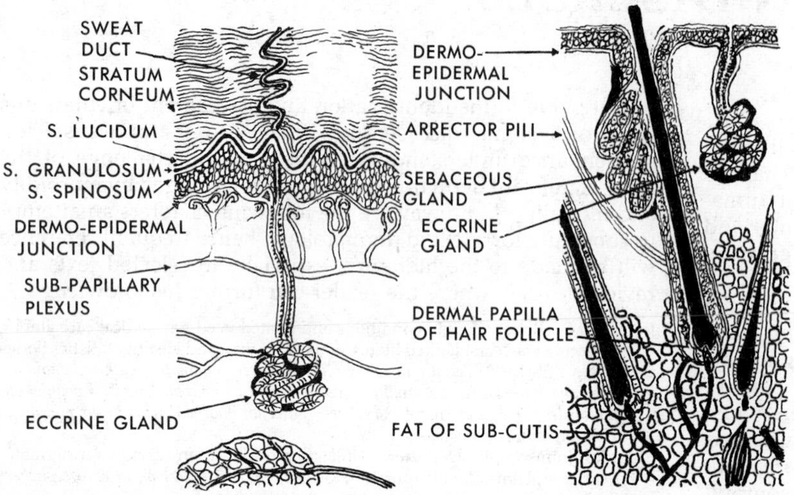

Figure 552–1. Structure of the skin.

suggest the label *stratum granulosum.* Eventually it will lose its nucleus to become part of the *stratum corneum.* In another 14 days, by wear and programmed replacement from beneath, it will be shed completely; this slough of skin is continuous and imperceptible in the normal individual, with a turnover time of four weeks from basal cell to extinction. Anatomically there is some variation. The stratum corneum has its greatest thickness on the palms and soles, for example, and in these areas epidermal turnover is prolonged.

The differentiation of the migratory epidermal cells involves the formation of one or more fibrous proteins known collectively as keratin. The process, complete in the stratum corneum, yields mature keratin, a system of filaments embedded in a continuous matrix within a thickened cell membrane. As the stratum corneum, keratin serves as a rate-limiting membrane affecting the passage of ions and molecules. It is the protective layer against harmful chemicals; it also admits selected substances, including topical allergens as well as topical therapy. It freely admits water, up to four times its weight, and it freely yields water to the environment as insensible perspiration. Transport across the membrane is enhanced by increased temperature, by the lipid solubility of the solute, and by increased hydration of the stratum corneum itself.

Pathologic processes that disorder the differentiation of epidermal cells toward keratin may manifest themselves as blocking the transport of insensible water, the admission of topical therapy, or even the clinical appearance of casings or scale, be it retained or overproduced keratin. Further, in the loss of the spinous adherence of cells at desmosomes, the intercellular spaces trap fluid to the consequent development of blisters.

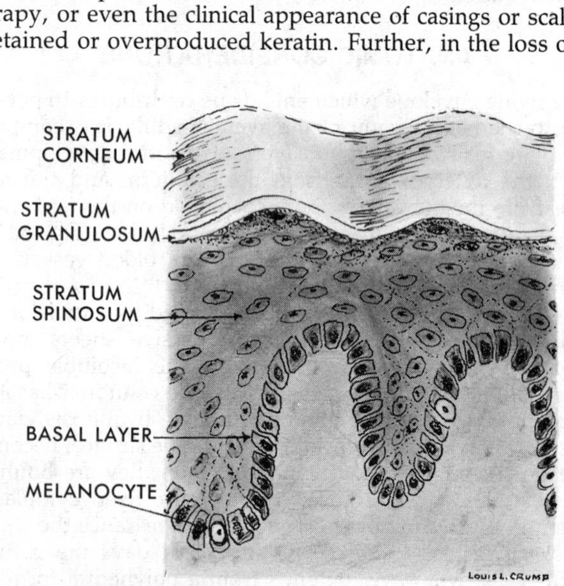

Figure 552–2. The stratified cellular epidermis.

Although the pathogenesis may vary, the disrupted cell is the keratinocyte—that general name for the epidermal cell derived from the basal layer. In the epidermis, however, there are also *melanocytes* which originate in the neural crest of the embryo and retain migratory capabilities in the adult. They transfer pigment to the epidermal cells through their dendritic processes. Malfunction can mean absence of pigment or pigment production to the extreme, both potential cosmetic disasters. Also present in the epidermis are Langerhans' cells, of long recognition, of debated origin and function, and of recent focus for their suspected role in contact dermatitis and delayed hypersensitivity. As dendritic nonkeratinocytes, probably originating from the mesenchyme, Langerhans' cells are found in the basal and suprabasal layers of the epidermis, and at times in the dermis. They can also be seen in stratified squamous epithelia as of the buccal and vaginal mucosa, and rather ubiquitously in lymph nodes, thymus, spleen, and other organs. Immunocompetent cells involved in the uptake and processing of antigenic material, they are the receptors for the initial cutaneous response to external antigens.

Beneath the epidermis is the principal mass of skin, the dermis, a mixture of fibrous protein and collagen embedded in mucopolysaccharide along with water, elastic fibers, nerves, blood vessels, lymph channels, glands, appendages, and a few cells, largely fibroblasts, mast cells, and histiocytes. Actually eccrine sweat glands and the pilosebaceous apparatus, although dermal in location, are of ectodermal origin and formed from embryonic invaginations into the mesoderm. Because the stratum corneum covers only the most superficial part, transport through these structures is more rapid. Undoubtedly the pilosebaceous and sweat glands contribute heavily to the transport of molecular substances through the skin.

MECHANICAL CONSIDERATIONS

The mechanical properties of skin are important from the standpoint of toughness and resistance to forces of disruption, to shearing, but also as they relate to wound healing, to the aging process, or to inherited disorders in which structural elements are defective. Strength and flexibility are significant attributes, and the extracellular components of the dermis are important contributors. *Collagen* fibers, for example, give high tensile strength, and their loose mesh permits the mobility of joints. The return of collagen to the unstressed state depends on the elastic restoring forces of *elastin.* In old age the degradation of the elastic fiber network leaves the collagen mesh without the support to restore fully its original configuration, and wrinkled skin is the surface evidence. The ground substance, which is less well understood, through its viscous and elastic properties, resists compression and accepts molding, thus serving to reduce point pressure on more sensitive skin structures.

PHYSIOLOGIC CONSIDERATIONS

The skin cannot survive without oxygen and nutrients. Although the prime provider role of blood vessels is dramatically underscored in its disruption, as with gangrenous toes and stubborn leg ulcers, the skin compared to other organs is low in metabolic requirements. Like the kidney, its blood flow is far in excess of nutritional need, and its vascular system is adapted to mechanisms that meet other demands such as the regulation of body heat. In normal and warm environments blood flow is greater in the digits and other acral skin areas, achieved in part through the arteriovenous shunt of the glomus body, a dermal vessel peculiar to the acral areas. At normal environmental temperatures and low work levels, dermal blood flow is the only thermoregulatory mechanism required to maintain a constant body temperature. Increase in the metabolic rate of the body will increase skin blood flow. Posterior hypothalamic centers in the brain control dermal blood flow through deep vasoconstrictor mechanisms of the sympathetic nervous system.

Apart from nutrition and thermal regulation, dermal blood vessels participate in the inflammatory response and demonstrate recognizable pathologic changes in specific diseases. Reacting to a noxious stimulus, transient vasoconstriction will be followed by dilatation with a ten-fold increase in blood flow, an increase in vessel permeability, and a consequent escape of fluid into the interstitial space. There is a relaxing of precapillary sphincters which become refractory to vasoconstrictor stimuli, and finally, initiation of the cellular response. With certain traumatic stimuli to normal skin in disease states, the dermal response may be a vascular proliferation or constriction, or even development of the complete lesion of the disease, the isomorphic response as seen in collagen diseases, psoriasis, and lichen planus.

SWEAT GLANDS

Eccrine

The thermoregulatory mechanism depends significantly on the eccrine sweat gland, which produces and transports to the skin surface a hypotonic solution for evaporation and cooling. Given sufficient thermal stimulation, an individual through his 2 to 3 million sweat glands can produce 2 to 3 liters of sweat per hour for a short interval. Each gland is a simple tubule with a coiled secretory segment deep in the dermis and a straight duct extending up to become spiraled terminally before it pierces the stratum corneum. It is well supplied with blood vessels, and, in its secretory part, with unmyelinated nerve endings, anatomically sympathetic but functionally parasympathetic.

Lesions develop with anatomic blockage of the sweat duct. A rupture in the mid-dermis nearer the secretory part stimulates little dermal response, although the trapped sweat may be visible in the skin. Like a deep millet seed, it is called descriptively *miliaria profunda.* Rupture more distally near the papillary plexus ensures proximity to blood vessels and nerve endings, which provokes redness and itching because of reactive dilatation of the capillaries and stimulation of the *c* fibers of the nerves. Clinically it is known as *miliaria rubra* or, more commonly, *prickly heat.* Inability of sweat to escape at the surface leaves a superficial drop of sweat with few symptoms, scattered dew drops in transparent casings; it is important only to be recognized for what it is—*miliaria crystallina.* In all physiologic entrapments of sweat the therapy is to reduce the activity of the gland, remove blockage at the duct orifice, and counteract the local irritant effects of escaped intradermal sweat. Cooling will reduce the need to sweat; mild keratolytics such as 1 per cent salicylic acid in alcohol will free the eccrine sweat pores of retained keratin and lipid, and anti-inflammatory agents such as topical steroids will reduce erythema and pruritus.

Sweat is formed not by passive filtration but by active metabolic processes, with lactate produced in the secretory segment and sodium resorbed in the ductal segment. Sweat appearing on the skin is usually lower in sodium and chloride and higher in lactate than interstitial fluid from which it is derived. The maximal capacity to resorb sodium is only one quarter the capacity to secrete. Hence at times of profuse sweating, significant amounts of sodium can be lost. True adaptation can be seen with repeated intense thermal stress, leading to a conservation of sodium through a mechanism that may involve increased adrenal aldosterone secretion and enhanced reabsorption in the ductal segment.

An increase in body heat arouses temperature-sensitive centers in the hypothalamus and serves as a potent stimulus for generalized sweating. Pyrogens raise the hypothalamic temperature threshold for inducing sweating, and fever is the consequence, the heat produced through shivering if the ambient temperature is low. When the receptor function returns to normal levels and body temperature is then perceived as too high, profuse sweating ensues.

The palms and soles have large eccrine sweat gland populations. Although they respond poorly to thermal stimulation, they do respond immediately and profusely to psychogenic stimuli. Palmar sweat as an index of emotional stress is used in the polygraph or lie-detector test.

The physical aspects of heat loss and retention have their obvious dramatic roles in the desert and polar regions, but they also have an important and certainly more extensive role in prophylactic skin care and management of dermal pathology. Heat may be lost or gained relative to environmental temperature by radiation, conduction, or convection. Ordinary metabolic heat from organs and muscle is transported by the blood to the skin, where it is lost through radiation and convection by adjustments in cutaneous circulation effecting perhaps small changes in skin surface temperature. The balance is maintained readily and without sweat. With excessive metabolic heat the regulated blood flow through skin is accelerated; the increased vascular surface area permits heat to be lost to the lower ambient temperature of the air, to colder solid or liquid surfaces as to rocks or lake water, and through the evaporation of water or sweat from the skin.

At rest in a 35° C, windy dry environment, an elevated body temperature will lose heat not by radiation or convection but through evaporation calculated as 150 grams of sweat per hour to remain stable. With exercise and consequent increase in metabolic heat, and with an extreme environmental temperature to 46° C, 830 grams of sweat per hour would be needed for stabilization. In a hot humid environment with evaporation restricted, profuse sweat drips rather than evaporating and the heat load is difficult to dissipate, with risk of severe hyperthermia, dehydration, and sodium depletion, which may be followed by collapse, failure of the eccrine apparatus, and fatal heat stroke; the victim's skin is flushed, warm, and dry. In hot environments it is vital to replace salt and water losses continuously and to promote cooling by evaporation with air currents, nonrestrictive clothing, and cool water immersion.

The conservation of body heat, less dramatic physiologically, is a more common phenomenon, since there is greater risk to life from unexpected or prolonged exposure to cold. Survival in water of 0° C unprotected is no more than 30 minutes. Actually one primary physiologic defense to cold, to shut down the cutaneous circulation, thus increasing the distance heat must be conducted to be lost at the surface, is inadequate for most environmental cold. We rely heavily on shelter and clothing. In pathologic conditions with inflammation, body heat loss can be impressive even with common protection at average temperatures, and the comfort of patients is compromised by their constant sense of chill. It is recognizing heat loss as it manifests the pathologic process and modifies the therapeutic management that is most important for our consideration in dermatology.

The Pilosebaceous-Apocrine Apparatus

The hair unit, including sebaceous and apocrine glands, develops in utero over the entire skin surface except the palms and soles. One would never see a furuncle, for example, an abscess of a hair follicle, on the palm, sole, or glans penis, unless the patient had had a skin graft from a hairy site. Before birth the apocrine portion of the hair-gland apparatus atrophies in most complexes, but persists as a full pilosebaceous-apocrine apparatus in the axillae and genital area, occasionally at the areolae of the breast, and about the umbilicus. The breast is actually a modified apocrine gland, as are the ceruminous glands of the ear and Moll's glands of the eyelid. At puberty apocrine glands enlarge to produce an oily, colorless substance, which remains odorless until bacterial decomposition results in a characteristic body odor. Individuals vary in the intensity of odor related to apocrine gland size and personal hygiene. Short chain fatty acids and ammonia are the major odorogenic products of bacterial degradation, but other unidentified substances in the sweat or on the skin could contribute to individual variations in the malodorous emanations.

A rare individual may have colored apocrine sweat, apocrine chromhidrosis, which can be axillary or exceptionally facial or, even more rarely, of the scalp, according to where vestigial apocrine glands are functional. Apart from concern and the need for reassurance, the nuisance of stained underclothing is a common complaint in those with axillary chromhidrosis. Most frequently yellow, the pigment can be green, blue, or blue-black and is attributed to one or more lipofuscins produced, for reasons unknown, within the apocrine gland. The staining must be distinguished from that resulting from surface pigments of corynebacteria or piedra, which thrive in the axilla and lend their pigment to colorless sweat after it leaves the sweat duct. The latter staining can be controlled with shaving and topical antimicrobial agents; true chromhidrosis cannot. Patients with ochronosis may stain axillary secretions or skin brown but have homogentisic acid in the urine.

As with eccrine sweat, apocrine secretions can be plugged, disrupting the duct, breaking into the dermis, and triggering intense pruritus with erythema. The problem, often provoked by emotional stimuli to apocrine excretion through adrenergic sympathetic discharge, is really an apocrine miliaria and is known as *Fox-Fordyce disease.* Usually involving the axillae, often the genital area, and occasionally the periareolar glands, the trapped apocrine sweat raises small discrete rounded lesions with a consequent relative apocrine anhidrosis. Therapy of variable success is aimed at reducing stimuli to apocrine sweating, limiting maceration from eccrine sweat, and counteracting the inflammatory response with topical and injectable steroids.

As distressing and persistent as apocrine miliaria may be, the severe disease of apocrine glands is the chronic, suppurative, and cicatricial problem known as *hidradenitis suppurativa.* It may involve the axillae exclusively, as it often does in women, or the anogenital area, or both; in some affected individuals it is associated with severe scarring acne, occasionally with cicatrizing perifolliculitis of the scalp, or a pilonidal cyst. Although an isolated axillary or inguinal lesion might be mistaken for an abscess, multiple lesions or recurrences, especially an associated acne or scalp problem, should suggest the diagnosis. Once made, vigorous antimicrobial therapy with topical preparations and systemic antibiotics is indicated to reduce smoldering infection and minimize sinus tract formation. Early surgery may reduce the number of glands at risk and abort a potentially devastating disease (Fig. 552–3).

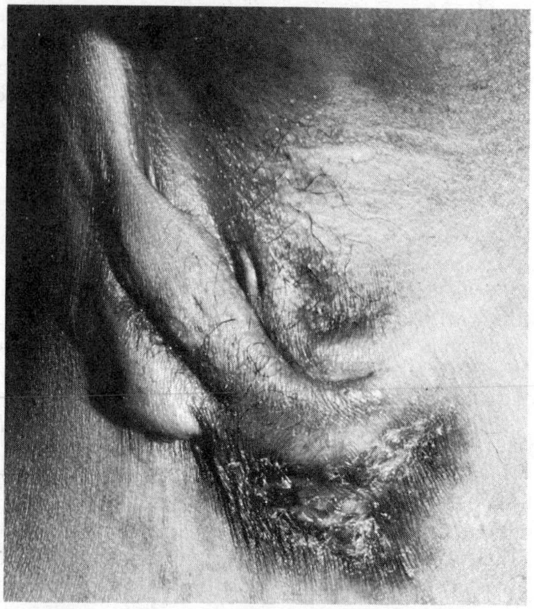

Figure 552–3. Hidradenitis suppurativa, axilla.

The *sebaceous gland* specialized for lipid synthesis is widely distributed over the body but concentrated in the scalp, face, upper back, and chest. Each hair follicle is associated with sebaceous glands, but the converse is not true. Some sebaceous glands without associated hairs open directly onto the surface and are known as sebaceous follicles; others, by reason of anatomic localization and modification, are singled out for special identification. In the buccal mucosa and at the vermilion border of the lip, for example, they are known as Fordyce's spots; around the female areola, as Montgomery's tubercles; at the prepuce, as Tyson's glands; and on the eyelids, as meibomian glands. As sebaceous glands they share in the pathophysiologic mechanisms to be considered; as normal anatomic structures they should not be confused with skin pathology.

The sebaceous gland depends upon and is extremely receptive to androgenic hormones. Maternal androgens ensure full development and function at birth. The vernix caseosa covering the neonate is mostly sebum. Normally the gland then atrophies until the child's pubertal hormones stimulate it once more. Sebaceous gland activity in children can result from congenital adrenal hyperplasia or anabolic hormone therapy as given in aplastic anemia. Disorders of androgen excess in adult women are associated with increased sebaceous gland activity. Androgen insufficiency in either sex such as hypogonadism or adrenal insufficiency is associated with decreased activity. Androgens increase the sebaceous gland size, increase the secretion of sebum, and increase sebaceous gland mitotic rate. Estrogens decrease gland size and secretion but do not decrease the mitotic rate. Their effect may be from the suppression of androgens primarily at sites of androgen synthesis rather than at the glandular level. In women, adrenal androgens in addition to gonadal androgens are a source of sebaceous stimulation. Progesterone in physiologic amounts has no effect, and the role of the pituitary is most likely indirect through tropic hormones. With severe caloric deprivation sebum secretion levels decrease.

The function of sebaceous gland lipid is in question. Although variously touted as a barrier to microbes or other hostile environment, as a regulator of percutaneous absorption, and as a vitamin D precursor, all these roles have been challenged. Further, skin conditions characterized by dry skin, such as ichthyosis or asteatosis, are allegedly associated with decreased sebum production, but without supporting data.

What is known is that sebaceous gland maturation, which begins at age eight to ten and continues through adolescence, remains fairly unchanged through adult life until it decreases some time past the fifth decade in women and the seventh decade in men. Patients with Parkinson's disease and postmenopausal women with breast cancer have statistically higher rates of sebum secretion than the average. Because the distribution of sebum levels overlaps with normal values, an individual reading has limited diagnostic importance.

The final portion of the pilosebaceous apparatus to be considered is the hair, and any understanding of hair implies some knowledge of its *growth cycle* and *pattern*. *Hair growth* can be reckoned in three phases: *telogen* when it is resting in its cornified sac, *anagen* when it is actively growing, and *catagen* when it is involuting. Throughout telogen, the resting hair is high in the follicle at the level of the arrector pili muscle, a stubby hair bulb resembling a club, and is inactive mitotically. When anagen begins, there is a burst of mitosis and downward growth. The newly formed hair shaft dislodges the old resting hair bulb, the club hair. With a hand lens a fallen or plucked hair can be determined from root inspection as having been resting or actively growing. Catagen is the brief respite when mitosis ceases and the hair pulls upward in the dermis and hair shaft to become a club hair. In the adult most hairs, 85 per cent, are in anagen at any given time, 14 per cent in telogen, and 1 per cent in catagen.

Hair growth cycles vary with *hair type*, of which there are several in humans. Vellus hair is fine, soft, short, nonpigmented, and common to "nonhairy" areas of the body. Its anagen phase is short and telogen long. A terminal hair is coarse, long, pigmented, and located in "hairy" areas—scalp, beard, eyebrow, eyelash, axilla, and pubes. The ratio of the duration of anagen to telogen in terminal hairs varies. It is short and equal for eyebrows, but for scalp hair anagen is long, two to six years, and telogen short, about three months. Hair length depends upon duration of active growth compared to that of resting.

Acute disease, high fever, and gross metabolic illness can all markedly affect the hair cycle. Classic postfebrile hair loss tends to be diffuse, with the loss first noted two to three months after the fever. The suggested mechanism is that the altered physiologic state stuns the actively growing follicles into a resting state. Following the ordinary physiologic pattern, the hair rests for three months, then is shed at the time new growth begins, a phenomenon called *telogen effluvium*. Excessive hair fall may continue over a month or more. Stress as from anesthesia, normal delivery, or psychic shock may do the same. Malabsorption or the serious malnutrition of kwashiorkor often has an associated severe hair loss. Debilitated chronically ill patients may lose hair, too, but more often they merely note change in texture. Depletion of dietary protein, anemia, and iron deficiency can be correlated with damaged hair shafts, suggesting insults insufficient to trigger the resting phase but enough to deform the hair. Complete disruption can follow more severe deprivation.

Interference with essential amino acid incorporation, as suggested for the effect of thallium ingestion, leads to a fracture of the hair shaft within the follicle. Once used for depilation in the therapy of scalp fungus, hair shedding occurs about one week after treatment. In an unsuspected (or intended) ingestion of rat poison containing thallium, hair loss should be anticipated, a so-called *anagen effluvium*, since the fall occurs during the active phase of the follicle cycle. Similar alopecias are seen with the antimitotic agents used in chemotherapy. Hair fall following exposure to X-irradiation occurs at a dose of no more than 300 R because of the exquisite sensitivity of the germinal layers of the hair follicle. Only growing hairs are affected; hence scalp and beard where most hairs are in anagen show the greatest fall, which occurs spontaneously in two weeks and regrows in two to three months. Permanent epilation depends on dose; 1200 R or so is usually required for permanent destruction of the hair follicles of the scalp. The damage can be dose related, for if mitosis is merely impaired, not halted, the hair shaft may not be disrupted but merely narrowed, as with methotrexate therapy for psoriasis or colchicine for gout. Heparin and coumarin, although they, too, show some mitotic inhibition, have their full effect through shunting anagen follicles into telogen until occasionally as many as half the follicles are at rest. At two to three months after the initiation of anticoagulant therapy, hair will fall; the cosmetic significance of the alopecia will depend upon the original density of hair growth and the percentage of follicles in telogen.

In many instances hair loss may be anticipated or its cause immediately identified. Even with the sparse or absent scalp hair of congenital ectodermal defects, the diagnosis is apparent from the history, perhaps reinforced by pedigree, and the physician feels no compulsion to justify the defect. With alopecia areata, however, there is a difference. Of obscure etiology, it is a problem of increased incidence in patients with autoimmune disease, Addison's disease, diabetes mellitus, or vitiligo. It commonly presents as one or two small circumscribed bald areas, usually of the scalp, which may not progress but in some few patients will increase in size, coalesce, and extend until all scalp hair is lost (alopecia totalis) or all body hair (alopecia universalis). Exclamation point hairs, 3 mm or so in length and tapered toward the skin surface, are diagnostic if present. As hair regrows it may, at first, be devoid of pigment; even the alopecic skin itself may share in the pigment loss. Most patients with alopecia areata will do well; four out of five will get full regrowth of hair. Initially the course is unpredictable but deserves guarded optimism. However, when the alopecia is extensive, recurs, is associated with nail dystrophy, or lasts more than a year, the prognosis for recovery is not good.

In the instances of hair loss cited thus far, the scalp, on inspection, appears as normal skin devoid of some or all hair. There is no scarring. When inflammatory and infiltrative diseases affect the scalp so as to produce hair loss, the basic lesion is grossly evident. The hair is lost because of the pathologic process disrupting and perhaps destroying the hair follicle. This is true even with traction alopecia when the pull of hair styles or the self-plucking of hairs, consciously or unconsciously as in trichotillomania, leads to the permanent damage of the hair follicles and occasionally their destruction.

As to *growth pattern*, the hair follicles common to both sexes that produce the same type of hair in pre- and postpubertal individuals are not hormone dependent. Others, common to both sexes, are androgen dependent, such as the conversion of vellus to terminal hair in the axillae, the lower pubic triangle, and the temporal area of the scalp. In males responding to higher concentration of androgens there is a conversion from vellus to terminal hair in the follicles of the beard, ears, nasal tip, sternum, and upper pubic triangle. At the same time on a genetic basis some terminal hair may change to vellus in the vertex and frontal regions of the scalp, with slow recession of the anterior hair line to produce male pattern baldness. Similar pattern loss occurs in women but rarely progresses to the total bare crown seen in men. In both, hereditary factors influence the time of onset, pattern, and severity, with androgen playing an undisputed role. Castration interrupts pattern baldness in males, and masculinizing diseases of women produce baldness subject to genetic predisposition.

Hypertrichosis and Hirsutism

Excessive hair growth may be genetically determined, as in a nevus, or from repeated local trauma, as with weights carried on the shoulders. It may be generalized and appear after encephalitis or with the onset of multiple sclerosis. It is seen in dermatomyositis and is induced by drugs such as phenytoin. Although the reason for the increased hair may be obscure, an association can be made with a genetic determinant or recognized problem.

Hirsutism, however, a term used mainly for the excessive growth of coarse terminal hair occurring in women in the adult male distribution, is more of a diagnostic challenge. In most, the hair growth is idiopathic without underlying pathology. Genetic and racial differences are considerable, and their recognition may help differentiate a familial problem from an underlying masculinizing process. If there is no menstrual abnormality, no male pattern balding, no increase in muscle mass or deepening of the voice, and a normal pelvic examination, the problem should probably not be pursued further. On the other hand, diffuse vellus hairs occurring suddenly over the face of women past 40 should arouse suspicion of underlying malignancy.

Aging and Actinic Damage

With age, the epidermis thins and the skin appendages atrophy. Hair becomes sparse and sebaceous secretions decrease, with consequent susceptibility to dryness, chapping, and fissuring. The dermis diminishes with loss of elastic and collagen fibers—hence loss of elasticity and support for dermal vessels easily visualized and readily ruptured (senile purpura).

Sunlight exposure wreaks far greater destruction on the skin than time itself, however, as the contrast between covered and exposed skin clearly shows, even in the skin of the elderly. It intensifies and augments the aging process. Sun-damaged skin is thin, wrinkled, and variably hyperpigmented with fine thread-like telangiectatic vessels and small erythematous scaling patches of actinic keratoses. Yellow papules in a reticulated pattern may occur on the nose and forehead. Comedones and follicular cysts appear in the periorbital region. The back of the neck becomes thickened. Histologically collagen is replaced by amorphous or granular material of slightly basophilic stain on hematoxylin and eosin preparation. Called elastotic, it gives its name to the clinical observation of thinning and sagging, senile elastosis.

553. THE EXAMINATION OF THE SKIN

The traditional approach to the medical patient is to elicit the chief complaint and elaborate the history before seeking supportive clinical findings. The dermatologist on the contrary looks first, with an eye trained to see and recognize, his hand lens being more important than his stethoscope. He has the advantages of concurrent review—the history of the present illness often being written for him in the skin—markers of genetic predisposition, and even something of the patient's physiologic age and exposure to the elements and to actinic radiation. It is all there: the ectoderm and the mesoderm; the blood vessels and the nerves; the collagen, the elastin, the ground substance. It is there and sharing, perhaps, in an inflammatory, metabolic, or even neoplastic change that is widespread in the body but comes to focus first in the skin. Dermatology is a visual specialty, and its excitement derives from the direct and patent entry into general medicine that the skin provides, and from the clarity with which pathologic processes can be assessed and followed. It is a showcase for reaction patterns and for responses to therapy.

For the examination of the skin, to see *what* is there and *all* that is there is the only cardinal rule. Good lighting is essential. Nonglaring north light is best for both lesion configuration and true color, but a mix of fluorescent bulbs to simulate daylight is acceptable. It can never be too bright, but the capability of side lighting in a darkened room is also useful for detecting minimally raised and depressed lesions.

The skin should be observed from head to toe in a routine repetitive way so that no orifice or appendage is overlooked. For the writer, the horizontal patient completely disrobed and covered with a sheet is easiest to examine in a systematic way. In the *supine* position the frontal scalp is examined first, then the face, with special attention to the eyes (conjunctiva, iris and pupil, eyelids), followed by the ears, nose, lips, mouth (observing mucosa and dentition), pharynx, neck, thorax, abdomen, genital area, anterior legs, and then the fingernails, forearms, and arms, anterior and posterior. With the patient changed to the *prone* position and the knees flexed, the feet, toenails, and webs can be examined easily, next the posterior aspect of the legs, the perianal and sacral area, the back, lower and upper, nuchal area, and then the full scalp to complete the round. By uncovering only limited areas of the body at a time the patient is mostly covered and comfortable throughout the examination. If the presenting complaint has been only a finger wart, the surprised patient is usually reassured that his integument has been assessed for present or potential pathology and good preventive medicine has been practiced.

After having surveyed the entire skin surface, *generalized observation* warrants first notation. A blue man with argyria, the result of silver deposits in sweat glands and elastic fibers, may present with a fungus infection. Although the pigmentation may be untreatable and permanent, it nonetheless is an important part of his dermatologic assessment. So, too, is the *pattern of a problem.* Skin change following a dermatome distribution is significant. At a distance a segmental color change over the thorax might suggest a diagnostic differential between herpes zoster and nevus, but on close inspection viral vesicles would resolve the diagnosis. The limitation of the specific viral lesions to a dermatome makes the presumptive diagnosis. It underscores the importance of the pattern of appearance—important for description and the diagnostic process, as well as for the record for others to interpret.

The examiner, then, must be aware of the whole skin and the pattern of the problem before focusing on specific lesions. He will have noted signs of aging, trauma, pigment response, general turgor, nutrition, and hygiene. He will attempt to assess the pathology he notes with reference to configuration and anatomic location. Distribution may follow innervation, as in the dermatome, or vascular patterns, as in the reticulated changes in mottled skin of chilled swimmers, cutis marmorata. The pathology may be localized or generalized, perhaps universal, involving the entire integument, including hair and nails. Most important, the examiner will try to assess what physical change has occurred in the skin. Is it flushed or blanched? If red, is it the hot bright red of infection or the cool blue red of a connective tissue disorder? He will attempt to make a microscopic judgment and decide whether the skin surface is normal or thickened, raised or flat, infiltrated with cells and at what level, filled with fluid, filled with pus, freely movable, bound down, atrophic, excoriated, or ulcerated.

Often the consultation request proffers dermatologic terms that bear no relation to the lesion described. It is far better to call an urticarial lesion a hive, or a lesion resembling a mosquito bite, than to define it as an erythematous papule, which is interpreted differently by the indoctrinated. Terms are useful in descriptive interchange, but if they defeat the honest analysis of the pathophysiologic process, their value is lost.

Despite this conviction, it is necessary to provide some guide to the description of pathologic changes in skin (Fig. 553–1). A defined lesion that leaves the epidermis and dermis unchanged except in color is a *macule.* Stroking the lesion and adjacent normal skin with eyes closed resolves any doubt; the macule cannot be distinguished. If the surface is raised in a circumscribed way by an infiltrate of cells or change in anatomic thickness, the lesion is a *papule* and should be further described as rounded or flat-topped, perhaps as angular, smooth, or verrucuous (the roughness of a wart), and by color. If penetration of the process into the dermis gives greater substance and depth, the lesion is *nodular* rather than papular. Either may be a sac for entrapped cellular debris and secretions, a *cyst,* suspected by the palpation of a soft center.

For wheals or hives, edema in the upper dermis produces raised rounded or plateau-like evanescent lesions known as *urticaria,* which, according to size, may be ordinary or giant. Trapped fluid in the skin produces a *vesicle* if the blister is less than 0.5 cm, a *bulla* if larger. The anatomic level of the fluid and its cellular content will affect translucency and stability. Significant vesicles may be so numerous as to become confluent and indistinguishable as vesicles, presenting instead as a weeping denuded area. Superficial bullae also rupture easily and in the mouth are rarely seen intact. Ones that occur more deeply, such as friction blisters, can persist, and some may be so overlayered with skin that it is difficult to distinguish them from a papule. When the fluid-filled sac contains abundant neutrophils, with or without bacteria, it is considered a *pustule*. If it occurs anatomically related to a pilosebaceous apparatus, it is a follicular pustule, usually conical, and with a protruding hair.

When skin is abnormal and raised over a relatively large but circumscribed area, the term *plaque* is used. If the skin surface is denuded, it may just be a superficial *erosion;* if the defect penetrates into the dermis, it is an *ulcer*. Coagulated blood elements can provide a *crust* for such lesions. When the deeper ones heal, there will be scar, pink and vascularized at first, then *atrophic,* i.e., white and avascular. Healing could occur with an exuberant pink raised hypertrophic scar that subsequently flattens or perhaps persists as a fibrous, rubbery cicatrix, a *keloid*. Even without recognized injury the skin may become depressed, with the normal skin markings and appendages diminished or effaced. Such *atrophy* can be part of a pathologic process or may result from such topical therapy as steroids.

In contrast to atrophic change, the skin in certain conditions may be thickened with accentuation of the normal epidermal pattern, as is caused by rubbing, *lichenification;* or the thickness may be from *scale,* flaking keratin, that may be loose or adherent, thick as an oyster shell (ostraceous), or fine as cigarette paper; scale may be dry or greasy and slough in a localized desquamation or generalized exfoliation.

Finally, the descriptive process will reflect pigment, its presence or absence, and the vascular changes that affect skin color,

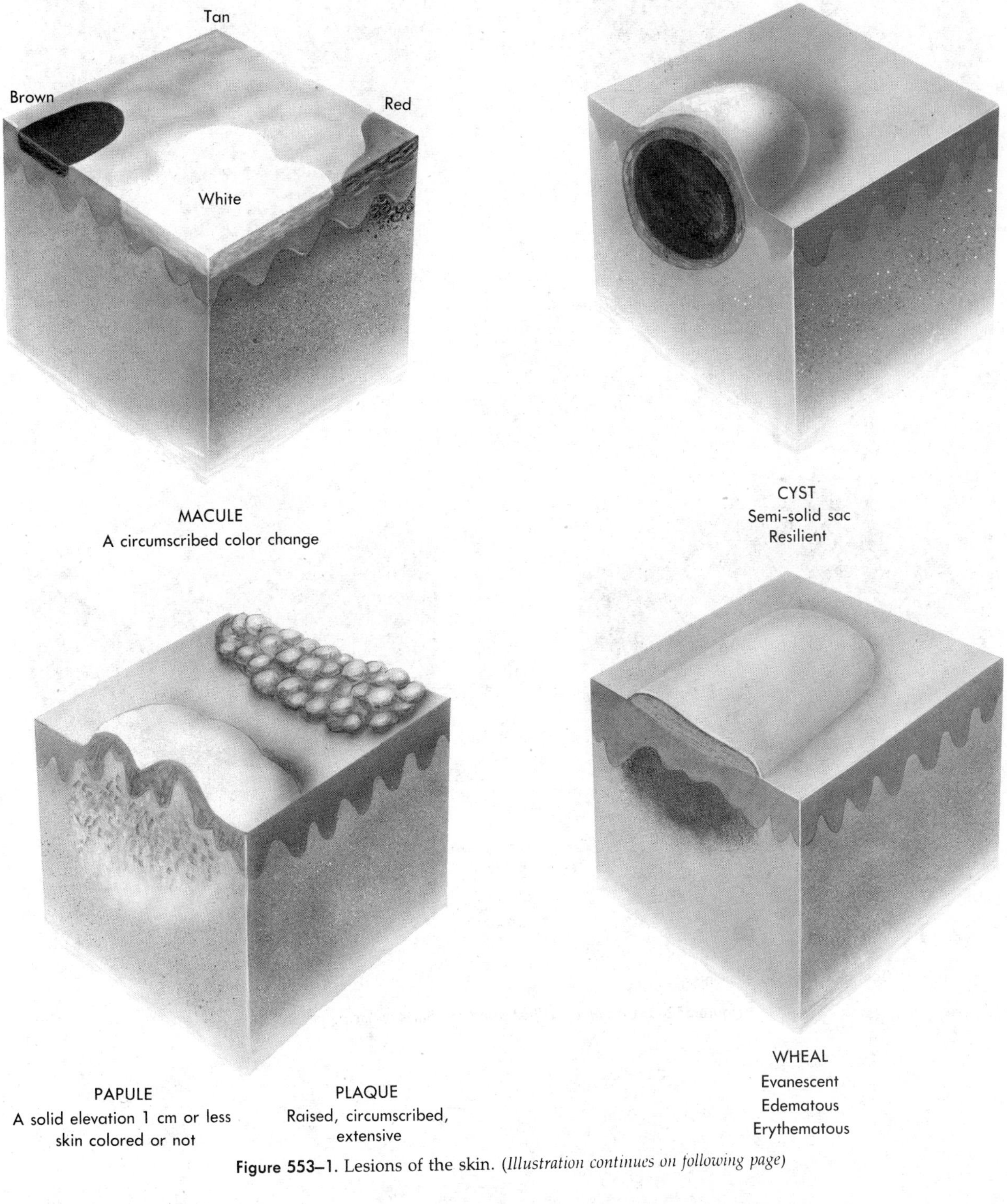

Figure 553–1. Lesions of the skin. *(Illustration continues on following page)*

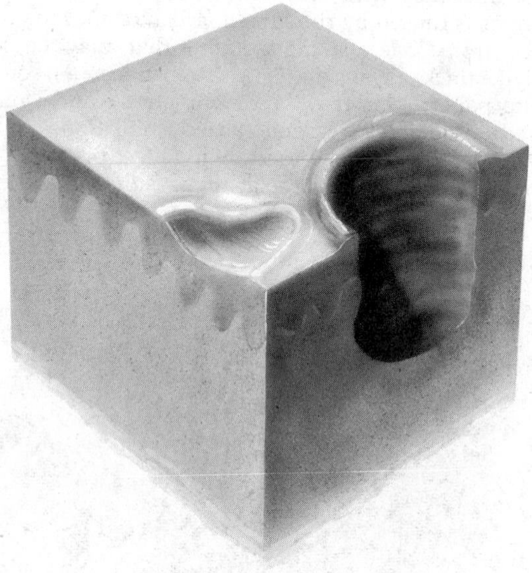

EROSION
Superficial denudation

ULCER
Defect penetrates dermis

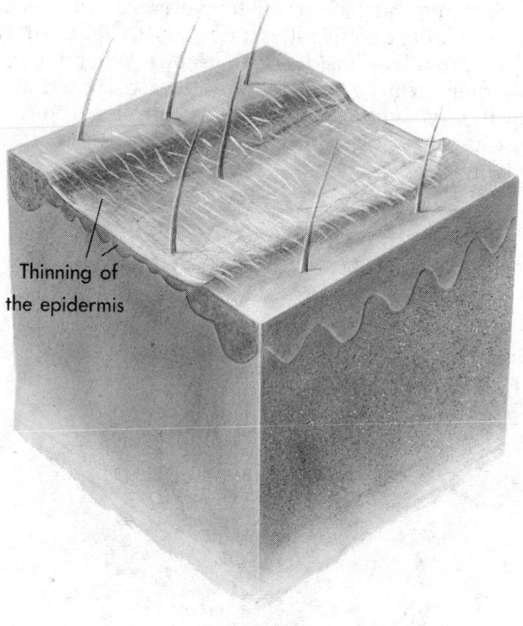

ATROPHY

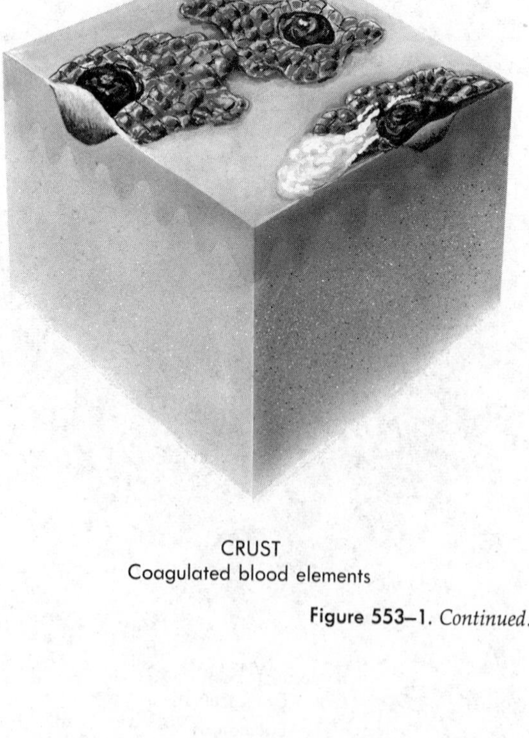

CRUST
Coagulated blood elements

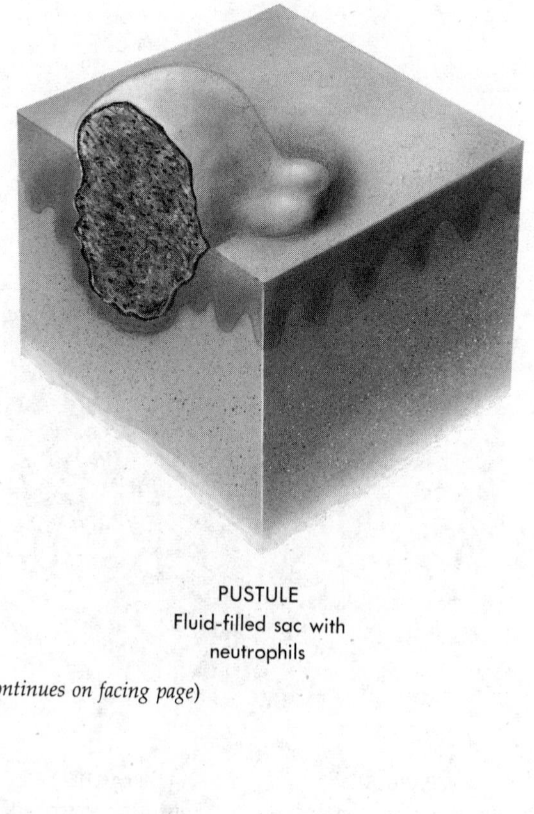

PUSTULE
Fluid-filled sac with
neutrophils

Figure 553–1. *Continued. (Illustration continues on facing page)*

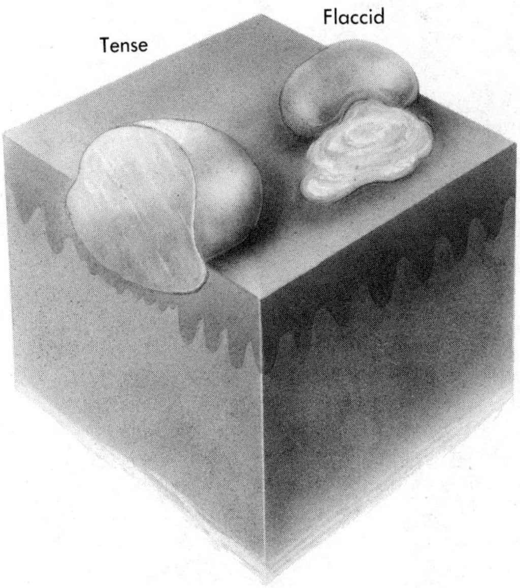

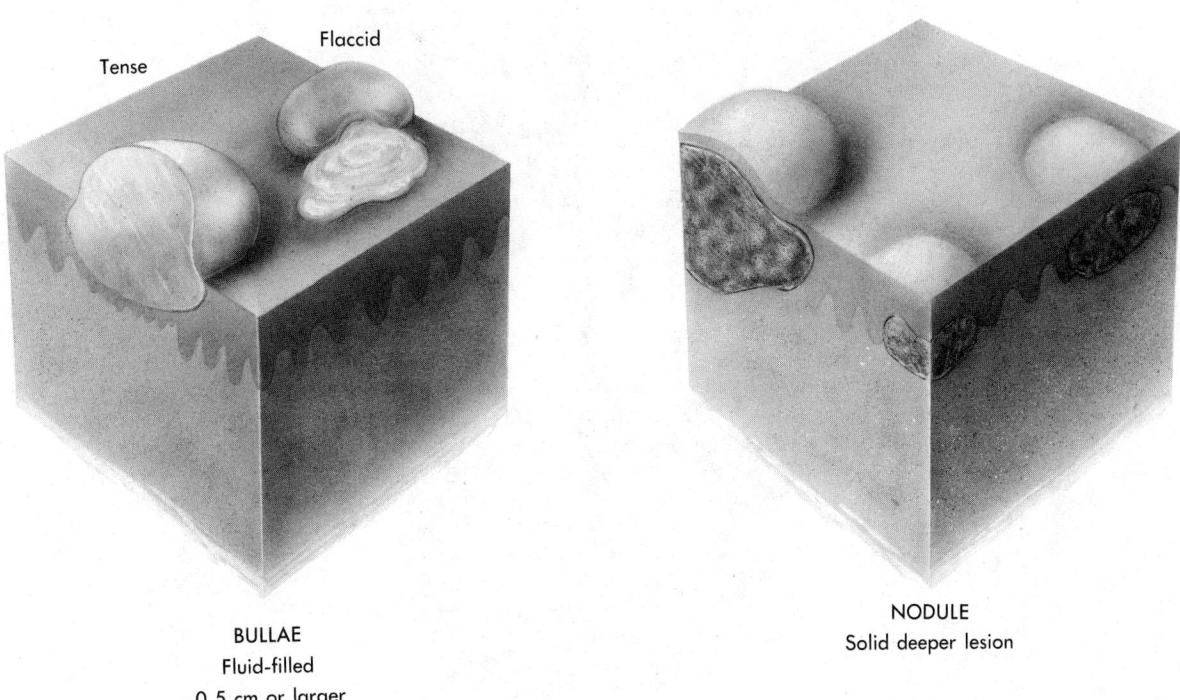

BULLAE
Fluid-filled
0.5 cm or larger

NODULE
Solid deeper lesion

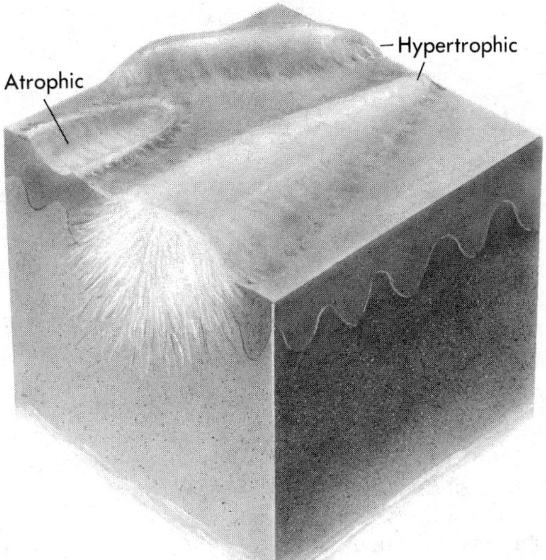

SCAR

Figure 553–1. *Continued. (Illustration continues on following page)*

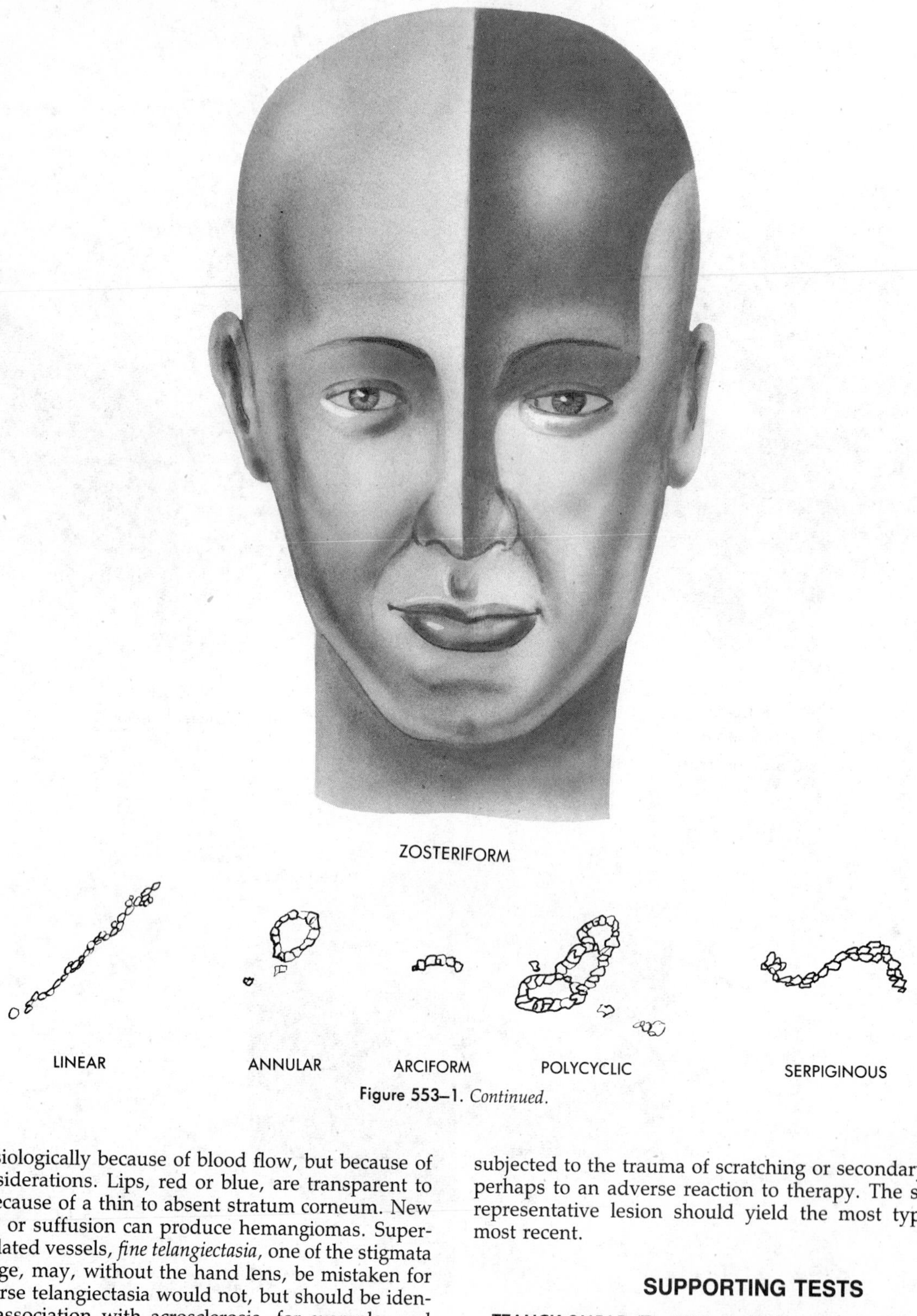

Figure 553–1. *Continued.*

not only physiologically because of blood flow, but because of anatomic considerations. Lips, red or blue, are transparent to blood color because of a thin to absent stratum corneum. New vessel growth or suffusion can produce hemangiomas. Superficial wispy dilated vessels, *fine telangiectasia*, one of the stigmata of solar damage, may, without the hand lens, be mistaken for erythema; coarse telangiectasia would not, but should be identified for its association with acrosclerosis, for example, and roentgen damage where it is found with atrophy and pigmentary change. The trick is to see what is present in the skin without prejudice and to tabulate the data without premature interpretation.

With the distribution of lesions noted and their pattern of arrangement determined, whether in a dermatome (zosteriform) or linear (/), annular (○), arciform (∩), polycyclic (∞), or serpiginous (~), the individual lesion can be assessed according to the broad description given. The eye may detect different kinds of lesions which in fact may be the same at different stages of development, or a primary lesion that has been subjected to the trauma of scratching or secondary infection or perhaps to an adverse reaction to therapy. The search for the representative lesion should yield the most typical and the most recent.

SUPPORTING TESTS

TZANCK SMEAR (Fig. 553–2). If the primary lesion is a vesicle or bulla, a rapid cytologic examination known as the Tzanck test can be helpful. The vesicle or bulla is unroofed with a sterile scissors and the base curetted lightly with the blunt side of a scalpel. A smear is made and stained with Wright's or Giemsa's stain to reveal the multinucleated epidermal giant cells of a viral infection or the rounded acantholytic cells devoid of their intercellular bridges, a phenomenon present in certain blistering diseases and in viral vesicles as well, but not in friction blisters or burns or in the vesicles of contact dermatitis.

THE KOH TEST AND CULTURE. Should the primary problem be a circumscribed scaling dermatitis of the sort that suggests a

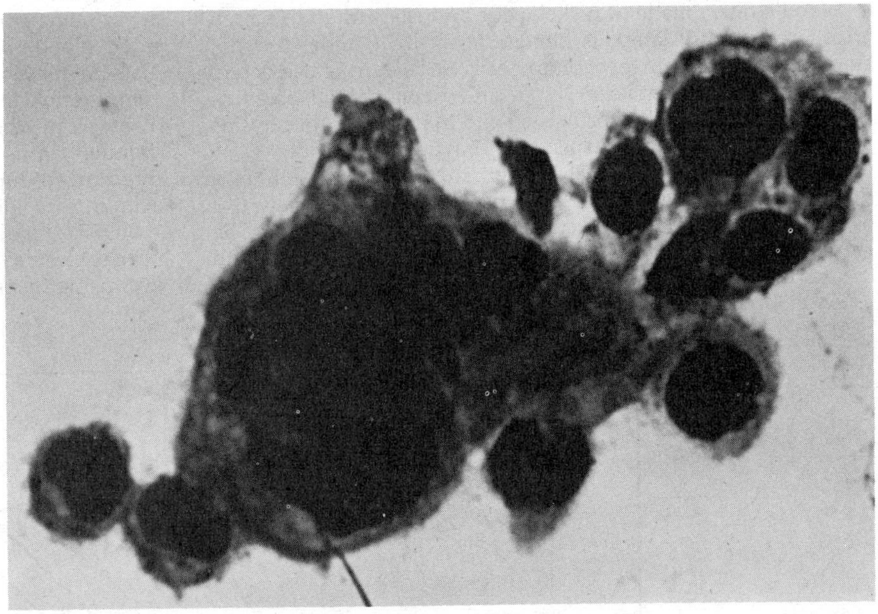

Figure 553–2. Positive Tzanck smear, herpes simplex.

diagnosis of fungus, a very simple examination for the presence of mycelia should be done. After heating a sample of scale with 10 per cent potassium hydroxide to dissolve the keratin (and a drop of methylene blue to improve visualization), fungal elements, if present, can be observed by direct microscopic examination (Fig. 553–3). The scale should be cultured in Sabouraud's medium to establish the identity of the fungus involved. If repeated attempts to visualize hyphae and grow fungus are negative, the diagnosis of mycotic infection is certainly in question.

WOOD'S LIGHT. Examination under long wave ultraviolet light will be helpful in detecting hair and skin infected with fungi that fluoresce at 360 nm; it is important for diagnosis and for plucking infected hairs for culture.

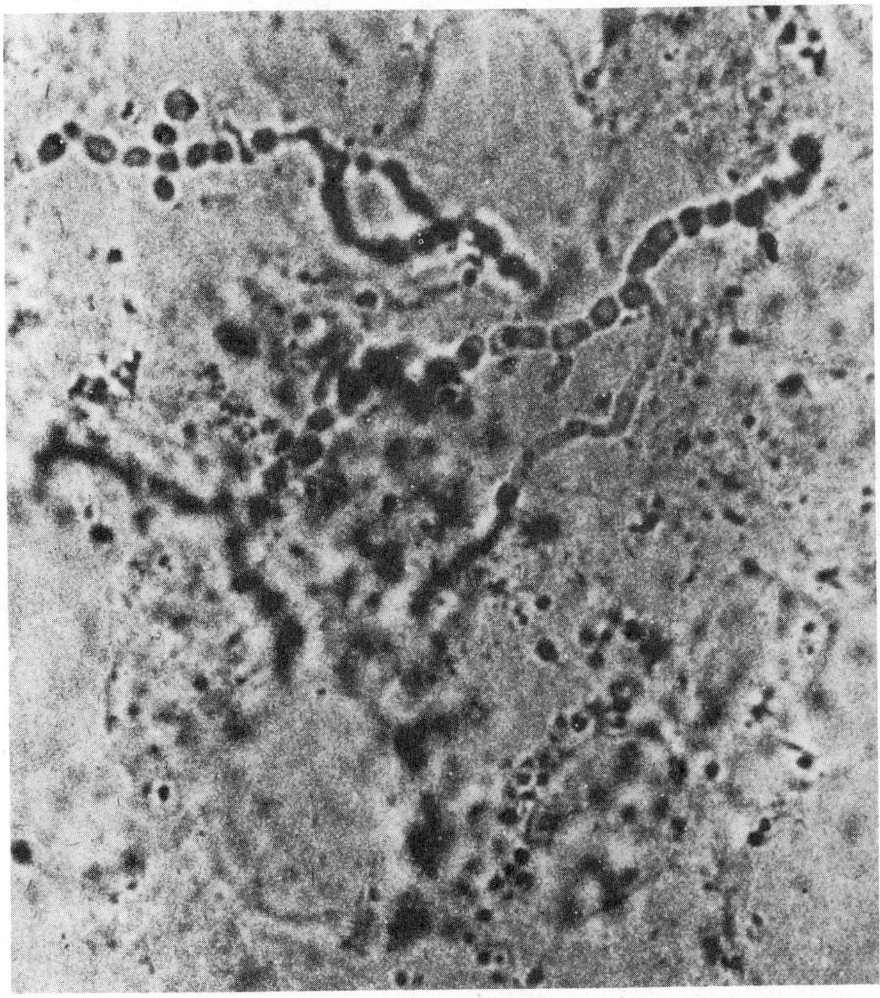

Figure 553–3. KOH preparation, high power.

Wood's filter, made of nickel oxide and silica fitted to a high pressure mercury lamp, is opaque to all light under 320 nm and above 400 nm. Inspection under Wood's light is also useful in differentiating between hypo- and depigmented areas of skin, an important diagnostic clue, and in detecting porphyrins in the urine of patients suspected of having porphyria.

BACTERIOLOGIC CULTURES. When the primary lesion is a pustule, bacteriologic cultures should be taken, especially if it is suspected that a micrococcus may be the etiologic agent. The nephritogenic strains of the *Streptococcus* are associated with glomerulonephritis, and certain strains of *Staphylococcus pyogenes* as well as the *Streptococcus* can produce a severe infection with bright erythema and extensive desquamation.

DIASCOPY. If it is unclear whether the redness of a macule is erythema from dilated capillaries or the purpura of extravasated blood, observation under firm pressure through clear glass or plastic will reveal the difference. The purpura is not compressible to pallor. Pressure with a glass slide is also useful in detecting the "apple jelly" glassy fawn-colored papules of granulomatous disease such as occur in the mycobacterial infections of lupus vulgaris and swimming pool granuloma, or even in sarcoidosis and lymphoma.

BIOPSY. Of all that may be done to aid the assessment of the primary lesion, the very best is to re-examine it with the clinical eye, using magnification greater than the hand lens, and to see

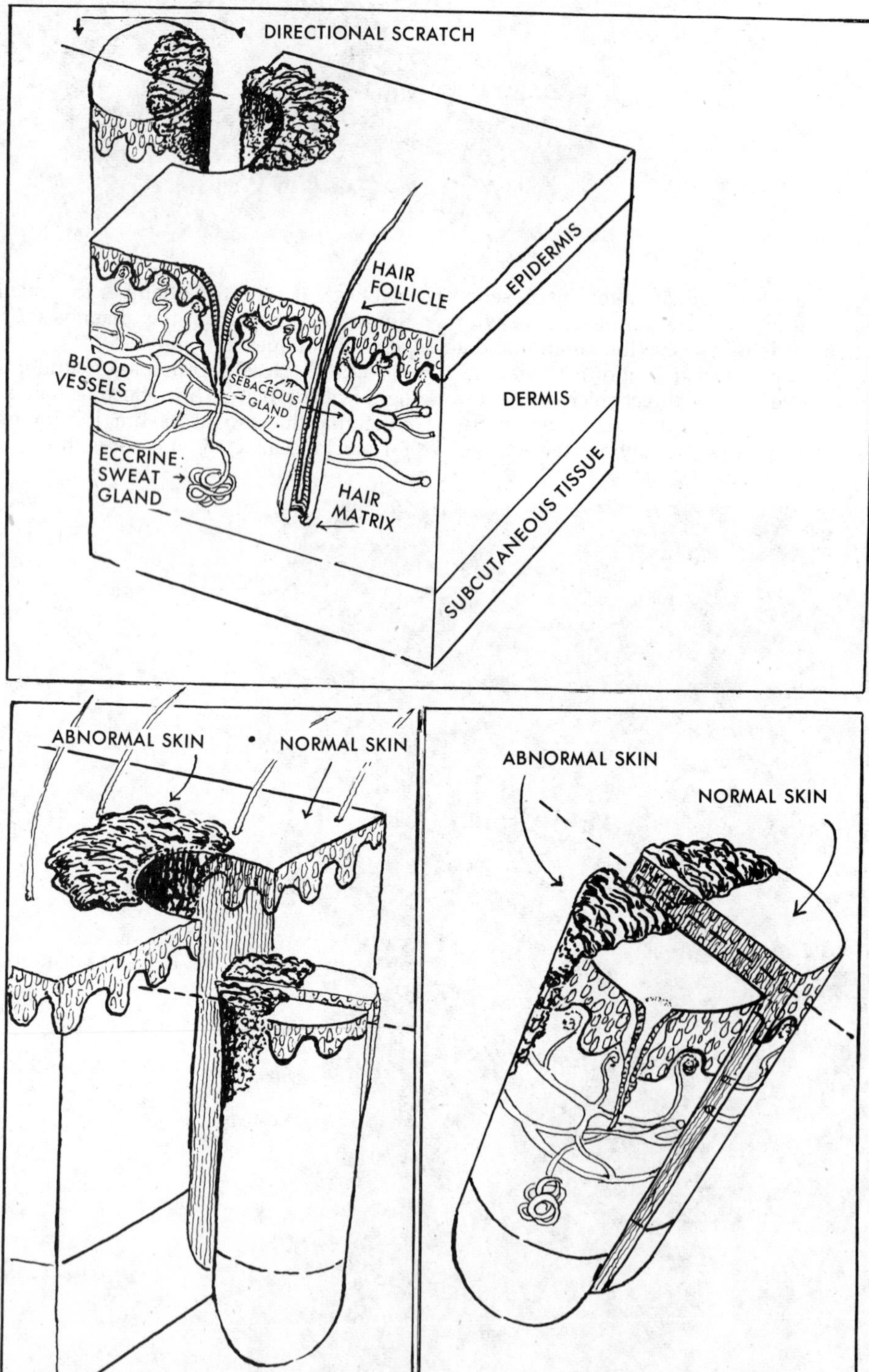

Figure 553–4. Punch biopsy of the skin.

it in cross-section. The biopsy has no magic other than the wonderment of seeing precisely what is going on at every level of the skin. For this to be pertinent, we must be looking at a representative lesion, and for best comparisons we should see it against the patient's normal skin for that area.

For the most complete histopathologic assessment, especially if for reasons of concern or cosmetics the lesion is to be removed, an elliptical excision is best. One procedure removes the lesion, secures tissue for diagnosis, and leaves a defect easily sutured. Of greater speed and ease is the punch biopsy, which at 2 mm is hardly more than a venipuncture but permits adequate tissue to be removed and examined. After anesthetizing the site with deep rather than superficial infiltration to avoid histologic distortion, a tubular blade bears through the skin by slight rotary motion, clockwise and back, to the depth of the subcutis. By light external pressure with a curved iris scissors astride the plug, the specimen lifts without the distorting pressure of forceps and can be easily clipped at its base through the loose subcutaneous tissue. The plug gently lifted to absorbent paper attaches upright, the fat adherent to the paper, the epidermis on top. Such orientation and some detailed instruction for fixing and sectioning is needed by even the most experienced technician who is unaccustomed to handling small specimens.

To enhance the value of the biopsy by contrast with normal tissue, the excision should, if possible, cut through normal and abnormal tissue, but here the laboratory will need a diagram (Fig. 553–4), and in addition a prebiopsy directional scratch on the skin sample made with a scalpel to establish the direction for histopathologic sectioning. Rotating the sections 90 degrees could provide all lesion or, most distressing, all normal skin.

For the punch biopsy suturing is not necessary for hemostasis; a Gelfoam plug to fill the defect or Monsel's solution (ferric subsulfate solution) on an applicator stick will suffice, but the cosmetic result will not be as fine as with a suture. Anatomic location and convenience of suture removal will influence the choice.

554. PRINCIPLES OF THERAPY

Before considering more detailed diagnostic formulations, it is possible to look at therapy as it seeks to correct the pathologic situation observed. Specific metabolic changes and cell infiltrates, as with lymphomas, will require a particular treatment regimen for management, but, apart from these, there is a broad group of pathologic changes that can be reversed and symptoms alleviated by therapeutic maneuvers directed toward restoration to the normal state.

The skin that is undergoing an *inflammatory* response with coalescent allergic or viral vesicles, so that it quite figuratively "weeps," requires a reduction of heat and a drying of the serous ooze through evaporation and coagulation of serum proteins. Superimposed infection will require antimicrobial therapy; debridement may be indicated. All of this can be accomplished with the wet dressing.

WET DRESSINGS

OPEN WET DRESSINGS. The prototype is a piece of undyed finely woven cloth, cotton or linen, thoroughly wet with clear water, wrung out so as not to drip, and then applied to the skin. Considered solely for its physical effects, the water evaporates, cooling and drying the underlying skin. As the cloth dries and is removed to be reimmersed, it cleanses. To get maximal benefit from evaporation, the dressing should not be more than a layer or two thick and should be changed every 15 to 30 minutes, depending on the ambient temperature and humidity. If permitted to dry completely and become adherent, the debriding effect will be greater, perhaps damaging. Remoistening the dressing in place may be needed to facilitate removal.

The wet dressing described can be initiated anywhere, even on a camping trip. In ordinary practice, however, the effectiveness of the wet dressing can be enhanced by medications added to the water. A mild protein precipitant, aluminum acetate, serves to coagulate bacterial and serum protein. As a 5 per cent preparation it is known as Burow's solution, and it must be further diluted for use. Appropriate concentrations, indications, and modes of prescribing various medications are shown for convenience in Table 554–1. If infection is a complication, potassium permanganate or silver nitrate should be in the wet dressing, but with precautions; potassium permanganate is a poison and must be kept from children's reach. Both preparations stain the skin and everything else they touch. Patient compliance will be improved by forewarnings. To use rubber gloves to protect nails from becoming brown, for example, and to use disposable containers for mixing solutions and plastic liners for sinks and tubs if porcelain is old or porous will reduce the burden of therapy. One further caution concerns the maneuver of removing the wet dressing to reimmerse the cloth rather than basting on new solution. Although important to enhance the cleansing effect, it is absolutely essential with potassium permanganate and silver nitrate, in which evaporation can permit the solute to increase in the dressing to concentrations sufficient to cause irritation or chemical burn.

The question is often raised about the use of antimicrobial agents in wet dressings. Apart from the risk of sensitization which limits the topical use of penicillin and neomycin, the quantities needed for adequate concentration in the dressing would make their use exceedingly inefficient and wasteful. The same might be said for enzymic preparations for debridement. Although the physical effects of the wet dressing would be helpful to reduce erythema and free tissue, the manipulations of the wet dressings would deactivate the enzymes prematurely. When required, they are best used separately as creams or gels.

Wet dressings, if needed at all, are needed three to four hours a day divided according to the patient's schedule. Although best split into four to five treatments of equal duration, two or three ten-minute dressings with the balance in the evening or whenever the patient is free are preferable to one solid four-hour block in the evening. Use of long narrow wrappers the length of a forearm or whole leg, just wide enough to circumvent it once, pinned top, bottom, and in between, obviates winding as with an Ace bandage, and hence is fast. Knowing that the dressing can be secured and ordinary work continued gives the patient a sense of release from an imprisoning routine. Dermatologic treatments can be time consuming and a nuisance; patients would much rather swallow a pill. The physician's attention to convenience and realistic scheduling may mean the difference between treatment and no treatment.

TABLE 554–1. USE OF WET DRESSINGS

Condition	Ingredient	Effect	Prescribed	Prepared Preparation H_2O	Approximate Final Concentration
Eczematous	A1Ac (Burow's solution)	Protein coagulation	Tablets or powder packets	1 tab/packet 500 ml 1 tab/packet 1000 ml	1:20 1:40
Mild infection	$AgNO_3$	Antimicrobial (especially gram-negative)	10% stock solution 25% stock solution	10 ml 1000 ml 5 ml 1000 ml	1:1000 1:800
Infection	$KMnO_4$	Antimicrobial	Tab 300 mg	1 tab 1500 ml 1 tab 3000 ml	1:5000 1:10,000

BATHS AND SOAKS. Should the need for wet dressings be extensive—head to toe or even half that—it requires little imagination to sense the chilling experience of lying naked under a wet sheet. It matters little that the initial temperature of the wet dressing was warm. Actually the solution need be of no set temperature. It should neither chill nor scald and is best at a temperature that the patient finds comfortable. However, evaporation from a wet dressing over an extensive surface of inflamed skin will soon cause chill. The useful alternative is to immerse the total body in water of selected temperature which permits regulated cooling; if starch powders are added to the bath, there will be an after-film and a drying effect. With infections potassium permanganate can be added to the tub. To protect against undissolved crystals burning the skin, tablets crushed with a hammer in fibrous paper should be dissolved in a small container and the solution decanted into the bath. When infection or necrotic debris is a problem in a limited area, such as the draining sinus tracts of a diabetic toe, foot immersion in appropriate medication serves as a limited therapeutic bath. Because there is the mechanical need to force the solution to the depths of the tract, such irrigation is difficult to achieve except with immersion. The same can be said for the treatment of pilonidal cysts and for many anogenital problems.

CLOSED WET DRESSINGS. The need for the open wet dressing or immersion soak will diminish as inflammation subsides, lesions dry, and draining infection is controlled. Further, not all lesions are benefited by cooling and drying. A patient with much retained keratin of the palms or soles or even generalized scaling may need maceration rather than drying. Another with an early abscess may need heat to focalize the infection. For these problems the *open* wet dressing can be covered with an impervious material to induce maceration and heat retention and to enhance penetration of a specific medication; it thereby becomes known as a *closed* wet dressing, prescribed because of need for its physical effects. Compared to the open dressing, its use is infrequent. However, it can be inadvertently created when a fastidious nurse or patient covers the open wet dressing with plastic to protect the bedclothing or furniture. The routine instructions for open wet dressings should include a warning about covering with plastic. Although it is unlikely that any significant harm has come from the extended or untimely use of open wet dressings, the inadvertent or injudicious use of occlusion can lead to a phenomenon in which a pruritic papular eruption occurs at the site of active dermatitis and then distally in body folds, and may even progress to become generalized. Unfortunately termed "autosensitization," the phenomenon is nonetheless very real.

TOPICAL THERAPY

In the general approach to therapy, wet dressings are but the beginning. Topical medications are the mainstay. Their array can be bewildering if some basic principles of selection are overlooked. They must be sorted out by active ingredients, but equal importance must be given to the vehicle that contains the active preparation.

BASES. Topicals vary in their base from lotions, through creams, to ointments. Beginning at one side of the spectrum with the simplest shake lotion, talc in water, there is a progression of relative concentrations of oil and water bases in the first of which water is the continuous phase with dispersed oil droplets. These are the water-washable bases, easy to apply and easy to wash away. They are nongreasy and vanish into the skin. As the oil-water ratio reverses and oil becomes the continuous phase with water dispersed, the preparation is more lubricating, leaves a film on the skin, and is cosmetically less elegant. At the far end of this spectrum is 100 per cent inert oil such as mineral oil or petrolatum.

Confusion about bases derives from mislabeling as lotions preparations that are other than powder and water, and from forgetting that the fluid state has little to do with the composition of the base. Water in oil and oil in water bases may pour or not. The same is true with inert oil. Mineral oil pours; petrolatum does not. A cream may be either an oil in water (water-washable) or water in oil; an ointment may be water in oil or inert oil. Both cream and ointment must be further defined if a prescription is to be compounded. Writing for the right medication in an unspecified inert oil base may result in having a preparation in mineral oil streaming down the patient's face.

BASE SELECTION. The selection of the base depends on the need for its physical properties. A powder in water such as the classic calamine lotion permits evaporation and cooling with some drying from the powder, suggestive surely of an open wet dressing. Petrolatum by contrast conserves heat, promotes maceration, and recalls completely the closed wet dressing. The inert oil has one additional role that may be overlooked, that of protection. One would not swim the English Channel without a covering of grease.

In between these two extremes there is a spectrum of possibilities permitting some cooling but adding lubrication. Choice will weigh need and cosmetic acceptance. When a medication is to be applied to the face or scalp, a greasy base would be unsightly and underutilized. If it is an antimicrobial, for example, known to penetrate better in an ointment base, the physician will nonetheless opt for a vanishing cream, recognizing the value of compliance and preferring therapy with less penetration over no therapy at all.

Having made a judgment about the base required, a separate selection is made for the active ingredients. Some compromises may be required. Steroids, for example, may be needed and a lotion base indicated, but because lotions are easily spilled and too lavishly applied, the same steroid in a nonpouring water-washable base may prove as effective and more economical. Similarly, when lubrication is needed, the ointment base of a steroid may serve just as well without the steroid and at a fraction of the cost. In such a situation a steroid cream used sparingly and rubbed well into the skin can be overlayered with a lubricating ointment for better utilization of both.

TOPICAL STEROIDS. Although specific medications will be included under consideration of the specific diseases, some of broad use are more conveniently considered together—for example, the steroids. It is difficult to imagine dermatology without them. As topical therapy their local anti-inflammatory action is a major stroke toward restoration of the skin to normal. By vasoconstriction they halt the edema and cellular infiltrates that contribute to pruritus and local discomfort. By breaking the itch-scratch cycle with its consequent tissue damage, they permit healing. By modifying the full effect of the antigen-antibody complexes in delayed hypersensitivity reactions, they abort the intensity of the inflammatory response and permit the situation to defuse over time with the erosion of the antigen. Here, they are curative in the sense that they erase the effects of the reaction until the reaction no longer occurs. When steroids alleviate the symptoms of a specific infection, as with some yeasts and fungi, they are not curative and infection will persist unless overcome by the host's defenses. The same is true with certain opportunistic organisms that overtake an area of active dermatitis. The response of the dermatitis to steroids with consequent restoration of the skin may discourage the invader. With more aggressive organisms and in the immunocompromised patient eradication will depend on specific antimicrobial therapy.

Hydrocortisone is the "Model A" of topical steroids. In a 1 per cent concentration it is still a useful preparation and continues to serve as a norm for comparing potency of the subsequently synthesized fluorinated corticosteroids, powerful anti-inflammatory agents at concentrations as low as 0.01 per cent. Less potent than the fluorinated steroids, prednisolone and methylprednisone are also less frequently used; concentration for concentration, they are more effective than hydrocortisone.

The adverse effects reported with steroids relate almost

exclusively to the fluorinated compounds, no doubt because of their high potency and because of their frequent use under occlusion (an impervious dressing analogous to the closed wet dressing which enhances absorption). Epidermal and dermal atrophy can be a pronounced adverse effect; decreased collagen synthesis and reduced stromal support for blood vessels lead to telangiectasia, purpura, and striae. A perioral dermatitis has also been reported with the fluorinated steroids, as well as aggravation of facial erythema, restricting absolutely the extended use of these compounds for the face. Further, the provoking of elevated intraocular pressure warrants a strong proscription against the prolonged application of any topical steroids near the eyes.

The reality of systemic absorption of topical steroids presents an additional hazard. Lowering of the plasma cortisol level is seen with as little as 20 per cent of the body under occlusion. The risk of rebound after discontinuing steroids in those skin diseases characterized by the phenomenon cannot be overlooked. Despite all side effects, steroids, systemically and topically, are supremely useful therapy, saving life and the quality of life.

Systemic steroids are used for three major groups of dermatologic patients. First are the severely ill with a life-threatening disease known to be responsive to corticosteroids. Initial doses will be high, 80 to 100 mg of daily prednisone or equivalent; if response is poor, the dose may be doubled. In the second group are those with an acute but severe self-limiting problem which the steroids will control or suppress during a predicted activity. Intermediate doses of 40 to 60 mg of prednisone will be initiated, and a planned but *supervised* taper would be extended over one to two weeks. Last are the patients with chronic problems who because of exacerbation or other stresses need a respite. For them the doses will be low, no more than 15 to 20 mg of prednisone, with a concurrent focus on increased supportive topical therapy so that the systemic treatment can be phased out.

SUNSCREENS. Although topical protection from ultraviolet light might be considered under photosensitivity, the carcinogenic and aging effects of actinic radiation for all skin, but especially for skin with little or no protective melanin, warrant placement here to emphasize a general usefulness as good preventive medicine. Its recommendation should be adjunctive to sun avoidance. Selecting activities, clothing, and times of the day to reduce the opportunity and intensity of ultraviolet light exposure is the best protection. Precautions are equally important on cloudy days.

The action of topical photoprotectives is to reduce penetration of photoactive nonionizing radiation to the viable epidermal cells beneath the keratin. Such protection can be achieved by absorbing or reflecting the radiation potentially damaging to normal, light-complexioned skin or abnormal skin peculiarly sensitive to light. No sunscreen enhances tanning. Rather, if an incomplete block, it permits melanin production relative to the radiation transmitted and the inherent capacity of the partially protected skin to respond.

Most sunscreens are designed to protect against the shorter burning rays of ultraviolet light in the wavelength range of 290 to 320 nm, UVB. Most effective for this is p-aminobenzoic acid used as a 5 per cent concentration in 50 to 70 per cent ethyl alcohol. Other non-PABA chemical sunscreens such as the benzophenones and cinnamates are also useful, although the protection factor may not be as high. If protection is required against the longer wavelengths of UVA, 320 to 400 nm, or visible light, 400 to 760 nm, then physical sunscreens are needed such as titanium dioxide, zinc oxide, kaolin, or iron oxide—all available as heavy creams or pastes. Unfortunately, such opaque protectors are not nearly so acceptable as the clear and milky lotions that protect against UVB. Because certain photodermatoses are evoked by UVA, even visible light, and because UVA may also contribute to skin aging and carcinogenesis, the physical sunscreens have a significant role for selected patients.

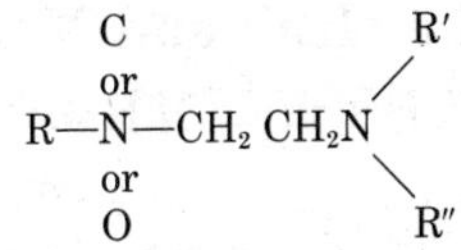

Figure 554–1. The three antihistamine linkages.

ANTIHISTAMINES. Before leaving the general considerations of dermatologic therapy, antihistamines deserve mention. Used often for their soporific and tranquilizing effect, they are still helpful in blocking one or more of the effects of histamine. No one antihistamine blocks all the effects. Those antagonists for the histamine H_2-receptor can be arranged biochemically in three major groups according to the linkage of their side arm through a C or N or O (Fig. 554–1). The selection of an effective agent for a given patient may be from any one group (Table 554–2) or from a combination of groups, but is unlikely to be enhanced by combining antihistamines within the group. If response to one antihistamine is minimal or poor, another from another group should be added or substituted. Evidence that blood vessels of human skin have H_2 as well as H_1-receptors has led to the evaluation of an H_2-receptor antagonist such as cimetidine in combination with an H_1-antagonist, and the combination has proved effective in the treatment of some cases of chronic urticaria unresponsive to standard antihistamines.

555. THE DIFFERENTIAL DIAGNOSIS

With the primary lesion assessed, a representative site biopsied, and perhaps general therapy initiated to reduce discomfort, the dermatologic diagnosis, if not immediately obvious, can be elaborated. There are broad classifications and wide-ranging considerations which help frame a diagnostic grid so that a reasonable differential can be narrowed. The skin has only a finite number of ways to respond, and many diagnoses have predilections for selected anatomic areas, suggesting their identity by their location. Further, the bulk of dermatologic problems is distributed among no more than a dozen diagnoses, so the framework need not be too cumbersome.

In the examination of the skin, noting the pattern of lesions has been stressed, but the value of the pattern has not been exploited. With a look to commonly encountered problems by anatomic region it is possible to check the supporting evidence that might be expected in a given diagnosis.

TABLE 554–2. SELECTED ANTIHISTAMINES GROUPED BY MOLECULAR LINKAGE

Carbon	Nitrogen	Oxygen
Alkylamines	**Ethylenediamines**	**Ethanolamines**
Chlorpheniramine (DL mixture) (Chlor-Trimeton)	Tripelennamine (Pyribenzamine)	Diphenhydramine (Benadryl)
Chlorpheniramine (D form) (Polaramine)	Pyrilamine (Neo-Antergan)	Bromodiphenhydramine (Ambodryl)
Parabromdylamine (Dimetane)		Dimenhydrinate (Dramamine)
		Carbinoxamine Maleate (Clistin)
Piperazines	**Phenothiazines**	
Meclizine (Bonamine)	Promethazine (Phenergan)	
Hydroxyzine (Atarax)		

The Head and Neck

SEBORRHEIC DERMATITIS

In the scalp, if there is scale and erythema but no evidence of atrophy or hair follicle disruption, the most likely diagnosis is that of seborrheic dermatitis. There may be pattern baldness and the complaint of hair thinning, but the observed pathology is a greasy scale, covering a yellow-red marginated base. The problem is common; it is shared by 12 million Americans, of whom 5.5 million have it severely enough to warrant medical consultation. Although usually a problem limited to the scalp or perhaps by extension to the retroauricular fold, it can involve the eyebrows and skin between, the eyelids in blepharitis, or the pinna in otitis externa, as well as the alae nasi, axillae, anterior thorax, periumbilical area, and genital area with focus in the crural and intergluteal folds. Obese patients with a predisposition to seborrheic dermatitis can have severe erythema and maceration in all intertriginous areas. An occasional individual can progress to a generalized exfoliative dermatitis.

The differential diagnosis in the adult is fairly limited. If scalp scaling is severe, laminated, and adherent, psoriasis must be considered. In fact, seborrheic dermatitis of such severity may be a forme fruste of psoriasis. Axillary and genital erythema raise the question of infection of the body folds with *Candida albicans* or *Corynebacterium*, but the presence of scalp lesions and the inability to demonstrate causative organisms support the diagnosis of seborrheic dermatitis. Even with positive routine cultures as for *Candida*, characteristic scalp lesions and other stigmata of seborrheic dermatitis (periumbilical erythema and scale) may suggest the diagnosis. Unresponsiveness to antiseborrheic therapy and discreteness of lesions would suggest the possibility of histiocytosis. In fact, the high prevalence of seborrheic diathesis may extend features of seborrheic dermatitis to an associated eruption. Lupus erythematosus has been observed in a seborrheic distribution with a greasiness to the lupus scale. Present, too, however, were atrophy, telangiectasia, and follicular plugging, classic for lupus erythematosus but not part of seborrheic dermatitis. In Parkinson's disease in which sebaceous glands are enlarged and sebum production is increased, seborrheic dermatitis is frequently a problem. Although treatment with L-dopa lowers sebum production, there is not always correlation of the degree of sebum suppression and neurologic improvement. Seborrheic dermatitis has been noted unilaterally in association with neurologic lesions, and with sympathetic nerve regeneration it has disappeared.

The tendency to develop seborrheic dermatitis in those genetically predisposed cannot be altered, but its manifestations can be suppressed, often by a simple acceptable routine. To reduce risk of progression and to delay hair fall, active treatment ought to be encouraged. Therapy should control inflammation and scaling, thereby reducing pruritus and oiliness. Medicated shampoos containing antimicrobial agents and salicylic acid may be all that is needed. Frequent shampooing is important, daily at first, although it need not always be with the medicated preparation. Topical steroid in lotion bases applied to the scalp two or three times daily will reduce erythema. If scale is marked, however, no medication will penetrate; warm oil soaks under plastic occlusion with or without salicylic acid will loosen the scale.

Once control has been achieved and the scalp appears normal, therapy may be reduced gradually until a minimal maintenance is determined: topical steroids every other day or less often; medicated shampoos alternating with regular shampoos in a determined repetitive pattern. As a rule, maintenance requirements will increase in winter.

For seborrheic dermatitis of areas other than the scalp, a similar routine is effective. The maceration of scale in body folds obviates the need for oil occlusion. In fact, warmth and erythema may suggest wet dressings as an initial therapy. These, combined with topical steroid, will usually control the problem, but ultraviolet light, cautiously administered, often hastens resolution.

It is also important to recognize conditions associated with seborrheic dermatitis. Severe *acne vulgaris*, for example, is always associated with some seborrheic dermatitis and so is *acne rosacea*.

ACNE

Diagnostically, acne will not be a problem. Its stigmata have become a hallmark of adolescence, and the advertising media have brought into sharp focus the characteristic erythematous papules and pustules of the pilosebaceous apparatus, the comedones open and closed (blackheads and whiteheads). When acne appears suddenly and for the first time in the 30-year-old or menopausal woman, everyone is surprised, the diagnosis is doubted, and there is uneasiness about underlying pathology. Newer investigative techniques that permit assessment of blood levels of free testosterone and dehydroepiandrosterone sulfate indicate that these may be elevated in such patients. At the present time, however, unless there are other clinical indications of virilization or endocrine dysfunction, the diagnosis of acne should merely be a challenge to active and adequate therapy, not to hormonal evaluation.

This is not to take acne lightly as a diagnosis. So prevalent in the second decade as to be considered almost a normal physiologic phenomenon, acne vulgaris defaces youth at a most vulnerable and insecure time. Further, it can persist throughout life and be severe and disfiguring, as in the conglobate form, causing marked morbidity and debility. Even severe cases that resolve can leave such destructive scarring that the psychologic burden never lifts.

There is other acne that is aggravated or perhaps frankly caused by oil, such as mechanics experience in their work, and by medications such as halogens and systemic steroids. Industrial exposure to the chlorinated hydrocarbons will almost invariably produce acne in exposed workers (chloracne). For these, improving the environment, removing the oil, discontinuing the bromides or iodides, or reducing the steroid dosage will be therapeutically advantageous. However, in most instances treating acne successfully relies on patient compliance derived mostly from an understanding of the pathophysiologic process. The patient should know that the aim of therapy is to foster the free drainage of the pilosebaceous unit, to avoid rupture, and to limit bacterial growth. The hydrolysis of the triglycerides of sebum by cutaneous bacteria yields fatty acids which have an inflammatory effect on the follicle, and which then, with its disruption, pass into the surrounding tissue as a primary irritant. The abnormality in acne is at the follicular dyskeratosis that plugs the duct. Comedones, open and closed, must be dislodged, and surface bacteria, especially *Corynebacterium acnes*, suppressed.

The patient should be instructed in the need for simple cleansing every four to six hours to stun bacteria and discourage their logarithmic growth. Washing with soap will do, or a mild alcohol preparation carried or kept in a locker may be used. A topical antimicrobial preparation should be applied twice daily, benzoyl peroxide 5 or 10 per cent, for example, or the antimicrobial clindamycin, tetracycline, or erythromycin 1 or 2 per cent in an alcohol base. Plugged follicles will respond to topical retinoic acid, presumably through the labilization of lysosomes in the keratinizing cells of the follicles. A brisk erythematous response is often induced that may necessitate a reduction in the concentration or frequency of application of the vitamin A acid. Further, the concern for enhanced damage from solar radiation, or the possibility of a co-carcinogenic effect as suggested by experiments in hairless albino mice, contraindicates its use in summer or in light-complexioned individuals. For these as for all patients with acne, the mechanical removal of comedones and the incision and drainage of pustules and cysts foster resolution.

Systemic broad-spectrum antimicrobials in low to moderate

doses given over long periods have proved a useful management for more severe acne, and, contrary to the expectations of some, have not been complicated by microbial resistance or superinfections. The tetracyclines, although commonly used, carry risk of dental discoloration, photosensitivity, and even pregnancy through drug interaction with oral contraceptives. Because they are incorporated into growing bones and teeth, they should not be prescribed from the fourth fetal month through age 12. There is also the possibility of subsequent mobilization from bone under stress, as in pregnancy, with consequent risk of maternal hepatitis or fetal absorption. All patients of the childbearing age should be cautioned if prolonged therapy is anticipated. Photosensitivity, impossible to predict, must be considered in the event of untoward reaction. Erythromycin is a useful alternative; compared to tetracycline, gastrointestinal distress may be more prevalent with erythromycin, but ingestion with meals and consumption of supplemental *Lactobacillus* as from yogurt reduce such symptoms. More severe acne may require more extensive surgical procedures, higher doses of antimicrobials, intralesional steroid, or even systemic steroid. Estrogens have been used in selected women with stubborn severe acne with good results, but used as cyclic estrogen progestin therapy they have all the attendant risk of anovulatory preparations given for contraception. X-ray has no part in the management of acne. The question of diet is invariably raised, but there is no evidence to support a role for diet as either cause or aggravation. Of proven value in cystic acne but with risk not fully assessed, oral isotretinoin (13-*cis*-retinoic acid and a probable metabolite of vitamin A) alters sebaceous gland differentiation, reducing sebum production in ways not clear but not as an antiandrogen. Within four weeks after treatment is begun, erythema and pustules are reduced. When treatment is stopped, usually after four months, sebum production returns toward pretreatment levels, yet the cystic acne continues in remission or even improves. The clinical toxic effects are similar to those of vitamin A, are dose dependent in incidence and severity, and are reversible when therapy is stopped. This includes pseudotumor cerebri or benign intracranial hypertension manifest by papilledema, headache, nausea, vomiting, and visual disturbances, which warrant an immediate stop to therapy and a neurologic assessment. Laboratory abnormalities seem limited to occasional elevations of liver function test results that return to pretreatment levels even as therapy is continued, and to elevations in blood lipids, especially triglycerides, that return to pretreatment levels after therapy. Current studies of treatment of dyskeratoses indicate the possibility of greater hepatic dysfunction with the prolonged use of isotretinoin over a period of years. Of primary importance is the fact that isotretinoin is teratogenic. Patients must not conceive while on therapy or for a month or more thereafter. Nor are blood banks to accept blood for transfusion from patients on isotretinoin therapy lest a recipient be or become pregnant. Clearly a useful adjunct for the treatment of recalcitrant persistent cystic acne, isotretinoin should not be prescribed without thoughtful review, detailed explanation, strict contraception, and close clinical and laboratory monitoring.

ACNE ROSACEA

Characteristically appearing in the central one third of the face, acne rosacea occurs more commonly in women of 30 to 50 years, but more severely in men; it can be seen in both sexes at any age. Comedones are lacking, and the acne pustules are associated with telangiectasia and persistent flush; spices, alcohol, hot drinks, and temperature extremes that foster flushing aggravate the condition. Rhinophyma (Fig. 555–1) is associated with longstanding rosacea, but ocular involvement (blepharitis, conjunctivitis, episcleritis, and keratitis) can be far more serious. Therapy as outlined for acne vulgaris can be helpful for the pustular component of rosacea, but the flush and telangiectasia remain. Foods and situations that provoke flushing should be avoided. For both acne vulgaris and acne rosacea, control of the seborrheic dermatitis is important for management.

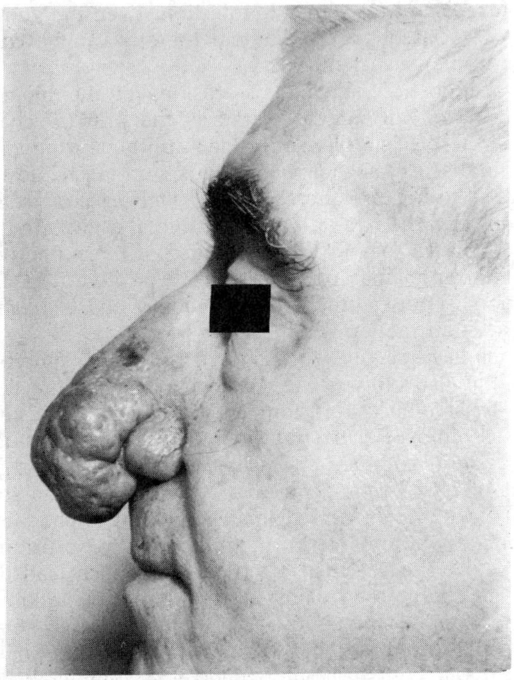

Figure 555–1. Rhinophyma.

LESIONS OF THE MOUTH

Pathology of the buccal mucosa and lips is often overlooked unless the patient offers a specific complaint or corroborative evidence is sought for a suspected diagnosis based on a distant lesion. When oral inspection is routine and the mucosa under dentures never excluded, a wide range of normal and pathologic change will be recognized.

Pigmentation, for example, most marked on the gingiva, buccal mucosa, hard palate, tongue, and soft palate, has an intensity commensurate with that of the skin and increases from childhood to adult life. Racial variation is considerable. Melanocytic nevi, usually compound, and less common in the mouth than on the skin, can be seen in all races, but most often in blacks. Exogenous pigment can be deposited from the silver amalgam of dental fillings through an accidental tattoo or by diffusion. A dark blue-black lesion of the lip, which might be deeply placed pigment but blanches on diascopy, is a benign phlebectasia. Relatively common past middle life, phlebectasia of the oral mucosa, tongue, and scrotum can be associated with similar lesions of the jejunum and may be a cause of gastrointestinal bleeding.

Vascular nevi of the lips and buccal mucosa are recognized from infancy or childhood. They can cause obstructive problems as well as bleeding because of friability. The less obvious punctate telangiectasia of Osler-Rendu-Weber disease is not often seen before puberty, but almost always involves the mucous membranes occurring in the mouth, nasal septum, nasopharynx, and throughout the gastrointestinal tract. The lesions of the tongue are diagnostic, for within the fungiform papillae is a single, dilated vessel that may lead to an expanded papilla.

The most common problems of the mouth, however, derive from infection and trauma. Periodontal and periapical disease are associated not only with bacteremia but also with local erosions and, in the most severe form, with acute necrotizing ulcerative gingivitis. Attention to oral hygiene, the removal of bacterial plaque, and the massaging of gingivae will restore tissue turgor and resistance to infection. Even the gum hypertrophy associated with phenytoin therapy can be controlled with scrupulous cleansing.

The diagnostic challenge of erosions of the mouth must include in the differential diagnosis the primary chancre of syphilis, herpes simplex infection, aphthous stomatitis, the blistering diseases such as pemphigus, and mechanical trauma as from ill-fitting prostheses. *Extragenital chancres* are not uncommon, and the lips and adjacent buccal cavity are the most common places to find them. Because of the numerous nonsyphilitic treponemas of the mouth, a positive dark field examination is not definitive of infection with *T. pallidum* and serologic confirmation is required.

Lesions of *herpes simplex, Herpesvirus hominis,* subtype 1 primarily, but also subtype 2 especially if a primary infection, may have extensive buccal erosions with gingivostomatitis and systemic symptoms. Recurrent lesions, which can be intraoral but are much more common on the lips, usually present as grouped vesicles of 1 to 3 mm; a positive Tzanck smear will show the multinucleated giant cells. Some 85 per cent of patients report prodromal symptoms of burning, tingling, or pruritus a few hours before the vesicular eruption. With such lead time, an attack may be aborted using topical steroid or 5-iodo-2-deoxyuridine applied frequently, every hour or two. Once the vesicles have erupted, the clinical infection, although short-lived, runs its course. Drying agents and antimicrobial preparations to thwart secondary bacterial infection should limit the problem to five to seven days. Acyclovir, which inhibits the multiplication of herpes simplex virus types 1 and 2, reduces morbidity in primary infections and viral shedding but not morbidity in recurrences. Because of the emergence of resistant virus, the use of acyclovir should be reserved for life-threatening herpetic infections, primary or secondary, which occur in the immunocompromised host.

Aphthous stomatitis or canker sores are recurrent, painful ulcerations of the oral mucosa. Although aphthae can be the first clinical manifestation of pernicious anemia and perhaps of folic acid or iron deficiency, most recurrent aphthae are of unknown cause. They are more common in women, and familial occurrence of a severe variety has been reported. An association between jejunal mucosal abnormalities and aphthae is suggested. Immunoglobulins, i.e., IgE-bearing lymphocytes, are reportedly increased.

No specific treatment is available for aphthae, but topical anesthetics such as viscous lidocaine or the antihistamine diphenhydramine held in the mouth just before mealtime, numb the pain and ease alimentation. Suspensions of antibiotic such as tetracycline, 250 mg per 5 ml held against the sores for two minutes before swallowing four or five times per day, promote healing. The antibiotic can be combined with the diphenhydramine. Steroids in the dental preparation Orabase are difficult to keep in place. To concentrate steroid locally, a cortisone tablet, 5 mg whole or halved, can dissolve in the ulcer; intralesional steroid can be injected. Such therapy can be used for all painful erosions of the mouth when anesthesia, infection control, and reduction of the inflammatory response will promote healing. It will be of benefit for oral erosions of the blistering diseases while the diagnosis is being elaborated, and will ease the discomfort of mechanical erosions from dentures and bridges while the cause is being corrected.

Friable white tissue, with or without erosion but along the bite line, suggests a chewing of the cheek and consequent damage to the mucosa. Lacy infiltrates or friable mucosa away from the bite line may suggest lichen planus, lupus erythematosus, or perhaps a white sponge nevus; the distinction from leukoplakia is difficult but important, and the lesion needs assessment. Stigmata of disease elsewhere are helpful; a biopsy is in order, but may not be definitive. The microscopic study, however, can rule out epithelial dysplasia. Requiring equally close surveillance and perhaps biopsy is smoker's palate, a papular, gray-white, palatal mucosa, the result of inflamed, plugged salivary glands, each papule bearing the red dot of a ductal orifice. The process seen in habitual pipe smokers is precancerous, but may show regression if smoking is stopped.

Any lesion of the buccal mucosa or lips that is not identified, especially one that is enlarging or eroded, should be biopsied. Actinic damage involves the lips, the lower more than the upper, with characteristic atrophy and fine scale and occasionally induration. Malignant change must always be suspect. Angular stomatitis, fissuring at the labial commissures, may be associated with *Candida albicans* infection, but most often is the result of chronic irritation with bacterial and yeast infection, opportunistic and secondary. The redundancy of tissue with aging but more with the gum and bone resorption of the edentulous, aggravated perhaps by ill-fitting prostheses, leads to chronic ulceration. When sleeping, such patients frequently salivate to macerate further one commissure or both.

Intensive topical therapy should reduce secondary infection with appropriate antimicrobial agents, the inflammation with steroid, and the risk of continuing irritation by sealing with a protective film such as zinc oxide paste, at least at night. If the defect is slow to respond, a biopsy should be taken; chronic ulcerations predispose to malignant change. If the physical fact of redundancy precludes healing, surgical revision is indicated.

The Thorax

In the course of the regional examination, note is constantly made of the isolated pigmentary lesions (see Ch. 556) and the stigmata of aging and actinic exposure (see Ch. 552). The present larger focus is the pattern of appearance of eruptions.

DRUG ERUPTION

Symmetrical, scaling, erythematous macules or papules on the thorax, if of sudden onset, would suggest a drug eruption (Fig. 555–2). Itching need not be present but would support the impression.

PITYRIASIS ROSEA

Should the lesions be oval with a collarette of fine scale and follow skin cleavage lines (Fig. 555–3), the diagnosis of pityriasis rosea is likely. In this self-limited eruption, which is not uncommon and is often seen in young adults, there is occasionally recognition of a larger antecedent lesion, the herald patch. Usually on the trunk it can be several centimeters in size, erythematous, and scaling. It is often mistaken for fungus; the negative KOH test result would correct that error. When the generalized eruption appears, the immediate reflex of the knowing examiner is to look again at the pharynx and palms lest luetic lesions be overlooked. Secondary syphilis is always in the differential diagnosis, and a serologic test should be obtained; but without systemic symptoms, coryza, or palmar and plantar lesions, syphilis is an unlikely cause of the eruption. Pityriasis rosea lasts six to eight weeks; although most patients are asymptomatic, one in five will complain of pruritus.

LICHEN PLANUS

Lichen planus, of characteristic color but sparse scale must, nevertheless, be included in the differential diagnosis of scattered scaling lesions of the thorax, especially if there are lesions on the flexor aspect of the wrists, lower legs, or genitalia. Most often the typical polygonal flat-topped papule with a lilac hue and, on close inspection, the delicate whitish lines of Wickham's striae can be found. The classic lesion is diagnostic, and the histology supports the diagnosis. Mouth lesions are seen in half the patients, a lacy white network involving the buccal mucosa and lips. Ulcerative, erosive, hypertrophic, and atrophic variants have been described, and lichen planus–like eruptions have been induced by certain drugs, heavy metals,

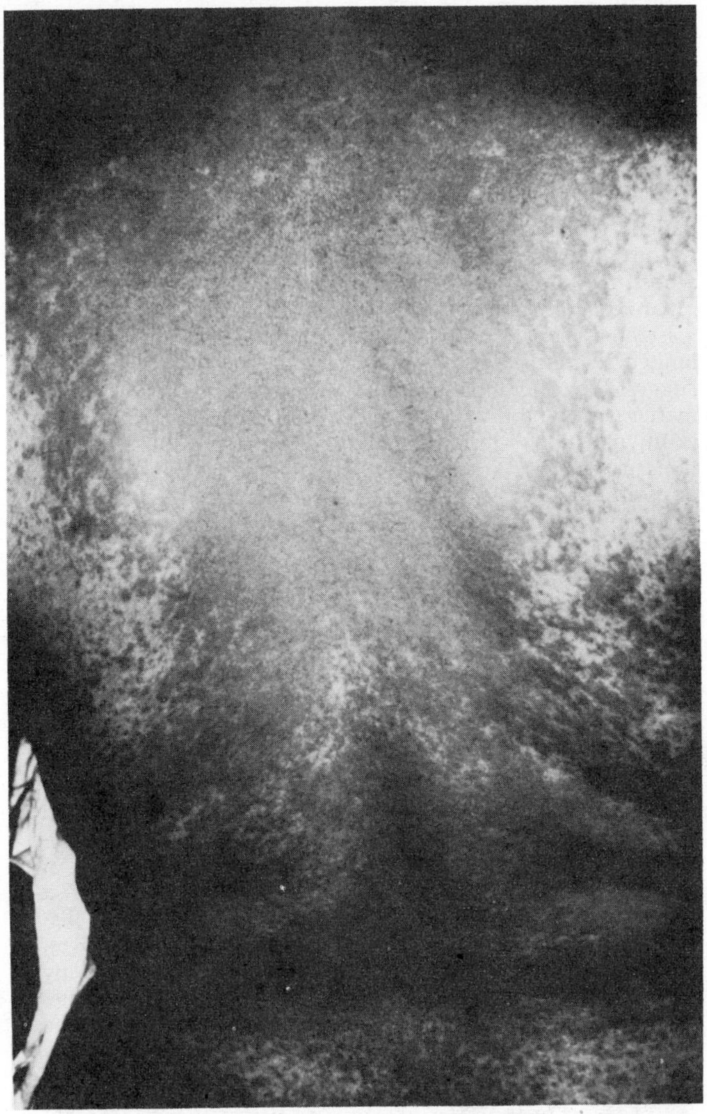

Figure 555–2. Drug eruption.

and color photo developers. The drugs include streptomycin, methyldopa, gold, phenothiazine, and the antimalarials chloroquine and quinacrine.

The etiology remains obscure, but the known association with drugs and chemicals and the observation of deficiency of glucose-6-phosphate dehydrogenase in lichen planus skin support a hypothesis that certain susceptible enzyme-deficient individuals respond to various chemicals and other environmental factors with lichen planus–like lesions. Eruptions resembling lichen planus have also been observed with polymyositis and lymphoma.

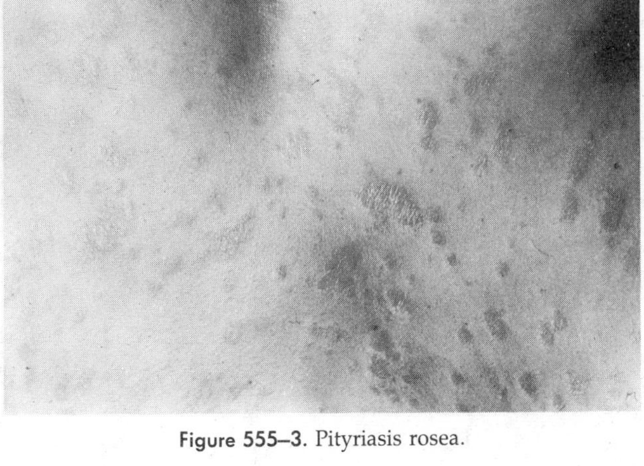

Figure 555–3. Pityriasis rosea.

PSORIASIS

Psoriasis, although classically presenting with plaques over the elbows and knees, can appear suddenly over the thorax as small, scattered papulosquamous lesions described as guttate. If these are the first manifestations of the disease, the finding of supporting stigmata may be essential. Characteristic silvery micaceous scale would be a helpful clue, and so, too, would be severe scaling of the scalp. Pitting of the fingernails with lifting and flaring is supportive, and a change suggestive of an oil droplet underneath the nail is pathognomonic. Nails can be greatly thickened. Historical or current evidence of scaling plaques of the elbows or knees, erythema or fissuring of the intergluteal fold, and associated arthritis of the distal interphalangeal joints all leave the diagnosis hard to challenge. In severe cases much of the skin may be involved (Fig. 555–4). In some there can be erosive, inflammatory joint disease, usually polyarticular and occasionally severe, even mutilating. Appearing in 4.5 per cent of psoriatic patients with no serologic evidence of lupus erythematosus or rheumatic factors, it is recognized as psoriatic arthritis.

In the United States more than one million people have psoriasis, and of these more than 11 per cent have experienced disability of such severity as to compromise employment and effectiveness. The disease can begin at any age and has its peak appearance in the third decade. Its severity, course, and remissions are unpredictable. It is inherited in a pattern still unclear. There are studies relating two HLA antigens and psoriasis. One, Bw17, is a useful genetic marker for that group of psoriatic patients with a high rate of affected relatives and a mean age of onset under 20 years (18.2 years). Those with HLA-B13 have little heritable tendency and milder disease.

Patients whose psoriasis requires therapy, or patients who demand it, are usually referred to a dermatologist, for, in general, physicians do not appreciate the discomfort and dis-

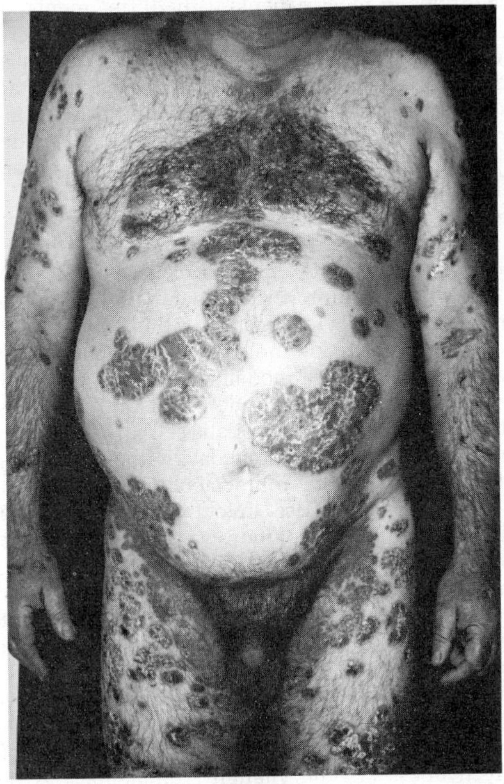

Figure 555–4. Psoriasis.

figurement of the disease and the potential for severity, arthritis, generalized exfoliation, or even death. Lesions are often dismissed as untreatable, or sometimes are subjected to an overkill with systemic therapy and attendant significant side effects. Systemic corticosteroids, for example, can induce prompt resolution of psoriatic lesions, but suppression requires ever-increasing doses. When therapy is tapered, there is a rebound phenomenon, with extension of lesions possibly to exfoliation. If systemic steroids are used for other valid reasons in patients with psoriasis, the risk of aggravated psoriasis should be recognized and weighed in the decision for initiating therapy.

Psoriasis is without cure but is responsive to treatments which can induce remission of many months to years and maintenance therapy that can help sustain the remission. Corticosteroids applied topically under occlusion or given intralesionally promote blanching and flattening of lesions. If the impetus to remit is enhanced by the use of tar and ultraviolet light through the Goeckerman regimen, the chance of steroid rebound will lessen and a true remission may be realized. Black coal tars are applied directly to the skin in sufficient amounts to penetrate, and then are wiped clean so as not to filter out the long range ultraviolet light, which evokes a phototoxic reaction. Increasing exposures to ultraviolet light are given on a set schedule—as often as twice daily for inpatients, perhaps once or twice weekly for outpatients. The duration of exposure is pushed to tolerance of erythema but not burn, lest the Koebner phenomenon, the isomorphic response by which tissue injury induces new lesions, activate a psoriatic flare. Within three to four weeks the most extensive psoriasis is usually resolved. Continuing use of light and tar, alone or together if possible, at reduced intervals helps preserve the favorable response. Variations of the Goeckerman method have included the use of anthralin paste with dressings after the baths and light.

Long wave ultraviolet light (UVA) has also been used from a high intensity source through photosensitization with oral psoralens which potentiate the effect of light. Experience with PUVA (psoralens plus UVA) suggests good resolution of the psoriatic lesions in most patients with 20 treatments, but with a need for maintenance therapy in a significant percentage. Treatment requires traveling to a center and risk of burn or eye damage from normal sunlight before and after therapy until the psoralen is metabolized. The importance of long-term assessment is recognized because of the laboratory inducement of skin malignancies and cataracts in albino mice on high dose psoralens and intense exposure to UVA. In fact, from the multicenter study where PUVA has been on protocol, there are data to show an increased prevalence of cutaneous malignancy, with more squamous cell carcinoma relative to basal cell carcinoma. Whether such tumor will follow the more benign course of actinically induced malignancy rather than the biologic aggressiveness of radiation-induced tumor remains to be seen.

The effect of the topical modalities utilizing ultraviolet light is believed to be through mitotic arrest and the consequent return toward normal of the psoriatic cell turnover time, which is at an accelerated three to four days rather than the normal 27 to 28 days. Surely the antimetabolites have this effect on mitosis and thereby induce involution of psoriatic lesions. Arsenic used as Fowler's solution was an early cellular poison for psoriasis, and its previous use in a given patient is an important historical fact to alert the examiner to search for sequelae of arsenic ingestion. Aminopterin, amethopterin or methotrexate, and azaribine have also been used for therapy, methotrexate being the most widely used and the only one still accepted. Its prescription in psoriasis is limited to grave situations and to rigid guidelines set by the Psoriasis Task Force, National Program for Dermatology. Of less risk and of promising effectiveness are the vitamin A analogues. A new oral aromatic retinoid etretinate on protocol in the United States and available in Germany causes psoriatic lesions to enlarge and disappear. Clinical toxic effects are similar to those of vitamin A and laboratory abnormalities similar to those experienced with isotretinoin.

Because patient care is so often fragmented among specialists and because not all patients appreciate the gravity of therapy, it is important for any physician to inquire about every treatment regimen prescribed for his patient. The psoriasis in a patient with clear skin on methotrexate may escape detection. In the same way the dermatologist should know if the patient whose skin cancer he is about to curette and electrodesiccate is on anticoagulation and has a pacemaker.

Isolated psoriatic lesions, especially if circinate, and psoriasis limited to the seborrheic areas such as axillae or groin may suggest the differential diagnosis of fungus infection. For that matter, so would the "herald patch" of pityriasis rosea. If there is any question, scrapings should be taken for KOH examination and culture. Not uncommonly, ubiquitous organisms are opportunistic. Patients *can* have two diagnoses, but the KOH test result and cultures sooner or later must support the clinical impression of fungus.

FUNGUS INFECTIONS

Scaling lesions of the thorax, with macular patches of all sizes and shapes, varying in color from white to tan to brown, represent *tinea versicolor* (Fig. 555–5). Extending sometimes to the neck, face, and arms, it is asymptomatic and is usually just a cosmetic bother. Wood's light examination aids visualization because of skin pigment change and because of the brick-red fluorescence of the causative organism, *Malassezia furfur (Pityrosporon orbiculare)*, which is not readily cultured. Scraping of the lesion removes scale and leaves normal skin beneath. Direct microscopic examination of the scale shows short hyphal filaments and grape-like clusters of budding forms (Fig. 555–6). The therapy prescribed is usually the common fungicides. Any preparation with sodium thiosulfate, haloprogin, or tolnaftate, for example, is useful, as is clotrimazole or miconazole. The

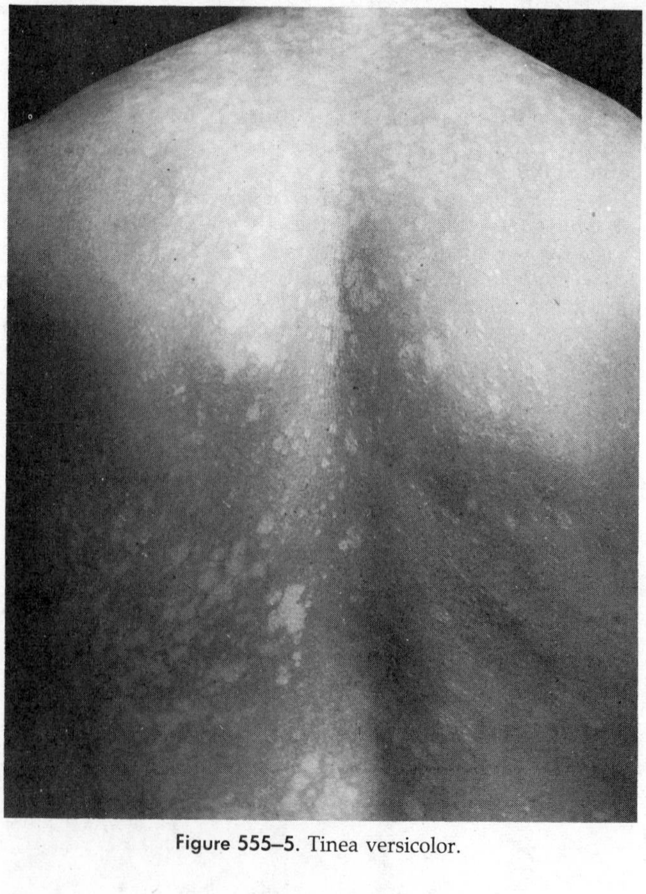

Figure 555–5. Tinea versicolor.

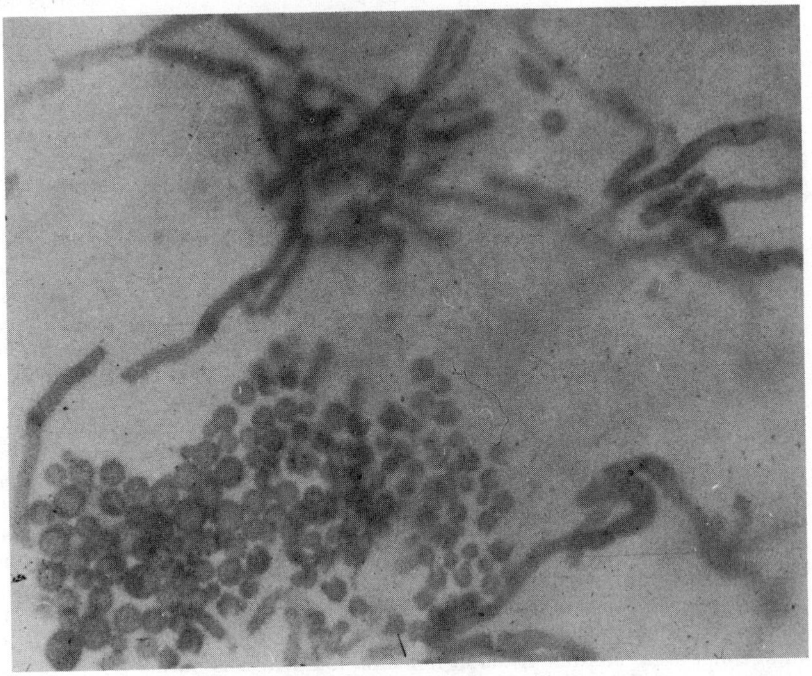

Figure 555–6. *Malassezia furfur.*

problem tends to recur, but can be prevented by daily scrubs with a keratolytic antimicrobial soap. No systemic therapy is indicated.

In general, if scaling lesions show hyphal elements and the appropriate cultures are positive but if another diagnosis is still suspected, the basic problem may not be fungus. A course of antifungal therapy should resolve the question; if it is a secondary invader, it will disappear, leaving the underlying pathology.

Traditionally, fungus is considered anatomically, from head to foot. Tinea capitis, so common to children, is hardly ever seen in adults except for a rare *Trichophyton tonsurans* infection. Occasionally parents of children with infected scalps can have glabrous or smooth, nonhairy skin involvement, having come in contact with the child's infection, but such anthropophilic fungi provoke little in tissue reaction. Animal fungi by contrast can stimulate a brisk reaction. From the broken hair "black dot" infection of *T. tonsurans* the spectrum extends through the red scaling dermatophytosis of groin and foot characteristic of *Trichophyton* and *Epidermophyton* infections to the boggy, bumpy tumefaction, raised, red, and tender, of a *Microsporum* infection such as *M. gypseum, M. canis,* or even *M. audouini.* These kerions resemble bacterial abscesses and initially can be misdiagnosed and mistreated. The importance of the direct and immediate examination for fungus by the KOH preparation cannot be overemphasized.

Scaling lesions of the trunk or body folds, if KOH-positive for hyphal elements, are tinea until proved otherwise. In areas where fungus has been associated with the continued maceration of wet clothing, as from occupation or wet swim trunks, plaques and nodules may develop; the history of maceration is important. Therapy which can be specific topically and systemically is less effective when good local care is neglected. Tub baths for adequate cleansing, removal of wet garments promptly, and use of drying powders can all be helpful.

Scaling lesions of the hands and feet offer a wider differential, since contact and chronic irritant dermatitis are so common. The differential diagnosis will be considered below. Persistent inflammation of nail beds and the presence of psoriatic lesions in the nail plate can deform nails without fungal infection. However, the opportunities for fungi to infect macerated keratin further the confusion. Scrapings for fungal study should be taken from glabrous skin and nails as well as finger and toe webs. Too often oral griseofulvin is prescribed for scaling lesions without benefit of confirmatory KOH examination and culture. Rarely it may be considered for a therapeutic trial despite negative test results but never without them. It is useful against most dermatophytes but inactive against deep fungi and *Candida* species. It works best for fungal infection of the scalp, trunk, or groin.

When griseofulvin is given as 1 gram per day after a fatty meal to enhance absorption, pruritus, if a symptom, should disappear in 24 to 48 hours. Glabrous skin involvement should clear in seven to fourteen days. Dystrophic, infected nails, however, will require continuing therapy for as long as the pregriseofulvin keratin is retained, i.e., as long as it takes for replacement—three to four months for fingernails, six months or longer for toenails. Interrupting therapy will permit reinfection from retained infected keratin. Even throughout constant therapy and thereafter, a topical antifungal agent should be used.

The lengthy duration of required treatment should give the physician pause about committing a patient to a half year or more of a medication that can have unpleasant neurologic, hematologic, and gastrointestinal side effects. Further, once cleared, the chance of reinfection is considerable because of the ubiquitous organisms and the selected inability of some individuals to resist such infections.

A useful alternative to prolonged treatment is to clear glabrous skin with a short oral course of griseofulvin while instituting a vigorous topical program that ideally will contain the infection in the nails and keep the skin free of disease. Should there be a relapse at a future date, the oral course can be repeated. Most mild to moderate tinea infections require only topical medication such as tolnaftate, haloprogin, miconazole, or clotrimazole.

YEAST INFECTIONS

Yeast infections of the skin mimic fungal infections as in the groin, but most often the erythema is a bit brighter, the scale is more macerated, and there will be telltale satellite lesions at the periphery of the patch. When *Candida* infects webs or paronychia—a common hazard of the prolonged water immersion experienced by bartenders and janitors—or when it involves the mouth or vagina as a sequela of systemic antimicrobial therapy, perhaps a signal of diabetes—the lesions are more characteristic. The erythematous base is often raw with a cheesy exudate, and there may be pruritus, but more often tenderness and pain occur.

Therapy to reduce erythema and itching is helpful in initiating symptomatic relief, and eradication of the underlying predisposing factors is mandatory, but specific topical anticandidal medications, such as nystatin, amphotericin, or the broader-spectrum clotrimazole, are also indicated and would be prescribed, as might be expected, in a water-washable or lotion base, never occlusive. The sexual partner of a patient with balanitis or vulvovaginitis should be alerted to the possibility of infection and treated if the patient's problem is slow to clear or recurrent. Vaginal suppositories of nystatin are available, as well as oral suspension for direct application to mouth lesions.

Candida albicans is usually the infecting species, but several others of the same genus, *Candida tropicalis,* for example, may be the agent under predisposing conditions, especially with paronychial infections. Since they are common organisms of the gastrointestinal tract, the chance for reinfection with *Candida* organisms is ever present. Precautions should include adequate cleansing and drying of the body folds routinely but especially after defecation, and the adding of an anticandidal preparation to any topical antibacterial medication that is to be used in the anogenital area. Neither nystatin nor amphotericin B is sufficiently absorbed from the gastrointestinal tract to be of value as systemic therapy; but taken orally, either agent will reduce the *Candida* population of the intestine. This may be indicated if topical control fails in the vulvovaginitis of *Candida*-induced pruritus among those on contraceptives or long-term antimicrobial therapy. Stubborn *Candida* infections respond well to the new oral antimicrobial agent ketoconazole, but risk of hepatotoxicity should limit its use to recalcitrant problems.

Despite the tendency to chronicity and recurrence, and despite the acute discomfort of the active infection, most candidiasis is responsive to therapy. Occasionally severe infection can have quite generalized erythematous crusting and be associated with horny excrescences on granulomatous bases. Labeled chronic mucocutaneous candidiasis, this intractable infection may appear at birth or early childhood and may be associated with endocrinopathy such as hypoparathyroidism, hypoadrenalism, and diabetes, or with congenital thymic disorders affecting lymphocyte function and cell-mediated immunity. There are data to suggest that chronic mucocutaneous candidiasis results from a deficiency of migration inhibitory factor or from the presence of an inhibitor to this factor or other mediator of delayed hypersensitivity. Despite endocrinopathy and the compromised immune status in the presence of severe extensive mucocutaneous infection, systemic candidiasis develops rarely—all the more surprising because in general medicine systemic manifestations of *Candida* infection are not that unusual.

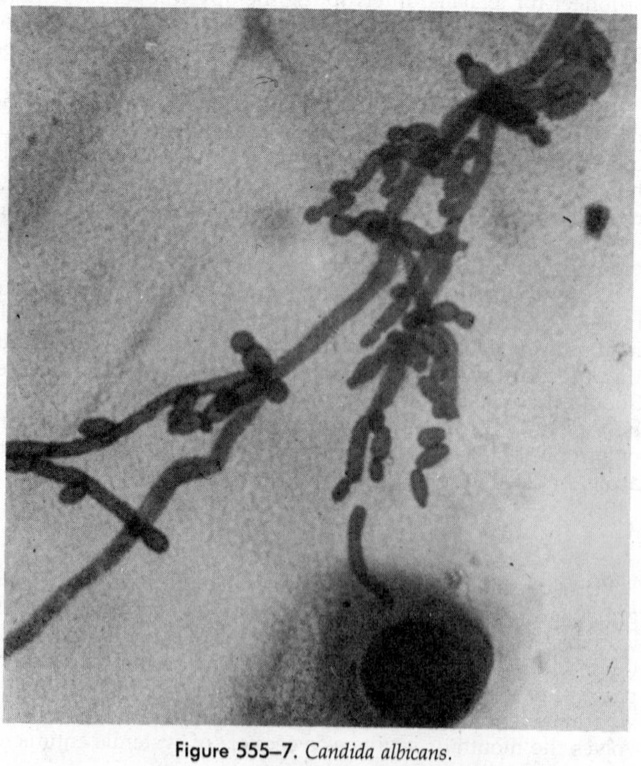

Figure 555–7. *Candida albicans.*

In systemic infection, bronchopulmonary and pulmonary candidiasis are the most common manifestations seen as complications of chronic primary pulmonary disease, especially in the diabetic or those on systemic corticosteroids or antimicrobial agents. Candidemia, with or without seeding, is a complication of surgery associated with prolonged use of indwelling catheters, and of those conditions requiring long-term therapy with immunosuppressive agents and antimetabolites.

Because of the frequent finding of *Candida* in and on the body, establishing *Candida* as a cause of a particular problem requires the demonstration of budding yeasts and filaments in the scraping or biopsy from the lesion in question (Fig. 555–7), a generous and repeated growth of the organism or culture, and a fit of the lesions to what might be anticipated for a *Candida* infection.

Dermatitis of the Hands and Feet

The problem of redness and scaling of the hands and feet can be exasperating to clinician and patient alike. Hands and feet have similar and sympathetic reaction patterns. A dermatitis on one may produce an "id" on the other. Both are subjected to trauma and both are exposed to abundant contactants, greater in variety on the hands perhaps, but greater in intensity on the feet in their enclosed pressure casings.

Thus far, a consideration of psoriasis and of fungus has included hands and feet, but the differential has not been extended for those from whom no fungus could be isolated and no stigmata of psoriasis identified. Erythema and scale of long standing, a chronic dermatitis, might mean a continuing contact dermatitis or the late manifestations of atopic dermatitis, or perhaps might be part of an ill-defined group of reaction patterns that are quite characteristic in their manifestations but of obscure etiology.

CONTACT DERMATITIS

Of all the dermatitides of the hands and feet, contact dermatitis is perhaps the most important. Irritants and allergic sensitizers commonly involve hands and feet. If the offending substance can be identified, avoidance or protection can restore a patient to normal. If the problem is ignored or the offender escapes detection and the dermatitis smolders, a chronicity is established that may totally disable the patient.

Any dermatitis that presents acutely with erythema and vesicles warrants intense restorative therapy and an undaunted search for the cause. Plants and airborne contactants can leave their linear vesicles or exposure pattern as a clue; the distribution in a hand or foot problem may not be that revealing. Nonetheless, history taking and patch testing may narrow the field. Screening trays are available to test to common allergens, to medications, to the components of shoes, and to cosmetics, and for every patient it is possible to test with the part of his own environment that is suspect, a part of the lining of a shoe, as an example. For hands rather than feet, photosensitivity may be checked to establish if the minimal erythema dose for the individual is lowered or if a photo-contact reaction can be demonstrated in association with medications or soaps.

If the offending irritant or allergen is identified, the source of the patient's exposure and other occult and unsuspected sources can be established to ensure protection. Fisher's text is the definitive reference for elaborating a suspected contact dermatitis and then sorting out the cross-reactions and tabulating where the allergen is to be found. Contact dermatitis placed first in prevalence among 75,000 consecutive visits to the Skin and Cancer Clinic of New York University. There were 11,100 visits for contact and an additional 4600 for chronic dermatitis of obscure etiology. The importance of recognition and identification cannot be overstated.

ATOPIC DERMATITIS

In that same pool of diagnoses atopic dermatitis placed seventh, a disease determined by heredity and characterized by a lower threshold to pruritus. With scratching, the skin becomes spongiotic and weeps, the eczematous form seen more often in the young. At any age rubbing can produce lichenification with accentuation of skin markings. Across the United States, 0.7 per cent of the population has this inherited diathesis of sufficient severity that a physician's consultation is warranted. Most cases contributing to the burden of the problem occur in infancy or childhood. After a period of quiescence from age two or three, it can recur in late childhood, in adolescence, or in early adult life, tending to localize in flexural areas of the neck, antecubital and popliteal folds, often about the eyelids, behind the ears, and at the wrists. Of those who are afflicted in adulthood, occasionally to the fifth decade, chronic hand and foot eczema is a common expression of the problem. At any age, a pruritic dermatitis in the "atopic distribution" should raise the possibility of the diagnosis. Such patients will have a personal history of atopic dermatitis and a personal or family history of atopy, asthma, hay fever, or perhaps urticaria, which is part of the complex but of more obscure relationship.

The atopic diathesis is manifest in the skin by a blanching response to injections of acetylcholine or methacholine, in contrast to normal skin in which vasodilatation results in erythema. The skin of the atopic has been shown to contain up to 60 times the concentration of acetylcholine of skin in nonatopic rashes, as well as an excess of cholinesterase. Sweat glands in the atopic have an increased sensitivity to acetylcholine rather like that produced by a partial beta receptor blockade. Atopic skin also differs from normal in its exquisite sensitivity to epinephrine and norepinephrine. In fact the "grainy" skin of patients with atopic dermatitis has been ascribed to a permanent state of piloerection mediated by norepinephrine.

The role of allergy in atopic dermatitis is not completely elaborated. Immediate urticarial reactions to skin tests with common antigens are frequently observed. The skin-sensitizing antibody can be transferred by serum to another subject and has been identified as a distinct immunoglobulin, IgE. Some patients with atopic dermatitis will have excessive serum levels of IgE but with little correlation between the serum level and the severity of the dermatitis. Further, high levels of IgE have been reported in nonatopic conditions. T-cell function is said to be deficient in atopic dermatitis, whether depressed by elevated IgE levels or de novo with the IgE rise in response to reacting B cells.

The major implications of these documented facts are that atopic skin responds to slight trauma with vasoconstriction and pruritus, leading to a weeping vesicular dermatitis acutely, and then more chronically to dry lichenified skin. Wet dressings, if indicated, will physically reduce erythema and weeping, and topical steroids and systemic antihistamines will alter the pruritus and inflammatory response. Dry or lichenified skin may suggest lubrication, but the inability to sweat may be aggravated by occlusive lubricants which, with retained heat, may increase pruritus. Should secondary pyogenic or fungal infection be present, specific therapy may be needed to control it. Restoring the integrity of the skin will thwart opportunistic organisms.

One major risk of atopic dermatitis derives from the depression of T-cell function which makes the patient more susceptible to widespread viral infection with vaccinia, herpes simplex, and, of less concern, molluscum contagiosum and verruca vulgaris. Even without active dermatitis, infection with herpes simplex can lead to a generalized vesicular eruption with high fever and significant mortality. With the control of variola, there is no longer a public health requirement for vaccination, which is absolutely contraindicated in the atopic patient and all close contacts. Protection from latent herpes simplex virus is not so easy to achieve.

Any acute flare in the dermatitis of an atopic should be inspected closely for vesicles. If they are present, to differentiate viral vesicles from the eczematous process of atopy, a Tzanck smear should be done in search of multinucleated giant cells indicative of viral infection. If such cells are found, the patient warrants close assessment and continued expectant observation. Widespread infection can occur; its severity will dictate therapy. Corticosteroids, topically and systemically, would be contraindicated because of the risk of viral dissemination, but all other topical therapy to promote resolution of the atopic dermatitis should be undertaken. Specific therapy with idoxuridine has not proved to be of much help with cutaneous infection. Acyclovir intravenously is effective and safe for the patient but should be used only if the severity of the problem warrants the risk of evoking resistant strains of herpes simplex virus, which are occurring with ever increasing frequency. Because contained viral infections can also occur in the atopic, all that may be needed is good supportive care.

Infection with the virus of verruca vulgaris or with molluscum contagiosum, even though generalized, merely requires a good topical regimen. Although some physicians would anesthetize and curette all lesions from the start, a trial of salicylic acid in flexible collodion or plaster, with self-peeling or paring by the patient, is less traumatic with less risk of scar. Destroying the epidermal cells in which the virus lives is all that is needed, but repetition and persistence are required to ensure extinction. The diagnosis of both these viral problems is usually obvious once one has seen a common verruca or an umbilicated shiny flesh-colored papule from which a core can be easily shelled. Both verruca vulgaris and molluscum contagiosum are seen most commonly in children, and both can be seen as venereal problems in young adults, but they are of greatest challenge and concern when widespread in the immunosuppressed patient or the atopic individual.

One further risk borne by the severe atopic is that of developing cataracts, which may be minimal or blinding. Occurring most frequently in the second and third decades, they are a serious complication of the atopic diathesis and may be further aggravated by corticosteroid therapy.

Canales L, Middlemas RO III, Louro JM, South MA: Immunological observations in chronic mucocutaneous candidiasis. Lancet 2:567, 1969. *Of interest for pedigree and for the focused study of an immune deficiency disease through the detailed assessment of one patient.*

Chilgren RA, Quie PG, Meuwissen HJ, Hong R: Chronic mucocutaneous candidiasis: Deficiency of delayed hypersensitivity, and selective local antibody defect. Lancet 2:688, 1977. *An update and further focus on delayed hypersensitivity.*

Farber EM, Cox AJ (eds.): Psoriasis: Proceedings of the Second International Symposium. New York, Yorke Medical Books, 1977. *The latest research and ruminations on psoriasis are published after each International Symposium.*

Fisher A: Contact Dermatitis. 2nd ed. Philadelphia, Lea & Febiger, 1973. *The cookbook for detecting the offending allergen in contact dermatitis.*

Fredriksson T, Petersson U: Severe psoriasis: Oral therapy with new retinoid. Dermatologica 157:238, 1978. *The dawn of a new era in the treatment of psoriasis.*

Montes LF, Pittman CS, Moore WJ, Taylor CG, Cooper MD: Chronic mucocutaneous candidiasis. JAMA 221:156, 1972. *The spontaneous clearing of resistant mucocutaneous candidiasis present from infancy after the detection and treatment of hypothyroidism at age seven is of interest for the implications for delayed hypersensitivity and anergy.*

556. SIGNIFICANT DERMATOLOGIC SIGNS OF DISEASE

In assessing the skin for pathology the diagnostic range extends to systemic implications of cutaneous signs. The integument nourished by blood with a markedly elevated bilirubin is a dramatic indicator of pathology. Because serologic tests can detect preclinical icterus, the clinical fact of jaundice loses its edge. However, there is an array of metabolic substances, abnormal or in excess of normal, that settle in the skin and await recognition. Lipids and amyloid are good examples. Pathologic processes such as vasculitis can affect both viscera and skin, and malignancy can extend or metastasize to both. There are also physiologic symptoms of pruritus or weakness and skin changes of ichthyosis or weeping dermatitis that relate to occult malignancy and respond to therapy directed at the malignancy. But most curious of all are the congenital aberrations and pigmentary hallmarks associated with specific systemic disease in an established but obscure relationship.

The purpose of the present chapter is to review these various skin stigmata so that they may be identified by the examiner, providing him with some broad indications of the kinds of problems with which they may be associated. Then, grouped with a special organ system as the key, selected skin signs are tabulated and ranked for potential value in suspecting or establishing a diagnosis (see Tables 556–4 to 556–7).

Acanthosis Nigricans

A brown-black velvety skin change, verrucous and creased, and localized in the axillae, nuchal folds, or groin is readily recognized as acanthosis nigricans (Fig. 556–1). Blending into normal adjacent skin, it is characteristically bilateral and symmetrical. Affecting any body fold and favoring flexural surfaces, it may rarely be generalized. Histologically there is epidermal thickening and folding over a hypertrophic papillary layer. Because acanthosis nigricans can occur with malignancy, with hormonal dysfunction, or as an inherited disorder, it is a clinical sign of note; yet neither the clinical nor the histologic appearance helps in the differential diagnosis of associated pathology.

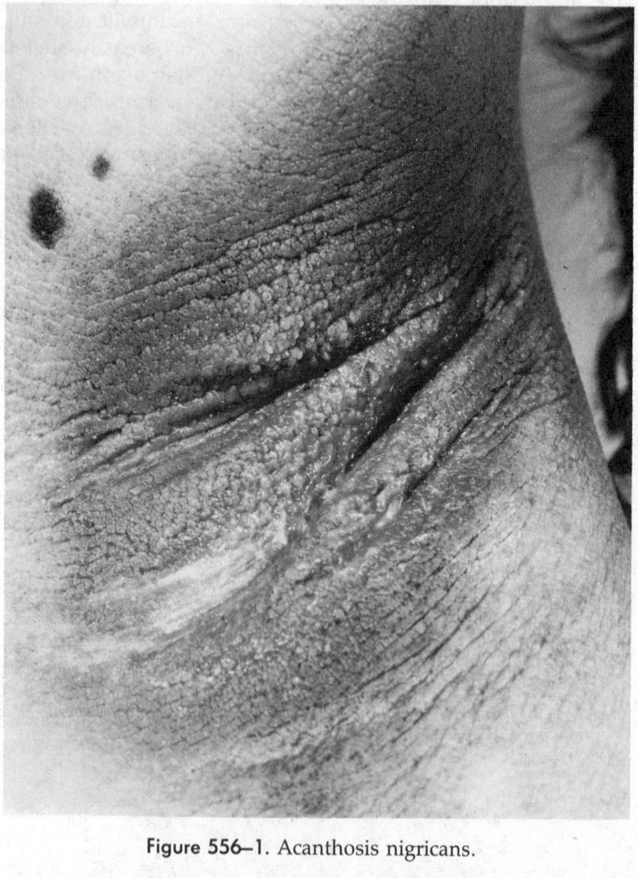

Figure 556–1. Acanthosis nigricans.

When found with visceral malignancy, usually an adenocarcinoma, the acanthosis nigricans has been labeled "malignant," a poor choice of terminology, for the skin change is in no way malignant.

Unassociated with malignancy, acanthosis nigricans is found with developmental, hormonal, and metabolic pathology, and after the administration of certain drugs and hormonal agents. In the inherited form benign cutaneous changes are considered nevoid genodermatoses present from birth or childhood with the possibility of spread or intensification at puberty. In the juvenile idiopathic type with cushingoid obesity, the onset is frequently at puberty. Acanthosis nigricans is found with adrenal insufficiency, Cushing's syndrome, acromegaly, Stein-Leventhal syndrome, and various pituitary and hypothalamic tumors or other lesions involving the base of the brain. It has been postulated that a pituitary peptide hormone secreted under hypothalamic control may stimulate papillary dermal hypertrophy. Crude preparations of MSH have been shown to induce acanthosis nigricans in a patient with melanoma, with MSH-like peptides the most likely agent. Diethylstilbestrol, corticosteroids, and nicotinic acid have also been implicated in the cutaneous phenomenon, and there are reports of appearance and disappearance correlated with the use of oral contraceptives. In insulin-resistant diabetes associated acanthosis nigricans tends to remit as the glucose intolerance lessens. Correlation is made with the antibody titer to insulin receptors.

Although there is no local therapy for acanthosis nigricans, the early recognition of the cutaneous sign, especially in the adult, warrants an immediate and thorough search for underlying pathology, especially tumor. The associated malignancies tend to be aggressive and rapidly fatal. Extension of the acanthosis nigricans is an ominous sign.

Banuchi SR, Cohen L, Lorinca AL, Morgan J: Acanthosis nigricans following diethylstilbestrol therapy: Occurrence in patients with childhood muscular dystrophy. Arch Dermatol 109:545, 1974. *Development of acanthosis nigricans in two of six children receiving diethylstilbestrol for childhood muscular dystrophy brings into question the role of estrogens in this uncommon disorder.*

Givens JR, Kerber IJ, Wiser WL, Andersen RN, Coleman SA, Fish SA: Remission of acanthosis nigricans associated with polycystic ovarian disease and a stromal luteoma. J Clin Endocrinol Metab 38:347, 1974. *The study of a case in which the suppression of luteinizing hormone and the hyperandrogenism associated with improvement of the acanthosis nigricans is important in light of the above.*

Kahn CR, Flier JS, Bar RS, Archer JA, Gorden P, Martin MM, Roth J: Syndromes of insulin resistance and acanthosis nigricans: Insulin receptor disorders in man. N Engl J Med 294:739, 1976. *Another link of hormonal abnormalities and circulating antibodies to acanthosis nigricans.*

Lerner AB: On the cause of acanthosis nigricans. N Engl J Med 281:706, 1969. *Hypothesizes that acanthosis nigricans is caused by the release of a peptide from either the pituitary gland or a nonpituitary neoplasm.*

Nordlund JJ, Lerner AB: Cause of acanthosis nigricans (letter). N Engl J Med 293:200, 1975. *Proof of the hypothesis cited above was demonstrated in a patient with melanoma.*

Ichthyosis

An integument that is rough and dry with retained scale but free of erythema suggests a "fish skin" designation (Fig. 556–2). On close inspection there may be fine scale with keratin-plugged follicles, or large polyhedral scales loosely adherent. The palms and soles may be normal, or may be thickened with accentuation of normal creases.

INHERITED. If the condition has been present from birth or childhood, perhaps only clinically apparent in dry winter months, the diagnosis is likely to be one of the *ichthyosiform dermatoses,* an inherited disorder in which excessive amounts of keratin are retained at the skin surface. Through an analysis of clinical and anatomic findings as well as a consideration of the cellular kinetics and genetic aspects, distinctions are made among the four more common types, of which ichthyosis vulgaris is the most common (Table 556–1). These ichthyoses

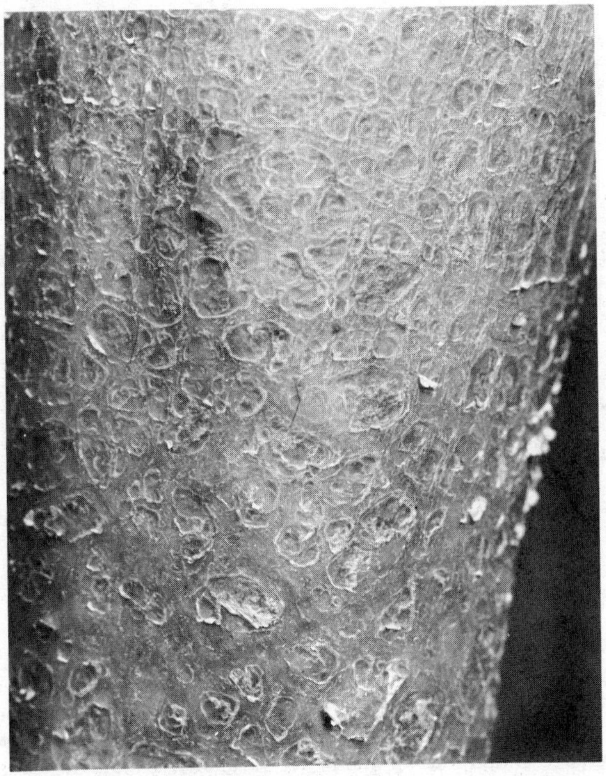

Figure 556–2. Ichthyosis.

are important to be recognized for what they are and to be differentiated from the ichthyosis-like dermatoses of abnormal lipid metabolism and the acquired ichthyosis of malignancy. Recently a biochemical deficiency of steroid sulfatase and aryl sulfatase C has been found underlying X-linked ichthyosis.

METABOLIC. Except for an inherited metabolic disorder as in Refsum's disease, the ichthyosis of abnormal lipid metabolism will appear later in life and be associated temporally with a drug that inhibits lipid synthesis, such as the butyrophenones or triparanol. So too, the dryness and scale of hypothyroidism, which may have a yellow cast because of carotenemia; it will appear with the disease and be supported by laboratory evidence of decreased thyroid function.

MALIGNANCY. The onset of ichthyosis in an adult without drug inducement or metabolic disorder is of grave significance, suggesting an underlying malignant process. Hodgkin's disease is found most frequently, but also other lymphomas, multiple myeloma, and carcinoma of the breast. As with *acanthosis nigricans*, the regression and recurrence of the tumor may be reflected in the activity of the dermatosis.

For those attuned to this significant cutaneous sign, the question of possible malignancy is often raised when the observation is of minimal dryness and polyhedral scale over the legs, arms, or abdomen of the older patient. Winter dryness at any age, but especially in the lipid-deprived skin of the elderly, is prone to pruritus and ichthyosiform change. If the problem is mild, limited, and historically of long standing or winter occurrence, the dermatosis observed is probably not a sign of tumor and should respond to simple lubrication. More intensive therapy would be to increase environmental moisture and free retained keratin with special lubricants, especially those containing urea, 15 to 30 per cent.

Frost P, Van Scott EJ: The ichthyosiform dermatoses. Classification based on anatomical and cellular kinetic observations. Arch Dermatol 94:113, 1966. *A classic sorting among recognized dermatological entities to separate and group by clinical and histologic data as well as cellular kinetics.*

Steinberg D, Vroom FQ, Engel WK, Cammermeyer J, Mize CE, Avigan J: Refsum's disease—a recently characterized lipoidosis involving the nervous system. Combined Clinical Staff Conference at the NIH. Ann Intern Med 66:365, 1967. *Although Refsum's disease is a rare inherited syndrome, it underscores the association of ichthyosis with multiple congenital ectodermal defects and a disturbance of lipid metabolism.*

Acquired Erythrodermas

ICHTHYOSIFORM

Generalized dryness and scaling with erythema in a universal distribution may be total body psoriasis. The plaque-like quality of the lesions is no longer discerned, but nail stigmata and severe scalp involvement, as well as an antecedent diagnosis of psoriasis, may aid the differential. An explosive ichthyosiform erythroderma may be a manifestation of mycosis fungoides (see Ch. 557.5).

Localized ichthyosiform or psoriasiform erythroderma may be of equal significance. *Bowen's disease*, a sharply demarcated red-brown plaque moderately thickened with scale, loose or adherent, is sometimes misdiagnosed as psoriasis. It commonly occurs on covered areas of the body, and since it can be a sequela of arsenic ingestion, patients treated in the past with Fowler's solution for psoriasis may have both psoriasis and Bowen's disease. They may also have the stigmata of arseniasis: arsenical keratoses, discrete hyperkeratotic papules of the palms and soles, plus the raindrop hyperpigmentation over the thorax. Bowen's disease is a cutaneous premalignancy, and the diagnosis can be established by biopsy. Although most Bowen's disease remains as intraepidermal carcinoma in situ for many years, it may transform into invasive squamous cell carcinoma. Any unremitting erythematous scaling lesion of long duration, especially if slowly enlarging, should be regarded with suspicion.

PAGET'S DISEASE

Paget's disease is another example. A sharply defined plaque of erythema, often eczematous with crusting or even erosion, it can be psoriasiform. Classically of the breast, it involves the nipple and areola unilaterally, perhaps only a portion, and is associated with underlying malignancy, most often a ductal adenocarcinoma. It appears usually, but not exclusively, in women; the mean age is 55 years. Extramammary Paget's disease, frequently of the anogenital area, occurs in both sexes at about the same age, but more often in women. It is without the invariable association of malignancy, which is found in less than half the patients. The malignancies that do occur derive most often from cutaneous apocrine structures.

Histologically Paget cells lie within the epidermis. Large round cells with large nuclei and abundant cytoplasm, they can be confused with nevus cells and those of Bowen's disease, although mucin stains are helpful in the differential. The histopathology is definitive and underscores the importance of biopsy for any persistent psoriasiform or eczematous lesion anywhere, but especially of the breast. In the patient with skin that is otherwise normal, the lesion of Paget's disease is obvious

TABLE 556–1. COMMON ICHTHYOSIFORM DERMATOSES

	Inheritance	Onset	Distribution	Clinical Associations	Kinetics
Lamellar ichthyosis	Autosomal recessive	Birth	Body, palms, soles	Ectropion	Increased
Epidermolytic hyperkeratosis	Autosomal dominant	Birth	Predominant flexural involvement	Blisters	Increased
X-linked ichthyosis (steroid sulfatase deficiency)	X-linked	Birth	Trunk	Corneal opacities	Normal
Ichthyosis vulgaris	Autosomal dominant	Childhood	Spares flexural areas	Atopy	Normal

and the course clear. It is the patient with other psoriasiform and eczematous dermatitis who is at risk of having Paget's disease overlooked. Any suspicious lesion of the areola should be treated intensively for a week or two with high potency steroid; if the skin does not return to normal, the lesion should be biopsied.

ACRODERMATITIS ENTEROPATHICA

This condition is occasionally misdiagnosed as psoriasis, and more often as candidiasis because of periorificial dermatitis, but it can present with reddened ichthyosiform plaques. It is a persistent dermatitis about the mouth, with acral involvement that begins as vesicles but is soon crusted, thickened, and perhaps superinfected with bacteria or *Candida,* and may be associated with diarrhea. The symptoms are due to zinc deficiency and are seen when there is hyperalimentation without attention to trace metal supplements in the course of malabsorptive disorders, but the disorder is of greater interest as an inherited defect. With its onset in childhood and poor prognosis without therapy, the adult form of acrodermatitis enteropathica, even if not controlled, will have been identified. Two thirds of patients have a family history of the disease, and an autosomal recessive inheritance is suggested. The affected children tend to be slow in growth and development, and to have a deficiency in cell-mediated immunity. They are reported to have increased IgA and deficient or "absent" thymus, and to lack germinal centers and plasmacytosis of lymph nodes and spleen. In the bowel, in the fasting state, jejunal cytoplasmic inclusions are found by electron microscopy. Plasma zinc levels are low, but also decreased are serum lipids and arachidonic acid. Prostaglandin synthesis is defective. Zinc supplements will dramatically reverse all clinical manifestations of the disease within a few days, even in adult patients plagued with the disease from childhood. Abnormalities of the intestinal mucosa were noted to revert to normal on oral zinc therapy.

Although it is not clear that the defect in zinc uptake is the primary lesion, prostaglandin "zinc-binding ligand" is necessary for zinc absorption. Aspirin, which inhibits prostaglandin synthesis, impairs zinc absorption in rats. Arachidonic acid, decreased in acrodermatitis enteropathica, is known to be a prostaglandin precursor. There is the further evidence of clinical benefit from a dietary supplement of zinc or prostaglandin. Curiously, human milk has PGE_2 as a zinc ligand; cow's milk has none, fitting the frequently observed onset of the disease at weaning. Because calcium ingestion can impede zinc absorption in the gastrointestinal tract, as can soy milk protein, the prescribing of zinc supplements should include precautions about calcium, soy proteins, and aspirin.

Evans GW, Johnson PE: Defective prostaglandin synthesis in acrodermatitis enteropathica (letter). Lancet 1:52, 1977. *A succinct assessment of the recognized role of zinc and prostaglandin in acrodermatitis enteropathica, the report of the isolation of a low-molecular weight zinc binding ligand from human milk, and the neat conclusion that the zinc-prostaglandin complex in human milk explains the observed clinical efficacy of human breast milk in the treatment of acrodermatitis enteropathica.*

Hirsch FS, Michel B, Strain WH: Gluconate zinc in acrodermatitis enteropathica. Arch Dermatol 112:475, 1976. *From clinical observations of two patients much is deduced about the effectiveness and best use of gluconate zinc.*

Kelly R, Davidson GP, Townley RRW, Campbell PE: Reversible intestinal mucosal abnormality in acrodermatitis enteropathica. Arch Dis Child 51:219, 1976. *The reassurance of the documented reversibility of the pathology of the intestinal mucosa was an important impetus to further the search for more effective therapy.*

Michaelson G: Zinc therapy in acrodermatitis enteropathica. Acta Derm Venereol 54:377, 1974. *The search is always for the cause, but without finding it the course may be altered. After 18 years of difficult and discouraging management of acrodermatitis enteropathica, an observed low serum zinc value suggested treatment with zinc sulfate with prompt and impressive good results.*

EXFOLIATIVE ERYTHRODERMA

When the skin is normal rather than thickened but generally red with fine scale, the term exfoliative erythroderma (Fig. 556–3) is used. It can be the eventuality of any extensive eruption; when seen, of itself, it gives few clues to the etiology. Drug allergy, contact dermatitis, an eczematous process, seborrheic dermatitis or psoriasis, the lymphomas and leukemias, or any extensive inflammatory insult to the skin may be the cause. Older patients are more predisposed to the phenomenon, and it is most difficult to clear in them; it may smolder for months or years.

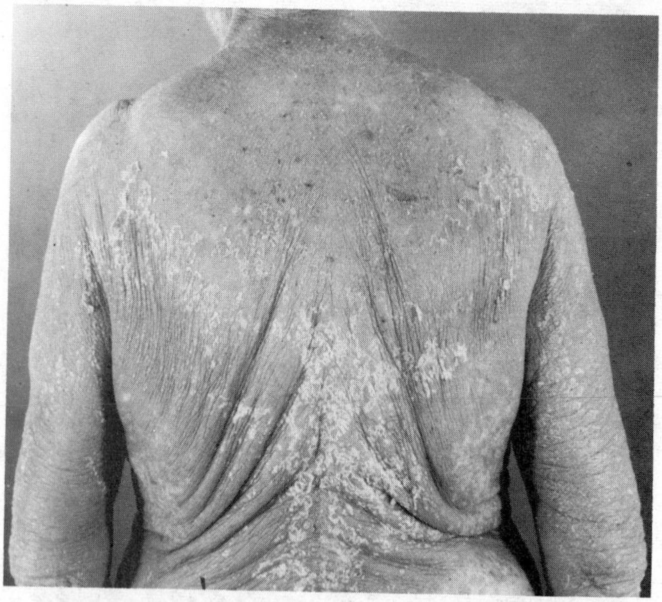

Figure 556–3. Exfoliative erythroderma.

The best treatment is prevention. Any acute dermatitis of whatever etiology should be quieted with wet dressings and topical steroids, with antihistamines or other sedation, and with rest. The specific cause should be sought, although it may remain obscure. If the eruption continues to progress, systemic steroids or immune suppression should be considered. If generalized exfoliation has occurred, initial efforts should be conservative and supportive, but systemic therapy will probably be needed.

PHOTOSENSITIVITY

The skin of the normal individual will react to sunlight in a range of responses that are modified by pigmentary protection, geographic location, solar and solstice time, and duration of exposure. The data derived would be a base line of normal and predictable responses, however varied or unpleasant, from no reaction through erythema to blistering; cumulatively one could anticipate actinic damage (see Ch. 552) and malignancy (see Ch. 557). Here, however, consideration is given only to responses that deviate from the normal as modified by genetic, chemical, allergic, or nutritional factors.

The patient with an abnormal light reaction could present with an exaggerated sunburn in a patterned exposure with the outline of protective clothing, but more often there is merely the subtle sparing of the submental area of the chin or the eyelids, perhaps with accentuation at the "V" of the neck. Frequently the lesions are not as diffuse as a burn but are characterized by papules or urticaria, or even an eczematous response.

To sort out the etiology, light must be suspected from historical or physical evidence and from any recognized predisposition to sun sensitivity. Seasonal recurrences, especially in the spring or early summer, would arouse suspicion. The evoked reaction may be to light alone, to light in association with abnormal metabolites as in the porphyrias, or to light plus chemicals and medications applied to the skin or ingested.

Light Alone

Adverse reactions to light alone are rare and may all have a genetic predisposition. *Xeroderma pigmentosum,* for example, inherited as an autosomal recessive problem, has a defect in DNA repair or replication. The light-exposed skin undergoes severe early solar damage with erythema, spotty pigmentation, atrophy, and neoplasm. From infancy there is photophobia and a prolonged erythematous response to sun. In albinism, too, there is photophobia and increased sun sensitivity, but the skin, except for lacking the protective shield of pigment, is normal. Repair is normal. The defect in the tyrosinase function of the melanocyte leaves the albino with a sunburn susceptibility comparable to that of the lightest-complexioned Celt.

But more than an exaggerated response to sun damage, light alone can evoke a polymorphous light eruption. Common among certain North American Indians, and reported in families and identical twins, it is without indication of genetic factors in most patients. As the name polymorphous photodermatitis implies, the eruption is a mixture of papules and vesicles which may become confluent. It occurs at any age but usually has its onset in young adulthood with no evidence of sex predisposition or protection from melanin; it is seen in a range of patients of all races from the lightly to the heavily pigmented. Pursuing a chronic course, it flares each spring until some sun tolerance develops in summer. Selected sun protection and topical steroids are the mainstay of therapy.

Light Plus

METABOLITES. With the porphyrias, of which there are at least seven types, light reacts with circulating porphyrins present in the cutaneous tissue to produce both acute and chronic change. The onset of photosensitivity in childhood and the associated severe scarring, hair loss, and discolored teeth readily suggest the diagnosis of congenital erythropoietic porphyria. Even the milder symptoms of burning, edema, and waxy scars of congenital erythropoietic protoporphyria will suggest light as a damaging factor. The manifestations of photosensitivity in the adult onset porphyrias are more subtle, however. The appearance of skin fragility with bullae and erosions localized to the dorsa of the hands, possibly involving the forehead or scalp of the balding older patient, is frequently missed as a sign of porphyria cutanea tarda (Fig. 556–4). Such patients excrete urinary uroporphyrins and some coproporphyrins and

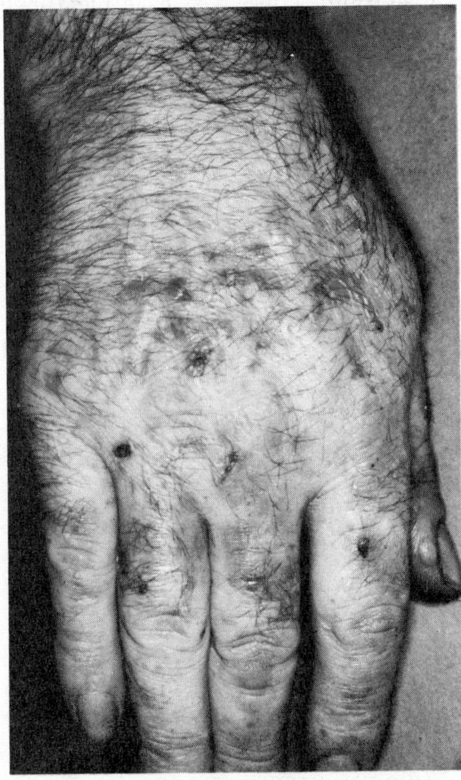

Figure 556–4. Porphyria cutanea tarda.

can be shown to be photosensitive to those wavelengths of light which the porphyrin molecule absorbs best: 400 to 410 nm in the blue-violet region, and 500 to 600 nm in the orange. Their sun-exposed skin becomes prematurely aged, with associated hypertrichosis characteristically found at the outer canthus of the eyes. Therapy by phlebotomy to reduce hepatic iron stores and porphyrin production, and the use of sun screens to filter out the damaging light rays give most patients with acquired porphyria sustained remissions from the dermatologic manifestations of the disease.

Photosensitivity is also observed with the aminoacidurias. In Hartnup disease, for example, in which there is a transport defect of tryptophan, with hydroxykynureninuria and tryptophanuria, minimal exposure to sun can lead to erythema, edema, and even vesiculation. At least for Hartnup disease, the eruption is associated with a cellular deficiency of nicotinamide. As in nutritional pellagra, high doses of nicotinamide improve the dermatitis. The observation that patients deficient in nicotinamide excrete increased amounts of certain porphyrins and indican has led to the suggestion for all these photosensitivity responses that sunlight induces photochemical reactions in the skin that lead to tissue destruction and antigen formation.

EXOGENOUS AGENTS. Of even greater diagnostic challenge are the many phototoxic and photoallergic reactions encountered. *Phototoxicity* occurs without recognized immune mechanisms. It is the kind of reaction seen in patients receiving systemic antimicrobial therapy such as Declomycin or sulfonamides; dyes such as acridine, methyl violet, or eosin; psychotherapeutic drugs such as phenothiazine; the sulfonylurea hypoglycemic agents; the thiazide diuretics; and the antifungal agent griseofulvin. Upon exposure to light there is burning, followed by prompt erythema and edema reaching a maximum intensity in 12 to 24 hours, and then by desquamation and hyperpigmentation. The initial reaction is common to a large number of people upon first exposure. The sensitivity will not persist, and future exposure to ultraviolet light will be normal.

Photoallergy differs in that reactions, although occasionally prompt and urticarial, can appear after 24 hours or more. They occur in only a small number of exposed individuals, are often persistent, and show cross-photosensitization; with photo patch testing there may be flares at previous reaction sites. Few oral ingestants contribute to the phenomenon, although sulfanilamide, sulfadiazine, and sulfisoxazole have been implicated as being both phototoxic and photoallergic. The bulk of photoallergy is through topical exposure, whether airborne or applied, and such reactions should be known as *photoallergic contact dermatitis.* It is postulated that light acts upon the offending chemical to form a haptene that binds protein, accounting for persistence and recurrence.

Therapy for all photodermatitis is the treatment for burn and contact dermatitis. With phototoxicity, if there is merely marked erythema, or if the reaction is noted early, topical steroids with occlusion will encourage vasoconstriction and reduce the overall intensity of the reaction. With photoallergy antihistamine may be helpful. Whether phototoxic or photoallergic, the offending agent must be sought to be identified and avoided, along with its cross-reactants.

Brodthager H: Polymorphous light eruption. *In* Urbach F (ed.): The Biologic Effects of Ultraviolet Radiation. Oxford, Pergamon Press, 1969. *A review of the physical effects of ultraviolet light.*

Cleaver JE: Defective repair replication of DNA in xeroderma pigmentosum. Nature 218:652, 1968. *The problem of radiation-induced malignancy came into sharper focus with the demonstration of a defect in DNA repair replication by fibroblasts from patients with xeroderma pigmentosum.*

Cleaver JE: Xeroderma pigmentosum: Variants with normal DNA repair and normal sensitivity to ultraviolet light. J Invest Dermatol 58:124, 1972. *Following the above, however, the reporting of variants of xeroderma pigmentosum, with the classic predisposition to cutaneous malignancy but with fibroblasts indistinguishable from normal cells in repair replication, would caution against inferences about DNA repair and carcinogenesis.*

Urbach F, Davies RE, Forbes PD: Ultraviolet radiation and skin cancer in man. *In* Montagna W (ed.): Advances in Biology of Skin Carcinogenesis. Oxford, Pergamon Press, 1966. *The basics for ultraviolet radiation and cutaneous malignancy in man.*

Light-Sensitive Diseases

Lupus erythematosus, known for its photosensitivity, is characterized by the isomorphic response whereby exposure to sunlight will evoke lesions of lupus erythematosus in the skin. In the patient with recognized disease the untoward response will be accepted and skin lesions, however mildly erythematous or urticarial, will be clinically identified as the disease. In a patient without antecedent diagnosis, however, an urticarial response to sunlight may be overlooked as a first manifestation of a collagen disease. Persistence of the hive, bluing of the erythema, development of scale, and follicular plugging should suggest the diagnosis, and histopathologic evidence should support it.

Pigmentary Disturbances

Color changes in the skin and mucous membrane are common and occasionally important. The wide range of normal hues and markings that racial diversity confers makes it necessary to review continuously the full array of normal possibilities through attention to the multiple banal lesions in every patient examined.

Melanin contributes significantly to the color of eyes, hair, and skin. It is most conspicuous in its heavy concentration or total absence. Brown to black eumelanin is a high molecular weight, relatively insoluble polymer, a polyquinone. In man it is derived from the phenolic precursors tyrosine and 3,4-dihydroxyphenylalanine (dopa). Tyrosinase, a copper-containing enzyme, catalyzes the oxidation of tyrosine in the cytoplasm of the melanocyte. Formed melanin is then transferred to keratinocytes; thus skin color derives from pigment in the epidermal cells as well as the melanocytes. When deep in the skin, melanin can appear blue or slate colored because of light scatter of the Tyndall effect.

Although melanocyte distribution is varied throughout the body, with twice higher concentrations in the skin of the head and forearms than in the rest of the skin (excepting the scrotum and foreskin), there are no differences in distribution or total numbers among races. Genotypic variations that underlie racial differences are within the ultrastructure of the melanocyte relating to the production and distribution of melanosomes following ultraviolet light irradiation or other stimulation. In situations in which generalized pigmentation is induced, the pigment pattern will reflect the melanocyte concentration.

HYPERPIGMENTATION

Ephelides

Increased concentrations of melanin may be localized or diffuse. The circumscribed melanoses commonly observed include *ephelides* or freckles, the small flat macules of less than 0.5 cm that first appear on sun-exposed areas at about age four and tend to fade in later life. Long wave ultraviolet light, 300 to 400 nm, will darken them. The melanocytes of ephelides are not increased in number but are more arborized and more active in melanin production.

Lentigines

These small flat macular lesions resemble ephelides clinically but are histologically distinct because of increased numbers of normal-appearing melanocytes. Evoked by aging and solar damage, they come in later life—so-called "liver spots," the *senile lentigo.*

A separate group unrelated to light, in fact occasionally involving mucous membranes, appearing at any age and genetically determined, is the *nevoid lentigines.* Associated with inherited syndromes such as the "leopard" syndrome and Moynihan's syndrome, they are present from birth and are found with a wide range of defects and mental retardation. In Peutz-Jeghers syndrome, the perioral mucous membrane and digital lentigines are associated with small bowel polyps, especially of the jejunum. These histologically distinct hamartomas arising from the muscularis mucosae have little malignant propensity in the small bowel, but when also present in the colon the risk of malignancy is increased.

Freckles of the axillae, especially when seen with irregular hyperpigmented mottling of the skin elsewhere, are known as Crowe's sign of neurofibromatosis. The pigment changes are believed to be a variant of café-au-lait spots, the large tan uniformly pigmented macules that may be present at birth anywhere on the skin or may appear later. Café-au-lait spots larger than 1.5 cm and more numerous than six are suggested as presumptive evidence of neurofibromatosis. They are also seen in other neurocutaneous syndromes such as tuberous sclerosis. In Albright's syndrome the circumscribed hypermelanotic macules may appear in a linear, rarely segmental pattern on one side or the other without crossing the midline. They occur on the forehead, nuchal and sacral areas, and buttocks. Their distribution rather than their clinical appearance or histology distinguishes them from the café-au-lait lesions of neurofibromatosis.

Pigmented Nevi

Pigmented nevi, often called moles, are formed of clusters of melanocytes and are rarely present from birth. They are divided clinically and histologically into four groups: the nevus spilus, and junctional, compound, and dermal nevi or moles. The nevus spilus (Fig. 556–5) is a small oval macule from tan to dark brown or black, usually of uniform color. Hyperpigmentation of the keratinocyte is intense, and there may be elongation of the rete ridges. The melanocytes are normal, not nested. Histologic differentiation is also used for the further classification of the moles or nevi, often called nevus cell nevi to distinguish them from the epidermal and connective tissue nevi. Junctional nevi have nevus cell nests above the basement membrane, compound nevi have them in both the epidermis and dermis, and intradermal nevi have them in the dermis

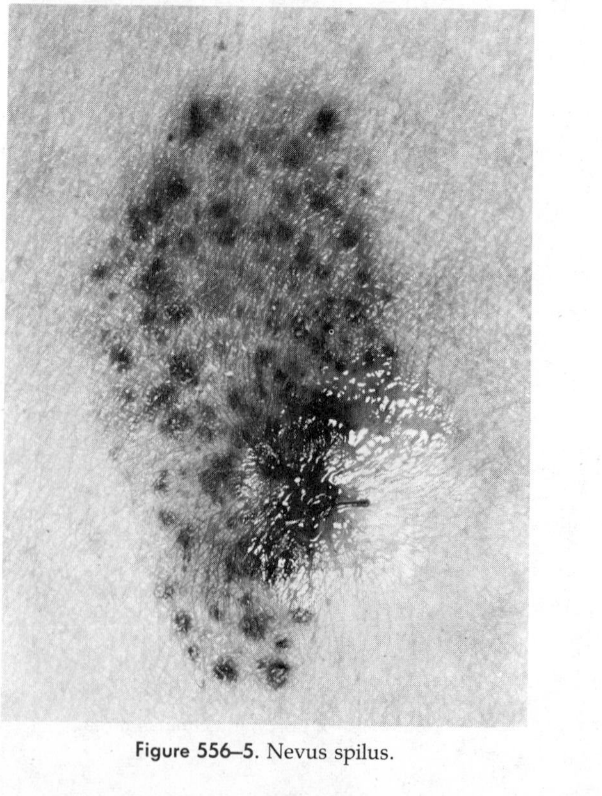

Figure 556–5. Nevus spilus.

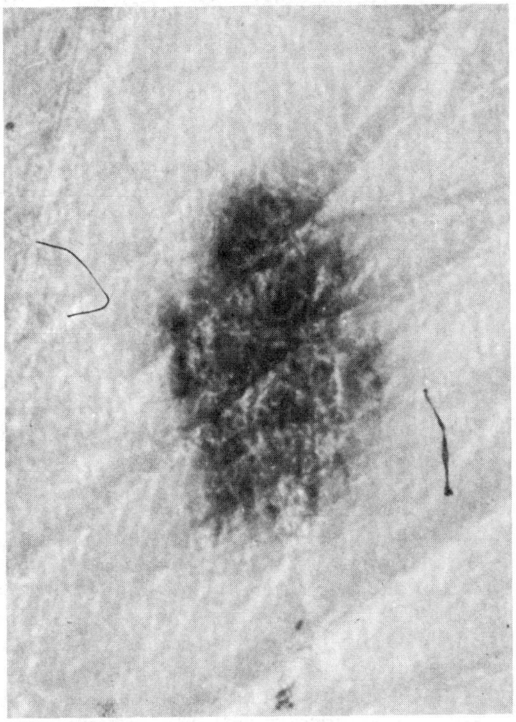

Figure 556–6. Junctional nevus.

alone. Junctional nevi tend to be flat and pigmented, dark brown to black, with the pigment orderly and the skin markings preserved (Fig. 556–6). Compound and intradermal nevi (Fig. 556–7) may be dome shaped, polypoid, or even verrucoid. They may be deeply pigmented but mostly are light or even skin colored.

Occasionally a depigmented area may develop around a nevus cell nevus, sometimes with eventual obliteration of the nevus. Occurring primarily in children and young adults, the *"halo nevus"* has been associated with vitiligo and noted in melanoma.

Not nevi but sometimes confused with them are *seborrheic keratoses,* the benign keratotic tumor of aging. Their distribution, growth, and depth of pigment are sunlight related, and their numbers can be legion. Beginning as yellow to light brown flat lesions with a verrucous or velvety surface, they can develop from less than 1 cm to several centimeters, become dark brown with a greasy keratotic scale, and assume a "tacked on" appearance.

Their importance is in differentiating them from nevi or not overlooking a changing nevus among them; also, they have been reported in their explosive appearance or sudden enlargement to be associated with underlying malignancy (the sign of Leser-Trélat).

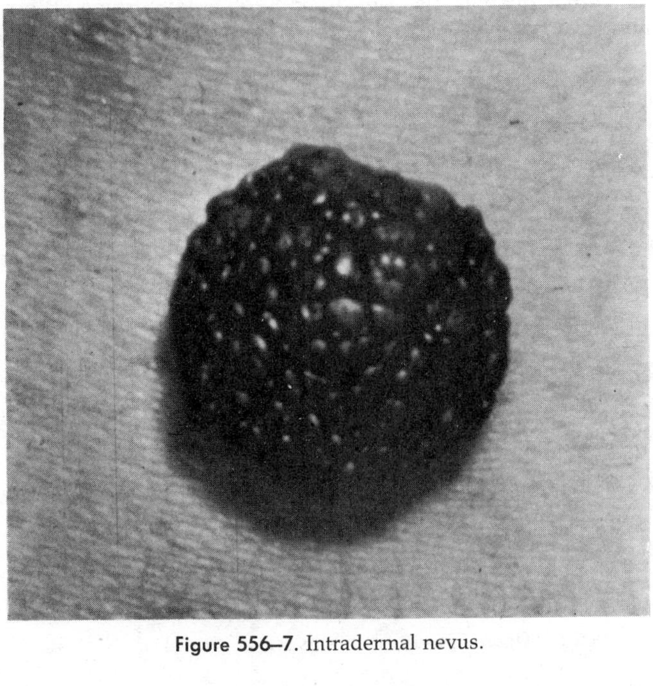

Figure 556–7. Intradermal nevus.

Pigment in Patterns

Whorls of pigmentation, zebra stripes, and angular flecks and sprays, occurring in no known neural or anatomic configuration and crossing the midline, should suggest *incontinentia pigmenti* (Fig. 556–8). The macules are dark brown or slate colored and intensely pigmented in childhood. With gradual fading they leave few dermatologic residua in later adult life. However, the patterned pigmentation should warn the examiner of the possibility of ectodermal defects and the need for genetic counseling. Although incontinentia pigmenti is of unknown etiology, the evidence suggests genetic transmission of the disease as an autosomal dominant with expression mainly in females or as an X-linked trait lethal for males. It presents with an inflammatory vesicobullous phase with little or no pigment change, and evolves either through a verrucous papillomatous phase or directly to the distinctive pigmentation. One or more of the stages may be present at birth or may begin in the first weeks of life. Despite the extent of the inflammatory lesion, the patient is afebrile. There may be pronounced eosinophilia of the blood and vesicle fluid.

The importance of recognizing the pigmentary stigma is the identification of a significant genodermatosis and the association of the diagnosis with other ectodermal abnormalities in 60 per cent of patients. Eyes, teeth, central nervous system, and cutaneous appendages are affected. Eye problems include strabismus, nystagmus, blue sclerae, optic atrophy, exudative chorioretinitis, papillitis, congenital retinal folds, and retrobulbar glioma. With the dental abnormalities, permanent dentition is compromised. There are impacted and missing teeth, pegged

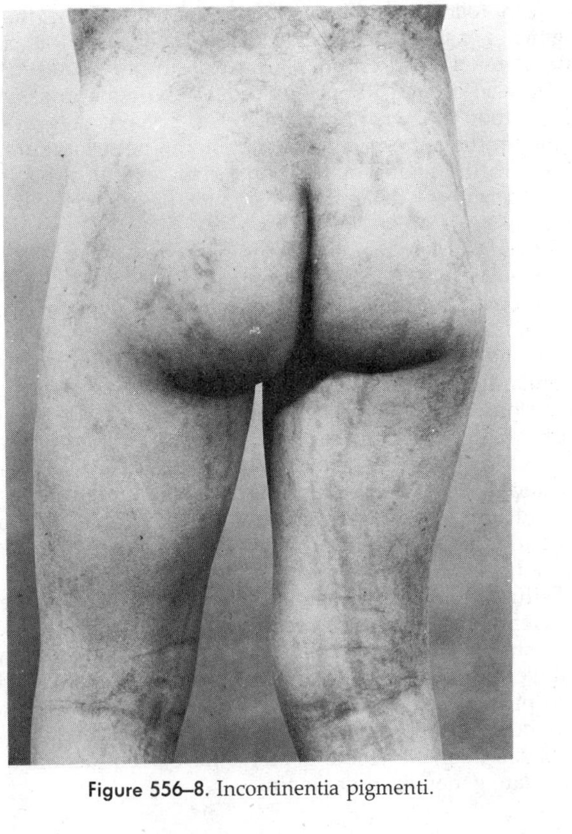

Figure 556–8. Incontinentia pigmenti.

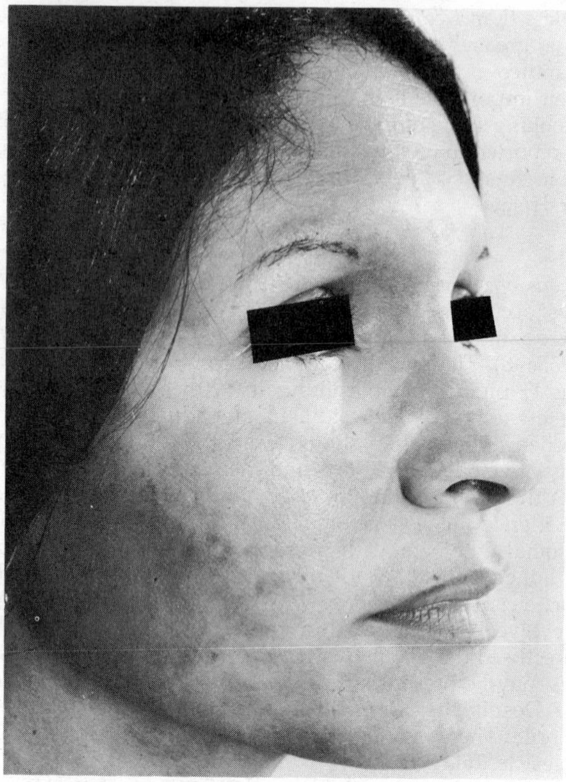

Figure 556–9. Melasma.

teeth, and malformed crowns. Neurologically, seizures and spastic paralysis are seen, and there may be mental retardation, deafness, and homonymous hemianopsia. Occasionally there are cardiac abnormalities and skeletal deformities, including syndactyly and shortened extremities.

Other Hyperpigmentations

Blotchy pigmentation of the skin without discrete lesions may be seen following inflammation, especially if the individual pigments easily. Thus it may follow trauma such as cuts and burns, generalized eruptions, or exposure to photosensitizers. It can also occur without antecedent erythema in a mask-like distribution known as *melasma* (Fig. 556–9). Aggravated by sunlight, the patterned pigmentation can be seen in pregnancy and with the taking of oral contraceptives, but it is also seen in men without laboratory evidence of abnormal hormonal levels.

Generalized hyperpigmentation is often associated with abnormalities of the endocrine system but can also be related to nutritional, metabolic, or chemical factors and to drugs. In primary adrenocortical insufficiency the pituitary activity increases in response to the decreased cortisol. With melanocyte-stimulating hormone (MSH) elaborated in excess by the pituitary along with the corticotropin (ACTH), there is consequent darkening of the skin. An MSH-producing tumor of the pituitary would have the same effect. If increased ACTH were also produced, the stimulation of the adrenal might make the initial clinical impression that of Cushing's syndrome. Without appreciation for the central lesions the adrenals might be removed.

Diffuse melanosis is seen in the cachectic and with metabolic problems such as hemochromatosis and biliary cirrhosis. It has been noted with inorganic arsenical poisoning and with a number of drugs, including busulfan and long-term high dose chlorpromazine. In malignancies such as melanoma, melanin may be deposited directly in the dermis. With certain tumors, as of the lung, MSH-like peptides have been identified which stimulate generalized darkening.

HYPOPIGMENTATION

Localized

In assessing a circumscribed area of leukoderma, the distinction between hypomelanosis and amelanosis is crucial and should be confirmed by Wood's light examination, which shows the amelanotic lesion as ivory white. If by historical data it can be determined that normal amounts of pigment were never present in the lesion, a developmentally determined nevoid lesion is suggested as distinct from the progressive pigmentary losses of varying cause.

Tuberous Sclerosis

A polygonal hypomelanosis, an ovoid lesion rounded at one end and tapered at the other like the leaf of a mountain ash, is seen from birth in 85 per cent of patients with tuberous sclerosis (Fig. 556–10). Found in the skin over trunk and limbs, the lesions range in size from a few millimeters to several centimeters. They appear before the other skin signs and can be of signal value in the differential diagnosis of seizures. By age four, 90 per cent of patients will have developed *adenoma sebaceum*—actually angiofibromas without sebaceous gland involvement. Clinically these are red-pink nodules with a smooth surface found at the nasolabial folds, over the cheeks and chin, and occasionally on the forehead and scalp. In the lumbosacral area the shagreen patch, a circumscribed area of subepidermal fibrosis, is almost always found. Skin-colored and slightly raised, it resembles studded leather. The ungual fibromas, soft pink papules growing out from the nail bed, are the fourth skin sign of tuberous sclerosis and appear first at puberty. Intraoral fibromas are also seen, and there can be increased pigmentation as manifested in bronzing of the skin and café-au-lait macules.

Because the classic triad of tuberous sclerosis, the seizures, mental retardation, and adenoma sebaceum, is so emphasized, the importance of subtle signs pathognomonic of the diagnosis is sometimes ignored.

DEPIGMENTATION

Partial Albinism

Areas of amelanosis in otherwise normal skin have a limited differential diagnosis. In partial albinism or piebaldism, the lack of pigment is unchanged from birth with melanocytes absent in the white areas. It is inherited as a simple autosomal dominant; there is frequently an associated white forelock. In contrast with vitiligo, there are often normally pigmented macules in hypomelanotic areas. Piebaldism associated with perceptual deafness is considered Woolf's syndrome. When there is also lateral displacement of inner canthi and of lacrimal

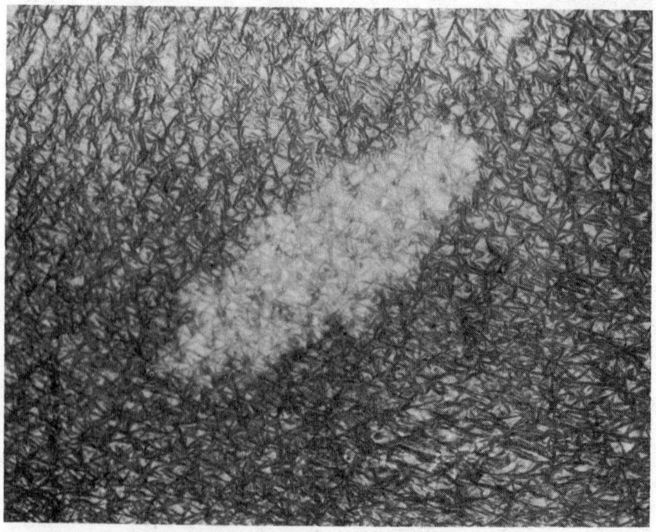

Figure 556–10. Tuberous sclerosis ash leaf.

puncta, prominence of the nasal root and the medial eyebrows, and heterochromic irides, it is considered Waardenburg's syndrome with a neural crest abnormality proposed as the cause.

Vitiligo

Vitiligo can be present from infancy but usually is not. Half the patients note the onset before the third decade. Pigment is lost in exposed areas, about body orifices, over pressure points, and from the axillae, genitalia, hair, and nevi (halo nevus). Occurring in 0.5 per cent of the population of the United States, vitiligo is inherited as an autosomal dominant trait with variable expression. Familial early graying is frequently found. Melanocytes, present from birth, persist in the vitiliginous areas for a time but eventually disappear. Autoimmune mechanisms have been suggested for the melanocyte destruction, and also the failure to protect against toxic intermediates generated during melanogenesis.

Individuals with vitiligo are usually healthy, but the prevalence of vitiligo is higher than expected among patients with diseases suspected of autoimmune pathogenesis: pernicious anemia, thyroid dysfunction, Addison's disease, and alopecia areata. Circulating antibody for gastric parietal cell antigens, thyroglobulin, and adrenal antigens has been demonstrated in patients with vitiligo, with and without endocrine pathology or pernicious anemia. In adult onset diabetes, vitiligo is encountered five times more frequently than in controls. Further, a number of ocular syndromes with uveitis, as well as gastritis, gastric cancer, IgA deficiency, and melanoma, are reported with vitiligo.

When vitiligo is *universal* and includes the hair, eye color remains. Even without a history of pigment loss, such a totally depigmented patient is readily distinguished from the albino. There is no photophobia. Biopsy would also differentiate between the two, for melanocytes are present in normal numbers in the albino; the pathology is in the enzyme tyrosinase which is defective or absent.

Albinism

Albinism, an inherited defect in melanin synthesis, affects skin, hair, and eyes to varying degrees according to the completeness of the defect, permitting classification of at least six types of oculocutaneous albinism and three of ocular albinism (Table 556–2). Skin and eye color may be diluted over a considerable range, with some individuals having yellow or yellow-brown hair with pigmented irides and some tanning on sun exposure. Eye symptoms may be minimal. Related to the severity of the defect and to the intensity and frequency of actinic exposure, the cumulative dosage of radiation will produce cutaneous malignancy. In a Nigerian study, no albino over the age of 20 was without such change.

Neurofibromas

Clinical neurofibromatosis of the skin (Fig. 556–11) is no diagnostic challenge. With its multiple skin-colored pedunculated tumors and subcutaneous nodules along nerve sheaths, the cosmetic disfigurement is vivid and remembered. If the disease is early, or not fully expressed, or even without the disease at all, an individual may have a solitary neurofibroma, an organoid overgrowth of Schwann cells and endoneurium that presents clinically as a smooth, flesh-colored, dome-shaped papule, soft to firm, looking rather like an intradermal nevus. A doughy feel and the ability to invaginate the lesion could aid the differential diagnosis. When seen in association with the café-au-lait spots (Fig. 556–12) and axillary freckles as described above, the diagnosis should be made.

Neurofibromatosis of von Recklinghausen is a dominantly inherited disorder with systemic manifestations in the nervous system, bone, and soft tissues as well as skin. Half the cases are sporadic, presumably representing new mutations, but once expressed they will transmit the disease as a mendelian dominant. It occurs in one of 3000 births and has a prevalence of 0.04 per cent.

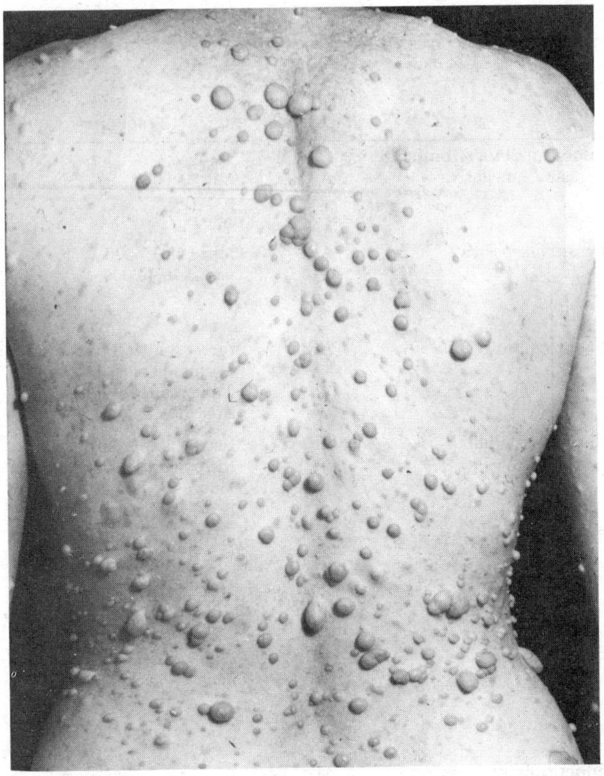

Figure 556–11. Neurofibromatosis—von Recklinghausen's disease.

The pigmentary stigmata of neurofibromatosis can be present at birth, and 90 per cent of patients with the disease will have them. The tumors, with rare exceptions, begin to develop after birth but before puberty, becoming more numerous throughout life. They may arise in all tissues, including bone and lung, in which they cause cystic lesions. Bone lesions, occurring in half the patients, are quite variable, and may represent growth

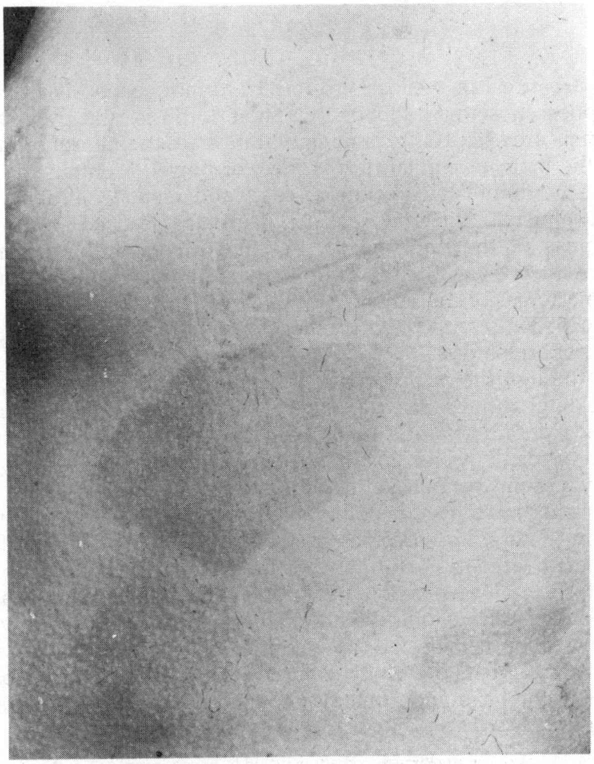

Figure 556–12. Café-au-lait spot.

TABLE 556–2. ALBINISM

	Inheritance	Frequency	Skin		Hair		
			Color	Pigmented Nevi Freckles		Color	Red Reflex
Oculocutaneous Albinism							
Tyrosinase-negative	AR*	1 in 34,000	pink/wte	none	white	gray-blue	present
Tyrosinase-positive	AR	blk: 1 in 15,000 wte: 1 in 40,000	wte-cream	present	wte-yellow red-darkens	blue-yellow brown	present but may be absent in dark races
Yellow-mutant	AR	rare—Amish, Polish, German-American; Blacks (American, Ceylonese, African)	wte at birth, slgt tan pos	present	wte-birth red/yellow 6 mos	blue at birth; darkens	present
Hermansky-Pudlak syndrome	AR	rare—cases from Puerto Rico; Southern Holland; Madras	cream-lgt normal	present	wte-red dk brown	blue-gray to brown	wte—present blk—absent
Cross-McKusick-Breen syndrome (oculocerebral hypopigmentation syndrome)	AR	extremely rare—3 in Amish family	pink/wte	present	wte-lt yel	gray-blue	?, cataracts
Chédiak-Higashi syndrome	AR	rare in most countries; none in blacks	pink/wte	present	blond-dk brown-steel gray	blue to brown	present but diminishes with time
Oculocutaneous Albinoidism	AD†		pink/wte	?	wte blond	blue	present
Ocular Albinism							
Vogt	X-linked	uncommon	normal	present	normal	blue	
Forsius-Eriksson	X-linked	less common	normal	present	normal	blue	
Autosomal recessive	AR	10 families	normal	present	normal	blue	present

*AR = Autosomal recessive.
†AD = Autosomal dominant.

disturbances as well as erosion by tumor. Scoliosis, severe kyphoscoliosis with gibbus formation, lordosis, and pseudoarthrosis are seen. Of greater significance are the neurofibromas in the brain or cranial nerves, eye, or bowel. Mental capacity may be diminished by the disease, and mental deficiency is not unusual. Bilateral acoustic neuromas lead to deafness; gliomas of the optic nerve present with exophthalmia and decreased visual acuity. There may be nodules of the iris and hamartomas of the retina.

In patients with pheochromocytoma, 5 to 10 per cent have neurofibromatosis.

Although the quality of life is severely compromised in von Recklinghausen's disease, the prognosis for survival is fairly good. Mesenteric and colonic neurofibroma may cause obstruction or result in bleeding. There is risk of malignancy—5 to 16 per cent in various series. The malignant tumors may be neurofibrosarcomas, histologically malignant nonmetastasizing brain tumors, liposarcomas, rhabdomyosarcomas, or undifferentiated sarcomas. The dangers for patients with neurofibromatosis are hypertension and sudden enlargement of a tumor. Blood pressure should be checked regularly and tumors with growth spurts biopsied. In younger patients, or those with limited numbers of lesions, continuing excisions of neurofibromas of the head and arms may contain the cosmetic disfigurement.

Crowe FW: Axillary freckling as a diagnostic aid in neurofibromatosis. Ann Intern Med 61:1142, 1964. *A subtle cutaneous sign of note.*

Fienman NL, Yakovac WC: Neurofibromatosis in childhood. J Pediat 76:339, 1970. *Underscoring the possibility and importance of early detection for counseling and because of the risk of malignancy.*

Person JR, Perry HO: Recent advances in phakomatoses. Int J Dermatol 17:1, 1978. *An excellent review.*

Schenkein I, Beuker ED, Helson L, Axelrod F, Dancis J: Increased nerve-growth-stimulating activity in disseminated neurofibromatosis. N Engl J Med 290:613, 1974. *This brief report is important for its observations and for provoking the challenging editorial that appeared in the same issue, cited below.*

Snyder SH: Nerve growth in neurofibromatosis (editorial). N Engl J Med 290:626, 1974.

Pseudoxanthoma Elasticum

A change in the skin of the neck and axilla that is reticular and sometimes telangiectatic, with small 1- to 3-mm tan-yellow papules resembling chicken skin, should bring pseudoxanthoma elasticum to mind. The problem is an inherited disorder of elastic tissue, occurring in both autosomal recessive and autosomal dominant forms that involve the skin, vascular system, and eyes. The earliest histologic change is the deposits of calcium on elastic fibers that seem otherwise normal. Fragmentation of these fibers in the skin, blood vessels, and Bruch's membrane produces the characteristic clinical features. Prevalence rates are estimated at 0.001 to 0.006 per thousand, and females are affected more frequently than males.

The skin lesions develop in the second decade or later and are progressive. Characteristically seen at the sides of the neck, in axilla, and in groin, they may be found in the flexural areas

TABLE 556–2. ALBINISM *(Continued)*

Eyes					Hair Bulb Incubation (Tyrosine)	Defect	Melanosome Maturation by Stage	Complications or Associated Problems
Nystagmus	*Photophobia*	*Visual Acuity*	*Pigment in Fundus*	*Other*				
Oculocutaneous Albinism								
marked	severe	legally blind	none	—	negative	no tyrosinase	I–unmelanized II	skin malignancy basal cell ca squamous cell ca
present but less	present but variable	severe defect in children; may improve with age	none; some with age	pigment cartwheel pupil, limbus	positive	no access of enzyme to tyrosine	I, II, some III, rare IV	skin malignancy basal cell ca squamous cell ca
present but variable	present but variable	marked defect; may improve with age	none; some with age	pigment cartwheel effect	neg to pos ?	unknown ? pheomelanogenesis	I, II, III	unknown
present but variable	present, may be severe	normal or slight decrease	none; some with age	may have pigment cartwheel	positive	pleiotropic effect—single gene mutation	I, II, III	storage-pool defect platelets; ceroid-like material in RE system, oral mucosa, urine
marked	—	blind	?, cataracts	?, cataracts	weakly positive	decreased melanocytes	I, II, III, IV	oligophrenia, athetosis, severe mental retardation
absent or slight	absent or slight	normal or slight decrease	some; increase with age	normal or cartwheel effect	positive	giant melanosomes, lethal defect in leukocytes	I, II, III, IV	infections; hematologic and neurologic abnormalities; lymphoreticular malignancy
no	no	normal or slight decrease	punctate		positive	unknown	unknown	none
present	severe	marked decrease	reduced		positive			
latent	absent or slight	color blind			positive			
present	severe	marked decrease			positive			

of arms and legs or about the umbilicus, and may involve the breast and penis or even the mucosal surfaces of the mouth, vagina, rectum, and stomach. Initially, and in mild cases, the small papules are best seen in stretched skin. In some, the lesions may have a serpiginous distribution with points of perforation. Eventually, there will be thickening of the skin and redundancy with exaggerated folds.

The combination of skin and eye changes is found most often (60 per cent); eye changes only are found in 30 per cent; skin changes only are found least frequently (10 per cent). Nearly all patients (80 per cent) have some vascular abnormality. This condition is presented in detail in Ch. 202.

Altman LK, Fialkow PJ, Parker F, Sagebiel RW: Pseudoxanthoma elasticum, an underdiagnosed genetically heterogenous disorder with protean manifestations. Arch Intern Med 134:1048, 1974. *A fine summary review with a clinical and histologic study of nine probands and the detection of seven previously unrecognized cases, underscoring the subtle and unsuspected presence of this disorder.*

McKee PH, Cameron CHS, Archer DB, Logan WC: A study of four cases of pseudoxanthoma elasticum. J Cut Pathol 4:146, 1977. *A light and electron microscopic focus on the histologic changes of pseudoxanthoma elasticum in an effort to elucidate its pathogenesis. Data support the theory that the basic lesion lies within the elastic fiber.*

Pope FM: Historical evidence for the genetic heterogeneity of pseudoxanthoma elasticum. Br J Dermatol 92:493, 1975.

Nodose Lesions of the Leg

The differential diagnosis of tender erythematous nodules of the lower legs is not so much of the lesion itself, which is a reaction pattern, but of the number of significant diagnoses that are characterized by such lesions. The cutaneous nodules vary in size, number, and location, appear suddenly or gradually, and disappear over weeks or months with or without scar or ulceration. They are sorted out according to their onset, course, distribution, and associations.

ERYTHEMA NODOSUM

Appearing acutely is the classic erythema nodosum, recognized as a clinical entity since 1798 and associated with a variety of infections and drug reactions. It is considered a hypersensitivity vasculitis; the ordinary presentation is of bilateral pretibial red nodules, occasionally with lesions of the extensor aspect of the arms. Rare in children and the elderly, it is most common between 15 and 23 years and is found in females three times more often than in males. According to the country and prevailing infections, it will be reported with tuberculosis, leprosy, sarcoid, streptococcal pharyngitis, pertussis, measles, primary atypical pneumonia, lymphogranuloma venereum, gonorrhea, syphilis, and also the superficial and deep fungus infections. It is seen in chronic ulcerative colitis and, less frequently, in regional enteritis or as a reaction to drugs such as iodides, bromides, sulfonamides, arsphenamine, contraceptives, and others.

The onset is often associated with fever and arthralgia, and occasionally with gastrointestinal upsets. It is a self-limited disease with a three- to five-week course and resolution without scarring. Recurrences and relapses occur in fewer than 10 per cent of patients. Any hematologic or roentgenographic abnormalities observed would be those of the underlying disease, to

Text continues on page 2266.

TABLE 556–3. CUTANEOUS LESIONS IN INFECTIOUS DISEASE

	Cutaneous Lesion	Systemic Component	Agents
Viral Diseases			
Rubella	Faint flush in 25%; centripetal spread of small, irregular pink macules and papules; petechiae on soft palate	Fever, malaise, headache, sore throat, adenopathy, mild respiratory infection, arthritis in adult women	Myxovirus
Varicella	Centrifugal spread of maculopapular lesions which vesiculate; may have mucosal lesions	Fever, malaise, pruritus	Herpesvirus
Variola	Erythematous macular eruption becomes vesicular with umbilication; most prominent in bathing trunk area; rash may be petechial	Fever, headache, vomiting	Poxvirus variolae
Hand, foot, and mouth disease	Vesicular eruption on margins of palms, soles, dorsa of hands, feet, lips, and buccal mucosa	Fever, malaise, abdominal pain	Coxsackievirus A5, A16, A10
Rubeola	Erythematous maculopapules; spreads from head to trunk to limbs; Koplik spots, blue-gray to white areas on tonsils may be seen	Fever, malaise, coryza, conjunctivitis, photophobia, adenopathy, encephalitis	Myxovirus
Bacterial Diseases			
Rheumatic fever	Subcutaneous nodules over bony prominences; erythema marginatum on trunk and limbs; erythema papillatum on flexor surfaces	Fever, carditis, chorea, arthritis	Group A hemolytic *Streptococcus*
Scarlet fever	Red pharynx with large tonsils, white exudate; 1 to 2 mm papules spread from neck to feet; rash most prominent in body folds	Fever, sore throat, lymphadenopathy, hematuria	Group A beta-hemolytic *Streptococcus*
Gonococcemia	Vesiculopustular lesions on extremities; may be purpuric	Fever, migratory arthritis, tenosynovitis, bacteremia (endocarditis)	*Neisseria gonorrhoeae*
Meningococcemia	Vesiculopustular lesion, which may be petechial on extremities or trunk, purpura fulminans	Myalgia, fever, encephalitis, hypotension, vomiting, septic arthritis, pericarditis, endocarditis, pneumonia, bacteremia	*Neisseria meningitidis*
Bacterial Diseases (*Continued*)			
Bacterial endocarditis	Petechiae, subungual splinter hemorrhages, Osler's nodes on fingers, hands, toes; Janeway lesions (palms and soles)	Fever, murmur, splenomegaly, bacteremia	Several, including viridans streptococci, *Staphylococcus*
Typhoid fever	1 to 3 mm slightly raised pink papules in groups of 10 to 20 lesions on upper part of abdomen and lower part of chest or midback (rose spots)	Headache, fever, aching, constipation	*Salmonella typhi*
Bartonellosis	Soft, round, hemangiomatous nodules and papules on neck, hands, and extensor surfaces	Fever, myalgias, malaise, headache, gastrointestinal irritability, anemia	*Bartonella bacilliformis*
Tularemia	Red, tender papule develops into vesiculopustule and then necrotic ulcer—usually on hand; some have maculopapular or petechial exanthem	Headache, malaise, myalgias, fever, adenopathy (regional)	*Francisella tularensis*
Diphtheria	Primary: cutaneous—tender pustular lesion to ulcer with gray membrane; does not extend below fascia, bluish rolled margins on lower extremities; secondary: infection of wound—purulent exudate or superinfection of eczematized skin; pharynx gray-white, pseudomembrane on tonsils	Fever, myocarditis, polyneuritis, croup, malaise, sore throat, dyspnea	*Corynebacterium diphtheriae*
Anthrax	95% have papule to vesicle with brawny gelatinous nonpitting edema surrounding the area (usually exposed surface)	Fever, malaise, pulmonary symptoms	*Bacillus anthracis*
Ritter's disease (SSSS)	Intense erythema of face and body, profuse desquamation, leaving raw, red, moist surface; bullae may be present	Refusal of feeding, vomiting, diarrhea, hypotension	Staphylococci phage type 71

Table continues on facing page.

TABLE 556–3. CUTANEOUS LESIONS IN INFECTIOUS DISEASE (*Continued*)

	Cutaneous Lesion	Systemic Component	Agents
Rickettsial Diseases			
Rocky Mountain spotted fever	Centripetal spread of maculopapular eruption; may become purpuric (initially on palms and soles)	Fever, chills, headache, myalgia, arthralgia, splenomegaly, hypotension, myocarditis	*Rickettsia rickettsii*
Boutonneuse fever	Tache noir—site of tick bite, small ulcer with black center and red halo; generalized red, maculopapular eruption; involves palms and soles	Fever, headache, regional lymphadenopathy	*R. conorii*
Epidemic typhus	Pink macules initially in axilla, to trunk, to extremities; may become petechial	Fever, chills, headache, malaise, weakness	*R. prowazekii*
Endemic typhus	Maculopapular eruption, primarily on trunk; does not become purpuric	Fever, chills, headache, malaise, nausea and vomiting	*R. mooseri*
Fungal Diseases			
Blastomycosis	Verrucous lesion with central healing and a serpiginous border on one side on exposed surfaces; small ulcers; 25% mucous (oral or nasal) lesions—only one half of these from a contiguous skin lesion	Fever, anorexia; bone, pulmonary, cerebral, liver, spleen, adrenal, and gastrointestinal tract may be involved	*Blastomyces dermatitidis*
Cryptococcosis	10–15% have cutaneous lesions; papules or nodules with surrounding erythema, also ulcers, pustules, and purple plaques	Pulmonary, one third renal involvement; 80% meningitis	*Cryptococcus neoformans*
Mucormycosis	Orbital, nasal sinus, or oropharyngeal form; red to gangrenous skin or mucosal changes with purulent drainage and swelling	Local pain, proptosis, CNS involvement	Phycomycetes
Fungal Diseases (*Continued*)			
Actinomycosis	25% cervicofacial; swelling over lower face or neck with indurated draining lesion; 15% thoracocutaneous lesion or subcutaneous abscess; 60% abdominal sinus or abscess	Osteomyelitis	*Actinomyces israelii*
Disseminated coccidioidomycosis	Subcutaneous cellulitis, abscesses, draining sinus tracts	Fever, malaise, chest pain, cough, anorexia, pulmonary fibrosis	*Coccidioides immitis*
Paracoccidioidomycosis	Painful ulcerative lesions—usually on face; abscesses with sinus tract	Cough, chest pain; bone, adrenal, CNS, and spleen involved	*Paracoccidioides brasiliensis*
Mycobacterial Diseases			
Tuberculosis	Lupus vulgaris (90% on head and neck), scrofuloderma—usually in cervical area; tuberculosis verrucosa cutis	Pulmonary, bone, and more widespread	*Mycobacterium tuberculosis*
Leprosy	Hypopigmented, slightly erythematous macules; nodules mainly on face; loss of eyebrows and lashes; raised hypopigmented plaques	Thickened peripheral nerves; sensory abnormalities	*Mycobacterium leprae*
Treponemal Disease			
Syphilis	Primary: chancre, eroded papule—usually on genitalia; secondary: erythematous macules and papules diffuse and on palms and soles, alopecia, condylomata lata; tertiary: locally destructive, partial spontaneous healing	Primary: adenopathy; secondary: malaise, fever, headache, adenopathy; tertiary: cardiac, neurologic involvement	*Treponema pallidum*

TABLE 556-4. CUTANEOUS LESIONS ASSOCIATED WITH GASTROINTESTINAL DISEASE

Diseases	Lesion and Description	Gastrointestinal Disorders and Symptoms	Other
Disorders Associated with Gastrointestinal Bleeding			
Degos' disease	Pink papules → small white scar with peripheral telangiectasias; spares palms, soles, and face	Cramps, vomiting, enteritis, bowel perforation, hemorrhage	CNS involvement
Osler-Weber-Rendu syndrome	Telangiectasias (multiple), especially upper half of body	Hemorrhage, hepatic arteriovenous anastomoses, hepatomegaly, cirrhosis	Epistaxis
Syndrome of phlebectasia of jejunum, oral cavity, and scrotum	Fordyce lesions (scrotum), caviar spots (tongue), phlebectasia (buccal mucosa and lips)	Hemorrhage and ulcer symptoms	
Blue rubber bleb disease	Cutaneous hemangiomas (predominantly on trunk and arms)	Hemorrhage; lesions involve liver and spleen	Lesions in CNS, lung, kidney, adrenal
Ehlers-Danlos syndrome	Easy bruising, fragile skin, pseudotumors at pressure points, stretchability of skin	Hiatal hernia, diverticula, rupture of bowel, hemorrhage	Pneumothorax, CNS bleeding, hyperextensible joints
Pseudoxanthoma elasticum	1- to 3-mm yellowish papules in plaques associated with telangiectasia, especially on neck and flexures; soft lax skin in folds at neck, axilla, umbilicus, face, antecubital fossa, groin	Hemorrhages	Angioid streaks of retina; vascular abnormalities, hypertension
Kaposi's sarcoma	Dark blue–purple macules → nodules initially on extremities; also hands, ears, nose	10% visceral involvement, hemorrhage, perforation, intestinal obstruction	Epidemic variety associated with AIDS
Henoch-Schönlein purpura	Erythematous macules which become papules, urticarial, purpuric, or necrotic (external aspects of limbs, buttocks, and occasionally face)	75% of patients > 2 years old have abdominal complaints: colic, vomiting, diarrhea, melena, hematemesis	Arthritis; renal involvement; fever
Polyarteritis nodosa	Tender nodules in groups along superficial arteries—may be cutaneous or subcutaneous; purpuric plaques, gangrene, Osler's nodes, and splinter hemorrhages have been noted	Pain, peritonitis; infarcts in bowel, liver, spleen; hemorrhage, pancreatitis, steatorrhea, gangrene of bowel	Multisystem: hypertension, myocardial infarction, renal thrombosis; neurologic—encephalopathy, convulsions, neuritis; arthralgia; myopathy
Disorders Associated with Gastrointestinal Polyposis			
Gardner's syndrome	Epidermal and sebaceous cysts, inclusion cysts; primarily on face and scalp	45% incidence of malignancy of colonic polyps	Osteomas, desmoid tumors
Peutz-Jeghers-Touraine syndrome	2- to 5-mm brown-black macules on lips, face, buccal mucosa, hands	Polyps with predilection for jejunum and ileum (malignancy proximal to ligament of Treitz)	
Cronkhite-Canada syndrome	Diffuse hyperpigmentation affecting palms, volar surface of fingers, face, and neck; alopecia (patchy → complete); dystrophic nails	Diarrhea, acquired polyps of gastrointestinal tract	
Disorders Associated with Dysphagia			
Scleroderma	Raynaud's, tense, smooth, hardened, and bound-down skin, starting with hands → upper extremities, face, trunk; cutaneous calcification; resorption of terminal phalanges; matlike telangiectasias	Dysphagia, malabsorption	Pulmonary fibrosis, arthritis
Plummer-Vinson syndrome	Angular stomatitis, brittle nails, koilonychia, atrophic tongue	Dysphagia due to strictures in esophagus	Anemia, iron deficiency
Epidermolysis bullosa	Trauma results in blisters which heal with scarring	Dysphagia due to strictures in esophagus	
Behçet's disease	Recurrent oral and genital ulcerations; pyoderma of groin and genitalia; sterile pustules at puncture sites	Dysphagia	Photophobia, uveitis, CNS abnormality

Table continues on facing page.

TABLE 556–4. CUTANEOUS LESIONS ASSOCIATED WITH GASTROINTESTINAL DISEASE (*Continued*)

Diseases	Lesion and Description	Gastrointestinal Disorders and Symptoms	Other
Disorders Associated with Diarrhea or Malabsorption			
Carcinoid	Flushing and patchy cyanosis and telangiectasia on face and upper trunk; hyperpigmented, hyperkeratotic lesions on legs, trunk, forearms, without hyperkeratosis on forehead, back, wrists, thighs	Diarrhea, metastatic lesions of carcinoid	Asthma, valvular heart disease, arthritis
Ulcerative colitis	3 to 34% have skin lesions; pyoderma gangrenosum (1 to 10%), purpura, aphthae, erythema nodosum, erythema multiforme, perianal fistula, and abscess (10 to 20%), pyostomatitis vegetans	Diarrhea, hemorrhage	Arthritis
Systemic mastocytosis	Flushing (secondary histamine release); generalized multiple reddish-brown or yellow macules, papules or nodules, or erythroderma	Symptoms in 23%—abdominal pain, cramps, diarrhea	(Mast cell leukemia is a possible complication)
Hartnup disease	Dry, scaly, well-marginated, affecting light-exposed area; stomatitis and glossitis	Diarrhea	Cerebral ataxia; renal aminoaciduria
Acrodermatitis enteropathica	Alopecia, pustular eruption around orifices and bullous or verrucous on extremities	Diarrhea	Zinc deficiency
Dermatitis herpetiformis	Papular and vesicular lesions with severe pruritus over extensor surfaces; symmetrical, chronic with recurrences; mucous membranes clear	Gluten enteropathy	
Reiter's syndrome	Mucocutaneous lesions, 80% keratosis blennorrhagica of palms and soles; hyperkeratosis of scalp; onycholysis, shedding and dystrophies of nails; scrotal and penile erosions; balanitis circinata sicca	Dysentery may precede other symptoms	Nonspecific urethritis, conjunctivitis, asymmetric arthritis
Crohn's disease	20% (15 to 50%) perineal ulceration with fistula formation; occasional pyoderma gangrenosum; 20% abdominal wall sinuses	Diarrhea, obstruction, perforation	Arthritis, iritis
Dermatogenic enteropathy	Erythroderma due to psoriasis, eczema or other etiology	Steatorrhea (malabsorption)	
Malabsorption syndrome	90% stomatitis; 50% angular stomatitis, purpura, petechiae; 10 to 20% have dermatitis, either erythematous or scaling like seborrheic dermatitis or psoriasis; in others, eczema, ichthyosis, asteatosis; alopecia, Beau's lines in nails, koilonychia; hyperpigmentation: melasmic, addisonian, or pellagroid	Diarrhea	
Pellagra	Hard, rough, cracked blackish and brittle epidermis of fingers, face, neck (Casal's necklace), dorsa of hands, arms, feet; fissures on palms and soles; earlier, may have blisters	Diarrhea; 50% achlorhydria	Dementia
Disorders Associated with Liver Disease			
Laennec's cirrhosis	Spider angiomas in 75%; palmar erythema; men—sparse axillary, pubic, and pectoral hair; Dupuytren's contracture; purpura; opaque white nails in 25%	Cirrhosis, hemorrhage from esophageal varices	Ascites, varices, testicular atrophy, gynecomastia
Biliary cirrhosis	Jaundice, melanotic hyperpigmentation generalized but more prominent on exposed areas; xanthelasma; tuberous xanthomas over extensor and pressure areas; flat xanthomas in palmar creases and scars	Biliary cirrhosis	Pruritus
Total lipoatrophy	Loss of subcutaneous fat; hypertrichosis, xanthomas, axillary and inguinal folds, associated with hyperpigmentation and linear epidermal thickenings (in congenital form)	Hepatic failure hematemesis, hepatomegaly	↑ Bone growth; diabetes; hyperlipemia; enlarged genitalia; renal, neurologic, and cardiac disorders
Hemochromatosis	15 to 20% gingival, palatal, buccal, and conjunctival hyperpigmentation—pigment most noticeable on flexures; loss of pubic and axillary hair	Cirrhosis	Diabetes, hypogonadism
Symptomatic porphyria	Bullous lesions on exposed parts of body; milia; hypertrichosis; onycholysis; conjunctival injection	Chronic liver dysfunction	
Disorders Associated with Pancreatic Disease			
Necrolytic migratory erythema	Symmetrical dermatitis initially eczematous over perineum, buttocks, and extremities → central blister with crusting, followed by hyperpigmentation, stomatitis	Glucagon-secreting tumor of pancreas	Weight loss, depression, anemia
Weber-Christian disease	Tender subcutaneous nodules on upper thighs and buttocks which resolve with depressed atrophic areas	Ileus, perforation	Fever, malaise
Nodular fat necrosis	Recurrent crops of red, painful, inflammatory subcutaneous nodules 0.5 to 5 cm initially on legs, especially lower; in 2 to 3% of patients with pancreatic disease, heal without atrophy	Pancreatitis or pancreatic neoplasm	Fever, eosinophilia, synovitis
Grey Turner's sign	Bruise-like discoloration of skin of left flank	Pancreatitis or other abdominal hemorrhage	
Cullen's sign	Bruise around umbilicus	Acute pancreatitis or ruptured common bile duct or perforated duodenal ulcer	
Miscellaneous Disorders			
Familial angioedema	Recurrent swelling of skin and mucous membranes	Nausea, vomiting, colic	Urinary symptoms, deficient in C1 esterase inhibitor
Familial Mediterranean fever	40% (8 to 45%) have erysipelas-like erythema on feet or lower legs	95 to 98% have abdominal pain	Fever, chest pain, arthralgia, renal amyloidosis
Acanthosis nigricans	Gray-brown to black pigmentation with thickened skin covered by small papillomas over axilla, sides of neck, groin, anogenital region; thickened palms; nails may be brittle or ridged	Gastric adenocarcinoma	Endocrinopathy Insulin resistance

TABLE 556–5. DISEASES WITH RENAL AND CUTANEOUS MANIFESTATIONS

Diseases	Cutaneous Manifestations	Renal Manifestations	Other
Tumors			
Hypernephroma	Solitary vascular lesions—tend to be pedunculated	Hypernephroma	
Tuberous sclerosis	60 to 70% skin lesions; adenoma sebaceum; periungual fibroma, shagreen patch, ash leaf spots, poliosis	Benign renal hamartomas, hematuria	Mental retardation (60–70%), epilepsy (70%), eye lesions (8 to 40%), rhabdomyoma
Anomalies of Development			
Oral-facial-digital syndrome	Short upper lip; hypertrophied frenula of lips and tongue; multilobed tongue; clefts of hard and soft palate; sparse hair; numerous milia	Polycystic kidneys	Polycystic liver; 50% mentally retarded; dental caries; brachydactyly and syndactyly
Neurofibromatosis	Neurofibromas, nodules in relation to peripheral nerves; 5 to 15% sarcomatous change in neurofibroma; café-au-lait spots; axillary freckles; oral tumors	60% oligophrenia; defect of renal tubules; osteomalacia; renal artery stenosis	Spinal deformities, endocrine and neurologic abnormalities, hypertension
Metabolic Disorders			
Sarcoidosis	Lupus pernio, plaques, maculopapular eruptions, erythema nodosum	25% hypercalciuria; nephrocalcinosis; polyuria, nocturnal polydipsia; 1 to 3% renal failure	Anemia, joint pain, adenopathy, CNS involvement, pulmonary fibrosis
Metastatic calcinosis	Nodules or plaques from 0.5 to 5 cm symmetrically on extremities and trunk—discharge of chalk-like material from lesions	Deposits in kidney of Ca^{++}	Blood vessels of muscles, stomach, lungs, and large blood vessels have deposits of Ca^{++}
Systemic amyloidosis, urticaria, and deafness syndrome	Urticaria	Nephropathy secondary to amyloid	Chills, malaise, deafness
Gout	Subcutaneous nodules, pink and most common on helix of ear, bursae of elbow, digits of hands and feet; chalky drainage	Renal calculi	
Cold agglutinins	Acrocyanosis	Hematuria	Anemia; may be associated with *Mycoplasma* pneumonia, reticulosarcoma, or lymphoma
Multiple myeloma	Plasmacytoma, petechial bleeding at perianal and periocular sites	Proteinuria, nephrolithiasis	Anemia; 10 to 20% amyloid; bone destruction; frequent infection; neuropathy
Diabetes mellitus	Necrobiosis lipoidica diabeticorum, granuloma annulare, carotenemia, lipodystrophy, frequent cutaneous infections	Kimmelstiel-Wilson disease; papillary necrosis	Heart, vascular, neurologic disease
Fabry's disease	Dry skin, dark red or black macule or papule in groups, especially on thighs, scrotum, and periumbilical	Hypertension, albuminuria, hematuria, uremia	Coronary artery disease, cerebrovascular attacks, eye lesions
Alcaptonuria	Skin discoloration (bluish-black) of nose tip, ear, extensor tendons, and costochondral junctions	Renal disease accelerates other abnormal findings; homogentisic acid in urine	Arthropathy
Hartnup disease	Stomatitis, glossitis; dry scaly eruption in light-exposed areas	Aminoaciduria	Diarrhea, cerebellar ataxia, psychiatric problems
Familial Mediterranean fever	40% erysipelas-like erythema	Death from renal amyloidosis	Fever, abdominal and chest pain, arthralgia, synovitis
Glomerulitis			
Hypersensitivity angiitis	Palpable purpura, urticaria, necrotic ulcerations	Necrotizing glomerular nephritis	Cardiac, neurologic, pulmonary, and joint involvement
Henoch-Schönlein purpura	See Table 556–4	40% microscopic hematuria (worse in adults)	Edema of feet and hands; polyarthritis; abdominal pain; fever, headache, anorexia
Scleroderma	See Table 556–4	Hypertension; 60% have abnormal BUN and creatinine	Arthritis, edema of hands; dysphagia; pulmonary fibrosis; malabsorption
Systemic lupus erythematosus	70 to 85% cutaneous lesions—butterfly erythema; maculopapular rash primarily above waist; chronic discoid lesions; alopecia; mucosal ulcers; periungual erythema; bullae; ecchymoses	50% renal disease (proteinuria-hematuria); 10% have nephrotic syndrome	Fever, fatigue, arthritis, pericarditis, neurologic involvement, pleural involvement
Polyarteritis nodosa	See Table 556–4	Cortical infarction, glomerulosclerosis, thrombosis	Malaise, fever, weight loss, abdominal pain, neurologic and cardiac involvement, arthralgia, myopathy
Nail-patella syndrome	Nails absent or hypotrophic	Chronic glomerulonephritis, renal dysplasia	Skeletal abnormalities; decrease in size or absence of patella
Wegener's granulomatosis	Early—papulonecrotic or vesicular lesions, symmetrically distributed over elbows, knees, buttocks; Later—erythematous, purpuric or vesicular lesions become generalized and oral ulcerations appear	Focal necrotizing glomerulitis, renal failure	CNS involvement; destruction of paranasal sinus, nasopharynx, and lung
Miscellaneous Disorders			
Osler-Weber-Rendu syndrome	Telangiectasias on upper half of body	Hematuria	Hemorrhages, epistaxis; cirrhosis of liver, arteriovenous anastomoses
Pseudoxanthoma elasticum	Yellow papules 1 to 3 mm in confluent plaques on neck and flexures; skin soft and lax	Hypertension from involvement of renal arteries	Gastrointestinal hemorrhage, circulatory abnormalities, arterial degeneration
Partial lipodystrophy	Loss of subcutaneous fat from face spreading downward	Nonspecific renal abnormalities; increased incidence	
Erythema multiforme	Erythematous macules, bullae, and target lesions symmetrical on distal extremities	Transient albuminuria	Infections or allergies possibly related
Sickle cell disease	Leg ulcers at early age; increased pigment in lower leg	Acute pyelonephritis, hematuria	Fever, abdominal pain, osteomyelitis, bone pain
Congenital ichthyosis, mental retardation, dwarfism, and renal impairment	Nonbullous congenital ichthyosiform erythroderma, most marked on back and extensor surfaces	Elevated BUN and creatinine, 50% of glomerular filtration rate	Mental retardation, dwarfism

TABLE 556–6. CUTANEOUS LESIONS IN DISORDERS WITH A HEMATOLOGIC COMPONENT

Diseases	Cutaneous Lesions	Hematologic Component	Other
Fanconi's syndrome	85% generalized olive-brown pigmentation most prominent on lower trunk, in flexures, and on neck with macules of hyper- and hypopigmentation	Hypoplastic anemia, neutropenia, thrombocytopenia, increased incidence of leukemia	Short broad hands, microcephaly, mental retardation, hypogonadism, aplasia of radii
Dyskeratosis congenita	Nail dystrophy; reticulate gray-brown pigmentation of neck, thighs, trunk; face and hands, atrophic skin; bullae on hands and feet secondary to trauma; leukoplakia on mucous membranes	Myeloid aplasia, refractory anemia, pancytopenia, blood dyscrasias, possible Fanconi's anemia	Dental abnormalities; mental and physical growth retarded
Sickle cell anemia	Leg ulcers at early age; increased pigment of lower leg	Anemia with typical red cells	Fever, abdominal pain, bone osteomyelitis
Cold agglutinin syndrome	Acrocyanosis, ulceration, gangrene	Anemia (hemolytic)	Hematuria, may be associated with *Mycoplasma* pneumonia, lymphoma, or reticulosarcoma
Gardner-Diamond syndrome	Recurrent painful erythematous and purpuric lesions	Autoerythrocyte sensitization	Psychiatric disturbances may be present
Chédiak-Higashi syndrome	Light color hair, skin, retinas, and translucent irides	Lethal defect in leukocytes	Frequent infections
Job's syndrome	Red, scaly, crusted lesions over scalp, ears, periorbital, skin, groin; cold staphylococcal abscesses	Defect in polymorphonuclear neutrophil function	Recurrent pneumonia; liver, spleen, and lymph nodes enlarged
Leukemia cutis	Erythroderma, papules, nodules, nonspecific infection, purpura, urticaria	Chronic lymphocytic leukemia most common type to develop lesions (11% of patients with acute myeloblastic or monocytic leukemia, as compared to 1.3% of acute lymphoblastic leukemia, developed leukemia cutis)	
Sézary's syndrome	Pruritus and generalized erythroderma, dystrophic nails, alopecia; thickening and convolution of skin, especially on face	Variant of mycosis fungoides or leukemia form of it	Adenopathy
Systemic mastocytosis	See Table 556–4	Mast cell leukemia	23% flushing, diarrhea, abdominal pain
Pernicious anemia	Glossitis, vitiligo, cheilitis (pallor, hyperpigmentation, jaundice)	Anemia, B_{12} deficiency	
Plummer-Vinson syndrome	Koilonychia, glossitis, cheilitis	Microcytic hypochromic anemia	Dysphagia, cancer of upper gastrointestinal tract
Methemoglobinemia	Violet or brownish skin color	Intrinsic defect in red cell enzyme of altered structure of hemoglobin	Inherited, acquired from medications (dapsone)
von Willebrand's disease	Albinism; ecchymoses or hematomas	Deficiency of factor VIII (long bleeding time)	
Polycythemia	Ruddy cyanosis; erythromelalgia; gangrene	May be primary or secondary; primary associated with elevated red blood cells, white blood cells, platelets; secondary with elevated red blood cells	Splenomegaly in primary form
Congenital erythropoietic porphyria	Photosensitivity and vesiculobullous eruption in light-exposed areas; hypertrichosis, alopecia; scarring marked	Hemolytic anemia; fluorescence of red blood cells	Splenomegaly; erythrodontia; nausea and vomiting on exposure to sunlight
Erythropoietic protoporphyria	Photosensitivity resulting in swelling and erythema and burning sensation; may have vesicular eruption in center of face with small scars; skin over knuckles thickened	High concentration of protoporphyrin in red blood cells—may have fluorescence of red blood cells	Cholecystitis, cholelithiasis
Paroxysmal cold hemoglobinuria	Pain and acrocyanosis; urticaria	Hemolysis on warming	Seen in syphilis, viral infections; chills, fever, aching, asthma
Multiple myeloma	Plasmacytoma; petechial bleeding at perianal, periocular areas	Plasma cell leukemia (eventual anemia, thrombocytopenia)	Proteinuria, nephrolithiasis, amyloidosis, bone destruction, neuropathies, frequent infections
Strawberry hemangioma (multiple)	Most common on head; superficial lesions red; deeper components dark blue or purple; grow rapidly after birth; ulceration and spontaneous involution.	May have thrombocytopenia	Cardiac hypertrophy due to high output; neurologic manifestations of lesions in CNS
Systemic lupus erythematosus	See Table 556–5	Anemia, thrombocytopenia	Fever, fatigue, arthritis, renal disease; serositis, neurologic disease

TABLE 556–7. DISEASES WITH BOTH CUTANEOUS AND RHEUMATIC COMPONENTS

Diseases	Cutaneous Lesions	Rheumatic Component	Other
Stevens-Johnson syndrome	Vesiculobullous and urticarial lesions; target lesions on mucous membranes and distal extremities	Arthralgias	Fever, malaise, nausea, vomiting, myalgias, chest pain, sore throat, eye involvement
Reiter's syndrome	See Table 556–4	Asymmetric arthritis of weight-bearing joints; tendinitis, fasciitis, ankylosing spondylitis	Urethritis, conjunctivitis (dysentery)
Behçet's disease	See Table 556–4	Arthralgia, noninflammatory joint effusions	Iritis or uveitis, fever, malaise, phlebitis, gastrointestinal ulcers, pericarditis, neurologic involvement
Rocky Mountain spotted fever	See Table 556–3	Arthralgia	Fever, chills, myalgia, headache
Gonococcemia	See Table 556–3	Migratory arthritis, tenosynovitis, septic arthritis	Fever, pharyngitis, urethritis
Rubella	See Table 556–3	Arthritis noted in adult women—elbows, knees, phalangeal joints, wrists	Fever, malaise, headache, sore throat, adenopathy
Meningococcemia	See Table 556–3	Septic arthritis	Myalgia, fever, hypotension, pneumonia, pericarditis, endocarditis
Diseases Associated with Hypersensitivity States			
Henoch-Schönlein purpura	See Table 556–4	Polyarthritis—knees, elbows, ankles, hands	Fever, anorexia, headache, abdominal pain; edema of hands and feet in children; 40% microscopic hematuria
Serum sickness	90% of skin lesions in this syndrome are urticarial; morbilliform and scarlatiniform eruptions are less common; rarely erythema multiforme, erythema nodosum	Arthralgias and arthritis; migratory distal large joints	Fever, lymphadenopathy
Hypersensitivity angiitis	See Table 556–5	May be associated with rheumatoid arthritis	Kidneys, lungs, gastrointestinal tract, heart, peripheral nerves; also affected by angiitis
Polyarteritis nodosa	See Table 556–4	Arthralgia	50% fever, malaise, weight loss, abdominal pain, hemiplegia, polyneuritis, renal, cardiac, gastrointestinal involvement
Erythema nodosum	Tender erythematous nodules on lower legs	Arthralgia	Fever, chills, malaise
Miscellaneous			
Psoriasis	Silvery scales on erythematous plaques; most common on scalp, knees, elbows	1–32% have arthritis, erosive polyarticular joint disease	
Reticulohistiocytoma	Small, firm, pink moderately pruritic papules or nodules on hands, face, scalp, ears, lips, trunk	Destructive polyarthritis with shortening of fingers	May involve lymph nodes, marrow, and endocardium
Sarcoidosis	See Table 556–5	50% polyarthralgia	70% of those with skin lesions have intrathoracic involvement
Systemic lupus erythematosus	See Table 556–5	Migratory arthritis (small joints of hands, wrists, elbows, shoulders, knees, and ankles)	Renal, cardiac, neurologic complications
Erythema elevatum diutinum	Multiple nodules and plaques on extensor surfaces of extremities; may resemble xanthomas but most are purple-red	Associated polyarthritis	
Scleroderma	See Table 556–4	Resorption of bone, dissociation of terminal phalanges	Pulmonary fibrosis, malabsorption, dysphagia
Ehlers-Danlos syndrome	See Table 556–4	Hyperextensibility of joints	Gastrointestinal bleeding, rupture of bowel

which the therapy should be directed. In more than a quarter of the cases, however, no etiology can be determined.

The histopathologic changes in the skin are nonspecific and are completely reversible. The venous walls can be edematous and the fat lobules show disintegration, but there is no leukocytoclastic or lymphocytic angiitis.

ACUTE FEBRILE NEUTROPHILIC DERMATOSIS

The same is true of the rare, self-limiting acute febrile neutrophilic dermatosis of Sweet. Characterized by high persistent fever with painful nodules and plaques occurring asymmetrically over the extremities, face, and neck, it is often noted to follow an upper respiratory infection and is considered a probable hypersensitivity reaction. However, it has also been observed with unsuspected malignancy, especially acute myelogenous leukemia, and as such may be considered a cutaneous marker of malignant change or immunologic dysfunction. The disease is reported most in middle-aged women, in whom it is associated with leukocytosis and an elevated sedimentation rate. Histopathologic examination of the skin lesions shows vasodilatation and endothelial swelling, with infiltration of polymorphonuclear leukocytes in the upper and mid-dermis. There is no suppuration and no scarring.

NODULAR LIQUEFYING PANNICULITIS

In this condition, by contrast, there are foci of fat necrosis with preservation of cell membranes but with basophilic granular changes of the cytoplasm, as well as loss of nuclear staining in the fat septum to produce characteristic ghost-like cells. The recurrent crops of red painful nodules 0.5 to 5 cm, which appear on the legs but occasionally elsewhere, can be noted to soften and drain a viscous aseptic material as evidence of fat liquefaction. Associated with pancreatitis or occasionally with acinous adenocarcinoma of the pancreas, the fat necrosis has been attributed to the action of the pancreatic enzyme lipase on the subcutaneous fat. Occurrences may be associated with episodes of abdominal pain, polyarthritis, and fever. The problem is rare. The differential diagnosis is that of other nodular lesions of the leg rather than Weber-Christian disease, a nonsuppurative panniculitis in which the nodular lesions are primarily on the trunk and thighs, and are associated with fever and recurrence.

ERYTHEMA INDURATUM

This chronic recurring nodular vasculitis of the lower legs is not rare, at least in Europe or Japan. It is found predominantly in women from the teens to old age; there are peak appearances in adolescence and at the menopause. Histologically panniculitis and vasculitis are seen, along with a granulomatous reaction that may be nonspecific or tuberculoid.

The lesions occur mostly on the posterior rather than anterior aspect of the lower legs and, rarely, on the thighs. The nodules, painful to pressure, may ulcerate with subsequent scarring, or resorb, leaving an atrophic depressed surface. Traditionally associated with tuberculosis, active disease is hardly ever found. Most observers now designate a group of nodose lesions as nodular vasculitis and distinguish between those associated with tuberculous infection (erythema induratum of Bazin) and those not.

The usual course of the problem is protracted and subject to remission and exacerbations. If there is antecedent or current evidence of tuberculosis infection, antituberculous therapy may be beneficial.

Cutaneous Correlations with Specific Organ Systems

Throughout Ch. 556, the focus has been on the lesion observed to identify and differentiate it from similar clinical presentations. Since multiple etiologies can generate the same lesion, a further focus is directed to the manifestations of internal malignancy in Ch. 557. Here, we will redistribute the dermatologic manifestations according to infection and disorders of specific systems. Infectious disease produces a variety of cutaneous responses, some primary, many secondary. They are grouped in Table 556–3* according to the etiologic agent, whether viral, bacterial, rickettsial, or fungal. The progression of lesions is indicated where applicable. In Table 556–4* are the gastrointestinal problems associated with dermatologic diagnoses and lesions that may have as a complication gastrointestinal bleeding or polyposis, or that may be associated with dysphagia or diarrhea, or with hepatic or pancreatic disease. In the same way renal, hematologic, and rheumatic disorders are presented, with a synopsis of the skin pathology, in Tables 556–5 to 556–7*, respectively. The data given are not all discussed in the text, but the standard general dermatologic references cited in Ch. 551 will provide depth of detail.

---

*Tables 556–3 to 556–7 were compiled with Dr. Virginia Fallon-Pellicci.

557. SELECTED SIGNIFICANT DERMATOLOGIC DIAGNOSES

The Blistering Diseases

The concentrated accumulation of fluid in the skin sufficient to replace the pre-existent tissue structure and produce a visible vesicle or bulla can be the result of forces as divergent as friction and infection, or may be from causes completely obscure. For blisters of unknown etiology categorization yields to microscopic morphologic grouping and to further sorting according to the clinical expression of disease. It is among these, the blisters known to be other than infectious, chemical, or traumatic, that the searchlight of immunofluorescence has been disclosing immune complexes to correlate with clinical disease and its course. Antibodies, circulating and tissue-fixed, whether cause or effect of the observed pathology, are important indicators that must be fully assessed.

In this chapter we shall assume that historical information and close observation will have enabled the examiner to identify blisters associated with solar and thermal burn, with infections such as herpes simplex, or with vesicants such as cantharidin used in the treatment of warts but found in certain stinging insects and flies. It is the differential diagnosis of the one or several blisters on a fairly normal base that is to be considered. In the physical examination, the distribution of the lesions and any extension to mucous membranes or eyes would have been noted. The tenseness of the bulla would have been assessed to estimate the morphologic depth of cleavage and whether this split is easily revealed or extended by light pressure or rubbing as one would skin a ripe peach (Nikolsky's sign).

Bullae that are flaccid on normal-appearing skin which is easily denuded, favoring a truncal location with associated mouth erosions, should suggest pemphigus. If the bullae are few and unroofed so that only superficial erosions are observed, there will still be a history of blisters. The presence of an erythematous base or of other nonbullous papular to urticarial lesions might mean erythema multiforme. Taut preserved bullae are found in pemphigoid and dermatitis herpetiformis, although in the latter the more common presentation is vesicular with marked pruritus and a characteristic distribution over the extensor aspect of the limbs, the shoulders, and the buttocks. The further diagnostic assessment and the support from biopsy and immunofluorescence studies are shown in Table 557–1, which is best perused after a review of the specific diseases.

PEMPHIGUS

Pemphigus is a cluster of blistering entities characterized histologically by acantholysis (see Ch. 553) with resultant fluid accumulation within bullae, and immunologically by the unexplained presence of circulating autoantibodies to an intercellular epidermal antigen. Of unknown etiology, it is found throughout the world, in both sexes, and in all races, with a reported higher incidence in Jews. The onset commonly occurs between 40 and 60 years. It has been seen in children and in families as fogo selvagem, or Brazilian wildfire, and in patients undergoing penicillamine therapy for rheumatoid arthritis. Such penicillamine-induced pemphigus, temporally related to treatment, is indistinguishable from spontaneous pemphigus clinically, histopathologically, or by immunofluorescence. Broadly, and according to the intraepidermal level of the acantholytic blister, pemphigus is divided into suprabasilar pemphigus vulgaris and, if more superficial and just under the corneum, subcorneal pemphigus foliaceus.

Pemphigus vulgaris, which had a 95 per cent mortality before the advent of steroids, can still present acutely and run a swiftly fatal course despite therapy. More often it is a controlled but chronic problem of varying severity. Occasionally it remains localized for months with lesions of the mouth or scalp, perhaps axilla or groin; within a year or so it can be predicted to become generalized. Those presenting with mouth lesions tend to have a poorer prognosis, and some 30 to 40 per cent of all those diagnosed will succumb to the disease or side effects of therapy. The Nikolsky sign is present in uninvolved as well as involved skin, and areas readily traumatized become sloughed. When this extends to the pharynx and larynx, hoarseness is a clinical sign. In general, lesions tend to favor the seborrheic areas—the scalp; the periocular, paranasal, and perioral areas; the presternum; the mid-back; the area around the umbilicus; and the groin. Denuded intertriginous lesions may tend to become vegetative through heaped peripheral collarettes of epidermis and crust, lending a descriptive name to the clinical subdivision of *pemphigus vegetans.* It is further classified into Neumann and Hallopeau types; the former affects younger patients, and the latter tends to follow a more benign course. Noted for pustules extending peripherally, both these pemphigus variants are characterized by vegetative lesions containing eosinophilic abscesses. Both variants can be fatal.

Pemphigus foliaceus is a milder disease, with finer, smaller lesions and more crust and scale; it almost always spares the mouth. It affects mainly the older patient, occasionally children, and is believed to occur in a localized variant as pemphigus

TABLE 557–1. THE BLISTERING DISEASES: CORRELATIONS WITH HISTOLOGY AND IMMUNOFLUORESCENCE

	Pemphigus	Pemphigoid	Erythema Multiforme	Dermatitis Herpetiformis
Histology				
Blister	Intraepidermal	Subepidermal	At basal layer	Subepidermal
Special	Acantholysis	Eosinophils predominate in papillary dermis	Vacuolar alteration at basal layer, necrotic keratinocytes	Neutrophils at tips of dermal papillae
Tzanck test	Acantholytic cells	Negative	Negative	Negative
Immunofluorescence				
Indirect	Positive—intercellular*	Positive—basement membrane	Negative	Negative
Direct	Positive—intercellular	Positive—basement membrane	Negative	Positive—granular deposits in papillary dermis, less often along basement membrane
Treatment	Corticosteroids Immunosuppressives Cyclophosphamide Azathioprine Gold	Corticosteroids ?Immunosuppressives	Supportive ?Corticosteroids	Sulfones Gluten-free diet

*Antibody levels correlate with disease activity.

erythematosus and as an endemic problem in Brazil, where it affects immigrants as well as Brazilians. In the era before steroids some 40 per cent succumbed.

Therapy for pemphigus includes corticosteroids, immunosuppressives, and gold in combinations which will vary according to the form and severity of the disease and the current persuasion of the practitioner. For active widespread disease, most will treat initially with high dose steroids (100 to 150 mg of prednisone or equivalent) to suppress the disease; if there is failure to respond, the dosage will be increased, perhaps doubled. When no new bullae form for several days, a slow taper is begun by first gradually reducing to zero the dosage for alternate days. If it is clear that prolonged or high dose corticosteroid therapy will be required, many elect to begin immunosuppressive therapy from the start: methotrexate, azathioprine,* or cyclophosphamide.* Gold therapy,* too, is being used with new interest, and in some patients is reported to be effective even without initial corticosteroid control. Of note is the unexplained but beneficial effect of ACTH infusion on those whose disease is uncontrolled by more than 200 mg of prednisone or equivalent. The management of pemphigus also includes therapeutic baths, protective ointments and powders, and intralesional injection of corticosteroids when bullae are few. Disease activity can be correlated with the titer of indirect immunofluorescent intercellular antibody.

A benign suprabasilar acantholytic disease is Hailey-Hailey disease, an incompletely penetrant autosomal dominant genodermatosis also known as *benign familial chronic pemphigus.* Small flaccid vesicles are noted about the neck and in body folds where they are aggravated by heat and humidity. The disease is rarely widespread and rarely involves the mouth. Two of three patients will have a family history of the problem. All can expect prolonged spontaneous remission.

PEMPHIGOID

Pemphigoid is a chronic and comparatively benign blistering disease in which subepidermal bullae *without* acantholysis present clinically as large, tense, irregular blisters frequently on an erythematous base. It is often associated with or preceded by pruritus and an urticarial, perhaps eczematous eruption. Serum IgG antibody to basement membrane of skin, capable of fixing complement, occurs at the site of pathologic change and suggests an autoimmune pathogenesis. However, the disease cannot be transferred passively and, unlike pemphigus vulgaris, antibody levels do not correlate with disease activity.

Pemphigoid is a problem of the elderly; it is chronic and subject to exacerbations and remissions. Lesions, which may occur anywhere, favor the abdomen, groin, inner aspect of the thighs, and flexor aspect of the forearms. Mucosal lesions occur but are small; they heal readily with minor discomfort and, unlike pemphigus vulgaris, are no threat to nutrition.

In *benign mucosal pemphigoid* subepidermal bullae without acantholysis form on the mucous membranes, less often the skin, with the possibility of severe residual scarring. Women are afflicted twice as often as men, but both may have involvement of the conjunctivae as well as the oral cavity, pharynx, larynx, esophagus, genitalia, and anus. Secondary fibrous bands may lead to dysphagia, hoarseness, blindness, and stenotic anogenital orifices. Response to steroid therapy—topical, intralesional, and systemic—is poor.

*Investigational drugs for this purpose.

Lever WF, Schaumburg-Lever G: Immunosuppressants and prednisone in pemphigus vulgaris. Therapeutic results obtained in 63 patients between 1961 and 1975. Arch Dermatol 113:1236, 1977. *A review of treatment results of a series of 63 patients over a decade and a half. Important to know for the assessment of therapy and outcome.*

Penneys NS, Eaglstein WH, Frost P: Management of pemphigus with gold compounds. A long-term follow-up report. Arch Dermatol 112:185, 1976. *The place of gold in the management of pemphigus is still debated, but a review of long-term follow-up is important.*

Rosenberg FR, Sanders S, Nelson CT: Pemphigus: A 20-year review of 107 patients treated with corticosteroids. Arch Dermatol 112:962, 1976. *Again in the consideration of long-term management for a chronic problem, experience with a therapeutic modality over years is helpful.*

DERMATITIS HERPETIFORMIS

Dermatitis herpetiformis is grouped with the blistering diseases. It can occasionally have bullae, but presents most often with intense pruritus and with excoriated papules or grouped vesicles in classic distribution over buttocks, shoulders, elbows and knees, and sometimes scalp, face, and ears. Histologically papillary microabscesses occur with aggregates of neutrophils leading to dermoepidermal separation and widespread destruction of the basement membrane. Direct immunofluorescent staining of uninvolved paralesional skin is positive at the dermoepidermal junction. Although IgG and IgM may be identified, as well as complement at the tips of the dermal papillae, IgA is the immunoglobulin most predominant; in fact, without it the diagnosis of dermatitis herpetiformis is in question. Since IgA does not fix complement by the direct pathway beginning with C1q, some other mechanism is necessary to implicate IgA. There is rather convincing evidence to suggest activation of the alternative pathway of complement through IgA aggregates, not unlike that which is known to occur in myeloma. Conventional complexes have been demonstrated, but circulating immunoglobulin and significant serum complement levels have not been detected.

Dermatitis herpetiformis appears between the second and fifth decades. It occurs in men twice as often as women. Of special interest, however, is its association with malabsorptive enteropathy. As in celiac disease, disaccharidase and dipeptidase activities are decreased, and there is villous atrophy of the small intestine most apparent in the proximal jejunum. In patients diagnosed as having dermatitis herpetiformis with IgA deposits at the dermoepidermal junction of the skin, 19 of 23 had total or partial villous atrophy. As in the celiac syndrome they had autoantibodies to thyroid, reticulin, and parietal cells, as well as atrophic gastritis and overt pernicious anemia. Comparisons of histocompatibility indicate that HLA antigens A1 and B8 have a high frequency in dermatitis herpetiformis when contrasted to normals, and even higher in adult celiac disease. No correlation can presently be made with HLA type and the presence or absence of intestinal involvement from the data at hand, but to identify villous atrophy may take more than one biopsy.

Whether dermatitis herpetiformis is a reaction pattern and whether the activity and extent of skin lesions can be correlated with observed enteropathy are not yet known. Three reports in as many years which document jejunal lymphoma complicating a clinical dermatitis herpetiformis, characterized by IgA skin deposits and intestinal villous atrophy, warrant careful consideration. Further, the riddle of antireticulin antibody titers and the degree of villous atrophy must be solved. There is a cross-reactivity reported between fraction III of gluten and reticulin. However, the anticipated favorable response to the gluten-free diet, important in the management of celiac disease, has not been noted consistently in dermatitis herpetiformis and is challenged. In a match of diet, HLA type, and mucosal abnormality in a series of 44 patients, 22 with celiac disease and 22 with dermatitis herpetiformis, milk antibody titer was used as an index of mucosal abnormality. It was similar in both groups, but antigluten antibody was consistently higher in celiac disease, suggesting that the antigluten response may not be part of the enteropathy of dermatitis herpetiformis. One patient with both diseases finds that her dermatitis herpetiformis is not benefited by the gluten-free diet that controls her celiac disease.

The classic case of dermatitis herpetiformis is not difficult to diagnose, and at its onset the severe pruritus and paucity of lesions might be confused only with scabies, which the telltale burrow and mite would differentiate. Halogens have been known to aggravate the disease or even to provoke it, and thus may provide a clue. A skin patch test with 20 per cent KI is frequently positive and has been known to induce characteristic lesions with IgA deposition. One last and perhaps definitive test is the therapeutic response to sulfapyridine or diaminodiphenylsulfone, each of which has a dramatic beneficial effect that suppresses pruritus and lesions in 12 to 24 hours. The individual dose required to maintain the patient must be titrated. The end-point is surprisingly sharp. Because the medications must be continued for long periods, there is considerable risk of hematologic or perhaps carcinogenic effects (sulfone), or hepatic and renal side effects (sulfa); hence treatment must be monitored closely.

Baker PG, Palmer RK: Autoantibodies in patients with coeliac disease and dermatitis herpetiformis. Lancet 1:750, 1976. *The study of the immune response in patients with celiac disease and dermatitis herpetiformis provides another means of differentiating between the two and another step toward elaborating the pathogenesis of both.*

Charlesworth EN, Backe JT, Garcia RL: Iodide-induced immunofluorescence in dermatitis herpetiformis. Arch Dermatol 112:555, 1976. *The observed provocation of immunofluorescent histologic findings under an epidermal patch test of potassium iodide gives a further piece of the puzzle in this disease related to celiac disease and gluten sensitivity but by contrast aggravated by iodides.*

Fausa O, Larsen TE, Husby G, Thune P: Gastro-intestinal investigations in dermatitis herpetiformis. Acta Derm Venereol 55:203, 1975. *A further effort to distinguish between dermatitis herpetiformis and celiac disease on the basis of gastrointestinal studies.*

O'Donoghue DP, Lancaster-Smith M, Johnson GD, Kumar PJ: Gastric lesion in dermatitis herpetiformis. Gut 17:185, 1976. *A closer focus at the gastric pathology and the presence of parietal cell antibody in the sera.*

Scott BB, Losowsky MD: Gluten antibodies in coeliac disease and dermatitis herpetiformis. Gut 17:398, 1976. *Gluten antibody levels, being higher in coeliac disease than in dermatitis herpetiformis, suggested a fundamental difference in the immunologic abnormality.*

Silk DBA, Mowat NAC, Riddell RH, Kirby JD: Intestinal lymphoma complicating dermatitis herpetiformis. Br J Dermatol 96:555, 1977. *Perhaps more than chance.*

HERPES GESTATIONIS

Should an extremely pruritic vesiculobullous disease occur in pregnancy, the most likely diagnosis is *herpes gestationis*. If the pregnancy is early and unsuspected, the grouped vesicles and intense pruritus might suggest dermatitis herpetiformis, but the lesions lack symmetry and pigmentation, are frequently bullous and occasionally urticarial, and resemble erythema multiforme more than any other diagnosis. Histopathologically they are subepidermal bullae with abundant eosinophils indistinguishable from those of bullous pemphigoid. The possibility of a toxic or allergic reaction to fetal or placental protein or their metabolites, or to hormones, has been considered but remains unproved. With exacerbations and remission the disease is likely to persist throughout the pregnancy and perhaps into the puerperium, especially if the onset is just ante partum. It can recur with the menses for a year or more after delivery and is likely to recur with subsequent pregnancies.

The problem for the mother is only one of discomfort, but for the fetus it is significant, with threat of abnormalities or death. Recent experience with successful outcome using systemic steroids would give a more optimistic, although guarded, prognosis.

Pruritus in pregnancy with erythematous papules in the absence of blisters may represent the rare papular dermatitis of Spangler that is generalized, intensely pruritic, difficult to control, and also associated with fetal risk. In the more benign prurigo gestationis of Besnier, without threat to the fetus, the pruritic papules occur mostly over the extremities in the last trimester and are usually amenable to topical therapy. In the differential diagnosis both conditions suggest drug eruptions and excoriations from other causes of pruritus, rather than any of the blistering diseases. Perhaps the most common pruritic disease of pregnancy, often misdiagnosed as a drug eruption or even erythema multiforme, is the *pruritic urticarial papules and plaques of pregnancy* (PUPPP), an intensely pruritic eruption characterized by erythematous urticarial plaques and papules that present on the abdomen and extend to the thighs, buttocks, and occasionally the arms, beginning in the third trimester. The histology is that of a superficial, occasionally mid-dermal perivascular and lymphocytic infiltrate with some edema of the papillary dermis. The response of symptoms to topical steroids is usually quite adequate and the eruption disappears at delivery, although it may recur. There is no risk to the infant.

ERYTHEMA MULTIFORME

Erythema multiforme is a reaction pattern in the skin and mucous membranes, an angiitis which in the upper corium leads to symptomless erythematous lesions, perhaps edematous or bullous, that darken with age, leaving the concentric rings of an "iris" or "target" lesion. Acute appearances and recurrences have been associated with recognized infections such as herpes simplex and, more recently, *Mycoplasma pneumoniae*, as well as with vaccinations, drugs, malignancy, deep x-ray therapy, and even infectious mononucleosis, but a third of the cases defy explanation. The expression of erythema multiforme may range from minor disease with a few scattered lesions to major illness with extensive bullous erosions, life-threatening fever, and prostration. The syndrome described and named erythema exudativum multiforme by Hebra in 1866 was not familiar to Stevens and Johnson, who reported "a new eruptive fever with stomatitis and ophthalmia" in 1922, giving their names to the extreme expression of the disease.

In the severe form, erythema multiforme can be associated with mild prodromal symptoms suggestive of an upper respiratory infection that would be unremarkable except for the very sudden and dramatic eruption that ensues. The eyes are involved almost as often as the mouth and vagina. Endoscopy reveals erosions of the esophagus and colon, leading to gastrointestinal symptoms. Nephritis and uremia may be a further complication. Its course lasts two to four weeks or longer, and is prone to recur. Although systemic steroids are usually used in severe cases, the improvement is not as prompt as expected in steroid-responsive blistering diseases and can be questioned. An underlying cause of erythema multiforme must always be sought, particularly with recurrent disease. Although most patients are between 10 and 30, in those over 50 years old a search for malignancy is warranted.

TOXIC EPIDERMAL NECROLYSIS

This eruption resembles scalded skin and may not be in the clinical differential of classic erythema multiforme, but the reaction pattern is analogous. Both diseases probably represent part of a continuous disease spectrum. Toxic epidermal necrolysis has a prodrome followed by the appearance of erythema and the loss of skin in sheets, with a threat of death and liability of recurrence. Two forms are recognized: one occurring mainly in young children with associated staphylococcal infections of phage Type 71, and the other affecting adults or older children and associated with drugs or other infections and conditions. When toxic epidermal necrolysis is induced by staphylococcal toxins, the epidermal cleavage is in the malpighian or granular layer, in contrast to the subepidermal split of toxic epidermal necrolysis from other causes. The prognosis is good. It is now separately labeled the staphylococcal scalded skin syndrome (SSSS), the histology reflecting the effect of toxin on the intercellular region of the lower granular layer without significant cytotoxic change in adjacent cells. The usefulness of corticosteroids and antimicrobial agents in the course of the epidermal change has not been demonstrated; but with the delay in developing a humoral response to staphylococcal toxin, and risk of contagion, specific prompt antimicrobial therapy is indicated. In toxic epidermal necrolysis of other causes, the epidermal cleavage occurs just above or at the basal layer as a result of basal cell disintegration. Although nonstaphylococcal infections, immunizations, and vaccinations have been implicated, the reaction is more often precipitated by drugs such as the sulfonamides, phenylbutazone, penicillin, hexametaphosphate, tetracycline, mithramycin, barbiturates, aspirin, amidopyrine, procaine, phenolphthalein, allopurinol, dapsone, gold salts, and hydantoin. Even a gin and tonic has caused toxic epidermal necrolysis, presumably from the quinine, and it has been reported following inhalation of acrylonitrile, a pesticide. Since the full thickness of the epidermis is separated in toxic epidermal necrolysis, the serum loss is greater and the prognosis is more guarded. Unlike staphylococcal scalded skin syndrome the mucous membranes are often involved, and associated membranoproliferative glomerulonephritis has been noted.

The clear histologic distinction between staphylococcal scalded skin syndrome and toxic epidermal necrolysis of other causes makes the biopsy an important diagnostic tool for differentiation and prognosis. By using the Nikolsky sign to advantage, skin peeled from a fresh wound of staphylococcal scalded skin syndrome shows, on frozen section, the stratum corneum with focally adherent granular cells. The Tzanck smear from the denuded base has broad cells with a low nucleus-to-cytoplasm ratio. In toxic epidermal necrolysis the full thickness of the epithelium is found on the frozen peeled specimen and the Tzanck preparation shows inflammatory cells, basal cells, and a high nucleus-to-cytoplasm ratio. Further, direct immunofluorescent staining in toxic epidermal necrolysis has shown intercellular fixation of immunoglobulins and complement at the basal cell layer, suggesting that drugs bind to intercellular epidermal protein and that the basal cells are the site of damage. Therapy is supportive with close attention to fluid balance, but corticosteroids or even renal dialysis may be required.

Mucocutaneous Lymph Node Syndrome (Kawasaki's Disease)

A recently recognized entity, first reported in 1967 in children, but now documented in adults, the mucocutaneous lymph node syndrome is included here because of the ocular and conjunctival involvement, the mucous membrane erythema and erosions, and the severe prostration with fever, rash, and lymphadenopathy. Of obscure etiology and unresponsive to recognized therapy, it can be associated with myocardial involvement and death from coronary artery occlusion.

Of epidemic prevalence in Japan, where more than 10,000 cases have been recorded, the diagnostic criteria of the syndrome have been met by children the world over—Hawaii, North America, England, Greece, Korea—and now by adults. Of the 633 American cases reported to the Center for Disease Control by 1981, the mean age was 4.2 years, ranging from 7 months to 27 years. Those affected present with ulcerative gingivitis, rhinitis, and fever which can last one to two weeks. There is acute nonsuppurative enlargement of cervical lymph nodes. On the third day or so of illness, a generalized macular eruption appears with intense bright erythema and edema of the palms and soles, followed by desquamation of the skin of fingers and toes. Proteinuria, pyuria, diarrhea, aseptic meningitis, and mild icterus may be observed, with leukocytosis and a shift to the left, slight anemia, and perhaps an elevated transaminase. Thrombocytosis even to 1 million platelets is seen. There are complaints of photophobia and arthralgia. The diagnosis is made only when a patient has five of the following six criteria: fever for more than five days, conjunctival injection, mouth lesions, desquamation of the peripheral extremities, erythematous rash, and lymph node enlargement. Diligent search for causative microorganisms and detailed study of paired serologic specimens have been unrewarding.

Although the course is usually benign and self-limited, sudden death has been reported in 1 to 2 per cent of patients; electrocardiograms have suggested myocarditis or pericarditis in 70 per cent of cases. Further, abnormal coronary angiograms were noted in more than half of 20 patients studied three weeks to four years after their illness. With a view of preventing coronary aneurysm, several treatment schedules were assessed, including steroids alone, with anticoagulants, with aspirin, and then aspirin and antibiotics alone. The steroid-treated group fared significantly less well and, from these data, steroids are contraindicated.

Darby CP, Kyong CU: Mucocutaneous lymph node syndrome. JAMA 236:2295, 1976. *Alerting the United States to clinical "findings" observed and reported primarily but not exclusively in Japan.*

Kato H, Koike S, Yokoyama T: Kawasaki disease: Effect of treatment on coronary artery involvement. Pediatrics 63:175, 1979. *A further review with additional cases.*

Kawasaki T, Kosaki F, Okawa S, Shigematusu I, Yanagawa HL: A new infantile acute febrile mucocutaneous lymph node syndrome (MLNS) prevailing in Japan. Pediatrics 54:271, 1974. *The initial report in the American literature.*

Melish ME, Hicks RV, Reddy V: Kawasaki syndrome: Update. Hosp Prac 17:99, 1982. *Kawasaki's disease may be more prevalent than first supposed.*

Behçet's Disease

So often considered in the differential diagnosis of erythema multiforme because of oral and genital erosions with inflammatory ocular disease, Behçet's disease should be mentioned here although it is reviewed in depth in Ch. 464. A chronic and frequently multisystem disease, it is characterized by the triad cited and often by joint and bowel disease, with vasculitis important to the pathogenesis. Of uncommon occurrence despite alleged under-reporting, it appears regularly in the differential diagnosis of aphthae, recurrent severe herpes simplex, and Reiter's syndrome. The variability in expression of the entity, however, and the lack of minimal criteria or specific diagnostic tests for irrefutable identification leave clinical considerations unconfirmed.

Oral and genital ulcerations are usually the first symptoms, followed within days, months, or years by the uveitis and other clinical signs that may express an associated thrombophlebitis or vasculitis. Fever, malaise, and arthralgia are usually present during periods of active disease. The ocular pathology produces the most disability.

The mucosal lesions may be superficial erosions or deep punched-out ulcers, with necrosis leading to pain, with dysphagia and fetor if of the mouth, and to perforation of the labia minora in the genital area. If the colon is involved, discrete mucosal ulcers can be observed with intervening normal bowel; thus it is differentiated from the continuous inflammatory change of ulcerative colitis.

Cutaneous lesions occur in some 80 per cent of cases: follicular pustules, furuncles, inflammatory dermal nodules, acneiform lesions, cellulitis, and other forms of pyoderma. Of interest, and perhaps of diagnostic significance, sterile pustules occur after intradermal injection of normal saline or even a needle prick. The histology of induced sterile pustules shows mild to intense perivascular round cell infiltrates at 24 hours, with an occasional cluster of polymorphonuclear leukocytes. On immunofluorescent study, no deposits of immunoglobulins, complement, fibrinogen, or albumin are noted, although circulating alpha$_2$ globulin, gamma globulin, IgA, IgG, and IgM have been elevated.

Therapy for the basic disease process is probably not helpful. Corticosteroids systemically and topically may reverse some of the inflammatory processes, but the condition is known for its natural clinical fluctuations. Immunosuppressive therapy, azathioprine and cyclophosphamide, is used to reduce the need of corticosteroids.

Mast Cell Disease

Mast cell disease is a group of entities of which the common denominator is the spindle-shaped, dendritic connective tissue mast cell which aggregates in excessive numbers in the skin and occasionally in other organs. Symptoms relate to the pharmacologic effect of the histamine released by the degranulated mast cell and to the disruption of the organ structure and strength, as in bones, by mast cell infiltrates.

Several schemata distinguish among the clinical manifestations of mastocytosis. The cells may appear in the skin alone, or with systemic involvement, rarely as systemic infiltrates without skin lesions. The classic mast cell infiltrate appears as a small, discrete, reddish brown pigmented macule that becomes hive-like when stroked (Darier's sign), the released histamine having provoked a wheal. Such *urticaria pigmentosa* is the most common form of mastocytosis, occurring primarily in children, with half the patients clearing and almost all improving before adult life. Occasionally in infants there may be a single nodular lesion, a larger aggregate of cells known as a *mastocytoma*. Stroking for urtication can induce systemic effects of flushing and colic, with sufficient local edema to produce vesicles and bullae. Rarely is there *diffuse mastocytosis* with the skin so widely infiltrated as to become thickened, doughy, and lichenified. When the diffuse form is seen in children or when the urticaria pigmentosa has its onset in adulthood, noncutaneous organ involvement must be suspected. Any tissue where the mast cell is found can be affected. The central nervous system is thus excluded, leaving bone, liver, spleen, and gastrointestinal tract as sites of predilection in *systemic mastocytosis* (see Ch. 438). Here the associated macular lesions of the skin may acquire persistent telangiectasia, or may become more papular, suggestive of leukemia cutis. A small percentage of patients with systemic mastocytosis actually develop leukemia, which can be mast cell leukemia but is usually not.

Urticaria pigmentosa without systemic involvement accounts for 90 per cent of persons affected with mast cell disease. These and the balance of patients with systemic mastocytosis demonstrating cutaneous involvement all have skin lesions readily recognized by the trained eye and provable by biopsy. The nests of mast cells are diagnostic. When selecting a lesion for histology, however, care must be taken lest the granules be discharged and thus rendered invisible by stroking or other manipulation prior to biopsy. Brisk skin cleansing must be avoided, and anesthesia should be injected at a distance and deeply. After fixation in 10 per cent formalin or absolute alcohol and staining with Giemsa, toluidine blue, or methylene blue, the characteristic basophilic metachromatic granules will be seen in the cytoplasm of the mast cell.

The symptomatology of mast cell disease varies with the site and extent of organ involvement. If it is confined to the skin, more than half the patients are asymptomatic. A third or so complain of pruritus, flushing, and headache often induced by the mechanical degranulation of the mast cell, as with hot baths and exercise, or by the pharmacologic degranulation, as with codeine and aspirin. In more extensive involvement patients may experience diarrhea and peptic ulcer, usually without acid hypersecretion.

Those mast cell lesions present at birth or appearing in childhood and limited to the skin have an excellent prognosis. In fact mast cell disease confined to skin and bone is compatible with life and minimal morbidity. Solitary lesions can be excised. Therapy otherwise relates to symptomatology, the avoidance of maneuvers and situations that lead to mast cell degranulation, or the selection of time for such discharge when it interferes least with the patient's life style and can be anticipated with antihistamine coverage.

Malignancy

Skin can undergo malignant change, and it can support the metastatic malignant growth of other organs. Even more, it can respond to the systemic presence of malignancy in ways that challenge the implication of the malignant cell and process. Considered here are the common *cutaneous malignancies*, often radiation induced; then *mycosis fungoides*, an uncommon neoplastic disease but a distinct histopathologic and clinical entity first manifested in the skin; Kaposi's sarcoma because of its recent epidemic presentation with the acquired immune deficiency syndrome; and finally *melanoma*.

THE COMMON CUTANEOUS MALIGNANCIES

The individual at highest risk for developing skin cancer is the light-complexioned, blue-eyed freckler who has had considerable ultraviolet light exposure, whether geographically determined or influenced by occupation and avocation. The effect of such natural radiation will be augmented by any x-irradiation ever received, or by any exposure to carcinogens such as the oral inorganic arsenicals or to chronic cutaneous infection, ulceration, or burn.

Basal Cell Epithelioma

The most common cancer of the skin by far is the basal cell epithelioma, which affects the white population but rarely blacks or Orientals. The prevalence in the United States is 3.9 per 1000, or 757,000 cases. The average patient is over 40 years of age, but basal cell epithelioma can be seen in young adults or even children. Men are more often affected than women (2.2:1.7). The clinical lesion is a raised nodule with a pearly translucent border showing telangiectatic vessels (Fig. 557–1). It may be ulcerated and, more rarely, pigmented. Some lesions remain unchanged for years; others can be ulcerated and invasive from the first clinical observation. When removed completely by any destructive measure—excision, desiccation and curettage, even x-ray—the subsequent morbidity of the enlarging eroding lesion is thwarted. Proximity to sensitive structures and the capacity to burrow compel early recognition.

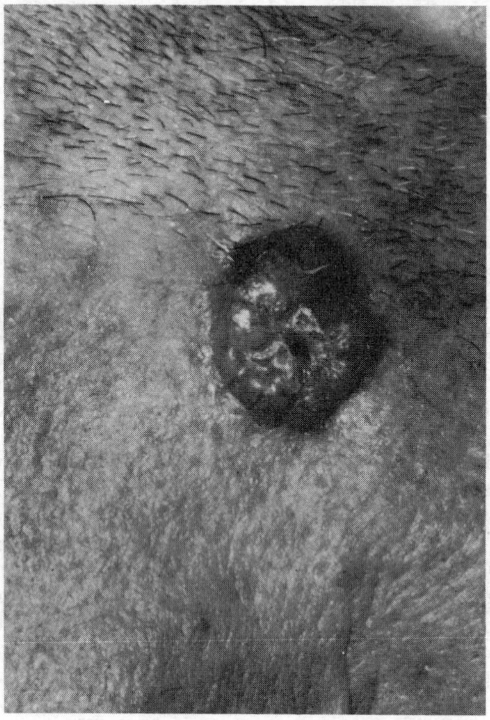

Figure 557–1. Basal cell epithelioma.

The clinical diagnosis is readily confirmed by biopsy. Therapy should be selected to ensure removal with minimal cosmetic compromise and without increasing risk through long-term radiation effects. X-ray therapy, for example, which induces cutaneous malignancy in 15 to 20 years and augments all other radiation effects, should be reserved for the feeble and elderly. Recurrent lesions, or those proximal to the eye, at the inner canthus, for example, where neither should normal tissue be sacrificed nor risk of recurrence permitted, are best treated by the microscopically monitored removal of the last malignant cell through the tedious staging of Mohs' chemosurgery; fixed or frozen tissue is charted, and each shaved specimen is checked for the persistence of the readily recognized basophilic cell.

Basal cell epitheliomas usually appear singly, but may not, and the individual who has developed one is prone to develop others. The areas most struck by sunlight in the erect individual are the surfaces prone to actinic damage and consequent cutaneous malignancy: cheeks, forehead, and nasolabial fold. Certain basal cell lesions, such as the sclerosing waxy morphea type occurring on the head and neck or the superficial spreading type seen on the trunk, may confound the inexperienced, but biopsy will usually be definitive. Nevoid tumors such as trichoepithelioma can occasionally be confused with keratotic basal cell epithelioma, especially if solitary. Multiple basal cell tumors appearing in childhood should alert the observer to the basal cell nevus syndrome and its associated abnormalities of skin, bone, central nervous system, eye, and gonads.

Squamous Cell Carcinoma

Induced by the same factors as basal cell epithelioma but with a fraction of the prevalence, squamous cell carcinoma arises in the light-exposed areas from keratinizing epidermal cells. The typical patient is more than 60 years old and male with a history of considerable sun exposure (Fig. 557–2). The tumors arising on sun damaged skin are, when compared to other squamous cell carcinoma, less aggressive, and less likely to metastasize, except perhaps for those of the ear and lip which, even when small, can metastasize to local lymph nodes. Squamous cell tumors induced by x-ray or arsenicals, or arising in burn scars, or in chronic granulomas such as lupus vulgaris, are of greater concern and have a poorer prognosis. Commencing in chronic ectodermal change as they do, they may go unnoticed or unappreciated until extensive and metastatic. Ordinarily squamous cell carcinoma appears as a slowly enlarging nodule with an inflamed, indurated base growing more rapidly than a basal cell tumor. Therapy is urgent complete removal. The prognosis is guarded for lesions of the lip, especially of the vermilion border, and for all lesions with metastases. Patients treated for cutaneous malignancy must be assessed periodically for recurrence and for new tumor. Those who have had one skin cancer are at risk of developing others even when the initiating factors are not apparent. They should be cautioned about this and about the need for surveillance, as well as the harmful effects of continued sun exposure.

MYCOSIS FUNGOIDES
(Cutaneous T-Cell Lymphoma)

Mycosis fungoides is a chronic fatal disease of the reticuloendothelial system, a T-cell lymphoma which initially and primarily involves skin but can involve lymph nodes and viscera. It is distinguishable from Hodgkin's disease and other malignant lymphomas. Clinically there is an erythematous pretumor stage which progresses to thickened, indurated, plaque-like lesions, and ultimately tumor. The early premycotic stage may last from months to years, with scaling and erythema persisting to the end; uncommonly, the presenting complaint can be a tumefaction. The disease is not rare, accounting for perhaps 1 per cent of deaths from lymphoma; it occurs in all races, usually in those from 40 to 60 years, but has been seen in teenagers.

A psoriasiform or eczematous dermatitis, chronic, persistent, and pruritic, that is not caused by drug or contactant should bring mycosis fungoides into the differential diagnosis. Fixed giant hive-like lesions or plaques are further clinical indicators, as is lymphadenopathy. Often, histopathologic confirmation of the diagnosis is delayed for years past the clinical impression of mycosis fungoides. Biopsies from plaques or tumors, however, provide the histologic features that establish the diagnosis: Pautrier's microabscesses, atypical cells nested within the epidermis; an infiltrate of atypical mononuclear cells; and hyperchromatic larger cells with irregular nuclei, the "mycosis cells." After the appearance of tumor, lymphadenopathy, or ulceration, the median survival is less than two to five years; with the appearance of all three, the median survival is less than one year.

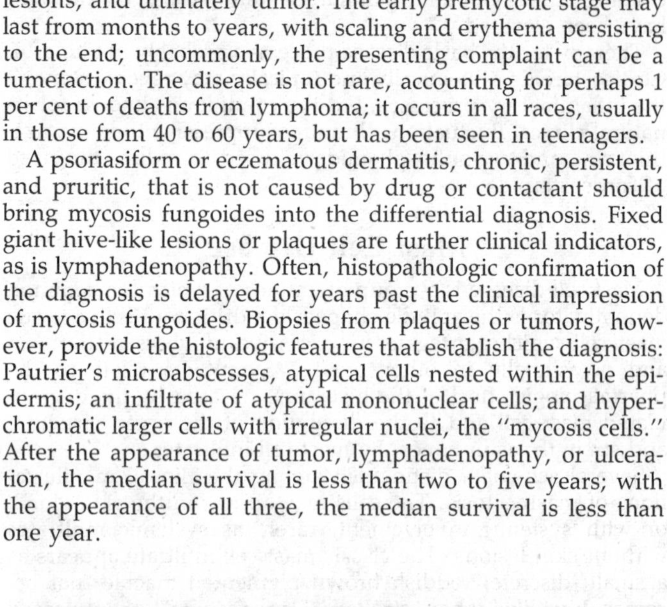

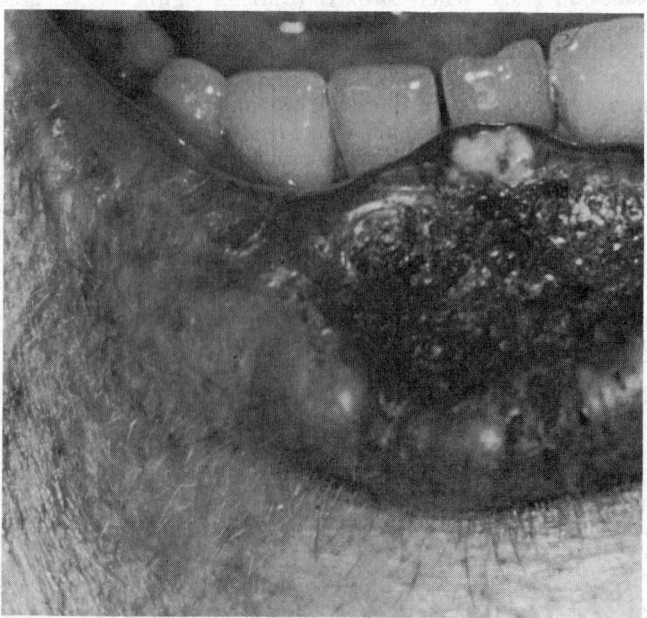

Figure 557–2. Squamous cell carcinoma.

Extracutaneous dissemination of mycosis fungoides, once thought rare, is no longer considered uncommon; visceral involvement is noted in two thirds of patients (61 to 82 per cent) at autopsy. Lung, liver, and spleen are the more common sites, but nearly every organ or tissue may be involved with atypical cells. Any lymph node involvement indicates the likelihood of spread to other extracutaneous sites. Staging for prognosis will have impetus as treatment protocols are developed. However, one third of patients who succumb to mycosis fungoides have disease limited to the skin.

Therapy for this uniformly fatal disease has been palliative. Pruritus, dermatitis, and tumor are treated at each stage as they appear. Corticosteroids have been used, as well as chemotherapeutic agents such as cyclophosphamide and chlorambucil, and also the antimetabolites azaribine and methotrexate. Bleomycin is a promising cytotoxic antibiotic because of its concentration in the skin (and lung). Electron beam therapy is of advantage for the remission of lesions if not the disease, as is conventional x-ray and, more recently, a simultaneous combined treatment with x-irradiation plus chemotherapy. Skin painting with nitrogen mustard or by intralesional injection has given favorable results, as have psoralens with high intensity ultraviolet light. To date, however, no protocol or series has been adequate to provide the definitive data for the proper treatment of this devastating disease.

No consideration of mycosis fungoides is complete without mention of Sézary's syndrome. Probably a variant of mycosis fungoides, it is characterized by an extensive exfoliative erythroderma with intense pruritus, lymphadenopathy, and large mononuclear cells in the skin and blood. Elevated leukocyte counts are found in most patients; all have a lymphocytosis, with atypical cells varying in size from 10 to 20 μ recognized as Sézary cells by their folded, lobulated nucleus and rim of PAS-positive, diastase-resistant cytoplasm. A "small cell" variant has been described. Studies of the ultrastructure of these abnormal lymphocytes have identified them in cutaneous infiltrates of mycosis fungoides. In Sézary's syndrome these abnormal thymus-derived cells constitute more than 40 per cent of purified lymphocyte fractions from the peripheral blood. In patients affected, immune mechanisms are generally not impaired.

Although Sézary's syndrome might be looked upon as the erythrodermatous phase of mycosis fungoides, it does not respond well to palliative therapy, even electron beam irradiation. Reduction of the intravascular neoplastic T-cells by leukapheresis to effect a mobilization and reduction of tissue infiltrates gives a new and innovative but not yet fully assessed approach to the management.

Edelson RL (ed.): Cutaneous T-cell lymphoma (special issue). J Dermatol Surg Oncol 6:357, 1980. *An excellent review.*

Epstein EH, Levin DL, Croft JD, Lutzner MA: Mycosis fungoides. Survival, prognostic features, response to therapy and autopsy findings. Medicine 51:61, 1972. *An important reference point for weighing the value and morbidity of therapy.*

Thomas LE, Rappaport H: Mycosis fungoides and its relationship to other malignant lymphomas. *In* Rebuck JW, et al. (eds.): The Reticuloendothelial System. Baltimore, Williams & Wilkins Company, 1975.

Van Scott EJ, Haynes HA: Cutaneous lymphoma. *In* Fitzpatrick TB (ed.): Dermatology in General Medicine. New York, McGraw-Hill Book Company, 1971, pp 556–573.

KAPOSI'S SARCOMA

Into the same limelight of uncommon but lethal cutaneous tumor has moved Kaposi's sarcoma, with new and fascinating connections to second primary malignancies and opportunistic infections that implicate reduced immune competence and the possible role of infectious agents and environmental factors. A rare neoplasm of multifocal origin, Kaposi's sarcoma presents as red-purple to blue-brown macules, plaques, and nodules of the skin and other organs. The cutaneous lesions may be firm or compressible, solitary or numerous, and may even appear initially as a dusky stain, especially about the toes.

Reporting an "idiopathic multiple pigmented sarcoma" of the skin, Moritz Kaposi in 1872 recognized that these round-cell and spindle-cell sarcomas were also to be found in viscera and seemed to occur predominantly in older men, leading to their demise. In Europe and North America, where it is more frequently seen among Jews and those of Mediterranean descent, the lesions commonly affect the lower extremities, are indolent, and often are associated with chronic lymphedema, indicating tumor infiltration of the lymphatics. Men are affected 10 to 15 times more often than women, are usually in their seventh decade, and have an average survival time of approximately 10 years, although some live much longer. The incidence of such Kaposi's sarcoma variously reported for the United States is less than 0.1 per 100,000 population and fewer than 0.02 per cent of all malignancies.

In tropical Africa, however, there is an endemic belt at an altitude of 1200 to 1500 meters where the disease accounts for 3 to 9 per cent of all malignancies, afflicting the black population while sparing white people and Indians. It is found among the young with a peak incidence in the first decade, with most patients less than 20 years of age, and with survival of less than three years. Visceral rather than cutaneous involvement and marked lymphadenopathy are the predominant clinical signs in these African children, who exhibit a unique form of Kaposi's sarcoma found in no other population.

The selective geographic distribution of the lymphadenopathic type of Kaposi's sarcoma is remarkably similar to that of Burkitt's lymphoma. With the electron microscopic studies that affirm an association between cytomegalovirus and Kaposi's sarcoma, another parallel is made with Burkitt's lymphoma, the malignancy so closely linked to the Epstein-Barr virus. In the acquiring of Kaposi's sarcoma, therefore, it would seem that infectious agents and immune status are of significance, as well as genetic and environmental factors. Kaposi's sarcoma has been observed to complicate systemic lupus erythematosus being treated with immunosuppression and to appear along with tumors of lymphoreticular origin in the immunosuppressed recipients of renal transplants. It is known to coexist with other primary malignancies. However, its appearance as an aggressive lethal tumor in the young male homosexual without underlying disease is the stunning observation of grave concern. Those affected have a mean age in the fourth decade. Their skin lesions are generalized in distribution and are smaller, softer, and lighter in color than the classic firm, indurated lesions of the legs. Mucous membrane tumors or symptomatic visceral or lung lesions may appear before the hemorrhagic sarcomas of the skin. Average survival time from onset of the disease is less than two years.

Such fulminant Kaposi's sarcoma is appearing alone or with *Pneumocystis carinii* pneumonia and other opportunistic infections in increasing numbers in a population comprising male homosexuals and drug abusers with geographic clustering in New York and California, a population that has experienced a variety of sexually transmitted diseases and demonstrates the presence of antibodies to cytomegalovirus implicated as a causal agent in the induction of the immunosuppressed state (see Ch. 430). The documented infectivity of contaminated blood products and seminal fluid has extended the risk to transfusion recipients and the heterosexual partners of bisexual individuals. Among those cases reported to the CDC since June, 1981, Kaposi's sarcoma was the presenting disease in almost half. A small painless red nodule of the skin, easily overlooked, can signal a profoundly compromised immune state and grave prognosis. There is no adequate therapy.

Friedman-Kien A, Laubenstein L, Rubenstein P, Buimovici-Klein E, Marmor M, Stahl R, Springland I, Soo Kim K, Zollar-Pazner S: Disseminated Kaposi's sarcoma in homosexual men. Ann Intern Med 96:693, 1982.

Hardwood A, Osoba D, Hofstader S, Goldstein M, Cardella C, Holecek M, Kunynetz R, Giammarco R: Kaposi's sarcoma in recipients of renal transplants. Am J Med 67:759, 1979.

Hardy M, Goldfarb P, Levine S, Dattner A, Muggia F, Levitt S, Weinstein E: De novo Kaposi's sarcoma in renal transplantation. CA 38:144, 1976.

Haverkos HW, Curran JW: The current outbreak of Kaposi's sarcoma and

opportunistic infections. CA 32:330, 1982. *Impressive data and review of the challenge of why these diseases are occurring now and in the population afflicted.*
Hymes K, Cheung T, Greene J, Prose N, Marcus A, Ballard H, William D, Laubenstein L: Kaposi's sarcoma in homosexual men—a report of eight cases. Lancet 2:98, 1981.
Klein M, Pereira F, Kantor I: Kaposi sarcoma complicating systemic lupus erythematosus treated with immunosuppression. Arch Dermatol 110:602, 1974.
Myers B, Kessler E, Levi J, Pick A, Rosenfeld J, Israel P: Kaposi sarcoma in kidney transplant recipients. Arch Intern Med 133:307, 1974.
Safai B, Good RA: Kaposi's sarcoma: A review and recent developments. CA 31:2, 1981. *An excellent review of the facets that suggest Kaposi's sarcoma as a potential model for a virus-associated human cancer.*
Safai B, Mike V, Giraldo G, Beth E, Good R: Association of Kaposi's sarcoma with second primary malignancies. CA 45:1472, 1980.

MELANOMA

Melanoma is a neoplasm of melanocytes that has the potential for invasion and metastasis. It contributes little to the burden of cutaneous malignancy by case load (fewer than 3 percent of new skin cancers), but by mortality it accounts for two thirds of the deaths from skin cancer, and at an appreciably young age. In fact, those who develop any malignancy between ages 35 and 40 are at greater risk only for cancer of the lung, breast, or cervix.

Along with other skin cancer, melanoma shows a currently increasing incidence, highest in Caucasians, and influenced adversely by ultraviolet light exposure as judged by the anatomic distribution of lesions and by occupational and geographical factors. As with other skin cancers, patients who develop melanoma are apt to have a light complexion and light-colored eyes, and to sunburn readily. They may have a family predisposition to the development of melanoma, or they may have had one primary melanoma which places them at greater risk of having a second primary.

Three out of four melanomas that develop in the skin undergo progressive change over an extended period from not less than six months to many years, thereby providing the informed examiner with a prolonged opportunity to recognize and remove surgically the potentially lethal lesion for probable cure. Change in texture, color, or size of a pre-existing nevus arouses suspicion of melanoma, but even without such signs there are clinical characteristics that make a pigmented lesion suspect. Any brown-black spot with areas of red or red-purple, plus white, whether gray-white or pink-white, and blue, should be examined histopathologically. There is further suspicion of melanoma if the borders of the lesion are irregular, appear notched or smudged, and have pigment streaming from the pigmented edge. Of grave concern is the lesion with a surface that is elevated or ulcerated and devoid of skin markings.

Regarding all melanotic lesions with red, white, and blue as possible melanoma and hence in need of definitive histopathologic diagnosis, one may gather a few vascular lesions and a rare pigmented basal cell epithelioma, but would also net a significant number of early melanomas when most are at a curative stage. This underscores the importance of examining the entire integument carefully, in good light, and with hand lens magnification, for all suspicious pigmented lesions. It presumes confidence in recognizing the common benign pigmented lesions of the skin reviewed in Ch. 556.

Primary cutaneous melanoma can be classified according to clinicohistologic type, the level of invasion, the thickness of the lesion, and the density of the inflammatory response. With the establishment of criteria for sorting among the various clinical presentations, realistic comparisons can be made, prognoses given, and the value of therapeutic measures assessed. Clinically, several types are recognized and the histology correlated.

Lentigo maligna (Fig. 557–3) begins as a small tan macular lesion, a circumscribed precancerous melanosis, the melanotic freckle of Hutchinson. Usually a lesion of the elderly, it can occur in the 20's. Over years, or even decades, it may enlarge by lateral growth, with the margins becoming irregular and the color modified to brown-black and pink-white. Eventually there will be dermal invasion, the vertical growth phase, associated with a papular or nodular surface. Melanotic freckles are mostly seen on the face but may occur anywhere on the skin where there has been significant sunlight exposure. The radial growth phase of 5 to 7 cm and measured in years provides the long lead time for therapy before active malignant invasion. Unfortunately, the benignity of appearance and the confusion of the smaller early lesion with a solar lentigo often delay definitive treatment until size alone precludes simple excision.

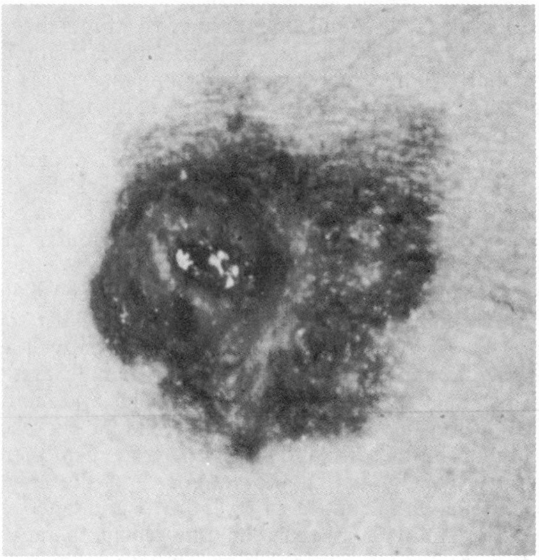

Figure 557–3. Lentigo maligna.

Superficial spreading melanoma occurs in younger individuals; it may appear anywhere in the body, characteristically on the upper back in both sexes and on the legs of women (Fig. 557–4). Fairly regular in outline, sometimes notched, lesions range in color from tan to black, often with the telltale mix of red, white, and blue. Initially barely palpable, these, too, become papular or nodular with the vertical growth phase.

Nodular melanoma, as might be suspected from the terminology, does not have a discernible radial growth phase but, from the first, is observed as a nodule or plaque, dark brown or black, with a gray or blue cast (Fig. 557–5). It is invasive from the start, and the prognosis is never as good as with other melanomas. Further, the nodular variety can occasionally be amelanotic and extremely difficult to diagnose clinically.

The clinicohistologic grouping recognizes an *acral lentiginous melanoma* of the palms, soles, and terminal phalanges, which is similar in its benign clinical appearance to *lentigo maligna melanoma,* but which, like it and like *superficial spreading melanoma,* can develop a vertical growth phase. It also distinguishes nodular melanoma of the mucous membranes, occurring more frequently in blacks and Orientals, and a miscellaneous group of melanomas that arise in various nevi, the central nervous system, and the viscera.

In all melanomas there is correlation between the depth of the histologic invasion and the prognosis. Clark and his coworkers have designated intraepidermal malignancy as Level I, invasion of the papillary dermis as Level II, filling the papillary dermis and impinging upon but not invading the reticular dermis as Level III, reaching into the reticular dermis as Level IV, and reaching into the subcutaneous tissue as Level V. Correlated with these levels is an increasing mortality: 8.3 per cent for Level II; 35.2 per cent for Level III: 46.1 per cent for Level IV; and 52 per cent for Level V. Breslow measures depth of tumor invasion with an ocular micrometer and finds 100 per cent five-year survival in those with a melanoma depth less than 0.75 mm; 74 per cent with a depth of 0.76 to 1.50 mm; 79 per cent at 1.51 to 2.25 mm; 44 per cent at 2.26 to 3.0

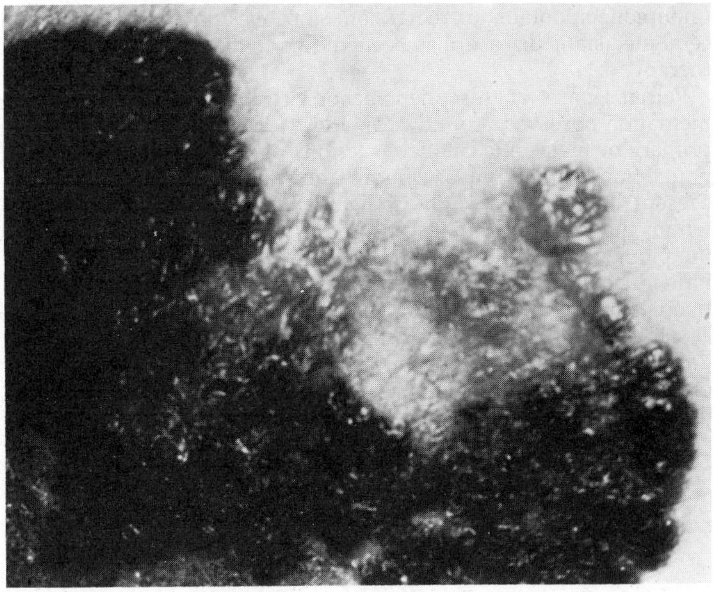

Figure 557–4. Superficial spreading melanoma.

mm; and 22 per cent at depths over 3 mm. Current histopathologic reporting gives both Clark levels and Breslow measurements, useful for clinical correlations, cooperative studies, and predictive value. There is also a difference in survival according to the clinical type of melanoma, with lentigo maligna melanoma having the longest survival, followed by superficial spreading melanoma, and, poorest, nodular melanoma.

Prognosis, in addition to a consideration of the type of melanoma, its size, and depth of invasion, is also dependent on the age and sex of the patient, the anatomic location of the tumor, and the presence or absence of metastases and of pigment. With similar lesions women fare better than men, and lesions of the leg or of the head or neck permit longer survival than those of the trunk. Absence of pigment portends a poor prognosis. So may pregnancy, although this is not certain for a given patient. In a study of women with melanoma there was no indication of benefit to the melanoma patient from termination of the pregnancy, oophorectomy, adrenalectomy, or hypophysectomy. Survival of those with localized disease was unchanged when compared to nonpregnant melanoma patients at the same stage. Those with nodal disease and pregnant did less well. They and those whose lesions had been activated during gestation should be cautioned against subsequent pregnancies.

The question of melanoma arising in pre-existing nevi is always posed. Congenital nevi account for fewer than 0.1 per cent of the nevi of the average young adult, but they are usually larger than acquired nevi and, since present from birth, are likely to be identified by the patient or his family. The risk of malignant change in such nevi is probably proportional to the numbers of aggregated melanocytes—hence the size of the lesion. Giant pigmented congenital nevi (the giant hairy or bathing trunk nevi) have an incidence of malignant change variously reported from 15 to 42 percent. Although melanoma is rare before puberty, almost half of those occurring in childhood arise in such giant congenital nevi. However, of all patients who develop melanoma, only one in four will recall a pre-existing pigmented lesion present from childhood, a figure supported by the 20 per cent of melanoma lesions that have histologic evidence of associated nevus.

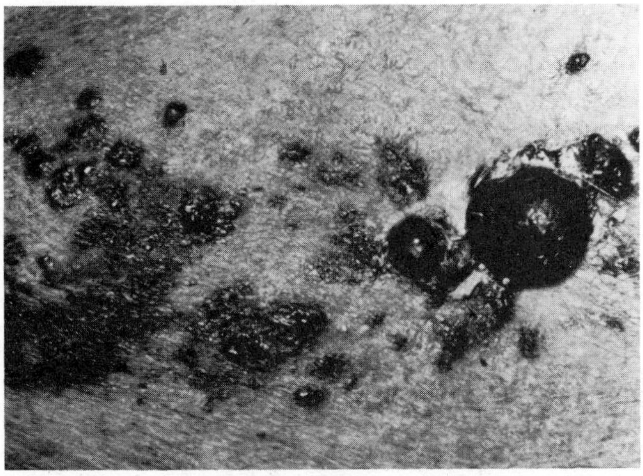

Figure 557–5. Nodular melanoma.

The removal of giant congenital nevi is indicated for malignant risk as well as cosmetic disfigurement, but often it is not surgically feasible. For small congenital nevi there are no data to support significant risk. If one accepts the relationship of size to risk, such aggregates of melanocytes must pose greater risk per unit area than normal skin. There is probably value in considering the removal of all congenital nevi larger than 1 cm after weighing the possibility of cosmetic disfigurement and such factors as complexion, eye color, and anatomic location.

When the sheer number of observed nevi preclude prophylactic excision and there is great variability among the nevi, the patient may well have the "B-K mole syndrome," characterized by myriad heritable melanocytic nevi and grave risk of multiple primary melanomas. One patient had six. In 25 individuals with one or more primary cutaneous melanoma, all from six families, 17 were examined and 15 had the syndrome. The prototypic "mole" is 1 cm in diameter, irregular in outline, and haphazardly colored tan, brown, black, and pink. Although appearing flat, it has a small palpable dermal component. These dysplastic nevi may be as few as 10 or more than 100, concentrating in a horsecollar distribution but found on the extremities as well. Unlike the ordinary noncongenital nevus, they appear later in childhood and after age 35. When observed in a group of four or five there is a striking difference among them, but it is by their histology with their atypical melanocytes that they can be identified. The melanomas that arise are biologically aggressive.

Melanoma, capable of persisting for years before active metastatic spread, can signal its presence by metastases with the primary lesion undiscoverable. In such cases (15 per cent in two large series) the occult primary melanoma may have undergone spontaneous regression, since melanoma, even visceral metastatic disease, has been known to disappear without therapy.

Perhaps parts of this phenomenon are the areas of depigmentation observed around nevi, and occasionally around the primary or metastatic cutaneous lesions of patients with melanoma. Such leukoderma is clinically indistinguishable from that present in halo nevi of the individual *without* melanoma, in whom the depigmentation can progress to the obliteration of the pigmented nevus clinically and histopathologically. In such individuals, free of malignancy, circulating anti-melanoma antibodies have been reported.

With suspected melanoma, an unequivocal diagnosis is mandatory. Clinical diagnoses can be quite wrong, and histopathologically certain pigmented lesions such as the Spitz nevus (benign juvenile melanoma) can be misread or confused with melanoma. A biopsy must be done and the histology reviewed.

The suspected lesion should be excised with a 5- to 10-mm border and penetration to the subcutaneous fat. If the size of the lesion precludes simple excision, an incisional biopsy is justified without concern over dissemination of tumor.

With confident histologic confirmation, a wide surgical excision is indicated. With a lesion less than 1 mm in depth, a 1-cm margin around the lesion is adequate. Depending upon the type and level of penetration of the tumor, further surgery or therapy may be suggested. Systemic and regional chemotherapy have been used and, more recently, immunotherapy with vaccinia and BCG.

Clark WH Jr, Reimer RR, Greene M, Ainsworth AM, Mastrangelo MJ: Origin of familial malignant melanomas from heritable melanocytic lesions: "B-K mole syndrome." Arch Dermatol 114:732, 1978. *The dysplastic nevus is another signal in our early warning system for melanoma.*

Day CL Jr, Mihm MC Jr, Sober AJ, Fitzpatrick TB, Malt RA: Narrower margins for clinical stage I malignant melanoma. N Engl J Med 306:479, 1982.

Kopf AW, Bart RS, Rodriguez-Sains, BA: Malignant melanoma: A review. J Dermatol Surg Oncol 3:41, 1977. *A thorough review.*

Mihm MC Jr, Fitzpatrick TB, Brown MML, Raker JW, Malt RA, Kaiser JS: Early detection of primary cutaneous malignant melanoma. A color atlas. N Engl J Med 289:989, 1973. *The ABC's of early detection.*

Part XXVI
OCCUPATIONAL AND ENVIRONMENTAL MEDICINE

558. PRINCIPLES OF OCCUPATIONAL MEDICINE

Charles E. Becker

Occupational medicine is concerned with the physical and emotional safety and health of workers. It encompasses issues of public concern, particularly the quality of air and water, the degree of environmental pollution, and the complex mosaic of legal, economic, social, and ethical questions that are raised whenever human action produces human disorders.

Among the 100 million workers in the United States today, approximately 100,000 deaths per year are attributed to the workplace. Yet there are only 8000 physicians whose self-determined primary specialty is occupational medicine, and only 800 of these have subspecialty board certification. Primary-care internists, family physicians, and emergency physicians constitute the "front line" for identification of work-related disorders, therefore, and must learn to target the medical history and to recognize classic signs and symptoms of occupational and environmental disorders.

Occupational medicine deals almost exclusively with diagnosis and prevention, not treatment. The diagnosis of an occupational disease may be difficult, since occupational diseases (1) may simulate many other disorders, (2) often lack unique pathology, and (3) may be marked by a long latency period between exposure and the manifestation of the disease.

Problems from chemical contamination do not always remain exclusively in the workplace; they may extend into the community: polychlorinated biphenyls (PCBs) in Japan; dioxin in Seveso, Italy; radiation exposure at Three Mile Island; mercury contamination in Minamata Bay; lead pollution in cities and around smelting plants; and nervous system, liver, and reproductive toxicity from chlordecone (Kepone) in Virginia. These events give rise to important political, social, and economic considerations that emphasize the need for specialized training in occupational medicine.

Competency in occupational medicine is best acquired from a base of general training in internal medicine, with extended knowledge and experience in epidemiology, industrial hygiene, and toxicology. The relationship between workplace-environmental exposures and disease centers on four basic concepts: recognition, prevention, exacerbation, latent manifestation. Workplace-associated diseases are presumed to be preventable when recognized and fully understood. Since the signs and symptoms of occupational diseases may be identical to those of many other diseases, a high level of suspicion is required for the recognition that allows prevention. Rather than causing an illness, occupational environmental conditions may, in fact, exacerbate or compound a pre-existing condition. For example, a patient with toxicity from aminoglycoside antibiotics may have additional otologic injury from loud noises occurring at work. Although some environmental and occupational diseases become manifest acutely, many have a long latency period and may extend from the workplace into the family or society and thus pose important considerations in diagnostic and preventive strategies.

In occupational medicine there are four basic categories of hazard: physical, biologic, psychologic, and chemical. Physical hazards may include vibration, heat, noise, radiation, and trauma. Occupational injuries account for approximately 14,000 deaths, 245 million lost work days, and $25 billion in direct and indirect costs annually in the United States. Biologic hazards include the well-known occupational risks of hepatitis or tuberculosis, for example. Psychologic hazards of stress and work-shift changes are complex and will be discussed subsequently. Chemical hazards involve exposure to solvents, dusts, vapors, and gases. It is important here to distinguish between toxicity and hazard. *Toxicity* is the inherent capability of a material to cause injury to a living cell. *Hazard* is the chance of a resultant injury from use of such a material in a given setting. Asbestos, for example, is a useful fire retardant construction material with known basic toxicity that may become hazardous during repair or demolition work or fire, which may cause its release into the air.

In occupational medicine one is also concerned with the difference between exposure and dose. Exposure is determined by surveillance of the environment with the knowledge that a toxic agent(s) has had the potential of being delivered into the body. For example, environmental measurements of lead can provide an index of exposure. Dose, however, can be assessed only by biologic monitoring of blood, urine, and hair, and indices of enzyme systems that may be affected. In the case of lead, the total dose delivered is dependent on the amount that is respirable and the amount absorbed from the gastrointestinal tract.

This chapter outlines some of the basic concepts and a few selected disorders encompassed in occupational medicine. Other chapters in this section describe at length occupational diseases of the lung (Ch. 559) and of the skin (Ch. 561) and a variety of chemical and physical sources of injury. Some chapters in other parts of the book contain useful information related to the discipline: toxic nephropathies (Ch. 81.3), epidemiology of cancer (Ch. 170), painful back and painful shoulders (Ch. 458 and 459), and neuropathies associated with the workplace (Ch. 565).

THE OCCUPATIONAL-ENVIRONMENTAL HISTORY

"When you come to a patient's house, you should ask him what sort of pains he has, what caused them, how many days he has been ill, whether the bowels are working and what sort of food he eats." So said Hippocrates in his work, *Affections*. I may venture to add one more question: "What occupation does he follow?" (*Diseases of Workers*, Preface, Bernardino Romazzini [1633–1714]).

Table 558–1 lists key elements of an occupational and environmental history that may be added to the data base collected on all patients. In every problem-oriented assessment of a current illness, individual problem lists should include such questions concerning the occupational health history as, Are symptoms associated with work, or do they improve during vacations and weekends? Are other workers similarly affected? Is there or has there been direct exposure to dust, fumes, and chemicals? Have there been work-related injuries? Is periodic testing and medical surveillance or routine industrial hygiene sampling of the workplace performed? A careful work history should include a chronologic list of all previous jobs with a reasonably detailed description of the work site, the scope of a typical work day, and such pertinent factors as protective equipment, ventilation, and pre-employment examinations.

A specific listing of the total number of days missed on each job and the reasons for the absences may be useful. Has a worker compensation claim been filed in the past? Does the worker perform additional jobs, i.e., is he or she moonlighting? A patient may not relate work to health, and so the physician should obtain initially, on each examination, specific answers to common occupational problems, for example, Have you ever been exposed to loud noises, excessive vibration, or heat? Do you work with asbestos? Have you been exposed to radioactive chemicals? Have you had previous chemical exposure? During the military, what were your duties?

TABLE 558–1. KEY ELEMENTS OF AN OCCUPATIONAL AND ENVIRONMENTAL HISTORY

Present illness (for each element of problem list)
- Symptoms related to work
- Other employees similarly affected
- Current exposure to dusts, fumes, chemicals, biologic hazards
- Prior first report of work injury

Work history

Description of all prior jobs; typical work day; change in work process

Work site
- Ventilation; medical and industrial hygiene surveillance; employment examinations; protective measures
- Union health and safety; moonlighting; days missed work last year, why; prior worker compensation claims

Past history
- Exposure to noise, vibration, radiation, chemicals, asbestos

Environmental history
- Present and prior home and work locations
- Jobs of "significant others"
- Hazardous wastes/spills exposure
- Air pollution
- Hobbies: painting, sculpture, welding, woodworking
- Home insulation-heating
- Home and work cleaning agents
- Pesticide exposure
- Do you wear seat belts?
- Do you have firearms at home or work?

Review of systems

Specific emphasis
- Shift changes; boredom; reproductive history

The environmental health history should include information about industries located in the neighborhood, exposure to hazardous waste or toxic spills, jobs of the spouse, degree of air pollution, and types of hobbies and recreational activities that also may contribute to health-related problems, such as painting, sculpturing, welding, or woodworking.

In addition, it may be important to elicit a description of home insulation or heating as well as exposure to cleaning agents and insecticides. Special questions should be directed toward unique workplace problems such as working hours and job schedule (Do these affect your sleep pattern? Are you bored on the job?). The reproductive history is essential: the number of miscarriages, children, stillbirths, previous pregnancies; difficulty in conceiving; and changes in libido and menses.

Signs and Symptoms of Occupational and Environmental Disorders

Because occupational and environmental diseases have a long latency and may be synergistic with other causes for disease, the clinician should always consider that the signs and symptoms may be caused by occupational or environmental conditions. Sometimes it may be useful to identify all the signs and symptoms that could be associated with disease of the environment or the workplace. A useful handbook by Daugaard provides such a guide to signs and symptoms of both acute and chronic occupational diseases compiled from standard works on toxicology and occupational medicine. For instance, knowledge of exposure to certain substances may implicate or suggest the cause: chlorinated hydrocarbons and acne, arsenic and thallium and alopecia; solvent exposure and anosmia; chlorinated hydrocarbons and arrhythmias; and aniline dyes and bladder or other cancers.

Reproductive hazards, noise–induced hearing abnormalities, and work-shift changes will be discussed as important occupational entities not covered specifically by other chapters in this section.

REPRODUCTIVE HAZARDS

Seven per cent of all newborns in the United States have birth defects, approximately 70 per cent of which are of unknown cause. The relationship between exposure to environmental and occupational agents and consequent development of male and female reproductive abnormalities is an area of intense study and interest. Animal studies have demonstrated the transmission to subsequent generations of chemically induced abnormalities of sperm and at a rate determined by mendelian principles. These observations have sparked interest in predicting and thereby preventing reproductive hazards from environmental agents. Short-term bioassays for mutagenesis, such as the Ames test, have been used to screen for teratogenic agents to predict reproductive outcome. These relatively inexpensive and rapid initial screening tests of chemicals can be performed in animals or bacteria. Agents encountered in the environment or the workplace can clearly cause reproductive hazards, i.e., testicular toxicity of dibromochloropropane (DBCP) recognized in California chemical workers in 1977. Male workers with sterility suffered no systemic illness and were working in an environment that was alleged to be safe. Previous laboratory tests in animals had suggested reproductive hazards from this chemical. The controversy surrounding this event sparked great interest in this subject. To date, the following environmental and occupational agents have been shown to cause adverse reproductive effects in men: anesthetic gases, carbon disulfide, diethylstilbestrol, toluene diamine, ethylene dibromide, chlordecone, and ionizing radiation. A much stronger data base is required to assess environmental effects on pregnancy outcome, spontaneous abortion, and stillbirth.

NOISE-INDUCED HEARING LOSS

More than five million people in the United States have noise-induced hearing loss. This most common form of hearing loss is associated with damage to, and loss of, hair cells in the organ of Corti. Early or moderately advanced, noise-induced hearing loss is associated with normal hearing in the low frequencies but gradually increasing loss of hearing at higher frequencies (with a maximum of 3,4, or 6 kHz). There may be some return toward normal function at 8 kHz. The audiometric shape of this curve is not pathognomonic because other otologic disorders, e.g., that caused by aminoglycoside antibiotic therapy, can result in an identical audiogram. Some of the hearing loss attributed to aging (presbycusis) may be due to the nearly ubiquitous noise pollution in modern society. Epidemiologic studies suggest that aging individuals in a nonindustrialized society have much better hearing preservation than older Americans. Major individual differences in susceptibility to noise-induced hearing loss occur. Men are much more susceptible to noise-induced hearing loss than women. Smoking and lack of skin pigmentation may also be risk factors for noise-induced hearing loss. Hearing impairment from occupational and environmental factors is a major and entirely preventable public health problem.

WORK SHIFT CHANGES

Twenty per cent of American workers work evenings or nights. In some industries, such as automobile production, petrol chemicals, and textile manufacturing, shift workers number nearly 50 per cent. There is growing evidence to suggest clinically significant health effects from shift work. Twenty per cent of workers are unable to tolerate shift work, tolerance for which also diminishes with increasing age. Daily physiologic variations known as circadian rhythms are distorted by shift work, which in turn alters the quality of sleep and causes important disturbances of the gastrointestinal tract and other organs. Diabetes mellitus and epilepsy may be aggravated by shift work, and the risk of accidents may be increased. Shift workers tend to have an increased number of subjective health complaints in general and may have enhanced risk factors complicating management of other medical disorders.

CONCLUSIONS

Strictly speaking, all diseases that are not genetic in origin are "environmental." Even genetic disorders are not totally endogenous, since they most frequently alter the ability of the host to accommodate to the environment. Broadly conceived, even the infectious diseases and nutritional disorders are environmental in origin. In practice, however, the term *environmental medicine* is used in a much more restrictive sense to reflect the chemical and physical hazards to which an individual is exposed and the injuries that may result from that exposure. Occupational medicine is that subset of environmental medicine directly concerned with the hazards of the workplace. The following chapters will describe in greater detail some of the specific hazards and injuries incident to modern occupations. The topics selected cannot be inclusive, since the boundaries of occupational and environmental medicine are indistinct, merging into the traditional domains of internal medicine, epidemiology, toxicology, surgery, orthopaedics, and many other clinical and basic science disciplines.

Daugaard J: Symptoms and Signs in Occupational Disease: A Practical Guide. Copenhagen, Munksgaard, 1978. *A thorough catalog of symptoms and signs of occupationally related conditions.*

Lauwerys RR: Industrial chemical exposure: Guidelines for biological monitoring. Davis, Calif., Biomedical Publications. *A paperback book with a practical guide to methods of assessment of exposure to toxic chemicals.*

Levy BS, Wegman TH: Occupational Health: Recognizing and Preventing Work-Related Disease. Boston, Little, Brown and Company, 1983. *A useful and easy-to-read paperback text by multiple authors encompassing a broad curriculum of occupational medicine; limited bibliography.*

Rom WN: Environmental and Occupational Medicine. Boston, Little Brown and Company, 1983. *A hard-bound, detailed text, well referenced, with strong emphasis on occupational lung disorders.*

559. OCCUPATIONAL LUNG DISEASE

Robert J. Mason

The air we exhale is cleaner than the air we inhale. The 15,000 liters of air we inhale per day to meet our metabolic needs contains a heterogeneous aerosol of dusts, vapors, and microorganisms. The net result is that people living in an urban environment inhale about 2 mg of dust each day. Of course, cigarette smokers and people who work in certain dusty environments inhale more. Elaborate protective mechanisms for filtering air and clearing deposited particles have evolved to protect the delicate alveolar-capillary membrane; in certain occupational settings, however, the defenses are inadequate and occupational pulmonary disease develops. The major factors that determine if disease will occur are the biologic properties of the inhaled material, the dose of the inhaled material (concentration and duration of exposure), and the defenses of the individual (genetic, physical, immunologic, concurrent illness).

Because of the diversity of industrial dusts and vapors, there can be a variety of clinical presentation for occupational pulmonary diseases (Table 559–1). The clinical presentation of almost all nonoccupational pulmonary diseases can be mimicked by an occupational disease. The key to diagnosis of occupational pulmonary disease is suspicion by the examining physician and an appropriate occupational history. The major problem is that the relation of the occupation to the illness may not be obvious: (1) There may be a long delay between initial exposure and impairment of pulmonary function or development of a carcinoma. (2) Symptoms may not occur at work. In some forms of occupational asthma, for example, the main symptoms occur after work, especially at night. (3) Exposure alone does not itself necessarily prove the etiology of the disease. Workers who have been exposed to an occupational hazard may have a nonoccupationally related disease.

TABLE 559–1. DIVERSITY OF OCCUPATIONAL PULMONARY DISEASES

Interstitial parenchymal disease
Asbestosis, coal workers' pneumoconiosis, silicosis, berylliosis, hypersensitivity pneumonitis
Pulmonary edema
Smoke inhalation, acute toxic fumes (NO_2, chlorine)
Pleural disease
Asbestos-related plaques and effusions, mesothelioma
Bronchitis
Grain dust, heavy dust exposures (coal workers)
Asthma
Toluene diisocyanate, platinum salts, formalin, flour, cotton dust, western red cedar
Bronchogenic carcinoma
Uranium, asbestos, chromates, nickel, chloromethyl ether
Infectious disease
Anthrax (wood sorters, imported hides)
Coccidioidomycosis (construction workers, archeologists)
Mycobacterial disease (silicosis)
Psittacosis (pet shop owners, taxidermists)
Echinococcus (sheep and dog handlers)
Q fever (tanners and sheep handlers)

It is important to differentiate occupational pulmonary diseases from other pulmonary diseases in order to provide specific treatment and to assist in obtaining financial compensation for the patient when warranted. Removal of the patient from the hazardous environment may be the only treatment that reduces symptoms or prevents deterioration. When an occupational pulmonary disease is diagnosed, fellow workers need to be notified and their status evaluated, and preventive measures need to be applied as appropriate. An index case of an occupationally related disease should be thought of conceptually as a case of tuberculosis so that appropriate public health measures are instituted and the conditions of the patient's working colleagues are evaluated.

Our major efforts should be directed toward preventing occupational diseases, but the means of prevention and the establishment of safe levels of exposure are difficult and complex. This is because individuals vary in their susceptibility to adverse effects, because it may take many years to assess the effect of a given exposure, and because establishment of levels of exposure has major economic consequences. Epidemiologic surveys can provide data for establishing exposure levels that should pose minimal risk for the general population. It is, however, the sensitive individual who is most adversely affected. How can these sensitive individuals be identified, how should they be advised, and should the standards be set low enough to avoid any risk even to sensitive individuals? Only a few traits of sensitive individuals are known, for example, bronchial hyper-reactivity for some types of occupational asthma, and cigarette smoking for most forms of occupationally related bronchogenic cancer. Ways of identifying sensitive individuals for different occupational hazards are needed so that the relative risks are known, the patients advised, and appropriate standards set.

Dosman JA, Cotton DJ: Occupational Pulmonary Disease; Focus on Grain Dust and Health. New York, Academic Press, 1980. *The proceedings of an international symposium on grain dust and health. Excellent introductory chapters on general occupational pulmonary disease by the leaders in this field. The discussion of grainhandlers' respiratory diseases forms the bulk of the text, but the problems are pertinent to all other forms of occupational pulmonary disease.*

Hunter D: The Diseases of Occupations. London, Hodder and Stroughton, 1978. *A wonderful historic perspective and a wealth of clinical information presented in a delightful style.*

Parkes WR: Occupational Lung Disorders. London, Butterworths, 1982. *An excellent, comprehensive, well-referenced text.*

Weil H, Ziskind MM: Occupational pulmonary diseases. *In* Fishman AP (ed.): Pulmonary Diseases and Disorders. New York, McGraw-Hill Book Company, 1980, pp 754–792. *Well written and well referenced, the next stop for additional reading on almost any aspect of occupational pulmonary disease.*

DEPOSITION AND CLEARANCE OF INHALED MATERIALS

DEPOSITION. The site of deposition is the most likely area for initial injury and production of symptoms. In general, this depends upon the aerodynamic size of the inhaled particles, the anatomy of the respiratory system, and the breathing pattern of the individual.

The first barrier for inhaled materials during quiet breathing is the nose, which removes essentially all particles larger than 10 μ. However, during exercise, because of the increased volume of ventilation and mouth breathing, up to 20 per cent of particles 10 to 20 μ in diameter pass the nose, mouth, and pharynx and are deposited in the large airways. This is an important consideration for workers in strenuous occupations in dusty environments or for exercising atopic children during pollen season. The second site of deposition is the ciliated epithelium of large and small airways. The number of particles deposited increases at high flow rates, during rapid shallow breathing, or in areas of disease, e.g., bronchiectasis. As the inhaled air passes into smaller and smaller bronchioles the rate of flow decreases and particles sediment. The third site of deposition is the alveolar surface, where deposition is by diffusion, aided by the relatively long residence time of the suspended particles and short distance to the alveolar wall. Slow, deep breathing favors alveolar deposition. The *respirable fraction* consists of particles (from 0.5 to 5 μ) that are most likely to be deposited in alveoli or very small airways and produce parenchymal lung disease. Particles larger than 10 μ are usually removed by the upper airway, and therefore they are considered more innocuous and less pathogenic. How then do asbestos fibers, which may be 25 μ long, penetrate so deeply into the lung? The explanation is that their site of deposition is based on aerodynamic diameter and not length.

CLEARANCE. Pulmonary clearance can be divided into three phases, depending on where the particles are deposited. (1) Particles that lie on the mucous blanket over the ciliary epithelium are normally cleared rapidly, within an hour. The cilia propel the mucus toward the pharynx, and the particles are swallowed or expectorated. This process could be severely impaired by viral infections that damage ciliated cells, extensive squamous metaplasia, genetic defects in ciliary function (ciliary dyskinesis syndromes), or alterations in the physical properties of mucus. (2) Particles deposited in the alveolar region distal to the ciliated airways are ingested by macrophages and then over a period of hours to days the particle-laden macrophages move to the small airways and are transported up the ciliary escalator. (3) Free particles that traverse the respiratory epithelium are ingested by interstitial macrophages and cleared by unknown pathways over months to years. Some ingested particles stay in the interstitium in the lung parenchyma, some are transported to regional lymph nodes, and others eventually make their way back to the airways and are cleared by the ciliated epithelium. The rate of clearance from the interstitium is thought to be dependent on the solubility of the ingested material. The rate of clearance is much slower in smokers than in nonsmokers. The ultimate fate of and tissue reaction to different dusts are determined mainly by the interaction of the dusts and the macrophages, but the precise cellular mechanisms and host factors that facilitate clearance or stimulate fibrosis are unknown.

Brain JD, Valberg PA: Deposition of aerosol in the respiratory tract. Am Rev Respir Dis 120:1325, 1979.

DIAGNOSIS AND ASSESSMENT OF HAZARDS

HISTORY. A detailed occupational history is the key to the diagnosis of an occupationally related illness (Table 558–1). People change jobs frequently. Furthermore, there may be a long interval between exposure and disease, especially for development of lung cancer. Therefore, all part-time and full-time jobs and hobbies must be recorded, preferably by recording the first job and then listing all subsequent jobs chronologically. Attention must be given to precisely what kind of job the worker did, which hazardous agents were present, whether they were in high or low concentration, whether or not protective clothing or masks were used, whether the workplace was monitored for exposure levels, and whether or not other workers developed similar illnesses. A useful clue for occupational asthma or bronchitis is the abatement of symptoms during vacations away from the job. Some work-related diseases may not be obvious. A nine-month exposure to asbestos in a shipyard during World War II may account for the mesothelioma or bronchogenic carcinoma arising 30 years later. Hobbies can also be important, e.g, pigeon breeding can lead to hypersensitivity pneumonitis, archeology to coccidioidomycosis, furniture and bathtub refinishing to occupational asthma. Exposure may also be indirect. Asbestos-related illness has been reported in family members exposed to work clothes of an asbestos worker and in households near asbestos-manufacturing plants. Similarly, sensitive individuals may be affected by very low concentrations of toluene diisocyanate originating from a neighborhood plant.

ROENTGENOGRAPHIC TECHNIQUES. Chest roentgenographs are especially useful for evaluating parenchymal and pleural disease. The standard description of abnormalities is based on the ILO U/C classification. Its purpose is to convey assessment of roentgenographs in a standard way for epidemiologic studies and not to make an etiologic assessment in terms of type of dust, fibrosis, or infection. Parenchymal opacities are assessed for size, shape, profusion, and extent. Newer radiographic techniques such as computed axial tomography are useful in individual cases for defining specific abnormalities such as pleural disease after asbestos exposure.

PULMONARY FUNCTION TESTING. Pulmonary function tests are useful for detailed assessment of an individual patient and for epidemiologic investigations of population groups. The detailed pulmonary function studies of an individual patient are, in general, the same for occupational or nonoccupational disease. The only major exception is for patients with suspected occupational asthma. In this case, specific bronchial provocation tests can be done under careful supervision in a defined laboratory environment to evaluate sensitivity to particular substances (see below). Individual patients can also be assessed for bronchoconstriction before, during, and after work. This type of testing has been useful for evaluating byssinosis. Because symptoms may occur only at work during strenuous exertion, evaluation should be carried out not only when the patient is at rest but also during exercise.

Simple measurement of FEV (forced expiratory volume in one second) has proven to be reproducible, sufficiently sensitive to detect clinical disease, and predictive for identifying patients who are likely to get progressive disease. Tests of small airways disease and maldistribution, i.e., flow at low lung volumes, comparison of flow volume curves during exhalation of helium-oxygen mixtures and air, and the single-breath nitrogen test, are more sensitive, but additional studies will be required to document their utility. Pre-employment and serial pulmonary function studies will help identify workers with pre-existing disease and those who develop abnormalities that antedate symptoms. In general, individuals who show evidence of disease the earliest are the ones likely to develop progressive disease and should be advised about their disease and alternative employment.

PATHOLOGY. Most occupational diseases can be diagnosed without biopsy. If biopsy is necessary, an open lung biopsy is preferred so that the types of dust retained in the lung can be identified by chemical analysis or by newer techniques of energy-dispersive x-ray analysis and x-ray diffraction.

ASSESSMENT OF HAZARDS. The description of the job usually identifies the offending substance, but direct measurements of the air the worker breathes will help quantitate the hazard and ensure that control measures are effective. Particulates are usually collected by filtration and weighed; vapors can be measured continuously. Federal and private organizations have established threshold limit values for different substances based on a time-weighted average concentration for an 8-hour working day, 40-hour working week, and a 40-year working span. Threshold limit values do not address the problems of high peak levels of short duration or the sensitive individual.

DISEASES PRODUCED BY INORGANIC MATERIALS

Coal Worker's Pneumoconiosis

DEFINITION. Coal worker's pneumoconiosis (CWP) is the parenchymal lung disease produced by the deposition of coal dust and the host response to the retained dust. Classification is based on roentgenographic appearance. Simple CWP is based on the profusion of small, round opacities up to 1 cm in diameter; complicated CWP is defined by the presence of one or more opacities greater than 1 cm in diameter. In addition to parenchymal disease, inhalation of coal dust also causes industrial bronchitis (see below).

OCCUPATIONAL EXPOSURE. Although first reported in the nineteenth century, lung disease associated with coal mining did not become a major occupational pulmonary disease until the 1930's, when machinery for underground mining was developed. The development of simple CWP is related to the dust exposure and the amount of coal dust retained in the lungs. The highest dust concentrations occur at the coal face, where the coal is cut and detached, and dust levels fall progressively as the coal is transported to the surface. Workers who cut into rock strata or work on the shuttle car system, which uses sand on the rails to improve traction, are exposed to silica as well as coal dust. The current dust standard is 2 mg per cubic meter. A recent study of United States miners reported a prevalence of 10 per cent simple CWP and 0.4 per cent complicated CWP. These studies are difficult to interpret because some of the severely affected miners have left the trade and because the prevalence data relate to exposure levels 20 to 30 years ago, which were much higher than the current standard. The economics of energy production and the large supply of unmined coal ensure that CWP will remain a clinical problem for many years.

In the 1977 Black Lung Benefits Reform Act, total disability is defined as inability to do regular work in or around the mine or coal preparation facility due to breathing impairment caused by pneumoconiosis. Total disability may be determined on the basis of roentgenographic evidence, pulmonary function impairment, or both. As a result, coal workers may be compensated for chronic airway obstruction due to cigarette smoking at a much higher rate than are workers in other industries with chronic airway obstruction.

PATHOLOGY AND PATHOGENESIS. ***Simple Coal Worker's Pneumoconiosis.*** The distinctive lesion of simple coal worker's pneumoconiosis is the *coal macule*, discrete, small, black nodules that are typically more profuse in the upper lobes. These lesions consist of dust-laden macrophages, fibroblasts, extracellular dust, and cell debris and a loose collection of reticulin fibers. These macules are sometimes associated with focal centrilobular emphysema (localized dilatation of the respiratory bronchioles) but are not thought to produce clinically significant respiratory impairment.

Complicated Coal Worker's Pneumoconiosis. Rarely the macules enlarge and coalesce to produce large, rubbery aggregates of black tissue greater than 1 cm in diameter, typically in a posterior segment of an upper lobe or the superior segment of a lower lobe. Progressive massive fibrosis, arbitrarily defined as a lesion with a diameter exceeding 3 cm, may result from one or more of four factors: (1) the presence of silica in addition to the coal dust, (2) a very high concentration of coal dust, (3) typical or atypical mycobacterial infections, and (4) poorly defined immunologic host factors. Some patients have antinuclear antibodies, high levels of rheumatoid factor, and antibodies to lung connective tissue components.

CLINICAL MANIFESTATIONS. *Simple CWP* produces no signs or symptoms. Diagnosis is made roentgenographically. Lesions progress very slowly; side-by-side comparisons are usually useful only if the chest films were obtained at least five years apart. Pulmonary function abnormalities are minimal. It takes about 30 years of underground mining to produce even a small decrease in FEV_1. The single-breath diffusing capacity is normal. The major determinant for pulmonary function abnormalities in coal miners is the presence or absence of cigarette smoking.

Complicated CWP may produce dyspnea on exertion and may progress to severe respiratory insufficiency due to obstructive and restrictive lung disease, cor pulmonale, pulmonary hypertension, and right ventricular failure. Rare patients have melanoptysis, which is the sudden coughing up of a small amount of jet black fluid. *Caplan's syndrome* is the association of large, peripheral, round lung opacities in coal miners with rheumatoid arthritis. The nodules may increase in size rapidly, e.g., within a few weeks, may cavitate, and are usually associated with active joint disease, high titers of rheumatoid factor, and the presence of subcutaneous nodules. However, the pulmonary nodules may appear before the clinical manifestation of rheumatoid arthritis. The nodules, which may appear up to ten years before joint disease, resemble nodules of rheumatoid lung disease; both have a center of necrotic tissue and a surrounding cellular zone of epithelial cells, lymphocytes, plasma cells, and other inflammatory cells. Vasculitis is commonly associated. Compared to progressive massive fibrosis, the nodules contain relatively little dust. Syndromes similar to that described by Caplan for coal workers have been described in patients with silicosis and asbestosis. The pathogenesis of Caplan's syndrome is thought to be an interaction, as yet undefined, of rheumatoid lung disease with the inhaled dust and its cellular response.

Coal dust can also produce chronic bronchitis that is manifested by cough and sputum production but minimal changes in pulmonary function. The bronchitic symptoms vary directly in relation to dust exposure, but there is poor correlation to radiographic category of parenchymal lung disease (CWP). The bronchitis ceases after the worker leaves the dusty environment. Cigarette smoking is thought to be at least five times more important than coal dust in producing airway obstruction.

DIAGNOSIS AND DIFFERENTIAL DIAGNOSIS. The diagnosis of CWP is based on the history of exposure and radiographic abnormalities. Simple CWP does not produce breathlessness, and, therefore, symptomatic patients with simple CWP should be studied for nonoccupational pulmonary disease. Patients with progressive massive fibrosis and associated mycobacterial infection may have minimal fever, weight loss, or other constitutional symptoms. Diagnosis of mycobacterial infection is made by sputum examination, culture, and occasionally biopsy. Patients respond to standard treatment regimens. The incidence of lung cancer is not increased in patients with simple or complicated CWP. Progressive massive fibrosis may be difficult to distinguish from bronchogenic carcinoma, especially if serial chest films are not available. Features that favor progressive massive fibrosis are the variable radiodensity of the lesion, irregular opacities at the periphery, calcification within the lesion, and a recent history of expectoration of jet black fluid if cavitation is present.

TREATMENT, PROGNOSIS, AND PREVENTION. The presence of simple CWP is not a sufficient reason for someone who has worked in the mines for many years to discontinue mining. However, a documented increase in the size of the opacities or presence of complicated CWP should exclude the worker from all dusty trades. When the exposure ceases, simple CWP will remain stable or decrease, but complicated CWP may progress. Prevention of CWP can be achieved only by dust control.

Morgan WKC, Lapp NL: Respiratory disease in coal miners. Am Rev Respir Dis 113:531, 1976. *A detailed, comprehensive review.*

Morgan WKC, Lapp NL, Seaton D: Respiratory disability in coal miners. JAMA 243:2401, 1980. *Pulmonary impairment and black lung legislation.*

Silicosis

DEFINITION. Silicosis is the parenchymal lung disease produced by inhalation of respirable particles of crystalline silica, SiO_2, and the tissue reaction to the retained dust. Quartz is the most common form of crystalline silica in nature; cristobalite and tridymite are other forms of crystalline silica, which occur rarely in nature but are produced by heating quartz in smelting and steel making or by heating diatomite, an amorphous form of silica. Silicates such as asbestos, kaolin, and talc are less fibrogenic and produce different pneumoconioses.

OCCUPATIONAL EXPOSURE. Silicosis occurs in workers in numerous occupations, including mining, quarrying, tunneling, stone cutting, sandblasting, and foundry work. The most tragic exposure in the United States was during the excavation of a tunnel at Gauley Bridge, West Virginia, in the 1930's, when 476 workers died of silicosis, and another 1500 contracted the disease. Since that time dust control and substitution of other abrasives for sand have decreased the incidence of fulminant disease.

PATHOLOGY AND PATHOGENESIS. The rate of development of clinical disease is dependent on the amount of inhaled silica. Three forms of silicosis can be distinguished: (1) chronic silicosis, in which exposure extends for more than 15 years before symptoms and radiographic changes occur; (2) accelerated silicosis, in which changes occur in 5 to 15 years; and (3) acute silicosis, in which changes occur within 5 years.

Chronic silicosis is characterized by small, silica-containing, upper lobe nodules composed of concentric swirls of hyalinized collagen, which is surrounded by a cellular capsule composed of macrophages, plasma cells, and fibroblasts. Hilar lymph nodes may contain similar nodules. Massive conglomerate lesions form by coalescence of the smaller nodules and may obliterate or distort some of the conducting airways and vasculature. The lesions seldom cavitate in the absence of tuberculosis.

Accelerated silicosis, which is seen in sandblasters, is similar to chronic silicosis but progresses more rapidly, commonly to massive fibrosis. Typical and atypical mycobacterial infections are frequent. In *acute silicosis*, which is rare, there is an eosinophilic coagulum in the alveolar spaces that stains with the periodic acid–Schiff stain and appears similar to alveolar proteinosis.

The good correlation between the fibrogenic potential of different types of silica in vivo and the cytotoxic effects of these dusts on macrophages in vitro suggests the following mechanism. Free silica is ingested by the macrophage but tends to disrupt its phagolysosome and is released extracellularly. More macrophages are recruited to the area of inflammation, and the cycle is slowly repeated. Collagen is formed and then becomes hyalinized. Macrophages produce factors that stimulate fibroblast proliferation and collagen formation. The precise role of these macrophage factors in the pathogenesis of silicosis is still unknown.

CLINICAL MANIFESTATIONS. Simple and complicated silicosis are defined radiographically as described for coal worker's pneumoconiosis. Simple silicosis generally produces no signs or symptoms; when people with simple silicosis cough and produce sputum, these symptoms can usually be attributed to cigarette smoking or inhalation of other dust. In complicated silicosis, dyspnea on exertion, recurrent infections, weight loss, and general weakness are frequent. The physical findings correlate with the severity of the complicated silicosis.

Radiographic studies in simple silicosis show nodules predominantly in the upper lung fields, which may become calcified. In complicated silicosis, large masses develop that may appear as an "angel's wing" pattern. As the fibrosis proceeds and lesions contract, adjacent areas of lung become overexpanded and appear radiolucent. Pleural reactions over the dense conglomerate lesions are frequent. The hilar lymph nodes are commonly enlarged and may develop the typical egg shell calcification of silicosis (Fig. 559–1).

Pulmonary function is normal in simple silicosis. As the disease progresses, restrictive, obstructive, and mixed types of abnormalities occur. The vital capacity, single-breath diffusion capacity, and compliance are reduced. Hypoxia occurs initially during exercise and later at rest. Because of the wide spectrum of clinical and radiographic disease, there is also a wide spectrum of pulmonary function abnormalities.

DIAGNOSIS AND DIFFERENTIAL DIAGNOSIS. The diagnosis of silicosis is based on a history of inhalation of respirable free silica and radiographic abnormalities. The major clinical problems are infectious complications and the possibility of concurrent collagen vascular disease. There is no increase in cancer of the lung. Historically the most important infectious complication was tuberculosis. Recently half of the mycobacterial infections have been reported to be caused by atypical organisms, either *Mycobacterium kansasii* or *M. avium intracellulare*, depending on the geographic area. Fungal, nocardial, and pyogenic bacterial infections also occur frequently. In the accelerated silicosis of sandblasters, more than 40 per cent of the individuals have antinuclear antibodies, and about 10 per cent have clinical manifestations of collagen vascular diseases such as rheumatoid arthritis, scleroderma, and systemic lupus erythematosus. It is uncertain if patients with accelerated disease should be treated with anti-inflammatory or immunosuppressive drugs with the hope of preventing progression of their lung disease. The link between the inflammatory and heightened immune response and subsequent fibrosis is unknown, but is potentially a site for treatment.

Coalescence of nodules and enlarging opacities may indicate spontaneous progression of silicosis, a complicating infectious process, or coexisting carcinoma. Because of expanding lesions, a history of mixed dust exposure, or the suspicion of infectious disease, carcinoma, or sarcoidosis, an open lung biopsy may be required. Silica can be seen as doubly refractile particles with polarized light. In mixed dust exposure, energy dispersive x-ray analysis can identify silicon and elements associated with silicates (calcium, magnesium, and iron).

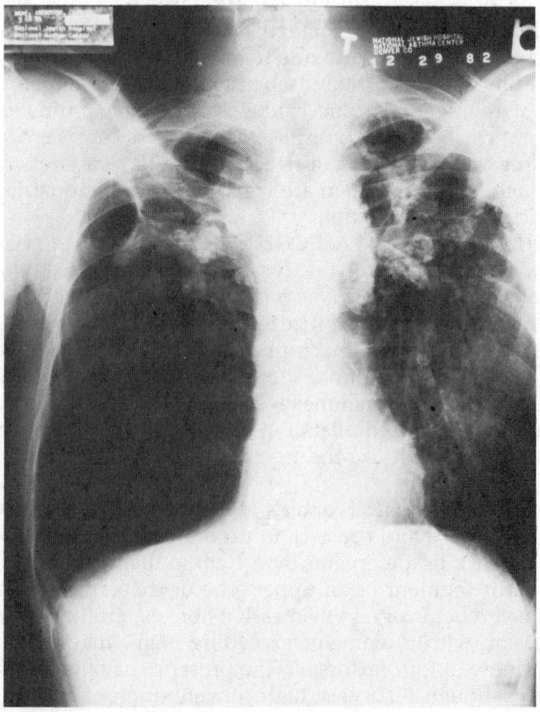

Figure 559–1. Patient with silicosis, classic egg shell lymph node calcification, and multiple cavities in the right upper lobe due to *Mycobacterium avium intracellulare* infection. Note the upper lung zone fibrosis, retraction, and secondary overdistention of the lower lobes.

Treatment, Prognosis, and Prevention. There is no proven treatment for silicosis. As in other forms of pneumoconiosis, the earlier the symptoms or radiographic abnormalities appear, the worse the prognosis. If symptoms occur within ten years of exposure, progression is likely, and the prognosis is grim. Preemployment examination should include a tuberculin skin test and chest film. Patients with silicosis and a positive tuberculin reaction should be treated for at least a year with isoniazid. Patients with active tuberculosis should be treated with standard drugs. In areas where *M. kansasii* is common the initial regimen should include three drugs (Ch. 298). Short-course therapy should be avoided, and treatment regimens should be longer than those for patients without silicosis. Prevention of silicosis is by avoiding dust exposure and by substitution when possible. For example, "sandblasting" is now commonly performed with metal grit and coal ash instead of sand.

Dauber JH: Silicosis. *In* Fishman AP (ed.): Update: Pulmonary Diseases and Disorders. New York, McGraw-Hill Book Company, 1982, pp. 149–166. *Excellent summary of pathogenesis.*
Ziskind M, Jones RN, Weill H: Silicosis. Am Rev Respir Dis 113:643, 1976.

Asbestos-Related Diseases

DEFINITIONS. Inhalation of asbestos fibers can produce fibrosis and tumors. The most common disease is interstitial pulmonary fibrosis, which is termed asbestosis. Asbestos fibers may also produce benign pleural effusions and fibrosis, pleural plaques, mesotheliomas of pleura and peritoneum, lung cancer, and cancers of the gastrointestinal tract. The types of disease, especially pleural disease, depend on the type of fiber. Asbestos fibers, a group of naturally occurring fibrous silicates of different chemical composition, are classified as serpentine (chrysotile) or amphibole (crocidolite, amosite, and anthophyllite). Chrysotile is a magnesium silicate, forms soft, flexible, curly fibers, accounts for over 90 per cent of the world's asbestos production, and rarely produces mesotheliomas. The amphiboles form straight, brittle fibers, have a greater potential for penetrating deep into the lung, and are more likely to produce pleural disease. Some amphiboles (e.g., crocidolite) are strongly implicated in the induction of mesotheliomas; others (e.g., anthophyllite) are associated with a high frequency of pleural plaques but not mesotheliomas. In general, increased fiber length (over 10 μ) is associated with increased fibrogenicity and oncogenicity. Since different types of asbestos tend to produce different asbestos-related diseases, the exposure to different types of fibers should be defined and recorded as completely as possible.

OCCUPATIONAL EXPOSURE. The major occupational exposures to asbestos occur in mining, milling, work in shipyards, insulation work, demolition of old buildings, construction, and production of asbestos cement. Two worker groups that have had high exposure to respirable asbestos and a high prevalence of disease are insulation and shipyard workers. During World War II, more than two million people were employed in U.S. shipyards, and, because of the long interval (20 to 40 years) between exposure and the development of disease, many of these individuals have only recently come to medical attention. Not only is there a long latent period, but the exposure may be brief or indirect. Workers exposed to amosite for only 6 to 12 months have an increased incidence of lung cancer. People who live near manufacturing plants or who handled clothing of asbestos workers have been reported to get asbestosis and mesotheliomas.

The incidence of asbestos-related diseases should decrease as dust control measures and work practices improve. The current threshold limit value is 2 fibers per cubic centimeter as a time-weighted average for eight hours. Much of our data on the incidence of disease are from insulation and shipyard workers who were employed from 1930 to 1950 when it is estimated that the level of exposure may have been as high as 50 to 500 fibers per cubic centimeter. It is difficult, therefore, to predict exactly how much the current standards will reduce the incidence of disease. In the past when exposure levels were high, the dose was the major determinant in production of disease. With the low current levels of exposure, host factors may become more important than the actual dose in predicting who will develop disease.

PATHOLOGY AND PATHOGENESIS. Asbestos produces interstitial fibrosis and pneumonitis, predominantly in the lower lobes. Because of the large individual variation in response among workers, host factors for amplifying or suppressing the fibrotic response are likely to be very important. Similarly, host factors may regulate movement of fibers within the lung parenchyma and the rate of dissolution of inhaled fiber, which may be important in the pathogenesis of parenchymal and pleural disease.

Ferruginous bodies are the pathologic hallmark of asbestos exposure. These bodies, which are 2 to 5 μ wide and 20 to 150 μ long, usually contain an amphibole fiber as a core, surrounded by an exterior composed of protein and iron pigments. The core can also be a different silicate or even a vegetable fiber. The presence of ferruginous bodies indicates past exposure to asbestos, but it does not establish the etiology of disease. Up to 50 per cent of urban dwellers have ferruginous bodies in their lungs at autopsy. However, the number of fibers found correlates with the intensity of the past exposure and therefore the presence of disease. Fibers can be collected by bronchoalveolar lavage.

Pleural reactions occur in two independent types: (1) a diffuse exudative reaction that involves both pleural surfaces and may eventually obliterate the pleural space and (2) discrete pleural plaques on the parietal pleura. Benign pleural effusions are commonly the first manifestation of asbestos-related pulmonary disease and occur within ten years of initial exposure. The pathology of the exudative lesion is not distinctive and accounts for some "idiopathic" pleural effusions. The pleural plaques are discrete, raised white lesions that occur over the lower ribs and diaphragm and are not associated with pleural adhesions. These plaques are composed of relatively acellular collagenous connective tissue, which contains uncoated asbestos fibers, mostly amphiboles, and may calcify.

Malignant mesotheliomas of the pleura are bulky, slow-growing tumors that spread by local extension and enclose the lung and mediastinum and present clinically with the symptoms of chest wall pain and weight loss (see Ch. 68). They vary histologically and can be difficult to diagnose even with an open pleural biopsy, because some of these tumors appear like metastatic adenocarcinomas. There is a high incidence in insulation workers and a low incidence in Canadian miners of chrysotile asbestos. Miners of a thinner type of crocidolite in Northwest Cape, South Africa, have a higher incidence of mesothelioma than miners of a thicker type of crocidolite in the Transvaal. These epidemiologic features imply that thin, straight fibers with a small aerodynamic diameter are most likely to penetrate deep into the lung and produce mesotheliomas. Mesotheliomas are not associated with cigarette smoking.

CLINICAL MANIFESTATIONS. Asbestosis presents like other forms of pulmonary fibrosis. The first symptoms are dyspnea on exertion and a nonproductive cough. Symptoms usually develop several years after radiographic changes appear. On physical examination, patients have end-inspiratory, crisp crackles that are heard best over the lower lobes. In advanced disease, clubbing of the fingers may be present.

Radiologic studies in asbestosis reveal small linear opacities in the lower lung fields as the initial abnormalities. These may extend to the pleura and resemble Kerley B lines. As the disease progresses the lung volumes decrease, and there is distortion of the pulmonary architecture. Pleural plaques, fibrosis, or effusions may also be present. Pleural plaques can be best seen on oblique views, but care must be used to differentiate true plaques from companion shadows that are produced by muscle attachments in normal individuals. The extent of the pleural disease is best detemined with computed tomography (Fig. 559–2).

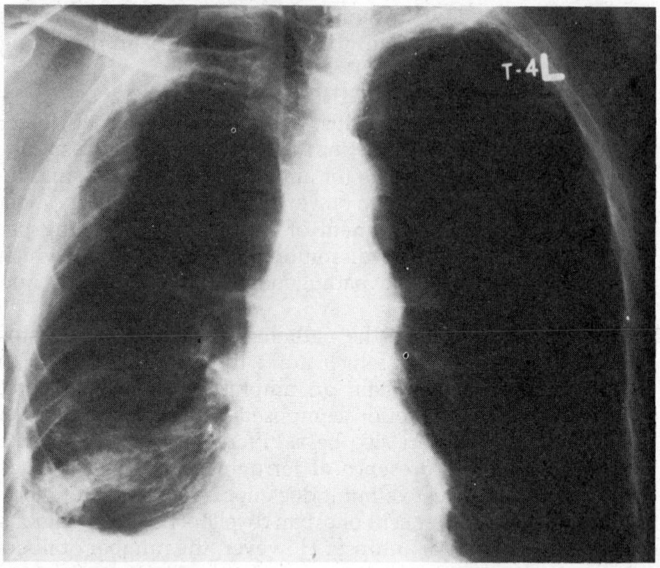

Figure 559–2. Patient with asbestosis and linear parenchymal marking, pleural calcifications, and an extensive right pleural reaction. There is also some pericardial calcification.

Pulmonary function tests classically show restrictive patterns typical of pulmonary fibrosis. The lung volumes, compliance, and single-breath diffusing capacity are all reduced. Because of the high prevalence of cigarette smoking in asbestos workers and the distortion of the airways in advanced disease, airway obstruction may also be present. Although asbestos can produce peribronchial inflammation and fibrosis, asbestos is not thought to produce clinically significant obstructive lung disease in the absence of obvious restriction and distortion of lung architecture.

DIAGNOSIS. The diagnosis of asbestosis requires a history of exposure and radiographic evidence of parenchymal lung disease, especially linear opacities in the lower lung fields. Patients usually also have dyspnea on exertion, end-inspiratory rales over the lower lobes, radiographic evidence of pleural disease, and pulmonary function impairment. If a biopsy is necessary to exclude other interstitial lung diseases or for other medical reasons, it should be an open lung biopsy, and the tissue should be examined for coated and uncoated fibers. Fibers can also be recovered and quantitated in bronchoalveolar lavage fluid.

Patients with asbestos exposure have an increased incidence of lung, laryngeal, and gastrointestinal cancer. Cigarette smoking together with asbestos exposure increases the risk of developing lung cancer about 60-fold over nonexposed, nonsmoking controls. In individuals not exposed to asbestos, smoking alone increases the risk about tenfold. The risk of lung cancer in nonsmoking asbestos workers is much smaller than in smokers, but it is greater than the risk in nonsmoking, nonexposed controls. The diagnosis of lung cancer is made by standard cytologic procedures and biopsy. The cell types of bronchogenic cancer due to asbestosis and cigarette smoking are not different from the cell types of other types of lung cancer. It remains to be shown how effective analysis of prospective serial roentgenograms and sputum cytology will be for detection and management of lung cancer in patients with asbestosis or a history of heavy exposure to asbestos.

TREATMENT, PROGNOSIS, AND PREVENTION. Asbestosis and its related diseases are for the most part not treatable. Most effort has to be made to prevent the diseases by reducing exposure and by encouraging workers to refrain from cigarette smoking. Those who work with asbestos should give up smoking; those who are young and cannot stop smoking should avoid trades that entail exposure to asbestos. It would be helpful to be able to identify those individuals who are likely to develop pulmonary fibrosis. Unfortunately the only available clue to those who will develop clinical asbestosis is the appearance of radiographic abnormalities during their working life. Workers who have an abnormal chest film when they leave their trade are the ones who are most likely to develop severe asbestosis.

Aisner J, Wiernik P (eds.): Asbestos related neoplasms. Semin Oncol 8:241, 1981. *Thorough discussion of pathogenesis, pathology, natural history, and options for therapy and palliation.*

Becklake M: Asbestos-related fibrosis of the lungs (asbestosis) and pleura. *In* Fishman AP (ed.): Update: Pulmonary Diseases and Disorders. New York, McGraw-Hill Book Company, 1982, pp 167–192. *A complete current review.*

Craighead JE, Mossman BT: The pathogenesis of asbestos associated diseases. N Engl J Med 306:1446, 1982.

Selikoff IJ, Hammond EC (eds.): Health hazards of asbestos exposure. Ann NY Acad Sci Vol. 330, 1979. *A wealth of information. The article by Hammond et al. on asbestos exposure, cigarette smoking, and death rates provides first data on possible carcinogenic effect of asbestos in nonsmokers (four cases).*

Disease Caused by Other Silicates

Nonasbestos silicates may also produce pneumoconioses. Talc, a hydrous magnesium silicate, may produce pulmonary fibrosis and pleural plaques. The pulmonary lesions tend to be more nodular than those seen in asbestosis. Talc is commonly extracted from rock that also contains silica and asbestos. Therefore, miners usually have exposure to mixed dusts. The particle size of talc used for cosmetics is large, 10 to 40 μ, and therefore personal use is unlikely to produce pneumoconiosis. Talc is found in pulmonary granulomas in intravenous drug abusers. Other silicates, i.e., kaolin, slate, and portland cement, rarely produce lung disease in the absence of free silica.

Disease Caused by Hard Metals and Other Inorganic Dusts

Dusts containing elements with high atomic numbers absorb roentgen rays and produce dramatic radiographic abnormalities. Most of these dusts are considered nonfibrogenic and produce minimal symptoms or pulmonary function abnormalities. Progressive disease strongly suggests mixed dust exposure that includes silica. The classic examples are *stannosis* (from tin oxide) and *baritosis* (from barium sulfate). Iron oxides accumulate in lungs of arc welders and hematite miners and, in the absence of inhalation of quartz or asbestos, produce abnormal chest films but minimal fibrosis or functional impairment.

Beryllium Disease

Beryllium disease differs from other occupational pulmonary diseases in that beryllium and its compounds become distributed throughout the body and produce a systemic illness. The acute fulminant form, caused by brief intense exposure, is characterized by bronchiolitis, pneumonia, and pulmonary edema. The mortality is as high as 10 per cent. The chronic form, which begins 5 to 15 years after exposure, presents as diffuse granulomatous pneumonitis, which progresses to pulmonary fibrosis and respiratory insufficiency. The hilar nodes may calcify.

Beryllium disease was initially associated with the manufacture of fluorescent lights, but this form of exposure ceased after beryllium was removed from fluorescent lights in 1949. Currently, exposures occur in the milling of beryllium metal alloys, which are used in the aerospace industry, in the manufacture of x-ray tubes, and in nuclear physics. Beryllium is quite toxic at even low concentration, and disease has been reported in people who handled clothes of exposed workers.

The diagnosis is made by the history of exposure and by demonstration of a granulomatous tissue reaction. Noncaseating granulomas may be found in skin, liver, spleen, and lymph nodes as well as in the lungs. Tissue and urine can be analyzed for beryllium content, though the concentration of beryllium in the urine indicates exposure only and does not correlate well with disease activity. Lymphocyte transformation in vitro by beryllium salts has been reported to differentiate beryllium disease from simple exposure and from other granulomatus diseases. However, beryllium disease remains difficult to differentiate from sarcoidosis (Ch. 67). Involvement of the uvea, salivary glands, or central nervous system strongly favors the diagnosis of sarcoidosis. Prolonged treatment with glucocorticoids is useful in suppressing beryllium disease in many patients.

Metal Fume Fever

Metal fume fever is a benign, self-limited, acute illness produced by inhalation of fumes of the metals zinc, copper, and magnesium. The syndrome occurs in people who weld galvanized metals in an enclosed, poorly ventilated space. Several hours after exposure, workers experience cough, dry throat, and tightness in the chest. These symptoms are followed by fever, chills, myalgias, and leukocytosis. The illness lasts only one day. Tolerance develops, and the worker may return to the same job without recurrence. However, the syndrome may recur after exposure following a layoff.

DISEASES PRODUCED BY ORGANIC MATERIALS

Hypersensitivity Pneumonitis

Inhalation of organic dusts produces inflammation in the lung parenchyma (hypersensitivity pneumonitis) or obstructive disease of the conducting airways (occupational asthma and bronchitis). Hypersensitivity pneumonitis, also termed extrinsic allergic alveolitis, will be discussed only briefly in this section because it is discussed in detail in Ch. 62. The classic example of hypersensitivity pneumonitis is *farmer's lung disease,* which is produced by inhalation of *Micropolyspora faeni* or *Thermoactinomyces vulgaris* in dust from moldy hay. Symptoms of chill, nonproductive cough, dyspnea, and malaise occur four to eight hours after exposure. Physical findings include fever, tachypnea, tachycardia, and rales. Evidence of obstructive airway disease such as wheezing or prolonged expiration is typically absent. The chest roentgenogram reveals bilateral, irregular parenchymal infiltrates. Patients with a chronic form of hypersensitivity pneumonitis may have pulmonary fibrosis and respiratory failure without a clear history of episodic disease. Other examples of hypersensitivity pneumonitis include *bagassosis* (from dried sugar cane), *suberosis* (from cork dust), *sequoiosis* (from redwood saw dust), *cheese washer's lung* (from moldy cheese), and *pigeon breeder's lung* (from bird droppings). The pathogenesis involves both humoral and cell-mediated immunity (type III and IV immunologic reactions). Patients have precipitating IgG against the pertinent fungal or avian antigens. Diagnosis is made by history, serum precipitins, Arthus skin reaction, in vitro lymphocyte transformation and lymphokine production, and occasionally by bronchial provocation tests or open lung biopsy. Treatment is by avoidance of the antigen when possible and with glucocorticoids when necessary.

Syndromes related to air treatment systems are common and have been lumped under the term *humidifier fever.* In some instances the clinical presentation is a classic hypersensitivity pneumonitis with fever, infiltrates, and identification of a source of aerosolization of *Micropolyspora faeni* or thermophilic actinomyces. However, in other cases the presentation is more like occupational asthma with cough, wheeze, chest tightness, and fever, but no pulmonary infiltrate. In these latter cases the causative agents include ameba, protozoa, fungi, and bacteria that have contaminated water for aerosolization. The successful treatment usually requires thorough cleaning of the air conditioning system and ducts.

Diseases produced by inhalation of toxic gas (e.g., chloride, sulfur dioxide, ammonia) are discussed in Ch. 560.

Occupational Asthma

DEFINITION. Asthma is broadly defined as a disease characterized by increased responsiveness of the airways to various stimuli and manifested by slowing of forced expiration that changes in severity either spontaneously or as a result of therapy (see Ch. 59). This definition allows for numerous syndromes that all result in bronchoconstriction but that may

TABLE 559–2. TYPES OF OCCUPATIONAL ASTHMA*

Material	Industry	Etiology: *IgE*	Etiology: *Other*	Onset of Typical Reaction
Animal dander	Veterinarians Laboratory workers	+	0	Immediate only
Green coffee bean	Food industry	+	0	Immediate only
Enzymes from *Bacillus subtilis*	Detergent industry	+	?	Immediate and late
Complex salts of platinum	Metal refining	+	?	Immediate and late
Flour, grain	Bakers, grain handlers	+	?	Immediate and late
Toluene diisocyanate (TDI)	Polyurethane industry	?	+	Dual and late
Western red cedar	Saw mills	?	+	Dual and late
Resin core solder	Electronics industry	0	+	Dual and late
Formalin	Medical	0	+	Immediate and late
Cotton dust	Cotton mills (byssinosis)	0	+	Late

*The cause and mechanisms of different types of occupational asthma are still being investigated and remain speculative.

The time of onset of reactions varies for different workers in a given industry, and it is likely that the precise combination of mechanisms that cause the airway obstruction will also vary for individual workers within a given industry.

The onset of reaction is immediate if it occurs within 30 minutes and late if it occurs after 30 minutes, usually 2 to 6 hours after exposure. Dual reactions include both immediate and late components. The type of reactions of patients with asthma due to western red cedar, toluene diisocyanate, and liquid core solder fluxes is similar in that about half have late reactions, half dual reactions, and less than 10 per cent immediate reactions only.

+ = probable; ? = possible; 0 = unlikely.

be produced by a variety of factors mediated through different mechanisms. In Table 559–2 there is a list of a few of the different forms of occupational asthma; a more complete list and description of the individual types of occupational asthma can be found in the references. Occupational asthma occurs in two different population groups. One group has pre-existing asthma that is exacerbated by an occupational dust or fume, and the other group has no previous history of asthma and first develops symptoms after the occupational exposure. Patients with known asthma tend to leave the industry if they become severely symptomatic. If their symptoms are mild they remain in the work force and may account for some of the heterogeneity in clinical studies. Individuals with pre-existing asthma are likely to be more sensitive, may have different clinical manifestations, and may react differently to components in the occupational fumes or dusts than individuals without pre-existing asthma.

OCCUPATIONAL EXPOSURE. Patients with immediate reactions can usually identify the offending agents, which may include both particulate dusts and gaseous fumes. For those with delayed reactions, identification of the offending material may be much more difficult. The sensitization and cause of the respiratory disease may not originate in the actual workplace of the patient. There have been reports of toluene diisocyanate produced in one factory affecting sensitive individuals in a neighboring workplace.

PATHOGENESIS. The pathogenesis of most cases of occupational asthma, especially the kinds with delayed symptoms, is not known. At least four different mechanisms for producing occupational asthma have been suggested:

1. *Production of specific IgE (or perhaps a sensitizing IgG) against an inhaled antigen.* The sensitization will usually occur within

one year of exposure; the affected individual is likely to be atopic; and exposure to the antigen evokes immediate symptoms, which are produced by a type I immunologic reaction, and in some individuals, a late reaction as well. Prick skin tests and the radioallergosorbent tests are almost always positive. Examples of asthma produced by this mechanism include baker's asthma and reactions to animal dander, green coffee beans, and castor beans.

2. *Direct damage to the airway epithelium and stimulation of irritant receptors that produce bronchospasm through parasympathetic reflexes.* Damage to the airway epithelium might allow penetration of inhaled materials into the submucosa, which would enhance their immunologic and inflammatory effects, and induction of nonspecific bronchial hyper-reactivity to other inhaled dusts and fumes. Viral infections and ozone have been shown to produce transient bronchial hyper-reactivity to histamine in normal subjects. Bronchial hyper-reactivity is considered to explain in part how acute episodic asthma can develop into a more persistent, chronic form that produces symptoms even in the absence of the sensitizing agent. Examples of reactions that could be caused by epithelial damage and inflammation include those due to toluene diisocyanate, platinum salts, western red cedar, formalin, resin core soldering flux, and aminoethyl ethanolamine.

3. *Production of substances that are generated slowly or are slow to react,* i.e., production of leukotrienes, platelet-activating factor (PAF), C5a and C3a for immune complex reactions and complement activation, and other chemotactic factors for polymorphonuclear leukocytes.

4. *The pharmacologic properties of the inhaled material,* i.e., release of mediators from mast cells (cotton dust), complement activation (western red cedar), or increased parasympathetic tone by inhibition of acetylcholinesterase (organic phosphate insecticides).

A great deal more investigation is necessary to define the precise mechanisms in different forms of occupational asthma.

CLINICAL MANIFESTATIONS. In general, the symptoms of cough, sputum production, and chest tightness are more common than wheezing. Cough is a symptom of airway irritation or obstruction, and patients with persistent cough, especially one that decreases when the worker has been away from work for three or four days, should be examined for the possibility of occupational asthma. In recording the history, it is important to identify all symptoms, and for each symptom to determine at what time of day, during what type of work, and where in the workplace the symptom occurs. Patients with immediate reactions can usually identify the eliciting substance. The symptoms occur at work and increase during the working day. Patients with late reactions may have symptoms that occur only after work, especially at night. Sometimes the only clue that these late symptoms are work related is that they decrease after the person is away from the workplace for several weeks.

Physical examination away from work may be normal. It is important to examine the patient at work or while symptoms are present for signs of airway obstruction. Some agents produce dermatitis, e.g., platinum salts and formalin. Chest roentgenograms are normal except for diseases that can progress to chronic obstructive lung disease, e.g., byssinosis.

DIAGNOSIS AND DIFFERENTIAL DIAGNOSIS. The diagnosis is made by history, pulmonary function tests, and immunologic tests. It is important to establish if the symptoms are only work related, because, if they are, the diagnosis is established, and the possibility of prevention by changing jobs can be strongly considered.

Pulmonary function studies are extremely useful for establishing the diagnosis. Routine spirograms obtained away from work may be normal. However, evaluations before, during, and after work may be diagnostic. The most important diagnostic tools are a peak flowmeter and a symptom diary. In general, measurements that allegedly determine the extent of small airway function and distribution of inspired air (frequency dependence of dynamic lung compliance, single-breath nitrogen test with determination of the alveolar plateau and closing volume, and comparison of maximal expiratory flow curves during exhalation of helium and air) show abnormalities before the FEV_1 is abnormal. However, the clinical importance and predictive value of these tests will have to await additional studies in patients with occupational asthma. Most patients with occupational asthma show bronchial hyper-reactivity to histamine or methylcholine, but it is not known if the hyper-reactivity is a cause or a result of the occupational disorder. Results of this test may be positive in an individual whose baseline studies are normal. However, byssinosis and toluene diisocyanate asthma have been reported not to show bronchial hyper-reactivity to histamine.

A specific bronchial provocation test is the single most diagnostic test. For this test the patient performs his exact work with actual industrial materials under careful supervision in a controlled laboratory setting, and measurements of pulmonary function are serially recorded. Inhalation challenges can also be performed with aerosolized material or in an environmental chamber. Bronchial provocation tests with inert substances (lactose) and with different types of dusts found in the work environment can help identify the inciting factor and exclude nonspecific bronchial hyper-reactivity. Extreme care must be used in selecting the doses of inhaled materials, and observation of the patient should be extended to cover late reactions. In patients with late or complex reactions and for substances for which there is no satisfactory skin test or antigen for the radioallergosorbent assay, bronchial provocation may be the only means of making the diagnosis with certainty, e.g., toluene diisocyanate.

Prick skin tests are useful for evaluating immediate hypersensitivity, but there are many false positive findings and perhaps some false negative ones.

TREATMENT, PROGNOSIS, AND PREVENTION. As in other forms of occupational disease, prevention has priority over treatment. Sometimes symptoms disappear if the worker moves to another area of the workplace and does different work. If this is not satisfactory, the worker may have to change jobs. Symptoms can be relieved by treating the airway obstruction with beta adrenergic agonists, theophylline, or cromolyn, but the disease will likely persist. It is not known if the long-term prognosis of those whose symptoms are controlled medically and who remain exposed to the sensitizing material is different from those who move to a new environment. In a few patients, such as those with baker's asthma, the symptoms disappear with time, perhaps because a blocking antibody (IgG) is produced. In some occupations, prevention can be achieved by changing the process or eliminating the antigen (detergents that contain proteases from *Bacillus subtilis*).

Bernstein IL: Occupational asthma. Clin Chest Med 2:255, 1981. *Review of clinical types, diagnosis, and therapy.*

Boushey HA, Holtzman MJ, Sheller JR, Nadel JA: Bronchial hyperreactivity. Am Rev Respir Dis 121:389, 1980. *A detailed state-of-the-art review of an important mechanism in occupational asthma.*

INDUSTRIAL BRONCHITIS

Although most bronchitis is still attributable to cigarette smoking, prolonged exposure to high levels of dust can produce industrial bronchitis. Two population groups that are clinically affected are coal workers and grain handlers. In coal workers, large particles (5 to 10 μ) are thought to be deposited on the epithelium of the proximal airways and to produce clinical bronchitis that only slightly decreases the FEV_1, does not produce emphysema, has no effect on life expectancy, and remits after the dust exposure is gone. In grain handlers, the cause and long-term effect of the clinical bronchitis is not as well characterized because the disease is more complex. A variety of components of grain dust (grain antigens, fungal antigens, grain weevils, mites, animal antigens, and bacterial endotoxins as well as inert dust) have been implicated in the production of symptoms, and these components probably elicit more of an inflammatory and immunologic reaction in the chronic bronchitis of grain handlers that the reaction produced by coal dust.

Morgan WKC: Industrial bronchitis. Br J Indust Med 35:285, 1978. *Detailed discussion of a complex issue.*

OCCUPATIONALLY RELATED LUNG CANCER

Certain minerals and chemicals are associated with a high incidence of lung cancer. There is a long delay (15 to 25 years) between exposure and the development of clinical cancer. But it is not known how to identify those individuals who are most likely to develop lung cancer or how clinically useful serial chest films and sputum cytology are in the detection and subsequent course of lung cancer. Materials that are thought to be responsible for the development of lung cancer include arsenic, asbestos (lung cancer and mesothelioma), carbonyl nickel (squamous cell carcinoma), chloromethyl ethers (oat cell carcinoma), chromates, coal tars, emissions from coke ovens, mustard gas, uranium, and other sources of radiation (oat cell carcinoma). The concept that specific occupational exposures are associated with specific cell types of lung cancer is controversial. The assessment of causality for lung cancer in patients who smoke cigarettes and have an occupational exposure is one of the most vexing problems for compensation.

Frank AL: Occupational Lung Cancer. *In* Harris CC (ed.): Pathogenesis and Therapy of lung cancer. New York, Marcel Dekker, Inc., 1978, pp 25–51.

560. PHYSICAL, CHEMICAL, AND ASPIRATION INJURIES OF THE LUNG

James D. Crapo

The lung has an extremely large and delicate surface exposed to the environment. Extensive defense mechanisms exist to protect the lung from inhaled pathogens and toxic substances. Under normal conditions, air is fully humidified and warmed to body temperature and all large particulate substances are cleared by the upper airways. These defenses are not adequate to handle many physical and chemical substances that cause lung injury. This chapter deals with a variety of lung injuries that are initiated by external factors rather than being due to an intrinsic defect or failure of the respiratory system and its defenses.

PHYSICAL DISORDERS

Thermal Injuries

About 25 per cent of patients with major burns have pulmonary complications, and these complications now account for the majority of burn-related deaths. Thermal injury to the lung is associated with three groups of complications: (1) *Immediate reaction*—direct thermal injury to upper airways, leading to upper airway obstruction, carbon monoxide poisoning, and smoke inhalation (potent bronchoconstrictors and edemagenic substances). (2) *Adult respiratory distress syndrome* (ARDS) developing 24 to 48 hours after the thermal injury. (3) *Late onset pulmonary complications,* which include pneumonia, atelectasis, thromboembolism, and chest-wall restriction caused by circumferential thoracic burns.

Few burns actually cause thermal injury to the lung parenchyma; the large capacity of the upper airways to humidify and modify the temperatures of inhaled air protects the alveolar tissue. Exceptions are steam burns and explosions in an enclosed space.

The initial symptoms are tachypnea, cough, dyspnea, wheezing, cyanosis, hoarseness, and stridor (an ominous sign). During the next 12 to 48 hours the patient may become increasingly hypoxic; lung compliance may decrease, and pulmonary edema may develop in the presence of normal pulmonary capillary

wedge pressure. Roentgenograms of the chest may show no significant changes or a pattern of diffuse, patchy infiltrates. The major complication is infection, usually caused by *Pseudomonas aeruginosa* or *Staphylococcus aureus*. The lung defenses against infection are compromised by thermal injury to the airway epithelium and often by an endotracheal or tracheostomy tube. The pathway of infection may be either by inhalation of airborne organisms or by hematogenous spread from the burn.

The constituents of smoke are potent mucosal irritants and bronchoconstrictors and contribute to the upper and lower lung lesions. Typical constitutents of smoke include oxides of nitrogen, sulfur and lead, ammonia, hydrochlorides, chlorine, and aldehydes. Acrolein, found in wood smoke, is a potent mucosal irritant which contributes to upper airway obstruction and to pulmonary edema. Carbon monoxide poisoning from inhaled smoke is discussed in Chemical Injury to the Lung.

The adult respiratory distress syndrome commonly develops 24 to 48 hours after the initial symptoms subside. The causes of adult respiratory distress syndrome in the burn patient are controversial, but possibilities include a chemical pneumonitis caused by constituents in smoke, a circulating burn toxin, disseminated intravascular coagulation, microembolism, or central neurogenic pulmonary edema. The extent of surface thermal injury does not correlate with the degree of respiratory distress that subsequently develops.

Late onset pulmonary burn complications—atelectasis, thromboembolism, and pneumonia—are discussed in Ch. 61, 65, and 260 to 266, respectively.

THERAPY. Carbon monoxide poisoning and upper airway obstruction are the most immediate life-threatening complications in the patient presenting with major burns or with the history of smoke or steam inhalation. The patient should be closely observed for evidence of these complications and given high levels of inspired oxygen. Fiberoptic bronchoscopy may help detect laryngeal and tracheobronchial inflammation and evidence of smoke contamination in the lower airways. Arterial blood gases should be monitored and prompt intubation or tracheostomy performed if evidence of significant airway obstruction develops. Corticosteroids may be helpful to treat edema of the upper airways, but must be used with caution since one of the major complications of both skin and lung thermal injury is infection. Prophylactic antibiotics are of no value in preventing pneumonia and may predispose to infection with resistant organisms. Careful pulmonary toilet, humidification, and sterile suctioning should be used to reduce the risk of pneumonia. Repeated bronchoscopy is often necessary to remove mucous plugs and thereby prevent segmental atelectasis and infection.

Crapo RO: Smoke-inhalation injuries. JAMA 246:1694, 1981. *A review of the clinical presentation and treatment of smoke inhalation injuries.*
Pruitt BA, Goodwin CW: Current treatment of the extensively burned patient. Surg Annu 15:331, 1983. *A general review of the approach to the burned patient; 97 references.*
Trunkey DD: Inhalation injury. Surg Clin North Am 58:1133, 1978. *A detailed review of pulmonary damage caused by smoke inhalation; 16 references.*

Radiation Injury (See also Ch. 562)

The predominant factors determining the incidence of radiation pneumonitis are the total radiation dose, the number of fractions, and the duration of time over which the total dose is given. Some chemotherapeutic drugs may potentiate damage from radiation. A total lung dose of less than 2000 rads generally is not associated with severe radiation pneumonitis, whereas a total dose in excess of 4000 rads, even if distributed over as many as 30 fractions, has virtually a 100 per cent risk of radiation pneumonitis.

HISTOPATHOLOGIC CHANGES. The reaction of the lung to radiation injury can be divided into three phases: (1) The acute phase, occurring one to two months after radiation, is characterized by vascular damage, congestion, edema, and mononuclear cell infiltration. Alveolar Type II cells and alveolar macrophages are increased in number. (2) The subacute phase occurs two to nine months later. The alveolar walls become infiltrated with mononuclear inflammatory cells and fibroblasts. (3) The chronic or fibrotic phase generally occurs more than nine months after irradiation. Capillary sclerosis and alveolar fibrosis are its predominant histologic features.

CLINICAL PRESENTATION. Signs of bronchial irritation may appear immediately after radiation therapy and/or evidence of esophagitis shortly thereafter, but patients may have no symptoms for 6 to 12 weeks, at which time mild cough appears. If large volumes of lung have been irradiated, or if high radiation doses over short periods have been given, dyspnea, tachypnea, and fever, sometimes high and spiking, can develop. These symptoms can be extremely severe, and will either progress to severe dyspnea and death or gradually subside, leaving varying degrees of respiratory impairment resulting from chronic lung fibrosis. The permanent changes of fibrosis take 6 to 24 months to evolve, and then usually remain stable after two years if no further exposure occurs. Auscultation of the chest is usually normal, although rales, signs of consolidation, and rubs may be found. Clubbing does not develop after radiation injury. Laboratory findings include a mild leukocytosis and an increased erythrocyte sedimentation rate. If the irradiated area is extensive, arterial hypoxemia may be found. Radiographic changes generally appear one to three months following treatment. After therapeutic thoracic irradiation the affected areas are generally demarcated by a sharp edge limited to the margins of the portal of irradiation and have a "ground glass appearance"—a hazy increase in density with indistinct pulmonary markings. In the later phases of the radiation injury, fibrosis and contraction of the irradiated region are the predominant radiographic findings.

Pulmonary function testing shows no change until clinical symptoms appear, at which time a restrictive ventilatory defect is present. Capillary sclerosis is associated with a decrease in blood flow to the affected region and a decrease in carbon monoxide transfer capacity. Severe radiation injury is associated with a decrease in lung compliance and hypoxemia.

Complications of radiation pneumonitis include small pleural effusions and occasionally spontaneous pneumothorax. The cough may be severe enough to cause rib fractures.

The differential diagnosis of acute radiation pneumonitis is usually complicated by the immunocompromised state of many of the patients, by the presence of bacterial, fungal, and protozoan pneumonias, particularly *Pneumocystis carinii*, or by the signs and symptoms of the neoplasm being treated. Radiation pneumonitis has not been documented in parts of the lung outside the radiation portal.

TREATMENT. The best management of radiation pneumonitis is to avoid it when possible. The patient who develops radiation pneumonitis requires supportive care, including medication for cough suppression and often oxygen delivered by nasal catheter or mask for hypoxemia. Corticosteroids (prednisone, 1 mg per kilogram of body weight) are effective at the start of pneumonitis. On occasion the response may be dramatic, with complete resolution of symptoms within 24 hours. Corticosteroids should be tapered as rapidly as possible. There is no evidence that corticosteroids given at the time of irradiation have any protective effect. They are also ineffective in the late fibrotic phases of the disease.

Antibiotics have been tried both prophylactically and when pneumonitis develops. There is no evidence that this treatment modifies the clinical course; therefore antibiotic therapy should be reserved for patients in whom the findings suggest significant infection to be present. Since the lesion involves occlusion and thrombosis of many small blood vessels, anticoagulation has been suggested but without experimental evidence of its effectiveness.

Catane R, Schwade JG, Turris AT, Webber BL, Muggia FM: Pulmonary toxicity after radiation and bleomycin: A review. Radiat Oncol Biol Phys 5:1513, 1979. *The synergistic effects of these two agents are reviewed; 32 references.*

Gross NJ: Pulmonary effects of radiation therapy. Ann Intern Med 86:81, 1977. *An excellent and thorough review with 112 references.*

Disorders of the Lung Caused by Barometric Pressure

Altitude

The major physiologic effects of reduced atmospheric pressure are due to the resulting low partial pressure of oxygen. At 10,000 feet (3048 meters) the alveolar PO_2 is approximately 60 mm Hg, and some individuals will manifest impairment of recent memory, judgment, and the ability to perform complex calculations, and demonstrate an increased heart rate and increased pulmonary ventilation. The time required for these symptoms to begin is partially related to age, physical fitness, and acclimatization. At 12,000 feet (3658 meters) the alveolar PO_2 is 52, and dyspnea, headache, nausea, and decreased visual acuity may occur. At 18,000 feet (5486 meters) the alveolar PO_2 is 40, and unacclimatized individuals will lose consciousness after several hours of exposure. At 22,000 feet (6706 meters) the alveolar PO_2 is 30, and almost all acutely exposed individuals become unconscious after sufficient time. The rapid change in physiologic functions that begins to occur at about 10,000 feet is due to the shape of the oxygen-hemoglobin dissociation curve, which has a steep downslope below a PO_2 of approximately 60 mm Hg. A small drop in PO_2 below this level results in a relatively large decrease in arterial saturation.

In general, commercial aircraft cabins are maintained at a pressure greater than or equal to that encountered at 8000 feet so that no supplemental oxygen is required. Some patients with reduced cardiac reserve or with chronic obstructive lung disease may have difficulty tolerating even a small drop in arterial oxygen saturation and may require supplemental oxygen during flights. Aircraft regulations require that the flight crew receive supplemental oxygen when the cabin pressure drops below that at 10,000 feet, and that passengers receive supplemental oxygen should the cabin pressure drop below that at 15,000 feet.

ACUTE MOUNTAIN SICKNESS. This syndrome occurs in unacclimated persons who rapidly ascend to a high altitude. Symptoms can occur at altitudes as low as 7000 to 8000 feet in particularly susceptible individuals, usually those in poor physical condition, and during a rapid ascent requiring significant physical exertion. The symptoms are headache, exertional dyspnea, malaise, anorexia, nausea, vomiting, diarrhea, and abdominal pain. Judgment may be impaired. Inability to sleep is a common problem. Cyanosis, Cheyne-Stokes breathing, and tachycardia are commonly present. In untreated individuals, these signs and symptoms subside gradually over a period of several days. The treatment is oxygen therapy or descent to a lower altitude. The disorder is thought to be related to an increase in ventilation stimulated by hypoxia and resulting in hypocapnia and respiratory alkalosis. Acetazolamide, 250 mg every eight hours prior to and during the ascent to altitude, can prevent symptoms, presumably by increasing renal excretion of bicarbonate and reducing the extent of the respiratory alkalosis. Furosemide, 80 mg every 12 hours, has also produced relief of symptoms.

CHRONIC MOUNTAIN SICKNESS (MONGE'S DISEASE). Chronic mountain sickness occurs in people living at high altitudes, usually at over 14,000 feet, for many years. These "highlanders" have a blunted respiratory drive in response to hypoxia and have a lower minute ventilation at high altitudes than do those who normally reside at lower altitudes. Chronic mountain sickness is characterized by what appears to be an exaggerated adaptive response to altitude. This includes erythrocytosis with hemoglobin levels as high as 25 grams per deciliter, a decreased minute ventilation with an elevated PCO_2, low arterial oxygen saturation, and an impaired sensitivity of the respiratory center to hypoxia. Clinical manifestations are similar to those of polycythemia rubra vera and include cyanosis, dyspnea, cough, palpitations, headache, giddiness, muscular weakness, pain in the extremities, sensory and motor changes, and episodic stupor. The only therapy is to move the patient to a lower altitude. Subacute forms of this illness also occur in which the marked cyanosis and alveolar hypoventilation are absent. A similar syndrome, brisket disease, has been described in cattle.

HIGH ALTITUDE PULMONARY EDEMA. Acute pulmonary edema is a potentially fatal complication of rapid ascent to altitudes of greater than 9000 feet. The mechanism is unknown, but clearly hypoxia is the provoking cause. Symptoms begin after 6 to 36 hours at high altitude and may follow an episode of acute mountain sickness. Rales, cyanosis, orthopnea, and hemoptysis commonly develop unless oxygen is administered or the patient is rapidly moved to a lower altitude.

At autopsy the lungs are typically heavy, congested, and edematous and have hyaline membranes in the small airways and alveoli. The cause of hyaline membrane formation is not known; this is not a characteristic finding in death caused by other forms of hypoxia. During a large military airlift in India, approximately 6 of each 1000 persons flown to an altitude of 11,500 feet developed this syndrome.

Hemodynamic studies have shown elevations of the pulmonary artery pressure with a normal pulmonary venous pressure. The pulmonary edema may be due to an increase in pulmonary capillary pressure in small regions of the pulmonary capillary bed, or to increased permeability in lung capillaries.

Increased Barometric Pressure

Pressure increases approximately 1 atmosphere for each 33 feet of descent in water. Direct body contact with increased barometric pressure under water is most commonly encountered during breathhold diving, when continuous consumption of oxygen and production of CO_2 lead to hypoxia and hypercapnia. The increasing serum carbon dioxide concentration causes an almost irresistible drive to breathe. Since hypoxia is a mild stimulation for ventilation, it is relatively easy to continue holding one's breath in the presence of profound hypoxia. A common hazardous error made by swimmers is to hyperventilate prior to a dive in an effort to increase the time of breath holding. This depletes the body of carbon dioxide stores, but does not significantly increase oxygen stores. In these circumstances hypoxia can cause unconsciousness before accumulation of carbon dioxide forces the termination of the dive. This is thought to account for many deaths in swimming pools. Decompression during ascent from a breathhold dive can cause a marked fall in alveolar Po_2, leading to the diver's losing consciousness just as the surface is reached.

DECOMPRESSION SICKNESS. Decompression sickness was first described in the last century in caisson workers in tunnel construction, where compressed air was used to exclude water and mud. The increase in military, commercial, and sport diving has made decompression sickness a relatively common clinical problem. When ordinary air is breathed under increased ambient pressure, inert gas, commonly nitrogen, dissolves in tissue and blood, reaching saturation equilibrium at the greater partial pressures. Upon rapid decompression to sea level, the inert gas may come out of solution to form intravascular bubbles. The onset of symptoms tends to be gradual, beginning minutes to hours after the termination of a dive. Manifestations include "bends" (deep pain in joints, aggravated by exercise), pruritus, cyanosis, substernal chest pain, dyspnea, nonproductive cough, evidence of spinal cord injury, confusion, blurred vision, visual field defects, paralysis, dysphasia, headache, vertigo, and seizures. In severe cases the symptoms may rapidly progress to shock and death. Symptoms of mild or early decompression sickness resemble and are often confused with acute alcohol intoxication.

The treatment of decompression sickness is recompression with a gradual return to sea level pressures over a period of days to weeks. Recompression decreases bubble size and permits their gradual resorption during the "ascent" to surface pressures.

Air embolism can occur in scuba divers who ascend without exhaling. Intrapulmonary gas expands and the high pressure may rupture a portion of the lung and introduce gas into the systemic circulation, mediastinum, pleura, or subcutaneous tissues. Gas bubbles may form arterial emboli to the brain and result in sudden unconsciousness, focal or generalized seizures, visual field loss or blindness, weakness, paralysis, hypoesthesia, or confusion. The therapy is rapid recompression similar to that employed to treat decompression sickness. Gas embolism has been reported during ascents of as little as 2.2 meters and is thought to be one of the most common causes of accidental death in divers.

THERAPEUTIC HYPERBARIC OXYGEN. Hyperbaric oxygen has been clearly proven to be beneficial in treating only a limited number of illnesses: acute carbon monoxide poisoning, acute cyanide poisoning, clostridial myonecrosis, decompression sickness, air embolism, and osteoradionecrosis. The hazards of oxygen toxicity limit the dose of oxygen that can be delivered by hyperbaric techniques. Central nervous system toxicity, usually in the form of convulsions, occurs at oxygen pressures greater than 2.5 atmospheres if the exposure is maintained for a sufficient length of time. Thus, hyperbaric oxygen therapy is limited to a maximum of two to three atmospheres of oxygen and durations of no more than one to three hours.

Kidd DJ, Elliott DH: Decompression disorders in divers. *In* Bennett PB, Elliott DH (eds.): The Physiology and Medicine of Diving and Compressed Air Work. Baltimore, Williams & Wilkins Company, 1975, pp 471–495. *A good text and a good chapter on the problems encountered in decompression.*

Singh I, Khanna PK, Srivastava MC, Lal M, Roy SB, Subramanyam CSV: Acute mountain sickness. N Engl J Med 280:175, 1969. *A good review.*

Strauss RH: Diving medicine. Am Rev Respir Dis 119:1001, 1979. *A comprehensive state-of-the-art review on all aspects of diving medicine.*

CHEMICAL INJURY TO THE LUNG

Toxic Inhaled Gases

A large number of gases and chemicals, to which exposures most frequently occur in an industrial setting, can cause both an acute and sometimes a chronic injury to the respiratory system.

A few agents cause an *"asthma-like" reaction* with cough, chest pain, and wheezing. Toluene di-isocyanate and other isocyanates (liberated as gas during the reaction of isocyanates with polyol in the manufacture of polyurethane foams), aluminum soldering flux, and platinum salts are typical examples. Reaginic and precipitating antibodies against platinum salts and soldering flux have been found in symptomatic individuals, suggesting an immunologic basis for the reaction. An allergic basis for the reaction to toluene di-isocyanate has not been demonstrated. The symptoms usually subside after removal from exposure; however, chronic lung injury may occur if the exposure is prolonged.

A number of highly irritating gases cause an *acute chemical pneumonitis.* Such gases include chlorine (used in the chemical and plastic industries and to disinfect water), ammonia (used in refrigeration), sulfur dioxide (used in paper manufacture and smelting of sulfide containing ores), ozone (generated in welding and in photochemical smog), nitrogen dioxide (released from decomposed corn silage), and phosgene (used in production of aniline dyes).

The prototype for injury of this type is *silo-filler's disease* (nitrogen dioxide). During the initial exposure there may be no symptoms, there may be tracheobronchitis with cough and shortness of breath, or there may be the immediate onset of acute pulmonary edema. Signs of ocular and oropharyngeal mucous membrane irritation may be present. The symptoms may rapidly progress, but commonly the initial symptoms resolve and are followed by a period of minimal symptoms (cough) lasting up to 48 hours. Fever, myalgias, dyspnea, and progressive hypoxemia then occur and the radiographic picture is that of pulmonary edema. These severe symptoms may resolve only to recur two to five weeks later and may lead to progressive pulmonary insufficiency with a picture of bronchiolitis obliterans. Treatment with corticosteroids (prednisone, 1 mg per kilogram per day) may dramatically improve the acute illness. Bronchodilators, mechanical ventilation, and supplemental oxygen may be necessary. Since there may be a period of temporary improvement following the initial exposure, observation for a period of 48 hours is advisable.

The clinical response caused by each irritant gas varies, but appears to be closely related to the degree of acute irritation it causes and to its water solubility. The less irritating gases, such as ozone and the oxides of nitrogen, phosgene, mercury, and nickel carbonyl, can be inhaled for prolonged periods of time and thereby cause injury throughout the respiratory system. Highly irritating and soluble gases, such as ammonia and hydrochloric acid, are less likely to be inhaled deeply and tend to result in immediate injury to the upper airways and have potential for obstruction secondary to mucosal edema. Less soluble gases, such as chlorine, cadmium, zinc chloride, osmium tetroxide, and vanadium, can cause injury to the entire tracheobronchial tree and do not commonly present with upper airway obstruction. Bronchiolitis and pulmonary edema are common, ultimately leading to bronchiolitis obliterans. The long-term consequences vary with the gas. Cadmium, for example, can cause diffuse emphysema and severe airway obstruction but only minimal fibrosis.

Different mechanisms are involved in the injury caused by these gases. Most of them cause injury by acting as a strong acid, a strong base, or an oxidant. Gases of chemicals that are strong acids or bases in water solution, such as hydrogen chloride, sulfuric acid, sulfur dioxide, and ammonia, tend to react more in the upper airways where they change tissue pH and thereby cause cell damage.

Chester EH, Kaimal PJ, Payne CB, Kohn PM: Pulmonary injury following exposure to chlorine gas. Chest 72:247, 1977. *Discussion of the response of two patients and a review of literature suggest that corticosteroid therapy may be beneficial.*

Horvath EP, doPico GA, Barbee RA, Dickie HA: Nitrogen dioxide-induced pulmonary disease. J Occup Med 20:103, 1978. *A well-written report of five cases and a review of the literature.*

Summer W, Haponik E: Inhalation of irritant gases. Clin Chest Med 2:273, 1981. *A comprehensive review of gases that are toxic to the lung; 74 references.*

Pulmonary Oxygen Toxicity

Oxygen is used in extremely high concentrations in large numbers of patients in intensive care units, often with endotracheal intubation and mechanical ventilation. The toxic effects of hyperoxic atmospheres may not infrequently outweigh the potential therapeutic benefits. Superoxide, an unstable free radical produced by the single electron reduction of oxygen, is produced as a normal byproduct of oxidative metabolism in almost every plant and animal tissue that uses oxygen as an electron sink. Superoxide dismutase is a protective enzyme that catalyzes the dismutation and therefore the detoxification of the superoxide free radical. If not scavenged by superoxide dismutase, this free radical can react with hydrogen peroxide to form the hydroxyl free radical (OH•) and free radical chain reactions can be initiated, resulting in the destruction of cell lipids and proteins. This "free radical injury" is the presumed chemical basis for oxygen toxicity (Fig. 560–1).

In the adult the major target tissue of oxygen injury is the pulmonary capillary endothelium. Other body organs are protected by the consumption of oxygen and the characteristics of the binding of oxygen to hemoglobin. The mixed venous Po_2 is maintained at about 40 to 50 torr even when the patient is breathing 100 per cent oxygen.

At autopsy the lungs are atelectatic, congested, and edematous and have hyaline membranes. The most serious injury appears to be destruction of the capillary bed with resultant interstitial and alveolar edema, hypoxemia, and sometimes death. Alveolar epithelium is also injured, causing hyperplasia of Type II cells. An acute tracheobronchitis also occurs, and histologic changes have been found in the ciliated epithelium and Clara cells in the small airways.

The typical presentation in the adult is that of an acutely ill patient who is receiving oxygen in high concentrations and mechanical ventilation for a lung injury that makes the onset of pulmonary oxygen toxicity difficult to detect. Lung compliance progressively falls; the patient develops tachypnea, substernal pain, and increased cough. The alveolar-arterial oxygen gradient gradually widens with progressive hypoxemia. Increasing concentrations of oxygen are needed to maintain adequate oxygenation of arterial blood, and the cycle progresses to pulmonary edema, respiratory failure, and death.

The earliest symptoms of oxygen toxicity are due to acute tracheobronchitis. A dry, hacking cough and substernal pain may occur within six to twelve hours while breathing pure oxygen. Nausea, vomiting, and paresthesias follow. Vital capacity decreases, and there is an increase in the respiratory rate.

The flow of tracheal mucus decreases after short exposures

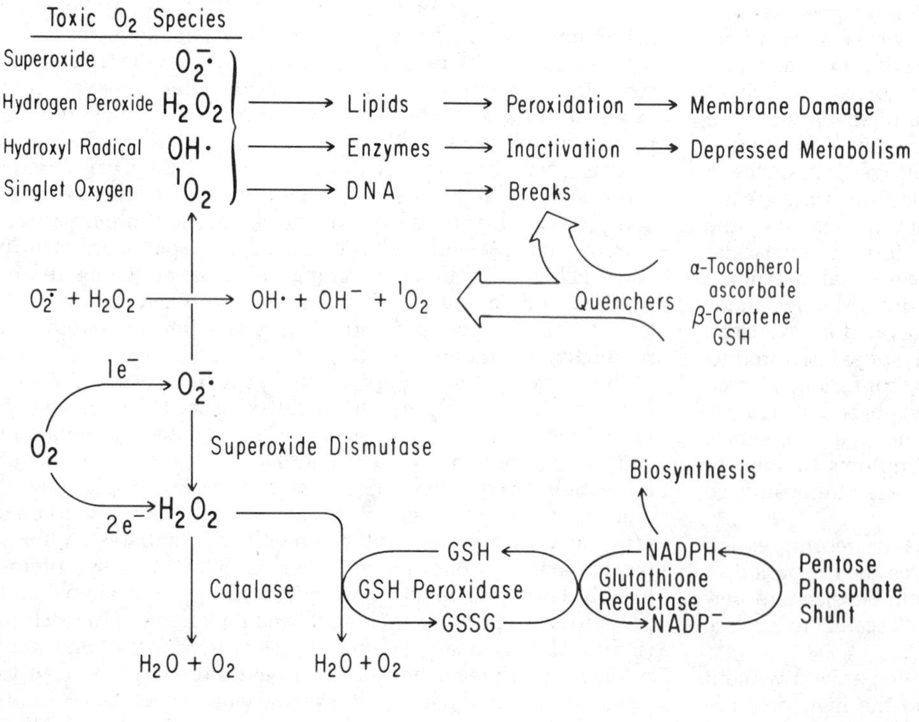

Figure 560–1. Toxic oxygen species and antioxidant defense systems. The incomplete reduction of oxygen produces superoxide and/or hydrogen peroxide. These species can react together in the presence of metal salts to form the hydroxyl radical and singlet oxygen. Free radical chain reactions can be initiated in lipid membranes, with enzymes and DNA also attacked by these reactive O_2 species. Quenchers interact with the oxygen species or with oxidized tissue components to block further tissue oxidation and to terminate free radical chain reactions. The antioxidant defense systems, superoxide dismutase, catalase, and glutathione peroxidase, function to detoxify superoxide and hydrogen peroxide, thus preventing the formation of other toxic O_2 species and the subsequent reactions with tissue. Glucose-6-phosphate dehydrogenase is the rate limiting enzyme in the pentose phosphate shunt and thereby controls the availability of NADPH. This cofactor is essential both for the reduction of glutathione and for the biosynthetic pathways critical for repair processes. Net tissue injury represents the balance between the rate of production of partially reduced oxygen species, the rate at which these species are scavenged, and the rate of repair of any injury that occurs.

to excess oxygen, probably reflecting functional injury of airway epithelium. These patients are therefore more susceptible to mucus impaction and to infection caused by failure to clear inhaled pathogens adequately.

The only proven therapy is prevention of the insult by using high oxygen concentrations judiciously. Corticosteroids have no proven benefit and may actually enhance the lung injury caused by hyperoxia. It is usually impossible clinically to distinguish early oxygen toxicity because of the severity of the original lung insult. The physician often faces a dilemma in which increasing concentrations of oxygen are essential for immediate survival but its administration contributes to deterioration of the patient a short time later. Alternative methods to improve tissue oxygen delivery without using high inspired partial pressures of oxygen should be used whenever possible. These include transfusion of packed red cells to raise the serum hemotocrit to even supranormal levels, measures to improve cardiac output, and measures to decrease the tissue oxygen demand by reducing fever or intense agitation.

The safe maximal concentration of oxygen is not known. Many recommend the range of 40 to 50 per cent oxygen as safe because little injury has been demonstrated in normal animals or human volunteers breathing 40 to 50 per cent oxygen for prolonged periods. The diseased lung may be more susceptible to oxygen injury, however. Rather than identify an arbitrary oxygen concentration that should not be exceeded, rational therapy is to use only enough oxygen to provide adequate arterial blood saturation—an arterial P_{O_2} of 60 torr. Patients should not continuously be given 40 to 50 per cent oxygen under the assumption that this concentration is harmless. If the patient survives oxygen toxicity, some residual damage to the lung parenchyma may remain, with septal fibrosis replacing areas where the pulmonary capillary bed was destroyed by the hyperoxia.

Crapo JD, Barry BE, Foscue HA, Shelburne J: Structural and biochemical changes in rat lungs occurring during exposures to lethal and adaptive doses of oxygen. Am Rev Respir Dis 122:123, 1980. *A detailed description of oxygen-induced injury in experimental animals.*

Deneke SM, Fanburg BL: Normobaric oxygen toxicity of the lung. N Engl J Med 303:76, 1980. *A comprehensive and well-written review.*

Frank L, Massaro D: Oxygen toxicity. Am J Med 69:117, 1980. *A current review with an excellent discussion of current and future studies aimed at modifying oxygen injury.*

Freeman BA, Crapo JD: Free radicals and tissue injury. Lab Invest 47:412, 1982. *A review of the mechanisms of production of free radicals and their role in tissue injury; 173 references.*

Carbon Monoxide Poisoning

Carbon monoxide is commonly produced by internal combustion engines, by poorly vented heating devices, and by gas refrigerators. Lower levels can exist in automobile repair shops, in areas in high automobile traffic density, and in arc welding. Natural gas is free of carbon monoxide, but its incomplete combustion by a faulty heating apparatus can produce carbon monoxide. The most common source of human exposure to carbon monoxide is smoking; cigarette smokers commonly have carboxyhemoglobin concentrations of 3 to 8 per cent. Endogenous carbon monoxide is normally produced from cleavage of the α-methylene bridge in the catabolism of heme, which results in a normal blood carboxyhemoglobin concentration of 0.5 to 0.8 per cent.

Carbon monoxide injures by causing tissue hypoxia. Carbon monoxide has an affinity for hemoglobin which is 218 times greater than that of oxygen. Thus, even small amounts of inspired carbon monoxide will have profound effects on the oxygen-carrying capacity of blood. An alveolar carbon monoxide tension of 0.5 torr and an arterial oxygen tension of 100 torr will produce blood concentrations of 50 per cent carboxyhemoglobin and 50 per cent oxyhemoglobin. In addition, carbon monoxide shifts the oxyhemoglobin saturation curve to the left and changes its shape, resulting in a further decrease in oxygen unloading in tissues.

The clinical picture of carbon monoxide poisoning is dependent upon the blood concentration of carboxyhemoglobin. Levels of less than 10 per cent carboxyhemoglobin produce few clinical symptoms. At 10 to 30 per cent carboxyhemoglobin, headaches and nausea occur and there may be mild dysfunction of the central nervous system with decreased visual acuity and impaired cognitive functions. Thirty to 40 per cent carboxyhemoglobin is associated with severe headaches, dyspnea on exertion, dizziness, nausea, vomiting, dimness of vision, ataxia, and possible collapse. Levels greater than 50 per cent carboxyhemoglobin cause tachypnea, convulsions, coma, and death from profound shock and respiratory and cardiovascular failure.

The diagnosis is confirmed by the determination of blood carboxyhemoglobin concentration. Carboxyhemoglobin has a characteristic cherry red color which can produce the classic bright red skin color in patients poisoned by carbon monoxide. This is in fact rare during life and is seen most often after death.

TREATMENT. The patient must be immediately removed from the contaminated environment. The specific therapy is administration of oxygen. Breathing normal air will result in a 50 per cent clearance of blood carbon monoxide in approximately five hours. Administration of 100 per cent oxygen at sea level will achieve a 50 per cent reduction of carboxyhemoglobin in 80 minutes, whereas oxygen at 3 atmospheres of pressure will achieve the same clearance in approximately 25 minutes. The use of 95 per cent oxygen–5 per cent carbon dioxide will hasten oxygenation, largely by lowering the pH (Bohr effect). In the acutely ill patient the presence of metabolic acidosis is a contraindication to further reductions in pH by administration of carbon dioxide. The level of carboxyhemoglobin is not the sole determinant of the need for therapy. Patients with neurologic abnormalities should be considered for treatment with hyperbaric oxygen even if carboxyhemoglobin levels are low.

Patients who do not become comatose usually recover without permanent sequelae. Among those who survive more severe intoxication, some have residual neurologic symptoms such as seizures, dysphasia, parkinsonism, or mental impairment. Some resolution of neurologic symptoms will occur over a period of weeks, and maximal recovery should be expected within two years of the acute episode.

Dinman BD: The management of acute carbon monoxide intoxication. J Occup Med 16:662, 1974. *A good clinical review.*

Jackson DL: Accidental carbon monoxide poisoning. JAMA 243:772, 1980. *A brief review of the effects and treatment of carbon monoxide poisoning.*

Unsworth IP: Acute carbon monoxide poisoning. Anaesth Intens Care 2:329, 1974. *A good discussion of the management of patients with carbon monoxide toxicity.*

ASPIRATION-RELATED INJURIES

Injury to the respiratory system by aspiration can be categorized by the nature of the aspirate: (1) *Infectious material.* Contamination of the lungs by aspiration of oropharyngeal bacterial flora is discussed in Ch. 63. (2) *Toxic or inflammatory substances.* Aspiration of gastric acid is the most commonly occurring example in an adult population; hydrocarbon aspiration occurs predominantly in children but is encountered in adults. Both these injuries can cause fulminant illness. By contrast, lipids (mineral oil, vegetable and animal fats) most often provoke a chronic inflammatory reaction. (3) *Inert matter.* The injury of drowning is predominantly secondary to asphyxia. Food particles can cause a fibrotic, granulomatous lesion or, if large enough to occlude the larynx or trachea, sudden death by asphyxiation ("café coronary").

Aspiration Pneumonitis

Aspiration pneumonitis refers to the caustic injury to the respiratory system caused by gastric acid. This is in contrast to "aspiration pneumonia," an infectious process caused by the contamination of the tracheobronchial tree by oropharyngeal flora. Aspiration of gastric acid can occur during vomiting or during regurgitation, and in the latter instance the event may go unnoted—i.e., "silent aspiration." The normal protective mechanisms of the upper airway include epiglottic closure during deglutition, glottic closure on contact with solids or fluids, the cough reflex, and the esophageal sphincters. Altered states of consciousness, anesthesia and surgery, neuromuscular disease, gastrointestinal disease, and medical devices (nasogastric tubes or uncuffed tracheostomy tubes) impair these defenses. The use of low pressure, high volume cuffs on endotracheal tubes serves to reduce the high incidence of aspiration of gastric contents in patients with predisposing disorders.

The main factors determining the extent of illness caused by gastric acid aspiration are as follows: (1) *pH of the aspirate.* The acidity of the material is the most important cause of lung injury, with a critical pH $\leq$ 2.5 inducing severe pneumonitis from acid aspiration. (2) *The presence of food particles.* Aspiration of gastric foodstuff has been shown to cause a severe pneumonitis and peribronchial inflammatory reaction in the absence of a low pH. (3) *Volume of the aspirate.* Aspiration of more than 0.4 ml per kilogram of body weight of gastric acid is sufficient to cause pneumonitis. (4) *Distribution of the aspirate.* Many patients who aspirate immediately begin to cough, which may expel the aspirate and thereby partially protect the lung from injury or may enhance dispersion of the acid over a greater area and turn a potentially localized lesion into a diffuse one. (5) *Contamination of the gastric contents with fecal matter,* as in intestinal obstruction. Such a soiling of the tracheobronchial tree is associated with a marked increase in mortality, but death presumably ensues from infection, not from acid injury.

PATHOPHYSIOLOGY. After intratracheal instillation, acid is rapidly distributed in the lungs, and can reach the pleura in 12 to 18 seconds. It is rapidly neutralized by bronchial secretions; in less than 30 minutes the pH at the bronchial surface will have returned to normal. The acid causes a chemical burn of the bronchi, bronchioles, and alveolar walls, with subsequent exudation of fluid into the lungs. Plasma volume may decrease by as much as 35 per cent in severe injury without fluid replacement, and cardiac output and systemic arterial blood pressure may fall. Pulmonary capillary wedge pressure is normal or low, indicating a nonhydrostatic cause of the pulmonary edema. The characteristics of phospholipids in the alveolar surface lining layer (surfactant) are altered, causing increased surface forces, and promoting early airway and alveolar closure. Lung compliance decreases secondary to the increase in interstitial fluids and the alteration of surface forces. These disturbances of airways, alveoli, and vascular elements cause profound imbalance of the normal ventilation-perfusion relationships. Hypoxemia is invariably present and usually severe. Increased right-to-left shunting is commonly present.

CLINICAL MANIFESTATIONS. Some patients aspirate a large volume of gastric acid and almost immediately become apneic and hypotensive and die. More commonly a patient aspirates stomach contents and, with various amounts of coughing, survives the initial crisis, but later develops a fulminant illness marked by dyspnea, cough, and pink, frothy sputum. Alternatively aspiration may be secondary to regurgitation and not accompanied by immediate coughing and agitation. With this so-called silent aspiration the patient presents with acute respiratory failure but with no obvious reason for the precipitous deterioration in function. Within two to five hours after aspiration of gastric acid, tachypnea, rales, and rhonchi occur, and wheezing, cyanosis, and hypotension may be present. Fever of 38 to 39° C in the first 36 hours occurs in about 50 per cent of patients.

Laboratory tests are nonspecific. A moderate leukocytosis with left shift develops early. Arterial blood gases, the best variable to follow, show hypoxemia, and the arterial oxygen tension does not reach predicted levels after the patient has been breathing 100 per cent oxygen for several minutes, indicating increased right-to-left shunting of blood. The arterial P_{CO_2} may be slightly elevated, normal, or mildly reduced, and pH will vary reciprocally. Abnormalities on chest roentgenograms are extremely variable, and there is no characteristic pattern. Extent of radiographic abnormalities does not correlate with clinical outcome. Although the distribution of the acid in some cases is preferentially to areas dependent at the time of aspiration, frequently the abnormalities are diffuse, presumably from enhanced dispersion of the acid during coughing. On radiographs taken early in the course, the majority of patients have perihilar or basilar infiltrates, usually bilateral or multicentric, with bilaterally symmetrical infiltrates in only about 40 per cent of cases. Pleural effusions and cavitation of infiltrates are not seen in uncomplicated cases. Bronchoscopic findings are diagnostic if food particles or gastric debris is seen in the trachea or bronchi. Subsegmental mucosal erythema in a suspected case is a supportive but not diagnostic finding.

The key to the accurate diagnosis of aspiration pneumonitis is a high index of suspicion for this entity in any patient with an abrupt respiratory deterioration, especially a patient with a condition that places him at increased risk of gastric acid aspiration. The differential diagnosis includes cardiogenic pulmonary edema, pulmonary embolus, bacterial pneumonia, and many of the causes of the adult respiratory distress syndrome such as sepsis, hypotension, amniotic fluid embolism, and increased intracranial pressure.

TREATMENT. Treatment of the individual whose aspiration was witnessed begins with the prompt establishment of an adequate airway. The airway should be suctioned to remove any particulate matter. A single lavage of 10 ml of saline may be used; larger volumes have been shown to increase the extent of injury in rabbits. Intratracheal instillation of sodium bicarbonate or of steroids is of no value.

General supportive measures include fluid replacement with crystalloid or colloid solution. Supplemental oxygen is given to maintain Pa_{O_2} >60 torr. Bronchodilators (intravenous aminophylline) may help. Associated pulmonary edema is not cardiogenic in origin and is usually associated with intravascular volume depletion. Therefore, there is no place for the routine use of digitalis or diuretics.

Antibiotics should not be used prophylactically for acid aspiration since they do not reduce morbidity or mortality and they increase the risk of subsequent infection with a resistant organism. The acid-damaged respiratory tract has an increased susceptibility to bacterial infection. In a patient who has been improving after aspiration, new deterioration, especially after the first three days, with increasing fever, leukocytosis, worsening hypoxemia, new infiltrates on chest x-ray, and the production of purulent sputum is suggestive of a secondary bacterial pneumonia. Management of the patient who has aspirated gastric contents that had been contaminated with fecal matter would include the early use of antibiotics providing activity against anaerobes and gram-negative organisms.

The role of systemic corticosteroids in aspiration pneumonitis is controversial. There have been no controlled human trials. Early anecdotal reports supported their use, but more recent retrospective and prospective but uncontrolled series totaling approximately 250 patients have failed to show any improvement in morbidity or mortality.

Positive-pressure ventilation is helpful, particularly when it is initiated early after the aspiration. Arterial oxygen tensions improve and mortality rates decrease with its use. Positive end-expiratory pressure (PEEP) to improve oxygenation has been beneficial in other forms of adult respiratory distress syndrome and is commonly used in the management of gastric acid aspiration. Caution should be used in applying PEEP, since in the acid-injured lung a marked increase in lung extravascular water content can occur, especially if PEEP >15 cm water is applied.

Aspiration pneumonitis carries a high mortality rate despite treatment, and because it largely occurs in a defined population at increased risk, efforts should be made at prevention. Elevation of the head of the bed will retard regurgitation. In intubated patients placement of a nasogastric tube to keep the stomach decompressed should be considered. Aspiration may occur even in the presence of a cuffed endotracheal tube. Elective general anesthesia should be given with the stomach empty, after at least a 12-hour fast. If anesthesia must be undertaken with a full stomach, consideration should be given to rapid induction and intubation while employing cricoid pressure. In recognition of the critical role of the degree of acidity of the aspirate, the pH of gastric contents can be raised by a single dose of cimetidine (300 to 400 mg orally two to four hours before surgery, given with minimal water) or by a single 10 ml dose orally of antacid, best given after premedication.

OUTCOME. Mortality from aspiration pneumonitis is high, reaching 28 to 62 per cent of cases. Factors associated with highest risk of death are age greater than 50 years, the early development of shock or apnea, severe and prolonged hypoxemia, pH of gastric contents ≤ 1.75 at the time of aspiration, and the development of secondary bacterial pneumonia. Most but not all survive the early moments. After the initial deterioration (24 to 36 hours), some then show steady improvement, with radiographic resolution within a week. Some have a second episode of deterioration, an event which should suggest a new problem such as bacterial infection, pulmonary embolism, heart failure, or another aspiration. Still others pursue a relentlessly worsening course to death. Few data exist regarding long-term clinical follow-up, but it is thought that pulmonary fibrosis of varying degrees ensues in some of these patients.

Newman GE, Effman EL, Putman CE: Pulmonary aspiration complexes in adults. Curr Prob Diagn Radiol 11(4):1–47, 1982. *A thorough review of the mechanisms, diagnosis, and treatment of aspiration; 65 references.*

Schwartz, DJ, Wynne JW, Gibbs CP, Hood CI, Kuck EJ: The pulmonary consequences of aspiration of gastric contents at pH values greater than 2.5. Am Rev Respir Dis 121:119, 1980. *Aspiration of gastric food particles will cause a severe pneumonitis in dogs even when the pH is 5.9.*

Drowning

Drowning accounts for about 7000 deaths annually in the United States, mostly in children and young adults. It is one of the three leading causes of accidental death. Pathophysiologically, drowning can be of four types: (1) *"Wet" drowning*—initial laryngospasm but early relaxation and subsequent aspiration of copious amounts of fluid. The majority of drownings are of this sort. (2) *"Secondary" drowning*—death occurs 15 minutes to 72 hours after extraction from the water, and is due to a form of adult respiratory distress syndrome. (3) *"Dry" drowning*—asphyxiation secondary to intense glottic spasm which persists beyond the point of apnea, so that when the muscles relax, no water is aspirated. This accounts for 10 to 20 per cent of drownings. (4) *Immersion syndrome*—cardiac arrest secondary to the intense parasympathetic discharge of the diving reflex.

The most important consequences of near-drowning are severe hypoxemia and metabolic acidosis. The difference between fresh water and salt water near-drowning appears to be of little significance. Life-threatening electrolyte disturbances caused by water aspiration in humans are rare, and the salt content of the aspirate is relatively unimportant. Hypoxemia is caused by occlusion of airways with fluid and particulate debris in the water, by changes in surfactant activity, by direct injury to the alveolar septa, and by bronchospasm. There is a marked increase in right-to-left shunting and an increase in physiologic dead space. Severe metabolic acidosis develops in most cases, presumably secondary to anaerobic metabolism in the asphyxiating victim, especially with the violent struggling that normally occurs. Cardiac arrhythmias, conduction disturbances, and central nervous system injury can occur in this setting. Cerebral edema is far more common than actual brain infarction.

Autopsies of drowned persons demonstrate wet, heavy lungs with varying amounts of hemorrhage and edema and some disruption of alveolar walls. In about 70 per cent, vomitus, sand, mud, and aquatic vegetation have been aspirated. Specimens from victims dying from "secondary drowning" show desquamation of alveolar epithelial cells, hemorrhage, hyaline membrane formation, acute inflammatory infiltrates, and foreign body reactions to particulate matter. Cerebral necrosis and edema are seen; changes of acute tubular necrosis are found sometimes in the kidneys.

CLINICAL MANIFESTATIONS, TREATMENT, AND OUTCOME OF NEAR-DROWNING. The initial appearance of the patient can vary widely, from coma to agitated alertness. Cyanosis, coughing, and the production of frothy pink sputum are common. Tachypnea, tachycardia, and a low grade fever in the first few hours are seen if the patient did not become hypothermic during submersion. Rales, rhonchi, and, less often, wheezes are heard. Neurologic signs vary between patients and can fluctuate in any given patient but usually derive from bihemispheric cerebral dysfunction. Signs of associated trauma should be sought.

Laboratory studies reveal mild hypokalemia, hypernatremia, and hyperchloremia, none of life-threatening magnitude. There may be a moderate leukocytosis. Hematocrit (Hct) and hemoglobin usually are normal on first measurement; in fresh water aspiration the Hct sometimes falls slightly in the first 24 hours. An increase in serum free hemoglobin is seen more often, without significant changes in Hct. Rarely the picture of disseminated intravascular coagulation has been reported in near-drowning. Arterial blood gases, usually obtained after preliminary resuscitation, show severe hypoxemia and metabolic acidosis. The most common electrocardiographic changes are sinus tachycardia and nonspecific S-T segment and T wave changes, which revert to normal within hours; however, other, more ominous abnormalities may occur—ventricular arrhythmias, complete heart block, or myocardial infarction. The chest x-ray may be normal initially in spite of severe respiratory disturbances. It often shows patchy infiltrates, and sometimes a classic pulmonary edema pattern is seen.

Treatment of the near-drowning victim begins with the establishment of an adequate airway and, if necessary, emergency cardiopulmonary resuscitation. Oxygen in high concentrations is necessary, since hypoxemia is present in essentially all victims. Even the patient who quickly becomes apparently normal should be hospitalized for 24 hours to watch for a subsequent picture of adult respiratory distress syndrome. During transportation to a hospital, supplemental oxygen should be continued, and precautions taken for potential cervical spine injury and other critical trauma.

In the hospital, subsequent therapy is dictated largely by the arterial blood gases and the degree of respiratory failure. Continuous positive airway pressure or PEEP is particularly helpful. Prophylactic antibiotics have not been shown to be beneficial. The use of corticosteroids for the pulmonary lesions of near-drowning remains controversial, and there have been no controlled prospective human studies of that therapy; animal models and retrospective studies in man have failed to demonstrate any benefit.

If there is evidence of cerebral edema, intracranial pressure (ICP) monitoring can be used to guide therapy. In the event of increased ICP, PEEP should be minimized, since it increases ICP. Hyperventilation to maintain a Pa_{CO_2} of 25 to 30 torr will decrease cerebral blood flow and ICP. Mannitol or glycerol should be used. Corticosteroids (e.g., dexamethasone, 16 mg intravenously initially, then 4 mg intravenously every four hours) are beneficial for the central nervous system injury. Seizures, shivering, or random nonpurposeful movements can increase ICP and should be aborted with pancuronium bromide. If these maneuvers fail to lower ICP, then barbiturates (e.g., pentobarbital, 3 mg per kilogram) every hour intravenously to obtain a serum level of 2.5 to 4 mg per deciliter can be tried.

Outcome in near-drowning is best judged by the neurologic status. The shorter the interval between extraction from the water to first spontaneous gasp, the better the prognosis for recovery without chronic neurologic sequelae, which include mental subnormality, minimal brain dysfunction, spastic quadriplegia, extrapyramidal syndromes, optic and cerebral atrophy, and peripheral neuromuscular damage. Between 5 and 20 per cent of children who survive near-drowning have such residual deficits. Survival without neurologic damage is better in children who are hypothermic when recovered, and occurs even after 40 minutes of submersion. Similar information regarding adults is lacking.

Conn AW, Edmonds JF, Barber GA: Near-drowning in cold fresh water: Current treatment regimen. Can Anaesth Soc J 25:259, 1978. *This paper describes a treatment protocol designed to minimize brain edema, including deliberate hypothermia, hyperventilation, muscle paralysis, barbiturates, and corticosteroids.*

Hoff BH: Multisystem failure: A review with special reference to drowning. Crit Care Med 7:310, 1979. *An excellent, thoroughly complete review of the evaluation and care of the nearly drowned patient with attention to all critical organ systems.*

Modell JH, Graves SA, Ketover A: Clinical course of 91 consecutive near-drowning victims. Chest 70:231, 1976. *Clinical details from this study refute the importance of a distinction between fresh vs. salt water immersion and provide guidelines for assessment.*

Redding JS: Drowning and near drowning. Can the victim be saved? Postgrad Med 74:85, 1983. *A review of current therapy.*

Hydrocarbon Pneumonitis

Hydrocarbon pneumonitis results from the direct toxic effects of volatile hydrocarbons on the respiratory epithelium and vasculature. It occurs in individuals who have ingested the hydrocarbons, but results almost exclusively from aspiration into the respiratory tract rather than from absorption from the gastrointestinal tract and systemic distribution. It does not occur from "sniffing" the compounds. The problem occurs most often in children, particularly below the age of five years, in whom it is usually accidental. It is an uncommon problem in adults, occurring most often in industrial accidents, in patients attempting suicide, in siphoning of gasoline, and in uninformed alcoholics seeking an ethanol substitute.

Different hydrocarbons cause respiratory injury of varying extent, the critical parameters being the viscosity and volume of the aspirate. The lower the viscosity or the larger the volume, the worse the lesion. Being lipid solvents, all these compounds are directly toxic to respiratory tissues. The lungs of children dying from hydrocarbon pneumonitis demonstrate hemorrhage, pulmonary edema, atelectasis, hyaline membrane formation, and necrosis of airway epithelium and alveolar septa. In animal models the acute inflammation begins to resolve by the third day, and is followed by a proliferative response of alveolar lining cells, an increase in intra-alveolar macrophages, and a mononuclear cell infiltration in perivascular and peribronchiolar tissues. By six weeks there is partial clearing of these changes, although the alveolar walls remain thickened. These compounds have systemic toxicity, and in fatal cases degenerative changes in the liver and kidneys have been seen.

CLINICAL MANIFESTATIONS. Aspiration usually occurs at the time of hydrocarbon ingestion. There may be choking and coughing, with a burning sensation in the mouth and throat. A history of vomiting after hydrocarbon ingestion is obtained in less than half the patients. Dyspnea, tachypnea, tachycardia, and high fever quickly ensue. Sputum may be bloody. Lethargy is common, but more severe disturbances of consciousness such as confusion, coma, and seizures also occur. Auscultation is frequently normal, but rales and rhonchi may be present.

The chest radiograph is particularly helpful, since even before auscultation becomes abnormal, infiltrates frequently occur, developing as quickly as 20 to 30 minutes after aspiration of some types of hydrocarbons but later in others. The distribution of the multiple, fluffy, ill-defined infiltrates is preferentially in the dependent areas of the lungs, predominantly on the right side, but occurs bilaterally in about one fourth of cases. Some patients present a picture of bilateral perihilar infiltrates, a "pulmonary edema" pattern. Pleural effusions, pneumothorax, and pneumomediastinum occur but are uncommon. Pneumatoceles can form later, especially in children.

Laboratory tests give nonspecific results. A moderate leukocytosis with left shift is common. Arterial hypoxemia of various degrees develops owing to shunting and to ventilation-perfusion mismatching.

The differential diagnosis is that of respiratory distress of abrupt onset, frequently in a patient with an impaired sensorium at the time of presentation. In the adult this is often an alcoholic. Gastric acid aspiration, an intracranial catastrophe, cardiogenic pulmonary edema, pulmonary embolism, and acute bacterial pneumonia can all present similarly. The correct diagnosis requires the history of hydrocarbon ingestion or aspiration. The diagnosis is also suggested by the odor of the patient's breath and by extensive radiographic abnormalities in a patient with a clear chest by auscultation.

TREATMENT. Emesis to remove residual hydrocarbons is contraindicated. Gastric lavage by nasogastric tube may induce vomiting and should be performed only in the patient who has ingested a large volume of hydrocarbons and then only after placement of a cuffed endotracheal tube. Supplemental oxygen should be given to maintain Pa_{O_2} >60 torr. Mechanical ventilation and PEEP may be necessary. There are no data to show that the routine use of antibiotics modifies the course. The use of systemic corticosteroids is supported by anecdotal reports of improvement after their use in children and adults. Prednisone, 1 mg per kilogram per day, or its equivalent should be used during the acute illness, with termination as the patient improves.

OUTCOME. Hydrocarbon pneumonitis in adults is rare, so that morbidity and mortality estimates are not available. In children death occurs in as many as 10 per cent of cases, but most children have a prompt clinical recovery. Bronchiectasis, recurrent bronchitis, and/or pulmonary fibrosis ensue in an unknown portion of cases. After recovery from the initial illness, children frequently are asymptomatic and have normal chest examinations and radiographs. However, pulmonary function abnormalities suggestive of small airway (<2 mm diameter) disease have been found in asymptomatic patients as late as 8 to 14 years after the hydrocarbon pneumonitis.

Gurwitz D, Kattan M, Levison H, Culham JAG: Pulmonary function abnormalities in asymptomatic children after hydrocarbon pneumonitis. Pediatrics 62:789, 1978. *This study of 17 children several years after hydrocarbon pneumonitis demonstrated obstructive changes in small airways that may predispose to later clinically important respiratory diseases.*

Lipoid Pneumonia

Lipoid pneumonia is a chronic inflammatory reaction of the lungs that results from the aspiration of vegetable, animal, or most commonly mineral oils. This material differs greatly from the excessive accumulation of endogenous lipids in the lungs occurring in fat embolism, cholesterol pneumonitis, pulmonary alveolar proteinosis, and the lipid storage diseases.

The most frequently implicated agent is a mineral oil, which is used as a laxative and to reduce dysphagia, either in clear liquid form or as petroleum jelly. Mineral oil is bland and when introduced into the pharynx can enter the bronchial tree without eliciting the cough reflex. It also mechanically impedes the ciliary action of the airway epithelium. Risk of mineral oil aspiration is increased in the debilitated or senile patient, in those having neurologic disease that interferes with deglutition, and in patients with esophageal disease. Mineral oil taken as nose drops to relieve nasal dryness has caused lipoid pneumonia, and in earlier years was a frequent cause of the illness. Smoking blackfat tobacco, a Kentucky tobacco to which mineral oils are added for flavoring and as humectants, has caused lipoid pneumonia. Inhalation of mineral oil mists by airplane and automobile mechanics has been implicated as a cause of the problem. Aspiration of vegetable (e.g., castor, olive) or animal (e.g., cod liver oil, milk, butter, egg yolk) fats has been an infrequent cause.

Mineral oils, which are relatively inert, cannot be hydrolyzed in the body and provoke a chronic inflammatory reaction which may not become clinically overt until years later. The fat is emulsified in the alveolar spaces, where macrophages accumulate and phagocytize it. Some macrophages disintegrate, releasing their lysosomal enzymes and fat. The alveolar septa become thickened and edematous, containing lymphocytes and lipid-laden macrophages. Oil droplets are seen in the pulmonary lymphatics and hilar nodes. Later, fibrosis develops and the normal lung architecture is effaced. It is usual in a single specimen to find both the early inflammatory and the later fibrotic picture, in keeping with repetitive aspirations over many months or years. If nodular, the lesion may grossly resemble tumor and is called a paraffinoma.

CLINICAL MANIFESTATIONS, DIAGNOSIS, AND TREATMENT. Most patients are asymptomatic, coming to a physician's attention because of an abnormal chest radiograph, or the lesion is found unexpectedly at autopsy. When patients are symptomatic, the complaints are nonspecific, with cough and exertional dyspnea being the most frequent. Chest pain (sometimes pleuritic), hemoptysis, fever (usually low grade), chills, night sweats, and weight loss may occur. The physical examination may be completely normal, or fever, tachypnea, dullness on percussion of the chest, bronchial or bronchovesicular breath sounds, rales, and rhonchi may be found. Clubbing is rare. Cor pulmonale uncommonly develops.

The erythrocyte sedimentation rate may be prolonged. In mild lipoid pneumonia arterial blood gases may be normal at rest but show hypoxemia after exercise. In more severe disease, resting hypoxemia, hypocapnia, and mild respiratory alkalosis develop. Pulmonary function testing reveals a restrictive ventilatory defect; static compliance of the lungs is decreased. The only specific laboratory finding is the presence in sputum of macrophages with clusters of vacuoles 5 to 50 μ in diameter that stain deep orange with Sudan IV, and extracellular droplets that similarly stain.

Radiographically, the earliest abnormalities are air space infiltrates, unilateral or bilateral, localized or diffuse, but most often in the dependent portions of the right lung. Air bronchograms may be seen. Hilar adenopathy and pleural reaction are rare. As fibrosis develops, there is volume loss and the appearance of linear and nodular infiltrates. A solid lesion may develop which closely resembles bronchogenic carcinoma.

The differential diagnosis is extensive, particularly in the late phase when multiple other causes of pulmonary fibrosis must be considered. Sarcoidosis, mycobacterial and fungal infection, chronic hypersensitivity pneumonitis, primary lung carcinoma, bronchiectasis, pneumoconiosis, pulmonary alveolar proteinosis, and pulmonary hemosiderosis are some of the major diseases that are a part of the differential diagnosis. The key to the correct diagnosis before biopsy is the history of chronic use of an oil or a lipid-based product, orally or intranasally, or an occupational exposure to oil mists. The presence of lipid-laden macrophages in the sputum confirms the diagnostic impression.

Once the diagnosis has been made and the aspiration stopped, the subsequent course is variable. Some patients will have no change in symptoms. Others will have improvement in some or all parameters, whereas a few patients continue to deteriorate with worsening pulmonary function and cor pulmonale.

Discontinuation of the use of the offending lipid is essential. Since the only way the body can dispose of mineral oil is by expectoration, the patient should be instructed in coughing exercises to be performed many times each day for months. Expectorants have not been shown to help. Systemic corticosteroids are recommended by some: prednisone, 40 mg orally each day at the beginning and then decreased to 10 mg daily until stabilization of clinical and radiographic signs (which might involve months of therapy). The use of steroids has been based on improvements seen in a very few patients in uncontrolled, anecdotal trials. The rationale has been that the cellular reaction, rather than the oil itself, is the destructive factor. Because of the well-recognized side effects from prolonged use of systemic corticosteroids, their use for lipoid pneumonia should be limited to those patients who have significant symptoms, and then for as brief a period as possible, to "buy time" while decreasing the lipid burden by expectoration.

Blöndal T, Hartvig P, Bengtsson A, Wilander E: An unnecessary case of paraffin oil pneumonia. Acta Med Scand 213:227, 1983. *The problems in diagnosis of mineral oil pneumonia are illustrated in a current case report.*

Heckers H, Melchar FW, Dittmar K, Knorpp K, Nekarda K: Long-term course of mineral oil pneumonia. Lung 155:101, 1978. *This case report documents persistence of oil in expectorated sputum for months after stopping the oil use and the sequential improvement in physiologic parameters.*

561. OCCUPATIONAL DISEASES OF THE SKIN

Edward A. Emmett

Occupational skin diseases are a group of heterogeneous conditions that share a common occupational etiology. They account for about one half of reported occupational disease in the United States. Occupational contact dermatitis, the prototypical disorder, makes up about 95 per cent of all occupational skin disease; infections, about 2.5 per cent; and a large number of different, infrequent diseases, the remainder. The relative frequency of each of these diseases in any location depends largely on the pattern of industrialization.

Almost all occupational skin disease is due to external contact with chemical, physical, and biologic agents. The cause is often multifactorial. In relatively few instances are systemically (rather than locally) absorbed agents responsible.

OCCUPATIONAL CONTACT DERMATITIS

DEFINITION. Occupational contact dermatitis is an erythematous or eczematous response of the skin as a result of local contact with one or more irritating, allergenic, or photosensitizing chemical agents.

ETIOLOGY. Many chemicals from a wide variety of classes—alkalies, acids, volatile organic solvents, metallic salts, organic prepolymers, and many others—are capable of inducing contact dermatitis. The cause is often multifactorial; in addition to one or more chemicals, friction, abrasion, changes in temperature and humidity, and ultraviolet radiation may play a role. Superinfection may occur. Severe and persistent occupational contact dermatitis is more frequent in those with an atopic diathesis.

INCIDENCE AND PREVALENCE. Workers' compensation reports put the incidence in the United States at about 1.4 per 1000 full-time workers per year, although, because of substantial under-reporting, the true incidence is estimated to be from 10 to 50 times higher.

EPIDEMIOLOGY. The incidence of occupational contact dermatitis is generally highest in the agricultural and manufacturing industries. The highest risks occur in poultry dressing plants, meat packing plants, fabrication of rubber products, leather tanning and finishing, manufacture of ophthalmic goods, plating and polishing, production of frozen fruits and vegetables, internal combustion engine manufacture, machining operations, and in canning and curing of seafoods, but virtually no industry is immune.

PATHOGENESIS. Contact dermatitis may result from direct local irritation, cell-mediated immune reactions, or photosensitivity.

Direct local irritation may be immediate, as in irritation from strong acids or alkalies, or may be delayed and occur only after repeated or prolonged local application as cumulative insult dermatitis. The latter can occur from one or more relatively mildly irritating substances that are termed marginal irritants.

Allergic contact dermatitis occurs as a result of sensitization to specific haptens through a process of cell-mediated immunity. The hapten combines with protein in the skin to form a complete antigen that is processed and presented to T lymphocytes by epidermal Langerhans cells, specialized macrophages that form an intraepidermal network. Among the most frequent allergens are poison ivy/oak; rubber additives, particularly accelerators and antioxidants; monomers of plastics and resins, such as epoxies, acrylates, and diisocyanates; nickel, chromium salts; paraphenylenediamine and derivatives; and formaldehyde. There are many more possible allergens; the number of substances reported to cause allergic contact dermatitis is very large.

Chemical photosensitivity results from the photochemical excitation of an ultraviolet (UV)-absorbing molecule with resultant tissue damage. In a photoirritant reaction there is direct damage to cellular components, for example, when psoralens in the presence of long UV bind covalently to DNA. Coal tar pitch, certain aromatic dyes, and UV absorbers used in printing processes also cause photoirritation. In the rarer photoallergic reaction, photochemical alteration of the inciting chemical forms an allergen in the skin, leading to a cell-mediated immune reaction.

A major part of the resistance to environmental chemicals is provided by the epidermal barrier in the stratum corneum. Damage to this barrier by trauma, inflammation, or skin disease or by altering barrier conditions, for example by occlusion, seems to play an important role in the development of contact dermatitis.

CLINICAL MANIFESTATIONS. The clinical presentation is dominated by dermatitis that is confined, at least initially, to the region of contact. The morphology varies according to the concentration and duration of the exposure, the pathogenesis, and individual constitutional differences, although there is much overlap. Acute irritant dermatitis is characterized by erythema (perhaps by edema), papules and vesicles, or in the more extreme instance by one or more large bullae filled with purulent fluid. Postinflammation hyperpigmentation and hypopigmentation may occur; necrosis may leave scars. The cause of acute irritant dermatitis is usually obvious because of the rapidity with which the reaction develops.

Cumulative insult dermatitis may develop only after a long period of contact. On the hands it tends to start under rings or watchbands and to be somewhat patchy in distribution. Individual susceptibility is probably important. Initially, drying and fissuring may be seen with subsequent development of an eczematous response with papules and vesicles. Excoriations and lichenification are frequent if the process persists. Relapse may occur on relatively brief exposure to mild irritants, even when the dermatitis is clinically healed, especially if the epidermal barrier has not yet been reestablished.

Allergic contact dermatitis most often presents as an acute or chronic eczematous reaction with erythema, papules and vesicles, scaling, and pruritus. Characteristically there is a latent period of at least seven to ten days before the development of dermatitis following first exposure to the allergen. Recurrence usually occurs 24 to 72 hours after an eliciting exposure. Certain allergens, for example, epoxy resin monomers, have a tendency to produce severe acute reactions with significant edema.

Localization is important for diagnosis. Over 90 per cent of occupational contact dermatitis involves the hands, sometimes in conjunction with other sites. Where the eruption is due to contact with objects or contaminated surfaces, the pattern of contact will determine localization. Reaction to immersion of the hands in liquids generally involves the dorsum of the hands and palmar aspects of the wrists. Photosensitivity reaction on exposed sites may be distinguished from airborne contact dermatitis by the relative sparing of shaded areas such as the eyelids or behind the ears.

DIAGNOSIS. A good occupational history is the cornerstone of diagnosis. It is most useful to get a description of the worker's daily activities, including nonoccupational activities, with particular attention to contact of the skin with chemicals. The localization of the eruption at its onset, initial appearance of lesions, nature of progression, and circumstances of remissions and recurrences are important to the determination of occupational etiology. A personal or family history or both will confirm the presence of atopy, in which there is increased susceptibility to irritants, changes in heat and humidity, and other factors. A complete examination of the skin will help rule out dermatoses other than contact dermatitis, including id reactions of the hands secondary to dermatophytosis of the feet. Allergic contact dermatitis is confirmed by diagnostic patch testing; photoallergy, by photopatch testing. Patch testing is relatively easy to perform, but the interpretation requires skill. There is no clinically useful confirmatory test for irritant contact dermatitis.

Other information may be necessary to make a precise diagnosis and formulate appropriate management. Toxicity information on industrial compounds can be obtained from Material Safety Data Sheets, which reveal the composition and properties of industrial materials. Recent regulations in the United States make these available to most employees and their physicians. A visit by the physician to the workplace allows the physician to view the work firsthand. If such a visit is made, opportunity for skin contact with hazardous agents should be explored as well as the use of protective measures.

Epidemologic surveys to establish the prevalence of dermatitis in workers at similar jobs and industrial hygiene surveys to characterize the nature and amount of chemical exposure may occasionally be helpful. Public health authorities, university centers for occupational and environmental health, and sometimes concerned employers may be able to assist in such investigations.

TREATMENT. Symptomatic treatment is similar to that for dermatitis of other types. Acute contact dermatitis is treated with cold wet dressings of Burow's solution. Systemic steroids in rapidly tapering doses are indicated in severe acute widespread disabling eruptions; topical steroids and emollients, for dry and chronic eczema. Superinfection requires appropriate systemic antibiotics. Antihistamines may be given for sedation and are mildly antipruritic. The patient should be given careful instruction to avoid casual exposures, and should be alerted to the fact that even when the skin has apparently healed the barrier may not have returned to normal. A temporary or permanent change of job tasks may be necessary. If a permanent job change is necessary, vocational rehabilitation should be considered. Some states require reporting of occupational diseases.

PROGNOSIS. The prognosis of occupational contact dermatitis is surprisingly poor, especially if effective treatment is not given early and if the dermatitis is prolonged. The reasons for this are not entirely clear; however, surveys have shown that a high percentage of individuals still have dermatitis several years later, in many cases despite a change of employment. Those with atopy appear to have the worst prognosis. In allergic contact dermatitis the prognosis is dependent on the ease with which the allergen can be avoided.

PREVENTION. Preventive measures serve both to prevent recurrences and to halt the development of novel disease. These include elimination or substitution for strong irritants and sensitizers; education of workers as to skin care; avoidance of overly harsh skin cleansers; prompt reporting and treatment of dermatitis; engineering controls to minimize skin contact with potential hazards; appropriate impervious protective clothing; good personal hygiene with rapid effective removal of contaminants; and counseling of individuals with predisposing conditions, such as atopy, regarding career selection.

OTHER OCCUPATIONAL DERMATOSES

A relatively large number of other dermatoses can result from occupational exposure. In large part, management is dependent upon diagnostic recognition and on discontinuing further exposures, using measures outlined above.

Chemical burns result from corrosive agents that produce necrosis, ulceration, and subsequent scarring. Prompt removal of these agents (such as strong acids, alkalies, phenol, alkyl metal compounds, and metal chlorides) from skin, eyes, and mucous membranes is essential. Water is generally best for removal; quicklime, tin tetrachloride, and titanium tetrachloride should be removed with mineral oil. Specific antidotes are few; these include topical or injected calcium gluconate for hydrofluoric acid burns.

Urticaria may occur from local contact or systemic absorption with agents that elicit an immediate hypersensitivity reaction or directly release histamine and other vasoactive substances.

Fiberglass dermatitis causes intense pruritus; there may be no visible changes or it may be accompanied by excoriations, pinpoint petechial papules, or both. Microscopy of a cellophane tape stripped from the skin, which had been treated with 10 per cent potassium hydroxide, reveals the fibers.

Relatively deep indolent *ulcers* of skin and mucous membranes result from contact with arsenic, chromates, and lime.

Chemical acne and folliculitis may result from contact with greases and oils, coal tar pitch, creosote, and a number of cosmetics (acne cosmetic) and from ingestion of bromides, iodides, and isoniazid. These forms of acne typically commence with comedones or inflammatory papules.

Chloracne is due to halogenated aromatic compounds with specific molecular shape, including dioxin and related chlorinated aromatic hydrocarbons. The illness is characterized by small straw-colored cysts and comedones that first involve the malar crescent and behind the ear and may not spread beyond these areas. Inflammatory pustules, abscesses, and large cysts may be seen in severe cases. Chloracne is the first and most constant finding in chronic dioxin poisoning. More variable findings may include porphyrinuria, hyperpigmentation, hypertrichosis, central and peripheral nervous system effects, alteration of lipid metabolism, and mild hepatotoxicity. Experimentally observed effects include teratogenicity, immunosuppression, and tumor induction.

Cutaneous granulomas occur as slightly erythematous grouped flesh-colored papules, with or without inflammatory changes, from foreign body reactions at the site of contact with talc and silica or as an immunologic response to beryllium and zirconium.

Chemical leukoderma, which may mimic vitiligo but which is confined to the areas of skin contact, may result from a number of phenols and catechols, including hydroquinone, monobenzyl, and monomethyl ethers of hydroquinone (used as rubber additives) and *p*-tertiary butyl and amyl phenols (in disinfectants).

Basal and squamous cell carcinomas and keratoacanthomas result from prolonged exposures to ultraviolet radiation, ionizing radiation, polycyclic aromatic hydrocarbons (including coal tar pitches and related products), and arsenic. Exposures to arsenic may be associated with various internal malignant neoplasms.

INFECTIONS AND INFESTATIONS

The development of infections and infestations frequently depends on occupational factors, individual susceptibility, and the geographic distribution of the causal organism. Occupational associations include the following:

Viral. Herpes simplex (dentists, medical personnel), milkers' nodules and papular stomatitis (veterinarians, milk handlers), orf (farmers, shepherds, abattoir workers), viral warts (butchers), Rift Valley fever (shepherds).

Bacterial. Staphylococcal infections of hands (abattoir workers and butchers), erysipeloid (fish, fowl, rabbit, and pig handlers), anthrax (wool, hair, and hide handlers), tularemia (farmers), nontuberculous mycobacterial infections (aquarium workers and pet shop attendants). Bacterial and yeast infections and tinea versicolor are prominent with heat, humidity, occlusion, and lack of hygiene.

Fungal. Dermatophyte infections are more frequent in farm workers, surveyors, zoo attendants, animal care technicians, and certain others. Particular examples include tinea verrucosum (farmers); infection due to *Trichophyton rubrum* (miners), *Microsporum canis* (pet shop workers), *Trichophyton violaceum* (wrestlers), and *Candida albicans* (those in wet work, particularly those in contact with sugar and fruit); sporotrichosis (mine workers); chromomycosis (agricultural workers); and actinomycosis (agricultural workers).

Protozoal. South American leishmaniasis (foresters).

Helminths. Creeping eruption (plumbers, gardeners, farm workers in the tropics), ankylostomiasis (miners), schistosomiasis and cercarial dermatitis (rice planters and canal workers).

In addition, bites and stings of arthropods and other creatures are common in those who work out of doors and in certain other occupations.

Emmett EA: Occupational skin disease. J Allergy Clin Immunol 72:649, 1983. *A brief review of important occupational dermatoses with current references and emphasis on the approach to a patient with suspected occupational skin disease.*

Maibach HI, Gellin GA: Occupational and Industrial Dermatology. Chicago, Yearbook Medical Publishers, 1982. *A multiauthor text that broadly covers occupational dermatoses and dermatotoxicology and describes the skin diseases of a number of specific occupations.*

562. RADIATION INJURY

Theodore L. Phillips

DEFINITIONS

Radiation injury may be defined as any somatic or genetic disruption of function or form caused by electromagnetic waves or accelerated particles. Common sources of such injury include ultraviolet radiation from the sun and man-made sources, microwave radiations from radar and ovens and other appliances, high-intensity ultrasound and ionizing radiations from natural and man-made sources.

Ultraviolet radiation, produced by the sun, is largely absorbed by the atmosphere of the earth. It has very short penetration in tissue and is thus of concern only for exposed body surfaces. It causes injury through direct chemical effects in molecules with high absorbance for the given wavelength. Ultrasound and microwave radiations exert their effects through the generation of heat during absorption.

Radiations with wavelengths shorter than light have an additional property, the ability to displace electrons from their normal orbits with production of charged particles. As these particles traverse tissue, they form ions and free radicals that then react with biologically important molecules, leading to cell injury and death. The ability of the high-energy ray to penetrate and cause large amounts of biologic damage after deposition of small amounts of energy makes it of concern to the physician.

Ionizing radiations, both natural and man made, are of two types: (1) photons or waves and (2) accelerated particles. The *photons* do not cause direct injury but cause damage through the interactions that occur with orbital electrons that become charged particles in tissue. Ionizing photons, called gamma rays, are given off by many types of nuclear decay. Man-made ionizing rays, called x-rays, occur when an accelerated electron is stopped rapidly in a dense material.

Accelerated particles include protons from solar radiation, heavy nuclei in cosmic rays, and beta and alpha particles given up in nuclear decay. These particles are charged and cause direct ionization. Neutrons are also given off in nuclear decay and are found in cosmic radiation. They cause damage through secondary reactions in tissue in which protons are produced, which then cause ionization.

Radiation dose is defined in terms of energy deposition. Previously the unit was the rad, 100 ergs per gram, but it is now the *gray* (abbreviated *Gy*), defined as equal to 100 rads or 1 joule per kilogram. Radioactivity is defined in terms of the rate of decay or disintegration. The *curie,* a unit based on the radioactivity of a gram of radium, is still used, but in the new SI unit system the unit is the *bequerel.* Because radiations differ in the density of the ionization they cause, the biologic effects vary. Densely ionizing radiations, such as heavy particles and neutrons, will have greater biologic effects. Thus the *rem* is a unit used for safety considerations in which a "quality factor" is applied to a quantity similar to a centigray (one hundredth of a gray).

Absorption of charged particles and their range in tissue are determined by their charge and mass. Particles with high charge and mass give up their energy rapidly and penetrate only short distances, unless they are of extremely high energy. Photons are absorbed exponentially by electron or nuclear interactions, and thus some radiation can penetrate long distances. Because photons diverge as they leave the source, the dose will decrease as the square of the distance from the source, as it does for light.

Injury from radiation may be either thermal (dealt with elsewhere in this book) or ionizing. Ionizing radiation injury expressed within a few hours or days is termed acute.

Low radiation doses that do not produce acute or delayed organ dysfunction are termed low level. Such small doses (1 gray or less) can produce genetic and carcinogenic effects in the population and are also of great concern.

ETIOLOGY

BIOLOGY OF ULTRAVIOLET RADIATION. Very short wave light photons are capable of generating chemical changes in DNA and other molecules, the most important of which is the production of pyrimidine dimers. Although they may be excised and repaired, if unrepaired these lesions lead to reproductive cell death and desquamation after skin irradiation. Ultraviolet exposure also causes immediate effects such as vasodilatation and erythema. The short penetration and the absorption by melanin limit human injury to the superficial layers of the skin.

CELLULAR BIOLOGY OF IONIZING RADIATIONS. When the electrons generated by photons or charged particles traverse a cell they cause the formation of ion pairs in both cell water and the DNA. During such events, radicals are formed with unpaired outer electrons. These radicals react with DNA or occur in the DNA itself. A radical may be repaired by reduction with SH groups or fixed by oxidation or electron transfer. If a free radical persists, it leads to a break in the DNA molecule. Single-strand breaks are generally repaired, but if two occur side by side a double-strand break occurs. Unrepaired double-strand breaks lead to chromosome aberrations that can be lethal to the cell or cause mutations and carcinogenesis.

Chromosome injury is expressed at the time of cell division. Most mammalian cells die of mitotic death. Deletions and dicentric chromosomes lead to loss of genetic information at each cell division. Some cells survive a few divisions but will be incapable of sustained reproduction. Intermitotic death occurs in some lymphocytes and gonadal cells, even after low radiation doses, but most cells will survive 10 to 30 Gy with no obvious damage until mitosis occurs. Intermitotic death is poorly understood but may be related to interference with RNA synthesis in cells with scant cytoplasmic organelles.

DOSE-RESPONSE RELATIONSHIPS. The percentage of cells that will survive after exposure to ionizing radiation decreases logarithmically with dose. There are two components to the injury, reparable and irreparable. Low-level effects are generally less than one would expect based on observations at high doses. Cells can repair radiation damage very effectively. Repair is primarily of single- and double-strand DNA breaks and requires only a few hours to complete.

The radiation dose required to reduce survival to 10 per cent is quite uniform in mammalian cells. The most sensitive cells require 1 Gy (100 rads) to reduce survival to 10 per cent and the most resistant about 3 Gy. Changes in sensitivity by a factor of 3 occur under hypoxia and as cells traverse the mitotic cycle.

INCIDENCE AND PREVALENCE

BACKGROUND RADIATION. Both ionizing and ultraviolet radiations are ubiquitous in the universe because of the fusion processes in stars. Gamma rays, x-rays, and highly energetic particles are emitted by stars and by nuclear decay of isotopes produced by stellar processes. On the earth, radiation comes from isotopes in the ground and construction materials and from the sun and other sources in space. The dose of radiation that one receives from this natural radiation depends on the altitude and the geologic nature of the region. Most people receive annually between 40 and 90 units known as millirems, which are one hundred thousandth of a Gy. Frequent flights at high altitude can cause a large increase in this dose. Such exposures do not cause clinically detectable syndromes, but may add to the incidence of genetic diseases and cancer.

MEDICAL EXPOSURE. Shortly after the discovery of x-rays by Röntgen in 1895 and the subsequent discovery of radioactivity, the first medical injuries occurred. The early workers were unaware of the cell-killing properties of the rays until damage to hands, eyes, and bone marrow was evident. After World War II the full hazards of radiation exposure were recognized, and exposures were strictly limited. Currently injury of the acute and chronic types is rare after medical exposure of personnel, but is of course a major side effect of radiation therapy.

Radiation is used in the treatment of 50 to 60 per cent of patients with malignant disease, and thus 300,000 to 400,000 patients are exposed and will be seen annually by general physicians as well as radiation oncologists. Although every precaution is taken to avoid clinically important late or delayed effects, acute reactions to radiation therapy are common. Since most tumors require doses for cure close to organ tolerance, the risk of injury is always present.

Injury due to inadvertent or accidental exposure of medical radiation workers is uncommon, but occasional cases will be seen either to the whole body or to hands or face during equipment repair or operational accidents. Workers and patients, as well as the general public, are also exposed to low-level radiation either while obtaining diagnostic studies or working in medical radiation environments. Permissible exposures have been reduced to 5 rem for workers and 500 millirem annually for the public, with half that exposure highly recommended. These rules keep medical exposure to the population as a whole to less than half the background level.

INDUSTRIAL AND MILITARY EXPOSURE. High-level radiation to the largest populations occurred at the Hiroshima and Nagasaki fission weapon explosions in World War II. Although most casualties were due to blast and burns, 40 to 50 per cent of the survivors had radiation injury. Frequent medical evaluations of this population have identified late effects, including several hundred cases of leukemia and other malignant diseases. Atomic weapons testing has led to inadvertent exposure of 300 or more persons, with about 25 per cent showing clinically detectable effects. The fallout from nuclear tests has also added a few millirem to the universal annual background radiation exposure.

Ingestion or inhalation of long-lived isotopes is also potentially injurious. About 5000 persons have been exposed to radium ingestion, and at least 400 malignant tumors have occurred, with increased incidence in the sinuses and in bone. Inhalation of plutonium and other alpha emitters is also a potential problem in the nuclear industry.

EPIDEMIOLOGY

Radiation injury is not caused by a vector, and the source and nature of the exposure should be obvious. It is not always so, however, and epidemiologic techniques are required. Persons may be exposed at work or in the environment without awareness, and clinical symptoms must be identified for an exposure to be suspected. In other cases psychologically deranged persons may have access to radioactive materials and ingest them or expose themselves but deny the exposure.

It is extremely important to determine the nature of the exposure and reconstruct the dose distribution to predict the level of the injury and the required treatment. In addition, the relationship between low-level exposures and subsequent genetic and carcinogenic effects can be learned only by careful dosimetry and long-term clinical follow-up.

PATHOGENESIS

CELL KINETICS AND RADIATION EFFECTS. A few cell types express injury and cell death that will be observed within a few hours after exposure because of intermitotic death. Most cells will live until one or more mitoses have passed. Most cells do not die in mitosis, although failure of cell separation due to dicentric chromosomes can be lethal. They will live out their normal life span, and their injury will become apparent only when depopulation occurs, since the dying cells cannot be replaced because of mitotic death.

Some cells, such as mature muscle cells and neurons, do not normally divide and will persist for many years after radiation exposure. Other cells, such as the functional stromal cells in the renal tubules and the liver, are replaced slowly, and eventually depopulation will occur. The capillary system exhibits slow replacement of the endothelial cells. The number of patent capillaries is slowly reduced after radiation doses of 5 Gy or more, which leads to secondary depletion of the nondividing cells such as neurons.

SPECIFIC TISSUE RADIOBIOLOGY. The tissues of the body can be divided into those critical to life and those whose injury by radiation may cause morbidity but is not fatal. The critical tissues for survival are discussed below. The doses quoted are for single exposure to high-energy photons. Because of sublethal damage repair, doses two to four times higher are required for the same effect after fractionated exposures.

Bone Marrow. Because of the short life span and rapid renewal of most peripheral blood and marrow cells, this organ shows the most evident and acute clinical syndrome. Small lymphocytes die an intermitotic death with depletion in a few hours. Depletion of platelets and granulocytes is maximal at three weeks. The normal survival of red blood cells is about 100 days so depletion is late. There is a dynamic balance among the declining numbers of mature cells living out their lives, delay in replacement because of a reduced stem cell pool and regeneration.

The marrow will regenerate after a single exposure up to 6 Gy and can be repopulated by transplantation after doses up to 10 Gy. Above that dose, damage to the vascular supply prevents regeneration.

Intestine. The mature surface and villus cells of the intestinal mucosa are replaced by the division of cells in the crypts that migrate up the villus. In contrast to this rapid renewal system, the muscular wall contains a slowly renewing capillary network. Doses as low as 1 Gy can reduce crypt cell survival to 50 per cent but histopathologically detectable injury requires 10 Gy or more. After 15 Gy the cell kill in the crypt is sufficient to cause complete loss of the villus and in some cases denudation. At this dose, depopulation peaks in four to eight days; regeneration by the surviving crypt cells is complete two weeks after exposure. Higher local doses will cause these acute changes, but will also lead to late injury in the muscular layer and serosa due to capillary injury; this late injury results in fibrotic responses and obstruction.

Central Nervous System. There are no rapid renewal systems in the CNS, but the glial cells and the endothelial cells cycle slowly and can show injury. The neurons are not injured except secondarily or by doses of 50 Gy or more. Very large exposures of 15 to 50 Gy can produce acute functional changes and, at the highest doses, immediate death. After 15 Gy, changes begin in four to five months and develop further over one to two years. There is focal necrosis and calcification, demyelinization, and gliosis, especially in the white matter.

Skin. After exposure to 3 to 9 Gy the skin may show transient vasodilatation, cessation of mitosis in the basal layer, and thinning of the prickle cell layer. At doses above 20 Gy, denudation and ulceration occur before repopulation begins from either surviving basal cells or cells at the periphery of the exposed area. Although there is usually healing to a normal-appearing epidermis, the cells of the hair follicles and sweat glands are often completely destroyed and will not regenerate if the dose was more than 10 to 15 Gy. Late vascular damage expression can cause a second wave of ulceration as well as telangiectasis.

Lung. In the lung, both the type II pneumocytes and the capillary cells as well as the mucosal cells of the bronchial tree are slowly regenerating. About 90 days after a dose of 10 Gy, acute pneumonitis will occur with capillary occlusion and endothelial cell loss. It is preceded by depletion of surfactant and type II cells. Secondary influx of alveolar macrophages is seen. This acute phase is followed over the ensuing nine months by replacement of the vessels and alveoli by collagen. Acute pneumonitis is reversible only at the lowest dose, 8 to 11 Gy in a single exposure.

Heart. The cardiac muscle cells do not proliferate; therefore, almost all radiation changes occur primarily in the endothelium of the capillaries. Four to six months after exposure to 15 Gy or more the capillaries become occluded, with dose-related reduction in their number. This can lead to loss of the muscle cell as well if all four or even three of the capillaries that surround each muscle cell are lost. At similar doses there is also injury to the pericardium with effusion and fibrotic thickening of the wall.

Liver. The hepatocytes are normally replaced very slowly, but injury to the liver can induce a wave of cell division. There is also continuous replacement of the sinusoidal endothelium in the lobules. Six weeks after 10 Gy, central lobular occlusion occurs with secondary hepatocyte loss and portal hypertension.

Kidney. After 10 Gy there is a reduction in the number of tubule cells and a flattening in the tubule lining. Whole nephrons are lost over a period of 4 to 18 months after exposure. At the same time the endothelium is lost, and many capillaries are occluded. At one year and beyond, damage in the glomerulus, with loss of foot processes and thickening of the basement membrane, can be seen. All of these processes may progress over as long as ten years. Secondary hypertension is common.

Gonads. In contrast to most other tissues there is little sparing of gonadal injury during fractionated exposure, making the gonads quite sensitive to complete depopulation of the reproductive cells. Sterilization can occur after as little as 5 to 10 Gy, and prolonged hypospermia after a few Gy. The hormone-secreting cells of the gonads are much more resistant, but, of course, ovarian hormone secretion is dependent on ovulation and is obliterated by sterilization.

CARCINOGENESIS AND MUTAGENESIS. Much smaller doses than those discussed above will cause changes in some of the chromosomes in all exposed tissues. At a dose of 1 Gy, half of the cells may contain at least one abnormal chromosome. Most of the injuries are deletions or will be expressed at mitosis as dicentrics or rings. Many, but not all, of these will result in reproductive cell death. Although radiation does not cause extensive sister chromatid exchanges, it does cause point mutations as well as deletions and rearrangements, all of which can be mutagenic and in some cases carcinogenic. Thus even one hundredth of a Gy can cause a small number of mutations that will lead to expression as malignant disease or abnormal offspring if a large enough population is observed.

CLINICAL MANIFESTATIONS

ACUTE WHOLE-BODY EXPOSURES. The classic acute whole-body radiation syndrome is usually seen after reactor accidents, malfunction of large treatment or research accelerators or industrial irradiation facilities, and after nuclear explosions. It is also seen after total-body irradiation for bone marrow transplantation and treatment of cancer.

The initial symptoms relate directly to the radiation dose. After 2 Gy of high-energy photons, about half of the patients will exhibit nausea and vomiting two to six hours after exposure, and after 3 Gy the incidence is 100 per cent. With doses above 3 Gy the syndrome may be divided into three types:

1. The *hematologic syndrome* occurs in patients receiving up to 10 or 12 Gy. At these doses, although the small intestine is affected, there is usually little or no diarrhea and the bowel is not denuded. The chief effects are in the bone marrow, although patients surviving the acute phase can develop lung or renal injury months to years later. In the hematologic syndrome the patient will experience the prodromal symptoms of nausea and vomiting in most serious cases, often associated with malaise and weakness. These symptoms subside over the first 24 hours and may be followed by salivary gland swelling. If the dose has been less than 5 Gy there will then be a quiescent period of two to three weeks. At that point, depopulation of the marrow and the resultant granulocyte and platelet suppression will lead to infection and hemorrhage. Purpura, petechiae, and fevers are common. Skin erythema and desquamation can occur, particularly if local areas of higher dose exist. Epilation occurs if the patient survives, but is temporary. If the dose is 3 Gy or below, recovery is usual and can occur at doses up to 5 or 6 Gy with medical support.

2. The *gastrointestinal syndrome* occurs at doses of 13 to 30 Gy. When the dose exceeds that needed to denude the small bowel, the gastrointestinal syndrome will occur before the hematologic syndrome, and since it is usually fatal, will be dominant. After initial symptoms similar to the hematologic syndrome, a brief asymptomatic period will ensue, although malaise and diarrhea may be persistent. Five to seven days after exposure, severe diarrhea and fluid loss occur, followed by infection with enteric bacteria. It is not possible to survive this syndrome, even with modern bone marrow transplantation techniques.

3. The *cardiovascular–central nervous system syndrome* occurs at doses greater than 20 to 30 Gy and is uniformly fatal. After 20 to 50 Gy the patient will experience immediate nausea, vomiting, and diarrhea. This is followed rapidly by ataxia, sweating, prostration, and shock. Huge doses, such as 30 to 500 Gy, can cause immediate death, which is due to generalized CNS dysfunction.

LOCAL OR REGIONAL RADIATION INJURY. The clinical syndromes following whole-body irradiation are all associated with acute effects that subside within two months of exposure. Local or regional exposures to very high doses can occur without immediate death, however, and thus late effects can be seen. The signs and symptoms to be expected after local or regional radiation exposure can be deduced from the pathogenesis section and will be summarized here.

Local irradiation of the bone marrow usually leads to no detectable clinical syndrome. The peripheral white and red cell counts will be depressed, but more than half the marrow must be exposed to doses greater than 4 Gy before any clinical symptoms similar to the acute whole body syndrome will occur. With doses over 10 Gy in a single exposure or 25 Gy fractionated exposure there will be prolonged aplasia of the marrow in the irradiated area. This will lead to clinical symptoms of marrow aplasia if additional radiation exposure, infection, or cytotoxic chemotherapy takes place.

Abdominal irradiation can lead to signs and symptoms from the liver, kidney, and small bowel. The stomach and colon can be injured by doses over 50 Gy of fractionated radiotherapy. Radiation hepatopathy results in ascites six to eight weeks after the exposure with other signs of portal hypertension. Renal injury leads to edema and proteinuria six to eight months later. Hypertension, occasionally severe, can be seen one to ten years after exposure, as can the symptoms of renal failure. The acute small-bowel or gastrointestinal syndrome can occur after abdominal exposure, but it is usually not fatal after local exposures. Delayed injury to the small bowel results in signs of intestinal obstruction or occasional malabsorption or diarrhea. Gastric irradiation produces signs of hypochlorhydria, and at 15 Gy can lead to large ulcers of the greater curvature.

Local radiation of the CNS predominantly produces late signs. Whole-brain irradiation with 10 Gy in a single exposure causes edema with transient nausea and vomiting. Doses of 15 Gy to 20 Gy can be fatal in 6 to 18 months with generalized dementia. More focal irradiation can produce a mass lesion with focal signs, headache, and vomiting.

Injury to the skin results from almost all local or regional exposures. This leads to transient erythema the first day. After three weeks, erythema, dry desquamation, or moist desquamation can occur. Epidermolysis and chronic ulceration occur early after a single exposure of over 25 Gy and with more delayed onset after 18 Gy. The subcutaneous tissues are also damaged. The skin may be ulcerated and heal at first, but reulcerate 2 to 20 years later because of progressive fibrosis and vascular damage in the subcutaneous tissue.

Thoracic irradiation can lead to symptoms due to either cardiac or pulmonary damage. Pulmonary damage is first seen three to four months after a single exposure or six weeks to two months after fractionated exposure. The patient experiences fever, dyspnea, and cyanosis. If the acute phase is survived, there will be chronic signs of pulmonary constriction and fibrosis. Somewhat higher doses cause acute pericarditis with symptoms similar to viral pericarditis with fever, malaise, and some dyspnea about 7 to 24 months after irradiation. Paradoxical pulse and cardiac tamponade with large effusions can be seen. Myocardial infarcts and chronic myocarditis are sometimes seen.

Gonadal irradiation in the male rarely leads to symptoms. Oligospermia will occur after low doses and aspermia after higher doses about six weeks after exposure. The duration will depend on the dose, but can be as long as two years. Ovarian effects usually occur by the next cycle and result in amenorrhea, which is rarely reversible, after doses of 5 Gy in a single exposure or 20 Gy in fractionated exposures.

SYSTEMIC EXPOSURE TO RADIONUCLIDES. Systemic radioisotopes cause symptoms and signs similar to external exposure, if one takes into account the distribution of the isotope and the dose to each organ. In each case there is whole-body exposure and specific-organ exposure that depends on concentration of the isotope in the organ and the nature and energy of the radioactivity. Ingestion of ^{131}I, for example, leads to whole-body exposure and high doses in normal thyroid. There can be symptoms of nausea and vomiting and the hematologic syndrome, followed by hypothyroidism and pharyngitis. Plutonium, usualy present in the air, concentrates in the pulmonary macrophages, causing local fibrosis and malignant disease. For each isotope, it is necessary to know the distribution to predict the symptoms.

DELAYED EFFECTS OF LOW-LEVEL EXPOSURE. These effects are purely genetic and carcinogenic. If an exposure does not lead to sterilization, genetic damage can persist in the sperm or egg. Experiments have shown point mutations in mice, but they have been difficult to prove in humans because of the background of about 10 per cent spontaneous abortions. Carcinogenesis occurs, and the symptoms will be related to the organ in which the tumor develops.

DIAGNOSIS

General Principles

It is essential that any facility likely to deal with radiation injuries have a trained team on call. The physician should obtain a clear history of the exposure, including the nature of the radiation, the distance from the source, and any documentation such as monitors or badges and witnesses. A preliminary

TABLE 562–1. SYMPTOMS, THERAPY AND PROGNOSIS AFTER RADIATION INJURY IN MAN

Dose range	0–1 Gy	1–2 Gy	2–6 Gy	6–10 Gy	10–20 Gy
Therapeutic needs	None	Observation	Specific treatment	Possible treatment	Palliative
Vomiting	None	5–50%	3 Gy = 100%	100%	100%
Time delay, nausea, and vomiting	—	3 hr	2 hr	1 hr	30 min
Main organ damaged	None	Lymphocytes	Bone marrow	Bone marrow	Small bowel
Symptoms and signs	—	Mod. leukopenia	Leukopenia, purpura, hemorrhage, epilation	Leukopenia, purpura, hemorrhage, epilation	Diarrhea, fever, electrolyte imbalance
Critical period	—	—	4–6 wk	4–6 wk	5–14 days
Therapy	Psychotherapy	Observation	Transfusion granulocytes, platelets; antibiotics	Transfusion; antibiotics; bone marrow transplant	Fluids and salts; possible marrow transplant
Prognosis	Excellent	Excellent	Guarded	Guarded	Poor
Lethality	None	None	0–80%	80–100%	100%
Time of death	—	—	2 months	1–2 months	2 wk
Cause of death	—	—	Infection, hemorrhage	Hemorrhage, infection	Enteritis, infection

estimate of the dose should be made from the history as well as the symptoms. Symptoms of malaise, nausea, and vomiting indicate an exposure over 1 Gy, and occur in all patients who have been exposed to 3 Gy or more (Table 562–1).

The physical examination should pay particular attention to the skin, conjunctiva, mucous membranes, and salivary glands. After high local doses there may be acute erythema. A patient who comes in two to three weeks after exposure may show signs of infection or hemorrhage.

Laboratory tests include an immediate complete blood count with differential count. The total lymphocyte count directly reflects the dose received in whole-body exposures within 24 hours. Elevation of the granulocyte count can occur transiently at 24 to 48 hours. If possible, a lymphocyte culture should be done by a cytogeneticist to determine the number of chromosome aberrations, which allows calculation of the dose received. Pulmonary function tests are useful after thoracic irradiation, as are lung scans and chest roentgenograms. Hematologic counts are essential one to three weeks after exposure to follow the pancytopenia and to direct therapy. In the gastrointestinal syndrome there may be findings of dehydration and electrolyte imbalances.

Specific Findings

WHOLE-BODY EXPOSURE. The granulocyte count may rise transiently to 10,000 or more 24 to 48 hours after exposure, while the lymphocyte count falls close to zero with doses of 3 Gy or more. The granulocyte count hits a nadir at four weeks and then returns toward normal at eight weeks. The lymphocyte count may remain low for many years.

LOCAL OR REGIONAL EXPOSURE. Clinical findings after such exposure vary widely and reflect the injury to the specific organ involved. CNS damage will be reflected in an abnormal neurologic examination, signs of edema, and enhancing areas on the CT scan months to years after irradiation. The cerebrospinal fluid is generally normal.

Radiation injury to the thorax is usually detected on the chest roentgenogram. Initially there are areas of patchy or confluent pneumonitis that conform to the shape of the exposed area. This progresses to stranded fibrosis and retraction toward the apex, hilum, or mediastinum. Cardiac injury may lead to transient ECG abnormalities, pericarditis with effusion detectable on ultrasound scans, and signs of myocardial ischemia.

Abdominal exposure leads to changes detectable in function tests for kidney and liver. High doses to the pancreas can lead to diabetes and a decrease in pancreatic enzymes. Chronic diarrhea can occur; it is due to malabsorption and bile salt irritation.

SYSTEMIC EXPOSURE TO RADIOISOTOPES. Large doses of gamma ray–emitting isotopes can cause symptoms and signs similar to those seen in the acute whole-body syndrome or local skin or mucosal injury. The most important diagnostic tests that must be obtained are radioactivity counts and spectroscopy to establish the nature of the isotope(s) and the predicted dose and its localization. Urine and blood samples and, if possible, a whole-body count in a suitable counter should be obtained.

GENETIC OR MUTAGENIC EFFECTS. The low doses usually associated with these effects do not cause changes in standard laboratory tests. Lymphocyte cultures are very sensitive and can predict the size of the exposure and the risk. Sperm counts will reflect the dose to the testis but not the genetic damage.

TREATMENT

ACUTE WHOLE-BODY EXPOSURE. The initial symptoms of whole-body exposure can be treated with antiemetics, and the profound weakness seen at doses above 3 Gy can be reduced by a short course of intravenous corticosteroids. Further therapy is not needed for patients who have received 2 Gy or less. Above that and up to 10 Gy, survival is possible with active medical management. Support similar to that used for the pancytopenic leukemia patient is needed at the higher doses. This includes reverse isolation or life-island type of support. Antibiotics should be used if the granulocyte count is below 1000 per microliter or if there is infection, in which case granulocyte transfusions should be used as well. Platelet transfusions should be given if the platelet count is below 10,000 per microliter. The diarrhea seen at lower doses is usually mild but may require intravenous fluid and electrolyte replacement.

Bone marrow transplantation can be a useful adjunct at doses of 5 Gy or more. Bone marrow samples and peripheral blood for tissue typing should be obtained early, before depletion occurs. Techniques similar to those used for leukemia should be employed (Ch. 156).

Exposures above 10 Gy, which will lead to the gastrointestinal or CNS syndromes, are uniformly fatal. Palliative support is indicated with fluids and the treatment of infection or hemorrhage.

LOCAL OR REGIONAL EXPOSURE. The most common injury requiring treatment will be in the skin. Dry or moist desquamation occurs and can be ameliorated by cleansing with an antibacterial soap. Crusts should be soaked off and the open areas dressed with petroleum jelly or bacitracin ointment. Large areas can benefit from temporary use of lanolin closed dressings, which should be changed daily; the area should be washed before each redressing (Table 562–2).

Most other local injuries cannot be treated specifically. The electrolyte imbalances seen with nausea and vomiting must be corrected. Severe hypokalemia can occur. Radiation pneumonitis can be reversed at borderline doses with prednisone 60 mg per day tapered over the ensuing month. The acute symptoms of pericarditis can be relieved by aspirin or other anti-inflammatory agents. Delayed effects of doses of 20 Gy or more may require skin grafts, resection of necrotic bone, and other surgical procedures, including resection of necrotic brain tissue.

SYSTEMIC EXPOSURE TO RADIONUCLIDES. After the victim has been given urgent first aid and decontaminated if there is

TABLE 562–2. ORGAN DAMAGE, DYSFUNCTION, TREATMENT AND PROGNOSIS AFTER LOCAL IRRADIATION

Organ	Acute Lesion	Delayed Lesion	Clinical Signs	Treatment	Prognosis
Bone marrow	Pancytopenia	Vascular occlusion Myelofibrosis	Infection Hemorrhage	Antibiotics Transfusion	Good if % of total marrow irradiation small
Intestine	Flattened villi	Fibrosis, obstruction	Diarrhea	Fluid, electrolyte acute Resection for obstruction	Good for acute Obstruction can be fatal
CNS	Edema	Necrosis	Headache Focal neurologic	Resection	Poor
Skin	Desquamation	Ulcer, necrosis	Pain, oozing	Cleansing, ointments, graft	Fair
Lung	Pneumonitis	Fibrosis	Cough, fever, cyanosis Dyspnea	Corticosteroids	Good Good at low dose Good if small volume
Heart	Pericarditis	Carditis	Fever, dyspnea	Anti-inflammatory, pericardiocentesis	Fair
Liver	Central venous thrombosis	Fibrosis	Ascites	Diuretics	Fair
Kidney	Tubular degeneration	Fibrosis	Proteinuria Hypertension, renal failure	Dialysis Transplant	Fair

surface contamination, the dose and nature of the exposure should be determined, making use of a whole-body counter if possible. Large body burdens should be treated by specific methods designed to remove the isotope or block uptake. After iodine exposure, stable iodine should be given as 5 drops of potassium iodide. One gram of soluble phosphate should be given to patients ingesting ^{32}P. Radium ingestion can be treated with magnesium sulfate or epsom salts, 10 grams in 100 ml of water. Strontium exposure is treated with 100 ml of aluminum phosphate gel.

Pulmonary exposures can be treated by bronchial lavage, expectorants, and DTPA (diethylenetriaminepentaacetic acid) aerosol mist. DTPA products are available from the United States Department of Energy for experimetal use and cause chelation of heavy metals.

Gastrointestinal absorption can be reduced with use of mild laxatives. Sodium alginate and aluminum hydroxide gel may reduce strontium uptake.

Certain heavier isotopes, including plutonium, americium, yttrium, lanthanum, cerium, scandium, zinc, and other fission products can be partially removed from the body by DTPA (0.5 to 1 gram given intravenously as soon as possible after exposure and repeated once in 250 ml of normal saline).

PROGNOSIS

ACUTE RADIATION SYNDROMES. Survival with little or no treatment outside good hygiene and treatment of infections can be expected after exposures to 3 Gy or less. Between 3 and 6 Gy, effective therapy with antibiotics, platelets, and granulocytes allows a high survival rate. Leukemic patients show 80 per cent survival after 10 Gy whole-body exposure at a dose rate of 4 Gy per hour when bone marrow transplantation is used. The use of all available methods will allow a high rate of survival after 5 Gy and some survival after acute exposures to 10 Gy. Survival has not been achieved in those patients exhibiting the gastrointestinal or CNS syndromes, probably because irreversible lung, kidney, and marrow damage have occurred.

LOCAL RADIATION EFFECTS. Acute skin reactions usually heal completely. If the exposure has been over 20 Gy, late ulceration can be expected. Most delayed radiation injury is irreversible and slowly progressive as depopulation of stromal and capillary cells occurs.

SYSTEMIC EXPOSURE. The prognosis will depend on the whole-body dose and the nature of the isotope. Large whole-body doses will result in a prognosis similar to that for whole-body external exposure. Thyroid ablation will occur after 50 to 100 millicuries of ^{125}I, and bone marrow ablation after smaller doses of ^{32}P.

GENETIC AND MUTAGENIC EFFECTS. Estimates of the risk of genetic and mutagenic effects are based on extrapolations from higher doses, generally 1 Gy or more, and are thus subject to the dose-response model used. Current best estimates place the additional risk of death from cancer at 77 to 226 per million persons per cumulative centigray of exposure. The risks are higher in the pediatric population and are much higher in the fetus and embryo, particularly in the first trimester.

PREVENTION

Because radiation injury always has an irreversible component, prevention is essential. The largest population exposure is from natural background and can be limited only by moving to a location with low background at low altitude.

The largest controllable additional exposure is medical. This can be limited by careful selection of diagnostic tests. Optimum techniques, collimation, and shielding of the gonads must be employed. The design of facilities must limit the exposure to public and monitored personnel to less than recommended levels. Proper training of workers using radiation is essential. Radiation treatment must be carried out by highly skilled specialists who limit the dose to tumor areas as much as possible.

Hall EJ: Radiation and Life. Elmsford NY, Pergamon Press, 1976. *An introductory overview of radiation in the environment for the student and lay person.*

Hall EJ: Radiobiology for the Radiologist. 2nd ed. Hagerstown, MD, Harper & Row, 1978. *The best introductory text on the biologic effects of radiation for the medical worker.*

Johns HE, Cunningham JR: The Physics of Radiology. 4th ed. Springfield, IL, Charles C Thomas, 1983. *The most comprehensive text in the field of medical radiation physics.*

Principles and General Procedures for Handling Emergency and Accidental Exposures of Workers. ICRP publication 28, Annals of the ICRP 2:1, 1978. *Detailed instructions and useful references for physicians who may be required to deal with victims of accidental exposure.*

Protection Against Ionizing Radiation from External Sources Used in Medicine. ICRP Publication 33, Annals of the ICRP 9:1, 1982. *The basic international manual that sets dose limits, protection standards, and monitoring standards. Essential for anyone employing radiation equipment.*

Shapiro J: Radiation Protection—A Guide for Scientists and Physicians. 2nd ed. Cambridge, Mass., Harvard University Press, 1981. *The standard text for those using ionizing radiations in medicine, with particular emphasis on radionuclides. Covers biology, physics, and protection aspects.*

Thames HD, Withers HR, Peters LJ, et al.: Changes in early and late radiation responses with altered dose fractionation: Implications for dose-survival relationships. Int J Radiation Oncol Biol Phys 8:219, 1982. *A detailed review of the factors influencing acute and late radiation injury. Some background in radiobiology needed.*

The Effects on Populations of Exposures to Low levels of Ionizing Radiations. Washington, National Academy of Sciences—National Research Council, 1980. *A detailed presentation and analysis of radiation exposure information and the incidence of malignancy induction with projections for large populations.*

563. ELECTRIC INJURY

Basil A. Pruitt, Jr.

INCIDENCE AND PREVALENCE. Electricity produces a spectrum of injury ranging from sudden death caused by cardiopulmonary arrest to immediate tissue injury and necrosis caused by transformation of electric energy into heat. Delayed organ damage may also occur; its pathogenesis is incompletely defined. The number of electric injuries occurring annually in the United States and other industrialized countries has paralleled the use of electricity. It is estimated that in the United States more than 1100 deaths occur from high voltage electricity and up to 300 from lightning injury each year. The incidence of electric injury is unknown, but the percentage of patients with high voltage electric injury admitted to burn centers in this country ranges from 0.04 to 6.7 per cent.

PATHOGENESIS. The effects of electricity on tissue depend upon current, voltage, type of current, i.e., direct or alternating and the frequency of the latter, pathway of the current, duration of contact, and environmental conditions. High-tension is arbitrarily defined as voltage above 1000, apparently because the likelihood of sudden death and remote tissue injury is much less with lower voltage. However, any voltage above 40 should be considered potentially dangerous. In general, alternating current is considered more dangerous than direct current, in part because of the tetanic effect of the former, which may "lock" the patient to the source of electricity, and its likelihood of producing cardiac and/or pulmonary arrest. Injurious tissue effects decrease as the frequency of alternating current increases above 60 cycles per second, which is extremely dangerous to the heart and respiratory center. The points of contact and the current pathway through the body are important in determining tissue damage; passage of current through the heart or respiratory center is particularly dangerous. Current flow from a hand to the feet of only 100 ma is capable of producing ventricular fibrillation. The longer the duration of passage of the electric current, the greater will be the tissue damage, emphasizing the need for rapid separation of the victim from the source of electricity. Environmental conditions influence the resistance at the point of contact; dry thickened palmar skin is more resistant to the passage of current than is similar thickness skin when moistened by perspiration or other liquid.

In high voltage electric injury, heat is the principal mediator of tissue damage, and such damage is related to both voltage and duration of application. Because all body tissues and fluids are conductive, the body should be considered as a volume conductor. Heat is produced in this conductor as a function of voltage drop and current flow per unit cross-sectional area, i.e., current density. This characteristic accounts for the rarity of major injury to the trunk and the frequency of severe injury to the digits and extremities in high-tension electric injury. The skin is severely injured and chars at the points of contact, where current density is highest. Charring of the skin may also occur from arcing across flexor surfaces of joints, and arcing can also ignite the patient's clothing and thereby produce associated flame burns. Below 1000 volts, when arcing and contact point charring occur, resistance rises rapidly and limits subsequent current passage and tissue heating; in this sense, such electric injury is self-limiting. Above 1000 volts, arcing is intense, and relatively constant levels of current are maintained with an associated marked increase in tissue destruction. The heated tissue cools unevenly, the superficial portions cooling more rapidly than the deeper portions. Since tissue injury caused by thermal energy depends upon both temperature and duration of exposure, the deeper tissues are more liable to severe injury. These characteristics of tissue as a volume conductor and a volume radiator influence surgical treatment in patients with high voltage electric injury.

Low voltage direct current may also produce tissue damage, and focal injury has occurred at the contact sites of ground plates used with electrosurgical devices. Prolonged application of direct current of as little as 3 volts to such grounding plates can cause tissue injury either directly or as a result of electrolysis of the conductive materials used to ensure contact of the grounding plates and the skin surface.

CLINICAL MANIFESTATIONS. Cardiopulmonary arrest is relatively common in patients who have sustained high voltage electric injuries. Cardiac arrhythmias may occur after resuscitation and persist for a variable period thereafter or develop as late as 24 to 48 hours post-injury. The risk of renal failure is also great in patients with electric injury for two reasons. First, the extent of deep tissue injury may not be appreciated, which leads to underestimation of fluid needs, inadequate resuscitation, and oliguria. Second, the deep tissue injury may liberate myoglobin, which may precipitate in the renal tubules unless a brisk urinary output is maintained. Hyperkalemia may also occur as a result of extensive tissue destruction and reach sufficient levels to interfere with cardiac function.

The effects of electric injury on the deep tissues of a limb may produce sufficient edema beneath the investing fascia of an involved muscle compartment to impair nutrient blood flow and to reduce flow to distal unburned tissue, requiring fasciotomy to relieve pressure and restore circulation.

BURNS OF THE ORAL COMMISSURE IN CHILDREN. Burns of the oral commissure are frequently sustained by children, usually less than three years of age, as a consequence of sucking on the end of a live extension cord or biting the cord of a light or small appliance. Although these burns often have the pearly white appearance of an avascular full thickness burn and initially appear to be significantly deforming, most heal with minimal cosmetic defects when treated conservatively with periodic debridement of only nonviable tissue. Following spontaneous healing, residual functional or cosmetic defects can be repaired electively.

REMOTE ORGAN INJURY. Instances of intestinal perforation, focal pancreatic necrosis, focal gallbladder necrosis, and direct liver injury have been reported, but are uncommon.

Deficits of cerebral, cerebellar, spinal cord, and peripheral nerve function may be evident immediately following electric injury or may be delayed in onset. In all patients with high voltage electric injury, a thorough neurologic examination must be performed on admission and at scheduled intervals thereafter, and any nerve deficits must be fully documented. Return of function following direct nerve damage is uncommon. In general, immediate and early deficits involving nerves not directly injured (motor nerves appear to be more sensitive to current injury than sensory nerves) show spontaneous resolution. Late appearing peripheral nerve deficits may be part of a polyneuritic syndrome involving nerves far removed from the points of electric contact. The immediate symptoms of spinal cord injury are considered to result from direct neuronal insult and are more often transient than are those of later onset, which are more apt to be permanent. Spinal cord deficits of delayed onset may take the form of quadriplegia, hemiplegia, or localized nerve deficits with signs of ascending paralysis, transverse myelitis, or an amyotrophic-lateral-sclerosis-like syndrome.

Delayed hemorrhage from moderate to large-sized blood vessels has occurred in many patients with high voltage electric injury and is ascribed by some to "arteritis" caused by electric injury per se. It has been our experience that such hemorrhage has occurred only when debridement has been inadequate or when the vessel wall underwent desiccation and necrosis secondary to exposure following debridement.

Fractures of long bones may result from falls following the electric shock, and compression fractures of vertebral bodies may result from tetanic contractions of the paraspinous muscles. Both types of fractures should be ruled out by indicated roentgenograms.

The opinions or assertions contained herein are the private views of the author and are not to be construed as official or as reflecting the views of the Department of the Army or the Department of Defense.

DELAYED ORGAN DAMAGE. Recurrent gastrointestinal dysfunction has been reported within 12 to 18 months following high voltage electric injury in up to three fourths of such patients. Cataracts are common sequelae of high voltage electric injury and are most frequent in patients in whom the contact point has been on the head or neck. The formation of such cataracts may be quite rapid or may occur three or more years following high voltage electric injury.

TREATMENT. Cardiopulmonary resuscitation must be begun immediately in any patient with cardiopulmonary arrest following electric injury. All patients who have sustained high voltage electric injury should undergo continuous electrocardiographic (ECG) monitoring for at least 48 hours beyond the last ECG evidence of dysrhythmia, if such occurs. In those patients with high urinary hemochromogen concentrations, an hourly urinary output of 75 to 100 ml should be maintained. If the patient remains oliguric despite the administration of more than the estimated fluid resuscitation needs or the hemochromogens do not clear promptly, 12.5 grams of mannitol should be added to each liter of intravenous fluid given until the pigment has cleared from the urine. Hyperkalemia should be treated by administration of hypertonic glucose, insulin, calcium salts, ion exchange resins, or hemodialysis, depending upon its severity (Ch. 76).

The clinical indications for fasciotomy and surgical exploration of a limb include stony hardness of a muscle compartment to palpation, cyanosis of distal unburned skin, impaired capillary refilling of distal unburned skin or nails, and absent or diminished pulsatile flow in distal arteries on ultrasonic flowmeter examination. If large vessel pulses are intact but significant deep tissue injury is otherwise indicated by clinical signs, arteriography is helpful in determining the need for operation. Arteriographic evidence of large vessel thrombosis merely confirms clinical findings, but luminal irregularity, "beading," or narrowing may be identified in severely injured vessels that will subsequently be occluded by thrombosis, when the arteriogram is performed early following injury. Moreover, "pruning" (a decrease in the density of muscular nutrient arteries in a limb) helps define the level of amputation needed to remove muscle that has sustained inapparent but irreversible damage. ^{133}Xenon wash-out studies have also been used to assess the need for amputation. Muscle flow of less than 1 ml per minute per 100 grams of tissue has been proposed as the level below which amputation is required. An intramuscular compartment pressure of greater than 30 mm Hg, as measured by a wick-type catheter, has also been used as an indication for the need of immediate post-injury wound decompression. Technetium-99m pyrophosphate scintigraphy performed within 24 hours following injury has been suggested as a means to determine the extent of muscle damage, i.e., frankly necrotic tissue showed no perfusion and uninjured tissue showed normal perfusion, while areas of increased uptake of the radioactive material showed variable degrees of partial necrosis requiring operative exposure and debridement of a variable amount of tissue. Since repeated debridement was often required in patients in whom the scintigraphic findings of partial necrosis were present, the clinical reliability, accuracy, and usefulness of that diagnostic method remain uncertain.

Tissue damaged by high voltage electric injury should be explored as soon as the patient is hemodynamically stable. The viability of vital structures and deep muscle is assessed, with necrotic tissue debrided to reduce the risk of infection and eliminate a source of hyperkalemia. Extensive muscle necrosis and destruction of vital structures, such as nerves, tendons, and vessels, speak for amputation at a level proximal to the area of tissue death. Operative wounds following debridement or amputation are left open, and the patient is rescheduled for exploration of the wounds 24 to 72 hours later, at which time further debridement of any residual necrotic tissue is carried out. If no, or only minimal, debridement is required, the amputation wound can be closed by a sausage type of delayed primary closure.

Vascularized free muscle flaps may be used for immediate coverage of deep electric injuries in which the tissues exposed following debridement, e.g., bone or tendon, do not have sufficient blood supply to support a skin graft.

In those patients in whom electric injury is confined to the skin and subcutaneous tissue, bacterial control is best achieved by the use of Sulfamylon burn cream, the active ingredient of which (mafenide acetate) can diffuse into the nonviable tissue to exert its antimicrobial action.

LIGHTNING INJURY. A lightning bolt may have a voltage in the neighborhood of 1 billion volts and induce currents ranging from 12,000 to 200,000 amperes. Its duration is characteristically brief, ranging from one hundredth to one thousandth of a second. The temperature in a lightning bolt may be as high as 30,000° K, but dissipates in a few microseconds. Cardiopulmonary arrest is common in patients struck by lightning and may be secondary to either asystole or fibrillation. Immediate cardiopulmonary resuscitation is life-saving in such patients, and persistent or recurrent ECG abnormalities are rare, although later signs of acute myocardial damage have been reported. Recovery of lightning-struck patients who have apparently been without signs of life for 15 or more minutes speaks for the immediate institution of cardiopulmonary resuscitation. Coma and neurologic deficits are common immediately after injury, but may resolve in a matter of hours. Myoglobinuria, although infrequent, is treated as described previously. The cutaneous burns are characteristically superficial and present a "splashed-on" appearance of arborescent and spidery character. Signs of vasoconstriction and mottling of the skin, previously considered characteristic of lightning injury, typically relent with adequate resuscitation. Prompt treatment of the sequelae of lightning injury, including immediate cardiopulmonary resuscitation, has significantly decreased the mortality associated with this injury, and two thirds of lightning-injured patients now survive.

Apfelberg DB, Masters FW, Robinson DW: Pathophysiology and treatment of lightning injuries. J Trauma 14:453, 1974. *Four cases of lightning injury are discussed with the clinical manifestations of this injury related to the pathophysiologic changes caused by lightning.*

Holliman CJ, Saffle JR, Kravits M, Warden GD: Early surgical decompression in the management of electrical injuries. Am J Surg 144:733, 1982. *The management of electric burns of the extremities is detailed, and the use of radionuclide scanning in assessing extent of muscle injury is described.*

Hunt JL, Mason AD Jr, Masterson TS, Pruitt BA Jr: The pathophysiology of acute electric injuries. J Trauma 16:335, 1976. *The experimental studies reported confirm that an electric injury is simply a thermal burn. The fact that tissue acts as a volume conductor is identified, as is the self-limiting nature of electric injury.*

Levine NS, Atkins A, McKell DW Jr, Peck SD, Pruitt BA Jr: Spinal cord injury following electric accidents; case reports. J Trauma 15:459, 1975. *Report of two patients with spinal cord injury following electric injury with a review of the spectrum and natural history of the neurologic sequelae of high voltage injury.*

Pruitt BA Jr: The burn patient: I. Initial care. *In* Ravitch MM (ed.): Current Problems in Surgery. Chicago, Year Book Medical Publishers, 1979, pp 43–52. *A thorough description of techniques of diagnosis and treatment of high voltage electric injury.*

Sances A Jr, Myklebust JB, Larson SJ, Darin JC, Swiontek T, Prieto T, Chilbert M, Cusick JF: Experimental electrical injury studies. J Trauma 21:589, 1981. *Experimental studies of electric injury relate tissue damage to voltage, current flow, and tissue characteristics, including cross-sectional area.*

564. DISORDERS DUE TO HEAT AND COLD

James P. Knochel

To maintain a normal body temperature requires that heat gain equal heat loss. Heat is produced by metabolism or gained from the environment. Thermoregulation is heavily dependent upon blood flow to cutaneous vessels. Cutaneous flow is regulated by hypothalamic centers. Vasoconstriction reduces and vasodilatation increases delivery of heated blood to the skin. Heat is exchanged between the skin and the environment by radiation, conduction, or convection. If heat loss is inadequate by these means, active sweating begins, and cooling occurs by vaporization of sweat. If heat gain is necessary, metabolic heat production rises by a voluntary increase of physical activity or involuntarily by shivering. Body heat thus produced is retained by cutaneous vasoconstriction. *Acclimatization,* a term defining critical cardiovascular, endocrine, exocrine, and other physiologic adaptations to heat stress, requires one to two weeks to develop. Such adaptations permit one to work comfortably and safely under conditions of heat stress that were previously intolerable.

DISORDERS DUE TO HEAT

HEAT CRAMPS. Workers who sweat profusely and replace sweat losses with water but inadequate salt may experience excruciating muscle cramps. They are more common in acclimatized and physically fit men whose bodies are able to produce voluminous quantities of sweat. The cramps tend to occur in muscles used while working and often do not appear until the person relaxes after work. Cooling the muscles during a cold shower is likely to bring on an attack. Cramps in the abdominal wall may suggest a perforated viscus. Mild hyponatremia is a consistent finding. Severe cramps may cause rhabdomyolysis and modest serum elevations of muscle enzymes (creatine phosphokinase). Salted liquids taken orally or saline given intravenously leads to rapid improvement. Heat cramps are preventable by replacement of sweat with a solution containing about 2.5 grams (one-half teaspoon) NaCl per liter of water, or merely by increasing dietary salt intake.

HEAT EXHAUSTION. Heat exhaustion is a common disorder that occurs after sustained heat stress of three or more days. Its cause is water or salt depletion or both.

Primary water loss heat exhaustion is particularly dangerous since it increases the risk of heat stroke. This form is seen most often in the elderly, infirm, obtunded, or very young who are unable to communicate their thirst. It is also seen in active persons who take salt supplements without adequate water. Deliberate efforts should be made to ensure water intake by patients in nursing homes where summertime room temperatures are often too high to prevent progressive, subtle dehydration. Symptoms of heat exhaustion resulting from predominant water loss include intense thirst, fatigue, weakness, anxiety, and impaired judgment. Signs may include dehydration, hyperventilation, paresthesias, tetany, agitation, hysteria, muscular incoordination, and psychotic behavior. Body temperature may rise to 38.9°C. Delirium, rising temperature, coma, and frank heatstroke may occur in advanced cases. Laboratory findings include hemoconcentration, hypernatremia, and oliguria.

Salt depletion heat exhaustion occurs mainly in unacclimatized persons in whom losses of thermal sweat are replaced with water but not adequate salt. Dehydration, weight loss, and thirst are absent in the pure form. Sweating and urinary output remain normal. Prominent symptoms include profound weakness, fatigue, severe headache, giddiness, and muscle cramps. In some patients, anorexia, myalgia, nausea, vomiting, and diarrhea may masquerade as a viral illness. Such patients appear haggard, with pale, clammy skin. Hypotension and tachycardia are common. Fever is notably absent.

Treatment of heat exhaustion should be individualized, depending upon symptoms and findings. Since kidney function is usually normal, most patients can be treated with lightly salted fluids, rest, and elimination of heat stress. Hypernatremic dehydration should be treated with isotonic dextrose at a rate sufficient to reduce serum sodium about 2 mEq per liter per hour. It is seldom necessary to administer hypertonic salt solutions to patients with hyponatremic heat exhaustion.

HEATSTROKE. Heatstroke is a catastrophic illness requiring immediate treatment for survival. It is convenient to subclassify heatstroke into two forms, classic and exertional.

Classic heatstroke occurs especially in the poor, the elderly, the chronically ill, alcoholics, patients with advanced heart disease, and the obese. Hot, humid weather of three or more days' duration usually precedes epidemics of this disorder. Deaths due to myocardial infarction and congestive heart failure in patients with cardiovascular disease increase sharply during heat waves because of increased demands placed upon the heart by heat stress. Certain medications also increase the propensity to develop heatstroke. These include drugs that depress sweating (anticholinergics, beta blockers, antihistamines), diuretics, and drugs that may increase heat production (amphetamines, neuroleptics). Rarely, patients with classic heatstroke may recall a prodrome resembling heat exhaustion or cessation of sweating. Once sweating stops, body temperature mounts and collapse soon follows. Typical findings include profound central nervous system dysfunction, especially coma or bizarre behavior; hot, dry, flushed skin; and hyperpyrexia. Rectal temperature exceeds 40.6°C and may reach 44°C or more. Hypotension is common. It is probably due to redistribution of blood from the central to the peripheral circulation since it often responds to cooling alone. Convulsive seizures, fasciculations, and muscle rigidity are absent until active cooling is under way.

Exertional heatstroke is more likely to develop in laborers, farmers, military recruits, football players, long distance runners, and those who work in boiler rooms or foundries. They display physical findings in the acute phase similar to those of patients with classic heatstroke, with one common exception: About half of these patients continue to sweat. If this occurs, the skin may be deceptively cool despite a high core temperature.

Other major differences between classic and exertional heatstroke become apparent from laboratory measurements. In the classic form, respiratory alkalosis is usual, and circulatory collapse may cause modest increases of lactate, a particularly ominous sign. In contrast, *lactic acidosis* is the rule in exertional heatstroke, may exceed 20 mmol per liter, and is not a foreboding finding in this condition. Although serum creatine phosphokinase activities may be slightly increased in classic heatstroke (usually not greater than 1000 to 2000 IU per liter), clinically important rhabdomyolysis is exceptionally rare unless heatstroke occurs in an individual who has a pre-existing myopathy, such as a chronic alcoholic. Major *rhabdomyolysis* and its associated complications such as hyperkalemia, hyperphosphatemia, hypocalcemia out of proportion to hypoalbuminemia, hyperuricemia, and myoglobinuria are almost invariable findings in exertional heatstroke. Both forms of heatstroke may be complicated by *hemorrhage* (resulting from *disseminated intravascular coagulation,* fibrinolysis, clotting factor deficiency due to hepatic injury, or *thrombocytopenia* due to bone marrow injury); *jaundice; acute renal failure; pancreatitis; brain damage; peripheral neuropathy; myocardial necrosis and arrhythmias;* and pulmonary capillary damage with *adult respiratory distress syndrome.* Hypokalemia in heatstroke usually results from respiratory alkalosis, but it may represent potassium deficiency in those who have performed hard work in the heat for one or two weeks. Hypoglycemia may also occur.

Treatment of heatstroke depends upon anticipation, prompt recognition, and rapid cooling. The importance of educating paramedical personnel, nurses, athletes, coaches, and trainers to prevent, accurately recognize, and initiate immediate cooling cannot be overestimated. Common mistakes include administration of fluids to comatose patients or delay of cooling.

Proper emergency management includes removal from direct sunlight, removal of clothing, wetting the body surface, and fanning to move air and thereby promote vaporization. When such simple measures are undertaken on the spot, some victims awaken. Most require aggressive cooling in the hospital. A thermistor probe temperature device should be inserted high in the rectum to ensure recording of core temperature.

Conventional cooling techniques include immersion in ice water while the skin is rubbed briskly or placing the patient on a stretcher, rubbing the skin with ice bags while keeping the skin wet, and moving air over the skin to promote vaporization of the water. Rapid cooling by ice water immersion may cause cutaneous vasoconstriction, shivering, and convulsions. Current experimental studies suggest that immersion in cool water (11°C) may facilitate cooling with equal speed by avoiding cutaneous vasoconstriction.

Hypotension often responds to cooling alone, but if it persists, 0.5 liter of normal saline should be infused. If additional quantities are necessary, one must guard against circulatory congestion. Hypotension not responding to such quantities of saline suggests myocardial injury or serious rhabdomyolysis, and vasopressor support may be necessary. The stomach should be emptied, since vomiting and aspiration often occur during cooling. Cooling should be stopped when core temperature reaches 39°C to avoid progressive hypothermia.

Steroids are unnecessary. Hypokalemia and hypophosphatemia are very common in the acute phase but usually resolve quickly without treatment. Glucose may be necessary for hypoglycemia. Although lactic acidosis usually responds to volume expansion, if it persists in the absence of hypotension, 44 to 88 mEq of $NaHCO_3$ may be helpful. Other complications described earlier should be anticipated, and appropriate measures taken as necessary.

MALIGNANT HYPERTHERMIA. This rare but serious disorder, representing an idiosyncratic reaction to general anesthesia, is discussed in Ch. 538.

MINOR DISORDERS RELATED TO HEAT STRESS. *Heat edema* is a transient, benign disorder that occurs during initial exposure to hot weather. It appears to result from aldosterone-mediated salt and water retention (a physiologic adaptation) and usually disappears spontaneously with continued heat exposure. It seldom, if ever, requires treatment. Diuretics should not be administered. *Miliaria* (heat rash) is caused by sweat gland occlusion. Its medical importance is enhanced, since it may impair sweat formation and evaporative heat loss.

Heat syncope occurs when a healthy person squats for a minute and then suddenly stands, upon which a sensation of transient dizziness or visual blurring may occur. Such symptoms are exaggerated by salt and water losses induced by sweating and by heat-induced vasodilatation of the superficial blood vessels and may cause syncope in an individual unacclimatized to heat. When acclimatization occurs, the associated retention of salt and water corrects the problem. Besides syncope, findings usually include slight tachycardia and moist skin. Fever is absent. Recovery occurs rapidly if the patient is allowed to remain supine. Removal from the heat and administration of lightly salted liquids are helpful.

Hart GR, Anderson RJ, Crumpler CP, Shlkin A, Reed G, Knochel JP: Epidemic classical heat stroke: Clinical characteristics and course of 28 patients. Medicine 61:189–197, 1982. *A detailed presentation of classic heatstroke, emphasizing the important roles of medications that impair heat loss and pre-existent disease in its pathogenesis. It also presents a detailed analysis of laboratory abnormalities commonly observed in this illness.*

Jones TS, Liang AP, Kilbourne EM, et al.: Morbidity and mortality associated with the July 1980 heat wave in St. Louis and Kansas City, Mo. JAMA 247:3327–3331, 1982. *A report illustrating increased death rates during heat waves.*

Knochel JP: Environmental heat illness. Arch Intern Med 133:841–864, 1974. *A general review of heat stress injuries and description of exertional heatstroke.*

Knochel JP, Reed G: Disorders of heat regulation. *In* Maxwell MH, Kleeman CR, Narins RG (eds.): Clinical Disorders of Fluid and Electrolyte Metabolism. 4th ed. New York. McGraw-Hill Book Company. In press. *A review of environmental heat illness, pharmacologic and endocrine hyperthermia, malignant hyperthermia, and hypothermic disorders.*

HYPOTHERMIA

Hypothermia, defined as a core temperature of less than 35°C, is a medical emergency that occurs in both temperate and cold environments. Its prompt recognition is critical to avoid serious morbidity or death. When body temperature declines, heat production increases by shivering, and heat loss is reduced by decreasing cutaneous blood flow. Reduction of core temperature decreases the rate of chemical reactions so that cooling proceeds until a new equilibrium is established between the body and its environment.

TABLE 564–1. CAUSES OF HYPOTHERMIA

Exposure plus:
I. Central nervous system disease
Brain tumor, injury, seizure
Cord transection
Hypoglycemia
Thiamin deficiency
Uremia
Hepatic failure
II. Interference with vasoconstriction
Drugs
Alcohol
Phenothiazines
Sepsis
Erythroderma
III. Interference with muscle movement
Paralysis, paresis
Extremes of age
Drugs
Alcohol
Phenothiazines
Hypothyroidism
IV. Mixed causes
Starvation
Adrenal insufficiency
Hypothyroidism
Hypopituitarism

From Fitzgerald FT, Jessop C: Accidental hypothermia: A report of 22 cases and review of the literature. Adv Intern Med 27:127, 1982. Reprinted with permission.

As hypothermia develops, cerebral blood flow declines. The resulting fall in nutrient availability is offset by a reduction in brain metabolism. This fall in metabolic demand permits successful cerebral resuscitation of hypothermic patients even after prolonged periods of anoxia and circulatory arrest.

PATHOGENESIS. The causes of hypothermia seen in clinical practice are summarized in Table 564–1. Advanced age, disorders causing hypometabolism, central nervous system disease, malnutrition, a variety of drugs, and exposure commonly cause hypothermia. In elderly persons, hypothermia, hyperventilation, hypotension, and thrombocytopenia are common signs of bacteremia and sepsis.

CLINICAL MANIFESTATIONS. A decline in mental status, ataxia, tremulous speech, and hyperreflexia appear as temperature falls to about 32°C. At lower temperatures, hyporeflexia, stupor, dysarthria, and sluggish pupillary responses appear. Shivering usually stops below 32°C. Muscle rigidity becomes prominent. Established hypothermia reduces heart rate, blood pressure, peripheral vascular resistance, cardiac output, and central venous presure. Creatine phosphokinase (MB isoenzyme) may increase with severe hypothermia without evidence of myocardial infarction, suggesting myocardial cellular damage. Cardiac arrhythmias are very common. Atrial arrhythmias are usually benign. Ventricular ectopic beats may herald ventricular fibrillation, an imminent danger if core temperature becomes less than 28°C. Stimulation, such as urethral catheterization, movement, endotracheal intubation, and vascular catheterization, also predisposes to the development of this arrhythmia. Osborn waves, characterized by a widening of the base of the QRS complex and J point deflection, are the most characteristic ECG findings. They can be seen with hypothermia from any cause and do not herald the onset of ventricular fibrillation. Early tachypnea and respiratory alkalosis are replaced by progressive hypoventilation. Advancing hypothermia leads to carbon dioxide retention and respiratory acidosis. Shivering increases lactic acid production and hypoxia in muscles and may cause severe lactic acidosis.

In early hypothermia, hypokalemia may be caused by respiratory alkalosis. Additional cooling corrects hypokalemia by reducing sodium-potassium transport. During therapeutic rewarming, sodium-potassium exchange accelerates, such that hypokalemia may become important and contribute to arrhythmias. Hypophosphatemia may also occur during the recovery phase of hypothermia.

TREATMENT. Significant hypothermia is a medical emergency. When it is suspected, an estimate of core temperature should be obtained, by inserting a thermistor probe high into the rectum. Esophageal temperature probes are difficult to place properly and may precipitate ventricular arrhythmias or fibrillation.

Airway patency must be insured in comatose patients and steps taken to prevent aspiration of gastric contents. A large intravenous catheter should be inserted, and thiamin and glucose given immediately in appropriate situations. Stimulation of the patient should be minimized to avoid precipitating ventricular fibrillation. Blood pressure, pulse, temperature, electrocardiogram, neurologic status, and urine output should be monitored frequently during rewarming.

A warming rate of about 0.5°C per hour is generally accepted as optimal. Most shivering patients will spontaneously rewarm at a rate equal to or greater than this. *Passive* rewarming and blankets for hemodynamically stable, moderately hypothermic patients is ideal. This method will allow a rise of 0.5 to 1°C per hour if the initial core temperature is greater than about 27°C. It is especially effective in patients with acute hypothermia without underlying disease. *Active* rewarming becomes necessary in patients with severe hypothermia or cardiopulmonary arrest or both. This is especially important in patients with ventricular fibrillation or asystole because the hypothermic myocardium is resistant to mechanical or pharmacologic intervention until temperatures are above 28°C to 30°C.

"Rewarming shock" and accentuated lactic acidosis have been most commonly encountered with active external rewarming techniques, i.e., heat applied to the surface of the body with hot water bottles or immersion in warm water. To avoid these problems, rapid rewarming of core blood has been attempted by several means in patients with severe hypothermia or cardiac arrest. Most patients with hypothermia will tolerate warm intravenous fluids and heated oxygen. If rapid rewarming is required, peritoneal lavage with solutions warmed to about 40°C is effective.

Supportive measures may be very important. Because of the wide diversity of electrolyte derangements in hypothermic patients, no general recommendations can be made regarding fluid management other than warming the fluid to 37 to 40°C before administration. Plasma volume expanders may be given if the central venous pressure is low. Oxygen and bicarbonate should be given if serious metabolic acidosis exists. Subsequent metabolic alkalosis and its adverse effects on oxyhemoglobin dissociation, calcium, and ventricular irritability must be avoided. As patients are rewarmed, metabolic acidosis may worsen as lactate is washed out of previously hypoxic tissues. Recognition and treatment of this phenomenon are important to reduce the risk of ventricular fibrillation and cardiovascular collapse. Severe respiratory impairment with significant carbon dioxide retention should be treated with assisted ventilation. Ventilatory adjustments should be made with respect to reduced carbon dioxide production. Hypoglycemia should be suspected in any patient with hypothermia. Hyperglycemia should be treated only if severe and potentially life threatening. Vasopressors should be avoided if possible because of their ability to induce ventricular arrhythmias. Drugs with significant myocardial depressing effects such as quinidine and propranolol should be avoided. Thyroxine should be given only if significant hypothyroidism is suspected.

Fitzgerald FR, Jessop C: Accidental hypothermia: A report of 22 cases and review of the literature. Adv Intern Med 27:127, 1982. Reuler JB: Hypothermia: Pathophysiology, clinical settings, and management. Ann Intern Med 89:519, 1978. *These two articles are excellent clinical reviews of hypothermia as seen in medical practice, with discussions of differential diagnosis, clinical manifestations, and treatment.*

Wong KC: Physiology and pharmacology of hypothermia. West J Med 138:227, 1983. *This is a recent general overview of the physiologic consequences of hypothermia, with 74 references.*

565. TRACE METAL POISONING

Donald B. Louria

Many trace elements, both metals and nonmetals, are capable of causing human disease. In some cases poisoning is a consequence of workplace exposure. In others the disease results from use of prescription or nonprescription medicines or as an adverse effect of medical procedures such as hemodialysis or insertion of prosthetic devices. Occasionally trace element poisoning results from attempts at suicide or homicide. Increasingly the source of poisoning is the food we eat, the liquids we drink, or the air we breathe; some soil or water has naturally high concentrations of potential toxins such as arsenic, but more often the environmental contamination is man made.

Over the past few decades, increased awareness of the health consequences of industrial substances, more stringent federal and state regulations, and fear of lawsuits have resulted in a healthier workplace. On the other hand, technologic advances have increased the use of trace elements, often with inadequate safety precautions until adverse effects are recognized. Furthermore, the majority of the potentially exposed work force is employed by small industries that may not have plant physicians or insist on proper worker protection.

We know a great deal about overwhelming exposure that results in acute illness, but our knowledge of the subtle consequences of chronic, low level trace element exposure is still grossly inadequate. This is well illustrated by lead exposure. Acute lead poisoning in children or adults is readily diagnosed, but we are only beginning to understand the consequences of increased body lead burdens in the absence of the anemia, colic, or clinically apparent encephalopathy.

The interrelationships between and among trace elements are also poorly understood. For example, copper smelter workers are exposed not only to copper but also to lead, zinc, arsenic, gold, silver, cadmium, and mercury; in these workers pneumonitis or other acute illnesses may result from two or more metals acting in concert. In other instances excesses or deficits of a trace element may act indirectly by inducing deficiency or toxicity of another trace element.

LEAD

ETIOLOGY. In the past lead poisoning was ascribed to pica (abnormal ingestion) among children living in dilapidated houses with peeling layers of lead-based paints. In the last two decades lead intoxication has occurred with increasing frequency in less socioeconomically deprived areas of the cities, as well as in more affluent suburbs. This may in part be related to environmental contamination from leaded gasoline; several studies relate environmental lead contamination to traffic density patterns. Contaminated soil is also a well-described source of lead.

In the United States, hundreds of occupations entail potentially significant exposure. Lead and other metal smelter workers or miners, welders, storage battery workers, and pottery makers are particularly heavily exposed. Workers in auto manufacturing, ship building, paint manufacture, and printing industries are also at substantial risk.

Lead-soldered kettles and cans and lead-glazed pottery can release lead when acidic fluids are stored or cooked in them. Demolition workers and those employed in firing ranges have become poisoned from intensive aerosol exposure. The concentration of lead in printing inks is significant; poisoning even occurred after repeated burning of newspapers and magazines in a fireplace. In the southern United States, moonshine whiskey is an important cause of poisoning. The stills are connected with lead solder, and old lead-containing radiators are used as condensers; 20 to 90 per cent of moonshine samples contain lead in the potentially toxic range.

In past centuries lead was added to wine to sweeten it, a deception that was eventually made punishable by death; recently, addition of lead to aphrodisiacs and various herbal and folk medicines has resulted in poisoning. Retained bullets can result in lead poisoning, especially if host metabolic changes favor lead mobilization or if a joint is involved, since synovial fluid appears to be a good solvent for lead.

Gasoline sniffing for hedonistic purposes can produce lead poisoning; the organic tetraethyl lead appears to have a proclivity for the nervous system.

In a sense we are all lead poisoned; prior to the industrial revolution the total body burden of lead was about 2 mg, whereas currently in industrialized societies the whole body content is about 200 mg. One hundred and fifty to 250 μg per day is ingested, 5 to 10 per cent of which is absorbed; in children the percentage is higher and absorption is facilitated by iron, calcium, magnesium, and perhaps zinc deficiency. Aerosol exposure is especially likely to result in poisoning, since approximately 40 per cent of inhaled lead is absorbed.

CLINICAL MANIFESTATIONS. The major toxic effects of lead are referable to the abdomen, the blood, and the nervous system.

Gastrointestinal Tract. The exact pathogenesis of lead colic remains uncertain; in part it appears to be due to a direct effect of lead on smooth muscle. The crampy, diffuse, often intractable abdominal pain may be accompanied by nausea, vomiting, anorexia, constipation, or occasionally diarrhea. The pain may be confined to the epigastric, periumbilical, or other areas of the abdomen and may simulate a variety of surgical and nonsurgical diseases. Lead-induced megacolon has been reported.

Blood. Lead interferes with a variety of red cell enzyme systems, including delta-aminolevulinic acid dehydratase and ferrochelatase. The former is needed for the conjugation of levulinic acid to form porphobilinogen; the latter facilitates the incorporation of iron into protoporphyrin IX (see Fig. 134–3). The red cell abnormalities include punctate basophilic stippling and clover leaf morphology. Anemia is frequent and may be normocytic normochromic, owing to decreased red cell life span, or microcytic hypochromic.

Nervous System. Either the brain or peripheral nerves may be involved. The CNS symptoms at first are vague and are often mistakenly disregarded; these manifestations include irritability, incoordination, memory lapses, labile affect, sleep disturbances, restlessness, listlessness, paranoia, headache, lethargy, and dizziness. In more serious cases manifestations include syncopal-like attacks, disorientation, flaccidity, more intense headache, severe mental impairment, ataxia, vomiting, cranial nerve palsies, localized neurologic signs, psychosis, somnolence, seizures, blindness, and coma. Severe lead encephalopathy is not restricted to children. Occasionally the brain manifestations mimic a space-occupying lesion. The cerebrospinal fluid may show an increased protein content, a modest pleocytosis (predominantly lymphocytic), and rarely diminished glucose levels. Papilledema has been reported, as have grayish deposits surrounding the optic disc and optic atrophy. Frank encephalopathy is an ominous prognostic sign in regard to both mortality and persistent brain damage. Most children who experience two or more bouts of clinically evident encephalopathy have neurologic residua.

The peripheral nerve involvement, seen more often in adults than in children, is almost always exclusively motor and involves muscle groups used extensively. Wrist drop and foot drop are seen most often; the former, depending on type of occupation, may be asymmetrical and there may be paresthesias.

The spinal cord may also be involved, manifestations having some similarity to those of amyotrophic lateral sclerosis.

Tetraethyl lead poisoning causes euphoria, nervousness, insomnia, hallucinations, convulsions, and sometimes frank psychosis.

The question of subtle brain damage in the absence of clinical evidence of encephalopathy remains controversial. Some studies suggest that inordinate body burdens of lead may result in mentation difficulties, emotional lability, intelligence and memory deficits, impaired psychomotor function, and behavioral aberrations in both children and adults, even in the absence of overt evidence of poisoning.

Other Clinical Manifestations. In adults the kidneys are often involved (see Ch. 81.3), the characteristic lesion being interstitial nephritis; as the disease progresses, glomerular filtration rate falls. In children, Fanconi's syndrome, characterized by glycosuria, aminoaciduria, and phosphaturia, may occur transiently; and occasionally, asymptomatic renal failure supervenes. Lead poisoning appears to be responsible for some cases of renal failure associated with either gout or hypertension.

Occasionally arrhythmias and cardiomegaly have been reported as have abnormalities of liver function. A gingival blue, blue-black, or gray line is found in up to 20 per cent of adult patients but is infrequent in children.

Lead readily crosses the placenta and is thought to be responsible for an increased incidence of spontaneous abortion and miscarriage. Some studies suggest lead poisoning may result in hypospermia and other sperm abnormalities. Teratogenic effects occur in lead-treated animals, but congenital abnormalities have not been convincingly documented in man. Lead exposure may also result in transient chromosomal breakage.

DIAGNOSIS. The interference with delta-aminolevulinic acid dehydratase results in marked increase in delta-aminolevulinic acid in the urine. Urinary coproporphyrin levels are also increased. Lead interferes with incorporation of iron into heme and zinc then replaces the iron to form zinc protoporphyrin (ZPP). The latter or its hydrolysis product erythrocyte protoporphyrin (EP) can be measured rapidly fluorometrically; both EP and ZPP are reliable indicators of lead poisoning. False-positive EP and ZPP elevations occur in patients suffering from iron deficiency anemia or erythropoietic protoporphyria. Table 565–1 lists some indications of undue lead absorption.

Blood aminolevulinic acid dehydratase activity can also be measured directly. Blood lead levels are readily determined by atomic absorption spectrophotometry or anodic stripping voltometry; specimens can be obtained by either venipuncture or finger stick; the latter technique suffers from low specificity because of skin contamination. Urine lead concentrations can also be measured; if concentrations are normal, increased body burdens can still be detected by measuring urinary lead excretion after administration of calcium disodium edetate (Table 565–2). In children a blood level of 60 μg per deciliter or greater is considered evidence of definite lead poisoning; and concentrations of 30 μg per deciliter or greater, evidence of excessive absorption. For adults, who show less enzyme inhibition at a given blood lead concentration, the permissible industrial concentration is currently up to 50 μg per deciliter.

Additional industrial exposure should probably not be permitted if blood levels exceed 50 μg per deciliter or if there is any increase in EP or ZPP.

TREATMENT. Three agents are used that form tight complexes with lead and thus promote its elimination from tissues (Table

TABLE 565–1. POSITIVE SCREENING TESTS INDICATING UNDUE LEAD ABSORPTION

Whole blood lead	Children	> 30 μg/dl
	Adults	> 40 μg/dl
Whole blood erythrocyte protoporphyrin or zinc protoporphyrin	Children	> 50 μg/dl
	Adults	> 70 μg/dl
Urine delta-aminolevulinic acid		> 3 mg/m²/24 hours
Reduction in erythrocyte delta-aminolevulinic acid dehydratase activity		< 15–20% of normal activity

TABLE 565–2. $CaNa_2$ EDTA LEAD MOBILIZATION TEST

	Children	Adults
Normal premobilization test	< 100 µg/day	< 150 µg/day
	Normal	
Post-$CaNa_2$ EDTA 50 mg/kg IM or IV or 500–1000 mg/m^2 (children); or 1 gm IM* × 2, 12 hours apart (adults)	< 1 µg Pb/mg $CaNa_2$ EDTA† administered over 24-hour collection period	< 650 µg/day
	Increased Body Burden	
	> 1 µg Pb/mg $CaNa_2$ EDTA administered	> 1000 µg/day

*Procaine must be used with intramuscular injections.
†EDTA = edetate.

565–3). Dimercaprol (British anti-lewisite, BAL) is given in oil intramuscularly; calcium disodium edetate (calcium versenate) can be given either intramuscularly or intravenously; and D-penicillamine is administered by mouth. Chelation should be undertaken only after careful consideration in those with milder evidences of poisoning, because each of the agents is associated with potentially severe adverse effects. Occasionally chelation may be complicated by acute renal failure. Because most of the body lead is stored in the bones, clinical improvement and reduction in blood lead levels (or reduction in EP or ZPP) may be followed by increases in blood lead concentrations and clinical evidence of repoisoning owing to mobilization of lead from bone. In such cases chelating agents should again be administered.

Treatment is ordinarily successful in extra-CNS disease, but is not predictably effective in patients with encephalopathy. Various degrees of mentation deficits may remain in both children and adults. Among adults the frequency of residual brain deficits is not clearly established.

Batuman V, Landy E, Maesaka JK, Wideen RP: Contribution of lead to hypertension with renal impairment. N Engl J Med 309:17, 1983.

Batuman V, Maesaka JK, Haddad B, et al: The role of lead in gout nephropathy. N Engl J Med 304:520, 1981. *These two articles present reasonably compelling evidence that renal dysfunction associated with either hypertension or gout may be related to lead intoxication in a small but important percentage of such cases.*

Browder AA, Joselow MM, Louria DB: The problem of lead poisoning. Medicine 52:121, 1973. *A thorough review with 150 references.*

Chisholm JJ Jr, Barltrop D: Recognition and management of children with increased lead absorption. Arch Dis Child 54:249, 1979. *An updated summary of environmental aspects, pathogenesis, and treatment of lead poisoning.*

Needleman HL, Gunnoc C, Leviton A, et al.: Deficits in psychologic and classroom performance of children with elevated dentine lead levels. N Engl J Med 300:689, 1979. *This important, although controversial, article gives substantial support for the notion that subtle lead poisoning can result in significant psychosocial defects. Based on comparison of 58 children with high dentine levels and 100 with low levels.*

Wedeen RP, Maesaka JK, Weiner B, et al.: Occupational lead nephropathy. Am J Med 59:630, 1975. *This meticulous assessment of glomerular and tubular function in six asymptomatic and two symptomatic adults strongly suggests that lead-induced nephropathy in occupationally exposed adults occurs far more frequently than previously recognized.*

Whitfield CL, Ch'ien LT, Whitehead JD: Lead encephalopathy in adults. Am J Med 52:289, 1972. *Twenty-three adults exposed to moonshine developed encephalopathy, manifestations ranging from confusion to coma, seizures, and death. This article emphasizes that encephalopathy can be a major problem in adults. Chelation therapy appeared to be effective.*

TABLE 565–3. CHELATION REGIMENS

	Children*	Adults*	Duration
$CaNa_2$ EDTA	50 mg/kg/day IM† or IV, or 1500 mg/m^2/24 hours (severe disease); 500–1000 mg/m^2/day (mild-moderate intoxication)	1.0 gram IV in 5% dextrose twice daily, or 2.0 grams/day IM in divided doses; longer-term, 1 gram IM 3 × per week† until lead burden reduced to satisfactory levels	Three to five days
BAL	3 mg/kg/dose IM, or 500–1000 mg/m^2/24 hours IM	2.5 mg/kg/dose IM	Two days if with $CaNa_2$ EDTA; three days if used alone
	(Given in divided doses every four hours first day, every six hours thereafter)		
Penicillamine	30 mg/kg/day PO	1.0–1.5 grams/day PO	Until blood lead and FEP‡ levels approach normal

*$CaNa_2$ EDTA and BAL are used together for severe illness.
†Procaine must be used for IM injections of $CaNa_2$ EDTA.
‡FEP, free erythrocyte protoporphyrin.

MERCURY

ETIOLOGY. Mercury has been used for at least 2000 years. At present more than 60 occupations involve mercury exposure. These include chloralkali work; manufacture of pesticides, insecticides, and fungicides; manufacture of mercury-containing instruments, lamps, neon lights, batteries, paper, paint, dye, electrical equipment, and jewelry; and dentistry.

In addition to occupational or industrial exposure, poisoning has resulted from inadvertent contamination of grains by mercury-containing pesticides; and accidental or intentional ingestion or injection of elemental mercury or mercury-containing compounds. In the past mercury was administered medicinally as a component of cathartics, teething powders, and anthelmintics. Mercury compounds are now rarely used as diuretics.

CLINICAL MANIFESTATIONS AND TREATMENT. The biologic effects, tissue distribution, and toxicity of mercury depend on the form in which it is introduced into the body. Mercury possesses a strong affinity for sulfhydryl, amine, phosphoryl, and carboxyl groups and inactivates a wide variety of enzymes. Mercury poisoning can be conveniently divided into four categories.

Metallic Mercury. Elemental mercury is a liquid at environmental temperatures but vaporizes with agitation as well as gentle heating. Bulk mercury is used in dental amalgams; up to 10 per cent of dental offices have been found to have excessive mercury vapor levels; and accidental spillage has occurred occasionally in homes or offices. The greatest exposure to metallic mercury is in industry. Heavy aerosol exposure to mercury produces chills, fever, cough, chest pain, and hemoptysis; roentgenograms show diffuse pulmonary infiltrates. Inhaled elemental mercury is readily absorbed from the alveoli; thereafter the target tissue is the brain. With mild exposure the manifestations are likely to be subtle and diagnosis difficult. Insomnia, nervousness, impaired judgment, memory deficits, emotional lability, headache, fatigue, loss of sexual drive, and depression are early manifestations and are often mistakenly ascribed to psychogenic causes. These symptoms have been referred to as micromercurialism. Abdominal cramps, dermatitis, and diarrhea may also occur, and the victim may complain of a metallic taste. As the poisoning becomes more severe, persistent involuntary tremors of the extremities are noted. Thereafter other signs of mercury poisoning may appear, including amblyopia, polyneuropathy, erythroderma, acrodynia, swollen gums with a blue line around the teeth, sialorrhea, and paresthesias. The major manifestation of mercury vapor exposure may be renal damage, including the nephrotic syndrome. A clinical picture simulating the mucocutaneous lymph node syndrome (Kawasaki's) has also been described.

Blood and urine levels may be unreliable, and clear evidence of poisoning may be documented only after administration of drugs that augment mercury excretion in the urine.

In most cases improvement occurs after removal from exposure or treatment with either dimercaprol (BAL) or N-acetyl penicillamine.

The effects of ingestion of even large amounts of metallic mercury range from no clinical disturbance to local gastrointestinal irritation to central nervous system damage. Aspiration of liquid mercury is also usually benign, although roentgenologic visualization of mercury globules may be evident for many years. After intravenous injection of mercury there may be no abnormalities other than roentgenologic densities or an illness ranging from mild to lethal with hepatic, renal, lung, and central nervous system dysfunction.

The wide range of clinical findings after elemental mercury exposure appears to relate in part to the rate of oxidation to mercuric salts and the rapidity of their subsequent excretion through the kidneys, saliva, and urine.

Inorganic Mercury. Exposure to $HgCl_2$ and Hg_2Cl_2 occurs primarily in industry and results from ingestion. $HgCl_2$ is far more toxic than Hg_2Cl_2. The major manifestations are renal and include proteinuria, granular casts in the urinary sediment, and pyuria from tubular damage. In some cases severe oliguria, and even anuria, may occur. Additionally, diarrhea, abdominal pain, hepatic dysfunction, and lesser evidences of central nervous system disease may be found (micromercurialism). Rhabdomyolysis with striking muscle enzyme elevation and acrodynia have also been reported. In this type of mercury poisoning BAL or penicillamine is usually effective.

Organomercurials with Rapid Metabolism to Inorganic Mercury. Included are phenyl and methoxyethyl mercury salts found in diuretics and fungicides. Toxicity is limited and usually renal.

Short Chain Alkyl Mercury Compounds. Methyl mercury is far more toxic than ethyl or diethyl mercury; the latter produces primarily renal abnormalities.

Methyl mercury is well absorbed from the intestinal tract, is widely distributed in the body, readily passes through the placenta into the fetus and also into breast milk. About 10 per cent localizes in the brain, and the ensuing damage is largely irreversible. Major epidemics have resulted from industrial contamination of water with subsequent biotransformation of elemental and inorganic mercury into methyl mercury, followed by ingestion by fish and then by man. Other epidemics have resulted from use of grains contaminated by organic mercurial pesticides or animal ingestion of seeds treated with mercury. The epidemics in the Minamata and Niigata regions of Japan, Iraq, Guatemala, Pakistan, and the United States have resulted in a high death rate and an appalling residue of permanent brain damage. In addition to the milder symptoms listed under elemental mercury poisoning, central nervous system manifestations include severe paresthesias, dysarthria, ataxia, visual field constriction, hearing loss, blindness, microcephaly, spasticity, paralysis, and coma. Some of the children of methyl mercury–poisoned mothers show various degrees of cerebral palsy–like abnormalities and mental retardation, and some die.

Chang LW: Neurotoxic effects of mercury—a review. Environ Res 14:329, 1977. *A very useful review with good clinical-pathologic correlations.*

Elhassani SB: The many faces of methylmercury poisoning. J Toxicol Clin Toxicol 19:875, 1982–1983. *A very nice, thorough review with 133 references.*

Joselow MM, Louria DB, Browder AA: Mercurialism: Environmental and occupational aspects. Ann Intern Med 76:119, 1972. *A useful summary with 149 references.*

Magos L: Mercury and mercurials. Br Med Bull 31:241, 1975. *A concise, valuable summary of the clinical manifestations and tissue localization after exposure to different chemical forms of mercury.*

ARSENIC

ETIOLOGY. Arsenic is ubiquitous in nature; it is present in the earth's crust in concentrations of 2 to 5 parts per billion. It is found in inordinately high concentrations in some well waters, particularly in Taiwan. It is used in the glass, pigment, and bronze-plating industries; in wood preservation; in a variety of metal alloys; in veterinary medicines; in some herbicides, insecticides, and rodenticides; in fire salts to produce multicolored flames; and by farmers and vintners. American industry uses about one half of the world's production of arsenic trioxide. Arsenic poisoning has also resulted from using certain herbal preparations and from the ingestion of illegal (moonshine) whiskey.

Elemental arsenic is not toxic even if ingested in substantial dosage. There are three toxic forms of arsenic: pentavalent salts, trivalent salts, and arsine gas. The arsenic in the earth's crust and in most foods is in the pentavalent form. Trivalent arsenic, which is far more toxic, accumulates in the body more readily than the pentavalent form. Arsenic gas (arsine) is extraordinarily toxic; it is formed by the hydrolysis of metallic arsenide or by the action of acids or nascent hydrogen on arsenical compounds, especially in the refining of certain metals. Arsine can be liberated in sewage plants, and in one small cluster of cases eight children were poisoned while cleaning out a cattle dip in Australia.

CLINICAL MANIFESTATIONS. The toxic potential of arsenicals relates to their ability to combine with sulfhydryl groups and thereby interfere with multiple enzyme systems. The evidences of *acute toxicity* are generally similar in those poisoned by either the respiratory or the gastrointestinal route, but the onset of clinical illness is much more rapid after arsine gas exposure, usually appearing within one to twelve hours. The initial manifestations usually include nausea, vomiting, weakness, colicky abdominal pain, and profuse diarrhea. The patient may complain of a metallic taste and there may be a garlic odor to the breath, but the latter is not pathognomonic of arsenic poisoning, occurring also in selenium, tellurium, and phosphorus poisonings. In arsine poisoning there may be a temperature elevation of up to 39° C.

Because arsenic preferentially binds to red blood cells, hemolytic anemia and hemoglobinuria occur early and red cell ghosts may be seen in the peripheral blood. Leukopenia occurs frequently, but in some cases moderate leukocytosis is found and both monocytosis and eosinophilia have been described.

Shortly after the initial red cell binding, arsenic can be found in liver, spleen, heart, kidneys, brain, and intestinal tract. Skin, nails, and hair do not contain arsenic until two to four weeks after exposure.

Other manifestations that may occur in the first week include jaundice, hematuria, hepatomegaly with hepatic enzyme abnormalities; electrocardiographic abnormalities; a cardiomyopathy that can be lethal; evidence of encephalopathy, including headache, irritability, delusions, and hallucinations; and respiratory muscle paralysis. Renal failure may occur consequent to the hemoglobinuria or as a result of cortical necrosis. Megaloblastic changes may be seen in the bone marrow. Optic neuritis with visual field constriction has been reported after pentavalent arsenic exposure.

The most prominent manifestation after the first week of illness is symmetrical polyneuropathy. At first sensory manifestations predominate, the patient complaining of a burning sensation in a stocking-glove distribution. Motor involvement follows almost immediately with diminished or absent reflexes and severe weakness. Prolonged encephalopathy and/or psychosis have been reported in a few instances.

In cases of subacute poisoning, Aldrich-Mees lines (transverse white bands) may be seen in the nails; like the garlic odor, these may be seen in other trace element intoxications. Erythroderma and exfoliative dermatitis may also supervene.

Chronic exposure is associated with several abnormalities. The most characteristic of these are the cutaneous lesions, particularly hyperpigmentation (arsenic melanosis) and hyperkeratoses located primarily on the palms and soles. Alopecia and so called raindrop depigmentation may also occur. In about 5 to 10 per cent of those chronically exposed, skin cancers appear after latent periods of 5 to more than 25 years; these tend to be multiple, are situated mainly on the trunk and upper extremities, and show either intraepithelial squamous cell (Bowen's disease) or basal cell morphology on histologic examination. In the United States the most frequent cause of such skin lesions in past years was the medicinal use of Fowler's solution, an inorganic trivalent arsenical. Currently most cases arise after occupational exposure, but a small number have been ascribed to chronic exposure to well water with high arsenic content.

Epidemiologic studies on gold ore miners, vineyard workers, laborers in sheep dip factories, and smelter workers show a clear increase in the incidence of squamous cell carcinoma of the lung, the risk of bronchogenic cancer correlating with the intensity and duration of arsenic trioxide exposure.

Several types of liver disease may occur; these include postnecrotic cirrhosis, hepatocellular carcinoma, and hemangioendothelioma. Additionally, portal fibrosis and/or sinusoidal collagenosis may be found, and this can lead to a form of noncirrhotic portal hypertension with splenomegaly and esophageal varices but normal hepatic artery wedge pressure. Like the skin cancers, the liver abnormalities may occur many years after exposure to arsenic has been discontinued, and the exposure period can have been relatively brief.

A severe form of peripheral arteriosclerosis in Taiwan called blackfoot disease has been attributed to chronic arsenic exposure, but the data are currently inconclusive. Arsenic exposure is also thought to induce chromosomal aberrations, but the significance of these abnormalities is not clear.

DIAGNOSIS. If the diagnosis is suspected, there is a qualitative urine test (Gutzeit test) employing sulfuric acid, zinc, and silver nitrate. Arsenic concentrations can be measured in blood, urine, hair, or nails by atomic absorption spectrophotometry or neutron activation techniques.

TREATMENT. The treatment of choice is dimercaprol (BAL), but it should be given within the first 24 hours after exposure. If the BAL is given later, it is less likely that improvement will be observed, and in most cases the peripheral neuropathy is refractory to treatment. Exchange transfusion shortly after the onset of acute illness has also been reported to be beneficial.

The neuropathy and renal failure may slowly resolve completely, or there may be residual abnormalities that range from mild to severe.

Gerhardt RE, Crecelius EA, Hudson JB: Moonshine-related arsenic poisoning. Arch Intern Med 140:211, 1980. *Twelve cases of arsenic poisoning are reviewed; in one half, illicit whiskey appeared to be the source.*

Schoolmeester WL, White DR: Arsenic poisoning. South Med J 73:198, 1980. *A fine comprehensive review with 102 references. Includes ten illustrative case reports.*

TRACE ELEMENTS WHOSE TOXICITY IS IN LARGE PART ASSOCIATED WITH HEMODIALYSIS

ZINC. The normal adult body zinc content is 1.5 to 3.0 grams. Daily intake ranges from 5 to 35 mg. Zinc is bound to metallothioneins synthesized in the liver and is excreted by both the urine and the gastrointestinal tract. Particularly high concentrations are found in the uveal tract, choroid plexus, and prostate; substantial amounts are also found in bone, brain, skeletal muscles, and other tissues of the eye.

Zinc has a strong affinity for red cells and plasma proteins. Consequently there is no loss across dialysis membranes; instead, blood zinc concentrations may increase markedly during hemodialysis. There appear to be two well-documented zinc sources: adhesive plaster (containing zinc oxide) used to prevent dialysis coils from unwinding, and the water of the dialysis fluid. Even if water has an initially low zinc content, galvanized iron pipes or tanks may release substantial amounts. This can be prevented by using deionized water or by reverse osmosis. Zinc may also be taken by mouth for a variety of reasons or may be administered intravenously.

The manifestations of zinc toxicity do not necessarily correlate well with plasma or whole blood zinc levels. Nausea, vomiting, anorexia, lethargy, irritability, abdominal pain, and anemia are the most frequent manifestations. The mechanisms responsible for the anemia are not well understood, but in many cases the anemia may be microcytic and associated with evidence of copper deficiency. Zinc can decrease copper absorption in the gut and also promote urinary copper excretion. Fever may accompany zinc toxicity. Other manifestations may include diarrhea, muscle pain, hyperamylasemia with or without pancreatitis, intestinal bleeding, thrombocytopenia, oliguria, hypotension, and renal failure with tubular necrosis. Injection of large amounts of zinc has resulted in death. Intestinal manifestations may supervene after either orally or parenterally induced zinc intoxication.

Welders, smelter workers, and solderers are exposed to aerosolized zinc and may experience zinc fume fever, characterized by chills, fever, myalgias, a metallic taste, cough, nausea, lethargy, and occasionally hemoptysis. There may be diffuse roentgenologic infiltrates and pulmonary dysfunction. Ordinarily all manifestations disappear rapidly after cessation of exposure. If more prolonged pulmonary dysfunction occurs, it is thought to result from the effects of other metals to which the workers are simultaneously exposed.

ALUMINUM. First described in 1972, aluminum-induced dialysis dementia is an often fatal disease. The tap water is usually to blame. Some waters naturally contain high concentrations of aluminum. In other cases aluminum sulfate had been added to the community water supply to remove organic materials. In still other cases the dialysis fluid appeared to be less responsible than aluminum-containing gels administered by mouth to reduce phosphate levels. However, if oral aluminum hydroxide is administered to nondialyzed patients suffering from renal failure, the encephalopathy syndrome occurs very rarely. Dialysis encephalopathy occurs only after repeated dialyses, usually spanning at least several months. Use of parenteral nutrition solutions containing aluminum can also be followed by aluminum poisoning.

Early manifestations include malaise, memory loss, and a characteristic speech disturbance. As the disease progresses, dysarthria, asterixis, myoclonic twitches, dementia, somnolence, and seizures occur. The electroencephalogram shows slowing, together with bursts of delta activity and high voltage, symmetric spikes. Among those who die, aluminum levels are markedly increased in the gray matter.

Other manifestations include anemia, myalgias, proximal myopathy, and severe skeletal pain caused by profound osteodystrophy that is unresponsive to vitamin D and is followed by fractures. Aluminum is deposited at the calcified bone-osteoid junction and bone formation is impaired.

Although frequently lethal, in some cases the encephalopathy has regressed after intake of oral aluminum is stopped or the aluminum content of the dialysis water is reduced or following renal transplantation. Treatment with deferoxamine, which complexes with aluminum, may be beneficial.

It has been suggested that Alzheimer's disease and other types of senile dementia may be related to brain aluminum deposition, but available data are unconvincing.

Those involved in aluminum processing or manufacturing, pottery or explosive making, or welding may be exposed to aluminum aerosols. Pulmonary granulomas, fibrosis, and in some cases postfibrosis emphysema may supervene. In bauxite smelters this is known as Shaver's disease.

COPPER. Since the late 1960's, copper tubing in dialysis equipment has been known to release copper when exposed to acid water. Copper levels may also be inordinately high in the dialysis water if the water is supplied through copper plumbing. Copper is a potent red cell poison, damaging cell membranes and inhibiting a variety of red cell enzymes. Major manifestations of toxicity include hemolysis and gastrointestinal disturbances. Nausea, vomiting, diarrhea, abdominal pain, fever, chills, hemolytic anemia, jaundice, hemoglobinuria, and severe myalgias all occur frequently. Myoglobinemia, necrotizing pancreatitis, and hepatic necrosis may also occur. There may be profound leukocytosis.

Copper poisoning during dialysis is fortunately readily avoidable, since copper is no longer a component of the tubing.

Copper poisoning may also occur after intentional or accidental ingestion. There may be a metallic taste, vomiting, and abdominal pain. In more severe cases hematemesis, melena, hepatic necrosis, and shock supervene.

In Wilson's disease rapid increases in circulating copper concentrations may be followed by acute hemolytic anemia.

These exposed to metallic copper industrially may develop transient pulmonary manifestations (metal fume fever). These disappear rapidly when exposure is stopped.

COBALT. Patients with renal failure may have elevated tissue cobalt levels. In a small number of cases, cardiomegaly and myocardial dysfunction have been attributed to the myocardial cobalt content. In some cases cobaltous chloride has been given by mouth to patients on maintenance hemodialysis to combat anemia. This has been associated with increased blood and myocardial cobalt levels and suggestive evidence of cardiomyopathy.

In the past cobalt had been used to increase red cell production. Toxicity included nausea, vomiting, anorexia, tinnitus, peripheral neuropathy, goiter resulting from blockage of iodine uptake, neurogenic deafness, hyperlipidemia, optic atrophy, and renal tubular damage.

Cobalt was added to beer in the 1960's as a foam stabilizer. This resulted in extraordinary cardiomyopathy, often accompanied by pericardial effusion. Mortality from heart failure or arrhythmias ranged from 5 to 47 per cent (see Ch. 51).

Persons exposed to cobalt industrially may occasionally develop cardiomyopathy. Workers exposed to finely powdered cobalt may also develop pulmonary interstitial fibrosis and cor pulmonale. Cobalt is often a component of alloys that are used in joint prostheses. Cases have been reported of joint pains, spontaneous dislocation of the prosthesis, and bone necrosis starting nine months to four years postoperatively, apparently caused by a reaction to the cobalt in the alloy.

OTHER METALS. In one group of dialysis patients *nickel* toxicity occurred when nickel leached from a stainless steel water heater tank into the dialysis fluid. Manifestations included nausea, vomiting, weakness, and headache. Symptoms developed within a few hours after dialysis and disappeared within 48 hours.

Tissue *tin* concentrations, especially in the liver, are increased in patients undergoing hemodialysis. However, tin levels are even higher in uremic patients who have not been dialyzed. No definite clinical disease has been associated with these increased body tin burdens.

Patients undergoing maintenance hemodialysis are often treated with *iron* for anemia. In such patients parenteral and occasionally oral iron administration may be followed by hemosiderosis and occasionally hemochromatosis. Serum ferritin concentrations exceed 500 ng per milliliter. A proximal myopathy has been described. The severity of the tissue iron overload and the likelihood of hemochromatosis may be related to the histocompatibility antigens A-3, B-7, and B-14. Iron overload has been complicated by porphyria cutanea tarda and by a variety of infections, including those due to species of *Yersinia* and *Vibrio* and to the yeast *Trichosporon cutaneum*. Treatment with deferoxamine may reduce the body iron burden.

Aggett PJ, Harrison JT: Current status of zinc in health and disease states. Arch Dis Child 54:909, 1979. *This is a superb review with 110 references. Only a small section is devoted to toxicity.*

Bogden JD, Oleske JM, Weiner B, et al.: Elevated plasma zinc concentrations in renal dialysis patients. Am J Clin Nutr 33:1088, 1980. *A careful study of two dialysis units that demonstrates clearly significant leakage of zinc from some coils.*

Manifold IH, Platts MM, Kennedy A: Cobalt cardiomyopathy in a patient on maintenance haemodialysis. Br Med J 2:1609, 1978. *A 17-year-old woman given oral cobalt for anemia.*

O'Hare JA, Callaghan NM, Murnaghan DJ: Dialysis encephalopathy. Clinical, electroencephalographic and interventional aspects. Medicine 62:129, 1983. *A marvelous summary article and a careful analysis of 14 patients who developed encephalopathy 16 to 92 months after starting dialysis.*

Ott SM, Maloney NA, Klein GL, et al: Aluminum is associated with low bone formation in patients receiving chronic parenteral nutrition. Ann Intern Med 98:910, 1983. *The toxicity of aluminum to bone is clearly shown in 14 patients receiving casein hydrolysate.*

Petrie JJB, Row PG: Dialysis anaemia caused by subacute zinc toxicity. Lancet 1:1178, 1977. *Ten patients on home dialysis were studied; nine developed anemia from zinc released from galvanized iron piping.*

Sandstead HH: Trace elements in uremia and hemodialysis. Am J Clin Nutr 33:1501, 1980. *A very good review article in which the author urges caution in ascribing the dialysis encephalopathy syndrome solely to aluminum.*

Taylor A, Marks V: Cobalt: A review. J Hum Nutr 32:165, 1978. *A nice review with 73 references.*

Webster JD, Parker TF, Alfrey A, et al.: Acute nickel intoxication by dialysis. Ann Intern Med 92:631, 1980. *Nausea, vomiting, weakness, and headache were the predominant manifestations among 37 patients. Symptoms remitted three to thirteen hours after dialysis was concluded.*

CADMIUM

ETIOLOGY. Over 10 million pounds of cadmium are used industrially every year in the United States. The metal is a component of alloys; it is used in the manufacture of electrical conductors and in electroplating; and it is present in ceramics, pigments, dental prosthetics, plastic stabilizers, and storage batteries. It is also a byproduct of zinc smelting and is used in the photographic, rubber, motor, and aircraft industries. Smelters, metal processing furnaces, and the burning of coal and oil are responsible for much of the cadmium in air.

CLINICAL MANIFESTATIONS. *Acute intoxication* from cadmium fumes produces a characteristic clinical picture. Four to ten hours after exposure dyspnea, cough, and substernal discomfort supervene, often accompanied by prominent myalgias and fatigue. In more severe cases wheezing, hemoptysis, and progressive dyspnea caused by pulmonary edema may occur.

In most cases, the pulmonary manifestations resolve rapidly but pulmonary function abnormalities may not disappear for months; in these cases vital capacity is reduced and there is a restrictive defect. Occasionally pulmonary edema is lethal. Autopsy and experimental studies show alveolar cell metaplasia and proliferation of Type II pulmonary cells.

Ingestion of large amounts of cadmium results in nausea, vomiting, and abdominal pain, often accompanied by weakness, prostration, and myalgias. The onset of the gastroenteritis occurs one half to five hours after ingestion and lasts for less than 24 hours.

Chronic cadmium exposure by aerosol for at least ten years has resulted in emphysema in a small number of cases. The emphysema is not accompanied by bronchitis and may appear many years after industrial exposure has stopped. Workers exposed for at least ten years also may suffer olfactory nerve damage; in some cases this progresses to total anosmia. The most frequent long-term consequence of aerosol or oral exposure is proteinuria. After prolonged and heavy contact, cadmium urinary excretion continues for years and is associated with damage to the proximal tubule. The major urinary protein is a low molecular weight β_2 microglobulin.

On occasion the proteinuria may be accompanied by glycosuria and aminoaciduria. Only infrequently is the proteinuria and tubular damage followed by progressive renal failure. An exception to the relatively benign course of the renal damage is the disease in Japan known as itai-itai (ouch-ouch), which affected almost exclusively multiparous women of ages 40 to 70 who lived in an area contaminated by industrial cadmium waste. Manifestations included striking back and joint pains, a waddly gait, osteomalacia, bone deformities, and fractures, all presumably secondary to cadmium-induced renal tubular damage. The occurrence of the disease primarily in middle-aged multiparous women remains unexplained; presumably concomitant nutritional deficiencies played an important role. In other areas of Japan greater cadmium intake produced no such manifestations.

Animal studies have suggested that cadmium administration can produce hypertension; there is no satisfactory evidence documenting an association of cadmium with hypertension in man. Some studies on workers exposed to cadmium have suggested an increased risk of lung or prostatic carcinoma, but the data are not convincing.

One of the most intriguing aspects of cadmium distribution in the body is its relation to metallothioneins, low molecular weight metal binding proteins with high cysteine content. The cadmium appears to induce production of the proteins in the liver and kidneys and probably in the intestines. The thioneins may act to prevent absorption of ingested cadmium and may play a role in storage and detoxification of cadmium in the liver and kidneys, the two tissues of maximal cadmium concentrations.

Brenner I: Cadmium toxicity. World Rev Nutr Diet 32:165, 1978. *Interactions with calcium, zinc, copper, and selenium are emphasized. Additionally there is a detailed analysis of the role of metallothioneins. Contains 183 references.*

Lauwery RR, Roels AA, Buchet JP, Bernard A, Stanescu D: Investigations on the lung and kidney function of workers exposed to cadmium. Environ Health Persp 28:137, 1979. *Three epidemiologic studies were conducted on more than 200 workers. The kidney was affected to a much greater extent than the lungs. Both tubular and glomerular aberrations were found, mainly in persons with substantially increased blood and urine cadmium concentrations.*

NICKEL

ETIOLOGY. Nickel is used widely industrially in various alloys, iron shell castings, ball bearings, and heart and joint prostheses. It is also used in nickel plating; as a catalyst; in magnetic tapes, dyes, and paints; and in acrylic plastics. It is found in petroleum and coal, in diesel fuels, and in soil and air. Municipal incinerators may contribute to the ambient air nickel concentrations.

Nickel is a potent contact allergen; the most frequent adverse effect for man is nickel dermatitis, which may be both persistent and severe. Serious systemic reactions have occurred in allergic persons given fluids intravenously through a nickel-containing needle. Prosthetic heart and joint valves have failed because of a reaction to the nickel in the prosthesis. In cases of recalcitrant nickel dermatitis, restriction in dietary nickel may be helpful.

CLINICAL MANIFESTATIONS AND TREATMENT. By far the most toxic of the nickel compounds is nickel carbonyl, created by a reaction between nickel and carbon monoxide. Industrial aerosol exposure is followed immediately by headache, drowsiness, substernal pain, nausea, and vomiting. This is followed by a latent period of one to five days, after which the victim experiences fever, chills, dyspnea, a feeling of chest tightness, cough that is sometimes productive of blood-tinged sputum, muscle pains, weakness, and fatigue. Hepatic enzyme concentrations may be considerably elevated. In severe cases cyanosis, progressive respiratory difficulties, and convulsions ensue, and death may follow in 4 to 23 days. At autopsy the lungs show hemorrhage, atelectasis, fibroblastic proliferation, and hyaline membrane formation. The treatment of choice is diethyl dithiocarbamate (Dithiocarb); dimercaprol (BAL) is an alternative but less effective therapeutic agent. Although overwhelming pneumonitis caused by nickel carbonyl is now rare, milder pulmonary toxicity in occupations such as welding probably occurs quite commonly and goes unrecognized under the general rubric of metal fume fever. Nickel exposure may also be followed by Löffler's syndrome.

CARCINOGENESIS. Nickel is considered a potent respiratory tract carcinogen. Studies of nickel refinery workers in the 1950's showed a fivefold increase in risk of lung cancer and a 150-fold increase in the risk of nasal cancer. Recent studies also indicate a substantially increased risk of larynx cancer. Among one group of Norwegian nickel workers, one third of all cancers involved the lungs and an additional 10 per cent involved the sinuses. Those occupations most at risk among nickel workers are roasting, smelting, and electrolysis. Workers developing lung, laryngeal, and nasal cancers have usually been exposed for at least ten years. Biopsies of nasal mucosa show potentially precancerous epithelial dysplasia in a substantial percentage of nickel workers. The cancer risk is so great that workers heavily exposed for over ten years should probably have annual nasal mucosa biopsies as well as sputum cytologic studies and roentgenologic examinations every four to six months in an attempt at secondary prevention. The incidence of respiratory tract cancer in nickel workers is dependent on both the extent of nickel exposure and the effects of cocarcinogens, in particular cigarette tobacco. Some data suggest that nickel in tobacco may play a role in cigarette-induced lung cancer and that nickel compounds attached to asbestos fibers may contribute to the neoplastic potential of asbestos; conversely, asbestos contamination of nickel may augment nickel carcinogenicity.

Sunderman FW Jr: A review of the metabolism and toxicity of nickel. Ann Clin Lab Sci 7:377, 1977. *An excellent review by one of the world's leading authorities (with 177 references).*

Sunderman FW Sr: Efficacy of sodium diethyldithiocarbamate (Dithiocarb) in acute nickel carbonyl poisoning. Ann Clin Lab Sci 9:1, 1979. *The data presented strongly suggest that this is currently the agent of choice.*

OTHER TOXIC METALS

Thallium

ETIOLOGY AND PATHOGENESIS. Thallium is used in optical lenses, jewelry, low temperature thermometers, semiconductors, luminescent tubes, dyes and pigments, scintillation counters, and fireworks. It forms a stainless alloy with silver, a corrosion-resistant alloy with lead, and may be a byproduct of lead and zinc production. In some areas it is still a component of rodenticides, pesticides, and insecticides. Thallium can enter the body through the respiratory tract, gastrointestinal tract, or skin. Like many other trace metals thallium has a strong affinity for sulfhydryl groups and thus interferes with many enzyme systems. Additionally, it enters the cell, exchanging for intracellular potassium.

CLINICAL MANIFESTATIONS. Poisoning can be acute and overwhelming after suicidal ingestion or it can be chronic and subtle. In acute poisoning manifestations include nausea, vomiting, abdominal pain, diarrhea that may be bloody, insomnia, myalgias, fever, hyperhidrosis, excessive thirst, delirium, seizures, coma, and respiratory failure. At least 10 per cent of acutely poisoned persons die.

Among those who survive at least a week or in those exposed to smaller amounts of thallium, the most predictable manifestations are a combined sensory and motor, often painful, peripheral neuropathy and alopecia. Although the head alopecia is total, the facial, axillary, and pubic hair are spared as is the inner one third of the eyebrows. Motor manifestations may predominate, and the ascending, predominantly motor paralysis may mimic Guillain-Barré syndrome. Abdominal colic, nausea, and vomiting occur frequently in both the acute and subacute forms of thallium toxicity and may so dominate the clinical picture that a diagnosis of acute appendicitis is made. Other manifestations of subacute intoxication include dementia, headache, fatigue, sleep disorders, intractable thirst, hallucinations, blindness caused by optic neuritis, impotence, amenorrhea, a blue discoloration of the gingivae, centrilobular hepatic necrosis, renal tubular necrosis, orthostatic hypotension, and myoclonic twitches. Multiple cranial nerves may be involved, but the eighth nerve is almost always spared. The electrocardiogram may show arrhythmias and changes similar to those associated with hypokalemia.

DIAGNOSIS. Thallium can be measured in blood and urine, but blood levels are often deceptively low even during clinically apparent poisoning. Since thallium is excreted in the urine, thallium determinations on 24-hour specimens are more reliable. A qualitative urine test is available. Urine is mixed with 0.4 per cent sodium bismuth in 20 per cent nitric acid and 10 per cent sodium iodide; if thallium is present, a red precipitate forms.

In some cases there is no history of occupational, environmental, or intentional exposure. Unexplained abdominal pain, neurologic abnormalities, and alopecia suggest the diagnosis.

TREATMENT. Treatment consists of hemodialysis, which can remove up to half the thallium body burden, potassium, forced diuresis, and administration of Prussian blue. Prussian blue, given by mouth, absorbs thallium so that fecal thallium concentrations increase. The half-life of thallium in the body is about one month, and repeated dialyses are usually needed. Hemoperfusion may also help. During potassium administration thallium is displaced from its intracellular site, and this may cause transient exacerbations of clinical manifestations. Barbiturates may increase the severity of the disease, and their use should be avoided.

PROGNOSIS. As many as 30 per cent of those poisoned suffer some residual effects. The neuropathy may persist for many months before resolving, and some are left with variable amounts of dementia, neuropathy, ataxia, visual impairment, and myoclonus.

Selenium

ETIOLOGY. Selenium is well absorbed from both the gastrointestinal tract and the lungs. The amount normally ingested varies markedly, depending on the local soil selenium content and on the geographic provenance of foods consumed. Grains, pork, kidney, seafoods, garlic, mushrooms, radishes, beef, egg yolk, and chicken frequently contain substantial amounts of selenium. The element is widely used in pigment, glass, electronics, ceramics, and steel industries.

CLINICAL MANIFESTATIONS. Both deficiency and toxicity syndromes are well described in animals. Deficiency, resulting from foraging on grains grown in soil deficient of selenium, produces white muscle disease, a diffuse, often severe myopathy. Excess caused by chronic ingestion of grains containing more than 10 parts per million of selenium results in two syndromes, alkali disease and the staggers. The former is milder and is characterized by anemia, emaciation, alopecia, and hoof deformity. The staggers is manifested by visual difficulties, anemia, liver cell degeneration, paralysis, and respiratory failure. In sheep, excessive selenium intake can produce severe cardiomyopathy.

In man a *selenium deficiency syndrome* has not been clearly defined. However, in the Republic of China diffuse cardiomyopathy has been associated with low soil and blood selenium levels, and the incidence of the disease allegedly has been strikingly reduced by selenium supplementation.

Selenium toxicity syndromes in man can be divided into acute and chronic poisoning. Subjects with inordinate exposure to selenium fumes experience one or more of the following abnormalities: intestinal disturbances, giddiness, apathy, lassitude, pallor, nervousness, depression, hair and nail loss, a garlic odor to the breath, and a metallic taste. Sore throat, dyspnea, and cough may also be noted. Symptoms usually disappear after removal from the occupational exposure. Among those ingesting excessive selenium the following symptoms and signs have been reported: nausea, vomiting, anorexia, fatigue, sore throat, emotional lability, a metallic taste, a garlic odor to the breath, a bronze color to the skin, hepatic dysfunction, and diffuse dermatitis. Increased selenium burdens may be associated with an increased prevalence of dental caries.

EPIDEMIOLOGY. Subacute and chronic selenium toxicity will likely be seen with an increasing frequency because selenium is being promoted as a nonprescription supplement. Epidemiologic data suggest an inverse relationship between selenium blood levels and the incidence of certain cancers, particularly of the intestinal tract. In experimental studies oral selenium in dosage of 0.1 to 2.0 parts per million diminishes the frequency of or delays the appearance of a variety of spontaneous or induced tumors.

In experimental animals selenium potentiates the immune response. Additionally, it is being used without adequate documentation in patients with cystic fibrosis on the assumption that the disease is related in part to selenium deficiency. There are as yet no convincing data to recommend that selenium supplements be taken by ostensibly healthy adults as a cancer preventive or as an immunopotentiator.

Manganese

Manganese toxicity occurs primarily in miners who have been exposed to manganese dioxide aerosols for prolonged periods. The manifestations, known as manganic madness, are limited to the central nervous system. The manganese is concentrated primarily in the basal ganglia and cerebellum accounting for the extrapyramidal Parkinson-like facies, the rigidity, and the difficulty in walking. Other manifestations include compulsive behavior (including singing, dancing, fighting, and running), explosive and involuntary laughter, headache, muscular weakness, tremors, dystonia, hypotonia, retropulsion and propulsion, dementia, speech disturbances, irritability, hypersomnia, and memory defects. In some cases psychosis may be the dominant feature. There is no effective therapy. After removal from manganese exposure or following attempts to reduce the body manganese load by treatment with calcium versenate or L-dopa, the mental aberrations usually improve but the neurologic abnormalities persist. Manganese contamination of dialysates or ingestion has been associated with abdominal pain, liver dysfunction, and evidence of pancreatitis.

Barium

Barium compounds are used in printing; in the production of paints, glass, paper, leather, soap, and rubber; in ceramics, plastic, steel, oil, textile, and dye industries; as fuel additives; and in insecticides, rodenticides, and depilatories. There are two major adverse effects. After accidental or intentional ingestion of large amounts, abdominal pain, vomiting, and increased peristalsis occur. If enough is absorbed, potassium is displaced intracellularly resulting in profound hypokalemia, which in turn may produce flaccid paralysis, potentially dangerous cardiac arrhythmias, renal failure, and respiratory paralysis. Treatment consists of administration of potassium and forced diuresis to promote barium excretion.

The other adverse effect from contact with barium is a benign pneumoconiosis that may supervene after one or more years of aerosol exposure. Chest roentgenograms show extensive, very dense, bilateral nodules up to 4 to 5 mm in diameter. There is no prominent fibrosis and no clinically significant disease; the nodules often regress after occupational exposure is stopped.

Boron

There are few reports of boron toxicity. Ingestion of boric acid can result in nausea, vomiting, diarrhea, anemia, seizures, a variety of skin eruptions characterized by intense erythema, desquamation, and exfoliation, and striking alopecia. Additionally, occupational aerosol exposure to diborane (B_2H_6) in high energy fuels can produce acute pulmonary edema that resolves after the exposure is discontinued.

Antimony

Industrial antimony toxicity is very rare, as are intentional ingestion or inadvertent poisoning from release of antimony from inexpensive enamelware. Manifestations of acute poisoning include nausea, abdominal pain, weakness, headache, vomiting, diarrhea, myalgias, and circulatory collapse. Gaseous SbH_3 (stibine) is as toxic as arsine, producing CNS toxicity and hemolysis. After antimonial injection for medicinal purposes, adverse effects include nausea, vomiting, cough, and muscle and joint pain. Hepatic dysfunction can occur, as can cardiac arrhythmias, including Adams-Stokes syndrome. Antimony is also considered one of the metals capable of causing metal fume fever.

Chromium

Chromium is used extensively in metal and galvanizing industries and in the manufacture of dyes, enamel, and paints. There is substantial epidemiologic evidence that chromate exposure is associated with an increased incidence of lung cancer. Additionally, chromium-exposed workers may show evidence of proximal renal tubule dysfunction and may suffer nasal septum perforations.

Molybdenum

In animals molybdenum produces diarrhea, anemia, alopecia, diminished growth, and bone and joint abnormalities. No clearly defined molybdenum toxicity syndrome has been reported in man.

Platinum

The major adverse effects observed in platinum workers are allergic pulmonary reactions, including bronchial asthma.

Plutonium

In experimental models, plutonium, because of its radioactivity, is a potent carcinogen. Workers have been generally well protected, and it seems unlikely that occupational exposure will be found to be a major problem. Some still controversial epidemiologic studies have suggested that accidental community exposure has resulted in an increase in frequency of certain cancers and fetal malformations.

Tellurium

Used particularly in rubber, metallurgic, and electronics industries, tellurium can cause giddiness, headache, nausea, a metallic taste, and a garlic smell to the breath. In animals tellurium causes neuropathy, but this has not been convincingly demonstrated in man.

Tin

Tin can be released into beverages or foods from tin cans; ingestion can produce nausea, vomiting, abdominal pain, and diarrhea. Such toxicity occurs infrequently. Additionally, there have been occasional reports of encephalopathy following industrial exposure to organic tin compounds; this was characterized by headache, vomiting, visual defects, and paresis. Aerosol exposure to tin may result in stannosis, a mild pneumoconiosis in which there may be dense bilateral infiltrates but usually no pulmonary dysfunction.

Vanadium

Vanadium is used in alloys and in the steel and chemical industries. Its inhalation can result in neurasthenia, anorexia, vertigo, throat pain, nasal irritation (even nasal hemorrhage), and acute bronchitis characterized by a cough that is sometimes accompanied by a whoop. The nasal mucosa of vanadium-exposed workers shows vascular hyperemia and round cell infiltration.

Doig AT: Baritosis: A benign pneumoconiosis. Thorax 31:30, 1976. *Nine cases are described. Despite dense infiltrates, no significant clinical disease or physiologic abnormalities occurred.*

Ghezzi R, Bozza Marrubini M: Prussian blue in the treatment of thallium intoxication. Vet Human Toxicol 21 (Suppl):64, 1979. *Five cases of rodenticide poisoning are reported. Clinical manifestations are summarized. Prussian blue increased fecal thallium and effected clinical improvement.*

Gordon AS, Prichard JS, Freedman MH: Seizure disorders and anemia associated with chronic borax intoxication. Can Med Assoc J 108:719, 1973. *Two infants poisoned by use of pacifiers dipped in borax.*

Louria DB, Joselow MM, Browder AA: The human toxicity of certain trace elements. Ann Intern Med 76:307, 1972. *A review of 12 metals with 154 references.*

Nordberg GF: Factors influencing metabolism and toxicity of metals: A consensus report. Environ Health Persp 25:3, 1978. *This marvelous analysis covers the toxicity and interactions with other metals of arsenic, cadmium, lead, and mercury. Highly recommended. Contains 312 references.*

Saddique A, Peterson CD: Thallium poisoning: A review. Vet Hum Toxicol 25:16, 1983. *A very good review indeed, with 48 references.*

Thallium poisoning. Clinical Conferences of the Johns Hopkins Hospital. Johns Hopkins Med J 142:27, 1978. *A single case accompanied by an excellent discussion of clinical manifestations and treatment.*

Yang G, Wang S, Zhou R, et al: Endemic selenium intoxication of humans in China. Am J Clin Nutr 37:872, 1983. *An extraordinary disease characterized by nail and hair loss and probably by skin and nervous system abnormalities was first described in Hubei Province of China. Stony coal with very high selenium content was the source, the incidence of the disease reaching almost 50 per cent in heavily affected villages.*

Part XXVII
LABORATORY REFERENCE RANGE VALUES OF CLINICAL IMPORTANCE

566. REFERENCE RANGES AND LABORATORY VALUES OF CLINICAL IMPORTANCE*

Norbert W. Tietz

Reference ranges are valuable guidelines for the clinician, but they should not be regarded as absolute indicators of health and disease. There are several reasons for using reference ranges with caution, some of which are listed in Ch. 20. Most importantly, values for "healthy" individuals often overlap significantly with values for persons afflicted with disease. In addition, laboratory values may vary significantly because of methodological differences and mode of standardization. This is especially true for immunological tests, which utilize antibodies that may have different characteristics. As a result, laboratory values in individual institutions may differ from those listed in this chapter.

The values in this chapter are primarily for adults in the fasting state. Values for other age groups, when included, are clearly identified.

All laboratory values are given in conventional and international units. In general, the international units given conform to the SI system (Système International d'Unités). However, in some cases the recommendations of the International Union of Pure and Applied Chemistry (IUPAC) and the Commission on World Standards of the World Association of Societies of Pathology (COWS of WASP) are used, since it is felt that these have found wider acceptance in clinical laboratories and offer advantages over the units recommended in the SI system.

Throughout this chapter we have used the prefixes for units as approved by the CGPM (Conférence Générale des Poids et Mésures), 1964, and the International Congress of Clinical Chemistry, 1966. The pertinent prefixes denoting the decimal factors are listed below.

PREFIXES DENOTING DECIMAL FACTORS

Prefix	*Symbol*	*Factor*
mega	M	10^6
kilo	k	10^3
hecto	h	10^2
deka	da	10^1
deci	d	10^{-1}
centi	c	10^{-2}
milli	m	10^{-3}
micro	μ	10^{-6}
nano	n	10^{-9}
pico	p	10^{-12}
femto	f	10^{-15}

*The material in this chapter was partially extracted from: *Clinical Guide to Laboratory Tests,* NW Tietz, ed.: Philadelphia, W. B. Saunders Company, 1983. The main contributors are RV Blanke and RA Blouin: Drugs and Toxicology; C Hougie: Coagulation; HP Lehmann: International Units; J Leonard: Endocrinology; W Mertz and RV Blanke: Trace Metals; DA Nelson: Hematologhy; SE Ritzmann: Proteins; and HE Sauberlich: Vitamins. A portion of the values was generated in the clinical laboratories of the University of Kentucky Medical Center. Other sources are listed under references for this chapter.

ABBREVIATIONS

For convenience and to preserve space we have used standard abbreviations commonly used in laboratory medicine. Less common abbreviations and some nonstandard abbreviations are given below.

AU	Arbitrary Units
BMD	Boehringer Mannheim Diagnostics, Inc.
EU	Ehrlich Unit
G-D	General Diagnostics
GPIMH	Guinea Pig Intestinal Mucosal Homogenate
ICSH	International Committee for Standardization in Hematology
IFA	Immunofluorescent Assay
IRP-2-hMG	2nd International Reference Preparation of Human Menopausal Gonadotropin
IU	International Unit (of hormone activity)
NEFA	Nonesterified Fatty Acids (Free Fatty Acids)
Occup.	Occupational
P-5′-P	Pyridoxal-5′-Phosphate
RIA	Radioimmunoassay
RID	Radialimmunodiffusion
RT	Room Temperature
U	International Unit (of enzyme activity)
WHO	World Health Organization

ACKNOWLEDGMENT. We thankfully acknowledge the assistance of Nancy M. Logan, B.A., and Susan C. Blandford in the preparation of this material.

Beutler E: Hemolytic Anemia in Disorders of Red Cell Metabolism. New York, Plenum Publishing Company, 1978.
Brown SS, Mitchell FL, Young DS (eds.): Chemical Diagnosis of Disease. Amsterdam, Elsevier/North-Holland Biomedical Press, 1979.
Conn HF, Conn RB (eds.): Current Diagnosis. 6th ed. Philadelphia, W. B. Saunders Company, 1980.
Gilman AG, Goodman L, Gilman A (eds.): The Pharmacological Basis of Therapeutics. 6th ed. New York, The Macmillan Company, 1980.
Henry JB (ed.): Todd-Sanford-Davidsohn Clinical Diagnosis and Management by Laboratory Methods. 16th ed. Philadelphia, W. B. Saunders Company, 1979.
Mabry C, Tietz NW: Tables of normal laboratory values. *In* Nelson WE, Vaughan VC, McKay RJ, Behrman RE (eds.): Nelson Textbook of Pediatrics. 12th ed. Philadelphia, W. B. Saunders Company, 1983.
Miale JB: Laboratory Medicine: Hematology. 5th ed. St. Louis, C. V. Mosby Company, 1977.
Tietz NW (ed.): Fundamentals of Clinical Chemistry. 2nd ed. Philadelphia, W. B. Saunders Company, 1976.
Tietz NW, Blackburn RH (eds.): Reference Ranges and General Information. Clinical Laboratories, A. B. Chandler Medical Center, University of Kentucky, Lexington, Kentucky, 1984.
Tietz NW (ed.): Clinical Guide to Laboratory Tests. Philadelphia, W. B. Saunders Company, 1983.
Williams WJ, Beutler E, Erslev AJ, Rundles RW: Hematology. 2nd ed. New York, McGraw-Hill Book Company, 1977.

CLINICAL CHEMISTRY, TOXICOLOGY, SEROLOGY

Test	Specimen	Reference Range	Reference Range (International Units)
Acetoacetate			
Semiquantitative	Serum or plasma (fluoride/oxalate)	Negative (< 3 mg/dL)	Negative (< 0.3 mmol/L)
	Urine	Negative	Negative
Acetone			
Semiquantitative	Serum or plasma (fluoride or oxalate)	Negative (< 3 mg/dL)	Negative (< 0.5 mmol/L)
Quantitative		0.3–2.0 mg/dL	0.05–0.34 mmol/L
Semiquantitative	Urine	Negative	Negative
Adrenocorticotropic hormone (ACTH)	Plasma (EDTA)	Adult 0800 h: 25–100 pg/mL 1800 h: < 50 pg/mL	 25–100 ng/L < 50 ng/L
Adrenocorticotropic Hormone Stimulation Test (Prolonged Infusion) *Dose: 500 μg Cortrosyn/d × 3*	Urine, 24 h	17–KGS: 2- to 4-fold rise 17–KS: 2-fold rise 17–OHCS: 2- to 5-fold rise Cortisol: 25–50 μg/dL	17–KGS: 2- to 4-fold rise 17–KS: 2-fold rise 17–OHCS: 2- to 5-fold rise Cortisol: 0.7–1.4 μmol/L
Adrenocorticotropic Hormone Stimulation Test (Rapid Test) *Dose: 250 μg Cortrosyn IM*	Serum; fasting, 30 and 60 min after stimulation	Cortisol Baseline: > 5.0 μg/dL After Cortrosyn: 2× baseline	 Baseline: < 0.14 μmol/L After Cortrosyn: 2× baseline
Alanine Aminotransferase (ALT, GPT)	Serum	*U/L* Newborn/Infant: 5–28 Adult: 8–20 > 60 y, M: 7–24 F: 7–16	*U/L* 5–28 8–20 7–24 7–16
Albumin			
Nephelometric, colorimetric	Serum	Adult: 3.5–5.0 g/dL > 60 y: 3.4–4.8 g/dL Avg. ~ 0.3 g/dL higher in ambulatory individuals	35–50 g/L 34–48 g/L Avg. ~ 3 g/L higher in ambulatory individuals
Nephelometric, rate	CSF	10–30 mg/dL	100–300 mg/L
	Urine	< 80 mg/d at rest < 150 mg/d ambulatory	< 80 mg/d < 150 mg/d
Aldolase	Serum	*U/L* 1.0–7.5 (30°C) 0.3–3.0 (at bed rest) 1.5–12.0 (37°C)	*U/L* 1.0–7.5 (30°C) 0.3–3.0 (at bed rest) 1.5–12.0 (37°C)
Aldosterone	Plasma (heparin, EDTA) or serum	*ng/dL* 3–11 y: 5–70 11–15 y: < 5–50 Adult, *average sodium diet* supine: 3–10 upright, F: 5–30 M: 6–22 2–3× higher during pregnancy; adrenal vein: 200–800 *Low sodium diet:* value increases 2- to 5- fold; Florinef suppression: < 4 ng/dL ACTH or angiotensin stimulation, 1 h: 2- to 5-fold increase	*nmol/L* 0.14–1.9 < 0.14–1.4 0.08–0.3 0.14–0.8 0.17–0.61 5.5–22 < 0.1 nmol/L

CLINICAL CHEMISTRY, TOXICOLOGY, SEROLOGY (*Continued*)

Test	Specimen	Reference Range	Reference Range (International Units)
	Urine, 24 h	*Total Urinary Na nmol/d* / *Plasma Renin activity ng AI/mL/h* / *Urinary aldosterone μg/d* < 20 / 5–24 / > 35–80 50 / 2–7 / 13–33 100 / 1–5 / 5–24 150 / 0.5–4 / 3–19 200 / / 1–16 250 / / 1–13 (assuming normal serum Na, K, and extracellular vol)	*Urinary aldosterone nmol/d* > 97–220 36–91 14–66 8–53 3–44 3–36
δ-Aminolevulinic Acid (δ-ALA)	Serum	15–23 μg/dL; lower in children	1.1–1.8 μmol/L
	Urine	1.3–7.0 mg/d	9.9–53.4 μmol/d
Ammonia Nitrogen *Resin or enzymatic*	Serum or plasma (Na-heparin)	*μg N/dL* Newborn: 90–150 < 1 mo: 29–70 Adult: 15–45	*μmol N/L* 64–107 21–50 11–32
	Urine, 24 h	140–1500 mg/d	10–107 mmol/d
Amobarbital	Serum	Therap. conc.: 1–5 μg/mL Toxic conc.: > 10 μg/mL	4–22 μmol/L > 44 μmol/L
Amylase *(Beckman; BMD)*	Serum	Adult: 25–125 U/L > 70 y: 20–160 U/L	25–125 U/L 20–160 U/L
	Urine, timed specimen	1–17 U/h	1–17 U/h
Androstenedione	Serum	*ng/dL(mean ± 1SE)* *M* / *F* Cord: 85 ± 27 / 93 ± 28 1–3 mo: 34 ± 11 / 19 ± 4 Adult: 107 ± 25 / 151 ± 38	*nmol/L (mean ± 1 SE)* *M* / *F* 2.9 ± 0.94 / 3.2 ± 1.0 1.2 ± 0.4 / 0.66 ± 0.14 3.74 ± 0.87 / 5.27 ± 1.33
Angiotensin I	Peripheral venous plasma (KEDTA)	11–88 pg/mL	11–88 ng/L
Angiotensin II	Plasma (KEDTA)	Arterial blood: 2.4 ± 1.2 ng/dL Venous blood: 50–75% of arterial blood concentration	24 ± 12 ng/L Fraction of arterial blood conc.: 0.50–0.75
Anion Gap **[Na − (Cl^- + HCO_3^-)]**	Plasma (heparin)	7–14 mmol/L	7–14 mmol/L
Antidiuretic Hormone–Water Deprivation Stimulation Test (Miller Test)	Serum (0600 h) and hourly urine for osmolality; when urine osmolality plateaus after fluid restriction, measure serum osmolality and ADH	Max. urine osmolality before vasopressin admin. more than serum osmolality; at end of test, serum osmolality: < 300 mOsmol/kg; urine osmolality: > 500 mOsmol/kg; ADH levels: see table under hADH; 1 h after vasopressin admin. < 5% increase in urine osmolality over previous specimen	
Antihyaluronidase Titer (AH Titer)	Serum	≤ 128 units/mL	≤ 128 units/mL
Antistreptolysin-O Titer (ASO Titer)	Serum	≤ 166 Todd Units; 170–330 Todd Units in school-aged children	
α_1-Antitrypsin	Serum	Newborn: 145–270 mg/dL Adult: 78–200 mg/dL	1.45–2.70 g/L 0.78–2.00 g/L
Arsenic	Whole blood (heparin)	*μg/dL* 0.2– 6.2 Chronic poisoning: 10–50 Acute poisoning: 60–93	*μmol/L* 0.03–0.82 1.33–6.65 7.98–12.37
	Urine, 24 h	5–50 μg/d	0.067–0.665 μmol/d
Ascorbic Acid, see *Vitamin C*			
Aspartate Aminotransferase (AST, SGOT, 30°C)	Serum	*U/L* Infant: 15–60 Adult: 8–20 < 60 y, M: 11–26 F: 10–20 With P-5′-P: 12–29	*U/L* 15–60 8–20 11–26 10–20 12–29

CLINICAL CHEMISTRY, TOXICOLOGY, SEROLOGY *(Continued)*

Test	Specimen	Reference Range	Reference Range (International Units)
Base Excess	Whole blood (heparin)	*mmol/L* Newborn: (−10)–(−2) Infant: (−7)–(−1) Child: (−4)–(+2) Adult: (−2)–(+3)	*mmol/L* (−10)–(−2) (−7)–(−1) (−4)–(+2) (−2)–(+3)
Bicarbonate	Serum	Art.: 21–28 mmol/L Ven.: 22–29 mmol/L	Art.: 21–28 mmol/L Ven.: 22–29 mmol/L
Bile Acids, Total	Serum, fasting Serum, 2 h postprandial	0.3–2.3 μg/mL 1.8–3.2 μg/mL	0.74–5.64 μmol/L 4.41–7.84 μmol/L (conv. factor based on cholic acid, M.W. 408.6)
	Feces	120–225 mg/d	294–551 μmol/d
Bilirubin *Total*	Serum	*Premature mg/dL* / *Full Term mg/dL* Cord: < 2.0 / < 2.0 0–1 d: < 8.0 / < 6.0 3–5 d: < 16.0 / < 12.0 Thereafter: < 2.0 / 0.2–1.0	*Premature* / *Full Term* (*μmol/L*) < 34 / < 34 < 137 / < 103 < 274 / < 205 < 34 / 3.4–17.1
	Urine	Negative	Negative
Conjugated (direct)	Serum	0–0.2 mg/dL	0–3.4 μmol/L
C-Peptide	Serum	*ng/mL* Adult: ≤ 4.0 > 60y, M: 1.5–5.0 F; 1.4–5.5	*μg/L* ≤ 4.0 1.5–5.0 1.4–5.5
C-Reactive Protein	Serum	Cord blood: 10–350 ng/mL Adult: 68–8200 ng/mL	10–350 μg/L 68–8200 μg/L
Calcium, Ionized (iCa)	Serum, plasma or whole blood (heparin)	*mg/dL* Cord 5.5 ± 0.3 Newborn, 3–24 h: 4.3–5.1 24–48 h: 4.0–4.7 Adult: 4.48–4.92 or 2.24–2.46 mEq/L 2.25–2.60 mEq/L >60 y:	*mmol/L* 1.37 ± 0.07 1.07–1.27 1.00–1.17 1.12–1.23 1.13–1.30
Calcium, Total	Serum	*mg/dL* Child: 8.8–10.8 Adult: 8.4–10.2 M, > 60 y: 8.4–10.0	*mmol/L* 2.2–2.70 2.1–2.55 2.1–2.50
	Urine, 24 h	*Ca in Diet* / *mg/d* Free Ca: 5–40 Low to average: 50–150 Average (20 mmol/d): 100–300	*mmol/d* 0.13–1.0 1.25–3.8 2.5–7.5
	CSF	2.1–2.7 mEq/L or 4.2–5.4 mg/dL	1.05–1.35 mmol/L 1.05–1.35 mmol/L
	Feces	Avg.: 0.64 g/d	16 mmol/d
Carbon Dioxide, Partial Pressure (P_{CO_2}), at sea level	Whole blood (heparin)	*mm Hg* Newborn: 27–40 Infant: 27–41 Adult, M: 35–48 F: 32–45	*kPa* 3.6–5.3 3.6–5.5 4.7–6.4 4.3–6.0
Carbon Dioxide, Total (T_{CO_2})	Serum, plasma (heparin)	*mmol/L* Cord: 14–22 Newborn: 13–22 Infant: 20–28 Child: 20–28 Adult: 22–28 > 60 y: 23–31	*mmol/L* 14–22 13–22 20–28 20–28 22–28 23–31
Carbon Monoxide	Whole blood (EDTA)	Nonsmokers: < 2% HbCO Smokers: < 10% HbCO Toxic: > 20% HbCO Lethal: > 50% HbCO	*HbCO Fraction:* < 0.02 < 0.10 >0.20 > 0.5

CLINICAL CHEMISTRY, TOXICOLOGY, SEROLOGY *(Continued)*

Test	Specimen	Reference Range		Reference Range (International Units)
Carboxyhemoglobin, see *Carbon Monoxide*				
Carcinoembryonic Antigen (CEA)	Serum	Nonsmokers:	0–3.0 ng/mL	0–0.3 μg/L
		Smokers:	0–5.0 ng/mL	0–5.0 μg/L
β-Carotene	Serum		*μ/dL*	*μmol/L*
		Infant:	20–70	0.37–1.30
		Child:	40–130	0.74–2.42
		Adult:	60–200	1.12–3.72
Carotene Absorption Test	Serum	Increase by ≥ 35 μg/dL		Increase by ≥ 0.65 μmol/L
Catecholamines,	Urine, 24 h			
HPLC		< 110 μg/d		< 650 nmol/d (conv. factor based on norepinephrine, M.W. 169.18)
Fluorometric		< 280 μg/d		< 1655 nmol/d
Catecholamines, Fractionated	Urine, 24 h			
		Norepinephrine	*μg/d*	*nmol/d*
		1–4 y:	0–29	0–170
		4–10 y:	8–65	47–380
		10–15 y:	15–80	89–470
		Adult:	0–100	0–590
		Epinephrine	*μg/d*	*nmol/d*
		1–4 y:	0–6.0	0–33
		4–10 y:	0–10.0	0–55
		10–15 y:	0.5–20	2.7–110
		Adult:	0–15	0–82
		Dopamine	*μg/d*	*nmol/d*
		1–4 y:	40–260	260–1700
		> 4 y:	65–400	425–2610
Catecholamines, Free	Plasma (EDTA and sodium metabisulfite)		*pg/ml*	*pmol/L*
		Epinephrine, random:	< 88	< 480
		Norepinephrine, random:	104–548	615–3240
		Dopamine, random:	< 136	< 888
Cerebrospinal Fluid Pressure	CSF	50–180 mm water		50–180 mm water
Cerebrospinal Fluid Volume	CSF	Child:	60–100 mL	0.06–0.10 L
		Adult:	100–160 mL	0.1–0.16 L
Ceruloplasmin	Serum		*mg/dL*	*mg/L*
RID		Newborn:	1–30	10–300
		6 mo–1 y:	15–50	150–500
		1–12 y:	30–65	300–650
		Thereafter:	15–60	150–600
Chloride	Serum or plasma (heparin)	98–106 mmol/d		98–106 mmol/d
	CSF	118–132 mmol/L		118–132 mmol/L
	Urine, 24 h		*mmol/d*	*mmol/d*
		Infant:	2–10	2–10
		Child:	15–40	15–40
		Thereafter:	110–250	110–250
		(vary greatly with Cl intake)		
	Sweat		*mmol/L*	*mmol/L*
		Normal (homozygote):	3–35	0–35
		Marginal:	30–60	30–60
		Cystic fibrosis:	60–200	60–200
Cholesterol, Total	Serum or plasma (EDTA)		*mg/dL*	*mmol/L*
		Cord:	45–100	1.17–2.59
		Newborn:	53–135	1.37–3.50
		Infant:	70–175	1.81–4.53
		Child:	120–200	3.11–5.18
		Adolescent:	120–210	3.11–5.44
		Adult:	140–310	3.63–8.03
		Recommended (desirable) range for adults:	140–220	3.63–5.70

CLINICAL CHEMISTRY, TOXICOLOGY, SEROLOGY (*Continued*)

Test	Specimen	Reference Range	Reference Range (International Units)
Chorionic Gonadotropin, β-Subunit (β-HCG)	Serum or plasma (EDTA)	*mIU/mL* M, and nonpregnant female: <3.0 F, postconception, 7–10 d: > 3.0 30 d: 100–5000 40 d: > 2000 10 wks: 50,000–140,000 > 16 wks: 10,000–50,000 Trophoblastic disease: > 100,000	*mIU/mL* < 3.0 > 3.0 100–5000 > 2000 50,000–140,000 10,000–50,000 > 100,000
Complement			
Total hemolytic complement activity	Plasma (EDTA)	75–160 U/mL or > 33% of plasma CH_{50}	75–160 kU/L or fraction of plasma CH_{50}: > 0.33
Total complement decay rate (functional)	Plasma (EDTA)	~ 10–20% Deficiency: > 50%	*Fraction decay rate* ~ 0.10–0.20 > 0.50
Classic pathway components:		*mg/dL*	*mg/L*
C1q	Serum	6.5 ± 0.7	65 ± 7
C1r	Serum	2.5–3.8	25–38
C1s (C1 esterase)	Serum	2.5–3.8	25–38
C2	Serum	2.8 ± 0.6	28 ± 6
C3 (β_1 C-globulin)	Serum	80–155	800–1550
C4 (β_1 E-globulin)	Serum	13–37	130–370
C5 (β_1 F-globulin)	Serum	6.4 ± 1.3	64 ± 13
C6	Serum	5.6 ± 0.8	56 ± 8
C7	Serum	4.9–7.0	49–70
C8	Serum	4.3–6.3	43–63
C9	Serum	4.7–6.9	47–69
Alternative pathway components:			
C4 binding protein	Serum	18–32	180–320
Factor B (C3 proactivator)	Serum	20–45	200–450
Properdin	Serum	2.8 ± 0.4	28 ± 4
Regulatory proteins			
β_1H-globulin (C3b inactivator accelerator)	Serum	56.1 ± 7.8	561 ± 78
C1 inhibitor (esterase inhibitor)	Plasma (EDTA)	17.4–24.0	174–240
C1 inhibitor by complement decay rate (functional)	Plasma (EDTA)	~ 10–20% Deficiency: >50%	*Fraction decay rate* ~ 0.10–0.20 > 0.50
C3b inactivator (KAF)	Serum	4.0 ± 0.7 mg/dL	40 ± 7 mg/L
S protein	Serum	41.8–60.0 mg/dL	418–600 mg/L
Copper	Serum	*μg/dL* Birth-6 mo: 20–70 6 y: 90–190 Adult, M: 70–140 F: 80–155 Pregnancy at term: 118–302	*μmol/L* 3.14–10.99 14.13–29.83 10.99–21.98 12.56–24.34 18.53–47.41
	Erythrocytes (heparin)	90–150 μg/dL	14.13–23.55 μmol/L
	Urine, 24 h	15–30 μg/d	0.24–0.47 μmol/d
Coproporphyrin	Urine, 24 h	34–234 μg/d	51–351 nmol/d
	Feces, 24 h	< 30 μg/g dry wt 400–1200 μg/d	< 45 nmol/g dry wt 600–1800 nmol/d
Corticobinding Globulin (CBG), see *Transcortin*			
Corticosterone	Serum or plasma (heparin, EDTA, or oxalate)	0.13–2.3 μg/dL	3.75–66 nmol/L
Cortisol	Serum or plasma (heparin)	0800 h: 5–23 μg/dL 1600 h: 3–15 μg/dL 2000 h: ≤ 50% of 0800 h	138–635 nmol/L 82–413 nmol/L Fraction of 0800h: ≤ 0.50
Cortisol, Free	Urine, 24 h	*μg/d* Child: 2–27 Adolescent: 5–55 Adult: 10–100	*nmol/d* 5.5–74 14–152 27–276

CLINICAL CHEMISTRY, TOXICOLOGY, SEROLOGY *(Continued)*

Test	Specimen	Reference Range	Reference Range (International Units)
Creatine Kinase (CK)			
Total, 30°C	Serum	*U/L* Newborn: 10–200 Adult, M: 12–80 F: 10–55 > 60 y, M: 20–110 F: 16–80 > 70 y, M: 22–90 F: 16–80 Ambulatory, M: 25–90 F: 10–70 Higher after exercise	*U/L* 10–200 12–80 10–55 20–110 16–80 22–90 16–80 25–90 10–70
Isoenzymes	Serum	Fraction 2 (MB) < 4–6% of total (method dependent)	Fraction of total: < 0.04–0.06
Creatinine *Jaffe, kinetic or enzymatic*	Serum or plasma	*mg/dL* Cord: 0.6–1.2 Child: 0.3–0.7 Adult, M: 0.6–1.2 F: 0.5–1.1	*μmol/L* 53–106 27–62 53–106 44–97
Jaffe, manual	Serum or plasma	0.8–1.5 mg/dL	70–133 μmol/L
	Urine, 24 h	*mg/d/kg* Child; 8–22 Adult, M: 14–26 F: 11–20 Declines with age to 10 mg/kg/d at age 90	*μmol/d/kg* 71–195 124–230 97–177
		or: *mg/d* M: 800–1800 F: 600–1600	*mmol/d* 7–16 5.3–14.0
Creatinine Clearance (Endogenous)	Serum or plasma, and urine	< 40 y, M: 97–137 mL/min/1.73m² F: 88–128 mL/min/1.73m² Decreases ~ 6.5 mL/min/1.73 m² per decade	0.93–1.32 mL/s/m² 0.85–1.23 mL/s/m²
Dehydroepiandrosterone Sulfate (DHEA-SO_4)	Serum or plasma (heparin or EDTA)	*μg/mL* Newborn: <300 1–4 d: <20 Child: 0.60–2.54 Adult, M: 1.99–3.34 F, Premeno-pausal: 0.82–3.38 Postmeno-pausal: 0.11–0.61 Pregnancy, Term: 0.23–1.17	*μmol/L* <780 <52 1.6–6.6 5.2–8.7 2.1–8.8 0.3–1.6 0.6–3.0
11-Deoxycortisol (Compound S)	Plasma (heparin, EDTA or oxalate)	*μg/dL* < 1 without metyrapone > 7 after metyrapone	*nmol/L* *< 30* *> 200*
Dexamethasone Suppression Test (Standard)			
Low dose, adult: 0.5 mg q 6 h × 8	Serum, 0800 h Control, day 2, day 3	Cortisol: suppression on day 3 to < 50% of baseline or to < 5 μg/dL	Cortisol: suppression on day 3, fraction of baseline: < 0.50 or < 138 nmol/L
	Urine, 24 h Day 1, 2, and 3	17-KGS: suppression on day 2 to < 7.5 mg/d	17-KGS: suppression on day 2 to < 26 μmol/d
		17-OHCS: suppression on day 2 to < 4.5 mg/d	17-OHCS: suppression on day 2 to < 12.4 μmol/d
		Free cortisol: < 50% of baseline	Free cortisol: fraction of baseline, < 0.50
High dose, adult: 2.0 mg q 6 h × 8		Cortisol, 17-KGS, 17-OHCS: suppression on day 3 to < 50% of baseline	Cortisol, 17-KGS, 17-OHCS: suppression on day 3, fraction of baseline: < 0.50

CLINICAL CHEMISTRY, TOXICOLOGY, SEROLOGY *(Continued)*

Test	Specimen	Reference Range		Reference Range (International Units)
Dexamethasone Single Dose Overnight Suppression Test				
Dose: 1 mg orally at 2300 h or 2400 h	Serum for cortisol, 0800 h following morning	Suppression to 5–10 μg/dL or to < 50% of baseline		Suppression to 138–276 nmol/L or fraction of baseline: < 0.50
			ng/mL	*nmol/L*
Digoxin	Serum, plasma (heparin, EDTA); collect at least 12 h after dose	Therap. conc.,		
		CHF:	0.8–1.5	1.0–1.9
		Arrhythmias:	1.5–2.0	1.9–2.6
		Toxic conc.,		
		Adult:	> 2.5	> 3.2
		Child:	> 3.0	> 3.8
Estradiol	Serum or plasm (heparin *or EDTA*)		*pg/mL*	*pmol/L*
		Adult, M:	8–36	29–132
		F,		
		Follicular:	10–90	37–330
		Midcycle:	100–500	370–1835
		Luteal:	50–240	184–880
		Postmenopausal:	10–30	37–110
	Urine, 24 h		*μg/d*	*nmol/d*
		Adult, M:	0–6	0–22
		F,		
		Follicular:	0–3	0–11
		Ovulatory peak:	4–14	15–51
		Luteal:	4–10	15–37
		Postmenopausal:	0–4	0–15
Estriol (E_3), Free	Serum	*Weeks of gestation*	*μg/L*	*nmol/L*
		25–28:	3.5–12.5	12–43.3
		30–32:	4.5–16.0	16–55.5
		34:	5.5–18.5	19–64.2
		36:	7.0–25.0	24–86.8
		37:	8.0–28.0	28–97.2
		38:	9.0–32.0	31–111
		39:	10.0–34.0	35–118
		40–41:	10.5–25.0	36–86.7
Estriol (E_3), Total	Serum		*ng/mL*	*nmol/L*
		Pregnancy (wks),		
		24–28:	30–170	104–590
		28–32:	40–220	140–760
		32–36:	60–280	208–970
		36–40:	80–350	280–1210
		Adult, M and non-pregnant F:	<2	<7
	Urine, 24 h		*mg/d*	*μmol/d*
		Pregnancy (wks),		
		30:	6–18	21–62
		35:	9–28	31–97
		40:	13–42	45–146
		Decrease of > 40% of previous value suggests fetus at risk		Fraction of previous value of < 0.60 suggests fetus at risk
Estrogens, Total	Serum		*pg/mL*	*ng/L*
		M:	40–115	40–115
		F, cycle-days,		
		1–10:	61–394	61–394
		11–20:	122–437	122–437
		21–30:	156–350	156–350
		Prepubertal and postmenopausal:	≤40	≤40
			μg/d	*μg/d*
	Urine, 24 h	M:	5–25	5–25
		F,		
		Preovulation:	4–25	4–25
		Ovulation:	28–100	28–100
		Luteal peak:	22–80	22–80
		Pregnancy, term:	< 45,000	< 45,000
		Postmenopausal:	< 10	< 10
Estrogen Receptor Assay (ERA)	0.5–1 g tissue		*fmol/mg protein*	*nmol/kg protein*
		Negative:	< 3.0	< 3.0
		Borderline positive:	3–10	3–10
		Positive:	> 10.0	> 10.0

CLINICAL CHEMISTRY, TOXICOLOGY, SEROLOGY *(Continued)*

Test	Specimen	Reference Range	Reference Range (International Units)
Estrone (E_1)	Serum	*pg/mL*	*pmol/L*
		M, Pubertal stage,	
		I: 11	41
		II: 16	59
		III: 21	78
		Adult: 30–170	111–630
		F, Pubertal stage,	
		I: 0–29	0–107
		II: 10–35	37–130
		III: 15–45	55–166
		IV: 20–80	74–296
		Follicular: 20–150	74–555
	Urine, 24 h	*µg/d*	*nmol/d*
		Adult, M: 3–8	11–30
		F,	
		Ovulatory peak: 11–31	41–115
		Luteal: 10–23	37–85
		Postmenopausal: 1–7	3.7–26.0
Ethanol	Serum, whole blood (oxalate)	*mg/dL*	*mmol/L*
		Toxic: 50–100	10.9–21.7
		Depression of CNS: > 100	> 21.7
		Fatalities reported: > 400	> 86.8
Fat, Fecal	Feces, 72 h	*g/d*	*g/d*
		Infant, breast-fed: < 1	< 1
		0–6 y: < 2	< 2
		Adult: < 7	< 7
		Adult (fat-free diet): < 4	< 4
Fatty Acids, Nonesterified (Free)	Serum or plasma (heparin)	*mg/dL*	*mmol/L*
		Adult: 8–25	0.30–0.90 (conv. factor based on oleic acid, M.W. 282.47)
		Child and obese adult: < 31	< 1.10
Fatty Acids, Total	Serum	190–420 mg/dL	7–15 mmol/L
Ferritin	Serum	*ng/mL*	*µg/L*
		Newborn: 25–200	25–200
		1 mo: 200–600	200–600
		2–5 mo: 50–200	50–200
		6 mo–15 y: 7–140	7–140
		Adult, M: 15–200	15–200
		F: 12–150	12–150
α_1-Fetoprotein	Serum	Adult: < 30 ng/mL	< 30 µg/L
		Mean: 2.6 ± 1.6 (1 SD) ng/mL	2.6 ± 1.6 (1 SD) µg/L
		Fetal: peak of 200–400 mg/dL in first trimester	Peak of 2–4 g/L in first trimester
		1 y: < 30 ng/mL	< 30 µg/L
	Amniotic fluid	*mg/dL*	*mg/L*
		Weeks / *median* / *± 2 log SD*	*median* / *± 2 log SD*
		11–12 / 2.4 / 1.0–5.0	24 / 10–50
		13–14 / 2.3 / 1.3–4.1	23 / 13–41
		15–16 / 1.8 / 0.9–3.5	18 / 9–35
		17–18 / 1.5 / 0.6–3.3	15 / 6–33
		19–20 / 1.0 / 0.5–2.5	10 / 5–25
		21–25 / 0.7 / 0.4–1.4	7 / 4–14
		26–30 / 0.6 / 0.3–1.0	6 / 3–10
		31–35 / 0.2 / 0.05–0.7	2 / 0.5–7.0
		36–40 / 0.1 / 0.02–0.3	1 / 0.2–3.0
Fibrinogen, see *Hematology section*			
FIGLU *Dose: 5 g histidine q 4 h × 3*	Urine, 24 h, after initial dose of histidine	< 35 mg/d	< 200 µmol/d
Folate	Serum	1.8–9 ng/mL	4.1–20.4 nmol/L
		> 60 y: 1.8–12 ng/mL	4.1–27.2 nmol/L
	Erythrocytes (EDTA)	150–450 ng/mL packed cells	340–1020 nmol/L packed cells
		< 60 y: 95–500 ng/mL packed cells	215–1132 nmol/L packed cells
Folate Absorption Test	Urine, 24 h	45 ± 7% of dose	Fraction of dose: 0.45 ± 0.07

CLINICAL CHEMISTRY, TOXICOLOGY, SEROLOGY *(Continued)*

Test	Specimen	Reference Range	Reference Range (International Units)
Follicle-Stimulating Hormone (FSH)	Serum or plasma (heparin)	*mIU/mL*	*IU/L*
		Adult, M: 4–25	4–25
		F,	
		Premenopausal: 4–30	4–30
		Midcycle peak: 10–90	10–90
		Pregnancy: low to undetectable	low to undetectable
		Postmenopausal: 40–250	40–250
	Urine, 24 h	*IU/d (IRP-2-hMG)*	*IU/d (IRP-2-hMG)*
		Birth-1 y, F: < 0.5–1.4	< 0.5–1.4
		1–8 y, M: < 0.5–4.5	< 0.5–4.5
		F: < 0.5–4.0	< 0.5–4.0
		9–10 y, M: 1–5	1–5
		F: 1–4	1–4
		11–12 y, M: 1.5–5	1.5–5
		F: 1–8	1–8
		13–14 y, M: 2–12	2–12
		F: 1–10	1–10
		Adult, M: 4–18	4–18
		F: 3–12	3–12
		Higher in males > 60 y	Higher in males > 60 y
Free Thyroxine Index (FT_4I)	Serum	*FT_4 Index* 1.2–5.0	
with normalized T_3RU		1–3 d: 9.3–26.6	
		1–4 wk: 7.6–20.8	
		1–4 mo: 7.4–17.9	
		4–12 mo: 6.1–14.5	
		1–6 y: 5.7–13.3	
		6–10 y: 5.5–10.0	
		> 10 y: 5.5–10.0	
		Borderline low: 4.8	
		Borderline high: 14.0	
Free Triiodothyronine, see *Triiodothyronine, Free*			
Fructose	Serum	1–6 mg/dL	55.5–333.0 μmol/L
	Urine	< 60 mg/d	< 333 μmol/d
Gastric Secretion Rate	Total gastric contents, six 15 min spec.	BAO: 0–5 mmol/h	0–5 mmol/h
		PAO: 5–20 mmol/h (post pentagastrin)	5–20 mmol/h (post pentagastrin)
		BAO/PAO: 0.20	0.20
Gastrin	Serum	< 60 y: < 100 pg/mL	< 100 ng/L
		> 60 y: upper 15% of population: 100–800 pg/mL	upper 15% of population: 100–800 ng/L
Gastrin-Calcium Infusion Stimulation Test	Serum	Gastrin: Slight or no increase Z.E. syndrome: > 450 pg/mL	Gastrin: Slight or no increase Z.E. syndrome: > 450 ng/L
Gastrin-Secretin Stimulation Test	Serum, fasting, at 15 min intervals for 1 h	No response or slight suppression	No response or slight suppression
IV dose: 5 U secretin/kg		Z.E. syndrome: Increase > 110 pg/mL if base level 80–500 pg/mL; increase > 1400 pg/mL if basal level is high	Z.E. syndrome: Increase > 110 ng/L if base level 80–500 ng/L; increase > 1400 ng/mL if basal level is high
Glucose	Serum	*mg/dL*	*mmol/L*
		Cord: 45–96	2.5–5.3
		Premature: 20–60	1.1–3.3
		Neonate: 30–60	1.7–3.3
		Newborn,	
		1 d: 40–60	2.2–3.3
		> 1 d: 50–80	2.8–4.4
		Child: 60–100	3.3–5.5
		Adult: 70–105	3.9–5.8
		> 60 y: 80–115	4.4–6.4
	Whole blood (heparin)	Adult: 65–95	3.6–5.3
	CSF	Adult: 40–70	2.2–3.9
Quantitative, enzymatic	Urine	< 0.5 g/d	< 2.8 mmol/d
Qualitative	Urine	Negative	Negative

CLINICAL CHEMISTRY, TOXICOLOGY, SEROLOGY *(Continued)*

Test	Specimen	Reference Range	Reference Range (International Units)
Glucose, 2 h Postprandial	Serum	< 120 mg/dL Diabetes: see *Glucose Tolerance Test, Oral*	<6.7 mmol/L
Glucose Tolerance Test (GTT) with Cortisone *Dose: 50 mg, 8.5 and 2 h before test*	Plasma (fluoride oxalate); fasting, 1, 1½, 2 h after glucose ingestion	*Glucose* *mg/dL* Fasting: 70–105 1 h: < 200 1½ h: < 200 2 h: < 140	*mmol/L* 3.9–5.8 < 11 < 11 < 7.8
Glucose Tolerance Test (GTT), *Oral*	Serum	*mg/dL* Adult, *Normal* *Diabetic* Fasting: 70–105 > 140 60 min: 120–170 ≥ 200 90 min: 100–140 ≥ 200 120 min: 70–120 ≥ 140	*mmol/L* *Normal* *Diabetic* 3.9–5.8 > 7.8 6.7–9.4 ≥ 11 5.6–7.8 ≥ 11 3.9–6.7 ≥ 7.8
IV	Serum	5 min: ~ 250 mg/dL 90 min: at or below fasting concentration or K = > 1.5%	5 min: ~13.9 mmol/L
γ-Glutamyltransferase (GGT), 37°C, ***aca***	Serum	M: 9–50 U/L F: 8–40 U/L	M: 9–50 U/L F: 8–40 U/L
Glycerol, Free	Plasma	3–10 y: 0.56–2.14 mg/dL 11–80 y: 0.29–1.72 mg/dL	0.061–0.232 mmol/L 0.032–0.187 mmol/L
Gold	Serum	< 10 μg/dL Therap. range: 38–500 μg/dL	< 0.51 μmol/L Therap. range: 1.93–25.40 μmol/L
	Urine, 24 h	< 1 μg/d	< 5 nmol/d
Gonadotropins, see *Pregnancy Tests* and *Chorionic Gonadotropin, β-subunit*			
Growth Hormone (HGH, Somatotropin)	Serum or plasma (EDTA, heparin)	*ng/mL* Cord: 10–50 Newborn: 10–40 Child: < 1–10 (occasional values up to 20) Adult, M: < 2 F: < 10 > 60 y, M: 0.4–10 F: 1–14	*μg/L* 10–50 10–40 < 1–10 < 2 < 10 0.4–10 1–14
Growth Hormone–Arginine Stimulation Test *Dose, adult: 30 g arginine HCl IV within 30 min; child: 0.5 g/kg*	Serum, fasting, 30 min intervals for 2 h	Fasting: < 5 ng/mL; rise to > 7 ng/mL during test (peak range 8–35 ng/mL) at 30–60 min	Fasting: < 5 μg/L; rise to > 7 μg/L during test (peak range 8–35 μg/L) at 30–60 min
Growth Hormone–Glucagon Stimulation Test *Dose: 1 mg glucagon IM or SC*	Serum, fasting, then hourly for 3–4 h	> 7 ng/mL after stimulation or > 5 ng/mL rise above baseline	> 7 μg/L after stimulation or > 5 μg/L rise above baseline
Growth Hormone–L-Dopa Stimulation Test *Dose, adult: 500 mg L-dopa, orally; child: 10 mg/kg*	Serum, fasting, 30, 60, 90, 120, and 180 min after L-dopa	Peak: > 7 ng/mL or > 5 ng/mL rise above baseline	> 7 μg/L or > 5 μg/L rise above baseline
Haptoglobin, see *Hematology section*			
HDL-Cholesterol (HDLC)	Serum or plasma (EDTA)	*mg/dL* *M* *F* Mean, adult: 45 55 Cord: 5–50 5–50 < 19 y: 30–65 30–70 20–29 y: 30–70 30–75 40+ y: 30–70 30–85 Values for blacks, ~ 10 mg/dL higher *HDLC, % of total cholesterol:* *CHD Risk* *M* *F* Dangerous: < 7 < 12 High: 7–15 12–18 Average: 15–25 18–27 Below average: 25–37 27–40 Protection probable: > 37 > 40	*nmol/L* *M* *F* 1.17 1.42 0.13–1.30 0.13–1.30 0.78–1.68 0.78–1.81 0.78–1.81 0.78–1.94 0.78–1.81 0.78–2.20 *Fraction HDLC of total cholesterol* *M* *F* < 0.07 < 0.12 0.07–0.15 0.12–0.18 0.15–0.25 0.18–0.27 0.25–0.37 0.27–0.40 > 0.37 > 0.40

CLINICAL CHEMISTRY, TOXICOLOGY, SEROLOGY *(Continued)*

Test	Specimen	Reference Range	Reference Range (International Units)
Hemoglobin A_{1c}	Whole blood (heparin, EDTA or oxalate)		
Electrophoresis		5.6–7.5% of total Hb	Fraction of Hb: 0.056–0.075
Column		6–9% of total Hb	Fraction of Hb: 0.06–0.09
Homovanillic Acid (HVA)	Urine, 24 h	Child: 3–16 μg/mg creatinine Adult: < 15 mg/d	1.9–10 mmol/mol creatinine < 82 μmol/d
17-Hydroxycorticosteroids (17-OHCS)	Urine, 24 h	*mg/d* 0–1 y: 0.5–1.0 Child: 1.0–5.6 Adult, M: 3.0–10.0 F: 2.0–8.0 or: 3–7 mg/g creatinine	*μmol/d* 1.4–2.8 2.8–15.5 8.2–27.6 5.5–22 or: 0.9–2.5 mmol/mol creatinine (conv. factor based on hydrocortisone, M.W. 362)
5-Hydroxyindole Acetic Acid (5-HIAA)			
Qualitative	Fresh random urine	Negative	Negative
Quantitative	Urine, 24 h	2–8 mg/d	10.5–42 μmol/d
17-Hydroxyprogesterone (17-OHP)	Serum	*ng/mL* M, Pub. stage I: 0.1–0.3 Adult: 0.2–1.8 F, Pub. stage I: 0.2–0.5 Follicular: 0.2–0.8 Luteal: 0.8–3.0 Postmenopausal: 0.04–0.5	*nmol/L* 0.3–0.9 0.6–5.4 0.6–1.5 0.6–2.4 2.4–9.0 0.12–1.5
Immunoglobulin A (IgA)	Serum	*mg/dL* Cord: 0–5 Newborn: 0–2.2 4–6 mo: 3–82 6 mo–2 y: 14–108 2–6 y: 23–190 6–12 y: 29–270 12–16 y: 81–232 Adult: 76–390	*mg/L* 0–50 0–22 30–820 140–1080 230–1900 290–2700 810–2320 760–3900
Immunoglobulin D (IgD)			
RID	Serum	Newborn: None detected Adult: 0–8 mg/dL	None detected 0–0.44 μmol/L
Immunoglobulin E (IgE)			
RID	Serum	*IU/mL* Adult: 0–380 < 60 y, M: 0–250 F: 0–175	*kIU/mL* 0–380 0–250 0–175
Immunoglobulin G (IgG)			
Nephelometric	Serum	*mg/dL* Cord: 760–1700 Newborn: 700–1480 ½–6 mo: 300–1000 6 mo–2 y: 500–1200 2–6 y: 500–1300 6–12 y: 700–1650 12–16 y: 700–1550 Adult: 600–1600 (higher in blacks)	*g/L* 7.6–17 7–14.8 3–10 5–12 5–13 7–16.5 7–15.5 6–16
	CSF	0.5–5 mg/dL	5–50 mg/L
Immunoglobulin G/Albumin Ratio	CSF and serum	0.3–0.6	0.3–0.6
Immunoglobulin G Synthesis Rate	CSF and serum	(−9.9) to (+3.3) mg/d	(−9.9) to (+3.3) mg/d

CLINICAL CHEMISTRY, TOXICOLOGY, SEROLOGY (*Continued*)

Test	Specimen	Reference Range	Reference Range (International Units)
Immunoglobulin M (IgM)	Serum	*mg/dL* Cord: 4–24 Newborn: 5–30 ½–6 mo: 15–109 6 mo–2 y: 43–239 2–6 y: 50–199 6–12 y: 50–260 12–16 y: 45–240 Adult: 40–345 Results vary with std. preparation	*mg/L* 40–240 50–300 150–1090 430–2390 500–1990 500–2600 450–2400 400–3450
	CSF	0–1.3 mg/dL	0–13 mg/L
Insulin (12 h Fasting)	Serum	*μIU/mL* Newborn: 3–20 Adult: 6–24 < 60 y: 6–35	*mIU/L* 3–20 6–24 6–35
Insulin with Oral Glucose Tolerance Test	Serum	*Min* *Insulin, μIU/mL* 0: 6–24 30: 25–231 60: 18–276 120: 16–166 180: 4–38	*mIU/L* 6–24 25–231 18–276 16–166 4–38
Insulin Tolerance Test			
Dose: 0.1–0.15 U/kg IV	Serum	*Glucose:* Decrease ~50% of the fasting level by 30 min and return to normal fasting limits by 90–120 min *HGH:* Increase of > 5 ng/mL within 60 min of hypoglycemia or > 20 ng/mL *Cortisol:* Increase of > 6 μg/dL with peak of > 20 μg/dL	Fractional decrease in glucose ~0.50 of the fasting level by 30 min and return to normal fasting limits by 90–120 min *HGH:* Increase of > 5 μg/L within 60 min of hypoglycemia or > 20 μg/mL Cortisol: Increase of > 165 nmol/L with peak of > 552 nmol/L
Intrinsic Factor, see *Vitamin* B_{12} *Intrinsic Factor*			
Inulin Clearance Test	Serum and urine	*Mean (±2 SD) mL/min* M / F 20–29 y: 132 (90–174) / 119 (84–156) 30–39 y: 128 (88–168) / 116 (82–150) 40–49 y: 120 (78–162) / 114 (82–146) 50–59 y: 110 (68–152) / 104 (66–142) 60–69 y: 97 (57–137) / 94 (58–130) 70–79 y: 82 (42–122) / 83 (45–121) 80–89 y: 67 (39–105) / 67 (39–105)	
Iron	Serum	*μg/dL* Newborn: 100–250 Infant: 40–100 Child: 50–120 Adult, M: 50–160 F: 40–150	*μmol/L* 17.90–44.75 7.16–17.90 8.95–21.48 8.95–28.64 7.16–26.85
Iron-Binding Capacity, Total (TIBC)	Serum	*μg/dL* Infant: 100–400 Thereafter: 250–400	*μmol/L* 17.90–71.60 44.75–71.60
Iron Saturation	Serum	20–55%	Fraction of iron saturation 0.20–0.55
17-Ketogenic Steroids (17-KGS)	Urine, 24 h	*mg/d* 0–1 y: < 1.0 1–10 y: < 5 11–14 y: < 12 Adult, M: 5–23 F: 3–15 > 70 y, M: 3–15 F: 3–13	*μmol/d* < 3.5 (conv. factor based on DHEA, M.W. 288) < 17 < 42 17–80 10–52 10–52 10–45
Ketone bodies			
Qualitative	Serum Urine, random	Negative (0.5–3.0 mg/dL) Negative	Negative (5–30 mg/L) Negative

CLINICAL CHEMISTRY, TOXICOLOGY, SEROLOGY (*Continued*)

Test	Specimen	Reference Range	Reference Range (International Units)
17-Ketosteroids (17-KS), Total			
		mg/d	*μmol/d*
Zimmerman reaction	Urine, 24 h	14 d–2 y: < 1	< 3.5 (conv. factor based on DHEA, M.W. 288)
		2–6 y: < 2	< 7
		6–10 y: 1–4	3.5–14
		10–12 y: 1–6	3.5–21
		12–14 y: 3–10	10–35
		14–16 y: 5–12	17–42
		Adult,	
		M, 18–30: 9–22	31–76
		M, > 30: 8–20	28–70
		F: 6–15	21–52
		Decreases with age	Decreases with age
Chromatography	Urine, 24 h	Adult, M: 5.0–12.0	Adult, M: 17–42
		F: 3.0–10.0	F: 10–35
LDL-Cholesterol (LDLC)	Serum or plasma (EDTA)	*mg/dL*	*mmol/L*
		M / *F*	*M* / *F*
		Cord blood: 10–50 / 10–50	0.26–1.30 / 0.26–1.30
		0–19 y: 60–140 / 60–150	1.55–3.63 / 1.55–3.89
		20–29 y: 60–175 / 60–160	1.55–4.53 / 1.55–4.14
		30–39 y: 80–190 / 70–170	2.07–4.92 / 1.81–4.40
		40–49 y: 90–205 / 80–190	2.33–5.31 / 2.07–4.92
		50–59 y: 90–205 / 90–220	2.33–5.31 / 2.33–5.70
		60–69 y: 90–215 / 100–235	2.33–5.57 / 2.59–6.09
		≥ 70 y: 90–190 / 95–215	2.33–4.92 / 2.46–5.57
		Recommended (desirable) range for adults: 65–175 mg/dL	1.68–4.53
L-Lactate	Whole blood (heparin)	*mg/dL*	*mmol/L*
		Venous: 4.5–19.8	0.5–2.2
		Arterial: 4.5–14.4	0.5–1.6
		Inpatients,	
		Venous: 8.1–15.3	0.9–1.7
		Arterial: < 11.3	< 1.25
Lactate Dehydrogenase (LDH), 30°C			
		U/L	*U/L*
Total (L → P)	Serum	Newborn: 160–450	160–450
		Neonate: 300–1500	300–1500
		Infant: 100–250	100–250
		Child: 60–170	60–170
		Adult: 45–90	45–90
		> 60 y: 55–100	55–100
		150–320	150–320
Total (P → L)	CSF	~ 10% of serum value	~ 0.10 fraction of serum value
Isoenzymes Electrophoresis (Agarose)	Serum	%	*Fraction of total:*
		Fraction 1: 14–26	0.14–0.26
		Fraction 2: 29–39	0.29–0.39
		Fraction 3: 20–26	0.20–0.26
		Fraction 4: 8–16	0.08–0.16
		Fraction 5: 6–16	0.06–0.16
Lactate/Pyruvate Ratio	Whole blood (heparin)	10/1	10/1
Lead	Whole blood (heparin)	*μg/dL*	*μmol/L*
		Child: < 30	< 1.45
		Adult: < 40	< 1.93
		Toxic: ≥ 100	≥ 4.83
	Urine, 24 h	< 80 μg/L	< 0.39 μmol/L
Lipase	Serum		
Tietz method		< 1.0 unit/mL	< 278 U/L
BMD turbidimetric		Adult: 10–150 U/L	10–150 U/L
		> 60 y: 18–180 U/L	18–180 U/L
Lithium	Serum, plasma, whole blood (heparin, EDTA)	Therap. conc.: 0.6–1.2 mEq/L	0.6–1.2 mmol/L
		Toxic conc.: > 2 mEq/L	> 2 mmol/L

CLINICAL CHEMISTRY, TOXICOLOGY, SEROLOGY (*Continued*)

Test	Specimen	Reference Range	Reference Range (International Units)
Luteinizing Hormone (LH)	Serum or plasma (heparin)	*mIU/mL* M, 10–13 y: 4–12 12–17 y: 6–16 15–18 y: 7–19 Adult: 6–23 F, 9–14 y: 2.0–14.0 12–18 y: 3.0–29.0 F, Follicular phase: 5–30 Midcycle: 75–150 Luteal: 3–30 Postmenopausal: 30–130	*IU/L* 4–12 6–16 7–19 6–23 2.0–14.0 3.0–29.0 5–30 75–150 3–30 30–130
	Urine	*IU/d* 11–13 y: 0.48–11.28 13–15 y: 2.6–27.6 15–17 y: 4.6–24.0 Adult, M: 13–60 F, Follicular phase: 7.2–23.5	*IU/d* 0.48–11.28 2.6–27.6 4.6–24.0 13–60 7.2–23.5
Lysozyme	Serum, plasma (EDTA)	5–15 μg/mL	5–15 mg/L
Magnesium	Serum	1.3–2.1 mEq/L higher in females during menses	0.65–1.05 mmol/L
	Urine, 24 h	6.0–10.0 mEq/d	3.00–5.00 mmol/d
Mercury	Whole blood (EDTA)	< 5.0 μg/dL	< 0.25 μmol/L
	Urine, 24 h	< 20 μg/L Toxic: > 150 μg/L	< 0.1 μmol/L > 0.75 μmol/L
Metanephrine, Total	Urine, 24 h	*μg/mg creatinine* < 1 y: 0.001–4.60 1–2 y: 0.27–5.38 2–5 y: 0.35–2.99 5–10 y: 0.43–2.70 10–15 y: 0.001–1.87 15–18 y: 0.001–0.67 Adult: 0.05–1.20	*mmol/mol creatinine* 0.0006–2.64 0.15–3.09 0.20–1.72 0.25–1.55 0.0006–1.07 0.0006–0.38 0.03–0.69
Methanol	Whole blood (fluoride/oxalate)	< 0.15 mg/dL Toxic: > 20 mg/dL	< 0.05 mmol/L > 6.24 mmol/L
	Urine	Occup. exposure: < 5.0 mg/dL	< 1.6 mmol/L
	Breath	< 0.8 ppm Occup. exposure: > 2.5 ppm	< 0.02 mmol/L > 0.08 mmol/L
Metyrapone (Metopyrone) Stimulation Test	Serum	11-Deoxycortisol: > 7.0 μg/dL Cortisol: < 8 μg/dL	11-Deoxycortisol: > 200 nmol/L Cortisol: < 220 nmol/L
Dose, adult: 750 mg q 4 h × 6; child: 300 mg/m²	Urine, 24 h	17-KGS: 2.5- to 3-fold rise, but at least 10 mg/d 17-KS: > 2× base level 17-OHCS: 3–5× base level	17-KGS: 2.5- to 3-fold rise but at least 35 μmol/d* 17-KS: > 2× base level 17-OHCS: 3–5× base level *(conv. factor based on DHEA, M.W. 288)
Single-Dose Metyrapone Test *Dose: 30 mg/kg orally with milk or snack at midnight*	Serum for 11-deoxycortisol determination at 0800 h following morning	> 7 μg/dL	> 200 nmol/L
Microsomal Antibodies, Thyroid, see *Thyroid Microsomal Antibodies*			
Myelin Basic Protein	CSF	< 4 ng/mL	< 4 μg/L
Myoglobin	Serum	*μg/mL ± 1 SD* M: 49 ± 17 F: 35 ± 14 Increases slightly with age	*μg/mL* 49 ± 17 35 ± 14
	Urine, random	Negative	Negative
Nitrogen, Total	Feces	Infant: 0.11–0.52 g N/d Adult: < 2 g N/d	7.9–37 mmol N/d < 143 mmol N/d

CLINICAL CHEMISTRY, TOXICOLOGY, SEROLOGY *(Continued)*

Test	Specimen	Reference Range	Reference Range (International Units)
Normetanephrine, Total	Plasma (EDTA and sodium metabisulfite)	Normotensive: 1.2 ng/mL ± 0.1 (SEM)	6.5 nmol/L ± 0.55
Osmolality	Serum	Child, adult: 275–295 mOsmol/kg	
	Urine, random	50–1400 mOsmol/kg, depending on fluid intake After 12 h fluid restriction: > 850 mOsmol/kg	
	Urine, 24 h	~ 300–900 mOsmol/kg	
Oxalate	Serum	1–2.4 µg/mL Ethylene glycol poisoning: > 20 µg/mL	11–27 µmol/L Ethylene glycol poisoning: > 228 µmol/L
	Urine, 24 h	8–40 µg/d Ethylene glycol poisoning: > 150 µg/d	90–456 µmol/L Ethylene glycol poisoning: > 1710 µmol/d
Oxygen, Partial Pressure (Po_2)	Whole blood (heparin), arterial	83–100 mm Hg (decreases with age and high altitude)	11–14.4 kPa
Oxygen Saturation	Whole blood (heparin), arterial	95–99%	Fraction saturated: 0.95–0.99
Po_2, see *Oxygen, Partial Pressure*			
Pentobarbital	Serum, plasma (heparin, EDTA); collect at trough conc.	*µg/mL* Therap. conc., hypnotic: 1–5 Therap. coma: 20–50 Toxic conc.: > 10	*µmol/L* 4–22 88–221 > 44
pH	Whole blood (heparin), arterial	7.35–7.45 Must be corrected for body temperature	H^+ concentration: 36–44 nmol/L
	Urine, random	Newborn/neonate: 5–7 Thereafter: 4.5–8 (average ~ 6)	0.1–10 µmol/L 0.01–32 µmol/L (average ~ 1.0 µmol/L)
Phenobarbital	Serum, plasma (heparin, EDTA); collect at trough conc.	µg/mL Therap. conc.: 15–40 Toxic conc., slowness, ataxia, nystagmus: 35–80 Coma with reflexes: 65–117 Coma without reflexes: > 100	*µmol/L* 65–172 151–345 280–504 > 430
Phenytoin (Dilantin)	Serum, plasma (heparin, EDTA); collect at steady-state trough conc.	Therap. conc.: 10–20 µg/mL Toxic conc.: > 20 µg/mL	40–79 µmol/L > 79 µmol/L
Phosphatase, Acid			
Prostatic (RIA)	Serum	< 3.0 ng/mL	< 3.0 µg/L
Roy, Brower, and Hayden, 37°C		0.11–0.60 U/L	0.11–0.60 U/L
Phosphatase, Alkaline *(p-nitrophenyl phosphate, carbonate buffer, 30°C)*	Serum	*U/L* Infant: 50–165 Child: 20–150 Adult: 20–70 > 60 yr: 30–75	*U/L* 50–165 20–150 20–70 30–75
Bowers and McComb, 30°C		25–90 U/L	25–90 U/L
IFCC, 30°C		M: 30–90 U/L F: 20–80 U/L	30–90 U/L 20–80 U/L
Phosphorus, Inorganic	Serum	*mg/dL* Cord: 3.7–8.1 Child: 4.5–5.5 Thereafter: 2.7–4.5 > 60 y, M: 2.3–3.7 F: 2.8–4.1	*nmol/L* 1.2–2.6 1.45–1.78 0.87–1.45 0.74–1.2 0.90–1.3
	Urine, 24 h	Adult, On diet containing 0.9–1.5 g P and 10 mg Ca/kg: < 1.0 g/d On nonrestricted diet: 0.4–1.3 g/d	Adult, On diet containing 29–48 mmol P and 0.25 mmol Ca/kg: < 32 mmol/d On nonrestricted diet: 13–42 mmol/d

CLINICAL CHEMISTRY, TOXICOLOGY, SEROLOGY *(Continued)*

Test	Specimen	Reference Range	Reference Range (International Units)
Porphobilinogen (PBG)			
Quantitative	Urine, 24 h	0–2.0 mg/d	0–8.8 μmol/d
Qualitative	Urine, fresh random	Negative	Negative
Potassium	Serum	*mEq/L*	*mmol/L*
		Newborn: 3.7–5.9	3.7–5.9
		Infant: 4.1–5.3	4.1–5.3
		Child: 3.4–4.7	3.4–4.7
		Thereafter: 3.5–5.1	3.5–5.1
	Plasma (heparin)	3.5–4.5 mmol/L	3.5–4.5 mmol/L
	Urine, 24 h	25–125 mEq/d; varies with diet	25–125 mmol/d; varies with diet
Pregnancy Tests			
Chorionic Gonadotropin (HCG) Tube Test			
Qualitative	Serum or urine	Negative Positive by 4th–8th d after expected menstrual period	Negative Positive by 4th–8th d after expected menstrual period
Semi-quantitative		Peak values up to 120,000 mIU/mL	Peak values up to 120,000 IU/L
Chorionic Gonadotropin, (β-HCG), see *Chorionic Gonadotropin, β-Subunit*			
Radio Receptor Assay (RRA); Qualitative	Serum	Negative; pregnancy can be detected 10 d after conception	Negative; pregnancy can be detected 10 d after conception
Pregnanediol	Urine, 24 h	*mg/d*	*μmol/d*
		< 2 y: < 0.1	< 0.3
		6–9 y: < 0.5	< 1.6
		M, 10–15 y: 0.1–0.7	0.3–2.2
		Adult: 0.6–1.5	1.9–4.7
		F, 10–15 y: 0.1–1.2	0.3–3.7
		Adult,	
		Follicular: < 1.0	<3.1
		Luteal: 2–7	6.2–22
		Postmenopausal: 0.2–1.0	0.6–3.1
		Week of pregnancy:	
		16: 5–21	16–65
		20: 6–26	19–81
		24: 12–32	37–100
		28: 19–51	59–160
		32: 22–66	69–206
		36: 13–77	41–240
		40: 23–63	72–197
Pregnanetriol	Urine, 24 h	*mg/d*	*μmol/d*
		2 wk–2 y: 0.02–0.2	0.06–0.6
		2–5 y: < 0.5	< 1.5
		5–15 y: < 1.5	< 4.5
		> 15 y: < 2.0	< 5.9
Pregnenolone	Serum	Adult: 0.3–2 ng/ml	0.9–6.3 nmol/L
Progesterone	Serum	*ng/mL*	*nmol/L*
		M, Pubertal stage I: 0.11–0.26	0.35–0.83
		Adult: 0.12–0.3	0.38–1
		F, Pubertal stage I: 0–0.3	0–1
		II: 0–0.46	0–1.5
		III: 0–0.6	0–2
		IV: 0.05–13.0	0.16–41
		Follicular; 0.02–0.9	0.06–2.9
		Luteal: 6.0–30.0	19–95
Progesterone Receptor Assay (PRA)	Tumor tissue	*fmol/mg protein*	*nmol/kg protein*
		Normal, or benign and non-responsive tumor: ≤ 5	≤ 5
		Positive: > 10	> 10
Prolactin (hPRL)	Serum	*ng/mL*	*μg/L*
		Adult, M: < 20	< 20
		F,	
		Follicular phase: <23	< 23
		Luteal phase: 5–40	5–40
		Pregnancy,	
		1st trimester: < 80	<80
		2nd trimester: < 160	<160
		3rd trimester: < 400	< 400
		Newborn: > 10-fold adult levels	

CLINICAL CHEMISTRY, TOXICOLOGY, SEROLOGY (*Continued*)

Test	Specimen	Reference Range	Reference Range (International Units)
Protein			
Total	Serum	*g/dL* Premature: 3.6–6.0 Newborn: 4.6–7.0 ≥ 3 y: 6.0–8.0 Ambulatory: 6.4–8.3 Recumbent: 6.0–7.8 > 60 y: slight lower (~0.2) ~ 0.5 g higher in ambulatory patients	*g/L* 36.0–60.0 46.0–70.0 60.0–80.0 64.0–83.0 60.0–78.0 ~ 2 ~ 5 g higher in ambulatory patients
Electrophoresis		*g/dL* Albumin, Adult: 3.5–5.0 > 60 y: 3.7–4.7 α_1-Globulin, Adult: 0.1–0.3 > 60 y: 0.2–0.5 α_2-Globulin, Adult: 0.6–1.0 > 60 y: 0.5–1.1 β-Globulin, Adult: 0.7–1.1 > 60 y: 0.5–1.2 γ-Globulin, Adult: 0.8–1.6 > 60 y: 0.6–1.6	*g/L* 35–50 37–47 1–3 2–5 6–10 5–11 7–11 5–12 8–16 6–16
Total	Urine, 24 h	1–14 mg/dL 50–80 mg/d at rest < 250 mg/d after intense exercise	10–140 mg/L 50–80 mg/d at rest < 250 mg/d after intense exercise
Electrophoresis		*Average % of Total Protein* Alb. 37.9 α_1 27.3 α_2 19.5 β 8.8 γ 3.3	*Fraction of Total* 0.379 0.273 0.195 0.088 0.033
Total	CSF		
Column		Lumbar: 8–32 mg/dL	80–320 mg/L
Turbidimetry		Lumbar, Adult: 15–45 mg/dL Newborn: 40–120 mg/dL	 150–450 mg/L 400–1200 mg/L
Electrophoresis		*% of Total* Prealbumin: 2–7 Albumin: 56–76 α_1-Globulin: 2–7 α_2-Globulin: 4–12 β-Globulin: 8–18 γ-Globulin: 3–12	*Fraction of Total* 0.02–0.07 0.56–0.76 0.02–0.07 0.04–0.12 0.08–0.18 0.03–0.12
Electrophoresis	Synovial fluid	Albumin: 63 α_1-Globulin: 7 α_2-Globulin: 7 β-Globulin: 9 γ-Globulin: 14 Fibrinogen: 0	0.63 0.07 0.07 0.09 0.14 0
Protoporphyrin	Whole blood (heparin or EDTA) Feces, 24 h	< 50 μg/dL RBC ≤ 60 μg/g dry wt or < 1500 μg/d	< 0.89 μmol/L RBC ≤ 0.11 mmol/kg dry wt or < 2.67 μmol/d
Pyruvic Acid	Whole blood (heparin)	0.3–0.9 mg/dL	0.03–0.10 mmol/L
Renal Plasma Flow (RPF)	Plasma and urine	M: 560–830 mL/min F: 490–700 mL/min or: 390 mL/min/m² body surface > 40 y: decreases ~ 75 mL/decade	
Renin	Plasma (EDTA)	*Normal sodium diet:* *ng/h/mL ± 1 SE* Supine: 1.6 ± 1.5 Standing (4 h): 4.5 ± 2.9 *Low sodium:* Supine: 3.2 ± 1.1 Standing (4 h): 9.9 ± 4.3	 *μg/h/L ± 1 SE* 1.6 ± 1.5 4.5 ± 2.9 3.2 ± 1.1 9.9 ± 4.3

CLINICAL CHEMISTRY, TOXICOLOGY, SEROLOGY *(Continued)*

Test	Specimen	Reference Range	Reference Range (International Units)
Riboflavin (Vitamin B_2)	Urine, random, fasting	*μg/g creatinine* Adult: 80–269 Pregnancy: 90–120	*μmol/mol creatinine* 24–81 27–36
Salicylates	Serum, plasma (heparin, EDTA); collect at trough conc.	Therap. conc.: 150–300 μg/mL Toxic conc.: > 300 μg/mL	1086–2172 μmol/L > 2172 μmol/L
Schilling Test (Intrinsic Factor Test) *Dose: 0.5– 1.0 μCi ^{58}Co-Vitamin B_{12}*	Urine, 24 h	> 7.5% of dose	Fraction of dose: 0.075
Secobarbital	Serum	Therap. conc.: 1–2 μg/mL Toxic conc.: > 5 μg/mL	4.2–8.4 μmol/L > 21.0 μmol/L
Sediment	Urine, fresh random		
Casts		Hyaline: occasional (0–1) casts/hpf RBC: not seen WBC: not seen Tubular epithelial: not seen Transitional and squamous epithelial: not seen	Hyaline: occasional (0–1) casts/hpf RBC: not seen WBC: not seen Tubular epithelial: not seen Transitional and squamous epithelial: not seen
Cells		RBC: 0–2/hpf WBC, Adult, M: 0–3/hpf F and child: 0–5/hpf Epithelial: few; more frequent in newborn Bacteria, Unspun: no organisms/oil immersion field Spun: < 20 organisms/hpf	RBC: 0–2/hpf WBC, M: 0–3/hpf F and child: 0–5/hpf Epithelial: few; more frequent in newborn Bacteria, Unspun: no organisms/oil immersion field Spun: < 20 organisms/hpf
Semen Analysis (Sperm Count)	Ejaculate	Volume: 2–6 mL Sperm count: > 20 million/mL Motility: > 50% Morphology: ≥ 60% normal forms	Volume: 0.002–0.006 L Sperm count: > 20 × 10^9/L Motility: Fraction of total: > 0.50 Morphology: Fraction of total: ≥ 0.60 normal forms
Sodium	Serum or plasma (heparin)	*mEq/L* Newborn: 134–146 Infant: 139–146 Child: 138–145 Thereafter: 136–146	*mmol/L* 134–146 139–146 138–145 136–146
	Urine, 24 h	40–220 mEq/d (diet dependent)	40–220 mmol/d
	Sweat	10–40 mEq/L	10–40 mmol/L
Specific Gravity	Urine, random	Adult: 1.002–1.030 After 12 h fluid restriction: > 1.025	Adult: 1.002–1.030 After 12 h fluid restriction: > 1.025
	Urine, 24 h	1.015–1.025	
Testosterone, Free	Serum	*ng/dL* — *% of total* *(mean ± 1 SE)* Cord, M: 1.0±0.4 — 2.9±0.6 F: 0.89±0.29 — 3.0±0.5 1–15 d, M: 0.8±0.8 — 1.3±0.2 F: 0.14±0.06 — 1.2±0.2 Prepubertal, M: 0.04±0.01 — 0.7±0.2 F: 0.04±0.01 — 0.7±0.1 Adult, M: 7.9±2.3 — 1.4±0.3 F: 0.31±0.07 — 0.9±0.2	*pmol/L* — *% of total* *(mean ± 1 SE)* 34.7±14 — 0.029±0.006 31±10 — 0.03±0.005 27.8±27.8 — 0.013±0.002 4.9±2 — 0.012±0.002 1.4±0.3 — 0.007±0.002 1.4±0.3 — 0.007±0.001 274±80 — 0.014±0.003 10.8±2.4 — 0.009±0.002

Test	Specimen	Reference Range	Reference Range (International Units)
Testosterone, Total	Serum	*ng/dL*	*nmol/L*
		Prepubertal,	
		M: 6.6 ± 2.5	0.23 ± 0.09
		F: 6.6 ± 2.5	0.23 ± 0.09
		Adult, M: 572 ± 135	19.8 ± 4.7
		F: 35 ± 10	1.3 ± 0.3
	Urine	*Pubertal stage* — *μg/kg body weight*	*nmol/kg body weight*
		I, M: 0.25	0.87
		F: 0.16	0.55
		II, M: 0.34	1.18
		F: 0.16	0.55
		III, M: 0.37	1.28
		F: 0.16	0.55
		μg/d	*nmol/d*
		20–50 y,	
		M: 50–135	173–470
		F: 2–12	7–42
		< 50 y,	
		M: 40–60	139–210
		F: 2–8	7–28
Thiopental	Serum, plasma (heparin, EDTA); collect at trough conc.	*μg/mL*	*μmol/L*
		Therap. conc.,	
		Hypnotic: 1.0–5.0	4.1–20.7
		Therap. coma: 30–100	123.9–413
		Anesthesia: 7–130	29–537
		Toxic conc.: > 10	> 41
Thyroglobulin (Tg)	Serum	< 50 ng/mL	< 50 μg/L
Thyroid Antibodies	Serum	Adult: ≤ 1:10 dilution Child: ≤ 1:4	Adult: ≤ 1:10 dilution Child: ≤ 1:4
Thyroid Microsomal Antibodies	Serum	Nondetectable (hemagglutination) or < 1:10 (IFA)	Nondetectable (hemagglutination) or < 1:10 (IFA)
Thyroid-Stimulating Hormone (hTSH)	Serum or plasma	*μIU/mL*	*mIU/L*
		Cord: 3–12	3–12
		Child: 4.5 ± 3.6	4.5 ± 3.6
		Adult: 2–10	2–10
		> 60 y, M: 2–7.3	2–7.3
		F: 2–16.8	2–16.8
Thyroid-Stimulating Hormone—Response to TRH	Serum	30 min after stimulation: *μU/mL*	30 min after stimulation: *mIU/L*
		Child: 11–35	Child: 11–35
		Adult, M: 15–30	Adult, M: 15–30
		F: 20–40	F: 20–40
Thyroid Uptake of Radioactive Iodine	Activity over thyroid gland	2 h: < 6% 6 h: 3–20% 24 h: 8–30%	Fractional uptake: 2 h: < 0.06 6 h: 0.03–0.20 24 h: 0.08–0.30
Thyroid Uptake of $^{99m}TcO_4^-$	Activity over thyroid gland	Uptake ratio: < 1.15 in euthyroid	< 1.15
Thyrotropin-Releasing Hormone	Plasma	5–60 pg/mL	50–60 ng/L
Thyrotropin-Releasing Hormone Stimulation Test *Dose, adult: 500 μg TRH IV*	Serum	TSH within 30 min, < 40y: > 6 μIU/mL rise > 40 y, M: > 2 μIU/mL rise hPRL: 3– to 5–fold rise above baseline (diminishes with age)	TSH within 30 min, < 40 y: > 6 μIU/mL rise > 40 y, M: > 2 μIU/mL rise hPRL: 3– to 5–fold rise above baseline (diminishes with age)
Thyroxine (T_4), Total	Serum	*μg/dL*	*nmol/L*
		Cord: 8–13	103–167
		Newborn: 11.5–24	148–310
		Neonate: 9–18	116–232
		Infant: 7–15	90–194
		1–5 y: 7.3–15	94–194
		5–10 y: 6.4–13.3	83–172
		Thereafter: 5–12	65–155
		> 60 y, M: 5.0–10.0	65–129
		F: 5.5–10.5	71–135
		Pregnancy, last 5 mo: 6.1–17.6	79–227
Thyroxine-Binding Globulin (TBG)	Serum	15.0–34.0 μg/mL	15.0–34.0 mg/L
Thyroxine Ratio, Effective (ETR)		0.86–1.13	0.86–1.13
Thyroxine, Free (FT_4)	Serum	0.8–2.4 ng/dL	10–31 pmol/L

CLINICAL CHEMISTRY, TOXICOLOGY, SEROLOGY *(Continued)*

Test	Specimen	Reference Range	Reference Range (International Units)
Thyroxine Index, Free, see *Free Thyroxine Index*			
Thyroxine/TBG Ratio	Serum	0.2–0.5 T_4 (μg/dL)/TBG (μg/mL)	2.7–6.4 T_4 (nmol/L)/TBG (mg/L)
Transferrin	Serum	Adult: 220–400 mg/dL > 60 y: 180–380 mg/dL	2.20–4.0 g/L 1.80–3.80 g/L
Transketolase			
Ribose/sedoheptulose, 37°C	Whole blood (heparin)	9–12 μmol/h/mL whole blood 2.1–2.4 μmol/h/10^9 red cells	150–200 U/L whole blood 0.035–0.040 nU/red cell
Trigylcerides (TG)	Serum, after ≥ 12 h fast	*mg/dL*: M, F Cord blood: 10–98, 10–98 0–5 y: 30–86, 32–99 6–11 y: 31–108, 35–114 12–15 y: 36–138, 41–138 16–19 y: 40–163, 40–128 20–29 y: 44–185, 40–128 30–39 y: 49–284, 38–160 40–49 y: 56–298, 44–186 50–59 y: 62–288, 55–247 Values decrease slightly above age 60 Levels for blacks: 10–20 mg/dL lower *Recommended* (desirable) levels for adults: M: 40–160 mg/dL F: 35–135 mg/dL	*mmol/L*: M, F 0.11–1.11, 0.11–1.11 0.34–0.97, 0.36–1.12 0.35–1.22, 0.40–1.29 0.41–1.56, 0.46–1.56 0.45–1.84, 0.45–1.45 0.50–2.09, 0.45–1.45 0.55–3.21, 0.43–1.81 0.63–3.37, 0.50–2.10 0.70–3.25, 0.62–2.79 (conv. factor based on triolein, M.W. 885) Values decrease slightly above age 60 Levels for blacks: 0.11–0.23 mmol/L lower *Recommended* (desirable) levels for adults: M: 0.45–1.81 mmol/L F: 0.40–1.53 mmol/L
Triiodothyronine (T_3-RIA)	Serum	*ng/dL* Cord: 30–70 Newborn: 75–260 1–5 y: 100–260 5–10 y: 90–240 10–15 y: 80–210 Thereafter: 115–190 > 60 y, M: 105–175 F: 108–205	*nmol/L* 0.46–1.08 1.16–4.00 1.54–4.00 1.39–3.70 1.23–3.23 1.77–2.93 1.62–2.69 1.66–3.16
Triiodothyronine, Free	Serum	*mean pg/dL* Cord: 130 ± 10 (SE) 1–3 d: 410 ± 20 6 wk: 400 ± 20 Adult (20–50 y): 230–660	*mean pmol/L* 2.00 ± 0.15 (SE) 6.31 ± 0.31 6.16 ± 0.31 3.54–10.10
Triiodothyronine Index, Free	Serum	1–5 y: 165 5–10 y: 150 10–15 y: 130	
Triiodothyronine Resin Uptake Test (T_3RU)	Serum	Newborn: 25–37% Adult: 24–34% > 60 y: 23–32%	Fractional uptake: Newborn: 0.25–0.37 Adult: 0.24–0.34 > 60 y: 0.23–0.32
Triolein-^{131}I Absorption Test	Plasma	> 1.7% of administered dose/L after 4–6 h	Fraction of administered dose: > 0.017/L
Dose: 50 μCi in milk	Feces, 72 h	< 5% of administered dose in 72 h specimen	Fraction of administered dose: < 0.05/72 h
Tubular Reabsorption of Phosphate (TRP)	Urine, 4 h (0800–1200 h) and serum	82–95%	Fraction reabsorbed: 0.82–0.95
Urea Nitrogen	Serum or plasma	*mg/dL* Cord: 21–40 Premature (1 wk): 3–25 Newborn: 4–12 Infant/child: 5–18 Adult: 7–18 > 60 y: 8–21 Higher after high protein intake	*mmol urea/L* 3.5–6.6 0.5–4.2 0.7–2.0 0.8–3.0 1.2–3.0 1.3–3.5
	Urine	12–20 g/d	200–333 mmol urea/d
Urea Nitrogen/Creatinine Ratio	Serum	12/1 to 20/1 Varies with diet and methods used	12/1 to 20/1

Test	Specimen	Reference Range	Reference Range (International Units)
Uric Acid			
Phosphotungstate	Serum	*mg/dL*	*μmol/L*
		Adult, M: 4.5–8.2	268–488
		F: 3.0–6.5	178–387
		> 60 y, M: 4.2–8.0	250–476
		F: 3.2–7.3	190–434
Uricase		Child: 2.0–5.5	119–327
		Adult, M: 3.5–7.2	208–428
		F: 2.6–6.0	155–357
	Urine, 24 h	*mg/d*	*mmol/d*
		Free purine diet	
		M: < 420	< 2.48
		F: slightly lower	
		Low purine diet,	
		M: < 480	< 2.83
		F: < 400	< 2.36
		High purine diet: < 1000	< 5.90
		Average diet: 250–750	1.48–4.43
Urinary Sediment, see *Sediment*			
Urobilinogen	Urine, 2 h	0.1–0.8 EU/2 h	0.1–0.8 EU/2 h
	Urine, 24 h	0.5–4.0 EU/d	0.5–4.0 EU/d
	Feces	75–275 EU/100 g	770–2750 EU/kg
		74–400 EU/d	75–400 EU/d
		40–280 mg/d	67–473 μmol/d
Uroporphyrin	Urine, 24 h	< 50 μg/d	< 60 nmol/d
	Feces, 24 h specimen	10–40 μg/d	12–48 nmol/d
	Erythrocytes (heparin or EDTA)	Negative	Negative
Vanillylmandelic Acid (Vanilmandelic Acid)	Urine, 24 h	*mg/d*	*μmol/d*
		Newborn: < 1.0	< 5.1
		Infant: < 2.0	< 10.1
		Child: 1–5	5.1–25.3
		Adolescent: 1–5	5.1–25.3
		Thereafter: 2–7	10.1–35.4
		or 1.5–7 μg/mg creatinine	or 0.86–4 mmol/mol creatinine
Viscosity	Serum	1.10–1.22 Centipoise	1.10–1.22 Centipoise
Vitamin A	Serum	30–65 μg/dL	1.05–2.27 μmol/L
Vitamin A Tolerance Test	Serum	3 and/or 6 h: 200–600 μg vit. A/dL	7–21 μmol/L
Dose: 5000 U vit. A in oil/kg orally			
Vitamin B_2, see *Riboflavin*			
Vitamin B_6	Plasma (EDTA)	3.6–18 ng/mL	14.6–72.8 nmol/L
Vitamin B_{12}	Serum	100–700 pg/mL	74–516 pmol/L
		> 60 y: 110–800 pg/mL	81–590 pmol/L
Vitamin B_{12} Intrinsic Factor	Gastric juice	50–400% enhancement of $^{57}Co-B_{12}$ uptake by GPIMH	Fractional increase in $^{57}Co-B_{12}$ uptake by GPIMH: 0.50–4.00
Vitamin C	Plasma (oxalate, heparin, or EDTA)	0.6–2.0 mg/dL	34–114 μmol/L
	Buffy coat (heparin)	20–53 μg/10^8 WBC	11.4–30.1 amol/cell
Vitamin C Saturation Test	Urine, 24 h	60–80% of test dose excreted	Fraction test dose excreted: 0.60–0.80
Vitamin D_3, 25-hydroxy	Plasma (heparin)	Summer: 15–80 ng/mL	37.4–200 nmol/L
		Winter: 14–42 ng/mL	34.9–105 nmol/L
Vitamin D_3, 1.25–dihydroxy	Serum	25–45 pg/mL	60–108 pmol/L
Vitamin E	Serum	5.0–20 μg/mL	11.6–46.4 μmol/L
Xylose Absorption Test	Whole blood (Na-fluoride)	*mg/dL*	*mmol/L*
		Child, 1 h (5 g dose): > 20	> 1.33
		Adult, 2 h (25 g dose): > 25	> 1.67
	Urine, 5h	Child: 16–33% of ingested dose	Fraction ingested dose: 0.16–0.33
		Adult, *g/5 h*	*mmol/5 h*
		5 g dose: > 1.2	> 8.00
		25 g dose: > 4.0	> 26.64
		> 65 y: > 3.5	> 23.31

HEMATOLOGY AND COAGULATION

Test	Specimen	Reference Drugs	Reference Range (International Units)
Activated Partial Thromboplastin Time (APTT)	Whole blood (Na citrate); remove plasma immediately	25–35 s (differs with method)	25–35 s
Microtechnique (Miale)	Capillary blood (siliconized micropipets; Na citrate)	Infant: < 90 s Reaches adult levels by 2–6 mo	< 90 s
Bleeding Time (BT)			
Ivy	Blood from skin pucture	Normal: 2–7 min Borderline: 7–11 min	2–7 min 7–11 min
Simplate (G-D)		2.75–8 min	2.75–8 min
Blood Volume	Whole blood (heparin)	M: 52–83 mL/kg F: 50–75 mL/kg	M: 0.052–0.083 L/kg F: 0.050–0.075 L/kg
Bone Marrow, Differential Count	Bone marrow aspirate	*% (mean)*	*Number fraction (mean)*
Myeloblasts		0.3–5.0 (2.0)	0.003–0.05 (0.02)
Promyelocytes		1.0–8.0 (5.0)	0.01–0.08 (0.05)
Myelocytes: Neutrophilic		5.0–19.0 (12.0)	0.05–0.19 (0.12)
Eosinophilic		0.5–3.0 (1.5)	0.005–0.03 (0.015)
Basophilic		0.0–0.5 (0.3)	0.00–0.005 (0.003)
Metamyelocytes		13.0–32.0 (22.0)	0.13–0.32 (0.22)
Polymorphonuclear neutrophils		7.0–30.0 (20.0)	0.07–0.30 (0.20)
Polymorphonuclear eosinophils		0.5–4.0 (2.0)	0.005–0.04 (0.02)
Polymorphonuclear basophils		0.0–0.7 (0.2)	0.00–0.007 (0.002)
Lymphocytes		3.0–17.0 (10.0)	0.03–0.17 (0.10)
Plasma cells		0.0–2.0 (0.4)	0.00–0.02 (0.004)
Monocytes		0.5–5.0 (2.0)	0.005–0.05 (0.02)
Reticulum cells		0.1–2.0 (0.2)	0.001–0.02 (0.002)
Megakaryocytes		0.03–3.0 (0.1)	0.0003–0.03 (0.001)
Pronormoblasts		1.0–8.0 (4.0)	0.01–0.08 (0.04)
Normoblasts		7.0–32.0 (18.0)	0.07–0.32 (0.18)
Clot Lysis, 37°C	Whole clotted blood	48–72 h	48–72 h
Clot Retraction			
Screen	Whole blood (no anticoagulant)	Retraction begins at 1 h, maximum at 24 h	Retraction begins at 1 h, maximum at 24 h
Clotting Time			
Lee-White, 37°C	Whole blood (no anticoagulant)	5–8 min	5–8 min
Clotting Time, Plasma	Plasma (citrate)	Platelet-rich plasma: 100–150 s	Platelet-rich plasma: 100–150 s
Differential Count, see *Bone Marrow Differential Count; Leukocyte Differential Count;* and *Synovial Fluid Differential Count*			
Eosinophil Count	Whole blood (EDTA); capillary blood	50–350 cells/μL (mm³)	50–350 × 10⁶ cells/L
Erythrocyte Count (RBC Count)	Whole blood (EDTA)	*millions of cells/μL (mm³)* 2–14 y: 3.7–5.2 Adult M: 4.3–5.9 F: 4.0–5.2	*× 10¹² cells/L* 3.7–5.2 4.3–5.9 4.0–5.2
Erythrocyte Sedimentation Rate (ESR)			
Westergren, modified	Whole blood (EDTA)	*mm/h* Child: 0–10 Adult: M, < 50 y: 0–15 > 50 y: 0–20 F, < 50 y: 0–20 > 50 y: 0–30	*mm/h* 0–10 0–15 0–20 0–20 0–30
Wintrobe		Child: 0–13 Adult: M, 0–9 F, 0–20	0–13 0–9 0–20
Zeta (ZSR)		41–54%	41–54 AU

HEMATOLOGY AND COAGULATION (*Continued*)

Test	Specimen	Reference Drugs	Reference Range (International Units)
Ferritin, see *Chemistry section*			
Fibrin Degradation Products			
Agglutination (Thrombo-Wellco test)	Whole blood; special tube containing thrombin and proteolytic inhibitor	< 10 μg/mL	< 10 mg/L
	Urine: 2 mL in special tube (see above)	< 0.25 μg/mL	< 0.25 mg/L
Staphylococcal clumping	Whole blood, collected with thrombin and ϵ-aminocaproic acid	< 10 μg/mL	< 10 mg/L
Fibrin Lysis Time	Plasma	> 60 min	> 60 min
Fibrinogen	Plasma (Na citrate)	200–400 mg/dL	2.00–4.00 g/L
Glucose-6-phosphate Dehydrogenase (G-6-PD) in Erythrocytes	Whole blood (ACD, EDTA, or heparin)	12.1 ± 2.09 U/g Hb (1 SD)	0.78 ± 0.13 MU/mol Hb (1 SD)
WHO and ICSH methods			
Haptoglobin (Hp)	Serum; avoid hemolysis		
RID		83–267 mg/dL	830–2670 mg/L
Hemoglobin-binding capacity		40–180 mg Hb/dL	6.20–27.90 μmol Hb/L
Nephelometry		26–185 mg/dL	260–1850 mg/L
Hematocrit (HCT, Hct) *Calculated from MCV and RBC (electronic displacement or laser)*	Whole blood (EDTA)	*% of packed red cells (V red cells/V whole blood × 100)*	*Volume fraction (V red cells/V whole blood)*
		1–3 d (cap): 45–67	0.45–0.67
		2 mo: 28–42	0.28–0.42
		6–12 y: 35–45	0.35–0.45
		12–18 y, M; 37–49	0.37–0.49
		F: 36–46	0.36–0.46
		18–49 y, M: 41–53	0.41–0.53
		F: 36–46	0.36–0.46
Hemoglobin (Hb)	Whole blood (EDTA)	*g/dL*	*mmol/L* (conv. factor based on hemoglobin, M.W. 64,000)
		1–3 d (cap): 14.5–22.5	2.25–3.49
		2 mo: 9.0–14.0	1.40–2.17
		6–12 y: 11.5–15.5	1.78–2.40
		12–18 y, M: 13.0–16.0	2.02–2.48
		F: 12.0–16.0	1.86–2.48
		18–49 y, M: 13.5–17.5	2.09–2.71
		F: 12.0–16.0	1.86–2.48
	Plasma (heparin, ACD, or EDTA)	1–4 mg/dL	0.16–0.62 μmol/L
	Serum	< 3 mg/dL with butterfly setup and 18 g needle	< 0.47 μmol/L with butterfly setup and 18 g needle
	Urine, fresh, random	Negative	Negative
Hemoglobin Electrophoresis	Whole blood (EDTA, citrate or heparin)		*Mass fraction*
		HbA > 95%	HbA > 0.95
		HbA_2 1.5–3.5%	HbA_2 0.015–0.035
		Lower in infants < 1 y	
		HbF < 2%	HbF < 0.02
Hemoglobin F *Alkali denaturation (White)*	Whole blood (EDTA)	*% HbF*	*Mass fraction HbF*
		1 day: 77.0 ± 7.3	0.77 ± 0.073
		6 mo: 4.7 ± 2.2	0.047 ± 0.022
		Adult: < 2.0	< 0.020
Hemoglobin H (HbH)	Whole blood (ACD, EDTA, or heparin)	No precipitation at 40 min	No precipitation at 40 min
Isopropanol precipitation			
Leukocyte Count (WBC Count)	Whole blood (EDTA)	*× 1000 cells/μL (mm^3)*	*Cells × 10^9/L*
		Birth: 9.0–30.0	9.0–30.0
		24 h: 9.4–34.0	9.4–34.0
		1 mo: 5.0–19.5	5.0–19.5
		1–3 y: 6.0–17.5	6.0–17.5
		4–7 y: 5.5–15.5	5.5–15.5
		8–13 y: 4.5–13.5	4.5–13.5
		Adult: 4.5–11.0	4.5–11.0
	CSF	0–5 mononuclear cells/μL	0–5 × 10^6 cells/L

HEMATOLOGY AND COAGULATION (*Continued*)

Test	Specimen	Reference Drugs	Reference Range (International Units)
Leukocyte Differential Count	Whole blood (EDTA)	*%* *Cells/μL (mm³)*	*Number fraction* *Cells × 10⁶/L*
Myelocytes		0 0	0 0
Neutrophils-'bands'		3–5 150-400	0.03–0.05 150–400
Neutrophils-'segs'		54–62 3000–5800	0.54–0.62 3000–5800
Lymphocytes		25–33 1500–3000	0.25–0.33 1500–3000
Monocytes		3–7 285–500	0.03–0.07 285–500
Eosinophils		1–3 50–250	0.01–0.03 50–250
Basophils		0–0.75 15–50	0–0.0075 15–20
Leukocyte Differential Count	CSF	*%*	*Number fraction*
Lymphocytes		62 ± 34	0.62 ± 0.34
*Monocytes**		36 ± 20	0.36 ± 0.20
Neutrophils		2 ± 5	0.02 ± 0.05
Histocytes		Rare	Rare
Ependymal cells		Rare	Rare
Eosinophils		Rare	Rare
*Includes pia-arachnoid mesothelial cells			
Mean Corpuscular Hemoglobin (MCH)	Whole blood (EDTA)	*pg/cell*	*fmol/cell*
		0.5–6 y: 23–30	0.36–0.46
		6–18 y: 25–35	0.39–0.54
		Adults 26–34	0.40–0.53
Mean Corpuscular Hemoglobin Concentration (MCHC)	Whole blood (EDTA)	*% Hb/cell or gHb/dL RBC* Adult and child: 31–36	*mmol Hb/L RBC* 4.81–5.58
Mean Corpuscular Volume (MCV)	Whole blood (EDTA)	*fL (μm³)*	*fL*
		1–3 d (cap): 95–121	95–121
		0.5–2 y: 70–86	70–86
		6–12 y: 77–95	77–95
		12–18 y, M: 78–98	78–98
		F: 78–102	78–102
		18–49 y, M: 80–100	80–100
		F: 80–100	80–100
Methemoglobin (MetHb)	Whole blood (EDTA, heparin, or ACD)	0.06–0.24 g/dL or 0.78 ± 0.37% of total Hb	9.3–37.2 μmol/L 0.008 ± 0.0037 (mass fraction)
Partial Thromboplastin Time (PTT)	Whole blood (Na citrate)		
Nonactivated		60–85 s (Platelin)	60–85 s
Activated		25–35 s (differs with method)	25–35 s
Plasma Volume	Plasma (heparin)	M: 25–43 mL/kg F: 28–45 mL/kg	M: 0.025–0.043 L/kg F: 0.028–0.045 L/kg
Platelet Count (Thrombocyte Count)	Whole blood (EDTA)	× *10³/μL (mm³)*	× *10⁹/L*
		Newborn: 84–478	84–478
		(After 1 wk, same as adult)	
		Adult: 150–400	150–400
Prothrombin Consumption (PCT, Serum Prothrombin Time)	Whole blood (no anticoagulant)	>30 s or >80% consumed in 1 h	>30 s >0.80 (fraction consumed)
Prothrombin Time	Whole blood (Na citrate)		
One-stage (Quick)		In general: 11–15 s (varies with type of thromboplastin)	11–15 s
		Newborn: prolonged by 2–3 s	prolonged by 2–3 s
Two-stage modified (Ware and Seegers)		18–22 s	18–22 s
RBC Count, see *Erythrocyte Count*			
Red Cell Volume	Whole blood (heparin)	M: 20–36 mL/kg F: 19–31 mL/kg	M: 0.020–0.36 L/kg F: 0.019–0.031 L/kg
Reticulocyte Count	Whole blood (EDTA, heparin, or oxalate)	Adult: 0.5–1.5% of erythrocytes or 25,000–85,000 cells/uL (mm³)	0.005–0.015 (number fraction) 25,000–85,000 × 10⁶ cells/L
Sulfhemoglobin	Whole blood (EDTA, heparin, or ACD)	≤ 1.0% of total Hb	< 0.010 of total Hb (mass fraction)

HEMATOLOGY AND COAGULATION (*Continued*)

Test	Specimen	Reference Drugs	Reference Range (International Units)
Synovial Fluid Differential Count	Synovial fluid		
		%	*Number fraction*
Polymorphonuclear cells		0–25	0–0.25
Monocytes		0–71	0–0.71
Lymphocytes		0–78	0–0.78
Clasmatocytes		0–26	0–0.26
Unclassified		0–21	0–0.21
Synovial cells		0–12	0–0.12
Thrombin Time	Whole blood (Na citrate)	Control time ± 2 s when control is 9–13 s	Control time ± 2 s when control is 9–13 s
Thromboplastin Time, activated, see *Activated Partial Thromboplastin Time (APTT)*			

Index

Note: In this index, the expression "vs." has been used to denote "differential diagnosis." Italics indicate illustration and t indicates tables.

AA protein, in amyloid diseases, 1169–1170
Abdomen, acute. See *Acute abdomen.*
  distention of, in malabsorption syndromes, 722
Abdominal abscess, 1584
Abdominal angina, 757–758
Abdominal aorta, coarctation of, 346
Abdominal aortic aneurysm, 347–348
  and back pain, 2061
  diagnosis in, 348
  prognosis in, 348
  surgical treatment of, 348
Abdominal epilepsy, 2151
Abdominal irradiation, as radiation injury, 2300
Abdominal pain, 646–647
  from muscle contraction, 2064
  in gastrointestinal disease, 464
Abetalipoproteinemia, 732, 1115–1116
Abortion, chromosome abnormality and, 141
Abscess. See also specific sites.
  abdominal, 789
  amebic, 1800
  amebic liver, 830
  anorectal, 785
  brain, 2111–2114
  cerebellar, 2113
  dental, 663
  epidural, 1549
    acute, vs. transverse myelitis, 2139
    cerebral, 2115
  spinal, 2116–2117
  extradural, cerebral, 2115
  mycobacterial, 1633
  perinephric, 619, 623
Absence attacks, 2150, 2152
  atypical, 2152
  petit mal, 2152
Absence status, 2153
Absorption, disorders of. See *Malabsorption syndromes.*
Acanthamoeba, 1801
Acanthocytosis, 732
Acanthosis nigricans, 1086, 1322, 2250, *2250*, *2263*
Acatalasia, 1158
  genetic factor in, 1158
Accelerated idioventricular rhythm, 313
  electrocardiography in, 313, *313*
Accelerated particles, 2297
Accidents
  epidemiology of, 36
  mortality statistics of, *35*t, 36
  prevention of, 36–37
Acetaldehyde, 53
Acetaldehyde dehydrogenase, 51
Acetaminophen
  for fever, 1473
  for pain, 2051
  hepatotoxicity of, 822
  nephrotoxicity of, 592–593
  poisoning from, 88
Acetazolamide
  in epilepsy, 2159
  in heart failure, 209
Acetoacetate, serum or plasma, reference values for, 2316
Acetohexamide, 1329
Acetone, serum or plasma, and urine, reference values for, 2316
Acetylcholine, 90, 91, 1243
  and atopic diathesis, 2249
  gastric secretion and, 681–682, 683
Acetylcholine receptors, 93
  antibodies to, in myasthenia gravis, 2211, 2213
N-Acetylgalactosamine-6-sulfatase deficiency, 1148
N-Acetylglucosaminyl phosphotransferase, 1149
Acetylstrophanthidin, 203
Achalasia, 672
  radiography in, 673, *673*
  treatment of, 674
Achlorhydria, with pernicious anemia, 897
Achoff nodules, 1529, *1529*
Achondroplasia, 1466
Acid(s). See also names of specific acids.
  gastric secretion of, abnormal, in peptic ulcer, 683
  role of, in gastrointestinal reflux disease, 669
  volatile, input and output of, 536
Acid maltase deficiencies, 2205
Acid mucopolysaccarides. See *Glycosaminoglycam storage.*
Acid phosphatase
  reference values for, 2336
  tartrate-resistant, in Gaucher's disease, 1117
Acid-base balance
  in coma, 1979
  in uremia, 550–551, *551*
  kidney in regulation of, 498–499, 499t
Acid-base balance disorders, 535–544
  anion gap in, 538–539
  bicarbonate metabolism in, 535–544
  CO_2 production and elimination in, 536
  definition of, 537–538, *538*
  pH plasma/CSF disequilibrium and, 537
  physiologic considerations in, 535–537
  renal bicarbonate processing in, 536–537
  types of, 538
Acid-base relationships, equations for, *465*, 466
Acidemia, 536
Acidosis, 499, 536. See also *Lactic acidosis; Metabolic acidosis; Respiratory acidosis.*
  in shock, 213, 220
  renal, in interstitial nephritis, 591
  renal tubular, 541
  with blood transfusion, 940
Aciduria. See also *Aminoaciduria(s)*
  argininosuccinic, 131t, 1130
  L/glyceric, 1108, 1109
  glycolic, 1108, 1109
  methylmalonic, 132
  orotic, 131
    hereditary, 1145
Aclasis, diaphyseal, 1466
Acne rosacea, 2243
  in seborrheic dermatitis, 2242
Acne vulgaris, 2242–2243
  chemical, 2297
  in seborrheic dermatitis, 2242
  vitamin A in, 1207
Acodermatitis enterohepatica, 1209
Acoustic neurilemoma, 2162t
Acoustic schwannoma, 2162t
Acquired immunodeficiency syndrome (AIDS), 1071, 1482, 1706, 1716, 1765, 1855, 1861–1863, 2142–2143
  blood transfusion and, 939, 1862
  clinical manifestations of, 1862
  dementia with, 1863
  diagnosis of, 1863
  drug abuse and, 1862
  epidemiology of, 1862
  etiology of, 1861–1862
  hepatitis immunization and, 46
  homosexuality and, 1862, 1863
  immune response in, 1862
  in Haitians, 1862
  in hemophilia, 1862
  Kaposi's sarcoma with, 1861, 1862, 1863
  opportunistic infection with, 1861, 1862–1863
  pathogenesis of, 1862
  Pneumocystis carinii pneumonia with, 1861, 1862
  prognosis in, 1863
  protozoan infection and, 1794, 1796, 1797, 1802
  treatment of, 1863
Acral lentiginous melanoma, 2274
Acrocyanosis, 356
  vs. Raynaud's phenomenon, 354–355, 356
Acrodermatitis enteropathica, 2256, *2263*
Acromegaly, 1261–1262, *1261*
  bromocriptine in, 1262
  cancer and, 1079
  clinical features of, 1261
  differential diagnosis of, 1262
  laboratory studies in, 1262
  neuropathy with, 2194
  pathogenesis in, 1262
  therapy for, 1262
    radiation, 1260
    surgery, 1260
  with arthritis, 1958
  with cancer, 1079
Acropachy, thyroid, 1283
Acrylamide, poisoning by, autonomic dysfunction in, 2027
ACTH. See also Adrenocorticotropic hormone.
  function of, 1307
  in epilepsy, 2159
  in gout, 1141
  in multiple sclerosis, 2146
  pituitary, in Cushing's disease, 1313
  vs. glucocorticosteroid therapy, 115–116
ACTH/Endorphin system, in septic shock, 1474
ACTH syndrome, ectopic, 1313–1316

Actinic damage, and aging, 2232
Actinobacillus actinomycetemcomitans, 1612, 1613
Actinomyces, 1612
Actinomycetoma, 1773
Actinomycin D, 1098
Actinomycosis, 1612–1613
abdominal, 1612
antibiotic therapy in, 1613
cervicofacial, 1612, 1613
clinical manifestations of, 1612–1613
diagnosis of, 1613
disseminated, 1612–1613
epidemiology of, 1612
pathogenesis of, 1612
pathology of, 1612
thoracic, 1612
treatment of, 1613
Activated charcoal, in poisoning, 87
Activated partial thromboplastin time, 1031
in pulmonary embolism, 430
reference values for, 2337
Actomyosin, 1030
Acuity, visual, testing of, 2033
Acupuncture, for pain, 2053
Acute abdomen, 796–799
computed tomography in, 798
differential diagnosis of, 796–798
laboratory diagnosis of, 797
physical findings in, 797
radiography in, 797
radionuclide imaging in, 797–798
ultrasonography in, 797–798
Acute leukemias. See topics under *Leukemia*.
Acute petroleum distillates, poisoning by, 88
Acyclovir
in herpes simplex encephalitis, 2127
in herpes simplex virus infection, 1717, 2244
in herpes zoster, 2129
in herpesvirus infection, 10
Addison's disease, 518, 527
ACTH stimulation test in, 1311
chronic vs. acute, 1310–1311, 1312
clinical manifestations of, 1310–1311, 1311t
depression in, 2011
diagnosis of, 1311–1312
etiology of, 1310
genetic factor in, 1310
glucocorticoids in, 1312
histocompatibility antigen in, 1310
hyperkalemia in, 534
hyperpigmentation in, 1311
immune response in, 1310
metyrapone test in, 1311
mineralocorticoids in, 1312
prognosis in, 1313
protocol for surgery, 1313t
treatment of, 1312–1313, 1312t
Adenine arabinoside in herpesvirus infection, 109
in varicella, 1723
Adenine phosphoribosyltransferase deficiency, 132, 1144
Adenocarcinoma(s)
esophageal, 674
gallbladder, 863
of colon, 764–765
of large intestine, 761
prostatic, 1378
pulmonary, 439t
Adenohypophysis, 1251. See also *Anterior pituitary*.
Adenoid cystic carcinoma of lung, 445
Adenoma(s). See under specific type.
Adenoma sebaceum, 2256
in tuberous sclerosis, 2085
Adenomatosis, multiple endocrine, 1405
Adenopathy. See specific types.
Adenosine deaminase deficiency, 132, 1144–1145, 1478
with severe combined immunodeficiency disorder, 1859–1860
Adenosine triphosphate
erythrocyte integrity and, 907
in hypophosphatemia, 1164–1165
synthesis of, in shock, 216–217
Adenosylcobalamin, 895
Adenoviral disease, 1705–1706
acute, of acute central nervous system, *2122*, 2123
epidemiology of, 1705
immune response in, 1705, 1706
in children, 1705
microbiology of, 1705
vaccine for, 1706
Adenylate cyclase, 91
hormonal (in)activation of, 1224–1225, *1225*
Adie's tonic pupil, 2035
Adolescence, 15. See also *Puberty*.
aggression in, 19
identity formation in, 19
psychosocial development in, 18–19
restructuring relationships in, 19
sexual behavior in, 19
stages of, 18
Adrenal(s). See also *Adrenal cortex*.
anatomy of, 1300
congenital hyperplasia of, 1395–1397, *1396t*
lipoid, 1357–1358
virilizing, 1363–1365
insufficiency of, hypercalcemia and, 1450
primary, hyperpigmentation in, 2256
neoplasms of, and Cushing's syndrome, 1314
Adrenal androgens
measurement of, 1310
production regulation of, 1305
Adrenal cortex, 1300–1320
development of, 1300
function of, 1300
hyperfunction in, 1369
hypofunction in, 1310–1313
in Cushing's syndrome, 1313–1317
in primary aldosteronism, 1317–1319
structure of, 1300
Adrenal medulla, 90
neural crest tumors of, 1410–1412
sympathetic nervous system and, 1408–1413
Adrenal steroid hormones, 1300–1307. See also specific compounds.
actions of, 1305–1307
assays of, 1307–1310
function assessment of, 1307–1310
metabolism of, 1302–1303
variable rates for, 1303
plasma binding of, 1302
plasma concentrations of, 1301–1302, 1301t
production rates for, 1301–1302, 1301t
production regulation of, 1303–1305
synthesis of, 1300–1302, *1301*
synthesis of, inhibition of, 1302
Adrenalectomy, in breast cancer, 1403–1404
Adrenergic antagonists, 93–95
alpha. See *Alpha-adrenergic blocking agents*.
beta. See *Beta-adrenergic blocking agents*.
in tetanus, 1581
Adrenergic nerves, blood pressure and, 273, 275
Adrenergic neuron-blocking agents
in hypertension, 279
in Raynaud's disease, 355
Adrenergic receptors, 91–95, 92t, 221, 222t
alpha, 91–92, 92t
beta, 91–92, 92t
physiologic regulation of, 92–93
radioligand binding studies of, 92
Adrenocortical insufficiency. See also *Addison's disease*.
adrenocorticotropic hormone in, 1310–1312
primary vs. secondary, 1310, *1312*
secondary, 1311–1313
treatment of, 1312–1313, 1312t
Adrenocorticosteroids. See also names of specific agents.
in epilepsy, 2159
Adrenocorticotropic hormone, 1252–1253. See also *ACTH*.
function tests of, 1254–1255
immunoassays for, 1307
in adrenocortical insufficiency, 1310–1312
in cancer, 1077
in Cushing's syndrome, 1313–1317
in ectopic ACTH syndrome, 1313–1316
in hypopituitarism, 1256, 1257
in pituitary tumor, 1264–1265
plasma, reference values for, 2316
production regulation of, 1303–1304
circadian rhythms and, 1303–1304, 1307
feedback inhibition of, 1304
with islet cell tumor, 1351
Adrenocorticotropic hormone stimulation test, 1308–1309, 1311
reference values for, 2316
Adrenogenital syndromes, 131
Adrenoleukodystrophy, 2148
Adriamycin, 338–339. See also *Doxorubicin*.
Adult celiac disease. See *Celiac disease, adult*.
Adult respiratory distress syndrome, 456, 457t, 472–473, *473*, 477, 1594
after pulmonary thermal inury, 2287
with acute pancreatitis, 774
with pulmonary hypertension, 261
Adulthood, in life cycle, 20–21
crises of, 21
issues, changes, and stages of, 20
Adverse drug reactions, 82–84. See also names of specific agents and diagnoses.
Aedes, 1752
Aedes aegypti, 1737, 1750, 1752
Aedes africanus, 1752
Aerobic bacteria, 1584
Aerobic exercise, 41
Aerophagia, 706
Afferent loop syndrome, after gastric surgery, 693
Afibrinogenemia, 1050–1051
Aflatoxins, 39, 783
hepatocellular carcinoma and, 850
AFP. See *Alpha*$_1$-fetoprotein.
African hemorrhagic fever, 1757
African tick typhus, 1682
African trypanosomiasis, 1780–1783
blood films in, 1782
chemotherapy for, 1782
clinical features of, 1781–1782
control of, 1783
diagnosis of, 1782
epidemiology of, 1780–1781
etiology of, 1780
follow-up in, 1782–1783
immune response in, 1781
pathogenesis of, 1781
pathology of, 1781

African trypanosomiasis (*Continued*)
prognosis in, 1783
prophylaxis for, 1783
relapse in, 1782–1783
serology of, 1782
treatment of, 1782–1783
vector in, 1780–1782
Agammaglobulinemia, 132
common variable, 1856
with immunoglobulin-bearing B lymphocytes, 1856
X-linked, 1855–1856, *1856*
Aganglionosis, congenital, 711–712
Age factor, 15
in atherosclerosis, 281
in bacterial meningitis, 1552
in congenital defects, 145, 147, 149
in hypertension, 267
in laboratory results, 63
in mutations, 118–119
Aged and aging, 15, 22–26. See also *Geriatrics.*
actinic damage and, 2232
and disorders of taste, 2032
and parkinsonism, 2070
cellular physiology and, 24
drug therapy and, 25, 27
drug therapy for, 78
genetic factor in, 24
Gompertz concept of, 23–24, *24*
immunology and, 24
institutionalization vs. home care, 25
physiologic vs. pathologic changes during, 22–23
psychosocial factors in, 24–25, 27–28
sexuality and, 21
survival statistics, 22, *22*
theories of, 24
Agenesis. See specific types.
Ageusia, 2032
Agglutination tests
in crypto coccosis, 1766
in histoplasmosis, 1760
in rheumatoid arthritis, 1915
in rickettsial disease, 1676
in sporotrichosis, 1767
Agglutinin(s), cold, 2264t
syndrome of, 2265t
Aggression, in adolescence, 19
Agnosia, 1996
Agoraphobia, and anxiety, 2009
Agraphia, 1994
Agriculture, recombinant DNA research in, 133
AIDS. See *Acquired immuno-deficiency syndrome.*
Air, chemical injury from. See *Occupational lung disease.*
Air embolism, with blood transfusion, 939
Air pollution
asthma and, 393
in bronchogenic carcinoma, 440
interstitial lung disease and, 407–408, 408t, 410, 417–418, 419
Airway(s)
artificial, 467
diseases of. See also *Respiratory disease.*
with interstitial lung disease, 416
in coma, 1977
in drug poisoning, 1980
maintenance of, 458, 467
Airway(s) obstruction, 397
above tracheal bifurcation, 403
below tracheal bifurcation, 403
causes of, 456
Airway(s) obstruction (*Continued*)
forced expiration measurement in, 397, 400–402
localized, 403–404, *404*
pathophysiology of, 397, *397*
respiratory failure management in, 471
Akathisia
in drug-induced parkinsonism, 2071
with tardive dyskinesia, 2076
Akinesia, definition of, 2069
Akinetic seizures, and syncope, 1986
δ-ALA. See *δ-Aminolevulinic acid.*
Alanine aminotransferase, 1203
serum, reference values for, 2316
Alaria americana, 1819
Albinism, 2257
classification of, *2258*
partial, 951, 2256–2257
Albinoidism, oculocutaneous, *2258*
Albright's syndrome, 1384, 1465, 2254
Albumin
administration of, in hemorrhage, 884
from recombinant DNA research, 133
serum, in acute viral hepatitis, 814
in liver disease, 810
in nephrotic syndrome, 579
serum, CSF, and urinary, reference values for, 2316
Albumin solutions, iso-oncotic, 520
Alcaptonuria, 1128, *2264*
genetic factor in, 1128
radiography in, 1128
Alcohol. See also *Alcohol intake* and *Ethanol.*
and neurologic disorders, 2064–2067
and sleep disorders, 1989, *1988*
withdrawal from, and anxiety, 2009
vs. schizophrenia, 2004
Alcohol dehydrogenase, 51, 52, 53
Alcohol dependence. See *Alcoholism.*
Alcohol intake. See also *Ethanol.*
abuse syndromes, 50
and headache, 2056
blood alcohol level (BAL) and, 51
cancer and, 1070
excessive episodic, 53
extent of, 50
hemochromatosis and, 1161, 1162
hyperlipidemia and, 38
in gastrointestinal disease, 645–646
peptic ulcer and, 684, 689
problem drinking, 53–54
vitamin deficiencies and, 1198
Alcohol intoxication
acute, 51–52
and ataxia, 2045
and syncope, 1986
"driving while intoxicated," 51
hangovers and, 52
Alcoholic cardiomyopathy, 336
Alcoholic cerebellar degeneration, 2066
Alcoholic cerebral atrophy, 2066
Alcoholic hallucinosis, 54
Alcoholic ketoacidosis, 540, 1336
treatment of, 541
Alcoholic liver disease, 835–837
cirrhosis with, 837
diagnosis of, 836
etiology of, 836
fatty liver with, 836
hepatitis with, 836–837
incidence of, 835–836
pathogenesis of, 836
treatment of, 837
Alcoholic myopathy, 2066, 2210
Alcoholics, myoglobinuria in, 2210
Alcoholics Anonymous, 53
Alcoholism, 50, 52–54. See also *Alcohol intake.*
and Wernicke's encephalopathy, 2064–2065, *2065*
addictive cycle of, 52
blackouts with, 53
central pontine myelinolysis in, 2066–2067
chronic pancreatitis and, 775, 777
clinical course of, 53
congenital defects and, 146
diagnosis of, 53
ethanol tolerance and, 52
genetic factor in, 52
highway fatalities and, 55
malnutrition and, 54, 55t
mortality and, 55
niacin deficiency in, 1201
pancreatitis and, 771
physical dependence in, 52–53
predisposing factors in, 52
problem drinking, 53
prognosis in, 54–55
psychologic dependence in, 52
psychopathology of, 52
psychosocial factor in, 52
pyridoxine deficiency and, 1203
related illnesses, 54, 55t
sideroblastic anemia and, 892
thiamin deficiency and, 1198
treatment of, 53–54
vitamin A and, 1207
withdrawal convulsions with, 54
withdrawal symptoms with, 53, 54
Aldolase, serum, reference values for, 2316
Aldomet. See *Methyldopa.*
Aldosterone, 163
kidney and, 1307
measurement of, 1309–1310
metabolism of, 1302–1303
production regulation of, 1304
plasma or serum, and urinary, reference values for, 2316
renal hydrogen ion secretion and, 499
sodium balance and, 497
synthesis of, 1301
Aldosterone antagonists, in heart failure, 209
Aldosterone-renin-angiotensin system, in pregnancy, 626
Aldosteronism
hypertension in, 1317–1319
primary, 531, 1317–1319
adrenal cortex in, 1317–1319
aldosteronism-producing adenoma in, 1317
bilateral adrenal hyperplasia in, 1317
clinical presentation in, 1318
diagnosis of, 1318–1319, *1318*
hypokalemia in, 1317, 1318–1319
medical therapy for, 1319
plasma renin in, 1318, 1319
surgery for, 1319
treatment of, 1319
secondary, 1319
Alexia, 1994
Alginic acid-antacid in gastroesophageal reflux disease, 671
Alimentary system. See *Gastrointestinal system.*
Aliquorrhea, 2166
Alkalemia, 536
Alkaline phosphatase
in acute viral hepatitis, 814
in liver disease, 809
Alkali therapy. See under specific diagnoses.

Alkalosis, 499, 536. See also *Metabolic alkalosis; Respiratory alkalosis.*
posthypercapneic, 542
Alkeran. See *Melphalan.*
Alkylating agents, 1095–1097, *1096t.* See also names of specific agents.
leukemia and, 987
Allele(s), 117, 121
alpha$_1$-antitrypsin deficiency and, 832
B27, in spondylarthropathies, 1918
Allelic exclusion, 1847
Allergic alveolitis, extrinsic, 2285
Allergic angiitis, and allergic granulomatosis, 1941
Allergic contact dermatitis, 2296
Allergic encephalomyelitis, experimental, 2140
Allergic granulomatosis, and allergic angiitis, 1941
Allergic purpura, 1038–1039
Allergic rhinitis, 1867–1870
antihistamines in, 1869
clinical manifestations of, 1867–1868, *1869*
diagnosis of, 1868–1869
etiology of, 1867
immune response in, 1867
immunoglobulin E in, 1867
immunotherapy in, 1870
incidence of, 1867
mast cell in, 1867
pathogenesis of, 1867, *1868*
perennial, 1868
prevalence of, 1867
seasonal, 1867–1868
topical corticosteroids in, 1869–1870
treatment of, 1869
Allergy. See also *Hypersensitivity and related topics.*
and atopic dermatitis, 2249
and contact dermatitis, 2248
aspergillosis syndromes, 1771
asthma from, 390–392
eosinophil in, 391
glucocorticosteroid therapy for, 113
pericarditis with, 342
with blood transfusion, 939
Alloantibodies, hemolysis and, 908
Allodermanyssus sanguineus, 1683
Allopurinol, 999
as nephrotoxin, 602
in acute leukemia, 990
in gout, 1142
in hyperuricosuria, 633
in non-Hodgkin's lymphoma, 999
Alopecia(s), 2231
Alpha-adrenergic agonists, in shock, 222–223, 222t
Alpha-adrenergic antagonists, 95
side effects of, 95
Alpha-adrenergic blocking agents, in primary pulmonary hypertension, 263–264
Alpha-adrenergic receptor antagonists, in shock, 223
Alpha-adrenergic receptor blocking agents, in hypertension, 279
Alpha-adrenergic receptors, 91–92, 92t
Alpha$_1$-Antitrypsin, 1056
serum, reference values for, 2317
Alpha$_1$-Anitrypsin deficiency, 1103, 1104
genetic factor in, 832
in chronic obstructive pulmonary disease, 400
in emphysema, 400
liver disease and, 824, 832
Alpha-chain disease, 1021
Alpha$_1$-fetoprotein (AFP), 146, 148, 1075
in hepatocellular carcinoma, 850, 851
serum or amniotic fluid, reference values for, 2323
Alpha-1, 4-glucosidase deficiency, 1106–1107
Alpha-mercaptopropionylglycine, 633
Alphaviral fevers, 1740
epidemiology of, 1740
vector in, 1740
Alport's syndrome, 132, 627–628
kidney disease and, 506
Alstrom's syndrome, 1172
Altered consciousness, neurologic examination in, 1977, *1977*
lung disorders due to, 2288–2289
polycythemia and, 966–967
Aluminum
in osteoporosis, 1456
osteomalacia and, 1428
toxicity of, in hemodialysis, 1428
Aluminum hydroxide antacids, phosphate and, 1427
Alveolar-arterial oxygen tension, 455
Alveolar-capillary block syndrome, 377
Alveolar proteinosis, 416–417
Alveolar ventilation, maintenance of, 459
Alveolitis, extrinsic allergic, 417–418, 2285
aspergillosis in, 1771
Alzheimer's disease, 27–28, 1999–2000
and memory failure, 1997, 1999
differential diagnosis of, 2000
etiology of, 1999
management of, 2000
pathology of, 1999
pathophysiology of, 1999
Alzheimer's Disease and Related Dementias Association, 28
Amanita, 783
Amanitine, 783
Amantadine
and atopic dermatitis, 2248
for influenza, 110, 1704–1705
in parkinsonism, 2072
Amaurosis, 2033. See also *Blindness.*
Amaurosis fugax, 2096, 2097, 2098
Amblyopia, 2033
nutritional, 2066
Amblyopia ex anopia, 2035
Amebiasis, 1799–1801
clinical manifestations of, 1800
diagnosis of, 1800
epidemiology of, 1799
pathogenesis of, 1800
pathology of, 1800
prevention of, 1801
prognosis in, 1801
radiography in, 1800
serology in, 1800
stool examination, 1800
treatment of, 1800–1801, 1801t
Amebic abscess(es), 1800
hepatic, 830
Amebic colitis. See *Amebiasis.*
Amebic meningoencephalitis, 1801
Amebicide, in liver abscess, 830
Amelanosis, 2256
Amenorrhea
galactorrhea with, 1399
"postpill," 1389
primary, 1386, 1386t
secondary, 1389, 1390
Amenorrhea-galactorrhea syndrome, 1263–1264
Amenorrhea traumatica, 1386
Amentia, vs. dementia, 1998
American Academy of Clinical Toxicology, 85
American Association of Poison Control Centers, 85
American Board of Medical Toxicology, 85
American trypanosomiasis. See *Chagas' disease.*
Amidopyrine, 954–955
Amikacin
clearance of, 76
dosage of, and data on, 101t
Amiloride, in heart failure, 209
Amine(s). See names of specific amines.
Amino acid(s)
absorption of, 720–721
analogues of, 1220
derivatives of, 1220
in cystinuria, 611–613
in renal hyperaminoacidurias, 610–611
Amino acid metabolism, 1120–1132, 1121t, 1125t
in liver disease, 805
Aminoacidopathies
acquired, 1121t–1125t
hereditary, 1121t–1125t
Aminoaciduria, 486
branched-chain, 1130
in Friedreich's ataxia, 2083
photosensitivity in, 2253
γ-Aminobutyric acid, 1243
Aminoglutethimide
in breast cancer, 1403–1404
in Cushing's syndrome, 1316, 1317
Aminoglutethimide, steroid therapy and, 1303
Aminoglycosides, 106, 1586
as nephrotoxins, 596
dosage of, and data on, 101t
in septic shock, 1475–1476
neuromuscular block due to, 2215
pharmacologic parameters of, 70t
serum and urinary, reference values for, 2317
δ-Aminolevulinic acid, 1153, 1154, 1155, 1156
Aminophylline
in respiratory failure, 460
in asthma, 395
Aminorex epidemic, 261, 262
Amiodarone, 326
Amitriptyline
for pain, 2052
in migraine, 2055
in parkinsonism, 2073
in postherpetic neuralgia, 2064
in tension headache, 2057
Ammonia nitrogen, serum or plasma and urinary, reference values for, 2317
Ammonium chloride tolerance test, 510
Amnesia, 1996–1997
antegrade, 2170
in Alzheimer's disease, 1999
in Korsakoff's syndrome, 2065
post-traumatic, 2170
retrograde, 2170
transient global, vs. syncope, 1986
with vertebral-basilar ischemia, 2098, *2098*
Amnestic strokes, 2095
Amnestic syndrome, Korsakoff's, 2065
Amniocentesis, 136–137
for chromosome abnormality diagnosis, 141, 144
for congenital defect diagnosis, 146, 148–149
pregnancy loss and, 136
Amobarbital, serum, reference values for, 2317
Amobarbital sodium, in hysteria, 2015

Amodiaquine, in malaria, 1779, 1780
AMP, cyclic. See *Cyclic adenosine monophosphate.*
Amphetamine(s), abuse of, 2021–2022
  poisoning by, 88
Amphetamine intoxication,chronic, vs. schizophrenia, 2004
Amphotericin, 913
Amphotericin B, 1759
  as nephrotoxin, 598
  in aspergillosis, 1770, 1771
  in blastomycosis, 1763
  in coccidioidomycosis, 1762
  in cryptococcosis, 1766
  in cutaneous leishmaniasis, 1791
  in histoplasmosis, 1761
  in kala azar, 1789
  in mucormycosis, 1772
  in paracoccidioidomycosis, 1765
Ampicillin
  as nephrotoxin, 596t, 597
  in listeriosis, 1611
Amputation, phantom limb pain in, 2064
Amrinone therapy, for heart failure, 204
Amyl nitrite, abuse of, 2024
Amylase, serum, and urinary, reference values for, 2317
Amylase excretion, in pancreatitis, 772–773
Amyloid(s), 1168–1169
  AA, 1169
  AL, 1170
  senile cardiac, 1170
Amyloid arthropathy, 1955
Amyloid angiopathy, intracerebral hemorrhage with, 2105
Amyloid diseases, 1168–1172
  chemical classification of, 1168–1169, 1169t
  inherited, autonomic dysfunction in, 2027
Amyloid neuropathy, 2195
Amyloidosis(es), 735
  AA, 1169–1170
  AL, 1170
  cardiac, 337
  clinical manifestations of, 1171
  congo red binding in, 1168, 1170, 1171
  deposit sites in, 1169, 1170
  diagnosis of, 1171
  familial, 1170–1171
    epidemiology of, 1170–1171
    types of, 1170–1171
    classification of, 1021, 1021t
  immunocytic (primary), 1021–1022
  hereditary, 2195
  kidney disease and, 506
  liver disease and, 833
  multiple myeloma with, 1170, 1171
  nonhereditary, 2195
  pathogenesis of, 1169–1171
  prognosis in, 1171
  rheumatoid arthritis with, 1169
  senile, 1170
  treatment of, 1171
  with ankylosing spondylitis, 1920
  with familial Mediterranean fever, 1167–1168, 1169, 1171
  with Fanconi's syndrome, 615
  with inflammatory joint disease, 1169
Amyloidosis, urticaria, and deafness syndrome, systemic, *2264*
Amylophagia, 889
Amyotrophic lateral sclerosis, 672, 2079–2080
  possible viral cause of, 2137
  vs. cervical spondylosis, 2184
  vs. myasthenia gravis, 2213
Amyotrophy, diabetic, 2193
Anaerobic bacteria, 1583–1586
  gram-negative bacilli, 1583
  gram-positive cocci, 1583
  gram-positive non-spore-forming bacilli, 1583
  in enteric infection, 1593
Anaerobic infection, 1583–1586
  antimicrobial agents in, 1586
  characteristics of, 1583
  diagnosis of, 1585
  facultative organisms in, 1584
  immune response in, 1584
  intra-abdominal, 1584
  of female genital tract, 1585
  of head and neck, 1585
  of skin and soft tissue, 1585
  oxidation-reduction potential in, 1583
  pathogenesis of, 1583–1584
  pleuropulmonary, 1584–1585
  prognosis in, 1586
  treatment of, 1585–1586
  virulence factors in, 1584
Anagen, 2231
Anal fissure, 785–786
Anal malignancy, 786
Analbuminemia, 132
Analgesic(s). See also names of specific agents.
  for back pain, 2063
  for dying patient, 33, 33t
  for pain, 2050
  in postherpetic neuralgia, 2064
  in sinus headache, 2058
  nephropathy and, 592–593
  toxic nephropathy and, 506
Analgesic agents, 2051–2052, *2051*
  in myofascial pain syndrome, 2064
Anaphylactic shock, 1871
Anaphylactoid purpura, 1038–1039
Anaphylactoid reaction(s), 1870
  agents causing, 1871t
  with blood transfusion, 939
Anaphylaxis, 1870–1872
  aspirin and, 1239
  clinical features of, 1871
  differential diagnosis of, 1872
  epinephrine in, 1872
  etiology of, 1871, 1871t
  immune response in, 1870, 1871
  immunoglobulin E in, 1870, 1871
  in drug reaction, 83
  insect sting and, 1872–1874
  pathogenesis of, 1871
  penicillin and, 1871, 1872
  prevention of, 1872
  treatment of, 1872
Anasarca in right ventricular failure, 198
Ancylostoma braziliense, 1821
Ancylostoma caninum, 1821
Ancylostoma duodenale, 1820–1821
Androgen(s), 1365–1367. See also specific compounds.
  adrenal, 1305
  deficiency of, 1369–1370
  in cancer chemotherapy, 1101t
  in gynecomastia, 1400–1401
  synthesis of, 1301
  target area dysfunction of, 1359–1362, *1360, 1361, 1362*
Androgen insensitivity
  complete, as disorder of androgen-dependent target area, 1360–1361
  partial, as disorder of androgen-dependent target area, 1360–1361
Androgen therapy, in aplastic anemia, 881
Androstenedione, 1301
  measurement of, 1310
  serum, reference values for, 1317
Anemia, 870–876. See also specific diagnoses, e.g., *Aplastic anemia; Cooley's anemia; Hemolytic iron deficiency anemia; Hypochromic anemia; Megaloblastic anemia; Normochromic normocytic anemia; Pernicious anemia.*
  acute posthemorrhagic, 883–884, 883t
  after gastric surgery, 692–693
  blood loss in, 872–873
  bone marrow examination in, 876, 876t
  cancer and, 1074
  cardiac output in, 872
  chronic disease and, 891–892
  compensation for, 871–872
  definition of, 871
  differential diagnosis of, 872–873
  drug-induced, 873, 873t
  endocrine factor in, 884
  genetic factor in, 872
  Heinz body, 1023
  hematocrit in, 871, 872
  hemogram in, 874–875
  hemolysis in, 873
  immune response in, 874
  in chronic myelogenous leukemia, 977
  laboratory data in, 874–876
  leukocytes in, 875
  macrocytosis in, 875, 875t
  microcytosis in, 875, 875t
  nonhematologic organ dysfunction and, 873–874, 874t
  of chronic disease, 873
  oxyhemoglobin dissociation curve in, 872
  pathophysiologic classification of, 871, 871t
  patient evaluation in, 872–876
  peripheral blood smear in, 876, 876t
  physical examination in, 874, 874t
  plasma volume alterations in, 871–872
  platelets in, 875
  progenitor cell failure and, 876–882
  red cell indices in, 875
  red cell mass in, 871
  reticulocytosis in, 875
  sickle cell, 2265. See also *Sickle cell syndromes.*
  sideroblastic, 892–893, *892*
  stool examination in, 875
  symptom onset with, 872
  systemic disorder with, 873
  toxins and, 873
  with dialysis, 562
  with uremia, 552, 556
Anesthesia
  definition of, 2047
  general, catastrophic reaction to, 2206
  local, in myofascial pain syndrome, 2064
Anesthetics
  allergy to, 1886
  as nephrotoxins, 602
  fluorocarbon, diabetes insipidus and, 1269
Aneurysm(s). See also specific sites.
  of abdominal aorta, 347–348
  with vasculitis, 2104
"Angel dust," abuse of, 2023–2024
Angiitis
  granulomatous, 2129
  hypersensitivity, 595, *2264*
  necrotizing, neuropathy with, 2196
Angina pectoris, 284–288
  aortic regurgitation and, 284
  aortic stenosis and, 284
  atherosclerosis and, 284

Angina pectoris (*Continued*)
beta-adrenergic blocking agents in, 94, 287
calcium-channel blocking agents in, 287
cigarette smoking and, 287
clinical classification of, 285–286, 285t
clinical diagnosis of, 285
coronary artery disease and, 285, 287
diagnostic tests in, 286
angiography, 285, 286
coronary arteriography, 286
echocardiography, 286
electrocardiography, 285, 286
scintigraphy, 286
ventriculography, 286
exercise and, 287
medical management of, 286–287
mitral regurgitation and, 284
nitrates in, 286
nitroglycerin in, 286
oxygen delivery and, 284
pathophysiology of, 284–285
prognosis in, 287, 298
rest pain with, 284, 285
S-T segment response in, 285, 286
stable, 285, 287
stress testing in, 285, 286
surgical management of, 285, 287
bypass grafting, 298–300
patient selection for, 298–299
coronary artery angioplasty, 287
coronary artery revascularization, 286, 287
unstable, 285
variant, 285–286
ventricular hypertrophy and, 284
with myocardial infarction, 289, 294
Angiodysplasia, gastrointestinal, 761
Angioedema. See also *Urticaria-angioedema.*
familial, *2263*
hereditary, 1854, 1865, 1866
vibratory, 1864–1865
Angiography. See also specific diagnoses.
cardiac, 186
cerebral, in cerebral atherothrombotic disease, 2101
in epilepsy, 2156
in herpes simplex encephalitis, 2127
coronary artery, 186, *187*
digital subtraction technique of, 64, *64*, 512–513
in angina pectoris, 285, 286
in asymmetric septal hypertrophy, 331
in congenital valvular aortic stenosis, 236–237
in insulinoma, 1346, *1346*
in pancreatic cancer, 779
in pericardial constriction, 344–345
in pulmonary embolism, 429–430
in subarachnoid hemorrhage, 2107
in tetralogy of Fallot, 233
pulmonary, 383
renal, 512, 513
spinal, in back pain, 2063
superior vena caval, 383
visceral, 654–655, *655*
Angioimmunoblastic lymphadenopathy, 996
Angiokeratomas, 1116
Angiopathy(ies)
amyloid, intracerebral hemorrhage with, 2105
congophilic, intracerebral hemorrhage with, 2105
nonarteriosclerotic, pathologic processes due to, *2093*
Angioplasty. See also *Percutaneous transluminal angioplasty.*
Angiostrongyliasis, 1826–1827
Angiostrongylus cantonensis, 1826
Angiostrongylus costaricensis, 1827
Angiotensins, 163
Angiotensin I, plasma, reference values for, 2317
Angiotensin II, 1305
plasma, reference values for, 2317
Angiotensin conversion inhibition, in primary pulmonary hypertension, 265
Angiotensin-converting enzyme
inhibitors of, in hypertension, 278–280
serum, in sarcoidosis, 432, 436–437
Anhidrosis, 2028
Animal(s)
marine, poisoning by, 1843–1845
poisonous, 782–783
Anion gap, 538–539
in metabolic acidosis, 539–541
plasma, reference values for, 2317
Anisakiasis, 1824
Anisocoria, essential, 2035
Ankle
clonus of, in striatonigral degeneration, 2079
swelling of, in immunocytic amyloidosis, 1021
Ankylosing spondylitis, 454, 1919–1920
and back pain, 2061
diagnosis of, 1919
extraskeletal involvement in, 1919–1920
immune response in, 1919
pathology of, 1919
prevalence of, 1919
prognosis in, 1920
treatment of, 1920
uveitis and, 2220
with interstitial lung disease, 414
Anopheles freeborni, 1776
Anorchia, 1372
Anorectal abscess, 785
Anorectal fistulas, 785
Anorexia, 646
Anorexia nervosa, 1188–1191, *1188*, 1250, 1387–1388
clinical manifestations of, 1189
endocrine factor in, 1188, 1189
epidemiology of, 1188
genetic factor in, 1188
gonadotropin releasing hormone in, 1250
hypothalamus in, 1188–1189
in males, 1189
pathogenesis of, 1188–1189
prognosis in, 1190
psychopathology of, 1188–1189
puberty and, 1189
refeeding effects in, 1189, 1190
treatment of, 1189–1190
nursing care in, 1190
psychotherapy in, 1190
Anosmia, 2031
Antabuse, 53
Antacids
for acute gastritis, 678
in hydrochloric acid neutralization, 689, 689t
in peptic ulcer, 689, 690
Antagonists, adrenergic, 93–95. See also names of specific agents.
Anterior pituitary, 1251–1266. See also *Pituitary* and *Posterior pituitary.*
anatomy of, 1251
cell types of, 1251–1252
embryology of, 1251
hormones of, 1252–1524, 1252t. See also specific hormones.
corticotropin-related peptides, 1252–1253, 1252t
Anterior pituitary (*Continued*)
hormones of, function tests for, 1254–1255
glycoproteins, 1252t, 1253
somatomammotropic, 1252t, 1253
hyperfunction of, 1261–1266
hyperprolactinemia and, 1263–1264, 1263t
in Cushing's syndrome, 1313–1317
tumors of, 1259–1260, 1387–1388, 2163
ACTH-secreting, 1264–1265
adenoma, 1259–1260
basophilic, 1264–1265
clinical features of, 1259
computed tomography in, 1259–1260, 1259
craniopharyngioma of, 1259–1260
diagnosis of, 1259–1260
differential diagnosis of, 1260
follicle-stimulating hormone secretion by, 1266
FSH/LH secretion by, 1266
gonadotropin secretion by, 1266
headache in, 2059
hormone-secreting, 1261–1266
impotence and, 2030
radiation therapy for, 1260
radiography in, 1259–1260, *1259*
surgery for, 1260
thyroid-stimulating hormone secretion by, 1266
treatment of, 1260
treatment outcome in, 2166
visual fields in, 1260
Anterograde amnesia, 1996
Anthracyclines, 1097–1098
cardiac damage from, 1098
in acute myelogenous leukemia, 991
Anthraquinone, 783
Anthrax, 1606–1608
antibiotic therapy in, 1607
clinical manifestations of, 1607
cutaneous, 1606, 1607
diagnosis of, 1607
epidemiology of, 1606
etiology of, 1606–1607
gastrointestinal, 1606–1607
industrial vs. agricultural, 1606
inhalation, 1606, 1607
pathogenesis of, 1606–1607
prevention of, 1607
prognosis in, 1607
toxin, 1607
treatment of, 1607
Anthrax vaccine, 1607
Anthropometric measurements
in nutritional assessment, 1180–1182
midarm muscle circumference, 1181t, 1182
triceps skinfold thickness, 1180–1182, 1181t
weight/height statistics, 1180, 1180t
Anthropometrics, criteria for, 1181t
Antiamebic agents, 1800–1801, 1801t
Antiarrhythmic drugs, 322–326. See also specific agents.
pharmacokinetics of, 322–323
Antibiotic(s), 96. See also specific agents.
antitumor, 1097–1098
hypersensitivity reactions to, 107–108, 107t
hypokalemia and, 533
in brucellosis, 1616
in hearing loss, 2040
in leptospirosis, 1668
in ulcerative colitis, 754–755
interstitial lung disease and, 418
oral nonabsorbable, 991
therapeutic window of, 75t
topical, 108
toxic reactions to, 107–108, 107t

Antibiotic prophylaxis
in infectious disease, 1483
in infective endocarditis, 1542, 1542t
Antibiotic therapy
for relapsing fever, 1664
in actinomycosis, 1613
in anthrax, 1607
in bartonellosis, 1618
in chronic bronchitis, 399
in gonorrhea, 1646t, 1647–1648
in infective endocarditis, 1540–1541, 1540t
in listeriosis, 1611
in pneumococcal pneumonia, 1503, 1503t
in psittacosis, 1672
in rat bite fever, 1666
in relapsing fever, 1664
in *Salmonella* infection, 1592
in salpingitis, 1643, 1648
in staphylococcal infection, 1550
in tetanus, 1580
in trachoma, 1670
in tropical phagedenic ulcer, 1665
in tularemia, 1605
pseudomembranous colitis and, 1576
Antibodies, 1846. See also *Immunoglobulin(s)*.
antineutrophil, 957
gram-negative bacteria and, 1595
monoclonal, 1849
Antibody deficiency disorder, 1855–1858, 1856t
with near-normal immunoglobulins, 1858
Antibody-dependent cellular cytotoxicity, 1851
Anticancer agents, 1091–1100. See also names of specific agents.
as nephrotoxins, 602
Anticholinergic agents
abuse of, 2024
in asthma, 395
in athetosis, 2077
in parkinsonism, 2072
in spasmodic torticollis, 2078
in torsion dystonia, 2078
ocular side effects of, 2225
poisoning from, 88
Anticholinesterase drugs, 95–96
in myasthenia gravis, 2213
Anticoagulants, 1057–1058
circulating, 1057
in infective endocarditis, 1541
in kidney disease, 505
in renal artery embolism, 623
in renal vein thrombosis, 624
in threatened stroke, 2100
in thrombophlebitis, 364–365
vitamin K deficiency and, 1052
Anticoagulation therapy, intracranial hemorrhage and, 2104
Anticonvulsants
as nephrotoxins, 601–602
vitamin D metabolism and, 1427, 1429–1430
Antidepressants
drug distribution and, 80
for pain, 2052
in depression, 2013
in tension headache, 2057
Antidiarrheal drugs, in Crohn's disease, 747
Antidiuretic hormone, 494–495, 1266–1273
drug effects on activity of, 1268, 1268t
in fluid volume disorders, 517
in osmolality disorders, 524–525
nonosmotic regulation of release of, 1268
osmotic regulation of release of, 1267–1268
physiologic effects of, 1266–1267
release pathology, 1268
secretion of, 1266, *1266*
Antidiuretic hormone (*Continued*)
syndrome of inappropriate production of, 522, 526, 527–528
syndrome of inappropriate secretion of, 1079, 1268
Antidiuretic hormone–water deprivation stimulation test, serum, reference values for, 2317
Antidotes, in accidental poisoning, 87
Antiepileptic drugs
selection of, 2158–2159, *2158*
side effects of, 2159
Antiestrogen therapy, in breast cancer, 1404
Antifolates, 1093–1094
Antifungal agents, dosage of and data on, 101t
Antifungal therapy, 1759
for coccidioidomycosis, 1762
for histoplasmosis, 1761
Anti-GBM glomerulonephritis, 575–576
membranous nephropathy and, 583
plasma exchange therapy in, 576
with and without pulmonary hemorrhage, 576
Antigen(s)
carcinoembryonic, 1075
colon cancer and, 768
in breast cancer, 1402
in pancreatic cancer, 778
serum, reference values for, 2319
oncofetal, 1075–1076
HLA. See *Human leukocyte antigen.*
T cell recognition of, 1850
Antigen-presenting cells, 1850
Antigenic drift, in influenza virus, 1701
Antigenic shift, in influenza virus, 1701
Antigentic variation, in influenza virus, 1700–1701
Antiglomerular basement membrane antibody disease, 502
Antihistamines
abuse of, 2024
in allergic rhinitis, 1869
in skin disease, 2241, *2241*
in urticaria-angioedema, 1866
Antihuman thymocyte globulin, 1026
Antihyaluronidase titer, serum, reference values for, 2317
Antihypertensive agents, 276–278, 277t
distribution of, 80
Antihypertensive therapy, dialysis with, 561
Anti-inflammatory agents
as nephrotoxins, 602
glucocorticosteroids as, 112–113
in peptic ulcer, 684, 689
Antilymphocyte globulin, in aplastic anemia, 879
Antimalarial agents, 1778–1780
in rheumatoid arthritis, 1916
resistance to, 1778–1779
sites of action of, 1780
Antimetabolites, 1093–1095
Antimicrobial agents
as nephrotoxins, 596–598
broad-spectrum, in acne, 2242
in anaerobic infection, 1586
in brain abscess, 2113
in respiratory failure, 461
in shigellosis, 1596
in tropical sprue, 737
in urinary tract infection, 621–622
in Whipple's disease, 735
in whooping cough, 1570
neuromuscular block caused by, 2215
use in wet dressings, 2239
Antimicrobial prophylaxis, for rheumatic fever, 1532–1533
Antimicrobial therapy, 96–108. See also specific agents.
bacterial resistance factor in, 97–98, 100t
bacterial susceptibility factor in, 97–98, 99t
combination, 102–103, 102t
drug mechanisms in, 97t
duration of, 106
failures with, 106–107
general principles of, 96–97
hepatic failure and, 101t, 102
identification of infecting agent for, 97
in bacterial meningitis, 1555–1556
in Crohn's disease, 747
in meningococcal disease, 1561
in rickettsial disease, 1676
pharmacologic factors in, 98, 100, 101t
reactions to, 107–108, 107t
renal failure and, 101t, 102
Antimitochondrial antibodies, in primary biliary cirrhosis, 838
Antimony
in cutaneous leishmaniasis, 1791
in kala azar, 1789
Antimony toxicity, 2314
Antimuscarinic drugs, in peptic ulcer, 688
Antineoplastic agents, interstitial lung disease and, 418
Antinuclear antibodies in liver disease, 811
rheumatic disease and, 1909, 1909t, 1910t
α_2-Antiplasmin, 1056
Antipsychotic agents, and parkinsonism, 2071
and tardive dyskinesia, 2075–2076
Antipyretics, 1472
Antiribonucleoprotein, 1909
Antischistosomal therapy, 1812, 1813, 1814, 1815
Antiseizure drugs, therapeutic window of, 75t
Antispasmodics, in threatened stroke, 2100
Antistreptolysin O test, 1520, 1521, 1522, 1524, 1528, 1531
Antistreptolysin O titer, serum, reference values for, 2317
Antithrombin, 1043–1044
Antithrombin III, 1056
Antithrombotic drugs, in threatened stroke, 2100
Antithymocyte globulin, in aplastic anemia, 879, 881
Antithyroglobulin antibodies, 1280
Antithyroid agents, 1284–1285
Antithyroid antibodies, 1280, 1281
Antituberculosis drugs, 1624–1625
as nephrotoxins, 597–598
dosage of, and data on, 101t
Antitubular basement membrane antibody disease, 502–503
Antitumor antibiotics, 1097–1098
Antiviral therapy, 108–111
biologic agents for, 111
chemotherapeutic agents in, 108–111
Antrectomy
complications of, 692
with truncal vagotomy, 691–692
Ants, 1837–1838
Anus, disease of, 785–786
Anxiety, 1, 2008–2011
in right ventricular failure, 199
Aorta
aging effects upon, 347
arteriosclerosis of, 347
coarctation of. See *Coarctation of aorta.*
disease of, 345–353
congenital, 346
heredofamilial, 346–347
increased dimensions of, 347–348

Aorta (*Continued*)
pulmonary artery communication defect and, 231–232
traumatic disease of, 348, *349*
Aortic aneurysm(s), 347
abdominal, 347–348
arteriosclerotic, 347
congenital, 346
dissecting, 350–351, 2092
syphilitic, 349–350
Aortic arch syndrome, 352–353
Aortic insufficiency, in late syphilis, 1655
Aortic occlusion, 353
Aortic pulmonary septal defect, 232
Aortic regurgitation, 254–255, 254t
angina pectoris and, 284
bacterial endocarditis prophylaxis in, 255
cardiac catheterization in, 255
clinical course of, 254
diagnosis of, differential, 255
echocardiography in, 255
electrocardiography in, 255
laboratory studies in, 255
radiography in, 255
etiology of, 254
left ventricular hypertrophy in, 254–255
medical therapy of, 255
pathologic physiology of, 254
pathology of, 254
physical examination in, 254–255
rheumatic fever and, 254
surgical therapy of, 255
valve replacement in, 255
with ventricular septal defect, 231
Aortic root, and right heart, communication shunts between, 232–233
Aortic stenosis, 252–254
angina pectoris and, 284
bacterial endocarditis prophylaxis with, 253
bicuspid valve with, 252
cardiac catheterization in, 253
clinical course of, 252
clinical features of, 252–253
congenital valvular, 236–237
angiography in, 236–237
cardiac catheterization in, 236–237
echocardiography in, 236
electrocardiography in, 236
radiography in, 236
stress testing in, 236
surgery for, 237
diagnosis of, differential, 253
echocardiography in, 253
electrocardiography in, 253
laboratory studies in, 253
radiography in, *168*, 253
etiology of, 252
medical therapy of, 253
myocardial oxygen consumption in, 252
pathologic physiology of, 252
pathology of, 252
physical examination in, 252–253
rheumatic fever and, 252
subvalvular (discrete), 237
supravalvular, 237
surgical treatment of, 253–254
symptoms of, 252
valve replacement in, 253–254
with coronary artery disease, 252
with heart failure, 252
Aortic valve, bicuspid, 236
Aortitis, 352–353
Aortography, 383
in dissecting aneurysm of aorta, 350–351, *351*
Apathy, in Huntington's disease, 2074
Apatite crystal deposition disease, 1950
Aphasia, 1993–1995, *1994*
Broca's, 1994
global, 1994
vs. dysarthria, 1994
Wernicke's, 1994
Aphasia syndrome, acquired epileptic, 2155
Aphthous fever, 1711–1712
Aphthous stomatitis, involving mouth, 2244
Aphthous ulcers, 664, *664*
Aplastic anemia, 877–882
chloramphenicol and, 877–878
classification of, 877
clinical description of, 879
physical examination in, 879
constitutional, 877
cyclophosphamide in, 878–879
diagnosis of, 879–880
bone marrow findings in, 879
differential, 880, 880t
Ham's test in, 879
marrow culture studies in, 880
peripheral blood findings in, 879
sucrose hemolysis test in, 879
drug-related, 877–878
environmental toxins and, 878
Epstein-Barr virus and, 878
etiology of, 877–878, 877t, 878t
genetic factor in, 878
hepatitis and, 878
idiopathic, *868*
immune response and, 878–879
in trigeminal neuralgia, 2059
infections and, 878–879
management of, 880–881
androgen therapy in, 881
antilymphocyte globulin in, 879, 881
bone marrow transplantation in, 878–879, 880, 881, 1026–1027, *1026*
HLA donor typing for, 880
immunosuppression in, 879–879, 881
platelet counts in, 880, *880*
prednisone in, 880, *880*, 881
transfusions for, 880
myelophthisic, 881–882, *882t*
parvovirus and, 878
pathogenesis of, 878–879
preleukemia and, 878
prognosis in, 881
serum immunoglobulins in, 879
unicellular, 877
Apnea
after head injury, 2170
and sleep disorders, 1990, *1988*
apocrine chromhidrosis, 2230
Apocrine glands, 2230
Apoprotein E deficiency, 1112
Apo-retinol binding protein, 1206
Apparent volume of distribution, and drug intake, 70–71, 70t, 71t
Appendicitis, 796–799
calculi with, 796
clinical findings in, 796
differential diagnosis of, 796–798
etiology of, 796
laboratory findings in, 796
pelvic, 796
retrocecal, 796
treatment of, 798
surgery in, 798–799
Apraxia, 1995–1996
APUD cells, 1230
Ara-C. See *Cytosine arabinoside.*
Arachidonic acid
cyclooxygenase pathway, 1237–1239, *1238*
function of metabolites and, 1239
Arachidonic acid (*Continued*)
in prostaglandin synthesis, 1226
lipoxygenase pathway and, 1239–1240, *1240*
metabolic pathways and, 391, *392*
metabolism of, *1238*, 1866
urticaria-angioedema and, 1866
oxygenation products of, 1237–1241
biosynthetic regulation of, 1240, *1240*
pharmacologic inhibition of, 1240
Arachidonic acid metabolites, in rheumatic disease, 1900
Arachnid(s), disease carried by, 1833, 1833t
Arachnidism, necrotic, 1837
Arachnodactyly. See *Marfan's syndrome.*
Arboviruses (arthropod-borne viruses), 1736–1750, 1736t
clinical syndromes from, 1736–1348, 1736t, 1742t
in acute central nervous system infections, *2122*, 2123
Areflexia, in Friedreich's ataxia, 2083
Arenavirus(es), in acute central nervous system infections, 1736, *2122*, 2123
Arenavirus hemorrhagic disease, 1756–1757
Argentine hemorrhagic fever, 1756–1757
Arginase deficiency, 1130
L-Arginine, 1255
Arginine vasopressin, 1079, 1266
Argininosuccinase deficiency, 1130
Argininosuccinate synthetase deficiency, 1130
Argininosuccinic aciduria, 131t, 1130
Argyll Robertson pupils, 2035
Arm, middle of, measurement of muscle circumference, 1181t, 1182
Armadillo disease, 2216
Arnold-Chiari malformation, 2084, 2187, 2188
Arrhythmias, 300–329. See also specific classes.
as late complication of cardiac surgery, 242
automaticity vs. re-entry in, 304–305, *305*
beta-adrenergic antagonists in, 94
cardiac catheterization in, 186
context factor and, 304
drug therapy of, 322–326
electrocardiography in, 301, *303*
etiology of, 304
hemodynamic consequences of, 304
His bundle recordings of, 301–304, *302*, *303*
in digitalis toxicity, 203–204
in shock, 212, 220–221
mechanisms of, 304–305, *305*
pacemakers for, 326–327, *326*, *327*
supraventricular vs. ventricular, 305
surgical treatment of, 328–329
with myocardial infarction, 292
Arsenic
as nephrotoxin, 601
blood and urinary, reference values for, 2317
poisoning with, 2310–2311
Arterial aneurysms, 2103
Arterial baroreflex, 272–273
Arterial blood gases, 378–381, *379*, *381*
impaired diffusion and, 379–380
in respiratory dysfunction, 464–465
right-to-left shunting and, 380–381
significance of, 381
ventilation-perfusion mismatching and, 380
Arterial carbon dioxide tension, 536–538
Arterial embolism, vs. arteriosclerosis obliterans, 359
Arterial hypertension. See *Hypertension.*
Arterial occlusion
myoglobinuria in, 2210
sudden, 361–362

Arterial oxygen tension, 455, *455*
Arterial pH, 535–538
  in respiratory dysfunction, 464–465, *465*, 466
Arterial pressure, 162
  autoregulation and, 162
Arterial pressure monitoring
  in critical care management, 474
  in shock, 219
Arterial system, 160
Arterial thrombosis, sudden, 361
Arteriography
  bronchial, 383
  cerebral, in subdural empyema, 2115
  in arteriosclerosis obliterans, 359
  in subarachnoid hemorrhage, 2107
  renal, 512
Arterioles, retinal, in amaurosis fugax, 2096, *2096*
Arteriosclerosis
  and parkinsonism, 2071
  diet and, 38
  of aorta, 347
  of extracranial arteries to brain, 2091
  retinal changes in, 2223
Arteriosclerosis obliterans, 358–360
  clinical manifestations of, 359
  diagnosis of, 359
    arteriography in, 359
  intermittent claudication in, 359, 360
  pathology of, 358
  pathophysiology of, 358–359
  prognosis in, 360
  treatment of, 359–360
    percutaneous transluminal angioplasty in, 360
    prostaglandin E_1 in, 360
    surgery for, 360
    sympathectomy in, 360
  vs. arterial embolism, 359
  with diabetes mellitus, 358, 359
Arteriosclerotic aneurysm, 359
Arteriosclerotic-hypertensive hemorrhage, 2104
  spontaneous intracranial, 2108
Arteriovenous fistula, 362
Arteriovenous malformations, 2104
  hemorrage from, prognosis in, 2107
  spinal, 2187
  treatment of, 2107
  with aneurysm, 2103
Arteritis
  cranial, 2057
  giant cell, 1946–1947
  granulomatous, 2129
  Takayasu's, 2093
  temporal (cranial), 1946–1947
Artery(ies). See names of specific artery(ies).
Artery of Adamkiewicz, surgical damage to, 2138
Artery-to-artery emboli, and stroke, 2095, *2095*
Arthritis
  acromegaly with, 1958
  associated diseases, 1957–1958
  bacterial, 1922–1923
  familial Mediterranean fever with, 1958
  fungal, 1924
  gonococcal, 1646, 1648, 1923
  hemochromatosis with, 1957
  hemoglobinopathy with, 1957
  hypergammaglobulinemia with, 1958
  hyperlipoproteinemia with, 1957–1958
  hyperparathyroidism with, 1958
  in rheumatic fever, 1529
  juvenile chronic, 1917
  meningococcal, 1560
Arthritis (*Continued*)
  psoriatic, 2245
  pyogenic, in bacterial endocarditis, 1554
  rheumatoid, 1911–1917. See also *Rheumatoid arthritis.*
  sarcoidosis with, 1957
  septic, vs. osteomyelitis, 1568
  sickle cell disease with, 1957
  staphylococcal septic, 1546
  syphilitic, 1924
  tuberculous, 1628, 1923
  uveitis and, *2220*
  viral, 1923
  vs. parkinsonism, 2071
  Whipple's disease with, 1958
  with acute rheumatic fever, 1529–1530
  with gout, 1132, 1136–1137, *1137*, *1138*, 1140, 1141
Arthrography, 1910
Arthrogryposis, 1387
Arthrogryposis multiplex congenita, 2207
Arthropathy
  amyloid, 1955
  calcium crystal deposition causing, 1950–1951
  enteropathic, 1921
  juvenile chronic, 1921
  peripheral, 1921
  psoriatic, 1921–1922
  reactive, 1921
Arthropod(s), 1833–1840, 1833t
  biting, 1833–1837
  contact dermatitis and, 1840
  invasive, 1838–1840
  stinging, 1837–1838
Arthropod-borne viruses. See *Arboviruses.*
Arthroscopy, 1910–1911
Artificial airway, complications with, 476
Arylsulfatase B deficiency, 1148
Asbestos exposure, 48
  cancer and, 2284
  occupational, 2283
Asbestosis, 417, 2283, *2284*
  pleural disease with, 449
Asbestos-related diseases, 2283–2284
Ascariasis, 863, 1822–1823
  clinical manifestations of, 1823
  complications of, 1823
  diagnosis of, 1823
  epidemiology of, 1822
  etiology of, 1822
  pathology of, 1822–1923
  prevention of, 1823
  treatment of, 1823
Ascaris lumbricoides, 1822
Ascites, 787–788
  chylous, 788
  clinical features of, 787
  clinical manifestations of, 844
  diagnosis of, 844
    differential, 787–788, 788t
  fluid evaluation in, 787
  in right ventricular failure, 198
  management of, 844
  abdominal paracentesis in, 844
  diuretics in, 844
  peritoneovenous (LeVeen) shunt in, 844
  sodium intake in, 844
  pathogenesis of, 843–844, 843t
  pseudochylous, 788
  spontaneous bacterial peritonitis with, 844
  urine, 788
  with cirrhosis, 843–844
Ascorbic acid, 1204–1205. See also *Vitamin C.*
  biochemical function of, 1204
  dietary sources of, 1204
  for cancer, 1205
Ascorbic acid (*Continued*)
  for common cold, 1205
  immune response and, 1204, 1205
  nitrosoamines and, 1205
  physiology of, 1204
  requirements for, 1204
  structure of, 1204, *1204*
  toxicity of, 1205
Ascorbic acid deficiency, 1204–1205
  assay in, 1205
  treatment of, 1205
Aseptic meningitis, 2122. See also *Viral meningitis.*
Asiatic cholera. See *Cholera.*
ASO titer, serum, reference values for, 2317
L-Asparaginase, 1099–1100, *1100*
Aspartate aminotransferase, 1203
  serum, reference values for, 2317
Aspergillar bronchitis, 1770
Aspergillomas, 1770
Aspergillosis, 1479, 1770–1771
  allergic bronchopulmonary, 1770–1771
  antifungal therapy in, 1770–1771
  chronic necrotizing pulmonary, 1771
  diagnosis of, 1770–1771
  epidemiology of, 1770
  etiology of, 1770
  immune response in, 1770–1771
  immunosuppressive therapy and, 2142
  in transplant recipients, 2142
  opportunistic pulmonary, 1771
  skin test in, 1770
  syndromes of, 1770
  treatment of, 1770–1771
Aspergillus, 1538, 1770–1771
  as natural carcinogen, 39
Aspergillus flavus, 783, 1770
Aspergillus fumigatus, 1770
Aspergillus niger, 1770
Aspiration
  in liver abscess, 830
  laryngeal, 672
  "silent," 2292
Aspiration pneumonia, 1513–1516
  clinical presentation of, 1514–1515
  in hospitalized patient, 1514, 1515
  inciting materials in, 1513–1514
  laboratory findings in, 1515
  management of, 1516
  pathogenesis of, 1514
  radiography in, 1515
  therapy of, 1516
  vs. aspiration pneumonitis, 2291
Aspiration pneumonitis, 2291–2293
Aspiration-related injuries, 2291–2293
Aspirin
  absorption of, 80
  acute gastritis from, 677, 678
  allergy to, 1886
  anaphylaxis and, 1239
  fluid volume disorders and, 518
  hepatotoxicity associated with, 822
  in cyclooxygenase inhibition, 1239
  in fever, 1472, 1473
  in mastocytosis, 1888
  in pain, 2051
  in peptic ulcer pathogenesis, 684, 689–690
  in rheumatoid arthritis, 1916
  in tension headache, 2057
  in threatened stroke, 2100
  nephrotoxicity of, 592–593
  neutrophil adhesiveness and, 950
  platelet dysfunction and, 1030, 1031
  poisoning from, 87–88
  sensitivity to, asthma and, 393
  urticaria-angioedema and, 1866
Asplenia syndrome, 240

Asterixis, in metabolic brain disease, 1975
Asthenia, 2044
Asthma, 390–396
  airborne pollutants in, 393
  aspergillosis in, 1770–1771
  aspirin sensitivity and, 393
  classification in, 390, 390t
  clinical manifestations of, 393–394
  definition of, 390
  differential diagnosis of, 394
  extrinsic, 390–392, *391t*, *392*
  from allergy, 390–392
  intrinsic, 392–394, *393*
  laboratory findings in, 394
  mast cell receptors in, 391–392, *392*
  mediator-neurogenic mechanisms interaction in, 393, *393*
  mediators in, 390–392, 391t
  membrane receptor interactions in, 391–392, *392*
  nonallergic provocative stimuli and, 393
  occupational, 2285–2286, *2285*
  parasympathetic nervous system in, 392–393, *393*
  pathology of, 390
  pathophysiology of, 390–394, *391t*, *392*, *393*
  physical stimuli and, 393
  prevalence of, 390
  prognosis in, 396
  psychologic factors in, 393
Asthma treatment, 394–396
  acute attack management in, 395–396
    with theophylline, 395
    with corticosteroids, 395, 396
  anticholinergic agents in, 395
  beta-adrenergic receptor agonists in, 394–395
  calcium-channel receptor antagonists in, 395
  cromones in, 395
  glucocorticosteroid therapy for, 113
  long-term management of, 396
  methylxanthines in, 395
  sympathomimetic drugs in, 394
Asthmatic bronchitis, 397
  chronic, 397
  characteristics of, 2161, 2162
  malignant, 2162
Asymmetric septal hypertrophy, 330–331
  angiography in, 331
  cardiac catheterization in, 331
  echocardiography in, 330–331, *330*
  electrocardiography in, 330–331
Ataxia, 2044–2045
  cerebellar, in ataxia telangiectasia, 2086
  Friedreich's, 333, *2081*, *2082*, 2083
  in alcoholic cerebellar degeneration, 2066
  in olivopontocerebellar degeneration, 2083
  in spinal cord compression, 2062
  in spinocerebellar degenerations, 2080
  in vitamin B_{12} deficiency, 2067
  in Wernicke's encephalopathy, 2065
  inherited, *2082*
  locomotor, 2119–2120
  truncal, in olivopontocerebellar degeneration, 2084
  vs. vertigo, 2041
Ataxia telangiectasia, 143, 1860, 2086
  leukemia with, 987
Atelectasis, 404–405
  clinical manifestations of, 405
  diagnosis of, 405
  pathogenesis of, 404–405
  treatment of, 405
  types of, 404–405
Atherogenesis
  lipids and, 38
  lipoproteins and, 38
Atheroma
  of internal carotid artery, 2094
  predilection sites of, in extracranial arteries to brain, *2091*
Atheromatous debris
  in retinal arterioles, 2096
Atherosclerosis, 281–283
  angina pectoris and, 284
  chronic renal failure and, 551–552, 556
  epidemiology of, 156
  exercise and, 283
  glucose metabolism in, 282
  history of, 281
  hyperlipidemia and, 1115
  pathogenesis of, 283–284
  lipoproteins in, 282, 283
  pathology of, 281
  prevention of, 284
  regression of, 284
  risk factors in, 281–283, 288
    age, 281
    cigarette smoking, 47, 282
    genetic factors, 283
    glucose metabolism, 282
    hyperlipidemia, 282, 1115
    hypertension, 282
    obesity, 282–283
    personality, 283
    physical activity, 283
    sex, 281
  sites of, 281
  treatment of, 284
Atherothrombosis, cerebral arterial, syndromes of, 2094–2097
Atherothrombotic disease, cerebral, role of surgery in, 2100–2101
Atherothrombotic stroke, 2091
Athetosis, 2077
  definition of, 2069
Athetotic dystonia, 2077
Atonic seizures, 2153
Atopic dermatitis, 2249
Atopic diathesis, 1864
Atopic response mediators, 390–392
Atrial fibrillation, 311–312, 317
  electrocardiography in, 311–312, *312*, 317, *318*
Atrial flutter, 309–310
  electrocardiography in, 310, *310*, *311*
Atrial premature beats, 305–306
  electrocardiography in, 305–306, *305*, *306*
Atrial septal defect, 228–229
  complications of, 229
  diagnosis of, 228–229
  echocardiography in, 229
  electrocardiography in, 229
  natural history of, 229
  radiography in, *167*,169, 229
Atrial tachycardia, ectopic, 308–309
  electrocardiography in, 308–309, *309*, *310*
  treatment of, 229
Atrioventricular block, 289, 319–322
  electrocardiography in, 319–320, *320*, *321*
Atrioventricular dissociation, 322
  electrocardiography in, 322, *322*
Atrioventricular junctional rhythm, accelerated, 312
  electrocardiography in, 312, *312*
Atrioventricular junctional tachycardia, 313, 315–317
  electrocardiography in, 315–316, *316*
Atrioventricular node, 301
Atrioventricular premature junction beats, 306
Atrium, late complications of surgery of, 241–242
Atromid S. See *Clofibrate.*
Atropa belladonna, 783
Atrophy
  definition of, 2198
  in Wohlfart-Kugelberg-Welander disease, 2080
  olivopontocerebellar, 2083–2084, *2081*, *2082*
  optic, 2219
Atropine, 95
  abuse of, 2024
  in cardiopulmonary resuscitation, 482
Audiometry, in evaluation of hearing loss, 2038
Auditory evoked responses, in hearing loss, 2038
Auer rods, 988
Aura, in epilepsy, 2152
Austrian's syndrome, 1533
Autoerythrocyte sensitivity, 1039–1040
Autoimmune disease
  Addison's disease as, 1310
  diabetes mellitus as, 1322, 1325
  Hashimoto's thyroiditis as, 1293
  HLA system and, 1882–1883
  hypoglycemia as, 1347
  of thyroid gland, 1280, 1281
  rheumatoid arthritis as, 1912
  Sjögren's syndrome as, 1936–1937
  systemic lupus erythematosus as, 1924–1927, 1926t
Autoimmune factor, in Chagas' disease, 1784
Autoimmune hemolytic anemia, drug-induced, 911
Autoimmune hemolytic disease, 908–911
  cold-reacting antibodies and, 910–911, 910t
  IgG, warm-reacting antibodies and, 908–910
Autoimmune response
  hormones and, 1231
  in neutropenia, 957
Autoimmunity, in hemolytic anemia, 908–911
Automatisms, in epilepsy, 2152
Automobile accidents, 36
  drunken driving and, 55
  prevention of, 36
Autonomic nervous system
  blood pressure and, 273
  disorders of, 2027–2031
  in epilepsy, 2151
  in heart failure, 194–195
  in intracranial tumor, 2163
  organization of, 90–91
  pharmacologic principles and, 90–96
  physiology of, 90–91
  therapeutic interventions and, 91–96
Autosomal dominant traits, 118–119, *118*
Autosomal recessive disorders, 119, *119*
AV. See *Atrioventricular.*
Axial osteomalacia, 1428
Axonal degeneration, in alcoholic neuropathy, 2066
Axonopathy, distal, 2189
5–Azacytidine (5-azaC), 1095
  therapy with, 926
Azathioprine, 1095
  immunosuppression with, 1095
  in chronic active hepatitis, 826
  in Crohn's disease, 747
  inhibiting agents of, 81t
Azotemia, renal vs. extrarenal causes of, 554
Antegrade amnesia, 2170
Anterior cord syndrome, 2176

B27 allele, in spondylarthropathies, 1918
BCNU, in cancer chemotherapy, 1096–1097
B cell(s), 1846–1849. See also *T cell–B cell interaction.*
  disorders of, 1013–1014. See also *Plasma cell disorders.*

B cell(s) (*Continued*)
diversity of, 1846–1847
immunoglobulins of, 1013
in hairy cell leukemia, 984, 985
molecular genetics of, 1846–1847
mononuclear phagocyte interaction with, *948*, 949
ontogeny of, 1846–1847
proliferation of, in chronic lymphocytic leukemia, 980–981, 982
response control, 1847–1848, *1848*
B cell neoplasms, 992, 992t, 993, 993t
B-cell stimulating factor-p1, 1847
Babesia, 1798
Babesia divergens, 1798
Babesia microti, 1798, 1799
Babesiosis, 1798–1799
clinical manifestations of, 1798
diagnosis of, 1799
epidemiology of, 1798
hemolysis with, 913
immune response in, 1798–1799
prevention of, 1799
splenectomy and, 1798
therapy of, 1799
transfusion and, 1798, 1799
vector in, 1798, 1799
Bacille Calmette-Guérin vaccine, 1621
Bacillus(i)
acid-fast, 1620
aerobic gram-negative, and pneumonia, 1810–1813
tubercle, 1621
Bacillus anthracis, 1606
Bacillus cereus, 782
Back pain, 1955–1957, 2060–2063
computed tomography in, 2062
etiology of, 1955–1956, 1955t
history in, 1956
laboratory findings in, 1956
management of, 1957
myelography in, 2063
physical examination in, 1956
radiography in, 1956–1957
in multiple sclerosis, 2146
in trigeminal neuralgia, 2059
Bacteremia
gonococcal, 1646–1647
gram-negative, 1594–1595
antibodies with, 1595
management of, 1595
Hemophilus influenzae, 1564
in bacterial meningitis, 1553
nosocomial, 1488
Salmonella, 1591
staphylococcal, 1548–1549
with cirrhosis, 1593
Bacterial arthritis, 1922–1923
Bacterial endocarditis. See also *Endocarditis, infective.*
cerebral manifestations of, 2116
glomerulonephritis with, 573
proplylaxis for, 249, 251, 253, 255
Bacterial infection(s), 1494–1620
cutaneous lesions in, *2260*
neutrophil disorders and, 949–953
occupational, 2297
of central nervous system, 2111–2121
of liver, 828–829
Bacterial interference, in staphylococcal infection, 1550
Bacterial meningitis. See under *Meningitis, bacterial.*
Bacterial pneumonia, secondary, 1730
Bacterial prostatitis, 1375, 1376
Bacteriologic culture(s)
in skin disease, 2238
Bacteriophage cloning, 135, *136*
Bacteriuria, 484, 619
asymptomatic vs. symptomatic, 621–622
bacteriologic findings in, 620–621
epidemiology of, 621
of pregnancy, 621
role of instrumentation in, 621
significant, 620
Bacteroides, 1583, 1584, 1585, 1593, 1664
Bacteroides fragilis, 1583, 1584, 1584, 1586
Bacteroides melaninogenicus asaccharolyticus, 1583
Bagasossis, 2285
Baker's cyst, 364
BAL. See *Blood alcohol level.*
Balance, in Wernicke's encephalopathy, 2065
Balantidiasis, 1803
Balantidium coli, 1803
Baldness. See *Alopecia.*
Ballism, definition of, 2069
Balloon catheter(s), in cardiac catheterization, 474, 183–184, 474
Banti's syndrome, 842
Bantu hypokinetic heat disease, 335
Bárány rotation maneuver, 2041
Barbiturate(s)
acute poisoning by, 2020
ADH activity and, 1268t
in epilepsy, 2158, *2158*
short-acting, abuse of, 2019–2021
steroid therapy and, 1303
withdrawal from, and anxiety, 2009
Barbiturate coma in stroke treatment, 2101
Bare lymphocyte syndrome, 1860
Baritosis, 2284
Barium enema. See under specific diagnoses.
Barium salts, hypokalemic periodic paralysis and, 533
Barium swallow. See under specific diagnoses.
Barium toxicity, 2314
Barometric pressure, lung disorders due to, 2288–2289
Baroreceptor(s), 162
in shock, 214
in water balance, 524
Barr body, 120
Barrett's epithelium, 674
Bartonella bacilliformis, 1617
Bartonellosis, 1617–1618
clinical manifestations of, 1617
diagnosis of, 1617
culture in, 1617
epidemiology of, 1617
hemolysis with, 913
pathology of, 1617
prevention of, 1618
prognosis in, 1618
treatment of, 1618
antibiotic therapy in, 1618
vector in, 1617
Bartter's syndrome 487, 519, 532, 542, 613
captopril in, 613
genetic factor in, 613
prostaglandin synthetase inhibition in, 613
Basal cell carcinoma, 2297
Basal cell epithelioma, 2271–2272, *2272*
Basal forebrain syndrome, 1991–1992
Basal ganglia, *2068*
in movement disorders, 2068
Basal metabolic rate, 1280
Base excess, of blood, reference values for, 2318
Basedow's disease, 1281
Basilar artery, 2089–2090
dissection of, 2092
occlusion of, 2095
collateral blood supply and, 2091
Basilar artery migraine, 2054, 2098
Basilar impression, 2187, 2188
Basis pontis, atrophy of, in olivopontocerebellar degeneration, 2083
Basophils, 941
Bassen-Kornzweig syndrome, vs. Friedreich's ataxia, 2083
Bath(s), in skin disease, 2240
Battle fatigue, 2009
Battle's sign, in skull fracture, 2171
Battlefield injury, 1574
BCG. See *Bacille-Calmette-Guérin vaccine.*
Becker dystrophy, 2203, 2204
Bed frame, for spinal cord injury, 2177
Bed rest, in back pain, 2063
Bed bugs, 1835
Bee stings, 1837–1838
Beef tapeworm, 1806
eradication of, 1809
Beer potomania, 526
Behavioral disorders
in Huntington's disease, 2074
in postencephalitic parkinsonism, 2071
neuroendocrine system in, 1250
vs. epilepsy, 2156
Behavior modification, for obesity, 1196
Behavioral techniques, in pain, 2053
Behçet's disease, 1960–1962, 2220, *2262, 2266*, 2270–2271
clinical manifestations of, 1961
diagnostic criteria for, 1961, 1961t
epidemiology of, 1960
immune response in, 1960–1961
pathology of, 1961
possibility of viral role in, 2137
treatment of, 1961
immunosuppressive agents in, 1961
Bejel, 1661–1162
Belching, 649
Bell's palsy, 2129, 2197
taste disorders and, 2032
Benign prostatic hyperplasia, 1376–1377
differential diagnosis of, 1377
tratment of, 1377
Benzene, 878
leukemia and, 987
Benzimidazole(s)
in tapeworm infection, 1809
substituted in peptic ulcer, 689
Benznidazole
in Chagas' disease, 1785–1786
Benzodiazepine(s)
abuse of, 2019–2021
and sleep disorders, 1988–1989
in central nervous system depressant abuse, 2022
Berenil
in African trypanosomiasis, 1782
Berger's disease, 574–575, *574*
immunoglobulins in, 574–575, *574*
Beriberi, 335, 1199
Bernard-Soulier (giant platelet) syndrome, 1037
"Berry" aneurysms, 2103
treatment of, 2107
Beryllium disease, 2284–2285
Besnier, prurigo gestationis of, 2269
Beta-adrenergic agonists, in primary pulmonary hypertension, 263
Beta-adrenergic blocking agents, 93–95, 94t
in shock, 222–223, 222t
in angina pectoris, 287
in hyperthyroidism, 1285
in migraine, 2055
in myocardial infarction, 294, 295
side effects of, 94–95
Beta-adrenegic receptor(s), 91–92, 92t
Beta-adrenergic receptor agonists
in asthma, 394–395
in hypertension, 277–278

Beta-aminoisobutyricaciduria, 1145
Beta-aminoproprionitrile, 783
Beta-lactam antibiotic-resistant staphylococci, 1550
Beta-lactamase(s), 1584, 1586
Bethanechol, in gastroesophageal reflux disease, 671
Bezoar(s), 705
Bicarbonate, serum, reference values for, 2318
Bicarbonate metabolism
  in acid-base balance disorders, 535–544
  renal processing in, 536–537
Bicarbonate secretion, gastric mucosa integrity and, 683, 684
Bicarbonate space, 536
Bicarbonate therapy
  in metabolic acidosis, 541
  in renal tubular acidosis, 608–609
Bicuspid aortic valve, 236
Biguanides, 1329
Bile
  formation of, 851–852, *852*
  reflux of, in gastric ulcer, 683
Bile acid(s)
  deficiency of conjugated, 729, 731
  increased deconjugation, 729–731
  total, serum and feces, reference values for, 2318
Bile acid–binding resin therapy, 1112, 1114
Bile duct(s)
  bleeding into, 862
  cysts of, 862
  disease of, 851–865
  obstruction of, 862–863
  pancreatitis in obstruction of, 862
  parasitic infection of, 863
  sclerosing cholangitis of, 862
  structural abnormalities of, 862
  tumor of, 863–864
    clinical manifestations of, 864
    diagnosis of, 864
    prognosis in, 864
    treatment of, 864
Bile salts, 851–852, *852*
Bilharziasis. See also *Schistosomiasis.*
  intestinal, 1813–1814
    clinical manifestations of, 1813–1814
    diagnosis of, 1814
    pathology of, 1813–1814
    treatment of, 1814
  urinary, 1812–1813
    clinical manifestations of, 1812–1813
    diagnosis of, 1813
    pathology of, 1812–1813
    treatment of, 1813
Biliary cirrhosis, *2263*
  primary, 837–839
    antimitochondrial antibodies in, 838
    associated diseases of, 838
    clinical features of, 838, 838t
    diagnosis of, 838
    etiology of, 837–838
    immune response in, 837–838
    laboratory findings in, 838
    pathology of, 838
    treatment of, 838–839
  secondary, 839
    biliary obstruction and, 839
    laboratory tests in, 839
    surgery for, 839
Biliary tract
  fluke infection of, 1815–1817
  parasitic disease of, 827–828, 828t
  radiography of, 853–855
  radionuclide imaging of, 855
  stricture of, 861–862
Biliary tract (*Continued*)
  ultrasonography of, 854, *854*
Bilirubin
  binding of, to plasma proteins, 806
  chemistry of, 806
  conjugated, reference values for, 2318
  enterohepatic circulation of, 807
  formation of, 806
  hepatic transport of, 806–807
  in acute viral hepatitis, 814
  metabolism of, 806–807, *806*
    inherited disorders of, 807–808, 807t
  plasma concentration of, 807
  total, reference values for, 2318
Bioethics, 11
Biofeedback, in pain, 2053
Biologicals, biotechnology production of, 133
Biologic antiviral agents, 111. See also specific products.
Biologic science, 4–6
Biological agents, neuropathy due to, 2195, *2195*
Biopsy. See also under specific organs.
  bone marrow. See under *Bone marrow* and *Bone marrow biopsy*.
  cerebral, in herpes simplex encephalitis, 2127
  in skin disease, 2238–2239
  muscle, diagnostic use of, 2200–2201, *2200*
  renal, 514–575
Biotin, dietary allowance for, 1178
Bismuth
  as nephrotoxin, 600–601
  in peptic ulcer, 689
Biting midges, 1835
Biting mites, 1835–1836
B-K mole syndrome, 2275
Black flies, 1835
Black widow spider, 1836–1837
Blackwater fever, 1777
Bladder
  dysfunction of, in vitamin B_{12} deficiency, 2067
    treatment of, 2147
  in bilharziasis, 1812–1813
  transitional cell cancer of, 643–644
Bladder anomaly, 639
  urinary, disorders of, 2028–2030, *2029*
Bland diet, 1214
Blastomyces dermatitidis, 1762
Blastomycosis, 1762–1764
  clinical manifestations of, 1763
  cutaneous lesions in, *2261*
    culture in, 1763
  diagnosis of, 1763
    skin test in, 1763
  disseminated, 1763
  epidemiology of, 1762–1763
  etiology of, 1762
  immune response in, 1763
  pathogenesis of, 1763
  pathology of, 1763
  prognosis in, 1763–1764
  pulmonary, 1763
  treatment of, 1763–1764
    antifungal therapy in, 1763
Bleb disease, blue rubber, *2262*
Bleeding. See *Hemorrhage* and specific sites.
Bleeding diatheses, systemic, intracerebral hemorrhage in, 2104
Bleeding time, 1030–1031
  reference values for, 2337
Blenorrhea, inclusion, 2221
Bleomycin, 1097
  interstitial lung disease and, 418
  toxicity of, 1092
Blepharoconjunctivitis, 2220
Blepharospasm, 2078–2079
"Blind loop syndrome," 708, 730–731
Blindness. See also *Amaurosis.*
  cortical, 2034
  hysterical, 2014
  river, 1832–1833
Blistering diseases, 2267–2270, *2268*
Bloating, 649–650
Blood
  coagulation of. See *Coagulation disorders.*
  diseases of. See names of specific diseases.
  expectoration of. See *Hemoptysis.*
  lipids. See *Lipids, serum.*
  loss of. See *Hemorrhage(s).*
  purification of. See under *Dialysis* and *Hemodialysis*.
Blood alcohol level, 51
Blood cells, precursors of, 866–867
Blood coagulation, 1040–1058. See also specific diagnoses.
  disorders of, acquired, 1051–1058
    clinical features of, 1044
    genetic factors in, 1044–1051, 1045t
    laboratory assessment of, 1044
  extrinsic vs. intrinsic pathways of, 1040–1043, *1042*
  inhibition of, 1043–1044, 1056
  process of, 1040–1044, *1042*
  vitamin K and, 1208–1209
Blood flow
  cerebral, cardiac disease and, 2092
    in brain injury, 2172
    in classic migraine, 2054
    in common migraine, 2055
Blood groups, 937–938, 937t
"Blood patch," epidural, in intracranial hypotenson, 2167
Blood pressure. See also *Hypertension.*
  adrenergic nerves and, 273, 275
  arterial baroreflex and, 272–273
  autonomic nervous system and, 273
  circulatory dynamics and, 273–274
  emergency reduction of, 279
  fluid volume and, 273
  in altered consciousness, 1976
  in heart failure, 194–195
  maintenance mechanisms of, 272–274
  measurement of, 266–267
    in cardiovascular disease, 151–152
  norepinephrine and, 272, 275
  renin-angiotensin system and, 273, 275
  salt intake and, 273
  vascular autoregulation and, 273
Blood products, reactions to, 1866
Blood supply, to brain, 2087
Blood transfusion, 936–940
  ABO blood groups and, 937–938, 937t
  acidosis with, 940
  acquired immunodeficiency syndrome and, 939, 1862
  air embolism with, 939
  allergy with, 939
  anaphylactoid reactions with, 939
  bleeding tendency with, 939
  circulatory overload with, 939
  citrate intoxication with, 939–940
  compatibility testing for, 937–938
  contaminated blood for, 938–939
  cytomegalovirus infection and, 939
  disseminated intravascular coagulation in, 939
  emergency, 937–938
  graft-versus-host disease and, 940
  hazards of, 938–940, 938t
  hemolysis with, 938
  hepatitis and, 939, 939t
  hyperkalemia with, 940

Blood transfusion (*Continued*)
hypothermia with, 940
indications for, 936
in fluid volume depletion, 520
malaria and, 939
massive, 939–940
microaggregates with, 940
noncardiac pulmonary edema with, 939
nonhemolytic febrile reactions, 938
red blood cell components for, 936–937, 937t
red cell immunogens and, 937
Rh factor in, 937–938
syphilis and, 939
thrombocytopenic purpura after, 393
whole blood components for, 936
Blood urea nitrogen, 510
Blood vessels. See also names of specific vessels.
aging and, 22
of skin, 229
Blood volume
cardiovascular function and, 163
in heart failure, 163
reference values for, 2337
Bloom's syndrome, 143
leukemia with, 987
Blue-ringed octopus, 1843–1844
Blue rubber bleb disease, *2262*
Body fluid compartments, 515–516
Body fat. See *Obesity.*
Body form, changes during puberty, 17
Body image
disturbed in anorexia nervosa, 1188
in bulimia nervosa, 1190
Body plethysmography, 374
Body rocking, in tardive dyskinesia, 2076
Body temperature. See also *Fever* and *Hypothermia.*
extreme, in coma, 1976
normal, regulation of, hypothalamus and, 2025–2026
Body weight. See also *Obesity.*
during puberty, 17
hypertension and, 267–268
Boerhaave's syndrome, 677
Bolivian hemorrhagic fever, 1751t, 1756–1757
Bone, 1419–1422. See also entries under *Skeletal.*
density disorders of, 1463–1465
dynamics of, 1421
formation of, 1420–1421
function of, 1419
in acromegaly, 1261
in Marfan's syndrome, 1151
in neurofibromatosis, 2085
in sarcoidosis, 436, *436*
mass measurement of, 1422
matrix disorders of, 1428
mineral content measurement of, 1422
mineral homeostasis and, 1415–1423
Paget's disease of. See *Paget's disease of bone.*
parathyroid hormone and, 1434
resorption of, 1420–1421
staphylococcal infection of, 1546–1547
structure of, 1419–1420, *1420*
tuberculosis of, 1628
vitamin D and, 1423–1425, *1423*, 1424t
Bone disease
in uremia, 489
metabolic, 1421–1422
bone mass measurement in, 1422
mineral content measurement in, 1422
risk factors for, 1421–1422, 1421t
serum measurements in, 1422
Bone marrow
anatomy of, 869–870
compartments of, 953, *955*
in acute leukemia, 960
in anemia, 876, 876t
in chronic myelogenous leukemia, 978
in hairy cell leukemia, 985
in hemolysis, 901
in iron deficiency anemia, 890
in leukemoid reaction, 958–959
in megaloblastic anemia, 894
in polycythemia vera, 969–970
irradiation of, in radiation injury, 2300, 2302t
marrow cell release from, 869, 870, *870*
neutrophil production by, 953–954, *955*
radiobiology of, 2299
tumor cells in, 960
Bone marrow biopsy
in acute myelogenous leukemia, 989
in anemias, 876
aplastic, 879
in chronic lymphoctic leukemia, 982
in hairy cell leukemia, 985
in Hodgkin's disease, 1005
in polycythemia vera, 969–970
Bone marrow differential count, reference value for, 2337
Bone marrow transplantation, 1025–1028
clinical results in, 1026, *1026*
cyclosphosphamide with, 1026, 1027
for aplastic anemia, 1026–1027, *1026*
for leukemia, *1026*, 1027, *1027*
graft-versus-host disease with 1026, 1027
immune system in, 1026
immunosuppression in, 1026
in acute lymphoblastic leukemia, 990
in acute myelogenous leukemia, 991
in aplastic anemia, 878–879, 880, 881
in Chediak-Higashi disease, 952
in chronic granulomatous disease, 951
in chronic myelogenous leukemia, 979
in neutropenia, 957
in severe B thalassemia, 926
preparation for, 1026
principles of, 1025–1026
Bone tumor, 1466–1468
benign, 1467
classification of, 1466–1467
malignant, 1467
metastatic, 1467–1468
primary, 1466–1467
staging of, 1466–1467
Bonnevie-Ullrich-Turner syndrome, 1151
Bordetella bronchiseptica, 1569
Bordetella parapertussis, 1569
Bordetella pertussis, 1568
Bornholm disease, 1730–1731
Boron toxicity, 2314
Borrelia, 1662
microbiology of, 1662
Borrelia vincentii, 1664
Boston Collaboration Drug Surveillance Program, 82
Botulism, 781, 1577–1578, 2199
antitoxin for, 1578
foodborne, 1577–1578
immunization for, 43t, 46
infant, 1578
mouse assay in, 1578
neurologic examination in, 1578
neuromuscular block due to, 2215
prevention of, 1578
prognosis in, 1578
toxin of, 1577–1578
unclassified, 1578
wounds and, 1578
Bouchard's nodes, *1952*
Bourneville's disease, 2085
Boutonneuse fever, 1682
cutaneous lesions in, *2661*
Bowel. See also entries under *Intestine* and *Intestinal.*
dysfunction of, in vitamin B_{12} deficiency, 2067
irritable. See *Irritable bowel syndrome.*
resting of, total parenteral nutrition in, 1216
Bowel habits, change in, 648–649
Bowen's disease, 1086, 2251
Box jellyfish, 1843
Brachial neuritis, acute, 2197–2198
Brachial plexus neuropathy, idiopathic, 2197–2198. See also *Brachial neuritis, acute.*
Brachydactyly, type E, 145
Bradycardia, 317–322. See also specific diagnoses.
functional rhythm and, 319
Bradycardia-tachycardia syndrome, 318–319
electrocardiography in, 319, *319*
Bradykinesia
definition of, 2069
in juvenile Huntington's disease, 2074
in parkinsonism, 2070
Brain
arterial blood supply of, 2087
blood flow within, in common migraine, 2055
blood supply to, 2087
edema of, glucocorticosteroid therapy for, 112, 114
hemispheres of, language and, 1993–1995
hemorrhage of, intracranial, 2103–2111
imaging techniques for, 1968–1969
in Alzheimer's disease, 1999–2000
in cardiorespiratory arrest, 480
in right ventricular failure, 198–199
in Wernicke's encephalopathy, 2065
infectious processes of, and epilepsy, 2150
injury to 2170–2175
anxiety and, 2009
computed tomography in, 2173
severe, prognosis in, 1981–1983, *1981*, *1982*
metabolic disease of. See *Metabolic brain disease.*
opiate receptors of, 1234
subtentorial lesions of, 1972–1973
supratentorial lesions of, 1972
Brain abscess, 1585, 2111–2114
enteric bacteria in, 1593
computed tomography in, 2113, 2114t
hematogenous, 2112
metastatic, 2112
staphylococcal, 1547
with congenital heart disease, 228
Brain damage, prevention of, in intracranial hypertenson, *2167*
Brain death, prognosis in, 1981–1983, *1983*
Brain swelling, in bacterial mmeningitis, 1553
Brain tumor, and epilepsy, 2150
hemorrhage into, 2104
metastatic, treatment outcome in, 2166
Brainstem
auditory evoked potentials of, 1970
dysfunction of, and drop attacks, 2047
and sensory loss, 2048–2049
gliomas of, 2164
infarcts of, 672
injury to, 2171
and ataxia, 2045
lesion of, vs. syringomyelia, 2084

Brainstem (*Continued*)
paraneoplastic degeneration of, and vertigo, 2043
surgery on, in pain relief, 2053
vascular malformations of, in Hippel-Lindau disease, 2086
Branchio-oto-renal syndrome, 145
Breast(s)
development of, 1398
metastatic carcinoma of, and back pain, 2061
nonmalignant diseases of, 1398–1401
Paget's disease of, 1086
Breast cancer, 1402–1405
CAMF protocol for, 1092t
carcinoembryonic antigen in, 1402
clinical manifestations in, 1402
endocrine factor in, 1402
epidemiology of, 1402
estrogen receptor protein in, 1402–1403, 1403t
etiology of, 1402
genetic factor in, 1402
hypercalcemia and, 1448
in male, 1405
metastatic disease with, 1402, 1404–1405
pathology of, 1402
radiation exposure and, 1402
staging in, 1402
treatment of, 1403–1405, 1403t
adjuvant therapy in, 1405
aminoglutethimide in, 1403–1404
antiestrogen therapy in, 1404
cytotoxic agents in, 1404–1405
endocrine therapy in, 1403–1404
radiation therapy in, 1403, 1404–1405
surgery for, 1403
Breath tests
in malabsorption syndrome, 726
Bretylium, 326
"Bright plaques," in retinal arterioles, 2096
Brill-Zinsser disease, 1678
Briquet's syndrome, 2014
Broca's aphasia, 1994
Broca's area, 1993
Bromide intoxication, 2021
Bromocriptine
in acromegaly, 1262
in galactorrhea, 1399
in hyperprolactinemia, 1264
Bronchial adenoma, 444
Bronchial blebs and bullae, 405
Bronchial constriction, pathogenesis of, *391*
Bronchial provocation test, in occupational asthma, 2286
Bronchiectasis, 422–424
clinical manifestations of, 423
diagosis of, 423
etiology of, 422–423
pathogenesis of, 423
pathology of, 423
prognosis in, 423–424
treatment of, 423
Bronchiolitis obliterans, 2289
Bronchitis
aspergillary, 1770
asthmatic, 398–399
chronic, 396, 397, 398–399. See also *Chronic obstructive pulmonary disease.*
bronchial hygiene measures in, 399
clinical manifestations in, 398
cough in, 398
course of, 398
differential diagnosis of, 398–399
laboratory findings in, 398
obstructive, 397
pathogenesis of, 398
Bronchitis (*Continued*)
chronic, pathology of, 398
prevalence of, 398
prognosis in, 398
sputum in, 398
wheezing in, 398
treatment of, 399
antibiotic therapy in, 399
bronchodilator agents in, 399
corticosteroids in, 399
Hemophilus influenzae and, 1564
industrial, 2286–2287
pulmonary hypertension and, 259–260
viral, 1695–1696, 1696t
Bronchocentric granulomatosis, 416
Bronchodilator agents
in chronic bronchitis, 399
in respiratory failure, 460–461
Bronchogenic carcinoma, 439–444
air pollution in, 440
clinical manifestations of, 440–441, 440t
diagnosis of, 441–443
biopsy in, 443
bronchoscopy in, 442–443
pleural fluid cytology in, 443
radiography in, 441–442, *442*, 443
sputum cytology in, 442
environmental factors in, 440
etiology of, 439
host factors in, 439
local extension of, 440–441, *440*
mediastinoscopy in, 443
metastasis with, 441
pathogenesis of, 439
prognosis of, 443–444
staging of, 443, 443t
systemic effects of, 441
TNM classification for, 443, 443t
tobacco and, 439–440
treatment of, 443–444
chemotherapy in, 444
immunotherapy in, 444
radiation therapy in, 444
surgery in, 443–444
Bronchogenic cysts, 405–406
Bronchography, 383
Bronchopulmonary aspergillosis, 416
Bronchopulmonary dysplasia, 477
Bronchopulmonary sequestration, 405–406
Bronchoscopy, 388–389. See also under specific diagnoses.
in bronchogenic carcinoma, 442–443
in interstitial lung disease, 411
Bronchospasm
atopic response indicators in, 390–392
in chronic airways disease, 396–397
nonspecific stimuli for, 393
parasympathetic nervous system in, 392–393, *393*
Brown spider, bite of, 1836
Brown-Séquard's syndrome, 2048, 2061, 2176
characteristics of, 2182
Brucella, 1614–1617
Brucella abortus, 1614, 1615
Brucella agglutination test, 1616
Brucella canis, 1614, 1615
Brucella melitensis, 1614, 1615
Brucella suis, 1614, 1615
Brucellosis, 1614–1617
animal tissue and products and, 1614–1615
clinical manifestations of, 1615
diagnosis of, 1615–1616
antibody titer in, 1616
culture in, 1615–1616
serology in, 1616
skin test in, 1616
epidemiology of, 1614–1615
Brucellosis (*Continued*)
pathogenesis of, 1615
pathology of, 1615
prevention of, 1617
prognosis in, 1616–1617
relapse in, 1616
treatment of, 1616
antibiotics in, 1616
Brugia malayi, 1828
Brugia timori, 1828
Bruits. See also under specific diagnosis.
carotid, 2094
management of, 2101
Bruton's X-linked agammaglobulinemia, 1482
Bruxism, and sleep disorders, *1988*, 1990
Bubonic plaque, 1600, 1601
Buckthorn neuropathy, 2195
Budd-Chiari syndrome, 841–842
Buerger's disease. See *Thromboangiitis obliterans.*
Bulbar encephalitis, with cancer, 1082
Bulbar muscles, in amyotrophic lateral sclerosis, 2079–2080
Bulimia nervosa, 1190–1191
vomiting in, 1190, 1191
Bullae, 2232, 2267
Bumetanide, in heart failure, 209
Bundle of His. See *His bundle.*
Bunyavirus, 1736
in acute central nervous system infections, *2122*, 2123
Buphthalmos, in glaucoma, 2218
Burkitt-like lymphoma, 1862
Burkitt's lymphoma, 999–1000, 1778
clinical features of, 1000
diagnosis of, 1000
chromosomal abnormality in, 999–1000
epidemiology of, 999
etiology of, 999–1000
genetic factor in, 999–1000
management of, 1000
pathogenesis of, 999–1000
pathology of, 1000
prognosis in, 1000
staging system for, 1000
vs. Kaposi's sarcoma, 2273
Burkitt's tumor, 994
relapses in, 963
Burnett's syndrome, 1449
Burns
caustic, esophageal, 676–677
chemical, 2296
enteric bacterial infection with, 1593–1594
fluid volume depletion and, 519
pulmonary complications in, 2287
Burow's solution, 2239, *2239*
Bursitis, 1959
vs. osteomyelitis, 1568
vs. parkinsonism, 2071
Burst-promoting activity, 964
Buruli ulcer, 1633
Busulfan, 1096
in chronic myelogenous leukemia, 978, 979
interstitial lung disease and, 418
Bypass grafting. See also *Coronary artery revascularization.*
graft patency in, 299–300
in angina pectoris, 298–300
in coronary artery disease, 297–300
myocardial infarction with, 299
postoperative management in, 299
reoperation in, 300
results of, 299
surgical procedure for, 299
Bypass surgery
for heart failure, 210
for obesity, 1196

^{14}C glycinecholate measurement, 726
C peptide, in diabetes mellitus, 1323, 1325
  serum, reference values for, 2318
C peptide suppression test, in insulinoma, 1345, *1346*
^{14}C xylose measurement, 726
Cadmium, toxicity of, 599, 2312–2313
"Cafe coronary," 2291
Café-au-lait spot(s), 2254, *2257*
  in neurofibromatosis, 2085
Caffeine, peptic ulcer and, 684
Calabar swellings, 1830–1831
Calcinosis, metastatic, *2264*
Calciotropic hormone system, 1415–1416, *1415*, *1417*
Calcitonin, 1451
  in calcium homeostasis, 1415
  in cancer, 1079
  in medullary carcinoma of thyroid, 1452
  in osteoporosis, 1460
  in Paget's disease of bone, 1462
  therapy with, 1453
Calcitriol, in sarcoidosis, 438
Calcium
  absorption of, 721–722
  body fluid distribution of, 1418, *1418*
  deficiency of, 1427–1428, 1430, 1431
  dietary allowance for, 1178
  dietary requirement of, 1418–1419
  homeostasis, 1415–1416, *1415*
  hormone regulation of, 1415–1416, 1416t
  in hormone action mediation, 1225, *1226*
  intake of, 1214
    osteoporosis and, 1456
  ionized, reference values for, 2318
  metabolism of, 1166, 1418–1419, *1418*
    glucocorticoids and, 1306
    in shock, 216
    in uremia, 551
    kidney regulation of, 500
  plasma concentration, 1416–1417, *1417*
    phosphate plasma concentration and, 1418
  total, reference values for, 2318
  transport of, 1415, *1417*
Calcium channel receptor antagonists
  in asthma, 395
  in migraine, 2055
Calcium chloride, in cardiopulmonary resuscitation, 481–482
Calcium crystal deposition, arthropathy in, 1950–1951
Calcium oxalate, deposition of, 1950
Calcium pyrophosphate dihydrate crystal deposition disease, 1950
Calcium therapy, in osteoporosis, 1460
Calcium-channel blocking agent(s)
  in angina pectoris, 287
  in myocardial infarction, 294
  in primary pulmonary hypertension, 264–265
  in Raynaud's disease, 355
Calculus(i)
  appendiceal, 796
  renal, 628–633. See also *Kidney stones.*
  urinary tract, in cystinuria, 612–613
California encephalitis, 1747
  clinical features of, 1747–1748
  diagnosis of, 1748
  epidemiology of, 1747
  prevention of, 1748
  vector in, 1747
  virus in, 1747
Callosal apraxia, 1995
Calmodulin, 1225, *1226*
Caloric irrigation, of tympanum, in diagnosis of eye movements, 2036
Caloric tests, in evaluation of vertigo, 2041
Calorie intake. See also *Protein-calorie malnutrition; Protein-caloric supplementation.*
  in obesity, 1193
Calymmatobacterium granulomatis, 1649
CAMF protocol, for breast cancer, 1092t
cAMP. See *Cyclic adenosine monophosphate.*
Camurati-Engelmann disease, 1465
Cancer. See also *Carcinoma* and specific diagnoses and sites.
  acromegaly with, 1079
  adrenocorticotropic hormone in, 1077
  alcohol intake and, 1070
  anemia with, 1074
  anorexia with, 1073–1074
  asbestos exposure and, 2284
  ascorbic acid for, 1205
  biologic effects of, 1073–1074
  brain in, 1081–1082
  bulbar encephalitis with, 1082
  cachexia with, 1073–1074
  calcitonin in, 1079
  causes of, 1069–1073
  cell heterogeneity and, 1061
  cerebellum in, 1082
  chorionic gonadotropin in, 1079
  chromosome abnormalities in, 1061–1062
  cigarette smoking and, 48, 1069–1070
  classification of, 1063
    TNM system, 1063, 1063t
  continuing care in, 1065
  cranial nerves in, 1081–1082
  Cushing's syndrome with, 1077
  cutaneous manifestations of, 1084–1086, 1085t–1086t
  cytogenetics of, 1061–1062
  definitions for, 1059
  dementia in, 1081–1082
  depression in, 2011
  detection of, 1064
  diagnosis of, 1064–1065
    general evaluation in, 1064
    initial, 1064
  diet and, 39, 1071–1072
  disseminated intravascular coagulation with, 1074
  drug intake and, 1071
  endocrine factor in, 1077–1080
  environmental factor in, 1069–1073, 1070t
  eosinophilopoietin in, 1080
  epidemiology of, 1069–1073
  erythrocytosis with, 1074
  erythropoietin in, 1079–1080
  etiology of, 1060
  food preparation and preservation and, 39
  genetic factor in, 1066, 1072t, 1073
  growth hormone in, 1079
  growth hormone–releasing hormone in, 1079
  growth of, 1061, 1062, *1062*
  hematologic complications with, 1074
  histology of, 1061
  historical background for, 1059
  hormone secretion by, 1077, 1077t
  hypercalcemia and, 1078
  hyperparathyroidism with, 1078
  hypoglycemia and, 1079
  hypophosphatemia with, 1078–1079
  immunosuppression and, 1071
  ionizing radiation and, 1070
  Karnofsky scale of "performance status" in, 1063, 1064t
  management principles for, 1065–1066
  markers in, 1063, 1075–1076
    ectopic polypeptides as, 1076
    oncofetal antigens as, 1075–1076
    placental proteins as, 1076
Cancer (*Continued*)
  metastatic, 1061
    pain in, 2049
  mortality statistics for, 1059, 1059t, 1060t
  muscle disorders in, 1083
  nervous system effects in, 1081
  neuromuscular junction disorders in, 1083
  nonmetastatic nervous system effects in, 1081–1084, 1081t
  nutrition and, 1071–1072
  occupational exposures and, 1070–1071
  occurrence patterns of, 1069
  osteoclast activating factor in, 1078
  paraneoplastic syndromes with, 1073, 1073t
  parasites and, 1071
  parathormone in, 1078
  peripheral nerves in, 1082–1083
  pollution and, 1071
  prognosis in, 1063, 1063t
  proopiomelanocortin in, 1077
  prostaglandins in, 1078
  pruritus with, 1084, 1086
  radiation exposure and, 1070
  screening for, 1064
  skin, 2271–2272
  solar radiation and, 1070
  spinal cord in, 1082
  staging of, 1063
  supportive care for, 1065–1066
  taste disorders and, 2032
  therapeutic approach to, 1065
  thrombosis with, 1074
  tobacco use and, 48, 1069–1070
  Trousseau's syndrome with, 1074
  vasopressin in, 1079
  viruses and, 1071
  vitamin A and, 1207
  weakness in, 1083
Cancer chemotherapy, 1090–1100, 1090t. See also specific agents and classes.
  antineoplastic agents for, 1093–1100
  biochemical tests in, 1091
  carcinogenicity of, 1092–1093, 1093t
  cell cycle factor in, 1090
  combination, 1091–1092, 1092t
  drug interactions and, 1091–1092
  fractional kill hypothesis in, 1090
  heterogeneity factor in, 1090
  hormone receptors and, 1091
  in adjuvant therapy, 1093
  infertility and, 1093
  kinetic basis for, 1090–1091
  pharmacokinetic response to, determinants in, 1091
  plant products for, 1098–1099
  response assessment in, 1091
  response prediction with, 1090–1091
  strategies of, 1091–1093
  with radiation therapy, 1092–1093
Cancer therapy. See also *Cancer chemotherapy.*
  for metastasis, 1089–1090
  histologic grading and, 1087
  hormonal, 1100, 1101t
  immunotherapy for, 1100–1101, *1101*
  local-regional disease management in, 1088–1089
  palliation in, 1087
  principles of, 1086–1102
  radiation as, 1088–1089, 1088t, *1089t*
  staging and, 1087
  surgery in, 1088
  tumor classification and, 1087
  tumor growth rate and, 1087, 1090, *1090*
Candida, 1538, 1768
  infections with, 2247, *2248*
Candida albicans, 1768–1769
Candida endophthalmitis, 2221

Candida glabrata, 1768
Candida vaginitis, 1642
Candidiasis (candidosis), 1479, 1482, 1768–1770
  oral, 665, *665*
  chronic mucocutaneous, 1861
  clinical manifestations of, 1768–1769
  diagnosis of, 1769
    culture in, 1769
    serology of, 1769
    skin tests in, 1769
  epidemiology of, 1768
  etiology of, 1768
  immune response in, 1768
  mucocutaneous, 1768, 1769
    polyglandular deficiency with, 1408
  pathogenesis of, 1768
  pathology of, 1768
  prevention of, 1769
  prognosis in, 1769
  systemic, 1768–1769
  treatment of, 1769
  types of, 2247
Canicola fever, 1666
Canker sore, 664
Cannabis, abuse of, 2022–2023
Capillariasis, 1820
Capillary system, 161
Caplan's syndrome, 1915, 2281
Capoten. See *Captopril*.
Capreomycin, 1625
Capsular-thalamic hemorrhage
  external, 2108
  internal, 2108
Capsulitis, adhesive, 1955
Captopril
  in Bartter's syndrome, 613
  in heart failure, 206
  in hypertension, 278
  in primary pulmonary hypertension, 265
Carbamate, poisoning from, 89
Carbamazepine
  in epilepsy, 2158, *2158*
  in glossopharyngeal neuralgia, 2059
  in postherpetic neuralgia, 2129
  in trigeminal neuralgia, 2059
Carbamyl phosphate synthetase deficiency, 1129–1130
Carbenicillin, pharmacokinetic parameters of, 70t
Carbenoxolone, in peptic ulcer, 689
Carbidopa, in parkinsonism, 2072
Carbohydrate(s)
  absorption of, 721, 724, 725
  dietary allowances for, 1177
  metabolism of, disorders of, 1104–1109
    exercise and, 40
    hormone control factor in, 1228
    in chronic renal failure, 553, 557
    in diabetes mellitus, 1323
    in liver disease, 804
Carbon dioxide
  elimination of, 536
  partial pressure of, reference values for, 2318
  production of, 536
  total, reference values for, 2318
Carbon dioxide–diffusing capacity, abnormalities of, 377
Carbon monoxide, blood, reference values for, 2318
Carbon monoxide poisoning, 86, 2291
Carbon tetrachloride, as nephrotoxin, 603
Carbonic anhydrase inhibitor(s)
  in heart failure, 209
  metabolic acidosis and, 539
Carboxyhemoglobin. See *Carbon monoxide*.
Carbuncles, 1546
Carcinoembryonic antigen(s), 1075
  colon cancer and, 768
  in breast cancer, 1402
  in pancreatic cancer, 778
  serum, reference values for, 2319
Carcinogenesis, 2299
  natural agents of, 39
  natural inhibitors of, 39
  oncogenes in, 1968
Carcinoid, *2263*
  metastatic malignant, 738
Carcinoid syndrome, 1413–1414
  5-hydroxyindoleacetic acid in, 1414
  treatment of, 1414
Carcinoma. See also under *Cancer* and specific diagnoses.
  metastatic, of breast, and back pain, 2061
    thyroid, and back pain, 2061
    to eye, 2222
  squamous cell, 2272, *2272*
Carcinomatosis, meningeal, 2164
    treatment outcome in, 2166
Carcinomatous myopathy, 2210
Carcinosarcoma, of lung, 445
Cardiac. See also *Heart*.
Cardiac amyloidosis, 337
Cardiac arrhythmias. See *Arrhythmias*.
Cardiac catheterization, 183–188. See also specific diagnoses.
  capabilities of, 183
  cardiac output measurements by, 184–185
  heart valve study by, 184–185, *184*
  hemodynamic measurements with, 183, 184t
  in aortic regurgitation, 255
  in aortic stenosis, 253
  in asymmetric septal hypertrophy, 330–331
  in atrial septal defect, 229
  in cardiovascular disease, 154
  in congenital valvular aortic stenosis, 236–237
  in Eisenmenger syndrome, 241
  in mitral regurgitation, 251
  in mitral stenosis, 248
  in pericardial constriction, 344
  in primary pulmonary hypertension, 262
  in pulmonary stenosis, 235
  in pulmonary vein connection anomaly, 239
  in tetralogy of Fallot, 233
  in valvular heart disease, 245–246
  indications for, 183, 183t
  left heart, 184
  right heart, 183–184
  risks of, 186, 188
  special techniques for, 186, *187*, *188*
Cardiac death, sudden. See *Sudden cardiac death*.
Cardiac emboli, and stroke, *2095*, 2096
Cardiac glycosides, 201–203, 201t, 202t. See also specific agents.
  blood level determinations in, 204
  dosage schedules for, 201, 201t
Cardiac output, 161
  in anemia, 872
  in fluid volume disorders, 521
  in heart failure, 194–195
  in shock, 212, 219
  indicator-dilution techniques for, 191
  low vs. high failure, 190
  measurements of, by cardiac catheterization, 184–185
    in critical care management, 475
  venous return and, 162
  with gastrointestinal hemorrhage, 649
Cardiac sound(s), 152
Cardiac syncope, 1985, *1984*
Cardiac tamponade, 290
  with pericardial effusion, 343
Cardiogenic shock, 289, 291
Cardiology. See also specific diagnoses and procedures.
  approach to patient in, 150–154
Cardiomegaly, in Friedreich's ataxia, 2083
Cardiomyopathy, 329–339. See also specific diagnoses.
  alcoholic, 336
  Chagas', 1785
  classification of, 329, 329t
  cobalt-beer, 336
  familial, 332–333
  infective, 333–334
  inflammatory, 333–334
  nutritional, 335–337
  peripartum, 338
  sudden death and, 296, 297
Cardiopulmonary bypass, thrombocytopenia in, 1036
Cardiopulmonary resuscitation, 480–482
  administration of, 481–482, 481t
  atropine in, 482
  calcium chloride in, 481–482
  catecholamines in, 482
  closed chest compression in, 481
  direct-current cardioversion in, 481
  electrocardiography in, 481, 482
  epinephrine in, 481–482
  failure with, 482
  isoproterenol in, 482
  lidocaine in, 482
  outcome determinants of, 480–481
  oxygen therapy in, 481
  patient consent for, 479
  respiratory assistance in, 481
Cardiorespiratory arrest
  brain in, 480
  heart in, 480–481
  kidneys in, 481
  outcome determinants of, 480–481
  pathophysiology of, 480–481
  respiratory muscles in, 481
Cardiorespiratory system, in puberty, 17
Cardiovascular abnormalities, hemolysis and, 913–914
Cardiovascular disease, 150–367
  arterial pressure and pulses in, 151–152, *152*
  angiography in, 186, *187*
  auscultation in, 152
  blood pressure measurement in, 151–152
  cardiac catheterization in, 154, 183–188
  chest pain in, 150
  cigarette smoking and, 47, 157
  cyanosis in, 151
  data components for, 150–154
  diabetes mellitus and, 157–158
  diagnostic procedures in, 164–169
  dizziness in, 150–151
  echocardiography in, 153, 175–179, *175–179*
  edema in, 150
  electrocardiography in, 153, 169–175
  epidemiology of, 155–158
  hemoptysis in, 150
  history in, 150–151
  hypercholesterolemia and, 157–158
  hypertension and, 157–158
  laboratory examinations in, 152–154
    indications for, 154–155
  liver disease and, 835
  management approach to, 150–155
  mortality from, 156t, 157t
  nuclear imaging in, 179–182
  obesity and, 157–158

Cardiovascular disease (*Continued*)
  palpitation in, 150
  physical appearance in, 151
  physical examination in, 151–152
  precordial movements in, 152, *152*
  prevalence of, 155–158
  radiography in, 152–153, 164–169
  radionuclide imaging in, 153
  risk factors of, 156–158, *157*, 268, 268t, *269*
  shortness of breath in, 150
  venous pressure and pulse in, 151, *151*
  with ankylosing spondylitis, 1920
  with diabetes mellitus, 1340
Cardiovascular system. See also *Peripheral circulation.*
  blood volume effects on, 163
  control of, 158–164
  disturbances of, in tetanus, 1580
  function of, 158–164
  functional anatomy of, 158–164
  gastrointestinal hemorrhage and, 649
  heart failure in, 163–164
  hormone factor in control of, 1229
  in spinal cord injury, 2177
  in syphilis, 1655
  integrated function of, 161–164, *161*
  stress response of, 162–163
Cardioversion, 327–328
  complications of, 328
  contraindications to, 328
  direct current, for heart failure, 200, 210
  indications for, 328
  technique of, 327
Carditis, with acute rheumatic fever, 1530
Caries, dental, 663
Carmustine, in multiple myeloma, 1018
Carnitine deficiency, *2205*, 2206
Caroli's disease, 862
β-Carotene, 725, 1206
  serum, reference values for, 2319
Carotene absorption test, reference values for, 2319
Carotenoid(s), 1206, 1207
Carotid artery
  dissection of, 2092
  internal, atheroma of, 2094
    occlusion of, 2094
    stenosis of, 2094
  lesion of, asymptomatic, management of, 2101
  occlusion of, intracranial anastomoses and, 2091
Carotid artery disease, symptoms of, *2097*
Carotid artery ischemia, symptoms and signs of, 2097
Carotid arterectomy, and headache, 2056
Carotid body, 162
Carotid endarterectomy, in cerebral atherothrombotic disease, 2100
Carotid sinus massage, in tachycardia, 307–308
Carotid sinus syncope, 1984, *1984*
Carotidynia, 2056
Carpal tunnel syndrome, 1915, 1960, 2196–2197
Carpenter's syndrome, 1172
Carrion's disease, 1617
Cartilage
  articular, 1897
  degeneration of, 1892
CAT. See *Computed tomography.*
Cat scratch disease, 1618–1620
  clinical manifestations of, 1618–1619, 1619t
  diagnosis of, 1619–1620
    differential, 1620
    skin tests in, 1619
  epidemiology of, 1618
  lymphadenopathy with, 1618–1620, 1619t
  pathogenesis of, 1618
Cat scratch disease (*Continued*)
  prevention of, 1620
  transmission of, 1618
  treatment of, 1620
Catagen, 2231
Catamenial epilepsy, 2153
Cataplexy, and drop attacks, 2046
Cataract(s), 2217
  atopic diathesis and, 2249
  in diabetic retinopathy, 1338
Catecholamines, 91, 1220, 1243. See also specific agents.
  biologic actions of, 1409–1410
  biosynthesis of, 1408–1409, *1409*
  fractionated, reference values for, 2319
  free, reference values for, 2319
  hypertension and, 274–275
  in cardiopulmonary resuscitation, 482
  in heart failure, 201
  in hypertension, 1408
  in hypoglycemia, 1342–1343
  inhibiting agents of, 81t
  mechanisms of action of, 1223, 1224–1226
  mediators of action, 1224, 1224t
  metabolism of, 1409, *1409*
  receptors for, 1224
  sodium balance and, 494
  urinary, reference values for, 2319
Catfish, 1844
Catheterization
  bacteriuria from, 621
  cardiac. See *Cardiac catheterization.*
  Swan-Ganz, 183–184, 474–475, *475*
Cauda equina, pseudoclaudication of, in lumbar spondylosis, 2184
Causalgia, 2063
  definition of, 2047
Caustic burns, of esophagus, 676–677
Caustic compounds, poisoning from, 88
Cavernous sinus thrombosis, 2116
CCNU, in cancer chemotherapy, 1096t, 1097
CEA. See *Carcinoembryonic antigen.*
Cefoxitin, 1586
Celiac compression syndrome, 758
Celiac disease, 899
  adult, 724, 725, 732
  carcinoma with, 734
  clinical manifestations of, 733
  corticosteroids in, 733–734
  dermatitis herpetiformis with, 734, 2269
  diagnosis of, 733
  dietary management of, 733–734
  etiology of, 732–733
  genetic factor in, 733
  gluten sensitivity in, 732–734
  histology of, 732
  hyposplenism with, 734
  immune response in, 733
  lymphoma with, 734
  neurologic complications with, 734
  pathogenesis of, 732–733
  radiography in, 733
  small bowel ulceration with, 734
  treatment of, 733–734, *734*
Celiac sprue. See *Celiac disease, adult.*
Cell(s)
  APUD, 1230
  blood, precursors of, 866–867
  chief, 681
  division of, 138–139
  gastrin, 681
  Gaucher, 1117, *1117*, 1118
  kinetics of, radiation effects and, 2299
  Langerhans, 942, 1009, 2228
  mast, disease of, 2271
  Paget, 2251
  parietal, 681
  Sertoli, 1365–1366
Cell count, in bacterial meningitis, 1553
Cell-mediated immunity, in kidney disease, 504–505
Cellular immunodeficiency disorder, 1858–1859, 1858t
  with immunoglobulins, 1858–1859
  with purine nucleoside phosphorylase deficiency, 1859
Cellular physiology
  aging and, 22, 24
Cellular retinoic acid binding protein, 1206
Cellulitis
  gas-forming, 1575t
  Hemophilus influenza, 1564
  in heroin addiction, 2018
  nonclostridial crepitant, 1593
  synergistic necrotizing, 1575t
  vs. osteomyelitis, 1568
Centipedes, 1837
  disease carried by, 1833, 1833t
Central core disease, 2206, 2207
Central cord syndrome, 2176
Central hearing loss, 2039
Central nervous system
  acute poisoning of, 1979–1981
  arboviral infection of, 1742–1749, 1742t
  diseases of, bacterial, 2111–2121
    neuroendocrine system effects and, 1246–1250
    respiratory failure and, 457
  infections of, in immunocompromised host, 2141–2143
  irradiation of, as radiation injury, 2302t
    local, 2300
  radiobiology of, 2299
  tuberculosis of, 1629
  viral infections of, acute, 2122t
    slow, 2135–2138
Central nervous system depressants, abuse of, 2019–2021
Central nervous system stimulants, abuse of, 2021–2022
Central pontine myelinolysis, 2066–2067
Central venous pressure monitoring
  in critical care management, 474, 477–478
  in shock, 218
Central vertigo, 2042
Centronuclear myopathy, 2207
Cephalosporins, 104–105, 104t
  as nephrotoxin, 596–597
  dosage of, and data on, 101t
Cercarial dermatitis, 1811, 1812, 1815
Cerebellar abscess, 2113
Cerebellar ataxia, in ataxia telangiectasia, 2086
Cerebellar cortex, in ataxia telangiectasia, 2086
Cerebellar hematoma, treatment of, 2111
Cerebellar hemispheres, hemangioblastomas of, in Hippel-Lindau disease, 2086
Cerebellar hemorrhage, 2108, *2110*
  in Hippel-Lindau disease, 2086
Cerebellar mass lesion, in Hippel-Lindau disease, 2086
Cerebellar peduncles, in olivopontocerebellar degeneration, 2083
Cerebellopontine angle
  tumors of, 2164
    and ataxia, 2045
Cerebellum
  acute lateral dysfunction of, and asthenia, 2044
  alcoholic degeneration of, 2066
  atrophy of, in olivopontocerebellar degeneration, 2083
  disorders of, and sensory loss, 2049
  in ataxia telangiectasia, 2086

Cerebellum (*Continued*)
in cancer, 1082
in spinocerebellar degenerations, 2080
in striatonigral degeneration, 2079
paraneoplastic degeneration of, and vertigo, 2043
tumor of, and ataxia, 2045
vs. Friedreich's ataxia, 2083
Cerebral angiography
in cerebral atherothrombotic disease, 2101
in epilepsy, 2156
Cerebral arteriography, in subdural empyema, 2115
Cerebral artery(ies)
anterior, 2087
occlusion of, 2094
atherothrombosis of, symptoms of, 2094–2097
syndromes of, 2094–2097
major, anatomy of, 2087–2090
blood supply to, 2087–2090
mechanical interference with, and stroke, *2095*, 2096
middle, 2087, *2087*
infarction of, 2094
occlusion of, 2094
posterior, 2090
occlusion of, 2095
thromboembolism of, symptoms of, 2094–2097
syndromes of, 2094–2097
thrombosis of, coagulation abnormalities and, 2093
polycythemia and, 2093
thrombocytosis and, 2093
Cerebral atherothrombotic disease, surgery in, 2100–2101
Cerebral biopsy, in herpes simplex encephalitis, 2127
Cerebral blood flow
in brain injury, 2172
reduced, cardiac disease and, 2092
Cerebral chromomycosis, 1774
Cerebral cortex, in amyotrophic lateral sclerosis, 2080
vascular malformation of, in Sturge-Weber disease, 2085
Cerebral disorders, regional diagnosis of, 1991–1993
Cerebral edema
in infarction, 2090
in stroke, 2099, 2101
Cerebral epidural abscess, 2115
Cerebral extradural abscess, 2115
Cerebral hemisphere(s), arterial supply to, 2087, *2087, 2088*
in vitamin B_{12} deficiency, 2067
tumors of, 2163
Cerebral hemorrhage, hypertension with, 271
Cerebral infarction, 2090–2103
and gait disorders, 2045
treatment of, 2101
Cerebral ischemia, 2090–2103
causes of, 2090, *2090*
coagulation alterations and, *2093*
management of, 2099–2102
Cerebral malaria, 1778
Cerebral manifestations, of bacterial endocarditis, 2116
Cerebral vascular disease
and drop attacks, 2047
and epilepsy, 2150
Cerebral vasospasm, 2105
Cerebral venous thrombosis, and stroke, *2095*
Cerebritis, staphylococcal, 1547
Cerebrospinal fluid examination. See *Lumbar puncture* and specific diagnoses.
Cerebrospinal fluid otorrhea, in skull fracture, 2171
Cerebrospinal fluid pressure
high, 2167–2168
low, syndrome of, 2166–2167
reference values for, 2319
Cerebrospinal fluid rhinorrhea, in skull fracture, 2171
Cerebrospinal fluid volume, reference values for, 2319
Cerebrovascular diseases, 2086–2111
and vertigo, 2042–2043
Cerebrovascular malformations, 2104
Cerebrum
atrophy of, alcoholic, 2066
blood flow in, in classic migraine, 2054
in cancer, 1081–1082
Certificates of Need, 8
Ceruloplasmin, 1209
deficiency of, 1158, 1159–1160
serum, reference values for, 2319
Cervical cancer, lupus simplex virus infection and, 1716
Cervical disc, herniation of, 2183
Cervical mucus, hormonal regulation of, 1381
Cervical rib, 2197
Cervical spine
disease of, and ear pain, 2058
injury to, 2175, 2176
Cervical spondylosis, 2184
vs. vitamin B_{12} deficiency, 2067
Cervical vertigo, 2042
Cervicitis, sexually transmitted, 1643
Cesarean section, hospital-acquired infection and, 1490
Cestodes, 1804–1809
eradication of, 1809
life cycle of, 1805
morphology of, 1804–1805
Chagas' disease, 334–335, 672, 708, 1783–1786
acute, 1784, 1785
cardiac, 1784–1785, 1786
chronic, 1784, 1785
clinical presentation of, 1784
congenital, 1784
diagnosis of, 1785
blood films in, 1785
culture in, 1785
serology in, 1785
xenodiagnostic test in, 1785
digestive, 1785, 1786
epidemiology of, 1783–1784
etiology of, 1783
evolution of, 1785
immune response in, 1784
pathogenesis of, 1784
pathology of, 1784
prognosis in, 1785
prophylaxis for, 1786
treatment of, 1785–1786
vector in, 1873, 1786
Chancre(s), 1653, *1653*
extragenital, 2244
in trypanosomiasis, 1782
Chancroid, 1650
Charcot joint, 1339, 1958
in tabes dorsalis, 2119
Charcot-Leyden crystals, 388
Charcot-Marie-Tooth disease, 2199
Charcot's triad, 860
Chédiak-Higashi disease, 950, 951–952
antibiotic prophylaxis in, 952
bone marrow transplantation in, 952
genetic factor in, 951
neutrophils in, 952, *952*
Chédiak-Higashi syndrome, 1479, 1482, 1484, *2258, 2265*
Cheese washer's lung, 2285
Chelating agents, in poisoning, 87
Chelation therapy
in lead poisoning, *2309*
in thalassemia major, 922
Chemical acne, 2297
Chemical burns, 2296
Chemical folliculitis, 2297
Chemical injury, to lung, 2289–2291
Chemical leukoderma, 2297
Chemical photosensitivity, 2296
Chemical pneumonitis, acute, 2289
Chemicals
food poisoning and, 782
toxic, neuropathy due to, 2195
Chemistry, clinical, values of importance, 2317–2335
Chemistry tests, reference values for, 2316–2340
Chemoattractants, in rheumatic disease, 1900–1901, *1902*
Chemoreceptors, 162,
in shock, 214
Chemotactic factors, 943
Chemotherapeutic agent(s), as nephrotoxins, 596–598
Chemotherapy. See also specific agents and conditions.
for colon cancer, 768
for pancreatic cancer, 780
for pulmonary tuberculosis, 1624–1627
in bronchogenic carcinoma, 444
in herpes simplex virus infection, 1717
in Hodgkin's disease, 1006–1007, 1008t
in stomach cancer, 700
Chenodeoxycholate, 853, 861
Chest
computed tomography of, 382–383
flail, 454, 457
Chest pain, 370–371
diagnostic approach to, 371
mechanism of, 370
Chest radiography
inspiration-expiration views for, 382
special views and techniques for, 382–383
standard views for, 381–382
Chest wall, 453–454
abnormality of, respiratory failure management in, 470–471
disorders of, 370–371
injury of, respiratory failure and, 457
Cheyne-Stokes respiration in left ventricular failure, 196
Chickenpox. See *Varicella.*
Chief cells, 681
Chigger(s), 1835–1836
Chigger-borne rickettsiosis, 1684
Chikungunya, 1740
Chilblain(s), 358
Childhood, as part of life cycle, 15
immunization in, 42
Children
acute toxic encephalopathy of, 2141
tuberculosis in, treatment of, 1627
Chinese restaurant syndrome, 782, 2056
Chlamydia, 1668–1672
immune response to, 1669
immunotypes of, 1668
in pregnancy, 1670
microbiology of, 1668–1669
neonatal infection with, 1670–1671
Chlamydia psittaci, 1668, 1669, 1671
Chlamydia trachomatis, 1648, 1668, 1669, 1670, 1671
microbiology of, 1648
Chlamydial conjunctivitis, 2221
Chloracne, 2242, 2297

Chlorambucil, 1096, 1096t
 in chronic lymphocytic leukemia, 982–983
 in nephrotic syndrome, 580, 581
 in polycythemia vera, 971
Chloramine, 912
Chloramphenicol, 105, 1586
 aplastic anemia and, 877–878
 in typhoid fever, 1588–1589
 leukemia and, 987
Chlordiazepoxide
 in anxiety, 2010
 in cystinuria, 613
 in depression, 2013
Chloride
 excretion of, 510–511
 metabolism of, in uremia, 551
 reference values for, 2319
Chloridorrhea, congenital, 714
Chloroethylnitrosoureas, 1096–1097
Chloroquine
 in liver abscess, 830
 in malaria, 1778–1780
 ocular side effects of, 2225
 resistance to, 1778, 1779
Chlorosis, 889
Chlorpromazine
 hepatotoxicity of, 822–823
 in schizophrenia, 2004
Chlorpropamide, 1329
 ADH activity and, 1268, 1268t
Choking, in Huntington's disease, 2074
Cholangiography
 in jaundice, 812
 in pancreatic cancer, 779
 retrograde, 660
 transhepatic, percutaneous, 67, *67*, 656–657, *656*, 854–855
Cholangiohepatitis, oriental, 863
Cholangiopancreatography, retrograde, endoscopic, 656, *656*, 659–660, *659*, *660*, 854–855
Cholangitis
 diagnosis of, 860
 sclerosing, 862
 suppurative, 861
 treatment of, 860–861
 with choledocholithiasis, 859–861
Cholecalciferol, 1423
Cholecystectomy, 857
 postoperative syndrome of, 864–865
Cholecystitis
 acalculous, 857
 acute, 857–859
  cholecystectomy for, 858–859
  clinical manifestations of, 857
  complications of, 859
  diagnosis of, 857–858
   radiography in, 857
   radionuclide scanning in, 857–858
   ultrasonography in, 857
  fistula formation with, 859
  pathogenesis of, 857
  pathology of, 857
  perforation with, 859
  prognosis in, 859
  treatment of, 858–859, *858*
 chronic, 855–857
  cholecystectomy for, 857
  choledocholithiasis with, 856
  clinical manifestations of, 855–856
  complications of, 856–857
  diagnosis of, 856
   radiography in, 856
 emphysematous, 859
Cholecystography
 contrast media, nephrotoxicity and, 603
 oral, 854, *854*
Choledocholithiasis, 859–861
 cholangitis with, 859–861
 clinical manifestations of, 860
 diagnosis of, 860
 endoscopic sphincterotomy for, 861
 natural history of, 860, *860*
 retained stones in, 861
 surgery for, 861
 treatment of, 860–861
Cholera, 1598–1599
 chemical values in, 1598, 1598t
 clinical manifestations of, 1598–1599
 diagnosis of, 1599
 enterotoxin of, 1598
 epidemiology of, 1598
 pandemics of, 1598
 pathogenesis of, 1598
 prevention of, 1599
 prognosis in, 1599
 susceptibility to, 1598
 transmission of, 1598
 treatment of, 1599
 vaccine for, 1599
Cholestasis, recurrent, 808
Cholestatic hepatitis syndrome, 814
Cholesteatoma(s), intracranial, 2166
Cholesterol, 1221
 absorption of, 720
 cancer and, 39
 coronary heart disease and, 38
 excretion of, 1111
 hyperlipidemia and, 38
 in pericarditis, 345
 metabolism of, 1111
 total, reference values for, 2319
 transport of, 1109–1110
Cholesterol desmolase deficiency, 1357
Cholesterol gallstones, and oral contraceptives, 852
Cholesterolosis, 855
Cholestyramine, 79
 therapy with, 1112, 1114
Cholinergic agents, 95–96
 in myasthenia gravis, 2214
Cholinergic agonists, 95
Cholinergic antagonists, 95
Cholinergic receptor(s), 91–96
 ligand binding studies of, 93
Chondromatosis, synovial, 1960
Chondrosarcoma, 1467
Chorea, 2074–2075
 common causes of, *2074*
 definition of, 2069
 hereditary, 2074–2075
 in postencephalitic parkinsonism, 2071
 secondary, 2075
 senile, 2075
Chorea minor, 1530
Chorea-acanthocytosis, 2075
Choriocarcinoma, 1287
Choriomeningitis, lymphocytic, 1736, 2123, 2125
Chorionic gonadotropin
 in cancer, 1079
 serum or plasma, reference values for, 2320
Chorionic somatomammotropin, 1253
Chorionic villi, transcervical aspiration of, 144
Chorioretinitis, 2220
 cytomegalovirus, 2221
 in congenital neurosyphilis, 2120
 infectious, 2221
Christmas disease, 131
Chromhidrosis, apocrine, 2230
Chromium, 1210
 deficiency of, 1210
 dietary allowance for, 1179
 excess of, 1210
 toxicity of, 2314
Chromomycosis, 1773–1774
 cerebral, 1774
 clinical manifestations of, 1774
 cutaneous, 1773–1774
 cystic, 1774
 diagnosis of, 1774
 epidemiology of, 1774
 etiology of, 1774
 treatment of, 1774
Chromosome(s), 122–123
 banding of, 140, *140*
 breakage syndromes of, 143
 cell division and, 138–139
 deletion of, 140, *141*
 description of, 138
 disorders of, 138–144
  abortion and perinatal death from, 141
  amniocentesis in diagnosis of, 144
  autosomal, 142, *143*
  classes of, 140
  clinical features of, 142–143
  population load of, 141, 142t
 heritable fragile sites of, 144
 independent assortment of, 122–123
 indications for study of, 142–144
 injury to, 2298
 inversion of, 140, *141*
 nomenclature for, 139–140
 number abnormality of, 140, *141t*
 preparation methods for, 139, *139*
 Robertsonian translocation of, 140
 sex chromatin of, 141–142
  pattern of, 1368
 structure abnormality of, 140
 translocation of, 140, *141*
 variants in, 139
Chromosomal abnormality
 in acute leukemia, 987, 988
 in Burkitt's lymphoma, 999–1000
 in cancer, 1061–1062
 in chronic lymphocytic leukemia, 982
 in gonadal dysgenesis, 1386–1387
 in hairy cell leukemia, 985
 in hemophilia, 1045–1046
 in hermaphroditism, 1363
 in Klinefelter's syndrome, 1370–1371
 in male pseudohermaphroditism, 1354–1360, *1355*
 in seminiferous tubule dysgenesis, 1370–1371
 in Turner's syndrome, 1387
 XO/XY mosaicism, 1354–1355
 XX karyotype, 1361, 1362–1363, 1364
 XX/XY mosaicism, 1363
 XXY karyotype, 1370–1371, *1371*
 47 XXY karyotype, 1370
 46 XY complement, 1354, 1355, 1363
 46 XY karyotype, 1372
 XYY karyotype, 1371
Chronic disease
 lifestyle intervention in, 35
 risk factors for, 35
Chronic granulomatous disease, 950–951
 antibiotic prophylaxis for, 951
 bone marrow transplantation in, 951
 genetic factor in, 950
 neutrophils in, 950–951, *951*
Chronic leukemias. See topics under *Leukemia.*
Chronic obstructive pulmonary disease, 397, 399–403
 alpha-antitrypsin deficiency in, 400
 cigarette smoking and, 48–49, 400
 clinical manifestations of, 400
 cor pulmonale in, 400, 403
 course of, 401
 differential diagnosis of, 401–422
 edema with, 403

Chronic obstructive pulmonary disease (*Continued*)
emphysematous vs. bronchial types, 400, 401t
environmental control in, 402–403
forced expiration measurement in, 400–402
hypercapnia in, 403
influenza with, 1704
laboratory findings in, 400–401
osteoporosis and, 1458
pathogenesis of, 399–400
pathology of, 400
prevalence of, 399–400
prognosis of, 401
pulmonary hypertension and, 259–260
treatment of, 402
corticosteroids in, 402
oxygen therapy in, 402
physical therapy in, 402
surgical therapy for, 403
Chubby puffer syndrome, 1990
Chvostek's sign, 1444
Chylomicron formation, 720
Chylomicronemia syndrome, 1115
Chylothorax, pleural disease with, 449
Chyme transport, 713
Chymopapain injection, in herniated disc, 2184
Cigar smoking, 50
Cigarette smoking
and myocardial infarction, 294
angina pectoris and, 287
atherosclerosis and, 282
bronchogenic carcinoma and, 439–440
cancer and, 48, 1069–1070
cancer mortality from, 48
cardiovascular disease and, 47, 157
cessation of, 50
risk reduction relation to, 49
chronic bronchitis and, 398
chronic obstructive pulmonary disease and, 48–49, 400
emphysema and, 400
environmental contamination from, 49
erythrocytosis and, 963–964
health risks and, 47, 47t
low tar and nicotine cigarettes in, 49
pancreatic cancer and, 778
peptic ulcer and, 49, 684, 689
pregnancy and, 49
respiratory epithelial effects, 48
sex factor in, 49
smoke constituents in, 47
smoke dose in, risk relation of, 47
thromboangiitis obliterans and, 360, 361
with asbestos exposure, lung cancer and, 2284
Ciguatera fish poisoning, 782, 1844
Cimetidine, 81
in gastroesophageal reflux disease, 671
in peptic ulcer, 688, 690, 697
Cinchonism, 1779
Cineangiography. See *Angiography.*
Cingulotomy, for pain relief, 2053
Circadian rhythm
and sleep, 1987
in adrenal steroid regulation, 1303–1304, 1307
Circulation. See also *Peripheral circulation.*
cerebral, reduced, cardiac disease and, 2092
digitalis and, 201
in coma, 1977
in drug poisoning, 1980
time of, heart failure and, 194
Circulatory system, autoregulation of, in shock, 215
disorders of, drug therapy and, 77–78
Circulatory system (*Continued*)
fetal and neonatal, 225, 227
in shock, 212–216
Cirrhosis, 835–845. See also *Biliary cirrhosis.*
alcohol intake and, 835–837
anemia with, 884
bacteremia with, 1593
cardiac, 840
cryptogenic, 839–840
hepatitis B and, 839–840
etiology of, 835, 835t
hepatocellular carcinoma and, 850
hyponatremia in, 527
Laennec's, *2263*
liver transplantation in, 848
major sequelae of, 840–845
peritonitis with, 1593
portal hypertension and, 840–842
with ascites, 843–844
Cis-platinum, 1097
Citrovorum factor, 899
Citrullinemia, 131, 136, 1130
Cladosporium, 1774
Cladosporium trichoides, 1774
Claudication. See *Intermittent claudication.*
Climacteric, 21
male, 1374
Climate, influence on puberty, 18
Clindamycin, 105, 1586
in lung abscess, 421–422
Clinical medicine, 3–4
as boundless discipline, 3–4
learning strategies in, 3–4
patient-student relationship in, 4
peer relationships in, 4
uncertainty principle of, 3
Clofazimine, for leprosy, 1637–1638
Clofibrate, 1113, 1114
ADH activity and, 1268, 1268t
therapy with, 1115
Clomiphene, 1255
Clomiphene citrate, 1367
Clonazepam in epilepsy, *2158,* 2159
in myoclonus, 2077, 2158, *2158*
Clonidine
in hypertension, 278–279
in pheochromocytoma, 1411–1412
withdrawal of, 275
Cloning
bacteriophage, 135, *136*
molecular, 135–136
plasmid, 135, *136, 138*
Clonorchiasis, 1815–1816
acute, 1816
clinical manifestations of, 1816
diagnosis of, 1816
treatment of, 1816
Clonorchis sinensis, 863, 1815–1816
Clorazepate, in epilepsy, 2158, *2158*
Clostridia, 1573–1574
in soft tissue infection, 1574, 1575t
toxin of, 1573–1574
Clostridia enterotoxemias, 1575–1576
Clostridial disease, 1573–1576, 1573t
Clostridial myonecrosis, 1574, 1575t
Clostridium, 1586
Clostridium botulinum, 46, 781, 1574, 1577–1578
Clostridium difficile, 1574–1577
Clostridium perfringens, 781, 1573, 1574, 1575, 1576
Clostridium ramosum, 1573
Clostridium septicum, 1575
Clostridium sordellii, 1577
Clostridium tetani, 1574, 1579
Clot lysis, reference values for, 2337
Clot retraction, 1031
reference values for, 2337
Clotting factors, 1040–1044, 1041t
deficiencies of, 1044–1045, 1045t. See also specific factors and diagnoses.
genetic factors in, 1044–1051, 1045t
from recombinant DNA research, 133
in liver disease, 810
in nephrotic syndrome, 579
inhibition of, 1057–1058
Clotting time
plasma, reference values for, 2337
whole blood, reference values for, 2337
Clubbing, digital, in congenital heart disease, 227
in hypertrophic pulmonary osteoarthropathy, 941
in infective endocarditis, 1536t
Cluster headache, 2055–2056
Coagulation disorders
and cerebral artery thrombosis, 2093
and cerebral ischemia, *2093*
and stroke, *2095*
in bacterial meningitis, 1554
with ulcerative colitis, 753
Coagulation factors, deficiency of, 1030, 1031
Coagulation system, 1028
Coagulation values, clinically important, 2337–2340
Coal dust, occupational exposure to, 2281
Coal macule, 2281
Coal tar, in psoriasis, 2246
Coal worker's pneumoconiosis, 417, 2281
Coarctation of aorta, 237–238, 346
abdominal, 346
echocardiography in, 238
electrocardiography in, 238
hypertension with, 274
radiography in, 238
surgery for, 242
Cobalophilin, 896
Cobalt, 1211
Cobalt toxicity, 2312
Cobalt-beer cardiomyopathy, 336
Cocaine, abuse of, 2021–2022
Coccidia, 1803
Coccidioides immitis, 1761
Coccidioidomas, 1761
Coccidioidomycosis, 1761–1762
clinical manifestations of, 1761–1762
diagnosis of, 1762
culture in, 1762
serology in, 1762
disseminated, 1761–1762
epidemiology of, 1761
etiology of, 1761
immune response in, 1761, 1762
pathogenesis of, 1761
pathology of, 1761
prevention of, 1762
primary, 1761
prognosis in, 1762
treatment of, 1762
antifungal therapy in, 1762
Coccidiosis, 1803
Coccygodynia, 784
Codeine, for relief of pain, 2051, 2052
Coffee intake, pancreatic cancer and, 778
Coffin-Lowry syndrome, 146
Cognitive function, global deterioration of, in acquired immunodeficiency syndrome, 2142
Colchicine, 1140–1141
for familial mediterranean fever, 1168, 1171
Cold, common. See *Common cold.*
disorders due to, 2304, 2306–2307
vascular disease of extremities and, 357–358
Cold agglutinin disease, 910–911, 910t
Cold agglutinins, *2264*

Cold hemagglutinin syndrome, 1020, 2265t
Cold hemoglobinuria, paroxysmal, *2265*
Cold sore, 664
Colestipol therapy, 1112, 1114
Colistin, 106
Colitis
  amebic, 1800
  antibiotic-associated, 1575
  ischemia, 759–760, *760*
  pseudomembranous, 1576–1577
  ulcerative, 2263t
Colitis cystica profunda, 784
Collagen, 1894–1896
  fibrils of, 1894, *1895*
  genetic types of, 1895, 1895t
  synthesis of, 1895–1896, 1896t
Collagen disease
  myopathy in, 2210
  pulmonary hypertension and, 258, 261
  with interstitial lung disease, 413–414
Collagen fibers, 2228
Collagen vascular disease, retinopathy of, 2224
Colloid cysts, intracranial, treatment outcome in, 2166
Colon. See also under *Large intestine.*
  dietary fiber and, 709
  diverticulitis of. See *Diverticulitis.*
  endoscopy of, 661
  fluid transport in, 713
  functions of, 703, 708–709
  motility disorders of, 708–712
Colon cancer, 764–769
  benign adenoma and, 762
  clinical manifestations of, 767
  diagnosis of, 767–768
    carcinoembryonic antigens and, 768
    colonoscopy in, 661, 767–768
    proctoscopy in, 767
  dietary factor in, 764–765
  environmental factors in, 764–765
  epidemiology of, 761, 764
  etiology of, 764–765
  familial polyposis of colon and, 766, 769
  follow-up of, 768
  Gardner's syndrome and, 766, 769
  genetic factor in, 765–766, 769
  metastatic, 767
  pathology of, 766, *766*
  polyps and, 762
  prevention of, 768–769
  prior colon cancer or adenoma and, 765, 769
  prognosis in, 768
  risk factors for, 765t, 769, *769*
  screening for, 768–769, *769*
  susceptibility to, 765–766, 765t, *766*
  treatment of, 768
    chemotherapy in, 768
    radiation therapy in, 768
    surgery in, 768
  ulcerative colitis and, 753, *753*, 765, 769
Colon diverticula, 711
Colon polyp(s), 762–763, *762*
  clinical manifestations of, 762
  colon cancer and, 762
  colonoscopic polypectomy for, 762–763
  familial polyposis and, 763, *763*
  follow-up for, 762–763
  generalized juvenile polyposis and, 764
  genetic factor in, 763–764, *763*, *764*
  pathology of, 762
  treatment of, 762
Colonoscopy, fiberoptic, 661
Colony-forming unit–granulocyte, monocyte cell, 940
Colony-stimulating factor(s), 940, 954, 959
Colorado tick fever, 1740–1741
  clinical manifestations of, 1741
  diagnosis of, 1741
    serology in, 1741
  epidemiology of, 1740–1741
  etiology of, 1740
  prevention of, 1741
  vector in, 1740
Colorectal cancer. See *Colon cancer.*
Coma
  barbiturate, in stroke treatment, 2101
  definition of, 1971
  emergency management of, 1977–1979
  general causes of, 1971–1975, *1971*
  in drug poisoning, management of, 1980
  in encephalitis, 2125
  in rabies, 2133
  in subtentorial mass lesions, 1972
  in supratentorial mass lesions, 1972
  prognosis in, 1981–1983
Comatose patient, with head injury, transport of, 2172
Combat, and anxiety, 2009
Common acute lymphoblastic leukemia antigen, 988, 990
Common cold, 1691–1695
  ascorbic acid for, 1205
  clinical manifestations of, 1693–1694
  diagnosis of, 1694
    serology in, 1694
  epidemiology of, 1692–1693
  etiology of, 1691–1692t
  pathology of, 1693
  prevention of, 1694–1695
  treatment for, 1694
  vaccine for, 1694
  vitamin C and, 1694
Community medicine, 7–8
Complement, 1852–1855
  acquired abnormalities of, 1854
  activating pathways of, 1852–1853, *1852*, *1853*
  clinical measurements of, 1854
  effector pathways of, 1852–1853, *1853*
  in hemolysis, 908
  in urticaria-angioedema, 1865–1866
  inherited abnormalities of, 1853–1854, 1854t
  plasma and serum, reference values for, 2320
  protein components of, 1852, 1852t
Complement fixation test. See under specific diagnoses.
Complement fragment C5a, 943
Complement system
  in rheumatic disease, 1900
  in shock, 217–218
  primary deficiencies of, 1861
Complicated migraine, 2055
Compound F. See *Cortisol.*
Compound nevi, 2254
Compound S. See *11-Deoxycortisol.*
Compression neuropathy, 2196–2197
Computed tomography, 65, *65*
  in acute abdomen, 798
  in back pain, 2062
  in brain abscess, 2113, 2114t
  in brain injury, 2173
  in Cushing's syndrome, *1315*, 1316, *1316*
  in drop attacks, 2047
  in epilepsy, 2155
  in gastrointestinal disease, 652, *652*
  in headache, 2060
  in herpes simplex encephalitis, 2127
  in Hodgkin's disease, 1004–1005
  in hyperprolactinemia, 1263
  in insulinoma, 1346
  in intracranial hemorrhage, 2106–2107
Computed tomography (*Continued*)
  in intracranial tumors, 2164, *2165*
  in jaundice, 812
  in kidney tumor, 640–643, *642*
  in liver tumor, 851
  in mediastinal disease, 451, 451
  in multiple sclerosis, 2145, 2146
  in nervous system disease, 1968–1969
  in pancreatic cancer, 779
  in pancreatitis, 773, *773*, *774*, *775*, *777*
  in paravertebral tumors, 2185
  in pituitary tumor, 1259–1260, *1259*
  in renal cystic disease, 633–634, *634*
  in stroke, 2100
  in subarachnoid hemorrhage, 2057, 2106–2107
  in subdural empyema, 2115
  of chest, 382–383
  renal, *512*, 513
Concussion, 2170
Concussion-postconcussion amnesia, 1986
Conduction disturbance(s), as cardiac surgery complication, 241–242
Conductive hearing loss, 2038–2039
Condylomata acuminata, vs. condylomata lata, 1654
Condylomata lata, of secondary syphilis, *1653*, 1654
  vs. condylomata acuminata, 1654
Cone shells, venomous, 1844
Confabulation, in Korsakoff's syndrome, 2065
Confidentiality, in medical practice, 13
Confusional state, definition of, 1974
Congenital abnormality, rubella and, 44, 1709–1710, 1711
Congenital defects, 144–146. See also specific abnormalities.
  age factor in, 145, 147, 149
  alcoholism and, 146
  diabetes mellitus and, 146
  environmental factor in, 144t, 145
  etiology of, 144–145, 144t
  fetal surgery for, 146
  genetic counseling and, 147–149, *147*
  genetic factor in, 144–145, 145t
  health significance of, 145
  incidence of, 144
  multifactorial inheritance and, 145, 145t
  phenylketonuria and, 146
  prenatal diagnosis of, 146, 148–149
  prevention of, 146
  progeny risk and, 145–146, 145t
Congenital heart disease, 225–242
  complex malformations and, 241
  counseling in, 225
  cyanosis in, 227
  digital clubbing in, 227
  environmental factor in, 225, 226t–227t
  etiology of, 225
  fetal and neonatal circulations and, 225, 227
  genetic factor in, 225, 226t–227t
  hypoxemia in, 228
  obstructive lesions in, 233–235. See also specific diagnosis.
    regurgitant lesions with, 235–238
  polycythemia in, 228
  pulmonary hypertension and, 258
  shunt lesions in, 227, 228–233. See also specific defects.
    arterial hypoxemia in, 227–228
    brain abscess with, 228
    magnitude and direction of, 227
    paradoxical embolus with, 228
    pulmonary blood flow and, 227
    pulmonary hypertension with, 228
    squatting behavior with, 228

Congenital heart disease (*Continued*)
shunt lesions in, surgical complications in, with intra-atrial surgery, 241–242
with intraventricular surgery, 242
transposition defects in, 238–239
when "cured" in adult, 241–242
when "uncured" in adult, 240–241
Congo red binding, 1168, 1170, 1171
Congo virus, 1755
Congo-CHF virus, 1755
Congophilic angiopathy, intracerebral hemorrhage with, 2105
Conium maculatum, 783
Conjunctivitis, 2220
acute hemorrhagic, 1733–1734
adenovirus, 1705–1706
chlamydial, 2221
gonococcal, 2220–2221
Hemophilus, 1565
with trachoma, 1669–1670
Connective tissue, 1894–1898
elastic fibers of, 1894
extracellular matrices of, 1894–1896
Connective tissue diseases, 2222–2223
genetic factor in, 1146–1153
pericarditis and, 341–342
purpura with, 1039
Conn's syndrome, 1317
Consanguinity, 117, 119
Consciousness
altered, general management of, 1976–1977
impairment of, sustained, 1971–1979
loss of, after trauma, 2170–2171
brief, 1983–1986, *1983*, *1984*
Constipation, 648, 709–711
clinical manifestations of, 709
diagnosis of, 709
etiology of, 709, 710t
narcotic drugs and, 2050
pathogenesis of, 709
treatment of, 709–710
Constructional apraxia, 1995
Consumer Product Act, 86
Contact dermatitis, 2248–2249
allergic, 2296
arthropods and, 1840
photoallergic, 2253
Contact seizures, 2150
Continuous positive pressure ventilation, 459, 468, 477
Contracture(s), 2216
in aged, 29
in torsion dystonia, 2078
Contrast media
allergy to, 1886
as nephrotoxins, 602–603
iodinated, 1277
Conversion reaction, vs. syncope, 1986
Converting enzyme, 1305
Convulsion(s). See also *Seizures.*
febrile, 2154
generalized, in intracranial tumor, 2162
grand mal, 2153
in head injury, 2173
tonic-clonic, 2149, 2153
generalized, nonepileptic, 2157
secondarily generalized, 2152
with toxemia of pregnancy, 625, 626
Cooley's anemia, 921–923. See also *B thalassemia, severe.*
prenatal diagnosis of, 926
Coombs' test, 874, 908
COPD. See *Chronic obstructive pulmonary disease.*
Copper, 1209–1210
as nephrotoxin, 600
deficiency of, 1210
Copper (*Continued*)
dietary allowance for, 1179
erythrocyte, reference values for, 2320
erythropoiesis in, 1209
excess of, 1210
metabolism of, 1209–1210
in Wilson's disease, 1158–1160
serum, reference values for, 2320
toxicity of, 2311
urinary, reference values for, 2320
Coprolalia, in Gilles de la Tourette's syndrome, 2077
Coproporphyria, hereditary, 1155
Coproporphyrin, 1153, 1154, 1155, 1157
urinary and fecal, reference values for, 2320
Copropraxia, in Gilles de la Tourette's syndrome, 2077
Cor pulmonale
in chronic obstructive pulmonary disease, 400, 403
respiratory failure with, 461
Cor triatriatum, 235
Coral snakes, 1841–1843
Cordotomy, in pain relief, 2053
Cornea, protection of, in coma, 1979
transplant of, in Creutzfeldt-Jakob disease transmission, 2136
in rabies transmission, 2134
ulcers of, 2221
Coronary artery(ies)
angioplasty of, in angina pectoris, 287
percutaneous transluminal, 186, *186*, 300
arteriography of, 186, *187*
disorders of, 284–300. See also specific diagnoses.
pulmonary trunk anomaly of, 232–233
Coronary artery disease
angina pectoris and, 285, 287
bypass grafting in, 297–300
life expectancy with, 298, *298*
cholesterol and, 38
cigarette smoking and, 47, *47*
exercise and, 40
hypothyroidism and, 1290
medical vs. surgical management of, 300
mitral regurgitation and, 249, 250, 251
nuclear imaging in, 180–181
surgical treatment of, 297–300
with acute myocardial infarction, 288–289, *288*
with aortic stenosis, 252
Coronary artery fistula, 232
Coronary artery revascularization. See also *Bypass grafting.*
in angina pectoris, 286, 287
in myocardial infarction, 295
Coronary care unit, myocardial infarction management in, 294
Coronaviruses, in common cold, 1691–1694, 1694t
Corpus callosum, in Marchiafava-Bignami disease, 2067
section of, in epilepsy, 2159
Corpus luteum, *1379*, 1380, 1382
insufficiency of, 1388–1389
Corpus striatum, in striatonigral degeneration, 2079
Cortical blindness, 2034
Corticoreticular epilepsy, 2149
Corticosteroid(s). See also specific agents and classes.
for pulmonary tuberculosis, 1626
in adult celiac disease, 733–734
in allergic rhinitis, 1869–1870
in asthma, 395, 396
in chronic active hepatitis, 826
in chronic bronchitis, 399
Corticosteroid(s) (*Continued*)
in chronic lymphocytic leukemia, 982–983
in chronic obstructive pulmonary disease, 402
in Crohn's disease, 747
in glomerulonephritis, 577
in herpes zoster, 2129
in IgG-mediated autoimmune hemolytic anemia, 909
in ileojejunitis, 735
in infectious mononucleosis, 1721
in interstitial lung disease, 412
in lupus nephritis, 586
in multiple sclerosis, 2146
in nephrotic syndrome, 580, 581
in neutropenia, 957
in peptic ulcer pathogenesis, 684
in polymyositis, 1949–1950
in psoriasis, 2246
in respiratory failure, 461
in rheumatoid arthritis, 1916
in rickettsial disease, 1677
in sarcoidosis, 438–439
in shock, 221
in systemic lupus erythematosus, 1931
in ulcerative colitis, 754–755
in Whipple's disease, 735
neutrophil adhesiveness and, 950
ocular side effects of, 2225
systemic, in skin disease, 2241
urinary, 1308
Corticosteroid-binding globulin, 1302, 1307, 1308t
Corticosterone, serum or plasma, reference values for, 2320
Corticotroph(s), 1252
Corticotroph tumors, 1264–1265
clinical features of, 1264–1265
Corticotropin. See *Adrenocorticotropic hormone.*
Corticotropin-related peptides, 1252–1253
Corticotropin-releasing factor, 1241, 1242, 1244, 1254, 1303, 1304
in galactorrhea, 1399
stimulation test with, 1308, 1315
Cortisol, 112, 114
assay of, 1307–1308, 1308t
cortisone conversion of, 1302, *1303*
derivatives of, 1302, *1303*
free, reference values for, 2320
metabolism of, 1302, *1303*
radioimmunoassay of, 1307–1308, 1308t
regulation of, 1303
circadian rhythms and, 1303–1304, 1307
serum or plasma, reference values for, 2320
synthesis of, 1300–1301
urinary, 1308
Cortisol-secreting adenoma, 1313
Cortisone, derivatives of, 1302, *1303*
Corynebacterium diphtheriae, 1571
Costochondral disease, 370
Co-trimoxazole, in pneumocystosis, 1797
Cough, 368–369
complications of, 368
diagnostic approach to, 368–369
in chronic bronchitis, 398
mechanism of, 368
nonproductive, 368
productive, 368
treatment of, 369
Cough fracture, 368
Cough syncope, 368
Coumarin anticoagulants, vitamin K deficiency and, 1052
Councilman bodies, 1752
Counseling. See *Genetic counseling.*
Coxarthrosis, 1953
Coxiella, 1672, 1673
microbiology of, 1672

Coxiella burnetii, 1672, 1677, 1686
Coxsackieviruses, 1728, 1729t
  infection with, 2125
  paralytic poliomyelitis due to, 2131
Cramps, 2215–2216
  heat, 2305
  muscle, 2199
Cranial arteritis, 2057
Cranial dystonia, 2078–2079
Cranial nerve(s), abnormalities of, in bacterial meningitis, 1552
  damage to, in skull fracture, 2171
  hemorrhage into, from aneurysmal rupture, 2105
  lesions of, in diabetics, 2193
  tumors of, in neurofibromatosis, 2085
Cranial neuralgias, 2059
Cranial polyneuritis, parainfectious, and vertigo, 2043
Craniopharyngioma
  characteristics of, *2162*
  pituitary, 1259
  treatment outcome in, 2166
Craniovertebral junction, anomalies of, congenital, 2187–2188
C-reactive protein
  in rheumatic disease, 1908
  serum, reference values for, 2318
Creatine kinase
  in myocardial infarction, 291
  serum, reference values for, 2321
Creatinine
  concentration of, plasma, 509–510, *509*
  in acute renal failure, 546
  in chronic renal failure, 558, *558*
  in pregnancy, 625
  serum or plasma, and urinary, reference values for, 2321
Creatinine clearance, 71, 76–77, 509–510, *509*
  serum or plasma, and urine, reference values for, 2321
Cretinism, 131, 1275
  endemic, 1299
  sporadic, 1298
Creutzfeldt-Jakob disease, 2001, 2136
"Crib" death, 1990
Crigler-Najjar syndrome, 132, 808
Crimean hemorrhagic fever, 1751t, 1755–1756
Crisis, myasthenic, 2214–2215
Critical care, hospital-acquired infection and, 1486
Critical care management
  cardiac output measurements in, 475
  cardiopulmonary resuscitation in, 480–482
  central venous pressure monitoring in, 474, 477–478
  complications of, 476–478
  consent for cardiopulmonary resuscitation in, 479
  electrocardiographic monitoring in, 473–474
  hemodynamic monitoring in, 473–474, 475t
    complications of, 477–478
  life support systems termination in, 479–480
  mortality with, 479
  patient consent and, 479
  psychological factors in, 478
  pulmonary arterial pressure monitoring in, 474–475, 474t, *475*, 478
  respiratory monitoring in, 473
  systemic arterial pressure monitoring in, 474, 477
Critical care medicine, 463–482
  attributes of, 463, 463t
  ethical issues in, 479–480
  indications for, 479
  social issues in, 479–480
  value of, 479
Crohn's colitis, 740, 742, 743, 747
  vs. ulcerative colitis, 746, 746t, 752
Crohn's disease, 735–736, 740–748, *2263*
  age of onset in, 740, *740*
  antidiarrheal drugs in, 747
  antimicrobial therapy in, 747
  clinical presentation of, 742–743
  colonoscopy in, 661, 744
  corticosteroids in, 747
  diagnosis of, 743–744
    differential, 744–746
  emotional factor in, 741
  epidemiology of, 740, 741t
  etiology of, 741
  extraintestinal complications of, 744–745, 745t
  genetic factors in, 740–741
  growth retardation with, 744, 746–747
  hepatobiliary complications with, 744–745
  immune response in, 741
  immunosuppressive therapy in, 747
  infection in, 741
  inflammation mediators in, 741
  intestinal absorption in, 744
  local complications in, 744
  malabsorption syndrome and, 744
  nutrient-losing enteropathy with, 744
  nutritional complications of, 744
  nutritional management in, 746
  pathogenesis of, 741
  pathology of, 741–742, *742*
  proctosigmoidoscopy in, 744
  prognosis in, 747
  prostaglandins in, 741
  radiography in, 743–744, *743*
  stool examination in, 744
  sulfasalazine in, 747
  surgery for, 747
  treatment of, 746–747
  with kidney disease, 745
Crohn's ileitis, 742
Cromolyn, in mastocytosis, 1888
Cromones, in asthma, 395
Cronkhite-Canada syndrome, 764, *2262*
Cross-dependence, definition of, 2016
Cross-McKusick-Breen syndrome, *2258*
Croup, 1695–1696, 1696t, 1699
Crowe's sign of neurofibromatosis, 2254
Crush injuries, myoglobinuria due to, 2210
Crust, 2233
Cruveilhier-Baumgarten syndrome, 841, *841*
Cryoglobulinemia, essential, 587
  glomerular involvement in, 587
Cryptococcosis, 1765–1767
  antifungal therapy in, 1766
  clinical manifestations of, 1765–1766
  cultures in, 1766
  cutaneous lesions in, *2261*
  diagnosis of, 1766
  disseminated, 1765–1766
  epidemiology of, 1765
  etiology of, 1765
  immune response in, 1765, 1766
  immunosuppressive therapy and, 2142
  in transplant recipients, 2142
  pathogenesis of, 1765
  pathology of, 1765
  prevention of, 1766
  prognosis in, 1766
  pulmonary, 1765, 1766
  serology in, 1766
  serotypes of, 1765
  treatment of, 1766
Cryptococcus bacillispora, 1765
Cryptococcus neoformans, 1765
Cryptorchidism, 1369, 1373–1374
Cryptosporidiosis, 1803
Cryptosporidium, 1803
CT. See *Computed tomography*.
Cullen's sign, *2263*
Cumulative insult dermatitis, 2296
Curarization, in tetanus, 1580
Cushing's disease, 1264–1265
  depression in, 2011
  dexamethasone suppression in, 1265
  differential diagnosis of, 1265
  laboratory studies in, 1265
  pathogenesis of, 1265
  therapy of, 1265
    pharmacologic, 1265
    radiation, 1265
    surgery, 1265
Cushing's syndrome, 529, 1313–1317
  adrenal cortex in, 1313–1317
  adrenocorticotropic hormone in, 1313–1317
  anterior pituitary in, 1313–1317
  clinical features of, 1314–1315, *1314t*
  diagnosis of, 1315
    computed tomography in, *1315*, 1316, *1316*
    CRF testing in, 1315
    dexamethasone suppression test in, 1315
    plasma ACTH in, 1315
    ultrasonography in, 1316
    urine free cortisol test in, 1315
  etiology of, 1313–1316
  glucocorticoids in, 1313–1314
  hypertension and, 276
  Nelson's syndrome and, 1317
  pathogenesis of, 1313–1314
  pathology of, 1313
  pituitary adenoma in, 1313
  treatment of, 1316–1317
    drug therapy in, 1316–1317
    radiation therapy in, 1316
    surgery in, 1316–1317
  tumor localization in, 1316
  vascular purpura with, 1039
  with cancer, 1077
Cutaneous chromomycosis, 1773–1774
Cutaneous correlations with specific organ systems, 2267
Cutaneous granuloma, 2297
Cutaneous larva migrans, 1821–1822
Cutaneous leishmaniasis, 1790–1792
Cutaneous lesions
  diseases with, *2264*, *2266*
  in disorders with hematologic component, *2265*
  in gastrointestinal disease, 2262–2263
  in infectious disease, *2260–2261*
Cutaneous mucormycosis, 1772
Cutaneous nerve, lateral, of thigh, injury to, 2197
Cutaneous stimulation, in pain, 2052
Cutis hyperelastica. See *Ehlers-Danlos syndrome*.
Cutis laxa, 1151
Cyanide poisoning, 88
Cyanocobalamin, 895
Cyanosis
  in altered hemoglobin-oxygen affinity, 933
  in congenital heart disease, 227
  in right ventricular failure, 197
  methylene blue therapy for, 934–935
Cyclic adenosine monophosphate (cAMP), 91
  in hormone action mediation, 1224–1225, *1225*
  in intestine fluid transport, 714, *714*
Cyclocryotherapy
  in glaucoma, 2218
Cycloguanil pamoate, 1791
Cyclooxygenase, 1239
  inhibition of, 1237, 1239, *1240*
    pharmacologic, 1240
  pathway of, 1237–1239, *1238*

Cyclophosphamide, 1096, 1096t
  ADH activity and, 1268t
  in aplastic anemia, 878–879
  in multiple myeloma, 1017–1018
  in nephrotic syndrome, 580, 581
  in Wegener's granulomatosis, 1944–1945
  interstitial lung disease and, 418
  with bone marrow transplantation, 1026, 1027
Cycloserine, 1203, 1625, 1626
Cylindroma, of lung, 445
Cylinduria, 484
Cyst(s), 2232. See also specific types.
  bony, in neurofibromatosis, 2085
Cystathionine β-synthase deficiency, 1131
Cystic chromomycosis, 1774
Cystic fibrosis, 390, 424–425
  chronic pulmonary disease in, 424
  clinical manifestations of, 424–425, 424t, 425t
  diagnosis of, 425
  epidemiology of, 424
  genetic factors in, 424, 425
  liver disease and, 833
  pancreatic exocrine insufficiency in, 424–425
  pathogenesis of, 424
  prognosis in, 425
  treatment of, 425
Cysticercosis, human, 1806–1807
Cystinosis, 132
  in Fanconi's syndrome, 615
  kidney disease and, 506
Cystinuria, 611–613, 732
  chlordiazepoxide in, 613
  genetic factors in, 612
  glutamine in, 613
  kidney stones and, 630, 631
  mercaptopropionylglycine in, 613
  methionine intake in, 612
  penicillamine therapy in, 612–613
  treatment of, 633
  urinary tract calculi in, 612–613
Cystitis, 619
  Candida, 1769
  hemorrhagic, 1705
Cytarabine. See *Cytosine arabinoside.*
Cytochrome deficiency, *2205*
Cytochrome P-450, 1153, 1155
Cytogenetics, 138
  population, 141, 142t
Cytogenic abnormality, in chronic myelogenous leukemia, 975
Cytogenics, clinical, 142, 143
Cytomegalic inclusion disease, 1718
Cytomegalovirus, 1695
  morphology of, 1717
  pathogenesis of, 1718
  pathology of, 1718
  perinatal, 1718, 1719
  prenatal, 1718, 1719
  prevention of, 1719
  prognosis in, 1719
  serology in, 1719
  treatment of, 1719
Cytomegalovirus chorioretinitis, 2221
Cytomegalovirus infection, 1479, 1717–1719
  blood transfusion and, 939
  clinical manifestations of, 1718
  culture in, 1718–1719
  diagnosis of, 1718–1719
  epidemiology of, 1717–1718
  host factor in, 1718, 1719
  immunogen therapy for, 1719
Cytomegalovirus vaccine, 1719
Cytosine arabinoside, 1094–1095, *1094*
  in acute myelogenous leukemia, 991
Cytotoxic agents
  in breast cancer, 1404–1405
  in Paget's disease of bone, 1462
Cytotoxicity
  antibody-dependent, 1851
  T cell-mediated, 1850, *1851*
Cytotoxin antibody, in inflammation, 1902–1903
Cytoxan. See *Cyclophosphamide.*

Dacarbazine, 1099
Dacryocystitis, 2220
Dairy products, brucellosis and, 1614, 1615
Dane (HBV) particle, 816
Dapsone
  for leprosy, 1637–1638
  resistance to, 1638
Darier's sign, 1887, 1888
  in mast cell disease, 2271
Datura stramonium, 783
Daunomycin, 1097–1098
Dawson's encephalitis, 2136. See also *Panencephalitis, subacute sclerosing.*
DDS syndrome, in dapsone therapy of leprosy, 1637
De Toni-Debré-Fanconi syndrome, 1430
Deadly nightshade, 783
Deafness, hysterical, 2014
Death and dying, 30–34. See also *Sudden cardiac death.*
  analgesic measures in, 33, 33t
  at home, 34
  communication in, 31
  environmental control during, 33, 33t
  Gompertz concept of, 23–24, *24*
  inappropriate treatment in, 30–31
  last 24 hours, 34
  life prolongation and, 12
  pain relief and, 31–33, *31*
  physician role in, 2, 30
  quality of life factor in, 13
  symptom control and, 33–34
  terminal illness with, 30
  with dignity, 11
Decerebrate posturing, after brain injury, 2171
Decimal factors, prefixes denoting, 2315
Decompression sickness, 2289
Decongestants, in sinus headache, 2058
Decubitus ulcers, in aged, 29
Deep tendon reflex contraction time, 1280
Deferoxamine, 922
Degenerative joint disease. See *Osteoarthritis.*
Degos' disease, *2262*
Dehydration, 724
Dehydroepiandrosterone, 1301, 1310
  serum or plasma, reference values for, 2321
Dejerine-Landouzy dystrophy, 333
Delirium
  definition of, 1974
  general causes of, 1971–1975
Delirium tremens, 54
  impending, 54
"Delta sign," in intracranial venous thrombosis, 2093
Delusions
  and disorders of taste, 2032
  in manic-depressive psychosis, 2005
  in schizophrenia, 2002
  somatic, pain in, 2049
Demeclocycline
  diabetes insipidus with, 1269
  hyposthenuria with, 1269
Dementia, 25, 27–28, 1998–2001, *1998, 1999*
  and anxiety, 2009
  and incontinence, 2029
Dementia (*Continued*)
  dialysis, 2311
  in cancer, 1081–1082
  in Creutzfeldt-Jakob disease, 2136
  in gait disorder, 2045
  in Huntington's disease, 2074
  in Marchiafava-Bignami disease, 2067
  in parkinsonism, 2070, 2071
  in vitamin B_{12} deficiency, 2067
  vs. amentia, 1998
  with acquired immunodeficiency syndrome, 1863
Dementia paralytica, 2119
Demyelinating diseases, 2143–2149
  and vertigo, 2043
  vs. transverse myelitis, 2139
Demyelinating encephalitis, acute, 2139
Demyelination
  in alcoholic neuropathy, 2066
  in Friedreich's ataxia, 2083
Dendrite, in herpesvirus hominis keratitis, 2221
Dendritic cells, 949
Denervation hypersensitivity, 2179
Dengue, 1737–1738
  clinical manifestations of, 1737
  culture in, 1737
  diagnosis of, 1737
  epidemiology of, 1737
  etiology of, 1737
  prevention of, 1738
  serology in, 1737
  vector in, 1737
Dengue hemorrhagic fever, 1751t, 1754–1755
  clinical manifestations of, 1754
  diagnosis of, 1754
  epidemiology of, 1754
  etiology of, 1754
  pathogenesis of, 1754
  pathology of, 1754
  prognosis in, 1755
  treatment of, 1754–1755
Dengue shock syndrome, 1754
Dental abscess, 663
Dental caries, 663
Deoxycorticosterone, 1301, 1302
Deoxycorticosterone acetate, in aldosterone measurement, 1310
11-Deoxycortisol, 1300
  in hirsutism, 1397
  plasma, reference values for, 2321
Deoxyribonucleic acid (DNA)
  autosensitivity syndrome and, 1039–1040
  in genetic information transmission, 122–127
  in metabolic disease, 1103
  in mutations, 124–126
  mitochondrial, 123
  recombinant research involving, 132
    expectations of, 133–135
    gene therapy from, 134–135
    inheritable disease diagnosis and, 135–137
    molecular cloning in, 135–136
    prenatal diagnosis and, 136–137
    probes for, 136–137
    products from, 133
    technology of, 133
  replication of, 123
  structure of, 122, 123
  synthesis of, in megaloblastic anemia, 893–895
Deoxyribonucleic acid viruses, in acute central nervous system infections, *2122*, 2123
Dependence, narcotic drugs and, 2050
Depigmentation, 2256–2257

Depressants, central nervous system, abuse of, 2019–2021
Depression, 2011–2013
aging and, 25, 28
and headache, 2057
and memory loss, 1997
and sleep disorders, *1988*, 1989
in Addison's disease, 2011
in Huntington's disease, 2074
in manic-depressive psychosis, 2005
in parkinsonism, 2070
in vitamin B_{12} deficiency, 2067
metabolic, myoglobinuria in, 2210
vs. dementia, 1999
Depressive psychosis, and hysterical symptoms, 2013
De Quervain's thyroiditis, 1291
Dermacentor andersoni, in Colorado tick fever, 1741
Dermatan sulfate, 1148
Dermatitis
allergic contact, 2296
atopic, 2249
contact, 2248–2249
photoallergic, 2253
cumulative insult, 2296
fiberglass, 2297
of hands and feet, 2248–2249
papular, of Spangler, 2269
seborrheic, 2242
Dermatitis herpetiformis, *2263*, 2268–2269, *2268*
with adult celiac disease, 734
Dermatoarthritis, lipoid, 1959
Dermatogenic enteropathy, *2263*
Dermatologic disease, 2227–2275
with diabetes mellitus, 1340–1341
Dermatologic signs of disease, 2250–2267
Dermatomyositis, 672, 1947–1950, 2199, 2209
clinical manifestations of, 1948
in cancer, 1083
Dermatomyositis-polymyositis, 2209
Dermatosis
ichthyosiform, 2250, *2251*
occupational, 2296–2297
neutrophilic, acute febrile, 2266
Dermis, 2227, 2228
Dermographism, 1864
Deslanoside, 202–203
17,20-Desmolase deficiency, 1359
Developmental abnormalities
cutaneous and renal manifestations of, *2264*
hormone factor in control of, 1229
Devic's disease, 2147. See also *Neuromyelitis optica.*
vs. transverse myelitis, 2139
Devil's grip, 1730–1731
Dexamethasone, 114
dosage regimen of, 114
in cancer chemotherapy, 1101t
Dexamethasone suppression, in Cushing's disease, 1265
Dexamethasone suppression test(s), 1255, 1308, 1308t
in Cushing's syndrome, 1315
reference values for, 2321, 2322
Dextran(s), osmotic nephropathy and, 604
Dextran solution, 220
Dextran therapy, in hemorrhage, 884
Dextroamphetamine, in pain, 2052
Dextrocardia, 239–240
Diabetes, stress, in disorders of neurometabolic regulation, 1250
Diabetes insipidus, 518, 519, 1269–1273
acquired nephrogenic, 1269
clinical manifestations of, 1270
Diabetes insipidus (*Continued*)
diagnosis of, 1270–1272
familial nephrogenic, 1269
hormone therapy for, 1272
hypernatremia with, 1270
hypertonic encephalopathy with, 1270, 1272
hypophysectomy and, 1270
laboratory manifestations in, 1270
lithium treatment and, 2007
nephrogenic, 594, 595, 1269–1270, 1273
pituitary, 1269
polyuria with, 1270, 1272
treatment of, 1272
vasopressin test in, 1271–1272, *1271*
Diabetes mellitus, 738–739, 1320–1341, *2264*. See also specific complications.
C peptide in, 1323, 1325
caloric intake in, 1327–1328
carbohydrate metabolism in, 1323
cardiovascular disease and, 157–158, 1340
classification of, 1320, 1320t
complications of, with hyperglycemia, 1326–1327
congenital defects and, 146
dermatologic lesions with, 1340–1341
diagnosis of, 1320–1321
dietary fiber intake in, 1328
dietary management in, 1327–1328
dietary restrictions in, 1213
epidemiology of, 1321
gastric emptying disorder with, 705–706
genetic factors in, 1322–1323, 1324, 1325, 1326
glucagon in, 1323
glucose tolerance test in, 1320–1321
glycogen suppression in, 1332
hemoglobin glycosylation and, 1326, *1326*
histocompatibility antigen in, 1322–1323, 1325
hyperglycemia in, 1324, *1325*, 1326–1327
hypertriglyceridemia with, 1114
hypoglycemia-therapy relationship in, 1327, 1331–1332
immune response in, 1322, 1325
insulin metabolism and, 1323–1324, *1324*
insulin resistance in, 1323–1324, *1324*
insulin therapy in, 1330–1332
insulin-dependent, 1320, 1321
clinical presentation of, 1321
genetic factors in, 1324, 1325
immune response in, 1325
insulin therapy in, 1330
pathogenesis of, 1324–1325
virus factor in, 1324–1325
kidney disease and, 506, 616–619, *616*, *618*
microvascular complications in, 1326
noninsulin-dependent, 1320, 1321
clinical presentation of, 1321
insulin therapy in, 1330, 1331
metabolic abnormalities in, 1324, *1325*
oral hypoglycemic agents in, 1328–1329
pathogenesis of, 1323–1324, *1325*
nutrient intake in, 1328
oral hypoglycemic agents in, 1328–1329, *1329*
osteoporosis and, 1458
pathogenesis of, 1323–1325
polyol/myoinositol metabolism in, 1326
secondary, 1321–1322
sorbitol metabolism in, 1326–1327, *1326*
therapy research in, 1332
treatment of, 1326–1332
virus in, 1324–1325
vision complications in, 1337–1338
with arteriosclerosis obliterans, 358, 359
with obesity, 1194
Diabetic amyotrophy, 2193
Diabetic foot, 1339
Diabetic glomerulopathy, 616–619, *616*, *618*
advanced, 617
diagnosis of, 617
glomerular filtration rate in, 616–618, *616*
occult, 616
pathogenesis of, 617–618, *618*
pathophysiology of, 617–618, *618*
prognosis in, 618–619
treatment of, 618–619
Diabetic ketoacidosis, 537, 540, 1332–1337
clinical picture of, 1335
differential diagnosis, 1336
fed vs. fasted state and, 1332–1334, *1333*
fluid replacement in, 1335–1336
glucose homeostasis and, 1332–1334, *1333*
hyperglycemia in, 1334–1335, *1334*
insulin deficiency and, 1332–1334, *1334*
insulin therapy in, 1335
pathophysiology of, 1334–1335, *1334*
potassium metabolism in, 1335, *1335*
treatment of, 541, 1335–1336
Diabetic nephropathy, 1338–1339
dialysis in, 561
manifestations of, 1338–1339
pathology of, 1338
treatment of, 1338–1339
Diabetic neuropathy, 1339–1340, 2192–2193. See also *Neuropathies.*
and ataxia, 2044
asymmetric, 1339–1340
autonomic, 1340, 2027
classification of, 1339, 1339t
hyperglycemia and, 1326–1327, *1326*
lesions with, 1339
symmetric distal polyneuropathy, 1339
Diabetic retinopathy, 1337–1338, 2223–2224
cataracts in, 1338
cotton-wool (soft) exudates in, 1337
glaucoma in, 1338
hyperglycemia and, 1326
nonproliferative, 1337–1338
proliferative, 1338
waxy exudates in, 1337
Diagnosis, 57–68
in art of medicine, 3
procedure validity for, 8
studies for, 59
test sensitivity and specificity in, 59, 61
Dialysis, 559–563, 1012–1013
aluminum deposition and, 1428
cardiovascular stress during, 562
clinical use of, 560–561
complications of, 562, 562t
disequilibrium, 561
hospital-acquired infection and, 1486
hypertriglyceridemia with, 1114
in acute pancreatitis, 774
in acute renal failure, 548
in chronic renal failure, 550, 551, 552, 553, 556
in poisoning, 87
infection with, 562
initiation of, 561, 561t
limitations of, 563
pseudogout with, 562
renal cysts and, 635
renal osteodystrophy with, 562
routine management of, 561–562
serositis with, 562
technical aspects of, 559–561, *559*
tenosynovitis with, 562
time-averaged clearance with, 560, 560t
with anemia, 562
with pruritus, 562
Dialysis ascites, 562

Dialysis dementia, 562
  aluminum-induced, 2311
Diaphragm, 452–453
  eventration of, 453
Diaphragmatic flutter, 453
Diaphragmatic hernias, 452–453
Diaphragmatic paralysis, 453
Diaphyseal aclasis, 1466
Diarrhea, 648–649, 712–719
  antibiotics for, 719
  biopsy in, 716
  bismuth subsalicylate for, 19
  cholera and, 1598
  chronic, of unknown origin, 717–718
  clinical classification of, 715, 716t
  cutaneous disorders with, *2263*
  diagnosis of, 715–716, 715t
  epidemic, 1734–1735
  fecal incontinence as, 718
  fluid replacement in, 718
  fluid volume depletion and, 519
  functional, 717
  intestinal motility derangement in, 714–715
  intestinal parasites and, 716, 717
  ion absorption/ion secretion factor in, 714, *714*
  laboratory examination in, 715–717
  metabolic acidosis and, 540
  opiates for, 718–719
  osmotic, 714
  pathophysiology of, 714–715
  perianal discomfort with, 718
  postvagotomy, 692, 692t
  proctosigmoidoscopy in, 716
  secretory, 714, 714t
  shigellosis and, 1596
  stool examination in, 715–717
  therapy of, 718
  traveler's, 717, 718, 719
  vasoactive intestinal polypeptide and, 717
Diarrheogenic syndrome, 1349–1350
Diascopy, in skin disease, 2238
Diastematomyelia, 2187
Diazepam
  in athetosis, 2077
  in depressant abuse, 2020
  in multiple sclerosis, 2146
  in myofascial pain syndrome, 2064
  in pain, 2051
  in tension headache, 2057
  in tetanus, 1580
Diazoxide, in primary pulmonary hypertension, 263
Dicarboxylic aminoaciduria, 611
Dicroceliasis, 1816
Dicrocoelium dendriticum, 1816
Diet, 37–39. See also *Enteral nutrition; Nutrition; Parenteral nutrition.*
  arteriosclerosis and, 38
  cancer and, 39
  diabetes mellitus and, 1213. See also *Dietary management, in diabetes mellitus.*
  hypertension and, 38–39
  in hyperlipidemia, 38
  in nutritional assessment, 1180, 1180t
  in obesity, 1195–1196
  for carbohydrate, 1177
  for energy, 1174, 1177t
  for fat, 1177
  for fat-soluble vitamins, 1177
  for minerals, 1178–1179
  for protein, 1174–1175
  for water-soluble vitamins, 1178
  recommended, 1174–1179, 1175t–1176t
  United States goals for, 1179
Dietary factor(s)
  in cancer, 1071–1072
Dietary factor(s) (*Continued*)
    in cancer, of colon, 764–765
    of stomach, 697–698
  in kidney stones, 629, 630
  in peptic ulcer, 689
Dietary management
  in chronic renal failure, 557–558
  in diabetes mellitus, 1327–1328
  in inborn errors of metabolism, 131
  in myocardial infarction, 294
Dietary requirement, for calcium, 1418–1419
Diethylcarbamazine, in filariasis, 1827
Diethylstilbestrol, in cancer chemotherapy, 1101t
Diffuse sclerosis, 2147
DiGeorge's syndrome, 1858
Digital clubbing, in congenital heart disease, 227
Digital subtraction angiography, renal, 512–513
Digitalis, 220–204, 323
  in shock, 223–224
  intoxication by, 64, 783
  mechanism of action of, 200–201, *200*
  molecular bases of, 201
  toxicity of, 203–204
Digitalis therapy
  agent selection for, 201–203, 201t, 202t
  blood level determinations in, 204
  diagnostic agents for, 203
  dosage schedules for, 203
  in heart failure, 200
  in myocardial infarction, 204
  intravenous agents for, 202–203
  oral agents for, 201–202
  toxicity with, arrhythmias in, 203–204
    electrocardiography in recognition of, 203, 204
    lidocaine therapy for, 204
    potassium therapy for, 203–204
    recognition of, 203
    treatment of, 203–204
Digitoxin, 202. See also *Digitalis.*
  pharmacokinetic parameters of, 70t
Digoxin, 323
  clearance of, 76
  elimination of, 81
  for intravenous administration, 202
  for oral administration, 201–202
  loading dose of, 77
  overdose of, 73
  pharmacokinetic parameters of, 70t
  serum and plasma, reference values of, 2322
  therapeutic serum range for, 203, 204
Dihydrocodeine, in pain, 2052
Dihydrofolate reductase deficiency, hereditary, 132
Dihydrotestosterone, in male sexual differentiation, 1361–1362, *1361*
5α-Dihydrotestosterone, 1365
2,8-Dihydroxyadenine lithiasis, 1144
Diiodohydroxyquin, in liver abscess, 830
DiMauro's disease, *2205*, 2206
Dimercaprol, in mercury intoxication, 599
Dimethyltryptamine (DMT), abuse of, 2023–2024
Diphenylhydantoin. See *Phenytoin.*
2,3-Diphosphoglycerate, 1164
2,3-Diphosphoglyceric acid, 917, *917*
Diphosphonates, in Paget's disease of bone, 1462
Diphtheria, 1571–1573
  anterior nasal, 1572
  bronchial, 1572
  carriers of, 1571
  clinical manifestations of, 1572
Diphtheria (*Continued*)
  diagnosis of, 1572–1573
  epidemiology of, 1571
  etiology of, 1571
  immunization for, 43–44, 43t
  laryngeal, 1572
  pathogenesis of, 1571–1572
  pharyngeal, 1572
  prevention of, 1573
  tonsillar (faucial), 1572
  toxin of, 1571–1572
  treatment of, 1573
Diphtheria antitoxin, 1573
Diphtheria-tetanus-pertussis vaccine, 1573
Diphtheritic myocarditis, 334
Diphtheritic neuropathy, 2195
Diphyllobothrium latum, 1805–1806
Diphyllobothrium pacificum, 1805
Diplopia, 2198
  in intracranial hypertension, 2058
Dipsomania, 53
Dipylidium caninum, 1808
Dipyrroles, 873
Direct-current electroconversion. See also *Cardioversion.*
  for digitalis toxicity, 204
  for heart failure, 200, 210
  in cardiopulmonary resuscitation, 481
Dirofilariasis, 1831
Disaccharidase deficiency, 724
Disc. See under specific name.
Discography, in back pain, 2063
Disinfection, for hospital-acquired infection, 1491
Disodium cromoglycate, in asthma, 395
Disopyramide, 324
Dissecting aneurysm of aorta
  aortography in, 350–351, *351*
  electrocardiography in, 350
  history in, 350
  laboratory studies in, 350–351
  physical findings in, 350
  prognosis in, 351
  radiography in, 350
  treatment of, 351
Disseminated intravascular coagulation, 914, 1031, 1035, 1053–1055
  coagulation factors replacement in, 1054–1055
  diagnosis of, 1054
  heparin therapy in, 1055
  in blood transfusion, 939
  in shock, 216
  laboratory tests in, 1054
  platelet transfusion in, 1055
  treatment of, 1054–1055
Distal myopathy, 2204
Distributions of values, in test results, 62, *62*
Disulfiram, 53
Diuresis
  blood volume and, 163
  erythrocytosis and, 963–964
  in heart failure, 163–164
  osmotic, 519
  solute, 519
  postobstructive, 519
Diuretics. See under specific names and diagnoses.
  abuse of, 519, 613
  as nephrotoxins, 602
  characteristics of, 522t
  complications with, 210
  "dry" weight maintenance and, 207
  early distal tubule, 523
  hypercalcemia and, 1449
  hypokalemia and, 533
  in heart failure, 194–200, 207–210

Diuretics (*Continued*)
in hypertension, 277
in kidney stones, 632
late distal nephron, 523
loop, 522–523
metabolic acidosis and, 540
osmotic, 533
potassium-sparing, 534
proximal, 522
sodium and water restriction and, 207
sodium control system and, 207, *207*
thiaside, nephrotoxicity of, 602
Diverticula, duodenal, 708, 862
Diverticulitis, 799–800
clinical findings in, 799
diagnosis of, 799–800
differential, 800
radiography in, 799, *800*
treatment of, 800
surgical, 800
Diverticulosis, 800
lower gastrointestinal hemorrhage and, 794, 795
Diverticulosis coli. See *Colon diverticula.*
Diverticulum, Zenker's, 676
Dizziness, 2040–2043
DNA. See *Deoxyribonucleic acid.*
Dobutamine
in shock, 222
Dodge formula, 186
Donovan bodies, 1650
Donovanosis, 1649–1650
L-Dopa, 1203, 1255
Dopamine, 1220, 1243, 1408–1410
deficiency of, in parkinsonism, 2070
in shock, 222
Dopamine receptor(s), 92
agonists to, direct-acting, in parkinsonism, 2073
Doppler sonography, in stroke, 2100
Dose-response relationships, 2298
Down's syndrome, 145
leukemia with, 987
with leukemoid reaction, 960
Doxorubicin, 338–339, 1097–1098
in acute myelogenous leukemia, 991
in multiple myeloma, 1018
toxicity of, 1092
Doxycycline, in rickettsial disease, 1676, 1677
Dracunculiasis, 1828
Dracunculus medinensis, 1828
Dressing apraxia, 1995
Dressler's syndrome, 341
with myocardial infarction, 292
Drop attacks, 1046, 2153
computed tomography in, 2047
vs. syncope, 1986
with vertebral-basilar ischemia, 2097, *2097, 2098*
Drowning, 37, 2293–2294
Drowsiness, 33t
definition of, 1971
Drug(s). See also names and pharmacologic categories.
absorption of, 69–70
accumulation of, 72, *72*
administration routes of, 69–70, *69*
and disorders of taste, 2032
and impotence, 2030, *2030*
and muscle weakness, 2210
and parkinsonism, 2071
and vertigo, 2042
antidotes to, in coma, 1979
cutaneous side effects of, thoracic, 2244, *2245*
distribution of, 70–71, 70t, 71t
dose-dependent kinetics, 71t, 73
elimination of, 71–72
Drug(s) (*Continued*)
half-life of, 71–72, *72*
ocular side effects of, 2225
oral bioavailability of, 69–70
poisoning by, 1979–1981, *1978–1979*
transport of, *69*
Drug abuse, 2015–2024
acquired immunodeficiency syndrome and, 1862
poisoning from, 88
Drug addiction
definition of, 2015
infective endocarditis and, 1537
myoglobinuria in, 2210
Drug allergy, 1883–1886, 1884t–1885t
diagnosis of, 1885
incidence of, 1883
management of, 1886
mechanisms of, 1883
predisposing factors in, 1883
prevention of, 1885
Drug clearance, 71
drug therapy and, 76
in aged, 78
renal vs. nonrenal, 76–77, 76t
Drug intake, cancer and, 1071
Drug interaction(s), 79–82
decreased drug availability and, 79–80
distribution factor in, 80–81, *80*
enzyme induction factor in, 80, 81
factors in, absorption, 79–80
metabolism, 80, 81, 81t
renal excretion, 81
increased drug availability and, 80–81
plasma protein binding and, 80–81
Drug intoxication
and ataxia, 2045
and syncope, 1986
Drug reaction, 82–84
exaggerated response as, 82–83
genetic factor in, 82
identification of, 84
immunologic, 83–84, 83t
mechanisms of, 82
recognition of, 84
to antimicrobial therapy, 107–108, 107t
toxic, 83–84
Drug resistance, in tuberculosis, 1626
Drug therapy. See also *Drug interactions; Drug reaction.*
active metabolites and, 75, 77
circulatory system disorders and, 77–78
drug clearance data for, 76
elimination rate constant, 76, 76t
for aged, 25, 27, 78
for heart failure, 199–210
hepatic disease effects from, 77
laboratory test errors and, 62
loading doses of, 71, 77
maintenance doses in, 72–73
overdose management in, 73
plasma concentration in, 73–75
plasma concentration–clearance relation and, 76
principles of, 69–84
renal disease effects, 75–77, 76t, *77*
renal vs. nonrenal clearance and, 76–77, 77t
therapeutic window concept of, 74, *74,* 75t
Drug-induced neuropathies, 2195, *2195*
Drunkenness, and ataxia, 2045. See also *Alcohol intake; Alcohol intoxication.*
DTIC. See *Dacarbazine.*
Duchenne dystrophy, 137, 333, 2202
clinical picture in, 2204
diagnosis and age, 2199
features of, *2202*
signs in, 2200
Ductus, patency maintenance of, 1239
Dumping syndrome, 692, 692t, 705
Duncan's disease, 1858
Duodenal ulcer
cigarette smoking and, 49
epidemiology of, 685
genetic factor in, 683
hydrochloric acid secretion and, 683
mucosal defense defect and, 683–684
pepsin secretion and, 683
radiography in, 686, *686*
symptoms of, 685, 685t
treatment of, 690, 690t
Duodenum
diverticula of, 708, 862
tumors of, 702
Dural sinus thrombosis, 2115
Dwarf tapeworm, 1807
eradication of, 1809
Dwarfism
psychosocial, 1249
short-limbed, 1860–1861
zinc deficiency in, 1209
Dynorphin, 1234
Dysarthria, 2198
in Friedreich's ataxia, 2083
in myotonic dystrophy, 2203
in olivopontocerebellar degeneration, 2083
Dysautonomia
familial, 2194–2195
of Riley-Day, 2194–2195
reflex, in spinal cord injury, 2177
Dysbetalipoproteinemia, 1112–1113
genetic factor in, 1112
xanthomas in, 1112–1113
Dyschondroplasia, 1466
Dyscontrol, episodic, vs. epilepsy, 2157
Dysdiadochokinesia, in olivopontocerebellar degeneration, 2083
Dysesthesias
definition of, 2047, 2188
in multiple sclerosis, treatment of, 2147
Dysfibrinogenemia, 1051
acquired, 1053
Dysgeusia, 2032
Dyskeratosis congenita, *2265*
Dyskinesia, definition of, 2069
Dysmetria
in olivopontocerebellar degeneration, 2083
in spinocerebellar degenerations, 2080
Dysmyelination, diseases of, 2148
Dysosmia, 2031
Dyspepsia
functional, 687
in peptic ulcer, 685
Dysphagia, 667, 2198. See also *Eating, disorders of.*
cutaneous disorders with, *2262*
in esophagus cancer, 674
in gastroesophageal reflux disease, 669
transfer, 672
Dysphonia, spastic, in spasmodic torticollis, 2078
Dyspnea, 371–372
diagnostic approach to, 372
in left ventricular failure, 195–196
mechanism of, 371
patterns of, 371–372
Dysproteinemia, neuropathy with, 2195
Dystonia(s), 2077–2079
athetotic, 2077
classification of, *2078*
cranial, 2078–2079
definition, 2069
in drug-induced parkinsonism, 2071
in postencephalitic parkinsonism, 2071
segmental, in spasmodic torticollis, 2078
Dystonia musculorum deformans, 1077–2078

Dystrophy, definition of, 2198. See also specific dystrophy.
Dysuria, 2028–2030, *2029*

E rosettes, 992
Ear(s)
  and hearing disorders, 2037–2040
  disease of, and headache, 2059
  pain in, 2058–2059
    tumors and, 2058
Eastern equine encephalitis, 1745
  clinical features of, 1745
  diagnosis of, 1745
  epidemiology of, 1745
  pathology in, 1745
  serology of, 1745
  vaccine for, 1745
  vector in, 1745
  virus of, 1745
Eating, disorders of, hypothalamus and, 2026
Eaton-Lambert syndrome, 2215
Ebola virus, 1757
Ebstein's anomaly, 234
  echocardiography in, 234
  electrocardiography in, 234
  radiography in, 234
  surgery for, 234
Ecchymoses, 1030
Eccrine sweat glands, 2229–2230
Echinococcal hepatic cyst, 863
Echinococcosis, 1807–1808
Echinococcus granulosus, 1807, 1808
Echinococcus multilocularis, 1807
Echinococcus oligarthus, 1807, 1808
Echocardiography. See also *Ultrasonography.*
  Doppler signal for, 177–178, *179*
  in angina pectoris, 286
  in aortic regurgitation, 255
  in aortic stenosis, 253
  in asymmetric septal hypertrophy, 330–331, *330*
  in atrial septal defect, 229
  in cardiovascular disease, 153, 175–179, *175–179*
  in coarctation of aorta, 238
  in congenital valvular aortic stenosis, 236
  in Ebstein's anomaly, 234
  in Eisenmenger syndrome, 241
  in heart disease, 175–179, *175–179*
  in infective endocarditis, 1539
  in mitral regurgitation, 251
  in mitral stenosis, 248
  in patent ductus arteriosus, 232
  in pericardial constriction, 344
  in pericardial effusion, 343
  in pulmonary stenosis, 235
  in pulmonary vein connection anomaly, 239
  in subvalvular aortic stenosis (discrete), 237
  in supravalvular aortic stenosis, 237
  in tetralogy of Fallot, 233
  in tricuspid valve atresia, 234
  in valvular heart disease, 244–245, *245*
  M-mode, 175–178, *175, 176, 179*
  two-dimensional, 176–177, *176–178*
Echothiopate iodide, in ocular disorders, side effects of, 2226
Echoviruses, 1728–1729, 1729t
  infections with, 2125
    paralytic poliomyelitis due to, 2131
Eclampsia, 271, 834
Ecology, and medicine, 6
Ecthyma, 1525
Ectopia lentis, 1131
Ectopic ACTH syndrome, 1313–1316
Ectopic atrial tachycardia, 308–309
  electrocardiography in, 308–309, *309, 310*
Ectopic polypeptide hormones, 1076
Ectopic polypeptide proteins, 1076
Eczema vaccinatum, 1727
Eczematous dermatitis, 2251
EDCI, 1076
Edema
  cerebral, in infarction, 2090
    in stroke, 2099, 2101
  heat, 2306
  in acute glomerulonephritis, 570–571
  in nephrotic syndrome, 579
  in right ventricular failure, 198
  refractory, 210
  pulmonary, high altitude, 2290
  with chronic obstructive pulmonary disease, 403
Edrophonium, 95
  in myasthenia gravis, 2213, 2214
Ehlers-Danlos sydrome, 130, 346, 1104, 1149, 1150–1151, 1458, *2262,* 2266
  benign hypermobilie, 1150
  ecchymotic, 1150, 1151
  familial joint laxity, 1151
  fibronectin deficient, 1151
  genetic factor in, 1150
  gravis, 1150
  mitis, 1150
  occipital horn, 1150, 1151
  x-linked, 1150
Eicosapentaenoic acid, 1239
Eighth nerve, damage to, and ataxia, 2045
Eisenmenger syndrome, 241
  cardiac catheterization in, 241
  echocardiography in, 241
  electrocardiography in, 241
  radiography in, 241
Ejaculation, premature, 2030
Elastin, 2228
Elastorrhexis, systemic, 1152
Elastosis, senile, 2232
Elderly, gait disturbances in, 2046
Electric injury, 2303–2304
Electricity, stimulation with, in pain, 2053
Electrocardiography, 169–175. See also specific diagnosis.
  computer interpretation of, 173–174
  digitalis toxicity recognition by, 203, 204
  electrophysiology of, 170
  in angina pectoris, 285, 286
  in aortic regurgitation, 255
  in aortic stenosis, 253
  in arrhythmia, 301, *303*
  in asymmetric septal hypertrophy, 330–331
  in atrial septal defect, 229
  in cardiopulmonary resuscitation, 481, 482
  in coarctation of the aorta, 238
  in congenital valvular aortic stenosis, 236
  in dissecting aneurysm of aorta, 350
  in Ebstein's anomaly, 234
  in Eisenmenger syndrome, 241
  in hypertension, 270
  in hyperkalemia, 534–535
  in hypokalemia, 533
  in infective endocarditis, 1539
  in left ventricular failure, 197
  in mitral regurgitation, 251
  in mitral stenosis, 248
  in myocardial infarction, 290–291, *290, 291,* 294
  in patent ductus arteriosus, 231
  in pericardial constriction, 344
  in pericardial effusion, 343
  in pericarditis, 342
  in pulmonary stenosis, 235
Electrocardiography (*Continued*)
  in pulmonary vein connection anomaly, 239
  in respiratory disease, 389–390
  in shock, 218
  in tetralogy of Fallot, 233
  in tricuspid valve atresia, 234
  in valvular heart disease, 244
  interpretation of, 172–173, *172t, 173t*
  lead systems for, 170–171, *170t, 171*
  learning principles for, 171–172, *172*
  recording techniques for, 174–175
  stress testing and, 174–175
  waveforms for, 171, *171*
Electroconvulsive treatment, in manic-depressive psychosis, 2007
Electrodes, in pain relief, 2053
Electroencephalography, 1969–1970
  in altered consciousness, 1977
  in encephalitis, 2124
  in epilepsy, 2149, 2156
  in herpes simplex encephalitis, 2127
  in viral meningitis, 2124
  sensory evoked potentials with, 1969–1970
Electrolyte balance, in uremia, 549–551, 555–556
Electrolytes
  absorption of, 721, 724–725
  in uremia, 489
  management of, in head injury, 2173
  urinary, 510–511
Electromyography, 2201
  in amyotrophic lateral sclerosis, 2080
  in back pain, 2063
  in myopathies, 2200, *2200*
  in nervous system disease, *1969,* 1970, 1970t
  in polymyositis, 1949
  in Werdnig-Hoffman disease, 2080
  in Wohlfart-Kugelberg-Welander disease, 2080
  single-fiber, in myasthenia gravis, 2212, 2213
Electron microscopy, in myopathies, 2201
Electronystagmography, 2041
Electroshock, direct-current, in heart failure, 200
Elek's test, for diphtheria, 1572
Elimination rate constant, drug therapy and, 76, 76t
Embden-Meyerhof pathway, in hemolytic anemia, 904–905, *904*
Embolectomy, in pulmonary embolism, 430
Embolism
  with congenital heart disease, 228
  with myocardial infarction, 292
Embolus(i)
  artery-to-artery, and stroke, 2095, 2095
  cardiac, and stroke, *2095, 2096*
Emery-Dreifuss muscular dystrophy, 2203
EMG. See *Electromyography.*
Electron transport, disorders of, 2206
Emotional factor
  in anorexia nervosa, 1188–1189, 1190
  in Crohn's disease, 741
  in gastrointestinal disease, 645
  in Huntington's disease, 2074
  in hyperthyroidism, 1281
  in schizophrenia, 2002
  in ulcerative colitis, 748
Emphysema, 397. See also *Chronic obstructive pulmonary disease.*
  $alpha_1$-antitrypsin deficiency in, 400
  cigarette smoking and, 48–49, 400
  clinical manifestations of, 400
  pathology of, 400
  pulmonary hypertension and, 259–260

Empty sella syndrome, 1260
primary, 2168
Empyema, 1584–1585
staphylococcal, 1547
subdural, 2114–2115
spinal, 2117–2118
with pleural disease, 449
Enanthems, in mucocutaneous enteroviral disease, 1732
Encephalitis
acute demyelinating, 2139–2140, 2147
and parkinsonism, 2071
arbovirus infection and, 1736, 1742–1750, 1742t. See also specific diagnoses.
differential diagnosis of, 1743–1744
clinical features of, 1742–1743
pathogenesis of, 1743
pathology of, 1743
vectors in, 1742, 1742t, *1743*
as measles complication, 2140
bulbar, cancer and, 1082
California, 1747–1748. See also *California encephalitis.*
Dawson's, 2136
eastern equine, 1745. See also *Eastern equine encephalitis.*
etiologic agent in, frequency of, *2123*
herpes simplex, 1716, 2126–2128
Japanese, 1748. See also *Japanese encephalitis.*
mumps virus infection, 1712–1713
Murray Valley, 1748–1749
necrotizing, acute, 2126–2128. See *Herpes simplex encephalitis.*
postvaccinal, 1727
Rocio, 1748–1749
St. Louis, 1746–1747. See also *St. Louis encephalitis.*
subacute inclusion body, 2136
tick-borne, 1749. See also *Tick-borne encephalitis.*
Venezuelan equine, 1745–1746. See also *Venezuelan equine encephalitis.*
viral, 2122–2126
western equine, 1744–1745. See *Western equine encephalitis.*
Encephalomyelitis, 2122, 2126
acute disseminated, 2139–2140, 2147
allergic, experimental, 2140
immune-mediated, 2139. See also *Encephalomyelitis, acute disseminated.*
myalgic, benign, 2131
parainfectious, 2139. See also *Encephalomyelitis, acute disseminated.*
and vertigo, 2043
postinfectious, 2123, 2139. See also *Encephalomyelitis, acute disseminated.*
postvaccinal, 2140
with measles, 1708
zoster, 2129
Encephalopathy. See also *Hepatic encephalopathy.*
from radiation injury, 1083
hypertensive, 271, 2102
hypertonic, 1270, 1272
metabolic, 1973
toxic, of children, 2141
Wernicke's, 2064–2065, *2065*
Enchondromatosis, 1466
Endarterectomy, carotid, in cerebral atherothrombotic disease, 2100
Endarteritis
focal, in syphilis, 1651
infective, 1538–1539
End-expiratory pressure ventilation, in acute respiratory failure, 459
Endocardial cushion defect, 230
atrioventricular canal defect with, 230
ostium primium with, 230
Endocardial fibroelastosis, 332
Endocarditis
bacterial, cerebral manifestations of, 2116
vs. bacterial meningitis, 1554
in bacterial meningitis, 1554
in systemic candidiasis, 1769
infective, 1533–1542
acute bacterial, 1537, 1548
clinical features of, 1535–1536, 1536t
complications of, 1536–1537
culture in, 1539
culture-negative, 1538
cure rates in, 1538t
diagnosis of, differential, 1539
echocardiography in, 1539
electrocardiography in, 1539
laboratory tests in, 1539
radiography in, 1539–1540
drug addiction and, 1537
fungal, 1538
gram-negative bacterial, 1537–1538
gram-positive cocci in, 1533
immune response in, 1539
in infants and children, 1538
microbiology of, 1533–1534, 1534t
nosocomial, 1538
pathogenesis of, 1534–1535, *1534*
pathology of, 1534–1535
pre-existing cardiac lesions in, 1534, 1534t, 1535t
pregnancy and, 1538
prevention of, 1541–1542, 1542t
prognosis in, 1541
prophylaxis in, antibiotic, 1542, 1542t
prosthetic valvular involvement and, 1537
recurrent, 1539
risk of, cardiac lesions and, 1535t
sites involved in, 1535t
staphylococcal, 1547–1548
treatment of, 1540
anticoagulants, in, 1541
antibiotic therapy in, 1540–1541, 1540t
surgery in, 1541
vs. infective endarteritis, 1538–1539
marantic, 1534
Endocrine disorders
and impotence, 2030
depression in, 2011
myopathy in, 2210
neuropathy with, 2194
Endocrine factor
in anemia, 884
in cancer, 1077–1080
in hypoglycemia, 1342, 1342t
in liver tumor, 849
in postassium balance, 498
in shock, 214–215
in sodium balance, 494, 497
Endocrine glands. See also specific structures and disorders.
extraglandular influences on, 1229–1230
hyperfunction of, 1230
multiple syndromes, 1231
hypofunction of, 1229–1230
genetic factor in, 1229
multiple syndromes, 1231
iatrogenic disease of, 1230
nonhormonal abnormalities of, 1231
polyglandular disorders of, 1405–1408, 1406t, 1407t
Endocrine system
aging and, 23
disorders of, 1229–1231
Endocrine system (*Continued*)
disorders of, clinical assessment in, 1231–1233
history in, 1231
laboratory testing in, 1231–1233
physical examination in, 1231
treatment of, 1233
Endocrinology. See also specific substances and systems.
principles of, 1219–1233
"End-of-dose" effect, in levodopa therapy, 2073
Endogenous opioid peptides, 1234–1237
Endogenous pyrogen, 1471–1472
Endometrium, 1382
cancer of, 1393
Endomyocardial fibrosis, 337
Endophthalmitis, 2220, 2221
Candida, 2221
Endorphin(s), 1234, 1253
biosynthesis of, 1234–1235, *1234*
clinical research on, 1236–1237
in shock, 214–215
β-Endorphin, 1235–1237, 1253
clinical research on, 1236–1237
immunoassay of, 1307
physiologic effects of, 1235–1236
pituitary secretion of, 1236
Endoscopic retrograde cholangiopancreatography, in pancreatitis, 772, 773, *776*, *777*
Endoscopic retrograde pancreatography, in pancreas cancer, 779, *779*
Endoscopy. See also specific procedures.
fiberoptic, 658
future of, 662
in esophagus cancer, 674, 675
in peptic ulcer, 686
in stomach cancer, 699
Endosomes, 1227
Endotoxin, 1594–1595
Endotracheal intubation
complications with, 476
for ventilatory assistance, 467–468, 468t
in respiratory failure, 460
nosocomial pneumonia and, 1511
Energy
dietary allowances for, 1174, 1177t
metabolism of, disordered, *2205*
Enkephalin(s), 1234
biosynthesis of, 1235, *1235*
Enkephalinase, 1235
Entamoeba hartmanni, 1800
Entamoeba histolytica, 830, 1799–1800
Enteral nutrition, 1211–1214
bland diet for, 1214
liquid diet for, 1214
protein-calorie supplementation by, 1211–1213, *1212t,* 1213t
restrictive diets in, 1213, 1213t
supplementary components for, 1214, 1214t
therapeutic diets for, 1213–1214
Enteric bacteria
extraintestinal infection from, 1592–1595
management of, 1595
Enteric bypass, liver disease and, 834
Enteric fever, 1590
Enteritis
acute infectious, 737
radiation, 738
Enteritis necroticans, 1576
Enterobiasis, 1824–1825
cellophane tape test in, 1825
epidemiology of, 1824
pruritus ani in, 1825
treatment of, 1825
Enterobius (Oxyuris) vermicularis, 1824
Enterococcus, 1519
Enterocolitis, pseudomembranous, 1576–1577

Enteropathy
  dermatogenic, *2263*
  gluten-sensitive, 732–734
  malabsorptive, with dermatitis herpetiformis, 2269
  protein-losing, 739–740, *739t*
Enterovirus(es), 1728–1730. See also specific groups.
  and respiratory tract illness, 1734
  characteristics of, 1728–1729, 1728t
  enanthems in, 1732
  in acute central nervous system infections, *2122*, 2123
  newly recognized, 1729, 1729t
  nonpolio, 1728–1730
  paralytic poliomyelitis due to, 2131
Enteroviral disease, 1728–1734
  clinical manifestations of, 1729
  epidemiology of, 1729
  laboratory diagnosis of, 1729–1730
  mucocutaneous, 1732–1733
  myocarditis with, 1731–1732
  neurologic complications with, 1730
  nonpolio, 1729–1730, 1729t
  of eye, 1733–1734
  of respiratory tract, 1734
  paralysis with, 1730
  pathogenesis of, 1729
  pericarditis with, 1731–1732
  prevention of, 1730
  serology of, 1729–1730
Enthesopathy, 1891–1892
Entrapment neuropathy(ies), 2196–2197
  vs. paravertebral tumor, 2185
Enuresis, and sleep disorders, 1989–1990, *1988*
Envenomation
  marine animal, 1843–1845, 1843t, *1844*
  snake bite and, 1841–1842
Environment, cigarette smoke contamination of, 49
Environmental agents, neuropathy caused by, 2195, *2195*
Environmental and occupational medicine, 2277–2340
Environmental factor(s)
  in aplastic anemia, 878
  in bronchogenic carcinoma, 440
  in cancer, 1069–1073, 1070t
    of colon, 764–765
  in congenital defects, 144t, 145
  in congenital heart disease, 225, 226t–227t
  in death and dying, 33, 33t
  in falls, 28
  in hemolysis, 912–913
  in hemolytic anemia, 902, 907–915
  in hypertension, 267
  in infectious disease, 1483. See also *Hospital-acquired infection.*
  in puberty, 18
Environmental medicine, definition of, 2279
Environmental-occupational history, 2277–2278, *2278*
Enzyme activity, in myopathies, 2201
Enzyme defects, with gout, 1139
Enzyme deficiency
  dominate vs. recessive genetic disorders and, 119
  in hemolytic anemia, 904–907
  in inborn errors of metabolism, 127–132, 129t–130t
  in metabolic disease, 1103
Enzyme induction, drug interaction and, 80, 81
Enzyme measurement, in myocardial infarction, 291
Enzymic preparations, in wet dressings, 2239
Eosinophil(s), 941, 1011
  in allergy, 391
  in immune response, 1011, 1012
Eosinophil chemotactic factors of anaphylaxis, in rheumatic disease, 1900–1901
Eosinophil count, reference values for, 2337
Eosinophilia
  diseases associated with, 1011–1013, 1012t
  tropical, 1830
  with worm infection, 1804
Eosinophilic factors of anaphylaxis, 390
Eosinophilic fasciitis, 1935
Eosinophilic granulomatosis, 1009–1011
Eosinophilic syndromes, 1011–1013
Eosinophilopoietin, in cancer, 1080
Ependymoma
  characteristics of, *2162*
  spinal, 2186
Ephelides, 2254
Epidemic parotitis. See *Mumps.*
Epidermal necrolysis, toxic, 2270
Epidermis, 2227
Epidermolysis bullosa, *2262*
Epidermolytic hyperkeratosis, *2251*
Epidermophyton infections, 2247
Epididymo-orchitis, with mumps, 1713
Epidural abscess, 1549
  acute, vs. transverse myelitis, 2139
  cerebral, 2115
  spinal, 2116–2117
Epidural bleeding, myelopathy in, 2139
Epidural "blood patch," in intracranial hypotension, 2167
Epidural hematoma, spinal, 2187
Epiglottitis, *Hemophilus influenzae*, 1664
Epilepsia partialis continua, 2153, 2154
  viral role in, 2137
Epilepsy (epilepsies), 2149–2160. See also *Seizure(s).*
  abdominal, 2151
  and disorders of taste, 2032
  catamenial, 2153
  classification of, 2151, *2151*
  clinical manifestations of, 2151–2155
  diagnosis of, 2155–2157
    computed tomography in, 2155
  focal, viral role in, 2137
  in tuberous sclerosis, 2085
  limbic, 2154
  myoclonus in, juvenile, 2152, 2154
    progressive, 2153, 2154
  nonconvulsive, and drop attacks, 2047
  petit mal, 2154
  photosensitive, 2153
  post-traumatic, 2171
  psychomotor, 2154
    vs. schizophrenia, 2004
  psychosocial considerations in, 2160
  reflex, 2153
  resective surgery in, 2159
  rolandic, 2154
  sensory, vs. sensory ischemia, 2098
  sensory symptoms in, 2151
  sylvian, 2154
  temporal lobe, 2154
  tonic disturbances and, 2150
  treatment of, 2157–2160
    emergency, 2159–2160
Epileptic acquired aphasia syndrome, 2155
Epileptic focus, 2149
Epileptic myoclonus, juvenile, 2152, 2154
Epileptic syndromes, 2154–2155, *2154*
Epileptogenesis, 2149
Epiloa, 2085
Epinephrine, 90–91, 93, 1243, 1408–1410
  deficiency of, 1413
  in anaphylaxis, 1872
Epinephrine (*Continued*)
  in asthma, 394
  in cardiopulmonary resuscitation, 481–482
  in insect sting allergy, 1974
  in shock, 222
  neutrophil adhesiveness and, 950
Episcleritis, 2223
Epispadias, 639
Epithelioma, basal cell, 2271–2272, *2272*
Epizootic stomatitis, 1711–1712
Epstein-Barr virus, 994, 999, 1071, 1695, 1719–1721, 1858, 1905, 1909
  aplastic anemia and, 878
  in X-linked lymphoproliferative syndrome, 1720
  morphology of, 1719
Equilibrium, disorders of, 2040–2043
Erb dystrophy, 333
Ergocalciferol, 1423
Ergotamine tartrate
  in cluster headache, 2056
  in migraine, 2055
Erlenmeyer flask deformity, 1117
Erosion, of skin, 2233
Eructation, 649
Erysipelas, 1525
Erysipeloid, 1611–1612
  clinical manifestations of, 1611–1612
  culture in, 1612
  epidemiology of, 1611
  treatment of, 1612
Erysipelothrix rhusiopathiae, 1611–1612
Erythema, necrolytic migratory, *2263*
Erythema chronicum migrans, 1923–1924
Erythema elevatum diutinum, *2266*
Erythema induratum, 1962, 2267
Erythema marginatum, 1530
Erythema multiforme, *2264*, 2269–2270
  herpes simplex virus infection with, 1716
Erythema multiforme major, 1506
Erythema nodosum, 2258, 2266, *2266*
  with ulcerative colitis, 753
Erythema nodosum leprosum, 1634, 1636, 1637, 1638
Erythroblastosis
  hemoglobin synthesis and, 920, *920*
  passive immunization to, 43t
Erythroblastosis fetalis, 46
Erythrocyte(s)
  circulating mass, regulation of, 964
  drug binding of, 911
  hematologic values for, 871, 871t
  hemolysis from trauma of, 913–915
  in anemia, 875
  in hemolytic disorders, 901, 901t
  in sickle cell syndrome, 927, 929
  intracorpuscular abnormalities and, 907
  oxidative stress and, 907
  parasites of, 913
  precursors of, 866, *867*, 894
Erythrocyte glutathione reductase, 1200
Erythrocyte membrane, in hemolytic anemia, 902–904
Erythrocyte sedimentation rate, reference values for, 2337
Erythrocytosis, 933, 963–971
  causes of, 965, 965t
  clinical evaluation in, 965–966, *966*
  diuresis and, 963–964
  drug-induced, 967
  kidney disease and, 967
  mechanisms of, 964–965
  pathophysiology of, 965
  physiologically inappropriate, 967
  primary, 970
  relative, 963–964
  tobacco use and, 963–964

Erythroderma(s)
  acquired, 2251–2254
  exfoliative, 2252, *2252*
Erythroid burst-forming units, 868, 964
Erythroid colony-forming units, 868, 964
Erythroid precursor development, 866, *867*, *868*
Erythroid progenitors, 964–965
Erythromelalgia (erythermalgia), 356–357
Erythromycin, 105, 1586
  in acne, 2243
  in relapsing fever, 1664
Erythromycin estolate hepatotoxicity, 823
Erythroplakia, 666, *666*
Erythropoiesis, 964
  in copper, 1209
  in megaloblastic anemia, 894
  in polycythemia vera, 969, 970
  ineffective, 888
  intramedullary, 866
Erythropoietic porphyria(s), congenital, 2253, *2265*
Erythropoietic protoporphyria, *2265*
Erythropoietin, 501, 869, 964–965
  assay of, 965–966
  in cancer, 1079–1080
  in interstitial nephritis, 591
  in uremia, 489
Escherichia coli, pneumonia caused by, 1510
Esophageal bleeding, in gastroesophageal reflux disease, 669
Esophageal cancer, 674–675
  cigarette smoking and, 48
  dysphagia in, 674
  endoscopy in, 674, 675
  radiation therapy for, 675
  radiography in, 674, 675, *675*
  surgery for, 675
Esophageal colic, 668, 672–673
Esophageal motor disorders, 672–674
  diagnosis of, 673–674, *673t*
  manometry in, 673–674, 673t
  pathogenesis of, 672
  pharmacologic stimulation in, 674
  radiography in, 673, *673*
  symptoms of, 672–673
  treatment of, 674
Esophageal spasm, diffuse, 672, *673*
Esophageal stricture, 669, 672
Esophageal tumor, 674–675
Esophageal ulcer, 669–670, 672
Esophageal varices
  bleeding with, 794, 795
    control of, 842–843
  with portal hypertension, 842–843
Esophagitis
  after gastric surgery, 693
  bleeding with, 794
Esophagogastroduodenoscopy, 658–659
Esophagus
  caustic burns of, 676–677
  disease of, 667–677
    symptomatology of, 667–668
  diverticula of, 676
  infection of, 676
  injury of, 676–677
    caustic burns, 676–677
    from drugs, 677
    from trauma, 677
    from vomiting, 677
    perforation, 677
  rings of, 675–676, *676*
  webs of, 675–676
Espundia, 1790–1792
Essential tremor, 2073–2074
Estradiol, 1301
  in male, 1365, *1366*
  serum or plasma and urinary, reference values for, 2322
  16β-Estradiol, 1381
Estriol, 1301
  free, reference values for, 2322
  total, reference values for, 2322
Estrogen(s), 1381
  in acne, 2243
  in cancer chemotherapy, 1101t
  in gynecomastia, 1400–1401
  in male sexuality, 1366
  in postmenopausal therapy, 1393, 1395
  total, reference values for, 2322
Estrogen receptor(s), 1100
Estrogen receptor assay, reference values for, 2322
Estrogen receptor protein, in breast cancer, 1402–1403, 1403t
Estrogen therapy
  in hypopituitarism, 1258
  in osteoporosis, 1460
  in prostate cancer, 1378–1379
Estrone, 1301
  in male, 1365, *1366*
  serum and urinary, reference values for, 2323
Ethacrynic acid, in heart failure, 208–209
Ethambutol, 1625, 1626
  as nephrotoxin, 598
  ocular side effects of, 2225
Ethanol. See also *Alcohol.*
  absorption of, 50–51
  metabolism of, 51, *51*
  neuropharmacology of, 51
  pharmacology of, 50–51
  poisoning from, 88–89
  serum and blood, reference values for, 2323
  tolerance to, 52
Ethanol toxicity, 836
Ethics. See *Medical ethics.*
Ethionamide, 1625
Ethnic factor, in human heredity, 117
Ethosuximide, in epilepsy, 2158, 2158t
Ethyl chloride, in myofascial pain syndrome 2064
Ethylene glycol
  as nephrotoxin, 603–604
  poisoning from, 89
Etidronate, osteomalacia and, 1428
Eubacterium, 1583
Eumycetoma, 1773
Euthyroid dysalbuminemic hyperthyroxinemia, 1279, 1283
Evans' syndrome, 909
Ewing's sarcoma, 1467
Exanthems, 1733
  roseoliform, 1733
Exchange transfusion, in poisoning, 87
Excretory system, aging and, 22
Excretory urography, in kidney tumor, 639, 640
Exercise, 40–41
  angina pectoris and, 287
  atherosclerosis and, 283
  carbohydrate metabolism and, 40
  cardiac response to, 162–163
  coronary heart disease and, 40
  for obesity, 1196
  health benefits of, 40–41
  isometric, 162–163
  isotonic, 163
  myoglobinuria in, 2211
Exercise (*Continued*)
  osteoporosis and, 40–41
  physical working capacity and, 40
  plan for, 41
  psychological effects of, 41
  risks of, 41
  ventricular function curve and, 162–163, *163*
  weight control and, 41
Exertional headache, 2056
Exfoliative erythroderma, 2252, *2252*
Exhaustion, heat, 2305
Exophiala jeanselmei, 1774
Exophthalmos, 1281
  with Graves' disease, 1281, 1282, 1283, 1284, 1287
Expiratory positive airway pressure, 468
Exposure, vs. dose, in occupational medicine, 2277
External capsular–putaminal hemorrhage, 2108
Extracellular compartment fluid, 516–517
Extracellular fluid
  effective osmolality concept of, 523–524, *524*
  sodium balance and, 496, *496*
Extractable nuclear antigen, 1909
Extradural abscess, cerebral, 2115
Extradural hematoma, in skull fracture, 2171
Extradural spinal inflammatory diseases, 2186
Extradural spinal tumors, 2185–2186
Extradural vascular disease, spinal, 2187
Extramedullary spinal vascular lesions, intradural, 2187
Extramedullary spinal tumors, intradural, 2186
Extrapyramidal disorders, general characteristics of, 2068–2070
Extrapyramidal rigidity, vs. pyramidal spasticity, 2045–2046
Extrapyramidal system, in movement disorders, 2068–2069
Extremities
  lower, in amyotrophic lateral sclerosis, 2080
  vascular disease of, 353–366
  weakness of, in striatonigral degeneration, 2079
Eye(s). See also *Ocular; Optic.*
  carcinoma metastatic to, 2222
  diseases of, 2217–2226
    and headache, 2059
    enterovirus, 1733–1734
  in ankylosing spondylitis, 1919
  in brain injury, 2171
  in metabolic brain disease, 1975
  in sarcoidosis, 434
  in subtentorial mass lesions, 1972
  in supratentorial mass lesions, 1972
  in systemic candidiasis, 1768
  in toxoplasmosis, 1793–1794
  infection of, trachoma, 1669–1670
  medications and, 2225–2226
  movements of, in ataxia telangiectasia, 2086
    in Friedreich's ataxia, 2083
    in olivopontocerebellar degeneration, 2083
    in striatonigral degeneration, 2079
  neurologic disorders of, 2032–2037, *2032*, *2034*, *2036*
  non-rapid movement (NREM) of, and sleep, 1987
  rapid movement (REM) of, and sleep, 1987
  "raccoon," in skull fracture, 2171

Fabry's disease, 132, 332, 1116–1117, 1470, *2264*
genetic factor in, 1116
kidney disease and, 506
Face
atypical pain in, 2057
and ear pain, 2058
nevi of, in tuberous sclerosis, 2085
trauma to, brain abscess due to, 2112
Facets
of vertebral body malalignment of, 2187
tropism of, 2187
Facial nerve, neuralgia of, 2060
Facial paralysis, idiopathic, 2197. See also *Bell's palsy.*
Facial weakness, in myotonic dystrophy, 2203
Facioscapulohumeral muscular dystrophy, 2199, 2203
features of, *2202*
Factor IV deficiency, 1030
Factor V deficiency, 1050
Factor VII deficiency, 1049
Factor VIII, in von Willebrand's disease, 1048–1049
Factor VIII deficiency, 1030. See also *Hemophilia.*
Factor VIII inhibitors, 1057
Factor VIII therapy, in hemophilia, 1046–1047
Factor VIII–von Willebrand protein for von Willebrand's disease, 1048
Factor IX deficiency, 1049
Factor X (Stuart-Prower) deficiency, 1049–1050
acquired, 1053
Factor XI deficiency, 1049
Factor XII (Hageman factor) deficiency, 1048
Factor XIII deficiency, 1051
Fainting, 1983–1985. See also *Syncope.*
Falls, 28, 36–37
Familial Mediterranean fever, 345, 1167–1168, 1470
amyloidosis with, 1167–1168, 1169, 1171
attack in, 1167–1168
colchicine for, 1168, 1171
epidemiology of, 1167
genetic factor in, 1167
prognosis in, 1168
treatment of, 1168
with arthritis, 1958
Familial myoclonus, benign, 2153
Familial periodic paralysis. See also *Paralysis, periodic, familial.*
Familial polyposis of colon, 763, *763*
colon cancer and, 766, 769
Familial polyposis syndrome, endoscopy in, 661
Familial tremor, 2073–2074
Family history, in genetics, 117
Fanconi's anemia, 143
leukemia with, 987
Fanconi's syndrome, 487, 539, 594, 595, 602, 614, 615–616, 615t, *2265*
amyloidosis with, 615
cystinosis in, 615
genetic factor in, 615
25-hydroxycholecalciferol-1,25-dihydroxycholecalciferol conversion in, 615
kidney transplantation with, 615
multiple myeloma with, 615
with fructose intolerance, 615
with Lowe's syndrome, 615–616
with Sjögren's syndrome, 615
with Wilson's disease, 615
Fansidar
in malaria, 1779, 1780
resistance to, 1779, 1780
Farcy, 1609
Farmer's lung disease, 2285
Fasciculation(s), 2199
in amyotrophic lateral sclerosis, 2080
in Wohlfart-Kugelberg-Welander disease, 2080
Fasciola gigantica, 1817
Fasciola hepatica, 1816–1817
Fascioliasis, 1816–1817
acute, 1817
clinical manifestations of, 1817
diagnosis of, 1817
extrabiliary, 1817
treatment of, 1817
Fasciolopsiasis, 1818
Fasciolopsis buski, 1818
Fasting, 1184
Fat
absorption of, 719–720, 723
dietary allowances for, 1177
fecal, reference values for, 2323
tests for. See under specific diagnoses.
intraluminal digestion of, 719–720
Fat embolism syndrome, 431–432
clinical features of 432
oxygen therapy in, 432
pathogenesis of, 432
positive end-expiratory pressure in, 432
prognosis in, 432
treatment of, 432
Fat intake
cancer and, 39
hyperlipidemia and, 38
in restricted diet, 1213
Fat necrosis, nodular, *2263*
Fatigue, 2044
Fatty acids
nonesterified, reference values for, 2323
total, reference values for, 2323
Fatty liver, in alcoholic liver disease, 836
Favism, 906
Febrile convulsions, 2154
Fecal impaction, 784
Fecal incontinence, 718, 786
Federal regulations, 8
Feeding centers, 646
Feet, dermatitis of, 2248–2249
Felty's syndrome, 955, 956, 957, 1915
Female pseudohermaphroditism, 1363–1365
congenital adrenal hyperplasia and, 1363–1364
maternal androgens and, 1364–1365
Female sexual development
and precocious puberty, 1383–1385, 1384t, 1385t
at menarche, 1388–1391, 1389t
at menopause, 1391
at puberty, 1385–1388
fetal, and female pseudohermaphroditism, 1363–1365, 1365t
differential abnormalities in, 1363–1365
differentiation factors in, 1353–1354, *1354, 1366*
genital development in, 1352–1353, *1352*
genital differentiation in, 1386–1387
gonadal differentiation in, 1351–1352, *1351*
phenotypic differentiation in, 1352–1353
virilization in, 1364–1365
hermaphroditism in, 1387
pseudopuberty in, 1383–1385, 1384t, 1385t
maturation of, 17–18
Feminization, testicular, 128
Ferritin, 887, 888, 890, 919
serum, 1162
reference values for, 2323
Ferrochelatase deficiency, 1155
Ferrous sulfate, 890
Ferruginous bodies, in asbestos exposure, 2283
Fetal surgery, 146
α_1-Fetoprotein, serum or amniotic fluid, reference values for, 2323
Fetor hepaticus, 845
Fetoscopy, pregnancy loss and, 136
Fever, 1470–1473
antipyretics in, 1472
aphthous, 1711–1712
as "allergic" drug reaction, 83t
diagnosis of, 1472
endogenous pyrogen and, 1471–1472
factitious, 1470
genetic factor in, 1470
humidifier, 2285
in altered consciousness, 1976
in leptospirosis, 1667
in malaria, 1777
in measles, 1707
manifestations of, 1472–1473
metal fumes causing, 2285
of unknown origin, 1470
pathogenesis of, 1471–1473
patient evaluation with, 1470–1471
production mechanisms for, *1472*
prolonged, in bacterial endocarditis, 1554
prostaglandins in, 1472
thermoregulatory center and, 1471–1472
treatment of, 1473
acetaminophen in, 1473
aspirin in, 1472, 1473
viral, undifferentiated, 1737–1750
West Nile, 1738
with granulomatous diseases, 1470
with infection, 1470–1471
Fiber(s)
collagen, 2228
dietary, 709
muscle, continuous activity of, 2216
ring, in myotonic dystrophy, 2202
Fiber intake, 1214
cancer and, 39
hyperlipidemia and, 38
Fiberglass dermatitis, 2297
Fiberoptic endoscopy, 658, 661
Fibrin degradation products, reference values for, 2338
Fibrin lysis time, reference values for, 2338
Fibrinogen, 1043, 1044
in liver disease, 810
radioisotope-labeled, 363–364
reference values for, 2338
Fibrinogen disorders, 1050–1051
Fibrinolysis, 1055–1056
genetic factor in, 1055
inhibition of, 1056
localized, 1056
primary, 1056
secondary, 1055–1056
therapeutic, 1056
Fibrin-stabilizing factor, 1051
Fibrogenesis imperfecta ossium, 1428
Fibromatosis, mesenteric, 791
Fibromuscular hyperplasia, arterial, 2092
Fibrosclerosis, multifocal, 1963
Fibrosis
mediastinal, 1964
pulmonary, idiopathic, 412–413, *412*
retroperitoneal, 1963–1964
Fibrositis, 1960
Fibrous dysplasia, 1465–1466
polyostotic, 1465–1466, *1466*
Fick principle, 184–185
FIGLU, urinary, reference values for, 2323

Filariasis, 1827–1833. See also specific diagnoses.
diagnosis of, 1827
parasites in, 1827, 1827t
perstans, 1831
treatment of, 1827
vectors in, 1827, 1827t
Filobasidiella bacillispora, 1765
Filobasidiella neoformans, 1765
Fingers, clubbing of. See *Clubbing*.
Fires, injury from, 37
Fish, food poisoning from, 782–783
Fish tapeworm, 1805–1806
eradication of, 1809
Fistula(s). See under specific types.
Fits, uncinate, 2152
Fitz-Hugh–Curtis syndrome, 858, 1646
Fitzgerald trait, 1048–1049
Five-day fever, 1685
Flail chest, 454, 457
Flatus, 649, 650
Flaujeac trait, 1048–1049
Flavin adenine dinucleotide, 1199, 1200
Flavin mononucleotide, 1199, 1200
Flavivirus(es), 1736, 1749
tick-borne, 1755
Fleas, 1834
Fletcher trait, 1048
Flies, bloodsucking, 1835
Flavokinase, 1200
Fletcher trait, 1048
Floppy baby syndrome, 1578
Flucytosine, 1759
in cryptococcosis, 1766
Fludrocortisone, 114
Fluid(s)
cerebrospinal. See under *Cerebrospinal fluid pressure, Cerebrospinal fluid volume*, and *Lumbar puncture*.
management of, in head injury, 2173
Fluid balance, in right ventricular failure, 198
in tetanus, 1580
Fluid intake, in renal hypertension, 275
Fluid therapy
in hemorrhage, 884
in shock, 220
Fluid volume
blood pressure and, 273
Fluid volume disorders, 515–523
antidiuretic hormone in, 517
circulatory compromise in, 520–521
diagnosis of, 521
etiology of, 521, 521t
pathogenesis of, 521
treatment of, 521
external fluid balance regulation and, 516–518, *519*
fluid transfer among compartments and, 516
intake and output elements in, 517–518
intake limits and, 515, *516*
of depletion, 518–520
clinical manifestations of, 519–520
diagnosis of, 520
effector loss and, 518
etiology of, 518–519, 518t
extrarenal losses and, 519
output loss and, 519
pathogenesis of, 518–519
treatment of, 520
of excess, 521–523, 522t
diagnosis of, 522–523
etiology of, 521–522
hormone excess and, 522
pathogenesis of, 521–522
primary renal sodium retention and, 522
treatment of, 522–523
Fluid volume disorder (*Continued*)
physiologic considerations in, 515–518
prostaglandins and, 518
renin-angiotensin-alderosterone system in, 517–518
response variables in, 515, *516*
sensors and effectors in, 516–517, *517*, 518
volume repletion reaction in, 518
Flukes. See also *Trematodes;* specific diagnoses.
hermaphroditic, 1815–1819
eradication of, 1815
Fluorescent treponemal antibody absorption test, 1657
Fluoride, 1428
caries prevention and, 663
Fluoropyrimidines, 1094
Fluoroscopy, 382
digital subtraction, 64
in heart disease, 168, 169, *169*
5-Fluorouracil, in cancer chemotherapy, 1094
Fluoxymestrone, in cancer chemotherapy, 1101t
Fluphenazine, in postherpetic neuralgia, 2064
Flurane anesthetiics, as nephrotoxins, 602
Focal cerebral signs, in bacterial meningitis, 1553
Focal neuropathy. See also *Neuropathy, focal*.
definition of, 2188
Focal signs, in metabolic brain disease, 1975
Folate, serum or erythrocytic, reference values for, 2323
Folate absorption test, reference values for, 2323
Folate deficiency, 898–899
drug-induced, 899
megaloblastic anemia and, 893
pregnancy and, 899
specific syndromes, 899
therapy of, 899
Folic acid
absorption of, 721
chemical structure of, 898, *898*
dietary allowance for, 1178
metabolic aspects of, 898
nutritional aspects of, 898
Folic acid deficiency, 724
neutropenia and, 955
Folic acid therapy, 899
in tropical sprue, 737
Follicle-stimulating hormone, 1253, 1381, 1382
function tests of, 1255
in hypopituitarism, 1256, 1258
in male sexuality, 1365, 1366–1367, 1368, 1370
serum or plasma, reference values for, 2324
Folliculitis, chemical, 2297
Fonsecaea, 1774
Fonsecaea pedrosoi, 1774
Foot and mouth disease, 1711–1712
immunogen therapy for, 1712
vaccine for, 1711
virus serotypes, 1711
Fontan principles, 234
Food poisoning, 780–783
bacterial, 781–782
by *Bacillus cereus*, 782
by *Vibrio parahaemolyticus*, 782
chemical, 782
clostridial, 781–782, 1577–1578
etiology of, 781, 781t
from fish and shellfish, 782–783
from mushrooms, 783
from mycotoxins, 783
from plant alkaloids, 783
staphylococcal, 781
Food preparation
and preservation, cancer and, 39
botulism and, 1577–1578
Forced expiration measurement, in chronic obstructive pulmonary disease, 400–402
Fordyce's disease, 1116
Fordyce's spots, 2230
Forgetfulness, 28
Fort Bragg fever, 1666
Fossa, posterior, inflammation of, and ear pain, 2058
tumors of, 2164
Fox-Fordyce disease, 2230
Fractures
of skull, 2171
depressed, 2171
Fragile-X syndrome, 146
Framingham Heart Study, 156–157
Francisella tularenis, 1603–1606
microbiology of, 1604
Frank-Starling mechanism, 162, 163, 192, 194
Freckles, 2254
Free erythrocyte protoporphyrin, 890
Free T_3 index, 1278, 1279, 1283–1284, 1289, 1290, 1291
Free T_4 index, 1278, 1279, 1283–1284, 1289, 1290, 1291
Free thyroxine index, reference values for, 2324
Friedländer's pneumonia, 1509–1510
Friedreich's ataxia, 333, *2081*, *2082*, 2083
Frontal lobe(s), abscess of, 2113
disorders of, 1991–1992, *1991*
and gait disorders, 2045
surgical lesion in, for pain relief, 2053
tumors of, 2163
Frontal polar syndrome, 1992
Functional psychoses, 2001–2007
Frostbite, 357–358
Fructokinase deficiency, 1108
Fructose, serum and urinary, reference values for, 2324
Fructose intolerance
genetic factors in, 1108
hereditary, 1108
with Fanconi's syndrome, 615
Fructose-1-phosphate aldolase deficiency, 131, 1108
Fructosuria, 1108
genetic factors in, 1108
α-l-Fucosidase deficiency, 1116
Fugue states, vs. behavioral disturbances, 2157
Fukuhara syndrome, *2205*
Fulminant hepatic failure, 847
cutaneous lesions in, *2261*
Fungal diseases. See also *Mycoses;* specific diagnoses.
occupational, 2297
of liver, 828
of thorax, 2246–2247
Fungi, 1758
Fungizone. See *Amphotericin B*.
Furosemide
hypercalcemia and, 1449
in ascites, 844
in heart failure, 208–209
Furuncles, 1546
Fused pelvic kidney, 638
Fusiform aneurysms, 2103
Fusobacterium, 1583, *1583*

Gag reflex, in amyotrophic lateral sclerosis, 2080
Gait
in alcoholic cerebellar degeneration, 2066
in Friedreich's ataxia, 2083

Gait (*Continued*)
in Huntington's disease, 2074
in parkinsonism, 2070
in striatonigral degeneration, 2079
Gait apraxia, 1996
Gait disorders, 2045–2046
in parkinsonism-plus, 2071
Galactokinase deficiency, 131, 1105
genetic factors in, 1105
Galactorrhea, 1398–1399, 1398t. See also *Amenorrhea-galactorrhea syndrome.*
bromocriptine in, 1399
corticotropin-releasing factor in, 1399
hyperpolactinemic, 1398–1399
normoprolactinemic, 1263, 1398
prolactin in, 1398–1399
treatment of, 1399
thyrotropin-releasing hormone in, 1399
with amenorrhea, 1399
Galactose-1-phosphate uridyl transferase deficiency, 131, 1104–1105
Galactosemia, 616, 1104–1105
classic, 1104–1105
genetic factors in, 1104–1105
β-Galactosidase deficiency, 1148
α-Galactosidase-A deficiency, 1116
Galactosyltransferase, 1076
Galactosyltransferase isoenzyme II, in pancreatic cancer, 778
Galerina, 783
Gallbladder
adenoma of, 863
adenomyomatous hyperplasia of, 863
cancer of, 863
cholesterol polyps of, 863
diseases of, 851–865
empyema of, 857
hydrops of, 856
porcelain, 856–857
tumors of, 863
Gallium-67 scan(s)
in interstitial lung disease, 411
in sarcoidosis, 437
Gallop rhythm, in left ventricular failure, 196–197
Gallstone(s), 852–853. See also *Cholecystitis.*
acute cholecystitis with, 857–859
asymptomatic, 855
biliary obstruction with, 853
choledocholithiasis and, 859–861
cholesterol, 852–853
chronic cholecystitis, 855–857
dissolution of, 853, 861
epidemiology of, 852–853
obstructive jaundice with, 853
oral contraceptives and, 852
pancreatitis and, 771–772
radiography in, 854–855, *854, 855*
with Crohn's disease, 745
Gallstone ileus, 857, 859
Gambian sleeping sickness, 1780–1783, 1781t
Gamma chain disease, 1020–1021
Gamma globulin
cerebrospinal fluid, in multiple sclerosis, 2144, 2146
in rubella, 1711
Gamma-glutamylcysteine synthetase deficiency, 907
Gamma-glutamyltranspeptidase, in liver disease, 809–810
Gammopathy, monoclonal, 1022
Gangliocytoma, hypothalamic, 1247
Ganglioneuromatosis, 708
Ganglionic blocking agents, 96
Gangrene
gas, 1574, 1575t
infected vascular, 1575
Gangrene (*Continued*)
progressive synergistic, 1520
streptococcal, 1575t
Gardner-Diamond syndrome, *2265*
Gardnerella vaginalis infection, 1566
Gardner's syndrome, 763–764, *764*, 2262
colon cancer and, 766, 769
Gas(es)
intestinal, 649–650
toxic, inhalation of, 2289–2290
Gas dilution (washout) measurement, 374
Gas exchange
decreased inspired PO_2 and, 455
impaired diffusion, 455
normal vs. abnormal 454–455
right-to-left shunts and, 455
ventilation-perfusion imbalance in, 455
Gas gangrene, 1574, 1575t
Gasser's syndrome, 1035–1036
Gastrectomy
complications of, 692
subtotal, 691
malabsorption syndrome with, 737–738
Gastric acid, aspiration of, 1514, 2291
Gastric diverticula, 706
Gastric emptying, postoperative, 704–705
Gastric mucosa, 681
integrity maintenance of, 682–683, *682*
Gastric outlet obstruction, 704
with peptic ulcer, 695–696
Gastric polyps, endoscopy of, 659
Gastric secretion
control of, 681–682, *681*, 683
products of, 682
Gastric secretion rate, reference values for, 2324
Gastric surgery. See also specific procedures.
complications of, 692–693
Gastric ulcer(s)
bile reflux in, 683
cigarette smoking and, 49
endoscopy of, 658–659
epidemiology of, 685
genetic factor in, 683
hydrochloric acid secretion in, 683
mucosal defense defect in, 683–684
pancreatic juice reflux in, 683
pepsin secretion in, 683
radiography in, 686, *686*
stress and, 684
symptoms of, 685, 685t
treatment of, 690, 690t
Gastric varices
bleeding with, 794
with portal hypertension, 842–843
Gastric volvulus, 706
Gastrin
gastric secretion and, 681–682, 683
serum, in peptic ulcer, 686–687, 687t
in Zollinger-Ellison syndrome, 696
reference values for, 2324
Gastrin-calcium infusion stimulation test, reference values for, 2324
Gastrin cells, 681
Gastrinoma, 1349
Gastrin-secretin stimulation test, reference values for, 2324
Gastritis, 677–681
acute, 677–678, 678t
chemical agents in, 677
clinical manifestations of, 677–678
diagnosis of, 678
endoscopic findings in, 678
etiology of, 677
from aspirin, 677, 678
hematemesis with, 677, 678
hypochlorhydria and, 677, 678
natural history of, 678
stress and, 677, 678
Gastritis (*Continued*)
acute, treatment of, 678
antacids in, 678
after gastric surgery, 693
bleeding with, 794
chronic, 678–680, 678t
clinical manifestations of, 679
duodenal juice reflux in, 679
etiology of, 679
genetic factor in, 679
histologic classification of, 678–679
immune response in, 679
natural history of, 679
pernicious anemia and, 679, 680
treatment of, 679–680
type of, by location, 679
eosinophilic, 680
gastric surgery and, 680
giant hypertrophic, 680
granulomatous, 680
stomach cancer and, 698
Gastrocoides hominis, 1818
Gastrocolic reflex, 710
Gastroduodenal motility, disorders of, 704–706
Gastroenteritis, 680
allergic, 735
eosinophilic, 735
nonbacterial, acute infectious, 1734–1735
Salmonella-induced, 1590–1592
staphylococcal, 1545
viral, 1734–1735
Gastroesophageal reflux disease, 668–672
columnar epithelium in, 670, 672
complications of, 669–671, 672
diagnosis of, 669
esophageal histology in, 669, *670*
hiatal hernia in, 668
management of, medical, 671
surgical, 671–672
pathogenesis of, 668
pulmonary aspiration with, 670–671, 671t, 672
symptoms of, 668–669
treatment of, 671–672, 671t
Gastrointestinal bleeding, 649. See also *Gastrointestinal hemorrhage.*
cardiovascular responses to, 649
cutaneous disorders with, 2262
from esophageal varices, 842–843
iron deficiency and, 889
Gastrointestinal cancer, endoscopy in, 658–659
Gastrointestinal disease, 645–802. See also specific diagnoses and symptoms.
alcohol intake in, 645–646
angiography in, 654–655, *655*
computed tomography in, 652, *652*
cutaneous lesions with, 2262–2263
diagnostic imaging procedures in, 650–658
emotional factor in, 645
endoscopy in, 658–662
jaundice in, 650
nuclear magnetic resonance imaging in, 657–658, *657*
nutritional factor in, 646
pathophysiologic basis for symptoms of, 646–650
physical examination in, 646–650
radionuclide imaging in, 652–654, *653, 654*
stress in, 645
ultrasonography in, 650–651, *651*
with uremia, 552–553
Gastrointestinal fistulas, 731
Gastrointestinal hemorrhage, 792–796. See also *Gastrointestinal bleeding.*
acute mucosal lesions and, 794
angiodysplasia and, 794, 795

Gastrointestinal hemorrhage (*Continued*)
blood pressure in, 792
causes of, 794–795, 795t
determination of, 793–794
diagnostic approach to, 794–795
laboratory tests for, 791–792
lower, cause determination in, 793–794
colonoscopy in, 661
diverticulosis and, 794, 795
hemorrhoids and, 794
vascular malformations and, 794, 795
vs. upper, 792–793
malignant lesions and, 794, 795
oxygen therapy in, 792
pathophysiology of, 792
rapidity and magnitude of, 792
recognition of, 791–792, *791*
resuscitation in, 792
transfusion in, 792
upper, cause determination in, 793
endoscopy for, 659
peptic ulcer and, 693–694, 794
therapy for, 793
vs. lower, 792–793
Gastrointestinal motility, 702–704
clinical assessment of, 704
control of, 703–704
disorders of, 704–712. See also specific sites and disorders.
electrical and mechanical correlates of, 703
fasting, 703
postcibal, 703
spinal cord transection and, 712
Gastrointestinal mucormycosis, 1772
Gastrointestinal polyposis, cutaneous disorders with, *2262*
Gastrointestinal symptoms, in classic migraine, 2055
Gastrointestinal system
adenovirus infection of, 1705
aging and, 23
angiodysplasia of, 761
functions of, 702–704
in lead poisoning, 2308
in right ventricular failure, 198
in spinal cord injury, 2177
lower, inflammation of, colonoscopy in, 661
sphincters of, 703
vascular malformations of, 761
viral disease of, 1734–1735
Gastroparesis, 705
Gastroparesis diabeticorum, 705–706
Gaucher cell, 1117, *1117*, 1118
Gaucher's disease, 132, 1117–1118
acute neuronopathic type, 1118
chronic non-neuropathic type, 1118
diagnosis of, 1118
genetic factor in, 1117, 1118
juvenile type, 1118
Norrbotten type, 1118
prognosis in, 1118
treatment of, 1118
Gaussian distribution, 61, 62
Gay bowel syndrome, 1596
Gaze
abnormalities of, 2035–2036
conjugate, in Wernicke's encephalopathy, 2065
impaired, in striatonigral degeneration, 2079
Gelastic epilepsy, 2151
Gemfibrosil, 1113, 1114
Gemfibrosil therapy, 1115
Gene(s), 122
autosomal loci of, 126–127
chromosomes and, 122–123
frequency of, 121–122

Gene(s) (*Continued*)
information transmission, 122–127
linkage of, 136
map of, 126–127, *126*, 127t
mutations of, splicing phenomena in, 136
nucleotide structure of, 136
protein synthesis and, 123–124, *125*
Gene action, regulation of, 126
Gene mapping, 126–127, *126*, 127t, 136
Gene therapy
from recombinant DNA research, present capabilities of, 134
future work on, 134
overview of, 135
risks in, 134–135
technology of, 134
General paresis, 2119
Genetic code, 123, 124t
Genetic compounds, 131
Genetic counseling, 147–149, *147*
diagnosis in, 147
family history in, 147
follow-up of, 149
informative, 148
prenatal diagnosis in, 148–149
probability factor in, 147–148
referral in, 148
risk in, 147–148
supportive, 148
Genetic engineering
in inborn errors of metablism, 132
recombinant DNA research in, expectations from, 133
Genetic factor(s). See also *Chromosome abnormality; Inborn errors of metabolism;* and *Inheritance patterns.*
and manic-depressive psychosis, 2006
and panic disorder, 2010
and schizophrenia, 2003
family history and, 117
in acatalasia, 1158
in acute leukemia, 987
in Addison's disease, 1310
in aging, 24
in alcaptonuria, 1128
in alcoholism, 52
in alpha-antitrypsin deficiency, 832
in altered hemoglobin-oxygen affinity, 933
in amyloidosis, 1170–1171
in amyotrophic lateral sclerosis, 2080
in anemia, 872
in anorexia nervosa, 1188
in aplastic anemia, 878
in atherosclerosis, 283
in Bartter's syndrome, 613
in bilirubin metabolism disorders, 807–808, 807t
in blood coagulation disorders, 1044–1051, 1045t
in breast cancer, 1402
in Burkitt's lymphoma, 999–1000
in cancer, 1066, 1072t, 1073
in celiac disease, 733
in Chediak-Higashi disease, 951
in chronic gastritis, 679
in chronic granulomatous disease, 950
in chronic lymphocytic leukemia, 980
in chronic myelogenous leukemia, 976
in chronic nephropathy, 627–628
in clotting factor deficiencies, 1044–1051, 1045t
in colon cancer, 765–766, 769
in congenital defects, 144–145, 145t
cardiac, 225, 226t–227t
in connective tissue disorders, 1146–1153
in Crohn's disease, 740–741
in cystic fibrosis, 424, 425
in cystinuria, 612

Genetic factor(s) (*Continued*)
in diabetes mellitus, 1322–1323, 1324, 1325, 1326
in drug reaction, 82
in duodenal ulcer, 683
in dysbetalipoproteinemia, 1112
in Ehlers-Danlos syndrome, 1150
in erythrocyte abnormalities, 907
in Fabry's disease, 1116
in familial combined hyperlipidemia, 1113–1114
in familial hypercholesterolemia, 1112
in familial hypertriglyceridemia, 1113
in familial Mediterranean fever, 1167
in Fanconi's syndrome, 615
in febrile disease, 1470
in fibrinolysis, 1055
in fructose intolerance, 1108
in fructosuria, 1108
in galactokinase deficiency, 1105
in galactosemia, 1104–1105
in gastric ulcer, 683
in Gaucher's disease, 1117, 1118
in glycogen storage disease, 1106–1107
in glucose-6-phosphate dehydrogenase deficiency, 905–906, 951
in glucose-6-phosphate dehydrogenase variants, 961–963
in gout, 1132, 1133, 1139
in Graves' disease, 1281–1282
in Hartnup disease, 611
in hemochromatosis, 832–833, 1160–1161, *1161*
in hemoglobin H disease, 923
in hemolytic anemia, 902–907
in hemophilia, 1030, 1045–1046
in hemorrhagic disorders, 1030
in hereditary elliptocytosis, 904
in hereditary spherocytosis, 902, 903
in hereditary stomatocytosis, 904
in hermaphroditism, 1363
in histidinemia, 1129
in homocystinuria, 1131
in hormone deficiency, 1229
in Hunter's syndrome, 1148
in Huntingdon's disease, 2074
in hydroxyprolinemia, 1129
in hyperaminoaciduria, 1120
in hyperprolinemias, 1129
in hypoparathyroidism, 1443
in hypophosphatemia, 1430
in α-L-iduronidase deficiency, 1146
in iminoglycinuria, 611
in immunodeficiency disease, 1855
in interstitial lung disease, 416
in intestinal polyposis, 763–764, *763*, *764*
in kidney disease, 506
in Klinefelter's syndrome, 1370–1371
in Lawrence-Moon-Bardet-Biedl syndrome, 1172
in leprosy, 1634–1635
in lipoprotein disorders, 1111–1114, 1112t
in lipoprotein lipase deficiency, 1113
in liver disease, 832–833
in male pseudohermaphroditism, 1354–1360, *1355*
in maple syrup urine disease, 1130
in Marfan's syndrome, 1149
in medullary sponge kidney, 637
in megaloblastic anemia, 893–900
in Menkes' syndrome, 1210
in metabolic diseases, 1103–1104
in methemoglobinemia, 934–935
in mucopolysaccharidoses, 1146
in multiple organ system disease, 1172–1173
in nephronophthisis, 636–673
in neutropenia, 955, 957

Genetic factor(s) (*Continued*)
in neutrophil functional disorders, 950–953
in Niemann-Pick disease, 1119
in non-Hodgkin's lymphoma, 994
in osteogenesis imperfecta, 1151
in pancreatitis, 772
in partial combined immunodeficiency disorder, 1860–1861
in pentosuria, 1107
in pernicious anemia, 897
in phenylketonuria, 1126
in polycystic kidney disease, 634, 635
in porphyria, 1153–1154, 1155–1156, 1155t
in Prader-Willi syndrome, 1173
in primary hyperoxaluria, 1108
in pseudohypoparathyroidism, 1447
in pseudoxanthoma elasticum, 1152–1153
in puberty, 18
in pyrimidine metabolism disorders, 1145
in pyruvate kinase deficiency, 905
in Reiter's syndrome, 1920
in renal cell carcinoma, 641
in renal glycosuria, 614
in renal hyperaminoaciduria, 611
in renal phosphate wasting, 615
in rickets, 1427
in seminiferous tubule dysgenesis, 1370–1371
in severe combined immunodeficiency disorder, 1859, 1860
in sickle cell syndromes, 927
in spondylarthropathies, 1918–1919, 1918t
in stomach cancer, 698
in systemic lupus erythematosus, 1924–1927
in thalassemia, 920–921, 922–926
in thalassemia intermedia, 922–923
in thalassemia trait, 923
in tumor cell origin, 961–963
in Turner's syndrome, 1173
in ulcerative colitis, 748–749
in unstable hemoglobin disease, 932
in urea cycle disorders, 1129–1130
in urticaria-angioedema, 1864–1865
in von Willebrand's disease, 1047–1048
in Waldenström's macroglobulinemia, 1020
in Werdnig-Hoffmann disease, 2080
in Werner's syndrome, 1172
in Wilson's disease, 832, 1158–1159
in xanthinuria, 1142
monogenic disorders and, 117–118, 118t
pedigree analysis and, 117, *118, 119, 120*
Genetic heterogeneity, 131
Genetic load, 122
Genetics, 117–149. See also *Mutations.*
biochemistry of, 122–127
dominant vs. recessive expression in, 118
expressivity factor in, 118
gene frequency and, 121–122
homozygotes vs. heterozygotes in, 118
mendelian patterns of inheritance in, 117–118, *118, 119, 120*
of major histocompatibility complex, 1877–1883
phenotype differentiation in, 1352–1354, *1353*
polygenic inheritance in, 121, *121*
Geniculate ganglia, lesions of, and visual disorders, 2034
Geniculate ganglion herpes, and vertigo, 2043
Genital tract, mycoplasmal infection of, 1508
Genital ulcer syndrome, sexually transmitted, 1641
Genitalia
fetal, development of, 1352–1353, *1352*
differation error in, 1386
Genitalia (*Continued*)
herpes simplex virus infection of, 1715–1716
Genitourinary tract
in spinal cord injury, 2177
infection of, mycoplasmal, 1508–1509
sexually transmitted, 1641–1643
Ureaplasma, 1508–1509
tuberculosis of, 1628
Genome, 138
Genotype, 138
Gentamicin
as nephrotoxin, 596
therapeutic window of, 101t
Geophagia, 889
Geriatrics, 15. See also *Aged and Aging.*
acute illness management in, 27
dementia management in, 27–28
diagnostic tests in, 27
function assessment in, 27
history-taking in, 26
influenza immunization in, 44
long-term care decisions in, 29–30
management problems in, 25–30
physical examination in, 26–27
support system assessment in, 27, 29–30
terminal illness care in, 30
German measles. See *Rubella.*
Germinoma, of pineal gland, 1247, 1275
Gerontology, 22
Giant aneurysm, 2103
Giant platelet syndrome, 1037
Giardia lambia, 1802
Giardiasis, 1802–1803
clinical manifestations of, 1802
diagnosis of, 1802–1803
epidemiology of, 1802
etiology of, 1802
immune response in, 1802
pathogenesis of, 1802
treatment of, 1803
Gigantism, cerebral, 1249
Gilbert's syndrome, 132, 807–808
Gilchrist's disease, 1762–1764
Gilles de la Tourette's syndrome, 2077
Gingiva, necrotizing infections of, 1585
Gingivitis, acute necrotizing ulcerative, 663–664, *664*
Gingivostomatitis
from herpes simplex virus, 1715
primary herpetic, 664–665, *665*
Gland(s)
meibomian, 2230
sebaceous, 2230
sweat, 2229–2232
Tyson's, 2230
ultimobranchial, 1451
Glanders, 1609
diagnosis of, 1609
epidemiology of, 1609
treatment of, 1609
Glanzmann's disease, 1037
Glasgow coma scale, *2172*
Glaucoma, 2033, 2217–2218
and headache, 2059
angle-closure, 2218
buphthalmos in, 2218
congenital, 2218
in diabetic retinopathy, 1338
open angle, 2217–2218
secondary, 2218
Glaucomatous optic atrophy, 2219
Glioblastoma multiforme, characteristics of, 2161, 2162t
Glioma(s)
in neurofibromatosis, 2085
of brainstem, 2164
Glioma(s) (*Continued*)
of optic nerve, 2164
Global aphasia, 1994
Globoid cell leukodystrophy, 2148
Globulin(s)
gamma, cerebrospinal fluid, in multiple sclerosis, 2144, 2146
in rubella, 1711
immune, rabies, 2134
serum, in acute viral hepatitis, 814
in liver disease, 810
Glomangioma, 362–363
Glomerular basement membrane antibody disease, 502, *502*
Glomerular capillary permeability, 508
Glomerular filtration rate, 492–493, 509–510, *509*
cyclooxygenase inhibition and, 1239
in chronic renal failure, 549–551, 554, 555, 556
in diabetic glomerulopathy, 616–618, *616*
in pregnancy, 624–625, *625*
uremia and, 489
Glomerular sclerosis, focal, 580–585, *581*
Glomerular syndromes, 485–486, 485t
Glomerulitis, cutaneous and renal manifestations of, *2264*
Glomerulonephritic syndrome, with toxic nephropathy, 595
Glomerulonephritis, 485
acute, 545, 569–578. See also specific diagnoses.
diffuse, 485–486
edema in, 570–571
group A streptococcal pharyngitis and, 1519, 1520, 1521, 1522, 1525, 1526
hematuria in, 569, 571
hypertension in, 570
mild, 485
primary renal diseases and, 570t, 571–585
proteinuria in, 569, 571
renal function impairment in, 569–570
anti-glomerular basement membrane antibody-mediated, 502
chronic, 588
complement activation-associated, 504
corticosteroids in, 577
immune response in, 575–577, *576*, 583–584
membranoproliferative, 583–584, *584*
plasma exchange therapy in, 576, 577
post-streptococcal, 571–573, *572*
rapidly progressive, 575–578, 575t, *576*
corticosteroids in, 577
idiopathic, 577
immune response in, 575–577, *576*
plasma exchange therapy in, 576, 577
Glomerulotubular balance, 517–518
Glomerulus(i), 490, *491*, 492
capillary wall of, 490
circulating immune complex-mediated disease of, 503–504, 503t
disorders of, 569–589. See also specific diagnoses.
immune response in, 568–569, *569*, 570t
injury in, 568–569
systemic disease and, 585–589
mesangium of, 490
permselectivity of capillary wall, 493
Glomus tumor, 362–363
Glossitis, 665–666, 724, 725
Glossopharyngeal neuralgia, 2059–2060
Glossopharyngeal zoster, 2128
Glove-stocking pattern of cutaneous sensory loss, 2199
Glucagon
in diabetes mellitus, 1323, 1332
in hypoglycemia, 1342

Glucagon test, in insulinoma, 1345
Glucagonoma, 1350
  islet cell tumor with, 1350
  treatment of, 1350
Glucocerebrosidase deficiency, 1117–1118
Glucocorticoid(s), 1302
  actions of, 1305–1306
  calcium metabolism and, 1306
  cardiovascular system effects of, 1306
  function assessment of, 1307–1309
  gastrointestinal effects of, 1306
  hematologic effects of, 1306
  hyperlipidemia with, 1115
  immunologic responses to, 1306
  in Addison's disease, 1312
  in cancer chemotherapy, 1101t
  in Cushing's syndrome, 1313–1314
  in hypopituitarism, 1257–1258
  inflammatory responses to, 1306
  interhormonal relationships and, 1306
  metabolism of, 1302, *1303*
    intermediary, 1305–1306, *1305*
  molecular mechanisms of action of, 1306
  nervous system effects of, 1306
  osteoporosis and, 1460
  production regulation of, 1303–1304
  stimulation test and, 1308–1309
  stress and, 1306
Glucocorticoid suppression test(s), 1308–1309
  in hyperparathyroidism, 1441
Glucocorticosteroids, 111–116, 112t
  biochemistry of, 112
  mechanisms of action of, 112–113
  pharmacology of, 112
Glucocorticosteroid receptors, 112
Glucocorticosteroid therapy
  agent selection in, 114
  alternate-day, 115
  burst or intermittent, 114
  clinical applications of, 112–113
  complications of, 116, 116t
  daily, 114–115
  dosage regimen in, 114–116
  local vs. systemic, 113–114
  regimen design in, 113–116
  side effects of, 114, 115
  synthetic agents for, 114
  vs. ACTH therapy, 115–116
  withdrawal syndromes and, 116
Gluconeogenesis, 1342
Glucose
  cerebrospinal fluid, in bacterial meningitis, 1553
  in coma, 1977
  reference values for, 2324, 2325
Glucose metabolism, atherosclerosis and, 282
Glucose therapy, in fluid volume depletion, 520
Glucose tolerance factor, 1210
Glucose tolerance test, in diabetes mellitus, 1320–1321
  in hypoglycemia, 1343–1344, *1344*
  reference values for, 2325
Glucose-galactose, malabsorption of, 732
Glucose-6-phosphatase deficiency, 1106
Glucose-6-phosphate dehydrogenase, genetic types of, 961
  in erythrocytes, reference values for, 2338
  variants of, 128, 131
    Hektoen, 128
Glucose-6-phosphate dehydrogenase deficiency, 82, 131, 905–906, 1103
  drug-induced hemolysis with, 905, 906
  genetic factor in, 905–960, 987
  hemolysis prevention in, 906
  hemolysis with, 905–906
  malaria and, 905–906
  race factor in, 905–906
Glucosylceramide, 1117
Glucosylceramide-β-D-glucosidase, in Gaucher's disease, 1118
Glucosylceramide lipidosis, 1117–1118
β-Glucuronidase deficiency, 1148–1149
Glue, inhalation abuse of, 2024
Glutamine, in cystinuria, 613
γ-Glutamyltransferase, serum, reference values for, 2325
Glutathione metabolism, *904*
Glutathione peroxidase deficiency, 907
Glutathione reductase deficiency, 907
Glutathione synthetase deficiency, 907
Glutathionine peroxidase, 1210
Gluten-free diet, 733, 734
Gluten-sensitive enteropathy, 732–734
Glybenclamide, 1329
D-Glyceric dehydrogenase deficiency, 1108
Glycerol, free, reference values for, 2325
Glycogen phosphorylase, 1225
Glycogen storage diseases, 1105–1107
  genetic factor in, 1106–1107
  gout with, 1139
  hepatic forms of, 1106
    treatment of, 1106
  liver disease and, 833
  muscular forms of, 1106–1107
    treatment of, 1107
  prenatal diagnosis of, 1107
Glycogen storage myopathies, 2204–2205
Glycogenolysis, 1342
Glycolytic pathways, in hemolytic anemia, 904–905, *904*
Glycoprotein hormones, 1253
Glycosaminoglycan storage
  consequences of, 1146
  etiology of, 1146
Glycosphingolipidosis, 1116–1117
Glycosuria
  familial renal, 614
  renal, 614, *614*
Gnathostoma spinigerum, 1822
Gnathostomiasis, 1822
Goeckerman treatment of psoriasis, 2246
Goiter
  adolescent, 1288
  congenital, 1298
  endemic, 1298, 1299
    epidemiology of, 1299
    etiology of, 1298, 1299
    iodine deficiency and, 1299
    pathology of, 1298
    treatment of, 1299
  multinodular, 1298–1299
    clinical manifestations of, 1298
    laboratory diagnosis of, 1298–1299
    thyroid cancer and, 1299
    treatment of, 1299
  sporadic, 1298–1299
    etiology of, 1298
    pathology of, 1298
Gold
  as nephrotoxin, 600
  serum and urinary, reference values for, 2325
Gold salts, 600
  in rheumatoid arthritis, 1916
  interstitial lung disease and, 418
Gompertz concept, 23–24, *24*
Gonad(s)
  bipotential, 1351, *1351*
  development error and, 1386–1387
  differentiation in, 1351–1353
  normal development of, 1351–1352
  radiobiology of, 2299
Gonadal dysgenesis, 1354–1356, 1386–1387
  chromosome abnormality in, 1386–1387
  management of, 1355, 1356
Gonadal dysgenesis (*Continued*)
  mixed, 1355–1356, 1387
  pathophysiology of, 1355
  pure, 1387
Gonadal irradiation, 2300
Gonadotrophs, 1252
Gonodotropin(s)
  in Leydig cell agenesis (dysgenesis), 1356
  plasma, 1367
  urinary, 1367
Gonadotropin releasing hormone, 1241, 1242
  analogues of, 1247
  and hypothalmic-pituitary-gonadal axis, 1245
  and prolactin-secreting tumors, 1263
  in anorexia nervosa, 1250
  in male pubertal development, 1368
  in menstrual cycle, 1382
  in testicular function, 1367
  in tests for luteinizing hormone and follicle stimulating hormone deficiencies, 1255
  secretion of, in hypothalamic hypogonadism, 1248–1249
Gonococcal conjunctivitis, 2220–2221
Gonococcal infection, 1644–1648
Gonococcal ophthalmia neonatorum, 2221
Gonococcal perihepatitis, 858
Gonococcal urethritis, 1645
Gonococcemia, 1646–1647, *2266*
  cutaneous lesions in, *2260*
Gonorrhea
  anorectal, 784
  antibiotic therapy in, 1646t, 1647–1648
    resistance to, 1647
  arthritis with, 1646, 1648, 1923
  bacteremia with, 1646–1647
  disseminated gonococcal infection and, 1646–1647
  epidemiology of, 1644
  homosexuality and, 1645
  host factor in, 1645
  in children, 1646
  in females, 1645
  in males, 1645
  laboratory diagnosis of, 1647
    culture in, 1647
    serology in, 1647
  pathogenesis of, 1644–1645
  pharyngeal, 1645, 1647
  prevention of, 1648
  prophylaxis for, 1648
  rectal, 1645
  treatment of, 1646t, 1647–1648
Goodpasture's syndrome, 415, 576, 595
Gorlin formula, 185
Gout, 132, 1132–1142, *2264*
  acute attack of, 1135–1136, 1140–1141
  arthritis with, 1132, 1136–1137, *1137*, *1138*, 1140, 1141
  classification of, 1132, 1132t
  clinical manifestations of, 1136–1139
  diagnosis of, 1140, *1140*
    differential, 1140
  dietary factor in, 1141
  epidemiology of, 1132–1133
  genetic factor in, 1132, 1133, 1139
  history of, 1132
  hyperuricemia and, 1132, 1132t, 1133t
  kidney in, 1136
  nephropathy with, 1138
  pathogenesis of, 1133–1136
  pathology of, 1133–1136
  secondary, 1139–1140
  tophaceous, 132
  tophi in, 1136, 1137–1138, 1140
  treatment of, 1140–1142
    allopurinol in, 1142
    colchicine in, 1140–1141

Gout (*Continued*)
treatment of, idomethacin in, 1141
oxyphenbutazone in, 1141
phenylbutazone in, 1141
probenecid in, 1141
sulfinpyrazone in, 1141
uric acid urolithiasis in, 1136, 1138–1139
with enzyme defects, 1139
with glycogen storage disease, 1139
with hypoxanthine-guanine phosphoribosyltransferase deficiency, 1139
with phosphoribosylpyrophosphate synthetase deficiency, 1139
Gowers' sign, in Duchenne dystrophy, 2202
Gradenigo's syndrome, 2115
Graft-versus-host disease
blood transfusion and, 940
with bone marrow transplantation, 1026, 1027
Gram-negative bacteremia, 1594–1595
antibodies with, 1595
management of, 1595
Grand mal seizure(s), 2153
postictal stage, and syncope, 1986
Granular cell myoblastomas, of lung, 446
Granulocyte(s)
development of, 940
in chronic myelogenous leukemia, 977
kinetics of, 942
marginated granulocyte pool and, 942
morphology of, 940–941
precursors of, 866, 894
Granulocyte transfusion, in acute myelogenous leukemia, 991
Granulocytopenia, in uremia, 552
Granuloma(s)
classification of, 438t
cutaneous, 2297
mycobacterial, 1633
in sarcoidosis, 433, *433*
in secondary syphilis, 1651
intracranial, 2162t
midline, 1945–1946
Granuloma inguinale, 1649–1650
Granulomatosis
Wegener's, 1943–1945, *2264*
vs. orbital pseudotumor, 2222
Granulomatous angiitis, 2129
Granulomatous disease(s), 1484
diagnosis of, 1482
fever with, 1470
hypercalcemia and, 1449
Granulomatous neuropathy, 2196
Granulomatous thyroiditis, 1291
Granulopoiesis, 942
Graves' disease, 1281–1287. See also *Hyperthyroidism.*
differential diagnosis of, 1284
etiology of, 1281
euthyroid, 1283
exophthalmopathy with, 1281, 1282, 1283, 1284, 1287
free T_4 index of, 1283–1284
histocompatibility antigens in, 1282, 1284
immune response in, 1280, 1281
in pregnancy, 1286
incidence of, 1281–1282
pathogenesis of, 1281
pathology of, 1282
physical examination in, 1283
prognosis in, 1287
radioactive iodine uptake test in, 1284
radioisotope scan in, 1284
serum T_3/T_4 ratio in, 1283–1284
$T_3(T_4)$ suppression test in, 1284
thyroid storm in, 1286–1287, 1286t
thyrotropin-releasing hormone infusion test in, 1284
Graves' disease (*Continued*)
treatment of, 1284–1287
antithyroid drugs in, 1284–1285, 1286
beta-adrenergic blocking agents in, 1285
lithium in, 1286
radioiodine in, 1285–1286
surgery in, 1285
Graves' orbitopathy, 2221
Gravity, specific, reference values for, 2333
Great arteries. See *Transposition of great arteries.*
Grey Turner's sign, *2263*
Grief, stages of, 2011
Griseofulvin, in fungal infections, 2247
Grönblad-Strandberg syndrome, 1152
Growth, hormone control in, 1228
Growth abnormality, with Crohn's disease, 744, 746–747
Growth and development, normal, 15–19
somatic changes in, 16–18, *16*
Growth hormone, 1253–1254
function tests of, 1255
hypothalamic disorders of secretion of, 1249
idiopathic deficiency of, 1249
in cancer, 1079
in hypopituitarism, 1256–1257, 1258
in pituitary tumor, 1261–1262
in protein-calorie malnutrition, 1185
serum or plasma, reference values for, 2325
Growth hormone releasing factor, 1241, 1242, 1245–1246, 1247, 1249, 1255
in cancer, 1079
in pituitary tumor, 1262
with islet cell tumor, 1351
Growth hormone stimulation tests, 2325
Growth hormone therapy, in hypopituitarism, 1258
Guillain-Barré syndrome, 44, 457, 1746, 2189, 2190–2192, 2200
vs. hysteria, 2014
vs. paralytic poliomyelitis, 2131
Guinea worm disease, 1828
Gumma(s)
neurologic changes in, 2118
syphilitic, 2120
late benign, 1654–1655
Gustation, disorders of, 2031–2032
Guthrie bacterial inhibition assay, 1127
Gutzeit test, in arsenic poisoning, 2311
Gynecologic infection, anaerobic, 1585
Gynecomastia, 1400–1401, *1400*
androgens in, 1400–1401
classification of, 1400, 1400t
estrogens in, 1400–1401
false, 1401

Hageman factor, 1048
Hailey-Hailey disease, 2268
Hair
aging and, 23
excessive growth of, 2231. See also *Hirsutism.*
growth pattern of, 2231
normal growth of, 1395
type of, 2231
Hairy cell leukemia. See *Leukemia—hairy cell.*
Haitians, acquired immunodeficiency syndrome in, 1862
Hallucinations
in metabolic brain disease, 1974
in schizophrenia, 2002
Hallucinogenic drugs, and anxiety, 2009
Halo nevus, 2255, 2257
Halogenated hydrocarbons, poisoning from, 89
Haloperidol
in Gilles de la Tourette's syndrome, 2077
in Sydenham's chorea, 2075
Halopyrimidines, 1089
Halothane, hepatotoxicity from, 823
Hamartoma
of hypothalamus, 1247
of lung, 446
Hamartoma-angiomyolipoma, 641
Ham's test, 912
Hands
dermatitis of, 2248–2249
in osteoarthritis, 1952–1953, *1952*
Hand-foot-and-mouth-disease, 1733
cutaneous lesions in, *2260*
Handgun control, 37
Hand-Schüller-Christian disease, 1248
Handwashing, hospital-acquired infection and, 1491
Hangovers, 52
headache in, 2056
Hansen's disease, 1634–1639. See also *Leprosy.*
Hantaan virus, 1757
Haptocorrin, 896
Haptoglobin, reference values for, 2338
Hardy-Weinberg equation, 121–122
Hartmanella, 1801
Hartnup disease, 611, 732, 1201, *2263, 2264*
genetic factor in, 611
photosensitivity in, 2253
Hashimoto's thyroiditis, 1287, 1293–1294
immune response in, 1280, 1293
laboratory diagnosis of, 1293–1294
Hashish, abuse of, 2022–2023
Haverhill fever, 1665
Hawaii-like viral agents, 1734, 1735
HBV particle, 816
Head
injuries to, 2170–2175
and anxiety, 2009
transport in, 2172
skin diseases of, 2242–2243
trauma to, and epilepsy, 2150
Headache(s), 2054–2060, *2054*. See also under various types.
exertional, 2056
computed tomography in, 2060
in intracranial tumor, 2162
occipital, in central vertigo, 2042
tension, from skeletal muscle contraction, 2064
traction, 2057
vascular, 2054–2056
with vertebral-basilar ischemia, *2097*, 2098
Willis', 2098
Health Systems Agency, 8
Hearing
aging and, 23
disorders of, 2037–2040
Hearing loss
and vertigo, 2042
noise-induced, 2278
Heart
afterload performance of, 159–160
in shock, 212, *213*, 214, 223
aging and, 22
biopsy of, 186
conduction system of, anatomy of, 301
contractility of, 160
in shock, 212–214
energetics of, 194
functional assessment of, nuclear imaging in, 179–181, *179, 180*
functional anatomy of, 158–159
in altered consciousness, 1976
in cardiorespiratory arrest, 480–481
in Friedreich's ataxia, 2083
in sarcoidosis, 435–436

Heart (*Continued*)
  intracardiac recordings in, 301–304, *302, 303*
  irradiation of, *2302*
  left, output of, and syncope, *1984*, 1985
  malposition of, 239–240
  performance of, 159–160
    assessment of, 191–193, 191t, *192*
  preload performance of, 159–160
    in shock, 212, *213*, 223
  pressures and volumes of, 160, 160t
  radiography of, 152–153, 164–169, *165–169*
  radiology of, 2299
  right, and aortic root, communication shunts between, 232–233
    filling of, and syncope, 1983–1985, *1984*
  rupture of, with myocardial infarction, 292
  size of, 164, 168, *165*
  transplantation of, 210
  tumor of, 366–367
Heart block
  as late cardiac surgery complication, 242
  congenital complete, 240–241
  with myocardial infarction, 292
Heart disease
  and cerebral blood flow reduction, 2092
  angiography in, 186
  brain abscess with, 2112
  cardiac catheterization in, 183–188
  cardiac enlargement in, 164, *165*, 168
  congenital. See *Congenital heart disease*.
  coronary. See names of specific disorders.
  echocardiography in, 175–179, *175–179*
  electrocardiography in, 169–175
  fluoroscopy in, *168*, 169, *169*
  nuclear imaging in, 179–182
  pulmonary hypertension and, 258
  radiography in, 164–169, *165–169*. See also specific diagnoses.
  rheumatic, epidemiology of, 155
  syphilitic, 1655
  valvular, 242–256, *245*. See also under names of specific valves.
Heart failure, 163–164, 189–210. See also *Left ventricular failure; Right ventricular failure.*
  afterload factor in, 192
    reduction of, 205–207, 205t, 206t
  autonomic nervous system in, 194–195
  biochemical basis for, 194
  blood pressure in, 194–195
  blood volume and, 163
  cardiac dilatation in, 193, *193*
  cardiac output in, 191, 194–195
  cardiac output–cardiac load relation in management of, 199
  cardiopulmonary system effects of, 194–195
  cardiovascular system effects of, 163–164
  categories of, 189–190
  chronic compensatory mechanisms in, 193–194
  circulation time and, 194
  clinical manifestations of, 195–199
  congestive, 189
  contractility factor in, 192–193
    intrinsic, 192–193
  digitalis therapy in, 200
  diuresis in, 163–164
  drug interactions in, 200
  ejection factor in, 193
  Frank-Starling mechanism and, 192
  hemodynamics of, 191–193
  hypertrophy factor in, 193–194
  hyponatremia in, 527
  in infective endocarditis, 1536
  initiating mechanisms of, 189
  muscle performance in, 194
Heart failure (*Continued*)
  pathophysiologic interplay in, 190–195
  performance assessment in, 191–193, 191t, *192*
  peripheral vasoconstriction in, 195
  positive pressure breathing in, 200
  preload factor in, 192
  pressure overload in, 189
  pulmonary edema in, management of, 199–200
  radiography in, *168*, 169
  refractory edema in, 210
  relaxation and distensibility in, 194
  respiratory failure with, 461
  salt intake in, 163, 164
  stress response and, 163
  stress testing in, 195
  subcellular bases for contraction in, 190
  systolic time intervals in, 193
  tachycardia in, 194–195
  Valsalva maneuver in, 195
  venous hypertension and, 194
  ventricular end-diastolic pressure in, 191–192
  volume overload in, 189
  with aortic stenosis, 252
Heart failure management
  acetazolamide in, 209
  aldosterone antagonists in, 209
  amiloride in, 209
  amrinone therapy in, 204
  bumetanide in, 209
  captopril therapy in, 206
  carbonic anhydrase inhibitors in, 209
  catecholamines in, 201
  clinical, 199–210
  digitalis therapy in, 200. See also *Digitalis therapy*.
  direct current cardioversion for, 200, 210
  diuretics in, 194–200, 207–210
    agents for, 207–209, 208t
    administration patterns for, 208t
    combined therapy with, 209–210
    complications of, 210
  drug therapy for, 199–210
  ethacrynic acid in, 208–209
  furosemide in, 208–209
  hydralazine therapy in, 207
  nitrates in, 207
  nitroglycerin therapy in, 206
  nitroprusside therapy in, 205–206
  oxygen therapy in, 199
  phentolamine therapy in, 206
  phlebotomy in, 200
  prazosin therapy in, 207
  sedatives in, 199–200
  spironolactone in, 209
  surgical therapy in, 210
    cardiac transplantation, 210
  thiazides in, 207–208
  triamterene in, 209
  trimazosin therapy in, 207
  vasodilator therapy in, 205–207, *205*
    agent choice for, 205–207, 206t
    principles of, 205
Heart muscle, performance of, 194
Heart rate, 160, 161
  in heart failure, 193
  in shock, 212
Heart sounds, 152, 196
Heart valve, cardiac catheterization study of, 184–185, *184*
Heartburn, 667–668
  in gastroesophageal reflux disease, 668
Heat
  disorders due to, 2304–2306
Heat (*Continued*)
  local, in back pain, 2063
  prickly, 2229
    in myofascial pain syndrome, 2064
Heat cramps, 2305
Heat exhaustion, 2305
Heat stress, disorders related to, 2306
Heatstroke, 2305
Heavy chain diseases, 1020–1021
Heberden's nodes, 1952–1953, *1952*
Height, during puberty, 17
Heinz bodies, 905, 906
Heinz body anemia, 1023
Heinz body hemolytic disease, 932–933
Helminths, biology of, 1775
Helminthiasis(es), 1804
Helminthic disease, 1804–1833
  diagnosis of, 1775–1776
  epidemiology of, 1775
  host factor in, 1775
  occupational, 2297
  of intestine, 737
Hemangioblastomas, of cerebellar hemispheres, in Hippel-Lindau disease, 2086
Hemangioma
  capillary, in Sturge-Weber disease, 2085
  cavernous, 1035
  of liver, 849
  strawberry, multiple, *2265*
Hemarthrosis(es), 1030, 1958
Hematemesis, 668, 791, 792
  with acute gastritis, 677, 678
  with peptic ulcer, 694
Hematin, 1156–1157, *1157*
Hematochezia, 791, 792
Hematocrit
  age factor and, 871
  altitude and, 871
  in anemia, 871, 872
  normal values, 871t
  plasma volume alterations and, 871
  reference values for, 2338
  sex factor and, 871
Hematologic component, disorders with, cutaneous lesions in, *2265*
Hematologic diseases, 866–1058. See also specific diagnoses.
  retinopathy of, 2224
Hematologic values, of clinical importance, 2337–2340
Hematology
  aging and, 23
  diagnostic, 866
  of uremia, 552
  red blood cell values in, 871, 871t
Hematoma(s). See under specific types.
Hematomyelia, 2187
Hematopoiesis
  colony-stimulating activity and, 869
  kinetics of, 870
  progenitor cell therapy and, 869
  progenitors of, 867–869
    marrow failure and, 869
    maturation of, 867–868, *869*
    regulation of, 868–869
Hematuria, 484, 509
  in acute glomerulonephritis, 569, 571
Heme, 886
  biosynthesis of, 887, 888, 1153, *1154*, 1155–1156, 1155t
  in hemoglobin synthesis, 919–920
Hemiballism, 2075
Hemicrania, chronic paroxysmal, 2056
Hemiparesis, 2045
Hemiplegia, in postencephalitic parkinsonism, 2071

Hemiplegic migraine, 2055, 2098
Hemispherectomy, in epilepsy, 2159
Hemispheric abscess, 2113
Hemlock, 783
Hemobilia, 862–863
Hemochromatosis, 132, 1160–1163, *2263*
  alcohol intake and, 1161, 1162
  clinical manifestations of, 1161–1162
  diagnosis of, 1162
    differential, 1162
    epidemiology of, 1161
    genetic factor in, 832–833, 1160–1161, *1161*
  hepatomegaly with, 1161–1162
  HLA locus in, 1160–1163
  idiopathic, 1160
  in thalassemia major, 921, 922
  iron metabolism in, 1160–1163
  liver biopsy in, 1162
  liver disease and, 832–833
  pathogenesis of, 1161
  pathology of, 1161
  phlebotomy for, 1162–1163, *1163*
  prevention of, 1162
  prognosis in, 1163
  screening for, 1161, 1162
  secondary, 1163
  treatment of, 1162–1163, *1163*
  with arthritis, 1957
Hemodialysis, 559. See also *Dialysis.*
  clinical use of, 560–561
  in drug poisoning, 1980
  neutrophil adhesiveness and, 950
  routine management of, 561
  technical aspects of, 559, *560*
  time-averaged clearance with, 560, 560t
  trace element toxicity with, 2311–2315
Hemodynamic factors, and stroke, *2095*, 2096
Hemodynamic monitoring
  complications of, 477–478
  in critical care management, 473–474, 475t
Hemoglobin(s)
  adult (A), 915, 920, 921, 922, 923
  chromatin structure of, 918
  chromosomal arrangement of, 915, *916*
  drug toxicity and, 934, 935t
  fetal (F), 915, 920, 921, 922, 923
    hereditary persistency of, 925
    with mutations, 925–926
  function of, 917–918
  gene structure of, 918, *919*
  globin mRNA metabolism, 918
  globin mRNA structure, 918
  glycosylation of, 1326, *1326*
  heme prosthetic groups, 917
  M hemoglobins, 935, 935t
  normal values, 871t
  nucleotide sequences, 915
  oxygen binding, 917–918, *917*
  polypeptide chains, 915, *915*, 916–917, *916*
  protein synthesis and, 918–919
  reference values for, 2338
  structure of, 915–917, *915, 916*
  synthesis of, 915–917, 918–920, *919, 920*
    erythroblastosis and, 920, *920*
    iron accumulation and, 919–920
    selective gene expression and, 920
  unstable, 932–933, 932t
  with altered oxygen affinity, 933–934
Hemoglobin A_{1c}, blood, reference values for, 2326
Hemoglobin C disease, homozygous, 932
Hemoglobin electrophoresis
  in sickle cell syndromes, 930–931, *930*
  reference values for, 2338
Hemoglobin F, reference values for, 2338
Hemoglobin Gun Hill, 932
Hemoglobin H, reference values for, 2338
Hemoglobin H disease, 923
  genetic factor in, 923
Hemoglobin Kansas, 933
Hemoglobin Kempsey, 933
Hemoglobin M Hyde Park, 935
Hemoglobin SC disease, 930
Hemoglobinopathy(ies), 128
  mutation detection in, 137
  sickling, retinopathy of, 2224
  thalassemic, 924–925
  with arthritis, 1957
Hemoglobinuria
  march, 913
  paroxysmal cold, 911, *2265*
  paroxysmal nocturnal, 911–912
Hemolysis
  alloantibodies and, 908
  amphotericin-induced, 913
  antibodies in, 908
  bone marrow response with, 901
  cardiovascular abnormalities and, 913–914
  chemical-induced, 912–913
  chloramine-induced, 912
  cold agglutinins and, 910–911
  complement in, 908
  consequences of, 900–901
  Coombs' test in, 908
  copper-induced, 912
  diagnosis of, 901
  drug-induced, 907, 911
  extravascular destruction of, 900
  immune, 908
  indirect antiglobulin test in, 908
  innocent bystander, 911
  intracorpuscular abnormalities with, 902–907
  intravascular, 900
    in spider bites, 1837
  metabolic factor in, 913
  microcirculation disorders and, 914–915, 914t
  pathophysiology of, 900
  red cell parasites and, 913
  red cell trauma and, 913–915
  vascular lesions and, 914
  with bakesiosis, 913
  with bartonellosis, 913
  with blood transfusion, 938
  with malaria, 913
  without complement activation, 908
Hemolysis hypersplenism, sequestrational, 907–908
Hemolytic anemia(s), 873
  acquired, 907–915
    vs. congenital, 902
  autoimmunity in, 908–911
  classification of, 900, 900t
  cross-transfusion studies in, 902
  Embden-Meyerhof pathway in, 904–905, *904*
  environmental factor in, 902, 907–915
  enzyme deficiencies in, 904–907
  erythrocyte membrane abnormalities in, 902–904
  erythrocyte oxidative stress and, 907
  genetic factor in, 902–907
  glycolytic pathways in, 904–905, *904*
  hereditary elliptocytosis, 904
  hereditary spherocytosis, 902–904
  hereditary stomatocytosis, 904
  hexose monophosphate shunt pathway in, 905–907
  immune response in, 908–911
  primaquine and, 905, 906
  spur cell, 913
  treatment of, 901
Hemolytic disease, Heinz body, 932–933
Hemolytic disorders, 900–915
  clinical findings in, 901
  differential diagnosis of, 901
  laboratory findings in, 901
  red cell morphology in, 901, 901t
Hemolytic-uremic syndrome, 587–588, 1035–1036
Hemoperfusion, in poisoning, 87
Hemophilia, 131, 132, 1045–1047
  acquired immunodeficiency syndrome and, 1862
  carrier detection in, 1047
  chromosome abnormality in, 1045–1046
  clinical manifestations of, 1046
  diagnosis of, 1046
  factor VIII deficiency in, 1045–1047
  factor VIII therapy in, 1046–1047
  genetic factor in, 1030, 1045–1046
  prognosis in, 1047
  treatment of, 1046–1047
Hemophilia B, 1049
Hemophilus species, microbiology of, 1563, 1563t
Hemophilus aphrophilus infection, 1566
Hemophilus ducreyi, 1650
Hemophilus infection, 1563–1566
  diagnosis of, 1565
  prevention of, 1565
  resistance in, 1565
  treatment of, 1565
Hemophilus influenzae, 1551
Hemophilus influenzae infection, 1563–1566
  clinical manifestations of, 1564–1565
  epidemiology of, 1563
  immune response in, 1563–1564
  pathogenesis of, 1563
Hemophilus parainfluenzae infection, 1565–1566
Hemophilus vaginalis, 1566
Hemoptysis, 369–370
  diagnostic approach to, 369–370
  in left ventricular failure, 196
Hemorrhage. See also specific sites.
  anemia with, 883–884
  cerebral, hypertension with, 271
  clinical manifestations of, 883–884, 883t
  diagnosis of, 883–884
    fluid therapy in, 884
  hypertensive, differential diagnosis of, 2109–2110
  intestinal, intramural, 760
  intracranial. See *Intracranial hemorrhage*
  leukocytes with, 883–884
  of thalamic–internal capsule, 2108
  platelet count with, 883–884
  reticulocytosis with, 883
  splinter, in infective endocarditis, 1536t
  thalamic, 2109
  treatment of, 884
    albumin therapy in, 884
    dextran therapy in, 884
Hemorrhagic diathesis, in uremia, 552
Hemorrhagic disorders, 1028–1040
  diagnosis of, 1030, 1030t
  genetic factor in, 1030
Hemorrhagic fever, 1750–1758
  African, 1757
  arbovirus infection and, 1736
  arenavirus diseases as, 1756–1757
  Crimean, 1755–1756
  epidemiology of, 1750, 1751t
  from dengue viruses, 1754–1755
  tick-borne flavivirus diseases as, 1755
  vectors in, 1750, 1751t
  viruses in, 1750, 1751t
  with renal syndrome, 1757–1758
  yellow fever as, 1750, *1750*, 1752–1754

Hemorrhagic leukoencephalitis, acute, 2140–2141
Hemorrhagic retinopathy, 2225
Hemorrhoids, 785
  lower gastrointestinal hemorrhage and, 794
Hemosiderin, 888
Hemosiderosis, 1161
  in thalassemia major, 921
Hemostasis, 1028
  laboratory evaluation of, 1030–1031
  screening tests for, 1030, 1031t
Hemothorax, with pleural disease, 449
Henderson-Hasselbalch equation, 465, 536
Henoch-Schönlein purpura, 595, 1038–1039, 1939, 1958–1959, *2262, 2264, 2266*
  glomerular involvement in, 587
Heparan sulfate, 1148
Heparin, 1057
  in disseminated intravascular coagulation, 1055
  in pulmonary embolism, 430–431
  in thrombophlebitis, 364–365
Hepatic alcohol dehydrogenase, 51
Hepatic disease(s). See *Liver Disease.*
Hepatic encephalopathy, 845–848
  ammonia in, 845
  aromatic amino acids in, 845
  blood-brain barrier in, 845–846
  chronic liver disease with, 847–848
  diagnosis of, 846
  fulminant hepatic failure with, 847
  gamma-aminobutyric acid in, 845
  mercaptans in, 845
  neurologic manifestations of, 846, 846t
  neurotransmitters in, 845
  pathogenesis of, 845–846
  precipitating factors in, 846, 846t
  protein intake in, 846
  stages of, 846t
  treatment of, 846–847
    lactulose therapy in, 846
    neomycin in, 846–847
Hepatic enzymes, in drug interaction, 80, 81
Hepatic failure, antimicrobial therapy and, 101t, 102
Hepatitis
  acute viral, 813–820. See also *Hepatitis A; Hepatitis B; Hepatitis non-A non-B.*
    alkaline phosphatase in, 814
    bilirubin in, 814
    cholestatic hepatitis syndrome with, 814
    clinical findings in, 813–814
    complications in, 814
    diagnosis of, 818
      differential, 818
    etiology of, 813, 813t
    evolving to chronic hepatitis, 814
    extrahepatic manifestations of, 814
    hematology in, 814
    hypoglycemia in, 814
    in heroin addiction, 2018
    laboratory findings in, 813–814
    liver biopsy in, 818
    management of, 818–819
    massive hepatic necrosis with, 814
    pathology of, 813
    prevention of, 819
    prothrombin time in, 814
    serodiagnosis of, 814, 815, *815t*, 818
    serum albumin in, 814
    serum globulins in, 814
    transaminases in, 814
  and disorders of taste, 2032
  aplastic anemia and, 878
  blood transfusion and, 939, 939t
  chronic, 824–827
    active, 825–826
Hepatitis (*Continued*)
  chronic, active, azathioprine in, 826
      corticosteroids in, 826
      diagnosis of, 826
      drug-induced, 825
      extrahepatic manifestations of, 825
      liver biopsy in, 826
      prednisone in, 826
      serology of, 825–826
      treatment of, 826
    diagnosis of, 824, 825
    etiology of, 824, 824t
    lobular, 825
    management of, 825
    pathology of, 824
    persistent, 824–825
    transaminases in, 825, 826–827
  depression in, 2011
  immunization for, 46
  post-transfusion, 817–818
  with alcoholic liver disease, 836–837
Hepatitis A, 815
  epidemiology of, 815
  etiology of, 813, 813t
  immune serum globulin for, 819
  in hospital-acquired infection, 1492
  passive immunization to, 43t
  prevention of, 819
  serodiagnosis of, 815, 815t
Hepatitis A antibodies, 815
Hepatitis A virus, 815
Hepatitis B, 816–817, *817*
  chronic active, 825
  cryptogenic cirrhosis and, 839–840
  delta (δ)-agent infection with, 817
  dialysis with, 561
  epidemiology of, 816
  etiology of, 813, 813t
  hepatocellular carcinoma and, 850
  immune serum globulin for, 819–820
  in hospital-acquired infection, 1492
  passive immunization to, 43t
  prevention of, 819–820
  serodiagnosis of, 815t, 816, *816*, 817, *817*
Hepatitis B surface antigen, 46, 816, *817*, 827
Hepatitis B vaccine, 42t, 820
Hepatitis B virus, 816, *816*
Hepatitis non-A non-B, 817–818
  epidemiology of, 818
  etiology of, 813, 813t
  in hospital-acquired infection, 1492
  prevention of, 820
  serodiagnosis of, 817–818
Hepatocellular adenoma, 849
Hepatocellular carcinoma, 849–850, 850t
  aflatoxins and, 850
  alpha-fetoprotein in, 850, 851
  cirrhosis and, 850
  epidemiology of, 849–850
  hepatitis B and, 850
Hepatolenticular degeneration. See *Wilson's disease.*
Hepatomegaly, with hemochromatosis, 1161–1162
Hepatorenal syndrome, 844–845
Hepatosplenic bilharziasis, 1813–1814
Hepatosplenomegaly, in Niemann-Pick disease, 1119, 1120
Herbicides, poisoning from, 89
Hereditary elliptocytosis, 904
  genetic factor in, 904
Hereditary hemorrhagic telangiectasia See *Rendu-Osler-Weber syndrome.*
Hereditary multiple exostoses, 1466
Hereditary pyropoikilocytosis, 904
Hereditary spherocytosis, 902–904
  aplastic crises in, 902
Hereditary spherocytosis (*Continued*)
  blood smears in, 902, 903
  clinical manifestations of, 902, 902t
  diagnosis of, 903
  erythrocyte membrane abnormalities in, 902, 903, *903*
  genetic factor in, 902, 903
  laboratory abnormalities in, 902t
  pathogenesis of, 903
  splenectomy in, 903
  test for autohemolysis in, 903
  treatment of, 903–904
Hereditary stomatocytosis, 904
  genetic factor in, 904
Heredity
  and manic-depressive psychosis, 2006
  and schizophrenia, 2003
Heredofamilial neuromyopathic diseases, 332–333
Heritable disease. See *Inborn errors of metabolism.*
Hermansky-Pudlak syndrome, *2258*
Hermaphroditism
  chromosome abnormality in, 1363
  genetic factor in, 1363
  true, 1363, 1387
Herner's syndrome, 2035
Herniated disc syndrome, 1953, 2182–2184
Heroin, abuse of, 2016–2019
    myoglobinuria in, 2210
    pulmonary complications in, 2018
Heroin nephropathy, 582
Herpangina, 1732–1733
Herpes. See also specific diagnoses.
  oral, 664–665
Herpes gestationis, 2269
Herpes labialis, 664, 1716
Herpes ophthalmicus, 2128, 2129
Herpes simplex, involving mouth, 2244
Herpes simplex encephalitis, 2126–2128
  clinical manifestations of, 2126
  diagnosis of, 2126–2127
    cerebral biopsy in, 2127
    electroencephalogram in, 2127
  epidemiology of, 2126
  etiology of, 2126
  pathogenesis of, 2126
  pathology of, 2126
  prognosis of, 2127
  treatment of, 2127
    computed tomography in, 2127
Herpes simplex virus infection, 1714–1717
  chemotherapy in, 1717
  clinical manifestations of, 1715–1716
  congenital, 1716
  culture in, 1717
  diagnosis of, 1716–1717
  encephalitis from, 1716
  epidemiology of, 1714–1715
  homosexuality and, 1715
  host factor in, 1716
  in neonates, 1716
  meningitis from, 1716
  pathogenesis of, 1715
  pathology of, 1715
  prevention of, 1717
  primary, 1715–1716
  recurrence of, 1715, 1716
  serology in, 1717
  transmission of, 1714–1715
  treatment of, 1717
  with cervical cancer, 1716
  with erythema multiforme, 1716
Herpes simplex viruses, 2126
  morphology of, 1714
  proctitis from, 784
  thymidine kinase gene of, 134

Herpes simplex viruses (*Continued*)
types of, 1714, 1714t
vs. varicella-zoster virus, 2128, 2129
Herpes zoster, 1721, 1723–1724, 2128–2130, 2196
and ear pain, 2058
and neuralgia, 2060, 2064
and vertigo, 2043
clinical manifestations in, 1723–1724
cranial, 2128
culture in, 1724
diagnosis of, 1724
epidemiology of, 1723
etiology of, 1721
host factor in, 1723, 1724
ophthalmic, 2128, 2129
pain in, 2050
passive immunization to, 43t
pathogenesis of, 1723
pathology of, 1723
serology in, 1724
treatment of, 1724
Herpesvirus(es)
in acute central nervous system infections, *2122*, 2123
reactivation of, immunosuppression and, 2141
Herpesvirus hominis keratitis, 2221
Herpesvirus infections, 2125
chemotherapy for, 108–110
in hospital-acquired infection, 1492
Heterophile agglutinins of Paul-Bunnell-Davidson, 1720
Heterophyes heterophyes, 1818
Hexamethylmelamine, 1099, *1099*
Hexokinase deficiency, 905
Hexose monophosphate shunt pathway, in hemolytic anemia, 905–907
Hiatal hernia, in gastroesophageal reflux disease, 668
Hiccup, 453
Hidradenitis suppurativa, 2230
High blood pressure. See *Hypertension.*
High density protein–cholesterol, serum or plasma, reference values for, 2325
High molecular weight kininogen deficiency, 1048–1049
High-performance liquid chromatography, 1232
Hind-brain ischemia, 2098
Hippel-Lindau disease, 2086
Hirschsprung's disease, 145, 711–712
Hirsutism, 1395–1398, 2231–2232
androgen-dependent, 1395–1397, 1396t
androgen-independent, 1395, 1396t
11-deoxycortisol in, 1397
diagnosis of, 1397
17-hydroxyprogesterone in, 1396, 1397
idiopathic, 1395, 1397
prognosis in, 1397
testosterone in, 1395–1397
treatment of, 1397
Hirudiniasis, 1841
His bundle, 301
His bundle recording, 301–304, *302, 303*
Histamine, 1243–1244
gastric secretion and, 682, 683
in allergy, 390
in rheumatic disease, 1900
in shock, 214
Histamine (H_2) receptor antagonists, in peptic ulcer, 688, 697
in Zollinger-Ellison syndrome, 697
Histidase deficiency, 1129
Histidinemia, 1129
genetic factor in, 1129
Histidinuria, 611
Histiocytes, 1009
Histiocytic lymphoma, 995, 996
chemotherapy for, 998
Histiocytic neoplasms, 992–993, 992t, 993t
Histiocytosis X, 414–415, 1248
Histocompatibility antigen(s). See also *HLA system; Histocompatibility complex, major.*
in diabetes mellitus, 1322–1323, 1325
in Graves' disease, 1282, 1284
Histocompatibility complex, major, 1847
Histocompatibility restriction, 1849, *1850*
Histoplasma capsulatum, 1759, 1760
Histoplasmosis, 1759–1761
clinical manifestations of, 1760
chronic pulmonary, 1760
culture in, 1760
diagnosis of, 1760
serology in, 1760
skin test in, 1760
disseminated, 1760
epidemiology of, 1759
etiology of, 1759
immune response in, 1759, 1760
ocular, 1760
pathogenesis of, 1759–1760
pathology of, 1759–1760
prevention of, 1761
primary, 1760
prognosis in, 1761
reinfection in, 1760
treatment of, 1760–1761
antifungal therapy in, 1761
History, in geriatrics, 26
Histotopes, 1849
Histrionic personality, 2013
Hitzig zones, in tabes dorsalis, 2120
HLA. See *Human leukocytic antigen.*
Hodgkin's disease, 1000–1009
bone involvement with, 1003
clinical manifestations of, 1002
diagnostic evaluation of, 1004–1006
bone marrow biopsy in, 1005
computed tomography in, 1004–1005
lymphangiography in, 1005, *1005*
radiography in, 1004–1005, *1004, 1005*
epidemiology of, 1001
etiology of, 1000–1001
hepatic involvement with, 1003
histopathologic classification of, 1001–1002, 1002t
immune response in, 1000–1001, 1003
immunologic abnormalities with, 1003
infectious complications of, 1003
lymphadenopathy in, 1002, *1004*
mode of spread of, 1006
of lung, 444–445
pathogenesis of, 1000–1001
pathology of, 1001–1002
prognosis in, 1008
pulmonary involvement with, 1002
Reed-Sternberg cell in, 1000, 1001, *1001*
spinal cord compression with, 1003
staging in, laparoscopy for 660
laparotomy for, 1005–1006
system for, 1003–1004, 1003t
stomach involvement in, 700–701
superior vena caval obstruction with, 1002–1003
theories of
contiguity, 1006
susceptibility, 1006
treatment of, 1006–1008, 1008t
chemotherapy for, 1006–1007, 1008t
Hodgkin's disease (*Continued*)
treatment of, combined modality therapy for, 1007–1008, 1008t
radiation therapy for, 1006, 1007, 1008t
Hoesch test, 1156
Homeostasis, hormone control factor in, 1228
Homicide(s), 37
in narcotic-related deaths, 2018
Homocystinuria, 132, 347, 1131–1132, 1458
ectopia lentis in, 1131
genetic factor in, 1131
methionine, 1131
thromboembolism in, 1131
Homogentisic acid oxidase deficiency, 1128
Homosexual(s)
male, acquired immunodeficiency syndrome and, 1862, 1863
gonorrhea and, 1645
herpes simplex virus infection and, 1715
infectious proctitis in, 784
Kaposi's sarcoma in, 2273
shigellosis and, 1596
syphilis and, 1652
Homosexuality
in sexual development, 19
sexually transmitted disease and, 1639–1640
Homovanillic acid, urinary, reference values for, 2326
Homozygous Hb C disease, 932
"Honeymoon cystitis," 621
Hookworm disease, 1820–1821
clinical manifestations of, 1821
complications of, 1821
diagnosis of, 1821
epidemiology of, 1821
pathology of, 1821
prevention of, 1821
treatment of, 1821
Horder's spots, 1671
Hormone(s), 1219–1220. See also specific products.
agonists of, 1224
antagonists of, 1224
autoimmune response and, 1231
biosynthetic defects and, 1231
central nervous system effects on, 1222
chemical assays of, 1232
competitive protein-binding, 1232
deficiency syndromes, 1229–1230
dynamic testing of, 1233
excess syndromes, 1230–1231
free, 1222–1223
levels of, 1232
high-performance liquid chromatography and, 1232
hyporesponsiveness to, 1230
in cancer therapy, 1100, 1101t
in direct action indices, 1233
in intermediary metabolism control, 1228–1229
influences of extracellular substances on, 1222
integrated responses to, 1228–1229
measurement of, interpretation of, 1232–1233
metabolism of, 1223
physiologic response influences on, 1222
plasma binding of, 1222–1223
production rates of, 1232
production regulation of, 1221–1222, *1221*
radioimmunoassay and, 1231–1232
radioreceptor assays and, 1232
receptor abnormalities, 1230
release of, 1221
releasing hormones, 1222

Hormone(s) (*Continued*)
releasing hormones, action of, mechanisms of, 1223–1229
rapidity of, 1229
"second messenger" concept, and, 1226
selective sampling of, 1232
storage of, 1221
synthesis of, 1220–1221, *1220*
target cell for, 1219
sensitivity evaluation of, 1233
target organ of, insensitivity of, 1230
tissue hypersensitivity to, 1230–1231
transport of, 1222–1223
tumor production of, 1230
Hormone agonists, 1224
Hormone antagonists, 1224
Hormone receptors, 1223–1224. See also specific hormone classes.
internalization of, 1226–1227, *1227*
"spare," 1224
Horner's syndrome, 451
Horseshoe kidney, 638
Hospice, 30t
Hospital care, 7
Hospital-acquired infection, 1485–1492
anatomic sites of, 1485, 1485t
aspiration pneumonia as, 1514, 1515
cesarean section and, 1490
control of, disinfection in, 1491
employee health and, 1491–1492
handwashing and, 1491
infection control committee for, 1490
isolation procedures in, 1490, 1490t
sterilization in, 1491
surveillance data for, 1486–1487, 1486t
dialysis and, 1486
endocarditis as, 1538
epidemiology of, 1485–1486
high risk locations for, 1486
in critical care areas, 1486
inanimate environment in, 1490–1491
meningitis in, 1490
meningococcal, 1492
of bloodstream, 1488–1489
pneumonia and, 1487–1488, 1511–1513
postoperative, 1489–1490
prosthesis and, 1490
tuberculosis and, 1491–1492
urinary tract in, 1487
Hospitalization
protein-calorie malnutrition and, 1183, 1184, 1187, 1187t
septic shock and, 1473–1474, 1476
Host factor
defense systems and, 1477–1478, 1477t
defects in, 1477–1485, 1480t–1481t, 1482t
pathology of, 1478
in cytomegalovirus infection, 1718, 1719
in gonorrhea, 1645
in helminthic disease, 1775
in herpes simplex virus infection, 1716
in herpes zoster, 1723, 1724
in immune complex disease, 1876
in infectious disease, 1477–1485
in leishmaniasis, 1787
in malaria, 1777
in mumps, 1713
in protozoan disease, 1775
in rickettsial disease, 1672
in staphylococcal infection, 1544–1545
in syphilis, 1651–1652
in varicella, 1722, 1723
Host-parasite alterations, neurologic disorders with, 2138–2143
"Hot dog headache," 782
Howell-Jolly bodies, 1024
Human chorionic gondotropin, 1076
in male sexuality, 1366, 1369
Human leukocyte antigen
disease susceptibility and, 1881–1883, 1882t
in renal cell carcinoma, 641
Human leukocyte antigen system, 121, 1880–1883. See also *Major histocompatibility complex.*
autoimmune disease and, 1882–1883
population genetics and, 1881
Human placental lactogen, 1076
Human T cell leukemia/lymphoma virus, 987, 994, 1861–1862
Human T cell leukemia virus, 987, 993, 1071
Humanism, in art of medicine, 6, 57
Humidification, 458
Humidifier fever, 2285
Hunter's syndrome, 332, 347
genetic factor in, 1148
Huntington's disease, 2001, 2074–2075
behavior in, 2074
vs. striatonigral degeneration, 2079
vs. tardive dyskinesia, 2076, *2076*
Hurler's syndrome, 131, 332, 347, 1146–1148
Hurler-Scheie compound, 1148
Huxley hypothesis, 190
Hydatid disease. See *Echinococcosis.*
Hydatidiform mole, 1287
Hydralazine
in heart failure, 207
in hypertension, 278
in primary pulmonary hypertension, 263
interstitial lung disease and, 418
Hydrarthrosis, intermittent, 1959
Hydrocarbon pneumonitis, 2294
Hydrocarbons
as nephrotoxins, 604
poisoning from, 88
Hydrocephalic dementia, 2000
Hydrocephalus, 2169
and parkinson-dementia complex, 2071
communicating, and gait disorders, 2045
in ependymoma of spine, 2186
in neurofibromatosis, 2085
in syringomyelia, 2084
normal-pressure, 2105
otitic, 2093, 2168
Hydrocephalus ex vacuo, 2169
Hydrochloric acid
antacids in neutralization of, 689, 689t
gastric secretion of, inhibition of, 688–689, *688*
sex factor in, 682, 682t
in peptic ulcer, 682, 683
measurement of, 687
Hydrocortisone. See also *Cortisol.*
in respiratory failure, 461
topical, in skin disease, 2240
Hydrogen ion(s)
concentration of, in shock, 220
kidney secretion of, 499
Hydromorphone, in pain, 2052
Hydromyelia, 2084
Hydronephrosis, 604
ultrasonography of, 514
ureteropelvic junction obstruction in, 639
Hydropericardium, 345
Hydrops fetalis, 923
Hydrothorax
in right ventricular failure, 198
simple, 448
Hydroxocobalamin, 895
25-Hydroxycholecalciferol, conversion of, to 1,25-dihydroxycholecalciferol, in Fanconi's syndrome, 615
17-Hydroxycorticosteroids
urinary, 1308
reference values for, 2326
18-Hydroxycorticosterone, 1301
Hydroxycortisone hemisuccinate, in cancer chemotherapy, 1101t
Hydroxyethyl starch (hetastarch), 220
5-Hydroxyindoleacetic acid
in carcinoid syndrome, 1414
reference values for, 2326
11-Hydroxylase deficiency, 1396, 1397
11β-Hydroxylase deficiency, 1364
17-Hydroxylase deficiency, 1387
17α-Hydroxylase deficiency, 1358
21-Hydroxylase deficiency, 1363–1364, 1395, 1397
Hydroxylysine-deficient collagen disease, 1150–1151
Hydroxyprogesterone, in cancer chemotherapy, 1101t
17-Hydroxyprogesterone
in hirsutism, 1396, 1397
serum, reference values for, 2326
Hydroxyproline oxidase deficiency, 1129
Hydroxyprolinemia, 1129
genetic factor in, 1129
3β-Hydroxysteroid dehydrogenase; $\Delta^{5\text{-}4}$ isomerase deficiency, 1358
17β-Hydroxysteroid dehydrogenase deficiency, 1358–1359
2-Hydroxystilbamidine, in blastomycosis, 1763
Hydroxyurea
in chronic myelogenous leukemia, 978, 979
in polycythemia vera, 971
Hymenolepis diminuta, 1808
Hymenolepis nana, 1807
Hyoscyamine, abuse of, 2024
Hyperadrenocorticism, 1458
Hyperaldosteronism, 542
primary, 276, 529
secondary, 1319
Hyperaminoaciduria(s), 1120, 1121t, 1125t, 1126
genetic factor in, 1120
mechanisms of, 1120, *1126*
Hyperargininemia, 1130
Hyperbaric oxygen, therapeutic, 2289
Hyperbilirubinemia, 132
acquired, 808–809
cyclic premenstrual unconjugated, 808
diffuse hepatocellular injury and, 808
effective enythropoiesis and, 808
fasting, 808
hemolysis in, 808
postoperative, 808
shunt, 808
Hypercalcemia, 551, 1417, 1448–1451
benign familial, 1438
cancer and, 1078
chronic renal failure and, 1450
differential diagnosis of, 1437–1438, 1438t
diuresis for, 1450–1451
drug intake and, 1449
granulomatous diseases and, 1449
hyperthyroidism and, 1449
idiopathic, of infancy, 1450
immobilization and, 1450
in hyperparathyroidism, 1435–1442
kidney transplantation and, 1450
malignancy and, 1438, 1448–1449
nonparathyroid origin of, 1438t, 1448–1450
symptoms of, 1436
treatment of, 1450–1451
glucocorticosteroid therapy in, 112
hydration in, 1450–1451
with bronchogenic carcinoma, 441
with multiple myeloma, 1018–1019
Hypercalciuria
absorptive, 629–630, 631
hyperparathyroidism and, 631

Hypercalciuria (*Continued*)
  kidney stones and, 629–630, 631
  renal, 630, 631
  resorptive, 630, 631
  treatment of, 632
    orthophosphates in, 632–633
    sodium cellulose phosphate in, 632
    thiazides in, 632
Hypercapnia, 455, 457–458, 464–465, 543
  metabolic alkalosis and, 542
Hyperchloremia, 551
Hypercholesterolemia, 1115
  cardiovascular disease and, 157–158
  familial, 128, 132, 1103, 1104, 1112, 1115
  xanthomas in, 1112
Hypercortisolism, 1264–1265
Hyperdipsia, 2027
Hyperemesis gravidarum, 834
Hypereosinophilic syndrome, 960–961, 1011
Hyperesthesia, definition of, 2189
Hypergastrinemic syndromes, 687
Hyperglycemia
  diabetic neuropathy and, 1326–1327, *1326*
  hyperkalemia and, 534
  in diabetes mellitus, 1324, *1325*, 1326–1327
  in diabetic ketoacidosis, 1334–1335, *1334*
Hyperhidrosis, 2028
Hyperimmunoglobulinemia E syndrome, 1861
Hyperkalemia, 489, 530
  cardiac action potential and, 531–532, *532*
  clinical manifestations of, 534–535
  electrocardiography in, 534–535
  etiology of, 534, 534t
  in acute renal failure, 546
  in interstitial nephritis, 591
  pathogenesis of, 534
  potassium excess and, 534–535
  renal factor in, 534
  transcellular shifts in, 534
  treatment of, 535
  with blood transfusion, 940
  with uremia, 550, 555–556
Hyperkalemic periodic paralysis, 534, 2208
Hyperkeratosis, epidermolytic, *2251*
Hyperkinesia, definition of, 2069
Hyperlipidemia, 1109
  atherosclerosis and, 282, 1115
  diet and, 38
  diseases associated with, 1115
  familial combined, 1113, 1115
  inherited, 1470
Hyperlipoproteinemia(s), 132, 1108–1116
  with arthritis, 1957–1958
Hypermagnesemia, 1165–1166
  effects of, on cardiovascular system, 1165–1166
    on nervous system, 1165
Hypernatremia, 1250
  adequate water intake and, 529
  clinical manifestations of, 529
  diagnosis of, 529
  essential, 529, 1269
  etiology of, 528–529, 528t
  excessive water losses and, 529
  neurogenic, 2026
  osmotic diuresis and, 529
  pathogenesis of, 528–529
  treatment of, 529
  with diabetes insipidus, 1270
Hypernephromas, 488
Hyperostosis, endosteal, 1465
Hyperoxaluria, 738
  enteric, 631
  kidney stones and, 630, 631
  primary, 1108–1109
    genetic factor in, 1108
  treatment of, 633
Hyperparathyroidism, 1435–1443. See also *Hypercalcemia*.
  abnormal parathyroid tissue in, 1441
  cyclic AMP excretion in, 1441
  diagnostic investigations of, 1438–1441
    differential diagnosis of, 1437–1438
    glucocorticoid suppression test in, 1441
    parathyroid hormone assay in, 1439–1440, *1439*
    radiography in, 1437, *1437*, 1441
  epidemiology of, 1435
  etiology of, 1435
  hypercalcemia in, 1435–1442
  hypercalciuria and, 631
  kidney stones and, 630, 631, 632
  osteoporosis and, 1458
  pathology of, 1435–1436
  pathophysiology of, 1436
  physical signs of, 1436–1437
  primary, 539
  prognosis of, 1442
  renal osteodystrophy and, 557
  serum calcium in, 1438–1439, 1440, *1440*
  serum parathyroid hormone in, 1435
  symptoms of, 1436
  treatment of, 632, 1441–1442
    parathyroid tissue autotransplantation in, 1442
    surgery in, 1441–1442
    vitamin D therapy in, 1442
  uremia with, 553
  urine calcium in, 1440
  vitamin D in, 1436, 1439, 1440, 1441
  with arthritis, 1958
  with cancer, 1078
  with renal phosphate wasting, 614–615
Hyperpathia, definition of, 2047
Hyperphagia, 646
Hyperphenylalaninemia(s), 1126–1128
  malignant, 1127
  persistent, 1127
  variants of, 1127
Hyperphosphatasia, hereditary, 1465
Hyperphosphatemia, 1164, 1417
Hyperpigmentation, disorders of, 2254–2256
  generalized, 2256
Hyperplasia. See under specific types.
Hyperpnea, 372
Hyperproinsulinemia, familial, 128, 1322, 1323
Hyperprolactinemia, 1263–1264
  clinical features of, 1263
  computed tomography in, 1263
  differential diagnosis of, 1263, 1263t
  idiopathic, 1249, 1263
  laboratory studies in, 1263
  microadenoma with, 1263, 1264
  pathogenesis of, 1263–1264
  therapy of, 1264
    bromocriptine in, 1264
    surgery in, 1264
Hyperprolinemia(s), 1129
  genetic factor in, 1129
Hypersensitivity
  delayed-type, 1849
  denervation, 2179
  fever with, 1470
  in drug reaction, 83
  in respiratory disease, 385–386
  in sarcoidosis, 433
  pericarditis with, 342
Hypersensitivity angiitis, *2264*, *2266*
Hypersensitivity pneumonitis, 417–418, 2285
Hypersensitivity states, diseases with, cutaneous and rheumatic components of, *2266*
Hypersensitivity vasculitis, 1939–1940
  glomerular involvement in, 585
Hypersomnia, *1988*, 1989
Hypersplenism, 1024
Hypertelorism, 145–146
  hemolysis, sequestrational, 907–908
Hypertension, 266–280. See also *Blood pressure; Portal hypertension; Pulmonary hypertension; Venous hypertension*.
  acute intracranial, and loss of consciousness, 1986
  age factor in, 267
  atherosclerosis and, 282
  benign essential, 272
  blood pressure measurement and, 266–267
  body weight and, 267–268
  cardiovascular disease and, 157–158
  case finding in, 270
    catecholamines and, 274–275, 1408
    cerebral hemorrhage with, 271
  chronic renal failure and, 552, 556
  cigarette smoking and, 268, 268t
  clinical manifestations of, 269–270
  clinical syndromes of, 270–272
  Cushing's syndrome and, 276
  death from, 269
  definition of, 266
  detection of treatable causes in, 270
  dialysis in, 561
  diet and, 38–39
  electrocardiography in, 270
  encephalopathy with, 271
  environmental factor in, 267
  epidemiology of, 155–158, 267–268
  etiology of, 274–275
  headache in, 2056
  in acute glomerulonephritis, 570
  in pregnancy, 271, 625–626
  in primary aldosteronism, 1317–1319
  in renal artery stenosis, 275–276
  intracranial, 2058, 2093, 2167–2168
    benign, 2168. See also *Pseudotumor cerebri*.
    emergency treatment of, *2167*
    pathogenesis of, *2167*
  left ventricular failure with, 272
  malignant, 270–271
    ocular changes in, 2223
  mineralocorticoids and, 1317–1319
    excess of, 276
  obesity and, 267–268, 1194
  ocular, 2218
  oral contraceptives and, 276
  organ damage with, 269–270
  pathogenesis of, 272–274
  prognosis in, 280
  prospective epidemiologic studies of, 268
  racial factor in, 267
  radiography in, 270
  renal, 275–276
  retinal examination in, 270
  retinopathy in, 271, 272, 2223
  risk factors and, 268, 268t, *269*, 270
  risk reduction in, 276
  salt intake and, 38–39, 268
  screening for, 274
  sex factor in, 267
  systolic, 274
  treatment of, 276–280
    adrenergic neuron-blocking agents in, 279
    alpha-adrenergic receptor blocking agents in, 279
    angiotensin-converting enzyme inhibitors in, 278–280
    beta-adrenergic receptor blocking agents in, 94, 277–278
    diuretics in, 277

Hypertension (*Continued*)
treatment of, drug therapy for, 276–280, 277t
centrally acting drugs in, 278–279
combined drug treatment in, 279, 279t
emergency therapy, 279
therapeutic choices in, 279–280
therapy withdrawal, 279
vasodilators in, 278
with coarctation of aorta, 274
with pheochromocytoma, 1410
with urinary tract obstruction, 606
Hypertensive encephalopathy, 271, 2102
Hypertensive intracerebral hemorrhage, 2109–2110
Hypertensive-arteriosclerotic hemorrhage, 2104
intracerebral, 2108
Hyperthermia, 1471
diagnosis of, 1472
hypothalamus and, 2026
in metabolic brain disease, 1975
malignant, *2205*, 2206
myoglobinuria in, 2211
Hyperthryoidism, 739. See also *Graves' disease; Thyrotoxicosis.*
and impotence, 2030
apathetic (masked), 1282, 2210
clinical findings in, 1282–1283, 1282t
differential diagnosis of, 1284
emotional factors in, 1281
hypercalcemia and, 1449
in pregnancy, 1286
iodine-induced, 1299
laboratory diagnosis of, 1283–1284, *1283*
osteoporosis and, 1458
surgery for, 1285
thyroid storm in, 1286–1287, 1286t
thyroid-stimulating hormone–induced, 1287
treatment of, 1284–1287
antithyroid drugs in, 1284–1285, 1286
beta-adrenergic blocking agents in, 94, 1285
choice of therapy for, 1286
lithium in, 1286
radioiodine in, 1285–1286
Hypertrichosis, 2231–2232
Hypertriglyceridemia, 1113–1114
acute pancreatitis and, 772
diseases associated with, 1114
familial, 1113, 1115
management of, 1114
Hypertrophic pulmonary osteoarthropathy, with bronchogenic carcinoma, 441
Hyperuricemia
asymptomatic, 1142
classification of, 1132, 1132t
gout and, 1132, 1132t, 1133t
mechanisms of, 1133–1136, *1134, 1135*
with acute leukemia, 990
Hyperuricosuria
kidney stones and, 630, 631
treatment of, 633
Hyperuricosuric calcium oxalate stone diathesis, 630
Hyperventilation, 372
and epilepsy, 2153
and syncope, 1985
in altered consciousness, 1976
vs. vertigo, 2041
Hyperventilation syndrome, 2010
Hypervitaminosis D, 1424–1425
Hypesthesia, definition of, 2047
Hypnotics, abuse of, 2019–2021
Hypnotism, in pain, 2053
Hypoadrenocorticism, 739
Hypoaldosteronism, 1313
hyporeninemic, 518, 519, 531, 534, 540, 550–551, 591, 1313
Hypocalcemia, 551, 724, 1417, 1422
in hypoparathyroidism, 1443–1446
with hypomagnesemia, 1166
Hypocapnia, 465
Hypochlorhydria, acute gastritis and, 677, 678
Hypochromia, 889, 890
Hypochromic anemia, 885–893
classification of, 885, 885t
differential diagnosis of, 891
iron deficiency, 885–891
microcytic, 885, 885t
red cell indices in, 885, 885t
sideroblastic, 892–893, *892*
Hypocitraturia, treatment of, 633
Hypocitruria, kidney stones and, 630
Hypodermomycosis, 1774
Hypofibrinogenemia, 1050–1051
Hypogammaglobulinemia, 723, 738
in chronic lymphocytic leukemia, 982
transient, of infancy, 1858
with arthritis, 1958
Hypogeusia, 2032
Hypoglycemia(s), 1341–1348. See also *Insulinoma.*
and syncope, 1986
autoimmune response in, 1347
cancer and, 1079
catecholamines in, 1342–1343
caused by non-beta cell tumor, 1347
clinical evaluation of, 1342–1343, *1343*
glucose tolerance test in, 1343–1344, *1344*
mixed meal test in, 1343–1344, *1344*
diabetes mellitus therapy and, 1327, 1331–1332
diseases associated with, 1347
drug-induced, 1344
ethanol-induced, 1344
etiology of, 1342, 1342t
factitial, 1347
fasting, 1342–1343, 1344–1347
food-stimulated, 1342–1344
glucagon in, 1342
glucose homeostasis in, 1341–1342, 1342t
in acute viral hepatitis, 814
in glucocorticoid function testing, 1309
in malaria, 1779
physiology of, 1341–1342
Hypogonadism, 1172–1173, 1369–1373
hypogonadotropic, 1372–1373, 1387
familial, 1387
hypothalamic, 1248–1249
primary, 1370
secondary, 1372–1373
Hypokalemia, 725
cardiac action potential and, 532, *532*
chronic, polymyositis in, 2210
clinical manifestations of, 533
ECF-ICF shifts in, 533
electrocardiography in, 533
etiology of, 532–533, 532t
pathogenesis of, 532–533
potassium depletion and, 532–534
treatment of, 533–534
urine potassium concentration in, 511
with hypomagnesemia, 1166
Hypokalemic periodic paralysis, 533
in protein-calorie malnutrition, 1185
stimulation tests of, 1308–1309
Hypomagnesemia, 724, 1166–1167
causes of, 1166, 1166t
consequences of, 1166, 1166t
hypocalcemia with, 1166
Hypomagnesemia (*Continued*)
hypokalemia with, 1166
treatment of, 1166–1167
Hyponatremia, 525, 525t, 725, 1249
acute, 528
antidiuretic hormone excess and, 525–527, *527*
chronic, 528
clinical manifestations of, 527
diagnosis of, 527–528
diuretic-induced, 526
in acute renal failure, 546
in central pontine myelinolysis, 2066
in head injury, 2173
primary effector ADH excess and, 526
reduced sodium delivery to diluting segments and, 525–526
treatment of, 528
with volume disorders, 526–527, *527*
Hypoparathyroidism, 738, 1427, 1443–1446
clinical manifestations of, 1443–1444
cyclic AMP excretion in, 1443
diagnosis of, 1444–1445
etiology of, 1443
functional, 1443
genetic factor in, 1443
hypocalcemia in, 1443–1446
idiopathic, 1443
neonatal, 1443
neuromuscular effects of, 1443–1444
pathophysiology of, 1443
serum calcium in, 1443–1446
serum parathyroid hormone in, 1443, 1445
serum phosphate in, 1443, 1445
surgically induced, 1443
treatment of, 1445
vitamin D therapy in, 1445–1446
vitamin D metabolism in, 1443, 1445
Hypophosphatasia, 1428
Hypophosphatemia, 913, 1164–1165, 1417–1418, 1419, 1422
adenosine triphosphate in, 1164–1165
causes of, 1164, 1164t
2,3-diphosphoglycerate in, 1164
genetic factor in, 1430
moderate, 1164
respiratory alkalosis and, 1164, 1165
severe, 1164
consequences of, 1164–1165, 1164t
treatment of, 1164
with cancer, 1078–1079
X-linked, 1427
Hypophysectomy
diabetes insipidus and, 1270
in breast cancer, 1403
Hypopigmentation, disorders of, 2256
Hypopigmentation syndrome, oculocerebral, *2258*
Hypopituitarism, 1255–1259
clinical features of, 1256–1257
diagnosis of, 1257
differential, 1257
disease states with, 1255–1256, 1256t
fertility restoration in, 1258
hormone-specific features of, 1256–1257
primary vs. secondary, 1255–1256, 1256t
treatment of, 1257
estrogen therapy in, 1258
glucocorticoids in, 1257–1258
growth hormone therapy in, 1258
testosterone therapy in, 1258
thyroxin therapy in, 1258
Hypopyon, in Behçet's syndrome, 2220
Hypospadias, 639
Hyposplenism, pathophysiology of, 1024
Hyposmia, 2031

Hypotension
  intracranial, 2058, 2166–2167
  orthostatic, 1984–1985, *1984*
    in autonomic dysfunction, 2028
    in Wernicke's encephalopathy, 2065
  postural, 1412–1413, 1412t
Hypotensive shock, 1871
Hypothalamic hormones, structure of, 1242, *1242*
Hypothalamic hypogonadism, 1248–1249
  postpubertal, 1248–1249
  prepubertal, 1248
Hypothalamic hypothyroidism, 1249
Hypothalamic disorders, 2025–2027, *2025*
Hypothalamic-adrenal dysfunction, 1249
Hypothalamic-lactotroph-breast axis, 1246
Hypothalamic-pituitary-adrenal axis, glucocorticosteroid therapy and, 114, 116
  in adrenal steroid hormone production regulation, 1303–1304
Hypothalamic-pituitary-adrenocortical axis, 1244–1245
Hypothalamic-pituitary-gonadal axis, 1245
Hypothalamic-pituitary-ovarian axis, 1381, *1381*, 1382
Hypothalamic-pituitary-somatotroph axis, 1245–1246
Hypothalamic-pituitary-testis axis, 1366–1367, *1367*, 1368
Hypothalamic-pituitary-thyoid axis, 1245, 1278
Hypothalamus. See also specific hormones.
  action of, hormone mechanism of, 1244
  as thermoregulatory center, 1382
  diseases of, age factor in, 1246–1247, 1247t
    infiltrative, 1248
    inflammatory, 1248
  hormone secretion regulation by, 1242–1244
    neurotransmitters in, 1242–1244, *1243*,1244t
  hormones of, structure of, 1242, *1242*
  in anorexia nervosa, 1188–1189
  in fever pathogenesis, 1471–1472
  lesions of, and impotence, 2030
  neuroendocrine role of, 2025–2027
  pituitary interrelationships with, 1242, *1242*
  radiation-induced dysfunction of, 1248
  regional syndromes of, *2025*
  trauma to, 1248
  tumors of, 1247
    gangliocytoma, 1247
    hamartoma, 1247
Hypothermia, 2306–2307, *2306*
  hypothalamus and, 2025
  in altered consciousness, 1976
Hypothyroidism, 672, 1287–1291
  and impotence, 2030
  biochemical abnormalities in, 1289–1290
  causes of, 1288t
  clinical manifestations of, 1288–1289, 1288t
  coronary artery disease and, 1290
  differential diagnosis of, 1290
  drug-induced, 1288t
  epidemiology of, 1288
  etiology of, 1287–1288, 1288t
  free thyroxine index in, 1289, 1290, 1291
  hormone replacement in, 1290, 1290t
    withdrawal of, 1291
  hyperlipidemia with, 1115
  hypothalamic, 1249
  laboratory diagnosis of, 1289–1290, *1289*
    thyrotropin-releasing hormone infusion test in, 1289
  muscle weakness in, 2210
  neuropathy with, 2194
  pathology of, 1288
Hypothyroidism (*Continued*)
  primary, 1287
  prognosis in, 1291
  screening for, 1288
  secondary, 1288
  serum thyrotropin in, 1289
  therapy of, 1290–1291
  thyroid-stimulating hormone deficient, 1384
Hypotonia, in Huntington's disease, 2074
Hypoventilation, 379, 455, 464
  in altered consciousness, 1976
Hypovitaminosis D, 1424
Hypovolemia, 518
Hypoxanthine-guanine phosphoribosyltransferase deficiency, 1143
  gout with, 1139
Hypoxemia, 464
  in congenital heart disease, 228
Hypoxia, 457
  cerebral, vs. cerebral ischemia, 2090
  in shock, 213, 220
Hypsarrhythmia, 2153
Hysteria, 2013–2015
Hysterical gait, 2046
Hysterical personality, depression in, 2011
Hysterical seizures, vs. epilepsy, 2156

Iceland disease, 2131
I-cell disease, 1149
Ichthyosiform dermatoses, 2250, *2251*
Ichthyosiform erythrodermas, 2251
Ichthyosis, 2250–2251, *2251*
  congenital, syndrome of, *2264*
Ictus, 2149
Ideational apraxia, 1995
Identity concept, for adolescence, 19
Idiopathic pulmonary fibrosis, 412–413, *412*
  clinical manifestations of, 412–413
  differential diagnosis of, 413
  pathogenesis of, 413
  staging of, 413
  therapy of, 413
Idiotopes, 1850–1851
Idoxuridine, in herpesvirus infection, 109, 1717
α-L-Iduronidase deficiency, 1146, 1148
  genetic factor in, 1146
IgA. See *Immunoglobulin A.*
IgD. See *Immunoglobulin D.*
IgE. See *Immunoglobulin E.*
IgG. See *Immunoglobulin G.*
IgG-mediated autoimmune hemolytic anemia, 908–910
  clinical manifestations in, 908–909
  corticosteroids in, 909
  differential diagnosis of, 909
  immunosuppression in, 909
  laboratory findings in, 909
  prognosis in, 909–910
  splenectomy in, 909
  treatment of, 909
IgM. See *Immunoglobulin M.*
IgM cold agglutinins, 910–911
IgM-JFA test, for toxoplasmosis, 1794
Ileal bypass, 738
Ileal disease, 738
Ileal resection, distal, 738
Ileocolitis. See *Crohn's colitis.*
Ileojejunitis
  corticosteroids in, 735
  nongranulomatous, 735
Ileum, ulceration of, 801–802
Ileus, 706–707
  adynamic, vs. mechanical, 706–707
Ileus (*Continued*)
  clinical manifestations of, 707
  diagnosis of, 707
  etiology of, 706–707
  paralytic, 707
  pathophysiologic consequences of, 707
  treatment of, 707
Imaging techniques, 64–68. See also specific procedures.
  future developments in, 67–68
  historical perspective on, 64
Imerslund's syndrome, 1131
Iminoglycinuria, 611
  genetic factor in, 611
Imipramine, in anxiety, 2010
  in manic-depressive psychosis, 2006
Immersion foot, 357
Immobilization
  hypercalcemia and, 1450
  osteoporosis and, 1458
Immotile cilia syndrome, 390
Immune complex(es)
  in glomerular disease, 503–504, 503t
  in inflammation, 1903–1908
  in rapidly progressive glomerulonephritis, 577
  skin reactions and, 386
Immune complex disease, 1874–1877
  circulating immune complexes in, 1874–1876
    tissue deposition of, 1874–1876, *1875*
  host factor in, 1876
  pathogenesis of, 1974–1976
  with tissue-fixed antigen, 1874
Immune complex induced vasculitis, as "allergic" drug reaction, 83t
Immune globulin(s), 42, 43, 111
  for varicella, 46
  in hepatitis, 46
  in measles, 45
  rabies, 2134
Immune response, 1846–1852
  aplastic anemia and, 878–879
  ascorbic acid and, 1204, 1205
  drug-induced, 83–84, 83t
  eosinophils in, 1011, 1012
  in acquired immune deficiency syndrome, 1862
  in acute rheumatic fever, 1527–1528
  in Addison's disease, 1310
  in adenovirus disease, 1705, 1706
  in African trypanosomiasis, 1781
  in allergic rhinitis, 1867
  in anaerobic infection, 1584
  in anaphylaxis, 1870, 1871
  in anemia, 874
  in ankylosing spondylitis, 1919
  in aspergillosis, 1770–1771
  in babesiosis, 1798–1799
  in Behçet's disease, 1960–1961
  in blastomycosis, 1763
  in candidiasis, 1768
  in celiac disease, 733
  in Chagas' disease, 1784
  in chlamydial infection, 1669
  in chronic gastritis, 679
  in chronic lymphocytic leukemia, 980–981, 982
  in coccidioidomycosis, 1761, 1762
  in Crohn's disease, 741
  in cryptococcosis, 1765, 1766
  in diabetes mellitus, 1322, 1325
  in giardiasis, 1802
  in glomerulus disorders, 568–569, *569*, 570t
  in Graves' disease, 1280, 1281
  in group A streptococcal infection, 1521, 1522

Immune response (*Continued*)
in hairy cell leukemia, 985
in Hashimoto's thyroiditis, 1280, 1293
in hemolytic anemia, 908–911
in *Hemophilus influenzae* infection, 1563–1564
in histoplasmosis, 1769
in Hodgkin's diease, 1000–1001, 1003
in idiopathic thrombocytopenic purpura, 1033–1034
in infectious disease, 1477, 1478, 1479, 1482, 1483, 1484–1485
in infectious mononucleosis, 1719, 1720
in infective endocarditis, 1539
in influenza, 1700–1701, 1702, 1703, 1704
in kala azar, 1788, 1789
in leishmaniasis, 1787
in leprosy, 1634, 1635–1636
in leptospirosis, 1667
in malaria, 1777
in measles, 1706–1707
in membranoproliferative glomerulonephritis, 583–584
in membranous nephropathy, 582
in meningococcal disease, 1558
in minimal change nephrotic syndrome, 580
in mycoplasmal pneumonia, 1507, 1508
in mumps, 1713–1714
in neutropenia, 957
in paracoccidioidomycosis, 1764
in pernicious anemia, 897
in pneumocystosis, 1796, 1797
in polyarteritis nodosa, 1941, 1942
in polymyositis, 1947, 1948–1949
in primary biliary cirrhosis, 837–838
in protein-calorie malnutrition,1185
in pulmonary tuberculosis, 1622
in pyoderma, 1525
in rapidly progressive glomerulonephritis, 575–577, *576*
in Reiter's syndrome, 1920
in rheumatoid arthritis, 1904–1905, *1905*, 1912–1913
in rheumatic disease, 1898–1899, 1898t, 1902–1904, 1903t, 1904t, 1908–1909, 1909t, 1910t
in rickettsial disease, 1672–1674, 1676
in rubella, 1710, 1711
in schistosomiasis, 1810–1812
in secondary immunologic thrombocytopenia, 1034–1035
in Sjögren's syndrome, 1936–1937
in spondylarthropathies, 1918–1919, 1918t
in staphylococcal infection, 1544–1545
in stomach cancer, 699–700
in systemic lupus erythematosus, 1924–1927, 1926t
in systemic sclerosis, 1932, 1934
in thrombocytopenic purpura, 1032–1034
in toxic nephropathy, 594–595
in toxoplasmosis, 1792, 1793–1794, 1795
in tuberculosis, 1622
in ulcerative colitis, 748–749
in urticaria-angioedema, 1864
in varicella, 1722
in vasculitis, 1938, 1939
in Wegener's granulomatosis, 1944
macrophages in, 1851
major histocompatibility complex and, 1877–1880
non-Hodgkin's lymphoma and, 994
reconstitution of, 1484–1485
renal injury and, 501–505, *502*, 503t
with kidney transplantation, 564, 566, 567
with purine enzyme deficiencies, 1144–1145
Immune system, 1846–1852. See also *B cell; Complement; T cell.*
Immune system (*Continued*)
idiotype regulatory mechanism of, 1850–1851
in bone marrow transplantation, 1026
Immune system agents, from recombinant DNA research, 133
Immune system disease, 1846–1890. See also specific diseases.
Immune system neoplasms, 992–994. See also specific diagnoses.
classification of, 992, 992t, 993, 993t
diagnosis of, 993–994
differential, 994
pathology of, 993
staging systems for, 993–994
Immune-mediated encephalomyelitis, 2139
Immunity
altered, neurologic disorders with, 2138–2143
to malaria, 1777
Immunization, 42–46. See also *Vaccine(s)* and specific diseases
active vs. passive, 42, 42t, 43, 43t
available vaccines for, 45
diphtheria-tetanus-pertussis vaccine for, 1573
for travelers, 1493
hypersensitivity reactions to, 43
in pediatrics, 42
passive, for adults, 43t
Immunocompromised host, neurologic complications in, 2141–2143
Immunocytic amyloidosis, 1021–1022
clinical features of, 1021–1022
pathophysiology of, 1021
treatment of, 1022
Immunodeficiency, herpesvirus infection in, 1716
toxoplasmosis in, 1794
with multiple myeloma, 1016
Immunodeficiency disease(s). See also *acquired immunodeficiency syndrome; Cellular immunodeficiency disorder; Partial combined immunodeficiency disorder; Severe combined immunodeficiency disorder.*
complement abnormality and, 1854
from antibody deficiency, 1855–1858, 1856t
from cellular immunodeficiency, 1858–1859, 1858t
genetic factors in, 1855
partial combined, 1860–1861
primary, 1855–1861
severe combined, 132, 1859–1860
Immunoglobulin(s), 1846, 1848–1849, 1849t
classes of, 1848–1849, 1849t
deficiency of, in Friedreich's ataxia, 2083
gene organization and translocation in, 1846–1847, *1847*
idiotypes of, 1850–1851
in Berger's disease, 574–575, *574*
in hemolysis, 908
in multiple sclerosis, 2144
in plasma cell disorders, 1013, *1013*
in renal injury, 501–502, *502*
molecules of, 1846–1847, *1847*
of B cells, 1013
Immunoglobulin A
deficiency of, 1855t, 1856, 1857
with *Candida*, 1861
in dermatitis herpetiformis, 2268
in DiGeorge's syndrome, 1858
in Nezelof's syndrome, 1858
secretory component deficiency of, 1857
serum, reference values for, 2326
Immunoglobulin D, 1848, 1849t
serum, reference values for, 2326
Immunoglobulin E, 1848, 1849t
Immunoglobulin E (*Continued*)
in allergic rhinitis, 1867
in anaphylaxis, 1870, 1871
in atopic dermatitis, 2249
in DiGeorge's syndrome, 1858
in inflammation, 1902
in insect sting allergy, 1873
in Nezelof's syndrome, 1858
in urticaria-angioedema, 1864, 1865
levels of, in hyperimmunoglobulinemia, 1861
tests for, 1868–1869
serum, reference values for, 2326
Immunoglobulin G, 1848, 1849t
deficiency of, 1855t, 1856
in insect sting allergy, 1872–1873
in rheumatoid arthritis, 1912–1913
in rheumatic disease, 1908–1909
serum, reference values for, 2326
Immunoglobulin G/albumin ratio, reference values for, 2326
Immunoglobulin G index, of spinal fluid, in neurosyphilis, 2120
Immunoglobulin G synthesis rate, reference values for, 2326
Immunoglobulin M, 1848, 1849t
deficiency of, 1855t, 1856, 1857
elevated levels of, 1857–1858
in rheumatic disease, 1908–1909
selective deficiency of, 1857
serum, reference values for, 2327
Immunoglobulin mosaicism, 962
Immunology
aging and, 24
of sarcoidosis, 432–434
Immunosuppression
and central nervous system infections, 2141–2143
cancer and,1071
in aplastic anemia, 878–879, 881
in bone marrow transplantation,1026
in IgG-mediated autoimmune hemolytic anemia, 909
in measles, 1707
infections and, 1477–1478
listeriosis and, 1610
nocardiosis and, 1613, 1614
nosocomial pneumonia and,1511–1512
with kidney transplantation, 566, 567
Immunosuppressive agents
glucocorticosteroids as, 112–113
in Behçet's disease, 1961
in myasthenia gravis, 2213, 2214
in rheumatoid arthritis, 1916
Immunosuppressive therapy
and listerial meningitis, 2142
chronic, and central nervous system infection, 2142
for cancer, 1100, 1101t
in acute myelogenous leukemia, 991
in allergic rhinitis, 1870
in bronchogenic carcinoma, 444
in Crohn's disease, 747
in pemphigus, 2268
in whooping cough, 1570
Impedance, measurement of, in hearing loss, 2038
Impedance plethysmography, in thrombophlebitis, 364
Impetigo, streptococcal, 1524
Impetigo contagiosa, 1524
Impotence, 1374, 2030–2031, *2030*
aging and, 21
Inborn errors of metabolism, 127–132
amino acid mutations in, 128
deficient end-product replacement in, 131
definition of, 128
dietary management in, 131

Inborn errors of metabolism (*Continued*)
enzyme activity in, 132
enzyme deficiency in, 127–132, 129t–130t
etiology of, 128
gene location and, 127t
genetic engineering in, 132
genetic heterogeneity in, 131
marrow transplantation in, 132
metabolic inhibitors in, 132
mutant protein modification in, 132
mutant protein replacement in, 132
mutation types in, 128
nonenzymic protein defects in, 128
organ transplantation in, 132
pathogenesis of, 128, 130–131, 131t
polymorphism in, 130, 131t
prenatal diagnosis of, 136–137
protein deficiency in, 128, 130, 131t
recombinant DNA research in, 135–137
renal transplantation in, 132
storage substance depletion in, 131–132
treatment of, 131–132
Inclusion blenorrhea, 2221
Inclusion body encephalitis, subacute, 2136
Incontinence, 2029, *2029*
in aged, 28–29
Incontinentia pigmenti, 2255, *2255*
Indirect antiglobulin test, 908
Indirect fluorescent antibody test, for rickettsial disease, 1676
Indolamines, 1243
Indomethacin
for gout, 1141
in chronic paroxysmal hemicrania, 2056
in patent ductus arteriosus, 232
Industrial bronchitis, 2286–2287
Industrial pollution, interstitial lung disease and, 407–408, 408t, 410, 417–418
Infant. See *Neonate.*
Infantile paralysis, 2130–2132
Infantile spasms, 2153
Infarction
cerebral, 2090–2103
treatment of, 2101
lacunar, 2092
and stroke, *2095*, 2096
myocardial, and stroke, 2091, *2092*
"watershed," 2090, 2091
Infection(s)
complement abnormality and, 1853–1854
hospital-acquired, 1485–1492. See also *Hospital-acquired infection.*
in coma, 1979
myopathy in, 2210
occupational factors in, 2297
ocular, 2220–2221
of brain, and epilepsy, 2150
of paranasal sinus, brain abscess due to, 2112
of urinary tract, and back pain, 2061
parameningeal, 2111–2118
syphilitic, of central nervous system, 2118–2121
systemic, and back pain, 2061
thrombocytopenia in, 1036
viral, of nervous system, 2121–2138
Infectious disease(s), 1469–1774. See also specific diagnoses; *Hospital-acquired infection.*
anatomic defects and, 1478
antibiotic prophylaxis in, 1483
clinical manifestations of, 1478–1479
compromised host management in, 1483–1485
cutaneous lesions in, *2260–2261*
defense systems and, 1477–1485, 1477t, 1480t–1481t, 1482t
diagnosis of, 1482–1483, 1482t
Infectious disease(s) (*Continued*)
environmental factors in, 1483
fever with, 1470–1473
host factor in, 1477–1485
immune response in, 1477, 1478, 1479, 1482, 1483, 1484–1485
immunosuppression and, 1477–1478
inflammatory response in, 1477, 1478, 1479, 1483, 1484
introduction to, 1469–1470
laboratory evaluation in, 1482
leukocyte dysfunction in, 1478
leukopenia in, 1478, 1479, 1483
management of, 1483
meningococcal, in hospital-acquired infection, 1492
pathogenesis of, 1478
pathology of, 1478
phagocyte disorders in, 1477, 1478, 1479, 1482, 1484
physical barriers in, 1477, 1478
reticuloendothelial system in, 1477, 1478
spleen in, 1478
Infectious mononucleosis, 1719–1721
clinical manifestations of, 1720
corticosteroid therapy in, 1721
diagnosis of, 1720–1721
epidemiology of, 1719–1720
etiology of, 1719
immune response in, 1719, 1720
leukocytosis in, 1720
pathogenesis of, 1720
pathology of, 1720
prognosis in, 1721
serology in, 1720
treatment of, 1721
Infectious neuropathy, 2196
Infertility
cancer therapy and, 1093
female, 1388–1389
salpingitis and, 1643, 1645
male, 1372
treatment of, 1372
Infestations, occupational factors in, 2297
Inflammation
as host defense, 1477, 1478, 1479, 1483, 1484
cytotoxin antibody in, 1902–1903
immune complexes in, 1903–1904
immunoglobulin E in, 1902
immunologically mediated, 1902–1904, 1903t
macrophage evolution and, 946, *947*
management of, 1484
mononuclear leukocytes in, 1904, 1904t
Inflammation headache, 2057
Inflammatory autonomic neuropathy, acute, 2192
Inflammatory disease
intestinal, liver disease and, 834
joint, amyloidosis with, 1169
of spinal canal, 2186–2187
Inflammatory neuropathy, chronic relapsing, 2192
Inflammatory polyneuropathy, 2190–2192
acute, 2191–2192
chronic, 2192
Influenza, 1700–1705
amantadine in, 1704–1705
antigenic drift in, 1701, 1702
antigenic shift in, 1701, 1702
antigenic variation in, 1700–1701
chemotherapy for, 110
clinical findings in, 1703
complications with, 1703–1704
culture in, 1704
diagnosis of, 1704
Influenza (*Continued*)
epidemics of, 1700, 1701, 1702, *1701, 1702*
epidemiology of, 1700–1701
immune response in, 1700–1701, 1702, 1703, 1704
immunization for, 44
interferon in, 1703
microbiology of, 1700, *1700*
mortality from, 1702
pandemics of, 1700, 1702, *1702t*
pathogenesis of, 1702–1703
pathology of, 1702–1703
prevention of, 1704–1705
pulmonary complications in, 1703–1704
rimantadine in, 1704–1705
serology in, 1704
treatment of, 1704
with Reye's syndrome, 1704
Influenza vaccine, 42t, 1704–1705
Informed consent, 8, 12
Inhalant(s)
abuse of, 2024
deposition and clearance of, 2280
Injury. See also *Accidents; Violence.*
from falls, 36–37
from fires, 37
Inorganic dusts, diseases caused by, 2284
Inorganic materials, diseases produced by, 2281–2285
Inorganic mercury, 2310
Inositol-1,4,5-triphosphate, 1225
Insect(s), disease carried by, 1833, 1833t
Insect sting allergy, 1872–1874
clinical manifestations of, 1873
diagnosis in, 1873–1874
epidemiology of, 1872
epinephrine in, 1874
etiology of, 1872–1873
immunoglobulin E in, 1873
immunoglobulin G in, 1873
natural history of, 1873
pathogenesis of, 1873
skin tests in, 1873
treatment of, 1874
venom immunotherapy in, 1874
Insecticides, poisoning from, 89, 96
Insomnia, 1988–1989, *1988*
Institutionalization, for aged, 25
Insulin
in glucocorticoid function testing, 1309
in protein-calorie malnutrition, 1185
metabolism of, 1323–1324, *1324*
resistance to, 1323–1324, *1324*
serum, reference values for, 2327
Insulin clearance test, reference values for, 2327
Insulin hypoglycemia test, 1254, 1255
Insulin therapy
ECF-ICF shifts in, 533
in diabetic ketoacidosis, 1335
in diabetes mellitus, 1330–1332
complications of, 1331–1332
preparations for, 1330t
regimens for, 1330, 1331t
Insulin tolerance test, reference values for, 2327
Insulin with oral glucose tolerance test, reference values for, 2327
Insulin-like growth factor, 1254
Insulinoma, 1344–1347, 1349
angiography in, 1346, *1346*
C peptide suppression test in, 1345, *1346*
computed tomography in, 1346
diagnosis of, 1345–1346
glucagon test in, 1345
hypoglycemia with, 1344
localization of, 1346

Insulinoma (*Continued*)
plasma glucose in, 1345, *1345, 1346*
serum insulin in, 1345, *1345, 1346*
supervised fasting test in, 1345
tolbutamide test in, 1345, *1345*
treatment of, 1346–1347
ultrasonography in, 1346
Intact nephron hypothesis, 489
Integument, aging and, 23
Intellect, dysfunction of, in olivopontocerebellar degeneration, 2084
Intensive care, life prolongation and, 12
Intercostal neuritis, 370
Interferon, 111, 1703
in influenza, 1763
Interleukin(s), 949
in rheumatic disease, 1901
Interleukin-1, 1847
Interleukin-2, 1849
Intermittent claudication
clinical manifestations of, 359
in arteriosclerosis obliterans, 359, 360
Intermittent mandatory ventilation, 468
Intermittent positive pressure ventilation, 459, 468
Internal capsular–thalamic hemorrhage, 2108
Internuclear ophthalmoplegia, in multiple sclerosis, 2145
Interstitial fibrosis, pulmonary hypertension and, 259, 260
Interstitial lung disease, 406–419
activity assessment in, 412
air pollution and, 407–408, 408t, 410, 417–418, 419
airways disease with, 416
alveolitis with, 409–410
Interstitial lung disease
anatomy of, 406–407, *406, 407*
ankylosing spondylitis with, 414
antibiotics and, 418
antineoplastic agents and, 418
biopsy in, 411
bronchoscopy in, 411
clinical features of, 410–411
collagen-vascular disorders and, 413–414
corticosteroids in, 412
differential diagnosis of, 408
epidemiology of, 407–408, 407t, 408t, 409t
fibrosis in, 410
from drugs, 408, 408t, 418
from inhaled inorganic dusts, 408, 408t, 417
from inhaled organic dusts, 408, 408t, 417–418
genetic factors in, 416
history in, 410
impairment assessment in, 412
industrial pollution and, 407–408, 408t, 410, 417–418
infection and, 419
laboratory studies in, 410–411
mixed connective tissue disease with, 414
of unknown etiology, 407, 407t, 409t, 412–417
paraquat and, 419
pathogenesis of, 408–410, *409*
physical examination in, 410
polymyositis/dermatomyositis with, 414
progressive systemic sclerosis with, 414
pulmonary function tests in, 411
pulmonary vasculitis with, 416
radiation and, 419
radiography in, 411
rheumatoid arthritis with, 413–414
scintigraphy in, 411
Sjögren's syndrome with, 414
stages of, 411–412
Interstitial lung disease (*Continued*)
systemic lupus erythematosus with, 414
therapy of, 412
Intervertebral disc disease, 2182–2184
Intestinal aganglionosis, 145, 711–712
Intestinal disease, adenoviral, 1705
Intestinal flora, in extraintestinal infection, 1593
Intestinal hemorrhage, intramural, 760
Intestinal infarction
acute, 758–759, *758*
nonocclusive, 759
Intestinal ischemic syndromes
acute, 758–760
chronic, 757–758
Intestinal parasites, 737
diarrhea and, 716, 717
Intestinal polyposis, 763–764, *763, 764*
genetic factor in, 763–764, *763, 764*
Intestinal pseudo-obstruction, 707–708
clinical manifestations of, 708
diagnosis of, 708
etiology of, 708, 708t
pathogenesis of, 708
treatment of, 708
Intestine
absorption mechanisms of, 719–722, *719*
active vs. passive transport in, 719
fluid transport in, 712–713, *713*
cyclic AMP concentration and, 714, *714*
fluke infection of, 1815, 1818–1819
in angiostrongyliasis, 1827
in ascariasis, 1822–1823
in bilharziasis, 1813–1814
in trichinellosis, 1825–1826
in trichuriasis, 1824
inflammatory disease of, 740, 796–802. See also specific diagnoses.
irradiation of, *2302*
mesenteric circulation in, 756–767, *756, 757*
pseudo-obstruction of, 731
radiobiology of, 2299
tuberculosis of, 1628–1629
vascular disease of, 756–761
Intoxication
bromide, 2021
water, 2027
Intra-aortic balloon counterpulsation
in myocardial infarction, 291, 294
in shock, 224
Intracellular compartment fluid, 516
Intracerebral hematomas, after brain injury, 2172
Intracerebral hemorrhage, 2103
hypertensive, 2110
differential diagnosis of, 2109–2110
investigation of, 2110
subarachnoid hemorrhage with, 2103
treatment of, 2111
Intracranial disorders, vs. amyotrophic lateral sclerosis, 2080
Intracranial hematoma, after brain injury, 2171–2172
Intracranial hemorrhage, 2103–2111
computed tomography in, 2106–2107
epidural, myelopathy in, 2139
external capsular–putaminal, 2108
in subcortical white matter, 2109
internal capsular–thalamic, 2108
into brain tumor, 2104
intraventricular, 2103
lobar, 2109t
pontine, 2108, 2110t
putaminal, 2109t
spontaneous, causes of, *2103*
clinical manifestations of, 2108–2109, *2108, 2109*
Intracranial hemorrhage (*Continued*)
subarachnoid, 2103, 2105
and headache, 2057
spinal, 2187
intracerebral, vs. spinal subarachnoid hemorrhage, 2187
subdural, myelopathy in, 2139
thalamic, 2109t
Intracranial hypertension, 2167–2168
benign, 2168–2169
emergency treatment of, *2167*
pathogenesis of, *2167*
Intracranial hypotension, 2166–2167
Intracranial pressure
altered, 2058
in brain injury, 2172
increased, and drop attacks, 2047
increased, in encephalitis, 2125
"Intracranial steal," 2104
classification of, 2161, 2162t
Intracranial tumors, 2161–2166
congenital, 2162t
metastatic, 2162t
syndromes of, 2163–2164
vascular, 2162t
Intracranial venous infarction, hemorrhage with, 2105
Intracranial venous thrombosis, 2093
Intradermal nevus, 2254, *2255*
Intradural extramedullary spinal inflammatory diseases, 2186
Intradural extramedullary spinal tumors, 2186
Intradural extramedullary spinal vascular lesions, 2187
Intramedullary spinal infectious processes, 2187
Intramedullary spinal tumors, 2186
Intraocular pressure, in glaucoma, 2217
Intraocular tumors, 2222
Intraretinal microvascular anomalies, 2223
Intravascular coagulation, in kidney disease, 505
Intraventricular hemorrhage, definition of, 2103
Intrinsic factor, 896, 897
vitamin B_{12}, reference values for, 2336
Intrinsic factor test, urinary, reference values for, 2333
Intussusception, 705
Iodine
metabolism of, 1275–1276, *1276*
intrathyroidal, 1276
deficiency of, 1287
endemic goiter and, 1299
in infants, 1299
treatment of, 1299
Iodothyronine, deiodination of, 1277, 1277t, 1278
5′-Iodothyronine deiodinase, 1277
Ionizing radiation, 2297
cancer and, 1070
cellular biology of, 2298
Iridocyclitis, 2220
Iridotomy, laser, in glaucoma, 2218
Iritis, 2219
Iron
absorption of, 722, 724, 885–887, 888–889
bioavailability of, 886
body distribution of, 885, 885t
cellular uptake of, 887–888
dietary, 885–886, 888–889
dietary allowance for, 1179
erythrocyte turnover rate of, 888
ferrokinetics of, 888
in hemoglobin synthesis, 919–920
in serum, reference values for, 2327
macrophage activity and, 888

Iron (*Continued*)
marrow transit time of, 888
metabolism of, 885–888, *886*
in hemochromatosis, 1160–1163
plasma transport rate of, 888
storage of, 888
transport of, 886–887, *886*
Iron cycle, 885, *886*
Iron deficiency anemia, 885–891
blood loss in, 872
blood smear in, 890, *890*
bone marrow examination in, 890
clinical manifestations of, 889
decreased iron uptake and, 888–889
epidemiology of, 885, 886
increased iron loss and, 889
iron metabolism and, 885–888
iron therapy in, 890–891
laboratory findings in, 889–890
pathogenesis of, 888–889, 889t
prognosis in, 891
red cell indices in, 889–890
treatment of, 890–891
Iron salts, 886
poisoning from, 89
Iron saturation, serum, reference values for, 2327
Iron storage disease. See *Hemochromatosis.*
Iron toxicity, 2312
Iron-binding capacity, total, reference values for, 2327
Irradiation. See under specific sites of radiation injury.
Irritable bowel syndrome, 650, 710–711, 717
clinical features of, 710–711
pathophysiology of, 710
personality traits and, 710–711
stress and, 710
treatment of, 711
Isaac's syndrome, 2216
Ischemia
carotid, symptoms and signs of, 2097
cerebral, 2090–2103
causes of, 2090, *2090*
coagulation alterations and, *2093*
hind-brain, 2098
vertebral-basilar, symptoms and signs of, 2097
Ischemic attack, transient, 2090, 2097, *2097*, 2098
Ischemic heart disease, sudden death and, 296, 297
Ischemic necrosis, 1955
Ischemic neurologic disability, reversible, 2091, 2097, *2097*
Islets of Langerhans, 1348, *1348*
Isoniazid, 1203, 1624, 1626
hepatotoxicity from, 823
in tuberculosis chemoprophylaxis, 1622
Isonicotinic acid hydrazide, 892, 1201
Isopropanol precipitation, reference values for, 2338
Isoproterenol, 93
in asthma, 394
in cardiopulmonary resuscitation, 482
in primary pulmonary hypertension, 263
in shock, 222
Isospora belli, 1803
Isosporiasis, 1803
Isotonic saline solution, 220
Isotretinoin, in acne, 2243
Isovaleric acidemia, 1130
Isovaleryl-CoA dehydrogenase deficiency, 1130
Ixodes holocyclus, 1683

Jacksonian march, 2151
Janeway's lesions, in infective endocarditis, 1536t
Japanese encephalitis, 1748
clinical features of, 1748
diagnosis of, 1748
epidemiology of, 1748
pathology in, 1748
vaccine for, 1748
vector in, 1748
virus in, 1748
Japanese river fever, 1684
Jarisch-Herxheimer reaction, 1660, 1663, 1664
Jaundice
cholangiography in, 660, 812
computed tomography in, 812
diagnosis of, 812–813
idiopathic dyserythropoietic, 808
idiopathic recurrent, 1393
in gastrointestinal disease, 650
in leptospirosis, 1667
laparoscopy in, 660
liver biopsy in, 812
ultrasonography in, 812
JC virus, in progressive multifocal leukoencephalopathy, 2137
Jejunal diverticula, 731
Jejunal stricture, 731
Jejunoileal bypass, 736
for obesity, 1196
Jejunum, ulceration of, 801–802
Jellyfish, 1843
Jerks, myoclonic, 2152
Jimson weed, 783
Job's syndrome, 952, 1479, *2265*
Jod-Basedow phenomenon, 1299
Joint(s), Charcot, in tabes dorsalis, 2119
diarthrodial, 1896–1897, *1896*
disorders of, radiography in, 1909–1911
with ulcerative colitis, 753
function of, 1896–1898
in disease, 1897–1898
infection of, 1892
inflammation of, 1897–1898
staphylococcal infection of, 1546–1547
structure of, 1896–1898
trauma to, 1897
Jones criteria, in rheumatic fever diagnosis, 1531
Joseph's disease, 2079
Junctional nevus, 2254, *2255*
Juvenile paresis, 2120
Juvenile polyposis, generalized, 764

Kala azar, 1787–1790
clinical features of, 1788
complications of, 1788
culture in, 1788–1789
diagnosis of, 1788–1789
epidemiology of, 1787–1788
immune response in, 1788, 1789
pathology of, 1788
postrecovery dermatitis in, 1788
prevention of, 1790
serology of, 1788, 1789
skin tests in, 1788, 1789
treatment of, 1789–1790
vector in, 1787–1788, 1790
Kallikrein-kinin system, 501
Kallmann's syndrome, 1248, 1373
Kanamycin, 1625
Kaolin, 79
Kaposi's sarcoma, 1861, 1862, 1863, 2262, 2273
Karnofsky scale, 1063, 1064t
Kartagener's syndrome, 128, 239, 390, 423, 1104, 1478
Kasabach-Merritt syndrome, 1035
Katayama fever, 1811, 1815
Kawasaki's disease, 1940, 1941, 2270
Kawasaki's syndrome, 352
Kayser-Fleischer rings, 1159, 1160
Kearns-Sayre syndrome, 2204, *2205*
Keloid, 2233
Keratan sulfaturia, 1148
Keratin, 2228
Keratinocyte, 2228
Keratitis, 2220
in herpesvirus hominis, 2221
Keratoacanthomas, 2297
Keratoconjunctivitis, 1715
epidemic, 1706
Keratoconjunctivitis sicca, 2223
Keratoses, seborrheic, 2255
Kerley's lines, 197
Keshan disease, 1210
Ketamine, abuse of, 2023–2024
Ketaoacidosis. See also *Diabetic ketoacidosis.*
alcoholic, 1336
Ketoconazole, 1759
in blastomycosis, 1763
in coccidioidomycosis, 1762
in histoplasmosis, 1761
in paracoccidioidomycosis, 1765
17-Ketogenic steroids
urinary, 1308
reference values for, 2327
α-Ketoglutarate:glyoxylate carboligase deficiency, 1108
Ketone bodies, serum and urinary, reference values for, 2327
Ketonuria, branched-chain, 1130
17-Ketosteroids
urinary, 1310, 1367
total, reference values for, 2328
Kidney(s)
acid-base balance regulation and, 498–499, 499t
acidification capacity measurement and, 510
adaptive functional changes in, 489
agenesis of, 145, 638
anatomy of, 490
anomaly of, 638–639
of number, 638
of parenchyma, 638–639
of position, 638
of vasculature, 639
bicarbonate processing by, 536–537
biopsy of, 514–515, 514t
blood flow of, 492
blood supply of, 490
cell-mediated immunity and, 504–505
coagulation-induced injury of, 505
collecting ducts of, defects in, 487
complement activation-associated glomerulonephritis of, 504
computed tomography of, *512*, 513
concentrating and diluting ability measurement and, 510
ectopic, 638
distal tubular defects of, 487
glomerulus of, 490, *491*, 492
immune-mediated injury of, 501–505, *502*, 503t
in ankylosing spondylitis, 1920
in blood cell mass regulation, 501

Kidney(s) (*Continued*)
in calcium metabolism regulation, 500
in cardiorespiratory arrest, 481
in gout, 1136
in Hippel-Lindau disease, 2086
in hydrogen ion secretion, 499
in magnesium metabolism regulation, 500
in mineral homeostasis regulation, 499–500
in phosphorus metabolism regulation, 500
in plasma protein metabolism, 501
in right ventricular failure, 199
in sarcoidosis, 436
in systemic candidiasis, 1768–1769
infection-mediated injury of, 506
interstitium of, 491
irradiation of, *2302*
isolated tubular defects of, 486
juxtaglomerular apparatus of, 491
medullary sponge, 506, 637–638
mineralocorticoid action in, 1306–1307
neoplastic injury of, 507
nephron of, 490
obstructive injury of, 507
parathyroid hormone and, 1434
parenchymal injury of, 501–507
peritubular capillaries of, 492
potassium processing by, 530–531, *531*
potassium transport function of, 497–498, *498*
proximal tubular defects of, 486–487
radiography of, 511–514, *513*
radiobiology of, 2299
radionuclide imaging of, 514
sodium transport function of, 493–494, *493, 496*
supernumerary, 638
toxin-mediated injury of, 505–506, 505t
tubular transport functions of, 493–498, *493, 496, 498*
tubules of, 491
water excretion regulation by, 497
ultrasonography of, *512*, 513–514
vascular injury of, 507
Kidney disease, 483–644. See also specific diseases.
acid-base balance in, 535–544
Alport's syndrome and, 506
amyloidosis and, 506
anti-tissue antibody-mediated, 502–503, *502*
biochemical injury and, 506
blood coagulation disorders with, 1053
cardinal findings in, 483–490
circulating immune complex-mediated, 503–504, 503t
cystic, 506, 633–638
classification of, 634, 634t
diagnosis of, 633, *633, 634*
treatment of, 634
cystinosis and, 506
diabetes mellitus and, 506, 616–619, *616, 618*
drug therapy effects on, 76–77, 76t, *77*
erythrocytosis and, 967
Fabry's disease and, 506
fluid volume, 515–523
genetic factors in, 506
in pregnancy, 624–627
metabolic injury and, 506
obstructive nephropathy in, 604–607, 605t
of glomerulus, 568–589
osmolality and, 523–529
parenchymal, 485–488
postrenal, 488
potassium balance and, 530–535
prerenal, 485, 485t
tubular, 608–616
Kidney disease (*Continued*)
tubulointerstitial, 504, 589–604, 589t
urinary manifestations of, 484
vascular disorders of, 623–624
vs. paravertebral tumor, 2185
with Crohn's disease, 745
Kidney failure
anemia with, 884
in pregnancy, 626–627
Kidney function, 483–484, 491–501, 491t, 493–500
blood volume effects on, 163
endocrine regulation of, 483
exocrine, 483–484
glomerular filtration rate measurements and, 509–510, *509*
homeostatic function of, 493–500
in pregnancy, 624–625, *625*
investigations of, 507–515
leukocyte excretion rate measurement in, 509
leukocyturia and, 509
protein excretion measurement in, 507–509
urine red blood cell measurement and, 509
Kidney stones, 628–633
analysis of, 631
clinical manifestations of, 631
composition of, 628, 628t, *629*
cystinuria and, 630, 631
diagnosis of, 631
dietary factor in, 629, 630
2,8-dihydroxyadenine, 1144
diuretics in, 632
etiology of, 628–634, 629t
fluid intake in, 631
hypercalciuria and, 629–630, 631
hyperoxaluria and, 630, 631
hyperparathyroidism and, 630, 631, 632
hyperuricosuria and, 630, 631
hyperuricosuric calcium oxalate in, 631
hypocitruria and, 630
idiopathic diathesis and, 631
in gout, 1136, 1138–1139
pathogenesis of, 628–634, 629t
renal tubular acidosis and, 630, 631
struvite, 631, 633
surgery for, 633
treatment of, 631–633
thiazides for, 632
urinary tract infection and, 630–631
with Crohn's disease, 745
with ulcerative colitis, 753
Kidney transplantation
clinical aspects of, 566
complications of, 566–567
disease recurrence with, 567, 567t
historical perspective on, 563
hypercalcemia and, 1450
hypercortisolism and, 566–567
histocompatibility and, 564
immune responses and, 564, 566, 567
immunologic aspects of, 564
immunosuppression with, 566, 567
in irreversible renal failure, 559, 563–568
living vs. cadaver donor for, 563–564, *565*
patient survival with, 568
recipient characteristics for, 564
rejection mechanisms with, 564, 566, 567, 568
retransplantation criteria for, 568
transfusions with, 566
with Fanconi's syndrome, 615
Kidney tumor, 488, 639–644. See also specific tumors.
algorithm for, 640, *640*
benign, 641
Kidney tumor (*Continued*)
classification of, 639, 639t
computed tomography in, 640, 641–642, *642*, 643
excretory urography in, 639, 640
magnetic resonance imaging in, 640
malignant, 641–643
metastatic, 644
sarcoma, 644
transitional cell, 643
ultrasonography in, 640
Kinetic apraxia, 1995
Kinin(s)
in shock, 214
sodium balance and, 497
Kinin-forming system in rheumatic disease, 1901
Kissing bugs, 1835
Klatskin tumor, 863
Klebsiella pneumonia, 1509–1510
clinical manifestations of, 1509
complications of, 1510
epidemiology of, 1509
laboratory findings in, 1509–1510
pathology of, 1509
prognosis in, 1510
radiography in, 1510
treatment of, 1510
Klebsiella pneumoniae, 1509–1510
Kleine-Levin syndrome, 1989, *1988*, 2025
Klinefelter's syndrome, 145, 1370–1371, *1371*, 1401, 1405
chromatin-negative, 1371
chromosome abnormality in, 1370–1371
genetic factors in, 1370–1371
Klippel-Feil syndrome, 145, 1387, 2084, 2187
Knees, in osteoarthritis, 1953
Koebner phenomenon, in psoriasis, 2246
KOH test and culture, in skin disease, 2236, *2237*
Koplik's spots, in measles, 1707
Korean hemorrhagic fever, 1751t
Korsakoff's amnestic syndrome, 2065
Korsakoff's dementia, 27
Korsakoff's syndrome, 1199, 1997
Kostmann's neutropenia, 955, 956
Kostmann's syndrome, 960
Krebs-Henseleit urea cycle, 805
Kupffer cell, 942
Kuru, 2135
Kveim-Siltzbach skin test, 436
in sarcoidosis, 432
Kwashiorkor, 335, 1183, 1184, 1185
clinical manifestations of, 1186–1187
diagnosis of, 1186–1187
Kyasanur forest disease, 1749, 1751t, 1755
Kyphoscoliosis, 453–454, 457
Kyphosis, 2187

Laboratory medicine, standard abbreviations in, 2315
Laboratory tests, 59, 61–63
accuracy of, 61
biological vs. statistical norms in, 63
clinical judgment in, 63
discontinuous distributions and, 63
distribution of values in, 62, *62*
drug therapy and, 62
in myopathies, 2200
law of errors and, 61
limitations of, 61
nonparametric methods in, 62
normal range and, 62–63
precision of, 61

Laboratory tests (*Continued*)
results evaluation in, 61
screening battery of, 61
sensitivity of, 61
sources of error in, 61–62
specificity of, 61
use and interpretation of, 61–63
value in diagnosis, 59, 63
Laboratory values of clinical importance, 2315–2340
Labyrinth, destruction of, ataxia, 2045
Labyrinthitis, acute, 2042
β-Lactamase (penicillinase) plasmid, 1647
Lactase deficiency, 710, 732
L-Lactate, blood, reference values for, 2328
Lactate dehydrogenase, serum and CSF, reference value for, 2328
Lactate/pyruvate ratio, reference values for, 2328
Lactation, 1398
nonpuerperal, 1398, 1398t
Lactic acidosis, 540
treatment of, 541
Lactogen, placental, 1253
Lactose, in restricted diet, 1213
Lactotrophs, 1252
Lactulose therapy, in hepatic encephalopathy, 846
Lacunar infarction, 2092
and stroke, *2095*, 2096
Lacunar strokes, 2095
Laennec's cirrhosis, *2263*
Lafora progressive myoclonus epilepsy, 2154
Lagophthalmos, 1282
Lamellar ichthyosis, *2251*
Laminectomy, in pain relief, 2053
Landry-Guillain-Barré-Strohl syndrome. See *Guillain-Barré syndrome.*
Langerhans cell, 942, 1009, 2228
eosinophilic, granulomatosis, 1009–1011
multifocal, 1010
unifocal, 1009–1010
Language
disturbances of, 1993–1995, *1994*
in schizophrenia, 2002
Laparoscopy, 660
in salpingitis, 1643, 1645
Laplace law, 193, *193*
Large intestine
neoplasms of, 761–769
epidemiology of, 761
histologic type, 761
Larva migrans, cutaneous, 1821–1822
Laryngeal aspiration, 672
Laryngeal cancer, cigarette smoking and, 48
Laryngitis
tuberculous, 1629
viral, 1695–1696, 1696t
Larynx, disease of, and ear pain, 2058
Laser iridotomy, in glaucoma, 2218
Laser trabeculoplasty, in glaucoma, 2218
Lassa fever, 1751t, 1756–1757
Lateral medullary syndrome, 2095
Lateral sinus thrombosis, 2115
Latex agglutination test
in cryptococcosis, 1766
in histoplasmosis, 1760
in rheumotoid arthritis, 1915
in sporotrichosis, 1767
Lathyrism, 783
Lathyrus sativus, 783
Laurence-Moon-Bardet-Biedl syndrome, 1172–1173, 1370
genetic factor in, 1172
Laurence-Moon-Biedl syndrome, 1370
Laxatives, 710
Lazy leukocyte syndrome, 956
LDL-cholesterol, serum or plasma, reference values for, 2328
LE. See *Systemic lupus erythomatosus.*
Lead
as nephrotoxin, 598–599
blood, reference values for, 2328
Lead absorption, screening tests for, *2308*
Lead mobilization test, *2309*
Lead nephropathy, chronic, 599
Lead poisoning, 892–893, 2307, 2309
acute, 598
Lecithin-cholesterol acyltransferase deficiency, 1116
Lecithin: cholesterol acetyltransferase, in liver disease, 810–811
Leeches, 1841
Left bundle branch block, 290
Left heart disease, pulmonary hypertension and, 258
Left heart hypoplastic syndrome, 235
Left ventricle
angiography study of, 186
dilatation of, mitral regurgitation and, 249, 250, 251
end-diastolic pressure, 192
function assessment of, with nuclear imaging, 179–181, *180*
hypertrophy of, in aortic regurgitation, 254–255
inflow obstruction to, 234–235
Left ventricular failure, 290
Cheyne-Stokes respiration in, 196
clinical manifestations of, 195–197
dyspnea in, 195–196
electrocardiography in, 197
heart signs in, 196–197
hemoptysis in, 196
mechanism of, 189
orthopnea in, 196
paroxysmal nocturnal dyspnea in, 196
physical signs, 196–197
pulmonary edema in, 196
pulmonary function tests in, 197
pulmonary hypertension and, 258
pulmonary signs in, 197
radiography in, 197
symptoms of, 195–196
with hypertension, 272
Leg(s), in alcoholic myopathy, 2066
nodose lesions of, 2259
weakness of, in striatonigral degeneration, 2079
Legionnaires' disease, 1515–1519
Legionella species, 1516–1517
Legionellosis, 1516–1519
clinical manifestations of, 1517–1518
diagnosis of, 1518
epidemiology of, 1517
etiology of, 1516–1517
pathogenesis of, 1517
prevention of, 1518–1519
therapy of, 1518
Leishmania, 1786–1787
Leishmania braziliensis, 1787, 1790–1791
Leishmania donovani, 1787
Leishmania mexicana, 1787, 1790, 1791
Leishmania tropica, 1790
Leishman-Donovan bodies, 1786
Leishmaniasis, 1786–1792
cutaneous, 1790–1792
chronic relapsing, 1790
clinical manifestations of, 1790
complications of, 1790–1791
diagnosis of, 1791
culture in, 1791
serology in, 1791
skin tests in, 1791
Leishmaniasis (*Continued*)
diffuse cutaneous, 1787, 1790–1791
epidemiology of, 1790
lupoid (recidiva), 1790
Old World vs. New World, 1790
pathology of, 1790
post–Kala azar, 1788
prevention of, 1791–1792
treatment in, 1791
vectors in, 1790, 1791–1792
etiology of, 1786
host factor in, 1787
immune response in, 1787
mucocutaneous, 1790–1792
skin test in, 1787
vector in, 1786
visceral. See *Kala azar.*
Lennert's lymphoma, 996
Lennox-Gastaut syndrome, 2152, 2154
Lentigines, nevoid, 2254
Lentiginous melanoma, acral, 2274
Lentigo (lentigines), 2254
senile, 2254
Lentigo maligna, 2274, *2274*
Lepromatous neuropathy, vs. syringomyelia, 2084
Leprosy, 1634–1639, 2196
borderline, 1635, 1636
classification of, 1635, 1635t
clinical manifestations of, 1636
diagnosis of, 1637
skin biopsy in, 1637
epidemiology of, 1634
etiology of, 1635
genetic factor in, 1634–1635
histopathology of, 1635
immune response in, 1634, 1635–1636
immunopathology of, 1635–1636
lepromatous, 1634, 1635, 1636
pathogenesis of, 1635
prevention of, 1638–1639
prognosis in, 1638
prophylaxis for, 1638–1639
reactional states in, 1634, 1636, 1638
reversal reactions in, 1636–1637, 1638
susceptibility to, 1634–1635
treatment of, 1637–1638
clofazimine for, 1637–1638
dapsone for, 1637–1638
resistance to, 1638
multidrug therapy in, 1638
rifampin for, 1637–1638
transmission of, 1634–1635
tuberculoid, 1634, 1635, 1636
vs. syringomyelia, 2084
Leptomeningeal metastases, and vertigo, 2043
Leptomeninges, metastatic tumors of, 2186
Leptospira interrogans, 1666, 1667
Leptospirosis, 1666–1668
antibiotics in, 1668
clinical features of, 1667
diagnosis of, 1667–1668
culture in, 1668
epidemiology of, 1666
immune response in, 1667
laboratory features of, 1667
pathology of, 1666–1667
prevention of, 1668
prognosis in, 1668
serology in, 1668
therapy of, 1668
Leriche's syndrome, 353, 359
Lesch-Nyhan syndrome, 136, 137, 1143
Leser-Trélat, sign of, 2255
Letterer-Siwe syndrome, 1010, 1248
Leucine, 1201

Leucine aminopeptidase, in liver disease, 809–810
Leukemia
  and central nervous system infection, 2142
  bone marrow transplantation for, *1026*, 1027, *1027*
  etiology of, 986–987
  human T cell, 980
  leukemoid reaction differentiation, 958–959
  ocular manifestations of, 2220
  prolymphocytic, 982
  radiation exposure and, 986–987
  retinopathy in, 2224
  RNA viruses and, 987
Leukemia—acute, 986–992
  bone marrow examination in, 960
  chemical-induced, 987
  chromosomal abnormality with, 987, 988
  classification of, 987–989, 988t
  clinical manifestations of, 989
  congenital conditions with, 987
  differential diagnosis of, 989–990
  drug-induced, 987
  genetic factor in, 987
  hyperuricemia with, 990
  incidence of, 987
  laboratory findings in, 989
  pathophysiology of, 987
  remission in, 990, 991
  supportive care in, 991–992
  therapy for, 990–991
    allopurinol in, 990
  vs. leukemoid reaction, 960
  with neutropenia, 955
Leukemia—acute lymphoblastic, 986
  central nervous system prophylaxis in, 990
  chromosome abnormalities in, 988–989
  classification of, 987–989, 988t
  clinical findings in, 989
  cytoplasmic markers for, 988
  histochemistry of, 987–988
  incidence of, 987
  laboratory findings in, 989
  morphology of, 987–988
  prognosis in, 990
  relapse in, 990
  remission in, 990
  surface markers for, 988
  therapy for, 990
    bone marrow transplantation in, 990
    chemotherapy in, 990
    maintenance therapy in, 990
    radiation therapy in, 990
Leukemia—acute lymphocytic, clonal development in, 963
Leukemia—acute myelogenous, 986
  central nervous system prophylaxis in, 991
  chromosomal abnormalities in, 988–989
  classification of, 987–989, 988t
  clinical findings in, 989
  cytoplasmic markers for, 988
  histochemistry of, 987–988
  immunotherapy in, 991
  incidence of, 987
  laboratory findings in, 989
  morphology of, 987–988
  platelet transfusion in, 992
  prognosis in, 991
  remission in, 990, 991
  supportive care in, 991–992
  surface markers for, 988
  therapy for, 990–992
    bone marrow transplantation in, 991
    chemotherapy in, 991
    granulocyte transfusion in, 991
    oral nonabsorable antibiotics in, 991
Leukemia—acute nonlymphocytic, chromosomal abnormalities in, 962
Leukemia—chronic, 975–986
Leukemia—chronic lymphocytic, 980–984, 995
  B lymphocyte proliferation in, 980–981, 982
  chromosome abnormality in, 982
  clinical manifestations of, 981
  clonal basis for, 962
  diagnosis of, 982
    differential, 982
  epidemiology of, 980
  genetic factor in, 980
  hypogammaglobulinemia in, 982
  immune response in, 980–981, 982
  laboratory abnormalities in, 981–982
  lymphocytosis in, 982
  mechanisms of, 980–981
  pathogenesis of, 980–981
  prognosis in, 983
  staging in, 981, 981t
  T-cell variants of, 980, 981
  treatment of, 982–983
    chlorambucil in, 982–983
    corticosteroids in, 983
    radiation therapy in, 983
  vs. leukemoid reaction, 960
Leukemia—chronic myelogenous (myeloid, myelocytic, granulocytic), 975–980
  accelerated (blastic) phase therapy, 979
  acute leukostatic complications with, 979
  blast crisis in, 977, 978
  clinical manifestations of, 977
  cytogenetic abnormalities in, 961–962, 975
  diagnosis of, 977–978
    bone marrow in, 978
    cytogenetic analyses in, 978
    differential, 978
    Philadelphia chromosome in, 975–980
  epidemiology of, 975–976
  etiology of, 975
  genetic factor in, 976
  laboratory abnormalities in, 977
    anemia, 977
    granulocytes, 977
  mechanisms of, 976–977
  neutrophil abnormalities in, 950
  neutrophil alkaline phosphatase activity in, 978
  pathogenesis of, 976–977
  physical examination in, 977
  prognosis in, 979–980
  radiation exposure and, 975, 976
  remission in, 962
  residual normal stem cells in, 962
  staging system for, 980
  thrombotic complications with, 979
  treatment of, 978–979
    bone marrow transplantation, 979
    busulfan in, 978, 979
    chemotherapy for, 978, 979
    hydroxyurea in, 978
    radiation therapy in, 979
    splenomegaly in, 977, 978
    tumor lysis syndrome with, 979
Leukemia—chronic myeloid, vs. leukemoid reaction, 959–960, 959t
Leukemia—chronic neutrophilic, 978
Leukemia—hairy cell, 982, 984–986
  acid phosphatase reaction in, 984–985
  B cell lineage of, 984, 985
  chromosome abnormality in, 985
  clinical manifestations of, 985
  diagnosis of, 985
    bone marrow in, 985
    cell staining in, 984
    differential, 985
Leukemia—hairy cell (*Continued*)
  electron microscopy in, 984, *984*
  immune response in, 985
  pathogenesis of, 984–985
  prognosis in, 985–986
  treatment of, 986
    androgen therapy in, 986
    chemotherapy in, 986
    interferon in, 986
    splenectomy in, 986
Leukemia—eosinophilic, 1011
Leukemia cutis, *2265*
Leukemoid reaction(s), 958–961, 978
  abnormal blood cells in, 958–959
  bone marrow in, 958–959
  colony-growing research in, 961
  eosinophilic, 960–961
  leukemia differentiation from, 958–959
  leukocytosis in, 958
  neutrophil alkalilne phosphatase reaction in, 978
  vs. acute leukemia, 960
  vs. chronic lymphocytic leukemia, 960
  vs. chronic myeloid leukemia, 959–960, 959t
  vs. idiopathic myelofibrosis, 959t
  vs. polycythemia vera, 959t
  with chronic myelogenous leukemia, 978
Leukeran. See *Chlorambucil.*
Leukocoria, in retinoblastoma, 2222
Leukocytes
  dysfunction of, 1478
  in anemia, 875
  kinetics of, 942
  with hemorrhage, 883–884
Leukocyte count
  differential, reference values for, 2339
  total, reference values for, 2338
Leukocytosis
  in chronic myelogenous leukemia, 977
  in infectious mononucleosis, 1720
  in leukemoid reaction, 958
  in polycythemia vera, 969, 970
Leukoerythroblastic reaction, 978
Leukoderma, chemical, 2297
Leukodystrophy(ies), 2148–2149
  globoid cell, 2148
  metachromatic, 2148
  sudanophilic, 2148
Leukoencephalitis, acute hemorrhaging, 2140–2141
Leukoencephalopathy, progressive multifocal, 2137
  immunosuppressive therapy and, 2142
Leukopenia, 953–958
  drug-induced, 1479
  in viral hemorrhagic fever, 1753
  infectious disease in, 1478, 1479, 1483
  management of, 1483–1484
  severe combined immunodeficiency disorder with, 1860
Leukoplakia, 666, *666*
Leukotomy, frontal, for pain relief, 2053
Leukotriene(s), 390, 391, 946, 1237–1241
  formation of, *1240*
Leukotriene B_4, 943
Levamisole, 1484
Levocardia, isolated, 240
Levodopa
  in parkinsonism, 2072–2073
  in postencephalitic parkinsonism, 2071
Levorphanol, in pain, 2052
Leydig cell agenesis (dysgenesis), 1356
Lhermitte's sign, in vitamin B_{12} deficiency, 2067
Lice, 1833–1834

Lichen planus, 2244–2245
Lichenification, 2233
Licorice extracts, in peptic ulcer, 689
Liddle's syndrome, 533, 542, 614
Lidocaine, 324–325
  in cardiopulmonary resuscitation, 482
  in digitalis toxicity, 204
  in myofascial pain syndrome, 2064
  pharmacokinetic parameters of, 70, 70t, 71, 72, *72*
Life cycle,15
  stages of, 20
Life expectation, 22
Life span, 22
Lifestyle, chronic disease prevention and, 35
Life-support systems
  discontinuation of, 11
  termination of, 479–480
Light, skin reactions to, 2252
Light-sensitive disease, 2254
Lightning injury, 2304
Limb(s). See also *Extremities.*
  in amyotrophic lateral sclerosis, 2079–2080
Limb-girdle dystrophy, 2199, 2203
  features of, *2202*
Limbic epilepsy, 2154
Limbic seizures, 2152
Limb-kinetic apraxia, 1995
Lincomycin, 105
Linear tomography, of chest, 383
Linguatuliasis, 1840–1841
Lipase, serum, reference values for, 2328
Lipid(s). See also *Fat.*
  absorption of, 720
  atherogenesis and, 38
  disorders of, in Friedreich's ataxia, 2083
  in nephrotic syndrome, 579
  sebaceous gland, 2230
  serum, in liver disease, 810–811
Lipid metabolism, in liver disease, 804–805
Lipid storage myopathies, 2205–2207, *2205*
Lipoatrophy, 1963
  total, *2263*
Lipodystrophy, partial, *2264*
Lipoid dermatoarthritis, 1959
Lipoid pneumonia, 2294–2295
Lipolysis
  impaired, 720, 720t
  micelle formation and, 720, 720t
β-Lipoprotein, 1253
Lipoprotein lipase deficiency, 1113, 1115
  genetic factor in, 1113
  xanthomas in, 1113
Lipoprotein metabolism
  acquired disorders of, 1114–1115
  inborn errors of, 1111–1114, 1112t
  rare disorders of, 1115–1116
Lipoprotein metabolism disorders, 1109–1120
Lipoproteins. See also *Cholesterol; Triglyceride(s).*
  atherogenesis and, 38
  catabolism of, 1110–1111
  cigarette smoking and, 48
  function of, 1109–1110
  in atherosclerosis, 282, 283
  in liver disease, 810–811
  physical characteristics of, 1109, 1109t
  structure of, 1109–1110
  transport of, 1109–1110, *1110*
β-Lipotropin, 1303
Lipoxygenase pathway, 1239–1240, *1240*
Lips, lesions of, 2244
Liquid diet, 1214
Listeria monocytogenes, 1609–1611
  serotypes of, 1610
Listeriosis, 781, 1609–1611
  bacteremia with, 1610
  carriers of, 1610
  clinical manifestations of, 1610
  diagnosis of, 1610–1611
    culture in, 1611
  epidemiology of, 1609–1610
  immunosuppression and, 1610, 2142
  in neonates, 1609, 1610, 1611
  in transplant recipients, 2142
  pathogenesis of, 1610
  pathology of, 1610
  prevention of, 1611
  prognosis in, 1611
  treatment of, 1611
    antibiotic therapy in, 1611
Lithiasis. See under specific types.
Lithium
  ADH activity and, 1268, 1268t
  as nephrotoxin, 600
  diabetes insipidus and, 1269
  elimination of, 81
  hypercalcemia and, 1449
  in cluster headache, 2056
  in hyperthyroidism, 1286
  in manic-depressive psychosis, 2007
  neutrophil production and, 957
  pharmacokinetic parameters of, 70t
  serum, plasma, and blood, reference values for, 2328
Litigation. See *Medicolegal considerations.*
Livedo reticularis, 356
Liver. See also *Hepatic.*
  abscess(es) of. See *Liver abscess(es).*
  benign adenoma of, in oral contraceptive use, 1393
  bilirubin transport by, 806–807
  biopsy of, in jaundice, 812
  biotransformation by, 805–806
  carcinoma of, 849–850
  detoxification by, 805–806
  diseases of. See under *Liver disease.*
  enlargement of. See *Hepatomegaly.*
  fatty, in alcoholic liver disease, 836
  focal nodular hyperplasia of, 849, 1393
  in bilharziasis, 1813–1814
  in hydatid disease, 1807–1808
  in Reye's syndrome, 2141
  in right ventricular failure, 198
  in Wernicke's encephalopathy, 2065
  infection of, bacterial, 828–829
    fluke, 1815–1817
    fungal, 828
  irradiation of, *2302*
  metastasis to, 850
  radiobiology of, 2299
  transplantation of, 848
  tumors of. See *Liver tumor(s).*
Liver abscess(es), 829–830
  amebic, 830
    epidemiology of, 830
    drug therapy in, 830
    serodiagnosis in, 830
  pyogenic, 829–830, *830*
    antibiotics for, 829–830
    aspiration of, 829–830, *830*
Liver disease, 803–851. See also *Hepatic encephalopathy* and specific diagnoses.
  alcohol intake in, 835–837
  alpha-antitrypsin deficiency and, 824, 832
  amino acid metabolism in, 805
  amyloidosis and, 833
  anemia with, 884
  blood coagulation disorders with, 1052–1053
  carbohydrate metabolism in, 804
Liver disease (*Continued*)
  cardiovascular disease and, 835
  cutaneous disorders with, *2263*
  cystic fibrosis and, 833
  drug-induced, 820–824
    causative agents of, 822–824
    diagnosis of, 820–821
    histopathologic classification of, 821–822, 821t
    management of, 820–821
  drug reactions and, 83
  drug therapy effects in, 77
  enteric bypass and, 834
  genetic factor in, 832–833
  glycogen storage disease and, 833
  granulomatous, 830–831
    associations reported with, 831, 831t
    differential diagnosis of, 831
  hemochromatosis and, 832–833
  hepatic biopsy in, 811
  hepatic metabolism in, 804–806
  hepatorenal syndrome with, 844–845
  history in, 803
  inflammatory intestinal disease and, 834
  laboratory tests in, 809–811
    alkaline phosphatase in, 809
    antinuclear antibodies in, 811
    clotting factors in, 810
    fibrinogen in, 810
    gamma-glutamyltranspeptidase in, 809–810
    hematologic tests in, 811
    leucine aminopeptidase in, 809–810
    lipoproteins in, 810–811
    mitochondrial antibody in, 811
    muscle antibodies in, 811
    5′-nucleotidase in, 809–810
    prothrombin time in, 810
    screening tests for, 809
    serum albumin in, 810
    serum globulins in, 810
    serum lipids in, 810–811
    stool examination in, 811
    transaminases in, 809
    urinalysis in, 811
    urobilinogen in, 811
  laparoscopy in, 660
  lecithin:cholesterol acyltransferase in, 810–811
  lipid metabolism in, 804–805
  parasitic, 827–828, 828t
  physical examination in, 803–804
  pregnancy and, 834–835
  protein metabolism in, 805
  protoporphyria and, 833
  sarcoidosis and, 833
  total parenteral nutrition and, 834
  toxic, 820–824
  transplantation in, 848
  vitamin D metabolism and, 1426
  Wilson's disease and, 824, 832, 1159
  with Crohn's disease, 744–745
  with ulcerative colitis, 753–754
Liver tumor(s), 848–851
  angiosarcoma, 850
  benign, 849
  biopsy in, 851
  cholangiocarcinoma, 850
  computed tomography in, 851
  diagnosis of, 851
    computed tomography in, 851
    endocrine factor in, 849
    fibrolamellar carcinoma, 849
    hemangioma, 849
    hepatocellular adenoma, 849
    hepatocellular carcinoma, 849–850

Liver tumor(s) (*Continued*)
  diagnosis of, malignant, 849–850
    oral contraceptives and, 849
    radionuclide scanning in, 851
    ultrasonography in, 851
Living will, 30
Loa loa, 1830
Lobar hematoma, 2105
Lobar hemorrhage, 2109t
Lobe, frontal, abscess of, 2113
    tumors of, 2163
  occipital, tumors of, 2163
  parietal, tumors of, 2163
  temporal, tumors of, 2163
Lobotomy, frontal, for pain relief, 2053
Locked-in state, definition of, 1971
Lockjaw. See *Tetanus.*
Locomotor ataxia, 2119–2120
Löffler's endomyocardial disease, 1011
Löffler's fibroplastic endocarditis, 337–338
Löffler's syndrome, 1822
Loiasis, 1830–1831
Long-acting thyroid stimulator, 1281
Loop of Henle, 494–495
  defect of, 487
Louping ill, 1749
Lowe's syndrome, with Fanconi's syndrome, 615–616
Lucio's phenomenon, in leprosy, 1636
Luft's disease, *2205*, 2206
Lumbar disc, herniation of, 2183
Lumbar puncture, 1968, 1968t
  and intracranial hypertension, 2058
  in back pain, 2063
  in brain abscess, 2113
  in headache, 2060
  in pseudotumor cerebri, 2168, 2169
  in spinal epidural abscess, 2117
  in subarachnoid hemorrhage, 2106
  in subdural empyema, 2115
  intracranial hypotension after, 2167
Lumbar spine, injury to, 2175, 2176
Lumbar spondylosis, 2184
Lung(s). See also *Pulmonary* and *Respiratory.*
  abscess(es) of. See *Lung abscess(es).*
  benign tumors of, 446
  biopsy of, 389
  carcinoma of, asbestos exposure and, 2284
    cigarette smoking and, 48, *48*
    occupationally related, 2287
    uncommon, 445
  cheese washer's, 2285
  diffusing capacity of, 377
  fat embolism syndrome of, 431–432
  fluke infection of, 1815, 1817–1818
  gas exchange in, 378–381, *379*, *380*
  hamartoma of, 446
  host defenses of, 1495–1496
  hyperlucent, unilateral, 406
  in ascariasis, 1822–1823
  in hydatid disease, 1807–1808
  in sarcoidosis, 434, *435*t
  in shock, 216, 220
  in tropical eosinophilia, 1830
  injuries to, chemical, 2289–2291
    occupational, 2287–2295
    physical, 2287–2295
    radiation, 2287–2288
    thermal, 2287
  irradiation of, *2302*
  neoplasms of, 439–447
    metastatic, 445–446
    primary lymphoma, 444–445
    pseudolymphoma, 445
  parenchymal infiltration of, 456
  pigeon breeder's, 2285
  radiobiology of, 2299
  radionuclide imaging of, 385

Lung(s) (*Continued*)
  solitary nodule of, 446–447
  ultrasonography of, 385
  ventilation in, 372–376, *373*, *374*, *375*, *376*
Lung abscess(es), 419–422, 1584–1585
  classification of, 420, 421t
  clinical manifestations of, 420
  definition of, 419
  diagnosis of, 420–421
    bronchoscopy in, 421, 422
    clindamycin in, 421–422
    radiography in, 420, *421*
  epidemiology of, 420
  etiology of, 420
  pathogenesis of, 420
  prognosis of, 422
  treatment of, 421–422
    penicillins in, 421–422
Lung aeration abnormalities, 404–406
  equation for, 466–467
  localized, 405–406
    hypoaeration, 404–405
Lung disease
  barometric pressure and, 2288–2289
  farmer's, 2285
  occupational, 2279–2287, *2279*
Lung perfusion scan, 385
Lung volumes, 372–374, *373*
  measurement of, 374
Lupus erythematosus. See also *Systemic lupus erythematosus.*
  anticoagulants associated with, 1057
  photosensitivity in, 2254
  retinopathy in, 2224
Lupus erythematosus cell, 1927, 1929, 1930
  rheumatic disease and, 1909
Lupus erythematosus syndrome, drug-induced, 84
Lupus nephritis, 585–586, 586t
  classification of, 585–586
  corticosteroids in, 586
  serologic monitoring in, 586
  treatment of, 586–587
Lupus pernio, 434
Luteinizing hormone, 1253, 1381, 1382
  function tests, 1255
  in hypopituitarism, 1256, 1258
  in male sexuality, 1366–1367, 1368, 1370
    isolated deficiency of, 1373
    serum or plasma and urine, reference values for, 2329
Lutembacher's syndrome, 229–230
Lyme disease, 1923–1924
Lymph node(s)
  biopsy of, 389
  mucocutaneous, syndrome of, 2270
Lymphadenitis
  mycobacterial, 1632–1633
  tuberculous, 736–737, 1627–1628
Lymphadenopathy
  cervical, in infectious mononucleosis, 1720
  differential diagnosis of, 994
  immunoblastic, 415
  in toxoplasmosis, 1793
  with cat scratch disease, 1618–1620, 1619t
Lymphangiectasia, 737
Lymphangiogram, retroperitoneal, 997
Lymphangiography, in Hodgkin's disease, 1005, *1005*
Lymphangioleiomyomatosis, 416
Lymphangitis, 365–366
Lymphatic filariasis, 1828–1830
  clinical manifestations of, 1829
  diagnosis of, 1829
  epidemiology of, 1828
  pathology of, 1828–1829
  prevention of, 1830
  treatment of, 1829–1830

Lymphatic filariasis (*Continued*)
  vector in, 1828, 1830
Lymphedema, 366
Lymphoblastic lymphoma, 995
Lymphocyte(s), 1846
  macrophage interaction with, *948*, 949
  precursors of, 867
Lymphocytic choriomeningitis, 1736
  virus in, 2123, 2125
Lymphocytic infiltrative disorders, 415
Lymphocytic interstitial pneumonitis, 415–416, 445
Lymphocytic lymphoma, 995, 996–997
  chemotherapy for, 998, 999
  radiation therapy for, 997, 998, 999
Lymphocytic thyroiditis, 1291, 1292–1293, *1292*
Lymphocytosis, in chronic lymphocytic leukemia, 982
Lymphogranuloma venereum, 1648–1649
  clinical manifestations of, 1649
  diagnosis of, 1649
    culture in, 1649
    serology in, 1649
  epidemiology of, 1648
  pathogenesis of, 1648–1649
  pathology of, 1648–1649
  treatment of, 1649
    antibiotic therapy in, 1649
Lymphokines, 949, 1846, 1848
  in sarcoidosis, 433–434
Lymphoma(s). See also *Non-Hodgkin's lymphoma.*
  and central nervous system infection, 2142
  Burkitt's. See *Burkitt's lymphoma.*
  cell classes of, 992, 992t
  intestinal, 736
  Lennert's, 996
  lymphoblastic, 995
  lymphocytic, 995, 996–997
    chemotherapy for, 998, 999
    radiation therapy for, 997, 998, 999
  primary, of central nervous system, in acquired immune deficiency syndrome, 2142
  pulmonary, 444–445
  T-cell, cutaneous, 2272–2273
Lymphopenia, 958
Lymphopenic hypogammaglobulinemia, 132
Lymphoproliferative disorders, 962–963
Lyon hypothesis, 120
Lysergic acid diethylamide (LSD), abuse of, 2023–2024
Lysosomal enzymes, in rheumatic disease, 1901
Lysosomal releasing factor, in shock, 217
Lysosomal storage disease, 132, 1146
Lysozyme, 946
  serum and plasma, reference values for, 2329

M component, 1170
  immunoglobulin in, 1020
  in plasma cell disorders, 1013
M protein, 1521, 1522, 1527
Macrocytosis, in anemia, 875, 875t
α_2-Macroglobulin, 1056
Macroglobulinemia, Waldenström's. See *Waldenström's macroglobulinemia.*
Macrophage(s), 1851
  activated, 946
  tissue, 941–942, *941*, 945–946, 946t
    evolution at inflammation site, 946, *947*
    in sarcoidosis, 433
    lymphocyte interaction with, *948*, 949
Macule, 2232
  coal, 2281

Madura foot, 1773
Maduromycosis, 1773
Major histocompatibility complex. See *Histocompatibility antigen.*
Magnesium, 1210. See also *Hypermagnesemia; Hypomagnesemia.*
  dietary, 1165
  dietary allowance for, 1179
  ionized, 1165
  metabolism of, 1165, 1166
    in uremia, 551
    regulation of, kidney in, 500
  serum, concentration of, 1165
    reference values for, 2329
  urine, reference values for, 2329
Magnetic resonance imaging, in kidney tumor, 640
Major histocompatibility complex, 1877–1883. See also *HLA system.*
  class I gene products encoded by H-2K and H-2D, 1878, *1879t*
  class II gene products encoded by H-2K region, 1878–1880, 1879t, *1880*
  genetics of, 1877–1883
  HLA-A, B, and C regions, 1880–1881
  HLA-D region, 1881
  human system, 1880–1883, *1880*
  immune response and, 1877–1880
  mouse research in, 1877–1880, *1877, 1878, 1879t, 1880*
  T cell and, 1878–1880, *1880*
  tissue transplantation and, 1877
Malabsorption, cutaneous disorders with, *2263*
Malabsorption syndrome(s). 649, 719–740, *2263*. See also specific diagnoses.
  bacterial overgrowth in, 726
  bleeding diathesis in, 724
  breath tests in, 726
  carbohydrate absorption in, 725
  classification of, 722, 722t
  clinical manifestations of, 722–723, 723t
  defective intraluminal hydrolysis or solubilization in, 729
  diagnosis of, 725–729
  drug-induced, 739
  fecal fat measurement in, 725
  inadequate surface factor in, 736
  infection with, 737
  jejunal aspirate culture in, 726
  jejunal histology in, 727–729, *728*
  laboratory tests in, 725–729, 726t
  lymphatic obstruction and, 736–737
  management of, 729–740
  mucosal cell abnormality in, 732
  pancreatic function in, 725
  pathophysiology of, 723–725, 723t
  prognosis of, 740
  radiography in, 726–727, *727*
  serum carotene in, 725
  small intestine biopsy in, 728t, 729
  stool examination, 725
  therapeutic agents in, dosages for, 729, 730t
  tryptophan metabolites in, 726
  vitamin B_{12} absorption in, 727
  with chronic pancreatitis, 775
  with Crohn's disease, 744
  with multiple defects, 737–738
  with vitamin K deficiency, 1052
  D-xylose absorption in, 725
Malabsorptive enteropathy, with dermatitis herpetiformis, 2269
Malaria, 1776–1780
  antimalarial drugs for, 1778–1780
  asymptomatic, 1778
  blood transfusion and, 939
Malaria (*Continued*)
  chemoprophylaxis for, 1493, 1780
  clinical manifestations of, 1777–1778
  complications of, 1778, 1779
  control of, 1780
  diagnosis of, 1778
    blood film examination in, 1778
    serology in, 1778
  epidemiology of, 1776–1777
  etiology of, 1776
  glucose-6-phosphate dehydrogenase deficiency and, 905–906
  hemolysis with, 913
  host factor in, 1777
  immune response in, 1777
  pathogenesis of, 1777
  pathology of, 1777
  pregnancy and, 1778, 1780
  prevention of, 1780
  recrudescence in, 1778
  sickle cell trait and, 927, 1777
  thalassemia trait and, 923
  therapy bof, 1778–1780
  vector in, 1776–1777
    species differences of, 1776, 1776t
Malassezia furfur, infection with, 2246, *2247*
Male climacteric, 21
Male infertility, 1372
Male pseudohermaphroditism, 1354–1362, 1388
  dysfunction of, androgen-dependent target areas in 1359–1362, *1360, 1361, 1362*
  classification of, 1354t
  chromosome abnormality in, 1354–1360, *1355*
  genetic factor in, 1354–1360, *1355*
  testicular function disorders in, 1356–1359, 1357t
Male sexual development
  and XX males, 1362–1363
  at puberty, 1368–1369
    gonadotropin releasing hormone in, 1368
  climacteric in, 1374
  fetal, differentiation abnormalities in, 1353–1354, *1354*
    differentiation factors in, 1353–1354, *1354*, 1365, *1366*
    genetic control of, 1354
    genital development in, 1352–1353, *1352*
    gonadal differentiation in, 1351, *1351*
    phenotypic differentiation in, 1352–1354, *1353*
Male sexual function
  disorders of, 2030–2031, *2030*
    impotence and, 1374
Male sexuality, maturation of, 17–18
Malformations, arteriovenous, 2104
    with aneurysm, 2103
    cerebrovascular, 2104
Malignant changes in skin, 2271–2276
Malignant disease
  neuropathy with, 2195
  ichythosis in, 2251
Malingering
  vs. hysteria, 2013
  vs. syncope, 1986
Mallory-Weiss lesions, 677, 794
Malnutrition, 1179–1183. See also *Protein-calorie malnutrition.*
  clinical assessment in, 1181t, 1182
  dietary constituents in, 1184–1185
  in childhood, sequelae of, 1184–1185
  laboratory assessment in, 1182–1183, 1182t
  protein-calorie, hypothalamic-pituitary-adrenal axis in, 1185
Maltase, acid, deficiencies of, 2205
Malum coxae senilis, 1953
Mammography, 1402
Mania, in manic-depressive psychosis, 2006
Manic-depressive psychosis, 2005–2007
Manganese, 1210
  deficiency of, 1210
  poisoning with, 1210
Manganese toxicity, 2314
Mannitol, as nephrotoxin, 604
Mannose-6-phosphate residues, 1104
Manometry, in esophageal motor disorders, 673–674, 673t
Mansonella ozzardi infection, 1831
Mansonella perstans, 1831
Mansonella streptocerca, 1833
Mantoux test, 386, 1622–1623
Maple syrup urine disease, 1130
  genetic factors in, 1130
Marasmus, 1183, 1185
  clinical manifestations of, 1187
  diagnosis of, 1187
Marburg-Ebola disease, 1757
Marburg virus, 1757
March hemoglobinuria, 913
Marchiafava-Bignami disesae, 2067
Marfan's syndrome, 346, 1149, 1151, 1458
  genetic factors in, 1149
Marijuana, abuse of, 2022–2023
Marine animal poisoning, 1843–1845, 1843t, *1844*
Maroteaux-Lamy syndrome, 1148
Marrow neutrophil reserve, 956
Marrow transplantation, in inborn errors of metabolism, 132
Mast cell, 1887, *1887*. See also *Mastocytosis.*
  derived products, 1887t
  in allergic rhinitis, 1867
  in urticaria-angioedema, 1864, 1866
Mast cell disease, 2271
Mastocytosis, 739, 1887–1889, 2271
  clinical manifestations of, 1887–1888
  diagnosis of, 1888
  malignant, 1889
  pathophysiology of, 1888
  prognosis in, 1888–1889
  systemic, *2263, 2265*
  treatment of, 1888
Masturbation, 19
Matter, white, spongy degeneration of, 2148
Mayaro, 1740
Maximal inspiratory pressure, 464
McArdle's disease, 1107, 2205
McCune-Albright syndrome, 1369, 1407, 1465
Mean corpuscular hemoglobin, 875
  reference values for, 2339
Mean corpuscular hemoglobin concentration, 875
  reference values for, 2339
Mean corpuscular volume, 875
  reference values for, 2339
Measles, 1706–1709
  acute disseminated encephalomyelitis after, 2140
  antibody prophylaxis for, 1708
  atypical, 1708
  clinical manifestations in, 1707–1708, *1707*
  complications of, 1708
  culture in, 1708
  cutaneous lesions in, *2260*
  diagnosis of, 1708–1709, 1709t
    serology in, 1708
  epidemiology of, 1706–1707
  etiology of, 1706
  immune response in, 1706–1707
  immunization for, 43t, 44–45
  pathology of, 1707
  physiologic responses in, 1707
  prevention of, 1709
  prognosis in, 1709

Measles (*Continued*)
treatment of, 1709
Measles vaccine, 42t, 1707, 1709
Measles virus, in subacute sclerosing panencephalitis, 2136
Mebendazole
for ascariasis, 1823
for hookworm disease, 1821
in enterobiasis, 1825
in tapeworm infection, 1809
in trichinellosis, 1826
in trichuriasis, 1824
Mechlorethamine. See *Nitrogen mustard.*
Meckel's diverticulum, 708
Meclazine, in vertigo, 2043
Meconium ileus, 424, 425
Mediastinal disease
diagnosis of, 451–452
computed tomography in, 451, *451*
radiography in, 451, *451*
symptoms of, 451
Mediastinitis, 452
Mediastinoscopy, 389
in bronchogenic carcinoma, 443
Mediastinum, anatomy of, 451
tumor of, 452, *452*
Medicaid, 7
Medical care, 60
costs of, 8
Medical education, 2–4
clinical experience in, 3–4
in science, 2–3
Medical ethics, 9, 11–14
competency factor in, 12–13
confidentiality and, 13
economic considerations and, 13–14
external factors affecting, 13–14
indications for medical intervention and, 11–12
life prolongation and, 12
paternalism vs. autonomy in, 12–13
principle of beneficence in, 1–2
quality of life factor in, 13
research and, 13
Medical history, 58
Medical profession, 1–14. See also *Medical ethics.*
as art, 1–4
as science, 4–6
defensive aspects of, 8
definition of, 1
historical development of, 9–11
physician as nonphysician in, 4
practice patterns in, 7
public accountability and, 8
public service aspect of, 7–8
Medical record(s), in medical practice, 8
problem-oriented organization of, 60
values of, 60
Medical research, 8
Medical science, 4–6
historical development of, 5–6, 8
physician's role in, 6
Medicare, 7
Medicolegal considerations, in practice of medicine, 8
Mediterranean fever, familial, *2263, 2264*
Medulla, in ataxia telangiectasia, 2086
arterial supply of, 2089, *2089*
Medullary cystic disease, 506
Medullary sponge kidney, 506, 637–638
Medullary syndrome, lateral, 2095
Medulloblastoma, characteristics of, *2162*
Mefloquine, in malaria, 1779
Megacolon
congenital vs. acquired, 711–712, *712*
radiography in, 712, *712*
Megacolon (*Continued*)
toxic, 750, *751*
Megakaryocytes, 869
reduced, 1032
Megaloblastic anemia, 893–900
bone marrow in, 894
DNA synthesis in, 893–895
drug-induced, 899
erythrocytes in, 894
erythropoiesis in, 894
etiologic classification of, 893–894, 893t
folate deficiency and, 893, 898–899
folic acid deficiency and, 724
genetic factors in, 893–900
mechanism of, 894
pathogenesis of, 894–895
pathology of, 894–895
pathophysiology of, 894–895
unresponsive, 899
vitamin B_{12} deficiency and, 724, 893, 895–897
Megaloblasts, morphology of, 894
Megaloureter, 639
Megalourethra, 639
Megestrolacetate, in cancer chemotherapy, 1101t
Meibomian glands, 2230
Meigs' syndrome, 2078–2079
pleural involvement with, 449
vs. tardive dyskinesia, 2076, *2076*
Meiosis, 122, 138–139
Melanocytes, 2228
concentration of, pigment pattern and, 2254
Melanocyte-stimulating hormones, 1303
Melanoma
cutaneous, 2274–2276
malignant, intraocular, 2222
Melanosis, diffuse, 2256
Melarsoprol, in African trypanosomiasis, 1782, 1783
MELAS, *2205*
Melasma, 2256, *2256*
Melatonin, 1243
biosynthesis of, 1274, *1274*
Melena, 791, 792
with peptic ulcer, 694
Melioidosis, 1608–1609
acute septicemic, 1608, 1609
clinical manifestations of, 1608
diagnosis of, 1608
culture in, 1608
serology in, 1608
epidemiology of, 1608
in veterans, 1608
pathogenesis of, 1608
pathology of, 1608
prevention of, 1609
prognosis of, 1609
subacute (chronic), 1608, 1609
treatment of, 1608–1609
Melphalan, 1096, 1096t
in multiple myeloma, 1017–1018
Membrane toxin, and myoglobinuria, 2210
Memory
impairment of, 1996–1997
in delirium, 1974
in Alzheimer's diseae, 2000
Menadione, 1208
Menarche
as part of life cycle, 17–18, 1382
hormone therapy with, 1394–1395
normal and abnormal, 1385–1388
sex steroid hormones and ovarian function after, 1388–1391, 1389t
Mendelian inheritance, 117–118, *118, 119, 120*
Meniere's syndrome, 2039
and vertigo, 2042
tinnitus in, 2040
Meningeal carcinomatosis, 2164
treatment outcome in, 2166
Meningeal neoplasm, diffuse, 2164
Meninges, vascular malformation of, in Sturge-Weber disease, 2085
Meningioma(s)
intracranial, in neurofibromatosis, 2085
mesodermal, characteristics of, *2162*
of spinal cord, 2186
treatment outcome in, 2166
Meningitis
and headache, 2057
and listeriosis, 1609–1611
anthrax, 1607
aseptic, 2122
bacterial, 1551–1557
age factor in, 1552
antimicrobial therapy in, 1555–1556
clinical manifestations of, 1552–1553
clinical settings for, 1551–1552
complications of, 1554
diagnosis of, 1554
epidemiology of, 1551
etiology of, 1551, 1551t
laboratory diagnosis of, 1553
cerebrospinal fluid examinatiion in, 1553, 1556
cultures in, 1553
meningococcal, 1559, 1561, 1562
neonatal, 1552
neurologic findings in, 1552–1553
pathogenesis of, 1552
pathology of, 1552
prognosis in, 1555
recurrent, 1554–1555
treatment of, 1555–1556
chemical, vs. bacterial meningitis, 1554;
cryptococcal, immunosuppressive therapy and, 2142
in transplant recipients, 2142
enteric bacteria in, 1593
eosinophilic, *Angiostrongylus cantonensis* in, 1826
from herpes simplex virus infection, 1716
granulomatous, and vertigo, 2043
Hemophilus influenzae, 1564
in coccidioidomycosis, 1762
in mumps virus infection, 1712
listerial, in transplant recipients, 2142
meningococcal, vs. staphylococcal meningitis, 1547
Mollaret's, viral role in, 2137
serous, 2122, 2168. See also *Pseudotumor cerebri; Viral meningitis.*
staphylococcal, 1547
syphilitic, acute, neurologic changes in, 2118
symptomatic, 2119
tuberculous, 1629
viral, 1689t, 1690t, 2122–2126
with angiostrongyliasis, 1826
Meningocele, spinal, 2187
Meningococcal disease, 1557–1562
chemoprophylaxis in, 1562
clinical manifestations of, 1559–1561
complications of, 1561
course of, 1561
diagnosis of, 1561
epidemiology of, 1557–1558
etiology of, 1557
immune response in, 1558
immunization for, 45
immunity to, 1558
in hospital-acquired infection, 1492

Meningococcal disease (*Continued*)
  incidence of, 1557
  nosocomial transmission of, 1558
  pathogenesis of, 1559
  pathology of, 1559
  prevention of, 1562
  prognosis in, 1562
  treatment of, 1561–1562
    antimicrobial therapy in, 1561
Meningococcal vaccine, 42t, 1562
Meningococcemia, 1559–1560, *1560*, 1561–1562, *2266*
  cutaneous lesions in, *2260*
Meningoencephalitis, 2122. See also *Viral encephalitis.*
  amebic, 1801
  aspergillar, immunosuppressive therapy and, 2142
Meningomyelitis, syphilitic, vs. vitamin B_{12} deficiency, 2067
Meningomyelocele, and syringomyelia, 2084
Meningomyelopathy, and ataxia, 2044
Meningonemiasis, human, 1832
Meningovascular syphilis, 2119
  neurologic changes in, 2118
Menkes' syndrome, 1210
  genetic factor in, 1210
Menopause, 1381
  as part of life cycle, 21
  estrogen therapy and, 1393, 1395
  osteoporosis and, 1456–1457
  sex steroid hormones and ovarian function after, 1391
Menoquinone, 1208
Menstrual cycle, 1381, 1382t
  endometrium in, 1382
  gonadotropin releasing hormone in, 1382
  iron deficiency and, 889
  mechanism of, 1380
  toxic shock syndrome and, 1545
Mental changes, in intracranial tumor, 2163
Mental retardation, 146
  depression in, 2012
  in Sturge-Weber disease, 2086
  in tuberous sclerosis, 2085
Meperidine, in heart failure, 199
Mephenytoin, in epilepsy, *2158*, 2159
Mephobarbital, in epilepsy, *2158*, 2159
Meprobamate
  in myofascial pain syndrome, 2064
  in pain, 2051
Meralgia paresthetica, 2197
Mercaptopropionylglycine, in cystinuria, 613
6-Mercaptopurine, 1095, 1201
  in acute lymphoblastic leukemia, 990
  in Crohn's disease, 747
Mercurials, 599
Mercury
  as nephrotoxin, 599–600
  blood, reference values for, 2329
  inorganic, poisoning by, 2309–2310
Mescaline, abuse of, 2023–2024
Mesenteric artery, 756–757, *757*
  embolism of, 759, *759*
  occlusion of, 758–759, *758*
Mesenteric fibromatosis, 791
Mesenteric panniculitis, 790–791
Mesenteric venous thrombosis, 760
Mesenteritis, retractile, 790–791
Mesentery
  circulation of, 756–757, *756*, *757*
  cyst of, 791
  tumor of, 791
Mesentery disease, 790–791
  inflammatory, 790–791
Mesial temporal sclerosis, in epilepsy, 2150
Mesoblastic nephroma, 641
Mesocardia, 240
Mesodermal meningioma, characteristics of, *2162*
Mesothelioma
  malignant, in asbestos workers, 2283
  of pleura, 450
Metabolic acidosis, 465, 499, 519, 537, 538
  acid excretion reduction in, 540
  acidifying salts and, 540
  anion gap in, 539–541
  bicarbonate losses in, 539–540
  bicarbonate regeneration failure in, 540
  chronic, 1427
  diagnosis of, 541
  dilutional, 539
  drug intake and, 541
  etiology of, 539, 539t
  hyperchloremic, 540
    hyperkalemic, 610
    hypokalemic, 608, 609
    normokalemic, 610
  hyperkalemic, hyperchloremic, 540
  organic acid accumulation in, 540–541
  pathogenesis of, 539
  treatment of, 541
  with uremia, 550
  in acute renal failure, 546
Metabolic alkalosis, 465, 499, 537, 538, 542–543
  and mineralocorticoids, 542
  chronic, 533
  clinical features of, 543
  diagnosis of, 543
  etiology of, 542–543, 542t
  hypokalemic, hypochloremic, 537
  organic acids accumulation and, 542
  pathogenesis of, 542
  potassium depletion in, 542
  sodium chloride transport and, 542
  treatment of, 543
  urine chloride concentration in, 511
  volume contraction in, 542
Metabolic alterations, myoglobinuria in, 2210
Metabolic brain disease
  causes of, *1973*
  clinical features of, 1974–1975
  exogenous, 1973–1975
  laboratory evaluation of, 1975, *1975*
  physical examination in, *1974*
Metabolic depression, myoglobinuria in, 2210
Metabolic diseases, 1103–1173
  acquired, 1104
  altered DNA structure in, 1103
  altered protein function in, 1103
  cellular disturbances in, 1103–1104
  enzyme deficiencies in, 1103
  functional disturbances in, 1103–1104
  genetic factor in, 1103–1104
  membrane function in, 1103–1004
Metabolic disorders,
  and epilepsy, 2150
  cutaneous and renal manifestations of, *2264*
  neuroendocrine system in, 1250
Metabolic factor, in hemolysis, 913
Metabolic lesions, *1971*
Metabolic myopathies, definition of, 2204
Metabolism. See also *Inborn errors of metabolism; Carbohydrate(s), Lipid(s), Protein(s),* etc.
  hormone control factor in, 1228–1229
  oxidative, in Friedreich's ataxia, 2083
Metachromatic leukodystrophy, 2148
Metagonimus yokogawai, 1818
Metals
  as nephrotoxins, 598–601, 598t
  hard, diseases caused by, 2284
Metals (*Continued*)
  trace, poisoning from, 2307–2315
Metal fume fever, 2285
Metallic mercury poisoning, 2309
Metallothionein gene, 134
Metamorphopsia, 2033
Metamyelocyte(s), 940–941
Metanephrine, total, reference values for, 2329
Metastasis, enteric bacterial infection with, 1594
Metastatic tumors, neuropathy with, 2195
Methadone
  in opiate dependence, 2019
  in pain, 2052
Methanol
  blood, urinary, and breath, reference values for, 2329
  poisoning from, 89
Methemoglobin, reference values for, 2339
Methemoglobinemia, 932, 934–936, *2265*
  acquired, 935, 935t
  classification of, 934
  drug-induced, 934, 935, 935t
  genetic factor in, 934–935
  pathophysiology of, 934
  toxic, 935, 935t
  with abnormal hemoglobins, 935, 935t
  with defective methemoglobin reduction, 934
Methicillin, vs. nephrotoxin, 596t, 597
Methicillin-resistant staphylococci, 1550
Methimazole, 1284–1285
Methionine
  in homocystinuria, 1131
  intake of, in cystinuria, 612
Methisazone, for poxvirus infection, 110
Methotrexate, *1092*, 1093–1094
  as nephrotoxin, 602
  in acute lymphoblastic leukemia, 990
  in psoriasis, 2246
  interstitial lung disease and, 418
  toxicity of, 1092, 1094
Methotrimeprazine, in pain, 2052
Methoxyflurane, as nephrotoxin, 602
Methsuximide, in epilepsy, *2158*, 2159
6-Methyl hydroxyprogesterone, in cancer chemotherapy, 1101t
MethylCCNU, in cancer chemotherapy, 1096t, 1097
Methysergide
  in cluster headache, 2056
  in migraine, 2055
Methylated nucleosides, 1076
Methylcobalamin, 895
Methylcobalamin deficiency, 1131
Methyldopa
  hepatotoxicity of, 823
  in hypertension, 278
Methylene blue, 934–935
5,10-Methylenetetrahydrofolate reductase deficiency, 1131
Methylmalonic aciduria, 132
Methylmalonyl CoA mutase, 895
N-Methylnicotinamide, 1202
Methylprednisolone, 114
  dosage regimen for, 114
  in respiratory failure, 461
  topical, in skin disease, 2240
Methyltransferase, thymidylate synthetase and, 895, *895*
Methyxanthines, in asthma, 395
Metoprolol
  in angina pectoris, 287
  in essential tremor, 2074
Metorchis conjunctus, 1818
Metrifonate, in urinary bilharziasis, 1813

Metronidazole, 105, 1586, 1665
in Crohn's disease, 747
in giardiasis, 1803
in liver abscess, 830
Metyrapone
in Cushing's syndrome, 1316, 1317
stimulation test with, 1309
reference values for, 2329
Metyrapone test, in Addison's disease, 1311
Miconazole, 1759
in coccidioidomycosis, 1762
in paracoccidioidomycosis, 1765
Microadenomatosis, 696
Microaneurysms, in diabetic retinopathy, 2223
Microangiopathic hemolytic disorders, 914–915, 914t
Microcirculation
hemolytic disorders and, 914–915, 914t
in shock, 215–216, 223
Microcytosis, in anemia, 875, 875t
Microscopy, electron, in myopathies, 2201
Microsporum infections, 2247
Microvascular anomalies, intraretinal, 2223
Micturition, abnormalities of, 2028–2030, *2029*
Midarm muscle circumference, 1181t, 1182
Midbrain
arterial supply of, 2089, *2090*
in striatonigral degeneration, 2079
Middle age, as part of life cycle, 20
Mid-life crisis, 21
Migraine, 2054–2056
ergotamine tartrate in, 2055
"hemiplegic," 2098
late-life, and drop attacks, 2047
vs. tension headache, 2056
Migratory erythema, necrolytic, *2263*
Migratory polyarthritis, in rheumatic fever, 1529
Miliaria crystallina, 2229
Miliaria profunda, 2229
Miliaria rubra, 2229
Miliary tuberculosis, 1629–1630
Milk-alkali syndrome, 543, 1449
Milrinone, 204
Milwaukee shoulder, 1955
Mineral deficiency, in gastrointestinal disease, 646
Mineral homeostasis, kidney in regulation of, 499–500
Mineral metabolism, hormone factor in control of, 1229
Mineral oil, interstitial lung disease and, 418
Mineralocorticoids, 1302
actions of, 1306–1307
excess states, 1317–1320
function assessment and, 1309–1310
hypertension and, 276, 1317–1319
in Addison's disease, 1312
in renal tubular acidosis, 610
kidney and, 1306–1307
metabolic alkalosis and, 542
metabolism of, 1302–1303
production regulation and, 1304–1305, *1304*
Mineralocorticoid therapy, 114
Minerals
dietary allowance for, 1178–1179
homeostasis of, 1415–1426
Minimental status examination, in diagnosis of dementia, 1998–1999, *1999*
Minocycline, in rickettsial disease, 1676
Minoxidil, in hypertension, 278
Mirizzi's syndrome, 856
Mite-borne typhus, 1684
Mithracin. See *Mithramycin.*
Mithramycin
in multiple myeloma, 1019
in Paget's disease of bone, 1462
Mitochondrial myopathies, 2207
Mitomycin, 1098
Mitomycin C–induced hemolytic uremic syndrome, 914–915
Mitochondria, in shock, 216–217
Mitochondrial antibody, in liver disease, 811
Mitochondrial myopathies, 2205, *2205*
Mitosis, 122, 138
Mitotane
in Cushing's syndrome, 1316, 1317
steroid therapy and, 1303
Mitral commissurotomy, 249
Mitral insufficiency, acute, 289
Mitral regurgitation, 249–252, 249t
angina pectoris and, 284
clinical features of, 250
coronary artery disease and, 249, 250, 251
differential diagnosis of, 251
etiology of, 249
laboratory studies in, 251
cardiac catheterization in, 251
echocardiography in, 251
electrocardiography in, 251
radiography in, 251
medical treatment of, 251
mitral valve prolapse and, 249, 250, 251
pathology of, 249
physical examination in, 250–251
physiology off, 249–250
prophylaxis of bacterial endocarditis in, 251
rheumatic fever and, 249
surgical considerations in, 252
valve replacement in, 252
Mitral stenosis, 246–249
and stroke, 2092, *2092*
clinical features of, 246–247
congenital, 235
differential diagnosis of, 248–249
etiology of, 246
in Lutembacher's syndrome, 229–230
laboratory studies in, 248
cardiac catheterization in, 248
echocardiography in, 248
electrocardiography in, 248
radiography in, *168*, *169*, 248
medical treatment in, 249
pathology of, 246
physical findings in, 247–248
physiology of, 246
prophylaxis of bacterial endocarditis, 249
pulmonary hypertension and, 246–247, 248
rheumatic fever and, 246, 249
surgical treatment in, 249
valve replacement in, 249
Mitral valve
prolapse of, and stroke, 2092, *2092*
supravalvular ring above, 235
Mitral valve prolapse, 229
Mitral regurgitation and, 249, 250, 251
Mixed connective tissue disease, 1909, 1935
with interstitial lung disease, 414
Mol deficiency, 952
Molecular biology, 5
Molecular disease, concept of, 128
Moles. See *Pigmented nevi.*
Mollaret's meningitis, viral role in, possibility of, 2137
Molluscum contagiosum virus, infection with, 2249
Mollusks, food poisoning from, 783
Molybdenum, dietary allowance for, 1179
Molybdenum toxicity, 2314
Monckeberg's sclerosis, 358
Monge's disease, 2288–2289
Moniliasis, 665, *665*
Monoamine oxidase inhibitors
in anxiety, 2010
in manic-depressive psychosis, 2006–2007
Monamine oxidase inhibitors (*Continued*)
tyramine and, 274–275
Monoclonal antibodies, 961
Monoclonal gammopathies of undetermined significance, 1022
Mononeuropathy multiplex. See also *Neuropathy, Multifocal.*
definition of, 2188
Mononuclear leukocytes, in inflammation, 1904, 1904t
Monocyte(s), 941–942, *941*, 945–946
mature, 942
Monocytopenia, 958
Monogenic disorders, 117–118, *118t*
Monokines, 949
Mononuclear phagocyte(s), 942–949, 946–949
as scavengers, 946–948
differentiation of, 945
functions of, 946–949
ingestion by, 946–949
killing action of, 948–949, 948t
lymphocyte interaction with, *948*, 949
secretion of, 946, 947t
structure of, 945
Mononucleosis, infections, 1719–1712
Mono-octanoin, 861
Monosaccharides, malabsorption of, 732
Monosodium glutamate, and headache, 2056
Monosodium L-glutamate, 782
Montgomery's tubercles, 2230
Morbilli. See *Measles.*
Morphine
abuse of, 2016–2019
in heart failure, 199
in pain, 2052
terminal, 32, 32t
Morquio-like syndrome, with B-galactosidase deficiency, 1148
Morquio's syndrome, 1148
Mortality, Gompertz concept and, 23–24, *24*
Mortality statistics, 35t, 36
for accident, *35t*, 36
Mosaicism, 961
immunoglobulin, 962
Moschcowitz's syndrome, 1035
Mosquito(es), 1835
Mosquito-borne virus infections, 2125
Mossman fever, 1684
Motor apraxia, 1995
Motor dysfunction, in Friedreich's ataxia, 2083
Motor function
episodic loss of, 2046–2047
impairment of, in amyotrophic lateral sclerosis, 2080
in Werdnig-Hoffman disease, 2080
Motoneuron, lower, anatomy and physiology of, 2178
Motor neuron disease(s), 2079–2080
postpoliomyelitic, 2132
primary, vs. postpoliomyelitis motor neuron disease, 2132
Motor neuron signs, combinations of, 2199
Motor neuropathy
hereditary, 2194–2195
of proximal lower extremity, in diabetics, 2193
Motor symptoms, in epilepsy, 2151
Motor unit, definition of, 2198
Mountain sickness, acute, 2288–2289
Mouth. See also *Oral* entries.
cancer of, 666–667, *667*
erosions of, 2244
infections of, 2243
lesions of, 2243–2244
Movement, abnormal involuntary, in extrapyramidal disorders, 2068

Movement disorders, 2068
Moxalactam, 1586
Moyamoya, 2093
MPS storage diseases. See *Mucopolysaccaridoses* and names of specific syndromes.
Mu chain disease, 1021
Mucocutaneous candidiasis. See *Candidiasis.*
Mucocutaneous leishmaniasis, 1790–1792
Mucocutaneous lymph node syndrome, 1940, 1941, 2270
Mucoepidermoid tumor, of lung, 445
Mucopolysaccharide storage disease, 131
Mucopolysaccharidoses, 130, 132, 347, 1146–1149, 1147t. See also names of specific syndromes.
  genetic factor in, 1146
Mucormycosis, 1479, 1771–1773
  clinical manifestations of, 1772
  cultures in, 1772
  cutaneous, 1772
  cutaneous lesions in, *2261*
  diagnosis of, 1772
  disseminated, 1772
  epidemiology of, 1772
  etiology of, 1771–1772
  gastrointestinal, 1772
  pathogenesis of, 1772
  pathology of, 1772
  prognosis of, 1772–1773
  pulmonary, 1772
  rhinocerebral, 1772
  treatment of, 1772
Mucosa, buccal, damage to, 2244
Mucosal neuroma syndrome, 1407
Mucous membranes, in Wernicke's encephalopathy, 2065
Mucus secretion, in infection, 1478
Muir's (Torre's) syndrome, 766
Müllerian (paramesonephric) ducts, 1352
Müllerian dysgenesis, 1386
Müllerian inhibiting factor deficiency, 1356
Multicentric reticulohistiocytosis, 1959
Multiceps, 1808–1809
Multicystic kidney, congenital, 638
Multifocal leukoencephalopathy, progressive, 2137
Multifocal neuropathy. See also *Neuropathy, multifocal.*
  definition of, 2188
Multi-infarct dementia, 2000
Multiple endocrine deficiency–autoimmune–candidiasis, 1443, 1444
Multiple endocrine neoplasia syndrome, 1452
Multiple myeloma, 1014–1020, 2264, *2265*
  anion gap in, 539
  bone pain with, 1019
    M-component marker and, 1018
  chemotherapy for, 1017
  clinical manifestations of, 1016, 1016t
  clinical staging of, 1016–1017, 1017t
  clinicopathologic features of, 1014–1016, *1015*
  clonal development in, 962–963
  diagnosis of, 1016
  epidemiology of, 1014
  etiology of, 1014
  hypercalcemia and, 1448–1449, 1018–1019
  indolent, 1019
  infection in, 1019
  immunodeficiency with, 1016
  immunoglobulin G in, *1013*
  M-component immunoglobulin in, 1014, 1015, 1018
  myeloma cell mass in, 1014–1015
  osteolysis with, 1018–1019
  osteoporosis and, 1458
  pathophysiology of, 1014
Multiple myeloma (*Continued*)
  prognosis in, 1017–1019, 1017t
  radiation therapy for, 1019
  renal function in, 1015–1016, 1017, 1019
  solitary, 1019
  spinal cord compression in, 1019
  supportive care in, 1018–1019
  transfusion in, 1019
  treatment of, 1017–1019
  with amyloidosis, 1170, 1171
  with Fanconi's syndrome, 615
Multiple sclerosis, 672, 2143–2147
  and fatigue, 2044
  and vertigo, 2043
  computed tomography in, 2145, 2146
  monophasic disorders possibly related to, 2147–2148
  variants of, 2147–2148
  viral cause of, 2137
  vs. amyotrophic lateral sclerosis, 2080
  vs. Friedreich's ataxia, 2083
  vs. hysteria, 2014
  vs. transverse myelitis, 2139
  vs. vitamin B_{12} deficiency, 2067
  viral cause of, 2137
Multisystem degeneration, and parkinsonism, 2071
Mumps, 1712–1714
  clinical manifestations of, 1712–1713
  diagnosis of, 1713
    culture in, 1713
    serology in, 1713
  epidemiology of, 1712
  host factor in, 1713
  hyperimmune globulin in, 1713–1714
  immune response in, 1713–1714
  immunization for, 45
  orchitis with, 1374
  pathogenesis of, 1712
  pathology of, 1712
  prevention of, 1713–1714
  virus of, morphology of, 1712
Mumps vaccine, 42t, 1713–1714
Mumps virus, in acute central nervous system infections, 2122, 2123
Münchausen syndrome, 2013
Mural thrombus, and stroke, 2091, *2092*
  infections with, 2125
Murine toxin, 1600
Murray Valley encephalitis, 1748–1749
Mus musculus, 1683
Muscarinic cholinergic receptors, 93
Muscle(s)
  atrophy of, in amyotrophic lateral sclerosis, 2080
    in Werdnig-Hoffman disease, 2080
  biopsy of, diagnostic use of, 2200–2201, *2200*
  cramps in, 2199
  diseases of, 2198–2216
    differential diagnosis of, 2198–2201
    primary, vs. amyotrophic lateral sclerosis, 2080
  disorders of, differential diagnosis of, 2178–2182
    in cancer, 1083
  lesions of, characteristics of, 2179
  paralysis of, depolarizing, 534
  rigidity of, in tetanus, 1579
  skeletal, contraction of, and myofascial pain syndrome, 2064
Muscle antibodies, in liver disease, 811
Muscle contraction headache, 2056–2057
Muscle fiber activity, continuous, 2216
Muscle phosphorylase deficiency, 1107
Muscle relaxant drugs, in myofascial pain syndrome, 2064
Muscle tension syndrome, psychophysiologic, vs. paravertebral tumor, 2185
Muscle tone, alterations in, 2069
Muscular dystrophy(ies), 457, 2201–2204, 2199
  Becker, 2203, 2204
  classification of, 2202, *2202*
  congenital, of Fukuyama, 2207
  Duchenne, 137, 333, 2202
  Emery-Dreifuss, 2203
  facioscapulohumeral, 2199, 2203
  limb-girdle, 2199, 2203
  myotonic, 333, 1372, 2199
  ocular, 2203, 2204
  vs. polymyositis, *2209*
Muscular overactivity, syndromes of, 2215–2216
Musculature, of adolescent, 17
Musculoskeletal disease, 1891–1894. See also specific diagnoses.
Musculoskeletal system
  aging and, 23
  in sarcoidosis, 436
Mushroom poisoning, 783
Mutagenesis, 2299
Mutagens, naturally occurring, 39
Mutational load, 122
Mutation(s), 124–126, *126*. See also *Genetics; Inborn errors of metabolism.*
  age factor in, 118–119
  autosomal dominant traits and, 118
  autosomal recessive disorders and, 119
  enzyme deficiency and, 119
  frame-shift, 125
  gene splicing and, 136
  heteroallelic compounds and, 119
  in thalassemias, 923–926, *924*
  mis-sense, 125
  mutant allele in, 118
  nonhomologous crossing over, 125
  non-sense, 125
  point, 125
  polygenic inheritance and, 121, *121*
  prenatal diagnosis of, 136–137
  suppressor, 125
  synonymous, 125
  x-linked inheritance, 119–120, *120*
Mutism, 1995
Myalgia, 2199
  epidemic, 1730–1731
Myalgic encephalomyelitis, benign, 2131
Myasthenia gravis, 457, 2199, 2200, 2211–2215
  and asthenia, 2044
  bulbar, vs. hysteria, 2014
  congenital, 2212–2213
  crisis of, 2214–2215
  in cancer, 1083
  neonatal, 2212
  thymus and, 1889
Myasthenic syndrome, 2215. See also *Eaton-Lambert syndrome.*
  in cancer, 1083
Mycetoma, 1773
  clinical manifestations of, 1773
  diagnosis of, 1773
  epidemiology of, 1773
  etiology of, 1773
  pathogenesis of, 1773
  pathology of, 1773
  prognosis in, 1773
  treatment of, 1773
Mycobacteria, 1631
  infection from, in silicosis, 2282
Mycobacterial lymphadenitis, 1632–1633
Mycobacterioses, 1630–1639. See also *Leprosy; Tuberculosis.*
  clinical description of, 1632

Mycobacterioses (*Continued*)
disseminated, 1633
epidemiology of, 1631–1632
lymphadenitis and, 1632–1633
of skeletal system, 1633
of skin, 1633
of soft tissue, 1633
pathogenesis of, 1632
pulmonary, 1632
radiography in, 1632
treatment of, 1632, 1633
Mycobacterium avium–intracellulare, 1631
in acquired immune deficiency syndrome, 2142
Mycobacterium fortuitum–chelonei, 1631, 1632, 1633
Mycobacterium hemophilum, 1631, 1633
Mycobacterium kansasii, 1631, 1632, 1633
Mycobacterium leprae, 1634
Mycobacterium marinum, 1631, 1633
Mycobacterium scrofulaceum, 1631, 1632
Mycobacterium simiae, 1631, 1632
Mycobacterium szulgai, 1631, 1632
Mycobacterium tuberculosis, 1620, 1622
microbiology of, 1620–1621
Mycobacterium ulcerans, 1631, 1633
Mycobacterium xenopi, 1631, 1632
Mycoplasma
infection from, 1505–1509
of genitourinary tract, 1508–1509
of respiratory tract, 1505–1508
pathogenesis of, 1505
reproductive abnormality and, 1508–1509
treatment of, 1509
microbiology of, 1505–1508
Mycoplasma hominis, 1505, 1508–1509
Mycoplasma pneumoniae, in respiratory disease, 1505–1508
Mycoplasmal pneumonia, 1505–1508
cardiovascular system in, 1507
clinical course of, 1507
clinical presentation of, 1506, *1506*
complications of, 1506–1507
diagnosis of, 1507–1508
differential, 1508
epidemiology of, 1505–1506
immune response in, 1507, 1508
musculoskeletal system in, 1507
nervous system in, 1507
pathology of, 1507
prevention of, 1508
therapy for, 1508
Mycoses, 1758–1774. See also specific diagnoses.
antifungal therapy for, 1759
diagnosis of, 1759
serology of, 1759
skin tests in, 1759
endemic, 1758–1759
opportunistic, 1759
Mycosis fungoides, 2272–2273
Mycotic aneurysm, 1536, 2103
Mycotoxins, 783
Myelin, degeneration of, in vitamin B_{12} deficiency, 2067
disorders affecting, *2143*
formation of, 2143
Myelin basic protein, CSF, reference values for, 2329
in multiple sclerosis, 2144
Myelinolysis, central pontine, 2066–2067
Myelinopathy, 2189, *2190*
Myelitis, transverse, acute, 2138–2139
Myeloblast, 940
Myelocathexis, 956
Myelocyte(s), 940–941
Myelodysplasia, neutrophil abnormalities in, 950
Myelofibrosis, 959
chromosomal abnormality and, 962
idiopathic, vs. leukemoid reaction, 959t
postpolycythemia, 972–974
with myeloid metaplasia, 972–974
clinical features of, 973
course of, 973–974
laboratory data in, 973
pathogenesis of, 972–973
prognosis in, 974
treatment of, 974
Myelogenous leukemia. See *Leukemia—chronic myelogenous.*
Myelography
in back pain, 2063
in extradural spinal tumors, 2185
in spinal epidural abscess, 2117
Myeloid metaplasia
agnogenic, 972–974
with myelofibrosis, 972–974
Myeloid to erythroid ratio, 956, 957
Myeloma, multiple. See *Multiple myeloma.*
Myelomeningocele. See *Spina bifida.*
Myelopathy
from radiation injury, 1083–1084
subacute necrotizing, 2139
transverse, acute, 2148
Myeloperoxidase deficiency, 953
neutrophils in, 953
Myelophthisis, 881–882, 882t
Myelopoiesis, regulation of, 940
Myeloproliferative disorders, 961–962, 972–975, 978
Myelosuppression, in polycythemia vera, 971
Myiasis, 1839
Myleran. See *Busulfan.*
Myoadenylate deaminase deficiency, myopathy with, 1144
Myocardial depressant factors, in shock, 214, 217
Myocardial failure. See *Heart failure.*
Myocardial imaging
technetium-99m pertechnetate in, 286
thallium-201 in, 286
Myocardial infarction
acute, 288–295, *288*
angina pectoris with, 289
control of, 294
arrhythmias with, 292
cigarette smoking and, 294
complications of, 291–292, 293t
coronary artery disease with, 288–289, *288*
coronary artery revascularization in, 295
coronary care unit management of, 294
creatine kinase in, 291
dietary management in, 294
differential diagnosis of, 291
electrocardiography in, 290–291, *290*, *291*, 294
embolism with, 292
enzyme measurement in, 291
follow-up in, 294–295
heart block with, 292
history in, 289
infarct size containment in, 295, 295t
intra-aortic balloon counterpulsation in, 291, 294
mechanical disorders with, 291–292
mechanisms of, 288–289
pericarditis with, 292
physical examination in, 289–290
prognosis in, 293–294, 293t
pulmonary embolism with, 292
recognition of, 289–291
rehabilitation after, 294–295
risk factors in, 288
treatment of, 294–295
Myocardial infarction (*Continued*)
acute, beta-adrenergic blocking agents in, 294, 295
calcium-channel blocking agents in, 294
oxygen therapy in, 294
thrombolytic therapy in, 295
ventricular function in, 293
ventricular septal defect with, 299
and stroke, 2091, *2092*
cigarette smoking and, 47
digitalis therapy in, 204
Dressler's syndrome with, 292
fluid volume depletion in, 521
heart rupture with, 292
infarct measurement in, 292–293
nuclear imaging in, 182
pericarditis with, 341
risk factors in, 268
scintigraphy in, 291, 294
"shoulder-hand syndrome" with, 292
S-T segment response in, 290–291, 294
Myocardial ischemia, chest pain with, 371
Myocardial oxygen consumption, in aortic stenosis, 252
Myocardial revascularization. See *Bypass grafting; Coronary artery revascularization.*
Myocarditis, 333–334
bacterial, 334
diphtheritic, 334, 1572
drug-induced, 338–339
giant cell, 335
in Chagas' disease, 1784–1786
in diphtheria, 1571
neonatal, 1731–1732
puerperal, 338
radiation, 338
toxoplasma, 334
viral, 333–334
with Chagas' disease, 334–335
with enterovirus disease, 1731–1732
with trichinosis, 334
Myocardium. See also *Cardiomyopathy.*
oxygen consumption by, with digitalis, 201
oxygen requirements of, in shock, 213, 223
perfusion imaging of, 181–182, *182*
Myoclonic jerks, 2152
Myoclonic seizures, 2152
Myoclonus, 2076–2077
common forms of, *2077*
definition of, 2069
essential, 2153
familial, benign, 2153
in metabolic brain disease, 1975
juvenile epileptic, 2152, 2154
nocturnal, and sleep disorders, 1989
ocular, 2037
palatal, 2153
segmental, 2153
Myoclonus epilepsy, progressive, 2153, 2154
Myofascial pain syndrome, 2064
Myoglobin, serum and urine, reference values for, 2329
Myoglobinuria, 2199, *2205*
familial, 2206
in alcoholic myopathy, 2066
in heroin addicts, 2210
sporadic, 2210–2211
with potassium depletion, 533
Myoinositol, 1327
Myokymia, 2216
Myoneural junction, diseases of, 2179
Myopathy(ies), 2198–2216. See also specific myopathy.
acquired, 2209–2210
centronuclear, 2207
congenital, 2199, 2207
definition of, 2198
distal, 2204

Myopathy(ies) (*Continued*)
glycogen storage, 2204–2205
inherited, 2201–2209
lipid storage, 2205–2207, *2205*
metabolic, 2204
mitochondrial, 2205, *2205*, 2207
myoadenylate deaminase deficiency with, 1144
myotubular, 2207
nemaline, 2207
ocular, *2205*
respiratory failure and, 457
rod, 2207
sporadic, 2209–2216
with chronic renal failure, 553, 557
with uremia, 553
Myopericarditis, enteroviral, 1731, 1732
Myositis, 1892
with malignancy, 1947, 1948
Myositis ossificans, 2209
Myotonia, 2200
Myotonia congenita, 2207–2208
Myotonic dystrophy, 672, 1372, 2199, 2203, 2204
features of, *2202*
Myotubular myopathy, 2207
Myxedema, 1287–1291. See also *Hypothyroidism.*
idiopathic, 1287
infantile, 1298
pretibial, 1281, 1282
Myxedema coma, 1289
treatment of, 1290–1291, 1291t
Myxedema madness, 1288
Myxedema megacolon, 1289
Myxedema wit, 1288
Myxoma, cardiac, 366
Myxoviruses, in acute central nervous system infections, *2122*

NADH-methemoglobin reductase, 934, 935
NADPH oxidase, 950
Naegleria meningoencephalitis, 1801
Nail-patella syndrome, 628, *2264*
Nairovirus, 1736, 1755–1756
Narcolepsy, 1989, *1988*
Narcotic analgesics. See also names of specific agents.
for terminal pain, 32, 32t, 2052
side effects of, 33
Nasal cannula, for oxygen administration, 459
Nasal headache, 2058
Nasal prongs, for oxygen administration, 459
Nasal regurgitation, 672
Nasopharynx, disease of, and ear pain, 2058
National Clearinghouse of Poison Control Centers, 85
Natriuretic hormone, 550
sodium balance and, 497
Natural killer cells, 1851
Nausea and vomiting, in intracranial tumor, 2163
Near-drowning, 2293–2294
Necator americanus, 1820–1821
Neck
pain in, 2060–2063
skin diseases of, 2242–2243
Necrolysis, epidermal, toxic, 2270
Necrolytic migratory erythema, *2263*
Necrosis, fat, nodular, *2263*
Necrotizing angiitis
generalized, 1941
neuropathy with, 2196
Necrotizing fasciitis, 1575t
Necrotizing venulitis, 1865
Niemann-Pick disease, 1119–1120, 1119t
Neisseria gonorrhoeae, 1644
Neisseria meningitidis, 1551, 1557
serogroups of, 1557, 1558
Nelson's syndrome, 1264, 1317
Nemaline myopathy, 2207
Nematodes, 1819–1827
Nematodiases, primate, 1822
Neomycin, in hepatic encephalopathy, 846–847
Neonate
Chagas' disease in, 1784
Chlamydial infection in, 1670–1671
cytomegalovirus infection in, 1718
group B streptococcal infection in, 1526–1527
herpes simplex virus infection in, 1716
myocarditis in, 1731–1732
parainfluenza virus disease in, 1698–1699
respiratory syncytial virus infection in, 1696–1698
rubella in, 1710
seizures in, 2153
varicella in, 1722
Neoplasms. See also *Tumor(s)* and names of specific neoplasms.
clonal development and, 961–963
fever with, 1470
genetic factor in cell origin in, 961–963
meningeal, diffuse, 2164
multiple endocrine, 1405–1406
of spinal canal, 2184–2186
stem cell origin of, 961–963
Neostigmine, 95
in myasthenia gravis, 2213, 2214
Neovascular glaucoma, 2218
Nephritic syndrome, acute, 569–578. See *Glomerulonephritis, acute*
Nephritis
anti-GBM, 575
Nephritis, interstitial, 486, 589–592. See also names of specific disorders.
IgG-IgA, 574–575
acute allergic, 486
clinical findings in, 590
definition of, 589–590
endocrine factor in, 591
etiology of, 589–590
idiopathic, 590
laboratory findings in, 590–592
pathology of, 590
renal functional pathophysiology in, 591
lupus. See *Lupus nephritis.*
radiation, 604
shunt, 573–574
tubulointerstitial, chronic, 486
Nephroblastoma, 632–642
Nephrolithiasis, 487. See also *Calculus(i).*
Nephroma, mesoblastic, 641
Nephron, 490
transport defects of, 608, 608t
Nephronophthisis, 636–638
genetic factor in, 636–637
Nephropathy(ies)
analgesic-associated, 592–593
Balkan, 590
chronic genetic factor in, 627–628
gouty, 1138
heroin, 582
interstitial, 589–592. See also names of specific disorders.
definition of, 589–590
etiology of, 589–590
immunologic, 590
membranous, 582–583, *582*
motor, subacute, 1082
Nephropathy(ies) (*Continued*)
obstructive, 589, 604–607. See also *Urinary tract obstruction.*
etiology of, 604–605, 605t
pathophysiology of, 605, 605t
prostaglandins in, 605
osmotic, 604
reflux, 619
salt-losing, 550
toxic, 505–506, 505t, 594–604. See also names of specific toxic agents.
associated clinical syndromes, 595
concentration-dependent cytotoxicity in, 594
definition of, 594
immune response in, 594–595
incidence of, 594
pathogenetic mechanisms in, 594–595
susceptibility factor in, 594
Nephrotic syndrome, 485–488, 578–585. See also names of specific disorders.
complications of, 579
corticosteroids in, 580, 581
edema in, 579
hypercoagulability and, 579
hyperlipidemia in, 579, 1115
hypoalbuminemia in, 579
immune response in, 580, 582
lipiduria in, 579
minimal change, 579–580
pathophysiology of, 578–579
primary renal diseases and, 578t, 579–584
proteinuria in, 578–579
Nephrotoxins, 596–604, 596t. See also names of specific nephrotoxic agents.
antimicrobial agents as, 596–598
chemotherapeutic agents as, 596–598
hydrocarbons as, 604
metals as, 598–601, 598t
nephron dysfunction and, *596*
organic solvents as, 603–604
therapeutic agents as, 601–603
Nerve(s). See also under names of specific nerves.
biopsy of, in neuropathy, 2198
cranial. See *Cranial nerves* and names of specific nerves.
cutaneous, lateral, of thigh, injury to, 2197
injury to, 2196–2197, *2196*
optic. See *Optic nerve.*
peripheral. See *Peripheral nerves.*
Nerve block, in pain relief, 2053
Nerve plexus, lesions of, 2179
Nerve root(s)
compression of, and back pain, 2061–2062
disorders of, 2178–2182
lesions of, characteristics of, 2179
mechanical, 2177–2188
vs. peripheral nerve lesions, *2180–2181*
Nervous system
aging and, 23
autonomic. See *Autonomic nervous system.*
central. See *Central nervous system.*
diseases of, approach to, 1965
computed tomography in, 1968–1969
diagnostic principles in, 1965–1966
diagnostic procedures in, 1968–1971
electroencephalography in, 1969–1970
electromyography in, *1969*, 1970, 1971t
history in, 1966–1967
laboratory tests in, 1968
lumbar puncture in, 1968, 1968t
nerve conduction studies in, 1970
neurodiagnostic studies in, 1969–1970
neurologic examination in, 1967–1968
neuromuscular transmission studies in, 1971

Nervous system (*Continued*)
  diseases of, nuclear magnetic resonance imaging in, 1969
    peripheral, 2188–2198. See also *Peripheral neuropathy.*
    radiography in, 1968–1969
    sensory evoked potentials in, 1969–1970
  in lead poisoning, 2308
  in Wilson's disease, 1159
  infectious disorders of, 2111–2138
  inflammatory disorders of, 2111–2138
  radiation injury of, 1083–1084, 1083t
  viral infections of, 2121–2138
    slow, 2135–2138
Neural tube defects, 146
Neuralgia(s). See also *Pain*
  cranial, 2059
  glossopharyngeal, 2059–2060
  postherpetic, 2064
    management of, 2129
    psychotropic drugs in, 2064
  spreading, post-traumatic, 2063
  trigeminal, 2059, 2129
Neurilemoma, acoustic, *2162*
Neuritis. See also *Pain.*
  brachial, acute, 2197–2198
  in diphtheria, 1571
  optic, 2147
    retrobulbar, 2219
  peripheral. See also *Peripheral Neuropathy.*
    definition of, 2188
Neurocutaneous syndromes, 2084–2086
Neuroectodermal tumors, treatment outcome in, 2166
Neuroendocrine system, 1241–1251
  anatomy of, 1241
  central nervous system disorders and, 1246–1250
  in metabolic regulation disorders, 1250
  in puberty, 18
  inhibiting hormones of, 1242–1246
  regulation of, 1241–1246
  releasing hormones of, 1242–1246
Neuroendocrinology, 1215
Neurofibromas, 2257–2258
  characteristics of, *2162*
  spinal, 2186
Neurofibromatosis, 416, 2084–2085, 2257, *2257*, *2264*
  and back pain, 2061
  Crowe's sign of, 2254
  skin in, 2257, *2257*
Neurohormones, from recombinant DNA research, 133
Neurohypophyseal hormones, 1272 1272t
Neurohypophysis, 1266
Neuroleptic syndrome, malignant, 2206
Neurologic complications
  in heroin addiction, 2018
  in immunocompromised host, 2141–2143
Neurologic disability, ischemic, reversible, 2091, 2097, *2097*
Neurologic disease, virus infection in, slow or latent, possibility of, 2137
Neurologic disorders
  with host-parasite alterations unexplained, 2138–2143
  with immunity altered, 2138–2143
Neurologic disturbances, vs. epilepsy, 2156
Neurologic examination, in altered consciousness, 1977, *1977*
Neuromuscular block, unusual causes of, 2215
Neuromuscular disorders
  and myasthenia gravis, 2212
  respiratory failure management in, 470
Neuromuscular junction
  diseases of, 2198–2216
  disorders of, in cancer, 1083
Neuromuscular system disease, and respiratory failure, 457
Neuromuscular transmission studies, 1971
Neuromyasthenia, epidemic, 2131
Neuromyelitis optica, 2147
Neuromyotonia, 2216
Neuron(s)
  anatomy and physiology of, 2178
  loss of, in Friedreich's ataxia, 2083
  motor, disease of, postpoliomyelitis, 2132
      primary, vs. postpoliomyelitis, 2132
  peripheral, disorders of, 2194–2195
Neuronal pathways, function of, *2068*
Neuronopathy, 2189–2190
  postinfectious sensory, 2191–2192
Neuropathic joint disease, 1339, 1958
Neuropathy(ies)
  acute nerve injury and, 2196–2197
  amyloid, 2195
  anatomic classification of, 2189–2190
  autonomic, diabetic, 2193
    inflammatory, acute, 2192
  brachial plexus, idiopathic, 2197–2198
  buckthorn, 2195
  classification of, 2189–2190, *2189*
  compression, chronic, 2196–2197
  definition of, 2188
  diabetic, 2192–2193
  diphtheritic, 2195
  disease-specific, 2195–2196
  dying-back, 2189
  entrapment, 2196–2197
    vs. paravertebral tumor, 2185
  focal, 2190
    classification of, *2189*
    diabetic, *2192*, 2193
  granulomatous, 2196
  infectious, 2196
  inflammatory, autonomic dysfunction in, 2027
    chronic relapsing, 2192
    demyelinating, and ataxia, 2044
  motor, hereditary, 2194–2195
    proximal lower extremity, in diabetics, 2193
  multifocal, 2190
    classification of, *2189*
    definition of, 2188
    diabetic, *2192*, 2193
  nerve biopsy in, 2198
  optic, ischemic, 2219
  peripheral. See also *Peripheral neuropathy.*
    definition of, 2188
  radiation injury, 1084
  reversible, rapid, in diabetics, 2193
  sensory, hereditary, 2194–2195
    postinfectious, 2191–2192
    primary, distal, in diabetics, 2192–2193
  symmetrical, generalized, 2189–2190
  toxic, 2195
  trigeminal, 2198
  uremic, 2193–2194
  vs. myasthenia gravis, 2213
  with acromegaly, 2194
  with cancer, 1082–1083
  with chronic renal failure, 553, 557
  with dysproteinemia, 2195
  with endocrine diseases, 2194
  with hypothyroidism, 2194
  with malignant disease, 2195
  with necrotizing angiitis, 2196
  with rheumatoid arthritis, 2196
  with uremia, 553
Neuropeptides, 1244, 1244t
Neurophysin II, 1079
Neurosarcoidosis, 434–435
Neurosis, symptoms in, 2007–2015
Neurosyphilis, 1655, 2118–2121
  congenital, 2120
Neurotoxic shellfish poisoning, 783
Neurotransmitters, 90, 91. See also specific substances and receptors.
  biogenic amine, 1242–1244
  in hepatic encephalopathy, 845
  in movement disorders, 2068
  neuropeptides as, 1244, 1244t
  sympathetic vs. parasympathetic interventions and, *90*, 91
Neutropenia, 953–958
  acute leukemias with, 955
  antineutrophil antibodies in, 957
  benign, chronic, 955–956
  bone marrow examination in, 956
  bone marrow transplantation in, 957
  chemical toxins and, 957
  clinical evaluation of, 956–957
  clinical manifestations of, 956
  congenital, 955, 957
  corticosteroids in, 957
  cyclic, 956
  drug-induced, 954–955, 960
  etiology of, 954–956, 954t
  folic acid deficiency and, 955
  idiosyncratic, 954
  immune response in, 957
  infections with, 955
    management of, 957
  kinetic mechanisms of, 954, *955*
  Kostmann's, 955, 956
  lithium therapy and, 957
  neutrophil transfusion in, 957–958
  physical agent-induced, 954
  rheumatoid arthritis with, 955
  splenectomy for, 957
  splenomegaly with, 955
  sterile environment requirement for, 958
  treatment of, 957–958
  vitamin B_{12} deficiency and, 955
Neutrophil(s), 942–949
  adhesiveness alterations in, 950, 950t
  chemotaxis and, 943–944, *943*
    depression of, 950, 950t
  circulating pool of, 950
  degranulation process of, 944–945, *945*
  function of, 943–945
    disorders of, 949–953
      acquired, 950
      congenital, 950–953
      screening for, 950, 950t
    evaluation of, 949–950
  granules of, 945, 945t
    abnormality of, 953
  in Chediak-Higashi disease, 952, *952*
    in chronic granulomatous disease, 950–951, *951*
  in myelodysplasia, 950
  in myelogenous leukemia, 950
  in myeloperoxidase deficiency, 953
  ingestion by, 944, *944*
  killing action of, 944–945, *945*
  kinetics of, 866, *868*, 953–954
  marginated pool of, 950
  mobility disorders of, 952–953, 952t
  production of, 866, *868*
  respiratory burst activation of, 944, 945, *945*
  structure of, 943, *943*
  transfusion of, in neutropenia, 957–958
Neutrophil alkaline phosphatase reaction, 978
Neutrophil chemotactic factor, 390
Neutrophil-releasing factor, 954

Neutrophilia, 959–960
Neutrophilic dermatosis, febrile, acute, 2266
Nevoid lentigines, 2254
Nevus(i)
facial, in tuberous sclerosis, 2085
melanoma arising in, 2275
nevus cell, 2254
of mouth, 2243
pigmented, 2254–2255
Spitz, 2276
Nevus spilus, 2254, *2254*
Newborn. See *Neonate.*
Nezelof's syndrome, 1858–1859
N-formylated oligopeptides, 943
Niacin, 1201–1202
biochemical function of, 1201
deficiency of, 1201–1202, *2263*
dietary sources of, 1201
in lipid disorders, 1202
physiology of, 1201
recommended dietary allowances for, 1178
requirements of, 1201
structure of, 1201, *1201*
toxicity of, 1202
Nickel, 1211
poisoning by, 2313
Niclosamide, in tapeworm infection, 1809
Nicotinamide, 1201
Nicotine, ADH activity and, 1268, 1268t
Nicotinic acid, 1201
therapy with, 1112, 1114, 1115
Nicotinic receptors, 93
Nifedipine
in hypertension, 278
primary pulmonary, 264–265
in Raynaud's disease, 355
Nifurtimox, in Chagas' disease, 1785–1786
Night blindness, vitamin A deficiency, 1206, 1207
Nightmares, and sleep disorders, 1990, *1988*
Nikolsky's sign, 1545, 2267, 2270
in angina pectoris, 286
in heart failure, 207
in myocardial infarction, 294
Nitrites, 39
and gastric carcinoma, 697–698
and headache, 2056
Nitroblue tetrazolium test, 950, 1482
Nitrofurantoin, in interstitial lung disease, 418
Nitrofurazone, in African trypanosomiasis, 1783
Nitrogen, total, reference values for, 2329
Nitrogen balance, 1215
Nitrogen mustard, 1095–1096
Nitroglycerin
absorption of, 69
in angina pectoris, 286
in heart failure, 206
in shock, 223
Nitroimidazoles, 1089
Nitroprusside
in heart failure, 205–206
in primary pulmonary hypertension, 263
in shock, 223
Nitrosamines, 39
and gastric carcinoma, 697
ascorbic acid and, 1205
Nitrosoureas, 1096t
as nephrotoxins, 602
in interstitial lung disease, 418
Nitrous oxide
abuse of, 2024
vs. vitamin B_{12} deficiency, 2067
NMR. See *Nuclear magnetic resonance (imaging).*
Nocardia asteroides, 1613, 1614
Nocardia brasiliensis, 1773
Nocardiosis, 1613–1614
Nodose lesions, of leg, 2259
Nodular liquefying panniculitis, 2266
Nodular melanoma, 2274, *2275*
Nodule(s), 2232
Achoff, 1529, *1529*
of leg, 2259
subcutaneous in rheumatic fever, 1530
Noise-induced hearing loss, 2278
Non-A non-B hepatitis, 816
Nonbacterial thrombotic endocarditis, with bronchogenic carcinoma, 441
Nondominant posteroinferior parietal lobe syndrome, 1992
Non-Hodgkin's lymphoma, 985, 994–999
chemotherapy for, 997–998, 988t
classification of, 992t, 993, 993t, 995
clinical manifestations of, 996
clonal development in, 963
epidemiology of, 994
etiology of, 994
exploratory laparotomy in, 997
genetic factor in, 994
histiocytic, 995
immune response in, 994
infection with, 999
lymphoblastic, 995–996
lymphocytic, 995
mixed histiocytic-lymphocytic, 995
of lung, 444–445
pathology of, 994–995
pleomorphic, 995
prognosis in, 999
radiation exposure and, 994
radiation therapy for, 997, 998
retroperitoneal lymphangiogram in, 997
staging system for, 996–997, 996t, 998–999
treatment of, 997–999
undifferentiated, 995
uric acid nephropathy with, 999
Nonketotic hyperosmolar syndrome, 1336–1337
Nonsteroidal anti-inflammatory drugs
allergy to, 1886
in rheumatoid arthritis, 1916
Nontraumatic coma, prognosis in, 1981, *1981, 1982*
Nontropical sprue. See *Celiac disease.*
Noonan's syndrome, 1173, 1387
Norepinephrine, 90, 91, 93, 1243, 1408–1410
blood pressure and, 272, 275
in shock, 222
Normal range of laboratory values, 62–63
Normetanephrine, total, reference values for, 2330
Normochromic normocytic anemia, 882–885. See also *Anemia.*
acute posthemorrhagic, 883–884, 883t
classification of, 883, 883t
marrow response in, 883, 883t
with chronic renal insufficiency, 884
with cirrhosis, 884
with endocrine disorders, 884
with liver disease, 884
North American blastomycosis, 1762–1764
North Asian tick-borne rickettsiosis, 1682
Norubicin, in acute myelogenous leukemia, 991
Norwalk-like viral agents, 1734, 1735
Nosocomial infection, 1485–1492. See also *Hospital-acquired infection.*
Nuclear cytoplasmic asynchronism, 894
Nuclear cytoplasmic dissociation, 894
Nuclear imaging
heart function assessment with, 179–181, *179, 180*
Nuclear imaging (*Continued*)
in cardiology, 179–182
infarct-avid imaging, 182
myocardial perfusion studies with, 181–182, *182*
positron tomography for, 182
Nuclear magnetic resonance (imaging), 65–66, *66–67*
in gastrointestinal disease, 657–658, *657*
in intracranial tumors, 2164
in multiple sclerosis, 2145, 2146
in nervous system disease, 1969
5′-Nucleotidase, in liver disease, 809–810
Nursing homes, 25
Nutrients, biochemical indices for, 1182–1183, 1182t
Nutrition. See also *Diet.*
assessment of, 1179–1183
cancer and, 1071–1072
diseases of, 1174–1218. See also *Malnutrition* and *Undernutrition.*
in Crohn's disease, 746
in gastrointestinal disease, 646
in puberty, 18
in tetanus, 1580
in ulcerative colitis, 754
parenteral, total, in head injuries, 2173
Nutritional amblyopia, 2066
Nutritional assessment
anthropometric measurements in, 1180–1182
questionnaire for, 1180, 1180t
Nutritional diseases, 1174–1218. See also *Malnutrition* and *Undernutrition.*
Nutritional therapy. See also *Enteral nutrition; Parenteral nutrition.*
Nylen-Barany test, 2041
Nystagmus, 2036–2037, *2036*
in ataxia telangiectasia, 2086
in Friedreich's ataxia, 2083
in olivopontocerebellar degeneration, 2083
in striatonigral degeneration, 2079
in vestibular disorders, 2041
in Wernicke's encephalopathy, 2065

Obesity, 1191–1197
age factor in, 1192
and atherosclerosis, 282–283
and cardiovascular disease, 157–158, 1194
and hypertension, 267–268, 1194
anthropometric criteria for, 1181t
appetite suppression for, 1196
behavior modification for, 1196
body fat assessment in, 1192
bypass procedures for, 834
clinical manifestations of, 1194–1195
clinical types of, 1192
diabetes mellitus with, 1194
dietary management of, 1195–1196
differential diagnosis of, 1195
diseases associated with, 1194, 1195t
drug management of, 1196
endocrine sequelae of, 1193, 1193t, 1195
epidemiology of, 1192
etiology of, 1193, 1193t
exercise for, 1196
experimental, 1192
gastrointestinal symptoms with, 1194–1195
height/weight guidelines and, 1191t, 1192
hormonal disorders and, 1250
hypertrophic vs. hyperplastic, 1192, 1193t
hypothalamic, 1193, 1250, 2026
lifelong, 1192
measurement of, 1191–1192, 1191t

Obesity (*Continued*)
metabolic abnormalities with, 1193–1194, 1193t
obstetric risk with, 1195
pathogenesis of, 1192
pathophysiology of, 1192, 1193t
prevention of, 1197
prognosis in, 1196–1197
respiratory system in, 1194
surgery for, 1196
surgical risk with, 1195
treatment of, 1195–1196
triceps skinfold thickness and, 1192
Obstetric infection, anaerobic, 1585
Obstruction. See names of specific types.
Obtundation, definition of, 1971
Occipital lobe, tumors of, 2163
Occipital nerve, greater, neuralgia of, 2060
Occlusion
arterial, myoglobinuria in, 2210
basilar artery, 2095
carotid artery, 2094
cerebral artery, 2094
vertebral artery, 2095
vertebral-basilar circulatory system, 2095
Occupational agents, neuropathy due to, 2195, *2195*
Occupational dermatoses, 2296–2297
Occupational exposures, cancer and, 1070–1071, 2287
Occupational lung disease, 2279–2287, *2279*
Occupational medicine, 2277–2279
Occupational skin diseases, 2295–2297
Occupational-environmental history, 2277–2278, *2278*
Occupational-environmental medicine, 2277–2340
Ockelbo fever, 1740
Octopus, poisoning by, 1843–1844
Ocular. See also *Eye(s)* and *Optic.*
Ocular albinism, 2257, *2258*
Ocular bobbing, 2037
Ocular histoplasmosis, 1760
Ocular hypertension, 2218
Ocular infections, 2220–2221
trachomatous, 1667
Ocular inflammation, 2219–2220
Ocular medications, 2225–2226
Ocular movement, disturbances of, 2035–2037, *2036*
Ocular muscular dystrophy, 2203, 2204
Ocular myoclonus, 2037
Ocular myopathy, 2199, *2205*
Ocular palsy, in postencephalitic parkinsonism, 2071
Ocular paralysis, 2035
Ocular side effects of drugs, 2225
Ocular vascular disease, 2223–2225
Oculocerebral hypopigmentation syndrome, *2258*
Oculocutaneous albinism, 2257, *2258*
Oculocutaneous disorders, 2225
Oculogyric crisis, in secondary parkinsonism, 2071
Oculomotor nerve
apraxia of, 1996
paralysis of, 2213
Odynophagia, 667
Olfaction, disorders of, 2031
Oligodendroglioma, characteristics of, *2162*
Oligosaccharide N-acetyl-neuraminidase deficiency, 1149
Oligospermia, 1372
Oliguria, urine sodium concentration in, 511
Olivopontocerebellar degeneration, 2083–2084, *2081, 2082*
and parkinsonism, 2071
Ollier's disease, 1466
Omentum, disease of, 790–791
Omeprazole, in peptic ulcer, 689, 690
Omsk hemorrhagic fever, 1749, 1751t, 1755
"On-off" phenomenon, in levodopa therapy, 2073
Onchocerca volvulus, 1832
Onchocerciasis, 1832–1833
Oncofetal antigens, 1075–1076
Oncogenes, 1066–1069
in carcinogenesis, 1068
in DNA of human tumors, 1068
proto-oncogenes and, 1068
recombinant DNA research in, 133
viral, 1066–1067
Oncology, 1059–1102
One cistron–one polypeptide principle, 128
Onycholysis, 1283
O'nyong-nyong fever, 1740
Oophorectomy, in breast cancer, 1403
Oophoritis, with mumps, 1713
Operant conditioning, in pain relief, 2053
Ophthalmia neonatorum, gonococcal, 2221
Ophthalmic zoster, 2128, 2129
Ophthalmologic disorders, neurologic, 2032–2037, *2032, 2034, 2036*
Ophthalmoplegia
in central pontine myelinolysis, 2067
in progressive supranuclear palsy, 2071
in Wernicke's encephalopathy, 2065
internuclear, 2036
in multilple sclerosis, 2145
myopathic, 2203, 2204
Ophthalmoplegic migraine, 2055
Ophthalmoscopic examination, 2033
Opiate(s), abuse of, 2016–2019
psychopathology in, 2017
Opiate receptors, 1234, 1235
Opiate withdrawal syndrome, 2020
Opioid peptides, 1234–1237
physiologic and pathophysiologic effects of, 1235–1236
receptor mapping for, 1235
Opisthorchiasis, 1816
Opisthorchis felineus, 1816
Opisthorchis viverrini, 1816
Optiz-Frias syndrome, 145–146
Opsoclonus, in cancer, 1082
Opsonins, 944
Opsonization, 944, *944*
Optic chiasm, lesions of, 2034
Optic disc
atrophy of, 2219
in vitamin B_{12} deficiency, 2067
pallor of, 2219
Optic nerve
acute bilateral disease of, 2034
atrophy of, 2219
in olivopontocerebellar degeneration, 2084
in syphilis, 2119, 2120
primary, 2034
gliomas of, 2164
Optic neuritis, 2033, 2147
retrobulbar, 2219
compressive, 2221
ischemic, 2033, 2219
Optic tract, abnormalities of, 2034
Oral candidiasis, 665, *665*
Oral cavity. See also *Mouth* and specific structures.
cancer of, cigarette smoking and, 48
Oral contraceptives
and gallstones, 852
and hepatic tumor, 849
and hepatotoxicity, 823–824
and hypertension, 276
complications with, 1392–1393
folate absorption and, 899
Oral contraceptives (*Continued*)
thromboembolism with, 1393
Oral disease, 662–667
Oral hypoglycemic agents, in diabetes mellitus, 1328–1329, *1329*
Oral-facial-digital syndrome, *2264*
Orbital disease, 2221-2222
Orbital tumors, 2221-2222
Orchitis, 1374–1375
Organ injury, electric, 2303, 2304
Organ systems, specific, cutaneous correlations with, 2267
Organ transplantation
in inborn errors of metabolism, 132
rejection of glucocorticosteroid therapy for, 114
Organic materials, diseases produced by, 2285–2286
Organic solvents, as nephrotoxins, 603–604
Organomercurials, poisoning by, 2310
Organophosphates, poisoning from, 89
Orgasmic headache, 2056
Oriental sore, 1790–1792
Ornithine carbamyl transferase deficiency, 1130,1145
Ornithine carbamyl transferase deficiency, 1130, 1145
Ornithodorus, 1663
Ornithosis. See *Psittacosis.*
Oropharyngeal airway, in acute respiratory failure, 458
Orotic aciduria, 131
hereditary, 1145
Oroya fever, 1617
Orthophosphates, in hypercalciuria, 632–633
Orthopnea, 372
in left ventricular failure, 196
Orthostatic hypotension, 1984–1985, *1984*
idiopathic, 2027
in autonomic dysfunction, 2028
in Wernicke's encephalopathy, 2065
Osler-Weber-Rendu disease, 1040
punctate telangiectasia of, 2243
Osler-Weber-Rendu syndrome, *2262, 2264*
Osler's nodes, in infective endocarditis, 1536t
Osmolality
disorders of, antidiuretic hormone in, 524–525
cell volume regulation in, 524
hypertonic, 528–529, 528t
hypotonic, 525–528, 525t
physiologic considerations in, 523–525
sensory element in, 524
water repletion reaction in, 524–525, *524*
serum, reference values for, 2330
urinary, reference values for, 2330
Osmoreceptors, in water balance, 524
Osteitis deformans. See *Paget's disease.*
Osteitis fibrosa, 1429, 1453
parathyroid hormone in, 1453
phosphate in, 1453, 1455
plasma calcium in, 1453, 1454
vitamin D metabolism in, 1453, 1455
Osteitis fibrosa cystica, 1436
Osteoarthritis, 1951–1954
clinical manifestations of, 1952–1953, *1952*
differential diagnosis of, 1953–1954
etiologic classification of, 1951, 1951t, 1952
laboratory findings in, 1953
pathogenesis of, 1952
pathology of, 1952
radiography in, 1953
spinal, 1953
treatment of, 1954
Osteoarthropathy, hypertrophic, 1464–1465, 1959
Osteoblasts, 1420–1421
Osteocalcin, vitamin K and, 1209

Osteoclast(s), 1421
Osteoclast activating factor, in cancer, 1078
Osteocytes, 1421
Osteodystrophy. See also *Renal osteodystrophy.*
  in chronic renal failure, 553, 557
Osteogenesis imperfecta, 347, 1151–1152, 1458
Osteolysis, with multiple myeloma, 1018–1019
Osteomalacia, 1425–1431, 1453–1454
  aluminum-induced, 1428, 1456
  diagnosis of, 1428–1430
  etidronate and, 1428
  hypophosphatemic, 615
  pathogenesis of, 1425–1428, 1426t
    biochemical features of, 1429–1430
    bone matrix disorders and, 1428
    calcium deficiency and, 1427–1428
    histologic features of, 1430
    mineralization inhibition and, 1428, 1430, 1431
    phosphate homeostasis disorders and, 1427
    vitamin D disorders and, 1425–1427, 1429
  phenytoin and, 1428
  radiography in, 1429, *1429*
  renal failure and, 1429, 1430
  treatment of, 1430–1431
  tumor-induced hypophosphatemic, 1427
Osteomyelitis, 1546–1547, 1566–1568
  clinical manifestations of, 1567
  diagnosis of, 1567–1568
  epidemiology of, 1567
  etiology of, 1567
  in coccidioidomycosis, 1761
  pathogenesis of, 1567
  pathology of, 1567
  prevention of, 1568
  radiography in, 1567–1568, *1567*
  treatment of, 1568
Osteonecrosis, 1463
Osteopetrosis, 1464
Osteoporosis, 1395, 1422, *1422*, 1456–1460
  bone marrow disorders and, 1458
  calcium intake and, 1456
  calcium therapy for, 1460
  chronic obstructive pulmonary disease and, 1458
  classification of, 1457, 1457t
  clinical presentation of, 1458
  connective tissue disorders and, 1458
  diagnosis of, 1459
  drug therapy in, 1460
  endocrine diseases and, 1458
  epidemiology of, 1456
  exercise and, 40–41
  gastrointestinal diseases and, 1458
  glucocorticoids and, 1460
  idiopathic, 1457
  immobilization and, 1458
  involutional, 1457–1458, 1457t
  juvenile, 1457
  menopause and, 1456–1457
  pathophysiology of, 1456
  post-traumatic painful, 2063
  radiography in, 1458–1459, *1459*
  risk factors for, 1456–1457
  treatment of, 1459–1460
Osteosarcoma, 1467, *1467*
  causes of, 1463, 1463t
  cortical, 1464–1465
  focal, 1465
  trabecular, 1464
Ostium primum defect, 230
Ostium secundum defect, 228
  with ventrricular septal defects, 231
Otitic hydrocephalus, 2058, 2093, 2168
Otitis externa, malignant, 2116
Otitis media, 1585
  brain abscess due to, 2112
  Hemophilus influenzae, 1564
  serous, 1868
Otogenic brain abscess, 2112
Otorrhea, cerebrospinal, in skull fracture, 2171
Otosclerosis, 2038–2039
  tinnitus in, 2040
Ouabain, in heart failure, 203–204
Ovary(ies), 1379–1395
  anatomy of, 1379–1380, *1379*
  cyst of, 1384
  development of, 1351–1352
  dysfunction of, hormone therapy for, 1392–1395
  function–hormone production correlates of, 1381, *1381*
  hormones of, 1381–1383, 1382t
    at menarche, 1388–1391
    at menopause, 1391–1392
    at puberty, 1385–1388
    decreased production of, 1383, 1386–1388, 1389–1390, 1391, 1394–1395
    in infancy and childhood, 1383–1385
    increased production of, 1383–1385, 1388, 1389, 1391, 1394–1395
    measurement of, 1381
    normal vs. abnormal response to, 1383–1392
    target tissue response to, 1381–1383
  hypothalamic-pituitary function and, 1382
  in phenotype differentiation, 1353
  morphology-function correlates of, 1380–1381, *1380*
  resistance to gonadotropins of, 1387
  tumor of, 1391–1392, 1392t
  with hypothalamic-pituitary axis dysfunction, 1387–1388
Overdose, opiate, treatment of, 2018–2019
Ovulation, 1382
Oxalate
  serum, reference values for, 2330
  urinary, reference values for, 2330
Oxalosis, 132, 1108
Oxamniquine, in intestinal bilharziasis, 1814
Oxazolidinediones, as nephrotoxins, 601–602
Oxidative metabolism, in Friedreich's ataxia, 2083
Oxidative phosphorylation, in shock, 216
Oxycodone, in pain, 2051
Oxygen
  delivery of, in angina pectoris, 284
  hemoglobin binding of, 917–918, *917*
  partial pressure, reference values for, 2330
Oxygen saturation, blood reference values for, 2330
Oxygen therapy
  complications with, 476
  delivery systems for, 467
  hyperbaric, 2289
  in cardiopulmonary resuscitation, 481
  in chronic obstructive pulmonary disease, 402
  in cluster headache, 2056
  in fat embolism syndrome, 432
  in gastrointestinal hemorrhage, 792
  in heart failure, 199
  in myocardial infarction, 294
  in pulmonary hypertension, 259, 260, 261
  in respiratory failure, 458–459, 460
  in shock, 220
  toxicity with, 477
Oxygen-hemoglobin dissociation curve
  in anemia, 872
Oxygen-hemoglobin dissociation curve (*Continued*)
  in shock, 216
  of abnormal hemoglobins, 933–934
  polycythemia and, 967
Oxygenation
  equations related to, 465–466, *466*
  red cell mass and, 964, *964*
Oxyphenbutazone, for gout, 1141
Oxytocin, 1266, 1273
  in hypopituitarism, 1257

Pacemakers, 300, 326–327, *326*, *327*
Pachydermoperiostosis, 1465
Pachymeningitis, hypertrophic, neurologic changes in, 2118
Paget cells, 2251
Paget's disease
  of bone, 1461–1463, 2251–2252
    biochemical features of, 1462
    clinical features of, 1461
    epidemiology of, 1461
    etiology of, 1461
    pathology of, 1461
    radiography in, 1461–1462, *1462*
    surgery for, 1462–1463
    therapy of, 1462–1463
  of breast, 1086, 1402
Pain, 2049–2054, *2051*. See also *Neuralgia; Neuritis.*
  abdominal, in gastrointestinal disease, 646
  acupuncture in, 2053
  analgesic agents for, 2051–2052, 2051(t)
  back, lumbar puncture in, 2063
  behavioral techniques for, 2053
  cutaneous stimulation for, 2052–2053
  diagnosis of, 2049–2050
  frontal leukotomy for, 2053
  frontal lobotomy for, 2053
  head, 2054–2060, *2054*
  hydromorphone in, 2052
  hypnotism in, 2053
  hysterical, 2013
  in alcoholic neuropathy, 2066
  in dying patient, 31–33, *31*
  in herpes zoster, 1723
  in peripheral common pathway lesions, 2182
  in psychophysiologic disorders, 2049
  in spinal cord injury, 2177
  in syringomyelia, 2084
  laminectomy for, 2053
  levorphanol in, 2052
  management of, 33, 33t, 2050–2054, 2051t
  mechanisms of, 2047–2048
  meprobamate in, 2051
  methadone in, 2052
  methotrimeprazine in, 2052
  morphine in, 2052
  myofascial syndrome and, 2064
  neck and back, 2060–2063
  nerve blocks for, 2053
  of tabes, 2063
  phantom limb, 2064
  post-thoracotomy, vs. paravertebral tumor, 2185
  surgery for, 2053
  surgical lesion in thalamus for, 2053
  tranquilizers in, 2051, 2052
Palatal myoclonus, 2076, 2153
Palate, smoker's, 2244
Pallor, of disc, 2219
Palsy. See under specific types of palsy.
Pancoast's syndrome, 441

Pancreas
  carcinoma of, 777–780
    angiography in, 779
    carcinoembryonic antigen in, 778
    chemotherapy for, 780
    cholangiography in, 779
    cigarette smoking and, 778
    clinical manifestations of, 778
    coffee intake and, 778
    computed tomography in, 779
    diagnosis of, 659–660, 778–779, *780*
      differential, 779
    endoscopic retrograde pancreatography in, 779, *779*
    epidemiology of, 777–778
    fine needle aspiration cytology in, 779
    galactosyltransferase isoenzyme II in, 778
    in Zollinger-Ellison syndrome, 696, 697
    incidence of, 777–778
    pancreatography in, 659–660, *659*
    pathophysiology of, 778
    radiation therapy for, 780
    radiography in, 778
    serology in, 778, 778t
    stimulation tests in, 779
    surgery for, 779–780
    therapy of, 779–780
    ultrasonography in, 779
    vs. pancreatitis, 659
  disease of, cutaneous disorders with, *2263*
  exocrine function of, 771
  in Hippel-Lindau disease, 2086
  in malabsorption syndrome, 725
  insufficiency of, primary, 729, 731
    secondary, 729, 731
    with cystic fibrosis, 424–425
  islet cell tumor of, 1348–1351
    associated syndromes of, 1348–1350, 1349t
    diagnosis of, 1348
    hormone production by, 1349t, 1351
    pathology of, 1348
  islets of Langerhans of, *1348*
Pancreas divisum, 772
Pancreatic cholera syndrome, 717
Pancreatic juice, reflux of, in gastric ulcer, 683
Pancreatic oncofetal antigen, 1076
Pancreatic polypeptide, with islet cell tumor, 1351
Pancreatic pseudocyst, pleural involvement with, 449
Pancreaticoduodenotomy, 779–780
Pancreatitis, 771–777
  acute, 771–775
    alcoholism and, 771
    amylase excretion in, 772–773
    clinical presentation of, 772
    complications of, 774–775, 774t
    computed tomography in, 773, *773, 774, 775*
    dialysis in, 774
    drug intake and, 772
    endoscopic retrograde cholangiopancreatography in, 772, 773
    etiology of, 771–772, 771t
    gallstones and, 771–772
    hematocrit in, 773
    hypertriglyceridemia and, 772
    laboratory tests in, 772–773
    pathogenesis of, 771–772
    phlegmon with, 774
    postoperative, 772
    prognosis in, 773–774, 774t
    pseudocyst with, 774–775, *775*
    radiography in, 773
    recurrence of, prevention of, 775
    "rest" therapy for, 774
Pancreatitis (*Continued*)
  acute, surgery for, 774
    treatment of, 773–774
    ultrasonography in, 773, *773, 774, 775*
    vascular insufficiency and, 772
    with adult respiratory distress syndrome, 774
  bile duct obstruction with, 862
  chronic, 775–777
    alcoholism and, 775, 777
    clinical manifestations of, 775
    computed tomography in, 777
    diagnosis of, 777
    endoscopic retrograde cholangiopancreatography in, *776*, 777
    etiology of, 775
    exocrine deficiency treatment in, 777
    pain with, 775, 777
    pathophysiology of, 775
    prognosis in, 777
    pseudocysts with, 775
    surgery for, 777
    treatment of, 777
    ultrasonography in, 777
    with malabsorption syndrome, 775
  classification of, 771
  computed tomography in, 773, *773, 774, 775, 777*
  genetic factor in, 772
  hyperglycemia in, 773
  hyperlipemia in, 773
  hypocalcemia in, 773
  pleural involvement with, 449
  vs. pancreatic carcinoma, 659
  with mumps, 1713
Pancreatography, retrograde, 659–660
Pancytopenia, 875
  drug-induced, 960
  etiology of, 880t
  in hairy cell leukemia, 985
Pandemic, influenza, 1702, *1702*, 1702t
Pandysautonomia
  acute, 2027
  postinfectious, 2192
Panencephalitis
  rubella, progressive, 2136
  subacute sclerosing, 2136
Panendoscopy, 658–659
Panic attacks, 2009, 2010
  in psychedelic abuse, 2024
Panniculitis, 1962–1963
  liquefying, nodular, 2266
  lobular, 1962
  mesenteric, 790–791
  nodular, 1962
  septal, 1962–1963
  with vasculitis, 1962–1963
Panniculus adiposus, 2227
Pantothenic acid, dietary allowance for, 1178
Papilledema, 2219
  in intracranial tumor, 2162
  in pseudotumor cerebri, 2168
  intracranial hypertension and, 2167
  vs. optic neuritis, 2034, *2034*
Papillitis, 2147, 2219
Papilloma, of lung, 446
Papovaviruses, and progressive multifocal leukoencephalopathy, 2137
Pappataci fever, 1738–1739
Papular dermatitis of Spangler, 2269
Papule(s), 2232
  urticarial, in pregnancy, 2269
Paracoccidioides brasiliensis, 1764
Paracoccidioidomycosis, 1764–1765
  antifungal therapy for, 1764–1765
  clinical manifestations of, 1764
  culture in, 1764
  diagnosis of, 1764
Paracoccidioidomycosis (*Continued*)
  disseminated, 1764, 1765
  epidemiology of, 1764
  etiology of, 1764
  immune response in, 1764
  pathogenesis of, 1764
  pathology of, 1764
  prognosis in, 1765
  pulmonary, 1764
  serology in, 1764
  skin test in, 1764
  treatment of, 1764–1765
Paragonimiasis, 1817–1818
  clinical manifestations of, 1817–1818
  diagnosis of, 1818
  pathology of, 1817
  prevention of, 1818
  treatment of, 1818
Paragonimus westermani, 1817
Parahemophilia, 1050
Parainfectious encephalomyelitis, 2139–2140, 2147
Parainfluenza virus disease, 1698–1700
  clinical manifestations of, 1699
  epidemiology of, 1698–1699
  microbiology of, 1698
  serology in, 1699
  treatment of, 1699
Paralysis
  general, of insane, 2119
  in Guillain-Barré syndrome, 2191
  in myasthenia gravis, 2213
  infantile, 2130–2132
  periodic, 2200
    familial, 2208–2209
    hyperkalemic, 2208
    hypokalemic, 533
    vs. hysteria, 2014
  tick, 2215
  Todd's, 2149, 2151
  transient, 2047
  with enteroviral disease, 1730
Paralytic poliomyelitis, 2130–2132
Paralytic rabies, 2133
Paralytic shellfish poisoning, 783
Parameningeal infections, 2111–2118
  vs. bacterial meningitis, 1554
Paramyxoviruses, in acute central nervous system infections, 2122, *2122*
Paranasal sinus infection, brain abcess due to, 2112
Paraplegia, in vitamin B_{12} deficiency, 2067
Paraproteinemias
  platelet disorders in, 1038
  vascular purpura with, 1039
Paraguat
  in interstitial lung disease, 419
  poisoning from, 89
Parasellar diseases, 1260
Parasites
  cancer and, 1071
  hemolysis and, 913
  liver, 827–828, 828t
  macro- vs. microparasite, 1804
Parasite-host alterations, unexplained, neurologic disorders with, 2138–2143
Parasitic cysts, intracranial, characteristics of, *2162*
Parasomnia, 1989–1990, *1988*
Parasympathetic nervous system, 90
  in asthma, 392, 393, *393*
Parasympathetic neurons, anatomy and physiology of, 2178
Parathormone, in cancer, 1078
Parathyroid hormone, 1431–1435
  action of, 1433–1434, *1434*
  assay of, 1434–1435, 1439–1440, *1439, 1440*
  bone and, 1434

Parathyroid hormone (*Continued*)
  deficiency of, 1443–1446
  function of, 1433
  in calcium homeostasis, 500, 1415, 1418, 1419
  in magnesium metabolism, 500
  in osteitis fibrosa, 1453
  in phosphorus metabolism, 500
  in pseudohypoparathyroidism, 1446–1448
  kidney and, 1434
  secretion of, 1431–1433
  serum concentration of, 1433, *1433*, 1434–1435
  sodium balance and, 494
  structure of, 1431, *1432*
  synthesis of, 1431, *1432*
  uremia and, 551
Parathyroidectomy, 632
Paravertebral tumors, 2185
Parent-child relationships, 19
Parenteral nutrition, 1215–1218
  complications of, 1217–1218
  protein-calorie supplementation in, 1215–1217, 1215t
  total, 1215, 1216–1218
    in small intestine disease, 1216
    indications for, 1216
    nutrients for, 1216–1217, 1217t
    zinc deficiency in, 1209
Paresis
  general, 1656 2119
    general, neurologic changes in, 2118
  juvenile, 2120
Paresthesias
  definition of, 2047, 2188
  in alcoholic neuropathy, 2066
  in multiple sclerosis, 2145, *2145*
    treatment of, 2147
  in vitamin B_{12} deficiency, 2067
Parietal cells, 681
Parietal lobe
  disorders of, 1992
  tumors of, 2163
Parinaud syndrome, 1618–1619, 2036
Parkinsonism, 2070–2073
  and asthenia, 2044
  and fatigue, 2044
  autonomic dysfunction and, 2027
  classification of, *2070*
  physical therapy in, 2072
  postencephalitic, 2071
    vs. hysteria, 2014
  primary, 2070–2071
  secondary, 2071
  vascular, 2071
  vs. essential tremor, 2074
  viral cause of, possibility of, 2137
Parkinsonism-plus, 2071
Parlodel. See *Bromocriptine.*
Paromomycin, in tapeworm infection, 1809
Paronychia, candidal infection of, 2247, 2248
Parotitis, epidemic, 1712–1714
Paroxysmal atrial tachycardia, 312–313
Paroxysmal cold hemoglobinuria, 911, *2265*
Paroxysmal hypothermia, 2026
Paroxysmal nocturnal dyspnea, 372
  in left ventricular failure, 196
Paroxysmal nocturnal hemoglobinuria, 911–912
  clinical manifestations of, 912
  diagnosis of, 912
  pathophysiology of, 911–912
  prognosis in, 912
  treatment of, 912
Parrot fever, 1671–1672
Pars plana vitrectomy, in diabetic retinopathy, 2224
Partial combined immunodeficiency disorder, 1860–1861
  genetic factor in, 1860–1861
  with short-limbed dwarfism, 1860–1861
  with thrombocytopenia and eczema, 1860
  with thymoma, 1861
Partial nonprogressing stroke, 2097, 2097t
  investigation of, 2099
  treatment of, 2100
Partial thromboplastin time, reference values for, 2339
Particles, accelerated, 2297
Parvovirus, aplastic anemia and, 878
Passivity, in schizophrenia, 2002
Patella, clonus of, in striatonigral degeneration, 2079
Patent ductus arteriosus, 231–232
  birth weight factor in, 232
  closure of, 1239
  echocardiography in, 232
  electrocardiography in, 231
  indomethacin in, 232
  radiography in, 231–232
  surgery for, 232
  ventricular septal defect with, 231
Paterson-Kelly syndrome, 889
Pathways, peripheral common, 2178–2182
Patient
  as consumer, 7–8
  care of, 60
  description of, 1
  education of, 7
  expectations of, 1–2, 7
Patient-physician relationship, 1–2
  data-gathering and, 58
  essence of, 57
  in death and dying, 30
  medical education and, 4
  medical practice patterns in, 7
  patient preferences and, 12–13
  with aged, 25–26
Peak expiratory flow rate, 464
Peapicker's disease, 1666
Pectus excavatum, 454
Pediatrics. See *Neonate.*
Pediculosis, 1833–1834
Pediculus humanus capitis, 1678
Pediculus humanus corporis, 1685
Pediculus humanus humanus, 1662, 1678
Pedigree, 117, *118, 119, 120*
PEEP. See *Positive end-expiratory pressure.*
Pelger-Huet anomaly, 953
Pelizaeus-Merzbacher disease, 2148
Pellagra, 1201, 1202, *2263*
Pelvic inflammatory disease. See *Salpingitis.*
Pelvis, disease in, and back pain, 2061
Pemphigoid, 2268, *2268*
Pemphigus, 2267–2268, *2268*
Pendred's syndrome, 1298
D-Penicillamine, 1203
  as nephrotoxin, 601–602
  in cystinuria, 612–613, 633
  in rheumatoid arthritis, 1916
  in Wilson's disease, 1160
Penicillin(s), 103–104
  allergy to, 83, 1886
  anaphylaxis and, 1871, 1872
  antistaphylococcal, 103
  as nephrotoxins, 597
  broad-spectrum, 103–104
  dosage of, and data on, 101t
  for group A streptococcal infection, 1524, 1526
  in actinomycosis, 1613
  in brain abscess, 2113
  in lung abscess, 421–422
  in neurosyphilis, 2121
  oral desensitization protocol for, 1886, 1886t
Penicillin(s) (*Continued*)
  prophylaxis with, for acute rheumatic fever, 1532–1533
  renal clearance of, 75
  therapy with, for syphilis, 1658–1660, 1659t
    in anthrax, 1607
    in rat bite fever, 1666
    in tropical phagedenic ulcer, 1665
Penicillin G, 103
  pharmacokinetic parameters of, 70t
Penicillinase-producing gonococci, 1647
Pentamidine
  in African trypanosomiasis, 1783
  in kala azar, 1789
Pentamidine isethionate
  in pneumocystosis, 1797
Pentastomiasis, 1840–1841
Pentazocine
  abuse of, 2017–2018
  in pain, 2052
Pentobarbital, serum and plasma, reference values for, 2330
Pentosuria, 1107
Pepsin, in peptic ulcer pathogenesis, 682, 683
Pepsinogen, 682
Peptic ulcer, 681–697. See also *Duodenal ulcer; Gastric ulcer; Zollinger-Ellison syndrome.*
  alcohol intake and, 684, 689
  anti-inflammatory agents in, 684, 689
  bleeding with, 693–694
  caffeine and, 684
  cigarette smoking and, 49, 684, 689
  complications of, 693–696
  corticosteroids and, 684
  dietary factors in, 689
  differential diagnosis of, 687–688
  dyspepsia in, 685
  endoscopy in, 686
  epidemiology of, 684–685
  gastric acid secretion in, inhibition of, 688–689, *688*
    measurement of, 687
  gastric secretion products and, 682, 683
  histamine (H_2) receptor antagonists in, 688, 697
  hospitalization for, 690
  infectious agents in, 684
  laboratory studies in, 686–687
  long-term maintenance therapy for, 690
  management principles for, 689–691
  medical therapy for, 688–691
  mucosal defense defect in, 683–684
  mucosal defense enhancement in, 689
  obstruction with, 695–696
  pain in, 685
  perforation with, 694–695
  physical examination in, 685
  postoperative recurrence of, 693
  prostaglandin synthesis in, 684, 689
  radiography in, 685–686, *686*
  sedatives in, 690
  serum gastrin in, 686–687, 687t
  stress and, 684
  surgical therapy for, 691–693, *691*t
    complications of, 692–693
  symptoms of, 685–685t
  upper gastrointestinal hemorrhage and, 794
Peptococcus, 1583
Peptostreptococcus, 1583
Percentile estimates, 62
Perchlorate (CPO_4^-) discharge test, 1298
Percutaneous transhepatic cholangiography. See *Cholangiography.*
Percutaneous transluminal angioplasty, in arteriosclerosis obliterans, 360
Percutaneous transluminal coronary angioplasty, 300

Perfusion lung scan, in pulmonary embolism, 427–429, *428*
Periarteritis nodosa, 341
Pericardial constriction
angiography in, 344–345
cardiac catheterization in, 344
clinical manifestations of, 344
echocardiography in, 344
electrocardiography in, 344
laboratory findings in, 344
pathophysiology of, 344–345
treatment of, 345
Pericardial effusion, 343–344
cardiac tamponade with, 343
chylous, 345
clinical manifestations of, 343
echocardiography in, 343
electrocardiography in, 343
in right ventricular failure, 198
laboratory findings in, 343–344
pathophysiology of, 343
radiography in, *167,* 169
treatment of, 344
Pericardial tamponade, fluid volume depletion in, 521
Pericardiectomy, 345
Pericardiocentesis, 344
Pericarditis
acute, 339–343
bacterial, 340
clinical manifestations of, 342
differential diagnosis of, 342–343
electrocardiography in, 342
etiology of, 339–342, 340t
fungal, 341
infectious, 340–341
laboratory findings in, 342
chest pain with, 371
cholesterol, 345
connective tissue disorders and, 341–342
constrictive. See *Pericardial constriction.*
Hemophilus influenzae, 1564
idiopathic, 339–340
meningococcal, 1560
metabolic disorders and, 342
post-traumatic, 341
radiation injury and, 342
tuberculosis and, 1627
with allergy, 342
with enteroviral disease, 1731–1732
with hypersensitivity, 342
with myocardial infarction, 292, 341
with postpericardiotomy syndrome, 341
with uremia, 552, 556
Pericardium, disorders of, 339–345
congenital, 345
neoplastic, 345
Pericholangitis, 834
Perihepatitis, gonococcal, 858
Perinephric abscess, 619, 623
Periodontal disease, 663
Periodontitis, juvenile, 952, 952t
Peripheral circulation, 160–161
Peripheral disorders, sensory, 2048
Peripheral nerve(s)
diseases of, characteristics of, 2179
disorders of, 2179
in diabetics, 2193
vs. amyotrophic lateral sclerosis, 2080
vs. nerve root lesions, *2180–2181*
in cancer, 1082–1083
in vitamin B_{12} deficiency, 2067
Peripheral nervous system, diseases of, 2188–2198. See also *Peripheral neuropathy.*
Peripheral neuropathy, 724, 725. See also *Neuropathy(ies).*
definition of, 2188
Peripheral neuropathy (*Continued*)
in alcoholic cerebellar degeneration, 2066
in vitamin B_{12} deficiency, 2067
vs. syringomyelia, 2084
Peripheral vascular disease, cigarette smoking and, 48
Peripheral vertigo, causes of, 2941
Perirectal abscess, 1593
Peritoneal dialysis. See also *Dialysis.*
ambulatory, continuous, 563, 563t
clinical use of, 560–561
technical aspects of, 560
time-averaged clearance with, 560, 560t
Peritoneum
anatomy of, 786
disease of, 786–790
ascites with, 787–788, 788t
diagnosis of, 786–787
infections of, 788–789
physiology of, 786
primary mesothelioma of, 790
pseudomyxoma of, 790
secondary carcinomatosis of, 789–790
tumors of, 789–790
Peritonitis, 1584
bacterial, acute, 788–789
primary, 789
fungal, 789
granulomatous, 790
parasitic, 789
practolol in, 1964
spontaneous, 1593
tuberculous, 789, 1629
with cirrhosis, 1593
Peritonsillar abscess, 1523
Pernicious anemia, 897–898, 2265. See also *Anemia.*
achlorhydria with, 897
chronic gastritis and, 679, 680
genetic factors in, 897
immune response in, 897
incidence of, 897
juvenile, 897
stomach cancer and, 698
therapy of, 897–898
vitamin B_{12} therapy in, 897–898
Pernio, 358
Perphenazine, in Sydenham's chorea, 2075
Personality disorders, 2007–2015
Personality
in atherosclerosis, 283
in Huntington's disease, 2074
in irritable bowel syndrome, 710–711
in parkinsonism, 2070
Perstans filariasis, 1831
Pertussis. See *Whooping cough.*
Pes cavus, in Friedreich's ataxia, 2083
Petechiae, in infective endocarditis, 1536t
Petit mal, impulsive, 2152
Petit mal absences, 2152
Petit mal epilepsies, 2150, 2154
Petroleum distillates, poisoning from, 88
Peutz-Jeghers syndrome, 764
lentigines in, 2254
Peutz-Jeghers-Touraine syndrome, *2262*
pH. See also *Arterial pH; Hydrogen ion concentration.*
blood and urinary, reference values for, 2330
Phaeohyphomycosis, 1774
Phaeomycotic cyst, 1774
Phaeosporotrichosis, 1774
Phagocyte chemotaxis, 1477, 1479
Phagocytosis, in rheumatic disease, 1901–1902, *1902*
Phakomatoses, 2084–2086
Phalloidin, 783
Phantom limb pain, 2064
Pharmaceutical agents, neuropathy due to, 2195, *2195*
Pharmacodynamics, 69, *69*
drug interaction and, 81–82
plasma drug concentration and, 74, 75
Pharmacokinetics, 69, *69,* 70t
autonomic nervous system and, 90–96
circulatory system disorders and, 77–78
drug dose–dependent, 71t, 73
drug interaction and, 79–82
in aged, 78
plasma drug concentration and, 74
plasma protein binding and, 75
Pharyngitis
herpes simplex virus and, 1715
in infectious mononucleosis, 1720
lymphonodular, acute, 1733
plaque and, 1601
streptococcal, 781
group A, 1519, 1520, 1521, 1522–1523, 1524t, 1527–1528
diagnosis of, 1523
penicillin for, 1524, 1526
treatment of, 1524, 1526
viral, 1695–1696, 1696t
Pharyngoconjunctival fever, 1705
Pharynx
diverticulum of, 676
enterovirus infection of, 1732–1733
gonococcal infection of, 1645, 1647
in striatonigral degeneration, 2079
Phenacetin, nephrotoxicity of, 592–593
Phencyclidine, abuse of, 2023–2024
Phenelzine, in anxiety, 2010
Phenformin, 1329
Phenindione, as nephrotoxin, 601
Phenobarbital
in epilepsy, 2158, *2158*
inhibiting agents of, 81t
serum and plasma, reference values for, 2330
Phenothiazine
in pain, 2052
in schizophrenia, 2004
Phenotype, 138
differentiation of, 1352–1354, *1353*
Phenoxybenzamine, 95
Phentolamine, 91, 95
in heart failure, 206
in primary pulmonary hypertension, 263
in shock, 223
Phenylalanine, 131
metabolism of, 1126, *1126*
Phenylalanine hydroxylase, deficiency of, 1126, 1127
L-Phenylalanine mustard. See *Melphalan.*
Phenylbutazone, 81
as nephrotoxin, 602
for gout, 1141
in leukemia, 987
Phenylketonuria, 130, 131, 137, 1126–1127
congenital defects and, 146
genetic factors in, 1126
transient, 1127
Phenytoin, 325
ADH activity and, 1268t
as nephrotoxin, 601
folate absorption and, 899
for digitalis toxicity, 204
in epilepsy, 2158, *2158*
in trigeminal neuralgia, 2059
inhibiting agents of, 81t
osteomalacia and, 1428
pharmacokinetics of, 70t, 71, 73
serum and plasma, reference values for, 2330

Phenytoin (*Continued*)
  steroid therapy and, 1303
Pheochromocytoma, 274, 1410–1412
  alpha-adrenergic antagonists in, 95
  catecholamine measurements in, 1410–1411, *1411*
  clonidine in, 1411–1412
  epinephrine-releasing, 1410
  hypertension with, 1410
  in neurofibromatosis, 2085
  localization of, 1412
  neurofibromatosis and, 2258
  pathology of, 1410
  treatment of, 1412
Phialophora, 1774
Philadelphia chromosome, 959, 961–962, 972, 1061
  in chronic myelogenous leukemia, 975–980
Phlebectasia of jejunum, oral cavity, and scrotum, syndrome of, *2262*
Phlebotomus fever, 1738–1739
  clinical manifestations of, 1739
  epidemiology of, 1738–1739
  etiology of, 1738
  vector in, 1738–1739
Phlebotomus papatasi, 1738
Phlebotomus verrucarum, 1617
  in hemochromatosis, 1162–1163, *1163*
  in heart failure, 200
  in polycythemia vera, 970–971
Phobias, and anxiety, 2009
Phocanema decipiens, 1824
Phosphatase
  acid, reference values for, 2330
  alkaline, reference values for, 2330
Phosphate
  decreased absorption of, 1427
  homeostasis disorders and, 1427
  in osteitis fibrosa, 1453, 1455
  increased excretion of, 1427
  metabolism of, in uremia, 551
  nutritional deficiency of, 1427
Phosphatidylinositol, 1226
Phosphodiesterases, 1225
Phosphofructokinase, deficiency of, 1107
6-Phosphogluconate dehydrogenase, deficiency of, 907
Phosphoinositides, 1226
Phospholipids, in hormone action mediation, 1225–1226, *1226*
Phosphoribosylpyrophosphate synthetase, 1103
  deficiency of, with gout, 1139
Phosphorus. See also *Hyperphosphatemia; Hypophosphatemia.*
  dietary, 1164
  dietary allowance for, 1178–1179
  inorganic, reference values for, 2330
  metabolism of, 1163–1164, 1418–1419, *1419*
    kidney regulation of, 500
  plasma concentration of, 1417–1418, *1417*
  serum concentration of, 1163–1164
Phosphorus-32, in polycythemia vera, 971
Phosphorylase, deficiency of, 1106, 1107
Photoallergy, 2253
Photodermatitis, 2252, 2253
Photoprotectives, topical, 2241
Photosensitive epilepsy, 2153
Photosensitivity, 2252–2254
  chemical, 2296
Phototoxicity, 2253
Phycomycosis, 1771–1773
Physical disorders of lung, 2287–2289
Physical examination, 58–59
  in geriatrics, 26–27
Physical fitness, exercise and, 40
Physician. See also *Patient-physician relationship.*
Physician (*Continued*)
  abilities required of, 57–58, 57t
  as humanist, 6
  as nonphysician, 4
  as scientist, 6
  attitudes and habits of, 57
  data gathering by, 58–59
  diagnosis formulation by, 59
  dying patient and, 2
  education of, 2–4
  intellectual abilities of, 57–58
  medical care by, 60
  noncognitive abilities of, 57
  problem definition by, 59–60
  qualities of, 2
  role of, in death and dying, 30
  skills of, interpersonal, 57
    motor and technical, 57
  tasks required of, 58–60, 57t
Physiologic vertigo, 2041, *2041*
Phytolacca americana, 783
Pica, 889
Pick's disease, 2001
Pickwickian syndrome, 543, *1988*, 1989
Piebaldism, 2256
Pigeon breeder's lung, 2285
Pigmentation
  blotchy, 2256
  disturbances of, 2254–2257
  of mouth lesions, 2243
  of skin, 2233
  patterns of, 2225–2256
Pigmented nevi, 2254–2255
Pilocarpine iontophoresis sweat test, 425
Pilosebaceous-apocrine apparatus, 2230–2231
Pineal gland, 1273–1275
  abnormalities of, 1275
  anatomy of, 1273–1274, *1274*
  calcification of, 1275
  secretions of, 1274
  tumor of, 1247–1248, 1275, 2164
    characteristics of, *2162*
Pinealoma, 1247, 1275
  aberrant, 1369
Pinworm, 1824–1825
Pipe smoking, 50
Piperacillin, 1586
Piperazine citrate, for ascariasis, 1823
Pirenzipine, in peptic ulcer, 688
Piroplasmosis. See *Babesiosis.*
Pit vipers, 1841–1843
Pituitary. See also *Anterior pituitary; Posterior pituitary.*
  ablation of, for pain relief, 2054
  adenomas of, 2163
    characteristics of, *2162*
  anatomy of, 1251
  β-endorphin secretion of, 1236
  embryology of, 1251
  fetal, 1251
  hormone regulation by, 1244–1246
    hypophysiotropic hormone in, 1244–1246
    neurotransmitters in, 1244, 1244t
  hypothalamus and, 1242, *1242*
Pituitary apoplexy, 1256
Pityriasis rosea, 2244, *2245*
Pityrosporon orbiculare infection, 2246, 2247
Placebo effect, 2051
Placental alkaline phosphatase, 1076
Placental lactogen, 1253
Placental proteins, 1076
Plague, 1600–1602
  buboes of, 1601, 1602
  clinical features of, 1600–1601
  culture in, 1601–1602
  diagnosis of, 1601–1602
  epidemiology of, 1600
  etiology of, 1600
Plague (*Continued*)
  laboratory features of, 1601
  meningitis with, 1601
  pathogenesis of, 1600–1601
  prevention of, 1602
  prognosis in, 1602
  streptomycin in, 1602
  toxins in, 1600
  treatment of, 1602
  vaccine for, 1602
  vectors in, 1600–1602
Plants, poisonous, 89, 782–783
Plaque(s)
  bright, in retinal arterioles, 2096
  cutaneous, 2233
    in pregnancy, 2269
Plasma cell(s), 1013
Plasma cell disorders, 1013–1022
  immunoglobulins in, 1013, *1013*
  with M-component secretion, 1014, 1014t
Plasma drug concentration, 73–75
  active metabolites and, 75
  assay time and, 74–75
  interpretation of, 74–75
  pharmacodynamics and, 74, 75
  plasma protein binding and, 75
  therapeutic window concept and, 74, *74*, 75t
Plasma exchange
  in glomerulonephritis, 576, 577
  in myasthenia gravis, 2214
Plasma protein(s), renal metabolism of, 501
Plasma protein binding
  drug interaction and, 80–81
  pharmacokinetics and, 75
  plasma drug concentration and, 75
Plasma renin activity, 1309
Plasma therapy, in fluid volume depletion, 520
Plasma volume, reference values for, 2339
Plasmid cloning, 135, *136*, *138*
Plasmin, 1043, *1043*
Plasminogen, 1043, *1043*
Plasmodium, 1776–1780
Plasmodium falciparum, 1776–1780, 1776t
Plasmodium malariae, 1776–1779, 1776t
Plasmodium ovale, 1776–1780, 1776t
Plasmodium vivax, 1776–1780, 1776t
Plateau waves, and transient paralysis, 2047
Platelet(s), 1028–1030, *1029*
  acquired disorders of, 1037–1038
  aggregation of, 1031
  bone marrow release of, 1028
  drug-induced abnormalities of, 1030, 1030t, 1031
  in anemia, 875
  in polycythemia vera, 969
  in thrombocytopenia, 1031–1036
  laboratory evaluation of, 1030–1031
  precursors of, 866–867, *869*
  qualitative disorders of, 1037–1038
  release abnormalities of, 1037
  secretion of, 1028
  transfusions of, 1038
  vascular interaction of, 1028
Platelet antiaggregants, in threatened stroke, 2100
Platelet arachidonic acid, cyclooxygenase pathway of, 1028, *1029*
Platelet count
  reference values for, 2339
  with hemorrhage, 883–884
Platelet-activating factors, 390
Platinum, toxicity of, 601, 2314
Platybasia, 2188
Platypnea, 372
Plethysmography, body, 374
Pleura
  anatomy of, 447

Pleura (*Continued*)
biopsy of, 389
physiology of, 447
tuberculosis of, 1627
Pleural disease
asbestos exposure and, 2283
biopsy in, 448
diagnostic procedures for, 447
empyema with, 449
exploration in, 448
exudates in, 448, 448t
hemothorax with, 449
history in, 447
inflammation in, 448–449
physical examination in, 447
radiography in, 447
thoracentesis in, 447
transudates in, 447–448, 448t
tuberculous involvement in, 448
with chylothorax, 449
with pulmonary embolus and infarction, 449
Pleural effusion, 457
with pneumonia, 448–449
Pleural fluid, examination of, 388
Pleural neoplasm, 450
Pleurisy, 370
Pleurodynia, epidemic, 1730–1731
Pleuropulmonary infection, anaerobic, 1584
Plexus nerve, lesions of, 2179
Plummer's disease, 1281
Plummer-Vinson syndrome, 889, *2262*, *2265*
Plutonium toxicity, 2315
Pneumaturia, 484
Pneumococcal disease, immunization for, 44
Pneumococcal pneumonia, 1498–1504
antibiotics for, 1503, 1503t
clinical findings in, 1500–1501
complications of, 1503–1504
differential diagnosis of, 1501–1502, 1503t
epidemiology of, 1499
laboratory findings in, 1501
pathogenesis of, 1499–1500, 1499t
pathology of, 1500
prevention of, 1504
prognosis in, 1504
radiography in, 1501, *1502*
spread of, 1500
treatment of, 1502
vs. pulmonary infarction, 1502, 1503t
Pneumococcal vaccine, 42t, 1504
Pneumococcus(i), 1498
microbiology of, 1498–1499
Pneumoconiosis, 417
coal worker's, 417, 2281
Pneumocystis carinii, 1479, 1796
Pneumocystis carinii pneumonia, 1861, 1862
Pneumocystosis, 1796–1797
clinical manifestations of, 1796–1797
course of, 1797
diagnosis of, 1797
epidemiology of, 1796
immune response in, 1796, 1797
lung biopsy in, 1797
pathogenesis of, 1796
pathology of, 1796
prevention of, 1797
serology in, 1797
treatment of, 1797
Pneumomediastinum, 452
Pneumonia, 1494–1519. See also *Aspiration pneumonia;* Klebsiella *pneumonia; Mycoplasmal pneumonia; Pneumococcal pneumonia;* Pseudomonas *pneumonia.*
aerobic gram-negative bacilli and, 1510–1513
aspiration, 1584
vs. aspiration pneumonitis, 2291
Pneumonia (*Continued*)
bacterial, secondary, 1730
causative organisms in, 1495
coccidioidal, chronic, 1761
clinical presentation of, 1496–1497
diagnosis of, 1497–1498
enteric bacterial infection with, 1593–1594
eosinophilic, chronic, 415
fiberoptic bronchoscopy in, 1497–1498
Friedländer's 1509, 1510
giant-cell, 1708
Hemophilus influenzae, 1564
hospital-acquired infection and, 1487–1488, 1511–1513
Klebsiella, 1509–1510
lipoid, 2294–2295
lung host defenses in, 1495–1496
management of, 1497–1498
meningococcal, 1560
mixed viral and bacterial, 1703–1704
necrotizing, 1584–1585
nosocomial, 1487
pathogenesis of, 1495–1496
percutaneous transtracheal aspiration in, 1497
plague, 1601
pleural effusion with, 448–449
staphylococcal, 1547
streptococcal, 1524
tissue culture in, 1498
viral, primary, 1703
with nocardiosis, 1613
with rickettsial infection, 1677
Pneumonitis
aspiration, 2291–2293
chemical, acute, 2289
hydrocarbon, 2294
hypersensitivity, 417–418, 2285
in ascariasis, 1822–1823
lymphocytic interstitial, 415–416, 445
radiation, 2287
with psittacosis, 1671
Pneumothorax, 450, 457
PNS. See *Partial nonprogressing stroke.*
Podagra, 1140
Podophyllotoxins, 1099
Poikilothermia, hypothalamus and, 2025
Poison centers, 85
Poisoning, 37, 84–89. See also specific chemicals.
absorption in, prevention of, 86
acrylamide, autonomic dysfunction in, 2027
activated charcoal in, 87
antidotes in, 87
chelating agents in, 87
death from, 85, 85t
definition of, 84
diagnosis of, 85–86
dialysis in, 87
drug, *1978–1979*, 1979–1981
elimination enhancement in, 87
emesis induction in, 86
epidemiology of, 85
etiology of, 85
exchange transfusion in, 87
from marine animals, 1843–1845
from snake bites, 1841–1843
gastric lavage in, 87
hemoperfusion in, 87
incidence of, 85
metabolism inhibition in, 87
packaging regulations and, 86
prevention of, 85, 86
supportive measures in, 86
toxicologic analysis in, 86, 86t
treatment of, 86–89
Poisonous animals and plants, 89, 782–783
Pokeweed, 783
Poliomyelitis
acute anterior, 2130–2132
autonomic dysfunction in, 2027
immunization for, 42t, 45
nonparalytic, 2131
paralytic, 2130–2132
vaccine-associated paralysis in, 45
Poliovirus, 2130
Poliovirus vaccines, 42t, 2132
Pollution, cancer and, 1071
Polyamines, 1076
Polyarteritis, with pulmonary involvement, 1941
Polyarteritis nodosa, 1941–1943, *2262*, *2264*, *2266*
clinical manifestations of, 1941–1942, 1942t
course of, 1942
diagnosis of, 1941–1942
differential, 1943
glomerular involvement in, 585
immune response in, 1941, 1942
intracerebral hemorrhage with, 2105
laboratory findings in, 1942–1943
of childhood, 1941
pathology of, 1941
treatment of, 1943
Polyarthritis, migratory, in rheumatic fever, 1529
Polychondritis, relapsing, 1951
Polycystic kidney disease, 506, 634–635
adult, 487–488, 634–635
childhood, 634
genetic factors in, 634, 635
ultrasonography of, 514
Polycystic ovarian disease, 1388, 1389, 1395, 1397
Polycystic ovary syndrome, 1249
Polycythemia, 963–971, *2265*. See also *Polycythemia vera.*
altitude and, 966–967
alveolar hypoventilation and, 967
and cerebral artery thrombosis, 2093
autonomous vs. secondary proliferation in, 964–965
cardiopulmonary disease and, 967
classification of, 965–965t
dehydration and, 963
endogenous colony formation in, 965–966
erythropoietin assay in, 965–966
in congenital heart disease, 228
mechanism of, 964–965
myelofibrosis with, 972–974
oxygen-hemoglobin dissociation curve and, 967
pathophysiology of, 964–965
physiologically appropriate, 966–967
relative, 963–964
secondary, 966–968
treatment of, 968
with urinary tract obstruction, 606
Polycythemia vera
bone marrow in, 969–970
chlorambucil in, 971
chromosomal abnormalities in, 962
clinical manifestations of, 968–969
course of, 970
diagnosis of, 970, 970t
differential, 970
erythropoiesis in, 969, 970
hydroxyurea in, 971
laboratory data in, 969
leukocytosis in, 969, 970
myelosuppression in, 971
phlebotomy in, 970–971
phosphorus-32 in, 971
platelets in, 969
remission in, 962
residual stem cells in, 962

Polycythemia vera (*Continued*)
  stem cell disorder in, 968
  treatment of, 970–971
  vs. leukemoid reaction, 959t
Polydipsia, primary, 525, 1271
Polymorphism, 130, 131t
Polymorphonuclear neutrophil, 941
Polymorphous photodermatitis, 2253
Polymyalgia rheumatica, 1946, 1947, 1949, 1955
Polymyositis, 1947–1950, 2200
  childhood, 1947
  clinical manifestations of, 1948
  corticosteroids in, 1949–1950
  diagnosis of, 1947, 1949
  electromyography in, 1949
  immune response in, 1947, 1948–1949
  in cancer, 1083
  incidence of, 1947
  laboratory data in, 1948–1949
  pathogenesis of, 1947–1948
  pathology of, 1947–1948
  prognosis in, 1948
  treatment of, 1949–1950
  vs. muscular dystrophy, *2209*
  vs. myasthenia gravis, 2213
Polymyositis/dermatomyositis, with interstitial lung disease, 414
Polymyxin B, 106
Polymyxin E, 106
Polyneuritis, 457
  acute, vs. paralytic poliomyelitis, 2131
  classification of, *2189*
  cranial, and vertigo, 2043
    and asthenia, 2044
  definition of, 2188
  diabetic, 2192–2193
  inflammatory, 2190–2192
  postinfectious, 2190. See also *Guillain-Barré syndrome.*
  sensory, 2191–2192
  symmetrical, 2188
Polyol, 1326, 1327
Polyol/myoinositol metabolism, in diabetes mellitus, 1326
Polypectomy, colonoscopic, 762–763
Polypeptide hormone(s), 1220–1221
  action, of, 1223, 1224–1226
    mediators of, 1224, 1224t
  biosynthesis of, 1220, *1220*
  ectopic, 1076
  metabolism of, 1223
  receptors for, 1224
  transport of, 1222
Polypeptide proteins, ectopic, 1076
Polyposis, gastrointestinal, cutaneous disorders with, *2262*
Polyposis coli, colonoscopy in, 661–662, *662*
Polysplenia syndrome, 240
Polyuria
  acquired, 1269–1270
  with diabetes insipidus, 1270, 1272
Pompe's disease, 132, 332, 1107, 2205
Pons, arterial supply of, 2089, *2089*
Pontiac fever, 1516–1518
Pontine hemorrhage, 2108, *2110*
Population genetics, HLA system and, 1881
Poriomania, 2157
Pork tapeworm, 1806–1807
  eradication of, 1809
Porphobilin, 1156
Porphobilinogen, 1153, 1154, 1155, 1156
  urinary, reference values for, 2331
Porphyria(s), 907, 1103, 1153–1158
  biochemical characterization of, 1154
  carriers of, 1156, 1157
  classification of, 1154, 1154t
Porphyria(s) (*Continued*)
  clinical presentation of, 1156
  diagnosis of, 1156
  drug-induced, 1156, 1156t
  epidemiology of, 1154
  erythropoietic, congenital, 1154–1155, *2265*
  genetic factors in, 1153–1154, 1155–1156, 1155t
  hematin therapy in, 1156–1157, *1157*
  heme biosynthesis and, 1153, *1154*, 1155–1156, 1155t
  hepatic, 1155–1156
  intermittent, acute, 83, 1155
    vs. hysteria, 2014
  management of, 1156–1157
  neurologic features of, 1156
  photosensitivity in, 2253
  prognosis in, 1157
  screening for, 1156
  symptomatic, *2263*
  toxic, 1158
  variegate, 1155
Porphyria cutanea tarda, 1157–1158, 2253, *2253*
  differential diagnosis of, 1157
  genetic vs. environmental factors in, 1157
Porphyrin
  biosynthesis of, sideroblastic anemia and, 892
  tissue production of, 1153
Port-wine hemangioma, in Sturge-Weber disease, 2085
Portal hypertension, 840–843
  arteriovenous fistula with, 841
  cirrhosis and, 840–842
  clinical manifestations of, 841
  congenital hepatic fibrosis and, 842
  diagnosis of, 842
  esophageal and gastric varices with, 841, *841*, 842–843
  hepatic vein thrombosis with, 841–842
  idiopathic, 842
  inferior vena cava obstruction with, 842
  noncirrhotic portal fibrosis with, 842
  pathogenesis of, 840–841, 841t
  portal vein thrombosis with, 841
  portal-systemic collaterals in, 841
  portal-systemic shunts in, 843
  splenic vein thrombosis with, 841
  splenomegaly with, 841
  surgical therapy for, 843
  veno-occlusive disease with, 842
Portal vascular system, 1241
Portal venous system, 840
Portal-systemic encephalopathy, 845
Positive end-expiratory, pressure, 468, 477
  in fat embolism syndrome, 432
  ventilation and, 459
Positive pressure breathing, in heart failure, 200
Positron tomography, 182
Postcentral primary somatosensory cortex syndrome, 1992
Postcholecystectomy syndrome, 864–865
Postconcussive syndrome, 2174
  and fatigue, 2044
Posterior cord syndrome, 2176
Posterior fossa tumors, 2164
Posterior pituitary, 1266–1273
  anatomy of, 1266
  and, diabetes insipidus, 1269–1273
  antidiuretic hormone of, 1266–1268, *1266*, 1268t
  hypothalamic nuclei of, 1266
  oxytocin production of, 1273
  physiology of, 1266–1267
Postherpetic neuralgia, management of, 2129
Postinfectious encephalomyelitis, 2139–2140, 2147
Postinfectious pandysautonomia, 2192
Postinfectious sensory neuronopathy, 2191–2192
Postpericardiotomy syndrome, pericarditis with, 341
Postphlebitic syndrome, 364
Postpoliomyelitis motor neuron disease, 2132
Postprandial dumping syndrome. See *Dumping syndrome.*
Post-traumatic amnesia, 2170
Post-traumatic epilepsy, 2171
Post-traumatic headache, 2057
Post-traumatic vertigo, 2042
Postural hypotension
  hyperadrenergic, 1412, 1412t
  hypoadrenergic, 1412–1413, 1412t
Posture
  deformed, in parkinsonism, 2070
  in extrapyramidal disorders, 2068
  in Huntington's disease, 2074
Postvaccinal encephalomyelitis, 2140
Potassium
  deficiency of, 336
  excretion of, 510–511
  food content of, 1214, 1214t
  for digitalis toxicity, 203–204
  in adrenal steroid regulation, 1304, 1305
  in aldosterone regulation, 1305
  in diabetic ketoacidosis, 1335, *1335*
  metabolism of, in interstitial nephritis, 591
    in uremia, 549–550
  serum, reference values for, 2331
Potassium balance
  disorders of, 530–535
    excitable tissues and, 531–532, *532*
    ICF/ECF transport and, 530, 531
    physiologic considerations in, 530–532
  renal processing and, 530–531, *531*
  endocrine factors in, 498
  kidney regulation of, 497–498, *498*
Potassium depletion
  clinical manifestations of, 533
  gastrointestinal losses and, 533
  hypokalemia and, 532–534
  in metabolic alkalosis, 542
Potassium hydroxide examination
  in fungus infections, 2247
  in psoriasis, 2245
Potassium permanganate, in wet dressing, 2239, *2239*
Pott's disease, 1628
Powassan virus encephalitis, 1749
Poxvirus infection, chemotherapy for, 110
Prader-Willi syndrome, 1172–1173, 2207
Praziquantel
  for hermaphroditic fluke infection, 1815, 1816, 1817, 1818
  in oriental schistosomiasis, 1815
  in tapeworm infection, 1809
  in urinary bilharziasis, 1813
Prazosin, 95
  in heart failure, 207
Prealbumin, thyroxine-binding, 1279
Prednisolone, 114
  in skin disease, 2240
Prednisone
  dosage regimen for, 114, 115
  in acute lymphoblastic leukemia, 990
  in aplastic anemia, 880, *880*, 881
  in Bell's palsy, 2197
  in cancer chemotherapy, 1092, 1101t
  in chronic bronchitis, 399
  in chronic lymphocytic leukemia, 983
  in cluster headache, 2056
  in Crohn's disease, 747

Prednisone (*Continued*)
in idiopathic thrombocytopenic purpura, 1034
in nephrotic syndrome, 580, 581
in skin disease, 2241
Preeclampsia, 626
Pre-excitation syndrome, 315–317
electrocardiography in, 315–317, *316, 317*
Prefrontal polar syndrome, 1992
Pregnancy, 1380
acute fatty liver of, 834–835
acute kidney failure in, 626–627
aldosterone-renin-angiotensin system in, 626
bacteriuria with, 621
Chlamydia in, 1670
cholestasis of, 835
cigarette smoking and, 49
group B streptococcal infection in, 1526–1527
hypertension in, 271, 625–626
hyperthyroidism in, 1286
in sarcoidosis, 437
kidney disease in, 624–627
kidney function in, 624–625, *625*
liver disease in 834–835
malaria in, 1778, 1780
papules and plaques of, 2269
pulmonary tuberculosis in, 1626–1627
pyelonephritis with, 621
renal parenchymal disease in, 626
serum creatinine in, 625
syphilis in, 1659
toxemia of, 625–626
toxoplasmosis and, 1792, 1794, 1795
ulcerative colitis and, 755
Pregnancy tests, reference values for, 2331
Pregnanediol, urinary, reference values for, 2331
Pregnanetriol, urinary, reference values for, 2331
Pregnenolone, serum, reference values for, 2331
Prehormone, 1220
Prekallikrein deficiency, 1048
Preleukemic syndromes, 960
Presbycusis, 2039
Pressure
cerebrospinal fluid, high, 2167–2168
low, syndrome of, 2166–2167
intracranial, increased, in encephalitis, treatment of, 2125
Pressure-sensitive receptors, 162
Preventive medicine, 35–37
behavior modification in, 35
health maintenance examination and, 55, 55t
injury prevention in, 36–37
screening tests in, 56
Prickly heat, 2229
Primaquine
hemolytic anemia and, 905, 906
in malaria, 1779–1780
Primary care, 7
Primary pulmonary hypertension, captopril in, 265
Primidone, in epilepsy, 2158, *2158*
Prinzmetal's angina, 285–286, 287
Probenecid, in gout, 1141
Procainamide, 324
clearance of, 76
interstitial lung disease and, 418
loading dose of, 77
pharmacokinetics of, 70t, 72, *73*
therapeutic window for, 74, *74*
Procarbazine, 1099
interstitial lung disease and, 418
Prochlorperazine, in vertigo, 2043
Procollagen peptidase deficiency, 1150, 1151
Proctalgia fugax, 785
Proctitis, 784
infectious, 784
ulcerative, nonspecific, 784
Proctosigmoidoscopy, in diarrhea, 716
Professional Standards Review Organizations, 8
Progesterone, 1381
serum, reference values for, 2331
Progesterone receptor assay, reference values for, 2331
Progestin(s), in cancer chemotherapy, 1101t
Progestogen withdrawal test, 1382
Progressive diaphyseal dysplasia, 1465
Progressive multifocal leukoencephalopathy, 2137
immunosuppressive therapy and, 2142
Progressive rubella panencephalitis, 2136
Progressive supranuclear palsy, and parkinsonism, 2071
Progressive systemic sclerosis, with interstitial lung disease, 414
Prohormone, 1220
Prolactin, 1253, 1254, 1367, 1398
function tests of, 1255
in galactorrhea, 1398–1399
in hypopituitarism, 1257
in pituitary tumor, 1263–1264, 1263t
serum, reference values for, 2331
Prolactin-releasing factor, 1246
Prolactinomas, 1399
Proliferative disorders, clonal development and stem origin of, 961–963
Proline, metabolic disorders of, 1129
Promonocyte, 941–942
Promyelocyte, 940, *941*
Proopiomelanocortin, 1077
Propionibacterium acnes, 1583
Propranolol, 91, 93–95, 325
absorption of, 69
in angina pectoris, 287
in essential tremor, 2074
in hyperthyroidism, 1285
in myocardial infarction, 294
in shock, 223
Proprioception, 2047
Proprioceptive ataxia, 2044–2045
Propylthiouracil, 1277, 1284–1285
Prostacyclin, 1238
in Raynaud's disease, 355
in shock, 214
Prostaglandin(s), 1237–1241
biosynthesis of, 1237–1239, *1238*
endogenons pyrogen and, 1472
fluid volume disorders and, 518
functions of, 1239
gastric mucosa integrity and, 683, 684
in allergy, 390
in asthma, 391
in cancer, 1078
in Crohn's disease, 741
in obstructive neuropathy, 605
in peptic ulcer, 688, 689
in shock, 214
renal, 501
renal vasodilatory effects of, 518
sodium balance and, 497
synthesis of, 1225, *1226*
arachidonic acid in, 1226
in peptic ulcer, 684, 689
Prostaglandin D_2, 1238
Prostaglandin E_1
in arteriosclerosis obliterans, 360
in Raynaud's disease, 355
Prostaglandin E_2, 1238
as natriuretic, 1239
Prostaglandin F_2, 1239
Prostaglandin synthetase inhibition, in Bartter's syndrome, 613
Prostate, 1375–1379
benign hyperplasia of, 1376–1377
cancer of, 1377–1379
diagnosis of, 1378
endocrine therapy in, 1378–1379
epidemiology of, 1377
Prostate cancer
pathology of, 1378
staging in, 1378, 1378t
surgery for, 1378–1379
treatment of, 1378–1379
Prostatitis, 1375–1376
bacterial, 1375, 1376
enteric bacilli in, 1594
nonbacterial, 1375, 1376
Prosthesis, hospital-acquired infection of, 1490
Prosthetic valves, infective endocarditis with, 1537
Protein(s)
AA, in amyloid diseases, 1169–1170
absorption of, 720–721
cerebrospinal fluid, in bacterial meningitis, 1553
C-reactive. See *C-Reactive protein.*
dietary allowances for, 1174–1175
ectopic polypeptide, 1076
homeostasis of, 1184
intake of, dietary, 1184
restricted diet and, 1213
supplements to, 1214
metabolism of, impairment of, 723
in liver disease, 805
renal failure and, 489
uremia and, 489
myelin basic, in multiple sclerosis, 2144
reference values for, 2332
synthesis of, genes and, 123–124, *125*
transcription in, 123
translation in, 123
Protein C, 1043
deficiency of, 1050
Protein N, in pseudohypoparathyroidism, 1446
Protein S, 1043
Protein-calorie malnutrition, 1183–1188
clinical manifestations of, 1186–1187, 1186t
diagnosis of, 1186–1187
electrolytes in, 1185
endocrine factors in, 1185
epidemiology of, 1183–1184
growth hormone in, 1185
hospitalization and, 1183, 1184, 1187, 1187t
hypothalamic-pituitary-adrenal axis in, 1185
immune response in, 1185
insulin secretion in, 1185
metabolic factors in, 1184–1185
mineral deficiencies in, 1185
pathophysiology of, 1184–1186
prevention of, 1187
"sugar-baby," 1185
thyroid hormone in, 1185
treatment of, 1187
Protein-calorie supplementation, 1211–1213, *1212*t
commercial supplements for, 1213, 1213t
complications of, 1213
in enteral nutrition, 1211–1213
in parenteral nutrition, 1215–1217, 1215t
indications for, 1212
patient selection for, 1211–1212
supplement choice for, 1212–1213
table foods for, 1212–1213
Protein deficiency
in gastrointestinal disease, 646

Protein deficiency (*Continued*)
inborn errors of metabolism and, 128, 130, 131t
Protein-losing enteropathy, 723, 739–740, *739*t
Proteinosis, alveolar, 416–417
Proteinuria, 484, 507–509, 508t
altered renal hemodynamics and, 508–509
in acute glomerulonephritis, 569, 571
in nephrotic syndrome, 578–579
in pregnancy, 625, 626
increased glomerular permeability and, 508
overflow, 508
selective, 508
tubular, 508
Proteus, pneumonia from, 1513
Prothrombin, 1028
deficiency of, 1050
Prothrombin consumption, reference values for, 2339
Prothrombin time, 1031, 1044
in acute viral hepatitis, 814
in liver disease, 810
reference values for, 2339
Protoporphyria, 1155
erythropoietic, *2265*
liver disease and, 833
Protoporphyrin, 919–920
blood and fecal, reference values for, 2332
Protozoa, biology of, 1775
Protozoan disease, 1775–1804. See also specific diagnoses.
diagnosis of, 1775–1776
epidemiology of, 1775
host factor in, 1775
occupational, 2297
of intestine, 737
Protracted abstinence syndrome, in alcoholism, 53
"Prune-belly" syndrome, 639
Prurigo gestationis of Besnier, 2269
Pruritic urticarial papules and plaques of pregnancy, 2269
Pruritus
aquagenic, 1865
in chronic renal failure, 553–554, 557
in dermatitis herpetiformis, 2269
in pregnancy, 2269
with cancer, 1084, 1086
Pruritus ani, 786
in enterobiasis, 1825
Pseudo-Bartter's syndrome, 613
Pseudoclaudication, cauda equina, in lumbar spondylosis, 2184
Pseudodementia, 1999
Pseudogout, 1140, 1950
Pseudohermaphroditism. See *Female pseudohermaphroditism; Male pseudohermaphroditism.*
Pseudo-Hurler polydystrophy, 1149
Pseudohyperkalemia, 534
Pseudohypertrophy, muscular, 2199, 2200, 2202
Pseudohypoparathyroidism, 738, 1103, 1446–1448
brachymetacarpia with, 1447
calcium metabolism in, 1446–1448
cyclic AMP excretion in, 1446
diagnosis of, 1447–1448
genetic factors in, 1447
N protein in, 1446
parathyroid hormone in, 1446–1448
pathophysiology of, 1447
serum phosphate in, 1447, 1448
vitamin D in, 1446–1448
Pseudoincontinence, 2029
Pseudolymphoma, of lung, 445
Pseudomembranous enterocolitis, 1576–1577
Pseudomonas, 1594, 1608–1609
Pseudomonas aeruginosa, 1512, 1594
Pseudomonas infection, 1594
Pseudomonas mallei, 1609
Pseudomonas pneumonia, 1510–1513
clinical features of, 1512
laboratory findings in, 1512–1513
pathogenesis of, 1512
pathology of, 1512
predisposing factors to, 1512
prognosis in, 1513
treatment of, 1513
Pseudomonas pseudomallei, 1608
Pseudomyxoma peritonei, 790
Pseudoneutropenia, 956
Pseudopapilledema, 2168, 2219
Pseudopseudohypoparathyroidism, 1446–1448
Pseudopuberty
female, 1383–1385, 1384t, 1385t
factitious, 1384
heterosexual, precocious, 1383
isosexual, precocious, 1383
Pseudoseizures, vs. epilepsy, 2156
Pseudotumor, orbital, 2221–2222
Pseudotumor cerebri, 2168–2169
Pseudouridine, 1076
Pseudoxanthoma elasticum, 347, 1152–1153, *1152*, 2258–2259, *2262*, *2264*
Psilocin, abuse of, 2023–2024
Psilocybin, abuse of, 2023–2024
Psittacosis, 1671–1672
antibiotic therapy in, 1672
carriers in, 1671
clinical manifestations of, 1671
differential diagnosis of, 1672
epidemiology of, 1671
pathology of, 1671
pneumonitis with, 1671
serology in, 1671–1672
treatment of, 1672
Psoralens, in psoriasis, 2246
Psoriasiform erythroderma, 2251
Psoriasis, 2245–2246, *2245*, *2266*
arthropathy with, 1921–1922
Psoriatic arthritis, 2245
Psychedelics, abuse of, 2023–2024
Psychiatric disorders, 1975–1976
Psychic symptoms, in epilepsy, 2151
Psychogenic fatigue, 2044
Psychogenic impotence, 2030
Psychogenic unresponsiveness, *1971*
Psychology, normative indices in, 15
Psychometric studies, in epilepsy, 2156
Psychomotor activity, in metabolic brain disease, 1975
Psychomotor epilepsy, 2154
Psychomotor seizures, 2152
and syncope, 1986
Psychophysiologic disorders, pain in, 2049
Psychophysiologic muscle tension syndromes, vs. paravertebral tumor, 2185
Psychosis(es)
amphetamine, 2022
cocaine, 2022
depressive, and hysterical symptoms, 2013
functional, 2001–2007
manic-depressive, 2005–2007
schizophrenic, and hysterical symptoms, 2013
Psychotherapy
in pain, 2053
in schizophrenia, 2005
Pteroylmonoglutamic acid, 898
Ptosis
in myasthenia gravis, 2212
in myotonic dystrophy, 2203
Ptosis (*Continued*)
in Wernicke's encephalopathy, 2065
Puberty, 16–18. See also *Adolescence.*
anorexia nervosa and, 1189
biologic processes in, 16–18
environmental factors in, 18
female, 1383–1388
delayed, 1385–1386
genetic factors in, 18
isosexual, precocious, 1383
male, 1368
delayed, 1368
precocious, 1368–1369
neuroendocrine control of, 18
precocious, 1383–1385, 1384t, 1385t
somatic changes in, 16–18, *16*
Public health, 7–8
Puerperal myocarditis, 338
Puffer fish poisoning, 783
Pulmonary. See also *Lung(s)* and *Respiratory.*
Pulmonary angiography, in pulmonary embolism, 429–430
Pulmonary arterial hypertension, radiography in, 169
Pulmonary arterial pressure monitoring, in critical care management, 474–475, 474t, *475*, 478
Pulmonary arteriovenous fistula, 233, 455
Pulmonary artery
aortic communication defect and, 231–232
coronary artery origin from, 232–233
Pulmonary aspiration, 670–671, 672t, 672
Pulmonary blastoma, 445
Pulmonary blastomycosis, 1763
Pulmonary capillary wedge pressure, in shock, 211, 220
Pulmonary circulation, 377–378
normal hemodynamics of, 256–257, 256t
structure in, 257
Pulmonary complications, in heroin addiction, 2018
Pulmonary cryptococcosis, 1765–1766
Pulmonary disease
brain abscess with, 2112
mycobacterial, 1632
occupational, 2279–2287, *2279*
Pulmonary edema, 290
cardiogenic, 456
causes of, 456
high altitude, 2289
in heart failure, management of, 199–200
in left ventricular failure, 196
noncardiogenic, 456
respiratory failure management in, 472–473, *473*
Pulmonary embolism, 426–431, 456
anticoagulants in, 430, 431
arterial blood gases in, 427
clinical manifestations of, 426–427
death from, 426
diagnosis of, 427, 429t
electrocardiography in, 427
embolectomy in, 430
epidemiology of, 426
etiology of, 426
hypoxemia with, 426
mechanisms of, 426
pathology of, 426
perfusion lung scan in, 427–429, *428*
pleural disease with, 449
prevention of, 431
prognosis in, 431
pulmonary angiography in, 429–430
pulmonary hypertension and, 258–259
radiography in, 427–429, *428*
shock from, 426
thrombolytic therapy in, 430

Pulmonary embolism (*Continued*)
thrombophlebitis and, 363, 364
treatment of, 430–431
vena caval interruption in, 431
venography in, 429
ventilation scan in, 429
with myocardial infarction, 292
Pulmonary fibrosis
familial, 416
idopathic, 412–413, *412*
Pulmonary function
in asbestosis, 2284
in interstitial lung disease, 411
in left ventricular failure, 197
in occupational lung disease, 2280
in silicosis, 2282
Pulmonary hemorrhage, in anti-GBM glomerulonephritis, 576
Pulmonary hemosiderosis, idiopathic, 415
Pulmonary histoplasmosis, 1760
Pulmonary hypertension, 256–265, 290
alveolar hypoventilation in, 260–261
arterial vs. venous, 257
bronchitis and, 259–260
chest pain with, 371
chronic obstructive lung disease and, 259–260
clinical manifestations in, 257–258, 257t
collagen disease and, 258, 261
combined pathology in, 260
congenital heart disease and, 258
emphysema and, 259–260
heart disease and, 258
interstitial fibrosis and, 259, 260
mitral stenosis and, 246–247, 248
occlusive pulmonary vascular disease and, 258–259
oxygen therapy in, 259, 260, 261
primary, cardiac catheterization in, 262
clinical picture in, 262
diagnosis of, 262–263
drug therapy in, 263–265, 264t
pathophysiology of, 262
prognosis in, 265
treatment of, 263–265
unexplained, 261–265, 261t
anorectic agent Aminorex and, 261, 262
definition of, 261
general features of, 261
pathology of, 261–262
vasodilators in, 263–264t
pulmonary veno-occlusive disease and, 265
respiratory disorders and, 259–261
sarcoidosis and, 261
secondary, 258–261
with adult respiratory distress syndrome, 261
with congenital heart disease, 228
Pulmonary infarction, vs. pneumococcal pneumonia, 1502, 1503t
Pulmonary mucormycosis, 1772
Pulmonary oxygen toxicity, 2290, 2291
Pulmonary stenosis
balloon valvuloplasty for, 235–236
cardiac catheterization in, 235
echocardiography in, 235
electrocardiography in, 235
radiography in, 235
surgery for, 235–236
ventriculography in, 235
with intact ventricular septum, 235–236
Pulmonary thromboembolism, 456–457
Pulmonary tuberculosis, 1623–1627
chemotherapy for, 1624–1627
regimens of, 1625–1626
resistance to, 1626
Pumonary tuberculosis (*Continued*)
chemotherapy for, results of, 1625–1626
retreatment regimen in, 1626
clinical description of, 1623–1624
control of, 1621–1622
corticosteroids for, 1626
diagnosis of, 1623–1624
epidemiology of, 1621–1622
etiology of, 1620–1621
immune response in, 1622
in children, 1627
in pregnancy, 1626–1627
infectiousness reversal in, 1626
kidney function in, 1626
liver function in, 1626
pathogenesis of, 1621
pathology of, 1621
primary, 1623
radiography in, 1623–1624
reactivation of, 1623
recurrence of, 1623
skin tests in, 1622–1623, 1624
sputum examination in, 1624
stages of, 1621
treatment of, 1624–1627
Pulmonary valve, regurgitation defect of, 238
Pulmonary vascular disease
pulmonary hypertension and, 258–259
respiratory failure management in, 473
Pulmonary vasculitis, 456–457
Pulmonary vein, anomalous connection of, 239
Pulmonary vein stenosis, 235
Pulmonary veno-occlusive disease, pulmonary hypertension and, 265
Pulmonary venous hypertension, radiography in, 169
Pulmonary vessels, radiography of, 168–169, *167, 168*
Pulmonic regurgitation, 256
Pulmonic stenosis, 256
"uncured," in adult, 240
with transposition of the great arteries, 239
Pulmonic valve, absence of, 238
Pulseless disease, 2093
Pulsus alternans, 152, 289
in left ventricular failure, 197
Pulsus paradoxus, 152, 463
Punch biopsy, in skin disese, 2238, 2239
Punctate telangiectasia, involving mouth, 2243
Pupil(s)
abnormalities of, neurogenic, 2034–2035
in brain injury, 2171
Purine analogues, 1095, *1095*
Purine enzyme, deficiencies of, immune response with, 1144–1145
Purine metabolism, 1133–1134, *1134*
disorders of, 1132–1145
Purine nucleoside phosphorylase, deficiency of, 1145, 1859
Purpura, 1030. See also specific diagnoses.
anaphylactoid, 1038–1039
in plague, 1601
senile, 1039, 2232
vascular, 1038–1040, 1039t
Purpura simplex, 1039
Pustule, 2233
Putaminal hemorrhage, *2109*
external capsular–, 2108
Putrescine, 1076
Pyelography
antegrade, 512
intravenous, 511, *512*
retrograde, 511–512
Pyelonephritis, 619–623
acute, 486
vs. chronic, 619
chronic, 590
hypertension and, 275
in pregnancy, 621
treatment of, 622
Pyknodysostosis, 1464
Pyloric stenosis, 704
congenital hypertrophic, 704
Pyloroplasty, with truncal vagotomy, 691
Pyoderma, 1524–1525, 1524t
Pyoderma gangrenosum, with ulcerative colitis, 753
Pyomyositis, staphylococcal, 1549
Pyramidal spasticity, vs. extrapyramidal rigidity, 2045–2046
Pyrantel pamoate
for ascariasis, 1823
for enterobiasis, 1825
for hookworm disease, 1821
for trichinellosis, 1826
Pyrazinamide, 1625, 1626
Pyridine derivatives, 1201
2-Pyridone, 1202
Pyridostigmine, 95
in myasthenia gravis, 2214
Pyridoxal, 1202–1203
Pyridoxal-5-phosphate, 1202–1203
Pyridoxamine, 1202–1203
Pyridoxine, 1202–1204
biochemical function of, 1202–1203
deficiency of, 1109, 1203–1204
assay in, 1203
drug-induced, 1203
in alcoholism, 1203
treatment of, 1203–1204
dependency syndromes and, 1203–1204
dietary allowance for, 1178
dietary sources of, 1203
physiology of, 1203
requirements for, 1203
structure of, 1202–1203, *1202*
toxicity of, 1204
Pyrimethamine
in malaria, 1779, 1780
in toxoplasmosis, 1795
Pyrimidine metabolism, disorders of, 1145
Pyrimidine 5′-nucleotidase, deficiency of, 7909, 1145
Pyrosis. See *Heartburn.*
Pyruvate carboxylase, 1210
Pyruvate dehydrogenase deficiency, *2205*
Pyruvate kinase deficiency, 905
genetic factor in, 905
hemolysis in, 905
Pyruvate metabolism, disorders of, 2206
Pyruvic acid, blood, reference values for, 2332
Pyuria, 484
Pyrvinium pamoate, in enterobiasis, 1825

Q fever, 1677, 1686–1687
QRS complex, examination of, 173
in right bundle branch block, 174
normal, 171, *171*
Quadriparesis, spastic, in central pontine myelinolysis, 2067
Quality of life, 13
Quantal squander, 2216
Queensland tick typhus, 1682
Questran. See *Cholestyramine.*
Quinacrine, in giardiasis, 1803
in tapeworm infection, 1809

Quinazoline derivative, in primary pulmonary hypertension, 263–264
Quinidine, 323–324
  in malaria, 1779
  pharmacokinetic parameters of, 70t
Quinine
  in malaria, 179
  ocular side effects of, 2225
  resistance to, 1779
Quinlan, Karen Ann, 11
Quinsy, 1523
Quintan fever, 1685–1686

Rabies, 2132–2135
  dumb, 2133
  furious, 2133
  immunization for, 43t, 44
  paralytic, 2133
  prophylaxis of, 2134–2135
    postexposure, 44
Rabies immune globulin, 2134
Rabies vaccine, 42t, 2134
  and acute disseminated encephalomyelitis, 2140
Rabies virus, 2132
  fixed, 2133
Race factor
  in genetics, 117
  in glucose-6-phosphate dehydrogenase deficiency, 905–906
  in hypertension, 267
  in puberty, 18
  in sickle cell syndromes, 927
Radiation
  background, 2298
  exposure to. See *Radiation exposure.*
  interstitial lung disease and, 419
Radiation dose, 2297
Radiation enteritis, 738
Radiation enterocolitis, 800–801
Radiation exposure, 2298
  and cancer, 1070
    breast, 1402
  and leukemia, 975, 976, 986–987
  and non-Hodgkin's lymphoma, 994
  and thyroid tumor, 1294
  low-level, delayed effects of, 2300
  specific findings in, 2301
  whole-body, acute, 2299
Radiation injury, 2297–2302
  and pericarditis, 342
  local or regional, 2300
  to lung, 2287–2288
Radiation myocarditis, 338
Radiation nephritis, 604
Radiation pneumonitis, 2287
Radiation syndromes, acute, 2302
Radiation therapy
  enterocolitis with, 800–801
  in acromegaly, 1260
  in acute lymphoblastic leukemia, 990
  in breast cancer, 1403, 1404–1405
  in bronchogenic carcinoma, 444
  in cancer, 1088–1089, 1088t, *1089t*
  in chronic lymphocytic leukemia, 983
  in chronic myelogenous leukemia, 979
  in colonic cancer, 768
  in Cushing's syndrome, 1265, 1316
  in esophageal cancer, 675
  in gastric carcinoma, 700
  in Hodgkin's disease, 1006, 1007, 1008t
  in intracranial tumors, 2165
  in multiple myeloma, 1019
  in non-Hodgkin's lymphoma, 997, 998
  in pancreatic cancer, 780
Radiation therapy (*Continued*)
  in pituitary tumor, 1260
  in thyroid tumor, 1295, 1297
  nervous system inury by, 1083–1084, 1083t
  nitroimidazoles in, 1089
  radioprotectors in, 1089
  radiosensitizers in, 1089
  with cancer chemotherapy, 1092–1093
Radiculopathy, 1340
Radioactive iodine uptake, 1279, 1284
Radioallergosorbent test, 386
Radiobiology, tissue, specific, 2299
Radiography. See also *Chest radiography; Contrast media;* specific techniques.
  conventional, 64
  in achalasia, 673, *673*
  in acute abdomen, 797
  in acute cholecystitis, 857
  in acute pancreatitis, 773
  in adult celiac disease, 733
  in alcaptonuria, 1128
  in amebiasis, 1800
  in aortic regurgitation, 255
  in aortic stenosis, 253
  in aspiration pneumonia, 1515
  in atrial septal defect, 229
  in back pain, 1956–1957
  in biliary disease, 853–855
  in brain injury, 2173
  in bronchogenic carcinoma, 441–442, *442, 443*
  in cardiovascular disease, 152–153, 164–169
  in chronic cholecystitis, 856
  in coarctation of aorta, 238
  in congenital valvular aortic stenosis, 236
  in Crohn's disease, 743–744, *743*
  in dissecting aortic aneurysm, 350
  in diverticulitis, 799, *800*
  in Ebstein's anomaly, 234
  in Eisenmenger syndrome, 241
  in esophageal cancer, 674, 675, *675*
  in esophageal motor disorders, 673, *673*
  in gallstones, 854–855, *854, 855*
  in gastric carcinoma, 699, *699*
  in gastric lymphoma, 700–701
  in heart disease, 164–169, *164–169*
  in Hodgkin's disease, 1004–1005, *1004, 1005*
  in hyperparathyroidism, 1437, *1437*, 1441
  in hypertension, 270
  in infective endocarditis, 1539–1540
  in interstitial lung disease, 411
  in joint disease, 1909–1911
  in *Klebsiella* pneumonia, 1510
  in left ventricular failure, 197
  in lung abscess, 420, *421*
  in malabsorption syndrome, 726–727, *727*
  in mediastinal disease, 451, *451*
  in megacolon, 712, *712*
  in mitral regurgitation, 251
  in mitral stenosis, 248
  in mycobacterioses, 1632
  in nervous system disease, 1968–1969
  in nocardiosis, 1613
  in occupational lung disease, 2280
  in osteoarthritis, 1953
  in osteomalacia, 1429, *1429*
  in osteomyelitis, 1567–1568, *1567*
  in osteoporosis, 1458–1459, *1459*
  in Paget's disease, 1461–1462, *1462*
  in pancreatic cancer, 778
  in patent ductus arteriosus, 231–232
  in peptic ulcer, 685–686, *686*
  in pituitary tumor, 1259–1260, *1259*
  in pleural disease, 447
  in pneumococcal pneumonia, 1501, *1502*
  in pulmonary embolism, 427–429, *428*
Radiography (*Continued*)
  in pulmonary stenosis, 235
  in pulmonary tuberculosis, 1623–1624
  in pulmonary venous anomaly, 239
  in renal osteodystrophy, 1454–1455
  in respiratory disease, 381–385, *384*
  in rickets, 1428–1429, *1429*
  in routine health examination, 55
  in sarcoidosis, 434, *435t, 436*
  in tetralogy of Fallot, 233
  in tricuspid valve atresia, 234
  in ulcerative colitis, 751–752, *751, 752*
  in urinary tract infection, 621
  in valvular heart disease, 244
  interventional percutaneous pyeloureteral techniques in, 512
  multipurpose department of, 64, *64*
  of chest, 380–381, *384*
  of kidneys, 511–514, *513*
  of pulmonary vessels, 168–169, *167, 168*
  of thyroid gland, 1280, 1284
  of urogenital tract, 511–514, *513*
Radioiodine, in hyperthyroidism, 1285–1286
Radioisotope(s), exposure to, systemic, 2301
Radioisotope scan
  in pulmonary embolism, 427
  in sarcoidosis, 437
Radioligand binding, 92
Radiology. See also specific techniques.
  algorithmic approach to, 66–67
  financial considerations in, 67
  multipurpose department of, 64, *64*
Radionuclide(s), exposure to, systemic, 2300, 2301
Radionuclide imaging. See also *Radionuclide scanning.*
  extrapulmonary, 390
  in acute abdomen, 797–798
  in back pain, 2062
  in cardiovascular disease, 153
  in gastrointestinal disease, 652–654, *653, 654*
  of biliary tract, 855
  of kidney, 514
  of lung, 385
  of urogenital tract, 514
Radionuclide scanning. See also *Radionuclide imaging.*
  in acute cholecystitis, 857–858
  in brain abscess, 2113
  in hepatic tumor, 851
  in herpes simplex encephalitis, 2127
  in subdural empyema, 2115
Ramsay-Hunt syndrome, 1724, 2084, 2154
  and herpes zoster, 2129
  and vertigo, 2043
Ranitidine, in peptic ulcer, 688, 690, 697
Rash
  in measles, 1707
  in Rocky Mountain spotted fever, 1681
  in typhus fever, 1678
Rastelli procedure, 239
Rat bite fever, 1665–1666
Rattus norvegicus, 1679
Rattus rattus, 1679
Raynaud's disease, 353–356
  clinical manifestations of, 354
  diagnosis of, 354–355
  prognosis in, 355
  treatment of, 355
Raynaud's phenomenon, 353–356
  clinical manifestations of, 354
  diagnosis of, 354–355
  etiology of, 353–354
  in mycoplasmal pneumonia, 1507
  in systemic sclerosis, 1932, 1933
  pathophysiology of, 354

Raynaud's phenomenon (*Continued*)
  prognosis in, 355
  secondary, 354, 355
  treatment of, 355–356
  vs. acrocyanosis, 354–355, 356
Rebuck skin window, 950
Recombinant DNA, vaccine research and, 133
Recommended dietary allowances, 1174–1179, 1175t, 1176t
Rectal ulcer, 784
Rectum
  diseases of, 783–785
  gonococcal infection of, 1645
Red cell volume, reference values for, 2339
5α-Reductase deficiency, 1361–1362, 1388
Reductionism, 5
Reed-Sternberg cells, 993, 1000, 1001, *1001*
Referred pain, definition of, 2050
Reflex(es)
  deep tendon, in amyotrophic lateral sclerosis, 2080
  hyperactive, in spinal cord compression, 2062
  myotatic, in Werdnig-Hoffman disease, 2080
  postural, disturbances of, in parkinsonism, 2069–2070
Reflex epilepsy, 2153
"Reflex sympathetic dystrophies," 2063
Reflex syncope, 1983, *1984*
Refraction, errors of, and headache, 2059
  vs. neurologic abnormalities, 2033
Refsum's disease, 2083
Regan isoenzyme, 1076
Regional enteritis, 740, 742. See also *Crohn's disease.*
Regional ileitis, 740. See also *Crohn's disease.*
Regurgitation, 668
  in gastroesophageal reflux disease, 668–669
  nasal, 672
Rehabilitation, after stroke, 2101–2102
Reifenstein's syndrome, 1401
Reiter's disease, 2220
Reiter's syndrome, 1920–1921, *2263, 2266*
Relapsing fever, 1662–1664
  louse-borne, 1664
  tick-borne, 1664
Relaxation techniques, for pain, 2053
Renal. See also *Kidney(s).*
Renal abscess, 619, 622–623
Renal acidosis, in interstitial nephritis, 591
Renal adenoma, 641
Renal amyloidosis, 132
Renal artery(ies)
  anomaly of, 639
  embolism of, 623
  stenosis of, hypertension in, 275–276
    in neurofibromatosis, 2085
Renal calculi, 487, 628–633. See also *Kidney stones.*
Renal cell carcinoma, 488, 641–642, 641t
  computed tomography in, 641–642, *642*
  diagnosis of, 639–640, 640t
  HLA antigen in, 641
  genetic factor in, 641
  staging for, 642, 642t
  treatment of, 642
Renal colic, 487
Renal cysts, 487–488
  acquired, 636
  computed tomography in, 633–634, *634*
  cystic renal medullary complex in, 636–637
  dialysis and, 635
  in congenital multicystic kidney, 638
  in medullary sponge kidney, 637–638
  in polycystic disease, 634–635
  simple, 635–636
    isolated, 487
Renal cysts (*Continued*)
  ultrasonography of, 513–514
Renal disease. See *Kidney disease* and names of specific diseases.
Renal dysplasia, 638
Renal failure, 488–489. See also *Uremia.*
  acute, 488, 544–549
    chemical toxins and, 545
    clinical manifestations of, 546
    definition of, 544
    diagnosis of, 546–548, 546t
    dialysis in, 548
    etiology of, 544–545, 545t
    hyperkalemia in, 534
    incidence of, 545
    intrarenal, 545–547
    pathogenesis of, 545–546, *546*
    postrenal, 544–545, 547
    prerenal, 544, 547
    prevention of, 549
    prognosis in, 548–549
    renal function recovery with, 548–549
    serum creatinine in, 546
    sodium excretion and, 547, 547t
    survival with, 548
    treatment of, 548
    uremia with, 546
    urinary indices in, 547, 547t
    with toxic nephropathy, 595
  antimicrobial therapy and, 101t, 102
  chronic, 549–558
    aggravating factors in, management of, 555
    antibiotic therapy in, 555, 557t
    atherosclerosis and, 551–552, 556
    carbohydrate metabolism in, 553, 557
    cardiovascular abnormalities with, 551–552, 556
    clinical manifestations of, 549–554
    diagnosis of, 546
    dialysis in, 550, 551, 552, 553, 556
      initiation of, 561, 561t
    dietary management in, 557–558
    follow-up principles in, 558
    glomerular filtration rate in, 549–551, 554, 555, 556
    hypercalcemia and, 1450
    hyperkalemia in, 534
    hypertension and, 552, 556
    hypovolemia and, 519
    infection with, 552, 555, 557
    management of, 555–558
    metabolic acidosis in, 540, 557
    myopathy with, 553, 557
    neuropathy with, 553, 557
    osteomalacia and, 1429, 1430
    pathophysiology of, 549–554
    pruritus in, 553–554, 557
    serum creatinine in, 558, *558*
    transfusion in, 556–557
    treatable parenchymal disease in, 555, 555t
    uric acid metabolism in, 553, 557
    vitamin D metabolism and, 1426
    volume depletion in, management of, 555
    with toxic nephropathy, 595
  functional, 844–845
  irreversible, 559–568
    dialysis in, 559–563
    kidney transplantation in, 559, 563–568
    pathogenesis of, 489
    protein metabolism and, 489
    with urinary tract obstruction, 606
Renal glycosuria, 486
  genetic factor in, 614
Renal hyperaminoaciduria, 610–611, 611t
Renal hypertension, 275–276
Renal hypoperfusion, 485
Renal infarction, 623
Renal ischemia, 485
Renal manifestations of disease, *2264*
Renal medulla, microcystic disease of, 488
Renal oncocytoma, 641
Renal osteodystrophy, 489, 553, 1453–1456
  biochemical features of, 1453
  clinical manifestations of, 1454
  hyperparathyroidism and, 557
  parathyroidectomy for, 1455–1456
  radiography in, 1454–1455
  treatment of, 1455–1456
  vitamin D and, 557
  with dialysis, 562
Renal papillary necrosis, 622
Renal phosphate wasting, 486
  genetic factor in, 615
  with hyperparathyroidism, 614–615
Renal plasma flow, tests of, reference values for, 2332
Renal syndrome, in hemorrhagic fever, 1757
Renal transitional cell tumors, 488
Renal transplantation, in inborn errors of metabolism, 132. See also *Kidney transplantation.*
Renal tubular acidosis, 550–551, 594, 595, 608–610, 609t
  bicarbonate therapy in, 608–609
  distal, 609–610, 609t
    generalized, 610
    gradient-limited, 487, 533, 540
  glomerular insufficiency in, 610
  kidney stones and, 630, 631
  mineralocorticoids in, 610
  proximal, 487, 539, 608–609
  treatment of, 633
  type IV, 519
Renal tubules. See also *Renal tubular acidosis.*
  disorders of, 608–616
  dysfunction of, with toxic nephropathy, 595
  necrosis of, diuretic phase of, 519
Renal vein thrombosis, 624
  membranous nephropathy and, 583
Rendu-Osler-Weber syndrome, 233
Renin, 163
  plasma, assay of, 1309
    reference values for, 2332
  production regulation of, 1304
  release of, 1239
Renin-angiotensin system
  and blood pressure, 273, 275
  in adrenal hormone production, 1303, 1304–1305, *1304*
  in shock, 214
Renin-angiotensin-alderosterone system
  in fluid volume disorders, 517–518
  sodium balance and, 497
Reovirus, in acute central nervous system infections, *2122*, 2123
Reproductive abnormality, mycoplasmal infection and, 1508–1509
Reproductive hazards, environmental and occupational, 2278
Reproductive system, in puberty, 17–18
Research, medical ethics and, 13
Reserpine
  in Huntington's disease, 2075
  in parkinsonism, 2071
  in Raynaud's disease, 355
Reservoir mask, for oxygen administration, 459
Respiration, 368, 454
  carbon dioxide output in, 536, 537
  diffusion in, 376–377
  functions of, 372–381
  gas exchange in, 378–381, *379, 380*

Respiration (*Continued*)
in altered consciousness, 1976
in Werdnig-Hoffmann disease, 2080
perfusion in, 377–378
ventilation in, 372–376, *373*, *374*, *375*, *376*
Respiratory. See also *Lung(s)* and *Pulmonary*.
Respiratory acidosis, 465, 538, 543–544
acute, 543
chronic, 543
Respiratory alkalosis, 465, 538, 544
hypophosphatemia and, 1164, 1165
Respiratory assistance
complications of, 476
in cardiopulmonary resuscitation, 481
mechanical ventilation for, 468–470, 468t
complications of, 477
patterns of, 468
techniques of, 467–470
ventilator emergencies with, 468–469
ventilator weaning with, 469–470
ventilatory devices for, 467
Respiratory disease(s), 368–462. See also under names of specific diseases.
biopsy for, 389
bronchoscopy in, 388–389
chronic airways disorders in, 396–404
diagnostic procedures in, 381–390
electrocardiography in, 389–390
fat embolism syndrome, 431–432
hypersensitivity, 385–386
interstitial. See *Interstitial lung disease*.
mediastinal involvement in, 451–452
neoplasms, 439–447
pleural fluid examination in, 388
pleural involvement in, 447–450
pulmonary embolism, 426–431, *428*
radiography in, 381–385, *384*
sarcoidosis, 432–439, *433*, 434t, *435–437*, 438t
serologic tests in, 386
skin tests in, 385–386
sputum examination in, 387–388, *387*
viral, 1691–1706
with ankylosing spondylitis, 1919–1920
with cystic fibrosis, 424–425
Respiratory distress, in pneumocystosis, 1796
Respiratory distress syndrome, adult, after pulmonary thermal injury, 2287
Respiratory dysfunction
arterial blood gas measurements in, 464–465
arterial pH in, 464–465, *465*, 466
assessment of, 463–467
lung function measurements in, 463–464
patient behavior and, 463
shunting and, 464, *464*
Respiratory epithelium, cigarette smoking and, 48
Respiratory failure, 454–462
acute, 458–460
airway maintenance in, 458
alveolar ventilation maintenance in, 459
antimicrobials in, 461
bronchodilators in, 460–461
causes of, 456–457
chronic, 460–462
clinical manifestations of, 457–458
corticosteroids in, 461
critical care management of, 470–473
gas exchange in, 454–455
humidification in, 458
in airways obstruction, 471
in chest wall abnormality, 457, 470–471
in neuromuscular disorders, 470
in pulmonary edema, 456, 472–473, *473*
in pulmonary vascular disease, 456–457, 473
intubation-assisted ventilation in, 460
Respiratory failure (*Continued*)
neuromuscular system disorders and, 457
oxygen therapy in, 458–459, 460
pathophysiology of, 454–455
patient monitoring in, 460
pleural disease and, 457
postoperative complications with, 461–462
respiratory stimulants and, 461
right heart failure and, 455–456
secretion control in, 461
sedation and, 461
treatment of, 458–462
with airways obstruction, 456
with heart failure, 461
with parenchymal infiltration disease, 456
Respiratory function, calculation of variables in, 465–467, 465t, *466*
Respiratory infection, adenoviral, 1705
Respiratory monitoring, in critical care management, 473
Respiratory muscles, in cardiorespiratory arrest, 481
Respiratory rate, 463
Respiratory syncytial virus infection, 1696–1698
chemotherapy for, 110–111
Respiratory system. See also *Respiratory tract*.
aging and, 22–23
compliance of, 466–467
hormone factors in control of, 1229
muscle function testing of, 390
Respiratory tract. See also *Respiratory system*.
enteroviral disease of, 1734
meningococcal infection of, 1560
mycoplasmal infection of, 1505–1508
Rest, in myofascial pain syndrome, 2064
Restriction fragment length polymorphisms (RFLP), 137
Retardation. See *Mental retardation*.
Retention, of urine, 2029, *2029*
Reticular dysgenesis, 1860
Reticulocyte(s), in anemia, 875
Reticulocyte count, reference values for, 2339
Reticulocytosis, 875
with hemorrhage, 883
Reticuloendothelial system, in infectious disease, 1477, 1478
Reticuloendotheliosis, leukemia, 984–986
Reticulohistiocytoma, *2266*
Reticulum cell sarcoma, ocular, 2220
Retina
arterioles of, in amaurosis fugax, 2096, *2096*
arteriosclerotic changes in, 2223
disease of, bilateral, 2033
hemangioma of, in Hippel-Lindau disease, 2086
peripheral, neovascularization of, 2224
tears of, 2033
vascular occlusions of, 2224–2225
Retinal, 1206
Retinal artery, occlusion of, 2224
Retinal vein, occlusion of, 2225
Retinitis pigmentosa, 2168
Retinoblastoma, intraocular, 2222
Retinochoroiditis, in toxoplasmosis, 1793
Retinoic acid, 1206
Retinoids, 1206
Retinol, 1206. See also *Vitamin A*.
Retinopathy
diabetic, 1337–1338, 2223–2224
hemorrhagic, 2225
in hypertension, 271, 272
vascular, 2223–2224
venous stasis, 2225
Retrobulbar optic neuritis, 2219
in nutritional amblyopia, 2066
Retrograde amnesia, 1996
Retrolental fibroplasia, retinopathy of, 2224
Retropulsion, 2046
Retroviruses, oncogenes of, 1067, 1067t
Reversal reactions, in leprosy, 1636–1637, 1638
Reverse transcriptase, 123
Reversible ischemic neurologic disability, 2091, 2097, *2097*
investigation of, 2099
treatment of, 2100
"Rewarming shock," 2307
Reye's syndrome, 847, 1694, 1722, 2141
with influenza, 1704
Rh factor, in blood transfusion, 937–938
Rh immune globulin, 46
Rhabdomyolysis, 534, 2210
with potassium depletion, 533
Rhabdomyosarcoma, of orbit, 2222
Rhabdovirus, in acute central nervous system infections, *2122*
Rheumatic component, diseases with, *2266*
Rheumatic diseases. See also under names of specific diseases.
acute phase phenomena in, 1908
antinuclear antibodies and, 1909, 1909t, 1910t
categories of, 1891–1892, 1891t
chemoattractants in, 1900–1901, *1902*
C-reactive protein in, 1908
diagnostic procedures in, 1906–1911
immune response in, 1898–1899, 1898t, 1902–1904, 1903t, 1904t, 1908–1909, 1909t, 1910t
immunoglobulins in, 1908–1909
inflammation in, 1898–1902, 1898t
mediators of, 1900–1901
inflammatory cell accumulation in, 1901–1902, *1902*
laboratory tests in, 1892–1893
lupus erythematosus cell and, 1909
lysosomal enzymes in, 1901
management goals in, 1893
pathophysiology of, 1891–1892
patient counseling in, 1894
phagocytosis in, 1901–1902, *1902*
rheumatoid factors in, 1908–1909
sedimentation rate in, 1908
synovial fluid analysis in, 1906–1908, 1907t
synovial membrane histopathology in, 1908
tissue destruction in, 1899–1900
treatment of, 1893–1894
Rheumatic fever
acute, 1527–1533
arthritis with, 1529–1530
carditis with, 1530
clinical manifestations of, 1529–1530
course of, 1531
diagnosis of, 1531–1532, 1531t
epidemiology in, 1528
erythema marginatum in, 1530
etiology of, 1527
group A streptococcal pharyngitis and, 1519, 1520, 1521, 1522, 1526, 1527–1528
immune response in, 1527–1528
laboratory findings in, 1530–1531
pathogenesis of, 1527–1528
pathology of, 1528–1529
penicillin for, 1532
prevention of, 1532–1533
prognosis in, 1531
subcutaneous nodules with, 1530
Sydenham's chorea with, 1530
treatment of, 1532
aortic stenosis after, 252
aortic regurgitation after, 254
cutaneous lesions in, *2260*
mitral regurgitation after, 249
mitral stenosis after, 246, 249

Rheumatic fever (*Continued*)
tricuspid stenosis after, 255
Rheumatoid heart disease, epidemiology of, 155
Rheumatism
nonarticular, 1959–1960
palindromic, 1959
Rheumatoid arthritis, 1911–1917
and back pain, 2061
antimalarials in, 1916
as autoimmune disease, 1912
aspirin in, 1916
cardiac manifestations of, 1914–1915
clinical features of, 1913
corticosteroids in, 1916
course of, 1915
criteria for, 1911
differential diagnosis of, 1915
drug therapy for, 1916–1917
etiology of, 1911–1912
exercise in, 1916
extra-articular manifestations of, 1914–1915
gold salts for, 1916
immune response in, 1904–1905, *1905*, 1912–1913
immunoglobulin G in, 1912–1913
immunosuppressive agents in, 1916
infectious agents and, 1912
joint manifestations in, 1913–1914, *1914*
laboratory findings in, 1915
management of, 1915–1917
neurologic manifestations of, 1915
neuropathy with, 2196
nonsteroidal anti-inflammatory agents in, 1916
onset of symptoms in, 1913
ophthalmologic manifestations of, 1915
pain in, 2049
pathogenesis of, 1912–1913
pathology of, 1912
penicillamine in, 1916
pericarditis and, 341
pleural involvement with, 449
prognosis in, 1915
pulmonary manifestations of, 1915
rest in, 1916
salicylate therapy in, 1916
skin in, 1914
surgery for, 1916
synovitis with, 1899–1900, *1899*, 1904–1905, *1905*
tissue destruction in, 1904–1905, *1905*
with interstitial lung disease, 413–414
with neutropenia, 955
Rheumatoid arthritis nuclear antigens, 1905
Rheumatoid arthritis precipitin, 1905
Rheumatoid diseases, 2222–2223
Rheumatoid factors, 1904, 1912, 1913
in rheumatic disease, 1908–1909
Rhinitis, 1867–1870. See also *Allergic rhinitis.*
Rhinophyma, in acne rosacea, 2243, *2243*
Rhinorrhea, in skull fracture, 2171
Rhinoviruses, in common cold, 1691–1694, 1694t
Rhipicephalus sanguineus, 1682
Rhodesian sleeping sickness, 1780–1783, 1781t
Rib, cervical, 2197
Ribavirin, 1698
for respiratory syncytial virus infection, 110–111
Riboflavin, 1199–1201
biochemical functions of, 1199
deficiency of, 1200–1201
dietary sources of, 1199–1200
physiology of, 1199
recommended dietary allowance for, 1178
requirements for, 1199–1200
Riboflavin (*Continued*)
structure of, 1199, *1200*
urinary, reference values for, 2333
Ribonucleic acid (RNA), 122. See also *RNA.*
aminoacyl-tRNA, 123–124
in genetic information transmission, 122–126
messenger (mRNA), 123, 124
ribosomal (rRNA), 123, 124
structure of, 123
transfer (tRNA), 123–124
types of, 123
Ribosomes, 124
Rickets, 1425–1431
diagnosis of, 1428–1430
genetic factor in, 1427
pathogenesis of, 1425–1428, 1426t
biochemical features of, 1429–1430
bone matrix disorders and, 1428
calcium deficiency and, 1427–1428, 1430
histologic features of, 1430
mineralization inhibition and, 1428, 1430, 1431
phosphate homeostasis disorders and, 1427
vitamin D disorders and, 1425–1427, 1429
radiography in, 1428–1429, *1429*
treatment of, 1430–1431
vitamin D–dependent, 615, 1427, 1429
vitamin D–resistant, 615, 1427
Rickettsia akari, 1683
Rickettsia australis, 1682, 1683
Rickettsia canada, 1678
Rickettsia conorii, 1682
Rickettsia mooseri (typhi), 1678, 1679
Rickettsia prowazekii, 1678
Rickettsia rickettsii, 1680
Rickettsia sibirica, 1682
Rickettsia tsutsugamushi, 1684
Rickettsiae, 1672, 1673
microbiology of, 1672
Rickettsial diseases, 1672–1687. See also names of specific diseases.
antimicrobial therapy in, 1676
cardiovascular system in, 1677
clinical features of, 1674–1675, 1674t
complications with, 1677
corticosteroids in, 1677
culture in, 1675
cutaneous lesions in, *2261*
diagnosis of, 1674–1675, 1674t
epidemiology of, 1672, 1673t
host factor in, 1672
immune response in, 1672–1674, 1676
laboratory diagnosis of, 1675–1676
pathogenesis of, 1672–1674, 1674t
serology in, 1675–1676
tetracyclines in, 1676, 1677
treatment of, 1676–1677
vectors in, 1672–1673
Rickettsialpox, 1683–1684
clinical course of, 1683–1684
epidemiology of, 1683
vector in, 1683
Riedel's thyroiditis, 1294
Rifampin, 105, 597–598, 1624–1625, 1626
for leprosy, 1637–1638
hepatotoxicity of, 823
steroid therapy and, 1303
Rift Valley fever, 1739–1740
vaccine for, 1730
Right atrium, late surgical complications in, 242
Right bundle branch block, QRS complex in, 174
Right heart, aortic root communication defect in, 232–233
Right heart failure, respiratory failure and, 455–456
Right middle lobe syndrome, 405
Right ventricle
double outlet, 239
end-diastolic pressure in, 192
functional assessment of, with nuclear imaging, 179–181, *179*
late surgical complications in, 242
outflow tract reconstruction of, prosthesis for, 242
Right ventricular failure, 197–199, 289
mechanism of, 189
Rigidity
extrapyramidal, vs. pyramidal spasticity, 2045–2046
in juvenile Huntington's disease, 2074
muscular, in parkinsonism, 2069, 2070
in tetanus, 1579
Riley-Day syndrome, 2027
dysautonomia in, 2194–2195
Rimantadine, in influenza, 1704–1705
RIND. See *Reversible ischemic neurologic disability.*
Ring fibers, in myotonic dystrophy, 2202
Ringer's lactate solution, 220
Risk factor management, in threatened stroke, 2100
River blindness, 1832–1833
RNA. See also *Ribonucleic acid.*
RNA virus(es)
in acute central nervous system infections, *2122*, 2123
leukemia and, 987
skin infections from, 1706–1712
RNA-dependent DNA polymerase, 123
Rochalimaea quintana, 1672, 1673, 1685
Rocio encephalitis, 1748–1749
Rocky Mountain spotted fever, 1674, 1678, 1680–1682, *2266*
antibiotic therapy in, 1681
clinical course of, 1681
cutaneous lesions in, *2261*
epidemiology of, 1680
prevention of, 1681–1682
treatment of, 1681
vector in, 1680
Rod myopathy, 2207
Roentgenography. See *Radiography.*
Rolandic epilepsy, 2150, 2154
Romaña's sign, 1784, 1785
Romberg's sign, in tabes dorsalis, 2120
Roots, nerve. See *Nerve root(s).*
Ross River fever, 1740
Rotator cuff tears, 1954–1955
Rotaviruses, 1734–1735
Roth's spots
in infective endocarditis, 1536t
in ocular hemorrhage, 2224
Round cell sarcoma, 1467
Roundworm. See *Ascariasis.*
Roussy-Levy syndrome, vs. Friedreich's ataxia, 2083
Royal Free disease, 2131
Rubella, 1709–1711, *2266*
clinical manifestations of, 1710
complications of, 1710–1711
congenital, 1710, 1711
congenital abnormality from, 44, 1709–1710, 1711
cutaneous lesions in, *2260*
diagnosis of, 1711
epidemiology of, 1710
etiology of, 1710
gamma globulin in, 1711
immune response in, 1710, 1711
immunization for, 43t, 44
pathology of, 1711

Rubella (*Continued*)
  postnatal, 1710
  prevention of, 1711
  vaccine for, 1711
Rubella panencephalitis, progressive, 2136
Rubella virus, in chronic encephalitis, 2136
Rubeola. See *Measles*.
Rural typhus, 1684

Sabin-Feldman dye test, for toxoplasmosis, 1794
Saddleback fever, 1741
Sagittal sinus, superior, thrombosis of, 2116
St. Louis encephalitis, 1746–1747
  clinical features of, 1746–1747
  diagnosis of, 1747
  epidemiology of, 1746
  pathology in, 1746–1747
  prevention of, 1747
  vector in, 1746
  virus of, 1746
St. Vitus' dance, 1530, 2075
Salicylate(s), 1239
  in rheumatoid arthritis, 1916
  poisoning from, 87–88
  serum and plasma, reference values for, 2333
Salicylism, 541
Saline solution therapy, in fluid volume depletion, 520
Salmonella, microbiology of, 1589–1590
Salmonella infection, 1589–1592. See also *Typhoid fever*.
  antibiotic therapy in, 1592
  carriers of, 1590, 1591
  clinical manifestations of, 1591
  culture of, 1592
  diagnosis of, 1591–1592
  epidemiology of, 1590
  etiology of, 1589–1590
  pathogenesis of, 1590–1591
  pathology of, 1590
  prevention of, 1592
  prognosis of, 1592
  treatment of, 1592
Salmonella dublin, 1590
Salmonella gastroenteritis, 781
Salmonella paratyphi, 1590, 1591
Salmonella species, 1589↑| 1590
Salmonella typhi, 1587, 1588, 1589, 1590, 1591
Salmonella typhimurium, 1590, 1591
Salmonellosis, 1590–1592
Salpingitis
  antibiotic therapy in, 1643, 1648
  complications of, 1643, 1645–1646
  etiology of, 1643
  gonococcal, 1643, 1645
  infertility and, 1643, 1645
  laparoscopy in, 1643, 1645
  sexually transmitted, 1643
Salt intake
  blood pressure and, 273
  hypertension and, 38–39, 268
  in heart failure, 163, 164
  in renal hypertension, 275
Sand flies, 1835
Sandfly fever, 1738–1739
Sanfilippo's syndrome, 1148
Sarcocystis hominis, 1803
Sarcoidosis, 338, 345, 413, *413*, 432–439, 1248, 2196, *2264*, *2266*
  acute, vs. chronic, 438, 438t
  and myopathy, 2210
  angiotensin-converting enzyme in, 432, 436–437
  biochemistry of, 438
Sarcoidosis (*Continued*)
  bronchoalveolar lavage in, 437
  calcitriol in, 438
  clinical features of, 434–436, 434t
  clinical management of, 436
  corticosteroids in, 438–439
  criteria of activity for, 436–437
  differential diagnosis of, 438, 438t
  epidemiology of, 434
  etiology of, 432–433
  eyes in, 434
  gallium scan in, 437
  heart in, 435–436
  hypercalcemia and, 1449
  hypersensitivity in, 433
  immunology of, 432–434
  in childhood, 437–438
  kidney in, 436
  Kveim-Siltzbach skin test in, 432
  liver disease and, 833
  lungs in, 434, 435t
  musculoskeletal system in, 436
  nervous system in, 434–435
  pregnancy in, 437
  pulmonary hypertension and, 261
  radiography in, 434, *435*t, *436*
  radioisotope scan in, 437
  skin in, 434
  treatment of, 438–439
  with arthritis, 1957
Sarcoma
  combined modality therapy for, 1088, 1088t
  Kaposi's, 1861, 1862, 1863, 2262, *2262*, 2273, *2273*
  of lung, 445
  reticulum cell, ocular, 2220
Sarcoplasm, in myotonic dystrophy, 2202
Sarcosporidiosis, 1803–1804
Satiety centers, 646
Scabies, 1838–1839
Scalded skin syndrome, staphylococcal, 2270
Scale, 2233
Scaling lesions, thoracic, 2247
Scalp, seborrheic dermatitis of, 2242
Scapula, winging of, 2199
Scapulohumeral syndrome, 2204
Scapuloperoneal syndrome, 2199
Scar, 2233
Scarlet fever, 1522, 1523
  cutaneous lesions in, *2260*
Schatzki's ring, 675, 676, *676*
Scheie's disease, 131
Scheie's syndrome, 1148
Schilder's disease, 2147
Schilling test, 897
  in vitamin B_{12} deficiency, 2067
  reference values for, 2333
Schistosoma, 1809–1812
Schistosoma haematobium, 1809, 1810, 1811, 1812–1813
Schistosoma japonicum, 1809, 1810, 1811, 1814–1815
Schistosoma mansoni, 1809, 1810, 1811, 1813–1814
Schistosomiasis, 1809–1815
  acute, 1811, 1815
  cerebral, 1815
  chronic, 1815
  control of, 1812
  diagnosis of, 1812
  epidemiology of, 1810–1811
  etiology of, 1810
  immune response in, 1810–1812
  management of, 1812
  oriental, 1814–1815
    clinical manifestations of, 1815
    diagnosis of, 1815
    pathology of, 1815
Schistosomiasis (*Continued*)
  oriental, treatment of, 1815
  pathogenesis of, 1811
Schistosomiasis haematobia, 1812–1813
Schistosomiasis japonica, 1814–1815
Schistosomiasis mansoni, 1813–1814
Schizophrenia, 1002–1005
  and hysterical symptoms, 2013
Schizotrypanides, 1784
Schmidt's syndrome, 1290, 1310, 1407–1408
Schwannoma
  acoustic, 2162t
    treatment outcome in, 2166
Schwartzman-Sanarelli phenomenon, 505
Scintigraphy
  in angina pectoris, 286
  in interstitial lung disease, 411
  in myocardial infarction, 291, 294
  of joints, 1910
  of kidney, 514
  of lung, 385
Scleritis, 2223
Scleroderma. See *Systemic sclerosis*.
Sclerosing pseudotumor, of orbit, 2222
Sclerosis
  amyotrophic lateral, 2079–2080, 2137. See also *Amyotrophic lateral sclerosis*.
  diffuse, 2147
  glomerular, focal, 580–585, *581*
  mesial temporal, in epilepsy, 2150
  multiple. See *Multiple sclerosis*.
  progressive systemic, with interstitial lung disease, 414
  systemic. See *Systemic sclerosis*.
  transitional, 2147
  tuberous, 416, 2085, 2256, *2256*
Scoliosis, 2187
  in Friedreich's ataxia, 2083
Scombroid fish poisoning, 782–783
Scopolamine, abuse of, 2024
  in vertigo, 2043
Scorpion fishes, 1844
Scorpion sting, 1838
Scotomas, *2032*, 2033
Scrapie, 2135
Scrub typhus, 1684–1685
  clinical course of, 1684–1685
  epidemiology in, 1684
  prevention of, 1685
  serology in, 1684
  treatment of, 1685
  vector in, 1684
Scurvy, 1204–1205
  vascular purpura with, 1039
Sea snakes, venomous, 1844
Sebaceous glands, 2230
Seborrheic dermatitis, 2242
Seborrheic keratoses, 2255
Secobarbital, serum, reference values for, 2333
Secondary care, 7
Secretory component deficiency, 1857
Secundum atrial septal defect, 229
Secretin stimulation test, in Zollinger-Ellison syndrome, 696
Secretory diarrhea, 714, 714t
Sedative(s)
  and fatigue, 2044
  and sleep disorders, 1989
  for heart failure, 199–200
  in peptic ulcer, 690
  poisoning by, 1979–1980
Sediment, urinary, reference values for, 2333
Sedimentation rate, in rheumatic disease, 1908
Segmental dystonia, in spasmodic torticollis, 2078

Segmental myoclonus, 2153
Segregational load, genetic, 122
Seizure(s), 2149. See also *Epilepsy (epilepsies).*
  akinetic, and drop attacks, 2046
  and syncope, 1985–1986
  atonic, 2153
  classification of, 2151, *2151*
    therapeutic, *2157*
  contact, 2150
  convulsive, *2151*
  focal, *2151*
  generalized, 2149, 2151t, 2152–2153
    in coma, 1977
  hysterical, vs. epilepsy, 2156
  in bacterial meningitis, 1553
  in encephalitis, treatment of, 2125
  in head injury, 2173
  in hypertensive encephalopathy, 2102
  in metabolic brain disease, 1975
  local, *2151*
  myoclonic, 2152
    and drop attacks, 2046
  neonatal, 2153
  nonconvulsive, 2151t
  nonepileptic, 2157
  occurrence patterns of, 2153
  partial, 2149, 2150, 2151–2153, 2151t
  psychomotor, 2152
  temporal lobe, 1992–1993, 2152
  tonic, 2153
  unclassified, 2153
  unexplained, in depressant abuse, 2020
Selenium, 1208, 1210
  deficiency of, 1210
  dietary allowance for, 1179
  excess of, 1210
  toxicity of, 2314
Sella, empty, syndrome of, 2168
Sella turcica, tumors of, 2163
Seminiferous tubule dysgenesis, 1370–1371, *1371*
  chromosome abnormality in, 1370–1371
  genetic factors in, 1370–1371
Semen
  examination of, 1368
    reference values for, 2333
Semustine, as nephrotoxin, 602
Senecio longilobus, 783
Senile chorea, 2075
Senile elastosis, 2232
Senile hypothermia, 2025
Senile lentigo, 2254
Senile purpura, 2232
Senile tremor, 2073–2074
Sensation, loss of, hysterical, 2014
Sense perception, aging and, 23
Sensory disorder(s)
  cutaneous, glove-stocking pattern of, 2199
  in syringomyelia, 2084
  in Friedreich's ataxia, 2083
  localization, 2048–2049
Sensory epilepsy, vs. sensory ischemia, 2098
Sensory neuron
  lower, anatomy and physiology of, 2178
  peripheral, disorders of, 2194–2195
  hereditary, 2194–2195
Sensory organs, aging and, 23
Sensory pathways, major, 2047–2048
Septic shock, 221, 1473–1477
  ACTH-endorphin system in, 1474
  antibacterial therapy in, 1475–1476
  antiendotoxin antiserum in, 1476
  antishock therapy in, 1476
  clinical manifestations of, 1475, 1475t
  coagulation/kinin system activation in, 1474
  complement system activation in, 1474–1475
  complications of, 1474, *1474*
Septic shock (*Continued*)
  diagnosis of, 1475
  epidemiology of, 1473–1474
  gram-negative vs. gram-positive organisms in, 1474
  hospitalization and, 1473–1474, 1476
  hyperbaric oxygen in, 1476
  pathogenesis of, 1474–1475, 1474t
  prevention of, 1476
  prognosis in, 1476
  surgery in, 1476
  treatment of, 1475–1476, *1476*
Septic shock syndrome, 1549
Septicemia, clostridial, 1575
Sequoiosis, 2285
Serologic values of clinical importance, 2317–2335
Serositis, with dialysis, 562
Serotonin, 1243
  biosynthesis of, 1413–1414, *1413*
  in rheumatic disease, 1900
  in shock, 214
  with islet cell tumor, 1351
Serous meningitis, 2122, 2168. See also *Pseudotumor cerebri; Viral meningitis.*
Serratia pneumonia, 1511, 1513, 1570
Sertoli cell, 1365–1366
Sertoli-cell-only syndrome, 1371–1372
Serum reverse T_3 measurement, 1279
Serum sickness, 1866, 1903, *2266*
Severe combined immunodeficiency disorder, 1859–1860
  autosomal recessive, 1859–1860
  genetic factors in, 1859, 1860
  with adenosine deaminase deficiency, 1859–1860
  with leukopenia, 1860
  X-linked recessive, 1860
Sex. See also *Female sexual development; Male sexual development.*
  embryonic, differentiation disorders of, 1354–1365
    differentiation factors and, 1365, *1366*
    differentiation process of, 1351–1354, *1352*
    phenotypic differentiation in, 1352–1354
Sex chromatin, 1368
  types of, 141–142
Sex factor(s)
  in atherosclerosis, 281
  in autosomal dominant inheritance, 120
  in cigarette smoking, 49
  in hypertension, 267
  in laboratory results, 63
  in survival, 22, *22*
Sexual function, male, disorders of, 2030–2031, *2030*
Sexuality. See also *Female sexuality; Male sexuality.*
  aging and, 21
  female maturation and, 17–18
  identity factor in, 19
  male maturation and, 17–18
  of adolescents, 19
Sexually transmitted disease, 1639–1644. See also specific diagnoses.
  common syndromes with, 1640–1643
  epidemiology of, 1639
  homosexuality and, 1639–1640
  in females, 1641–1643
  in males, 1640–1641
  incidence of, 1640, 1640t
  infectious agents in, 1639, 1640t
Sézary's syndrome, 982, 996, *2265*, 2273
Sham feeding, 693
Shellfish poisoning, 782–783, 1844
Shift work, health effects from, 2278
Shigella, 1596
  prevention of, 1597
Shigella boydii, 1596, 1597
Shigella dysenteriae, 1596–1597
Shigella dysentery, 781
Shigella flexneri, 1596, 1597
Shigella sonnei, 1596, 1597
Shigellosis, 1596–1597
  antimicrobials in, 1596
  clinical manifestations of, 1596–1597
  culture in, 1597
  diagnosis of, 1597
  epidemiology of, 1596
  etiology of, 1596
  in custodial institutions, 1596
  in male homosexuals, 1596
  pathogenesis of, 1596
  pathophysiology of, 1596
  prognosis in, 1597
  treatment of, 1597
Shin-bone fever, 1685
Shingles. See *Herpes zoster.*
Shock, 211–225. See also *Septic shock.*
  acidosis in, 213, 220
  anaphylactic, 220
  alpha-adrenergic receptor antagonist in, 223
  arrhythmias in, 212, 220–221
  ATP synthesis in, 216–217
  autoregulatory vascular adjustment in, 215
  baroreceptors in, 214
  biochemistry of, 216–218
  calcium metabolism of, 216
  capillary permeability in, 215–216
  cardiac filling pressure in, 212
  cardiac output in, 212, 219
  causes of, 211, 211t
  chemoreceptors in, 214
  circulatory control in, 212–216
  circulatory system in, 214–216
  clinical findings in, 211, 211t
  compensated, 211
  complement system in, 217–218
  decompensated, 211
  disseminated intravascular coagulation in, 216
  electrocardiography in, 218
  endocrine factor in, 214–215
  endorphins in, 214–215
  heart rate in, 212
  histamine in, 214
  hydrogen ion concentration in, 220
  hypoxia in, 213, 220
  in bacterial meningitis, 1554
  irreversible, 211–212
  intra-aortic balloon counterpulsation in, 224
  intraorgan blood flow distribution in, 215
  kinins in, 214
  lysosomal-releasing factor in, 217
  management of, 219–224
  microcirculation in, 215–216, 223
  mitochondria in, 216–217
  monitoring in, arterial pressure, 219
    central venous pressure, 218
    hemodynamic, 218–219
    Swan-Ganz catheter, 218–219
  myocardial contractility in, 212–214
  myocardial depressant factors in, 214, 217
  myocardial ischemia and perfusion pressure in, 213
  myocardial oxygen demand in, 213, 223
  oncotic pressure in, 215–216
  oxidative phosphorylation in, 216
  oxyhemoglobin dissociation curve in, 216
  pathophysiology of, 211–212, *212*
  pre- and postcapillary resistance in, 215
  prostacyclin in, 214
  prostaglandins in, 214

Shock (*Continued*)
  pulmonary capillary wedge pressure in, 218, 219, 220
  pulmonary pathology in, 216, 220
  renin-angiotensin system in, 214
  "rewarming," 2307
  septic, 221
  serotonin in, 214
  spinal, after spinal cord injury, 2175
    in acute transverse myelitis, 2138
  thromboxane in, 214
  tissue perfusion in, 212–216, 213t
  treatment of, 218–224
    alpha-adrenergic agonists in, 222–223, 222t
    beta-adrenergic agonists in, 222–223, 222t
    corticosteroid therapy in, 221
    digitalis in, 223–224
    dobutamine in, 222
    dopamine in, 222
    epinephrine in, 222
    fluid therapy in, 220
    glucocorticosteroid therapy for, 112
    isoproterenol in, 222
    nitroglycerin in, 223
    nitroprusside in, 223
    norepinephrine in, 222
    oxygen therapy in, 220
    phentolamine in, 223
    propranolol in, 223
    surgical, 224
    sympathomimetic agents in, 221–222, 222t
    vasodilator therapy in, 223
    vasoconstriction therapy in, 223
  urinary output in, monitoring of, 219
  vasopressin in, 214
Shock lung, 216, 220
Shoulder pain, 1954–1955
  after stroke, 2102
Shoulder-hand syndrome, 1955, 2063
  with myocardial infarction, 292
Shunt, intracardiac. See also *Atrial septal defect; Ventricular septal defect*.
  intracardiac, cardiac catheterization study of, 185–186, *185*
Shy-Drager syndrome, 1413, 2027
  and parkinsonism, 2071
Sialidoses, 1149
Siberian tick typhus, 1682
"Sick role," and hysteria, 2013
Sick sinus syndrome, 318–319
Sickle cell anemia, *2265*
  clinical manifestations in, 929–930
  pain in, 2049
  vaso-occlusive crisis in, 929
Sickle cell disease(s), 132, 1104, *2264*
  prenatal diagnosis of, 136–137
  retinopathy of, 2224
  with arthritis, 1957
Sickle cell syndromes, 927–932
  clinical manifestations of, 929–931
  diagnosis of, 930–931, 930t
  epidemiology of, 927
  erythrocytes in, 927, 929
  genetic counseling in, 932
  genetic factors in, 927
  hemoglobin abnormality in, 927–929, *928*
  hemoglobin electrophoresis in, 930–931, *930*
  pathophysiology of, 927–929, *928*
  peripheral blood smear in, 931
  prenatal diagnosis in, 932
  prevention of, 932
  prognosis in, 931
  racial factors in, 927
  screening tests for, 930
  treatment of, 931
Sickle cell trait, clinical manifestations of, 929
  malaria and, 927, 1777
Sideroblastic anemia, 892–893, *892*
  acquired, 892–893
  alcoholism and, 892
  complicating other diseases, 892
  drug-induced, 892
  hereditary, 893
  idiopathic, refractory, 892
  porphyrin biosynthesis in, 892
  toxin-induced, 892–893
Siderosomes, 1024
Sigmoidoscopy, fiberoptic, 661
Silica, occupational exposure to, 2282
Silicates, diseases caused by, 2284
Silicon, 1211
Silicosis, 417, 2282–2283, *2282*
Silo-filler's disease, 2289
Silver nitrate, in wet dressing, 2239, *2239*
Simian virus 40, and progressive multifocal leukoencephalopathy, 2137
Simmonds' cachexia, 1188
Sinoatrial arrest, 318
Sinoatrial block, 318
  electrocardiography in, 318, *318*
Sinoatrial node, 300, 301
Sinus
  cavernous, thrombosis of, 2116
  dural, thrombosis of, 2115–2116
  lateral, thrombosis of, 2115–2116
  paranasal, aspergillosis of, 1771
    infection of, brain abscess due to, 2112
  sagittal, superior, thrombosis of, 2116
Sinus bradycardia, 317–318
Sinus headache, 2058
Sinus node, 301
Sinus tachycardia, electrocardiography in, 308, *309*
Sinus thrombosis, 2093
  and stroke, *2095*
Sinus venosus defect, 228
Sinusitis, 1585
  Hemophilus influenzae, 1565
Sipple's syndrome, 1406–1407
Sjögren's syndrome, 1915, 1936–1937, 2223
  clinical manifestations of, 1936–1937
  diagnosis of, 1937
  immune response in, 1936–1937
  pathogenesis of, 1936
  treatment of, 1937
  with Fanconi's syndrome, 615
  with interstitial lung disease, 414
Skeletal hyperostosis, idiopathic diffuse, 1953
Skeletal system
  deformities of, in Friedreich's ataxia, 2083
  Hemophilus influenzae infection of, 1564
  mycobacterioses of, 1633
  tuberculosis of, 1628
Skin
  abscesses of, in heroin addiction, 2018
  aging and, 23
  anatomic considerations and, 2227–2228
  biopsy of, in leprosy, 1637
  café au lait lesions of, in neurofibromatosis, 2085
  cancer of, 2271–2272
  diseases of, 2227–2275. See also *Dermatitis*.
    differential diagnosis of, 2241–2249
    pathophysiology of, 2227–2232
    pigmentary, 2254–2257
    radiation and, 2300
    signs of, 2250–2267
    soaks for, 2240
    therapeutic principles in, 2239–2241
    topical therapy in, 2240–2241
    with ulcerative colitis, 753
  examination of, 2232–2239
    tests in, 2236–2239
Skin (*Continued*)
  in disseminated coccidioidomycosis, 1761
  in neurofibromatosis, 2085
  in sarcoidosis, 434
  in spinal cord injury, 2177
  in systemic candidiasis, 1769
  irradiation of, as radiation injury, 2300, 2302
  lesions of, *2233–2236*
    in Wernicke's encephalopathy, 2065
    patterned arrangement of, 2236
  malignancy-associated lesions of, 1084–1086
  mechanical considerations in, 2228–2229
  mycobacterioses of, 1633
  occupational diseases of, 2295–2297
  physiologic considerations, 2229
  radiobiology of, 2299
  RNA virus infections of, 1706–1712
  scalded, syndrome of, staphylococcal, 2270
  staphylococcal infection of, 1546
  stimulation of, in pain, 2052
  streptococcal infections of, 1524–1525
  structure of, *2228*
  tumors of, in neurofibromatosis, 2085
Skin tests
  delayed reactions to, 386
  in respiratory disease, 385–386
Skull
  fracture of, 2171
    depressed, 2171
  trauma to, brain abscess due to, 2112
  tumors of, 2164
Sleep
  disorders of, 1986–1990
    classification of, 1988–1990, *1988*
    in manic-depressive psychosis, 2006
  hypothalamus and, 2025
Sleep apnea, 457
  syndromes of, *1988*, 1990
Sleeping sickness. See *African trypanosomiasis*.
Slow-reacting substance of anaphylaxis, 391–392
Slow viral infections of nervous system, 2135–2138
Small airways disease, 397
Small intestine
  bacterial overgrowth in, 729–731
  chyme transport in, 713
  diverticula of, 708
  fluid transport in, 713
  functions of, 703
  ischemia of, 735
  malabsorption syndrome and, 732–736
  motility disorders of, 706–708
  resection of, nutritional management in, 736
  secretions of, 713
  ulceration of, 801–802
  total parenteral nutrition in, 1216, 1216t
Small intestine neoplasm(s), 770
  clinical manifestations of, 770
  differential diagnosis of, 770
  epidemiology of, 770
  etiology of, 770
  pathology of, 770
  prevention of, 770
  prognosis in, 770
  risk factors in, 770
  therapy of, 770
Smallpox, 110
  case identification for, 1727
  clinical manifestations of, 1726
  cutaneous lesions in, *2260*
  diagnosis of, 1726–1727
  eradication of, 1724–1726
  pathogenesis of, 1726
  pathology of, 1726
  possible recurrence of, 1726

Smallpox (*Continued*)
vaccination for, 1725, 1727–1728
complications of, 1727–1728
contraindications for, 1727
primary, 1727
protection from, 1727
revaccination, 1727
risks of, 1727
storage reserves of, 1726
variola minor and, 1726
Smell, disorders of, 2031
Smoker's palate, 2244
Snakebites, 1841–1843
clinical effects of, 1841–1842, 1842t
epidemiology of, 1841
from venomous species, 1841, 1841t, 1842t
laboratory findings in, 1842
passive immunization to, 43t
pathogenesis of, 1841
treatment of, 1842–1843
antivenin for, 46
Snuff, 48
Soaks, in skin disease, 2240
Sodium
excretion of, 510–511
acute renal failure and, 547, 547t
food content of, 1214, 1214t
intake of, diuretics and, 207
sodium balance and, 495–496
metabolism of, in interstitial nephritis, 591
in uremia, 550, 556
reference values for, 2333
renal control system and, 207, *207*
Sodium balance
endocrine factors in, 494, 497
extracellular fluid and, 496, *496*
kidney regulation of, 493–498, *493*, *496*
kinins and, 497
natriuretic hormone and, 497
neurologic factor in, 497
prostaglandins and, 497
renin-angiotensin-aldosterone system and, 497
Sodium chloride, in metabolic alkalosis, 542
Sodium fluoride, in osteoporosis, 1460
Sodium nitrite, 782
Sodium transport, 721
Sodoku, 1665–1666
Soft tissue
mycobacterioses of, 1633
clostridia infection of, 1574, 1575t
Solar radiation, cancer and, 1070
Solution, Burow's, 2239, *2239*
Solvents, organic, abuse of, 2024
Somatomammotropic hormones, 1253–1254
Somatomedin A, 1254
Somatomedin C, 1254
Somatosensory evoked potentials, 1970
Somatostatin, 1278
Somatostatinoma, 1350
islet cell tumor with, 1350
Somatotrophs, 1252
Somatotropin. See *Growth hormone.*
Somatotropin release–inhibiting factor, 1241, 1242, 1245–1246
Somnolence, narcotic drugs and, 2050
Somogyi phenomenon, 1332
Sonography, Doppler, in stroke, 2100
Sorbitol, in diabetes mellitus, 1326–1327, *1326*
Sore throat, streptococcal, 1522–1523
South American blastomycosis, 1764
Spangler, papular dermatitis of, 2269
Sparganosis, 1805–1806
Spasms
habit, 2077
infantile, 2153
mobile, 2077
torsion, 2077–2078
Spasmodic torticollis, 2078
Spastic ataxia, 2045
Spastic dysphonia, in spasmodic torticollis, 2078
Spastic quadriparesis, in central pontine myelinolysis, 2067
Spasticity
in amyotrophic lateral sclerosis, 2080
in olivopontocerebellar degeneration, 2084
in spinal cord compression, 2062
in spinal cord injury, 2177
in striatonigral degeneration, 2079
pyramidal, vs. extrapyramidal rigidity, 2045–2046
vs. parkinsonism, 2069
Specific gravity, reference values for, 2333
Spectrin, 903
Speech therapy, after stroke, 2102
Sperm count, reference values for, 2333
Spermatogenesis, 1365
Spermidine, 1076
Spermine, 1076
Spherocytosis, hereditary, 1104
Sphincter of Oddi, stenosis of, 864
Sphingolipidoses, 130
Sphingomyelin lipidosis, 1119–1120, 1119t
Sphingomyelin storage disease, 1119–1120
indeterminate forms of, 1120
Sphingomyelinase, deficiency of, 1119, 1120
Spider bite(s), 1836–1837
passive immunization to, 43t
Spike-and-wave complex, in epilepsy, 2149
Spike wave stupor, 2153
Spina bifida, 145
and syringomyelia, 2084
Spina bifida occulta, 2187
Spinal canal
inflammatory diseases of, 2186–2187
neoplasms of, 2184–2186
stenosis of, 2187
vascular disorders of, 2187
Spinal cord
anomalies of, congenital, 2187–2188
compression of, and back pain, 2061
and bladder dysfunction, 2029
extradural, 2185
in multiple myeloma, 1019
inflammatory diseases and, 2186
intradural, 2186
vascular disorders and, 2187
vs. amyotrophic lateral sclerosis, 2080
vs. transverse myelitis, 2139
degeneration of, from vitamin B_{12} deficiency, vs. Friedreich's ataxia, 2083
disorders of, 2178–2182
and sensory loss, 2048
and drop attacks, 2046
in amyotrophic lateral sclerosis, 2080
in ataxia telangiectasia, 2086
in cancer, 1082
in vitamin B_{12} deficiency, 2067
injuries to, 2175–2177
beds for, 2177
neurologic syndromes with, 2176
rehabilitation after, 2177
intramedullary lesion of, vs. syringomyelia, 2084
lesions of, characteristics of, 2179
mechanical, 2177–2188
subacute necrotic destruction of, 1082
syringomyelia of, 2084
thoracic, in striatonigral degeneration, 2079
transection of, and bladder dysfunction, 2029
gastrointestinal motility and, 712
tumor of, vs. vitamin B_{12} deficiency, 2067
vascular malformations of, hemorrhage due to, 2187
Spinal epidural abscess, 2116–2117
Spinal epidural hematoma, 2187
Spinal kyphosis, 2187
Spinal nerves, tumors of, in neurofibromatosis, 2085
Spinal scoliosis, 2187
Spinal shock
after spinal cord injury, 2175
in acute transverse myelitis, 2138
Spinal subdural empyema, 2117–2118
Spine
anatomy and physiology of, and back pain, 2060–2061
anomalies of, congenital, 2187–2188
cervical, disease of, and ear pain, 2058
imaging techniques for, 1969
injuries to, 2175–2177
tuberculous destruction of, 1628
tumor of, vs. Friedreich's ataxia, 2083
Spinocerebellar degenerations, 2080–2084, *2081*, *2082*
Spinothalamic tract, destruction of, in pain relief, 2053
Spirillary fever, 1665–1666
Spirillum minus, 1665
Spirochetes, dark-field examination of, 1657
Spirometra, 1805
Spironolactone, in heart failure, 209
Spitz nevus, 2276
Spleen. See also specific diagnoses.
absence of, 240
anatomy of, 1023–1024, *1023*
colony-forming unit of, 868
functions of, 1023–1024
in infectious disease, 1478
multiple masses in, in cardiac anomaly, 240
platelet pool of, 1024
Splenectomy
babesiosis and, 1798
for neutropenia, 957
in hairy cell leukemia, 986
in hereditary spherocytosis, 903
in idiopathic thrombocytopenic purpura, 1034
in IgG-mediated autoimmune hemolytic anemia, 909
in thalassemia major, 922
indications for, 1025
postoperative infection and, 903
Splenic flexure syndrome, 710
Splenomegaly, 1024–1025
causes of, 1024–1025, 1024t
congestive, 1024–1025
diagnosis of, 1025
hyposplenism after, 1024
in chronic myelogenous leukemia, 977
in infectious mononucleosis, 1720
infiltrative, 1025
pathogenesis of, 1024–1025
reticuloendothelial hyperplasia and, 1024
splenectomy for, 1025
with neutropenia, 955
Spider bites, antivenin for, 46
Spondylarthritis, 1921
Spondylarthropathies, 1917–1922
genetic factors in, 1918–1919, 1918t
immune response in, 1918–1919, 1918t
types of, 1917–1918, *1918*
Spondylitis, ankylosing. See *Ankylosing spondylitis.*
tuberculous, 1628
Spondylolisthesis, 2187
Spondylosis, 2184
Spongy degeneration of white matter, 2148
Sporotrichosis, 1767–1768
culture in, 1767
diagnosis of, 1767
disseminated, 1767

Sporotrichosis (*Continued*)
epidemiology of, 1767
etiology of, 1767
lymphocutaneous, 1767
pathogenesis of, 1767
pathology of, 1767
prognosis of, 1768
pulmonary, 1767
serology of, 1767
treatment of, 1767–1768
Sporothrix schenckii, 1767
Spot(s)
café-au-lait, 2254, *2257*
Fordyce's, 2230
Roth, in ocular hemorrhage, 2224
Sprue, 732–734. See also *Celiac disease; Tropical sprue.*
collagenous, 734
immunodeficient, 1802
tropical, 737
Spur cell hemolytic anemia, 913
Sputum examination, 387–388, *387*
cultures for, 388
for cytology, 388
specimen collection for, 387
Squamous cell carcinoma, 2272, *2272*, 2297
Squander, quantal, 2216
S-T segment response in angina pectoris, 285, 286
in myocardial infarction, 290–291, 294
Stannosis, 2284
Staphylococcal infection, 1543–1551
antibiotic therapy for, 1550
bacterial interference in, 1550
carriers of, 1543–1544, 1550
clinical manifestations of, 1545–1549
culture in, 1549–1550
diagnosis of, 1549–1550
epidemiology of, 1543–1544
host factor in, 1544–1545
immune response in, 1544–1545
invasive, 1546–1549
microbial virulence of, 1544
of bone, 1546–1547
of joint, 1546–1547
of skin, 1546
pathogenesis of, 1544–1545
prevention of, 1550–1551
teichoic acid antibody assay in, 1550
toxin-produced disease, 1545–1546
treatment of, 1550
Staphylococcal scalded skin syndrome, 1545–1546, 2270
vs. toxic epidermal necrolysis, 1546
Staphylococcus(i)
bacteriology of, 1543
beta-lactam antibody-resistant, 1550
methicillin-resistant, 1550
Staphylococcus aureus, 781, 1534, 1543–1550
Staphylococcus epidermidis, 1543, 1545, 1546, 1547, 1549, 1550
Staphylococcus saprophyticus, 1547
Starvation, 1184
metabolic acidosis and, 540
Starling forces, 521–522, 524, 526
Starling's law of the heart, 212
Status epilepticus, 2153–2154
Status epilepticus,
major motor, 2153
emergency treatment of, 2160, *2160*
partial, complex, 2153
"Steal," intracranial, 2104
Steatorrhea, 725, 723
Stein-Leventhal syndrome, 1249
Stem cells, 940
in proliferative disorders, 961–963
residual normal, 962
Stem cells (*Continued*)
mitral, and stroke, 2092, *2092*
x-ray of, *167*, *168*, *169*
of internal carotid artery, 2094
tricuspid, 255–256
Stercoral ulcers, 784
Sterilization, for hospital-acquired infection, 1491
Steroids
in myasthenia gravis, 2213, 2214
in pemphigus, 2268
systemic, in skin disease, 2241
topical, in skin disease, 2240–2241
Steroid hormone(s), 1221, 1227–1228
action of, 1223, 1227–1228, *1227*
metabolism of, 1223
receptors for, 1227–1228, *1227*
transport of, 1222
Steroid sulfatase deficiency, *2251*
Stevens-Johnson syndrome, 1506, *2266*, 2269
Stiff man syndrome, 2216
Still's disease, 1917
adult-onset, 1917
Stimulants, central nervous system, abuse of, 2021–2022
Stingrays, 1844
Stokes-Adams attack, 2092
Stomach. See also *Gastric* entries.
acute dilatation of, 706
functions of, 702–703
physiology of, 681–683, *681*, *682*
Stomach cancer, 697–702
adenomatous, 701–702
after subtotal gastric resection, 698
benign, 701
blood group A and, 698
chemotherapy in, 700
clinical manifestations of, 698–699, 698t
diagnosis of, 687–688, 699–700
dietary factors in, 697–698
endoscopy in, 658, 699
epidemiology of, 697
etiology of, 697–698
extragastric signs of, 699
gastritis and, 698
genetic factor in, 698
immune response in, 699–700
incidence of, 698
leiomyomatous, 701
leiomyosarcomatous, 701
lymphomatous, 700–701
metastatic, 701
nitrates and, 697–698
nitrosamines and, 697
pathology of, 698
pernicious anemia and, 698
polyps and, 698
prevalence of, 698
prevention of, 700
prognosis in, 700
radiation therapy in, 700
radiography in, 699, *699*
surgery for, 700
treatment of, 700
Stomatitis
aphthous, involving mouth, 2244
epizootic, 1711–1712
ulcerative, 664
Stonefishes, 1844
Stool examination
in anemia, 875
in diarrhea, 715–717
in malabsorption syndrome, 725
Strabismus, 2035
Stratum corneum, 2228
Stratum germinativum, 2227
Stratum granulosum, 2228
Stratum spinosum, 2227
Strawberry hemangioma, multiple, *2265*
Street virus, 2132
Streptobacillary fever, 1665
Streptobacillus moniliformis, 1665
Streptocerciasis, 1833
Streptococcal disease, 1519–1542. See also specific diagnoses.
clinical classification of, 1519–1520, 1520t
group A infections of, 1519, 1520–1526
antistreptolysin O test in, 1520, 1521, 1522, 1524, 1525
carriers of, 1521–1522
epidemiology of, 1521–1522
epidemics of, 1520–1521, 1522
immune response in, 1521
M protein in, 1521, 1522, 1527
pathogenesis of, 1520–1521
prevention of, 1525–1526
prophylaxis of, 1525–1526
T antigens in, 1521
transmission of, 1521–1522
group B infections of, 1519, 1526–1527
sexual transmission of, 1526–1527
group C infections of, 1520
group D infections of, 1519
group G infections of, 1520
Streptococcal myonecrosis, 1575t
Streptococcus
brain abscess due to, 2112
classification of, 1519–1520
in infective endocarditis, 1533–1534
microbiology of, 1519
Streptococcus mutans, 1520
Streptococcus pneumoniae, 1498, 1533
Streptococcus pyrogenes, 1527
Streptokinase, 1056
in pulmonary embolism, 430
Streptomycin
as nephrotoxin, 596
in plague, 1602
in pulmonary tuberculosis, 1625, 1626
Streptozocin, as nephrotoxin, 602
Stress
acute gastritis and, 677, 678
cardiovascular system response to, 162–163
gastrointestinal disease and, 645
glucocorticoids and, 1306
irritable bowel syndrome and, 710
metabolic regulation disorders and, 1250
peptic ulcer and, 684
Stress diabetes, in disorders of neurometabolic regulation, 1250
Stress testing, 162–163
electrocardiography in, 174–175
in angina pectoris, 285, 286
in congenital valvular aortic stenosis, 236
in heart failure, 195
myocardial perfusion imaging with, 181–182, *182*
Stretch reflexes, hyperactive, in metabolic brain disease, 1975
Striatonigral degeneration, 2079
and parkinsonism, 2071
Stroke(s)
amnestic, 2095
atherothrombotic, 2091
cardiac thromboembolism and, 2091, *2092*
completed, 2091
course of, 2099
prognosis of, 2099
treatment of, 2101
computed tomography in, 2100
investigation of, 2099
lacunar, 2095
nonprogressing, partial, 2097
partial, nonprogressing, 2091, 2097, 2097t

Stroke(s) (*Continued*)
  prevention of, 2095
  progressing, 2091
  rehabilitation after, 2101–2102
  stroke volume in, 212, *213*
  threatened, pathogenesis of, 2095–2097, *2095*
    prognosis of, 2098
    treatment of, 2100
  thromboembolic, causes of, 2091, *2092*
  vascular, 2086
Stroke-in-evolution, 2091
Strongyloides, 1821
Strongyloides stercoralis, 1819–1820
Strongyloidiasis, 1819–1820
  clinical manifestations of, 1820
  diagnosis of, 1820
  epidemiology of, 1820
  etiology of, 1819–1820
  pathology of, 1820
  prevention of, 1820
  treatment of, 1820
Struma ovarii, 1287
Stupor
  definition of, 1971
  general causes of, 1971–1975, *1971*
  in subtentorial mass lesions, 1972
  in supratentorial mass lesions, 1972
  spike wave, 2153
Sturge-Weber disease, 2085–2086
  seizures in, 2150
Subacute inclusion body encephalitis, 2136. See also *Panencephalitis, subacute sclerosing*.
Subaortic stenosis
  hypertrophic, idiopathic, 330–331, *330*
  tunnel, 331
Subarachnoid hemorrhage, 2105
  and headache, 2057
  clinical features of, 2105
  computed tomography in, 2057, 2106–2107
  definition of, 2103
  intracerebral, vs. spinal subarachnoid hemorrhage, 2187
  intracerebral hemorrhage with, definition of, 2103
  laboratory investigation in, 2106
  prognosis in, 2107
  spinal, 2187
Subclavian vein thrombosis, 363
Subcortical white matter, hemorrhage in, 2109
Subcutaneous injection, abscesses with, 1593
Subcutaneous tissue disorders, 1962–1963
Subdiaphragmatic abscess, pleural involvement with, 449
Subdural bleeding, myelopathy in, 2139
Subdural empyema, 2114–2115
  computed tomography in, 2115
  spinal, 2117–2118
Subdural hematoma, chronic, in brain injury, 2174
Suberosis, 2285
Substantia nigra, in striatonigral degeneration, 2079
Subtentorial lesions, 1971, 1972–1973
Sucralfate, in peptic ulcer, 689, 690
Sucrase, deficiency of, 732
Sucrose hemolysis test, 912
Sudanophilic leukodystrophy, 2148
Sudden cardiac death, 296–297
  and ventricular arrhythmias, 296–297
  etiology of, 296
  high-risk patients for, 296–297
  pathogenesis of, 296
  prevention of, 297
Sudden infant death syndrome, 1990
Sudeck's atrophy, 2063
"Sugar-baby" protein-calorie malnutrition, 1185
Suicide, 37
  acute alcohol intoxication and, 51
  and depressant abuse, 2020
  attempted, by drug overdose, 1981
  in Huntington's disease, 2074
  in manic-depressive psychosis, 2006
  in narcotic-related deaths, 2018
  risk of, in depression, 2012
Sulfadiazine, in toxoplasmosis, 1795
Sulfasalazine, in Crohn's disease, 747
Sulfhemoglobin, reference values for, 2339
Sulfinpyrazone
  as nephrotoxin, 602
  in gout, 1141
Sulfite, allergy to, 1886
Sulfoiduronate sulfatase, deficiency of, 1148
Sulfonamide(s), 103
  as nephrotoxins, 597
  in malaria, 1779, 1780
  in nocardiosis, 1614
  in paracoccidioidomycosis, 1764–1765
  therapeutic window of, 101t
Sulfonylureas, 1328–1329, *1329*
Sulfhemoglobinemia, 935, 936
  drug-induced, 935t, 936
Sunlight, skin reactions to. See *Photosensitivity*.
Sunscreens, in skin disease prevention, 2241
Superior mesenteric artery syndrome, 761
Superior sagittal sinus thrombosis, 2116
Superior vena cava angiography, 383
Superoxide, 946
Superoxide dismutase, 1584
Suppressor-effector, 1850
Supratentorial lesions, *1971*, 1972
Supraventricular tachycardia, 316, *316*, *317*
Suramin, in African trypanosomiasis, 1782
Surgery
  for heart failure, 210
  for pain relief, 2053–2054
  for trigeminal neuralgia, 2059
Survival statistics, 22, *22*
Swallowing, in Werdnig-Hoffman disease, 2080
Swan-Ganz catheter, 183–184, 474–475, *475*
  for monitoring in shock, 218–219
  in adult respiratory distress syndrome, 474
Sweat chloride concentrations, 390
Sweat glands, 2229–2232
Sweating
  abnormalities of, 2028
  fluid volume depletion and, 519
Sweet, acute febrile neutrophilic dermatosis of, 2266
Swimmer's itch, 1811, 1812
Swyer-James (Macleod's) syndrome, 406
Sydenham's chorea, 1530, 2075
Sylvian epilepsy, 2150, 2154
Sylvest's disease, 1730–1731
Symblepharon formation, drug induced, 2225
Symmetrel. See *Amantadine*.
Symmetrical generalized neuropathy, 2189–2190. See also *Polyneuropathy*.
Symmetrical polyneuropathy. See also *Polyneuropathy*.
  definition of, 2188
Sympathectomy
  for thromboangiitis obliterans, 361
  in arteriosclerosis obliterans, 360
  in Raynaud's disease, 355–356
Sympathetic nervous system, 90
  adrenal medulla and, 1408–1413
Sympathetic neurons, lower, anatomy and physiology of, 2178
Sympathochromaffin system, 1408–1410
  physiology of, 1408–1410
Sympathomimetic agent(s)
  in respiratory failure, 460–461
  in shock, 221–222, 222t
Sympathomimetic amines, 93
Syncope, 1983–1985, *1984*
  psychomotor seizures and, 1986
  vs. drop attacks, 2046
  vs. epilepsy, 2156
  vs. vertigo, 2041
Syndrome of inappropriate antidiuretic hormone secretion, 1268
Synovial fluid, 1897
  differential count of, reference values for, 2340
  in rheumatic disease, 1906–1908, 1907t
Synovial membrane, in rheumatic disease, 1908
Synovial tumor, 1960
Synoviography, 1910
Synovitis, 1891, 1897, 1898
  crystal-induced, 1892
  in rheumatoid arthritis, 1904–1905, *1905*
  rheumatoid, 1899–1900, *1899*
  villonodular, pigmented, 1960
Synovium, 1899, *1899*
Syphilis, 1650–1661
  arthritis with, 1924
  blood transfusion and, 939
  cardiovascular, 1655
  case detection in, 1652
  chancre of, 1653, *1653*
  clinical manifestations of, 1653–1655, *1653*
  congenital, 1656–1657, 1658, 1659–1660
    serology in, 1658
  dark-field examination in, 1657
  deaths from, 1652
  diagnosis of, 1657
  differential diagnosis of, 1653, 1654
  epidemiology of, 1652
  etiology of, 1651
  false-positive tests in, 1658
  follow-up examinations in, 1660, 1660t
  general paresis with, 1656
  gumma of, 1654–1655
  history of, 1651
  homosexuality and, 1652
  host factor in, 1651–1652
  in pregnancy, 1659
  Jarisch-Herxheimer reaction in, 1660
  late (tertiary), 1654–1656, 1655t
  latent, 1654
  meningovascular, 1655–1656, 2118, 2119
  natural course of, 1652
  nervous system in, 1655–1656
  of central nervous system, 2118–2121
  pathogenesis of, 1651–1652
  prevention of, 1660–1661
  primary, 1653, *1653*
  relapsing, 1654
  secondary, 1653–1654, *1653*
  serology in, 1657–1658, 1657t, 2120–2121
    treatment schedules and, 1660, 1660t
  stages of, 1650–1651, 1652, 1653–1655, *1653*
  tabes dorsalis with, 1656
  treatment of, 1658–1660, 1659t
    for contacts, 1660
    penicillin for, 1658–1660, 1659t
  treponemal persistence in, 1660
  treponemal tests for, 1657–1658, 1660
  VDRL test in, 1657, 1658, 1660
Syphilitic aortitis, 348–350, *349*
Syphilitic heart disease, 348–350
  antisyphilitic treatment in, 350
Syphilitic meningitis
  acute, 2118

Syphilitic meningitis (*Continued*)
symptomatic, 2119
Syphilitic meningomyelitis, vs. vitamin B_{12} deficiency, 2067
Syphilitic tabes dorsalis, and ataxia, 2044
Syringobulbia, 2084
Syringomyelia, 2084
and sensory loss, 2048
Systemic elastorrhexis, 1152
Systemic lupus erythematosus, 341, 1909, 1924–1932, *2264, 2265, 2266*
cerebral hemorrhge with, 2105
classification criteria, 1925t
clinical manifestations of, 1927–1929, 1928t, 1931t
corticosteroids in, 1931
diagnosis of, 1930
drug-induced, 1925, 1926t, 1930
epidemiology of, 1924
etiology of, 1924–1925, *1926*
genetic factor in, 1924–1927
glomerular involvement in, 585–586, 586t
immune response in, 1924–1927, 1926t
laboratory findings in, 1929–1930
pathogenesis of, 1926–1927
pathology of, 1927
pleural involvement with, 449
treatment of, 1930–1931
with interstitial lung disease, 414
Systemic sclerosis, 341, 674, 731, 1932–1936, *2262, 2264, 2266*
clinical manifestations of, 1933–1934, 1933t
CREST syndrome variant in, 1933, 1934, 1935
diagnosis of, 1933–1934
differential diagnosis of, 1934, 1934t
immune response in, 1932, 1934
in Raynaud's phenomenon, 1932, 1933
laboratory findings in, 1934
pathogenesis of, 1932
pathology of, 1932–1933
treatment of, 1934–1935
Systemic side effects of topical ocular medications, 2225–2226

T cell(s)
antigen recognition by, 1850
cytotoxic, 1850, *1851*
idiotypic networks and, 1850–1851
in atopic dermatitis, 2249
in group A streptococcal disease, 1521
lymphocyte, 1849–1850
development of, 1849–1850
differentiation of, 1849, *1849*
helper, 1846, 1848, 1849, 1850
histocompatibility restrictions and, 1849, *1850*
"killer," 1849
suppressor, 1846, 1849, 1850
variants of, in chronic lymphocytic leukemia, 980, 981
major histocompatibility complex and, 1878–1880, *1880*
mononuclear phagocyte interaction with, *948*, 949
receptors, 1850
T cell–B cell interaction cognate (MHC restricted), 1848
T cell-derived–B cell growth factor, 1847
T cell growth factor, 949
T cell leukemia, human, 980
T cell lymphoma, cutaneous, 2272–2273
T cell neoplasms, 992, 992t, 993, 993t, 994
T_3 suppression test, 1279, 1284

Tabes dorsalis, 1656, 2119–2120. See also *Locomotor ataxia.*
autonomic dysfunction in, 2027
congenital neurosyphilis and, 2120
lightning pains in, 2063
neurologic changes in, 2118
syphilitic, and ataxia, 2044
Taboparesis, 2119
Tachycardia, 307–317. See also specific diagnoses.
carotid sinus massage in, 307–308
clinical examination for, 307
ectopic, 305
in Wernicke's encephalopathy, 2065
sinus, 308
ventricular, electrocardiography in, 313–315, *314, 315*
with gastrointestinal hemorrhage, 649
Taenia solium, 1806–1807
Taenia saginata, 1806
Takayasu's arteritis, 2093
Takayasu's syndrome, 346, 352–353, *352*
Tandem walking, in evaluation of vertigo, 2041
Tangier disease, 1116
Tapeworm, 1804–1809. See also *Cestodes*; specific diagnoses.
eradication of, 1809
Tar, in psoriasis treatment, 2246
Tardive dyskinesia, 2075–2076
in drug-induced parkinsonism, 2071
phenothiazines and, 2005
variants of, 2076
vs. chorea, 2069
Tarsal tunnel syndrome, 1915
Tartrate–inhibitable acid phosphatase, 1076
Tarui's disease, 2205
Taste, disorders of, 2031–2032
Tay-Sachs disease, enzyme replacement in, 132
Technetium-99m
in cardiology imaging, 179–180
in gastrointestinal imaging, 653–654, *653, 654*
Technetium-99m–labeled albumin scan, in pulmonary embolism, 427
Technetium-99m pertechnetate, in myocardial imaging, 286
Technetium-99m stannous pyrophosphate
in cardiology imaging, 182
in myocardial imaging, 291, 294
Teeth,
and ear pain, 2058
pain in, 2058
Tegretol. See *Carbamazepine.*
Teichoic acid antibody assay, in staphylococcal infection, 1550
Telangiectasia(s), 1116, 2236. See also *Ataxia telangiectasias*.
ataxia, 2086
punctate, involving mouth, 2243
Telecanthus-hypospadias, 145
Tellurium toxicity, 2315
Telogen, 2231
Telogen effluvium, 2231
Temperature, body. See also *Hyperthermia* and *Hypothermia*.
extreme, in coma, 1979
impaired sensation of, in syringomyelia, 2084
normal, 1471
regulation of, hypothalamus and, 2025–2026
Temporal lobe(s),
abscess of, 2113
disorders of, 1992–1993, *1992*
tumors of, 2163

Temporal lobe epilepsy, 2154
Temporal lobe seizures, 2152
Temporal sclerosis, mesial, in epilepsy, 2150
Temporomandibular joint, disorders of, and ear pain, 2058
Temporomandibular joint syndrome, 2057
Tendinitis
bicipital, 1954
calcific, 1954
Tennis elbow, 1959–1960
Tenosynovitis, 1959
tuberculous, 1628
Tension headache, 2056–2057
from skeletal muscle contraction, 2064
Teratoma, of pineal gland, 1275
Terminal deoxynucleotidyl transferase, 992
Tertiary care, 7
Testicular feminization, 1359–1360, *1360*, 1400
Testis(es), 1365–1375. See also specific disorders.
at puberty, 1368–1369
biopsy of, in evaluation of testicular function, 1367–1368
development of, 1351–1352
fetal, 1365
differentiation and development disorders of, 1354–1356, *1355*
function of, disorders of, 1356–1359, 1357t
evaluation of, 1367–1368
gonadal dysgenesis and, 1354–1356
gonadotropin unresponsiveness in, 1356
hormones of, 1365
hypothalamus-pituitary interaction and, 1366–1367, *1367*, 1368
in phenotypic differentiation, 1353, *1353*
in XY agonadism, 1356
Leydig cell agenesis (dysgenesis) in, 1356
regression of, 1356
tumor classification in, 1375t
germinal, 1375, 1375t
interstitial cell, 1369, 1375, 1375t
undescended, 1373–1374
vanishing testis syndrome and, 1356
Testosterone, 1301, 1365, 1366, 1381
biosynthesis of, deficiencies of, 1356–1359, *1357*t
free, reference values for, 2333
in hirsutism, 1395–1397
in male sexual differentiation, 1361–1362, *1361, 1362*
measurement of, 1310
plasma, 1367
total, reference values for, 2334
urinary, 1367
Testosterone therapy
in androgen deficiency, 1369–1370
in hypopituitarism, 1258
Tetanus, 1579–1582
airway management in, 1580
cardiovascular system in, 1580–1581
chemoprophylaxis for, 1582
clinical criteria of, 1579–1580
diagnosis of, 1580
epidemiology of, 1579
etiology of, 1579
immunization for, 43, 43t, 1580, *1581*, 1582
nervous system effects in, 1579
pathogenesis of, 1579
prevention of, 1582
prognosis in, 1582
prophylaxis for, *1581*, 1582
in wound management, 43
tetanic spasms in, 1579, 1580
toxins, 1579
treatment of, 1580
adrenergic blocking agents in, 1581
antibiotic therapy in, 1580

Tetanus (*Continued*)
treatment of, antitoxin in, 1580
curarization in, 1580
diazepam in, 1580
ventilatory support in, 1580
Tetanus immunoglobulin (human), 1580, *1581*, 1582
Tetany, 1443–1444, *1444*, 2216
treatment of, 1445
Tetrabenazine, in Huntington's disease, 2075
Tetracycline(s), 79, 105, 1586
as nephrotoxins, 597
for Rocky Mountain spotted fever, 1681
in acne, 2243
in brucellosis, 1616
in relapsing fever, 1664
in rickettsial disease, 1676, 1677
therapeutic window of, 101t
3,5,3′,5′-Tetraiodothyronine (T_4). See *Thyroxine.*
Tetralogy of Fallot, 233–234
angiography in, 233
cardiac catheterization in, 233
echocardiography in, 233
electrocardiography in, 233
radiography in, 169, 233
surgery for, 234
ventriculography in, 234
Tetrodon poisoning, 783
Tetrodotoxic fishes, 1844
Thalamic hemorrhage, *2109*
Thalamic syndrome, 2049
Thalamic–internal capsular hemorrhage, 2108
Thalamus
damage to, and sensory loss, 2049
in Korsakoff's syndrome, 2065
surgical lesion in, for pain relief, 2053
Thalassemias, 875, 920–927
5-azacytidine therapy in, 926
clinical classification of, 921t
epidemiology of, 921
genetic factor in, 920–921
genetics of, 923–926
molecular, 924–925
homozygous B, *867*
mutations in, 923–926, *924*
deletion, 925
globin stability and, 925
Hb F production with, 925–926
mRNA translation in, 925
polyadenylation in, 925
promoter, 924
splicing, 924–925
severe β, 921–923. See also *Cooley's anemia.*
bone marrow transplantation in, 926
experimental therapy of, 926
prenatal diagnosis of, 926
sickle β, 930
silent carriers of, 923
Thalassemia intermedia, 922–923
genetic factor in, 922–926
Thalassemia major, 921–922
β globin production in, 921
blood transfusions in, 921–922
chelation therapy in, 922
growth abnormality in, 921–922
iron overload in, 921–922
splenectomy in, 922
thalassemia trait in, 921
Thalassemia trait, 923
differential diagnosis of, 923
gene frequency in, 923
genetic factor in, 923
malaria and, 923
prenatal diagnosis of, 926
β-Thalassemic gene defects in, 136, 137, *137*
Thalidone diuretics, in hypokalemia, 2208
Thallium, as nephrotoxin, 601
Thallium toxicity, 2313–2314
Thallium-201, in myocardial imaging, 286, 291, 294
in cardiology, 181–182, *182*
Theophylline. See also *Aminophylline.*
in asthma, 395
inhibiting agents of, 81t
pharmacokinetic parameters of, 70t
poisoning from, 89
Therapeutic window concept, 74, *74*, 75t
Thermal injuries of lung, 2287
Therapy
medical, allocation of scarce resources in, 11
indications for, 11–12
Thermanesthesia, definition of, 2047
Thermhypesthesia, definition of, 2047
Thermoregulatory center, 1471
Thiabendazole
in strongyloidiasis, 1820
in toxocariasis, 1824
in trichinellosis, 1826
Thiamin, 1198–1199
biochemical function of, 1198
deficiency of, 1198–1199
assay in, 1199
in alcoholism, 1198
treatment of, 1199
dietary allowance for, 1178
dietary sources of, 1198
physiology of, 1198
requirements for, 1198
structure of, 1198, *1198*
toxicity of, 1199
Thiamin pyrophosphate, 1198
Thiamine
in coma, 1979
in Korsakoff's syndrome, 2065
in Wernicke's encephalopathy, 2065
Thiazide(s)
hypercalcemia and, 1449
in heart failure, 207–208
in kidney stones, 632
Thiazide diuretics
as nephrotoxins, 602
in hypokalemia, 2208
6-Thioguanine, 1095
Thiopental, serum and plasma, reference values for, 2334
Thiopurines, 1095
6-Thiopurine, immunosuppression with, 1095
Thioridazine, ocular side effects of, 2225
Thiourea derivatives, 1284–1285, 1286
Thirst
hypernatremia and, 529
hypothalamus and, 2026
regulation of, 1268
Thirst center, in water balance, 524
Thomsen's disease, 2207–2208. See also *Myotonia congenita.*
Thoracentesis, in pleural disease, 447
Thoracic disc, herniation of, 2183
Thoracic irradiation, 2300
Thoracic outlet syndrome, 2197
Thoracic spine, injury to, 2175, 2176
Thoracolumbar spinal injuries, 2176
Thoracotomy, pain after, vs. paravertebral tumor, 2185
Thorax, pain in, from muscle contraction, 2064
irradiation injury to, 2300
skin diseases of, 2244–2248
Thorn apple, toxicity of, 783
Thrombasthenia, 1030, 1031, 1037
Thrombin, 1028, 1030, 1043
Thrombin time, 1031
reference values for, 2340
Thromboangiitis obliterans, 360–361
clinical manifestations of, 360–361
diagnosis of, 361
epidemiology of, 360
pathology of, 360
prognosis in, 361
tobacco use and, 360, 361
treatment of, 361
sympathectomy for, 361
Thrombocyte count, reference values for, 2339
Thrombocythemia, essential (hemorrhagic), 974–975
Thrombocytopenia, 1028, 1030, 1031, 1036–1037
causes of, 1031t, 1032
dilutional, 1036
in cardiopulmonary bypass, 1036
in infection, 1036
platelets in, destruction of, 1032–1035
production of, 1032
sequestration of, 1036
survival of, vs. consumption, 1035–1036
secondary immunologic, 1034–1035
immune response in, 1034–1035
Thrombocytopenic purpura
drug-induced, 1032–1033, 1032t
idiopathic, 1033–1034
acute vs. chronic, 1033–1034
corticosteroids for, 1034
immune response in, 1033–1034
refractory, 1034
splenectomy in, 1034
treatment of, 1034
immune response in, 1032–1034
isoimmune neonatal, 1034
post-transfusion, 939, 1034
thrombotic, 1035
Thrombocytopoiesis, ineffective, 1032
Thrombocytosis, 1036–1037
and cerebral artery thrombosis, 2093
and stroke, *2095*
essential, 974–975
Thromboembolism
and oral contraceptives, 1393
cerebral arterial, symptoms of, 2094–2097
syndromes of, 2094–2097
Thrombolysis, 1056
Thrombolytic agents, from recombinant DNA research, 133
Thrombolytic therapy
in myocardial infarction, 295
in pulmonary embolism, 430
Thrombophlebitis, 363–365
anticoagulants in, 364–365
clinical manifestations of, 363
complications of, 364
diagnosis of, 363
differential, 364
impedance plethysmography in, 364
radioisotope-labelled fibrinogen in, 363–364
ultrasonography in, 364
venography in, 363
epidemiology of, 363
iliofemoral, 363
in heroin addicts, 2018
of calf, 363
pathogenesis of, 363
pathology of, 363
prophylaxis for, 364
pulmonary embolism and, 363, 364
septic, 363
treatment of, 364–365
with bronchogenic carcinoma, 441

Thromboplastin time, partial, 1044
Thrombopoietin(s), 869, 1028
Thrombosis
  cavernous sinus, 2116
  cerebral, and stroke, *2095*
  dural sinus, 2115–2116
  intracranial, 2093
  lateral sinus, 2115–2116
  sinus, 2093
  superior sagittal sinus, 2116
    and stroke, *2095*
Thrombotic microangiopathy, 587–588
Thrombotic thrombocytopenic purpura, 587–588, 914–915
Thromboxane, in shock, 214
Thromboxane A_2, 1237–1241
  biosynthesis of, 1238
Thrombus, mural, and stroke, 2091, *2092*
Thrush, 665, *665*, 1768
Thymectomy
  effects of, 1889
  in myasthenia gravis, 2213, 2214
Thymic hypoplasia, 1858
Thymidine kinase gene, 134
Thymidylate synthetase, methyltransferase and, 895, *895*
Thymolipoma, 1890
Thymoma, 1889–1890
  with partial combined immunodeficiency disorder, 1861
Thymus, 1889
  congenital hypoplasia of, 1889
  hyperplasia of, 1889
  in ataxia telangiectasia, 2086
  myasthenia gravis and, 1889
  tumors of, 1889–1890, 1890t
Thyroglobulin, 1276
  serum, concentration of, 1280
  reference values for, 2334
Thyroid acropachy, 1283
Thyroid antibodies, serum, reference values for, 2334
Thyroid cancer
  anaplastic, 1296
  clinical manifestations of, 1296–1297
  diagnosis of, 1296–1297
  familial, 1294
  follicular, 1295–1296
  medullary, 1296
  multinodular goiter and, 1299
  natural history of, 1295–1296
  papillary, 1295
  pathology of, 1295–1296
  radiation therapy for, 1297
  radioiodine therapy for, 1297
  solitary nodule in, 1296–1297
  surgery for, 1296–1297
  triiodothyronine in, 1297
  types of, 1295
Thyroid gland, 1275–1299
  anatomic evaluation of, 1280
  anatomy of, 1275
  autoimmune disease of, 1280, 1281
  basal metabolic rate and, 1280
  biopsy of, 1280
  deep tendon reflex contraction time and, 1280
  embryology of, 1275
  function of, regulation of, 1278, *1278*
    tests of, 1278–1281
      nonthyroidal illness and, 1280
  medullary carcinoma of, 1452
    calcitonin assay in, 1452
  metabolic indices for, 1280
  physical examination of, 1278
  physiology of, 1275–1278
  radioactive iodine uptake in, 1279, 1284
Thyroid gland (*Continued*)
  radiography of, 1280, 1284
  radioiosotope scan of, 1280, 1284
  regulation tests of, 1279
  thyrotropin-releasing hormone infusion test for, 1279, 1284, 1289
  ultrasonography of, 1280
Thyroid hormones, 1228
  assay of, 1278–1279
  circulating, 1276–1277, 1277t
  conversion regulation and, 1277, 1277t
  free T_4 (T_3) index of, 1278, 1279, 1283–1284, 1289, 1290, 1291
  in protein-calorie malnutrition, 1185
  kinetics of, 1277, 1277t
  mechanism of action of, 1223, *1227*, 1228, 1277–1278
  metabolism of, 1223
  receptors for, *1227*, 1228
  resin uptake test for, 1279
  serum concentrations of, 1278–1279, 1278t
  serum reverse T_3 measurement of, 1279
  structure of, 1275, *1276*
  synthesis of, 1276, *1276*
  T_3 suppression test of, 1279, 1284
  transport of, 1222
Thyroid microsomal antibodies, serum, reference values for, 2334
Thyroid preparations, 1290, 1290t
  withdrawal of, 1291
Thyroid-stimulating hormone, 1253
  function tests of, 1255
  in hypopituitarism, 1256, 1258
  serum or plasma, reference values for, 1279, 2334
  serum radioimmunoassay of, 1279
Thyroid-stimulating hormone–response to TRH, reference values for, 2334
Thyroid stimulating immunoglobulin, 1280, 1281
Thyroid storm, 1286–1287, 1286t
Thyroid tumor(s), 1294–1297
  benign, 1294–1295
  epidemiology of, 1294
  etiology of, 1294
  follicular adenoma, 1294–1295
  malignant, 1295–1297
  radiation exposure and, 1294
  radiation therapy for, 1295, 1297
  radioiodine therapy for, 1295, 1297
  surgery for, 1295, 1296–1297
  thyrotropin and, 1294
Thyroid uptake
  of radioactive iodine, reference values for, 2334
  of $^{99m}TcO_4$, reference values for, 2334
Thyroidectomy, 1285
Thyroiditis, 1291
  acute, 1291
  chronic, 1293–1294
  DeQuervain's, 1291
  giant cell, 1291
  granulomatous, 1291
    subacute, 1291
  Hashimoto's, 1287, 1293–1294
  subacute lymphocytic, 1291, 1292–1293, *1292*
  subacute nonsuppurative, 1291–1292
Thyrotoxicosis, 1281, *1281*
  and asthenia, 2044
  and periodic hypokalemic paralysis, 2209
  myasthenia gravis and, 2213
Thyrotrophs, 1252
Thyrotropin. See *Thyroid-stimulating hormone.*
Thyrotropin-displacing activity, 1280, 1281
Thyrotropin releasing hormone, 1241, 1242, 1245, 1246, 1249, 1250, 1255, 1278
Thyrotropin releasing hormone (*Continued*)
  in galactorrhea, 1399
  infusion test for, 1279, *1280*, 1284, 1289
  plasma, reference values for, 2334
Thyrotropin releasing hormone stimulation test, reference values for, 2334
Thyrotoxic myopathy, 2210
Thyroxin therapy, in hypopituitarism, 1258
Thyroxine, 1275. See also *Thyroid hormones.*
  free, in hypothyroidism, 1289, 1290, 1291
    reference values for, 2334
  total, reference values for, 2334
L-Thyroxine, for hypothyroidism, 1290
Thyroxine-binding globulin, 1276–1277, 1277t, 1278, 1279
  serum, reference values for, 2334
Thyroxine-binding prealbumin, 1276, 1279
Thyroxine index, reference values for, 2335
Thyroxine ratio, effective, reference values for, 2334
Thyroxine/TBG ratio, reference values for, 2335
TIA. See *Transient ischemic attack(s).*
Tic(s), 2077
  definition of, 2069
  in postencephalitic parkinsonism, 2071
Tic douloureux, 2059
Tick(s), 1836
Tick paralysis, 1836
  neuromuscular block due to, 2215
Tick-borne encephalitis, 1749
  vector in, 1749
  virus in, 1749
Tick-borne flavivirus disease, 1755
Tick-borne rickettsiae, 1680–1683
  Eastern hemisphere, 1682–1683
Tietze's syndrome, 370, 1960
Timed forced expiratory volume, 464
Tin toxicity, 2312, 2315
Tinea capitis, 2247
Tinea versicolor, 2245, *2246*
Tinnitus, 2037, 2040
Tissue(s), aging and, 22
Tissue radiobiology, specific, 2299
Tissue transplantation, major histocompatibility complex and, 187
TNM cancer staging system, 1063, 1063t
TNM classification. See under specific diagnoses.
Tobacco use, 46–50. See also *Cigarette smoking.*
  bronchogenic carcinoma and, 439–440
  cancer and, 1069–1070
  chewing in, 48
  cigar smoking in, 50
  erythrocytosis and, 963–964
  glossitis and, 666
  history of, 46–47
  leukoplakia/erythroplakia and, 666
  oral cancer and, 666
  pipe smoking in, 50
  thromboangiitis obliterans and, 360, 361
Tobramycin
  as nephrotoxin, 596
  therapeutic window of, 101t
Tocopherols, 1208
Tocotrienols, 1208
Todd's paralysis, 2149, 2151
Togaviruses, in acute central nervous system infections, *2122*, 2123
Tolazamide, 1329
Tolbutamide, 1329
  inhibiting agents of, 81t
Tolbutamide test, in insulinoma, 1345, *1345*
Tolerance
  drug, definition of, 2016
    narcotics and, 2050

Tolerance intervals, 62
Tolosa-Hunt syndrome, 2222
Toluene, abuse of, 2024
Tongue
atrophy of, in amyotrophic lateral sclerosis, 2080
in Werdnig-Hoffman disease, 2080
inflammation of, 665–666
Tongue worm, 1840
Tonic seizures, 2153
Tonic-clonic convulsions, 2153
nonepileptic, 2157
secondarily generalized, 2152
Tonometry, in glaucoma, 2218
Tonsil(s), tumor of, and glossopharyngeal neuralgia, 2060
Tonsillitis, and ear pain, 2058
Tophus, 1136, 1137–1138, 1140
Torsades de pointes, electrocardiography in, 315, *316*
Torsion dystonia, 2077–2079
Torticollis, spasmodic, 2078
Total parenteral nutrition, liver disease and, 834
Tourette's syndrome, 2077
Tourists. See *Travelers.*
Toxemia of pregnancy, 271, 625–626
blood pressure measurement in, 625
convulsions with, 625, 626
glomerular capillary endotheliosis and, 625
renal biopsy in, 626
Toxic disturbances, and epilepsy, 2150
Toxic epidermal necrolysis, vs. staphylococcal scalded skin syndrome, 1546
Toxic neuropathy, 2195
Toxic psychosis, definition of, 1974
Toxic shock syndrome, 221, 1545
and menstruation, 1545
Toxicity
acute amphetamine, 2022
acute cocaine, 2022
drug reaction and, 83–84
Toxicologic values of clinical importance, 2317–2335
Toxin(s)
membrane, and myoglobinuria, 2210
middle molecular weight, 554
Toxocara canis, 1823
Toxocara cati, 1823
Toxocariasis, 1823–1824
epidemiology of, 1823
treatment of, 1824
Toxoplasma, myocarditis and, 334
Toxoplasma gondii, 1792
Toxoplasmosis, 1792–1796
central nervous system, immunosuppressive therapy and, 2142
in acquired immune deficiency syndrome, 2142
clinical manifestations of, 1793–1794
congenital, 1794, 2221
diagnosis of, 1794–1795
culture in, 1794
differential, 1795
serology in, 1794–1795
epidemiology of, 1792–1793
histology in, 1795
immune response in, 1792, 1793–1794, 1795
ocular involvement in, 1793–1794
pathogenesis of, 1793
pathology of, 1793
pregnancy and, 1792, 1794, 1795
prevention of, 1795
therapy of, 1795
Trabeculoplasty, laser, in glaucoma, 2218
Trace elements, toxicity of, with hemodialysis, 2311–2315
Trace metal poisoning, 2307–2315
Trace metals deficiency, in gastrointestinal disease, 646
Trace minerals, 1209–1211
deficiency of, 1209–1211
dietary allowance for, 1179
Tracheobronchitis, 477
Tracheostomy, 458, 467
complications with, 476
Trachoma, 1669–1670, 2221
antibiotic therapy in, 1670
conjunctivitis with, 1669–1670
culture in, 1670
epidemiology of, 1669
in neonates, 1670–1671
prevention of, 1670
serology in, 1670
treatment of, 1670
Traction headache, 2057
Tranquilizers, in pain, 2051, 2052
Transaminases
in acute viral hepatitis, 814
in chronic hepatitis, 825, 826–827
in liver disease, 809
Transcobalamins, 896
Transcortin, 1302
Transferrin, 887–888, 890, 919
serum, reference values for, 2335
total iron-building capacity of, 887
Transferrin saturation, 1162
Transfusion. See also specific constituents.
babesiosis and, 1798, 1799
in chronic renal failure, 556–557
in gastrointestinal hemorrhage, 792
in malaria, 1779
platelet, 1038
with kidney transplantation, 566
Transient erythroblastopenia of childhood, 878
Transient global amnesia, 1997
Transient ischemia, and drop attacks, 2046
Transient ischemic attack(s), 2090, 2097, *2097*
and transient paralysis, 2047
and vertigo, 2043
differential diagnosis of, 2098
investigation of, 2099
treatment of, 2100
Transitional sclerosis, 2147
Transketolase, blood, reference values for, 2335
Transketolase activity coefficient, 1199
Transplantation. See under names of specific organs.
Transposition of great arteries, 238–239
isolated "simple," 238
surgery for, 238, 239
with pulmonic stenosis, 239
with ventricular inversion, 239
with ventricular septal defect, 238–239
Transverse myelitis, acute, 2138–2139
Transverse myelopathy, acute, 2148
Trauma
facial, brain abscess due to, 2112
headache following, 2057
hyperkalemia with, 534
skull, brain abscess due to, 2112
Traumatic unconsciousness, 2170
Travelers
diet of, 1493
health maintenance by, 1492–1494
immunization for, 1493
malaria chemoprophylaxis for, 1493
Traveler's diarrhea, 717, 718, 719, 1493–1494
Trematodes, 1809–1819
digenetic, 1815
Tremor(s)
definition of, 2069
Tremor(s) (*Continued*)
essential, 2073–2074
familial, 2073–2074
in metabolic brain disease, 1975
in parkinsonism, 2070
senile, 2073–2074
Trench fever, 1677, 1685–1686
clinical course of, 1685
culture in, 1685
epidemiology of, 1685
prevention of, 1686
serology in, 1685
treatment of, 1685–1686
Trench foot, 357
Treponema carateum, 1661
*Treponema pallidum,*1650, 1651
antibody tests for, 1657–1658
FTA-ABS test for, 1657–1658, 1660
IgMFTA-ABS test for, 1658
MHA-TP test for, 1657–1658
microbiology of, 1651
Treponema pertenue, 1661–1662
Treponemal tests, 1657
Treponematoses, nonsyphilitic, 1661–1662
Trepopnea, 372
Triamterene, in heart failure, 209
Triceps skinfold thickness, 1180–1182, 1181t
obesity and, 1192
Trichinella spiralis, 1825–1826
Trichinellosis, 1825–1826. See also *Trichinosis.*
clinical manifestations of, 1825–1826
diagnosis of, 1826
serology in, 1826
epidemiology of, 1825
pathogenesis of, 1825
pathology of, 1825
prevention of, 1826
treatment of, 1826
Trichinosis, 334. See also *Trichinellosis.*
Trichomonas vaginalis, 1642, 1803
Trichomoniasis, 1803
Trichophyton infection, 2247
Trichostrongyliasis, 1822
Trichostrongylus, 1822
Trichuriasis, 1824
epidemiology of, 1824
treatment of, 1824
Trichuris trichiura, 1824
Tricuspid insufficiency, 256, 289
Tricuspid stenosis, 255–256
rheumatic fever and, 255
Tricuspid valve
atresia of, 234
echocardiography in, 234
electrocardiography in, 234
radiography in, 234
surgery for, 234
Ebstein's anomaly of, 234
Tricyclic antidepressants
in anxiety, 2010
in chronic paroxysmal hemicrania, 2056
in Huntington's disease, 2075
in manic-depressive psychosis, 2006
in parkinsonism, 2073
Trifluorothymidine, in herpes simplex virus infection, 1717
Trifluridine, in herpesvirus infection, 109–110
Trigeminal nerve, in Sturge-Weber disease, 2085
Trigeminal neuralgia, 2059, 2129
Trigeminal neurilemoma, characteristics of, *2162*
Trigeminal neuropathy, 2198
Triglyceride(s)
absorption of, 720
lipoprotein lipase-mediated catabolism of, 1110–1111

Triglyceride(s) (*Continued*)
lipoprotein remnant catabolism and, 1111
medium-chain, in malabsorption syndrome, 731–732
metabolism of, 1110–1111
serum, reference values for, 2335
transport of, 1109–1110
Triglyceride storage disease, *2205*
Trihexyphenidyl, in torsion dystonia, 2078
Triiodothyronine
free, reference values for, 2335
in Raynaud's disease, 355
in thyroid cancer, 1297
serum, reference values for, 2335
Triiodothyronine index, free, reference values for, 2335
Triiodothyronine resin uptake test, reference values for, 2335
3,5,3'-Triiodothyronine (T_3), 1275. See also *Thyroid hormones.*
3,5,3'-Triiodothyronine (T_3) suppression test, 1279, 1284
Trimazosin therapy, in heart failure, 207
Trimethadione, in epilepsy, *2158*, 2159
Triolein-^{131}I absorption test, reference values for, 2335
Tripanosomiasis, American, 334–335
Tripelennamine, abuse of, 2018
Trisomy, autosomal, 142, *143*
Trisomy 21, 145
recurrence of, 146
Tropical eosinophilia, 1830
Tropical phagedenic ulcer, 1664–1665
antibiotic therapy in, 1665
diagnosis of, 1665
epidemiology of, 1664–1665
pathogenesis of, 1665
penicillin therapy in, 1665
treatment of, 1665
Tropical splenomegaly syndrome, 1778
Tropical sprue, 737, 899
antimicrobials in, 737
folic acid therapy in, 737
Troponin C, 1225
Trousseau's sign, 1444, *1444*
Truncal vagotomy
with antrectomy, 691
with pyloroplasty, 691
Truncus arteriosus, 232
Trypanosoma brucei, 1780
Trypanosoma cruzi, 1783, 1784
Trypanosomiases. See *African trypanosomiasis; Chagas' disease.*
Tryptophan, 1201, 1203, 1413–1414
Tryptophan load test, 1203
Tsetse fly, 1780–1781
Tsutsugamushi disease, 1684
Tubercle(s), Montgomery's, 2230
Tuberculin skin test, 386, 1622–1623, 1624
Tuberculomas, 1629
Tuberculosis, 1620–1630. See also *Pulmonary tuberculosis.*
abdominal, 1628–1629
arthritis with, 1923
bacille Calmette-Guérin vaccine in, 1621
chemoprophylaxis in, 1621–1622
clinical description of, 1623–1624
control of, 1621–1622
disseminated, 1629–1630
endobronchial, 1627
epidemiology of, 1621
etiology of, 1620–1621
extrapulmonary, 1627–1630
genitourinary, 1628
immune response in, 1622
immunity in, 1622
immunization for, 45–46
Tuberculosis (*Continued*)
in hospital-acquired infection, 1491–1492
intestinal, 736–737, 1628–1629
isoniazid in, 1621–1622
lymphatic, 1627–1628
Mantoux test in, 1622–1623
miliary, 1629–1630
pathogenesis of, 1621
pathology of, 1621
pericardial, 1627
pleural, 448, 1627
recurrence of, 1623
skeletal, 1628
tuberculin skin test in, 1622–1623, 1624
Tuberculous lymphadenitis, 736–737, 1627–1628
Tuberculous pericarditis, 340–341
Tuberous sclerosis, 416, 2085, 2256, *2256*
Tubular basement membrane antibody disease, 502–503
Tubular necrosis, acute, dialysis in, 561
Tubular reabsorption of phosphate, reference values for, 2335
Tularemia, 1604–1606
antibiotic therapy in, 1605
clinical manifestations of, 1605
complications of, 1605
diagnosis of, 1605
culture in, 1604
serologic diagnosis in, 1604
skin tests in, 1604
epidemiology of, 1604
pathology of, 1604–1605
prevention of, 1606
prognosis in, 1605–1606
transmission of, 1604–1605
treatment of, 1605
vectors of, 1603–1604
Tularemia vaccine, 1606
Tumor(s). See under specific organs and diagnoses.
Tumor lysis syndrome, 979
Tumor markers, 1075–1076
Tungiasis, 1839–1840
Tuning forks, in evaluation of hearing loss, 2038
Turcot's syndrome, 764
Turner's syndrome, 145, 237, 1173, 1387
chromosome abnormality in, 1387
genetic factor in, 1173
osteoporosis and, 1458
Tympanum, caloric irrigation of, in diagnosis of eye movements, 2036
Thyphoid fever, 1587–1589
carriers of, 1587, 1588
chloramphenicol in, 1588–1589
clinical manifestations of, 1587–1588
complications of, 1588
diagnosis of, 1588
cultures in, 1588
differential, 1588
Widal test in, 1588
epidemiology of, 1587
immunization for, 45
laboratory findings in, 1588
pathogenesis of, 1587
pathology of, 1587
prognosis in, 1589
prophylaxis for, 1589
relapse with, 1588
treatment of, 1588–1589
Typhoid vaccine, 1589
Typhus fever
epidemic louse-borne, 1678–1679
clinical course of, 1678–1679
cutaneous lesions in, *2261*
epidemiology of, 1678
Typhus (*Continued*)
epidemic louse-borne, prevention of, 1679
treatment of, 1679
vector in, 1678
murine (flea-borne), 1679–1680
clinical course of, 1680
epidemiology of, 1679
prevention of, 1680
treatment of, 1680
vector in, 1679
Typhus group disease(s), 1672, 1673t, 1674t, 1678–1680
vectors in, 1678
Typhus vaccine, 1679
Tyramine, monoamine oxidase inhibitors and, 274–275
Tyrosine, 1220
metabolism of, 1126, *1126*
Tyrosine kinase, in hormone action mediation, 126
Tyrosinemia, 616
Tyson's glands, 2230
Tzanck smear
in skin disease, 2236, *2237*
in toxic epidermal necrolysis, 2270

UDPG-4 epimerase deficiency, 1105
Ulcer. See also under specific types.
Buruli, 1633
corneal, 2221
decubitis, 29
dermal, 2233
duodenal, 683–685, *686*, 690
gastric, 683–685
peptic, 681–697
phagedenic, tropical, 1664–1665
Ulcerative colitis, 748–756, *2263*
age of onset in, 748, *748*
clinical manifestations of, 749–750
colon cancer and, 765, 769
course of, 740–750
diagnosis of, 750–752
colonoscopy in, 752
differential, 752
proctosigmoidoscopy in, 751
radiography in, 751–752, *751*, *752*
rectal biopsy in, 751
emotional factors in, 748
epidemiology of, 748
etiology of, 748
extraintestinal complications with, 753
extraintestinal manifestations of, 748
genetic factors in, 748–749
hepatobiliary complications of, 753–754
immune response in, 748–749
infection and, 748
local complications with, 752–753
nutritional management in, 754
pathogenesis of, 748
pathology of, 749, *749*, 750
pregnancy and, 755
prognosis in, 755–756
skin disorders with, 753
toxic megacolon with, 750, *751*
treatment of, 754
antibiotics in, 754–755
corticosteroids in, 754–755
surgery for, 754, 755
vs. Crohn's colitis, 746, 746t, 752
with coagulation disorders, 753
with colon cancer, 753, *753*
with joint disorders, 753
with kidney stones, 753
with visual disorders, 753

Ulcerative proctitis, 755
Ulnar palsy, 2197
Ultimobranchial gland, 1451
Ultrasonography, 65, *65*, 175. See also *Echocardiography.*
Doppler, in echocardiography, 177–178, *179*
in acute abdomen, 797–798
in acute cholecystitis, 857
in congenital defect diagnosis, 146, 148
in Cushing's syndrome, 1316
in gastrointestinal disease, 650–651, *651*
in insulinoma, 1346
in jaundice, 812
in kidney tumor, 640
in liver tumor, 851
in pancreatic cancer, 779
in pancreatitis, 773, *773*, *774*, *775*, 777
in thrombophlebitis, 364
of biliary tract, 854, *854*
of kidneys, *512*, 513–514
of lung, 385
of thyroid gland, 1280
Ultraviolet radiation, 2297
biology of, 2298
in psoriasis, 2246
Uncertainty principle, in practice of medicine, 3
Uncinate fits, 2152
Unconsciousness, traumatic, 2170
Undernutrition. See also *Malnutrition.*
epidemiology of, 1183–1184
indices of, 1186t
pathophysiology of, 1184
Unilateral hyperlucent lung, 406
Unstable hemoglobin disease
drug-induced, 932–933
genetic factor in, 932
representative hemoglobins in, 932, 932t
Unverricht-Lundborg progressive myoclonus epilepsy, 2154
Uranium, as nephrotoxin, 600
Urate
serum, 1133, 1133t
solubility factor and, 1133, 1133t
Urea, serum, in uremia, 554
Urea cycle, 1129, *1129*
disorders of, 1129–1130
genetic factors in, 1129–1130
Urea nitrogen, serum or plasma, reference values for, 2335
Urea nitrogen/creatinine ratio, reference values for, 2335
Ureaplasma infection
of genitourinary tract, 1508–1509
reproductive abnormalities and, 1508–1509
treatment of, 1509
Ureaplasma urealyticum, 1505, 1508–1509
Uremia
acid-base balance in, 550–551, *551*
acute, 488
anemia with, 552, 556
approach to patient with, 554–555, 555t
as catabolic disorder, 489
bone disorders in, 489
calcium metabolism in, 551
chloride metabolism in, 551
chronic, 488
complications of, 555–557
electrolyte balance in, 549–551, 555–556
electrolytes in, 489
erythropoietin in, 489
gastrointestinal disorders with, 552–553
glomerular filtration rate and, 489
granulocytopenia in, 552
hematologic abnormalities with, 552, 556
hemorrhagic diathesis in, 552
hyperkalemia with, 550, 555–556
Uremia (*Continued*)
hypertriglyceridemia with, 1114
infection with, 552, 555, 557
magnesium metabolism in, 551
metabolic acidosis with, 550
myopathy with, 553
neuropathy with, 553
osteodystrophy wih, 553, 557
peripheral neuropathy in, 489
phosphate metabolism in, 551
platelet function in, 1037–1038
pleural involvement with, 449
potassium metabolism in, 549–550
protein metabolism and, 489
renal biopsy in, 555
renal osteodystrophy in, 489
sodium metabolism in, 550, 556
toxin retention in, 554
treatable parenchymal disease in, 555, 555t
urea concentration in, 553
water metabolism and, 549–551, 555–556
with acute renal failure, 546
with hyperparathyroidism, 553
Uremic acidosis, 550
Uremic neuropathy, 2193–2194
Uremic pericarditis, 552, 556
Uremic pseudodiabetes mellitus, 553
Uremic syndrome, 914–915
in renal failure, 488–489
Ureter
anomalies of, 639
transitional cell cancer of, 643
Ureteral obstruction
at pelvic brim, 488
at ureteropelvic junction, 488
at ureterovesical junction, 488
bilateral, 544–545
Ureterocele, 639
Ureteropelvic junction obstruction, in hydronephrosis, 639
Ureterosigmoidostomy, metabolic acidosis and, 540
Urethra
anomalies of, 639
diverticuli of, 639
strictures of, 639
Urethral obstruction, renal failure and, 547
Urethral syndrome, sexually transmitted, 1642
Urethritis
differential diagnosis of, 1640–1641
gonococcal, 1645
sexually transmitted, 1640–1641, *1641*
Uric acid
serum, reference values for, 2336
synthesis of, 1134, *1135*
toxic nephropathy and, 506
Uric acid metabolism, in chronic renal failure, 553, 557
Uricosurics, as nephrotoxins, 602
Urinary antiseptics, 622
Urinary bladder, disorders of, 2028–2030, *2029*
Urinary incontinence, in aged, 28–29
Urinary output, in shock, 219
Urinary tract
anomalies of, congenital 638–639
calculi of, in cystinuria, 612–613
in bilharziasis, 1812–1813
tumors of, 639–644
urothelial, 643–644
Urinary tract infection, 619–623
and back pain, 2061
clinical manifestations of, 620
complications of, 622–623
diagnosis of, 620
microscopic examination in, 621
radiography in 621
Urinary tract infection (*Continued*)
enteric bacteria in, 1594
epidemiology of, 621
hospital-acquired, 1487
kidney stones and, 630–631
mycoplasmal, 1508
natural history of, 621
pathogenesis of, 619–620
prophylaxis for, 622
recurrent, 622
sexually transmitted, 1641–1643
staphylococcal, 1547
symptomatic, 621–622
treatment of, 621–622
antiseptic therapy for, 106
Ureaplasma in, 1508–1509
Urinary tract obstruction 605, 607, 605t
clinical manifestations of, 605–606, 606t
diagnosis in, 606–607
hypertension with, 606
infection in, 606
pathophysiology of, 605, 605t
polycythemia with, 606
postobstructive diuresis with, 606
renal failure with, 606
treatment of, 607
tubular dysfunction in, 606
Urination, abnormalities of, 2028–2030, *2029*
Urine
acidity measurement of, 510
concentration and dilution activity measurement, 510
cytology of, 484
electrolyte measurement of, 510–511
formation of, 483, 492–493
in kidney disease, 484
specific gravity of, 510
Urobilinogen
in liver disease, 811
urinary and fecal, reference values for, 2336
Urogenital tract
radiography of, 511–514, *513*
radionuclide imaging of, 514
Urography
adverse effects of, 513
excretory, 511, *512*, 513
Urokinase, 1056
Uroporphyrin, 1153, 1155, 1156, 1157
urinary, fecal, and erythrocytic, reference values for, 2336
Uroporphyrinogen, 1153, 1155
Urothelial tumors, 643–644
Ursodeoxycholate, 853
Urticaria, 2232, 2297
aquagenic, 1865
cholinergic, 1865
contact, 1865
heat, 1865
light, 1865
Urticaria-angioedema
arachidonic acid metabolism and, 1866
aspirin and, 1866
classification of, 1864, 1864t
clinical manifestations of, 1864
cold-induced, 1865
complement-mediated, 1865–1866
diagnosis of, 1866
differential, 1866
genetic factors in, 1864–1865
idiopathic, 1864
IgE-dependent,1864–1865
immune response in, 1864
immunoglobulin E in, 1864, 1865
incidence of, 1863–1864
laboratory findings in, 1866
mast cell in, 1864, 1866
pathogenesis of, 1864

Urticaria-angioedema (*Continued*)
pathology of, 1864
pressure, 1864
prevalence of, 1863–1864
prevention of, 1866
treatment of, 1866
Urticaria pigmentosa, 1887–1889, 2271
Urticarial papules and plaques, of pregnancy, 2269
Uterine bleeding, dysfunctional, 1386
Uveitis, 2219–2220
arthritis and, 2220
Uveoencephalitic syndrome, viral role in, 2137
Uveomeningitis, 2220

Vaccination, 42–46, 42t, 43t. See also *Immunization;* specific vaccines.
anthrax, 1607
central nervous system complications of, 2139–2141
diptheria, 42t, 43–44
diphtheria-tetanus-pertussis, 1573
eastern equine encephalitis, 1745
foot and mouth disease, 1711
hepatitis B, 42t, 46
influenza, 42t, 44
Japanese encephalitis, 1748
measles, 42t, 44–45, 1709
meningococcal, 42t, 45
mumps, 42t, 45, 1713
pertussis, 1570
pneumacoccal, 42t, 44
poliomyelitis, 42t, 45
poliovirus, 42t, 2132
rabies, 42t, 44, 2134
and acute disseminated encephalomyelitis, 2140
Rift Valley fever, 1740
rubella, 42t, 44, 1711
tetanus, 42t, 1582
tick-borne encephalitis, 1749
tuberculosis, 45–46
typhoid, 45
varicella, 46
Venezuelan equine encephalitis, 1745–1746
western equine encephalitis, 1744
Vaccinia virus, 1727–1728
Vaginal bleeding, cyclic, with infertility, 1388
Vaginal secretions, 1381
Vaginitis
Candida, 1642
differential diagnosis of, 1642t
mixed, 1643
sexually transmitted, 1642
Vaginosis, nonspecific, 1642–1643
Vagotomy
complications of, 692–693
incomplete, 693
proximal gastric, 692
truncal, 691–692
Vagovagal syncope, 1985, *1984*
Valproate, in myoclonus, 2077
Valproic acid, in epilepsy, 2158, *2158*
Valsalva maneuver, in heart failure, 195
Valsalva sinus, congenital aneurysm of, 232
Values, laboratory, of clinical importance, 2315–2340
Valve replacement
in aortic regurgitation, 255
in aortic stenosis, 253–254
in mitral regurgitation, 252
in mitral stenosis, 249
Valvular heart disease, 242–256, *245*
cardiac catheterization in, 245–246
echocardiography in, 244–245, *245*
Valvular heart disease (*Continued*)
electrocardiography in, 244
history in, 243
laboratory studies in, 244–246
physical examination in, 243–244
radiography in, 244
sudden death and, 296, 297
Vanadium, 1211
toxicity of, 2315
Vancomycin, 105–106
as nephrotoxin, 596
for pseudomembranous colitis, 1577
Vanillylmandelic acid, urinary, reference values for, 2336
Varicella, 1721–1723, 2128
clinical manifestations of, 1722
complications of, 1722
congenital abnormality and, 1722
cutaneous lesions in, *2260*
diagnosis of, 1722
culture in, 1722
serology in, 1722
epidemiology of, 1721
etiology of, 1721
host factor in, 1722, 1723
immune response in, 1722
immunization for, 46
maternal infection in, 1722
pathogenesis of, 1721–1722
pathology of, 1721–1722
prevention of, 1723, 2130
progressive, 1722
treatment of, 1722–1723
adenine arabinoside in, 1723
immune globulin in, 1723
vs. rickettsial pox, 1683
Varicella vaccine, 1723
Varicella-zoster virus, 1721, 2128
vs. herpes simplex virus, 2128, 2129
Varicocele, 1372
Varicose veins, 365
Variola. See *Smallpox.*
Variola virus, 1726
Vascular capacitance, in fluid volume disorders, 521
Vascular disease
ocular, 2223–2225
of extremities, 353–366. See also specific diagnoses.
cold damage and, 357–358
communication abnormality in, 362–363
lymphatic vessel disorders in, 365–366
organic arterial obstruction and, 358–360
smooth muscle abnormality in, 353–357
venous disorders and, 363–365
of spinal canal, 2187
Vascular headache, 2054–2056
and ear pain, 2058
Vascular malformations, lower gastrointestinal hemorrhage and, 794, 795
Vascular nevi, involving mouth,2243
Vascular occlusions, retinal, 2224–2225
Vascular parkinsonism, 2071
Vascular protheses, paraprothetic-enteric and aortoenteric fistulas with, 760–761
Vascular purpura, 1038–1040, 1039t
drug-induced, 1039
Vascular retinopathies, 2223–2224
Vascular stroke, 2086
Vasculitis, 1937–1941
and vertigo, 2043
aneurysms with, 2104
classification of, 1938–1939
clinical spectrum of, 1938t
hypersensitivity, 585, 1939–1940
immune response in, 1938, 1939
nodular, 1962
panniculitis with, 1962–1963
Vascular-interstitial fluid shifts, in fluid volume disorders, 521
Vasculopathies
intracerebral hemorrhage with, 2105
nonarteriosclerotic, 2092–2093
and stroke, *2095*, 2096
"Vasoactive" drugs, in threatened stroke, 2100
Vasoactive intestial polypeptide, 717, 1246
Vasoconstriction therapy, in shock, 223
Vasodepressor syncope, *1983*, 1984, *1984*
Vasodilators
arterial, 205
for heart failure, 205–207, *205*, 205t
in hypertension, 278
in primary pulmonary hypertension, 263–265, 264t
in Raynaud's disease, 355
in shock, 223
in threatened stroke, 2100
venous, 205
Vasomotor changes, in intracranial tumor, 2163
Vasopressin, 1239, 1266–1268, *1266*. See also *Antiduretic hormone.*
in cancer, 1079
in esophageal varices, 843
in hypopituitarism, 1257
in shock, 214
Vasospasm, cerebral, 2105
Vectorcardiogram, 174
Vegetative state, definition of, 1971
Vena caval interruption, in pulmonary embolism, 431
Venereal disease, infectious proctitis and, 784. See also *Sexually transmitted disease.*
Venereal Disease Research Laboratories test, 1657–1658, 1657t, 1660
Venezuelan equine encephalitis, 1745–1746
clinical features of, 1745–1746
diagnosis of, 1746
epidemiology of, 1745
pathology in, 1745–1746
prevention of, 1746
vaccine for, 1746
vector in, 1745
virus of, 1745
Venodilators, 164
Venography
in pulmonary embolism, 429
in thrombophlebitis, 363
renal, 512
Venom immunotherapy, in insect sting allergy, 1874
Venous congestion, in right ventricular failure, 197–198
Venous hypertension, heart failure and, 194
Venous infarction, intracranial, hemorrhage with, 2105
Venous return, cardiac output and, 162
Venous stasis retinopathy, 2225
Venous system, 160
Venous thrombosis
cerebral, and stroke, *2095*
intracranial, 2093
Ventilation, 372–376, *373, 374, 375, 376*
abnormalities of, 376
alveolar maintenance of, 459
distribution of, 375–376, *376*
disturbances in, 376
dynamic properties in, 374–375, *374, 375*
equations related to, 465
forced expiratory volume in, 374–375, *374*
forced vital capacity, 374–375, *374*
functional residual capacity in, 372–374
maximal expiratory flow rate in, 374–375, *374, 375*
obstructive disorders, 376, 376t

Ventilation (*Continued*)
regional, determination of, by radionuclide imaging, 385
residual volume in, 372–374
restrictive disorders of, 376, 376t
static properties of, 373–374
tidal volume in, 372–374
total lung capacity in, 372–374
vital capacity in, 372–374
Ventilation-perfusion mismatching, 464, *464*
Ventilation scan, in pulmonary embolism, 429
Ventilator(s)
mechanical, 459, 468–470
weaning from, 469–470
Ventricle(s). See also *Left ventricle* entries; *Right ventricle* entries.
function curve of, 162–163, *163*
late surgical complications, 242
single, 234
Ventricular arrhythmias, sudden death and, 296–297
Ventricular end-diastolic pressure, in heart failure, 191–192
Ventricular fibrillation, 315
Ventricular function, in myocardial infarction, 293
Ventricular function curve, 159, *159*
Ventricular hypertrophy, angina pectoris and, 284
Ventricular premature beats, 307
electrocardiography in, 307
Ventricular septal defect, 230–231, 289
cardiac catheterization study of, *185*
large, 230–231
ostium secundum defect with, 231
small, 230
with aortic regurgitation, 231
with left ventricular-right atrial shunt, 231
"uncured," in adult, 240
with patent ductus arteriosus, 231
with transposition of great arteries, 238–239
Ventricular tachycardia, 313–315
electrocardiography in, 313–315, *314*, *315*
Ventricular-atrial shunt, with ventricular septal defect, 231
Ventriculography
in angina pectoris, 286
in pulmonary stenosis, 235
in tetralogy of Fallot, 234
left, 186
Venturi mask, 459
Venulitis, necrotizing, 1865
Verapamil, 325–326
in hypertension, 278
in migraine, 2055
Verruca virus, infection with, 2249
Verruga peruana, 1617
Vertebrae, transitional, 2187
Vertebral artery(ies), 2089–2090
dissection of, traumatic and spontaneous, 2092
occlusion of, 2095
cerebral anastomoses and, 2091
Vertebral-basilar artery disease
ischemic symptoms of, *2097*
correlation with anatomic structures, *2098*
Vertebral-basilar circulatory system, occlusion of, 2095
Vertebral-basilar ischemia, symptoms and signs of, 2097
Vertigo, 2040–2043
peripheral, causes of, 2941
physiologic, 2041, *2041*
Vesicle(s), 2232
Vestibular ataxia, 2045
Vestibular disorders, vs. ataxia, 2045
Vestibular dysfunction, and drop attacks, 2047
Vestibular failure, 2046
Vestibular neuronitis, 2042
Vestibular system, disorders of, 2040–2043
Vestibular vertigo, causes of, 2041, *2041*
Vestibulopathy, peripheral, 2042
Vibrio cholerae, 1598–1599
Vibrio parahaemolyticus, 782
Vidarabine
in herpes simplex encephalitis, 2125, 2127
in herpes simplex virus infection, 1717
in herpes zoster, 2129
Vinblastine, 1098–1099
Vinca alkaloids, 1098
Vincent's infection. See *Gingivitis.*
Vincristine, 1098–1099
ADH activity and, 1268, 1268t
in acute lymphoblastic leukemia, 990
Vindesine, 1099
Violence
epidemiology of, 37
prevention of injury from, 37
VIPoma (vasoactive intestinal polypeptideoma, 1349–1350
islet cell tumor with, 1349
treatment of, 1349–1350
Viral capsid antigen, 1719
Viral disease(s), 1687–1758. See also specific diagnoses.
cutaneous lesions in, *2260*
diagnostics from recombinant DNA research in, 134
of respiratory tract, 1691–1706
Viral encephalitis, 2122–2126
Viral fevers, arthropod-borne, 1736–1750
Viral hemorrhagic fever, 1750–1758
Viral hepatitis. See entries under *Hepatitis*
Viral infections
and acute disseminated encephalomyelitis, 2140
and Reye's syndrome, 2141
central nervous system complications of, 2139–2141
latent, in neurologic diseases, 2137
mosquito-borne, 2125
occupational, 2297
of nervous system, 2121–2138
acute, 2122
chronic, 2122
latent, 2122
slow, 2122, 2135–2138
Viral meningitis, 2122–2126
etiologic agent in, 2123t
Virus(es), 1687–1691. See also specific categories.
arthropod-borne, central nervous system infection with, 1742t
California encephalitis, 1747
cancer and, 1071
clinical classification of, 1690–1691, 1690t
dengue, 1737–1738
eastern equine encephalitis, 1745
Epstein-Barr, in infectious mononucleosis, 1719–1721
families of, *1687*, 1688t
hemadsorption, 1698
herpes simplex, 2126
vs. varicella-zoster virus, 2128, 2129
in acute central nervous system infections, *2122*
in diabetes mellitus, 1324–1325
influenza, 1700–1705
Japanese encephalitis, 1748
leukemia and, 987
lymphocytic choriomeningitis, 2123
oncogenes of, 1066–1067
parainfluenza, 1698–1700
Virus(es) (*Continued*)
pathogenic classification of, 1689–1690, *1689*t, *1690*t
polio, 2130
rabies, 2132, 2133
respiratory syncytial, 1696–1698
rubella, 1710
St. Louis encephalitis, 1746–1747
taxonomy of, 1688–1689, 1688t
varicella-zoster, 1721–1724, 2128
Venezuelan equine encephalitis, 1745–1746
West Nile, 1738
western equine encephalitis, 1744
Virilization, ovarian function and, 1383, 1385t, 1386, 1387, 1388
Visceral abscesses, glomerulonephritis with, 574
Visceral disease, vs. paravertebral tumor, 2185
Visceral larva migrans, 1823
Visceral reflex syncope, 1984, *1984*
Viscosity, serum, reference values for, 2336
Vision
abnormalities of, in migraine, 2054
in nutritional amblyopia, 2066
in Wernicke's encephalopathy, 2065
loss of, binocular, 2033
in pseudotumor cerebri, 2168
neurologic disorders of, 2032–2037, *2032*, *2034*, *2036*
vitamin A and, 1206
Visna, 2135
Visual acuity
aging and, 23
testing of, 2033
Visual agnosia, 1996
Visual disorders, with ulcerative colitis, 753
Visual evoked potentials, 1969–1970
Visual evoked response, 1260
Visual field, defects of, *2032*, 2033
Visual symptoms, in multiple sclerosis, 2145, *2145*
Vital capacity, 463
Vitamin(s). See also names of specific vitamins.
as drugs, 1198
deficiencies of, 1197–1209
alcohol-induced, 1198
clinical development of, 1198
dietary factor in, 1197–1198
drug-induced, 1198
in gastrointestinal disease, 646
multiple, 1197
fat-soluble, absorption of, 720
toxicity from, 1198
Vitamin A, 1206–1207
biochemical function of, 1206
cancer and, 1207
deficiency of, 724, 1207
alcoholism and, 1207
assay in, 1207
in night blindness, 1206, 1207
treatment of, 1207
dietary allowances for, 1177
dietary sources of, 1206–1207
in acne, 1207
physiology of, 1206
requirements for, 1206–1207
serum, reference values for, 2336
structure of, 1206, *1206*
therapy with, hypercalcemia and, 1449
toxicity, 1207, 1465
Vitamin A tolerance test, reference values for, 2336
Vitamin B
in alcoholic cerebellar degeneration, 2066
in nutritional amblyopia, 2066
Vitamin B complex deficiency, 725

Vitamin B_1, 1198–119. See also *Thiamin*.
Vitamin B_2. See also *Riboflavin*.
urinary, reference values for, 2333
Vitamin B_6. See also *Pyridoxine*.
plasma, reference values for, 2336
Vitamin B_{12}
absorption of, 721, 727
chemical structure of, 895, *895*
deficiency of, 724, 896–897, 2067
and ataxia, 2044
megaloblastic anemia and, 893, 895–897
neurologic symptoms, 896
neutropenia and, 955
specific syndromes of, 897
dietary allowance for, 1178
ECF-ICF shifts in, 533
malabsorption of, 732
metabolic aspects of, 895–896
microbiologic assay of, 896
nutritional aspects of, 895–896
radioisotope dilution assay, 896
serum, reference values for, 2336
synthesis of, 895
therapy with, 896–897, *897*
in pernicious anemia, 897–898
in vitamin B_{12} deficiency, 2067
indications for, 898
Vitamin B_{12} binding proteins, 896, 896t
Vitamin B_{12} intrinsic factor, reference values for, 2336
Vitamin C. See also *Ascorbic acid*.
common cold and, 1694
dietary allowance for, 1178
nitrosamines formation and, 39
plasma and blood, reference values for, 2336
Vitamin C saturation test, reference values for, 2336
Vitamin D
abnormal metabolism of, 1426–1427
abnormal target tissue response, 1427
bioavailability of, 1423–1424
bone and, 1423–1425, *1423*, 1424t
decreased bioavailability of, 1425–1426
deficiency of, 724, 1424, 1429, 1430
dietary allowances for, 1177
excess, 1424–1425
in calcium homeostasis, 1415
in hyperparathyroidism, 1436, 1439, 1440, 1441
in hypoparathyroidism, 1443, 1445
in mineral homeostasis, 499
in osteitis fibrosa, 1453, 1455
in pseudohypoparathyroidism, 1446–1448
malabsorption of, 1426
metabolism of, 1424, 1424t
molecular forms of, 1423
nephrotic syndrome and, 1426
nutritional deficiency of, 1425–1426
renal osteodystrophy and, 557
serum measurement of, 1424
sunlight and, 1425
target tissue response, 1424
therapy with, 1430
hypercalcemia and, 1449
in hyperparathyroidism, 1442
in hypoparathyroidism, 1445–1446
in osteoporosis, 1460
toxicity of, 1425
Vitamin D-dependent rickets, 615
Vitamin D endocrine system, 1423–1424, *1423*
disorders of, 1425–1427
Vitamin D-resistant rickets, 615
Vitamin D_3, 25-hydroxy, plasma, reference values for, 2336
Vitamin D_3, 1,25-dihydroxy, serum, reference values for, 2336
Vitamin E, 1208
deficiency of, 724, 1208
dietary allowances for, 1177
dietary requirement for, 1208
physiology of, 1208
serum, reference values for, 2336
toxicity of, 1208
Vitamin K, 1208–1209
blood coagulation and, 1208–1209
deficiency of, 724, 1051–1052, 1208, 1209
anticoagulants and, 1052
coumarin, 1052
causes of, 1051, 1052
malabsorption syndromes with, 1052
of newborn, 1052
dietary allowances for, 1177
dietary sources of, 1208
function of, 1051
metabolism of, 1051–1052
osteocalcin and, 1209
physiology of, 1208–1209
Vitamin K-dependent clotting factor deficiencies, 1049–1050
Vitiligo, 2257
Vitrectomy, pars plana, in diabetic retinopathy, 2224
Vitritis, infectious, 2220
Vocalization, in Gilles de la Tourette's syndrome, 2077
Vogt-Koyanagi-Harada syndrome, 2220
viral role in, 2137
Voiding, abnormalities of, 2028–2030, *2029*
Volhynia fever, 1685
Vomiting
complications of, 648, *648*
disorders associated with, 648, 648t
esophageal injury from, 677
in bulimia nervosa, 1190, 1191
pathophysiology of, 704
quality of vomitus, 647
surreptitious, 613
types of, 647
von Gierke's disease, 1106
von Recklinghausen's disease, 2084–2085, 2257, *2257*
von Willebrand's disease, 1047–1048, *2265*
clinical manifestations of, 1048
diagnosis of, 1048
factor VIII in, 1048–1049
factor VIII–von Willebrand protein for, 1048
genetic factor in, 1047–1048
immunologic assay in, 1048
platelets in, 1037
treatment of, 1048
von Willebrand factor, 1047
VM-26, in cancer chemotherapy, 1099
VP-16, in cancer chemotherapy, 1099

Waardenburg's syndrome, 2257
Waldenström's macroglobulinemia, 982, 985, 995, 1020
chlorambucil in, 1020
clinical features of, 1020
clonal development in, 963
diagnosis of, 1020
genetic factors in, 1020
M-compound immunoglobulin in, 1020
pathophysiology of, 1020
plasmapheresis in, 1020
prognosis in, 1020
treatment of, 1020
Wallenberg's syndrome, 2049, 2095
War, and anxiety, 2009
Warfarin, 81
in pulmonary embolism, 430, 431
in thrombophlebitis, 364–365
inhibiting agents of, 81t
Wasps, 1837–1838
Wassermann test, 1657
Wasting, definition of, 2198
Water
absorption of, 721, 724–725
excretion of, kidney regulation and, 497
metabolism of, hormone factor in control of, 1229
in uremia, 549–551, 555–556
regulation of, central nervous system disorders of, 1249–1250
Water balance, hypothalamus and, 2026
Water intoxication, 2027
Water repletion reaction, 1268
"Watershed" infarction, 2090, 2091
Watson-Schwartz test, 1154, 1156
Weakness, 2044
facial, in myotonic dystrophy, 2203
in alcoholic neuropathy, 2066
in amyotrophic lateral sclerosis, 2080
in Guillain-Barré syndrome, 2191
in motor unit disorders, 2198
in multiple sclerosis, 2145, *2145*
in myasthenia gravis, 2215
in spinal cord compression, 2062
in Wohlfart-Kugelberg-Welander disease, 2080
of muscles, 2198
"Wearing-off" phenomenon, in levodopa therapy, 2073
Weber-Christian disease, 1962, *2263*
Wegener's granulomatosis, 1943–1945, *2264*
clinical manifestations of, 1944
diagnosis of, 1944
glomerular involvement in, 585
immune response in, 1944
pathology of, 1944
prognosis in, 1944–1945
treatment of, 1944
cyclophosphamide in, 1944–1945
vs. orbital pseudotumor, 2222
Weight. See *Body weight*.
Weight control exercise and, 41
in hyperlipidemia, 38
in obesity, 1195–1196
Weight loss
after gastric surgery, 692
in malabsorption syndromes, 722
Weight/height statistics, in anthropometric measurements, 1180, 1180t
Weil-Felix reaction, 1676
Weil's syndrome, 1667
Weksler Adult Intelligence Scale, in diagnosis of dementia, 1998–1999
Werdnig-Hoffmann disease, 2080, 2199, 2207
Wermer's syndrome, 1405–1406
Werner's syndrome, 1172
genetic factor in, 1172
Wernicke's aphasia, 1994
Wernicke's encephalopathy, 2064–2065, *2065*
balance in, 2065
Wernicke-Korsakoff syndrome, 1199
West Nile fever, 1738
culture in, 1738
diagnosis of, 1738
serology in, 1738
epidemiology of, 1738
etiology of, 1738
vector in, 1738
Western equine encephalitis, 1744
clinical features in, 1744
diagnosis of, 1744
serology in, 1744

Western equine encephalitis (*Continued*)
  epidemiology of, 1744
  etiology of, 1744
  pathology in, 1744
  prevention of, 1744
  treatment of, 1744
  vaccine for, 1744
  vector in, 1744
  virus of, 1744
West's syndrome, 2153
Wet dressings, in skin disease, 2239, *2239*, 2240
Whipple's disease, 734–735
  antimicrobials in, 735
  corticosteroids in, 735
  periodic acid–Schiff positive macrophages in, 728–729, *728*, 734–735
  with arthritis, 1958
Whipple's resection, in pancreatic carcinoma, 779–780
Whipple's triad, 1343, 1345
Whipworm, 1824
White matter
  spongy degeneration of, 2148
  subcortical, hemorrhage in, 2109
Whole-body radiation exposure, acute, 2299
Whooping cough, 1568–1570, 1705
  clinical manifestations of, 1569
  complications of, 1569
  diagnosis of, 1569–1570
  epidemiology of, 1569
  etiology of, 1568–1569
  immunization for, 1569, 1570
  immunotherapy in, 1570
  pathology of, 1569
  prevention of, 1570
  treatment of, 1570
    antimicrobials in, 1570
Williams syndrome, 237
Williams trait, 1048–1049
Willis' headache, 2098
Wilms' tumor. See *Nephroblastoma.*
Wilson's disease, 132, 487, 600, 912, 1158–1160, 1210
  copper metabolism in, 1158–1160
  diagnosis of, 1159–1160
  genetic factors in, 832, 1158–1159
  liver disease and, 824, 832, 1159
  nervous system in, 1159
  pathology of, 1159
  screening for, 1160
  treatment of, 1160
    penicillamine for, 1160
  with Fanconi's syndrome, 615
Winter vomiting disease, 1734–1735
Wiskott-Aldrich syndrome, 132, 1478, 1860
Withdrawal, from opiate addiction, 2017
Withdrawal syndrome
  general depressant, 2020
  opiate, 2017, 2020
Wohlfart-Kugelberg-Welander disease, 2080
Wolff-Parkinson-White syndrome, 234, 315, *316*, *318*, 331
Wolffian (mesonephric) ducts, 1352
Women
  cigarette smoking and, 49
  depression in, 2012
Wood's light, skin inspection with, 2237–2238
Woolf's syndrome, 2256
Word deafness, 1994
Worms. See also *Nematodes;* specific diagnoses.
  cestodes, 1804–1809
  filaria, 1827–1833
  flukes, 1809–1819
  infection with, 1804
  nematodes, 1819–1827
  tapeworms, 1804–1809
  trematodes, 1809–1819
Wound(s), tetanus prophylaxis in, 43
Wound infection, postoperative, 1489
Wuchereria bancrofti, 1828

Xanthine oxidase deficiency, 1142
Xanthinuria, 1142–1143
  genetic factor in, 1142
Xanthoma(s)
  dysbetalipoproteinemia, 1112–1113
  in hypercholesterolemia, 1112
  in lipoprotein lipase deficiency, 1113
Xenopsylla cheopis, 1679
Xeroderma pigmentosum, 2252
X-linked agammaglobulinemia, 1855–1856, *1856*
X-linked ichthyosis, *2251*
X-linked inheritance, 119–120, *120*
  dominant traits in, 120, *120*
  recessive traits in, 120, *120*
  sex-influenced autosomal dominant inheritance and, 120
X-linked lymphoproliferative syndrome, 1720, 1858
X-ray tomography, in back pain, 2062
Xylitol dehydrogenase deficiency, 1107
Xylocaine. See *Lidocaine.*
Xylose absorption test, reference values for, 2336
D-Xylose, absorption of, 725

Yaws, 1661–1662
Yeast infections
  thoracic, 2247
  vaginal. See entries under *Vaginitis.*
Yellow fever, 1750, *1750*, 1751t, 1752–1754
  clinical manifestations in, 1752–1753
  diagnosis of, 1753
Yellow fever (*Continued*)
  diagnosis of, culture in, 1753
    serology in, 1753
  epidemiology of, 1750, 1752
  jungle, 1750, 1752
  pathogenesis of, 1752
  pathology of, 1752
  prevention of, 1753–1754
  prognosis in, 1753
  treatment of, 1753
  urban, 1750, 1752
  vector in, 1750, 1752
  virus in, 1750
Yellow fever vaccine, 1753–1754
Yersinia enterocolitica, 1603
Yersinia species
  infection from, 1600–1603, 1921
  microbiology of, 1603
Yersinia pestis, 1600
  microbiology of, 1600
Yersinia pseudotuberculosis, 1603
  culture in, 1603
  epidemiology of, 1603
  treatment of, 1603
Y-linked inheritance, 120–121

Zebrafish, 1844
Zenker's diverticulum, 676
Zinc, 1209
  deficiency of, 1209
    in dwarfism, 1209
    parenteral nutrition and, 1209
  dietary allowance for, 1179
  metabolism of, 1209
  uptake of, in acrodermatitis enteropathica, 2252
Zinc toxicity, 2311
Zollinger-Ellison syndrome, 679, 681, 696–697, 1406
  clinical manifestations of, 696
  diagnosis of, 687, 696–697
  gastric acid secretion in, 696
  histamine (H_2) receptor antagonists in, 697
  pancreatic tumor in, 696, 697
  pathophysiology of, 696
  peptic ulcer with, 683, 686–687, 696
  secretin stimulation test in, 696
  serum gastrin in, 686–687, 696
  treatment of, 691, 697
Zona, 2128. See also *Herpes zoster.*
Zoonotic viruses, 1736
Zoster, 2128. See also *Herpes zoster.*
  segmental, immunosuppressive therapy and, 2142
Zoster encephalomyelitis, 2129
Zoster sine herpete, 2129
Zygomycosis, 1771–1773

The colophon on the front cover and spine is an abstraction which symbolizes the universal aspects of medicine. The circle represents the world. The stylized triangle in the upper area is the classic image of positive and negative forces—the Law of Life. The vertical line with the upper right staff suggests the staff of Æsculapius and Hermes, and the horizontal bar connects all three symbols into the total summation of medicine as Art and Science.